Taber's®
CYCLOPEDIC
MEDICAL
DICTIONARY

Edited by

CLAYTON L. THOMAS, M.D., M.P.H.

Visiting Scientist
Harvard University
School of Public Health

Director Emeritus of Medical Affairs
Tambrands Inc.

Dictionary Editor, F. A. Davis Company
Dena Ramras Vardara
Assistant Dictionary Editor, F. A. Davis Company
Elizabeth J. Egan
Dictionary Illustrator
Beth Anne Willert, M.S.

EDITION 17 ILLUSTRATED

Taber's

CYCLOPEDIC MEDICAL DICTIONARY

F.A. DAVIS COMPANY PHILADELPHIA

PRINTED IN THE UNITED STATES OF AMERICA

Last digit indicates print number 10 9 8 7 6 5 4 3

NOTE: As new scientific information becomes available through basic and clinical research, recommended treatments and drug therapies undergo changes. The author and publisher have done everything possible to make Taber's accurate, up to date, and in accord with accepted standards at the time of publication. The author, editors, and publisher are not responsible for errors or omissions or for consequences from application of the book, and make no warranty, expressed or implied, in regard to the contents of the book. Any practice described in this book should be applied by the reader in accordance with professional standards of care used in regard to the unique circumstances that may apply in each situation. The reader is advised always to check product information (package inserts) for changes and new information regarding dose and contraindications before administering any drug. Caution is especially urged when using new or infrequently ordered drugs.

Library of Congress Cataloging in Publication Data

Taber, Clarence Wilbur, 1870–1968
  Taber's Cyclopedic Medical Dictionary, edition 17.

  Medicine — Dictionaries I. Thomas, Clayton L., 1921–   . II. Title. III. Title: Cyclopedic medical dictionary. [DNLM: 1. Dictionaries, Medical. W 13 T113d]
R121.T144 1993   610′.3′21   62-8364
ISBN 0-8036-8313-8
ISBN 0-8036-8312-x (indexed)

DISTRIBUTORS

United States of America
F. A. DAVIS COMPANY
1915 Arch Street
Philadelphia, PA 19103

Atlanta, Georgia
J. A. MAJORS COMPANY
3770-A Zip Industrial Boulevard
P.O. Box 82686, 30354

Boston, Massachusetts
LOGIN BROTHERS NEW ENGLAND
2 Keith Way
Hingham, Massachusetts 02043

RITTENHOUSE BOOK DISTRIBUTORS, INC.
Sterling Road
South Lancaster, Massachusetts 01561

Chicago, Illinois
LOGIN BROTHERS BOOK COMPANY, INC.
1436 West Randolph Street, 60607

Cleveland, Ohio
LOGIN BROTHERS OHIO
1550 Enterprise Parkway
Twinsburg, Ohio 44087

Dallas, Texas
J. A. MAJORS COMPANY
P.O. Box 819074, 75381-9074

Houston, Texas
J. A. MAJORS COMPANY
8723 Knight Road, 77054

Los Angeles, California
J. A. MAJORS COMPANY — CALIFORNIA
1220 West Walnut Street
Compton, California 90220

New York, New York
LOGIN BROTHERS NEW JERSEY
4 Sperry Road
Fairfield, New Jersey 07006

Philadelphia, Pennsylvania
RITTENHOUSE BOOK DISTRIBUTORS, INC.
511 Feheley Drive
King of Prussia, Pennsylvania 19406

St. Louis, Missouri
MATTHEWS BOOK COMPANY
11559 Rock Island Court
Maryland Heights, Missouri 63043

Canada
LOGIN BROTHERS CANADA
324 Saulteaux Crescent
Winnipeg, Manitoba
R3J 3T2

Europe
WILLIAMS & WILKINS LTD.
Broadway House
2–6 Fulham Broadway
London SW6 1AA
England

Australia, New Zealand
MACLENNAN AND PETTY, PTY. LTD.
P.O. Box 425
Artarmon NSW 2064
Australia

Mexico & Central America
LIBRERIA INTERACADEMICA
S. A. de C.V.
Av Sonora 206
Col. Hipodromo
Mexico 06100, D.F.

Panama & South America
INTER-BOOK MARKETING SERVICE
Ruas das Palmeiras, 32-Apt. 701
22270 Rio De Janeiro
Brazil

India
JAYPEE BROTHERS MEDICAL PUBLISHERS
G/16 EMCA House
23/23 B Ansari Road
Darya Ganj, New Delhi 110 002
India

Southeast Asia
INFO-MED, LTD.
Room 1002, Allied Kajima Building
138 Gloucester Road
Wanchai
Hong Kong

CONTENTS

INTRODUCTION TO EDITION 17

Each time I revise this volume, I recall with pleasure its beginnings when Mr. Clarence Wilbur Taber originally provided what he was convinced was the need of nurses and those in allied health professions, as well as any intelligent layman, for assistance in coping with medical terminology. The success of the original edition, more than a half century ago, and all subsequent editions confirmed his convictions.

No doubt, the self-imposed mandate of the original editor was no more or less than that of myself: to provide a comprehensive, accurate source of information not only about words but also disease entities and biological and social concepts important to understanding medicine and its importance to both those who provide medical care and those who need it.

To reflect the ever-changing nature of medicine, over 2200 new terms have been added to the body of the dictionary in this edition. Included are: *age is not a diagnosis, Alice in Wonderland syndrome, burnout, "cookbook" medicine, defensins, gene therapy, intraosseous infusion, mass sociogenic illness, medical waste, Morbidity and Mortality Weekly Report, needle-stick injuries, prostate-specific antigen, reading machines for the blind, serum bank, sharps,* and *surrogate parenting.* The addition of new appendices introduces subjects such as Universal Precautions and Nursing Theory. Revisions to existing appendices provide updated information on topics such as Poisons, Drug Abuse, and Medical Emergencies.

An editor's efforts would amount to very little without the excellent leadership and managerial skill provided for the F.A. Davis Company by the team of Robert H. and Rob Craven and those directly involved in bringing the book to completion, i.e., Dena Ramras Vardara, Dictionary Editor, and Elizabeth J. Egan, Assistant Dictionary Editor. Furthermore, the excellent illustrations provided by Beth Anne Willert serve to enhance the value of Taber's to the reader.

Most important of all, my wife, Peggy, provides the support and inspiration for all of my efforts and thus enables me to edit this volume.

Clayton Lay Thomas, M.D., M.P.H.

SOURCES CONSULTED

The accuracy of a medical dictionary depends upon the editor's ability to stay abreast of the medical and scientific changes that dictate the need to add new words and to delete terms and concepts that are no longer valid or useful. This can be accomplished through constant alertness to the medical literature as well as the spoken words that herald advances in the biological sciences. To do this without comprehensive medical libraries and electronically accessed data banks would be virtually impossible. The Countway Library at the Harvard Medical School and the National Library of Medicine in Bethesda, Maryland and their staffs are of invaluable assistance in obtaining reference materials.

The several consultants in a number of disciplines important to the nursing and allied health fields have provided excellent materials and suggestions concerning this edition of Taber's. Those individuals are listed on the next page. We appreciate the quality and quantity of their assistance.

We acknowledge also *The Barnhart Dictionary Companion* (published by Springer-Verlag New York, Inc.) and the *Dictionary of the Rheumatic Diseases* (American College of Rheumatology, Glossary Committee), from which several entries were derived.

Clayton Lay Thomas, M.D., M.P.H.

CONSULTANTS

Tonia Dandry Aiken, RN, BSN, JD
Patricia Gauntlett Beare, RN, PhD
Carroll Conner Bouman, MS, RN
Kevin R. Brown, MD, MPH, EMT-P
Virginia B. Burggraf, RN, CMSN
Charles Christiansen, EdD, OTR, FAOTA
Lynn Allen Colby, MS, PT
Marilynn E. Doenges, BSN, MA, RN, CS
Jacqueline Fawcett, PhD, FAAN
Sara G. Fuller, PhD, RN, CPNP
Barbara A. Gylys, MEd, CMA-A

Diane Bronkema Hamilton, RN, PHD
Terence C. Karselis, MS, MT (ASCP)
Janet Ross Kerr, RN, PhD, (CANADA)
Carolyn Kisner, MS, PT
Thomas Kraker, MEd, RT(R)
Susan Lampe, RN, MS
Judith E. Meissner, RN, MSN
Mary Frances Moorhouse, RN, CCP, CCRN
Morris E. Weaver, PhD

(Material supplied by the consultants has been reviewed and edited by Clayton L. Thomas, M.D., Editor, with whom final responsibility rests for the accuracy of content.)

Taber's Feature-Finder

MAIN ENTRY — acetohexamide (ăs″e-tō-hĕks′ă-mīd). An orally administered hypoglycemic agent.

Caution: This drug should be used only in patients with diabetes of the non-insulin-dependent type who cannot be treated with diet alone and who are unwilling or unable to take insulin if weight reduction and dietary control fail. — **CAUTION**

ABBREVIATION — ADC. *anodal duration contraction; axiodistocervical.*

PRONUNCIATION — addict (ăd′ĭkt) [L. *addictus*, given over]. One physically or psychologically, or both, dependent on a substance, esp. alcohol or drugs. — **ETYMOLOGY**

Addison's Disease. [Thomas Addison, Brit. physician, 1793–1860] Disease resulting from deficiency in the secretion of adrenocortical hormones. SYN: *adrenocortical hypofunction; chronic hypoadrenocorticism.* — **BIOGRAPHICAL INFORMATION** — **SYNONYM**

SYMPTOMS — SYM: Increased pigmentation of skin and mucous membranes, irregular patches of vitiligo, black freckles over head and neck, weakness, fatigability, hypotension, nausea, vomiting, anorexia, weight loss, and sometimes hypoglycemia.

ETIOLOGY — ETIOL: Progressive destruction of the adrenal gland whether due to an infectious disease, such as tuberculosis, or infiltration by neoplastic tissue or hemorrhage into the gland.

TREATMENT — TREAT: Adrenocortical hormone therapy is dramatic in its effect and must be given promptly in adrenal crisis in order to prevent death. SEE: *adrenal; epinephrine.* — **CROSS REFERENCE**

PROGNOSIS — PROG: If untreated, the disease will continue a chronic course with progressive but usually relatively slow deterioration; in some patients the deterioration may be rapid. Patients treated properly have an excellent prognosis.

NURSING IMPLICATIONS — NURSING IMPLICATIONS: *Acute Adrenal crisis:* Monitor patient for dehydration, hypotension, hypoglycemia, hyperkalemia, petechial hemorrhages, somnolent state, and profound hypovolemic shock. SEE: *Nursing Diagnosis in Appendix.* — **NURSING DIAGNOSES CROSS REFERENCES**

additive (ăd′ĭ-tĭv). In pharmacology, the effect that one drug or substance contributes to the action of another drug or substance.

SUBENTRY — *a., food.* Substance added to food to increase its flavor, storage characteristics, color, aroma, or other qualities.

adduction (ă-dŭk′shŭn). Movement of a limb or eye toward median plane of body or, in case of digits, toward axial line of a limb. SEE: *abduction* for illus. — **ILLUSTRATION CROSS REFERENCE**

Not an actual page.
Only references to Nursing Diagnoses appear in color on text pages.

FEATURES AND THEIR USE

Taber's is more than just a medical dictionary. In addition to listing important health science terms, it covers concepts that are vital to the practitioner and student of Nursing and Allied Health. All who work in fields related to health care will find *Taber's Cyclopedic Medical Dictionary* a comprehensive resource tool.

1. **Vocabulary:** The vocabulary is updated to meet the ongoing needs of those in the Nursing and Allied Health professions. The editor, consultants, and F.A. Davis staff have researched and included new entries reflecting the many changes in the health care professions, approaches to patient care, and aspects of law and ethics.

2. **Definitions:** The definitions are written in encyclopedic style, offering a comprehensive understanding of the word or concept described. They stand out in a paragraph apart from supplemental material, making it easier to pinpoint the core information.

3. **Entry format:**
   Main entries are alphabetized letter by letter, regardless of spaces or hyphens that may occur between the words. A comma marks the end of an entry for alphabetical purposes; e.g., **ear, words pert. to** precedes **earache** as well as **ear dust.** For alphabetical purposes in eponymic terms, the **'s** is ignored, e.g., **Albini's nodules** precedes **albinism.** In some cases compound terms are listed under the adjective. Many words formerly hyphenated are now listed as one word (corticosteroid, gastrointestinal), and American rather than British forms are used.
   Subentries are listed under the noun they modify (such as *labor, premature* or *technician, emergency medical*), indented from the main entry, and printed in bold italic typeface.

4. **Pronunciation:** More than 95% of the main entries are spelled phonetically. Pronunciations are given as simply as possible with most long and short vowels marked diacritically and secondary accents indicated. *Diacritics* are marks over or under vowels. Only two diacritics are used in *Taber's:* the macron ⁻ showing the long sound of vowels, as the a in rāte, e in rēbirth, i in īsle, o in ōver, and u in ūnite; and the breve ˘ showing the short sound of vowels, as the a in ăpple, e in ĕver, i in ĭt, o in nŏt, and u in cŭt. *Accents* are marks used to indicate stress upon certain syllables. A single accent ' is called a primary accent. A double accent ″ is called a secondary accent; it indicates less stress upon a syllable than that given by a primary accent. This difference in stress can be seen in the word an″es-the′si-a.

5. **Etymology:** An etymology indicates the origin and historical development of a term. Etymologies for approx. 90% of the main entries are presented in brackets following the term. The major sources of medical terminology are Latin and Greek.

6. **Abbreviations:** Standard abbreviations for entries are included with the definition and also are listed alphabetically throughout the text. Additional abbreviations used for charting and prescription writing are listed in the Appendix. Nonmedical abbreviations used for convenience are listed on page xli.

7. **Synonyms:** Synonyms are listed at the end of the definition. Many synonymous terms have their own complete definitions to ease the facility of use. Related terms are indicated by a SEE or RS (related subject) reference. If numerous related terms are applicable, they appear as a separate entry titled *words pert. to.*

8. **Eponyms:** Included as main entries are the names of individuals who were the first to discover, describe, or popularize a concept, a microorganism, a disease, a syndrome, or an anatomical structure. A brief biography is included within these entries, appearing in brackets immediately following the pronunciation. Biographical information includes the person's medical designation, the country in which the person was born or worked, and the date of birth and death, if known.

9. **Masculine and feminine:** The masculine form of any noun or pronoun may be read and implied as the feminine or neuter, as the circumstances may make appropriate.

10. **Italics and boldface:** Synonymous terms and cross references are italicized, as are the Latin names for biological materials, including botanical and zoological specimens, and anatomical structures. The terms for which an abbreviation stands are italicized, as are some foreign words. Boldface type is used for all main entries and subentries, for headings used in tables, and to highlight Caution statements in the form of boldface lines above and below the text.

11. **Caution statements:** This notation is used to draw particular attention to clinically important information. The information is of much more than routine interest, and it should be considered when delivering medical care. These statements are further emphasized by boldface lines above and below the text.

12. **Cross references:** These are indicated in one of the following ways: (1) The notation "SEE:" followed by a term or terms in italics; (2) contained within a paragraph devoted to Related Subjects, abbreviated "RS:"; or (3) Nursing Diagnoses cross references, which appear highlighted in color at the end of entries as follows: SEE: *Nursing Diagnoses* in *Appendix.*

13. **Supplemental information:** Supplemental information is often included with the definition and is set apart by a paragraph indent. A heading will often appear with this information. This edition includes an *Index of Major Subheadings* listing the entries with the following headings: entries cross-referenced to Nursing Diagnosis appendix (see #17 below), nursing implications, caution, diagnosis, etiology, first aid, poisoning, prognosis, signs and symptoms, and treatment. Some other headings not included in the *Index of Major Subheadings* are: contraindications, differential diagnosis, examination, function, incompatibility, indications, pathology, physiology, and therapy.

14. **Illustrations:** This edition has over 200 illustrations, all of which use color to highlight and differentiate portions of the drawings. A list of illustrations appears on page xxxv.

15. **Tables:** This edition has over 75 tables located appropriately throughout the text. A list of tables appears on page xxxix. The entry to which the table is keyed appears in boldface on this list.

16. **Appendix:** Detailed information on measurement systems, conversion rules, and scientific notation are contained in the Appendix. Long tables that would interfere with finding words in the text are grouped in the Appendix.

   Updated tables in this edition include: Normal Ranges of Laboratory Values, Physical Constants of Elements, Required Daily Dietary Allowances, Poison Control Centers, and Poisons, Drug Abuse, and Medical Emergencies.

   In addition, this edition features several new appendices: Documentation Terms, Conceptual Models and Theories of Nursing, Nursing Organizations, and Universal Precautions.

   Once again, *Taber's* features *The Interpreter,* which contains questions and statements most often used during examination, in taking a patient's history, and in diagnosis, given in five languages: English, Spanish, Italian, French, and German. For convenience, *The Interpreter* is arranged in categories that deal with specific aspects of examination, history, and diagnosis, and a separate table of contents for the *The Interpreter* helps the reader to quickly locate each section.

17. **Nursing Diagnoses Appendix:** This appendix has also been updated through the 10th NANDA (North American Nursing Diagnosis Association) conference. It it divided into three sections: (1) Two lists of NANDA's nursing diagnoses, one organized by Doenges & Moorhouse Diagnostic Divisions, and one by Gordon's Functional Health Patterns; (2) Nursing diagnoses commonly associated with 296 diseases/disorders cross-referenced from the body of the dictionary; and (3) description of all NANDA-approved diagnoses through the 10th conference in alphabetical order. For each nursing diagnosis, *definition, related factors,* and *defining characteristics* descriptive categories are provided. See the *Quick View of Contents* on page 2482 for more explanation.

INDEX OF
MAJOR SUBHEADINGS

Many entries contain supplemental information under a special heading. The following index has been compiled to aid the reader in quickly locating information on: Nursing Implications, Caution, Diagnosis, Etiology, First Aid, Poisoning, Prognosis, Symptoms, and Treatment. In addition and for reader convenience, included is a listing of diseases/disorders which appear throughout the text and are cross referenced to their commonly associated Nursing Diagnoses in the Appendix.

xv

Nursing Implications

nutrition
tracheitis
tracheostomy
transient ischemic
attack
triage
trigeminal neuralgia
typhoid fever
unconsciousness
uricosuric agent
urinary calculi
urinary tract infection
vaginitis
varicose ulcers
varicose veins
vertigo
vomiting
warfarin sodium
x-ray

CAUTION

acetaminophen
acetohexamide
acid, boric
acid, folic
acid, hydrochloric
acid poisoning
adrenal crisis
aflatoxin
air syringe
airway
airway, oropharyngeal
alcoholism, acute
alkali poisoning
aminopyrine
amnesia, anterograde
amniocentesis
anabolic agents
antidote, universal
anti-G suit
antishock garment
anti-stain formulary
appendicitis, acute
arthritis, rheumatoid
aurotherapy
Balke test
bandage
bandage, Esmarch
bath, bubble
bath, steam
bed

bleeding, venous
blister
blood component
therapy
bowel movement
brain death
breast, self-examination
of
cardiopulmonary
resuscitation
cardioversion
catheter, condom
chancre
chemical peel of the skin
chin-left airway
technique
chloramphenicol
chlorpropamide
cocaine hydrochloride
poisoning, acute
coma
concussion of brain
constipation
containers, care and
handling of
cooking
Creutzfeldt-Jakob
disease
cryptosporidiosis
cyanoacrylate adhesives
delirium tremens
Demerol
diethylstilbestrol
diphtheria
disinfection of field of
operation
disulfiram
dog bite
dopamine hydrochloride
dressing, hot moist
eardrops
ear plug
eclampsia
edrophonium test
emetic
enuresis
erythropoietin
Esmarch's bandage
ether anesthesia
etretinate
excreta
exercise tolerance test
exfoliative dermatitis

eye
eyedrops
familial periodic
paralysis
fasting
febrile convulsions
feeding, tube
fever
finger, dislocation of
fire emergencies
flea infestation
fluid replacement
fluoridation
fluroxene
folic acid
fracture
fumigant
gasoline
gastric lavage
gelatin sponge,
absorbable
glaucoma
glove
gonorrhea
gray syndrome of the
newborn
heat, application of
heel puncture
hemofiltration
hemophilia
hemorrhage
hepatitis B
herpes genitalis
hyperbaric oxygen
therapy
hyperemesis gravidarum
hypertensive crisis
hypoacidity
hypodermic
hypoglycemic agents,
oral
hypothermia, accidental
ice bag
ice massage
injection
instruments, care and
sharpening of
insulin
insulin shock
intravenous treatment
iodoquinol
iron dextran injection
isopropyl alcohol

Caution

xix

erysipelas
erysipeloid
erythema
fecal impaction
fever
folliculitis decalvans
freckle
furunculus
gangrene
gastrectasia, gastrectasis
gastritis
gingivitis
glaucoma
glossoplegia
goiter
goiter, exophthalmic
gonorrhea
gout
granuloma inguinale
granulosis rubra nasi
gumboil
hay fever
headache
heart block
heart failure
hematuria
hemiplegia
hemoglobinuria
hemolytic disease of the
  newborn
hemophilia
hemorrhage, cerebral
hemorrhage, uterine
hemorrhagic
  nephrosonephritis
hernia
herpangina
heterophoria
hiccough, hiccup
hoarseness
hobnail liver
hyperactivity
hyperemesis gravidarum
hypergenitalism
hyperhidrosis
hyperinsulinism
hypermelanoses
hyperpnea
hyperptyalism
hypertension
hypertrichosis
hypoglycemia
hypomelanoses
hysteria

icterus, obstructive
idiopathic pulmonary
  fibrosis
impetigo contagiosa
inanition
incompetent palatal
  syndrome
incoordination
infection
influenza
kala-azar
keratitis
keratoderma
  blennorrhagica
keratosis, seborrheic
labyrinthitis
lactose intolerance
lagophthalmos,
  lagophthalmus
laryngitis, acute
  catarrhal
Leeuwenhoek's disease
Legionnaires' disease
leprosy
leptomeningitis
leukoencephalopathy,
  progressive multifocal
leukorrhea
Lhermitte's sign
lichen planus
Little's disease
liver, abscess of
liver, cirrhosis of
Lyme disease, Lyme
  arthritis
lymphadenitis
lymphadenitis,
  tuberculous
lymphangitis
lymphogranuloma
  venereum
macrocephalia
Madura foot
maduromycosis
malaria
mastitis
melanoma
Meniere's disease
meningitis, acute
  meningococcal
menorrhagia
migraine
miliaria
miosis

mole
molluscum contagiosum
moniliasis
mumps
myasthenia gravis
mydriasis
myocarditis
myositis
myxedema
nabothian cysts
necrosis
nephritis
neuralgia
neuralgia, trigeminal
neuritis
neuritis, multiple
neuritis, retrobulbar
nystagmus
obesity
odontoma, follicular
oligopnea
oliguria
onychia, piannic
ophthalmia neonatorum
orf
organic brain syndromes
organic psychoses
ornithosis
orthopnea
osteitis deformans
osteoarthropathy,
  hypertrophic
  pulmonary
osteomalacia
otosclerosis
pachymeningitis,
  hemorrhagic
pant
papilledema
paralysis, Bell's
paraplegia
paratyphoid fever
paresis
paronychia
pathological reaction to
  alcohol
pellagra
pelvic inflammatory
  disease
peptic ulcer
pericarditis
periostitis
peritonitis
peritonitis, acute diffuse

thiram poisoning
tincture of iodine
   poisoning
tin poisoning
toadstool poisoning
toluene poisoning
turpentine poisoning
verdigris poisoning
warfarin poisoning
xylene poisoning
zinc salts poisoning

PROGNOSIS
acne vulgaris
Addison's disease
AIDS
anaphylactic shock
angina pectoris
apoplexy
battered child syndrome
Bell's palsy
bronchi, foreign bodies in
bronchopneumonia
calculus, renal
calculus, vesical
cardiomyopathy,
   hypertrophic
cat scratch disease
chorea, Sydenham's
coccidioidomycosis
comedo
croup, membranous
cryptococcosis
cystic fibrosis
diabetes insipidus
diabetes mellitus
diphtheria
Ebola virus disease
eczema
Ehlers-Danlos syndrome
epilepsy
erysipelas
folliculitis decalvans
gas, vesicant
gonorrhea
heart, fatty
   degeneration of
heart, fatty infiltration of
heat exhaustion
hemolytic uremic
   syndrome
hemophilia
hydrocephalus

hype.
   pseudo..
idiopathic pulm..
   fibrosis
influenza
intussusception
leprosy
leukemia, acute
   myelogenous
leukemia, chronic
   myelogenous
leukemia, hairy cell
lichen planus
liver, abscess of
liver, acute yellow
   atrophy of
liver, amyloid
liver, cancer of
liver, cirrhosis of
lung, edema of
lung abscess
lung collapse
marasmus
measles
meningitis, acute
   meningococcal
Minamata disease
mumps
myasthenia gravis
myotonia congenita
neuralgia,
   sphenopalatine
papilledema
Parkinson's disease
pericarditis
peritonitis, acute diffuse
peritonitis, chronic
phenol poisoning
phenylketonuria
placenta previa
poisoning, potato
poliomyelitis, acute
   anterior
polyarteritis (nodosa)
polymyositis
prurigo
pyelonephritis
pyloric obstruction and
   dilatation
rabies
Raynaud's disease
Reiter's syndrome
Reye's syndrome
rickets

Symptoms

scu..
spasm o.
splenitis   ..
steatoma
stomach cancer
stomatitis parasitica
stomatitis, ulcerative
strabismus, paralytic
stroke
sycosis
Sydenham's chorea
Tay-Sachs disease
tetany
tonsillitis
trichinosis
typhoid fever
typhus
varicella
verruca
yellow fever

SYMPTOMS
abortion
abruptio placentae
abscess, brain
acapnia
acetaminophen
   poisoning
acetonemia
acne vulgaris
acromegaly
actinomycosis
Addison's disease
adult respiratory
   distress syndrome
   (ARDS)
aeroembolism
AIDS
alcoholism, acute
alcoholism, chronic
alkalosis, metabolic
alkalosis, respiratory
allergy
amebiasis
amyloid kidney
anaphylactic shock
anemia
anemia, pernicious

gangrene, moist
gas, lewisite
gas, lung irritant
gas, nose irritant
gas, vesicant
gasoline poisoning
gastrectasia, gastrectasis
gastritis, acute
gastritis, chronic
glanders
glossitis, acute
glottis, edema of
goiter, exophthalmic
gonorrhea
gout
granulosis rubra nasi
gumboil
gumma
hay fever
heart, dilatation of
heart, fatty
  degeneration of
heart, fatty infiltration of
heart, fibroid
heart failure
heat exhaustion
hematemesis
hematuria
hemlock poisoning
hemophilia
hemoptysis
hemorrhage
hemorrhage, cerebral
hepatic coma
heroin toxicity
herpangina
herpes genitalis
hip, dislocation of
hip, dislocation of,
  backward
hip, dislocation of,
  forward
hippocratic facies
histoplasmosis
Hodgkin's disease
human bite
hydropericardium
hydrothorax
hyperemesis gravidarum
hyperinsulinism
hyperopia
hyperthyroidism
hypertrophy,
  pseudomuscular

hypoglycemia
hypothermia, accidental
hypothyroidism
hysteria
icterus, hemolytic
icterus, obstructive
ileus
impetigo contagiosa
infection
inflammation
influenza
injury
ink poisoning
insulin shock
internal injury
interstitial cystitis
intestinal obstruction
iodine poisoning
iritis
iron poisoning
jejunum, inflammation
  of
keratitis, interstitial
keratoconjunctivitis,
  phlyctenular
keratosis pilaris
keratosis, seborrheic
knee, game
labyrinthitis
laryngitis, acute
  catarrhal
laryngitis, atrophic
laryngitis, chronic
laryngitis, syphilitic
laryngitis, tuberculous
laryngostenosis,
  occlusion
larynx, foreign bodies in
Lassa fever
leprosy
leptomeningitis
leukemia, chronic
  myelogenous
leukorrhea
lichen planus
Little's disease
liver, abscess of
liver, acute yellow
  atrophy of
liver, amyloid
liver, cancer of
liver, cirrhosis of
lung, edema of
lung abscess

lung collapse
lung collapse, hypostatic
lung collapse, passive
lymphadenia ossea
lymphadenitis
lymphadenitis,
  tuberculous
lymphangitis
lymphogranuloma
  venereum
lymphoma, non-
  Hodgkin's
malaria
manganese poisoning
marasmus
Marfan's syndrome
mastitis
mastoiditis
match poisoning
McArdle's disease
measles
meningitis, acute
  meningococcal
meningitis, tuberculous
meningoencephalitis
  due to Naegleria and
  Acanthamoeba
menopause
mercurialism
mercuric chloride
  poisoning
mercurous chloride
  poisoning
mercury poisoning
metal fume fever
migraine
miliaria
Minamata disease
molluscum contagiosum
mononucleosis,
  infectious
mountain fever
multiple sclerosis
mumps
myasthenia gravis
mycosis fungoides
myelitis
myocarditis
myotonia congenita
myxedema
narcotic poisoning
Necator americanus
neuralgia,
  sphenopalatine

neuralgia, trigeminal
neuritis
neuritis, intraocular
neuritis, multiple
neuritis, retrobulbar
nicotine poisoning, acute
nitrous oxide
odontoma, follicular
ophthalmia, sympathetic
opiate poisoning
orchitis
orchitis, syphilitic
orchitis, tuberculous
organic brain syndromes
organic dust toxic
    syndrome
ornithosis
Oroya fever
orthopnea
osteitis deformans
osteomalacia
osteomyelitis
oxalic acid poisoning
pachymeningitis,
    hemorrhagic
pancreatitis, acute
pancreatitis, acute
    hemorrhagic
pancreatitis, chronic
panniculitis
paralysis, Bell's
parathion poisoning
paratyphoid fever
paresis
Parkinson's disease
paronychia
paroxysmal cold
    hemoglobinuria
pediculosis capitis
pediculosis corporis
pediculosis pubis
peliosis
pellagra
pelvic inflammatory
    disease
peptic ulcer
perforation of stomach
    or intestine
pericarditis
pericarditis, fibrinous
periostitis
peritonitis, acute diffuse
peritonitis, chronic
pernio

Perthes' disease
pertussis
pharyngitis, acute
pharyngitis, chronic
phenol poisoning
phenylketonuria
phlebitis
phlegmasia alba dolens
phosphaturia
phosphorus poisoning
placenta previa
plague
pleurisy, diaphragmatic
pneumonia
pneumonia,
    desquamative
    interstitial
pneumopericardium
pneumothorax
pneumothorax,
    spontaneous
poison ivy dermatitis
pokeroot poisoning
poliomyelitis, acute
    anterior
polycythemia vera
polymer fume fever
potassium chromate
    poisoning
Pott's disease
pregnancy
progeria
prostate cancer
prostatism
pseudoangina
pseudocirrhosis
psittacosis
purpura, idiopathic
    thrombocytopenic
pyelonephritis
pyemia
pyloric obstruction and
    dilatation
rabies
ranula
Raynaud's disease
respiratory distress
    syndrome of the
    premature infant
retinal detachment
retinitis
Reye's syndrome
rheumatic fever
rhinitis, atrophic

rhinitis, chronic
    hypertrophic
rhinoscleroma
rickets
ringworm
rubella
scabies
scalenus syndrome
scarlet fever
sciatica and low back
    pain
scombroid poisoning
scurvy
scurvy, infantile
seasickness
sepsis, puerperal
serum rash
shock
sick sinus syndrome
silver nitrate poisoning
snow blindness
spasmus nictitans
spider bites or poisoning
spider bites or
    poisoning, black
    widow
spider bites or
    poisoning, brown
    recluse
spina bifida cystica
splenitis
sprain
sprain of ankle or foot
sprain of back
stomach cancer
stomatitis
stomatitis, catarrhal
stomatitis, mercurial
stomatitis parasitica
stomatitis, ulcerative
stramonium poisoning
stricture of urethra
stroke
sty(e)
subclavian steal
    syndrome
suffocation
sulfuric acid poisoning
superior vena cava
    syndrome
sycosis
symblepharon
synovitis
syphilis

syphilitic macules
syringomyelia
tabes dorsalis
tapeworm
Tay-Sachs disease
tenosynovitis crepitans
tetany
thromboangiitis
  obliterans
thrombosis
thrombosis, coronary
thyrotoxicosis
tincture of iodine
  poisoning
tinea
tin poisoning
toadstool poisoning
tongue-tie
tonsillitis, acute
toxemia
transient ischemic
  attack
trichiasis
trichinosis
Trichomonas vaginalis
tricuspid atresia
tugging, tracheal
tularemia
turpentine poisoning
typhoid fever
typhus
unconsciousness
undernutrition
uremia
urticaria
uterus, prolapse of
uterus, rupture of, in
  pregnancy
vaginitis
varicella
varicocele
varicose veins
wen
wound, bullet
wound, cellulitis of
yaws
yellow fever

TREATMENT
abetalipoproteinemia
abruptio placentae
abscess, brain
acathisia

acetaminophen
  poisoning
acne, cystic
acne vulgaris
acrodermatitis
  enteropathica
acrodynia
acromegaly
Actinomyces israelii
actinomycosis
Adams-Stokes syndrome
Addison's disease
adult respiratory
  distress syndrome
  (ARDS)
afibrinogenemia
afterpains
AIDS
alcoholism, acute
alcoholism, chronic
alcohol withdrawal
  syndrome
alkali poisoning
alkalosis, metabolic
alkalosis, respiratory
allergy
alopecia
amebiasis
amenorrhea
ammonia toxicity
anaphylactic shock
ancylostomiasis
anemia
anemia, pernicious
anetoderma
aneurysm, aortic
angel's trumpet
angina pectoris
angina, unstable
angioedema
anhidrosis
anthrax
aphthous ulcer
appendicitis
appendicitis, chronic
arc eyes
arevareva
ariboflavinosis
arsenic poisoning
arteriosclerosis
arteritis, temporal
arthritis
arthritis, gonorrheal
arthritis, rheumatoid

arum family poisoning
Ascaris lumbricoides
aspergillosis
aspirin poisoning
asteatosis cutis
asthenia,
  neurocirculatory
asthma
ataxia, locomotor
athlete's foot
attention deficit disorder
autonomic hyperreflexia
babesiosis
back pain
balanitis xerotica
  obliterans
balantidiasis
Barlow's disease
bartonellosis
bedbug
bedsore
bee sting
Behçet's syndrome
Bell's palsy
bends
beriberi
black eye
blastomycosis
blepharophimosis
  syndrome
blind loop syndrome
blister
blister, blood
boil
boric acid poisoning
botulism
botulism, infant
brass poisoning
breast cancer
bronchi, foreign bodies in
bronchiectasis
bronchitis, acute
bronchitis, chronic
bronchopneumonia
bronchospasm
brucellosis
bruxism
Buerger's disease
buphthalmia,
  buphthalmos
burn
burn, brush
burn, inhalation
burning mouth

enterotoxigenic
exfoliative dermatitis
familial periodic
  paralysis
fasciolopsiasis
febrile convulsions
fecal impaction
fever
fibroma, uterine
fibromyalgia
fire ant stings
fish poisoning
flames, inhalation of
flatus
flea bites
folliculitis decalvans
foot and mouth disease
Fordyce-Fox disease
fracture
fructose intolerance
fumes, nitric acid
furunculus
gallstone
gangrene, gas
Gardnerella vaginalis
  vaginitis
gas, lewisite
gas, lung irritant
gas, nose irritant
gas, tear
gas, vesicant
gas distention
gastritis, acute
gastritis, chronic
gastroesophageal reflux
gastroesophageal reflux,
  chronic
Gaucher's disease
Gilles de la Tourette's
  syndrome
gingivitis, acute
  necrotizing
glanders
glaucoma
glossitis, acute
gluten-induced
  enteropathy
gonorrhea
gout
granuloma inguinale
Grave's ophthalmopathy
Grover's disease
growing pains
Guillain-Barré

syndrome
gumboil
Haemophilus influenza
  type b infections
hay fever
headache
headache, postlumbar
  puncture
heatstroke
hematemesis
hemlock poisoning
hemochromatosis
hemolytic disease of the
  newborn
hemolytic uremic
  syndrome
hemophilia
hemoptysis
hemorrhage, cerebral
hemorrhage of knee
hemorrhage, stomach
hemorrhage, thigh
hemorrhage, uterine
hemorrhagic
  nephrosonephritis
hemorrhoid
hepatic coma
hepatitis, acute viral
hepatitis, amebic
hepatolenticular
  degeneration
hernia
heroin toxicity
herpangina
herpes genitalis
herpes simplex
herpes zoster
hiccough, hiccup
hip, dislocation of,
  backward
hip, dislocation of,
  downward
hip, dislocation of,
  forward
Hirschsprung's disease
histoplasmosis
Hodgkin's disease
hornet sting
human bite
hydrocephalus
hydronephrosis
hydropericardium
hyperemesis gravidarum
hypereosinophilic

syndrome, idiopathic
hyperhidrosis
hypertensive crisis
hyperthyroidism
hypertrophy,
  pseudomuscular
hyperventilation
hypoacidity
hypothermia, accidental
hypothyroidism
hysteria
ichthyosis
idiopathic pulmonary
  fibrosis
ileitis, regional
impetigo contagiosa
impotence, impotency
incontinence
influenza
insulin shock
interstitial cystitis
intestinal obstruction
iritis
irritable bowel syndrome
irritant poisons
kala-azar
Kawasaki disease
keloid
keratitis
keratoconjunctivitis
  sicca
keratosis pilaris
keratosis, seborrheic
kwashiorkor
lactase deficiency
  syndrome
lactose intolerance
Landouzy-Dejerine
  dystrophy
laryngitis, acute
  catarrhal
laryngitis, atrophic
laryngitis, chronic
laryngitis, syphilitic
laryngostenosis,
  occlusion
Lassa fever
lead encephalopathy,
  acute
lead poisoning, acute
lead poisoning, chronic
Leeuwenhoek's disease
Legionnaires' disease
leprosy

peritonitis, chronic
personality disorders
pertussis
Peyronie's disease
pharyngitis, acute
pharyngitis, chronic
pharyngoconjunctival
  fever, acute
phencyclidine
  hydrochloride
phenothiazine
phenylketonuria
pheochromocytoma
phimosis
phlegmasia alba dolens
phycomycosis
pinta
pityriasis rosea
placenta previa
plague
pneumocystis carinii
  pneumonia
pneumonia,
  desquamative
  interstitial
pneumonia, primary
  atypical
poisoning, arsenic
poisoning, lead
poisoning, potato
poison ivy dermatitis
pokeroot poisoning
polyarteritis (nodosa)
polycystic ovary
  syndrome
polycythemia vera
polymer fume fever
polymyositis
polyneuropathy, diabetic
postmyocardial
  infarction syndrome
post-term pregnancy
potbelly
Pott's disease
premenstrual tension
  syndrome
prickly heat
prostate cancer
prurigo
pruritus
pruritus ani
pseudogout
psoriasis
ptosis, abdominal

puerperal sepsis
pyelonephritis
pyemia
pyloric obstruction
  and dilatation
pyloric stenosis
quadriplegia
rabies
ranula
rash, diaper
Raynaud's disease
Raynaud's phenomenon
Recklinghausen's
  disease
Reiter's syndrome
relapsing fever
renal failure, acute
renal tubular acidosis
respiratory distress
  syndrome of the
  premature infant
respiratory failure, acute
restless legs syndrome
retinal detachment
retinitis
retinitis pigmentosa
Reye's syndrome
rheumatic fever
rhinitis, acute
rhinitis, allergic
rhinitis, atrophic
rhinitis, chronic
  hypertrophic
rhinoscleroma
rickets
rickets, renal
ringworm
Rocky Mountain
  spotted fever
rosacea
rubella
rupia
scabies
scalded skin syndrome,
  staphylococcal
scalenus syndrome
scar, painful
scarlet fever
Schatzki ring
schizophrenia
  (schizophrenic
  disorders)
sciatica and low back
  pain

scleroderma
scombroid poisoning
scorpion sting
scrofula
scrofuloderma
scrub typhus
scurvy
seasickness
seborrhea
sepsis, puerperal
septic shock
serum sickness
severe combined
  immunodeficiency
  disease
sexual dysfunction
shellfish, paralytic
  poisoning from
shingles
shock
sickle cell anemia
sick sinus syndrome
sinusitis, acute
  suppurative
sinusitis, chronic
  hyperplastic
sleep, disorders of
smoke poisoning
snore
social phobias
somatoform disorders
spasm
spasm of esophagus
spider bites or
  poisoning, black
  widow
spider bites or
  poisoning, brown
  recluse
sprain
sprain of ankle or foot
sprain of back
sprue, tropical
staphyloma, total
startle syndromes
stature, short
status sternuens
steatoma
sterility
stiff man syndrome
stingray
Stokes-Adams syndrome
stomach cancer
stomatitis, catarrhal

stomatitis, mercurial
stomatitis parasitica
stomatitis, ulcerative
strabismus, paralytic
strabismus sursum
   vergens
streptobacillus
   moniliformis
Strongyloides stercoralis
sty(e)
suffocation
sulfuric acid poisoning
sunburn
sunstroke
swelling
swimming pool
   granuloma
sycosis
Sydenham's chorea
symblepharon
syphilis
syphilis, endemic
syringomyelia
tabes dorsalis
tachycardia, sinus
Taenia lata
Taenia solium
Tay-Sachs disease
tellurium poisoning
temporomandibular
   joint syndrome
tennis elbow

tenosynovitis crepitans
tetanus
thoracic squeeze
thrombophlebitis
thrombosis
thrombosis, coronary
thyroid storm
tic douloureux
tincture of iodine
   poisoning
tinea
tin poisoning
tongue-tie
tonsillitis, acute
torticollis, spasmodic
toxic-allergic syndrome
toxic shock syndrome
toxoplasmosis
trachoma
transfusion syndrome,
   multiple
trench fever
trichiasis
trichinosis
Trichomonas vaginalis
Trichuris trichiura
trigger finger
trypanosomiasis,
   South American
tuberculosis
tularemia
typhoid fever

typhus
unconsciousness
uremia
urethritis, nonspecific
urticaria
uterus, prolapse of
uterus, rupture of, in
   pregnancy
uveitis
vaginitis
vaginitis, candidal
vaginitis, nonspecific
varicella
varicocele
varicose veins
verruca
vitiligo
vomiting
von Willebrand's disease
wasp sting
Weil's disease
wen
Whipple's disease
Wilson's disease
wound, bullet
wound, cellulitis of
wound, contused
wound, lacerated
yaws
yellow fever
Zollinger-Ellison
   syndrome

LIST OF ILLUSTRATIONS

Illustrations are listed according to the main entry or subentry they accompany. Information in parentheses indicates the aspect shown or additional material illustrated. In most cases, each drawing falls on the same page as the entry it illustrates; however, when there is no space on that page for the illustration, it will appear on the preceding or following page.

LIST OF TABLES

ABBREVIATIONS USED IN TEXT*

ABBR	abbreviation	Gr.	Greek
ABNORM	abnormalities	i.e.	id est (that is)
ADM	administration	INCOMPAT	incompatibility
ADVAN	advantages	IND	indications
Amerind	American Indian	L.	Latin
amt.	amount	LL.	Late Latin
ANAT	anatomy	MD.	Middle Dutch
approx.	approximately	ME.	Middle English
AS	Anglo-Saxon	Med. L.	Medieval Latin
Brit.	British	NA	Nomina Anatomica
C	centigrade	NF	National Formulary
CHEM	chemical	NL	New Latin
Chem. symb.	chemical symbol	OB	obstetrics
CLASSIF	classification	O.Fr.	Old French
CNS	central nervous system	PATH	pathology
COMP	composition	pert.	pertaining
CONTRA	contraindication	phys	physical; physiology
DEVELOP	development	pl.	plural
DIAG	diagnosis	POSTOP	postoperative
DIFF. DIAG	differential diagnosis	PREVENT	prevention
		PROG	prognosis
DISADV	disadvantages	PROPH	prophylaxis
e.g.	exempli gratia (for example)	q.v.	quod vide (which see)
		rel.	related; relating
EQUIP	equipment	RS	related subjects
esp.	especially	sing.	singular
ETIOL	etiology	Sp.	Spanish
Ex.	example	sp. gr.	specific gravity
EXAM	examination	SYM	symptoms
F	Fahrenheit	SYMB	symbol
F.A.	first aid	SYN	synonym
Fr.	French	THERAP	therapeutic; therapy
fr.	from	TREAT	treatment
FUNCT	function	USP	United States Pharmacopeia
Ger.	German		

---

* Medical and charting abbreviations appear in the Appendix.

A

α. Alpha, q.v., first letter of Greek alphabet.

Å. angstrom unit.

A₂. aortic second sound.

a. accommodation; ampere; anode; anterior; aqua; area; artery.

ā. ante [L., before].

a-, an- [Gr., not]. Prefix meaning without, away from, not.

A.A., a.a. achievement age; Alcoholics Anonymous; amino acid; arteriae.

aa [Gr. ana, of each]. Prescription notation meaning the stated amount of each of the substances is to be used in compounding the prescription.

A.A.A. American Academy of Allergists; American Association of Anatomists.

A.A.A.S. American Association for the Advancement of Science.

A.A.C.N. American Association of Critical-Care Nurses; American Association of Colleges of Nursing, which is concerned with academic aspects of nursing education.

A.A.F.P. American Academy of Family Practice.

A.A.G.P. American Academy of General Practice, former name of the American Academy of Family Practice.

AAL. anterior axillary line.

A.A.M.A. American Association of Medical Assistants.

A.A.M.D. American Association on Mental Deficiency.

A.A.M.I. Association for the Advancement of Medical Instrumentation.

AAMT. American Association for Medical Transcription.

A.A.N. American Academy of Nursing. An organization formed by the American Nurses' Association. Membership in this honorary association is an indication that the person selected has made a significant contribution to nursing. A member is titled Fellow of the American Academy of Nursing, abbreviated F.A.A.N.

A.A.N.A. American Association of Nurse Anesthetists.

A.A.N.N. American Association of Neurological Nurses.

A.A.O.H.N. American Association of Occupational Health Nurses.

A.A.P. American Academy of Pediatrics; American Association of Pathologists.

A.A.P.A. American Academy of Physician Assistants.

Aaron's sign (ăr′ŏns) [Charles D. Aaron, U.S. physician, 1866–1951]. Distress in region of heart or stomach upon pressure over McBurney's point, q.v., in appendicitis.

AARP. American Association of Retired Persons.

A.A.R.T. American Association for Respiratory Therapy.

AAS. atomic absorption spectroscopy.

AASECT. American Association of Sex Educators, Counselors, and Therapists.

ab. antibody.

ab- [L. ab, from]. Prefix meaning from, away from, negative, absent.

Abadie's sign (ă-bă-dēz′). 1. [Charles A. Abadie, Fr. ophthalmologist, 1842–1932] In exophthalmic goiter, spasm of the levator palpebrae superioris. 2. [Jean Abadie, Fr. neurologist, 1873–1946] In tabes dorsalis, insensibility to pressure over the Achilles tendon.

A band. In heart muscle, dark-staining segment of a myofibril fiber. SYN: anisotropic disk; transverse disk.

abandonment. The abandoning, without adequate warning, of a patient needing further medical care by the person responsible for that care.

abaptiston (ă″băp-tĭs′tŏn) [Gr. abaptistos, not dipped]. Trephine that cannot slip and injure the brain.

abarognosis (ăb″ăr-ŏg-nō′sĭs) [Gr. a-, not, + baros, weight, + gnosis, knowledge]. Loss of ability to sense weight. SEE: baragnosis.

abarthrosis (ăb-ăr-thrō′sĭs) [L. ab, from, + Gr. arthron, joint, + osis, condition]. A movable joint or point upon which bones move freely upon each other. SYN: diarthrosis.

abarticular [″ + articulus, joint]. At a distance from a joint.

abarticulation. 1. Dislocation of a joint. 2. Diarthrosis. SYN: abarthrosis.

abasia (ă-bā′zē-ă) [Gr. a-, not, + basis, step]. Motor incoordination in walking. Inability to walk due to impairment of coordination.

　a. -astasia. Lack of motor coordination with inability to stand or walk. SYN: astasia-abasia.

　a. atactica. Uncertain movements in walking.

　a., paralytic. Abasia in which the leg muscles are paralyzed.

　a., paroxysmal trepidant. Abasia caused by trembling and sudden stiffening of legs on standing, making walking impossible. May be related to hysteria.

　a., spastic. A., paroxysmal trepidant, q.v.

abasic (ă-bā′sĭk). Pert. to abasia. SYN: aba-

tic.

abate (ă-bāt′) [L. *ab*, from, + *battere*, to beat]. 1. To lessen or decrease. 2. To cease or cause to cease.

abatement (ă-bāt′mĕnt). Decrease in severity of pain or symptoms.

abatic (ă-băt′ĭk). Pert. to abasia. SYN: *abasic*.

abaxial, abaxile (ăb-ăk′sē-al, -sĭl) [L. *ab*, from, + *axis*, axis]. 1. Not in line of axis of the body or a part. 2. At opposite end of the axis of a part.

Abbé-Zeiss apparatus, counting cell hemocytometer [Ernst Abbé, Ger. physicist, 1840–1905; Carl Zeiss, Ger. optician, 1816–1888]. A device for counting blood cells in a specific quantity of blood.

Abbott′s method [Edville G. Abbott, U.S. orthopedic surgeon, 1871–1938]. Treatment of scoliosis by a series of plaster jackets.

Abbott-Miller tube [William Osler Abbott, U.S. physician, 1902–1943; Thomas Grier Miller, U.S. physician, b. 1886]. A double-channel intestinal tube used to relieve intestinal distention. Commonly called Miller-Abbott tube, q.v.

ABC. *antigen-binding capacity; airway, breathing, circulation* (mnemonic for assessing status of emergency patients).

abdomen (ăb-dō′mĕn, ăb′dō-mĕn) [L., belly]. [NA] The portion of the trunk located between the back, below the diaphragm, and including the lower portion of the abdominopelvic cavity. Contains the stomach, lower part of esophagus, small and large intestines, liver, gallbladder, spleen, pancreas, and bladder. A serous membrane, the peritoneum, lines this cavity, but not all of the organs in the abdomen are covered by this membrane. SEE: *abdominal quadrants* for illus.

   a., acute. An abnormal condition of the abdomen in which there is a sudden, abrupt onset of severe pain. It requires immediate evaluation and diagnosis, as it may indicate a need for immediate surgical intervention. SYN: *surgical abdomen.*

   a., boat-shaped. A., scaphoid, q.v.

   a., carinate. A., scaphoid, q.v.

   a., navicular. A., scaphoid, q.v.

   a. obstipum. Congenital shortness of the rectus abdominis muscle.

   a., pendulous. Condition in which the excessively relaxed anterior wall of the abdomen hangs down over the pubis.

   a., scaphoid. Condition in which the anterior wall is hollowed, presenting a sunken appearance as in emaciation and some cerebral diseases. SYN: *a., boat-shaped; a., carinate; a., navicular.*

   a., surgical. A., acute, q.v.

abdominal (ăb-dŏm′ĭ-năl). Pert. to the abdo-

men.

abdominal cavity. The cavity within the abdomen. It is lined with a serous membrane, the peritoneum, and contains the following organs: stomach with lower portion of esophagus, small and large intestines (except sigmoid colon and rectum), liver, gallbladder, spleen, pancreas, kidneys, and ureters. It is continuous with the pelvic cavity; the two constitute the abdominopelvic cavity. SEE: *abdominal quadrants* for illus.

abdominal crisis. Severe pain in the abdominal area. Usually refers to the pain that occurs during sickle cell anemia crisis or that results from syphilis.

abdominal decompression. Technique used in obstetrics to facilitate childbirth. The abdominal area is surrounded by an airtight chamber in which pressure may be intermittently decreased below atmospheric pressure. During labor pains, the pressure is decreased and the uterus is permitted to work more efficiently because the abdominal muscles are elevated away from the uterus.

abdominal examination. INSPECTION: Visual examination of the abdomen is most satisfactorily performed while patient is supine with thighs slightly flexed. In the healthy individual, the abdomen is of an oval form, marked by elevations and depressions corresponding to abdominal muscles, umbilicus, and in some degree by form of adjacent viscera. It is larger relative to size of chest in children than in adults; more rotund and broader inferiorly in females than in males.

   Alterations in shape resulting from disease are enlargement (which may be general and symmetrical as in ascites, or partial and irregular from tumors, hypertrophy of such organs as the liver and spleen, or distention of portions of intestines by gas) and retraction (as in extreme emaciation and in several forms of cerebral disease, esp. noticeable in tubercular meningitis of children).

   The respiratory movements of the abdominal walls bear a certain relation to movements of the thorax and are often increased when the latter are arrested and vice versa; thus, abdominal movements are increased in pleurisy, pneumonia, and pericarditis, but decreased or wholly suspended when disease causes abdominal pain or in peritonitis.

   The superficial abdominal veins are also at times visibly enlarged, indicating an obstruction to the flow of blood, either in the portal system (as in cirrhosis) or in the inferior vena cava.

   AUSCULTATION: Listening to sounds produced in the abdomen. Useful in diagnosing normal sounds produced by peristaltic action of intestines, aneurysm of abdominal aorta, fetal heart sounds, and vascular sounds from placenta. Intestinal sounds may be absent in paralytic ileus, q.v.

PERCUSSION: Patient should be placed in same position as for palpation, and percussion should be for the most part mediate. In exploring abdomen by means of percussion, finger should first be placed immediately below the xiphoid cartilage, pressed firmly down, and carried along the median line toward the pubes, striking it all the way, now forcibly, now gently. The different tones of stomach, colon, and small intestines will be distinctly heard. Percussion should then be made laterally, alternately to one side, then the other, until whole surface is percussed. Abdominal aneurysm gives dullness or flatness over it unless a distended intestine lies above it.

PALPATION: May be performed with tips of fingers, whole hand, or both hands; pressure may be slight or forcible, continuous or intermittent. To obtain greatest amount of information, place patient in supine position with head slightly raised and thighs flexed. The head is supported in order to relax the abdominal wall. It is sometimes necessary to place patient in standing position or leaning forward.

Palpation is of assistance in detecting size, consistency, and position of viscera, existence of tumors and swellings, and whether the tumors change position with respiration or are movable. Also ascertain whether tenderness exists in any portion of the abdominal cavity, if pain is increased or relieved by firm pressure, and if pain is accentuated by sudden release of firm pressure, i.e., rebound tenderness.

Impulse, if one exists, is systolic and expansive, although when situated high there also may be a slight diastolic movement. A thrill is rarely perceptible. Surface of tumor is usually rounded and smooth but may be nodular. Effusion of blood into surrounding tissues may produce lobulations.

abdominal gestation. Abdominal pregnancy. Extrauterine pregnancy in belly cavity.

abdominalgia (ăb-dŏm-ĭn-ăl'jē-ă) [L. *abdomen,* belly, + Gr. *algos,* pain]. Pain in the abdomen.

abdominal inguinal ring. The internal opening of the inguinal canal, bounded inferiorly by the inguinal ligament, medially by the inferior epigastric vessels, and above and laterally by the lower free border of the transversus abdominis muscle. SEE: *canal, inguinal; ring, abdominal; ring, inguinal; hernia.*

abdominal muscles. The group of four muscles which make up the abdominal wall, consisting of: 1. the external oblique, which is the most superficial muscle, whose fibers are directed downward and medially from the lower ribs to the linea alba and pelvis; 2. the internal oblique, whose fibers are directed upward and medially from the iliac crest and lumbodorsal fascia to the lower ribs; 3. the rectus abdominis, which is a vertically oriented muscle from the crest of the pubis to the cartilages of the 5th, 6th, and 7th ribs and xiphoid process; and 4. transversus abdominis, whose fibers are oriented transversely. These muscles participate in a variety of functions including flexion, side bending and rotation of the trunk, stabilization of the trunk in the upright posture, expiratory phase of respiration, coughing, and the Valsalva maneuver.

abdominal quadrants. Four parts or divisions of the abdomen determined by drawing imaginary vertical and horizontal lines through the umbilicus. The quadrants and their contents are:

Right upper quadrant (RUQ): right lobe of liver, gallbladder, part of transverse colon, part of pylorus, hepatic flexure, right kidney, and duodenum; *Right lower q. (RLQ):* cecum, ascending colon, small intestine, appendix, bladder if distended, right ureter, right spermatic duct in male; right ovary and right tube, and uterus if enlarged in female; *Left upper q. (LUQ):* left lobe of liver, stomach, transverse colon, splenic flexure, pancreas, left kidney, and spleen; *Left lower q. (LLQ):* small intestine, left ureter, sigmoid flexure, descending colon, bladder if distended, left spermatic duct in male; left ovary and left tube, and uterus if enlarged in female. SEE: illus.

abdominal reflexes. Contraction of the muscles of the abdominal wall upon stimulation of the overlying skin. Absence of these reflexes indicates damage to the pyramidal tract.

abdominal regions. The abdomen and its external surface are divided into nine regions by four imaginary planes: two horizontal, one at the level of the ninth costal cartilage (or the lowest point of the costal arch), and the other at the level of the highest point of the iliac crest; two vertical, through the centers of the inguinal ligaments (or through the nipples or through the centers of the clavicles) or curved and coinciding with the lateral borders of the two abdominal rectus muscles. SEE: *abdominal quadrants* for illus.

abdominal rings. The apertures in the abdominal wall. *External:* an interval in aponeurosis of external oblique muscle, just

RIGHT UPPER QUADRANT
LEFT UPPER QUADRANT
RIGHT LOWER QUADRANT
LEFT LOWER QUADRANT

UMBILICAL REGION
EPIGASTRIC REGION

RIGHT HYPOCHONDRIAC REGION
LEFT HYPOCHONDRIAC REGION
RIGHT LUMBAR REGION
LEFT LUMBAR REGION
RIGHT INGUINAL (ILIAC) REGION
LEFT INGUINAL (ILIAC) REGION

HYPOGASTRIC REGION (PUBIC)

ABDOMINAL QUADRANTS AND REGIONS

above and to outer side of crest of the pubic bone. *Triangular:* about one inch from base to apex and one-half inch transversely; provides passage for spermatic cord in the male and round ligament in the female. *Internal* or *deep:* situated in the transversalis fascia, midway between the anterior superior spine of ilium and symphysis pubis, ½ in. (1.8 cm) above Poupart's ligament; oval form, larger in the male. Surrounds spermatic cord in the male and round ligament in the female.

abdominal section. Abdominal incision for any operation on abdominal organs. SYN: *laparotomy,* q.v.

abdomino- (ăb-dŏm′ĭ-nō). Combining form rel. to the abdomen.

abdominocardiac reflex (ăb-dŏm″ĭ-nō-kăr′dē-ăk). A change in heart rate, usually a slowing, resulting from mechanical stimulation of abdominal viscera.

abdominocentesis (ăb-dŏm″ĭ-nō-sĕn-tē′sĭs) [L. *abdomen,* belly, + Gr. *kentesis,* puncture]. Puncture of the abdomen with an instrument for withdrawal of fluid from the abdominal cavity. SYN: *paracentesis, abdominal.*

abdominocystic [″ + Gr. *kystis,* bladder]. Pert. to the abdomen and bladder.

abdominodiaphragmatic breathing. A controlled breathing pattern using reciprocal action of the abdominal muscles for expiration and diaphragm for inspiration; frequently used to maintain control during exertion or regain control when in a state of dyspnea.

abdominogenital (ăb-dŏm″ĭ-nō-jĕn′ĭ-tăl). Pert. to the abdomen and genital organs.

abdominohysterectomy [″ + Gr. *hystera*, womb, + *ektome*, excision]. Removal of uterus through abdominal incision.

abdominohysterotomy (ăb-dŏm″ĭ-nō-hĭs-tĕr-ŏt′ō-mē) [″ + ″ + *tome*, incision]. Incision of the uterus through a surgical opening in the abdomen.

abdominoperineal. Concerning the abdomen and perineal area.

abdominoplasty. Plastic surgery on the abdomen.

abdominoscopy (ăb-dŏm″ĭ-nŏs′kŏ-pē) [″ + Gr. *skopein*, to examine]. Examination of the abdominal cavity and its contents by use of an endoscope. SEE: *peritoneoscopy*.

abdominoscrotal [″ + *scrotum*, bag]. Pert. to the abdomen and scrotum.

abdominoscrotal muscle. Cremaster muscle.

abdominothoracic (ăb-dŏm″ĭ-nō-thō-ră′sĭk) [″ + Gr. *thorax*, chest]. Pert. to the abdomen and thorax.

abdominothoracic arch. The costal arch; the anterior and lateral boundary between the line dividing the thorax and the abdomen.

abdominouterotomy (ăb-dŏm″ĭ-nō-ū-tĕr-ŏt′ō-mē) [″ + *uterus*, womb, + Gr. *tome*, incision]. Abdominohysterotomy, q.v.

abdominovaginal (ăb-dŏm″ĭ-nō-văj′ĭ-năl) [″ + *vagina*, sheath]. Pert. to the abdomen and vagina.

abdominovesical (ăb-dŏm″ĭ-nō-vĕs′ĭ-kăl) [″ + *vesica*, bladder]. Pert. to the abdomen and urinary bladder.

abducens (ăb-dū′sĕnz) [L., drawing away]. Pert. to drawing away from the median line of the body.

    a. labiorum. Muscle that elevates angle of mouth. SYN: *caninus muscle; levator anguli oris muscle*. SEE: *Muscles* in *Appendix*.

    a. oculi. Musculus rectus lateralis bulbi.

abducens muscle. Rectus lateralis muscle of eye, which moves the eyeball outward. SEE: *Muscles* in *Appendix*.

abducens nerve. Sixth cranial nerve; it innervates rectus lateralis muscle of eye. SEE: *cranial nerves*.

abducent (ăb-dū′sĕnt) [L. *abducens*, drawing away]. 1. Abducting, leading away from. 2. Abducens, q.v.

abducent nerve. Abducens nerve, q.v.

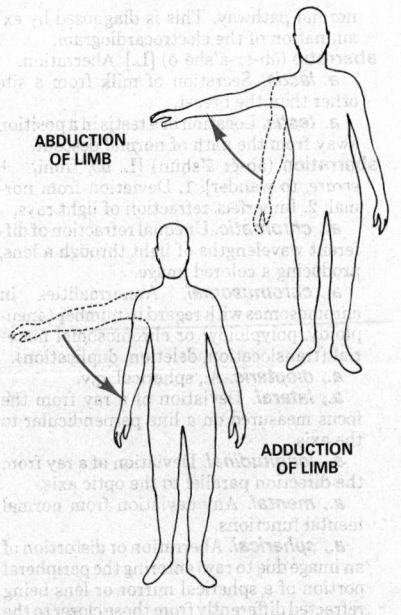

ABDUCTION OF LIMB

ADDUCTION OF LIMB

abduct (ăb-dŭkt′) [L. *abductus*, led away]. To draw away from the median plane of the body or one of its parts.

abduction (ăb-dŭk′shŭn). 1. The lateral movement of the limbs away from median plane of body, or the lateral bending of the head or trunk. SEE: illus. 2. The movement of the digits away from the axial line of a limb. 3. Outward rotation of the eyes.

abductor (ăb-dŭk′tor). A muscle that upon contraction draws a part away from median plane of body or axial line of an extremity. Opposite of adductor. SEE: *Muscles* in *Appendix*.

abenteric (ăb-ĕn-tĕr′ĭk) [L. *ab*, from, + Gr. *enteron*, intestine]. Rel. to or involving organs located outside the intestines.

Abernethy, John (ăb′ĕr-nē″thē). British surgeon, 1764–1831.

    A.'s fascia. A layer of areolar tissue separating the external iliac artery from the iliac fascia over the psoas muscle.

    A.'s sarcoma. A circumscribed, usually malignant, fatty tumor occurring principally on the trunk.

aberrant (ăb-ĕr′ănt) [L. *ab*, from, + *errare*, to wander]. Deviating from normal. SYN: *abnormal.*

aberrant conduction. In the electrical conduction system of the heart, the condition of the electrical stimulus traveling via an abnormal pathway. This is diagnosed by examination of the electrocardiogram.

aberratio (ăb-ĕr-ā′shē-ō) [L.]. Aberration.

   a. lactis. Secretion of milk from a site other than the breast.

   a. testis. Location of a testis in a position away from the path of normal descent.

aberration (ăb-ĕr-ā′shŭn) [L. *ab*, from, + *errare*, to wander]. 1. Deviation from normal. 2. Imperfect refraction of light rays.

   a., chromatic. Unequal refraction of different wavelengths of light through a lens, producing a colored image.

   a., chromosomal. Abnormalities in chromosomes with regard to number (aneuploidy, polyploidy) or chromosomal material (translocation, deletion, duplication).

   a., diopteric. A., spherical, q.v.

   a., lateral. Deviation of a ray from the focus measured on a line perpendicular to the axis.

   a., longitudinal. Deviation of a ray from the direction parallel to the optic axis.

   a., mental. Any deviation from normal mental functions.

   a., spherical. Aberration or distortion of an image due to rays entering the peripheral portion of a spherical mirror or lens being refracted differently from those closer to the center. Thus the peripheral rays are focused on the optical axis at a different point from the central rays.

abetalipoproteinemia (ā-bā″tă-lĭp″ō-prō′tēn-ē′mē-ă) [Gr. *a-*, not, + *beta* + *lipos*, fat, + *protos*, first, + *haima*, blood]. A rare inherited disease characterized by defective synthesis of apoprotein B, with resulting absence of chylomicrons, and very low and low-density lipoproteins in plasma. Clinically there is malabsorption, fat, ataxia, neuropathy, retinitis pigmentosa, and acanthocytosis of red blood cells.
   TREAT: Vitamin E.

abevacuation (ăb-ē-văk″ū-ā′shŭn) [L. *ab*, from, + *evacuare*, to empty]. 1. Abnormal evacuation, either excessive or deficient. 2. Metastases.

abeyance (ă-bā′ăns) [O. Fr.]. A temporary suspension of activity, sensation, or pain.

ABGs. *arterial blood gases.*

ability. Being able to accomplish a mental or physical task.

   a., verbal. Being able to use words, either spoken or written, to communicate in an effective manner.

abiogenesis (ăb-ē-ō-jĕn′ĕ-sĭs) [Gr. *a-*, not, + *bios*, life, + *genesis*, generation, birth]. Spontaneous generation of life; theoretical production of living from nonliving matter.

abiogenetic, abiogenous (ăb-ē-ō-jĕ-nĕt′ĭk, ăb-ē-ŏj′ĭ-nŭs). Pert. to spontaneous genera-

tion.

abiologic, abiological (ā-bī-ō-lŏj′ĭk, -ăl). Not related to biology or the science of life.

abiosis (ăb-ē-ō′sĭs) [Gr. *a-*, not, + *bios*, life, + *osis*, condition]. Absence of life.

abiotic (ăb-ē-ŏt′ĭk). Incompatible with life; not viable.

abiotrophy (ăb-ē-ŏt′rō-fē) [″ + ″ + *trophe*, nourishment]. Premature loss of vitality or degeneration of tissues and cells with consequent loss of endurance and resistance.

abirritant (ăb-ĭr′ĭ-tănt) [L. *ab*, from, + *irritare*, to irritate]. Relieving irritation; soothing.

abirritation (ăb″ĭr-rĭ-tā′shŭn). 1. Asthenia or atony. 2. Decreased response to stimuli.

ablactation (ăb-lăk-tā′shŭn) [L. *ab*, from, + *lactatio*, suckling]. Cessation of milk secretion; weaning.

ablate (ăb-lāt′) [L. *ablatus*, taken away]. To remove, esp. by excision.

ablatio (ăb-lā′shē-ō) [L., carrying away]. Ablation, removal, detachment.

   a. placentae. Premature detachment of a normally situated placenta; abruptio placentae, q.v. SEE: *placenta.*

   a. retinae. Detachment of retina. SEE: *retina.*

ablation (ăb-lā′shŭn) [L. *ab*, from, + *latus*, carried]. Removal of a part, as by incision.

-able. Suffix indicating ability or capacity for.

ABLEDATA. Computerized database of commercially available products for rehabilitation and independent living. For information, contact Newington Children's Hospital, 181 East Cedar Street, Newington, CT 06111. Telephone is (800)344-5405 or (203)667-5405.

ablepharia (ăb-lĕ-fā′rē-ă) [Gr. *a-*, not, + *blepharon*, eyelid]. Congenital absence of or reduction in size of the eyelids.

ablepharon (ă-blĕf′ă-rŏn). Ablepharia.

ablepharous (ă-blĕf′ă-rŭs). Without eyelids.

ablephary (ă-blĕf′ă-rē). Ablepharia.

ablepsia (ă-blĕp′sē-ă) [Gr. *a-*, not, + *blepein*, to see]. Lack of or loss of sight. Blindness.

abluent (ăb′lū-ĕnt) [L. *ab*, from, + *luens*, washing]. An agent possessing cleansing qualities, as a detergent.

ablution (ăb-lū′shŭn). A cleansing or washing.

abnormal (ăb-nor′măl) [L. *ab*, from, + *norma*, rule]. Deviating from normal. SYN: *aberrant.*

abnormality (ăb″nor-măl′ĭ-tē). Deviation from normal. SYN: *aberration.*

abocclusion (ăb″ō-kloo′zhŭn). Dentition in which the teeth of the mandible and the maxilla are not in contact.

aborad (ăb-ō′răd) [″ + *oris*, mouth]. Away

from the mouth.

aboral (ăb-ō′răl). Opposite to, or away from, the mouth.

abort (ă-bort′) [L. *abortare*, to miscarry]. 1. To expel an embryo or fetus prior to viability. 2. To arrest progress of disease. 3. To arrest growth or development. 4. To discontinue an effort or project before its completion.

abortifacient (ă-bor-tĭ-fā′shĕnt) [L. *abortio*, abortion, + *facere*, to make]. Anything used to cause or induce an abortion. SEE: *RU486*.

abortion (ă-bor′shŭn) [L. *abortio*]. The termination of pregnancy before the fetus reaches the stage of viability. The legal definition of viability differs from state to state, usually 20 to 24 weeks. Some premature neonates greater than 24 weeks or 500 gm are viable.

SYM: Abdominal cramps and bleeding from vagina, sometimes with clots and bits of tissue.

ETIOL: Among most common causes are faulty development of embryo, abnormalities of the placenta, endocrine disturbances, acute infectious diseases, severe trauma, and shock. Problems related to uterus, genetic factors, immunologic factors, use of certain drugs.

NURSING IMPLICATIONS: Evaluate and support patient's physical condition. Monitor vital signs, fluid status, and progress of patient. Observe character and amount of vaginal bleeding, being careful to preserve embryonic or fetal tissue. Evaluate onset, intensity, and location. Be alert for shock due to excessive blood loss; also monitor patient for development of infection or disseminated intravascular coagulation (DIC), q.v.

Assess and support the patient's psychological status, remaining with her to help allay anxiety. Be aware of the coping and defense mechanisms utilized, and be alert for responses such as anger, guilt, depression, sadness, happiness, or grief. Provide appropriate support for the patient. Patient may require long-term psychological and obstetrical counseling.

Following abortion, instruct patient to report excessive bleeding, pain, inflammation, or fever; avoid intercourse, tampons, and douching until follow-up examination in 2 weeks.

If the patient is to have surgical completion of the abortion, explain the procedure to her.

a., accidental. Abortion that occurs spontaneously.

a., ampullar. Tubal abortion occurring from the ampulla of the oviduct.

a., artificial. Abortion surgically induced.

a., complete. Abortion in which the complete products of conception have been expelled.

a., criminal. Illegal abortion.

a., elective. Abortion done at the request of the mother. It is not done for therapeutic reason(s).

a., habitual. Three or more consecutive spontaneous abortions.

a., imminent. Impending abortion characterized by bleeding and colicky pains that increase. Cervix is usually effaced and patulous.

a., incomplete. Abortion in which part of the products of conception has been retained in the uterus.

a., induced. Abortion brought on intentionally. Abortions may be induced by use of drugs, by use of suction or scraping of lining of uterus for removal of the products of conception, or by injection of sterile hypertonic solutions into the amniotic cavity. SEE: *curettage, uterine; RU486*.

a., inevitable. Abortion that cannot be halted.

a., infected. Abortion accompanied by infection of retained material with resultant febrile reaction.

a., missed. Abortion in which the fetus has died prior to the twentieth completed week of gestation but the products of conception are retained in the uterus for eight weeks or longer. This term implies that the diagnosis was erroneously delayed. The use of ultrasound permits diagnosis of a nonviable fetus prior to eight weeks following fetal death. Thus, to term such a condition "missed" abortion is incorrect.

a., nontherapeutic. Elective abortion, q.v.

a., septic. Abortion in which there is an infection of the products of conception and the endometrial lining of uterus.

a., spontaneous. Abortion occurring without apparent cause. SYN: *miscarriage*. SEE: *Nursing Diagnoses* in *Appendix*.

a., therapeutic. Abortion performed when the mental or physical health of the mother would be endangered by continuation of the pregnancy or when the fetus has a known condition incompatible with life.

a., threatened. The appearance of signs and symptoms of possible loss of fetus. Vaginal bleeding with or without intermittent pain is usually the first sign. If fetus is still alive and attachment to uterus has not been interrupted, pregnancy may continue. Absolute bedrest and sedation recommended, with avoidance of coitus, douches, stress, or cathartics.

a., tubal. 1. A spontaneous abortion in which the fetus has been expelled through the distal end of the uterine tube. 2. The escape of the products of conception into the peritoneal cavity by way of the uterine tube.

abortionist (ă-bor′shŭn-ĭst). One who performs an abortion.

abortive (ă-bor′tĭv) [L. *abortivus*]. 1. Preventing the completion of something. 2. Abortifacient; that which prevents the normal continuation of pregnancy.

abortus (ă-bor′tŭs) [L.]. An aborted fetus.

aboulia. SEE: *abulia.*

ABP. *arterial blood pressure.*

abrachia (ă-brā′kē-ă) [Gr. *a-*, not + L. *brachium,* arm]. Congenital absence of arms.

abrachiocephalia (ă-brā″kē-ō-sĕ-fā′lē-ă) [″ + ″ + *kephale,* head]. Congenital absence of arms and head.

abradant (ă-brăd′ĕnt). An abrasive.

abrade (ă-brād′) [L. *ab,* from, + *radere,* to scrape]. 1. To chafe. 2. To roughen or remove by friction.

abrasion (ă-brā′zhŭn) [″ + *radere,* to scrape]. 1. A scraping away of a portion of skin or of a mucous membrane as a result of injury or by mechanical means, as in dermabrasion for cosmetic purposes. SEE: *avulsion; bruise.* 2. The wearing away of the substance of a tooth. Normally occurs from mastication; may be accomplished by mechanical or chemical means.

abrasive. 1. Producing abrasion. 2. That which abrades.

abreaction (ăb″rē-ăk′shŭn) [″ + *re,* again, + *actus,* acting]. In psychoanalysis, release or discharge of emotional tension by consciously recalling or acting out a painful experience that had been either forgotten or repressed. Abreaction may allow this painful or consciously intolerable experience to become bearable because of the insight gained during the process. The method used to bring about abreaction is termed catharsis, q.v.

abruptio (ă-brŭp′shē-ō) [L. *abruptus*]. A tearing away from.

a. placentae. Premature detachment of normally situated placenta after the 20th week of gestation; ablatio placentae. SEE: *placenta.*

SYM: Hemorrhage, concealed or evident, or a combination of both. Pain may be constant, accompanied by a tetanic contraction if a large portion or all of the placenta separates; or there may be rhythmic uterine contractions as in labor. Increased fetal movements and changes in heart rate until fetus dies. Albumin in urine. Anemia.

ETIOL: Unknown. May be associated with toxemia, hypofibrinogenemia, and disseminated intravascular coagulation.

PATH: Extravasation of blood between placenta and uterine wall, occasionally between muscle fibers of the uterus. SEE: *Couvelaire uterus.*

TREAT: In mild cases, rest in bed. In severe cases, shock must first be combated. A soft and partially dilated cervix is an indication for immediate artificial rupture of membranes followed by natural or artificial induction of labor. If the fetus is alive and if the mother's cervix is firm and not dilated, cesarean section is the treatment of choice. If the uterus fails to contract after cesarean section, an immediate hysterectomy usually is necessary.

NURSING IMPLICATIONS: Be alert for and attempt to prevent the development of serious maternal and fetal complications, such as shock, disseminated intravascular coagulation (DIC), q.v., and fetal death. Monitor patient's vital signs and fetal baseline data, including fetal heart rate and rhythm changes, position, and degree of engagement. Assess vaginal blood loss by keeping a perineal pad count, and record character and amount of blood loss, fundal height, and uterine contractions or tetany. Administer prescribed fluids and medications. Provide noninvasive measures to increase patient comfort and calm reassurance to reduce anxiety. Prepare the patient for labor induction, delivery, or surgery as appropriate. SEE: *Nursing Diagnoses* in *Appendix.*

ABS. *absolute.*

abscess (ăb′sĕs) [L. *abscessus,* a going away]. A localized collection of pus in any part of the body which is the result of disintegration or displacement of tissue. SEE: *inflammation; pus; suppuration.*

a., acute. Abscess with local symptoms of inflammation, with fluctuation, and pointing; i.e., about to rupture; also pressure and constitutional symptoms. Inflammation becomes intensified with increased heat, redness, swelling, and edema. Pain becomes throbbing and greater, with impaired loss of function of the part. The tissue over the abscess becomes elevated, soft, and eventually fluctuant; becomes discolored and necrotic. The abscess decreases in size when the pus is evacuated. Pressure symptoms occur, according to size and location. In floor of mouth or neck, swelling may cause dyspnea and dysphagia. Constitutional symptoms vary from slight to high fever (fever may be absent in a well walled-off abscess) with chills and sweats if associated with pyemia and septicemia. Any or all general symptoms may be absent in deep-seated abscesses except possible anemia and eventual loss of weight and strength.

The abscess may "point," i.e., come to a head and rupture, or at that mature stage it may be drained by incising it. If an abscess is left untreated, it may spread, become encapsulated or even absorbed.

a., alveolar. Abscess about root of a tooth in alveolar cavity. Usually the result of necrosis and infection of dental pulp following dental caries. SYN: *a., apical alveolar.*

a., amebic. 1. Abscess occurring in the liver, developing as a complication of amebic dysentery. Caused by *Entamoeba histolytica.* 2. Abscess in the brain caused by *Entamoeba histolytica.*

a., anorectal. Abscess in the tissue near the rectum. SYN: *a., ischiorectal; a., perirectal.*

a., apical. Abscess at the apex of lung or at extremity of root of a tooth.

a., appendiceal, appendicular. Pus formation around an inflamed vermiform appendix.

a., arthrifluent. A wandering abscess, q.v., having origin in a diseased joint.

a., atheromatous. Softening in the wall of a blood vessel as the result of atherosclerosis.

a., axillary. Abscess or multiple abscesses in axilla.

a., Bartholin. Abscess of Bartholin's gland.

a., bicameral. Abscess with two pockets.

a., bile duct. Abscess of the bile duct. SYN: *a., cholangitic.*

a., bilharziasis. Abscess in an intestinal wall caused by *Schistosoma.*

a., biliary. Abscess of the gallbladder.

a., blind. Abscess with no external opening, such as a dental granuloma.

a., bone. A., Brodie's, q.v.

a., brain. Intracranial abscess; one involving the brain or its membranes. It is seldom primary but usually occurs secondary to infections of middle ear, nasal sinuses, face, or skull, or from contamination from penetrating wounds or skull fractures. It may also have a metastatic origin arising from septic foci in the lungs (bronchiectasis, empyema, lung abscess), in bone (osteomyelitis), or in the heart (endocarditis). Infection of nerve tissue by the invading organism results in necrosis and liquefaction of the tissue, with edema of surrounding tissues.

Brain abscesses may be acute, subacute, or chronic. Their clinical manifestations depend on part of brain involved, size, virulence of infecting organisms, and other factors. SYN: *a., cerebral; a., intracranial.* SEE: *Nursing Diagnoses* in *Appendix.*

SYM: Severe and persistent headache usually localized over infected area; fever,

vomiting, vertigo, malaise, sometimes irritability and other mental symptoms.

TREAT: Chemotherapy; surgical intervention may be required.

a., breast. A., mammary, q.v.

a., Brodie's. Suppuration of articular end of a bone, esp. the tibia. SYN: *a., bone.*

a., bursal. Abscess in a bursa.

a., canalicular. Abscess of breast discharging into the milk ducts.

a., caseous. Abscess in which the pus has a cheesy appearance.

a., cerebral. A., brain, q.v. SYN: *a., intracranial.*

a., cholangitic. Abscess of the bile duct.

a., chronic. Abscess with pus but without signs of inflammation; usually of slow development. Formed by liquefaction of tuberculous tissue. May occur anywhere in or on the body but more frequently in the spine, hips, genitourinary tract, and lymph glands. Symptoms may be very mild. Pain when present is caused by pressure upon surrounding parts. Tenderness often absent. Chronic septic changes accompanied by afternoon fever may occur. Amyloid disease may develop if the abscess persists for a prolonged period. SYN: *a., cold.*

a., circumscribed. Abscess limited or confined by surrounding tissue.

a., circumtonsillar. Abscess around the tonsil. SYN: *a., peritonsillar; quinsy.*

a., cold. A., chronic, q.v.

a., collar-button. Two pus-containing cavities, one larger than the other, connected by a narrow channel. SYN: *a., shirt-stud.*

a., deep. Abscess arising from below the deep fascia.

a., dental. Abscess beside a tooth, usually near the root.

a., dentoalveolar. Abscess in the alveolar process surrounding the root of a tooth.

a., diffuse. A collection of pus not circumscribed by a well-defined capsule.

a., dry. Abscess that disappears without pointing or breaking.

a., embolic. Abscess due to movement of infectious material from the site of an infection to another site.

a., emphysematous. Abscess containing air or gas. SYN: *a., tympanitic.*

a., endamebic; a., entamebic. A., amebic, q.v.

a., epidural. A., extradural, q.v.

a., epiploic. Abscess in the omentum.

a., extradural. Abscess on the dura mater.

a., fecal. Abscess containing feces. SYN: *a., stercoral.*

a., filarial. Abscess caused by filaria, q.v.

a., follicular. Abscess forming in a follicle.

a., frontal. Abscess in the frontal lobe of the brain.

a., fungal. Abscess caused by a fungus.

a., gangrenous. Abscess attended with gangrene of surrounding parts.

a., gas. A tympanitic abscess; one containing gas due to presence of gas-forming organisms such as *Clostridium perfringens.*

a., gingival. Abscess of the gum.

a., gravitation. A., wandering, q.v.

a., helminthic. Abscess due to the presence of a parasitic worm.

a., hemorrhagic. Abscess containing blood.

a., hepatic. Abscess of the liver, esp. an amebic abscess.

a., hot. A., acute, q.v.

a., hypostatic. A., wandering, q.v.

a., idiopathic. Abscess due to an unknown cause.

a., iliac. Abscess in the iliac region.

a., interloop. Collections of pus between the folded surfaces of the small and large intestines and their mesenteries. May be associated with bowel perforations or Crohn's disease.

a., intracranial. A., brain, q.v. SYN: *a., cerebral.*

a., intradural. Abscess within the layers of the dura mater.

a., intramammary. A., mammary, q.v. SYN: *a., breast.*

a., intramastoid. A mastoid process abscess of the temporal bone.

a., ischiorectal. Abscess in the ischiorectal fossa.

a., kidney. Abscess or multiple abscesses of renal cortex. SYN: *a., renal.*

a., lacrimal. Suppuration of a lacrimal gland or in a lacrimal duct.

a., lacunar. Abscess in the urethral lacunae.

a., lateral; a., lateral alveolar. Abscess in periodontal tissue.

a., liver. A., hepatic, q.v.

a., lumbar. Abscess in the lumbar region.

a., lung. Abscess occurring in the lung. SEE: *empyema.*

a., lymphatic. Abscess of a lymph node.

a., mammary. Abscess in the female breast, esp. one involving the glandular tissue. Usually seen during lactation or at time of weaning. SYN: *a., breast; a., intramammary.*

a., marginal. Abscess near the orifice of the anus.

a., mastoid. Suppuration of the mastoid portion of the temporal bone.

a., mediastinal. Suppuration in the mediastinum.

a., metastatic. Secondary abscess at a distance from focus of infection.

a., migrating. Abscess at a distance from focus of disease with pus along fascial sheaths of muscles. SYN: *a., wandering.*

a.'s, miliary. Multiple small embolic abscesses.

a., milk. Mammary abscess during lactation.

a., mother. Primary abscess giving rise to other abscesses.

a., multiple. Group of abscesses accompanying pyemia.

a., mycotic. Abscess caused by fungi.

a., nocardial. Abscess caused by *Nocardia.*

a., orbital. Suppuration in the orbit.

a., ossifluent. Abscess dependent on degeneration of bone tissue.

a., otic cerebral. Abscess of the brain originating in the ear.

a., palatal. Abscess in an upper lateral incisor, erupting toward the palate.

a., palmar. Purulent effusion into the tissues of the palm of the hand.

a., pancreatic. Abscess of pancreatic tissue, usually as a complication of acute pancreatitis or abdominal surgery.

a., parafrenal. Abscess on the side of the frenulum of the penis. Usually involves Tyson's gland.

a., parametric; a., parametritic. Abscess between the folds of the broad ligaments of the uterus.

a., paranephric; a., paranephritic. Abscess in the tissues around the kidney.

a., parapancreatic. Abscess in the tissues adjacent to the pancreas.

a., parapharyngeal. Abscess between the muscles of the pharynx and the deep cervical fascia.

a., parietal. Periodontal abscess arising in the periodontal tissue other than the orifice through which the vascular supply enters the dental pulp.

a., parotid. Abscess of parotid gland.

a., pelvic. Abscess of the pelvic peritoneum, esp. Douglas' pouch.

a., pelvirectal. Deep rectal abscess.

a., perianal. Abscess of the skin around the anus.

a., periapical. Periodontal abscess at the root apex of a tooth.

a., pericemental. Alveolar abscess not involving the apex of a tooth.

a., pericoronal. Abscess around the crown of an unerupted molar tooth.

a., peridental. Abscess of periodontal tissue.

a., perinephric. Abscess in tissue about the kidney. SYN: *a., perirenal.*

a., periodontal. Abscess arising in the periodontal tissue (structures of support for teeth).

a., peripleuritic. Abscess in the tissue surrounding the parietal pleura.

a., periproctic. Abscess in the areolar tissue about the anus. SYN: *a., perirectal.*

a., perirectal. A., periproctic, q.v.

a., perirenal. A., perinephric, q.v.

a., peritoneal. Abscess within the peritoneal cavity usually following peritonitis.

a., peritonsillar. Abscess of the tissue around the tonsillar capsule. SYN: *a., circumtonsillar; quinsy.*

a., periureteral. Abscess of area around a ureter.

a., periurethral. Abscess in tissue surrounding the urethra.

a., perivesical. Abscess in tissue around the urinary bladder.

a., phlegmonous. An acute abscess in the connective tissue.

a., pneumococcic. Abscess due to infection with pneumococci.

a., postcecal. Abscess situated behind the cecum. SYN: *a., retrocecal.*

a., postmammary. A., retromammary, q.v.

a., prelacrimal. Abscess of the lacrimal bone producing a swelling at inner canthus of eye.

a., premammary. Subcutaneous or subareolar abscess of the mammary gland.

a., primary. Abscess originating at point of infection.

a., prostatic. Abscess within the prostate gland.

a., protozoal. Abscess caused by a protozoon.

a., psoas. Abscess with pus descending in sheath of psoas muscle due to vertebral disease, usually of tuberculous origin.

a., pulmonary. Abscess of the lungs. Suppuration of lung tissue with one or more localized areas of necrosis resulting in pulmonary cavitation.

a., pulp. 1. A cavity discharging pus formed in the pulp of a tooth. 2. Abscess of the tissues of the pulp of a finger.

a., pyemic. A metastatic abscess, usually multiple, due to pyogenic organisms.

a., rectal. Abscess in the rectum.

a., renal. Abscess or multiple abscesses of the renal cortex. SYN: *a., kidney.*

a., residual. Abscess occurring from old inflammatory products at the site of an earlier abscess.

a., retrocecal. A., postcecal, q.v.

a., retromammary. Abscess between the mammary gland and the chest wall.

a., retroperitoneal. Abscess located between the peritoneum and the posterior abdominal wall.

a., retropharyngeal. Abscess of the

lymph nodes in the walls of the pharynx. It sometimes simulates diphtheritic pharyngitis.

a., retrovesical. Abscess behind the bladder.

a., root. Abscess of the root of a tooth. SYN: *a., apical.*

a., sacrococcygeal. Abscess over the sacrum and coccyx.

a., satellite. Secondary abscess arising from and located near the primary abscess.

a., scrofulous. Abscess due to tuberculous degeneration of bone or lymph nodes.

a., secondary. A., embolic, q.v.

a., septicemic. Abscess resulting from septicemia.

a.'s, shirt-stud. Two pus-containing cavities, one larger than the other, connected by a narrow channel. SYN: *a., collarbutton.*

a., spermatic. Abscess of the seminiferous tubules.

a., spinal. Abscess due to necrosis of a vertebra.

a., splenic. Abscess of the spleen.

a., stercoral; a., stercoraceous. Abscess containing feces. SYN: *a., fecal.*

a., sterile. Abscess from which attempts to culture microorganisms are in vain.

a., stitch. Abscess formed about a stitch or suture.

a., streptococcal. Abscess caused by streptococci.

a., subaponeurotic. Abscess beneath an aponeurosis or fascia.

a., subarachnoid. Abscess of the midlayer of the covering of the brain and spinal cord.

a., subareolar. Abscess underneath the areola of the mammary gland, sometimes draining through the nipple.

a., subdiaphragmatic. Abscess beneath the diaphragm. SYN: *a., subphrenic.*

a., subdural. Abscess beneath the dura of brain or spinal cord.

a., subepidermal. Abscess beneath the epidermis.

a., subfascial. Abscess beneath the fascia.

a., subgaleal. Abscess beneath the galea aponeurotica; i.e., the epicranial aponeurosis.

a., submammary. Abscess beneath the mammary gland.

a., subpectoral. Abscess beneath the pectoral muscles.

a., subperiosteal. Bone abscess below the periosteum.

a., subperitoneal. Abscess between the parietal peritoneum and the abdominal wall.

a., subphrenic. A., subdiaphragmatic,

q.v.

a., subscapular. Abscess between the serratus anterior and the posterior thoracic wall.

a., subungual. Abscess beneath the fingernail. May follow injuries with pins, needles, or splinters.

a., sudoriparous. Abscess of a sweat gland.

a., superficial. Abscess occurring above the deep fascia.

a., suprahepatic. Abscess in the suspensory ligament between the liver and the diaphragm.

a., sympathetic. Abscess arising some distance from the primary cause.

a., syphilitic. Abscess occurring in the tertiary stage of syphilis.

a., thecal. Abscess in a tendon sheath.

a., thymus. Abscess of the thymus.

a., tonsillar. Acute suppurative tonsillitis.

a., tooth. A., alveolar, q.v.

a., traumatic. Abscess caused by injury.

a., tropical. Amebic abscess of the liver.

a., tuberculous. A., chronic, q.v.

a., tubo-ovarian. Abscess involving both the fallopian tube and the ovary.

a., tympanitic. Abscess that contains air or gas.

a., tympanocervical. Abscess arising in the tympanum and extending to the neck.

a., tympanomastoid. A combined abscess of the tympanum and mastoid.

a., urethral. Abscess in the urethra.

a., urinary. Abscess caused by escape of urine into the tissues.

a., urinous. Abscess that contains pus and urine.

a., verminous. Abscess that is caused by or contains insect larvae or other animal parasites.

a., wandering. Abscess at a distance from focus of disease with pus along fascial sheaths of muscles. SYN: *a., migrating.*

a., warm. A., acute, q.v.

a., worm. Abscess caused by or containing worms.

abscissa (ăb-sĭs′ă) [L. *abscindere*, to cut off]. In a graph of a two-dimensional coordinate system wherein horizontal and perpendicular lines are crossed in order to provide a frame of reference, the abscissa is the horizontal line or x-axis. The ordinate, q.v., is the vertical line or y-axis. SEE: illus.

abscission (ăb-sĭ′zhŭn) [L. *abscindere*, to cut off]. Removal by excision.

absconsio (ăb-skŏn′sē-ō) [L.]. A cavity or fossa.

abscopal (ăb-skō′păl). Concerning the effect of radiation on tissues of the same person or organism at some distance from the actual radiation site or target.

absence (ăb′sĕnz). 1. Brief temporary loss of consciousness, as may occur in petit mal epilepsy, q.v. SYN: *absentia epileptica.* 2. Lack of development of a structure.

absence seizure. Seizure in which there is a sudden lapse of consciousness for 2 to 10 seconds. There is usually a blank facial expression that may be accompanied by certain movements such as repeated eye-blinking or lip-smacking. There is no convulsion or fall. The patient resumes activity as if the seizure had not occurred. The seizure may be induced by voluntary hyperventilation for 2 to 3 minutes. This type of attack is characteristic of petit mal epilepsy.

NURSING IMPLICATIONS: Document the time, duration, patient expression, and any repetitive movements noted during the seizure, and evaluate the patient's response following the seizure. Provide support, reassurance, patient education.

absentia epileptica (ăb-sĕn′shē-ă) [L., absence]. Momentary loss of consciousness. There is no convulsion but there may be transient stereotyped muscle movement. SEE: *absence seizure; epilepsy.*

abs. feb. L. *absente febre*, in the absence of fever.

Absidia (ăb-sĭd′ē-ă). Genus of pathogenic fungi of the order Phycomycetes and the family Mucoraceae. SEE: *phycomycosis.*

absinthe, absinth (ăb′sĭnth) [L. *absinthium*, wormwood]. A liquor containing oil of wormwood, anise, and other herbs. It is highly toxic, esp. to the nervous system.

absinthism (ăb′sĭn-thĭzm). Deterioration of the nerve centers following excessive use of absinthe.

absolute. Unrestricted, complete.

absolute alcohol. Ethyl alcohol with not more than 1% of water by weight.

absolute scale. Temperature scale in which zero is at the point of absolute zero, q.v. SYN: *Kelvin scale.*

absolute temperature. Temperature measured on the absolute scale, q.v.

absolute zero. The lowest possible temperature, $-273.15°$C or $-459.67°$F; equal to zero on the absolute scale.

absorb (ăb-sorb′) [L. *absorbere*, to suck in]. To take in, suck up, or imbibe. SEE: *absorption; adsorb; adsorption.*

absorbance (ăb-sor′băns). The ability of a material or tissue to absorb radiation.

a., photometric. A photometrically measured quantity that is directly proportional to the concentration of a substance in solution. Also given as $A = 2 - \log \%T$, where T is transmittance. SEE: *Beer's law.*

absorbefacient (ăb-sor′bĕ-fā′shĕnt) [″ + *facere*, to make]. Causing or that which causes absorption.

absorbent (ăb-sor'běnt). 1. A substance that absorbs. 2. Having the power to absorb.

absorptiometer (ăb-sorp"shē-ŏm'ĕ-tĕr) [L. *absorptio*, absorption, + Gr. *metron*, measure]. 1. Instrument for measuring thickness of a layer of liquid, drawn by capillary attraction, between glass plates. 2. Instrument for measuring the absorption of gas by a liquid.

absorptiometry, dual photon. Use of two sources of radiation of different energies to measure the density of a material, esp. bone. SEE: *bone densitometry*.

absorption (ăb-sorp'shŭn) [L. *absorptio*]. 1. The taking up of liquids by solids, or of gases by solids or liquids. 2. The taking up of light or of its rays by black or colored rays. 3. The taking up by the body of radiant heat, causing a rise in body temperature. 4. The reduction in intensity of an x-ray beam as it passes through a substance. 5. The passage of a substance through some surface of the body into body fluids and tissues, as the passage of ether through the respiratory epithelium of lungs into the blood during anesthesia, or passage of oil of wintergreen through the skin, the result of several processes: diffusion, q.v., filtration, q.v., osmosis, q.v.

RS: adsorption; chondrolysis; imbibition; osmosis; resorption.

a., colon. Water (important in the conservation of body fluids) and products of bacterial action are normally absorbed esp. in the ascending colon. Some nutrients and drugs are absorbed by the lower bowel. In the human, cellulose is not digested or absorbed but passes from the body as unchanged residue. SEE: *fiber*.

a., cutaneous. Absorption through the skin.

a., disjunctive. Separation of a slough by absorption of a layer of adjacent healthy tissue.

a., external. Absorption of material by the skin and mucous membrane.

a., mouth. Some substances, but no nutrients, can be absorbed from the mouth; some drugs, esp. alkaloids, can be absorbed through the oral mucosa.

a., parenteral. Absorption from a site other than the gastrointestinal tract.

a., pathologic. Absorption into the blood or lymph of substances normally excreted or of a product of disease processes, e.g., pus.

a., percutaneous. A., cutaneous, q.v.

a., protein. In the digestive process, proteins are hydrolyzed to their constituent amino acids in the walls of the intestines. They are transported via the portal vein to the liver and then into the general circulation and to the tissues. Each tissue synthesizes its own form of protein from the amino acids received from the blood.

a., small intestine. The most important absorption of products of digestion occurs in the small intestines, esp. the ileum. Products of digestion absorbed from the gastrointestinal tract pass into either blood or lymph. The mesenteric veins unite to form the portal vein and carry such blood to the liver; the mesenteric lymphatics are called lacteals because, during absorption of a fatty meal, the lymph they contain looks milky and is called chyle. The lacteals empty into the cisterna chyli and are joined by lymphatics from other parts of the body; the mixed lymph travels, via the thoracic duct, to the subclavian vein, where it empties into the bloodstream.

a., stomach. Absorption of water, alcohol, and some salts through the gastric mucosa.

absorption lines. In spectroscopy, q.v., dark lines of solar spectrum. SYN: *Fraunhofer's lines*, q.v.

absorption spectrum. Spectrum of absorption lines produced when light passes through and is partially absorbed by a substance.

absorptive (ăb-sorp'tĭv). Absorbent.

abstinence (ăb'stĭ-nĕns) [L. *abstinere,* to abstain]. Going without something voluntarily, esp. refraining from indulgence in food, alcoholic beverages, or sexual intercourse.

abstinence syndrome. Partial collapse resulting from withdrawal of alcohol, stimulants, and some opiates. SYN: *withdrawal syndrome.*

abstract (ăb'străkt, ăb-străkt') [L. *abstrahere,* to draw away]. 1. A preparation containing the soluble principles of a drug concentrated and mixed with lactose. 2. A summary or abridgment of an article, book, or address.

   a., discharge. A summary of the hospital or clinic record of a patient. Prepared after time of discharge.

abstraction (ăb-străk'shŭn). 1. Removal or separation of a constituent from a mixture or compound. 2. Absorption of the mind; inattention or absent-mindedness. 3. The process whereby thoughts and ideas are generalized and dissociated from particular concrete instances or material objects.

abterminal (ăb-tĕr'mĭ-năl) [L. *ab,* from, + *terminus,* end]. Away from an end and toward the center, said of electric currents in muscles.

abulia (ă-bū'lē-ă) [Gr. *a-,* not, + *boule,* will]. 1. Absence of or inability to exercise will power (or initiative) or to make decisions. 2. Syndrome of slow reaction, lack of spontaneity, and brief spoken responses. May be part of the clinical picture that accompanies infarction of a cerebellar vessel. SEE: *hypobulia.*

abuse (ă-būs') [L. *abusus,* using up]. Misuse; excessive or improper use.

   a., child. Emotional, physical, or sexual injury to a child. May be due to positive action or omission on the part of those responsible for the care of the child. SEE: *child abuse.*

   a., elder. Emotional, physical, or sexual injury, or financial exploitation of an elder. May be due to positive action or omission on the part of those responsible for the care of the elder. Elders may also be exploited by individuals and "philanthropic" organizations.

   a., sexual. SEE: *sexual abuse.*

   a., spouse. Emotional, physical, or sexual mistreatment of one's spouse.

   a., substance. An imprecise term for abuse of drugs, alcohol, or other substances that alter mood or behavior.

abused person. SEE: *frozen watchfulness.*

abutment (ă-bŭt'mĕnt) [Fr. *abouter,* to place end to end]. The tooth to which a partial denture is anchored.

ABVD. *adriamycin, bleomycin, vinblastine,* and *dacarbazine.* A combination of chemotherapy drugs.

A.C. *acromioclavicular; adrenal cortex; air conduction; alternating current; anodal closure; atriocarotid; auriculocarotid; axiocervical.*

Ac. Chem. symb. for the element actinium.

a.c. L. *ante cibum,* before meals.

acacia (ă-kā'shē-ă). NF. Gum arabic. A dried, gummy exudation from the tree *Acacia senegal.* Used as a suspending agent or vehicle in pharmaceutical or other industrial products.

acalculia (ă-kăl-kū'lē-ă) [Gr. *a-,* not, + L. *calculare,* to reckon]. A learning or speech disorder characterized by the inability to perform simple arithmetic operations.

acampsia (ă-kămp'sē-ă) [" + *kamptein,* to bend]. Inflexibility of a limb; rigidity, ankylosis.

acantha [Gr. *akantha,* thorn]. 1. The spine. 2. A vertebral spinous process.

acanthamebiasis (ă-kăn"thă-mē-bī'ă-sĭs). A very rare disease caused by free-living amebae that ordinarily are found in water, soil, and decaying vegetation. Two species, *Naegleria fowleri* and *Acanthamoeba,* can cause meningoencephalitis. SEE: *meningoencephalitis, primary amebic.*

   Species of *Acanthamoeba (A. polyphaga, A. castellani)* have been associated with lesions of the eye.

acanthesthesia (ă-kăn"thĕs-thē'zē-ă) [" + *aisthesis,* sensation]. A sensation as of a pinprick; a form of paresthesia, q.v.

Acanthia lectularia (ă-kăn'thē-ă lĕk-tū-lă'rē-ă). The bedbug. SYN: *Cimex lectularius.*

acanthiomeatal line. An imaginary line through the acanthion and external auditory meatus.

acanthion [Gr. *akanthion,* little thorn]. Tip of anterior nasal spine.

acantho- [Gr. *akantha,* thorn]. Combining form meaning thorn, spine.

Acanthocephala (ă-kăn"thō-sĕf'ă-lă) [" + *kephale,* head]. A class of wormlike entozoa related to the Platyhelminthes, including a few species parasitic in man.

acanthocephaliasis (ă-kăn"thō-sĕf-ă-lī'ă-sĭs). Infestation with Acanthocephala.

Acanthocheilonema perstans (ă-kăn"thō-kī"lō-nē'mă pĕr'stăns). *Dipetalonema perstans.* A species of filaria that infects wild or domestic animals and occasionally man. In man, the adult worm migrates to the subcutaneous tissue and produces a nodule. The adult worm may, rarely, be seen beneath the conjunctiva.

acanthocyte (ă-kăn'thō-sīt") [Gr. *akantha,*

thorn, + *kytos*, cell]. An abnormal erythrocyte that in wet preparations has protoplasmic projections so that the cell appears to be covered with thorns. SEE: *abetalipoproteinemia.*

acanthocytosis (ă-kăn″thō-sī-tō′sĭs) [″ + ″ + *osis*, condition]. Acanthocytes in the blood.

acanthoid (ă-kăn′thoyd) [″ + *eidos*, form, shape]. Thorny; spiny; of a spinous nature.

acanthokeratodermia (ă-kăn″thō-kĕr″ă-tō-dĕr′mē-ă) [″ + *keras*, horn, + *derma*, skin]. Hypertrophy of the horny portion of the skin of the palms of hands and soles of feet, and thickening of the nails.

acantholysis (ă-kăn-thŏl′ĭ-sĭs) [″ + *lysis*, dissolution]. Any disease of the skin accompanied by degeneration of the cohesive elements of the cells of the outer or horny layer of the skin.

   a. **bullosa.** Obsolete term for epidermolysis bullosa, q.v.

acanthoma (ăk″ăn-thō′mă) [″ + *oma*, tumor]. Benign tumor of the skin. Previously used to denote cancer of skin.

   a. **adenoides cysticum.** A cystic tumor, often familial, occurring on chest, face, and in axillary regions. Tumors contain tissues resembling sweat glands and hair follicles. SYN: *epithelioma adenoides cysticum.*

acanthopelvis, acanthopelyx (ă-kăn″thō-pĕl′vĭs, -pĕl′ĭks) [″ + *pelyx*, pelvis]. A prominent and sharp pubic spine on a rachitic pelvis.

acanthosis (ăk″ăn-thō′sĭs) [″ + *osis*, condition]. Increased thickness of prickle cell layer of skin.

   a. **nigricans.** Rare chronic inflammatory disease of skin in adults sometimes associated with cancer of some internal organ. Characterized by symmetrically distributed hard and soft papillary growths accompanied by hyperpigmentation and hyperkeratosis. SYN: *keratosis nigricans.*

acanthotic (ăk″ăn-thŏt′ĭk). Pert. to acanthosis.

acapnia (ă-kăp′nē-ă) [Gr. *akapnos*, smokeless]. Literally, absence of carbon dioxide, but term is used to indicate the presence of less than normal amount of carbon dioxide in blood and tissues; e.g., after voluntary overbreathing. SEE: *hyperventilation.*

   SYM: Depressed respiration, giddiness, paresthesia, cramps, involuntary contraction of fingers, occasionally convulsions.

acapnial (ă-căp′nē-ăl). Showing or pert. to acapnia.

acarbia (ă-kăr′bē-ă). Diminution of bicarbonate in the blood.

acardia (ă-kăr′dē-ă) [Gr. *a-*, not, + *kardia*, heart]. Congenital absence of the heart.

acardiac (ă-kăr′dē-ăk). Having no heart.

acardiacus (ă-kăr-dī′ă-kŭs). A parasitic twin without a heart, therefore utilizing the circulation of its twin. SYN: *acardius.*

acardiotrophia (ă-kăr″dē-ō-trō′fē-a) [″ + ″ + *trophe*, nutrition]. Atrophy of the heart.

acardius. Acardiacus, q.v.

acariasis (ăk″ă-rī′ă-sĭs) [L. *acarus*, mite, + Gr. *-iasis*, condition]. Any disease caused by a mite or acarid. SYN: *acarinosis; acaridiasis.*

   a., **demodectic.** Infection of hair follicles with *Demodex folliculorum.*

   a., **psoroptic.** Misnomer for psoroptic sarcoptidosis, which affects animals but is rarely seen in man. SEE *mange.*

   a., **sarcoptic.** Infestation with a burrowing mite, *Sarcoptes scabiei,* which deposits its eggs in the burrows. SEE: *scabies.*

acaricide (ă-kăr′ĭ-sīd) [″ + *caedere,* to kill]. 1. An agent that destroys acarids. 2. Destroying a member of the order Acarina.

acarid, acaridan (ăk′ă-rĭd, ă-kăr′ĭ-dăn) [L. *acarus,* mite]. A tick or mite; member of the order Acarina.

Acaridae. A family of mites that irritate the skin. SEE: *itch, grain; itch, grocer's.*

acaridiasis (ă-kăr″ĭ-dī′ă-sĭs) [″ + Gr. *-iasis,* condition]. Disease caused by a mite. SYN: *acariasis; acarinosis.*

Acarina (ăk″ă-rī′nă). An order of the class Arachnida that includes a large number of species of minute animals known as mites or ticks. Most are ectoparasites, with infestation causing local dermatitis with pruritus and sometimes systemic reactions. They also are vectors of a number of diseases. SEE: *Ixodidae; Sarcoptidae; scabies; tick.*

acarinosis (ă-kăr″ĭ-nō′sĭs) [L. *acarus,* mite, + Gr. *osis,* condition]. Disease caused by a mite. SYN: *acariasis; acaridiasis.*

acarodermatitis (ăk″ă-rō-dĕr″mă-tī′tĭs) [″ + Gr. *derma,* skin, + *itis,* inflammation]. Inflammation of skin caused by a mite.

acaroid (ăk′ă-royd) [″ + Gr. *eidos,* form, shape]. Resembling a mite.

acarology (ăk″ă-rŏl′ō-jē) [″ + Gr. *logos,* word, reason]. Study of mites and ticks.

acarophobia (ăk″ăr-ō-fō′bē-ă) [″ + Gr. *phobos,* fear]. Abnormal fear of small objects such as pins, needles, worms, mites, and other small insects.

Acarus (ăk′ăr-ŭs) [L., mite]. A genus of mites.

   A. **folliculorum.** *Demodex folliculorum,* q.v.

   A. **scabiei.** *Sarcoptes scabiei.* SEE: *scabies; Sarcoptidae.*

acarus [L.]. Any mite or tick.

acaryote (ă-kăr′ē-ōt) [Gr. *a-,* not, + *karyon,* nucleus]. Without a nucleus. SEE *eucaryote; prokaryote.*

acatalasia (ă"kăt-ă-lā'zē-ă). A rare inherited disease in which there is an absence of the enzyme catalase. The gingival and oral tissues are particularly susceptible to bacterial invasion with subsequent gangrenous changes and alveolar bone destruction.

acataleptic (ă-kăt"ă-lĕp'tĭk). 1. Deficient mentally. 2. Uncertain or doubtful.

acatamathesia (ă-kăt"ă-mă-thē'zē-ă) [Gr. *a-*, not, + *katamathesis*, understanding]. 1. Loss of ability to understand spoken words. 2. Inability to comprehend as a result of a brain lesion.

acataphasia (ă-kăt"ă-fă'zē-ă) [" + *kataphasis*, affirmation]. 1. Inability to verbalize thoughts coherently. This condition is due to a cerebral lesion. 2. A form of disordered speech in which statements are incorrectly formulated; individuals may use words that sound like the ones they mean to use but are not appropriate to their thoughts, or they may use totally inappropriate expressions.

acatastasia (ă-kăt-ăs-tā'zē-ă) [Gr. *akatastasis*, disorder]. Irregularity; deviation from normal.

acathexis (ă"kă-thĕks'ĭs) [Gr. *a-*, not, + *kathexis*, retention]. In psychoanalysis, lack of emotion toward a thing or idea that is unconsciously important to the individual.

acathisia (ă"kă-thĭz'ē-ă) [" + *kathisis*, sitting]. Inability to sit down because the thought of doing so causes severe anxiety. Patient has a feeling of restlessness and an urgent need of movement and complains of a feeling of muscular quivering. This symptom may appear as a complication of therapy with antipsychotic medications such as phenothiazines or reserpine. Also spelled akathisia or akatizia.

TREAT: If due to drugs, decrease or eliminate use of the medicine.

acaudal, acaudate (ā-kaw'dăl, -dāt) [" + L. *cauda*, tail]. Having no tail.

ACC. *anodal closure contraction.*

acc. *accommodation.*

accelerated idioventricular rhythm. ABBR: AIVR. An abnormal ectopic cardiac rhythm originating in the ventricular conducting system. This may or may not occur intermittently and is usually between 60 and 100 beats per minute.

acceleration (ăk-sĕl"ĕr-ā'shŭn) [L. *accelerans*, hastening]. 1. Increase in the rapidity of motion or function, as pulse or respiration. 2. Numerical expression of the rate of change in velocity for a given unit of time.

a., angular. Rate of change in velocity per unit of time during circular movement.

a., central. A., centripetal, q.v.

a., centripetal. Rate of change in velocity per unit of time while on a circular or curved course.

a., linear. Rate of change in velocity per unit of time while on a straight course.

a., negative. Decrease in the rate of change in velocity per unit of time.

a., positive. Increase in the rate of change in velocity per unit of time.

a., standard, of free fall. The rate of change in velocity of a freely falling body as it is acted upon by gravity to travel to the earth. It is 9.81 meters (32.17 feet) per second squared.

acceleration injury. Head injury caused when the head remains stationary and is hit by a moving object, such as a batter being hit in the head by a baseball.

acceleration-deceleration injury. Head injury caused when both the head and the object of collision are moving, such as a bicycle rider hitting a moving car.

accelerator (ăk-sĕl'ĕr-ā"tor). Anything that increases action or function. 1. In chemistry, a catalyst. 2. A device that speeds up charged particles to high energy levels to produce x radiation and neutrons.

accelerator nerves. Sympathetic nerves that contain fibers whose impulses increase rate and force of heartbeat. Postganglionic fibers arise principally in cervical and thoracic ganglia. SEE: *death*.

accelerator reflexes. Statokinetic reflexes, q.v.

accelerometer. An instrument that detects change in velocity of the object to which it is attached. The device may be designed to record the changes and indicate the direction(s) of the acceleration.

accentuation (ăk-sĕn"chū-ā'shŭn) [L. *accentus*, accent]. Emphasis.

acceptance. According to Dr. Elisabeth Kübler-Ross, the fifth and final stage of dying. Individuals who achieve this stage (not all do) come to terms with the impending death and await the end with quiet expectation.

acceptor (ăk-sĕp'tor) [L. *accipere*, to accept]. A compound that unites with a substance freed by another compound, called a donor, q.v.

a., hydrogen. A substance that combines with hydrogen and is reduced when a substrate is oxidized by an enzyme.

a., oxygen. A substance that combines with oxygen and is oxidized when a substrate is reduced by an enzyme.

access, medical. SEE: *medical access.*

accessorius (ăk"sĕs-ō'rē-ŭs) [L., supplementary]. Accessory, supplementary, as certain muscles, glands, nerves.

accessory (ăk-sĕs'ō-rē). Auxiliary; assisting. Term applied to a lesser structure that resembles in structure and function a similar organ, as the accessory pancreatic duct (of

Santorini) or accessory suprarenal glands. An organ or structure that assists other organs in performing their functions, as accessory reproductive organs.

accessory motion. Motions which accompany active motion and are necessary for normal motion, but which cannot be isolated voluntarily. The motions include joint play as well as motions in related joints such as upward rotation of the scapula when the arm is abducted. SYN: *accessory movement.*

accessory muscles of respiration. In labored breathing, use of muscles other than the diaphragm and intercostals. The sternocleidomastoid, spinal, neck, abdominal muscles, and even the platysma may be utilized. Their use is a sign of an abnormal breathing pattern.

accessory nerve. Motor nerve made up of a cranial and a spinal part that supplies the trapezius and sternomastoid muscles and pharynx. Accessory portion joins the vagus, to which it supplies its motor and some of its cardioinhibitory fibers. SYN: *eleventh cranial nerve; spinal accessory nerve.*

accessory sign. A nonpathognomonic sign.

accident (ăk′sĭ-dĕnt) [L. *accidens*, happening]. 1. An unexpected event. 2. An unforeseen occurrence of an unfortunate nature; a mishap. 3. An unexpected complicating event in the course of a disease or following surgery.

   a., cerebrovascular. ABBR: CVA. A sudden, unexpected interference in brain function resulting from a vascular disturbance such as cerebral hemorrhage, occlusion of a vessel by a thrombus or embolus, vasospasm, or vasodilation. SYN: *apoplexy; stroke* (def. 5).

   a., radiation. Undesired contact or excessive exposure to ionizing radiation.

   a., serum. An allergic reaction following the therapeutic introduction of a foreign serum into a hypersensitive individual. SEE: *anaphylaxis.*

accidental (ăk″sĭ-dĕn′tăl). Occurring suddenly, unexpectedly, inadvertently, under unforeseen circumstances.

accident-prone. Said of persons having an unusually high rate of accidents. The validity of this concept is questionable.

accipiter (ăk-sĭp′ĭ-tĕr) [L., a hawk]. A nose bandage with clawlike ends that spread over the face.

ACCI. *anodal closure clonus.*

acclimation, acclimatization (ăk-lĭ-mā′shŭn, ă-klī″mă-tĭ-zā′shŭn) [Fr. *acclimater,* acclimate]. The act of becoming accustomed to a different environment.

acclimatize (ăk-klī′mă-tīz). To become accustomed to a different environment.

accommodation (ă-kŏm″ō-dā′shŭn) [L. *ac-*

VISUAL ACCOMMODATION

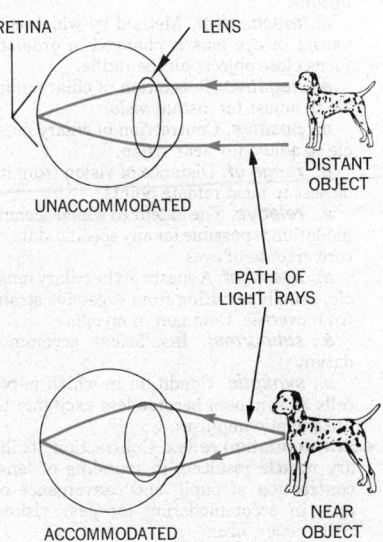

RETINA   LENS

UNACCOMMODATED

DISTANT OBJECT

PATH OF LIGHT RAYS

ACCOMMODATED

NEAR OBJECT

commodare, to suit]. ABBR: a; acc. 1. Adjustment or adaptation. 2. In ophthalmology, the term is applied to a phenomenon noted in receptors in which continued stimulation fails to elicit a sensation or response. 3. The adjustment of the eye for various distances whereby it is able to focus the image of an object on the retina by changing the curvature of the lens. In accommodation for near vision, the ciliary muscle contracts, causing increased rounding of the lens; the pupil contracts and the optic axes converge. These three actions constitute the accommodation reflex. The ability of the eye to accommodate decreases with age. SEE: illus.; *adaptation.*

   a., absolute. Accommodation of one eye independent of the other.

   a., amplitude of. The difference between refracting power of the eye when accommodating for near and far vision. It is measured in diopters (D) and normally diminishes progressively from childhood to old age. It is approximately 16 D at age 12, 6.5 D at age 30, and 1 D at age 50. SEE: *diopter.*

   a., binocular. Accommodation of both eyes jointly.

a., excessive. Greater-than-needed accommodation of the eye.

a., histologic. Change in cell form and function due to change in surrounding conditions.

a., mechanism. Method by which curvature of eye lens is changed in order to focus close objects on the retina.

a., negative. Relaxation of ciliary muscle to adjust for distant vision.

a., positive. Contraction of ciliary muscle to adjust for near vision.

a., range of. Distance of vision from its closest to most remote points.

a., relative. The extent to which accommodation is possible for any specific state of convergence of eyes.

a., spasm of. A spasm of the ciliary muscle, usually resulting from excessive strain from overuse. Common in myopia.

a., subnormal. Insufficient accommodation.

a., synaptic. Condition in which nerve cells at synapses become less excitable to presynaptic impulses.

accommodation reflex. Contraction of ciliary muscle resulting in rounding of lens, contraction of pupil, and convergence of eyes in accommodation for near vision. SYN: *reflex, near.*

accommodative iridoplegia (ă-kŏm′ō-dā″tĭv ĭr″ĭ-dō-plē′jē-ă). Noncontraction of pupils during accommodation.

accoucheur, accoucheuse (ă-koo-shŭr′, ă-koo-shĕz′) [Fr.]. An obstetrician or midwife.

accountability. Responsibility of health care professionals for the actions and judgments involved in patient care.

accreditation. The process of recognizing that a facility or institution has met established standards. In the United States, there are two types of educational accreditation, institutional and specialized. The former recognizes the institution for having facilities, policies, and procedures that meet accepted standards. The latter recognizes specific programs of study within institutions for having met established standards.

It is important to keep in mind that spurious claims of being accredited have been made by institutions.

Accredited Record Technician. ABBR: A.R.T. A person who, as a result of training and experience, is competent to process, maintain in a secure place, compile, and report information present in a patient's medical record. This is done according to regulatory requirements established by the health care facility to comply with medical, administrative, ethical, legal, and accreditation considerations.

accrementition (ăk″rē-mĕn-tĭsh′ŭn) [L. *ac-*

crescere, to increase]. Growth of tissues by addition of similar tissue.

accretio (ă-krē′shē-ō) [L.]. Adhesion of parts normally separate from each other.

a. cordis. Condition in which fibrous bands extend from external pericardium to surrounding structures, resulting in angulation and torsion of heart.

accretion (ă-krē′shŭn) [L. *accrescere,* accrue]. 1. Increase by external addition; accumulation. 2. The growing together of parts naturally separate. 3. Accumulation of foreign matter in a cavity.

acculturation. The process in which a member of one culture assumes the values, attitudes, and behavior of a second culture in order to become an accepted member of that culture.

accuracy. 1. The ratio of the error of measurement to the true value. 2. State of being free of error.

Accutane. SEE: *retinoic acid.*

ACD. *absolute cardiac dullness.*

AC/DC. Slang for a bisexual individual.

ACD sol. Citric acid, trisodium citrate, dextrose solution. Anticoagulant used when collecting blood for transfusions.

ACE. *adrenal cortical extract.*

Ace bandage. Trade name for an elastic bandage made of woven material.

acedia (ă-sē′dē-ă) [Gr. *a-,* not, + *kedos,* care]. Mental state of indifference, insensibility, lack of energy or emotion. SYN: *apathy.*

acellular. Not containing cells.

acenesthesia (ă-sĕn″ĕs-thē′zē-ă) [″ + *koinos,* common, + *aisthesis,* sensation]. Absence of a feeling of well-being, present in such disorders as hypochondriasis and neurasthenia.

acentric (ă-sĕn′trĭk) [″ + L. *centrum,* center]. Not central; peripheral.

A.C.E.P. *American College of Emergency Physicians.*

acephalia, acephalism (ă-sĕ-fā′lē-ă, ă-sĕf′ă-lĭzm) [″ + *kephale,* head]. A developmental disorder in which the head is absent.

acephalo- (ă-sĕf′ă-lō-) [Gr. *a-,* not, + *kephale,* head]. Combining form meaning without a head.

acephalobrachia (ă-sĕf″ă-lō-brā′kē-ă) [″ + ″ + *brachion,* arm]. A developmental anomaly in which head and arms are absent.

acephalocardia (ă-sĕf″ă-lō-kăr′dē-ă) [″ + ″ + *kardia,* heart]. Congenital absence of the head and heart.

acephalochiria (ă-sĕf″ă-lō-kĭ′rē-ă) [″ + ″ + *cheir,* hand]. Congenital absence of the head and hands.

acephalocyst (ă-sĕf′ă-lō-sĭst) [″ + ″ + *kystis,* bag]. A sterile hydatid cyst.

acephalogastria (ă-sĕf″ă-lō-găs′trē-ă) [″

+ " + *gaster,* stomach]. Congenital absence of the head, chest, and upper abdomen.

acephalopodia (ă-sĕf″ă-lō-pō′dē-ă) [" + " + *pous,* foot]. Congenital absence of the head and feet.

acephalorhachia (ă-sĕf″ă-lō-rā′kē-ă) [" + " + *rhachis,* spine]. Congenital absence of the head and vertebral column.

acephalostomia (ă-sĕf″ă-lō-stō′mē-ă) [" + " + *stoma,* mouth]. Congenital absence of the head; however, an opening resembling a mouth is present on the superior portion of the body.

acephalothoracia (ă-sĕf″ă-lō-thō-rā′sē-ă) [" + " + *thorax,* chest]. Congenital absence of the head and chest.

acephalus (ă-sĕf′ă-lŭs). A fetus lacking a head.

acerbity (ă-sĕrb′ĭ-tē) [L. *acerbus,* sharp]. Astringency combined with acidity.

acervuline (ă-sĕr′vū-lĭn) [L. *acervulus,* a little heap]. Aggregated, occurring in clusters.

acervuloma (ă-sĕr″vū-lō′mă) [" + *oma,* tumor]. Intracranial tumor containing psammoma bodies.

acervulus (ă-sĕr′vū-lŭs) [L.]. Sandy, gritty, sabulous.

   a. cerebri. Gritty matter filling the follicle of the pineal gland. SYN: *brain sand.*

acestoma (ă-sĕs-tō′mă) [" + *oma,* tumor]. The fresh granulations that later form a cicatrix.

acetabular (ăs″ĕ-tăb′ū-lăr). Pert. to the acetabulum.

acetabulectomy (ăs″ĕ-tăb″ū-lĕk′tō-mē) [L. *acetabulum,* a little saucer for vinegar, + Gr. *ektome,* excision]. Surgical removal of the acetabulum.

acetabuloplasty (ăs″ĕ-tăb′ū-lō-plăs″tē) [" + Gr. *plassein,* to form]. Surgical repair and reconstruction of the acetabulum.

acetabulum (ăs″ĕ-tăb′ū-lŭm) [L., a little saucer for vinegar]. 1. The rounded (cotyloid) cavity on the external surface of the innominate bone (os coxae or os innominatum) that receives head of femur. 2. The ventral sucker of the fluke.

acetal (ăs′ĕ-tăl). Chemical combination of an aldehyde with two molecules of alcohol.

acetaldehyde (ăs″ĕt-ăl′dĕ-hīd″). CH_3CHO. An intermediate in yeast fermentation and metabolism of alcohol. SYN: *acetic aldehyde.*

acetamide (ăs″ĕt-ăm′īd). CH_3CONH_2. Acetic acid amide, used in industry for synthesis of chemicals and as a solvent.

acetaminophen (ă-sĕt″ă-mĭn′ō-fĕn). USP. A synthetic drug with antipyretic and analgesic actions similar to aspirin, used in patients with sensitivity to aspirin. It does not have the anti-inflammatory or antirheu-

matic actions of aspirin. Trade names for acetaminophen include Tylenol and Datril.

Caution: Acute overdose may cause fatal hepatic necrosis.

acetaminophen poisoning. In therapeutic doses this drug is virtually nontoxic. In oral doses of greater than 140 mg/kg in adults, toxicity may occur. Doses of 10 to 25 grams or more in adults may be fatal. Estimate of amount of drug ingested may be determined from the plasma concentration. Values obtained 4 hours after ingestion of greater than 140 mg/kg will be associated with minimal hepatic toxicity in children or adults.

   SYM: Nausea, vomiting, drowsiness, pallor, shock, sweating, liver tenderness. Within 24 to 48 hours these signs subside, and evidence of liver damage appears. Symptoms include jaundice, liver tenderness, confusion, blood clotting abnormalities, and abnormal liver enzyme tests (aspartate amino transferase, AST; alanine amino transferase, ALT).

   TREAT: Gastric lavage to be done immediately, but protect airway. This is most effective if done within 4 hours of ingestion of the drug. A specific antidote, N-acetylcysteine, is given orally within 8 to 10 hours after ingestion in a dose of 140 mg/kg for the initial dose and then 70 mg/kg doses every 4 hours for 17 doses. SEE: *Poisons and Poisoning* in *Appendix.*

acetanilid (ăs″ĕ-tăn′ĭ-lĭd). A white powder or crystalline substance obtained by interaction of glacial acetic acid and aniline.

   ACTION/USES: Analgesic, antipyretic, and anti-inflammatory. Acute or chronic poisoning may develop due to prolonged administration or drug idiosyncrasy. Because of its toxicity, it is rarely used.

acetanilid poisoning. Symptoms are cyanosis due to formation of methemoglobin, cold sweat, irregular pulse, dyspnea, and unconsciousness. Sudden cardiac failure may occur.

   F.A.: In acute poisoning, analeptics such as caffeine, external heat, inhalation of oxygen, gastric lavage or emetics, artificial respiration, blood transfusion. If cyanosis is severe, give 1% methylene blue, 1 to 2 mg/kg body weight I.V. In chronic poisoning, stop use of drug; iron preparations for secondary anemia. SEE: *Poisons and Poisoning* in *Appendix.*

acetarsol, acetarsone (ăs″ĕ-tăr′sŏl, -sōn). An arsenic compound, acetylaminohydroxy-phenylarsonic acid. Contains 27% arsenic. Used in amebiasis and *Trichomonas vaginalis* infections.

acetate (ăs′ĕ-tāt). A salt of acetic acid.

acetazolamide (ăs″ĕt-ă-zŏl′ă-mīd). USP. A drug that inhibits the enzyme carbonic anhydrase. At one time it was used as a diuretic, but more effective drugs are now available. It has been used in treating epilepsy and to reduce intraocular pressure in managing glaucoma. Trade name is Diamox.

acetic (ă-sē′tĭk) [L. *acetum,* vinegar]. Pert. to vinegar; sour.

acetic acid. CH_3COOH. NF. An aqueous solution containing not less than 36% or more than 37% by weight of CH_3COOH. Used as a reagent, a caustic; sometimes taken internally. Vinegar contains 4% to 6% of this acid. SYN: *acid, ethanoic.*

    a.a., glacial. USP. A solution containing not less than 99.5% by weight of acetic acid.

acetic aldehyde. Acetaldehyde, q.v.

acetify (ă-sĕt′ĭ-fī) [″ + *fieri,* to become]. To produce acetic fermentation or vinegar.

acetimeter (ă-sĕ-tĭm′ĕ-tĕr) [″ + Gr. *metron,* measure]. An apparatus that determines the amount of acetic acid in fluid.

acetoacetic acid (ăs″ĕ-tō-ă-sē′tĭk). A ketone body formed when fats are incompletely oxidized, as in diabetes. May appear in the urine in starvation or inadequately treated diabetes mellitus. SYN: *diacetic acid.*

Acetobacter (ă-sē″tō-băk′tĕr) [L. *acetum,* vinegar, + Gr. *bakterion,* little rod]. A genus of nonpathogenic bacteria of the family Pseudomonadaceae.

    A. aceti. Species of *Acetobacter* that transforms wine or cider into vinegar. This produces a stringy substance in the liquid, called mother of vinegar.

acetolase (ă-sĕt′ō-lās). An enzyme that catalyzes conversion of alcohol into acetic acid.

acetohexamide (ăs″ĕ-tō-hĕks′ă-mīd). USP. An orally administered hypoglycemic agent.

Caution: This drug should be used only in patients with diabetes of the non-insulin-dependent type who cannot be treated with diet alone and who are unwilling or unable to take insulin if weight reduction and dietary control fail.

acetoin (ă-sĕt′ō-ĭn). The substance formed when glucose is fermented by *Enterobacter aerogenes.* After being oxidized to diacetyl, it provides the characteristic odor of butter.

acetone (ăs′ĕ-tōn). C_3H_6O. Dimethyl ketone, a colorless, volatile, inflammable liquid, miscible with water, useful as a solvent, and having a characteristic sweet, fruity, ethereal odor. Found in the blood and urine in diabetes, other metabolic disorders, and after lengthy fasting, produced when the fats are not properly oxidized due to inability to oxidize glucose in the blood. SEE: *acetoacetic acid; acidosis; ketone; ketonuria; ketosis; test, acetone.*

    a. in urine, test for. 1. Wet specially treated paper or stick with urine. If acetone is present, the paper will turn a certain color. These test papers or sticks are commercially available. 2. Take 5 ml of urine; add a few crystals of ammonium sulfate and dissolve; add a small crystal of sodium nitroprusside, and shake a little. Cover with a layer (about 2 ml) of strong ammonia. The presence of acetone is indicated by the formation of a purple ring between the layers of liquid. A commercially available tablet is also used for this test.

acetone bodies. Certain substances related to acetone. An example is acetoacetic acid, q.v. SYN: *ketone bodies,* q.v.

acetonemia (ăs″ē-tō-nē′mē-ă) [*acetone* + Gr. *haima,* blood]. Large amounts of acetone in blood.

    SYM: Abnormal excitement, gradual depression, acidosis.

acetonitrile (ăs″ĕ-tō-nī′trĭl). CH_3CN. Methyl cyanide, an ingredient of some commercially available nail care products. When ingested, it produces a toxic reaction similar to cyanide poisoning. The onset is delayed 9 to 12 hours or more. Also found in the urine of cigarette smokers. Treatment for poisoning is the same as for cyanide poisoning. SEE: *cotinine; cyanide poisoning.*

acetonuria (ăs″ĕ-tō-nū′rē-ă) [*acetone* + Gr. *ouron,* urine]. The presence of acetone and diacetic bodies in the urine, as in the ketosis of diabetes, starvation, etc., due to incomplete oxidation of fats. Preferred term is *ketonuria.* SEE: *acetone; acidosis; test, acetone.*

acetophenazine maleate (ăs″ĕ-tō-fĕn′ă-zĕn măl′ē-āt). USP. An antipsychotic drug of the phenothiazine group. Trade name is Tindal.

acetophenetidin (ăs″ĕ-tō-fĕ-nĕt′ĭ-dĭn). Previously used name for phenacetin, q.v.

acetosoluble (ăs″ĕ-tō-sŏl′ū-bl). Soluble in acetic acid.

acetous (ăs′ĕ-tŭs) [L. *acetum,* vinegar]. 1. Pert. to vinegar. 2. Sour in taste.

acetum (ă-sē′tŭm) [L.]. (pl. *aceta*) 1. Vinegar. 2. A drug dissolved in a weak vinegar solution.

acetyl (ăs′ĕ-tĭl, ă-sĕt′ĭl) [″ + Gr. *hyle,* matter]. CH_3CO, the univalent radical.

    a. CoA. Acetylcoenzyme A, q.v.

acetylation (ă-sĕt″ĭ-lā′shŭn). The introduction of one or more acetyl groups into an organic compound.

acetylcholine (ăs″ĕ-tĭl-kō′lēn). ABBR: ACh. An ester of choline occurring in various organs and tissues of the body. It is thought to play an important role in the transmission of nerve impulses at synapses and myoneural junctions. It is quickly destroyed by an enzyme, cholinesterase. Either excessive or deficient action of acetylcholine at the motor endplates may result in neuromuscular block. SEE: *cholinergic fibers.*

a. chloride. A salt of acetylcholine injected intramuscularly or subcutaneously as a parasympathetic stimulant. It lowers blood pressure by dilating peripheral vessels, and it relaxes smooth muscle spasms. Trade name is Miochol.

acetylcholinesterase (ăs″ĕ-tĭl-kō″lĭn-ĕs′tĕr-ās). ABBR: AChE. Enzyme that stops the action of acetylcholine. It is present in various body tissues, including muscles, nerve cells, and red blood cells.

acetylcoenzyme A. A condensation product of coenzyme A, q.v., and acetic acid.

acetylcysteine (ăs″ĕ-tĭl-sĭs′tē-ĭn). USP. Chemical substance that, when nebulized and inhaled, liquefies mucus and pus. Also used in the treatment of poisoning due to acetaminophen. Trade name is Mucomyst. SEE: *acetaminophen poisoning.*

acetylene (ă-sĕt′ĭ-lēn). C_2H_2. A colorless explosive gas with a garlic-like odor.

acetylsalicylic acid (ă-sē″tĭl-săl″ĭ-sĭl′ĭk). ABBR: ASA. Previously used name for aspirin, USP, q.v.

acetylsalicylic acid poisoning. SEE: *aspirin poisoning.*

acetyltransferase (ăs″ĕ-tĭl-trăns′fĕr-ās). Enzyme that is effective in the transfer of an acetyl group from one compound to another.

ACH. *adrenocortical hormone.*

ACh. *acetylcholine.*

achalasia (ăk″ă-lā′zē-ă) [Gr. *a-,* not, + *chalasis,* relaxation]. Failure to relax; said of muscles, such as sphincters, the normal function of which is a persistent contraction with periods of relaxation. SEE: *Nursing Diagnoses in Appendix.*

a. of the cardia. Failure of relaxation of the cardiac sphincter, resulting in difficulty in passage of foods to the stomach. In advanced cases, dysphagia is marked and dilation of the esophagus may occur. SYN: *cardiospasm.*

a., pelvirectal. Congenital absence of ganglion cells in distal large bowel, resulting in failure of colon to relax.

a., sphincteral. Failure of intestinal sphincters to relax.

AChE. *acetylcholinesterase.*

ache (āk) [AS. *acan*]. 1. A continued pain as distinguished from a sudden or spasmodic pain. May be dull or severe. 2. To suffer continued pain.

acheilia (ă-kī′lē-ă) [Gr. *a-,* not, + *cheilos,* lip]. Congenital absence of one or both lips.

acheiria (ă-kī′rē-ă) [″ + *cheir,* hand]. 1. Congenital absence of one or both hands. 2. Loss of sensation in, with accompanying sense of loss of, one or both hands. May result from temporary or permanent injury or malfunction of sensory mechanism, or may occur in hysteria. 3. Inability to determine to which side of the body a stimulus has been applied. SYN: *achiria.*

acheiropodia (ă-kī″rō-pō′dē-ă) [″ + ″ + *pous,* foot]. Congenital absence of hands and feet.

achievement age. The age of a person with regard to level of acquired learning. Determined by a proficiency test and expressed in terms of the chronological age of the average person showing the same level of attainment. SEE: *age.*

Achilles jerk (ă-kĭl′ēz) [Achilles, hero of the *Iliad,* whose vulnerable spot was his heel because it was from this part that he was suspended when immersed in the river Styx]. Achilles tendon reflex, q.v.

Achilles tendon. The tendon of the gastrocnemius and soleus muscles of the leg. SYN: *tendo calcaneus.*

Achilles tendon reflex. Plantar flexion, which is also called extension of the ankle, resulting from contraction of calf muscles following a sharp blow to the Achilles tendon. The variations and their significance correspond closely to those of the knee jerk. It is exaggerated in upper motor neuron disease and diminished or absent in lower motor neuron disease. The character of the response is influenced by the metabolic rate; thus, attempts have been made to use this reflex as an index of thyroid function. The value of such use is questionable.

achillobursitis (ă-kĭl″ō-bŭr-sī′tĭs) [*Achilles* + L. *bursa,* a pouch, + Gr. *itis,* inflammation]. Inflammation of the bursa lying over the Achilles tendon. SYN: *Albert's disease.*

achillodynia (ă-kĭl″ō-dĭn′ē-ă) [″ + Gr. *odyne,* pain]. Pain caused by inflammation between the Achilles tendon and bursa.

achillorrhaphy (ă-kĭl-or′ă-fē) [″ + Gr. *rhaphe,* seam, ridge]. Suture of Achilles tendon.

achillotenotomy (ă-kĭl″ō-tĕn-ŏt′ō-mē) [″ + Gr. *tenon,* tendon, + *tome,* incision]. Achillotomy, q.v.

achillotomy (ă-kĭl-ŏt′ō-mē) [″ + *tome,* incision]. Division of the Achilles tendon. SYN: *achillotenotomy.*

achiria (ă-kī′rē-ă) [Gr. *a-,* not, + *cheir,* hand]. Acheiria, q.v.

achlorhydria (ā″klor-hī′drē-ă) [″ + *chloros,* green, + *hydor,* water]. Absence of free hydrochloric acid in the stomach.

ETIOL: May be associated with gastric

carcinoma, gastric ulcer, pernicious anemia, adrenal insufficiency, chronic gastritis. SEE: *achylia*.

a., histamine-proved. Absence of free acid in gastric secretion even after subcutaneous injection of histamine hydrochloride.

achloropsia (ă-klō-rŏp′sē-ă) [″ + *chloros*, green, + *opsis*, vision]. Color blindness in which green cannot be distinguished. SEE: *deuteranopia*.

acholuria (ă-kō-lū′rē-ă) [″ + *chole*, bile, + *ouron*, urine]. Absence of bile pigments in urine in some forms of jaundice.

achondrogenesis (ă-kŏn″drō-jĕn′ĕ-sĭs) [Gr. *a-*, not, + *chondros*, cartilage, + *genesis*, generation, birth]. Failure of growth of bone, esp. the bones of the extremities.

achondroplasia (ă-kŏn″drō-plā′sē-ă) [″ + ″ + *plasis*, a molding]. Defect in the formation of cartilage at the epiphyses of long bones, producing a form of dwarfism; sometimes seen in rickets. SYN: *chondrodystrophy*.

achroma (ă-krō′mă) [″ + *chroma*, color]. An absence of color or normal pigmentation as in leukoderma, albinism, vitiligo.

achromasia (ăk″rō-mā′zē-ă) [Gr. *achromatos*, without color]. 1. Absence of normal pigmentation of the skin as in albinism, vitiligo, leukoderma. 2. Pallor. 3. The lack of the ability to be stained, said of cells or tissues.

achromate (ă-krō′māt) [Gr. *a-*, not, + *chroma*, color]. A person who is color blind.

achromatic (ăk″rō-măt′ĭk) [Gr. *achromatos*, without color]. 1. Lacking in color. 2. Not dispersing light into its constituent components. 3. Not containing or composed of chromatin. 4. Difficult to stain, with reference to cells and tissues.

achromatic lens. Lens that transmits light without separating the spectral colors.

achromatin (ă-krō′mă-tĭn). The weakly staining substance of a cell nucleus.

achromatism (ă-krō′mă-tĭzm″) [Gr. *a-*, not, + *chroma*, color, + *-ismos*, condition]. Colorlessness.

achromatocyte (ăk″rō-măt′ō-sīt) [Gr. *achromatos*, without color, + *kytos*, cell]. A decolorized red blood cell. SYN: *achromocyte; ghost corpuscle*.

achromatolysis (ă-krō″mă-tŏl′ĭ-sĭs) [″ + *lysis*, dissolution]. Dissolution of cell achromatin.

achromatophil (ā″krō-măt′ō-fĭl) [″ + *philos*, love]. A cell or tissue not stainable in the usual manner.

achromatopsia (ă-krō″mă-tŏp′sē-ă) [″ + *opsis*, vision]. Complete color blindness.

achromatosis (ă-krō″mă-tō′sĭs) [″ + *osis*, condition]. Condition of being without natural pigmentation. SEE: *achroma*.

achromatous (ă-krō′mă-tŭs). Without color.

achromaturia (ă-krō″mă-tū′rē-ă) [″ + *ouron*, urine]. Colorless or nearly colorless urine.

achromia (ă-krō′mē-ă) [Gr. *a-*, not, + *chroma*, color]. 1. Absence of color; pallor. 2. Achromatosis, q.v. 3. Condition in which erythrocytes have large central pale areas; hypochromia.

a., congenital. Albinism, q.v.

achromic (ă-krō′mĭk). Lacking color.

Achromobacter. A genus of gram-negative bacilli. They may be normal inhabitants of the lower gastrointestinal tract. May cause nosocomial infections.

achromocyte (ă-krō′mō-sīt) [″ + ″ + *kytos*, cell]. In a blood smear, large, pale, crescent-shaped cells produced from fragile red cells as the bloodfilm preparation is being made. SYN: *crescent bodies; selenoid cells*.

achromophil (ă-krō′mō-fĭl) [″ + ″ + *philos*, love]. Achromatophil, q.v.

achromotrichia (ă-krō″mō-trĭk′ē-ă) [″ + ″ + *trichia*, condition of the hair]. Lack of color or graying of the hair. SYN: *canities*.

a., nutritional. Grayness of hair due to dietary deficiency.

Achromycin (ăk″rō-mī′sĭn). Trade name for tetracycline, an antibiotic effective in treatment of many bacterial infections.

achroodextrin (ăk″rō-ō-dĕks′trĭn) [Gr. *achroos*, colorless, + *dextrin*]. One of the varieties of dextrin resulting from hydrolysis of starch.

achylia (ă-kī′lē-ă) [Gr. *a-*, not, + *chylos*, juice]. Absence of chyle or other digestive ferments.

a. gastrica. Complete absence or marked diminution in amount of gastric juice. SEE: *achlorhydria*.

a. pancreatica. Absence or deficiency of pancreatic secretion. Usually a manifestation of chronic pancreatitis.

achylosis (ă″kī-lō′sĭs). Achylia, q.v.

achylous (ă-kī′lŭs) [Gr. *achylos*, without chyle]. 1. Lacking in any kind of digestive secretion. 2. Without chyle.

acicular (ă-sĭk′ū-lăr) [L. *aciculus*, little needle]. Needle-shaped.

acid [L. *acidum*, acid]. 1. Any substance that liberates hydrogen ions (protons) in solution; a hydrogen ion donor. An acid reacts with a metal to form a salt, neutralizes bases, and turns litmus paper red. SEE: *alkali; base; indicator; pH*. 2. A sour substance. 3. The "street" or slang term for LSD, q.v.

a., acetic. CH$_3$COOH. Substance that gives sour taste to vinegar. Also used as a reagent and as a caustic. SYN: *a., ethanoic*.

a., acetic, dilute. Solution containing 6% pure acetic acid by weight.

a., acetic, glacial. USP. Solution containing not less than 99.5% of acetic acid by weight.

a., acetoacetic. CH_3COCH_2COOH. A ketone body formed when fats are incompletely oxidized. Appears in urine in abnormal amounts in starvation or inadequately treated diabetes. SYN: *a., acetylacetic; diacetic acid.*

a., acetylsalicylic. ABBR: ASA. The previously used name for aspirin, q.v.

a., adenylic. A nucleotide formed by condensation of adenosine and phosphoric acid. It is one of the hydrolytic products of nucleic acids and is present in muscle, blood corpuscles, yeast, and other nuclear material. SYN: *adenosine monophosphate.*

a., alginic. An organic acid obtained from species of marine algae. It is used as a pharmaceutical aid and as a thickening agent in food products.

a., amino. An organic acid containing one or more NH_2 (amino) groups and a COOH (carboxyl) group. Amino acids are the basic building blocks for all of the body's protein elements and are the end products of protein digestion or hydrolysis. Certain of these are essential in the human body for growth and repair of tissues. Oral preparations of essential amino acids may be used as dietary supplements. SEE: *amino acid.*

a., aminoacetic. NH_2CH_2COOH. A nonessential amino acid, q.v. SYN: *glycine.*

a., aminobenzoic. A., para-aminobenzoic, q.v.

a., aminocaproic. USP. A hemostatic drug. It is a specific antidote for an overdose of a fibrinolytic agent. Trade name is Amicar.

a., aminoglutaric. A., glutamic, q.v.

a., aminosalicylic. A., para-aminosalicylic, q.v.

a., aminosuccinic. A., aspartic, q.v.

a., arachidonic. SEE: *arachidonic acid.*

a., arsonic. An organic acid that contains the $AsO(OH)_2$ group.

a., arylarsonic. Arsonic acid combined with an aryl radical.

a., ascorbic. USP. $C_6H_8O_6$. A vitamin that occurs naturally in fresh fruits, esp. citrus fruits, and in fresh vegetables. Essential in maintenance of collagen formation, osteoid tissue of bones, and formation and maintenance of dentin. This essential vitamin is used as a dietary supplement and in the prevention and treatment of scurvy. Scurvy develops after approx. 3 months of ascorbic acid deficiency in the diet. The usefulness of large daily doses (1 to 5 gm or more a day) of this vitamin in preventing or treating the common cold in otherwise healthy persons has not been established although it may decrease the severity of symptoms. Continuous treatment with large doses can cause kidney stones. SYN: *vitamin C; vitamin, antiscorbutic.*

a., aspartic. $COOH \cdot CH(NH_2) \cdot CH_2 \cdot COOH$. A nonessential amino acid, q.v.; one of the products of pancreatic digestion. SYN: *a., aminosuccinic.*

a., barbituric. $C_4H_4N_2O_3$. A crystalline compound from which phenobarbital and other barbiturates are derived. SYN: *malonylurea.*

a., benzoic. USP. $C_7H_6O_2$. A white crystalline material having a slight odor. Used in keratolytic ointments and as a food preservative. Saccharin is a derivative of this acid.

a., bile. Any one of the complex acids that occur as salts in bile; e.g., cholic, glycocholic, and taurocholic acids. They give bile its foamy character, are important in the digestion of fats in the intestine, and are reabsorbed from the intestine to be used again by the liver.

a., boric. H_3BO_3. A white crystalline substance that in water forms a very weak acid solution poisonous to plants and animals. Soluble in water, alcohol, or glycerin. SEE: *boric acid.*

Caution: Because of its toxicity, the use of boric acid should be quite limited. It is particularly dangerous because it can be accidentally swallowed, esp. by children or used in food because of its resemblance to sugar.

---

a., butyric. C_3H_7COOH. An acid having a rancid odor; found in rancid butter, in cheese, perspiration, and cod liver oil.

a., carbolic. Phenol, q.v.

a., carbonic. H_2CO_3. An acid formed from carbon dioxide being dissolved in water.

a., carboxylic. Any acid containing the group COOH. The simplest examples are formic and acetic.

a., chaulmoogric. A cyclic unsaturated fatty acid in chaulmoogra oil, formerly used in treatment of leprosy (Hansen's disease).

a., cholic. An acid formed in the liver by hydrolysis of other bile acids. Important in digestion.

a., chromic. CrO_3. An escharotic sometimes used to remove warts.

a., citric. $C_6H_8O_7$. An acid prepared synthetically or from lemon or lime juice in form of colorless crystals or white crystalline powder. Soluble in water, ether, or alcohol. Used as a preventive of scurvy. Hydrous form is used as a flavoring agent or vehicle. SEE: *vitamin C.*

a., deoxyribonucleic. ABBR: D. Deoxyribonucleic acid, q.v.

a., desoxyribonucleic. Former spelling of deoxyribonucleic acid, q.v.

a., diacetic. A., acetoacetic, q.v.

a., 2,3-dihydroxypropanoic. A., glyceric, q.v.

a., ethanedioic. A., oxalic, q.v.

a., ethanoic. A., acetic, q.v.

a., ethylenediaminetetraacetic. ABBR: EDTA. A chelating agent that, in the form of its calcium or sodium salts, is useful in removing certain substances such as lead and digitalis from the body. SEE: *chelation.*

a., fatty. A carboxylic acid that can be combined with glycerol to form fats; the simplest members of the series are formic and acetic; most typical are stearic and palmitic. A saturated fatty acid has single bonds in its carbon chain, with the general formula $C_nH_{2n}O_2$. An unsaturated fatty acid has one or more double or triple bonds in its carbon chain. In human nutrition, it is felt that by decreasing the intake of saturated fatty acids, cholesterol content of the blood will be decreased.

a., folic. USP. $C_{19}H_{19}N_7O_6$. A member of the vitamin B complex. Found naturally in green plant tissue, liver, and yeast. When produced synthetically, it is identical with pteroylglutamic acid.

Caution: Folic acid should not be used in the treatment of pernicious anemia because it does not protect patients against the development of changes in the central nervous system that accompany this type of anemia.

a., formic. HCOOH. The first member of the monobasic fatty acid series. It is a much stronger acid than the others in the series. It occurs naturally in certain animal secretions and in muscle, but it may also be prepared synthetically. It is one of the irritants present in the sting of insects such as bees and ants. SYN: *a., methanoic.*

a., formiminoglutamic. $C_6N_2O_4H_{10}$. An intermediate product in the metabolism of histidine. Its increase in the urine after administration of histidine in patients with folic acid deficiency is the basis for the FIGLU excretion test.

a., gallic. $C_6H_2(OH)_3COOH$. A colorless crystalline acid. It occurs naturally as an excrescence on the twigs of trees, esp. oak trees, as a reaction to the deposition of gall ⸻p eggs. It is used as a skin astringent and ⸻ manufacture of writing inks and dyes. ⸻., 3,4,5-trihydroxybenzoic.

⸻ **curonic.** $CHO(CHOH)_4COOH$. ⸻ion product of glucose that is ⸻e urine. Toxic products (such as ⸻ menthol, and phenol) that have entered the body through the intestinal system are detoxified in the liver by conjugation with glucuronic acid. SYN: *a., glycuronic.*

a., glutamic. $COOH \cdot (CH_2)_2 \cdot CH(NH_2) \cdot COOH$. A nonessential amino acid formed during protein metabolism. SYN: *a., aminoglutaric.*

a., glyceric. $CH_2OH \cdot CHOH \cdot COOH$. An intermediate product of oxidation of fats. SYN: *a., 2,3-dihydroxypropanoic.*

a., glycocholic. $C_{26}H_{43}NO_6$. A bile acid yielding glycine and cholic acid on hydrolysis.

a., glycuronic. A., glucuronic, q.v.

a., hexadecanoic. A., palmitic, q.v.

a., homogentisic. An intermediate product of tyrosine catabolism; found in the urine in alkaptonuria. SYN: *alkapton.*

a., hydriodic. HI. In solution, it is used in various forms of chemical analyses. SYN: *hydrogen iodide.*

a., hydrochloric. HCl. An inorganic acid. Normally present in the gastric juice. It destroys fermenting bacteria that might cause intestinal tract disturbances. Five to 10 ml of a 10% solution of hydrochloric acid in 125 to 250 ml of water is used in treating hypoacidity or achlorhydria. SYN: *muriatic acid.*

Caution: When so used, it must be diluted accurately and sipped through a drinking straw. This will prevent the acid from damaging the teeth.

a., hydrocyanic. HCN. A colorless, extremely poisonous, highly volatile liquid. Occurs naturally in plants. It is obtained synthetically by several methods. Has many industrial uses: electroplating, fumigation, and production of dyes, pigments, synthetic fibers, and plastic. Exposure of man to 200 to 500 parts of acid per 1,000,000 parts of air for 30 minutes is fatal. It acts by preventing cellular respiration. SYN: *hydrogen cyanide; prussic acid.* SEE: *cyanide* in *Poisons and Poisoning* in *Appendix.*

a., hydrosuccinic. A., malic, q.v.

a., hydroxy. An acid containing one or more hydroxyl (OH) groups in addition to the carboxyl (COOH) group.

a., hydroxytoluic. A., mandelic, q.v.

a., imino. An acid formed as a result of oxidation of amino acids in the body.

a., inorganic. An acid containing no carbon atoms. SYN: *mineral acid.*

a., lactic. USP. A mixture of lactic acid, $C_3H_6O_3$, and lactic acid lactate, $C_6H_{10}O_5$, equivalent to a total of not less than 85% and not more than 90%, by weight, of $C_3H_6O_3$. Occurs in sour milk from fermentation of lactose and is formed in muscles during the metabolic changes that occur during strenuous exercise. Lactic acid milk (buttermilk or acidophilus milk) is administered to help prevent growth of putrefactive bacteria in the large intestine. SYN: *2-hydroxypropionic acid.*

a., linoleic. $C_{18}H_{32}O_2$. An unsaturated fatty acid, a dietary essential. First isolated from linseed oil but also found in corn oil. It is required for synthesis of prostaglandins. SYN: *a., linolic.*

a., linolenic. $C_{18}H_{30}O_2$. An unsaturated fatty acid, a dietary essential.

a., lysergic. $C_{16}H_{16}N_2O_2$. A crystalline substance derived from ergot. Its derivative, lysergic acid diethylamide, LSD, is a potent hallucinogen. SEE: *LSD.*

a., malic. $C_4H_6O_5$. Substance found in certain sour fruits such as apples and apricots. Active in aerobic metabolism of carbohydrate. SYN: *a., hydrosuccinic.*

a., malonic. $C_3H_4O_4$. A dibasic acid formed by oxidation of malic acid. Occurs in beets. Active in the tricarboxylic acid cycle in carbohydrate metabolism. Its inhibition of succinic dehydrogenase is the classic example of competitive inhibition.

a., mandelic. $C_8H_8O_3$. A colorless hydroxy acid, q.v. Its salt is used in urinary tract infections. SYN: *a., hydroxytoluic.*

a., methanoic. A., formic, q.v.

a., mineral. A., inorganic, q.v.

a., muriatic. A., hydrochloric, q.v.

a., nicotinic. $C_6H_5NO_2$. A member of the vitamin B complex. Occurs naturally in liver, yeast, milk, cheese, and cereals. Used for prevention and treatment of pellagra. SYN: *niacin.*

a., nitric. HNO_3. A strong corrosive acid prepared from sulfuric acid and a nitrate. It is used in manufacture of explosives and dyes and as a coagulant in testing urine for albumin (Heller's test).

a., nucleic. Any one of a group of high-molecular-weight substances found in the cells of all living things. They have a complex chemical structure formed of sugars (pentoses), phosphoric acid, and nitrogen bases (purines and pyrimidines). Most important are ribonucleic acid, q.v., and deoxyribonucleic acid, q.v.

a., 9-octadecenoic. A., oleic, q.v.

a., oleic. $C_{18}H_{34}O_2$. An unsaturated fatty acid found in most organic fats and oils. SYN: *a., 9-octadecenoic.*

a.'s, omega-3 fatty. A group of fatty acids contained in oils present in some saltwater fish. They have been used to attempt to reduce elevated levels of very low density lipoproteins and chylomicrons in plasma.

a., organic. An acid containing the carboxyl radical, COOH.

a., oxalic. $C_2H_2O_4$. The simplest dibasic organic acid. Its potassium or calcium salt occurs naturally in rhubarb, wood sorrel, and many other plants. It is the strongest organic acid and is poisonous. When properly diluted, it is effective in removing ink or rust stains from cloth. It is used also as a reagent. SYN: *a., ethanedioic.*

a., palmitic. $C_{16}H_{32}O_2$. A saturated fatty acid occurring as esters in most natural fats and oils. SYN: *a., hexadecanoic.*

a., pantothenic. $C_9H_{17}NO_5$. One of the B-complex vitamins.

a., para-aminobenzoic. ABBR: PABA. $NH_2C_6H_4COOH$. A member of the vitamin B complex. It is used as a dietary supplement, an antirickettsial drug, a reagent, and a sunscreening agent. It should not be used in persons known to be sensitive to sulfonamides. Inhibits bacteriostatic action of sulfonamides; hence, all but topical use is contraindicated during sulfonamide therapy. SYN: *aminobenzoic acid.*

a., para-aminosalicylic. ABBR: PAS. $C_7H_7NO_3$. A white or nearly white and practically odorless powder that darkens when exposed to air or light. An antituberculosis drug, the effectiveness of which is greatly enhanced when used in combination with streptomycin and isoniazid; it is believed to delay development of bacterial resistance. SYN: *aminosalicylic acid.*

a., pectic. An acid derived from pectin.

a., pentanoic. A., valeric, q.v.

a., perchloric. $HClO_4$. A colorless unstable liquid compound; the highest oxygen acid of chlorine.

a., phenic. Phenol, q.v.

a., phenylglycolic. A., mandelic, q.v.

a., phosphoric. An acid formed by oxidation of phosphorus, used as an alkaloidal reagent. The phosphoric acids are orthophosphoric acid, H_3PO_4; pyrophosphoric acid, $H_4P_2O_7$; metaphosphoric acid, HPO_3; and hypophosphoric acid, $H_4P_2O_6$. The salts of these acids are phosphates.

a., phosphorous. An oxygen acid of phosphorus. The phosphorous acids are orthophosphorous acid, $H_2(HPO_3)$; pyrophosphorous acid, $H_4P_2O_5$; metaphosphorous acid, HPO_2; and hypophosphorous acid, $H(H_2PO_2)$. The salts of these acids are phosphites.

a., phosphotungstic. $24WO_3 \cdot 2H_3PO_4 \cdot 48H_2O$. A trigonal crystalline organic acid, the water content of which may vary. Used in the form of its sodium salt in testing for alkaloids.

a., picric. $C_6H_2(NO_2)_3OH$. A yellow crystalline substance that precipitates proteins.

Used as a dye and a reagent. SYN: *trinitrophenol.*

a., prussic. A., hydrocyanic, q.v.

a., pteroylglutamic. A., folic, q.v.

a., pyruvic. $CH_3CO \cdot COOH$. An intermediate product of glycolysis in muscle tissues.

a., ribonucleic. ABBR: RNA. A substance found in cytoplasm and chromosomes. It assists in selection and synthesis of proteins from the amino acid sequences.

a., salicylic. USP. $C_7H_6O_3$. A substance that occurs as white needle-shaped crystals or as white crystalline powder. It is used as a local antiseptic or keratolytic agent.

a., saturated fatty. Fatty acid in which the carbon atoms are linked to other carbon atoms by single bonds. SEE: *a., unsaturated fatty; fatty acid.*

a., silicic. An acid containing silica, as H_2SiO_3, H_2SiO_4, or H_2SiO_6. When silicic acid is precipitated, silica gel is obtained.

a., stearic. NF. $C_{18}H_{36}O_2$. A monobasic fatty acid occurring naturally in plants and animals. Used in manufacture of soap and pharmaceutical products such as glycerin suppositories.

a., succinic. $COOH(CH_2)_2COOH$. An intermediate in carbohydrate metabolism.

a., sulfonic. An organic compound of the general formula SO_2OH derived from sulfuric acid by replacement of a hydrogen atom.

a., sulfosalicylic. A crystalline acid soluble in water or alcohol. Used as a reagent for precipitating proteins, as in testing for albumin in urine.

a., sulfuric. H_2SO_4. A colorless, corrosive, heavy liquid prepared from sulfur; used in the production of a great number of industrial products. It is rarely used in medicine. SYN: *vitriol, oil of.*

a., sulfurous. H_2SO_3. An inorganic acid. It is a powerful chemical reducing agent and is used commercially, esp. for its bleaching properties.

a., tannic. A glucoside prepared from oak galls and sumac that yields gallic acid and glucose on hydrolysis. SYN: *tannin,* q.v.

a., tartaric. $C_4H_6O_6$. Substance obtained from byproducts of wine fermentation. Widely used in industry in manufacture of carbonated drinks, flavored gelatins, dyes, and metals. Also used as a reagent.

a., taurocholic. A bile acid that yields cholic acid and taurine on hydrolysis.

a., trichloroacetic. $C_2HCl_3O_2$. A caustic crystalline substance.

a., 3,4,5-trihydroxybenzoic. A., gallic, q.v.

a., unsaturated fatty. Organic acid in which some of the carbon atoms are linked to other carbon atoms by double bonds, thus containing less than the maximum possible number of hydrogen atoms; for example, compare unsaturated oleic and linoleic acids with the saturated stearic acid. SEE: *a., saturated fatty; fatty acid.*

a., uric. $C_5H_4N_4O_3$. An important organic constituent of normal urine. Usually occurs in form of salts (urates).

a., valeric. $C_5H_{10}O_2$. An oily liquid of the fatty acid series, existing in four isomeric forms and having a distinctly disagreeable odor. SYN: *a., pentanoic.*

acidaminuria (ăs″ĭd-ăm″ĭ-nū′rē-ă) [L. *acidum,* acid, + *amine* + Gr. *ouron,* urine]. Excess of amino acids in urine.

acid-base balance. The mechanisms by which the acidity and alkalinity of body fluids are kept in a state of equilibrium so that the hydrogen ion concentration, q.v., of arterial blood is maintained at approx. pH 7.35 to 7.45. This is accomplished by action of buffer systems of the blood and the regulatory (homeostatic) functions of the respiratory and urinary systems. Disturbances in acid-base balance result in acidosis, q.v., or alkalosis, q.v. SEE: *pH.*

acidemia (ăs-ĭ-dē′mē-ă) [″ + Gr. *haima,* blood]. Excessive acidity of the blood due to an uncompensated reduction in circulating alkaline substances or uncompensated increase in circulating acid substances. The hydrogen ion concentration, q.v., of the blood increases, as reflected by a lowering of serum pH values. SEE: *acid-base balance; acidity; acidosis.*

acid fallout. Acid rain, q.v.

acid-fast. Not decolorized easily by acids after staining. Pert. to bacteria that after staining are decolorized by a mixture of acid and alcohol. The acid-fast bacteria retain the red dyes, but the surrounding tissues are decolorized. In clinical medicine, an example of this type of organism is *Mycobacterium tuberculosis.*

acidifiable (ă-sĭd′ĭ-fī″ă-bl) [″ + *fieri,* to be made, + *habilis,* able]. Capable of being transformed to produce an acid reaction.

acidification (ă-sĭd″ĭ-fĭ-kā′shŭn) [″ + *factus,* made]. Becoming sour; conversion into an acid.

acidifier (ă-sĭd′ĭ-fī″ĕr) [″ + *fieri,* to be made]. Substance that increases the acidity of that to which it is added or exposed.

acidify. To make a substance acid by adding acidic material.

acidimeter (ăs″ĭ-dĭm′ĕ-tĕr) [″ + Gr. *metron,* measure]. Instrument for testing the amount of free acid in a solution.

acidimetry (ăs″ĭ-dĭm′ĕ-trē). Determination of an acid's strength or of the acidity of a fluid.

acidity (ă-sĭd'ĭ-tē). 1. The quality of possessing hydrogen ions (protons). SEE: *acid; hydrogen ion; pH.* 2. Sourness.

  a. of stomach. Sourness due to fermentation of food in the stomach or over-secretion of acid.

  a., titratable. The amount of hydrogen ion excreted in the urine in a dihydrogen form.

acidocyte (ăs'ĭ-dō-sīt″) [L. *acidum,* acid, + Gr. *kytos,* cell]. Eosinophil; eosinophilic leukocyte, q.v.

acidocytopenia (ăs″ĭ-dō-sī″tō-pē'nē-ă) [″ + ″ + *penia,* lack]. Abnormal reduction of number of eosinophils in the blood.

acidocytosis (ăs″ĭ-dō-sī-tō'sĭs) [″ + ″ + *osis,* condition]. Abnormal increase in number of eosinophilic leukocytes in the blood.

acidophil(e) (ă-sĭd'ō-fĭl, -fīl) [″ + Gr. *philos,* love]. 1. Capable of being stained by acid stains such as eosin. Said of cells or parts of cells prepared for microscopic study. SYN: *acidophilic; acidophilous.* 2. An acid-staining cell of the anterior pituitary. 3. A bacterial organism that grows well in an acid medium.

acidophilic (ă-sĭd″ō-fĭl'ĭk). 1. Having affinity for acid or pert. to certain tissues and cell granules. 2. Pert. to a cell capable of being stained by acid stains, an eosinophil. SYN: *acidophilous.*

acidophilus milk (ăs″ĭ-dŏf'ĭ-lŭs). Milk fermented by *Lactobacillus acidophilus* cultures. SEE: *milk.*

acidoresistant (ăs″ĭ-dō-rĕ-zĭs'tănt). Acid-resisting; said about bacteria.

acidosic (ăs″ĭ-dō'sĭk). Characterized by acidosis.

acidosis (ăs″ĭ-dō'sĭs) [L. *acidum,* acid, + Gr. *osis,* condition]. Excessive acidity of body fluids due to an accumulation of acids (as in diabetic acidosis or renal disease) or an excessive loss of bicarbonate (as in renal disease). The hydrogen ion concentration, q.v., is increased, and thus the pH is decreased. SEE: *acid-base balance; acidemia; buffer; pH.*

  a., carbon dioxide. Acidosis resulting from carbon dioxide retention, as in drowning or decreased respiration.

  a., compensated. Acidosis in which the pH of body fluids has been returned to normal. Compensatory mechanisms maintain the normal ratio of bicarbonate to carbonic acid (approx. 20:1) in blood plasma, even though the bicarbonate level is decreased or the carbon dioxide level is elevated.

  a., diabetic. Acidosis occurring in advanced stages of uncontrolled diabetes mellitus due to accumulation of ketone bodies, q.v. SEE: *diabetic coma.*

  a., hypercapnic. A., respiratory, q.v.

  a., hyperchloremic. Acidosis in which there is an abnormally high level of chloride in the blood serum.

  a., lactic. Accumulation of lactic acid in the blood above normal range of 0.4 to 1.3 mmol/L. Blood lactate is increased in certain diseases and during exercise or hyperventilation; and secondary to administration of some drugs, e.g., oral hypoglycemic agents.

  a., metabolic. Acidosis resulting from increase in acids other than carbonic acid. Possible causes are excessive ingestion of acids or acid salts, ketosis, severe dehydration, diarrhea, vomiting, renal disease, impaired liver function.

  NURSING IMPLICATIONS: Monitor arterial blood gas values and fluid balance, utilizing an arterial line and indwelling urinary catheter as necessary. Monitor the patient's level of consciousness related to central nervous system depression, assessing for lethargy, drowsiness, headache, and liver damage. Assess for hyperventilation (a compensatory mechanism) and monitor for cardiac dysrhythmias. Assess for symptoms produced by associated gastrointestinal distress, such as nausea, vomiting, diarrhea, and abdominal pain. Administer prescribed I.V. fluids and other therapies such as oxygen and sodium bicarbonate, and evaluate patient's response and changes in arterial blood gas values. Be prepared to institute safety precautions for seizure activity. SEE: *Nursing Diagnoses* in *Appendix.*

  a., renal. Acidosis due to impaired kidney function. The acidosis is induced by excessive loss of bicarbonate or inability to excrete phosphoric and sulfuric acids.

  a., respiratory. Acidosis secondary to pulmonary insufficiency resulting in retention of carbon dioxide.

  NURSING IMPLICATIONS: Monitor the patient's arterial blood gas values and serum potassium level. Evaluate the patient's level of consciousness related to central nervous system depression, assessing for headache, restlessness, irritability, disorientation, blurred vision, depressed reflexes, and cardiac dysrhythmias. Prepare the patient for and assist with inhalation therapy or mechanical ventilation to decrease carbon dioxide levels, and provide prescribed therapies for associated hypoxemia and for underlying conditions.

acidotic (ăs″ĭ-dŏt'ĭk). Pert. to acidosis.

acid poisoning. Ingestion of a toxic acid. SEE: *acids* in *Poisons and Poisoning* in *Appendix.*

  F.A.: Dilute with large volumes of water. Give oral milk, egg white, magnesium oxide, milk of magnesia, lime water, or aluminum hydroxide gel. Avoid carbonates as neutralizers because, in the presence of strong acids, they will react to produce carbon dioxide gas. This may cause distention and rupture of the stomach. Give demulcents and morphine for pain.

Caution: The use of emetics and stomach tubes is dangerous.

acid-proof. Acid-fast, q.v.

acid rain. Rain that, in passing through the atmosphere, is contaminated with acid substances, esp. sulfur dioxide and nitrogen oxide. These pollutants are oxidized in the atmosphere to sulfuric acid and nitric acid. Rainwater is classed as being abnormally acid if the pH is below 5.6. Values as low as pH 2.4 were recorded in Scotland in 1974. Severe harmful effects on aquatic and plant life have been reported in the U.S., Canada, Scandinavia, and western Europe. SYN: *acid fallout.*

acid reflux test. Test for reflux of acid into the esophagus from the stomach. An electrode for detecting pH is placed in the stomach and a reading taken; then the electrode is withdrawn until it is in the esophagus. Normally, the pH will become more alkaline, i.e., rise, as the electrode is moved from the stomach into the esophagus. If there is acid reflux, the pH will be acid in both the stomach and esophagus.

acid salt. Salt formed when only a part of the hydrogen of an acid is replaced by a metal.

acidulate [L. *acidulus,* slightly acid]. To make somewhat sour or acid.

acidulous (ă-sĭd'ū-lŭs). Slightly sour or acid.

acidum (ăs'ĭ-dŭm) [L.]. Acid.

aciduria (ăs-ĭd-ū'rē-ă) [L. *acidum,* acid, + Gr. *ouron,* urine]. The condition of excessive acid in the urine.

aciduric (ăs''ĭ-dū'rĭk) ["" + *durare,* to endure]. Capable of growing in an acid medium, but preferring a slightly alkaline medium, as certain bacteria.

acies (ă'sē-ēz) [L., edge]. Margin or border.

acinar (ăs'ĭ-năr) [L. *acinus,* grape]. Rel. to or affecting an acinus, q.v.

acinesia (ăs''ĭ-nē'sē-ă) [Gr. *a-,* not, + *kinesis,* movement]. Akinesia, q.v.

acinesic, acinetic (ăs-ĭ-nē'sĭk, -nĕt'ĭk). Akinetic, q.v.

Acinetobacter (ăs''ĭ-nĕt''ō-băk'tĕr) [Gr. *akinetos,* immovable, + *bakterion,* rod]. A genus of microorganisms widely distributed in nature that are usually nonpathogenic. *Acinetobacter lwoffi* was previously known as *Mima polymorpha,* and *Acinetobacter anitratus* was previously known as *Herellea vaginicula.*

acini (ăs'ĭ-nī). Pl. of acinus.

aciniform (ă-sĭn'ĭ-form) [L. *acinus,* grape, + *forma,* shape]. Resembling grapes. SYN: *acinous.*

acinitis (ăs''ĭ-nī'tĭs) ["" + Gr. *itis,* inflammation]. Inflammation of glandular acini.

acinose (ăs'ĭ-nōs) [L. *acinosus,* grapelike]. Composed of acini.

acinous (ăs'ĭ-nŭs). Pert. to glands resembling a bunch of grapes, such as acini and alveolar glands. SYN: *aciniform.*

acinus (ăs'ĭ-nŭs) [L., grape] (pl. *acini*). [NA] Smallest division of a gland; a group of secretory cells surrounding a cavity.

A.C. joint. *acromioclavicular joint.*

ackee (ă'kē). Akee, q.v.

acladiosis (ăk-lăd''ē-ō'sĭs). An ulcerative skin disease believed to be due to fungi of the genus *Acladium.*

aclasis, aclasia (ăk'lă-sĭs, ă-klā'zē-ă) [Gr. *a-,* not, + *klasis,* a breaking away]. Abnormal tissue arising from and continuous with a normal structure, as in chondrodysplasia.

   a., diaphyseal. Imperfect formation of cancellous bone in cartilage between diaphysis and epiphysis.

acleistocardia (ă-klīs''tō-kăr'dē-ă) [Gr. *akleistos,* not closed, + *kardia,* heart]. Patent foramen ovale of the heart.

ACLS. *Advanced Cardiac Life Support.*

acme (ăk'mē) [Gr. *akme,* point]. 1. The highest point; peak. 2. The time of greatest intensity of a symptom or disease process.

acne (ăk'nē) [Gr. *akme,* point]. 1. An inflammatory disease of the sebaceous glands and hair follicles of the skin characterized by comedones, papules, pustules. Cysts and nodules may develop and scarring is common. Usually associated with seborrhea. 2. Acne vulgaris, q.v.

   a. atrophica. Acne with residual pitting and scarring.

   a., bromide. Characteristic acne caused by bromide.

   a. cachecticorum. A type of acne seen in debilitated patients.

   a. ciliaris. Acne that affects the edges of the eyelids.

   a. conglobata. Acne vulgaris with abscesses, cysts, and sinuses that leave scars.

   a., cystic. Acne with cysts containing keratin and sebum.

   TREAT: The vitamin A derivative, isotretinoin, has been effective in treating this condition. For Caution concerning its use, SEE: *isotretinoin.*

   a. fulminans. A rare type of acne in teenaged boys. Characterized by inflamed, tender, ulcerative, and crusting lesions of the upper trunk and face. It has a sudden onset and is accompanied by fever, leukocytosis, and an elevated sedimentation rate. About half of the cases have inflammation of several joints.

a., halogen. Acne due to exposure to halogens such as bromine, chlorine, or iodine.

a. indurata. Acne vulgaris with chronic, discolored, indurated surfaces.

a., keloid. Infection about the hair follicles at back of neck causing scars and thickening of skin.

a. keratosa. Acne vulgaris in which suppurating nodules crust over to form horny plugs. These occur at the corners of the mouth.

a. neonatorum. Acne in the newborn.

a. papulosa. Acne characterized by formation of papules with very little inflammation.

a., petroleum. Acne that may occur in those who work with petroleum and oils.

a. pustulosa. Acne with pustule formation and subsequent deep scars.

a. rosacea. Rosacea, q.v.

a., steroid. Acne caused by systemic or topical use of corticosteroid drugs.

a., summer. Acne that appears only in hot, humid climatic conditions or that is made much worse in such weather. Even though the exact cause is unknown, it is not caused by increased exposure to the sun's rays.

a., tropical. Severe acne caused by or aggravated by living in a hot, humid climate. Skin of the thorax, back, and legs is most commonly affected.

a. urticaria. An acneiform eruption of itching wheals.

a. varioliformis. Vesiculopustular folliculitis that occurs most commonly on temples and frontal margins of the scalp but may be seen on chest, back, or nose.

a. vulgaris. Common acne.

SYM: Either papules about comedones with black centers, or pustules, or hypertrophied nodules caused by overgrowth of connective tissue. In the indurative type, the lesions are deep-seated and cause scarring. Face, neck, and shoulders are common sites.

ETIOL: Unknown. Predisposing causes include hereditary or familial tendencies and disturbances in androgen-estrogen balance affecting activity of sebaceous glands. Acne begins at puberty. At that time the increased secretion of androgen in both males and females causes an increase in the size and activity of the pilosebaceous glands. Specific inciting factors may include food allergies, endocrine disorders, therapy with adrenal corticosteroid hormones, and psychogenic factors. Vitamin deficiencies, ingestion of halogens, and contact with chemicals such as tar and chlorinated hy-

drocarbons may be specific causative factors. The fact that bacteria are important once the disease is present is indicated by the successful results following antibiotic therapy. The lesions may become worse in females before the premenstruum.

TREAT: Local; systemic when indicated. Topical cleansing and peeling (keratolytic) agents and the use of tetracycline, but this drug should not be used during the last two trimesters of pregnancy, and not prior to age 12 in order to prevent tooth discoloration. Topical application of vitamin A acid is quite effective. Severe cystic acne, q.v., responds very well to orally administered isotretinoin, but because this drug is teratogenic, it cannot be used in women of childbearing age unless they are not sexually active or effective contraceptive use is guaranteed. Careful extraction of comedones and incision and drainage of cysts and pustules. Avoidance of conditions known to cause exacerbations. For Caution concerning use of isotretinoin, SEE: *isotretinoin.*

PROG: Obstinate and recurrent.

NURSING IMPLICATIONS: Instruct the patient to wash the skin thoroughly but to avoid intense scrubbing and excessive skin abrasion. Teach the patient to keep hands away from face and other sites of lesions, to limit the use of cosmetics, and to observe for, recognize and avoid causes of exacerbations. Explain the need to reduce sun exposure when vitamin A acid is prescribed. Provide emotional support and understanding, particularly if the patient is an adolescent.

acnegenic (ăk″nē-jĕn′ĭk) [Gr. *akme*, point, + *gennan*, to produce]. Causing or producing acne.

acneiform (ăk-nē′ĭ-form) [″ + L. *forma*, shape]. Resembling acne. Also spelled acneform.

acnemia (ăk-nē′mē-ă) [Gr. *a-*, not, + *kneme*, lower leg]. Wasting of the calves of the legs.

A.C.N.M. *American College of Nurse Midwives.*

A.C.O.G. *American College of Obstetricians and Gynecologists.*

aconite (ăk′ō-nīt) [Gr. *akoniton*]. The dried tuberous root of *Aconitum*, esp. *A. napellus* (monkshood) and *A. lycoctonum* (wolfsbane); a poisonous and very powerful alkaloid. Its action, which is due to the presence of two very potent alkaloids, was well known to the ancients. Aconite is believed to have been used as an arrow poison early in Chinese history and perhaps also by the inhabitants of ancient Gaul. Aconite is no longer used but is of historical interest.

aconitine (ă-kŏn′ĭ-tĭn). The active ingredient

in aconite.

acorea (ă-kō-rē′ă) [Gr. *a-*, not, + *kore*, pupil]. Absence of the pupil of the eye.

acoria (ă-kō′rē-ă) [″ + *koros*, satiety]. 1. Lacking in satisfaction after eating but not from hunger. 2. Gluttony. RS: bulimia; hyperorexia; polyphagia.

acormus (ă-kor′mŭs) [″ + *kormos*, trunk]. 1. Lack of a trunk. 2. A fetal abnormality consisting of a head and extremities without a trunk.

acousia (ă-koo′zē-ă) [Gr. *akousis*, hearing]. The hearing faculty. SYN: *acusis*.

acousmatamnesia [″ + *amnesia*, forgetfulness]. Inability to recall and identify sounds.

acoustic (ă-koos′tĭk) [Gr. *akoustikos*]. Pert. to sound or to the sense of hearing.

acoustic center. The hearing center in the brain located in the temporal lobe of the cerebrum.

acoustic meatus. The opening to the external or internal auditory canal.

acoustic nerve. A nerve consisting of two separate parts: vestibular and cochlear nerves, with superficial origin at junction of pons and medulla. SYN: *auditory nerve; eighth cranial nerve; vestibulocochlear nerve.*

PHYS: Special senses of hearing and equilibrium. Vestibular and cochlear nerves consist of special somatic afferent fibers. Cells of origin of vestibular nerve are bipolar and lie in the vestibular ganglion, peripheral branches terminating in receptors of semicircular ducts, saccule, and utricle. Cells of origin of cochlear nerve are bipolar and lie in the spiral ganglion, peripheral branches terminating in spiral organ of Corti. The two nerves become joined, enter the internal acoustic meatus with the facial nerve, and then separate.

acousticophobia (ă-koos″tĭ-kō-fō′bē-ă) [Gr. *akoustos*, heard, + *phobos*, fear]. Abnormal fear of loud sounds.

acoustic reflectometry. Diagnostic technique for the detection of middle ear effusion. Measures the level of sound transmitted and reflected from the middle ear to a microphone located in a probe tip placed against the ear canal opening and directed toward the tympanic membrane.

acoustic reflex threshold. A test to measure the intensity of a sound at which the stapedial muscle of the inner ear contracts. The test can be used to determine the presence of cochlear pathology and, therefore, is used in differentiating conductive from sensorineural hearing loss.

acoustics (ă-koos′tĭks). The science of sound, its production, transmission, and effects.

acoustic trauma. Injury to hearing by noise, esp. loud noise.

A.C.P. *American College of Physicians; American College of Pathologists.*

acquired (ă-kwīrd′) [L. *acquirere*, to get]. Not hereditary or innate.

acquired immune deficiency syndrome. ABBR: AIDS, q.v. SEE: *AIDS-related complex; Kaposi's sarcoma.*

acquisitus (ă-kwĭs′ĭ-tŭs) [L.]. Acquired.

A.C.R. *American College of Radiology.*

acral (ăk′răl) [Gr. *akron*, extremity]. Pert. to extremities.

acrania (ă-krā′nē-ă) [Gr. *a-*, not, + *kranion*, skull]. Partial or complete congenital absence of the cranium.

Acremonium (ăk″rē-mō′nē-ŭm). A genus of fungi, some of which are pathogenic.

acrid (ăk′rĭd) [L. *acer*, sharp]. Burning, bitter, irritating.

acridine (ăk′rĭ-dĭn). A coal tar hydrocarbon from which certain dyes are prepared.

acrimony (ăk′rĭ-mō″nē). [L. *acrimonia*, pungency]. Quality of being pungent, acrid, irritating.

acrisorcin (ăk-rĭ-sor′sĭn). USP. Chemical used in treating tinea versicolor. Trade name is Akrinol.

acritical (ā-krĭt′ĭ-kăl) [Gr. *a-*, not, + *kritikos*, critical]. Not marked by a crisis.

acro- (ăk′rō) [Gr. *akron*, extremity]. A combining form meaning extremity, top, extreme point.

acroagnosis (ăk″rō-ăg-nō′sĭs) [″ + *gnosis*, knowledge]. Absence of feeling of one's limb.

acroanesthesia (ăk″rō-ăn-ĕs-thē′zē-ă) [″ + *an-*, not, + *aisthesis*, sensation]. Lack of sensation in one or more of the extremities.

acroarthritis (ăk-rō-ăr-thrī′tĭs) [″ + *arthron*, joint, + *itis*, inflammation]. Arthritis of the hands or feet.

acroasphyxia (ăk″rō-ăs-fĭk′sē-ă) [″ + *asphyxia*, pulse stoppage]. Cold, pale condition of hands and feet; symptom of Raynaud's disease.

acroataxia (ăk″rō-ă-tăk′sē-ă) [Gr. *akron*, extremity, + *ataktos*, out of order]. Muscular incoordination involving, or limited to, the fingers and toes.

acroblast (ăk′rō-blăst) [″ + *blastos*, germ]. A part of the Golgi apparatus in the spermatid from which the acrosome arises.

acrobrachycephaly (ăk″rō-brăk″ĭ-sĕf′ă-lē) [″ + *brachys*, short, + *kephale*, head]. State of having an abnormally short head in the anterior-posterior diameter due to fusion of the coronal suture.

acrobystitis (ăk″rō-bĭs-tī′tĭs) [Gr. *akrobystia*, prepuce, + *itis*, inflammation]. Inflammation of the prepuce. SYN: *acro-*

posthitis; posthitis.

acrocentric (ăk″rō-sĕn′trĭk) [Gr. *akron,* extremity + L. *centrum,* center]. Pert. to a chromosome in which the centromere is located near one end. At metaphase it has the appearance of a wishbone.

acrocephalia (ăk″rō-sĕf-ā′lē-ă) [″ + *kephale,* head]. Acrocephaly, q.v. SYN: *oxycephalia.*

acrocephalic (ăk″rō-sĕ-făl′ĭk). Pert. to acrocephaly, q.v.

acrocephalosyndactylia, acrocephalosyndactyly (ăk″rō-sĕf″ă-lō-sĭn-dăk-tĭl′ē-ă, -sĭn-dăk′tĭl-ē) [″ + ″ + *syn,* together, + *daktylos,* a finger]. A congenital condition marked by a peaked head and webbed fingers and toes. SYN: *Apert's syndrome.*

acrocephaly (ăk″rō-sĕf′ă-lē) [Gr. *akron,* extremity, + *kephale,* head]. State of having a malformed cranial vault with a high or peaked appearance and a vertical index above 77. SYN: *oxycephaly.*

ETIOL: Premature closure of the coronal, sagittal, and lambdoidal sutures.

acrochordon (ăk″rō-kor′dŏn) [″ + *chorde,* cord]. A small outgrowth of epidermal and dermal tissue. Pedunculated, smooth or irregular, flesh-colored, benign tumors. These occur most often on the eyelids, neck, and axillae, but may be seen almost anywhere on the skin. Except for being unsightly, they are harmless, unless they become twisted on their pedicle. SYN: *fibroepithelial polyp; skin tag.*

acrocinesia, acrocinesis (ăk″rō-sĭn-ē′sē-ă, -sĭs) [″ + *kinesis,* movement]. Excessive movement of the extremities. SYN: *acrokinesia.*

acrokinetic (ăk″rō-sĭn-ĕt′ĭk). Showing excessive motion of the extremities.

acrocontracture (ăk″rō-kŏn-trăkt′ūr) [″ + L. *contrahere,* to draw together]. Contracture of the hands or feet.

acrocyanosis (ăk″rō-sī-ă-nō′sĭs) [″ + *kyanosis,* dark-blue color]. Cyanosis of the extremities. Acrocyanosis of the hands and feet may be normal in the infant within the first hour after birth.

ETIOL: Due to vasomotor disturbances. Seen in catatonia or hysteria.

acrodermatitis (ăk″rō-dĕr-mă-tī′tĭs) [″ + *derma,* skin, + *itis,* inflammation]. Dermatitis of the extremities.

    a. chronica atrophicans. Dermatitis of hands and feet that progresses slowly upward on the affected limbs.

    a. continua. An obstinate eczematous eruption confined to the extremities.

    a. enteropathica. Rare childhood disease with onset between 3 weeks and 18 months. May be fatal if untreated. The ge-

netically determined cause is malabsorption of zinc. Onset is insidious with failure to thrive, diarrhea, loss of hair, and development of vesiculobullous lesions, particularly around body orifices.

TREAT: Zinc sulfate given orally will abolish all clinical manifestations of the disease within a few days.

    a. hiemalis. A dermatitis occurring in winter, affecting the extremities. It tends to disappear spontaneously.

    a. perstans. A. continua, q.v.

acrodermatosis (ăk″rō-dĕr″mă-tō′sĭs) [Gr. *akron,* extremity, + *derma,* skin, + *osis,* condition]. Any skin disease that affects the hands and feet.

acrodolichomelia (ăk″rō-dŏl″ĭ-kō-mē′lē-ă) [″ + *dolichos,* long, + *melos,* limb]. Condition in which the hands and feet are abnormally long.

acrodynia (ăk″rō-dĭn′ē-ă) [″ + *odyne,* pain]. A disease of infants and young children caused by chronic mercury poisoning. It has a prolonged clinical course with various grades of severity. The child is listless, irritable, and no longer interested in play. The rash has several variations. Initially, the tips of the fingers and toes become pink, the hands and feet become pink but color shades off at the wrists and ankles. As the disease progresses, the skin of the extremities desquamates, there are profuse sweating and pruritus, and pain is excruciating in the hands and feet. Neurological symptoms with neuritis and mental apathy develop.

TREAT: Remove source of mercury; administer dimercaprol (BAL) antidote; supportive therapy. SYN: *pink disease.*

acrodysesthesia (ăk″rō-dĭs″ĕs-thē′zē-ă) [″ + *dys,* bad, + *aisthesis,* sensation]. Dysesthesia, q.v., in arms and legs.

acroesthesia (ăk″rō-ĕs-thē′zē-ă) [″ + *aisthesis,* sensation]. 1. Abnormal sensitivity of the extremities. 2. Pain in the extremities.

acrogeria (ăk″rō-jĕr′ē-ă) [″ + *geron,* old man]. A condition in which the skin of the hands and feet shows signs of premature aging.

acrognosis (ăk″rŏg-nō′sĭs) [″ + *gnosis,* knowledge]. Sensory perception of limbs.

acrohyperhidrosis (ăk″rō-hī″pĕr-hī-drō′sĭs) [″ + *hyper,* excessive, + *hidrosis,* sweating]. Excessive perspiration of hands and feet.

acrohypothermy (ăk″rō-hī″pō-thĕr′mē) [″ + *hypo,* below, + *therme,* heat]. Abnormal coldness of extremities.

acrokeratosis verruciformis (ăk″rō-kĕr″ă-tō′sĭs vĕ-roo′sĭ-for″-mĭs) [″ + *keras,* horn, + *osis,* condition; L. *verruca,* wart,

+ *forma,* form]. Hereditary disease of the skin characterized by warty growths on the extremities, principally on the backs of the hands and on the feet.

acrokinesia (ăk″rō-kĭn-ē′sē-ă) [″ + *kinesis,* movement]. Excessive motion of the extremities. SYN: *acrocinesia.*

acrolein (ăk-rō′lē-ĭn) [L. *acer,* acrid, + *oleum,* oil]. A volatile liquid produced by dry distillation of glycerin. SYN: *acrylaldehyde.*

acromacria (ăk″rō-măk′rē-ă) [Gr. *akron,* extremity, + *makros,* long]. Abnormal length of fingers. SYN: *arachnodactyly.* SEE: *Marfan's syndrome.*

acromastitis (ăk″rō-măs-tī′tĭs) [″ + *mastos,* breast, + *itis,* inflammation]. Inflammation of the nipple. SYN: *thelitis.*

acromegaly (ăk″rō-mĕg′ă-lē) [″ + *megas,* big]. A chronic disease of middle-aged persons characterized by elongation and enlargement of bones of the extremities and certain head bones, esp. frontal bone and jaws, accompanied by enlargement of nose and lips and thickening of soft tissues of the face. It is often associated with somnolence, moodiness, and decreased libido. SYN: *Marie's disease.*

SYM: Onset of the disease is so gradual that neither the patients nor their associates notice it. Early complaints include muscular pains, headache, sweating. Facial features are enlarged, and mandible and malar bones become prominent with protrusion of orbital ridge. Teeth become widely separated; hands and feet gradually enlarge. About one fourth of the patients will develop diabetes. As the disease progresses, muscular weakness becomes a serious feature, and visual impairment may progress to blindness.

ETIOL: Hyperfunction of the eosinophilic cells of the anterior lobe of the pituitary resulting in excess production of growth hormone. SEE: *somatostatin.*

TREAT: The dopamine agonist bromocriptine may be used with either x-ray therapy or surgical removal of pituitary gland.

acromelalgia (ăk″rō-mĕl-ăl′jē-ă) [Gr. *akron,* extremity, + *melos,* limb, + *algos,* pain]. Erythromelalgia, q.v.

acromelic (ăk″rō-mĕl′ĭk) [″ + *melos,* limb]. Pert. to the end of the extremities.

acrometagenesis (ăk″rō-mĕt″ă-jĕn′ĕ-sĭs) [″ + *meta,* beyond, + *genesis,* generation, birth]. Abnormal growth of extremities.

acromial (ă-krō′mē-ăl) [″ + *omos,* shoulder]. Rel. to the acromion.

acromial angle. The angle at the edge of the spine of the scapula where it ascends to become the acromion.

acromial process. The acromion, q.v.

acromial reflex. Flexion of forearm with internal rotation of hand resulting from quick blow upon acromion. Elicited in hyperkinetic states.

acromicria (ăk″rō-mĭk′rē-ă) [″ + *mikros,* small]. Congenital shortness or smallness of the extremities and face.

acromioclavicular joint (ă-krō″mē-ŏ-klă-vĭk′ū-lăr) [″ + *omos,* shoulder, + L. *clavicula,* small key]. An arthrodial joint between the acromion and the acromial end of the clavicle.

acromiocoracoid (ă-krō″mē-ŏ-kor′ă-koyd) [″ + ″ + *korax,* crow, + *eidos,* form, shape]. Pert. to the acromion and coracoid process.

acromiohumeral (ăk-rō″mē-ŏ-hū′mĕr-ăl) [″ + ″ + L. *humerus,* shoulder]. Pert. to the acromion and humerus.

acromion (ă-krō′mē-ŏn) [Gr. *akron,* extremity, + *omos,* shoulder]. [NA] The lateral triangular projection of the spine of the scapula that forms the point of the shoulder and articulates with the clavicle. SYN: *acromial process.* SEE: *acromioclavicular joint.*

acromioscapular (ă-krō″mē-ŏ-skăp′ū-lăr) [″ + ″ + L. *scapula,* shoulder blade]. Pert. to the acromion and scapula.

acromiothoracic (ă-krō″mē-ŏ-thō-răs′ĭk) [″ + ″ + *thorax,* chest]. Pert. to the acromion and thorax.

acromphalus (ăk-rŏm′făl-ŭs) [″ + *omphalos,* umbilicus]. 1. Center of navel. 2. Projection of umbilicus, as in beginning of umbilical hernia.

acromyotonia, acromyotonus (ăk″rō-mī-ŏ-tō′nē-ă, -ŏt′ŏ-nŭs) [″ + *mys,* muscle, + *tonos,* tension]. Myotonia of extremities causing spasmodic deformity.

acroneurosis (ăk″rō-nŭ-rō′sĭs) [Gr. *akron,* extremity, + *neuron,* nerve, + *osis,* condition]. Nervous disorder in the extremities.

acronym (ăk′rō-nĭm) [″ + *onym,* name]. Word formed by combining the first letter or letters of a name or a phrase.

Ex.: MASH for *M*obile *A*rmy *S*urgical *H*ospital.

acronyx (ăk′rō-nĭks″) [L. *acer,* sharp, + Gr. *onyx,* claw]. An ingrown nail.

acro-osteolysis (ăk″rō-ŏs″tē-ŏl′ĭ-sĭs) [Gr. *akron,* extremity, + *osteon,* bone, + *lysis,* dissolution]. 1. A familial disease in which there is dissolution of the tips of the extremities of young children. There is no history of trauma, and spontaneous amputation does not occur. Etiology unknown. 2. An occupational disease seen in workers who come in contact with vinyl chloride polymerization processes. Characterized by Raynaud's phenomenon, scleroderma-like skin changes, and x-ray evidence of bone destruction of the distal phalanges of the hands. Recovery follows removal from exposure. SEE: *Raynaud's disease.*

acropachy (ăk'rō-păk"ē) [" + *pachys,* thick]. Clubbing of fingers or toes.

acropachyderma (ăk"rō-păk"ē-dĕr'mă) [" + " + *derma,* skin]. Clubbing of the fingers, deformed long bones, and thickening of the skin of the scalp, face, and extremities.

acroparalysis (ăk"rō-pă-răl'ĭ-sĭs) [" + *paralyein,* to disable]. Paralysis of one or more extremities.

acroparesthesia (ăk"rō-păr-ĕs-thē'zē-ă) [" + *para,* abnormal, + *aisthesis,* sensation]. Sensation of prickling, tingling, or numbness in the extremities.

acropathology (ăk"rō-pă-thŏl'ō-jē) [" + *pathos,* disease, suffering, + *logos,* word, reason]. Pathology of disease of the extremities.

acropathy (ă-krŏp'ă-thē) [" + *pathos,* disease, suffering]. Any disease of the extremities.

acrophobia (ăk-rō-fō'bē-ă) [" + *phobos,* fear]. Morbid fear of high places.

acroposthitis (ăk"rō-pŏs-thī'tĭs) [Gr. *akroposthis,* prepuce, + *itis,* inflammation]. Inflammation of the prepuce of the penis. SYN: *acrobystitis; posthitis.*

acropustulosis, infantile. Cyclical eruption of pustules on the soles and feet of infants between 2 and 10 months of age. The pustules become vesicopapular, crust over, and heal within 7 to 10 days. A new crop appears in 2 to 3 weeks and they also heal. These periodic outbreaks occur for about 2 years and then stop.
ETIOL: Unknown, and symptomatic therapy is all that is required.

acroscleroderma (ăk"rō-sklĕr-ō-dĕr'mă) [Gr. *akron,* extremity, + *scleros,* hard, + *derma,* skin]. Hard, thickened skin condition of toes and fingers. SYN: *sclerodactylia.*

acrosclerosis (ăk"rō-sklĕr-ō'sĭs) [" + " + *osis,* condition]. A scleroderma of the upper extremities, sometimes extending to neck and face. Usually follows Raynaud's disease, q.v.

acrosome (ăk'rō-sōm) [" + *soma,* body]. The anterior end of the head of the spermatozoon.

acroteric (ăk"rō-tĕr'ĭk) [Gr. *akroterion,* summit]. Pert. to the outermost parts of the extremities, as the tips of the fingers.

acrotism (ăk'rō-tĭzm) [Gr. *a-,* not, + *krotos,* striking, + *-ismos,* condition]. Imperceptibility of the pulse.

acrotrophoneurosis (ăk"rō-trŏf"ō-nū-rō'sĭs) [Gr. *akron,* extremity, + *trophe,* nourishment, + *neuron,* nerve, + *osis,* condition]. Trophoneurosis of extremities

with trophic, neuritic, and vascular changes. Usually caused by prolonged immersion in water.

acryl(o)-. Combining form indicating acrylic.

acrylaldehyde (ăk"rĭl-ăl'dĕ-hīd). Acrolein, q.v.

acrylamide (ă-krĭl'ă-mīd). C_3H_5NO. The amide of acrylic acid.

acrylate (ăk'rĭ-lāt). A salt or ester of acrylic acid.

acrylic acid (ă-krĭl'ĭk). $CH_2:CH \cdot COOH$. A colorless corrosive liquid. Used in making acrylic polymers, q.v., and resins, q.v.

acrylic resin. General term for various polymers of acrylic acid and their esters. Some of these compounds are used medically as components of contact lenses and dental materials.

acrylonitrile (ăk"rĭ-lō-nī'trĭl). C_3H_3N. A toxic compound used in making plastics. SYN: *vinyl cyanide.*

A.C.S., ACS. *American Cancer Society; American Chemical Society; American College of Surgeons; anodal closing sound.*

A.C.S.M. *American College of Sports Medicine.*

act (ăkt). To accomplish a function; the accomplishment of a function.
  a., compulsive. The repetitive, ritualistic performance of an act. This may be done despite the individual's attempts to resist the act.
  a., impulsive. Sudden action caused by an abnormal impulse or desire.

ACTH. *adrenocorticotropic hormone,* a pituitary hormone that stimulates the cortex of the adrenal glands to produce adrenal cortical hormones. SEE: *cortisone.*

actin (ăk'tĭn). Protein derived from the actomyosin in muscle. In response to chemical changes in the tissue, actin may have a globular or an elongated form. This property is important in contracting and relaxing muscle tissue.

acting out. Expressing oneself through actions rather than speech.
  a.o., neurotic. 1. A form of transference, q.v., in which tension is relieved by responding to a situation as if it were the same situation that originally gave rise to the tension; a displacement of behavioral response from one situation to another. 2. In psychoanalysis, a form of displacement, q.v., in which the patient relives memories rather than expressing them verbally.

actinic (ăk-tĭn'ĭk) [Gr. *aktis,* ray]. 1. Pert. to radiant energy such as x-rays, ultraviolet light, sunlight, particularly the photochemical effects. 2. Pert. to the capability of radiant energy to produce chemical changes.

actinic burns. Burns caused by ultraviolet or

sun rays. Treatment as in dry heat burns. SEE: *burn.*

actinic dermatitis. Inflammation and erythema of the skin caused by exposure to radiation.

actinism (ăk'tĭn-ĭzm). That property of radiant energy that produces chemical changes, as in photography or heliotherapy.

actinium (ăk-tĭn'ē-ŭm) [Gr. *aktis,* ray]. SYMB: Ac. At. wt. 227; at. no. 89. A radioactive element.

actino- (ăk'tĭ-nō) [Gr. *aktis,* ray]. Combining form indicating a similarity to a ray or referring to radiation such as x-ray or electromagnetic radiation, e.g., light rays.

Actinobacillus (ăk''tĭ-nō-bă-sĭl'lŭs). Small gram-negative coccobacilli that affect mostly domestic animals, but *Actinobacillus actinomycetemcomitans* has been implicated in endocarditis in humans.

actinochemistry (ăk''tĭ-nō-kĕm'ĭs-trē) ['' + *chemeia,* chemistry]. Branch of chemistry concerned with the effects of light rays. SYN: *photochemistry.*

actinodermatitis (ăk''tĭn-ō-dĕr-mă-tī'tĭs) ['' + *derma,* skin, + *itis,* inflammation]. Dermatitis caused by exposure to radiation.

Actinomyces (ăk''tĭn-ō-ō-mī'sēz) ['' + *mykes,* fungus]. A genus of bacteria of the family Actinomycetaceae that contain gram-positive staining filaments. These bacteria cause various diseases in humans and animals.

   A. antibioticus. A species of *Actinomyces* from which the antibiotic actinomycin is obtained.

   A. bovis. A species of *Actinomyces* that causes actinomycosis (lumpy jaw) in cattle.

   A. israelii. A species of *Actinomyces* that causes actinomycosis in humans. One clinical form is called lumpy jaw due to the characteristic appearance of the swollen jaw produced by the infection.

   TREAT: Prolonged therapy with very large doses of penicillin G is required.

Actinomycetales (ăk''tĭ-nō-mī''sĕ-tā'lēz). An order of bacteria that includes the families Mycobacteriaceae, Actinomycetaceae, Actinoplanaceae, Dermatophilaceae, Micromonosporaceae, Nocardiaceae, and Streptomycetaceae.

actinomycete (ăk''tĭ-nō-mī'sēt). Any bacterium of the order Actinomycetales.

actinomycetic (ăk''tĭ-nō-mī-sĕt'ĭk). Pert. to *Actinomyces.*

actinomycetin (ăk''tĭn-ō-mī-sĕt'ĭn). A lytic substance obtained from *Actinomyces;* it destroys some gram-positive and gram-negative organisms.

actinomycin A (ăk''tĭn-ō-mī'sĭn). An antibacterial substance obtained from *Actinomyces antibioticus,* heat-stable and highly toxic, effective against gram-positive organisms. It is orange-colored and is soluble in alcohol and ether.

actinomycin B. Similar to actinomycin A but not soluble in alcohol. Not used clinically because of its toxicity.

Actinomycin D. Trade name for dactinomycin.

actinomycoma (ăk''tĭ-nō-mī-kō'ma) [Gr. *aktis,* ray, + *mykes,* fungus, + *oma,* tumor]. A tumor produced by actinomycosis, q.v.

actinomycosis (ăk''tĭn-ō-mī-kō'sĭs) ['' + '' + *osis,* condition]. A noncontagious bacterial disease in animals (lumpy jaw) and humans. Infection may be of the cervicofacial, thoracic, or abdominal regions, or may be generalized.

   SYM: Formation of slow-growing granulomas that later break down, discharging viscid pus containing minute yellowish (sulfur) granules.

   ETIOL: *Actinomyces bovis* in cattle; *Actinomyces israelii* in humans. This organism is normally present in the mouth. SEE: *nocardiosis.*

   TREAT: Prolonged administration of penicillin is usually effective. Tetracyclines are the second choice. Surgical incision and drainage of accessible lesions is helpful when combined with chemotherapy.

actinomycotic (ăk''tĭn-ō-mī-kŏt'ĭk). Pert. to actinomycosis.

actinon (ăk'tĭn-ŏn) [Gr. *aktis,* ray]. A radioactive isotope of actinium. SYN: *radon 219.*

actinoneuritis (ăk''tĭn-ō-nū-rī'tĭs) ['' + *neuron,* nerve, + *itis,* inflammation]. Inflammation of a nerve or nerves resulting from exposure to radium or x-rays.

actinophytosis (ăk''tĭ-nō-fī-tō'sĭs) ['' + *phyton,* plant, + *osis,* condition]. Infection due to *Actinomyces.*

actinotherapy (ăk''tĭn-ō-thĕr'ă-pē) ['' + *therapeia,* treatment]. Treatment of disease by rays of light, esp. actinic or photochemically active rays, or by x-rays or radium.

action (ăk'shŭn) [L. *actio*]. Performance of a function or process; in pathology, a morbid process.

   a., antagonistic. The ability of a drug or muscle to oppose or resist the action or effect of another drug or muscle. Opposite of synergistic action.

   a., astringent. Action in which the tissue cells are contracted or shrunk.

   a., bactericidal. Action that kills bacteria.

   a., bacteriostatic. Action that stops or prevents growth of bacteria without killing them.

   a., ball-valve. Intermittent obstruction of a passageway or opening so that the flow of fluid or air is prevented from moving in the normal direction and at the usual rate.

a., calorigenic. Heat produced by the metabolism of food.

a., capillary. The movement of fluid to a certain level in a small-diameter tube.

a., cumulative. Sudden increased action of a drug after several doses have been given.

a., drug. SEE: *drug action.*

a., reflex. Involuntary movement produced by sensory nerve stimulation.

a., sparing. The effect of a nonessential nutrient in the diet such that it decreases the requirement for an essential dietary substance.

Ex.: Protein is especially important for tissue growth and development in children. If protein intake is sufficient but caloric intake is inadequate, a protein deficiency will develop. In this situation, the addition of sufficient carbohydrates to the diet is said to spare the protein.

a., specific. The particular action of a drug on another substance or upon an organism or part of that organism.

a., specific dynamic. Stimulation of metabolic rate by ingestion of certain foods, esp. proteins.

a., synergistic. The ability of a drug or muscle to aid or enhance the action or effect of another drug or muscle. Opposite of antagonistic action.

a., thermogenic. Action of a food, drug, or physical agent to cause a rise in output of body heat.

a., trigger. The initiation of activity, physiological or pathological, that may have no relation to the action that started it.

action of arrest. The action of decreasing or slowing the function of an organ or cell or a chemical reaction.

action potential. The change in electrical potential of nerve or muscle fiber when stimulated.

activate (ăk′tĭ-vāt). 1. To make active. 2. To make radioactive.

activated partial thromboplastin time. ABBR: APTT. The time required for a fibrin clot to form after the activating factor, calcium, and a phospholipid have been added to the blood sample. The normal value ranges from 16 to 40 seconds. A prolonged time indicates a clotting factor deficiency or any one of a number of diseases or medications.

activator (ăk′tĭ-vā″tor). 1. A substance in the body that converts an inactive substance into an active agent, as the action of hydrogen ions on pepsinogen converting it to pepsin. 2. Any substance that specifically induces an activity, such as an inductor or organizer in embryonic development or a

trophic hormone.

active motion. Active range of motion, q.v.

active plate activator. A removable orthodontic appliance equipped to provide the force for tooth movement. May be used continuously or intermittently.

active principle. The chemical substance in a pharmaceutical preparation that is responsible for the therapeutic effects of the medicine. SEE: *drug action.*

active range of motion. ABBR: AROM. The range of movement of a joint that a patient is able to perform either without assistance or with active assisted motion, i.e., the examiner assists in the test of movement. SYN: *active motion.*

active transport. The movement by a cell membrane of molecules against a concentration or electrochemical gradient is accomplished by the process of active transport. This requires metabolic work. An example is the very low concentration of potassium ions in extracellular fluid. Other ions actively transported are sodium, calcium, hydrogen, iron, chloride, iodide, and urate. Several sugars and the amino acids are actively transported.

activins. A family of polypeptide growth factors which help regulate various biological functions, esp. fertility. SEE: *inhibin.*

activities of daily living. ABBR: ADL. The self-care, communication, and mobility skills required for independence in everyday living. The distinction is made between basic activities of daily living and ancillary but very important activities, such as telephone use, preparing meals, laundry, housecleaning, taking medicines, and handling finances. SYN: *independent living skills; daily living skills.*

NURSING IMPLICATIONS: Evaluate the patient's ability to perform ADLs and assist or arrange assistance as needed.

activities of daily living, index of. Developed by S. Katz and his colleagues. It assesses personal self-maintenance in the elderly and focuses on the unaided performance of six basic personal care activities: eating, toileting, dressing, bathing, transferring, and continence.

activity (ăk-tĭv′ĭ-tē). The production of energy or motion; the state of being active. Various conditions are described by the use of this word: enzyme activity describes the rate of influence of the enzyme on a particular system; extravehicular activity indicates the actions of space travelers while outside a space vehicle; radiation activity indicates the energy produced by a source of radiation.

a., optical. The rotation of the plane of polarized light when the light passes through a chemical solution.

a., purposeful. The goal-directed use of time, energy or attention that involves the active participation of the doer. Purposeful activity by humans often involves a social environment (others), a physical environment (objects, tools, and materials) and a process, which often culminates in a product.

activity analysis. A process used by occupational therapists to assess the psychosocial, psychodynamic, physical, or developmental characteristics of an activity in determining its utility as a therapeutic modality.

activity theory. A social theory of aging that stresses a continuation of role performances and asserts that the more active older persons are, the higher their life satisfaction and morale. According to this theory, older individuals find substitutes for former roles that they may have had to relinquish.

actomyosin (ăk″tō-mī′ō-sĭn). The combination of actin and myosin in a muscle. Upon muscle stimulation, these substances shorten without changing their volume and thus cause contraction of the muscle.

actual (ăk′chū-ăl) [L. *actus*, doing]. Real, existent.

actual cautery. Cautery acting by virtue of its heat and not chemically.

acufilopressure (ăk″ū-fĭ′lō-prĕsh″ūr) [L. *acus*, needle, + *filum*, thread, + *pressura*, pressure]. Acupressure, q.v., increased by a ligature.

acuity (ă-kū′ĭ-tē) [L. *acuere*, to sharpen]. Clearness, sharpness.

a., visual. Acuteness or sharpness of vision.

acuminate (ă-kū′mĭn-āt) [L. *acuminatus*, sharpened]. Conical or pointed.

acupressure (ăk′ū-prĕsh″ūr) [L. *acus*, needle, + *pressura*, pressure]. Compression of blood vessels by means of needles in surrounding tissues.

acupressure forceps. Spring-handled forceps for compressing blood vessels.

acupressure needles. Elastic needles for compressing blood vessels.

acupuncture (ăk′ū-pŭngk″chūr) [″ + *punctura*, puncture]. Technique for treating certain painful conditions and for producing regional anesthesia by passing long thin needles through the skin to specific points. The free ends of the needles are twirled or in some cases used to conduct a weak electric current. Anesthesia sufficient to permit abdominal, thoracic, and head and neck surgery has been produced by the use of acupuncture alone. The patient is fully conscious during the surgery. Acupuncture as a method of medical investigation (but not for anesthesia) has been known in the

Far East for centuries but received little attention in Western cultures until the early 1970s.

acus (ā′kŭs) [L., needle]. A surgical needle.

acusection (ăk″ū-sĕk′shŭn) [″ + *secare*, to cut]. Section by an electrosurgical needle.

acusis (ă-kūs′ĭs) [Gr. *akousis*, hearing]. SEE: *presbyacusis.*

acusticus (ă-kū′stĭ-kŭs) [Gr. *akoustikos*, hearing]. The acoustic nerve, q.v.

acute (ă-kūt′) [L. *acutus*, sharp]. 1. Sharp, severe. 2. Having rapid onset, severe symptoms, and a short course; not chronic.

acute care. Health care delivered to patients experiencing acute illness or trauma. Acute care generally occurs in a hospital or emergency room setting and is generally a short-term pattern of care in contrast to chronic care, which is long term.

acute confusional states. SEE: *confusional states, acute.*

acute mountain sickness. ABBR: AMS. Following a recent gain in altitude, the development of a headache, gastrointestinal symptoms such as anorexia, nausea, or vomiting, and fatigue, lassitude or weakness. This condition may occur in aviators and mountain climbers. SEE: *high altitude pulmonary edema.*

acutenaculum (ăk″ū-tĕn-ăk′ū-lŭm) [L. *acus*, needle, + *tenaculum*, holder]. A needle holder.

acute necrotizing ulcerative gingivitis. ABBR: ANUG. Trench mouth, q.v.

acute phase reactions. The increase in certain plasma proteins in response to almost any disease process that causes tissue damage. The blood sedimentation rate is influenced by these changes in plasma proteins, as is the synthesis of C-reactive protein. The reaction is induced by interleukin-1, interleukin-6, and tumor necrosis factor. This reaction is important in promoting the body defenses against microorganisms. SYN: *acute phase response.* SEE: *C-reactive protein; cytokines; IL-1; sedimentation rate; tumor necrosis factor.*

acute respiratory failure. SEE: *respiratory failure, acute.*

acute tubular necrosis. ABBR: ATN. Acute damage to the renal tubules usually due to ischemia associated with shock. SEE: *renal failure, acute.*

acute urethral syndrome. Syndrome experienced by women, characterized by acute dysuria, urinary frequency, and lack of significant bacteriuria; i.e., less than 10^{-5} organisms per ml of urine. Pyuria may or may not be present. The etiology of the syndrome is unknown, but it is important to attempt to determine whether or not a specific bacterial infection of the bladder or vagina is present and to treat appropriately.

NURSING IMPLICATIONS: The history of the illness is very important, including those events that cause an increase in symptoms, as well as those that decrease them. Also ask the degree of pain, location, whether it radiates, and the frequency and duration of discomfort. Instruct the patient in procedure for clean-catch, midstream urine specimen collection, and prepare the patient for vaginal examination.

acutorsion (ăk″ū-tor′shŭn) [″ + *torsio,* twisting]. Twisting of an artery with a needle to control hemorrhage.

acyanoblepsia (ă-sī″ă-nō-blĕp′sē-ă) [Gr. *a-,* not, + *kyanos,* blue, + *blepsis,* vision]. Inability to discern blue colors. SYN: *acyanopsia.*

acyanopsia (ă-sī″ă-nŏp′sē-ă). Acyanoblepsia, q.v.

acyanotic (ă-sī″ă-nŏt′ĭk) [″ + *kyanos,* blue]. Pert. to the absence of cyanosis.

acyclic (ă-sī′klĭk). 1. Without a cycle. 2. In chemistry, aliphatic, q.v.

acyclovir (ă-sī′klō-vĭr). An antiviral drug approved for use in herpes simplex infections of the genitals and herpes infections of the skin of immunocompromised patients. Trade name is Zovirax.

acyl (ăs′ĭl). In organic chemistry, the radical left when the hydroxyl group (OH) is removed from an organic acid.

acylation (ăs″ĭ-lā′shŭn). Incorporation of an acid radical into a chemical.

acystia (ă-sĭs′tē-ă) [″ + *kystis,* bladder]. Congenital absence of bladder.

acystinervia, acystineuria (ă-sĭs″tĭ-nĕr′vē-ă, -nū′rē-ă) [″ + ″ + *neuron,* nerve]. Defective nerve supply to or paralysis of the bladder.

AD. *anodal duration; average deviation.*

ad [L., to]. In prescription writing, ad indicates that a substance should be added to the formulation up to a specified volume.

ad- [L., to]. Prefix indicating adherence, increase, toward, as adduct.

-ad [L., to]. Suffix meaning toward, in direction of, as cephalad.

a.d. L. *auris dextra,* right ear.

A.D.A. *American Dental Association; American Diabetes Association; American Dietetic Association.*

A.D.A.A. *American Dental Assistants Association.*

adactylia, adactylism, adactyly (ă″dăk-tĭl′ē-ă, ă-dăk′tĭ-lĭzm, -lē) [Gr. *a-,* not, + *daktylos,* finger]. A congenital anomaly consisting of absence of digits of hand or foot.

adamantine (ăd″ă-măn′tĭn) [Gr. *adamantinos*]. Very hard; said of enamel of teeth.

adamantinoma (ăd″ă-măn″tĭ-nō′mă) [″ + *oma,* tumor]. A tumor of the jaw, esp. the lower one, arising from enamel-forming cells. May be partly cystic, partly solid, and may reach a large size. May be benign or of low-grade malignancy. SYN: *ameloblastoma.*

adamantoblast (ăd″ă-măn′tō-blăst) [Gr. *adamas,* hard surface, + *blastos,* germ]. An enamel-forming cell present only during tooth formation. SYN: *ameloblast.*

adamantoblastoma (ăd″ă-măn″tō-blăs-tō′mă) [″ + ″ + *oma,* tumor]. Overgrowth of an adamantoblast.

adamantoma (ăd″ă-măn-tō′mă) [Gr. *adamas,* hard surface, + *oma,* tumor]. Adamantinoma, q.v.

Adam's apple. The laryngeal prominence formed by the two laminae of the thyroid cartilage. SYN: *pomum adami; prominentia laryngea* [NA].

Adams-Stokes syndrome [Robert Adams, Irish physician, 1791–1875; William Stokes, Irish physician, 1804–1878]. Altered state of consciousness due to decreased flow of blood to the brain. Caused by any transient interference with cardiac output such as incomplete or complete heart block. The patient may be lightheaded or become completely unconscious and have convulsions.

TREAT: Place patient in recumbent position with legs elevated. Emergency use of cardiac pacemaker may be needed. Long-term treatment consists of implanting a demand-type cardiac pacemaker.

NURSING IMPLICATIONS: Monitor apical and radial pulse, blood pressure, and electrocardiogram. Note symptoms and their duration. Provide reassurance and support.

adaptation (ăd″ăp-tā′shŭn) [L. *adaptare,* to adjust]. 1. Adjustment of an organism to a change in internal or external conditions or circumstances. 2. Adjustment of the eye to various intensities of light, accomplished by changing size of pupil and accompanied by chemical changes occurring in the rods. 3. In psychology, a change in quality, intensity, or distinctness of a sensation that occurs after continuous stimulation of constant intensity. 4. In dentistry, the proper fitting of dentures or bands to the teeth, or closeness of a filling to walls of a cavity.

a., chromatic. A change in hue or saturation, or both, resulting from pre-exposure to light of other wavelengths.

a., dark. Adjustment of the eyes for vision in dim light. SYN: *scotopia.*

a., light. Adjustment of the eyes for vision in bright light. SYN: *photopia.*

adaptation model. SEE: *Appendix 23.*

adapted clothing. Garments designed with

special features, such as Velcro closures, to permit independent dressing by persons with physical disabilities.

adapter (ă-dăp′tĕr). 1. Device for joining one part of an apparatus to another part. 2. Device to facilitate connecting electrical supply cords to different receptacles. 3. Device for adapting one type of electrical supply source to the specific requirements of an instrument.

Ex.: An adapter is used to change a 120-volt alternating current to a 12-volt direct current.

adaptive device. Device specifically designed and fabricated with the purpose of permitting or assisting persons with disabilities to perform life tasks independently.

adaxial (ăd-ăk′sē-ăl) [L. *ad*, toward, + *axis*, axis]. Toward the main axis. Opposed to abaxial.

ADC. *anodal duration contraction; axiodistocervical.*

add. Prescription abbreviation meaning *let there be added.*

adde (ăd′ē) [L.]. Add, used as a direction in writing prescriptions.

addict (ăd′ĭkt) [L. *addictus*, given over]. One physically or psychologically, or both, dependent on a substance, esp. alcohol or drugs.

addiction (ă-dĭk′shŭn). Becoming involved, for a variety of reasons, in one of several forms of repetitive behavior, e.g., gambling, eating disorders, reckless driving, might be loosely referred to as addiction, but the term is best reserved to indicate addiction to narcotics, drugs of abuse, alcohol, and tobacco, q.v.

addiction to drugs, alcohol, and tobacco. Dependence, both physiological and emotional, upon alcohol, certain drugs of abuse noted for their effects on the central nervous system, and tobacco. True addiction is characterized by withdrawal symptoms upon discontinuing the substance. SYN: *drug dependence*. SEE: *addiction.*

Addis count method (ăd′ĭs) [Thomas Addis, Scot.-born U.S. physician, 1881–1949]. Method for counting the sediment (casts and cells) in a 12-hour urine sample.

Addison's disease [Thomas Addison, Brit. physician, 1793–1860]. Disease resulting from deficiency in the secretion of adrenocortical hormones. SYN: *adrenocortical hypofunction; chronic hypoadrenocorticism.*

SYM: Increased pigmentation of skin and mucous membranes, irregular patches of vitiligo, black freckles over head and neck, weakness, fatigability, hypotension, nausea, vomiting, anorexia, weight loss, and sometimes hypoglycemia.

ETIOL: Progressive destruction of the adrenal gland, whether due to an infectious disease, such as tuberculosis, or infiltration by neoplastic tissue or hemorrhage into the gland.

TREAT: Adrenocortical hormone therapy is dramatic in its effect and must be given promptly in adrenal crisis in order to prevent death. SEE: *adrenal; epinephrine.*

PROG: If untreated, the disease will continue a chronic course with progressive but usually relatively slow deterioration; in some patients the deterioration may be rapid. Patients treated properly have an excellent prognosis.

NURSING IMPLICATIONS: *Acute adrenal insufficiency (Addisonian crisis):* Assess for this life-threatening emergency due to an insufficiency of or a sudden decrease in adrenocortical hormones in patients with primary or secondary adrenocortical insufficiency experiencing the stress of infection, surgery, hemorrhage, or physical or psychological trauma, or the sudden withdrawal of replacement therapy. Also assess for in patients following adrenal or pituitary surgery or who have experienced sudden adrenal hemorrhage or pituitary destruction. Death may occur due to circulatory collapse. Monitor every ½ hour to 4 hours as necessary: blood pressure for hypotension (postural hypotension most likely), heart rate for tachycardia, fluid and electrolyte balance (including daily weight and urine output, measured hourly if necessary) for dehydration, hypoglycemia, hyponatremia, hyperkalemia, and profound hypovolemic shock. Patient may demonstrate headache, mental confusion, lassitude, and gastrointestinal symptoms such as nausea, vomiting, diarrhea and abdominal discomfort. Administer prescribed adrenocortical steroids, salt and fluid replacement. Protect the patient from exposure to stressors such as infection (using protective isolation), environmental noise, light, and temperature changes. Chronic maintenance therapy: Teach the patient about the need for lifelong replacement therapy and medical supervision. Instruct regarding self-administration of steroid therapy (two thirds in A.M.; one third in P.M.) and conditions requiring a temporary increase in dosage. Patient should always carry an emergency kit of 100 mg of I.M. hydrocortisone in the event oral medication cannot be taken. Explain the symptoms of over and under dosage and the course of action to take if either occurs. Teach the patient to increase fluid and salt replacement if perspiring, and to follow a diet high in sodium, carbohydrates and protein, with small frequent meals if hypoglycemia or anorexia occurs. Patients should wear or carry medical identification indicating disease problem and therapy. Because stress may precipitate a crisis, discuss stress management with the patient. SEE: *Medic Alert*. SEE: *Nursing Diagnoses* in *Appendix*.

addisonism (ăd′ĭ-sŭn-ĭzm″). Symptom complex resembling Addison's disease but not caused by disease of the suprarenal glands. There is abnormal skin pigmentation with debility. May be seen in pulmonary tuberculosis.

Addison's planes. Imaginary planes that divide the abdomen into nine regions to aid in the location of internal structures. SEE: *abdominal regions*.

addition (ă-dĭ′shŭn). In chemistry, a reaction in which two substances unite without loss of atoms or valence.

additive (ăd′ĭ-tĭv). In pharmacology, the effect that one drug or substance contributes to the action of another drug or substance. SEE: *synergism*.

　　a., food. Substance added to food for one or more of the following reasons: to maintain or impart a certain consistency to food, improve or maintain nutritive value, enhance palatability, produce light texture, control pH, or enhance flavor. Thus, food additives are used to keep bread mold-free and to help bread rise during baking, to color margarine, to prevent discoloration of some fruits, and to prevent fats and oils from becoming rancid.

　　Adding of these materials to foods is regulated by the U.S. Food and Drug Administration.

adducent (ă-dū′sĕnt) [L. *adducere*, to bring toward]. Causing adduction.

adduct (ă-dŭkt′) [L. *adductus*, brought toward]. To draw toward the main axis of body or a limb.

adduction (ă-dŭk′shŭn). Movement of a limb or eye toward median plane of body or, in case of digits, toward axial line of a limb. SEE: *abduction* for illus.

　　a., convergent-stimulus. Convergence of eyes upon fixation of gaze on an object at the near point of vision.

adductor (ă-dŭk′tor). A muscle that draws toward the medial line of the body or to a common center.

adductor reflex. Contraction of adductor muscles of the thigh upon applying pressure to, or tapping, medial surface of thigh or knee.

adelomorphous (ă-dĕl″ō-mor′fŭs) [Gr. *adelos*, not seen, + *morphe*, shape]. Having undefined form. Applied to the central cells of the gastric glands.

adenalgia (ăd″ĕn-ăl′jē-ă) [Gr. *aden*, gland, + *algos*, pain]. Pain in a gland. SYN: *ade-*

nodynia.

adenase (ăd′ĕ-nāz) [″ + *-ase*, enzyme]. Enzyme secreted by the pancreas, spleen, and liver that converts adenine, q.v., into hypoxanthine, q.v. SEE: *enzyme.*

adendric, adendritic (ă-dĕn′drĭk, ă″dĕn-drĭt′ĭk) [Gr. *a-*, not, + *dendrites*, rel. to a tree]. Without dendrites, as certain cells in spinal ganglia.

adenectomy (ăd″ĕn-ĕk′tō-mē) [Gr. *aden*, gland, + *ektome*, excision]. Excision of a gland.

adenectopia (ăd″ĕ-nĕk-tō′pē-ă) [″ + ″ + *topos*, place]. Malposition of a gland; a gland in a position other than its normal position.

adenia (ă-dē′nē-ă). Chronic inflammation and enlargement of a lymph gland.

adeniform (ă-dĕn′ĭ-form) [″ + L. *forma*, shape]. Glandlike in form.

adenine (ăd′ĕ-nīn). $C_5H_5N_5$. 6-aminopurine, a crystalline substance; one of the two purine bases of ribonucleic acid and deoxyribonucleic acid.

adenitis (ăd″ĕ-nī′tĭs) [″ + *itis*, inflammation]. Inflammation of lymph nodes or a gland.

adenization (ăd″ĕ-nĭ-zā′shŭn). Abnormal change into a glandlike structure.

adeno- [Gr. *aden*, gland]. Prefix denoting a gland.

adenoacanthoma (ăd″ĕ-nō-ăk″ăn-thō′mă) [″ + *akantha*, thorn, + *oma*, tumor]. Adenocarcinoma in which some cells have undergone squamous metaplasia.

adenoameloblastoma (ăd″ĕ-nō-ă-mĕl″ō-blăs-tō′mă) [″ + O. Fr. *amel*, enamel, + Gr. *blastos*, germ, + *oma*, tumor]. Benign tumor of the jaw, originating from ameloblast cells of forming teeth; an odontogenic tumor.

adenoblast (ăd′ĕ-nō-blăst) [″ + *blastos*, germ]. 1. Embryonic cells that produce glandular tissue. 2. Any tissue that produces secretory or glandular activity.

adenocarcinoma (ăd″ĕ-nō-kăr″sĭn-ō′mă) [″ + *karkinos*, crab, + *oma*, tumor]. A malignant adenoma arising from a glandular organ.

　　a., acinar. Adenocarcinoma in which the cells are in the shape of alveoli. SYN: *a., alveolar.*

　　a., alveolar. A., acinar, q.v.

adenocele (ăd′ĕ-nō-sēl″) [″ + *kele*, tumor, swelling]. A cystic tumor arising from a gland. A tumor of glandular structure.

adenocellulitis (ăd″ĕ-nō-sĕl″ū-lī′tĭs) [″ + L. *cella*, small chamber, + Gr. *itis*, inflammation]. Inflammation of a gland and adjacent cellular tissue.

adenocyst (ăd′ĕ-nō-sĭst″) [″ + *kystis*, sac]. A cystic tumor arising from a gland.

adenocystoma (ăd″ĕ-nō-sĭs-tō′mă) [″ + *kystis*, sac, + *oma*, tumor]. Cystic adenoma.

adenodynia (ăd″ĕ-nō-dĭn′ē-ă) [″ + *odyne*, pain]. Pain in a gland. SYN: *adenalgia*.

adenoepithelioma (ăd″ĕ-nō-ĕp″ĭ-thĕl-ē-ō′mă) [″ + *epi*, on, + *thele*, nipple, + *oma*, tumor]. Tumor consisting of glandular and epithelial elements.

adenofibroma (ăd″ĕ-nō-fī-brō′mă) [″ + L. *fibra*, fiber, + Gr. *oma*, tumor]. Tumor of fibrous and glandular tissue (connective tissue); frequently found in the uterus or breast.

adenofibrosis (ăd″ĕ-nō-fī-brō′sĭs) [″ + ″ + Gr. *osis*, condition]. Degeneration of tumor that contains fibrous connective tissue.

adenogenous (ăd″ĕ-nŏj′ĕ-nŭs) [″ + *gennan*, to produce]. Originating in glandular tissue.

adenohypophysis (ăd″ĕ-nō-hī-pŏf′ĭ-sĭs) [″ + *hypo*, under, + *phyein*, to grow]. The anterior lobe of the pituitary gland, q.v.

adenoid (ăd′ĕ-noyd) [″ + Gr. *eidos*, form, shape]. Lymphoid; having the appearance of a gland.

adenoidectomy (ăd″ĕ-noyd-ĕk′tō-mē) [″ + ″ + *ektome*, excision]. Excision of adenoids. SEE: *tonsillectomy*.

NURSING IMPLICATIONS: Carefully monitor the patient's vital signs and observe for symptoms of shock. Inspect the mouth and pharynx for bleeding, large clot formation, or oozing, and observe the patient for frequent swallowing, which indicates bleeding. Be certain clots are not obstructing oropharynx. Position the patient either prone with head to the side or in a lateral recumbent position to promote drainage. When the operative wound has healed sufficiently, encourage oral intake of cool fluids and soft foods. The patient should be instructed not to gargle until the surgical site has healed.

Young patients: In nonthreatening manner, assure child concerning routines and procedures; provide emotional support to child and family members; encourage parental presence. Evaluate for vomiting of partially digested swallowed blood. Monitor child's ability to swallow fluids offered. SEE: *Nursing Diagnoses in Appendix.*

adenoid hypertrophy. Enlargement of the pharyngeal tonsil occurring commonly in children. May result from infection of Waldeyer's ring, q.v., or may be congenital.

adenoiditis (ăd″ĕ-noyd-ī′tĭs) [″ + ″ + *itis*, inflammation]. Inflammation of adenoid tissue.

adenoids (ăd′ĕ-noyds). Lymphatic tissue forming a prominence on the wall of the pharyngeal recess of the nasopharynx. SEE:

pharyngeal tonsil.

adenoid tissue. The pharyngeal tonsil, q.v.; adenoids, q.v.

adenolipoma (ăd″ĕ-nō-lĭp-ō′mă) [″ + *lipos*, fat, + *oma*, tumor]. A benign tumor having glandular characteristics but composed of fat.

adenolymphitis (ăd″ĕ-nō-lĭm-fī′tĭs) [Gr. *aden*, gland, + L. *lympha*, lymph, + Gr. *itis*, inflammation]. Inflammation of a lymph gland. SYN: *lymphadenitis*, q.v.

adenolymphocele (ăd″ĕ-nō-lĭm′fō-sēl) [″ + ″ + Gr. *kele*, tumor, swelling]. Cystic dilatation of a lymph node from obstruction.

adenolymphoma (ăd″ĕ-nō-lĭm-fō′mă) [″ + ″ + Gr. *oma*, tumor]. A lymph gland adenoma.

adenoma (ăd″ĕ-nō′mă) [″ + *oma*, tumor] (pl. *adenomata*). A neoplasm of glandular epithelium.

    a., acidophil(ic). Tumor of the pituitary gland in which cells stain with acid dyes. Cause of acromegaly and gigantism. SYN: *a., eosinophil(ic).*

    a., basophil(ic). Tumor of the pituitary gland in which cells stain with basic dyes. Cause of Cushing's syndrome, q.v.

    a., chromophobe. Tumor of the pituitary gland composed of cells that do not stain readily. May cause pituitary deficiency or diabetes insipidus.

    a., eosinophil(ic). A., acidophil(ic), q.v.

    a., fibroid. Fibroadenoma, q.v.

    a., follicular. Adenoma of the thyroid.

    a., Hürthle cell. Tumor of the thyroid that contains mostly eosinophil-staining cells. These are called Hürthle cells and are usually benign.

    a., islet. Nonmalignant neoplasm of the pancreas sometimes containing beta cells. May be cause of hypoglycemia. SYN: *insuloma; a., langerhansian.*

    a., langerhansian. A., islet, q.v.

    a., malignant. Adenocarcinoma, q.v.

    a., papillary. Adenoma in which the alveoli of the adenoma are filled with fluid.

    a., pituitary. Adenoma of the pituitary gland.

    a., sebaceous. Enlarged sebaceous glands, esp. of the face.

    a. sebaceum. Benign, usually solitary growth on face developing from epithelium of sebaceous glands.

    a., tubular. Adenoma in the form of a tubular gland.

    a., villous. Large polyp of the mucosal surface of the large intestine.

adenomalacia (ăd″ĕ-nō-mă-lā′shē-ă) [Gr. *aden*, gland, + *malakia*, softening]. Glandular softening.

adenomatome (ăd″ĕ-nō′mă-tōm) [″ + *oma*, tumor, + *tome*, incision]. Instrument for removing adenoids.

adenomatosis (ăd″ē-nō-mă-tō′sĭs) [″ + *oma,* tumor, + *osis,* condition]. The condition of multiple glandular tissue overgrowths.

adenomatous (ăd″ē-nō′mă-tŭs). Pert. to adenomata.

adenomere (ăd′ē-nō-mēr″) [″ + *meros,* part]. The functional part of a gland.

adenomyoma (ăd″ē-nō-mī-ō′mă) [″ + *mys,* muscle, + *oma,* tumor]. Tumor containing glandular and smooth muscular tissue.

adenomyometritis (ăd″ē-nō-mī″ō-mĕ-trī′tĭs) [″ + ″ + *metra,* womb, + *itis,* inflammation]. A hyperplastic condition of the uterus caused by pelvic inflammation; grossly it resembles an adenomyoma.

adenomyosarcoma (ăd″ē-nō-mī″ō-săr-kō′mă) [″ + ″ + *sarx,* flesh, + *oma,* tumor]. Adenosarcoma that includes muscle tissue.

adenomyosis (ăd″ē-nō-mī-ō′sĭs) [″ + *mys,* muscle, + *osis,* condition]. Benign invasive growth of the endometrium into the muscular layer of the uterus.

adenopathy (ăd-ē-nŏp′ă-thē) [″ + *pathos,* disease, suffering]. Swelling and morbid change in lymph nodes; glandular disease.

adenopharyngitis (ăd″ē-nō-făr″ĭn-jī′tĭs) [″ + *pharynx,* throat, + *itis,* inflammation]. Inflammation of tonsils and pharyngeal mucous membrane.

adenophthalmia (ăd″ē-nŏf-thăl′mē-ă) [″ + *ophthalmos,* eye]. Inflammation of the meibomian gland, q.v.

adenosarcoma (ăd″ē-nō-săr-kō′mă) [″ + *sarx,* flesh, + *oma,* tumor]. Tumor with adenomatous and sarcomatous characteristics.

adenosclerosis (ăd″ē-nō-sklĕ-rō′sĭs) [″ + *sklerosis,* hardening]. Glandular hardening.

adenose (ăd′ē-nōs). Glandlike.

adenosine (ă-dĕn′ō-sēn). A nucleotide containing adenine and ribose.

   a. 3′,5′-cyclic monophosphate. ABBR: AMP. A cyclic form of adenosine. Its synthesis from adenosine triphosphate (ATP) is stimulated by an enzyme, adenylate cyclase (also called cyclic AMP synthetase). Adenosine 3′,5′-cyclic monophosphate is important in a wide variety of metabolic responses to cell stimuli.

   a. deaminase conjugated with polyethylene glycol. ABBR: ADA. A cytoplasmic enzyme used to treat severe combined immunodeficiency disease (SCID) due to ADA deficiency. Trade name is Pegademase.

   a. diphosphate, a. 5′-diphosphate. ABBR: ADP. A compound of adenosine containing two phosphoric acid groups.

This substance is produced during muscle contraction. It is reformed when the muscle relaxes.

   a. monophosphate, a. 5′-monophosphate. ABBR: AMP; 5′-AMP. Substance formed by condensation of adenosine and phosphoric acid. It is one of the hydrolytic products of nucleic acids and is present in muscle, red blood cells, yeast, and other nuclear material. SYN: *adenylic acid.*

   a. triphosphate. ABBR: ATP. A compound of adenosine containing three phosphoric acid groups. This substance is present in all cells, but particularly in muscle cells. When this substance is split by enzyme action, energy is produced. The energy of the muscle is stored in this compound.

adenosine triphosphatase (ă-dĕn″ō-sĭn trī-fŏs′fă-tās). ABBR: ATPase. Enzyme that splits adenosine triphosphate to yield phosphate and energy.

adenosis (ăd″ē-nō′sĭs) [Gr. *aden,* gland, + *osis,* condition]. Any disease of a gland, esp. of a lymphatic gland.

adenotome (ăd′ē-nō-tōm) [″ + *tome,* incision]. Device for excising a gland, esp. the adenoid glands.

adenotonsillectomy (ăd″ē-nō-tŏn″sĭl-lĕk′tō-mē) [″ + L. *tonsilla,* almond, + Gr. *ektome,* excision]. Surgical removal of the tonsils and adenoids.

adenous (ăd′ē-nŭs). Like a gland.

adenovirus (ăd′ē-nō-vī′rŭs). One of a group of closely related viruses that can cause infections of the upper respiratory tract. A large number have been isolated.

adenyl (ăd′ē-nĭl). The radical $C_5H_4N_5$—; present in adenine.

   a. cyclase. Enzyme present on most cell surfaces. It catalyzes the production of cyclic AMP (adenosine 3′,5′-cyclic monophosphate) from ATP (adenosine triphosphate).

adenylate cyclase (ă-dĕn′ĭ-lāt sī′klās). An enzyme important in the synthesis of adenosine 3′,5′-cyclic monophosphate (cyclic AMP) from adenosine triphosphate. SYN: *cyclic AMP synthetase.*

adenylic acid. Adenosine monophosphate, q.v.

adeps (ăd′ĕps) [L.]. Lard; omental hog fat. Used in preparation of ointments.

   a. benzoinatus. Benzoinated lard.

   a. lanae. Wool fat. Purified anhydrous lanolin from sheep wool. Used as an ointment base.

   a. lanae hydrosus. Hydrous wool fat; lanolin.

adermia (ă-dĕr′mē-ă) [Gr. *a-,* not, + *derma,* skin]. Congenital or acquired defect of or lack of skin.

adermogenesis (ă-dĕr″mō-jĕn′ĕ-sĭs) [″ +

" + *genesis,* generation, birth]. Imperfect development of skin.

ADH. *antidiuretic hormone* (vasopressin).

A.D.H.A. *American Dental Hygienists' Association.*

adherence, bacterial (ăd-hēr'ĕns). The property of bacteria that allows them to adhere to specific receptors that are present on some cells but not on others. If bacteria normally present in the intestinal tract did not have this ability, they would be washed out of the intestines.

adherent (ăd-hē'rĕnt) [L. *adhaerere,* to stick to]. Attached to, as of two surfaces.

adhesin. In conjugation of some bacteria, a protein on the cell surface that causes aggregation of cells.

adhesio (ăd-hē'zē-ō) [L. *adhaesio,* stuck to]. Adhesion.

adhesion (ăd-hē'zhŭn) [L. *adhaesio,* stuck to]. 1. A holding together or uniting of two surfaces or parts, as in wound healing. 2. A fibrous band holding parts together that are normally separated. 3. An attraction to another substance: thus, molecules or blood platelets adhere to each other or to dissimilar materials.

   a., abdominal. Adhesion in the abdominal cavity, usually involving the intestines. Caused by inflammation or trauma. If causing great pain or intestinal obstruction, adhesions are treated surgically.

   a., pericardial. Adhesion of the pericardial sac. If extensive, adhesions may lead to restriction of the normal movement of the heart. SEE: *pericarditis.*

adhesiotomy (ăd-hē''zē-ŏt'ō-mē) [L. *adhaesio,* stuck to, + Gr. *tome,* incision]. Surgical division of adhesions.

adhesive (ăd-hē'sĭv) [L. *adhaesio,* stuck to]. 1. Causing adhesion. 2. Sticky; adhering. 3. That which causes two bodies to adhere.

adhesive capsulitis. Adherence of folds in an articular capsule preventing normal joint play and causing restricted movement.

adhesive inflammation. Inflammation of serous membrane, making adhesions possible by formation of fibrin.

adhesive tape. USP. A fabric, film, or paper, one side of which is coated with an adhesive substance so that it remains in place after application to the skin. In general, there are two types of backings for the adhesive material: occlusive and nonocclusive. The former prevents air from going through the backing and the latter does not. The possibility of skin irritation when the occlusive type is used is increased, thus its use is rarely needed. SEE: *plaster, adhesive.*

   NURSING IMPLICATIONS: Prevent skin damage when removing tape by carefully peeling tape back following the direction of hair growth, holding skin taut behind tape removal edge. Evaluate skin for irritation. If the adhesive material has irritated the skin, do not use solvents to assist in removal. Some patients are allergic to certain adhesive agents; note signs of this and use hypoallergenic adhesive tape if indicated.

adiadochokinesia, adiadochokinesis (ă-dī''ă-dō''kō-kī-nē'sē-ă, -nē'sĭs) [Gr. *a-,* not, + *diadochas,* successive, + *kinesis,* movement]. 1. Inability to make rapid alternating movements. 2. In neurology, rapid antagonistic movements that cannot be carried out smoothly. Seen in cerebellar disease. RS: asynergia; dysmetria; gait.

adiaphoresis (ă-dī''ă-fō-rē'sĭs) [" + *diaphorein,* to perspire]. Deficiency or absence of sweat.

adiastole (ă''dī-ăs'tō-lē) [" + *diastole,* dilatation]. Imperceptibility of diastole, q.v.

Adie's syndrome (ā'dēz) [William John Adie, Brit. neurologist, 1886–1935]. A syndrome characterized by a tonic pupil that responds slowly or not at all to light, accompanied by slow constriction and relaxation in the change from near to distant vision, and impaired accommodation. The affected pupil is frequently larger than the normal pupil. Loss of certain deep tendon reflexes may also be present, but there are no other signs of CNS disease. SEE: *pupil, tonic.*

adipectomy (ăd''ĭ-pĕk'tō-mē) [L. *adeps,* fat, + Gr. *ektome,* excision]. Excision of fat or adipose tissue, usually a large quantity. SEE: *liposuction.*

adipic (ă-dĭp'ĭk). Rel. to adipose tissue, q.v.

adipo-, adip- [L. *adeps,* fat]. Combining forms pert. to fat. See also words beginning with lipo-, lip-.

adipocele (ăd'ĭ-pō-sēl'') [L. *adeps,* fat, + Gr. *kele,* tumor]. A hernia that contains fat or fatty tissue. SYN: *lipocele.*

adipocellular (ăd''ĭ-pō-sĕl'ū-lăr). Containing fat and cellular tissue.

adipocere (ăd'ĭ-pō-sēr'') [" + *cera,* wax]. A brown, waxlike substance composed of fatty acids and calcium soaps. It is formed in animal tissues that have been buried in a moist place. SYN: *grave wax.*

adipocyte (ăd'ĭ-pō-sīt) [" + Gr. *kytos,* cell]. Fat cell.

adipofibroma [" + *fibra,* fiber, + Gr. *oma,* tumor]. A fibroma and adipoma.

adipogenous, adipogenic (ăd''ĭ-pŏj'ĕn-ŭs, -pō-jĕn'ĭk) [" + Gr. *gennan,* to produce]. Inducing the formation of fat.

adipoid (ăd'ĭ-poyd) [L. *adeps,* fat, + Gr. *eidos,* form, shape]. Fatlike; lipoid.

adipokinesis (ăd''ĭ-pō-kĭ-nē'sĭs) [" + Gr. *kinesis,* movement]. 1. Metabolism of fat with production of free fatty acids. 2. Mobilization and metabolism of body fat.

adipokinetic action. The action of substances to promote formation of free fatty acids from body fat stores.

adipolysis (ăd″ĭ-pŏl′ĭ-sĭs) [″ + Gr. *lysis*, dissolution]. The hydrolysis or digestion of fat.

adiponecrosis (ăd″ĭ-pō-ně-krō′sĭs) [″ + Gr. *nekrosis*, state of death]. Necrosis affecting fatty tissue.

adipose [L. *adiposus*, fatty]. Fatty; pert. to fat.

adipose capsule. Perirenal fat.

adipose tissue. Connective or areolar tissue containing masses of fat cells.

adiposis (ăd″ĭ-pō′sĭs) [″ + Gr. *osis*, condition]. Abnormal accumulation of fat in the body. SYN: *corpulence; liposis; obesity.*

   a. cerebralis. Obesity due to intracranial disease, esp. of the pituitary.

   a. dolorosa. Scattered areas of painful cutaneous nodules or fat accumulations in menopausal women. SYN: *Dercum's disease.*

   a. hepatica. Fatty degeneration or infiltration of the liver.

adipositis (ăd″ĭ-pō-sī′tĭs) [L. *adiposus*, fatty, + Gr. *itis*, inflammation]. Infiltration of an inflammatory nature in and beneath subcutaneous adipose tissue.

adiposity (ăd″ĭ-pŏs′ĭ-tē). Excessive fat in the body. SYN: *adiposis; corpulence; obesity.*

adiposogenital dystrophy (ăd″ĭ-pō″sō-jĕn′ĭ-tăl dĭs′trō-fē) [″ + *genitalis*, genital, + Gr. *dys*, bad, disordered, + *trophe*, nourishment]. Combination of adiposity, impaired development of genital organs, and altered secondary sex characteristics. SYN: *Fröhlich's syndrome.*

   ETIOL: A disturbance of function or a tumor of the hypothalamus and pituitary gland.

adiposuria (ăd″ĭ-pō-sū′rē-ă) [″ + Gr. *ouron*, urine]. Fat in the urine. SYN: *lipuria.*

adipsia, adipsy (ă-dĭp′sē-ă, -sē) [Gr. *a-*, not, + *dipsa*, thirst]. Absence of thirst.

aditus (ăd′ĭ-tŭs) [L.]. An approach; an entrance.

   a. ad antrum. The recess of the tympanic cavity that leads from the epitympanic recess to the tympanic antrum.

   a. ad aquaeductum cerebri. The entrance to the sylvian aqueduct, situated at lower posterior angle of third ventricle of brain.

   a. laryngis. [NA] Upper aperture of the larynx.

adjunct (ăd′jŭnkt). An addition to the principal procedure or course of therapy.

adjuster. Device for holding together the ends of the wire forming a suture.

adjustment [L. *adjuxtare*, to bring together]. 1. Adaptation to a different environment; a person's relation to his or her environment

and inner self. 2. A change made to improve function or condition. Ex.: Changing the position of the lenses of a microscope in order to bring the object into focus.

adjustment disorder. A maladaptive reaction to an identifiable psychological or social stress that occurs within three months of the onset of the stressful situation. The reaction is characterized by impairment of function or symptoms in excess of what would be considered normal for that stress. The symptoms are expected to remit when the stress ceases; or, if the stress continues, then a new level of adaptation is achieved.

adjuvant (ăd′jū-vănt) [L. *adjuvans*, aiding]. 1. That which assists, esp. a drug added to a prescription to hasten or increase the action of a principal ingredient. 2. In immunology, a variety of substances, including inorganic gels such as alum, aluminum hydroxide, and aluminum phosphate, that increase the antigenic response.

   a., Freund's complete [Jules Thomas Freund, Hungarian-born U.S. immunologist, 1890–1961]. A water-in-oil emulsion in which an antigen solution is emulsified in mineral oil with killed mycobacteria to enhance antigenicity. The intense inflammatory response produced by this emulsion makes it unsuitable for use in humans.

   a., Freund's incomplete. A water-in-oil emulsion in which an antigen solution without mycobacteria is emulsified in mineral oil. On injection, this mixture induces a strong persistent antibody formation.

adjuvant therapy. In cancer therapy, the use of another form of treatment in addition to the primary surgical therapy.

ADL. *activities of daily living*, q.v.

Adler, Alfred. Austrian psychiatrist (1870–1937) who founded the school of individual psychology. SEE: *psychology, individual.*

ad lib. [L. *ad libitum*]. Prescription abbreviation meaning *at pleasure* or *as much as is wanted.*

Administration on Aging. ABBR: AoA. Located within the Department of Health and Human Services, the AoA is the principal agency having the responsibility to carry out the Older Americans Act of 1965. Its functions and duties include developing and conducting research in the field of aging, as well as coordinating and assisting federal, state, and local agencies in planning and developing programs for older persons.

A.D.N. *Associate Degree in Nursing.* A registered nurse who has completed an associate degree program in nursing.

ad nauseam (ăd naw′sē-ăm) [L.]. Of such degree or extent as to produce nausea.

adneural (ăd-nū′răl) [L. *ad*, to, + Gr. *neuron*, nerve]. Near or toward a nerve.

adnexa (ăd-nĕk′să) [L.]. Accessory parts of a structure.

   a., dental. Tissues surrounding the tooth; i.e., periodontal ligament and alveolar bone proper.

   a. oculi. Lacrimal glands.

   a. uteri. Ovaries and fallopian tubes.

adnexal (ăd-nĕk′săl). Adjacent or appending.

adnexal pain. SEE: *pain, adnexal.*

adnexitis (ăd″nĕk-sī′tĭs) [L. *adnexa,* appendages, + Gr. *itis,* inflammation]. Inflammation of the adnexa uteri.

adolescence (ăd″ō-lĕs′ĕns) [L. *adolescens*]. The period from the beginning of puberty until maturity. The onset of puberty and maturity is a gradual process and variable among individuals; thus, it is not practical to set exact age or chronological limits in defining the adolescent period.

adolescent (ăd″ō-lĕs′ĕnt). 1. Pert. to adolescence. 2. Young man or woman not fully grown.

adolescent turmoil. In psychoanalytic theory, the belief that adolescence is invariably accompanied by turmoil. This is no longer thought to be inevitable, or even the usual case.

adoption (ă-dŏp′shŭn) [L. *ad,* to, + *optare,* to choose]. The assumption of the responsibility of caring for a child by a person (or persons) who is not the natural parent. This usually requires a legal procedure.

adoral (ăd-ō′răl) [″ + *os,* mouth]. Toward or near the mouth.

ADP. *adenosine diphosphate.*

adrenal (ăd-rē′năl) [L. *ad,* to, + *ren,* kidney]. Originally used to indicate nearness to the kidney. Now used in reference to the adrenal gland or its secretions.

adrenal crisis. Acute adrenocortical insufficiency.

Caution: Death due to circulatory collapse will result unless the condition is treated promptly and vigorously by instituting corticosteroid therapy. The cause may be a hemorrhage into the adrenal cortex as a result of infection or it may occur at birth, resulting from trauma. In the adult, headache, lassitude, confusion, restlessness, vomiting, and shock progressing to death occur if the cortex is destroyed. Relative adrenal insufficiency can occur in patients for two to three months after discontinuation of adrenocortical hormone therapy. Sudden stress, such as surgery or trauma, can produce a subacute form of adrenal crisis in these patients. SEE: *Addison's disease; Waterhouse-Friderichsen syndrome.*

---

adrenalectomy (ăd-rē″năl-ĕk′tō-mē) [L. *ad,* to, + *ren,* kidney, + Gr. *ektome,* excision]. Excision of an adrenal gland.

ADRENAL GLANDS

ADRENAL GLAND

KIDNEY

ADRENAL GLAND

RENAL ARTERY

RIGHT KIDNEY

AORTA

URETER

INFERIOR VENA CAVA

NURSING IMPLICATIONS: Monitor vital signs, including central venous pressure (CVP) frequently. Administer hydrocortisone and other medications as directed. Observe for signs and symptoms of hypocorticism as well as infection. Reduce physical and psychological stress. Instruct those patients requiring lifelong replacement therapy. SEE: *Nursing Diagnoses* in *Appendix.*

adrenal gland. A triangular body covering the superior surface of each kidney. SYN: *suprarenal gland.* SEE: illus.

EMBRYOLOGY: The adrenal gland is essentially a double organ composed of an outer cortex and an inner medulla. The cortex arises in the embryo from a region of the mesoderm that also gives rise to the gonads, or sex organs. The medulla arises from ectoderm, which also gives rise to the sympathetic nervous system.

ANAT: The entire gland is enclosed in a tough connective tissue capsule from which trabeculae extend into the cortex. The cortex consists of cells arranged into three zones: the outer zona glomerulosa, the middle zona fasciculata, and the inner zona reticularis. The cells are arranged in a cordlike fashion. The medulla consists of chromaffin cells arranged in groups or anastomosing cords. The two adrenal glands are situated retroperitoneally, each embedded in perirenal fat above its respective kidney. In the adult, the average weight is 5 gm, and the range is 4 to 14 gm. The gland usually is heavier in males than in females.

PHYS: The adrenal medulla synthesizes and stores three catecholamines: dopamine, norepinephrine, and epinephrine. Dopamine's chief effects are dilation of systemic arteries, increased cardiac output, and increased flow of blood to the kidneys. The primary action of norepinephrine is to constrict the arterioles and venules with resultant increased resistance to blood flow, elevated blood pressure, and slowing of the heart. Epinephrine constricts vessels in the skin and splanchnic area, dilates vessels in skeletal muscle, increases heart activity, dilates the bronchi by relaxing bronchial musculature, increases level of glucose in the blood by stimulating the production of glucose from glycogen in the liver, increases the amount of fatty acid in the blood, and diminishes activity of the gastrointestinal system. The three catecholamines are also produced in other parts of the body.

The adrenal medulla is controlled by the sympathetic nervous system and functions in conjunction with it. It is intimately related to adjustments of the body in response to stress and emotional changes. Anticipatory states tend to bring about the release of norepinephrine. More intense emotional reactions, esp. those in response to extreme stress, tend to increase the secretion of both norepinephrine and epinephrine; epinephrine is important in mobilizing the physiological changes that occur in the "fight or flight" response to emergency situations.

The cortex secretes a group of hormones that vary in quantity and quality. They are all synthesized from cholesterol and contain the basic steroid nucleus perhydrocyclopentanophenanthrene. These compounds are grouped according to their chemical structure and biological activity as follows: glucocorticoids (cortisol, corticosterone), which act principally on carbohydrate metabolism; mineralocorticoids (aldosterone, dehydroepiandrosterone), which affect metabolism of the electrolytes sodium and potassium; androgens (17-ketosteroids), estrogens (estradiol), and progestins (progesterone), all three of which are important in the physiology of reproduction. There is considerable overlap in the biological activity of many of these compounds. SEE: *steroid.*

Almost all body systems are influenced by the action of adrenocortical hormones. Cortisol and cortisone are important in carbohydrate, water, muscle, bone, central nervous system, gastrointestinal, cardiovascular, and hematological metabolism. They are also important anti-inflammatory agents. The principal long-term effect of cortisone and cortisol is catabolic.

The 17-ketosteroids act principally as androgenic and anabolic agents. Aldosterone's principal action is to control sodium and potassium levels in the blood.

PATH: In the medulla, increased secretion of catecholamines occurs when a pheochromocytoma develops. In this condition, the patient develops hypertension, excessive sweating, paroxysmal attacks of blanching or flushing of the skin, tachycardia, headache, anorexia, weight loss, personality changes, signs of increased metabolism, constipation, and postural hypotension. Diagnosis may be confirmed by determining the level of catecholamines or their metabolic end products in the urine. SEE: *pheochromocytoma.*

In the cortex, when excess secretion of cortical hormones occurs, one of a variety of syndromes may result, depending upon which hormones or group of hormones are increased. If cortisol is increased, the signs of Cushing's syndrome result: obesity with striae and redistribution of fat to produce a "buffalo hump" and "moon face," muscle wasting, osteoporosis, decreased glucose tolerance, atherosclerosis, and systolic hypertension. If the androgens are increased, male sex characteristics are accentuated in the female with voice change, hirsutism, clitoral enlargement, and pronounced muscular development. Baldness and acne will develop in either sex with this condition. It is termed adrenogenital syndrome, q.v.

When aldosterone is elevated, hypertension, low serum potassium, elevated serum sodium, increased urine volume, and, rarely, edema will be present. This is called primary aldosteronism. SEE: *aldosteronism, primary.*

Adrenocortical deficiency may be acute or chronic. The chronic form is called Addison's disease and is characterized by anemia, sluggishness, weakness, weight loss, hypotension, sometimes hypoglycemia, nausea, vomiting, diarrhea, abnormal skin pigmentation, and mental changes. The acute form is called adrenal crisis, q.v. Adrenal crisis due to hemorrhage into the adrenal gland caused by meningococcal infection is called the Waterhouse-Friderichsen syndrome.

Adrenalin (ă-drĕn′ă-lĭn). Trade name for epinephrine, q.v.

adrenaline (ă-drĕn′ă-lēn). British designation for epinephrine, q.v.

adrenalinemia (ă-drĕn″ă-lĭn-ē′mē-ă) [L. *ad*, to, + *ren*, kidney, + Gr. *haima*, blood]. Epinephrine in the blood.

adrenalinuria (ă-drĕn″ă-lĭn-ŭ′rē-ă) [″ + ″ + Gr. *ouron*, urine]. Epinephrine in the urine.

adrenarche (ăd″rĕn-ăr′kē) [″ + ″ + Gr. *arche*, beginning]. Changes that occur at puberty resulting from effects of increased secretion of adrenocortical hormone. SEE: *menarche; pubarche.*

adrenergic (ăd-rĕn-ĕr′jĭk) [″ + ″ + Gr. *ergon*, work]. Term applied to nerve fibers that, when stimulated, release epinephrine at their endings. Includes nearly all sympathetic postganglionic fibers except those innervating sweat glands.

adrenergic neuron-blocking agents. Substances that inhibit transmission of sympathetic nerve stimuli regardless of whether alpha- or beta-adrenergic receptors are involved. SEE: *alpha-adrenergic receptor; beta-adrenergic receptor.*

adrenitis (ăd″rē-nī′tĭs) [″ + ″ + Gr. *itis*, inflammation]. Inflammation of the adrenal glands. SYN: *adrenalitis.*

adrenoceptive (ă-drē″nō-sĕp′tĭv) [″ + ″ + *recipere*, to receive]. Concerning the sites in organs or tissues that are acted upon by adrenergic transmitters.

adrenochrome (ăd″rē′nō-krōm) [″ + ″ + Gr. *chroma*, color]. A red pigment obtained by oxidation of epinephrine.

adrenocortical (ăd-rē″nō-kor′tĭ-kăl). Pert. to the adrenal cortex.

adrenocortical hormones. A group of hormones secreted by the adrenal cortex that are classified by biological activity into glucocorticoids, q.v., mineralocorticoids, q.v., androgens, q.v., estrogens, q.v., and progestins, q.v. SEE: *adrenal gland.*

adrenocorticotropic (ăd-rē″nō-kor″tĭ-kō-trŏp′ĭk) [″ + ″ + *cortex*, bark, + Gr. *tropikos*, turning]. Having a stimulating effect on the adrenal cortex.

adrenocorticotropic hormone. ABBR: ACTH. A hormone secreted by anterior lobe of the pituitary. It is essential to the growth, development, and continued function of the adrenal cortex. SYN: *corticotropin.*

adrenocorticotropin (ăd-rē″nō-kor″tĭ-kō-trŏp′ĭn). Adrenocorticotropic hormone, q.v.

adrenogenital (ăd-rē-nō-jĕn′ĭ-tăl) [″ + ″ + *genitalis,* genital]. Pert. to the adrenal glands and the genitalia.

adrenogenital syndrome. Condition caused by excess secretion of androgenic hormones by the adrenal gland or by excess medication with male hormones. In congenital forms, the female infant may be considered erroneously to be male and the male child will have accelerated growth and penile enlargement. In acquired forms, masculine secondary sex characteristics appear in the female, and there is precocious puberty in the male.

adrenogenous (ăd″rĕn-ŏj′ĕ-nŭs) [″ + ″ + Gr. *gennan,* to produce]. Originating in or produced by the adrenal gland.

adrenoleukodystrophy (ă-drē″nō-loo″kō-dĭs′trō-fē) [″ + ″ + Gr. *leukos,* white, + *dys,* bad, + *trephein,* to nourish]. A hereditary disease of children, transmitted as a sex-linked recessive trait. There is an abnormality of the white matter of the brain and atrophy of the adrenal glands. The mental and physical deterioration progresses to dementia, aphasia, apraxia, dysarthria, and blindness. There is no treatment, except symptomatic.

adrenolytic (ăd″rēn-ō-lĭt′ĭk) [L. *ad,* to, + *ren,* kidney, + Gr. *lysis,* dissolution]. Preventing or inhibiting the activity of adrenergic nerves. Interfering with the response of epinephrine.

adrenomegaly (ăd-rēn″ō-mĕg′ă-lē) [″ + ″ + Gr. *megas,* large]. Enlarged adrenal gland(s).

adrenomimetic (ă-drē″nō-mĭ-mĕt′ĭk) [″ + ″ + Gr. *mimetikos,* imitating]. Sympathicomimetic, q.v.

adrenopathy (ăd″rēn-ŏp′ă-thē) [″ + ″ + Gr. *pathos,* disease, suffering]. Any disease of the adrenal glands.

adrenosterone (ăd″rĕ-nŏs′tĕ-rōn). An androgenic hormone secreted by the adrenal cortex.

adrenotoxin (ăd-rē″nō-tŏk′sĭn) [″ + ″ + Gr. *toxikon,* poison]. A substance toxic to the adrenal glands.

adrenotropic (ăd-rē″nō-trŏp′ĭk) [″ + ″ + Gr. *tropikos,* turning]. Nourishing or stimulating to the adrenal glands with reference esp. to hormones that stimulate function of the adrenal glands.

Adriamycin. Trade name of doxorubicin, an antibiotic, antineoplastic drug.

ADS. *antidiuretic substance.*

Adson's maneuver. A test for thoracic outlet syndrome. The patient's arm is moved back into extension and external rotation with the elbow extended and forearm supinated. The radial pulse is palpated while the patient is asked to tuck his chin, side bend his head toward the opposite side and rotate his chin toward the side of the extended arm. The patient is then asked to inhale. A positive sign of numbness or tingling in the hand or diminished pulse indicates the brachial plexus or blood vessels are compromised at the site of the scalene muscle. SYN: *Adson test.*

adsorb. Attachment of a substance to the surface of another material. SEE: *absorb; absorption.*

adsorbate (ăd-sor′bāt). Anything that is adsorbed.

adsorbent (ăd-sor′bĕnt). A substance that leads readily to adsorption, such as activated charcoal or magnesia.

adsorption (ăd-sorp′shŭn) [L. *ad,* to, + *sorbere,* to suck in]. Adhesion by a gas or liquid to the surface of a solid.

adsternal (ăd-stĕr′năl) [″ + Gr. *sternon,* chest]. Near or toward the sternum.

adterminal (ăd-tĕr′mĭ-năl) [″ + *terminus,* boundary]. Toward extremity of any structure, as end of nerve or muscle.

adtorsion (ăd-tor′shŭn) [″ + *torsio,* twisted]. Convergent squint; inward rotation of both eyes.

adult (ă-dŭlt′) [L. *adultus,* grown up]. The fully grown and mature organism.

adulteration (ă-dŭl″tĕr-ā′shŭn) [L. *adulterare,* to pollute]. The addition or substitution of an impure or weaker, and usually cheaper, substance in a formulation or product.

adult foster care. ABBR: AFC. Long-term care for elderly individuals in an adult foster care facility. Typically, such a facility resembles a residence rather than a nursing home, and thus might have fewer regulations than in a nursing home.

adult onset G$_{M2}$ gangliosidosis. A slowly progressing disease caused by the gradual accumulation of the GM ganglioside in neurons due to defective hexosaminidase (Hex A). It is found among the Ashkenazi Jews and manifests with symptoms of psychosis or dementia. It may be referred to as adult onset Tay-Sachs disease.

adult respiratory distress syndrome (ARDS). A form of restrictive lung disease due to abnormal permeability of either the pulmonary capillaries or the alveolar epithelium. The condition is often found in patients whose lungs were initially normal but who have had some severe infection, trauma, or systemic illness. It commonly occurs in patients who are young and were previously healthy. ARDS affects an estimated 150,000 persons each year, and one half of these will die despite supportive therapy.

SYM: Dyspnea, tachypnea, tachycardia, diaphoresis, changes in level of consciousness; pink, frothy sputum; rhonchi.

TREAT: Vigorous efforts to maintain oxygen exchange. This is done by using assisted ventilation and oxygen. Antibiotics appropriate to the infecting organism.

NURSING IMPLICATIONS: Monitor patient's respiratory status, observe for inspiratory retractions of chest wall, use of accessory muscles of respiration, and dyspnea.

Assess ventilatory rate, depth, and rhythm, noting subtle changes. Auscultate for adventitious pulmonary sounds. Observe sputum volume and character, especially frothiness. Monitor patient's level of consciousness, cardiac rate and rhythm, blood pressure, arterial blood gas values, serum electrolyte levels, and chest x-ray results. Monitor fluid balance by measuring intake and output and daily weight. Maintain patent airway, suctioning as required. Provide oxygen therapy with continuous positive airway pressure (CPAP) or mechanically ventilate with positive end-expiratory pressure (PEEP) as prescribed. Provide adequate enteral or parenteral nutrition. Use intervention measures to prevent problems related to immobility. Provide emotional support to patient and family throughout the period of acute illness, the period of mechanical ventilation, and the recovery period, when patient is apt to be weak and fatigued. SEE: *Nursing Diagnoses* in *Appendix.*

advance (ăd-văns′) [Fr. *avancer,* to set forth]. To carry out the surgical procedure of advancement, q.v.

advance directive. A document prepared while an individual is alive and competent. It provides guidance to the health care team in the event the person is no longer capable of making decisions. The directive states the individual's preferences concerning life support measures and organ donation, and may give authority to another person to make decisions for the terminally ill patient who may be in a coma. A law, The Patient Self-Determination Act, mandating the responsibility of health care providers to develop written materials concerning advance directives, was enacted in the U.S. in December 1991. SEE: *living will.*

advanced cardiac life support. ABBR: ACLS. A procedure that includes basic life support (BLS), plus the use of adjunctive equipment to support ventilation, establishment of an I.V. fluid lifeline, drug administration, cardiac monitoring, defibrillation, control of cardiac arrhythmias, and postresuscitation care. ACLS requires the supervision and direction of a physician in person at the scene of the accident or emergency, or direct communication, or by an alternative method of communication previously defined by the physician, such as standing orders. SEE: *basic life support; cardiopulmonary resuscitation; emergency cardiac care.*

advanced trauma life support. ABBR: ATLS. Treatment measures necessary to stabilize a patient who has sustained serious injury.

advancement (ăd-văns′mĕnt) [Fr. *avancer*, to set forth]. Operation to remedy strabismus, by which the ocular muscle is severed and then attached at a point further removed from its origin.

a., capsular. Attachment of capsule of Tenon in front of its normal position.

adventitia (ăd″vĕn-tĭsh′ē-ă) [L. *adventicius*, coming from abroad]. The outermost covering of a structure or organ, such as the tunica adventitia or outer coat of an artery.

adventitious (ăd″vĕn-tĭsh′ŭs). 1. Acquired; accidental. 2. Arising sporadically. 3. Pert. to adventitia.

adverse effects. Adverse reactions, q.v.

adverse reactions. In pharmacology and therapeutics, the development of undesired side effects or toxicity caused by the administration of drugs. Onset of such reactions may be sudden or take days to develop. Early detection by use of laboratory tests is sometimes possible in the case of drugs that might adversely affect the blood-forming organs, the liver, or kidneys. It is important that all health care personnel be alert to the possibility of a patient's developing an adverse reaction to the drug or drugs administered. SYN: *adverse effects; drug interaction; drug reactions*.

adynamia (ăd″ĭ-nā′mē-ă) [Gr. *a-*, not, + *dynamis*, strength]. Weakness or loss of strength, esp. due to muscular or cerebellar disease. SYN: *asthenia; debility*.

adynamic (ăd″ĭ-năm′ĭk, ā-dī-năm′ĭk). Pert. to adynamia.

adynamic ileus. Intestinal obstruction resulting from lack of intestinal motility. This causes abdominal distention and interferes with postsurgical recovery, particularly from abdominal surgery.

NURSING IMPLICATIONS: Auscultate for bowel sounds in all four quadrants. Assess for increased abdominal distention by inspection, by measuring abdominal girth, and by percussing for tympanic note every 4 to 8 hours as necessary. Report nausea, vomiting, lack of passage of flatus, and change in bowel sounds. Prepare patient for diagnostic procedures. Promote bedrest in a quiet environment.

A.E. *above elbow;* term used to refer to the site of amputation of an upper extremity.

Aedes (ā-ē′dēs) [Gr. *aedes*, unpleasant]. A genus of mosquitoes belonging to the family Culicidae. Many species are troublesome pests and some are transmitters of disease.

A. aegypti. A species of *Aedes* that transmits yellow fever and dengue.

aeluropsis (ē″lū-rŏp′sĭs) [Gr. *ailouros*, cat, + *opsis*, vision]. Condition in which the eye or palpebral fissure is slanting toward the nose.

aer- (ĕr) [Gr. *aer*, air]. Combining form indicating relationship to gas or air.

aerated (ĕr′ā″tĕd). Containing air or gas.

aeration (ĕr″ā′shŭn). 1. Act of airing. 2. Process whereby carbon dioxide is exchanged for oxygen in blood in the lungs. 3. Saturation or charging of a fluid with gases.

aeriform (ĕr′ĭ-form) [″ + L. *forma*, shape]. Airlike; gaseous.

aero- (ĕr′ō). Combining form indicating relationship to air or gas.

Aerobacter (ĕr″ō-băk′tĕr) [″ + *bakterion*, little rod]. Previously used name for *Enterobacter aerogenes*, q.v.

aerobe (ĕr′ōb) [″ + *bios*, life] (pl. *aerobes*). A microorganism that is able to live and grow in the presence of oxygen.

a., facultative. A microorganism that prefers an environment devoid of oxygen but has adapted so that it can live and grow in the presence of oxygen.

a., obligate. A microorganism that can live and grow only in the presence of oxygen.

aerobic (ĕr-ō′bĭk). 1. Living only in the presence of oxygen. 2. Concerning an organism living only in the presence of oxygen.

aerobic exercise. Exercise during which the utilization of and metabolism of oxygen produces energy. Aerobic exercise is required for sustained periods of hard work and vigorous athletic activity. SEE: *anaerobic exercise*.

aerobic training. Exercise training for the purpose of attaining aerobic conditioning. No formula can be universally applied, but a general guideline is that aerobic conditioning will be obtained by normal, healthy persons who exercise three to five times a week for 20 to 30 minutes each time and at an intensity that produces a heart rate of 220 minus the age of the individual.

aerobiosis (ĕr″ō-bī-ō′sĭs) [″ + *biosis*, mode of living]. Living in an atmosphere containing oxygen.

aerocele (ĕr′ō-sēl) [″ + *kele*, tumor, swelling]. Distention of a cavity with gas.

aerocolpos (ĕr″ō-kŏl′pŏs) [″ + *kolpos*, vagina]. Distention of the vagina with air.

aerocoly (ĕr″ŏk′ō-lē) [″ + *kolon*, colon]. Distention of colon with gas.

aerocystoscopy (ĕr″ō-sĭs-tŏs′kō-pē) [″ + *kystis*, bladder, + *skopein*, to examine]. Examination with a cystoscope of the bladder distended by air.

aerodontalgia (ĕr″ō-dŏnt-ăl′jē-ă) [″ + *odous*, tooth, + *algos*, pain]. Pain in the teeth resulting from change in atmospheric pressure.

aerodontia (ĕr″ō-dŏn′shē-ă). Branch of dentistry concerned with the effect of changes in atmospheric pressure on the teeth.

aerodynamics (ĕr″ō-dī-năm′ĭks) [″ +

dynamis, force]. Science of air or gases in motion.

aeroembolism (ĕr″ō-ĕm′bō-lĭzm) [″ + *embolos,* plug, + *-ismos,* condition]. A condition in which nitrogen bubbles form in fluids and tissues of body during rapid ascent to high altitudes. Can also occur in skin diving or in hyperbaric oxygen therapy if return to sea level atmospheric pressure is too rapid.

SYM: Boring, gnawing pain in joints; itching of skin and eyelids; unconsciousness; convulsions; paralysis. Symptoms are relieved by recompression, i.e., return to lower altitudes or by placing patient in a hyperbaric pressure chamber. Even though oxygen by mask may be available, ascents above 25,000 feet should be avoided except in planes with pressurized cabins. SEE: *bends; caisson disease.*

aerogenesis (ĕr″ō-jĕn′ĕ-sĭs) [″ + *genesis,* generation, birth]. Formation of gas.

aerogenic, aerogenous (ĕr″ō-jĕn′ĭk, -ŏj′ĕn-ŭs). Gas forming.

aerogram (ĕr′ō-grăm″) [″ + *gramma,* something written]. Roentgenogram of an organ after it has been inflated or filled with air or gas.

aeromedical transportation. Air transportation of patients from a primary treatment area to a regional medical center or emergency hospital.

aerometer (ĕr-ŏm′ĕ-tĕr) [″ + *metron,* measure]. Device for measuring density of gases.

Aeromonas (ĕr″ō-mō′năs). Genus of bacteria found in natural water sources and soil. It is a gram-negative, non-spore-forming, motile bacillus. Aeromonads are commonly pathogenic for cold-blooded marine animals, and their importance in serious human diseases has been increasing, esp. in immunocompromised hosts. As opportunistic infections, Aeromonas infections may also occur in otherwise healthy hosts.

A. hydrophilia. A type of *Aeromonas* that has been found to be pathogenic for man. Organisms are sensitive to chloramphenicol, trimethoprim-sulfamethoxazole, and some quinolones.

aeroneurosis (ĕr″ō-nū-rō′sĭs) [Gr. *aer,* air, + *neuron,* nerve, + *osis,* condition]. A chronic functional nervous disorder affecting aviators, characterized by gastric distress, nervous irritability, insomnia, emotional instability, and increased motor activity.

aeroparotitis. Swelling of one or both parotid glands due to introduction of air into the glands. This may occur in those who play wind instruments; during vigorous nose blowing; and during too vigorous Valsalva's maneuver, q.v. SYN: *pneumoparotitis.*

aeropathy (ĕr-ŏp′ă-thē) [″ + *pathos,* disease, suffering]. Morbid condition caused by a marked change in atmospheric pressure, such as mountain fever, q.v., or caisson disease, q.v.

aeroperitoneum, aeroperitonia (ĕr″ō-pĕr″ĭ-tō-nē′ūm, -tō′nē-ă) [″ + *peritonaion,* peritoneum]. Distention of peritoneal cavity with gas.

aerophagia, aerophagy (ĕr″ō-fā′jē-ă, ĕr″ŏf′ă-jē) [″ + *phagein,* to eat]. Swallowing of air.

aerophilic, aerophilous (ĕr″ō-fĭl′ĭk, -ŏf′ĭ-lŭs) [″ + *philein,* to love]. Requiring air for growth and development. SYN: *aerobic.*

aerophobia (ĕr-ō-fō′bē-ă) [″ + *phobos,* fear]. Morbid fear of a draft or of fresh air.

aerophore (ĕr′ō-for) [″ + *phoros,* bearing]. A portable apparatus for inflating the lungs of stillborn or asphyxiated infants.

aerophyte (ĕr′-ō-fīt) [″ + *phyton,* plant]. A plant or vegetative organism that derives its sustenance from air.

aeroscope (ĕr′ō-skōp) [″ + *skopein,* to examine]. Device for examining visible particles in the air.

aerosinusitis (ĕr″ō-sī″nŭs-ī′tĭs) [″ + L. *sinus,* a hollow, + Gr. *itis,* inflammation]. Chronic inflammation of nasal sinuses due to changes in atmospheric pressure.

aerosis (ĕr-ō′sĭs) [″ + *osis,* condition]. Accumulation of gas in tissues.

aerosol (ĕr′ō-sŏl) [″ + L. *solutio,* solution]. A colloidal solution that is dispensed in the form of a mist.

aerosolization (ĕr″ō-sŏl″ī-zā′shŭn). Producing an aerosol.

aerosol therapy. The inhalation of aerosolized medicines, such as corticosteroids or mucolytic agents, in the treatment of pulmonary conditions such as asthma, bronchitis, and emphysema. SEE: *inhalation therapy.*

aerospace medicine. The branch of medicine concerned with the physiologic, pathologic, and psychologic problems man encounters in the environment of space. Previously called aviation medicine.

Aerosporin (ĕr″ō-spō′rĭn). Trade name for polymyxin B sulfate. SEE: *polymyxin.*

aerotaxis (ĕr″ō-tăk′sĭs) [Gr. *aer,* air, + *taxis,* arrangement]. Movement of organisms away from or toward air; said of aerobic and anaerobic bacteria.

aerotherapy (ĕr″ō-thĕr′ă-pē) [″ + *therapeia,* treatment]. The use of air in the treatment of disease, utilizing changes in composition and density. SEE: *decompression chamber; hyperbaric oxygen.*

aerothermotherapy (ĕr″ō-thĕr″mō-thĕr′ă-pē) [″ + *thermos,* heat, + *therapeia,* treatment]. Therapeutic use of hot air.

aerothorax (ĕr″ō-thō′răks) [″ + *thorax*, chest]. Pneumothorax, q.v.

aerotitis (ĕr-ō-tī′tĭs) [″ + *ot-*, ear, + *itis*, inflammation]. Inflammation of the ear, esp. the middle ear, due to failure of the eustachian tube to remain open during sudden changes in barometric pressure, as may occur while flying, diving, or working in a pressure chamber. SYN: *barotitis.*

aerotropism (ĕr-ŏt′rō-pĭzm) [″ + *trope,* a turn, + *-ismos*, condition]. The tendency of organisms, esp. bacteria and protozoa, to move toward (positive aerotropism) or away from (negative aerotropism) air.

aerourethroscope (ĕr-ō-ū″rē′thrō-skōp″) [″ + *ourethra,* urethra, + *skopein,* to examine]. An apparatus for visual examination of the urethra after dilatation by air.

aerourethroscopy (ĕr″ō-ū″rē-thrōs′kō-pē). Visual examination of the urethra when distended with air.

Aesculapius (ĕs″kū-lā′pē-ŭs). The Roman name for the god of medicine; son of Apollo and the nymph Coronis.

    A., staff of. A staff or crude stick with a snake wound around it. Snakes were sacred to Aesculapius because it was believed that they had the power to renew their youth by shedding their old skin and growing a new one. The staff of Aesculapius is used to signify the art of healing and is used by many medical organizations. SEE: *caduceus.*

aesthetics (ĕs-thĕt′ĭks) [Gr. *aisthesis,* sensation]. The philosophy or the theory of beauty and the fine arts. These concepts are especially important in dental restorations and in plastic and cosmetic surgery. Also spelled esthetics.

afebrile (ă-fĕb′rĭl) [Gr. *a-*, not, + L. *febris,* fever]. Without fever.

affect (ăf′fĕkt) [L. *affectus,* exerting influence on]. In psychology, the emotional reactions associated with an experience. SEE: *mood.*

    a., blunted. Greatly diminished emotional response to a situation or condition.

    a., flat. Virtual absence of emotional response to a situation or condition.

affection (ă-fĕk′shŭn). 1. Love, feeling. 2. Physical or mental disease.

affective (ă-fĕk′tĭv). Pert. to an emotion or mental state.

affective disorders. A group of disorders characterized by a disturbance of mood accompanied by a full or partial manic or depressive syndrome that is not caused by any other physical or mental disorder.

afferent (ăf′ĕr-ĕnt) [L. *ad,* to, + *ferre,* to bear]. Carrying impulses toward a center, as when a sensory nerve carries a message toward the brain; also said of certain veins and lymphatics. Opposite of efferent, q.v.

afferent nerves. Nerves that transmit impulses from the peripheral toward the central nervous system.

affidavit. A written or printed declaration or statement of facts, made voluntarily, that is confirmed by the person's oath or affirmation.

affiliation (ă-fĭl-ē-ā′shŭn) [L. *affiliare,* to take to oneself as a son]. 1. Membership in a larger organization. 2. Association. In nursing education, the administrative association of two hospitals or schools of nursing. This enables nurses to obtain specialized training and experience that might not otherwise be available to them.

affinity (ă-fĭn′ĭ-tē) [L. *affinis,* neighboring]. Attraction.

    a., chemical. Force causing certain atoms to combine with others to form molecules. SEE: *chemoreceptor.*

    a., elective. Force causing a substance to elect one substance rather than another with which to unite.

    a., selective. A., elective, q.v.

afflux (ăf′lŭks) [L. *ad,* to, + *fluere,* to flow]. Rush of blood to a part.

A fiber. A heavily medullated, fast-conducting nerve fiber.

afibrinogenemia (ă-fī″brĭn-ō-jĕ-nē′mē-ă) [Gr. *a-*, not, + L. *fibra,* fiber, + Gr. *gennan,* to produce, + *haima,* blood]. A rare blood disease characterized by the absence or decrease of fibrinogen in the blood plasma so that the blood is incoagulable; may be congenital or acquired. (The term "hypofibrinogenemia" more accurately describes the disease process.) The acquired type is due to one of several causes that can reduce the plasma concentration of fibrinogen. This has been observed in severe trauma and burns; following extensive surgery; in obstetric complications of abruptio placentae or retention of a dead fetus; in neoplastic disease; in hepatic cirrhosis; in leukemia; in sarcoidosis; and in polycythemia vera.

    TREAT: The clinical picture may develop suddenly. Administration of whole fresh blood and fibrinogen may prevent death from hemorrhage.

aflatoxicosis (ăf′lă-tŏk″sĭ-kō′sĭs). Poisoning caused by ingestion of peanuts or peanut products contaminated with *Aspergillus flavus* or other *A.* strains that produce aflatoxin, q.v. Farm animals and humans are susceptible to this toxicosis. SYN: *x-disease.*

aflatoxin (ăf′lă-tŏk′sĭn). A toxin produced by some strains of *Aspergillus flavus* and *A. parasiticus* that has a carcinogenic effect in experimental animals. It may be present in peanuts and other seeds contaminated with *Aspergillus* molds.

Caution: It is not practical to attempt to remove aflatoxin from contaminated food products in order to make them edible.

AFO. *ankle foot orthosis.*

AFP. *alpha-fetoprotein.*

afteraction. Continued reaction for some time after the stimulus ceases, particularly in nerve centers. In the sensory centers this action gives rise to aftersensations.

afterbirth. Placenta and membranes that are expelled after the birth of a child.

aftercare. 1. Care of a convalescent after conclusion of treatment in a hospital or mental institution. 2. The continuing program of rehabilitation designed to reinforce the effects of therapy and to help the patient adjust to his or her environment.

aftercataract. 1. Secondary cataract. 2. Development of an opacity of the lens capsule after cataract removal.

aftercurrent. Current produced in a tissue after electrical stimulation has ceased.

afterdischarge. The discharge of impulses from a reflex center after stimulation of the receptor has ceased. Results in prolongation of response.

aftereffect. A response occurring sometime after the original stimulus or condition has produced its primary effect.

afterhearing. Persistence of sensation of sound after the stimulus causing the sound has ceased.

afterimage. Image that persists subjectively after the cessation of stimulus. If colors are same as object, it is called positive; negative if complementary colors are seen. In the former case, the image is seen in its natural bright colors without any alteration; in the latter, the bright parts become dark, while dark parts are light.

    a., negative. Afterimage in which the colors and light intensity are reversed.

    a., positive. Afterimage in which the colors and light intensity are unchanged.

afterimpression. Aftersensation, q.v.

afterload. In cardiac physiology, the stress or tension that develops in the ventricular wall during systole. SEE: *preload.*

aftermovement. Persistent and spontaneous contraction of a muscle after a strong contraction against resistance has ceased. This is easily demonstrated by standing and forcibly pushing the arm against a wall while standing with the frontal plane perpendicular to the wall. When this is stopped and the patient has moved away from the wall, the arm will involuntarily adduct and be elevated. SYN: *Kohnstamm's phenomenon.*

afterpains. Uterine cramps due to contrac-

tion of uterus, occurring during first few days after childbirth; commonly seen in multiparae. Pains are more severe during nursing. The pains rarely last longer than 48 hours postpartum.

    TREAT: Analgesics, but do not use aspirin if there is a bleeding tendency. The earlier given, the less needed.

afterperception. Perception of a sensation after cessation of stimulus.

afterpotential wave. The wave produced after the action potential wave passes along a nerve. On the recording of the electrical activity, it will be either a negative or positive wave smaller than the main spike.

aftersensation. Sensation persisting after stimulus causing it has ceased.

aftertaste. Persistence of gustatory sensations after cessation of stimulus.

aftertreatment. Secondary treatment; that following primary treatment regimen. SEE: *aftercare.*

aftervision. Afterimage, q.v.

Ag [L. *argentum*]. Chem. symb. for the element silver.

against medical advice. ABBR: AMA. Said of a patient's decision to discontinue treatment or hospitalization even though advised by competent professional personnel to continue.

agamic (ă-găm'ĭk) [" + *gamos,* marriage]. 1. Reproducing asexually. 2. Asexual.

agammaglobulinemia (ă-găm"ă-glŏb"ū-lĭn-ē'mē-ă) [" + *gammaglobulin* + Gr. *haima,* blood]. A rare disease characterized by the virtual absence of all immunoglobulins from the blood plasma with resultant loss of the ability to produce immune antibodies, and the absence of natural blood group isoantibodies from the serum; may be congenital or acquired. The sex-linked congenital form is inherited like hemophilia as a sex-linked recessive characteristic and occurs only in male children. The non-sex-linked form occurs as an autosomal dominant characteristic. This latter form is quite rare.

agamogenesis (ăg"ă-mō-jĕn'ē-sĭs) [" + *gamos,* marriage, + *genesis,* generation, birth]. 1. Asexual reproduction. 2. Parthenogenesis, q.v.

agar (ā'găr, ăg'ăr) [Malay, gelatin]. 1. Seaweed belonging to the genus *Gelidium.* The source of agar-agar. 2. A dried mucilaginous product obtained from certain species of algae, especially of the genus *Gelidium.* It is unaffected by bacterial enzymes, hence widely used as a solidifying agent for bacterial culture media; also used as a laxative because of its great increase in bulk upon absorption of water. 3. A culture medium containing agar.

agar-agar. Agar (defs. 2 and 3), q.v.

agaric (ă-găr'ĭk) [Gr. *agarikon*, a sort of fungus]. Mushroom, esp. species of the genus *Agaricus*.

agastria (ă-găs'trē-ă) [Gr. *a-*, not, + *gaster*, stomach]. Absence of the stomach.

agastric (ă-găst'rĭk). Lacking an alimentary canal, as in certain animals such as tapeworms.

agathanasia (ăg"ă-thă-nā'zē-ă) [Gr. *aganthos*, good, + *thanatus*, death]. The concept of death with dignity, concerned with omitting actions and discontinuing procedures that maintain life beyond reasonable limits. Therapy to relieve excessive pain, even though such action might shorten the terminally ill patient's life, would be embodied in this concept. SEE: *"death with dignity"; euthanasia.*

AGC. *absolute granulocyte count.*

AgCl. Chem. symb. for silver chloride.

age [Fr. *age*, L. *aetas*]. 1. The time from birth to the present for a living individual as measured in units of time. 2. A particular period of life, as middle age or old age. 3. To grow old. 4. In psychology, the degree of development of an individual expressed in terms of the age of an average individual of comparable development or accomplishment.

   a., achievement. ABBR: A.A. Age of a person with regard to level of acquired learning; determined by a proficiency test and expressed in terms of the chronological age of the average person showing the same level of attainment.

   a., anatomical. An estimate of age as judged by the stage of development or deterioration of the body or tissue as compared with persons or tissues of known age.

   a., biological. One's present position in regard to the probability of survival. To determine biological age assessing and measuring the functional capacities of the life-limiting organ system, e.g., the cardiovascular system.

   a., bone. An estimate of biological age based on x-ray studies of the stage of development of ossification centers of the long bones of the extremities. SEE: *epiphysis.*

   a., chronological. ABBR: C.A. Age as determined by years since birth.

   a., developmental. An index of maturation expressed in months or years, which represents a value obtained by comparing performance with scaled norms for a particular age group. SEE: *age, achievement.*

   a., emotional. Judgment of age with respect to the stage of emotional development.

   a., functional. Defining age in terms of physical or functional capacity. Frequently, this term is applied to the aged.

   a., gestational. Age of embryo or fetus as timed from the date of onset of the last menstrual period.

   a., menarcheal. Elapsed time expressed in years from menarche.

   a., mental. ABBR: M.A. Age of a person with regard to mental ability, determined by a series of mental tests devised by Binet and expressed in terms of the chronological age of the average person showing the same level of attainment.

   a., physiological. Age as determined by functional ability as compared with persons of the same chronological age.

age, words pert. to: adolescence; age criteria in medicine; aging; age is not a diagnosis; Alzheimer's disease; chronologically enhanced; climacteric; geriatrics; maturation; menarche; menopause; puberty; senility; skin, tenting of.

aged (ājd', ā'jĕd). 1. To have grown older or more mature. 2. Persons who have grown old. SEE: *aging.*

ageism (āj'ĭzm) [Robert Butler, U.S. physician, who coined the term in 1968]. Discrimination against aged persons.

age is not a diagnosis. Being of a certain age, esp. of an age wherein deterioration of the mind and body is assumed to have taken place. Statistically and in general, the condition of persons in their 70s and 80s will be different in many respects from their condition in the 30s to 60s. Nevertheless, just because one has attained a certain chronological age is not, of itself, reason to believe an individual is mentally or physically infirm, incompetent, handicapped, or disabled. SEE: *aging; chronologically enhanced.*

agenesia, agenesis (ā"jĕn-ē'sē-ă, ă-jĕn'ē-sis) [Gr. *a-*, not, + *genesis*, generation, birth]. 1. Failure of an organ or part to develop or grow. 2. Lack of potency.

agenitalism (ă-jĕn'ĭ-tăl-ĭzm) [" + L. *genitalis*, genital, + Gr. *-ismos*, condition]. Absence of genitals.

agent (ā'jĕnt) [L. *agere*, to do]. Something that causes an effect; thus, bacteria that cause disease are said to be agents of the specific diseases they cause. A medicine would be classed as a therapeutic agent.

   a., sclerosing. A substance used to cause sclerosis, esp. of the lining of a vein. SEE: *varicose veins.*

Agent Orange. A defoliant that the U.S. military forces used extensively in the Vietnam War. It contained the toxic chemical dioxin as an unwanted and undesired contaminant. SEE: *dioxin.*

age of consent. The age at which a minor may legally engage in voluntary sexual intercourse or no longer require parental consent for marriage. Varies among states, usually between 13 and 18 years old.

agerasia (ā-jĕr-ā'sē-ă) [Gr. *a-*, not, + *geras*, old age]. Healthy, vigorous old age; youthful appearance of an old person.

age-specific. Data, especially in vital statistics and epidemiology, that are related to age.

ageusia, ageustia (ă-gū'sē-ă, ă-goos'tē-ă) [" + *geusis*, taste]. Absence, partial loss, or impairment of the sense of taste. SEE: *dysgeusia; hypergeusia; hypogeusia.*

ETIOL: May be due to disease of the chorda tympani or of the gustatory fibers; excessive use of condiments; effect of certain drugs; aging; or lesions involving sensory pathways or taste centers in the brain.

    a., central. Ageusia due to a cerebral lesion.

    a., conduction. Ageusia due to a lesion involving sensory nerves of taste.

    a., peripheral. Ageusia due to a disorder of taste buds of mucous membrane of tongue.

agger (ăj'ĕr) [L.]. (pl. *aggeres*) A small elevation or eminence; a mound.

    a. nasi. The ridge of the nose.

agglomerate (ă-glŏm'ĕ-rāt) [L. *ad*, to, + *glomerare*, to wind into a ball]. To congregate; to form a mass.

agglutinable (ă-gloo'tĭ-nă-bl) [L. *agglutinans*, gluing]. Capable of agglutination.

agglutinant (ă-gloo'tĭ-nănt). 1. Substance causing adhesion. 2. Causing union by adhesion, as in healing of a wound. 3. An antibody produced in the body in response to stimulation by an antigen (agglutinogen). SYN: *agglutinin.*

agglutination (ă-gloo"tĭ-nā'shŭn). 1. One type of antigen-antibody reaction in which a solid antigen clumps together with a soluble antibody. It requires a cell with antigenic markers close to the surface, available for interaction with the antibody. Often used in reference to transfusion reactions when antibodies attach the antigens on red blood cells of a different blood type, causing the cells to clump together, and for laboratory tests. 2. Adhesion of surfaces of a wound.

    a., direct. A test for the presence of a specific antibody performed by mixing a dilute antiserum with the antigen it is specific for. Ex.: Type A red blood cells are mixed with serum. If clumping occurs, the serum contains anti-A immunoglobulins.

    a., passive. Inert particles or cells with no foreign antigenic markers are coated with a known soluble antigen and mixed with serum. If agglutination occurs, an antibody to the antigen is present in the blood. Frequently, red blood cells are used as the carriers after they are washed to remove any known antibodies.

agglutinative (ă-gloo'tĭ-nā"tĭv). Causing or

capable of causing agglutination.

agglutinin (ă-gloo'tĭ-nĭn) [L. *agglutinans,* gluing]. The term used for antibodies, q.v., present in the blood that attach to antigens, q.v., on red blood cells, causing them to agglutinate or clump together. Agglutinins cause transfusion reactions when blood from a different group is given. These antibodies are present at birth and require no exposure to an antigen to be created since they are genetically determined. Used primarily in reference to laboratory tests of agglutination. SEE: *agglutinogen; antibody; antigen; blood groups; blood typing; isoagglutinin.*

    a., anti-Rh. An antibody produced in human plasma but sometimes produced in Rh-negative mothers bearing an Rh-positive fetus or in Rh-negative individuals who have received one or more transfusions of Rh-positive blood.

    a., cold. Agglutinin that acts only at low temperatures; present in the serum of patients with atypical pneumonia and in certain blood diseases.

agglutinogen (ă-gloo-tĭn'ō-jĕn) [L. *agglutinans,* gluing, + Gr. *gennan,* to produce]. The term used for the specific antigen that stimulates the recognition of an agglutinin, q.v., or antibody. Used primarily in reference to laboratory tests for testing for antibodies against specific blood types. SEE: *blood groups.*

    a.'s, A and B. Discovered by Karl Landsteiner in 1901, these two antigenic substances are found in the red blood cells of human beings and react with the alpha (anti-A) and beta (anti-B) isoagglutinins in the blood. The red corpuscles may contain A or B, both A and B, or neither A nor B agglutinogens. The four resulting blood groups are A, B, AB, and O, respectively. Blood groups are inherited according to Mendel's laws, q.v.

    a.'s, M and N. These two antigenic substances are found in the red corpuscles of human beings. Anti-M and anti-N agglutinins are rarely found in normal serum. The red blood cells may contain M or N, or both M and N agglutinogens, resulting in blood types M, N, or MN, respectively.

    a., Rh. A specific substance called the Rh factor, present in red cells. It was discovered in 1940 by Landsteiner and Wiener, who prepared anti-Rh serum by injecting red cells from Rhesus monkeys into rabbits or other animals. They found that the red cells of 85% of people of the Caucasian race will be agglutinated when in contact with anti-Rh. These persons are termed Rh-positive. The remaining 15% whose red cells are not agglutinated by anti-Rh are termed

Rh-negative. More than 25 blood factors are known to belong to the Rh system. Their importance in blood typing and blood type incompatibility between mother and fetus makes this blood group system second in importance only to the ABO group.

agglutinogenic, agglutogenic (ă-gloo″tĭ-nō-jen′ĭk, ă-gloo″tō-jĕn′ĭk). Producing agglutinins.

agglutinophilic (ă-gloo″tĭn-ō-fĭl′ĭk) [″ + Gr. *philos*, fond]. Readily agglutinating.

aggregate (ăg′rĕ-gāt) [L. *aggregatus*, collect]. 1. Total substances making up a mass. 2. To cluster or come together.

aggregation (ăg″rĕ-gā′shŭn). A clustering or coming together of substances.

   a., cell. Clumping together of blood cells, esp. platelets or red cells.

   a., familial. A cluster of the same disease in closely related families.

aggression (ă-grĕsh′ŭn) [L. *aggredi*, to approach with hostility]. 1. A forceful physical, verbal, or symbolic action. May be appropriate and self-protective, indicating healthy self-assertiveness, or it may be inappropriate. The behavior may be directed outward towards the environment or inward towards the self. 2. Activity performed in a forceful manner.

aging (āj′ĭng). Growing old, maturing. Progressive changes related to the passage of time. There is no precise method for determining the rate or degree of aging. In a study of 1500 persons age 100 years or more, it was determined that longevity is not inheritable; sexual activity is both good and feasible for the aged; the strain of child-rearing does not shorten life; the older person's offspring need not love him or her; and that one should work hard all during life, however long. SEE: *age is not a diagnosis; skin, tenting of.*

agitated depression. Depression accompanied by restlessness and increased psychomotor activity.

agitation (ăj″ĭ-tā′shŭn) [L. *agitare*, to drive]. 1. Excessive restlessness, increased mental and physical activity, esp. the latter. 2. Tremor. 3. Shaking of a container so that the contents are rapidly moved and mixed. 4. Severe motor restlessness, usually nonpurposeful, associated with anxiety.

agitographia (ăj″ĭ-tō-grăf′ē-ă) [″ + Gr. *graphein*, to write]. Writing with excessive rapidity, with unconscious omission of words and syllables.

agitophasia (ăj″ĭ-tō-fā′zē-ă) [″ + Gr. *phasis*, speech]. Excessive rapidity of speech, with slurring, omission, and distortion of sounds. SYN: *agitolalia.*

aglaucopsia, aglaukopsia (ă″glaw-kŏp′sē-ă) [Gr. *a-*, not, + *glaukos*, green, +

opsis, vision]. Green blindness; color blindness in which there is a defect in the perception of green. SEE: *color blindness.*

aglossia (ă-glŏs′ē-ă) [″ + *glossa*, tongue]. Congenital absence of the tongue.

aglossostomia (ă″glŏs-ō-stō′mē-ă) [″ + ″ + *stoma*, mouth]. Congenital absence of tongue and mouth opening.

aglutition (ă-gloo-tĭsh′ŭn) [″ + L. *glutire*, to swallow]. Difficulty in swallowing or inability to swallow.

aglycemia (ă″glī-sē′mē-ă) [″ + *glykys*, sweet, + *haima*, blood]. Lack of sugar in the blood.

aglycosuric (ă-glī″kō-sū′rĭk) [″ + ″ + *ouron*, urine]. Free from glycosuria.

agminate(d) (ăg′mĭ-nāt) [L. *agmen*, a crowd]. Aggregate; grouped in clusters.

agminated follicles. Aggregations of solitary follicles or groups of lymph nodes, principally in lower portion of small intestine. SYN: *Peyer's patches.*

agnathia (ăg-nā′thē-ă) [Gr. *a-*, not, + *gnathos*, jaw]. Absence of the lower jaw.

agnea (ăg′nē-ă) [″ + *gnosis*, knowledge]. Inability to recognize objects.

AgNO₃. Chem. symb. for silver nitrate.

agnogenic (ăg-nō-jĕn′ĭk) [″ + *gnosis*, knowledge, + *gennan*, to produce]. Of unknown origin or etiology.

agnosia (ăg-nō′zē-ă) [″ + *gnosis*, knowledge]. Loss of comprehension of auditory, visual, or other sensations although the sensory sphere is intact.

   a., auditory. Mental inability to interpret sounds.

   a., finger. Inability to identify fingers of one's own hands or of others.

   a., optic. Mental inability to interpret images that are seen.

   a., tactile. Inability to distinguish objects by sense of touch.

   a., visual object. SEE: *visual object agnosia.*

-agogue (ă-gŏg) [Gr. *agogos*, leading, inducing]. Suffix meaning a producer or leader.

agonad, agonadal (ă-gō′năd, ă-gōn′ă-dăl) [Gr. *a-*, not, + *gone*, seed]. Lacking gonads.

agonal (ăg′ō-năl) [Gr. *agon*, a contest]. Rel. to death or agony, e.g., agonal changes in tissue that occur after death.

agonist (ăg′ŏn-ĭst). 1. The muscle directly engaged in contraction as distinguished from muscles that have to relax at the same time; thus, in bending the elbow, the biceps brachii is the agonist and the triceps the antagonist, q.v. 2. In pharmacology, an agonist is a drug which binds to the receptor and stimulates the receptor's function. Drugs which mimic the body's own regulatory function are called agonists.

agony (ăg′ō-nē). 1. Extreme mental or physical suffering. 2. Death struggle.

agoraphobia (ăg″ō-ră-fō′bē-ă) [Gr. *agora*, marketplace, + *phobos*, fear]. Overwhelming symptoms of anxiety, often leading to a panic attack. This may occur in a variety of everyday situations (e.g., standing in line; eating in public; in crowds of people; on bridges or in tunnels; while driving) in which a person might have an attack and be unable to escape or get help, or suffer embarrassment. Panic attack symptoms often include rapid heartbeat, chest pain, difficulty breathing, gastrointestinal distress, faintness, dizziness, weakness, sweating, fear of loss of control or of going crazy, dying, or impending doom. People with these symptoms often avoid phobic situations, even to the point of staying at home for their entire lives.

-agra [Gr. *agra*, a seizure]. Suffix indicating sudden severe pain.

agranulocyte (ă-grăn′ū-lō-sīt) [Gr. *a-*, not, + L. *granulum*, granule, + Gr. *kytos*, cell]. A nongranular leukocyte.

agranulocytic (ă-grăn-ū-lō-sīt′ĭk). Pert. to agranulocytosis.

agranulocytosis (ă-grăn″ū-lō-sī-tō′sĭs) [″ + ″ + ″ + *osis*, condition]. An acute disease characterized by a deficit or absolute lack of granulocytic white blood cells (neutrophils, basophils, and eosinophils). SYN: *granulocytopenia.*

agranuloplastic (ă-grăn″ū-lō-plăs′tĭk) [″ + L. *granulum*, granule, + Gr. *plastikos*, formative]. Unable to form granular cells.

agranulosis (ă-grăn″ū-lō′sĭs). Agranulocytosis, q.v.

agraphesthesia. Inability to recognize letters or numbers drawn by the examiner on the skin. Patient's eyes are closed if this is done on skin visible to him. SEE: *graphesthesia.*

agraphia (ă-grăf′ē-ă) [″ + *graphein*, to write]. Loss of the ability to write. SYN: *logagraphia.* SEE: *aphasia, motor.*

   a., absolute. Complete inability to write.

   a., acoustic. Inability to write words that are heard.

   a., amnemonic. Inability to write sentences, although letters or words can be written.

   a., atactic. A., absolute, q.v.

   a., cerebral. Inability to express thoughts in writing.

   a., mental. A., cerebral, q.v.

   a., motor. Inability to write due to muscular incoordination.

   a., optic. Inability to copy words.

   a., verbal. Inability to write words although letters can be written.

agromania (ăg″rō-mā′nē-ă) [Gr. *agros*, field, + *mania*, frenzy]. Unreasonable desire for solitude or solitudinous wandering. Morbid desire to live in solitude or in the country.

agrypnocoma (ă-grĭp″nō-kō′mă) [Gr. *agrypnos*, sleepless, + *koma*, a deep sleep]. Coma in which the individual is partially awake as if in an extreme lethargic state; may be associated with muttering, delirium, and lack of sleep.

agrypnotic (ă″grĭp-nŏt′ĭk). 1. Afflicted with insomnia. 2. Causing wakefulness.

ague (ā′gū) [Fr. *aigu*, sharp, acute]. Originally used to indicate a chill or fever, esp. if due to malaria. Rarely used except colloquially.

agyria (ă-jī′rē-ă) [Gr. *a-*, not, + *gyros*, circle]. Incompletely developed convolutions of the cerebral cortex.

ah. *hypermetropic astigmatism.*

A.H.A. *American Heart Association; American Hospital Association.*

AHF. *antihemophilic factor*, coagulation factor VIII. SEE: *coagulation factors.*

AHG. *antihemophilic globulin*, coagulation factor VIII. SEE: *coagulation factors.*

Ahlfeld's sign (äl′fĕlts) [Friedrich Ahlfeld, Ger. obstetrician, 1843–1929]. Irregular uterine contractions after the third month of pregnancy. It is a presumptive sign of pregnancy.

A.I. *aortic insufficiency; artificial insemination; artificial intelligence; axioincisal.*

aichmophobia (ăk″mō-fō′bē-ă) [Gr. *aichme*, point, + *phobos*, fear]. Morbid fear of being touched by pointed objects or fingers.

A.I.D. *Agency for International Development; artificial insemination by donor* (heterologous insemination).

aid (ād). Assistance provided to a person, esp. one who is sick, injured, or troubled. SEE: *first aid.*

   a., hearing. A device, usually electronic, that amplifies sound to the level required to enable a hearing-impaired person to hear.

AIDS. *Acquired Immune Deficiency Syndrome.* The syndrome of opportunistic infections that occur as the final stage of infection by the human immunodeficiency virus (HIV). The virus attaches to the CD4 receptor on T4 lymphocytes, causing their destruction and a progressive loss of immune function. A retrovirus, HIV enters the cell, and infiltrates the cell's RNA, through which it transfers its own DNA to the cell's DNA by means of an enzyme, reverse transcriptase. The change in DNA prevents the cell from functioning normally; it only serves to create more HIV.

   In the very early period following infection, there may be signs of an acute, brief, nonspecific viral infection with fever, malaise, rash, arthralgias, and lymphadenopathy. After that, serologic evidence of AIDS appears. Most patients do not experience the viral syndrome. After this infection, the patient may remain an asymptomatic carrier and may remain so for years. The time from infection to clinical diagnosis varies from several years to more than a decade; but the time from infection to evidence of antibody formation is about 3 months but, in rare cases, persons known to have been infected with the virus and to have developed the disease have not produced antibodies.

Walter Reed Classification System: Stage 0: exposure. Stage 1: infection. Flulike syndrome characterized by fever, myalgia, malaise, lymphadenopathy; identification of HIV antibodies in blood (HIV+). Stage 2: chronic lymphadenopathy. Stage 3: T4 count less than 400. Stage 4: reduced delayed hypersensitivity (skin test) response to common allergens. Stage 5: complete anergy and appearance of chronic viral or fungal infections of mucous membranes. Stage 6: AIDS as defined by presence of opportunistic infections present in sites other than skin or mucous membranes. The length of time a patient stays in each stage is still relatively unclear.

In the U.S., AIDS is the leading cause of death in men and women who are under age 45 and in children 1 to 5 years of age. An estimated 100,000 Americans died in the 10-year period following the original report of cases in June 1981. Also, by that time an estimated one million persons were currently infected with the virus. It is estimated that the cost of treating everyone in the U.S. infected with HIV may reach $10.4 billion by 1994.

DIAG: Presence of antibodies to HIV in the blood is a sign of HIV infection. These antibodies do not destroy the virus, they simply serve as markers of infection. AIDS is diagnosed when opportunistic infections in sites other than the skin and mucous membranes are present. The original diagnostic criteria for AIDS has been revised so that it is less restrictive. This change is important to persons who do, indeed, have AIDS but did not meet the previous diagnostic criteria, and thus were denied certain medical and economic assistance. The revised criteria will include persons who have 200 or fewer CD4 cells or T cells per cubic mm of blood. (Normal level is about 1000 per cubic mm.)

SYM: Infections by opportunistic organisms, those that can be eliminated in people with healthy immune systems, are common because most of the causative organisms are present in humans all the time.

Infections common in stage 5 of HIV infection include:

1. *Candida albicans* (thrush); fungal infection of mouth or vagina.
2. Herpes simplex; fungal infection of mouth and anus.
3. Herpes varicella zoster (chickenpox); fungal infection of skin.

Opportunistic organisms and sites of infection characteristic of stage 6 (AIDS) include:

1. Cytomegalovirus: lungs, GI tract, eyes.
2. *Pneumocystis carinii* (PCP) (protozoa): lungs.
3. Cryptococcus (fungus): brain, liver, bone.
4. Toxoplasmosis (parasite): brain.
5. Cryptosporidiosis (parasite): GI tract.
6. Histoplasmosis (fungus): lungs, liver, bone marrow.
7. Salmonella (bacteria): GI tract.

Kaposi's sarcoma, normally a rather benign skin malignancy characterized by purple lesions, also appears in a virulent form in AIDS. SEE: *AIDS-related complex.*

MODE OF TRANSMISSION: HIV infection is spread by bodily secretions of the infected person coming in contact with the recipient's blood through a break in the skin or mucous membranes. Sexual intercourse, contaminated needles or blood transfusions, and placental transfer from mother to fetus are the most common means of transmission. In one series of children contracting AIDS from the nursing mother, the mode of transmission was most probably due to direct swallowing of blood from the traumatized nipples. Those mothers allowed nursing to continue well beyond the time the children had developed teeth. This permitted trauma to the nipples. In addition, there is increasing evidence that AIDS may be transmitted through breast milk.

HIGH-RISK GROUPS: In the United States, intravenous drug abusers, homosexuals, bisexuals, prostitutes and others with multiple sexual partners, the sexual partners of infected or at risk individuals, and those receiving multiple blood transfusions are at greatest risk. In other parts of the world, particularly Africa, heterosexuals and their partners are at highest risk. Blood is now routinely screened for the presence of HIV antibodies to minimize the risk to patients receiving blood transfusions.

PREVENTION: Educate public about HIV infection; encourage condom use, especially among teenagers and young adults and educate concerning hazard of using shared needles; educate heterosexuals, homosexuals and bisexuals to limit their number of sex partners; screen donated blood for HIV antibodies; avoid use of needles that are not sterile; educate people with AIDS concerning how to avoid infecting others. SEE: *condom, instructions for use; safe sex; Universal Precautions* in *Appendix.*

TREAT: Currently, multiple drugs are being tested against the HIV organism. AZT (azidothymidine) was the first FDA approved drug. Foscarnet is approved for treatment of cytomegalovirus retinitis which infects immunocompromised persons, including those with AIDS. Didanosine (DDI) is also approved for use in treating AIDS. It may be used alone or with AZT. Trade name is Videx. No drug has been found that eliminates or cures HIV infection.

PROG: Currently, scientists believe that all patients who are infected with HIV will progress to the AIDS stage and will die. The length of time between infection and death may be brief or many years. The time from infection to clinical signs is, on the average, 10 to 11 years. SEE: *sharps; Universal Precautions* in *Appendix.*

NURSING IMPLICATIONS: Follow CDC Universal Precautions for blood and body fluid as follows: eye protection; wear gloves (and gown) when hands (and clothing) could be in contact with patients' secretions or excretions; wear masks for anticipated respiratory contact with droplet secretions or spilled blood; avoid accidental skin punctures by careful handling of used needles; wash hands thoroughly using soap, friction, and flowing water; mark laboratory specimens "blood and body fluid precautions"; double-bag and identify contaminated linens, reusable equipment, disposables, and trash. Teach patients about the potential for the transmission of infectious agents to or from others by way of infectious blood or body fluids, emphasizing the importance of thorough handwashing and personal hygiene, along with specific measures to prevent oral, genital, or orogenital transmission. Provide supportive care related to fatigue, anorexia, and fever. Spend time with the patient to limit feelings of isolation and rejection. Provide psychological support to assist the patient in dealing with guilt, fear, anger, confusion, anxiety, or depression about the illness or the poor prognosis. Assist the patient to obtain social service support and funds for housing, food, and medication, for inpatient, outpatient, and hospice care.

Information about AIDS may be obtained in the U.S. by calling 1-800-342-2437. In Canada, call 1-800-668-AIDS in Ontario. SEE: *Nursing Diagnoses* in *Appendix.*

AIDS-dementia complex. Severe mental

changes, i.e., dementia, q.v., that may be associated with AIDS.

AIDS-related complex. ABBR: ARC. The group of clinical signs and symptoms associated with stages 1 to 5 of infection by human immunodeficiency virus (HIV): progressive lymphadenopathy, fatigue, intermittent fevers, weight loss greater than 10%, chronic or persistent intermittent diarrhea, night sweats, diminished delayed hypersensitivity (skin test) response to common allergens, presence of HIV antibodies in blood, decreased T4 lymphocyte count. SEE: *AIDS.*

A.I.H. *artificial insemination by husband* (homologous insemination).

ailment. A mild illness.

ailurophobia (ā-lū″rō-fō′bē-ă) [Gr. *ailouros,* cat, + *phobos,* fear]. Morbid fear of cats.

ainhum (ān′hŭm) [East African, to saw]. A fissured constriction around a digit; of unknown origin. Due to the constriction, the digit will eventually require amputation. Usually affects the fourth or fifth toes and less commonly other digits of the feet or hands. It is predominantly a disease of members of dark-skinned races. There is no specific treatment.

air (ār) [Gr. *aer,* air]. The invisible, tasteless, odorless mixture of gases surrounding the Earth. Clean air at sea level is made up of approximately 78% nitrogen and 21% oxygen by volume. The remaining constituents are water vapor, carbon dioxide, and traces of ammonia, argon, helium, neon, krypton, xenon, and other rare gases.

   a., alveolar. Air in the alveoli; that involved in the pulmonary exchange of gases between air and the blood. Its content is determined by sampling the last portion of a maximal expiration.

   a., complemental. Volume of air that can be inspired over and above the tidal air, q.v., by deepest possible inspiration. SYN: *inspiratory reserve volume.*

   a., dead space. Volume of air that fills the respiratory passageways and is not available for exchange of gases with the blood.

   a., dead space, mechanical. Dead space provided by artificial means, as with mechanical ventilation or the addition of plastic tubing to a ventilator circuit.

   a., functional residual. Volume of air left in the lungs at the end of a normal expiration. It is the sum of supplemental air, q.v., and residual air, q.v.

   a., liquid. Air liquefied by great pressure. It produces intense cold on evaporation.

   a., minimal. The small volume of air trapped in alveoli when lungs collapse with the thorax open; it is impossible to expel, even if lung is removed.

a., reserve. A., supplemental, q.v.

a., residual. The amount remaining in the lungs after the fullest possible expiration. About 1500 cc in the adult.

a., supplemental. Volume of air that can be expired after a normal expiration by fullest possible expiration. About 1600 cc in the adult. SYN: *expiratory reserve volume.*

a., tidal. Volume of air that flows in and out of the lungs with each normal respiration; average for adult male is about 500 cc.

air, words pert. to: "aer-" words; aspiration; atelectasis; expiration; inspiration; respiration; ventilation.

air bag. A system for providing passive restraint for occupants of automobiles the moment a collision occurs. The air bag inflates when the automobile or truck impacts something in front of it. It is estimated that 10,000 lives would be saved annually in the U.S. if every car and truck had air bags on both sides of the front seat. SEE: *passive restraint device.*

air bed. 1. Large inflated cushion used as a mattress. 2. A special bed that permits the patient actually to float on a cushion of air. SEE: *air-fluidized bed.*

air bronchogram sign. Radiographic appearance of an air-filled bronchus as it passes through an area of increased anatomic density as in pulmonary edema and pneumonia.

air cell. Air vesicle, q.v.

air conditioning. Use of special equipment to control, esp. to lower, temperature and humidity of the air while ensuring adequate ventilation.

air conduction. The conduction of sound to the inner ear via the pathway provided by the air in the ear canal.

air curtain. A current of air directed around a patient so that air that would normally circulate around and contaminate the patient is blocked by a curtain of air. Used in isolating patients from dustborne bacteria or allergens. SEE: *laminar air flow.*

air cushion. An airtight inflatable cushion.

air embolism [L. *embolismus*]. Obstruction of a blood vessel by an air bubble.

ETIOL: Air may enter a vessel postoperatively, during change of an intravenous set on a central line or by injection into a central line port or rupture of a central line balloon, during an intravenous injection if the syringe is not properly filled, or from intravenous tubing if fluid is permitted to flow through tubing from which air has not been evacuated. NOTE: A very small amount of air in the tubing or syringe will not cause symptoms.

NURSING IMPLICATIONS: When an embolism is suspected in the venous circulation (moving toward the heart), immediately turn the patient to the left side with head down to trap air in the right heart. Assess for sudden onset of dyspnea, hypotension, cyanosis, chest pain, hemoptysis, or decreasing level of consciousness. Stop the I.V. if air is still in the line; otherwise, slow the I.V. rate to keep vein open only, administer oxygen, and notify the patient's physician.

air flow, laminar. SEE: *laminar air flow.*

air-fluidized bed. A special bed consisting of a mattress filled with approx. 100 billion ceramic spheres that are suspended by a continual flow of warm air at the rate of approx. 40 cubic feet (1.13 cubic meters) per minute. This creates a surface that feels like a liquid, having a specific gravity of 1.3. The patient "floats" on the mattress with only minimal penetration. Because of the even distribution of weight, the bed is particularly useful in treating patients with burns or decubitus ulcers. Nursing care of the patient is greatly simplified because the patient can be moved by fingertip pressure.

air gap principle. A procedure used to decrease the amount of scattered radiation reaching the radiographic film by increasing the object-film distance.

air hunger. Shortness of breath marked by rapid, labored breathing. SEE: *dyspnea.*

airplane splint. An appliance usually used on ambulatory patients in the treatment of fractures of the humerus. It takes its name from the elevated (abducted) position in which it holds the arm suspended in air.

air pollution. Contamination of air by noxious substances, as from automobile exhaust, or industrial waste.

air sac. Air vesicle, q.v.

airsickness. Condition of giddiness, nausea, vomiting, headache, and often extreme drowsiness occurring during air flight. SEE: *seasickness.*

air splint. Type of splint used for immobilizing fractured or injured extremities. It is usually an inflatable cylinder, open at both ends, that becomes rigid when it is inflated and thus prevents the part confined in the cylinder from moving.

air swallowing. Voluntary or involuntary swallowing of air. It occurs involuntarily in infants as a result of improper feeding. In adults it occurs in neurasthenia or hysteria or when on a fluid diet. SYN: *aerophagia.*

air syringe. A syringe on a dental unit to deliver compressed air through a fine nozzle to clear or dry an area, or to evacuate debris from operative field.

Caution: Use of high pressure may injure the tissues.

air travel, patient precautions concerning.
Very few medical conditions preclude air travel but some conditions do require special considerations. Expansion of gas at cabin pressure may be a problem to those who have had recent abdominal surgery. Persons with difficulty with blocked sinuses or eustachian tubes should not fly until the condition has cleared up. Motion sickness can be controlled by medicines such as transdermal scopolamine. Patients with a recent history of myocardial infarction should not travel without their physicians' approval. Persons with impaired pulmonary function may need supplemental oxygen, depending upon their functional capacity. Those with an intestinal ostomy may need a larger bag because of gas expansion. If a person has had recent surgery involving the inner ear, they should not travel by air if there is any difficulty with equalizing air pressure between ambient air and the middle ear. If the jaws have been wired as part of the treatment for a jaw fracture, wire cutters must be carried in case motion sickness causes vomiting. Pregnant women will need their physicians' permission to travel during the last several weeks of their pregnancy and immediately after delivery. Diabetics will, of course, need a supply of insulin. Patients with infectious disease spread by the airborne route will not be allowed to fly.

air vesicle. Pulmonary alveolus; one of the terminal saccules of an alveolar duct where gases are exchanged in respiration.

airway. 1. Natural passageway for air to and from the lungs. 2. Device used to prevent or correct obstructed respiratory passage, esp. during anesthesia and during cardiopulmonary resuscitation, q.v. Maintaining the airway is, obviously, essential to the life of the patient. In an emergency situation, and esp. when the patient is unconscious or has a bilateral fracture of the lower jaw, there is a good possibility that the tongue will close the oropharyngeal airway. Methods for opening the airway are described in cardiopulmonary resuscitation, q.v.; chin-lift airway technique, head tilt, q.v.; and jawthrust technique. SEE: illus.

Caution: If a patient is unconscious or has an injury to the head and upper neck, assume there is spinal injury. To move the patient could cause paralysis by transection of the spinal cord. SEE: *jaw-thrust technique.*

    a., nasopharyngeal. A method of establishing an airway in a patient who is cooperative or unconscious. An active gag reflex may prevent the placing of a small, soft, flexible tube through the patient's nose into the nasopharynx. The tube should be equal in length to the distance from the nose to the ear lobe. It has a flange on the end remaining outside the nose to keep it from sliding into the pharynx. The tube may be used to transport air to the patient by use of a bag-valvemask attachment or directly by the resuscitator blowing into the tube as in mouth-to-mouth respiration assistance. The use of a one-way valve will protect the resuscitator against contamination from the patient. SEE: *Universal Precautions* in *Appendix.*

    a., oropharyngeal. A curved device for use in establishing an airway in an unconscious patient who does not gag when it is in place. Once the device is in place it extends through the mouth to the oropharynx. It is essential that the proper size airway be used. Air is delivered to the device by mouth-to-device method or by attaching a bag-valvemask and blowing into that. SEE: *cardiopulmonary resuscitation; Universal Precautions* in *Appendix.*

Caution: Do not move the head of an unconscious patient. To do so could cause paralysis.

A.K. *above knee;* term used to refer to the site of amputation of a lower extremity.

akaryocyte (ă-kăr′ē-ŏ-sīt″) [Gr. *a-*, not, + *karyon*, kernel, + *kytos*, cell]. A non-nucleated cell, such as an erythrocyte.

akaryote (ă-kăr′ē-ōt) [″ + *karyon*, kernel]. Akaryocyte, q.v.

akatamathesia (ă-kăt″ă-mă-thē′zē-ă) [″ + *katamathesis*, understanding]. The mental condition of being unable to understand.

akathisia (ăk″ă-thĭ′zē-ă) [″ + *kathisis*, sitting]. Acathisia, q.v.

akee (ăk′ē, ă-kē′) [Liberian]. The tropical tree *Blighia sapida.* Ingestion of the unripe fruit can cause severe hypoglycemia. Also spelled ackee.

akinesia (ā″kĭ-nē′zē-ă) [Gr. *a-*, not, + *kinesis*, movement]. Complete or partial loss of muscle movement. Also spelled acinesia.

    a. algera. Akinesia with intense pain caused by voluntary movement.

akinetic (ā″kĭ-nĕt′ĭk). 1. Pert. to akinesia. 2. Rel. to or characterized by amitosis.

Al. Chem. symb. for the element aluminum (British: aluminium).

NASOPHARYNGEAL AIRWAY

TILT HEAD BACK BEFORE INSERTING NASOPHARYNGEAL AIRWAY. INSERT THROUGH NOSTRIL, PAST THE PHARYNX INTO THE LARYNX AND TRACHEA TO MAINTAIN PATENCY OF AIRWAY

PHARYNX

NASOPHARYNGEAL AIRWAY

TRACHEA

ESOPHAGUS

OROPHARYNGEAL AIRWAY

TRACHEA

TONGUE

ESOPHAGUS

OROPHARYNGEAL AIRWAY

PHARYNX

TILT HEAD BACK BEFORE INSERTING OROPHARYNGEAL AIRWAY. TO MAINTAIN PATENCY INSERT DEVICE INTO PROPER POSITION TO HOLD TONGUE AWAY FROM POSTERIOR WALL OF PHARYNX

-al [L.]. 1. Suffix indicating connection with, as in abdominal, marginal. 2. In chemistry, it indicates an aldehyde.

ala (ā'lă) [L., wing] (pl. *alae*). 1. An expanded or winglike structure or appendage. 2. Axilla, q.v.

   a. auris. Protruding portion of the external ear. SYN: *auricle; pinna.*

   a. cerebelli. [NA] Winglike projection of central lobule of cerebellum. SYN: *a. lobuli centralis.*

   a. cinerea. Gray triangular prominence on the floor of the fourth ventricle. The autonomic fibers of the vagus nerve arise from the cells of the nucleus of this area. SYN: *triangle of the vagus nerve; trigonum nervi vagi.*

   a. cristae galli. [NA] Small projection on each side of the crista galli, q.v., of the ethmoid bone.

   a. lobuli centralis. A. cerebelli, q.v.

   a. major ossis sphenoidalis. [NA] Greater wing of the sphenoid bone.

   a. minor ossis sphenoidalis. [NA] Lesser wing of the sphenoid bone.

   a. nasi. [NA] Wing of the nose; broad portion forming the lateral wall of each nostril.

   a. of ethmoid. Small projection on each side of the ethmoid bone.

   a. of ilium. Broad, upper portion of the iliac bone.

   a. of sacrum. Broad projection on each side of the base of the sacrum.

   a. vomeris. [NA] Wing of the vomer; projection on each side of the superior border of the vomer.

alacrima (ā-lăk'rĭ-mă) [Gr. *a-*, not, + L. *lacrima*, tear]. Deficiency of or absence of tears. SYN: *dry eye.* SEE: *Sjögren's syndrome.*

Alagille syndrome. Arteriohepatic dysplasia with bile duct hypoplasia or paucity.

alalia (ă-lā'lē-ă) [" + *lalein*, to talk]. Loss of ability to speak due to defect or paralysis of the vocal organs. Aphasia, q.v.

   ETIOL: Due to organic brain disease or psychoneurosis.

alanine (ăl'ă-nēn). USP. A naturally occurring amino acid, $C_3H_7NO_2$. It is classed as being nonessential in human nutrition.

alanine aminotransferase. ABBR: ALT. Current term for serum glutamic pyruvic transaminase (SGPT).

alar (ā'lăr) [L. *ala*, wing]. 1. Pert. to or like a wing. 2. Axillary.

ALARA. *as low as reasonably achievable.*

alar artery. Branch of angular artery supplying tissues of ala nasi.

alar cartilage. Cartilage forming the broad lateral wall of each nostril.

alastrim (ă-lăs′trĭm) [Portuguese *alastrar*, to spread]. Mild form of smallpox with sparse rash and low-grade fever. SYN: *variola minor.*

alate (ā′lāt) [L. *ala*, wing]. Winged.

alba [L. *albus*, white]. 1. White. 2. White substance of the brain.

albedo (ăl-bē′dō) [L.]. Whiteness. Reflection of light from a surface.

    a. retinae. Reflections associated with retinal edema.

    a. unguium. White semilunar area near nail root. SYN: *lunula.*

Albers-Schönberg disease (ăl-bărs-shĕrn′bărg) [Heinrich Ernst Albers-Schönberg, Ger. roentgenologist, 1865–1921]. Excessive calcification of bones causing marblelike appearance.

Albert's disease [Eduard Albert, Austrian surgeon, 1841–1900]. Inflammation of the bursae lying over the Achilles tendon. SYN: *achillobursitis.*

albicans [L.] (pl. *albicantia*). 1. White or whitish. 2. Corpus albicans, q.v.

    a., corpus. [NA] A mass of fibrous tissue that replaces the regressing corpus luteum following rupture of the graafian follicle. It forms a white scar that gradually decreases in size and eventually disappears.

albidum (ăl′bĭ-dŭm) [L.]. White.

albidus (ăl′bĭ-dŭs) [L.]. White.

Albini's nodules (ăl-bē′nēz) [Giuseppe Albini, It. physiologist, 1830–1911]. Minute nodules on margins of mitral and tricuspid valves of the heart; sometimes seen in newborns.

albinism (ăl′bĭn-ĭzm) [L. *albus*, white, + Gr. *-ismos*, condition]. Congenital, nonpathological, partial or total absence of pigment in skin, hair, and eyes. Frequently accompanied by astigmatism, photophobia, and nystagmus because the choroid is not sufficiently protected from light as a result of lack of pigment.

albino (ăl-bī′nō). A person afflicted with albinism, q.v.

albinuria (ăl″bĭ-nū′rē-ă) [″ + Gr. *ouron*, urine]. Passing of white or colorless urine of low specific gravity. SYN: *achromaturia.*

albocinereous (ăl″bō-sĭn-ē′rē-ŭs) [″ + *cinereus*, gray]. Pert. to both white and gray matter of brain and spinal cord.

Albright's disease [Fuller Albright, U.S. physician, 1900–1969]. Polyostotic fibrous dysplasia, q.v., accompanied by café au lait macules and endocrine disorders, esp. precocious puberty in girls.

albuginea (ăl-bū-jĭn′ē-ă) [L. from *albus*, white]. A layer of firm, white, fibrous tissue forming the investment of an organ or part, as of the eye, testicle, ovary, or spleen. SYN: *tunica albuginea.*

    a. corporum cavernosorum. A strong, very elastic, white fibrous coat, forming a sheath common to both corpora cavernosa of the penis.

    a. oculi. Sclera, or tough white supporting covering of the eyeball.

    a. ovarii. The layer of firm fibrous tissue lying beneath the epithelial ovarian covering.

    a. testis. The thick, unyielding layer of white fibrous tissue lying under the tunica vaginalis.

albugineotomy (ăl″bū-jĭn″ē-ŏt′ō-mē) [*albuginea* + Gr. *tome*, incision]. Incision of tunica albuginea, esp. of the testis.

albugineous (ăl″bū-jĭn′ē-ŭs). Pert. to or resembling tunica albuginea.

albuginitis (ăl″bū-jĭn-ī′tĭs) [″ + Gr. *itis*, inflammation]. Inflammation of tunica albuginea.

albugo (ăl-bū′gō) [L.]. White opacity of the cornea.

albumen (ăl-bū′mĕn) [L.]. Albumin, q.v.

albumin (ăl-bū′mĭn) [L. *albumen*, white of egg]. One of a group of simple proteins widely distributed in plant and animal tissues; it is found in the blood as serum albumin, in milk as lactalbumin, and in the white of egg as ovalbumin. It is soluble in cold water; when coagulated by heat it is no longer dissolved by cold or hot water. In the stomach coagulated albumins are made soluble by peptase, being changed at the same time into albumoses and peptones. In general, albumins from animal sources are of higher quality than those from vegetable sources because animal proteins contain greater quantities of essential amino acids. SEE: *albumose; amino acid; peptone.*

    a., acid. Compound resulting from action of acid on albumin.

    a., alkali. Compound resulting from action of weak alkalies on albumin.

    a., blood. A., serum, q.v.

    a., circulating. Albumin present in body fluids.

    a., derived. Albumin changed by chemical action; albuminate.

    a., egg. White of an egg; ovalbumin.

    a., human. USP. Sterile solution of serum albumin obtained from healthy blood donors. Administered intravenously to restore blood volume. Trade names are Buminate, Albuminar, and Plasbumin.

    a., muscle. Form of albumin found in muscular tissue.

    a., native. Any albumin normally

present in an organism.

a., serum. The main protein found in the blood. SYN: *a., blood.*

a., urinary. Albumin in urine.

a., vegetable. Albumin in, or derived from, plant tissue.

albuminate (ăl-bū″mĭ-nāt). The compound formed when albumin combines with an acid or alkali (base).

albuminaturia (ăl-bū″mĭ-nă-tū′rē-ă) [L. *albumen*, white of egg, + Gr. *ouron*, urine]. Presence of albuminates in urine.

albuminiferous (ăl-bū″mĭn-ĭf′ĕ-rŭs) [″ + *ferre*, to bear]. Producing albumin.

albuminimeter (ăl-bū″mĭn-ĭm′ĕ-tĕr) [″ + Gr. *metron*, measure]. Instrument for measuring amount of albumin in urine.

albuminiparous (ăl-bū″mĭn-ĭp′ă-rŭs) [″ + *parere*, to bring forth, to bear]. Yielding albumin.

albuminocholia (ăl-bū″mĭ-nō-kō′lē-ă) [″ + Gr. *chole*, bile]. Albumin in the bile.

albuminogenous (ăl-bū″mĭn-ŏj′ĕ-nŭs) [″ + Gr. *gennan*, to produce]. Producing albumin.

albuminoid (ăl-bū′mĭ-noyd″) [″ + Gr. *eidos*, form, shape]. 1. Resembling albumin. 2. A protein.

albuminolysis (ăl-bū″mĭn-ŏl′ĭ-sĭs) [″ + Gr. *lysis*, dissolution]. Proteolysis; decomposition of protein.

albuminoptysis (ăl″bū-mĭn-ŏp′tĭ-sĭs) [″ + Gr. *ptyein*, to spit]. Albumin in sputum.

albuminoreaction (ăl-bū″mĭ-nō-rē-ăk′-shŭn) [″ + *re*, again, + *agere*, to act]. The presence (positive reaction) or absence (negative reaction) of albumin in the sputum. Positive reaction indicates inflammatory condition of lungs.

albuminorrhea (ăl-bū″mĭ-nō-rē′ă) [″ + Gr. *rhoia*, flow]. Presence of albumin in urine. SYN: *albuminuria*, q.v.

albuminose (ăl-bū′mĭn-ōs). 1. Albumose, q.v. 2. Albuminous, q.v.

albuminosis (ăl-bū″mĭ-nō′sĭs) [″ + Gr. *osis*, condition]. Abnormal increase of albumin in blood plasma.

albuminous (ăl-bū′mĭ-nŭs). Pert. to, resembling, or containing albumin.

albumin test. The most common type of albumin found in urine is serum albumin. Before testing, certain precautions must be observed: The specimen of urine must be fresh. The specimen must also be clear; the safest way to ensure this is to filter it through special filter paper. Because albuminuria can be caused by many different conditions, the results of tests require careful interpretation. Quantitative methods are also available.

There are many tests for albumin, but the usual ones are:

Acetic acid test: Over a Bunsen burner, heat the top inch (2.5 cm) of a test tube filled with urine. A cloudiness will occur, which may be due to phosphate or albumin. Add 2 to 3 drops of acetic acid. If the cloud disappears, it is due to phosphates; if it becomes intensified, albumin is present.

Heller's test: Pour about ½ in. (1.3 cm) of concentrated nitric acid in a test tube and overlay it carefully with the urine, using a pipette. If an opaque line appears at the junction of the fluids, albumin is present. The line may take a few minutes to develop. SEE: *Heller's test.*

Paper strip or tablet tests: There are several tests based on the principle that certain chemicals impregnated in paper or in tablet form will change color when exposed to protein-containing urine. Within certain limits, these tests are reliable and have the advantage of providing a result in a few seconds.

Sulfosalicylic acid test: Add 10 to 20 drops of sulfosalicylic acid to urine in a test tube. Albumin is shown as a white, cloudy precipitate. This may be carried out as a ring test, as in Heller's test.

albuminuretic [L. *albumen*, white of egg, + Gr. *ouretikos*, causing urine to flow]. Pert. to or causing albuminuria.

albuminuria (ăl-bū-mĭ-nū′rē-ă) [″ + Gr. *ouron*, urine]. Presence of readily detectable amounts of serum protein, esp. serum albumin but also serum globulin and others, in the urine. A common sign of renal impairment. It occurs in febrile states, malignant hypertension, congestive heart failure, nephrotic syndrome, and other kidney disorders. Its presence, however, is not always a sign of disease because it may be found in normal persons following vigorous exercise. SYN: *proteinuria.* SEE: *nephritis; nephrosis.*

a., cyclic. Presence of small amounts of albumin in the urine at regular diurnal intervals, esp. in childhood and adolescence.

a., digestive. Albuminuria following ingestion of certain foods.

a., extrarenal or accidental. Albuminuria due to contamination of urine with pus, chyle, or blood.

a., functional. Intermittent or temporary albuminuria not associated with a pathologic condition. SYN: *a., transient.*

a., intrinsic. Albuminuria resulting from intrinsic renal disease. SYN: *a., true.*

a., orthostatic. A., postural, q.v.

a., pathological. Albuminuria caused by a disease.

a., physiological. A., functional, q.v.

a., postural. Transient albuminuria in normal individuals who have remained in an erect position for a considerable length of time. SYN: *a., orthostatic.*

a., renal. Albuminuria caused by defective renal function, esp. of the glomeruli.

a., toxic. Albuminuria due to toxins generated within the body or poison from outside source.

a., transient. A., functional, q.v.

a., true. A., intrinsic, q.v.

albuminuric retinitis (ăl″bū-mĭ-nū′rĭk rĕt″ĭ-nī′tĭs). Inflammation of retina associated with chronic kidney disease, characterized by hazy retina, blurred disk margin, distention of retinal arteries, retinal hemorrhages, and white patches in the fundus, esp. the stellate figure at the macula. SEE: *retinitis.*

albumoscope (ăl-bū′mō-skōp) [″ + Gr. *skopein*, to examine]. An instrument for determining the presence of albumin in the urine.

albumose (ăl′bū-mōs). The intermediate chemical produced by digestion of proteins, converted by further digestion into peptone.

albumosemia (ăl″bū-mō-sē′mē-ă) [″ + Gr. *haima*, blood]. Presence of albumose in blood.

albumosuria (ăl″bū-mō-sū′rē-ă) [″ + Gr. *ouron*, urine]. Presence of albumose in urine.

albus [L.]. White.

Albuterol. Bronchodilator used in inhalation treatments.

Alcaligenes (ăl″kă-lĭj′ĭ-nēz). Genus of rod-shaped, gram-negative bacteria found in the intestinal tract of man, dairy products, and soil.

A. faecalis. Species of bacteria normally found in the intestinal tract of man. It has been associated with septicemia and epidemics of urinary tract infections.

Alcock's canal [Benjamin Alcock, Irish anatomist, b. 1801]. Pudendal canal; space in the external fascia of the ischiorectal fossa, above the tuberosity of the ischium, through which the internal pudendal artery, veins, and nerve pass.

alcohol (ăl′kō-hŏl) [Arabic *al-koh'l*, something subtle]. 1. A class of organic compounds formed from hydrocarbons by substituting one or more hydroxyl (OH) groups for a similar number of hydrogen atoms. 2. Ethyl alcohol, a colorless, volatile, flammable liquid of the formula C_2H_5OH. Its molecular weight is 46.07; boiling point 78.5°C. Present in fermented or distilled liquors, and is obtained, in its pure form, from grain by fermentation and fractionation distillation. The USP standard is a liquid that contains not less than 92.3% by weight of C_2H_5OH. SYN: *a., ethyl; a., grain; ethanol.*

ACTION/USES: Used in preparing essences, tinctures, extracts; manufacturing of ether, ethylene, and other industrial products; as a rubbing compound; as an antiseptic when in 70% solution. Arrests growth of putrefactive bacteria and is, therefore, used as a preservative of biological specimens and in certain patent medicines. Used in antifreeze products because of its low freezing point. Acts as a depressant to the nervous system when taken in excessive amounts. Used I.V. to stop premature labor. SEE: *alcoholism; Breathalyzer; fetal alcohol syndrome; hangover.*

a., absolute. Contains 99% alcohol and not more than 1% by weight of water.

a., cetyl. A white insoluble solid substance, $C_{16}H_{34}O$, used in manufacture of ointments.

a., dehydrated. Alcohol containing not less than 99.2% by weight of ethyl alcohol. This corresponds to 99.5% by volume of ethyl alcohol.

a., denatured. Alcohol rendered unfit for use as a beverage or medicine by addition of toxic ingredients. Used commercially as a solvent.

a., diluted. Alcohol containing not less than 41% and not more than 42% by weight of ethyl alcohol. Used as a solvent. SYN: *ethanol, diluted.*

a., ethyl. Ordinary or grain alcohol. SEE: *alcohol* (def. 2).

a., grain. Ethyl alcohol. SEE: *alcohol* (def. 2).

a., methyl. CH_4O. A colorless, volatile, flammable liquid obtained from distillation of wood. Even though its physical properties are similar to those of ethyl alcohol, it is not fit for human consumption. Poisoning with methyl alcohol can lead to blindness and death. It is used as a solvent, for fuel, as an additive for denaturing ethyl alcohol, as an antifreeze agent, and in the preparation of formaldehyde. SYN: *carbanol; methanol; a., wood.* SEE: *methyl alcohol* in Poisons and Poisoning in *Appendix.*

a., rubbing. USP. SEE: *rubbing alcohol.*

a., wood. A., methyl, q.v.

Alcohol, Drug Abuse, and Mental Health Administration. ABBR: ADAMHA. An agency of the United States government that is part of the National Institutes of Health within the Department of Health and Human Services. The agency administers grant programs supporting research, training, and service programs in alcoholism, drug abuse, and mental health.

alcoholic (ăl-kō-hŏl′ĭk) [L. *alcoholicus*]. 1. Pert. to alcohol. 2. One afflicted with alcoholism, q.v.

alcoholic blackout. An episode of forgetting all or part of what occurred during or following a period of alcohol intake.

alcoholic fermentation. The conversion of carbohydrates to alcohol through action of yeast.

alcoholic psychosis. Severe mental disorder caused by alcoholism. Included are pathological intoxication, delirium tremens, Korsakoff's psychosis, acute hallucinosis. SEE: *alcoholism, acute; delirium tremens; hallucinosis, acute alcoholic; intoxication; Korsakoff's syndrome.*

Alcoholics Anonymous. ABBR: A.A. An organization composed of alcoholics who are trying to help themselves and others abstain from alcohol by offering encouragement and discussing experiences, problems, feelings, techniques, etc. Similar groups, not associated with A.A., are available for families, esp. spouses, of alcoholics (Al-Anon) and for children of alcoholics (Ala-Teen). The organization has groups in most cities in the U.S. and can be contacted through its listings in telephone directories.

alcoholism (ăl′kō-hŏl-ĭzm) [Arabic *al-koh'l,* something subtle, + Gr. *-ismos,* condition]. Alcoholism is a chronic, progressive, and potentially fatal disease. It is characterized by tolerance and physical dependency or pathologic organ changes, or both — all the direct or indirect consequences of the alcohol ingested.

Alcoholism has been defined as having the following characteristics:
1. "Chronic and progressive" — physical, emotional, and social changes that develop are cumulative and progress as drinking continues.
2. "Tolerance" — brain adaptation to the presence of high concentrations of alcohol.
3. "Physical dependency" — withdrawal symptoms occur from decreasing or ceasing consumption of alcohol.
4. The person with alcoholism cannot consistently predict on any drinking occasion the duration of the episode or the quantity that will be consumed.
5. Pathologic organ changes can be found in almost any organ, but most often involve the liver, brain, peripheral nervous system, and the gastrointestinal tract.
6. The drinking pattern is generally continuous but may be intermittent, with periods of abstinence between drinking episodes.
7. Social, emotional, and behavioral symptoms and consequences of alcoholism result from the effect of alcohol on the function of the brain. The degree to which these symptoms and signs are considered deviant will depend upon the cultural norms of the society or group in which the person lives.

(Definition prepared by the National Council on Alcoholism/American Medical Society on Alcoholism, Committee on Definitions.)

DETECTION: The chemical carbohydrate deficient transferrin is of benefit as a marker for heavy alcohol use. It is elevated in alcoholics but not in those who are not heavy drinkers.

ETIOL: Unknown. Psychological, physiological, and sociological factors play an important part. The exhilaration factor is often the cause of intoxication in nonalcoholic individuals. Alcoholism is an illness and should be so treated. Even though it is accepted that a genetic factor is at work in the development of alcoholism, the precise genetic mechanism has not been determined.

a., acute. Acute intoxication with temporary mental disturbances and muscular incoordination.

Caution: When stupor or coma is observed in a patient who is suspected of being intoxicated by alcohol, other causes such as intracranial disease, insulin shock, etc., should also be considered. Acute alcoholism can cause death.

SYM: There may be motor instability (staggered gait, blurred or double vision, impaired reflex action); reduced mental function; increased pulse rate; decreased blood pressure; dilated pupils; flushing of skin; drowsiness or stupor.

TREAT: Coma due to alcohol is a medical emergency and requires vigorous therapy. I.V. fluids, intubation to prevent aspiration of vomitus, and oxygen inhalation may be required.

a., chronic. Pathological state from habitual use of alcohol in toxic amounts.

SYM: Malnutrition; vitamin deficiency; alcoholic cirrhosis of liver; gastritis; pancreatitis; and neurological disorders such as tremulousness, hallucinosis, seizures, delirium tremens, coma. Prolonged, excessive ingestion of alcohol is toxic to the cells of the liver. This may lead to cirrhosis and death. Alcoholism is, in some urban areas, the third most frequent cause of death in persons between the ages of 25 and 65. The effect of alcohol on the liver is independent of poor diet. Alcohol ingestion during pregnancy may cause congenital defects.

TREAT: Withdrawal of alcohol, tranquilizing drugs, adequate nutrition and rest; correction of vitamin deficiency, psychotherapy. SEE: *Alcoholics Anonymous; alcohol withdrawal syndrome; asterixis; Breath-*

alyzer; delirium tremens; hangover; hepatic coma; intoxication.

alcoholomania (ăl"kō-hŏl"ō-mā'nē-ă) [Arabic *al-koh'l*, something subtle, + Gr. *mania*, frenzy]. Abnormal craving for alcohol.

alcoholometer (ăl"kō-hŏl-ŏm'ē-tĕr) [" + Gr. *metron*, measure]. An instrument for measuring quantity of alcohol in a fluid.

alcoholophilia (ăl"kō-hŏl-ō-fil'ē-ă) [" + Gr. *philein*, to love]. Morbid craving for alcohol.

alcohol syndrome, fetal. Birth defects in infants born to mothers whose chronic alcoholism persisted during the gestation period. Shortly after birth, these infants may exhibit signs of alcohol withdrawal.

alcoholuria (ăl"kō-hŏl-ū'rē-ă) [" + Gr. *ouron*, urine]. Presence of alcohol in the urine.

alcohol withdrawal syndrome. The signs and symptoms produced when an individual with a high tolerance to alcohol suddenly decreases the amount of intake of alcohol. Included may be tremors or shakes of the hands; increased pulse, respirations, and temperature; anxiety, panic, any type of hallucination, and confusion. SEE: *delirium tremens.*

TREAT: Refer to treatment at *alcoholism, chronic.*

aldehyde (ăl'dĕ-hīd) [*alcohol dehyd*rogenatum]. 1. Oxidation product of a primary alcohol; has the characteristic group — CHO. 2. Acetaldehyde, CH_3CHO. Intermediate in yeast fermentation and alcohol metabolism. SYN: *acetic aldehyde.*

Alder-Reilly anomaly [Albert von Alder, Ger. physician, b. 1888; William Anthony Reilly, U.S. pediatrician, b. 1901]. Large dark leukocyte granules that stain lilac. They are composed of mucopolysaccharide deposits and are indicative of mucopolysaccharidosis, q.v.

aldolase (ăl'dō-lās). An enzyme present in skeletal and heart muscle and the liver; important in converting glycogen into lactic acid. Its serum level is increased in certain muscle diseases and in viral hepatitis.

aldopentose (ăl"dō-pĕn'tōs). A five-carbon sugar with the aldehyde, — CHO, group at the end. Arabinose is an aldopentose.

aldose. A carbohydrate of the aldehyde group (— CHO).

aldosterone (ăl-dŏs'tĕr-ōn, ăl"dō-stēr'ōn). The most biologically active mineralocorticoid hormone secreted by the adrenal cortex. Functions in regulation of metabolism of sodium, chloride, and potassium. SEE: *adrenal gland.*

aldosteronism (ăl"dō-stēr'ōn-ĭzm"). A condition in which the blood contains abnormally high levels of aldosterone. This causes retention of sodium, urinary loss of potassium, and alkalosis. The patient develops episodes of tetany, weakness, paralysis, hypertension, cardiac irregularity, polyuria, and polydipsia. SYN: *hyperaldosteronism.*

a., primary. Aldosteronism due to disorders of the adrenal gland. SYN: *Conn's syndrome.* SEE: *Nursing Diagnoses* in *Appendix.*

a., secondary. Aldosteronism due to extra-adrenal disorders.

aldrin (ăl'drĭn). A derivative of chlorinated naphthalene used as an insecticide. SEE: *dieldrin* in *Poisons and Poisoning* in *Appendix.*

alemmal (ă-lĕm'ăl) [Gr. *a-*, not, + *lemma*, husk]. Without a neurilemma, as a nerve fiber.

Aleppo boil. Cutaneous leishmaniasis, caused by infection with the parasite *Leishmania tropica.* Characterized by one or multiple ulcerations of the skin. SYN: *Delhi boil; Oriental sore.*

alertness. Being aware, attentive, and mentally functional. This condition is essential to the task of operating machines and machinery, including motor vehicles and airplanes. When alertness is absent, the individual may be drowsy or even unconscious. There are experimental devices for detecting lack of alertness in persons involved in critical jobs. These devices are intended to arouse or increase the alertness of the persons involved.

alethia (ă-lē'thē-ă) [" + *lethe*, forgetfulness]. Inability to forget; dwelling on the past.

aleukemia (ă-loo-kē'mē-ă) [" + *leukos*, white, + *haima*, blood]. Deficiency of leukocytes in the blood. The existence of leukopenia or aleukocytosis.

aleukemic leukemia (ă"loo-kē'mĭk). Acute myelogenous leukemia, q.v.

aleukocytosis (ă-loo"kō-sī-tō'sĭs) [" + *leukos*, white, + *kytos*, cell, + *osis*, condition]. Absence or extreme decrease of leukocytes in the blood.

aleuron, aleurone (ăl-oo'rŏn, -rōn) [Gr. *aleuron*, flour]. The protein granules present in the outer layer of the endosperm of cereal grain.

Alexander-Adams operation [William Alexander, Brit. surgeon, 1844–1919; James A. Adams, Scottish gynecologist, 1857–1930]. Surgery in which the round ligaments of the uterus are shortened and their ends sutured to the exterior abdominal ring. Used in treating uterine displacement.

alexia [Gr. *a-*, not, + *lexis*, word]. Loss of

the ability to read; word blindness. Not caused by loss of visual acuity.

ETIOL: Central nervous system lesion.

a., motor. Loss of the ability to read aloud while remaining able to understand what is written or printed.

a., musical. Loss of the ability to read music. It may be sensory, optic, or visual, but not motor.

a., optic or visual. Inability to understand what is written or printed.

alexithymia. A clinical feature common in post-traumatic stress disorder (PTSD) characterized by the inability to identify and articulate feelings. Often feelings are reported to the health care worker in the form of physical symptoms. Patients suffering from chemical dependency and somatoform disorders may also display alexithymia.

aleydigism (ă-lī'dĭg-ĭzm). Absence of function of Leydig cells, q.v., resulting in hypogonadism.

ALG. *antilymphocyte globulin.* SEE: *globulin, antilymphocyte.*

algae (ăl'jē) [L. *alga,* seaweed]. Plants belonging to the subphylum Algae of the phylum Thallophyta, the lowest division of the plant kingdom. They are nonparasitic plants without roots, stems, or leaves; they contain chlorophyll and vary in size from microscopic forms to massive seaweeds. They live in fresh or salt water or in moist places. Some serve as a source of food.

Ex.: kelp and Irish moss.

a., blue-green. Algae that grow in brackish water. Preparations of blue-green algae for medical use are not approved for sale in the U.S.

algesia (ăl-jē'zē-ă) [Gr. *algesis,* sense of pain]. Supersensitivity to pain. A form of hyperesthesia, q.v. SYN: *algesthesia.*

algesic (ăl-jē'sĭk). Painful. SYN: *algetic.*

algesichronometer (ăl-jē"zē-krō-nŏm'ĕ-tĕr) [" + *chronos,* time + *metron,* measure]. An instrument for measuring time taken to feel pain.

algesimeter (ăl"jē-sĭm'ĕ-tĕr) [" + *metron,* measure]. An instrument for measuring degree of sensitivity to pain. SYN: *algometer.*

algesthesia (ăl"jĕs-thē'zē-ă) [Gr. *algos,* pain, + *aisthesis,* sensation]. 1. Perception of pain. 2. Supersensitivity to pain. A form of hyperesthesia, q.v. SYN: *algesia.*

algetic (ăl-jĕt'ĭk). Painful. SYN: *algesic.*

-algia (ăl'jē-ă) [Gr.]. Suffix signifying pain.

algicide (ăl'jĭ-sīd) [L. *alga,* seaweed, + *caedere,* to kill]. Substance that destroys algae.

algid (ăl'jĭd) [L. *algidus,* cold]. Cold; chilly.

algid stage. Cold and cyanotic skin occurring in cholera and some other diseases.

alginate (ăl'jĭ-nāt). Any salt of alginic acid. It is derived from kelp, a type of seaweed. Used as a thickening agent in foods; and as a pharmaceutical aid. In dentistry, this irreversible hydrocolloid is used as a material for taking impressions.

alginic acid. SEE: *acid, alginic.*

algiomotor (ăl"jē-ŏ-mō'tor) [Gr. *algos,* pain, + L. *motor,* a mover]. Causing painful contraction of muscles, particularly pain during peristalsis.

algiomuscular (ăl"jē-ŏ-mŭs'kū-lăr) [" + L. *musculus,* muscle]. Algiomotor, q.v.

alglucerase. A drug prepared from the human placenta used in treating Type I Gaucher's disease, q.v.

algogenic (ăl-gō-jĕn'ĭk). 1. [" + *gennan,* to produce]. Causing pain. 2. [L. *algor,* cold, + Gr. *gennan,* to produce]. Lowering body temperature, esp. below normal.

algolagnia (ăl"gō-lăg'nē-ă) [Gr. *algos,* pain, + *lagneia,* lust]. Sexual satisfaction derived by experiencing pain or by inflicting pain on others.

a., active. Sadism.

a., passive. Masochism.

algolagnist (ăl-gō-lăg'nĭst). One who practices algolagnia.

algometer [" + *metron,* measure]. Instrument for measuring degree of sensitivity to pain. SYN: *algesimeter.*

algophobia (ăl"gō-fō'bē-ă) [" + *phobos,* fear]. Morbid fear of pain.

algor (ăl'gor) [L., cold]. 1. A chill. 2. The sensation of cold; cold.

a. mortis. The chill of death.

algorithm (ăl'gŏ-rĭthm). A formula or set of rules for solving a particular problem. In medicine, a set of steps used in diagnosing and treating a disease. Appropriate use of algorithms in medicine may lead to more efficient and accurate patient care as well as reducing costs.

algos (ăl'gŏs) [Gr.]. Pain.

alible (ăl'ĭ-bl) [L. *alibilis,* nutritive]. Nutritive.

Alice in Wonderland syndrome [Alice, from Lewis Carroll's *Alice in Wonderland*]. Perceptual distortions of space and size. This may be a symptom of neurologic involvement in infectious mononucleosis, and may be caused by hallucinogenic drugs.

alicyclic (ăl-ĭ-sī'klĭk). Having properties of both aliphatic (open-chain) and cyclic (closed-chain) compounds, q.v.

alien (āl'yĕn). 1. Strange, foreign, or contrary. 2. A stranger, foreigner, or outsider.

alienate (āl'yĕn-āt). To isolate, estrange, or dissociate.

alienation (āl"yĕn-ā'shŭn) [L. *alienare,* to make strange]. Isolation, estrangement, or dissociation, esp. from society.

alienia (ā"lī-ē'nē-ă) [Gr. *a-,* not, + L. *lien,* spleen]. Absence of the spleen.

aliform (ăl′ĭ-form) [L. *ala*, wing, + *forma*, shape]. Wing-shaped.

aliform process. Wing of the sphenoid bone.

alignment (ă-līn′měnt) [Fr. *aligner*, to put in a straight line]. 1. The act of arranging in a straight line. 2. The state of being arranged in a straight line. 3. In orthopedics, the placing of portions of a fractured bone into correct anatomical position. 4. In dentistry, bringing teeth into correct position. 5. In radiography, positioning the body part in proper relation to the radiographic film and x-ray tube to enable proper visualization of the object.

aliment (ăl′ĭ-měnt) [L. *alimentum*, nourishment]. Nutriment, food.

alimentary (ăl″ĭ-měn′tăr-ē) [L. *alimentum*, nourishment]. Pertaining to food or nutrition, or the digestive tract.

alimentary canal or tract. The digestive tube from the mouth to anus, including mouth or buccal cavity, pharynx, esophagus, stomach, small and large intestines, and rectum. Drugs administered orally are absorbed in the stomach or intestine, transported via the portal vein and through the liver before entering the general circulation; or they may be absorbed into the lacteals and enter the bloodstream by way of the thoracic duct of the lymphatic system. SEE: *digestive system* for illus.

alimentary duct. The thoracic duct, q.v., of the lymphatic system.

alimentation (ăl″ĭ-měn-tā′shŭn). The process of nourishing the body; it includes mastication, swallowing, digestion, absorption, and assimilation. SEE: *hyperalimentation; hypoalimentation; total parenteral nutrition.*

RS: absorption; anabolism; catabolism; digestion; food; metabolism; total parenteral nutrition.

a., artificial. Feeding, usually intravenous or by a nasal tube passed into the stomach, of patient unable to take nourishment normally. SEE: *total parenteral nutrition.*

a., forced. 1. Feeding of a patient unwilling to eat. 2. Forcing a person to eat a greater quantity than desired.

a., rectal. Feeding by means of nutrient enemas, q.v.

alimentotherapy (ăl″ĭ-měn″tō-thěr′ă-pē) [L. *alimentum*, nourishment, + Gr. *therapeia*, treatment]. Treatment of disease by dietary regulation. SYN: *dietotherapy.* SEE: *dietetics.*

alinasal [L. *ala*, wing, + *nasus*, nose]. Pert. to the alae nasi or wings of the nose.

alinement (ă-līn′měnt) [Fr. *aligner*, to put in a straight line]. Alignment, q.v.

aliphatic (ăl″ĭ-făt′ĭk) [Gr. *aleiphar, aleipha-*

tos, fat, oil]. Belonging to that series of organic chemical compounds characterized by open chains of carbon atoms rather than by rings.

aliquot (ăl′ĭ-kwŏt) [L. *alius*, other, + *quot*, how many]. A portion obtained by dividing the whole into equal parts without a remainder. A portion that represents a known quantitative relationship to the whole or to other portions.

alisphenoid (ăl-ĭ-sfē′noyd) [L. *ala*, wing, + Gr. *sphen*, wedge, + *eidos*, form, shape]. Pert. to the greater wing of the sphenoid bone.

alizarin (ă-līz′ă-rĭn) [Arabic *ala sara*, extract]. A red dye obtained from coal tar or madder.

alkalemia (ăl″kă-lē′mē-ă) [Arabic *al-qaliy*, ashes of salt wort, + Gr. *haima*, blood]. Excessive alkalinity of the blood due to a decrease in the hydrogen ion concentration or an increase in hydroxyl ions. The blood is normally slightly alkaline (pH 7.35 to 7.45).

alkalescence (ăl″kă-lěs′ens). 1. Slight alkalinity. 2. Process of becoming alkaline.

alkalescent (ăl″kă-lěs′ent). Alkaline or becoming alkaline.

alkali (ăl′kă-lī) [Arabic *al-qaliy*, ashes of salt wort]. A strong base, esp. the metallic hydroxides. Alkalies combine with acids to form salts; combine with fatty acids to form soap; neutralize acids; and turn litmus paper blue. SEE: *acid; base; pH;* words beginning with *alkal-.*

a., corrosive. Strongly corrosive metallic hydroxides most commonly of sodium, ammonium, and potassium, as well as carbonates. Because of their great combining power with water and their action on the fatty tissues, they cause rapid and deep destruction. They have a tendency to gelatinize tissue, turning it a somewhat grayish color and forming a soapy, slippery surface, accompanied by pain and burning. SEE: *corrosion; corrosive poisoning.*

alkalimeter (ăl″kă-lĭm′ě-těr) [″ + Gr. *metron*, measure]. Device for measuring degree of alkalinity of a mixture.

alkalimetry (ăl″kă-lĭm′ě-trē). Measurement of degree of alkalinity of a mixture.

alkaline (ăl′kă-līn). Pert. to or having the reactions of an alkali.

alkaline phosphatase. SEE: *phosphatase, alkaline.*

alkaline reserve. The amount of base in the blood, principally bicarbonates, available for neutralization of fixed acids (acetoacetate, β-hydroxybutyrate, and lactate). A fall in alkaline reserve is called acidosis; a rise, alkalosis. Normally, the carbon dioxide combining power of the venous plasma is 21 to 30 mEq/L and the carbon dioxide content of whole blood is 20 to 25 mEq/L.

alkaline salts. SEE: *hydrogen sulfide* in *Poisons and Poisoning* in *Appendix.*

alkaline tide. The increase in alkaline reserve and occasional occurrence of alkaline urine during gastric digestion.

alkalinity (ăl″kă-lĭn′ĭ-tē). State of being alkaline. SEE: *hydrogen ion.*

alkalinize (ăl′kă-lĭn-īz″). To make alkaline. SYN: *alkalize.*

alkalinuria (ăl″kă-lĭn-ū′rē-ă) [*alkali* + Gr. *ouron,* urine]. Alkaline urine. SYN: *alkaluria.*

alkali poisoning. Ingestion of an alkali.

F.A.: Large amounts of water by mouth; diluted vinegar or lemon juice. Then olive oil or milk and egg whites by mouth. Mild stimulants to prevent shock. Tracheotomy if necessary. If esophagus is known to be injured, it is imperative to use corticosteroid therapy beginning as soon as possible. It is advisable to use a broad-spectrum antibiotic if corticosteroids are used.

TREAT: Morphine is useful to allay pain. Rest, heat, quiet, and adequate fluid intake are imperative.

Caution: Avoid emetics, strong acids, and lavage.

---

alkali reserve. SEE: *alkaline reserve.*

alkalitherapy (ăl″kă-lĭ-thĕr′ă-pē) [″ + Gr. *therapeia,* treatment]. Therapeutic use of alkalies. SYN: *alkalotherapy.*

alkalization (ă″kă-lĭ-zā′shŭn). Process of making something alkaline.

alkalize (ăl′kă-līz). To make alkaline. SYN: *alkalinize.*

alkaloid (ăl′kă-loyd) [*alkali* + Gr. *eidos,* form, shape]. One of a group of organic alkaline substances obtained from plants. Alkaloids react with acids to form salts that are used for medical purposes.

Ex.: atropine, morphine, nicotine, quinine.

INCOMPAT: coffee (caffeine), tea (tannin).

a., synthetic. A synthetic substance similar to plant alkaloids.

alkalometry (ăl″kă-lŏm′ĕ-trē) [″ + Gr. *metron,* measure]. Determination of the alkali content of a substance.

alkalosis (ăl″kă-lō′sĭs) [″ + Gr. *osis,* condition]. Excessive alkalinity of body fluids due to accumulation of alkalies or reduction of acids. SEE: *acid-base balance.*

a., altitude. Alkalosis resulting from exposure to decreased oxygen content of air at high altitudes. This causes respiratory alkalosis. SEE: *a., respiratory.*

a., compensated. Alkalosis in which pH

of body fluids has been returned to normal. Compensatory mechanisms maintain the normal ratio of bicarbonate to carbonic acid (approx. 20 : 1) even though the bicarbonate level is increased.

a., hypochloremic. Metabolic alkalosis due to loss of chloride. Produced by severe vomiting.

a., hypokalemic. Metabolic alkalosis due to excess loss of potassium. May be caused by diuretic therapy.

a., metabolic. Alkalosis in which plasma bicarbonate is increased and there is a proportionate rise in the plasma concentration of CO_2. This is usually the result of increased loss of acid from the stomach or kidney; potassium depletion accompanying diuretic therapy; excessive alkali intake; or continued severe adrenal gland hyperactivity. SEE: *acid-base balance.*

SYM: There are no specific signs or symptoms; but if the alkalosis is severe, apathy, confusion, stupor, and tetany may develop as evidenced by a positive Chvostek's sign, q.v.

TREAT: Therapy for the primary disorder is essential. Administer saline solution I.V. and, in patients with hypokalemia due to diuretic therapy, potassium is administered. Only rarely will it be necessary to administer acidifying agents I.V.

NURSING IMPLICATIONS: Monitor arterial blood gas values, serum potassium level, and fluid balance. Assess patient for anorexia, nausea and vomiting, tremors, muscle hypertonicity, muscle cramps, tetany, Chvostek's sign, and mental confusion progressing to stupor and coma. Assess for compensatory hypoventilation and resultant hypoxia. Administer prescribed oxygen, oral or I.V. fluids, sodium chloride or ammonium chloride, potassium if hypokalemia is a factor, along with therapy prescribed for causative factor. Evaluate patient's response to therapy. Teach patient about dangers of excess sodium bicarbonate intake.

a., respiratory. Alkalosis with an acute reduction of plasma bicarbonate with a proportionate reduction in plasma CO_2.

SYM: Patients will develop paresthesias, numbness and tingling, carpopedal spasm, tetany, and will complain of feeling lightheaded.

ETIOL: Hyperventilation due to hypoxia, anxiety, fever, salicylate intoxication, exercise, or excessive mechanical assist to breathing, as could occur in a respirator.

TREAT: Therapy for the underlying cause. The immediate treatment for acute hyperventilation, especially in the type induced by anxiety, is increasing the CO_2 by having the patient rebreathe into a paper bag. Equally helpful is to have the patient breathe while one nostril is closed off and the mouth is kept closed; this is a simple and effective method of preventing or treating hyperventilation.

NURSING IMPLICATIONS: Identify patients at risk (experiencing pain, anxiety, hysteria, or other etiologic factors) and take preventive measures, having the hyperventilating patient breathe with mouth and one nostril closed or into a paper bag, or adjusting mechanical ventilation to reduce tidal volume or rate. Assess for hyperventilation, dry oral mucosa, numbness or tingling of nose, circumoral area and extremities, tetany and hyperreflexia, inability to concentrate and mental confusion leading to lethargy and coma. Monitor arterial blood gas values, vital signs, and neurologic status. In severe cases, monitor serum potassium levels (potassium moves into the cells as hydrogen ions move out in an attempt to compensate) and cardiac status for dysrhythmias. Administer prescribed therapy to treat causative factors. Provide reassurance to allay patient anxiety.

alkalotherapy (ăl″kă-lō-thĕr′ă-pē) [*alkali* + Gr. *therapeia*, treatment]. Therapeutic use of alkalies. SYN: *alkalitherapy*.

alkalotic (ăl″kă-lŏt′ĭk). Pert. to alkalosis.

alkaluria (ăl″kă-lū′rē-ă) [*alkali* + Gr. *ouron*, urine]. The condition of alkali in the urine. SYN: *alkalinuria*.

alkapton(e) (ăl-kăp′tŏn) [″ + Gr. *hapto*, to bind to]. Homogentisic acid; a yellowish-red substance sometimes occurring in urine as the result of the incomplete oxidation of tyrosine and phenylalanine.

alkaptonuria (ăl″kăp-tō-nū′rē-ă) [*alkapton* + Gr. *ouron*, urine]. A rare inherited disorder characterized by the excretion of large amounts of homogentisic acid in the urine, a result of incomplete metabolism of the amino acids tyrosine and phenylalanine. Presence of the acid is indicated by the darkening of urine on standing or when alkalinated and the dark staining of diapers or other linen. SEE: *ochronosis*.

alkene (ăl′kēn). A bivalent aliphatic hydrocarbon containing one double bond; formed by removal of two hydrogen atoms.

Ex.: When the ethane molecule

$$H-\underset{\underset{H}{|}}{\overset{\overset{H}{|}}{C}}-\underset{\underset{H}{|}}{\overset{\overset{H}{|}}{C}}-H$$

loses two hydrogen atoms, it becomes ethylene,

$$H-\overset{\overset{H}{|}}{C}=\overset{\overset{H}{|}}{C}-H$$

with a double bond between two carbons. These are also called unsaturated hydrocarbons.

Alkeran. Trade name for melphalan, an alkylating antineoplastic agent.

alkyl (ăl′kĭl). A hydrocarbon molecule from which one atom of hydrogen is absent. The resulting substances are called alkyl groups or alkyl radicals.

Ex.: The methane hydrocarbon molecule

$$H-\underset{\underset{H}{|}}{\overset{\overset{H}{|}}{C}}-H$$

becomes an alkyl radical, in this case the methyl radical, when it loses one hydrogen molecule,

$$H-\underset{\underset{H}{|}}{\overset{\overset{H}{|}}{C}}$$

In chemical formulae, hydrocarbon radicals are abbreviated R.

alkylate (ăl′kĭ-lāt). Provide therapy involving the use of an alkylating agent.

alkylating agent. A substance that introduces an alkyl radical into a compound in place of a hydrogen atom. Because these substances have the ability to interfere with cell metabolism and growth, they are used in treating certain types of malignancies.

alkylation (ăl″kĭ-lā′shŭn). A chemical process in which an alkyl radical replaces a hydrogen atom.

ALL. *acute lymphocytic leukemia.*

all- [Gr. *allos*, other]. Prefix meaning other, different, alternate. SEE: *allo-*.

allachesthesia (ăl″ă-kĕs-thē′zē-ă) [Gr. *allache*, elsewhere, + *aisthesis*, sensation]. Perception of tactile sensation as being remote from the actual point of stimulation.

allantochorion (ă-lăn″tō-kŏ′rē-ŏn). Fusion of the allantois and chorion into one structure.

allantoic (ăl″ăn-tō′ĭk). Pert. to the allantois.

allantoid [Gr. *allantos*, sausage, + *eidos*, form, shape]. 1. Sausage-shaped. 2. Pert. to the allantois.

allantoin (ă-lăn′tō-ĭn). $C_4H_6N_4O_3$. A white crystalline substance occurring in allantoic and amniotic fluids and as end product of purine metabolism in mammals other than primates. Also produced synthetically by oxidation of uric acid. At one time allantoin was used to promote wound healing.

allantoinuria (ă-lăn″tō-ĭn-ū′rē-ă) [*allantoin*

+ Gr. *ouron*, urine]. Allantoin in the urine.

allantois (ă-lăn'tō-ĭs) [Gr. *allantos*, sausage, + *eidos*, form, shape]. An elongated bladder developing from the hindgut of the fetus in mammals, birds, and reptiles. In mammals, it contributes to the development of the umbilicus and placenta. In birds and reptiles, it provides for the exchange of gases through the shell.

allayed (ă-lād'). Mitigated, q.v.

allele (ă-lēl', ă-lĕl') [Gr. *allelon*, of one another]. One of two or more different genes containing specific inheritable characteristics that occupy corresponding positions (loci) on paired chromosomes. A pair of alleles is usually indicated by a capital letter for the dominant and a lowercase letter for the recessive. An individual possessing a pair of identical alleles, either dominant or recessive, is said to be homozygous for this gene. The union of a dominant gene and its recessive allele produces a heterozygous individual for that characteristic. More than one inheritable characteristic may be present on the same pair of genes (alleles); e.g., the genes for blood type A, B, and O are at the same position on alleles. SYN: *allelic gene; allelomorph.*

     a., histocompatibility. One of many different forms of the histocompatibility gene. Each allele creates specific cell surface antigenic markers on cells. SEE: *histocompatibility antigens.*

allelic (ă-lĕl'ĭk). Pert. to alleles.

allelic gene. Allele, q.v.

allelomorph (ă-lē'lō-morf, ă-lĕl'ō-morf) [" + *morphe*, form]. Allele, q.v.

allelotaxis (ă-lē"lō-tăk'sĭs) [" + *taxis*, order]. Development of a part from several embryonic structures.

Allen-Doisy test (ăl'ĕn-doy'sē) [Edgar V. Allen, U.S. endocrinologist, 1892–1943; Edward A. Doisy, U.S. biochemist and physiologist, b. 1893]. Used to determine estrogen content. A spayed mouse is injected with the material being tested. The appearance of cornified cells on vaginal smear constitutes a positive reaction.

Allen-Doisy unit. The smallest amount of estrogen that will produce a characteristic change (appearance of cornified cells) in the vaginal epithelium of a spayed mouse. SYN: *mouse unit.*

allergen (ăl'ĕr-jĕn) [Gr. *allos*, other, + *ergon*, work, + *gennan*, to produce]. Any substance that causes manifestations of allergy. It may or may not be a protein or an antigen. Among common allergens are inhalants (dusts, pollens, fungi, smoke, perfumes, odors of plastics), foods (wheat, eggs, milk, chocolate, strawberries), drugs (aspirin, antibiotics, serums), infectious agents (bacteria, viruses, fungi, animal parasites), contactants (chemicals, animals, plants, metals), and physical agents (heat, cold, light, pressure, radiations). SEE: *allergy; antigen; sensitization; irritation.*

allergenic (ăl"ĕr-jĕn'ĭk). Producing allergy.

allergic (ă-lĕr'jĭk). Pert. to, sensitive to, or caused by an allergen.

allergic salute. The characteristic way children with allergic rhinitis wipe their noses by rubbing their noses with an upward movement of the hand.

allergist. A physician who specializes in diagnosing and treating allergies.

allergization (ăl"ĕr-jĭ-zā'shŭn). Introduction of a foreign substance into the body in order to bring about a state of sensitivity.

allergy (ăl'ĕr-jē) [Gr. *allos*, other, + *ergon*, work]. An acquired, abnormal immune response to a substance (allergen) that does not normally cause a reaction. Sensitization, or an initial exposure to the allergen, is required; subsequent contact with the allergen then results in a broad range of inflammatory responses. Allergic conditions include eczema, allergic rhinitis or coryza, hay fever, bronchial asthma, urticaria (hives), and food allergy. Allergens may be introduced by contact, ingested (e.g., food), inhaled (e.g., pollen), or injected (e.g., drugs). The hypersensitivity immune reactions of allergies are primarily governed by antibodies, but T cells may also be involved.

     TYPES: *Type I* (immediate) reactions are a local or systemic anaphylaxis (extremely rapid) inflammatory response to allergens mediated by immunoglobulin E (IgE). Local responses include urticaria (hives, allergic rhinitis), asthma, q.v., and angioedema, q.v. Systemic anaphylaxis is life-threatening. The allergen reaches the bloodstream, triggering a massive release of chemical mediators that produce severe bronchial obstruction, vasodilation, and increased vascular permeability, which can cause laryngeal or pulmonary edema, and shock, q.v.

     Type II (cytotoxic) reactions are antigen-antibody reactions mediated by IgG and IgM that cause transfusion reactions and many drug reactions. These reactions cause lysis of blood cells (erythrocytes, leukocytes, and platelets) due to the release of complement, q.v.

     Type III (immune complex) reactions occur when IgG or IgM antibodies attach to antigens, creating complexes that circulate in the blood. The complexes cause damage when they adhere to the walls of blood vessels, thus initiating an inflammatory response. Serum sickness, demonstrated by fever, joint and muscle pain, lymphadenopathy, and urticaria, is a Type III reaction that can occur in sensitized people after the administration of penicillins, sulfonamides, or antitoxins developed from animals (e.g., tetanus, snake venom, rabies).

Type IV (cell mediated) reactions are mediated by sensitized T lymphocytes, not antibodies. Contact dermatitis, one Type IV reaction, involves many common allergens, including rubber used in elastic materials, poison ivy, chromium in leather, and nickel used in costume jewelry. These combine with skin proteins, altering the normal self-antigens so that new, foreign antigens are created. Contact dermatitis is characterized by acute erythema, edema, itching, and scaling. Delayed hypersensitivity reactions (Type IV reactions) are used as a clinical tool in skin tests for sensitivity. Small amounts of an agent are placed on the skin; if the individual is sensitized to the substance and has a competent immune system, an inflammatory reaction will occur. The site of application is compared at the end of the test with a site exposed to a non-sensitizing substance such as a saline solution.

SYM: Local or systemic inflammatory responses demonstrated by redness, edema, and heat. Respiratory symptoms include wheezing, coughing, sneezing, and nasal congestion. Increased blood eosinophil levels (eosinophilia) are common.

ETIOL: Inherited tendency or acquired sensitivity over time to any substance that is recognized as a foreign antigen. The number of exposures necessary to produce enough antibodies to cause an allergic response varies. An allergy may occur the second time a person is exposed to a particular allergen or may not occur until years later when repeated exposures have produced sufficient antibodies or sensitized T cells.

TREAT: Delayed hypersensitivity demonstrated by skin testing is often used to determine those allergens to which the patient reacts. Many allergens can be eliminated from the environment (e.g., foods, animals). Antihistamines or corticosteroids may be prescribed to reduce symptoms. Desensitization, q.v., may be used to promote tolerance of allergens if allergic responses significantly interfere with lifestyle or are life-threatening.

RS: anaphylaxis; atopy; hay fever; hypersensitivity reactions; serum sickness; Arthus reactions; anergy.

NURSING IMPLICATIONS: Careful assessment to determine presence of any allergic reactions in past. Close observation during initial 20 minutes of blood adminis-

tration and following administration of drugs not previously used. Have diphenhydramine, epinephrine, or corticosteroids readily available if systemic anaphylaxis should occur. Teach patients how to identify and eliminate potential common allergens (e.g., household sprays and cleansers, animals, fabrics, foods) and how to identify allergic reaction. Occasionally, patients may need to have drugs for treatment of systemic anaphylaxis available at home.

a., atopic. An allergic reaction in which the predisposition to hypersensitivity to an allergen is inherited as part of one's genetic makeup.

a., contact. Hypersensitivity reaction following direct contact with an allergen to which the individual is sensitive.

a., drug. Hypersensitivity reaction to a drug.

a., food. SEE: *food allergies.*

allesthesia (ăl″ĕs-thē′sē-ă) [″ + *aisthesis,* sensation]. Perception of stimulus in the opposite limb from the one stimulated. SYN: *allochesthesia; allochiria.*

alliaceous (ăl″ē-ā′shŭs) [L. *allium,* garlic, + *-aceus,* of a specific kind]. Tasting like garlic or onions.

allied health professional. An individual who has received special training in one of the several fields of allied health such as laboratory, radiology, emergency medical care, physical therapy, dental hygiene, or occupational therapy. SEE: *emergency medical technician; paramedical personnel.*

alliesthesia (ăl″ē-ĕs-thē′sē-ă) [Gr. *allios,* changed, + *aisthesis,* sensation]. The perception of an external stimulus as pleasant or unpleasant depending upon internal stimuli. A particular stimulus may be perceived as pleasant at one time and unpleasant at another.

alliteration (ă-lĭt″ĕr-ā′shŭn) [L. *ad,* to, + *litera,* letter]. A speech disorder in which words beginning with the same consonant sound are used to excess.

allo- [Gr. *allos,* other]. Prefix indicating divergence, difference from, or opposition to the normal.

alloantigen (ăl″lō-ăn′tĭ-jĕn) [″ + *anti,* against, + *gennan,* to produce]. Isoantigen, q.v.

allobiosis (ăl″ō-bī-ō′sĭs) [″ + *bios,* life]. The altered responses produced in organisms exposed to environmental or physiological changes.

allochesthesia (ăl″ō-kĕs-thē′zē-ă) [Gr. *allache,* elsewhere, + *aisthesis,* sensation]. Allesthesia, q.v.

allochezia, allochesia (ăl″ō-kē′zē-ă, ăl″ō-kē′shē-ă) [Gr. *allos,* other, + *chezein,* to defecate]. Excretion of feces through an abnormal opening.

allochiria, allocheiria (ăl″ō-kī′rē-ă) [″ + *cheir,* hand]. Allesthesia, q.v.

allochroism (ăl-ōk′rō-ĭzm, ăl″ō-krō′ĭzm) [″ + *chroa,* color, + *-ismos,* condition]. Change in color.

allochromasia (ăl″ō-krō-mā′sē-ă). Change in color of hair or skin.

allocinesia (ăl″ō-sĭn-ē′sē-ă) [Gr. *allos,* other, + *kinesis,* movement]. Movement on side of body opposite to the one the patient has been requested to move. SEE: *allokinesis.*

allodiploidy (ăl″ō-dĭp′loy-dē) [″ + *diploe,* fold, + *eidos,* form, shape]. Possession of two sets of chromosomes, each from a different species. A hybrid is allodiploid.

allodynia (ăl″ō-dĭn′ē-ă). The condition in which an ordinarily painless stimulus, once perceived, is experienced as being painful.

alloeroticism (ăl″ō-ē-rŏt′ĭ-sĭzm). Alloerotism, q.v.

alloerotism (ăl″ō-ĕr′ō-tĭzm) [″ + *Eros,* god of love]. Sexual urges stimulated by and directed toward another person. Opposite of autoerotism.

alloesthesia. Allesthesia, q.v.

allogeneic, allogenic (ăl″ō-jĕ-nē′ĭk, ăl″ō-jĕn′ĭk). Having a different genetic constitution but belonging to the same species. SEE: *isogeneic.*

allograft (ăl′ō-grăft) [″ + L. *graphium,* grafting knife]. Transplant tissue obtained from the same species. The tissues that survive best are cornea, bone, artery, and cartilage. SYN: *homograft.* SEE: *autograft; heterograft.*

alloimmune (ăl″ō-ĭm-ūn′) [″ + L. *immunis,* safe]. Immunity to allogeneic antigens.

allokinesis (ăl″ō-kĭ-nē′sĭs) [″ + *kinesis,* movement]. Passive or reflex movement; involuntary movement.

allokinetic (ăl″ō-kĭ-nĕt′ĭk). Characterized by passive or reflex movement.

allolalia (ăl″ō-lā′lē-ă) [″ + *lalia,* talk]. 1. Speech defect or impairment, esp. due to a brain lesion. 2. A type of dysphasia in which words are spoken unintentionally, or inappropriate words are substituted for appropriate ones.

allomerism (ă-lŏm′ĕr-ĭzm) [″ + *meros,* part, + *-ismos,* condition]. Change in chemical constitution without a change in form. SEE: *allomorphism.*

allomorphism (ăl″ō-mor′fĭzm) [″ + *morphe,* form, + *-ismos,* condition]. Change in form without a change in chemical constitution. SEE: *allomerism.*

allongement (ăl-ŏnzh-mŏn′) [Fr., elongation]. Lengthening of a structure by surgical methods.

allopath (ăl′ō-păth). One who practices al-

lopathy, q.v.

allopathy (ăl″ŏp′ă-thē) [Gr. *allos,* other, + *pathos,* disease, suffering]. 1. System of treating disease by inducing a pathologic reaction that is antagonistic to the disease being treated. 2. A term erroneously used for the regular practice of medicine to differentiate it from homeopathy, q.v.

allophasis (ăl-ŏf′ă-sĭs) [Gr. *allos,* other, + *phasis,* speech]. Incoherent speech.

alloplasia (ăl″ō-plā′zē-ă) [″ + *plasis,* a molding]. Development of tissue at a location where that type of tissue would not normally occur. SYN: *heteroplasia.*

alloplasty (ăl′ō-plăs-tē) [″ + *plasis,* a molding]. 1. Plastic surgery using inert material. 2. In psychiatry, adaptation by altering the external environment rather than changing oneself. SEE: *autoplasty.*

alloploidy (ăl″ō-ploy′dē) [″ + *ploos,* fold, + *eidos,* form, shape]. State of having two or more sets of chromosomes derived from different ancestral species.

allopolyploidy (ăl″ō-pŏl′ē-ploy-dē) [″ + *polys,* many, + *ploos,* fold, + *eidos,* form, shape]. State of having more than two sets of chromosomes derived from different ancestral species.

allopsychic (ăl-ō-sī′kĭk) [″ + *psyche,* mind]. Pert. to mental processes in relation to the external environment.

allopsychosis [″ + ″ + *osis,* condition]. Derangement of perceptive powers.

allopurinol (ăl″ō-pū′rĭn-ŏl). USP. A drug that inhibits the enzyme xanthine oxidase. Because its action causes a reduction in both serum and urine levels of uric acid, allopurinol is used in the treatment of gout, q.v., and of renal calculi caused by uric acid.

Allergic response to this drug has been reported. Trade name is Zyloprim.

all-or-none law. In response to a stimulus, the heart will either contract to its greatest extent or will not contract at all. SYN: *Bowditch's law.*

allostery (ăl-ō-stĕr′ē) [Gr. *allos,* other, + *stereos,* shape]. In bacteria, alteration of a regulatory site on a protein changes its shape and activity. This change is important in altering the way the organism responds to its molecular environment.

allotherm (ăl′ō-thĕrm) [″ + *therme,* heat]. An animal whose body temperature varies according to the temperature of the environment. SYN: *poikilotherm.* SEE: *homotherm.*

allotransplantation (ăl″ō-trăns″plăn-tā′shŭn) [″ + L. *trans,* through, + *plantare,* to plant]. Grafting or transplantation of tissue from one individual into another of the same species.

allotriogeustia (ă-lŏt″rē-ō-jŭst′ē-ă, -gū′stē-

ă) [Gr. *allotrios*, strange, + *geusis*, taste].
Perverted appetite or sense of taste. SEE:
paragensia.

allotriophagy (ă-lŏt″rē-ŏf′ă-jē) [″ + *phagein*, to eat]. A perversion of appetite with ingestion of material not fit for food, as starch, clay, ashes, or plaster. SYN: *pica*.

allotriosmia. Incorrect identification of odors. SYN: *heterosmia*.

allotropic (ăl″ō-trŏp′ĭk) [Gr. *allos*, other, + *tropos*, direction]. 1. Pert. to the existence of an element in two or more distinct forms with different physical properties. 2. Altered by digestion so as to be changed in its nutritive value. 3. Indicating one who is concerned with the welfare and interests of others; i.e., not self-centered.

allotropism, allotropy (ă-lŏt′rō-pĭzm, -pē) [″ + *trope*, a turn, + *-ismos*, condition]. Existence of an element in two or more distinct forms with different physical properties.

allotype. Genetic variants of protein that occur in a single species. The serum from a person with one form of allotype could be antigenic to a member of the same species.

alloxan (ăl-ŏk′săn) [*allantoin* + *oxalic*]. $C_2H_2N_2O_4$. An oxidation product of uric acid. In experimental animals, it causes diabetes by destroying the islet cells of the pancreas.

alloy (ăl′oy, ă-loy′) [Fr. *aloyer*, to combine]. A metallic substance (e.g., brass) resulting from the fusion or mixture of two or more metals. Also, a substance (e.g., steel) formed from the fusion or mixture of a metal and a nonmetal. In dentistry, this is often an alloy containing mercury; this type of alloy is called an amalgam.

allyl (ăl′ĭl) [L. *allium*, garlic, + Gr. *hyle*, matter]. C_3H_5. A univalent unsaturated radical. It is present in garlic and mustard.

Alma-Ata Declaration. A declaration made in 1978 at the Conference on Primary Health Care in Alma-Ata, Russia. It stated that primary health care is the key to attaining health for all by the year 2000. Defined as essential to this were eight elements: education, food supply, safe water, maternal and child health including family planning, immunization, prevention and control of endemic diseases, appropriate treatment of common diseases and injuries, and provision of essential drugs.

alochia (ă-lō′kē-ă) [Gr. *a-*, not, + *lokhos*, pert. to childbirth]. Absence of lochia, the vaginal discharge following childbirth.

aloe (ăl′ō). USP. The dried juice of one of several species of plants of the genus *Aloe*. It is a component of compound benzoin tincture. Whether or not aloe has medical uses is controversial.

ALOPECIA AREATA

aloin (ăl′ō-ĭn). Yellow crystalline substance obtained from aloe, q.v.

alopecia (al″ō-pē′shē-ă) [Gr. *alopekia*, fox mange]. Absence or loss of hair, esp. of the head.
ETIOL: May result from physiologic changes as a part of the aging process; effects of serious illness; drugs; endocrine disorders; certain forms of dermatitis; hereditary factors; radiation.
TREAT: Treatment of seborrheic dermatitis, q.v., if present. Scalp baldness may be treated by surgical transplantation of hair follicles from another part of the body to the scalp.

a. adnata. A. congenitalis, q.v.

a. areata. Loss of hair in sharply defined patches usually involving the scalp or beard. SEE: illus.

a. capitis totalis. Complete absence of hair of the scalp.

a., cicatricial. Loss of hair due to formation of scar tissue.

a. congenitalis. Baldness due to absence of hair bulbs at birth.

a. follicularis. Baldness due to inflammation of the hair follicles of the scalp.

a. furfuracea. A. pityroides, q.v.

a. liminaris. Loss of hair along the hairline, both front and back, of the scalp.

a. liminaris frontalis. Loss of hair in the frontal area of the scalp of women between 15 and 20 years of age.

a., male pattern. Typical hair loss pattern of males in which the alopecia begins in the frontal area and proceeds until only a horseshoe area of hair remains in the back and temples. This loss is dependent upon the presence of the androgenic hormone, testosterone.

a. medicamentosa. Loss of hair due to administration of certain medicines, esp. those containing cytotoxic agents. SEE:

scalp tourniquet.

a. neurotica. Loss of hair following a disease or injury to the nervous system, and occurring at site of injury. SEE: *trichotillomania.*

a. pityroides. Loss of both scalp and body hair accompanied by desquamation of branlike scales. SYN: *a. furfuracea.*

a. prematura. Premature baldness.

a. senilis. Baldness of old age.

a. symptomatica. Loss of hair after prolonged fevers or during the course of a disease; may result from systemic or psychogenic factors.

a. totalis. Loss of hair from the entire body.

a. toxica. Loss of hair thought to be due to toxins of infectious disease.

a. universalis. A. totalis, q.v.

alpha (ăl′fă). First letter of the Greek alphabet, α. In chemistry, denotes first in a series of isomeric compounds, or position adjacent to a carboxyl group.

alpha-adrenergic blocking agent. A substance that interferes with the transmission of stimuli through pathways that normally allow sympathetic nervous excitatory stimuli to be effective. SEE: *beta-adrenergic blocking agent.*

alpha-adrenergic receptor. A site in autonomic nerve pathways wherein excitatory responses occur when adrenergic agents such as norepinephrine and epinephrine are released. SEE: *beta-adrenergic receptor.*

alpha-1 antitrypsin. An inhibitor of trypsin that may be deficient in patients who have emphysema.

alpha-fetoprotein. ABBR: AFP. An antigen present in the human fetus and in certain pathological conditions in the adult. The maternal serum level can be evaluated at 16 to 18 weeks of pregnancy to detect fetal abnormalities. Elevated levels indicate the possibility that neural tube defects (principally anencephaly or spina bifida) are present in the fetus. Decreased levels may indicate an increased risk of having a baby with Down syndrome. If an abnormal level of AFP is found, further tests such as ultrasound or amniocentesis, q.v., will need to be done. Elevated serum levels are found in adults with certain hepatic carcinomas or chemical injuries. Test results may be abnormal in persons with diabetes, multiple pregnancies, or obesity.

alpha-globulins. One of the serum globulins. SEE: *globulin, serum.*

alpha particles, rays. Radioactive, positively charged particles, two protons and two neutrons, ejected at high speeds in certain atomic disintegrations.

alpha-rhythm. In electroencephalography, rhythmic oscillations in electric potential occurring at an average rate of 10 per second. SYN: *alpha-wave.*

alpha-tocopherol. Vitamin E, q.v.

alpha-wave. Alpha-rhythm, q.v.

Alport's syndrome [Arthur Cecil Alport, S. African physician, 1880–1959]. Congenital glomerulonephritis associated with deafness and a decrease in large thrombocytes. Occasionally there are eye abnormalities such as cataract. There is no specific treatment for this disease, but renal dialysis or kidney transplantation may be of benefit. SEE: *macrothrombocytes.*

ALS. *amyotrophic lateral sclerosis* (also called Lou Gehrig's disease).

ALT. *alanine aminotransferase.*

alternans (awl-tĕr′nănz) [L. *alternare,* to alternate]. Alternation.

a., pulsus. Regular heart rhythm in which strong beats alternate with weak ones.

Alternaria (awl″tĕr-nā′rē-ă). A genus of fungi of the Dematiaceae family. The fungus can cause pneumonitis, and may cause wound or skin infections in immunocompromised patients. It has been implicated as the cause of pulmonary disease in wood pulp workers.

alternating current. ABBR: A.C. An electric current that reverses direction at regular intervals. SEE: *direct current.*

alternative medicine. Approaches to medical diagnosis and therapy that have not been developed by use of generally accepted methods of validating their effectiveness. Included are a great number of "systems," including manipulative medicine, ayurveda, shiatsu, hypnosis, biofeedback, acupuncture, acupressure, holistic medicine, macrobiotics, rolfing, Christian Science, reflexotherapy, homeopathy, aroma therapy, and faith healing. This is not to say that, were these methods subjected to scientific study, all of them would be found to be ineffective.

alternator. An electrical generator that produces alternating current.

alt. hor. L. *alternis horis,* every other hour.

altitude sickness. Symptoms produced by decreased oxygen in the environment. The symptoms may come on abruptly, as when an airplane ascends quickly to high altitude, or slowly, as in mountain climbing. The deficiency of oxygen causes headache, shortness of breath, malaise, decreased ability to concentrate, lack of judgment, lightheadedness, fainting, and if severe, may cause death. The initial symptom may be euphoria so that the individual is unaware of the cause of the difficulty. Adaptation to living at high altitudes is best accomplished over a period of weeks and months. SYN: *mountain sickness.* SEE: *bends; high-alti-*

tude hypoxia; pulmonary edema.

altretamine. A drug used for treating persistent or recurrent ovarian cancer.

altricious (äl-trĭsh'ŭs) [L. *altrix,* nourisher]. 1. Slow in developing. 2. Requiring long-term nursing care.

alum (ăl'ŭm) [L. *alumen*]. USP. 1. A double sulfate of aluminum and potassium or aluminum and ammonia. Strongly astringent, used topically as styptic. 2. Any of a group of double sulfates of a trivalent metal and a univalent metal.

    a., ammonia. Aluminum ammonia sulfate.

    a., potassium. Aluminum potassium sulfate.

aluminosis (ă-loo"mĭn-ō'sĭs) [" + Gr. *osis,* condition of]. Chronic inflammation of the lungs in alum workers due to alum particles in inspired air.

aluminum. SYMB: Al. At. wt. 26.9815; at. no. 13; sp. gr. 2.699. A silver-whitish metal used to filter low-energy radiation out of the x-ray beam.

    a. acetate. A salt formed by the reaction between aluminum sulfate and lead acetate. Its aqueous solution, known as Burow's solution, is used as a local astringent.

    a. ammonia sulfate. Ammonia alum; an astringent.

    a. hydroxide gel. USP. A white viscous suspension containing aluminum hydroxide and hydrated aluminum oxide; an antacid especially useful in treatment of peptic ulcer.

    a. potassium sulfate. Potassium alum; an astringent and styptic.

alveoalgia [L. *alveolus,* small cavity, + Gr. *algos,* pain]. Pain in the socket of a tooth. SEE: *socket, dry.*

alveobronchiolitis, alveobronchitis (ăl"vē-ō-brŏng"kē-ō-lī'tĭs, -brŏng-kī'tĭs) [L. *alveolus,* small hollow or cavity, + Gr. *bronchos,* windpipe, + *itis,* inflammation]. Inflammation of the bronchioles and pulmonary alveoli; bronchopneumonia, q.v.

alveolalgia (ăl"vē-ō-lăl'jē-ă) [" + Gr. *algos,* pain]. Pain in the alveolus of a tooth.

alveolar (ăl-vē'ō-lăr). Pert. to an alveolus, q.v.

alveolar air. Air in the pulmonary alveoli; that involved in the pulmonary exchange of gases. Its content is determined by sampling the last portion of a maximal expiration.

alveolar bone. Alveolar process, q.v.

alveolar-capillary block. Impaired ability of gases to pass through the pulmonary alveolar-capillary membrane.

alveolar duct. A branch of a respiratory bronchiole that leads to the alveoli of the lungs. SEE: *alveolus* for illus.

alveolar periosteum. The connective tissue surrounding the alveolar process of mandible or maxilla and contributing to its growth; in surgery, this later may be included with overlying tissues in a mucoperiosteal flap or full-thickness flap excision.

alveolar process. The part of the mandible and maxilla containing the tooth sockets.

alveolar proteinosis. Pulmonary alveolar proteinosis, q.v.

alveolate (ăl-vē'ō-lāt). Honeycombed; pitted.

alveolectomy (ăl"vē-ō-lĕk'tō-mē) [L. *alveolus,* small hollow or cavity, + Gr. *ektome,* excision]. Surgical removal of all or part of the alveolar process of mandible or maxilla; usually performed in treatment of neoplasms.

alveoli (ăl-vē'ō-lī) [L.]. Pl. of alveolus, q.v.

    a. dentales. [NA] Tooth sockets.

    a. pulmonis. [NA] Air cells of the lungs.

alveolitis (ăl"vē-ō-lī'tĭs) [" + Gr. *itis,* inflammation]. Inflammation of alveoli.

    a., allergic. A diffuse granulomatous lung disease caused by hypersensitivity to inhalation of organic dusts. Usually occurs in those whose hobby or occupation leads to heavy exposure to dust. SYN: *pneumonitis, hypersensitivity.* SEE: *farmer's lung; bagassosis.*

alveoloclasia (ăl-vē"ō-lō-klā'sē-ă) [" + Gr. *klasis,* fracture]. Destruction of a tooth socket.

alveolodental (ăl-vē"ō-lō-dĕn'tăl) [" + *dens,* tooth]. Pertaining to the alveolus of the tooth and to the tooth itself.

alveololingual (ăl-vē"lō-lĭng'gwăl) [" + *lingua,* tongue]. Concerning the alveolar process and tongue.

alveoloplasty (ăl-vē"ō-lō-plăs'tē) [" + Gr. *plassein,* to form]. Reconstruction of the alveolus by use of plastic surgery.

alveolotomy (ăl"vē-ō-lŏt'ō-mē) [" + Gr. *tome,* incision]. Surgical incision of the alveolus of a tooth.

alveolus (ăl-vē'ō-lŭs) [L., small hollow or cavity] (pl. *alveoli*). 1. A small hollow. 2. The socket of a tooth. 3. Air cell of the lungs. SEE: illus.; *canals of Lambert; pores of Kohn.* 4. One of the honeycombed depressions of the gastric mucous membrane. 5. A follicle of a racemose gland.

    a. dentalis. Tooth socket.

    a., pulmonary. One of the terminal saccules of an alveolar duct where gases are exchanged in respiration. SYN: *air vesicle; alveoli pulmonis* (pl.).

alveus (ăl'vē-ŭs) [L.]. A channel or groove.

    a. hippocampi. [NA] A layer of white matter covering ventricular surface of the hippocampus.

alymphia (ă-lĭm'fē-ă) [Gr. *a-,* not, + L. *lympha,* lymph]. Complete or partial deficiency of lymph.

alymphocytosis (ă-lĭm"fō-sī-tō'sĭs) [" + "

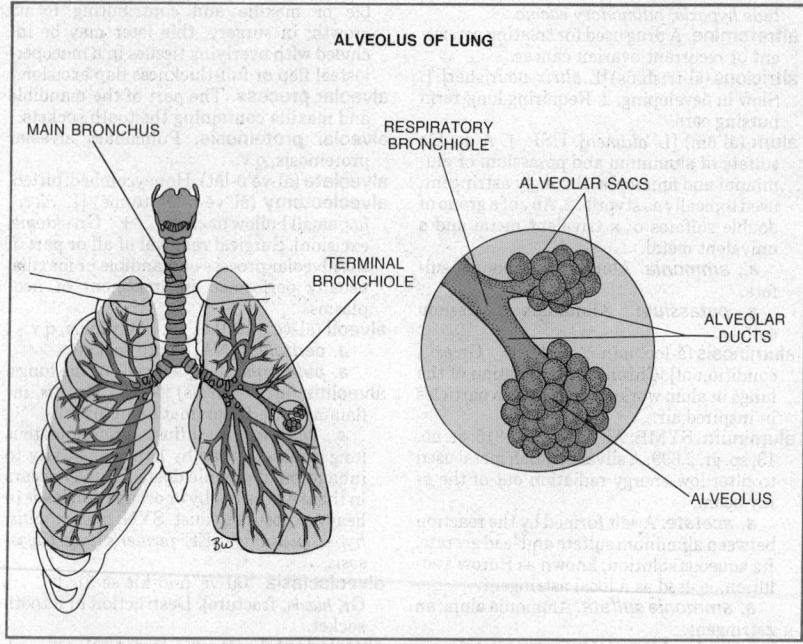

ALVEOLUS OF LUNG

MAIN BRONCHUS

RESPIRATORY
BRONCHIOLE

ALVEOLAR SACS

TERMINAL
BRONCHIOLE

ALVEOLAR
DUCTS

ALVEOLUS

+ Gr. *kytos,* cell, + *osis,* condition]. Decreased number or absence of lymphocytes in the blood.

alymphoplasia (ă″lĭm-fō-plā′zē-ă) [″ + ″ + Gr. *plasis,* a developing]. Failure of lymph tissue to develop.

　　a., thymic. A sometimes fatal disorder in which the thymus fails to develop, causing a deficiency of gamma globulin. There is deficiency of lymph tissue throughout the body.

Alzheimer's disease (ălts′hī-mĕrz) [Alois Alzheimer, Ger. neurologist, 1864–1915]. A chronic, organic mental disorder; a form of presenile dementia due to atrophy of frontal and occipital lobes. Onset is usually between ages 40 and 60. One study estimated a prevalence rate of 10.3% in persons over age 65. The estimate was 3% from ages 65 to 74; 18.7% for those aged 75 to 84; and 47.2% for those over 85 years. Involves progressive, irreversible loss of memory, deterioration of intellectual functions, apathy, speech and gait disturbances, and disorientation. Course may take from a few months to four or five years to progress to complete loss of intellectual function. SEE: *Pick's disease.* SEE: *Nursing Diagnoses in Appendix.*

NURSING IMPLICATIONS: Deter-

mine patient's needs for assistance with self-care and allow the person to be as independent as possible. If sleep disturbances occur, ensure that patient is sufficiently active and not sleeping during daytime hours. Observe for symptoms of urinary tract incontinence and illness. Ensure that environment is free of safety hazards and monitor activity to prevent accidents. Prevent frustration by ensuring that expectations are consistent with patient's ability to perform tasks. Treat patient with warmth and understanding and provide opportunities for verbalization of feelings. Provide support and understanding to patient's family and associates. Refer to available resources in locale, such as counseling, support groups, and respite care, if indicated.

Am. *mixed astigmatism; ametropia.* Chem. symb. for the element americium.

A.M.A. *American Medical Association.*

AMA. *against medical advice,* q.v.

amaas (ă′măs). A mild form of smallpox. SYN: *alastrim; variola minor.*

amacrine (ăm′ă-krĭn) [Gr. *a-,* not, + *makros,* long, + *is, inos,* fiber]. Lacking a long process.

amacrine cell. A modified nerve cell in the

retina that has short branches (dendrites) but no long process (axon). SEE: *neuron*.

amalgam (ă-măl'găm) [Gr. *malagma*, soft mass]. Any alloy containing mercury.

    a., dental. An alloy containing mercury, tin, silver, and copper that is used in dentistry to restore teeth. SEE: *amalgam, mercury in*.

amalgam, mercury in. About 50% of the amalgam used in dentistry is elemental mercury. Whether or not the amount of mercury absorbed is harmful or not is controversial. Dentists are of the opinion that the amount of mercury absorbed from food is much more than would be received from amalgams. This, too, is controversial.

amalgamate (ă-măl'gă-māt"). To make an amalgam.

amalgamation (ă-măl"gă-mā'shŭn). The process of mixing metallic particles with mercury to produce an amalgam. SYN: *trituration* (def. 3).

amalgamator (ă-măl'gă-mā"tor). A device that provides a mechanical means of amalgamation. This can also be done by hand using a mortar and pestle.

amanita (ăm"ă-nī'tă, -nē'tă) [Gr. *amanitai*, mushrooms]. Any of various mushrooms of the genus *Amanita*, e.g., *A. muscaria* and *A. phalloides*. Most are extremely poisonous. SEE: *Poisons and Poisoning* in *Appendix*.

amantadine hydrochloride (ă-măn'tă-dēn hī"drō-klor'īd). USP. An antiviral agent originally used for prophylaxis against certain strains of the influenza virus. Trade name is Symmetrel.

amastia (ă-măs'tē-ă) [" + *mastos*, breast]. Lack of breast development. SYN: *amazia*.

amaurosis (ăm"aw-rō'sĭs) [Gr., darkening]. Complete loss of vision, esp. that in which there is no apparent pathologic condition of the eye.

    a., albuminuric. Amaurosis caused by kidney disease.

    a., congenital. Amaurosis present at birth.

    a., diabetic. Amaurosis associated with diabetes.

    a., epileptoid. Sudden blindness following an epileptic seizure and lasting up to two weeks.

    a. fugax. Temporary loss of vision in one eye due to insufficient flow of blood to the retina. May last for up to 10 minutes. SYN: *blindness, transient*, q.v.

    a., lead. Amaurosis caused by lead poisoning.

    a. partialis fugax. Sudden transitory blindness with symptoms similar to migraine: nausea; vomiting; dizziness; and disturbances of vision.

    a., reflex. Amaurosis due to reflex action

caused by irritation of a remote part.

    a., saburral. Amaurosis in conjunction with acute gastritis.

    a., toxic. Amaurosis from optic neuritis caused by toxins that may be endogenous, such as in diabetes, or exogenous, as in alcohol or tobacco.

    a., uremic. Amaurosis caused by acute renal failure.

amaurotic (ăm-aw-rŏt'ĭk). Pert. to amaurosis or one afflicted with amaurosis.

amaxophobia [Gr. *amaxa*, a carriage, + *phobos*, fear]. Fear of riding in a vehicle.

amazia (ă-mā'zē-ă) [Gr. *a-*, not, + *mazos*, breast]. Lack of development of the breasts. SYN: *amastia*.

ambergris. An amorphous gray material formed in the intestinal tract of the sperm whale. It is vomited and usually found floating in the ocean. It is valuable because it is in demand for use in the manufacture of perfume.

ambi- [L. *ambi-*, on both sides]. Prefix indicating both or both sides; around; about.

ambidextrous (ăm"bĭ-dĕk'strŭs) [" + *dexter*, right]. Possessing the ability to work effectively with either hand.

ambient (ăm'bē-ĕnt) [L. *ambiens*, going around]. Surrounding.

    Ex.: Ambient temperature — the temperature in one's immediate location.

ambient noise. The entire amount of noise present in a given environment; Total noise from all sources.

ambiguous [L. *ambiguus*, to be uncertain]. To have several meanings or interpretations. In anatomy, being difficult to classify.

ambilateral (ăm"bĭ-lăt'ĕr-ăl) [L. *ambi-*, on both sides, + *latus*, side]. Pert. to both sides.

ambilevous (ăm-bĭ-lē'vŭs) [" + *laevus*, lefthanded]. Awkward in use of either hand. SYN: *ambisinister*.

ambiopia (ăm"bē-ō'pē-ă) [" + Gr. *ops*, eye]. Double vision. SYN: *diplopia*, q.v.

ambisexual (ăm"bĭ-sĕks'ū-ăl) [" + *sexus*, sex]. Pertaining to both sexes. SEE: *bisexual*.

ambisinister (ăm"bĭ-sĭn'ĭs-tĕr) [" + *sinister*, left]. Awkward in use of either hand. SYN: *ambilevous*.

ambitendency (ăm"bĭ-tĕn'dĕn-sē) [" + *tendere*, to stretch]. Ambivalence of the will. SEE: *ambivalence*.

ambivalence (ăm-bĭv'ă-lĕns) [" + *valentia*, strength]. Coexistence of contradictory feelings about an object, person, or idea.

ambivalent (ăm-bĭv'ă-lĕnt). Relating to or characterized by ambivalence.

ambivert (ăm'bĭ-vĕrt) [" + *vertere*, to turn]. An individual whose personality type falls between introversion and extroversion, possessing some tendencies of each.

amblyacousia (ăm″blē-ă-koo′sē-ă) [Gr. *amblys*, dull, + *akousis*, hearing]. Dullness of hearing.

amblychromasia (ăm″blē-krō-mā′sē-ă) [″ + *chroma*, color]. The state in which the cell nucleus stains faintly.

amblychromatic (ăm″blē-krō-măt′ĭk). Staining faintly.

amblyopia (ăm″blē-ō′pē-ă) [″ + *ops*, eye]. Reduction or dimness of vision, esp. that in which there is no apparent pathologic condition of the eye.

a., crossed. Amblyopia of one eye with hemianesthesia of the opposite side of the face. SYN: *a. cruciata.*

a. ex anopsia. Amblyopia resulting from disuse. Usually in one eye and associated with convergent squint or very poor visual acuity.

a., reflex. Amblyopia due to irritation of peripheral area.

a., toxic. Amblyopia due to effect of alcohol, tobacco, lead, drugs, or other toxic substances.

a., uremic. Dimness or loss of vision during a uremic attack.

amblyoscope (ăm′blē-ŏ-skōp″) [″ + ″ + *skopein*, to examine]. Instrument for stimulating vision in an amblyopic eye.

ambon (ăm′bŏn) [Gr., edge of a dish]. Elevated ring of fibrocartilage around the edge of a bone socket.

ambos (ăm′bōs) [Ger.]. Incus or anvil bone of the middle ear.

Ambu bag (ăm′bū). Proprietary name for a bag used to assist in providing artificial ventilation of the lungs. SEE: illus. at *bag-valve-mask.*

ambulance [L. *ambulare*, to move about]. A vehicle for transportation of the sick and injured, equipped and staffed to provide medical care during transit.

ambulant, ambulatory (ăm′bū-lănt, -lă-tō″rē). Able to walk, not confined to bed.

Ambu simulator. Proprietary name for a manikin used in teaching the technique of cardiopulmonary resuscitation.

Amcill. Trade name for ampicillin, q.v.

Ameba, Amoeba (ă-mē′bă). A genus of protozoa, class Sarcodina, found in soil and water; common name, ameba, q.v. Some are parasitic in man, but most of the parasitic species have been reclassified in the genus *Entamoeba*, q.v.

ameba, amoeba [Gr. *amoibe*, change] (pl. *amebae, amoebae; amebas, amoebas*). A minute, one-celled protozoan animal form of life found in soil and water. It constantly changes shape by sending out fingerlike processes of protoplasm (pseudopodia), by which it moves about and through which it obtains nourishment. It possesses an outer translucent substance called the ectoplasm; but the inner substance, endoplasm, is denser and contains a nucleus. It feeds by surrounding its food and enclosing it in the so-called food vacuole. Oxygen is absorbed from the surrounding water, and CO_2 is eliminated through the plasma membrane. Reproduction is by binary fission, in which the nucleus divides by mitosis. Some species of *Entamoeba*, q.v., are parasitic in man.

amebapore. A pore-forming protein released on a cell membrane by *Entamoeba histolytica*. This forms large pores in the target cell membrane, i.e., the cell the bacterium is attacking.

amebiasis (am″ē-bī′ă-sĭs) [″ + *-iasis*, state]. Infection with amebae, esp. *Entamoeba histolytica*. SEE: *amebapore.*

SYM: Many patients are asymptomatic. Disease is generally characterized by dysentery with diarrhea, weakness, and prostration. Nausea, vomiting, and pain may be present. One serious complication is amebic hepatitis.

ETIOL: *Entamoeba histolytica* is acquired by ingesting food or drink containing encysted forms.

DIAG: Cysts or trophozoites of *E. histolytica* in stools.

PATH: Small abscesses and, later, ulcers of mucous membrane of colon, sometimes resulting in perforation. Liver abscesses may result from amebae being carried to liver via portal vein.

TREAT: In acute amebiasis, metronidazole (Flagyl). Chloroquine and metronidazole are useful in liver abscess. Metronidazole should not be prescribed for pregnant patients. Repeated treatment at intervals for up to three months is necessary to assure the amebae have been eliminated.

For treatment of asymptomatic carriers of cysts, either iodoquinol or diloxanide furoate is suitable. These are available from the Drug Service, Centers for Disease Control, Atlanta, Georgia 30303. Phone number is (404) 639-3670.

a., hepatic. Infection of the liver by amebae, usually with abscess formation.

amebic (ă-mē′bĭk). Pert. to or caused by amebae.

amebic carrier state. State in which an individual harbors a form of pathogenic ameba but has no clinical signs of the disease.

amebic dysentery. Infection with *Entamoeba histolytica*. SEE: *amebiasis.*

amebic hepatitis. Amebic abscess of the liver.

amebicide, amebacide (ă-mē′bĭ-sīd) [Gr. *amoibe*, change, + L. *caedere*, to kill]. An agent that kills amebae.

amebiform (ă-mē'bĭ-form) [″ + L. *forma*, shape]. Shaped like an ameba.

amebocyte (ă-mē'bō-sīt″) [″ + *kytos*, cell]. A cell showing ameboid movements.

ameboid (ă-mē'boyd) [″ + *eidos*, form, shape]. Resembling an ameba.

ameboidism (ă-mē'boyd-ĭzm). 1. Amebalike movements. 2. Denoting a condition shown by certain nerve cells.

ameboid movement. Cellular movement much like that of an amoeba. A protoplasmic pseudopod, q.v., extends, and then the remaining cell contents flow into the pseudopod, which swells gradually. This type of movement allows cells such as leukocytes to move through very small openings. SEE: *diapedesis.*

ameboma (ăm″ē-bō'mă) [″ + *oma*, tumor]. Tumor composed of inflammatory tissue caused by amebiasis.

ameburia (ăm″ē-bū'rē-ă) [Gr. *amoibe*, change, + *ouron*, urine]. Presence of amebae in the urine.

amelanotic (ă″mĕl-ă-nŏt'ĭk). Lacking melanin; unpigmented.

amelia (ă-mē'lē-ă) [Gr. *a-*, not, + *melos*, limb]. Congenital absence of one or more limbs. SEE: *phocomelia.*

amelification (ă-mĕl″ĭ-fĭ-kā'shŭn) [O. Fr. *amel*, enamel, + L. *facere*, to make]. Formation of dental enamel by ameloblasts.

amelioration (ă-mēl″yō-rā'shŭn) [L. *ad*, to, + *melior*, better]. Improvement; moderation of a condition.

ameloblast (ă-mĕl'ō-blăst) [O. Fr. *amel*, enamel, + Gr. *blastos*, germ]. A cell from which tooth enamel is formed.

ameloblastoma (ă-mĕl″ō-blăs-tō'mă) [″ + ″ + *oma*, tumor]. A tumor of the jaw, esp. the lower one, arising from enamel-forming cells. May be partly cystic, partly solid, and may reach large size; of low-grade malignancy. SYN: *adamantinoma.*

amelodentinal [O. Fr. *amel*, enamel, + L. *dens, dent-*, tooth]. Pert. to both enamel and dentin.

amelogenesis (ăm″ē-lō-jĕn'ĕ-sĭs) [″ + Gr. *genesis*, generation, birth]. Formation of dental enamel.

amelus (ăm'ē-lŭs) [Gr. *a-*, not, + *melos*, limb]. Individual with congenitally absent arms and legs.

amenia (ă-mē'nē-ă) [Gr. *a-*, not, + *men*, month]. Amenorrhea, q.v.

amenorrhea (ă-mĕn″ō-rē'ă) [″ + ″ + *rhoia*, flow]. Absence or suppression of menstruation; normal before puberty, after menopause, and during pregnancy and lactation. SYN: *amenia.* SEE: *oligomenorrhea.*
ETIOL: The most common causes of abnormal amenorrhea are congenital abnormalities of the reproductive tract; metabolic disorders (obesity, malnutrition, diabetes); systemic diseases (syphilis, tuberculosis, nephritis); emotional disorders (excitement, anorexia nervosa); endocrine disorders, esp. those involving the ovaries, pituitary, thyroid, and adrenal glands; hormonal imbalance of estrogen, progesterone, or follicle-stimulating hormones.
TREAT: Underlying cause should be determined and corrected. If hormone deficiencies exist, substitutional therapy is recommended.
NURSING IMPLICATIONS: Encourage patient to seek medical attention if absence of menstruation is not related to pregnancy, menopause, or hormonal therapy. Ascertain if patient is also experiencing other symptoms. Indicate that there could be many reasons for this symptom and the importance of a thorough investigation to identify the problem.

a., dietary. Cessation of menstruation due to voluntary or involuntary (as in starvation) dietary restriction.

a., emotional. Amenorrhea resulting from shock, fright, hysteria.

a., exercise. A form of stress amenorrhea. Seen in those whose intense exercise program involves running approximately 100 miles (161 km) or more each week, or the equivalent rate and extent of energy output in other sports. Not all of those who participate in high-level-intensity sports will experience amenorrhea.

a., hyperprolactinemic. Amenorrhea due to an excessive secretion of prolactin by the pituitary. SEE: *prolactin.*

a., hypothalamic. Amenorrhea due to malfunction of the hypothalamus.

a., lactational. ABBR: LAM. The absence of menstrual periods during lactation. Fertility has been shown to be greatly reduced in women who breast feed for 6 to 12 months.

a., nutritional. A., dietary, q.v.

a., pathologic. Amenorrhea due to organic disease.

a., physiologic. Amenorrhea during prepuberty, pregnancy, lactation, and postmenopause periods; not related to organic disease.

a., postpartum. Amenorrhea that may last for only a month or two and would thus be within normal limits; or it may be permanent and thus abnormal. SEE: *Sheehan's syndrome.*

a., primary. Delay of menarche beyond age 18.

a., secondary. Cessation of menses in a woman who has previously menstruated.

a., stress. Cessation of menstruation due to mental or physical stress. Women in prisoner-of-war camps have experienced this type of amenorrhea. Some athletes who train intensively become amenorrheic. The physiology of this is not fully understood. It may be related to hormonal changes caused by stress or to the concomitant alteration in ratio of muscle to fat as training intensity increases.

amenorrheic (ă-měn″ō-rē′ĭk). Pert. to amenorrhea.

amentia (ă-měn′shē-ă) [L. *ab*, from, + *mens*, mind]. 1. Congenital mental deficiency; mental retardation, q.v. 2. Mental disorder characterized by confusion, disorientation, and occasionally stupor. SEE: *dementia*.

   a., nevoid. Sturge-Weber syndrome; congenital syndrome characterized by port-wine nevi along distribution of trigeminal nerve; angiomas of leptomeninges and choroid; intracranial calcifications; mental retardation; epileptic seizures; and glaucoma.

   a., phenylpyruvic. Mental retardation due to phenylketonuria, q.v.

Americaine. Trade name for benzocaine, q.v.

American Association of Retired Persons. ABBR: AARP. The largest voluntary association of older persons (retired or not) in the U.S., with a membership of almost 30 million. Its goal is to improve every aspect of living for persons aged 50 years or over. The association works with congress and state legislatures to represent the interest of older persons.

American Occupational Therapy Certification Board. ABBR: A.O.T.C.B. An independent agency recognized to certify the eligibility to practice of occupational therapists and occupational therapy assistants.

American Red Cross. A branch of the international philanthropic organization Red Cross Society. It provides humanitarian services for persons in the armed forces and their families. Another major function is to provide emergency aid during civil disasters such as floods and earthquakes. In addition, it funds and manages a great number of centers for collecting and processing blood and blood products.

American Sign Language. ABBR: ASL. A nonverbal method of communicating in which the hands and fingers are used to indicate words and concepts. Used by deaf or speech-impaired persons.

americium (ăm-ĕr-ĭsh′ē-ŭm). SYMB: Am. At no. 95; at. wt. of longest-lived isotope 243. A metallic radioactive element.

ametria (ă-mē′trē-ă) [Gr. *a-*, not, + *metra*, uterus]. Congenital absence of the uterus.

ametrometer (ăm″ē-trŏm′ē-tĕr) [*ametropia* + Gr. *metron*, measure]. Instrument for measuring degree of ametropia, q.v.

ametropia (ă″mě-trō′pē-ă) [Gr. *ametros*, disproportionate, + *ops*, eye]. Imperfect refractive powers of eye in which the principal focus does not lie on the retina. This causes hyperopia, myopia, or astigmatism, q.v.

AMI. *acute myocardial infarction.*

amicrobic (ă″mī-krō′bĭk) [Gr. *a-*, not, + *mikros*, small, + *bios*, life]. 1. Lacking microbes. 2. Not caused by microbes.

amidase (ăm′ĭ-dās). A deamidizing enzyme, q.v., one that catalyzes the hydrolysis of amides.

amide (ăm′īd). Any organic substance that contains the monovalent radical $-CONH_2$. It is usually formed by replacing the hydroxyl ($-OH$) group of the $-COOH$ by the $-NH_2$ group.

amido-. A prefix signifying the presence of the radical bond $CONH_2$.

amidulin (ă-mĭd′ū-lĭn) [Fr. *amidon*, starch]. Soluble starch.

amikacin sulfate. USP. An aminoglycoside antibiotic. Trade name is Amikin.

amimia (ă-mĭm′ē-ă) [Gr. *a-*, not, + *mimos*, mimic]. Loss of power to express ideas by signs or gestures.

   a., amnesic. Amimia in which signs and gestures can be made but their meaning is not remembered.

   a., ataxic. Amimia in which signs and gestures cannot be made because of nervous or muscular disorders.

amine (ă-mēn′, ăm′īn). Any one of a group of nitrogen-containing organic compounds that are formed when one or more of the hydrogens of ammonia have been replaced by one or more hydrocarbon radicals.

amino- (ă-mē′nō, ăm′ĭ-nō). Prefix denoting presence of an amino group (NH_2).

aminoacetic acid (ăm″ĭn-ō-ă-sē′tĭk). NH_2-CH_2COOH. A nonessential amino acid, q.v. SYN: *glycine.*

amino acid. One of a large group of organic compounds marked by presence of both an amino group (NH_2) and a carboxyl (COOH) group. Their basic formula is $NH_2-COOH-R$ in which R stands for any aliphatic or aromatic radical. They are amphoteric and exhibit properties marked by both the amino and carboxyl groups. They are the building blocks of which proteins are constructed and are the end products of protein digestion or hydrolysis.

Approximately 80 amino acids are found in nature; only 20 are necessary for human metabolism or growth but, because some are supplied by food and the others can be produced by the body, the ones that must be provided by food are called essential. These are histidine (essential for normal adult but amount required is not known), isoleucine, leucine, lysine, methionine, cysteine,

EXAMPLES OF AMINO ACIDS

SERINE	TYROSINE	GLYCINE
(structure)	(structure)	(structure)
ASPARTIC ACID	ARGININE	HISTIDINE
(structure)	(structure)	(structure)

phenylalanine, tyrosine, threonine, tryptophan, and valine. The nonessential amino acids are: alanine, aspartic acid, arginine, citrulline, glutamic acid, glycine, hydroxyglutamic acid, hydroxyproline, norleucine, proline, and serine.

Arginine, while nonessential for the adult, cannot be formed quickly enough to supply the demand in infants and thus is classed as essential in early life.

Some proteins contain all the essential amino acids and are called complete proteins. Examples are milk, cheese, eggs, and meat. Proteins that do not contain all the essential amino acids are called incomplete proteins. Examples are vegetables and grains. Amino acids pass unchanged through the intestinal wall and portal vein into the blood, then through the liver into the general circulation, from which they are absorbed by the tissues according to the specific amino acid needed by that tissue to make its own protein. Amino acids if not otherwise metabolized may be converted into urea. SEE: illus.; *deaminization; diges-*

tion; protein.

 a.a., essential. In human nutrition, amino acids that are required for growth and development and that cannot be produced by the body. They must be obtained from food.

 a.a., nonessential. Amino acids that can be produced by the body and are not required in the diet.

aminoacidemia (ă-mē″nō-, ăm″ĭ-nō-ăs″ĭ-dē′mē-ă) [*amino acid* + *Gr. haima,* blood]. Excess of amino acids in the blood.

amino acid group. The NH₂ group that characterizes the amines.

aminoacidopathies (ăm″ĭ-nō-ăs″ĭ-dŏp′ă-thēz) [″ + *Gr. pathos,* disease, suffering]. Various disorders of amino acid metabolism, of which there are nearly 100, including cystinuria, alkaptonuria, and albinism.

aminoaciduria (ă-mē″nō-, ăm″ĭ-nō-ăs″ĭ-dū′rē-ă) [″ + *Gr. ouron,* urine]. Excess amino acids in the urine.

aminobenzene (ă-mē″nō-, ăm″ĭ-nō-bĕn′zēn). C₆H₇N. The simplest aromatic amine, an oily liquid derived from benzene.

Used in manufacture of dyes for medical and industrial purposes. SYN: *phenylamine*.

aminobenzoic acid. USP. NH$_2$C$_6$H$_4$COOH. A drug used as a topical ultraviolet screening agent. Trade name is Pabanol. SYN: *paraaminobenzoic acid*.

aminocaproic acid. SEE: *acid, aminocaproic*.

aminoglutethimide (ăm″ĭ-nō-gloo-tĕth′ĭ-mīd). Chemical that interferes with the production of adrenocortical hormone. It has been used to decrease the hypersecretion of cortisol by adrenal tumors. It also has been used to treat cancer of the adrenal gland and breast cancer sensitive to adrenal hormone stimulation.

aminoglycoside. A chemical compound that is present in a number of antibiotics, some of which are derived from microorganisms and others are produced synthetically.

aminohippuric acid, sodium. USP. The sodium salt of aminohippuric acid. It is given intravenously to test renal blood flow and the excretory capacity of the renal tubules.

aminolysis (ăm″ĭ-nŏl′ĭ-sĭs) [*amine* + Gr. *lysis*, dissolution]. Metabolic transformation of amino-containing compounds by removing the amino group.

aminometradine (ăm″ĭ-nō-mĕt′ră-dēn). A nonmercurial diuretic given orally.

aminophylline (ăm-ĭ-nŏf′ĭ-lĭn, ăm″ĭ-nō-fĭl′ĭn). USP. C$_{16}$H$_{24}$N$_{10}$O$_4$. A mixture of theophylline and ethylenediamine. Used esp. in acute asthma that has not responded to epinephrine. Used also as a stimulant to the respiratory center and heart muscle, and as a diuretic. Trade names are Rectalad, Somophyllin, and Aminodur. SYN: *theophylline ethylenediamine*.

aminophylline poisoning. SEE: *Poisons and Poisoning in Appendix*.

aminopterin (ăm-ĭ-nŏp′tĕr-ĭn). A folic acid antagonist used in treatment of acute leukemia.

aminopurine (ăm″ĭ-nō-pū′rĭn). An oxidation product of purine. Includes adenine and guanine. SEE: *methyl purine; oxypurine*.

aminopyrine (ăm″ĭn-ō-pī′rĭn). An antipyretic and analgesic drug. It is not approved for use in the U.S. SYN: *amidopyrine*.

Caution: Because this drug may cause fatal agranulocytosis, it should not be used.

---

aminosalicylic acid. USP. C$_7$H$_7$NO$_3$. A white or nearly white and practically odorless powder that darkens when exposed to air or light. It is an antituberculosis drug, but its effectiveness is greatly enhanced when used in combination with streptomycin and isoniazid; it is believed to delay development of bacterial resistance. SYN:

para-aminosalicylic acid.

aminuria (ăm-ĭ-nū′rē-ă) [*amine* + Gr. *ouron*, urine]. Presence of amines in urine.

Amitid. Trade name for amitriptyline hydrochloride, q.v.

amitosis (ăm″ĭ-tō′sĭs) [Gr. *a-*, not, + *mitos*, a thread, + *osis*, condition]. Direct cell division; simple division of the nucleus and cell without the changes in the nucleus that characterize mitosis, q.v.

amitotic (ăm″ĭ-tŏt′ĭk). Rel. to or characterized by amitosis.

amitryptyline hydrochloride (ăm″ĭ-trĭp′tĭ-lēn). USP. Antidepressant available for either oral or intramuscular administration.

AML. *acanthiomeatal line; acute myelocytic leukemia*.

ammeter (ăm′mĕ-tĕr) [*ampere* + Gr. *metron*, measure]. An instrument, calibrated in amperes, that measures the strength of an electric current. SEE: *milliammeter*.

ammoaciduria (ăm″ō-ăs″ĭ-dū′rē-ă) [*ammonia* + *amino acid* + Gr. *ouron*, urine]. Abnormal amount of ammonia and amino acids in the urine.

ammonemia (ă-mō-nē′mē-ă) [*ammonia* + Gr. *haima*, blood]. Ammoniemia, q.v.

ammonia (ă-mō′nē-ă) [*Ammo*, Egyptian deity near whose temple it was originally obtained]. NH$_3$. An alkaline gas formed by decomposition of nitrogen-containing substances such as proteins and amino acids. Ammonia is converted into urea in the liver. It is related to many poisonous substances but also to the proteins and many useful chemicals. Dissolved in water, it neutralizes acids and turns litmus paper blue.

    a., aromatic spirit of. USP. A pungent solution of approx. 4% ammonium carbonate in 70% alcohol flavored with lemon, lavender, and myristica oil. It is used to elicit reflex stimulation of respiration and as "smelling salts" to stimulate persons who have fainted.

    a., blood. Ammonia in the blood. Increased values are found in liver failure. SEE: *ammoniemia*.

ammoniacal (ăm″ō-nī′ă-kăl). Having the characteristics of or pert. to ammonia.

ammonia intoxication. SEE: *ammonia toxicity*.

ammonia solution, diluted. A solution containing approx. 10 grams of ammonia per 100 ml of water.

ammonia solution, strong. A solution containing approx. 28% ammonia in water.

ammoniated (ă-mō′nē-āt′d). Containing ammonia.

ammonia toxicity. Ammonia is produced in the intestinal tract by bacterial action. After absorption it is transported to the liver, where it is metabolized. In diseases such as cirrhosis of the liver, the ammonia absorbed may be shunted past the liver. This results in an accumulation of ammonia in the blood (ammoniemia). The resulting developments, including alterations in consciousness, neurologic changes, abnormal electroencephalogram, and a flapping tremor (asterixis), are due at least in part to ammonia toxicity. SEE: *hepatic coma; Poisons and Poisoning in Appendix.*

TREAT: Directed to the prevention of production and absorption of ammonia in the intestinal tract; and by using enemas and antibiotics such as neomycin to prevent growth of the bacteria that produce ammonia in the intestinal tract. Limit protein in diet.

ammonia water. NH_4OH. Ammonium hydroxide.

ammoniemia (a-mō″nĭ-ē′mē-ă) [*ammonia* + Gr. *haima*, blood]. Excessive ammonia in the blood. Normally only faint traces of ammonia are found in the blood. Increased amounts are due to a pathologic condition such as impaired liver function. SYN: *ammonemia.* SEE: *ammonia toxicity.*

ammonium (ă-mō′nē-ŭm). The radical, NH_4^+, that forms salts analogous to those of alkaline metals.

a. alum. Aluminum ammonium sulfate, an astringent. SEE: *alum.*

a. carbonate. $(NH_4)_2CO_3$. Compound used in preparing aromatic ammonia spirit.

a. chloride. USP. NH_4Cl. Compound used as an expectorant and as an acidifier in treating acid-base balance.

a. hydroxide. NH_4OH. A solution of ammonia in water, used as a household cleaner and as a refrigerant. SEE: *Ammonia in Poisons and Poisoning in Appendix.*

a. thiosulfate. The chemical in fixing solution that removes unexposed silver bromide crystals from radiographic film during the development process.

ammoniuria (ă-mō″nē-ū′rē-ă) [″ + Gr. *ouron*, urine]. Excessive ammonia in the urine.

ammonotelic (ă-mō″nō-tēl′ĭk). Pert. to animals that excrete amino nitrogen in the form of ammonia. Included in this group are most aquatic vertebrates but not whales. SEE: *urea cycle; ureotelic; uricotelic.*

amnesia (ăm-nē′zē-ă) [Gr.]. A loss of memory. Often applied to episodes during which patients forget their identity, though they may conduct themselves properly enough, and following which no memory of the period persists. Such episodes are often hysterical and sometimes epileptic, while trauma, senility, alcoholism, and other or-

ganic reaction types account for a smaller number.

a., anterograde. Amnesia for events occurring after a precipitating event or medication.

Caution: This type of short-term memory loss may be induced in persons who use benzodiazepine drugs, e.g., triazolam, lorazepam, fluazepam, after ingesting alcohol to induce sleep.

---

a., auditory. Loss of memory for the meanings of sounds or spoken words. SYN: *aphasia, auditory; deafness, word.*

a., lacunar. Loss of memory for isolated events.

a., retroanterograde. A memory disorder in which present-day events are referred to the past and vice versa.

a., retrograde. Amnesia for events occurring before the precipitating trauma.

a., tactile. Inability to distinguish objects by sense of touch. SYN: *astereognosis.*

a., transient global. Transient amnesia that occurs in otherwise healthy persons. Onset is usually sudden and may last for a few hours. Remote memory is retained even though memory for recent events is absent. Recovery is usually rapid.

a., traumatic. Amnesia caused by sudden physical injury.

a., visual. Inability to remember the appearance of objects or to be cognizant of printed words.

amnesiac. A person who has amnesia.

amnesic (ăm-nē′sĭk). Pert. to amnesia.

amnesic aphasia. Loss of memory for words.

amnestic (ăm-nĕs′tĭk). Pert. to or causing amnesia.

amniocentesis (ăm″nē-ō-sĕn-tē′sĭs) [Gr. *amnion*, lamb, + *kentesis*, puncture]. Transabdominal puncture of the amniotic sac using a needle and syringe in order to remove amniotic fluid. The material obtained to be studied chemically and cytologically to detect genetic and biochemical disorders, maternal-fetal blood incompatibility, and, later in the pregnancy, to determine fetal maturity. The procedure also provides a means of transfusing the fetus with platelets or blood; and instillation of drugs for treating the fetus.

This procedure is usually performed no earlier than at 14 weeks' gestation. It is important that the analysis be done by persons expert in the fields of chemistry and cell culture. Cell cultures may require 30 days; and, if the test has to be repeated, the time required may be insufficient to allow corrective action. SEE: illus.

AMNIOCENTESIS

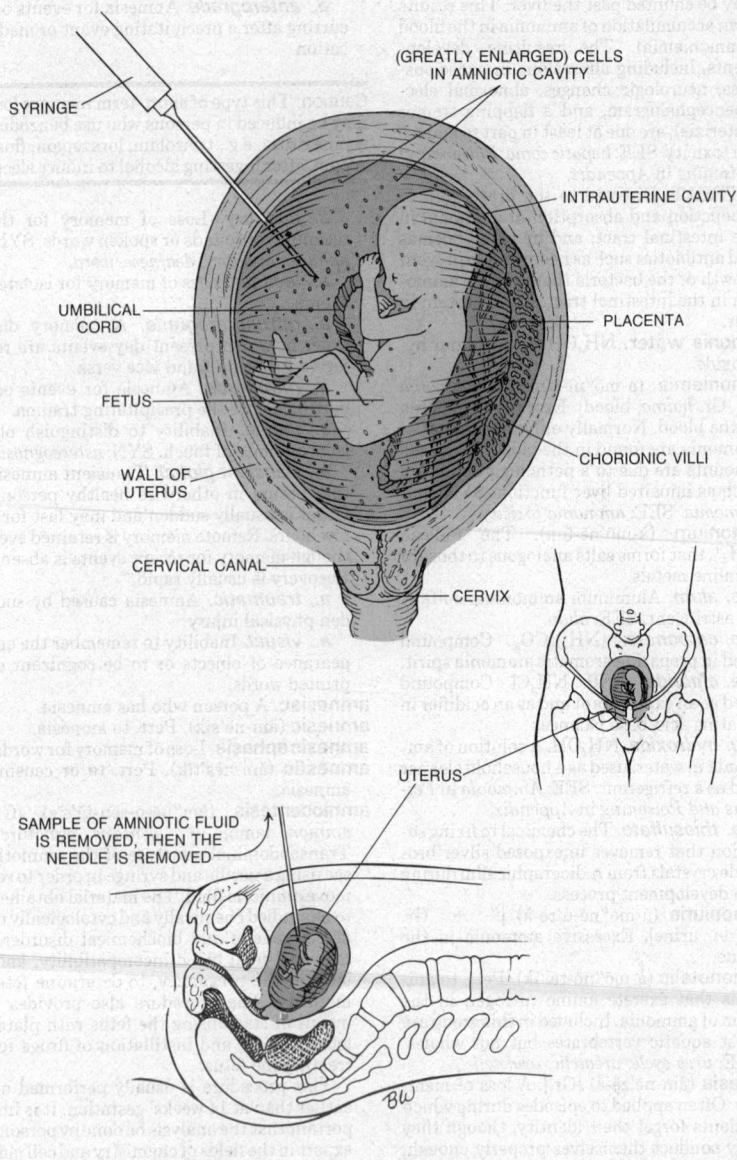

SYRINGE

(GREATLY ENLARGED) CELLS
IN AMNIOTIC CAVITY

INTRAUTERINE CAVITY

UMBILICAL
CORD

PLACENTA

FETUS

CHORIONIC VILLI

WALL OF
UTERUS

CERVICAL CANAL

CERVIX

UTERUS

SAMPLE OF AMNIOTIC FLUID
IS REMOVED, THEN THE
NEEDLE IS REMOVED

Caution: The procedure can cause abortion; and trauma to the fetus is possible.

NURSING IMPLICATIONS: Prepare the patient for what to expect during the procedure, and be certain that a consent form has been signed. Provide emotional support during the actual procedure. Prepare equipment for the tap, making sure that test tubes are amber colored or tape-covered to shield the fluid from light which could break down bilirubin. Obtain baseline vital signs and fetal heart sounds and palpate the fundus for fetal and uterine activity. Monitor these for 30 minutes prior to the procedure, throughout the procedure, and for 30 minutes post procedure. Assess the patient for lightheadedness, nausea, or diaphoresis as well as for anxiety, pain, and labor onset throughout the procedure, and have the patient rest on her left side following the procedure. Instruct the patient to be aware of and report effects indicative of complications, such as unusual fetal hyper- or hypoactivity, clear or bloody vaginal drainage, uterine contractions, abdominal pain, or fever and chills. SEE: *chorionic villus sampling; fetal monitoring, in utero.*

amniochorial, amniochorionic (ăm″nē-ō-kō′rē-ăl, -kō-rē-ŏn′ĭk). Relating to both amnion and chorion.

amnioclepsis (ăm″nē-ŏ-klĕp′sĭs) [″ + *kleptein*, to steal]. Gradual, unperceived loss of amniotic fluid.

amniogenesis (ăm″nē-ō-jĕn′ĕ-sĭs) [″ + *genesis*, generation, birth]. Formation of the amnion.

amniography [″ + *graphein*, to write]. Roentgenography of amniotic sac after injection of a radiopaque substance into the amniotic fluid. Used in diagnosing fetal abnormalities.

amnioinfusion (ăm″nē-ō-ĭn-fū′zhŭn). Injection of solutions into the amniotic fluid. Usually done to induce abortion.

amnion (ăm′nē-ŏn) [Gr. *amnion*, lamb]. The inner of the fetal membranes; a thin, transparent sac that holds the fetus suspended in the liquor amnii or amniotic fluid, q.v. The amnion grows rapidly at the expense of the extraembryonic coelom, and by the end of the third month it fuses with the chorion, forming the amniochorionic sac. Commonly called the bag of waters. SYN: *amniotic sac.* SEE: *oligohydramnios;* words beginning with *amnio-.*

    a. nodosum. Rounded or oval opaque elevations 1 to 6 mm in diameter in the placenta that are seen in the part of the amnion in contact with the chorionic plate and near the insertion of the cord into the placenta.

They are present in approx. 60% of pregnancies.

amnionitis (ăm″nē-ō-nī′tĭs) [″ + *itis,* inflammation]. Inflammation of the amnion.

amniorrhea (ăm″nē-or-rē′ă) [″ + *rhoia,* flow]. Escape of the amniotic fluid.

amnioscope (ăm′nē-ŏ-skōp) [Gr. *amnion,* lamb, + *skopein,* to examine]. Optical device for looking inside the amniotic cavity.

    a., suction. Amnioscope designed to allow suction to be applied so that it is held in place against the fetal scalp. This permits evacuation of the amniotic fluid from the area pressing against the scalp, thus leaving a clear field for sampling blood from that site.

amnioscopy. Direct visual examination of the fetus by use of an optical device that is inserted into the amniotic cavity via the abdominal wall.

amniote (ăm′nē-ōt). Any animal or group belonging to the Amniota, a major group of vertebrates, the members of which develop an amnion. Includes reptiles, birds, and mammals.

amniotic (ăm-nē-ŏt′ĭk). Pert. to the amnion.

amniotic band disruption sequence syndrome. A collection of fetal malformations associated with multiple fibrous strands of amnion that appear to develop or entangle fetal parts in utero. This leads to structural malformations and deformations and disruption of function. Defects associated with this condition include limb defects and amputations; abnormal dermal ridge patterns; simian creases; clubbed feet; craniofacial defects including cleft lip and palate; and visceral defects such as gastroschisis and omphalocele. Failure to understand the cause of this condition can lead to misdiagnosis and inappropriate family and genetic counseling. SEE: *multiple malformation syndromes.*

amniotic cavity. The fluid-filled cavity of the amnion, q.v.

amniotic fluid. Liquor amnii. The liquid or albuminous fluid contained in the amnion, q.v. This fluid is transparent and almost colorless. The liquid protects the fetus from injury, helps maintain an even temperature, prevents formation of adhesions between the amnion and the skin of the fetus, and prevents conformity of the sac to the fetus. The amniotic fluid is continually being absorbed and renewed at a rapid rate. About one third of the water in the amniotic fluid is replaced each hour.

amniotic fluid embolism. SEE: *embolism, amniotic.*

amniotic sac. Amnion, q.v.

amniotitis (ăm-nē-ŏ-tī′tĭs) [Gr. *amnion,* lamb, + *itis,* inflammation]. Inflammation of the amnion. SYN: *amnitis; amnionitis.*

amniotome (ăm′nē-ō-tōm) [″ + Gr. *tome*, incision]. Instrument for puncturing fetal membranes.

amniotomy (ăm″nē-ŏt′ō-mē). Surgical rupture of the fetal membranes. Done to induce or expedite labor. A digital amniotome, a small pointed instrument that fits over the tip of the finger, facilitates this procedure.

NURSING IMPLICATIONS: Explain the procedure to the patient, then correctly position and drape the site, and thoroughly cleanse the perineum. Before beginning procedure, monitor fetal heart rate and uterine contractions for baseline information and continue this throughout and following the procedure. Immediately listen to the fetal heart sounds because there is an increased risk of cord prolapse when an amniotomy is performed. When the physician has completed the amniotomy, assess the color and amount of amniotic fluid expelled. Test the fluid's pH with nitrazine paper if there is any question of its origin, i.e., the possibility that it is urine and not amniotic fluid.

amnitis (ăm-nī′tĭs). Inflammation of the amnion. SYN: *amniotitis; amnionitis.*

amobarbital (ăm″ō-bar′bĭ-tăl). USP. $C_{11}H_{18}N_2O_3$. An odorless, white, crystalline powder. Used as a sedative.

a. sodium. $C_{11}H_{17}N_2NaO_3$. An odorless, white, granular powder. Following administration, it is absorbed and inactivated rapidly in the liver. Used as a sedative.

A-mode (amplitude modulation) display. SEE: *ultrasound, A-mode.*

amodiaquine hydrochloride (ăm″ō-dī′ă-kwĭn). USP. An antimalarial drug similar in action to chloroquine. Trade name is Camoquin Hydrochloride.

amoeba (ă-mē′ba) [Gr. *amoibe,* change]. A one-celled protozoan animal form. SEE: *ameba.*

amok, amuck (ă-mŏk′, ă-mŭk′) [Malay, to engage furiously in battle]. A state of murderous frenzy.

amor (ă′mor) [L.]. Love, esp. sexual love.

amorphia, amorphism (ă-mor′fē-ă, ă-mor′fĭzm) [Gr. *a-,* not, + *morphe,* form]. State of being without definite form.

amorphous (ă-mor′fŭs). Without definite form.

amotio (ă-mō′shē-ō) [L. *amovere,* to move from]. A detachment.

a. retinae. Detached retina.

amoxicillin (ă-mŏks″ĭ-sĭl′ĭn). USP. A semisynthetic penicillin. Trade names include Amoxil, Polymox, Robamox, and Trimox.

Amoxil. Trade name for amoxicillin, q.v.

AMP. *adenosine monophosphate,* q.v.

amperage (ăm-pēr′ĭj). Strength of an electric current expressed in amperes.

ampere (ăm′pēr). ABBR: amp. Unit of intensity of electric current which is produced by 1 volt acting through resistance of 1 ohm. SEE: *electromotive force.*

ampere meter. Instrument denoting in amperes the strength of a current. SEE: *ammeter.*

amphetamine (ăm-fĕt′ă-mēn, -mĭn). A colorless liquid that volatilizes slowly at room temperature. It is a central nervous system stimulant. The preparation most commonly used is the sulfate, marketed in tablet or capsule form.

a. sulfate. USP. $(C_9H_{13}N)_2H_2SO_4$. A synthetic, white, crystalline substance that acts as a central nervous system stimulant. Used in treatment of narcolepsy and certain types of mental depression. Use of amphetamines to control appetite in treating obesity has not proved to be effective. Large doses are toxic, and prolonged use may cause drug dependence. Trade names are Benzedrine and Amphedrine.

amphetamine poisoning. SEE: *Poisons and Poisoning* in *Appendix.*

amphi- [Gr. *amphi,* on both sides]. Prefix indicating on both sides, on all sides, double. In chemistry, it denotes certain positions or configurations of molecules.

amphiarthrosis (ăm″fē-ăr-thrō′sĭs) [″ + *arthrosis,* joint]. A form of articulation in which the body surfaces are connected by cartilage; mobility is slight, but may be exerted in all directions. The articulations of the bodies of the vertebrae are examples.

amphiaster (ăm″fē-ăs′tĕr) [″ + *aster,* star]. Double star figure formed during mitosis, q.v. SYN: *diaster.*

Amphibia (ăm-fĭb′ē-ă) [Gr. *amphibios,* double life]. A class of cold-blooded animals that live on land and in water. They breathe through gills during their aquatic larval stage but breathe through lungs in their adult stage. Includes salamanders, frogs, and toads. SEE: *metamorphosis.*

amphibious (ăm-fĭb′ē-ŭs). Able to live both on land and in water.

amphiblastula (ăm″fē-blăs′tū-lă) [Gr. *amphi,* on both sides, + *blastula,* little sprout]. A form of blastula in which the blastomeres are of unequal size. Seen in sponges.

amphibolic (ăm″fĭ-bŏl′ĭk) [Gr. *amphibolia,* uncertainty]. 1. Having unknown or varying prognosis. 2. Possessing anabolic and catabolic activity.

amphicelous (ăm″fĭ-sē′lŭs) [Gr. *amphi,* on both sides, + *koilos,* hollow]. Concave on each end, as a vertebra.

amphicentric (ăm″fĭ-sĕn′trĭk) [″ + *ken-*

tron, center]. Centering or converging at both ends.

amphichroic, amphichromatic (ăm″fē-krō′ĭk, -krō-măt′ĭk) [″ + *chroma,* color]. 1. Turning red litmus paper blue, and blue, red. 2. Reacting as both an acid and an alkali. 3. Capable of exhibiting two colors.

amphicyte (ăm′fē-sīt) [″ + *kytos,* cell]. One of the cells enveloping the bodies of cerebrospinal ganglionic neurons.

amphidiarthrosis (ăm″fē-dī-ăr-thrō′sĭs) [″ + *diarthrosis,* articulation]. An articulation with amphiarthrosis and diarthrosis, such as that of the lower jaw.

amphimixis (ăm″fē-mĭks′ĭs) [″ + *mixis,* mingling]. Mixing of maternal and paternal germ cells in reproduction, thus giving hereditary characteristics from both parents.

amphitheater (ăm″fĭ-thē′ă-tĕr) [″ + *theatron,* theater]. An operating room with tiers of seats around it for students and other observers.

amphitrichate, amphitrichous (ăm-fĭt′rĭ-kāt, -kŭs) [″ + *thrichos,* hair]. Having a flagellum or flagella at both ends, said of microorganisms.

ampho- [Gr. *ampho,* both]. Prefix indicating both.

amphocyte (ăm′fō-sīt) [″ + *kytos,* cell]. A cell that stains with either acid or basic stains.

amphodiplopia (ăm-fō-dĭ-plō′pē-ă) [″ + *diploos,* double, + *ops,* vision]. Double vision in each eye. SYN: *amphoterodiplopia.*

Amphojel (ăm′fō-jĕl). A trade name for aluminum hydroxide gel, USP.

ampholyte (ăm′fō-līt) [″ + *electrolyte*]. Substance that acts as a base or an acid, depending upon the pH of the solution into which it is introduced.

amphoric (ăm-for′ĭk) [L. *amphoricus*]. Pert. to a sound as that caused by blowing across the mouth of a bottle; a resonance; a cavernous sound on percussion of a pulmonary cavity.

amphoricity (ăm″for-ĭs′ĭ-tē). The condition of producing amphoric sounds.

amphoriloquy (ăm″for-ĭl′ō-kwē) [L. *amphora,* jar, + *loqui,* to speak]. The presence of amphoric sounds in speaking.

amphorophony (ăm″for-ŏf′ō-nē) [Gr. *amphoreus,* jar, + *phone,* voice]. Amphoric voice sound.

amphoteric, amphoterous (ăm-fō-tĕr′ĭk, ăm-fŏt′ĕr-ŭs) [Gr. *amphoteros,* both]. Having the ability to react as both an acid and a base.

amphoteric compound. A compound that reacts as both an acid and a base.

amphotericin B (ăm″fō-tĕr′ĭ-sĭn). USP. An antibiotic agent obtained from a strain of *Streptomyces nodosus.* It is used in treat-

ment of deep-seated mycotic infections. The drug usually is administered parenterally. Trade name is Fungizone.

amphoteric reaction. Reaction in which a compound reacts as both an acid and a base.

amphoterism (ăm-fō′tĕr-ĭzm). State of reacting as both an acid and a base.

amphoterodiplopia (ăm-fŏt″ĕr-ō-dī-plō′pē-ă) [″ + *diploos,* double, + *ops,* vision]. Double vision in each eye. SYN: *amphodiplopia.*

amphotonic [″ + *tonos,* tone]. Pert. to or characterized by amphotony.

amphotony (ăm-fŏt′ō-nē). Hyperexcitability of both the sympathetic and parasympathetic nervous systems.

ampicillin (ămp″ĭ-sĭl′ĭn). USP. A semisynthetic penicillin; broad-spectrum antibiotic. Trade names include Amcill, Omnipen, Polycillin, and Principen.

   a. **sodium.** USP. Monosodium salt of ampicillin. Trade names include Omnipen-N, Polycillin-N, and Principen/N.

amplification (ăm″plĭ-fĭ-kă′shŭn) [L. *amplificatio,* making larger]. Enlargement, magnification, expansion.

amplifier (ăm′plĭ-fī″ĕr). That which enlarges, extends, increases, or makes more powerful. In electronics, a device for increasing the electric current or signal.

amplitude (ăm′plĭ-tūd) [L. *amplitudo*]. 1. Amount, extent, size, abundance, or fullness. 2. In physics, the extent of movement, as of a pendulum or sound wave. The maximum displacement of a particle, as that of a string vibrating, as measured from the mean to the extreme. 3. Magnitude of an action potential. 4. In radiography, the extent of tube travel during tomography.

amplitude modulation. Modification of the amplitude, esp. of a current used for muscle stimulation.

ampule (ăm′pūl) [Fr. *ampoule*]. A small glass container that can be sealed and its contents sterilized. This is a French invention for containing hypodermic solutions.

ampulla (ăm-pŭl′lä) [L., little jar] (pl. *ampullae*). [NA] Saclike dilatation of a canal or duct.

   a. **ductus deferentis.** An irregular and nodular dilatation of the vas deferens just before its junction with the excretory duct of the seminal vesicle.

   a. **of lacrimal duct.** Slight dilatation of the lacrimal duct medial to the punctum.

   a. **of rectum.** Slight dilatation of rectum proper just before continuing as anal canal. Also: *infraperitoneal portion of rectum proper.*

   a. **of semicircular canal.** A dilatation at end of semicircular canal that houses an ampulla of a semicircular duct.

a. of semicircular ducts. Dilatation of semicircular ducts near their junction with the utricle. In their walls are the cristae ampullares.

a. of uterine tube. The dilated distal end of a uterine tube terminating in a funnel-like infundibulum.

a. of vas deferens. Ampulla ductus deferentis, q.v.

a. of Vater. Papilla of Vater, q.v.

ampullitis (ăm″pŭl-lī′tĭs) [″ + Gr. *itis*, inflammation]. Inflammation of any ampulla, esp. of ductus deferens.

ampullula (ăm-pŭl′ū-lă) [dim. of L. *ampulla*]. A small dilatation, esp. of a lymph or blood vessel.

amputation (ăm″pū-tā′shŭn) [L. *amputare*, to cut around]. Removal, usually by surgery, of a limb, part, or organ.

NURSING IMPLICATIONS: In the immediate postoperative period, assess the patient's vital signs, and observe the stump (residual limb) dressing for bleeding at least every two hours. Help to prevent contracture formation by encouraging the patient to move and do range of motion exercises as well as muscle strengthening exercises as soon as ordered, postoperatively. Evaluate the cardiovascular status by checking proximal pulses, skin color, and temperature. Manage pain, as ordered, and prevent postoperative complications. Assist the stump to shrink by encouraging the patient to do stump conditioning exercises and by correct bandaging of the stump. Instruct the patient to massage the stump. Encourage the patient to verbalize anger and frustration, cope with grief, self-image, and life adjustments, and to deal with phantom limb pain. SEE: *Nursing Diagnoses* in *Appendix.*

a., congenital. Amputation of parts of the fetus in utero, formerly believed to be caused by constricting bands but now believed to be a developmental defect.

a., double-flap. Amputation in which two flaps of soft tissue are formed to cover the end of the bone.

a. in contiguity. Amputation at a joint.

a. in continuity. Amputation elsewhere than at a joint.

a., primary. Amputation performed before inflammation sets in.

a., secondary. Amputation performed during period of suppuration.

a., spontaneous. Nonsurgical separation of an extremity or digit. SEE: *ainhum.*

a., tertiary. Amputation performed after abatement of inflammatory reaction.

amputee (ăm″pū-tē′). One who has had an amputation, esp. of the arm(s) or leg(s).

A.M.R.A. *American Medical Record Association.*

Amsler grid [Marc Amsler, Swiss ophthalmologist, 1891–1968]. A grid of lines used in testing for macular degeneration, q.v. The grid is observed with each eye separately.

A.M.T. *American Medical Technologists.*

amuck, amok (ă-mŭk′) [Malay *amok*, furious attack]. State of murderous frenzy.

amusia (ă-mū′sē-ă) [Gr. *amousos*, unmusical]. Music deafness; inability to produce or appreciate musical sounds.

a., motor. Inability to produce musical sounds.

a., sensory. Music deafness. Inability to appreciate musical sounds.

a., vocal. Being unable to sing.

Amussat's operation (ăm′ū-săz) [Jean Z. Amussat, Fr. surgeon, 1796–1856]. Surgical formation of an artificial anus, by lumbar colotomy in ascending colon.

amychophobia (ă-mī″kō-fō′bē-ă) [Gr. *amyche*, scratch, + *phobos*, fear]. Morbid fear of being scratched; fear of the claws of any animal.

amyelencephaly (ă-mī″ĕl-ĕn-sĕf-ā′lē) [Gr. *a-*, not, + *myelos*, marrow, + *enkephalos*, brain]. Congenital absence of brain and spinal cord.

amyelia (ă-mī-ē′lē-ă) [″ + *myelos*, marrow]. Congenital absence of spinal cord.

amyelinic (ă-mī″ē-lĭn′ĭk). Not possessing a myelin sheath.

amyelus (ă-mī′ĕ-lŭs). An individual with congenital absence of the spinal cord.

amygdala (ă-mĭg′dă-lă) [L., almond] (pl. *amygdalae*). 1. A mass of gray matter in the anterior portion of the temporal lobe. It is thought that the structure plays an important role in arousal. 2. Obsolete term for the tonsil.

amygdalin (ă-mĭg′dă-lĭn). A bitter-tasting glycoside derived from the pit or other seed parts of several plants including almonds and apricots. Amygdalin, from which the poisonous hydrocyanic acid can be produced by enzymatic action, is the substance known in the U.S. as Laetrile. Amygdalin has no therapeutic or nutritional value. SEE: *Laetrile.*

amygdaline (ă-mĭg′dă-lĭn, -lĭn) [L. *amygdalinus*]. 1. Pert. to a tonsil. 2. Pert. to or shaped like an almond. SYN: *amygdaloid.*

amygdaloid (ă-mĭg′dă-loyd) [Gr. *amygdale*, almond, + *eidos*, form, shape]. Resembling a tonsil or an almond.

amygdaloid fossa. A depression that contains the tonsil.

amygdaloid tubercle. A projection from the middle cornu of the lateral ventricle, marking area of the amygdaloid nucleus.

amygdalolith (ă-mĭg′dă-lō-lĭth″) [″ + *lithos*, stone]. Stone in a distended crypt of a tonsil.

amygdalopathy (ă-mĭg″dă-lŏp′ă-thē) [″ + *pathos*, disease, suffering]. Any disease of a tonsil.

amygdalotome (ă-mĭg′dă-lō-tōm″) [″ + *tome*, incision]. Instrument for excision of a tonsil.

amyl (ăm′ĭl) [Gr. *amylon*, starch]. C_5H_{11}. A hypothetical univalent radical, nonexistent in a free state.

    a. nitrite. USP. $C_5H_{11}NO_2$. A volatile and highly flammable clear liquid. Used as a vasodilator, esp. for anginal pain.

amylaceous (ăm″ĭ-lā′shē-ŭs). Starchy.

amylase (ăm′ĭ-lās) [″ + -*asis*, colloid enzyme]. A class of enzymes that split or hydrolyze starch. Those found in animals are called α-amylases; those in plants are called β-amylases. SEE: *antiamylase; enzyme; macroamylase.*

    a., pancreatic. Amylopsin, q.v.

    a., salivary. Ptyalin, q.v.

    a., vegetable. Diastase, q.v.

amylasuria (ăm″ĭ-lās-ū′rē-ă) [″ + *ouron*, urine]. Increased amount of amylase in the urine. Occurs in pancreatitis.

amylemia (ăm″ĭ-lē′mē-ă) [″ + *haima*, blood]. Presence of starch in the blood.

amylodextrin [″ + *dexter*, right]. Soluble substance produced during the hydrolysis of starch into sugar.

amylodyspepsia (ăm″ĭ-lō-dĭs-pĕp′sē-ă) [″ + *dys*, bad, + *pepsis*, digestion]. Inability to digest starchy foods.

amylogenesis (ăm″ĭ-lō-jĕn′ē-sĭs) [″ + *genesis*, generation, birth]. The production of starch.

amylogenic (ăm″ĭ-lō-jĕn′ĭk) [″ + *gennan*, to produce]. Producing starch.

amyloid (ăm′ĭ-loyd) [Gr. *amylon*, starch, + *eidos*, form, shape]. 1. Resembling starch; starchlike. 2. A protein-polysaccharide complex having starchlike characteristics produced and deposited in tissues during certain pathological states. It is a homogeneous, highly refractile substance staining readily with Congo red. It is associated with a variety of chronic diseases, particularly tuberculosis, osteomyelitis, leprosy, Hodgkin's disease, and carcinoma.

amyloid degeneration. Degeneration of organs or tissues from deposition of amyloid. Structures are waxy and translucent, having hyaline appearance. Liver, spleen, and kidneys are usually involved, but any tissue may be infiltrated.

amyloid disease. Amyloidosis, q.v.

amyloid kidney. Enlarged, firm, smooth kidney usually associated with amyloid disease of spleen or liver.

    SYM: Face pale, waxy skin that may be edematous. Liver and spleen may also be enlarged; not tender to pressure. Diarrhea if intestines are involved. Albumin, hyaline, and waxy casts in urine.

amyloid nephrosis. A nephrotic syndrome from myeloid degeneration of kidney.

amyloidosis (ăm″ĭ-loy-dō′sĭs) [Gr. *amylon*, starch, + *eidos*, form, shape, + *osis*, condition]. A metabolic disorder marked by deposition of amyloid in organs and tissue. Thought to be the result of disordered function of the reticuloendothelial system and abnormal immunoglobulin synthesis. There is no known method of preventing formation of amyloid deposits except to control the primary disease with which it is associated. SYN: *amylosis.*

    a., lichen. A form of amyloidosis limited to the skin.

    a., localized. Amyloidosis in which isolated amyloid tumors are formed.

    a., primary. Amyloidosis not associated with a chronic disease.

    a., secondary. Amyloidosis associated with a chronic disease, such as tuberculosis, syphilis, Hodgkin's disease, rheumatoid arthritis, and with extensive tissue destruction. Spleen, liver, kidneys, and adrenal cortex most frequently involved.

amylolysis (ăm″ĭl-ŏl′ĭ-sĭs) [″ + *lysis*, dissolution]. Hydrolysis of starch into sugar in the process of digestion.

amylolytic (ăm″ĭl-ō-lĭt′ĭk). Pert. to or characterized by amylolysis.

amylolytic enzyme. An enzyme that hydrolyzes starch. SYN: *amylase.*

amylopectin (ăm″ĭl-ō-pĕk′tĭn). The insoluble component of starch. The soluble component is amidin. SYN: *amylin.*

amylophagia (ăm″ĭ-lō-fā′jē-ă) [″ + *phagein*, to eat]. Abnormal craving for starch.

amylopsin (ăm″ĭ-lŏp′sĭn) [″ + *opsis*, appearance]. Enzyme in pancreatic juice that hydrolyzes starch into achroodextrin and maltose. SYN: *amylase, pancreatic.* SEE: *digestion; duodenum; enzyme.*

amylose (ăm′ĭ-lōs) [Gr. *amylon*, starch]. A group of carbohydrates that includes starch, cellulose, and dextrin. SEE: *saccharose.*

amylosuria (ăm″ĭ-lō-sū′rē-ă) [″ + *ouron*, urine]. Amylose in the urine.

amylum (ăm′ĭ-lŭm) [Gr. *amylon*, starch]. Starch.

amyluria [″ + Gr. *ouron*, urine]. Starch in the urine.

amyosthenia (ă-mī″ŏs-thē′nē-ă) [Gr. *a-*, not, + *mys*, muscle, + *sthenos*, strength]. Weakness of muscles. SEE: *myasthenia.*

amyosthenic (ă-mī″ŏs-thĕn′ĭk). Pert. to muscular weakness. SYN: *amyasthenic.*

amyotonia (ă-mī″ō-tō′nē-ă) [″ + ″ + *tonos*, tone]. Deficiency or lack of muscular tone.

    a. congenita. A noninherited but sometimes familial disease characterized by absence of muscular development, with the lower extremities being the first involved. It is first apparent at, or shortly after, birth. SYN: *myotonia congenita; Oppenheim's disease.*

amyotrophia, amyotrophy (ă-mī″ō-trō′fē-ă, ă-mī-ŏt′rō-fē) [" + " + *trophe,* nourishment]. Muscular atrophy.

   a., progressive spinal. Progressive muscular atrophy.

amyotrophic (ă-mī″ō-trŏf′ĭk). Pert. to muscular atrophy.

amyotrophic lateral sclerosis. A syndrome marked by muscular weakness and atrophy with spasticity and hyperreflexia due to degeneration of motor neurons of spinal cord, medulla, and cortex. Even though prognosis is very poor, some patients have remained active for 10 to 20 years after the disease was diagnosed. If only cells of motor cranial nuclei in the medulla are involved, condition is called progressive bulbar palsy. There is no specific therapy; however, patients often benefit from referral to occupational or physical therapy, or both. Also called Lou Gehrig's disease. SYN: *motor neuron disease.* SEE: *Nursing Diagnoses in Appendix.*

   ETIOL: Unknown, but the possibility of the illness being associated with a specific genetic defect holds promise of determining the course of the disease. Once this is done, it might be possible to treat the genetic abnormality.

amyous (ăm′ē-ŭs) [" + *mys,* muscle]. 1. Weak; deficient in muscular strength. 2. Without muscle.

Amytal. Trade name for amobarbital, q.v.

Amytal Sodium. Trade name for amobarbital sodium, q.v.

amyxia (ă-mĭks′ē-ă) [" + *myxa,* mucus]. Absence or deficiency of mucus.

amyxorrhea (ă-mĭks-ō-rē′ă) [" + " + *rhoia,* flow]. Lack of normal secretion of mucus.

An. 1. Chem. symb. for actinon. 2. *anisometropia.* 3. *anode.* 4. *antigen.*

an- [Gr.]. A negative prefix indicating without or not.

A.N.A. *American Nurses' Association.* A professional nursing organization comprising state and local affiliates. It provides nurses with a mechanism to determine the functions, activities, and goals of their profession. SEE: *Code for Nurses.*

ana (ăn′ă). 1. [Gr.] ABBR: aa. Prescription term meaning *so much of each.* 2. *antinuclear antibody.*

ana-. A prefix used in words derived from Greek. It indicates up, against, or back.

anabolic (ăn″ă-bŏl′ĭk) [Gr. *anabolikos*]. Promoting or pert. to anabolism.

anabolic agents. Testosterone, or steroid hormones resembling testosterone, which stimulates anabolism (rather than catabolism) in the body. Anabolic steroids have been used, sometimes in large doses, by male and female athletes to improve performance, esp. in events requiring strength. This use has been judged to be illegal by various organizations that supervise sports, including the International Olympic Committee and the U.S. Olympic Committee. SEE: *doping; ergonomic aids.*

Caution: Indiscriminate use of anabolic agents is inadvisable because of the undesirable side effects they may produce, particularly in women, in which case hirsutism, masculinization, and clitoral hypertrophy may occur.

anabolin (ă-năb′ō-lĭn). A product of anabolism. SYN: *anabolite.*

anabolism (ă-năb′ō-lĭzm) [Gr. *anabole,* a building up, + *-ismos,* condition]. The building up of the body substance; the constructive phase of metabolism by which a cell takes from the blood the substance required for repair and growth, building it into a cytoplasm, thus converting a nonliving material into the living cytoplasm of the cell. Opposite of catabolism, the destructive phase of metabolism.

   RS: assimilation; catabolism; metabolism; nutrition; synthesis.

anabolite (ă-năb′ō-līt″). Any product of anabolism. SYN: *anabolin.*

anacamptics (ăn″ă-kămp′tĭks) [Gr. *anakamptein,* to bend back]. Study of reflection of light or sound.

anacamptometer (ăn″ă-kămp-tŏm′ĕ-tĕr) [Gr. *ana,* up, + *kamptos,* bent, + *metron,* to measure]. Device for measuring intensity of deep reflexes.

anacatesthesia (ăn″ă-kăt″ĕs-thē′zē-ă) [" + " + *aisthesis,* sensation]. A sensation of hovering.

anacidity (ăn″ă-sĭd′ĭ-tē) [Gr. *an-,* not, + L. *acidum,* acid]. Abnormal deficiency of acidity, esp. of hydrochloric acid in the gastric juice.

anaclasis (ă-năk′lă-sĭs) [Gr. *anaklasis,* reflection]. 1. Refraction or reflection of light. 2. Refraction of light in the interior of the eye. 3. Reflex action. 4. Refraction for therapeutic reasons. 5. Forcible movement of a joint in order to treat fibrous ankylosis.

anaclitic (ăn″ă-klĭt′ĭk). Leaning or depending on. In psychoanalysis, pert. to the dependence of an infant on the mother figure for care.

anaclitic depression. SEE: *depression, anaclitic.*

anacrotic (ăn″ă-krŏt′ĭk) [Gr. *ana,* up, +

krotos, stroke]. 1. Ascending or vertical upstroke of a sphygmogram. 2. Pert. to a pulse with more than one expansion of the artery. 3. Pert. to two heartbeats traced on the ascending line of a sphygmogram. SYN: *anadicrotic*. SEE: *pulse*.

anacrotic pulse. Pulse in which one or more small waves occur on ascending limb of tracing of pulse waves, as in aortic stenosis.

anacrotism (ă-năk′rō-tĭzm). Existence of a double beat on ascending line of sphygmogram. SYN: *anadicrotism*.

anacusia, anacusis, anakusis (ăn-ă-kū′sē-ă, -sĭs) [Gr. *an-*, not, + *akouein*, to hear]. Total deafness.

anadicrotic (ăn″ă-dī-krŏt′ĭk) [Gr. *ana*, up, + *dikrotos*, double beating]. 1. Pert. to a pulse with more than one artery expansion. 2. Pert. to two beats on the ascending line of a sphygmogram. SYN: *anacrotic*.

anadicrotism (ăn-ă-dĭk′rō-tĭzm). Existence of a double beat on ascending line of the sphygmogram. SYN: *anacrotism*.

anadidymus (ăn″ă-dĭd′ĭ-mŭs) [″ + *didymos*, twin]. A developmental abnormality in which the lower extremities of two fetuses are joined together.

anadipsia (ăn″ă-dĭp′sē-ă) [Gr. *ana*, intensive, + *dipsa*, thirst]. Intense thirst.

anadrenalism (ăn″ă-drē′năl-ĭzm) [Gr. *an-*, not, + *adrenal* + Gr. *-ismos*, condition]. Failure of the adrenal gland to function.

anadromous [Gr. *anadromos*, running upward]. Descriptive of fish that migrate from sea water to fresh water. SEE: *sushi*.

anaerobe (ăn′ĕr-ōb) [Gr. *an-*, not, + *aer*, air, + *bios*, life]. A microorganism that can live and grow in the absence of oxygen.

 a., facultative. Organism that prefers an oxygen environment but is capable of living and growing in its absence.

 a., obligatory. Organism that can live and grow only in absence of oxygen.

anaerobic (ăn″ĕr-ō′bĭk). 1. Pert. to an anaerobe. 2. Able to live without oxygen.

anaerobic exercise. Exercise during which the energy needed is provided without utilization of inspired oxygen. This type of exercise is limited to short bursts of vigorous activity. SEE: *aerobic exercise*.

anaerobiosis (ăn″ĕr-ō-b-ō′sĭs) [″ + *aer*, air, + *bios*, life, + *osis*, condition]. 1. Life in an oxygen-free atmosphere. 2. Functioning of an organ or tissue in absence of free oxygen.

anagen (ăn′ă-jĕn) [Gr. *ana*, up, + *genesis*, generation, birth]. Growing stage of hair development. SEE: *catagen; telogen*.

anakatadidymus (ăn″ă-kăt″ă-dĭd′ĭ-mŭs) [Gr. *ana*, up, + *kala*, down, + *didymos*, twin]. A congenital anomaly in which twins

are separated above and below but joined at the trunk.

anakré [African term for big nose]. Goundou, q.v.

anal (ā′năl) [L. *analis*]. Rel. to the anus or outer rectal opening.

anal canal. The terminal portion of the large intestine, its external aperture being the anus. This includes the internal and external sphincter muscles of the anus. The canal remains closed except during defecation and passage of flatus. It is about 1½ inches (3.8 cm) long. SEE: illus.

anal continence plug. A disposable device inserted in the anal canal to prevent anorectal incontinence. It is useful in incontinence involving both liquid and solid fecal material.

analepsis (ăn″ă-lĕp′sĭs) [Gr. *analepsis*, a taking up]. Gaining strength after an illness. Restoration to health.

analeptic (ăn″ă-lĕp′tĭk) [Gr. *analeptikos*, restorative]. 1. A drug that stimulates the central nervous system. 2. A restorative agent.

anal erotism. Localization of libido in the anal region. SEE: *anal stage*.

analgesia (ăn-ăl-jē′zē-ă) [Gr. *an-*, not, + *algos*, pain]. Absence of normal sense of pain.

 a. algera, a. dolorosa. Spontaneous pain with loss of sensibility in a part.

 a., paretic. Complete analgesia of upper limb in conjunction with partial paralysis.

 a., patient-controlled. SEE: *patient-controlled analgesia*.

analgesic (ăn″ăl-jē′sĭk). 1. Relieving pain. 2. A drug that relieves pain. SYN: *analgetic*.

analgesic nephropathy. SEE: *nephritis, analgesic*.

analgetic (ăn″ăl-jĕt′ĭk). 1. Relieving pain. 2. A drug that relieves pain. SYN: *analgesic*.

analgia (ăn-ăl′jē-ă) [″ + *algos*, pain]. State of being without pain.

analgic (ăn-ăl′jĭk). Without pain.

anal incontinence. Failure of the anal sphincter to prevent involuntary expulsion of gas, liquid, or solids from the lower bowel.

analog, analogue (ăn′ă-lŏg) [Gr. *analogos*, analogy, proportion]. 1. One of two organs in different species that are similar in function but different in structure. 2. In chemistry, a compound that is structurally similar to another.

analogous (ă-năl′ō-gŭs). Similar in function but different in origin or structure.

analogy (ă-năl′ō-jē) [Gr. *analogos*, analogy, proportion]. 1. Likeness or similarity between two things that are otherwise unalike. 2. In biology, similarity in function, but difference in structure or origin. Opposite of homology.

anal personality. In Freudian psychology, a

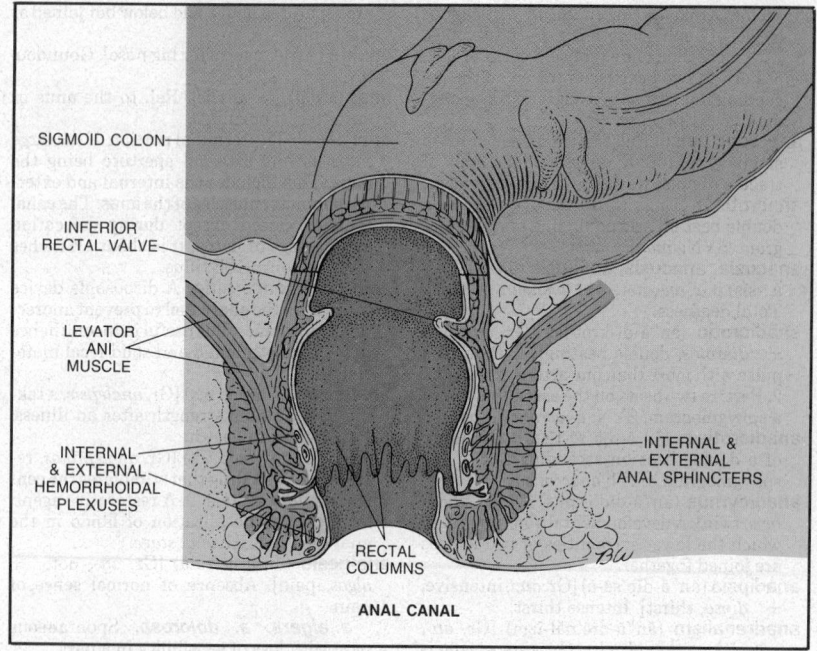

SIGMOID COLON

INFERIOR
RECTAL VALVE

LEVATOR
ANI
MUSCLE

INTERNAL
& EXTERNAL
HEMORRHOIDAL
PLEXUSES

INTERNAL &
EXTERNAL
ANAL SPHINCTERS

RECTAL
COLUMNS

ANAL CANAL

personality disorder characterized by excessive orderliness, stinginess, and obstinacy. If carried to an extreme, these qualities lead to the development of obsessive-compulsive type of behavior.

anal reflex. Contraction of anal sphincter following irritation of skin about anus. Reflex is lost in lesions of posterior columns of cord and is exaggerated in anal fissures.

anal stage. In Freudian psychology, the second phase of sexual development, from infancy to childhood, in which libido is concentrated in the anal region. In order of appearance, these phases are oral, anal, phallic, and genital.

analysand (ăn-ăl'ĭ-zănd). A patient who is being psychoanalyzed.

analysis (ă-năl'ĭ-sĭs) [LL. *ana,* up, back, + Gr. *lysis,* dissolution] (pl. *analyses*). 1. Separation of anything into its constituent parts. 2. In chemistry, determination of or separation into constituent parts of a substance or compound. 3. Treatment by a physician trained as a psychoanalyst.

    a., centrifugal. Any one of a group of devices used for chemical analysis that employs centrifugal force to quickly mix, transfer, and process a great number of samples.

    a., chromatographic. Analysis of substances on the basis of color reaction of the constituents as they are differentially absorbed on one of a variety of materials such as filter paper.

    a., cohort. The tabulation and analysis of morbidity or mortality rates in relation to the ages of a specific group of people (cohort), identified at a particular period of time and followed as they pass through different ages during part or all of their life span.

    a., colorimetric. Analysis by adsorption of a compound and the identification of its element by color.

    a., continuous-flow. A type of laboratory instrument that, prior to analyzing specimens, separates them by placing an air bubble between individual specimens as they are injected into a tube. Specimens are then analyzed as they flow along the tube.

    a., densimetric. Analysis by determination of the specific gravity (density) of a solution, and then estimation of the amount of solids.

    a., gastric. Analysis of the stomach contents to determine the concentration of free hydrochloric acid and combined (total) acid, presence or absence of lactic acid, presence or absence of occult blood, presence of pus, excessive mucus, and amount and types of bacteria.

a., qualitative. Determination of the nature of the elements in a substance.

a., quantitative. Determination of the quantity of each element in a substance.

a., spectrophotometric. Determination of materials in a compound by measuring amount of light they absorb in the infrared, visible, or ultraviolet regions of the spectrum.

a., volumetric. Quantitative analysis performed by the measurement of the volume of solutions or liquids.

analysis of variance. ABBR: ANOVA. A statistical technique for defining and segregating the causes of variability affecting a set of observations. Use of this technique provides a basis for analyzing the effects of various treatments or variables on the subjects or patients being investigated. In an experimental design in which several samples or groups are drawn from the same population, estimates of population variance between samples should differ from each other only by chance. ANOVA provides a method for testing the hypothesis that several random and independent samples are from a common, normal population.

analyst (ăn′ă-lĭst) [Fr. *analyse*, analysis]. 1. One who analyzes. 2. A practitioner of psychoanalysis. SYN: *psychoanalyst*.

analytic (ăn-ă-lĭt′ĭk) [Gr. *analytikos*]. Pert. to analysis.

analytical balance. A very sensitive scale used in chemical analysis.

analyze (ăn′ă-līz) [Fr. *analyse*, analysis]. To separate into parts or principles in order to determine the nature of the whole; examine methodically.

analyzer (ăn′ă-lī″zĕr). 1. Device used to determine the optical rotation produced when polarized light passes through a solution. 2. Any device that determines some characteristic of the object, chemical, or action being investigated. Thus there are devices for analyzing a voice; the breath for presence of certain chemicals such as alcohol; images; cells in a solution; and chemicals. SEE: *Breathalyzer*.

a., automated. A chemical instrument system designed to perform assays that were done, and may still be done, manually.

a., batch. A discrete automated chemical analyzer in which the instrument system sequentially performs a single test on each of a group of samples.

a., continuous flow. An automated chemical analyzer in which the samples and reagents are pumped continuously through a system of modules interconnected by tubing.

a., discrete. An automated chemical analyzer in which the instrument performs tests on samples that are kept in "discrete containers," in contrast to a continuous flow analyzer.

a., parallel. A discrete automated chemical analyzer which performs a single test on a group of samples, at practically the same time (actually, within milliseconds).

anamnesis (ăn″ăm-nē′sĭs) [Gr. *anamnesis*, recalling]. 1. Recollection; faculty of remembering. 2. That which is remembered. 3. The past medical history of a patient. SEE: *catamnesis*.

anamnestic (ăn″ăm-nĕs′tĭk). 1. Pert. to past medical history of patient. 2. Assisting the memory.

anamniotic [Gr. *an-*, not, + *amnion*, amnion]. Without an amnion.

anangioplasia (ăn-ăn″jē-ŏ-plā′sē-ă) [Gr. *an-*, not, + *angeion*, vessel, + *plassein*, to form]. Imperfect vascularization of a part.

anangioplastic (ăn-ăn″jē-ŏ-plăs′tĭk). Pert. to imperfect development of the vascular system.

anaphase (ăn′ă-fāz) [″ + *phainein*, to appear]. Stage in meiosis, q.v., and mitosis, q.v., between metaphase and telophase in which there is longitudinal bisection of chromosomes (the chromatids), which separate and move toward their respective poles.

anaphoresis (ăn″ă-fŏ-rē′sĭs) [″ + *phoresis*, bearing]. The flow of electropositive particles toward the anode (positive pole) in electrophoresis, q.v.

anaphoria (ăn″ă-for′ē-ă) [Gr. *ana*, up, + *phorein*, to carry]. Tendency of eyeballs to turn upward. SYN: *anatropia*.

anaphrodisia (ăn-ăf″rō-dĭz′ē-ă) [Gr. *an-*, not, + *aphrodisia*, sexual desire]. Diminished or absent desire for sex.

anaphrodisiac (ăn″ăf-rō-dĭz′ē-ăk). 1. Repressing sexual desire. 2. An agent that represses sexual desire.

anaphrodite (ăn-ăf′rō-dīt). Person with impairment or absence of sexual desire.

anaphylactia (ăn″ă-fĭ-lăk′shē-ă) [Gr. *ana*, up, + *phylaxis*, protection]. Anaphylaxis, q.v.

anaphylactic (ăn″ă-fĭ-lăk′tĭk). Pert. to or characterized by anaphylaxis, q.v.

anaphylactic shock. Systemic anaphylaxis that produces life-threatening changes in circulation and bronchioles consistent with shock, q.v. SEE: *allergy; anaphylaxis*.

SYM: Acute respiratory distress; hypotension; edema; rash; tachycardia; pale, cool skin; convulsions may be present; cyanosis.

If untreated, unconsciousness and death may be the outcome. Edema can be life-threatening if larynx is involved, since air flow is obstructed with even minimal swelling.

ETIOL: The result of a Type I, q.v., allergic or hypersensitivity reaction during which the allergen is absorbed into the blood directly or through the mucosa. Most common agents are contrast dyes used in diagnostic studies, and drugs. Chemical mediators released during the reaction cause constriction of the bronchial smooth muscle, vasodilation, and increased vascular permeability.

TREAT: Vasopressor agents, esp. epinephrine, antihistamines, corticosteroids; oxygen; I.V. fluids rapidly, if indicated. Epinephrine acts not only as a vasopressor but also to relax smooth muscles in the airway and to increase myocardial contractions. Endotracheal intubation and mechanical ventilation are often necessary.

PROG: Death may occur if emergency treatment is not given.

NURSING IMPLICATIONS: Careful assessment to determine if patient has any history of allergic reactions, particularly to drugs, blood, or contrast media. Close observation of patient at risk for reaction. Immediate emergency care at first sign of respiratory distress: establish an airway, provide oxygen, notify physician, and ensure epinephrine, corticosteroids, and other emergency drugs are readily available. Patients who are unable to avoid exposure to allergens should be certain they have emergency kits with them for treatment and that they know how to use the kits. Patients who have had any anaphylactic reaction should wear a Medic Alert tag.

anaphylactogenesis (ăn″ă-fī-lăk′tō-jĕn′ĕ-sĭs). The process of producing anaphylaxis.

anaphylactogenic (ăn″ă-fī-lăk′tō-jĕn′ĭk). 1. Producing anaphylaxis. 2. The agent producing anaphylactic reactions.

anaphylatoxin (ăn″ă-fī-lă-tŏk′sĭn). A substance composed of the C3 and C5 components of complement, q.v., that cause vasoactive mediators to be released from mast cells, promoting increased vascular permeability and the formation of edema during an anaphylactic reaction.

anaphylaxis (ăn″ă-fī-lăk′sĭs) [″ + phylaxis, protection]. One form of a Type I allergic or hypersensitivity reaction to an allergenic antigen, q.v., mediated by interactions between mast cells and immunoglobulin E (IgE), q.v., that produce the antigen-antibody reaction. SEE: anaphylactic shock.

a., active. Anaphylaxis resulting from injection of an antigen.

a., exercise-induced. Onset of anaphylaxis during exercise. It is more common in women than men. The cause is unknown. Treatment is that of anaphylaxis associated with an allergen.

a., heterologous. Passive anaphylaxis by transfer of serum from an animal of a different species.

a., homologous. Passive anaphylaxis by transfer of serum from an animal of the same species.

a., local. Local inflammatory reaction following repeated injections of antigenic material. Includes allergic rhinitis to animal dander or pollen, hives, and angioneurotic edema in which fluid accumulates in the eyelids, hands, and lips. SYN: Arthus reaction.

a., passive. Anaphylaxis induced by injection of serum from a sensitized animal into a normal one. After a few hours the latter becomes sensitized.

a., passive cutaneous. ABBR: PCA. A laboratory test of antibody levels in which serum from a sensitized individual is injected into the skin. Intravenous injection of an antigen accompanied by Evans blue dye at a later time reacts with the antibodies produced in response to the antigen, creating a wheal and blue spot at the site, indicating local anaphylaxis.

a., systemic. Involves systemic release of histamine and other chemical mediators, leading to respiratory and vascular changes that can result in life-threatening anaphylactic shock. SEE: allergy; anaphylactic shock.

anaplasia (ăn″ă-plā′zē-ă) [″ + plassein, to form]. Loss of cellular differentiation and function, characteristic of most malignancies.

anaplastic (ăn″ă-plăs′tĭk) [″ + plassein, to form]. Pert. to anaplasia.

anapnea (ăn″ăp-nē′ă) [Gr. anapnein, to breathe again]. 1. Respiration. 2. Regaining the breath.

anapneic (ăn″ăp-nē′ĭk). Pert. to anapnea or relieving dyspnea.

anapophysis (ăn″ă-pŏf′ĭ-sĭs) [Gr. ana, back, + apophysis, offshoot]. An accessory spinal process of a vertebra, esp. thoracic or lumbar vertebrae.

anarthria (ăn-ăr′thrē-ă) [Gr. an-, not, + arthron, joint]. Loss of motor power to speak distinctly. May be a result of a neural lesion or a muscular defect.

a. literalis. Stammering.

anasarca (ăn″ă-săr′kă) [Gr. ana, through, + sarkos, flesh]. Severe generalized edema, q.v. SYN: dropsy.

anasarcous (ăn″ă-săr′kŭs). Edematous.

anaspadias (ăn″ă-spā′dē-ăs) [″ + spadon,

a rent]. Congenital opening of urethra on dorsum of penis; or opening by separation of the labia minora and a fissure of the clitoris. SYN: *epispadias*.

anastole (ăn-ăs′tō-lē) [Gr.]. Shrinking away or retraction of the edges of a wound.

anastomose (ă-năs′tō-mōs) [Gr. *anastomosis*, opening]. 1. To communicate directly or by means of connecting two parts together, esp. nerves or blood vessels. 2. To make such a connection surgically.

anastomosis (ă-năs″tō-mō′sĭs) [Gr., opening] (pl. *anastomoses*). 1. A natural communication between two vessels; may be direct or by means of connecting channels. 2. The surgical or pathological connection of two tubular structures.

a., antiperistaltic. Anastomosis between two parts of the intestine such that the peristaltic flow in one part is opposite of that in the other.

a., arteriovenous. Anastomosis between an artery and a vein by which the capillary bed is bypassed.

a., crucial. An arterial anastomosis on the back of the thigh, formed by the medial femoral circumflex, inferior gluteal, lateral femoral circumflex, and first perforating arteries.

a., end-to-end. Anastomosis in which the ends of two structures are joined.

a., Galen′s. Anastomosis between the superior and inferior laryngeal nerves.

a., heterocladic. Anastomosis between branches of different arteries.

a., homocladic. Anastomosis between branches of the same artery.

a., Hyrtl′s. An occasional looplike anastomosis between right and left hypoglossal nerves in geniohyoid muscle.

a., intestinal. Surgical connection of two portions of the intestines. SYN: *enteroenterostomy*.

a., isoperistaltic. Anastomosis between two parts of the intestine such that the peristaltic flow in both parts is in the same direction.

a., precapillary. Anastomosis between small arteries just before they become capillaries.

a., Schmiedel′s. Abnormal communications between the vena cava and the portal system.

a., side-to-side. Anastomosis between two structures lying or positioned beside each other.

a., terminoterminal. Anastomosis between the peripheral end of an artery and the central end of the corresponding vein; and between the central end of the artery and peripheral end of the vein.

a., ureterotubal. Anastomosis between the ureter and the fallopian tube.

a., ureteroureteral. Anastomosis between two parts of the same ureter.

anastomotic (ă-năs″tō-mŏt′ĭk). Pert. to, or marked by, anastomosis.

anatomic (ăn″ă-tŏm′ĭk) [Gr. *anatome*, dissection]. Rel. to the anatomy or structure of an organism.

anatomical snuffbox. Snuffbox, anatomical, q.v.

anatomist (ă-năt′ō-mĭst). A specialist in the field of anatomy.

anatomy (ă-năt′ō-mē) [Gr. *anatome*, dissection]. 1. The structure of an organism. 2. The branch of science dealing with the structure of organisms. 3. Dissection or cutting apart.

a., applied. Application of anatomy to diagnosis and treatment, esp. surgical treatment.

a., comparative. Comparison of homologous structures of different animals.

a., descriptive. Description of individual parts of the body. SYN: *a., systematic*.

a., developmental. Embryology of the organism from the time of egg fertilization until adulthood is attained.

a., gross. Study of structures able to be seen with the naked eye. SYN: *a., macroscopic*.

a., macroscopic. A., gross, q.v.

a., microscopic. Study of structure by use of a microscope. SYN: *histology*.

a., morbid. Study of anatomical changes that occur in diseased tissues. SYN: *a., pathological*.

a., pathological. Study of the structure of abnormal, diseased, or injured tissue.

a., radiological. Anatomical investigation based on the radiological appearance of tissues and organs.

a., surface. Study of form and markings of the surface of the body, esp. as they relate to underlying tissues and organs.

a., systematic. A., descriptive, q.v.

a., topographic. Study of the structure and form of a portion of the body with particular emphasis on the relationships of the parts to each other.

a., x-ray. A., radiological, q.v.

anatoxic (ăn″ă-tŏks′ĭk) [Gr. *ana*, backward, + *toxikon*, poison]. Pert. to anatoxin.

anatoxin (ăn″ă-tŏks′ĭn). A toxin, q.v., that has been treated to destroy its toxicity but is still capable of inducing antibody formation on injection. SYN: *toxoid*.

anatricrotic (ăn″ă-trī-krŏt′ĭk) [Gr. *ana*, up, + *tresis*, three, + *krotos*, stroke]. Pert. to three beats on the ascending line of a sphygmogram.

anatricrotism (ăn″ă-trĭk′rō-tĭzm). Existence of three beats on the ascending line of a sphygmogram.

anatripsis (ăn″ă-trĭp′sĭs) [″ + *tripsis,* friction]. Therapeutic use of rubbing or friction massage.

anatriptic (ăn″ă-trĭp′tĭk) [″ + *tripsis,* friction]. 1. Pert to anatripsis. 2. An agent applied by rubbing.

anatropia (ăn″ă-trō′pē-ă) [″ + *trope,* a turning]. Tendency of eyeballs to turn upward. SYN: *anaphoria.*

Anavar. Trade name for oxandrolone, q.v.

anaxon(e) (ăn-ăk′sŏn) [Gr. *an-,* not, + *axon,* axis]. A nerve cell, as of the retina, having no axon.

A.N.C. *Army Nurse Corps.*

AnCC. *anodal closure contraction.*

anchor (ăng′ker) [Gr. *ankyra,* anchor]. A metal implant placed within alveolar bone to provide retention for a tooth crown, bridge, or denture anchorage.

anchorage (ăng′kĕr-ĭj). 1. Surgical fixation, as of prolapsed abdominal organs. 2. The part to which anything is fixed, as a tooth to which a bridge is fastened.

anchors. Various types of attachments for orthodontic tooth movement.

ancillary (ăn′sĭl-lār″ē) [L. *ancillaris,* handmaid]. Something that assists another action or effect but is not essential to the accomplishment of the action.

Ancobon. Trade name for flucytosine, q.v.

anconad (ăn′kō-năd) [Gr. *ankon,* elbow, + L. *ad,* to]. Toward the elbow.

anconagra (ăn″kŏn-ăg′ră) [″ + *agra,* a seizure]. Gout of the elbow.

anconal, anconeal (ăn′kō-năl, ăn-kō′nē-ăl). Pert. to the elbow.

anconal fossa, anconeal fossa. Fossa olecrani; the hollow on the distal end of the humerus in which the olecranon rests when the elbow is extended.

anconeus (ăn-kō′nē-ŭs) [Gr. *ankon,* elbow]. Short extensor muscle of forearm located on the back of the elbow. It arises from the back portion of the lateral epicondyle of the humerus, and its fibers insert on side of the olecranon and upper fourth of shaft of ulna. Extends forearm and abducts ulna in pronation of the wrist.

anconitis (ăn″kō-nī′tĭs) [″ + *itis,* inflammation]. Inflammation of the elbow joint.

ancrod. An enzyme purified from venom of a Malayan pit viper; used because of its anticoagulant effect. It may be as safe as heparin.

Ancylostoma (ăn″sĭl-ŏs′tō-mă) [Gr. *ankylos,* crooked, + *stoma,* mouth]. A genus of nematodes of the family Ancylostomatidae whose members are intestinal parasites and include the hookworms.

   A. braziliense. Species of hookworm infesting dogs and cats; may cause cutaneous larva migrans in man. SEE: *larva migrans, cutaneous.*

   A. caninum. Species of hookworm infesting dogs and cats; may cause cutaneous larva migrans in man. SEE: *larva migrans, cutaneous.*

   A. duodenale. Species of hookworm widely distributed in temperate regions. Commonly infests man, causing ancylostomiasis, q.v. SEE: *Necator americanus.*

Ancylostomatidae (ăn″sĭ-lŏs″tō-măt′ĭ-dē). A family of nematodes belonging to the suborder Strongylata. It includes the genera *Ancylostoma* and *Necator,* common hookworms of man.

ancylostomiasis (ăn″sĭ-lŏs-tō-mī′ă-sĭs) [Gr. *ankylos,* crooked, + *stoma,* mouth, + *-iasis,* condition]. Hookworm infestation, esp. *Ancylostoma duodenale* or *Necator americanus.* Common in tropical and semitropical areas where the effects of climate and poor sanitation bring the larvae in contact with bare skin, usually of the foot. Feces of infected individuals are the source of infection.

   The hookworm eggs hatch, and the larvae enter through the host's skin, causing inflammation, itching, and sometimes allergic reactions. They pass from the skin to the venous circulation to the lungs, where they migrate to the respiratory tree. If larvae are numerous, they may cause an eosinophilic pneumonia. Larvae travel up the bronchi and are finally swallowed, thus gaining entry to the intestinal tract. Larvae mature in the intestines, where they attach to the mucous membrane and suck blood from the host. The larvae secrete an anticoagulant that causes additional bleeding. They may cause nausea, colicky pains, and diarrhea. Loss of blood leads to anemia. In children, normal mental and physical growth is retarded. If untreated, larvae may live in the intestinal tract for as long as 30 years. However, most individuals lose the infection within 2 years. SYN: *hookworm disease.*

   TREAT: In severe cases it may be necessary to treat the severe anemia prior to ridding the patient of the parasites. Mebendazole and pyrantel pamoate are the drugs of choice for *Necator* and *Ancylostoma* infections. The latter has the advantage of single-dose administration. Nutritional supplementation including iron will be needed when anemia is severe. In some severe cases in children, blood transfusion may be needed.

ancyroid (ăn′sĭ-royd) [Gr. *ankyra,* anchor, + *eidos,* form, shape]. Shaped like the fluke of an anchor.

Andernach's ossicles (ŏn′dĕr-nŏks) [Johann Winther von Andernach, Ger. physician, 1487–1574]. Ossa suturarum; small bones found in cranial sutures. SYN: *wormian bones; sutural bones.*

Andersen's disease [Dorothy H. Andersen, U.S. pediatrician, 1901–1963]. Glycogen storage disease, type IV. SEE: *glycogen storage disease.*

Andral's decubitus (ăn'drăls) [Gabriel Andral, Fr. physician, 1797–1876]. Position assumed by patient lying on sound side during beginning stages of pleurisy.

andriatrics (ăn"drē-ăt'rĭks) [Gr. *andros,* man, + *iatreia,* medical treatment]. Study of diseases of men, esp. of male genital organs. SYN: *andrology.*

andro- [Gr. *andros,* man]. A prefix signifying man, male, or masculine.

androgalactozemia (ăn"drō-găl-ăk"tō-zē'mē-ă) [" + *gala,* milk, + *zemia,* loss]. Oozing of milk from a man's breast.

androgen (ăn'drō-jĕn) [Gr. *andros,* man, + *gennan,* to produce]. Substance producing or stimulating the development of male characteristics (masculinization), such as the hormones testosterone and androsterone, q.v.

androgenic (ăn"drō-jĕn'ĭk). Causing masculinization. SYN: *andromimetic.*

androgyne (ăn'drō-jīn) [" + *gyne,* woman]. A female pseudohermaphrodite. SYN: *androgynus.*

androgynoid (ăn-drŏj'ĭ-noyd) [" + " + *eidos,* form, shape]. A person possessing female gonads (ovaries) but secondary sex characteristics of a male (a female pseudohermaphrodite). Term is less commonly used for a person possessing male gonads (testes) but secondary sex characteristics of a female (a male pseudohermaphrodite).

androgynous (ăn-drŏj'ĭ-nŭs) [" + *gyne,* woman]. 1. Resembling or pert. to an androgynoid, q.v. 2. Without definite sexual characteristics.

androgynus (ăn-drŏj'ĭ-nŭs). A female pseudohermaphrodite. SYN: *androgyne.*

android (ăn'droyd) [" + *eidos,* form, shape]. Resembling a male; manlike.

andrology (ăn-drŏl'ō-jē) [" + *logos,* word, reason]. Study of diseases of men, esp. of the male genital organs. SYN: *andriatrics.*

andromimetic (ăn"drō-mĭ-mĕt'ĭk) [" + *mimetikos,* imitative]. Causing masculinization. SYN: *androgenic.*

andromorphous (ăn"drō-mor'fŭs) [" + *morphe,* form]. Resembling a male in physical structure and appearance.

andropathy (ăn-drŏp'ă-thē) [" + *pathos,* disease, suffering]. Any disease peculiar to the male.

androphilic (ăn"drō-fīl-ĭk) [" + *philos,* fond of]. Preferring humans; said of certain parasites.

androphobia (ăn"drō-fō'bē-ă) [" + *phobos,* fear]. Morbid fear of the male sex.

androstane (ăn'drō-stān). $C_{19}H_{32}$. A steroid hydrocarbon that is the precursor of androgenic hormones.

androsterone (ăn"drō-stēr'ōn, ăn-drŏs'tĕr-ōn). $C_{19}H_{30}O_2$. An androgenic steroid found in the urine. It is a metabolite of testosterone and androstenedione. It has been synthesized. As one of the androgens (male sex hormones), androsterone contributes to the characteristic changes of growth and development of the genitals and axillary and pubic hair, deepening of the voice, and development of the sweat glands in the male.

-ane. In chemistry, indicates a saturated hydrocarbon.

anecdotal evidence (ăn"ĭk-dōt'l) [Gr. *an,* not, + *ekdotos,* given out]. Evidence presented to support a scientific argument. It is of limited benefit because of being based on hearsay evidence rather than a systematic collection of data.

anecdotal records. Notes used in nursing education to document observed incidents of a student's clinical behavior related to attainment of clinical learning objectives. Such anecdotal notes have been upheld in court as documented evidence for failing a student; the notes have not been treated as hearsay evidence.

anechoic room. A room in which the boundaries are made so that all sound produced in the room is absorbed; i.e., not reflected.

Anectine. Trade name for succinylcholine chloride, q.v.

anelectrotonus (ăn"ĕl-ĕk-trŏt'ō-nŭs) [Gr. *ana,* up, + *elektron,* amber, + *tonos,* tension]. The state of diminished irritability of a nerve or muscle in region near the anode during the passage of an electric current.

Anel's operation (ă-nĕlz') [Dominique Anel, Fr. surgeon, 1679–1725]. Ligation of an artery immediately above and on proximal side of an aneurysm.

Anel's probe. A probe for the lacrimal and nasal ducts.

anemia (ă-nē'mē-ă) [Gr. *an-,* not, + *haima,* blood]. A reduction in the number of circulating red blood cells per cu mm, the amount of hemoglobin per 100 ml, or the volume of packed red cells per 100 ml of blood. It exists when hemoglobin content is less than that required to provide the oxygen demands of the body. Because variables such as lifestyle, residential altitude, age, and sex can influence red cell and hemoglobin concentration, it is not possible to state that anemia exists when the hemoglobin is less than a specific value. If the onset of anemia is slow, the body may adjust so well that there will be no functional impairment even though the hemoglobin may be less than 6 gm/100 ml of blood.

Anemia is not a disease; it is a symptom of various diseases. Anemia is classified on the basis of mean corpuscular volume (MCV) as microcytic (<80), normocytic (80–94), and macrocytic (>94); on the basis of mean corpuscular hemoglobin (MCH) as hypochromic (<27), normochromic (27–32), and hyperchromic (>32); and by etiological factors.

SYM: Pallor of skin, fingernail beds, and mucous membranes; weakness; vertigo; headache; sore tongue; drowsiness; general malaise; dyspnea; tachycardia; palpitation; angina pectoris; gastrointestinal disturbances; amenorrhea; loss of libido; slight fever.

ETIOL: Anemia may result from excessive blood loss, excessive blood cell destruction, or decreased blood cell formation. Anemia due to excessive blood loss results from acute or chronic hemorrhage. Anemia due to excessive blood cell destruction occurs in hemolytic diseases or hypersplenism. Anemia due to decreased blood formation may result from defective nucleoprotein synthesis (as in pernicious and other macrocytic anemias); deficiency of iron in the diet; inhibition of bone marrow (as in certain toxic states); loss of bone marrow; or bone marrow failure. SEE: *anemia of chronic disease; anemia, iron deficiency.*

TREAT: Treatment of anemia must be specific for the cause.

Anemia due to excessive blood loss: Acute blood loss: immediate measures to stop bleeding; restoration of blood volume by transfusion; measures to combat shock. Chronic blood loss: usually produces iron-deficiency anemia, q.v.

Anemia due to excessive blood cell destruction: Treatment of specific hemolytic disorder.

Anemia due to decreased blood cell formation: Deficiency states: replacement therapy to combat the specific deficiency; e.g., iron, vitamin B_{12}, folic acid, ascorbic acid. Disorders of bone marrow: if anemia is due to toxic state, removal of toxic agent may result in spontaneous recovery. SEE: *blood transfusion.*

NURSING IMPLICATIONS: Evaluate patient for signs and symptoms related to blood loss, inadequate erythropoiesis, or premature erythrocyte destruction. Carry out ordered diagnostic tests.

Rest: Assess patient for fatigue, and plan care and activity accordingly. Adjust the patient's activities of daily living according to their tolerance.

Mouth care: Evaluate patient daily for development of mouth lesions or ulcers. Alkaline mouthwashes are beneficial for patients who develop mouth ulcers; a sponge stick may be utilized instead of a toothbrush. Dental consultation may be required.

Diet: Encourage patients to eat by providing small portions of food of their preference. If the patient has mouth lesions, oral hygiene done before meals may help to increase appetite. In addition, provide appropriate nutritional counseling for the patient's individual dietary needs.

Medications: Teach the patient about the reasons for the medications, possible side effects, and correct dosage and administration of the medication. Patients receiving iron therapy should be aware that their stools will become black and that the medicine may cause constipation.

Patient education: Insure that the patient and family understand the cause of the anemia and the rationale behind the prescribed treatment. Teaching should also include the importance of following the prescribed rest and activity regimen, the prescribed diet, taking prescribed medications, prevention of infection, taking temperature regularly, and continuing with periodic blood tests and medical evaluations. SEE: *Nursing Diagnoses* in *Appendix.*

a., achlorhydric. A hypochromic, microcytic anemia associated with a lack of free hydrochloric acid in gastric juice.

a., addisonian. A., pernicious, q.v.

a., aplastic. Anemia caused by aplasia of bone marrow or its destruction by chemical agents (benzene, arsenic, nitrogen mustards) or physical factors (x-rays and other sources of ionizing radiation). An idiopathic form may occur.

a., blind loop. Megaloblastic anemia due to a blind loop or multiple diverticulosis of the jejunum, which becomes infected with bacteria. These organisms destroy vitamin B_{12}, thus causing anemia. May be treated surgically by removing diverticuli or blind loops or administering vitamin B_{12} and antibiotics. SEE: *a., megaloblastic.*

a., chlorotic. A microcytic, hypochromic anemia occurring in adolescent girls and young women, usually associated with dietary deficiency of iron and protein. SYN: *chlorosis; green sickness.* SEE: *a., iron-deficiency.*

a., congenital hemolytic. Inherited chronic disease characterized by hemolysis of blood cells, jaundice, and splenomegaly. SYN: *icterus, hemolytic; jaundice, hemolytic.*

a., Cooley's. Anemia resulting from inheritance of a recessive trait responsible for interference with hemoglobin synthesis. SYN: *thalassemia major,* q.v.; *a., erythroblastic.*

a., deficiency. Condition resulting from lack of an essential ingredient, such as iron or vitamins, in the diet or the inability of the intestine to absorb them. SYN: *a., nutritional.*

a., drepanocytic. A., sickle cell, q.v.

a., erythroblastic. Anemia resulting from inheritance of a recessive trait responsible for interference with hemoglobin synthesis. SYN: *thalassemia major,* q.v.; *Cooley's anemia.*

a., hemolytic. Anemia resulting from hemolysis of red blood cells. Is either acquired, as from the effects of toxic agents, congenital (familial), or from severe preeclampsia. SEE: *hemolytic uremic syndrome.*

a., hyperchromic. Anemia in which mean corpuscular hemoglobin concentration (MCHC) is greater than normal. The red blood cells are darker staining than normal.

a., hypersplenic. Condition resulting from excessive destruction of red blood cells in the spleen.

a., hypochromic. Anemia in which there is a hemoglobin deficiency and mean corpuscular hemoglobin concentration is less than normal.

a., hypoplastic. Term that has been used to describe aplastic anemia. If anemia due to failure of formation of red blood cells is meant, pure red blood cell aplasia is the term of choice.

a., iron-deficiency. Anemia resulting from a greater demand on the stored iron than can be supplied.

ETIOL: Inadequate iron intake, malabsorption of iron, chronic blood loss, pregnancy and lactation, intravascular hemolysis, or a combination of these factors.

Usually successfully treated with oral ferrous sulfate or ferrous gluconate and a well-balanced diet. Iron-deficiency anemia is probably the most common chronic disease of mankind. It is estimated that at least 18,000,000 people in the U.S. are iron deficient.

a., Jaksch's. Infantile pseudoleukemia; enlargement of spleen and lymph nodes accompanied by progressive anemia without leukemic changes in the blood.

a., macrocytic. Anemia marked by abnormally large erythrocytes.

a., Mediterranean. SEE: *thalassemia.*

a., megaloblastic. Anemia in which megaloblasts are found in the blood.

a., microcytic. Anemia with abnormally small erythrocytes.

a., myelopathic. Anemia caused by disruption, usually by metastasis, in bone marrow function.

a., normochromic. Anemia in which the red blood cells contain the normal amount of hemoglobin.

a., normocytic. Anemia in which size and hemoglobin content of red blood cells remain normal.

a., nutritional. A., deficiency, q.v.

a. of chronic disease. A misnomer in that chronic diseases, esp. those involving infection, are frequently associated with anemia, but many chronic diseases not related to inflammation are not associated with anemia. A more appropriate term would be anemia of chronic inflammation.

a., pernicious. A chronic, macrocytic anemia characterized by achlorhydria. Occurs most commonly in 40- to 80-year-old northern Europeans of fair complexion. It has, however, been reported in other races and ethnic groups. The disease is rare in blacks and Asians. SYN: *addisonian anemia.*

SYM: Weakness, sore tongue, paresthesias (tingling and numbness) of extremities, and gastrointestinal symptoms such as diarrhea, nausea, vomiting, pain; signs of cardiac failure may be present in severe anemia.

ETIOL: Failure of the stomach to secrete enough intrinsic factor to ensure intestinal absorption of vitamin B_{12}, the extrinsic factor. This is due to atrophy of the glandular mucosa of the fundus of the stomach and is associated with absence of hydrochloric acid.

TREAT: Intramuscular injection of vitamin B_{12}.

a., pure red cell aplasia. Anemia due to decreased production of red cells.

a., septic. Anemia due to severe infection.

a., sickle cell. A hereditary, chronic, hemolytic anemia characterized by presence of large numbers of crescent- or sickle-shaped red blood cells in the blood. Occurs almost exclusively in blacks. Due to a defect in the hemoglobin molecule. SYN: *a., crescent cell; a., drepanocytic.* SEE: *sickle cell anemia; sickle cell crisis.* SEE: *Nursing Diagnoses* in *Appendix.*

a., splenic. Enlargement of spleen due to portal or splenic hypertension with accompanying anemia, leukopenia, thrombocytopenia, and gastric hemorrhage. SYN: *Banti's syndrome; splenomegaly, congestive.*

a., traumatic cardiac hemolytic. Anemia caused by the rupture of the red blood cell membrane in patients who have had intracardiac plastic surgery involving placement of a prosthesis. Seen esp. in those whose aortic valve has been replaced.

anemic (ă-nē'mĭk). Pert. to anemia; deficient in red blood cells, in hemoglobin, or in volume of blood.

anemic hypoxia. Inadequate oxygenation due to reduction in amount or capability of hemoglobin to transport oxygen.

anemometer. In pulmonary function studies, a device for measuring the rate of flow of air through a tube. The rate that air flows into or out of the lung may be measured by using a calibrated anemometer.

anemophobia (ăn″ĕ-mō-fō'bē-ă) [Gr. *anemos,* wind, + *phobos,* fear]. Morbid fear of drafts or of the wind.

anencephalus (ăn″ĕn-sĕf'ă-lŭs) [Gr. *an-,* not, + *enkephalos,* the brain]. Congenital absence of brain and cranial vault, with the cerebral hemispheres completely missing or reduced to small masses. A condition that is incompatible with life.

anephrogenesis (ă-nĕf″rō-jĕn'ĕ-sĭs) [Gr. *a-,* not, + *nephros,* kidney, + *genesis,* generation, birth]. Congenital lack of kidneys.

anergasia (ăn″ĕr-gā'sē-ă) [Gr. *an-,* not + *ergon,* work]. Anergia; functional inactivity resulting from a structural lesion of the central nervous system.

anergastic reaction (ăn″ĕr-găs'tĭk). Disorder involving cerebral lesions or organic psychoses. Loss of memory and impairment of mental activity, function, or judgment.

anergia (ăn-ĕr'jē-ă) [″ + *ergon,* work]. Inactivity; lack of energy.

anergic (ăn-ĕr'jĭk). Sluggish; inactive. Deficient in energy; listless. SEE: *anergy.*

anergic stupor. Acute phase of dementia.

anergy (ăn'ĕr-jē). 1. Impaired or absent ability to react to common antigens administered through skin testing. 2. Lack of energy.

aneroid (ăn'ĕr-ŏyd) [Gr. *a-,* not, + *neron,* water, + *eidos,* form, shape]. Operating without a fluid, as an aneroid barometer that utilizes atmospheric pressure instead of a liquid, such as mercury.

anerythroplasia (ăn″ĕ-rĭth″rō-plā'zē-ă) [Gr. *an-,* not, + *erythros,* red, + *plasis,* a molding]. Absence of red blood cell formation in the bone marrow.

anerythroplastic (ăn″ĕ-rĭth″rō-plăs'tĭk). Rel. to or characterized by anerythroplasia.

anerythropsia (ăn″ĕ-rĭ-thrŏp'sē-ă) [″ + ″ + *opsis,* vision]. Inability to distinguish clearly the color red.

anesthecinesia, anesthekinesia (ăn-ĕs-thē″sĭn-ē'zē-ă, -kĭ-nē'zē-ă) [″ + *aisthesis,* sensation, + *kinesis,* movement]. Sensory and motor paralysis.

anesthesia (ăn″ĕs-thē'zē-ă) [″ + *aisthesis,* sensation]. Partial or complete loss of sensation with or without loss of consciousness as result of disease, injury, or administration of an anesthetic agent, usually by injection or inhalation.

STAGES: The first stage of pharmacologically induced general anesthesia includes preliminary excitement until voluntary control is lost. Because hearing is the last sense to be lost, content of conversation of operating room staff should be guarded during this stage. The second stage consists of loss of voluntary control. In the third stage there is entire relaxation, no muscular rigidity, and deep regular breathing.

SIGNS: The signs of depth of anesthesia, based on pupillary size, eye motion, and the character of respirations as originally described for ether, have been found to be unreliable and poorly correlated with the alveolar concentration of anesthetic. The types of medicines used for premedication as well as the type of anesthetic employed will influence the signs of anesthesia.

EMERGENCY MEASURES: Artificial respiration by anesthetist, injection of cardiac stimulant, inhalation of oxygen, injection of epinephrine into heart muscle. SEE: *cardiopulmonary resuscitation.*

a., audio. Anesthesia produced by sound; used by dentists to inhibit pain perception.

a., basal. 1. A level of unconsciousness that is just above the level of complete surgical anesthesia. The patient does not respond to verbal stimuli but does react to noxious stimuli, such as a pinprick. Basal anesthesia is useful in combination with local or regional anesthesia, making the patient unaware of the surgical experience. Commonly used in foot and hand surgery. 2. An anesthetic state of insensitivity produced by the administration of potent sedatives alone. 3. Any type of anesthetic state in which the patient is completely unconscious.

NURSING IMPLICATIONS: During emergence from general anesthesia, guard airway and monitor vital signs. Evaluate level of consciousness, status of protective reflexes, motor activity, and emotional state. Reorient patient to person, place, and time, repeating as necessary. Provide quiet area for patients who have received ketamine. For regional anesthesia, evaluate for sympathetic blockade by monitoring sensory response along with vital signs. Block will wear off from head to toe. Indications of sympathetic innervation return include stable vital signs and temperature, ability to vasoconstrict, perianal pinprick sensations, ability to plantar flex the foot against resistance, and ability to determine whether great toe is flexed or extended without seeing movement or position.

a., block. Regional anesthesia resulting from nerve blocking by injection of alcohol or other substance into or very near a nerve trunk. SYN: *a., conduction; a., neural.*

a., bulbar. Anesthesia produced by a lesion of the pons.

a., caudal. Anesthesia produced by insertion of a needle into sacrococcygeal notch and injection of local anesthetic into the epidural space.

a., central. Pathologic anesthesia due to a lesion of the central nervous system.

a., closed. Inhalation anesthesia technique in which the gases are rebreathed. This requires appropriate treatment of the exhaled gas in order to absorb the expired carbon dioxide and to replenish the oxygen and anesthetic gas or gases.

a., conduction. A., block, q.v.; a., neural, q.v.

a., crossed. Anesthesia of the side opposite to the site of the lesion.

a., dissociative. A type of anesthesia characterized by catalepsy, amnesia, and marked analgesia. The patient experiences a strong feeling of dissociation from the environment.

a. dolorosa. Pain in an anesthetized zone, as in thalamic lesions.

a., electric. Anesthesia induced by the use of an electric current.

a., endotracheal. Production of anesthesia by administering the inhaled gas via a tube that is passed through the trachea.

a., epidural. Anesthesia produced by injecting a local anesthetic agent into the peridural space of the spinal cord. SYN: *peridural anesthesia.*

a., frost. A., ice, q.v.

a., general. Anesthesia that is complete and affecting the entire body with loss of consciousness when the anesthetic acts upon the brain. This type of anesthesia is usually accomplished following administration of inhalation or intravenous anesthetics. Commonly used for surgical procedures.

a., Gwathmey's. Anesthesia induced by injecting an olive oil and ether solution into the rectum.

a., hypotensive. Anesthesia during which the blood pressure is lowered.

a., hypothermic. General anesthesia during which the body temperature is lowered.

a., hysterical. Bodily anesthesia occurring in hysteria.

a., ice. Local anesthesia produced by cooling the area. This can be accomplished by applying ice to the area or by applying a volatile liquid such as ethyl chloride to the area. SYN: *a., frost.*

a., infiltration. Local anesthesia produced by injecting the local anesthetic solution directly into the tissues, such as injection of procaine solution into the gums for dental procedures.

a., inhalation. General anesthesia produced by inhaling vapor or gas anesthetics such as ether, nitrous oxide, and methoxyflurane.

a., insufflation. Instillation of gaseous anesthetic materials into the inhaled air.

a., local. Anesthesia affecting a local area only, the anesthetic acting upon nerves or nerve tracts. Local anesthesia to facilitate placing a needle in the skin, i.e., as in a hypodermic injection, may be accomplished by applying an ice cube to the site for 10–30 seconds just prior to the needle stick. This affords anesthesia for a few seconds. A much longer period of anesthesia is produced by subcutaneous injection of bacteriostatic saline solution with benzyl alcohol. The anesthesia lasts for 2–5 minutes, providing sufficient time to allow surgical removal of skin tags, warts, and non-melanotic moles. SEE: *a., block; a., infiltration.*

a., mixed. General anesthesia produced by more than one drug, as nitrous oxide gas for induction followed by ether for maintenance of anesthesia.

a., neural. Injection of an anesthetic into a nerve or immediately around it (intraneural and paraneural). SYN: *a., block; a., conduction.*

a., neuroleptic. General anesthesia produced by the use of a neuroleptic agent such as droperidol, a narcotic analgesic, and nitrous oxide.

a., open. Application, usually by dropping, of a volatile anesthetic agent onto a gauze held over the nose and mouth.

a., peripheral. Local anesthesia produced by blocking a nerve with an appropriate agent.

a., primary. First stage of anesthesia, q.v., before unconsciousness.

a., pudendal. A type of local anesthesia used in obstetrics. The pudendal nerve on each side, near the spinous process of the ischium, is blocked.

a., rectal. General anesthesia produced by introduction of anesthetic agent into the rectum.

a., refrigeration. Anesthesia induced by lowering temperature of a part to near freezing by topical ethyl chloride spray or by immersion of the body or a part in a container of finely cracked ice.

a., regional. Nerve or field blocking, causing insensibility over a particular area. SEE: *a., block; a., infiltration.*

a., segmental. Anesthesia due to a pathological or surgically induced lesion of a nerve root.

a., sexual. Absence of sexual desire.

a., spinal. 1. Anesthesia resulting from disease or injury to conduction pathways of the spinal cord. 2. Anesthesia produced by injection of anesthetic into subarachnoid space of spinal cord.

a., splanchnic. Anesthesia produced by injecting an anesthetic agent into the splanchnic ganglion.

a., surgical. Depth of anesthesia at which relaxation of muscles and loss of sensation and consciousness are adequate for the performance of surgery.

a., tactile. Loss of sense of touch.

a., topical. Local anesthesia induced by application of an anesthetic directly to surface of area to be anesthetized.

a., traumatic. Loss of sensation resulting from injury to nerve.

a., twilight. State of light anesthesia. SEE: *twilight sleep.*

anesthesia, words pert. to: words beginning "anesthe-"; carbon dioxide; chloroform; cocaine; cyclopropane; ether; ethyl chloride; ethylene; halothane; labor; nitrous oxide; paraldehyde; procaine.

anesthesimeter (ăn-ĕs″thē-sĭm′ĕ-tĕr) [Gr. *an-*, not, + *aisthesis*, sensation, + *metron*, measure]. 1. Device that determines the quantity of anesthetic administered. 2. Device that measures the degree of loss of sensation in the skin.

anesthesiologist (ăn″ĕs-thē″zē-ŏl′ō-jĭst). A physician specializing in anesthesiology.

anesthesiology (ăn″ĕs-thē″zē-ŏl′ō-jē) [″ + ″ + *logos*, word, reason]. Science of anesthesia.

anesthetic (ăn″ĕs-thĕt′ĭk). 1. Pert. to or producing anesthesia. 2. Agent that produces anesthesia; subdivided into general and local, according to their action. SEE: *anesthesia.*

anesthetist (ă-nĕs′thĕ-tĭst). One who administers anesthetics, esp. for general anesthesia. May be a specially trained physician or nurse.

anesthetization (ă-nĕs″thĕ-tĭ-zā′shŭn). Induction of anesthesia.

anesthetize (ă-nĕs′thĕ-tīz). To induce anesthesia.

anethole (ăn′ĕ-thōl). Chemical present in oil of anise and in oil of fennel. Used as a flavoring agent.

anetoderma (ăn″ĕt-ō-dĕr′mă) [Gr. *anetos*,

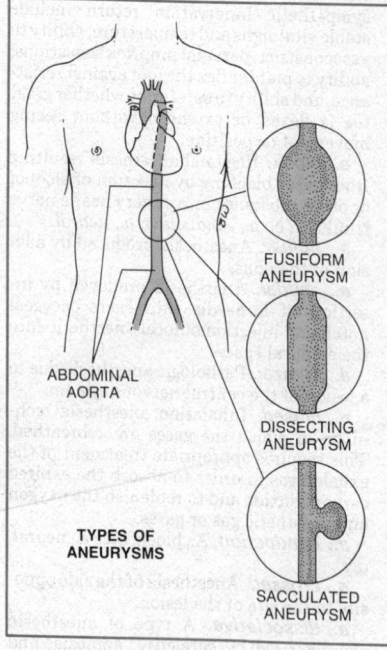

FUSIFORM ANEURYSM

ABDOMINAL AORTA

DISSECTING ANEURYSM

TYPES OF ANEURYSMS

SACCULATED ANEURYSM

relaxed, + *derma*, skin]. Localized laxity of the skin with protruding, saclike areas. These lesions are due to loss of normal skin elasticity. SYN: *macular atrophy,* q.v.

TREAT: Excision of cosmetically objectionable areas.

aneuploidy (ăn″ū-ploy′dē) [Gr. *an-*, not, + *eu*, well, + *ploos*, fold, + *eidos*, form, shape]. Condition of having an abnormal number of chromosomes for the species indicated.

aneurine hydrochloride (ă-nū′rĭn). Thiamine hydrochloride, vitamin B_1.

aneurysm (ăn′ū-rĭzm) [Gr. *aneurysma*, a widening]. Localized abnormal dilatation of a blood vessel, usually an artery. Due to congenital defect or weakness of the wall of the vessel. SEE: illus.

ETIOL: In the aorta, arteriosclerosis accompanied by hypertension is a cause, as is syphilis. Bacterial or mycotic infection and trauma are common causes of aneurysms in peripheral arteries.

a., aortic. Aneurysm affecting any part of the aorta.

SYM: Dyspnea, cough, sputum, dysphagia, congestion of head and neck. Inequality in the right and left radial pulses.

PATH: Pressure on trachea, esophagus,

veins, or nerves.
TREAT: Surgery.

a., arteriovenous. Aneurysm in which artery and vein become connected by a saccule.
SYM: Pain, expansile pulsation, bruit.
ETIOL: Usually traumatic, may be congenital.

a., atherosclerotic. Aneurysm due to degeneration or weakening of the arterial wall caused by atherosclerosis.

a., berry. Small saccular congenital aneurysm of a cerebral vessel. It communicates with the vessel by a small opening. Rupture of this type of aneurysm may cause bleeding severe enough to be fatal.

a., cirsoid. A dilatation of a network of vessels commonly occurring on the scalp. The mass may form a pulsating subcutaneous tumor. SYN: *a., racemose.*

a., compound. Aneurysm in which some of the layers of the vessel are ruptured and others dilated.

a., dissecting. Aneurysm in which the blood makes its way between the layers of a blood vessel wall, separating them; a result of necrosis of the medial portion of the arterial wall.

a., fusiform. Aneurysm in which all the walls of a blood vessel dilate more or less equally, creating a tubular swelling.

a., mycotic. Aneurysm due to bacterial infection.

a., racemose. A., cirsoid, q.v.

a., sacculated. Aneurysm due to the yielding of a weak area on one side of the vessel and not involving the entire circumference; usually due to trauma. It is attached to the artery by a narrow neck.

a., varicose. Aneurysm forming a blood-filled sac between an artery and a vein.

a., venous. Aneurysm of a vein.

aneurysmal (ăn″ū-rĭz′măl) [Gr. *aneurysma*, a widening]. Pert. to aneurysm.

aneurysmectomy (ăn″ū-rĭz-měk′tō-mē) [″ + *ektome*, excision]. Surgical removal of the sac of an aneurysm.

aneurysmoplasty (ăn″ū-rĭz′mō-plăs″tē) [″ + *plassein*, to form]. Surgical repair of an aneurysm.

aneurysmorrhaphy (ăn″ū-rĭz-mor′ă-fē) [″ + *rhaphe*, seam, ridge]. Surgical closure of the sac of an aneurysm.

aneurysmotomy (ăn″ū-rĭz-mŏt′ō-mē) [″ + *tome*, incision]. Incision of the sac of an aneurysm, allowing it to heal by granulation.

A.N.F. *American Nurses' Foundation.*

angel dust (PCP). "Street" or slang term for phencyclidine, q.v.

angel's trumpet [*Datura ruaveolens*]. A flowering shrub native to the southeastern U.S.

Portions of the plant are used for hallucinogenic effects. The flowers are made into a stew or tea, and the leaves are eaten. The flowers contain large quantities of the alkaloids atropine, hyoscyamine, and hyoscine. Ingestion of plant products produces intense thirst, visual disturbances, flushing, CNS hyperexcitability, sensory flooding, and a delirious incoherent state. This is followed by hyperthermia, tachycardia, hypertension, visual hallucinations, disturbed consciousness, clonus, and subsequent convulsions. If condition is untreated, death may occur.
TREAT: Gastric lavage, followed by 1 to 4 mg of I.V. physostigmine sulfate. This dosage should reverse the acute delirious state in one or two hours, but it may need to be repeated several times.

angel's wing. Posterior projection of the scapula usually caused by paralysis of the serratus anterior muscle. SYN: *scapula, winged.*

Angelucci's syndrome (ăn″jē-loo′chēz) [Arnaldo Angelucci, It. ophthalmologist, 1854–1934]. Great excitability, palpitation, and vasomotor disturbance associated with vernal conjunctivitis.

anger (ăng′er) [L. *angere*, anguish]. The basic emotion of extreme displeasure or exasperation in reaction to a person, a situation, or an object. Anger is instrumental in mobilizing and enhancing our ability to respond to adverse situations; and, for that reason, it may be essential to survival in certain circumstances. It has been suggested that anger may be a reaction to dying and that a patient's anger may be directed to friends or family and to those responsible for his or her medical care.

angi- (ăn′jē) [Gr. *angeion*, vessel]. Prefix meaning a blood or lymph vessel.

angiasthenia (ăn″jē-ăs-thē′nē-ă) [″ + *a-*, not, + *sthenos*, strength]. Loss of vascular tone.

angiectasia, angiectasis (ăn″jē-ĕk-tā′zē-ă, -ĕk′tă-sĭs) [″ + *ektasis*, stretching]. Dilation of a blood or lymph vessel.

angiectomy (ăn″jē-ĕk′tō-mē) [″ + *ektome*, excision]. Excision or resection of a blood vessel.

angiectopia (ăn″jē-ĕk′tŏ′pē-ă) [″ + *ektopos*, out of place]. Displacement of a vessel.

angiemphraxis (ăn″jē-ĕm-frăk′sĭs) [″ + *emphraxis*, stoppage]. Obstruction of a vessel.

angiitis (ăn″jē-ī′tĭs) [″ + *itis*, inflammation]. Inflammation of a blood or lymph vessel. SYN: *vasculitis.*

angina (ăn-jī′nă, ăn′jĭ-nă) [L. *angina*, quinsy, from *angere*, to choke]. 1. Angina pectoris, q.v. 2. Acute sore throat.

USUAL DISTRIBUTION AND REFERRAL OF PAIN IN ANGINA PECTORIS

ANGINA PECTORIS

a. decubitus. Attacks of angina pectoris occurring while in recumbent position.

a., intestinal. Abdominal pain caused by insufficient blood supply to the intestines. Usually occurs after eating.

a., Ludwig's. Submaxillary cellulitis; a deep infection of tissues of the floor of the mouth.

a. of effort. Angina pectoris with onset during exercise. SYN: exertion angina.

a. pectoris. Severe pain and a sensation of constriction about the heart. The condition is caused by a relative deficiency of oxygen supply to heart muscle. The pain typically radiates to the left shoulder and down the left arm, or, rarely, from the heart to the abdomen. Pain may also radiate to the back or to the jaw. SEE: illus.

SYM: Steady severe pain and feeling of pressure in region of the heart; great anxiety, fear of approaching death (angor animi), and fixation of the body; face pale, ashen, or livid; brow bathed in sweat. Dyspnea often noted; pulse variable, usually tense and quick. Blood pressure is raised during an attack. Cardiac arrhythmia may be present during angina. Attack may be of brief duration or last for a considerable period.

TREAT: During attack, inhalation of amyl nitrite or use of nitroglycerin sublingually. Nitroglycerin may be administered by using transdermal patches. Beta blocking drugs, e.g., propanolol, are effective in treating angina but their side effects may make it necessary to discontinue the drug. Calcium channel blockers such as nifedipine, verapamil, or diltiazem, are used in treating angina. Avoidance of excitement; physical rest.

PROG: May be grave. Attacks may be intermittent, and with proper rest and care, recovery is possible. SEE: *angina, silent; angina, stable; angina, unstable; angina, variant; myocardial ischemia; percutaneous transluminal coronary angioplasty.*

NURSING IMPLICATIONS: Monitor and record pattern of pain, including time of onset, duration, location and radiation, intensity, and precipitating circumstances. Evaluate cardiopulmonary status, administer medications and oxygen as ordered, and note response. It is important to remain with the patient and provide emotional support during the episode. Teach patient how to use the prescribed form of nitroglycerin for anginal attacks, and the importance of seeking immediate medical attention if three doses at 5-minute intervals have failed to provide relief. SEE: *Nursing Diagnoses* in *Appendix*.

a., Prinzmetal's. A., variant, q.v.

a., silent. Decreased supply of oxygen to the heart muscle, but pain is absent. Approximately 10% to 20% of patients with diabetes mellitus and coronary artery disease have silent angina; also, a similar percentage of patients with acute myocardial infarctions have silent angina, i.e., infarctions that cause no pain.

a., stable. Angina that occurs with exercise and is predictable. Usually promptly relieved by rest or nitroglycerin.

a., unstable. Angina that has changed to a more frequent and more severe form. It can occur during rest and may be an indication of impending myocardial infarction. TREAT: Unstable angina should be treated as a medical emergency and the patient hospitalized without delay.

a., variant. Angina pectoris occurring during rest. It is not preceded by exercise or increase in heart rate. These patients have normal exercise potential when the angina is not present. ETIOL: Coronary artery spasm. SYN: *Prinzmetal's angina.*

a., Vincent's. SEE: *Vincent's angina.*
anginal (ăn'jĭ-nal). Pert. to angina.
anginiform (ăn-jĭn'ĭ-form) [L. *angina*, quinsy, + *forma*, having the form of].

Mimicking or resembling angina, especially angina pectoris.

anginoid (ăn′jĭ-noyd) [″ + Gr. *eidos*, form, shape]. Resembling angina, esp. angina pectoris.

anginophobia (ăn″jĭ-nō-fō′bē-ă) [″ + Gr. *phobos*, fear]. Morbid fear of an attack of angina pectoris.

anginose (ăn′jĭ-nōs) [L. *angina*, quinsy]. Pert. to or resembling angina.

anginous (ăn′jĭ-nŭs). Resembling angina. SYN: *anginose.*

angio- (ăn′jē-ō) [Gr. *angeion*, vessel]. A combining form denoting a seed, vessel, or something contained within a vessel.

angioataxia (ăn″jē-ō-ă-tăk′sē-ă) [″ + *ataktos*, out of order]. Variability in arterial tonus.

angioblast (ăn′jē-ō-blăst) [″ + *blastos*, germ]. 1. The earliest tissue arising from mesenchyme cells of the embryo, from which blood vessels develop. 2. A cell that participates in vessel formation.

angioblastoma (ăn″jē-ō-blăs-tō′mă) [″ + ″ + *oma*, tumor]. Tumor of particular blood vessels of the brain, or of the meninges of the brain.

angiocardiogram (ăn″jē-ō-kăr′dē-ō-grăm) [″ + *kardia*, heart, + *gramma*, something written]. Serial x-rays of the heart taken immediately after intravenous injection of a radiopaque dye.

angiocardiography (ăn″jē-ō-kăr″dē-ŏg′ră-fē) [″ + ″ + *graphein*, to write]. Roentgenography of the heart and great vessels after intravenous injection of a radiopaque solution.

angiocardiokinetic (ăn″jē-ō-kăr″dē-ō-kĭ-nĕt′ĭk) [″ + ″ + *kinesis*, movement]. Causing movement (contraction or dilation) of heart and blood vessels.

angiocardiopathy (ăn″jē-ō-kăr″dē-ŏp′ă-thē) [″ + ″ + *pathos*, disease, suffering]. Disease of the blood vessels of the heart.

angiocarditis (ăn″jē-ō-kăr-dī′tĭs) [″ + ″ + *itis*, inflammation]. Inflammation of the heart and large blood vessels.

angiocavernous (ăn″jē-ō-kăv′ĕr-nŭs) [″ + L. *caverna*, cavern]. Rel. to angioma cavernosum, q.v.

angiocholecystitis (ăn″jē-ō-kō″lē-sĭs-tī′tĭs) [″ + *chole*, bile, + *kystis*, bladder, + *itis*, inflammation]. Inflammation of gallbladder and bile vessels.

angiocholitis (ăn″jē-ō-kō-lī′tĭs) [″ + ″ + *itis*, inflammation]. Inflammation of biliary vessels. SYN: *cholangitis.*

angiodystrophia (ăn″jē-ō-dĭs-trō′fē-ă) [″ + *dys*, bad, + *trophe*, nourishment]. Faulty nutrition of vessels.

angioedema (ăn″jē-ō-ē-dē′mă) [″ + *oi-*

dema, swelling]. A condition characterized by development of urticaria and edematous areas of skin, mucous membranes, or viscera. It is usually benign when limited to the skin. The reaction may be immunoglobulin E dependent with associated atopic diathesis, specific antigen sensitivity to foods, drugs, stings, or molds; or physical reaction of the skin to cold, light, pressure, or exercise. The condition may also be complement mediated as in hereditary angioedema, necrotizing vasculitis, or serum sickness reactions to blood products. SYN: *angioneurotic edema.*

TREAT: Antihistamines and sympathomimetic agents for symptomatic relief. If the disease is related to complement, attenuated androgens or epsilon-aminocaproic acid can prevent or treat attacks, respectively.

angioendothelioma (ăn″jē-ō-ĕn″dō-thē″lē-ō′mă) [″ + *endon*, within, + *thele*, nipple, + *oma*, tumor] (pl. *-mata* or *-mas*). A tumor consisting of endothelial cells, commonly occurring as single or multiple tumors of bone.

angiofibroma (ăn″jē-ō-fī-brō′mă) [″ + L. *fibra*, fiber, + Gr. *oma*, tumor] (pl. *-mas* or *-mata*). A tumor consisting of fibrous tissue.

angiogenesis (ăn″jē-ō-jĕn′ĕ-sĭs) [″ + *genesis*, generation, birth]. Development of blood vessels.

angiogenic (ăn″jē-ō-jĕn′ĭk) 1. Pert to angiogenesis. 2. Of vascular origin.

angiogenic factors. A group of polypeptides that act in one of two ways: to stimulate vascular endothelial cells to move or divide; or to act indirectly by mobilizing host cells, such as macrophages, to release endothelial growth factors. These factors are found in tumors in which new vessels are being formed and in normal tissues in which new vessels are not being formed. The importance of these factors in both tumors and other pathological conditions is unclear.

angioglioma (ăn″jē-ō-glī-ō′mă) [Gr. *angeion*, vessel, + *glia*, glue, + *oma*, tumor]. A mixed angioma and glioma.

angiogram (ăn′jē-ō-grăm) [″ + *gramma*, something written]. Serial roentgenography of a blood vessel taken in rapid sequence following the injection of a radiopaque substance into the vessel. This technique has been used to define the size and shape of various veins and arteries of organs and tissues.

    a., aortic. Angiogram of aorta. Used in diagnosing aneurysms or presence of tumors that contact and deform the aorta.

    a., cardiac. Angiogram of the heart. Used to determine the size and shape of the cavities of the heart and the condition of the valves.

a., cerebral. Angiogram of blood vessels of the brain.

angiograph (ăn′jē-ō-grăf″) [″ + *graphein*, to write]. A variety of sphygmograph.

angiography (ăn″jē-ŏg′ră-fē). 1. A description of blood vessels and lymphatics. 2. Roentgenography of blood vessels after injection of radiopaque substance. 3. Recording the movements of the arterial pulse by use of a sphygmograph.

a., aortic. Angiography of the aorta and its branches.

a., cardiac. Angiography of the heart and coronary arteries.

a., cerebral. Angiography of the vascular system of the brain.

a., coronary. Angiography of the coronary vessels of the heart. This can provide useful information about the adequacy of blood supply to the myocardium.

a., digital subtraction. Use of a computer technique to investigate arterial blood circulation. A reference image is obtained by use of fluoroscopy. Then a contrast medium is injected intravenously. Another film is produced from the fluoroscopic image, and then the computer technique "subtracts" the image produced by surrounding tissues, and the third image is an enhanced view of the arteries.

a., peripheral. Angiography of the vessels of the extremities.

a., pulmonary. Angiography of the pulmonary vessels.

a., selective. Angiography in which a catheter is introduced directly into the vessel to be visualized.

a., vertebral. Selective angiography of the vertebrobasilar system.

angiohyalinosis (ăn″jē-ō-hī-″ă-lĭn-ō′sĭs) [Gr. *angeion*, vessel, + *hyalos*, glass, + *osis*, condition]. Hyaline degeneration of the walls of blood vessels.

angiohypertonia (ăn″jē-ō-hī″pĕr-tō′nē-ă) [″ + *hyper*, over, + *tonos*, act of stretching, tension]. Spasm of blood vessels, esp. arteries. SYN: *angiospasm; vasospasm.* SEE: *hypertension.*

angiohypotonia (ăn″jē-ō-hī″pō-tō′nē-ă) [″ + *hypo*, under, + *tonos*, act of stretching, tension]. Angioparalysis; angioparesis; vascular dilatation. SEE: *hypotension.*

angioid (ăn′jē-oyd) [″ + *eidos*, form, shape]. Resembling a blood vessel.

angioid streaks. Dark, wavy, anastomosing striae lying beneath retinal vessels.

angiokeratoma (ăn″jē-ō-kĕr″ă-tō′mă) [″ + *keras*, horn, + *oma*, tumor]. A skin disorder occurring chiefly on feet and legs, characterized by formation of telangiectases or warty growths accompanied by

thickening of the epidermis along the course of dilated capillaries.

angiokinetic (ăn″jē-ō-kĭ-nĕt′ĭk) [″ + *kinesis*, movement]. Pert to constriction and dilation of blood vessels. SYN: *vasomotor.*

angioleukitis (ăn″jē-ō-loo-kī′tĭs) [″ + *leukos*, white, + *itis*, inflammation]. Inflammation of lymphatics.

angiolipoma (ăn′jē-ō-lĭp-ō′mă) [″ + *lipos*, fat, + *oma*, tumor]. A mixed angioma and lipoma.

angiolith (ăn′jē-ō-lĭth) [″ + *lithos*, stone]. Calcareous deposit in wall of a blood vessel.

angiology (ăn″jē-ŏl′ō-jē) [″ + *logos*, word, reason]. The science of the blood vessels and lymphatics.

angiolymphitis (ăn″jē-ō-lĭm-fī′tĭs) [″ + L. *lympha*, lymph, + *itis*, inflammation]. Inflammation of the lymphatics. SYN: *lymphangitis.*

angiolysis (ăn″jē-ŏl′ĭ-sĭs) [″ + *lysis*, dissolution]. Obliteration of blood vessels, as in the umbilical cord when it is tied just after birth.

angioma (ăn″jē-ō′mă) [″ + *oma*, tumor]. A form of tumor, usually benign, consisting principally of blood vessels (hemangioma) or lymph vessels (lymphangioma). Considered to be remnants of fetal tissue misplaced or undergoing disordered development. SEE: *choristoma; epithelioma; hamartoma; nevus.*

a., capillary. Congenital, superficial hemangioma appearing as irregularly shaped, red discoloration of otherwise normal skin. Due to overgrowth of capillaries.

a. cavernosum. Congenital hemangioma appearing as an elevated dark-red tumor, ranging in size from a few mm to several cm. It may pulsate; commonly involves the subcutaneous or submucous tissue and consists of blood-filled vascular spaces. It is nonmalignant, and small ones may disappear without therapy.

a., senile. Hemangioma common in elderly persons due to weakening of capillary walls; consists of a compressible mass of blood vessels. SYN: *spot, ruby.*

a., serpiginous. A skin disorder characterized by appearance of small, red, vascular dots arranged in rings; due to proliferation of capillaries.

a. simplex. A., capillary, q.v.

a., spider. SEE: *spider nevus.*

a., stellate. Hemangioma in which numerous telangiectatic vessels radiate from a central point. Commonly associated with hepatic disease, hypertension, and pregnancy. SYN: *spider nevus.*

a., telangiectatic. Angioma composed of abnormally dilated blood vessels.

a. venosum racemosum. Swelling associated with severe varicosities of superficial veins.

angiomalacia (ăn"jē-ō-mă-lă'sē-ă) [Gr. *angeion*, vessel, + *malakia*, softness]. Softening of blood vessel walls.

angiomatosis (ăn"jē-ō-mă-tō'sĭs) [" + *oma*, tumor, + *osis*, condition]. Condition of multiple angiomas.

   a., bacillary. An infectious disease causing proliferation of small blood vessels in the skin and visceral organs of patients with human immunodeficiency virus infection and other immunocompromised hosts. The causative agent is thought to be an uncharacterized rickettsia-like organism closely related to *Rochalimaea quintana.* SYN: *epitheloid angiomatosis.* SEE: *cat scratch disease.*

angiomatous (ăn"jē-ō'mă-tŭs). Resembling an angioma.

angiomegaly (ăn"jē-ō-měg'ă-lē) [" + *megas*, large]. Enlargement of blood vessels, esp. in the eyelid.

angiometer (ăn"jē-ŏm'ě-těr) [" + *metron*, measure]. Instrument for measuring tension and diameter of blood vessels.

angiomyocardiac (ăn"jē-ō-mī"ō-kăr'dē-ăk) [" + *mys*, muscle, + *kardia*, heart]. Pert. to blood vessels and cardiac muscle.

angiomyolipoma (ăn"jē-ō-mī"ō-lĭ-pō'mă) [" + " + *lipos*, fat, + *oma*, tumor]. Nonmalignant growth containing vascular, fatty, and muscular tissues.

angiomyoma (ăn"jē-ō-mī-ō'mă) [" + " + *oma*, tumor]. Tumor composed of blood vessels and muscle tissue. SYN: *glomus tumor.*

angiomyoneuroma (ăn"jē-ō-mī"ō-nū-rō'mă) [" + " + *neuron*, nerve, + *oma*, tumor]. Painful, benign tumor of the arteriovenous anastomoses of the skin. SYN: *glomangioma.*

angiomyosarcoma (ăn"jē-ō-mī"ō-săr-kō'mă) [" + " + *sarx*, flesh, + *oma*, tumor]. Tumor composed of blood vessels, muscle tissue, and connective tissue.

angioneurectomy (ăn"jē-ō-nū-rěk'tō-mē) [" + *neuron*, nerve, + *ektome*, excision]. Excision of vessels and nerves.

angioneuromyoma (ăn"jē-ō-nū"rō-mī-ō'mă) [" + " + *mys*, muscle, + *oma*, tumor]. Glomangioma, q.v. SEE: *angiomyoneuroma.*

angioneurotic edema. Angioedema, q.v.

angioneurotomy (ăn"jē-ō-nū-rŏt'ō-mē) [" + " + *tome*, incision]. Cutting of vessels and nerves.

angionoma (ăn"jē-ō-nō'mă) [Gr. *angeion*, vessel, + *nome*, ulcer]. Ulceration of a vessel.

angioparalysis (ăn"jē-ō-pă-răl'ĭ-sĭs) [" + *paralyein*, loosen, dissolve]. Vasomotor relaxation of blood vessel tone.

angiopathology (ăn"jē-ō-pă-thŏl'ō-jē) [" + *pathos*, disease, suffering, + *logos*, word, reason]. Morbid changes in diseases of the blood vessels.

angiopathy (ăn-jē-ŏp'ă-thē). Any disease of blood vessels or lymph vessels. SYN: *angiosis.*

angiophacomatosis, angiophakomatosis (ăn"jē-ō-făk"ō-mă-tō'sĭs) [" + *phakos*, lens, + *oma*, tumor, + *osis*, condition]. Retinocerebral hemangiomatosis, Hippel's disease, q.v., or von Hippel-Lindau disease.

angioplasty (ăn'jē-ō-plăs"tē) [" + *plassein*, to form]. Altering the structure of a vessel, either by a surgical procedure or by dilating the vessel using a balloon inside the lumen. SEE: *percutaneous transluminal coronary angioplasty.*

   a., laser coronary. The use of laser energy to vaporize an atherosclerotic plaque in a diseased coronary vessel. SEE: *percutaneous transluminal coronary angioplasty.*

angiopoiesis (ăn"jē-ō-poy-ē'sĭs) [" + *poiein*, to make]. The process of forming blood vessels.

angiopoietic (ăn"jē-ō-poy-ĕt'ĭk). Pert. to or causing the formation of vessels.

angiopressure (ăn'jē-ō-prěsh"ŭr). Pressure applied to a blood vessel to arrest hemorrhage.

angiorrhaphy (ăn"jē-or'ă-fē) [" + *rhaphe*, seam, ridge]. Suture of a vessel, esp. a blood vessel.

angiorrhexis (ăn"jē-or-ěk'sĭs) [" + *rhexis*, rupture]. Rupture of a vessel, esp. a blood vessel.

angiosarcoma (ăn"jē-ō-săr-kō'mă) [" + *sarx*, flesh, + *oma*, tumor]. Malignant neoplasm originating from blood vessels. SYN: *hemangiosarcoma.*

angiosclerosis (ăn"jē-ō-sklě-rō'sĭs) [" + *sklerosis*, hardening]. Hardening of the walls of the vascular system.

angioscope (ăn'jē-ō-skōp) [" + *skopein*, to examine]. A microscope for studying capillary vessels.

angioscotoma (ăn"jē-ō-skō-tō'mă) [" + *skotoma*, darkness]. The defect produced in the visual field by the shadows of the retinal blood vessels.

angiosis (ăn"jē-ō'sĭs) [Gr. *angeion*, vessel, + *osis*, condition]. Any disease of blood vessels or lymph vessels. SYN: *angiopathy.*

angiospasm (ăn'jē-ō-spăzm) [" + *spasmos*, a convulsion]. Spasmodic contraction of blood vessels. May cause cramping of muscles or intermittent claudication.

angiospastic (ăn"jē-ō-spăs'tĭk). Pert. to angiospasm.

angiostenosis (ăn"jē-ō-stě-nō'sĭs) [" + *stenoein*, to make narrow, + *osis*, condition]. Narrowing of a vessel, esp. a blood vessel.

angiosteosis (ăn″jē-ŏs″tē-ō′sĭs) [″ + *osteon,* bone, + *osis,* condition]. Calcification of a vessel.

angiostomy (ăn″jē-ŏs′tō-mē) [″ + *stoma,* mouth]. Operation making artificial fistulous opening into a blood vessel.

angiostrophy (ăn″jē-ŏs′trō-fē) [″ + *strophe,* twist]. Twisting the cut end of a blood vessel to arrest bleeding.

angiotelectasis (ăn″jē-ō-tĕl-ĕk′tă-sĭs) [″ + *telos,* end, + *ektasis,* stretching out]. Dilatation of terminal arterioles.

angiotenic (ăn″jē-ō-tĕn′ĭk) [″ + *teinen,* to stretch]. Characterized by or caused by distention of blood vessels.

angiotensin (ăn″jē-ō-tĕn′sĭn). A vasopressor substance that is produced when renin is released from the kidney. Renin is formed by the juxtaglomerular apparatus of the kidney. SEE: *apparatus, juxtaglomerular.*

   a. I. Physiologically inactive form of angiotensin; precursor of angiotensin II, q.v.

   a. II. Physiologically active form of angiotensin; powerful vasopressor and stimulator of aldosterone production and secretion.

   a. amide. A vasoconstrictor drug.

angiotensinogen (ăn″jē-ō-tĕn-sĭn′ō-jĕn). A serum globulin fraction formed in the liver; converted to angiotensin as a result of hydrolysis by renin.

angiotitis (ăn″jē-ō-tī′tĭs) [″ + *otos,* ear, + *itis,* inflammation]. Inflammation of blood vessels of the ear.

angiotome (ăn′jē-ō-tōm″) [Gr. *angeion,* vessel, + *tome,* incision]. Any segment of the embryonic vascular system.

angiotomy (ăn″jē-ŏt″ō-mē). Sectioning of blood vessels.

angiotonic (ăn″jē-ō-tŏn′ĭk) [″ + *tonos,* tension]. Increasing arterial tension.

angiotonin (ăn″jē-ō-tŏn′ĭn). Former name for angiotensin, q.v.

angiotribe [″ + Gr. *tribein,* to crush]. A forceps designed for application of a strong, crushing force to a tissue containing an artery. This is done in order to control hemorrhage.

angiotrophic (ăn″jē-ō-trŏf′ĭk) [″ + *trophe,* nourishment]. Pert. to nutrition of blood vessels or lymph vessels.

angle (ăng′gl) [L. *angulus*]. 1. The figure or space outlined by the diverging of two lines from a common point or by the meeting of two planes. 2. A projecting or sharp corner.

   a., acromial. Angle formed by junction of lateral and posterior borders of the acromion.

   a., acute. Angle less than 90°.

   a., alpha. Angle formed by intersection of visual line with optic axis.

   a., alveolar. Angle between the horizontal plane and a line drawn through the base of the nasal spine and the middle point of the alveolus of the upper jaw.

   a., biorbital. Angle formed by the meeting of the axes of the orbits.

   a., cardiophrenic. The medial, inferior corner of the pulmonary cavity bordered by the heart and diaphragm.

   a., carrying. Angle made at the elbow by extending the long axis of the forearm and the upper arm. This obtuse angle is more pronounced in the female than in the male.

   a., cavity. Angle formed by two or more walls of a cavity preparation in restorative dentistry.

   a., cephalometric. Angle formed by intersecting anthropometric lines used in studies of the skull and for diagnosis of orthodontic problems.

   a., cerebellopontine. Angle formed by junction of the cerebellum and pons.

   a., costal. Meeting point of the lower border of the false ribs with the axis of the sternum.

   a., costophrenic. The lateral, inferior corner of the pulmonary cavity bordered by the ribs and diaphragm.

   a., craniofacial. Angle formed by the basifacial and basicranial axes at the midpoint of the sphenoethmoidal suture.

   a., facial. Angle made by lines from the nasal spine and external auditory meatus meeting between the upper middle incisor teeth.

   a., flat. Angle between two lines that join at an angle of almost 180°.

   a., gamma. Angle between the line of vision and the optic axis.

   a., gonial. Angle of the mandible.

   a., metafacial. Angle between the base of the skull and the pterygoid process.

   a., obtuse. Angle greater than 90°.

   a., occipital. Angle formed at the opisthion by the intersection of lines from the basion and from the lower border of the orbit.

   a. of convergence. Angle between the visual axis and the median line when an object is looked at.

   a. of incidence. Angle between a ray striking a surface and a line drawn perpendicular to the surface at the point of incidence.

   a. of iris. Angle between the cornea and iris at the periphery of the anterior chamber of the eye.

   a. of jaw. Angle formed by junction of the posterior edge of the ramus of the mandible and the lower surface of the body of the mandible.

a. of Louis. SEE: *a., sternal.*

a. of mandible. A. of jaw, q.v.

a. of Treitz. Sharp curve at the duodenojejunal junction.

a., ophryospinal. Angle formed at the anterior nasal spine by intersection of lines drawn from the auricular point and the glabella.

a., optic. A., visual, q.v.

a., parietal. Angle formed by the meeting of a line drawn tangent to the maximum curve of the zygomatic arch and a line drawn tangent to the end of the maximum frontal diameter of the skull. If these lines are parallel, the angle is zero; if they diverge, a negative angle is formed.

a., pontine. A., cerebellopontile, q.v.

a., pubic. Angle formed by junction of the rami of the pubes.

a., right. Angle of 90°.

a., sphenoid. Angle formed at the top of the sella turcica by intersection of lines drawn from the nasal point and the tip of the rostrum of the sphenoid.

a., sternal. Angle formed by junction of the manubrium and the body of the sternum.

a., venous. Angle formed by junction of the internal jugular and subclavian veins.

a., visual. Angle formed by lines drawn from the nodal point of the eye to the edges of the object viewed.

Angle's classification [Edward Hartley Angle, U.S. dentist, 1855–1930]. SEE: *malocclusion.*

angophrasia (ăn″gō-frā′zē-ă) [Gr. *anchein*, to choke, + *phrasis*, utterance]. Drawling, choking speech in paralytic dementia.

angor (ăng′gor) [L., strangling]. Violent distress, as in angina pectoris.

angor animi (ăng′gor ăn′ĭ-mē) [″ + L. *animus*, soul]. The feeling that one is dying, as may occur in connection with angina pectoris.

angstrom unit (ŏng′strŭm) [Anders J. Ångström, Swedish physicist, 1814–1874]. SYMB: Å. ABBR: A.U. An internationally adopted unit of measurement of wave length; equal to 10^{-10} meter, or 0.1 nanometer. Used especially to specify radiation wavelengths. SYN: *angstrom.*

angular (ăng′gū-lăr) [L.]. Having corners or angles.

angular artery. The artery at the inner canthus of the eye; facial artery.

angulation (ăng″ū-lā′shŭn). Abnormal formation of angles by tubular structures such as the intestine, a blood vessel, or ureter.

angulus [L.]. Angle.

anhedonia (ăn″hē-dō′nē-ă) [Gr. *an-*, not, + *hedone*, pleasure]. Lack of pleasure in acts that are normally pleasurable. SEE: *hedonism.*

anhedonic (ăn″hē-dŏn′ĭk). Pert. to anhedonia.

anhidrosis (ăn″hī-drō′sĭs) [″ + *hidros*, sweat]. Diminished or complete absence of secretion of sweat. May be generalized or localized, temporary or permanent, accompanying disease conditions or may be a congenital anomaly. SYN: *anidrosis.*

TREAT: Treatment of cause or accompanying conditions. Soft, nonirritating clothing; bland, soothing ointments and lubricants for skin. Air conditioning provides comfort in most instances.

anhidrotic (ăn″hī-drŏt′ĭk). 1. Inhibiting or preventing perspiration. 2. Agent that inhibits or prevents perspiration. SYN: *anidrotic; antihidrotic; antiperspirant; antisudorific.*

anhistic, anhistous (ăn-hĭs′tĭk, -hĭs′tŭs) [″ + *histos*, tissue]. Seemingly without structure.

anhydrase (ăn″hī′drās) [″ + *hydor*, water, + *-ase*, enzyme]. Enzyme that promotes the removal of water from a chemical compound.

anhydration (ăn-hī′drā′shŭn) [″ + *hydor*, water]. Removal of water from a substance. SYN: *dehydration*, q.v.

anhydride (ăn-hī′drīd) [Gr. *an-*, not, + *hydor*, water]. Compound formed by removal of water from a substance, esp. from an acid.

anhydrochloric (ăn-hī-drō-klō′rĭk) [″ + ″ + *chloros*, green]. Lacking hydrochloric acid.

Anhydron. Trade name for cyclothiazide, q.v.

anhydrous (ăn-hī′drŭs) [″ + *hydor*, water]. Lacking water.

anianthinopsy (ăn-ē-ăn′thĭn-ŏp″sē) [″ + *ianthinos*, violet, + *opsis*, vision]. Inability to recognize violet or purple.

anicteric (ăn″ĭk-tĕr′ĭk) [″ + *ikteros*, jaundice]. Without jaundice.

anidrosis (ăn-ĭ-drō′sĭs) [″ + *hidros*, sweat]. Anhidrosis, q.v.

anidrotic (ăn-ĭ-drŏt′ĭk). Anhidrotic, q.v.

anileridine (ăn″ĭ-lĕr′ĭ-dēn). USP. A narcotic analgesic similar to meperidine (Demerol).

aniline (ăn′ĭ-lĭn) [Arabic *an-nil*, the indigo plant]. C_6H_7N. The simplest aromatic amine, an oily liquid derived from benzene. Used in manufacture of dyes for medical and industrial purposes. Aniline has antipyretic action but is too toxic to use as a medicine. SYN: *aminobenzene; phenylamine.*

aniline poisoning. SEE: *Poisons and Poisoning* in *Appendix.*

anilingus [L. *anus* + *lingere*, to lick]. Oral stimulation of the anus by use of the tongue or lips. SEE: *cunnilingus.*

anilism (ăn′ĭl-ĭzm) [Arabic *an-nil*, the indigo

plant, + Gr. -*ismos*, condition]. Chronic aniline poisoning. SEE: *aniline* in *Poisons and Poisoning* in *Appendix*.

SYM: Cardiac block, weakness, intermittent pulse, vertigo, muscular depression, cyanosis.

anima (ăn′ĭ-mă) [L., soul]. 1. Soul. 2. According to Jung, an individual's inner self as distinguished from the external personality (persona). 3. Also according to Jung, anima refers to the feminine inner personality present in men, as opposed to animus, which refers to the masculine inner personality present in women.

animal (ăn′ĭ-măl) [L. *animalis,* living]. 1. A living organism that requires oxygen and organic foods, is incapable of photosynthesis, has limited growth, and is capable of voluntary movement and sensation. 2. Any animal other than man. 3. Pert. to or from an animal. 4. A person who is beastlike.

   a., cold-blooded. An animal whose body temperature varies according to the temperature of the environment. SYN: *allotherm; poikilotherm.*

   a., control. In medical research involving use of animals, an animal that is not treated, but is housed and cared for under the same conditions as the treated animal(s). SEE: *control,* def. 2.

   a., warm-blooded. An animal whose body temperature remains constant regardless of the temperature of the environment. SYN: *homotherm.*

animal companions. For some persons, having an animal companion in the home seems to be a health-promoting factor. There is evidence that patients with animal companions survived after heart attacks or angina longer than did those without such companions.

animalcule (ăn″ĭ-măl′kūl) [L. *animalculum,* little animal]. Any microscopic animal organism. A protozoan.

animation (ăn-ĭ-mā′shŭn) [L. *animus,* soul]. State of being alive or active.

   a., suspended. Temporary cessation of vital functions with loss of consciousness; state of apparent death.

animatism (ăn′ĭ-mă-tĭzm). Belief that everything in nature, animate and inanimate, contains a spirit or soul.

animi agitatio (ăn′ĭ-mē ă-jĭ-tā′shē-ŏ) [″ + *agitare,* to turn over]. Mental agitation.

animism (ăn′ĭ-mĭzm). Attribution of spiritual qualities and mental capabilities to inanimate objects.

animus [L., breath, mind, soul]. 1. An animating or energizing motive or intention. 2. A feeling of bitter hostility; grudge. 3. According to Jung, the masculine inner personality present in women. SEE: *anima*.

anion (ăn′ĭ-ŏn) [Gr. *ana,* up, + *ion,* going]. An ion carrying a negative charge; it is attracted by, and travels to, the anode (positive pole). Opposite of cation. Examples are acid radicals and corresponding radicals of their salts. SEE: *electrolyte; ion.*

anion channel. Channels in red blood cells that cross the cell membrane. Chloride ions (Cl^-) and bicarbonate ions (HCO_3^-) are exchanged via these channels.

anion exchange. SEE: *resin, ion-exchange.*

anion gap. A concept used to estimate electrolyte (anion and cation) levels in the serum and conditions that influence them. The anion gap ranges from 8 to 18 mEq per liter in normal patients. This is estimated by subtracting the sum of the anions chloride and bicarbonate ($Cl^- + HCO_3^-$) from the sum of the cations sodium and potassium ($Na^+ + K^+$). Because the potassium cation is low in serum, the anion gap is calculated by the formula $Na^+ - (Cl^- + HCO_3^-)$.

anionic (ăn″ĭ-ŏn′ĭk). Containing or pert. to anions.

anionic detergent. A chemical substance with disinfectant properties due to the presence of an active, negatively charged chemical group. May be natural or synthetic.

aniridia (ăn″ĭ-rĭd′ē-ă) [Gr. *an-,* not, + *iris,* rainbow, iris]. Congenital absence of all or part of the iris. SYN: *irideremia.*

anisakiasis (ăn″ĭs-ā-kī′ă-sĭs). Disease of human gastrointestinal tract accompanied by intestinal colic, fever, and abscesses, caused by eating uncooked fish containing larval nematodes of the family Anisakidae.

aniseikonia (ăn-ĭs-ī-kō′nē-ă) [Gr. *anisos,* unequal, + *eikon,* image]. A condition in which the size and shape of the ocular image of one eye differ from those of the other. SYN: *anisoiconia.*

anise oil. Volatile oil obtained from distillation of the dried ripe fruit of *Pimpinella anisum,* or star anise, *Illicium verum.* It is used as a flavoring substance.

anismus. Excessive contraction of the external sphincter of the rectum.

aniso- (ăn-ī′sō) [Gr. *anisos,* unequal]. Prefix meaning unequal, asymmetrical, or dissimilar.

anisoaccommodation (ăn-ī″sō-ă-kŏm″mŏ-dā′shŭn) [″ + L. *accommodare,* to suit]. Difference in ability of the eyes to accommodate. SEE: *accommodation.*

anisochromatic (ăn-ī″sō-krō-măt′ĭk) [″ + *chroma,* color]. Not of uniform color.

anisocoria (ăn-ī″sō-kō′rē-ă) [″ + *kore,* pupil]. Inequality of the size of the pupils; may be congenital or associated with aneurysms, head trauma, diseases of the nervous system, brain lesion, paresis, or locomotor ataxia.

anisocytosis (ăn-ī″sō-sī-tō′sĭs) [″ + *kytos*, cell, + *osis*, condition]. Condition in which there is excessive inequality in size of cells, esp. erythrocytes.

anisogamy (ăn″ī-sŏg′ă-mē) [″ + *gamos*, marriage]. Sexual fusion of two gametes of different form and size.

anisognathous (ăn″ī-sŏg′nă-thŭs) [″ + *gnathos*, jaw]. Having an upper jaw wider than the lower one.

anisoiconia (ăn-ī″sō-ī-kō′nē-ă) [″ + *eikon*, image]. Condition in which ocular image in one eye is different in size and shape from that of the other. SYN: *aniseikonia*.

anisokaryosis (ăn-ī″sō-kăr″ē-ō′sĭs) [″ + *karyon*, nucleus, + *osis*, condition]. Unequal size of the cell nuclei.

anisomastia (ăn-ī-sō-măs′tē-ă) [″ + *mastos*, breast]. Condition in which breasts are markedly unequal.

anisomelia (ăn-ī″sō-mē′lē-ă) [″ + *melos*, limb]. Condition in which paired limbs are noticeably unequal.

anisometrope (ăn-ī″sō-mĕt′rōp) [Gr. *anisos*, unequal, + *metron*, measure, + *ops*, vision]. One afflicted with anisometropia.

anisometropia (ăn-ī″sō-mĕ-trō′pē-ă). Condition in which refractive power of the eyes is unequal.

anisometropic (ăn-ī″sō-mĕ-trŏp′ĭk). Pert. to or characterized by anisometropia.

anisonormocytosis (ăn-ī″sō-nor″mō-sī-tō′sĭs) [″ + L. *norma*, rule, + Gr. *kytos*, cell, + *osis*, condition]. Condition in which the total number of leukocytes is normal but the proportion of different types is abnormal.

anisophoria (ăn″ī-sō-fō′rē-ă) [″ + *phoros*, bearing]. Eye muscle imbalance so that the horizontal visual plane of one eye is different from that of the other.

anisopia (ăn″ī-sō′pē-ă) [″ + *ops*, vision]. Condition in which the visual power of the eyes is unequal.

anisosthenic (ăn-ī″sŏs-thĕn′ĭk) [″ + *sthenos*, strength]. Of unequal strength, said of paired muscles.

anisotonic (ăn-ī″sō-tŏn′ĭk) [″ + *tonos*, act of stretching, tension]. Pert. to a solution not isotonic as compared with another.

anisotropal (ăn″ī-sŏt′rō-păl) [″ + *tropos*, a turning]. 1. Not equal in every direction. 2. Unequal in power of refraction. SYN: *anisotropous*.

anisotropic (ăn-ī″sō-trŏp′ĭk). Having different optical properties in different directions, as have certain crystals; double polarizing power.

anisotropous (ăn-ī-sŏt′rō-pŭs). 1. Not equal in every direction. 2. Unequal in refractive power. SYN: *anisotropal*.

ankh (ăngk) [Egyptian, *life*]. A figure resembling a cross but with an oval on each side in place of the arms. In ancient Egypt, a symbol of life.

ankle (ăng′kl) [AS. *ancleow*]. 1. The joint between the leg and foot; the articulation of the tibia, fibula, and talus. The ankle is a hinge joint. 2. In popular usage, the region of this joint, including the tarsus and lower end of leg. SEE: *foot* for illus.

ankle bone. The talus, q.v.

ankle clonus. Repetitive extension-flexion movement of muscles of ankle, associated with increased muscle tonus. Commonly a symptom of corticospinal disease.

NURSING IMPLICATIONS: Keep patient's foot at a right angle to the horizontal plane of the body. This may be accomplished by using a foot splint. If the splint is removed, avoid dorsiflexion of the foot to prevent movement of the ankle, clonus, or spasm. When the involved joint is moved, it should be moved slowly and evenly. Do not grasp the extremity, but rather support it with the palms. If the joint is exercised, it should be done when the joint is warm and relaxed.

a.c. reflex. Reflex elicited by quick, vigorous dorsiflexion of the foot while the knee is held in a flexed position, resulting in repeated clonic movement of the foot so long as it is maintained in dorsiflexion.

ankle foot orthosis. ABBR: AFO. Any of a class of splints for the foot, commonly made of lightweight thermoplastic splinting material, which are fitted to provide stability and prevent deformities.

ankle jerk. Contraction of calf muscles resulting in extension of the foot following application of a brisk tap to the Achilles tendon.

ankle joint. The ankle, q.v.

ankylo- (ăng′kĭ-lō) [Gr. *ankylos*, crooked]. Prefix meaning crooked, bent, a fusion or growing together of parts.

ankyloblepharon (ăng″kĭ-lō-blĕf′ăr-ŏn) [″ + *blepharon*, eyelid]. Adhesion of the edges of upper and lower eyelids. SYN: *blepharosynechia*.

ankylochilia (ăng″kĭ-lō-kī′lē-a) [″ + *cheilos*, lip]. Adhesion of the upper and lower lips.

ankylocolpos (ăng-kĭ-lō-kŏl′pŏs) [″ + *kolpos*, vagina]. Imperforation or atresia of the vagina.

ankylodactylia (ăng-kĭ-lō-dăk-tĭl′ē-a) [″ + *daktylos*, finger]. Adhesion of two or more fingers or toes.

ankyloglossia (ăng″kĭ-lō-glŏs′sē-ă) [″ + *glossa*, tongue]. Abnormal shortness of frenum of tongue. SYN: *tongue-tie*.

ankylopoietic (ăng″kĭ-lō-poy-ĕt′ĭk) [Gr. *an-*

kyle, stiff joint, + *poiein,* to form]. 1. Indicating the presence of ankylosis. 2. Causing ankylosis.

ankyloproctia (ăng″kĭ-lō-prŏk′shē-ă) [Gr. *ankylos,* crooked, + *proktos,* anus]. Stricture or imperforation of the anus.

ankylosed. Fixed; stiffened; held by adhesions; affected with ankylosis, q.v.

ankylosed tooth. A deciduous tooth which is submerged and out of occlusion because it is attached to another tooth or the alveolar bone by a bridge of cementum.

ankylosis (ăng″kĭ-lō′sĭs) [Gr. *ankyle,* stiff joint, + *osis,* condition]. Immobility of a joint.

ETIOL: May be congenital (sometimes hereditary), or it may be the result of disease, trauma, surgery, or contractures resulting from immobility.

NURSING IMPLICATIONS: If ankylosis is created surgically, maintain immobilized joint until bone has healed (usually 6 to 12 weeks); maintain correct body alignment. If nonsurgical ankylosis, maintain the joint in a functional position, utilize splints for patients with spastic muscles, and initiate passive range of motion exercises to affected joints. Prevent immobility-induced contractures that can result in ankylosis. This is done by putting joints through normal range of motion passively whenever an individual is unable to exercise joints actively.

a., artificial. The surgical fixation of a joint.

a., bony. The abnormal union of the bones of a joint. SYN: *a., true.*

a., dental. A condition characterized by the loss of tooth movement due to the fusion of the root cementum with the adjacent alveolar bone.

a., extracapsular. Ankylosis caused by rigidity of parts outside a joint.

a., false. A., fibrous, q.v.

a., fibrous. Ankylosis due to the formation of fibrous bands within a joint. SYN: *a., false; a., ligamentous.*

a., intracapsular. Ankylosis due to undue rigidity of structure within a joint.

a., ligamentous. A., fibrous, q.v.

a., true. A., bony, q.v.

Ankylostoma (ăng″kĭ-lŏs′tō-mă). *Ancylostoma,* q.v.

ankylostomiasis (ăng″kĭ-lō-stō-mī′ă-sĭs). Ancylostomiasis, q.v.

ankylotia (ăng″kĭ-lō′shē-ă) [Gr. *ankylos,* crooked, + *ot-,* ear]. Stricture or imperforation of external auditory meatus of ear.

ankylotome (ăng′kĭl-ō-tōm, ăng-kĭl′ō-tōm) [″ + *tome,* incision]. An instrument for cutting the frenulum of the tongue in tongue-tie.

ankylurethria (ăng″kĭl-ū-rē′thrē-ă) [″ + *ourethra,* urethra]. Stricture or imperforation of the urethra.

anlage (ŏn′lŏ-jhă) [Ger., a laying on]. The first accumulation of cells in an embryo that constitutes the beginning of an organized tissue, organ, or part. SYN: *primordium.*

annatto (ă-nŏ′tō) [Cariban]. Yellowish-red coloring matter obtained from the pulp of *Bixa orellana,* a tropical tree. The material is used in coloring foods.

annealing (an-nēl′ĭng) [AS. *anaelan,* to burn]. Softening a material, such as glass, metal, or wax, by heating and cooling to remove internal stresses and make it more easily adapted or swaged, as in preparation of materials for restorative dentistry.

annectent (ă-nĕk′tĕnt) [L. *annectens,* tying or binding to]. Linked; connected; joined.

Annelida (ă-nĕl′ĭ-dă). The phylum that includes earthworms, leeches, and other segmented worms. Some annelids serve as intermediate hosts for parasitic worms.

annexa (ă-nĕks′ă) [L. *annectere,* to tie or bind to]. Accessory parts of a structure. SYN: *adnexa.*

annexitis (ă-nĕks-ī′tĭs) [″ + Gr. *itis,* inflammation]. Inflammation of adnexa uteri. SYN: *adnexitis.*

annular (ăn′ū-lăr) [L. *annulus,* ring]. Circular; ring-shaped, e.g., annular ligament of the elbow.

annulorrhaphy (ăn″ū-lor′ă-fē) [″ + Gr. *rhaphe,* seam, ridge]. Closure of a hernial ring by suture.

annulus (ăn′ū-lŭs) [L.] (pl. *annuli*). A ring-shaped structure; a ring. Also spelled anulus, q.v.

anococcygeal (ā″nō-kŏk-sĭ′jē-al) [L. *anus,* anus, + Gr. *kokkyx,* coccyx]. Rel. to both anus and coccyx.

anococcygeal body. The muscle and fibrous tissue lying between the coccyx and anus.

anococcygeal ligament. A band of fibrous tissue joining the tip of the coccyx with the external sphincter ani.

anodal (ăn-ō′dăl) [Gr. *ana,* up, + *hodos,* way]. Pert. to the anode, q.v.

anodal closure contraction. ABBR: ACC. Contraction of muscles at anode on closure of circuit.

anodal opening contraction. Contraction of the muscles at the anode when the electrical circuit is open.

anode (ăn′ōd) [Gr. *ana,* up, + *hodos,* way]. The positive pole of an electrical source. In radiography, the target of the x-ray tube. SEE: *cathode.*

anodmia (ăn-ŏd′mē-ă) [Gr. *an-,* not, + *odme,* stench]. Loss of the sense of smell. SYN: *anosmia.*

anodontia (ăn″ō-dŏn′shē-ă) [″ + *odous,*

tooth]. Absence of teeth. SYN: *edentia.*

anodyne (ăn'ō-dīn) [" + *odyne,* pain]. A drug that relieves pain. SYN: *analgesic; antalgesic.*

anodynia (ăn"ō-dĭn'ē-ă). Cessation or absence of pain.

anogenital. Concerning the anal and genital areas.

anomaloscope (ă-nŏm'ă-lō-skōp") [Gr. *anomalos,* irregular, + *skopein,* to examine]. Device for detecting color blindness.

anomalous (ă-nŏm'ă-lŭs) [Gr. *anomalos,* uneven]. Irregular; deviating from or contrary to normal.

anomaly (ă-nŏm'ă-lē) [Gr. *anomalia,* irregularity]. Deviation from normal. SYN: *birth defect; congenital anomaly.*

 a., congenital. Intrauterine development of an organ or structure that is abnormal with reference to form, structure, or position. SYN: *birth defect.*

anomia (ă-nō'mē-ă) [Gr. *a-,* not, + *onoma,* name]. Inability to remember names of objects.

anomie (ăn'ō-mē) [Fr. from Gr. *anomia,* lawlessness]. A term coined by the French sociologist Emile Durkheim (1858–1917) to indicate a condition similar to alienation. The individual feels there has been a disintegration of his or her norms and values. Durkheim felt such individuals were prone to take their lives because of the anxiety, isolation, and alienation that they experience.

anonychia (ăn-ō-nĭk'ē-ă) [Gr. *an-,* not, + *onyx,* nail]. Absence of the nails.

anoperineal (ā"nō-pĕr-ĭ-nē'ăl). Rel. to both the anus and perineum.

Anopheles (ă-nŏf'ē-lēz) [Gr. *anopheles,* harmful, useless]. A genus of mosquitoes belonging to the family Culicidae, order Diptera. It is a vector of *Plasmodium,* the causative agent of malaria, and may be involved in the transmission of causative agent of dengue, filariasis, and possibly other diseases. Of the almost 100 species of Anopheles, only a few are capable of transmitting the causative organism of malaria. SEE: *malaria.*

anophthalmia (ăn-ŏf-thăl'mē-ă) [Gr. *an-,* not, + *ophthalmos,* eye]. Congenital absence of one or both eyes.

anopia (an-ō'pē-ă) [" + *ops,* eye]. 1. Anophthalmia. 2. Anophoria.

anoplasty (ā'nō-plăs"tē) [L. *anus,* anus, + Gr. *plassein,* to form]. Plastic surgery of the anus.

Anoplura (an-ō-ploo'ră) [Gr. *anoplos,* unarmed, + *oura,* tail]. An order of insects composed of the sucking lice. SEE: *louse; pediculosis.*

anopsia (ăn-ŏp'sē-ă) [Gr. *an-,* not, + *opsis,* sight]. 1. Hyperphoria. 2. Inability to use the vision, as in those confined in the dark, or

from disuse of an eye in strabismus, or resulting from cataract, or in refractive errors.

anorchia. Anorchism, q.v.

anorchidism (ăn-or'kĭ-dĭzm"). Anorchism.

anorchism (ăn-or'kĭzm) [" + *orchis,* testicle, + *-ismos,* condition]. Congenital absence of one or both testes. SYN: *anorchidism.*

anorectal (ā-nō-rĕk'tăl). Pert. to both the anus and rectum.

anorectic, anorectous (ăn-ō-rĕk'tĭc, -tŭs) [Gr. *anorektos,* without appetite for]. Having no appetite.

anorexia (ăn-ō-rĕk'sē-ă) [Gr. *an-,* not, + *orexis,* appetite]. Loss of appetite. Seen in depression, malaise, commencement of fevers and illnesses, also in disorders of alimentary tract, esp. of stomach, and as a result of alcoholic excesses and drug addiction, esp. cocaine. Many medicines and medical procedures have the undesired side effect of causing malaise with concurrent anorexia.

 NURSING IMPLICATIONS: Provide patient with oral hygiene before and after eating. Determine patient's food preferences and offer only those. Provide small, frequent meals or slightly smaller meals with between-meal and bedtime nutritional snacks. Keep patient areas free of odors. Provide quiet atmosphere for meals. Encourage family and friends to bring favorite home-cooked meals, and to join patient for meals. Warn others that mealtime conversation should be on pleasant topics and should not address the patient's food intake or lack thereof. Document actual intake, indicating particular foods, amount eaten, and approximate nutrient intake.

 RS: acoria; ageusia; bulimia; hyperorexia; nausea; parageusia; parorexia; pica; polyphagia; pyrosis; taste.

 a. nervosa. Occurs most commonly in females between the ages of 12 and 21 but may occur in older women and men.

 Diagnosis is made by the following criteria: Intense fear of becoming obese. This does not diminish as weight loss progresses. The patient claims to feel fat even when emaciated. A loss of 25% of original weight may occur. No known physical illness accounts for the weight loss. There is a refusal to maintain body weight over a minimal normal weight for age and height.

 Psychiatric therapy in a hospital is usually required if patient refuses to eat. The patient may need to be fed parenterally. SEE: *bulimia.* SEE: *Nursing Diagnoses* in *Appendix.*

 NURSING IMPLICATIONS: Monitor patient's vital signs and fluid and electrolyte balance (intake, output, daily weight, and laboratory values). It may be necessary to check patient's body orifices for secreted weights prior to weighing. Offer small, frequent meals and nutritionally complete fluids. Explain edema or bloating if present. If tube feeding or parenteral nutrition is required, explain procedure to patient. Calmly recognize patient's need for nutrition, and avoid arguments about food or weight by patient. Monitor patient's exercise and other activities, to be sure food intake is not being negated by vomiting, catharsis, or excessive exercise. Encourage patient to express feelings freely, supporting patient's assertiveness. Assist others in dealing with their feelings about patient and patient's behavior, and instruct them not to discuss food or weight with the patient. Assist patient in obtaining continued support by referring them to the national support and information organizations. SEE: *Appendix, Helpline Resources in the U.S.*

anorexigenic (ăn″ō-rĕk″sĭ-jĕn′ĭk) [″ + ″ + *gennan*, to produce]. Causing loss of appetite.

anorgasmy (ăn-or-găz′mē) [″ + *orgasmos*, swelling]. Failure to experience orgasm during either sexual intercourse or masturbation.

anorthography (ăn″or-thŏg′ră-fē) [″ + *orthos*, straight, + *graphein*, to write]. Agraphia, esp. motor agraphia; loss of power to express oneself in writing. SEE: *agraphia.*

anorthopia (ăn″or-thō′pē-ă) [″ + ″ + *ops*, eye]. 1. Vision in which straight lines do not appear straight; symmetry and parallelism not properly perceived. 2. Strabismus.

anoscope (ā′nō-skōp) [L. *anus*, anus, + Gr. *skopein*, to examine]. Speculum for examining the anus and lower rectum.

anosigmoidoscopy (ā″nō-sĭg″moy-dŏs′kō-pē) [″ + Gr. *sigmoeides*, shaped like Greek S, + *skopein*, to examine]. Direct visual examination of the anus, rectum, and colon by use of an endoscope.

anosmatic (ăn-ŏz-măt′ĭk) [Gr. *an-*, not, + *osme*, smell]. Lacking the sense of smell.

anosmia (ăn-ŏz′mē-ă). Loss of the sense of smell. SYN: *anodmia.*

anosmic, anosmous (ăn-ŏz′mĭk, -mŭs). 1. Lacking the sense of smell. 2. Odorless.

anosognosia (ăn-ō-sŏg-nō′zē-ă) [″ + ″ + *gnosis*, knowledge]. The apparent denial, unawareness of, or failure of recognition of one's own neurological defect.

anosphrasia (ăn-ŏs-frā′zē-ă) [Gr. *an-*, not, + *osphresis*, smell]. Absence of or imperfect sense of smell.

anospinal (ā″nō-spī′năl) [L. *anus* + *spina*, thorn]. Pert. to the anus and spinal cord, or to the center in the spinal cord that controls the contraction of the anal sphincter.

anostosis (ăn-ŏs-tō′sĭs) [Gr. *an-*, not, + *osteon*, bone, + *osis*, condition]. A defective formation or development of bone; failure to ossify.

anotia (ăn-ō′shē-ă) [″ + *ours*, ear]. Congenital malformation with absence of the ears.

anotropia (ăn″ō-trō′pē-ă) [Gr. *ana*, up, + *trope*, a turning]. Tendency of the eyes to turn upward and away from the visual axis.

ANOVA. Term used in statistics for *analysis of variance.* SEE: *analysis of variance.*

anovaginal (ā″nō-văj′ĭ-năl). Pert. to the anus and vagina.

anovarism (ăn-ō′văr-ĭzm) [Gr. *an-*, not, + LL. *ovarium*, ovary, + Gr. *-ismos*, condition]. Absence of ovaries.

anovesical (ā″nō-vĕs′ĭ-kl) [L. *anus*, anus, + *vesica*, bladder]. Rel. to both the anus and urinary bladder.

anovular, anovulatory (ăn-ŏv′ū-lăr, ăn-ŏv′ū-lă-tō″rē) [Gr. *an-*, not, + LL. *ovarium*, ovary]. Not accompanied by production of and discharge of an ovum.

anovular cycle. Menstrual cycle in which ovulation is absent.

anoxemia (ăn-ŏk-sē′mē-ă) [″ + *oxygen* + Gr. *haima*, blood]. Insufficient oxygenation of the blood. SEE: *hypoxemia; respiration.*

anoxia (ăn-ŏk′sē-ă) [″ + *oxygen*]. Without oxygen. Term is often used incorrectly to indicate hypoxia, q.v.

a., altitude. Anoxia due to insufficient oxygen content of inspired air at high altitudes.

a., anemic. Anoxia due to decrease in hemoglobin concentration or number of erythrocytes in the blood.

a., anoxic. Anoxia due to disordered pulmonary mechanisms of oxygenation. May be due to reduced oxygen supply, respiratory obstruction, reduced pulmonary function or inadequate respiratory movements.

a., histotoxic. Anoxia due to inability of the tissues to utilize oxygen. SEE: *cyanide.*

a., hypokinetic. A., stagnant, q.v.

a., stagnant. Anoxia due to insufficient peripheral circulation, as occurs in cardiac failure, shock, arterial spasm, and thrombosis.

anoxic (ăn-ŏks′ĭk). Pert. to or caused by a general lack of oxygen, and characterized by a generally subnormal oxygen tension of the blood.

ansa (ăn′să) [L., a handle] (pl. *ansae*). [NA] In anatomy, any structure in the form of a loop or arc.

a. cervicalis. [NA] Formerly called ansa hypoglossi. A nerve loop in the neck formed by fibers from the first three cervical nerves.

a. hypoglossi. [NA] A. cervicalis, q.v.

a. lenticularis. [NA] Tortuous fiber tract from the globus pallidus, extending around the internal capsule, to the ventral thalamic nucleus.

a. nervorum spinalium. [NA] Connecting loops of nerve fibers between the anterior spinal nerves.

a. peduncularis. [NA] Complex fiber tract from the anterior temporal lobe, extending around the internal capsule, to the mediodorsal thalamic nucleus.

a. sacralis. Nerve loop connecting the sympathetic trunk with the coccygeal ganglion.

a. subclavia. [NA] Nerve loop that passes anterior and inferior to the subclavian artery, connecting the middle and inferior cervical sympathetic ganglia.

anserine bursitis. SEE: *bursitis, anserine.*

ANSER system. A group of questionnaires for evaluating developmental dysfunction in children.

A.N.S.I. *American National Standards Institute.*

ansiform (ăn'sĭ-form) [L. *ansa,* a handle, + *forma,* shape]. Shaped like a loop.

ant- [Gr.]. Prefix denoting opposed to, counteracting, against.

ant. Small, social insect of the order Hymenoptera, and family Formicidae, distributed worldwide. Ants live in highly organized groups and have within their colonies members that specialize in performing specific tasks.

Antabuse (ăn'tă-būs"). Proprietary name for disulfiram. Administered orally in treatment of alcoholism. Ingestion of alcohol following taking of drug causes severe reactions including nausea and vomiting and may endanger the life of the patient. SEE: *Poisons and Poisoning* in *Appendix.*

antacid (ănt-ăs'ĭd) [Gr. *anti,* against, + L. *acidum,* acid]. An agent that neutralizes acidity, esp. in the stomach and duodenum. Ex.: aluminum hydroxide; magnesium oxide. SEE: *peptic ulcer.*

antagonism (ăn-tăg'ō-nĭzm") [Gr. *antagonizesthai,* to struggle against]. Mutual opposition or contrary action, as between muscles or medicines.

a., microbiological. The inhibition of one bacterial organism by another. This mechanism is one of the most important host defenses against microbial pathogens.

antagonist (ăn-tăg'ō-nĭst). That which counteracts the action of something else, as a muscle or drug. Opposite of synergist.

a., dental. The tooth in the opposite arch with which a tooth occludes in function.

a., drug. Drugs which prevent receptor stimulation. A drug that is an antagonist has an affinity for a cell receptor, and, by

binding to it, the cell is prevented from responding.

a., muscular. A muscle that opposes the action of the prime mover and produces a smooth movement by balancing the opposite forces.

a., narcotic. A drug that prevents or reverses the action of a narcotic. SEE: *nalorphine.*

antalgesic (ănt-ăl-jē'sĭk) [Gr. *anti,* against, + *algos,* pain]. A drug that relieves pain. SYN: *analgesic; anodyne.*

antalgic (ănt-ăl'jĭk). Antalgesic, q.v.

antalkaline (ănt-ăl'kă-lĭn, -lĭn) [" + *alkaline*]. An agent that neutralizes alkalinity.

antaphrodisiac (ănt"ăf-rō-dĭz'ē-ăk) [" + *aphrodisiakos,* sexual]. An agent that depresses sexual desire. SYN: *anaphrodisiac.*

antasthenic (ănt"ăs-thĕn'ĭk) [" + *astheneia,* weakness]. 1. Relieving weakness; strengthening, invigorating. 2. Agent that strengthens, relieves weakness.

antasthmatic (ănt"ăz-măt'ĭk) [" + Gr. *asthma,* panting]. 1. Preventing or relieving asthma. 2. Agent that prevents or relieves an asthma attack.

antatrophic (ănt"ă-trō'fĭk) [" + *atrophia,* atrophy]. Preventing or curing atrophy.

antazoline phosphate (ăn-tăz'ō-lēn). USP. An antihistamine used in dilute solution to treat allergic conjunctivitis. A component of the trade name preparation Vasocon-A.

ante- [L.]. Prefix meaning before.

antebrachium (ăn"tē-brā'kē-ŭm) [L. *ante,* before, + *brachium,* arm]. [NA] The forearm.

antecardium (ăn"tē-kăr'dē-ŭm) [" + Gr. *kardia,* heart]. The area on the anterior surface of the body overlying the heart and the lower part of the thorax. SYN: *precordia; precordium.*

antecedent (ăn"tē-sē'dĕnt) [L. *antecedere,* to precede]. Something that comes before something else; a precursor.

a., plasma thromboplastin. ABBR: PTA. Blood coagulation factor XI. SYN: *Christmas factor.* SEE: *coagulation factors.*

ante cibum (ăn'tē sē'bŭm) [L.]. ABBR: a.c. Used in prescription writing to indicate *before meals.*

antecubital (ăn"tē-kū'bĭ-tăl) [" + *cubitum,* elbow]. In front of the elbow; at the bend of the elbow.

antecubital fossa. Triangular area lying anterior to and below the elbow, bounded medially by the pronator teres and laterally by the brachioradialis muscles. SYN: *cubital fossa.*

antecurvature (ăn"tē-kŭr'vă-tŭr") [" + *curvatura,* bend]. Bending forward abnormally. SYN: *anteflexion.*

antefebrile (an"tē-fē'brĭl, -fē'brĭl, -fĕb'rĭl) [L.

ante, before, + *febris*, fever]. Before the development of fever. SYN: *antepyretic.*

anteflect (ăn'tē-flĕkt) [" + *flectere*, to bend]. To bend or cause to bend forward.

anteflexion (ăn″tē-flĕk'shŭn). The abnormal bending forward of part of an organ, esp. of the uterus at its body and neck. SEE: *anteversion.*

antegrade (ăn'tē-grād). Moving forward or in the same direction as the flow.

antelocation (ăn″tē-lō-kā'shŭn) [" + *locare*, to place]. Forward displacement of an organ.

antemetic (ănt″ē-mĕt'ĭk) [Gr. *anti*, against, + *emetikos*, emetic]. 1. Preventing or alleviating nausea and vomiting. 2. Agent that prevents or moderates nausea and vomiting. SYN: *antiemetic.*

ante mortem (ăn'tē mor'tĕm) [L.]. Before death.

ante mortem statement. Declaration of the individual made immediately preceding death. SYN: *deathbed statement,* q.v.

antenatal (ăn″tē-nā'tăl) [" + *natus*, born]. Occurring before birth. SYN: *prenatal.*

antenatal diagnosis. Diagnostic procedures done to determine the health and genetic status of the fetus. Methods include amniocentesis, chorionic villus sampling, cell culture, biochemical methods, nonstress testing, oxytocin challenge test, biophysical profile, amnioscopy, amniography, and ultrasound.

antenatal surgery. Surgical procedure done on the fetus prior to delivery. This type of surgery is done only at certain medical centers. SEE: *amnioscopy; embryoscopy.*

Antepar. Trade name for piperazine citrate, q.v.

antepartal; ante partum (ăn″tē-păr'tăl, -tŭm) [L.]. Before the onset of labor, used with reference to the mother.

antepyretic (ăn″tē-pī-rĕt'ĭk) [L. *ante*, before, + Gr. *pyretos*, fever]. Before the development of fever. SYN: *antefebrile.*

anterior [L.]. Before or in front of. In anatomical nomenclature, refers to the ventral or abdominal side of the body.

anterior chamber. Aqueous chamber of eye. Bounded in front by cornea, behind by iris and lens. SEE: *eye.*

anterior drawer sign or test. With the knee flexed to a right angle, there is increased anterior glide of the tibia in anterior cruciate ligament rupture. SEE: *posterior drawer sign.*

anterior horn cell. A large nerve cell in the anterior horn of the spinal cord. The axon of the cell is an efferent fiber innervating a muscle.

antero- [L.]. Prefix denoting anterior, front, before.

anteroexternal (ăn″tĕr-ō-ĕks-tĕr'năl) [L. *antero*, anterior, + *externus*, outside]. In anatomy, located to the front and laterally.

anterograde [" + *gradior*, to step]. Moving frontward.

anteroinferior [" + *inferior*, below]. In front and below.

anterointernal (ăn″tĕr-ō-ĭn-tĕr'năl) [" + *internus*, within]. In anatomy, located to the front and to the inner side.

anterolateral [" + *latus*, side]. In front and to one side.

anteromedial [" + *medius*, middle]. In front and toward the center.

anteroposterior [" + *posterior*, rear]. Passing from front to rear.

anterosuperior [" + *superior*, above]. In front and above.

anteversion (ăn″tē-vĕr'zhŭn) [" + *vertere*, to turn]. 1. A tipping forward of an organ as a whole, without bending. SEE: *anteflexion.* 2. Excessive anterior angulation of the neck of the femur, i.e., femoral neck anteversion, leading to excessive internal rotation of the femur. Normal value for femoral neck anteversion is approximately 15 degrees. Any increase in this anterior angulation is called femoral anteversion.

anteverted (an″tē-vĕrt'ĕd). Tipped forward.

anthelix (ănt'hē-lĭks, ăn'thē-lĭks) [Gr. *anti*, against, + *helix*, coil]. Curved prominence of the external ear parallel to and in front of the helix. SYN: *antihelix.*

anthelmintic, anthelminthic, antihelmintic (ănt″hĕl-mĭn'tĭk, -thĭk, ăn″tī-hĕl-mĭn'tĭk) [" + *helmins*, worm]. An agent that destroys parasitic intestinal worms.

Anthemis (ăn'thĕm-ĭs). 1. A genus of aromatic flowering plants. 2. Camomile; chamomile; dried blossoms of *Anthemis nobilis.* A bitter tonic; an antispasmodic.

anthemorrhagic (ănt″hĕm-ō-răj'ĭk) [" + *haima*, blood, + *rhegnynai*, to burst forth]. Agent for preventing or arresting hemorrhage. SYN: *antihemorrhagic.*

anthocyanin (ăn″thō-sī'ă-nĭn) [Gr. *anthos*, flower, + *kyanos*, a blue substance]. Any one of a group of reddish-purple pigments occurring in flowers.

Anthomyia (ăn″thō-mī'yă) [" + *myia*, fly]. A genus of fly of the order Diptera, related to the housefly. Larvae sometimes infest man.

 A. canicularis. A small black housefly, whose larvae may infest the human intestine after accidental ingestion, often resulting in gastrointestinal disturbances.

anthophobia (ăn″thō-fō'bē-ă) [" + *phobos*, fear]. Morbid dislike or fear of flowers.

anthracene (ăn'thră-sēn). $C_{14}H_{10}$. A hydrocarbon obtained from distilling coal tar. Used in manufacturing dyes.

anthracia (an-thrā'sē-ă) [Gr. *anthrax*, coal, carbuncle]. Presence of carbuncles.

anthracoid (an'thră-koyd) [" + *eidos*, form, shape]. Resembling or pert. to anthrax.

anthracometer (ăn"thră-kŏm'ĕ-ter) [" + *metron*, measure]. An instrument for measuring the amount of combustion products in the air.

anthraconecrosis (ăn"thrā-kō-nĕ-krō'sĭs) [" + *nekrosis*, state of death]. Gangrene in which tissue becomes dry and black.

anthracosilicosis (ăn"thrā-kō-sil"ĭ-kō'sĭs) [" + L. *silex*, flint, + Gr. *osis*, condition]. A form of pneumoconiosis in which carbon and silica deposits accumulate in the lungs due to breathing coal dust. SYN: *coal worker's pneumoconiosis.* SEE: *anthracosis; silicosis.*

anthracosis (ăn-thrā-kō'sĭs) [" + *osis*, condition]. Accumulation of carbon deposits in the lungs due to breathing smoke or coal dust. SYN: *black lung.*

Anthra-Derm. Trade name for anthralin, q.v.

anthralin (ăn'thră-lĭn). USP. A synthetic hydrocarbon used in ointment form for treating various skin diseases including fungal infections and eczema. Trade names are Anthra-Derm and Drithocreme.

anthrax (ăn'thrăks) [Gr., coal, carbuncle]. Acute, infectious disease caused by *Bacillus anthracis,* usually attacking cattle, sheep, horses, and goats. Man contracts it from contact with animal hair, hides, or waste.

SYM: Disease may attack lungs (woolsorter's disease) or the loose connective tissue, giving rise to malignant edema, necrosis of mediastinal lymph nodes, and pleural effusion. This is followed by respiratory distress, cyanosis, shock, and coma. More commonly anthrax occurs in form of a pustule called anthrax boil or malignant pustule. This cutaneous form will exhibit redness, vesiculation and induration with central ulceration, and development of a black eschar. Rarely, the disease may occur in intestinal tract. If untreated, anthrax may be fatal.

ETIOL: *B. anthracis.* Workers who handle wools, hides, and brushes are commonly affected.

TREAT: Penicillin or tetracyclines. Erythromycin is also effective for most strains.

NURSING IMPLICATIONS: Educate individuals at risk about the prevention, transmission, and course of anthrax. For patients with inhalation anthrax, monitor vital signs and provide respiratory support as ordered. For cutaneous anthrax, keep lesions clean and covered with sterile dressings. Provide frequent oral hygiene and skin care. Encourage oral fluid intake and offer frequent, small, nutritious meals. Maintain isolation precautions: mask and gown, handwashing, and incineration of contaminated materials. Control hyperpyrexia with appropriate nursing and prescribed medical therapies. SEE: *Universal Precautions* in *Appendix.*

anthropo- [Gr. *anthropos*, man]. Prefix denoting relationship to man or human life.

anthropobiology (ăn"thrō-pō-bī-ŏl'ō-jē) [" + *bios*, life, + *logos*, word, reason]. Study of the biology of man and the great apes.

anthropogeny (ăn"thrō-pŏj'ĕ-nē) [" + *gennan*, to produce]. Origin and development of man.

anthropoid (ăn'thrō-poyd) [" + *eidos*, form, shape]. 1. Resembling man. 2. An ape.

anthropological baseline. An imaginary line that passes from the lower border of the orbit to the superior margin of the external auditory meatus.

anthropology (ăn"thrō-pŏl'ō-jē) [" + *logos*, word, reason]. The scientific study of man. Included are investigation of man's origin and development of physical, cultural, religious, and social attributes.

anthropometer (ăn"thrō-pŏm'ĕ-tĕr) [" + *metron*, measure]. Device for measuring the human body and its parts.

anthropometry (ăn-thrō-pŏm'ĕt-rē). Science of measuring the human body. Includes craniometry, osteometry, skin fold evaluation for subcutaneous fat estimation, and height and weight measurements. Usually performed by an anthropologist.

anthropomorphism (ăn"thrō-pō-mor'fĭzm) [" + *morphe*, form, + *-ismos*, condition]. Attributing human qualities to nonhuman organisms or objects.

anthropophilic (ăn"thrō-pō-fil'ĭk) [" + *philein*, to love]. Preferring man, said of parasites that prefer a human host rather than other animals. SYN: *androphilic.*

anthropozoonoses (ăn"thrō-pō-zō"ō-nō'sēs) [" + *zoon*, animal, + *nosis*, disease]. Infectious diseases acquired by man from vertebrate hosts of the causative agents. Included are rabies and trichinosis.

anti- [Gr.]. Prefix meaning against.

antiadrenergic (ăn"tē-ă-drĕn-ĕr'jĭk) [Gr. *anti*, against, + L. *ad*, to, + *ren*, kidney, + Gr. *ergon*, work]. Preventing or counteracting adrenergic action.

antiagglutinin (ăn"tē-ă-gloo'tĭ-nĭn). A specific antibody opposing the action of an agglutinin.

antiamebic (ăn"tē-ă-mē'bĭk) [" + *amoibe*, change]. A medicine used to prevent or treat amebiasis.

antianaphylaxis (ăn"tē-ăn-ă-fĭ-lăks'ĭs) [" + *ana*, away from, + *phylaxis*, protection]. Prevention of anaphylaxis. Usually attained by administering repeated doses of the sensitizing substance too small to cause an anaphylactic reaction. SYN: *desensitization.*

antiandrogen (ăn″tē-ăn′drō-jĕn) [″ + *androgen*]. Substance that acts to inhibit or prevent the action of an androgen.

antianemic (ăn″tē-ă-nē′mĭk). Preventing or curing anemia.

antibody (ăn″tē-ăn′tĭ-bŏd-ē) [″ + *antibody*]. An antibody specific for, and produced in response to the administration of, another antibody.

antitoxin (ăn″tē-ăn″tĭ-tŏk′sĭn) [″ + *antitoxin*]. An antibody, produced in response to the administration of an antitoxin, that counteracts the effect of the antitoxin.

antiapoplectic (ăn″tē-ăp″ō-plĕk′tĭk). Preventing or relieving apoplexy.

antiarrhythmic (ăn″tē-ă-rĭth′mĭk) [″ + *a-*, not, + *rhythmos*, rhythm]. A drug or physical force that acts to control or prevent cardiac arrhythmias.

antiarthritic (ăn″tē-ăr-thrĭt′ĭk) [″ + *arthritikos*, gouty]. Relieving arthritis.

antibacterial (ăn″tĭ-băk-tē′rē-ăl). Destroying or stopping the growth of bacteria.

antibiosis (ăn″tĭ-bī-ō′sĭs) [″ + *bios*, life]. The association or relationship between two organisms wherein one is harmful to the other.

antibiotic (ăn″tĭ-bī-ŏt′ĭk). 1. Destructive to life. 2. Pert. to antibiosis. 3. Any of a variety of natural or synthetic substances that inhibit growth of or destroy microorganisms. Used extensively in treatment of infectious diseases in plants, animals, and man. The first antibiotic to be used clinically was germicidin, isolated by René Dubos and used initially in 1939 to treat bacterial infections in cattle. That report predated the initial clinical use of penicillin. SEE: *antimicrobial drugs* for table.

 a., bacteriocidal or bactericidal. Antibiotic that kills microorganisms.

 a., bacteriostatic. Antibiotic that inhibits growth of microorganisms.

 a., broad-spectrum. Antibiotic that is effective against a wide variety of microorganisms.

antibiotic resistant. Strains of bacteria that have become resistant to the action of antibiotics, or were never sensitive to them.

antibody (ăn″tĭ-bŏd″ē). Complex glycoproteins produced by B lymphocytes in response to the presence of an antigen, q.v. Antibodies, all of which are immunoglobulins, may combine with specific antigens to destroy or control them, providing protection against most common infections. Al-

most all antibodies except natural antibodies, e.g., antibodies to different blood types, are created by B cells linking with a foreign antigen on the surface of an invading organism.

Antibodies neutralize or destroy antigens in several ways. They can directly lyse the antigen, neutralize toxins released by bacteria, opsonize the antigen or form a complex to stimulate phagocytosis, promote antigen clumping (agglutination), or prevent the antigen from adhering to host cells. SYN: *immunoglobulin.* SEE: *antigen; autoantibody; cytokines; immunoglobulin.*

 a., antireceptor. An antibody that acts against the receptor on a cell rather than on the cell itself.

 a., blocking. Antibody that combines with an antigen and specifically blocks its ability to produce sensitizing reactions.

 a., cross-reacting. Antibody that reacts with antigens functionally similar to its specific antigen.

 a., fluorescent. Antibody reaction made visible by incorporating a fluorescent dye into the antigen-antibody reaction and examining the specimen with a microscope equipped for fluorescent microscopy.

 a., maternal. Antibody produced by the mother and transferred to the fetus in utero.

 a., monoclonal. SEE: *monoclonal antibodies; hybridoma.*

 a., natural. Antibody present in a person without known exposure to the specific antigen, such as an anti-A antibody in a person with B blood type; may be the result of unknown, accidental exposure.

antibody combining site. The particular area on an antibody molecule to which part of an antigen links, creating an antigen-antibody reaction. SEE: *antibody; antigen; antigenic determinant.*

antibody therapy. The use of antibodies to treat patients with immunodeficiency. This is done by using parenteral immune globulin.

antibrachium (ăn″tĭ-brā′kē-ŭm). Antebrachium; the forearm.

antibromic (ăn″tĭ-brō′mĭk) [Gr. *anti*, against, + *bromos*, smell]. 1. Deodorizing. 2. A deodorant.

antiburnscar garment. A carefully fitted garment of material with calibrated stretch characteristics worn to provide uniform pressure over burn graft sites in order to reduce scarring during healing.

anticarcinogenic. A substance or action that prevents or delays tumor formation.

anticardium (ăn″tĭ-kăr′dē-ŭm). Antecardium; the area on the anterior surface of the body overlying the heart and the lower part of the thorax. SYN: *precordia; precordium.*

anticariogenic. A substance or action that interferes with the development of dental caries.

anticarious (ăn″tĭ-kā′rē-ŭs) [″ + *caries,* decay]. Preventing decay of teeth.

anticatarrhal (ăn″tĭ-kă-tăr′ăl) [″ + L. *catarrhus,* catarrhal]. Relieving catarrh.

anticholagogue (ăn″tĭ-kŏl′ă-gŏg) [Gr. *anti,* against, + *chole,* bile, + *agein,* to lead forth]. Medicine used to decrease secretion of bile.

anticholinergic (ăn″tĭ-kō″lĭn-ĕr′jĭk). 1. Impeding the impulses of cholinergic, esp. parasympathetic, nerve fibers. 2. An agent that blocks parasympathetic nerve impulses. Effects include dry mouth and blurred vision, and are side effects seen with use of phenothiazine and tricyclic antidepressant drug therapy. SYN: *parasympatholytic.*

anticholinesterase (ăn″tĭ-kō-lĭn-ĕs′tĕr-ās). Substance that opposes the action of cholinesterase.

anticipate (ăn-tĭs′ĭ-pāt) [L. *ante,* before, + *capere,* to take]. 1. To occur prior to the usual time of onset of a particular illness or disease, said of an event, sign, or symptom. 2. In nursing and medicine, to plan in order to be prepared for other than the routine or fully expected.

anticipatory grief. Grief experienced prior to the impending death of a loved one.

anticipatory guidance. Information concerning normal expectations of age group or disease entity in order to provide support for coping with problems before they actually arise.

anticlinal (ăn″tĭ-klī′năl) [Gr. *anti,* against, + *klinein,* to incline]. Inclined in opposite directions.

anticoagulant (ăn″tĭ-kō-ăg′ū-lănt) [″ + L. *coagulans,* forming clots]. 1. Delaying or preventing blood coagulation. 2. Agent that prevents or delays blood coagulation.

　a. citrate dextrose solution. USP. Anticoagulant used for storing whole blood.

　a. citrate phosphate dextrose solution. USP. Anticoagulant used for storing whole blood.

　a. heparin solution. USP. Anticoagulant used for storing whole blood.

　a. sodium citrate solution. USP. Anticoagulant used for storing whole blood.

　a., warfarin sodium. SEE: *warfarin sodium.*

anticoagulant therapy. Use of drugs that interfere with blood coagulation to prevent diseases that are caused by venous thrombosis, e.g., myocardial infarction, and to help prevent systemic embolism in patients with atrial fibrillation. The principal adverse reaction to these drugs is bleeding.

Thus, control of the dose and monitoring the effects on the clotting mechanism are essential. SEE: *warfarin sodium.*

anticodon (ăn″tĭ-kō′dŏn). A triple arrangement of bases on transfer ribonucleic acid (tRNA) that complements the corresponding triplet on messenger ribonucleic acid (mRNA).

anticonvulsant (ăn″tĭ-kŏn-vŭl′sănt) [″ + L. *convulsio,* pulling together]. 1. Preventing or relieving convulsions. 2. Agent that prevents or relieves convulsions.

anticytotoxin. Something that opposes the action of a cytotoxin. SEE: *cytotoxin.*

antidepressant (ăn″tĭ-dē-prĕs′sănt). Anything, medicine or other mode of therapy, that acts to prevent, cure, or alleviate mental depression.

antidiabetic (ăn″tĭ-dī″ă-bĕt′ĭk). 1. Preventing or relieving diabetes. 2. Agent that prevents or relieves diabetes.

antidiarrheal (ăn″tĭ-dī-ă-rē′ăl). Substance used to prevent or treat diarrhea.

antidiuretic (ăn″tĭ-dī-ū-rĕt′ĭk) [″ + *dia,* intensive, + *ouresis,* urination]. 1. Lessening urine secretion. 2. Drug that decreases urine secretion.

antidiuretic hormone. ABBR: ADH. Vasopressin, q.v.

antidotal (ăn″tĭ-dō′tăl). Acting as or pert. to an antidote.

antidote (ăn′tĭ-dōt) [Gr. *antidoton,* given against]. A substance that neutralizes poisons or their effects.

　a., chemical. Antidote that reacts with the poison to produce a harmless chemical compound. For example, table salt precipitates silver nitrate and forms silver chloride. Chemical antidotes should be used sparingly, and after their use the stomach contents should be removed by gastric lavage because they may produce serious results if allowed to remain in the stomach.

　a., mechanical. Antidote that prevents absorption of the poison. Includes fats, oils, milk (casein coagulum), whites of eggs, finely divided charcoal, fuller's earth, or mineral oil. (Fats and oils are not to be used in treating phosphorus, camphor, aspidium, and cantharides poisonings.)

　a., physiologic. Antidote that produces physiological effects opposite to the effects of the poison; e.g., sedatives are given for convulsants and stimulants are given for hypnotics. These should not be given without physician's definite instructions.

　a., universal. Antidote that is given orally and is effective against a great number of toxic substances. There is, of course, no truly "universal" antidote.

　Two parts activated charcoal, one part tannic acid, and one part magnesium oxide.

(The charcoal absorbs; the tannic acid precipitates metals, alkaloids, and some glucosides; and the magnesium oxide neutralizes acids.) Give orally by dissolving 5 tsp (approx. 25 ml) of the mixture in 4 oz (120 ml) of warm water. After the patient has swallowed the antidote, the stomach contents should then be removed by gastric lavage within a few minutes. Treatment may be repeated.

Caution: Do not use gastric lavage in patients who have ingested caustics. The stomach or esophagus may be ruptured by introduction of the tube.

---

antidromic (ăn″tĭ-drŏm′ĭk) [Gr. *anti,* against, + *dromos,* running]. Denoting nerve impulses traveling in the opposite direction from normal.

antidysenteric (ăn″tĭ-dĭs″ĕn-tĕr′ĭk). 1. Preventing or relieving dysentery. 2. Agent that prevents or relieves dysentery.

antiemetic (ăn″tĭ-ē-mĕt′ĭk) [″ + *emetikos,* inclined to vomit]. 1. Preventing or relieving nausea and vomiting. 2. Agent that prevents or relieves nausea and vomiting.

antienzyme (an″tĭ-ĕn′zīm). Substance that opposes the action of an enzyme.

antiepileptic (ăn″tĭ-ĕp″ĭ-lĕp′tĭk). 1. Opposing epilepsy. 2. Any procedure or therapy that combats epilepsy.

antiestrogen (ăn″tĭ-ĕs′trō-jĕn). Substance that blocks or modifies the action of estrogen.

antifebrile (ăn″tĭ-fē′brĭl, -fē′brīl, -fĕb′rĭl) [″ + L. *febris,* fever]. 1. Reducing fever. 2. Agent that reduces fever. SYN: *antipyretic.*

antifibrinolysin (ăn″tĭ-fī″brĭ-nŏl′ĭ-sĭn) [″ + L. *fibra,* fiber, + Gr. *lysis,* dissolution]. Substance that counteracts fibrinolysis.

antifungal (ăn″tĭ-fŭng′găl). 1. Destroying or inhibiting the growth of fungi. 2. Agent that destroys or inhibits the growth of fungi.

antigalactic (ăn″tĭ-gă-lăk′tĭk). 1. Preventing or diminishing the secretion of milk. 2. Agent that prevents or diminishes the secretion of milk.

antigen (ăn′tĭ-jĕn) [Gr. *anti,* against, + *gennan,* to produce]. A protein marker on the surface of cells that identifies the cell as "self" or "non-self"; identifies the type of cell, e.g., skin, kidney; stimulates the production of antibodies, q.v., by B lymphocytes that will neutralize or destroy the cell if necessary; and stimulates cytotoxic responses by granulocytes, monocytes, and lymphocytes.

Antigens on the body's own cells are called autoantigens, q.v. Antigens on all other cells are called foreign antigens.

Matching certain types of tissue antigens is essential for the success of an organ transplant. Inflammation, q.v., occurs when neutrophils, monocytes, and macrophages encounter an antigen from any source during bodily injury. The antigen may be foreign, or an autoantigen that has been damaged and, therefore, appears to be foreign. Reactions to antigens by T and B cells are part of the specific immune response, q.v. SEE: *autoantigen; cytokines; histocompatibility antigens.*

a. ′s, histocompatibility. SEE: *histocompatibility locus antigens.*

a., H-Y. A histocompatibility antigen located on the cell membrane. It has a primary role in determining the sexual differentiation of the male embryo.

a., prostate-specific. SEE: *prostate-specific antigen.*

a., soluble. An antigen present in a liquid (aqueous) substance.

a., specific. The property of mature B and T lymphocytes that enables them to respond to specific foreign antigens entering the body. Antigen specificity requires mature B and T cells that have been previously exposed to the antigen and, therefore, are able to recognize it again and respond by neutralizing or destroying it. The exact process by which B lymphocytes become capable of recognizing and responding to antigens is unknown. Development of antigen specificity by T cells requires macrophage processing, q.v., of the antigen for recognition.

a., tumor-specific. Antigens produced by certain tumors. These appear on the tumor cells but not on normal cells derived from the same tissue.

antigen-antibody reaction. The combination of an antigen with its specific antibody. May result in agglutination, precipitation, neutralization, complement-fixation, or increased susceptibility to phagocytosis. The antigen-antibody reaction forms the basis for B cell mediated immunity, q.v.

antigenic (ăn-tĭ-jĕn′ĭk). Capable of causing the production of an antibody.

antigenic determinant. The specific area of an antigen that binds with an antibody combining site, q.v., and determines the specificity of the antigen-antibody reaction. SEE: *antigen.*

a.d., epitope. The simplest form of an antigenic determinant within a complex antigenic marker. The epitope links with a paratope, one area of an antibody combining site, q.v.

antigenic drift. A change in the protein marker or antigen, q.v., on an organism. As a result, the body's previous immune response to the organism must change. This is frequently seen in the influenza virus as it changes its antigenic make-up from year to year.

antigenicity. The condition of being able to produce an immune response to an antibody.

antigen presenting cell. Cells that break down antigens and display their fragments on surface receptors next to major histocompatibility complex (MHC), q.v., molecules. This presentation is necessary for some T lymphocytes that are unable to recognize soluble antigens. Macrophages are the primary antigen presenting cell. SEE: *macrophage processing.*

antigen processing. The series of activities that occur when a protein is recognized by the body as foreign, culminating in the production of a specific antibody or cytotoxic cell response. SEE: *antigen; macrophage processing.*

antiglobulin (ăn″tĭ-glŏb′ū-lĭn). Substance that opposes the action of globulin.

antiglobulin test. A test for the presence of antibodies against the Rh factor on red blood cells. Antiglobulin antiserum produced in rabbits is mixed with serum containing Rh positive red blood cells. If anti-Rh antibodies have coated the red cells, the cells will agglutinate or clump together. SYN: *Coombs' test.*

antigoitrogenic (ăn″tĭ-goy″trō-jĕn′ĭk) [″ + L. *guttur*, throat, + Gr. *gennan*, to produce]. Preventing the formation of a goiter.

antigonorrheic (ăn″tĭ-gŏn″ō-rē′ĭk). 1. Curing gonorrhea. 2. Agent that cures gonorrhea.

anti-G suit [″ + *G*, gravity]. Garment designed to produce uniform pressure on the lower extremities and abdomen. Normally the suit is used by aviators to help prevent pooling of blood in the lower half of the body during certain flight maneuvers. The garment has also been used in treating severe forms of postural hypotension. The suit's usefulness in treating shock is questionable. SEE: *MAST.*

Caution: This garment is contraindicated in congestive heart failure, cardiogenic shock, and penetrating chest trauma.

---

antihelix (ăn″tĭ-hē′lĭks) [″ + Gr. *helix*, coil]. Inner curved ridge of the external ear parallel to the helix.

antihemolysin (ăn″tĭ-hĕ-mŏl′ĭ-sĭn). Substance that opposes the action of hemolysin.

antihemophilic factor. USP. ABBR: AHF. Blood coagulation factor VIII. Trade names are Antihemophilic Globulin, Hemofil, He-

mofil F, and Profilate. SEE: *coagulation factors.*

Antihemophilic Globulin (AHG). Trade name for antihemophilic factor (AHF), q.v.

antihemorrhagic (ăn″tĭ-hĕm-ō-răj′ĭk). 1. Preventing or arresting hemorrhage. 2. Agent that prevents or arrests hemorrhage.

antihidrotic (ăn″tĭ-hī-drŏt′ĭk) [″ + *hidrotikos*, sweating]. 1. Preventing or decreasing perspiration. 2. Agent that prevents or decreases perspiration. SYN: *anhidrotic; antiperspirant; antisudorific.*

antihistamine (ăn″tĭ-hĭs′tă-mēn, -mĭn). Drug that opposes the action of histamine. Many of the first antihistamines were noted for their side effects of drowsiness and dry mouth. Antihistamines are now available which have fewer side effects, e.g., terfenadine (short-acting) and astemizole (long-acting). Trade names are Seldane and Hismanal, respectively. SEE: *histamine.*

antihistamine poisoning. SEE: *Poisons and Poisoning* in *Appendix.*

antihistaminic (ăn″tĭ-hĭs″tă-mĭn′ĭk). 1. Opposing the action of histamine. 2. Agent that opposes the action of histamine.

antihormone. A substance that interferes with the action of a hormone.

antihydropic (ăn″tĭ-hī-drŏp′ĭk) [Gr. *anti*, against, + *hydropikos*, dropsical]. 1. Relieving generalized edema. 2. Agent that relieves generalized edema.

antihypercholesterolemic (ăn″tĭ-hī″pĕr-kō-lĕs″tĕr-ŏl-ē′mĭk) [″ + *hyper*, above, + *chole*, bile, + *stereos*, solid, + *haima*, blood]. 1. Preventing or controlling elevation of the serum cholesterol level. 2. Agent that prevents or controls elevation of the serum cholesterol level.

antihypertensive (ăn″tĭ-hī″pĕr-tĕn′sĭv) [″ + ″ + L. *tensio*, tension]. 1. Preventing or controlling high blood pressure. 2. Agent that prevents or controls high blood pressure.

antihypnotic (ăn″tĭ-hĭp-nŏt′ĭk). 1. Preventing or inhibiting sleep. 2. Agent that prevents or inhibits sleep.

anti-icteric (ăn″tĭ-ĭk-tĕr′ĭk) [″ + *ikteros*, jaundice]. 1. Preventing or relieving jaundice. 2. Agent that prevents or relieves jaundice.

anti-infectious (ăn″tĭ-ĭn-fĕk′shŭs). Counteracting infection.

anti-inflammatory (ăn″tĭ-ĭn-flăm′ă-tō-rē). 1. Counteracting inflammation. 2. Agent that counteracts inflammation.

antiketogenesis (ăn″tĭ-kē-tō-jĕn′ĕ-sĭs) [″ + *ketone* + Gr. *gennan*, to produce]. The prevention or inhibition of formation of ketone bodies. During starvation, diabetes, and certain other conditions, the metabolism of the ketone bodies, β-hydroxybutyric acid, acetoacetate, and acetone, is decreased; thus they accumulate in the blood. Providing increased carbohydrates in the diet or intravenously will help to prevent or treat this. Carbohydrates are therefore antiketogenic. In ketonemia due to diabetes, both insulin and carbohydrates are required in order to permit the metabolism of carbohydrate to proceed at a rate that would control ketone formation.

antiketogenetic, antiketogenic (ăn″tǐ-kē″tō-jě-nět′ĭk, -jěn′ĭk). Pert. to antiketogenesis.

antilactase (ăn″tǐ-lăk′tās) [″ + *lac*, milk, + *-ase*, enzyme]. Substance that opposes the action of lactase.

antilipemic (ăn″tǐ-lǐ-pē′mĭk). 1. Preventing or counteracting the accumulation of fatty substances in the blood. 2. Agent that prevents or counteracts the accumulation of fatty substances in the blood.

Antilirium. Trade name for physostigmine salicylate, q.v.

antilithic (ăn″tǐ-lǐth′ĭk) [″ + *lithos*, stone]. 1. Preventing or relieving calculi. 2. Agent that prevents or relieves calculi.

antiluetic (ăn″tǐ-loo-ět′ĭk) [Gr. *anti*, against, + L. *lues*, pestilence]. 1. Curing or relieving syphilis. 2. Agent that cures or relieves syphilis. SYN: *antisyphilitic*.

antilymphocyte serum (ăn″tǐ-lǐm″fō-sĭt′). ABBR: ALS. Serum developed in animals containing antibodies directed against lymphocytes that promotes some degree of immunosuppression when injected into a patient. The antibodies do not affect the activities of other white blood cells. Used to reduce rejection of transplanted organs or other tissue such as skin grafts. May cause excessive immunosuppression. SEE: *monoclonal antibodies*.

antilysin (ăn-tǐ-lī′sĭn). Antibody that opposes the action of lysin.

antilysis (ăn-tǐ-lǐ′sĭs) [″ + *lysis,* dissolution]. Prevention or inhibition of lysis due to the action of antilysin.

antilyssic (ăn-tǐ-lĭs′ĭk) [″ + *lyssa*, frenzy]. Preventing or curing rabies. SYN: *antirabic*.

antilytic (ăn-tǐ-lĭt′ĭk). Pert. to antilysis.

antimalarial (ăn″tǐ-mă-lā′rē-ăl). 1. Preventing or relieving malaria. 2. Agent that prevents or relieves malaria. SYN: *antipaludian*.

antimere (ăn″tǐ-mēr) [″ + *meros,* a part]. One of corresponding parts of the body on opposite sides of the long axis.

antimetabolite (ăn″tǐ-mě-tăb′ō-līt). 1. A substance, structurally similar to a metabolite, that opposes the action of or replaces a metabolite. It is believed that certain antibiotics are effective because they act as antimetabolites. 2. A class of antineoplastic drugs used to treat cancer. Antimetabolites are structurally similar to vitamins, coenzymes, or other substances essential for growth and division of normal and neoplastic cells. These drugs are most effective against rapidly growing tumors. A drug-induced block of DNA synthesis occurs when the cells take in the antimetabolite rather than the necessary nutrient or enzyme.

antimetropia (ăn″tǐ-mě-trō′pē-ă) [″ + *metron*, measure, + *ops,* eye]. An ocular disorder in which each eye has a different error of refraction.
   Ex.: One eye may be hyperopic; the other, myopic.

antimicrobial (ăn″tǐ-mī-krō′bē-ăl). 1. Destructive to or preventing the development of microorganisms. 2. Agent that destroys or prevents the development of microorganisms.

antimicrobial drugs. Chemical substances that either kill microorganisms or prevent their growth. SEE: table.

antimicrobic (ăn″tǐ-mī-krō′bĭk) [″ + *mikros*, small, + *bios,* life]. Antimicrobial.

Antiminth. Trade name for pyrantel pamoate, q.v.

antimitotic (ăn″tǐ-mī-tŏt′ĭk). Interfering with or preventing mitosis.

antimonial (ăn″tǐ-mō′nē-ăl). Pert. to or containing antimony.

antimony (ăn′tǐ-mō″nē). SYMB: Sb. At. wt. 121.75; at. no. 51. Stibium; a crystalline metallic element. Its compounds are used in alloys and medicines and may form poisons.

antimony poisoning. SYM: Acrid metallic taste. Cardiac and arterial depression; sweating and vomiting about 30 minutes after ingestion. In large doses, it causes irritation of lining of alimentary tract, resembling arsenic poisoning.
   F.A.: Vomiting caused by the poison may be sufficient. Gastric lavage with 1% sodium bicarbonate solution. BAL (British antilewisite) is effective, esp. if the poisoning is due to a trivalent form such as tartar emetic. Otherwise, treat symptomatically. SEE: *arsenic* in *Poisons and Poisoning* in *Appendix*.

antimuscarinic. Opposing the action of muscarine or agents that act like muscarinics. Atropine and scopolamine are antimuscarinic drugs.

antimycotic (ăn″tǐ-mī-kŏt′ĭk) [Gr. *anti*, against, + *mykes,* fungus]. Inhibiting or preventing the growth of fungi.

antinarcotic (ăn″tǐ-năr-kŏt′ĭk) [″ + *narkotikos,* benumbing]. 1. Opposing the action of a narcotic. 2. Agent that opposes the action of a narcotic.

antinatriuresis (ăn″tǐ-nā″trǐ-ū-rē′sĭs) [″ + L. *natrium*, sodium, + Gr. *ouresis*,

Antimicrobial Drugs

This list of generic antimicrobial, antiviral, and antifungal drugs can only be considered representative of the types currently available. Some are no longer used clinically but are of historical interest.

acyclovir	clarithromycin	lincomycin	phenethicillin
amantadine	clindamycin	lomefloxacin	piperacillin
amdinocillin	clotrimazole	mafenide acetate	polymyxin B
amikacin sulfate	cloxacillin	meclocycline	primaquine
p-aminosalicylic acid	colistimethate	methacycline	pyrimethamine
amoxicillin	cyclacillin	methenamine	rifampin
amphotericin B	cycloserine	mandelate	rimantadine
ampicillin	dapsone	methicillin	rosoxacin
azlocillin	demeclocycline	metronidazole	sisomicin
aztreonam	dicloxacillin	mezlocillin	spectinomycin
bacitracin	dideoxycilidine	miconazole	streptomycin
carbenicillin	dideoxyinosine	minocycline	sulfabenzamide
cefaclor	dirithromycin	monensin	sulfacetamide
cefadroxil	doxycycline	moxalactam	sulfacytine
cefamandole	epitillin	nafcillin	sulfadiazine
cefepime	erythromycin	nalidixic acid	sulfadoxine
cefmetazole	ethambutol	natamycin	sulfasalazine
cefonicid	ethionamide	neomycin	sulfisoxazole
cefoperazone	fleroxacin	netilmicin	sulfomyxin
ceforanide	floxacillin	nifurpirinol	teicoplanin
cefotaxime	fluconazole	nitrofurantoin	tetracycline
cefotetan	flucytosine	norfloxacin	ticarcillin
cefoxitin	foscarnet	novobiocin	tobramycin
cefsulodin	furazolidone	nystatin	tolnaftate
ceftazidime	ganciclovir	oleandomycin	triacetin
ceftizoxime	gentamicin	ormetoprim	trifluridine
ceftriaxone	griseofulvin	oxacillin	trimethoprim
cefuroxime	haloprogin	oxytetracycline	trimethoprim-
cephalexin	hydroxystilbamidine	paromomycin	sulfamethoxazole
cephalothin	idoxuridine	penicillin	trisulfapyrimidine
cephapirin	imapenem	penicillin G	troleandomycin
cephradine	interferon-d	benzathine	undecylenic acid
chloramphenicol	interferon-d (gamma)	penicillin G	vancomycin
chlortetracycline	isoniazid	potassium	vidarabine
cinoxacin	kanamycin	penicillin G procaine	viomycin
ciprofloxacin	ketoconazole	penicillin V	zidovudine

making water]. Decreasing the excretion of sodium in the urine.

antinauseant (ăn″tĭ-naw′sē-ănt). 1. Preventing or relieving nausea. 2. Agent that prevents or relieves nausea.

antineoplastic (ăn″tĭ-nē″ō-plăs′tĭk). 1. Preventing the development, growth, or proliferation of malignant cells. 2. Agent that prevents the development, growth, or proliferation of malignant cells.

antinephritic (ăn″tĭ-nĕ-frĭt′ĭk). 1. Preventing or relieving inflammation of the kidneys. 2. Agent that prevents or relieves inflammation of the kidneys.

antineuralgic (ăn″tĭ-nū-răl′jĭk) [″ + *neuron*, nerve, + *algos*, pain]. 1. Relieving neuralgia. 2. Agent that relieves neuralgia.

antineuritic (ăn″tĭ-nū-rĭt′ĭk). 1. Preventing or relieving inflammation of a nerve. 2. Agent that prevents or relieves inflammation of a nerve.

antinuclear (ăn″tĭ-nū′klē-ăr). Having an affinity for or reacting with the nucleus of a cell.

antinuclear antibodies. ABBR: ANA. A group of antibodies that react against normal components of the cell nucleus. These antibodies are present in a variety of immunologic diseases, including systemic lupus erythematosus, progressive systemic sclerosis, Sjögren's syndrome, scleroderma, polymyositis, dermatomyositis; and in persons taking hydralazine, procainamide, or isoniazid. In addition, ANA is present in some normal individuals.

antiodontalgic (ăn″tē-ō″dŏn-tăl′jĭk) [″ + *odous*, tooth, + *algos*, pain]. 1. Relieving toothache. 2. Agent that relieves toothache.

anti-oncogene. A gene that inhibits or prevents the growth of tumor cells. SEE: *oncogene*.

antiovulatory (ăn″tē-ŏv′ū-lă-tō″rē). Inhibiting or preventing ovulation.

antioxidant (ăn″tē-ŏk′sĭ-dănt). Agent that prevents or inhibits oxidation.

antioxidation (ăn″tē-ŏk″sĭ-dā′shŭn). Prevention or inhibition of oxidation.

antipaludian (ăn″tĭ-pă-loo′dē-ăn). 1. Preventing or curing malaria. 2. Agent that prevents or cures malaria. SYN: *antimalarial*.

antiparalytic (ăn″tĭ-păr-ă-lĭt′ĭk). Relieving paralysis.

antiparasitic (ăn″tĭ-păr-ă-sĭt′ĭk). 1. Destructive to parasites. 2. Agent that destroys parasites.

antipathic (ăn″tĭ-păth′ĭk) [Gr. *anti*, against, + *pathein*, to feel]. Antagonistic.

antipathy (ăn-tĭp′ă-thē). 1. Feeling of strong aversion. 2. Antagonism.

antipedicular (ăn″tĭ-pē-dĭk′ū-lăr). Effective against pediculosis, said of a medicine or procedure.

antiperiodic (ăn″tĭ-pē-rē-ŏd′ĭk) [″ + *periodos*, a circle]. Preventing regular recurrences of a disease or symptoms, as in malaria.

antiperistalsis (ăn″tĭ-pĕr″ĭ-stăl′sĭs) [″ + *peri*, around, + *stalsis*, constriction]. Reversed peristalsis; a wave of contraction in the gastrointestinal tract moving toward the oral end. In the duodenum it is associated with vomiting; in the ascending colon it occurs normally. SEE: *peristalsis*.

antiperistaltic (ăn″tĭ-pĕr″ĭ-stăl′tĭk). 1. Pert. to antiperistalsis. 2. Impeding peristalsis.

antiperspirant (ăn″tĭ-pĕr′spī-rănt). 1. Inhibiting perspiration. 2. Substance that inhibits perspiration. SYN: *anhidrotic; antihidrotic; antisudorific*.

antiphagocytic (ăn″tĭ-făg-ō-sĭt′ĭk). Preventing or inhibiting phagocytosis.

antiphlogistic (ăn″tĭ-flō-jĭs′tĭk) [″ + *phlogistos*, on fire]. 1. Preventing or relieving inflammation. 2. Agent that prevents or relieves inflammation.

antiplasmin (ăn″tĭ-plăz′mĭn). Substance that opposes the action of plasmin.

antiplastic (ăn″tĭ-plăs′tĭk) [″ + *plassein*, to form]. 1. Preventing or inhibiting wound healing. 2. Agent that prevents or inhibits wound healing by preventing formation of granulation tissue.

antiplatelet (ăn″tĭ-plāt′lĕt). 1. Destructive to platelets. 2. Agent that destroys platelets.

antipodal (ăn-tĭp′ō-dăl) [Gr. *antipous*, with feet opposite]. Located at opposite positions.

antipraxia (ăn″tĭ-prăk′sē-ă). Functions or symptoms antagonistic to each other.

antiprostaglandin (ăn″tĭ-prŏs″tă-glăn′dĭn). Drug that acts to interfere with prostaglandin activity. Such drugs are used in treating arthritis and dysmenorrhea.

antiprostatitis (ăn″tĭ-prŏs″tă-tī′tĭs). Inflammation of Cowper's gland.

antiprotease (ăn″tĭ-prō′tē-ās). Substance that interferes with proteolysis.

antiprotozoal (ăn″tĭ-prō″tō-zō′ăl). Destructive to protozoa.

antipruritic (ăn″tĭ-proo-rĭt′ĭk). 1. Preventing or relieving itching. 2. Agent that prevents or relieves itching.

antipsoriatic (ăn″tĭ-sō″rē-ăt′ĭk) [Gr. *anti*, against, + *psora*, itch]. 1. Preventing or relieving psoriasis. 2. Agent that prevents or relieves psoriasis.

antiputrefactive (ăn″tĭ-pū″trĕ-făk′tĭv). Preventing putrefaction.

antipyogenic (ăn″tĭ-pī-ō-jĕn′ĭk) [″ + *pyon*, pus, + *gennan*, to produce]. 1. Preventing or inhibiting pus formation. 2. Agent that prevents or inhibits pus formation. SYN: *antipyic*.

antipyresis (ăn″tĭ-pī-rē′sĭs) [″ + *pyretos*, fever]. Use of antipyretics.

antipyretic (ăn-tĭ-pī-rĕt′ĭk). 1. Reducing fever. 2. Agent that reduces fever. SYN: *antifebrile*.

antipyrotic (ăn″tĭ-pī-rŏt′ĭk) [″ + *pyrotikos*, burning]. 1. Promoting the healing of burns. 2. Agent that promotes the healing of burns.

antirabic (ăn″tĭ-rā′bĭk). Preventing or curing rabies. SYN: *antilyssic*.

antirachitic (ăn″tĭ-ră-kĭt′ĭk) [″ + *rachitis*, rickets]. 1. Helping to cure rickets. 2. Agent for treating rickets.

antirheumatic (ăn″tĭ-roo-măt′ĭk). 1. Preventing or relieving rheumatism. 2. Agent that prevents or relieves rheumatism.

antiricin (ăn″tĭ-rī′sĭn). Agent that opposes the action of ricin.

antiscabietic (ăn″tĭ-skā″bē-ĕt′ĭk) [Gr. *anti*, against, + L. *scabies*, itch]. 1. Preventing or relieving scabies. 2. Agent that prevents or relieves scabies.

antiscorbutic (ăn″tĭ-skor-bū′tĭk) [″ + L. *scorbutus*, scurvy]. 1. Preventing or relieving scurvy. 2. Agent that prevents or relieves scurvy.

antiseborrheic (ăn″tĭ-sĕb″ō-rē′ĭk). 1. Counteracting or effectively treating seborrhea. 2. Agent that counteracts or effectively treats seborrhea.

antisecretory (ăn″tĭ-sē-krē′tō-rē). 1. Inhibiting secretory activity of a gland or organ. 2. Agent that inhibits secretory activity of a gland or organ.

antiself. The reaction of antibodies or lymphocytes with antigens present in the host.

antisepsis (ăn″tĭ-sĕp′sĭs) [″ + *sepsis*, putrefaction]. The prevention of sepsis by preventing or inhibiting the growth of causative microorganisms.

antiseptic (ăn″tĭ-sĕp′tĭk). 1. Rel. to antisepsis. 2. Agent capable of producing antisepsis.

Chemically, antiseptics may be inorganic, such as the mercury preparations, or organic, such as carbolic acid (phenol). Oxidizing disinfectants liberate oxygen when in contact with pus or organic substances. When in use they should be washed away and replaced frequently to help remove pus, blood, and other substances. Different types of bacteria are sensitive to different antiseptics. SEE: *disinfectant* (table).

RS: asepsis; disinfectant; deodorant; germicide; sterilization.

antiserum (ăn″tĭ-sē′rŭm). Serum that contains antibodies for a specific antigen; may be of human or animal origin. SYN: *serum, immune.*

  a., monovalent. Antiserum containing antibodies specific for one antigen.

  a., polyvalent. Antiserum containing antibodies specific for more than one antigen.

antishock garment. A special garment that can be quickly placed on a patient in shock. The device contains inflatable compartments that, when filled with air, compress the lower extremities and abdominal area. This compression helps to prevent pooling of blood and fluids in the tissues. The value of this garment in treating shock is questionable. Also known as MAST, *military antishock trousers.*

  NURSING IMPLICATIONS: Fill inflatable compartments from the bottom upward. Do not remove garment until venous access and fluid resuscitation are initiated. Deflate compartments from top to bottom, evaluating frequently for increasing hypotension. SEE: *anti-G suit.*

Caution: This garment is contraindicated in congestive heart failure, cardiogenic shock, and penetrating chest trauma.

---

antisialagogue (ăn″tĭ-sī-ăl′ă-gŏg) [Gr. *anti*, against, + *sialon*, saliva, + *agogos*, drawing forth]. An agent, such as atropine, that lessens or prevents production of saliva.

antisialic (ăn″tĭ-sī-ăl′ĭk). 1. Inhibiting the secretion of saliva. 2. Agent that inhibits the secretion of saliva.

antisocial (ăn″tĭ-sō′shăl). Pert. to a person whose outlook and actions are socially negative and whose behavior is repeatedly in conflict with what society perceives as the norm. SEE: *asocial.*

antisocial personality disorder. SEE: *personality, antisocial.*

antispasmodic [″ + *spasmos*, convulsion]. 1. Preventing or relieving spasm. 2. Agent that prevents or relieves spasm. SEE: *spasm.*

anti-stain formulary. A formula that is effective in removing stains from various materials. An anti-stain formulary for removing stains from bed linens and other cotton fabrics is as follows:

Blood: Soak in cold water, then wash in lukewarm soap solution. For old stains, soak in 1% ammonia solution and then launder.

Chocolate or cocoa: Allow hot water to run through stained fabric; then wash in hot soap solution. Use Javelle water, q.v., to bleach if necessary.

Cosmetics: Nail polish, lipstick, or rouge —ordinary washing; stubborn stains remaining can be removed by acetone, followed by warm chlorine bleach.

Feces: Soak in cold water, rinse, then wash with soap and hot water. Use a brush to scrub.

Fruit stains: Stretch stained article over a basin and pour boiling water directly over the spot until it disappears. If this fails, use Javelle water, q.v., rinsing between each application.

Grass stains: Use alcohol, then wash with household baking soda and hot water. Put in the sun to bleach.

Ink: If fresh, immerse in cold or tepid water or skimmed milk. Old ink stains respond well to lemon juice, salt, and sunlight. Whatever is used, the material should be rinsed thoroughly after using to remove all the solution.

Iodine: Soapy water, ammonia solution, and hot water rinse.

Iron rust: Use lemon juice and salt; expose to the sunlight. For firm fabrics, use strong solution of oxalic acid. Rinse very thoroughly.

Meat juices: Same as for blood.

Mercurochrome: Pour hot water through the material. Acid alcohol does very well, or equal parts of Dakin's solution, q.v., and 5% acetic acid (vinegar).

Mildew: If fresh, use strong soapsuds and hang in the sunlight. If an old stain, use Javelle water, q.v., rinse thoroughly, and repeat the washing if indicated.

Paints, varnishes: Turpentine or benzol (use only in a well-ventilated area). If old stain, soak well in grease to soften, then apply turpentine or the other solutions. Chloroform dissolves lacquer paint stains.

Acetone sponged on fabric removes varnish. Shellac is soluble in 50% solution of alcohol.

Caution: Chloroform is toxic and should be used only in a very well-ventilated area.

Perspiration: Wash in strong soap solution and dry in sunlight.

Picric acid: If fabric will not be harmed, boil in dilute sodium hydroxide solution for one-half hour and bleach in Javelle water, q.v.

Scorch: Apply hydrogen peroxide to the area, then rub well while the material is soaked in strong soap solution. Dry in sunlight.

Silver salts: If not too old, silver stains can be removed by sodium thiosulfate (photographer's hypo).

Tea or coffee: If fresh, pour boiling water through it. If old, soak in borax before pouring boiling water over it.

Urine: Soak in boiling water, then pour 5% Lysol solution over it.

antistaphylococcic (ăn″tĭ-stăf″ĭ-lō-kŏk′sĭk) [Gr. *anti*, against, + *staphyle*, bunch of grapes, + *cocci*, bacteria]. Destructive to staphylococci.

antistreptococcic (ăn″tĭ-strĕp″tō-kŏk′sĭk). Destructive to streptococci.

antistreptolysin (ăn″tĭ-strĕp-tŏl′ĭ-sĭn). Antibody that opposes the action of streptolysin, a hemolysin produced by streptococci.

antisudoral (ăn″tĭ-soo′dor-ăl) [″ + L. *sudor*, sweat]. Inhibiting or preventing perspiration. SYN: *anhidrotic; antihidrotic; antiperspirant.*

antisudorific (ăn″tĭ-soo″dor-ĭf′ĭk). 1. Inhibiting or preventing perspiration. 2. Agent that prevents or inhibits perspiration. SYN: *anhidrosis; antihydrosis; antiperspirant.*

antisyphilitic (ăn″tĭ-sĭf″ĭ-lĭt′ĭk) [″ + L. *syphiliticus*, pert. to syphilis]. 1. Curing or relieving syphilis. 2. Agent that cures or relieves syphilis. SYN: *antiluetic.*

antitabetic (ăn″tĭ-tă-bĕt′ĭk) [″ + L. *tabes*, wasting away]. 1. Preventing or relieving tabes dorsalis. 2. Agent that prevents or relieves tabes dorsalis.

antithenar (ăn-tĭth′ĕn-ăr) [″ + *thenar*, palm]. The eminence on ulnar side of the palm, formed by the muscles of the little finger. SYN: *hypothenar eminence.*

antithrombotic (ăn″tĭ-thrŏm-bŏt′ĭk). Interfering with or preventing thrombosis or blood coagulation.

antithyroid (ăn″tĭ-thī′royd) [″ + *thyreoeides*, thyroid]. 1. Preventing or inhibiting the functioning of the thyroid gland. 2. Agent that prevents or inhibits the functioning of the thyroid gland.

antitonic (ăn″tĭ-tŏn′ĭk) [″ + *tonos*, tone]. Diminishing tonicity.

antitoxic (ăn″tĭ-tŏk′sĭk) [″ + *toxikon*, poison]. Neutralizing a poison, esp. a bacterial toxin. SEE: *antitoxin.*

antitoxic serum. Serum that contains antitoxin, q.v.

antitoxigen (ăn″tĭ-tŏk′sĭ-gĕn) [″ + ″ + *gennan*, to produce]. Antigen that stimulates the production of antitoxin. SYN: *antitoxinogen.*

antitoxin (ăn″tĭ-tŏk′sĭn). Antibody produced in response to and capable of neutralizing a specific biologic toxin.

Ex.: diphtheria antitoxin, gas-gangrene antitoxin, and tetanus antitoxin, which counteract the toxins produced by the diphtheria, gas-gangrene, and tetanus bacteria. Antitoxins are used for prophylactic and therapeutic purposes. SEE: *antivenin.*

antitoxinogen (ăn″tĭ-tŏk-sĭn′ō-jĕn) [Gr. *anti*, against, + *toxikon*, poison, + *gennan*, to produce]. Antigen that stimulates production of antitoxin. SYN: *antitoxigen.*

antitragicus (ăn″tĭ-trăj′ĭ-kŭs). A small muscle in the pinna of the ear.

antitragus (ăn″tĭ-trā′gŭs) [″ + L. *tragus*, goat]. [NA] A projection on the ear of the cartilage of the auricle in front of the tail of the helix, posterior to the tragus.

antitrichomonal. 1. Resistant to or lethal to trichomonads. 2. A medicine effective in treating trichomonal infections.

antitrismus (ăn″tĭ-trĭs′mŭs) [″ + *trismos*, grinding]. A condition in which the mouth cannot close because of tonic spasm. SEE: *trismus.*

antitrypsin (ăn″tĭ-trĭp′sĭn). A substance that inhibits the action of trypsin.

a., alpha 1-. A low-molecular-weight glycoprotein that inhibits proteolytic enzymes. Deficiency of this enzyme in the serum is associated with early-onset emphysema in some and liver disease in others. There is no specific therapy, but liver transplant may be of benefit in those with liver disease.

antitryptic (ăn″tĭ-trĭp′tĭk). Inhibiting the action of trypsin.

antituberculotic (ăn″tĭ-too-bĕr′kū-lŏt″ĭk). Inhibiting the spread or progress of tuberculosis in the body.

antitussive (ăn″tĭ-tŭs′ĭv) [Gr. *anti*, against, + L. *tussis*, cough]. 1. Preventing or relieving coughing. 2. Agent that prevents or relieves coughing.

a., centrally acting. Agent that depresses medullary centers, thus suppressing the cough reflex.

antiuratic (ăn″tĭ-ū-răt′ĭk) [″ + L. *uras*, urate]. 1. Preventing the precipitation of urates. 2. Substance that inhibits or prevents formation of urates.

antivaccinationist (ăn″tĭ-văk″sĭ-nā′shŭn-ĭst). One who is opposed to vaccination.

antivenene (ăn″tĭ-vĕn′ēn). Antivenin.

antivenereal (ăn″tĭ-vĕ-nē′rē-ăl). Preventing or curing venereal diseases.

antivenin (ăn″tĭ-vĕn′ĭn). Serum that contains antitoxin specific for an animal or insect venom. Antivenin is prepared from immunized animal sera and is used in the treatment of poisoning by animal or insect venom. SYN: *antivenene; antivenom.*

    a., black widow spider. Antitoxic serum obtained from horses immunized against venom of the black widow spider (*Latrodectus mactans*). Specific in treatment of bites of black widow spider. Available from Merck Sharp & Dohme, West Point, PA 19486.

    a., (Crotalidae) polyvalent. USP. Antisnakebite serum obtained from serum of horses immunized against venom of four types of pit vipers: *Crotalus atrox, C. adamanteus, C. terrificus,* and *Bothrops atrox* (family Crotalidae). Specific in treatment of bites of these snakes.

antivenom (ăn″tĭ-vĕn′ŏm). Antivenin.

antivenomous (ăn″tĭ-vĕn′ŏ-mŭs). Opposing the action of venom.

Antivert. Trade name for meclizine hydrochloride, q.v.

antiviral (ăn″tĭ-vī′răl). Opposing the action of a virus.

antiviral resistance. The developed resistance of a virus to specific antiviral therapy.

antivitamin. A vitamin antagonist; one of a group of substances, natural or synthetic, that opposes the action of certain vitamins.

antivivisection (ăn″tĭ-vĭv″ĭ-sĕk′shŭn). Opposition to the use of live animals in experimentation. SEE: *vivisection.*

antixenic (ăn″tĭ-zē′nĭk) [Gr. *anti,* against, + *xenos,* strange]. Pert. to living tissue reaction to any foreign substance.

antixerotic (ăn″tĭ-zē-rŏt′ĭk) [″ + *xerosis,* dryness]. Preventing dryness of the skin.

antizymotic (ăn″tĭ-zĭ-mŏt′ĭk) [″ + *zymosis,* fermentation]. Agent that prevents or arrests fermentation.

    Ex.: alcohol; salicylic acid.

antra (ăn′tră) [L.]. Pl. of antrum, q.v.

antral (ăn′trăl). Pert. to an antrum.

antrectomy (ăn-trĕk′tō-mē) [L. *antrum,* cavity, + Gr. *ektome,* excision]. Excision of the walls of an antrum.

antritis (ăn″trī′tĭs) [″ + Gr. *itis,* inflammation]. Inflammation of an antrum, esp. the maxillary sinus.

antro- [L. *antrum,* cavity]. Prefix denoting relationship to an antrum.

antroatticotomy (ăn″trŏ-ăt″ĭ-kŏt′ō-mē) [″ + *atticus,* attic, + Gr. *tome,* incision].

Operation to open the maxillary sinus and the attic of the tympanum.

antrobuccal (ăn″trŏ-bŭk′ăl) [″ + *bucca,* cheek]. Concerning the maxillary sinus and the cheek.

antrocele (ăn′trŏ-sēl) [″ + Gr. *kele,* tumor, swelling]. Fluid accumulation in a cyst in the maxillary sinus.

antroduodenectomy (ăn″trŏ-dū″ŏ-dĕ-nĕk′tō-mē) [″ + *duodeni,* twelve, + Gr. *ektome,* excision]. Surgical removal of the pyloric antrum and the upper portion of the duodenum.

antronasal (ăn″trŏ-nā′zăl) [″ + *nasalis,* nasal]. Rel. to the maxillary sinus and nasal fossa.

antrophore (ăn′trŏ-for) [″ + Gr. *phorein,* to carry]. A medicated bougie, q.v., for local treatment of any accessible cavity or canal.

antroscope (ăn′trŏ-skōp) [″ + Gr. *skopein,* to examine]. An instrument for visual examination of a cavity, esp. the maxillary sinus.

antroscopy (ăn-trŏs′kŏ-pē). Visual examination of a cavity, esp. the maxillary sinus, using an antroscope.

antrostomy (ăn-trŏs′tō-mē) [″ + Gr. *stoma,* mouth]. Operation to form an opening in an antrum.

antrotome (ăn′trŏ-tōm) [″ + Gr. *tome,* incision]. An instrument used to perform antrotomy.

antrotomy (ăn″trŏt′ō-mē). Cutting through an antral wall.

antrotympanic (ăn″trŏ-tĭm-păn′ĭk) [L. *antrum,* cavity, + Gr. *tympanon,* drum]. Rel. to the mastoid antrum and the tympanic cavity.

antrotympanitis (ăn″trŏ-tĭm″păn-ī′tĭs) [″ + ″ + *itis,* inflammation]. Chronic inflammation of tympanic cavity and mastoid antrum.

antrum (ăn′trŭm) [L., cavity] (pl. *antra*). [NA] Any nearly closed cavity or chamber, esp. in a bone.

    a. auris. External acoustic meatus.

    a. cardiacum. The thoracic portion of the esophagus, functionally the superior portion of the stomach.

    a., duodenal. The duodenal cap, a dilatation of duodenum near pylorus and seen during digestion.

    a., gastric. Distal non-acid-secreting segment of the stomach or pyloric gland region that produces the hormone gastrin.

    a., mastoid; a. mastoideum. [NA] Cavity in the mastoid portion of the temporal bone. SYN: *a., tympanic.*

    a., maxillary. The maxillary sinus; a cavity in the maxillary bone communicating with the middle meatus of the nasal cavity.

    a. of Highmore. A., maxillary, q.v.

a., puncture of. Puncture made in maxillary sinus by placing trocar through sinus wall. Entry is from the nasal cavity. Instrument enters from near floor of nose, approx. 1½ in. (3.8 cm) from external opening. Pus is then drained. SYN: *antrotomy.*

NURSING IMPLICATIONS: Irrigate antrum as ordered. The physician may order the antrum to be irrigated with a solution such as warm normal saline. Follow hospital procedure for the irrigation. Carefully note and describe the character of drainage in the solution return. Apply ice packs for edema and pain. As healing progresses, warm compresses may be used. Evaluate for the development of complications such as chills, fever, nausea, vomiting, facial or periorbital edema, visual disturbances, or personality changes.

a., pyloric; a. pyloricum. [NA] Bulge in the pyloric portion of the stomach along the greater curvature on distention.

a., tympanic; a.tympanicum. A., mastoid, q.v.

ANTU. Alpha-naphthylthiourea, a powerful rat poison.

Antuitrin S. Trade name for chorionic gonadotropin, human, q.v.

Anturane. Trade name for sulfinpyrazone, q.v.

anuclear (ă-nū'klē-ăr). Lacking a nucleus, said of erythrocytes.

ANUG. *acute necrotizing ulcerative gingivitis.* SEE: *trench mouth.*

anulus (ăn'ū-lŭs) [L.] (pl. *anuli*). [NA] A ring-shaped structure; a ring. Also spelled annulus.

a. abdominalis. A. inguinalis profundus, q.v.

a. femoralis. Femoral ring; the abdominal opening of the femoral canal.

a. fibrosus. The tough outer portion of the intervertebral disk.

a. inguinalis profundus. Deep inguinal ring; the opening in the fascia transversalis for the ductus deferens in the male or the round ligament in the female. SYN: *a. abdominalis.*

a. inguinalis superficialis. Superficial inguinal ring; the opening in the external oblique muscle for the ductus deferens in the male and the round ligament in the female.

a. tympanicus. Tympanic ring; part of the temporal bone forming a ring at the inner end of the external auditory canal.

a. umbilicalis. Opening in the abdominal wall of a fetus through which the umbilical vessels pass.

a. urethralis. Elevated muscular ring surrounding the opening of the bladder into the urethra. SYN: *sphincter, bladder.*

anuresis (ăn-ū-rē'sĭs) [Gr. *an-*, not, + *our-*

esis, urination]. Absence of urination. SEE: *anuria.*

anuretic (ăn-ū-rĕt'ĭk). Pert. to anuresis, q.v.

anuria (ăn-ū'rē-ä) [" + *ouron,* urine]. Absence of urine formation. SEE: *anuresis.*

anus (ā'nŭs) [L.]. [NA] The outlet of the rectum lying in the fold between the buttocks.

a., artificial. Opening into the bowel formed by colostomy.

a., imperforate. Condition in which the anus is closed.

a., vulvovaginal. Congenital anomaly in a female in which the anus is imperforate but there is an opening from the rectum to vagina.

anvil (ăn'vĭl) [AS. *anfilt*]. Middle ossicle of ear. SYN: *incus.* SEE: *ear* for illus.

anxiety (ăng-zī'ĕ-tē). A feeling of apprehension, worry, uneasiness, or dread, esp. of the future.

Everyone has been anxious at some time. Anxiety is the normal reaction to that which is threatening to one's body, lifestyle, values, or loved ones. A certain amount of anxiety is normal and stimulates the individual to purposeful action. Excess anxiety interferes with efficient functioning of the individual. SEE: *anxiety neurosis.*

NURSING IMPLICATIONS: Assess for level of anxiety (mild, moderate, severe, panic), recognizing related physical characteristics, e.g., sympathetic nervous system arousal, and effects on patient's perceptual field and ability to learn and solve problems. Also assess the coping and defense mechanisms the patient is using and the surrounding circumstances. Anxiety can be communicated, so remain calm and do not allow the patient's anxiety to unduly affect you. The presence of a calm, caring nurse in a quiet, controlled atmosphere helps to prevent escalation of the patient's anxiety, and can actually reduce anxiety by providing feelings of connection and stability and lessening feelings of isolation. At lower anxiety levels, assist the patient to identify and reduce or remove stressors, if possible; anxiety may be in response to an unknown or unconscious threat. Provide outlets for the patient's excess energy. Establish a trusting relationship that encourages the patient to express feelings and concerns, expectations and needs. Explore previously used effective behaviors to see if they can be used in the present situation, and encourage the patient to solve problems. Avoid offering false reassurance. At higher levels of anxiety focus care on reducing environmental and other stimuli. Use clear, simple validating statements, repeating as necessary, and reinforce reality if distortion is evident. Attend to patient's physical needs and encourage physical activity to utilize patient's energies.

a., free-floating. Anxiety unrelated to an identifiable condition, situation, or cause.

anxiety disorders. A group of psychiatric disorders characterized principally by anxiety. Phobias of various types are included along with panic, obsessive-compulsive disorder, posttraumatic stress disorder, and anxiety states. SEE: *Nursing Diagnoses* in *Appendix.*

anxiety neurosis. A mental disorder characterized by excessive anxiety that is not restricted to specific situations or objects and is often associated with somatic symptoms. This disorder must be differentiated from normal anxiety, which occurs in realistically threatening situations.

Anxiety neurosis may be manifested when an individual without organic disease, during clear consciousness, complains of palpitation, heart pain, dyspepsia, constriction of the throat, bandlike pressure about head, or cold, sweaty, tremulous extremities. SEE: *effort syndrome.*

anxiolytic (ăng″zī-ō-lĭt′ĭk) [L. *anxietas,* anxiety, + Gr. *lysis,* dissolution]. Counteracting or diminishing anxiety. This may be done by drug, social, or psychiatric therapy.

A.O.A. *Alpha Omega Alpha,* an honorary medical fraternity in the U.S.; *American Osteopathic Association.*

AoA. *Administration on Aging.*

A.O.C. *anodal opening contraction.*

AOD. *adult-onset diabetes mellitus.* SEE: *diabetes, non-insulin-dependent.*

A.O.R.N. *Association of Operating Room Nurses.*

aorta (ā-or′tă) [L. from Gr. *aorte*] (pl. *aortas, -tae*). [NA] The main trunk of the arterial system of the body. It is about 3 cm in diameter at its origin in the upper surface of the left ventricle. It passes upward as the ascending aorta, turns backward and to the left (arch of the aorta) at about the level of the fourth thoracic vertebra, and then passes downward as the descending aorta, which is divided into the thoracic and abdominal aorta. The latter terminates at its division into the two common iliac arteries. At the point of origin from the ventricle, the aorta contains three valves. These open when the heart beats and close when the blood flow momentarily ceases at the end of systole. SEE: illus.

The divisions of the aorta are as follows:

Ascending aorta (two branches): Two coronary arteries (right and left) provide blood supply to the myocardium.

Aortic arch (three branches): The innominate artery divides into the right subcla-

vian artery, which provides blood from the right arm and other areas, and right common carotid artery, which supplies the right side of the head and neck. The left common carotid artery supplies the left side of the head and neck. The left subclavian artery provides blood for the left arm and portion of the thoracic area.

Thoracic aorta: Two or more bronchial arteries provide blood for bronchi. Four or five esophageal arteries provide blood to the esophagus. Pericardial arteries supply the pericardium. Nine pairs of intercostal arteries supply blood for intercostal areas. Mediastinal branches supply lymph glands and the posterior mediastinum. Superior phrenic arteries supply the diaphragm.

Abdominal aorta: The celiac artery supplies the stomach, liver, and spleen. The superior mesenteric artery supplies all of the small intestine except the superior portion of the duodenum. The inferior mesenteric artery supplies all of the colon and rectum except the right half of the transverse colon. Middle suprarenal branches supply the adrenal (suprarenal) glands. Renal arteries supply the kidneys, ureters, and adrenals. Testicular arteries supply testicles and ureter. Ovarian arteries (correspond to internal spermatic arteries of the male) supply the ovaries, part of ureters, and uterine tubes. Inferior phrenic arteries supply the diaphragm and esophagus. Lumbar arteries supply lumbar and psoas muscles and part of the abdominal wall musculature. The middle sacral artery supplies the sacrum and coccyx. Right and left common iliac arteries supply lower pelvic and abdominal areas and the lower extremities.

aortal (ā-or′tăl). Pert. to the aorta.

aortalgia (ā″or-tăl′jē-ă) [L. from Gr. *aorte,* aorta, + *algos,* pain]. Pain in the aortic area.

aortarctia (ā″or-tărk′shē-ă) [″ + L. *arctare,* to narrow]. Aortic narrowing. SEE: *coarctation.*

aortectasia (ā″or-tĕk-tā′zē-ă) [″ + *ek,* out, + *tasis,* a stretching]. Dilatation of the aorta.

aortectomy (ā″or-tĕk′tō-mē) [″ + *ektome,* excision]. Excision of part of the aorta.

aortic (ā-or′tĭk). Pert. to aorta or its orifice in the left ventricle of the heart.

aortic balloon pump. SEE: *phase-shift balloon pumping.*

aortic murmur. An abnormal, soft sound heard on auscultation; may be due to obstruction or regurgitation. Symptom of aortic valvular disease. SEE: *Auscultation* under *heart.*

aortic opening. 1. Path through the diaphragm for the aorta. 2. Posterior opening

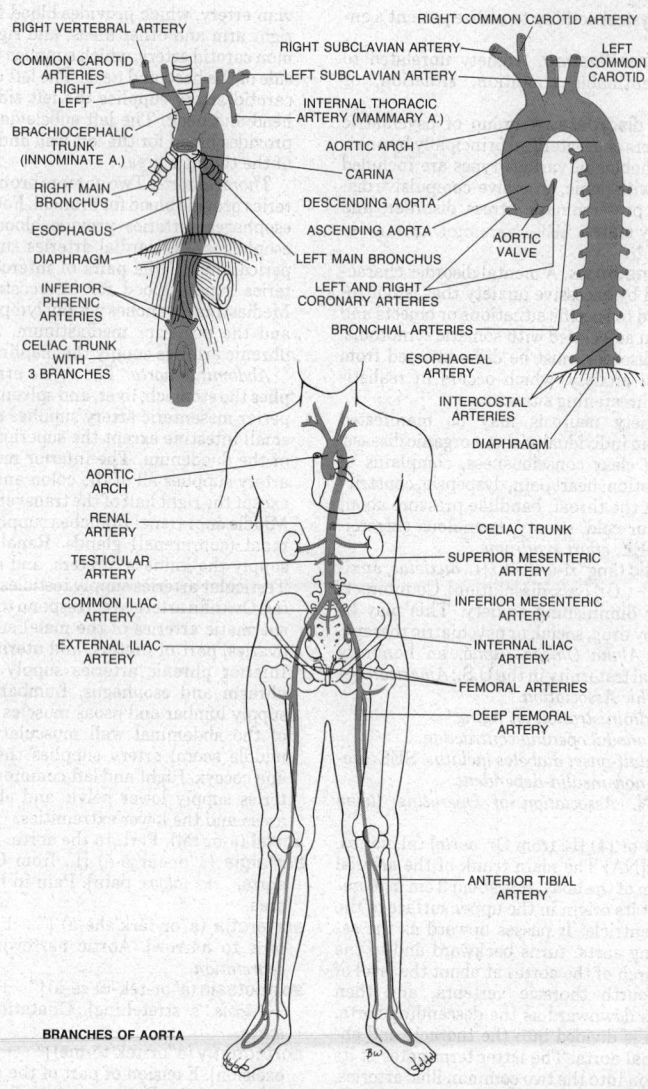

RIGHT VERTEBRAL ARTERY

COMMON CAROTID ARTERIES
RIGHT
LEFT

BRACHIOCEPHALIC TRUNK (INNOMINATE A.)

RIGHT MAIN BRONCHUS

ESOPHAGUS

DIAPHRAGM

INFERIOR PHRENIC ARTERIES

CELIAC TRUNK WITH 3 BRANCHES

RIGHT COMMON CAROTID ARTERY

RIGHT SUBCLAVIAN ARTERY

LEFT SUBCLAVIAN ARTERY

LEFT COMMON CAROTID

INTERNAL THORACIC ARTERY (MAMMARY A.)

AORTIC ARCH

CARINA

DESCENDING AORTA

ASCENDING AORTA

LEFT MAIN BRONCHUS

AORTIC VALVE

LEFT AND RIGHT CORONARY ARTERIES

BRONCHIAL ARTERIES

ESOPHAGEAL ARTERY

INTERCOSTAL ARTERIES

DIAPHRAGM

AORTIC ARCH

RENAL ARTERY

TESTICULAR ARTERY

COMMON ILIAC ARTERY

EXTERNAL ILIAC ARTERY

CELIAC TRUNK

SUPERIOR MESENTERIC ARTERY

INFERIOR MESENTERIC ARTERY

INTERNAL ILIAC ARTERY

FEMORAL ARTERIES

DEEP FEMORAL ARTERY

ANTERIOR TIBIAL ARTERY

BRANCHES OF AORTA

in the diaphragm.

aortic regurgitation. Leakage of the blood from the aorta through the aortic valve back into the left ventricle after the ventricular contraction is completed. SYN: *insufficiency, aortic.*

ETIOL: Diseases of the heart or aortic valves with defects or weakness of heart muscle.

aortic stenosis. Narrowing of aorta or its orifice due to lesions of the wall with scar formation. Due to infection as in rheumatic fever, or embryonic anomalies. Hypertrophy of the heart is a common result. SYN: *aortostenosis.* SEE: *Nursing Diagnoses* in *Appendix.*

aortic valve. The valve between the left ventricle and the ascending aorta that prevents regurgitation of blood back into the left ventricle. It is composed of three segments, each of which is called a semilunar cusp. The valve is open during ventricular systole and closed during diastole.

aortitis (ā-or-tī′tis) [L. from Gr. *aorte*, aorta, + *itis*, inflammation]. Inflammation of the aorta. Associated with syphilis as well as other diseases in which vascular changes have taken place. A common cause of aortic aneurysm.
SYM: Possible cough, cyanosis, dyspnea, cardiac asthmatic attacks, hemoptysis.

aortoclasia (ā″or-tō-klā′zē-ä) [″ + *klasis*, a breaking]. Aortic rupture.

aortocoronary (ā-or″tō-kor′ō-nā-rē). Pert. to both the aorta and the coronary arteries.

aortocoronary bypass. Surgical procedure for establishing a shunt so blood may pass from the aorta to a branch of a coronary artery in order to bypass an obstruction. This procedure involves a vascular prosthesis, usually obtained from one of the saphenous veins. SYN: *coronary artery bypass surgery.*

aortogram (ā-or′tō-grăm″) [″ + *gramma*, something written]. The roentgenogram record of aortography.

aortography (ā″or-tog′ră-fē) [L. from Gr. *aorte*, aorta, + *graphein*, to write]. Roentgenography of aorta after injection of contrast fluid.

   a., retrograde. Aortography by injection of contrast fluid into the aorta by means of one of its branches, and thus against the direction of the blood flow.

   a., translumbar. Aortography by injection of contrast fluid into the abdominal aorta through a needle inserted into the lumbar area near the level of the 12th rib.

aortoiliac (ā-or″tō-ĭl′ē-ăk). Pert. to both the aorta and the iliac arteries.

aortolith (ā-or′tō-lĭth) [″ + *lithos*, stone]. Calcareous deposit in the aortic wall.

aortomalacia (ā-or″tō-mă-lā′shē-ä) [″ + *malakia*, softness]. Softening of the walls of the aorta.

aortopathy (ā″or-tŏp′a-thē) [″ + *pathos*, disease, suffering]. Any aortic disease.

aortoplasty. Surgical repair of the aorta.

aortoptosia, aortoptosis (ā″or-tŏp-tō′zē-ä, -sĭs) [″ + *ptosis*, a dropping]. Downward displacement of abdominal aorta.

aortorrhaphy (ā″or-tor′ă-fē) [″ + *rhaphe*, seam, ridge]. Suture of the aorta.

aortosclerosis (ā-or″tō-sklĕr-ō-sĭs) [″ + *skleros*, hard]. Aortic sclerosis.

aortostenosis (ā-or″tō-stĕn-ō′sĭs) [″ + *stenosis*, a narrowing]. Narrowing of aorta on its orifice due to lesions of the wall with scar formation, infection as in rheumatic

fever, or embryonic anomalies. Hypertrophy of the heart is a common result. SYN: *aortic stenosis.*

aortotomy (ā″or-tŏt′ō-mē) [″ + *tome*, incision]. Incision of the aorta.

AOS. *anodal opening sound.*

aosmic (ā-ŏz′mĭk) [Gr. *a-*, not, + *osme*, smell]. Without odor.

A.O.T.A. *American Occupational Therapy Association.*

A.O.T.C.B. *American Occupational Therapy Certification Board.*

A.O.T.F. *American Occupational Therapy Foundation.*

A.P. *anteroposterior.*

A.P.A. *American Pharmaceutical Association; American Physiotherapy Association; American Psychiatric Association.*

APACHE II. Acronym for *acute physiology and chronic health evaluation.* A severity of disease classification system.

apallesthesia (ä-păl″ĕs-thē′zē-ä) [″ + *pallein*, to tremble, + *aisthesis*, sensation]. Inability to sense vibrations. SYN: *pallanesthesia.* SEE: *pallesthesia.*

apancreatic (ä-păn″krē-ăt′ĭk). 1. Caused by absence of the pancreas. 2. Pert. to noninvolvement of the pancreas.

aparalytic (ä-păr″ă-lĭt′ĭk) [Gr. *a-*, not, + *paralyein*, to loosen]. Marked by lack of paralysis.

aparathyrosis (ä-păr″ä-thī-rō′sĭs) [″ + *para*, near, + *thyreos*, an oblong shield, + *osis*, condition]. Parathyroid deficiency.

apareunia (ā″păr-ū′nē-ä) [″ + *pareunos*, lying with]. Inability to accomplish sexual intercourse. SEE: *dyspareunia.*

aparthrosis (ăp″ăr-thrō′sĭs) [Gr. *apo*, from, + *arthron*, joint, + *osis*, condition]. 1. A joint that moves freely in any direction, such as the shoulder joint. SYN: *diarthrosis.* 2. Dislocation of a joint.

apastia (ä-păs′tē-ä) [Gr., fasting]. Abnormal refusal to eat.

apathetic (ăp″ă-thĕt′ĭk) [″ + *pathos*, disease, suffering]. Indifferent; without interest. SYN: *apathic.*

apathic (ä-păth′ĭk). Indifferent. SYN: *apathetic.*

apathism (ăp′ă-thĭzm) [″ + *pathos*, disease, suffering, + *-ismos*, condition]. Slowness to react to stimuli. Opposite of erethism, q.v.

apathy (ăp′ă-thē) [Gr. *apatheia*]. Indifference; insensibility; lack of emotion.

apatite (ăp′ă-tīt″) [Ger. *Apatit*, "the deceptive stone"]. A mineral containing calcium and phosphate ions and a univalent anion in a specific ratio.

A.P.C. *aspirin, phenacetin,* and *caffeine,* common ingredients in various headache and cold tablets. Phenacetin is no longer felt to be suitable for use in any form.

APE. *anterior pituitary extract.*

ape. Large, nonhuman primate.

apeidosis (ăp″ī-dō′sĭs) [Gr. *apo*, away, + *eidos*, form, shape]. Slow modification or disappearance of the clinical and histological characteristics of a disease.

apellous (ă-pĕl′ŭs) [Gr. *a*-, not, + L. *pellis*, skin]. 1. Lacking skin. 2. Lacking foreskin; circumcised.

apenteric (ăp″ĕn-tĕr′ĭk) [Gr. *apo*, from, + *enteron*, intestine]. Outside the intestine. SYN: *abenteric.*

apepsia (ă-pĕp′sē-ă) [Gr. *a*-, not, + *pepsis*, digesting]. Cessation of digestion.

apepsinia (ă″pĕp-sĭn′ē-ă). Absence of pepsin in the gastric juice.

aperient (ă-pēr′ē-ĕnt) [L. *aperiens*, opening]. A very mild laxative.

aperiodic. Occurring other than periodically.

aperistalsis (ă″pĕr-ĭ-stăl′sĭs) [Gr. *a*-, not, + *peri*, around, + *stalsis*, constriction]. Absence of peristalsis.

apéritif (ă-pĕr″ĭ-tēf′) [L. *aperire*, to open]. An alcoholic beverage, such as wine, taken before a meal to stimulate the appetite.

aperitive (ă-pĕr′ĭ-tĭv). 1. Stimulating the appetite. 2. Aperient, q.v.

Apert's syndrome (ă-pärz′) [Eugene Apert, Fr. pediatrician, 1868–1940]. A congenital condition marked by a peaked head and webbed fingers and toes. Oral manifestations include cleft palate or uvula, prognathic mandible with maxillary hypoplasia resulting in extreme malocclusion.

apertura (ăp″ĕr-tū′ră) [L.] (pl. *aperturae*). [NA] An opening.

aperture (ăp′ĕr-chūr″). An orifice or opening, especially to anatomical or bony spaces or canals.

apex (ā′pĕks) [L., tip] (pl. *apices*). [NA] The pointed extremity of a conical structure.

　　a. of the lung The superior, subclavicular portion of the lung.

　　a., root. The end of the root of a tooth.

apex beat. In systole, the movement of the apex of the left ventricle against the chest wall. Felt in the 5th left intercostal space, approx. 3 ½ in. (8.9 cm) from the middle of the sternum, about 1 in. (2.5 cm) within a line drawn down from the middle of the clavicle parallel with the sternum (the mammary line). Generally may be detected by inspection or palpation; when these fail, may be localized by auscultation. If the patient is in a recumbent position, the apex beat may be detected 1 in. (2.5 cm) or more higher. When the body is inclined to the left, the beat may be detected in or outside the mammary line. During forced inspiration, it may become imperceptible or be found below its usual place. During forced expiration, the beat becomes more forcible and may be found above its usual place. The patient, as a rule, should be examined in erect or sitting position while breathing quietly.

ABNORM: Deformity of chest may cause displacement in any direction.

Weak apex beat: may be noted in healthy persons at rest, in heart failure, pericardial effusion, emphysema, shock, or collapse.

Changes in force and extent: may be increased by hypertrophy of heart, excited action of heart from exercise or drugs, reflex irritation, excitement, or disease (as exophthalmic goiter).

Displacement to the left: may result from hypertrophy and dilatation of the heart (down and to the left); pneumothorax on the right; pericardial effusion (up and to left); chronic diseases of left lung and pleura associated with retraction, as fibroid tuberculosis and pleural adhesions; abdominal tumors and effusions (up and to left); pressure of a pleural effusion on the right side (up and to left).

Displacement to right: may be caused by chronic disease of the right lung or pleura associated with retraction; pneumothorax on the left; pressure of a pleural effusion on the left side.

Displacement downward: may result from hypertrophy and dilatation of heart, chiefly the left ventricle; pressure of solid growths in upper mediastinum; aneurysm of aortic arch; enlargement of liver, causing traction through central tendon of diaphragm.

Precordial prominence: may result from deformity, enlargement of heart, pericardial effusions.

apexcardiogram. Graphic record of the movements of the chest wall produced by the apex beat.

apexigraph, apexograph (ā-pĕks′ĭ-grăf, -ō-grăf) [L. *apex*, tip, + Gr. *graphein*, to write]. An instrument for determining location and size of apex of a tooth root.

apex murmur. Murmur over the apex of the heart.

Apgar score [Virginia Apgar, U.S. anesthesiologist, 1909–1974]. System of scoring infant's physical condition one minute and five minutes after birth. The heart rate, respiration, muscle tone, response to stimuli, and color are each rated 0, 1, or 2. The maximum total score is 10. Those with low scores require immediate attention if they are to survive. The test may be repeated at 5 or more minutes after birth in order to judge recovery of infants with low scores. A low score at one minute is a sign of asphyxia and the need for immediate assisted ventilation. A low score at five minutes is an index of the

Apgar Score

Sign	Score 0	Score 1	Score 2
Heart rate	Absent	Slow (less than 100)	Greater than 100
Respiratory effort	Absent	Slow, irregular	Good; crying
Muscle tone	Limp	Some flexion of extremities	Active motion
Reflex irritability	No response	Grimace	Cough or sneeze
Color	Blue, pale	Body pink; extremities blue	Completely pink

possibility of death. SEE: table.

A.P.H.A. *American Public Health Association.*

aphacia (ă-fā'sē-ă). Aphakia, q.v.

aphacic (ă-fā'sĭk). Aphakic, q.v.

aphagia (ă-fā'jē-ă) [Gr. *a-*, not, + *phagein*, to eat]. Inability to swallow.

aphakia (ă-fā'kē-ă) [" + *phakos*, lentil]. Absence of the crystalline lens of the eye.

aphakic (ă-fā'kĭk). Pert. to aphakia.

aphalangia (ă"fă-lăn'jē-ă) [" + *phalanx*, closely knit row]. Absence of fingers or toes.

aphanisis (ă-făn'ĭ-sĭs) [Gr. *aphaneia*, disappearance]. Fear or apprehension that sexual potency will be lost.

aphasia (ă-fā'zē-ă) [Gr. *a-*, not, + *phasis*, speaking]. Absence or impairment of the ability to communicate through speech, writing, or signs, due to dysfunction of brain centers. It is considered to be complete or total when both sensory and motor areas are involved. SEE: *alalia.*

    a., **amnesic.** Loss of memory for words.

    a., **anomic.** Inability to name objects.

    a., **ataxic.** A., motor, q.v.

    a., **auditory.** Inability to understand spoken words. SYN: *amnesia, auditory; deafness, word.*

    a., **Broca's.** A., motor, q.v.

    a., **conduction.** Aphasia due to lesion of conduction path between motor and speech centers.

    a., **expressive.** A., motor, q.v.

    a., **fluent.** Aphasia in which words are easily spoken but those used are incorrect and may be unrelated to the content of the other words spoken.

    a., **gibberish.** Utterance of meaningless phrases.

    a., **global.** Aphasia involving failure of expression and perception of language as well as other means of communication.

    a., **jargon.** Communication that results in the use of jargon or disconnected words.

    a., **mixed.** Combined sensory and motor aphasia.

    a., **motor.** Aphasia in which patients know what they want to say but cannot say it. Inability to coordinate muscles controlling speech. May be complete or partial. Broca's area is disordered or diseased. SYN: *a., ataxic; a., expressive.*

    a., **nominal.** Inability to name objects.

    a., **optic.** Inability to call name of an object recognized by sight without the aid of sound, taste, or touch; a form of agnosia, q.v.

    a., **receptive.** A., sensory, q.v.

    a., **semantic.** Inability to understand meaning of words.

    a., **sensory.** Inability to understand spoken words if auditory word center is involved (auditory aphasia), or the written word if visual word center is affected (visual aphasia). If both centers are involved, patient will not understand spoken or written word.

    a., **syntactic.** Loss of proper grammatical construction.

    a., **traumatic.** Aphasia caused by head injury.

    a., **visual.** Inability to understand the written word. SYN: *word blindness.*

    a., **Wernicke's.** A., sensory, q.v.

aphasic, aphasiac (ă-fā"zĭk, ă-fā'zē-ăk). Pert. to aphasia.

aphasiologist (ă-fā"zē-ŏl'ō-jĭst) [Gr. *a-*, not, + *phasis*, speaking, + *logos*, word, reason]. Person who studies the pathology of language and the production of speech and written language.

aphemia (ă-fē'mē-ă) [" + *pheme*, speech]. 1. Loss of the power to speak. SYN: *aphasia, motor.* 2. Loss of the power to speak distinctly. SYN: *anarthria.*

aphephobia (ăf"ĕ-fō'bē-ă) [Gr. *haphe*, touch, + *phobos*, fear]. Morbid fear of being touched.

apheresis (ă-fĕr'ē-sĭs) [Gr. *aphairesis*, separation]. Technique of separating blood into components. These components may be further processed for special purposes such as removing toxic or unwanted substances from the blood. The technique is quite expensive. SYN: *pheresis.*

aphonia (ă-fō′nē-ă) [Gr. *a-*, not, + *phone*, voice]. Inability to produce speech sounds from larynx. Not caused by a brain lesion. May occur in chronic laryngitis.

ETIOL: Disease of vocal cords, paralysis of laryngeal nerves, pressure on recurrent laryngeal nerve; or it may be functional due to hysteria or psychiatric causes.

a., hysterical. Aphonia due to hysteria. There is no organic defect.

a. paranoica. Obstinate silence in the mentally ill.

a., spastic. Aphonia resulting from spasm of vocal muscles, esp. that initiated by efforts to speak.

aphonogelia (ă-fō″nō-jē′lē-ă) [″ + *phone*, voice, + *gelos*, laughter]. Inability to laugh out loud.

aphose (ăf′ōz) [″ + *phos*, light]. A subjective visual perception of darkness, or of a shadow.

aphrasia (ă-frā′zē-ă) [″ + *phrasis*, speech]. Inability to speak or understand phrases.

aphrodisiac (ăf″rō-dĭz′ē-ăk). An agent that stimulates sexual desire.

aphthae (ăf′thē) [Gr. *aphtha*, small ulcer]. Small ulcers on a mucous membrane of the mouth, as in thrush.

a., Bednar's. Whitish ulceration of the posterior hard palate in infants.

a., cachectic. Lesions formed beneath the tongue; accompanied by severe constitutional symptoms.

aphthoid (ăf′thoyd). Resembling aphthae.

aphthongia (ăf-thŏn′jē-ă) [Gr. *a-*, not, + *phthongos*, voice]. Inability to speak due to spasm of muscles controlling speech.

aphthosis (ăf-thō′sĭs) [Gr. *aphtha*, small ulcer, + *osis*, condition]. Any condition characterized by aphthae.

aphthous (ăf′thŭs) [Gr. *aphtha*, small ulcer]. Pert. to, or characterized by, aphthae. Typical in recurrent stomatitis.

aphthous ulcer. Solitary or multiple ulcers of the oral cavity that tend to recur. These lesions are usually less than 0.5 cm in diameter, are painful, and may last for two weeks. Ulcers that persist for longer than two weeks should be biopsied in order to rule out cancer.

ETIOL: Unknown, but an autoimmune basis is suspected. Exposure to certain foods, or fever or mental stress, may precede these lesions.

TREAT: Application of topical tetracycline several times a day will relieve pain and shorten healing time. Application of a topical anesthetic or a protective paste, such as Orabase, will provide symptomatic relief and make it possible to eat without pain. SYN: *canker sore; stomatitis, aphthous.* SEE: *cold sore.*

apical (ăp′ĭ-kal, ā′pĭ-kal) [L. *apex*, tip]. Pert. to the apex of a structure.

apical heave. In children, visible heaving of the chest over the apex of the heart. This indicates left ventricular hypertrophy. SEE: *substernal thrust.*

apicectomy (ăp″ĭ-sĕk′tō-mē) [L. *apex*, tip, + Gr. *ektome*, excision]. 1. Excision of the apex of the petrous portion of the temporal bone. 2. Former term for apicoectomy, q.v.

apices (ā′pĭ-sēz, ăp′ĭ-sēz) [L.]. Pl. of apex.

apicitis (ăp-ĭ-sī′tĭs) [L. *apices*, tips, + Gr. *itis*, inflammation]. Inflammation of an apex, esp. apex of lung or the root of a tooth.

apicoectomy (ăp-ĭ-kō-ĕk′tō-mē) [L. *apex*, tip, + Gr. *ektome*, excision]. Excision of the apex of a tooth root.

apicolocator (ā″pĭ-kō-lō′kă-tor) [″ + *locare*, to place]. Instrument for locating apex of the root of a tooth.

apicolysis (ăp″ĭ-kŏl′ĭ-sĭs) [″ + Gr. *lysis*, dissolution]. Artificial collapse of the apex of a lung by making an opening through the anterior chest wall.

NURSING IMPLICATIONS: Explain the procedure to the patient; at the same time, assess the patient for symptoms of anxiety, and provide emotional support. During and after the procedure, assess for symptoms indicative of a tension pneumothorax, such as increased pulse and respirations, cyanosis, and marked dyspnea. Also assess for symptoms of a mediastinal shift, such as cyanosis, severe dyspnea, distended neck veins, increased pulse and respiratory rate, and excessive, uncontrollable coughing.

Following the procedure, the patient is usually positioned on the affected side.

apicostomy (ăp″ĭ-kŏs′tō-mē) [L. *apex*, tip, + Gr. *stoma*, mouth]. Surgical removal of the mucoperiosteum and bone in order to expose the apex of the root of the tooth.

apicotomy (ăp″ĭ-kŏt′ō-mē) [L. *apex*, tip, + Gr. *tome*, incision]. Incision of an apical structure.

apinealism (ă-pĭn′ē-ăl-ĭzm) [Gr. *a-*, not, + L. *pinea*, pine cone, + Gr. *-ismos*, condition]. Absence of pineal gland.

apiphobia [L. *apis*, bee, + phobia]. Unrealistic fear of bees.

A.P.L. Trade name for chorionic gonadotropin, human, q.v.

aplanatic lens (ă″plă-năt′ĭk lĕnz) [Gr. *a-*, not, + *planetos*, wandering]. A lens that corrects spherical aberration.

aplasia (ă-plā′zē-ă) [″ + *plasis*, a developing]. Failure of an organ or tissue to develop normally.

a. axialis extracorticalis congenita. Congenital defect of the axon formation on the surface of the cerebral cortex.

a. cutis congenita. Defective development of localized area of skin, usually on the scalp. Area is usually covered by a thin, translucent membrane.

a., gonadal. Congenital absence of gonadal tissue.

aplastic (ă-plăs′tĭk) [″ + *plastikos*, shaped]. Pert. to aplasia; having deficient or arrested development.

aplastic anemia. Anemia caused by deficient red cell production due to disorders of bone marrow.

ETIOL: 40% to 70% of the cases are idiopathic; most common in adolescents and young adults. Exposure to chemical and antineoplastic agents, and ionizing radiation can result in aplastic anemia; chronic renal failure; and infiltration of the bone marrow by cells that are not normally present there; can interfere with normal blood production. Examples: metastatic carcinoma, miliary tuberculosis. A congenital form has been described.

NURSING IMPLICATIONS: Give the patient and the family an opportunity to discuss matters of concern and provide emotional support. Assist to understand measures to prevent infection and the importance of adequate rest. Encourage compliance with prescribed medical regimen and regular follow-up. Explain side effects of drugs and transfusion. In acute phase, carry out prescribed treatment, observe for signs of infection or hemorrhage and ensure a restful environment. Explain the reasons for reverse isolation if this is instituted. SEE: *protective isolation.*

Apley's scratch test. A test to functionally assess range of motion of the shoulders. The patient reaches over his head with one hand and behind his back with his other hand and is then asked to scratch his back. This is a quick method of testing abduction and lateral rotation of one shoulder and adduction and medial rotation of the other shoulder.

A.P.M.A. *American Podiatric Medical Association.* Formerly called the American Podiatry Association.

apnea (ăp-nē′ă) [″ + *pnoe*, breathing]. Temporary cessation of breathing. May result from reduction in stimuli to the respiratory center, as in overbreathing, in which carbon dioxide content of the blood is reduced; from failure of respiratory center to discharge impulses, as when the breath is held voluntarily; or during Cheyne-Stokes respiration.

It is a serious symptom, esp. in such conditions as arteriosclerosis, meningitis, coma, heart and kidney diseases, and also following an injury to the brain in which concussion results. Sometimes Cheyne-Stokes respiration is noticed in perfectly healthy children and in the aged during profound sleep. SEE: *apnea monitoring; Cheyne-Stokes respiration; sleep apnea* under *sleep, disorders of; sudden infant death syndrome.*

a., sleep. SEE: *sleep apnea* under *sleep, disorders of.*

apnea alarm mattress. A mattress that is designed to sound an alarm when the infant lying on it ceases to breathe. SEE: *apnea monitoring; sudden infant death syndrome.*

apnea monitoring. Monitoring the respiratory movements, especially of infants. This may be done by use of an apnea alarm mattress, q.v.; or use of devices to measure thoracic and abdominal movement of the infant as well as heart rate. SEE: *sudden infant death syndrome.*

apneic oxygenation. The supplying of oxygen to the upper airway of patients who are not breathing.

apneumatic (ăp″nū-măt′ĭk) [Gr. *a*-, not, + *pneuma*, air]. 1. Free of air, as in a collapsed lung. 2. Pert. to a procedure done in the absence of air.

apneumatosis (ăp″nū-mă-tō′sĭs) [″ + ″ + *osis*, condition]. Noninflation of air cells of lung; congenital atelectasis.

apneumia (ăp-nū′mē-ă) [″ + *pneumon*, lung]. Congenital absence of the lungs.

apneusis (ăp-nū′sĭs). Abnormal respiration marked by sustained inspiratory effort. Caused by surgical removal of the upper portion of the pons.

apo- (ăp′ō) [Gr. *apo*, from]. Prefix denoting separation or derivation from.

apo(a). Abbreviation for apolipoprotein(a).

apocamnosis (ăp″ō-kăm-nō′sĭs) [Gr. *apokamnein*, to grow weary]. Weariness; easily induced fatigue.

apochromatic lens (ăp″ō-krō-măt′ĭk). A lens that corrects both spherical and chromatic aberrations.

apocrine (ăp′ō-krēn, -krĭn, -krĭn) [Gr. *apo*, from, + *krinein*, to separate]. Denoting secretory cells that contribute part of their protoplasm to the material secreted. SEE: *eccrine; holocrine; merocrine.*

apocrine sweat glands. Sweat glands located in the axillae and pubic region that open into hair follicles rather than directly onto the surface of the skin as do eccrine sweat glands, q.v. They appear after puberty and are better developed in women than in men. The characteristic odor of perspiration is produced by the action of bacteria on the material secreted by the apocrine sweat glands. SEE: *sweat gland.*

apocrustic (ăp″ō-krŭs′tĭk) [Gr. *apokroustikos*, able to ward off]. 1. Astringent and repellent. 2. An astringent and repellent agent.

apodal (ă-pō'dăl) [Gr. *a-*, not, + *pous*, foot]. Lacking feet.

apodemialgia (ăp"ō-dē"mē-ăl'jē-ă) [Gr. *apodemia*, away from home, + *algos*, pain]. An abnormal desire to leave home; wanderlust. Opposite of nostalgia.

apodia (ă-pō'dē-ă) [Gr. *a-*, not, + *pous*, foot]. Congenital absence of one or both feet.

apoenzyme (ăp-ō-ĕn'zīm). The protein portion of an enzyme. SEE: *holoenzyme; prosthetic group.*

apoferritin (ăp"ō-fĕr'ĭ-tĭn). A protein that combines with iron to form ferritin. It is not found in the body except attached to iron.

apogee (ăp'ō-jē) [Gr. *apo*, from, + *gaia*, earth]. The climax or period of greatest severity of a disease.

apokamnosis (ăp"ō-kăm-nō'sĭs). Apocamnosis, q.v.

apolar (ă-pō'lăr) [Gr. *a-*, not, + *polos*, pole]. Without poles or processes. Some nerve cells are apolar.

apolepsis (ăp"ō-lĕp'sĭs) [Gr. *apolepsis*, a leaving off]. 1. Cessation of a function. 2. Retention or suppression of an excretion or secretion.

apolipoprotein. The nonlipid protein portion of a lipoprotein. The apolipoproteins are classified according to their function into five major groups with subclasses in some groups. They are apolipoproteins B100, A-I, A-II, B, and E.

Apolipoproteins bind to specific enzymes on cell membranes and transport the lipoproteins to their sites of metabolism. SEE: *lipoprotein.*

apomorphine (ăp"ō-mor'fēn) [Gr. *apo*, from, + *morphine*]. A morphine derivative prepared by removal of one molecule of water from the morphine molecule.

 a. hydrochloride. A grayish white powder that becomes green on exposure to water or air. Emetic; sometimes valuable in cases of poisoning when gastric lavage cannot be employed. In small doses it may be used as an expectorant.

aponeurology (ăp"ō-nū-rŏl'ō-jē) [" + *neuron*, nerve, tendon, + *logos*, word, reason]. The branch of anatomy dealing with aponeuroses.

aponeurorrhaphy (ăp"ō-nū-ror'ă-fē) [" + " + *rhaphe*, seam, ridge]. Suture of an aponeurosis.

aponeurosis (ăp"ō-nū-rō'sĭs) [" + *neuron*, nerve, tendon] (pl. *aponeuroses*). A flat fibrous sheet of connective tissue that serves to attach muscle to bone or other tissues. May sometimes serve as a fascia, q.v.

 a., epicranial. Fibrous membrane connecting the occipital and frontal muscles. SYN: *galea aponeurotica.*

 a., lingual. Connective tissue sheet of the tongue to which lingual muscles attach.

 a., palatine. Connective tissue sheet of the soft palate to which palatal muscles attach.

 a., pharyngeal. Sheet of connective tissue lying between the mucosal and muscular layers of the pharyngeal wall. SYN: *fascia, pharyngobasilar.*

 a., plantar. Sheet of connective tissue investing the muscles of the sole of the foot. SYN: *fascia, plantar.*

aponeurositis (ăp"ō-nū-rō-sī'tĭs) [" + " + *itis*, inflammation]. Inflammation of an aponeurosis.

aponeurotic (ăp"ō-nū-rŏt'ĭk) [" + *neuron*, nerve, tendon]. Pert. to an aponeurosis.

aponeurotome (ăp"ō-nū'rō-tōm) [" + " + *tome*, incision]. Surgical instrument for cutting an aponeurosis.

aponeurotomy (ăp"ō-nū-rŏt'ō-mē). Incision of an aponeurosis.

aponia (ă-pŏn'ē-ă) [Gr. *a-*, not, + *ponos*, toil, pain]. 1. Abstaining from exertion. 2. Absence of pain.

aponic (ă-pŏn'ĭk). 1. Rel. to aponia. 2. Relieving pain or fatigue.

apophyseal, apophysial (ăp"ō-fĭz'ē-ăl) [Gr. *apo*, from, + *physis*, growth]. Pert. to an apophysis.

apophysis (ă-pŏf'ĭ-sĭs) [Gr. *apophysis*, offshoot] (pl. *apophyses*). [NA] A projection, esp. from a bone; an outgrowth without an independent center of ossification.

 Ex.: A tubercle.

 a., basilar. Basilar process of the occipital bone.

 a., lenticular. Lenticular process of the incus, which articulates with the stapes.

 a. of Ingrassia. Smaller wing of sphenoid bone.

 a. of Rau, a. raviana. Anterior process of malleus.

 a., temporal. Mastoid process of the temporal bone.

 a., vertebral. Superior and inferior articular process of the vertebral arches.

apophysitis (ă-pŏf"ĭ-sī'tĭs) [Gr. *apo*, from, + *physis*, growth, + *itis*, inflammation]. Inflammation of an apophysis.

apoplectic (ăp"ō-plĕk'tĭk) [Gr. *apoplektikos*, crippled by stroke]. Pert. to apoplexy.

apoplectiform (ăp"ō-plĕk'tĭ-form) [Gr. *apoplexia*, stroke, + L. *forma*, form]. Resembling apoplexy. SYN: *apoplectoid.*

apoplectoid (ăp"ō-plĕk'toyd) [" + *eidos*, form, shape]. Resembling apoplexy. SYN: *apoplectiform.*

apoplexia (ăp"ō-plĕk'sē-ă) [Gr. *apoplessein*, to cripple by a stroke]. Apoplexy, q.v.

 a. uteri. Sudden hemorrhage from the uterus.

apoplexy (ăp'ŏ-plĕk"sē) [Gr. *apoplessein*, to cripple by a stroke]. 1. Copious effusion of blood into an organ, as abdominal apoplexy; pulmonary apoplexy. 2. Sudden loss of consciousness followed by paralysis caused by hemorrhage into brain; formation of an embolus or thrombus that occludes an artery; or rupture of an anterocerebral artery causing subarachnoid hemorrhage. SYN: *cerebrovascular accident; stroke*, q.v. SEE: *cerebrovascular accident*.

SYM: Acute onset with unconsciousness and stertorous respiration due to paralysis of portion of the soft palate; expiration puffs out the cheeks and mouth. Pupils sometimes unequal, the larger one being on the side of the hemorrhage. Paralysis usually involves one side of the body, with eyeballs turned away from the affected side, skin covered with clammy sweat, surface temperature of skin is often subnormal; speech may be disordered or impossible. Onset more gradual if caused by a thrombosis, q.v.

F.A.: In hospital or at home keep patient, if conscious, quiet and sitting up or lying down with head and shoulders elevated. This will help to prevent aspiration of saliva. Loosen clothing, esp. around the neck. Do not give stimulants. Apply cooling applications to head and neck.

PROG: Depends upon symptoms. Often poor.

a., esophageal. SEE: *esophageal apoplexy*.

apoptosis (ă-pŏp-tō'sĭs, ă-pō-tō'sĭs) [Gr. *apo*, from, + *ptosis*, a dropping]. Disintegration of cells into membrane-bound particles that are then phagocytosed by other cells. The process may be important in limiting growth of tumors.

aporepressor (ăp"ō-rē-prĕs'or). A protein, the synthesis of which is directed by a regulator gene, that functions only when bound with specific low-molecular-weight compounds called corepressors.

aposia (ă-pō'zē-ă) [Gr. *a-*, not, + *posis*, drink]. Absence of thirst. SYN: *adipsia*.

aposthia (ă-pŏs'thē-ă) [Gr. *a-*, not, + *posthe*, foreskin]. Congenital absence of the prepuce.

apotemnophilia (ăp"ō-tĕm"nō-fĕl'ē-ă) [Gr. *apo*, away, + *temnein*, to cut, + *philein*, to love]. A form of paraphilia characterized by the individual requesting amputation of an extremity for erotic reasons.

apothanasia (ăp"ō-thă-nā'zē-ă) [Gr. *apo*, away, + *thanatos*, death]. Prolongation of life.

apothecaries' weights and measures. An outdated and obsolete system of weights and measures formerly used by physicians and pharmacists based on 480 grains = 1 ounce and 12 ounces = 1 pound. Has been replaced by the metric system, q.v. SEE: *Weights and Measures* in Appendix.

apothecary (ă-pŏth'ĕ-kā-rē) [Gr. *apotheke*, storing place]. A druggist or pharmacist. In England and Ireland, one licensed by the Society of Apothecaries of London or the Apothecaries' Hall of Ireland as an authorized physician and dispenser of drugs.

apothem, apotheme (ăp'ō-thĕm, -thēm) [Gr. *apo*, from, + *thema*, deposit]. The brown precipitate that appears when vegetable decoctions or infusions are exposed to the air or are boiled a long time.

apotripsis (ăp"ō-trĭp'sĭs) [Gr. *apotribein*, to abrade]. Removal of corneal scar or opacity.

apparatus (ăp"ă-rā'tŭs, -răt'ŭs) [L. *apparare*, to prepare]. 1. A number of parts acting together in the performance of some special function. 2. A group of structures or organs that work together to perform a common function. 3. A mechanical device or appliance used in operations and experiments.

a., acoustic. Auditory apparatus; the anatomical structures essential for hearing.

a., biliary. Structures concerned with secretion and excretion of bile. Includes liver, gallbladder, and hepatic, cystic, and common bile ducts.

a., dental. The tooth and its supporting tissues.

a., Golgi. SEE: *Golgi apparatus*.

a., juxtaglomerular. Thickened portion of an afferent arteriole near each glomerulus in the cortex of a kidney. Consists of modified smooth muscles that acquire a clear swollen appearance. The function is to monitor glomerular blood flow and, in a feedback relation, to produce renin. SEE: *angiotensin*.

a., lacrimal. The tear-secreting gland and the lacrimal duct, which provides the passageway for the tears from the eye to the nasal cavity. SEE: *lacrimal apparatus* for illus.

a., masticatory. The teeth, jaws, muscles of mastication, and the temporomandibular joints constitute the masticatory apparatus for chewing.

a., respiratory. The respiratory system.

a., sound-conducting. Those parts of the acoustic apparatus that transmit sound.

a., sound-perceiving. Those parts of the acoustic apparatus that are essential for the perception of sounds.

a., urogenital. The genitourinary system.

a., vocal. The collection of organs that produce sounds and thus speech phonation.

apparent [L. *apparens*, appearing]. 1. Obvious and easily seen, not disguised or hidden. 2. Seeming, from initial appearance or evidence, to be obvious and clear, but later examination or evidence will prove the initial impression or opinion to be erroneous.

appearance. The visible presentation of an object.

appendage (ă-pĕn′dĭj). Anything attached or appended to a larger or major part, as a tail or a limb. SEE: *appendix*.

　　a., atrial. A small muscular pouch attached to each atrium of the heart.

　　a., auricular. A., atrial, q.v.

　　a.'s of the eye. The eyelid, eyelashes, eyebrow, lacrimal apparatus, and conjunctiva.

　　a.'s of the fetus. The amnion, chorion, and umbilical cord.

　　a.'s of the skin. The nails, hair, sebaceous and sweat glands.

　　a., uterine. The ovaries, fallopian tubes, and uterine ligaments.

appendalgia (ăp″ĕn-dăl′jē-ă) [L. *appendere,* hang to, + Gr. *algos,* pain]. Pain in lower right quadrant in region of vermiform appendix.

appendectomy (ăp″ĕn-dĕk′tō-mē) [″ + Gr. *ektome,* excision]. Surgical removal of the vermiform appendix.

　　a., incidental. Removal of the appendix at the time of another surgical procedure in the abdominal cavity.

appendical, appendiceal (ă-pĕn′dĭ-kăl, ăp-ĕn-dĭs′ē-ăl). Pert. to an appendix.

appendical reflex. Tenderness at McBurney's point accompanied by rigidity, considered a reflex expression by way of sympathetic cerebrospinal arc.

appendicectasis (ă-pĕn″dĭ-sĕk′tă-sĭs) [L. *appendere,* hang to, + Gr. *ektasis,* a stretching]. Dilatation of the vermiform appendix.

appendicectomy (ă-pĕn″dĭ-sĕk′tō-mē) [″ + Gr. *ektome,* excision]. Surgical removal of the appendix.

appendices (ă-pĕn′dĭ-sēz). Pl. of appendix, q.v.

appendicitis (ă-pĕn″dĭ-sī′tĭs) [L. *appendere,* hang to, + Gr. *itis,* inflammation]. Inflammation of the vermiform appendix. It generally occurs in the young, most often between ages 15 and 25, and very rarely before the 5th year or after the 50th. More common in males than in females. The disease may be acute, subacute, or chronic. When this diagnosis is considered in the adult female, it must be differentiated from pain associated with ovulation (mittelschmerz, q.v.), ruptured ectopic pregnancy, and pelvic inflammatory disease.

　　TREAT: Surgical removal of the appendix. From 10% to 30% of appendices removed will be normal. SEE: *Nursing Diagnoses in Appendix.*

　　a., acute. SYM: Abdominal pain, usually severe and generally throughout the abdomen, followed by nausea and vomiting; localization of pain in the right lower quadrant of abdomen with tenderness and rigidity over right rectus muscle or McBurney's point; fever usually rising within several hours, 99° to 101°F (37.2° to 38.3°C); pulse increasing with temperature; patient lying on back with right lower extremity frequently flexed to relieve muscle tension; leukocytosis present shortly after onset. In mild cases symptoms begin to subside on the second day. A well-defined abscess usually develops 24 to 72 hours after the onset of symptoms and may be palpable in the right ileocecal region.

　　NURSING IMPLICATIONS: *Preop:* Carefully assess the patient for signs and symptoms that will assist in the diagnosis of appendicitis, such as elevated temperature; nausea or vomiting; onset, intensity, and location of pain; rebound tenderness; constipation or diarrhea; and an elevated white blood cell count. The patient should be placed in a position of comfort. Prepare the patient physically and emotionally for surgery.

Caution: No cathartics or enemas should be administered to a patient with suspected appendicitis. Heating pads should never be used because of possibility of causing a rupture of the appendix.

Postop: Position the patient comfortably (Fowler's position if the patient had a ruptured appendix or peritonitis). Administer prescribed medications to keep the patient comfortable. Change patient's position, have patient cough and breathe deeply, and encourage early ambulation to prevent respiratory complications. Observe the dressing for presence of any bleeding or drainage. Closely monitor I.V. fluids, and measure and record the patient's intake and output.

　　a., chronic. May follow an acute attack leaving a cicatricial narrowing of the lumen of the appendix, or adhesions.

　　SYM: Gastric indigestion, frequently simulating a gastric ulcer, duodenal ulcer, or gallbladder disease. Tenderness manifested in the right lower abdomen.

　　TREAT: Surgical.

　　a., gangrenous. When inflammation is extreme, blood vessels are blocked in the mesentery, circulation to appendix is cut off, and diffuse peritonitis ensues.

appendicoenterostomy (ă-pĕn″dĭk-ō-ĕn″tĕr-ŏs′tō-mē) [L. *appendere,* hang to, + Gr. *enteron,* intestine, + *stoma,* mouth]. 1. Appendicostomy, q.v. 2. The establishment of an anastomosis between appendix and intestine.

appendicolithiasis (ă-pĕn″dĭ-kō″lĭ-thī′ă-sĭs) [″ + Gr. *lithos*, stone, + *-iasis*, state]. Formation of calculi in the vermiform appendix.

appendicolysis (ă-pĕn″dĭ-kŏl′ĭ-sĭs) [″ + Gr. *lysis*, dissolution]. Operation that frees appendix from adhesions. This is done by slitting the serosa at its base.

appendicopathy (ă-pĕn″dĭ-kŏp′ă-thē) [″ + Gr. *pathos*, disease, suffering]. Any disease of the vermiform appendix.

   a. oxyurica. Lesion of the appendical mucosa supposedly due to oxyurids (intestinal parasitic worms).

appendicostomy (ă-pĕn″dĭ-kŏs′tō-mē) [″ + Gr. *stoma*, mouth]. Operation in which an opening is made in the vermiform appendix for the purpose of irrigating the cecum and colon.

appendicular (ăp″ĕn-dĭk′ū-lăr) [L. *appendere*, to hang to]. 1. Pert. to an appendix. SYN: *appendiceal*. 2. Pert. to the extremities, as opposed to axial, which pertains to the head and trunk.

appendicular skeleton. The bony structure that makes up the shoulder girdle, upper extremities, pelvis, and lower extremities.

appendix (ă-pĕn′dĭks) [L.] (pl. *appendixes, appendices*). [NA] An appendage, esp. the appendix vermiformis. SEE: *digestive system* and *omentum* for illus. SYN: *appendage.*

   a., atrial. A small muscular pouch attached to each atrium of the heart.

   a., auricular. A., atrial, q.v.

   a., ensiform. The lowest portion of the sternum. SYN: *a., xiphoid; xiphoid process.*

   a. epididymidis. [NA] A cystic structure attached to the epididymis, a vestigial remnant of the mesonephric duct.

   a. epiploica. One of numerous pouches of peritoneum, filled with fat and attached to the colon.

   a. testis. [NA] Small bladderlike structure at upper end of testis, a vestigial remnant of cephalic portion of müllerian duct.

   a., ventricular. Saccule, laryngeal, q.v.

   a. vermiformis. [NA] A worm-shaped process projecting from the blind end of the cecum and lined with a continuation of the mucous membrane of the cecum. SYN: *processus vermiformis; vermiform appendix.*

   a., vesicular. A cystic structure attached to the fimbriated end of the uterine tube. It is a vestigial remnant of the mesonephric duct.

   a., xiphoid. The xiphoid process; small, lowest portion of the sternum. SYN: *a., ensiform; xiphoid process.*

apperception (ăp″ĕr-sĕp′shŭn) [L. *ad*, to,

+ *percipere*, to perceive]. The perception and interpretation of sensory stimuli; awareness of the meaning and significance of a particular sensory stimulus as modified by one's own experiences, knowledge, thoughts, and emotions.

apperceptive (ăp″ĕr-sĕp′tĭv). Pert. to apperception.

appersonification. Identifying, perhaps unconsciously, with another person and impersonating him or her.

appestat (ăp′ĕ-stăt) [L. *appetitus*, longing for, + Gr. *states*, stand]. Area of brain (probably in the hypothalamus) that is thought to control appetite and food intake.

appetite (ăp′ĕ-tīt) [L. *appetitus*, longing for]. Strong desire, especially for food. Appetite is differentiated from hunger in that the latter is an uncomfortable sensation caused by lack of food, whereas appetite is a pleasant sensation based on previous experience that causes one to seek food for the purpose of tasting and enjoying.

   a., perverted. Desire to eat unnatural and indigestible substances such as paint or laundry starch. SYN: *pica.*

appetite, words pert. to: acoria; anorexia; apositia; bulimia; dysorexia; hyperorexia; parageusia; pica; polyphagia; taste; weight; set point.

appetizer (ăp′ĕ-tī″zĕr). That which promotes appetite.

applanation (ăp″lă-nā′shŭn) [L. *ad*, toward, + *planare*, to flatten]. Abnormal flattening, esp. of the corneal surface.

applanometer (ăp″lă-nŏm′ĕ-tĕr) [″ + *planum*, plane, + Gr. *metron*, measure]. Device for measuring intraocular pressure. SEE: *tonometer.*

apple, Adam's. The laryngeal prominence formed by the two laminae of the thyroid cartilage.

apple packer's epistaxis. Nosebleed due to handling packing trays containing certain dyes.

apple picker's disease. Bronchitis resulting from a fungicide used on apples.

apple sorter's disease. Contact dermatitis caused by chemicals used in washing apples.

appliance (ă-plī′ăns). 1. In dentistry, a device used to provide or facilitate a particular function, such as artificial dentures; device used to correct bite. 2. A device for influencing a specific function, e.g., a cane, crutch or walker to assist walking, or an appliance to discourage thumb sucking. SEE: *penile prosthesis; prosthesis.*

applicator (ăp′lĭ-kā″tor) [L. *applicare*, to attach]. Device, usually a slender rod with a pledget of cotton on the end, for making local applications.

apposition (ăp″ō-zĭ′shŭn) [L. *ad*, toward,

+ *ponere*, to place]. 1. Condition of being positioned side by side or fitted together. SYN: *contiguity*. 2. The adding of one substance to another one as one layer of tissue upon another. 3. Developing by means of accretion as would be the case in bone or dental cementum formation.

approach (ă-prōch'). Surgical procedures for exposing an organ or tissue.

approximal (ă-prŏk'sĭ-măl) [" + *proximus*, nearest]. Contiguous; next to.

approximate (ă-prŏk'sĭ-māt) [" + *proximare*, to come near]. To place or bring objects close together.

apraxia (ă-prăk'sē-ă) [Gr. *a-*, not, + *praxis*, action]. 1. Inability to perform purposive movements although there is no sensory or motor impairment. 2. Inability to use objects properly.

    a., akinetic. Inability to carry out spontaneous movements.

    a., amnesic. Inability to produce a movement on command because the command is forgotten, although the ability to perform the movement is present.

    a., constructional. Inability to draw or construct two- or three-dimensional forms or figures and impairment in the ability to integrate perception into kinesthetic images.

    a., developmental. Disorder of motor planning and execution occurring in developing children; thought to be due to central nervous system immaturity.

    a., dressing. Inability to dress due to patient's deficient knowledge of the spatial relations of his or her body.

    a., ideational. Misuse of objects due to inability to perceive their correct use. SYN: *a., sensory.*

    a., motor. Inability to perform movements necessary to use objects properly, although the names and purposes of the objects are known and understood.

    a., sensory. A., ideational, q.v.

apraxic. Pert. to or characterized by apraxia.

Apresoline Hydrochloride. Trade name for hydralazine hydrochloride, q.v.

aproctia (ă-prŏk'shē-ă) [Gr. *a-*, not, + *proktos*, anus]. Absence or imperforation of anus.

apron (ā'prŏn) [O. Fr. *naperon*, cloth]. 1. Outer garment covering front of the body for protection of clothing during surgery, during certain nursing procedures, while working with plaster of paris, etc. 2. Part of the body resembling an apron.

    a., Hottentot. Abnormally long labia minora. SYN: *velamen vulvae.*

    a., lead. Garment worn in radiography to prevent radiation exposure to the trunk of the body.

aprosody (ă-prŏs'ō-dē) [Gr. *a-* not, + *prosodia*, voice modulation]. Absence of normal variations of pitch, rhythm, and stress in the speech.

aprosopia (ăp"rō-sō'pē-ă) [" + *prosopon*, face]. Congenital defect in which part or all of the face is absent.

aprotes. Chemical substances that are either cations such as sodium, calcium, potassium, and magnesium that carry a positive charge; or anions such as chloride and sulfate that carry a negative charge. These chemicals are unable to donate or accept protons; thus they are not acids, bases, or buffers. SEE: *buffer.*

APT. *alum-precipitated toxoid.*

A.P.T.A. *American Physical Therapy Association.*

aptitude (ăp'tĭ-tūd). Inherent ability or skill in learning or performing physical or mental endeavors.

aptitude test. A mental or physical (or both) test designed to evaluate skill or ability to perform certain tasks or assignments.

APT test. In infants, a method of differentiating swallowed maternal blood in the stool from gastrointestinal bleeding from the infant. The blood could be swallowed during delivery or from a bleeding nipple fissure. To test: 1. Rinse a bloody stool or diaper until a pink supernatant is obtained. 2. Centrifuge the supernatant and remove the top fluid. 3. To 5 parts of the solution removed add 1 part of 0.25 normal (1%) sodium hydroxide. Within 1 to 2 minutes, a color reaction takes place. A yellow-brown color indicates the blood originated from the mother; a persistent pink color indicates the blood is from the fetus. It is advisable to test control specimens from both the fetus and the infant. SEE: *swallowed blood syndrome.*

aptyalia, aptyalism (ăp"tē-ā'lē-ă, ăp-tē'ă-lĭzm, ă-tī'ă-lĭzm) [" + *ptyalon*, saliva]. Absence or deficiency of secretion of saliva. SYN: *asialia; dry mouth; oligosialia; xerostomia.*

    ETIOL: Disease (mumps, typhoid fever); dehydration; effect of drugs; x-ray irradiation; old age; obstruction of salivary ducts; Sjögren's syndrome, in which there is deficient function of lacrimal, salivary, and other glands.

APUD cells. *amine precursor uptake and decarboxylation* cells. A class of cells that produces hormones such as insulin, ACTH, glucagon, and thyroxin; and amines, including dopamine, serotonin, and histamine. These cells are involved in multiple endocrine neoplasia Types I and II, q.v.

apudoma [from *APUD cells*]. A tumor of APUD cells, q.v.

apulmonism (ă-pool'mŏn-ĭzm) [Gr. *a-*, not,

+ L. *pulmo,* lung, + Gr. *-ismos,* condition]. Congenital absence of part or all of a lung.

apus (ā'pŭs) [" + *pous,* foot]. A person who has apodia, congenital absence of the feet.

apyetous (ă-pī-'ĕ-tŭs) [" + *pyesis,* suppuration]. Nonsuppurative, nonpurulent. SYN: *apyogenous.*

apyknomorphous (ă-pĭk"nō-mor'fŭs) [" + *pyknos,* thick, + *morphe,* form]. Not pyknomorphous; pert. to a cell that does not stain deeply because its stainable material is not compact.

apyogenous (ă-pī-ŏj'ĕn-ŭs) [" + *pyon,* pus, + *genos,* origin]. Not producing pus.

apyretic (ā-pī-rĕt'ĭk) [" + *pyretos,* fever]. Without fever. SYN: *afebrile.*

apyrexia (ā-pī-rĕks'ē-ă) [" + *pyrexis,* feverishness]. Absence of fever.

apyrogenetic, apyrogenic (ā"pī-rō-jĕ-nĕt'ĭk, -jĕn'ĭk) [" + " + *genos,* origin]. Not causing fever.

AQ. *achievement quotient.*

aq. L. *aqua,* water.

aqua (awk'wă) [L. *aqua*] (pl. *aquae*). Water. ABBR: a.; aq.

   a. aerata. Carbonated water.

   a. ammonia. NH₄OH. Ammonium hydroxide.

   a. calcariae. Lime water.

   a. camphorae. Camphor water.

   a. destillata. Distilled water.

   a. fervens. Hot water.

   a. fontana. Spring water.

   a. fortis. Weak nitric acid.

   a., medicated. An aqueous solution of a volatile substance. Usually contains only a comparatively small percentage of the active drug. Many are merely water saturated with a volatile oil. They are used more as vehicles and to give odor and taste to solutions.

   a. oculi. The fluid (aqueous humor) of the eye.

   a. pura. Pure water.

   a. purificata. Purified water.

   a. regia. Nitrohydrochloric acid water (20% nitric acid and 80% hydrochloric acid). SYN: *nitromuriatic acid.*

   a. rosea. Rose water.

   a. sterilisata. Sterilized water.

   a. tepida. Lukewarm water.

Aquamephyton. Trade name for phytonadione (vitamin K), q.v.

aquanaut (ă'kwă-nawt). An individual who works underwater, esp. researchers in deepsea environments, usually for an extended length of time.

aquaphobia (ăk"wă-fō'bē-ă) [" + Gr. *phobos,* fear]. Abnormal fear of water. SEE: *hydrophobia.*

Aquaplast. A type of low temperature, thermoplastic splinting material principally

used for making upper extremity orthoses.

aquapuncture (ăk"wă-pŭngk'chūr) [" + *punctura,* puncture]. Subcutaneous injection of water, as to produce counterirritation.

Aquatensen. Trade name for methyclothiazide, q.v.

aquatic. 1. Pert. to water. 2. Inhabiting water.

aqueduct (ăk'wĕ-dŭkt") [" + *ductus,* duct]. Canal or channel. SYN: *aqueductus.*

   a., cerebral. Canal in the midbrain connecting the third and fourth ventricles. SYN: *aqueductus cerebri.*

   a., vestibular. Small passage reaching from the vestibule to the posterior surface of the temporal bone's petrous section.

aqueductus (ăk"wĕ-dŭk'tŭs). [NA] A canal or channel. SYN: *aqueduct.*

   a. cerebri. [NA] Canal in the midbrain connecting the third and fourth ventricles. SYN: *aqueduct, cerebral.*

   a. cochleae. Canal connecting subarachnoid space and the perilymphatic space of the cochlea.

   a. Fallopii. Canal for facial nerve in the temporal bone.

   a. Sylvii. A. cerebri, q.v.

   a. vestibuli. [NA] Small passage reaching from the vestibule to the posterior surface of the temporal bone's petrous section.

aqueous (ā'kwē-ŭs) [L. *aqua,* water]. 1. Of the nature of water; watery. 2. Aqueous humor, q.v.

aqueous chambers. Anterior and posterior chambers of the eye, which contain the aqueous humor.

aqueous humor. Transparent liquid contained in the anterior and posterior chambers of the eye. Produced by the ciliary processes, it passes from the posterior to the anterior chamber, and then to the venous system by way of the canal of Schlemm.

aquiparous (ăk-wĭp'ă-rŭs) [" + *parere,* to bring forth, to bear]. Producing water.

AR. *achievement ratio; alarm reaction.*

Ar. Chem. symb. for the element argon.

ara-A. Vidarabine, q.v.

arabinose (ă-răb'ĭ-nōs). Gum sugar, a pentose obtained from plants. Sometimes found in urine. SYN: L-*arabinose.*

arabinosuria (ă-răb"ĭ-nō-sū'rē-ă) [*arabinose* + Gr. *ouron,* urine]. Arabinose in the urine.

Ara-C. Cytarabine, an antineoplastic drug of the antimetabolite class.

arachidonic acid (ă-răk"ĭ-dŏn'ĭk). The essential fatty acid, 5,8,11,14-eicosatetraenoic acid, formed from unsaturated acids of plants. It is a precursor of prostaglandins.

   An essential fatty acid present in peanut It is metabolized in the body via two pri pal pathways to produce a group of c cals called eicosanoids. Included in these are prostaglandins, thromboxane, and leukotrienes. Synthesis of prostaglandins and thromboxane is directly inhibited by nonsteroidal, anti-inflammatory agents such as salicylates, indomethacin, and ibuprofen. Corticosteroids inhibit formation of arachidonic acid from phospholipases.

arachnid (ă-răk'nĭd). A member of the class Arachnida.

Arachnida (ă-răk'nĭ-dă) [Gr. *arachne*, spider]. A class of the Arthropoda, including the spiders, scorpions, ticks, and mites.

arachnidism (ă-răk'nĭd-ĭzm) [" + *eidos*, form, shape, + -*ismos*, condition of]. Systemic poisoning from spider bite. SYN: *arachnoidism.*

arachnitis (ă″răk-nī′tĭs) [" + *itis*, inflammation]. Inflammation of the arachnoid membrane. SYN: *arachnoiditis.*

arachnodactyly (ă-răk″nō-dăk′tĭl-ē) [" + *dactylos*, finger]. Spider fingers; a state in which fingers and sometimes toes are abnormally long, slender, and curved. SYN: *acromacria; dolichostenomelia.* SEE: *Marfan's syndrome.*

arachnoid (ă-răk'noyd) [" + *eidos*, form, shape]. 1. Resembling a web. 2. Arachnoid membrane; arachnoidea, q.v.

   a., cranial. Arachnoidea encephali, q.v.

   a., spinal. Arachnoidea spinalis, q.v.

arachnoidea (ă-răk-noyd′ē-ă). [NA] A thin, delicate membrane, the intermediate membrane that encloses the brain and spinal cord. It is separated from the pia mater, the inner membrane, by the subarachnoid space and from the dura mater, the outer membrane, by the subdural space. SYN: *arachnoid membrane.*

   a. encephali. The part of the arachnoidea enclosing the brain. SYN: *arachnoid, cranial.*

   a. spinalis. The part of the arachnoidea enclosing the spinal cord. SYN: *arachnoid, spinal.*

arachnoidism (ă-răk′noyd-ĭzm) [Gr. *arachne*, spider, + *eidos*, form, shape, + -*ismos*, condition]. Systemic poisoning from spider bite. SYN: *arachnidism.* SEE: *spider bites or poisoning.*

arachnoiditis (ă-răk″noyd-ī′tĭs) [" + *eidos*, form, shape, + *itis*, inflammation]. Inflammation of the arachnoid membrane. SYN: *arachnitis.*

arachnoid membrane. Arachnoidea, q.v.

arachnoid villi. Body, pacchionian, q.v.

arachnolysin (ă-răk-nŏl′ĭ-sĭn) [" + *lysis*, dissolution]. The hemolysin present in spider venom.

arachnophobia (ă-răk″nō-fō′bē-ă) [" + *phobos*, fear]. Morbid fear of spiders.

Aralen Hydrochloride. Trade name for

chloroquine hydrochloride, q.v.

Aralen Phosphate. Trade name for chloroquine phosphate, q.v.

Aramine. Trade name for metaraminol bitartrate, q.v.

Aran-Duchenne disease (ăr-ŏn′dū-shĕn). SEE: *Duchenne-Aran disease.* SYN: *progressive muscular atrophy.*

araneous (ă-rā′nē-ŭs) [L. *aranea*, cobweb]. Resembling a cobweb.

Arantius' body, nodule (ăr-ăn′shē-ŭs) (pl. *Arantii*) [Julius Caesar Arantius, It. anatomist and physician, 1530–1589]. Small nodule at center of each of the aortic valve cusps. SYN: *noduli valvularum aortae.*

arbor. A structure resembling a tree with branches.

arborescent (ăr″bor-ĕs′ĕnt) [L. *arborescere*, to become a tree]. Branching; treelike.

arborization (ăr″bor-ĭ-zā′shŭn) [L. *arbor*, tree]. Ramification; branching, esp. terminal branching of nerve fibers and capillaries. SEE: *nerve.*

arbor vitae (ăr′bor vī′tē) [L. *arbor*, tree, + *vita* life]. 1. A treelike structure; a treelike outline seen in a section of the cerebellum. 2. A tree or shrub of the genus *Thuja* or *Thujopsis.* 3. A series of branching ridges within the cervix of the uterus. SYN: *plica palmatae.*

arboviruses (ăr″bō-vī′rŭs-ĕs) [*arthropodborne viruses*]. A large group, more than 250, of viruses that multiply in both vertebrates and arthropods such as mosquitoes and ticks. They are known to cause diseases such as yellow fever and viral encephalitis. SEE: *arenaviruses; Togaviridae.*

ARC. *AIDS-related complex*, q.v. SEE: *AIDS.*

arc (ărk) [L. *arcus*, bow]. A curved line; a portion of a circle.

   a., reflex. The path followed by a nerve impulse to produce a reflex action. The impulse originates in a receptor at the point of stimulation, passes through an afferent neuron or neurons to a reflex center in the brain or spinal cord, and from the center out through efferent neurons to the effector organ, where the response occurs. SEE: illus.

arcade (ăr-kād). Any anatomic structure composed of a series of arches.

   a., Flint's. The arteriovenous anastomoses at the bases of the pyramids of the kidney.

arcanum (ăr-kā′nŭm) [L. *arcanum*, a secret] (pl. *arcana*). Secret remedy.

arcate (ăr′kăt) [L. *arcatus*, bow-shaped]. Arched, bow-shaped.

arc eyes. Burn of eyes caused when welders fail to wear protective eye shields while welding or following extended periods of welding even though protective eye gear was

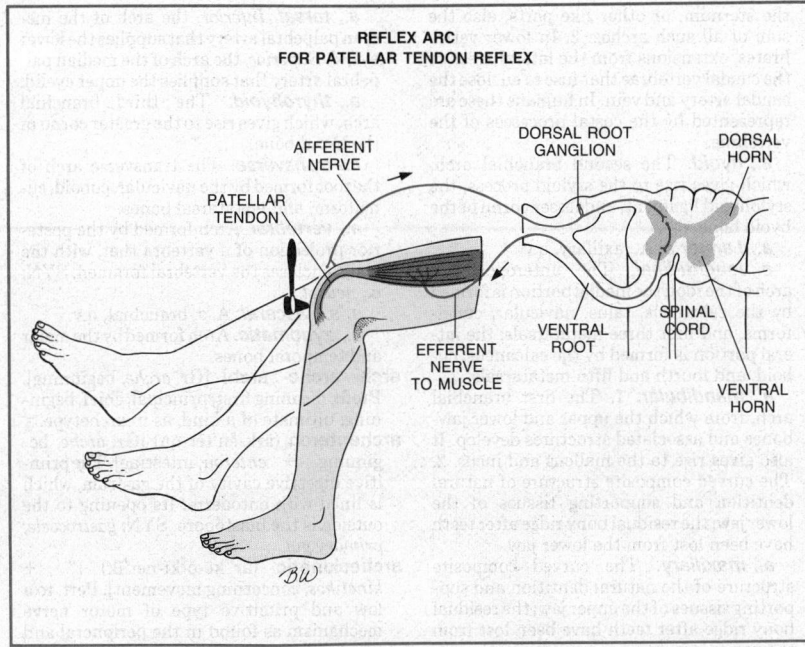

REFLEX ARC
FOR PATELLAR TENDON REFLEX

AFFERENT NERVE

PATELLAR TENDON

DORSAL ROOT GANGLION

DORSAL HORN

EFFERENT NERVE TO MUSCLE

VENTRAL ROOT

SPINAL CORD

VENTRAL HORN

worn.

TREAT: Irrigation of eye with copious amounts of sterile saline may be necessary for several hours in addition to instillation of anti-inflammatory eye drops and other medications.

arch [L. *arcus*, a bow]. Any anatomic structure of a curved or bowlike outline.

a., abdominothoracic. The lower boundary of the front of the thorax.

a., alveolar. Arch of the alveolar process of either jaw.

a., aortic; a. of the aorta. Proximal curved part of the aorta, at about the level of the fourth thoracic vertebra. The innominate, left common carotid, and left subclavian arteries arise from the aortic arch.

a.'s, aortic. A series of six pairs of vessels that develop in the embryo and connect the aortic sac with the dorsal aorta. During the fifth to seventh weeks, the arches undergo transformation, some persisting as functional vessels, others persisting as rudimentary structures, and some disappearing entirely.

a., axillary. An anomalous muscular slip across the axilla, between the pectoralis major and latissimus dorsi muscles. SYN:

a., Langer's; Langer's muscle.

a.'s, branchial. A series of arches that bear the gills in lower vertebrates, and in higher vertebrates play an important role in the development of the head and neck. First is the mandibular; second, the hyoid. The third, fourth, and fifth are transitory. SYN: *a.'s, gill; a.'s, visceral.*

a., carotid. The third aortic arch, which provides the common carotid artery.

a., costal. Arch formed by the ribs.

a., crural. The inguinal ligament, which extends from the anterior superior iliac spine to pubic tubercle. SYN: *a., femoral; Poupart's ligament.*

a., deep crural. A band of fibers arching in front of sheath of femoral vessels; the downward extension of the transversalis fascia.

a., dental. Arch formed by the alveolar process and teeth on either jaw.

a., femoral. A., crural, q.v.

a., glossopalatine. The anterior pillar of the fauces, q.v.; one of two folds of mucous membrane extending from the soft palate to the sides of the tongue.

a., hemal. 1. Arch formed by the body and processes of a vertebra, a pair of ribs and the sternum, or other like parts; also the sum of all such arches. 2. In lower vertebrates, extensions from the lateral areas of the caudal vertebrae that fuse to enclose the caudal artery and vein. In humans these are represented by the costal processes of the vertebrae.

a., hyoid. The second branchial arch, which gives rise to the styloid process, the stylohyoid ligament, and lesser cornu of the hyoid bone.

a., Langer's. A., axillary, q.v.

a., longitudinal. The anteroposterior arch of the foot; the medial portion is formed by the calcaneus, talus, navicular, cuneiforms, and first three metatarsals; the lateral portion is formed by the calcaneus, cuboid, and fourth and fifth metatarsals.

a., mandibular. 1. The first branchial arch, from which the upper and lower jawbones and associated structures develop. It also gives rise to the malleus and incus. 2. The curved composite structure of natural dentition and supporting tissues of the lower jaw; the residual bony ridge after teeth have been lost from the lower jaw.

a., maxillary. The curved composite structure of the natural dentition and supporting tissues of the upper jaw; the residual bony ridge after teeth have been lost from the upper jaw.

a., nasal. Arch formed by the nasal bones and by the nasal processes of the maxilla.

a., neural. A., vertebral, q.v.

a.'s of Corti. A series of arches made up of the rods of Corti.

a.'s of foot. The instep of the foot formed by longitudinal arch and transverse arch, q.v.

a., palmar. *Deep,* an arch formed in the palm by the communicating branch of the ulnar and the radial artery. *Superficial,* an arch in the palm forming the termination of the ulnar artery.

a.'s, pharyngeal. A.'s, branchial, q.v.

a., pharyngopalatine. The posterior pillar of the fauces, q.v.; one of two folds of mucous membrane extending from the soft palate to the sides of the pharynx.

a., plantar. Arch formed by the external plantar artery and deep branch of the dorsalis pedis artery.

a., pubic. Arch formed by the rami of the ischia.

a., pulmonary. The fifth aortic arch on the left side. It becomes the pulmonary artery.

a., superciliary. A curved process of the frontal bone lying just above the orbit and subjacent to the eyebrow.

a., supraorbital. A bony arch formed by the upper margin of the orbit.

a., tarsal. *Inferior,* the arch of the median palpebral artery that supplies the lower eyelid. *Superior,* the arch of the median palpebral artery that supplies the upper eyelid.

a., thyrohyoid. The third branchial arch, which gives rise to the greater cornu of the hyoid bone.

a., transverse. The transverse arch of the foot formed by the navicular, cuboid, cuneiform, and metatarsal bones.

a., vertebral. Arch formed by the posterior projection of a vertebra that, with the body, encloses the vertebral foramen. SYN: *a., neural.*

a.'s, visceral. A.'s, branchial, q.v.

a., zygomatic. Arch formed by the malar and temporal bones.

arch-, arche-, archi- [Gr. *arche,* beginning]. Prefix meaning first, principal, chief, beginning, ultimate of a kind, as in archetype.

archenteron (ärk-ĕn'tĕr-ŏn) [Gr. *arche,* beginning, + *enteron,* intestine]. The primitive digestive cavity of the gastrula, which is lined with entoderm. Its opening to the outside is the blastopore. SYN: *gastrocoele; primary gut.*

archeokinetic (är"kē-ō-kī-nĕt'ĭk) [" + *kinetikos,* concerning movement]. Pert. to a low and primitive type of motor nerve mechanism as found in the peripheral and ganglionic nervous systems. SEE: *paleokinetic.*

archetype (är'kĕ-tīp) [" + *typos,* model]. 1. Original type, from which other forms have developed by differentiation. 2. An ideal or perfect anatomical type. Used as a theoretical standard in judging other individuals.

archiblast (är'kĭ-blăst) [" + *blastos,* a germ, bud]. The outer layer that surrounds the germinal vesicle.

archiblastic (är"kĭ-blăs'tĭk). Derived from, or pert. to, the archiblast.

archiblastoma (är"kĭ-blăs-tō'mă) [" + *blastos,* germ, + *oma,* tumor]. Tumor of archiblastic tissue.

archigaster (är'kĭ-găs"tĕr) [" + *gaster,* belly]. The primitive embryonic alimentary canal.

archinephron (är"kĭ-nĕf'rŏn) [" + *nephros,* kidney]. Primordial kidney, an organ of the embryo. SYN: *mesonephros; wolffian body.*

archineuron (är-kĭ-nū'rŏn) [" + *neuron,* nerve, tendon]. The central cell of the cerebral cortex and all its processes. The nervous impulse that is transmitted to initiate physiological function originates in the archineuron.

archipallium (är"kĭ-păl'ē-ŭm) [" + L. *pallium,* a cloak]. Olfactory cortex, older than neopallium.

archiplasm (är'kĭ-plăzm) [" + LL. *plasma,*

form, mold]. 1. The most primitive living substance. 2. The substance of the fertilized ovum.

archistome (ăr'kĭ-stōm) [" + *stoma*, mouth]. Invagination of blastula making a little opening into the archenteron. SYN: *blastopore*.

architectural barrier. Any limitation in the design of facilities that restricts the access of persons with disabilities and limited mobility, including those using wheelchairs.

architis (ăr-kī'tĭs) [Gr. *archos*, anus, + *itis*, inflammation]. Inflammation of the anus; proctitis.

archo- [Gr. *archos*, rectum]. Prefix denoting relationship to the rectum or anus.

arch width. The measured distance between the canines, bicuspids, and the first molars. These distances establish the shape and size of the dental arch.

arciform (ăr'sĭ-form) [L. *arcus*, bow, + *forma*, shape]. Bow-shaped; shaped like an arc. SYN: *arcuate*.

arctation (ărk-tā'shŭn) [L. *arctatus*, pressing together]. Stricture of any canal opening.

arcuate (ăr'kū-āt) [L. *arcuatus*, bowed]. Bowed, shaped like an arc. SYN: *arciform*.

arcuation (ăr-kū-ā'shŭn). A bending; curvature.

arcus (ăr'kŭs) [L. *arcus*, a bow] (pl. *arcus*). An arch, q.v.

  a. alveolaris mandibulae. The arch formed by the alveolar process of the body of the mandible.

  a. alveolaris maxillae. [NA] The arch formed by the alveolar process of the maxilla.

  a. dentalis. Dental arch.

  a. juvenilis. Opaque ring about the periphery of the cornea similar to arcus senilis but occurring in young individuals. May be due to hypercholesterolemia, corneal irritation or inflammation, or the result of a congenital anomaly.

  a. plantaris. [NA] The plantar arch.

  a. senilis. Opaque white ring about periphery of the cornea, seen in aged persons. Due to deposit of fat granules in cornea or to hyaline degeneration.

ARD. *acute respiratory distress.*

ardanesthesia (ăr″dăn-ĕs-thē′zē-ă) [L. *ardor*, heat, + Gr. *an-*, not, + *aisthesis*, sensation]. Inability to feel heat. SYN: *thermanesthesia*.

ardor (ăr'dor) [L., heat]. Burning; great heat.

  a. urinae. A burning sensation during urination.

  a. veneris. Sexual desire.

ARDS. *adult respiratory distress syndrome.*

area (ā'rē-ă) [L. *area*, an open space] (pl. *areas, areae*). 1. A circumscribed space; one having definite boundaries. 2. Part of an organ that performs a specialized function.

  a., acoustic. A., vestibular, q.v.

  a., association. Area of the cerebral cortex that is not sensory or motor, in the usual meaning of those terms. Thought to be a region in which higher mental processes are mediated.

  a., auditory. The hearing center of cerebral cortex located in the floor of the lateral fissure and surfacing on the dorsal surface of the superior temporal gyrus. It receives auditory fibers from the medial geniculate body.

  a., body surface. The area covered by the skin. It is usually expressed in square meters. The surface area (S) may be calculated by multiplying 0.007184 times the weight (W) in kilograms raised to the 0.425 power and the height (H) in centimeters raised to the 0.725 power. Thus:

$$S = 0.007184 \times W^{0.425} \times H^{0.725}$$

SEE: *rule of nines.*

  a., Broca's. SEE: *Broca's area.*

  a.'s, Brodmann's. The division of the cerebral cortex into 47 areas. This was originally done on the basis of cyto-architectural characteristics, but the areas are now differentiated and classified with respect to their different functions.

  a. germinativa. Area of germination of the ovum.

  a., Kiesselbach's. Area of anterior portion of nasal septum. Because of its abundant supply of capillaries, it is a common site of nosebleed.

  a., macular. Area of the retina that functions in central vision.

  a., mitral. Area over the apex of the heart, where mitral valve sounds are heard.

  a., occipital. Portion of brain below the occipital bone.

  a. pellucida. Clear central portion of area germinativa of the earliest stages of the embryo.

  a., Rolando's. Area situated in anterior central convolution in front of fissure of Rolando in each hemisphere. Governs motor acts of the body.

  a., silent. Any cortical area in the brain that upon stimulation produces no detectable motor activity or sensory phenomenon, and in which a lesion may occur without producing detectable motor or sensory abnormalities.

  a., vestibular. Fundus of the internal auditory meatus. SYN: *a., acoustic.*

areata, areatus (ă″rē-ā′tă, ă″rē-ā′tŭs). Occurring in circumscribed areas or patches.

areflexia (ă″rē-flĕk′sē-ă) [Gr. *a-*, not, + L. *reflectere*, to bend back]. Absence of reflexes.

arenaceous (ăr″ĕ-nā′sē-ŭs) [L. *arenaceus,* sandy]. Resembling sand or gravel. SYN: *arenoid.*

arenation (ă″rĕ-nā′shŭn) [L. *arena,* sand]. A sand bath or application of hot sand.

arenaviridae. Arenaviruses, q.v.

arenaviruses (ă″rē-nă-vī′rŭs-ĕs) [″ + *virus,* poison]. A group of viruses once classed as causing disease by being arthropod-borne. This method of transmission is not obligatory. The principal viruses in this group are lymphocytic choriomeningitis virus (LCM virus) and Lassa virus. The LCM virus rarely infects man, but when it does, the disease is usually a mild form of meningitis. The Lassa virus causes a highly contagious, severe febrile illness and may be fatal. SEE: *Lassa fever.*

arenoid (ăr′ē-noyd) [″ + Gr. *eidos,* form, shape]. Resembling sand or gravel. SYN: *arenaceous.*

areola (ă-rē′ō-lă) [L. *areola,* a small space] (pl. *areolae*). 1. A small space or cavity in a tissue. 2. A circular area of different pigmentation, as around a wheal, around the nipple of the breast, or the part of the iris around the pupil.

    a. mammae. [NA] The pigmented area surrounding the nipple.

    a. papillaris. A. mammae, q.v.

    a., second. A pigmented area surrounding the areola mammae during pregnancy.

    a. umbilicalis. A pigmented area surrounding the umbilicus.

areolar (ă-rē′ō-lăr). Rel. to an areola.

areolar glands. Large modified sweat glands lying beneath the areola of the breast with ducts opening on its surface. They secrete a lipoid material that lubricates the nipple. SYN: *glands, Montgomery's.*

areolar tissue. Loose connective tissue that occupies the interspaces of the body.

areolitis (ăr″ē-ō-lī′tĭs) [″ + Gr. *itis,* inflammation]. Inflammation of mammary areola.

arevareva (ăr-ē″vă-rā′vă) [Tahitian, skin rash]. Severe skin disease characterized by scales and accompanied by general debility. SEE: *kava.*

    ETIOL: Thought to be caused by excess use of kava, an intoxicating beverage.

    TREAT: Discontinuation of use of kava.

ARF. *acute respiratory failure; acute renal failure.*

Arfonad. Trade name for trimethaphan camsylate, q.v.

argamblyopia (ăr″găm-blē-ō′pē-ă) [Gr. *argos,* idle, + *amblus,* dulled, + *ops,* eye]. Reduction in vision as a result of not using the eye.

Argasidae (ăr-găs′ĭ-dī) [Gr. *argeeis,* shining]. Family of soft ticks usually infecting birds, but may attack man, causing severe pain and fever.

argentaffin, argentaffine (ăr-jĕnt′ă-fĭn) [L. *argentum,* silver, + *affinis,* associated with]. Denoting cells that react with silver salts, thus taking a brown or black stain.

argentaffinoma (ăr″jĕn-tăf″ĭ-nō′mă) [″ + ″ + Gr. *oma,* tumor]. An argentaffin cell tumor that may arise in intestinal tract, bile ducts, pancreas, bronchus, or ovary. These tumors secrete serotonin and may produce the carcinoid syndrome, q.v. SYN: *carcinoid.*

argentum (ăr-jĕn′tŭm) [L.]. SYMB: Ag. At. wt. 107.868; at. no. 47. Silver.

arginase (ăr′jĭ-nās). Enzyme of the liver that catalyzes the hydrolysis of arginine, forming urea and ornithine.

arginine (ăr′jĭ-nēn, -nĭn) [L. *argentum,* silver]. USP. $C_6H_{14}N_4O_2$. Crystalline basic amino acid obtained from decomposition of vegetable tissues, protamines, and proteins. Also prepared synthetically. It is a guanidine derivative, yielding urea and ornithine on hydrolysis. SEE: *amino acid.*

    a. glutamate. The L(+) —arginine salt of L(+) —glutamic acid. It has been used in treating ammonia intoxication due to severe liver insufficiency.

    a. hydrochloride. L(+) —arginine salt of hydrochloric acid. It has been used to treat ammonia intoxication due to severe liver insufficiency.

    a., suberyl. A combination of suberic acid and arginine. It forms a portion of the molecule of various bufotoxins (toad poisons).

argininosuccinic acid (ăr″jĭ-nĭ″nō-sŭk-sĭn′ĭk). A compound intermediate in the synthesis of arginine. Formed from citrulline and aspartic acid.

argininosuccinicaciduria (ăr″jĭn-ĭn-ō-sŭk-sĭn″ĭk-ăs-ĭ-dū′rē-ă). Hereditary metabolic disease caused by excessive excretion, and thus deficiency, of argininosuccinase, an enzyme required to metabolize argininosuccinic acid. Clinical evidence of this defect includes mental retardation, friable tufted hair, convulsions, ataxia, liver disease, and epilepsy.

argon (ăr′gŏn) [Gr. *argos,* inactive]. SYMB: Ar. At. wt. 39.948; at. no. 18. An inert gas composing approx. 1% of the atmosphere.

Argyll Robertson pupil (ăr-gīl′ rŏb′ĕrt-sŏn) [Douglas Argyll Robertson, Scottish ophthalmologist, 1837–1909]. More properly the name of a symptom often present in paralysis and locomotor ataxia (due to syphilis), in which the light reflex is absent but there is no change in the power of contraction during accommodation. Usually bilateral.

argyria, argyriasis (ăr-jĭr′ē-ă, ăr″jĭ-rī′ă-sĭs) [Gr. *argyros,* silver]. Bluish discoloration of skin and mucous membranes resulting from prolonged administration of silver. SYN: *argyrism; argyrosis.*

argyric (ăr-jĭr′ĭk). Pert. to silver.

argyrism (ăr′jĭr-ĭzm) [Gr. *argyros,* silver]. Argyria, q.v.

Argyrol (ăr′jĭ-rŏl). Trade name for mild silver protein. Used as an antiseptic in infections of the eye, nose, and throat and for urethral irrigations.

argyrophil (ăr-jī′rō-fĭl) [″ + *philos,* fond]. Denoting cells that bind with silver salts, which can then be reduced to produce a brown or black stain.

argyrosis (ăr″jĭ-rō′sĭs) [″ + *osis,* condition]. Argyria, q.v.

arhinia. Arrhinia, q.v.

arhythmia. Arrhythmia, q.v.

Arias-Stella reaction [Javier Arias-Stella, Peruvian pathologist, b. 1924]. An endometrial gland cell abnormality consisting of hyperchromatic nuclei, which may be present in normal or ectopic pregnancy. It is not a sign of endometrial adenocarcinoma.

ariboflavinosis (ă-rī″bō-flā″vĭn-ō′sĭs) [Gr. *a-,* not, + *riboflavin* + Gr. *osis,* condition]. Condition arising from a deficiency of riboflavin in the diet.

SYM: Lesions on the lips; stomatitis and, later, fissures in the angles of the mouth; seborrhea around the nose; vascularization of cornea.

TREAT: Riboflavin, given orally.

Aristocort. Trade name for triamcinolone, q.v.

Aristocort Acetonide. Trade name for triamcinolone acetonide, q.v.

Aristocort Forte Parenteral. Trade name for triamcinolone diacetate, q.v.

aristogenics (ă-rĭs″tō-jĕn′ĭks) [Gr. *aristos,* best, + *gennan,* to produce]. The science that deals with the genetic and prenatal influences affecting the expression of certain characteristics in offspring. SYN: *eugenics.*

Aristospan. Trade name for triamcinolone hexacetonide, q.v.

arithmetic mean. In statistics, the number obtained by adding all of the values listed in a group and dividing by the total number of values in the group. SYN: *average.*

arkyochrome (ăr′kē-ō-krōm) [Gr. *arkys,* net, + *chroma,* color]. A nerve cell in which the stainable substance is arranged in a network.

arkyostichochrome (ar″kē-ō-stĭk′ō-krōm) [″ + *stichos,* row, + *chroma,* color]. A nerve cell in which the stainable material is arranged both as a network and in parallel lines.

Arlidin. Trade name for nylidrin hydrochloride, q.v.

arm [AS]. 1. In anatomy, the upper extremity from shoulder to elbow. 2. In popular usage, the entire upper extremity, from shoulder to hand. SEE: illus.

a., bird. Atrophy of the forearm muscles.

a., brawny. Hard, swollen arm after removal of a breast, due to lymphedema.

a., Saturday-night. A form of paralysis of the brachial plexus, sometimes seen in intoxicated persons.

ETIOL: Sleeping in a chair, with the arm hanging over the back of the chair while the head rests on the shoulder or arm.

arm, carrying angle. The angle between the long axis of the upper and lower arm. This angle is nearly straight in the male and is increased in the female, i.e., in the female the lower part of the arm will deviate away from the body more than is the case in the male. This is a secondary sex characteristic.

arm, words pert. to: axilla; "brachio-" words; brachium; forearm; humerus; radius; ulna.

armamentarium (ăr″mă-měn-tā′rē-ŭm) [L. *armamentum,* implement]. The total equipment of a physician or institution, such as instruments, drugs, books, supplies.

armature (ăr′mă-tūr) [L. *armatura,* equipment]. 1. In biology, a structure that serves to protect or is used to attack a predator, e.g., a stinger. 2. A part of an electrical generator, consisting of a coil of insulated wire mounted around a soft iron core.

armature, biological [Term coined by Mortimer Lorber, U.S. physician, in 1991]. The connective-tissue-rich aggregate of larger ducts, vessels, and autonomic nerves that in many mammalian exocrine glands serves as an internal framework whose function of support, and often anchorage, resembles that of the armature within a clay sculpture.

arm board. 1. Board placed under and attached to the arm for stabilization during I.V. administration. 2. Device attached to the sides of a wheelchair to permit support or positioning of the arm, especially for persons with upper extremity paralysis. SYN: *arm trough.*

armpit. Axilla, q.v.

Arneth, Joseph (ăr′nāt). German physician, 1873–1955.

A.'s classification of neutrophils. A classification of polymorphonuclear neutrophils based on the number of lobes (one to five) in the nucleus. Termed Stages 1 to 5, respectively.

A.'s formula. The normal ratio of various types of polymorphonuclear neutrophils based on the number of lobes (one to five) in the nucleus.

Arnold, Friedrich. German anatomist, 1803–

UPPER ARM
(ANTERIOR VIEW)

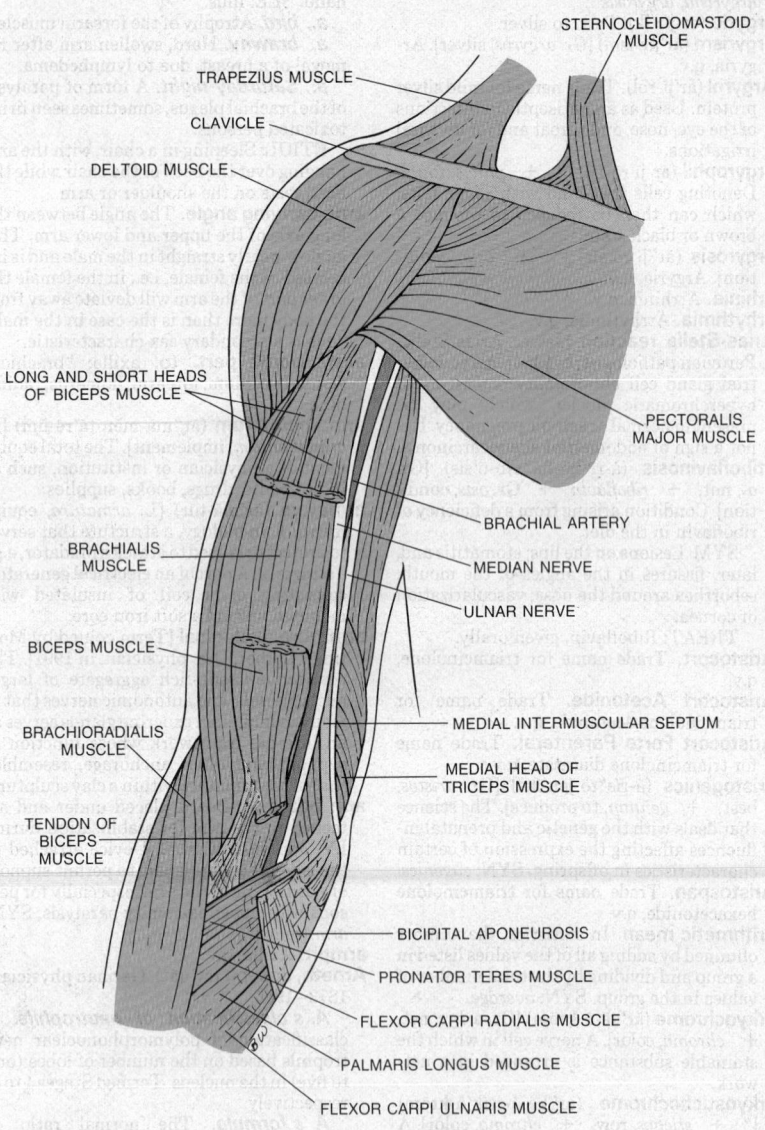

STERNOCLEIDOMASTOID
MUSCLE

TRAPEZIUS MUSCLE

CLAVICLE

DELTOID MUSCLE

LONG AND SHORT HEADS
OF BICEPS MUSCLE

PECTORALIS
MAJOR MUSCLE

BRACHIAL ARTERY

BRACHIALIS
MUSCLE

MEDIAN NERVE

ULNAR NERVE

BICEPS MUSCLE

MEDIAL INTERMUSCULAR SEPTUM

BRACHIORADIALIS
MUSCLE

MEDIAL HEAD OF
TRICEPS MUSCLE

TENDON OF
BICEPS
MUSCLE

BICIPITAL APONEUROSIS

PRONATOR TERES MUSCLE

FLEXOR CARPI RADIALIS MUSCLE

PALMARIS LONGUS MUSCLE

FLEXOR CARPI ULNARIS MUSCLE

1890.
A.'s canal. Passage in the temporal bone for lesser superficial petrosal nerve.
A.'s ganglion. Otic ganglion.
A.'s nerve. Auricular branch of the vagus nerve. SEE: *cough, reflex.*
Arnold-Chiari deformity (ăr'nōlt-kē'ă-rē) [Julius Arnold, Ger. pathologist, 1835–1915; Hans Chiari, Austrian pathologist, 1851–1916]. A condition in which the inferior poles of the cerebellar hemispheres and the medulla protrude through the foramen magnum into the spinal canal. It is one of the causes of hydrocephalus and is usually accompanied by spina bifida cystica and meningomyelocele.
AROM. *active range of motion.*
aroma (ă-rō'mă) [Gr. *aroma*, spice]. An agreeable odor.
aromatic (ăr″ō-măt'ĭk). 1. Having an agreeable odor. 2. Belonging to that series of organic chemical compounds in which the carbon atoms form closed rings (as in benzene) as distinguished from the aliphatic series, in which the carbon atoms form straight or branched chains.
aromatic ammonia spirit. Solution consisting of 34 gm of ammonium carbonate in 1000 ml diluted ammonia solution, fragrant oils, alcohol, and purified water. Used as antacid and carminative. It acts as a reflex stimulant when its vapor is inhaled.
aromatic compounds. Ring or cyclic compounds related to benzene, many having a fragrant odor.
aromatic elixir. A flavoring agent used in preparing medicines.
arousal. 1. Alertness, state of being prepared to act. 2. Erotic excitement.
arousal level. In testing a newborn's behavior, the level of arousal is important. These levels are deep sleep; sleep with rapid eye movements; drowsy state; a quiet, alert state; an awake and active state; and a state of active, intense crying. The infant is capable of the most responsive and complex interactions with the environment in the quiet and alert states. SEE: *psychomotor and physical development of infant.*
arrachement (ă-răsh-mŏn') [Fr., extraction]. Pulling out the capsule in a membranous cataract through a corneal incision.
array (ă-rā'). Systematic listing or presentation of items or components.
array detector. A photodetector used in some spectrophotometers consisting of hundreds of photodiodes in a linear arrangement (array) and used to sense the complete visible spectrum.
arrectores pilorum (ă″rĕk-tō′rĕz pĭl-ō′rŭm) [L. *arrectores*, raisers, + *pilus*, hair] (sing. *arrector pili*). Involuntary muscle fibers

arising in the skin and extending down to connect with the hair follicles on the side toward which the hair slopes. After certain stimuli including cold or fright, they contract, straighten the follicles, and raise the hairs, resulting in "gooseflesh" or cutis anserina.
arrest (ă-rĕst′). Stoppage, particularly the cessation of motion of a part normally in motion.
  a., cardiac. Cessation of the heartbeat. SEE: *cardiopulmonary resuscitation.*
  a., epiphysial. Arrest of growth of long bones.
  a., pelvic. Condition in which the presenting part of the fetus becomes fixed in the maternal pelvis.
  a., respiratory. Cessation of spontaneous respirations.
  a., sinus. Condition in which the sinus node of the heart does not initiate impulses for heartbeat. If this condition persists, it is usually treated by implanting a permanent cardiac pacemaker. SEE: *pacemaker, cardiac, artificial.*
arrhenoblastoma (ă-rē″nō-blăs-tō′mă) [Gr. *arren*, male, + *blastos*, germ, + *oma*, tumor]. An ovarian tumor that secretes male sex hormone and thus causes secondary male sex characteristics (virilization) in the female.
arrhinia (ă-rĭn′ē-ă) [Gr. *a-*, not, + *rhis*, nose]. Congenital absence of the nose.
arrhythmia (ă-rĭth′mē-ă) [″ + *rhythmos*, rhythm]. Irregularity or loss of rhythm, esp. of the heartbeat. SYN: *dysrhythmia.*
  a., cardiac. Irregular heart action caused by physiological or pathological disturbances in discharge of cardiac impulses from the sinoatrial node or their transmission through conductile tissue of the heart. SEE: *bradycardia; cardioversion; pacemaker, cardiac, artificial; sick sinus syndrome; tachycardia.* SEE: *Nursing Diagnoses in Appendix.*
  a., sinus. Cardiac irregularity characterized by an increased heart rate during inspiration and decrease in heart rate on expiration. This arrhythmia has no clinical significance except in older patients, in which case it may occur in coronary artery disease.
arrhythmic (ă-rĭth′mĭk). Pert. to or characterized by loss of rhythm.
A.R.R.T. *American Registry of Radiologic Technologists.*
arseniasis (ăr″sĕ-nī′ă-sĭs) [L. *arsenium*, arsenic, + *-iasis*, condition]. Chronic arsenic poisoning. SYN: *arsenicolism.*
arsenic (ăr′sĕ-nĭk) [L. *arsenicolum*]. SYMB: As. At. wt. 74.922; at. no. 33; sp. gr. 5.73. A metallic element of grayish-white color,

very poisonous, used in the manufacture of dyes and medicines.

Arsenic may be present in soil, water, and air as a common environmental toxicant. Minute traces of arsenic are found in vegetables and animal forms of life and are present in eggs. Many household and garden pesticides contain various forms of arsenic. All of these are toxic if ingested or inhaled in sufficient quantity. An accumulation of arsenic in the body will cause disorders of alimentary tract, nausea, vomiting, diarrhea, dehydration, neuritis, and paralysis of wrist and ankle muscles. SEE: *Poisons and Poisoning* in *Appendix*.

a. trioxide. As_2O_3. A white powder used at one time internally in form of a 1% solution. Its toxicity makes it unsafe to use.

arsenic, words pert. to: acetarsone; arsphenamine; tryparsamide.

arsenical (är-sĕn'ĭ-kăl). 1. Pert. to or containing arsenic. 2. A drug containing arsenic.

arsenicolism (är-sĕn'ĭ-kăl-ĭzm) [L. *arsenicum*, arsenic, + Gr. *-ismos*, condition of]. Chronic arsenic poisoning. SYN: *arseniasis*.

arsenicophagy (är″sĕn-ĭ-kŏf′ă-jē) [″ + *phagein*, to eat]. Habitual eating of arsenic.

arsenic poisoning. Morbid condition produced by ingestion of arsenic.

SYM: In acute poisoning, may appear in a few minutes or, when taken with solid food, may not appear for many hours. Metallic taste and odor of garlic on breath, burning pain throughout gastrointestinal tract, vomiting and purging, dehydration, shock syndrome, coma, convulsions, paralysis, death.

F.A.: Lavage stomach with copious amounts of water. If this cannot be done, induce vomiting. Administer dimercaprol (British antilewisite) immediately.

TREAT: After first aid, maintain fluid and electrolyte balance. Morphine for pain. Treat for shock and pulmonary edema. Blood transfusion may be required because of hemolysis. SEE: *Poisons and Poisoning* in *Appendix*.

arsenium (är-sē′nē-ŭm) [L.]. Arsenic.

arsenoresistant (är-sĕn″ō-rē-zĭs′tănt) [L. *arsenium*, arsenic, + *resistare*, to withstand]. Resistant to arsenic compounds.

arsenotherapy (är″sĕ-nō-thĕr′ă-pē) [″ + Gr. *therapeia*, treatment]. Treatment with arsenic and its compounds.

arsenous (är′sĕ-nŭs) [L. *arsenium*, arsenic]. Of the nature of, or pert. to, arsenic or its compounds, esp. those containing arsenic in its lower valency. SYN: *arsenical*.

arsenous hydride. Arsine, q.v.

arsine (är′sĭn). A very poisonous gas used in chemical warfare. SYN: *arsenous hydride*.

arsphenamine (ärs-fĕn′ă-mēn). A light yellow powder containing about 30% arsenic. Formerly used in treatment of syphilis. SYN: *salvarsan*.

A.R.T. *Accredited Record Technician.*

Artane. Trade name for trihexyphenidyl hydrochloride, q.v.

artefact (är′tĕ-făkt) [L. *ars*, art, + *factus*, made]. SEE: *artifact*.

arterectomy (är″tĕ-rĕk′tō-mē) [Gr. *arteria*, artery, + *ektome*, excision]. Excision of an artery or arteries.

arteria (är″tē′rē-ă) (pl. *arteriae*). Artery, q.v.

arterial (är-tē′rē-ăl). Pert. to one or more arteries.

arterial bleeding. Bleeding from an artery. Blood is bright red and comes in spurts. Arrest by applying pressure on proximal side of vessel (nearest heart).

arterial blood gases. ABBR: ABGs. Literally, any of the gases present in blood. Clinically, the determination of levels of oxygen, O_2, and carbon dioxide, CO_2, in the blood. These gases are important in diagnosing and treating disturbances of acid-base balance. Values are usually expressed as the partial pressure of the gas; i.e., $PaCO_2$ and PaO_2. Several other blood chemistry values are important in managing acid-base disturbances; included would be the levels of the bicarbonate ion, HCO_3^-; blood pH; sodium; potassium; and chloride. These data are then used to calculate the anion gap, q.v.

arterial circulation. Movement of blood through the arteries. It is maintained by the pumping of the heart and influenced by the elasticity and extensibility of arterial walls, peripheral resistance in the areas of small arteries, and the quantity of blood in the body. SEE: *circulation*.

arterial line. A hemodynamic monitoring system consisting of a catheter in an artery connected to pressure tubing, a transducer, and an electronic monitor. Used to measure systemic blood pressure and to provide ease of access for the drawing of blood for study of gases present. Considered to be more accurate than conventional methods utilizing venous blood.

arterial varix. An enlarged and tortuous artery.

arteriectasis, arteriectasia (är″tē-rē-ĕk′tă-sĭs, -ĕk-tā′zē-ă) [″ + *ektasis*, a stretching out]. Arterial dilatation.

arteriectomy (är″tĕ-rē-ĕk′tō-mē) [″ + *ektome*, excision]. Surgical removal of a part of an artery.

arterio- [Gr. *arteria*, artery]. Combining form indicating relationship to an artery.

arteriocapillary (är-tē″rē-ō-kăp′ĭ-lăr″ē) [″ + L. *capillus*, like hair]. Pert. to both arteries and capillaries.

arteriocapillary fibrosis. Sclerosis of capillaries and arterioles.

arteriofibrosis (ăr-tē″rē-ō-fī-brō′sĭs) [″ + L. *fibra,* fiber, + Gr. *osis,* condition]. Arteriocapillary fibrosis.

arteriogram (ăr″tē-rē-ō-grăm) [″ + *gramma,* something written]. Roentgenogram of an artery after injection of a radiopaque dye.

arteriography (ăr″tē-rē-ŏg′ră-fē) [″ + *graphein,* to write]. 1. Roentgenography of arteries after injection of a radiopaque dye. 2. Description of arteries.

arteriola (ăr-tē″rē-ō′lă) [L.] (pl. *arteriolae*). [NA] Small artery; an arteriole.

> ***a. macularis inferior.*** [NA] The inferior macular arteriole, which supplies the macula retinae of the eye.
>
> ***a. macularis superior.*** [NA] The superior macular arteriole, which supplies the macula retinae of the eye.
>
> ***a. medialis retinae.*** [NA] The medial arteriole of the retina.
>
> ***a. nasalis retinae inferior.*** [NA] Inferior nasal arteriole of the retina.
>
> ***a. nasalis retinae superior.*** [NA] Superior nasal arteriole of the retina.
>
> ***a. recta.*** [NA] One of the small arteries of the kidney that supply the renal pyramids.
>
> ***a. temporalis retinae inferior.*** [NA] Inferior temporal artery of the retina.
>
> ***a. temporalis retinae superior.*** [NA] Superior temporal artery of the retina.

arteriole (ăr-tē′rē-ōl) [L. *arteriola*] (pl. *arterioles*). A minute artery, esp. one that, at its distal end, leads into a capillary. SYN: *arteriola.*

arteriolith (ăr-tē′rē-ō-lĭth) [″ + Gr. *lithos,* stone]. An arterial calculus.

arteriolitis (ăr-tēr″ē-ō-lī′tĭs) [″ + Gr. *itis,* inflammation]. Inflammation of the arteriolar wall.

arteriology (ăr-tē″rē-ŏl′ŏ-jē) [″ + Gr. *logos,* word, reason]. Science of arteries, usually combined with study of other vessels, as in angiology, q.v.

arteriolonecrosis (ăr-tē″rē-ō″lō-nĕ-krō′sĭs) [″ + Gr. *nekros,* corpse, + *osis,* condition]. Destruction of an arteriole.

arteriolosclerosis (ăr-tē″rē-ō″lō-sklĕ-rō′sĭs) [L. *arteriola,* small artery, + Gr. *sklerosis,* hardening]. Thickening of the walls of the arterioles with loss of elasticity and contractility.

arteriolosclerotic (ăr-tē″rē-ō″lō-sklĕ-rŏt′ĭk). Pert. to or characterized by arteriolosclerosis.

arteriomotor (ăr-tē″rē-ō-mō′tor) [Gr. *arteria,* artery, + L. *movere,* to move]. Causing changes in interior diameter of arteries by dilatation and constriction.

arteriomyomatosis (ăr-tē″rē-ō-mī″ō-mă-tō′sĭs) [″ + *mys,* muscle, + *oma,* tumor, + *osis,* condition]. Thickening of arterial walls due to overgrowth of muscle fibers.

arterionecrosis (ăr-tē″rē-ō-nĕ-krō′sĭs) [″ + *nekros,* corpse, + *osis,* condition]. Arterial necrosis.

arteriopathy (ăr″tē-rē-ŏp′ă-thē) [″ + *pathos,* disease, suffering]. Any disease of the arteries.

arterioplasty (ăr-tē″rē-ō-plăs′tē) [″ + *plassein,* to form]. Repair or reconstruction of an artery.

arteriopressor (ăr-tē″rē-ō-prĕs′or) [″ + L. *pressura,* force]. Causing increased arterial blood pressure.

arteriorrhaphy (ăr-tē″rē-or′ă-fē) [″ + *rhaphe,* seam, ridge]. Arterial suture.

arteriorrhexis (ăr-tē″rē-ō-rĕk′sĭs) [″ + *rhexis,* rupture]. Rupture of an artery.

arteriosclerosis (ăr-tē″rē-ō-sklĕ-rō′sĭs) [″ + *sklerosis,* to harden]. Term applied to a number of pathological conditions in which there are thickening, hardening, and loss of elasticity of the walls of arteries. This results in altered function of tissues and organs. Changes may occur in the intima, media, or both. In the Western world, this condition is the leading cause of death and serious morbidity. The terms arteriosclerosis and atherosclerosis are used interchangeably.

SYM: Symptoms may include intermittent claudication; changes in skin temperature, intensity of pulse; headache; dizziness; or memory defects depending on the organ system involved.

ETIOL: Cause is unknown. Some risk factors include age; familial predisposition; sedentary lifestyle; hypertension; increased blood lipids, particularly cholesterol and triglycerides; obesity; cigarette smoking; diabetes mellitus; inability to cope with stress; family history of early-onset atherosclerosis; and the male sex (at ages 35 to 44, the death rate for white males is six times that of white females).

TREAT: Regular exercise; diet low in saturated fatty acids; abstaining from use of tobacco; general moderation in all things to reduce or avoid stress; therapy for treatable diseases such as obesity, diabetes, and hypertension if any of these are present.

NURSING IMPLICATIONS: Assist the patient to modify risk factors associated with arteriosclerosis. Cigarette smoking should be discontinued, sedentary activity patterns changed, emotional stress reduced, obesity controlled, saturated fat intake reduced to control triglyceride and cholesterol levels, and hypertension and diabetes mellitus treated and controlled. Insure adequate rest periods. Encourage regular exercise of a type and extent appropriate to the patient's health.

a., hypertensive. Arteriosclerosis resulting from hypertension.

a., medial. Arteriosclerosis of the peripheral arteries with calcium deposits in the media. SYN: *a., Mönckeberg's.*

a., Mönckeberg's. A., medial, q.v.

a., nodular. Arteriosclerosis due to formation of fibrous plaques in the intima.

a. obliterans. Arteriosclerosis in which the lumen of the artery is completely occluded.

a., senile. Arteriosclerosis accompanying old age.

arteriosclerotic (ăr-tē″rē-ō-sklĕ-rŏt′ĭk). Pert. to or characterized by arteriosclerosis.

arteriospasm (ăr-tē′rē-ō-spăzm″) [Gr. *arteria*, artery, + *spasmos*, a convulsion]. Arterial spasm.

arteriostenosis (ăr-tē″rē-ō-stĕ-nō′sĭs) [″ + *stenosis*, act of narrowing]. Narrowing of the lumen of an artery, either temporary or permanent.

arteriostosis (ăr-tē″rē-ŏs-tō′sĭs) [″ + *osteon*, bone, + *osis*, condition]. Calcification of an artery.

arteriostrepsis (ăr-tē″rē-ō-strĕp′sĭs) [″ + *strepsis*, a twisting]. Twisting of divided end of an artery to arrest hemorrhage.

arteriosympathectomy (ăr-tē″rē-ō-sĭm″pă-thĕk′tō-mē) [″ + *sympatheia*, suffer with, + *ektome*, excision]. Removal of arterial sheath containing fibers of sympathetic nerve.

arteriotomy (ăr″tē-rē-ŏt′ō-mē). Surgical division or opening of an artery.

arteriotony (ăr-tē″rē-ŏt′ō-nē) [″ + *tonos*, tension]. Blood pressure; intra-arterial blood tension.

arteriovenous (ăr-tē″rē-ō-vē′nŭs) [″ + L. *vena*, a vein]. Rel. to both arteries and veins.

arterioversion (ăr-tē″rē-ō-vĕr′shŭn) [″ + L. *versio*, a turning]. Eversion of arterial wall to arrest hemorrhage from open end.

arteritis (ăr″tĕ-rī′tĭs) [″ + *itis*, inflammation]. Inflammation of an artery. SEE: *endarteritis, polyarteritis.*

a., cranial. A., temporal, q.v.

a., giant cell. A., temporal, q.v.

a., granulomatous. A., temporal, q.v.

a. nodosa. Widespread inflammation of adventitia of small and medium-sized arteries with impaired function of the involved organs. SYN: *periarteritis nodosa; polyarteritis nodosa.*

a. obliterans. Inflammation of intima of artery causing occlusion of the lumen. SYN: *endarteritis obliterans.*

a., rheumatic. Inflammation of small arteries resulting from rheumatic fever.

a., rheumatoid. Inflammation of arteries associated with rheumatoid arthritis.

a., temporal. A relatively common chronic inflammation of large arteries, usually the temporal, occipital, or ophthalmic arteries, accompanied by presence of giant cells. Causes thickening of intima with narrowing and eventual occlusion of lumen. Occurs in elderly persons.

SYM: Headache; tenderness over the affected artery; visual loss; facial pain.

ETIOL: Unknown, but there is a genetic predisposition.

TREAT: Corticosteroids. SYN: *a., cranial; a., giant cell; a., granulomatous.*

artery (ăr′tĕr-ē) [Gr. *arteria*, windpipe] (pl. *arteries*). One of the vessels carrying blood from the heart to the tissues. The ancients believed that air circulated through them, from which supposition the name, artery, was derived.

The arteries carry the oxygenated blood from the left ventricle of the heart to all parts of the body. There are two major divisions, pulmonary and systemic. The pulmonary artery carries the venous blood from the right ventricle to the lungs. The systemic division begins with the aorta and carries arterial blood from the left ventricle to the various parts of the body. SEE: *aorta* and *coronary artery disease* for illus.

ANAT: The arteries have three coats: the inner, tunica intima, or serous; the outer, tunica adventitia, or white fibrous; and the middle, tunica media, or yellow fibrous. SEE: *Arteries in Appendix.*

a., coiled. A., spiral, q.v.

a., distributing. A., muscular, q.v.

a., elastic. Artery in which elastic tissue is predominant in the tunica intima and tunica media. Elastic arteries include the aorta and its larger branches (innominate, common carotid, subclavian, and common iliac) — vessels that conduct blood to the muscular arteries.

a., end. Artery whose branches do not anastomose with those of other arteries, e.g., arteries to brain and spinal cord.

a., muscular. Artery with smooth muscle tissue in its wall, esp. the tunica media, by means of which the flow of blood to tissues can be regulated through contraction and relaxation. These arteries also contract spastically when injured, thus preventing excessive loss of blood.

a., sheathed. The terminal portion of a pulp artery in the spleen. It has distinctive thickenings in its walls.

a., spiral. The coiled terminal branch of a uterine artery. It supplies the superficial two thirds of the endometrium, and in a pregnant uterus, it empties into intervillous spaces, supplying blood that bathes the chorionic villi at the placental site.

a., terminal. A., end, q.v.

artery, words pert. to: adventitia; aneurysm; angina pectoris; arteriosclerosis; circulation; endarteritis; hypertonia; hypotonia; intima; lumen; media; mesarteritis; periarteritis; sclerosis.

arthral (ăr′thrăl). Pert. to a joint.

arthralgia (ăr-thrăl′jē-ă) [Gr. *arthron*, joint, + *algos*, pain]. Pain in a joint.

    a. saturnina. Joint pain resulting from lead poisoning.

arthrectomy (ăr-thrĕk′tō-mē) [″ + *ektome*, excision]. Excision of a joint.

arthresthesia (ăr″thrĕs-thē′zē-ă) [″ + *aisthesis*, sensation]. Joint sensibility; the perception of articular motions.

arthritic (ăr-thrĭt′ĭk). 1. Pert. to arthritis. 2. A person afflicted with arthritis.

arthritides (ăr-thrĭt′ĭ-dēz). Pl. of arthritis.

arthritis (ăr-thrī′tĭs) [″ + *itis*, inflammation] (pl. *arthritides*). Inflammation of a joint, usually accompanied by pain, swelling, and, frequently, changes in structure.

    ETIOL: Arthritis may result from or be associated with a number of conditions including infection (gonococcal, tuberculous, pneumococcal); rheumatic fever; ulcerative colitis; trauma; neurogenic disturbances such as tabes dorsalis; degenerative joint disease such as osteoarthritis; metabolic disturbances such as gout; neoplasms such as synovioma; hydrarthrosis; para- or periarticular conditions such as fibromyositis, myositis, or bursitis; various other conditions such as acromegaly, psoriasis, Raynaud's disease. SEE: *bursitis; rheumatism.*

    TREAT: Patients often benefit from referral to occupational or physical therapy, or both.

    a., acute secondary. Arthritis caused by osteitis. Severe pain, redness, and swelling.

    a., acute suppurative. Purulent distention of synovial sac; a serious form.

    a., allergic. Arthritis following ingestion of food allergens or occurring in serum sickness.

    a., atrophic. A., rheumatoid, q.v.

    a. deformans. A., rheumatoid, q.v.

    a., degenerative. A., osteo-, q.v.

    a., gonorrheal. Arthritis due to gonorrheal infection. Usually attacks knee joint; during acute stage, several joints may be affected.

    TREAT: Penicillin, parenterally, in an appropriate dose for 10 to 14 days. If organism is resistant to penicillin, substitute appropriate antibiotic.

    a., gouty. Arthritis caused by gout, q.v.

    a., hypertrophic. A., osteo-, q.v.

    a., juvenile rheumatoid. Chronic, inflammatory, systemic disease which may cause joint or connective tissue damage and visceral lesions throughout the body. Affects juveniles with onset prior to age 16. Complete remission occurs in 75% of patients. SYN: *Still's disease.*

    NURSING IMPLICATIONS: Nursing care is essentially as for adult with rheumatoid arthritis, with the following special concerns: aspirin dosage is based on child's body surface area; braces or splints may be needed to prevent or diminish joint contractures or deformities; sunglasses for photophobia related to iridocyclitis. Assist the parents in encouraging the child's independence and participation in school and social activities that do not increase joint pain or cause undue fatigue. Encourage adequate rest and sleep and a nutritious diet. Instruct the child and family about the disease process, its pathology, symptoms, treatment, and the expected course. SEE: *Nursing Diagnoses* in *Appendix.*

    a., neurogenic. A., neurotrophic, q.v.

    a., neurotrophic. Arthritis accompanying or following diseases of the nervous system. Occurs in tabes dorsalis and syringomyelia. SEE: *Charcot's joint.*

    a., osteo-. A chronic disease involving the joints, esp. those bearing weight. Characterized by degeneration of articular cartilage, overgrowth of bone with lipping and spur formation, and impaired function. SYN: *a., degenerative; a., hypertrophic; degenerative joint disease.*

    a., palindromic. Transient recurrent arthritis, of unknown etiology, of large joints.

    a., psoriatic. A form of arthritis that may develop after psoriasis has developed. The exacerbations and remissions of arthritic symptoms parallel those of psoriasis.

    a., rheumatoid. A chronic systemic disease characterized by inflammatory changes in joints and related structures that result in crippling deformities. SEE: illus.

    ETIOL: The specific cause is unknown, but it is generally believed that the pathological changes in the joints are related to an antigen-antibody reaction that is poorly understood. Environmental and familial factors are of doubtful importance. Onset may vary, but usually occurs in middle age.

    TREAT: There is no specific therapy. If the condition is severe and painful, bedrest may be required for a short time. The salicylates, such as aspirin and sodium salicylate, are the most commonly used drugs in treating rheumatoid arthritis. Aspirin in high doses is as effective as other nonsteroidal anti-inflammatory drugs (NSAIDs) and are much less expensive. However, aspirin can

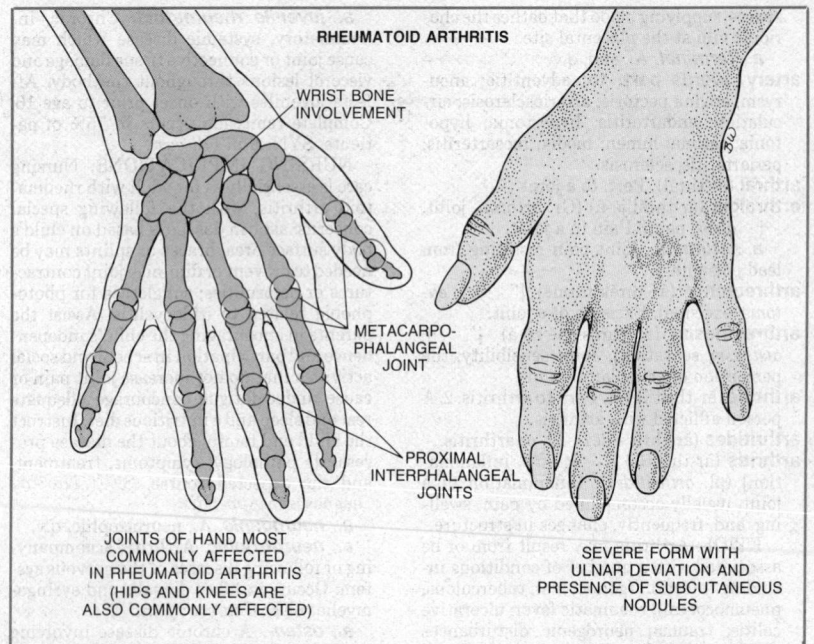

RHEUMATOID ARTHRITIS

WRIST BONE INVOLVEMENT

METACARPO-PHALANGEAL JOINT

PROXIMAL INTERPHALANGEAL JOINTS

JOINTS OF HAND MOST COMMONLY AFFECTED IN RHEUMATOID ARTHRITIS (HIPS AND KNEES ARE ALSO COMMONLY AFFECTED)

SEVERE FORM WITH ULNAR DEVIATION AND PRESENCE OF SUBCUTANEOUS NODULES

cause serious gastrointestinal bleeding. Gold compounds, nonsteroidal anti-inflammatory agents such as naproxen, indomethacin, and ibuprofen, and corticosteroids (for short-term anti-inflammatory use only) are also used in treatment. Even though NSAIDs help to control pain, they do not alter the course of the disease. Intra-articular injection of certain corticosteroids is useful in treating acute inflammation of synovial tissue of one or two painful joints. This local treatment is effective for up to 21 days and may be used to allow a patient to remain ambulatory. Local or systemic use of corticosteroids does not cure the basic disease process or prevent the progression of pathological changes in the joint.

Caution: Long-term use of corticosteroids is contraindicated due to the development of undesired side effects.

The use of exercise and physical therapy is important in maintaining range of motion of the affected joints. Until the inflammatory response has subsided, passive exercise is employed to prevent contractures. When inflammation has subsided, active exercise is used to maintain muscle strength and range of motion. A variety of self-help devices are available for patients with severe limitation of joint movement, thus enabling these patients to remain self-sufficient. The use of surgical procedures such as arthroplasty, e.g., total joint replacements, has been effective in very severe forms of rheumatoid arthritis.

NURSING IMPLICATIONS: Evaluate patient for symptoms of joint inflammation, such as redness, swelling, pain, and reduced mobility of joints. Also evaluate for fatigue, irritability, and temperature elevation. Inflamed joints should be splinted as ordered to prevent contractures and maintain range of motion with gentle passive exercise. When inflammation has subsided, use warm baths or soaks to joints before active range of motion. Administer ordered medications, evaluate response, and teach patient about side effects that should be reported. Explain rationale for short-term use of corticosteroids and need for tapering dosage rather than abrupt discontinuance. Encourage total body rest and adequate nutrition. Provide information on self-help devices and support groups. SEE: *Nursing*

Diagnoses in *Appendix.*

a., suppurative. Inflammation of a synovial membrane with purulent effusion into the joint capsule; usually due to bacterial infection. SYN: *synovitis, purulent.*

a., syphilitic. Arthritis occurring in secondary and tertiary stages of syphilis; characterized by tenderness, swelling, and limitation of motion.

a., tuberculous. Tuberculosis of a joint.

arthro- [Gr. *arthron,* joint]. Prefix pert. to joints.

arthrocace (är-thrŏk'ă-sē) [" + *kake,* badness]. Infected cavity of a joint.

arthrocele (är'thrō-sēl) [" + *kele,* tumor, swelling]. 1. Hernia of a synovial membrane, penetrating the capsule of a joint. 2. Any joint swelling.

arthrocentesis (är"thrō-sĕn-tē'sĭs) [" + *kentesis,* a puncture]. Puncture of a joint space by using a needle. Usually done in order to remove accumulated fluid from the joint.

NURSING IMPLICATIONS: Prepare patient for procedure by explaining what will be done and what discomfort to expect. Obtain equipment, position and drape patient, and assist operator to cleanse and anesthetize site, collect specimens, or administer medication. Dress site and teach patient about required follow-up care, including symptoms to report and activity restrictions.

arthrochondritis (är"thrō-kŏn-drī'tĭs) [" + *chondros,* cartilage, + *itis,* inflammation]. Inflammation of an articular cartilage.

arthroclasia (är"thrō-klā'zē-ă) [" + *klasis,* a breaking]. Artificial breaking of adhesions of an ankylosed joint to provide movement.

arthrodesis (är-thrō-dē'sĭs) [" + *desis,* binding]. The surgical immobilization of a joint; artificial ankylosis.

arthrodia (är-thrō'dē-ă) [Gr.]. A type of synovial joint that permits only simple gliding movement within narrow limits imposed by ligaments.

arthrodynia (är"thrō-dĭn'ē-ă) [Gr. *arthron,* joint, + *odyne,* pain]. Pain in a joint.

arthrodysplasia (är"thrō-dĭs-plā'zē-ă) [" + *dys,* bad, + *plassein,* to form]. An hereditary condition characterized by deformity of various joints.

arthroempyesis (är"thrō-ĕm-pī-ē'sĭs) [" + *empyesis,* suppuration]. Suppuration in a joint. SYN: *arthrempyesis.*

arthroendoscopy (är"thrō-ĕn-dŏs'kō-pē) [" + *endon,* within, + *skopein,* to examine]. Inspection of interior of a joint by using an endoscope.

arthrogram (är'thrō-grăm) [" + *gramma,* something written]. Visualization of a joint

by radiographic study after injection of a contrast medium into the joint space.

arthrography (är-thrŏg'ră-fē) [" + *graphein,* to write]. 1. A description of the joints. 2. Roentgenography of a joint.

arthrogryposis (är"thrō-grĭ-pō'sĭs) [" + *grypos,* curved, + *osis,* condition]. Fixation of a joint in a flexed or contracted position. May be due to adhesions in or around the joint.

a. multiplex congenita. Generalized fixation or ankylosis of joints that is present at birth. May be due to a variety of changes in the spinal cord, muscles, or connective tissue.

arthrokinematics. Description of the movement of the bone surfaces within a joint when a bone moves through a range of motion.

arthrokleisis (är"thrō-klī'sĭs) [" + *kleisis,* a closure]. Ankylosis or fixation of a joint produced naturally or surgically.

arthrolith (är'thrō-lĭth) [" + *lithos,* stone]. Calculous deposit in a joint.

arthrology (är-thrŏl'ō-jē) [Gr. *arthron,* joint, + *logos,* word, reason]. The science of joints.

arthrolysis (är-thrŏl'ĭ-sĭs) [" + *lysis,* dissolution]. The operation of restoring mobility to an ankylosed joint.

arthromeningitis (är"thrō-mĕn"ĭn-jī'tĭs) [" + *meninx,* membrane, + *itis,* inflammation]. Inflammation of a synovial membrane. SYN: *synovitis.*

arthrometer (är-thrŏm'ĕ-tĕr) [" + *metron,* measure]. Instrument for measuring the degree of movement of a joint. SYN: *goniometer.*

arthroneuralgia (är"thrō-nū-răl'jē-ă) [" + *neuron,* nerve, + *algos,* pain]. Pain in or around a joint.

arthropathology (är"thrō-pă-thol'ō-jē) [" + *pathos,* disease, + *logos,* word, reason]. The pathology of joint disease.

arthropathy (är-thrŏp'ă-thē) [" + *pathos,* disease, suffering]. Any joint disease.

a., Charcot's. SEE: *Charcot's joint.*

a., inflammatory. An inflammatory joint disease; arthritis.

a., Jaccoud. A form of chronic arthritis that may occur after several attacks of rheumatic fever. It is thought to be distinct from rheumatoid arthritis.

arthrophyte (är'thrō-fīt) [Gr. *arthron,* joint, + *phyton,* growth]. Abnormal growth in joint cavity.

arthroplasty (är'thrō-plăs"tē) [" + *plassein,* to form]. The operative procedure of reshaping or reconstructing a diseased joint. This may be done to alleviate pain, to permit normal function, or to correct a developmental or hereditary joint defect. The procedure may require use of an artificial joint.

NURSING IMPLICATIONS: Postoperatively, the patient may be placed in traction or may require other immobilization devices such as splints, pillows, or casts. Position the patient as prescribed. Monitor patient for blood loss, thromboembolism, or infection. Perform frequent neurovascular checks on the involved extremity. Assist the patient with prescribed exercise and activity. Take appropriate measures to prevent dislocation of the prosthesis. Provide emotional support and encouragement for the patient during the rehabilitation period. SEE: *Nursing Diagnoses* in *Appendix.*

arthropneumoroentgenography (är″thrō-nū″mō-rĕnt-gĕn-ŏg′rä-fē) [″ + *pneuma,* air, + *roentgenography*]. X-raying of joint after injecting a gas such as sterile air or helium into the joint space. SEE: *arthrogram.*

arthropod (är′thrō-pŏd). A member of the phylum Arthropoda.

Arthropoda (är-thrŏp′ō-dä) [″ + *pous,* foot]. A phylum of invertebrate animals characterized by bilateral symmetry, a hard, jointed exoskeleton, segmented bodies, and jointed paired appendages. Includes the crustaceans; insects; myriapods; arachnids; and similar forms. It is the largest animal phylum, containing over 700,000 species. Many are of medical importance as causative agents of disease, as vectors, or as parasites.

arthropyosis (är″thrō-pī-ō′sĭs) [″ + *pyosis,* suppuration]. Suppuration of a joint.

arthrosclerosis [Gr. *arthron,* joint, + *sklerosis,* a hardening]. Stiffening or hardening of the joints, esp. in the aged.

arthroscope (är′thrō-skōp) [″ + *skopein,* to examine]. An endoscope for examining interior of a joint.

arthroscopy (är-thrŏs′kō-pē). Direct joint visualization by means of an arthroscope.

NURSING IMPLICATIONS: *Preop:* Prepare patient by explaining procedure and discomfort that may be experienced. Ascertain that an informed consent form has been signed by patient, answering any questions and correcting misconceptions. Provide usual physical preparation based on orthopedic surgeon's protocol and on type of anesthesia to be employed.

Postop: Monitor vital signs until stable, and provide fluids via I.V. route or by mouth, depending on anesthetic patient received. Assess dressings for drainage, documenting presence of any drainage devices and their contents. Reinforce or replace bandage using aseptic technique. Teach patient about prescribed exercises and activity or ambulation restrictions, stressing

weight-bearing concerns and use of crutches if knee joint was involved. Instruct patient regarding use of ice as an analgesic and to prevent swelling. Explain that the joint will feel sore, sometimes with grinding sensations for a few days, depending upon extent of procedure. Instruct patient to report any unusual drainage, redness, joint swelling, or a "mushy" feeling in the joint, severe or persistent pain, or fever, as these may indicate infection, effusion, or hemarthrosis. SEE: *Nursing Diagnoses* in *Appendix.*

arthrosis (är-thrō′sĭs) [″ + *osis,* condition]. 1. Joint. 2. Joint affection caused by trophic degeneration.

arthrospore (är′thrō-spor) [″ + *sporos,* a seed]. A bacterial spore formed by segmentation.

arthrosteitis (är″thrŏs-tē-ī′tĭs) [″ + *osteon,* bone, + *itis,* inflammation]. Inflammation of the bony structures of a joint.

arthrostenosis (är″-thrō-stĕ-nō′sĭs) [″ + *stenos,* narrow]. Pathological narrowing of a joint.

arthrostomy (är-thrŏs′tō-mē) [″ + *stoma,* mouth]. The surgical formation of a temporary opening into a joint for drainage purposes.

arthrosynovitis (är″thrō-sĭn″ō-vī′tĭs) [″ + L. *synovia,* joint fluid, + Gr. *itis,* inflammation]. Inflammation of synovial membrane of a joint.

arthrotome (är′thrō-tōm) [″ + *tome,* incision]. Knife for making incisions into a joint.

arthrotomy (är-thrŏt′ō-mē). Cutting into a joint.

arthrous (är′thrŭs) [Gr. *arthron,* joint]. Jointed or pert. to a joint.

arthroxesis (är-thrŏk′sĭ-sĭs) [″ + *xexis,* scraping]. Scraping of diseased tissue from a joint.

Arthus reaction or phenomenon (är-toos′) [Nicholas Maurice Arthus, Fr. bacteriologist, 1862–1945]. A local necrotic lesion that forms as the result of a severe local inflammatory reaction that occurs at site of injection of an antigen in a previously sensitized individual. Arthus reactions are a form of Type III hypersensitivity reactions producing an antigen-antibody immune complex, q.v., and are the cause of occupational pneumonitis or alveolitis in certain individuals.

artichoke factor. Chlorogenic acid, cynarin, and other substances found in artichokes that make water and some foods taste sweet if ingested within a few minutes after eating artichokes.

articular (är-tĭk′ū-lär) [L. *articularis*]. Pert. to articulation.

articulate (ăr-tĭk'ū-lāt, -lăt) [L. *articulatus,* jointed]. 1. To join together as a joint. 2. In dentistry, the arrangement of teeth on a denture. 3. Clearly spoken. 4. To enunciate clearly.

articulated (ăr-tĭk'ū-lāt'd). State of articulation or of being jointed.

articulatio (ăr-tĭk"ū-lā'shē-ŏ) [L.]. The site of union or junction of two bones.

articulation. 1. The place of union between two or more bones; a joint. It is classified as being immovable (synarthrosis), slightly movable (amphiarthrosis), or freely movable (diarthrosis). Cartilage, or fibrous or soft tissue, lines the opposing surfaces of all joints. 2. The relative position of the tongue and palate necessary to produce a given sound. 3. Enunciation of words and sentences. 4. The movement of articulating surfaces through their available joint play or range of motion, used to determine joint mobility or as a technique for treating joint pain.

a., apophyseal. The joint between the superior and the inferior articulating processes of the vertebrae.

a., articulator. The use of a mechanical device to simulate the action of the temporomandibular joint when placing teeth in complete dentures or partial removable dentures so that they articulate properly.

a., confluent. Speech in which syllables are run together.

a., dental. The contact relationship between upper and lower teeth when moving against each other or into or out of centric position.

articulator (ăr-tĭk'ū-lā'tor). Device used in dentistry for maintaining casts of the teeth in a precise and natural relationship.

articulo mortis (ăr-tĭk'ū-lō" mor'tĭs) [L.]. At the time of death.

articulus (ăr-tĭk'ū-lŭs) [L.]. 1. A knuckle or a joint. 2. A segment.

artifact, artefact (ăr'tĭ-făkt, ăr'tĕ-făkt) [L. *ars,* art, + *facere,* to make]. 1. Anything artificially produced. 2. In histology and radiography, any structure or feature produced by the technique used and not occurring naturally. 3. In electronics, the appearance of a spurious signal not consistent with results expected by the signal being studied. Ex.: In medical electronics, an electrocardiogram might contain artifacts produced by a defective machine, electrical interference, patient movement, or loose electrodes.

artificial (ăr"tĭ-fish'ăl). Not natural; formed in imitation of nature.

artificial assists. General term indicating various means of supporting bodily functions.

Ex.: artificial limb, crutch, cardiac pacemaker, or respirator.

artificial heart transplant. A device designed to be implanted in the patient, the purpose of which is to assist the action of the heart, or to replace it. Efforts to perfect such a device continue.

artificial hyperemia. Bringing blood to the superficial tissues by means of counterirritation, such as may be produced by cupping or acupuncture.

artificial impregnation. Artificial insemination, q.v.

artificial insemination. ABBR: AI. Mechanical placement of semen containing viable spermatozoa into the vagina.

a.i., donor. ABBR: AID. Artificial insemination of a woman with sperm from an anonymous donor. This procedure is generally done in cases in which the husband is sterile. SEE: *Universal Precautions* in *Appendix.*

a.i., husband. ABBR: AIH. Use of a husband's sperm to artificially inseminate his wife.

artificial intelligence. ABBR: AI. There is no general agreement about the precise meaning of this term. One definition indicates that AI is "programming computers to function in ways that, if observed in human beings, would be regarded as intelligent." Another definition states "AI is the study of ways in which computers can be made to perform cognitive tasks at which, at present, people are better." SEE: *Turing test.*

artificial kidney transplant. Efforts to perfect a device for implanting in a patient for the purpose of taking over kidney function are experimental.

artificial pneumothorax. Artificial introduction of air into pleural cavity. Oxygen, nitrogen, or filtered atmospheric air is used.

artificial respiration. Maintenance of respiratory movements by artificial means. SEE: *cardiopulmonary resuscitation.*

artisan's cramp. A spasmodic affection of the muscles induced by prolonged work requiring delicate coordination and occurring only in performance of that particular work. Most apt to occur in writing, piano playing, sewing, and telegraphing. SEE: *writer's cramp.*

arum family poisoning. A genus of house plants (including dieffenbachia, caladium and philodendron) that are poisonous because they contain calcium oxalate crystals. Ingestion causes irritation, pain, burning, and swelling of the affected areas.

TREAT: Wash the area with water. Apply ice to area by chewing it. If pain is severe, corticosteriods are of benefit.

aryepiglottic (ăr″ē-ĕp″ĭ-glŏt′ĭk) [Gr. *arytaina*, ladle, + *epi*, upon, + *glottis*, back of tongue]. Pert. to the arytenoid cartilage and epiglottis.

aryl-. Prefix denoting a radical derived from an aromatic hydrocarbon.

    a. group. In chemistry, a radical group of the aromatic or benzene series.

arytenoid (ăr″ĭ-tē′noyd) [Gr. *arytaina*, ladle, + *eidos*, form, shape]. 1. Resembling a ladle or pitcher mouth. 2. Rel. to the arytenoid cartilage, gland, ligament, or muscle.

arytenoidectomy (ăr″ĭ-tē″noyd-ĕk′tō-mē) [″ + ″ + *ektome*, excision]. Excision of arytenoid cartilage.

arytenoiditis (ăr-ĭt″ē-noy-dī′tĭs) [″ + ″ + *itis*, inflammation]. Inflammation of arytenoid cartilage or muscles.

arytenoidopexy (ăr″ĭ-tĕ-noy′dō-pĕk″sē) [″ + ″ + *pexis*, fixation]. Surgical fixation of the arytenoid muscle or cartilage.

AS. L. *auris sinistra*, left ear; *aortic stenosis*.

As. 1. *astigmatic; astigmatism*. 2. Chem. symb. for the element arsenic.

ASA. *acetylsalicylic acid*. SYN: *aspirin*.

asafetida, asafoetida (ăs-ă-fĕt′ĭd-ă) [L. *asa*, gum, + *foetida*, smelly]. A gum resin, obtained from the roots of *Ferula asafoetida*, with characteristic strong odor and garlic taste. Even though this substance is no longer used in medicine, it is of historical interest. In the early part of the 20th century, it was used as a carminative and as an amulet to ward off disease. Used in Asia as a condiment and food flavoring, and as an animal repellent in veterinary medicine.

ASAHP. *American Society of Allied Health Professions*.

ASAP. *as soon as possible*. SEE: *stat*.

asaphia (ă-săf′ē-ă, ă-să′fē-ă) [Gr. *asapheia*, obscurity]. Inability to speak distinctly.

asbestiform (ăs-bĕs′tĭ-form) [Gr. *asbestos*, unquenchable, + L. *forma*, appearance]. Having structure similar to asbestos.

asbestos (ăs-bĕs′tŏs) [Gr. *asbestos*, unquenchable]. Fibrous, incombustible form of magnesium and calcium silicate used to make insulating materials.

asbestos bodies. A beaded, dumbbell-shaped body formed when a macrophage engulfs asbestos fibers.

asbestosis (ăs″bĕ-stō′sĭs) [″ + *osis*, condition]. Lung disease, a form of pneumonoconiosis, q.v., resulting from protracted inhalation of asbestos particles. Exposure to asbestos has been associated with the later development of cancer of the lung, including bronchogenic carcinoma, and especially mesothelioma. The latency period may be 20 years or more.

ascariasis (ăs″kă-rī′ă-sĭs) [Gr. *askaris*, pinworm, + *-iasis*, condition of]. Condition resulting from infestation by *Ascaris lumbricoides*, q.v.

ascaricide (ăs-kăr′ĭ-sīd) [″ + L. *cidus*, killing]. 1. Drug that kills ascaris worms. 2. That which kills ascaris worms.

ascarides (ăs-kăr′ĭ-dēz). Pl. of *Ascaris*, q.v.

Ascaris (ăs′kă-rĭs) (pl. *ascarides*). A genus of nematodes, roundworms, belonging to the superfamily Ascaridoidea. They inhabit the intestines of invertebrates.

    A. lumbricoides. A species of *Ascaris* that lives in the human intestine. Eggs are passed with the feces and require at least two weeks' incubation in the soil before they become infective. After being swallowed, the eggs hatch in the intestinal tract and the larvae enter the venous circulation, pass to the lungs, from which they migrate up the respiratory passages and are swallowed, and reach their site of continued residence, the jejunum. In a 1- to 2-year life span, the female is capable of producing 200,000 eggs per day. The eggs are passed with the feces, and a new cycle is started. Children up to the age of 12 to 14 are likely to be infected. Intestinal obstruction may be a complication in children under 6 years of age.

    TREAT: *Pyrantel pamoate* is the drug of choice. Mebendazole is also effective. No drug is useful during the pulmonary phase of the infection.

ascaris. A worm of the genus *Ascaris*.

Aschheim-Zondek test (ăsh′hĭm-tsŏn′dĕk) [Selmar Aschheim, Ger. gynecologist, 1878–1965; Bernhardt Zondek, Ger.-born Israeli obstetrician-gynecologist, 1891–1966]. A test for pregnancy in which the patient's urine is injected subcutaneously into immature female mice.

Aschner's phenomenon, reflex, sign (ăsh′nĕrz) [Bernhard Aschner, Austrian gynecologist, 1883–1960]. Slowing of the pulse following pressure applied to the eyeball or the carotid sinus. Sometimes used to slow the heart during attacks of supraventricular tachycardia. May also be used as a diagnostic test for angina pectoris. Slowing of the heart produced by this reflex may relieve anginal pain. SYN: *oculocardiac reflex*.

Aschoff, Ludwig (ăsh′ŏf). German pathologist, 1866–1942.

    A.'s bodies. A.'s nodules, q.v.

    A.'s cells. Large cells with basophilic cytoplasm and a large vesicular nucleus often multinucleated. Characteristic of Aschoff's nodules.

    A.'s nodules. Small nodules composed of cells and leukocytes found in the interstitial tissues of the heart in rheumatic myocarditis.

asci (ăs′ī). Pl. of ascus.

ascia (ăs′ē-ă, ăs′kē-ă) [L. *ascia*, ax]. A form of

spiral bandage with each turn overlapping the previous one for a third of its width.

ascites (ă-sī′tēz) [Gr. *askitēs* from *askos*, a leather bag]. The accumulation of serous fluid in the peritoneal cavity. SEE: *edema.*

ETIOL: Interference in venous return as occurs in cardiac disease, obstruction of flow in vena cava or portal vein; obstruction in lymphatic drainage; disturbance in electrolyte balance as occurs in sodium retention, depletion of plasma proteins, or cirrhosis of the liver.

NURSING IMPLICATIONS: Evaluate respiratory effort, appetite and food intake, fluid intake and output, and weight. Measure abdominal girth, marking site for future measurement. Assist with paracentesis, evaluating vital signs, weight, girth, and obtain serum protein, sodium, and potassium levels pre- and post-procedure.

a. chylosus. Chyle in the ascitic fluid, usually resulting from rupture of thoracic duct.

ascitic (ă-sĭt′ĭk). Pert. to ascites.

ascitic fluid. Clear and pale straw-colored fluid occurring in ascites, sp. gr. 1.005 to 1.015.

Ascoli's reaction, test (ăs-kō′lēz) [Alberto Ascoli, It. serologist, 1877–1957]. Precipitation test for anthrax. Used for detection of anthrax bacilli in animal hides and meat.

Ascomycetes (ăs″kō-mī-sē′tēz) [Gr. *askos*, leather bag, + *mykes*, fungus]. The sac fungi; the largest class of Eumycetes, the true fungi (of the phylum Thallophyta). Organisms in this group are characterized by possession of a saclike sporangium (ascus, q.v.) in which ascospores are developed. Includes the true yeasts, blue molds, and penicillin.

ascorbic acid (ăs-kor′bĭk) [Gr. *a-*, not, + L. *scorbutus*, scurvy]. USP. Vitamin C. It occurs naturally and can be synthesized. SEE: *acid, ascorbic; vitamin C.*

ascospore (ăs′kō-spor) [Gr. *askos*, leather bag, + *sporos*, seed]. A spore produced within an ascus or spore sac.

ascus (ăs′kŭs) [Gr. *askos*, leather bag] (pl. *asci*). A saclike spore case within which ascospores, typically eight, are formed; characteristic of the Ascomycetes, q.v.

-ase. A suffix used in forming the name of an enzyme. It is added to the name or a part of the name of the substance upon which it acts; e.g., lipase, which acts on fats (lipids).

asepsis (ā-sĕp′sĭs) [Gr. *a-*, not, + *sepesthai*, to decay]. Sterile; a condition free from germs, infection, and any form of life. SEE: *antisepsis; sterilization.*

aseptic (ā-sĕp′tĭk). Rel. to asepsis; free from septic matter.

aseptic-antiseptic [Gr. *a-*, not, + *sepsis,*

decay, + *anti,* against, + *sepsis,* decay]. Both aseptic and antiseptic.

aseptic technique. Method used to prevent contamination in procedures where a sterile field is required. Instruments are sterilized or disinfected. Personnel wear sterile gloves and clean caps and masks. SEE: *Universal Precautions* in *Appendix.*

Asepto syringe. Trade name for a type of syringe with a bulb top and blunt-tipped end. Generally used for aseptic irrigation of wounds.

asexual (ā-sĕk′shū-ăl) [″ + L. *sexualis,* having sex]. Without sex; nonsexual.

asexualization (ā-sĕk″shū-ăl-ĭ-zā′shŭn). Sterilization by ablation of the ovaries or testes.

ash (ăsh) [AS. *aesc,* ash]. Incombustible powdery residue of a substance that has been completely incinerated.

ASHD. *arteriosclerotic heart disease.*

Asherman's syndrome [Joseph G. Asherman, Czech. physician, b. 1889]. Intrauterine adhesions. These may cause amenorrhea.

asialia (ă″sī-ā′lē-ă, ā″sē-ā′lē-ă) [Gr. *a-*, not, + *sialon,* spittle]. Failure to secrete or deficiency of saliva. SYN: *aptyalism.*

Asiatic cholera. An acute infectious epidemic disease. SEE: *cholera.*

asiderosis (ā″sĭd-ĕ-rō′sĭs) [″ + *sideros,* iron, + *osis,* condition]. Deficiency of iron reserve in the body.

ASIS. *anterior superior iliac spine.* Radiographic palpation point on the skin on each side of the front of the pelvis.

ASLO. *antistreptolysin-O.*

as low as reasonably achievable. ABBR: ALARA. In radiology, a program of radiation protection in which personnel attempt to keep their exposure to ionizing radiation at an absolute minimum.

A.S.M.T. *American Society for Medical Technology.*

asocial (ā-sō′shĭl). 1. Withdrawn from society. 2. Inconsiderate of the needs of others.

asoma (ā-sō′mă) [Gr. *a-*, not, + *soma,* body]. Deformed fetus with an imperfectly formed trunk and head.

asonia (ă-sō′nē-ă) [″ + L. *sonus,* sound]. Tone deafness.

asparaginase (ăs-păr′ă-jĭn-āz). An antineoplastic agent derived from the bacterium *Escherichia coli.*

asparagine (ăs-păr′ă-jĭn). Aminosuccinic acid, a nonessential amino acid.

Asparagus (ă-spăr′ă-gŭs) [Gr. *asparagos*]. A genus of liliaceous herbs.

aspartame (ă-spăr′tām). An artificial sweetener synthesized from two amino acids, aspartic acid and phenylalanine. It is 180 times sweeter than sugar. It is unsuitable for use in cooking because its flavor is changed when heated. Trade names are Equal and NutraSweet.

aspartate aminotransferase. ABBR: AST. Current term for serum glutamic-oxaloacetic transaminase (SGOT).

aspartic acid. COOH·CH(NH₂)·CH₂·COOH. A nonessential amino acid, q.v.; one of the products of pancreatic digestion.

aspastic (ă-spăs′tĭk) [Gr. a-, not, + spastikos, having spasms]. Nonspastic.

aspecific (ă-spē-sĭf′ĭk). Not specific.

aspect (ăs′pĕkt) [L. aspectus, a view]. 1. That part of a surface facing in any designated direction. 2. Appearance, looks.

aspergillin (ăs″pĕr-jĭl′ĭn). 1. A pigment produced by Aspergillus niger, q.v. 2. An inappropriate name applied to a number of antibiotic substances produced by various species of Aspergillus.

aspergillosis (ăs″pĕr-jĭl-ō′sĭs) [aspergillus + Gr. osis, condition]. Aspergillus infection in the tissues or on any mucous surface marked by inflammatory granulomatous lesions. This condition may develop in the bronchi, lungs, aural canal, skin, or the mucous membranes of the eye, nose, or urethra. It may extend through the various viscera, producing mycotic nodules in the lungs, liver, kidney, and other organs. The disease is not transmissible from human to animals or animals to human.

TREAT: Amphotericin B. At construction sites, application of 8-copper quinolate may control fungal growth on inanimate objects.

   a., aural. A form of otomycosis, q.v.

   a., pulmonary. Disease of the lungs caused by Aspergillus.

Aspergillus (ăs″pĕr-jĭl′ŭs) [L. aspergere, to sprinkle]. A genus of Ascomycetes, including several species of the molds, some of which are pathogenic. The principal pathogenic species is A. fumigatus, although others (A. flavus, A. nidulans, and A. niger) may be pathogenic. SEE: aspergillosis.

   A. clavatus. A species found in soil and manure. Its cultures yield the antibacterial substance clavacin.

   A. concentricus. A species once thought to be the cause of tinea imbricata ringworm.

   A. flavus. A mold found on corn, peanuts, and grain.

   A. fumigatus. Found in soil and manure, this fungus is the common cause of aspergillosis in man and birds. It has been found in the ear, nose, and lungs.

   A. glaucus. A bluish mold found on dried fruit.

   A. nidulans. A species common in soil, causing one form of white mycetoma.

   A. niger. A pathogenic form with black spores, frequently present in the external auditory meatus. Causes otomycosis.

   A. ochraceus. A species that produces the characteristic odor of brewing coffee.

   A. versicolor. A species that produces a toxin similar to aflatoxin.

aspermatic (ă-spĕr-măt′ĭk) [Gr. a-, not, + sperma, seed]. Pert. to aspermatism.

aspermatism (ă-spĕr′mă-tĭzm) [″ + ″ + -ismos, condition of]. Absence or nonemission of semen. SYN: aspermia. SEE: azoospermia.

aspermatogenesis (ă-spĕr″mă-tō-jĕn′ĕ-sĭs) [″ + ″ + genesis, generation, birth]. Nonfunction of the sperm-producing system of the testicles.

aspermia (ă-spĕr′mē-ă) [″ + sperma, seed]. Lack of, or failure to ejaculate, semen.

aspermous (ă-spĕr′mŭs). Pert. to aspermia. SYN: aspermatic.

asperous (ăs′pĕr-ŭs) [L. asper, rough]. Uneven; having minute elevations.

aspersion (ăs-pĕr′zhŭn) [L. aspersio, sprinkling]. Sprinkling an affected part with water; a form of hydrotherapy, q.v.

asphalgesia (ăs″făl-jē′zē-ă) [Gr. asphe-, self, + algos, pain]. A burning sensation sometimes felt on touching certain articles during hypnosis.

asphyctic, asphyctous (ăs-fĭk′tĭk, -tŭs) [Gr. a-, not, + sphyxis, pulse]. 1. Pert. to, or affected with, asphyxia. 2. Without pulse.

asphyxia (ăs-fĭk′sē-ă) [″ + sphyxis, pulse]. Condition caused by insufficient intake of oxygen.

SYM: In general, symptoms include dyspnea, cyanosis, rapid pulse, impairment of senses, mental disturbances; in extreme cases, convulsions, unconsciousness, and death.

ETIOL: *Extrinsic causes:* Choking; toxic gases; exhaust gas (principally carbon monoxide); electric shock; drugs; anesthesia; traumatic asphyxia; crushing injuries of chest; compression of chest; injury of respiratory nerves or centers; diminution of oxygenation of environment; drowning. *Intrinsic causes:* Hemorrhage into lungs or pleural cavity; foreign bodies in throat; swelling of air passages; diseases of air passages; ruptured aneurysm or abscess; edema of the lung; cardiac deficiency; tumors such as goiter; pharyngeal and retropharyngeal abscesses. *Other causes:* Paralysis of the respiratory center; paralysis of respiratory muscles; anesthesia; pneumothorax; narcotic drugs; electrocution; child abuse.

F.A.: Artificial respiration, q.v.

   a., autoerotic. A., sexual, q.v.

   a. carbonica. Suffocation from inhalation of coal or water gas, or carbon monoxide.

a., fetal. Asphyxia occurring in a fetus; results from interference in placental circulation or from premature separation of placenta, as in abruptio placentae.

a. livida. Asphyxia in which the skin is cyanotic from lack of oxygen in blood.

a., local. Asphyxia in which a limited portion of the body is involved, such as the fingers, hands, toes, or feet due to insufficient blood supply. One of the symptoms usually associated with Raynaud's disease, q.v.

a. neonatorum. Respiratory failure in the newborn.

a. pallida. Asphyxia in which difficulty in breathing is accompanied by weak and thready pulse, pale skin, and absence of reflexes.

a., sexual. Some individuals apply a makeshift noose (or hangman's knot) around the neck and stand so that they are partially suspended from the rope to which the noose is attached. By lowering the body slightly, the noose tightens and cerebral hypoxia results. This is done during masturbation in order to heighten the intensity of orgasm. If the hypoxia is allowed to be present for more than a few moments, the person may become unconscious and will die if the suspending noose is not released by another person.

Cerebral hypoxia may enhance orgasm. Aviators and mountain climbers have experienced this without use of a noose around the neck, and not necessarily while masturbating. SYN: *a., autoerotic.*

asphyxial (ăs-fĭk′sē-ăl). Pert. to asphyxia; asphyctic.

asphyxiant (ăs-fĭk′sē-ănt). An agent, esp. any gas, that will produce asphyxia.

asphyxiate (ăs-fĭk′sē-āt). To cause asphyxiation or asphyxia.

asphyxiation (ăs-fĭk″sē-ā′shŭn). A state of asphyxia or suffocation. Act of producing asphyxia. SEE: *asphyxia.*

aspidium (ăs-pĭd′ē-ŭm) [Gr. *aspidion,* little shield]. The root and stalk of *Dryopteris filixmas* (male fern) or *D. marginalis* (marginal fern). Used medicinally in form of oleoresin.

a. oleoresin. Extract of male fern; male fern oleoresin.

USE: As an anthelmintic in treatment of tapeworm infestation of intestines. Care should be taken that it is not administered with an oil, since absorption may occur.

aspirate (ăs′pĭ-rāt) [L. *ad,* to, + *spirare,* to breathe]. 1. Aspiration; to draw in or out by suction. 2. A sound like that of the letter *h.*

aspiration (ăs-pĭ-rā′shŭn). 1. Drawing in or out as by suction. Foreign bodies may be aspirated into the nose, throat, or lungs on inspiration. 2. The withdrawing of a fluid from a cavity by means of suction with an instrument called an aspirator. Cavities most commonly aspirated are pericardial, peritoneal, pleural and thecal (lumbar puncture). The object of aspiration is to remove fluid or air from an affected area such as in pleural effusion, pneumothorax, ascites, or an abscess; or to obtain specimens such as blood from a vein or serum from the spinal canal.

EQUIP: Disinfecting solution for the skin; local anesthetic; two aspirating needles with the aspirating apparatus as indicated; utensil for receiving the fluid and a sterile receptacle for the specimen; sterile sponges, towels, basins; sterile gloves, face masks, and gowns; sterile forceps; surgical dressings as the case may require, stimulant ordered if indication arises.

NURSING IMPLICATIONS: Prevent pathologic respiratory aspiration by positioning the unconscious patient to protect the airway and promote evacuation of mucus or vomitus, and by suctioning the nasopharynx as necessary. The patient should be draped to ensure privacy and to be kept warm. Provide support during the procedure. Carefully observe the type and amount of any drainage or material that is aspirated.

aspirator (ăs′pĭ-rā-tor). Apparatus for evacuating fluid contents of a cavity. Varieties are piston pump, compressible rubber tube, rubber bulb, and siphon, a trocar and cannula, and hypodermic needle and syringe.

a., dental. The apparatus for removing water, saliva, blood, or tissue debris from the oral cavity by suction.

aspirin (ăs′pĕr-ĭn). USP. ABBR: ASA. $C_9H_8O_4$. Acetylsalicylic acid. A derivative of salicylic acid. It occurs as white crystals or powder. It is one of the most widely used analgesics and antipyretics. Also, because it is widely available, it is often misused and is one of the most frequent causes of accidental poisoning in children. Prolonged use will cause gastrointestinal irritation and bleeding in some individuals.

aspirin poisoning. In acute poisoning, signs vary with increasing doses from mild lethargy and hyperpnea to coma and convulsions. Sweating, dehydration, hyperpnea, hyperthermia, and restlessness may be present with moderate doses. In chronic poisoning, tinnitus, skin rash, bleeding tendency, weight loss, and mental symptoms may be present. Aspirin poisoning in very young infants may produce very few signs and symptoms other than dehydration or hyperpnea.

TREAT: Repeated gastric lavage with activated charcoal. I.V. fluids for dehydra but do not overload the system. Use enough I.V. fluids to establish good rate, i.e., 3 to 4 ml/kg/hr of urine flow. Just as important as I.V. fluid therapy is alkalinization of urine by administering bicarbonate. The goal is a urine pH of 8 or higher. Also, after urine flow is established, add potassium 30 mEq/L of administered fluid. After serum potassium levels reach 5 mEq/L, discontinue potassium. If alkalinization of the urine is not accomplished, hemodialysis may be needed. Treat tachycardia with appropriate drug. SEE: *salicylates* in *Poisons and Poisoning* in *Appendix*.

asplenia (ă-splē'nē-ă) [Gr. *a-*, not, + L. *splen*, spleen]. Absence of the spleen.

asplenia syndrome. A developmental disorder originating prior to the 5th fetal week. The vascular structures on the left side, including the spleen, are absent.

asporogenic (ăs"pō-rō-jĕn'ĭk) [" + *sporos*, seed, + *gennan*, to produce]. Not reproducing by spores.

asporous (ă-spō'rŭs). Having no spores.

A.S.R.T. *American Society of Radiologic Technologists.*

assault (ă-sawlt') [L. *assultus*, having assailed]. 1. The threat of unlawful touching of another. 2. The willful attempt to harm someone. SEE: *battery*.

  a., sexual. Sexual intercourse against the will of the victim. SEE: *rape*.

assay (ă-sā', ăs'ā) [O. Fr. *assai*, trial]. The analysis of a substance or mixture to determine its constituents and the relative proportion of each.

  a., biological. Estimation of strength of a drug or substance by comparing its effects in test animals to a reference standard. SYN: *bioassay*.

assessment, nursing. SEE: *nursing assessment*.

assident (ăs'ĭ-dĕnt) [L. *assidere*, to sit by]. A term applied to symptoms to indicate they are usually but not invariably present with a certain disease.

assimilable (ă-sĭm'ĭ-lă-bl) [L. *ad*, to, + *similare*, to make like]. Capable of assimilation.

assimilate (ă-sĭm'ĭ-lāt). To absorb digested food.

assimilation (ă-sĭm"ĭ-lā'shŭn). 1. The processes whereby the products of digestion are converted into the chemical substances of the body tissues, first passing through the lacteals and blood vessels; transformation of ̶d into living tissue. The constructive ̶e of metabolism, i.e., anabolism. 2. In ̶ology, the absorption of newly per- ̶'nformation into the existing subjec- ̶cious structure. ̶One who aids or supports.

  a., dental. SEE: *dental assistant*.

assisted circulation. Use of a mechanical device to augment or replace the action of the heart in pumping blood.

assisted death. Helping an individual who wants to die to do so. This may take the form of counseling or by actually providing the means and instruments for allowing the person to act to commit suicide. The legal and moral questions concerning such acts, esp. if the assisting person is a physician or someone involved in medical care, are debatable. SEE: *assisted suicide; euthanasia*.

assisted suicide. The rendering of assistance to a person who wants to end his or her life but is not able to do this alone. This may be due to a physical disability or lack of knowledge of how to accomplish suicide. Whether or not physicians should become involved in helping patients commit suicide is debatable. Physicians or other medical care personnel who do assist a patient who wishes to take his or her life may be considered in the U.S. legal system to have murdered the patient. Some state governments have legalized this procedure. SEE: *assisted death; euthanasia*.

associated movements. Synchronous correlation of two or more muscles or muscle groups that, though not essential for the performance of some function, normally accompany it, as the swinging of arms accompanies normal walking. Associated movements are characteristically lost in cerebellar disease.

association [L. *ad*, to, + *socius*, companion]. 1. Joining or uniting; coordination with another idea or structure; relationship. In psychiatry, association refers in particular to the interrelationship of the conscious and unconscious ideas. 2. In genetics, the occurrence together of two characteristics at a frequency greater than would be predicted by chance. 3. In clinical epidemiology the relationship of the occurrence of two events, but evidence that the event being investigated actually causes the second condition is lacking; e.g., malaria occurs in warm climates with proper breeding conditions for certain types of mosquitoes, but those conditions are *associations*. The actual *cause* is the malaria parasite.

  a., controlled. An idea suggested by a word uttered by the physician. SYN: *a., induced*. SEE: *association test*.

  a., free. In psychoanalysis, the uninhibited and uncensored oral expression of ideas as they arise in the patient's mind.

  a., induced. The idea expressed when the physician gives a stimulus word. SYN: *a., controlled*. SEE: *association test*.

association areas. Areas of the cerebral cortex that are connected to motor and sensory areas of the same side, to similar areas on the other side, and to other regions of the brain, as the thalamus. They serve to integrate the simpler motor and sensory functions.

association center. Center controlling associated movements.

association neuron. A neuron that transmits impulses from afferent to efferent neurons.

association of ideas. The linking together in a memory chain of two or more ideas, associated by some similarity or relationship, or by both having been experienced at the same time.

association test. Test in which the patient is given a word (stimulus word) and replies immediately with another word (reaction word) suggested by the first. The words chosen and the time taken in responding (association time) may be indicative of the patient's mental condition.

association time. SEE: *association test.*

assonance (ăs'ŏ-năns) [L. *assonans,* answering with same sound]. 1. Similarity of sounds in words or syllables. 2. Abnormal tendency to use alliteration.

assumption of risk. A doctrine of law whereby the plaintiff assumes the risk of medical treatment or procedures and may not recover damages for injuries sustained as a result of the known and described dangers.

AST. *aspartate aminotransferase.*

Ast. *astigmatism.*

astasia (ă-stā'zē-ă) [Gr. *a-,* not, + *stasis,* stand]. Inability to stand or sit erect due to motor incoordination.

   a. **-abasia.** A form of hysterical ataxia, q.v., with incoordination and inability to stand or walk although all leg movements can be performed while sitting or lying down.

astatine (ăs'tă-tēn, -tīn) [Gr. *astatos,* unstable]. SYMB: At. At. no. 85; at. wt. 210. A radioactive element. May be of use in treatment of hyperthyroidism.

asteatosis (ăs"tē-ă-tō'sĭs) [Gr. *a-,* not, + *stear,* tallow, + *osis,* condition]. Any disease condition in which there is persistent scaling of the skin, suggesting scantiness or absence of sebaceous secretion.

   a. **cutis.** A dry, fissured condition of the skin with a deficient sebaceous secretion.

   ETIOL: Symptomatic form: senility or systemic disorders that give rise to trophic changes in the nervous system. Local form may be caused by frequent contact with irritants.

   TREAT: Removal of underlying cause. Local application of oils and fats.

aster (ăs'tĕr) [Gr., star]. The stellate rays forming around the dividing centrosome during mitosis.

astereognosis (ă-stĕr"ē-ŏg-nō'sĭs) [Gr. *a-,* not, + *stereos,* solid, + *gnosis,* knowledge]. Inability to recognize objects or forms by touch.

asterion (ăs-tē'rē-ŏn) [Gr., starlike] (pl. *asteria*). A craniometric point at junction of the lambdoid, occipitomastoid, and parietomastoid sutures.

asterixis (ăs"tĕr-ĭk'sĭs) [Gr. *a-,* not, + *sterixis,* fixed position]. Abnormal muscle tremor consisting of involuntary jerking movements, esp. in the hands. Also seen in tongue and muscle groups of foot. May be due to various diseases that interfere with brain metabolism. When due to hepatic coma, asterixis is called "liver flap" or "liver tremor." SYN: *tremor, flapping.* SEE: *alcoholism; hepatic coma.*

asternal (ā-stĕr'năl) [" + *sternon,* chest]. 1. Not connected with the sternum. 2. Having no sternum.

asternia (ā-stĕr'nē-ă). Congenital absence of the sternum.

asteroid (ăs'tĕr-oyd) [Gr. *aster,* star, + *eidos,* form, shape]. Star-shaped.

asthenia (ăs-thē'nē-ă) [Gr. *asthenes,* without strength]. Lack or loss of strength; debility. Any weakness, but esp. one originating in muscular or cerebellar disease. SYN: *adynamia.*

   a., **neurocirculatory.** A psychosomatic disorder characterized by mental and physical fatigue, dyspnea, giddiness, precordial pain and palpitation, esp. on exertion. SYN: *neurosis, cardiac.* SEE: *chronic fatigue syndrome.*

   ETIOL: Unknown but occurs in individuals who are under conditions of stress. It is common among soldiers in combat.

   TREAT: Removal from stress situation and psychotherapy.

asthenic (ăs-thĕn'ĭk). 1. Weak; pert. to asthenia. 2. Body habitus characterized by a narrow, shallow thorax, long thoracic cavity, and a short abdominal cavity.

asthenobiosis (ăs-thē"nō-bī-ō'sĭs) [Gr. *asthenes,* without strength, + *bios,* life, + *osis,* condition]. Condition of reduced biological activity of an animal, resembling hibernation but not related to temperature or humidity.

asthenocoria (ăs-thē"nō-kō'rē-ă) [" + *kore,* pupil]. A sluggish pupillary light reflex.

asthenometer (ăs"thĕ-nŏm'ĕ-ter) [" + *metron,* measure]. An instrument for determining muscular strength or weakness.

asthenope (ăs'thĕ-nōp) [" + *opsis,* power of sight]. An individual who is affected with asthenopia, q.v.

asthenopia (ăs″thē-nō′pē-ă). Weakness or tiring of eyes accompanied by pain, headache, and dimness of vision.

SYM: Pain in or around eyes; headache, usually aggravated by use of eyes for close work; fatigue; vertigo; reflex symptoms as nausea, twitching of facial muscles, migraine.

a., accommodative. Asthenopia due to strain of ciliary muscles.

a., muscular. Asthenopia caused by weakness of extrinsic ocular muscles.

a., nervous. Asthenopia of hysteric or neurasthenic origin.

a., photogenous. Asthenopia caused by excessive or improper illumination.

asthenopic (ăs″thē-nŏp′ĭk). Rel. to asthenopia.

asthenospermia (ăs″thē-nō-spĕr′mē-ă) [″ + *sperma*, seed]. Loss or reduction of motility of spermatozoa in semen. Associated with infertility.

asthenoxia [″ + *oxygen*]. Deficient oxygenation of waste products.

asthma (ăz′mă) [Gr., panting]. A disease caused by increased responsiveness of the tracheobronchial tree to various stimuli. The result is paroxysmal constriction of the bronchial airways. Clinically, there is severe dyspnea accompanied by wheezing. Between attacks the patient may be quite comfortable. In some cases the attacks become continuous, a condition called status asthmaticus, and may be fatal. No age is exempt, but asthma occurs most frequently in childhood or early adulthood. The patient may assume a "hunched forward" position in an attempt to get more air. Other allergic disorders may coexist. Recurrence and severity of attacks are greatly influenced by secondary factors, by mental or physical fatigue, by exposure to fumes, by endocrine changes at various periods in life, and by emotional situations.

Asthma is the leading cause of chronic illness in childhood. It is estimated to occur in 5% to 10% of children at some time during their development. Prior to puberty, twice as many boys as girls have asthma; the attack rate is equal in adults. SYN: *chronic desquamating eosinophilic bronchitis.*

ETIOL: *Extrinsic causes:* Allergens inhaled in the air (pollen, mold spores, animal dander, or dust) or infections of the respiratory tract. Occasionally foods (eggs, shellfish, or chocolate) or drugs (aspirin) may precipitate an attack. This type of asthma involves immunoglobulin E (IgE) and is also termed reagin-mediated. *Intrinsic causes:* In some cases asthma develops in persons with allergies of unknown etiology. It may be precipitated by infection of the upper or lower respiratory tracts.

TREAT: Avoid all sources of indoor inhalant factors such as house dust, danders, molds, tobacco smoke, and strong odors. In dry, cold weather, humidified air should be maintained. Acute attacks may be relieved by a number of drugs such as epinephrine, ephedrine, cromolyn sodium, aminophylline, or beta-adrenergic stimulants, e.g., albuterol, terbutaline, or pirbuterol. Also, the short-term use of aerosol corticosteroids is effective for newly-diagnosed mild asthma. If this medication is used, it is important to follow the directions concerning controlling the dose. Use of bronchodilator aerosols are effective and have the advantage of utilizing much less medicine than would be needed by injection. For persistent asthma (status asthmaticus), the use of adrenocortical hormones plus continuous oxygen, I.V. fluids if patient is dehydrated, and continuation of bronchodilator therapy. Careful monitoring of blood gases, pH, and ECG is indicated. Sedation is indicated but should be used only if the patient is carefully monitored. Even though use of adrenocortical hormones may provide dramatic relief, these hormones should be used only as long as is necessary to control the acute asthmatic attack. Prolonged use of these hormones may lead to the development of serious side effects. The use of sedatives and expectorants is sometimes necessary. In all cases, effort should be made to control causative factors including the component of the disease due to emotional disturbance, esp. in the intrinsic group. Elimination of antigen, or countermeasures, such as immunization, desensitization, or hyposensitization, are desirable. For asthma due to infection of respiratory tract, antibiotics should be used to control infection or prevent recurrence. SEE: *bronchoalveolar lavage.*

NURSING IMPLICATIONS: Assess ventilatory rate and effort; determine the inspiratory–expiratory ratio, presence and timing of wheezing, use of ancillary muscle groups and retractions, and other symptoms indicative of respiratory fatigue or distress. Position the patient to ease ventilatory effort and facilitate ventilation. Monitor vital signs and mental status for anxiety, irritability, and reduced level of consciousness. Administer humidified air or oxygen as prescribed, monitoring arterial blood gas values if the situation warrants. Remain with the patient, providing a calm atmosphere and reassurance that the measures taken will improve breathing. Assess for symptoms of dehydration and provide increased oral fluids in frequent small amounts to help thin inspissated respiratory secretions. Document characteristics of sputum. Administer prescribed medications, such as oral or inhaled beta-adrenergics or steroids, oral, subcutaneous, or intravenous epinephrine, and evaluate patient's response. When acute attack has subsided, teach patient breathing exercises (such as floppy-lipped breathing and working during expiration) to increase respiratory efficiency. Instruct the patient and family about eliminating allergens, and teach them measures to take at home to prevent or decrease the severity of future asthmatic attacks. Assist the patient in identifying and reducing stressors associated with the attacks, such as emotional stress, fatigue, exercise, and cold air. SEE: *Nursing Diagnoses* in *Appendix.*

a., bronchial. Allergic asthma. Common form of asthma due to hypersensitivity to an allergen.

a., cardiac. This condition, more properly termed paroxysmal nocturnal dyspnea, consists of attacks of shortness of breath which usually occur at night and awaken the patient. This is due to advanced forms of heart failure associated with elevations of pulmonary venous and capillary pressures. SEE: *heart failure, congestive.*

a., exercise-induced. SEE: *exercise-induced asthma.*

a., extrinsic. Asthma due to some environmental factor, usually allergic.

a., intrinsic. Asthma assumed to be due to some endogenous cause because no external cause can be found.

asthmagenic. Producing asthma.

asthmatic (ăz-măt'ĭk) [L. *asthmaticus*]. Pert. to or of the nature of asthma.

astigmatic (ăs″tĭg-măt'ĭk). Pert. to or afflicted with astigmatism.

astigmatism (ă-stĭg'mă-tizm) [Gr. *a-*, not, + *stigma*, point, + *-ismos*, condition of]. ABBR: As. or Ast. Form of ametropia, q.v., in which the refraction of a ray of light is spread over a diffuse area rather than being sharply focused on the retina. Due to differences in curvature in various meridians of the cornea and lens of the eye.

ETIOL: Exact cause is unknown. Some types show a familial pattern.

a., compound. Astigmatism in which both horizontal and vertical curvatures are involved.

a., index. Astigmatism resulting from inequalities in refractive indices of different parts of the lens.

a., mixed. Astigmatism in which one meridian is myopic and the other hyperopic.

a., simple. Astigmatism along one meridian only.

astigmatometer (ăs″tĭg-mă-tŏm'ĕ-tĕr) [″ + *stigma*, point, + *metron*, measure]. An instrument for measuring astigmatism.

astigmatoscope (ăs″tĭg-măt'ō-skōp) [″ + ″ + *skopein*, to examine]. Instrument for detecting and measuring astigmatism.

astigmatoscopy (ă-stĭg″mă-tŏs'kō-pē). Use of the astigmatoscope.

astigmia (ă-stĭg'mē-ă). Astigmatism, q.v.

astigmometer (ăs″tĭg-mŏm'ĕ-tĕr). Astigmatometer, q.v.

astigmoscope (ăs-tĭg'mō-skōp). Astigmatoscope, q.v.

astomatous, astomous (ăs-tōm'ă-tŭs, ăs'tō-mŭs) [Gr. *a-*, not, + *stoma*, mouth]. Without a mouth or oral aperture; as certain protozoa.

astomia (ă-stō'mē-ă). Congenital absence of the mouth.

astragalectomy (ăs″trăg-ă-lĕk'tō-mē) [*astragalus* + Gr. *ektome*, excision]. Surgical removal of the talus (astragalus).

astragalus (ă-străg'ă-lŭs) [Gr. *astragalos*, ball of the ankle joint]. Obsolete term for the talus of the ankle. SEE: *talus.*

astraphobia (ăs-tră-fō'bē-ă) [Gr. *astrape*, the heavens, + *phobos*, fear]. Fear of thunder and lightning.

astrict (ă-strĭkt') [L. *astringere*, to bind fast]. To contract or constrict, as the action of an astringent. To compress, as an artery in a hemorrhage.

astriction (ă-strĭk'shŭn). Action of astringent.

astringent (ă-strĭn'jĕnt) [L. *astringere*, to bind fast]. 1. Drawing together, constricting, binding. 2. An agent that has a constricting or binding effect, i.e., one that checks hemorrhages or secretions by coagulation of proteins on a cell surface. The principal astringents are salts of metals such as lead, iron, zinc (ferric chloride, zinc oxide); permanganates; and tannic acid. SEE: *styptic.*

astro- [Gr. *astron*, star]. Prefix indicating relationship to a star, or star-shaped.

astrobiology. Study of extraterrestrial life.

astroblast (ăs'trō-blăst) [″ + Gr. *blastos*, germ]. A cell that gives rise to an astrocyte. It develops from spongioblasts derived from embryonic neuroepithelium.

astroblastoma (ăs″trō-blăs-tō'mă) [″ + ″ + *oma*, tumor]. A Grade II astrocytoma, q.v., composed of cells with abundant cytoplasm and two or three nuclei.

astrocyte (ăs'trō-sīt) [″ + *kytos*, cell]. A star-shaped neuroglial cell with many branching processes.

astrocytoma (ăs″trō-sī-tō'mă) [″ + ″ + *oma*, tumor]. Tumor of the brain or spinal cord composed of astrocytes. They are graded according to the prognosis.

a., malignant. A tumor of the brainstem, cerebellum, spinal cord, or the white matter of the cerebral hemispheres. Onset is typically in the fifth decade of life. Prognosis after treatment by surgery, radiation, or other means, is poor, in that few survive more than two years.

astroglia (ăs-trŏg'lē-ă) [" + *glia,* glue]. Astrocytes making up neuroglial tissue.

astrokinetic motions (ăs"trō-kĭ-nĕt'ĭk) [" + *kinesis,* movement]. Pert. to movements of the centrosome.

astrophobia (ăs"trō-fō'bē-ă) [" + *phobos,* fear]. Morbid fear of stars and celestial space.

astrosphere (ăs'trō-sfēr) [" + *sphaira,* sphere]. A group of fibrils or fine rays that radiate from the centrosome (microcentrum) of the dividing cell. SYN: *aster.*

astrostatic (ăs"trō-stăt'ĭk) [" + *statikos,* standing]. Pert. to astrosphere in its resting condition.

asyllabia (ă"sĭl-ā'bē-ă) [Gr. *a-,* not, + *syllabe,* syllable]. A form of alexia, q.v., in which the patient recognizes letters but cannot form syllables or words.

asylum (ă-sī'lŭm) [Gr. *asylon,* sanctuary]. An institution for the care of the mentally ill, esp. those who are so severely handicapped as to be unable to care for themselves or would be a hazard to self or society if they were not institutionalized.

asymbolia (ā-, ă-sĭm-bō'lē-ă) [Gr. *a-,* not, + *symbolon,* a sign]. Inability to comprehend words, gestures, or any type of symbol. Asemia, q.v., is the more generally accepted term for this condition. SEE: *aphasia.*

asymmetry (ă-sĭm'ē-trē) [" + *symmetria,* symmetry]. Lack of symmetry.

asymphytous (ă-sĭm'fĭ-tŭs) [" + *symphysis,* a growing together]. Separate or distinct; not grown together.

asymptomatic (ā"sĭmp-tō-măt'ĭk) [" + *symptoma,* occurrence]. Without symptoms.

asynchronism (ă-sĭn'krō-nĭzm) [" + *syn,* together, + *chronos,* time, + *-ismos,* condition of]. 1. The failure of events to occur in time with each other as they usually do. 2. Incoordination.

asynclitism (ă-sĭn'klĭ-tĭzm) [" + *synklinein,* to lean together, + *-ismos,* condition of]. An oblique presentation of the fetal head in labor.

a., anterior. Anterior parietal presentation. SYN: *Naegele's obliquity.*

a., posterior. Posterior parietal presentation. SYN: *Litzmann's obliquity.*

asyndesis (ă-sĭn'dē-sĭs) [Gr. *a-,* not, + *syn,* together, + *desis,* binding]. Mental defect in which related thoughts cannot be

assembled to form a comprehensive concept.

asynechia (ă"sĭ-nĕk'ē-ă) [" + *synecheia,* continuity]. Lack of continuity of structure in an organ or tissue.

asynergia, asynergy (ă-sĭn-ĕr'jē-ă, ă-sĭn'ĕr-jē) [" + Gr. *synergia,* cooperation]. Lack of coordination among parts or organs normally acting in unison. In neurology, lack of coordination between muscle groups. Movements are jerky and in sequence instead of being made together. Seen in cerebellar diseases.

asynovia (ă-sĭn-ō'vē-ă) [" + *syn,* with, + *oon,* egg]. Lack, or insufficient secretion, of synovial fluid of a joint.

asyntaxia (ă"sĭn-tăk'sē-ă) [" + *syntaxis,* orderly arrangement]. Failure of proper development of the embryo.

asystematic (ă-sĭs"tĕ-măt'ĭk) [" + LL. *systema,* arrangement]. Not systematic; not limited to one system or set of organs.

asystole, asystolia (ă-sĭs'tō-lē, ă"sĭs-tō'lē-ă) [" + *systole,* contraction]. Cardiac standstill; absence of contractions of the heart.

asystolic cardiac rhythm. In the ECG, the tracing appears as a flat (isoelectric) line during cardiac arrest.

At. Chem. symb. for the element astatine.

Atabrine Hydrochloride (ăt'ă-brĭn). Trade name for quinacrine hydrochloride, q.v.

atactic (ă-tăk'tĭk) [Gr. *ataktos,* irregular]. Incoordinate, irregular, as muscular incoordination, esp. in aphasia. SYN: *ataxic.*

atactiform (ă-tăk'tĭ-form) [" + L. *forma,* form]. Similar to ataxia.

ataractic (ăt"ă-răk'tĭk) [Gr. *ataraktos,* quiet]. 1. Of or pert. to ataraxia. 2. A drug that produces ataraxia, q.v.; a tranquilizer.

Atarax. Trade name for hydroxyzine hydrochloride, q.v.

ataraxia, ataraxy (ăt"ă-răk'sē-ă, -sē) [Gr. *ataraktos,* quiet]. A state of complete mental calm and tranquility, esp. without depression of mental faculties or clouding of consciousness.

atavism (ăt'ă-vĭzm) [L. *atavus,* ancestor, + Gr. *-ismos,* condition]. The appearance of a characteristic presumed to have been present in some remote ancestor; due to chance recombination of genes or environmental conditions favorable to their expression in the embryo. SYN: *throwback.*

atavistic (ăt-ă-vis'tĭk). Pert. to atavism.

ataxia (ă-tăk'sē-ă) [Gr., lack of order]. Defective muscular coordination, esp. that manifested when voluntary muscular movements are attempted.

a., alcoholic. Ataxia due to a loss of proprioception, in chronic alcoholism.

a., Briquet's. Hysterical ataxia accompanied by skin and leg muscle anesthesia.

a., Bruns'. Condition resulting from bilateral lesions of the frontal lobes. Stance and gait are affected, and there is a tendency to fall or stagger backwards.

a., bulbar. Ataxia due to a lesion in the medulla oblongata or pons.

a., cerebellar. Ataxia due to cerebellar disease.

a., choreic. Lack of muscular coordination seen in persons with chorea.

a., Friedreich's. An inherited degenerative disease with sclerosis of the dorsal and lateral columns of the spinal cord. Accompanied by ataxia, speech impairment, lateral curvature of the spinal column, and peculiar swaying and irregular movements, with paralysis of the muscles, esp. of the lower extremities. Onset in childhood or adolescence.

a., hereditary cerebellar. Disease of late adolescence caused by atrophy of cerebellum. Characterized by ataxic gait, hesitating and explosive speech, nystagmus, and sometimes optic neuritis. SYN: *a., Marie's.*

a., hereditary spinal. A., Friedreich's, q.v.

a., hysterical. Ataxia of leg muscles due to hysteria.

a., locomotor. Degeneration of the dorsal columns of the spinal cord and sensory nerve trunks, due to infection of the central nervous system with *Treponema pallidum*, the causative organism of syphilis. SYN: *tabes dorsalis.*

SYM: Postural instability, esp. when eyes are closed, and a staggering wide-base gait are characteristic. Pain and paresthesias are common, esp. lightning pains, described as sharp, stabbing, and paroxysmal. Ankle and knee reflexes are diminished or lost. Other symptoms characteristic of tertiary stage of syphilis, q.v. SEE: *gait.*

TREAT: Penicillin. Therapy may arrest disease but complete cure is rare.

a., Marie's. A., hereditary cerebellar, q.v.

a., motor. Inability to perform coordinated muscle movements.

a., sensory. Ataxia resulting from interference in conduction of sensory responses, esp. proprioceptive impulses from muscles. Becomes aggravated when eyes are closed. SEE: *a., spinal.*

a., spinal. Ataxia due to spinal cord disease.

a., static. Loss of deep sensibility causing inability to preserve equilibrium in standing.

a. -telangiectasia. A degenerative brain disease of children characterized by a specific immunologic dysfunction and progressive cerebellar degeneration, telangiectasis

of the bulbar conjunctiva, and increased tendency to experience malignancy. It is transmitted as an autosomal recessive. Death usually occurs in adolescence or early adulthood. Parents should be informed that subsequent children have a 25% risk of having this condition. SYN: *Louis-Bar syndrome.*

ataxiagram (ă-tăk'sē-ă-grăm) [Gr. *ataxia*, lack of order, + *gramma*, something written]. Ataxiagraph record or tracing.

ataxiagraph (ă-tăk'sē-ă-grăf) [" + *graphein*, to write]. Instrument for measuring the degree and direction of swaying in ataxia.

ataxiameter (ă-tăk"sē-ăm'ĕ-tĕr) [" + *metron*, measure]. Apparatus measuring ataxia.

ataxiamnesia (ă-tăk"sē-ăm-nē'zē-ă) [" + *amnesia*, forgetfulness]. Condition with ataxia and amnesia.

ataxiaphasia (ă-tăk"sē-ă-fā'zē-ă) [" + *phasis*, speech]. Inability to arrange words into sentences. Also spelled *ataxaphasia.*

ataxic, ataxial (ă-tăk'sĭk, ă-tăk'sē-ăl). Pert. to, or marked by, ataxia.

ataxophobia (ă-tăk"sō-fō'bē-ă) [" + *phobos*, fear]. Morbid dread of disorder or untidiness.

A.T.B.C.B. *Architectural and Transportation Barriers Compliance Board.* A federal agency charged with enforcing legislation requiring federal buildings and transportation facilities to be accessible to persons with disability.

atelectasis (ăt"ĕ-lĕk'tă-sĭs) [Gr. *ateles*, imperfect, + *ektasis*, expansion]. 1. Condition in which lungs of a fetus remain unexpanded at birth. May be partial or total. 2. A collapsed or airless condition of the lung. May be caused by obstruction by foreign bodies, hypoventilation as occurs secondary to pain in fractured ribs and in patients being ventilated with inadequate tidal volumes, mucous plugs or excessive secretions, or by compression from without as by tumors, aneurysms, or enlarged lymph nodes. It sometimes is a complication following abdominal operations. A special chronic form, designated middle lobe syndrome, results from compression of the middle lobe bronchus by surrounding lymph nodes. SEE: *canals of Lambert; pores of Kohn.*

NURSING IMPLICATIONS: Inspect for dyspnea, inspiratory retractions, and diaphoresis. Percuss lung fields for dullness, auscultate for decreased breath sounds, also for tachycardia. Provide respiratory toilet, and incentive spirometry or IPPB treatments as prescribed. Prevent occurrence postoperatively by encouraging deep breathing and coughing, frequent repositioning, and by administering analgesia to relieve pain and facilitate ventilatory effort. Assist patient to mobilize and clear secretions. Provide emotional support.

atelencephalia (ăt-ĕl″ĕn-sĕ-fā′lē-ă) [Gr. *ateleia*, incompleteness, + *enkephalos*, brain]. Congenital anomaly with imperfect development of the brain. Also spelled *ateloencephalia*.

atelia (ă-tē′lē-ă) [Gr. *ateleia*, incompleteness]. Imperfect or incomplete development.

ateliosis (ă-tē″lē-ō′sĭs) [Gr. *a-*, not, + *teleios*, complete, + *osis*, condition]. A form of infantilism due to pituitary insufficiency, in which growth is arrested without deformity. The voice and face may resemble those of a child.

ateliotic (ă-tē″lē-ŏt′ĭk). Pert. to or characterized by atelia.

atelo- (ăt′ĕ-lō) [Gr. *ateles*, imperfect]. Prefix denoting imperfect or incomplete.

atelocardia (ăt″ĕ-lō-kăr′dē-ă) [″ + *kardia*, heart]. Congenital incomplete development of the heart.

atelocephaly (ăt″ĕ-lō-sĕf′ă-lē) [″ + *kephale*, head]. Incomplete development of the head.

atelocheilia (ăt″ĕ-lō-kī′lē-ă) [″ + *cheilos*, lip]. Incomplete development of the lip.

atelocheiria (ăt″ĕ-lō-kī′rē-ă) [″ + *cheir*, hand]. Incomplete development of the hand.

ateloencephalia (ăt″ĕ-lō-ĕn″sĕ-fā′lē-ă). Atelencephalia.

ateloglossia (ăt″ĕ-lō-glŏs′ē-ă) [″ + *glossa*, tongue]. Incomplete development of the tongue.

atelognathia (ăt″ĕ-lŏg-nā′thē-ă) [″ + *gnathos*, jaw]. Incomplete development of the jaw.

atelomyelia (ăt″ĕ-lō-mī-ē′lē-ă) [″ + *myelos*, marrow]. Incomplete development of the spinal cord.

atelopodia (ăt″ĕ-lō-pō′dē-ă) [″ + *pous*, foot]. Incomplete development of the foot.

ateloprosopia (ăt″ĕ-lō-prō-sō′pē-ă) [″ + *prosopon*, face]. Incomplete development of the face.

atelorhachidia (ăt″ĕ-lō-rā-kĭd′ē-ă) [″ + *rhachis*, spine]. Incomplete development of the spinal cord.

atelostomia (ăt″ĕ-lō-stō′mē-ă) [″ + *stoma*, mouth]. Incomplete development of the mouth.

athelia (ă-thē′lē-ă) [Gr. *a-*, not, + *thele*, nipple]. Congenital absence of the nipples.

athermic, athermous (ă-thĕr′mĭk, -mŭs) [″ + *therme*, heat]. Without fever or rise of temperature.

athermosystaltic (ă-thĕr″mō-sĭs-tăl′tĭk) [″ + ″ + *systaltikos*, drawing together].

Not contracting due to action of heat or cold, said of skeletal muscle.

atherogenesis (ăth″ĕr-ō-jĕn′ĕ-sĭs) [Gr. *athere*, porridge, + *genesis*, generation, birth]. Formation of atheromata in the walls of arteries.

atheroma (ăth″ĕr-ō′mă) [″ + *oma*, tumor] (pl. *atheromata*). Fatty degeneration or thickening of the walls of the larger arteries occurring in atherosclerosis, q.v. SEE: *arteriosclerosis*.

atheromatosis (ăth″ĕr-ō″mă-tō′sĭs). Generalized atheromatous disease of the arteries.

atheromatous (ăth″ĕr-ō′mă-tŭs). Pert. to atheroma.

atheronecrosis (ăth″ĕr-ō″nĕ-krō′sĭs) [″ + *nekros*, corpse, + *osis*, condition]. Necrosis or degeneration accompanying arteriosclerosis, q.v.

atherosclerosis (ăth″ĕr-ō″sklĕ-rō′sĭs) [″ + Gr. *sklerosis*, hardness]. The most common form of arteriosclerosis, q.v.

athetoid (ăth′ĕ-toyd) [Gr. *athetos*, unfixed, changeable, + *eidos*, form, shape]. Resembling or affected with athetosis.

athetosis (ăth-ĕ-tō′sĭs) [″ + *osis*, condition]. A condition in which slow, irregular, twisting, snakelike movements occur in the upper extremities, esp. in the hands and fingers. These involuntary movements prevent sustaining the body, esp. the extremities, in one position. All four limbs may be affected or the involvement may be unilateral. The symptoms may be due to one of several diseases, including encephalitis, cerebral palsy, hepatic encephalopathy, drug toxicity, Huntington chorea, and as an undesired side effect of prolonged treatment of parkinsonism with levodopa.

Types of athetosis: Athetosis with spasticity—muscle tone fluctuates between normal and hypertonic; there is frequently moderate spasticity in the proximal parts and athetosis more distally. Modified primitive spinal reflex patterns are often present.

Athetosis with tonic spasms—muscle tone fluctuates between hypotonus and hypertonus. Excessive extension or flexion is evident. There are strong postural asymmetry and frequent spinal or hip abnormalities or deformities.

Choreoathetosis—muscle tone fluctuates from either hypotonic to normal or hypotonic to hypertonic. There are extreme ranges of motion. Deformities are rare, but subluxation of the shoulder and finger joints often occurs.

Pure athetosis—this type is much rarer than others. Muscle tone fluctuates between hypotonus and normal. Deformities are rare. Twitches and jerks of muscles or individual muscle fibers are seen. Characterized by slow, writhing, involuntary movements that are more proximal than distal.

NURSING IMPLICATIONS: Assess muscle tone, joint range of motion, involuntary movements, and joint deformities. Evaluate interference with activities of daily living and self-image. Provide emotional support and acceptance, informing the patient of available support services and groups.

athlete's foot. A fungus infection of the foot caused by various dermatophytes, esp. *Trichophyton rubrum*, *T. mentagrophytes*, and *Epidermophyton floccosum*, which invade the "dead" outer layers of the skin. SYN: *dermatophytosis; tinea pedis*.

TREAT: Careful attention to hygiene is important. The feet, esp. between the toes, should be carefully dried after bathing. Loose macerated skin should be gently removed and a bland drying powder applied. Shoes that provide good ventilation and socks that absorb moisture are important treatment adjuncts. Going barefoot in suitable climates will be of benefit. Severe cases should be treated with griseofulvin, but most subacute or chronic cases will respond to one of several fungicidal medications such as 2% miconazole cream, 1% clotrimazole cream or lotion, or Whitfield's tincture (3% salicylic acid, 6% benzoic acid in 70% alcohol).

NURSING IMPLICATIONS: Teach the patient to practice scrupulous foot care, washing the feet daily and drying thoroughly with special attention to areas between the toes. Encourage application of prescribed powder or medications. Reinforce the importance of keeping the feet as dry as possible, wearing well-ventilated shoes and absorbent socks. SEE: *Nursing Diagnoses in Appendix.*

athletic trainer. A person who, as a result of training and experience, is capable of working with athletes and their environment to help prevent injuries, advise them concerning appropriate equipment, recognize and evaluate injuries, administer emergency treatment, and determine if specialized medical care is required. The athletic trainer is also involved as part of the health care team in rehabilitating those who have experienced sports injuries. In many instances, the first member of the health care team an injured athlete encounters is an athletic trainer. It is important that the trainer be prepared to act to ensure that the best possible treatment and management are provided. In some states in the U.S., athletic trainers must be licensed in order to practice. SEE: *training, athletic.*

athrepsia, athrepsy (ă-thrĕp′sē-ă, -sē) [Gr. *a-*, not, + *threpsis*, nourishment]. Malnutrition, marasmus, q.v.

Athrombin-K. Trade name for warfarin potassium, q.v.

athyroidemia (aĭh″ĭ-roy-, ă-thī″roy-dē′mē-ă) [″ + ″ + ″ + *haima*, blood]. Absence of thyroid hormone from the blood.

athyroidism (ă-thī′roy-dĭzm) [″ + ″ + ″ + *-ismos*, condition of]. Suppression of thyroid secretions, or absence of the thyroid gland; hypothyroidism.

atlantad (ăt-lăn′tăd). Toward the atlas.

atlantal (ăt-lăn′tăl). Pert. to the atlas.

atlantoaxial (ăt-lăn″tō-ăk′sē-ăl) [Gr. *atlas*, a support, + L. *axis*, a pivot]. Pertaining to the atlas, the first cervical vertebra, and the axis, the second cervical vertebra.

atlantodidymus (ăt-lăn″tō-dĭd′ĭ-mŭs) [″ + *didymus*, twin]. Atlodidymus, q.v.

atlanto-occipital (ăt-lăn″tō-ŏk-sĭp′ĭ-tăl) [″ + L. *occipitalis*, occipital]. Pertaining to the atlas and the occipital bones.

atlas (ăt′lăs) [Gr.]. [NA] The first cervical vertebra by which the head articulates with the occipital bone, so called because of Atlas, the Greek god who was supposed to support the world on his shoulders.

atloaxoid (ăt″lō-ăk′soyd) [″ + L. *axis*, a pivot, + Gr. *eidos*, form, shape]. Pert. to the atlas and axis.

atlodidymus (ăt-lō-dĭd′ĭ-mŭs) [″ + Gr. *didymos*, twin]. A malformed fetus with one body and two heads.

ATLS. *advanced trauma life support.*

atm. *atmosphere; atmospheric.*

atmo- [Gr. *atmos*, vapor or steam]. Prefix indicating rel. to steam or vapor.

atmosphere (ăt′mŏs-fĕr) [″ + *sphaira*, sphere]. 1. The gases surrounding the earth. 2. Climatic condition of a locality. 3. In physics, pressure of the air upon the earth at mean sea level, approx. 14.7 lb/sq in. (101325 pascals or 760 torr). 4. In chemistry, any gaseous medium around a body.

   a., standard. The pressure of air at sea level when the temperature is 0°C (32°F). This is equal to 14.7 lb/sq in., or 760 torr, or 101325 pascals (newtons per square meter). SYN: *standard atmosphere.*

atmospheric (ăt″mŏs-fĕr′ĭk). Pert. to the atmosphere.

ATN. *acute tubular necrosis.*

at. no. *atomic number.*

ATNR. *asymmetrical tonic neck reflex.*

atom (ăt′ŏm) [Gr. *atomos*, indivisible]. The smallest part of an element. The atom consists of the nucleus, which contains protons and neutrons, and surrounding electrons. The nucleus is positively charged, and this determines the atomic number of an element. A large number of entities in the atomic nucleus have been identified, and the search for others continues. Dimensions of atoms are of the order of 10^{-8} cm. SEE: *atomic theory; electron.*

a., tagged. An atom that has been made radioactive so that its course may be followed in the body. SYN: *radioactive tracer.*

atomic (ă-tŏm′ĭk). Pert. to an atom or atoms.

atomic number. ABBR: at. no. Number of protons in the nucleus of an atom.

atomic theory. 1. Theory that all matter is composed of atoms. 2. Theories pert. to the structure, properties, and behavior of the atom.

atomic weight. ABBR: at. wt. The relative weight of an atom as compared with the standard carbon atom isotope with a mass of 12. Therefore, carbon has an at. wt. of 12; oxygen, 16; hydrogen, 1.008; and nitrogen, 14.008.

atomization (ăt″ŏm-ĭ-zā′shŭn). Converting a fluid into spray or vapor form. SEE: *nebulizer; vaporizer.*

atomize (ăt′ŏm-īz). To reduce a liquid to the form of a spray or a vapor.

atomizer (ăt′ŏm-ī-zĕr). Apparatus for changing jet of liquid to a spray.

atonic (ă-tŏn′ĭk) [Gr. *a*, not, + *tonos*, stretching]. Without normal tension or tone.

atonicity (ăt-ō-nĭs′ĭ-tē). State of being atonic, or without tone.

atony (ăt′ō-nē) [″ + *tonos*, stretching]. Debility; or lack of normal tone or strength.

a., gastric. Lack of muscle tone in stomach and failure to contract normally, causing a delay in movement of food out of stomach. Secondary to certain diseases.

atopen (ăt′ō-pĕn) [″ + *topos*, place]. An allergen, exciting cause of atopy, q.v.

atopic (ă-tŏp′ĭk). 1. Pert. to atopy. 2. Displaced; malpositioned.

atopognosis (ă-tŏp″ŏg-nō′sĭs) [″ + *topos*, place, + *gnosis*, knowledge]. Inability to locate a sensation of touch or feeling.

atopy (ăt′ō-pē) [Gr. *atopia*, strangeness]. A Type I hypersensitivity or allergic reaction for which there was a genetic predisposition. Differs from normal hypersensitivity reactions to various allergies that are not genetically determined. The basis for the predisposition lies in the histocompatibility genes. The child of two parents with the atopic allergy has a 75% chance of developing similar symptoms; if one parent is affected, the child has a 50% chance of developing the atopy. Hay fever and asthma are two of the most commonly inherited allergies; contact dermatitis and gastrointestinal reactions also may be inherited. As with all Type I hypersensitivity reactions, IgE is the primary

antibody involved. SEE: *allergy; immunity; reagin.*

atoxic [Gr. *a-*, not, + *toxikon*, poison]. Nonpoisonous.

ATP. *adenosine triphosphate.*

ATPase. *adenosine triphosphatase.*

atraumatic (ā″traw-măt′ĭk) [Gr. *a-*, not, + *traumatikos*, relating to injury]. Not causing trauma or injury. SEE: *needle, atraumatic.*

atresia (ă-trē′zē-ă) [″ + *tresis*, a perforation]. Congenital absence or closure of a normal body opening or tubular structure.

a., anal; a. ani. Imperforate anus.

a., aortic. Congenital closure of the aortic valvular opening into the aorta.

a., biliary. Closure or absence of some or all of the major bile ducts.

a., duodenal. Congenital closure of a portion of the duodenum.

a., esophageal. Congenital failure of the esophageal tube to develop.

a., follicular. Normal death of the ovarian follicle following failure of the ovum to be fertilized.

a., intestinal. Congenital closure of any part of the intestine.

a., mitral. Congenital closure of the mitral valve opening.

a., prepyloric. Congenital closure of the pyloric end of the stomach.

a., pulmonary. Congenital closure of the pulmonary valve between the right ventricle and the pulmonary artery.

a., tricuspid. Congenital closure of the tricuspid valve between the right atrium and ventricle.

a., urethral. Absence or closure of the urethral orifice or canal.

a., vaginal. Congenital closure or absence of the vagina.

atresic (ă-trē′zĭk). Pert. to atresia.

atreto- (ă-trē′tō) [Gr. *atretos,* imperforate]. Prefix signifying absence of an opening.

atria (ā′trē-ă). Pl. of atrium, q.v.

atrial (ā′trē-ăl). Pert. to the atrium.

atrial fibrillation. ABBR: AF. Irregular and rapid discharge from multiple ectopic atrial foci cause randomized quivering of the atria with no real atrial systole to force blood into the ventricles and enhance cardiac output, and no real atrial diastole. Impulses are transmitted through the A-V node at irregular intervals, causing an irregularly irregular ventricular response, often very rapid when untreated. The apical impulse varies in strength and stroke volume as well as rhythm; thus some beats are not transmitted to peripheral sites, resulting in a pulse deficit.

Patients with chronic atrial fibrillation are at risk of cerebral emboli from dislodged mural thrombi, so anticoagulants are usually prescribed. The cardiac arrhythmia is recognized from the lack of P waves, irregularly irregular ventricular complexes, and wavy baseline.

ETIOL: May occur in normal persons, esp. during stress or exercise, in acute alcoholism, and post surgery. May be present in persons with cardiopulmonary disease who develop acute hypoxia, increased CO_2 (hypercapnia), or metabolic disorders. Persistent AF usually occurs in patients with rheumatic heart disease, mitral valve disease, hypertension, or thyrotoxicosis.

NURSING IMPLICATIONS: Evaluate apical-radial pulses for pulse deficit. Evaluate patient for evidence of forward cardiac failure (fatigue, activity intolerance) and backward failure (pulmonary congestion, neck vein distention, anorexia, peripheral edema, and weight gain). Instruct patient concerning optimal physical function by utilizing frequent rest periods and the need to restrict sodium intake, and instruct concerning the prescribed drug(s).

atrial flutter. A cardiac arrhythmia originating in the atrial muscle cells characterized by rapid (approximately 300 times per minute) regular atrial activity and usually regular ventricular response of varying rates (usually a factor of 300).

atrial natriuretic factor. A hormone secreted by the atrial tissue of the heart in response to an increase in blood pressure. The hormone influences blood pressure, blood volume, and cardiac output. It also stimulates the excretion of salt in the urine. These actions serve to reduce the workload of the heart.

atrichia (ă-trĭk'ē-ă) [Gr. *a-*, not, + *thrix*, hair]. 1. Absence of hair. 2. Lacking cilia or flagella.

atrichosis (ă-tri-kō'sĭs) [" + " + *osis*, condition]. Congenital absence of hair.

atrichous (ă-trĭk'ŭs). 1. Without flagella. 2. Without hair.

atrionector (ăt″rē-ō-nĕk'tor) [L. *atrium*, corridor, + *nector*, connector]. Sinoatrial node.

atrioseptopexy (ă″trē-ō-sĕp'tō-pĕk″sē) [" + *saeptum*, a partition, + Gr. *pexis*, fixation]. Plastic surgical repair of an interatrial septal defect.

atriotome (ā'trē-ō-tōm) [" + Gr. *tome*, incision]. Instrument used in surgically opening the cardiac atrium.

atrioventricular (ā″trē-ō-vĕn-trĭk'ū-lăr) [" + *ventriculus*, ventricle]. Pert. to both atrium and ventricle.

atrioventricular bundle. A bundle of modified cardiac muscle fibers that forms a part of the impulse-conducting system of the heart. It extends from the atrioventricular (A-V) node a short distance in the intraventricular septum, then divides into two branches that supply fibers to the two ventricles. SYN: *bundle of His.*

atrioventricular (A-V) junction. Cardiac tissue surrounding the A-V node, including the bundle of His, which can function automatically.

atrioventricularis communis (ā″trē-ō-vĕn-trĭk″ū-lā′rĭs kŏ-mū′nĭs). Persistence of the common atrioventricular canal. A congenital anomaly of the heart in which the division of the common atrioventricular canal in the embryo fails to occur. This causes atrial septal defect and atrioventricular valve incompetence.

atriplicism (ă-trĭp'lĭ-sĭzm). Poisoning due to eating one form of spinach, *Atriplex littoralis.*

atrium (ā'trē-ŭm) [L., corridor] (pl. *atria*). A chamber or cavity communicating with another structure.

a. of ear. Portion of the tympanic cavity lying below the malleus; the tympanic cavity proper.

a. of heart. The upper chamber of each half of the heart. The right atrium receives deoxygenated, dark red blood from the entire body (except lungs) through the superior and inferior venae cavae and coronary sinus; the left atrium receives oxygenated red blood from the lungs through the pulmonary veins. Blood passes from the atria to the ventricles through the atrioventricular orifices. In the embryo, the atrium is a single chamber that lies between the sinus venosus and the ventricle.

a. of lungs. The space at the end of an alveolar duct that opens into the alveoli, or air sacs, of the lungs.

Atromid-S. Trade name for clofibrate, q.v.

atrophia (ă-trō'fē-ă) [Gr.]. Wasting; a decrease in size of an organ or tissue. SYN: *atrophy.*

atrophic (ă-trō'fĭk). Pert. to, or marked by, atrophy.

atrophie blanche. SEE: *livedoid vasculitis.*

atrophied (ăt'rō-fēd). Wasted. Afflicted with atrophy.

atrophoderma (ăt″rō-fō-dĕr'mă) [Gr. *a-*, not, + *trophe*, nourishment, + *derma*, skin]. Atrophy of the skin.

atrophodermatosis (ăt-rō″fō-dĕr-mă-tō′ sĭs) [" + " + " + *osis*, condition]. Any skin disease in which cutaneous atrophy is a prominent symptom.

atrophy (ăt'rō-fē) [Gr. *atrophia*]. 1. A wasting; a decrease in size of an organ or tissue. 2. To undergo or cause atrophy.

ETIOL: May result from death and resorption of cells, diminished cellular proliferation, pressure, ischemia, malnutrition, decreased activity, or hormonal changes.

a., acute yellow. Extensive necrosis of liver cells with jaundice, mental disturbances, and cutaneous hemorrhages. A complication of hepatitis.

SYM: Early central nervous system symptoms before jaundice sets in; slow onset; some fever with nausea and vomiting; black vomit; malaise.

a., brown. Atrophic tissue that has a yellowish-brown appearance rather than its normal color. Seen principally in the heart and liver of aging persons. The pigmentation is due to the presence of lipofuscin, which is known as the "wear and tear" pigment associated with aging. Its presence in tissue is a sign of free radical injury. SEE: *lipofucsin; radical, free.*

a., compression. Atrophy due to constant pressure on a part.

a., correlated. Wasting of a part following destruction of a correlated part.

a., Cruveilhier's. Atrophy of the spinal muscles.

a., healed yellow. Postnecrotic cirrhosis of the liver.

a., Hoffmann's. SEE: *Werdnig-Hoffmann disease.*

a., Landouzy-Déjérine. A hereditary form of progressive muscular dystrophy with onset in childhood or adolescence. Characterized by atrophic changes in muscles of shoulder girdle and face, inability to raise arms above the head, myopathic facies, eyelids that remain partly open in sleep; and inability to whistle or purse lips. SYN: *dystrophy, Landouzy-Déjérine.*

a., muscular. Atrophy of muscle tissue, esp. due to lack of use or denervation.

a., myelopathic. Muscular atrophy resulting from a lesion of the spinal cord.

a., myotonic. Myotonia congenita, q.v.

a. of disuse. Atrophy from failure to exercise a part normally.

a., optic. Atrophy of the optic disk resulting from degeneration of the second cranial (optic) nerve.

a., pathologic. Atrophy that results from the effects of disease processes.

a., peroneal muscular. A hereditary disease characterized by atrophy of muscles supplied by peroneal nerves, progressing slowly to the muscles of hands and arms. SYN: *Charcot-Marie-Tooth disease,* q.v.

a., physiologic. Atrophy that occurs as a result of the normal aging processes in the body.

Ex.: Atrophy of embryonic structures; atrophy of childhood structures upon reaching maturity, as the thymus; atrophy of structures in cyclic phases of activity, as the corpus luteum; atrophy of structures following cessation of functional activity, as the ovary and mammary glands; and atrophy of structures with aging.

a., postmenopausal vaginal. SEE: *vaginal atrophy, postmenopausal.*

a., progressive muscular. Chronic disease marked by progressive wasting of the motor cells of the spinal cord; the muscular atrophy begins with the extremities and ultimately causes death from paralysis of muscles of respiration. SYN: *Duchenne-Aran disease.* SEE: *dystrophy, progressive muscular; sclerosis, amyotrophic lateral.*

a., Sudeck's. [Paul Herman Martin Sudeck, Ger. surgeon, 1866–1938]. Acute atrophy of a bone at the site of injury. Probably due to reflex local vasospasm.

a., trophoneurotic. Atrophy due to disease of the nerves or nerve centers supplying the affected muscles.

a., unilateral facial. Progressive atrophy of one side of the facial tissues.

atropine sulfate (ăt′rō-pēn sŭl′fāt). USP. Salt of an alkaloid obtained from belladonna. It is a parasympatholytic agent and counteracts effects of parasympathetic stimulation. Used prior to the administration of a general anesthetic agent to inhibit salivation and secretions of the respiratory tract. The use of relatively nonirritating anesthetics has decreased the need of atropine for that purpose.

atropine sulfate poisoning. SYM: Dryness of mouth; thirst; burning pain in throat; dry, hot, and flushed skin; hyperpyrexia; palpitations; restlessness; excitement; delirium.

F.A.: Lavage with slurry of activated charcoal or 1% tannic acid. Pilocarpine will make patient more comfortable, but barbiturates are required to control excitement. SEE: *Poisons and Poisoning* in *Appendix.*

atropinism, atropism (ăt′rō-pĭn-ĭzm, -pĭzm). Atropine poisoning.

atropinization (ăt-rō″pĭn-ĭ-zā′shŭn). Administration of atropine until desired pharmacologic effect is achieved.

Atropisol. Trade name for atropine sulfate, q.v.

attachment (ă-tăch′mĕnt). 1. A device or other material affixed to something else. 2. In dentistry, a plastic or metal device used for retention or stabilization of a dental prosthesis, such as a partial denture.

a., epithelial. The mechanism by which the surrounding soft tissue is attached to the calcified tooth root.

attack (ă-tăk′) [Fr. *attaquer*, join]. 1. The onset of an illness or symptom, usually dramatic, e.g., a heart attack or an attack of gout. 2. An assault.

attendant. A paramedical hospital employee who assists in the care of patients.

attending. The person having primary responsibility for a patient.

attention [L. *attendere*, to wait upon]. Directing or concentrating one's consciousness on only one object or an internal or external stimulus.

attention deficit disorder. ABBR: ADD. The American Psychiatric Association describes this as a disease of infancy and childhood characterized by developmentally inappropriate inattention, impulsivity, and hyperactivity. The children do not persist with tasks and problems, and they have difficulty organizing and completing work. Their school work is performed impulsively and is sloppy; and is full of oversights such as omissions, insertions, and misrepresentation of easy items. The children appear not to listen or not to have heard what was said. The hyperactivity component is characterized by the children being unable to sit still and by excessive running or climbing. The activity tends to be haphazard, poorly organized, and not goal-directed. All of the symptoms vary with situation and time. Also, the condition may exist without the hyperactivity component.

The onset in half of the cases is prior to age four and may occur in 3% of children. It is six to nine times more common in boys than girls.

A variety of names have been applied to this disorder: hyperkinetic syndrome; hyperactive child syndrome; minimal brain damage; minimal brain dysfunction; minimal cerebral dysfunction. SYN: *hyperactive syndrome.*

TREAT: Careful attention to home, social, and school environmental factors that contribute to the child's difficulties. Establish routines and goals, and praise the child when either they are achieved or a reasonable effort is made. Medications that have been of benefit include methylphenidate, dextroamphetamine, and magnesium pemoline.

attention reflex. Change in size of pupil when attention is suddenly fixed. SYN: *Piltz's reflex.*

attenuant (ă-tĕn'ū-ănt) [L. *attenuare*, to thin]. 1. Diluting, making thin or weak. 2. An agent that thins the blood.

attenuate (ă-tĕn'ū-āt). To render thin or make less virulent.

attenuated (ă-tĕn'ū-āt'd). 1. Diluted. 2. Pert. to reduced virulence of pathogenic microorganism.

attenuation (ă-tĕn″ū-ā'shŭn). 1. Dilution. 2. Lessening of virulence. This may be accomplished with bacteria and viruses by heating, drying, treating with chemicals, passing through another organism, or culturing under unfavorable conditions. 3. The change (decrease) in a beam of radiation as it passes through matter. 4. In acoustics, the reduction in sound intensity of the initial sound source as compared with the sound intensity at a point away from the source.

Attenuvax. Trade name for measles virus vaccine, live, q.v.

attic (ăt'ĭk) [L. *atticus*]. The cavity of the middle ear or the portion lying above the tympanic cavity proper. SYN: *recess, epitympanic.* SEE: *ear; tympanum.*

attic disease. Chronic suppurative inflammation of the attic of the ear.

atticitis (ăt″ĭ-sī'tĭs) [L. *atticus*, attic, + Gr. *itis*, inflammation]. Inflammation of the attic of the ear.

atticoantrotomy (ăt″ĭ-kō-ăn-trŏt'ō-mē) [″ + Gr. *antron*, cave, + *tome*, incision]. Surgical opening of the attic and mastoid antrum of the ear.

atticotomy (ăt″ĭ-kŏt'ō-mē) [″ + Gr. *tome*, incision]. Surgical opening of tympanic attic of the ear.

attitude [LL. *aptitudo*, fitness]. 1. Bodily posture or position assumed, esp. with reference to position of limbs. A particular attitude is often a symptom of disease or abnormal mental state, e.g., the stereotyped position assumed by catatonics or theatric expression seen in hysteria. 2. Behavior toward a person, group, thing, or situation representative of conscious or unconscious mental views developed through cumulative experience.

   a., crucifixion. Position in which body is rigid with arms at right angles to long axis of body. Seen in catatonia.

   a., defense. Position automatically assumed to avert pain.

   a., fetal. Position of the fetus with respect to maternal anatomical landmarks.

   a., forced. Abnormal position due to disease or contractures.

   a., frozen. Stiffness of gait, seen in amyotrophic lateral sclerosis.

   a., illogical. Peculiar attitudes caused by disease.

   a., passional. Theatric or dramatic gestures and expressions of face and figure assumed by hysteric patients.

   a., stereotyped. Position taken and held for a long period, seen frequently in mental diseases.

atto [Danish, *atten*, eighteen]. SYMB: a. In SI units, a prefix indicating 10^{-18}.

attolens (ă-tōl'ĕnz) [L.]. Raising or lifting up.

attraction (ă-trăk'shŭn) [L. *attrahere*, to draw toward]. Force, act, or process that causes bodies to approach each other.

   a., capillary. The force by which liquids rise in fine tubes or through pores of loose material.

a., chemical. The tendency of atoms of one element to unite with those of another to form compounds.

a., molecular. The tendency of molecules with unlike electrical charges to attract each other. SEE: *adhesion; cohesion.*

attrahens. To bring toward.

attribute [L. *attributus*, character, reputation]. A quality or characteristic of animate or inanimate objects, e.g., adaptability is an attribute of living organisms.

attrition (ă-trĭsh'ŭn) [L. *attritio*, a rubbing against]. 1. Wearing away by friction or rubbing. 2. Any friction that breaks the skin. 3. Wearing away, as of teeth, in the course of normal use.

at. wt. *atomic weight.*

atypia (ā-tĭp'ē-ă) [Gr. *a-*, not, + *typos*, type]. The state of not conforming to a standard or regular type.

atypical (ā-tĭp'ĭ-kăl) [" + *typikos*, pert. to type]. Deviating from the normal; not conforming to type.

A.U. *angstrom unit; aures unitas*, both ears; *auris uterique*, each ear.

Au [L. *aurum*]. Chem. symb. for the element gold.

Aub-Dubois table (awb-dū-boy') [Joseph C. Aub, U.S. physician, 1890–1973; Eugene F. Dubois, U.S. physician, 1882–1959]. Table of normal basal metabolic rates according to age.

audible. Capable of being heard.

audible sound. Sound containing frequency components between 15 and 15,000 Hz (cycles per second).

audile (aw'dĭl). 1. Pert. to hearing. 2. Individual who retains more of what is heard than information received through other forms of communication. 3. In psychoanalysis, one whose mental images are auditory. SEE: *motile; visile.*

audioanesthesia (aw"dē-ō-ăn"ĕs-thē'zē-ă) [L. *audire*, to hear, + Gr. *an-*, not, + *aisthesis*, sensation]. Anesthesia or analgesia produced by sound; used by dentists to help prevent perception of pain.

audiogenic (aw-dē-ō-jĕn'ĭk) [" + Gr. *genesis*, generation, birth]. Originating in sound.

audiogram (aw'dē-ō-grăm") [" + Gr. *gramma*, something written]. Record of the audiometer. SEE: illus.

audiologist. A specialist in the evaluation, habilitation, and rehabilitation of persons with disorders of hearing function.

audiology (aw"dē-ŏl'ō-jē) [" + Gr. *logos*, word, reason]. The study of hearing disorders through identification and evaluation of hearing loss, and the rehabilitation of persons with hearing loss, esp. that which

cannot be improved by medical or surgical means.

audiometer (aw"dē-ŏm'ĕ-tĕr) [" + Gr. *metron*, measure]. An instrument for testing hearing.

audiometry (aw"dē-ŏm'ĕ-trē). Testing of the hearing sense. SEE: *spondee threshold.*

a., averaged electroencephalic. A method of testing the hearing of children who cannot be adequately tested by conventional means. The test is based on the electroencephalogram's being altered by perceived sound without the requirement of behavioral response. Thus the test may be done while an autistic, severely retarded, or hyperkinetic child is asleep or sedated. SEE: *auditory evoked response.*

a., evoked response. Use of computer-aided technique to average the brain's response to latency of auditory stimuli. Auditory brain stem evoked response (ABER) is one form of this type of audiometry. This method of testing hearing ability is used in individuals, esp. children, who cannot be tested in the usual manner.

audit. In medical care facilities, an official examination of the record of all aspects of patient care. This is done by trained staff, who are not usually affiliated with the institution. The purpose of an audit is to be able to compare the quality of care provided with accepted standards.

audition (aw-dĭ'shŭn) [L. *auditio*, hearing]. Hearing.

a., chromatic. Condition in which certain color sensations are aroused by sound stimuli.

a., colored. Condition in which color sensation is perceived when certain sounds reach the ear.

a., gustatory. Condition in which certain taste sensations are aroused by sound stimuli.

a., mental. Recollection of a sound based on previous auditory impressions.

audito-oculogyric reflex (aw"dĭt-ō-ŏk"ū-lō-jĭ'rĭk). The sudden turning of the head and eyes in direction of an alarming sound.

auditory (aw'dĭ-tō"rē) [L. *auditorius*]. Pert. to the sense of hearing.

auditory brain stem evoked response. ABBR: ABER. SEE: *brain stem auditory evoked responses.*

auditory bulb. The membranous labyrinth and cochlea.

auditory canal. One of the two canals associated with the structures of each ear. They are the external auditory canal, leading from the external auditory meatus to the tympanic membrane, length less than 1 in. (2.5 cm); and the internal auditory canal, leading from the structures of the inner ear

AUDIOGRAM
LEFT EAR

A PRESBYACUSIS. AIR AND BONE CONDUCTION ARE EQUALLY AFFECTED.

B SEVERE MIXED HEARING LOSS.

C MODERATELY SEVERE MIXED HEARING LOSS.

D PURE AIR CONDUCTION LOSS BECAUSE OF UNCOMPLICATED OTOSCLEROSIS.

E NORMAL AUDIOGRAM.

< LEFT EAR BONE CONDUCTION, RIGHT EAR MASKED

X LEFT EAR AIR CONDUCTION

to the internal auditory meatus and the cranial cavity, for the transmission of the nerves of hearing and equilibrium.

auditory epilepsy. Epilepsy in which the attack is precipitated by certain sounds. SEE: *epilepsy.*

auditory evoked response. Response to auditory stimuli as determined by a method independent of the individual's subjective response. The electroencephalogram has been used to record response to sound. By measuring intensity of sound and presence of response, one can test the acuity of hearing of psychiatric patients, persons who are asleep, and children too young to cooperate in a standard hearing test. SEE: *audiometry, averaged electroencephalic.*

auditory muscles. The tensor tympani and stapedius muscles. SEE: *Muscles* in *Appendix.*

auditory nerve. The 8th cranial nerve; it is a sensory nerve with two sets of fibers: cochlear nerve (hearing) and vestibular nerve (equilibrium), the latter having three branches, the superior, inferior, and middle branches. SYN: *vestibulocochlear nerve.*

auditory ossicles. The bones of the middle ear. SEE: *ear* for illus.

auditory placode. The embryonic thickenings of the epithelial layer, which become the inner ear of the embryo.

auditory reflex. Any reflex produced by stimulation of the auditory nerve, esp. blinking of the eyes upon the sudden unexpected production of a sound.

auditory teeth. Toothlike projections in the cochlea.

auditory tube. Eustachian tube, q.v.

Auenbrugger's sign (ow-ĕn-broog'ĕrz) [Leopold Joseph Auenbrugger, Austrian physician, 1722–1809]. Epigastric prominence due to marked pericardial effusion.

Auerbach's plexus (ow'ĕr-bǎks) [Leopold Auerbach, Ger. anatomist, 1828–1897]. A plexus of sympathetic nerve fibers situated between the longitudinal and circular fibers of the muscular coat of the stomach and intestines. SYN: *plexus myentericus.*

Auer's bodies (ow'ĕrz) [John Auer, U.S. physician, 1875–1948]. Rod-shaped structures present in the cytoplasm of myeloblasts, myelocytes, and monoblasts. They are pathognomic of leukemia.

Aufrecht's sign (owf'rĕkhts) [Emanuel Aufrecht, Ger. physician, 1844–1933]. Diminished breathing sound heard above the jugular fossa indicative of tracheal stenosis.

augment (awg-mĕnt') [L. *augmentum,* increase]. To add to or increase.

augmentation (awg″mĕn-tā'shŭn). The act, process, or condition of augmenting.

Ex.: Adding to or increasing the action of

a muscle; the enhancement of the action of a drug.

  a., breast. SEE: *mammaplasty, augmentation.*

augmentative communication. The use of technological systems, usually involving microcomputers, for improving or enabling disabled persons to have the ability to communicate.

augnathus (awg-nā'thŭs) [Gr. *au,* again, + *gnathos,* jaw]. Fetus with a double lower jaw.

aura (aw'rǎ) [L., breeze]. A subjective sensation preceding a paroxysmal attack. In epilepsy the aura may precede the attack by several hours or only by a few seconds. Epileptic aura may be of a psychic nature or sensory with olfactory, visual, auditory, or taste hallucinations. In migraine the aura immediately precedes the attack and consists of ocular sensory phenomena.

aural (aw'rǎl) [L. *auris,* the ear]. 1. Pert. to the ear. 2. Pert. to an aura.

aural polyp. SEE: *polyp, aural.*

aurantiasis cutis (aw″rǎn-tī'ǎ-sĭs kū'tĭs) [L. *aurantium,* orange, + Gr. *-iasis,* condition of; L. *cutis,* skin]. Yellow pigmentation of skin due to ingesting excessive amount of foods that contain carotene, such as carrots, oranges, and squash. SEE: *carotenemia.*

Aureomycin (aw″rē-ō-mī'sĭn). Trade name for the antibiotic chlortetracycline hydrochloride, q.v.

auriasis (aw-rī'ǎ-sĭs) [L. *aurum,* gold, + Gr. *-iasis,* condition of]. 1. Gray patches of skin discoloration after administration of gold. 2. Deposition of gold in tissues. SYN: *chrysiasis.*

auric (aw'rĭk) [L. *aurum,* gold]. Pert. to gold.

auricle (aw'rĭ-kl). Auricula, q.v.

auricula (aw-rĭk'ū-lǎ) [L., little ear] (pl. *auriculae*). 1. [NA] The portion of the external ear not contained within the head; the pinna. 2. A small conical pouch forming a portion of the right and left atria of the heart. Each projects from the upper anterior portion of each atrium. 3. An obsolete term for the atrium of the heart.

auricular (aw-rĭk'ū-lǎr). Rel. to the auricle of the ear.

auriculare (aw-rĭk″ū-lā'rē) (pl. *auricularia*). A craniometric point at center of opening of external auditory canal.

auriculocervical nerve reflex (aw-rĭk″ū-lō-sĕr'vĭk'l) [L. *auricula,* little ear, + *cervicalis,* pert. to the neck]. Congestion of ear on same side upon stimulation of distal end of the divided auriculocervical nerve. SYN: *Snellen's reflex.*

auriculocranial (aw-rĭk″ū-lō-krā'nē-ǎl) [″ + *cranialis,* pert. to the skull]. Concerned with the ear and the cranium.

auriculopalpebral reflex (aw-rĭk″ū-lō-păl′pĕb-răl) [″ + *palpebra*, eyelid]. Closure of the eye resulting from tactile or thermal stimulation of the external auditory meatus or deeper portions of canal up to the tympanum. SYN: *Kisch's reflex*.

auriculotemporal (aw-rĭk″ū-lō-tĕm′pŏ-răl) [″ + *temporalis*, pert. to the temples]. Pert. to the ear and area of the temple.

auriform (aw′rĭ-form) [L. *auris*, ear, + *forma*, shape]. Ear-shaped.

auris (aw′rĭs) [L.]. The ear.

  a. dextra. Right ear.

  a. externa. External ear (pinna and external auditory meatus).

  a. interna. Internal ear (semicircular canals, vestibule, cochlea).

  a. media. Middle ear (tympanum).

  a. sinistra. Left ear.

auriscalp, auriscalpium (aw′rĭ-skălp, aw″rĭ-skăl′pē-ŭm) [″ + *scalpere*, to scrape]. 1. Scraping instrument used to remove foreign matter from ear. 2. Earpick.

auriscope (aw′rĭ-skōp) [″ + Gr. *skopein*, to examine]. Instrument for making an ear examination. SYN: *otoscope*.

aurotherapy (aw″rō-thĕr′ă-pē) [L. *aurum*, gold, + Gr. *therapeia*, treatment]. Treatment of disease by administration of gold salts; used in the treatment of rheumatoid arthritis, autoimmune bullous disease, esp. pemphigus vulgaris. The advisability of using gold in treating rheumatoid arthritis is controversial. SYN: *chrysotherapy*.

Caution: Side effects, including toxicity to the kidneys and bone marrow, are important. The patient will need frequent monitoring of blood and urine.

aurum (aw′rŭm) [L.]. Gold.

auscult (aws-kŭlt′). Auscultate, q.v.

auscultate (aws′kŭl-tāt) [L. *auscultare*, listen to]. To examine by auscultation.

auscultation (aws″kŭl-tā′shŭn). Process of listening for sounds within the body, usually to sounds of thoracic or abdominal viscera, in order to detect some abnormal condition, or to detect fetal heart sounds. The technique is also helpful in diagnosing vascular abnormalities such as arteriovenous fistulae. SEE: *percussion.*

  PROCEDURE: The chest should be draped with a loose-fitting garment that can easily be moved aside to allow the stethoscope to be placed directly against the skin. When chest is covered with hair, moisten hair because it may produce friction sounds, resembling rales. Auscultate all over chest anteriorly and posteriorly, on full inspiration, full expiration, and after coughing. In comparing the two sides, auscultate sym-

metrical parts. Patient should be relaxed. Position of examiner is important, and should be situated so that his or her vascular sounds cannot be confused with those of the patient.

  a., immediate. Auscultation in which ear is applied directly to bared or thinly covered surface.

  a., mediate. Auscultation in which sounds are conducted from the surface to ear through an instrument such as a stethoscope.

auscultatory (aws-kŭl′tă-tō″rē). Pert. to auscultation.

auscultatory percussion. Auscultation at the same time percussion is made.

auscultoplectrum (aws-kŭl″tō-plĕk′trŭm) [L. *auscultare*, listen to, + Gr. *plektron*, hammer]. Instrument used for both auscultation and percussion.

Austin Flint murmur [Austin Flint, U.S. physician, 1812–1886]. A presystolic or late diastolic heart murmur best heard at the apex of the heart. It is present in some cases of aortic insufficiency and is thought to be due to the vibration of the mitral valve caused by the backward-flowing blood from the aorta meeting the blood flowing in from the left auricle.

Australia antigen. An antigen present in the sera of patients with viral hepatitis, but rarely present in patients with infectious hepatitis. This antigen is also found in normal populations in the tropics and southeast Asia. It was first isolated in the serum of an Australian aborigine. SYN: *hepatitis B surface antigen.*

autacoid (aw′tă-koyd) [Gr. *autos*, self, + *akos*, remedy, + *eidos*, form, shape]. 1. A term originally used by the British physiologists Edward Shäfer and Sharpey-Shafer as a substitute for the word *hormone.* 2. A term used to describe prostaglandins and related compounds that are formed rapidly, act, and then decay or are destroyed enzymatically.

autarcesis (aw-tăr′sĭ-sĭs, aw″tăr-sē′sĭs) [″ + *arkein*, to ward off]. Resistance to infection through natural immunity.

autarcetic (awt″ăr-sĕt′ĭk). Pert. to autarcesis.

autism (aw′tĭzm) [Gr. *autos*, self, + *-ismos*, condition]. Mental introversion in which the attention or interest is fastened upon the patient's own ego. A self-centered mental state from which reality tends to be excluded.

  a., infantile. A syndrome appearing in childhood with symptoms of self-absorp-

tion, inaccessibility, aloneness, inability to relate, highly repetitive play and rage reactions if interrupted, predilection for rhythmical movements, and many language disturbances.
ETIOL: Unknown.

auto- [Gr. *autos*, self]. Prefix meaning self.

autoactivation (aw″tō-ăk″tĭ-vā′shŭn) [″ + L. *agere*, to act]. Gland activation by its own secretion.

autoagglutination (aw″tō-ă-gloo″tĭ-nā′shŭn) [″ + L. *agglutinare*, adhere to]. Agglutination, or clumping of red blood cells, in response to an autotransfusion, the transfusion of an individual's own blood which has been removed by phlebotomy or during surgery.

autoagglutinin (aw″tō-ă-glū′tĭ-nĭn). Substance present in an individual's blood that agglutinates that person's red blood cells.

autoamputation (aw″tō-ăm″pū-tā′shŭn). Spontaneous amputation of a part or limb. SEE: *ainhum.*

autoanalysis (aw″tō-ă-năl′ĭ-sĭs) [″ + *analyein*, break down]. Patient's own analysis of mental state underlying patient's mental disorder.

Autoanalyzer (aw″tō-ăn′ă-līz″ĕr). Trade name of a device for performing analytic tests on a large number of laboratory specimens. The testing is done automatically with the specimens being tested sequentially.

autoantibody (aw″tō-ăn′tĭ-bŏd″ē) [″ + *anti*, against, + AS *bodig*, body]. ABBR: AAb. An antibody, produced by B cells in response to an altered "self" antigen on one type of the body's own cells, that attacks and destroys these cells. Autoantibodies are the basis for autoimmune diseases such as rheumatoid arthritis and diabetes mellitus. Several theories exist as to why autoantibodies are formed. The most commonly accepted theory proposes that a virus or direct trauma damages the antigen, changing its appearance. Consequently, B cells see it as "non-self" or foreign, and antibodies are produced for its destruction. SEE: *antibody; antigen; autoimmunity; immunoglobulin.*

autoantigen (aw″tō-ăn′tĭ-jĕn) [″ + ″ + *gennan*, to produce]. A substance that stimulates the production of antibodies in the individual from which it was derived.

autoantitoxin (aw″tō-ăn″tĭ-tŏk′sĭn) [″ + ″ + *toxikon*, poison]. Antitoxin produced by the body itself.

autoblast (aw′tō-blăst) [″ + *blastos*, germ]. Independent cell, as a protozoa.

autocatalysis (aw″tō-kă-tăl′ĭ-sĭs) [″ + *katalysis*, dissolution]. Increase in the rate of a chemical reaction resulting from products that are produced in the reaction acting as catalysts. SEE: *catalyst.*

autocatharsis (aw-tō-kă-thăr′sĭs) [″ + *katharsis*, a cleansing]. A form of psychotherapy in which patients in discussing their own problems gain an insight into their mental difficulties.

autocatheterization. Catheterization of oneself, esp. urinary catheterization.

autochthonous (aw-tŏk′thō-nŭs) [Gr. *autos*, self, + *chthon*, earth]. 1. Found where developed, as in the case of a blood clot or a calculus. 2. Pert. to a tissue graft to a new site on the same individual.

autochthonous infections. Infections due to organisms normally present in the patient's body. These may occur when host defenses are compromised.

autocinesia, autocinesis (aw″tō-sĭ-nē′sē-ă, -nē′sĭs) [″ + *kinesis*, movement]. Voluntary movement. SYN: *autokinesis.*

autoclasis (aw″tŏk′lă-sĭs) [″ + *klasis*, a breaking]. Destruction of a part from internal causes.

autoclave (aw′tō-klāv) [″ + L. *clavis*, a key]. Apparatus for sterilization by steam pressure, usually at 250°F (121°C) for a specified length of time. SEE: *sterilization.*

autocrine factor. A growth factor produced by the cell, most probably in response to a virus. This factor is important in the development of malignancies.

autocrine system. The secretion of a cell that acts to influence only its own growth. SEE: *paracrine.*

autocystoplasty (aw″tō-sĭs′tō-plăs″tē) [″ + *kystis*, bladder, + *plassein*, to mold]. Plastic repair of bladder with grafts from patient's own body.

autocytolysis (aw″tō-sī-tŏl′ĭ-sĭs). Self-digestion or self-destruction of cells.

autodermic (aw″tō-dĕr′mĭk) [″ + *derma*, skin]. Pert. to one's own skin, esp. rel. to dermatoplasty with patient's own skin.

autodigestion (aw″tō-dī-jĕs′chŭn) [″ + L. *dis*, apart, + *gerere*, to carry]. Digestion of tissues by their own secretion, such as digestion of the stomach wall by gastric juice, which occurs in certain stomach disorders.

autodiploid (aw″tō-dĭp′loyd) [″ + *diploe*, fold, + *eidos*, form, shape]. Having two sets of chromosomes; caused by redoubling the chromosomes of the haploid cell.

autodrainage (aw″tō-drān′ĭj) [″ + AS *dreahnian*, drain]. Drainage of a cavity by the fluid passing through a channel made in patient's own tissues.

autoecholalia (aw″tō-ĕk-ō-lā′lē-ă) [″ + *echo*, echo, + *lalia*, babble]. Repetition of the last portion of one's own statements.

autoecic (aw-tē′sĭk) [″ + *oikos*, house]. Pert. to parasite that goes through its entire life cycle in one organism.

autoerotism (aw″tō-ē-rŏt′ĭsm) [Gr. *autos*, self, + *erotikos*, rel. to love]. Sexual arousal by one's own body or sexual gratification using one's own body, as in masturbation.

autoexamination (aw″tō-ĕg-zăm″ĭ-nā′shŭn) [″ + L. *examinare*, to examine]. Self-examination. SEE: *breast, self-examination of.*

autofundoscope (aw″tō-fŭn′dō-skōp) [″ + L. *fundus*, bottom, + Gr. *skopein*, to examine]. Apparatus for autoexamination of retinal vessels of the eye.

autogenesis (aw-tō-jĕn′ĕ-sĭs) [″ + *genesis*, generation, birth]. Abiogenesis; self-production; origin within the organism.

autogenetic, autogenic (aw-tō-jĕ-nĕt′ĭk, aw-tō-jĕn′ĭk). Pert. to self-production or autogenesis.

autogenous (aw-tŏj′ĕ-nŭs). 1. Self-producing; originating within the body. 2. Denoting a vaccine from a culture of the patient's own bacteria.

autograft (aw′tō-grăft) [″ + L. *graphium*, grafting knife]. A graft transferred from one part of a patient's body to another.

autohemagglutination (aw″tō-hĕm″ă-glū″tĭ-nā′shŭn). Agglutination of one's own red cells.

autohemic (aw″tō-hē′mĭk) [″ + *haima*, blood]. Done with one's own blood.

autohemolysin (aw″tō-hē-mŏl′ĭ-sĭn) [″ + ″ + *lysis*, dissolution]. Antibody acting on corpuscles of individual in whose blood it is formed.

autohemolysis (aw″tō-hē-mŏl′ĭ-sĭs). Hemolysis of a person's blood corpuscles by the person's own serum.

autohemotherapy (aw″tō-hē″mō-thĕr′ă-pē) [″ + *haima*, blood, + *therapeia*, treatment]. Treatment by withdrawal and injection intramuscularly of patient's own blood.

autohypnosis (aw″tō-hĭp-nō′sĭs). Self-induced hypnosis.

autoimmune disease (aw″tō-ĭm-mūn′) [″ + L. *immunis*, safe]. A disease produced when the body's normal tolerance of its own antigenic markers on cells disappears. Autoantibodies (AAbs) are produced by B lymphocytes and attack normal cells whose surface contains a "self" antigen or autoantigen (AAg) causing destruction of tissue. Diabetes mellitus, in which AAbs attack the insulin-producing cells of the pancreas, is one autoimmune disease. Others include rheumatoid arthritis, caused by inflammatory changes in the connective tissue of joints, and multiple sclerosis, caused by AAb destruction of the myelin sheath covering nerves. Hemolytic anemia, some forms of glomerulonephritis, myasthenia gravis, chronic thyroiditis, Reiter's syndrome, insulin-dependent diabetes mellitus, Graves' disease, and systemic lupus erythematosus are also considered to be autoimmune diseases. SEE: *autoimmunity.*

autoimmune theory. A physiological theory of aging, originally proposed by Dr. Ray Walford. Aging occurs because antibodies develop, attack, and destroy the normal cells in the body. According to this theory, defects occur in the body's autoimmune system so that it cannot distinguish itself from foreign structures.

autoimmunity (aw″tō-ĭm-mū′nĭ-tē). The loss of normal tolerance by the immune system of "self" antigens (autoantigens) on the surface of the body's cells. B cells are activated to produce autoantibodies (AAbs) against these autoantigens (AAgs), causing the destruction of normal tissue. Exactly why leukocytes do not normally react with "self" antigens is not known. It is theorized that, as the fetus develops, B and T cells circulating in the blood are exposed to all of the antigens on newly formed cells. Consequently, they become tolerant of each new antigen, and do not respond to them. Several theories seek to explain the loss of the immune system's normal acceptance of "self" antigens. The most popular theory argues that AAbs are formed when antigens on cells are damaged by viruses or trauma, changing their appearance so that they appear foreign. Autoantigens may also combine in some way with foreign antigens, thus changing their appearance and stimulating B cell activity. The sequestered antigen theory holds that AAgs are separated from the blood during development of the fetus. When injury causes contact with B cells in the blood, AAbs are formed. Another theory proposes that a decrease in T8 (CD4) cell activity stimulates AAb production. Other theories hold that defective genes or abnormal B cells cause the autoimmune problems. SEE: *autoantibody; antigen; autoimmune disease.*

autoinfusion (aw″tō-ĭn-fū′zhŭn) [Gr. *autos*, self, + L. *in*, into, + *fundere*, to pour]. Forcing blood from extremities to body core by applying Esmarch bandages, q.v.

autoinoculation (aw″tō-ĭn-ŏk″ū-lā′shŭn) [″ + L. *inoculare*, to ingraft]. Inoculation by use of organisms obtained from another part of the body.

autointoxication (aw″tō-ĭn-tŏk″sĭ-kā′shŭn) [″ + L. *in*, into, + Gr. *toxikon*, poison]. A condition caused by poisonous substances produced within the body. SYN: *toxicosis, endogenic.*

autoisolysin (aw″tō-ī-sŏl′ĭ-sĭn) [″ + *isos*, equal, + *lysis*, dissolution]. An antibody that causes dissolution of cells of the subject from which it was obtained. It also causes lysis of cells of other animals of the same species.

autokeratoplasty (aw″tō-kĕr′ă-tō-plăs″tē) [″ + *keras*, horn, + *plassein*, to form]. Corneal grafting using tissue from the patient's other eye.

autokinesis (aw″tō-kĭ-nē′sĭs) [″ + *kinesis*, movement]. Voluntary movement. SYN: *autocinesia*.

a., visual. The illusion that an object in space, esp. during the night, moves as one continues to look at it. Thus, an aviator looking at a distant light may perceive that the light has moved, even though it is stationary.

autokinetic (aw″tō-kĭ-nĕt′ĭk). Being able to move voluntarily.

autolesion (aw′tō-lē″zhŭn) [″ + L. *laedere*, to wound]. Self-inflicted injury.

autologous (aw-tŏl′ō-gŭs) [″ + *logos*, word, reason]. Indicating something that has its origin within an individual, esp. a factor present in tissues or fluids.

autologous blood transfusion. Transfusion of blood that has either been donated by the patient in advance of surgery or collected from the surgical site during the procedure. Use of the patient's own blood, rather than blood from a donor, prevents possible exposure to the AIDS virus and other bloodborne diseases.

autolysate (aw-tŏl′ĭ-sāt) [″ + *lysis*, dissolution]. Specific product of autolysis.

autolysis (aw-tŏl′ĭ-sĭs). 1. The self-dissolution or self-digestion that occurs in tissues or cells by enzymes in the cells themselves, such as occurs after death and in some pathological conditions. 2. Hemolysis of blood cells occurring as a result of the action of an animal's own serum or plasma.

autolysosomes. The lysosomes that enable digestion of injured portions of the cell in which they are located.

autolytic (aw″tō-lĭt′ĭk). Pert. to autolysis. SEE: *enzyme*.

automatic [Gr. *automatos*, self-acting]. Spontaneous; involuntary.

automatic implanted ventricular defibrillator. Cardioversion device surgically implanted in patients who are at high risk for sudden cardiac death from ventricular arrhythmias. Device is capable of automatically cardioverting the arrhythmia.

automatism (aw-tŏm′ă-tĭzm) [″ + *-ismos*, condition of]. 1. Automatic actions or behavior without conscious volition or knowledge. The subject, though amnesic, appears normal to an observer, but the real personality is latent during a secondary state or period of automatism, usually a hysterical

trance. Such patients are not responsible for their acts and must not be left alone. They may carry out complicated acts without remembering having done so. 2. The spontaneous activity of cells or tissues, as the movement of cilia or the contraction of smooth muscles in tissues or organs removed from the body.

autonomic (aw-tō-nŏm′ĭk) [Gr. *autos*, self, + *nomos*, law]. 1. Self-controlling; functioning independently. 2. Rel. to the autonomic nervous system.

autonomic hyperreflexia. A condition commonly seen in patients with injury to the upper spinal cord. It is caused by massive sympathetic discharge of stimuli from the autonomic nervous system. It may be triggered by distention of the bladder or colon; catheterization of or irrigation of the bladder; cystoscopy; or transurethral resection. SYN: *autonomic dysreflexia*.

SYM: Sudden hypertension, bradycardia, sweating, severe headache, and gooseflesh.

TREAT: Ganglionic blocking agents such as mecamylamine hydrochloride, USP, or trimethaphan camsylate, USP.

NURSING IMPLICATIONS: Place patient in sitting position to decrease blood pressure, monitoring pressure and other vital signs and patient symptoms until episode is resolved. Drain urinary bladder by catheterization or check for kinking or obstruction of indwelling catheter, irrigating with no more than 30 ml of sterile normal saline solution. If catheter remains obstructed, remove and insert new catheter immediately. Check rectum for impaction, using a local anesthetic ointment for lubrication and for anesthesia if necessary to remove an impaction. Remove any other stimuli that may be triggering response. Obtain urine specimen for culture because infection may be a cause. Administer medication prescribed to reduce blood pressure. Provide calm atmosphere and emotional support throughout. Educate patient about complication and actions to prevent and alleviate it.

autonomic nervous system. This portion of the nervous system is inappropriately named because rather than being truly "autonomic," it is intimately responsive to changes in somatic activities. The part of the nervous system that is concerned with control of involuntary bodily functions. It regulates the function of glands, esp. the salivary, gastric, and sweat glands, and the adrenal medulla; smooth muscle tissue; and the heart. The autonomic nervous system may act on these tissues to reduce or slow activity or to initiate their function.

It is divided into the sympathetic or thoracolumbar system and the parasympathetic or craniosacral system. The *sympathetic system* is made up of the paired ganglionated sympathetic trunk; its connections (rami communicantes) with the thoracic and lumbar parts of the spinal nerve; the large and small splanchnic nerves; and certain ganglia in the abdomen (e.g., the mesenteric ganglia). The *parasympathetic system* consists of certain fibers of some cranial nerves, such as the motor fibers of the vagus, and of other fibers connected with the sacral part of the spinal cord. SEE: illus.

FUNCT: Stimulating sympathetic fibers usually produces vasoconstriction in the part supplied, general rise in blood pressure, erection of the hairs, gooseflesh, pupillary dilation, secretion of small quantities of thick saliva, depression of gastrointestinal activity, and acceleration of the heart. In general, these activities occur in emergencies such as fright and are associated with the expenditure of energy as a response to the need to flee, fight, or to be frightened. They are mediated through the release of a transmitter agent, norepinephrine.

Stimulating parasympathetic nerves generally produces vasodilation of the part supplied, general fall in the blood pressure, contraction of the pupil, copious secretion of thin saliva, increased gastrointestinal activity, and slowing of the heart. SEE: *nervous system*.

EXAM: The following tests will help to evaluate the state of the autonomic nervous system. Serial measurement of blood pressure and body temperature with respect to diurnal variation. Test of sweating by painting an area of the skin with iodine and dusting the area with starch; the areas without autonomic function will fail to turn dark. Parasympathetic function may be tested by instilling a 2% solution of methacholine into one conjunctival sac. This produces constriction of the pupil in patient with parasympathetic disorders. If parasympathetic supply to the bladder is impaired, there will be incomplete emptying and urinary retention.

autonomous (aw-tŏn'ō-mŭs). Independent of external influences.

autonomy (aw-tŏn'ō-mē) [Gr. *autos,* self, + *nomos,* law]. Functioning independently.

autophagia, autophagy (aw"tō-fā'jē-ă, aw-tŏf'ă-jē) [" + *phagein,* to eat]. 1. Biting oneself. 2. Self-consumption by a cell.

autophagocytosis. The digestion within a cell of portions of individual cell organelles or mitochondria that have been injured or

have atrophied. This digestive process is essential if the cell is to survive. SEE: *endocytosis; heterophagocytosis; phagolysosome; phagosome; pinocytosis.*

autophil (aw'tō-fĭl) [" + *philein,* to love]. Person having a sensitive autonomic nervous system.

autophilia (aw-tō-fĭl'ē-ă). Narcissism, q.v. Self-love.

autophobia (aw"tō-fō'bē-ă) [" + *phobos,* fear]. 1. A psychoneurotic fear of being alone. 2. Abnormal fear of being egotistical.

autophony (aw-tŏf'ō-nē) [" + *phone,* voice]. The vibration and echolike reproduction of the patient's own voice, breath sounds, and murmurs; usually due to diseases of the middle ear and auditory tube.

autoplasmotherapy (aw"tō-plăs"mō-thĕr'ă-pē) [" + LL. *plasma,* form, mold, + *therapeia,* treatment]. Treatment by injecting patient's own blood plasma.

autoplastic (aw"tō-plăs'tĭk) [" + *plassein,* to form]. Pert. to autoplasty, q.v.

autoplasty (aw'tō-plăs"tē). Plastic surgery using grafts from the patient's body.

autoploidy (aw"tō-ploy'dē). Autopolyploidy, q.v.

autopolyploidy (aw"tō-pŏl'ē-ploy"dē) [" + *polys,* many, + *ploos,* fold, + *eidos,* form, shape]. The condition of having more than two complete sets of chromosomes.

autoprecipitin (aw"tō-prē-sĭp'ĭ-tĭn) [Gr. *autos,* self, + L. *praecipitare,* to cast down]. Precipitin active against serum of animal in which it was formed.

autopsy (aw'tŏp-sē). Postmortem examination of the organs and tissues of a body to determine cause of death or pathological conditions. SYN: *postmortem examination.*

a., psychological. An attempt to determine what, if any, emotional or psychological factors caused or contributed to an individual's having taken his or her own life.

autopsychic (aw"tō-sī'kĭk) [" + *psyche,* soul]. Aware of one's own personality.

autopsychosis (aw"tō-sī-kō'sĭs) [" + *psyche,* soul]. Mental disease in which patients' ideas about themselves are disordered.

autoradiogram. Autoradiograph, q.v. SYN: *radioautogram.*

autoradiograph (aw"tō-rā'dē-ŏ-grăf). The radiograph formed by radioactive materials present in the tissue or individual. This is made possible by injecting radiochemicals into the person or tissue and then exposing x-ray film by placing the individual or tissue adjacent to the film.

autoradiography. Use of autoradiographs in investigating certain diseases. SYN: *radioautography.*

autoregulation (aw"tō-rĕg"ū-lā'shŭn). Con-

182

AUTONOMIC NERVOUS SYSTEM

trol of an event such as blood flow through a tissue (e.g., cardiac muscle) by alteration of the tissue. Thus, if not enough blood is flowing through a tissue, certain changes occur to cause an increase; if the flow is too great, another change will cause a decrease.

autoreinfusion (aw″tō-rē-in-fū′zhŭn) [″ + L. *re*, back, + *in*, into, + *fundere*, to pour]. Intravenous injection of patient's blood that has been collected from a site in which bleeding had occurred, such as the abdominal or pleural cavity. SEE: *autologous blood transfusion.*

autosensitization (aw″tō-sĕn″sĭ-tĭ-zā′shŭn). Becoming sensitized to one's own cells, fluids, or tissues.

autosepticemia (aw″tō-sĕp″tĭ-sē′mē-ă) [″ + *septos*, rotten, + *haima*, blood]. Septicemia from poisons existing within the organism.

autoserodiagnosis (aw″tō-sē″rō-dĭ-ăg-nō′sĭs) [″ + L. *serum*, whey, + Gr. *dia*, through, + *gnosis*, knowledge]. Diagnosis through serum from patient's blood.

autoserotherapy (aw″tō-sē″rō-thĕr′ă-pē) [″ + ″ + Gr. *therapeia*, treatment]. Treatment by hypodermic injection of patient's own blood serum.

autoserous (aw″tō-sē′rŭs). Pert. to autoserum q.v.

autoserum (aw″tō-sē′rŭm). Serum obtained from patient's own blood or cerebrospinal fluid to be reinjected into the patient.

autosite (aw′tō-sīt) [Gr. *autos*, self, + *sitos*, food]. The fairly normal member of asymmetrical conjoined twins, the other twin being dependent on the autosite for its nutrition.

autosmia (aw-tŏz′mē-ă) [″ + *osme*, smell]. Awareness of the odor of one's own body.

autosomatognosis (aw″tō-sō″mă-tŏg-nō′sĭs) [″ + *soma*, body, + *gnosis*, knowledge]. The feeling that a part of the body that has been removed is still present. SEE: *phantom limb.*

autosome (aw′tō-sōm) [″ + *soma*, body]. Any of the chromosomes other than the sex (X and Y) chromosomes. SEE: *chromosome.*

autosplenectomy (aw″tō-splĕn-ĕk′tō-mē) [″ + *splen*, spleen, + *ektome*, excision]. Multiple infarcts of the spleen that cause it to become fibrotic and nonfunctioning. Seen in sickle cell anemia, q.v.

autostimulation (aw″tō-stĭm″ū-lā′shŭn). 1. In immunology, stimulation of oneself by substances present in that person. 2. Stimulating or motivating oneself.

autosuggestibility (aw″tō-sŭg-jĕs″tĭ-bĭl′ĭ-tē) [″ + L. *suggerere*, to suggest]. Peculiar lack of resistance to any suggestion that may be offered by oneself.

autosuggestion (aw″tō-sŭg-jĕs′chŭn). The acceptance of an idea or thought arising from within one's own mind bringing about some physical or mental action or change.

autotemnous (aw″tō-tĕm′nŭs) [″ + *temnein*, to divide]. Pert. to cells propagating by spontaneous division.

autotherapy (aw″tō-thĕr′ă-pē) [″ + *therapeia*, treatment]. 1. Self-treatment. 2. Treatment of disease by administering patient's own pathological tissues, i.e., purulent material, usually as autogenous vaccine.

autotomography (aw″tō-tō-mŏg′ră-fē) [″ + Gr. *tome*, incision, + *graphein*, to write]. Radiographic tomography in which the structure under examination is moved during exposure; used instead of moving the x-ray tube and film.

autotopagnosia (aw″tō-tŏp-ăg-nō′zē-ă) [″ + *topos*, place, + *a-*, not, + *gnosis*, knowledge]. Inability to orient various parts of body correctly. Occurs in lesions of the thalamoparietal pathways of the cortex.

autotoxemia, autotoxicosis (aw″tō-tŏk-sē′mē-ă, aw″tō-tŏk″sĭ-kō′sĭs) [″ + *toxikon*, poison, + *haima*, blood; ″ + *toxikon*, poison, + *osis*, condition]. Self-poisoning due to absorption of a toxic substance generated within the body.

autotoxin (aw″tō-tŏk′sĭn). Poison generated within the body upon which it acts.

autotransfusion (aw″tō-trăns-fū′zhŭn) [″ + L. *trans*, across, + *fundere*, pour]. A method of returning the patient's own extravasated blood to the circulation. Blood that is shed into the peritoneal cavity during surgery, by a ruptured ectopic pregnancy or ruptured spleen, is collected during operation and transfused immediately into the circulation of the patient.

autotransplantation (aw″tō-trăns″plăn-tā′shŭn) [″ + ″ + *plantare*, to plant]. Surgical transfer of a piece of tissue from one part of the body to another part.

autotrophic (aw″tō-trō′fĭk) [″ + *trophe*, nourishment]. Self-nourishing; pert. to green plants and bacteria, which form protein and carbohydrate from inorganic salts and carbon dioxide; capable of growing in absence of organic compounds.

autotuberculin (aw″tō-tū-bĕr′kū-lĭn) [″ + L. *tuberculum*, a small swelling]. Tuberculin prepared from cultures of patient's own sputum.

autovaccination (aw″tō-văk″sĭ-nā′shŭn) [″ + *vacca*, cow]. 1. Vaccination with autogenous vaccine or autovaccine. 2. A vaccination resulting from virus or bacteria from a sore of a previous vaccination, as may occur following scratching the sore of a smallpox vaccination and subsequent transfer of the virus to a break in the skin elsewhere.

autovaccine (aw″tō-văk′sēn). Vaccine prepared from virus developed in the patient's own body.

autoxidation (aw″tŏk-sĭ-dā′shŭn) [″ + *oxys*, acid, + *gennan*, to produce]. Spontaneous combining of a substance with oxygen.

auxiliary (ăwg-zĭl′ē-ār-ē) [L. *auxiliarius*, help]. 1. Providing additional aid. 2. A person who aids.

   a., dental. Includes all persons who assist the dentist: dental hygienists, chair-side assistants, and radiology or laboratory technicians.

auxin [Gr. *auxe*, increase]. Plant-sprout hormone promoting growth in plant cells and tissues.

auxocyte (awk′sō-sīt) [Gr. *auxanu*, to increase, + *kytos*, cell]. Early growth stage of a spermatocyte, oocyte, or sporocyte.

auxotroph (awk′sō-trŏf) [″ + *trophe*, nutrition]. A mutant or other organism needing a specific factor for growth different from that required by the parent organism.

A-V. *atrioventricular.*

availability. In nutrition, the extent to which a nutrient is present in a form that can be absorbed and utilized.

avalanche theory [Fr. *avaler*, to descend]. Theory that nervous impulses are reinforced and thereby become more intense as they travel peripherally.

avalvular (ă-văl′vū-lăr). Without valves.

avascular (ă-văs′kū-lăr) [Gr. *a-*, not, + L. *vasculum*, little vessel]. Lacking in blood vessels or having a poor blood supply, said of tissues such as cartilage.

avascularization (ă-văs″kū-lăr-ĭ-zā′shŭn). Expulsion of blood from tissues, esp. the extremities, as by use of Esmarch bandage, q.v.

Avazyme. Trade name for chymotrypsin, q.v.

A-V block. A condition in which the depolarization impulse is delayed or blocked at the A-V node or a more distal site, as in the A-V bundle or bundle branches. A-V block can be partial or complete block. Divided into three subgroups: first-, second-, and third-degree A-V block. Second-degree block is further divided into Wenckebach or Mobitz I and Mobitz II, q.v.

A-V bundle. A bundle of fibers of the impulse-conducting system of the heart. From its origin in the A-V node, it enters the interventricular septum, where it divides into two branches whose fibers pass to the right and left ventricles respectively, the fibers of each trunk becoming continuous with the Purkinje fibers of the ventricles. SYN: *bundle of His.*

Avellis' paralysis syndrome [Georg Avellis, Ger. laryngologist, 1864–1916]. Paralysis of half of the soft palate, pharynx, and larynx and loss of pain, heat, and cold sensations on opposite side.

Aventyl Hydrochloride. Trade name for nortriptyline hydrochloride, q.v.

average. SEE: *arithmetic mean.*

aversion therapy. A form of behavior in which an undesired stimulus, e.g., drinking alcohol, is presented to the patient at the same time as an unpleasant or painful stimulus. The goal is to have the individual associate the undesired stimulus with the unpleasant one and thus discontinue the former.

avian. Concerning birds.

aviation medicine. The branch of medicine concerned with diseases and pathologic conditions resulting from, or incident to, air travel. SYN: *aerospace medicine.*

aviation physiology. The branch of physiology that deals with conditions encountered by man in high altitudes, as in aircraft flights, mountain climbing, or in space vehicles. The principal factors dealt with are hypoxia, extreme temperature and radiation, effects of forces of acceleration and deceleration, weightlessness, motion sickness, enforced inactivity, and disturbance of biological rhythm.

avidin (ăv′ĭ-dĭn) [L. *avidus*, greedy]. A protein isolated from raw egg white. Said to be an inhibitor of biotin, thereby causing a deficiency in biotin. Formerly called vitamin H.

avidity. 1. Eagerness; having a strong attraction for something. 2. Concerning the ability of antibodies to bind to antigens.

avirulent (ă-vĭr′ū-lĕnt) [Gr. *a-*, not, + L. *virus*, poison]. Without virulence.

avitaminosis (ā-vī″tă-mĭ-nō′sĭs) [″ + *vitamin* + *osis*, condition]. Disease due to lack of vitamins in the diet; a deficiency disease. SEE: *vitamin.*

avitaminotic (ā-vī-tăm-ĭn-ŏt′ĭk). Pert. to or affected with avitaminosis.

avivement (ă-vēv-mŏn′) [Fr.]. Surgical trimming of wound edges prior to suturing them together.

Avlosulfon. Trade name for dapsone, q.v.

Avogadro's law (ŏv-ō-gŏd′rōs) [Amadeo Avogadro, It. physicist, 1776–1856]. Equal volumes of gases contain equal numbers of molecules, pressure and temperature being the same.

Avogadro's number. Number of molecules, 6.0221367×10^{23}, in one gram-molecular weight of a compound.

avoidance (ă-voyd′ăns). The conscious or unconscious effort to escape from situations or events perceived by the individual to be threatening to personal comfort, safety, or well-being.

avoirdupois measure (ăv″ĕr-dĕ-poyz′) [Fr.,

to have weight]. A system of weighing or measuring articles in which 7000 grains equal 1 pound.

To find the capacity of a vessel or space in gallons, divide the contents in cubic inches by 231 for liquid gallons, or by 268.8 for dry gallons. To convert gallons to cubic inches, multiply the given number of liquid gallons by 231. The dry gallon (half-peck) contains 268.8 cu in. Six dry gallons are equal to nearly seven liquid gallons. The bushel contains 2150.42 cu in. (35,240.0 cu cm) and is a cylindrical measure 18.5 in. (47 cm) in diameter and 8 in. (20.3 cm) deep. Measures of capacity are all cubic measures. The number of pounds in a bushel depends upon the density of the article contained therein. SEE: *apothecaries' measure; metric system; Troy weight; Weights and Measures in Appendix.*

avulsion (ă-vŭl'shŭn) [Gr. *a-*, not, + L. *vellere*, to pull]. A tearing away forcibly of a part or structure. If surgical repair is necessary, merely apply a sterile dressing while waiting for surgery to be done. If fingers, toes, feet, or hands are completely avulsed, they may be successfully rejoined to the body if prompt and expert surgical care is available.

axanthopsia (ăk"săn-thŏp'sē-ă) [" + *xanthos*, yellow, + *opsis*, vision]. Yellow blindness.

axenic (ă-zĕn'ĭk) [" + *xenos*, stranger]. Germfree, as pert. to animals, or pure, as pert. to cultures or microorganisms. Sterile.

axial (ăk'sē-ăl) [L. *axis*, axle]. Situated in or pert. to an axis.

axial line. A line running in the main axis of the body or part of it. The axial line of the hand runs through the middle digit; the axial line of the foot runs through the second digit.

axial skeleton. Head and trunk.

axifugal (ăks-ĭf'ū-găl) [" + *fugere*, to flee]. Receding from the axis. SYN: *centrifugal.*

axilemma (ăk"sĭ-lĕm'ă) [" + Gr. *lemma*, husk]. The plasma membrane of an axon.

axilla (ăk-sĭl'ă) [L. *axilla*] (pl. *axillae*). [NA] The armpit.

axilla conformer. A splint designed to prevent adduction contractures following severe burns to the axilla region.

axillary (ăk'sĭ-lār-ē). Pert. to the axilla.

axillofemoral bypass graft (ăk"sĭl-ō-fĕm'or-ăl). The surgical establishment of a connector between the axillary artery and the common femoral arteries. A synthetic artery graft is used and implanted subcutaneously. This technique is used in treating patients with insufficient blood flow to the legs.

axio- (ăk'sē-ō) [L. *axis*, axle]. Combining form indicating relationship of the term that follows to an axis. In dentistry, the long axis of the tooth is referred to by this term.

axiobuccal (ăk"sē-ō-bŭk'kăl) [L. *axis*, axle, + *bucca*, cheek]. Concerning the angle formed by the long axis of the tooth and the buccal walls of a cavity of the tooth.

axioincisal (ăk"sē-ō-ĭn-sī'zăl) [" + *incisor*, a cutter]. Concerning the angle formed by the long axis of the tooth and the incisal walls of a cavity in the tooth.

axiolabial (ăk"sē-ō-lā'bē-ăl) [" + *labialis*, pert. to the lips]. Concerning the angle formed by the long axis of the tooth with the labial walls of a cavity in the tooth.

axiolingual (ăk"sē-ō-lĭng'gwăl) [" + *lingua*, tongue]. Concerning the angle formed by the long axis of the tooth and the lingual walls of a cavity in the tooth.

axiomesial (ăk"sē-ō-mē'zē-ăl) [" + Gr. *mesos*, middle]. Concerning the angle formed by the long axis of a tooth and the mesial walls of a cavity in the tooth.

axio-occlusal (ăk"sē-ō-ō-klū'zăl) [" + *occlusio*, closure]. Concerning the angle formed by the long axis of the tooth and the occlusal walls of a cavity in the tooth.

axioplasm (ăk"sē-ō-plăzm) [" + LL. *plasma*, form, mold]. Neuroplasm of an axis cylinder.

axiopulpal (ăk"sē-ō-pŭl'păl) [" + *pulpa*, pulp]. Concerning the angle formed by the long axis of a tooth and the pulpal walls of a cavity in the tooth.

axipetal (ăk-sĭp'ĕt-ăl) [L. *axis*, axle, + *petere*, to seek]. Directed toward the axis. SYN: *centripetal.*

axis [L.] (pl. *axes*). 1. A real or imaginary line that runs through the center of a body or about which a part revolves. 2. [NA] The second cervical vertebra or epistropheus, which bears the odontoid process (dens) about which the atlas rotates.

   a., basicranial. Axis connecting the basion and gonion.

   a., basifacial. Axis from subnasal point to gonion.

   a., binauricular. Axis between the two auricular points.

   a., cardiac. A graphic representation of the main conduction vector of the heart, determined through measurements of direction and amplitude of the complexes in several of the twelve leads on a twelve-lead electrocardiogram. Normal axis is zero to +90°.

   a., celiac. Axis between the celiac artery and abdominal aorta.

   a., cerebrospinal. Central nervous system.

   a., condylar. Axis through the two condyles of the mandible about which movement takes place when the mouth opens.

SYN: *hinge a.; transverse mandibular a.*

a., frontal. Imaginary line running from side to side in the frontal plane, about which side-to-side movement occurs. Also called coronal axis.

a., hinge. A projected line connecting the condyles of the mandible. When the mandible starts to move, it rotates around this imaginary line. SYN: *mandibular a.*

a., neural. Central nervous system.

a., optic. A line that connects the anterior and posterior poles of the eye.

a., principal. In optics, a line that passes through the optical center or nodal point of a lens perpendicular to the surface of the lens.

a., sagittal. Imaginary line running anterior-posterior, about which frontal plane motion occurs.

a., visual. A line passing from object of vision directly through center of cornea and lens to the fovea.

axis cylinder. An axon (def. 2), q.v.

axis deviation. Cardiac axis which is not normal. Left axis deviation is $-1°$ to $-89°$. Right axis deviation is $+91°$ to $-90°$. This condition is usually indicative of cardiac disease.

axis traction. Traction made on the fetus in the direction of the long axis of the birth canal.

axo- [Gr. *axon*, axis]. Prefix pert. to axis or axon.

axodendrite (ăk″sō-děn′drīt) [″ + *dendron*, tree]. Process given off from a nerve cell axon (not an axis cylinder).

axofugal (ăk-sŏf′ū-găl) [″ + L. *fugere*, to flee]. Axifugal, q.v.

axolemma (ăk″sō-lěm′ă) [″ + *lemma*, husk]. Axis cylinder sheath of a nerve fiber. SYN: *axilemma.*

axolysis (ăk-sŏl′ĭ-sĭs) [″ + *lysis*, dissolution]. Destruction of the axis cylinder of a nerve.

axometer (ăk-sŏm′ĕ-tĕr) [″ + *metron*, measure]. Measuring device for use in adjusting the frames of glasses so that the lenses are suitable for the optic axes of the eyes.

axon, axone (ăk′sŏn, -sōn) [Gr. *axon*, axis]. 1. A process of a neuron that conducts impulses away from the cell body. Typically, one arising from a portion of the cell devoid of Nissl granules, the axon hillock. Axons may possess either or both of two sheaths (myelin sheath and neurilemma) or neither. Axons are usually long and straight, and most end in synapses in the central nervous system or ganglia or in effector organs (e.g., motor neurons). They may give off side branches or collaterals. An axon with its sheath(s) constitutes a nerve fiber. 2. A nerve cell process that resembles an axon in structure, specifically the peripheral process of a dorsal root ganglion cell (sensory neuron) that functionally and embryologically is a dendrite, but structurally is indistinguishable from an axon. SYN: *axis cylinder.* SEE: *nerve; neuron.*

axoneme (ăk′sŏn-nēm) [″ + *nema*, thread]. Axial thread of a chromosome.

axoneuron (ăk-sō-nū′rŏn) [″ + *neuron*, nerve]. A nerve cell of the cerebrospinal system.

axonometer (ăk-sō-nŏm′ĕ-tĕr) [″ + *metron*, measure]. Device for determining the axis of astigmatism.

axonotmesis (ăk″sŏn-ŏt-mē′sĭs) [″ + *tmesis*, incision]. Nerve injury that damages the nerve tissue without actually severing the nerve.

axon reflex. SEE: *reflex, axon.*

axopetal (ăk-sŏp′ĕ-tăl) [″ + L. *petere*, to seek]. Conducted along an axon toward a cell body of a neuron.

axoplasm (ăk′sō-plăzm) [″ + LL. *plasma*, form, mold]. The cytoplasm (neuroplasm) of an axon that encloses the neurofibrils.

axospongium (ăk-sō-spŏn′jē-ŭm) [″ + *spongos*, sponge]. The fine fibrillar network of the axon substance of a nerve cell.

Ayerza's syndrome (ŏ-yĕr′thŏz) [Abel Ayerza, Brazilian physician, 1861–1918]. A condition characterized by dyspnea, chronic cyanosis, erythrocytosis, enlargement of spleen and liver, and hyperplasia of bone marrow. Polycythemia usually results from pulmonary insufficiency.

ayurvedic medicine (ā′yŭr-vă′dĭc) [Sanskrit *ayus*, lifespan, life, + *veda*, knowledge, science]. An ancient Hindu medical system. Its goal is to improve health by harmonizing mind and body. It utilizes herbal remedies, massage therapy, yoga, and pulse diagnosis.

A modern revival of this system is known as Maharishi Ayur-Veda and has been directed by Maharishi Mahesh Yogi. Some of its advertising practices have been questionable.

Az. *azote.*

azalein (ă-zā′lē-ĭn) [L. *azalea*, azalea). A red dye.

Azapen. Trade name for methicillin sodium, q.v.

azathioprine (ā″ză-thī′ō-prēn). USP. A chemical substance that is cytotoxic and is used for immunosuppression. Trade name is Imuran.

azo-. Prefix indicating the presence of —N:N— group in a chemical structure. This group is usually connected at either end with carbon atoms. SEE: *azo compounds.*

azo compounds. Organic substances that

contain the azo group. An example is azobenzene, $C_6H_5N:NC_6H_5$. They are related to aniline and include important dyes and indicators. SEE: *indicator* for table.

azoic (ă-zō'ĭk) [Gr. *a-*, not, + *zoe*, life]. Containing no living organisms.

Azolid. Trade name for phenylbutazone, q.v.

azoospermia (ă-zō-ō-spĕr'mē-ă) [" + *zoon*, animal, + *sperma*, seed]. Absence of spermatozoa in the semen.

Azorean disease (ā-zor'ē-ăn). A form of hereditary ataxia present in Portuguese families whose ancestors lived in the Azores. It is a degenerative disease of the nervous system. Symptoms vary but may include gait ataxia, limitation of eye movements, widespread muscle fasciculations, mild cerebellar tremor, loss of reflexes in lower limbs, and extensor plantar reflex response.

azotation (ăz"ō-tā'shŭn). Nitrogen absorption from the air.

azote (ăz'ōt) [" + *zoe*, life]. Nitrogen.

azotemia (ăz"ō-tē'mē-ă) [" + " + *haima*, blood]. Presence of nitrogenous bodies, esp. urea in increased amounts, in the blood. SEE: *uremia*.

Azotobacter (ă-zō"tō-băk'tĕr). Rod-shaped, gram-negative, nonpathogenic soil and water bacteria that fix atmospheric nitrogen. The single genus of the family Azotobacteraceae.

azoturia (ăz"ō-tū'rē-ă) [" + " + *ouron*, urine]. An increase in nitrogenous compounds, esp. urea, in urine.

Azulfidine. Trade name for sulfasalazine, q.v.

azure lunulae (ăz'ŭr loo'nū-lē) [O. Fr. *azur*, blue, + L. *lunula*, little moon]. Blue discoloration of the base, or lunulae, of the fingernails. May be seen in patients with hepatolenticular degeneration (Wilson's disease). Blue discoloration of the entire nail may be present in argyria and following therapy with quinacrine hydrochloride.

azurophil(e) (ăz-ū'rō-fĭl) [" + Gr. *philein*, to love]. Staining readily with azure dye.

azurophilia (ăz"ū-rō-fĭl'ē-ă). Condition in which some blood cells have azurophil granules.

azygography (ăz"ĭ-gŏg'ră-fē) [Gr. *a-*, not, + *zygon*, yoke, + *graphein*, to write]. Radiographic visualization of the azygos veins by use of I.V. radiopaque solution.

azygos (ăz'ĭ-gŏs) [" + *zygon*, yoke]. Occurring singly, not in pairs.

azygos vein. A single vein arising in the abdomen as a branch of the ascending lumbar vein. It passes upward through the aortic hiatus of the diaphragm into the thorax, then along the right side of the vertebral column to the level of the fourth thoracic vertebra, where it turns and enters the superior vena cava. In the thorax, it receives the hemiazygos, accessory azygos, and bronchial veins, as well as the right intercostal and subcostal veins. In cases of obstruction to the inferior vena cava, the azygous vein is the principal vein by which blood can return to the heart.

azygous (ăz'ĭ-gŭs). Single, not paired.

azymia (ā-zĭ'mē-ă) [" + *zyme*, ferment]. State of being without a ferment or enzyme.

azymic, azymous (ā-zĭ'mĭk, -mŭs, ăz'ĭ-mŭs). 1. Unfermented or unleavened. 2. Denoting the absence of an enzyme.

B

β. Beta, second letter of the Greek alphabet. SEE: *beta*.

B. 1. Chem. symb. for the element boron. 2. *Bacillus; Balantidium; barometric; base; bath; behavior; buccal.*

B.A. *Bachelor of Arts.*

Ba. Chem. symb. for the element barium.

Babbitt metal (băb'ĭt) [Isaac Babbitt, U.S. inventor, 1799–1862]. Antifriction alloy of copper, antimony, and tin used occasionally in dentistry.

babble. To talk excessively, at length, perhaps irrationally, and in effect to say nothing of importance or pertinence to the situation.

Babcock's operation (băb'kŏks) [William Wayne Babcock, U.S. surgeon, 1872–1963]. Extirpation of the saphenous vein. One way of treating varicose veins.

Babcock's test [Stephen Moulton Babcock, U.S. chemist, 1843–1931]. Test to determine the amount of fat in milk by centrifuging equal parts of milk and sulfuric acid.

Babès-Ernst granules (bă'băz-ĕrnst) [Victor Babès, Rumanian bacteriologist, 1854–1926; Paul Ernst, Ger. pathologist, 1859–1937]. Metachromatic granules.

Babesia (bă-bē'zē-ă) [Victor Babès]. A genus of the order Haemosporidia that consists of parasites found in the blood of cattle, sheep, horses, dogs, and other vertebrate animals. They are transmitted by ticks. They infest red blood cells, bringing about their destruction with resulting hemoglobinuria.

B. bigemina. The causative organism of Texas fever in cattle.

B. bovis. The causative organism of hemoglobinuria and jaundice (red-water fever) in cattle.

babesiosis (bă-bē-zē-ō'sĭs). A rare, often severe, and sometimes fatal disease of man caused by an intraerythrocytic protozoan, *Babesia microti,* and perhaps other *Babesia* species. The disease, transmitted by ticks, occurs mostly in the northeastern U.S., esp. on the islands off the coast of New England, e.g., Martha's Vineyard and Nantucket. Severe forms are most likely to occur in persons over age 40 and those with a nonfunctioning spleen or no spleen. In rare cases the infection is transmitted by blood transfusion from an asymptomatic carrier. The incubation period may be from weeks to months.

SYM: Fever, chills, drenching sweats, myalgia, arthralgia, nausea and vomiting, and hemolytic anemia.

DIAG: Presence of parasite in red blood cells and by serologic studies. On the blood smear it may be difficult to differentiate the parasites from the malaria organism, *Plasmodium falciparum.*

TREAT: Quinine and clindamycin have been effective. Exchange transfusion may be needed in asplenic patients in whom a large proportion of their red blood cells contain parasites.

babies, boarder. SEE: *boarder babies.*

Babinski's reflex (bă-bĭn'skēz) [Joseph Babinski, Fr. neurologist, 1857–1932]. Dorsiflexion of the great toe on stimulating the sole of the foot. Normally, when the lateral aspect of the sole of the relaxed foot is stroked, the great toe is flexed. If the toe extends instead of flexes and the outer toes spread out, Babinski's reflex is present. This occurs in lesions of the pyramidal tract. Babinski's reflex is normally present in infants under the age of six months. Care must be taken to avoid interpreting voluntary extension of the toe as Babinski's reflex.

Babinski's sign. Loss of or diminished Achilles tendon reflex in sciatica.

baby [ME. *babie*]. Lay term for an infant.

b., battered. Baby or child whose body provides evidence of physical abuse such as bruises, cuts, scars, fractures, or abdominal visceral injuries that have occurred at various times in the past. SEE: *battered child syndrome.*

b., blue. Newborn child with cyanosis. This may be caused by anything that prevents proper oxygenation of the blood, esp. a congenital anomaly that permits blood to go directly from the right to the left side of the heart without going through the lungs.

b., collodion. Newborn covered with a collodion-like layer of desquamated skin. May be due to ichthyosis vulgaris.

baby boom. The increase in births from 1946 through 1964, i.e., post World War II.

baby bottle syndrome. Decay of primary teeth in older infants and toddlers related to taking a bottle of punch or other sweet liquid to bed and retaining the liquid, which creates massive caries. SYN: *bottle mouth syndrome; bottle caries.*

Baby Doe regulations. Federal, state, and hospital policies insuring that handicapped infants will receive life-saving treatment without regard to the quality of life.

bacampicillin hydrochloride. USP. An antibacterial drug.

bacca (băk'ă) [L.] (pl. *baccae*). A berry.

bacciform (băk'sĭ-form) [″ + *forma,*

form]. Berry-shaped; coccal.

Bacid. Trade name for lactobacillus acidophilus, q.v.

Bacillaceae (băs-ĭ-lā′sē-ē). A family (order Eubacteriales) of rod-shaped cells that can produce endospores. Usually gram-positive, commonly found in soil. Genera of family are *Bacillus* and *Clostridium*.

bacillar, bacillary (băs′ĭl-ăr, băs′ĭl-ăr-ē). 1. Pert. to or caused by bacilli. 2. Rodlike.

bacille Calmette-Guérin (bă-sēl′). An organism of the strain *Mycobacterium bovis*, rendered completely avirulent by long-term cultivation on bile-glycero-potato medium. Used in BCG vaccine, q.v., in prevention of human tuberculosis.

bacillemia (băs-ĭ-lē′mē-ă) [L. *bacillus*, rod, + Gr. *haima*, blood]. The presence of bacilli in the circulating blood.

bacilli (bă-sĭl′ī). Pl. of bacillus.

bacilliform (bă-sĭl′ĭ-form) [″ + *forma*, form]. Resembling a bacillus in shape.

bacillophobia (băs″ĭ-lō-fō′bē-ă) [″ + Gr. *phobos*, fear]. Morbid fear of bacilli.

bacillosis (băs″ĭ-lō′sĭs) [″ + Gr. *osis*, infection]. Infection by bacilli.

bacilluria (băs″ĭ-lū′rē-ă) [″ + Gr. *ouron*, urine]. Bacilli in the urine. SEE: *clean-catch method*.

Bacillus (bă-sĭl′ŭs) [L.]. A genus of bacteria belonging to the family Bacillaceae. All species are rod-shaped, sometimes occurring in chains. They are spore-bearing, aerobic, motile or nonmotile; most are gram-positive and nonpathogenic. One well-known species pathogenic to man is *B. anthracis*.

    B. anthracis. An aerobic, spore-forming bacillus pathogenic to man and domestic animals, being the causative agent of anthrax, q.v.

    B. cereus. An aerobic spore-forming bacillus that may be an opportunistic invader in immunocompromised patients.

    B. stearothermophilus. Species of bacillus that produce heat-resistant spores. These are used to test for steam autoclave effectiveness.

    B. subtilis. The common hay bacillus, which has a close resemblance to *B. anthracis*. Generally, it is considered nonpathogenic, but it occasionally causes conjunctivitis in man. It is often found as a contaminant of laboratory specimens.

    B. thuringiensis. A species of bacillus that is rarely pathogenic.

bacillus (pl. *bacilli*). 1. Any rod-shaped microorganism. 2. A rod-shaped microorganism belonging to the class Schizomycetes. SEE: *Bacillus; bacteria*.

    b., acid-fast. Bacillus not readily decolorized by acids or other means when stained.

Bacillus species. ABBR: Bacillus spp. All of

Use of a footrest relieves swayback.

Bend the knees and hips, not the waist.

Hold heavy objects close to you.

Never bend over without bending the knees.

HOW TO STAY ON YOUR FEET WITHOUT TIRING YOUR BACK

Adapted from "Your Back and How to Care for It," Copyright 1965, Schering Corporation, Bloomfield, N.J.

the species of Bacillus.

bacitracin (băs-ĭ-trā′sĭn). USP. An antibiotic substance obtained from a strain of *Bacillus subtilis*. Its antibacterial actions are similar to those of penicillin, including gram-positive cocci and bacilli and some gram-negative organisms. Because of its toxicity when used parenterally, bacitracin is usually applied topically in ointment form.

    b., zinc. The zinc salt of bacitracin, used in topical antibacterial ointments.

back. 1. The dorsum. 2. The posterior region of the trunk from neck to pelvis.

    Misuse of the back is common among those whose duties include care of the sick. Therefore, it is important to learn basic concepts in care of the back. SEE: illus. (*How to Stay on Your Feet Without Tiring Your Back*).

backbone. The vertebral column; spinal column, q.v. SEE: *vertebra*.

backcross. In genetics the pairing of a first filial generation hybrid with an organism whose genotype is identical to the parental strain.

backflow. Abnormal backward flow of fluids.

background radiation. Total radioactivity from cosmic rays, natural radioactive materials, and whatever other radiation may be in a specific area.

back pain. Any pain in the back. Usually characterized by dull, continuous pain and tenderness in the muscles or their attachments in the lower lumbar, lumbosacral, or sacroiliac regions. Pain is often referred to the leg, following the distribution of the sciatic nerve.

ETIOL: Infection or abnormality in another part of the body such as uterine or prostatic disorders; disorders of the vertebral column such as intervertebral disk abnormality; local disturbances such as lumbar or sacral fractures, lumbosacral strain or sprain; structural inadequacies of supporting ligaments of the spinal column; muscle injury, spasm, myositis, or inflammation of fascial attachments; psychogenic factors.

TREAT: Treat specific primary cause. General treatment includes allowing time for the condition to improve without specific therapy such as surgery. Important in this phase are measures to allay pain and discomfort, such as analgesics, preferably salicylates or other nonsteroidal anti-inflammatory agents, muscle relaxants, heat, whirlpool. Tender areas or trigger points may be anesthetized by local infiltration with 1% procaine or topical application of ethyl chloride spray. Special measures to relax tense muscles and improve blood flow are helpful. Orthopedic supports and strapping if necessary in special cases. Physical therapy utilizing appropriate therapeutic exercises to retrain muscles and balance forces in the pelvis and spine. After the acute attack, several activities are especially good for the back: brisk walking, bicycling and swimming. All of these involve minimal impact and they do not put the back into an awkward position. Psychotherapy when necessary, esp. in excessive muscle tension resulting from emotional disturbances.

Most patients will not need surgical intervention, but some conditions, such as herniated disk, persistent pain upon vertebral column rotation, overgrowth of bone that causes narrowing of the spinal canal (lumbar stenosis), and spondylolisthesis may need surgery.

backrest. An adjustable device for supporting the back in bed.

backscatter. In radiation physics, the deflection of ionizing radiation from the target back more than 90 degrees.

backup. Anything that serves to replace a function or system that fails.

bacteremia (băk-tĕr-ē′mē-ă) [Gr. *bakterion*,

rod, + *haima*, blood]. Bacteria in the blood. SEE: *sepsis.*

bacteria (băk-tē′rē-ă) [Gr. *bakterion,* rod] (sing. *bacterium*). Any microorganism of the class Schizomycetes. SEE: *gram-negative; gram-positive; Gram's method.*

There are three principal forms of bacteria. *Spherical* or *ovoid:* When appearing singly, they are called micrococci; when in pairs, diplococci; when in irregular clusters, staphylococci; when in chains, streptococci; cocci that remain adherent after splitting successively in two or three perpendicular directions from square or cubical groups known as sarcinae. *Rod-shaped:* Known as bacilli. When the rods are somewhat oval, they are called coccobacilli; when attached end to end forming a chain, streptobacilli. *Spiral:* When the spiral organisms are rigid, they are called spirilla; when flexible, spirochetes; when forming curved rods, vibrios. SEE: illus.

Most bacteria are relatively constant in form in growing cultures. But in old cultures or cultures grown under adverse environmental conditions, aberrant forms appear.

It has been estimated that each of us carries 10^{14} bacteria in and on our bodies, and that all the total population of our planet excretes 10^{22} bacteria in feces per day.

CHARACTERISTICS: *Mutation:* Most bacteria, like all living organisms, have the ability to adapt to environmental changes or to potentially lethal agents, e.g., antibiotics. Thus, an organism that originally was sensitive to a specific antibiotic can mutate so that it loses the sensitivity. SEE: *bacterial resistance.*

Size: An average rod-shaped bacterium measures about 1 micrometer in diameter by 4 micrometers in length. They vary considerably in size from less than 0.5 to 1.0 micrometer in diameter to 10 to 20 micrometers in length in some of the longer spiral forms.

Motility: Some bacteria are incapable of movement (all cocci), but most bacilli and spiral forms exhibit independent movement. The power of locomotion depends on the possession of one or more flagella, slender whiplike appendages. Bacteria having no flagella are called atrichous; those having a flagellum at one end, monotrichous; those having flagella at each end, amphitrichous; those having a tuft at one end, lophotrichous; those having flagella protruding from all surfaces of the cell, peritrichous.

Capsules: Many bacteria possess a capsule, a layer of slimy mucoid substance that surrounds each cell. The presence of a cap-

BACTERIAL FORMS

DIPLOCOCCI   STAPHYLOCOCCI   STREPTOCOCCI

BACILLI   COCCOBACILLI   SARCINAE

SPIROCHETES   SPIRILLA   VIBRIOS

sule is associated with the virulence of certain pathogenic forms.

Spores: Certain species of the rod-shaped bacteria have the ability to develop an encysted or resting stage known as a spore or endospore. The size, shape, and position of the spore within the cell are characteristic of particular species. Spores are terminal if formed at the end of a cell, central if formed at the center, subterminal if formed between the center and end. Spore formation is common among the bacilli but does not usually occur in the cocci or spiral forms. Bacterial spores are remarkably resistant to heat, drying, and the action of disinfectants.

Reproduction: Binary fission is the usual mode of reproduction. Budding, branching, filamentous growth, and the development of conidia also occur.

Colony formation: A group of bacteria growing in one place is called a colony. A colony is usually composed of the descendants of a single cell. Colonies differ in shape, size, color, texture, type of margin, and other characteristics. Each species of bacteria has a characteristic type of colony formation. Sometimes a single species may produce two types of colonies: one the smooth or S-type, the other the rough or R-type. Sometimes colonies contain clear

spots and have a moth-eaten appearance. Such colonies are called plaques and are thought to be due to the lytic action of bacteriophages.

Food requirements: Bacteria possess no chlorophyll, and therefore cannot carry on photosynthesis. A few can obtain their energy from inorganic substances. These are termed autotrophic and include many of the soil bacteria. The majority derive their nourishment from organic material and are termed heterotrophic. If they live on living organisms, they are called parasites; if their food is from nonliving organic matter, they are called saprophytes. If bacteria produce disease in their host, they are pathogenic. Most bacteria can be pathogenic in some circumstances.

Oxygen requirements: Most bacteria require free or atmospheric oxygen. These are called aerobes. Bacteria living in the absence of atmospheric oxygen are called anaerobes. Those showing a preference for free oxygen and yet capable of living in its absence are called facultative anaerobes; those that grow only in the absence of oxygen are called obligate anaerobes.

Temperature requirements: Most bacteria grow best at moderate temperatures. These are called mesophilic. Cold-loving bacteria, which thrive in temperatures between 0° and 30°C (32° and 86°F), are called psychrophilic; those that thrive in high temperatures between 40° and 70°C (104° and 158°F) are called thermophilic. The optimum temperature for most saprophytes is around 25°C, for most pathogens, 37°C.

ACTIVITIES: *Enzyme production:* Bacteria produce enzymes that act on complex food molecules, breaking them down into simpler materials capable of assimilation. Carbohydrases act on sugars, breaking them down to alcohol and carbon dioxide, a process called fermentation. Proteolytic enzymes bring about the decomposition of proteins with the formation of ill-smelling products, a process called putrefaction. Putrefaction is the decomposition of organic substances, esp. nitrogenous substances, in the absence of air and with resulting unpleasant odors. Decay is the gradual decomposition of organic matter exposed to air by bacteria and fungi. Bacteria are the principal agents of decay and putrefaction.

Toxin production: Many bacteria produce poisonous substances called toxins. There are two types: exotoxins, which diffuse from the bacterial cell into the surrounding medium, and endotoxins, which are liberated only when the bacterial cell dies and disintegrates. Bacteria well known for their toxin production are the diphtheria, staphylococcal, tetanus, and botulinus organisms.

Miscellaneous: Some bacteria produce pigments; some produce light, thus appearing luminescent at night. Many chemical substances are produced as a result of bacterial activity, among them acids, gases, alcohol, aldehydes, ammonia, carbohydrates, and indole. Pathogenic forms produce hemolysins, leukocidins, coagulases, and fibrolysins. Soil bacteria play an important role in various phases of the nitrogen cycle (nitrification, nitrogen fixation, and denitrification).

METHODS OF STUDYING: Principal methods used in the study of bacteria follow:

(1) Examination of unstained bacteria in a hanging-drop preparation. Dark-field illumination is necessary to see extremely small forms.

(2) Staining methods include general stains, differential stains, stains for special bacteria, and stains for specific parts. Of the differential stains, Gram's method and staining for acid-fast bacteria are widely used. Bacteria fall into three groups: gram-positive bacteria (those that retain the stain); gram-negative bacteria (those that are decolorized by alcohol); and acid-fast bacteria (those that, when stained with cer-

tain dyes, retain the stain even when treated with an acid).

(3) In cultural methods, the bacteria are grown on various culture media, and under certain specific conditions; e.g., increased CO_2, presence or absence of oxygen. In synthetic media, the exact composition of the medium is known; in nonsynthetic media, the constituents are uncertain and unreliable. Media, on the basis of consistency, may be liquid (nutrient broth, milk, blood serum); liquefiable solid, which consists of liquid media made solid by addition of gelatin or agar-agar; and nonliquefiable solid (potato, carrots, starch paste).

(4) Animal inoculation.

(5) Immunological methods including immunofluorescence. This technique involves staining bacteria on smears or in tissues with fluorescein-containing reagents. After this process the preparation is rinsed to remove the unbound fluorescein and then examined with a suitable light microscope equipped with special filters and incident light source. The fluorescent-stained cells are readily apparent as yellow-green masses. SEE: *polymerase chain reaction.*

(6) Sterilization methods. Sterilization is the process of rendering any material free of living microorganisms. It may be accomplished by physical or chemical means. Physical agents employed are heat, light, ionizing radiation, and filtration. Sterilization may be accomplished in a flame; in a hot-air oven (150° to 170°C for one hour); in streaming steam (100°C for 20 min or longer); by steam under pressure (10 to 15 lb or 4.5 to 6.8 kg) in an autoclave (121°C for 20 min); or by ionizing radiation. Ultraviolet light is destructive to bacteria, as are certain gases such as ethylene oxide, methyl bromide, and hydrogen cyanide. Sudden exposure of some organisms to a large and virtually instantaneous reduction of pressure may be lethal. This causes the organisms to explode or rupture.

Chemical agents that inhibit bacterial growth are called antiseptics and their action is described as being bacteriostatic; those that kill bacteria are called germicides or bactericides. Among disinfectants are strong acids and alkalies, metallic salts (bichloride of mercury), halogens (chlorine, iodine), oxidizing agents (hydrogen peroxide), organic compounds (phenol, formaldehyde, salicylic acid), and other substances such as boric acid. Substances used in the treatment of diseases caused by bacteria are called chemotherapeutic agents, such as antibiotics. They include the sulfonamide compounds and the antibiotics.

b., antibody-coated. Bacteria that, due

to the specific antigen-antibody response they have produced in the body, become coated with those antibodies. The presence of these antibodies on bacteria may be detected by use of direct immunofluorescence.

bacterial adherence. The process of attachment of bacteria to tissue cells. Some bacteria need to adhere to cells in order to colonize a site and cause infection.

bacterial plasmids. SEE: *plasmids.*

bacterial resistance. Development of resistance to a drug by an organism previously susceptible to it. This has been manifested by pathogenic organisms (as gonococci, streptococci, staphylococci, and tubercle bacilli) to various chemotherapeutic drugs, and occurs both in vitro and in vivo. It may be due to appearance of resistant mutant strains, development of alternate metabolic pathways, decomposition of the drug, or unknown factors. SEE: *antiviral resistance; transfer factor.*

bacterial synergism. The interaction of indigenous flora to allow a strain of bacteria to become pathogenic when it would normally be harmless.

bacterial vaginosis. SEE: *vaginosis, bacterial.*

bactericidal (băk″tĕr-ĭ-sī′dăl). Destructive to or destroying bacteria.

bactericide (băk-tĕr′ĭ-sīd) [Gr. *bakterion,* rod, + L. *caedere,* to kill]. An agent that destroys bacteria, but not necessarily their spores.

bactericidin. Anything lethal to bacteria.

bacterid (băk′tĕr-ĭd). Any skin rash caused by bacterial toxins or bacteria. The bacterial infection is usually remote from the rash.

bacteriemia (băk-tĕr-ē-ē′mē-ă) [″ + *haima,* blood]. Bacteremia, q.v.

bacterio- (băk-tē′rē-ō). Prefix pert. to bacteria.

bacterioagglutinin (băk-tē″rē-ō-ă-gloo′tĭ-nĭn) [″ + L. *agglutinans,* gluing]. An antibody in serum that causes agglutination, or clumping, of bacteria in vitro.

bacteriocidal (băk″tĕr-ē-ō-sī′dăl). Bactericidal, q.v.

bacteriocin (băk-tē′rē-ō-sĭn). Protein produced by certain bacteria that exerts a lethal effect on closely related bacteria. In general, bacteriocins are more potent but have a narrower range of activity than antibiotics. SEE: *colicin.*

bacteriocinogen (băk-tē″rē-ō-sĭn′ō-gĕn). A plasmid that produces bacteriocin.

bacteriogenic (băk-tē″rē-ō-jĕn′ĭk) [″ + *gennan,* to produce]. 1. Caused by bacteria. 2. Producing bacteria.

bacteriohemagglutinin (băk-tē″rē-ō-hĕm″ă-gloo′tĭ-nĭn) [″ + *haima,* blood, + L. *agglutinans,* gluing]. A hemagglutinin

formed in the body by bacterial action.

bacteriohemolysin (băk-tē″rē-ō-hē-mŏl′ĭ-sĭn) [″ + ″ + *lysis,* dissolution]. A hemolysin formed in the body by bacterial action.

bacterioid (băk-tĕr′ē-oyd) [″ + *eidos,* form, shape]. Resembling bacteria.

bacteriologic, bacteriological [″ + *logos,* word, reason]. Pert. to bacteriology.

bacteriologist. An individual with academic training in the field of bacteriology.

bacteriology. Science that deals with bacteria.

bacteriolysin (băk-tē″rē-ōl′ĭ-sĭn) [″ + *lysis,* dissolution]. A substance, esp. an antibody produced within the body of an animal, that is capable of bringing about the lysis of bacteria.

bacteriolysis (băk-tē″rē-ōl′ĭ-sĭs). The destruction or dissolution of bacteria.

bacteriolytic (băk-tē″rē-ō-lĭt′ĭk). Pert. to bacteriolysis.

bacteriophage (băk-tē′rē-ō-fāj″) [Gr. *bakterion,* rod, + *phagein,* to eat]. A virus that infects bacteria. Bacteriophages are widely distributed in nature, having been isolated from feces, sewage, and polluted surface waters. They are regarded as bacterial viruses, the phage particle consisting of a head composed of either RNA or DNA and a tail by which it attaches to host cells. SYN: *phage.*

bacteriophytoma (băk-tē″rē-ō-fī-tō′mă) [″ + *phyton,* plant, + *oma,* tumor]. A tumorlike growth caused by bacteria.

bacterioprecipitin (băk-tē″rē-ō-prē-sĭp′ĭ-tĭn). Precipitin produced in the body by the action of bacteria.

bacterioprotein (băk-tē″rē-ō-prō′tē-ĭn). Any of the proteins within the cells of bacteria.

bacteriopsonin (băk-tē″rē-ŏp′sō-nĭn). An opsonin, q.v., acting on bacteria.

bacteriosis (băk-tē″rē-ō′sĭs) [″ + *osis,* condition]. Any disease caused by bacteria.

bacteriostasis (băk-tē″rē-ōs′tă-sĭs) [″ + *stasis,* standing still]. The arrest of bacterial growth.

bacteriostatic (băk-tē-rē-ō-stăt′ĭk). Inhibiting or retarding bacterial growth.

bacteriotoxic (băk-tē″rē-ō-tŏk′sĭk). 1. Toxic to bacteria. 2. Due to bacterial toxins.

bacteriotoxin (băk-tē″rē-ō-tŏk′sĭn) [″ + *toxikon,* poison]. Toxin specifically produced by or destructive to bacteria.

bacteriotropin (băk-tē″rē-ŏt′rō-pĭn) [″ + *tropos,* a turn]. An opsonin or a substance that enhances the ability of phagocytes to engulf bacteria.

bacteristatic. Inhibiting the growth of bacteria. SEE: *bactericidal.*

bacterium (pl. *bacteria*). A general term for unicellular microscopic organisms under the kingdom of prokaryotes. Except for mycoplasmas (not really bacteria) they have a rigid cell wall. They are classed with respect to their motility, reaction to staining with particular dyes; and with respect to their pathogenicity for other living organisms including man. Fungi, algae, protozoa, and viruses are not bacteria.

bacteriuria (băk-tē″rē-ū′rē-ă) [Gr. *bakterion*, rod, + *ouron*, urine]. Presence of bacteria in the urine.

  b., significant. Concentration of pathogenic bacteria in the urine of 10^5 per ml or greater.

bacteroid (băk′tĕr-oyd) [″ + *eidos*, form, shape]. 1. Resembling a bacterium. 2. A structurally modified bacterium.

Bacteroides (băk-tĕr-oyd′ēz). A genus of non-spore-forming, gram-negative rods, anaerobic bacteria occurring normally in digestive, respiratory, and genital tracts, frequently found in necrotic tissue, and often in the blood following infections. Some species are pathogenic and may be implicated in peritonitis and peritoneal abscesses. *Bacteroides* are the most common bacteria in the colon, where they outnumber *Escherichia coli* by at least 100 to 1. The species most commonly encountered is *B. fragilis*.

Bactocill. Trade name for oxacillin sodium.

bad breath. Halitosis, q.v. Offensive odor of the breath. Its origin may be in the mouth or nose, lungs, blood, or digestive tract. Many individuals have bad breath due to drying of the oral mucosa. On awakening, those who snore or sleep with their mouths open may have particularly noticeable bad breath. If bad breath is due to an ingested food, such as onions or garlic, local therapy with a mouthwash will be of no benefit because the odor is present in the blood and is excreted from the lungs. In almost all other cases, the cause may be treated by attending to decayed teeth and by careful oral hygiene. SYN: *halitosis.*

bad news, giving. It is inevitable that health care professionals will have to deliver bad news to a patient. There is no set formula for how to do this because each situation is different. The more insight you have into the patient, the better prepared you will be to try to provide reassurance, positive thinking, and planning for the future. Essential to this process will be feedback from the patient during this encounter. You will be able to tell whether the information you are supplying is helping the patient to cope with the problem. There may come a point in which the glazed look of the patient is sure evidence that nothing more you say will be heard. In that case, return later. In all of this interchange, the information given must be realistic but not overly optimistic or pessimistic. Nevertheless, it is important to provide a basis for hope, to emphasize all of the positive aspects of the patient's condition, and to assure the patient that all that is possible will be done to ameliorate the condition and to help the patient cope.

bag [ME. *bagge*]. A sack or pouch.

  b., Douglas. SEE: *Douglas bag.*

  b. of waters. The amnion, q.v. The membrane enclosing the liquor amnii and the fetus. It refers sometimes to that portion of the membrane protruding into the os uteri. It is the inner embryonic membrane, the chorion being the outer envelope.

  b., Politzer's. Soft rubber bag for inflation of middle ear. SEE: *aerotitis.*

bagassosis (băg-ă-sō′sĭs) [Sp. *bagazo*, husks, + Gr. *osis*, condition]. A form of hypersensitivity pneumonitis, q.v., due to inhalation of bagasse dust, the moldy, dusty fibrous waste of sugar cane after removal of the sugar-containing sap. The dust contains antigens from thermophilic actinomycetes.

bag lady, bag man. Impoverished, homeless, usually elderly persons in urban areas who are seen carrying all their possessions in shopping bags or carts.

bag-valve-mask resuscitator. Manually operated resuscitator consisting of a bag reservoir, a one-way flow valve, and a face mask capable of ventilating a nonbreathing patient. Commonly known as an Ambu bag. SEE: illus.

baker [AS. *bacan*, cook by dry heat]. Two or more electric lamps mounted in semicircular containers used for applying heat to various parts of the body. Called electric light bakers.

Baker's cyst [William M. Baker, Brit. surgeon, 1839–1896]. Synovial cyst (pouch) arising from the synovial lining of the knee. It occurs in the popliteal fossa.

baker leg. Knock-knee; genu valgum.

BAL. *British anti-lewisite.* Trade name for dimercaprol, a compound used as an antidote in poisoning from heavy metals. SEE: *dimercaprol.*

balance (băl′ăns) [L. *bilanx*]. 1. Scale; a device for measuring weight. 2. A state of equilibrium; condition in which the intake and output of substances such as water and nutrients are approx. equal. SEE: *homeostasis.* 3. The ability to maintain the center of gravity over the base of support as in standing balance.

  b., acid-base. Normal balance between acid and base production and excretion in body, resulting in a stable concentration of hydrogen ions in the body fluids.

  b., analytical. A very sensitive scale.

  b., electrolyte. Condition in which elec-

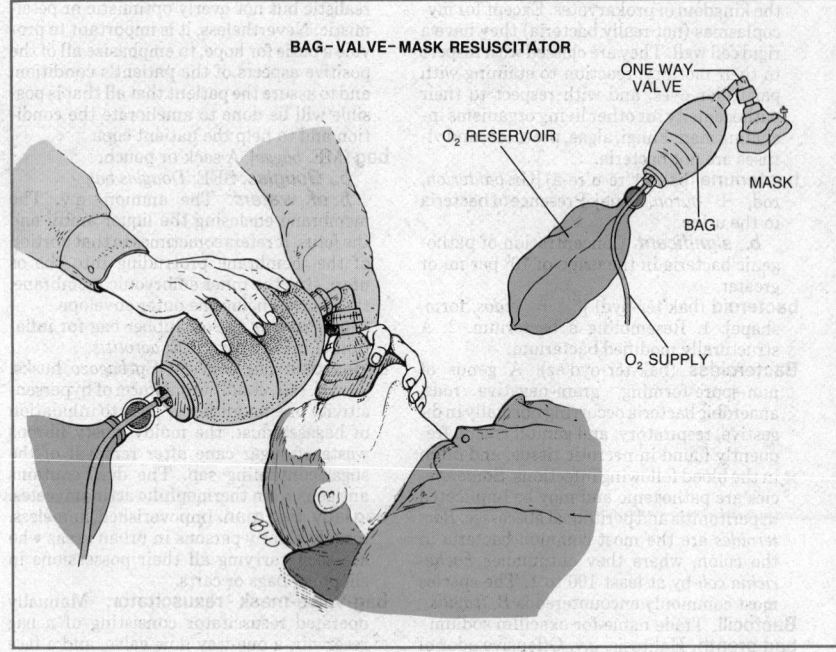

BAG-VALVE-MASK RESUSCITATOR

ONE WAY VALVE

O_2 RESERVOIR

MASK

BAG

O_2 SUPPLY

trolytes, esp. sodium and potassium, are maintained in suitable concentrations for cellular and metabolic processes.

b., fluid. Balance between intake and excretion of fluids, esp. water, in the body.

b., nitrogen. Body state in which intake of nitrogen in protein foods is equal to nitrogen output, principally through loss of nitrogenous substances in the urine and feces.

balance beam. In occupational therapy and physical therapy, a device, usually consisting of a narrow beam elevated several inches from the floor, used for assessing and training balance and motor coordination.

balance board. Device, usually consisting of a padded platform mounted on a curved base, commonly used in therapy with children having CNS deficits. Designed to facilitate the development of appropriate equilibrium-related postural reflexes.

balanic (bă-lăn′ĭk) [Gr. *balanos*, glans]. Pert. to the glans clitoridis or glans penis.

balanitis (băl-ă-nī′tĭs) [″ + *itis*, inflammation]. Inflammation of the skin covering the glans penis.

b. xerotica obliterans. Pathological condition of the skin of the penis. There are sclerotic and atrophic patches that can

cause narrowing of the urinary meatus and phimosis. The cause is thought to be chronic balanoposthitis.

TREAT: Symptomatic and may be of little benefit.

balano- (băl′ă-nō) [Gr. *balanos*, glans]. Combining form pert. to the glans penis or the glans clitoridis.

balanocele (băl′ă-nō-sēl″) [″ + *kele*, tumor, swelling]. Protrusion of the glans penis through a rupture of the prepuce.

balanoplasty (băl′ă-nō-plăs″tē) [″ + *plassein*, to form]. Plastic surgery of glans penis.

balanoposthitis (băl″ă-nō-pŏs-thī′tĭs) [″ + *posthe*, prepuce, + *itis*, inflammation]. Balanitis, q.v.

balanopreputial (băl″ă-nō-prē-pū′shē-ăl). Pert. to glans penis and prepuce.

balanorrhagia (băl″ă-nŏ-rā′jē-ă) [″ + *rhegnynai*, burst forth]. Balanitis with pus formation.

balantidial (băl-ăn-tĭd′ē-ăl). Pert. to *Balantidium*, a genus of protozoa.

balantidiasis (băl″ăn-tĭ-dī′ă-sĭs). Infection caused by infestation with *Balantidium coli*.

SYM: Abdominal pain, diarrhea, vomiting, weakness, and loss of weight.

TREAT: Tetracyclines, metronidazole,

or paromomycin.

Balantidium (băl-ăn-tĭd′ē-ŭm) [Gr. *balantidion,* a bag]. A genus of ciliated protozoa. A number of species are found in the intestines of both vertebrates and invertebrates.

B. coli. A species of *Balantidium* that is the largest protozoon parasitic of man. It lives in the large intestine and is the cause of balantidiasis. It is a normal parasite of hogs.

balanus (băl′ă-nŭs) [Gr. *balanos,* glans]. The glans penis or glans clitoridis.

baldness [ME. *ballede,* without hair]. Lack of or partial loss of hair on head. SEE: *alopecia.*

b., male pattern. Baldness in the male due to influence of the male hormone testosterone. Onset of baldness is also related to age in that hair loss increases with age. Genetic predisposition is also a factor, and baldness does not usually occur in males having no familial tendency to become bald. The use of minoxidil has helped stimulate growth of hair in some individuals.

Balint's syndrome [Rudolph Balint, Hungarian physician, 1874–1929]. Inability to scan the peripheral visual field and to grasp an object under visual guidance, and visual inattention. Usually due to bilateral occipitoparietal lesions of the brain.

Balkan frame. A framework that fits over the bed. Suspended from the frame and connected through ropes and pulleys are weights used to produce desired continuous traction while permitting freedom of motion, thus maintaining desired immobilization of the part being treated.

Balke test [Bruno Balke, contemporary Ger.-born U.S. physician]. A test to determine maximum oxygen utilization. The subject walks on a flat (0% grade) treadmill at a constant rate of 3.5 miles/hour for 2 min. The treadmill is inclined 1% each successive minute until the subject is exhausted and unable to continue. Oxygen utilization is measured throughout the test.

Caution: The test is not suitable for individuals who have impairment of their musculoskeletal, cardiovascular, or respiratory systems.

---

ball. A spherically shaped object.

b., hair. Mass of hair that has accumulated in the intestine or stomach. SYN: *trichobezoar.*

b. of foot. The padded portion of the anterior extremity of the sole of the foot.

b. of thumb. Thenar eminence of the thumb.

b. thrombus. A round blood clot, esp. one in the heart. SEE: *thrombus.*

ball-and-socket joint. Synovial joint in which one rounded bone head moves within

a concavity of another bone. SYN: *enarthrosis.*

ball bearing feeder. Device attaching to the arms of wheelchairs that is designed to provide active assistance for upper extremity function. SYN: *mobile arm support.*

ballism, ballismus (băl′ĭzm, bă-lĭz′mŭs) [Gr. *ballismos,* jumping about]. 1. Condition characterized by jerking, twisting movements seen in chorea. 2. Obsolete term for paralysis agitans.

ballistics (bă-lĭs′tĭks) [Gr. *ballein,* to throw]. Science of the motion and trajectory of missiles such as bullets, bombs, rockets, and guided missiles.

ballistocardiograph (bă-lĭs″tō-kär′dē-ō-grăf) [″ + *kardia,* heart, + *graphein,* to write]. Mechanism for measuring and recording the impact caused by the discharge of blood from the heart at each beat and the resulting recoil. The minute movements of the body with each heartbeat are recorded as they are transmitted to the special platform that supports the subject.

balloon [It. *ballone,* great ball]. 1. To expand, dilate, or distend, as expanding a cavity by filling it with air or water in a bag. 2. A flexible, expandable object that can be placed inside a vessel or cavity to expand it or at the end of a catheter in order to help prevent its removal. SEE: *catheter; percutaneous transluminal coronary angioplasty.*

balloon bezoar. SEE: *bezoar, balloon.*

ballooning. The distention of a cavity, as the vagina, by air, etc., for examination.

balloon tamponade, nasal. SEE: *epistaxis; nosebleed* for illus.

ballottable (bă-lŏt′ă-bl). Capable of showing the ballottement phenomenon. SEE: *ballottement.*

ballottement (băl-ŏt-mŏn′) [Fr. *balloter,* to toss about]. A palpatory technique used in detecting or examining a floating object in the body, such as an organ or fetus. Used in examining the abdomen esp. when ascites is present. Applied particularly to a diagnostic maneuver in pregnancy. The rebound of the fetus or a fetal part, when displaced by a light tap of the examining finger through the vagina.

ball-valve action. Action of a mass, such as a pedunculated cyst or thrombus, moving to open and close the passageway of a tube or chamber, thus causing intermittent obstruction. A ball-valve thrombus may form in the heart and cause repeated blockage of an opening connecting two chambers of the heart.

balm [Gr. *balsamon,* balsam]. 1. A balsam. 2. A soothing or healing ointment.

b. of Gilead. 1. Mecca balsam from *Commiphora opobalsamum,* probably Biblical myrrh. 2. Balsam fir, source of Canadian balsam. 3. Poplar bud resin.

balneology (băl-nē-ŏl′ō-jē) [L. *balneum*, bath, + Gr. *logos*, word, reason]. The science of baths and bathing.

balneotherapy, balneotherapeutics (băl″nē-ō-thĕr′ă-pē, -thĕr″ă-pū′tĭks) [″ + Gr. *therapeia*, treatment]. The use of baths in treatment of disease.

balsam (bawl′săm) [Gr. *balsamon*, balsam]. A fragrant, resinous, oily exudate from various trees and plants. Balsams are resins combined with oil. They are used in topical preparations to treat irritated skin or mucous membrane.

b. of Peru. A dark-brown, viscid, resinous liquid obtained from the bark of the tree *Myroxylon perierae* or *M. balsamum*.

Balser's fatty necrosis (băl′zĕrs) [W. Balser, 19th-century Ger. physician]. Gangrenous pancreatitis with fatty necrotic areas in interlobular tissue and sometimes in pericardial fat and bone marrow.

Baltimore Longitudinal Study of Aging. An investigation initiated in 1958 for the purpose of examining aging in healthy, upper middle class persons with regard to certain physiological and psychological variables.

bamboo spine. Roentgenogram of the spine in ankylosing spondylitis that resembles the stalk of the bamboo plant.

Bancroft's filariasis [Joseph Bancroft, Brit. physician, 1836–1894]. A filarial infection caused by *Wuchereria bancrofti*. SEE: *elephantiasis*.

band. 1. A cord or tapelike tissue that connects or holds structures together. SEE: *bundle; ligament; tract.* 2. Any appliance that encircles or binds the body or a limb. 3. Segment of a myofibril. 4. Metal strip or seamless band for attaching orthodontic appliances to teeth.

bandage [ME. *bande*, a band]. 1. A piece of soft, usually absorbent gauze or other material applied to a limb or other part of the body as a dressing. 2. To cover by wrapping with a piece of gauze or other material.

Bandages are of various types and materials and are used to hold dressings in place, apply pressure to a part, immobilize a part, obliterate cavities, give support to an injured area, and aid in checking hemorrhages. Types of bandages include roller, triangular, four-tailed, many-tailed (Scultetus), quadrangular, elastic (elastic knit, rubber, synthetic, or combinations of these), adhesive, elastic adhesive, newer cohesive bandages under various proprietary names, impregnated bandages (plaster of paris, waterglass [silica], starch), and stockinet. Use of a self-adhering, form-fitting roller bandage facilitates bandaging by eliminating the special techniques needed when ordinary gauze roller bandages are used. SEE: *sling*; illus.

Caution: When bandaging, do not allow skin of one part to be held against the skin of another part, as severe skin infection can result.

b., abdomen. A single wide cravat or several narrow ones that are used to hold dressing in place or to exert a moderate pressure.

b., Ace. Trade name for a woven elastic bandage available in various widths and lengths. Provides uniform support, yet permits areas such as joints to move without loosening the bandage.

b., adhesive. Bandage made of adhesive tape, q.v.

b., amputation-stump. An elastic bandage applied to the stump (residual limb) after amputation in order to control postoperative edema and shape the residual limb. The elastic bandage is applied in a recurrent or figure-of-eight fashion with more pressure applied to the distal than to the proximal portion of the limb.

b., ankle. Bandage in which one loop is brought around the sole of foot and the other around the ankle and secured in front or on the side.

b., axilla. Bandage with a spica-type turn starting under the affected axilla, crossing over the shoulder of the affected side, and making the long loop under the opposite armpit.

b., back. (Triangular) Open bandage to the back. This is applied the same as the chest bandage, the point being placed above the scapula of the injured side.

b., Barton. Double figure-of-eight bandage for the lower jaw.

b., breast. (Roller) Suspensory bandages and compresses for the breasts.

b., butterfly. Adhesive bandage used in place of sutures to hold wound edges together.

b., buttocks. T or double-T bandage or open triangle bandage for the buttocks.

b., capeline. Bandage applied to the head or shoulder or to a stump like a cap or hood.

b., chest. (Roller) Figure-of-eight (spica), many-tailed (Scultetus), or triangular (open-chest) bandage for the chest.

b., circular. Bandage applied in circular turns about a part.

b., cohesive. Material that has an intense power of sticking to itself but not to other substances. Used to bandage fingers, extremities, etc., or to build up pads.

b., cravat. Triangular bandage folded to

TYPES OF BANDAGES

FIGURE-OF-EIGHT   RECURRENT   SPIRAL REVERSE

BANDAGE OF SHOULDER   RECURRENT B. OF HEAD

TRIANGULAR BANDAGE OF ELBOW, AND ARM

TYPES OF BANDAGES

BARTON

BUTTERFLY STRIPS

PILLOW SPLINT

ANKLE STRAPPING

WRIST BANDAGE

form a band around the injured part. This is done by pulling the point over toward the base, folding the base over the point, and then folding again. This makes a bandage wide enough to cover a large knee. When folded a second time, it is wide enough to make the cravat bandage of the elbow. Folded a third time, it could be used in making a figure-of-eight for the foot, ankle, hand, wrist, or head. It is an effective bandage in arresting hemorrhages and in retaining splints and dressings. The center of the cravat should be laid against the affected part, the ends of the cravat carried around the limb and tied over the center of the base. When used to retain splints, it should be tied on the outer side of the limb and against the splint, thus preventing the knot from irritating the skin. When used to retain a dressing in the axilla, the center of the cravat should be placed under the arm and the ends carried upward and crossed over the shoulder and tied in the axillary space of the opposite side, thus forming a figure-of-eight. The cravat can also be used as a sling when only a simple support is needed.

In using cravats for ties or splints, care should be taken so that the knots do not pass over and press unduly on the surface of the limb. Knots should be placed where they are easily found and not subject to pressure; the ends should be neatly tucked in. All knots should be square or reef knots.

b., cravat elbow. Bandage in which one bends the elbow about 45° and places center of bandage over point of elbow. Then one brings one end around forearm and the other end around upper arm, pulls tight, and ties.

b., cravat, for clenched fist. Hand bandage to arrest bleeding or to produce pressure. The wrist is placed on the center of the cravat, one end is brought around over the fist and back to the starting point, and the same procedure is then repeated with the other end. The two ends are pulled tight, twisted, and carried around the fist again so that pressure is placed on the flexed fingers.

b., cravat, for fracture of clavicle. Bandage in which one first puts a soft pad 2 × 4 in. (5.1 × 10.2 cm) in the forepart of the axilla. A sling is made by placing the point of the open bandage on the affected shoulder, the hand and wrist laid on it and directed toward the opposite shoulder, the point brought over and tucked underneath the wrist and hand. The ends are then lifted and the bandage is laid flat on the chest, the covered hand is carried up on the shoulder, the ends are brought together in the back and tied, the tightness being decided by how

high the shoulder should be carried. A cravat bandage is then applied horizontally above the broad part of the elbow and tied over a pad on the opposite side of the chest. Tightening this cravat pushes out the shoulder.

b., cravat, sling. Bandage used for support of the hand and in fracture of the upper arm. The wrist is laid upon the center of the cravat bandage, the forearm being held at right angle, and the two ends are carried around the neck and tied. SEE: *binder.*

b., crucial. SEE: *b., T.*

b., demigauntlet. Bandage that covers the hand but leaves the fingers uncovered.

b., ear. (Roller) T bandage for the ear. A piece is sewn across the right angle of the T bandage.

b.'s, elastic. Bandages that have the property of stretching and hence making compression when correctly applied. Usually made of special weaves or of material incorporating rubber. Applied over swollen extremities or joints, on the chest in empyema, on fractured ribs, or for supporting varicose veins, etc.

b., Esmarch. 1. Triangular bandage, q.v. 2. Rubber bandage wrapped about an extremity, after elevation, from its periphery toward the heart to force blood out of the extremity prior to operation or to increase circulating blood. On removal for surgery, a proximal band is left in place to prevent blood from returning to the extremity.

Caution: If bandage is applied too tightly or for a prolonged period, tissue damage may occur.

---

b., eye. Bandage for retaining dressings. The simple roller bandage for one eye or the monocle or crossed bandage. The binocular or crossed bandage for both eyes is 2 in. × 6 yd (5.1 cm × 5.49 meters).

b., figure-of-eight. Bandage in which the turns cross each other like the figure eight. Used to retain dressings or to exert pressure for joints (or to leave joint uncovered), to fix splints for the foot or hand, for the great toe, and for sprains or hemorrhage.

b., finger. Roller bandage with oblique fixation at wrist.

b., foot. (Triangular) Bandage in which the foot should be placed on the triangle with the base of the bandage backward and behind the ankle; the apex is carried upward over the top of the foot. The ends are brought forward, folded once or twice, crossed and carried around the foot, and tied on top.

b., forearm. (Triangular) Open sling bandage for support of the forearm.

b., four-tailed. A strip of cloth with each

end split into two. Tails used to cover prominences such as elbow, chin, nose, knee.

b., Fricke's. Special bandage for supporting and immobilizing the scrotum.

b., groin. (Special) Bandage that is most easily applied with the patient standing or lying on a pelvic rest. A spica bandage encircles the trunk and the crossing is placed either anteriorly or laterally. To bandage both groins, the double spica is used. Such a double bandage is used principally in applying a plaster cast.

b., hand. (Roller, 1 in. or 2.5 cm wide). Demigauntlet bandage for the hand to hold a dressing on the back of the hand. For thumb and hand, the ascending spica of the thumb, with spiral of the hand, is used. A triangular bandage for open bandage of the hand. A descending spica is used for the thumb and figure-of-eight bandage for amputation stump or clenched fist.

b., head. Single recurrent roller capeline or skull cap bandage. The double roller recurrent bandage is used for the scalp. Any of the quadrants of the skull may be bandaged. Use triangular or shawl bandage for open bandage of the head.

In another form of head bandage, place center of narrow cravat under chin, bring ends to top of head, and tie single knot. Have patient or an assistant hold ends and separate knot, which forms two loops. Place one low on back of head and bring the other forward over forehead, eyes, or chin as necessary. Adjust so it is symmetrical and tie ends on top of head.

b., heel. Triangular bandage used for the heel.

b., hip. (Triangular) In an open bandage of the hip, a cravat bandage or other band is tied around the waist; the point of another bandage is slipped under and rolled or pinned directly above the position of the wound. The base is rolled up, the ends carried around the thigh, crossed, and tied.

b., immovable. Bandage for immobilizing a part.

b., impregnated. Wide-meshed bandage used to make molds or immobilize parts of the body. Material is impregnated with substances such as plaster of paris, which are applied wet and harden after drying.

b., knee. The knee cravat, the triangular, and the figure-of-eight bandages are used.

b., knotted. Bandage used to exert pressure on a compress or pad over a bleeding wound.

b., leg. Bandage applied by fixing the initial end by a circular or oblique fixation at the ankle or with a figure-of-eight of the foot and ankle.

b., Maisonneuve's. Plaster-of-paris bandage made of folded cloth held in place by other bandages.

b., many-tailed. Bandage with split ends used for trunk and limbs. A piece of roller to which slips are stitched in an imbricated fashion. SEE: *b., four-tailed; b., Scultetus.*

b., Martin's. Roller bandage of rubber used to make pressure on an extremity as for varicose veins, and for exsanguination, as Esmarch bandage, q.v.

b., neck. (Roller) *Neck spica:* Bandage 2½ in. × 8 yd (6.4 cm × 7.3 meters). *Bandage following thyroid gland surgery:* Roller bandage 2½ in. × 9 yd (6.4 cm × 8.2 meters). *Adhesive plaster bandage for thyroidectomy:* Used to hold dressing on wound in place. Apply a small dressing to center of strip and then apply to back of neck. *Special bandage:* A double-loop bandage of the head and neck made by using a figure-of-eight turn.

b., oblique. Bandage applied obliquely to a limb, without reverses.

b., plaster. Bandage stiffened with a paste of plaster of paris, which sets and becomes very hard.

b., postoperative. (Dressing) A simple divergent or convergent spica bandage.

b., pressure. Bandage for applying pressure, usually used to stop hemorrhage.

b., protective. Bandage that covers a part or keeps dressings in place.

b., quadrangular. A towel or large handkerchief, folded variously and applied as a bandage of head, chest, breast, or abdomen.

b., recurrent. Bandage over the end of a stump.

b., reversed. Bandage applied to a limb in such a way that the roller is inverted or half twisted at each turn so as to make it fit smoothly.

b., roller. A long strip of soft material, usually from ½ to 6 in. (1.3 to 15.2 cm) wide and 2 to 5 yd (1.83 to 4.57 meters) long, rolled on its short axis. When rolled from both ends to meet at center, it is called a double-headed roller.

b., rubber. Roller bandage of rubber used for pressure as in swollen parts for immobilization.

b., Scultetus. Many-tailed bandage. A succession of interlocking, overlapping bands originally used to enclose a rigid support against a fractured extremity but now used without the splint or impregnated as a supporting bandage of the abdomen or lower extremity. SEE: *binder, Scultetus,* for illus.

b., shoulder. Open bandage of the shoulder: Spica bandage. Shoulder and neck: Shawl bandage of both shoulders and neck.

b., spica. Bandage in which a number of

figure-of-eight turns are applied, each a little higher or lower, overlapping a portion of each preceding turn so as to give an imbricated appearance. For breast, shoulder, limbs, thumb, great toe, and hernia at the groin. For support, to exert pressure, or to retain dressings.

b., spiral reverse. Technique of twisting, in its long axis, a roller bandage on itself at intervals during application to make it fit more uniformly. These reverse folds may be necessary every turn or less, depending on contour of part being bandaged.

b., suspensory. Bandage for supporting any part but esp. the breast or scrotum.

b., T. Bandage shaped like the letter T. For the perineum and, in certain cases, for the head.

b., tailed. Bandage with ends split.

b., toe. Small bandage, about 2 in. (5.1 cm) wide.

b., triangular. A 36- to 42-in. (232- to 271-cm) square, usually muslin cut diagonally, making two triangular bandages. Frequently used in first aid. SYN: *b., Esmarch* (def. 1). SEE: *triangular bandage* for illus.

b., Velpeau. A special immobilizing roller bandage that incorporates the shoulder, arm, and forearm.

bandage roller. A device for rolling bandages.

banding. Use of chemicals to stain chromosomes so that the characteristic bands may be visualized.

Bandl's ring (bǎn'd'ls) [Ludwig Bandl, Ger. obstetrician, 1842–1892]. Ringlike thickening and indentation at the junction of the upper and lower uterine segments that obstruct delivery of the fetus. SEE: *retraction ring.*

bandwidth. In electronics the range of frequencies within which performance with respect to some characteristic falls within specified limits.

bandy leg. Bowleg. SYN: *genu varum.*

bank. A stored supply of body fluids or tissues for use in another individual, e.g., blood bank, eye bank, kidney bank, tissue bank.

b., sperm. Repository for storage of semen so that it may be used for artificial insemination. In some banks the specimen is frozen. SEE: *Universal Precautions* in *Appendix.*

Banthine. Trade name for methantheline bromide, USP. An anticholinergic.

Banting, Sir Frederick Grant. Canadian scientist, 1891–1941; co-discoverer of insulin, with Charles Herbert Best and John J. R. Macleod in 1922. Nobel laureate 1923.

Banti's syndrome (bǎn'těz) [Guido Banti, It. physician, 1852–1925]. A syndrome combining anemia, splenic enlargement, hemorrhages, and ultimately cirrhosis of liver.

Considered secondary to portal hypertension.

bar. A metal piece attaching two or more units of a removable dental prosthesis.

bar, median. Contractures or constrictions of vesical neck of the bladder caused by benign hypertrophy or fibrosis of the prostate. This may cause obstruction to the flow of urine from the bladder.

baragnosis bǎr-ǎg-nō'sǐs) [Gr. *baros*, weight, + *a-*, not, + *gnosis*, knowledge]. Inability to estimate weights. Indicative of parietal lobe lesion. Opposite of barognosis. SYN: *abarognosis.*

Bárány's caloric test [Robert Bárány, Austrian physician and physiologist, 1876–1936. Won Nobel prize in medicine in 1914]. Vestibular function is evaluated by irrigating the ear canal with either warm or cold water. Normally, when warm water is used, rotatory nystagmus toward the irrigated ear is observed. When cold water is used, the normal response is rotatory nystagmus away from the irrigated ear. If vestibular function is impaired, the response may be absent or diminished. If one ear is normal and the other is not, a comparison between the two may be made.

barber's itch. 1. An affection of the face due to infection of hair follicles and associated glands by staphylococci. Characterized by formation of papules and pustules. SYN: *folliculitis barbae.* 2. A dermatomycosis caused by a fungus, *Microsporum lanosum* or *Trichophyton mentagrophytes*, *T. violaceum*, or *T. purpureum.* SYN: *tinea barbae.*

barbital (bǎr'bǐ-tǎl). 5,5-diethylbarbituric acid, a crystalline powder and derivative of barbituric acid. Used as a hypnotic and sedative, it is habit forming.

b., sodium. The soluble monosodium salt of barbital. Has same properties as barbital but because of greater solubility, it is more rapidly absorbed.

barbital poisoning. SEE: *barbiturates* in *Poisons and Poisoning* in *Appendix.*

barbiturates (bǎr-bǐt'ū-rǎts, bǎr-bǐ-tū'rǎts). A group of organic compounds derived from barbituric acid. All derivatives depress the central nervous system and depress respiration, affect heart rate, and decrease blood pressure and temperature. These drugs can be habit forming. For sedative action, these drugs have been replaced by safer drugs such as benzodiazepines.

Ex.: Amytal, Pentothal, phenobarbital, Seconal. SEE: *Poisons and Poisoning* in *Appendix.*

barbotage (bǎr-bō-tŏzh') [Fr. *barboter*, to dabble]. Repeated injection and withdrawal of fluid, as in gastric lavage, or the administration of an anesthetic into the subarachnoid space by alternate injection of anesthetic and withdrawal of cerebrospinal fluid into the syringe.

barbula hirci (băr′bū-lă hĭr′sī) [L. *barbula,* little beard, + *hircus,* goat]. 1. Hairs present on the ears. 2. Axillary hair.

barefoot doctor. In the People's Republic of China, persons trained to administer medical care in locations where there is a shortage of physicians.

baresthesia (băr-ĕs-thē′zē-ă) [Gr. *baros,* weight, + *aisthesis,* sensation]. Sense of weight or pressure; pressure sense.

baresthesiometer (băr″ĕs-thē″zē-ŏm′ĕ-tĕr) [″ + ″ + *metron,* measure]. Instrument for determining sensitivity to weight or pressure.

bariatrics (băr″ē-ă′trĭks) [″ + *iatrike,* medical treatment]. Branch of medicine dealing with prevention, control, and treatment of obesity.

barium (bă′rē-ŭm). SYMB: Ba. At. wt. 137.373; at. no. 56. A soft metallic element of the alkaline earth group.

   b. sulfate. USP. A radiopaque barium compound used in roentgenography of the gastrointestinal tract. Trade names are Barosperse and Esophotrast.

barium compounds. Compounds containing barium and suitable diluents or additives. Used to color fireworks and, in the form of insoluble barium sulfate, to visualize the hollow viscera in roentgenography. Poisoning occasionally occurs when the soluble salts are used accidentally in place of the insoluble sulfate. SEE: *Poisons and Poisoning* in *Appendix.*

barium enema. Use of barium sulfate as an enema to facilitate x-ray and fluoroscopic examination of the colon.

   PROCEDURE: Careful preparation of the patient will greatly increase the chances of the test to produce useful information. The patient is given the following written instructions with a careful explanation to ensure compliance. 1. A minimum-residue diet must be followed for all meals for two days prior to the test. 2. Two nights prior to the test, 60 ml (2 oz) of milk of magnesia must be taken in 120 ml (4 oz) of water at bedtime. 3. On the day before the test, a clear liquid diet must be taken for all meals. 4. At 5 P.M. on the day before the test, 60 ml (2 oz) of castor oil must be taken. 5. At 10 P.M. on the day before the test, a cleansing enema consisting of 1500 ml (50 oz) of lukewarm water must be given. 6. On the day of the test, only clear liquids are allowed for meals. SEE: *diet, minimum residue.*

   b.e., double contrast. A technique of barium enema x-ray study of the large intestine in which air is insufflated into the rectum and colon. This technique is thought to be much more effective in demonstrating pathologic lesions of the large intestine than is ordinary barium enema.

barium meal. Use of ingested barium sulfate to visualize the outline of the esophagus, stomach, and small intestines during x-ray or fluoroscopic examination. Also called *upper G.I. series.*

   PROCEDURE: If the test does not follow a barium enema, the patient should receive nothing by mouth after midnight on the night preceding the test. No food or liquids should be taken by mouth until the last roentgenogram is taken. If the test is done within a few days after a barium enema examination, it is important to be sure the colon is free of barium, which could interfere with visualization of the stomach and intestines. A cleansing enema and 60 ml (2 oz) of milk of magnesia in 120 ml (4 oz) of water the evening prior to the test will remove residual barium from the colon.

barium swallow. Radiographic examination of the esophagus during and after introduction of a contrast medium consisting of barium sulfate. Structural abnormalities of the esophagus and vessels such as esophageal varices may be diagnosed by use of this technique.

barium test. Nonspecific term for any test involving use of barium sulfate as a radiopaque material for outlining anatomical areas such as the esophagus and other portions of the intestinal tract by use of radiographic or fluoroscopic examinations. SEE: *barium enema; barium meal.*

bark [Old Norse *börkr*]. 1. The outer cover of stems, branches, roots, and main trunks of trees and woody plants. 2. A particular kind of bark used in medicine.

   Ex.: cascara sagrada, cinchona, wild cherry.

Barlow's disease [Sir Thomas Barlow, Brit. physician, 1845–1945]. A deficiency disease due to lack of vitamin C (ascorbic acid). Occurs in both breast-fed and bottle-fed babies who fail to receive adequate supplementary quantities of vitamin C. Occurs usually between 6 and 12 months of age. SEE: *scurvy, infantile.*

   TREAT: Vitamin C. Then adequate daily intake of fruit juices (orange, grapefruit, tomato).

Barlow's test. Assessment maneuver designed to detect subluxation or dislocation of the hip. The examiner adducts and then extends the legs with his fingers over the heads of the femurs. A dysplastic joint will be felt to dislocate as the femur leaves the acetabulum.

baro- [Gr. *baros,* weight]. Prefix indicating

weight, heaviness.

barognosis (băr-ŏg-nō'sĭs) [" + *gnosis*, knowledge]. The ability to estimate weights. Opposite of baragnosis.

barograph. A device used to measure and record changes in atmospheric pressure.

baroreceptor (băr"ŏ-rē-sĕp'tor). A sensory nerve ending that is stimulated by changes in pressure. Baroreceptors are found in the walls of the atria of the heart, vena cava, aortic arch, and carotid sinus.

baroreflexes (băr"ŏ-rē'flĕk-sĕs) [" + L. *reflexus*, bent back]. Reflexes mediated or activated through a group of nerves located in various blood vessels in the intrathoracic and cervical areas and in the heart and its great vessels. They are sensitive to mechanical changes produced when the pressure inside the vessel to which they are attached is altered. The response is called a baroreflex. Because the nerve groups are stimulated by mechanical rather than chemical means, they are called mechanoreceptors.

baroscope (băr'ŏ-skōp) [" + *skopein*, to examine]. Instrument that registers changes in the density of air.

barosinusitis (băr"ŏ-sī"nū-sī'tĭs) [Gr. *baros*, weight, + L. *sinus*, curve, + Gr. *itis*, inflammation]. Pain in and inflammation of one or more of the nasal sinuses due to one's having ascended or descended to a different altitude. This could occur while one is flying at a time when the outlet from a sinus is blocked. SEE: *aerotitis; barotitis.*

barostat. A receptor sensitive to alteration of pressure and which provides feedback stimuli to counteract the alterations. Such a feedback system is present in the part of the carotid sinus sensitive to changes in blood pressure.

barotaxis (băr"ŏ-tăk'sĭs) [" + *taxis*, turning]. Stimulation of cells by altering the pressure of the atmosphere.

barotitis (băr"ŏ-tī'tĭs) [" + *otos*, ear, + *itis*, inflammation]. Inflammation of the ear due to sudden changes in barometric pressure such as occur during flying. Closure of the eustachian tube due to upper respiratory infection prevents the middle ear from adjusting to pressure changes encountered during flight. SYN: *aerotitis; bag, Politzer's.*

barotrauma (băr"ŏ-traw'mă) [" + *trauma*, wound]. Any injury caused by a change in atmospheric pressure between a potentially closed space and the surrounding area. SEE: *aerotitis; barosinusitis; barotitis; bends; caisson disease.*

barotropism (băr-ŏt'rŏ-pĭzm) [" + *trope*, turning]. Barotaxis, q.v.

Barr body [Murray L. Barr, Canadian anatomist, b. 1908]. Sex chromatin mass seen within the nuclei of normal female somatic cells. According to the Lyon hypothesis, one of the two X chromosomes in each somatic cell of the female is genetically inactivated. The Barr body represents the inactivated X chromosome.

barrel chest. A condition of increased anteroposterior chest diameter caused by increased functional residual capacity due to air trapping from small airway collapse in patients with chronic obstructive pulmonary disease, i.e., chronic bronchitis and emphysema.

barren [O. Fr. *barhaine*, unproductive]. Sterile; incapable of producing offspring.

barrier [O. Fr. *barriere*]. An obstacle, impediment, obstruction, boundary, or separation.

b., blood-brain. Barrier that exists between circulating blood and the brain, preventing certain damaging substances from reaching brain tissue and cerebrospinal fluid. It consists of either the perivascular glial membrane or the vascular endothelium or both.

b., placental. Barrier provided by placental tissues, between the fetal and maternal circulation. Substances of small size, excluding blood cells, may traverse this barrier.

b., primary radiation. Wall or partition constructed to serve as a shield against direct exposure to x-rays.

b., secondary radiation. Wall or partition constructed to serve as a shield against scattered or leakage of x-rays.

barrier-free design. An approach to the design of living environments that emphasizes accessibility by persons with physical disability.

barrier layer cell. An optical sensor sometimes used in colorimeters. SYN: *photovoltaic cell.*

Bartholin's abscess (băr'tō-lĭnz) [Caspar Bartholin, Dan. anatomist, 1655–1738]. An abscess that develops when Bartholin's glands become occluded in an acute inflammatory process.

Bartholin's cyst. Cyst commonly formed in chronic inflammation of Bartholin's glands, q.v. Carcinoma is rare.

Bartholin's ducts. Large ducts of the sublingual salivary gland. They parallel Wharton's duct, q.v.

Bartholin's gland. A small compound mucous gland, situated one in each lateral wall of the vestibule of the vagina, near the vaginal opening at the base of the labia majora.

bartholinitis (băr"tō-lĭn-ī'tĭs) [*Bartholin* + Gr. *itis*, inflammation]. Inflammation of Bartholin's gland.

Barton, Clara. U.S. nurse, 1821–1912. Founder of the American National Red

Cross, she aided the wounded in the Civil War. Contemporary of Florence Nightingale, q.v.

Bartonella (băr″tō-něl′ă) [A. L. Barton, S. Amer. physician, 1871–1950]. A genus of the family Bartonellaceae.

B. bacilliformis. Motile gram-negative bacillus; the cause of bartonellosis.

bartonellosis (băr″tō-něl-ō′sĭs) [*Bartonella* + Gr. *osis,* condition]. A disease caused by infection with *Bartonella bacilliformis,* transmitted by female sandflies *(Phlebotomus).* The first clinical stage is noneruptive and is called Oroya fever, a severe febrile, hemolytic anemia. The second stage is eruptive and is called verruga peruana. It is marked by the appearance of small tumors on the skin and mucous membranes. SYN: *Carrion's disease.*

TREAT: Responds to several antibiotics, but ampicillin or chloramphenicol has the added advantage of being effective against *Salmonella,* which may be present as a secondary infection.

Bartter's syndrome [Frederic Crosby Bartter, U.S. physician, 1914–1983]. Hyperplasia of the juxtaglomerular cells of the kidney, hypokalemic alkalosis, and hyperaldosteronism without a rise in blood pressure. It usually occurs in children and may be accompanied by dwarfism. Etiology is unknown. Some cases have responded to therapy with prostaglandin inhibitors.

Baruch's law (băr′ooks) [Simon Baruch, Ger.-born U.S. physician, 1840–1921]. Theory that water has a sedative effect when its temperature is the same as that of the skin and a stimulating effect when it is below or above the skin temperature.

bary- [Gr. *barys,* heavy]. Prefix indicating heavy, dull, hard.

baryglossia (băr-ĭ-glŏs′ē-ă) [Gr. *barys,* heavy, + *glossa,* tongue]. Slow, thick utterance of speech.

barylalia (băr-ĭ-lā′lē-ă) [″ + *lalia,* speech]. Indistinct, husky speech due to imperfect articulation.

baryphonia (băr″ĭ-fō′nē-ă) [″ + *phone,* voice]. 1. Heavy, thick quality of the voice. 2. Barylalia, q.v.

basad (bā′săd) [Gr. *basis,* base, + L. *ad,* toward]. Toward the base.

basal (bā′săl). 1. Pert. to the base. 2. Of primary importance.

basal ganglia. Four masses of gray matter located deep in the cerebral hemispheres—caudate, lentiform, and amygdaloid nuclei and the claustrum. The caudate and lentiform nuclei and the fibers of the internal capsule that separate them constitute the corpus striatum.

basal lamina. Basement lamina, q.v.; base-

ment membrane.

basal metabolic rate. ABBR: BMR. The metabolic rate as measured under so-called basal conditions: 12 hours after eating, after a restful sleep, no exercise or activity preceding test, elimination of emotional excitement, and in a comfortable temperature. It is usually expressed in terms of Cal. (kilocalories) per square meter of body surface per hour. The use of this test is no longer justified due to the availability of better tests of thyroid function. SEE: *thyroid function tests.*

basal metabolism. The amount of energy needed for maintenance of life when the subject is at digestive, physical, and emotional rest.

basal ridge. An eminence on the lingual surface of the incisor teeth, esp. the upper ones. It is situated near the gum. SYN: *cingulum* (def. 2).

basal temperature chart. A daily chart of temperature obtained upon awakening. Some women are able to predict the time of ovulation by carefully analyzing the character and rhythm of the temperature chart. This information and other data can be used to establish that the woman is ovulating. Use of this method to control conception by predicting time of ovulation is unreliable in most cases. SEE: *conception;* illus.

base [Gr. *basis,* base]. 1. The lower part of anything; the supporting part. 2. The principal substance in a mixture. 3. Any substance that combines with hydrogen ions (protons); a hydrogen ion acceptor. Strong bases feel slippery and are corrosive to human tissues.

Ex.: sodium hydroxide (NaOH) (lye or caustic soda); potassium hydroxide (KOH) (caustic potash).

Whether an unknown chemical compound is a base or acid may be determined by the color produced when it is added to a solution containing an indicator, q.v. SYN: *alkali,* q.v. SEE: *acid; pH.*

b., cavity, or b., cement. In dentistry, the lining material placed in a cavity preparation, such as zinc phosphate, zinc oxide-eugenol, or calcium hydroxide along with small amounts of other medicinal or adhesive materials.

b., denture. That part of the denture made of metal, resin, or both, that supports the artificial teeth and rests on abutment teeth or the residual alveolar ridge.

b. of radiographic film. A layer of polyester or other suitable material that supports the film emulsion.

baseball finger. Condition resulting from violent backward dislocation of the terminal phalanx onto the dorsum of the middle pha-

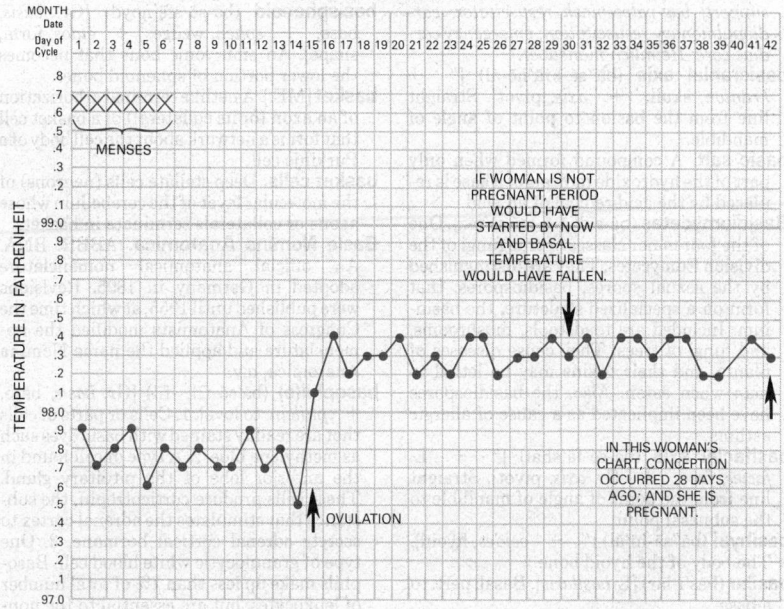

BASAL BODY TEMPERATURE CHART

MONTH
Date
Day of Cycle: 1 2 3 4 5 6 7 8 9 10 11 12 13 14 15 16 17 18 19 20 21 22 23 24 25 26 27 28 29 30 31 32 33 34 35 36 37 38 39 40 41 42

TEMPERATURE IN FAHRENHEIT

MENSES

IF WOMAN IS NOT PREGNANT, PERIOD WOULD HAVE STARTED BY NOW AND BASAL TEMPERATURE WOULD HAVE FALLEN.

IN THIS WOMAN'S CHART, CONCEPTION OCCURRED 28 DAYS AGO; AND SHE IS PREGNANT.

OVULATION

lanx, as when a finger is struck on its tip when extended. SYN: *mallet finger.* SEE: hammer finger.

Basedow's disease (băz′ē-dōz) [Karl A. von Basedow, Ger. physician, 1799–1854]. Graves' disease; exophthalmic goiter, q.v.

baseline (bās′līn). A known or initial value with which subsequent determinations of what is being measured can be compared, e.g., baseline temperature or blood pressure.

basement lamina [Gr. *basis,* base, + L. *lamina,* thin plate]. Preferred term for a thin layer of delicate noncellular material of a fine filamentous texture underlying the epithelium. Its principal component is collagen. SYN: *basement membrane; hyaline membrane.*

basement membrane. Basement lamina, q.v.

base pair. In the double-stranded helical arrangement of DNA, the connecting chemicals, i.e., base pairs, are either an adenine-thymine pair or a guanine-cytosine pair. These base pairs connect the helical strands of DNA like the edges of a spiral staircase.

baseplate (bās′plāt). A temporary, preformed shape made of wax, metal, or acrylic resin which represents the base of a denture; used in assessing the relations of maxillary-

mandibular teeth or for placement of artificial teeth in denture preparation.

basi-, basio- [Gr. *basis,* base]. Prefixes denoting base or basion.

basial (bā′sē-ăl) [L. *basialis*]. Pert. to the basion.

basiarachnoiditis (bā″sē-ă-răk″noy-dī′tĭs) [Gr. *basis,* base, + *arachne,* spider, + *eidos,* form, shape, + *itis,* inflammation]. Inflammation of the arachnoid membrane at base of brain.

BASIC. *Beginner's All-Purpose Symbolic Instruction Code.* A widely used programming language. Frequently used on personal and small business computer systems.

basic. 1. In chemistry, possessing properties of a base. 2. Fundamental.

basic life support. ABBR: BLS. The phase of cardiopulmonary resuscitation (CPR) and emergency cardiac care (ECC) that either (1) prevents circulatory or respiratory arrest or insufficiency by prompt recognition and early intervention or by early entry into the emergency care system (ECS) or both; or (2) externally supports the circulation and respiration of a victim of cardiac arrest through CPR. When cardiac or respiratory arrest occurs, BLS can and should be initiated by any person present who is familiar with CPR. SEE: *advanced cardiac life support; bag-valve-mask resuscitator; cardiopulmonary resuscitation; emergency cardiac care; Heimlich maneuver.*

basicranial axis (bā″sē-krā′nē-ăl) [″ + *kranion*, skull, + *axis*, pivot]. Straight line from the basion to point of angle of mandible.

basic salt. A compound formed when only part of the hydroxide radicals of a base is replaced by the acid radical of an acid.

Basidiomycetes (bă-sĭd″ē-ō-mī-sē′tēz). One of the four major classes of true fungi of the division Eumycetes. They are distinguished by the sexual spores, basidiospores, that form on a specialized structure, the basidium. Included are toadstools, mushrooms, and fungi of trees. They cause diseases of plants, and their toxins may be lethal to man when eaten. Also, the basidiospores have been implicated as a cause of allergic asthma.

basifacial axis (bā-sē-fā′shăl) [″ + L. *facies*, face, + Gr. *axis*, pivot]. Straight line from the point of angle of mandible to the subnasal point.

basihyal (bā″sē-hī′ăl) [″ + *oeides*, hyoid]. The body of the hyoid bone.

basilar (băs′ĭ-lăr) [L. *basilaris*]. Basal; pert. to a base.

basilateral (bā″sē-lăt′ĕr-ăl) [″ + L. *lateralis*, pert. to the side]. Both lateral and basilar.

basilemma (bā″sē-lĕm′ă) [Gr. *basis*, base, + *lemma*, husk]. The basement membrane.

basilic (bă-sĭl′ĭk) [L. *basilicus*]. Prominent, important.

basilic vein. Large vein on inner side of biceps of the arm just above the elbow. Usually chosen for intravenous injection or withdrawal of blood.

basiloma (băs-ĭ-lō′mă) [Gr. *basis*, base, + *oma*, tumor]. Basal cell carcinoma.

basin. An open, bowl-like container for holding liquids. It may be of special shape to fit around a structure.

> *b., emesis.* A kidney-shaped basin that can fit close to the neck so vomitus may be collected without soiling the bed linens.

basio- [Gr. *basis*, base]. Prefix denoting base or basion.

basioccipital bone (bā″sē-ŏk-sĭp′ĭ-tăl) [″ + L. *occiput*, head]. Basilar process of occipital bone.

basion (bā′sē-ŏn). Midpoint of anterior border of the foramen magnum.

basiphobia (bā″sē-fō′bē-ă) [Gr. *basis*, a stepping, + *phobos*, fear]. Fear of walking.

basirhinal (bā-sē-rī′năl) [Gr. *basis*, base, + *rhis*, nose]. Pert. to base of brain and nose.

basis (bā′sĭs) [L., Gr.] (pl. *bases*). [NA] Base of a structure or organ.

basisphenoid (bā-sē-sfē′noyd) [Gr. *basis*, base, + *sphen*, wedge, + *eidos*, form, shape]. An embryonic bone that becomes the lower portion of sphenoid bone.

basket [ME.]. A netlike terminal arborization of an axon (or its collateral) of a basket cell that forms a network about the cell body of a Purkinje cell.

basket cells. Deep stellate cells (neurons) of the molecular layer of the cerebellum whose axons or collaterals terminate in baskets.

Basle Nomina Anatomica. ABBR: BNA. An official anatomical nomenclature adopted in Germany in 1895. Revisions were published until 1955, at which time the Congress of Anatomists modified the nomenclature and applied the name Nomina Anatomica, q.v.

basophil(e) (bă′sō-fĭl, -fīl) [Gr. *basis*, base, + *philein*, to love]. 1. Cells or parts of cells that are readily stained with basic dyes such as methylene blue. 2. A type of cell found in the anterior lobe of the pituitary gland. These cells produce corticotropin, the substance that stimulates the adrenal cortex to secrete adrenal cortical hormone. 3. One type of granulocytic white blood cell. Basophils make up less than 1% of total number of leukocytes, but are essential to the nonspecific immune response to inflammation, q.v., because of their important role in releasing histamine and other chemicals that act on blood vessels. SEE: *blood cell* for illus.

basophilia (bā-sō-fĭl′ē-ă). 1. A pathological condition in which basophilic erythrocytes are found in the blood. 2. Condition in which there are a high number of basophilic leukocytes in the blood.

basophilic (bā-sō-fĭl′ĭk). Pert. to the staining characteristics of various cells.

basophilism (bā-sŏf′ĭ-lĭzm). Condition characterized by excessive numbers of basophils.

> *b., pituitary.* A clinical syndrome (Cushing's syndrome) characterized by basophilic invasion or adenoma of the pituitary gland. SYN: *Cushing's syndrome,* q.v.

basophobia (băs-ō-fō′bē-ă) [Gr. *basis*, a stepping, + *phobos*, fear]. 1. Abnormal fear of walking. 2. Emotional inability to stand or walk in the absence of muscle disease.

bass deafness. Deafness to bass notes.

Bassini's operation (bă-sē′nēz) [Edoardo Bassini, It. surgeon, 1844–1924]. A specific surgical procedure for inguinal hernia.

bastard [O. Fr. *batard*]. 1. One born out of wedlock; illegitimate, q.v. 2. Not genuine; irregular.

bath [AS. *baeth*]. The medium and method of cleansing the body or any part of it, or treating it therapeutically as with air, light,

Bath Temperatures

Room Temperature		Water Should Be	
F	C	F	C
Below 76°	24.4°	94–96°	34.4–35.6°
Above 76°	24.4°	92–94°	33.3–34.4°
Hot summer days		90°	32.2°

Bath Temperatures for Treating Hyperthermia or Hyperpyrexia

Rectal Temperature		Water Should Be	
F	C	F	C
103°	39.4°	90°	32.2°
104°	40°	86°	30°
104.5°	40.3°	82°	27.8°
105°	40.6°	76°	24.4°
105.5°	40.8°	60–70°	15.6–21.1°

vapor, or water. The temperature of the cleansing bath for a bed patient should be about 95°F (35°C) with a room temperature of 75° to 80°F (23.9° to 26.7°C). SEE: table.

THERAP. EFFECT: Warm and hot baths and applications act to soothe both the mind and the body. Thus they tend to calm and relax a nervous, agitated patient. Gradually elevated hot tub and vapor baths relax all the muscles of the body. Hot baths relax tissues, including the capillaries of the skin, drawing blood from the deeper tissues, and also help to relieve pain and stimulate nerves. Cold baths and applications abstract heat and stimulate reaction, esp. if followed by brisk rubbing of the skin. Cold contracts small blood vessels when applied locally. SEE: *hydrotherapy*.

b., acid. Bath consisting of 5 oz (150 ml) hydrochloric acid or 1 gal (3.8 L) vinegar added to 30 gal (114 L) water.

b., air. Therapeutic use of air, warmed or vaporized, on the nude body.

b., alcohol. Application of alcohol to the patient as a stimulant and defervescent in dilute form.

b., alkaline. Eight oz (227 gm) of sodium bicarbonate or washing soda added to 30 gal (114 L) of water.

b., alum. Use of alum in washing solution as an astringent.

b., antipyretic. Bath in cool water (65° to 75°F or 18.3° to 28.9°C). The patient

should not be cooled to the point of shivering, as this indicates excessive heat loss.

b., aromatic. Bath to which some volatile oil or perfume or some herb is added.

b., astringent. Bathing in liquid containing an astringent.

b., bed. Bath for a patient confined to bed.

NURSING IMPLICATIONS: Assemble all required equipment; ensure appropriate room temperature and that there are no drafts. Shield patient, remove top covers and replace with bath blanket. Assess patient's ability to bathe self. The patient is expected to perform all or part of the bath, with the nurse bathing the patient only if the patient is unable or not permitted to do so. Water temperature for bath should be 110° to 120°F (43.3° to 48.1°C). The entire body, including the perineal area and genitalia, must be bathed and dried. Only one body area should be washed at a time, then rinsed thoroughly and dried. The patient should remain covered except for the area being bathed. Change bath water as often as necessary to maintain temperature or permit thorough rinsing. After the bath is completed, apply lotion to the skin. After completing the bath, the patient should have oral hygiene, hair combed, and a clean gown applied. Bathing of obese patients may be facilitated by drying crevices with a hand-held hair dryer.

b., bland. Bath containing substances such as starch, bran, or oatmeal for the relief of skin irritation; an emollient bath.

b., blanket. Bath in which wet pack and blankets are used.

b., box. Bath in which patient's entire body except the head is completely enclosed in a box.

b., bran. Bath in which one places bran (2 to 3 lb or 907 gm to 1.4 kg) in a muslin bag and soaks it in hot water 15 min, then adds bag and hot water to bath water (30 gal, 95°F, or 114 L, 35°C), using bag as a washing-sponge.

b., brine. B., saline, q.v.

b., bubble. Bath in which the water contains many small bubbles produced mechanically as by an air pump or chemically by bubble bath preparations.

Caution: Perfumes used in bubble baths are frequently the cause of vaginitis and skin irritation, esp. in children.

b., carbon dioxide. An effervescent saline bath consisting of water, salts, and CO_2. The natural CO_2 baths are known as Nauheim baths.

b., cold. Bath in water at a temperature

below 65°F (18.3°C).

b., colloid. B., emollient, q.v.

b., continuous. Bath administered for an extended period but seldom for longer than several hours. Used in treating hypothermia or hyperthermia, certain skin diseases, and in the past in treating some types of mental disorders, esp. agitation.

b., contrast. Bath used for hands or feet. Fill two large basins or pails of sufficient depth with water, one as hot and the other as cold as the patient can stand. Change or add hot and cold water frequently to keep temperatures same as in beginning. Put part to be treated in hot water for one minute, then into cold for one-half minute, then again into hot water. Repeat for prescribed length of time, ending with cold water.

b., earth. Bathing in warmed earth or sand.

b., emollient. Bath used for irritation and inflammation of skin and after erysipelas. SEE: *b., glycerin; b., oatmeal; b., powdered borax; b., starch.*

b., foam. Tub bath in which an extract of a saponin-containing vegetable fiber has been added. Oxygen or carbon dioxide is driven through this mixture to form foam.

b., foot. Immersion of feet and legs to a depth of 4 in. (10 cm) above ankles in water at 98°F (36.7°C).

b., full. Bath in which the whole body except the head is immersed in water.

b., glycerin. Bath consisting of 10 oz (300 ml) of glycerin added to 30 gal (114 L) water.

b., herb. Full bath to which is added a mixture of 1 to 2 lb (454 to 907 gm) of herbs such as chamomile, wild thyme, or spearmint tied in a bag and boiled with 1 gal (3.8 L) of water.

b., hip. B., sitz, q.v.

b., hot. Tub bath with the water covering the body to a little above the nipple level. The temperature is gradually raised from 98°F (36.7°C) to desired degree, usually to 108°F (42.2°C).

b., hot air. Exposure of entire body except head to hot air in a bath cabinet.

b., hyperthermal. Bath in which the whole body except the head is immersed in water from 105° to 120°F (40.6° to 48.9°C) for one to two minutes.

b., kinetotherapeutic. Bath given for underwater exercises of weak or partially paralyzed muscles.

b., lukewarm. Bath in which patient's body except head is immersed in water from 94° to 96°F (34.4° to 35.6°C) for 15 to 60 minutes.

b., medicated. Bath to which substances such as bran, oatmeal, starch, sodium bicarbonate, Epsom salts, pine products, tar, sulfur, potassium permanganate, and salt are added.

b., milk. Bath taken in milk for emollient purposes.

b., mud. The use of mud in order to apply moist heat.

b., mustard. Stimulative hot foot bath consisting of a mixture of 1 tablespoon (15 ml) of dry mustard in a quart (946 ml) of hot water added to a pail or large basin filled with water of 100° to 104°F (37.8° to 40°C).

b., Nauheim. Bath in which the body is immersed in warm water through which carbon dioxide is bubbled.

b., needle. Bath in which water is forcibly sprayed on the body in fine jet streams.

b., neutral. Bath in which no circulatory or thermic reaction occurs, temperature 92° to 97°F (33.3° to 36.1°C).

b., neutral sitz. Same as sitz bath, q.v., except temperature is 92° to 97°F (33.3° to 36.1°C) or for foot bath 104° to 110°F (37.8° to 40°C), duration 15 to 60 minutes.

b., oatmeal. Bath consisting of 2 to 3 lb (907 gm to 1.4 kg) oatmeal added to 30 gal (114 L) water.

b., oxygen. Bath given by introducing oxygen into the water through a special device that is connected to an oxygen tank or through generation of oxygen by chemical means.

b., paraffin. The limb is repeatedly immersed in warm paraffin 104° to 150°F (37.8° to 65.6°C) and quickly withdrawn until it is encased in layers of the material. Paraffin may be applied with paintbrush for larger joints. Used when there is need to apply topical heat to traumatized or inflamed areas.

b., powdered borax. Bath consisting of ½ lb (227 gm) added to 30 gal (114 L) water; 5 oz (150 ml) glycerin may be added.

b., saline. Bath given in artificial seawater made by dissolving 8 lb (3.6 kg) of sea salt or a mixture of 7 lb (3.2 kg) of sodium chloride and ½ lb (227 gm) of magnesium sulfate in 30 gal (114 L) of water. SYN: *b., salt; b., seawater.*

b., sauna. A hot, humid atmosphere created in a small enclosed area by pouring water on heated rocks.

b., seawater. B., saline, q.v.

b., sedative. A prolonged warm bath. A continuous flow of water as well as an air cushion or back rest may be used.

b., sheet. Bath given by wrapping the patient in a sheet previously dipped in water 80° to 90°F (26.7° to 32.2°C), and by rubbing the whole body with vigorous strokes on the sheet.

b., shower. Water sprayed down upon

the body from an overhead source.

b., sitz. Immersion of thighs, buttocks, and abdomen below the umbilicus in water. In a hot sitz bath the water is first 92°F (33.3°C) and then elevated to 106°F (41.1°C).

b., sponge. Bath in which patient is not immersed in a tub but washed with a washcloth or sponge.

b., starch. Bath consisting of 1 lb (454 gm) of starch mixed into cold water, with boiling water added to make a solution of gluelike consistency, then added to 30 gal (114 L) of water.

b., steam. Bath given in a chamber into which steam under low pressure is allowed to escape. Best form of application is that in which subject sits in cabinet or lies in box with head outside.

Caution: Temperature must be controlled carefully to avoid burning the patient.

---

b., stimulating. Bath that increases cutaneous blood flow. SEE: *b., cold; b., mustard; b., saline.*

b., sun. Exposure of all or part of the nude body to sunlight.

b., sweat. Bath given to induce perspiration.

b., towel. Bath given by applying towel dipped in water 60° to 70°F (15.6° to 21.1°C) to arms, legs, and anterior and posterior surfaces of trunk, removing towel, and drying parts.

b., whirlpool. Continuous localized jets of water at a temperature of 105° to 120°F (40.6° to 48.9°C) agitate the water into which the body or a part of it is immersed.

bathophobia (băth″ō-fō′bē-ă) [Gr. *bathos,* deep, + *phobos,* fear]. Abnormal fear of depths. Commonly refers to fear of height or of looking down from a high place.

bathyanesthesia (băth-ē-ăn″ĕs-thē-′zē-ă) [″ + *an-,* not, + *aisthesis,* sensation]. Loss of deep sensibility.

bathycardia (băth″ē-kăr′dē-ă) [″ + *kardia,* heart]. Low position of the heart in the thorax due to anatomical conditions rather than disease.

bathyesthesia (băth″ē-ĕs-thē′zē-ă) [″ + *aisthesis,* sensation]. A consciousness or sensibility of parts of the body beneath the skin.

bathyhyperesthesia (băth-ē-hī″pĕr-ĕs-thē′zē-ă) [″ + *hyper,* above, + *aisthesis,* sensation]. Excessive sensitivity of muscular tissues and deep body structures.

bathyhypesthesia (băth″ē-hīp″ĕs-thē′zē-ă) [″ + *hypo,* under, + *aisthesis,* sensation]. Impairment of sensitivity in muscular tissues and other deep structures of body.

battered child syndrome. Physical violence inflicted upon a child by adults, usually one or both of the parents or guardians, often under circumstances that make it appear that the injury was accidental. Clinical findings: bruises, scratches, burns, hematomas, and fractures of long bones, ribs, or skull. Poor skin hygiene and some degree of malnutrition also may be present. SEE: *Nursing Diagnoses* in *Appendix.*

ETIOL: Most parents or guardians of abused children have a history of being so treated as a child.

DIAG: Most distinguishing feature is variation in stages of healing of bone lesions seen in roentgenogram, indicating injuries incurred at different times.

PROG: Variable. Death rate is high, and surviving children often suffer from longterm physical and mental injuries, and will possibly become abusive parents. In domestic situations in which a child is abused, it is important to examine other children and infants living in the same home because about 20% of them will have signs of physical abuse. That examination should be done without delay in order to attempt to prevent further abuse of children in that home. SEE: *child abuse; shaken baby syndrome.*

battered woman syndrome. A pattern of repeated physical assault of a woman by her spouse. Typically, the pattern begins with verbal abuse and progresses to increasingly violent physical abuse. Death can occur. Estimates indicate that over one million women a year are victims. Shelters for battered women are available in many cities. Frequently, women are afraid to report this type of abuse because they feel trapped in the relationship. Women from any socioeconomic level may be affected.

battery [Fr. *battre,* to beat]. 1. Device for generating electric current by chemical action. 2. A series of tests, procedures, or diagnostic examinations given to or done on a patient. 3. The unlawful touching of another which is without consent, justification or excuse. In legal medicine, battery occurs if a medical or surgical procedure is performed without proper consent. SEE: *assault; sexual harassment.*

Battle sign [William Henry Battle, Brit. surgeon 1855–1936]. Bogginess of the temporal or postauricular region of the head. This indicates fracture of the basilar area of the skull.

Baudelocque's diameter (bōd-lŏks′) [Jean Louis Baudelocque, Sr., Fr. obstetrician, 1746–1810]. Distance between the depression just beneath the last lumbar vertebra and the margin of the symphysis pubis. The external conjugate diameter of the pelvis.

Baudelocque's method. In obstetrics, manipulation to convert a fetal face presentation into a vertex presentation.

baud rate (bawd) [named for Jean M. Émile Baudot, French engineer, 1845–1903]. A unit of telegraphic signaling speed. In computers, it is used to indicate the rate of transmission of data from a computer to a distant site by use of a special device, usually attached to a telephone, called a modem. A baud is one pulse per second.

Baumé scales (bō-mā′) [Antoine Baumé, Fr. chemist, 1728–1805]. Hydrometer scales for determination of the specific gravity of liquids.

bay (bā). An anatomical recess or depression filled with liquid.

Bayes' theorem [Thomas Bayes, Brit. mathematician, 1702–1761]. This theorem, published posthumously in 1764, is concerned with analyzing the probability that a patient may be considered to have a certain diagnosis or disease when it is known that the patient has certain attributes such as an abnormal test. It is usually known how frequently that particular attribute is present in the population considered to have the specific disease.

Bayley Scales of Infant Development. A standardized test battery used to provide information about the developmental status of children aged 2 to 30 months. The battery is designed to indicate motor, mental and behavioral levels based on performance and parental reports.

bayonet leg. Backward dislocation of tibia and fibula at the knee joint.

Bazin's disease (bă-zăz′) [Antoine P. E. Bazin, Fr. dermatologist, 1807–1878]. Chronic skin disease occurring in young adult females. Characterized by hard cutaneous nodules that break down to form necrotic ulcers that leave atrophic scars. The disease is almost invariably preceded by tuberculosis. Nevertheless, the etiological relationship to that disease is debated. SYN: *erythema induratum.*

B cell mediated immunity. The result of the specific immune response, q.v. Protection against infection or reinfection by common organisms, e.g., streptococci and staphylococci, is provided by B lymphocytes. B cells are stimulated by direct contact with a foreign antigen and differentiate into plasma cells, q.v., that produce antibodies, q.v., against the antigen, and memory cells that enable the body to quickly produce these antibodies if the same antigen appears at a later time. B cell differentiation is also stimulated by interleukin-2 (IL-2), q.v., secreted by T4 cells, and by foreign antigens processed by macrophages. SYN: *humoral immunity.* SEE: *antibody; B cells; specific immune response; T cell mediated immunity; vaccination.*

B cells. Lymphoid stem cells from the bone marrow that migrate to and become mature antigen-specific cells in the spleen and lymph nodes. Many immature B cells are found in the spleen which, because of the large amount of blood passing through it, provides many chances for the B cells to become exposed to new antigens, promoting their differentiation into functional cells. Each mature B lymphocyte is capable of being stimulated by a specific antigen entering the body. After the B cell comes in contact with the antigen, it changes into a plasma cell or a memory cell. Plasma cells produce antibodies, q.v., that destroy the invading cell. Memory cells are available to quickly produce antibodies if the same antigen appears again. All B cells are antigen-specific and respond to only one foreign protein.

The antigen-antibody reaction is part of the specific immune response. It is the basis for vaccination and plays a major role in defending against infection from common organisms. SYN: *B lymphocytes.* SEE: *antibody; antigen; cytokines; immunoglobulins; plasma cells; T cells; vaccination.*

BCG. *bacille Calmette-Guérin.*

BCG vaccine. A form of tuberculosis vaccine. A freeze-dried preparation of a live, attenuated strain of *Mycobacterium bovis (bacille Calmette-Guérin).* Used in children for immunization against tuberculosis, but its efficacy is questionable. BCG vaccine is indicated in an infant who is tuberculin-negative and resides in a household in which repeated exposure to untreated or ineffectively treated cases of tuberculosis occurs. Also used to prevent recurrence of bladder tumors. It is instilled in the bladder when so used. SEE: *bacille Calmette-Guérin.*

b.d. L. *bis die,* twice a day.

bdellometer (dĕl-ŏm′ĕ-tĕr) [Gr. *bdella,* leech, + *metron,* measure]. Mechanical substitute for a leech. SEE: *leech.*

Bdellovibrio [″ + *vibrio*]. A parasite on bacteria that invades the bacteria by forming a hole in the cell wall. It lives and reproduces inside the cell.

B.E. *below elbow,* term used to refer to the site of amputation of an upper extremity; *barium enema.*

Be. Chem. symb. for the element beryllium.

beaded (bĕd′ĕd). Referring to disjointed colonies along the inoculation line in a streak or stab.

beads, rachitic. Visible swelling where the

ribs join their cartilages, seen in rickets. SYN: *rachitic rosary.*

beaker (bē'kĕr). Glass vessel with wide mouth for mixing or holding liquids.

beam. 1. In nuclear medicine and radiology, a group of atomic particles traveling a parallel course. 2. Isoelectric line of an oscilloscope. 3. Part of an analytical balance to which the weighing pans are attached. 4. A long, slender piece of wood, metal, or plastic resin that serves as a support in some part of a dental appliance.

beard. The hair on the face and throat.

bearing down. The expulsive effort of a parturient woman in second stage of labor. The Valsalva maneuver is utilized, causing increased pressure against the uterus by increasing intra-abdominal pressure.

beat [AS. *beatan,* to strike]. A pulsation or throb as of contraction of the heart or the passage of blood through a vessel.

   b., apex. Impulse of the heartbeat felt by the hand when held over the fifth intercostal space in left midclavicular line.

   b., artificially paced. Heartbeat stimulated by an artificial pacemaker.

   b., capture. Ventricular contraction responding to an impulse from the sinus that reaches the atrioventricular node at a time at which the node is nonrefractory.

   b., dropped. The absence of a ventricular contraction of the heart.

   b., ectopic. Heartbeat beginning at a place other than sinoatrial node.

   b., escape. Heartbeat that occurs after a prolonged pause, or failure of the sinus node to stimulate the heart to contract.

   b., forced. Extrasystole brought on by artificial heart stimulation.

   b., premature. Heartbeat that arises from a site other than the sinus node and occurs early in the cardiac cycle before the expected sinus beat.

Beau's lines (bōz) [Joseph Honoré Simon Beau, Fr. physician, 1806–1865]. White lines across the fingernails, usually a sign of systemic disease. May be due to trauma, coronary occlusion, hypercalcemia, or skin disease. The lines are visible until the affected area of the nail has grown out and been trimmed away.

Bechterew's (also Bekhterev's) reflex (bĕk'tĕr-ĕvs) [Vladimir Mikhailovich von Bechterew, Russ. neurologist, 1857–1927]. 1. Contraction of facial muscles due to irritation of nasal mucosa. 2. Dilatation of pupil on exposure to light. 3. Contraction of lower abdominal muscles when skin of inner surface of thigh is stroked.

Beck's triad. Signs seen with pericardial tamponade, consisting of hypotension, distended neck veins and muffled heart sounds.

beclomethasone dipropionate. USP. A corticosteroid drug. Trade names are Vancenase and Beclovent inhaler.

becquerel (bĕk'rĕl) [Antoine Henri Becquerel, French physicist, 1852–1908]. SYMB: Bq. An SI-derived unit of measure of activity of a radionuclide equal to one spontaneous nuclear transition per second. It is equal to 3.7×10^{10} curies. SEE: *curie; SI Units* in *Appendix.*

bed [AS. *bedd*]. 1. A supporting structure or tissue. 2. A couch or support for the body during sleep.

   Making an occupied bed: Assemble all necessary articles, placing clean linens on back of chair at bedside. Tell the patient what you are going to do; check temperature of room and adjust windows if necessary. Loosen all bedclothes; remove all but one blanket. Hang on back of chair. Remove top sheet from under remaining blanket. Place in laundry bag or fold and place on seat of chair to form receiver for dirty linens. Turn patient away from you if possible, and ensure safety by placing chair or bedrail for security. Bottom sheet is also folded in neat, flat folds to center of bed.

   Place clean bottom sheet on exposed half of mattress, folding neatly to center creases. Tuck top of sheet under head of mattress; miter corner and tuck under mattress to foot of bed. Sheet must cover mattress completely. Place clean sheet with center crease to patient's back. Fold top of clean sheet and tuck securely under mattress. Help patient to roll toward you under blanket to clean side of bed. Again ensure safety. Proceed to other side of bed. Remove soiled bottom sheet and place on first piece of soiled linen on chair. Pull through clean bottom sheet and rubber sheet. Proceed as for first side, tightening sheet to avoid any wrinkles. Ask patient to raise buttocks if possible.

   Remove pillows and pillow cases; replace cases with clean ones. Pull mattress to head of bed; replace pillows and adjust to patient's comfort. Place clean top sheet, wide hem to top, over blanket; draw blanket out from under sheet and replace with top of blanket well over patient's shoulders. Put on spread and turn top hem of sheet over spread at least 8 in. (20 cm). Remake foot of bed, allowing sufficient room for feet and toes of patient to move freely.

   Remove soiled linens from room. Avoid shaking bedclothes in order to prevent spreading dust, a possible source of infection. Place patient's signal or call device in proper and convenient place, straighten room, and evaluate comfort and appearance carefully.

Caution: Special drainage and irrigation tubes must be handled carefully in order not to disturb their function or placement or to cause the patient pain.

---

b., air. Bed inflated with air. Also, a special bed that literally floats the patient on a cushion of air that comes from holes in a special mattress. Used in burn cases and to prevent bedsores.

b., air-fluidized. SEE: *air-fluidized bed.*

b., capillary. A network of capillaries.

b., circular. Special bed that allows a patient to be turned end-over-end while held between two frames. This permits turning the patients without disturbing them by turning the two frames inside a circular apparatus that holds the ends of the frames. Useful in treating paralyzed or immobilized patients. Trademark: Circ-O-Lectric bed.

b., float. Bed in which the patient is supported either on a water mattress or on minute ceramic beads with air flowing through them. This type of bed is particularly useful in treating decubitus ulcers and burn patients.

b., flotation. Bed in which the patient reclines in a hollow, flexible, mattress-shaped device that is filled with water. This enables equal distribution of pressure on the body. Used in treating and preventing decubiti.

b., fracture. Bed for patients who have fractures.

b., Gatch. Adjustable bed that provides elevation of the back and knees.

b., hydrostatic. B., water, q.v.

b., kinetic. Bed that constantly turns patients side to side through 270°. Used to prevent the hazards of immobility in patients requiring bedrest over long periods of time, as in multiple trauma and some neuromuscular diseases. SYN: *Roto-Bed. SEE: Circ-O-Lectric bed.*

b., metabolic. Bed arranged to facilitate collecting the feces and urine of a patient so that metabolic rate can be calculated.

b., nail. The skin at tip of digit that lies beneath a nail.

b., open. Bed that is available for assignment to a patient.

b., recovery. Bed prepared to receive patient immediately following an operative procedure requiring anesthesia. Usually a portable bed or stretcher.

b., surgical. Bed equipped with a mechanism by which the head or the foot of the bed can be raised or lowered independently of each other.

b., tilt. SEE: *table, tilt.*

b., water. A rubber mattress filled with water. Used for prevention of bedsores. SEE: *b., flotation.*

bed blocking. Placing bedblocks under legs of bed to raise one end.

Foot of bed raised: In shock; bleeding from lower limbs; edema of lower limbs, vulva, or scrotum; to retain enema; when weight is used on lower limbs; in reduction of inguinal hernia.

Head of bed raised: To drain abdomen or pelvis; to aid respiration; in treatment for bleeding from head, neck, or upper chest; in treatment of congestive heart failure.

bed blocks. Blocks of sturdy material, usually wood, for placement under either the two lower or upper bed legs in order to elevate the respective end of the bed.

bed board. A firm board placed beneath the mattress of a bed. This prevents the mattress from sagging. Used to treat some persons with back difficulties. SEE: *back board.*

bedbug. An insect, *Cimex lectularius* of the family *Cimicidae,* the saliva of which contains an irritating substance that causes a purpuric reaction or an urticarial wheal. The adult bugs are about 4 to 5 mm in length and survive for up to a year without feeding and at low temperature. The female ingests 0.0185 ml of blood each feeding, the male 0.015 ml. Bedbugs can be a cause of anemia in infants. There is much speculation but no proof that bedbugs transmit diseases to humans, either through bites or infected feces.

TREAT: Antipruritic lotions containing phenol, camphor, and menthol.

CONTROL: Largely a matter of cleanliness. In heavy infestations, use appropriate insecticide, spraying furniture, mattresses, floors, baseboards, walls.

NOTE: Use of wooden frames for beds provides a nesting and breeding site for these insects.

bedfast. Unable or unwilling to leave the bed; bedridden.

bedlam [From Hospital of St. Mary of Bethlehem, pronounced Bedlem in ME.]. 1. An asylum for the insane. 2. Any place or situation characterized by a noisy uproar.

Bednar's aphthae [Alois Bednar, physician in Vienna, 1816–1888]. Infected, traumatic ulcers appearing on hard palate of infants. Usually caused by sucking infected objects.

bedpan [AS. *bedd,* bed, + *panna,* flat vessel]. A pan-shaped device placed under a bedridden patient for collecting and containing fecal and urinary excreta.

NOTE: In general, the use of a bedpan is uncomfortable and, because of the awkwardness of the position, requires more exertion on the patient's part than using a bedside toilet. Thus patients who are recovering from myocardial infarction and others should not be forced to use a bedpan if it is possible to move them from their bed to a bedside toilet.

bedrest. 1. Device for propping up patients in bed. 2. The confining of a patient to bed for rest.

bedridden. Unable or unwilling to leave the bed; bedfast.

bedsore [AS. *bedd*, bed, + *sare*, open wound]. Pressure sore; ischemic necrosis and ulceration of tissue, esp. over a bony prominence. Due to pressure from prolonged confinement in bed or from a cast or splint. The stages correspond to tissue layers. First stage consists of skin redness. The second stage shows redness, edema, and induration. In the third stage, the skin becomes necrotic, with exposure of fat. In the fourth stage, necrosis extends through the skin and fat to muscle; further fat and muscle necrosis characterize the fifth stage. In the sixth stage, bone destruction begins, progressing ultimately to osteomyelitis. SYN: *decubitus.*

Emaciated, weak, or elderly patients and those who must remain in one position because of orthopedic or similar problems are esp. likely to develop bedsores. Bedsores are located in areas over bony prominences that are thinly covered with flesh, as the end of the spine, buttocks, heels, elbows, shoulder blades, and back of the head and ears in children.

PREDISPOSING CAUSES: Any factor that interferes with the circulation of the blood and mobility of the patient; prolonged fever; emaciation; obesity; paralysis; old age; poor nutrition; poorly made beds or those containing irritating bits of debris; lack of cleanliness; bruising; infrequent change of positions; cardiac diseases, nephritis, diabetes, or anemia.

TREAT: Prevention is easier than a cure; prophylactic measures in keeping the bed dry and clean; relieving the pressure as soon as the first signs of redness appear and reporting this occurrence to the nurse in charge or attending physician at once; use of the prescribed medication as directed by the physician. Thorough drying of skin after baths and gentle massage for stimulation of circulation; frequent change of position of patient if possible; maintenance of proper nutrition; chemical or surgical debridement of ulcers; use of sheepskin, or substitute, under vulnerable area; placing patient on special air bed, q.v., or flotation bed, q.v.

bedwetting. Enuresis, q.v.

BEE. basal energy expenditure. SEE: *energy expenditure, basal.*

bee. Insects of the order Hymenoptera and superfamily Apoidea. Included is the common honeybee, *Apis mellifera,* which produces honey and beeswax. SEE: *propolis.*

Beer's law. The basic law that is the foundation for all absorption photometry, and predicts the linear relationship between the absorbance (A) of a solution and its concentration (c). Given as:A = ebc; where A = absorbance, e = molar absorptivity; b = cell path (distance), and c = concentration.

Beer's operation [Georg Joseph Beer, Ger. ophthalmologist, 1763–1821]. Flap operation for cataract or artificial pupil.

bee sting [AS. *beo,* bee, + *stingan,* to pierce]. Injury resulting from bee's venom. The stinger, which is barbed, usually remains in the wound. Pain, mottled redness, and edema result.

TREAT: Application of fairly strong household ammonia or baking soda paste. Remove stinger if present. If pain is severe, injection of 2% procaine solution. Antihistamines help to relieve discomfort.

NOTE: Some individuals are hypersensitive to bee venom and may suffer severe anaphylactic reactions leading to death. In such cases immediate subcutaneous or intravenous administration of epinephrine is indicated.

beeswax (bēz'wǎks). Yellow wax obtained from honeycomb of bees. A purified form is used in ointments.

beeturia (bēt-ū'rē-ǎ). Pink to deep red color of urine that sometimes follows eating of beets.

behavior [ME. *behaven,* to hold oneself in a certain way]. 1. The manner in which one acts; the actions or reactions of individuals under specific circumstances. 2. Any response elicited from an organism.

behavioral science. The science concerned with all aspects of behavior.

behavioral system model. SEE: *Appendix 23.*

behaviorism. A theory of conduct that regards normal and abnormal behavior as the result of conditioned reflexes quite apart from the concept of will. It does not apply to conditions resulting from organic disease.

behavior patterns, types A and B. *Type A* behavior pattern is characterized by the individual being overly concerned with time deadlines and achieving self-determined goals. In addition, these persons are aggressive, usually anxious. The importance of this type of behavior pattern in coronary artery disease, hypertension, and peptic ulcer may be considerable, but scientific proof of this possibility is difficult.

Type B behavior pattern is best defined by the absence of the factors present in type A behavior pattern. SEE: *coronary heart disease; heart disease risk factors.*

behavior therapy. Various techniques used to change maladaptive behaviors, based on principles of learning theory. Cigarette smoking, eating disorders and alcohol abuse are commonly treated through techniques of behavior therapy, which may include the use of positive reinforcement, aversive conditioning, discrimination, and modeling.

Behçet's syndrome (bā'sĕts) [Hulusi Behçet, Turkish dermatologist, 1889–1948]. A multisystem, chronic recurrent disease characterized by ulceration of the mouth and genitalia, iritis, uveitis, arthritis, and thrombophlebitis. The joint pain usually comes later in the history of the disease than the ulcers of the mouth and genitalia. Iritis frequently is accompanied by conjunctivitis, episcleritis, keratitis, retinal thrombophlebitis, and optic atrophy. The central nervous system, heart, and intestinal tract may be involved. The disease is found worldwide, but is most common in the eastern Mediterranean and eastern Asia. In these areas it occurs mostly in young men and is a leading cause of blindness. In the Western world it is less severe and affects men twice as frequently as women and is not a leading cause of blindness. The period between attacks is irregular, but may be as short as days or as long as years. Needle punctures provoke inflammatory skin lesions, and for that reason should be avoided.

TREAT: Immunosuppressive therapy, e.g., chlorambucil, is helpful. Corticosteroids are useful in controlling serious inflammation until the immunosuppressive agents begin to have an effect. The immunosuppresive agent azathioprine has been found to prevent progression of Behçet's syndrome.

bejel (bĕj'ĕl). A nonvenereal form of syphilis endemic in Arab countries; it particularly affects children.

bel (bĕl). A unit of measurement of the intensity of sound. It is expressed as a logarithm of the ratio of two sounds of acoustic intensity, one of which is fixed or standard; the ratio is expressed in decibels, q.v.

belch [AS. *baelcan*, to eructate]. Escape of gas from the stomach through the mouth; to eructate.

belching. Raising of gas from the stomach and expelling it through the mouth and nose. In order for belching to occur, first there is an increase in gastric pressure; then the lower esophagus sphincter relaxes to allow equalization of pressure in the stomach and esophagus; then relaxation of the upper esophagus sphincter allows the gas to escape through the pharynx and mouth. SEE: *water brash.*

ETIOL: Gastric fermentation; air swallowing; drinking carbonated beverages or eating gas-containing foods.

belemnoid (bē-lĕm'noyd) [Gr. *belemnon*, dart, + *eidos*, form, shape]. Dart-shaped; styloid.

Bell, Sir Charles. Scottish physiologist and surgeon, 1774–1842.

    B.'s law. Fact that anterior spinal nerve roots contain only motor fibers and posterior roots only sensory fibers. SYN: *Bell-Magendie's law.*

    B.-Magendie's law. Bell's law, q.v.

    B.'s nerve. Long thoracic nerve; nervus thoracicus longus [NA].

    B.'s palsy. Unilateral facial paralysis of sudden onset. The cause is unknown but is presumed to involve swelling of the seventh (facial) nerve due to immune or viral disease, resulting in ischemia and compression of the nerve at the point where it leaves the bony tissue. Characterized by weakness of the entire half of the face followed by paralysis. The patient cannot control salivation or lacrimation, and in severe cases cannot close the eye on the affected side. Facial expression is distorted.

TREAT: Protection of exposed eye by temporary patching or use of methylcellulose drops. Corticosteroids, such as oral prednisone 60 to 80 mg/day for 1 week, which are then reduced over the second week, may decrease acute pain.

PROG: Partial facial paralysis is usually resolved within several months. Likelihood of complete recovery after total paralysis varies from 20% to 90%.

belladonna (bĕl"ă-dŏn'ă) [It., beautiful lady]. USP. An anticholinergic. *Atropa belladonna,* a poisonous plant with reddish flowers and shining black berries. Source of various alkaloids, including atropine and scopolamine. Used mainly for sedative and spasmolytic effects on gastrointestinal tract.

    b. leaf. Powder from dried leaf and flowering top of *Atropa belladonna Linné* or *A. belladonna acuminata.* An anticholinergic agent, it is used generally in tincture form though the dry extract in tablet form may be used.

belladonna and atropine poisons. These include stramonium, hyoscyamus, scopolamine, belladonna, and atropine. SEE: *atropine* in *Poisons and Poisoning* in *Appendix.*

Bellini's tubule (bĕ-lē'nēz) [Lorenzo Bellini, It. anatomist, 1643–1704]. The straight connecting tubule of the kidney.

bell-metal resonance. A metallic sound heard in pneumothorax when a coin placed on the chest wall is struck by another coin.

Bellocq's cannula (bĕl-ŏks') [Jean Jacques Bellocq, Fr. surgeon, 1732–1807]. An instrument for drawing in a plug through nostril and mouth to control epistaxis.

belly [AS. *baelg*, bag]. 1. The abdomen or abdominal cavity. 2. The fleshy, central portion of a muscle.

bellyache. Colic, gastralgia.

belly button. Umbilicus, q.v.; navel.

belonephobia (bĕl″ō-nĕ-fō′bē-ă) [Gr. *belone*, needle, + *phobos*, fear]. Morbid fear of sharp-pointed objects.

belonoid (bĕl′ō-noyd) [″ + *eidos*, form, shape]. Needle-shaped.

belonoskiascopy (bĕl″ō-nō-skī-ăs′kō-pē) [″ + *skia*, shadow, + *skopein*, to examine]. Subjective retinoscopy by means of shadows and movements to determine refraction.

Benadryl (bĕn′ă-drĭl). Trade name for diphenhydramine hydrochloride, USP, an antihistaminic agent.

Bence Jones protein [Henry Bence Jones, Brit. physician, 1814–1873]. Protein that occurs in urine of patients with multiple myeloma and occasionally in patients with other diseases of the reticuloendothelial system. When urine samples are heated to 50° to 60°C, a precipitate forms. It disappears when the urine is boiled and reappears when the urine cools.

Bender's Visual Motor Gestalt test. [Lauretta Bender, N.Y. psychiatrist, b. 1897] A test in which the subject copies a series of patterns. The results vary with the type of psychiatric disorder present.

Bendopa. Trade name for levodopa.

bendroflumethiazide (bĕn″drō-floo″mĕ-thī′ă-zīd). USP. A thiazide-type diuretic. Trade name is Naturetin.

bends. Painful condition in limbs and abdomen caused by bubbles of nitrogen in blood and tissues as a result of rapid reduction of air pressure. Also, this condition may develop when a person ascends too rapidly after having been exposed to increased pressure while deep sea diving.

TREAT: Restore pressure by placing patient in a hyperbaric chamber and slowly returning to ambient pressure. SEE: *caisson disease; decompression illness; hyperbaric chamber.*

benediction hand. Paralysis in the intrinsic muscles of the hand innervated by the ulnar nerve resulting in marked flexion of the joints of the 4th and 5th digits so that the hand resembles the Pope giving a blessing. SYN: *bishop's hand; papal hand.*

Benedict's solution (bĕn′ĕ-dĭkts) [Stanley R. Benedict, U.S. chemist, 1844–1936]. A solution used to test for presence of sugar. To 173 gm sodium or potassium citrate and 100 gm anhydrous sodium carbonate (dissolved in 700 ml water) is added 17.3 gm crystalline copper sulfate that has been dissolved in 100 ml of water. Sufficient water is added to the mixture to make 1000 ml. SEE: *Benedict's test.*

Benedict's test. Add 8 drops of clear urine (filtered if necessary) to a test tube containing 5 ml of Benedict's solution, q.v. Boil from 1 to 2 minutes, agitating the test tube during this time, and then allow it to cool undisturbed. Formation of red, yellow, olive green, or green precipitate indicates presence of sugar.

Benedikt's syndrome [Moritz Benedikt, Austrian physician, 1835–1920]. Hemiplegia with oculomotor paralysis and clonic spasm or tremor on opposite side. It is caused by lesions that damage the third nerve and involve the nucleus ruber and corticospinal tract.

benefit. 1. Something that promotes health. 2. Term for service stipulations of an insurance policy, esp. a medical policy.

Benemid. Trade name for probenecid.

benign (bē-nīn′) [L. *benignus*, mild]. Not recurrent or progressive. Opposite of malignant.

benign forgetfulness. A memory defect characterized by the inability to immediately recall a name or date, but the item, whether recent or remote, is eventually recalled.

benign positional vertigo. SEE: *vertigo, benign positional.*

benign prostatic hypertrophy. ABBR: BPH. Enlargement of the prostate gland, a condition commonly seen in males over 50. It is a progressive condition and can cause obstruction of the urethra with interference in urine flow. Surgical resection of the portion of the gland encroaching on the urethra may be necessary. Approx. 350,000 men will undergo surgery each year for BPH.

Surgery may be delayed by using balloon dilatation of the prostate. The technique involves placing a balloon catheter in the distal urethra. The balloon is inflated by injecting dilute contrast media at high pressure. The balloon is left in place for about 10 minutes and then the pressure is released. Even though this procedure may help to relieve the symptoms of BPH, it is not known how long the improvement will last. SEE: *Nursing Diagnoses in Appendix.*

Bennett double-ring splint. Metal splint that slips on the finger and limits hyperextension of the proximal interphalangeal joint.

bentonite (běn′tŏn-īt) [Fort Benton, U.S.]. A hydrated aluminosilicate that forms a thick, slippery substance when water is added. Used as a suspending and clarifying agent. It may be heat-sterilized.

Bentyl. Trade name for dicyclomine hydrochloride.

benzaldehyde (běn-zăl′dě-hīd). A pharmaceutical flavoring agent derived from oil of bitter almond.

benzalkonium chloride (běnz″ăl-kō′nē-ŭm klō′rĭd). NF. An antimicrobial preservative. White or yellowish-white thick gel. Usually has a mild aromatic odor. In aqueous solution it has a bitter taste. Used as a detergent and germicide. Trade names are Zephiran Chloride, Roccal, and Hyamine 3500.

Benzedrine (běn′zě-drēn). Trade name for amphetamine sulfate.

benzene, benzin, benzine (běn′zēn, běn-zēn′, běn′zĭn) [benz(oin) + Gr. ene, suffix used in chemistry to denote unsaturated compound]. C_6H_6. A volatile liquid, immiscible with water and able to dissolve fats, that is used as a solvent. It is the simplest member of the aromatic series of hydrocarbons, and it is used in the synthesis of innumerable dyes and drugs. The phenyl radical, C_6H_6, will be recognized in the formulae for phenol, dimethylaminoazobenzene (see under azo compounds), and benzoic acid. SYN: benzol. SEE: benzene and b. hexachloride in Poisons and Poisoning in Appendix.

benzestrol (běn-zěs′trŏl). USP. A synthetic estrogenic substance used orally.

benzethonium chloride (běn″zě-thō′nē-ŭm). USP. A synthetic quaternary ammonium detergent compound used as a disinfectant and antiseptic agent. It is incompatible with soap. Trade names are Hyamine 1622 and Phemerol Chloride.

benzidine (běn′zĭ-dĭn). Compound used as a test to determine traces of blood in feces.

Prepare benzidine solution as follows: to a saturated solution of benzidine in glacial acetic acid add equal volume of 3% hydrogen peroxide and about 1 ml of the suspected material. Appearance of a blue color indicates presence of blood.

A diet consisting of milk, crackers, and rice should be adhered to for at least 48 hours prior to the test. This permits clearing of the intestinal tract of iron-containing foods so that feces can be tested for blood.

benzoate (běn′zō-āt). A salt of benzoic acid.

benzocaine (běn′zō-kān). USP. Local anesthetic, ethyl aminobenzoate, used topically. Trade name is Americaine.

benzodiazepine (běn″-zō-dī-ăz′ě-pēn). A chemically similar group of psychotropic drugs with potent hypnotic and sedative action; used predominantly as antianxiety and sleep-inducing drugs. Side effects of these drugs may or may not be of importance in a patient. They include impairment of psychomotor performance; amnesia; euphoria; dependence; and rebound, i.e., the return of symptoms, transiently worse than before treatment, upon discontinuation of the drug. Treatment with benzodiazepines should not exceed four months.

benzoic acid. USP. $C_7H_6O_2$. A white crystalline material having a slight odor. Used in keratolytic ointments, and as a food preservative. Saccharin is a derivative of this acid.

benzoin (běn′zoyn, -zō-ĭn) [Fr. benjoin]. USP. A balsamic resin obtained from various species of a tree, Styrax, esp. S. benzoin or S. paralleloneuris. Used as a stimulant expectorant, as an inhalant in laryngitis and bronchitis, or as a protective coating for ulcers, etc. It is also used as a solution applied to the skin to prepare the site for application of adhesives, esp. adhesive tape.

benzol. Benzene.

benzonatate (běn-zō′nă-tāt). USP. Medicine chemically related to procaine that is used in anticough preparations. Trade name is Tessalon.

benzoylpas calcium. USP. An antibacterial drug used as a tuberculostatic.

benzoyl peroxide. USP. A keratolytic agent. Trade names are Benoxyl and Persadox.

benzthiazide (běnz-thī′ă-zīd). USP. A diuretic agent. Trade names are Aquatag and Exna.

benztropine mesylate (běnz′trō-pēn). USP. An antiparasympathomimetic agent usually used with other drugs in treating parkinsonism. Trade name is Cogentin.

benzyl. The hydrocarbon radical of benzyl alcohol and various other compounds.

   b. benzoate. USP. An aromatic, clear, colorless oily liquid with a sharp, burning taste. Used as a topical scabicide. Trade name is Benylate.

benzylpenicillin procaine (běn″zĭl-pěn-ĭ-sĭl′ĭn). Penicillin G procaine.

Bérard's aneurysm (bā-rärz′) [Auguste Bérard, Fr. surgeon, 1802–1846]. An arteriovenous aneurysm in the tissues surrounding the injured vein.

Béraud's valve (bā-rōz′) [Bruno J.J. Béraud, Fr. surgeon, 1823–1865]. Fold of mucous membrane of the lacrimal sac at the junction of the lacrimal duct. SYN: Krause's valve.

berdache (běr-dăsh′) [Fr.]. An individual of a definite sex, male or female, who assumes the status and role of the opposite sex and who is viewed by the community as being of one physiologic sex but as having assumed the status and role of the opposite sex.

Transvestism is not synonymous with berdache, nor is homosexual behavior necessarily a component of this condition.

bereavement. The expected reactions of grief and sadness upon learning of the loss of a loved one.

beriberi (bĕr′ē-bĕr′ē) [Singhalese *beri*, weakness]. A disease caused by deficiency of thiamine in diet. Characterized by peripheral neurologic, cerebral, and cardiovascular abnormalities. Early deficiency produces fatigue, irritation, poor memory, sleep disturbances, precordial pain, anorexia, abdominal discomfort, and constipation. Endemic in Asia, the Philippines and other islands of the Pacific, and formerly in rice-growing sections of the U.S. SYN: *neuritis, dietetic; neuritis, endemic.*

ETIOL: Subsistence on highly polished rice, which has lost all thiamine content through the milling process. Secondary deficiency can arise from decreased absorption, impaired absorption, or impaired utilization of thiamine.

TREAT: Oral or parenteral administration of thiamine; establishment of a properly balanced diet.

Berkefeld filter (bĕr′kĕ-fĕld) [Wilhelm Berkefeld, Ger. manufacturer, 1836–1897]. A filter of diatomaceous earth designed to allow virus-size particles to pass through.

berkelium (bĕrk′lē-ŭm) [U. of California at Berkeley, where first produced]. SYMB: Bk. At. wt. of best-known isotope is 247; at. no. 97. A transuranium element.

berloque dermatitis (bĕr′lŏck) [Fr., charm for a watch or bracelet]. SEE: *dermatitis, berlock, or d., berloque.*

Bernard's duct (bĕr-närz′) [Claude Bernard, Fr. physiologist, 1813–1878]. An accessory pancreatic duct; ductus pancreaticus accessorius [NA].

Bernard's glandular layer. Inner layer of cells lining acini of pancreas.

Bernstein test [Lionel Bernstein, U.S. physician, b. 1923]. Test to reproduce the pain of heartburn. This is done by swallowing a dilute solution (0.1 N) hydrochloric acid. This is compared with infusing normal saline into the esophagus. The latter does not cause heartburn.

Bertin, columns of (bĕr′tăn) [Exupère Joseph Bertin, Fr. anatomist, 1712–1781]. Renal cortical columns supporting the blood vessels in the kidneys. The part that separates the medullary pyramids. Also called *columnae renales* [NA].

Bertin's ligament. Iliofemoral ligament.

berylliosis (bĕr″ĭl-lē-ō′sĭs) [*beryllium* + Gr. *osis*, condition]. Beryllium poisoning, usually of the lungs. The beryllium particles cause fibrosis and granulomata at any site,

whether inhaled or accidentally introduced into or under the skin.

beryllium (bĕ-rĭl′ē-ŭm) [Gr. *beryllos*, beryl]. SYMB: Be. At. wt. 9.0122; at. no. 4; sp. gr. 1.848. A metallic element.

bestiality (bĕs-tē-ăl′ĭ-tē) [L. *bestia*, beast]. The use of animals for the purpose of sexual enjoyment. Animals used include snakes, poultry, and nonhuman mammals. SYN: *zooerasty.*

beta (bā′tă). 1. Second letter of Gr. alphabet, written β. 2. Used as a prefix to chemical words to note isomeric variety or position in compounds of substituted groups.

beta-adrenergic agent. Synthetic or natural drugs that stimulate beta (sympathetic) receptors.

beta-adrenergic blocking agent. A substance that interferes with the transmission of stimuli through pathways that normally allow sympathetic nervous inhibiting stimuli to be effective.

These agents are used in treating hypertension, angina, certain cardiac arrhythmias, and postmyocardial infarction. They may also be helpful in preventing migraine, and treating stage fright and benign essential tremor. SYN: *beta blocker.*

beta-adrenergic receptor. A site in autonomic nerve pathways wherein inhibitory responses occur when adrenergic agents such as norepinephrine and epinephrine are released.

beta cells. 1. Basophilic cells in the anterior lobe of pituitary that give a positive periodic acid stain reaction. 2. Cells of the islets of Langerhans of the pancreas that secrete insulin.

betacism (bā′tă-sĭzm) [Gr. *beta*, the letter b, + *-ismos*, condition]. Speech defect giving the *b* sound to other consonants.

Betadine. Trade name for povidone-iodine, a topical anti-infective.

betaine hydrochloride (bē′tă-ĭn) [L. *beta*, beet]. A colorless crystalline substance containing 23% hydrochloric acid. It is obtained from an alkaloid found in the beet and other plants. Used orally as a source of hydrochloric acid in treating hypochlorhydria.

beta-lactamase resistance. Term used to describe microorganisms that produce the enzyme beta-lactamase, also called penicillinase, and thus have the ability to resist the action of certain types of antibiotics, including some but not all forms of penicillin.

Betalin S. Trade name for thiamine hydrochloride.

betamethasone (bā″tă-mĕth′ă-sōn). USP. A synthetic glucocorticoid that has the pharmaceutical actions of cortisone. Various preparations and dose forms including an ointment or cream for topical ap-

plication are available. Trade name is Ce-
lestone.

Betapar. Trade name for meprednisone.

beta particles, rays. Negatively charged
particles emitted by radium; more penetrating than alpha rays. Absorbed by 1 mm lead
or 0.6 mm platinum. SEE: *electron.*

beta subunit. Glycoprotein hormones containing two different polypeptide subunits
designated α and β chains. Analysis of the
units of these hormones, e.g., follicle-stimulating, luteinizing, chorionic gonadotropin,
and thyrotropin, enables early diagnosis of
such conditions as pregnancy and ectopic
pregnancy.

betatron (bā'tă-trŏn). A circular electron accelerator that produces either high-energy
electrons or x-rays.

betazole hydrochloride (bā'tă-zōl). USP. An
isomer of histamine. It is used intramuscularly to attempt to stimulate gastric secretion. Contraindicated in persons who have
atopic allergy. Trade name is Histalog.

bethanechol chloride (bĕ-thā'nĕ-kŏl). USP.
Cholinergic drug used in treating paralytic
ileus and also in treating urinary retention
not caused by organic disease. Trade names
are Urecholine and Duvoid.

Bethesda system. A system of reporting
cervical/vaginal diagnoses. The results
given use specific descriptive diagnoses and
include information on human papilloma
virus-associated cellular changes and low-
grade squamous intraepithelial lesions. Information concerning the adequacy of the
material sent for evaluation is also provided.
SEE: *Papanicolaou test.*

Betz cells [Vladimir A. Betz, Russ. anatomist,
1834–1894]. A form of giant pyramidal cell
in the cortical motor area of the brain. The
axons of these cells are included in the pyramidal tract.

bevel (bĕv'ĕl). 1. A surface slanting from the
horizontal or vertical. 2. In dentistry, to produce a slanting surface in the enamel margins of a cavity preparation, named according to the surface resulting.

bezoar (bē'zor) [Arabic *bazahr*, protecting
against poison]. A hard mass of entangled
material sometimes found in the stomachs
and intestines of animals and man as a hairball (trichobezoar), hair and vegetable fi-
berball (trichophytobezoar), and foodball
(phytobezoar).
    b., balloon. An inflated ballon that is left
in the stomach as an artificial bezoar. This
experimental technique is used in treating
obesity.

BFP. *biologically false positive.*

Bi. Chem. symb. for the element bismuth.

bi- (bī) [L. *bis*, twice]. Prefix indicating two,
double, twice.

biarticular (bī"ăr-tĭk'ū-lăr) [" + *articulus,*
joint]. Pert. to two joints; diarthric; for example, temporomandibular joints.

bias (bī'ŭs). In experimental medicine, statistics, and epidemiology, any effect or interference at any stage of an investigation
tending to produce results that depart systematically from the true value. The reasons
this may occur include selection bias, response bias, or observer bias.

bibasic (bī-bā'sĭk) [" + Gr. *basis,* founda-
tion]. Pert. to an acid with two hydrogen
atoms replaceable by bases to form salts.

bibliomania (bĭb"lē-ō-mā'nē-ă) [Gr. *biblion,*
book, + *mania,* madness]. Obsession
with the collecting of books.

bibliotherapy (bĭb"lē-ō-thĕr'ă-pē) [" +
therapeia, treatment]. A nonphysical, psychotherapeutic technique in which the patient is induced to read books. Used in treating mental illness.

bibulous (bĭb'ū-lŭs) [L. *bibulus,* from *bibere,*
to drink]. Possessing the ability to absorb
moisture.

bicameral (bī-kăm'ĕr-ăl) [L. *bis,* twice, +
camera, a chamber]. Having two cavities or
chambers.

bicapsular (bī-kăp'sū-lăr) [" + *capsula,*
container]. Having two capsules.

bicarbonate (bī-kăr'bō-nāt). Any salt containing the HCO_3^- (bicarbonate) anion.
SEE: *carbonic acid.*
    b., blood. Bicarbonate in the blood. The
amount present is an indicator of the alkali
reserve.

bicellular (bī-sĕl'ū-lăr) [" + *cellularis,* little
cell]. 1. Composed of two cells. 2. Having two
chambers or compartments.

biceps (bī'sĕps) [" + *caput,* head]. A muscle with two heads.
    b. brachii. Muscle of the upper arm, hav-
ing two heads. Flexes arm and forearm and
supinates hand.
    b. femoris. One of the hamstring mus-
cles lying on posterior lateral side of thigh.
Flexes knee and rotates it outward.

biceps reflex. Normal contraction of biceps
muscle when tendon is percussed.

Bichat, Marie François X. (bē-shä'). French
physiologist and anatomist, 1771–1802.
Founder of scientific histology and pathological anatomy.
    B.'s canal. The subarachnoid canal,
which extends from the third ventricle to
the middle of Bichat's fissure and carries the
veins of Galen.
    B.'s fat ball. Mass of fat behind the buc-
cinator muscle. SYN: *sucking pad.*
    B.'s fissure. The horseshoe fissure sepa-
rating the cerebrum from the cerebellum.
    B.'s ligament. Lower fasciculus of the
posterior sacroiliac ligament.

BICONCAVE LENS

BICONVEX LENS

B.'s tunic. The tunica intima of the blood vessels.

bichloride of mercury (bī-klō′rīd). $HgCl_2$. Corrosive mercuric chloride; a crystalline salt. SEE: *mercuric chloride; mercuric chloride poisoning; mercuric chloride* in *Poisons and Poisoning* in *Appendix*.

bicipital (bī-sĭp′ĭ-tăl) [L. *biceps*, two heads]. 1. Pert. to a muscle having two heads. 2. Having two heads.

BiCNU. Trade name for carmustine, q.v.

biconcave (bī-kŏn′kāv) [L. *bis*, twice, + *concavus*, concave]. Concave on each side, esp. as a type of lens. SEE: illus.

biconvex (bī-kŏn′vĕks) [″ + *convexus*, rounded raised surface]. Convex on two sides, esp. as a type of lens. SEE: illus.

bicornate, bicornis (bī-kor′nāt, -nĭs) [″ + *cornutus*, horned]. Having two processes or hornlike projections.

bicornis uterus. Anomalous uterus resulting from incomplete union of the müllerian ducts. May be double or single organ with two horns.

bicoronal (bī″kō-rō′năl) [″ + Gr. *korone*, crown]. Pert. to the two coronas.

bicorporate (bī-kor′pŏ-rāt) [″ + *corpus*, body]. Having two bodies.

bicuspid (bī-kŭs′pĭd) [″ + *cuspis*, point]. Having two cusps or projections or having two cusps or leaflets.

bicuspid tooth. Premolar tooth; a permanent tooth with two cusps on the grinding surface and a flattened root. There are four premolars in each jaw, two on either side between the canine and molars. SEE: *tooth*.

bicuspid valve. Valve between the left atrium and left ventricle of the heart. SYN: *mitral valve*. SEE: *heart*.

bicycle ergometer. Stationary bicycle used in determining the amount of work performed by the rider.

b.i.d. L. *bis in die*, twice daily.

bidet (bē-dā′) [Fr., a small horse]. A basin designed so that one may sit astride it. Attachments allow a stream of water to flow over the genital and perineal area. Thus a bidet provides an excellent means of cleaning the perineum.

biduous (bĭd′ū-ŭs) [L. *bis*, twice, + *dies*, a day]. Continuing for two days.

Bielschowsky disease (bē″ĕl-shō′skē) [Max Bielschowsky, Ger. neuropathologist, 1869–1940]. Early juvenile type of cerebral sphingolipidosis.

bifacial (bī-fā′shē-ăl) [″ + *facies*, face]. Having similar opposite surfaces.

bifid (bī′fĭd) [″ + *findere*, to cleave]. Cleft or split into two parts.

bifid spine. Congenital fissure of vertebral column. SYN: *spina bifida cystica*, q.v.

bifid tongue. Cleft tongue.

bifocal (bī-fō′kăl) [″ + *focus*, hearth]. Having two foci, as bifocal eyeglasses.

bifocal glasses. Eyeglasses that combine two lenses with different refracting powers, one for distant and one for near vision. Often prescribed for presbyopia, q.v. SEE: *glasses, trifocal*.

bifurcate, bifurcated (bī′fŭr-kāt[′d], bī-fŭr′kāt[′d]) [″ + *furca*, fork]. Having two branches or divisions; forked.

bifurcation (bī-fŭr-kā′shŭn). 1. A separation into two branches; the point of forking. 2. The anatomical area where roots divide in a multirooted tooth.

bigemina (bī-jĕm′ĭ-nă) [L.]. Pl. of bigeminum.

bigeminal (bī-jĕm′ĭ-năl) [L. *bigeminum*, twin]. Double, paired.

bigeminal pulse. Pulse in which two beats follow each other in rapid succession, each group of two separated by a longer pause. The initial beat is regarded as the normal one and is usually of greater intensity than the second one. Detection of this type of irregular pulse should alert one to look for its cause, which may be one of several forms of heart disease.

bigeminum (bī-jĕm′ĭ-nŭm) [L.] (pl. *bigem-*

ina). A bigeminal body.

bigeminy (bī-jĕm′ĭ-nē). The condition of occurring in pairs, esp. bigeminal pulse, q.v.

b., junctional. Cardiac arrhythmia in which every other beat is a junctional ectopic or premature junctional contraction.

b., nodal. B., junctional, q.v.

b., ventricular. Cardiac arrhythmia in which every other beat is a ventricular ectopic or premature ventricular contraction.

bi-ischial. Concerning both ischial tuberosities.

bilabe (bī′lāb) [L. *bis*, twice, + *labium*, lip]. Thin, long device equipped with a hinged lower jaw. It is introduced into the bladder via the urethra for the purpose of removing small calculi from the bladder.

bilateral (bī-lăt′ĕr-ăl) [″ + *latus*, side]. Pert. to, affecting, or rel. to two sides.

bilateral carotid body resection. ABBR: BCBR. A rarely used method of treating carotid sinus syncope. The carotid body is removed bilaterally. SEE: *syncope, carotid sinus.*

bilateralism (bī-lăt′ĕr-ăl-ĭzm) [″ + ″ + Gr. *-ismos*, condition]. Bilateral symmetry, q.v.

bilateral symmetry. Symmetry of paired organs or an organism whose right and left halves are mirror images of each other or in which a median longitudinal section divides the organism into equivalent right and left halves. SYN: *bilateralism.*

bilayer. A two-component layer.

b., lipid. The outer membrane of most cells includes two layers of lipid molecules. These are arranged so that one part of each molecule is soluble in water and is hydrophilic; the other is water-insoluble and is hydrophobic. The membrane is virtually impermeable to water and water-soluble substances, such as ions, glucose, and urea; but fat-soluble substances, such as oxygen, carbon dioxide, and alcohols, can freely cross it. SEE: *cell* for illus.

bile (bīl) [L. *bilis*, bile]. A secretion of the liver. It is a thick, viscid fluid that has a bitter taste and passes from the bile duct of the liver into the common bile duct and then into the duodenum as needed. The bile from the liver is straw colored, while that from the gallbladder varies from yellow to brown and green.

Bile also is stored in the gallbladder, drawn upon as needed, and discharged into the duodenum. Contraction of the gallbladder is brought about by a hormone, cholecystokinin-pancreozymin, produced by the duodenum, its secretion being stimulated by the entrance of fatty foods into the duodenum. Added to water, bile decreases surface tension, giving a foamy solution favoring

the emulsification of fats and oils; this action is due to the bile salts, mainly sodium glycocholate and taurocholate.

COMP: Bile pigments (principally bilirubin, q.v., and biliverdin, q.v.) are responsible for the variety of colors observed. In addition, bile contains cholesterol, lecithin, mucin, and other organic and inorganic substances.

FUNCT: Its importance as a digestive juice is due to its emulsifying action, which facilitates the digestion of fats in the intestines by pancreatic steapsin, plus a further effect of the bile salts, which form compounds with the fatty acids and are necessary for their absorption. Bile also stimulates peristalsis. Normally the ejection of bile occurs only during duodenal digestion. Bile is both an antiseptic and a purgative. About 800 to 1000 ml/24 hr are secreted in the normal adult. SEE: *gallbladder.*

PATH: Interference with the flow of bile produces jaundice, resulting in unabsorbed fats being found in the feces. In such instances, fats should be restricted in the diet. Gallstones also may be produced in the gallbladder when the free flow of bile from the gallbladder is impeded.

TESTS: There are several methods of testing for bile in the urine.

Gmelin's test: A depth of 1 in. (2.5 cm) of concentrated nitric acid is carefully overlaid with the sample of urine. Bile is present when there is a play of colors at the junction of the fluids. This test also can be carried out by pouring some urine onto blotting or filter paper and then placing a drop of concentrated nitric acid on the moist paper. From the spreading edge of the drop of acid, a ring of various colors will develop in which green predominates and forms the outer band.

Iodine test: Pour urine into a test tube to a depth of 1 in. (2.5 cm), and carefully overlay it with dilute tincture of iodine. A bright green ring will appear at the junction of the fluids if bile is present.

RS: "bili-" words; "chol-" words; stercobilin; urobilin.

b., cystic. Bile stored in the gallbladder. It is concentrated as compared with hepatic bile.

b., hepatic. Bile secreted by the liver cells. It is collected in the bile ducts and flows to the gallbladder.

bile acids. Complex acids, of which cholic, glycocholic, and taurocholic acids are examples, and which occur as salts in bile. They give bile its foamy character, are important in the digestion of fats in the intestine, and are reabsorbed from the intestine to be used again by the liver. This circulation of bile acids is called the enterohepatic circulation.

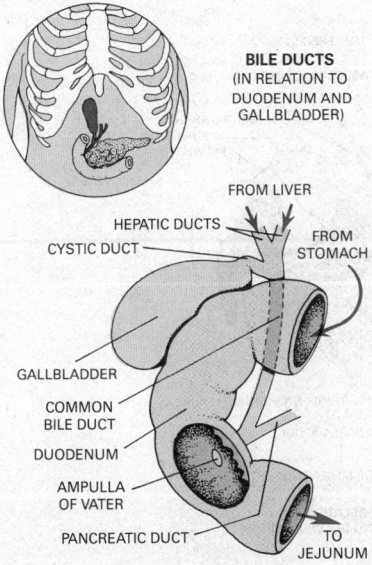

BILE DUCTS
(IN RELATION TO
DUODENUM AND
GALLBLADDER)

FROM LIVER

HEPATIC DUCTS

CYSTIC DUCT

FROM
STOMACH

GALLBLADDER

COMMON
BILE DUCT

DUODENUM

AMPULLA
OF VATER

PANCREATIC DUCT

TO
JEJUNUM

In Hay's test for bile acids, some urine is placed in a watchglass and a little powdered sulfur is sprinkled on the surface. If bile acids are present, the sulfur sinks because of the lowering of the surface tension by the bile salts.

bile ducts. Intercellular biliary passages conveying the bile from the liver to the hepatic duct, which joins the duct from the gallbladder (cystic duct) to form the common bile duct (ductus choledochus), and which enters the duodenum about 3 in. (7.6 cm) below the pylorus. SEE: illus.; *duct, common bile; duct, cystic; duct, hepatic; gallbladder.*

bile pigments. Complex, highly colored substances found in bile derived from hemoglobin. They impart brown color to intestinal contents and feces. Van den Bergh's test, q.v., is used to detect the type of bilirubin, q.v., in the blood serum.

Ex.: bilirubin, biliverdin.

bile salts. Alkali salts of bile sodium glycocholate and sodium taurocholate.

Bilharzia (bĭl-hăr′zē-ă) [Theodor Maximilian Bilharz, Ger. helminthologist, 1825–1862]. Former name for *Schistosoma,* the human blood fluke. SEE: *Schistosoma.*

bilharzial, bilharzic (bĭl-hăr′zē-ăl, -zĭk). Pert. to *Bilharzia* (*Schistosoma*).

bilharziasis (bĭl″hăr-zī′ă-sĭs). Schistosomiasis, q.v. SEE: *Bilharzia.*

bili- [L. *bilis*]. Prefix pert. to bile.

biliary (bĭl′ē-ār-ē). Pert. to bile.

biliary calculus. A stone formation in any of the biliary passages or in the gallbladder. SYN: *cholelith; gallstone.*

biliary colic. Pain caused by the pressure or passing of gallstones.

biliary tract. The organs and ducts that participate in the secretion, storage, and delivery of bile into the duodenum. SEE: illus.; *bile ducts; gallbladder; liver.*

bilicyanin (bĭl″ĭ-sī′ă-nĭn) [L. *bilis,* bile, + *cyaneus,* blue]. A blue or purple pigment, an oxidation product of biliverdin.

biliflavin (bĭl″ĭ-flă′vĭn) [″ + *flavus,* yellow]. A yellow pigment derived from biliverdin.

bilifulvin (bĭl″ĭ-fŭl′vĭn) [″ + *fulvus,* tawny]. Bilirubin mixed with other substances.

bilifuscin (bĭl″ĭ-fŭs′ĭn) [″ + *fuscus,* brown]. A dark brown pigment from bile and gallstones.

biligenesis (bĭl″ĭ-jĕn′ĕ-sĭs) [″ + Gr. *genesis,* generation, birth]. The formation of bile.

biligenetic, biligenic (bĭl″ĭ-jĕn-ĕt′ĭk, -jĕn′ĭk) [″ + Gr. *gennan,* to produce]. Forming bile.

bilihumin (bĭl″ĭ-hū′mĭn) [″ + *humus,* earth]. A dark insoluble residue that may remain after applying solvents to bile or gallstones.

bilineurine (bĭl″ĭ-nū′rĭn) [″ + Gr. *neuron,* nerve]. Choline, q.v.

bilious (bĭl′yŭs) [L. *bilosus*]. 1. Pert. to bile. 2. Afflicted with biliousness.

bilious fever. Fever with vomiting of bile.

biliousness (bĭl′yŭs-nĕs). 1. A symptom of a disordered condition of the liver causing constipation, headache, loss of appetite, and vomiting of bile. 2. Excess of bile.

biliprasin (bĭl″ĭ-prā′sĭn) [L. *bilis,* bile, + Gr. *prason,* green]. In bile, green pigment similar to biliverdin.

bilirachia (bĭl-ĭ-rā′kē-ă) [″ + Gr. *rhachis,* spine]. Presence of bile in the spinal fluid.

bilirubin (bĭl-ĭ-roo′bĭn) [″ + *ruber,* red]. $C_{33}H_{36}O_6N_4$. The orange-colored or yellowish pigment in bile. It is carried to the liver by the blood. It is produced from hemoglobin of red blood cells by reticuloendothelial cells in bone marrow, in the spleen, and elsewhere. It is changed chemically in the liver and excreted in the bile via the duodenum. As it passes through the intestines, it is converted into urobilinogen by bacterial enzymes, most of it being excreted through the feces. If urobilinogen passes into the circulation, it is excreted through the urine or re-excreted in the bile. The accumulation of bilirubin leads to jaundice in many cases, esp. to physiologic jaundice of the newborn.

    b., *direct.* Bilirubin conjugated by the liver cells to form bilirubin diglucuronide, which is water-soluble.

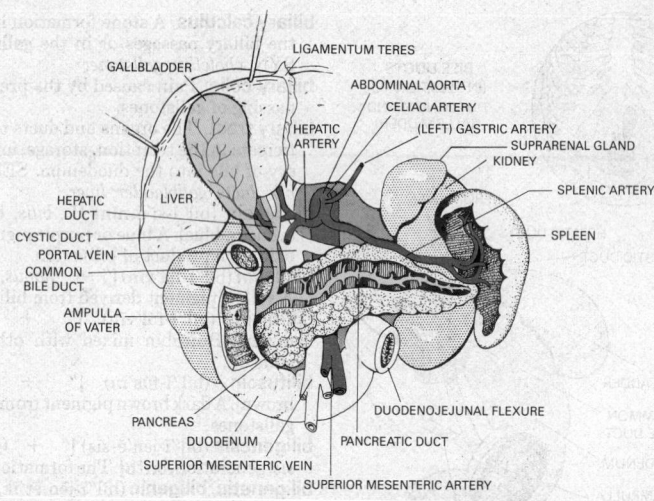

LIGAMENTUM TERES
GALLBLADDER
ABDOMINAL AORTA
CELIAC ARTERY
HEPATIC ARTERY
(LEFT) GASTRIC ARTERY
SUPRARENAL GLAND
KIDNEY
SPLENIC ARTERY
HEPATIC DUCT
LIVER
SPLEEN
CYSTIC DUCT
PORTAL VEIN
COMMON BILE DUCT
AMPULLA OF VATER
DUODENOJEJUNAL FLEXURE
PANCREAS
DUODENUM
PANCREATIC DUCT
SUPERIOR MESENTERIC VEIN
SUPERIOR MESENTERIC ARTERY

**BILIARY TRACT (IN RELATION TO
LIVER, PANCREAS, AND DUODENUM)**

b., indirect. Unconjugated bilirubin that is present in the blood. It is fat-soluble.

bilirubinate (bĭl-ĭ-roo′bĭn-āt). A salt of bilirubin.

bilirubinemia (bĭl″ĭ-roo-bĭn-ē′mē-ă) [″ + *ruber,* red, + Gr. *haima,* blood]. Presence of bilirubin in blood. Bilirubin is normally present in small amounts. However, in certain pathological conditions in which excessive destruction of red blood cells occurs, or in which there is interference with bile excretion, the amount is increased. In the newborn infant with erythroblastosis fetalis and greatly elevated bilirubin, exchange transfusion may be required.

bilirubinuria (bĭl″ĭ-roo-bĭn-ū′rē-ă) [″ + ″ + Gr. *ouron,* urine]. Presence of bilirubin in urine.

biliuria (bĭl-ĭ-ū′rē-ă). Presence of bile in the urine.

biliverdin (bĭl-ĭ-vĕr′dĭn) [″ + *viridis,* green]. $C_{33}H_{34}O_6N_4$. A greenish pigment in bile formed by the oxidation of bilirubin.

billion [Fr. *bi,* two, + *million,* million]. 1. In the U.S., billion is a number equal to 1 followed by 9 zeros (1,000,000,000) or (10^9). 2. In Europe, billion is a number equal to 1 followed by 12 zeros (10^{12}), i.e., bi-million, or twice the number of zeros in a million (10^6).

Billroth's operation(s) [Christian Albert Theodor Billroth, Austrian surgeon, 1829–1894]. Gastrectomy.

Billroth I: Excision of the pylorus of the stomach with anastomosis of the upper portion of the stomach to the duodenum.

Billroth II: Subtotal excision of the stomach with closure of the proximal end of the duodenum and side-to-side anastomosis of the jejunum to the remaining portion of the stomach.

bilobate (bī-lō′bāt) [L. *bis,* twice, + *lobus,* lobe]. Having two lobes.

bilobular (bī-lŏb′ū-lăr). Having two lobules.

bilocular (bī-lŏk′ū-lăr) [″ + *loculus,* cell]. 1. Having two cells. 2. Divided into compartments.

bimanual (bī-măn′ū-ăl) [″ + *manus,* hand]. With both hands, as in bimanual palpation.

bimanual examination. SEE: *pelvic examination.*

bimaxillary (bī-măk′sĭ-lĕr″ē) [″ + *maxilla,* jawbone]. Pert. to or afflicting both jaws.

bimodal (bī-mō′dăl) [″ + *modus,* mode]. Pert. to a graphic presentation that contains two peaks.

binary (bī′năr-ē) [L. *binarius,* of two]. 1. Composed of two elements. 2. Separating into two branches.

binary acid. Acid containing hydrogen and one other element.

binary code. SEE: *binary system.*

binary digit. One of two digits, usually 0 or 1, used in a binary system of enumeration.

binary gas. A toxic gas composed of two ingredients, neither of which is toxic by itself.

Used in chemical warfare.

binary system. A numbering system particularly well suited to use by computers. All of the information placed into a computer is in binary form, i.e., numbers made up of zeros and ones (0's and 1's). In this system each "place" in a binary number represents a power of 2; i.e., the number of times 2 is to be multiplied by itself. Ex.: the binary number 1000 indicates that the first zero to the right is 1×2^0 which is zero; the next zero to the left indicates 0×2^1 and, again, that is zero; the next zero represents 0×2^2 (i.e., 2×2) but again the value is zero; the one in the next, and last, place to the left represents 1×2^3 or $1 \times 2 \times 2 \times 2$, or 8. The numerical value is the sum of each of these calculations; in this case this is 8. Next, calculate the value of 101010. The first zero to the right from the initial example will be equivalent to zero; the next digit to the left, a one, indicates 1×2^1 which is 2; the next digit, a zero, represents 0×2^2 (i.e., $0 \times 2 \times 2$) or zero; the next digit, a one, represents 1×2^3 (i.e., $1 \times 2 \times 2 \times 2$) which is 8; the next digit, a zero, indicates 0×2^4 and, again, zero times something is zero; the next and last digit is a one and stands for 1×2^5 (i.e., $1 \times 2 \times 2 \times 2 \times 2 \times 2$) which is 32. Again, we add all of these values and find that the number 101010 in binary notation is equal to 42 (i.e., $32 + 8 + 2$).

binaural (bĭn-aw'răl) [L. *bis*, twice, + *auris*, ear]. Pert. to both ears.

binauricular (bĭn″aw-rĭk′ū-lăr) [″ + *auricula*, little ear]. Binaural; pert. to both auricles of the ear.

bind. 1. To fasten, wrap, or encircle with a bandage. 2. In chemistry and immunology, the uniting, i.e., bonding, or adherence of one molecule or chemical entity to another. Examples would be the joining of a toxin to an antitoxin; or a hormone to its receptor on the surface of a cell.

binder (bīnd′ĕr) [AS. *bindan*, to tie up]. 1. A broad bandage most commonly used as an encircling support of abdomen or chest. 2. In dental materials, a substance that holds a mixture of solid particles together. SEE: *bandage*.

b., abdominal. A wide band fastened snugly about the abdomen for support.

b., chest. A broad band used for encircling the chest to apply heat, dressings, or pressure, and for supporting the breasts. Improved by using shoulder straps to keep the binder from slipping.

b., double-T. A horizontal band about the waist to which two vertical bands are attached in back, brought around leg, and again fastened to horizontal band. Holds dressings about perineum or genitalia, esp. in males.

SCULTETUS BINDER

A MULTIPLE-TAIL BINDER APPLIED SEQUENTIALLY STARTING AT THE END SHOWN. EACH TAIL IS PULLED FIRM AND THEN OVERLAPPED BY THE NEXT ONE. THEY MAY BE HELD IN PLACE BY SAFETY PINS OR ADHESIVE TAPE. THIS BINDER IS UNSUITABLE FOR USE ON THE CHEST DUE TO MOVEMENT DURING BREATHING

b., obstetrical. A broad bandage encircling entire abdomen from ribs to pelvis, affording support.

b., Scultetus [Johann Schultes (Scultetus), Ger. surgeon, 1595–1645]. A many-tailed binder applied around the abdomen so the ends overlap each other as if they were roof shingles. It is used to hold dressings in place and to support abdominal muscles postoperatively. SEE: illus.

b., T. Two strips of material fastened together resembling a T, used as a bandage to hold a dressing on perineum of women.

b., towel. A towel encircling abdomen or chest with ends pinned together.

Binder's syndrome. Syndrome related to facial growth, with hypoplasia of the maxillae and nasal bones resulting in a flattened face, elongated nose, and smaller maxillary arch with crowding of the teeth and malocclusions. SYN: *maxillonasal syndrome; maxillonasal dysostosis.*

binocular (bĭn-ŏk′ū-lăr) [L. *bis*, twice, + *oculus*, eye]. Pert. to both eyes.

binocular vision. Normal vision involving simultaneous use of both eyes.

binomial (bī-nō′mē-ăl) [″ + *nomen*, name]. In mathematics and statistics, an equation containing two variables.

binotic (bĭn-ŏt'ĭk) [" + Gr. *ous*, ear]. Pert. to or having two ears. SYN: *binaural*.

binovular (bĭn-ŏv'ū-lăr) [" + *ovum*, egg]. Derived from or pert. to two ova. SYN: *biovular*.

binuclear, binucleate (bī-nū'klē-ăr, -āt) [" + *nucleus*, kernel]. Having two nuclei.

bio- [Gr. *bios*, life]. Prefix indicating relationship to life.

bioactive. Affecting living tissues.

bioassay (bī"ō-ăs'ā) [" + O. Fr. *asaier*, to try]. In pharmacology, the determination of the strength of a drug or substance by comparing its effect on a live animal or an isolated organ preparation to the effect of a standard preparation.

bioastronautics (bī"ō-ăs"trō-naw'tĭks). Study of the effects of space travel on living plants and animals.

bioavailability (bī"ō-ă-văl"ă-bĭl'ĭ-tē). The rate and extent to which an active drug or metabolite enters the general circulation, thereby permitting access to the site of action. Bioavailability is determined either by measurement of the concentration of the drug in body fluids or by the magnitude of the pharmacologic response.

biocatalyst (bī-ō-kăt'ă-lĭst) [" + *katalyein*, to dissolve]. An enzyme; a biochemical catalyzer.

biocenosis (bī"ō-sĕn-ō'sĭs) [" + *koinos*, shared in common, + *osis*, condition]. An ecological unit or community.

biochemical marker. Any biochemical compound such as antigen, antibody, abnormal enzyme, or hormone that is sufficiently altered in a disease to serve as an aid in diagnosis or in predicting susceptibility to the disease.

biochemistry [" + *chemeia*, chemistry]. The chemistry of living things; the science of the chemical changes accompanying the vital functions of plants and animals.

biochemorphology (bī"ō-kĕ-mor-fŏl'ō-jē) [" + " + *morphe*, shape, + *logos*, word, reason]. Science of the relationship between chemical structure and biological action. SEE: *stereochemistry*.

biocide (bī'ō-sīd) [" + L. *caedere*, to kill]. A substance, esp. a pesticide or antibiotic, capable of destroying living organisms.

bioclimatology (bī"ō-klī-mă-tŏl'ō-jē) [" + *klima*, climate, + *logos*, word, reason]. Study of the relationship of climate to life.

biocolloid (bī"ō-kŏl'oyd) [" + *kollodes*, glutinous]. A colloid from animal, vegetable, or microbial tissue.

biodegradable. Susceptible to degradation by biological processes, such as bacterial or enzymatic action.

biodegradation (bī"ō-dĕg"rĕ-dā'shŭn). The

breakdown of organic materials into simple chemicals by biochemical processes. Also called biological degradation.

biodynamics (bī"ō-dī-năm'ĭks) [Gr. *bios*, life, + *dynamis*, force]. The science of the force or energy of living matter.

bioelectronics (bī"ō-ē"lĕk-trŏn'ĭks). Study of the transfer of electrons between molecules in biological systems.

bioenergetics (bī"ō-ĕn"ĕr-jĕt'ĭks). Study of energy transfer and relationships between all living systems.

bioequivalent. The property of having the same biological effects of that to which a medicine was compared.

biofeedback. A training program designed to develop one's ability to control the autonomic (involuntary) nervous system. After learning the technique, the patient may be able to control heart rate, blood pressure, and skin temperature or to relax certain muscles. The patient learns by using monitoring devices that sound a tone when changes in pulse, blood pressure, brain waves, and muscle contractions occur. Then the patient attempts to reproduce the conditions that caused the desired changes.

biofilm. A moist film that covers surfaces, esp. those of implanted devices, including catheters. This film consists of bacteria imbedded in a film of adhesive polymer. Bacteria within the film may be protected from the action of antibiotics. It can be seen with a scanning electron microscope.

biogenesis (bī"ō-jĕn'ĕ-sĭs) [" + *genesis*, generation, birth]. Accepted theory that life can originate only from pre-existing life and never from nonliving material.

biogenetic. Pert. to biogenesis.

biogenic amines. A group of chemical compounds, most of which are important in neurotransmission. Included are norepinephrine, histamine, serotonin, and dopamine.

biogerontology. The study of three primary aspects of life: aging, longevity, and death. Also referred to as biological gerontology.

biohazard. Anything that is harmful or potentially harmful to man, other species, or the environment.

bioinequivalent. Not being equivalent to that to which a drug is compared.

bioinstrument. A device placed in the body to record or transmit data from the individual.

biokinetics (bī"ō-kī-nĕt'ĭks) [" + *kinetikos*, moving]. The study of growth changes and movements in developing organisms.

biologic, biological [" + *logos*, word, reason]. Pert. to biology.

biological armature. SEE: *armature, biological*.

biological degradation. The breakdown of

organic materials into simple chemicals by biochemical processes.

biological mother. The individual who actually gave birth to the child. This term would not apply to an individual who provided the uterus for the gestation of a fertilized ovum obtained from a donor. SEE: *birth mother; surrogate parenting.*

biological response modifiers. A vague term for any form of therapeutic intervention that will modify the host reponse to various diseases.

biological rhythms. SEE: *clock, biological.*

biologicals. General term applied to medicinal compounds that are prepared from living organisms and their products. Includes serums, vaccines, antigens, and antitoxins.

biological warfare. ABBR: BW. Warfare in which disease-producing microorganisms, toxins, or organic biocides are deliberately used to destroy, injure, or immobilize livestock, vegetation, or human life.

Ex.: anthrax, brucellosis, plague. SEE: *chemical warfare.*

biologic fitness. SEE: *fitness, biologic.*

biologic half-life. The time required to reduce the concentration of a drug in the blood, plasma, or serum by 50%. This is a measure of the rate of drug distribution and elimination. SEE: *half-life; pharmacokinetics.*

biologist. A specialist in biology.

biology (bī-ŏl′ō-jē) [Gr. *bios*, life, + *logos*, word, reason]. Science of life and living things.

biology, radiation. SEE: *radiation biology.*

bioluminescence (bī″ō-loo″mĭ-nĕs′ĕns) [″ + L. *lumen*, light]. Emission of visible light from living organisms. The best known example is the cold light produced by fireflies. SEE: *luciferase.*

biolysis (bī-ŏl′ĭ-sĭs) [″ + *lysis*, dissolution]. Chemical decomposition of living tissue by the action of living organisms.

biolytic (bī-ō-lĭt′ĭk). Pert. to biolysis. Capable of destroying life.

biomagnetometry. Experimental use of multichannel computerized scanning instruments for obtaining noninvasive spatial and temporal data on the electrical activity of the body. The technique has considerable promise for investigating epilepsy, stroke, migraine, mental disorders, schizophrenia, and language disorders.

biomass (bī′ō-măs) [″ + L. *massa*, mass]. All of the living organisms in a specified area.

biome (bī′ōm) [″ + *oma*, mass]. The totality of living organisms in a specified ecological area.

biomechanics (bī″ō-mě-kăn′ĭks). The application of mechanical forces to living organisms and the investigation of the effects of the interaction of force and the body or system. Includes forces that arise from within and outside the body. SEE: *kinesiology.*

biomedical. Biological and medical; pert. to application of natural sciences to the study of medicine.

biomedical engineering. Application of the principles and practices of engineering science to biomedical research and health care.

Ex.: Development of devices such as cardiac pacemakers, hearing aids, and sophisticated artificial limbs and joints.

biometeorology (bī″ō-mē″tē-or-ŏl′ō-jē) [″ + *meteoros*, raised from off the ground, + *logos*, word, reason]. Study of the effects of meteorology on all forms of life.

biometrics (bī″ō-mĕt′rĭks). Study of the application of mathematics and statistics to the analysis and solution of problems in the fields of biology and other life sciences.

biometry (bī-ŏm′ĕ-trē) [″ + *metron*, measure]. 1. Application of statistics to biological science. 2. Computation of life expectancy.

biomicroscope (bī″ō-mī′krŏ-skōp). A microscope used with a slit lamp for viewing segments of the living eye.

bion (bī′ŏn) [Gr. *bios*, life]. Any living organism.

bionics (bī-ŏn′ĭks). Study of biological functions and mechanisms and the application of these findings to the design of machines, esp. computers.

bionomics (bī″ō-nŏm′ĭks) [″ + *nomos*, law]. Ecology, q.v.

bionomy (bī-ŏn′ō-mē). The science pert. to life processes. SEE: *ecology; physiology.*

biophagism, biophagy (bī-ŏf′ă-jĭzm, -ă-jē) [″ + *phagein*, to eat]. Absorbing or obtaining nourishment from living matter.

biophotometer (bī″ō-fō-tŏm′ĕ-tĕr) [″ + *photos*, light, + *metron*, measure]. Device for evaluating visual adaptation to the dark. Used to determine presence or absence of vitamin A deficiency.

biophysics (bī″ō-fĭz′ĭks) [″ + *physikos*, natural]. Application of physical laws to biological processes and functions.

biopsy (bī′ŏp-sē) [″ + *opsis*, vision]. Excision of a small piece of living tissue for microscopic examination. The tissue may be obtained by use of a syringe and needle. Usually performed to attempt to establish a diagnosis.

b., aspiration. Removal of tissue by use of a needle and syringe.

b., brush. Removal of tissue for investigation by use of a brush.

b., liver. Removal of tissue from the liver by use of a large bore needle that permits removal of a core of tissue.

228

b., muscle. Removal of muscle tissue for microscopic examination and chemical analysis.

b., needle. Removal of tissue by use of a needle. Usually it is attached to a syringe.

b., punch. Removal of a small bit of tissue by use of a hollow punch.

biopsychosocial. Biological, psychological and social; pertaining to the application of knowledge from the biological and behavioral sciences to solve human problems.

biopterin (bī-ŏp'tĕr-ĭn). The chemical 2-amino-4-hydroxy-6-(1,2-hydroxypropyl) pteridine, important in metabolizing phenylalanine. A deficiency of this is a rare cause of phenylketonuria.

bioremediation. Conversion of hazardous wastes and pollutants into harmless materials by the action of microorganisms.

biorhythms (bī'ō-rĭth"ŭms) [" + *rhythmos,* rhythm]. Cyclic phenomena that occur with established regularity in living organisms.

Ex.: circadian rhythms, the sleep cycle, the menstrual cycle. SEE: *clock, biological.*

bios (bī'ŏs) [Gr., life]. 1. Organic life. 2. A group of substances (including inositol biotin, and thiamine) necessary for the most favorable growth of some yeasts.

biosafety level. ABBR: BSL. A system for classifying the safety precautions required for those working with dangerous microorganisms. The lowest level applies to work places in which nonpathogenic organisms are involved, and the highest level involves highly infectious organisms for which there are no cures or vaccines.

bioscience (bī'ō-sī'ĕns) [Gr. *bios,* life, + L. *scientia,* knowledge]. Life science.

biosensor [Gr. *bio,* life, + sensor]. A device that senses and analyzes biological information. This may be simple temperature, blood pressure, or heart rate or more sophisticated determination of chemicals and enzymes in body fluids. The device may be used in the laboratory or placed within the body.

-biosis (bī-ōs'ĭs). Combining form indicating mode of life.

biospectrometry (bī"ō-spĕk-trŏm'ĕ-trē) [" + L. *spectrum,* image, + Gr. *metron,* measure]. Use of a spectroscope to determine the amounts and kinds of substances in tissues.

biospectroscopy (bī"ō-spĕk-trŏs'kō-pē) [" + " + Gr. *skopein,* to examine]. Examination of tissue by use of a spectroscope.

biosphere (bī'ō-sfēr") [" + *sphaira,* ball]. That portion of the earth that supports ecological systems.

biostatics (bī"ō-stăt'ĭks) [" + *statikos,* standing]. Science of the relationship of structure to function.

biostatistics. Application of statistical processes and methods to the analysis of biological data. SEE: *morbidity rates; vital statistics.*

biosynthesis (bī"ō-sĭn'thĕ-sĭs) [" + *synthesis,* a putting together]. The formation of chemical compounds by a living organism.

biota (bī-ō'tă) [Gr. *bios,* life]. Combined and total animal and plant life in an area.

biotaxis, biotaxy (bī"ō-tăk'sĭs, -sē) [" + *taxis,* arrangement]. 1. The selecting and arranging activity of living cells. 2. Systematic classification of living organisms.

Biot's breathing (bē-ōz') [Camille Biot, Fr. physician, b. 1878]. Breathing characterized by several short breaths followed by long irregular periods of apnea. Seen in patients with increased intracranial pressure. SEE: *Cheyne-Stokes respiration.*

biotechnology. The application of biological systems and organisms to technical and industrial processes. This broad definition includes such ancient endeavors as the use of yeast in preparing bread for baking, and such modern concepts as genetic engineering.

biotelemetry (bī"ō-tĕl-ĕm'ĕ-trē) [Gr. *bios,* life, + *tele,* distant, + *metron,* measure]. Recording biological events such as temperature, heart rate, ECG, and EEG in subjects remote from the investigator. This is done by transmitting and receiving by telephone or other electronic methods.

biotics (bī-ŏt'ĭks) [Gr. *biotikos,* living]. The science that deals with the functions of life.

biotin (bī'ō-tĭn). A component of the vitamin B complex formerly designated as vitamin H. This water-soluble, heat-sensitive substance is essential for the metabolism of fat and carbohydrates. Present in many foods, but liver, kidney, milk, egg yolks, and yeast are particularly rich sources. Deficiency states have been reported in humans and experimental animals when the diet contains large amounts of raw egg white. This is due to a biotin antagonist, avidin, in the egg white that renders the biotin in the diet unavailable. Children with biotin deficiency have retarded mental and physical development, alopecia, impaired immunity, and anemia.

biotoxin (bī-ō-tŏk'sĭn) [Gr. *bios,* life, + *toxikon,* poison]. A toxin produced by or found in a living organism.

biotransformation. The chemical alterations that a substance undergoes in the body.

biotype (bī'ō-tīp) [" + *typos,* mark]. 1. Individuals possessing the same genotype. 2. In microbiology, the former name for biovar. SEE: *biovar.*

biovar [*biological variation*]. In microbiology, a term for variants within a species. These are usually distinguished by certain biochemical or physiological characteristics.

biovular twins [L. *bis*, twice, + *ovum*, egg]. Twins from two separate ova.

bipara (bĭp'ă-ră) [" + *parere*, to bring forth, to bear]. A woman who has given birth for the second time to an infant or infants, alive or dead, weighing 500 gm or more. SYN: *secundipara*.

biparasitic (bī"păr-ă-sĭt'ĭk) [" + Gr. *para*, beside, + *sitos*, food]. Pert. to a parasite living upon another parasite.

biparental (bī"pă-rĕn'tăl) [" + *parere*, to bring forth, to bear]. Derived from two parents, male and female.

biparietal (bī"pă-rī'ĕ-tăl). Concerning the parietal bones or their eminences.

biparous (bĭp'ă-rŭs). Producing two ova or offspring at one time.

bipartite patella. The developing patella that matures from two centers rather than one. This usually congenital condition causes no symptoms but may be mistaken for a fracture.

biped (bī'pĕd) [" + *pes*, foot]. An animal with two feet.

bipenniform (bī-pĕn'ĭ-form) [" + *penna*, feather, + *forma*, shape]. Muscle fibers that come from each side of a tendon in the manner in which barbs come from the central shaft of a feather.

biperforate (bī-pĕr'fŏ-rāt) [" + *perforatus*, pierced with holes]. Having two openings or perforations.

biperiden (bī-pĕr'ĭ-dĕn). USP. An anticholinergic drug used in treating parkinsonism. Trade name is Akineton.

biplane. Existing in two different planes.

bipolar (bī-pōl'ăr) [" + *polus*, a pole]. 1. Having two poles or processes. 2. Pert. to the use of two poles in electrotherapeutic treatments. The term *biterminal* should be used when referring to an alternating current. 3. A two-poled nerve cell.

bipolar affective disorder. A disorder in which the patient exhibits both manic and depressive episodes.

biramous (bī-rā'mŭs) [" + *ramus*, a branch]. Possessing two branches.

bird-breeder's lung. Attacks of chills, fever, and cough with shortness of breath in persons closely associated with birds such as pigeons and parakeets. In some patients the onset is slow rather than acute. The symptoms are due to antigenic substances in the bird's excreta. Symptoms usually subside when exposure to the excrement ceases. SYN: *pigeon breeder's disease*. SEE: *psittacosis*.

birefractive, birefringent (bī"rē-frăk'tĭv,

-frĭn'jĕnt) [" + *refrangere*, to break up]. Splitting a ray of light in two. SEE: *refraction*.

birth [Old Norse *burdhr*]. Act of being born; passage of a child from the uterus.

     b., complete. The instant of complete separation of the body of the infant from that of the mother, regardless of whether the cord or placenta is detached.

     b., cross. Labor with fetus lying transversely across the uterus.

     b., dry. Birth following premature rupture of the fetal membranes.

     b., live. An infant showing one of the three evidences of life (breathing, heart action, movements of a voluntary muscle) after complete birth.

     b., multiple. Birth of two or more offspring produced in the same gestation period.

     b., premature. Birth of a fetus sometime after it is developed enough to survive but before reaching 5.5 lb (2500 gm) in weight. This weight standard applies only to Western and European populations. SEE: *prematurity*.

birth canal. The canal through which the fetus passes in birth, comprising the cervix, vagina, and vulva.

birth center. Nonhospital facility for providing family-oriented maternity care for women judged to be at low risk of experiencing obstetrical complications.

birth certificate. A legal written record of the birth of a child, required by law throughout the United States.

birth control. Prevention of implantation of the ovum, or of birth, by temporary or permanent measures. Temporary birth control methods include contraceptive pills (i.e., steroid hormones), the condom, intrauterine devices (IUD), the rhythm method, vaginal sponge, foam, the diaphragm, the cervical cap, and spermicides. Sterilization in men is performed by vasectomy, and female sterilization is performed by tubal ligation. Sterilization is usually permanent but it is possible to reverse the process. SEE: *abortion; contraceptive; RU486.*

birth control pill. A class of medicines taken in pill form to control conception. They contain synthetic forms of estrogen and progesterone or synthetic progesterone alone. SYN: *the pill.* SEE: *contraceptive.*

birth defect. A congenital anomaly.

birthing chair. A specially designed chair used during childbirth. The mother is in a sitting or semireclining position and is more comfortable than if in the usual supine position. In addition, the process of labor is facilitated by this position.

birth injury. Injury sustained by the neonate

during the birth process.

birthmark. Nevus; a congenital discoloration of a circumscribed area of the skin, due to pigmentation or to a vascular tumor.

birth mother. The biological mother, q.v. SEE: *surrogate parenting.*

birth palsy. Paraplegia or hemiplegia due to birth injury.

birth parent(s). The biological parent(s) of a child. SEE: *surrogate parenting.*

birth rate. The number of live births in one year for each 1000 persons in the population.

birth trauma. Otto Rank's term to describe what he considered the basic source of anxiety in human beings, the birth process. The importance of this concept is controversial.

birth weight. The weight of the newborn. Normal weight of the newborn is between 2.5 kg (5.5 lb) and 4.5 kg (10 lb). Birth weight is an important index of maturation and chance for survival. Weight of less than 2.5 kg is associated with an increased chance of death in the perinatal period. Medical advances have increased the chance of survival of newborns of 2.0 kg or more.

bisacodyl (bĭs-ăk′ō-dĭl; bĭs″ă-kō′dĭl). USP. A cathartic drug that acts by its direct effect on the colon. May be administered orally or by rectal suppository. Trade names are Dulcolax and Theralax.

bisacromial (bĭs″ă-krō′mē-ăl) [L. *bis,* twice, + Gr. *akron,* point, + *omos,* shoulder]. Pert. to the two acromial processes.

bisection (bī-sĕk′shŭn) [″ + *sectio,* a cutting]. Division into two parts by cutting.

bisexual (bī-sĕks′ū-ăl) [″ + *sexus,* sex]. 1. Hermaphroditic; having imperfect genitalia of both sexes in one person. 2. An individual who is sexually attracted to others of either sex. SEE: *heterosexual; homosexual; lesbian.*

bisferious (bĭs-fĕr′ē-ŭs) [″ + *ferire,* to beat]. Having two beats; dicrotic.

bishydroxycoumarin (bĭs″hī-drŏk″sē-koo′mă-rĭn). Previously used name for dicumarol, USP, q.v.

bisiliac (bĭs-ĭl′ē-ăk) [″ + *ilium,* ilium]. Pert. to the two iliac crests or any corresponding iliac structures.

bis in die [L.]. Twice in a day. ABBR: b.d.; b.i.d.

bismuth (bĭz′mŭth) [Ger. *Wismuth,* white mass]. SYMB: Bi. At. wt. 208.980; at. no. 83. A silvery metallic element. Its compounds are used as a protective for inflamed surfaces. Its salts are used as an astringent, and in treatment of diarrhea.

   b. subcarbonate. An odorless, tasteless powder used as an antacid, astringent, and protective.
   INCOMPAT: Sulfides, acids, acid salts.
   b. subgallate. A bright yellow powder

without odor or taste. First introduced for treatment of skin diseases. General use is the same as bismuth subnitrate.

   b. subnitrate. USP. Heavy white odorless powder. Used as an astringent, protective, antiseptic.
   INCOMPAT: Acids, tannins, and sulfides.

bismuth colloids. Several bismuth compounds that are effective in treating peptic ulcers. They act in an acid medium by inhibiting the action of pepsin and reacting with the proteins in the ulcer crater to form a barrier that prevents the diffusion of acid into the area. SEE: *peptic ulcer.*

bismuth poisoning. Poisoning due to ingestion of bismuth.
   SYM: Metallic taste, foul breath, fever, gastrointestinal irritation, bluish line at gum margin, ulcerative process of gums and mouth, headache, renal tubular damage.
   F.A.: Removal of source of bismuth; gastric lavage; high enemas; respiratory support; chelation therapy with BAL.

bisulfate (bī-sŭl′fāt). An acid sulfate in which a monovalent metal and a hydrogen ion are combined with the sulfate radical. SEE: *disulfate.*

bit. Abbreviation for *binary digit.* Computers work with binary numbers made up of zeros and ones (0's and 1's). A bit is a single number in a binary digit. SEE: *binary system; byte.*

bite (bīt) [AS. *bitan,* to bite]. 1. To cut with the teeth. 2. Puncture or tearing of the skin by the teeth, as by an animal. SEE: *bites or stings.* 3. In dentistry, the angle and manner in which the upper and lower teeth meet.
   b., balanced. Balanced occlusion of the teeth.
   b., close, closed. Bite in which lower incisors lie behind upper incisors.
   b., end-to-end. Bite in which incisors of both jaws meet along cutting edge when jaw is closed.
   b., open. Bite in which a space exists between the upper and lower incisors when the mouth is closed.
   b., over-. Bite in which upper incisors overlap lower ones when jaws are closed.
   b., under-. Condition in which lower incisors pass in front of upper incisors upon closing the mouth.

bitelock. Device used in dentistry for retaining bite rims outside the mouth in the same position they were inside the mouth.

bitemporal (bī-tĕm′pō-răl) [L. *bis,* twice, + *temporalis,* pert. to a temple]. Pert. to both temples or temporal bones.

biteplate (bīt′plāt). Dental device used to correct or diagnose malocclusion. It is worn in the palate, usually on a temporary basis.

bites or stings. Injuries in which body surfaces are torn by insects or animals, resulting in abrasions, punctures, or lacerated wounds. SEE: *dog bite; human bite; rabies; snake bite.*

SYM: May be evidence of a wound, usually surrounded by a zone of redness and swelling, often accompanied by pain, itching, or throbbing. Often become infected and may contain specific noxious materials such as bacteria, toxins, viruses, or venom.

F.A.: If the wound is suspected of containing poison, apply tourniquet first. Wash with saline solution thoroughly; apply dry sterile dressing. Administer appropriate antitetanus therapy. Treatment for shock may be needed.

Some insect bites or stings contain an acid substance resembling formic acid and consequently are relieved by topically applied alkalies, as ammonia water or baking soda paste. For intense local pain, injection of local anesthetic may be required. Systemic medication may be needed for generalized pain.

Others, such as the stings of the bee, wasp, and hornet, contain unknown organic substances for which there is no specific antidote. Remove the stinger if one is present. At the site of bites or stings by poisonous spiders, esp. the black widow, q.v., scorpions, tarantulas, and poisonous fish, a firm bandage should be applied promptly. Intravenous calcium gluconate given very slowly is specific for controlling muscle pain due to black widow spider bite. It is also effective in relieving muscular cramps due to contact with jellyfish or Portuguese man-of-war.

Sea urchin spines break off in the skin and cause irritation. Remove the spines as soon as possible; surgical methods are not usually necessary. The spines can be softened and dissolved by vinegar, and the affected area can be soaked two to three times a day. If this treatment plus wet vinegar dressings does not effect a cure, surgical intervention will be required. The spines are radiopaque and thus may be located radiologically if they have migrated to deep tissue.

For jellyfish and other stings the local application of a meat tenderizer containing papain is an effective treatment. A slurry of the powder is applied as quickly as possible to the affected area. Demerol or morphine may be required for control of pain.

A stingray injures by penetrating the skin with the barb in its tail. This causes intense pain, local swelling, nausea, vomiting, weakness, and perhaps shock. Treat symptomatically, cleanse wound thoroughly, and remove all foreign material. Soak site of wound in hot water 113° to 140°F (45° to 60°C) for 30 to 60 minutes. Surgical debridement and closure of wound. SEE: *black widow; scorpion; spider, brown recluse; tarantula.*

bitewing radiograph. A type of radiograph that shows the crowns and upper third of the roots of upper and lower teeth; made by using a dental film packet with a bitewing or tab that holds the film in place when the jaws are closed on the bite tab. Also called interproximal radiograph.

Bitot's spots (bē'tōz) [Pierre A. Bitot, Fr. physician, 1822–1888]. Triangular, shiny, gray spots on the conjunctiva seen in vitamin A deficiency.

bitrochanteric (bī"trō-kăn-tĕr'ĭk). Concerning both greater trochanters of the two femurs.

bitter (bĭt'ĕr) [AS. *biter*, strong]. Having a disagreeable taste.

bituminosis (bī-tū"mĭ-nō'sĭs). A form of pneumoconiosis from dust of soft coal.

biuret (bī'ū-rĕt) [L. *bis*, twice, + *urea*]. A crystalline decomposition derivative of urea.

biuret test. A method for measuring protein in the serum. The presence of biuret can be detected by the addition of sodium hydroxide and copper sulfate solutions to the sample. A rose to violet coloring indicates the presence of protein, and a pink and finally blue color indicates the presence of urea.

bivalent (bī-vā'lĕnt) [" + *valens*, powerful]. 1. Having a valence of two; having a combining power of two atoms of hydrogen. 2. In cytology, a structure consisting of two paired homologous chromosomes, each split into two sister chromatids during meiosis.

biventer (bī-vĕn'tĕr) [" + *venter*, belly]. A part or organ such as a muscle with two bellies; pert. to several muscles.

biventral (bī-vĕn'trăl). Digastric; with two bellies.

bizygomatic (bī"zī-gō-măt'ĭk). Concerning the most prominent point on each of the two zygomatic arches.

Bjerrum's screen (byĕr'oomz) [Jannik P. Bjerrum, Dan. ophthalmologist, 1827–1892]. Tangent plane consisting of a large square of black cloth with a central mark for fixation, used for mapping the field of vision, esp. central and paracentral scotomata.

Bjerrum's sign. A sickle- or comet-shaped blind spot usually found in central zone of the visual field. Seen in glaucoma.

B.K. *below knee,* term used to refer to the site of amputation of a lower extremity.

Bk. Chem. symb. for the element berkelium.

black (blăk) [AS. *blaec*]. 1. Devoid of color or reflecting no light. 2. Marked by dark pigmentation.

black death. An acute, severe infection appearing in a bubonic or pneumonic form, caused by the bacillus *Yersinia pestis.* This term was applied to the condition in the Middle Ages when massive epidemics occurred in Europe. The infection is characterized by an abrupt onset with chills and fever. SEE: *bubonic plague; plague; plague, pneumonic.*

black eye. Bruising, discoloration and swelling of the eyelid and tissue around the eye due to trauma.

TREAT: Application of ice packs during the first 24 hours will inhibit swelling. Hot compresses after the first day may aid absorption of the fluids that produce discoloration. Topically applied leeches have been used to extract the pigment from the traumatized area. SEE: *leech.*

blackhead. A plug of dried, usually dark colored sebum in a sebaceous gland. SYN: *comedo.*

black lung. Lay term for the chronic lung disease or pneumoconiosis found in coal miners. SYN: *coal worker's pneumoconiosis.*

black measles. A severe type of measles in which the eruption is dark in color due to an effusion of blood into the skin. Also called hemorrhagic measles.

blackout. 1. Sudden loss of consciousness. This may occur while coughing, following nocturnal urination, or while swallowing in patients who have esophageal disease. SEE: *postural hypotension.* 2. Temporary loss of consciousness. In aviators, temporary or transient loss of vision or consciousness is usually due to a fall of blood pressure in the head. This is caused by the centrifugal force experienced in high-speed aircraft maneuvers that produce positive G forces. SEE: *alcoholic blackout; red-out.*

black vomit. Vomit that appears black due to the presence of blood that has been in the stomach and has been acted upon by gastric juices. Usually seen in yellow fever and other conditions in which blood collects in the stomach.

blackwater fever. Hemoglobinuria following chronic falciparum malaria infection.

SYM: Sudden onset, fever, tender and enlarged liver and spleen, dark urine, epigastric pain, vomiting, jaundice, sudden shock.

black widow. A species of poisonous spider, *Latrodectus mactans,* found in the United States. Its bite causes severe abdominal cramps. An antivenin is available for I.V. use after an appropriate skin test. For acute pain and muscle contraction, give 10 ml of calcium gluconate I.V. or I.M. and repeat as necessary. The very young and patients over 60 should be hospitalized if they have signs of a heavy dose of venom. SEE: *bites or stings; spider, black widow.*

bladder (blăd′dĕr) [AS. *blaedre*]. A membranous sac or receptacle for a secretion, as the gallbladder, q.v. Commonly used to designate the urinary bladder. SEE: *b., urinary; genitourinary system; urinary tract* for illus.

b., atony of. Inability to urinate due to lack of muscular tone. It is frequently seen after traumatic deliveries or after the use of epidural anesthesia.

b., autonomous. Bladder in which there is interruption in both afferent and efferent limbs of reflex arcs. Bladder sensations absent; dribbling constant; residual urine large in amount.

b., exstrophy of. Congenital eversion of the urinary bladder. The abdominal wall fails to close and the inside of the bladder may be seen to protrude through the abdominal wall.

b., hypertonic. 1. Bladder with excessive muscular tone. 2. Increased muscular activity of the bladder.

b., irritable. State of the bladder marked by increased frequency of contraction with an associated desire to urinate.

b., nervous. Bladder condition characterized by a constant desire to urinate without the power to do so completely.

b., neurogenic. Any dysfunction of the urinary bladder from lesions of central nervous system or nerves supplying the bladder.

b., spastic. Neurogenic bladder due to complete transection of the spinal cord above the sacral segments.

b., urinary. The muscular, membranous, distensible reservoir for the urine that receives urine from the kidneys through the ureters and that discharges urine from the body through the urethra. Its function is that of a reservoir for urine. SYN: *vesica urinaria* [NA]. SEE: *Sioux alarm.*

ANAT: The lower portion, continuous with the urethra, is called the neck; its upper tip, connected with the umbilicus by the median umbilical ligament, is called the apex. The region between the two openings of the two ureters and the urethra is the trigone. The wall of the bladder consists of an inner mucous layer of transitional epithelium, a muscular coat of smooth muscle, the outer layer comprising the detrusor urinae, and a fibrous layer. On its free superior surface is a layer of peritoneum. The bladder is supported by numerous ligaments. Blood is supplied by the superior, middle, and inferior vesical arteries and numerous veins and lymphatics; and it is innervated with nerves derived from the third and fourth sacral nerve by way of the hypogastric plexus.

The bladder is situated in the anterior inferior portion of the pelvic cavity. In the female it lies in front of the anterior wall of the vagina and the uterus, and in the male it lies in front of the rectum. It has a storage capacity in health of 500 ml (about 34 oz) or more. In disease states it may be greatly distended. A frequent cause of distention of the bladder in elderly males is interference with urination due to hypertrophy of the prostate gland, which surrounds the urethra and neck of the bladder. SEE: *urinary tract* for illus.

PHYS: An average of 40 to 50 oz (about 1.2 to 1.5 L) of urine is secreted within a 24-hour period. This value is quite dependent upon amount of fluid ingested and loss of fluid through exhalation, sweat, and the bowels. Inability to empty the bladder is known as retention and may require catheterization. Sphincter muscles are part of the mechanism that controls retention within the bladder.

The force of urination is much greater in the child than in the adult because the bladder is more nearly an abdominal than pelvic organ in the child. Thus the child's abdominal muscles help to expel the urine.

EXAM: *Palpation:* The bladder cannot be palpated when empty. When full it appears as a tumor in the hypogastric region that, on palpation, is smooth and oval.

Percussion: When it is distended with urine, the rounded superior margin is easily made out by observing the tympanic sound of the intestines on one hand and dull sound of the bladder on the other.

bladder drill. Technique used in treating stress urinary incontinence in women. It consists of investigating the patient and requiring that the urine be passed hourly. The patient charts the number of times of urination, intervals between urination, and volume of urine passed. She also notes the degree and frequency of incontinence. The intervals between urinations are gradually increased. SYN: *bladder training.*

bladder training. Bladder drill, q.v.

bladder worm. A larval form of tapeworm with a rounded cyst or bladder into which a scolex is invaginated. The bladder worm of *Taenia solium* (pork tapeworm) encysts in muscles of pigs; that of *T. saginata* (beef tapeworm) in muscles of cattle. SYN: *cysticercus.*

Blalock-Hanlon procedure. Surgical creation of an atrial septal defect or enlargement of the foramen ovale in the infant with transposition of the great arteries. Useful in improving oxygenation until total repair is undertaken.

blanch (blănch). 1. To lose color, esp. of the face, usually suddenly and in the context of being frightened or saddened. 2. To briefly scald a vegetable or nut-fruit in order to facilitate removal of the skin, peel, or covering. 3. To bleach.

blanch test, blanching test. Circulation test performed by applying and then quickly releasing pressure to a fingernail or toenail. The nailbed should lose color and return to normal within two seconds or less. Used to verify the presence of adequate circulation in conditions that may compromise circulation to extremities and in critical illness. SYN: *capillary nail refill test.*

bland [L. *blandus*]. Soothing, mild.

bland diet. A diet designed to buffer gastric acidity by providing meals of palatable, non-irritating foods. Content of diet includes milk, cream, prepared cereals, gelatin, soup, rice, butter, crackers, eggs, lean meats, fish, cottage cheese, custards, tapioca, cookies, and plain cake. Multivitamins may be a necessary adjunct.

IND: Gastritis, peptic ulcer, hiatus hernia.

Blandin's glands (blŏn-dănz′) [Philippe F. Blandin, Fr. surgeon, 1798–1849]. Small glands deeply placed on each side of the frenulum of the tongue near the apex. SYN: *Nuhn's glands.*

blanket, hypothermia. SEE: *hypothermia blanket.*

blast [AS. *bloest,* a puff of wind]. A violent movement of air such as accompanies the explosion of a shell or bomb; a violent sound, as the blast of a horn.

-blast [Gr. *blastos,* germ]. A combining form used as a suffix indicating an immature stage in cellular development; e.g., erythroblast, hematoblast.

blastema (blăs-tē′mă) [Gr. *blastema,* sprout]. Immature material from which cells and tissues are formed.

blastid (blăs′tĭd) [Gr. *blastos,* germ]. The clear space marking site of the organizing nucleus in the impregnated ovum.

blast injury. Injury as a result of a sudden increase or decrease in ambient pressure, e.g., sudden decrease in pressure as would occur if the pressure inside an aircraft flying at high altitude were to be decreased; or if pressure is suddenly increased due to an explosion.

blasto- [Gr. *blastos,* germ]. Prefix indicating germ or bud.

blastocele, blastocoele (blăs′tō-sēl) [″ + *koilos,* hollow]. The cavity in the blastula, q.v., of the developing embryo.

blastochyle (blăs′tō-kīl) [″ + *chylos,* juice]. Fluid contained in the blastocele.

blastocyst (blăs′tō-sĭst) [″ + *kystis,* bag]. Stage in the development of a mammalian embryo that follows the morula. It consists of an outer layer of trophoblast to which is attached an inner cell mass. The enclosed cavity is the blastocele. The whole is called blastodermic vesicle or blastocyst. At this stage, implantation in the endometrium (lining of the uterus) occurs.

blastocyte (blăs'tō-sīt) [" + *kytos*, cell]. An undifferentiated embryonic cell.

blastocytoma (blăs-tō-sī-tō'mă) [" + " + *oma*, tumor]. Blastoma, q.v.

blastoderm (blăs'tō-děrm) [" + *derma*, skin]. A disk of cells (germinal disk or blastodisk) that develops on the surface of the yolk in an avian or reptilian egg from which the embryo develops; also applied to the embryonic disk of mammalian embryos, a disk of cells lying between the yolk sac and the amniotic cavity from which the embryo develops. From the blastoderm, the three germ layers (ectoderm, mesoderm, and endoderm) arise.

blastodermic vesicle. A blastocyst, q.v.

blastodisk (blăs'tō-dĭsk) [" + *diskos*, disk]. Flat disk of embryonic cells on the surface of the yolk of the ovum. Formed from the blastomeres.

blastogenesis (blăs"tō-jĕn'ĕ-sĭs) [" + *genesis*, generation, birth]. 1. Multiplication by budding. 2. Transmission of characteristics by the germ plasm.

blastokinin (blăs"tō-kī'nĭn). A globulin found in the uterine lumen of some mammals near the time of blastocyst implantation.

blastolysis (blăs-tŏl'ĭ-sĭs) [" + *lysis*, dissolution]. Lysis or destruction of a germ cell or a blastoderm.

blastoma (blăs-tō'mă) [" + *oma*, tumor] (pl. *blastomata*). A neoplasm composed of immature, undifferentiated cells derived from the blastema of an organ or tissue.

blastomere (blăs'tō-mēr) [" + *meros*, a part]. One of the cells resulting from the cleavage of a fertilized ovum.

blastomerotomy (blăs"tō-mēr-ŏt'ō-mē) [" + " + *tome*, incision]. Destruction of blastomeres.

Blastomyces (blăst-ō-mī'sēz) [Gr. *blastos*, germ, + *mykes*, fungus]. A genus of yeastlike budding fungi pathogenic to humans. At room temperature the genus grows as a mycelial (fungal) form and at body temperature as a yeastlike form.

    B. brasiliensis. Fungus causing South American blastomycosis. This organism and disease are also called *Paracoccidioides brasiliensis* and paracoccidioidomycosis respectively.

    B. dermatitidis. Pathogen that causes North American blastomycosis, a rare fungus infection in man.

blastomycete (blăs"tō-mī'sēt). Any organism of the genus *Blastomyces*.

blastomycosis (blăs"tō-mī-kō'sĭs) [" + *mykes*, fungus, + *osis*, condition]. Infection caused by inhalation of the conidia of *Blastomyces dermatitidis.* This rare fungus infection may produce inflammatory lesions of skin (cutaneous form) or lungs, or a generalized invasion of skin, lungs, bones, central nervous system, kidneys, liver, and spleen. Also called Gilchrist's disease.

    TREAT: Amphotericin B or ketoconazole.

blastopore (blăs'tō-por) [" + *poros*, passageway]. In the embryo of mammals, the small opening into the archenteron made by invagination of the blastula.

blastospore (blăs'tō-spor) [" + *sporos*, seed]. A spore formed by budding from a hypha, as in yeast.

blastula (blăs'tū-lă) [L.] (pl. *blastulae*). An early stage in the development of an ovum, consisting of a hollow sphere of cells enclosing a cavity, the blastocele. In large-yolked eggs, the blastocele is reduced to a narrow slit. In mammalian development, the blastocyst or blastodermic vesicle corresponds to the blastula of lower forms.

Blatta (blăt'ă) [L.]. A genus of insects (that includes the cockroaches) of the order Orthoptera.

    B. germanica. The German cockroach or croton bug.

    B. orientalis. The Oriental cockroach, also known as the black beetle, a common European house pest.

bleaching. Use of an oxidizing chemical to remove stain or discoloration from a tooth.

bleaching powder. Chlorinated lime or calcium hypochlorite.

bleb (blĕb). Elevation of the epidermis, irregularly shaped. A blister or a bulla. May vary in size from less than 1 cm to as much as 5 to 10 cm; it may contain serous, seropurulent, or bloody fluid. A primary skin lesion. May occur in dermatitis herpetiformis, pemphigus, and syphilis. SEE: *bulla.*

bleeder [AS. *bledan*, to bleed]. 1. One whose ability to coagulate blood is either deficient or absent. Thus, small cuts and injuries lead to profuse bleeding. Such a person may be treated with one of several blood fractions to assist in arresting bleeding following trauma. SEE: *hemophilia.* 2. A small artery that has been cut or torn.

bleeder's disease. Hemophilia, q.v., a congenital blood condition marked by inability of blood to coagulate. SEE: *coagulation, blood.*

bleeding [AS. *bledan*, to bleed]. 1. Emitting blood, as from an injured vessel. 2. Process of emitting blood, as a hemorrhage or the operation of letting blood.

Normally, when plasma of the blood is exposed to air, it changes to allow fibrin to form. This entangles the corpuscles and forms a blood clot. SEE: *blood, clotting of; coagulation factors; hemorrhage.*

b., arterial. Bleeding in spurts of bright red blood.

F.A.: Pressure with fingers at nearest pressure point between it and heart. Locate artery and apply digital pressure above it until bleeding stops or until the artery is ligated. SEE: table.

b., breakthrough. Intermenstrual bleeding, esp. that which occurs during use of progestational agents.

b., occult. Inapparent bleeding, esp. that which occurs into the intestines and can be detected only by chemical tests of the feces.

b., venous. Continuous flow of dark red blood.

F.A.: May be controlled by firm continuous pressure applied directly to the bleeding site. If bleeding is from an area over soft tissues, hold a large but compact bandage firmly against the bleeding point.

Caution: A tourniquet should not be used. If the bleeding is over a bony area, as in the case of a ruptured varicose vein of the leg, a coin held firmly against the vein will provide immediate control of the blood loss. The patient should then be seen by a physician as soon as possible.

---

bleeding time. Time required for blood to stop flowing from a small wound or pinprick. This test is done using one of several techniques. Depending on the method used, the time may vary from 1 to 3 minutes (Duke method) or from 1 to 9 minutes (Ivy method). The Duke method consists of timing the cessation of bleeding after the ear lobe has received a standardized puncture. The Ivy method is done in a similar manner following puncture of the skin of the forearm. The validity of this test to predict clinically significant bleeding has been questioned.

blenn-, blenno- [Gr. *blennos*, mucus]. Combining form meaning mucus or pert. to it.

blennadenitis (blĕn″ăd-ĕ-nī′tĭs) [″ + *aden*, gland, + *itis*, inflammation]. Inflammation of mucous glands.

blennemesis (blĕn-ĕm′ĕ-sĭs) [″ + *emesis*, vomiting]. Vomiting of mucus.

blennogenic, blennogenous (blĕn″ō-jĕn′ĭk, blĕn-ŏj′ĕ-nŭs) [″ + *gennan*, to produce]. Secreting mucus.

blennoid (blĕn′oyd) [″ + *eidos*, form, shape]. Like mucus; mucoid.

blennophthalmia (blĕn″ŏf-thăl′mē-ă) [″

+ *ophthalmos*, eye]. 1. Catarrhal conjunctivitis. 2. Gonorrheal ophthalmia.

blennorrhagia (blĕn″ō-rā′jē-ă) [″ + *rhegnynai*, to break forth]. A discharge from mucuos membranes.

blennorrhea (blĕn″ō-rē′ă) [Gr. *blennos*, mucus, + *rhoia*, flow]. Any discharge from mucous membranes. SYN: *blennorrhagia.*

b., inclusion. Inflammation of conjunctiva in newborn. Caused by a filterable virus, *Chlamydia trachomatis*, that forms cytoplasmic inclusion bodies in the epithelial cells.

b. neonatorum. Gonococcal conjunctivitis in the newborn.

blennothorax (blĕn″ō-thō′răks) [″ + *thorax*, chest]. Accumulation of mucus in bronchial tubes or alveoli.

blennuria (blĕn-ū′rē-ă) [″ + *ouron*, urine]. Presence of mucus in the urine.

Blenoxane. Trade name for bleomycin sulfate, USP.

bleomycin (blē-ō-mī′sĭn). Any one of a group of antitumor agents produced by *Streptomyces verticillus.*

b., sulfate, sterile. USP. Bleomycin used in treating various carcinomas of the skin, head, neck, and lungs, as well as testicular tumors. Trade name is Blenoxane.

blepharadenitis (blĕf″ăr-ăd-ĕ-nī′tĭs) [Gr. *blepharon*, eyelid, + *aden*, gland, + *itis*, inflammation]. Inflammation of the meibomian glands.

blepharal (blĕf′ăr-ăl). Pert. to an eyelid.

blepharectomy (blĕf″ă-rĕk′tō-mē) [″ + *ektome*, excision]. Surgical excision of all or part of an eyelid.

blepharedema (blĕf″ăr-ĕ-dē′mă) [″ + *oidema*, swelling]. Edema of the eyelids causing swelling and a baggy appearance.

blepharism [″ + *-ismos*, condition]. Twitching or blinking of the eyelids.

blepharitis (blĕf″ăr-ī′tĭs) [″ + *itis*, inflammation]. Ulcerative or nonulcerative inflammation of the edges of the eyelids involving hair follicles and glands that open onto the surface.

SYM: Eyelids red, tender, and sore with sticky exudate and scales on the edges; lids may become inverted with lashes falling out and epiphora, q.v., occurring. Styes and meibomian cysts are associated with the condition.

ETIOL: In ulcerative type, bacterial infection usually by staphylococci; in nonulcerative type, cause is often unknown. May be due to allergy, exposure to dust, smoke, or irritating chemicals.

NURSING IMPLICATIONS: Keep the scalp, eyebrows, and eyelids clean. Bathe eyelids with warm saline solution to remove

Arrest of Arterial Bleeding*

For Wounds of the Face

Artery	Course	Bone Against Which Pressure Is Applied	Spot to Apply Pressure
Temporal	Upward ½ in. (13 mm) in front of ear	Temporal bone	Against bony prominence immediately in front of the ear or on temple
Facial	Upward across the jaw diagonally	Lower part of lower maxilla	An inch (2.5 cm) in front of angle of lower jaw
Carotid	From outer upper edge of sternum to angle of jaw	Cervical vertebrae	Deep down and backward an inch (2.5 cm) to the side of the prominence of the windpipe

For Wounds of the Upper Extremity

Artery	Course	Bone Against Which Pressure Is Applied	Spot to Apply Pressure
Subclavian	Across middle of first rib to armpit	First rib behind clavicle	Deep down and backward over center of clavicle against first rib (depress the shoulder first)
Axillary	Downward across outer side of armpit to inside of humerus	Head of humerus	High up in the armpit against upper part of humerus
Brachial	Along inner side of humerus under edge of biceps muscle	Shaft of humerus	Against shaft of humerus by pulling aside and gripping biceps, pressing tips of fingers deep down against the bone

For Wounds of the Lower Extremity

Artery	Course	Bone Against Which Pressure Is Applied	Spot to Apply Pressure
Femoral	Down the thigh from the pelvis to the knee from a point midway between iliac spine and symphysis pubis to inner side of end of femur at knee joint	Brim of pelvis	Against brim of pelvis, midway between iliac spine and symphysis pubis
Femoral		Shaft of femur	High up on the inner side of the thigh, about 3 in. (7.6 cm) below brim of pelvis, over the line given in the direction of the knee
Posterior Tibial	Downward to foot in hollow just behind the prominence of inner ankle	Inner side of tibia, low down above ankle	For wounds in the sole of the foot, against the tibia in center of the hollow behind the inner ankle

* Adapted from Hilda M. Gration, R.N.

any drainage or crusts. When prescribed ointment is applied, first cleanse eyelids, and then apply ointment to lid margins beginning at the inner and working toward the outer canthus of the eye. Teach the patient how to apply warm compresses for removal of crusts and scales and to apply prescribed sulfonamide or antibiotic ointment. In-

struct patient to keep hands away from eyes and to wash hands before and after eye care.

b. angularis. Blepharitis in which medial angle of the eye is involved with blocking of openings of lacrimal ducts.

b. ciliaris. Inflammation affecting the ciliary margins of the eyelids.

b. marginalis. B. ciliaris, q.v.

b. parasitica. Blepharitis caused by parasites such as mites or lice.

b., seborrheic. A nonulcerative form of blepharitis in which waxy scales form on the eyelids. Usually associated with seborrheic dermatitis of the surrounding skin.

b. squamosa. Chronic blepharitis with scaling.

b. ulcerosa. Blepharitis with ulceration.

blepharo- [Gr. *blepharon*, eyelid]. Prefix pert. to the eyelid.

blepharoadenitis (blĕf″ăr-ō-ăd″ĕ-nī′tĭs) [″ + *aden*, gland, + *itis*, inflammation]. SEE: *blepharadenitis*.

blepharoadenoma (blĕf″ăr-ō-ăd-ĕ-nō′mă) [″ + ″ + *oma*, tumor]. Adenoma or glandular tumor of eyelid.

blepharoatheroma (blĕf″ăr-ō-ăth″ĕ-rō′mă) [″ + *athere*, thick fluid, + *oma*, tumor]. Sebaceous cyst of an eyelid.

blepharochalasis (blĕf″ăr-ō-kăl′ă-sĭs) [″ + *chalasis*, relaxation]. Hypertrophy of skin of the upper eyelid due to loss of elasticity following edematous swellings such as in recurrent angioneurotic edema of lids. The skin may droop over the edge of the eyelid when the eyes are open.

blepharochromhidrosis (blĕf″ă-rō-krōm-hĭ-drō′sĭs) [″ + *chroma*, color, + *hidros*, sweat, + *osis*, condition]. Colored sweat, usually of a bluish color, from the eyelids.

blepharoclonus (blĕf″ă-rōk′lō-nŭs) [″ + *klonos*, tumult]. Clonic spasm of the muscles that close the eyelids (orbicularis oculi).

blepharoconjunctivitis (blĕf″ă-rō-kŏn-jŭnk″tĭ-vī′tĭs) [″ + L. *conjungere*, to join together, + Gr. *itis*, inflammation]. Inflammation of eyelids and conjunctiva.

blepharodiastasis (blĕf-ă-rō-dī-ăs′tă-sĭs) [″ + *diastasis*, separation]. Excessive separation of eyelids, causing eye to open wide.

blepharoncus (blĕf″ă-rŏn′kŭs) [″ + *onkos*, tumor]. Tumor of the eyelid.

blepharopachynsis (blĕf″ă-rō-pă-kĭn′sĭs) [″ + *pachynsis*, thickening]. Abnormal thickening of the eyelid.

blepharophimosis syndrome (blĕf″ă-rō-fī-mō′sĭs) [″ + *phimosis*, narrowing]. Narrowing of slit between eyelids, ptosis usually with poor movement of the upper eyelid, and defective skin creases. Also an abnormal fold of skin extending from the lower lid into the medial canthal area. These give a sleepy appearance. When this occurs in families, there may be impaired fertility in the female.

TREAT: Surgical for the lid difficulties.

blepharoplast (blĕf″ă-rō-plăst). A minute mass of chromatin in a cell, forming the base of a flagellum. Morphologically it is identical to a centriole. SYN: *basal body*.

blepharoplasty (blĕf′ă-rō-plăs″tē). Plastic surgery upon the eyelid.

blepharoplegia (blĕf″ă-rō-plē′jē-ă) [Gr. *blepharon*, eyelid, + *plege*, a stroke]. Paralysis of an eyelid.

blepharoptosis (blĕf″ă-rō-tō′sĭs) [″ + *ptosis*, a dropping]. Drooping of the upper eyelid.

blepharopyorrhea (blĕf″ă-rō-pī-ō-rē′ă) [″ + *pyon*, pus, + *rhoia*, flow]. Purulent material flowing from the eyelid.

blepharorrhaphy (blĕf″ă-ror′ă-fē) [″ + *rhaphe*, seam, ridge]. Reducing length of or obliterating palpebral fissure by stitching margins of eyelids. May be required to prevent damage to the cornea. SYN: *tarsor-rhaphy*.

blepharorrhea (blĕf″ă-rō-rē′ă) [″ + *rhoia*, flow]. Discharge from the eyelid.

blepharospasm (blĕf′ă-rō-spăsm) [″ + *spasmos*, a convulsion]. A twitching or spasmodic contraction of the orbicularis oculi muscle due to habit spasm, eyestrain, or nervous irritability.

b., essential. Blepharospasm that cannot be attributed to any cause. It may be so severe as to be virtually debilitating. Surgical therapy has helped some of these patients. Botulinum toxin A injected into the muscles that control the spasm has been of benefit. This may be effective for 2 to 3 months and then the treatment will need to be repeated.

blepharosphincterectomy (blĕf″ă-rō-sfink″tĕr-ĕk′tō-mē) [″ + *sphinkter*, a constrictor, + *ektome*, excision]. Excision of part of the orbicularis palpebrarum to relieve pressure of eyelid on cornea.

blepharostat (blĕf′ă-rō-stăt) [″ + *histanai*, cause to stand]. Device for separating the eyelids during an operation.

blepharostenosis (blĕf″ă-rō-stĕn-ō′sĭs) [″ + *stenosis*, act of narrowing]. Narrowing of the palpebral slit through inability to open the eye normally.

blepharosynechia (blĕf″ă-rō-sĭ-nē′kē-ă) [″ + *synecheia*, a holding together]. Adhesion of the edges of the upper eyelid to the lower. SYN: *ankyloblepharon*.

blepharotomy (blĕf-ă-rŏt′ō-mē) [″ + *tome*, incision]. Surgical incision of eyelid.

blepsopathia (blĕp″sō-păth′ē-ă) [Gr. *blepsis*, sight, + *pathos*, disease, suffering]. Neurasthenia caused by excessive eyestrain.

Bleuler, Eugen [1857–1939]. Swiss psychiatrist known for his important studies in schizophrenia.

blind [AS.]. 1. Without the sense of sight. 2. In medical research, a situation in which one group of patients will receive the therapy and another group will be given another type of therapy or a placebo and another (control) group could remain untreated but followed in the same manner as the other group(s). In such studies, it is the practice that physicians treating and following the patients do not know which groups received which therapy. The treating physicians are said to be "blinded." The study is designed in this manner in order to attempt to prevent the treating physicians from being influenced, i.e., biased in their judgment of the efficacy or failure of the therapy administered or of the placebo effect(s).

blinded. SEE: *blind,* def. 2.

blind loop syndrome. A condition caused by intraluminal growth of bacteria in the upper portion of the small intestine. Conditions that are associated with this syndrome are anatomical lesions that lead to stasis of such as diverticula or surgically created blind loops; diseases that are associated with motor function of the small intestine; and any condition that decreases gastric acid secretion. This leads to malabsorption, q.v. The syndrome is diagnosed by the clinical signs and symptoms of malabsorption and the use of breath tests, q.v., for detecting overgrowth of bacteria in the intestine.

TREAT: Antimicrobial therapy and nutritional support. Tetracyclines may be ineffective due to bacterial resistance.

blindness. Amaurosis; inability to see. The leading causes of blindness in the U.S. are cataract, glaucoma, and age-related macular degeneration. SEE: *amblyopia ex anopsia.*

b., amnesic color. Inability to remember names of colors seen.

b., color. Absence of or defect in the perception of color. SEE: *color blindness.*

b., cortical. Blindness resulting from a lesion of visual area of cerebral cortex.

b., day. Inability to see in daylight; hemeralopia.

b., eclipse. Blindness due to burning the macula while viewing an eclipse without using protective lenses.

b., hysterical. Partial or total blindness associated with attacks of hysteria and occurring in absence of any organic defect.

b., legal. A degree of loss of visual acuity that prevents a person from performing work requiring eyesight. In the U.S. this is defined as corrected visual acuity of 20/200 or less, or visual field of 20° or less in the better eye. In the U.S. in 1978 there were an estimated 498,000 blind persons. It is estimated there are 20 to 40 million blind people worldwide.

b., letter. Inability to understand the meaning of letters; a form of aphasia.

b., night. Nyctalopia; inability to see at night.

b., psychic. Sight without recognition due to brain lesion.

b., river. SEE: *onchocerciasis.*

b., snow. Blindness resulting from glare of sunlight upon the snow. May result in photophobia and conjunctivitis, the latter resulting from effects of ultraviolet radiations. Usually temporary.

b., solar. Blindness, eclipse, q.v.

b., transient. Temporary blindness in one or both eyes. The onset is usually sudden. May be caused in both eyes by any condition that temporarily interferes with maintenance of blood pressure in the ophthalmic arteries, such as migraine; carotid artery insufficiency; temporal arteritis; retinal artery spasm caused by hypertensive encephalopathy, uremia, or eclampsia; optic neuritis; glaucoma; and hysteria. SYN: *amaurosis fugax.*

b., word. Inability to understand written or printed words.

blindness, words pert. to: ablepsia; acatamathesia; achloropsia; "achro-" words; acritochromacy; aglaukopsia; amaurosis; amaurotic; amblyopia; amblyopia ex anopsia; aphemesthesia; axanthopsia; blind spot; braille; hemeralopia; hemiachromatopsia; hemianopia; meropia; nyctamblyopia; nyctalopia; nyctotyphlosis; Optacon; tritanopia; xanthocyanopia.

blind sight. The ability to see that occurs in persons who are blind because of a brain lesion rather than damage to the eye. It is manifested by their being able to reach for and track an object. These individuals apparently do not know they can see.

blind spot. 1. Physiological scotoma situated 15° to outside of visual fixation point; corresponds to point where optic nerve enters the eye (optic disk), a region devoid of rods and cones. SYN: *optic disk.* 2. In psychiatry, the inability of an individual to have insight into his or her own personality.

blink. To open and close the eye involuntarily. To wink rapidly, esp. in response to being surprised or startled, or in response to an object closely approaching the eye without warning.

blink reflex. Automatic closing of the eyes in response to a sudden movement of an object toward the eyes.

blister [MD. *bluyster,* a swelling]. 1. A collection of fluid below or within the epidermis. 2. To form a blister.

TREAT: Cleanse area with mild soap; apply protective dressing. Unless a blister is painful or interferes with function due to its size, it should not be punctured. If the blister does need to be punctured, do this aseptically and leave the skin in place. Apply sterile pressure bandage. Later, after about two days, debride if necessary.

Caution: If infection develops, treat as for any other wound, including tetanus prophylaxis or booster as required.

---

b., blood. Small subcutaneous or intracutaneous extravasation of blood due to rupture of blood vessels.

TREAT: Apply a firm dressing with moderate pressure to aid in stopping extravasation and hasten absorption. In some cases it is desirable to puncture aseptically and aspirate.

b., fever. Herpes simplex of lip.

b., fly. Blister produced by application of cantharides to the skin.

bloated (blōt'ĕd) [AS. *blout*]. Swollen or distended beyond normal size as by serum, water, or gas.

bloating. Abdominal distress of distention caused by abnormal intestinal motility and not to excess gas. Therapy for this troublesome symptom is rarely effective.

block [MD. *blok*, trunk of a tree]. 1. An obstruction or stoppage. 2. A method of regional anesthesia used to stop the passage of sensory impulses in a nerve, nerve trunk, dorsal root of a spinal nerve, or spinal cord, thus depriving a patient of sensation in the area involved. SEE: *anesthesia*. 3. To obstruct any passageway or opening.

b., air. A leakage of air from the respiratory passageways and its accumulation in connective tissues of the lungs, there forming an obstruction to the normal flow of air.

b., atrioventricular. A heart block in which impulses are impeded at or below the atrioventricular (A-V) node. SYN: *A-V block*.

b., bite. 1. A wedge of sturdy material used to maintain space between the two jaws. 2. A film holder held between the teeth for stable retention of the film packet during dental radiology.

b., ear. Blockage of auditory tube to the middle ear. May result from trauma, infection, or an accumulation of cerumen.

b., field. Regional anesthesia in which a limited operative area is walled off by an anesthetic.

b., heart. Interferences with the heart's contraction, causing dissociation of the atrial and ventricular rhythms. Due to failure of the contractile impulses to pass through the conductile tissue (atrioventricular node and bundle of His). SEE: *heart block*.

b., mandibular. Regional anesthesia of lower face and mandibular tissues by infiltration of the mandibular division of the trigeminal nerve.

b., neuromuscular. A disturbance in transmission of impulses from motor endplate to a muscle. May be caused by an excess or deficiency of acetylcholine or by drugs that act to simulate the action of an excess or deficiency of acetylcholine.

b., paravertebral. Infiltration of stellate ganglion with a local anesthetic.

b., second division. Regional anesthesia of upper face and maxillary tissues by infiltration of the maxillary division of the trigeminal nerve.

b., sinoatrial. Heart block in which there is interference in the passage of impulses between the sinus node and the atria.

b., spinal. Blockage in the flow of cerebrospinal fluid within the spinal canal.

b., ventricular. Interference in the flow of cerebrospinal fluid between the ventricles or from the ventricles through the foramina to the subarachnoid space.

blockade (blŏk-ād'). Prevention of the action of something, such as the effect of a drug or of a body function.

b., adrenergic. Inhibition of responses to adrenergic sympathetic nerve impulses and to agents such as epinephrine.

b., cholinergic. Inhibition of cholinergic nerve stimuli or cholinergic agents.

blocker. A drug that acts by preventing the normal action of a system or cell receptor.

blocking. 1. Obstructing; the arrest of passage through. 2. In psychoanalysis, a sudden break in free association as a defense against unpleasant ideas.

blocking factors. Substances present in the serum of tumor-bearing animals that are capable of blocking the ability of immune lymphocytes to kill tumor cells.

blood [AS. *blod*]. The cell-containing fluid that circulates through the heart, arteries, veins, and capillaries and carries nourishment, electrolytes, hormones, vitamins, antibodies, heat, and oxygen to the tissues and taking away waste matter and carbon dioxide. SEE: *erythropoietin.*

COMP: Human blood is composed of fluid (plasma) in which are suspended red and white corpuscles, platelets, and fat globules and a great variety of chemical substances including carbohydrates, proteins, hormones, and gases such as oxygen, carbon dioxide, and nitrogen. Blood consists of approx. 22% solids and 78% water. SEE: *blood cell* for illus.

Expressed in metric units, an adult

weighing 70 kg has a blood volume of about 5 L or 70 ml/kg of body weight. The blood specific gravity varies from 1.048 to 1.066, the corpuscles being heavier and plasma lighter than this. Blood is of slightly higher specific gravity in men than in women. Specific gravity is higher after exercise and at night.

In passing through the lungs the blood gives up carbon dioxide; after leaving the heart it is carried to the tissues as arterial blood, and then returned to the heart. It moves in the aorta at an average speed of 30 cm/second, and it makes the circuit of the vascular system in about 20 seconds. It constitutes approximately 7% to 8% of the body weight. The pH of the blood is from 7.35 to 7.45. SEE: *blood count; circulation; corpuscle; plasma; platelet.*

FUNCT: Provides nutrition and respiration for all tissues; transportation of waste from the tissues to the excretory organs; chemical and thermal regulation and coordination of the body; defense against infection through the action of antibodies, q.v., and phagocytes, q.v.

Formation: Red blood cells are produced at the rate of approx. 2,400,000 each second. The fact that each red blood cell lives for approx. 120 days keeps the number of red cells at a level concentration.

Characteristics: Blood has a distinctive, somewhat metallic, odor. Arterial blood is bright red or scarlet and usually pulsates as it issues from a cut artery. Venous blood is dark red or crimson and flows steadily as it comes from a cut vein.

b., clotting of. SEE: *coagulation, blood.*

b., cord. A specimen of blood obtained from the umbilical cord vein or artery of the fetus.

b., defibrinated. Whole blood from which fibrin was separated during the clotting process. If whole blood is stirred, the stringy elastic fibrin comes out on the stirrer; it can be washed until white. The remaining thick, red blood can no longer clot and is called defibrinated blood. If it is centrifuged, the clear liquid that now appears in the upper half of the centrifuged tube is called serum; this differs from plasma chiefly in that it does not contain fibrinogen (the precursor of fibrin). The corpuscles are in the lower portion of the tube. SEE: *buffy coat.*

b., occult. The presence of blood in such small quantities that it is not apparent to the eye. Thus blood may be present in feces but of such color and consistency as to be unnoticed by the patient. Usually detected only by chemical tests or by microscopic or spectroscopic examination. SEE: *benzidin*

test.

b., sludged. Blood in which red corpuscles have massed together in the smaller blood vessels, and block or slow the blood flowing through the vessels.

RS: erythrocyte; leukocyte.

b., synthetic. ABBR: S.B. Experimental effort to produce blood made either by use of chemicals or by genetic engineering techniques is progressing. Synthetic blood would be free of the potential of acting as a carrier of an infectious agent such as the AIDS virus (HIV) or that of hepatitis B.

b., transfusion of a single unit. In general, a patient who receives only a single unit of blood is in no more need of a blood transfusion than the donor. Nevertheless, administration of a single unit may be indicated in elderly surgical patients with coronary disease; and in patients who have an acute blood loss of several units, but are stabilized by use of one unit. Also, if at surgery or during bleeding from the intestinal tract, a single unit controls the bleeding, then a single unit is justified. Nevertheless, it is important to remember that each blood transfusion has the potential of being infectious with HIV or hepatitis B virus, or both. SEE: *autologous blood transfusion; blood transfusion; blood component therapy; transfusion reactions.*

b., unit of. Approximately one pint (473 ml) of blood. The usual amount available for use in transfusion.

b., vessels. Veins, arteries, and capillaries.

blood bank. The place where whole blood and certain derived components are processed, typed, and stored until needed for transfusion. Blood is mixed with adenine-supplemented citrate phosphate dextrose and is stored at 4°C (39°F). Heparin may be used as a preservative. Banked blood should be used as soon as possible because the longer it is stored, the fewer red blood cells survive in usable form. Ninety percent of the red cells survive up to 14 days of storage, but only 70% remain after 24 days. SEE: Caution at *blood component therapy.*

blood-brain barrier. A barrier membrane between circulating blood and the brain, preventing certain damaging substances from reaching brain tissue and cerebrospinal fluid. SEE: *membrane, glial.*

blood cell. Minute body in the blood. There are several principal types: erythrocytes or red blood corpuscles, leukocytes or white blood corpuscles, and platelets. SEE: illus.; *blood.*

blood cell casts. Masses of red cells molded by the renal tubules, the blood originating

TYPES OF CELLS PRESENT IN BLOOD

BASOPHILS   EOSINOPHILS   NEUTROPHILS
└─────────────────── GRANULATED ───────────────────┘

┌── UNGRANULATED ──┐

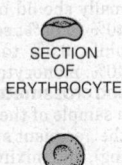

SECTION
OF
ERYTHROCYTE

ERYTHROCYTE

MONOCYTES   LYMPHOCYTES   PLATELETS SHOWN WITH LARGER
                                RED BLOOD CELLS
                                (ERYTHROCYTES)

from the glomeruli. Abnormal microscopic body in the urine composed of coagulated serum covered with red blood cells.

blood clot. Coagulated mass of blood. SYN: *coagulum.* SEE: *blood, clotting of.*

blood coagulation. SEE: *coagulation, blood.*

blood component therapy. Blood is a mixture of a great number of components including cellular and noncellular constituents. Except in the case of acute hemorrhage, the transfusion of whole blood is rarely needed. Instead, transfusion of specific blood components is indicated. Use of a component rather than whole blood permits several patients to benefit from a single blood donation. Components used in clinical medicine include packed or sedimented red blood cells; leukocyte-poor red blood cells; frozen glycerolized red blood cells (RBCs); thawed deglycerolized RBCs; washed RBCs; whole blood; whole blood, heparinized; granulocytes; platelets; plasma and plasma fractions. The latter include antihemophilic factor (factor VIII); prothrombin complex (factors VII, IX, and X); gamma globulin; and albumin. SEE: *blood transfusion.*

Caution: It is mandatory that appropriate measures be taken to prevent transmission of hepatitis B virus and human immunodeficiency virus (HIV) as a result of the use of blood or blood component therapy. SEE: *Universal Precautions* in *Appendix.*

blood corpuscles. The solid or cellular elements in the blood. SYN: *blood cell.* SEE: *erythrocyte; leukocyte.*

blood count. Enumeration of the red corpuscles and the leukocytes per cu mm of whole blood. A blood count indicates the number of these cells. The differential blood count tells the percentage of the various white cells in each 100 cells counted. Normally in each cu mm of blood there is an average of 5 million erythrocytes in the male and 4.5 million in the female. Prolonged exposure to high altitude increases the number. The leukocytes average 5000 to 10,000/cu mm. Platelets average 150,000 to 400,000/cu mm by direct counting method. A special chamber is filled with blood and the cells are visualized under the microscope and then counted. The type of fluid used to dilute the blood depends upon whether the white or red cells are to be counted. Hemoglobin and hematocrit are determined from samples of whole blood.

   b.c., differential. A blood count determined by microscopic examination of a very thin layer of blood on a glass slide after it has been suitably stained in order to demonstrate the morphology of the various cells. The number and variety of white cells in each 200 counted are obtained. Also, even though the red cells are not counted by this method, their shape, size, and color can be evaluated. Some blood diseases and inflammatory conditions may be recognized in this way. In a differential count, the varieties of the leukocytes and their percentages normally should be: neutrophils (segmented), 40% to 60%; eosinophils, 1% to 3%; basophils, 0.5% to 1%; lymphocytes, 20% to 40%; monocytes, 4% to 8%.

blood crossmatching. The process of mixing a sample of the donor's red blood cells with the recipient's serum (major crossmatching), and mixing a sample of the recipient's blood with the donor's serum (minor crossmatching). It is done before transfusion to determine compatibility of blood.

blood donor. One who gives blood to be used for transfusion.

blood doping. SEE: *doping, blood; erythrocyte reinfusion.*

blood dust. Minute colorless bodies in the blood, particles of the blood corpuscle. SYN: *hemoconia.*

blood gas analysis. Chemical analysis of the blood for the concentration of oxygen and carbon dioxide. This may be done on arterial or venous blood; the specimen may be obtained from an arm vein or by use of a catheter extending from a peripheral vein to the heart. The blood sample is usually collected in a heparinized vacuum tube with care being taken to assure that the specimen is not exposed to air. SEE: *blood gases.*

blood gases. During metabolic processes, oxygen is utilized and carbon dioxide is produced. Levels of these gases vary in response to certain disease conditions. It is therefore important to analyze the blood for these gases in order to be able to evaluate the extent of the deviation of acids and bases from the normal. In order to be able to institute appropriate therapy, information obtained from those values is analyzed with respect to other laboratory results and the clinical condition. SEE: *acidosis; alkalosis.*

blood groups. A genetically determined system of antigens located on the surface of the erythrocyte. There are a number of human blood group systems; each system is determined by a series of two or more genes that are allelic or closely linked on a single autosomal chromosome. The ABO system (discovered in 1901 by Landsteiner) is of prime importance in blood transfusions. The Rhesus (Rh) system is esp. important in obstetrics. There are about 30 Rh antigens.

   The population can be phenotypically divided into four ABO blood groups: A, B, AB, and O. Individuals in A group have the A antigen on the surface of their red cells; B group has the B antigen on red cells; AB group has A and B antigens on red cells; and O group has neither A nor B antigens on red cells. The individuals in each group have in their sera the corresponding antibody, also called an agglutinin, q.v., to the red cell antigens that they lack. Thus, a group A person has in the blood serum the anti-B antibody; group B has anti-A antibodies; group AB has no antibodies for A and B; and group O individuals have anti-A and anti-B antibodies in their sera.

   Blood group factors are important in clinical medicine because of the interaction of the antigens on cells with their agglutinin(s) in the serum.

   Ex.: destruction of red cells transfused from either a group A or group B donor to a group O recipient — the anti-A and anti-B agglutinins in the recipient's serum would react with the A or B antigens on the donor's red cells.

   Analysis of blood groups is important in identifying blood stains for medicolegal purposes, for genetic and anthropological studies, and in determining the probability of fatherhood in disputes involving claimed or disclaimed paternity. SEE: *Rh blood factor.*

bloodless. Without blood.

bloodletting. Removal of blood from the body as a therapeutic measure, usually by venipuncture. This technique is used in treating hemochromatosis, polycythemia vera, and in infants born with elevated hematocrits.

blood levels. The concentration of anything, but especially a drug, in the plasma, serum, or blood.

blood platelets. Small, colorless bodies in circulating blood, averaging about 3 microns in diameter. They tend to agglutinate into small clusters in shed blood. Platelets may originate from giant bone marrow cells (megakaryocytes). They play an important role in clotting through release of thrombokinase, which, in the presence of calcium, reacts with prothrombin to form thrombin.

   The normal number of platelets in circulating blood in adults is about 150,000 to 400,000/cu mm. Reduction below normal is called thrombocytopenia. In certain forms of hemophilia, blood platelets are abnormally stable and fail to release thrombokinase, thus increasing coagulation time.

blood poisoning. A vague term usually used to indicate the presence of large numbers of bacteria in the circulating blood. SEE: *pyemia; septicemia; toxemia.*

blood pressure. As popularly used, the pressure, determined indirectly, existing in the large arteries at the height of the pulse wave; the systolic intra-arterial pressure. More generally, the pressure exerted by the blood on the wall of any vessel. This pressure reaches its highest values in the left ventricle during systole. It decreases in the arterial system as the distance from the heart increases, and is lower in capillaries than in the arteries. The systolic arterial blood pressure rises during activity or excitement and falls during sleep. In the normal, relaxed, sitting adult, it may be as low as 100 or as high as 140 mm of mercury (Hg).

The following findings in adults are considered abnormal: systolic pressure persistently above 140; diastolic pressure persistently above 90. When either the systolic pressure is 160 or more or the diastolic pressure is 115 or above, the elevation is considered severe. Blood pressure varies with age, sex, altitude, muscular development, and according to states of mental and physical stress and fatigue. Usually it is lower in women than in men, low in childhood, and higher in elderly individuals. SEE: *b.p., chronic low; b.p., normal.*

RS: diastole; hypertension; hypotension; pulse pressure; systole.

   b.p., central. Blood pressure in the heart chambers, in a great vein, or close to the heart. If determined in a vein, it is termed central venous blood pressure; if in the aorta or a similar large artery close to the heart, it is designated central arterial blood pressure.

   b.p., chronic low. In general, if a person is healthy, low blood pressure is harmless and may be associated with long life. SEE: *hypotension; hypotension, orthostatic.*

   b.p., diastolic. Blood pressure during the relaxation phase between heartbeats, normally about 80 mmHg. It is dependent primarily upon the elasticity of the arteries and peripheral resistance, which in turn is dependent upon caliber of arterioles and capillaries.

   b.p., direct measurement of. Determining the blood pressure in one of several arteries. Done by placing a sterile needle or small catheter inside an artery and having the blood pressure transmitted through that system to a suitable recorder. As the blood pressure fluctuates, the changes are recorded graphically.

   b.p., indirect measurement of. A simple external method for measuring blood pressure.

   Palpation method: The same arm, usually the right, should be used each time the pressure is measured. The arm should be raised to heart level if the patient is sitting, or kept parallel to the body if the patient is recumbent. The patient's arm should be relaxed and supported in a resting position. Exertion during the examination could result in a higher blood pressure reading. Either a mercury-gravity or aneroid-manometer type of blood pressure apparatus may be used. The blood compression cuff should be the width and length appropriate for the size of the subject's arm; narrow (2.5 to 6 cm) for infants and children and wide (13 cm) for adults. The inflatable bag encased in the cuff should be 20% wider than one-third the circumference of the limb used. The deflated cuff is placed evenly and snugly around the upper arm so that its lower edge is about one inch above the point of the brachial artery where the bell of the stethoscope will be applied. While feeling the radial pulse, inflate the cuff until the pressure is about 30 mm above the point where the radial pulse was no longer felt. Deflate the cuff slowly and record as accurately as possible the pressure at which the pulse returns to the radial artery. Systolic blood pressure is determined by this method; diastolic blood pressure cannot be determined by this method.

   Auscultatory method: Begin as above. After inflating the cuff until the pressure is about 30 mm above the point where the radial pulse disappears, place the bell of the stethoscope over the brachial artery just below the blood pressure cuff. Then deflate the cuff slowly, about 2 to 3 mmHg per heartbeat. The first sound heard from the artery is recorded as the systolic pressure. The point at which sounds are no longer heard is recorded as the diastolic pressure. For convenience the blood pressure is recorded as figures separated by a slant. The systolic value is recorded first.

   Ex.: 120/80 indicates systolic pressure of 120 and diastolic of 80.

Sounds heard over the brachial artery change in quality at some point prior to the point the sounds completely disappear. Some physicians consider this the diastolic pressure. This value should be noted when recording the blood pressure by placing it between the systolic pressure and the pressure noted when the sound disappears. Thus, 120/90/80 would indicate a systolic pressure of 120 with a first diastolic sound change at a pressure of 90 and a final diastolic pressure of 80. The latter pressure would be the point of disappearance of all sounds from the artery. When the values are so recorded, the physician may use either of the last two figures as the diastolic pressure. When the change in sound and the disappearance of all sound coincide, the result should be written as follows: 120/80/80.

b.p., mean. Half of the sum of systolic and diastolic values. For a normal person in good health, about 100 mmHg.

b.p., negative. Blood pressure is less than atmospheric pressure as in the great veins near the heart.

b.p., normal. In healthy young persons, 100 to 140 mmHg systolic and 60 to 90 mmHg diastolic. Loss of resilience in the vascular tree and physiological changes of age must be considered when levels above 140 systolic or above 90 diastolic are obtained in apparently healthy older persons.

b.p., systolic. The greatest force caused by the contraction of the left ventricle of the heart.

blood pressure monitor. A device that automatically obtains and usually records the blood pressure at certain intervals. The apparatus may use the direct or indirect method of determining pressure. In some models, an alarm or light signal is activated if the pressure rises or falls to abnormal levels.

blood pressure monitoring, ambulatory. Technique of providing a portable device worn by the patient for automatic inflation and deflation of a blood pressure cuff and recording the blood pressure. The machines may be programmed to obtain readings at frequent or occasional intervals.

bloodshot. Local congestion of the smaller blood vessels of a part, as when the vessels of the conjunctiva are dilated and visible.

blood shunting. A condition in which blood, by going through an abnormal pathway or bypass, does not travel its normal route. May occur when an arteriovenous fistula forms or in congenital anomalies of the heart in which the blood passes from the right atrium or ventricle directly to the left atrium or ventricle respectively, through a defect in the wall (septum) that normally separates the atria and ventricles.

blood smear. Drop of blood spread thin on a slide for purpose of examination.

Procedure: Clean glass with alcohol, rinse in warm water, and wipe clean with lint-free towel or lens paper. Slide must be grease-free. Place a small drop of blood on the slide. Bring the end of another slide (spreader slide) against first slide at a 45° angle and pull it back against drop of blood so that the drop will spread between the point of contact of the two slides. Then push spreader slide forward against the first slide and the blood will form an even smear. The smear must be thin. Dry slide by waving in air. Do not heat.

Stain: A common method is to cover the blood smear with Wright's stain. Allow to stand 2 min. Add an equal amount of distilled water or buffer solution, mixing uniformly. Let stand 5 min. Gently wash off stain. Allow to dry. If permanent slide is desired, apply balsam or methacrylate and apply a glass cover slip.

bloodstream. The blood that flows through the circulatory system of an organism.

blood sugar. Sugar in the form of glucose, normally 60 to 100 mg/100 ml of blood. It rises after a meal to as much as 150 mg/100 ml of blood but this may vary. SEE: *glucose.*

blood test. A test to determine the chemical, physical, or serological characteristics of the blood or some portion of it.

blood transfusion. The replacement of blood or one of its components. Effective and safe transfusion therapy requires a thorough understanding of the clinical condition being treated. This is essential in order to determine whether or not a transfusion of whole blood or one of the blood components is indicated. Also it is contraindicated to add an extra load on the circulation of a patient whose cardiovascular system is already severely compromised. Most patients require blood components rather than whole blood. SEE: *autologous blood transfusion; blood component therapy; blood, transfusion of a single unit; Universal Precautions in Appendix; transfusion, exchange; transfusion reactions.*

NURSING IMPLICATIONS: Identify patient from hospital identification band or blood bank band. Patient's blood type, and the RH and blood type, Rh and compatibility of unit of blood to be administered should be checked by two health care professionals before administration. Check the unit's expiration date and time. If it is outdated, do not use. Retrieve blood from blood bank refrigerator immediately prior to administration. Blood should not be stored in other than blood bank refrigerators, and cannot be returned to blood bank refrigerator storage if its temperature exceeds 50°F (10°C). This will occur within approx. 30 minutes of removal from storage. Check and document patient's vital signs before initiating transfusion. Administer through approved blood filter, preferably piggybacked through physiologic saline solution on a Y set. No other I.V. solutions should be infused with blood because of possible incompatibility. Initiate blood flow rate to limit intake in first 15 minutes to no more than 50 ml, and remain with patient for this time period, assessing for and teaching patient to report any adverse reactions such as back or chest pain, hypotension, increase in temperature of more than 1.8°F (1°C), chills, pain at the infusion site, tachycardia, tachypnea, wheezing, cyanosis, urticaria, or rashes. If any of these should occur, stop the transfusion, keep the vein open with physiologic saline solution, and notify the patient's physician and the blood bank. If incompatibility is suspected, return the blood and set to the blood bank and obtain samples of the patient's blood and urine. If no symptoms occur in the first 15 minutes, increase the transfusion rate to the time ordered or run as fast as the patient's condition permits. Once the transfusion starts, the blood should be administered within 4 hours to maintain its biological effectiveness and limit the risk of bacterial growth. Monitor blood pressure and patient response every 30 minutes throughout the transfusion and 30 minutes afterwards, observing stated precautions. Blood should not be administered through a central line unless an approved in-line warming device is used. A warmer also should be used whenever multiple transfusions place the patient at risk for hypothermia, which can lead to dysrhythmias and cardiac arrest.

   b.t., autologous. SEE: *autologous blood transfusion.*

blood typing. The method used to determine various factors when blood is tested according to blood group systems such as ABO, MN, or Rh-Hr.

blood urea nitrogen. ABBR: BUN. Nitrogen in the blood in the form of urea. The normal concentration is 9 to 25 mg/ml. The level of urea in the blood provides a rough estimate of kidney function. An increase in the blood urea nitrogen level usually indicates decreased renal function.

blood vessels. The veins, arteries, and capillaries.

blood warmer. Device for warming banked blood to body temperature prior to using it for transfusion.

bloody sweat. Excretion of blood or blood pigment through the sweat gland. SYN: *hemathidrosis.*

bloody weeping. Hemorrhage from conjunctiva.

blotch. A blemish, spot, or area of discoloration on the skin.

blotting methods. Various techniques for analyzing a tiny portion of the primary structure of genomic material (DNA or RNA).

   b.m., Northern [name given to distinguish it from Southern blot]. A blot analysis

technique for analyzing a small portion of RNA.

   b.m., Southern [E. M. Southern, contemporary Brit. physician]. A blot analysis technique used in molecular genetics to analyze a very small portion of human genomic material, DNA.

   b.m., Western [name given to distinguish it from Southern blot]. Technique for analyzing protein antigens. SYN: *immunoblotting.*

blowfly. One of a number of genera of flies belonging to the family Calliphoridae. Most are scavengers, their larvae living in decaying flesh or meat although occasionally they may live in decaying or suppurating tissue. However, one species, the screw-worm fly, *Callitroga hominivorax,* attacks living tissue, laying its eggs in the nostrils or open wounds of the host domestic animals or humans, giving rise to myiasis, q.v.

blowpipe. A tube through which a gas or current of air passed under pressure, being directed upon a flame. It is employed to concentrate and intensify the heat of the flame.

BLS. *basic life support.*

blue [O. Fr. *bleu*]. 1. A primary color of the spectrum; sky color; azure. 2. Cyanotic.

blue baby. SEE: *baby, blue.*

bluebottle flies. Flies of the family Calliphoridae. They breed in dung or the flesh of dead animals.

Blue Cross. A nonprofit medical care insurer in the U.S. The insurance is mostly for hospital services. SEE: *Blue Shield.*

Blue Shield. A nonprofit medical care insurer in the U.S. The insurance is for that part of medical care provided by health care professionals. SEE: *Blue Cross.*

Blumberg's sign (blŭm′bĕrgs) [Jacob Moritz Blumberg, Ger. surgeon and gynecologist, 1873–1955]. The occurrence of a sharp acute pain when the examiner presses his or her hand over McBurney's point and then releases the hand pressure suddenly. This sign is indicative of peritoneal inflammation. SYN: *rebound tenderness.*

Blumenbach's clivus (bloo′mĕn-bawks) [Johann F. Blumenbach, Ger. physiologist and anthropologist, 1752–1840]. Sloping part of sphenoid bone behind posterior clinoid processes.

blush [AS. *blyscan,* to be red]. Redness of the face and neck due to vasodilation caused by emotion or heat. Blushing may also be associated with certain diseases, including carcinoid syndrome, pheochromocytoma, and Zollinger-Ellison syndrome.

B lymphocytes. B cells, q.v.

B.M.A. *British Medical Association.*

B-mode (brightness mode) display. In ultrasonography, imaging dots on the screen indicate echoes. The brighter the dot relative to the background, the greater the strength of the echo.

B.M.R. *basal metabolic rate.*

B.M.S. *Bachelor of Medical Science.*

BMT. *bone marrow transplant.*

BNA. *Basle Nomina Anatomica,* an anatomical nomenclature adopted by the German Anatomical Society in 1895, at Basel, Switzerland. It includes some 4500 terms. SEE: *Nomina Anatomica.*

board. 1. A flat, long piece of a substance, such as wood or firm plastic. SEE: *bed board.* 2. A corporate or governmental body, such as a board of directors or a board of health.

    b., back. A stiff board placed on a stretcher so that the patient's back is kept flat. Used when a spinal injury is suspected.

board certification. In medicine this process denotes that an individual practitioner has met standards above and beyond those of admission to licensure and has passed specialty examinations in the field. The various medical professional organizations establish their standards and administer their board certification examinations. Individuals successfully completing all requirements are called Fellows, such as Fellow of the American College of Surgeons (F.A.C.S.) or Fellow of the American College of Physicians (F.A.C.P.). Board certification status may be required by a hospital for admission to the medical staff or to determine the rank of a staff member; e.g., general staff member, associate staff, or full attending status.

board certified. In medicine this designation signifies that a physician has successfully completed the requirements of a particular specialty or subspecialty and has passed the certification examinations administered by the specialty board. By this method, an individual becomes a certified specialist in a particular field of medicine.

board eligible. In medicine the designation in the board certification process which signifies that a physician has completed all of the requirements for admission to the medical specialty board certification examination.

boarder babies. Children who live in hospitals because there is no one available to care for them.

Boas' point (bō'ăz) [Ismar I. Boas, Ger. physician, 1858–1938]. A tender spot left of the 12th dorsal vertebra in patients with gastric ulcer.

Bochdalek's ganglion (bŏk'dăl-ĕks) [Victor Bochdalek, Czech. anatomist, 1801–1883]. Ganglion of plexus of dental nerve in the maxilla above the canine tooth.

bode plot (bōd). A graph used to describe the frequency-gain characteristics of an electronic amplifier.

Bodo (bō'dō). A genus of the Bodonidae, flagellate protozoa often found in stale feces or urine and sometimes in the urinary bladder. Nonpathogenic.

body [AS. *bodig*]. 1. Soma; the physical part of man as distinguished from mind and spirit. 2. The trunk. 3. The principal mass of any structure. 4. The largest or most important part of any organ.

    EXAM: The nude body is examined and both sides are compared. Physical examination is made by inspection, palpation, manipulation, mensuration, auscultation, q.v., and use of the sense of smell. Physical examination should also include observation of the body as the person walks and goes through the various ranges of motions of the trunk, neck, and extremities. Chemical and microscopic examination may be made of the blood, sputum, feces, urine, cerebrospinal fluids, and other fluids of the body. Radiological studies also may be used.

    b., acetone. Ketone bodies. One of a number of substances that increase in the blood as a result of faulty fat metabolism. Among them are β-hydroxybutyric acid, acetoacetic acid, and acetone. They are increased in persons with untreated or inadequately controlled diabetes mellitus and are the primary cause of acidosis. They may also occur in other metabolic disturbances.

    b., amygdaloid. Almond-shaped gray matter in the lateral wall and roof of the third ventricle of the brain.

    b., aortic. One of two small bodies that are located in the arch of the aorta and contain the endings of the aortic nerve. They respond to oxygen concentration in the blood and to changes in blood pressure.

    b., asbestosis. Minute bodies formed by the deposition of various salts and minerals around an asbestos particle. These may be found in the sputum, lung, or feces.

    b.'s, Aschoff. Microscopic foci of fibrinoid degeneration and granulomatous inflammation found in interstitial tissues of the heart in rheumatic fever.

    b., Barr. Sex chromatin mass that represents the genetically inactivated X chromosome found in somatic cells of normal females. SEE: *Barr body.*

    b., basal. Small granule usually present at the base of a flagellum or a cilium in protozoa. SYN: *granule, basal.*

    b., carotid. Flat structure at the bifurcation of the common carotid artery. Contains cells that respond to changes in concentration of oxygen in the blood and to changes in blood pressure, thus aiding in regulating circulation.

    b., chromaffin. One of a number of bodies composed principally of chromaffin cells, q.v., that lie serially arranged along both sides of the dorsal aorta and in the kidney, liver, and gonads. They are ectodermal in origin, having the same origin as cells of the sympathetic ganglia. SYN: *paraganglia*.

b.'s, chromophilous. Large granular bodies in nerve cells, demonstrated by selective staining. SYN: *b.'s, Nissl; granule, Nissl.*

b., ciliary. A structure directly behind the iris of the eye. It secretes the aqueous humor and contains the ciliary muscle that changes the shape, and thus the refractive power, of the lens by tightening and relaxing the tension on the lens. SEE: *eye* for illus.

b., coccygeal. An arteriovenous anastomosis at the tip of the coccyx formed by the middle sacral artery. Also called glomus coccygeum [NA].

b.'s, Donovan. The common name for the causative organism, *Calymmatobacterium granulomatis*, of granuloma inguinale, q.v.

b., foreign. An object present at a site where it would not normally or naturally be present.

b., geniculate, lateral. One of two bodies forming elevations on the lateral portion of the posterior part of the thalamus. Each is the termination of afferent fibers from the retina, which it receives through the optic nerves and tracts.

b., geniculate, medial. One of two bodies lying in the posterior part of the dorsal thalamus. Each receives fibers from the acoustic center of the medulla and from the inferior colliculus through the brachium.

b., Heinz. SEE: *Heinz bodies.*

b., Hensen's. Modified Golgi net found in the hair cells of the organ of Corti.

b., inclusion. Nonliving substances in the protoplasm of a cell. Seen in disease caused by virus infections.

b., ketone. One of a number of substances that increase in the blood as a result of faulty fat metabolism. Among them are β-hydroxybutyric acid, acetoacetic acid, and acetone. They increase in persons with untreated or inadequately controlled diabetes mellitus and are the primary cause of acidosis. They may also occur in other metabolic disturbances.

b.'s, Leishman-Donovan. Small bodies found in the spleen and liver of victims of kala-azar or dum-dum fever. Now known to be *Leishmania donovani,* causative organism of the disease. They are found both within and outside of living cells and in circulating blood.

b., malpighian. 1. Renal corpuscle consisting of a glomerulus enclosed in Bowman's capsule. 2. Lymph nodule found in the spleen.

b., mammillary. Rounded body of gray matter found in the diencephalon. It forms a rounded eminence projecting into the anterior portion of the interpeduncular fossa. Their nuclei constitute an important relay station for olfactory impulses.

b., medullary. The deeper white matter of the cerebellum enclosed within the cortex.

b.'s, Negri. Inclusion bodies found in the cells of the central nervous system of animals infected with rabies. They are acidophilic masses appearing in large ganglion cells or in cells of the brain, esp. those of the hippocampus and cerebellum. Their presence is considered conclusive proof of rabies.

b.'s, Nissl. Large granular bodies in nerve cells, demonstrated by selective staining. They are absent in the axon and axon hillock. They show changes under various physiological conditions and in pathological conditions may dissolve and disappear (chromatolysis). SYN: *b., chromophilous; granules, Nissl.*

b., olivary. Rounded mass located in the anterolateral portion of the medulla oblongata. Consists of a convoluted sheet of gray matter enclosing white matter. SYN: *oliva.*

b., pacchionian. Arachnoid granulation. Numerous small ovoid or villuslike projections of the arachnoid membrane of the brain. They may project into the superior sagittal sinus as arachnoid villi or press against the outer dura and grow into the inner plate of the cranium, forming ovoid depressions. SYN: *arachnoid villi; granulation, arachnoidal.*

b., perineal. Mass of tissue that separates the anus from the vestibule and the lower part of the vagina. SEE: *perineum* for illus.

b., pineal. Glandlike structure in the brain, shaped like a pine cone, and located in a pocket near the splenium of the corpus collosum. It appears to be the major site of melatonin biosynthesis in most mammals and in humans, but the effect of melatonin on the body and the exact function of the pineal body remain unknown. SYN: *pineal gland.*

b., pituitary. The hypophysis; pituitary gland, q.v.

b., polar. Small cell produced in oogenesis resulting from the divisions of the primary and secondary oocytes.

b., postbranchial. One of two bodies that develop from the posterior wall of the 4th pharyngeal pouch. They become incorporated into the thyroid gland. SYN: *ultimobranchial body.*

b., psammoma. Laminated calcareous body seen in certain types of tumors, sometimes associated with chronic inflammation.

b.'s, quadrigeminal. Four rounded projections from the roof of the midbrain. SYN: *colliculus superior et inferior* [NA].

b., restiform. The inferior cerebellar peduncles. Two bands of fibers that connect the medulla with the cerebellum.

b., striate. The corpus striatum, composed of the cordate and lenticular nucleoli of the brain.

b., trachoma. Mass of cells present as an inclusion body in the conjunctival epithelial cells of individuals with trachoma.

b., vertebral. Short column of bone forming the weight-supporting portion of a vertebra. From its dorsolateral surfaces project the roots of the arch of a vertebra.

b., vitreous. Jellylike substance within the eye that fills the space between the lens and the retina. It is colorless, structureless, and transparent. Nevertheless, it may contain minute particles called floaters, q.v.

b., wolffian. Mesonephros or middle kidney of the embryo.

body cavities. The thorax, abdomen, cranium, and pelvis.

body composition. Quantitation of the various components of the body, esp. of the fat, water, protein, and bone mineral. Determination of the specific gravity of the body is done to estimate the percent fat. This may be calculated by various methods, including underwater weighing, which determines the density of the individual; use of radioactive potassium, ^{40}K; measuring the total body water by dilution of tritium; and use of various anthropometric measurements such as height, weight, and skin fold thickness at various sites. None of these methods is free of the potential for error. Underwater weighing is useful but may provide misleading information when used in analyzing body composition of highly trained athletes. The obese person has a lower body density than does the lean person, because the specific gravity of fat tissue is less than that of muscle tissue. The fat content for young men will vary from about 5% to 27% and for women from about 18% to 35%.

body fluids. Total body water in humans varies from 50% of the body weight in obese individuals to 70% in the non-obese. The principal compartments for body fluids are intracellular and extracellular. A much smaller segment, the transcellular, includes fluid in the tracheobronchial tree, the gastrointestinal tract, the bladder, cerebrospinal fluid, and the aqueous humor of the

eye. The chemical composition of fluids in the various compartments is carefully regulated. SEE: *acid-base balance.*

body image. 1. The subjective image or picture people have of their physical appearance based on their own observations and the reaction of others. 2. The conscious and unconscious perception of one's body at any particular time.

body language. The unconscious use of posture, gestures, or other forms of nonverbal expression in communication. SEE: *kinesics.*

body mass index. ABBR: BMI. An index for estimating obesity. The weight in kilograms is divided by the height in meters squared, i.e.,

$$\frac{W}{H^2}$$

It is important to take age into consideration when interpreting these values because a high level in a young person is more likely to indicate obesity than in an old one. SYN: *Quatelet index.* SEE: *obesity; ponderal index.*

Technical definitions specify obesity in adult males as having a BMI of greater than 27.8 kg/m²; and for females, 27.3 kg/m². Being underweight is specified for adult males as having a BMI of less than 20.7 kg/m²; and for females, 19.1 kg/m².

body mechanics. Application of kinesiology to use of the body in daily life activities and to the prevention and correction of problems related to posture and lifting.

body odor. The presence of an unusual odor arising from the skin. This odor is usually unpleasant and may come from any site, including the perineal area, navel, and armpits. Underarm odor is the result of bacterial action on the apocrine sweat glands in the axillae. The malodorous chemicals produced are isomers of 3-methyl-2-hexanoic acid. Because apocrine glands are more plentiful in the axillae of men than in women, men will in general be more malodorous than women. SEE: *halitosis.*

"body packer" syndrome. The ingestion of multiple small packages, usually containing drugs of abuse, for the purpose of transporting them illegally. In cases where the packages contain cocaine, rupture of them has caused death due to the inadvertent overdose.

body rocking. Rhythmic, purposeless body movement seen in individuals, whether adults or infants, who are bored, lonely, mentally subnormal, or disturbed. It is also seen in some blind children.

body section radiography. Radiological examination of specific layers of the body, blurring out overlying and underlying anatomical structures.

body snatching. Robbing a grave of its body. Done in the past to obtain bodies for anatomical study in medical schools.

body surface area. The surface area of the body expressed in square meters. It may be calculated when the height and weight of a subject are known by using a standard formula. Body surface area is an important measure in calculating pediatric dosages, in the management of burn patients, and in determining radiation doses. Nomograms for accurately determining body surface area are available for both pediatric and adult patients. SEE: illus.; *area, body surface; burns; rule of nines.*

body type. Classification of the human body according to muscle and fat distribution. SEE: *ectomorph; endomorph; mesomorph; somatotype.*

Boeck's sarcoid (bĕks) [Caesar P. M. Boeck, Norwegian dermatologist, 1845–1917]. Former name for sarcoidosis, q.v.

Boerhaave syndrome (boor′hă-vĕ) [Hermann Boerhaave, Dutch physician, 1668–1738]. Complete, spontaneous rupture of the esophagus usually associated with violent retching or vomiting. SEE: *Mallory-Weiss syndrome.*

boil [AS. *byl,* a swelling]. A furuncle, an acute circumscribed inflammation of the subcutaneous layers of the skin, gland, or hair follicle. The deeper tissue inflammation is so severe that blood clots in the vessels and forms a "core." This is the cause of the acuteness of the pain; the "core" is ultimately expelled or reabsorbed. Boils are most commonly due to a localized infection with staphylococci.

    TREAT: Protect from irritation; apply moist heat intermittently. Keep skin scrupulously clean and avoid injury or trauma to involved region. Bedrest may be necessary in severe cases. After lesions are fluctuant, surgical incision and drainage may be desirable. The area around draining abscesses should be protected by an antibiotic ointment to prevent new lesions on surrounding areas. If lesions are large and located on the face, an appropriate antibiotic should be used systematically to prevent possible complications such as meningitis or septicemia.

boiling. Process of vaporization of a liquid. Boiling water destroys most microorganisms (but may not kill spores and some viruses); toughens and hardens albumin in eggs; toughens, i.e., denatures, fibrin and dissolves tissues in meat; bursts starch granules; and softens cellulose in cereals and vegetables.

boiling point. The degree of heat required to bring a liquid to a boil, which varies according to the chemicals present in different liquids. Water boils at 212°F (100°C) under ordinary conditions, at sea level. To kill most vegetable forms of microorganisms, water should be boiled 30 minutes. Aeration (pouring from one vessel to another) will overcome the flat taste of boiled water.

bolometer (bō-lŏm′ĕ-tĕr) [Gr. *bole,* a ray, + *metron,* measure]. 1. Device for measuring the force of the heartbeat apart from blood pressure. 2. An instrument for gauging minute degrees of radiant heat.

bolus (bō′lŭs) [L., from Gr. *bolos,* a lump]. 1. A mass of masticated food ready to be swallowed. 2. A rounded preparation of medicine for oral ingestion. 3. A concentrated mass of a diagnostic substance given rapidly intravenously, such as an opaque contrast medium, or an intravenous medication.

    b., alimentary. The mass of masticated food in the esophagus that is ready to be passed into the stomach.

bombesin (bŏm′bĕ-sĭn). A neuropeptide present in the gut and brain tissue of humans. It is also present in the increased concentrations in cell cultures of small cell carcinomas of the lung.

bond. A force that binds ions or atoms together. It is represented by a line drawn from one molecule or atom to another as in H–O–H.

    b., hydrogen. The chemical linkage of hydrogen to other chemicals, esp. nitrogen and oxygen.

bonding. In dentistry, using an adhesive or cement to hold a covering to a stained or damaged tooth. Also used in orthodontic appliances to hold them in place by using an adhesive applied directly to the enamel of teeth.

bonding, male-male or female-female. Nonsexual feeling of love, respect, and communality of individuals for each other. Persons can experience these feelings with dignity and without regard to the societally dictated impression that all such relationships are homosexual.

bonding, mother-infant. The very important emotional and physical attachment, i.e., bond, between infant and mother that is initiated in the first hour or two after normal delivery of a baby who has not been dulled by anesthetic agents or drugs. It is believed that the stronger this bond, the greater the chances of a mentally healthy infant-mother relationship in both the short- and long-term periods following childbirth. Because of this it is further believed that initial contact between mother and infant should be in the delivery room

250

Nomogram for the Assessment of body Surface Area*

Source: Lentner, C (ed): Geigy Scientific Tables, ed 8. Ciba Geigy, Basle, Switzerland, 1981.

*The body surface area is given by the point of intersection with the middle scale of a straight line joining height and weight.

Nomogram for the Assessment of body Surface Area* *(Continued)*

Height

Body surface

Mass

*The body surface area is given by the point of intersection with the middle scale of a straight line joining height and weight.

BONE

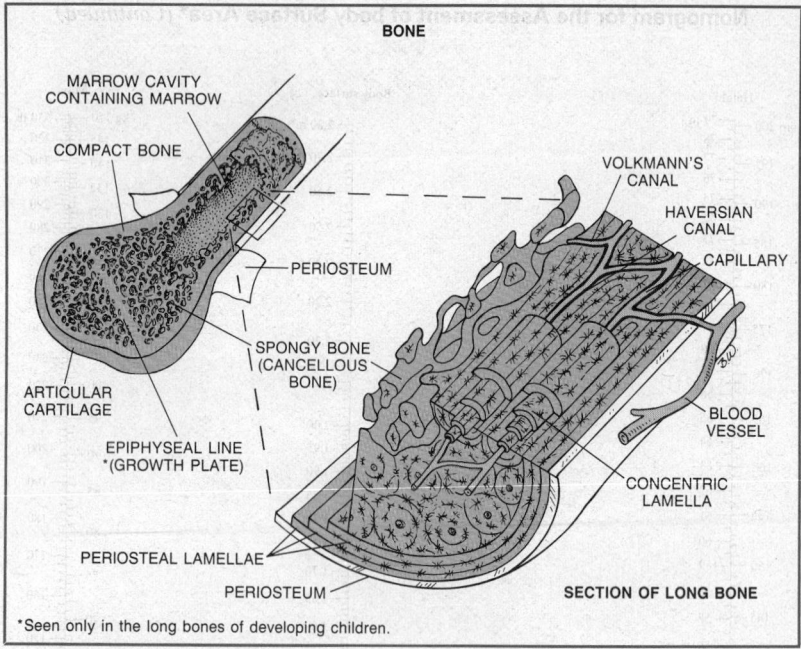

MARROW CAVITY
CONTAINING MARROW

COMPACT BONE

VOLKMANN'S
CANAL

HAVERSIAN
CANAL

CAPILLARY

PERIOSTEUM

SPONGY BONE
(CANCELLOUS
BONE)

ARTICULAR
CARTILAGE

BLOOD
VESSEL

EPIPHYSEAL LINE
*(GROWTH PLATE)

CONCENTRIC
LAMELLA

PERIOSTEAL LAMELLAE

PERIOSTEUM   SECTION OF LONG BONE

*Seen only in the long bones of developing children.

and that this contact should be for as long as possible in the first hours after birth.

bone [AS. *ban*, bone]. 1. Osseous tissue, a specialized form of dense connective tissue consisting of bone cells (osteocytes) embedded in a matrix made up of calcified intercellular substance. SEE: illus. (*Bone*). 2. An individual unit of the skeleton. SYN: *os.* SEE: illus. (*Relationship of Bones to Abdominal and Pelvic Areas*); *cell* for illus.

Bones provide shape and support for the body of vertebrates. They also serve as storage sites for mineral salts, and play an important role in providing in the marrow a site for the formation of blood cells. Bone consists of about 50% water and 50% solid matter, the solids being chiefly cartilage hardened by impregnation with inorganic salts, esp. carbonate and phosphate of lime. In old age there is a tendency for bones to become osteoporotic and to break easily. This condition is esp. likely to develop in women. They surround and protect some vital organs, and give points of attachment for the muscles, serving as levers and making movement possible. The outer surface is less porous than the inner and is called the compact tissue; the more porous portion is

called cancellous tissue. The compact tissue is tunneled by a central canal containing marrow and fine branching canals. Small blood vessels and lymphatics for the maintenance and repair of bone tissue run in these canals. This is known as the haversian system. The exterior covering of the bone, or periosteum, serves to extend the blood supply to the bone. According to their shape, bones are classified as flat, irregular, long, and short. SEE: *osteoporosis.*

For depressions, openings, and cavities in bones: SEE: *antrum* (nearly enclosed cavity); *canal; fissure* (slitlike opening); *foramen* (opening for blood vessels and nerves); *fossa* (concavity); *groove; meatus* (tubelike passage or opening; canal); *sinus* (air cavity within a bone; or groove lodging a blood sinus); *sulcus* (groove).

For processes (enlargements or protrusions) of bones: SEE: *crest* (a ridge); *condyle* (rounded process for articulation); *head* (rounded end of a bone separated from body by a constricted region, the neck); *spine* (pointed process); *trochanter* (very large process); *tubercle* (small rounded process); *tuberosity* (large rounded process). SEE: *osteoporosis.*

RELATIONSHIP OF BONES TO ABDOMINAL AND PELVIC AREAS

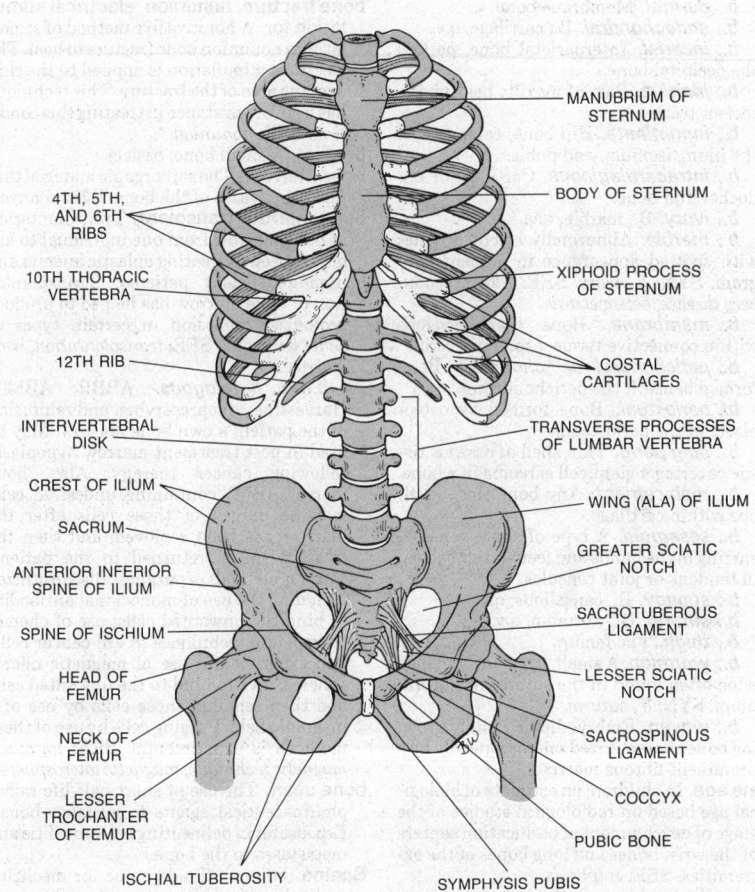

MANUBRIUM OF STERNUM

BODY OF STERNUM

XIPHOID PROCESS OF STERNUM

COSTAL CARTILAGES

TRANSVERSE PROCESSES OF LUMBAR VERTEBRA

WING (ALA) OF ILIUM

GREATER SCIATIC NOTCH

SACROTUBEROUS LIGAMENT

LESSER SCIATIC NOTCH

SACROSPINOUS LIGAMENT

COCCYX

PUBIC BONE

SYMPHYSIS PUBIS

4TH, 5TH, AND 6TH RIBS

10TH THORACIC VERTEBRA

12TH RIB

INTERVERTEBRAL DISK

CREST OF ILIUM

SACRUM

ANTERIOR INFERIOR SPINE OF ILIUM

SPINE OF ISCHIUM

HEAD OF FEMUR

NECK OF FEMUR

LESSER TROCHANTER OF FEMUR

ISCHIAL TUBEROSITY

For names of principal bones: SEE: *skeleton*.

b., alveolar. The bony tissue or process of the maxilla or mandible that supports the teeth.

b., ankle. The astragalus or talus, q.v.

b., breast. The sternum, q.v.

b., brittle. Abnormal brittleness of bones.

b., cancellous. A spongy bone in which the matrix forms connecting bars and plates, partially enclosing many intercommunicating spaces filled with bone marrow.

b., cartilage. Endochondral bone that develops from cartilage.

b., cavalry. Localized bony formation in adductor magnus femoris, sometimes seen in horseback riders. SYN: *riders' bone*.

b., collar. The clavicle.

b., compact. Dense hard bone with microscopic spaces.

b., cotyloid. Bone that during development forms a part of medial portion of the acetabulum. It fuses with the pubis.

b., cranial. Bone of the cranium or brain case.

b., dermal. Membrane bone.

b., endochondral. B., cartilage, q.v.

b., incarial. Interparietal bone, part of the occipital bone.

b., incisive. Part of maxilla bearing the incisor teeth.

b., innominate. Hip bone, composed of the ilium, ischium, and pubis.

b., intracartilaginous. Cartilage or endochondral bone.

b., ivory. B., marble, q.v.

b., marble. Abnormally calcified bones with spotted appearance in a roentgenogram. SYN: *b., ivory.* SEE: *Albers-Schönberg disease; osteopetrosis.*

b., membrane. Bone that develops within connective tissue, esp. in the skin.

b., perichondral or -chondrial. Bone formed beneath the perichondrium.

b., periosteal. Bone formed by osteoblasts of the periosteum.

b., ping pong. Thin shell of osseous tissue covering a giant cell sarcoma in a bone.

b., replacement. Any bone that develops within cartilage.

b., sesamoid. A type of short bone occurring in the hands and feet and embedded in tendons or joint capsules.

b., spongy. B., cancellous, q.v.

b., sutural. B., wormian, q.v.

b., thigh. The femur.

b., wormian. A small, irregularly shaped bone often found in the sutures of the cranium. SYN: *b., sutural.*

b., woven. Embryonic or rapidly growing bone characterized microscopically by a prominent fibrous matrix.

bone age. In children, an estimate of biological age based on radiological studies of the stage of development of ossification centers of the wrist bones and long bones of the extremities. SEE: *epiphysis.*

bone cell. A nucleated cell occupying a separate lacuna of bone. SEE: *osteoblast; osteoclast; osteocyte.*

bone cyst. A cystic bone tumor.

bone densitometry. Method of determining the density of bone by use of radiographic techniques. The use of dual photon absorptiometry will provide density data of the axial skeleton with a precision of 2% to 3%. Used in testing for degree of osteoporosis. SEE: *absorptiometry, dual photon.*

bone graft. A piece of bone taken from the pa-

tient that is used to take the place of a removed bone or a bony defect at another site. SEE: *graft; prosthesis.*

bone implant. The use of implanted materials to repair bone or to cover implanted objects such as artificial hips or tooth implants.

bone fracture, nonunion. SEE: *nonunion.*

bone fracture, nonunion, electrical stimulation for. A noninvasive method of stimulating a nonunion bone fracture to heal. The electrical stimulation is applied to the skin over the area of the fracture. This technique has been of assistance in treating this condition. SEE: *nonunion.*

bonelet. A small bone; ossicle.

bone marrow. The soft organic material that fills the cavities of the bone. SEE: *marrow.*

bone marrow transplant. Transplantation of bone marrow from one individual to another. Used in treating aplastic anemia and immunodeficient patients. Transplantation of bone marrow has helped to produce prolonged remission in certain types of acute leukemia. SEE: *transplantation, bone marrow.*

b.m.t., autologous. ABBR: ABMT. Harvesting, cryopreserving, and reinfusion of the patient's own bone marrow. May be used in post treatment marrow hypoplasia following cancer therapy. Also, bone marrow (BM) containing undesired cells may be purged of those cells after the marrow has been removed; and then the treated BM is returned to the patient. Various methods of purging cells are utilized including the use of monoclonal antibodies to bind the unwanted cells; use of chemotherapeutic techniques to kill cancer cells; and experimental use of magnetic microspheres, q.v., to bind to the unwanted cells and then separate those cells by use of a magnetic field. Purging cells by use of these methods is experimental. SEE: *immunomagnetic technique; magnetic microspheres.*

bone scan. The use of short half-life radiopharmaceutical agents to visualize bones. Esp. useful in delineating osteomyelitis and metastases to the bone.

Bonine (bō'nēn). Trade name for meclizine hydrochloride, USP, an agent used for prevention and treatment of motion sickness and vomiting.

bony. Resembling or of the nature of bone. SYN: *osseous.*

booster (boo'stĕr). An additional dose of an immunizing agent to increase the protection afforded by the original series of injections. The booster is given some months or years after the initial immunization.

boot. A special shoe or bandage for covering the foot, ankle, and lower leg.

borate (bō′rāt). Any basic salt of boric acid.
SEE: *Poisons and Poisoning* in *Appendix*.

borated. Anything to which borax has been added.

borax (bor′ăks) [L., from Arabic, from Persian *burah*]. Sodium borate. Its chief use is as a detergent and water softener; also a weak antiseptic.

borborygmus (bor″bō-rĭg′mŭs) [Gr. *borborygmos*, rumbling in the bowels] (pl. *borborygmi*). A gurgling, splashing sound normally heard over the large intestine; caused by passage of gas through the liquid contents of the intestine.

PATH: Its absence may indicate paralytic ileus, or obstruction of the bowels due to torsion, volvulus, or strangulated hernia.

border (bor′dĕr). The outer part or edge; boundary.

b., brush. A brushlike structure found on the free surface of epithelial cells in the proximal convoluted portion of a renal tubule. The microvilli that form the border greatly increase the exposed surface area of the cell.

b., striated. A modified layer of the surface protoplasm of columnar epithelial cells lining the intestine. It consists of regular, perpendicular striations containing minute protoplasmic processes.

b., vermilion. The red boundary of the lips which represents the highly vascular, hyalinized, keratinized epithelial covering between the outer skin and the moist oral mucosa of the mouth.

borderline. An incomplete state, as in a borderline diagnosis, in a patient who has some of the requirements for a definite diagnosis but not enough for certainty; a condition judged numerically, e.g., high blood pressure, in which the value is close to a hypertensive level but not at a level to be clearly a case of hypertension.

borderline personality. SEE: *personality, borderline.*

Bordetella (bor″dĕ-tĕl′lă) [Jules Bordet, Belg. physician, bacteriologist, and physiologist, 1870–1961]. A genus of Brucellaceae bacteria that are hemolytic gram-negative coccobacilli. Some species are parasitic and pathogenic in warm-blooded animals, including humans.

B. pertussis. The causative agent of whooping cough. First isolated by Bordet and Gengou. Formerly called *Haemophilus pertussis.*

boredom. Feeling of tiredness or depression because of lack of activity or challenging and meaningful stimuli.

boric acid. H_3BO_3. An odorless white crystalline powder containing boron, it is obtained by condensation and evaporation from certain mineral salts. It is used as a mild antiseptic solution, esp. for the eyes, mouth, and bladder.

boric acid poisoning. Boric acid is highly poisonous when taken internally.

SYM: Nausea, vomiting, diarrhea, convulsions, central nervous system depression, livid skin rash, shock.

TREAT: Induce vomiting with ipecac administration; wash out stomach. Give saline cathartic and large volumes of water. Dialysis may be required if poisoning is severe. SEE: *Poisons and Poisoning* in *Appendix*.

borism. Symptoms caused by internal use of borax or boron compounds. Includes dry skin, eruptions, and gastric disturbances.

Bornholm disease (born′hōm) [named for the Danish island Bornholm]. An epidemic disease caused by coxsackie B virus. Characterized by sudden onset of pain in chest and fever. SYN: *pleurodynia, epidemic.*

boroglycerin (bor″ō-glĭs′ĕr-ĭn). $C_3H_5BO_3$. A compound formed when boric acid and glycerin are heated together.

boroglycerol (bor″ō-glĭs′ĕr-ŏl). Boroglycerin, q.v.

boron [*borax* + carb*on*]. SYMB: B. At. wt. 10.81; at. no. 5. A nonmetallic element, found only as a compound such as boric acid or borax, q.v.

Borrelia (bor-rē′lē-ă). A genus of spirochetes, some of which are causative agents for relapsing fevers and Lyme disease in humans. Though classed as bacteria, spirochetes are quite different in their physical appearance from most bacteria in that they have a spiral shape.

B. burgdorferi. The cause of Lyme disease, q.v.

B. duttonii. Causative agent for tickborne relapsing fever in Central and South America.

B. recurrentis. Causative agent of louseborne relapsing fever.

borreliosis. Any of several diseases, all of which are arthropod-borne, caused by Borrelia, q.v.

boss [O. Fr. *boce*, a swelling]. A round circumscribed swelling or growth. Thus a boss is present when a tumor becomes large enough to produce swelling.

bosselated (bŏs′ĕ-lāt-ĕd). Marked by numerous bosses.

bossing. Prominence of the forehead.

Boston arm. A type of prosthesis for persons who have had an arm amputated above the elbow. The arm, which operates by means of a small battery-driven motor, obeys signals received from electric energy produced by movement of the remaining muscle groups. This allows control of elbow function with respect to direction and strength of motion.

Boston brace. A low-profile plastic thoraco-lumbosacral orthosis (spinal jacket) with no metal suprastructure, used to treat mild to moderate lower thoracic and lumbar scoliosis.

Botallo's duct (bō-tăl′ŏz) [Leonardo Botallo, It. anatomist, 1530–1600]. Ductus arteriosus, q.v.

botany (bŏt′n-ē) [Gr. *botanikos,* pertaining to plants]. The study of plants; a division of biology.

botfly (bŏt′flī) (pl. *botflies*). Insect belonging to the order Diptera of the family Oestridae. Parasitic to mammals, esp. horses and sheep. Human infestation is rare.

botryoid (bŏt′rē-oyd) [Gr. *botrys,* bunch of grapes, + *eidos,* form, shape]. Resembling a bunch of grapes. SYN: *staphyline.*

botuliform (bŏt-ū′lĭ-form) [L. *botulus,* sausage, + *forma,* shape]. Shaped like a sausage.

botulin (bŏt′chū-lĭn). The neurotoxin responsible for botulism, q.v. It is not destroyed by the action of gastric or intestinal secretions.

botulinic acid. A toxin found in putrid sausage.

botulism (bŏt′ū-lĭzm) [″ + Gr. *-ismos,* condition]. A severe form of food poisoning from food containing the botulinus toxins A, B, C, D, E, F, and G, produced by *Clostridium botulinum.* This organism is found in the soil and in the intestinal tract of domestic animals. Cases of human botulism are usually associated with development of the bacteria under anaerobic conditions in raw, improperly canned or otherwise preserved foods, esp. meats (as ham and sausage) and nonacid vegetables (as string beans). The toxin is a powerful exotoxin. It is thermolabile, losing its toxic properties when exposed to temperature of 80°C (176°F) for 30 minutes or boiling at 100°C (212°F) for 10 minutes. The toxin has a selective action on the central nervous system. In fatal cases, cardiac and respiratory paralysis occur through involvement of the medullary centers. The fatality rate in the United States is 20% to 35%.

Botulinum toxin A has been used in treating dysphasias, stuttering, strabismus, and blepharospasm, q.v.

SYM: Fatigue, weakness, dizziness, blurred or double vision, headache, and digestive complaints, as nausea, vomiting, diarrhea, and abdominal pain. Progresses to paralysis of the central nervous system and of the cardiac and respiratory systems.

TREAT: It is important to administer trivalent (ABE) antitoxin as soon as the condition is suspected and prior to the onset of neurological symptoms. The antitoxin is available from the state or local health department or the Bacterial Diseases Division, Centers for Disease Control, Atlanta, GA 30333, (404) 639-3670 during the day or (404) 639-2888 at night. Do not withhold treatment while waiting for results of laboratory tests. SEE: *botulinum toxin* in *Poisons and Poisoning* in *Appendix.*

b., infant. An infectious form of botulism first recognized in 1976. Most cases occur in infants less than one year of age.

SYM: Constipation, lethargy, listlessness, poor feeding, ptosis, loss of head control, difficulty in swallowing, hypotonia, generalized weakness, and respiratory insufficiency.

The disease may be mild or severe. It is thought to cause 5% of the cases of sudden infant death syndrome (SIDS).

TREAT: Careful supportive care.

Bouchut's respiration (boo-shooz′) [Jean A. E. Bouchut, Fr. physician, 1818–1891]. Respiration in which expiration is longer than inspiration, seen in children with bronchopneumonia and asthma.

Bouchut's tubes. A set of tubes used for intubation of the larynx.

bougie (boo′zhē) [Fr. *bougie,* candle]. A slender, flexible instrument for exploring and dilating tubal organs, esp. the male urethra.

bouillon (boo-, bool-yŏn′) [Fr.]. Clear broth made from meat. Used in foods and as a culture medium for bacteria.

bound. 1. In chemistry, the holding in combination of one molecule by another. SEE: *bind,* def. 2. 2. Contained, not free.

bouquet (boo-kā′) [Fr., nosegay]. A cluster or bunch of structures, esp. of blood vessels.

bourdonnement (boor-dōn-mŏn′) [Fr.]. A humming sound; tinnitus.

boutonnière (boo-tŏn-yār′) [Fr., buttonhole]. 1. Incision through perineum behind an impervious stricture. 2. Buttonhole-like opening in a membrane.

boutonnière deformity. Contractures of hand musculature characterized by proximal interphalangeal joint flexion and distal interphalangeal joint hyperextension.

boutons terminaux (boo-tŏn′ tĕr-mĭ-nō′) [Fr., terminal buttons]. Bulblike expansions at the tips of axons that come into synaptic contact with the cell bodies of other neurons.

bovine (bō′vīn) [L. *bovinus*]. Pert. to cattle.

bovine somatotropin A. An experimental growth hormone used to increase milk production in cows.

bowel [O. Fr. *boel,* intestine]. The intestine.

bowel movement. Evacuation of feces. Number of bowel movements varies in normal individuals, some having a movement after each meal, others one in the morning and one at night, and still others only one in several days. Thus, to say that the healthy person must have at least one bowel movement a day in order to maintain health is unreasonable and not based on factual evidence. SYN: *defecation; flatus.*

Caution: Persistent change in bowel habits may be a sign of a malignant growth in the gastrointestinal tract and for that reason should be investigated thoroughly.

NURSING IMPLICATIONS: Obtain history of patient's usual bowel habits and document any change. Ask patient about and inspect stool for color, characteristics, odor, shape, consistency, and the presence of any unusual coatings or contents (mucus, blood, fat). Provide privacy for patient to move bowels, simulating usual situation as closely as possible. Ventilate area or use deodorant spray after bowel movement to limit patient's embarrassment and reduce discomfort of other patients sharing area. Burning several matches in the area will help to remove malodors. Teach patient about the importance of screening stool for occult blood, and about use of diet and activity to help prevent constipation.

bowleg (bō'lĕg). A bending outward of the lower limb. SYN: *bandy leg; genu varum.* SEE: *rickets.*

Bowman's capsule (bō'mǎns) [Sir William Bowman, Brit. physician, 1816–1892]. The renal or malpighian corpuscle. It consists of a visceral layer closely applied to the glomerulus and an outer parietal layer. It functions as a filter in the formation of urine. SEE: *kidney* for illus.

Bowman's glands. The olfactory glands. Branched tubuloalveolar glands located in the lamina propria of the olfactory membrane. The glands produce mucus that keeps the olfactory surface moist.

Bowman's membrane. Thin homogeneous membrane separating corneal epithelium from corneal substance. SYN: *lamina, anterior elastic.*

box. A container or receptacle. It may be made of almost any material. SEE: *snuffbox, anatomical.*

boxing. In dentistry, the building up of vertical walls, usually in wax, around the impression to produce the desired size and form of the base of the cast, and to preserve certain landmarks of the impression.

box-note. In emphysema, a hollow sound heard on percussion.

box splint. Splint for fractures below the knee.

Boyer's bursa (bwă-yāz') [Baron Alexis de Boyer, Fr. surgeon, 1757–1833]. A bursa

anterior to the thyrohyoid membrane.

Boyer's cyst. A painless and gradual enlargement of the subhyoid bursa.

Boyle's law [Robert Boyle, Brit. physicist, 1627–1691]. Law stating that at a constant temperature, the volume of a gas varies inversely with the pressure. SEE: *Charles' law; Gay-Lussac's law.*

Bozeman-Fritsch catheter (bŏz'mǎn-frĭtch) [Nathan Bozeman, U.S. surgeon, 1825–1905; and Heinrich Fritsch, Ger. gynecologist, 1844–1915]. Double-lumen uterine catheter with several openings at tip.

B.P. *blood pressure; British Pharmacopoeia.*

b.p. *boiling point.*

BPD. *biparietal diameter; bronchopulmonary dysplasia.*

BPH. *benign prostatic hypertrophy.*

Bq. *becquerel.*

Br. 1. *Brucella.* 2. Chem. symb. for the element bromine.

brace (brās). 1. Any one of a great variety of devices, used in orthopedics, for holding joints or limbs in place. 2. Colloquial term for temporary dental prostheses used to align or reposition teeth.

brachia (brā'kē-ă). Pl. of brachium.

brachial (brā'kē-ăl) [L. *brachialis*]. Pert. to the arm.

brachial artery. Main artery of arm. Continuation of the axillary artery on the inside of the arm. SEE: illus.

brachialgia (brā″kē-ăl'jē-ă) [L. *brachialis,* brachial, + Gr. *algos,* pain]. Intense pain in the arm.

brachialis (brā″kē-ăl'ĭs) [L. *brachialis,* brachial]. A muscle of the arm lying immediately under the biceps brachii.

brachial plexus. Network of lower cervical and upper dorsal spinal nerves supplying the arm, forearm, and hand. SEE: *Nerve Plexuses* in *Appendix.*

brachial veins. The veins that accompany the brachial artery.

brachiocephalic (brā″kē-ō-sĕ-făl'ĭk) [L. *brachium,* arm, + Gr. *kephale,* head]. Pert. to the arm and head.

brachiocrural (brā″kē-ō-kroo'răl) [″ + *cruralis,* pert. to the leg]. Pert. to the arm and thigh.

brachiocubital (brā″kē-ō-kū'bĭ-tăl) [″ + *cubitus,* forearm]. Pert. to the arm and forearm.

brachiocyllosis (brā″kē-ō-sĭl-ō'sĭs) [″ + Gr. *kyllosis,* a crooking]. Abnormal curvature of the arm.

brachioradialis (brā″kē-ō-rā″dē-ă'lĭs) [″ + *radialis,* radius]. A muscle lying on the lateral side of the forearm. SEE: *Muscles* in *Appendix.*

brachium (brā'kē-ŭm) [L., arm, from Gr.

BRACHIAL ARTERY

AXILLARY ARTERY

ANTERIOR HUMERAL
CIRCUMFLEX ARTERY

POSTERIOR HUMERAL
CIRCUMFLEX ARTERY

PROFUNDA BRACHIAL ARTERY
(POSTERIOR BRANCH)
(ANTERIOR BRANCH)

ULNAR
ARTERY

BRACHIAL
ARTERY

SUPRATROCHLEAR
ARTERY

RADIAL ARTERY

ULNAR ARTERY

COMMON INTEROSSEOUS
ARTERY

DEEP PALMAR ARCH

SUPERFICIAL PALMAR ARCH

METACARPAL ARTERY

DIGITAL ARTERY

RIGHT ANTERIOR ARM

brakhion, shorter, hence "upper arm" as opposed to longer forearm] (pl. *brachia*). [NA] 1. The upper arm from shoulder to elbow. 2. Anatomical structure resembling an arm.

    b. conjunctivum. The superior cerebellar peduncle. SEE: *peduncle, cerebellar, superior.*

    b. pontis. The middle cerebellar peduncle. SEE: *peduncle, cerebellar, middle.*

brachy- [Gr. *brachys*, short]. Prefix for short.

brachybasia (brăk-ē-bā′sē-ă) [″ + *basis*, walking]. A slow shuffling gait seen in partial paraplegia. SEE: *gait.*

brachycardia (brăk-ē-kăr′dē-ă) [″ + *kardia*, heart]. Slowness of heart action. SYN: *bradycardia.*

brachycephalic, brachycephalous (brăk″ē-sĕ-făl′ĭk, -sĕf′ă-lŭs) [″ + *kephale*, head]. Having a cephalic index of 81.0 to 85.4. This is considered to be a short head, but is not necessarily abnormal, as this index falls within the standard range of variation among humans.

brachycheilia (brăk″ē-kī′lē-ă) [″ + *cheilos*, lip]. Condition of having abnormally short lip or lips.

brachydactylia (brăk″ē-dăk-tĭl′ē-ă) [″ + *daktylos*, finger]. Abnormal shortness of the fingers and toes.

brachygnathia (brăk-ĭg-nā′thē-ă) [″ + *gnathos*, jaw]. Abnormal shortness of the lower jaw.

brachymetropia (brăk″ē-mĕ-trō′pē-ă) [″ + *metron*, measure, + *opsis*, sight]. Myopia; nearsightedness.

brachymorphic (brăk″ē-mor′fĭk) [″ + *morphe*, form]. Shorter and broader than usual, with reference to body type.

brachyphalangia (brăk″ē-fă-lăn′jē-ă) [″ + *phalanx*, closely knit row]. Shortness of a bone or bones of a finger or toe.

brachystasis (brā-kĭs′tă-sĭs) [″ + *stasis*, standstill]. Condition in which a muscle does not relax upon contracting but maintains its shortened state.

brachytherapy (brăk″ē-thĕr′ă-pē) [″ + *therapeia*, treatment]. In radiation therapy, the use of implants of radioactive materials such as radium, cesium, iridium, or gold at the site. It is in contrast to teletherapy.

bracket. A support of wood, metal, or some durable material. In dentistry, a variety of specific brackets used in orthodontic appliances.

Bradford frame [Edward H. Bradford, U.S. orthopedic surgeon, 1848–1926]. An oblong frame, about 7 × 3 feet (2.13 × 0.91 meters), made of 1 in. (2.5 cm) pipe covered with canvas strips that run from one side of the frame to the other and are movable. Used for patients with fractures or disease of the hip or spine, thus permitting the patient to uri-

nate and defecate without moving the spine or changing position.

brady- [Gr. *bradys*, slow]. Prefix indicating slow.

bradyacusia (brăd″ē-ă-koo′sē-ă) [″ + *akouein*, to hear]. Abnormally low hearing acuity.

bradyarrhythmia (brăd″ē-ă-rĭth′mē-ă) [″ + *a-*, not, + *rhythmos*, rhythm]. Slow and irregular heartrate.

bradycardia (brăd″ē-kăr′dē-ă) [″ + *kardia*, heart]. A slow heartbeat characterized by a pulse rate that is under 60 beats per minute. SEE: *arrhythmia; tachycardia.*

    b., sinus. A slow sinus rhythm with an atrial rate below 60 beats per minute in an adult, 70 beats per minute in a child, or 100 beats per minute in a fetus.

bradycrotic (brăd″ē-krŏt′ĭk) [″ + *krotos*, pulsation]. Pert. to slowness of pulse.

bradydiastole (brăd″ē-dī-ăs′tō-lē) [″ + *diastole*, dilatation]. Prolongation of the diastolic pause, as in myocardial lesions.

bradyecoia (brăd″ē-ē-koy′ă) [Gr. *bradyekoos*, slow to hear]. Partial deafness.

bradyesthesia (brăd″ē-ĕs-thē′zē-ă) [″ + *aisthesis*, sensation]. Slowness of perception.

bradyglossia (brăd″ē-glŏs′ē-ă) [″ + *glossa*, tongue]. Abnormal slowness of speech. SYN: *bradylalia; bradyphrasia.*

bradykinesia (brăd″ē-kĭ-nē′sē-ă) [″ + *kinesis*, movement]. Extreme slowness of movement.

bradykinin (brăd″ē-kī′nĭn). A plasma kinin. SEE: *kinin.*

bradylalia (brăd″ē-lā′lē-ă) [″ + *lalein*, to talk]. Slowness of speech. SYN: *bradyglossia; bradyphrasia.* SEE: *speech.*

bradylexia (brăd″ē-lĕks′ē-ă) [Gr. *bradys*, slow, + *lexis*, word]. Abnormal slowness of reading not attributable to lack of intelligence. SEE: *dyslexia.*

bradylogia (brăd″ē-lō′jē-ă) [″ + *logos*, word, reason]. Slow speech due to mental impairment.

bradyphagia (brăd″ē-fā′jē-ă) [″ + *phagein*, to eat]. Abnormal slowness in eating.

bradyphrasia (brăd″ē-frā′zē-ă) [″ + *phrasis*, utterance]. Slowness of speech; seen in some types of mental disease.

bradyphrenia [″ + Gr. *phren*, mind]. Decreased speed of thought and information processing. Seen in some forms of dementia.

bradypnea (brăd″ĭp-nē′ă, brăd″ĭ-nē′ă) [″ + *pnoe*, breathing]. Abnormally slow breathing.

bradyrhythmia (brăd″ē-rĭth′mē-ă) [″ + *rhythmos*, rhythm]. 1. Slowness of heart or pulse rate. 2. In electroencephalography, slowness of brain waves (1 to 6 per sec).

bradyspermatism (brăd-ē-spĕr′mă-tĭzm) [″

+ *sperma*, semen + *-ismos*, condition]. Abnormally slow ejaculation of semen.

bradysphygmia (brăd″ē-sfĭg′mē-ă) [″ + *sphygmos*, pulse]. Abnormally slow pulse.

bradystalsis (brăd″ē-stăl′sĭs) [″ + *stalsis*, constriction]. Abnormal slowness of peristalsis.

bradytachycardia (brăd″ē-tăk″ē-kăr′dē-ă) [″ + *tachys*, swift, + *kardia*, heart]. Increased heart rate alternating with slow rate. SEE: *sick sinus syndrome*.

bradyteleokinesis [″ + Gr. *telein*, complete, + *kinesis*, movement]. The cessation or slowing of a movement prior to completing its intended action.

bradyuria (brăd″ē-ū′rē-ă) [″ + *ouron*, urine]. Slowness in passing urine.

braille (brāl) [Louis Braille, blind Fr. educator, 1809–1852]. A system of reading and writing that enables the blind to see by using their sense of touch. Raised dots, which represent numerals and letters of the alphabet, can be identified by the fingers. SEE: *Optacon; Braille Alphabet* in *Appendix*.

brain (brān) [AS. *braegen*]. A large soft mass of nerve tissue contained within the cranium. Cranial portion of the central nervous system. SYN: *encephalon*.

ANAT: The brain is composed of neurons (nerve cells) and neuroglia or supporting cells. The brain consists of gray and white matter. Gray matter is composed principally of nerve cell bodies and is concentrated in the cerebral cortex and the nuclei and basal ganglia. White matter is composed of nerve cell processes, which form tracts connecting various parts of the brain with each other.

The brain consists of five parts: the cerebrum, cerebellum, pons varolii, medulla oblongata, and midbrain. The weight of the brain and spinal cord is about 1350 to 1400 gm, of which 2% is the cord. The cerebrum represents about 85% of the weight of the brain. *Lobes:* Frontal, parietal, occipital, temporal, insular. *Glands:* Pituitary, pineal. *Membranes:* Meninges, consisting of the dura mater (external), arachnoid (middle), and pia mater (internal). *Nerves:* Cranial. SEE: illus. (*Brain*); *Cranial Nerves* in *Appendix; cranial nerves* for illus.

Subdivisions of the brain are (1) diencephalon, q.v., including the epithalamus, thalamus, and hypothalamus (optic chiasma, hypophysis, tuber cinereum, and maxillary bodies); (2) myelencephalon, q.v., including the corpora quadrigemina, tegmentum, crura cerebri, and the medulla oblongata; (3) metencephalon, q.v., including the cerebellum and pons; (4) telencephalon, q.v., including the rhinencephalon, corpora striata, and cerebrum (cerebral cortex).

Ventricles: The cavities of the brain are the first and second lateral ventricles, which lie in the cerebral hemispheres, the third ventricle of the diencephalon, and the fourth ventricle of the medulla. The first and second communicate with the third by the interventricular foramina, the third with the fourth by the cerebral canal (aqueduct of Sylvius), the fourth with the subarachnoid spaces by the two foramina of Luschka and the foramen of Magendie. The ventricles are filled with cerebrospinal fluid, which is formed by the choroid plexuses in the walls and roofs of the ventricles. SEE: illus. (*Vascular Anatomy of Brain*).

PHYS: The brain is the primary center for regulating and coordinating body activities. Sensory impulses are received through afferent nerves; these register as sensations, which are the basis for perception. It is the seat of consciousness, thought, memory, reason, judgment, and emotion. Motor impulses are discharged through efferent nerves to muscles and glands initiating activities. Through reflex centers automatic control of body activities is maintained. The most important reflex centers are the cardiac, vasomotor, and respiratory centers, which regulate circulation and respiration. SEE: *central nervous system; spinal cord.*

brain death. Cessation of brain function. Criteria for concluding that the brain has died include lack of response to stimuli; absence of all reflexes; absent respirations; isoelectric electroencephalogram for at least 30 minutes that will not change in response to sound or pain stimuli. The patient may be kept alive by life-support devices, but death is the inevitable outcome.

Caution: Some drugs, including barbiturates, methaqualone, diazepam, mecloqualone, meprobamate, and trichloroethylene can produce short periods of isoelectric encephalograms. It is important to exclude hypothermia as the cause of apparent brain death.

---

brain edema. An increase in brain volume due to an increase in its water content. It is caused by a variety of conditions but the mechanisms are several, including increased permeability of brain capillary endothelial cells; swelling of brain cells associated with hypoxia or water intoxication; and interstitial edema resulting from obstructive hydrocephalus. SYN: *brain swelling.*

brain fever. Meningitis.

brain graft. An experimental technique of transplanting brain cells into the brain. This type of therapy has promise, but is used only experimentally.

BRAIN

LATERAL ASPECT

PARIETAL LOBE

OCCIPITAL LOBE

FRONTAL LOBE

TEMPORAL LOBE

CEREBELLUM

PONS

MEDULLA OBLONGATA

SPINAL CORD

MENINGES

VENOUS SINUS OF DURA MATER

BONE OF SKULL

ARACHNOIDAL GRANULATION

DURA MATER

ARACHNOID

SUBARACHNOID SPACE

BLOOD VESSELS

PIA MATER

NEUROGLIAL MEMBRANE SEPARATING THE BLOOD VESSELS FROM THEIR PIAL SHEATH

CEREBRAL CORTEX

PIAL SHEATHS SURROUNDING CEREBRAL VESSELS

SUPERIOR SAGITTAL SINUS

CEREBRUM

ARACHNOIDAL GRANULATION

BONE OF SKULL

CORPUS CALLOSUM

CISTERNA SUPERIOR

CEREBELLUM

SUBARACHNOID SPACE

CHOROID PLEXUS OF LATERAL VENTRICLE

CHOROID PLEXUS OF 3RD VENTRICLE

PITUITARY GLAND

SPHENOID BONE

PONS

MEDULLA OBLONGATA

SPINAL CORD

MEDIAL ASPECT

VASCULAR ANATOMY OF BRAIN

VENTRAL VIEW

- OLFACTORY BULB
- MIDDLE CEREBRAL ARTERY
- ANTERIOR COMMUNICATING ARTERY
- POSTERIOR COMMUNICATING ARTERY
- INTERNAL CAROTID ARTERY
- SUPERIOR CEREBELLAR ARTERY
- POSTERIOR CEREBRAL ARTERY
- BASILAR ARTERY
- ANTERIOR INFERIOR CEREBELLAR ARTERY
- VERTEBRAL ARTERIES
- POSTERIOR INFERIOR CEREBELLAR ARTERY

LATERAL VIEW

BRANCHES OF ANTERIOR CEREBRAL ARTERY

BRANCHES OF POSTERIOR CEREBRAL ARTERY

MIDDLE CEREBRAL ARTERY

MEDIAL VIEW

ANTERIOR CEREBRAL ARTERY

POSTERIOR CEREBRAL ARTERY

MIDDLE CEREBRAL ARTERY

brain implant. Transplantation of tissue into the brain in an attempt to treat a disease. Implanting tissue from the adrenal gland into the caudate nucleus (of the nondominant side of the brain) has been done experimentally to treat Parkinson's disease.

Brain's reflex [Walter Russell Brain, Brit. physician, 1895–1966]. Extension of flexed arm on assuming quadrupedal posture.

brain sand. Laminated bodies consisting principally of phosphates, carbonates of calcium, and magnesium found in the pineal body.

brain scan. Use of radioactive isotopes injected into the circulation to detect abnormalities in structure and function of the brain.

brain stem. The stemlike part of the brain that connects the cerebral hemispheres with the spinal cord. Comprises the medulla oblongata, the pons, and the midbrain.

brain stem auditory evoked potential. ABBR: BAEP. Study of brain (ECG) waves during sound stimuli. Used to determine threshold of sound required to produce a brain stem response. This provides an objective measure of hearing acuity. SEE: *auditory evoked response; evoked responses; somatosensory evoked responses; visual evoked responses.*

brainstorm. 1. Sudden idea. 2. Temporary outburst of mental excitement; often maniacal, esp. in paranoia.

brain swelling. Brain edema, q.v.

brain tumor. Term usually used inexactly to describe any intracranial mass — neoplastic, cystic, inflammatory (abscess), or syphilitic. Treatment methods include surgery, radiation, and chemotherapy. Experimentally, immunologic therapy has been investigated, as has hyperthermia and laser photoactivation. None of these has reached the point of being clinically useful. SEE: *neoplasm; tumor.* SEE: *Nursing Diagnoses* in *Appendix.*

SYM: The general symptoms are those due to an increase in intracranial pressure such as headache, changes in the retina such as choked disk recognized by ophthalmoscopic examinations, and vomiting (without nausea). Mental changes (esp. dullness), epileptiform convulsions, and giddiness are often general but may be localized signs. In addition, history and cranial radiological studies are of great value. The injection of air into the ventricles prior to x-ray examination is known as pneumoventriculography.

In general, neoplasms of the brain do not metastasize to other parts of the body. They contain almost no blood vessels and may produce pain or other sensations. The most malignant ones in childhood are gliomas, q.v.

brainwashing. Intense psychological indoctrination, usually political, for the purpose of displacing the individual's previous thoughts and attitudes with those selected by the regime or person inflicting the indoctrination.

bran. The outer coating or husk of cereal grains, such as wheat or oats, produced as a by-product of milling these grains. Because some of the cellulose in bran is indigestible, it may be used to add bulk to the diet and thus be of assistance in preventing and treating constipation. SEE: *fiber, dietary.*

branch. In anatomy, a subdivision arising from a main or larger portion, esp. of an artery, vein, nerve, or lymphatic vessel.

branchial (brăng′kē-ăl) [L. *branchia*, gills]. Pert. to or resembling gills of a fish or a homologous structure in higher animals.

branchial arches. Five pairs of arched structures that form the lateral and ventral walls of the pharynx of the embryo. They are partially separated from each other externally by the branchial clefts and internally by the pharyngeal pouches. The fifth arch is rudimentary. They play an important role in the formation of structures of the face and neck. The first is the mandibular arch, the second the hyoid arch. SYN: *visceral arches.*

branchial clefts. A series of openings between the embryonic branchial arches. They become functional gill slits in fish.

branchial grooves. A series of furrows separating the embryonic branchial arches. They are homologous to the branchial clefts of fish and amphibians.

branchial muscles. Muscles that develop from the mesoderm of the embryonic branchial arches. Include most muscles of face and neck.

branchiogenic, branchiogenous (brăng″kē-ō-jĕn′ĭk, brăng″kē-ŏj′ĕ-nŭs) [L. *branchia*, gills, + Gr. *gennan*, to produce]. Having origin in a branchial cleft.

branchioma (brăng″kē-ō′mă) [″ + Gr. *oma*, tumor]. A tumor derived from the branchial epithelium.

branchiomeric (brăng″kē-ō-mĕr′ĭk) [″ + Gr. *meros*, part]. Of or pert. to the branchial arches.

Brandt-Andrews maneuver. Technique for expressing the placenta from the uterus during the third stage of labor. One hand puts gentle traction on the cord while the other is used to press the anterior surface of the uterus backward. SEE: *Credé's method.*

brandy. An alcoholic liquid obtained by the distillation of fermented fruit, esp. grapes, usually containing 50% ethyl alcohol by volume. Used medically as a tonic, peripheral vasodilator, and as a sedative.

Branhamella (Neisseria) catarrhalis (brăn"hă-mĕl'ă). Species of *Neisseria* found in the upper respiratory tract. They may be mistaken for meningococci.

brash. A burning sensation in the stomach sometimes accompanied by belching of sour fluid. SYN: *heartburn; pyrosis.*

  b., water. SEE: *water brash.*

brass poisoning. Poisoning due to the inhalation of fumes of zinc and zinc oxide with destruction of tissue in the respiratory passage. Rarely fatal.

  SYM: Dryness and burning in respiratory tract; cough; headache; chills.

  TREAT: Entirely symptomatic. Inhalations of humidified air make patient more comfortable.

brawny induration. Pathological hardening and thickening of tissues, usually due to inflammation.

Braxton Hicks sign [John Braxton Hicks, Brit. gynecologist, 1823–1897]. Intermittent painless uterine contractions that may occur every 10 to 20 minutes. They occur after the third month of pregnancy. These contractions do not represent true labor pains but are often so interpreted. The sign is not present in every pregnancy. Also called Hicks sign.

Brazelton Neonatal Assessment Scale [T. Berry Brazelton, American pediatrician, b. 1918]. Scale for evaluating the behavior and responses of the newborn infant. It is based on four dimensions: interaction with the environment; motor processes including motor responses, general activity level, and reflexes; control of physiologic state as determined by reaction to a distinct stimulus such as a rattle, bell, light, or a pinprick; and response to stress as judged by tremulousness, startle reaction, and change in skin coloration. The test has been used as late as one week after birth to demonstrate alteration in the infant's behavior due to drugs administered to the mother while the infant was in utero.

break. 1. In orthopedics, a fracture. 2. To interrupt continuity in a tissue or electric circuit or channel of flow or communication.

breakbone fever. An acute febrile disease characterized by sudden onset, with headache, fever, prostration, joint and muscle pain, lymphadenopathy, and a rash that appears simultaneously with a second temperature rise following an afebrile period. Causative agent is a Group B arbovirus. SYN: *dengue.*

breakdown, nervous. SEE: *nervous breakdown.*

breast [AS. *breost*]. 1. The upper anterior aspect of the chest. 2. Mammary gland, a compound alveolar gland consisting of 15 to 20 lobes of glandular tissue separated from each other by interlobular septa. Each lobe is drained by a lactiferous duct that opens on the tip of the nipple. The mammary gland secretes milk used for nourishment of the infant. SEE: *lactiferous glands; milk;* illus.

DEVELOP: During puberty, estrogens from the ovary stimulate growth and development of the duct system. During pregnancy, progesterone secreted by the corpus luteum and placenta acts synergistically with estrogens to bring the alveoli to complete development. Following parturition, prolactin (luteotrophin) in conjunction with adrenal corticoids initiates lactation, and oxytocin from the posterior pituitary induces ejection of milk. Sucking or milking reflexly stimulates both milk secretion and discharge of milk.

CHANGES IN PREGNANCY: First 6 to 12 weeks, there are fullness and tenderness, erectile tissues develop in nipples, nodules are felt, pigment is deposited around the nipple (primary areola) (in blondes the areolae and nipples become darker pink and in brunettes they become dark brown and in some cases even black), and a few drops of fluid may be squeezed out. Next 16 to 20 weeks, the secondary areola shows small whitish spots in pigmentation due to hypertrophy of the sebaceous glands, the so-called glands of Montgomery.

NURSING IMPLICATIONS: Most complications of the puerperal period may be prevented by proper care. Prenatally, this involves toughening the nipple and areolar area by massage during the third trimester. During nursing, the nipple and surrounding tissue must be properly positioned in the infant's mouth because sucking on the nipple may cause erosion, soreness, and cracking. If the nipple appears retracted, the mother may roll it gently between her fingers until it becomes erect.

The infant will begin nursing for several minutes' duration from either breast. The time is gradually increased according to tolerance of the mother's nipples. When lactation is well established, the infant takes 10 to 15 minutes to empty the breasts. Engorgement may be prevented by nursing on demand from birth; but, if it occurs, applying hot wet compresses and expressing milk manually help to soften the areola so that the infant can grasp the nipple. Breast massage and more frequent and longer feedings are also helpful. The breasts should be washed daily with water, and in the first few weeks may also be washed and dried after each feeding to remove any remaining milk and help prevent soreness. A nonalcoholic

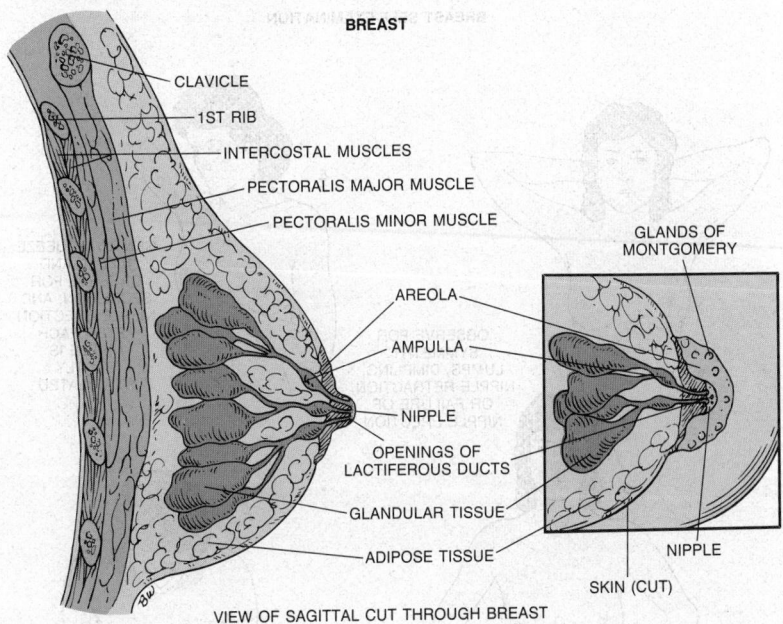

BREAST

CLAVICLE
1ST RIB
INTERCOSTAL MUSCLES
PECTORALIS MAJOR MUSCLE
PECTORALIS MINOR MUSCLE
GLANDS OF MONTGOMERY
AREOLA
AMPULLA
NIPPLE
OPENINGS OF LACTIFEROUS DUCTS
GLANDULAR TISSUE
ADIPOSE TISSUE
NIPPLE
SKIN (CUT)

VIEW OF SAGITTAL CUT THROUGH BREAST

lubricant (lanolin, petroleum jelly) may be rubbed gently into the nipple area; however, if the infant rejects the nipple, the lubricant must be washed off before feeding. Exposure to air for 20 to 30 minutes after feeding helps dry the nipple. If cracking occurs, further measures are warranted, including use of a heat lamp or sunlight after feedings and limiting sucking time to five minutes on each breast with use of a pacifier to meet infant sucking needs. A sterile nipple shield can be tried during nursing but should be discontinued if it does not control discomfort or if it results in infant frustration. It may help to begin nursing from the breast that feels best. The mother should be encouraged to persist with breast feeding as soreness usually subsides in a few days. Leaking may be controlled by pressing the palm of the hand firmly over the leaking nipple or by crossing the arms firmly across the breasts. A well-fitted brassiere that supports the breasts in an upward and inward position should be worn. The cups may be lined with soft pads to absorb released milk, but plastic should be avoided because it permits retained moisture to soften and macerate the nipple.

b., chicken. Deformity in which the chest protrudes, caused by rickets or obstructed respiration in infancy. SYN: *pigeon breast.*

b., self-examination of. ABBR: BSE. Technique that enables a woman to detect changes in her breasts. The examination should be done after the menstrual period, as normal physiologic changes that may confuse results occur in the premenstrual period. This method of self-examination is esp. useful in the early detection of breast cancer.

The use of all available means to diagnose and treat breast cancer without delay cannot be overemphasized. It is estimated that 135,000 women develop breast cancer annually, and 42,000 will die each year from this disease. The annual mortality rate is about 23 per 100,000 of the female population. Every person caring for female patients should be familiar with the method of self-examination of the breast. Women esp. should know this technique in order to be able to examine themselves as well as to instruct others.

Self-examination of the breast should be done once a month soon after the completion of the menstrual period and on a monthly basis after menopause. If any ab-

BREAST SELF-EXAMINATION

1. OBSERVE FOR SYMMETRY, LUMPS, DIMPLING, NIPPLE RETRACTION, OR FAILURE OF NIPPLE ERECTION

4. GENTLY SQUEEZE NIPPLE AND OBSERVE FOR SECRETION, AND NIPPLE ERECTION AFTER EACH NIPPLE IS GENTLY STIMULATED

6. WHILE LEANING FORWARD, OBSERVE BREASTS AS THEY ARE REFLECTED IN MIRROR TO DETECT IRREGULARITY, RETRACTED AREAS, NIPPLE RETRACTION ESPECIALLY ON ONE SIDE ONLY

FEEL FOR NODES, IRREGULARITY, AND TENDERNESS BOTH IN BREASTS AND AXILLARY AREAS normality, a lump, or thickening is discovered, see your physician immediately.

Technique: (SEE: illus.) 1. Stand before a mirror. Inspect both breasts for anything unusual, such as any discharge from the nipples, puckering, dimpling, or scaling of the skin.

The next two steps are designed to emphasize any change in the shape or contour of your breasts. As you do them, you should be able to feel your chest muscles tighten. 2. Watching closely in the mirror, clasp your hands behind your head and press hands forward. 3. Next, press hands firmly on hips and bow slightly toward the mirror as you pull your shoulders and elbows forward.

Some women perform the next step in the shower. Fingers glide over soapy skin, making it easy to concentrate on the texture underneath. 4. Raise your left arm. Use three or four fingers of your right hand to explore your left breast firmly, carefully, and thoroughly. Beginning at the outer edge, press the flat part of your fingers in small circles, moving the circles slowly around the breast. Gradually work toward the nipple. Be sure to cover the entire breast. Pay special attention to the area between the breast and the armpit, including the armpit itself. Feel for any unusual lump or mass under the skin. 5. Gently squeeze the nipple and look for a discharge. Repeat the examination on your right breast.

6. Other women perform steps 4 and 5 lying down. If you wish to, lie flat on your back, left arm over your head and a pillow or folded towel under your left shoulder. This position flattens the breast and makes it easier to examine. Use the same circular motion described earlier. Repeat on your right breast.

You might want to try both positions — standing and lying down — to see which is more comfortable for you. However, the most important point is to perform a breast examination each month. SEE: NOTE under *breast cancer; mammography.*

Caution: Even though BSE is an important adjunct to early detection of breast changes, it is not as accurate as mammography.

---

breast cancer. Malignant neoplasm of the breast. Breast cancer is the leading cause of death in women between the ages of 30 and 50, and is second only to heart disease as a cause of death in women over 50. Approximately one woman in 10 will develop breast cancer in her lifetime. About 1000 men develop breast cancer each year.

Risk factors in order of importance include: patient's mother had bilateral breast cancer diagnosed prior to menopause; close relative who developed breast cancer but was menopausal; over age 50 and nulliparous or experienced pregnancy for the first time after age 30; history of chronic breast disease, especially epithelial hyperplasia; exposure to ionizing radiation of more than 0.5 Gy (50 rad) during adolescence; and obesity. Early menarche, late menopause, and menstrual cycle irregularity also increase the chances of breast cancer development. Artificial menopause prior to age 35 and childbearing prior to age 18 provide some protection from breast cancer.

DIAG: About 90% of the cases of breast masses are discovered by breast self-examination (BSE) or accidentally by the patient. The remainder are detected by physical examination by a health professional or by screening techniques, such as mammography. Positive diagnosis can be made only by obtaining tissue for microscopic examination.

NOTE: BSE is a useful procedure and should not be neglected, but mammography should also be performed because it can detect a much smaller suspicious lesion than can be felt by use of BSE.

TREAT: The type of treatment, whether surgical, chemotherapeutic, or a combination of the two, is determined by the extent of the disease and the patient's age. SEE: *breast, self-examination of; cathepsin-D; mammography.*

breast feeding, drugs and. Maternal medications may be secreted in breast milk. It is important that the nursing mother take no medicines without first discussing whether or not the medicine will be present in her milk and whether or not it is harmful to the nursing infant.

breast implant. Implantation of a foreign substance in the breast area for augmentation or as a cosmetic prosthesis for women who have had a mastectomy. In some cases, use of silicone materials has caused unfavorable results.

breast pump. A manual or electric pump used to draw milk from the female breast.

breast stimulation. Stimulation of the breast has been used to increase uterine contractions in patients with ruptured membranes and when uterine contractions are absent or rare. The stimulus causes an increase in oxytocin, q.v., production.

breath (brĕth) [AS. *braeth,* odor]. The air inhaled and exhaled in act of respiration.

DIAG: *Foul odor (os fetor):* May indicate neglect of mouth or teeth; improper diet; constipation; mouth breathing; lack of exercise; use of drugs, alcohol, or tobacco. It also depends upon the food ingested and may indicate stomatitis, necrosis of jaw, caries of teeth, tonsillitis, diphtheria, gangrene and abscess of the lungs, fetid bronchitis, bronchiectasis, pyothorax, catarrh, diabetes, kidney disease, and other disorders. Mouthwashes and gargles are ineffective in removing the odor if os fetor is due to systemic causes or ingestion of food such as garlic. *Urinous odor*: Indicates uremia. *Sweetish odor* (that of ripe apples): Found in diabetes mellitus, esp. during coma. This sweet odor is due to the excretion of acetone in the breath. This condition develops quickly in infants and children who have gone several hours without food. SEE: *breath tests*.

Rattling and shortness of breath: Edema; presence of fluids in the air passages. *Sighing breath*: Air hunger; occurs in internal hemorrhage. Therefore be alert to the development of this symptom following abdominal surgery and in typhoid fever.

b., liver. The characteristic odor of the breath that accompanies severe liver disease. It has been described as "mousy."

b., uremic. The "fishy" or ammoniacal breath odor characteristic of individuals with uremia.

Breathalyzer (brĕth'ă-lĭ-zĕr). Apparatus used to analyze specific contents of expired air. One such device is used to test for presence of alcohol in expired air in order to determine whether or not a person is legally intoxicated.

breath-holding. Stopping of breathing voluntarily or involuntarily. May be seen in children who use this to attempt to control the behavior of their parents.

breath-holding attacks. A benign condition that always has its onset with crying. The young child stops breathing, becomes cyanotic, the limbs become rigid and extended, and consciousness may be lost. This is followed by the body becoming limp, resumption of respirations and, after a few seconds, the child is fully alert. This pattern of behavior disappears spontaneously prior to school age.

breathing. Act of inhaling and exhaling air. SEE: *chest; respiration*.

b., asthmatic. Harsh breathing with a prolonged wheezing expiration heard all over the chest.

b., bronchial. Harsh breathing with a prolonged high-pitched expiration that sometimes has a tubular quality. Heard in consolidation of lung tissue.

b., Cheyne-Stokes. SEE: *Cheyne-Stokes respiration*.

b., cog-wheel. Respiratory murmur, not continuous but broken into waves, not indicative of any special disease but frequently observed in bronchitis and in incipient tuberculosis.

b., continuous positive-pressure. A method of mechanically assisted pulmonary ventilation. A device administers air or oxygen to the lungs under a continuous pressure that never returns to zero. SYN: *ventilation, continuous positive-pressure*.

b., intermittent positive-pressure. A mechanical method for assisting pulmonary ventilation employing a device that administers air or oxygen for the inflation of the lungs under positive pressure. Exhalation is usually passive. SYN: *ventilation, intermittent positive-pressure*.

b., Kussmaul. SEE: *Kussmaul's breathing*.

b., shallow. Type of breathing that occurs in acute pulmonary disease. Noted when chest walls are thick, in the old and feeble, in emphysema, in pleural effusion, in incipient tuberculosis, in painful conditions of the chest such as fractured ribs, pleurodynia and early pleurisy, and in pulmonary edema.

breath test for lactase deficiency. The measurement of hydrogen in the breath after ingestion of 50 grams of lactase. SEE: *lactase deficiency syndrome*.

breath tests. A variety of tests wherein specific substances in the breath are detected in order to help explain metabolic changes.

breech [AS. *brec*, buttocks]. The nates, or buttocks.

breech presentation. A common abnormality of delivery where the fetal buttocks present rather than the head. SEE: *presentation, breech*.

breeze. A movement of air.

bregma (brĕg'mă) [Gr., front of head] (pl. *bregmata*). That point on the skull where the coronal and sagittal sutures join. The anterior fontanel in the fetus and young infant.

bregmatic. Pert. to the bregma.

bregmocardiac reflex (brĕg″mō-kăr'dē-ăk) [Gr. *bregma*, front of head, + *kardia*, heart]. Reduced heart rate following pressure on posterior fontanel.

Breisky's disease (brī'skēz) [August Breisky, Ger. gynecologist, 1832–1889]. Atrophic disease affecting the female external genitalia, seen most often in older women. Characterized by severe itching and a white marblelike appearance of the skin, frequently with excoriations. Without medical intervention, the skin may undergo malignant degeneration. SYN: *kraurosis vulvae; leukoplakia vulvae*.

Brenner's tumor [Fritz Brenner, Ger. pathologist, 1877–1969]. A benign fibroepithelioma of the ovary.

Breokinase. Trade name for urokinase.

Brethine. Trade name for terbutaline sulfate.

brevicollis (brĕv″ĭ-kŏl′ĭs) [L. *brevis*, short, + *collum*, neck]. Shortness of the neck.

brevilineal (brĕv-ĭ-lĭn′ē-ăl) [L. *brevis*, short, + *linea*, line]. Shorter and broader than usual, with reference to body type. SYN: *brachymorphic.*

Brevital Sodium. Trade name for methohexital sodium.

Bricanyl. Trade name for terbutaline sulfate.

bridge (brĭj) [AS. *brycg*]. 1. Narrow band of tissue. 2. Dental appliance replacing missing teeth that is attached to adjacent teeth for support. SYN: *fixed partial denture.*

b. of nose. Upper portion of the external nose formed by the junction of the nasal bones.

bridgework (brĭj′work). A partial denture held in place by attachments other than clasps.

b., fixed. Partial plates held by crowns or inlays cemented to the natural teeth.

b., removable. Partial plates held by clasps that permit their removal.

bridle (brī′dl). In anatomy, a frenum.

Bright's disease [Richard Bright, Brit. physician, 1789–1858]. A vague and obsolete term for disease of the kidneys. Usually refers to nonsuppurative inflammatory or degenerative kidney diseases characterized by proteinuria and hematuria and sometimes by edema, hypertension, and nitrogen retention. SEE: *nephritis.*

brightness gain. The increase in the intensity of an image in a fluoroscopic intensifier.

brim. 1. An edge or margin. 2. Brim of pelvis. Superior aperture of the lesser or true pelvis; the inlet. Formed by the iliopectineal line of the innominate bone and the sacral promontory. Oval-shaped in the female; heart-shaped in the male.

Briquet's syndrome [Paul Briquet, Fr. physician, 1796–1881]. A personality disorder in which alcoholism and somatization disorder occur.

brisement (brēz-mŏn′) [Fr., crushing]. Breaking, by forcible means, of anything, as of an ankylosis.

Brissaud's reflex (brĭs-sōz′) [Edouard Brissaud, Fr. physician, 1852–1909]. Contraction of tensor fasciae latae muscle following stroking or tickling of sole of foot. A component of the extensor plantar response.

Bristamycin. Trade name for erythromycin stearate.

British antilewisite. ABBR: BAL. Trade name for dimercaprol, a compound used as an antidote in poisoning due to heavy metals such as arsenic, gold, and mercury.

British Pharmacopoeia. ABBR: B.P. The standard reference on drugs and their preparations used in Great Britain.

British thermal unit. ABBR: BTU. Amount of heat necessary to raise the temperature of 1 lb of water from 39°F to 40°F. One BTU is equal to 252 calories or 1055 joules.

brittle diabetes. Diabetes in which regulation of the insulin dosage is difficult because of the unpredictable variation in insulin sensitivity and a tendency toward ketosis. This type of diabetes is particularly prone to be present in individuals whose diabetes developed during childhood.

broach (brōch) [ME. *broche*, pointed rod]. 1. A dental instrument used for enlarging a root canal or for removing the pulp. 2. Technique of preparing the intramedullary canal of a bone by using a cutting device. This is done in preparation for a prosthetic replacement.

Broadbent's sign [Sir William Henry Broadbent, Brit. physician, 1835–1907]. A visible retraction of the left side and back in the region of the 11th and 12th ribs synchronous with the cardiac systole in adhesive pericarditis.

Broca's area (brō′kăs) [Pierre Paul Broca, Fr. anatomist, anthropologist, neurologist, and surgeon, 1824–1880]. Area of the left hemisphere of the brain at the posterior end of the inferior frontal gyrus. It contains the motor speech area and controls movements of tongue, lips, and vocal cords. Loss of speech may follow hemorrhage into this area. SYN: *motor speech area.* SEE: *aphasia, motor.*

Brodie's abscess [Sir Benjamin Collins Brodie, Brit. surgeon, 1783–1862]. An abscess of the head of a bone, esp. of the head of the tibia.

SYM: May be aching pains in area, followed by slight swelling and tenderness on movement. Symptoms less acute but similar to osteomyelitis.

ETIOL: It is usually of tubercular origin or from subacute staphylococcal infection.

brom-, bromo- [Gr. *bromos*, stench]. Prefixes indicating presence of bromine.

bromelain (brō′mĕ-lān). Proteolytic enzyme present in the pineapple plant. Is effective as a meat tenderizer. The enzyme will clot milk. Trade name is Ananase.

bromide (brō′mīd) [Gr. *bromos*, stench]. A binary compound of bromine combined with an element or a radical. It is a central nervous system depressant, and overdosage can cause serious mental disturbance.

bromide poisoning. Poisoning due to an overdose of bromide.

SYM: Prompt vomiting; abdominal pain,

respiratory and eye irritation if inhaled; or corrosion of mouth and intestinal tract if swallowed. Cyanosis, tachycardia, and shock.

F.A.: If inhaled, oxygen; provide respiratory support and treat pulmonary edema. If ingested, induce emesis with ipecac, perform gastric lavage, and treat shock. SEE: *Poisons and Poisoning* in *Appendix.*

bromidrosiphobia (brō″mĭ-drō-sĭ-fō′bē-ă) [″ + *hidros,* sweat, + *phobos,* fear]. Abnormal fear of personal odors, accompanied by hallucinations.

bromidrosis, bromhidrosis (brō″mĭ-drō′sĭs). Sweat that is fetid or offensive due to bacterial decomposition. It occurs mostly on feet, groin, and axillae.

NURSING IMPLICATIONS: Daily periodic cleansing with soap and water, thorough rinsing and drying, use of deodorants, and frequent changes of clothing as needed.

RS: anhidrosis; chromidrosis; uridrosis.

bromine (brō′mēn, -mĭn) [Gr. *bromos,* stench]. SYMB: Br. At. wt. 79.904; at. no. 35. Liquid nonmetallic element. It is obtained from natural brines from wells and sea water. Its compounds are used in medicine and photography. SEE: *bromide.*

bromism, brominism (brō′mĭzm, brō′mĭn-ĭzm) [″ + *-ismos,* condition]. Poisoning resulting from prolonged use of bromides. SEE: *bromides* in *Poisons and Poisoning* in *Appendix.*

bromocriptine mesylate (brō″mō-krĭp′tēn). USP. An ergot derivative that suppresses secretion of prolactin. It has been used to stimulate ovulation in the galactorrhea-amenorrhea syndrome. It is used in treating acromegaly. It is of limited usefulness in treating parkinsonism. Trade name is Parlodel.

bromoderma (brō″mō-dĕr′mă) [″ + *derma,* skin]. Acnelike eruption due to allergic sensitivity to bromides.

bromodiphenhydramine hydrochloride (brō″mō-dī″fĕn-hī′dră-mēn). USP. An antihistamine; also has sedative properties. Trade name is Ambodryl Hydrochloride.

bromoiodism (brō″mō-ī′ō-dĭzm) [″ + *ioeides,* violet colored, + *-ismos,* condition]. Poisoning from bromine and iodine or their compounds.

bromomenorrhea (brō″mō-mĕn-ō-rē′ă) [″ + *men,* month, + *rhoia,* flow]. Menstrual discharge characterized by an offensive odor.

brompheniramine maleate (brōm″fĕn-ĭr′ă-mēn). USP. An antihistamine. Trade name is Dimetane.

Brompton's cocktail [Brompton Chest Hospital, England]. A mixture of cocaine, morphine, and antiemetics used to alleviate pain and induce euphoria, esp. in patients with cancer.

bronchadenitis (brŏng″kăd-ĕ-nī′tĭs) [Gr. *bronchos,* windpipe, + *aden,* gland, + *itis,* inflammation]. Inflammation of bronchial glands.

bronchi (brŏng′kī) [L.] (sing. *bronchus).* [NA] The two main branches leading from the trachea to the lungs, providing the passageway for air movement. The trachea divides opposite the 3rd thoracic vertebra into the right and left main bronchi. The point of division is called the carina tracheae [NA] and is the site where foreign bodies too large to enter either bronchus would rest after passing through the trachea. The right bronchus is shorter and more vertical than the left one. After entering the lung each bronchus divides further and terminates in bronchioles. SEE: illus.

b., foreign bodies in. The presence of any foreign material in the bronchi may cause various diseases, large objects leading to collapse of the lung. Beans, nuts, or seeds may cause pneumonia, bronchitis, or lung abscess. Foreign bodies usually are aspirated into the right bronchus because it has a less acute angle compared with the left.

SYM: Immediate choking and gagging. Later, symptoms of bronchitis, atelectasis, pneumonia, or lung abscess. Small metal bodies may produce no symptoms.

TREAT: Removal through bronchoscope.

PROG: Good if removed before complications occur. Better in case of metallic objects than in those consisting of vegetable matter.

bronchi, words pert. to: alveobronchitis, "bronch-" words; mesobronchitis; rales.

bronchial (brŏng′kē-ăl). Pert. to the bronchi or bronchioles.

bronchial crises. Paroxysms of coughing in locomotor ataxia.

bronchial glands. Mucous or mixed glands in the bronchi or bronchioles.

bronchial tree. Bronchi and bronchial tubes.

bronchial tubes. The smaller divisions of the bronchi.

bronchial washing. Irrigation of one or both bronchi in order to collect cells for cytologic study or to help cleanse the bronchi.

bronchiarctia (brŏng″kē-ărk′shē-ă) [Gr. *bronchos,* windpipe + L. *arctare,* to compress]. Bronchial tube stenosis. SYN: *bronchiostenosis.*

bronchiectasis (brŏng″kē-ĕk′tă-sĭs) [″ + *ektasis,* dilatation]. Chronic dilatation of a bronchus or bronchi, with a secondary infection that usually involves the lower portion of the lung. Dilatation may be in an isolated segment or spread throughout the bronchi.

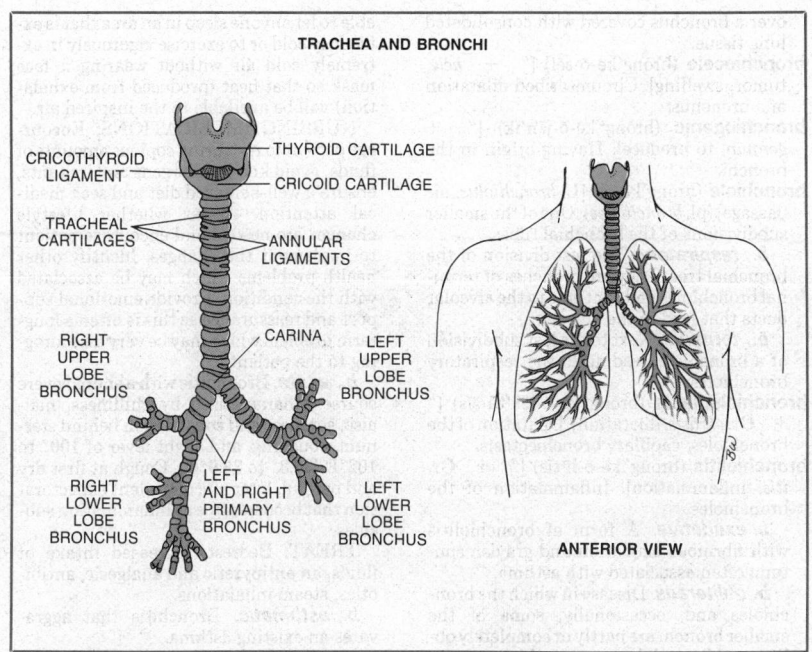

TRACHEA AND BRONCHI

CRICOTHYROID LIGAMENT

THYROID CARTILAGE

CRICOID CARTILAGE

TRACHEAL CARTILAGES

ANNULAR LIGAMENTS

RIGHT UPPER LOBE BRONCHUS

CARINA

LEFT UPPER LOBE BRONCHUS

RIGHT LOWER LOBE BRONCHUS

LEFT AND RIGHT PRIMARY BRONCHUS

LEFT LOWER LOBE BRONCHUS

ANTERIOR VIEW

SYM: Cough, dyspnea, expectoration of foul secretion, esp. in the morning or when changing position. On standing, sputum separates into three layers: a bottom one that is thick and contains pus cells; a middle layer of greenish fluid; and an upper layer of froth.

ETIOL: Acquired or congenital, on one or both sides of chest. Acquired bronchiectasis usually secondary to obstruction or infections, as bronchopneumonia, chronic bronchitis, tuberculosis, whooping cough.

TREAT: Antibiotics for treatment and prophylaxis, and postural drainage. Resection of affected areas in selected patients. Aerosols for bronchodilation in bronchospasm. SEE: *postural drainage.*

NURSING IMPLICATIONS: Assess the patient for presence of increasing severity of respiratory distress. Increase oral fluids and use a humidifier or vaporizer to help thin inspissated secretions. Teach and encourage the patient to breathe deeply and cough effectively. Teach patient and family to perform chest physiotherapy for involved lobes, including proper positioning for postural drainage, percussion, and vibration several times daily, especially in the early morning, ½ hour before meals, and at bedtime. Suction the oropharynx if the patient is unable to clear airway. Provide frequent oral hygiene to remove foul-smelling secretions and help prevent anorexia. Teach the patient disposal of secretions. Encourage well-balanced, high-protein meals and adequate rest to promote tissue healing. Instruct the patient to avoid air pollutants and people with upper respiratory infections; if indicated, recommend self-help groups to assist in stopping cigarette smoking. Administer and teach the patient and family about the need for prescribed medications, such as antibiotics, bronchodilators, and expectorants. Teach the patient not to take over-the-counter drugs without physician approval.

b., saccular. Dilated bronchi are of saccular or irregular shape. Proximal third to fourth branches of the bronchi are severely dilated and end blindly with extensive collapse.

b., varicose. Dilated bronchi resemble varicose veins; irregular dilatation and constriction as seen in cystic fibrosis.

bronchiloquy (brŏng-kil′ō-kwē) [" + L. *loqui*, to speak]. Unusual vocal resonance over a bronchus covered with consolidated lung tissue.

bronchiocele (brŏng′kē-ō-sēl) [″ + *kele,* tumor, swelling]. Circumscribed dilatation of a bronchus.

bronchiogenic (brŏng″kē-ō-jĕn′ĭk) [″ + *gennan,* to produce]. Having origin in the bronchi.

bronchiole (brŏng′kē-ōl) [L. *bronchiolus,* air passage] (pl. *bronchioles*). One of the smaller subdivisions of the bronchial tubes.

b., respiratory. The last division of the bronchial tree. They are branches of terminal bronchioles and continue to the alveolar ducts that lead to the alveoli.

b., terminal. Next to the last subdivision of a bronchiole, leading to the respiratory bronchioles.

bronchiolectasis (brŏng″kē-ō-lĕk′tă-sĭs) [″ + Gr. *ektasis,* dilatation]. Dilatation of the bronchioles; capillary bronchiectasis.

bronchiolitis (brŏng″kē-ō-lī′tĭs) [″ + Gr. *itis,* inflammation]. Inflammation of the bronchioles.

b. exudativa. A form of bronchiolitis with fibrinous exudation and grayish sputum; often associated with asthma.

b. obliterans. Disease in which the bronchioles and, occasionally, some of the smaller bronchi are partly or completely obliterated by nodular masses which contain granulation and fibrotic tissue.

b., vesicular. Bronchopneumonia, q.v.

bronchiolus (brŏng-kē′ō-lŭs) [L.] (pl. *bronchioli*). [NA] Bronchiole; one of the smaller subdivisions of the bronchial tubes.

bronchiospasm (brŏng′kē-ō-spăzm) [Gr. *bronchos,* windpipe, + *spasmos,* a convulsion]. Spasmodic contraction of the bronchial tubes.

bronchiostenosis (brŏng″kē-ō-stĕn-ō′sĭs) [″ + *stenosis,* act of narrowing]. Narrowing of the bronchial tubes. SYN: *bronchiarctia.*

bronchitis (brŏng-kī′tĭs) [″ + *itis,* inflammation]. Inflammation of mucous membrane of the bronchial tubes. SEE: *Nursing Diagnoses* in *Appendix.*

ETIOL: Infectious agents such as viruses, esp. influenza virus, or pyogenic organisms such as various species of *Streptococcus, Pneumococcus, Staphylococcus,* and *Haemophilus.* Infection often preceded by the common cold. Predisposing factors are exposure, chilling, fatigue, and malnutrition. Acute bronchial irritation may also be caused by various physical and chemical agents such as dusts and fumes. Allergic factors may be of importance.

NOTE: Even though the pathway of air to the bronchi and lungs is capable of warming inspired cold air, there are limits beyond which this system fails. Thus it is inadvisable to let anyone sleep in an area that is extremely cold or to exercise vigorously in extremely cold air without wearing a face mask so that heat (produced from exhalation) will be available to the inspired air.

NURSING IMPLICATIONS: Encourage patient to rest, drink copious amounts of fluids, avoid known allergens and irritants, ensure a well-balanced diet and seek medical attention. Assess whether lifestyle changes are needed and encourage patient to implement the changes. Identify other health problems which may be associated with the condition. Provide emotional support and reassurance as this is often a long-term problem which may be very discouraging to the patient.

b., acute. Bronchitis with a short, severe course. Characterized by chilliness, malaise, soreness and constriction behind sternum, coughing, and slight fever of 100° to 102°F (37.8° to 38.9°C). Cough at first dry and painful, later mucopurulent expectoration that becomes free as inflammation subsides.

TREAT: Bedrest, increased intake of fluids, an antipyretic and analgesic, antibiotics, steam inhalations.

b., asthmatic. Bronchitis that aggravates an existing asthma.

b., chronic. Bronchitis characterized by increased mucus secretion by the tracheobronchial tree. The productive cough is usually present for at least three months of two consecutive years. The diagnosis can be made only if bronchopulmonary diseases such as bronchiectasis, tuberculosis, and tumor have been excluded. The predominant pathological change is hypertrophy and hyperplasia of the mucus-secreting glands of the trachea, bronchi, and bronchioles.

TREAT: It is important to have the patient who smokes stop smoking. Change of climate and occupation may be indicated but may be impossible due to social and economic circumstances. If infection is present, appropriate antibiotics should be administered.

b., plastic. Bronchitis characterized by violent cough and paroxysms of dyspnea in which casts of the bronchial tubes are expectorated.

b., putrid. Chronic form of bronchitis with foul-smelling sputum.

b., vegetal. Bronchitis resulting from lodging of foods of vegetable origin in the bronchus.

bronchium (brŏng′kē-ŭm) [Gr. *bronchos*] (pl. *bronchia*). One of the subdivisions of the bronchus, smaller than the bronchus and larger than the bronchioles.

broncho-, bronch- [Gr. *bronchos*, windpipe].
Prefix rel. to the bronchi.

bronchoadenitis (brŏng″kō-ăd″ĕ-nī′tĭs) ["
+ *aden*, gland, + *itis*, inflammation].
Bronchadenitis, q.v.

bronchoalveolar (brŏn″kō-ăl-vē′ō-lăr) ["
+ *alveolus*, small hollow]. Concerning the
bronchi and alveoli.

bronchoalveolar lavage. Introduction, by
use of a fiberoptic bronchoscope, of sterile
saline into the lung in order to remove secretions, cells, and protein from the lower respiratory tract. The fluid is usually used to
treat cystic fibrosis, pulmonary alveolar
proteinosis, severe asthma with bronchial
obstruction due to mucus plugging; and for
obtaining materials for diagnostic purposes.

bronchoblennorrhea (brŏng″kō-blĕn″ŏ-
rē′ä) [" + *blennos*, mucus, + *rhoia*,
flow]. Chronic bronchitis in which sputum
is copious and thin.

bronchocele (brŏng′kō-sēl) [" + *kele*,
tumor, swelling]. A localized dilatation of a
bronchus.

bronchoconstriction (brŏng″kō-kŏn-strĭk′
shŭn) [" + L. *constringere*, to draw to-
gether]. Constriction of the bronchial tubes.

bronchodilatation (brŏng″kō-dĭl-ă-tā′shŭn)
[" + L. *dilatare*, to open]. Dilatation of a
bronchus.

bronchoedema (brŏng″kō-ě-dē′mä) [" +
oidema, swelling]. Edematous swelling of
the mucosa of the bronchial tubes, reducing
size of air passageways and inducing dyspnea.

bronchoesophageal (brŏng″kō-ě-sŏf″ă-
jē′ăl) [" + *oisophagos*, esophagus]. Concerning the bronchus and the esophagus.

bronchofiberscope (brŏng″kō-fī′bĕr-skōp)
[" + L. *fibra*, fiber, + Gr. *skopein*, to
examine]. A fiberoptic endoscope for visual
examination of the bronchi.

bronchogenic (brŏng-kō-jĕn′ĭk) [" + *gennan*, to produce]. Having origin in the bronchus.

bronchogram (brŏng′kō-grăm) [" +
gramma, something written]. An x-ray of
the lung obtained during bronchography,
q.v.

bronchography (brŏng-kŏg′ră-fē) [" +
graphein, to write]. An x-ray of the lung, or a
portion of it, after a radiopaque substance
has been instilled into the trachea or bronchial tree.

broncholith (brŏng′kō-lĭth) [" + *lithos*,
stone]. A calculus in the bronchus.

broncholithiasis (brŏng″kō-lĭth-ī′ă-sĭs) ["
+ *lithos*, stone, + *-iasis*, state]. Bronchial inflammation or obstruction caused by
calculi in the bronchi.

bronchomotor (brŏng″kō-mō′tor) [" + L.
motus, moving]. Causing change of caliber
of the bronchi.

bronchomycosis (brŏng″kō-mī-kō′sĭs) ["
+ *mykes*, fungus, + *osis*, condition].
Any fungus infection of the bronchi or bronchial tubes, usually caused by fungi of the
genus *Candida*.

bronchopathy (brŏng-kŏp′ă-thē) [" +
pathos, disease, suffering]. Any pathological
condition involving the bronchi or bronchioles.

bronchophony (brŏng-kŏf′ō-nē) [" +
phone, voice]. The voice as heard over a normal bronchus by use of a stethoscope.

bronchoplasty (brŏng′kō-plăs″tē) [" +
plassein, to form]. Surgical repair of a bronchial defect.

bronchoplegia (brŏng″kō-plē′jē-ă) [" +
plege, stroke]. Paralysis of the muscles of the
walls of the bronchial tubes.

bronchopleural (brŏng″kō-ploor′ăl) [" +
pleura, side, rib]. Pert. to the bronchi and
the pleural cavity.

bronchopneumonia (brŏng″kō-nū-mō′nē-
ă) [" + *pneumonia*, lung inflammation].
Inflammation of the terminal bronchioles
and alveoli. SEE: *pneumonia*.

SYM: Cough and expectoration; respiration short and shallow from 50 to 75
breaths/minute. Cyanosis may ensue. Nostrils dilate with each inspiration, and in
children the temperature reaches 103° to
105°F (39.4° to 40.6°C). Before death, the
temperature may go as high as 108°F
(42.2°C) with a pulse of 140. Duration of the
fever, 2 to 3 weeks. Improvement may be
followed by increased severity as new
patches form.

In the aged, many of these symptoms are
absent. There are a slight cough and little
sputum, and fever of 100° to 101°F (37.8° to
38.3°C) may or may not be in evidence.
Weakness, sore throat, chills, and chest
pain may be present. The elderly and bedridden are esp. susceptible.

ETIOL: May be caused by various types
of pneumococci; Group A hemolytic streptococcus; *Klebsiella pneumoniae;* various
staphylococci; and *Francisella tularensis*.
May also be caused by other pathogenic
bacteria and viruses, rickettsias, and fungi.

TREAT: Bedrest, increased intake of
fluids, analgesics for pain, antibiotics, soft
diet, oxygen for cyanosis. Treatment of
shock if it occurs.

PROG: Depends principally upon time at
which treatment is initiated, recovery generally occurring more quickly in those
treated during the first three days. Also
prognosis more favorable for those under
50; unfavorable for the very young and very
old. Mortality greatly reduced by use of antibiotics.

COMPLICATIONS: Lung abscess, atelectasis, empyema, pericarditis, and paralytic ileus.

NURSING IMPLICATIONS: Carefully monitor the patient for any changes in the type and amount of respiratory distress, particularly frequency and type of cough, dyspnea, and chest pain. Restlessness and apprehension are also symptoms of respiratory distress and should be noted. Also promote lung expansion and aeration through turning and changing the patient's position frequently, and having the patient cough and breathe deeply 8 to 10 times each hour. The use of spirometry, which allows the patient to know the values obtained, provides incentive. The patient may receive humidified oxygen; if so, guidelines for care of the patient receiving oxygen therapy should be followed.

Monitor arterial blood gas values, maintain patent airway and adequate oxygenation, administering supplemental oxygen for PaO_2 of less than 55 to 60 mmHg. Assisted mechanical ventilation may be necessary. Note the character and amount of sputum produced and collect specimens as required. Teach patient to sneeze and cough into disposable tissue and provide plastic bag for disposal. Prevent pneumonia by encouraging annual vaccination for high-risk individuals, advising against the indiscriminate use of antibiotics which may allow colonization by resistant organisms and suggest avoidance of others with respiratory infections. Also encourage deep breathing, coughing, and position changes for all bedfast or postoperative patients.

Early ambulation is helpful, but the patient must be allowed to rest and encouraged not to become overly fatigued.

The patient should have good oral hygiene, may need or prefer small, frequent feedings (to decrease the possibility of abdominal distention), and will need increased protein in addition to good nutrition in order to assist with the resolution of the pneumonia and to promote healing. Hyperthermia is prevented through environmental temperature control, antipyretic administration as ordered, and tepid sponge baths in addition to increased oral fluids (unless contraindicated). SEE: *Nursing Diagnoses* in *Appendix.*

bronchopulmonary (brŏng″kō-pŭl′mō-nă-rē) [Gr. *bronchos,* windpipe, + L. *pulmonarius,* pert. to lung]. Pert. to bronchi and lungs.

bronchopulmonary dysplasia. Iatrogenic chronic lung disease that develops in premature infants following a period of intensive respiratory therapy.

bronchopulmonary lavage. Washing out or irrigation of the bronchi and bronchioles in order to remove tenacious secretions.

bronchorrhagia (brŏng″kor-ā′jē-ă) [″ + *rhegnynai,* to break forth]. Bronchial hemorrhage.

bronchorrhaphy (brŏng-kor′ă-fē) [″ + *rhaphe,* seam, ridge]. Suturing of a wound of the bronchus.

bronchorrhea (brŏng-kō-rē′ă) [″ + *rhoia,* flow]. Abnormal secretion from the bronchial mucous membrane, sometimes very offensive.

bronchorrhoncus (brŏng″kor-ŏn′kŭs) [″ + *rhonchos,* snore]. A bronchial rale.

bronchoscope (brŏng′kō-skōp) [″ + *skopein,* to examine]. An endoscope designed to pass through the trachea to allow visual inspection of the tracheobronchial tree. The device is also designed to permit the passage of an instrument that can be used to obtain tissue for biopsy or to remove a foreign body from the tracheobronchial tree.

bronchoscopy (brŏng-kŏs′kō-pē). Examination of the bronchi through a bronchoscope.

bronchosinusitis (brŏng″kō-sī″nŭs-ī′tĭs) [″ + L. *sinus,* a hollow, + Gr. *itis,* inflammation]. Infection of bronchi and sinus at the same time.

bronchospasm (brŏng′kō-spăzm) [″ + *spasmos,* a convulsion]. Abnormal narrowing with obstruction of the lumen of the bronchi due to spasm of the peribronchial smooth muscle. Clinically this is accompanied by coughing and wheezing. Bronchospasm is present in persons with asthma or bronchitis or both.

TREAT: Use of active bronchodilator, corticosteroids.

bronchospirochetosis (brŏng″kō-spī″rō-kē-tō′sĭs) [″ + *speira,* coil, + *chaite,* wavy hair, + *osis,* condition]. Hemorrhagic bronchitis; bronchopulmonary spirochetosis resulting from spirochetes.

bronchospirometer (brŏng″kō-spī-rŏm′ĕ-tĕr) [″ + L. *spirare,* to breathe, + Gr. *metron,* measure]. An instrument for determining the volume of air inspired from one lung and for collecting air for analysis.

bronchostaxis (brŏng″kō-stăk′sĭs) [″ + *staxis,* dripping]. Hemorrhage from the walls of a bronchus.

bronchostenosis (brŏng″kō-stĕn-ō′sĭs) [″ + *stenosis,* act of narrowing]. Stenosis of a bronchus.

bronchostomy (brŏng-kŏs′tō-mē) [″ + *stoma,* mouth]. Surgical formation of an opening into a bronchus.

bronchotomy (brŏng-kŏt′ō-mē) [″ + *tome,* incision]. Surgical incision of a bronchus, the larynx, or trachea.

bronchotracheal (brŏng″kō-trā′kē-ăl) [″

+ *trachea*, rough]. Pert. to both bronchi and trachea.

bronchovesicular (brŏng″kō-vĕ-sĭk′ū-lăr) [″ + L. *vesicula*, a tiny bladder]. Pert. to bronchial tubes and alveoli with special reference to sounds intermediate between bronchial or tracheal sounds and alveolar sounds.

bronchus (brŏng′kŭs) [Gr. *bronchos*, windpipe] (pl. *bronchi*). One of the two large branches of the trachea. The trachea proper terminates at the level of the 4th dorsal vertebra. SEE: *bronchi*.

Bronkaid Mist. Trade name for epinephrine, USP.

Bronkephrine. Trade name for ethylnorepinephrine hydrochloride, USP.

Bronkosol. Trade name for isoetharine.

brontophobia (brŏn″tō-fō′bē-ă) [Gr. *bronte*, thunder, + *phobos*, fear]. Abnormal fear of thunder.

bronzed skin. Seen in chronic adrenocortical insufficiency, i.e., Addison's disease. Also seen in hemochromatosis, some cases of diabetes mellitus, and cirrhosis of the liver.

brood capsule. Cystlike bodies that develop within a hydatid cyst of *Echinococcus granulosus*.

brooding. Anxiety and pondering about a trivial and unhappy event or matter.

broth [ME.]. 1. A nutrient drink made from meat, such as bouillon, usually served hot. 2. A liquid medium made from meat. It is used in making bacterial culture media.

brow. The forehead.

brown atrophy. Atrophy of organs such as the liver and heart, particularly noticeable in aging patients or in those with severe malnutrition or cachexia due to cancer. This is caused by the deposition of lipofuscin, q.v., in the affected organs.

brown baby syndrome. Dark grayish brown color due to the skin of an infant undergoing phototherapy for hyperbilirubinemia. This condition may last for months but is not known to produce permanent harm.

brownian movement (brow′nē-ăn) [Robert Brown, Brit. botanist, 1773–1858]. Oscillatory movement of particles resulting from chance bombardment by molecules moving at high velocities.

brown recluse spider. SEE: *spider, brown recluse.*

Brown-Séquard's syndrome (brown′sā-kärz′) [Charles E. Brown-Séquard, Fr. physician, 1817–1894]. Hemisection of the spinal cord with the following neurological changes: 1. Paralysis on the same side as the lesion, loss of position and vibratory sense, and ataxia. 2. Loss of pain and temperature sensitivity on the side opposite the lesion.

brow presentation. Condition in which the brow or face of the infant comes first on presentation in labor; makes vaginal delivery almost impossible. Cesarean section is frequently needed if the presentation cannot be altered. SEE: *presentation, brow,* for illus.

Brucella (broo-sĕl′ă) [Sir David Bruce, Brit. physician and bacteriologist, 1855–1931]. A genus of coccobacilli. It is nonmotile, aerobic, gram-negative, and pathogenic to humans, and it causes undulant fever and abortion in cattle, hogs, and goats. SEE: *brucellosis.*

brucellar. Pert. to *Brucella.*

brucellin (broo-sĕl′ĭn). An extract of a suspension of any species of *Brucella.* Injected intradermally, it may be of assistance in diagnosing brucellosis.

brucellosis (broo″sĕl-ō′sĭs) [*Brucella* + Gr. *osis*, condition]. A widespread infectious febrile disease affecting principally cattle, swine, and goats, but sometimes affecting other animals, including humans. It is caused by bacteria of the genus *Brucella*, several species being involved: *B. melitensis* and *B. suis*, the cause of brucellosis in goats and swine respectively, and *B. abortus*, the cause of contagious abortion in cattle, dogs, and other domestic animals. The organisms are intracellular parasites. In humans it is called brucellosis or Malta fever, q.v., and is caused by any of the three species.

TREAT: For the disease in adult humans, combined tetracycline for 4 to 6 weeks and streptomycin for the first two weeks of the tetracycline therapy. Doxycycline is also effective. In children the use of tetracycline may cause staining of developing teeth.

Bruch's membrane (brooks) [Karl W. L. Bruch, Ger. anatomist, 1819–1884]. A glassy membrane of the uvea of the eye lying between the choroid membrane and the pigmented epithelium of the retina. SYN: *lamina basalis of the choroid; vitreous lamella.*

brucine (broo′sēn, broo′sin) [J. Bruce, Scot. explorer in Africa, 1730–1794]. A poisonous alkaloid from *Strychnos nux vomica* and other *Strychnos* species. Similar to but less powerful than strychnine, q.v.

Bruck's disease (brooks) [Alfred Bruck, Ger. physician, b. 1865]. A rare disease characterized by muscle atrophy and skeletal disorders such as multiple fractures and ankyloses.

Brudzinski sign. Flexion of the hips when the neck is flexed from a supine position; present in children with meningitis. SEE: *Kernig's sign; meningitis.*

bruise (brooz) [O. Fr. *bruiser*, to break]. An injury with diffuse effusion into subcutaneous tissue and in which skin is discolored but not broken. A contusion, q.v.

b. of head, chest, and abdomen. May

be associated with internal injuries. SEE: *ecchymosis.*

SYM: Pain, swelling, tenderness, discoloration.

NURSING IMPLICATIONS: Collect data regarding the exact cause and location of the injury. Assess for possible additional injuries dependent on the specific location of the original injury. Cleanse skin abrasions thoroughly. A frequent (hourly) neurological exam should be done on any patient who has or may have sustained a head injury.

b., stone. Bruise of the bottom of the foot, usually seen in children who walk barefoot on stones.

bruissement (broo-ēs-mŏn') [Fr., droning noise]. A purring sound heard upon auscultation.

bruit (brwē, broot') [Fr., noise]. An adventitious sound of venous or arterial origin heard on auscultation.

b., carotid. SEE: *carotid bruits.*

b., placental. A purring or blowing noise originating in the pregnant uterus due to fetal circulation of blood. It is synchronous with the maternal pulse.

Brunner's glands (brŭn'ĕrz) [Johann C. Brunner, Swiss anatomist, 1653–1727]. Compound glands of the duodenum and upper jejunum. They are embedded in the submucous tissue and lined with columnar epithelium. They are similar to the pyloric glands of stomach. They secrete a clear, alkaline mucinous solution. SYN: *glands, duodenal.*

brush. Tufts of hair or bristles set in a handle.

b., tooth-. SEE: *toothbrush and toothbrushing.*

brush border. Hollow microvilli on the free surface of specialized cells in the renal tubules and intestinal epithelium.

Brushfield spots [T. Brushfield, Brit. physician, 1858–1937]. Gray or pale yellow spots sometimes present at the periphery of the iris of children with Down syndrome, q.v.

brushing. 1. A technique of tactile stimulation using small, electrically rotated brushes over selected dermatomes to elicit muscular responses in the rehabilitation of persons with central nervous system damage. 2. Cleaning with a brush; e.g., toothbrushing.

bruxism (brŭk'sĭzm) [Gr. *brychein,* to grind the teeth, + *-ismos,* condition]. Grinding of the teeth, esp. in children, during sleep. If untreated, bruxism can damage teeth and the temporomandibular joint. In severe cases the teeth are worn down due to attrition.

ETIOL: Psychological stress or abnormalities of tooth occlusion are the principal causes.

TREAT: If condition is due to psychological causes, reduce tension, anxiety, and stress. The teeth should be treated for caries, malocclusion, or periodontal disease. Occlusal guards for the teeth may be of benefit.

Bryant's traction [Sir Thomas Bryant, Brit. surgeon, 1828–1914]. Traction applied to the lower leg with the force pulling vertically. Used esp. in treating fractures of the femur in children.

Bryrel. Trade name for piperazine citrate.

B.S. *Bachelor of Science; Bachelor of Surgery.*

BSE. *breast self-examination.* SEE: *breast, self-examination of,* for illus.

B.S.N. *Bachelor of Science in Nursing.* The degree conferred on a registered nurse who has completed a baccalaureate degree in nursing.

BTE work simulator [Trademark, Baltimore Therapeutic Equipment Company]. A mechanical device with interchangeable handles that simulates the work demands of many jobs and can objectively measure the work output of the user. This device is widely used in rehabilitation settings which evaluate and train injured workers for return to employment.

BTU. *British thermal unit.*

bubo (boo'bō) [Gr. *boubon,* groin, swollen gland] (pl. *buboes*). An inflamed, swollen or enlarged lymph node often exhibiting suppuration, occurring commonly after infective disease due to absorption of infective material. Nodes most commonly affected are those of the groin and axilla.

b., axillary. Bubo in the axilla or armpit.

b., indolent. Bubo in which suppuration does not occur.

b., inguinal. Bubo in the region of the groin.

b., pestilential. Bubo occurring in bubonic plague.

b., venereal. Bubo resulting from a venereal disease. SEE: *lymphogranuloma venereum.*

bubonadenitis (boo-bŏn-ăd-ĕ-nī'tĭs) [" + *aden,* gland, + *itis,* inflammation]. Inflammation of an inguinal gland.

bubonic plague [" + L. *plaga,* stroke, wound]. An acute, infectious disease associated with a high fatality rate. Called the black death in the Middle Ages. SEE: *plague.*

ETIOL: Caused by *Yersinia pestis,* which is usually from infected rats and ground squirrels, and is transmitted to human beings by bite of the rat flea. It is characterized by enlargement of lymphatic glands and severe toxic symptoms, accompanied by intense adenitis or pneumonia.

bucardia (bū-kăr′dē-ă) [Gr. *bous*, ox, + *kardia*, heart]. Severe hypertrophy of the heart. Cor bovinum.

bucca (bŭk′ă) [L., cheek] (pl. *buccae*). [NA] The cheek; fleshy portion of side of face.

buccal (bŭk′ăl). Pert. to the cheek or mouth.

buccal cavity. The mouth.

buccal fat pad. The corpus adiposum or sucking pad, q.v., an encapsulated mass of fat lying superficial to the buccinator muscle. It is well developed in infants and is thought to aid in the act of sucking. SYN: *sucking pad.*

buccal glands. Small saliva-secreting glands situated in the mucous membranes of the mouth.

buccinatolabialis (bŭk″sĭn-ă-tō-lā″bē-ă′lĭs) [L. *buccinator*, trumpeter, + *labialis*, pert. to the lips]. The buccinator and orbicularis oris considered as a single muscle.

buccinator (bŭk′sĭn-ā-tor). The muscle of the cheek. SEE: *Muscles* in *Appendix.*

buccoaxiocervical (bŭk″kō-ăk″sē-ō-sĕr′vĭ-kăl). The angle formed by the intersection of the buccal, axial, and cervical walls of a cavity in a tooth.

buccocervical (bŭk″kō-sĕr′vĭ-kăl). Concerning the buccal surface and cervical margin of a tooth.

buccodistal (bŭk″kō-dĭs′tăl). Concerning the buccal and distal surfaces of a tooth.

buccogingival (bŭk″kō-jĭn′jĭ-văl). Concerning the buccal and gingival surfaces of a tooth.

buccolabial (bŭk″kō-lā′bē-ăl). Concerning the buccal and labial surfaces of a tooth.

buccolingual (bŭk″kō-lĭng′gwăl). Concerning the buccal and lingual surfaces of a tooth.

buccomesial (bŭk″kō-mē′zē-ăl). Concerning the buccal and mesial surfaces of a tooth.

bucco-occlusal (bŭk″kō-ō-kloo′săl). Concerning the buccal and occlusal surfaces of a tooth.

buccopharyngeal (bŭk″kō-fă-rĭn′jē-ăl). Concerning the mouth and pharynx.

buccopulpal (bŭk″kō-pŭl′păl). Concerning the buccal and pulpal surfaces of a tooth.

buccoversion (bŭk″kō-vĕr′zhŭn) [L. *bucca*, cheek, + *versio*, turning]. A tooth that twists in a buccal direction.

buccula (bŭk′ū-lă) [L., a little cheek]. A fold of redundant fatty tissue under the chin. Known as a double chin.

Buck's extension [Gurdon Buck, U.S. surgeon, 1807–1877]. An apparatus consisting of a weight and pulley for applying extension to a limb by attaching it so force will be applied in the long axis of the extremity.

Buck's traction. Traction of the lower extremity applied in line with the long axis of the leg. The force is applied to adhesive tape attached to the skin.

Bucky diaphragm [Gustav P. Bucky, Ger.-born U.S. roentgenologist, 1880–1963]. A grid that is suspended immediately beneath the radiographic table. It is constructed so that the effects of backscatter and secondary radiation are eliminated when radiographs of dense structures are taken.

buclizine hydrochloride (bū′klĭ-zēn). An antihistamine used to treat motion sickness. Trade name is Vibazine.

bud [ME. *budde*, to swell]. 1. In anatomy, a small structure resembling a bud of a plant. 2. In embryology, a small protuberance or outgrowth that is the anlage or primordium of an organ or structure.

 b., taste. An ovoid body embedded in the stratified epithelium of the tongue and also found sparingly on the epiglottis and soft palate. Buds contain the sensory receptors for taste. SEE: *taste cells.*

 b., tooth. The earliest evidence of tooth development. SEE: *enamel organ.*

budding. A method of asexual reproduction in which a budlike process grows from the side or end of the parent and develops into a new organism, which in some cases remains attached and in others separates and lives an independent existence. It is common in lower animals (sponges, coelenterates) and plants (yeasts, molds).

Buerger's disease (bŭr′gĕrz) [Leo Buerger, U.S. physician, 1879–1943]. Thromboangiitis obliterans, q.v.

 SYM: Paresthesia of the foot or pain confined to one toe. Easy fatiguability. Cramps in legs not to be confused with those occurring in the aged. Legs give out, esp. when walking. Ulceration or moist gangrene may set in; amputation may be necessary.

 TREAT: Absolute and continued abstinence from tobacco in all forms is extremely important. Avoid excessive use of affected limb, exposure to temperature extremes, trauma, use of drugs that diminish blood supply to extremities, and fungus infections. If gangrene, pain, or ulceration is present, complete bedrest is advised; if these are absent, patient should walk for 30 min twice daily. For arterial spasm, blocking of the sympathetic nervous system by injection of various drugs or by sympathectomy may be done.

 NURSING IMPLICATIONS: Instruct patient to avoid tight or restrictive clothing, and to avoid sitting or standing in one position for prolonged periods. Patient should not walk barefoot, and shoes and stockings should be carefully fitted. Teach patient to protect extremity from temperature extremes. Explain desired actions and side effects of prescribed medications, and evaluate patient response to therapy. Instruct patient to avoid use of over-the-counter drugs without physician approval. Teach Buerger exercises if prescribed. Encourage participation in support groups to stop smoking. Inspect, and teach patient to inspect tissues for injury, and to report any and all injuries to physician for treatment. SEE: *exercise, Buerger's postural.*

bufa-, bufo- (bū′fã, bū′fō) [L. *bufo,* toad]. Combining form indicating origin from or association with toads.

buffalo hump. Deposition of excess fat in lower midcervical and upper thoracic area of the back. Usually due to excessive adrenocortical hormone production or therapy.

buffer (bŭf′ĕr) [ME. *buffe,* to deaden shock of]. 1. A substance, esp. a salt of the blood, tending to preserve original hydrogen-ion concentration of its solution, upon adding an acid or base. 2. A substance tending to offset reaction of an agent administered in conjunction with it.

   b., blood. Buffer present in the blood. The principal buffers are carbonic acid, carbonates and bicarbonates, monobasic and dibasic phosphates, and proteins. Hemoglobin is an important protein buffer.

buffy coat. Light stratum of blood seen when the blood is centrifuged or allowed to stand in a test tube. The red blood cells settle to the bottom and, between the plasma and the red blood cells, a light-colored layer contains mostly white blood cells. Platelets are at the top of this coat; the next layers, in order, are lymphocytes and monocytes; granulocytes; and reticulocytes.

bufotoxin [L. *bufo,* toad, + Gr. *toxikon,* poison]. A general term for any toxin present in the skin of a toad.

bug. A lay term applied loosely to any small insect or arthropod; more specifically a member of the order Hemiptera, which includes the squash bug, chinch bug, and bedbug. They have sucking mouth parts, incomplete metamorphosis, and two pairs of wings, the fore pair being half membranous. Bugs of medical importance include the following:

   b., assassin. A member of the family Reduviidae. Many are predaceous; others are blood-sucking. *Panstrongylus, Triatoma,* and *Rhodnius* are vectors of trypanosome diseases (Chagas' disease) in humans. SEE: *trypanosomiasis.*

   b., bed-. A member of the family Cimicidae, esp. of the genus *Cimex.* SEE: *bedbug.*

   b., kissing. Several species of the family Reduviidae. *Melanolestes picipes* is the common kissing bug, or black corsair.

   b., red. The larvae of mites of the family Trombiculidae, commonly called chiggers,

q.v.

buggery. Sodomy, q.v.

bulb [L. *bulbus,* bulbous root; Gr. *bolbos*]. Any rounded or globular structure.

   b., aortic. Dilated portion of the truncus arteriosus in the embryo that gives rise to the roots of aorta and pulmonary arteries.

   b., duodenal. Upper duodenal area just beyond pylorus.

   b., hair. Expanded portion at the lower end of the hair root.

   b. of the eye. The eyeball, q.v.

   b. of the urethra. Posterior portion of the corpus spongiosum found between the two crura of the penis.

   b. of the vestibule. Vaginal bulb or bulbus vestibuli, q.v.

   b., olfactory. Anterior enlargement of the olfactory tract.

   b., terminal, of Krause. Encapsulated sensory nerve ending similar in structure to the corpuscles of Pacini. SYN: *corpuscle of Golgi-Mazzoni.*

bulbar. Pert. to or shaped like a bulb.

bulbar paralysis. Paralysis due to changes in motor centers of the oblongata. SEE: *paralysis.*

bulbiform (bŭl′bĭ-form) [″ + *forma,* shape]. Shaped like a bulb.

bulbitis (bŭl-bī′tĭs) [″ + Gr. *itis,* inflammation]. Inflammation of the urethra in its bulbous portion.

bulbocavernosus (bŭl″bō-kăv″ĕr-nō′sŭs) [″ + *cavernosus,* hollow]. A muscle ensheathing the bulb of the penis in the male or covering the bulbus vestibuli in the female. Also called in the male, ejaculator urinae or accelerator urinae; in the female, sphincter vaginae.

bulbocavernosus reflex. Contraction of bulbocavernosus muscle on percussing dorsum of penis.

bulboid (bŭl′boyd) [″ + Gr. *eidos,* form, shape]. Shaped like a bulb.

bulbomimic reflex (bŭl″bō-mĭm′ĭk) [″ + Gr. *mimikos,* imitator]. Contraction of facial muscles following pressure on eyeball.

bulbonuclear (bŭl″bō-nū′klē- är) [″ + *nucleus,* kernel]. Pert. to the nuclei in the medulla oblongata.

bulbospongiosus (bŭl″bō-spŏn″jē-ō′sŭs). One of the three voluntary muscles of the penis. It acts to empty the canal of the urethra after urination and to assist in erection of the corpus cavernosum urethrae. The anterior fibers contribute to penile erection by contracting to compress the deep dorsal vein of the penis.

bulbospongiosus reflex. Contraction of bulbospongiosus muscle on percussing dorsum of penis.

bulbourethral glands (bŭl″bō-ū-rē′thrăl) [″

+ Gr. *ourethra*, urethra]. Cowper's glands. Two small glands, one on each side of the prostate gland, each with a duct about 1 in. (2.5 cm) long, terminating in the wall of the urethra. They secrete a viscid fluid forming part of the seminal fluid. SEE: *prostate; urethra.*

bulbous (bŭl'bŭs) [L. *bulbus*]. Bulb-shaped; swollen; terminating in an enlargement.

bulbus [L.; Gr. *bolbos*]. Bulb, q.v.

b. corpus spongiosum. Bulb of the urethra. A bulbous swelling of the corpus spongiosum penis at the base of the penis.

b. vestibuli. [NA] Two oval masses of erectile tissue lying beneath the vestibule and resting on the urogenital diaphragm. They are homologous to the bulbus spongiosum penis of the male.

bulimia (bū-lĭm'ē-ă) [L.]. Excessive and insatiable appetite.

b. nervosa. A disorder which includes the following characteristics: recurrent episodes of binge eating, self-induced vomiting and diarrhea, excessive exercise, strict dieting or fasting, and an exaggerated concern about body shape and weight. SYN: *bulimorexia.* SEE: *anorexia nervosa.*

bulimic. Pert. to bulimia.

bulk. In nutrition a substance that absorbs water while in the intestinal tract. The increased mass, i.e., bulk, helps to stimulate peristalsis. Bulk materials are used to treat constipation.

bulla (bŭl'lă) [L., a bubble] (pl. *bullae*). A large blister or skin vesicle filled with fluid; a bleb, q.v. SEE: *pompholyx.*

b. ethmoidalis. [NA] A rounded projection into the middle meatus of the nose underneath the middle turbinated bone, formed by an anterior ethmoid cell.

b. ossea. The dilated portion of the bony external meatus of the ear. SEE: *pompholyx.*

bullet wound. Puncture wound from a bullet. SEE: *wound, bullet.*

bullous (bŭl'ŭs) [L. *bulla*, bubble]. Having the nature of a bulla, q.v.

BUN. *blood urea nitrogen.*

bundle. A group of fibers. SYN: *fasciculus,* q.v.; *fasciola.*

b., Arnold's. The frontopontile tract. It passes from the cerebral cortex of the frontal lobe through the internal capsule and cerebral peduncle to the pons.

b., atrioventricular. Bundle of fibers of the impulse-conducting system of the heart. From its origin in the A-V node, it enters the interventricular septum, where it divides into two branches whose fibers pass to the right and left ventricles respectively, the fibers of each trunk becoming continuous with the Purkinje fibers of the ventricles. SYN: *A-V bundle; bundle of His.* SEE: *heart*

block.

b. of His. B., atrioventricular, q.v.

b. of Türck. The temporopontinus tract. Fibers pass from the cerebral cortex of temporal lobe and terminate in the pons.

bundle branch block. ABBR: BBB. A defect in the heart's electrical conduction system in which there is failure of conduction down one of the main branches of the bundle of His. SEE: *heart block.*

b.b.b., left. ABBR: LBBB. Defect in the conduction system of the heart in which the left bundle does not conduct impulses normally.

b.b.b., right. ABBR: RBBB. Defect in the conductive system of the heart in which the right bundle does not conduct impulses normally.

bundling. A mandatory system of drug distribution involving monitoring and reporting side effects to the U.S. Food and Drug Administration.

bunion (bŭn'yŭn). Inflammation and thickening of the bursa of the joint of the great toe, usually associated with marked enlargement of the joint and lateral displacement of the toe.

ETIOL: Heredity; degenerative bone or joint diseases such as arthritis; the wearing of tight-fitting shoes and high heels which force toes together and displace weight onto the forefoot.

Bunnell block. An orthotic device prescribed following surgical repair of flexor tendon hand injuries to prevent flexion at joints proximal to the one being exercised during the rehabilitation regimen.

Bunsen burner (bŭn'sĕn) [Robert W. E. von Bunsen, Ger. chemist, 1811–1899]. A gas burner with an adjustment by which the air holes at the bottom of the tube can be closed or opened. If the holes are closed, the flame burns yellow and gives light but a relatively small amount of heat. By adjusting the air intake, a blue flame is produced. This is the hottest, most efficient and smokeless flame that can be produced by the burner.

Bunyaviridae (bŭn"yă-vĭr'ĭ-dē). A family of viruses that includes a large group of arthropod-borne viruses. Diseases caused by these viruses include certain types of encephalitis, some types of hemorrhagic fevers, phlebotomus fever, and Rift Valley Fever.

buphthalmia, buphthalmos (būf-thăl'mē-ă, -mōs) [Gr. *bous*, ox, + *ophthalmos*, eye]. Condition of infantile glaucoma resulting in uniform enlargement of eye, particularly the cornea. Disease may stop spontaneously or continue until it produces blindness. SEE: *glaucoma; hydrophthalmos.*

TREAT: Iridectomy, sclerotomy, miotics.

bur, burr (bŭr). A device that rotates at high speed and is so designed and held in a special tool to enable dentist to cut by grinding the tooth, bone, or previous restorations.

Burdach's tract (boor′dăks) [Karl F. Burdach, Ger. physiologist, 1776–1847]. Continuation of the dorsolateral column of the spinal cord into the medulla oblongata. SYN: *cuneate fasciculus.*

buret, burette (bū-rĕt′) [Fr.]. A special hollow glass tube usually with a stopcock at the lower end. It is marked so that the amount of liquid released through the outlet will be known. Used in chemical analysis to measure the amount of liquid reagent used.

Burkitt's lymphoma [Denis P. Burkitt, Ugandan physician, b. 1911]. A highly undifferentiated lymphoblastic lymphoma that involves sites other than the lymph nodes and reticuloendothelial system. It is rare in the United States and most common in Central Africa, where the distribution suggests that environmental and climatic factors, such as insect vectors, are determinants. There is a strong association of this disease with the Epstein-Barr virus.

burn [AS. *baernan,* to burn]. Tissue injury resulting from excessive exposure to thermal, chemical, electrical, or radioactive agents. The effects vary according to the type, duration, and intensity of the agent and part of body involved. The effects may be local, resulting in cell injury or death, or both local and systemic, involving primary shock (that occurs immediately after the injury and is rarely fatal) or secondary shock (that develops insidiously following severe burns and is often fatal). Burns are usually classified as:

First degree (minimal depth in skin): Superficial burns, damage being limited to outer layer of the epidermis. Characterized by erythema, hyperemia, tenderness, and pain. No vesiculation.

Second degree (superficial to deep partial thickness of skin): Burns in which damage extends through the epidermis and into the dermis but not of sufficient extent to interfere with regeneration of epidermis. If secondary infection results, the damage from a second-degree burn may be equivalent to that of a third degree. Vesicles usually present.

Third degree (full thickness of skin including tissue beneath skin): Burns in which both epidermis and dermis are destroyed with damage extending into underlying tissues. Tissues may be charred or coagulated. SEE: illus.

COMPLICATIONS (in burns and scalds): Sloughing, gangrene, erysipelas, nephritis, pneumonia, or intestinal disturbances. Sudden attacks of rigor, vomiting, rise of temperature, and convulsions are all suspicious symptoms. A superficial burn covering a large part of the body is more serious than a small, deep one, unless important nerves and blood vessels are involved. If two thirds of the skin is destroyed, death may be expected, even in a burn of the first degree. Shock must always be anticipated regardless of degree of burn.

PRECAUTIONS: Never allow a person whose clothing is burning to run. The individual should lie down and roll. If possible, wrap the individual in a rug, blanket, or anything within reach and smother the flames. Be careful not to allow the individual to inhale the smoke. Cut away the clothing, taking care not to pull any portion of the skin away. Do not open any blisters, as this increases the chance for infection. All burned patients must receive appropriate tetanus prophylaxis.

NOTE: In severe, widespread burns, it is imperative that the patient be transferred to a burn center as soon as practical.

TREAT: The principal points in the initial care of burn patients include immediate evaluation of respiratory system for evidence of respiratory distress or smoke inhalation injury; cardiovascular status; percent of body burned and depth of burns; evaluation of other injuries. Immediate therapy of respiratory distress by use of endotracheal intervention and mechanical ventilation with positive end-expiratory pressure and supplemental oxygen. Volume resuscitation with Ringer's lactate solution calculated as follows: 4 ml/kg of body weight for each percent of body surface area burned. Administer half of this amount during first 8 hours after the burn. Insert nasogastric tube for gastric decompression and Foley catheter to monitor urinary output. Be aware that a stress ulcer (Curling's) may develop in the stomach. SEE: *ulcer, Curling's.*

Emergency Wound Care: Clean burned areas; gently remove old devitalized tissues with aseptic techniques; apply topical antimicrobial agent to all second and third degree burns; cover burns with closed dressing; keep patient warm. If there are circumferential third degrees burns of extremities, assess need for decompressive escharotomies. Do not apply ice or cold dressings because of the risk of hypothermia. Diagnosis of organism causing infection either of the burn sites or systemic infection is followed by appropriate antibiotic therapy and surgical excision of necrotic tissue. Use of artificial skin may be helpful in immediately closing the wound and in improving the quality of the resulting skin cover.

Nutritional therapy is instituted without

BURNS

9% (ENTIRE HEAD AND NECK)

18% (FRONT)

18% (BACK)

RULE OF NINES

9%

9%

1%

18%

18%

ADULT PERCENTAGES

18%

18% (BACK)

9%

9%

1%

13.5%

13.5%

PERCENTAGES IN A CHILD

CLASSIFICATION OF BURNS

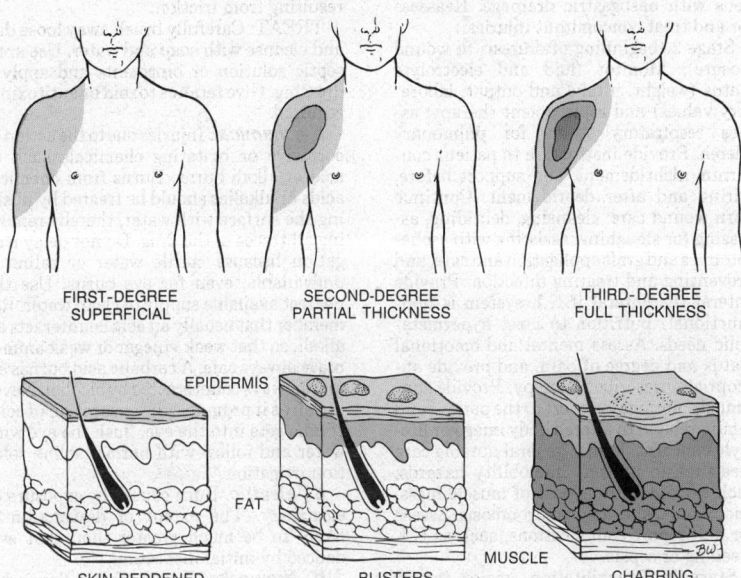

FIRST-DEGREE
SUPERFICIAL

SECOND-DEGREE
PARTIAL THICKNESS

THIRD-DEGREE
FULL THICKNESS

EPIDERMIS

FAT

MUSCLE

SKIN REDDENED

BLISTERS

CHARRING

delay. SEE: *Burn Care Resources* in *Appendix.*

NURSING IMPLICATIONS: Emergency care: Establish a patent airway, flush chemical contact areas, initiate an I.V. line, remove easily separated clothing and soak adherent clothing thoroughly. Cover burn wounds to prevent shock, fluid and heat loss, and pain. Assess for shock symptoms and quickly assess extent of burns using rule of nines, q.v.; assess for concomitant injuries. Transport to burn center as appropriate and available.

Stage 1 (injury onset to full resuscitation): Maintain a patent airway and provide adequate ventilation and oxygenation; monitor arterial blood gas values; assess for inhalation injury and respiratory distress, initiate mechanical ventilation if required. Carefully removing soaked adherent clothing and initial dressings, assess depth and extent of burns, repeating assessment periodically. Weigh patient and begin fluid replacement therapy according to an established formula to manage fluid shift to tissue spaces, fluid loss, and shock. Monitor serum electrolyte levels, urinary output, and vital signs. Initiate aseptic wound care; administer prescribed tetanus prophylaxis and antibiotics; and provide pain relief and emotional support. Assess G.I. function and prevent or manage gastric dilatation and ileus with nasogastric drainage. Reassess for and treat concomitant injuries.

Stage 2 (beginning of diuresis to wound closure): Monitor fluid and electrolyte status (weight, intake and output, laboratory values) and replacement therapy; assess respiratory status for pulmonary edema. Provide instruction to patient concerning debridement, and support before, during and after debridement. Continue burn wound care: cleansing, debriding, assessing for sloughing, assisting with escharotomies and graft application and care, and preventing and treating infection. Provide enteral (parenteral if G.I. system is nonfunctional) nutrition to meet hypermetabolic needs. Assess mental and emotional status and degree of pain, and provide appropriate prescribed therapy. Provide continued emotional support to the patient and family related to altered body image or lifestyle concerns. Utilize general nursing care measures to prevent immobility hazards, such as contractures, loss of muscle mass, pneumonia, and venous thrombosis. Assess for and report complications, such as G.I. bleeding or sepsis.

Stage 3: Rehabilitation (major wound closure to return to optimal physical and psychological function): Continue interventions to heal remaining wounds, protect healed wounds. Use individually fitted elastic garments to prevent hypertrophic scar formation, and exercise to promote full joint range-of-motion. While providing adequate rest, encourage patient to increase activity tolerance and endurance. Promote physical and emotional independence, and support patient and family through resumption of vocational and social functioning. Explain that further cosmetic and reconstructive surgery may be required. Inform patient and family about available support groups and services. SEE: *Nursing Diagnoses* in *Appendix.*

b., acid. Burn caused by exposure to corrosive acids such as sulfuric, hydrochloric, and nitric.

F.A.: Wash with large volumes of water; apply dilute alkalies such as baking soda (sodium bicarbonate) paste, soap solution dressing, and chalk paste. Follow by application of a bland oil or ointment.

b., alkali. Burn caused by caustic alkalies such as lye, caustic potash (potassium hydroxide), and caustic soda (sodium hydroxide).

SYM: Painful lesion of skin often associated with gelatinization of tissue.

F.A.: Wash with large volumes of water. Dress with bland ointments.

b., brush. A combined burn and abrasion resulting from friction.

TREAT: Carefully brush away loose dirt and cleanse with soap and water. Use antiseptic solution or ointments and apply a dressing. Give tetanus toxoid or antitoxin if required.

b., chemical. Injuries due to the action of corrosive or irritating chemicals such as acid or alkali burns. Burns from chemical acids or alkalies should be treated by flushing the surface with water, thereby removing all traces of the drug. Do not delay irrigation because sterile water or saline is unavailable, even for eye burns. Use the nearest available supply of clean water. Remember that usually an acid counteracts an alkali, so that weak vinegar or weak ammonia is always safe. A carbolic acid burn is almost always counteracted by alcohol. Never use oil as it promotes the absorption of acid. If lime gets into the eye, flush the eye with water and follow with normal saline solution irrigation.

b., electric. Burn caused by exposure to electricity. The extent of destruction is likely to be much greater than that evidenced by initial inspection.

b., fireworks. Injury from fireworks; usually a burn, often with embedded foreign bodies and a high incidence of infection and tetanus, which should be prevented by meticulous care of injury and use of antitetanus serum.

b., flash. A burn resulting from an explosive blast such as occurs from ignition of highly inflammable fluids, or in war from a high-explosive shell or a nuclear blast.

b., gunpowder. Burn resulting from exploding gunpowder. It is often followed by tetanus, which should be prevented by administration of antitetanus serum and meticulous care of injury area.

b., inhalation. Burn in which flames or very hot gases have been inhaled. Suspect in all patients with facial burns or with singed nose hairs or elevated carboxyhemoglobin greater than 5 in arterial blood gases. Major complication is airway obstruction from edema of air passages. SYN: *respiratory burn.*

TREAT: Usual treatment is early intubation and ventilatory management with high oxygen levels and positive end-expiratory pressure or constant positive airway pressure.

b. of eye. Burn of eyeball due to contact with chemical, thermal, electrical, or radioactive agents.

F.A.: Wash immediately with the nearest available supply of water. Do not delay because water is not sterile or cool. Irrigation may need to be continued for hours if burn is due to lye.

b., radiation. Burn resulting from overexposure to radiant energy as from roentgen rays, radium emanations, sunlight, or nuclear blast.

b., respiratory. Burn in which the respiratory tract is injured, as from inhalation of hot gases. SYN: *inhalation burn.*

b., thermal. Burn resulting from contact with fire, hot objects, or fluids.

b., x-ray. SEE: *b., radiation.*

Burnett's syndrome [Charles Hoyt Burnett, U.S. physician, 1913–1967]. Milk-alkali syndrome, q.v.

burning foot syndrome. A sensation of burning of the sole of the foot. Occurs in certain vitamin deficiencies and in patients with chronic renal failure, due to build-up of toxic waste products.

burning mouth syndrome. Sensation of burning of the oral mucosa. The mucosa is normal. The pain is present upon awakening and becomes worse as the day goes on. A variety of conditions may cause this including tongue thrusting, diabetes, Candida infections, inadequate saliva, allergy, and psychological factors such as anxiety or depression.

TREAT: Therapy for the causative condition(s).

burnish (bĕr'nĭsh). To condense or polish a metal surface by smooth metal instrument; e.g., in dentistry, a gold filling.

burnisher (bĕr'nĭsh-ĕr). An instrument with a blade or nib for smoothing the margins of a dental restoration.

burnout. 1. Rendering unserviceable by excessive heat. 2. Condition resulting from chronic job stress. Characterized by physical and emotional exhaustion and sometimes physical illness. Frustration from a perceived inability to end the stresses and problems associated with this lack of power in the job contribute to the individual's loss of concern for patients or good job performance. Nurses are especially prone to burnout, particularly those working in highly stressful conditions.

b., radiographic. Loss of radiographic detail by excessive exposure.

b., wax. Removal of an invested wax pattern from a mold by heating, thereby preparing the mold for casting metal. SYN: *inlay burnout.*

Buro-sol Concentrate. Trade name for aluminum acetate topical solution.

Burow's solution [Karl August von Burow, Ger. surgeon, 1809–1874]. Solution of aluminum acetate. Used in dermatology as a drying agent for weeping skin lesions.

burr. SEE: *bur.*

burrow (bŭr'rō). A tunnel made in the skin by the itch mite, *Sarcoptes scabiei.*

burrowing. The formation of a subcutaneous tunnel made by a parasite or of a fistula or sinus containing pus.

bursa (bŭr'să) [Gr., a leather sack] (pl. *bursae*). 1. A padlike sac or cavity found in connecting tissue usually in the vicinity of joints. It is lined with synovial membrane and contains a fluid, synovia, that acts to reduce friction between tendon and bone, tendon and ligament, or between other structures where friction is likely to occur. 2. A blind sac or cavity.

b., Achilles. Bursa located between the tendon of Achilles and the calcaneus.

b., adventitious. Bursa not usually present but that develops in response to friction or pressure.

b., olecranon. Bursa at the elbow joint lying between olecranon process and the skin.

b., omental. The lesser peritoneal cavity; the cavity of the great omentum. It communicates with the greater or true peritoneal cavity via the vestibule and epiploic foramen.

b., patellar. One of several bursae located in the region of the patella. Includes the suprapatellar, infrapatellar, and prepatellar bursae. Some communicate with the cavity of the knee joint.

b., pharyngeal. Small, median, blind sac found in lower portion of the pharyngeal tonsil.

b., subacromial. Large bursa lying between the acromion and coracoacromial ligament above and the insertion of the supraspinatus muscle below. Also known as subdeltoid bursa.

bursae (bŭr'sē). Pl. of bursa, q.v.

bursal (bŭr'săl). Pert. to a bursa.

bursalis (bŭr-săl'ĭs) [L., pert. to a bursa]. Obturator internus muscle.

bursectomy (bŭr-sĕk'tō-mē) [Gr. _bursa,_ a leather sack, + _ektome,_ excision]. Excision of a bursa.

bursitis (bŭr-sī'tĭs) [" + _itis,_ inflammation]. Inflammation of a bursa, esp. those located between bony prominences and muscle or tendon, as the shoulder and knee. Common forms include painful shoulder (SEE: _bursa, subacromial_), miner's or tennis elbow (SEE: _bursa, olecranon_), housemaid's knee (prepatellar bursitis), and bunion, q.v. SEE: _Nursing Diagnoses_ in _Appendix._

TREAT: Rest and immobilization of affected part during acute stage. Active mobilization as soon as acute symptoms subside will help to prevent adhesions. Analgesics, heat, and diathermy are helpful. Injection of local anesthetics or cortisone into bursa may be required. In chronic bursitis, surgical removal of calcification may be necessary.

NURSING IMPLICATIONS: Encourage patient to rest and to restrict movement of the affected part if there are pain and loss of range of motion of a joint. Medical evaluation should be done if pain and loss of function are severe and do not improve with rest. Physical therapy may be needed.

b., anserine. Inflammation of the sartorius bursa located over the medial side of the tibia just below the knee. This causes pain upon climbing stairs.

bursolith (bŭr'sō-lĭth) [" + _lithos,_ stone]. A calculus formed in a bursa.

bursopathy (bŭr-sŏp'ă-thē) [" + _pathos,_ disease, suffering]. Any pathological condition of a bursa.

bursotomy (bŭr-sŏt'ō-mē) [" + _tome,_ incision]. Incision of a bursa.

bursula (bŭr'sū-lă) [L., little sack]. A small bursa.

b. testium. The scrotum.

Burton's line (bŭr'tŏns) [Henry Burton, Brit. physician, 1799–1849]. A blue line along the margin of the gingiva visible in chronic lead poisoning.

bus (bŭs). In electronics, one or more conductors over which information from one or

more sources is transmitted to one or more destinations.

bush tea disease. Veno-occlusive disease of the liver due to ingesting of pyrrolidizine alkaloids present in some herbal teas.

busulfan (bū-sŭl'făn). USP. An antineoplastic agent used in treating chronic granulocytic leukemia. Trade name is Myleran.

butacaine sulfate (bū'tă-kān). USP. A topical local anesthetic. Trade name is Butyn Sulfate.

butamben (bū-tăm'bĕn). USP. An anesthetic agent that is used topically. It is poorly and slowly absorbed and thus does not cause systemic toxicity. Trade name is Butesin.

butane (bū'tān). C_4H_{10}. A gaseous, inflammable hydrocarbon derived from petroleum.

Butazolidin (bū"tă-zōl'ĭ-dĭn). Trade name for phenylbutazone, USP, used in treatment of acute rheumatic disease. It has a potent anti-inflammatory action.

Butisol Sodium (bū'tĭ-sōl sō'dē-ŭm). Trade name for butabarbital sodium, USP, a sedative and hypnotic.

butt [ME. _butte,_ end]. To join the ends of two objects together.

butterfly. 1. Anything shaped like a butterfly. 2. An adhesive bandage used in place of sutures to hold wound edges together.

butterfly rash. Skin rash of both cheeks joined by an extension across the bridge of the nose. Seen in systemic lupus erythematosus, esp. after the patient's face has been exposed to sunlight. Also seen in seborrheic dermatitis, tuberous sclerosis, q.v., and dermatomyositis, q.v. SEE: _lupus erythematosus._

buttocks (bŭt'ŭks) [AS. _buttuc,_ end]. The external prominences posterior to the hips. Formed by the gluteal muscles and underlying structures. SYN: _nates._

button (bŭt'n). 1. An anatomical or pathological structure that resembles a button. 2. A medical device shaped like a button.

button aid. An adaptive aid permitting button closure by persons with the functional use of only one extremity.

buttonhole. A straight cut through the wall of a cavity.

button suture. Suture in which threads are passed through buttons on the surface and tied to prevent thread from cutting through or into underlying tissue.

butylene (bū'tĭ-lēn). A hydrocarbon gas, C_4H_8.

butyraceous (bū"tĭ-rā'shŭs) [L. _butyrum,_ butter]. Containing or resembling butter.

butyrate (bū'tĭ-rāt). A salt of butyric acid.

butyric acid (bū-tĭr'ĭk) [L. _butyrum,_ butter]. C_3H_7COOH. A fatty acid derived from butter but rare in most fats. It is a viscid liquid with a rancid odor. Used in disinfectants, emulsifying agents, and pharmaceuticals.

butyrin (bū′tĭr-ĭn). A soft, yellow semiliquid fat that is present in butter.

butyroid (bū′tĭ-royd) [″ + Gr. *eidos,* form, shape]. Having the appearance or consistency of butter.

butyrometer (bū″tĭ-rŏm′ĕ-tĕr) [″ + Gr. *metron,* measure]. Device for estimating amount of butterfat in milk.

butyrophenone (bū″tĭ-rō-fē′nōn). A class of chemicals, some of which are useful in treating mental disorders. One, haloperidol, USP, is particularly useful in treating Gilles de la Tourette's syndrome.

butyrous (būt′ĭ-rŭs). Of butterlike consistency.

Byler's disease. An inherited disorder in which infants develop cholestatic jaundice and, gradually, cirrhosis. A high incidence of retinitis pigmentosa is associated with this disease, and mental retardation is frequently seen in the children. Death from liver disease occurs by adolescence.

bypass. A means of circumvention; a shunt. It is surgically possible to install an alternate route for the blood to bypass an obstruction if a main or vital artery such as the abdominal aorta or a coronary artery becomes obstructed. The various procedures are named according to the arteries involved.

Ex.: coronary artery, aortoiliac, or femoropopliteal bypasses. The heart itself may be bypassed by providing an extracorporeal device to pump blood while a surgical procedure is being done on the heart.

bysma (bĭs′mä) [Gr., plug]. A plug or tampon.

byssinosis (bĭs″ĭ-nō′sĭs) [Gr. *byssos,* cotton, + *osis,* condition]. Pneumoconiosis of cotton, flax, and hemp workers. Characterized by wheezing and tightness in the chest, it is caused by the inhalation of dust and foreign materials contained therein, including bacteria, mold, and fungi. The disease does not occur in textile workers who work with cotton after it is bleached. Symptoms are usually more pronounced at the beginning of each work week than later on. SEE: *pneumonoconiosis.*

byssocausis (bĭs″ō-kaw′sĭs) [″ + *kausis,* burning]. Cauterization by moxa; moxibustion, q.v.

byssoid (bĭs′oyd) [″ + *eidos,* form, shape]. Consisting of a filamentous fringe, the filaments being of unequal length.

byte (bīt). Computers work with binary numbers made up of zeros and ones (0's and 1's). A bit, q.v., is a single number in a binary digit. Bits used by a computer are grouped into larger units. A group of eight bits is called a byte. SEE: *binary system; bit.*

C

C. 1. Chem. symb. for the element carbon. 2. *kilocalorie* (when capitalized) and *calorie* (if not capitalized); *Celsius* (scale or thermometer); *centigrade*; L. *centum*, one hundred; *circa*, about; *clonus; closure; compound; congius* (gallon); L. *cum*, with. In handwritten notes or medical charts, this is usually written c̄.

^{14}C. Radioactive carbon.

CA 125. An antigen produced by tissues derived from coelomic epithelium. It is associated with various epithelial cancers, including ovarian cancer. It may be used experimentally to assess response to treatment in women with known ovarian cancer.

Ca. 1. Chem. symb. for the element calcium. 2. *cathode.*

CABG. *coronary artery bypass graft.*

Cabot's ring bodies (kăb′ŏts). [Richard C. Cabot, U.S. physician, 1868–1939] Blue-staining threadlike inclusions in the red blood cells in severe anemia. They may appear as rings, figures-of-eight, or twisted. Their origin is unknown.

cac-, caci-, caco- [Gr. *kakos*, bad]. Prefix denoting bad or diseased.

CaC₂. Calcium carbide.

cacanthrax (kăk-ăn′thrăks) [″ + *anthrax*, carbuncle]. Anthrax.

cacao (kă-kā′ō, kă-kaw′ō) [Mex.-Sp. from Nahuatl *cacahuatl*, cacao beans]. 1. Seed of *Theobroma cacao* used to prepare cacao butter (theobroma oil), chocolate, and cocoa. 2. A reddish to brown powder prepared from the roasted ripe seeds of *Theobroma cacao* (family Sterculiaceae), having a chocolate odor and taste. Used in a syrup base, as a flavoring vehicle for certain medications, in beverages, and confections.

cachectic (kă-kĕk′tĭk) [Gr. *kakos*, bad, + *hexis*, condition]. Pert. to cachexia.

cachectins. Tumor necrosis factors, q.v.

cachet (kă-shā′) [Fr., a seal]. Two concave pieces of wafer (rice paper) between which medicine is placed. The margins of the wafer are sealed together. Used for administering medicines with an unpleasant taste. It is swallowed whole.

cachexia (kă-kĕks′ē-ă) [Gr. *kakos*, bad, + *hexis*, condition]. A state of ill health, malnutrition, and wasting. It may occur in many chronic diseases, certain malignancies, and advanced pulmonary tuberculosis.

NURSING IMPLICATIONS: Monitor patient's response to activity to prevent fatigue. Encourage frequent rest periods and space activities based upon patient's response. Provide oral hygiene. Supply high-calorie, high-nutrient, concentrated soft foods and fluids to reduce effort required in eating. Reposition patient frequently to promote ventilatory excursions, mobilize secretions, and prevent skin breakdown. Inspect skin and protect tissues from pressure, using flotation pads and mattresses and other assistive devices. Handle patient gently, supporting joints when moving, to prevent pain and pathologic fractures. Monitor elimination to prevent retention of urine or stool, and to protect skin integrity and patient's self-esteem if incontinence is present. Offer assistance to patient and family in coping with feelings about change in body image, illness state, and approaching death. SEE: *decubitus ulcer; death.*

c., cancerous. Cachexia caused by a cancerous condition.

c. hypophysiopriva. Symptoms resulting from total loss of function of the pituitary gland.

c., lymphatic. Cachexia caused by Hodgkin's disease of the lymph nodes.

c., malarial. Cachexia due to chronic malaria.

c., pituitary. Group of symptoms caused by atrophy of pituitary gland, including emaciation, premature aging, atrophy of genitals with loss of secondary sex characteristics, and lowering of basal metabolic rate. SYN: *Simmonds' disease.*

c., strumipriva. Cachexia due to removal of the thyroid gland.

cachinnation (kăk-ĭ-nā′shŭn) [L. *cachinnare*, to laugh aloud]. Excessive, inappropriate, loud laughter. May be associated with schizophrenia.

CaCl₂. Calcium chloride; a bleaching powder.

caco-, cac-, caci- [Gr. *kakos*, bad]. Prefix denoting bad or diseased.

CaCO₃. Calcium carbonate; chalk.

CaC₂O₄. Calcium oxalate.

cacodylate (kăk′ō-dĭl-āt). A salt of cacodylic acid.

cacogenesis (kăk″ō-jĕn′ĕ-sĭs) [″ + *genesis*, generation, birth]. Any abnormal development or growth.

cacogenic (kăk″ō-jĕn′ĭk). Pert. to cacogenesis.

cacogeusia (kăk″ō-gū′sē-ă) [″ + *geusis*, taste]. The presence of an unpleasant taste in the mouth.

cacoplastic (kăk″ō-plăs′tĭk) [″ + *plastikos*, formed]. 1. Pert. to or causing morbid growth. 2. Incapable of normal development or formation.

cacorhythmic (kăk″ō-rĭth′mĭk) [″ +

rhythmos, rhythm]. Showing irregularity of rhythm.

cacosmia (kă-kŏz'mē-ă) [" + *osme,* smell]. 1. An unpleasant odor. 2. Subjective perception of a disagreeable odor. SYN: *kakosmia.* SEE: *hallucination, olfactory; parosmia.*

cacotrophy (kăk-ŏt'rō-fē) [" + *trophe,* nourishment]. Malnutrition.

cacumen (kăk-ū'mĕn) [L. *cacumen,* summit] (pl. *cacumina*). 1. Anterior portion of the superior vermis of the cerebellum. SYN: *culmen.* 2. The top or apex of a plant.

CAD. *coronary artery disease; computer-assisted design.*

cadaver (kă-dăv'ĕr) [L. *cadere,* to fall, die] (pl. *cadavera*). A dead body; a corpse. Term usually applied to a body used for dissection.

cadaveric (kă-dăv'ĕr-ĭk). Pert. to a dead body.

cadaverine (kă-dăv'ĕr-ĭn). A malodorous substance, pentamethylenediamine, produced by the bacterial decomposition of proteins. May occur in the urine in cystinuria.

cadaverous (kă-dăv'ĕr-ŭs). Resembling, esp. having the color or appearance of, a corpse.

cadence (kā'dĕns). Rhythmic movement or beat as in marching or dancing.

cadmiosis (kăd-mē-ō'sĭs). A form of pneumoconiosis, q.v., due to inhalation of tissue reaction to cadmium dust.

cadmium (kăd'mē-ŭm) [Gr. *kadmia,* earth]. SYMB: Cd. At. wt. 112.40; at. no. 48; sp. gr. 8.65. A metallic element present in zinc ores. It is a soft, bluish-white metal and is used industrially in electroplating and in atomic reactors. Its salts are poisonous. SEE: *Poisons and Poisoning* in *Appendix.*

caduceus (kă-dū'sē-ŭs) [L., a herald's wand]. In mythology, the wand or staff that belonged to Apollo. It was given to Hermes or Mercury. It consists of two serpents entwined around a staff, surmounted by two wings. Used as the medical insignia of certain groups such as the U.S. Army Medical Corps. Even though it is sometimes used to symbolize the medical profession, the staff of Aesculapius, q.v., Roman god of medicine, is usually considered to be the more appropriate symbol.

caelotherapy (sē"lō-thĕr'ă-pē) [L. *caelum,* heaven, + Gr. *therapeia,* treatment]. Therapy utilizing religion or religious symbols.

café au lait macules. Pale brown areas of increased melanin in the skin. The sites are usually 0.8 to 8 in. (2 to 20 cm) in diameter with irregular borders. They appear in infancy and tend to disappear with age. These macules are common and can occasionally be markers for systemic disease including neurofibromatosis.

Cafergot. Trade name for a combination of caffeine and ergotamine tartrate.

caffeine (kăf'ēn, kă-fēn'). USP. $C_8H_{10}N_4O_2$. An alkaloid present in coffee, chocolate, tea, many "cola" drinks, cocoa, and over-the-counter medicines such as Anacin, Excedrin, No-Doz, and Vivarin. The amount of caffeine received when coffee, decaffeinated coffee, tea, and cola drinks are ingested varies with respect to the strength of the preparation of brewed coffee or tea as well as the size of the container used for dispensing these beverages. Caffeine in 180 ml (6 oz) of coffee varies from 110 to 150 mg; in decaffeinated coffee, from 2 to 5 mg; and from 20 to 46 mg in 150 ml (5 oz) of tea. The caffeine in cola drinks has been found to range from 30 to 60 mg in a 360 ml (12 oz) serving; but caffeine-free cola drinks are available.

The pharmacologic action of caffeine includes: central nervous system stimulation; stimulates gastric acid and pepsin secretion; elevates free fatty acids in plasma; acts as a diuretic; increases basal metabolic rate; decreases total sleep time; and may increase blood sugar level. In athletic endeavors caffeine is considered to be an ergogenic aid in that it tends to enhance endurance and improves reaction time. The possibility that caffeine contributes to cardiovascular disease, various cancers, and birth defects has been investigated. These studies have not provided definitive answers.

SYM: The toxic effects of large doses of caffeine include insomnia, restlessness, and excitement as early signs; later, this may progress to mild delirium. Tachycardia, extrasystoles, and hyperpnea also may be present.

c. and sodium benzoate. A mixture of equal parts of caffeine and sodium benzoate. Used as a CNS stimulant.

c. and sodium salicylate. A mixture of caffeine with sodium salicylate, containing about 52% caffeine. Combines action of caffeine, q.v., and salicylate. SEE: *salicylate, sodium.*

c., citrate. A mixture of equal parts of caffeine and citric acid. Used as a CNS stimulant.

caffeine intoxication. Following ingestion of excess caffeine, usually in excess of 250 mg, the onset of at least five of the following will be experienced: symptoms of restlessness, nervousness, excitement, insomnia, flushed face, diuresis, gastrointestinal disturbance, muscle twitching, rambling flow of thought and speech, tachycardia or arrhythmia, periods of inexhaustibility, or psychomotor agitation. In addition, evidence of other physical or mental disorders such as anxiety disorder must be ruled out. SYN: caffeinism. SEE: *aminophylline* in *Poisons and Poisoning* in *Appendix*.

caffeinism (kăf′ĕn-ĭzm). Caffeine intoxication, q.v.

Caffey, John (kăf′fē). U.S. pediatrician, 1895–1966.

C.'s disease. Infantile cortical hyperostosis.

cage, Faraday. A room or space entirely enclosed within a wire mesh to prevent electromagnetic interference with electronic devices.

cage, thoracic. The soft tissue and bones enclosing the thorax.

CAH. *congenital adrenal hyperplasia.*

C.A.H.E.A. *Committee on Allied Health Education and Accreditation.*

CAI. *computer assisted instruction.*

cainotophobia (kī-nō″tō-fō′bē-ă) [Gr. *kainotes*, novelty, + *phobos*, fear]. Fear of novelty. SYN: *cenotophobia*.

caisson disease (kā′sŏn) [Fr. *caisse*, a box]. A condition that develops in divers subjected to rapid reduction of air pressure after coming to the surface following exposure to compressed air. The cause is nitrogen bubbles in the tissue spaces and small blood vessels. Symptoms appear when a diver is exposed to a depth of 30 feet (9.1 meters) or greater for sufficient time for the tissues to be saturated with nitrogen, and then ascends to the surface rapidly; or when an aviator ascends rapidly in an unpressurized aircraft from sea level to 18,000 feet (5486 meters) or higher.

SYM: Deep boring, usually constant pain in joints; itching or burning of the skin; burning sensation in lungs and coughing; and a variety of neurological signs.

TREAT: Recompression and then slow decompression. This is done in a special hyperbaric chamber. SYN: *decompression illness*. SEE: *bends*.

caked breast. Accumulation of milk in the secreting ducts of the breast following delivery. SEE: *breast*.

Cal. *large Calorie.* Also abbr. C. One large Calorie is equal to 1000 calories. A large Calorie may be noted by capitalizing the initial letter of the word or by using kilocalorie (abbr. kcal). This measure of heat or energy is used to indicate the amount of heat that can be provided by food; and by the energy expressed in Calories required for physical activity. SYN: *kcal*. SEE: *calorimeter*.

cal. *small calorie.* Also abbr. c. When a small calorie is indicated the initial letter should not be capitalized, to differentiate from a kilocalorie or large Calorie. SEE: *Cal.*

calamine (kăl′ă-mīn). USP. A pink powder, containing zinc oxide with small amt. of ferric oxide. Used externally in various skin conditions as a protective and astringent, as an ointment, or as a lotion.

calamus scriptorius [L.]. Inferior portion of the floor of the fourth ventricle of the brain. It is shaped like a pen and lies between the restiform bodies.

calcaneal, calcanean (kăl-kā′nē-ăl, -ăn) [L. *calcaneus*, heel]. Pert. to the calcaneus, the heel bone.

calcaneoapophysitis (kăl-kā′nē-ō-ă-pŏf″ē-zī′tĭs) [″ + Gr. *apophysis*, offshoot, + *itis*, inflammation]. Pain and inflammation of the posterior portion of the calcaneus at the place of insertion of the Achilles tendon.

calcaneocuboid (kăl-kā″nē-ō-kū′boyd) [″ + Gr. *kubos*, cube, + *eidos*, form, shape]. Concerning the calcaneum and cuboid bone.

calcaneodynia (kăl-kā″nē-ō-dĭn′ē-ă) [″ + Gr. *odyne*, pain]. Pain in the heel.

calcaneofibular (kăl-kā″nē-ō-fĭb′ū-lăr) [″ + *fibula*, pin]. Concerning the calcaneum and fibula.

calcaneonavicular (kăl-kā″nē-ō-nă-vĭk′ū-lăr) [″ + *navicula*, boat]. Concerning the calcaneum and navicular bone.

calcaneoscaphoid (kăl-kā″nē-ō-skă′foyd) [″ + Gr. *skaphe*, skiff, + *eidos*, form, shape]. Concerning the calcaneum and scaphoid bone.

calcaneotibial (kăl-kā″nē-ō-tĭb′ē-ăl) [″ + *tibia*, shinbone]. Concerning the calcaneum and tibia.

calcaneum (kăl-kā′nē-ŭm) [L. *calcaneus*, heel] (pl. *calcanea*). Calcaneus.

calcaneus (kăl-kā′nē-ŭs) [L.] (pl. *calcanei*). 1. [NA] The heel bone, or os calcis. It articulates with the cuboid bone and with the talus. 2. Talipes calcaneus.

calcanodynia (kăl″kăn-ō-dĭn′ē-ă) [″ + Gr. *odyne*, pain]. Pain in the heel when standing or walking; calcaneodynia.

calcar (kăl′kăr) [L., a spur]. A spurlike process.

c. avis. [NA] Lower of two elevations on inner wall of posterior horn of lateral ventricle of brain. SYN: *hippocampus minor*.

c. femorale. A bony spur that strengthens the femoral neck.

c. pedis. The heel.

calcareous (kăl-kā′rē-ŭs) [L. *calcarius*, of lime]. Of the nature of lime; chalky.

calcarine (kăl′kăr-ĭn) [L. *calcar*, spur]. Spur-shaped.

calcariuria (kăl-kăr″ē-ū′rē-ă) [L. *calcarius*, of lime, + Gr. *ouron*, urine]. Presence of calcium lime salts in the urine.

calcaroid (kăl′kăr-oyd) [L. *calcar*, spur, + Gr. *eidos*, form, shape]. Deposit in brain tissue that resembles calcification.

calcemia (kăl-sē′mē-ă) [L. *calx*, lime, + Gr. *haima*, blood]. Increased calcium in the blood.

calcic (kăl'sĭk) [L. *calcarius*]. Pert. to calcium or lime.

calcicosis (kăl″sĭ-kō'sĭs) [L. *calx*, lime, + Gr. *osis*, infection]. Pneumoconiosis caused by inhaling dust from limestone (marble).

calciferol (kăl-sĭf'ĕr-ŏl). Vitamin D₂. A synthetic vitamin D. It has the most vitamin D activity of those substances derived from ergosterol. Used for prophylaxis and treatment of vitamin D deficiency, rickets, and hypocalcemic tetany. SYN: *ergocalciferol.*

calciferous (kăl-sĭf'ĕr-ŭs) [″ + *ferre*, to carry]. Containing calcium, chalk, or lime.

calcific (kăl-sĭf'ĭk) [″ + *facere*, to make]. Forming or composed of lime.

calcification (kăl″sĭ-fĭ-kā'shŭn). Process in which organic tissue becomes hardened by the deposition of lime salts in the tissues.

   c., arterial. Deposition of calcium in walls of arteries.

   c., metastatic. Calcification of soft tissue with transference of calcium from bone, as in osteomalacia and disease of the parathyroid glands.

   c., Mönckeberg's. Calcium deposit in the media of arteries.

calcific tendinitis. Deposition of calcium in chronically inflamed tendon, esp. the tendons of the shoulder.

calcigerous (kăl-sĭj'ĕr-ŭs) [″ + *gerere*, to bear]. Containing calcium or lime salts.

Calcimar. Trade name for calcitonin.

calcination (kăl″sĭ-nā'shŭn) [L. *calcinare*, to char]. Drying by roasting to produce a powder.

calcine (kăl'sĭn). To expel water and volatile materials by heating to a high temperature. Lime is formed from limestone in this manner by the removal of carbon dioxide.

calcinosis (kăl″sĭ-nō'sĭs) [L. *calx*, lime, + Gr. *osis*, condition]. Condition marked by abnormal deposition of lime salts in tissues.

   c. circumscripta. Subcutaneous calcification.

calcipectic (kăl″sĭ-pĕk'tĭk) [″ + Gr. *pexis*, fixation]. Pert. to calcipexis, q.v.

calcipenia (kăl″sĭ-pē'nē-ă) [″ + Gr. *penia*, poverty]. Calcium deficiency in body tissues and fluids.

calcipexis, calcipexy (kăl″sĭ-pĕk'sĭs, -pĕk'sē) [″ + Gr. *pexis*, fixation]. Fixation of calcium in body tissues.

calciphylaxis (kăl″sĭ-fĭ-lăk'sĭs) [″ + Gr. *phylaxis*, protection]. A state of induced tissue sensitivity characterized by calcification of tissue when challenged by an appropriate stimulus.

calciprivia (kăl″sĭ-prĭv'ē-ă) [″ + *privus*, without]. Deficiency or absence of calcium.

calcitonin (kăl″sĭ-tō'nĭn). Hormone from the thyroid gland in man important in bone and

calcium metabolism. In other mammals, it is produced by the ultimobranchial bodies, which become fused with the thyroid; for that reason, it formerly was designated thyrocalcitonin.

calcitriol. A metabolite of vitamin D that promotes the absorption of calcium and phosphate in the intestines and their deposition in bone tissue.

calcium (kăl'sē-ŭm) [L. *calx*, lime]. SYMB: Ca. At. wt. 40.08; at. no. 20. Silver-white metallic element, a major component of limestone.

   Lime, CaO, is its oxide. Calcium phosphate constitutes 75% of body ash and about 85% of mineral matter in bones. SEE: "*calci-*" words.

   FUNCT: Calcium must be carried by the blood in solution in order to be available for bone growth and metabolism. Unless certain activating substances, such as vitamin D, are present, increased calcium intake does not affect the tissues or blood calcium. The secretions of the parathyroid glands are a factor in the utilization of calcium, making it possible for the blood to carry dissolved calcium. Even though some foods may influence calcium absorption, none of these is believed to be of importance in persons whose intake of calcium is typical for the diet of individuals living in the U.S.

   Calcium is of great importance in blood coagulation; gives firmness and rigidity to bones and teeth; is important in acid-base balance; is essential for lactation; is important in activating enzymes; is essential for the function of nerves and muscles, including the myocardium, and for maintaining the permeability of membranes.

   Calcium is taken into the body as a constituent of various foods. While much of it may prove insoluble and escape absorption, some of it passes through the intestine into the blood, where it can be measured by chemical tests. Its level in the serum is normally 8.5 to 10.5 mg/dl. Low blood calcium causes tetany with muscular twitching, spasms, and convulsions. Blood deprived of its calcium will not clot; and it is essential for the curdling of milk.

   Calcium is deposited in the bones but can be mobilized again to keep the blood level constant when there is a period of insufficient intake. At any given time the body of an adult contains about 700 gm of calcium phosphate; of this, 120 gm are the element calcium. Ordinarily an adult takes in 0.8 gm of calcium per day. During pregnancy, 1.3 gm of calcium a day will be required.

   SOURCES: *Excellent:* beans; cauliflower; chard; cheese; cream; egg yolk; kale; milk; molasses; rhubarb. *Good:* almonds; beets;

bran; cabbage; carrots; celery; chocolate; dates; figs; kohlrabi; lemons; lettuce; oranges; oysters; parsnips; pineapples; raspberries; rutabagas; shellfish; spinach; turnips; walnuts; watercress.

DEFICIENCY: Symptoms are brittle bones, poor development of bones and teeth, dental caries, rickets, tetany, heart atony, hyperirritability, excessive bleeding. Laboratory error and variation may be the causes of inaccurate or inconsistent values in evaluating the calcium level. SEE: *osteoporosis; Recommended Daily Dietary Allowances* in *Appendix.*

c. carbonate, precipitated. $CaCO_3$. USP. Precipitated chalk. A fine, white, tasteless and odorless powder. Used as an antacid and as an antidote to corrosive acid poisoning.

c. chloride. $CaCl_2 \cdot 2H_2O$. USP. A deliquescent salt occurring as translucent crystals having a sharp saline taste. Used to raise the calcium content of the blood in disorders resulting from lack of sufficient calcium, such as in hypocalcemic tetany. Used in solution and administered intravenously. SYN: *calcium chloride dihydrate.*
INCOMPAT: Ephedrine.

c. cyclamate. A non-nutritious sweetening agent. SEE: *cyclamate.*

c. disodium edetate. Substance used to bind certain metallic ions in the body. Used in treating poisoning due to those metals.

c. gluconate. USP. A granular or white powder without odor or taste. Its actions and uses are the same as those of calcium chloride. More pleasant to taste and nonirritating when administered orally or intramuscularly in a 10% solution.

c. glycerophosphate. Calcium salt of glycerophosphoric acid. Used as a dietary supplement and in formulating drugs.

c. hydroxide. USP. $Ca(OH)_2$. 1. A white powder used in preparing calcium hydroxide solution, which is used as an astringent applied to the skin and mucous membranes. In solution it is called lime water. Used in dentistry as cavity liner or a pulp capping material under a layer of zinc phosphate. It has the effect of inducing tertiary dentin formation for bridging or root closure, but may be related to a chronic pulpitis and pulp necrosis after pulp capping. SYN: *lime, slaked.*

c. lactate. USP. A white, odorless, and nearly tasteless powder, less irritating than the chloride. Used orally or parenterally as an alternative to calcium gluconate.

c. levulinate. USP. Soluble white powder used when intravenous administration of calcium is required.

c. mandelate. Calcium salt of mandelic

acid. Used in treating urinary tract infections.

c. oxalate. A calcium-containing substance present in urine in crystalline form. It is a constituent of some renal calculi.

c. oxide. A corrosive and easily pulverized mineral occurring as a hard white or grayish-white mass. Used as a germicide and disinfectant.

c. pantothenate. USP. One of the B complex vitamins. SEE: *vitamin B complex.*

c. phosphate, precipitated. A white, amorphous powder used as an antacid in treatment of gastric hyperacidity.

c. saccharin. A non-nutritious sweetening agent. SEE: *saccharin.*

c. sulfate. A white powder that absorbs water. Used in making plaster of paris, q.v.

c., total serum. The sum of the diffusible and nondiffusible calcium in the blood serum.

c. tungstate. Fluorescent material used for radiological imaging; used in intensifying screens.

calcium-45 (^{45}**Ca**). A radioactive isotope of calcium. It has a half-life of 164 days.

calcium channel antagonists. Calcium entry blockers, q.v.

calcium entry blockers. A group of drugs that act by slowing the influx of calcium ions into muscle cells resulting in decreased arterial resistance and decreased myocardial oxygen demand. They are used in treating angina hypertension and supraventricular tachycardia, but may cause hypotension; thus, it is important to monitor blood pressure during the initial treatment period. These drugs have not been shown to provide protection against coronary artery disease. Drugs that have this function include nicardipine, nifedipine, verapamil, and diltiazem. SYN: *calcium channel antagonists; calcium channel blockers.*

Calcium Disodium Versenate. Trade name for edetate calcium disodium.

calciuria (kăl″sē-ū′rē-ă) [″ + Gr. *ouron,* urine]. Presence of calcium in the urine.

calcophorous (kăl-kŏf′or-ŭs) [″ + Gr. *phoros,* bearing]. Containing or producing lime or any salts of calcium.

calcospherite (kăl″kō-sfē′rīt) [″ + Gr. *sphaira,* sphere]. One of many small calcareous bodies found in tumors, nervous tissue, the thyroid, and prostate.

calculary (kăl′kū-lā-rē) [L. *calculus,* pebble]. Pert. to a calculus.

calculi (kăl′kū-lī). Pl. of calculus, q.v.

calculifragous (kăl″kū-lĭf′ră-gŭs) [″ + *frangere,* to break]. Breaking of calculi.

calculogenesis (kăl″kū-lō-jĕn′ē-sĭs) [″ + Gr. *genesis,* generation, birth]. Formation of calculi.

calculosis (kăl"kū-lō'sĭs) [" + *osis*, condition]. Formation of or tendency to form calculi.

calculous (kăl'kū-lŭs). Like a calculus.

calculus (kăl'kū-lŭs) [L., pebble] (pl. *calculi*). Commonly called stone; any abnormal concretion within the animal body. A calculus is usually composed of mineral salts. These pathological concretions can occur in the kidneys, ureters, bladder, or urethra, and are usually formed of crystalline urinary salts held together by viscid organic matter. SEE: *gallstone; kidney stone*.

ETIOL: abnormal function of the parathyroid glands; disordered uric acid metabolism as in gout; excessive intake of milk and alkali. The cause of most kidney stones is unknown.

c., biliary. Cholelith, q.v.; gallstones, q.v., composed almost entirely of excessive blood pigment, some with calcium deposits. SEE: *gallbladder*.

c., dental. Calcified deposits on teeth and located on subgingival, supragingival, or occlusal surfaces. SEE: *dental plaque; tartar*.

c., hemic. Calculus formed of coagulated blood.

c., pancreatic. Calculus in the pancreas, q.v., formed of calcium carbonate with other salts and inorganic materials.

c., renal. Calculus in the kidney. SYN: *nephrolith, urolith*.

SYM: Blockage of urine flow from kidney. If the ureter is blocked by the stone, sudden, severe, and paroxysmal renal colic with chills, fever, hematuria, and frequency of urination.

TREAT: Relief of pain, force fluids unless passage is completely blocked by the calculus. Smooth muscle relaxants help in passing the stone and relieving pain. If the stone is preventing urine flow or if the stone continues to grow and cause infection, surgery must be performed. Alternatively, the stone may be disintegrated ultrasonically. SEE: *extracorporeal shock-wave lithotriptor; kidney stone removal, laser treatment for*.

PROG: Serious if allowed to continue untreated.

c., salivary. Calculus in salivary duct. Usually affects duct of submandibular gland.

SYM: Obstructs flow of saliva, causing severe pain and swelling of gland, esp. while eating.

TREAT: Removal of stone by surgery.

c., urinary. Calculus in any part of the urinary system. SEE: *calculus, renal.* SEE: *Nursing Diagnoses* in *Appendix*.

c., vesical. Calculus in the bladder.

SYM: Increased frequency of urination, pain, and diurnal hematuria increased by exercise.

TREAT: Use of an analgesic and an antispasmodic if necessary; adequate fluid intake. Special urological, ultrasonic, or surgical procedure if stone is large or impacted. SEE: *extracorporeal shock-wave lithotriptor*.

PROG: Stone is usually small enough to pass through urethra.

calculus, words pert. to: "calcu-" words; "chol-" words; gravel; "lith-" words.

calefacient (kăl"ē-fā'shĕnt) [L. *calere*, to be warm, + *facere*, to make]. Conveying or that which conveys a sense of warmth when applied to a part of the body.

calf (kăf) [AS. *cealf*]. The fleshy muscular back part of the leg below the knee formed by the gastrocnemius and soleus muscles.

caliber (kăl'ĭ-bĕr) [Fr. *calibre*, diameter of bore of gun]. The diameter of any orifice, canal, or tube.

calibration (kăl-ĭ-brā'shŭn). 1. Determination of the accuracy of an instrument by comparing the information or measurement provided with that of a known standard or an instrument known to be accurate. 2. Measuring the size of anything, esp. the diameter of vessels or the caliber of an orifice.

calibrator (kăl'ĭ-brā-tor). Instrument for measuring the inside diameter of tubes or orifices.

caliceal (kăl"ĭ-sē'ăl) [Gr. *kalyx*, cup of a flower]. Concerning a calix.

calicectasis (kăl"ĭ-sĕk'tă-sĭs) [" + *ektasis*, dilatation]. Dilatation of the renal calyx.

calices. Pl. of calix, q.v.

caliculus (kă-lĭk'ū-lŭs) [L., small cup]. A cup-shaped structure.

c. gustatorius. [NA] A taste bud. SEE: *taste buds*.

c. ophthalmicus. [NA] The optic cup.

caliectasis (kăl"ē-ĕk'tă-sĭs) [Gr. *kalyx*, cup of a flower, + *ektasis*, dilatation]. Dilatation of the renal calyx. SYN: *calicectasis*.

californium (kăl"ĭ-for'nē-ŭm) [Named for California, the state and university where it was first discovered in 1950]. SYMB: Cf. At. wt. 251; at. no. 98. A chemical element prepared by bombardment of curium with alpha particles. It has properties similar to dysprosium.

caligo (kă-lī'gō) [L., darkness]. Dimness of vision.

caliper(s) (kăl'ĭ-pĕr) [Fr. *calibre*, diameter of bore of gun]. Instrument for measuring diameters of solids such as those of chest or pelvis.

calisthenics (kăl"ĭs-thĕn'ĭks) [Gr. *kalos*, beautiful, + *sthenos*, strength]. An exercise program that emphasizes development of gracefulness, suppleness, and range of motion and the strength required for such movement.

calix (kā'lĭks) [Gr. *kalyx*, cup of a flower] (pl. *calices*). [NA] Any cuplike organ or cavity. SYN: *calyx*.

Calliphora vomitoria (kă-lĭf'ĕr-ă). Common blowfly whose larvae sometimes cause myiasis disorders.

callisection [L. *callus*, hardened, insensitive, + *sectio*, a cutting]. Vivisection under anesthesia.

callomania (kăl"ō-mā'nē-ă) [Gr. *kalos*, beautiful, + *mania*, madness]. 1. Belief in one's own beauty; a delusion of the insane. 2. Unrealistic attraction to something only because of its beauty.

callosal (kă-lō'săl) [L. *callus*, hardened skin]. Pert. to the corpus callosum.

callosity, callositas (kă-lŏs'ĭ-tē, -ĭ-tăs) [L. *callosus*, hard]. Circumscribed thickening and hypertrophy of the horny layer of the skin. May be oval or elongated, gray or brown, slightly elevated, with smooth burnished surfaces; they appear on flexor surfaces of hands and feet. Caused by friction, pressure, or other irritation. SYN: *callus*.

TREAT: Temporary removal by salicylic acid or careful shaving. Permanent removal only by elimination of cause.

callosomarginal (kă-lō"sō-măr'jĭ-năl) [L. *callus*, hardened skin, + *margo*, margin]. Pert. to the corpus callosum and marginal gyrus; marking the sulcus between them.

callosum (kă-lō'sŭm) [L. *callosus*, hard]. The great commissure of the brain between the cerebral hemispheres. SYN: *corpus callosum*.

callous (kăl'ŭs). Hard, like a callus.

callus (kăl'ŭs) [L., hardened skin]. 1. Hypertrophied thickening of circumscribed area of horny layer of skin. SYN: *callosity*. 2. The osseous material woven between ends of a fractured bone that is ultimately replaced by true bone in the healing process. SEE: *porosis*.

  c., definitive. The exudate, found between two ends of a fractured bone, that develops into true bone.

  c., provisional. Temporary deposit between ends of a fractured bone that is reabsorbed when true bone develops.

calmative (kă'-, kăl'mă-tĭv). 1. Sedative; soothing. 2. An agent that acts as a sedative.

Calmette's reaction (kăl-mĕtz') [Albert Leon Charles Calmette, Fr. bacteriologist, 1863–1933]. Ophthalmic reaction, q.v.

calmodulins. Intracellular proteins that combine with calcium and activate a variety of cellular processes.

calomel (kăl'ō-mĕl) [Gr. *kalos*, beautiful, + *melas*, black]. Mercurous chloride.

calor (kā'lor) [L., heat]. 1. Heat. 2. Moderate heat of fever. One of the four classic signs of

inflammation, the others being rubor (redness), tumor (swelling), and dolor (pain).

calorescence (kăl"or-ĕs'ĕns). In physics, the conversion of invisible nonluminous rays of heat to incandescent rays.

Calori's bursa (kăl-ō'rēz) [Luigi Calori, It. anatomist, 1807–1896]. Bursa found between arch of aorta and trachea.

caloric (kă-lor'ĭk) [L. *calor*, heat]. Rel. to heat or to a calorie.

caloricity (kăl"or-ĭs'ĭ-tē). Power of developing and maintaining body heat.

calorie (kăl'ō-rē) [L. *calor*, heat]. A unit of heat. A calorie may be equated to work or to other units of heat measurement. To convert small calories to joules multiply by 4.1855. SEE: table.

  c., gram. C, small.

  c., kilogram. C, large.

  c., large. ABBR: C, Cal, or kcal. The amount of heat needed to change temperature of one kilogram of water from 14.5°C to 15.5°C. Commonly employed in metabolic studies. When writing of human nutrition the large or kilogram calorie is used. It is always capitalized in order to distinguish it from a small calorie. SYN: *c., kilogram*.

  c., small. ABBR: c, cal. The amount of heat needed to change temperature of one gram of water one degree centigrade. SYN: *c., gram; microcalorie*.

calorifacient (kă-lor"ĭ-fā'shĕnt) [L. *calor*, heat, + *faciens*, making]. Producing heat.

calorific (kăl"ō-rĭf'ĭk). Producing heat.

calorigenic (kă-lor"ĭ-jĕn'ĭk) [" + Gr. *gennan*, to produce]. Pert. to production of heat or energy.

calorimeter (kăl"ō-rĭm'ĕ-tĕr) [" + Gr. *metron*, measure]. Instrument for determining the amount of heat exchanged in a chemical reaction or by the animal body under specific conditions.

  c., bomb. Apparatus for determination of potential food energy. Heat produced in combustion is measured by the amount of heat absorbed by a known quantity of water in which the calorimeter is immersed.

  c., respiration. Apparatus for determination of heat production produced from exchange of respiratory gases.

calorimetry (kăl"ō-rĭm'ĕ-trē). Determination of heat loss or gain.

caloripuncture (kăl"ō-rĭ-pŭnk'chūr). Use of heated needles in cauterization by puncture. SYN: *ignipuncture*.

calory. Calorie.

calvaria (kăl-vā'rē-ă) [L., skull]. [NA] The domelike superior portion of the cranium, composed of the superior portions of the frontal, parietal, and occipital bones. Also called skull cap; cranium, q.v.; skull.

Calvé-Perthes disease (kăl-vā'pĕr'tās)

Recommended Daily Caloric and Protein Allowances*†

Designed for the maintenance of good nutrition of practically all healthy people in the U.S.

	Age (years)	Weight‡ kg	Weight‡ lb	Height‡ cm	Height‡ in.	Protein gr	Average Energy Allowance (kcal)§
Infants	0.0–0.5	6	13	60	24	13	650
	0.5–1.0	9	20	71	28	14	850
Children	1–3	13	29	90	35	16	1300
	4–6	20	44	112	44	24	1800
	7–10	28	62	132	52	28	2000
Males	11–14	45	99	157	62	45	2500
	15–18	66	145	176	69	59	3000
	19–24	72	160	177	70	58	2900
	25–50	79	174	176	70	63	2900
	51+	77	170	173	68	63	2300
Females	11–14	46	101	157	62	46	2200
	15–18	55	120	163	64	44	2200
	19–24	58	128	164	65	46	2200
	25–50	63	138	163	64	50	2200
	51+	65	143	160	63	50	1900
Pregnant	1st trimester					60	+0
	2nd trimester					60	+300
	3rd trimester					60	+300
Lactating	1st 6 months					65	+500
	2nd 6 months					62	+500

Source: Adapted from Recommended Daily Allowances, Food and Nutrition Board, National Academy of Sciences, National Research Council, Washington, D.C. Revised 1990.

* For complete table, SEE: *Appendix.*

† The allowances, expressed as average daily intakes over time, are intended to provide for individual variations among most normal persons as they live in the U.S. under usual environmental stresses. Diets should be based on a variety of common foods in order to provide other nutrients for which human requirements have been less well defined.

‡ Weights and heights of Reference Adults are actual medians for the U.S. population of the designated age. The use of these figures does not imply that the height-to-weight ratios are ideal.

§ Kilojoules (kJ) = 4.1855 × kcal.

[Jacques Calvé, Fr. orthopedist, 1875–1954; Georg C. Perthes, Ger. surgeon, 1869–1927]. Disorder characterized by aseptic necrosis of the epiphysis of the head of the femur.

calvities (kăl-vĭsh'ē-ēz) [L. *calvus*, bald]. Baldness; alopecia, q.v.

calx (kălks) [L.]. 1. Lime. 2. [NA] The heel.

    c. chlorinata. Chlorinated lime. Used as a deodorant and disinfectant.

calyces. Pl. of calyx.

calyciform (kă-lĭs'ĭ-form) [Gr. *kalyx*, cup of a flower, + L. *forma*, shape]. Cup-shaped.

Calymmatobacterium granulomatis (kă-lĭm″mă-tō-băk-tē′rē-ŭm). The organism, a gram-negative bacillus, that causes granuloma inguinale. Presence of Donovan bodies in lesions is diagnostic.

calyx (kā′lĭx) [Gr. *kalyx*, cup of a flower] (pl. *calyces*). Any cuplike organ or cavity. SYN: *calix* [NA].

camera (kăm′ĕr-ă) [Gr. *kamara*, vault]. In anatomy, a chamber or cavity.

    c. anterior bulbi. [NA] The anterior chamber of the eye between the cornea and the iris.

    c. posterior bulbi. [NA] Posterior chamber of the eye between the iris and the lens.

camisole (kăm′ĭ-sōl) [Fr., little shirt]. A straitjacket.

camomile. The flowering heads of the plant *Anthemis nobilis.* Used in bitters to improve appetite and digestion. Also spelled chamomile.

Camoquin Hydrochloride. Trade name for amodiaquine hydrochloride.

CAMP. *cyclic adenosine monophosphate.*

camphor (kăm′for) [Malay, *kapur*, chalk]. USP. A gum obtained from an evergreen

tree native to China and Japan.
 ACTION/USES: Topically, as 0.1% preparation, as an antipruritic.

camphorated. Combined with or containing camphor.

camphorated oil. Liniment containing camphor.

camphoromania (kăm-for-ō-mā'nē-ă) [" + Gr. *mania*, madness]. Abnormal craving for camphor.

camphor poisoning. SEE: *Poisons and Poisoning* in *Appendix*.

campimeter (kămp-ĭm'ĕ-tĕr) [L. *campus*, field, + Gr. *metron*, measure]. Device for measuring field of vision.

campimetry (kămp-ĭm'ĕ-trē). Measurement of field of vision. SYN: *perimetry* (def. 2).

campospasm (kăm'pō-spăzm). Camptocormia.

camptocormia (kămp"tō-kor'mē-ă) [Gr. *kamptos*, bent, + *kormos*, trunk]. Deformity characterized by habitual flexion of trunk forward when individual is erect. SYN: *camptospasm*.

camptodactylia (kămp"tō-dăk-tĭl'ē-ă) [" + *dactylos*, finger]. Permanent flexion of fingers or toes.

camptomelic dwarfism. Condition in which infants have craniofacial anomalies, defects of the ribs, and scapular hypoplasia. The cause is unknown, and death usually occurs in the neonatal period.

camptospasm (kămp'tō-spăzm) [" + *spasmos*, spasm]. Camptocormia.

Campylobacter (kăm'pĭ-lō-băk'tĕr) [Gr. *kampylos*, curved, + *bakterion*, little rod]. A genus of bacteria consisting of gram-negative, non-spore-forming, spirally curved, motile rods. One or both ends of the cell have a single polar flagellum.

 C. fetus. Species with several subspecies that can cause disease in man as well as animals.

 C. jejuni. A subspecies of *C. fetus* formerly called *Vibrio fetus*. It can cause an acute enteric disease characterized by diarrhea, abdominal pain, malaise, fever, nausea, and vomiting. The disease is usually self-limiting. Treatment consists of fluid and electrolyte replacement and treatment with the antibiotic to which the organism is sensitive.

 C. pylori. Previously used name for *Helicobacter pylori*.

Canadian Nurses' Association. ABBR: CNA. Official national organization for the professional nurses from the ten provinces of Canada and the Northwest Territories. All services provided by the organization are offered in English and French.

Canadian Nurses' Association Testing Service. ABBR: CNATS. An organization affiliated with the Canadian Nurses' Association responsible for administering the nursing licensure examination to graduates of approved schools of nursing. Successful completion of the examination qualifies the candidate as a registered nurse. Analogous to National Council Licensure Examination (NCLEX) in the U.S.

canal (kă-năl') [L. *canalis*, channel]. A narrow tube, channel, or passageway. SEE: *duct; foramen; groove; space.*

 c., adductor. A triangular space lying beneath the sartorius muscle and between the adductor longus and vastus medialis muscles. It extends from the apex of the femoral triangle to the popliteal space and transmits the femoral vessels and the saphenous nerve. Also called Hunter's canal.

 c., Alcock's. Canalis pudendalis [NA]. A canal on the pelvic surface of the obturator internus muscle formed by the obturator fascia. It transmits the pudendal vessels and nerve. SYN: *c., pudendal.*

 c., alimentary. The digestive tract from mouth through the intestine.

 c.'s, alveolar. Canales alveolares [NA]. Canals in the maxilla that transmit the posterior superior alveolar blood vessels and nerves to the upper teeth. SYN: *c.'s, dental.*

 c., alveolar, inferior. C., mandibular.

 c., anal. Canalis analis [NA]. The terminal portion of the rectum opening at the anus.

 c., auditory, external. The external auditory meatus; transmits sound waves.

 c., auditory, internal. Canal in the petrous portion of the temporal bone that transmits the acoustic and facial nerves and the acoustic artery.

 c., birth. Parturient canal; passageway through which the fetus passes in parturition; specifically, the cervix, vagina, and vulva.

 c., carotid. Canalis caroticus [NA]. A canal in the petrous portion of the temporal bone that transmits the interior carotid artery and the interior carotid plexus of sympathetic nerves.

 c., central. Canalis centralis [NA]. A small canal lying in the center of the spinal cord extending from the fourth ventricle to the conus medullaris. Contains cerebrospinal fluid.

 c., cervical. Canalis cervicis uteri [NA]. Canal in the cervix of the uterus extending from the internal to external os.

 c., cochlear, spiral. Canalis spiralis cochleae [NA]. A part of the bony labyrinth of the ear. A spiral tube about 30 mm long making two and three-quarters turns about a central bony axis, the modiolus. Contains the scala tympani, scala vestibuli, and cochlear duct.

c., condylar. Canalis condylaris [NA]. A canal in the occipital bone for passage of the emissary vein from the transverse sinus. Opens anterior to the occipital condyle.

c., craniopharyngeal. Canal in the fetal sphenoid bone that contains the stalk of Rathke's pouch.

c.'s dental. Alveolar canals.

c.'s, ethmoidal. Two grooves running transversely across the lateral mass of the ethmoid bone to the cribriform plate that lie between ethmoid and frontal bones. The anterior ethmoidal canal transmits the anterior ethmoidal vessels and the nasociliary nerve; the posterior ethmoidal canal transmits the posterior ethmoidal vessels and nerve.

c., facial. Canalis facialis [NA]. A canal in the internal acoustic meatus of the temporal bone that transmits the facial nerve.

c., femoral. Canalis femoralis [NA]. The medial division of the femoral sheath. It is a short compartment about 1.5 cm long, lying behind the inguinal ligament. Contains some lymphatic vessels and a lymph node.

c., gastric. A longitudinal groove on the inner surface of the stomach following the lesser curvature. Extends from esophagus to pylorus.

c.'s, haversian. Minute canals found in compact bone that contain blood and lymph vessels, nerves, and sometimes marrow, each surrounded by lamellae of bone constituting a haversian system. SEE: *bone*.

c., hyaloid. Canalis hyaloideus [NA]. A canal in the vitreous body of the eye extending from the optic papilla to the central posterior surface of the lens. It serves as a lymph channel. In the fetus the canal contains the hyaloid artery. This normally disappears six weeks prior to birth.

c., hypoglossal. Canalis hypoglossi [NA]. Canal in the occipital bone that transmits the hypoglossal nerve and a branch of the posterior meningeal artery.

c., incisive. Canalis incisivus [NA]. A short canal in the maxillary bone leading from the incisive fossa in the roof of the mouth to the floor of the nasal cavity. Transmits the nasopalatine nerve and the branches of the greater palatine arteries to the nasal fossa.

c., infraorbital. Canalis infraorbitalis [NA]. Canal in the maxilla lying in the floor of the orbit that transmits the infraorbital nerve and artery. It terminates anteriorly at the infraorbital foramen.

c., inguinal. Canalis inguinalis [NA]. A narrow, somewhat elongated opening in the lower lateral portion of the abdominal wall, extending from the abdominal (internal) inguinal ring to the subcutaneous (external) inguinal ring. It is an oblique passageway about 1½ in. (3.8 cm) long and in the male serves to transmit the spermatic cord and the ilioinguinal nerve and in the female the round ligament of the uterus and the ilioinguinal nerve. It forms a channel through which an indirect inguinal hernia descends.

c., intestinal. The alimentary canal from stomach to anus.

c., lacrimal. The lacrimal duct.

c., mandibular. Canalis mandibulae [NA]. Canal in the mandible that transmits the inferior alveolar blood vessels and nerve to the teeth.

c., maxillary. C.'s, alveolar.

c., medullary. The marrow cavity of long bones.

c., nasolacrimal. Canal lying between the lacrimal bone and the inferior nasal conchae. Contains the nasolacrimal duct.

c., Nuck's. A persistent peritoneal pouch that accompanies the round ligament of the uterus through the inguinal canal.

c., nutrient. An opening on the surface of compact bone through which blood vessels gain access to the medullary cavity of long bones.

c., obturator. An opening in the obturator membrane of the hip bone that transmits the obturator vessels and nerve.

c.'s of Lambert. In the lung, bronchioalveolar communications. These may be of assistance in preventing atelectasis. SEE: *pores of Kohn*.

c., optic. Foramen through which the optic nerve passes.

c., pharyngeal. Canal between sphenoid and palatine bones for transmission of branches of sphenopalatine vessels.

c., portal. The connective tissue (continuation of Glisson's capsule) and its contained vessels (interlobular branches of hepatic artery, portal vein, and bile duct and lymphatic vessel) located between adjoining liver lobules.

c., pterygoid. Canalis pterygoideus [NA]. Canal of the sphenoid bone transmitting pterygoid vessels, artery, and nerve.

c., pterygopalatine. Canalis palatinus major [NA]. Canal lying between maxillary and palatine bones that transmits descending palatine nerves and artery.

c., pudendal. C., Alcock's.

c., pulp. The central cavity of a tooth filled with pulp. Contains blood vessels and sensory nerve endings.

c., root. The passageway in the root of a tooth. The nerve and blood vessels pass through the canal.

c., sacral. Canalis sacralis [NA]. Cavity within the sacrum, a continuation of the vertebral canal.

c., Schlemm's. Space or series of spaces at the junction of the sclera and the cornea of the eye into which aqueous humor is drained from the anterior chamber through the pectinate villi.

c.'s, semicircular, bony. Canals located in the bony labyrinth of the internal ear and enclosing the three semicircular ducts (superior, posterior, and lateral) that open into the vestibule. They are enclosed within the petrous portion of the temporal bone.

c.'s, semicircular, membranous. Semicircular ducts. SEE: *duct, semicircular.*

c., spinal. C., vertebral.

c., spiral, cochlear. C., cochlear, spiral.

c., spiral, of the modiolus. Canalis spiralis modioli [NA]. A series of irregular spaces that follow the course of the attached margin of the osseous spiral lamina to the modiolus. They provide for the transmission of filaments of the cochlear nerve and blood vessels. The spiral ganglion lies in the spiral canal.

c., uterine. The cavity of the uterus.

c., uterocervical. The cavity of the cervix of the uterus.

c., uterovaginal. The combined cavity of the uterus and vagina.

c., vaginal. The cavity of the vagina.

c., vertebral. Canalis vertebralis [NA]. The cavity formed by the foramina of the vertebral column. It contains the spinal cord and its meninges.

c.'s, Volkmann's. Small canals found in bone through which blood vessels pass from the periosteum. They connect with the blood vessels of haversian canals or the marrow cavity.

canalicular (kăn″ă-lĭk′ū-lăr) [L. *canalicularis*]. Pert. to a canaliculus.

canaliculus (kăn″ă-lĭk′ū-lŭs) [L.] (pl. *canaliculi*). A small channel or canal. In bone or cementum, radiating out from lacunae and anastomosing with canaliculi of neighboring lacunae.

canalis (kă-nā′lĭs) [L., channel] (pl. *canales*). Canal.

canalization (kăn″ăl-ī-zā′shŭn). Formation of channels in tissue.

canavanine (kă-năv′ă-nĭn). An amino acid originally isolated from soybean meal. It prevents growth of some bacteria.

cancellated (kăn′sĕ-lāt″ĕd) [L. *cancellus*, lattice]. Reticulated; lattice-like structure.

cancelli (kăn-sĕl′ī). Pl. of cancellus. Reticulations forming spongy tissue of bones.

cancellous (kăn′sĕl-ŭs). Having a reticular or latticework structure, as the spongy tissue of bone.

cancellus (kăn-sĕl′ŭs) [L.] (pl. *cancelli*). An osseous plate of which cancellous bone is

composed; any structure arranged as a lattice.

cancer (kăn′sĕr) [G. *karkinos*, crab]. Cancers, of which there are an estimated 200 different kinds, have the properties of uncontrolled growth of cells derived from normal tissues, and of being able to kill the host by the spread of cells from the site of origin to distant sites or by local spread. Cancers that arise in epithelial tissues are called carcinomas; and those from mesenchymal tissues, are classed as sarcomas. Leukemias are also classed as malignant growths.

Cancer incidence and deaths in the U.S. by site and sex are shown in the accompanying illustration based on 1990 projections. More than 900,000 new cases of cancer are diagnosed annually in the U.S., and there are 600,000 deaths from cancer each year. It was estimated that 117,000 deaths from cancer in 1978 could have been prevented by earlier diagnosis and treatment. In the last 40 years in the U.S., the cancer death rate has declined in women and increased in men.

SYM: The important warning signals of cancer are: unusual bleeding or discharge from any internal or external body site; a lump or thickening in any area but esp. the breast; a sore that does not heal; a change in bowel or bladder habits; hoarseness or persistent cough; indigestion or difficulty in swallowing; change in size or shape or appearance of a wart or mole; unexplained loss of weight. These are the major signs of cancer, and, once any one of them is observed in oneself or in a patient, it should be brought to a physician's attention without delay.

ETIOL: Unregulated, disorganized proliferation of cell growth may be stimulated by various chemicals, viruses, and physical agents such as ionizing radiation and ultraviolet light. Cancer may be caused by the use of cytotoxic agents used to treat cancer. A number of agents are specific carcinogens, notably the chemicals contained in tobacco products. Other lifestyle factors such as high dietary fat intake and low fiber intake may be important contributors to the development of cancer in humans.

DIAG: Depending on the site, diagnosis is made by various means, the most important being biopsy, q.v.; use of devices for visualization of hollow organs; roentgenography including computerized axial tomography (CAT); mammography; ultrasound; cytology such as the Papanicolaou test, q.v.; and palpation for lumps. Some of these techniques and devices will demonstrate an increase in the size or change in the shape of an organ, but such alteration may be due to ei-

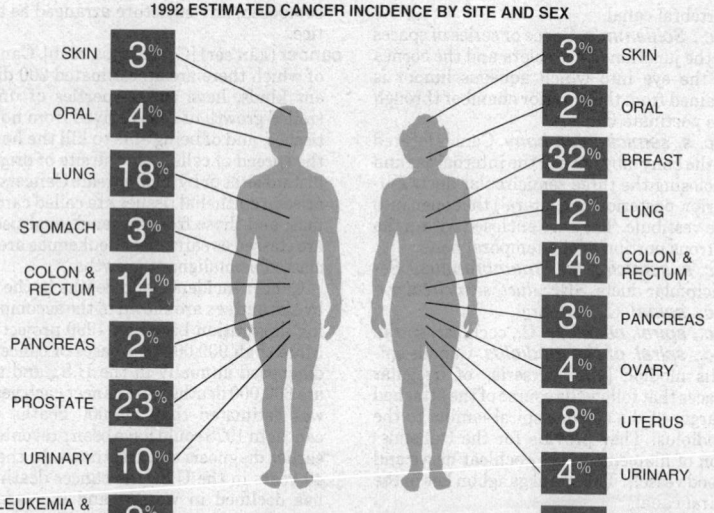

1992 ESTIMATED CANCER INCIDENCE BY SITE AND SEX

Male		Female	
SKIN	3%	3%	SKIN
ORAL	4%	2%	ORAL
		32%	BREAST
LUNG	18%	12%	LUNG
STOMACH	3%	14%	COLON & RECTUM
COLON & RECTUM	14%	3%	PANCREAS
PANCREAS	2%	4%	OVARY
PROSTATE	23%	8%	UTERUS
URINARY	10%	4%	URINARY
LEUKEMIA & LYMPHOMAS	9%	7%	LEUKEMIA & LYMPHOMAS
ALL OTHER	14%	11%	ALL OTHER

Excluding nonmelanoma skin cancer and carcinoma in situ of uterine cervix.

1992 ESTIMATED CANCER DEATHS BY SITE AND SEX

Male		Female	
SKIN	1%	1%	SKIN
ORAL	2%	1%	ORAL
		19%	BREAST
LUNG	34%	22%	LUNG
STOMACH	3%	12%	COLON & RECTUM
COLON & RECTUM	11%	5%	PANCREAS
PANCREAS	4%	5%	OVARY
PROSTATE	12%	4%	UTERUS
URINARY	5%	3%	URINARY
LEUKEMIA & LYMPHOMAS	9%	9%	LEUKEMIA & LYMPHOMAS
ALL OTHER	19%	19%	ALL OTHER

Cancer Statistics, 1992, American Cancer Society, New York, N.Y.

ther a benign or malignant growth.

There are various cancer staging systems to help delineate the extent and prognosis of tumors. An example of one of these is the tumor, node, metastasis system (TNM). Numbers are added to each category to indicate degree of dissemination. SEE: *cancer staging;* table *(American Cancer Society Recommendations for Cancer Detection).*

TREAT: Surgery, chemotherapy, q.v.; hormone therapy; radium; and radiotherapy are recognized effective methods of treatment of patients with cancer. Application of proper method or a combination of methods is necessary for effective therapy. Therefore, early diagnosis is the most important factor. SEE: *Karnofsky scale.*

NURSING IMPLICATIONS: It is important when working with the patient with cancer that all members of the health team work in collaboration with each other as well as with the patient and family. Provide knowledge of the disease process, its progress, treatment, and outcome for the patient and family. Identify and support patient and family coping mechanisms and allow for and encourage verbalization of feelings and fears, particularly with relation to death and dying.

Physical care should include maintenance of fluid and electrolyte balance and nutritional status, maintenance of elimination as well as personal hygiene, decreasing effects of immobilization, and facilitating comfort. Also strive to decrease the patient's fears of helplessness, avoid giving false hope, and provide the patient and family with realistic reassurance about pain control.

Emotional support provided by nurses depends on their personal experiences and philosophies about life and death. It is essential for nurses who work with patients with terminal illnesses to be aware of their own fears and feelings related to death and dying. SEE: *Nursing Diagnoses* in *Appendix.*

c., bone. A malignancy of bone tissue. Primary bone tumors are rare in adults. They are seen most frequently in children and adolescents. Secondary or metastatic bone tumors are far more common. Tumors arising in other areas of the body which metastasize to the bones most often spread to areas such as the spine and pelvis.

c., hard. Cancer composed of fibrous tissue. SYN: *carcinoma, scirrhous.*

c., lip. An epithelioma of the lower lip usually seen in men or smokers.

c., scirrhous. C., hard.

cancer, words pert. to: adenocarcinoma; brain tumor; carcinoma; epithelioma;

Hodgkin's disease; hospice; leukemia; polyp; sarcoma; scirrhus; tumor.

cancer cell. Cell present in neoplasm possessing characteristics that differentiate it from normal tissue cells; such as degree of anaplasia, irregularity in shape, indistinctness of cell outline, nuclear size, changes in structure of nucleus and cytoplasm, increased number of mitoses, and ability to metastasize.

cancer, chemoprevention of. The use of certain foods and drugs to prevent the progression of preneoplastic conditions and some neoplastic states. This subject is the object of extensive investigations.

cancer clusters. The occurrence of a rare type of cancer in a small geographic area and in much greater number than could be expected through chance alone.

cancer detection, American Cancer Society recommendations for. SEE: table.

cancer grading and staging. The standardized procedure for expressing cancer cell differentiation, called grading; and extent of dissemination of the cancer, called staging. This procedure is of great assistance in comparing the results of various forms of therapy. Cancer is graded on the differentiation of the tumor cells and the number of mitoses present. These are thought to be correlated with the ability of the tumor to grow and spread. Some cancers are graded I to IV, the latter being the most anaplastic and having the least resemblance to normal tissue.

Cancers are staged with respect to their size, amount of local spread (metastases), and whether or not blood-borne metastasis has occurred. There are two major staging systems; the TNM for judging size of primary tumor (T); evidence of regional extension (N); and evidence of metastases (M). Another system classifies cancers as Stage 0 to IV based on the size of the tumor and its spread.

cancericidal (kăn″sĕr-ĭ-sī′dăl) [L. *cancer,* crab, + *cidus,* killing]. Lethal to malignant cells.

cancerigenic (kăn″sĕr-ĭ-jĕn′ĭk) [″ + Gr. *gennan,* to produce]. Causing cancer. SYN: *carcinogenic.*

cancer of cervix. SEE: *cervix, cancer of.*

cancerogenic (kăn″sĕr-ō-jĕn′ĭk) [″ + Gr. *gennan,* to produce]. Carcinogenic.

cancerophobia [″ + Gr. *phobos,* fear]. Unreasonable fear of cancer.

cancerous. Pert. to malignant growth.

cancer, person-years of life lost due to. The difference between the age of death of a person due to cancer and the life expectancy of the individual if death from cancer had not occurred. In 1984, in the U.S., 6,881,281

American Cancer Society Recommendations for Cancer Detection*

What	To Detect	Who	When
Sigmoidoscopy (examination of colon/rectum)	Colorectal cancer	Everyone over 50	After 2 negative exams 1 year apart, perform every 3 to 5 years
Test for blood in stools	Colorectal cancer	Everyone over 50	Annually
Digital rectal examination	Rectal cancer	Everyone over 40	Annually
Pap test (microscopic examination of cells)	Cervical cancer	Women 20 to 65; younger women who are sexually active	After 2 negative exams 1 year apart, perform at least every 3 years†
Pelvic examination	Reproductive system cancers in women	All women over 20	Every 3 years for women 40 and under; yearly thereafter
Endometrial (uterine) tissue sample	Uterine cancer	Women at high risk‡	At menopause
Breast self-examination	Breast cancer	Women over 20	Every month
Breast physical examination	Breast cancer	All women over 20	Every 3 years for women 40 and under; yearly thereafter
Mammography (breast x-ray)	Breast cancer	All women over 35	Baseline — between ages 35 and 40; every 1 to 2 years between ages 40 and 49; yearly thereafter
Health counseling and cancer checkup	Thyroid, testes, prostate, ovary, lymph node, mouth and skin cancer	Everyone over 20	Every 3 years ages 20 to 40; yearly after age 40

Source: American Cancer Society; used with permission.

* The American Cancer Society recommends that healthy adults have these screening tests periodically as indicated and immediately if suspicious symptoms appear. In addition, many experts recommend yearly chest x-rays for mature smokers.

† The American College of Obstetrics and Gynecology disagrees. It recommends a *yearly* Pap test.

‡ High-risk women have histories of infertility, obesity, failure to ovulate, abnormal uterine bleeding, or estrogen therapy.

person-years of life were lost due to cancer deaths. The average years of life lost per person dying from cancer in 1984 was 15.2 years.

cancra (kăng′krä). Pl. of cancrum.

cancriform (kăng′krĭ-form) [″ + *forma*, appearance]. Having the appearance of cancer.

cancroid (kăng′kroyd) [″ + Gr. *eidos*, form, shape]. 1. Like a cancer. 2. A type of keloid, q.v. 3. Epithelioma, q.v.

cancrum (kăng′krŭm) [L. *cancer*, crab, creeping ulcer] (pl. *cancra*). A rapidly spreading ulcer.

   c. nasi. Gangrenous inflammation of nasal membranes.

   c. oris. Trench mouth, q.v.

   c. pudendi. Ulceration of vulva.

candela (kăn-děl′ä) [L. *candela*, candle]. SYMB: cd. The SI base unit of luminous intensity.

candicidin (kăn″dĭ-sĭ′dĭn). USP. Antibiotic produced by certain species of *Streptomyces*.

Candida (kăn′dĭ-dä) [L. *candidus*, glowing white]. A genus of yeastlike fungi that develop a pseudomycelium and reproduce by budding. Commonly part of the normal flora of the mouth, skin, intestinal tract, and vagina. One of the most common causes of vaginitis in women of reproductive age. Formerly called *Monilia.*

C. albicans. A small, oval budding fungus that is the primary etiologic organism of moniliasis (candidiasis). Formerly called *Monilia albicans.*

candidemia. Cells from the yeast Candida in the blood.

candidiasis (kăn″dĭ-dī′ă-sĭs). Infection of the skin or mucous membrane with any species of *Candida,* but chiefly *Candida albicans,* q.v. Usually localized in skin, nails, mouth, vagina, vulva, bronchi, or lungs, but may invade the bloodstream.

SYM: Oral lesions consist of painless white plaques which are adherent and discrete on the oral and pharyngeal mucosa, including the tongue. Skin lesions are red, macerated, and usually in intertriginous areas. Other sites include the nails (paronychia), the penis (balanitis), and the anus (pruritus ani). Invasive systemic infections may be present in any organ, including the brain, heart, kidneys, and eyes. The symptoms produced in systemic infections depend on the extent of the infection and the organ(s) affected.

TREAT: Mucous membrane or skin infections may be treated with oral nystatin, ketoconazole, or clotrimazole. Systemic infections are treated with amphotericin B. If the central nervous system is involved, flucytosine is used in conjunction with amphotericin B. Some strains of *Candida albicans* are resistant to flucytosine. Vaginal candidiasis may be treated with butoconazole, clotrimazole, miconazole, nystatin, terconazole, or tioconazole. All are effective; however, pregnant patients should consult their physician prior to taking or applying these drugs.

NURSING IMPLICATIONS: Assess for erythematous, papular skin rash; red, swollen nailbeds; cream-colored pseudomembranous patches on mucous membranes; white or yellow vaginal discharge with pruritus. Teach patient procedures and use of prescribed drugs. Patient with recurrent vaginal infection should have partner examined and treated simultaneously to prevent reinfection.

candle [L. *candela*]. A solid mass of combustible material such as tallow or wax in which a wick is imbedded. When the wick is lit, the wax burns slowly to produce heat and light. Candles are used in bacteriology, where they are placed lighted in an airtight jar and allowed to extinguish themselves. In so doing,

an atmosphere containing approximately 10% carbon dioxide is produced. This CO_2 concentration is required for culturing certain organisms, particularly *Neisseria gonorrhoeae.*

cane. A slender stick held in the hand and used for support during walking.

canescent (kă-nĕs′ĕnt) [L. *canus,* gray]. Gray in color.

cane sugar. Sucrose. Table sugar obtained from sugar cane. SEE: *saccharose.*

canine (kā′nīn) [L. *caninus,* dog]. 1. Pert. to a dog. 2. A canine tooth; the four teeth, also known as the eyeteeth (upper and lower), between the incisors and molars. SEE: *dentition* for illus.

canities (kăn-ĭsh′ē-ēz) [L., gray hair]. Congenital (rare) or acquired whiteness of the hair. The acquired form may develop rapidly or slowly and be partial or complete. SYN: *achromatrichia.*

c. unguium. Gray or white streaks in nails. SYN: *leukonychia.*

canker sore (kăng′kĕr) [L. *cancer,* crab, creeping ulcer]. Ulceration of the mouth and lips. SEE: *aphthous ulcer.*

cannabis (kăn′ă-bĭs) [Gr. *kannabis,* hemp]. The dried flowering tops of the *Cannabis sativa* (hemp) plant. Tetrahydrocannabinols produce euphoric effects when ingested or smoked. Cannabis preparations are used experimentally to alleviate symptoms of severe glaucoma. SYN: *marijuana,* q.v.

cannibalism. The human consumption of the flesh of human beings. SEE: *kuru.*

cannula (kăn′ū-lă) [L., a small reed]. A tube or sheath enclosing a trocar, the tube allowing the escape of fluid after withdrawal of the trocar from the body.

c., nasal. Tubing used to deliver oxygen at levels from 1 to 6 liters per minute. Tubing extends approximately 1 cm into each naris and is connected to a common tube, which is then connected to the oxygen source. Used in situations, as in cardiac disease, where a low-flow, small-percentage oxygen therapy is desirable. Exact percentage of oxygen delivered to patient varies with respiratory rate and other factors.

cannulate (kăn′ū-lāt). To introduce a cannula through a passageway.

cannulation of large veins. Technique of providing access to the venous circulation by placing a flexible cannula in one of the large veins, usually the femoral or subclavian. The cannula is used to provide a means of hyperalimentation or fluid replacement in treating patients in shock. When the subclavian vein is used, pneumothorax is a possible complication.

canthal (kăn′thăl) [Gr. *kanthos,* angle]. Pert. to a canthus.

cantharidal (kăn-thăr'ĭ-dăl) [Gr. *kantharis*, beetle, + *eidos*, form, shape]. Pert. to or containing cantharides.

cantharides (kăn-thăr'ĭ-dēz) (sing. *cantharis*). Dried insects of the species *Cantharis vesicatoria*. Formerly used externally as a counterirritant and vesicant, and internally for its supposed aphrodisiac effect. It is no longer used. Poisonous if taken internally in large doses. SYN: *Spanish fly*.

Cantharis (kăn'thă-rĭs). A genus of beetles, *C. vesicatoria*, known as Spanish fly. SEE: *cantharides*.

canthectomy (kăn-thĕk'tō-mē) [Gr. *kanthos*, angle, + *ektome*, excision]. Excision of a canthus.

canthi (kăn'thī). Pl. of canthus.

canthitis (kăn-thī'tĭs) [" + *itis*, inflammation]. Inflammation of a canthus.

cantholysis (kăn-thŏl'ĭ-sĭs) [" + *lysis*, dissolution]. Incision of an optic canthus of an eye to widen the palpebral slit.

canthoplasty (kăn'thō-plăs"tē) [" + *plassein*, to form]. Plastic surgery of an optic canthus. Enlargement of palpebral fissure by division of the external canthus.

canthorrhaphy (kăn-thor'ă-fē) [" + *rhaphe*, seam, ridge]. Suturing of a canthus.

canthotomy (kăn-thŏt'ō-mē) [" + *tome*, incision]. Surgical division of a canthus.

canthus (kăn'thŭs) [Gr. *kanthos*, angle] (pl. *canthi*). The angle at either end of the slit between the eyelids; the external canthus or commissura palpebrarum lateralis [NA], and the internal canthus or commissura palpebrarum medialis [NA].

Cantil. Trade name for mepenzolate bromide.

CaO. Calcium oxide, quicklime, calx.

Ca(OH)₂. Calcium hydroxide; slaked lime.

C.A.O.T. *Canadian Association of Occupational Therapists.*

cap (kăp) [LL. *cappa*, hood]. 1. A covering. SYN: *tegmentum*. 2. First part of the duodenum. SYN: *pyloric cap.* 3. The protective covering of the developing tooth. 4. The artificial covering of a tooth. Used for cosmetic reasons. SEE: *enamel organ.* 5. [L.] *capiat*, let him take.
   c., cradle. Seborrhea of the scalp seen in infants.
   c., knee. Bone in front of the knee. SYN: *patella.*

capacitance (kă-păs'ĭ-tăns) [L. *capacitas*, holding]. 1. State of being able to store an electric charge. 2. Ratio of the charge transferred from one to the other of a pair of conductors to the potential difference between the conductors.

capacitation (kă-păs"ĭ-tā'shŭn). Making something have the capacity to evolve; e.g., the process of the sperm becoming capable of fertilization.

capacitor (kă-păs'ĭ-tor). Electronic device for storing electric charges.

capacity. 1. The potential ability to contain, or to hold the power to do something. 2. Cubic content. 3. Ability to perform mentally. 4. Measure of the electrical output of a generator.

CAPD. *continuous ambulatory peritoneal dialysis.* SEE: *peritoneal dialysis.*

Capdepont-Hodge syndrome. Hereditary condition resulting in defective formation and calcification of dentin, resulting in misshapen teeth of blue or brown appearance. SYN: *dentinogenesis imperfecta.*

capeline (kăp'ĕ-lĭn) [Fr., a hat]. A bandage used for the head, or the stump of an amputated limb. SEE: *bandage, head.*

Capgras' syndrome. [Jean Marie Joseph Capgras, Fr. psychiatrist, 1873–1950]. The patient's delusion that a close relative or friend has been replaced by an impostor. SYN: *"illusion of doubles."*

capillarectasia (kăp"ĭ-lă-rĕk-tā'sē-ă) [L. *capillaris*, hairlike, + Gr. *ektasis*, dilatation]. Dilatation of capillary vessels.

Capillaria (căp"ĭ-lār'ē-ă). A genus of parasitic nematodes.
   C. philippinensis. Species of roundworm discovered in the Philippines. It causes severe diarrhea, malabsorption, and enteric protein loss in man; mortality is high.

capillariasis (kăp"ĭ-lă-rī'ă-sĭs) [*Capillaria* + Gr. *-iasis*, condition]. A disease, first described in 1968, due to infestation of the small bowel with the roundworm *Capillaria philippinensis.* Reported from northern Luzon in the Philippine Islands.
   TREAT: Thiabendazole.

capillaries (kăp'ĭ-lă"rēz). Pl. of capillary.

capillariography (kăp"ĭ-lār"ē-ŏg'ră-fē) [L. *cappillaris*, hairlike, + Gr. *graphein*, to write]. Radiographic examination of the capillaries after injection of a contrast medium.

capillaritis (kăp"ĭ-lār-ī'tĭs) [" + Gr. *itis*, inflammation]. Inflammation of the capillaries. SYN: *telangiitis.*

capillarity (kăp"ĭ-lăr'ĭ-tē). A surface tension effect, seen by the elevation or depression of a liquid at the point of contact with a solid, as in capillary tubes. SYN: *capillary attraction.*

capillaropathy (kăp"ĭ-lăr-ŏp'ă-thē) [" + Gr. *pathos*, disease]. Capillary disorders or disease.

capillaroscopy (kăp"ĭ-lăr-ŏs'kŏ-pē) [" + Gr. *skopein*, to examine]. Examination of capillaries for diagnostic purposes.

capillary (kăp'ĭ-lār"ē) [L. *capillaris*, hairlike] (pl. *capillaries*). 1. Any of the minute blood vessels, averaging 0.008 mm in diameter, carrying blood and forming the capillary system. Capillaries connect the ends of the smallest arteries (arterioles) with the beginnings of the smallest veins (venules). 2. Pert. to a hair; hairlike.

c.'s, arterial. Very small vessels that are the terminal branches of the arterioles or metarterioles.

c.'s, bile. Intercellular biliary passageways that convey bile from liver cells to the interlobular bile ducts.

c.'s, blood. Minute blood vessels that convey blood from the arterioles to the venules and form an anastomosing network that brings the blood into intimate relationship with the tissue cells. Their wall consists of a single layer of squamous cells called endothelium through which oxygen diffuses to the tissue and products of metabolic activity enter the bloodstream. They average about 8 microns in diameter, but are capable of being constricted so as to have almost no lumen at all.

c.'s, lymphatic. The smallest lymphatic vessels. They are thin-walled tubes forming a dense network in most tissues of the body. They differ from blood capillaries in that they are generally slightly larger in diameter. They collect interstitial fluid; thus the composition of the lymph will vary with respect to the tissue being drained. Intestinal lymphatics will contain fatty materials during digestion; those from the liver will contain proteins. Lymph capillaries unite to form larger lymphatic vessels, which drain into lymph nodes drained by efferent lymph vessels, which flow via the thoracic duct into the venous blood system at the junction of the left internal jugular and subclavian veins.

c.'s venous. Minute vessels that convey blood from a capillary network into the small veins or venules.

capillary attraction. Capillarity, q.v.

capillary nail refill test. Used as a quick, gross estimate of state of perfusion and in estimating extent of dehydration. It is measured from when the patient's nail turns pale after it is depressed until it becomes pink again. Normal range is two seconds or less. SYN: *nail blanch test; turgor, skin.*

capillary permeability. Ability of substances to diffuse through capillary walls into the tissue spaces. Influenced by hypoxia, adrenocortical hormone, and the concentration of calcium ions in the blood.

capillus (kă-pĭl′ŭs) [L., a hair] (pl. *capilli*). 1. A hair, esp. of the head. 2. A filament. 3. A hair's breadth.

capital [L. *capitalis*]. Pert. to the head.

capitate (kăp′ĭ-tāt) [L. *caput,* head]. Head-shaped; having a rounded extremity.

capitation fee (kăp″ĭ-tā′shŭn). Amount paid a physician annually from each patient in a medical group plan.

capitatum (kăp″ĭ-tā′tŭm). Os capitatum [NA]. Third bone in distal row of carpus; i.e., the wrist. SYN: *os magnum.*

capitellum (kăp″ĭ-tĕl′ŭm) [L., small head]. The round eminence at lower end of the humerus articulating with radius; its radial head. SYN: *capitulum humeri* [NA].

capitula [L.]. Pl. of capitulum.

capitular (kă-pĭt′ū-lăr). Pert. to a capitulum.

capitulum (kă-pĭt′ū-lŭm, kă-pĭch′ū-lŭm) [L., small head] (pl. *capitula*). [NA] A small, rounded articular end of a bone.

c. fibulae. The proximal extremity or head of the fibula; articulates with tibia.

c. humeri. [NA] Rounded prominence at distal end of humerus. Articulates with the radius. SYN: *capitellum.*

c. mallei. In the middle ear, the head or large rounded extremity of the malleus; bears facet for the incus.

c. stapedis. The head of the stapes; articulated with lenticular process of incus of the middle ear.

Caplan's syndrome [Anthony Caplan, Brit. physician, 1907–1976]. Rheumatoid arthritis with progressive massive fibrosis of the lung in coal miners and in other pneumoconioses. SYN: *rheumatoid pneumoconiosis.*

capnography. Continuous recording of the level of carbon dioxide in expired air in mechanically ventilated patients.

capnophilic (kăp-nō-fĭl′ĭk) [Gr. *kapnos,* smoke, + *philein,* to love]. Describing bacteria that grow best in an atmosphere containing carbon dioxide.

capotement (kă-pōt-mŏn′) [Fr.]. Splashing sound that may be heard when the dilated stomach contains air and fluid.

Capoten. Trade name for captopril, q.v.

capping (kăp′ĭng). 1. Placing a protective substance over the exposed pulp of a tooth. 2. Placing an artificial crown on a tooth for cosmetic purposes. 3. In immunology, the aggregation of living B lymphocytes that have reacted with fluorescein-labeled antiimmune globulin cells to form a polar cap.

capreomycin sulfate. USP. A tuberculostatic drug. Trade name is Capastat Sulfate.

capsicum (kăp′sĭ-kŭm). Cayenne pepper; dried ripe fruit of Capsicum species. Used as a carminative, stimulant, and rubefacient.

capsid (kăp′sĭd). Protein covering around the central core of a virus particle. The capsid, which develops from protein units called protomers, protects the nucleic acid in the core of the virus particle from the destructive enzymes in biological fluids and promotes attachment of the virus to susceptible cells.

capsitis (kăp-sī'tĭs) [L. *capsa,* box, + Gr. *itis,* inflammation]. Capsulitis of crystalline lens.

capsomer (kăp'sō-mĕr) [" + Gr. *meros,* part]. Short ribbons of protein that make up a portion of the capsid viral particle.

capsula [L., little box] (pl. *capsulae*). [NA] A sheath or continuous enclosure around an organ or structure.

   c. articularis. [NA] Capsule of a joint.

   c. bulbi. Tenon's capsule, q.v.

   c. fibrosa perivascularis. Glisson's capsule.

   c. glomeruli. [NA] Bowman's capsule; malpighian capsule.

   c. lentis. [NA] Crystalline lens capsule of the eye.

capsulae (căp'sū-lē) [L.]. Pl. of capsula, q.v.

capsular. Pert. to a capsule.

capsular pattern. Characteristic pattern of proportional limitation of passive range of motion of a joint that suggests the presence of arthritis in that joint. (Ex: the capsular pattern of the glenohumeral joint, in order of most restriction, is: lateral rotation, abduction, and medial rotation.)

capsulation. Enclosure in a capsule.

capsule [L. *capsula,* little box]. 1. Capsula, q.v. 2. A special container made of gelatin. Size is for a single dose of a drug; the enclosure prevents the patient from tasting the drug.

   c., articular. A two-layered sleeve or covering for a synovial joint. The inner layer is synovial and the outer is fibrous.

   c., auditory. Embryonic cartilaginous capsule enclosing the developing ear.

   c., bacterial. The membrane that surrounds some bacterial cells. It is a loose gel-like structure that, in pathogenic bacteria, helps to protect against phagocytosis.

   c., Bowman's. The glomerular capsule of the kidneys.

   c., cartilage. The layer of matrix that forms the innermost portion of the wall of a lacuna enclosing a single cell or a group of cartilage cells. It is basophilic.

   c., Glisson's. An outer capsule of fibrous tissue which covers the liver, its ducts, and its vessels. SYN: *capsula fibrosa perivascularis* [NA].

   c., glomerular. Bowman's capsule, q.v.

   c., joint. The fibrous tissues enclosing a joint.

   c., lens. A transparent structureless membrane that surrounds and encloses the lens of the eye.

   c., nasal; c., optic; c., otic. Cartilaginous capsules that develop in the embryonic skull to enclose each of the paired sense organs — nasal cavity, eyes, and ears, respectively.

   c. of kidney. Fat-containing connective tissue surrounding the kidney.

   c. of Tenon. A thin fibrous sac enveloping the eyeball, forming a socket in which it rotates.

   c., renal. Fibrous capsule surrounding the kidney.

   c., suprarenal. A tough connective tissue capsule that encloses the adrenal gland.

   c., temporomandibular joint. Fibrous covering of the synovial joint between the skull and mandible on each side of the head.

capsulectomy (kăp"sū-lĕk'tō-mē) [L. *capsula,* little box, + Gr. *ektome,* excision]. Surgical removal of a capsule.

capsulitis (kăp"sū-lī'tĭs) [" + Gr. *itis,* inflammation]. Inflammation of a capsule.

capsulociliary (kăp"sū-lō-sĭl'ē-ĕr-ē) [" + *ciliaris,* pert. to the eyelashes]. Pert. to capsule of lens and ciliary structures.

capsulolenticular (kăp"sū-lō-lĕn-tĭk'ū-lăr) [" + *lenticularis,* pert. to a lens]. Concerning the capsule of the eye and the lens.

capsuloplasty (kăp'sū-lō-plăs"tē) [" + Gr. *plassein,* to mold]. Plastic surgery of a capsule, esp. one of a joint.

capsulorrhaphy (kăp"sū-lor'ă-fē) [" + Gr. *rhaphe,* seam, ridge]. Suture of a joint capsule or of a tear in a capsule.

capsulotome (kăp'sū-lō-tōm") [" + Gr. *tome,* incision]. Instrument for incising the capsule of the crystalline lens.

capsulotomy (kăp"sū-lŏt'ō-mē). Cutting of the capsule of crystalline lens.

captopril. A drug that blocks the conversion of angiotensin I to angiotensin II. It is used in diagnosing renovascular hypertension that can be alleviated by surgery. In addition, it is useful in lowering the blood pressure of most patients with hypertension, in treating congestive heart failure, and in treating the vascular and renal crises that may occur in scleroderma. Trade name is Capoten.

capture. In atomic physics the joining of an elementary particle such as an electron, or neutron with the atomic nucleus.

   c., ventricular. The normal response of the ventricle of the heart to the electrical impulse from the electrical conducting system.

caput (kā'pŭt, kăp'ŭt) [L.] (pl. *cap'ita*). [NA] 1. The head. 2. The chief extremity of an organ.

   c. medusae. Plexus of dilated veins about the umbilicus seen in one form of cirrhosis of the liver (Cruveilhier-Baumgarten syndrome) indicating portal vein obstruction. It may be seen in newborns.

   c. succedaneum. Swelling produced on the presenting part of the fetal head during labor. It may be mistaken for the bag-of-waters. It recedes within 2 to 3 days.

ETIOL: Effusion of serum into cellular tissue of exposed scalp through venous interference from pressure.

Carafate. Trade name for sucralfate.

caramel (kăr′ă-mĕl, kär′mĕl). NF. Flavoring and coloring agent made by heating sugar or glucose to 180° to 200°C until it forms a uniform dark brown, thick mass. Most of the sweet taste is destroyed by this process.

carbachol (kär′bă-kŏl). USP. Drug with action similar to acetylcholine. Used to produce miosis during eye surgery. Trade names are Miostat and Isopto Carbachol.

carbamazepine (kăr-bă-măz′ĕ-pēn). Drug used for treatment of trigeminal neuralgia and temporal lobe epilepsy; used in psychiatry as a mood-stabilizing drug in bipolar affective disorder. Trade name is Tegretol.

carbamide (kăr′bă-mīd, kär-băm′īd). CO(NH)₂. Urea in an anhydrous, sterile powder form.

carbaminohemoglobin (kär-băm′′ĭ-nō-hē′′mō-glō′bĭn). Chemical combination of carbon dioxide and hemoglobin.

carbarsone (kär′bär-sōn). USP. A white, crystalline, odorless powder; contains about 28% arsenic, having a chemical structure resembling tryparsamide. Used as an antiamebic agent. Trade name is Carb-O-Sep.

carbenicillin indanyl sodium (kär′′bĕn-ĭ-sĭl′ĭn). USP. A semisynthetic antibiotic of the penicillin group. Trade name is Geocillin.

carbidopa (kär′′bĭ-dō′pă). USP. Drug used with levodopa in treating parkinsonism.

carbinoxamine maleate (kär′′bĭn-ŏk′să-mēn). USP. An antihistamine that acts by blocking histamine receptors. Trade name is Clistin.

Carbocaine. Trade name for mepivacaine hydrochloride.

carbohydrase (kär′′bō-hī′drās). One of a group of enzymes (such as amylase and lactase) that hydrolyze carbohydrates.

carbohydrate (kär′′bō-hī′drāt) [L. *carbo,* carbon, + Gr. *hydor,* water]. A group of chemical substances, including sugars, glycogen, starches, dextrins, and celluloses, that contain only carbon, oxygen, and hydrogen. Usually the ratio of hydrogen to oxygen is 2:1. It is estimated that glucose and its polymers (including starch and cellulose) represent the most abundant organic chemical compounds on earth, surpassing in quantity even the great stores of fuel hydrocarbons beneath the earth's crust.

Carbohydrates are one of the three classes of nutrients. Green plants utilize the sun's energy to combine carbon dioxide and water to form carbohydrates. Most plant carbohydrates (celluloses) are unavailable for direct metabolism by vertebrates. However, the bacteria present in some vertebrates' intestinal tracts break down cellulose to molecules that can be absorbed. Man's intestinal tract lacks the enzyme that splits cellulose into sugar molecules, but humans do split starch into maltose by means of their salivary and pancreatic amylase enzymes.

CLASSIF: Carbohydrates are grouped according to the number of carbon atoms they contain and how many of the basic types are combined into larger molecules. The most common simple sugars, monosaccharides, contain five or six carbon atoms and are called pentoses and hexoses, respectively. Two monosaccharides linked together are called a disaccharide. A series or chain of monosaccharides or disaccharides is called a polysaccharide. Ribose is the most important pentose; glucose, fructose, and galactose are the most important hexoses in human metabolism. The disaccharide sugars present in the diet are maltose (2 D-glucose molecules), sucrose or cane sugar (glucose and fructose), and lactose or milk sugar (D-glucose and D-galactose). These sugars are split and eventually converted to glucose by the action of enzymes. The two important polysaccharides are starch and glycogen, the latter of which is called animal starch. The basic monosaccharide building-block for both of these large polymers is glucose. Dietary starch and glycogen are metabolized first to glucose and then to CO_2 and water in the human. SEE: table.

COMP: All carbohydrates contain only carbon, hydrogen, and oxygen molecules.

FUNCT: Carbohydrates are a basic source of energy; stored in the body as glycogen in virtually all tissues but principally in the liver and muscles. From these sites they can be mobilized, making these stores an important source of reserve energy.

DIGESTION AND ABSORPTION: Cooked but not raw starch is broken down by salivary amylase to disaccharide. Both cooked and raw starch are split in the small intestine by pancreatic amylase. Disaccharides cannot be absorbed until they have been separated into glucose molecules by enzymes present in the brush border of cells lining the intestinal tract. Glucose and galactose are the actively absorbed sugars. Fructose is absorbed by diffusion. SEE: table.

METABOLISM: Although very complex at the molecular level, the metabolism of carbohydrates can be explained as follows. Carbohydrates are absorbed in the form of glucose, galactose, or fructose. These monosaccharides are available for direct utilization in energy production, or they may be stored after conversion to glycogen. The

Classification of Important Carbohydrates

Classification	Examples	Some Properties
Monosaccharides $(C_8H_{10}O_5) \cdot H_2O$ or $C_6H_{12}O_6$	Glucose Fructose	Crystalline, sweet, very soluble, readily absorbed
Disaccharides $(C_6H_{10}O_5)_2 \cdot H_2O$ or $C_{12}H_{22}O_{11}$ hydrolyzed to simple sugars	Sucrose Lactose Maltose	Crystalline, sweet, soluble, digestible Present in milk
Polysaccharides $(C_6H_{10}O_5)_n$ composed of many molecules of simple sugars. (Since polysaccharides can be composed of various numbers of monosaccharides and disaccharides, n refers to an unknown number of these groups.)	Starch Dextrin Cellulose Glycogen	Amorphous, little or no flavor, less soluble. Vary in solubility and digestibility.

Digestion of Carbohydrates

Enzyme	Found in	Carbohydrates Digested	End Product
Sucrase (invertase)	Intestine	Sucrose	Glucose and fructose
Maltases	Intestine and mucosal cells of intestine	Maltose	Two D-glucose
Lactase	Intestine	Lactose	D-glucose and D-galactose
Salivary amylase	Saliva (mouth)	Cooked starch, glycogen, and dextrins	Maltose
Pancreatic amylase	Pancreas	Raw and cooked starch and glycogen	Maltose

glycogen is available for metabolism to glucose whenever there is need for reserve energy. SEE: *muscle metabolism.*

SOURCES: Carbohydrates are present in food in digestible and indigestible forms. Those that can be utilized are an important source of energy. Those that can't be utilized, usually some form of cellulose, are beneficial in adding bulk to the diet. Whole grains, vegetables, legumes (peas and beans), tubers (potatoes), fruits, honey, and refined sugar are excellent sources of carbohydrate. Calories derived from sugar and candy have been termed empty calories because these foods lack essential amino acids, vitamins, and minerals. SEE: *fiber, dietary.*

NUTRITION: Carbohydrates contain 4.1 Cal/gm and are esp. useful as a source of energy. As indicated, however, some forms are virtually devoid of dietary essentials other than calories.

carbohydrate deficient transferrin. A chemical that is of use as a marker for alcohol abuse. The compound is elevated in those who are chronic heavy drinkers, but is not present in nondrinkers. SEE: *alcoholism.*

carbohydrate loading. Dietary manipulation for the purpose of enhancing amount of glycogen stored in muscle tissue. Used by athletes prior to high-intensity endurance events such as competing in a marathon foot race. Phase I is begun 7 days prior to competition. It depletes glycogen from specific muscles used in the event by exercising to exhaustion while participating in the sport for which one is preparing. The glycogen exhaustion is maintained by a high-fat, high protein diet for 3 days. It is important that 100 grams of carbohydrate be included in this phase in order to prevent ketosis, q.v. Phase II consists of a high-carbohydrate diet of at least 1000 to 2000 kcal for 3 days. This is called the supersaturation phase because the goal is to enhance glycogen storage. Synthesis of glycogen is facilitated by the extended period of depletion in Phase I. Carbohydrates used should be complex ones, e.g., those present in grain-derived food such as bread and pasta, rather than simple carbohydrate-containing items such as candy and soft drinks. Phase III begins on the day of the event. Any type of food may be eaten up to 4 to 6 hours prior to competition. Food eaten from that time up to the time of competition is a matter of individual preference.

carbolism (kăr′bŏl-ĭzm). Poisoning by carbolic acid. SEE: *phenol*.

carbolize (kăr′bŏl-īz). To add or mix with carbolic acid.

carboluria (kăr″bō-lū′rē-ă) [″ + *oleum*, oil, + Gr. *ouron*, urine]. Phenol in the urine.

carbon [L. *carbo*, carbon]. SYMB: C. At. wt. 12.0111; at. no. 6. This nonmetallic element is the characteristic constituent of organic compounds.

Carbon occurs in two pure forms, diamond and graphite, and in impure form in charcoal, coke, and soot. Its compounds are constituents of all living tissue. Carbon combines with hydrogen, nitrogen, and oxygen to form the basis of all organic matter. Organic carbon compounds provide energy in foods.

carbon-14. SYMB: ^{14}C. Radioactive isotope of carbon with a half-life of 5600 years. It is used as a tracer in metabolic studies and in archeology to date materials containing carbon.

carbonate (kăr′bŏn-āt) [L. *carbo*, carbon]. Any salt of carbonic acid.

   c. of soda. Sodium carbonate used commercially in crude form, as washing soda. The free alkali present is irritating and in strong concentrations has the effect of sodium hydroxide, q.v.

carbon dioxide. USP. CO_2. A colorless gas, heavier than air. Produced in the combustion or decomposition of carbon or its compounds. It is the final metabolic product of carbon compounds present in food. The body eliminates CO_2 through the lungs, in urine, and in perspiration. It is also given off by decomposition of vegetable or animal matter or formed by alcoholic fermentation as in rising bread. It is necessary to all plant life and is absorbed directly from the air.

In small quantities (up to about 5%) in inspired air, it stimulates respiration; in greater quantities, it produces an uncomfortable degree of mental activity with confusion. Although not toxic in low concentration, it can cause death by suffocation. Great amounts are added to the atmosphere daily, but because it is used by green plants,

the air content is kept down to about 0.03%. Approx. one sq. meter of leaf surface can absorb the carbon dioxide from 2500 L of air in one hour. It is estimated that an acre of trees uses 4½ tons (4082 kg) of CO_2 a year. SEE: *capnography; carbon dioxide solid therapy.*

carbon dioxide combining power. This test, done in blood serum, is a determination of the amount of carbon dioxide that the blood serum can hold in chemical combination. It is a test of the buffer capacity of the blood.

The blood serum CO_2 determination is used to help measure the degree of acidosis or alkalosis. Carbon dioxide in aqueous solution forms a weak acid (H_2CO_3), and the amount of this acid that the blood serum can take up is a measure of its reserve power to prevent the occurrence of acidosis. The normal amount is 50 to 70 ml/dl of blood (usually expressed as 50 to 70 volumes %). Values below 50 indicate acidosis, above 70 alkalosis.

carbon dioxide inhalation. CO_2 (5% to 7½%), mixed with oxygen for inhalation, stimulates breathing the same way as increased CO_2 production during exercise. Inhalation of oxygen and CO_2 is used as an accessory during artificial respiration and as a continuation of resuscitation after spontaneous breathing has returned. Also used to stimulate respiration in patients with pulmonary diseases.

carbon dioxide poisoning. CO_2 gas is most commonly used in carbonated drinks. Commercially it is used in its solidified form to make dry ice. Poisoning is rarely fatal unless the patient is in a closed space. It is a profound respiratory stimulant.

   SYM: Extremely deep breathing; sensation of pressure in the head; ringing in ears; acid taste in mouth; slight burning in nose. Within a short time, respiration almost ceases and patient becomes unconscious.

   TREAT: Remove to fresh air, administer artificial respiration, oxygen inhalation.

carbon dioxide solid therapy. Solid carbon dioxide (CO_2 snow) is used for therapeutic refrigeration. Solid CO_2 has a temperature of −80°C. Application to skin 1 to 2 seconds causes superficial frostbite, 4 to 5 seconds a blister, 10 to 15 seconds superficial necrosis, 15 to 45 seconds ulceration. Used mostly for removal of certain nevi and warts, occasionally for telangiectasia.

carbonemia (kăr″bō-nē′mē-ă) [L. *carbo*, carbon, + Gr. *haima*, blood]. Excess accumulation of carbonic acid in the blood.

carbonic. Pert. to carbon.

   c. acid. H_2CO_3. Acid resulting from mixture of carbon dioxide and water.

   c. anhydrase. An enzyme that catalyzes

union of H_2O and CO_2 to form carbonic acid or reverse action. Present in red blood cells.

carbonize (kär′bŏn-īz). To char or convert into charcoal.

carbon monoxide. CO. An insidious poisonous gas. A colorless, tasteless, odorless gas, it gives no warning of its presence; it is widely distributed as the result of imperfect combustion and oxidation. It is found in the exhaust gas from all internal combustion engines used in most motor-powered vehicles. It is present in illuminating gas and results from the inefficient and incomplete combustion of coal. It is found in sewers, cellars, and mines.

Smoking tobacco increases the CO content of the blood, thus interfering with the transport of oxygen in the blood. This in turn also decreases the individual's ability to see at night.

carbon monoxide (CO) poisoning. Poisoning can occur from small amounts of CO inhaled over a long period of time or from large amounts inhaled in a short time. For example, riding in a closed automobile or parking in an automobile with motor running may cause death from the inhalation of these noxious fumes from leaking exhausts and exhaust heaters. Another cause of death is the operation of a gasoline motor in an enclosed area such as a closed garage or basement. Poisoning from CO is produced as a result of a chemical combination of this gas with the hemoglobin of the blood, thus preventing the blood from carrying oxygen to the tissues. Because this combination is relatively stable, patients may need prolonged periods of oxygen administration in addition to artificial respiration.

The affinity of CO for hemoglobin is more than 200 times as great as that of oxygen. Therefore exposure to CO causes a marked reduction in the ability of the blood to transport oxygen. SEE: *Poisons and Poisoning* in *Appendix*.

SYM: The symptoms of CO poisoning are somewhat variable. Respiration is deep and difficult. Carboxyhemoglobin (COHb), which is the substance formed when carbon monoxide combines with hemoglobin, is cherry red in color. Thus the tissues and skin of individuals with CO poisoning and a carboxyhemoglobin level of 30% or greater are much pinker than normal. Their appearance has been described as "cherry red." The pulse may be slowed initially but it soon becomes increased. There may be pounding of the heart; dizziness is frequent; muscular function may be so weakened as to cause inability to stand. There may be ringing in the ears, throbbing in the temples, headache, faintness and nausea, and dilated pupils. A patient who is breathing when found usually recovers when brought into fresh air and given stimulants. SEE: table.

TREAT: Immediately remove the person from exposure to CO. Using a tight-fitting mask, administer 100% oxygen, under pressure (hyperbaric) if possible. Use artificial respiration if indicated. Keep the patient absolutely quiet and immobile in order to reduce the body's oxygen requirements. If cerebral edema develops, give 50 ml of 50% glucose I.V. and prednisone 1 mg/kg I.V. every 4 hours as needed. If hypotension is present, this should be corrected; monitor cardiac function and treat altered function as indicated. A sedative such as diazepam may be needed if patient becomes excited during recovery.

COMPLICATIONS: When such patients recover, they often have some nervous system involvement including various types of paralysis, blindness, interference with sensation, muscular spasms, or twitchings for an indefinite period of time. Most of these complications disappear in time, but occasionally they remain permanently.

carbon tetrachloride (tĕt″rä-klō′rīd). CCl_4. A clear, colorless liquid with ethereal odor resembling chloroform; not flammable. Although having narcotic and anesthetic properties resembling chloroform, it is too toxic to be suitable as an anesthetic. In general, this substance is too toxic for any medical use. Inhalation of a small quantity has been known to produce death. The mechanism of injury is acute atrophy of the liver and kidney.

carbon tetrachloride poisoning. Toxic effects due to prolonged inhalation.

SYM: Irritation of eyes, nose, and throat; headache; confusion; central nervous system depression; ventricular fibrillation; visual disturbances; nausea; anorexia.

F.A.: Remove clothes contaminated with carbon tetrachloride. Oxygen inhalation and artificial respiration. Lavage with saline solution. Leave saline cathartic in stomach. SEE: *Poisons and Poisoning* in *Appendix*.

carbonuria (kär″bō-nū′rē-ä) [L. *carbo*, carbon, + Gr. *ouron*, urine]. The presence or excretion of carbon compounds in the urine.

carbonyl (kär′bŏn-ĭl) [″ + Gr. *hyle*, matter]. The divalent radical CO, characteristic of aldehydes and ketones.

carboplatin. A cytotoxic, platinum-containing drug used in treating ovarian cancer. SEE: *cisplatin*.

Carbowax. Trade name for preparations of polyethylene glycols.

carboxyhemoglobin (kär-bŏk″sē-hē″mō-glō′bĭn) [″ + Gr. *oxys*, acid, + *haima*,

Toxic Symptoms of Carbon Monoxide

Carbon Monoxide Concentration		Response
Percent CO in Air	Parts Per Million	
0.005	50	No apparent toxic symptoms.
0.01	100	Can be tolerated for several hr without symptoms.
0.02	200	Possible mild frontal headache in 2–3 hr.
0.08	800	Headache, dizziness, and nausea in 45 min; collapse and possible unconsciousness in 2 hr.
0.16	1600	Headache, dizziness, and nausea in 20 min; collapse and possible death in 2 hr.
0.32	3200	Headache and dizziness in 5–10 min; unconsciousness and possible death in 10–15 min.
0.64	6400	Headache and dizziness in 1–2 min; possible death in 10–15 min.
1.28	12,800	Immediate unconsciousness; possible death in 1–3 min.

Source: Adapted from Hamilton, A and Hardy, H: Industrial Toxicology, ed 3. Publishing Sciences Group, Littleton, MA, 1974.

blood, + L. *globus,* sphere]. Compound formed by carbon monoxide and hemoglobin in poisoning by carbon monoxide.

carboxyl (kăr-bŏk′sĭl). The characteristic group (COOH) of organic carboxylic acids, e.g., formic acid (HCOOH) and acetic acid (CH₂COOH).

carboxylase (kăr-bŏk′sĭ-lās). An enzyme that catalyzes the removal of the carboxyl group (COOH) from amino acids; an enzyme found in brewer's yeast that catalyzes the decarboxylation of pyruvic acid with the production of acetaldehyde and carbon dioxide. In the body, this requires the presence of vitamin B₁ (thiamine), which acts as a coenzyme.

carboxylation. In chemistry the replacement of hydrogen by a carboxyl (—COOH) molecule.

carboxylic acids. A group of organic acids that contain the carboxylic acid, —COOH group.

carboxylmethylcellulose sodium. USP. Chemical used as a pharmaceutic aid and as a food additive.

carbuncle, carbunculus (kăr′bŭng″k'l, kăr″bŭng′kū-lŭs) [L. *carbunculus,* small glowing ember]. A circumscribed inflammation of the skin and deeper tissues that terminates in a slough and suppuration and is accompanied by marked constitutional symptoms.

SYM: It is characterized by a painful node, at first covered by tight reddened skin that later becomes thin and perforates, discharging pus through several openings. Also fever, leukocytosis, and sometimes prostration. Most commonly found on nape of neck, on upper back or on buttocks.

ETIOL: Staphylococci. Predisposing factors the same as in furuncle, q.v. Diabetics are particularly susceptible.

TREAT: Antibiotics given systemically are usually effective. Incision and drainage when lesion is about to point or come to a head. Keep covered with warm compresses to promote blood supply to the area.

NURSING IMPLICATIONS: Use sterile technique when changing dressings. Dressings should be changed frequently to facilitate drainage and promote healing. All contaminated equipment should be disinfected, and all soiled dressings disposed of properly. Teach the patient and family to avoid contact with wound drainage and prevent spread of bacteria by proper handwashing, disinfecting of contaminated linens and equipment, and disposal of dressings in impermeable bags. SEE: *Universal Precautions* in *Appendix.*

carbuncular. Pert. to a carbuncle.

carbunculosis (kăr-bŭng″kū-lō′sĭs) [″ + Gr. *osis,* condition]. Appearance of several carbuncles in succession.

carbutamide (kăr-bū′tă-mīd). An oral hypoglycemic agent.

carcass (kăr′kăs). A dead body. Usually applied to nonhuman bodies.

carcinoembryonic antigens (kăr″sĭn-ō-ĕm″brē-ŏn′ĭk). ABBR: CEA. A class of antigens normally present in the fetus. Originally isolated from colon tumors, they were thought erroneously to be specific for those tumors. If the previously elevated CEA level returns to normal after surgery, removal of the colonic tumor is thought to be complete.

carcinogen (kăr′sĭn-, kăr-sĭn′ō-jĕn). Any substance or agent that produces or increases the risk of developing cancer in humans or lower animals.
  c., chemical. Chemical substance capable of causing cancer.

carcinogenesis (kăr″sĭ-nō-jĕn′ĕ-sĭs) [Gr. *karkinos,* crab, + *genesis,* generation, birth]. The production or origin of cancer.

carcinogenic (kăr″sĭ-nō-jĕn′ĭk). Producing cancer.

carcinoid (kăr′sĭ-noid) [″ + *eidos,* form, shape]. A tumor derived from the argentaffin cells in the intestinal tract, bile ducts, pancreas, bronchus, or ovary. These tumors secrete serotonin (5-hydroxytryptamine) and other vasoactive substances.

carcinoid syndrome. A syndrome produced by metastatic carcinoid tumors that secrete excessive amounts of serotonin. Serotonin is metabolized to 5-hydroxyindoleacetic acid (5-HIAA).
  SYM: Include one or more of the following: brief episodes of flushing, esp. of the face and neck; tachycardia; facial and periorbital edema; hypotension; intermittent abdominal pain with diarrhea; valvular lesions of the heart; loss of weight; hypoproteinemia; signs of pellagra. The latter symptom is due to the body's available tryptophan, which is the precursor of serotonin, being used for serotonin production instead of for manufacture of niacin and protein.
  DIAG: Clinical presentation and greatly increased excretion of 5-HIAA in urine; some foods, e.g., bananas, pineapples, tomatoes, walnuts, avocados, and certain drugs can cause an increased level of this chemical.
  TREAT: Surgery, except in the case of an isolated tumor, is not indicated. High-protein diet with nicotinamide supplement to prevent pellagra. Serotonin antagonist for control of diarrhea and malabsorption. Somatostatin and its analogues have been effective in inhibiting flushing and diarrhea and in reversing the hypotension.

carcinolysis (kăr″sĭ-nŏl′ĭ-sĭs) [Gr. *karkinos,* crab, + *lysis,* dissolution]. Destruction of carcinoma cells.

carcinolytic (kăr″sĭ-nō-lĭt′ĭk). Destructive to cancer cells.

carcinoma (kăr″sĭ-nō′mă) [″ + *oma,* tumor]. A new growth or malignant tumor that occurs in epithelial tissue. These neoplasms tend to infiltrate and give rise to metastases. It may affect almost any organ or part of the body and spread by direct extension or through lymphatics or the bloodstream. Etiology is unknown. SYN: *cancer.* SEE: *cancer.*

  c., alveolar cell. A type of carcinoma of the lung.
  c., basal cell. A malignancy of the skin that rarely metastasizes. Typically, it begins as a small, shiny papule that is difficult to distinguish from other causes of discrete dermatitis. The lesion enlarges to form a whitish border around a central depression or ulcer that may bleed. When the lesion reaches this stage, it is often called a rodent ulcer.
  TREAT: After biopsy, the removal method used is determined by the size, location, and appearance of the lesion.
  c., bronchogenic. A malignant lung tumor that originates in the bronchi. The most common type of bronchogenic tumors are squamous cell or epidermoid. Oat cell and adenocarcinoma are the next most common tumors.
  ETIOL: Usually associated with history of cigarette smoking.
  TREAT: Surgery is the most effective treatment. More than one-half of the tumors are advanced and inoperable when diagnosed. The prognosis for patients with bronchogenic carcinoma is very poor. The five-year survival rate is less than 10%.
  c., chorionic. Tumor containing cells characteristic of the chorion of the embryo. Occurs in the testis, ovary, and other parts of the body. SYN: *choriocarcinoma.*
  c., cylindrical. Carcinoma of glands usually of entodermal origin including adenocarcinoma and carcinoma simplex. Cells are nearly cylindrical in shape.
  c., embryonal. Malignant teratoma.
  c., epidermoid. Tumor on a surface such as the skin. Usually of two types: one a wartlike growth, slow-growing, mildly malignant; the other a flat and rapidly infiltrating neoplasm.
  c., giant cell. Carcinoma characterized by presence of giant cells.
  c., glandular. Carcinoma of cells of the secreting variety. SEE: *adenocarcinoma.*
  c. in situ. ABBR: CIS. Malignant cell changes in the epithelial tissue that do not extend beyond the basement membrane.
  c., lipomatous. Carcinoma of fatty tissue.
  c., medullary. Carcinoma that is soft because of the predominance of cells and in which there is little fibrous tissue.
  c., melanotic. Carcinoma containing melanin.
  c., mucinous. Carcinoma in which the glandular tissue secretes mucin.
  c., oat cell. A poorly differentiated tumor of the bronchus that contains small oat-shaped cells.
  c. of cervix. SEE: *cervix, cancer of.*

c., scirrhous. A form of cylindrical carcinoma with a firm, hard structure.

c., squamous-cell. A form of epidermoid carcinoma principally of squamous cells.

carcinomatophobia (kăr″sĭ-nō″mă-tō-fō′bē-ă) [Gr. *karkinos,* crab, + *oma,* tumor, + *phobos,* fear]. Morbid fear of carcinoma.

carcinomatosis (kăr″sĭ-nō″mă-tō′sĭs) [″ + ″ + *osis,* condition]. The condition of having widespread dissemination of carcinoma in the body.

carcinophilia (kăr″sĭ-nō-fĭl′ē-ă) [″ + *philos,* love]. Having affinity for cancer cells.

carcinosarcoma (kăr″sĭ-nō-săr-kō′mă) [″ + *sarx,* flesh, + *oma,* tumor]. A malignant tumor containing the elements of both carcinoma and sarcoma.

c., embryonal. Wilms' tumor, q.v.

carcinosis (kăr″sĭ-nō′sĭs) [″ + *osis,* condition]. Carcinomatosis, q.v.

cardamom, cardamon [Gr. *kardamomon*]. Dried ripe fruit of an herb, *Elettaria repens* or *E. cardamomum,* used as an aromatic and carminative.

Cardarelli's sign (kăr″dă-rĕl′lēz) [Antonio Cardarelli, It. physician, 1831–1926]. Pulsating movement of the trachea to one side; may be present with aneurysm of the aorta.

Cardene. Trade name for nicardipine, q.v.

cardia (kăr′dē-ă) [Gr. *kardia,* heart]. Upper orifice of stomach connecting with the esophagus.

cardiac (kăr′dē-ăk) [L. *cardiacus*]. 1. Pert. to the heart. 2. Pert. to the cardia.

cardiac arrest. Sudden cessation of functional circulation. SEE: *cardiopulmonary resuscitation.*

cardiac arrhythmia. SEE: *arrhythmia.*

cardiac atrophy. Fatty degeneration of the heart.

cardiac catheterization. Passage of a tiny plastic tube into the heart through a blood vessel. Samples of blood are withdrawn for testing; blood pressure and cardiac output are measured. Used in diagnosis of heart disorders and anomalies.

NURSING IMPLICATIONS: *Precatheterization:* Prepare the patient physically and emotionally for the procedure, using procedural and sensation messages. Assess for allergies and premedicate with antihistamines as required.

During catheterization: Assist with procedure per agency protocol. Monitor pressures and cardiac rhythm and assist with hemodynamic studies. Provide for patient comfort and safety, assessing changes in emotional status, level of consciousness, and verbal and nonverbal responses, to help determine patient's response to procedure and need for reassurance or medication to prevent vasovagal reactions or coronary artery spasm. Assess for complications: cardiac dysrhythmia or allergic reaction to contrast medium.

Postcatheterization: Provide emotional support to patient and answer questions. Monitor cardiac rhythm until stable. Monitor vital signs (including apical pulse for one full minute and temperature) every 15 minutes for the first 1 to 2 hours, then every hours for 4 hours or until stable. Avoid taking blood pressure in arm used for insertion of catheter. Maintain pressure dressing over entry site (30 minutes for brachial site, then replace with ace bandage; 4 to 6 hours with sandbag for femoral site) and keep involved extremity extended, cautioning patient to avoid flexion or hyperextension for 12 hours for femoral site or 24 hours for brachial site. Maintain patient on bedrest per protocol, usually 2 to 3 hours for brachial site or 6 hours for femoral site, or until fluid balance is restored, as angiographic contrast medium causes osmotic diuresis. Assess dressings for bleeding and be alert for patient complaint of increasing dressing tightness as this may indicate hematoma formation. Assess the neurovascular status of involved extremity, particularly distal to the cannulation site, as arterial thrombosis is the most frequent complication. Assess for complications such as pericardial tamponade, myocardial infarction, pulmonary embolism, stroke, congestive heart failure, cardiac dysrhythmia, infection, and thrombophlebitis. Resume preoperative medication regimen and manage post-procedural pain, reporting unusually severe site or extremity pain or onset of chest discomfort. Patient must be driven home, and have responsible adult in attendance until following morning. Provide the patient and family with written discharge instructions, explaining that patient should report to physician occurrence of any of the following symptoms: new bleeding or swelling at the entry site, increased tenderness, redness, draining or pain at the entry site, fever, any changes in color, temperature or sensation in the extremity utilized. Patient may take acetaminophen or other non-aspirin analgesic every 3 to 4 hours as needed for pain. Entry site should be covered with an adhesive bandage for 24 hours, or until stitches, if present, are removed, usually within 6 days. Shower is permitted day following procedure, tub bath 48 hours following procedure. Patient is to avoid strenuous activity for 24 hours. Provide patient with information regarding follow-up appointment date and time. SEE: *Nursing Diagnoses* in *Appendix.*

cardiac compensation. The ability of the heart through its reserve power to compensate for impaired functioning of its valves.

cardiac cycle. The period from the beginning of one beat of the heart to the beginning of the succeeding beat, including the *systole*, contraction of the atria and ventricles propelling the blood onward, and the *diastole*, the period during which the cavities are being refilled with blood. The atria contract immediately before the ventricles. The ordinary cycle lasts 0.8 second with the heart beating approx. 60 to 85 times a minute in the adult at rest. The atrial systole lasts 0.1 second; the ventricular systole 0.3 second, and the diastole 0.4 second; thus even though the heart seems to be working continuously, it actually rests for a good portion of each cardiac cycle.

RS: circulation; diastole; heart; systole.

cardiac failure. Condition resulting from inability of the heart to pump sufficient blood to meet the needs of the body. SEE: *heart failure*.

cardiac hypertrophy. Enlargement of the heart. SEE: *heart, hypertrophy of*.

cardiac insufficiency. Inadequate cardiac output due to failure of the heart to function properly, as in valvular deficiency.

cardiac massage. SEE: *cardiopulmonary resuscitation*.

cardiac monitor. SEE: *monitor, cardiac*.

cardiac output. The amount of blood discharged from the left or right ventricle per minute. For an average adult at rest, cardiac output is approx. 3.0 L per square meter of body surface area each minute. Cardiac output is determined by multiplying the stroke volume by the heart rate. SYN: *volume, minute*.

cardiac plexus. Plexus cardiacus [NA]. The nerve plexus at the base of the heart made up of branches of the vagus nerves and sympathetic trunks. Afferent nerves from this plexus provide the nerve supply to the heart.

cardiac reflex. Reflex in which the response is a change in cardiac rate. Stimulation of sensory nerve endings in the wall of the carotid sinus by increased arterial blood pressure reflexly slows the heart (Marey's law); stimulation of vagus fibers in the right side of the heart by increased venous return reflexly increases heart rate (Bainbridge's reflex).

cardiac reserve. The capacity of the heart to increase cardiac output and raise blood pressure above basal pressure to meet body requirements.

cardialgia (kăr″dē-ăl′jē-ă) [Gr. *kardia*, heart, + *algos*, pain]. Pain at the pit of the stomach or region of the heart, usually occurring in paroxysms.

cardiaortic (kăr″dē-ā-or′tĭk) [″ + *aorte*, aorta]. Pert. to the heart and aorta.

cardiasthenia (kăr″dē-ăs-thē′nē-ă) [″ + *astheneia*, weakness]. Type of neurasthenia with predominance of cardiac symptoms.

cardiasthma (kăr″dē-ăz′mă) [″ + *asthma*, panting]. Dyspnea due to heart disease.

cardiectasia, cardiectasis (kăr″dē-ĕk-tā′sē-ă, -ĕk′tă-sĭs) [″ + *ektasis*, dilatation]. Dilatation of the heart.

cardiectomy (kăr″dē-ĕk′tō-mē) [″ + *ektome*, excision]. Excision of the cardiac end of the stomach.

Cardilate. Trade name for erythrityl tetranitrate.

cardinal [LL. *cardinalis*, important]. Of primary importance, as in the cardinal symptoms: temperature, pulse, respiration.

cardio- [Gr. *kardia*, heart]. Prefix pert. to the heart.

cardioaccelerator (kăr″dē-ō-ăk-sĕl′ĕr-ā-tor) [″ + L. *accelerare*, to hasten]. That which increases the rate of the heartbeat.

cardioactive (kăr″dē-ō-ăk′tĭv) [″ + L. *activus*, acting]. Acting upon the heart.

cardioangiography (kăr″dē-ō-ăn″jē-ŏg′ră-fē) [″ + *angeion*, vessel, + *graphein*, to write]. Angiocardiography, q.v.

cardioangiology (kăr″dē-ō-ăn″jē-ŏl′ō-jē) [″ + ″ + *logos*, word, reason]. The science of the heart and blood vessels.

cardioaortic (kăr″dē-ō-ā-or′tĭk) [″ + *aorte*, aorta]. Pert. to the heart and the aortic artery.

cardiocatheterization (kăr″dē-ō-kăth″ĕ-tĕr-ĭ-zā′shŭn). Cardiac catheterization, q.v.

cardiocele (kăr′dē-ō-sēl) [″ + *kele*, tumor, swelling]. A herniation or protrusion of the heart through an opening in the diaphragm, or through a wound.

cardiocentesis (kăr″dē-ō-sĕn-tē′sĭs) [″ + *kentesis*, puncture]. Surgical incision or puncture of the heart.

cardiochalasia (kăr″dē-ō-kă-lā′zē-ă) [″ + *chalasis*, relaxation]. Relaxation of the muscles of the cardiac sphincter of the stomach.

cardiocirrhosis (kăr″dē-ō-sĭr-rō′sĭs) [″ + *kirrhos*, orange-yellow, + *osis*, condition]. Cirrhosis of the liver, and heart disease.

cardiodiaphragmatic (kăr″dē-ō-dī″ă-frăg-măt′ĭk). Concerning the heart and the diaphragm.

cardiodilator (kăr″dē-ō-dī′lā-tor) [″ + L. *dilatare*, to enlarge]. Device for dilating the cardia of the gastroesophageal junction.

cardiodynamics (kăr″dē-ō-dī-năm′ĭks). Science of forces involved in propulsion of blood from heart to tissues and back to heart.

cardiodynia (kăr″dē-ō-dĭn′ē-ă) [Gr. *kardia*, heart, + *odyne*, pain]. Pain in the region of the heart.

cardioesophageal. Concerning the junction of the esophagus and the stomach.

cardioesophageal reflux. SEE: *gastroesophageal reflux.*

cardiogenesis (kăr″dē-ō-jĕn′ĕ-sĭs) [″ + *genesis*, generation, birth]. Formation and growth of the embryonic heart.

cardiogenic (kăr″dē-ō-jĕn′ĭk) [″ + *gennan*, to produce]. Having origin in the heart itself.

cardiogenic shock. Failure to maintain blood supply to the circulatory system and tissues because of inadequate cardiac output. SEE: *shock.*

cardiogram (kăr′dē-ō-grăm″) [″ + *gramma*, something written]. A graph of the electrical activity of the heart muscle. Made with an electrocardiograph machine. SYN: *electrocardiogram.*

cardiograph (kăr′dē-ō-grăf″) [″ + *graphein*, to write]. A device for registering the electrical activity of the heart muscle.

cardiographic (kăr″dē-ō-grăf′ĭk). Pert. to cardiography.

cardiography (kăr″dē-ŏg′ră-fē). The recording and study of the electrical activity of the heart.

cardiohepatic (kăr″dē-ō-hĕ-păt′ĭk) [″ + *hepatos*, liver]. Pert. to the heart and liver.

cardiohepatomegaly (kăr″dē-ō-hĕp″ă-tō-mĕg′ă-lē) [″ + ″ + *megas*, large]. Enlargement of the heart and liver.

cardioinhibitory (kăr″dē-ō-ĭn-hĭb′ĭ-tō-rē) [″ + L. *inhibere*, to check]. Inhibiting action of the heart.

cardiokinetic (kăr″dē-ō-kĭ-nĕt′ĭk) [″ + *kinesis*, movement]. Pert. to that which excites heart action.

cardiokymography. ABBR: CKG. The x-ray method of recording the outline of the heart as it beats. Its usefulness in clinical medicine has not been shown.

cardiolipin (kăr″dē-ō-lĭp′ĭn) [″ + *lipos*, fat]. Previously used term for diphosphatidylglycerol, q.v.

cardiolith (kăr′dē-ō-lĭth″) [″ + *lithos*, stone]. A concretion or calculus in the heart.

cardiologist (kăr-dē-ŏl′ō-jĭst) [″ + *logos*, word, reason]. A physician specializing in treatment of heart disease.

cardiology (kăr-dē-ŏl′ō-jē). The study of the heart.

cardiolysin (kăr″dē-ŏl′ĭ-sĭn) [″ + *lysis*, dissolution]. A lysin acting on heart muscle.

cardiolysis (kăr-dē-ŏl′ĭ-sĭs). Operation for separation of adhesions constricting the heart in adhesive mediastinopericarditis. Involves resection of the ribs and sternum over the pericardium.

cardiomalacia (kăr″dē-ō-mă-lā′shē-ă) [Gr. *kardia*, heart, + *malakia*, softening].

Softening of the heart muscle.

cardiomegaly (kăr″dē-ō-mĕg′ă-lē) [″ + *megas*, large]. Hypertrophy of the heart. SYN: *megacardia.*

cardiomotility (kăr″dē-ō-mō-tĭl′ĭ-tē) [″ + L. *motilis*, moving]. The ability of the heart to move.

cardiomyoliposis (kăr″dē-ō-mī″ō-lĭp-ō′sĭs) [″ + *mys*, muscle, + *lipos*, fat, + *osis*, condition]. Fatty degeneration of the heart.

cardiomyopathy (kăr″dē-ō-mī-ŏp′ă-thē) [″ + ″ + *pathos*, disease, suffering]. ABBR: CMP. Disease of the myocardium, esp. due to primary disease of the heart muscle. SEE: *myocarditis.*

  c., alcoholic. Disease of the heart muscle due to alcohol consumption.

  c., congestive. Cardiomyopathy associated with enlargement of the left ventricle of the heart and congestive heart failure.

  c., constrictive. SEE: *c., restrictive.*

  c., hypertrophic. A common disorder of heart muscle characterized by asymptomatic hypertrophy of the intraventricular septum. The disorder may be present in neonates. In some patients, the disease is transmitted genetically. The cause of the disease is unknown.

  SYM: Congestive heart failure, dyspnea, fatigue, chest pain similar to angina, dizziness, syncope. In addition, the ECG is usually abnormal, as is the chest roentgenogram and echocardiogram. Many children with the disease are asymptomatic, except for a heart murmur.

  TREAT: Symptomatic treatment of dyspnea and chest pain. Calcium entry blockers, particularly verapamil. Cardioversion for arrhythmias. Surgery may be indicated in patients who do not respond to conservative therapy.

  PROG: The disease may have a long, benign course or may result in sudden death while exercising.

  c., parasitic. Cardiomyopathy due to infection of cardiac muscle with parasitic organisms.

  c., primary. Cardiomyopathy in which the origin, i.e., cause, is unknown.

  c., restrictive. Disease of the heart muscle associated with lack of flexibility of the ventricular walls of the heart. SEE: *pericarditis.*

  c., secondary. Any cardiomyopathy (CMP) in which either the cause is known or it is associated with a well-defined systemic disease. Included will be CMP associated with inflammation, toxic chemicals, metabolic abnormalities, and inherited disorders of muscles.

cardiomyopexy (kăr″dē-ō-mī′ō-pĕk″sē) [″

+ " + *pexis,* fixation]. Surgical fixation of a vascular tissue such as pectoral muscle to the cardiac muscle and pericardium in order to improve blood supply to the myocardium.

cardiomyotomy. Surgical therapy for achalasia, q.v. The muscles surrounding the cardioesophageal junction are cut but the underlying mucous membrane is left intact.

cardionecrosis (kăr″dē-ō-nĕ-krō′sĭs) [″ + *nekros,* dead, + *osis,* condition]. Necrosis of heart tissue.

cardionecteur, cardionector (kăr″dē-ō-nĕk′tĕr) [″ + L. *nektor,* joiner]. The conduction system of the heart: the sinoatrial node in which the stimulus for atrial contraction arises; the bundle of His, which transmits the impulse from the atrium to the atrioventricular node, which stimulates ventricular contraction.

cardionephric (kăr″dē-ō-nĕf′rĭk) [″ + *nephros,* kidney]. Pert. to the heart and kidney.

cardioneural (kăr″dē-ō-nū′răl) [″ + *neuron,* nerve]. Pert. to nervous control of the heart.

cardioneurosis (kăr″dē-ō-nū-rō′sĭs) [″ + ″ + *osis,* condition]. Functional neurosis with cardiac symptoms.

cardiopathy (kăr″dē-ŏp′ă-thē) [″ + *pathos,* disease, suffering]. Any disease of the heart.

cardiopericarditis (kăr″dē-ō-pĕr″ĭ-kăr-dī′tĭs) [″ + *peri,* around, + *kardia,* heart, + *itis,* inflammation]. Inflamed myocardium and pericardium.

cardiophobia (kăr″dē-ō-fō′bē-ă) [″ + *phobos,* fear]. Morbid fear of heart disease.

cardiophone (kăr′dē-ō-fōn) [″ + *phone,* voice]. Device, esp. a stethoscope, for listening to sound of the heart.

cardioplasty (kăr″dē-ō-plăs′tē) [″ + *plassein,* to form]. Operation on the cardiac sphincter of the stomach to relieve cardiospasm.

cardioplegia (kăr″dē-ō-plē′jē-ă) [″ + *plege,* stroke]. Intentional arrest of cardiac function by use of cold, electrical stimuli, or medication in order to greatly decrease the need of the myocardium for oxygen. This is done during surgery requiring cardiopulmonary bypass.

cardiopneumatic (kăr″dē-ō-nū-măt′ĭk) [″ + *pneuma,* air]. Pert. to the heart and lungs.

cardiopneumograph (kăr″dē-ō-nū′mō-grăf) [″ + ″ + *graphein,* to write]. Device for recording motion of heart and lungs.

cardioptosis (kăr″dē-ŏp-tō′sĭs) [″ + *ptosis,* a dropping]. Prolapse of the heart.

cardiopulmonary (kăr″dē-ō-pŭl′mō-nĕr-ē) [″ + L. *pulmo,* lung]. Pert. to both the heart and lungs.

cardiopulmonary arrest. Sudden cessation of functional ventilation and circulation. SEE: *cardiopulmonary resuscitation.*

cardiopulmonary resuscitation. ABBR: CPR. ASSESSMENT: An individual capable of administering emergency medical care to a person who is apparently unconscious must determine immediately the state of consciousness, cardiac and pulmonary function, and be certain CPR is required. If trauma to the head and neck has been sustained or if patient is unconscious, assume there is spinal injury and do not move the victim unless absolutely necessary. Movement of an individual with a neck injury could cause paralysis. If the individual cannot be roused, institute *basic life support* (BLS) by calling for help in order to activate the *emergency medical care* (EMC) system.

The victim is then carefully placed in a supine position on a firm, flat surface. Be certain that the head is not elevated and that the arms are alongside the body. Kneel at the level of the victim's shoulder and *open airway.* The head is tilted back and the chin lifted up unless spinal injury is present or suspected. In that case, move the spine as little as possible by using the jaw-thrust technique, q.v., for opening the airway. This will prevent the tongue and glottis from obstructing the airway. If liquid or solid material is visible in the mouth, remove it. If dentures are present and interfere with resuscitation, remove them. Next assess *breathing* by listening for breath signs while maintaining an open airway, and watch for rise and fall of the chest. If this does not happen, the victim is breathless. This assessment should require no more than 3 to 5 seconds.

The goal of CPR is to provide oxygen quickly to the brain, heart, and other vital organs until appropriate, definitive medical treatment can restore normal heart and pulmonary function. Rescue breathing is begun using mouth-to-mouth technique. The rescuer gently pinches the victim's nose closed, using the hand on the victim's forehead in order to prevent air from escaping through the nose during the time the lung is being inflated. The rescuer takes a deep breath and seals his or her lips around the outside of the victim's mouth, creating an airtight seal; then gives two full breaths, each taking 1 to 1½ seconds. The rescuer inhales air in between each ventilation and makes certain that the chest rises. Using too much air too swiftly may result in increased pharyngeal pressure and allow air to enter the stomach. If signs of adequate ventilation, i.e., chest rising and feeling the escape of air during exhalation, are not present, then reposition the head and repeat rescue breathing. If this does not result in ventilation, proceed with the Heimlich maneuver, q.v., for clearing the airway of a foreign body.

Caution: In order to prevent transmission of disease from patient to those administering CPR, a bag-valve-mask or other suitable device should be used in place of mouth-to-mouth technique.

Next assess *circulation* by checking the pulse in the carotid artery. This is done in 5 to 10 seconds by locating the groove between the trachea and the strap muscles of the neck. Press gently to avoid compressing the artery. If pulse is present but there is no breathing, rescue breathing should be initiated at a rate of one per 5 seconds (12 per minute). If there is no pulse, the diagnosis of cardiac arrest is confirmed and external chest compression is begun after the initial two breaths. This consists of serial, rhythmic applications of pressure over the lower half of the sternum. In order to reduce the chance of rib fracture, it is important that the heels of the hands be properly placed over the middle of the sternum just above the notch where the ribs meet the sternum in the middle of the lower part of the chest. The fingers may be either extended or interlaced, but must not be pressed against the lateral chest wall. Proper compression is accomplished by locking the elbows in position, with the rescuer's arms extending straight up from the chest with the shoulders directly over the chest. This will cause the thrust of each external chest compression to be straight down on the sternum. It is depressed 1.5 to 2.0 in. (3.8 to 5.0 cm) for the normal-sized adult. For a child, the chest is depressed 1.0 to 1.5 in. (2.8 to 3.8 cm); for an infant, the chest is depressed 0.5 to 1.0 in. (1.3 to 2.54 cm). The chest compression pressure is released completely to allow blood to flow into the heart. The chest should return to its normal position after each compression. The rate of compression should be a minimum of 80 per minute and up to 100 per minute if possible for an adult or child, but at least 100 per minute for an infant. Pressure should be released for the same amount of time required for compression. This is necessary in order to allow the air administered to leave the lungs.

While these maneuvers are being continued, it is imperative that efforts to activate the emergency medical system (EMS) be made, but do not interrupt CPR for more than 7 seconds. This is done by calling or having someone call the local emergency telephone number, 911, if available. The person contacting the EMS should provide full details concerning the location of the emergency, the phone number from which the call is being made, the nature of the emergency, the number of persons who need help, and what aid is being given to the victim(s). Lay persons being instructed in CPR should utilize the one-rescuer technique. If trained professionals arrive at the scene, they will proceed with two-rescuer CPR and advanced cardiac life support (ACLS), q.v., as appropriate for the situation. One rescuer does ventilation while the second does external chest compressions at the same rate as for one-person CPR. When the compressor becomes fatigued, the rescuers exchange positions. It is important that the victim's condition be monitored to assess the effectiveness of the rescue effort. Do this by checking the pulse during chest compression; to determine whether or not spontaneous breathing has returned, stop chest compression for 5 seconds at about the end of the first minute and every few minutes thereafter. SEE: illus.; table; *advanced cardiac life support; basic life support; emergency cardiac care; jaw-thrust technique for establishing the airway; Universal Precautions* in Appendix.

cardiopuncture [" + L. *punctura,* piercing]. Surgical puncture of the heart. SYN: *cardiocentesis.*

cardiopyloric (kăr″dē-ō-pī-lor′ĭk) [" + *pyloros,* gatekeeper]. Pert. to the cardiac and pyloric ends of the stomach.

cardiorenal (kăr″dē-ō-rē′năl) [Gr. *kardia,* heart, + L. *renalis,* pert. to kidney]. Pert. to both the heart and kidneys.

cardiorrhaphy (kăr″dē-or′ă-fē) [" + *rhaphe,* seam, ridge]. Suturing of the heart muscle.

cardiorrhexis (kăr″dē-ō-rĕk′sĭs) [" + *rhexis,* rupture]. Rupture of the heart.

cardiosclerosis (kăr″dē-ō-sklĕ-rō′sĭs) [" + *sklerosis,* hardening]. Hardening of the cardiac tissues and arteries.

cardiospasm (kăr′dē-ō-spăzm) [" + *spasmos,* a convulsion]. Disordered motor function of the distal end of the esophagus and failure of the esophageal orifice (cardia) of the stomach to relax. Thus, the word is a misnomer in that failure of relaxation (achalasia) and absence of esophageal motility (aperistalsis) are the pathological processes involved.

SYM: Substernal fullness, dysphagia, regurgitation, esp. at night.

ETIOL: Due to absence or injury of ganglion cells in Auerbach's plexus.

CARDIOPULMONARY RESUSCITATION

OPEN AIRWAY BY RAISING CHIN AND TILTING HEAD BACKWARD FROM CHEST. THIS FORCES EPIGLOTTIS AND TONGUE AWAY FROM AIRWAY

ARROWS INDICATE RELAXED TONGUE OCCLUDING AIRWAY

MAINTAIN HEAD TILT AND CHIN RAISED. LISTEN FOR BREATH, OR IT CAN BE FELT

MAINTAIN HEAD TILT, CHIN RAISED POSITION. INFLATE LUNGS WHILE HOLDING NOSE CLOSED

IF MOUTH IS HELD CLOSED LUNGS MAY BE INFLATED BY BLOWING THROUGH PATIENT'S NOSE

IF TRACHEOSTOMY IS PRESENT INFLATE LUNGS BY BLOWING THROUGH STOMA

TREAT: Bland semisolid foods warmed to body temperature are of some help, but dilatation of the esophageal sphincter will allow the esophagus to drain by force of gravity. It may be possible to do this mechanically; if not, surgical myotomy may be required.

cardiosphygmograph (kăr″dē-ō-sfĭg′mō-grăf) [″ + *sphygmos*, throb, + *graphein*, to write]. Instrument for graphically recording movements of the heart and pulse.

cardiosymphysis (kăr″dē-ō-sĭm′fĭ-sĭs) [″ + *symphysis*, growing together]. Medias-

INITIAL APPROACH TO PATIENT WHO MAY NEED CARDIOPULMONARY RESUSCITATION

QUESTION PATIENT TO
DETERMINE RESPONSIVENESS

IF NO RESPONSE TO
QUESTIONS, IMMEDIATELY
CALL FOR HELP AND
ASSISTANCE

POSITION PATIENT FOR ACCESS
TO FACE AND ANTERIOR CHEST

tinopericarditis.

cardiotachometer (kăr″dē-ō-tăk-ŏm′ĕ-tĕr)
[Gr. *kardia*, heart, + *tachos*, speed, +
metron, measure]. Instrument for measuring the heart rate over a long period of time.

cardiotherapy (kăr″dē-ō-thĕr′ă-pē) [″ +
therapeia, treatment]. The treatment of

cardiac diseases.

cardiothyrotoxicosis (kăr″dē-ō-thī″rō-tŏk″
sĭ-kō′sĭs) [″ + *thyreos*, shield, + *toxikon*, poison, + *osis*, condition]. Heart
disease due to disease of the thyroid gland,
usually hyperthyroidism.

cardiotomy (kăr″dē-ŏt′ō-mē) [″ + *tome*,

EXTERNAL CHEST COMPRESSION

THE RESCUER'S BACK IS MOVED UP AND DOWN
SUFFICIENT TO DEPRESS THE STERNUM
1½ to 2 INCHES (3.8 to 5 CM)
AND THEN RELEASED

SHOULDERS
DIRECTLY
OVER
STERNUM

ELBOWS
LOCKED
AND ARMS
KEPT STIFF

PROPER POSITION OF
HAND OVER LOWER
PORTION OF STERNUM
NOT OVER ABDOMEN

incision]. Incision of the heart.

cardiotonic (kăr″dē-ō-tŏn′ĭk) [″ + *tonos*, tone]. Increasing tonicity of the heart. Various drugs, including digitalis, are cardiotonic. SEE: *inotropic*.

cardiotoxic (kăr″dē-ō-tŏk′sĭk) [″ + *toxikon*, poisoning]. Having a poisonous effect upon the heart.

cardiovalvulitis (kăr″dē-ō-văl″vū-lī′tĭs) [″ + L. *valvula*, valve, + Gr. *itis*, inflammation]. Inflammation of valves of the heart.

cardiovalvulotome (kăr″dē-ō-văl′vū-lō-tōm″) [″ + ″ + Gr. *tome*, incision]. Instrument for excising part of a valve, esp. the mitral valve.

cardiovascular (kăr″dē-ō-văs′kū-lăr) [″ + L. *vasculum*, small vessel]. Pert. to the heart and blood vessels.

cardiovascular reflex. 1. Sympathetic increase in heart rate when increased pressure in, or distention of, great veins occurs. 2. Reflex vasoconstriction resulting from reduced venous pressure.

cardiovasology (kăr″dē-ō-văs-ŏl′ō-jē) [″ + L. *vas*, vessel, + Gr. *logos*, word, reason]. Science of the heart and blood vessels. SYN: *cardioangiology*.

cardioversion (kăr′dē-ō-vĕr″zhŭn) [″ + L. *versio*, a turning]. Synchronized electric shock used to terminate cardiac arrhythmias. Unlike defibrillation, which is an unsynchronized shock, cardioversion is timed to avoid the T wave of the cardiac cycle. In the conscious patient, sedation may be required prior to the procedure.

Caution: Cardioversion should not be used in sinus tachycardia or arrhythmias (other than ventricular fibrillation) caused by digitalis toxicity. It should be used only in emergency situations when potassium administration and other measures have failed. The cardioverter may induce lethal ventricular fibrillation unresponsive to further electrical shocks.

NURSING IMPLICATIONS: Explain procedure to the patient and provide support throughout. Start an I.V. infusion; attach the patient to the ECG monitor and record 12-lead ECG. Chest electrodes are placed to provide tall R waves while not interfering with paddle placement. The patient is placed in a supine position and adequately ventilated. The recorder is turned on to document the cardioversion and demonstrate the patient's post-treatment rhythm. The patient should be observed for skin burns, rhythm disturbances, respiratory problems, hypotension, and changes in the ECG's ST segment.

cardioverter (kăr′dē-ō-vĕr″tĕr). Electrical device used to administer electrical shocks to the heart when electrodes are placed on the chest wall. Useful in emergency treatment of cardiac arrhythmias such as ventricular tachycardia. Changing the arrhythmia to normal sinus rhythm is called

Basic Cardiac Life Support Standards

Former Standard	Present Standard	Rationale
Training of rescuers One- and two-person CPR	Lay rescuers: One-person CPR only. If present, second lay rescuer should call for professional help. If first rescuer tires, second may provide relief. Professional rescuers (nurses, physicians, emergency medical technicians): Both one- and two-person CPR	One-person CPR improves performance and retention of skills. Two-person CPR may be confusing and has not been used often. Two-person CPR: Less fatiguing; performance may be extended over longer time periods.
Opening airway (establishing breathlessness) Head tilt/chin lift and jaw thrust	Lay rescuers: Head tilt/chin lift only Professional rescuers: Both head tilt/chin lift and jaw thrust	Head tilt/chin lift is safe, effective, simple, and easy to learn. Though effective, jaw thrust is tiring and technically difficult.
After establishing breathlessness (victim over 1 year of age) Four quick "staircase" breaths	Two slow breaths of 1 to 1½ seconds each. After delivering first breath, pause to inhale before delivering second.	Slower breaths prevent air entrapment between breaths. Decreased air pressure minimizes risk of opening the esophagus and creating gastric distention with possible regurgitation and aspiration. Pause allows rescuer to increase lung volume, enabling more oxygen delivery to lungs.
After establishing breathlessness (infant victim) Four quick, full puffs of air	Same as above (two slow breaths of 1–1½ seconds each; pause between breaths)	Same as above
After establishing complete airway obstruction Four back blows and four abdominal thrusts (Heimlich maneuver)	The abdominal thrust is the only recommended technique for removal of a foreign body causing airway obstruction in victims over 1 year of age. The chest thrust remains the approved technique for obese persons and women in late pregnancy.	Exclusive use of abdominal thrusts is more effective and safer than back blows alone or back blows in combination with abdominal thrusts.

Basic Cardiac Life Support Standards *(Continued)*

Former Standard	Present Standard	Rationale
	Due to risk of abdominal injury, the combination of chest thrusts and back blows remains accepted protocol in infant victims under 1 year of age.	
Near-drowning victims No clear guidelines available. Instruction usually in rescue breathing or CPR. Some emphasis on clearing lower airway of water before onset of CPR.	Start rescue breathing as soon as possible. Perform abdominal thrusts only if a foreign object appears to be obstructing the airway or if victim does not respond to mouth-to-mouth ventilation. If necessary, start CPR after abdominal thrusts have been performed.	The necessity of clearing lower airway of aspirated water has not been proved. Attempts to remove water from airway by nonsuctioning techniques are unnecessary and may be dangerous by causing ejection of gastric contents and subsequent aspiration.
After establishing lack of pulse (infant victim) Compress victim's sternum at nipple line with two or three fingers.	Compress victim's sternum one fingerwidth below nipple line with two or three fingers.	Recent studies demonstrate that an infant's heart lies lower in the chest (in relation to external landmarks) than previously believed.
External chest compression, one-person CPR 60–80 external chest compressions per minute	80–100 external chest compressions per minute	Rapid chest compressions increase blood flow from the heart. Increase in intrathoracic pressure promotes blood flow from the thoracic cavity to the brain and heart.
Delivering breaths, two-person CPR One breath on the upstroke of every fifth chest compression, no pause in chest compressions	One breath of 1–1½ seconds *during a pause* after every fifth chest compression. Pause may be shorter.	Slower breaths minimize risk of gastric distention, regurgitation, and aspiration.

cardioversion, q.v.

    c., automatic implantable. An implantable device for detecting and terminating ventricular tachycardia or fibrillation.

carditis (kär-dī′tĭs) [″ + *itis,* inflammation]. Inflammation of the heart muscles. Usually involves two of the following: pericardium, myocardium, or endocardium.

    c., Coxsackie. Carditis or pericarditis that may occur in infections with enteroviruses of the Coxsackie groups, and also echovirus groups.

    c., rheumatic. Carditis occurring in conjunction with rheumatic fever.

Cardrase. Trade name for ethoxzolamide.

care, long-term. A term referring to a range of care services from health to social services for individuals experiencing chronic physical or mental impairments, or both, in order to maintain continuity from one discipline or institution to another. The goal is to maintain an optimal level of functioning and insure utilization of the patient's potential.

care, medical. The use of medical skill to benefit a patient.

care, primary medical. The medical care of a person at the initial time and place the patient presents. The provision of this service is usually accomplished in a physician's office, in an outpatient clinic, or in the emergency department of a hospital.

care, respite. Provision of short-term care to older persons in the community for the purpose of giving caregivers a temporary relief from their responsibilities. This service also may be available for persons who care for severely handicapped children.

care, secondary medical. Medical care of a patient by a physician acting as a consultant. The provider of primary medical care usually refers the patient for this level of care.

care, tertiary medical. Medical care of a patient in a facility staffed and equipped to administer comprehensive care. In the usual situation, this level of care is provided in a large hospital to which the patient has been referred or transferred.

caregiver. One who provides care to a dependent or partially dependent patient. In an acute care setting, the caregiver is most often a professional; however, in the home-care situation this person is often a family member. Care of caregivers is a focus of nurses, social workers, and other health care providers who manage chronic patients. Generally caregivers are in need of emotional support and comfort due to the extreme stress of their lives. SEE: *burnout*.

C.A.R.F. *Commission on Accreditation of Rehabilitation Facilities*.

caries (kăr′ēz, kăr′ĭ-ēz) [L., rottenness]. Gradual decay and disintegration of soft, or bony tissue, or a tooth. If the decay is allowed to progress, the surrounding tissue will become inflamed and an abscess will form.

Ex.: chronic abscess; tuberculosis; and bacterial invasion of teeth. In caries, the bone disintegrates by pieces, while in necrosis large masses of bone are discharged.

    c., arrested. The state in which a carious lesion appears not to progress between dental examinations.

    c., bottle mouth. Extensive caries and discoloration of the teeth that can be observed in children from 19 months to 4 years of age who have had prolonged bottle feedings.

    c., cervical. Caries involving the neck of the tooth, slightly above or below the junction between root cementum and the enamel crown.

    c., classification of. G.V. Black's classification of dental caries according to the part of the tooth involved: Class I occlusal; Class II interproximal, commonly at the dentinoenamel junction; Class III interproximal surfaces not involving incisal surfaces; Class IV interproximal but involving an incisal surface; Class V faciocervical area.

    c., dental. Decay of the teeth. A progressive decalcification of the enamel and dentin of a tooth. The etiological factors are not fully known but attention to diet by minimizing intake of refined carbohydrates and good dental hygiene prevent growth of bacteria that play a role in promoting the development of caries. Proper brushing of the teeth is effective in preventing and removing dental plaque, q.v., in all areas except from the areas between the teeth and in deep fissures. Use of dental floss or tape will remove plaque from between adjacent tooth surfaces; and deep pits and fissures may be sealed by application of resins to those areas. The sealant may need to be replaced periodically. Early detection and dental restorations offer the best form of control once caries has formed. Topical application of fluoride promotes resistance to dental caries if applied during the stage of tooth formation. Teeth will be less likely to develop caries if appropriate amounts of fluoride are ingested while the teeth are developing. It is important that excess fluoride not be ingested because greater amounts than required (about one mg each day) will cause mottling of the teeth. Fluoride in the diet does not obviate the need for topical application of fluoride to the teeth. SEE: *plaque, dental;* illus.

    c., necrotic. A diseased condition in which masses of bone lie in a suppurative cavity.

    c., radiation. Dental caries that develops as an undesired side effect of treatment of malignancies of the oral cavity with ionizing radiation.

    c., rampant. A sudden onset of widespread caries that affects most of the teeth in the mouth and quickly penetrates to the dental pulp.

    c. sicca. Dry tuberculosis of ends of bones and joints unaccompanied by fluid or swelling.

    c., spinal. Caries of the vertebrae, usually tuberculous. SYN: *Pott's disease*.

carina (kă-rī′nă) [L., keel of a boat] (pl. *carinae*). A structure with a projecting central ridge.

    c. nasi. Olfactory nasal sulcus, q.v.

    c. tracheae. [NA] Ridge at lower end of trachea separating openings of the two bronchi.

    c. urethralis. Ridge extending posteriorly from the urethral orifice and continuous with the anterior column of the vagina.

carinae (kă-rī′nē) [L.]. Pl. of carina.

carinate (kăr′ĭ-nāt) [L. *carina*, keel of a boat].

DENTAL CARIES

CARIES

ENAMEL

CROWN

PULP AND
PULP CAVITY

CEMENTUM

DENTIN

ROOT
CANAL

ACID BREAKS DOWN THE ENAMEL
THAT COVERS THE CROWN OF
THE TOOTH

CARIES
LESION

DECAY PENETRATES THE DENTIN,
THE LAYER UNDER THE ENAMEL

CARIES NOW
COMMUNICATES
WITH THE
PULP

THE CAVITY, IF NOT REPAIRED,
SPREADS INTO THE PULP OF THE
TOOTH. THIS MAY CAUSE INFLAMMATION
AND AN ABSCESS. THEN THE TOOTH
MAY HAVE TO BE EXTRACTED.

Keel-shaped; possessing a conspicuous central ridge.

caring behaviors. Behaviors evidenced by nurses in caring for patients.

NURSING IMPLICATIONS: The following are the 10 highest ranked caring behaviors, derived from nursing literature, then selected by nurses as evident in caring situations with patients: attentive listening, comforting, honesty, patience, responsibility, providing information so the patient can make an informed decision, touch, sensitivity, respect, calling the patient by name.

cariogenesis (kăr″ē-ō-jĕn′ĕ-sĭs) [L. caries, rottenness, + Gr. genesis, generation, birth]. The formation of caries. SEE: caries, dental.

cariogenic (kā″rē-ō-jĕn′ĭk) [″ + Gr. gennan, to produce]. Conducive to caries formation.

carious (kā′rē-ŭs). 1. Affected with or rel. to caries. 2. Having pits or perforations.

carisoprodol (kăr″ĭ-sō-prō′dŏl). USP. A drug that relaxes muscles by acting on the central nervous system. Trade names are Rela and Soma.

carminative (kăr-mĭn′ă-tĭv) [L. carminativus, cleanse]. An agent that helps to prevent gas formation in the gastrointestinal tract.

carmustine. An antineoplastic drug. Trade name is BCNU.

carnal (kăr′năl) [L. carnalis, flesh]. Rel. to the desires and appetites of the flesh; sensual.

carnal knowledge. A phrase used in medicolegal cases to denote sexual intercourse.

carneous (kăr′nē-ŭs) [L. carneus, fleshy]. Fleshy.

carnitine (kăr′nĭ-tĭn). A chemical, γ-trimethylamine-β-hydroxybutyrate, that is important in metabolizing palmitic and stearic acids. It has been used therapeutically in treating myopathy due to carnitine deficiency.

carnivore (kăr′nĭ-vor). An animal that primarily eats meat, particularly an animal of the order Carnivora, which includes cats, dogs, and bears.

carnivorous (kăr-nĭv′ō-rŭs) [L. carnivorus]. Flesh eating.

carnophobia (kăr″nō-fō′bē-ă) [″ + Gr. phobos, fear]. Abnormal aversion to meat.

carnose (kăr′nōs). Having the consistency of or resembling flesh.

carnosine (kăr′nō-sĭn). A chemical substance, β-alanylhistidine, present in muscle. Its function is unknown.

carnosity (kăr-nŏs′ĭ-tē) [L. carnositas, fleshiness]. An excrescence resembling flesh; a fleshy growth.

carotenase (kăr-ŏt′ĕ-nās) [Gr. karoton, carrot]. An enzyme that converts carotene into vitamin A. SYN: carotinase.

carotene (kăr′ō-tēn) [Gr. *karoton*]. A yellow crystalline pigment present in various plant and animal tissues. It is abundant in yellow vegetables (carrots, squash, corn). Carotene, which exists in several forms, is the precursor of vitamin A. It is stored in and converted to vitamin A in the liver.

carotenemia (kăr″ō-tě-nē′mē-ă) [″ + *haima*, blood]. Carotene in the blood characterized by yellowing of the skin (pseudojaundice). Carotenemia can be distinguished from true jaundice by the lack of yellow discoloration of the conjunctivae in carotenemia. It is a benign condition. SYN: *carotenosis*.

carotenoid (kă-rŏt′ĕ-noyd) [″ + *eidos*, form, shape]. 1. One of a group of pigments (as carotene, q.v.) ranging in color from light yellow to red-hued, widely distributed in plants and animals. The possibility that some carotenoids may be of benefit in treating cancer is being investigated. 2. Resembling carotene.

carotenosis [″ + *osis*, condition]. Carotenemia, q.v.

carotic (kă-rŏt′ĭk) [Gr. *karos*, deep sleep]. 1. Carotid. 2. Resembling stupor; stupefying.

caroticotympanic (kă-rŏt″ĭ-kō-tĭm-păn′ĭk). Concerning the carotid canal and the tympanic cavity, i.e., middle ear.

carotid (kă-rŏt′ĭd) [Gr. *karos*, deep sleep]. 1. Pert. to the right and left common carotid arteries, both of which arise from the aorta, and are the principal blood supply to the head and neck. Each of these two arteries divides to form external and internal carotid arteries. 2. Pert. to any carotid part, as carotid sinus.

carotid body. A flat structure at the bifurcation of the common carotid artery. Contains cells that respond to changes in concentration of oxygen in the blood and to changes in blood pressure.

carotid bruits. Murmurs heard in the cervical area that do not disappear with venous compression, are maximal over the carotid bifurcation, and are not due to transmitted cardiac murmurs. The presence of asymptomatic carotid bruits increases with advanced age, but is not associated with increased risk for stroke in elderly patients. In addition, carotid bruits may spontaneously disappear without sequelae.

carotid endarterectomy. A surgical technique for removing intra-arterial obstructions of the lower cervical portion of the internal carotid artery. The technique was developed in the hope of preventing some strokes. Except in cases of severe stenosis with multiple transient ischemic attacks (TIA), the technique is not considered to be of benefit. SEE: *transient ischemic attacks*.

carotid sinus. A dilated area at the bifurcation of the common carotid artery that is richly supplied with sensory nerve endings of the sinus branch of the vagus nerve. These, when stimulated by distention of the vessel wall brought about by a rise in blood pressure, bring about reflex vasodilation and a slowing of the heart rate.

carotid siphon. The S-shaped terminal portion of the internal carotid artery that is the origin of most of the arteries to the brain.

carotidynia (kăr-ŏt″ĭ-dĭn′ē-ă) [″ + *odyne*, pain]. Pain elicited by pressure on the common carotid artery. Also spelled carotodynia.

carotinase. Carotenase.

carotinemia. Carotenemia.

carpal [Gr. *karpalis*]. Pert. to the carpus or wrist.

carpal boss. A bony growth on the dorsal surface of the third metacarpocarpal joint.

carpale (kăr-pā′lē) [Gr. *karpos*]. Any wrist bone.

carpal spasm. Involuntary contraction of the muscles of the hand. SEE: *tetany*.

carpal tunnel. The canal in the wrist bounded by osteofibrous material through which the flexor tendons and the median nerve pass.

carpal tunnel syndrome. Paresthesias, pain, or numbness affecting some part of the median nerve distribution of the hand(s), i.e., palmar side of thumb, index finger, and radial half of the ring finger, and radial half of the palm. The paresthesias and pain may radiate into the arm. There may be a history of cumulative trauma to the wrist, e.g., in carpenters, rowers, or those who regularly use vibrating tools or machinery.

TREAT: Rest, including avoidance of that which aggravates the symptoms. This may require intermittent splinting of the wrist in order to relieve tension on the median nerve. Analyze the patient's job requirements and provide recommendations for modified tools, or a change in job assignment. Instruct patient to avoid tension on the median nerve. Injections of corticosteroids under the actual tunnel, but not the median nerve. Surgery is required in the majority of cases. However, cortisone injection into the painful site or use of nonsteroidal anti-inflammatory drugs may eliminate the symptoms. SEE: *repetitive motion injury*.

NURSING IMPLICATIONS: Medical evaluation of the severity of the problem and underlying cause should be encouraged. If a splint is prescribed to relieve symptoms, teach patient how to apply and assist to determine how to modify lifestyle to minimize problem. If surgery is carried out on an outpatient basis, discuss bathing and other activities of daily living which may pose problems for the patient. Alert patient to symptoms indicative of complications and encourage to come for follow-up care. SEE: *Nursing Diagnoses in Appendix.*

carpectomy (kăr-pĕk'tō-mē) [" + *ektome,* excision]. Excision of the carpus or portion of it.

carphenazine maleate (kăr-fĕn'ă-zēn). USP. A tranquilizer of the phenothiazine class. Trade name is Proketazine.

carphologia, carphology (kăr-fō-lō'jē-ă, -fŏl'ō-jē) [Gr. *karphos,* dry twig, + *legein,* to pluck]. Involuntary picking at bedclothes, seen esp. in febrile or exhaustive delirium of the low muttering type. A grave symptom in cases of extreme exhaustion or approaching death. SYN: *floccillation.*

carpo- [Gr. *karpos*]. Prefix pert. to the carpus.

carpometacarpal [" + *meta,* beyond, + *karpos,* wrist]. Pert. to both the carpus and metacarpus.

carpopedal (kăr"pō-pĕd'ăl) [" + L. *ped,* foot]. Pert. to both the wrist and foot.

carpopedal spasm. Spasm of the hands and feet, sometimes seen in laryngismus stridulus, q.v., and in the hyperventilation syndrome. It is caused by hypocalcemia and commonly encountered during hyperventilation because the lowered carbon dioxide alters the level of ionized calcium. SEE: *hyperventilation, tetany.*

carpoptosis (kăr"pŏp-tō'sĭs) [" + *ptosis,* a falling]. Wrist drop.

carpus (kăr'pŭs) [L.]. [NA] The eight bones of the wrist joint. SEE: *skeleton; wrist.*

carrageen, carragheen (kăr'ă-gēn). Irish moss. Dried red alga, *Chondrus crispus,* from which the substance carrageenan, or carragheenan, is obtained. It is used as a demulcent and thickening agent in medicines and foods.

Carrel-Dakin treatment (kăr-ĕl'dā'kĭn) [Alexis Carrel, Fr.-U.S. surgeon, 1873–1944; Henry D. Dakin, U.S. chemist, 1880–1952]. Method of wound irrigation first utilized in 1915. The wound is intermittently irrigated with Dakin's solution, q.v.

carrier [O. Fr. *carier,* to bear]. 1. A person who harbors a specific pathogenic organism in the absence of discernible symptoms or signs of the disease and who is potentially capable of spreading the organism to others. 2. That which carries anything, as an insect such as a fly that passively carries infectious organisms. 3. A substance that, when combined with another substance (transport substance), is capable of passing through cell membranes as occurs in active transport mechanisms. SEE: *CDC blood and body fluids precautions; fomes; isolation; microorganisms; vector; communicable disease* for

table. 4. A heterozygote; one who carries a recessive gene together with its normal allele. 5. An instrument or apparatus for transporting something. In dentistry, amalgam carrier.

CLASSIFICATION: *Infection by animal carriers:* Some microorganisms may be carried from animal to man by direct contact, indirect transfer, or by intermediary hosts.

Airborne infection: Pathogenic organisms in the respiratory tract, discharged from the mouth or nose, may be borne on the air and settle on food, clothing, walls, and floors. If they are of the type that resists drying for a long period, they may remain virulent until transmitted to another person. Coughing, sneezing, and expectorating may be responsible for droplet infection.

Contact infection: This is the result of transmission from person to person as in kissing, coming in contact with those afflicted with communicable diseases or with utensils handled by one with an infection.

Food-borne infection: Bacteria may be transported by food. Root and salad vegetables may carry bacteria from the soil or from manure used as fertilizer. Cooking provides safeguards by destroying microorganisms on food.

Human carriers: Some parasites may live in or upon the body of persons who themselves do not suffer from the parasites but may carry them to others. Carriers may be asymptomatic contact carriers (those who never show symptoms), incubationary carriers (those in whom the infection is starting but has not completed the incubation period), and convalescent carriers (those who have recovered but still harbor the organism causing their disease).

Insect vectors: An insect may act as a physical carrier, as the tick that may transmit the organism causing Rocky Mountain spotted fever, or one may act as an active intermediate host, such as the Anopheles mosquito, which transmits malaria.

Prenatal infection: This is the result of the fetus being infected from the mother's bloodstream or from contiguity with the maternal membranes.

Soil-borne infection: Soil-borne, spore-forming organisms commonly enter the body through wounds as in tetanus and gas gangrene.

Water-borne infection: Organisms producing typhoid, dysentery, cholera, and amebic infections may be carried through a water supply or in public pools used for bathing. These organisms may pass into the water from the feces of an infected person and be communicated to others.

c., active. A person who harbors a pathogenic organism for a considerable period following recovery from disease due to the organism.

c., convalescent. One who harbors an infective organism during recovery from the disease caused by the organism.

c., genetic. One whose chromosomes contain a pathologic mutant gene that may be transmitted to offspring. In some cases such as Tay-Sachs disease, this can be detected prenatally by a laboratory test done on amniotic fluid.

c., healthy. One who harbors an infectious organism but does not succumb to the disease.

c., incubatory. One who harbors and spreads an infectious organism during the incubation period of a disease.

c., intermittent. One who is capable of spreading infectious organisms at intervals.

c., passive. C., healthy.

carrier-free (kăr'ē-ĕr-frē). A radioactive isotope that is not attached to a carrier.

Carrion's disease (kăr-ē-ōnz') [Daniel A. Carrion, a Peruvian student who lost his life after voluntarily taking an injection, 1850 – 1885]. An infectious disease occurring in the valleys of the Andes Mountains in Peru, Chile, Bolivia, and Columbia. It appears in an acute febrile anemic stage followed in several weeks by a nodular skin eruption. Caused by *Bartonella bacilliformis* transmitted by the sandfly. SYN: *bartonellosis.*

carrying angle, arm. SEE: *arm, carrying angle.*

car sickness. Sickness induced by riding in cars. A form of motion sickness, q.v.

cartilage (kăr'tĭ-lĭj) [L. *cartilago,* gristle]. A specialized type of dense connective tissue consisting of cells embedded in a ground substance or matrix. The matrix is firm and compact, rendering it capable of withstanding considerable pressure or tension. Cartilage has a bluish-white or gray color and is semi-opaque; it has no nerve or blood supply of its own. The cells lie in cavities called lacunae. They may be single or in groups of two, three, or four.

Cartilage constitutes a part of the skeleton in adults, occurring in the costal cartilages of the ribs, the nasal septum, in the external ear and lining the eustachian tube, in the wall of the larynx, in the trachea and bronchi, between bodies of the vertebrae, and covering the articular surfaces of bones. It forms the major portion of the embryonic skeleton, providing a model in which most bones develop.

c., articular. Hyaline cartilage covering the articular surfaces of bones.

c., costal. Cartilage connecting the true ribs and the sternum.

c., fibrous. Cartilage containing visible collagenic fibers. SYN: *fibrocartilage.*

c., hyaline. A bluish-white glassy translucent cartilage. The matrix appears homogeneous although it contains collagenous fibers forming a fine network. The walls of the lacunae stain intensely with basic dyes. Hyaline cartilage is flexible and slightly elastic. Its surface is covered by the perichondrium except on articular surfaces. Found in articular cartilage, in costal cartilages, in septum of the nose, in larynx and trachea.

c., semilunar. One of the interarticular cartilages of the knee joint.

c., thyroid. The largest cartilage of the larynx, a shield-shaped cartilage that forms the prominence known as the Adam's apple.

c., yellow. A network of yellow elastic fibers, holding cartilage cells, and pervading intercellular substance. Found in the epiglottis, the external ear, and the auditory tube. It strengthens them and maintains their shape.

cartilage, words pert. to: "cartilag-" words; "chondr-" words; cricoid.

cartilaginification (kăr″tĭ-lă-jĭn″ĭ-fĭ-kā′shŭn) [″ + *facere,* to make]. Cartilage formation or chondrification; the development of cartilage from undifferentiated tissue.

cartilaginoid (kăr″tĭ-lăj′ĭ-noyd) [″ + Gr. *eidos,* form, shape]. Resembling cartilage.

cartilaginous (kăr″tĭ-lăj′ĭ-nŭs). Pert. to or consisting of cartilage.

cartilago (kăr″tĭ-lă′gō) [L.] (pl. *cartilagines*). [NA] Cartilage.

caruncle (kăr′ŭng-kl) [L. *caruncula,* small flesh]. A small fleshy growth.

c., lacrimal. Caruncula lacrimalis [NA]. Caruncle found on the conjunctiva near the inner canthus. A small reddish elevation at the medial angle of the eye.

c., sublingual. Protuberance on each side of the frenulum of the tongue, containing the openings of the ducts from the submandibular and sublingual salivary glands.

c., urethral. A small, red, papillary growth, highly vascular, sometimes found in the urinary meatus in females. It is characterized by pain on urination and is very sensitive to friction.

caruncula (kăr-ŭng′kū-lă) [L.] (pl. *carunculae*). [NA] A tiny, fleshy protuberance. SYN: *caruncle.*

c. hymenales. [NA] Small irregular nodules representing remains of the hymen. SYN: *caruncula myrtiformes.*

Carvallo's sign [J. M. Rivero-Carvallo, contemporary Mexican physician]. An increase in intensity of the presystolic murmur heard in patients with tricuspid stenosis during inspiration, and its decrease during expiration. This is best demonstrated with the patient in an erect position.

carver. A knife or other instrument used for fashioning or shaping an object. In dentistry, artificial teeth or dental restorations.

   c., amalgam. A small, sharp instrument of varying shape used to carve or contour amalgam for interdental occlusion.

   c., wax. A blunt instrument of varying shape to heat and carve or shape wax patterns.

cary-, caryo- [Gr. *karyon*, nucleus]. A combining form meaning nucleus. SEE: words beginning with *kary-, karyo-.*

Casal necklace [Gaspar Casal, Sp. physician, 1691–1759]. Bilaterally symmetrical lesions of the neck which represent a portion of the skin's involvement in pellagra, q.v. The lesions start out as erythemas and progress to vesiculation and crusting.

cascade (kăs-kād'). The continuation of a process through a series of steps; each step initiates the next step until the final step is reached. The action may or may not become amplified as each step progresses. SEE: *citric acid cycle.*

cascara sagrada (kăs-kăr'ă să-grä'dă). USP. The dried bark of *Rhamnus purshiana*, a small tree grown on western U.S. coast, and in parts of South America. The main ingredient in aromatic cascara sagrada fluid extract, a cathartic.

case [L. *casus*, happening]. 1. An occurrence of disease; incorrectly used to refer to a patient. 2. An enclosing structure.

caseate (kā'sē-āt) [L. *caseus*, cheese]. To undergo cheesy degeneration, as in certain necroses.

caseation (kā"sē-ā'shŭn). 1. Process of conversion of necrotic tissue into a granular amorphous mass resembling cheese. 2. Precipitation of casein during coagulation of milk.

case control. In epidemiology, a study in which index cases are matched to comparison cases in an attempt to discover risk factors or exposure.

case-control study. An investigative technique used in epidemiology. Cases are those individuals who have the disease or illness being investigated, and controls are those individuals who do not have the disease. The frequency of occurrence of possible causes of the disease in the two groups is then obtained and the data analyzed for possible differences. An example would be to obtain a group of patients who had developed a disease such as cancer and then to choose individuals from the same population who did not have the disease. The first

such study involved an investigation of chimney sweeps in England who developed cancer of the scrotum. The hypothesis was that something peculiar to their occupation led to a higher incidence of cancer than was prevalent in the general population.

casefinding. Actively seeking to identify persons who have disease.

case history. The complete medical, family, social, and psychiatric history of a patient up to the time of admission for the present illness.

casein (kā'sē-ĭn) [L. *caseus*, cheese]. The principal protein in milk; present in milk curds. It supplies all of the amino acids necessary for growth and development. When coagulated by rennin or acid, it becomes one of the principal ingredients of cheese. SEE: *caseinogen.*

caseinogen (kā-sē-ĭn'ō-jĕn) [" + Gr. *gennan*, to produce]. The principal protein, from which casein is derived, in milk. It is the substance in solution, and casein is the result of its precipitation. Its conversion into casein is the essential process in the curdling of milk.

case law. Opinions or decisions made by the courts.

case management. An individualized approach to obtaining the needed services for a patient by using a case manager to link the patient to direct service providers. It is a particularly valuable approach to meeting the service needs of the homebound elderly.

caseous (kā'sē-ŭs). 1. Resembling cheese. 2. Pert. to transformation of tissues into a cheesy mass.

CaSO₄. Calcium sulfate.

Casoni's reaction (kă-sō'nēz) [Tomaso Casoni, It. physician, 1880–1933]. Appearance of a wheal surrounded by an erythematous zone following intradermal injection of sterile hydatid fluid. A sensitive test for presence of hydatid cysts resulting from infection with *Echinococcus granulosus.* The test gives 40% false-positive results.

cassava. A group of perennial herbs of the genus *Manihot.* The plant is one of the most efficient converters of solar energy to carbohydrate. The root of *M. esculenta* provides an excellent source of starch and it has the ability to thrive in poor, dry, acid soils. In order to be suitable for eating, the root is processed by one of several methods to remove or control the amount of cyanide present. Tapioca is made from cassava.

cassette (kă-sĕt') [Fr., little box]. A flat, lightproof box with an intensifying screen in it, for holding x-ray film or a case for film or magnetic tape.

cast [ME. *casten*, to carry]. 1. A solid mold of a part, usually applied in situ for immobiliza-

CASTS

SHORT ARM CAST
FOR IMMOBILIZING
THE WRIST

ARM CAST WITH
SUSPENSION

SHORT LEG
CAST FITTED
WITH HEEL

tion as in fractures, dislocations, and other severe injuries. Most often made of plaster of paris, sodium silicate, starch, or dextrin that is rubbed into crinoline, then soaked in water, carefully applied to the immobilized part, and allowed to harden. SEE: illus. 2. In dentistry, a positive copy of tissues of the jaw over which denture bases may be made. To make an accurate metallic reproduction of a wax pattern of a dental appliance, tooth crown, or inlay cavity preparation. 3. Pliable or fibrous material shed in various pathological conditions, the product of effusion. It is molded to the shape of the part in which it has been accumulated. According to source, casts are classified as bronchial, intestinal, nasal, esophageal, renal, tracheal, urethral, and vaginal; as to constituents, classified as bloody, fatty, fibrinous, granular, hyaline, mucous, and waxy.

NURSING IMPLICATIONS: Monitor neurovascular status distal to cast, and report and teach patient to report deterioration in sensory or motor abilities, e.g., paresthesias, paralysis, diminished pulses, pallor, coldness, or pain. Also report pain or burning under the cast, identifying the region involved. Be prepared to bivalve or re-

move the cast as necessary to relieve pressure. Teach the patient not to place anything inside a cast to relieve itching, but that relief of this often can be obtained by application of cold, well-sealed ice bag to cast. Teach patient how to protect cast from injury, any prescribed exercises or activity limitations, and use of any required assistive devices such as slings, crutches, or cane. SEE: *Nursing Diagnoses* in *Appendix*.

   c., blood. Urinary cast composed principally of red blood cells.

   c., body. Cast used to immobilize the spine. It may extend from the thorax to the groin.

   c., bronchial. Cast seen in sputum of patients with asthma and some with bronchitis.

   c., epithelial. Cast containing cells from inner lining of uriniferous tubules. Seen in acute nephritis.

   c., fatty. Any cast made up of fat globules.

   c., fibrinous. Yellow-brown cast seen in acute nephritis.

   c., granular. Dark urinary cast of granular substance; usually a degenerative form of a hyaline or waxy cast.

c., hyaline. Urinary cast made up of homogenous protein.

c., pseudo-. Epithelial cells swollen and held in groups, resembling casts. Alkaline urine has a tendency to dissolve casts.

c., pus. Leukocyte cast found in urine in suppuration of kidney.

c., urinary. Cast found in the urine formed from protein precipitates in the renal tubules. SEE: *mucoprotein, Tamm-Horsfell.*

c., uterine. Cast from the uterus passed in exfoliative endometritis or membranous dysmenorrhea.

c., waxy. Light yellowish, well-defined urinary cast with tendency to split transversely, found in some cases of amyloid degeneration and advanced nephritis.

Castellani's paint (kăs-těl-ăn'ēz) [Aldo Castellani, It. physician, 1878–1971]. Paint used as a disinfectant for skin and in treatment of fungus infections of the skin. Composed of phenol, resorcinol, basic fuchsin, boric acid, and acetone.

Castle's intrinsic factor [William Bosworth Castle, U.S. physician and educator, 1897–1990]. A substance secreted by the stomach, essential for the absorption of cyanocobalamin (vitamin B_{12}; extrinsic factor). Absence of intrinsic factor causes pernicious anemia.

castor oil. USP. A fixed oil expressed from the seed of the plant *Ricinus communis.* Used externally as an emollient and internally as a cathartic. In the digestive tract it is hydrolyzed to ricinoleic acid, which acts as an irritant type of laxative. Trade name is Neoloid.

castrate (kăs'trāt) [L. *castrare*, to prune]. 1. To remove the testicles or ovaries. SEE: *spay.* 2. One who has been castrated.

castrated. Rendered incapable of reproduction by removal of the testicles or ovaries.

castration (kăs-trā'shŭn). 1. Excision of the testicles or ovaries. 2. Destruction or inactivation of the gonad.

c., female. Removal of the ovaries. SYN: *oophorectomy; spaying.*

c., male. Removal of the testes. SYN: *orchiectomy.*

c., parasitic. Destruction of the gonads by parasitic organisms early in life. It may result from direct infestation of the gonad or indirectly from effects of infestation in other parts of the body.

castration anxiety or complex. Anxiety about the possibility of injury to or loss of the testicles or ovaries.

casualty (kăz'ū-ăl-tē) [L. *casualis*, accidental]. 1. Accident causing injury or death. 2. Person injured or killed in an accident. 3. Serviceman captured, missing, injured, or killed.

casuistics (kăz-ū-ĭs'tĭks) [L. *casus,* chance]. 1. Analysis of records of clinical cases in order to establish the general characteristics of a disease. 2. The determination of right and wrong in moral questions by application of ethical principles to a particular case.

cat. Any member of the Felidae family, including lions, leopards, wildcats, and esp. the domesticated cat, *Felis catus.* SEE: *cat scratch disease.*

cata- [Gr. *kata,* down]. Prefix indicating down or downward, against, or according to.

catabasis (kă-tăb'ă-sĭs) [Gr. *kata,* down, + *basis,* going]. The decline of a disease.

catabatic (kăt-ă-băt'ĭk). Pert. to catabasis, q.v.

catabolic (kăt″ă-bŏl'ĭk). Pert. to catabolism.

catabolic illness. Rapid weight loss with loss of body fat and muscle mass that frequently accompanies short-term, self-limiting conditions such as infection or injury. This condition may be associated with diabetic ketoacidosis, multiple organ system failure, and chemotherapy or radiation therapy for cancer.

TREAT: Reduce inflammation, provide appropriate nutrients, and administer growth factors to enhance protein synthesis.

catabolin (kă-tăb'ō-lĭn). Catabolite.

catabolism (kă-tăb'ō-lĭzm) [Gr. *katabole,* a casting down, + *-ismos,* condition]. The destructive phase of metabolism, the opposite of anabolism. Catabolism includes all the processes in which complex substances are converted into simpler substances, usually with the release of energy. SEE: *anabolism; metabolism.*

catabolite (kă-tăb'ō-līt). Any product of catabolism. SYN: *catabolin.*

catacrotic (kăt″ă-krŏt'ĭk) [″ + *krotos,* beat]. Indicating the downstroke of pulse tracing interrupted by an upstroke.

catacrotism (kă-tăk'rō-tĭzm) [″ + ″ + *-ismos,* condition]. A pulse with one or more secondary expansions of the artery following the main beat.

catadicrotic (kăt″ă-dī-krŏt'ĭk) [″ + *dis,* twice, + *krotos,* beat]. Manifesting one or more secondary expansions of a pulse on the descending limb of the tracing.

catadicrotism (kăt″ă-dī′krō-tĭzm) [″ + ″ + ″ + *-ismos,* condition]. Two minor expansions following the main beat of an artery.

catadioptric (kăt″ă-dī-ŏp′trĭk) [″ + *diopsesthai,* to see through]. Pert. to refraction and reflection of light simultaneously.

catagen (kăt'ă-jĕn) [″ + *gennan,* to produce]. Intermediate phase of hair-growth cycle that falls after the growth or anagen stage and before the resting or telogen phase.

catagenesis (kăt″ă-jĕn′ĕ-sĭs) [″ + *genesis*, generation, birth]. Retrogression or involution.

catalase (kăt′ă-lās). An enzyme present in almost all cells. It catalyzes the decomposition of hydrogen peroxide to water and oxygen.

catalepsy (kăt′ă-lĕp″sē) [Gr. *kata*, down, + *lepsis*, seizure]. A condition seen in psychotic patients wherein there is generalized diminished responsiveness usually characterized by a trancelike state. Doctors and nurses should keep in mind that even though the patient is in a trance, conversations may be heard. Therefore one's actions toward and talk about such patients should be the same as if they were fully conscious.

cataleptic. Pert. to catalepsy.

cataleptiform (kăt-ă-lĕp′tĭ-form) [″ + *lepsis*, seizure, + L. *forma*, shape]. Having the form of catalepsy.

cataleptoid (kăt″ă-lĕp′toyd) [″ + ″ + *eidos*, form, shape]. Resembling or simulating catalepsy.

catalysis (kă-tăl′ĭ-sĭs) [Gr. *katalysis*, dissolution]. The speeding up of the rate of a chemical reaction by a catalyst, q.v.

catalyst (kăt′ă-lĭst). A substance that speeds up the rate of a chemical reaction without itself being permanently altered in the reaction. Catalysts are effective in small quantities and are not used up in the reaction, i.e., they can be recovered unchanged.

Ex.: hydrochloric acid, which catalyzes the hydrolysis of sucrose; ptyalin, which catalyzes the hydrolysis of starch. SYN: *catalyzer.*

catalytic (kăt-ăl-ĭt′ĭk) [Gr. *katalysis*, dissolution]. Pert. to catalysis, q.v.

catalyze (kăt′ă-līz) [Gr. *katalysis*, dissolution]. To cause catalysis.

catalyzer (kăt′ă-lī-zĕr). A catalyst, q.v.

catamenia (kăt-ă-mē′nē-ă) [Gr. *kata*, according to, + *men*, month]. Cyclic process of the flow of menstrual blood from the uterus. SYN: *menses; menstruation.*

catamenial (kăt″ă-mēn′ē-ăl). Pert. to the menses or catamenia.

catamnesis (kăt-ăm-nē′sĭs) [Gr. *kata*, down, + *mneme*, memory]. A patient's medical history, after treatment; follow-up history. SEE: *anamnesis.*

cataphasia (kăt-ă-fā′zē-ă) [″ + *phasis*, speech]. A speech disorder causing an involuntary repetition of the same word.

cataphoresis (kăt″ă-fō-rē′sĭs) [Gr. *kata*, down, + *phoresis*, being carried]. The transmission of electronegative ions or drugs into the body tissues or through a membrane by use of an electric current.

cataphoria (kăt″ă-fō′rē-ă) [″ + *pherein*, to bear]. Tendency of visual axes to incline below the horizontal plane.

cataphoric. Pert. to cataphora or cataphoresis.

cataphrenia (kăt″ă-frē′nē-ă) [″ + *phrein*, mind]. A type of dementia that usually resolves in recovery.

cataplasia, cataplasis (kăt″ă-plā′zē-ă, kă-tăp′lă-sĭs) [″ + *plassein*, to form]. Atrophic change in tissues or cells.

cataplasm (kăt′ă-plăzm) [L. *cataplasma*]. A poultice, q.v.

cataplectic (kăt-ă-plĕk′tĭk) [″ + *plexis*, stroke]. Pert. to cataplexy.

cataplexy, cataplexia (kăt′ă-plĕks-ē, kăt-ă-plĕk′sē-ă). The brief, sudden loss of muscle control brought on by strong emotion or emotional response, such as a hearty laugh, excitement, surprise, or anger. Even though this may cause collapse, the patient remains fully conscious. The episode will last from a few seconds to as much as two minutes. Once the condition begins, it usually continues but may be less severe with age. About 70% of patients with narcolepsy, q.v., will also have cataplexy.

TREAT: Imipramine hydrochloride is of benefit.

Catapres. Trade name for clonidine hydrochloride.

cataract (kăt′ă-răkt) [L. *cataracta*, waterfall]. Opacity of lens of eye or its capsule or both. Varieties are capsular, polar, lamellar, nuclear, cortical, morgagnian, congenital, infantile, traumatic, diabetic, senile. An estimated 1.25 million people worldwide are blinded by cataracts each year. SEE: illus.

STAGES: Incipient stage (spoke-shaped opacities, cloudlike opacities, opacity of cortex or nucleus). Stage of swelling or immature stage (swollen lens, shallow anterior chamber). Mature stage (lens shrinks due to loss of fluid and becomes opaque, anterior chamber regains its normal depth, no shadow thrown by iris or lens with focal illumination). Hypermature stage (lens becomes either solid and shrunken or soft and liquid).

SYMP: At first, the visual image is distorted, particularly during night driving or in very bright light. As the cataract progresses, severe visual impairment develops.

ETIOL: Common form is result of the aging process; other forms may be congenital or caused by infection, injury, exposure to radiation, adrenal cortical hormones taken for long periods, ultraviolet radiation, or cataracts may occur as a complication of diabetes. Premature development of cataracts has been linked to cigarette smoking.

TREAT: Surgical removal of lens except

CATARACT

RETINA
TENDON OF LATERAL RECTUS MUSCLE
CONJUNCTIVA
CHOROID
CILIARY BODY
IRIS
SCLERA
ANTERIOR CHAMBER
OPTIC NERVE
CORNEA
LENS
CATARACT
POSTERIOR CHAMBER
POSTERIOR CAPSULE OF LENS
CENTRAL ARTERY AND VEIN OF RETINA
TENDON OF MEDIAL RECTUS MUSCLE
VITREOUS BODY
CILIARY PROCESSES
CATARACT

in presence of associated inflammation. The most frequently used treatment is surgical removal of the cataract and implantation of a plastic lens. This technique, involving either local or general anesthesia, may be used in patients of virtually any age. SEE: *phacoemulsification.*

NURSING IMPLICATIONS: *Preop:* Prepare patient for postoperative need to have eye bandaged.

Postop: Modern surgical technology does not require rigid adherence to the practice of immobilization of the head. Care should be taken to prevent increases in intraocular pressure, so the patient should be instructed not to sneeze, cough, or bend from the waist. Rapid movements should be avoided. The patient may turn to the unoperated side (if a unilateral repair). Control nausea and vomiting. Observe patient for sudden eye pain and other symptoms of hemorrhage. The patient should be oriented to the environment and the nurse should spend time talking with the patient at intervals to decrease the effects of sensory deprivation; use touch as a means of communication. All persons entering the room should be certain the patient knows they are in the room in order to prevent startling the patient. The patient

should receive prescribed analgesics as needed, and be out of bed as allowed by the physician. Teach family to keep patient areas unobstructed and free of hazards and to aid patient independence and safety.

Check the operative site for any drainage or symptoms of infection. Instruct the patient and family in the correct technique for administration of eye drops, as well as in the need for an eye shield or eyeglasses for protection as ordered by the physician. SEE: *Nursing Diagnoses* in *Appendix.*

c., capsular. Cataract of opacity of the capsule.

c., hypermature. Overripe cataract, q.v.

c., immature. An early cataract, too poorly developed to require therapy.

c., lenticular. Cataract occurring in the lens.

c., morgagnian. A fluid cataract with a hard nucleus.

c., nuclear. Cataract in which the central portion of the lens is opacified.

c., overripe. Stage following a mature cataract in which lens solidifies and shrinks.

c., radiation. Cataract that occurs due to exposure to radiation, especially from sunlight.

c., ripe. Mature cataract.

c., senile. Cataract of old persons.

cataractogenic (kăt″ă-răk″tō-jĕn′ĭk) [L. *cataracta,* waterfall, + Gr. *gennan,* to produce]. The causation of or formation of a cataract.

catarrh (kă-tăr′) [Gr. *katarrhein,* to flow down]. Term formerly applied to inflammation of mucous membranes, esp. of head and throat.

c., dry. Severe spells of coughing with little or no expectoration. Generally seen in the old in association with emphysema or asthma.

catarrhal (kă-tăr′ăl). Of the nature of or pert. to catarrh.

catatonia (kăt-ă-tō′nē-ă) [″ + *tonos,* tension]. 1. A phase of schizophrenia in which the patient is unresponsive. The tendency to assume and remain in a fixed posture and inability to move or talk are characteristic of this phase. 2. Stupor.

catatonic. Stuporous; pert. to catatonia.

catatricrotic (kăt″ă-trī-krŏt′ĭk) [″ + *treis,* three, + *krotos,* beat]. Manifesting a third impulse in the descending stroke of the sphygmogram.

catatricrotism (kăt″ă-trī′krō-tĭzm). Condition in which the pulse shows a third impulse in the descending stroke of a pulse tracing.

catatropia (kăt″ă-trō′pē-ă) [″ + *tropos,* turning]. Having both eyes turned downward.

catchment area. Geographical area defining the portion of a population served by a designated medical facility.

cat-cry syndrome. SEE: *cri du chat syndrome.*

catecholamines (kăt″ē-kōl′ă-mēns). Biologically active amines, epinephrine and norepinephrine, derived from the amino acid tyrosine. They have marked effect on the nervous and cardiovascular systems, metabolic rate, temperature, and smooth muscle. SEE: *serotonin.*

catelectrotonus (kăt″ē-lĕk-trŏt′ō-nŭs) [″ + *elektron,* amber, + *tonos,* tension]. The state of increased excitability produced in a nerve or muscle in the region near the cathode during the passage of an electric current.

catenating (kăt′ĕn-āt″ĭng) [L. *catena,* chain]. 1. Concerning a disease that is linked with another. 2. Formation of a series of symptoms. SEE: *concatenation.*

catenation. SEE: *concatenation.*

catenoid (kăt′ē-noyd) [″ + Gr. *eidos,* form, shape]. Chainlike; pert. to protozoan colonies whose individuals are joined end to end.

caterpillar sting. More than 50 species of butterfly and moth larvae possess urticating hairs that contain a toxin. Contact with these hairs can cause numbness and swelling of the infected area, severe radiating pain, localized swelling, enlarged regional lymph nodes, nausea, and vomiting. Even though shock and convulsions may occur, no deaths have been reported. The disease is self-limiting. The larva of the flannel moth, *Megalopyge opercularis,* known as the puss caterpillar or *woolly worm,* is frequently the cause of this sting, particularly in the southern U.S. The "fuzz" from these larvae can be transported by wind.

TREAT: Local application of moist soaks, and antihistamines.

catfish sting. Toxic and allergic reaction due to exposure to the venom contained in venomous glands at the base of fins of the catfish.

TREAT: Immediate immersion of the stung part in water as hot as the patient can stand for one hour or until pain is controlled. Tetanus prophylaxis if needed.

catgut. Sheep's intestine twisted for use as an absorbable ligature.

c., chromic. Catgut treated with chromium trioxide. This enhances the strength of the suture material.

catharsis (kă-thăr′sĭs) [Gr. *katharsis,* purification]. 1. Purgative action of the bowels. 2. The freudian method of freeing the mind by recalling from the patient's memory those events or experiences that were the exciting causes of a psychoneurosis. SEE: *abreaction.*

cathartic (kă-thăr′tĭk) [Gr. *kathartikos,* purging]. An active purgative, producing bowel movements.

Ex.: cascara sagrada; castor oil. SEE: *purgative.*

cathepsin-D (kă-thĕp′sĭn). An estrogen-induced lysomal protease. The level in blood may be a predictor of early recurrence and death in breast cancer patients whose lymph nodes were negative for evidence of metastasis.

cathepsis (kă-thĕp′sĭs) [Gr. *kathepsis,* boiling down]. In living tissues, synthesis or hydrolysis of proteins; in dead tissues, autolysis of proteins.

catheresis (kăth-ĕ-rē′sĭs) [Gr. *kathairesis,* destruction]. 1. Weakness resulting from medication. 2. Weak action.

catheter (kăth′ĕ-tĕr) [Gr. *katheter,* something inserted]. A tube passed through the body for evacuating or injecting fluids into body cavities. Made of elastic, elastic web, rubber, glass, metal, or plastic. SEE: illus.

c., arterial. Catheter inserted into an artery to measure pressure or to remove blood.

c., balloon. A double-lumened catheter in which a balloon surrounds the catheter. The balloon may be expanded by injecting

TYPES OF CATHETERS

ROUND TIP

WHISTLE TIP

FOLEY TRIPLE LUMEN
(SELF RETAINING)

DRAINAGE
AIR
IRRIGATION

CROSS SECTION

air, saline, or contrast medium. SEE: *tuboplasty, transcervical balloon; percutaneous transluminal coronary angioplasty.*

   c., cardiac. A long, fine catheter esp. designed for passage through the lumen of a blood vessel into the chambers of the heart. SEE: *cardiac catheterization.*

   c., central. Catheter inserted into a central vein or artery for diagnostic or therapeutic purposes or both.

   c., central venous. Catheter inserted into the superior vena cava to permit intermittent or continuous monitoring of central venous pressure and to facilitate obtaining blood samples for chemical analysis.

   c., condom. A specially designed condom that includes a catheter attached to the end. The catheter carries urine to a collecting bag. Its use prevents the male patient with urinary incontinence from soiling clothes or bed linens.

Caution: Continual use of this device may cause excoriation of the skin of the penis.

   c., double-channel. Catheter providing for inflow and outflow.

   c., elbowed. Catheter that has an acute bend near the beak. Used in patients with enlarged prostate. SYN: *c., prostatic.*

   c., eustachian. Catheter passed into eustachian tube through nasal passages.

   c., female. A short catheter, about 5 in. (12.7 cm) in length, used to pass into the bladder of the female.

   c., Foley. A urinary tract catheter that has a balloon attachment at one end. After the catheter is inserted, the balloon is filled with sterile water. Thus the catheter is prevented from leaving the bladder until the balloon is emptied.

   c., indwelling. Any catheter that is allowed to remain in place in a vein, artery, or body cavity.

   c., intra-aortic. SEE: *intra-aortic balloon counterpulsation.*

   c., intravenous. Catheter inserted into a vein to administer fluids or medications or to measure pressure.

   c., Karman. Catheter used for suction curettage of the uterus.

   c., male. Catheter used to pass into the bladder of the male. Catheter is 12 to 13 in. (30.5 to 33 cm) long.

   c., pacing. Catheter for insertion into a vein or the pulmonary artery that contains wires or leads for providing electrical stimuli from an external cardiac pacemaker.

   c., prostatic. Catheter, 15 to 16 in. (38 to 40.6 cm) long, with a short elbowed tip designed to pass prostatic obstruction. SYN: *c., elbowed.*

   c., pulmonary artery. Catheter inserted into the pulmonary artery to measure pulmonary artery pressures, pulmonary capillary wedge pressure, and cardiac output.

   c., self-retaining. Bladder catheter that remains in place due to its design, e.g., a Foley catheter.

   c., suprapubic. A urinary catheter closed drainage system. It is inserted through the skin, about 2.5 cm above the symphysis pubis, into the distended bladder. This is usually done under general anesthesia. If it is to remain in place, it is sutured to the abdominal skin.

   c., Swan-Ganz. SEE: *Swan-Ganz catheter.*

   c., Tenckhoff peritoneal. A catheter placed into the peritoneal cavity through the anterior abdominal wall. It is left in for an extended period and is used for peritoneal dialysis. SEE: *dialysis, continuous ambulatory peritoneal.*

   c., triple-lumen. A central catheter containing three separate channels or passageways.

   c., vertebrated. Catheter is in sections to be fitted together, so that it is flexible.

   c., winged. Catheter with little flaps at each side of beak to aid in retaining it in the bladder.

catheter fever. Rise in temperature caused by a urinary tract infection following passage of a catheter or urethral bougie.

catheterization (kăth″ĕ-tĕr-ĭ-zā′shŭn) [Gr. *katheterismos*]. Use or passage of a catheter.

   c., cardiac. The passage of a catheter into the heart through an arm vein and blood vessels leading into the heart for the purpose of obtaining cardiac blood samples, detecting abnormalities, and determining intracardiac pressure. SEE: *cardiac catheterization.*

   c., urinary bladder. Introduction of a

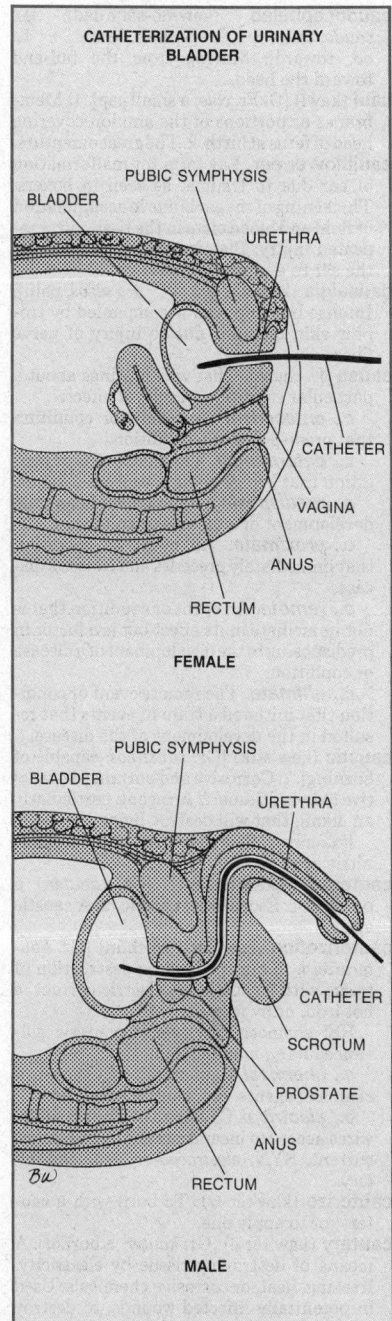

CATHETERIZATION OF URINARY BLADDER

PUBIC SYMPHYSIS
BLADDER
URETHRA
CATHETER
VAGINA
ANUS
RECTUM

FEMALE

PUBIC SYMPHYSIS
BLADDER
URETHRA
CATHETER
SCROTUM
PROSTATE
ANUS
RECTUM

MALE

catheter through the urethra into the bladder for withdrawal of urine. SEE: illus.

NURSING IMPLICATIONS: Explain procedure and reason for catheterization to the patient. Assemble necessary equipment, and properly position and drape the patient. Follow hospital procedure for insertion of the catheter. Maintain sterile technique. After insertion of an indwelling catheter, connect it to a closed straight drainage system. Document the procedure results and the patient's response in the nurse's progress notes.

Female: Patient should be in a supine position with knees flexed and apart, and with the feet flat against each other (frog position). Pillows may be placed under the head and shoulders to relax abdominal muscles.

Male: Patient should be in a supine position with legs extended. Care should be taken following the procedure to return the prepuce to its normal position to prevent any subsequent swelling.

c., self-. Male and female patients may be instructed in the technique of clean intermittent self-catheterization. The method is quite similar to that of the clean-catch method, q.v., except a catheter is used. The patient will need instruction in order to understand their own anatomy and physiology, and how to be certain the catheter is clean and how it is washed and stored after use. Self-catheterization will need to be done 3 or 4 times each day. It allows patients to be free of indwelling catheters and may permit return to normal activities of daily living.

catheterize (kăth'ĕ-tĕr-īz). To pass or introduce a catheter into a part, usually indicating catheterization of bladder.

cathexis (kă-thĕk'sĭs) [Gr. *kathexis*, retention]. The emotional or mental energy used in concentrating on an object or idea.

cathodal (kăth'ō-dăl) [Gr. *kathodos*, downward path]. Pert. to the cathode.

cathode (kăth'ōd). ABBR: ca. 1. The negative electrode from which electrons are emitted. Opposite of the anode or positive pole. 2. In a vacuum tube, the electrode that serves as the source of the electron stream.

cathode stream. Negatively charged electrons sent out as particles from the cathode in discharges through the vacuum. They move in a straight line and, upon hitting solid matter, produce roentgen rays.

cathodic (kă-thŏd'ĭk). 1. Pert. to a cathode. 2. Proceeding outwardly or efferently as applied to a nerve impulse.

cation (kăt'ī-ŏn) [Gr. *kation*, descending]. An ion with a positive charge of electricity. It is attracted by and travels to the cathode (negative pole). Opposite of anion. SEE: *ion.*

cation exchange. The transfer of cations between those in a liquid medium and those in a solid polymer. The polymer is termed the cation exchanger. Application of this technique is involved in ion-exchange chromatography.

catlin (kăt'lĭn). Surgical knife with double edges.

catoptric (kă-tŏp'trĭk) [Gr. *katoptrikos*, reflecting]. Pert. to reflected light or mirrors.

catoptrophobia (kăt″ŏp-trō-fō'bē-ă) [Gr. *katoptron*, mirror, + *phobos*, fear]. Morbid fear of mirrors or of breaking them.

CAT scan. Computerized axial tomography scan. SEE: *tomography, computerized.*

cat scratch disease. A febrile disease characterized by lymphadenitis, thought to be transmitted by cats. A few days after a minor scratch a pustule develops at the site. Regional lymphadenopathy develops within about 2 weeks, but may be as long as 2 months. Fever, malaise, headache and anorexia accompany the lymphadenopathy.

ETIOL: Not definitely proven, but an uncharacterized rickettsia-like organism, closely related to *Rochalimaea quintana* is thought to be the causative organism, as is *Bartonella bacilliformis.* Also, this organism probably causes bacillary angiomatosis. SEE: *angiomatosis, bacillary.*

TREAT: Aminoglycosides and I.V. gentamicin have been of benefit in shortening the course of the disease.

PROG: Excellent. SEE: *Nursing Diagnoses* in *Appendix.*

cat's eye pupil. A slitlike pupil.

cat's eye reflex. SEE: *reflex, cat's eye.*

Caucasian. Pert. to the white race.

caucasoid. Person with the physical characteristics of the white race.

cauda (kaw'dă) [L.] (pl. *caudae*). [NA] A tail or tail-like structure.

   c. epididymidis. [NA] The inferior portion of the epididymis that is continuous with the ductus deferens.

   c. equina. [NA] The terminal portion of the spinal cord and the roots of the spinal nerves below the first lumbar nerve.

   c. helicis. [NA] A pointed process extending inferiorly from the helix of the auricular cartilage of the ear.

   c. pancreatis. [NA] The tail of the pancreas.

   c. striati. Tail-like posterior extremity of the corpus striatum.

caudad (kaw'dăd) [L. *cauda*, tail, + *ad*, toward]. Toward the tail; in a posterior direction.

caudal (kawd'ăl) [L. *caudalis*]. 1. Pert. to any tail-like structure. 2. Inferior in position.

caudate (kaw'dāt) [L. *caudatus*]. Possessing a tail.

caudocephalad (kaw-dō-sĕf'ă-lăd) [L. *cauda*, tail, + Gr. *kephale*, head, + L. *ad*, toward]. Moving from the tail-end toward the head.

caul (kawl) [O. Fr. *cale*, a small cap]. 1. Membranes or portions of the amnion covering head of fetus at birth. 2. The great omentum.

cauliflower ear. Lay term for malformation of ear due to trauma, as seen in boxers. Thickening of the ear is due to accumulation of fluid and blood clots in the tissue after repeated injury. Plastic surgery may restore the ear to a normal shape.

causalgia (kaw-săl'jē-ă) [″ + *algos*, pain]. Intense burning pain accompanied by trophic skin changes, due to injury of nerve fibers.

cause [L. *causa*]. That which brings about a particular condition, result, or effect.

   c., antecedent. An event or condition that predisposes to a condition.

   c., determining. The final event or condition that brings about a cause.

   c., predisposing. That which favors the development of a disease or condition.

   c., proximate. An event or condition that immediately precedes and causes a disease.

   c., remote. An event or condition that is not immediate in its effect but is a factor in predisposing to the development of a disease or condition.

   c., ultimate. The remote event or condition that initiated a train of events that resulted in the development of the disease.

caustic (kaw'stĭk) [Gr. *kaustikos*, capable of burning]. 1. Corrosive and burning; destructive to living tissue. 2. An agent, particularly an alkali, that will destroy living tissue.

   Ex.: silver nitrate, potassium hydroxide, nitric acid.

cauterant (kaw'tĕr-ănt) [Gr. *kauter*, a burner]. 1. Escharotic; caustic. 2. A caustic agent.

cauterization (kaw″tĕr-ĭ-zā'shŭn) [Gr. *kauteriazein*, to burn]. Cautery; destruction of tissue with a caustic, an electric current, a hot iron, or by freezing.

   RS: chemocautery; electrocautery; galvanocautery; moxibustion.

   c., chemical. Cauterization by the use of chemical agents, esp. caustic substances.

   c., electrical. Cauterization by platinum wires heated to incandescence by an electric current. SYN: *electrocautery; galvanocautery.*

cauterize (kaw'tĕr-īz). To burn with a cautery, or to apply one.

cautery (kaw'tĕr-ē) [Gr. *kauter*, a burner]. A means of destroying tissue by electricity, freezing, heat, or corrosive chemicals. Used in potentially infected wounds; to destroy excess granulation tissue. Thermocautery consists of red-hot or white-hot object, usually piece of wire or pointed metallic instrument, heated in a flame or with electricity (galvanocautery, electrocautery).

cava (kā'vă). 1. A hollow area or a body cavity. 2. Vena cava.

caval (kā'văl). Pert. to the vena cava.

cavalry bone. Rider's bone; bony deposit in the adductor muscles of the thigh.

cavern (kăv'ĕrn). A cavity caused by a disease process.

cavernitis (kăv″ĕr-nī'tĭs) [L. *caverna*, hollow, + Gr. *itis*, inflammation]. Inflammation of the corpus cavernosum of the penis.

cavernoma (kăv″ĕr-nō'mă) [″ + Gr. *oma*, tumor]. A cavernous angioma. SEE: *hemangioma*.

cavernositis (kăv″ĕr-nō-sī'tĭs) [″ + Gr. *itis*, inflammation]. Inflammation of the corpus cavernosum.

cavernous (kăv'ĕr-nŭs) [L. *caverna*, a hollow]. Containing hollow spaces.

cavitary (kăv'ĭ-tā″rē). Pertaining to a cavity.

cavitation [L. *cavitas*, hollow]. Formation of a cavity. May occur as a normal process as in the formation of the amnion in human development or pathologically as in the development of cavities in lung tissue in pulmonary tuberculosis.

cavitis (kă-vī'tĭs) [″ + Gr. *itis*, inflammation]. Inflammation of a vena cava.

cavity (kăv'ĭ-tē) [L. *cavitas*, hollow]. A hollow space, such as a body organ or the hole in a tooth produced by caries.

  c., abdominal. Cavity of the peritoneum between the diaphragm and pelvis, containing all the abdominal organs.

  c., alveolar. A tooth socket.

  c., amniotic. Fluid-filled cavity around the developing embryo.

  c., articular. The synovial cavity of a joint.

  c., body. In vertebrates, the space between the body wall and the visceral organs. SYN: *coelom*.

  c., buccal. Cavity of the mouth.

  c., cotyloid. The acetabulum.

  c., cranial. Cavity of the skull, which contains the brain.

  c., dental. A hole in a tooth caused by dental caries.

  c., glenoid. A shallow concavity on the lateral surface of the head of the scapula that receives the head of the humerus.

  c., oral. Mouth or buccal cavity. Includes the vestibule and oral cavity proper.

  c., pelvic. Cavity of the pelvis. Includes the major pelvic cavity, which lies between the iliac fossa and above the iliopectineal lines, and the minor pelvic cavity, which lies below the iliopectineal lines or the inlet of the pelvis.

  c., pericardial. Space between the epicardium (visceral pericardium) and the parietal pericardium.

  c., peritoneal. The potential space between the parietal peritoneum lining the body wall and the visceral peritoneum forming surface layer of visceral organs.

  c., peritoneal, lesser. The omental bursa.

  c., pleural. The potential space between the parietal pleura and visceral pleura.

  c., pulp. Cavity in a tooth containing dental pulp and nerve termination.

  c., Rosenmüller's. Cavity on either side of the openings of the eustachian tube.

  c., serous. Space between two layers of serous membrane.

  Ex.: pleural, pericardial, and peritoneal cavities.

  c., splanchnic. One of the cavities of the body, such as the cranial, thoracic, and abdominal cavities, that contain important organs. SYN: *visceral cavity*.

  c., tympanic. Cavity of the middle ear.

  c., uterine. Cavity of the body of the uterus.

cavity classification. Any method of arranging the cavities or lesions of teeth into groups that can be recognized and described. Carious lesions are usually named for the surface of the tooth affected (labial, buccal, or occlusal), the type of tooth surface involved (pit and fissure or smooth surface), and by an accepted numbering designation. SYN: *caries classification*.

cavity preparation. An artificial cavity prepared in the tooth for the purpose of restoring the tooth by use of appropriate dental materials.

cavum (kā'vŭm) [L. *cavus*, a hollow]. [NA] A cavity or space.

  c. abdominis. [NA] The abdominal cavity.

  c. conchae. [NA] The inferior portion of the cavity of the auricle of the ear. It leads to the external acoustic meatus.

  c. mediastinale. The mediastinum.

  c. medullare. [NA] The medullary cavity of a long bone.

  c. oris. [NA] The oral cavity.

  c. pelvis. [NA] The pelvic cavity.

  c. septi pellucidi. An abnormal dilatation or increase in the space in the septum pellucidum of the brain. It is thought to be a characteristic pathological change seen in boxers who have experienced a great number of blows to the head.

  c. trigeminale. The space between the two layers of the dura mater of the brain in which the trigeminale ganglion is located. SYN: *space, Meckel's*.

c. tympani. [NA] The middle ear cavity.

c. uteri. [NA] The cavity of the uterus.

cavus (kā'vŭs) [L., hollow]. Condition of exaggerated height of arch of foot. SYN: *talipes cavus.*

cayenne pepper (kī-ĕn', kā-ĕn'). Capsicum, q.v.

C bar. Curved part of a hand splint that maintains the thumb web space.

CBC. *complete blood count.*

C.C. *chief complaint; Commission Certified,* with reference to certification of stains by the Biological Stain Commission.

cc. *cubic centimeter.*

CCl₃·CHO. Chloral.

CCl₄. Carbon tetrachloride.

CCNU. Code name for a chemotherapeutic agent used in treating certain neoplastic conditions. Also called *lomustine.*

CCPD. *continuous cycling peritoneal dialysis.*

CCRN. Registered trademark indicating certification by the American Association of Critical-Care Nurses Certification Corporation.

C.C.U. *coronary care unit.*

Cd. Chem. symb. for the element cadmium.

CD4. A protein on the surface of cells that normally helps the body's immune system combat disease. AIDS virus attaches itself to the protein to attack white blood cells. SEE: *AIDS.*

CDC. *Centers for Disease Control.*

CDH. *congenital dislocation of the hip.*

CD receptors. Receptors specific to mature T lymphocytes that are responsible, along with major histocompatibility complex (MHC) genes, q.v., for the recognition of antigens. CD2, CD3, and CD4 receptor molecules have been identified. CD4 receptors on T4 lymphocyte are the sites to which the human immunodeficiency virus (HIV) binds, producing infection. SEE: *AIDS.*

Ce. Chem. symb. for the element cerium.

cebocephalus (sē"bō-sĕf'ă-lŭs) [Gr. *kebos,* monkey, + *kephale,* head]. Fetus with a monkey-like head.

cecal (sē'kăl) [L. *caecalis,* pert. to blindness]. 1. Pert. to cecum. 2. Blind, terminating in a closed extremity.

cecectomy (sē-sĕk'tō-mē) [L. *caecum,* blindness, + Gr. *ektome,* excision]. Surgical removal of the cecum.

cecitis (sē-sī'tĭs) [" + Gr. *itis,* inflammation]. Inflammation of the cecum.

cecocolopexy (sē"kō-kō-lō'pĕk"sē) [" + Gr. *kolon,* colon, + *pexis,* fixation]. Surgical fixation of the colon and the cecum.

cecocolostomy (sē"kō-kō-lŏs'tō-mē) [" + " + *stoma,* mouth]. Colostomy consisting of joining of the cecum to the colon.

cecoileostomy (sē"kō-ĭl"ē-ŏs'tō-mē) [" + *ileum,* ileum, + Gr. *stoma,* mouth]. Sur-

gical formation of anastomosis between the cecum and the ileum.

Cecon. Trade name for ascorbic acid.

cecopexy (sē'kō-pĕk"sē) [" + Gr. *pexis,* fixation]. Surgical fixation of the cecum to the abdominal wall.

cecoplication (sē"kō-plĭ-kā'shŭn) [" + *plica,* fold]. Reduction of a dilated cecum by making a fold in its wall.

cecoptosis (sē"kŏp-tō'sĭs) [" + Gr. *ptosis,* a dropping]. Falling displacement of the cecum.

cecosigmoidostomy (sē"kō-sĭg"moyd-ŏs'tō-mē) [" + Gr. *sigmoeides,* shaped like Gr. letter S, + *stoma,* mouth]. Surgical formation of a communication between the cecum and sigmoid.

cecostomy (sē-kŏs'tō-mē) [" + Gr. *stoma,* mouth]. Surgical formation of an artificial opening into the cecum.

cecotomy (sē-kŏt'ō-mē) [" + Gr. *tome,* incision]. Incision into the cecum.

cecum (sē'kŭm) [L. *caecum,* blindness]. A blind pouch or cul-de-sac that forms the first portion of the large intestine, located below the entrance of the ileum at the ileocecal valve. It averages about 6 cm in length and 7.5 cm in width. At its lower end is the vermiform appendix.

Cedilanid. Trade name for lanatoside C.

Cedilanid-D. Trade name for deslanoside.

Cefadyl. Trade name for cephapirin sodium.

cefamandole nafate. USP. An antibacterial drug. Trade name is Mandol.

cefoxitin sodium. USP. An antibacterial drug.

Celbenin. Trade name for methicillin sodium.

-cele [Gr. *kele,* tumor, swelling; *koilia,* cavity]. Suffix indicating a swelling or tumor.

Celestone. Trade name for betamethasone.

celiac (sē'lē-ăk) [Gr. *koilia,* belly]. Rel. to the abdominal regions.

celiac artery. The first branch of the abdominal aorta. Branches supply the stomach, liver, spleen, duodenum, and pancreas.

celiac disease. Intestinal malabsorption syndrome characterized by diarrhea, malnutrition, bleeding tendency, and hypocalcemia.

TREAT: Gluten-free diet that may have to be continued for an indefinite period. SEE: *gluten-free diet; gluten-induced enteropathy.*

celiac plexus. Sympathetic plexus lying near the origin of celiac artery. SEE: *Nerve Plexuses* in *Appendix.*

celiectomy (sē"lē-ĕk'tō-mē) [" + *ektome,* excision]. 1. Surgical removal of an abdominal organ. 2. Excision of celiac branches of vagus nerve.

celiocentesis (sē"lē-ō-sĕn-tē'sĭs) [" +

kentesis, puncture]. Puncture of the abdomen.

celiocolpotomy (sē″lē-ō-kōl-pŏt′ō-mē) [″ + *kolpos,* vagina, + *tome,* incision]. Surgical incision of the vagina through the abdominal wall.

celioenterotomy (sē″lē-ō-ĕn″tĕr-ŏt′ō-mē) [″ + *enteron,* intestine, + *tome,* incision]. Incision in the abdominal wall to gain access to the intestines.

celiogastrostomy (sē″lē-ō-găs-trŏs′tō-mē) [″ + *gaster,* stomach, + *stoma,* mouth]. Incision in the abdominal wall for making a gastric fistula. SYN: *laparogastrostomy.*

celiogastrotomy (sē″lē-ō-găs-trŏt′ō-mē) [Gr. *koilia,* belly, + *gaster,* stomach, + *tome,* incision]. Incision into the stomach through the abdominal wall.

celiohysterectomy (sē″lē-ō-hĭs-tĕr-ĕk′tō-mē) [″ + *hystera,* uterus, + *ektome,* excision]. Removal of uterus through the abdomen.

celiohysterotomy (sē″lē-ō-hĭs″tĕr-ŏt′ō-mē) [″ + ″ + *tome,* incision]. Opening into the uterus through an abdominal incision.

celioma (sē-lē-ō′mă) [″ + *oma,* tumor]. An abdominal tumor.

celiomyalgia (sē″lē-ō-mī-ăl′gē-ă) [″ + *mys,* muscle, + *algos,* pain]. Rheumatic pain in muscles of the abdomen.

celiomyomectomy (sē″lē-ō-mī″ō-mĕk′tō-mē) [″ + ″ + *oma,* tumor, + *ektome,* excision]. Cutting of muscular tissue via an abdominal incision.

celiomyomotomy (sē″lē-ō-mī″ō-mŏt′ō-mē) [″ + ″ + ″ + *tome,* incision]. Incision of muscles of the abdomen.

celiomyositis (sē″lē-ō-mī″ō-sī′tĭs) [″ + ″ + *itis,* inflammation]. Inflammation of muscles of the abdomen.

celioparacentesis (sē″lē-ō-păr″ă-sĕn-tē′sĭs) [″ + *para,* beside, + *kentesis,* puncture]. Puncture of the abdomen for purposes of tapping or drainage.

celiopathy (sē″lē-ōp′ă-thē) [″ + *pathos,* disease, suffering]. Any disease of the abdomen.

celiorrhaphy (sē″lē-or′ă-fē) [″ + *rhaphe,* seam, ridge]. Suture of wound in the abdominal wall. SYN: *laparorrhaphy.*

celiosalpingectomy (sē″lē-ō-săl″pĭn-jĕk′tō-mē) [″ + *salpinx,* tube, + *ektome,* excision]. Removal of the fallopian tubes through an abdominal incision.

celioscope (sē′lē-ō-skōp) [″ + *skopein,* to examine]. An endoscope for visual examination of a body cavity.

celioscopy (sē″lē-ŏs′kō-pē). Examination of a body cavity through a celioscope.

celiotomy (sē″lē-ŏt′ō-mē) [″ + *tome,* incision]. Surgical incision into the abdominal

cavity.

c., vaginal. Incision into the abdomen through the vagina.

celitis (sē-lī′tĭs) [″ + *itis,* inflammation]. Abdominal inflammation. SYN: *peritonitis.*

cell [L. *cella,* a chamber]. 1. A small enclosed or partly enclosed cavity such as an air cell. 2. A mass of protoplasm containing a nucleus or nuclear material. It is the unit of structure of all animals and plants. SEE: illus.

Cells and the products of cells make up all the tissues of the body. All functional activities of the body are carried on by cells, and their structure and form are closely correlated with their functions. Cells arise only from pre-existing cells, new cells arising by cell division. Growth and development result from the increase in numbers of cells and the differentiation of cells into different types of tissues. Specialized germ cells, the spermatozoa and ova, contain in their nuclei the genes for hereditary characteristics.

Meiosis, q.v., is one type of cell division, in which two successive divisions of the nucleus of germ cells produce cells that contain half the number of chromosomes present in somatic cells. *Mitosis,* q.v., is the other type of cell division, in which each daughter cell contains the same number of chromosomes as the parent cell. SEE: *cell division* for illus.

Cell inclusions include nutrient substances (fat droplets, glycogen and protein granules); chromophilic substance (Nissl bodies); pigment granules (melanin); crystals of various substances; and secretory granules. Also present in the cytoplasm are submicroscopic bodies, once called microsomes, demonstrated by differential centrifugation. They are small fragments of the endoplasmic reticulum and contain particles of ribonucleoprotein (ribosomes). Thus, microsomes should be called ribosomes. Ribosomes are important in protein synthesis within the cell.

STRUCTURE: When a typical cell is fixed and stained, it exhibits a centrally located nucleus surrounded by cytoplasm.

Nucleus: The nucleus possesses a nuclear membrane that encloses clear karyoplasm. One or more densely staining bodies, the nucleoli, usually are present.

Cytoplasm: This includes the cell protoplasm lying outside the nucleus. Its outermost layer constitutes the cell membrane, which forms the limiting membrane of the cell. Within the ground substance of the cytoplasm is the ergastoplasm (granular endoplasmic reticulum), which contains ribonucleoprotein, a substance that can be identified only by use of the electron microscope. Ribonucleoprotein is important in protein synthesis.

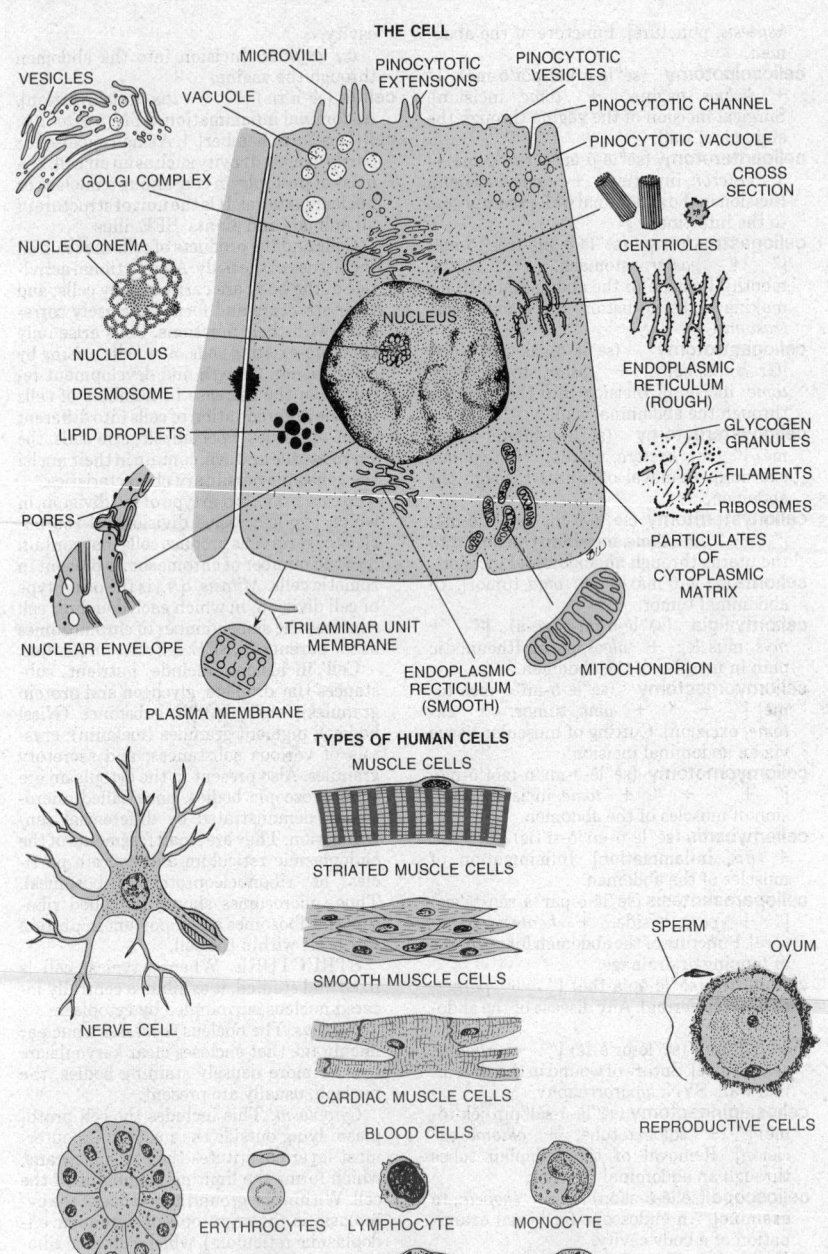

THE CELL

MICROVILLI
PINOCYTOTIC EXTENSIONS
PINOCYTOTIC VESICLES
PINOCYTOTIC CHANNEL
PINOCYTOTIC VACUOLE

VESICLES
VACUOLE
CROSS SECTION
CENTRIOLES

GOLGI COMPLEX
NUCLEOLONEMA
NUCLEUS
ENDOPLASMIC RETICULUM (ROUGH)

NUCLEOLUS
DESMOSOME
GLYCOGEN GRANULES
FILAMENTS
RIBOSOMES

LIPID DROPLETS
PARTICULATES OF CYTOPLASMIC MATRIX

PORES
NUCLEAR ENVELOPE
TRILAMINAR UNIT MEMBRANE
PLASMA MEMBRANE
ENDOPLASMIC RECTICULUM (SMOOTH)
MITOCHONDRION

TYPES OF HUMAN CELLS

MUSCLE CELLS

STRIATED MUSCLE CELLS

SMOOTH MUSCLE CELLS

NERVE CELL

CARDIAC MUSCLE CELLS

SPERM
OVUM

REPRODUCTIVE CELLS

BLOOD CELLS

ERYTHROCYTES
LYMPHOCYTE
MONOCYTE

GLAND CELL

NEUTROPHIL
EOSINOPHIL
BASOPHIL

A cell may produce other cells, and it has the power of exercising the vital processes of life. Cells of one tissue differ from those of other tissues, depending upon their function. Those of one tissue in man are very similar to those of corresponding tissues in other vertebrates.

c., acidophil. Cell with an affinity for staining with acid dyes.

c., acinar. Cell present in the acinus of an acinar gland, as those of the pancreas.

c., adipose. A fat cell.

c., adventitial. A macrophage along a blood vessel, together with perivascular undifferentiated cells associated with it.

c.'s, alpha. Cells of the anterior lobe of the pituitary and the pancreas. In the latter they are the source of glucagon.

c., ameloblast. The cell which produces the enamel rods of the tooth crown.

c.'s, argentaffin. Cells found in the epithelium of the digestive tract (stomach, intestine, appendix). Cytoplasm of the cells contains granules that stain selectively with silver.

c., B. SEE: *B cells.*

c., band. The developing leukocyte at a stage at which the nucleus is not segmented.

c., basal. A type of cell in the basal layer of the epidermis.

c., basket. 1. A branching basal or myoepithelial cell of the salivary and other glands. 2. Certain cells of the cerebellar cortex in which Purkinje cells rest.

c., basophil. Cell with an affinity for staining with basic dyes.

c.'s, beta. 1. Insulin-secreting cells of the pancreas that constitute the bulk of the islets of Langerhans. 2. Basophil cells of the anterior lobe of the pituitary.

c.'s, Betz. Large pyramidal cells of the motor area of cerebral cortex.

c., bipolar. A neuron with two processes — an axon and a dendrite. Found in retina of eye and in cochlear and vestibular ganglia of the acoustic nerve.

c., blast. A newly formed cell of any type. Large numbers of blast cells in the peripheral blood indicate high level of bone marrow production of the particular cell, e.g., lymphoblast (lymphocyte), monoblast (monocyte).

c., blood. Any type of nucleated or non-nucleated cell normally found in the blood or blood-forming tissues.

c.'s, capsule. Cells forming a single layer about the cell bodies of sensory neurons of spinal ganglia. SYN: *amphicytes; satellite cells.*

c., castration. An enlarged and vacuolated basophil cell seen in the pituitary in gonadal insufficiency or following castra-

tion.

c., cementoblast. The cell which produces the cementum layer which covers the tooth root and provides attachment for the supporting periodontal ligament.

c.'s, cementocyte. The cells trapped within cementum which, by their metabolic activity, maintain cementum as a living calcified tissue.

c., centroacinar. Duct cell of the pancreas more or less invaginated into the lumen of an acinus.

c.'s, chief. 1. Cells of the parathyroid gland that secrete the hormone. 2. Secretory cells that line the gastric glands and secrete pepsin or its precursor. 3. Chromophobe cells of the pituitary.

c.'s, chromaffin. Chromium-staining cells found in the adrenal medulla and other epinephrine-containing cells.

c., cleavage. Cell that results from mitosis or splitting of the fertilized ovum.

c.'s, clue. SEE: *clue cells.*

c., columnar. An epithelial cell with height greater than width.

c., cone. Cell in the retina whose scleral end forms a cone that serves as a light receptor. Vision in bright light, color vision, and acute vision depend upon functioning of the cones. SEE: *c., rod.*

c., cuboid. Cell with height about equal to width and depth.

c., daughter. Any cell formed from the division of a mother cell.

c., endothelial. A flat cell making up the lining of the vessels and endocardium.

c., epithelial. Cell forming epithelial surfaces of membranes and skin.

c., ethmoidal. One of several cavities that honeycomb the lateral masses of the ethmoid bone, forming a part of the paranasal air sinuses. SYN: *ethmoid sinus.*

c., fat. Cell in which fat is stored. SYN: *adipocyte; lipocyte.*

c.'s, foam. Cells that contain vacuoles. They are lipid-filled reticuloendothelial cells.

c., ganglion. 1. Any neuron whose cell body is located within a ganglion. 2. Neuron of the retina of the eye whose cell body lies in the ganglion cell layer. The axons of ganglion cells form the fibers of the optic nerve.

c., giant. 1. Large cell often with many nuclei found in bone marrow. They are thought to give rise to blood platelets. SYN: *megakaryocyte.* 2. Any large cell whether it contains one or multiple nuclei.

c., glia. C., neuroglia.

c., goblet. Epithelial cell containing a large globule of mucin that is distended like a goblet.

c., Golgi's. SEE: *Golgi's cells or neurons.*

c.'s, granule. Certain small neurons of the cerebrum and cerebellum that contain granules.

c., gustatory. A neuroepithelial cell or taste cell of a taste bud.

c., HeLa. A strain of cells that have been continuously cultured from a patient's carcinoma of the cervix. Named for the first two letters of the patient's first and last names, Henrietta Lacks. The cultured cells are used to study the growth of other cells including viruses.

c., horizontal. A neuron of the inner nuclear layer of the retina. The axons of these cells run horizontally and serve to connect various parts of the retina.

c.'s, Hürthle. Large eosinophil-staining cells occasionally present in the thyroid gland.

c., hybridoma. SEE: *hybridoma.*

c., interstitial. One of the many cells found in connective tissue of the ovary and the seminiferous tubules of the testes, accounting for their internal secretion.

c.'s, islet. Cells of the islet of Langerhans of the pancreas.

c., juxtaglomerular. Cell of the juxtaglomerular apparatus of the kidney. These granular cells are thought to produce renin.

c., Kupffer. A fixed phagocytic cell found in the sinusoids of the liver.

c., L.E. Abbreviation for *lupus erythematosus,* q.v., cell. A mature neutrophilic polymorphonuclear leukocyte that contains the phagocytosed nucleus of another cell. It is characteristic but not diagnostic of lupus erythematosus. SEE: *L.E. cell.*

c.'s, Leydig's. The interstitial cells of the testes.

c., littoral. Macrophage found in the sinuses of lymphatic tissue.

c., lutein. Cell of the corpus luteum of the ovary that contains fatty granules of a yellowish color. Granulose lutein cells are hypertrophied follicle cells; these lutein (paralutein) cells develop from the theca interna.

c., mast. Cell found in connective tissue of vertebrates that contains heparin and histamine.

c.'s, mastoid. The air cells in the mastoid process of the temporal bone.

c.'s, memory. Cells derived from B lymphocytes that have the ability to quickly recognize a foreign antigen to which the body has been previously exposed. They stimulate production of plasma cells to produce the appropriate antibody. SEE: *B cells; lymphocyte.*

c.'s, microglia. Neuroglial cells of mesodermal origin present in the brain and spinal cord.

c., mother. Any type of cell that divides and gives rise to two or more cells. The latter are called daughter cells.

c., mucous. Cell that secretes mucus found in mucus-secreting glands.

c., myeloma. Cell present in the bone marrow of patients with multiple myeloma.

c.'s, natural killer. SEE: *natural killer cells.*

c., nerve. Special cell of nerves that have processes extending from the cell body. One process, the axon, transmits nerve impulses, and the other, the dendrite, receives impulses and transmits them to the cell body.

c.'s, neuroglia. Non-nerve cells of the supporting tissue of the central nervous system and the retina of the eye. Includes astrocytes, oligodendrocytes, and microglia.

c., Niemann-Pick. A foamy, lipid-filled cell present in the spleen and bone marrow in Niemann-Pick's disease.

c., odontoblast. The cell which produces the dentin of the tooth and is responsible for the sensitivity of and metabolism of dentin in the tooth.

c., olfactory. Special cell of the olfactory mucosa that has a combined neuroepithelial function.

c., osteoblast. The mesodermal cell which produces the bone matrix and forms bone layer by layer on its surface.

c., osteocyte. The type of cell trapped within bone matrix and, by its metabolic activity, maintains bone as a living tissue.

c., oxyntic. Parietal cell of the stomach. In the human, hydrochloric acid, q.v., is formed in these cells.

c., parent. C., mother.

c.'s, phalangeal. Cells that support the hair cells of the organ of Corti. They form several rows of outer phalangeal cells (Deiters' cells) and a single row of inner phalangeal cells.

c., pigment. Any cell that normally contains pigment granules.

c.'s, plasma. Cells derived from lymphoid elements. They are found in lymphoid tissue and the cellular connective tissue of the intestinal tract. They are important in antibody, q.v., production in that they are capable of secreting all classes of immunoglobulin, q.v. SEE: *B cells; lymphocytes; T cells.*

c., prickle. Cell possessing spinelike protoplasmic processes that connect with similar processes of adjoining cells. Found in the stratum germinativum of the epidermis.

c.'s, primordial. Original germ cells that in the embryo migrate to the gonadal ridge, where they form all of the germ cells.

c., Purkinje's. Cell of the cerebral cortex

of the brain with dendrites extending into the molecular layer and axons that go to the white matter of the cerebellum.

c., pus. A leukocyte present in pus. Cells of this type are often degenerated or necrotic.

c., pyramidal. Nerve cell of the cerebral cortex.

c., red. The erythrocyte of the blood, the principal purpose of which is to transport oxygen to the cells of the body. The hemoglobin that the red cell contains is oxygenated in the lungs, and the oxygen contained in the arterial system is released to the tissues throughout the body.

c., reticular. Undifferentiated cell of the spleen, bone marrow, and lymphatic tissue that has the potential to develop into one of several types of connective tissue cells or into macrophages.

c.'s, reticuloendothelial. Reticular or endothelial cells of the reticuloendothelial system, q.v.

c., Rieder. Myeloblast that may be present in acute leukemia, possessing a lobulated or double nucleus.

c., rod. Cell in the retina of the eye whose scleral end is long and narrow, forming a rod, a sensory element of the eye. Rods are stimulated by dim light. SEE: *c., cone.*

c.'s, rosette. Nuclear material surrounded by phagocytes. These cells occur frequently in blood in which L.E. cells are present. Rosette cells are not diagnostic of lupus erythematosus. SEE: *E rosette; L.E. cell.*

c.'s, Rouget. Cells with branching processes that, in a frog, surround the walls of a capillary. They are capable of contracting upon stimulation.

c.'s, satellite. 1. Flat epithelium-like cells forming the inner portion of a double-layered capsule that covers a neuron. 2. Neuroglial cells enclosing the cell bodies of neurons in spinal ganglia.

c., segmented. Segmented neutrophil, i.e., one with a nucleus of two or more lobes connected together by slender filaments.

c., sensory. Cell that when stimulated gives rise to nerve impulses that are conveyed to the central nervous system.

c.'s, septal. Cells attached to or in the septa of the lungs. They function in some animals as macrophages.

c., Sertoli. Supporting tissue cell of the seminiferous tubules of the testicle. Spermatids attach to these cells until they become mature spermatozoa.

c., sickle. An abnormal erythrocyte shaped like a sickle. SEE: *anemia, sickle cell.*

c., signet-ring. Vacuolated cell with the nucleus off center. Mucus-secreting adeno-

carcinomas usually contain these cells.

c., somatic. A body cell rather than a germ cell.

c., spider. An astrocyte.

c., squamous. Flat scalelike epithelial cell.

c., stellate. Star-shaped cell with processes extending out from it.

c.'s, Sternberg-Reed; c.'s, Reed-Sternberg. Giant multinucleated cells seen in Hodgkin's disease.

c., stipple. Red blood cell that contains small basophilic-staining dots. Seen in lead poisoning, malaria, severe anemia, and leukemia.

c.'s, sympathicotrophic. Large epithelial cells occurring in groups in the hilus of the ovary. Thought to be chromaffin cells.

c.'s, sympathochromaffin. Chromaffin cells of ectodermal origin present in the fetal adrenal gland. Sympathetic and medullary cells arise from them.

c., T. SEE: *T cells.*

c., target. Erythrocyte with a rounded central area surrounded by a clear ring lightly stained, and this in turn surrounded by a dense ring of peripheral protoplasm. Present in certain blood disorders.

c., tart. Phagocytes that have ingested unaltered nuclei of cells. These nuclei are observed unchanged within the phagocytic cell.

c., taste. Cell of a taste bud.

c., totipotent. Undifferentiated embryonic cell that has the potential for developing into any type of cell.

c., Touton giant. SEE: *Touton cells.*

c., Türk's irritation. Cell resembling a plasma cell, found in cases of severe anemia or chronic infection.

c., Tzanck. A degenerated cell from the keratin layer of the skin. It is not connected to adjacent cells. Seen in pemphigus.

c., undifferentiated. Cell resembling an embryonic cell in that it has not demonstrated a change into a mature cell of any type.

c., visual. Rod or cone cell of the retina.

c., wandering. A macrophage capable of ameboid movement.

c., white. Any one of the leukocytes of the blood.

c.'s, zymogenic. Chief cells or enzyme-producing cells of the gastric glands.

cell bank. Facility for keeping cells frozen at extremely low temperatures. These cells are used for investigating hereditary diseases, human aging, and cancer. Collections of banked cells are kept by the National Institutes of Health (Human Genetic Mutant Cell Repository and the Aging Cell Repository) and at the Cornell Institute for Medical Research.

cell counter, electronic. Electronic instrument employed for the purpose of blood cell counting, employing either an electrical resistance or optical gating technique. SEE: *flow cytometry.*

cell culture. The growth of cells in vitro, q.v., for experimental purposes. The cells proliferate but do not organize into tissue.

cell cycle. The series of events that occur during the growth and development of a cell. SEE: *cell division* for illus.

cell division. The fission of a cell. SEE: *meiosis; mitosis;* illus.

cell-free. Pert. to fluids or tissues that contain no cells or in which all of the cells have been disintegrated by laboratory treatment.

cell growth cycle. The order of physical and biochemical events that occur during growth of cells. In tissue culture studies, the cyclic changes are divided into specific periods or phases: the DNA synthesis or S period; the G_2 period or gap; the M or mitotic period; and the G_1 period.

cell kill. In antineoplastic therapy, the number of malignant tumor cells destroyed by a treatment.

cell kinetics. The study of cells and their growth and division. Study of these factors has led to understanding of cancer cells and has been useful in developing chemotherapeutic methods.

cell mass. In embryology, the mass of cells that develops into an organ or structure.

cell mediated immunity. SEE: *immunity, cell mediated.*

cell membrane. The membrane that encloses the cell. Composed of proteins, lipids, and carbohydrates. SEE: illus.

cellobiose (sĕl″ō-bī′ōs). A disaccharide resulting from the hydrolysis of cellulose.

cellophane (sĕl′ō-fān). Thin, transparent, waterproof sheet of cellulose acetate. Used as a dialysis membrane.

cell organelle. Any of the structures in the cytoplasm of a cell. Includes the cell membrane, mitochondria, endoplasmic reticulum, Golgi complex, ribosomes, lysosomes, nucleus, and centriole. SEE: *organelle* for illus.

cell receptor. SEE: *receptor.*

cell sorting. A technique used to separate cells with a surface antigen from those without it. SEE: *flow cytometry.*

cellucidal (sĕl″ū-sī′dăl) [L. *cella,* a chamber, + *caedere,* to kill]. Destructive to cells.

cellula (sĕl′ū-lă) [L., little cell] (pl. *cellulae*). [NA] 1. A minute cell. 2. A small compartment.

cellular (sĕl′ū-lăr). Pert. to, composed of, or derived from cells.

cellular immunity. T-cell mediated immune functions requiring cell interactions; e.g., graft rejection, or destruction of infected cells.

cellulase (sĕl′ū-lās). An enzyme that converts cellulose to cellobiose. Present in some microorganisms and marine life.

cellulifugal (sĕl″ū-lĭf′ū-găl) [″ + *fugere,* to flee]. Extending or moving away from a cell.

cellulipetal (sĕl″ū-lĭp′ĭ-tăl) [″ + *petere,* to seek]. Extending or moving toward a cell.

cellulite. A nontechnical term for subcutaneous deposits of fat, esp. in the buttocks, legs, and thighs.

cellulitis (sĕl-ū-lī′tĭs) [″ + Gr. *itis,* inflammation]. Inflammation of cellular or connective tissue, spreading as in erysipelas. An infection in or close to the skin is usually localized by the body defense mechanisms. However, if inflammation spreads through the tissue, the process is called cellulitis.

c., pelvic. Inflammation of the parametrium, q.v. May occur in puerperal fever or septic conditions of the uterus and appendages. SYN: *parametritis.*

cellulofibrous (sĕl″ū-lō-fī′brŭs) [″ + *fibra,* fiber]. Both cellular and fibrous.

cellulose (sĕl′ū-lōs) [L. *cellula,* little cell]. Plant fiber; a fibrous form of carbohydrate, $(C_6H_{10}O_5)_n$, constituting the supporting framework of plants. It is present in plants including cotton and trees. It is composed of a great number of glucose units. When ingested, it stimulates peristalsis and aids in intestinal elimination. When ingested by humans, cellulose provides no nutrient value because it is not chemically changed or absorbed in digestion; it remains a polysaccharide, q.v.

Some foods that contain cellulose are: apples, apricots, asparagus, beans, beets, bran flakes, broccoli, cabbage, celery, mushrooms, oatmeal, onions, oranges, parsnips, prunes, spinach, turnips, wheat flakes, whole grains, whole wheat bread. SEE: *fiber, dietary.*

c., oxidized. USP. Cellulose that has been oxidized by nitrogen dioxide and is made to resemble cotton or gauze. Used to arrest bleeding by direct application to site of hemorrhage.

c., sodium, carboxymethyl. USP. A hydrophilic cellulose derivative used as a bulk-forming type of laxative. It is also used as a food additive for the purpose of thickening various types of prepared foods. ABBR: CMC.

cellulotoxic (sĕl″ū-lō-tŏk′sĭk) [″ + Gr. *toxikon,* poison]. 1. Poisonous to cells. 2. Caused by cell toxins.

cell wall. Cell membrane. Plant cells are en-

CELL DIVISION

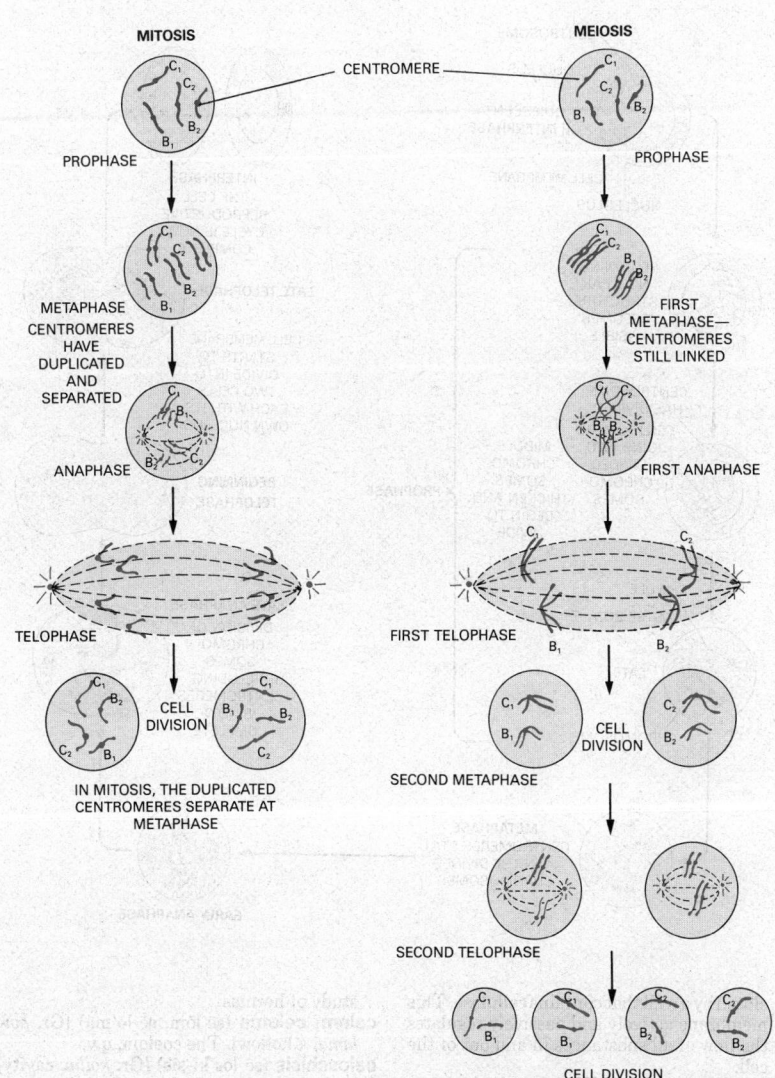

MITOSIS

MEIOSIS

CENTROMERE

PROPHASE

PROPHASE

METAPHASE
CENTROMERES
HAVE
DUPLICATED
AND
SEPARATED

FIRST
METAPHASE—
CENTROMERES
STILL LINKED

ANAPHASE

FIRST ANAPHASE

TELOPHASE

FIRST TELOPHASE

CELL
DIVISION

CELL
DIVISION

IN MITOSIS, THE DUPLICATED
CENTROMERES SEPARATE AT
METAPHASE

SECOND METAPHASE

SECOND TELOPHASE

CELL DIVISION

IN MEIOSIS, THE CENTROMERES ARE NOT
DUPLICATED AND SEPARATED UNTIL THE
SECOND TELOPHASE

CELL DIVISION—MITOSIS
(SEQUENCE OF ANIMAL CELL REPRODUCTION)

CENTROSOME

NUCLEUS

QUIESCENT
OR **INTERPHASE**

CELL MEMBRANE

NUCLEOLUS

BEGINNING:
NUCLEAR
STRUCTURE
BECOMES
VISIBLE

CENTROSOME
HAS DIVIDED

CENTROMERE
JOINS TWO
DIVIDED
CHROMO-
SOMES

MIDDLE:
CHROMO-
SOMES
THICKEN AND
BEGIN TO
DIVIDE

PROPHASE

SPINDLE

ASTER BODY

LATE

CHROMOSOME

METAPHASE
CENTROMERES STILL
JOIN THE DIVIDED
CHROMOSOMES

EARLY ANAPHASE

INTERPHASE
THE CELL
REPRODUCTIVE
CYCLE IS NOW
COMPLETE

LATE TELOPHASE

CELL MEMBRANE
STARTS TO
DIVIDE INTO
TWO CELLS
EACH WITH ITS
OWN NUCLEUS

**BEGINNING
TELOPHASE**

LATE ANAPHASE
DIVISION OF
CHROMO-
SOMES
INCLUDING
CENTROMERES
IS NOW
COMPLETE

closed by a wall that contains cellulose. This membrane actively and passively regulates the flow of all substances in and out of the cell.

celo-. 1. [Gr. *kele*, tumor, swelling]. A combining form meaning tumor or hernia. 2. [Gr. *koilia*, cavity]. A combining form meaning cavity.

celology (sē-lŏl'ō-jē) [Gr. *kele*, tumor, swelling, + *logos*, word, reason]. The surgical study of hernias.

celom, celoma (sē'lŏm, sē-lō'mă) [Gr. *koiloma*, a hollow]. The coelom, q.v.

celoschisis (sē-lŏs'kĭ-sĭs) [Gr. *koilia*, cavity, + *schisis*, fissure]. Congenital fissure of the abdominal wall.

celoscope (sē'lō-skōp) [" + *skopein*, to examine]. Device for visual examination of a body cavity.

celosomia (sē-lō-sō'mē-ă) [" + *soma*,

CELL MEMBRANE/PLASMA MEMBRANE

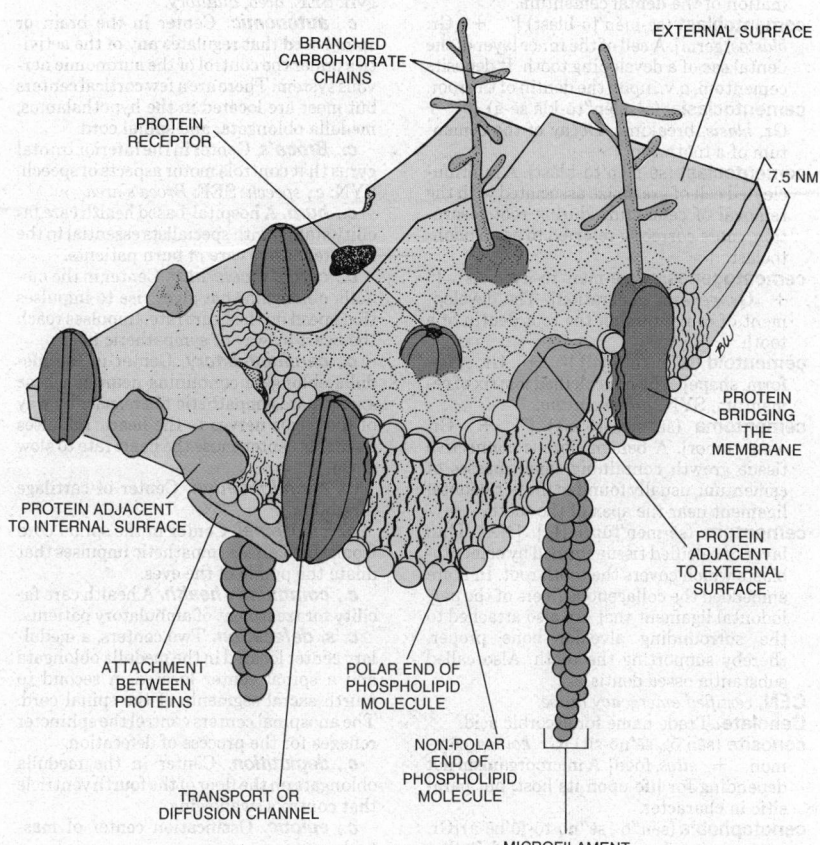

EXTERNAL SURFACE

BRANCHED
CARBOHYDRATE
CHAINS

PROTEIN
RECEPTOR

7.5 NM

PROTEIN
BRIDGING
THE
MEMBRANE

PROTEIN ADJACENT
TO INTERNAL SURFACE

PROTEIN
ADJACENT
TO EXTERNAL
SURFACE

ATTACHMENT
BETWEEN
PROTEINS

POLAR END OF
PHOSPHOLIPID
MOLECULE

NON-POLAR
END OF
PHOSPHOLIPID
MOLECULE

TRANSPORT OR
DIFFUSION CHANNEL

MICROFILAMENT

SCHEMATIC DEPICTION OF CELL MEMBRANE/PLASMA MEMBRANE

body]. Congenital fissure of sternum with
herniation of fetal viscera.

celozoic [" + *zoon*, animal]. Inhabiting the
intestinal cavity of the body, said of parasitic protozoa.

Celsius scale (sĕl'sē-ŭs) [Anders Celsius,
Swedish astronomer, 1701–1744]. A temperature scale on which the boiling point of
water is 100° and the melting point of ice is
0°. This is the official scientific name of the
temperature scale that is also known as centigrade. SEE: *Miscellaneous Units of Measurement* in *Appendix*.

cement (sē-mĕnt'). 1. Any material that
when prepared in the appropriate manner
hardens into a firm mass. 2. The process of
causing two objects to stick together as
would be the case in using an adhesive to join
a gold inlay to the cavity of a tooth; also
serves to insulate the pulp from metallic fillings. 3. The material used to make one substance adhere to another.

cementicle (sē-mĕn'tĭ-kl). Small calcified
area in the periodontal membrane of the
root of a tooth.

cementitis (sē"mĕn-tī'tĭs) [L. *cementum*, cement, + Gr. *itis*, inflammation]. Inflammation of the dental cementum.

cementoblast (sē-měn'tō-blăst) [" + Gr. *blastos*, germ]. A cell of the inner layer of the dental sac of a developing tooth. It deposits cementum, q.v., upon the dentin of the root.

cementoclasia (sē-měn"tō-klā'sē-ă) [" + Gr. *klasis*, breaking]. Decay of the cementum of a tooth root.

cementoclast (sē-měn'tō-klăst). A multinucleated cell of great size associated with the removal of cementum during root resorption, more correctly referred to as an odontoclast.

cementogenesis (sē-měn"tō-jěn'ě-sĭs) [" + Gr. *genesis*, generation]. The development of cementum on the root dentin of a tooth.

cementoid (sē"měn'toyd) [" + Gr. *eidos*, form, shape]. The noncalcified matrix of cementum. SYN: *precementum*.

cementoma (sē"měn-tō'mă) [" + Gr. *oma*, tumor]. A benign fibrous connective tissue growth containing small masses of cementum, usually found in the periodontal ligament near the apex of the tooth.

cementum (sē-měn'tŭm) [L.]. [NA] Thin layer of calcified tissue formed by cementoblasts which covers the tooth root. In it are embedded the collagenous fibers of the periodontal ligament that are also attached to the surrounding alveolar bone proper, thereby supporting the tooth. Also called substantia ossea dentis.

CEN. *certified emergency nurse.*

Cenolate. Trade name for ascorbic acid.

cenosite (sěn'ō-, sē'nō-sīt) [Gr. *koinos*, common, + *sitos*, food]. A microorganism not depending for life upon its host, but parasitic in character.

cenotophobia (sěn"ō-, sē"nō-tō-fō'bē-ă) [Gr. *kainotes*, novelty, + *phobos*, fear]. Pathological aversion to new things and new ideas. SYN: *cainotophobia.*

cenotype (sē'nō-, sěn'ō-tīp) [" + *typos*, a type]. An original type; term used in ontogeny and cytology.

censor (sěn'sěr) [L. *censor*, judge]. In psychoanalysis, a psychic inhibition that prevents abhorrent unconscious thoughts or impulses from seeking objective expression unless in a form unrecognized at the conscious level.

centenarian. A person over the age of 100.

center (sěn'těr) [L. *centrum*, center]. 1. Middle point of a body. 2. A group of nerve cells within the central nervous system that controls a specific activity or function. 3. A facility specializing in a particular service.

   c., apneustic. Center in the brain stem that regulates breathing.

   c., auditory. Center for hearing in the anterior gyri of the transverse temporal gyri. SEE: *area, auditory.*

   c., autonomic. Center in the brain or spinal cord that regulates any of the activities under the control of the autonomic nervous system. There are a few cortical centers but most are located in the hypothalamus, medulla oblongata, and spinal cord.

   c., Broca's. Center in the inferior frontal gyrus that controls motor aspects of speech. SYN: *c., speech.* SEE: *Broca's area.*

   c., burn. A hospital-based health care facility staffed with specialists essential to the comprehensive care of burn patients.

   c., cardioaccelerator. Center in the medulla oblongata that gives rise to impulses that speed up the heart rate. Impulses reach the heart by way of sympathetic fibers.

   c., cardioinhibitory. Center in the medulla oblongata containing neurons whose axons, parasympathetic fibers, pass by way of the vagus nerves to the heart. Impulses from this center cause the heart rate to slow down.

   c., chondrification. Center of cartilage formation.

   c., ciliospinal. Center in the spinal cord from which arise sympathetic impulses that dilate the pupils of the eyes.

   c., community health. A health care facility for treatment of ambulatory patients.

   c.'s, defecation. Two centers, a medullary center located in the medulla oblongata and a spinal center located in second to fourth sacral segments of the spinal cord. The anospinal centers control the sphincter reflexes for the process of defecation.

   c., deglutition. Center in the medulla oblongata on the floor of the fourth ventricle that controls swallowing.

   c., epiotic. Ossification center of mastoid process.

   c., feeding. An area in the ventrolateral nucleus of the hypothalamus that originates signals to the cerebral cortex that stimulate eating. SEE: *c., satiety; weight; set point.*

   c., germinal. Area in lymph node tissue that responds in a specific manner to antigenic stimulation.

   c., gustatory. Cerebral center that is supposed to control taste. SYN: *taste area.*

   c.'s, heat-regulating. Two centers, a heat loss center and a heat-production center, located in the hypothalamus. They regulate body temperature.

   c., higher. 1. Center in the cerebrum from which impulses based on conscious sensations, wishes, or desires are initiated. 2. Center in any portion of the brain, in contrast to one in the cord.

   c., independent living. A center provided in the community for coordinating services for persons with disability. These services would include counseling, training, assistance with devices, and respite care.

c., lower. Center in the brain, stem or spinal cord.

c., medullary. Area in the brain stem that regulates respiratory activity.

c., micturition. Center controlling reflexes of urinary bladder. Located in second to fourth and fourth to sixth sacral segments of the cord; higher centers are present in medulla oblongata, hypothalamus, and cerebrum.

c., motor cortical. Area in the frontal lobe, the origin of impulses for voluntary movements.

c., neighborhood health. Community health center, q.v.

c., nerve. One of many centers in cerebrospinal or ganglionic systems originating or controlling certain functions.

c., ossification. Spot where ossification begins in bones.

c., pneumotaxic. Center in the pons that rhythmically inhibits inspiration.

c., psychocortical. One of the centers of cerebral cortex concerned with voluntary muscular movements.

c., reflex. Region within the brain or spinal cord where connections (synapses) are made between afferent and efferent neurons of a reflex arc.

c., respiratory. Region in the medulla oblongata that controls respiratory movements. It consists of inspiratory, expiratory, and pneumotaxic centers.

c., satiety. An area in the ventromedial hypothalamus that modulates the stimulus to eat by sending inhibitory impulses to the feeding center. Blood glucose and insulin level influence the activity of the satiety center. SEE: *c., feeding; weight, set point.*

c., speech. Center in the inferior frontal gyrus that controls motor aspects of speech.

c., suicide prevention. A health care facility dedicated to attempting to prevent suicide by counseling and crisis intervention.

c., taste. C., gustatory.

c., temperature. C., thermoregulatory.

c., thermoregulatory. One of the temperature-regulating centers in the hypothalamus.

c., vasoconstrictor. Center in the medulla that brings about the constriction of blood vessels.

c., vasodilator. Center located in the medulla oblongata that brings about vasodilation of blood vessels.

c., vasomotor. Center through which the diameter of blood vessels is controlled; the vasoconstrictor and vasodilator centers.

c., visual. Center in the brain that receives visual information transmitted from the retina.

c., Wernicke's. Area in the dominant hemisphere of the brain that functions to recall, recognize, and interpret words and other sounds in the process of using language.

c., word. Area in the dominant hemisphere of the brain that functions to recognize and perceive spoken or written words.

Centers for Disease Control. ABBR: CDC. Division of the U.S. Public Health Service, in Atlanta, Georgia, for investigation and control of various diseases, esp. those that have epidemic potential. Telephone number is (404) 639-3311.

centesis (sĕn-tē′sĭs) [Gr. *kentesis,* puncture]. Puncture of a cavity.

centigrade (sĕn′tĭ-grād) [L. *centum,* a hundred, + *gradus,* a step]. ABBR: C. 1. Having 100 degrees. 2. Pert. to a thermometer divided into 100°. The boiling point of water is 100° and the freezing point is 0°. The official scientific name for the centigrade scale is Celsius. SEE: *thermometer.*

centigram (sĕn′tĭ-grăm) [″ + Gr. *gramma,* a small weight]. A measure of weight; the hundredth part of a gram; 0.15432 gr. SEE: *metric system; Metric System* in *Appendix.*

centiliter (sĕn′tĭ-lē-tĕr) [″ + Gr. *litra,* measure of wt.]. One-hundredth part of a liter (1 liter equals approx. 33 fluid ounces); 10 ml. SEE: *metric system.*

centimeter (sĕn′tĭ-mē-tĕr) [″ + Gr. *metron,* measure]. ABBR: cm. Unit of length in metric system, q.v. One-hundredth part of a meter. To convert centimeters to inches, multiply by 0.3937. To convert inches to centimeters, multiply by 2.54.

centimorgan. ABBR: cM. One one-hundredth of a morgan. A measure of genetic distance and indicates the likelihood of crossover of two loci on a gene.

centinormal (sĕn″tĭ-nor′măl) [″ + *norma,* rule]. One-hundredth part of the normal, as the strength of a solution.

centipede (sĕn′tĭ-pēd″) [″ + *pes,* foot]. An arthropod of the subclass Chilopoda characterized by an elongated flattened body of many segments, each with a pair of jointed legs. The first pair of appendages are hooklike claws bearing openings of ducts from poison glands. The bites of large tropical centipedes may cause severe local and sometimes general symptoms, but they are rarely fatal.

centipoise (sĕn′tĭ-poyz). A unit of viscosity one one-hundredth of a poise. SEE: *poise.*

centrad (sĕn′trăd) [Gr. *kentron,* center, + L. *ad,* toward]. Toward the center.

central (sĕn′trăl). 1. Situated at, or rel. to, a

center. 2. Principal or controlling.

central core disease. A rare form of benign familial polymyopathy characterized by hypotonia, delay in walking, and muscle weakness that does not progress. When stained in certain ways and studied microscopically, there is a central area of the muscle fibers that does not stain; thus, the name.

central I.V. line. SEE: *catheter, central venous; central line.*

central line. A venous access device inserted into and kept in the vein in order to maintain a route for administering fluids and medicines or for gaining access to the heart for obtaining information about pressures in the venous circulation. Having the line open permits venous access at a later time when the veins might be collapsed and thus difficult to enter. SEE: *catheter, central venous; central I.V. line.*

central nervous system. ABBR: CNS. Brain and spinal cord, with their nerves and end organs that control voluntary and involuntary acts. Includes parts of the brain governing consciousness and mental activities; parts of brain, spinal cord, and their sensory and motor nerve fibers controlling skeletal muscles; and end organs of the body wall. SEE: *autonomic, parasympathetic,* and *sympathetic nervous systems; brain* and *cranial nerves* for illus.

COMP: Nerve tissue that forms the brain, spinal cord, and the nerves from both. Tissue is made up of gray and white matter. Gray matter is composed of cells of nervous tissue, while the white matter is composed of nerve fibers from the cells. White matter in the brain and cord carries messages or impulses from the body or outside world to the cells or gray matter.

central venous pressure. ABBR: CVP. The pressure within the superior vena cava; it reflects the pressure under which the blood is returned to the right atrium. The normal range is between 5 and 10 cm H_2O (2 to 8 mmHg). A high CVP indicates circulatory overload (as in congestive heart failure), whereas a low CVP indicates reduced blood volume (as in hemorrhage or fluid loss). CVP can be estimated by examination of the cervical veins or dorsal veins of the hand if the neck and hand are at the level of the heart. Those veins will be well filled if CVP is normal or high, and the veins will tend to be collapsed if the pressure is low.

centration. Ability of the preschool child to focus or center attention on only one aspect or characteristic of a situation at a time. First described by Piaget.

centre. Center.

centri- [L. *centrum,* center]. Combining form indicating something is located near to or in the center.

centriciput (sĕn-trĭs'ĭ-pŭt) [" + L. *caput,* head]. The central part of the upper surface of the skull between the occiput and sinciput.

centrifugal (sĕn-trĭf'ū-găl) [" + L. *fugere,* to flee]. Receding from the center. SYN: *axifugal.* SEE: *centrifuge.*

centrifugal force. The force that impels a thing, or parts of it, outward from the center of rotation. SEE: *centrifuge.*

centrifuge (sĕn'trĭ-fūj). A device that spins test tubes at high speeds. Thus, centrifugal force, q.v., causes the heavy particles in the liquid in the tubes to settle to the bottom and the lighter liquid to go to the top. When unclotted blood is centrifuged, the plasma goes to the top and the heavy red cells go to the bottom of the tube. The white blood cells are heavier than the plasma but lighter than the red blood cells. Therefore they form a thin layer between the red blood cells and the plasma. SEE: *buffy coat.*

   c., human. Device for the accommodation of a human subject being rotated while suspended from a long arm. It is used to investigate the ability of subjects to withstand positive G forces.

centrilobular (sĕn"trĭ-lŏb'ū-lăr). Concerning the center of a lobule.

centriole (sĕn'trē-ōl). A minute organelle consisting of a hollow cylinder closed at one end and open at the other, found in the cell center or attraction sphere of a cell. Preceding mitosis it divides, forming two daughter centrioles (diplosomes). During mitosis the centrioles migrate to opposite poles of the cell, and each forms the center of the aster to which the spindle fibers are attached. SEE: *mitosis.*

centripetal (sĕn-trĭp'ĕ-tăl) [" + L. *petere,* to seek]. Directed toward the axis. SYN: *axipetal.*

centrocyte (sĕn'trō-sīt) [" + *kytos,* cell]. A cell with single and double hematoxylin-stainable granules of varying size in its protoplasm.

centrodesmus (sĕn-trō-dĕz'mŭs) [Gr. *kentron,* center, + *desmos,* a band]. The matter connecting the two centrosomes in a nucleus during mitosis.

centrolecithal (sĕn"trō-lĕs'ĭ-thăl) [" + *lekithos,* yoke]. Pert. to an egg, esp. an ovum, with the yolk centrally located.

centromere (sĕn'trō-mēr) [" + *meros,* part]. A constricted region of a chromosome that divides the chromosome into two arms.

centrosclerosis (sĕn"trō-sklĕ-rō'sĭs) [" + *sklerosis,* a hardening]. Filling of the bone marrow space with bone tissue.

centrosome (sĕn'trō-sōm) [" + *soma,* body]. A region of the cytoplasm of a cell usually lying near the nucleus, containing in its center one or two centrioles, the diplosome. SEE: *mitosis*.

centrosphere (sĕn'trō-sfēr) [" + *sphaira*, sphere]. The cytoplasm of the centrosome.

centrostaltic (sĕn"trō-stăl'tĭk) [" + *stellein*, send forth]. Pert. to a center of motion.

centrum (sĕn'trŭm) [L.] (pl. *centra*). 1. Any center, esp. an anatomical one. 2. Body of a vertebra.

   c. semiovale. Mass of white matter at center of each cerebral hemisphere.

   c. tendineum. Central tendon of the diaphragm.

cephalad (sĕf'ă-lăd) [Gr. *kephale*, head, + L. *ad*, toward]. Toward the head.

cephalalgia (sĕf-ă-lăl'jē-ă) [" + *algos*, pain]. Headache, pain in the head. A symptom of numerous diseases and disorders. SEE: *headache*.

cephalalgic (sĕf-ăl-ăl'jĭk). Of the nature of cephalalgia.

cephalea (sĕf-ă-lē'ă) [Gr. *kephale*, head]. Cephalalgia.

cephaledema (sĕf"ăl-ĕ-dē'mă) [" + *oidema*, swelling]. Edema of the head.

cephalexin (sĕf"ă-lĕk'sĭn). USP. An analogue of the antibiotic cephalosporin. Effective against gram-positive and gram-negative organisms. Trade name is Keflex.

cephalhematocele (sĕf"ăl-hē-măt'ō-sēl) [" + *haima*, blood, + *kele*, tumor]. A bloody tumor communicating with the dural sinuses.

cephalhematoma (sĕf"ăl-hē"mă-tō'mă) [" + " + *oma*, tumor]. A subcutaneous swelling containing blood, often found on the head of a baby several days after birth when delivery was accompanied by use of forceps. The swelling disappears within two to three months.

cephalic (sĕ-făl'ĭk) [L. *cephalicus*]. 1. Cranial; pert. to the head. 2. Superior in position.

cephalic index. An arbitrary measure of cranial capacity. Derived from the division of the maximal length of the head into the value of the maximal breadth multiplied by 100.

cephalocaudal pattern of development. Principle of maturation that motor development, control, and coordination progress from the head to the feet.

cephalocele (sĕf'ă-lō-sēl) [" + *kele*, hernia]. Protrusion of the brain from the cranial cavity.

cephalocentesis (sĕf"ă-lō-sĕn-tē'sĭs) [" + *kentesis*, puncture]. Surgical puncture of cranium.

cephalodynia (sĕf"ă-lō-dĭn'ē-ă) [" + *odyne*, pain]. Pain in the head. SYN: *cephalalgia; headache*.

cephaloglycin (sĕf"ă-lō-glī'sĭn). An analogue

of the antibiotic cephalosporin.

cephalogyric (sĕf"ă-lō-jī'rĭk) [" + *gyros*, a turn]. Of or pert. to rotation of the head.

cephalohemometer (sĕf"ă-lō-hē-mŏm'ĕ-tĕr) [" + *haima*, blood, + *metron*, measure]. Instrument for determining changes in intracranial blood pressure.

cephalomenia (sĕf"ă-lō-mē'nē-ă) [" + *men*, month]. Vicarious menstruation from the nose or head.

cephalomeningitis (sĕf"ă-lō-mĕn"ĭn-jī'tĭs) [" + *meninx*, membrane, + *itis*, inflammation]. Inflammation of the cerebral meninges.

cephalometer (sĕf-ă-lŏm'ĕ-tĕr) [" + *metron*, measure]. 1. Device for measuring the head. 2. In radiology, use of a device that maintains the head in a certain position for radiographic examination and measurement.

cephalometry (sĕf"ă-lŏm'ĕ-trē). Measurement of the head of living persons using certain bony points directly or by tracing radiographs made using well-established planes for linear and angular measurements. Used in dentistry to assess growth and to determine orthodontic or prosthetic treatment plans.

cephalomotor (sĕf"ă-lō-mō'tor) [Gr. *kephale*, head, + L. *motus*, motion]. Pert. to movements of the head.

cephalone (sĕf'ă-lōn) [" + *on*, being]. A mentally retarded individual with a large head.

cephalonia (sĕf"ă-lō'nē-ă). A condition marked by mental retardation and enlargement of the head.

cephalopathy (sĕf"ă-lŏp'ă-thē) [" + *pathos*, disease, suffering]. Any disease of the head or brain.

cephalopelvic (sĕf"ă-lō-pĕl'vĭk). Concerning the fetal head and the maternal pelvis; esp. the size of the pelvic outlet through which the fetal head will pass during delivery.

cephaloplegia (sĕf"ă-lō-plē'jē-ă) [" + *plege*, stroke]. Paralysis of muscles of the head or neck or both.

cephalorhachidian (sĕf"ă-lō-ră-kĭd'ē-ăn) [" + *rhachis*, spine]. Pert. to the head and spine.

cephaloridine (sĕf"ă-lor'ĭ-dēn). An analogue of the antibiotic cephalosporin C.

cephaloscope (sĕf'ă-lō-skōp) [" + *skopein*, to examine]. Device for auscultation of the head.

cephalosporin (sĕf"ă-lō-spor'ĭn). General term for a group of antibiotic derivatives of cephalosporin C. Cephalosporin C is obtained from the fungus *Cephalosporium*.

cephalothin sodium (sĕf'ă-lō-thĭn"). USP. A semisynthetic analogue of the antibiotic cephalosporin C. Trade name is Keflin.

cephalothoracic (sĕf″ă-lō-thō-răs′ĭk) [″ + *thorakos*, chest]. Concerning the head and thorax.

cephalothoracopagus (sĕf″ă-lō-thō″ră-kŏp′ă-gŭs) [″ + ″ + *pagos*, thing fixed]. A double fetus joined at the head and thorax.

cephalotome (sĕf′ă-lō-tōm) [″ + *tome*, incision]. Instrument for cutting the head of the fetus to facilitate delivery.

cephalotomy (sĕf-ă-lŏt′ō-mē). Cutting the fetal head to facilitate delivery.

cephalotrypesis (sĕf″ă-lō-trĭp-ē′sĭs) [″ + *trypesis*, a boring]. Removing a portion of bone from the skull. SYN: *trephination.*

cephapirin sodium (sĕf-ă-pī′rĭn). USP. An antibiotic similar to cephalothin. Trade name is Cefadyl.

Cephulac. Trade name for lactulose.

ceptor (sĕp′tor) [L. *receptor*, receiver]. General term for a nerve ending that, upon being stimulated, passes the stimulus on to the cell to which the ceptor is attached.

  c., chemical. Ceptor that initiates chemical reactions in the body.

  c., contact. Ceptor that receives stimuli contributed by direct physical contact.

  c., distance. Ceptor that perceives stimuli remote from the immediate environment.

cera (sē′ră) [L.]. Wax.

  c. alba. White wax.

  c. flava. Yellow wax.

ceramics, dental [Gr. *keramos*, potter's clay]. The use of porcelain or porcelain-type materials in dental work.

ceramide (sĕr′ă-mīd). A class of lipids that do not contain glycerol. They are derived from a sphingosine. Glycosphingolipids, q.v., and sphingomyelins, q.v., are derived from ceramides.

  c. oligosaccharides. A class of glycosphingolipids.

ceramodontia (sē-răm″ō-dŏn′shee-ă) [Gr. *keramos*, potter's clay, + *odous*, tooth]. Dental ceramics.

cerate ceratum (sē′rāt) [L. *ceratum*]. A medicinal formulation for topical use containing wax and of such consistency that it may be spread easily at ordinary temperature upon muslin or similar material with a spatula, and yet not so soft as to liquefy and run when applied to the skin. Rarely prescribed.

ceratocele (sĕr′ă-tō-sēl) [Gr. *keras*, horn, + *kele*, hernia]. Hernia of Descemet's membrane through outer layer of the cornea. SYN: *keratocele.*

ceratotome (sē-răt′ō-tōm) [″ + *tome*, incision]. A knife for division of the cornea.

cercaria (sĕr-kā′rē-ă) [Gr. *kerkos*, tail] (pl. *cercariae*). A free-swimming stage in the development of a fluke or trematode. Cercar-iae develop within sporocysts or rediae that parasitize snails or bivalve mollusks. They emerge from the mollusk and either enter their final host directly or encyst in an intermediate host that is ingested by the final host. In the latter case, the encysted tailless form is known as a metacercaria. SEE: *fluke; trematode.*

cercaricide. Lethal to cercaria.

cerclage (sār-klŏzh′) [Fr., hooping]. Encircling tissues with a ligature, wire, or loop.

  c., cervical. The use of ligatures around the cervix uteri to treat cervical incompetence during pregnancy. This helps to prevent spontaneous abortion.

Cercomonas (sĕr-kŏm′ō-năs) [Gr. *kerkos*, tail, + *monas*, unit]. A genus of free-living, flagellate protozoa. May be present in stale specimens of feces or urine. Not pathogenic.

cercomoniasis (sĕr″kō-mō-nī′ă-sĭs). Infestation with *Cercomonas intestinalis.*

cercus (sĕr′kŭs) [L., tail] (pl. *cerci*). A hairlike structure.

cerea flexibilitas (sē′rē-ă flĕk″sĭ-bĭl′ĭ-tăs) [L. *cera*, wax, + *flexibilitas*, flexibility]. A cataleptic state in which limbs retain any position in which they are placed. Characteristic of catatonic patients. SEE: *catalepsy.*

cereals [L. *cerealis*, of grain]. Edible seeds or grains.

  COMP: All cereals are similar in composition. The carbohydrates are the principal nutrient present and protein is next. Cereals contain 70% to 80% carbohydrate in the form of starch; and 8% to 15% protein. Vitamin B complex is abundant in wheat germ. Many cereals are of high fiber content.

cerebellar (sĕr-ĕ-bĕl′ăr) [L., little brain]. Pert. to the cerebellum.

cerebellifugal (sĕr″ĕ-bĕl-ĭ-fū′găl) [″ + *fugere*, to flee]. Extending or proceeding from the cerebellum.

cerebellipetal (sĕr″ĕ-bĕl-lĭp′ĭ-tăl) [″ + *petere*, to seek]. Extending toward the cerebellum.

cerebellitis (sĕr″ĕ-bĕl-ī′tĭs) [″ + Gr. *itis*, inflammation]. Inflammation of the cerebellum.

cerebellospinal (sĕr″ĕ-bĕl-ō-spī′năl) [″ + *spina*, thorn]. Pert. to the cerebellum and spinal cord.

cerebellum (sĕr-ĕ-bĕl′ŭm) [L.]. [NA] A portion of the brain forming the largest portion of the rhombencephalon. It lies dorsal to the pons and medulla oblongata, overhanging the latter. It consists of two lateral cerebellar hemispheres and a narrow medial portion, the vermis. It is connected to the brain stem by three pair of fiber bundles, the inferior, middle, and superior peduncles. The cerebellum is involved in synergic control of skeletal muscles and plays an important role in the coordination of voluntary muscular movements. It receives afferent impulses and discharges efferent impulses but does not serve as a reflex center in the usual sense; however, it may reinforce some reflexes and inhibit others.

Even though the cerebellum does not initiate movements, it interrelates with many brain stem structures in executing a variety of movements, including maintaining proper posture and balance; walking; running; fine voluntary movements as required in writing, dressing, eating, and playing musical instruments; and smooth tracking movements of the eyes. The cerebellum controls the property of movements, such as speed, acceleration, and trajectory.

cerebral (sĕr′ĕ-brăl, sĕ-rē′brăl) [L. *cerebrum*, brain]. Pert. to the cerebrum.

cerebral anoxia. Lack of oxygen supply to the brain. Usually due to cardiopulmonary arrest, q.v. If nothing is done to treat this condition, irreversible anoxic damage to the brain will begin after 4 to 6 minutes and sooner in some cases. If basic resuscitation measures are begun before the end of this period, the onset of cerebral death may be postponed. SEE: *cardiopulmonary resuscitation; hypoxia.*

cerebral hemorrhage. The result of rupture of a sclerosed or diseased blood vessel in the brain. Often associated with high blood pressure.

RS: apoplexy; hemiplegia; stroke.

cerebral palsy. SEE: *palsy, cerebral.*

cerebral palsy feeder. A mechanical device operated by simple gross movements; designed to permit independent eating by persons with severe motor control difficulties.

cerebration (sĕr″ĕ-brā′shŭn) [L. *cerebratio*, brain activity]. Mental action of the brain.

cerebrifugal (sĕr″ĕ-brĭf′ū-găl) [L. *cerebrum*, brain, + *fugere*, to flee]. Away from the brain; pert. to efferent nerve fibers.

cerebripetal (sĕr″ĕ-brĭp′ĕ-tăl) [″ + *petere*, to seek]. Proceeding toward the cerebrum, as nerve fibers or impulses.

cerebroid (sĕr′ĕ-broyd) [″ + Gr. *eidos*, form, shape]. Resembling brain tissue.

cerebromedullary (sĕr″ĕ-brō-mĕd′ū-lā-rē). Pert. to the brain and spinal cord. SYN: *cerebrospinal.*

cerebromeningitis (sĕr″ĕ-brō-mĕn″ĭn-jī′tĭs) [″ + Gr. *meninx*, membrane, + *itis*, inflammation]. Inflammation of the cerebrum and its membranes.

cerebropathy (sĕr-ĕ-brŏp′ă-thē) [″ + *pathos*, disease, suffering]. Any disease of the brain, esp. the cerebrum.

cerebrophysiology (sĕr″ĕ-brō-fĭz-ē-ŏl′ō-jē) [″ + Gr. *physis*, nature, + *logos*, word,

reason]. Physiology of the brain.

cerebropontile (sĕr″ĕ-brō-pŏn′tĭl) [″ + *pons*, bridge]. Pert. to the cerebrum and pons varolii.

cerebropsychosis (sĕr″ĕ-brō″sī-kō′sĭs) [″ + *psyche*, soul, mind, + *osis*, condition]. Any mental disorder due to a cerebral lesion.

cerebrosclerosis (sĕr″ĕ-brō″sklĕ-rō′sĭs) [″ + Gr. *sklerosis*, hardening]. Hardening of the brain, esp. of the cerebrum.

cerebroside (sĕr′ĕ-brō-sĭd″). A lipid or fatty substance present in nerve and other tissues.

cerebrosidosis (sĕr″ĕ-brō″sī-dō′sĭs). Form of lipoidosis with kerasin in the fatty cells. SEE: *Gaucher's disease.*

cerebrospinal (sĕr″ĕ-brō-spī′năl) [″ + *spina*, thorn]. Referring to the brain and spinal cord, as the cerebrospinal axis.

cerebrospinal axis. The central nervous system.

cerebrospinal fluid. A water cushion protecting the brain and spinal cord from physical impact. Usually shrinking or expanding of the cranial contents is balanced quickly by increase or decrease in the amount of this fluid.

FORMATION: The fluid is formed by the choroid plexuses of the lateral and third ventricles, that of the lateral ventricles passing through the foramen of Monro to the third ventricle, and through the aqueduct of Sylvius to the fourth ventricle. Here it may escape through the central foramen of Magendie or the lateral foramen of Luschke into the cisterna magna, and so over the brain and cord surfaces, occupying the subarachnoid spaces. It is absorbed by the arachnoid villi and through the perineural lymph spaces of both brain and cord.

CHARACTERISTICS: The fluid is watery, clear, and colorless. Normally the initial pressure of spinal fluid in a recumbent adult, as determined by spinal puncture, is equivalent to 70 to 180 ml of water. Amount in normal adult is 100 to 140 ml. Sp. gr.: 1.003 to 1.008. Total cell count in adults is 0 to 10/ml; in children 0 to 20/ml (cells should be counted at once); total protein 20 to 45 mg/dl; and glucose 0 to 75 mg/dl. Its concentration and alkaline reserve are similar to those of the blood. It does not clot on standing. Although the choroid plexuses can reflect certain blood constituents (e.g., iodides), changes in blood sugar, chloride, or urea will manifest themselves quickly in the fluid as well. Otherwise, changes take place largely subsequent to secretion. Turbidity suggests an excessive cell count. If due to red blood cells, centrifugation will show a red deposit.

Formation of a web after a clear fluid has been allowed to stand is characteristic of tuberculous meningitis (rarely other inflammatory reactions). Cerebrospinal fluid usually shows a yellowish discoloration when containing blood from the subarachnoid spaces (in contrast to blood from trauma of puncture), although for a few days the cells may not be entirely disintegrated. A similar appearance may result from a spinal block above the point of puncture, the fluid spontaneously coagulating due to an excessive albumin content. Total protein is increased in infections (as meningitis, brain abscess, tabes dorsalis), various types of hemorrhage or thrombosis, virus diseases (as encephalitis, anterior poliomyelitis, lymphocytic meningitis), and conditions such as chronic alcoholism. Cell count increases esp. in tuberculous meningitis, epidemic encephalitis, lymphocytic choriomeningitis, poliomyelitis (several days after onset), syphilis of central nervous system, and certain types of tumors of the spinal cord or brain. SEE: *blood-brain barrier; lumbar puncture.*

cerebrospinal ganglia. Sensory ganglia on the roots of cranial and spinal nerves.

cerebrospinal nerves. Cranial nerves, q.v., and spinal nerves, q.v.

cerebrospinal puncture. A puncture for the collection of cerebrospinal fluid. It may be collected from spaces around the spinal cord (lumbar puncture), from the cisterna magna (cisternal puncture), or in infants with open fontanelles (by ventricular puncture).

cerebrotomy (sĕr″ĕ-brŏt′ō-mē) [″ + Gr. *tome,* incision]. 1. Incision of the brain to evacuate an abscess. 2. Dissection of the brain.

cerebrovascular (sĕr″ĕ-brō-văs′kū-lăr) [″ + *vasculum,* vessel]. Pert. to the blood vessels of the brain, esp. to pathological changes.

cerebrovascular accident. ABBR: CVA. A general term most commonly applied to cerebrovascular conditions that accompany either ischemic or hemorrhagic lesions. These conditions are usually secondary to atherosclerotic disease, hypertension, or a combination of both. Also called apoplexy, stroke, or "a shock."

TREAT: Supportive measures as needed, including maintaining airway, oxygen therapy, prevention of hypothermia or hyperthermia, and provision of nutritional and fluid requirements. Physical therapy must be instituted immediately or as soon as possible to help insure that sensorimotor function is improved or restored.

NURSING IMPLICATIONS: *During initial attack:* Insure maintenance of a patent airway by positioning patient in a prone position or with head turned to the side; loosen clothing at throat. Keep patient warm and quiet. Monitor vital signs and neurological status frequently. Arrange for tests to be carried out expeditiously. Provide support to patient and family.

During convalescence: Assess the patient's neurological status to detect changes or complications. Monitor fluid balance and nutritional status, providing enteral (or parenteral if G.I. system is nonfunctional) nutrition until patient is able to eat. Assess swallowing ability and assist in determining time for initiation of oral foods and fluids. Assess bowel status daily, initiating bowel training and providing fluids, fiber, and stool softeners to prevent constipation and need for enemas. Assess bladder function, initiating bladder training and keeping patient clean and dry if incontinent. Do not encourage use of an indwelling catheter, as this may result in urinary tract infection and delay patient's recovery. Maintain correct body alignment, taking care to prevent external hip rotation and foot drop, also shoulder and hip subluxation. Carry out range-of-motion exercises to maintain joint mobility, and encourage the patient to actively exercise joints as ability permits to maintain muscle strength and mass. Reposition patient frequently and avoid placing on weakened or paralyzed side, inspecting skin and massaging and cushioning pressure areas to prevent tissue breakdown. Position distal parts of extremities higher than proximal areas to encourage venous return. Assess respiratory status, auscultating for adventitious sounds, and encourage deep breathing and coughing to prevent respiratory complications. Provide support and encouragement to patient and family as patient works to retrain muscles and regain lost function. Collaborate with physical therapist regarding mobilization techniques. Encourage all communication attempts and collaborate with speech therapist, following prescribed treatment plan. Recognize and help family to understand emotional lability, and provide emotional support to patient and support persons. Establish with the patient and family a plan to promote the patient's physical, intellectual, and communicative abilities and to regain lost functions in order to facilitate independence. Encourage them to utilize and participate in available support services and groups. Physical therapy, as prescribed, is one of the most important parts of the immediate and long-range program for rehabilitation of the patient. SEE: *Nursing Diagnoses* in *Appendix.*

cerebrum (sĕr′ĕ-brŭm, sĕr-ē′brŭm) [L.]. The

largest part of the brain, consisting of two hemispheres separated by a deep longitudinal fissure. The hemispheres are united by three commissures — the corpus callosum and the anterior and posterior hippocampal commissures. The surface of each hemisphere is thrown into numerous folds or convolutions called gyri, which are separated by furrows called fissures or sulci.

EMBRYOLOGY: The cerebrum develops from the telencephalon, the most anterior portion of the prosencephalon or forebrain.

STRUCTURE: Each cerebral hemisphere consists of three primary portions — the rhinencephalon or olfactory lobe, the corpus striatum, and the pallium or cerebral cortex. The cortex is a layer of gray matter that covers the surface of each hemisphere. The part covering the rhinencephalon (phylogenetically the oldest) is called archipallium; the larger nonolfactory cortex is called neopallium. Within the cerebrum are two cavities, the lateral ventricles (right and left), and the rostral portion of the third ventricle. The white matter or medullary substance of each hemisphere consists of three kinds of fibers: commissural fibers, which pass from one hemisphere to the other; projection fibers, which convey impulses to and from the cortex; and association fibers, which connect various parts of the cortex within one hemisphere.

Basal ganglia: Masses of gray matter deeply embedded within each hemisphere. They are the caudate, lentiform, and amygdaloid nuclei and the claustrum. *Fissures and sulci:* Lateral cerebral fissure (of Sylvius), central sulcus (of Rolando), parietooccipital fissure, calcarine fissure, cingulate sulcus, collateral fissure, sulcus circularis, longitudinal cerebral fissure. *Gyri:* Superior, middle, and inferior frontal gyri; anterior and posterior central gyri; superior, middle, and inferior temporal gyri; cingulate, lingual, fusiform, and hippocampal gyri. *Lobes:* Principal lobes are frontal, parietal, occipital, temporal, and central (insula or island of Reil).

PHYS: The cerebrum is concerned with sensations or the interpretation of sensory impulses; and all voluntary muscular activities. It is the seat of consciousness and the center of the higher mental faculties such as memory, learning, reasoning, judgment, intelligence, and the emotions.

On the basis of function, several areas have been identified and located. Among them are motor projection areas, which give rise to fibers carrying efferent impulses to effector organs, the skeletal muscles; sensory projection areas, which receive impulses from sense organs or sensory receptors by way of the brain stem, including the somesthetic (visual, auditory, gustatory, and olfactory) areas; and association areas, which are concerned with the higher mental faculties.

Cerespan. Trade name for papaverine hydrochloride.

cerium (sē'rē-ŭm) [L.]. SYMB: Ce. At. wt. 140.12; at. no. 58. A metallic element obtained from the rare earths.

ceroid (sē'royd). A fatty pigment present in various tissues.

ceroma (sē-rō'mă) [L. *cera*, wax, + Gr. *oma*, tumor]. A waxy tumor that has undergone amyloid degeneration.

ceroplasty (sē'rō-plăs"tē) [" + Gr. *plassein*, to mold]. Manufacture of anatomical models and pathological specimens in wax.

certifiable (sĕr"tĭ-fī'ă-b'l). 1. Pert. to infectious diseases that must be reported or registered with the health authorities. 2. In forensic medicine, a term applied to a mentally incompetent individual who requires the care of a guardian or institution.

certification (sĕr"tĭfĭ-kā'shŭn). 1. A legal document prepared by an official body that indicates a person or institution has met certain standards; or that the person has completed a prescribed course of instruction or training. 2. The completion of a form indicating the cause of death. 3. The legal process based on medical evidence of declaring a person insane or mentally incompetent. SEE: *commitment.*

certified emergency nurse. ABBR: CEN. Nurses who have been admitted to take the examination administered by the Board of Certification of Emergency Nursing and have passed that exam. In order to maintain certification as a CEN, a nurse must pass the examination every four years.

certify [L. *certus*, certain, + *facio*, to make]. 1. Declaration concerning the sanity of an individual. 2. To report certain specified diseases to public health authorities.

ceruloplasmin (sĕ-roo"lō-plăz'mĭn). A glycoprotein, blue in color, to which the majority of the copper in the blood is attached. It is decreased in Wilson's disease, q.v.

cerumen (sĕ-roo'mĕn) [L. *cera*, wax]. The waxlike, soft brown secretion found in the external canal of the ear. SEE: *ear wax.*

ceruminal (sĕ-roo'mĭ-năl). Pert. to the cerumen.

ceruminolysis (sĕ-roo"mĭ-nŏl'ĭ-sĭs). The dissolution or disintegration of cerumen in the external ear canal.

ceruminolytic agent (sĕ-roo"mĭ-nō-lĭt'ĭk). An agent that dissolves cerumen in the external ear canal. Obstruction of the ear canal with cerumen can cause itching, pain, and temporary conductive hearing loss. Removal of the obstruction manually with a blunt curette or loop or by irrigation should be the first approach to treatment. Cerumen solvents are not always recommended because they often do not solve the problem and frequently cause maceration of skin of the canal and allergic reactions.

ceruminosis (sĕ-roo″mĭ-nō′sĭs) [″ + Gr. *osis*, condition]. Excessive secretion of cerumen.

ceruminous (sĕ-roo′mĭ-nŭs). Pert. to cerumen.

ceruminous glands. Modified sweat glands in the skin lining the external auditory canal that secrete cerumen.

ceruse (sē′roos) [L. *cerussa*]. The basic carbonate of lead; white lead formerly used in paint.

cervical (sĕr′vĭ-kăl) [L. *cervicalis*]. 1. Of, pert. to, or in the region of the neck. 2. Pert. to the cervix of an organ, as the cervix uteri.

cervical cap. Device made of a flexible material that is shaped to provide a covering for the uterine cervix. Used to prevent conception.

cervical intraepithelial neoplasia. ABBR: CIN. Dysplasia of the basal layers of the squamous epithelium of the uterine cervix. This may progress to involve deeper layers of the epithelium. Grades 1, 2, or 3 represent increasing progression of the pathological process. Grade 3 (CIN 3) represents carcinoma in situ. CIN 3 is also classed stage 0 of cancer of the cervix. SEE: *cervix, cancer of.*

cervical nerves. First eight spinal nerves. SEE: *skeleton; spinal nerves.*

cervical plexus. A plexus formed by loops joining the anterior rami of the first four cervical nerves. It receives communicating rami from the sympathetic ganglia. SEE: *Nerve Plexuses* in *Appendix.*

cervical ribs. SEE: *rib, cervical.*

cervical spondylosis. Degenerative arthritis, osteoarthritis, of the cervical vertebrae and related tissues. If severe, it may cause pressure on nerve roots with subsequent pain or paresthesia in the arms.

cervical vertebrae. First seven bones of the spinal column. SEE: *skeleton.*

cervicectomy (sĕr″vĭ-sĕk′tō-mē) [L. *cervix*, neck, + Gr. *ektome*, excision]. Removal of the cervix uteri.

cervices. Pl. of cervix.

cervicitis (sĕr-vĭ-sī′tĭs) [″ + Gr. *itis*, inflammation]. Inflammation of the cervix uteri.

cervico- (sĕr′vĭ-kō) [L. *cervix*]. Prefix pert. to the neck or to the neck of an organ.

cervicobrachial (sĕr″vĭ-kō-brā′kē-ăl) [″ + Gr. *brachion*, arm]. Pert. to the neck and arm.

cervicocolpitis (sĕr″vĭ-kō-kŏl-pī′tĭs) [″ + Gr. *kolpos*, vagina, + *itis*, inflammation]. Inflammation of the cervix and vagina.

cervicodynia (sĕr″vĭ-kō-dĭn′ē-ă) [″ + Gr. *odyne*, pain]. A pain or cramp of the neck; cervical neuralgia.

cervicofacial (sĕr″vĭ-kō-fā′shē-ăl) [″ + *facies*, face]. Pert. to the neck and face.

cervicovaginitis (sĕr″vĭ-kō-văj″ĭ-nī′tĭs) [″ + *vagina*, sheath, + Gr. *itis*, inflammation]. Inflammation of the cervix of the uterus and the vagina.

cervicovesical (sĕr″vĭ-kō-vĕs′ĭ-kăl) [″ + *vesica*, bladder]. Pert. to the cervix uteri and bladder.

cervix (sĕr′vĭks) [L.] (pl. *cervices*). [NA] The neck or a part of an organ resembling a neck. SEE: words beginning with *cervico-*.

c., cancer of. Malignant neoplasm of the cervix of the uterus. Annually, it causes 5% of the cancer deaths in women. It may occur at any age, beginning at puberty. The mortality rate increases with age.

SYM: Absent except in advanced cases.

ETIOL: A precise cause is unknown, but the risk factors include: early age at first intercourse; multiple sexual partners; promiscuous male sexual partners, esp. those whose previous wife has cervical cancer. It is suspected that an oncogenic factor, most probably a virus, is transmitted sexually, and the human papilloma virus is thought to be an important factor.

In the past, it was thought that cervical malignancies did not occur in celibate women, esp. nuns. There is little evidence to support this. Thus, when a celibate woman has symptoms suggestive of cervical cancer, that diagnosis should be considered.

DIAG: Periodic Papanicolaou tests beginning after the individual becomes sexually active; colposcopy.

COURSE: The disease begins insidiously and may progress slowly or rapidly through the earliest change of dysplasia of the squamous epithelium of the cervix through the various grades of cervical intraepithelial neoplasm (CIN), to carcinoma in situ, to the four stages of carcinoma of the cervix, i.e., stages 0 through IV.

TREAT: Radiation, surgery or cytotoxic agents. SEE: *cervical intraepithelial neoplasia; colposcopy; Papanicolaou test.*

c. uteri. Neck of the uterus. The lower part from the internal os outward to the external os. It is rounded and conical in shape, and a portion protrudes into the vagina. It is about 1 in. (2.5 cm) long, penetrated by the cervical canal, through which the fetus and menstrual flow escape. It may be torn in childbirth, esp. in the primigravida.

Deeper tears may occur in manual dilatation and use of forceps; breech presentation also may be a cause. Laceration may be single, bilateral, stellate, or incomplete. Tears are repaired by suturing in order to prevent hemorrhage and later complications.

c. vesicae. Neck of the bladder.

c.e.s. *central excitatory state.*

cesarean hysterectomy (sē-sār′ē-ăn) [L. *caesarea,* cut]. Cesarean section, q.v., immediately followed by hysterectomy.

cesarean section. Removal of the fetus by means of an incision into the uterus, usually by way of the abdominal wall. May be performed by extraperitoneal or intraperitoneal abdominal route. There are several varieties of cesarean section, differing mainly in the technique employed. The most frequent indication for cesarean section is fetopelvic (also called cephalopelvic) disproportion. Either the fetus is too large to be delivered through the pelvic outlet, the pelvis is abnormally small, or there is a combination of these factors. Some physicians feel that a breech presentation of the fetus is best handled by cesarean section. It is not necessarily true that once a patient has had a cesarean section all subsequent deliveries must be done in this manner.

NURSING IMPLICATIONS: *Preop:* Because approximately 20% of births in the U.S. are by cesarean section, all expectant parents should be encouraged to give some thought to their preferences should this method become necessary for them, thus lessening many otherwise negative feelings. Concerns include, but are not limited to, anesthetic choices, presence of family or friend in recovery area, and physical contact or holding of the healthy newborn by the mother. The couple should also view a film of preparation for and delivery by section. If cesarean section is the choice, physical preparation is carried out by the nurse in accordance with established protocol. The patient should be informed about what to expect. The father or partner should be included in the experience if at all possible. If the father or partner chooses not to be present, or if this is not possible, attempts should be made to involve this person in the immediate care of the newborn and in the post delivery concerns for the mother.

Postop: Monitor vital signs and ensure a patent airway, suctioning and administering oxygen as necessary and prescribed. Assess dressing and perineal pad for bleeding every 15 minutes times 4, then every 30 minutes, then every hour, then every 4 hours, as prescribed for specific patient. Gently palpate fundus for firmness and avoid incision, and administer intravenous oxytocin as prescribed. Carry out routine

postoperative care and positioning for general anesthesia if used, or assess level of regional anesthesia until sensation has returned completely. Monitor intake and output, reporting blood-tinged urine, keep patient comfortably warm, and assess for and manage pain and nausea. Provide opportunity for and encourage parent-infant interaction and attachment. Encourage deep breathing, coughing, and repositioning to facilitate ventilation and mobilization of secretions. When bowel sounds are present, encourage oral fluids and foods to facilitate voiding and normal bowel activity. Monitor urinary output and bowel movements. Conduct usual postpartal instruction regarding fundus, lochia, perineal care, breast and nipple care, infant care, and care of incision. Instruct patient and partner about activity restrictions after discharge. Answer any questions about this cesarean section experience, and about concerns for future pregnancies and deliveries, i.e., vaginal versus repeat section. Reinforce positive feelings, but be sure to allow verbalization of negative ones, assisting in dealing with deviations from expectations and disappointments. SEE: *Nursing Diagnoses* in *Appendix.*

c.s., cervical. Surgical removal of the fetus, placenta, and membranes through an incision in the portion of the uterus just above the cervix.

c.s., classic. Cesarean section in which the fetus, placenta, and membranes are removed surgically by an incision through the abdominal and uterine walls.

c.s., extraperitoneal. Surgical removal of the fetus, placenta, and membranes through an incision into the lowest portion of the anterior aspect of the uterus. This approach does not entail entering the peritoneal cavity.

c.s., low transverse. Surgical removal of the fetus, placenta, and membranes through a transverse incision into the lower uterine segment. Use of this incision is associated with a decreased incidence of maternal and fetal mortality and morbidity in future pregnancies.

c.s., postmortem. Surgical removal of the fetus from the uterus immediately after maternal death.

cesarotomy (sēz″ă-rŏt′ō-mē) [″ + Gr. *tome,* incision]. Cesarean section, q.v.

cesium (sē′zē-ŭm) [L. *caesius,* sky blue]. SYMB: Cs. At. wt. 132.905; at. no. 55. A metallic element. It has a number of isotopes; radioactive isotope ^{137}Cs, which has a half-life of 30 years, is used therapeutically for irradiation of cancerous tissue.

cesspool. Colloquial term for *septic tank,* q.v.

Cestan-Chenais syndrome (sĕs-tăn′shĕn-ā') [Raymond Cestan, Fr. neurologist, 1872–1934; Louis J. Chenais, Fr. physician, 1872–1950]. A neurological disorder produced by a lesion of the pontobulbar area of the brain.

Cestoda (sĕs-tōd'ă) [Gr. *kestos*, girdle]. A subclass of the class Cestoidea, phylum Platyhelminthes, which includes the tapeworms, having a scolex and a chain of segments (proglottids).
Ex.: Taenia. Intestinal parasites of man and other vertebrates.

cestode (sĕs'tōd) [" + *eidos*, form, shape]. A tapeworm; a member of the Cestoda family.

cestodiasis (sĕs"tō-dī'ă-sĭs) [" + " + -*iasis*, condition]. Infestation with tapeworms. SEE: *Cestoda; tapeworm.*

cestoid (sĕs'toyd) [" + *eidos*, form, shape]. Like a tapeworm.

Cestoidea (sĕs-toy'dē-ă). A class of flatworms of the phylum Platyhelminthes. Includes the tapeworms.

Cetacort. Trade name for hydrocortisone.

Cetamide. Trade name for sulfacetamide sodium.

Cetane. Trade name for ascorbic acid.

cetyl alcohol. A white insoluble solid substance, $C_{16}H_{34}O$, used in manufacture of ointments.

cetylpyridinium chloride. USP. An antiinfective agent used topically and as a preservative in the manufacture of drugs. Trade names are Ceepryn and Cepacol.

CF. *Christmas factor; citrovorum factor.*

Cf. Chem. symb. for the element californium.

C.F.T. *complement fixation test.*

C.G.S. *centimeter-gram-second,* a name given to a system of units for length, weight, and time.

CH₄. Methane; marsh gas.

C₂H₂. Acetylene.

C₂H₄. Ethylene.

C₆H₆. Benzene.

Chaddock's reflexes (chăd'ŏks) [Charles G. Chaddock, U.S. neurologist, 1861–1936]. 1. Extension of great toe when the outer edge of the dorsum of the foot is stroked. Present in disease of the corticospinal tract. 2. Flexion of wrist and fanning of fingers when tendon of palmaris longus muscle is pressed.

chafe (chāf) [O. Fr. *chaufer*, to warm]. To injure by rubbing or friction.

chafing (chāf'ĭng). A superficial inflammation that develops when skin is subjected to friction from clothing or adjacent skin as may occur at the axilla, groin, anal region, or between digits of hands and feet or at the neck or wrists. Erythema, maceration, and sometimes fissuring occur. Bacterial or mycotic infection may result secondarily. SYN: *erythema intertrigo.*

Chagas' disease (chăg'ăs) [Carlos Chagas, Braz. physician, 1879–1934]. Trypanosomiasis, American, q.v.

chagoma. An erythematous swelling following the bite of the parasite that transmits trypanosomiasis. SEE: *trypanosomiasis, American.*

chain (chān) [O. Fr. *chaine*, chain]. 1. A related series of events or things. 2. In bacteriology, bacterial organisms strung together. 3. In chemistry, the linkage of atoms together in a straight line or in a circle or ring. The ring or straight-line structures may have side chains branching off from the main compound.
   c., food. SEE: *food chain.*
   c., heavy. The large polypeptide chains of antibodies. SEE: *heavy chain disease.*
   c., light. Small polypeptide chains of antibodies.

chaining (chān'ĭng). A behavioral therapy process whereby reinforcement is given for behaviors related to established behavior. Also called *chained reinforcement.*

chain of custody. In legal medicine, the procedure or protocol for assuming that the material obtained for diagnosis has been taken from the named patient, is properly labeled, and has not been tampered with en route to the laboratory.

chain of survival concept. In emergency and critical care medicine, the concept that more people could survive sudden cardiac arrest when a particular sequence of events occurs as rapidly as possible. This sequence is: (1) recognition of early warning signs, (2) activation of the emergency medical system, (3) basic cardiopulmonary resuscitation, (4) defibrillation (if needed), (5) intubation, and (6) intravenous administration of needed medications. Conceptually, each of these interventions is regarded as a link in a chain, and that weakness in any link lessens the chance of survival. SEE: *airway, nasopharyngeal; airway, oropharyngeal; cardiopulmonary resuscitation.*

chair, birthing. SEE: *birthing chair.*

chalasia (kă-lā'zē-ă) [Gr. *chalasis*, relaxation]. Relaxation of sphincters.

chalazion (kă-lā'zē-ŏn) [Gr. *khalaza*, hailstone] (pl. *chalazia, -zions*). Small, hard tumor analogous to sebaceous cyst developing on the eyelids, formed by distention of a meibomian gland with secretion. SYN: *meibomian cyst.* SEE: *steatoma.*

chalcosis (kăl-kō'sĭs) [Gr. *chalkos*, copper, + *osis*, condition]. 1. Chronic poisoning from copper. 2. Copper deposits in lungs and tissues.

chalice cell (chăl'ĭs) [Gr. *kalyx*, cup of a flower]. Crateriform shell remaining after mucus has been discharged from an epithelial cell. SYN: *goblet cell; cell, mucous.*

chalicosis (kăl-ĭ-kō′sĭs) [Gr. *chalix*, limestone, + *osis*, condition]. Pneumoconiosis associated with the inhalation of dust produced by stone cutting.

chalinoplasty (kăl′ĭ-nō-plăs″tē) [Gr. *chalinos*, corner of mouth, + *plassein*, to mold]. Plastic surgery of the mouth and lips, esp. of corners of the mouth.

challenge (chăl′ĕnj). In immunology, administration of a specific antigen to an individual known to be sensitive to that antigen in order to produce an immune response.

chalone (kăl′ōn) [Gr. *chalan*, to relax]. A poorly defined substance that acts to regulate certain intracellular activity, including cell division.

chamber (chăm′bĕr) [Gr. *kamara*, vault]. Compartment or closed space.

   c., altitude. SEE: *c., low pressure.*

   c., anterior. Space between the cornea and iris of the eye.

   c., aqueous. Anterior and posterior chambers of the eye, containing the aqueous humor.

   c., Boyden. Chamber used to measure chemotaxis. Cells are placed on one side of a membrane and chemotactic material on the other. The number of cells migrating to the filter quantitates the chemotactic effect.

   c., hyperbaric. An airtight enclosure strong enough to withstand high internal pressure. Used to expose animals, humans, or an entire surgical team to increased air pressure. SEE: *hyperbaric oxygen therapy.*

   c., low pressure. Chamber designed to simulate high altitudes by exposing humans or animals to low atmospheric pressure. Such studies are essential for simulated flights into the atmosphere and space.

   c., posterior. In the eye, the space behind the iris and in front of the vitreous body. It is occupied by the lens, its zonules, and the aqueous humor. SEE: *eye,* illus. of; *chamber, anterior.*

   c., pressure. C., hyperbaric, q.v.

   c., pulp. That part of the pulp cavity contained within the crown of the tooth. It is continuous with root canals.

   c., vitreous. Cavity behind the lens in the eye containing the vitreous humor.

chamomile, camomile (kăm′ē-mīl) [Gr. *khamaemelon*, earth apple]. Flowers of the *Anthemis* yielding a bluish volatile oil and a bitter infusion.

chancre (shăng′kĕr) [Fr., ulcer]. A hard, syphilitic primary ulcer, the first sign of syphilis, appearing approx. two to three weeks after infection. SEE: *syphilis.*

   SYM: Begins as a painless erosion or papule that ulcerates superficially. Generally single; sometimes multiple. Has a scooped-out appearance due to level or sloping edges that are adherent. It has a shining red or raw floor. Induration persists. Slightly purulent secretion. Heals without leaving scar. May appear at almost any site including mouth, penis, urethra, hand, toe, eyelid, conjunctiva, vagina, or cervix.

Caution: During the chancre stage, the condition is highly contagious and the chancre itself contains many spirochetes. Discovery of these organisms in the chancre is the basis for the positive dark-field test for syphilis. Syphilis may occur, however, without a chancre developing.

---

   c., hard. Primary lesion of syphilis. SYN: *hunterian chancre.* SEE: *chancre; syphilis.*

   c., simple. A nonsyphilitic venereal ulcer. SYN: *chancroid; c., soft.*

   c., soft. C., simple, q.v.

   c., true. The primary lesion of syphilis, q.v. SEE: *chancre.*

chancroid (shăng′kroyd) [″ + Gr. *eidos*, form, shape]. A highly infectious nonsyphilitic venereal ulcer. It is caused by *Haemophilus ducreyi* (also called Ducrey's bacillus), a gram-negative bacillus. SYN: *chancre, simple.*

   SYM: Begins with pustule or ulcer, multiple, abrupt edges, rough floor, yellow exudate, purulent secretion, sensitive and inflamed. Scar remains. Rapid progress. May affect the penis, urethra, vulva, or anus. Multiple lesions may develop by autoinoculation. Types include transient, phagedenic, giant, and serpiginous.

   INCUB: Approx. three to five days.

   TREAT: Ceftriaxone or erythromycin.

chancrous (shăng′krŭs). Pert. to or of the nature of chancre.

change, fatty. SEE: *fatty change.*

change of life. The menopause, q.v.; climacteric, q.v.

channel [L. *canalis,* a waterpipe]. 1. A conduit, groove, or passageway through which a variety of materials may flow. 2. In cell biology, a passageway in the cell membrane through which materials may pass. The opening is open or closed, depending upon the molecular interaction between the material and the opening. SEE: *calcium entry blockers.*

chapped (chăpt) [ME. *chappen*]. Inflamed, roughened, fissured, as from exposure to cold.

character (kăr′ăk-tĕr). 1. The total qualities, esp. those of the personality, thought, and morality, as evidenced from an individual's speech, writings, and actions, that distinguish one person from another. 2. The feature or characteristic of an organism or individual that results from the expression of the genetic information received, i.e., inherited, from the parents.

c., acquired. Trait or quality that was not inherited but is the result of environmental influence.

c., anal. Personality type that is the result of the persistence of the anal or excretory stage of development into adulthood. Such persons are frequently compulsive with respect to neatness, obstinacy, and frugality. Although not a precise definition of a mental disorder, the term "anal character" is useful in describing the behavior of affected individuals.

c., dominant. In genetics, a trait that is manifest even though it was present in only one gene.

c., primary sex. Inherited trait directly concerned with the reproductive tract.

c., recessive. In genetics, a trait that does not develop or appear unless it was present in the genes received from both parents.

c., secondary sex. Trait peculiar to either sex but not concerned with the reproductive tract. Voice quality, facial hair, and body fat distribution are examples.

c., sex-conditioned. Genetic trait carried by both sexes but expressed or inhibited by the sex of the individual.

c., sex-limited. Trait present in only one sex even though the gene responsible is present in both sexes.

c., sex-linked. Trait transmitted only on the sex-determining chromosome.

characteristic (kăr″ăk-tĕr-ĭs′tĭk). 1. The trait or character that is typical of an organism or individual. 2. In logarithmic expressions, the number to the left of the decimal point, as distinguished from the mantissa, which is the number to the right of the decimal point.

characteristic radiation. X radiation produced by the shifting of electrons within an atom to another orbit.

characterize. To mark, identify, or describe the attributes of something. This is done to facilitate distinguishing an individual or material from other examples of similar individuals or materials.

charbon (shăr-bŏn′) [Fr., coal]. Infection with *Bacillus anthracis.* SYN: *anthrax.*

charcoal (chär′kōl) [ME. *charcole*]. Activated charcoal, USP, very fine powder prepared from soft charred wood.

ACTIONS/USES: In treating persons who have ingested poisons, activated charcoal is given orally as a suspension in water, using 8 ml of diluent per gram of charcoal. For infants this may be given by using a nippled bottle. The dose is 1 to 2 grams/kg of

body weight. If the amount of toxic substance ingested is known, administer an amount of charcoal equivalent to 10 times the amount of toxin. Superactivated charcoal (SuperChar) is two or three times more effective than activated charcoal. Charcoal should be administered as soon as possible after intake of the toxic substance. It is contraindicated in patients who have ingested corrosive chemicals. Ionized chemicals such as acids, alkalis and salts of cyanide, iron and lithium are not well absorbed by charcoal.

c., superactivated. A type of charcoal used in treating poisoning. It is several more times as effective as activated charcoal. Trade name is SuperChar. SEE: *charcoal.*

Charcot's joint (shär-kōz′) [Jean M. Charcot, Fr. neurologist, 1825–1893]. A type of diseased joint associated with tabes dorsalis, syringomyelia, or other conditions involving disease or injury to the spinal cord, characterized by hypermobility. Decalcification of bone on joint surfaces occurs accompanied by overgrowth of bone about margins. Pain is usually absent, although there are exceptions. Deformity and instability of the joint are characteristic.

Charcot-Leyden crystals (shär-kō′lī′dĕn) [Charcot; Ernest V. von Leyden, Ger. physician, 1832–1910]. Colorless, hexagonal, double-pointed and often needlelike crystals found in the sputum in asthma and bronchial bronchitis or in the feces in ulceration of the intestine, esp. amebiasis.

Charcot-Marie-Tooth disease [Charcot; Pierre Marie, Fr. neurologist, 1853–1940; Howard Henry Tooth, Brit. physician, 1856–1925]. A form of progressive neural muscular atrophy, a disease with hereditary tendencies characterized by progressive weakness of distal muscles of the arms and feet. The muscles atrophy, reflexes are lost, foot drop develops, and there is loss of cutaneous sensations. Usually develops in childhood but may occur in adults; more common in males. Its cause is unknown. SYN: *atrophy, peroneal muscular.*

Charcot's triad. The combination of nystagmus, intention tremor, and scanning speech. It is frequently associated with multiple sclerosis.

charge. 1. In electricity, the amount of electrical force present. 2. To add electrical energy to a battery. 3. The cost to the patient of a medical service or hospitalization.

c., customary and reasonable. The usual cost of a specific service to a patient. The term is used in the medical insurance industry to determine the amount the provider will be reimbursed for a specific service or procedure.

charlatan (shăr'lă-tăn) [It. *ciarlatano*]. A pretender to special knowledge or ability, as in medicine. SYN: *quack*.

charlatanry (shăr'lă-tăn-rē). Undue pretension to knowledge or skill that is not possessed. SYN: *quackery*.

Charles' law (shărl) [Jacques A. C. Charles, Fr. physicist, 1746–1823]. At constant pressure, a given amount of gas will expand its volume in direct proportion to the absolute temperature. SYN: *Gay-Lussac's law*. SEE: *Boyle's law*.

charleyhorse. Pain and tenderness in the fibromuscular tissue of the thighs usually due to muscle strain or tear. Characterized by sudden onset and aggravation upon movement. SYN: *fibromyositis*.

    F.A.: Relief can be obtained from rest, local applications of cold, gentle massage, and aspirin.

chart [L. *charta*, paper]. 1. A simple form or sheet of paper for recording the course of a patient's illness. Includes records of temperature, pulse, respiratory rate, blood pressure, urinary and fecal output, and doctors' and nurses' notes. 2. To record on a graph the sequence of events such as vital signs. SEE: *charting*. 3. The complete clinical record of a patient, including physical and psychosocial state of health as well as results of diagnostic tests. Plans for meeting the needs of the patient are also included. SEE: *problem-oriented medical record*. 4. To record the clinical, radiographic, and forensic findings of the teeth and surrounding tissues.

    c., dental. A diagrammatic representation of the teeth of the mouth on which the clinical and radiographic findings can be recorded, often including the restorations present, decayed surfaces, missing teeth, and periodontal conditions.

charta (kär'tă) [L.]. Preparation intended principally for external application, made either by saturating paper with medicinal substances or by applying the latter to the surface of the paper by the addition of some adhesive liquid.

charting. The process of making a tabulated record of the progress of the patient during the hospital stay; a clinical record. Record information about the patient and the treatment. The physician needs detailed information that the nurse or others may contribute through observation of and contact with the patient. These notes, containing details of the patient's reactions and progress, aid the physician in making a diagnosis. Almost any member of the professional health-care team may be responsible for providing and recording information concerning the patient's therapy, course, and progress. Verbal reports are not sufficient; they take time and may be misunderstood.

    NOTE: Procedures for charting may be different for various hospitals. The system specified by each hospital should be used. Written documentation is considered legal evidence. It must be promptly made, dated, clear, concise, and legible. Use authorized abbreviations. Correct mistakes by making note of the mistaken entry and correction. If an entry is made late, place it in the chart just after the most recent entry; be certain it is dated and provides the time the entry was made. Slang should not be used. SEE: *Charting* in *Appendix; nursing process; problem-oriented medical record*.

    GENERAL RECORDS: *Blood pressure:* Record is usually kept on sheet with temperature, pulse, and respiration record. *Diet:* If patient is on regular diet, it is sufficient to chart breakfast, dinner, and supper, but when on any other diet, chart exactly what the patient is given at each meal and the amount of food actually eaten. The amount of liquids taken (not "Water p.r.n."); hours of giving; kind of diet (full, light, soft, liquid, special); appetite. *Discharge or death:* Discharge or death of patient with hour and date of same and the name of the individual who ordered discharge or who pronounced the patient dead.

    Fluids: Hours of giving; kind; amount. *Heat:* Chart by whose order heat is applied to an unconscious patient, who executed the order, for how long heat was applied, and what method was used. *Infant feeding:* The formula should be charted the first time; afterward, amount given, and, if regurgitated, approximate the amount. *Laboratory:* Hour; kind of specimen; by whom taken; by whom ordered (not necessary in case of routine urine specimen on admission); by which method specimen was sent to the laboratory. SEE: *chain of custody*.

    Dressings: Change of dressings on wounds and the amount and character of drainage (remark "Specimen Saved" if this has been done); hour; by whom; stitches or drains removed; patient's reaction if pained or shocked by dressing. *Drugs:* Any unfavorable reaction from drugs or treatments. Chart time when drugs or treatments are administered. All medicines, treatments, preparation, etc., are to be charted by the nurse who administers them whether in charge of the patient or not. Confine name of medicine, dose and route of administration, and frequency to the prescribed column. When administering soluble salts or medicines dispensed in liquid form, state dose actually administered, not the amount of solution. Any unusual therapeutic action or idiosyncrasy resulting from a drug should be recorded.

Nursing care: Hour; baths and shampoos; alcohol rubs and decubitus dressing; special mouth care; sitting up for first time; out of bed for first time; walking for first time; narcotics (treatments are also charted, but as treatments). *Operations:* Name of operation; preparation; preoperative medication if given by nurse or in ward; hour of going to O.R.; hour of going to and leaving recovery room or intensive care unit (ICU); hour of return to room; condition on return to room; hour of recovery from anesthetic; condition every half hour for next three or four hours, depending on state patient is in and severity of operation. Recovery room or ICU staff members will record treatment and condition while patient is in their care.

Personal care: Baths, personal hygiene, and patient's reactions to these. For women, record menstruation and type of menstrual protection used. *Physician:* Record physician's visit. Physician's orders must be recorded as well as the time they are written and carried out. *Physical therapy:* Hour of going for treatment and hour of return; condition of patient. *Postoperative:* Changing position of postoperative patients should be recorded under "Remarks." Record passive and active exercise of patient. *Specimens:* Record the taking of specimens of blood, exudates, transudates, etc., for examination. The result will be shown by the report of the pathologist. *Surgical preparations:* The signature of the nurse who does surgical preparations should appear after "Preliminary preparation of field of operation." Observe the same rule for narcotics.

Symptoms: Accurate description of all symptoms, i.e., character of pulse and respiration, mental state, description of pain, and nature of any discharge. The remarks should be appropriate and accurate. Subjective as well as objective symptoms should be recorded. *Time:* Everything relating to the patient's progress should be charted as it occurs. Record the hour with all statements on charts. Record on the first line of the sheet the day, date of admission, whether the patient walked in or was admitted by ambulance, and condition of patient. Four-hour graphic charts are kept for all surgical and obstetrical cases the first three days (usually at 8, 12, and 4, around the clock), and for all patients whose temperature is above normal. The temperature, pulse, and respirations of all other patients are charted appropriately according to the requirements of the institution.

Treatments: Hour of giving; nature of treatment; by whom given; patient's reac-

tion. *X-ray:* Hour; to radiology room or portable at bedside; return from radiology room; condition of patient.

Visits of clergyman (especially important in case of Roman Catholic patients): Hour; name of clergyman; rite performed.

Miscellaneous: Any sudden or marked change in patient's condition; notification of patient's relatives and clergyman. Special charts are also provided for certain purposes such as the temperature, pulse, and respiration chart; anesthesia chart generally kept by the anesthetist; blood-pressure chart used in conditions apt to affect the blood pressure; intake and output charts used in all patients with fluid and electrolyte imbalance; and laboratory records usually filed with the patient's chart. If any laboratory records have been made and not filed with the chart, their existence should be noted on the clinical chart at the time made and also upon the final page of the chart.

PHYSICAL SYMPTOMS: *Appetite:* Good, poor, special likes or dislikes. *Convulsions:* Type, duration, consciousness lost; note fecal or urinary incontinence; was patient injured during convulsion or in fall that came with convulsion; aura. *Defecation:* (see Excretions; Feces; Urine in this entry). *Diaphoresis* (perspiration): State whether slight, moderate, or profuse. *Emesis:* Amount, color, odor, consistency of the vomitus, and manner of ejecting. (See Vomiting in this entry.)

Enemas: Results and unusual appearances, distention before or after, describe results fully. Note whether or not flatus was expelled with the return of the enema. Chart the solution, strength, temperature, and amount used. Also douches and irrigations.

Excretions: Time, character, and other facts. *Feces:* Enema or natural movement; amount; consistency; color; abnormal odor; abnormal constituents. Defecation accompanied by pain or tenesmus.

General appearance: Color; posture; rash; mood; mental state. *Hemorrhages, discharges:* Description. When unusual, save specimens for examination. *Nausea:* Accompanied by vomiting; following certain foods, drugs, or treatments. *Nerves:* All symptoms of nervousness or excitability. *Pain:* Location; time of onset; character; sharp, dull, burning, grinding, throbbing; duration (constant, how long); intermittent; intervals.

Pathological conditions: Vomiting, convulsions. Record time of onset, duration, severity, general appearance of patient before, during, and after the attack. In convulsions it is important to record the localization of the convulsive motion if present, and whether or not the patient was incontinent; and if the patient fell, what, if any, injury was sustained and what treatment was provided. Temperature, pulse, and respiration (TPR) immediately after, and what was done to relieve condition. Explanation as to the cause if known. *Pulse:* Rate: beats per minute. Character: full, bounding, weak, thready, faint. Rhythm: regular, irregular, intermittent. *Respiration:* Rate per minute. Character: deep, shallow, difficult, easy, labored, quiet, stertorous, Cheyne-Stokes. Rhythm: regular, irregular, gasping.

Sleep: Hours of sleeping during the day as well as the night. If impossible to estimate accurately, approximate it and note that it is an approximation. Time and amount. Sleepwalking, nightmares, or talking in sleep should be recorded. *Temperature:* Indicate whether taken by mouth, rectum, or axilla; degree; following chill or treatment. If temperature is quite high and patient does not appear to have fever of that extent, take temperature again but remain at bedside to be sure patient is not placing thermometer against some hot object.

TPR: Taken as ordered. The nurse charts the TPR and general condition of the patient before going to the operating room, and the pulse and respiration with general condition upon return from the operating room. *Unconsciousness or coma:* Time of onset; conditions associated with or that caused onset; appearance of patient while in coma; medicines or treatment given while in coma; duration. *Unusual conditions:* Chart these such as appearance of blood, twitching, convulsions, coma, drowsiness, lethargy, unconsciousness.

Urine: State time of voiding, amount, color and appearance, whether voided or per catheter. Note time of beginning 24-hour specimen collection; when bladder is emptied for the purpose, this specimen is sent to laboratory for qualitative test. Note time of completion of collecting a 24-hour specimen; note amount on chart and on laboratory label. Send specimen to the laboratory for all patients remaining in the hospital overnight. A check mark may be used in the urine column when patient uses lavatory or defecates. At all other times the amount of urine is to be charted (totaled every 12 hours). Record if urination is accompanied by pain or burning; any abnormal appearance; specimen to laboratory.

Vomiting: Cause; forcible or projectile; vomitus amount, color, odor, consistency, any unusual constituents.

MENTAL SYMPTOMS: Calmness; cheerfulness; delirium (kind); depression (degree); apparent effect of visitors, etc.; de-

lusions and on what subjects; hallucinations; illusions and on what subjects; temper fits; willingness to cooperate; worry.

Visitors: Reaction to visitors and mood change after visitors depart. Especially important in depressed and psychiatric patients.

c., dental. Recording on a chart the clinical findings within the mouth; while examining each tooth and probing the gingival sulcus, the noting of the restorations present, missing teeth, periodontal pocket depth, and conditions of all soft tissues.

chartula (kăr′tū-lă) [L., small piece of paper]. A paper folded to form a receptacle containing a dose of medicinal substance.

chasma (kăz′mă) [Gr., a cleft]. An opening, gap, or wide cleft.

chaude-pisse (shōd-pēs′) [Fr.]. A burning sensation during urination, esp. in acute gonorrhea.

chaulmoogra oil, chaulmugra, chaulmaugra (chŏl-moo′grŭ, chŏl-mŏ′grŭ) [Bengali *caulmugra*]. A vegetable oil used in treatment of leprosy and some dermatoses. Though generally replaced by sulfones in treatment of leprosy, chaulmoogra oil is still used in endemic areas because of its availability and low cost.

Chaussier's areola (shō-sē-āz′) [François Chaussier, Fr. physician, 1746–1828]. Indurated tissue around the lesion of a malignant pustule.

chavicine (chăv′ĭ-sēn). A yellow, oily ingredient of black pepper.

CHB. *complete heart block.*

Ch.B. *Bachelor of Surgery;* used mostly in the United Kingdom.

CHD. *congenital hip dislocation; congenital heart disease; coronary heart disease.*

check [O. Fr. *eschec*]. 1. To slow down or arrest the course of. 2. To verify.

check bite. A sheet of hard wax used to make an impression of teeth to check articulation.

check-up. General term for visit to a physician for a physical examination.

Chédiak-Higashi syndrome (shē′dē-ăk-hē-gă′shē) [M. Chédiak and O. Higashi, contemporary French and Japanese physicians, respectively]. A lethal metabolic disorder, inherited as an autosomal recessive, in which neutrophils contain peroxidase-positive inclusion bodies. Partial albinism, photophobia, and pale optic fundi are clinical features. Children usually die by the age of 5 to 10 of a lymphoma-like disease.

cheek [AS. *ceace*]. 1. Side of face forming lateral wall of mouth below eye. SYN: *bucca.* 2. The buttock.

cheekbone. The malar bone, q.v.; os zygomaticum [NA]; zygomatic bone.

cheek retractor. Device that encloses the

cheek at the angle of the mouth for properly exposing operating field.

cheilectomy (kī-lĕk'tō-mē) [Gr. *cheilos*, lip, + *ektome*, excision]. 1. Surgical removal of abnormal bone around a joint in order to facilitate joint mobility. 2. Surgical removal of a lip.

cheilectropion (kī"lĕk-trō'pē-ŏn) [" + *ektrope*, a turning aside]. Eversion of the lip.

cheilitis (kī-lī'tĭs) [" + *itis*, inflammation]. Inflammation of the lip.

   c. actinica. Irritation of lips resulting from exposure to sunlight.

   c. exfoliativa. Seborrheic dermatitis of the lips.

   c. glandularis. Disorder of the lips resulting from hypertrophy of mucous glands and their ducts. SYN: *myxadenitis labialis.*

   c. venenata. Dermatitis of the lips resulting from chemical irritants present in lipsticks, lip cream, and various other materials.

cheilognathopalatoschisis (kī"lō-nā"thō-păl-ă-tŏs'kĭ-sĭs) [" + *gnathos*, jaw, + L. *palatum*, palate, + Gr. *schisis*, a splitting]. Developmental anomaly in which there is a cleft in the hard and soft palate, upper jaw, and lip.

cheilophagia (kī"lō-fā'jē-ă) [" + *phagein*, to eat]. Habit of biting one's own lip.

cheiloplasty (kī'lō-plăs"tē) [" + *plassein*, to form]. Plastic operation upon the lips.

cheilorrhaphy (kī-lor'ă-fē) [" + *rhaphe*, seam, ridge]. Surgical repair of a cleft lip.

cheiloschisis (kī-lŏs'kĭ-sĭs) [" + *schisis*, a splitting]. Harelip.

cheilosis (kī-lō'sĭs) [" + *osis*, condition]. Morbid condition of lips with reddened appearance and fissures at the angles, seen frequently in deficiency of vitamin B complex, esp. riboflavin.

cheilostomatoplasty (kī"lō-stō-măt'ō-plăs"tē) [" + *stoma*, mouth, + *plassein*, to form]. Plastic surgery and restoration of the mouth.

cheilotomy, chilotomy (kī-lŏt'ō-mē) [" + *tome*, incision]. Excision of part of the lip.

cheirognostic (kī"rŏg-nŏs'tĭk) [Gr. *cheir*, hand, + *gnostikos*, knowing]. 1. Able to distinguish left from right side of body. 2. Able to perceive which side of the body is being stimulated.

cheirology (kī-rŏl'ō-jē) [" + *logos*, word, reason]. Communication by use of the hands and fingers. SYN: *dactylology.*

cheirospasm (kī'rō-spăsm) [" + Gr. *spasmos*, a convulsion]. Writer's cramp; spasm of the muscles of the hand.

chelate (kē'lāt) [Gr. *chele*, claw]. 1. In chemistry, to combine with a ring structure much as a claw would grasp an object, said of the ion of a metal. 2. In toxicology, to use a compound to enclose or grasp a toxic substance and make it nonactive and thus nontoxic.

chelating agent. A drug that is used to chelate, q.v., substances, esp. toxic chemicals in the body.

chelation (kē-lā'shŭn) [Gr. *chele*, claw]. Combining of metallic ions with certain heterocyclic ring structures so that the ion is held by chemical bonds from each of the participating rings. When this structure is diagrammed it appears that the metallic ion is being held by a claw. Calcium disodium edetate, q.v., is a chelating agent.

cheloid (kē'loyd) [Gr. *kele*, tumor, swelling, + *eidos*, form, shape]. Keloid.

chemabrasion (kĕm-ă-brā'shŭn). Use of a chemical to destroy superficial layers of skin. Technique may be used to treat scars, tattoos, or abnormal pigmentation. SYN: *chemexfoliation.*

chemexfoliation (kĕm'ĕks-fō'lē-ā"shŭn). Chemabrasion, q.v.

chemical [Gr. *chemeia*, chemistry]. Pert. to chemistry.

Chemical Abstract Service. ABBR: CAS. A branch of the American Chemical Society that maintains a registry of chemicals, active ingredients used in drugs, and food additives. Each chemical is assigned a permanent CAS number through which current data can be traced.

chemical bond. SEE: *bond.*

chemical change. A change in which a substance breaks up or combines with other substances to make new substances with new properties or characteristics.

   Ex.: Oxygen and hydrogen combine to form water. Sodium (a metal) and chlorine (a gas) combine to form sodium chloride, or common salt. Glucose ($C_6H_{10}O_5$) is metabolized to carbon dioxide (CO_2) and water (H_2O). Oxygen combines with hemoglobin when the hemoglobin in the blood comes into contact with the oxygen in the air in the alveoli of the lungs to form oxyhemoglobin. The difference can be seen by comparing the bright scarlet color of the arterial blood containing oxyhemoglobin with the very dark red color of the venous blood containing reduced hemoglobin.

chemical compound. 1. A substance consisting of two or more chemical elements in definite proportions and in chemical combination and for which a chemical formula can be written, as in water (H_2O) or salt (NaCl). 2. A substance that can be separated by chemical means into simpler substances.

chemical disasters. The accidental release of large amounts of chemicals. The effects suffered by the people in the area are determined by the toxicity of the chemical, its speed in spreading, its composition (liquid, solid, or gaseous state), and the spill site, esp. with respect to proximity to a water supply or buildings. The major effect may be due to the chemical itself or to a resulting fire or explosion. In general, the medical care facilities of the area are most probably not capable of caring for hundreds or thousands of casualties. SEE: *chemical warfare.*

chemical element. 1. Element. 2. Any chemical compound or substance composed of chemical elements. SEE: *Physical Constants of the Elements* in *Appendix.*

chemical peel of the skin. The use of chemicals to erode the superficial layers of the skin. Used to treat acne, skin wrinkles, and blemishes. SEE: *dermabrasion; Retin-A.*

Caution: This technique can be dangerous. It must be done under the supervision of a person skilled in this type of therapy.

---

chemical reflex. Any reflex action initiated by a chemical stimulus.

chemical warfare. The tactics and technique of conducting warfare by use of toxic chemical agents. The chemicals include nerve gases; agents that cause temporary blindness, paralysis, hallucinations, or deafness; eye and lung irritants; blistering agents, including mustard gas; defoliants; and herbicides. SEE: *biological warfare.*

chemiluminescence (kĕm″ĭ-loo″mĭ-nĕs′ ĕns). Cold light or light produced as a result of a chemical reaction and without the production of heat, e.g., the light produced by certain bacteria, fungi, and fireflies. SEE: *luciferase.*

chemise (shĕ-mēz′) [LL. *camisa,* linen shirt]. Surgical dressing consisting of a square bandage tied around a catheter passing through the center of the bandage.

chemist (kĕm′ĭst). One trained in chemistry.

chemistry [Gr. *chemeia,* chemistry]. Science dealing with the molecular and atomic structure of matter and of the composition of substances — their formation, decomposition, and the various transformations that they may undergo.

    c., analytical. Chemistry concerned with the detection of the presence of chemical substances (qualitative analysis) or the determination of the amounts of substances present (quantitative analysis) in a compound.

    c., biological. Chemistry of living things, involving all the chemical processes that take place within an organism, such as the digestion of food, anabolism, and catabolism. SYN: *biochemistry.*

    c., general. Study of the entire field of chemistry with emphasis on fundamental concepts or laws.

    c., inorganic. Chemistry of compounds not containing carbon.

    c., medicinal. SEE: *chemistry, pharmaceutical.*

    c., nuclear. Radiochemistry or the study of changes that take place within the nucleus of an atom, esp. when the nucleus is bombarded by electrons, neutrons, or other subatomic particles.

    c., organic. Chemistry of carbon compounds.

    c., pathological. Study of chemical changes induced by disease processes, e.g., changes in the chemistry of organs and tissues; blood; secretions; or excretions.

    c., pharmaceutical. Chemistry of medicines, their composition, synthesis, analysis, storage, and actions.

    c., physical. Theoretical chemistry or that concerned with fundamental laws underlying chemical changes and the expression of these laws mathematically.

    c., physiological. Study of the chemical nature of living matter and the changes occurring in the metabolic activities of plants and animals.

chemobiotic (kē″mō-bī-ŏt′ĭk). Combination of an antibiotic with a chemotherapeutic agent.

chemocautery (kĕm″ō-kaw′tĕr-ē) [Gr. *chemeia,* chemistry, + *kauterion,* branding iron]. Cauterization by chemical agents.

chemoceptor (kĕm′ō-sĕp-tĕr). A chemoreceptor, q.v.

chemocoagulation (kē″mō-kō-ăg″ū-lā′ shŭn) [″ + L. *coaglutio,* coagulation]. Coagulation brought about by chemical agents.

chemodectoma (kē″mō-dĕk-tō′mä) [″ + *dektikos,* receptive, + *oma,* tumor]. Tumor of the chemoreceptor system. SEE: *paraganglioma.*

chemokinesis. The accelerated random locomotion of cells, usually in response to chemical stimuli.

chemoluminescence (kē″mō-loo″mĭ-nĕs′ ĕns). A chemical reaction that produces light. SYN: *chemiluminescence.* SEE: *luciferase.*

chemolysis (kē-mŏl′ĭ-sĭs) [″ + *lysis,* dissolution]. Destruction by chemical action.

chemonucleolysis (kĕm″ō-nū-klē-ŏl′ĭ-sĭs). Method of dissolving a herniated nucleus pulposus, q.v., by injection of the enzyme chymopapain into it. The use of this procedure is controversial, and is considered to be contraindicated for use in patients with a herniated lumbar disk in which the nucleus pulposis protrudes through the annulus.

chemopallidectomy (kē″mō-păl″ĭ-dĕk′tō-mē) [″ + L. *pallidum,* globus pallidus, + Gr. *ektome,* excision]. Destruction of a portion of the globus pallidus of the brain by use of a chemical.

chemoprevention of cancer. SEE: *cancer, chemoprevention of.*

chemoprophylaxis (kē″mō-prō″fī-lăk′sĭs). Use of a drug or chemical to prevent a disease, e.g., the taking of an appropriate medicine to prevent malaria.

chemopsychiatry (kē″mō-sī-kī′ă-trē). Use of drugs in treating psychiatric illnesses.

chemoreceptor (kē″mō-rē-sĕp′tor) [″ + L. *recipere*, to receive]. A sense organ or sensory nerve ending (as in a taste bud) that is stimulated by and reacts to certain chemical stimuli and that is located outside of the central nervous system. Chemoreceptors are found in the large arteries of the thorax and neck (carotid and aortic bodies), the taste buds, and in the olfactory cells of the nose. SEE: *carotid body; taste buds.*

chemoreflex (kē″mō-rē′flĕks) [″ + L. *reflectere*, to bend back]. Reflex resulting from chemical stimulus.

chemoresistance (kē″mō-rē-zĭs′tăns). Specific resistance of a body cell or microorganism to the effect of a drug.

chemosensitive (kē″mō-sĕn′sĭ-tĭv). Reacting to the action of a chemical or change in chemical composition.

chemosensory (kē″mō-sĕn′sō-rē). Detection of a chemical by sensory means, esp. by odor detection.

chemoserotherapy (kē″mō-sē″rō-thĕr′ă-pē). Combined use of a drug and serum in treating disease.

chemosis (kē-mō′sĭs) [Gr. *cheme*, cockleshell, + *osis*, condition]. Edema of conjunctiva about the cornea.

chemosmosis (kē″mŏs-mō′sĭs). Chemical reaction through a semipermeable membrane.

chemosterilant (kē″mō-stĕr′ĭ-länt). 1. Chemical that kills microorganisms. 2. Chemical that produces sterility, usually of the male, in organisms such as insects.

chemosurgery. Destruction of tissue by use of chemical compounds.

chemosynthesis (kē″mō-sĭn′thē-sĭs). The formation of a chemical compound from other chemicals or agents. In biological systems, this involves metabolism.

chemotactic (kē″mō-tăk′tĭk). Pert. to chemotaxis.

chemotaxis (kē″mō-tăk′sĭs) [Gr. *chemeia*, chemistry, + *taxis*, arrangement]. The movement of additional white blood cells to an area of inflammation in response to the release of chemical mediators by neutrophils, monocytes, and injured tissue. SYN: *chemotropism.*

chemothalamectomy (kē″mō-thăl-ă-mĕk′tō-mē). Chemical destruction of a part of the thalamus of the brain.

chemotherapeutic index. The ratio of the toxicity of a drug, expressed as maximum tolerated dose/kg of body weight to the minimal curative dose/kg of body weight. This index is utilized in judging the safety and effectiveness of drugs used in treating parasitic conditions.

chemotherapy (kē″mō-thĕr′ă-pē) [″ + *therapeia*, treatment]. In the treatment of disease, the application of chemical reagents that have a specific and toxic effect upon the disease-causing microorganism. SEE: *Nursing Diagnoses* in *Appendix.*

    c., combination. In antineoplastic drug therapy, the use of two or more drugs to treat malignant disease.

chemotic (kē-mŏt′ĭk). Pert. to chemosis.

chemotropism (kē-mŏt′rō-pĭzm) [″ + *tropos*, a turning]. Ability or impulse to progress or turn in a certain direction due to the influence of certain chemical stimuli, as the root of a plant toward its food supply.

chenodeoxycholic acid. A drug that is given orally to dissolve cholesterol gallstones.

chenopodium oil (kĕn-ō-pō′dē-ŭm) [Gr. *chen*, goose, + *pous*, foot]. Oil of American wormseed. A pale-yellow, volatile oil with pungent, irritating odor.

    ACTION/USES: Antihelmintic against hookworm.

cherophobia (kē″rō-fō′bē-ă) [Gr. *chairein*, to rejoice, + *phobos*, fear]. Morbid fear of and aversion to gaiety.

cherry-red spot. A red spot in each retina. Seen in Tay-Sachs disease, q.v.

cherubism (chĕr′ū-bĭzm). Cherubic appearance of the face of a child due to infiltration of the jaw, esp. the mandible, with masses of vascular fibrous tissue containing giant cells.

chest [AS. *cest*, a box]. The thorax.

    MENSURATION: The object of measuring the chest is to determine the comparative bulk of the two sides and the amount of expansion and retraction accompanying inspiration and expiration of the two sides. The points of measurement are between the spinous processes behind and the median line in front on the level of the 6th costosternal articulation. The right side is from ½ inch to 1 inch (1.3 to 2.5 cm) larger than the left. When a pleural cavity is distended with air or fluid, the measurement of the affected side may exceed that of the healthy side by 2 or 3 inches (5.6 to 7.6 cm); after removal of the fluid there may be an equal diminution in the measurement of the affected side, as compared with the healthy one. In unilateral emphysema, the total difference between the fullest inspiration and fullest expiration on the affected side will scarcely exceed ¹⁄₁₆ inch (1.6 mm), while on the other side there may be a difference of 2 or 3 in. (5.6 to 7.6 cm).

PALPATION: Serves to detect any thoracic tenderness, edema, friction fremitus, or rales. Edema of chest walls is recognized by pitting when pressure is made with finger; it may be observed in empyema and in certain types of heart failure.

The friction sound of pleurisy and harsh, sonorous rales can be detected sometimes by palpation. Thoracic tenderness is observed in pleurisy, pneumonia associated with pleurisy; pleurodynia, intercostal neuralgia (confined to certain spots); fracture of the ribs; and in contusion and inflammation of the pleural surfaces.

PERCUSSION: Place finger being used as a pleximeter firmly against chest and preferably parallel to ribs. Make finger that is used as plexor strike the one on chest perpendicularly, fix forearm, and use no more force than can be obtained from a gentle swing of the wrist. Percuss all parts of chest anteriorly and posteriorly, during both inspiration and expiration. In comparing sides be sure to percuss corresponding parts.

Normal resonance: On the right side, pulmonary resonance extends from half an inch to an inch (1.3 to 2.5 cm) above the clavicle, downward to upper border of 6th rib in front, and to a line drawn through the 10th spinous process posteriorly. On the left side, pulmonary resonance extends from a half inch to an inch (1.3 to 2.5 cm) above the clavicle downward within the mammary line to the 10th rib, and posteriorly to a line drawn through the 10th spinous process.

Cracked pot sound: Modified tympany can be simulated by percussing over the cheek when mouth is partially open. May be heard normally over the chest of a crying infant. In the adult it usually indicates a cavity that has a free communication with a bronchus. Best detected by keeping ear near open mouth of patient while percussing.

Dullness or flatness: Recognized in tuberculous condition, pneumonic consolidation, pleural effusions of all kinds; collapse of lung, congestion and edema of lung, enlargement of liver or spleen (at base), and neoplastic growths in the lung. It is important to determine the extent of movement of the diaphragm. To do this have the patient hold breath in deep inspiration while in a sitting position. Then quickly percuss the chest on both sides posteriorly to find and mark the lowest point of pulmonary resonance. Repeat this while the patient holds breath following complete expiration. On both sides of the chest the top and bottom marks should be from ¾ to 2½ in. (2 to 6 cm)

apart. The top line on the right is usually 1 to 2 cm higher than the left due to the presence of the liver below the right diaphragm. Diseases that interfere with aeration of the lungs or that paralyze the diaphragm will cause the normal movement of the diaphragm to be altered.

Hyperresonance: Observed in pneumothorax, lung collapse, tuberculous or bronchiectatic cavities, emphysema, lowered pulmonary tension in the initial stage of pneumonia and above a pleural effusion (Skoda's resonance), flatulent distention of the stomach or colon frequently observed over the left base.

Tympanitic note: A hollow drumlike sound, like that normally obtained by percussing the larynx or empty stomach. The conditions mentioned under Hyperresonance are also capable of producing tympany.

Pitch: Depends largely upon the volume of air and the tension of walls of cavity, and upon size of opening that communicates with the cavity. The less the air, the greater the tension; the smaller the opening, the higher the pitch of the note. In beginning tuberculous consolidation, the note over the affected apex is higher pitched. Normally the note over the right apex is higher pitched than that over the left.

RS: breathing; fremitus; resonance; respiration; pectus excavatum; "thoraco-" words.

c., emphysematous. Chest characteristic of advanced emphysema. The thorax is short and round; the anterior-posterior diameter is often as long as the transverse diameter; ribs are horizontal; the angle formed by divergence of the costal margin from the sternum is very obtuse or quite obliterated. Often termed barrel-shaped.

c., flail. Condition of the chest wall due to multiple fractures of the rib cage; it moves paradoxically, i.e., in with inspiration and out during expiration.

c., flat. Deformity of chest in which the anterior-posterior diameter is short, the thorax long and flat, and ribs oblique. The scapula is prominent; spaces above and below clavicles are depressed. Angle formed by divergence of the costal margins from the sternum is very acute.

c., funnel. Pectus excavatum, q.v.

c., pigeon. Condition of the chest in which sides are considerably flattened and sternum prominent. The sternal ends of the ribs are enlarged or beaded, and this characteristic has given rise to the term rachitic rosary. Often a circular construction of the thorax at level of the xiphoid cartilage. Due to obstruction of infantile respiration or to rickets.

chest drainage. Placement of a drainage tube in the chest cavity, usually in the pleural space. Used to drain air, fluid, or blood from the pleural space in order to permit the compressed and collapsed lung to expand. The tube is connected to a system that produces suction. This not only helps to remove the material from the pleural space, but also prevents air from being sucked into the space.

chestnut, horse. The inedible seed pod of the horse chestnut or buckeye tree *(Aesculus hippocastanum)*. The nut contains a glucoside, aesculin, that is toxic. The young twigs and sprouts of *A. hippocastanum* are also toxic. Symptoms of aesculin poisoning include muscle twitching, weakness, incoordination, dilated pupils, vomiting, diarrhea, stupor, and paralysis. Other species of chestnuts are edible.

chest prominences and depressions. An unnatural prominence or depression is often observed over the lower part of the sternum and is generally congenital. The term funnel breast or shoemaker's breast (because it may result from pressure of tools) has been applied to the sternal depression. The correct term is pectus excavatum.

A unilateral or local depression may be caused by consolidation, cavity, or pleurisy with fibrous adhesions.

A unilateral or local prominence may be due to pleurisy with effusion; pneumothorax, hydrothorax, hemothorax; aneurysm or tumor; compensatory emphysema resulting from impairment of the opposite lung; cardiac enlargements (left side); enlargements of abdominal organs, esp. liver and spleen.

chest P.T. *chest physical therapy.*

chest regions. Anterior, posterior, and lateral. *Anterior divisions* (R. and L.): clavicular, infraclavicular, and supraclavicular, mammary and inframammary, upper and lower sternal. *Posterior divisions* (R. and L.): scapular, infrascapular, interscapular, and suprascapular. *Lateral divisions:* Axillary and infra-axillary.

chest thump. A sharp blow to the chest in the precordial area. Done to attempt restoration of normal heart beat in patients with cardiac arrest or ventricular tachycardia.

Cheyne-Stokes respiration (chān′stōks′) [John Cheyne, Scot. physician, 1777 – 1836; William Stokes, Irish physician, 1804 – 1878]. A common and bizarre breathing pattern characterized by a period of apnea lasting 10 to 60 seconds followed by gradually increasing depth and frequency of respirations. It accompanies depression of frontal lobe and diencephalic dysfunction. This condition may be present as a normal finding in children. SEE: *respiration, Cheyne-Stokes,* for illus.

CHF. *congestive heart failure.*

Chiari's deformity (kē-är′ēz). SEE: *Arnold-Chiari deformity.*

Chiari-Frommel syndrome (kē-är′ē-frŏm′mĕl) [Hans Chiari, Austrian pathologist, 1851 – 1916; Richard Julius Ernst Frommel, Ger. gynecologist, 1854 – 1912]. Persistent lactation and amenorrhea following childbirth. It is due to the continued secretion of prolactin and decreased gonadotropin production. A pituitary adenoma may or may not be present.

chiasm, chiasma (kī′ăzm, kī-ăz′mă) [Gr. *khiasma,* cross]. A crossing or decussation.

   c., optic. An incomplete crossing of the optic fibers (the outer fibers not crossing each other); the point of crossing of the fibers of the optic nerves.

chickenpox. An acute viral disease with mild constitutional symptoms (headache, fever, malaise) followed by an eruption appearing in crops and characterized by macules, papules, vesicles, and crusting. Chickenpox and herpes zoster are different manifestations of infection with the same virus. SYN: *varicella,* q.v. SEE: *varicella; varicella-zoster immune globulin.*

chief complaint(s). The symptom or group of symptoms that represents the primary reason(s) for a patient's seeking health care.

chiggers (chĭg′ĕrs). Redbugs. The six-legged larvae of mites of the family Trombiculidae, order Acarina of the class Arachnida. They are parasitic on insects, various vertebrates, and man. Eggs are laid on the ground and hatch in about 12 days, after which they attach to host at first opportunity. They attach themselves to the surface of the skin and inject a salivary secretion that dissolves the surrounding tissue, producing a wheal with intense itching and severe dermatitis. A tubular structure, a stylostome, is developed that is used in ingesting the semidigested tissue debris. The mites do not feed on blood. The most common species attacking humans in North America is *Trombicula alfreddugesi.* The irritation is the result of sensitization to the injected saliva. To prevent being infested when exposed, wear clothes that completely cover the skin and are tight at the neck and arms, and stuff pant legs into shoes with high tops. Certain chemical compounds such as diethyltoluamide (Off) will repel chiggers. SEE: *Tunga.*

   TREAT: Proprietary preparations are available that, when applied to the affected area, asphyxiate the mite. One of these, Kwell, contains hexachlorohexane. Benzyl benzoate ointment and gamma benzene hexachloride are also effective.

chigoe infestation. Infestation of a parasite of dogs, pigs, and barefooted humans by the flea *Tunga penetrans.* In humans the usual sites of invasion are the spaces between the toes, where the burrowing female swells and causes a painful open sore.

TREAT: The gravid flea is removed, using a sterile needle. The site is treated with tincture of iodine, which is toxic to the remaining fleas and eggs.

chikungunya virus. A mosquito-borne virus that causes a denguelike disease with hemorrhagic complications.

chilblain (chĭl′blān) [AS. *cele,* cold, + *blegen,* to puff]. A form of cold injury characterized by localized erythema and sometimes blistering. The affected area itches, may be painful, and may progress to crusted ulcerations. The cause is thought to be prolonged constriction of arterioles in reaction to exposure to cold and dampness. SYN: *pernio.*

NURSING IMPLICATIONS: Evaluate patient for circulatory insufficiency. Instruct concerning need to protect susceptible areas from cold exposure.

child [AS. *cild,* child]. Any human between infancy and puberty. SEE: *pediatrics.*

child abuse. Emotional, physical, or sexual injury to a child. Also seen after instances of severe disruption in the process of parental attachment. May be due to positive action or omission on the part of those responsible for the care of the child. In domestic situations in which a child is abused, it is important to examine other children and infants living in the same home because about 20% of them will have signs of physical abuse. That examination should be done without delay in order to attempt to prevent further abuse of children in that home. Do not allow infant or child to remain in the hostile environment where the abuse occurred. To fail to do this may be disastrous for the child. SEE: *battered child syndrome; shaken baby syndrome.*

NURSING IMPLICATIONS: Determine the nature of physical abuse. Assess child's level of consciousness, reaction and size of pupils, and vital signs. Systematically inspect and palpate all parts of the body for signs of injury. Provide reassurance and support to the child and allow for expression of feelings and concerns.

childbearing. The act of carrying and being delivered of a child.

    c., delayed. SEE: *elderly primigravida.*

childbed. Period during and immediately subsequent to parturition. SYN: *puerperium.*

childbed fever. Puerperal sepsis.

childbirth. The process of giving birth to a child. SYN: *labor; parturition.*

    c., natural. The delivery of a fetus without the use of analgesics, sedatives, or anesthesia. Termed natural because this method was the only approach to childbirth prior to the development of modern obstetrical techniques. Natural childbirth is accomplished by having the woman, and often the spouse, go through a training period months prior to actual delivery. This training is called psychoprophylactic preparation for childbirth. More recently, natural childbirth has come to include a more noninterventionist approach, with less reliance on technology and a greater reliance on emotional support during labor and delivery, as appropriate. SEE: *Lamaze; psychoprophylactic childbirth.*

    c., prepared. A term referring to the mother, and often to the father, of the baby who has been educated about childbirth, anesthesia, and analgesia during labor. The mother may opt to have natural childbirth or to receive medications or regional anesthesia. SEE: *childbirth, natural; Lamaze technique or method; psychoprophylactic childbirth.*

child neglect. Failure by those responsible for caring for a child to provide for the child's nutritional, emotional, and physical needs.

childproof. Description of articles so designed as to be harmless to children, esp. medicine containers that children cannot open.

chilectropion (kī″lĕk-trō′pē-ŏn) [Gr. *cheilos,* lip, + *ektrope,* turning out]. Eversion of the lip. SYN: *cheilectropion.*

chilitis (kī-lī′tĭs) [″ + *itis,* inflammation]. Inflammation of the lips. SYN: *cheilitis,* q.v.

chill (chĭl) [AS. *cele,* cold]. An attack of shivering accompanied by the sensation of coldness and pallor of the skin produced by involuntary contraction of many muscle groups. It may be due to a disturbance in the temperature-regulating centers of the hypothalamus. Chills accompany various diseases, esp. malaria and pneumococcal pneumonia, and are coarse or fine, diffuse, or trembling. SEE: *windchill factor.*

SYM: A real chill is ushered in by extreme sensation of cold; shivering; chattering of the teeth and, in extreme cases, a marked tremor of the entire body followed by a rapidly rising temperature.

ETIOL: Infections or diseases (as malaria, pneumococcal pneumonia, bacteremia); parasites in blood; bacterial vaccines; and transfusion reactions. Postoperative chills or chills in puerperium are indicative of infection.

NURSING IMPLICATIONS: Make patient comfortable by applying blankets and putting in a warm (not hot) environment. Provide warm drinks when patient is able to tolerate them or when permitted by physician. Take patient's temperature and then retake it 20 to 30 minutes after the chill has subsided. Record the duration and severity of the chill. Question the patient about related signs and symptoms. Observe vital signs and evaluate for signs of septic shock.

c., nervous. A tremor accompanied by a chilly sensation but not with fever. It may follow severe pain or extreme nervousness. It usually passes quickly and seldom is serious.

chilo-, cheilo- [Gr. *cheilos*, lip]. Prefix denoting relationship to the lip.

chiloangioscopy (kī″lō-ăn″jē-ŏs′kō-pē) [″ + *angeion*, vessel, + *skopein*, to examine]. Microscopic examination of the circulation in the lip.

Chilomastix mesnili (kī″lō-măs′tĭks měs-nĭl′ē). A species of Mastigophora. A protozoon that is considered a presumptive parasite in the intestines.

chimera (kī-mē′rä). In human biology, the mixing of the blood (and blast cells) of embryos of double-egg twins so that even though each twin originally had a different blood group, each now has a mixed group.

chimney sweeps' cancer. Epithelioma of the scrotum. Due to chronic irritation by coal soot. SEE: *cancer.*

chimpanzee (chĭm-păn′zē). An intelligent ape native to parts of Africa. Because of its similarity to man, it is used in experimental medicine.

chin [AS. *cin*, chin]. Point of the lower jaw; region below lower lip. SYN: *mentum* [NA].

China clay. Kaolin, q.v.

Chinese restaurant syndrome. A group of transient symptoms that some persons develop after eating food containing a considerable amount of monosodium glutamate.

SYM: Burning sensation, headache, facial pressure, perspiration, and chest pain.

chin jerk. Reflex contraction of muscles of mastication on suddenly depressing the jaw.

chin-lift airway technique, head-tilt. A method of opening the airway of an unconscious patient by elevating the chin and tilting the head. This provides the maximum opening of the airway, esp. in unconscious patients in whom the tongue is blocking the airway. This is done by using the fingertips to bring patient's chin forward and support the lower jaw. The patient's head will also be tilted by this maneuver. The maneuver can be completed by applying gentle pressure to

the patient's forehead with the other hand. The patient's mouth must be kept open; however, do not use the thumb for this purpose. SEE: *airway; bag-valve-mask; cardiopulmonary resuscitation; jaw-thrust technique for establishing the airway; Universal Precautions* in *Appendix.*

Caution: This technique is not to be used in patients with neck or spinal injuries.

---

chin reflex. Clonic movement resulting from percussing or stroking lower jaw.

chip. A small fragment of something.

chiragra (kī-răg′rä) [Gr. *cheir*, hand, + *agra*, seizure]. Pain in the hand.

chiralgia (kī-răl′jē-ä) [″ + *algos*, pain]. Pain in the hand of nontraumatic or neuralgic origin.

c. paresthetica. Numbness and pain in the hand, esp. in the region supplied by the radial nerve.

chirognostic (kī″rŏg-nŏs′tĭk) [″ + *gnostikos*, knowing]. Having the ability to distinguish the right from the left, or the side of the body being stimulated.

chirokinesthesia (kī″rō-kĭn″ĕs-thē′zē-ä) [″ + *kinesis*, movement, + *aisthesis*, sensation]. Subjective perception of motions of the hand.

chiromegaly (kī″rō-měg′ă-lē) [″ + *megas*, large]. Enlargement of the hands, wrists, or ankles.

chiroplasty (kī′rō-plăs″tē) [″ + *plassein*, to form]. A plastic operation on the hand.

chiropodist (kĭ-rŏp′ō-dĭst, kī-) [″ + *pous*, foot]. Obsolete term for podiatrist. SEE: *podiatry.*

chiropody (kĭ-rŏp′ō-dē). Obsolete term for treatment of disorders of the feet. SEE: *podiatrist.*

chiropractic (kī″rō-prăk′tĭk) [Gr. *cheir*, hand, + *prattein*, to do]. System of health care based on the premise that the relationship between structure and function in the human body is a significant health factor and that such relationships between the spinal column and the nervous system are important, since the normal transmission and expression of nerve energy are essential to the restoration and maintenance of health. (Adapted from definition supplied by the American Chiropractic Association.)

chiropractor. A person certified and licensed to provide chiropractic care.

chirospasm (kī′rō-spăzm) [″ + *spasmos*, spasm]. Spasmodic affection of muscles of hand; writer's cramp.

chisel (chĭs′l). A beveled-edge steel cutting instrument used in dentistry and orthopedics.

chi-square (kī-skwār). A statistical test to determine the similarity of the number of occurrences being investigated to the expected occurrences. The symbol for chi-square is χ^2.

chitin (kī'tĭn) [Gr. *chiton*, tunic]. A white, horny substance in outer covering of body of invertebrates such as crabs. Also occurs in some fungi.

chitinous (kī'tĭ-nŭs). Pert. to or composed of chitin.

Chlamydia (klă-mĭd'ē-ă) [Gr. *chlamys*, cloak]. A genus of microorganisms that are intracellular parasites. They cause a wide variety of diseases in man and animals.

  C. trachomatis. This organism causes a great variety of diseases, including genital infections in males and females. In industrialized countries *C. trachomatis* is the most common sexually transmitted pathogen, causing an estimated 3 million new infections annually. The specific diseases caused by *C. trachomatis* include 35% to 50% of cases of nonspecific urethritis, q.v.; neonatal inclusion conjunctivitis, q.v.; lymphogranuloma venereum, q.v.; psittacosis (ornithosis), q.v.; pneumonia, q.v.; and trachoma, q.v.

  Chlamydial infections may cause pelvic inflammatory disease in women and this may result in infertility. The pregnant woman with such an infection can transmit the disease to her infant during the birth process.

  C. psittaci. This organism causes disease mostly in birds and lower mammals. Humans are occasionally accidental hosts. In humans, the illness is either influenza-like or a serious pneumonic disease. SEE: *psittacosis.*

chloasma (klō-ăz'mă) [Gr. *chloazein*, to be green]. Pigmentary skin discolorations, usually those occurring in yellowish-brown patches or spots.

  SYM: Areas rounded or oval with ill-defined margins; light yellow to black. In those due to external factors, pigmentation develops only at site of irritation or beyond.

  c., gravidarum. Brownish pigmentation of the face, often occurring in pregnancy. It usually disappears after delivery. Also seen in some persons who take progestational agents for birth control. SYN: *mask of pregnancy.*

  c., idiopathic. Chloasma caused by external agents such as sun, heat, mechanical means, and x-rays.

  c., symptomatic. Chloasma caused by various diseases, such as syphilis or cancer.

  c. traumaticum. Skin discolorations following trauma.

  c. uterinum. Chloasma of pregnancy and other uterine conditions.

chloracne (klor-ăk'nē). A generalized acneiform dermatitis that may occur in persons exposed to chemicals containing chlorine.

chloral (klō'răl) [Gr. *chloras*, green]. 1. An oily liquid having a bitter taste. 2. Chloral hydrate.

chloral hydrate. USP. Colorless, transparent crystals having aromatic, slightly acrid odor, and having a caustic, faintly bitter taste; soluble in alcohol and water. Trade names are Noctec and SK-Chloral Hydrate.

  ACTION/USES: As a sedative and hypnotic. Most commonly used to induce sleep as it allows almost normal sleep pattern in most patients.

chloral hydrate poisoning. Depresses and eventually paralyzes the central nervous system. Can be toxic to the liver. There may be nausea and vomiting due to gastric irritation. Pulse is feeble, respirations are shallow and irregular; lassitude; weakness; dizziness; sleep.

  F.A.: Maintain airway; use cuffed endotracheal tube if necessary. Assisted respiration may be required. Induce emesis. If this is not accomplished, administer a slurry of activated charcoal and remove by suction through the same tube used to instill the charcoal. Trendelenburg position, I.V. glucose. If overdose was administered by enema, give an activated charcoal cleansing enema. SEE: *Poisons and Poisoning* in *Appendix.*

chlorambucil (klō-răm'bū-sĭl). USP. A cytotoxic agent used in treating chronic lymphocytic leukemia, Hodgkin's disease, and certain lymphomas. Trade name is Leukeran.

chloramines (klō'ră-mĭns). Organic chlorine compounds that decompose slowly, liberating chlorine. Used extensively in dairies, food manufacturing establishments, and as a germicide.

  Ex.: chloramine-T; dichloramine-T.

chloramphenicol (klō"răm-fĕn'ĭ-kŏl). USP. An antibiotic originally isolated from *Streptomyces venezuelae.* It is now made synthetically. It is a broad-spectrum agent and is especially useful in typhoid fever (for which it is the antibiotic of choice) and other infections caused by *Salmonellae*, and in rickettsial infections. Trade names are Chloromycetin and Chloroptic. SEE: *gray syndrome of the newborn.*

Caution: Certain blood dyscrasias may follow the use of chloramphenicol, esp. in neonates; consequently it should not be used indiscriminately or for minor infections. If used for prolonged periods, careful blood checks should be made. Be sure to read the literature that comes with each package of this medicine prior to deciding to use it rather than another antibiotic.

chlorate (klō′rāt). A salt of chloric acid. SEE: *potassium chlorate; Poisons and Poisoning* in *Appendix*.

chlorbutanol. Chlorobutanol, q.v.

chlorbutol. Chlorobutanol, q.v.

chlorcyclizine hydrochloride. Official name for the hydrochloride of 1-(*p*-chloro-α-phenylbenzyl)-4-methylpiperazine, an antihistamine. Trade name is Perazil.

chlordane (klor′dān). A poisonous substance used as an insecticide. SEE: *Poisons and Poisoning* in *Appendix*.

chlordiazepoxide hydrochloride (klor″dī-ăz″ĕ-pŏk′sīd). USP. A benzodiazepine derivative used in treating anxiety, alcohol withdrawal syndrome, and as a premedication in anesthesia. Trade names are A-poxide, Chlordiazachel, Librium, and Murcil.

chloremia (klō-rē′mē-ă) [Gr. *chloros,* green, + *haima,* blood]. Increased chloride in the blood.

chlorhexidene gluconate (klor-hĕk′sĭ-dēn). A topical anti-infective agent. Trade name is Hibiclens.

chlorhydria (klor-hī′drē-ă) [″ + *hydor,* water]. Excess of hydrochloric acid in the stomach.

chloride (klō′rīd) [Gr. *chloros,* green]. A binary compound of chlorine; a salt of hydrochloric acid. Blood serum contains 100 to 110 mEq/L (350 to 390 mg/dl), principally as sodium chloride. Chloride levels are elevated in nephritis, eclampsia, anemia, and cardiac disease; decreased in fevers, diabetes, and pneumonia.

chloridemia (klō″rĭ-dē′mē-ă) [″ + *haima,* blood]. Chlorides in the blood.

chloride poisoning. SEE: *barium salts* in *Poisons and Poisoning* in *Appendix*.

chloridimeter (klor-ĭ-dim′ĕ-tur). An instrument for determining the amount of chloride in a body fluid.

chloriduria (klō″rĭ-dū′rē-ă) [″ + *ouron,* urine]. Excess of chlorides in urine.

chlorinated (klō′rĭn-ā-tĕd). Impregnated with chlorine.

chlorinated lime. Calcium hypochlorite and calcium chloride; widely used in solution as a bleach and as an antiseptic.

chlorination (klō″rĭ-nā′shŭn). Treatment of water by addition of chlorine and its compounds for the killing of bacteria. For effective disinfection, a concentration of 0.5 to 1 part of chlorine per million parts of water is necessary.

chlorine (klō′rēn) [Gr. *chloros,* green]. SYMB: Cl. At. wt. 35.453; at. no. 17. A highly irritat-

ing gas destructive to the mucous membranes of the respiratory passages. It is very poisonous and excessive inhalation may cause death. Chlorine is an active bleaching agent and germicide. Both of these effects are due to its oxidizing powers. It is used extensively in the disinfection of water supplies and in treatment of sewage.

FUNCT: Chlorine is found combined with sodium in the blood and exercises some influence upon metabolism, helps to maintain osmotic pressure, and aids in the regulation and stimulation of muscular action. The body fluids contain 0.85% salt concentration. The inorganic salts keep in solution proteins of the blood, milk, and other secretions. Chlorine is present in the hydrochloric acid of the gastric juice. It aids digestion, activates enzymes, and is essential to normal gastric secretion.

chlorine preparations. Preparations used for disinfecting. Compounds (hypochlorites) such as Dakin's solution or Javelle water are very effective as germicides. As a disinfecting agent in washing dishes and utensils used by infected patients, 1/10 of 1% solution should be used; the dishes should then be washed well in soap and hot water and rinsed well, or boiled and then washed well.

For disinfection of the stools of patients, 5% or even stronger solutions may be used for ½ hour or longer. The covered container is set aside while the solution acts. Dakin's solution is nonirritating and is used as a wound disinfectant, but it must be carefully prepared daily and used only when fresh.

chlorite (klō′rīt). A salt of chlorous acid; used as a disinfectant and bleaching agent.

chlorobutanol (klō-rō-bū′tă-nŏl). Colorless crystals with camphor odor and taste. SYN: *chlorbutanol; chlorbutol.*

USES: Antiseptic and local anesthetic used in dentistry, and as a preservative in many pharmaceuticals.

INCOMPAT: Decomposed by alkalies and should not be mixed with borax or carbonates. Soluble in ether, chloroform, and volatile oils.

chloroform (klō′rō-form) [Gr. *chloros,* green, + L. *forma,* form]. CHCl₃. A heavy, clear, colorless liquid with strong etherlike odor, formed by the action of chlorinated lime on methyl alcohol. At one time chloroform was administered by inhalation to produce anesthesia, but this usage is obsolete.

chloroformism (klō′rō-form″ĭzm). The habit of inhaling chloroform for pleasure.

chloroleukemia (klō″rō-loo-kē′mē-ă) [″ + *leukos,* white, + *haima,* blood]. Leukemia with chlorosis.

chloroma (klō-rō′mă) [″ + *oma,* growth]. A

greenish sarcoma of the periosteum of cranial bones; green cancer.

Chloromycetin (klō″rō-mī-sē′tĭn). Trade name for chloramphenicol, USP, q.v.

chloropenia (klō″rō-pē′nē-ă) [″ + *penia*, poverty]. Deficiency in chlorine. SYN: *hypochloremia.*

chloropenic (klō″rō-pēn′ĭk). Deficient in chlorine.

chlorophane (klō′rō-fān) [″ + *phainein*, to show]. A green-yellow pigment in the retina.

chlorophenothane (klō″rō-fĕn′ō-thān). An insecticide, better known as DDT, q.v., that is quite effective but should not be used because of its toxicity to various animals.

chlorophyll, chlorophyl (klō′rō-fĭl) [″ + *phyllon*, leaf]. The green pigment in plants that accomplishes photosynthesis. Essential in the utilization of that energy is combining carbon dioxide (CO_2) and carbohydrate according to the following scheme: 6 $CO_2 + 6 H_2O + light \rightarrow C_6H_{12}O_6 + 6 O_2$. Thus, the primary source of energy in our planet is the light absorbed by chlorophyll. Four forms of chlorophyll (a, b, c, and d) occur in nature.

chloropia, chloropsia (klō-rō′pē-ă, klō-rŏp′sē-ă) [″ + *opsis*, vision]. Viewed objects have a green hue. A sign of digitalis toxicity.

chloroplast, chloroplastid (klō′rō-plăst, klō″rō-plăs′tĭd) [″ + *plastos*, formed]. Small, round, green bodies found in the cells of leaves and stems of plants that are important in the process of photosynthesis. They possess a stroma and contain four pigments: chlorophyll a, chlorophyll b, carotene, and xanthophyll.

chloroprivic (klō″rō-prĭv′ĭk) [″ + L. *privare*, to deprive of]. Lack of, or due to loss of, chlorides.

chloroprocaine hydrochloride (klō″rō-prō′kān). USP. A local anesthetic more potent and less toxic than procaine. Trade name is Nesacaine.

chloroquine hydrochloride (klō′rō-kwĭn). USP. $C_{18}H_{26}ClN_3 \cdot 2HCl$. A white crystalline powder used for its antimicrobial action, esp. in the treatment of malaria. It is useful also in amebic dysentery complicated by liver abscess and in treating lupus erythematosus. Trade name for chloroquine phosphate, USP, is Aralen Phosphate; trade name for chloroquine hydrochloride, USP, is Aralen Hydrochloride.

chlorosis (klō-rō′sĭs) [″ + *osis*, condition]. A form of iron-deficiency anemia. SEE: *anemia, iron-deficiency.*

chlorothiazide sodium (klō″rō-thī′ă-zīd). USP. An effective diuretic. Administered orally. Trade name is Sodium Diuril.

chlorotic (klō-rŏt′ĭk). Of the nature of or afflicted with chlorosis.

chlorotrianisene (klō″rō-trī-ăn′ĭ-sēn). USP. $C_{23}H_{21}ClO_3$. A synthetic estrogen that is about one-eighth as potent as diethylstilbestrol. It is little used because it accumulates in fat tissue. Trade name is TACE.

chlorpheniramine maleate (klor″fĕn-ĭr′ă-mēn). USP. An antihistamine that may be used orally or by injection. It is available under a number of trade names, including Chlor-Trimeton and Teldran.

chlorphenoxamine hydrochloride (klor″fĕn-ŏk′să-mēn). USP. Drug used in treating parkinsonism. Trade name is Phenoxene.

chlorpromazine (klor-prō′mă-zēn). USP. A tranquilizing agent, it is used primarily in its hydrochloride form in major and minor psychotic states. Trade name for chlorpromazine hydrochloride is Thorazine.

chlorpromazine poisoning. SEE: *Poisons and Poisoning* in *Appendix.*

chlorpropamide (klor-prō′pă-mĭd). USP. An oral hypoglycemic agent of the sulfonylurea class. Trade name is Diabinese.

Caution: This drug should be used only in patients with diabetes of the insulin-independent type who, if weight reduction and dietary control fail, cannot be treated with diet alone and who are unwilling or unable to take insulin.

chlorprothixene (klor-prō-thĭks′ēn). USP. Drug used in treating mental illness. Trade name is Taractan.

chlortetracycline hydrochloride (klor″tĕt-ră-sī′klēn). USP. A golden-colored antibiotic isolated from a strain of *Streptomyces aureofaciens.* It is a broad-spectrum antibiotic, inhibiting growth of or destroying some strains of streptococci, staphylococci, pneumococci, rickettsiae, and viruses. Trade name is Aureomycin.

chlorthalidone (klor-thăl′ĭ-dōn). USP. An effective diuretic. Trade name is Hygroton.

Chlor-Trimeton. Trade name for chlorpheniramine maleate.

chlorzoxazone (klor-zŏk′să-zōn). A muscle relaxant. Trade name is Paraflex.

Ch.M. *chirurgiae magister*, Master of Surgery.

choana (kō′ă-nă) [Gr. *choane*, funnel] (pl. *choanae*). A funnel-shaped opening, esp. one of the posterior nares, the communicating passageways between the nasal fossae and the pharynx.

choanoid (kō′ăn-oyd) [″ + *eidos*, form, shape]. Shaped like a funnel.

choke [ME. *choken*]. To prevent respiration by compression or obstruction of the larynx or trachea.

choked disk. Edema of the optic disk. SEE: *papilledema.*

chokes. Respiratory symptoms such as substernal distress, paroxysmal cough, tachypnea, or asphyxia, which may occur in decompression illness, esp. in cases of aeroembolism resulting from exposure to pressure lower than atmospheric. SEE: *caisson disease.*

choke-saver. Commercial name for a curved tweezer-like forceps, usually made of plastic, for inserting into the throat of a person choking. The device is used to grasp and remove the food from the obstructed airway. SEE: *Heimlich maneuver.*

choking [ME. *choken*, to suffocate]. Obstruction within respiratory passage or constriction about the neck, interfering with breathing and circulation of brain. May also result from spasm of the larynx induced by an irritating gas. SEE: *Emergency Measures* for *choking on food; Heimlich maneuver.*

SYM: Face purple; eyes protrude; arms thrown about; coughing; constriction and injury about neck; cyanosis; dizziness; unconsciousness.

choking on food. Inadequately chewed food may be inhaled inadvertently. The most commonly involved is a piece of meat or other solid food. The usual result is panic accompanied by inability to speak, cyanosis, and fainting. Lay persons in the vicinity may assume the patient is having a heart attack.

EMERGENCY MEASURES: For complete airway obstruction, evidenced by inability to speak, using the fingers or curved forceps, reach into the throat, dislodge the obstruction, and remove it. It may be possible to forcibly eject the food by quickly and forcibly compressing the abdomen and lower chest (the Heimlich maneuver). This maneuver consists of (1) wrapping your arms around the victim's waist from behind; (2) making a fist with one hand and placing it against the victim's abdomen between the navel and rib cage; (3) clasping your fist with your free hand and pressing in with a quick forceful upward thrust. Repeat several times if necessary. This will produce sudden air pressure on the object. If an object is lodged in the throat and breathing is possible, interference should be limited until professional aid is available. Emergency cricothyroidotomy may be needed. SEE: *Heimlich maneuver.*

cholagogue (kō′lă-gŏg) [Gr. *chole*, bile, + *agein*, to lead forth]. An agent that increases the flow of bile into the intestine, i.e., a choleretic, or cholecystagogue.

Cholan-DH. Trade name for dehydrocholic acid.

cholangiectasis (kō-lăn″jē-ĕk′tă-sĭs) [″ + *angeion*, vessel, + *ektasis*, dilatation]. Dilation of bile ducts.

cholangiocarcinoma (kō-lăn″jē-ō-kăr″sĭ-nō′mă) [″ + ″ + *karkinos*, crab, + *oma*, tumor]. Malignancy of the bile ducts.

cholangioenterostomy (kō-lăn″jē-ō-ĕn″tĕr-ŏs′tō-mē) [″ + ″ + *enteron*, intestine, + *stoma*, mouth]. Surgically produced communication between a bile duct and the intestine.

cholangiogastrostomy (kō-lăn″jē-ō-găs-trŏs′tō-mē) [″ + ″ + *gaster*, stomach, + *stoma*, mouth]. Surgical formation of a communication between a bile duct and the stomach.

cholangiography (kō-lăn″jē-ŏg′ră-fē) [″ + ″ + *graphein*, to write]. Radiographic examination of the bile ducts.

cholangiole (kō-lăn′jē-ōl) [″ + ″ + *ole*, dim. suffix]. The small terminal portion of the bile duct.

cholangiolitis (kō-lăn″jē-ō-lī′tĭs) [″ + ″ + ″ + Gr. *itis*, inflammation]. Inflammation of the bile ducts. This occurs in various forms of hepatitis.

cholangioma (kō-lăn-jē-ō′mă) [″ + *angeion*, vessel, + *oma*, tumor]. A tumor of the bile ducts.

cholangiostomy (kō″lăn-jē-ŏs′tō-mē) [″ + ″ + *stoma*, mouth]. Surgical formation of a fistula into the gallbladder.

cholangiotomy (kō″lăn-jē-ŏt′ō-mē) [″ + ″ + *tome*, incision]. Incision of an intrahepatic bile duct for removal of gallstones.

cholangitis (kō″lăn-jī′tĭs) [″ + *angeion*, vessel, + *itis*, inflammation]. Inflammation of the bile ducts.

cholanopoiesis (kō″lă-nō-poy-ē′sĭs) [Gr. *chole*, bile, + *ano*, upward, + *poiesis*, making]. Synthesis of cholic acid in the liver.

cholate (kō′lāt). Any salt or ester of cholic acid.

cholecalciferol (ko″lē-kăl-sĭf′ĕr-ōl). USP. Vitamin D_3; an antirachitic, oil-soluble vitamin occurring as white, odorless crystals.

cholecyst (kō′lē-sĭst) [″ + *kystis*, bladder]. The gallbladder.

cholecystagogue (kō″lē-sĭs′tă-gŏg) [″ + ″ + *agogos*, leader]. Drug or action that causes emptying of the gallbladder.

cholecystalgia (kō″lē-sĭs-tăl′jē-ă) [″ + ″ + *algos*, pain]. Biliary colic.

cholecystangiography (kō″lē-sĭs″tăn-jē-ŏg′ră-fē) [″ + ″ + *angeion*, vessel, + *graphein*, to write]. Radiographic examination of the gallbladder and bile ducts after injection of a contrast medium.

cholecystectasia (kō″lē-sĭs-tĕk-tā′zē-ă) [″ + ″ + *ektasis*, dilatation]. Dilatation of the gallbladder.

cholecystectomy (kō″lē-sĭs-tĕk′tō-mē) [″ + ″ + *ektome*, excision]. Excision of a gallbladder.

NURSING IMPLICATIONS: *Preop:* Prepare patient for surgery physically and psychologically and for possible postoperative discomfort. Teach the patient about pain assessment and management, expected postoperative therapies and restrictions, and deep-breathing, coughing, and mobility exercises and techniques.

Postop: Monitor vital signs every 2 to 4 hours; assess dressing and any wound or nasogastric drainage tubes, noting patency, character, and volume of drainage. Place patient in semi-Fowler's position to facilitate drainage. Assess pain and G.I. and urinary function. Administer prescribed analgesics and antiemetics as required, and encourage voiding. Monitor fluid and electrolyte balance, and administer prescribed fluid therapy and electrolyte therapy. Encourage deep breathing, coughing, and early ambulation. Assess peripheral circulation and promote venous return, using leg exercises and elastic stockings or pneumatic leg dressings as prescribed. Assess skin and sclerae for jaundice. Provide discharge teaching to patient and family regarding return appointment date and time, wound care, restrictions on operating a motor vehicle and avoidance of heavy lifting or straining for prescribed period. Explain the importance of daily exercise, such as walking. Explain that diet is not restricted; however, patient may be more comfortable limiting intake of fats and gas-forming foods. SEE: *Nursing Diagnoses* in *Appendix.*

c., laparoscopic. Surgical removal of the gallbladder by use of lights, video monitors, scissors, and other instruments inserted in the abdominal cavity through small incisions in the abdominal wall. Use of this technique minimizes the time spent in the hospital and recovery period. The abdominal scars are minimal.

cholecystenterorrhaphy (kō″lē-sĭs-tĕn″tĕr-or′ă-fē) [″ + ″ + *enteron,* intestine, + *rhaphe,* seam, ridge]. Suture of gallbladder to intestinal wall.

cholecystenterostomy (kō″lē-sĭs-tĕn″tĕr-ŏs′tō-mē) [″ + ″ + *enteron,* intestine, + *stoma,* mouth]. Surgical establishment of a connection between the gallbladder and the small intestine.

cholecystic (kō″lē-sĭs′tĭk). Pert. to the gallbladder.

cholecystitis (kō″lē-sĭs-tī′tĭs) [Gr. *chole,* bile, + *kystis,* bladder, + *itis,* inflammation]. Inflammation of the gallbladder.

SYM: In acute cholecystitis there is fever, gradually developing or sudden pain in upper abdomen, nausea, vomiting, visible but mild jaundice in about 20% of patients. Frequently pain is referred to back or right shoulder. Approx. 10% of patients do not have pain.

ETIOL: Acute cholecystitis is caused by the chemical irritation due to obstruction of the cystic duct preventing the outflow of bile from the gallbladder. However, not all patients with gallstones experience cholecystitis.

TREAT: In acute cholecystitis, cholecystectomy; if this is not possible, draining of gallbladder (cholecystostomy) followed by cholecystectomy at a later date.

NURSING IMPLICATIONS: Assess patient for nausea, vomiting, increased pulse and respiratory rate, flatulence, right upper quadrant pain, and food intolerance. Withhold oral fluids and maintain I.V. therapy during acute episode. Provide for patient comfort and administer ordered medicines for pain relief. If surgery is to be performed, prepare the patient physically and emotionally. Nutrition education includes instructions on the advisability of losing weight if the patient is obese.

cholecystnephrostomy (kō″lē-sĭst″nē-frŏs′tō-mē) [″ + *kystis,* bladder, + *nephros,* kidney, + *stoma,* mouth]. Making a surgical anastomosis of the gallbladder into the renal pelvis.

cholecystocolostomy (kō″lē-sĭs″tō-kō-lŏs′tō-mē) [″ + ″ + *kolon,* colon, + *stoma,* mouth]. Making a surgical passage from the gallbladder to colon.

cholecystocolotomy (kō″lē-sĭs″tō-kō-lŏt′ō-mē) [″ + ″ + ″ + *tome,* incision]. Surgical incision into the gallbladder and colon.

cholecystoduodenostomy (kō″lē-sĭs″tō-dū″ō-dē-nŏs′tō-mē) [″ + ″ + L. *duodeni,* twelve, + Gr. *stoma,* mouth]. Surgical formation of a passage from the gallbladder to duodenum.

cholecystogastrostomy (kō″lē-sĭs″tō-găs-trŏs′tō-mē [″ + ″ + *gaster,* belly, + *stoma,* mouth]. Surgical formation of a passage from the gallbladder to the stomach.

cholecystogram (kō″lē-sĭs′tō-grăm) [″ + ″ + *gramma,* something written]. A radiographic picture of the gallbladder.

cholecystography (kō″lē-sĭs-tŏg′ră-fē) [″ + ″ + *graphein,* to write]. Examination of the gallbladder by radiographic study.

cholecystoileostomy (kō″lē-sĭs″tō-īl-ē-ŏs′tō-mē) [″ + *kystis,* bladder, + L. *ileum,* ileum, + Gr. *stoma,* mouth]. Forming a communication between the gallbladder and ileum.

cholecystojejunostomy (kō″lē-sĭs″tō-jĕ-jū-nŏs′tō-mē) [″ + ″ + L. *jejunum,* empty, + Gr. *stoma,* mouth]. Forming a communication between the gallbladder and jejunum.

cholecystokinin-pancreozymin. A hormone secreted into the blood by the mucosa of the upper small intestine. It stimulates gallbladder contraction and secretion of pancreatic enzymes. SEE: *Zollinger-Ellison syndrome.*

cholecystolithiasis (kō″lē-sĭs″tō-lĭ-thī′ă-sĭs) [″ + ″ + *lithos,* stone, + *-iasis,* condition]. Gallstones in the gallbladder.

cholecystolithotripsy (kō″lē-sĭs″tō-lĭth′ō-trĭp″sē) [″ + ″ + ″ + *tripsis,* a rubbing]. Crushing of a gallstone in the unopened gallbladder.

cholecystomy (kō″lē-sĭs′tō-mē) [Gr. *chole,* bile, + *kystis,* bladder, + *tome,* incision]. Cholecystotomy.

cholecystopathy (kō″lē-sĭs-tŏp′ă-thē) [″ + ″ + *pathos,* disease, suffering]. Any gallbladder affection.

cholecystopexy (kō″lē-sĭs′tō-pĕk″sē) [″ + ″ + *pexis,* fixation]. Suturing the gallbladder to the abdominal wall.

cholecystoptosis (kō″lē-sĭs-tō-tō′sĭs) [″ + ″ + *ptosis,* a dropping]. Downward displacement of the gallbladder.

cholecystorrhaphy (kō″lē-sĭs-tor′ă-fē) [″ + *kystis,* bladder, + *rhaphe,* seam, ridge]. Suturing of the gallbladder.

cholecystostomy (kō″lē-sĭs-tŏs′tō-mē) [″ + ″ + *stoma,* mouth]. Surgical formation of an opening into the gallbladder through the abdominal wall.

cholecystotomy (kō″lē-sĭs-tŏt′ō-mē) [″ + ″ + *tome,* incision]. Incision of the gallbladder through the abdominal wall for removal of gallstones.

choledochal (kō-lē-dŏk′ăl) [″ + *dochos,* receptacle]. Rel. or pert. to the common bile duct.

choledochectasia (kō-lĕd″ō-kĕk-tā′zē-ă) [″ + ″ + *ektasis,* distention]. Distention of the common bile duct.

choledochectomy (kō-lĕd″ō-kĕk′tō-mē) [″ + ″ + *ektome,* excision]. Excision of a portion of the common bile duct.

choledochitis (kō″lē-dō-kī′tĭs) [″ + ″ + *itis,* inflammation]. Inflammation of the common bile duct.

choledochoduodenostomy (kō-lĕd″ō-kō-dū-ō-dē-nŏs′tō-mē) [″ + ″ + L. *duodeni,* twelve, + Gr. *stoma,* mouth]. Surgical communication between the common bile duct and duodenum.

choledochoenterostomy (kō-lĕd″ō-kō-ĕn-tĕr-ŏs′tō-mē) [″ + ″ + *enteron,* intestine, + *stoma,* mouth]. Surgical passage between the common bile duct and intestine.

choledochography (kō-lĕd″ō-kŏg′ră-fē) [″ + *dochos,* receptacle, + *graphein,* to write]. X-ray examination of the bile duct following administration of a radiopaque substance.

choledochojejunostomy (kō-lĕd″ō-kō-jē-jū-nŏs′tō-mē) [″ + ″ + L. *jejunum,* empty, + Gr. *stoma,* mouth]. Surgical joining of the common bile duct to the jejunum of the small intestine.

choledocholith (kō-lĕd′ō-kō-lĭth″) [″ + ″ + *lithos,* stone]. Calculus, or stone, in the common bile duct.

choledocholithiasis (kō-lĕd″ō-kō-lĭ-thī′ă-sĭs) [″ + ″ + *lithos,* stone, + *-iasis,* condition]. Calculi in the common bile duct.

choledocholithotomy (kō-lĕd″ō-kō-lĭth-ŏt′ō-mē) [″ + ″ + ″ + *tome,* incision]. Removal of a gallstone through an incision of the bile duct.

choledocholithotripsy (kō-lĕd′ō-kō-lĭth″ō-trĭp-sē) [″ + ″ + ″ + *tripsis,* a crushing]. Crushing of a gallstone in the common bile duct.

choledochoplasty (kō-lĕd′ō-kō-plăs″tē) [Gr. *chole,* bile, + *dochos,* receptacle, + *plassein,* to form]. Operation for repair of the common bile duct.

choledochorrhaphy (kō-lĕd″ō-kor′ă-fē) [″ + ″ + *rhaphe,* seam, ridge]. Suturing the severed ends of the common bile duct.

choledochostomy (kō-lĕd″ō-kŏs′tō-mē) [″ + ″ + *stoma,* mouth]. Surgical formation of an opening into the common bile duct through the abdominal wall.

choledochotomy (kō″lĕd-ō-kŏt′ō-mē) [″ + ″ + *tome,* incision]. Surgical incision of the common bile duct.

choledochus (kō-lĕd′ō-kŭs) [″ + *dochos,* receptacle]. The common bile duct. SYN: *ductus choledochus* [NA].

choleic (kō-lē′ĭk). Cholic; pert. to the bile.

cholelith (kō′lē-lĭth) [″ + *lithos,* stone]. A biliary concretion of gallstone.

cholelithiasis (kō″lē-lĭ-thī′ă-sĭs) [″ + ″ + *-iasis,* condition]. Formation or presence of calculi or bilestones in the gallbladder or common duct. The stones may or may not cause symptoms. SEE: *Nursing Diagnoses* in *Appendix.*

SYM: Digestive disturbances; heaviness in right hypochondrium; tenderness on pressure over gallbladder. Gallstone colic when a stone obstructs the bile duct. Pain may radiate to back and right shoulder. Colic usually manifest when stomach is empty. Jaundice if flow of bile is obstructed. Pain may be associated with vomiting and sweating. If distended, the gallbladder is palpable.

TREAT: Cholecystectomy; in very poor-risk patients, cholecystostomy. Lithotripsy has been used to disintegrate stones so that they are small enough to pass.

cholelithic (kō″lē-lĭth′ĭk). Pert. to or caused by biliary calculus.

cholelithotomy (kō″lē-lĭ-thŏt′ō-mē) [″ + *lithos,* stone, + *tome,* incision]. Removal of gallstones through a surgical incision.

cholelithotripsy, cholelithotrity (kō″lē-lĭth′ō-trĭp-sē, kō″lē-lĭ-thŏt′rĭ-tē) [″ + ″ + *tripsis,* a crushing]. Crushing of a biliary calculus.

cholemesis (kō-lĕm′ĕ-sĭs) [″ + *emein,* to vomit]. Bile in the vomitus.

cholemia (kō-lē′mē-ă) [″ + *haima,* blood]. Bile or its pigments in the blood.

cholepathia (kō″lē-păth′ē-ă) [″ + *pathos,* disease]. Disease of the bile duct.

    c. spastica. Spasmodic contraction of biliary ducts.

choleperitoneum (kō″lē-pĕr″ĭ-tō-nē′ŭm) [″ + *peri,* around, + *teinein,* to stretch]. Bile in the peritoneum.

cholepoiesis (kō″lē-poy-ē′sĭs) [″ + *poiein,* to make]. The formation of bile.

cholera (kŏl′ĕr-ă) [L. *cholera,* bilious diarrhea]. An acute infection involving the entire small bowel, characterized by profuse watery diarrhea and vomiting, which produces severe loss of fluids and electrolytes, muscular cramps, oliguria, dehydration, and collapse. SYN: *Asiatic cholera.*

    SYM: Four stages are usually described as follows:

    Invasion: At the conclusion of the incubation period there is malaise, headache, diarrhea, and anorexia. Headache and slight fever are present. May last a few days and then subside. This is termed the cholerine stage. Sometimes this stage is missing entirely.

    Evacuation: Purging, violent vomiting, and muscular cramps. Stools loose, copious, and watery, and the flecks of mucus present a typical rice-water appearance. Sometimes there are particles of blood and mucus. Vomiting is severe and persistent; the material expelled may also resemble rice water. Muscular cramps commonly start in extremities; involve calves of legs; and later even arms, hands, feet, and trunk. Thirst is unquenchable, and hiccough sometimes develops. Signs of physical depression soon terminate in collapse. Duration of this stage is 2 to 12 hours, seldom more.

    Stage of Collapse: Almost complete arrest of circulation; eyes sunken; cheeks hollow; nose pinched; skin dry and wrinkled; body surface cold and covered with clammy sweat; breath cool; temperature in axilla 85° to 95°F (29.4° to 35°C), while in the rectum it may be 103°F (39.4°C) or more. Respirations quickened, pulse weak, systolic blood pressure decreased; urine output diminished or absent; diarrhea and cramps may continue. The mind usually is clear until shortly prior to death, when coma develops.

Stage lasts from few hours to one or two days, and generally ends in death. Cause of death is dehydration and electrolyte imbalance.

    Stage of Reaction: Sometimes, even when death seems imminent, surface temperature begins to rise, vomiting ceases, bowel evacuations become less frequent and more feculent, and convalescence follows. Complete recovery may ensue in from one to two weeks. Occasionally, typhoid symptoms set in, temperature goes to 106° to 107°F (41.1° to 41.7°C), and outcome is fatal. Sometimes in this stage, an erythemal eruption or one of the urticarial type appears, particularly on extremities. Such eruptions have no special significance.

    ETIOL: Causative organism *Vibrio cholerae* (also called *Vibrio comma,* cholera bacillus, comma bacillus, Koch's bacillus), which is a short, curved, motile, gram-negative rod producing a potent endotoxin that interferes with cellular metabolism. It is a mucolytic enzyme. Transmission is through water, milk, or other foods contaminated with excreta of patients or carriers.

    INCUB: A few hours to four to five days.

    TREAT: Vigorous replacement of fluid and electrolytes by intravenous administration of a 2-to-1 mixture of normal saline and ⅙ molar sodium lactate. If patient is in shock, give 100 ml/kg of body weight and less if shock is not present. The fluid should be given rapidly until blood pressure returns to normal. Children will require additional potassium. Fluids also should be given *ad lib* by mouth. Tetracycline given early in the disease is effective in killing the causative organism.

    PROPH: Cholera vaccine. Following the initial two or three injections, booster doses should be administered every six months if the person remains in an endemic area. If traveling in an area where cholera exists, do not drink unboiled or untreated water, do not add ice to beverages, do not eat raw or partially cooked fish or shellfish, do not eat uncooked vegetables or fruits you have not peeled yourself, do not assume bottled water is safe, and swim only in chlorinated swimming pools. Seek medical attention immediately if diarrhea or a febrile illness develops.

    c. sicca. A term sometimes applied to a fulminating variety of cholera that occurs without vomiting or diarrhea.

choleragen (kŏl′ĕr-ă-gĕn). The potent enterotoxin produced by *Vibrio cholerae.* It acts on the mucosal cells of the small bowel to cause increased secretion of chloride and bicarbonate into the intestine.

choleresis (kŏl-ĕr-ē′sĭs, kō-lĕr′ĕ-sĭs) [Gr.

chole, bile, + *hairesis,* removal]. The secretion of bile by the liver.

choleretic (kŏl-ĕr-ĕt′ĭk). 1. Stimulating excretion of bile by the liver. 2. Any agent that increases excretion of bile by the liver.

choleric (kŏl′ĕr-ĭk). Irritable; quick-tempered without apparent cause.

choleriform (kŏl-ĕr′ĭ-form) [L. *cholera,* + *forma,* shape]. Resembling cholera.

cholerigenous, cholerigenic (kŏl-ĕr-ĭj′ĕn-ŭs, kŏl″ĕr-ĭ-jĕn′ĭk) [″ + Gr. *gennan,* to produce]. Giving rise to cholera.

cholerine (kŏl′ĕr-ĭn). A mild form or initial stages of Asiatic cholera.

choleroid (kŏl′ĕr-oyd) [″ + Gr. *eidos,* form, shape]. Resembling cholera.

choleromania (kŏl″ĕr-ō-mā′nē-ă) [″ + Gr. *mania,* madness]. Madness occasionally seen in cholera.

cholerophobia (kŏl″ĕr-ō-fō′bē-ă) [″ + Gr. *phobos,* fear]. Morbid fear of acquiring cholera.

cholestasia (kō″lē-stā′zē-ă) [Gr. *chole,* bile, + *stasis,* stoppage]. Arrest of the bile excretion.

cholestatic. Pert. to or caused by cholestasia.

cholesteatoma (kō″lē-stē″ă-tō′mă) [″ + *steatos,* fat, + *oma,* tumor]. An epithelial pocket or cystlike sac filled with keratin debris. Can occur in the meninges, central nervous system, and bones of skull, but is most common in the middle ear and mastoid area. The cystic process, which is filled with a combination of epithelial cells and cholesterol, most commonly enlarges to occlude the middle ear. Enzymes formed within the sac cause erosion of adjacent bones, including the ossicles, and destroy them. Cholesteatomas are divided into congenital, primary acquired, and secondary acquired.

cholesteremia, cholesterolemia (kō-lĕs″tĕ-rē′mē-ă, kō-lĕs″tĕr-ōl-ē′mē-ă) [″ + *stereos,* solid, + *haima,* blood]. The presence of excess cholesterol in the blood. SYN: *hypercholesterolemia.*

cholesterin (kō-lĕs′tĕr-ĭn). Cholesterol, q.v.

cholesterinemia (kō-lĕs″tĕr-ĭn-ē′mē-ă). Cholesteremia.

cholesterinuria (kō-lĕs″tĕr-ĭn-ū′rē-ă) [″ + *stereos,* solid, + *ouron,* urine]. Presence of cholesterol in the urine.

cholesterohydrothorax (kō-lĕs″tĕr-ō-hī″drō-thō′răks) [″ + ″ + *hydor,* water, + *thorax,* chest]. An effusion in the pleural cavity of fluid that contains cholesterol.

cholesterol (kō-lĕs′tĕr-ŏl) [″ + *stereos,* solid]. $C_{27}H_{45}OH$. A monohydric alcohol. A sterol widely distributed in animal tissues and occurring in the yolk of eggs, various oils, fats, nerve tissue of the brain and spinal cord, the liver, kidneys, and adrenal glands.

It can be synthesized in the liver and is a normal constituent of bile. It is the principal constituent of most gallstones. It is important in metabolism, serving as a precursor of various steroid hormones, e.g., sex hormones, adrenal corticoids.

In most individuals an elevated blood level of cholesterol constitutes an increased risk of developing coronary heart disease (CHD). Scientific evidence has established that lowering definitely elevated blood cholesterol (specifically, blood levels of low density lipoprotein cholesterol) will reduce the risk of heart attacks due to CHD.

Risk categories and recommended actions are included in the accompanying table.

Age	Moderate Risk	High Risk
20–29	>200 mg/dl	>220 mg/dl
30–39	>220 mg/dl	>240 mg/dl
≥40	>240 mg/dl	>260 mg/dl

Cholesterol levels may be decreased by several factors, including: diet, e.g., decrease total fat in diet, decrease percent of fat in diet derived from cholesterol and saturated fats; avoid smoking; avoid anabolic steroids.

Drugs used for control of cholesterol include lovastatin, niacin, gemfibrozil, clofibrate, probucol, and bile-acid resins (cholestyramine, colestipol).

If the recommendations are followed, in the U.S. an estimated 20% to 25% of adults will need treatment. SEE: tables; *coronary heart disease; heart disease, ischemic.*

cholesteroluria (kō-lĕs″tĕr-ŏl-ū′rē-ă) [″ + ″ + *ouron,* urine]. Presence of cholesterol in urine.

cholesterosis (kō-lĕs-tĕr-ō′sĭs) [″ + ″ + *osis,* condition]. Cholesterol deposition in excessive amounts.

cholestyramine resin (kō″lē-stī′ră-mĭn). USP. An ion-exchange resin used to treat itching associated with jaundice. It acts by lowering the level of bile acids in the serum. Trade name is Questran.

choletelin (kō-lĕt′ĕl-ĭn) [″ + *telos,* end]. Yellow pigment that is the oxidation product of bilirubin.

choletherapy (kō″lē-thĕr′ă-pē) [″ + *therapeia,* treatment]. Use of bile salts as a medicine.

choleuria (kō″lē-ū′rē-ă) [″ + *ouron,* urine]. Bile in urine.

choleverdin (kō″lē-vĕr′dĭn) [″ + L. *viridis,* green]. Green pigment appearing in gallstones and in urine in jaundice. SYN: *biliverdin.*

cholic acid (kō′lĭk). The sodium salt of conjugated taurocholic or glycocholic acid.

choline (kō′lĭn, -lēn) [Gr. *chole,* bile].

Major Contributors of Saturated Fatty Acids (SFA) in the American Diet

Ranked* Food Items	% Dietary SFA Calories†	Average Daily Calories Now‡
1. Hamburgers, cheeseburgers, meatloaf	9.3	26
2. Whole milk, whole-milk beverages	9.1	25
3. Cheeses (excluding cottage cheese)	7.3	20
4. Beef steaks, roasts	7.3	20
5. Hot dogs, ham, luncheon meats	7.0	20
6. Doughnuts, cookies, cake	4.8	13
7. Eggs	4.5	13
8. Pork (includes chops, roasts)	4.0	11
9. Butter	3.7	10
10. White bread, rolls, crackers, etc.	3.2	9
Total	60.2%	167 cal

Source: Reprinted with permission from Dr. W. Virgil Brown and *Cholesterol and Coronary Disease . . . Reducing the Risk,* Vol 1, No 5, p 4., June 1987.
* Ten food groups, in rank order, found to contribute the most saturated fatty acid to the diet (National Health and Nutrition Examination Survey II, 1976–1980). These ten items make up over 60% of saturated fatty acids for the average American.
† Percentage of total SFA provided by each group.
‡ SFA calories from each group, assuming an intake of 2,000 kcal/day with 14% of calories (280) from SFA.

Specific Steps to Reduce Saturated Fatty Acid*

1. Select lean cuts of meat, trim visible fat, and broil or grill.
2. Reduce daily portions of meat.
3. Reduce consumption of processed meats (e.g., hot dogs, luncheon meat, sausage).
4. Remove skin from poultry before cooking.
5. Use skimmed milk or 1% low-fat milk and dairy products made from skimmed milk.
6. Eliminate butter and substitute vegetable-oil margarine.
7. Reduce consumption of fatty cheeses; find low-fat substitutes.
8. Reduce consumption of egg yolks; use substitutes with little saturated fat.
9. Avoid foods containing coconut and palm oil; read labels.
10. Choose fish as a substitute for poultry or lean meat.

Source: Reprinted with permission from Dr. W. Virgil Brown and *Cholesterol and Coronary Disease . . . Reducing the Risk,* Vol 1, No 5, p 3., June 1987.
* If these guidelines are adopted on a daily basis, the saturated fat content of the American diet can be markedly reduced.

Cholesterol Risk Categories and Recommendations

Total Cholesterol Level	Recommendation
Desirable level Less than 200 mg/dl	Recheck cholesterol level every 5 years.
Borderline high 200 to 239 mg/dl	Dietary control of cholesterol in diet. Recheck cholesterol level annually.
Borderline high with risk factors Family history of premature coronary heart disease; cigarette smoking; hypertension; low level of high-density lipoprotein; diabetes; history of stroke; severe obesity.	For men with one risk factor, women with two risk factors, or anyone with coronary heart disease, determine level of low-density lipoprotein and initiate stringent dietary program for lowering cholesterol; further treatment with drugs if necessary.
High 240 mg/dl or higher	Same as above.

$C_5H_{15}NO_2$. An amine, widely distributed in plant and animal tissues. It is a constituent of lecithin and other phospholipids. It is essential in normal fat and carbohydrate metabolism. A deficiency leads to lipoidosis of the liver. It is also involved in protein metabolism, serving as a methylating agent, and it is a precursor of acetylcholine.

cholinergic (kō″lĭn-ĕr′jĭk) [″ + *ergon*, work]. 1. Nerve endings that liberate acetylcholine. 2. An agent that produces the effect of acetylcholine.

cholinergic fibers. They include all preganglionic fibers, all postganglionic parasympathetic fibers, postganglionic sympathetic fibers to the sweat glands, and efferent fibers to skeletal muscle.

cholinesterase (kō″lĭn-ĕs′tĕr-ās). Any enzyme that catalyzes the hydrolysis of choline esters, such as acetylcholinesterase, which catalyzes the breakdown of acetylcholine to acetic acid and choline. Cholinesterases are inhibited by physostigmine (eserine).

cholinoceptive (kō″lĭn-ō-sĕp′tĭv) [″ + L. *receptor*, receiver]. Concerning sites on cells that are acted on by cholinergic transmitters.

cholinolytic (kō″lĭn-ō-lĭt′ĭk) [″ + *lysis*, dissolution]. A drug or chemical that blocks the action of acetylcholine.

cholinomimetic (kō″lĭ-nō-mĭ-mĕt′ĭk) [″ + *mimetikos*, imitating]. Acting in the same way as acetylcholine.

cholochrome (kō′lō-krōm) [″ + *chroma*, color]. Any bile pigment.

chologenic (kō″lō-jĕn′ĭk) [″ + *gennan*, to produce]. Producing or stimulating the production of bile.

cholohemothorax (kō″lō-hĕm″ō-thō′răks) [″ + *haima*, blood, + *thorax*, chest]. Presence of bile and blood in the thorax.

chololith (kŏl′ō-lĭth) [″ + *lithos*, stone]. A gallstone; biliary calculus.

chololithiasis (kŏl″ō-lĭth-ī′ăs-ĭs) [″ + ″ + *-iasis*, state]. Presence of concretions in the gallbladder. SYN: *cholelithiasis*.

cholorrhea (kŏl″ō-rē′ă) [″ + *rhoia*, flow]. Excessive secretion of bile.

Choloxin. Trade name for dextrothyroxine sodium.

choluria (kō-lū′rē-ă) [″ + *ouron*, urine]. Bile salts in the urine.

chondral (kŏn′drăl) [Gr. *chondros*, cartilage]. Pert. to cartilage.

chondralgia (kŏn-drăl′jē-ă) [″ + *algos*, pain]. Pain in or around a cartilage.

chondralloplasia (kŏn″drăl-ō-plā′zē-ă) [″ + *allos*, other, + *plassein*, to form].

Presence of cartilage in abnormal places.

chondrectomy (kŏn-drĕk′tō-mē) [″ + *ektome*, excision]. Surgical excision of a cartilage.

chondric (kŏn′drĭk) [Gr. *chondros*, cartilage]. Pert. to cartilage.

chondrification (kŏn-drĭ-fĭ-kā′shŭn) [″ + L. *facere*, to make]. Conversion into cartilage.

chondrigen (kŏn′drĭ-jĕn) [″ + *gennan*, to produce]. Basal substance of cartilage and corneal tissue, which turns into chondrin on boiling. Also spelled *chondrogen*.

chondrin (kŏn′drĭn) [Gr. *chondros*, cartilage]. Gelatin-like matter obtained by boiling cartilage.

chondritis (kŏn-drī′tĭs) [″ + *itis*, inflammation]. Inflammation of cartilage.

chondroadenoma (kŏn″drō-ăd-ē-nō′mă) [″ + *aden*, gland, + *oma*, tumor]. Cartilaginous tissue in an adenoma.

chondroangioma (kŏn″drō-ăn-jē-ō′ma) [″ + *angeion*, vessel, + *oma*, tumor]. Cartilaginous elements in an angioma.

chondroblast (kŏn′drō-blăst) [″ + *blastos*, germ]. A cell that forms cartilage.

chondroblastoma (kŏn″drō-blăs-tō′mă) [″ + ″ + *oma*, tumor]. A benign neoplasm in which the cells resemble cartilage cells and the tumor appears to be cartilage.

chondrocalcinosis (kŏn″drō-kăl″sĭn-ō′sĭs) [″ + L. *calx*, lime, + Gr. *osis*, condition]. Pseudogout; chronic recurrent arthritis clinically similar to gout. The crystals found in synovial fluid are calcium pyrophosphate dihydrate and not urate crystals. The most commonly involved joint is the knee.

chondroclast (kŏn′drō-klăst) [″ + *klastos*, broken into bits]. A giant cell involved in the absorption of cartilage.

chondrocostal (kŏn″drō-kŏs′tăl) [″ + L. *costa*, rib]. Pert. to the ribs and costal cartilages.

chondrocranium (kŏn-drō-krā′nē-ŭm) [″ + *kranion*, head]. The cartilaginous embryonic cranium before ossification.

chondrocyte (kŏn′drō-sīt) [″ + *kytos*, cell]. A cartilage cell.

chondrodermatitis nodularis chronica helicis. Growth of nodules on the helix of the ear.

chondrodynia (kŏn″drō-dĭn′ē-ă) [″ + *odyne*, pain]. Pain in or about a cartilage.

chondrodysplasia (kŏn″drō-dĭs-plā′zē-ă) [″ + Gr. *dys*, + *plasis*, a molding]. Disease, usually hereditary, resulting in disordered growth. Characterized by multiple exostoses of growth of the epiphyses, esp. of the long bones, metacarpals, and phalanges. SYN: *dyschondroplasia; Ollier's disease.*

chondrodystrophy (kŏn″drō-dĭs′trō-fē) [″ + ″ + *trophe*, nourishment]. Achondroplasia, q.v.

chondroendothelioma (kŏn″drō-ĕn″dōthē″lē-ō′mă) [″ + *endon*, within, + *thele*, nipple, + *oma*, tumor]. An endothelioma that contains cartilage.

chondroepiphysitis (kŏn″drō-ĕp″ĭ-fĭz-ī′tĭs) [″ + *epiphysis*, a growing on, + *itis*, inflammation]. Inflammation of the epiphyseal portion of the bone and the attached cartilage.

chondrofibroma (kŏn″drō-fī-brō′mă) [″ + L. *fibra*, fiber, + Gr. *oma*, tumor]. A mixed tumor with elements of chondroma and fibroma.

chondrogen (kŏn′drō-jĕn) [Gr. *chondros*, cartilage, + *gennan*, to produce]. Basal substance of cartilage and corneal tissue, which turns into chondrin on boiling. Also spelled *chondrigen.*

chondrogenesis (kŏn″drō-jĕn′ĕ-sĭs) [″ + *genesis*, generation, birth]. Formation of cartilage.

chondrogenic (kŏn″drō-jĕn′ĭk). Forming cartilage.

chondroid (kŏn′droyd) [″ + *eidos*, form, shape]. Resembling cartilage; cartilaginous.

chondroitin (kŏn-drō′ĭ-tĭn). Substance present in connective tissue, including the cornea and cartilage.

chondrolipoma (kŏn-drō-lĭp-ō′mă) [″ + *lipos*, fat, + *oma*, tumor]. Cartilaginous and fatty tissue tumor.

chondrology (kŏn-drŏl′ō-jē) [″ + *logos*, word, reason]. The science of cartilages.

chondrolysis (kŏn-drŏl′ĭ-sĭs) [″ + *lysis*, dissolution]. The breaking down and absorption of cartilage.

chondroma (kŏn-drō′mă) [″ + *oma*, tumor]. A cartilaginous tumor of slow growth. It may occur wherever there is cartilage. It causes no pain.

chondromalacia (kŏn-drō-măl-ā′shē-ă) [″ + *malakia*, softness]. Softness of the articular cartilage, usually involving the patella.

chondromatosis (kŏn″drō-mă-tō′sĭs) [″ + *oma*, tumor, + *osis*, condition]. Formation of multiple chondromas of the hands and feet.

chondromatous (kŏn-drŏm′ă-tŭs) [″ + *oma*, tumor]. Pert. to chondroma, or tumor of a cartilage.

chondromucin (kŏn″drō-mū′sĭn). Chondromucoid, q.v.

chondromucoid (kŏn″drō-mū′koyd) [″ + L. *mucus*, mucus, + Gr. *eidos*, form,

shape]. A basophilic glycoprotein present in interstitial substance of cartilage.

chondromucoprotein (kŏn″drō-mū″kōprō′tē-ĭn) [″ + ″ + *protos*, first]. The ground substance, i.e., the fluid or solid material that occupies the space between the cells and fibers of cartilage.

chondromyoma (kŏn″drō-mī-ō′mă) [″ + *mys*, muscle, + *oma*, tumor]. Myoma and cartilaginous neoplasm combined.

chondromyxoma (kŏn″drō-mĭks-ō′mă) [″ + *myxa*, mucus, + *oma*, tumor]. Chondroma with myxomatous elements.

chondromyxosarcoma (kŏn-drō-mĭk″sōsär-kō′mă) [″ + ″ + *sarx*, flesh, + *oma*, tumor]. A cartilaginous and sarcomatous tumor.

chondro-osseus (kŏn″drō-ŏs′ē-ŭs) [″ + L. *osseus*, bony]. Composed of cartilage and bone.

chondro-osteodystrophy (kŏn″drō-ŏs″tēō-dĭs′trō-fē) [″ + *osteon*, bone, + *dys*, bad, + *trophe*, nourishment]. Developmental deformity of the epiphyses. This produces dwarfism, kyphosis, and pigeon breast.

chondropathology (kŏn″drō-pă-thŏl′ō-jē) [Gr. *chondros*, cartilage, + *pathos*, disease, + *logos*, word, reason]. Pathology of disease of cartilages.

chondropathy (kŏn-drŏp′ă-thē). Any disease of cartilage.

chondroplasia (kŏn″drō-plā′zē-ă) [″ + *plassein*, to mold]. Formation of cartilage.

chondroplast (kŏn′drō-plăst). A cell that forms cartilage. SYN: *chondroblast.*

chondroplasty (kŏn′drō-plăs″tē) [″ + *plassein*, to mold]. Plastic or reparative surgery on cartilage.

chondroporosis (kŏn″drō-pō-rō′sĭs) [″ + *poros*, passage]. The porous condition of pathological or normal cartilage during ossification.

chondroproteins (kŏn-drō-prō′tē-ĭns). [″ + *protos*, first]. A group of glucoproteins found in cartilage, tendons, and connective tissue.

chondrosarcoma (kŏn-drō-săr-kō′mă) [″ + *sarx*, flesh, + *oma*, tumor]. Cartilaginous sarcoma.

chondrosin (kŏn′drō-sĭn). Material produced when chondroitin sulfate is hydrolyzed.

chondrosis (kŏn-drō′sĭs) [″ + *osis*, condition]. The development of cartilage.

chondrosternal (kŏn″drō-stĕr′năl) [″ + *sternon*, chest]. Pert. to sternal cartilage.

chondrosternoplasty (kŏn″drō-stĕr′nōplăs″tē) [″ + ″ + *plassein*, to mold]. Surgical correction of a deformed sternum.

chondrotome (kŏn′drō-tōm) [″ + *tome,* incision]. Device for cutting cartilage.

chondrotomy (kŏn-drŏt′ō-mē). Dissection or surgical division of cartilage.

chondroxiphoid (kŏn″drō-zĭ′foyd) [″ + *xiphos,* sword, + *eidos,* form, shape]. Concerning the sternum and the xiphoid process.

Chondrus [L., cartilage]. A genus of red algae that includes *Chondrus crispus,* the source of carrageenan, a mucilaginous substance used as an emulsifying agent. Commonly called Irish moss or carrageen.

choosing death. The choice of an individual to die, esp. in the case of choosing to withdraw from chronic dialysis with no medical reason for withdrawing. In one study, stopping dialysis in this situation was three times more common in patients treated at home than in those treated at dialysis centers. SEE: *death; death with dignity; do not attempt to resuscitate; suicide.*

Chopart's amputation (shō-pärz′) [François Chopart, Fr. surgeon, 1743–1795]. Disarticulation at the midtarsal joint.

chorda (kor′dă) [Gr. *chorde,* cord] (pl. *chordae*). A cord or tendon.

   c. dorsalis. The notochord.

   c. gubernaculum. Embryonic structure forming a part of the gubernaculum testis in the male and the round ligament in the female.

   c. obliqua. The oblique ligament, an oblique cord that connects the shafts of the radius and ulna. Extends from the lateral side of the tubercle of the ulna to a point just below the radial tuberosity.

   c. tympani. [NA] Branch of the facial nerve that leaves the cranium through the stylomastoid foramen, traverses the tympanic cavity and joins a branch of the lingual nerve. Efferent fibers innervate the submandibular and sublingual glands; afferent fibers convey taste impulses from anterior two thirds of the tongue.

   c. umbilicalis. Umbilical cord connecting fetus and placenta.

   c. vocalis. Vocal folds of the larynx.

   c. willisii. One of several fibrous cords across the superior longitudinal sinus of the brain.

chordae tendineae (kor′dē tĕn-dĭn′ē-ē). [NA] Small tendinous cords that connect the free edges of the atrioventricular valves to the papillary muscles.

chordal (kor′dăl). Pert. to a chorda, esp. the notochord.

Chordata (kor-dā′tă) [LL., notochord]. A phylum of the animal kingdom including all animals that have a notochord during their development. Includes all vertebrates.

chordee (kor-dē′) [Fr., corded]. Painful downward curvature of the penis on erection. Occurs in congenital anomaly (hypospadia) or in urethral infection such as gonorrhea. SEE: *Peyronie's disease.*

chorditis (kor-dī′tĭs) [Gr. *chorde,* cord, + *itis,* inflammation]. Inflammation of the spermatic or vocal cord.

   c. nodosa. Formation of small whitish nodules on one or both vocal cords in individuals who misuse their voice.

   SYM: Hoarseness, inability of singers to produce the desired sounds.

   TREAT: Voice rest. Surgical removal of nodules if they do not respond to conservative therapy.

chordoma (kor-dō′mă) [″ + *oma,* tumor]. Rare tumor that occurs any place along the vertebral column. Composed of embryonic nerve tissue and vacuolated physaliform cells. The neoplasm may cause death because of the damage of the expanding tissue and the surgical inaccessibility of the tumor.

chordotomy (kor-dŏt′ō-mē) [″ + *tome,* incision]. Division of a portion of the spinal cord to relieve pain.

chorea (kō-rē′ă) [Gr. *choreia,* dance]. A nervous condition marked by involuntary muscular twitching of the limbs or facial muscles.

   c., acute. Sydenham's chorea, q.v.

   c., Bergeron's. SEE: *c., electric.* SYN: *Dubini's disease.*

   c., chronic. C., Huntington. SYN: *chronic progressive hereditary chorea.*

   c., electric. A rare form of chorea characterized by sudden involuntary contraction of a group of muscles. This causes violent movements as if the patient had been stimulated by an electric current.

   c., epidemic. Dancing mania; uncontrolled dancing. Manifest in the 14th century in Europe. SYN: *choreomania; choromania; dancing mania.*

   c., gravidarum. A form of Sydenham's chorea seen in some pregnant women, usually in those who have had chorea before, esp. in their first pregnancy. SEE: *c., Sydenham's.*

   c., Henoch's. A form of progressive electric chorea.

   c., hereditary. Huntington chorea, q.v.

   c., Huntington. A disease of the central nervous system that usually has its onset between 30 and 50 years of age, but can begin at any age. It is transmitted as an autosomal dominant trait with complete penetrance. The patient has progressive dementia with bizarre involuntary movements characteristic of chorea. Emotional disturbances may precede the onset of chorea, but they are not diagnostic. Included are mania, hallucinations, paranoia, irritability, eccentricity, hostility, apathy, and depression. Suicide may occur. As the intellect fails, memory and attention span deteriorate. The chorea may be controlled by use of reserpine and tetrabenazine, but their side effects outweigh their benefit. Haloperidol is also of use in treating chorea, but the smallest dose possible should be used to help prevent tardic dyskinesia. There is no effective therapy for the mental deterioration. Emotional changes can be treated, as can depression and psychosis. As dementia progresses, the patient loses the ability to cope with the activities of daily living and develops fecal and urinary incontinence. SYN: *Huntington disease.*

c., hyoscine. Movements simulating chorea and sometimes accompanied by delirium, seen in acute hyoscine intoxication.

c., mimetic. Chorea due to imitative movements.

c. minor. C., Sydenham's.

c., posthemiplegic. Chorea affecting partially paralyzed muscles subsequent to a hemiplegic attack.

c., senile. Mild, usually benign disorder of the elderly marked by chorea-like movements but not associated with mental disorder.

c., Sydenham's. A disease, usually of childhood, commonly occurring between 5 and 15 years of age or during pregnancy; more females than males are affected. Usually associated with rheumatic fever. Characterized by involuntary purposeless contractions of the muscles of the trunk and extremities; anxiety; impairment of memory and sometimes of speech. SYN: *c. minor; Saint Vitus' dance.*

TREAT: Rest of body and mind. The child should remain in school unless the chorea is so severe as to make this inadvisable. Protection against injury in severe cases. Sedation may be needed if chorea is severe.

PROG: Recovery usually in course of 6 to 10 weeks. Relapses not infrequent, esp. in pregnancy. A possible sequel is chronic chorea. Rare complication is death from heart disease.

choreal (kō-rē′al, kō′rē-ăl). Pert. to chorea.

choreic (kō-rē′ĭk). Pert. to or of nature of chorea.

choreiform (kō-rē′ĭ-form) [Gr. *choreia,* dance, + L.*forma,* form]. Of the nature of chorea.

choreoathetoid (kō″rē-ō-ăth′ĕ-toyd) [″ + *athetos,* not fixed, + *eidos,* form, shape]. Concerning choreoathetosis, q.v.

choreoathetosis (kō″rē-ō-ăth″ĕ-tō′sĭs) [″ + ″ + *osis,* condition]. Type of athetosis frequently seen in cerebral palsy, charac-

terized by extreme range of motion, jerky involuntary movement more proximal than distal, and fluctuating muscle tone from hypotonia to hypertonia.

choreomania (kō″rē-ō-mā′nē-ă) [″ + *mania,* madness]. Dancing mania. Seen in the Middle Ages. SYN: *chorea, epidemic.*

chorioadenoma (kō″rē-ō-ăd″ĕn-ō′mă) [Gr. *chorion,* outer membrane enclosing an embryo, + *aden,* gland, + *oma,* tumor]. Adenoma of the chorion.

c. destruens. A type of hydatidiform mole in which the chorionic villi penetrate the myometrium.

chorioallantois (kō″rē-ō-ă-lăn′tō-ĭs). In embryology, the membrane formed by the union of the chorion and allantois. In the human embryo, this develops to form the placenta.

chorioamnionitis (kō″rē-ō-ăm″nē-ō-nī′tĭs) [″ + *amnion,* lamb, + *itis,* inflammation]. Inflammation of the membranes that cover the fetus.

chorioangioma (kō″rē-ō-ăn-jē-ō′mă) [″ + *angeion,* vessel, + *oma,* tumor]. A vascular tumor of the chorion.

choriocapillaris (kō″rē-ō-kăp-ĭl-lā′rĭs) [Gr. *choroeides,* resembling a membrane, + L. *capillaris,* hairlike]. Capillary layer of choroid.

choriocarcinoma (kō″rē-ō-kăr″sĭ-nō′mă) [Gr. *chorion,* chorion, + *karkinoma,* cancer]. An extremely rare, very malignant neoplasm, usually of the uterus but sometimes at site of ectopic pregnancy. Though actual cause is unknown, it may occur following hydatid mole, a normal pregnancy, or abortion.

TREAT: The response of this cancer to methotrexate, USP, or actinomycin therapy may be dramatic. Complete remissions for over 10 years have been observed.

choriocele (kō′rē-ō-sēl) [Gr. *choroeides,* resembling a membrane, + *kele,* tumor, swelling]. A protrusion of the choroid coat of the eye through a defective sclera.

chorioepithelioma (kō″rē-ō-ĕp″ĭ-thē″lē-ō′mă). Choriocarcinoma.

choriogenesis (kō″rē-ō-jĕn′ĕ-sĭs) [Gr. *chorion,* chorion, + *genesis,* generation, birth]. Formation of the chorion.

chorioid (kō′rē-oyd). Choroid.

choriomeningitis (kō″rē-ō-mĕn″ĭn-jī′tĭs) [″ + *meninx,* membrane, + *itis,* inflammation]. Cerebral meningitis with cellular infiltration of the meninges.

c., lymphocytic. An acute central nervous system disease of viral origin characterized by flu-like symptoms (fever, malaise, headache) sometimes followed by acute septic meningitis.

chorion (kō′rē-ŏn) [Gr.]. An extraembryonic

membrane that, in early development, forms the outer wall of the blastocyst. It is formed from the trophoblast and its inner lining of mesoderm. From it develop chorionic villi, which establish an intimate connection with the endometrium, giving rise to the placenta. SEE: *placenta* and *umbilical cord* for illus.; *trophoblast.*

c. frondosum. The outer surface of the chorion. Its villi contact the decidua basalis. This is the placental portion of the chorion.

c. laeve. The smooth, nonvillous portion of the chorion.

chorionepithelioma (kō″rē-ŏn-ĕp″ĭ-thē″lē-ō′mă) [″ + *epi,* on, + *thele,* nipple, + *oma,* tumor]. Choriocarcinoma, q.v.

chorionic (kō-rē-ŏn′ĭk). Pert. to the chorion.

chorionic plate. In the placenta, that portion of the chorion attached to the uterus.

chorionic villi. The vascular projections from the chorion.

chorionic villus sampling. ABBR: CVS. Procedure for obtaining a sample of the chorionic villi by use of a catheter inserted into the cervix and into the outer portion of the membranes surrounding the fetus. Microscopic and chemical examination of the sample obtained is of assistance in prenatal evaluation of the chromosomal, enzymatic and DNA status of the fetus. The sample is usually obtained between 9 to 12 weeks following the last menstrual period. This is prior to the time amniocentesis may be done. The chance of having a successful pregnancy outcome is less after CVS than after amniocentesis, q.v. In addition, the accuracy of data obtained from CVS is lower than that obtained from amniocentesis.

chorionitis (kō″rē-ŏn-ī′tĭs) [″ + *itis,* inflammation]. Inflammation of the chorion.

chorioretinal (kō″rē-ō-rĕt′ĭ-năl). Concerning the choroid and retina of the eye.

chorioretinitis (kō″rē-ō-rĕt″ĭn-ī′tĭs) [Gr. *chorioeides,* skinlike, + L. *rete,* network, + Gr. *itis,* inflammation]. Inflammation of the choroid and retina.

chorista (kō-rĭs′tă) [Gr. *choristos,* separated]. An error of development in which tissues have grown in a displaced position. These tissues are histologically normal.

choristoma (kō-rĭs-tō′mă) [″ + *oma,* tumor]. A neoplasm due to overdevelopment of embryonic rudiments in sites where the tissues are not normally found.

choroid (kō′royd) [Gr. *chorioeides,* skinlike]. Dark brown vascular coat of the eye between the sclera and retina, extending from ora serrata to optic nerve. Consists of blood vessels united by connective tissue containing pigmented cells and is made up of five layers: suprachoroid; layer of large vessels; layer of medium-sized vessels; layer of cap-

illaries; lamina vitrea (homogeneous membrane placed next to pigmentary layer of retina). It is a part of the uvea or vascular tunic of the eye.

choroideremia (kō-roy-dĕr-ē′mē-ă) [″ + *eremia,* destitution]. A hereditary primary choroidal degeneration transmitted as an X-linked trait. In males, the earliest symptom is night blindness followed by constricted visual field and eventual blindness. In females, the condition is nonprogressive and vision is usually normal.

choroiditis (kō″royd-ī′tĭs) [″ + *itis,* inflammation]. Inflammation of the choroid.

c., anterior. Choroiditis in which outlets of exudation are at the choroidal periphery.

c., areolar. Choroiditis in which inflammation spreads from around the macula lutea.

c., central. Choroiditis in which exudation is limited to the macula.

c., diffuse. Choroiditis in which the fundus is covered with spots.

c., exudative. Choroiditis in which the choroid is covered with patches of inflammation.

c., metastatic. Choroiditis due to embolism.

c., suppurative. Choroiditis in which suppuration occurs.

c., Tay's. A familial condition characterized by degeneration of the choroid, esp. in the region about the macula lutea. Occurs in aged persons.

choroidocyclitis (kō-roy″dō-sĭk-lī′tĭs) [Gr. *chorioeides,* skinlike, + *kyklos,* a circle, + *itis,* inflammation]. Inflammation of the choroid coat and ciliary processes.

choroidoiritis (kō-royd″ō-ī-rī′tĭs) [″ + *iris,* iris, + *itis,* inflammation]. Inflammation of the choroid coat and iris.

choroidopathy (kō″roy-dŏp′ă-thē) [″ + *pathos,* disease, suffering]. Any disease of the choroid.

choroidoretinitis (kō-royd″ō-rĕt″ĭn-ī′tĭs) [″ + L. *rete,* network, + Gr. *itis,* inflammation]. Inflammation of the choroid and retina.

choroid plexus. A highly vascularized area protruding into the lateral ventricle of the brain. Similar areas are present in the third ventricle. These structures secrete cerebrospinal fluid.

Christian name. An individual's given name. SEE: *surname.*

Christian Science. A system of religious teaching based on Christian Scientists' interpretation of Scripture. Founded in 1866 by Mary Baker Eddy. The system emphasizes full healing of disease by mental and spiritual means because a major belief is that cause and effect are mental.

Christian-Weber disease. SEE: *Weber-Christian disease.*

Christmas disease [*Christmas,* family name of the first patient with the disease who was studied]. A form of hemophilia in males resulting from plasma thromboplastin component (PTC or Factor IX) deficiency. Transmitted as an X-linked trait. SYN: *hemophilia B.*

Christmas factor. ABBR: CF. Plasma thromboplastin component (PTC). A thromboplastin activator present in blood plasma.

chromaffin (krō-măf′ĭn) [Gr. *chroma,* color, + L. *affinis,* having affinity for]. 1. Staining readily with chromium salts. 2. Denoting pigmented cells forming medulla of the adrenal glands and the paraganglia.

chromaffin cells. Cells such as those of the adrenal medulla that contain granules that stain brown when cells are stained with a fluid containing potassium bichromate.

chromaffinoma (krō″măf-ĭ-nō′mä) [″ + ″ + Gr. *oma,* tumor]. A chromaffin cell tumor. SYN: *paraganglioma.*

chromaffinopathy (krō″măf-ĭn-ŏp′ă-thē) [″ + ″ + Gr. *pathos,* disease]. Any disease of chromaffin tissue.

chromaffin reaction. The turning brown of cytoplasmic granules containing epinephrine when subjected to stains containing chromium salts. Such granules stain green with ferric chloride, yellow with iodine, and brown with osmic acid.

chromaffin system. The mass of tissue forming paraganglia and medulla of suprarenal glands, which secretes adrenalin and stains readily with chromium salts. Similar tissue is found in the organs of Zuckerkandl, and in the liver, testes, ovary, and heart. SEE: *adrenal gland.*

chromaphil (krō′mă-fĭl) [″ + *philein,* to love]. Pert. to a histological element or cell that stains readily with chromium salts. SYN: *chromaffin.*

chromate (krō′māt) [Gr. *chromatos,* color]. A salt of chromic acid. SEE: *potassium chromate.*

chromatic (krō-măt′ĭk). Pert. to color.

chromatid (krō′mă-tĭd) The two halves into which a chromosome is longitudinally divided during mitosis and meiosis. They are held together at the centromere and migrate to opposite poles of the dividing cell at anaphase.

chromatin (krō′mă-tĭn) [Gr. *chroma,* color]. A deeply staining substance present in the nucleus of a cell that contains the genetic material. It is a deoxyribonucleic acid attached to a protein structure base.

    c., sex. SEE: *Barr body.*

chromatin-negative. Lacking the sex chromatin; characteristic of nuclei in cells of normal human males. SEE: *Barr body.*

chromatinolysis (krō″mă-tĭn-ŏl′ĭ-sĭs) [″ + *lysis,* dissolution]. 1. Destruction of chromatin. 2. The emptying of a cell, bacterial or other, by lysis.

chromatinorrhexis (krō″mă-tĭn-or-rĕk′sĭs) [″ + *rhexis,* rupture]. Splitting of chromatin.

chromatin-positive. Having the sex chromatin (the Barr body, q.v.); characteristic of nuclei in cells of normal human females.

chromatism (krō′mă-tĭzm) [″ + *-ismos,* condition]. 1. Unnatural pigmentation. 2. Chromatic aberration.

chromatogenous (krō″mă-tŏj′ĕn-ŭs) [″ + *gennan,* to produce]. Causing pigmentation or color.

chromatogram (krō-măt′ō-grăm) [″ + *gramma,* something written]. Record produced by chromatography.

chromatography (krō″mă-tŏg′ră-fē) [″ + *graphein,* to write]. A method of separating two or more chemical compounds in solution by virtue of their being removed from the solution at different rates when percolated down a column of a powdered absorbent or passed across the surface of an absorbent paper.

    c., adsorption. Chromatography accomplished by applying the material to be tested to one end of a sheet or column containing a solid. As the material moves, the various constituents adhere to the surface of the particles of the solid at different distances from the starting point in accordance with their chemical characteristics.

    c., column. A form of adsorption chromatography wherein the adsorptive material is packed into a column.

    c., gas. Chromatography wherein the gases to be separated from each other are adsorbed as they pass over the appropriate solids.

    c., gas-liquid. ABBR: GLC. Chromatographic analysis wherein a gas moves over a liquid, and chemical substances are separated by their different adsorption rates on the liquid.

    c., high-performance liquid. ABBR: HPLC. Application of high pressure to liquid chromatography technique in order to increase the speed of separation and to enhance resolution.

    c., paper. Chromatography in which paper strips are used as the porous solid medium.

    c., partition. Chromatography in which substances in solution are separated by being exposed to two immiscible solvents. The immobile solvent is located between the spaces of an inert material such as starch, cellulose, or silica. The substances move with the mobile solvent as it passes down the column at a rate governed by their partition coefficient.

c., thin layer. ABBR: TLC. Chromatography involving the differential adsorption of substances as they pass through a thin layer or sheet of cellulose or some other inert compound.

chromatoid (krō'mă-toyd) [Gr. *chroma*, color, + *eidos*, form, shape]. Staining in the same manner as chromatin.

chromatokinesis (krō"mă-tō-kī-nē'sĭs) [" + *kinesis*, movement]. The movement of chromatin during the division of a cell.

chromatolysis (krō"mă-tŏl'ĭ-sĭs) [" + *lysis*, dissolution]. Dissolution of chromophil substance (Nissl bodies) in neurons in certain pathological conditions, or following injury to the cell body or axon.

chromatometer (krō-mă-tŏm'ĕt-ĕr) [" + *metron*, measure]. A scale of colors for testing color perception.

chromatophil, chromatophilic (krō'mă-tō-fĭl", krō"mă-tō-fĭl'ĭk) [" + *philein*, to love]. Staining easily.

chromatophore (krō-măt'ō-for) [" + *phoros*, bearing]. A pigment-bearing cell.

chromatopsia (krō"mă-tŏp'sē-ă) [" + *opsis*, vision]. Abnormally colored vision.

chromatoptometry (krō"măt-ŏp-tŏm'ĕ-trē) [" + *optos*, visible, + *metron*, measure]. Measurement of color perception.

chromatosis (krō"mă-tō'sĭs) [" + *osis*, condition]. 1. Pigmentation. 2. The pathological deposition of pigment in any part of the body where it is not normally present or excessive deposition where it is present.

chromaturia (krō-mă-tū'rē-ă) [" + *ouron*, urine]. Abnormal color of the urine.

chromesthesia (krō"mĕs-thē'zē-ă) [" + *aisthesis*, sensation]. The association of color sensations with words, taste, smell, or sounds.

chromicize (krō'mĭ-sīz). To impregnate with chromium or its salts.

chromidiosis (krō-mĭd-ē-ō'sĭs). Movement of chromatin and nuclear substance from nucleus to the cytoplasm of the cell.

chromidium (krō-mĭd'ē-ŭm) [" + *-idion*, a dim. termination] (pl. *chromidia*). An extranuclear granule seen in the cytoplasm of a cell.

chromidrosis, chromhidrosis (krō"mĭd-rō'sĭs) [" + *hidros*, sweat]. Excretion of colored sweat. Red sweat may be due to an exudation of blood into the sweat glands or to microorganisms in those glands.

SYM: Localized in eyelids, breasts, axillae, genitocrural regions; occasionally on hands and limbs. It is grayish, bluish, violaceous, brownish; it collects on skin, giving a greasy, powdery appearance to parts.

ETIOL: May be due to ingestion or absorption of certain substances, as pigment-producing bacteria. May be caused by certain disorders of metabolism.

TREAT: Relief of underlying condition.

RS: anhidrosis; bromidrosis; hidrosis; hyperhidrosis; uridrosis.

chromium (krō'mē-ŭm) [L., color]. SYMB: Cr. At. wt. 51.996; at. no. 24. A very hard, metallic element. It is an essential trace element required for normal glucose metabolism.

chromium poisoning. SYM: A disagreeable taste in the mouth, pain, diarrhea, collapse, and cramping. If fatal, death is due to uremia.

TREAT: Chalk, magnesia, and other weak alkalies to neutralize its acid effects. Wash out stomach and give cathartics, analgesics for pain.

chromoblast (krō'mō-blăst) [Gr. *chroma*, color, + *blastos*, germ]. An embryonic cell that becomes a pigment cell.

chromocenter (krō'mō-sĕn"tĕr) [" + *kentros*, middle]. Irregular clumps of chromatin material seen in the nuclei of cells that are not dividing. SYN: *karyosome*.

chromocystoscopy (krō"mō-sĭs-tŏs'kō-pē) [" + *kystis*, bladder, + *skopein*, to examine]. Determination of functional activity of kidneys and bladder by use of dyes.

chromocyte (krō'mō-sīt) [" + *kytos*, cell]. Any colored cell.

chromocytometer (krō"mō-sī-tŏm'ĕt-ĕr) + " + *metron*, measure]. Instrument for determining the hemoglobin in red blood corpuscles.

chromodacryorrhea (krō"mō-dăk"rē-ō-rē'ă) [" + *dacryon*, tear, + *rhoia*, flow]. Flow of blood-stained tears.

chromogen (krō'mō-jĕn) [" + *gennan*, to produce]. Any principle that may be changed into coloring matter.

chromogenesis (krō"mō-jĕn'ĕ-sĭs) [" + *genesis*, generation, birth]. Production of pigment.

chromogenic (krō"mō-jĕn'ĭk). Pigment-producing.

chromolipoid (krō"mō-lĭp'oyd) [" + *lipos*, fat, + *eidos*, form, shape]. Any lipoid that is pigmented. SYN: *lipochrome*.

chromolysis (krō-mŏl'ĭ-sĭs) [" + *lysis*, dissolution]. Dissolution of chromophil substance (Nissl bodies) in neurons in certain pathological conditions, or following injury to the cell body or axon. SYN: *chromatolysis*.

chromomere (krō'mō-mēr) [Gr. *chroma*, color, + *meros*, part]. 1. One of a series of chromatin granules found in a chromosome. 2. A highly refractile purple granule that forms the central portion of a blood platelet.

chromometer (krō-mŏm'ĕ-tĕr) [" + *metron*, measure]. Device for determining the pigment in a substance.

chromometry (krō-mŏm'ĕt-rē). The estimation of coloring matter in the substance examined.

chromomycosis (krō"mō-mī-kō'sĭs) [" + *myxa*, mucus, + *osis*, condition]. A chronic fungal infection of the skin marked by itching and warty plaques on the skin and subcutaneous swellings of feet, legs, and other exposed areas. Various fungi have been implicated, including *Phialophora verrucosa*, *P. pedrosoi*, *P. compacta*, and *Cladosporium carrionii*. Some of these are also called *Fonsecaea pedrosoi* and *F. compacta*.

chromoparic (krō-mō-pär'ĭk) [" + L. *parere*, to produce]. Producing color. Usually refers to bacteria that color their immediate surroundings. SYN: *chromogenic*.

chromopexic, **chromopectic** (krō"mō-pĕk'sĭk, -pĕk'tĭk) [" + *pexis*, fixation]. Pert. to fixation of coloring matter, as the liver function in forming bilirubin.

chromophane (krō'mō-fān) [" + *phainein*, to show]. Retinal pigment.

chromophil(e) (krō'mō-fĭl, -fīl) [" + *philein*, to love]. 1. Any structure that stains easily. 2. One of two types of cells present in pars distalis of the pituitary gland. It is considered a secretory cell.

chromophilic, **chromophilous** (krō-mō-fĭl'ĭk, krō-mŏf'ĭl-ŭs). Staining readily.

chromophobe (krō'mō-fōb) [" + *phobos*, fear]. Any cell or tissue that stains either poorly or not at all. A type of cell found in pars distalis of the pituitary gland.

chromophobia (krō"mō-fō'bē-ă). Condition of staining poorly.

chromophobic (krō-mō-fō'bĭk). Resistant to staining.

chromophore (krō'mō-for) [" + *pherein*, to bear]. Any chemical that when present in a cell that has been prepared properly displays color.

chromophoric (krō"mō-for'ĭk) [" + *pherein*, to bear]. Pert. to or bearing color.

chromophose (krō'mō-fōz) [" + *phos*, light]. A subjective sensation of a spot of color in the eye. SYN: *centrophose*.

chromophytosis (krō"mō-fī-tō'sĭs) [" + *phyton*, plant, + *osis*, condition]. Tinea versicolor, q.v.

chromoplasm (krō'mō-plăzm) [" + LL. *plasma*, form, mold]. Chromatin, q.v.

chromoplastid [" + *plastos*, formed]. Colored plastids other than chloroplasts present in plant cells.

chromoprotein (krō"mō-prō'tē-ĭn) [" + *protos*, first]. One of a group of conjugated proteins consisting of a protein combined with hematin or another colored, metal-containing, prosthetic group.

Ex.: Hemoglobin; hemocyanin; chlorophyll; flavoproteins; cytochromes.

chromopsia [" + *opsis*, vision]. Chromatopsia, q.v.

chromoptometer (krō"mŏp-tŏm'ĕ-tĕr) [" + *opsis*, sight, + *metron*, measure]. Instrument for determining keenness of color vision.

chromoradiometer [" + L. *radius*, ray, + Gr. *metron*, measure]. An instrument for measuring penetrative power of roentgen rays.

chromoscope (krō'mō-skōp) [" + *skopein*, to examine]. Instrument for determining color perception.

chromoscopy (krō-mŏs'kō-pē). Examination for color perception.

chromosomal breakage. The break of a chromosome. When this occurs, the two fragments may rejoin or a fragment may rejoin another broken chromosome. Unrepaired chromosome breaks may be associated with Fanconi's anemia, ataxia-telangiectasia, and Bleum's syndrome.

chromosomal map. SEE: *gene map*.

chromosome (krō'mō-sōm) [Gr. *chroma*, color, + *soma*, body]. A linear thread in the nucleus of a cell. It contains the DNA, which transmits genetic information. Chromosomes stain deeply with basic dyes and are esp. conspicuous during mitosis. They contain the genes or hereditary determiners. The normal number of chromosomes is constant for each species, being 46 in man (23 pairs in all somatic cells). These constitute the diploid number. In the formation of the gametes (ovum and spermatozoon) the number is reduced to one half (haploid number), i.e., the ovum and sperm each contain 23, or one of each of the 23 pairs. Of these, 22 are considered autosomes and one is the sex chromosome (X or Y). At fertilization, the chromosomes from the sperm unite with the chromosomes from the ovum. This random union determines the sex of the embryo. The female sex chromosome from the ovum may contribute only an X to the embryo. The male sex chromosome may contribute an X or a Y to join with the chromosome derived from the ovum. Thus the embryo may have XX in its sex chromosome, in which case a female would develop; or XY, in which case a male would develop. SEE: *Barr body; gene; heredity; karyotype;* illus.

c., accessory. An unpaired sex chromosome. SEE: *c., sex*.

c.'s, banded. Special staining of chromosomes delineates bands of various width on the regions or loci of the chromosomes.

KARYOTYPE OF PAIRS OF HUMAN
CHROMOSOMES OF MALE AND FEMALE

MALE

FEMALE

THIS ILLUSTRATION DEPICTS
A COMPLETE MALE OR FEMALE
KARYOTYPE DEPENDING UPON
WHETHER THE MALE 23D OR
FEMALE 23D CHROMOSOME
IS PRESENT

This facilitates analyzing and investigating chromosomes.

   c., bivalent. A double chromosome resulting from the conjugation of two homologous chromosomes in synapsis, which occurs during the first meiotic division.

   c.'s, giant. Extremely large chromosomes seen in the salivary glands and in other organs and tissues of insects.

   c., Philadelphia; c., Ph¹. An abnormality of chromosome 22 characterized by a shortening of its long arms. This anomaly is found in many patients with chronic leukemia.

   c., sex. One of two chromosomes, the X and Y chromosomes, concerned with the determination of sex in humans and which carry the genes for sex-linked characters.

   c., somatic. An autosome.

   c., X. One of a pair of female-determining chromosomes (XX) present in the somatic cells of all human females. Characteristics transmitted on the X chromosome are said to be X-linked or sex-linked.

c., Y. The male member of a pair of human chromosomes (XY) present in the somatic cells of all human males. The only characteristic that is thought to be on the Y chromosome is the trait for hairy ears.

chromotherapy (krō″mō-thĕr′ă-pē) [Gr. *chroma,* color, + *therapeia,* treatment]. The use of colored light in the treatment of disease.

chromotoxic (krō″mō-tŏk′sĭk) [″ + *toxikon,* poison]. Caused by toxic action on the hemoglobin.

chromotrichia (krō″mō-trĭk′ē-ă) [″ + *thrix,* hair]. Coloration of the hair.

chromotropic (krō″mō-trŏp′ĭk) [″ + *tropikos,* turning]. 1. Being attracted to color. 2. Attracting color.

chromoureteroscopy (krō″mō-ū-rē″tĕr-ŏs′kō-pē) [″ + *oureter,* ureter, + *skopein,* to examine]. Inspecting orifices of ureters after giving a substance to dye the urine.

chronaxie (krō′năk-sē) [Gr. *chronos,* time, + *axia,* value]. A number expressing the sensitivity of a nerve to electrical stimulation. It is the minimum duration, measured in milliseconds, during which a current of prescribed strength must pass through a motor nerve in order to cause contraction in the associated muscle; the strength of direct current (the rheobasic voltage) that will just suffice if given an indefinite time is first determined, and exactly double this strength is taken for the final determinations.

chronaximeter (krō″năk-sĭm′ĕt-ĕr) [″ + ″ + *metron,* measure]. Device for measuring chronaxie.

chronic [Gr. *chronos,* time]. 1. Of long duration. 2. Designating a disease showing little change or of slow progression. Opposite of acute.

chronic bacterial prostatitis. ABBR: CBP. Inflammation of the prostate due to longstanding bacterial infection. Clinical symptoms of fever, pain, and dysuria may be relatively mild as compared to acute infection. Therapy depends upon the causative organism and in addition to antibiotics may involve treatment of prostatic hypertrophy.

chronic desquamating eosinophilic bronchitis. Asthma, q.v.

chronic fatigue syndrome. ABBR: CFS. A somewhat vague illness that may follow symptoms of acute viral infection. It is characterized by severe, prolonged exhaustion. The disease is not new; it has been termed fabricula, neuresthenia, epidemic neuromyasthenia, Iceland disease, and epidemic myalgic encephalitis. The cause is unknown. Diagnosis is difficult because of the problems encountered in attempting to define fatigue, and the tendency to confuse CFS with other types of illnesses. Diagnosis is established when the two major criteria, the new onset of severe relapsing fatigue that persists for at least 6 months and the symptoms cannot be explained on any other basis, are present and at least 8 of the following are present: mild fever; sore throat; unexplained muscle weakness; myalgia; generalized fatigue for at least 24 hours following previously tolerated exercise; generalized headache; migratory arthralgia; neuropsychologic symptoms such as photophobia, forgetfulness, excessive irritability, confusion, inability to concentrate, or depression; sleep disturbance; and onset of the major criteria in a period of hours or days. Treatment is symptomatic.

chronic granulomatous disease. Congenital disease, characterized by polymorphonuclear leukocytes that are able to ingest but unable to kill certain bacteria. It occurs mostly in children. Twenty percent of cases reported are in girls. Evidence for X-linked, i.e., sex-linked, inheritance is present in most boys but not in girls with the disease. Carrier females rarely experience severe bacterial infections. Death is due to chronic and recurrent infections. SEE: *nitroblue tetrazolium test.*

TREAT: There is no specific therapy. Prolonged antibiotic therapy helps prevent infection. Bone marrow transplantation has been tried experimentally.

chronicity (krŏn-ĭs′ĭt-ē). State of being chronic.

chronic obstructive lung disease. ABBR: COLD. Disease process that causes decreased ability of the lungs to perform their function of ventilation. Diagnostic criteria include history of persistent dyspnea on exertion with or without chronic cough and less than one half of normal predicted maximum breathing capacity. Diseases that cause this are chronic bronchitis, pulmonary emphysema, chronic asthma, and chronic bronchiolitis. Also called chronic obstructive pulmonary disease. SEE: *emphysema.* SEE: *Nursing Diagnoses* in *Appendix.*

chrono- [Gr. *chronos,* time]. Combining form indicating a relationship to time or timing.

chronobiology (krŏn″ō-bī-ŏl′ō-jē) [Gr. *chronos,* time, + *bios,* life, + *logos,* word, reason]. Study of the timing characteristics of life processes to attempt to describe the factors that influence biological rhythms; and the influence of biological rhythms on life processes. SEE: *circadian; clock, biological.*

chronognosis (krŏn″ŏg-nō′sĭs) [″ + *gnosis,* knowledge]. Subjective realization of the passage of time.

chronograph (krŏn'ō-grăf) [" + *graphein*, to write]. Device for recording short intervals of time.

chronological (krŏn"ō-lŏj'ĭ-kăl) [" + *logos*, word, reason]. Occurring in natural sequence according to time.

chronologically enhanced. Euphemism for having attained the status or condition of being elderly or aged.

chronopharmacology. A method used in pharmacokinetics which describes the diurnal changes in plasma drug concentrations.

chronophobia. Fear of time or its perceived duration, esp. in prisoners.

chronoscope (krŏn'ō-skōp) [" + *skopein*, to examine]. Device for measuring extremely short intervals of time.

chronotaraxis (krō-nō-tăr-ăk'sĭs) [" + *taraxis*, without order]. Being unable to orient oneself with respect to time.

chronotropic (krŏn"ō-trŏp'ĭk) [" + *tropikos*, turning]. Influencing rate of occurrence of an event, such as the heartbeat. SEE: *inotropic*.

chronotropism [" + " + *-ismos*, condition]. Interference with periodic events such as the heartbeat.

    c., negative. Modifying rate by decreasing it.

    c., positive. Modifying rate by increasing it.

chrysarobin (krĭs"ă-rō'bĭn) [Gr. *chrysos*, gold, + Brazilian *araraba*, bark]. A mixture of neutral principles obtained from goa powder, which is deposited in the wood of Araroba, a leguminous tree of South America. It is used topically, as an ointment, for treatment of certain skin disorders.

chrysiasis (krĭ-sī'ă-sĭs). Deposition of gold in living tissues as in gold therapy. SYN: *auriasis*.

chrysoderma (krĭs"ō-dĕr'mă) [" + *derma*, skin]. Discoloration of the skin due to deposition of gold.

chrysotherapy (krĭs"ō-thĕr'ă-pē) [" + *therapeia*, treatment]. Use of gold compounds as a medicine. This practice is still employed in treating rheumatoid arthritis.

Chvostek's sign (vŏs'tĕks) [Franz Chvostek, Austrian surgeon, 1835–1884]. Spasm of facial muscles following a tap on one side of the face over the area of the facial nerve. Seen in tetany, q.v.

chylangioma (kī"lăn-jē-ō'mă) [Gr. *chylos*, juice, + *angeion*, vessel, + *oma*, tumor]. Tumor of intestinal lymph vessels containing chyle.

chyle (kīl) [Gr. *chylos*, juice]. The milklike, alkaline contents of the lacteals and lymphatic vessels of the intestine, consisting of the products of digestion and principally absorbed fats. It is carried by the lymphatic vessels to the cisterna chyli and then by way of the thoracic duct to the left subclavian vein, where it enters the bloodstream. A large quantity is formed in 24 hours.

    RS: achylia; cisterna chyli; oligochylia; receptaculum chyli; secretion.

chylemia (kī-lē'mē-ă) [" + *haima*, blood]. Chyle in the peripheral circulation.

chylifacient (kī"lĭ-fā'shĕnt) [" + L. *facere*, to make]. Forming chyle.

chylifaction, chylification (kī-lĭ-făk'shŭn, kī-lĭ-fī-kā'shŭn). The formation of chyle.

chylifactive (kī-lĭ-făk'tĭv). Forming chyle; chylifacient.

chyliferous (kī-lĭf'ĕr-ŭs) [" + L. *ferre*, to carry]. Carrying chyle.

chyliform (kī'lĭ-form) [" + L. *forma*, shape]. Resembling chyle.

chylocele (kī'lō-sēl) [" + *kele*, tumor, swelling]. Distention of the tunica vaginalis testis with infused chyle.

chyloderma (kī"lō-dĕr'mă) [" + *derma*, skin]. Lymph accumulated in the enlarged lymphatic vessels and thickened skin of the scrotum. SYN: *elephantiasis, scrotal*.

chylology (kī-lŏl'ō-jē) [" + *logos*, word, reason]. The study of chyle.

chylomediastinum (kī"lō-mē"dē-ăs-tī'nŭm) [" + L. *mediastinum*, median]. Chyle in the mediastinum.

chylomicron (kī"lō-mī'krŏn) [" + *mikros*, small]. Small particle of fat in the blood after digestion and absorption of fat in food. Perceptible under a microscope.

chylopericardium (kī"lō-pĕr"ĭ-kăr'dē-ŭm) [" + L. *peri*, around, + Gr. *kardia*, heart]. Chyle in the pericardium.

chyloperitoneum (kī"lō-pĕr"ĭ-tō-nē'ŭm) [" + *peritonaion*, peritoneum]. Effused chyle in peritoneal cavity.

chylophoric (kī"lō-for'ĭk) [" + *phoros*, bearing]. Conveying chyle; chyliferous.

chylopneumothorax (kī"lō-nū"mō-thō'răks) [" + *pneumon*, air, + *thorax*, chest]. Chyle and air in the pleural space.

chylopoiesis (kī"lō-poy-ē'sĭs) [" + *poiesis*, production]. Formation of chyle and its absorption by lacteals in the intestines. SYN: *chylification*.

chylorrhea (kī"lō-rē'ă) [Gr. *chylos*, juice, + *rhoia*, flow]. Escape of chyle due to rupture of the thoracic duct.

chylothorax [" + *thorax*, chest]. Chyle in pleural cavities.

chylous (kī'lŭs). Pert. to or of the nature of chyle.

chyluria (kī-lū'rē-ă) [" + *ouron*, urine]. Presence of chyle or fat globules in the urine.

chymase (kī'mās). An enzyme in gastric juice that accelerates the action of the pancreatic

the lens by tightening and relaxing the tension on the lens zonule. SEE: *eye* for illus.

ciliary ganglion. A ganglion lying in the posterior part of the orbit. Receives preganglionic fibers through the oculomotor nerve from the Edinger-Westphal nucleus of the midbrain. From it six short ciliary nerves pass to the eyeball. Postganglionic fibers innervate the ciliary muscle, sphincter of the iris, and the smooth muscles of blood vessels of these structures, and also the cornea.

ciliary glands. A form of sweat glands of the eyelid. SEE: *glands, Moll's.*

ciliary muscle. Smooth muscle forming a part of the ciliary body of the eye. Contraction pulls the choroid forward, lessening tension on fibers of the zonula (suspensory ligament), thereby allowing the lens, which is elastic, to assume a more spherical shape; thus accommodation for near vision is accomplished.

ciliary nerves, long. Two or three branches of the nasal nerves supplying the ciliary muscle, iris, and cornea.

ciliary nerves, short. Several branches of the ciliary ganglion supplying the ciliary muscle, iris, and tunics of the eyeball.

ciliary processes. About 70 folds arranged meridionally so as to form a circle. They have the same structure as the rest of the choroid and secrete nutrient fluids that nourish neighboring parts, as cornea, lens, vitreous body. They also serve as points of attachment for the suspensory ligament of the lens.

ciliary reflex. Normal contraction of pupil in accommodation of vision from distant to near.

Ciliata (sĭl″ē-ă′tă). A class of Protozoa characterized by the presence of cilia.

ciliate (sĭl′ē-āt) [L. *cilia*, eyelids]. Ciliated.

ciliated (sĭl′ē-ā-tĕd). Possessing cilia.

ciliated epithelium. Epithelium with hairlike processes on the surface. They wave actively only in one direction. Present in the respiratory tract and fallopian tubes.

ciliectomy (sĭl″ē-ĕk′tō-mē) [″ + Gr. *ektome*, excision]. Excision of a portion of the ciliary body or ciliary border of the eyelid.

ciliogenesis (sĭl″ē-ō-jĕn′ĕ-sĭs). Formation of cilia.

ciliospinal (sĭl″ē-ō-spī′năl) [″ + *spinalis*, pert. to a spine]. Pert. to the ciliary body and spinal cord.

ciliospinal center. Spinal cord center that controls dilation of the pupil.

ciliospinal reflex. Dilation of the pupil following stimulation of the skin of the neck by pinching or scratching the skin.

ciliostatic (sĭl″ē-ō-stăt′ĭk) [″ + Gr. *statos*, placed]. Interfering with or preventing movement of the cilia.

ciliotomy (sĭl″ē-ŏt′ō-mē) [″ + Gr. *tome*, incision]. Surgical cutting of the ciliary nerve.

ciliotoxicity. The action of anything that interferes with ciliary motion.

cilium (sĭl′ē-ŭm) [L.]. [NA] Sing. of cilia.

cillosis (sĭl-ō′sĭs) [L.]. Spasmodic twitching of the eyelid.

cimbia (sĭm′bē-ă) [L.]. Slender band of white fibers crossing the ventral surface of a cerebral peduncle.

cimetidine. USP. A drug that is a histamine H_2 receptor antagonist; represents a new class of pharmacological agents. It inhibits gastric secretions and is indicated for treatment of gastric and duodenal ulcers. Trade name is Tagamet. SEE: *peptic ulcer.*

Cimex lectularius (sī′mĕks lĕk-tū-lă′rē-ŭs). The bedbug. An insect belonging to the order Hemiptera. SYN: *Acantha lectularia.* SEE: *bedbug.*

cimicosis (sĭm″ĭ-kō′sĭs). Itching due to the bite of a bedbug.

CIN. *cervical intraepithelial neoplasia.*

cinchona (sĭn-kō′nă, -chō′nă) [Sp. *cinchon*, Countess of Cinchon]. The dried bark of the tree cinchona, the source of quinine. SEE: *quinine.*

cinchonism (sĭn′kŏn-ĭzm) [″ + Gr. *-ismos*, condition]. Poisoning from cinchona or its alkaloids. SYN: *quininism.*

cinchophen (sĭn′kō-fĕn). Light yellow powder with slightly bitter taste. It frequently produces serious side effects, e.g., a fatal form of hepatitis. At one time it was used in treating gout, but it is seldom used in contemporary medical therapy.

cinclisis (sĭn′klĭ-sĭs) [Gr. *kinklisis*, a wagging]. Swift spasmodic movement of any part of the body.

cincture sensation (sĭnk′chūr) [L. *cinctura*, girdle]. Sensation of a tight girdle about the waist. SYN: *zonesthesia.*

cine- [Gr. *kinesis*, movement]. Combining form indicating a relationship to movement.

cineangiocardiography (sĭn″ē-ăn″jē-ō-kăr″dē-ŏg′ră-fē) [Gr. *kinesis*, movement, + *angeion*, vessel, + *kardia*, heart, + *graphein*, to write]. Continuous photographic record of the blood vessels by use of fluoroscopy. A radiopaque agent is injected just prior to the study.

  c., radionuclide. The use of a scintillation camera to record and project the image of a radioisotope as it travels through the heart and great vessels.

cinecystourethrogram (sĭn-ĕ-sĭs″tō-ū-rē′thrō-grăm). Motion picture record of radiological investigation of the urinary bladder and urethra when they are filled with and are emptying themselves of a radiopaque medium.

cinefluorography (sĭn″ē-floo″or-ŏg′rā-fē). Motion pictures of images produced by fluoroscopic examination.

cinematics (sĭn″ē-măt′ĭks) [Gr. *kinema*, motion]. Science of motion; kinematics.

cinematoradiography (sĭn″ē-măt-ō-rā″dē-ŏg′rā-fē) [″ + L. *radius*, ray, + Gr. *graphein*, to write]. Radiography of an organ in motion.

cinemicrography (sĭn″ē-mī-krŏg′rā-fē) [Gr. *kinesis*, movement, + *mikros*, small, + *graphein*, to write]. Motion picture record of the object seen through the use of a microscope.

cineplastics (sĭn″ē-plăs′tĭks) [″ + *plassein*, to form]. Formation of muscles in a stump after amputation so that it is possible to impart motion and direction to an artificial limb.

cineraceous (sĭn-ē-rā′shŭs) [L. *cinis*, ashes]. Like ashes.

cineradiography (sĭn″ē-rā″dē-ŏg′rā-fē) [Gr. *kinesis*, movement, + L. *radius*, ray, + Gr. *graphein*, to write]. Motion picture record of images produced during fluoroscopic examination.

cinerea (sĭn-ē′rē-ă) [L. *cinereus*, ashen-hued]. Gray matter of the brain or spinal cord.

cinereal (sĭn-ē′rē-ăl). Pert. to the cinerea.

cineritious (sĭn″ĕr-ĭsh′ŭs) [L. *cineritius*, ashen]. Ashen-gray colored.

cinesi- [Gr. *kinesis*, movement]. Prefix rel. to motion. SEE: words beginning with *kinesi-*.

cineurography (sĭn″ē-ū-rŏg′rā-fē) [Gr. *kinesis*, movement, + *ouron*, urine, + *graphein*, to write]. Use of cineradiography to obtain motion picture of the urinary tract.

cingulotomy (sĭn′gū-lŏt″ō-mē) [L. *cingulum*, girdle, + Gr. *tome*, incision]. Surgical excision of the anterior half of the cingulate gyrus of the brain. May be done to alleviate intractable pain.

cingulum (sĭn′gū-lŭm) [L., girdle] (pl. *cingula*). [NA] 1. A band of association fibers in the cingulate gyrus extending from the anterior perforated substance posteriorly to the hippocampal gyrus. 2. A convexity on the cervical third of the lingual aspect of incisors and canines. SYN: *basal ridge*.

cinnamic acid. A white insoluble powder derived from cinnamon, q.v. It is used as a flavoring agent in cooking and in the preparation of perfumes and medicines.

cinnamon. A volatile oil derived from the bark of *Cinnamomum zeylanicum*. It is used as a flavoring agent in preparing pharmaceutical products, and in cooking.

cinoxacin. USP. An antibacterial drug. Trade name is Cinobac.

CinQuin. Trade name for quinidine sulfate.

circa (sĭr′kă) [L.]. ABBR: c. About. Used before dates or figures that are approximate.

circadian (sĭr″kă-dē′ăn, sĭr-kă′dē-ăn) [L. *circa*, about, + *dies*, day]. Pert. to events that occur at approximately 24-hour intervals, such as certain physiological phenomena. SEE: *clock, biological; night work, maladaption to.*

circinate (sĕr′sĭ-nāt) [L. *circinatus*, made round]. Circular.

circle [L. *circulus*, a little ring]. Any ring-shaped structure.

   c. of diffusion. One or more circles on projection plane of an image not in focus of the lens of the eye.

   c. of Willis. Union of the anterior and posterior cerebral arteries (branches of the carotid), forming an anastomosis at the base of the brain. SEE: *Willis' circle* for illus.

Circ-O-Lectric bed. A bed designed to allow the patient's position to be changed from supine to prone by rotating the bed through 180° by use of electromechanical rotation.

circuit (sĕr′kĭt) [L. *circuire*, to go around]. 1. Course or path of an electric current. 2. The path followed by a fluid circulating in a system of tubes or cavities. 3. The path followed by nerve impulses in a reflex arc from sensory receptor to effector organ.

circular [L. *circularis*]. 1. Shaped like a circle. 2. Recurrent.

circulation [L. *circulatio*]. Movement in a regular or circular course.

   c., bile salts. Circulation of the sodium glycocholate and taurocholate found in hepatic bile, which pass with it into the duodenum and then into the intestine, where they are absorbed along with the fats.

   c., blood. Circulation in which the blood leaving the left ventricle enters the aorta, from which it is pumped into the various large arteries. It thus reaches the coronary arteries of the heart itself and the arteries of the head, body wall, abdominal viscera, and extremities. Passing through the various capillary systems, it is gathered into veins, of which there are two collecting systems: (1) Most veins empty their blood into the superior and inferior venae cavae. (2) The veins from the stomach, pancreas, spleen, and intestine unite to form the portal vein, which runs to the liver. In the latter, it breaks up into a new capillary system, which drains through the hepatic veins into the vena cava inferior. The combined blood of the venae cavae and the coronary veins enters the right atrium, passes through the right ventricle, and is forced out into the pulmonary artery. The pulmonary capillary system drains by way of the pulmonary veins into the left atrium and thence into the left ventricle.

   c., collateral. Circulation that is established through an anastomosis between two vessels supplying or draining two adjacent vascular areas. This enables the blood to bypass an obstruction in the larger vessel that supplies or drains the two areas or will enable blood to flow to or from a tissue even though the principal vessel involved may be obstructed.

c., coronary. Circulation through the muscular tissue of the heart. Blood leaves the aorta through the right and left coronary arteries, which supply the myocardium. Blood passes through capillaries and is collected in veins, most of which empty into the coronary sinus, which opens into the right atrium. A few of the small veins open directly into the atria and ventricles. SEE: illus.

c., extracorporeal. Circulation of blood outside the body. This may be through an artificial kidney or a heart-lung device.

c., fetal. Circulation through the fetus. Blood, oxygenated in the placenta, passes through the umbilical vein and ductus venosus to the inferior vena cava and thence to the right atrium of the fetus, from which it may follow one of two courses—through the foramen ovale to the left atrium and then through the aorta to the tissues, or through the right ventricle, pulmonary artery, and ductus arteriosus to the aorta and then to the tissues. In either case the blood bypasses the lungs, which are not functioning before birth. Blood is returned to the placenta through the umbilical arteries, which are continuations of the hypogastric arteries. At birth or shortly after, the ductus arteriosus and the foramen ovale close, establishing normal circulation. Failure of either to occur may give rise to a blue baby. SEE: *ductus arteriosus, patent; fetal circulation* for illus.

c., lymph. Lymph is formed from the tissue fluid that fills the tissue spaces of the body. It is collected into lymph capillaries, which carry the lymph to the larger lymph vessels. These converge to form one of two main trunks, the right lymphatic duct and the thoracic duct. The right lymphatic duct drains the right side of the head, neck, and trunk and right upper extremity; the thoracic duct drains all the remaining portion of the body. It has its origin at the cisterna chyli, which receives the lymphatics from the abdominal organs. It courses upward through the diaphragm and thorax and empties into the left subclavian artery near its junction with the left interior jugular vein. The right lymphatic duct empties into the right subclavian vein. Along the course of lymph vessels there are lymph nodes, which function as filtering structures. They filter out bacteria and particulate substances, thus preventing their entrance into the bloodstream. Lymph flow is maintained by difference in pressure at the two ends of the system. Important accessory factors aiding the flow of lymph are breathing movements and muscular activities.

c., portal. Circulation in which blood from the systemic arteries is supplied to the abdominal organs and is collected into the portal vein, through which the blood enters the liver. It passes into sinusoids, which lead to central veins of the lobules and eventually to the hepatic veins, which empty into the inferior vena cava. A portal system also exists in the circulation between the hypothalamus and the hypophysis (anterior pituitary). The hypothalamus releases hormone-releasing factors into the blood, where they are carried to the hypophysis and the appropriate hormone released.

c., pulmonary. Circulation in which the venous blood received into the right atrium passes through the tricuspid valve into the right ventricle. From there it passes into the pulmonary artery, which divides into two branches, one going to each lung. (This is the only instance in which an artery contains venous or dark blood deficient in oxygen.) The artery branches in the lung into capillaries, and here, by means of the hemoglobin in the red corpuscles, the blood takes up oxygen from the inspired air. Red arterial blood returns to the heart by the four pulmonary veins, two from each lung entering the left atrium. (This is the only instance in which veins contain fully oxygenated blood.)

c., systemic. General circulation through the whole body except the lungs.

c., venous. Circulation of the blood via the veins.

circulation rate. The minute volume or output of the heart per minute. In an average-sized adult with a pulse rate of 70, the amount is about three liters per square meter of body surface each minute.

circulation time. The time required by a particle of blood to make the complete circuit of both the systemic and pulmonary systems. Circulation time is determined by injecting a substance into a vein and timing its reappearance in arteries at the point of injection. This procedure necessitates that the blood with the contained substance passes through veins to the heart and through the right atrium and ventricle, through the pulmonary circuit to the lungs, and back through the left atrium and ventricle, and then out through the aorta and arteries to the place where detected. Dyes such as fluorescein and methylene blue or substances

CIRCULATION OF BLOOD THROUGH HEART AND MAJOR VESSELS

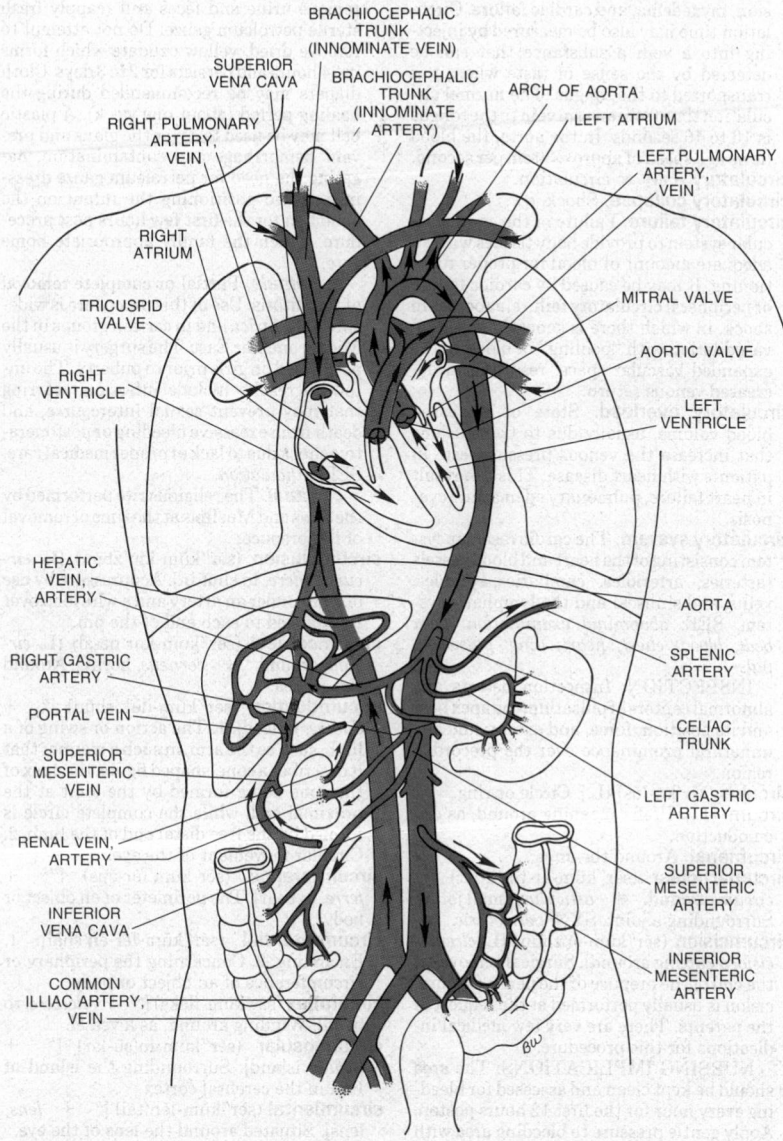

BRACHIOCEPHALIC TRUNK (INNOMINATE VEIN)

BRACHIOCEPHALIC TRUNK (INNOMINATE ARTERY)

SUPERIOR VENA CAVA

RIGHT PULMONARY ARTERY, VEIN

RIGHT ATRIUM

TRICUSPID VALVE

RIGHT VENTRICLE

HEPATIC VEIN, ARTERY

RIGHT GASTRIC ARTERY

PORTAL VEIN

SUPERIOR MESENTERIC VEIN

RENAL VEIN, ARTERY

INFERIOR VENA CAVA

COMMON ILLIAC ARTERY, VEIN

ARCH OF AORTA

LEFT ATRIUM

LEFT PULMONARY ARTERY, VEIN

MITRAL VALVE

AORTIC VALVE

LEFT VENTRICLE

AORTA

SPLENIC ARTERY

CELIAC TRUNK

LEFT GASTRIC ARTERY

SUPERIOR MESENTERIC ARTERY

INFERIOR MESENTERIC ARTERY

such as potassium ferrocyanide or histamine have been used as tracers. Average circulation time is 18 to 24 seconds.

Circulation time is reduced in anemia and hyperthyroidism; increased in hypertension, myxedema, and cardiac failure. Circulation time may also be measured by injecting into a vein a substance that can be detected by the sense of taste when it is transported to the tongue. The normal circulation time from an arm vein to the tongue is 10 to 16 seconds. In the aorta, the blood flows at a speed of approx. 30 cm per second.

circulatory. Pert. to circulation.

circulatory collapse. Shock, q.v.

circulatory failure. Failure of the cardiovascular system to provide body tissues with an adequate amount of blood for proper functioning. It may be caused by cardiac failure or peripheral circulatory failure, as occurs in shock, in which there is general peripheral vasodilation with "pooling" of blood in the expanded vascular space, resulting in decreased venous return.

circulatory overload. State of increased blood volume, usually due to transfusions that increase the venous pressure, esp. in patients with heart disease. This can result in heart failure, pulmonary edema, and cyanosis.

circulatory system. The cardiovascular system consisting of the heart and blood vessels (arteries, arterioles, capillaries, venules, veins, and sinuses) and the lymphatic system. SEE: *abdominal examination; apex beat; blood; chest; heart; lung; pulsation; pulse.*

INSPECTION: Inspection detects any abnormal centers of pulsation; the apex beat and its position, force, and extent; and any unnatural prominence over the precordial region.

circulus (sĕr′kū-lŭs) [L.]. Circle or ring.

circum- [L.]. Prefix meaning around, as circumduction.

circumanal. Around the anus.

circumarticular (sĕr″kŭm-ăr-tĭk′ū-lăr) [L. *circum,* around, + *articulus,* small joint]. Surrounding a joint. SYN: *periarthric.*

circumcision (sĕr″kŭm-sĭ′zhŭn) [L. *circumcisio,* a cutting around]. Surgical removal of the end of the prepuce of the penis. Circumcision is usually performed at the request of the parents. There are very few medical indications for this procedure.

NURSING IMPLICATIONS: The area should be kept clean and assessed for bleeding every hour for the first 12 hours postop. Apply gentle pressure to bleeding area with a folded gauze pad. If bleeding is not controlled, continue intermittent pressure, notify physician, and prepare for blood vessel

ligation. Sterile petroleum gauze is usually applied to the penis after circumcision and is left in place for 24 hours; it is replaced if it becomes dislodged before that time period is up. Wash penis gently at diaper change to remove urine and feces and reapply fresh sterile petroleum gauze. Do not attempt to remove dried, yellow exudate which forms in 24 hours and persists for 2 to 3 days. Cloth diapers may be recommended during the healing period (about one week). A plastic bell may be used to cover the glans and prevent hemorrhage and contamination, negating the need for petroleum gauze dressings. Avoid positioning the infant on the abdomen for the first few hours post procedure. Teach the family appropriate home care.

c., female. Partial or complete removal of the clitoris. Use of this procedure is widespread in Africa and in certain groups in the Middle and Far East. The surgery is usually performed on girls prior to puberty. The untoward results include infection, scarring that may prevent sexual intercourse, and death from excessive bleeding or postoperative shock due to lack of proper medical care. SEE: *infibulation.*

c., ritual. The religious rite performed by the Jews and Muslims at the time of removal of the prepuce.

circumclusion (sĕr″kŭm-klū′zhŭn) [L. *circumcludere,* to shut in]. Acupressure by use of a pin under an artery and a wire loop over it, attached to each end of the pin.

circumcorneal (sĕr″kŭm-kor′nē-ăl) [L. *circum,* around, + *corneus,* horny]. Around the cornea.

circumduction (sĕr″kŭm-dŭk′shŭn) [″ + *ducere,* to lead]. 1. The action or swing of a limb, such as the arm, in such a manner that it describes a cone-shaped figure, the apex of the cone being formed by the joint at the proximal end, while the complete circle is formed by the free distal end of the limb. 2. Circular movement of the eye.

circumference (sĕr-kŭm′fĕr-ĕns) [″ + *ferre,* to bear]. The perimeter of an object or body.

circumferential (sĕr″kŭm-fĕr-ĕn′shăl). 1. Encircling. 2. Concerning the periphery or circumference of an object or body.

circumflex (sĕr′kŭm-flĕks) [″ + *flectere,* to bend]. Winding around, as a vessel.

circuminsular (sĕr″kŭm-ĭn′sū-lăr) [″ + *insula,* island]. Surrounding the island of Reil in the cerebral cortex.

circumlental (sĕr″kŭm-lĕn′tăl) [″ + *lens,* lens]. Situated around the lens of the eye.

circumnuclear (sĕr″kŭm-nū′klē-ăr) [″ + *nucleus,* kernel]. Surrounding the nucleus.

circumocular (sĕr″kŭm-ŏk′ū-lăr) [″ +

oculus, eye]. Surrounding the eye.

circumoral (sĕr″kŭm-ō′răl) [L. *circum*, around, + *os*, mouth]. Encircling the mouth.

circumoral pallor. White area around the mouth contrasting vividly with color of face, seen esp. in scarlet fever.

circumorbital (sĕr″kŭm-or′bĭt-ăl) [″ + *orbita*, orbit]. Around an orbit.

circumpolarization (sĕr″kŭm-pō″lăr-ĭ-zā′shŭn) [″ + *polaris*, polar]. The rotation of a ray of polarized light.

circumrenal (sĕr″kŭm-rē′năl) [″ + *renalis*, pert. to kidney]. Around or about the kidney.

circumscribed (sĕr′kŭm-skrībd) [″ + *scribere*, to write]. Limited in space by that which is drawn around or confines an area.

circumstantiality (sĕr″kŭm-stăn″shē-ăl′ĭ-tē) [L. *circum*, around, + *stare*, to stand]. Disturbance in the associative thought and speech processes in which the patient digresses into unnecessary details and inappropriate thoughts prior to communicating the central idea. It is observed in schizophrenia, obsessional disturbances, and certain cases of dementia.

circumvallate (sĕr″kŭm-văl′āt) [″ + *vallare*, to wall]. Surrounded by a wall or raised structure.

circumvallate papillae. V-shaped row of papillae at base of tongue.

circumvascular (sĕr″kŭm-văs′kū-lăr) [″ + *vasculum*, vessel]. Perivascular; around a blood vessel.

cirrhosis (sĭ-rō′sĭs) [Gr. *kirrhos*, orange yellow, + *osis*, condition]. A chronic disease of the liver characterized by formation of dense perilobular connective tissue, degenerative changes in parenchymal cells, alteration in structure of the cords of liver lobules, fatty and cellular infiltration, and sometimes development of areas of regeneration. In addition to the clinical signs and symptoms inherent in the cause of the cirrhosis, those due to cirrhosis are the result of loss of functioning liver cells and increased resistance to flow of blood through the liver (portal hypertension). When severe enough, this leads to ammonia toxicity, q.v. SEE: *hepatic coma*.

ETIOL: May be due to various factors such as nutritional deficiency (lack of proteins, choline, or methionine), poisons (including alcohol, carbon tetrachloride, phosphorus), or previous inflammation caused by a virus or bacterium. SEE: *esophageal varices; liver; liver flap; Müller maneuver*.

TREAT: Therapy depends upon the cause and severity of the disease.

NURSING IMPLICATIONS: Assess patient for anorexia, indigestion, nausea and vomiting, constipation or diarrhea, dull abdominal aching pain; for bleeding tendencies and hemorrhage from esophageal varices; for "mousy" breath, pruritus, extreme skin dryness, poor tissue turgor, abnormal pigmentation, spider angiomas, palmar erythema, and jaundice. Also assess for symptoms of progressive hepatic encephalopathy, including lethargy, behavioral or personality changes, slurred speech, asterixis, i.e., "liver flap," peripheral neuritis, paranoia, hallucinations, mental dullness, and coma. Patient may also show limited thoracic expansion related to hepatomegaly or ascites, and endocrine changes such as menstrual irregularities, testicular atrophy, gynecomastia, and loss of chest and axillary hair. Monitor known bleeding site frequently, applying direct pressure to site if bleeding occurs. Weigh the patient daily and measure abdominal girth to monitor ascites, also assess ankles and sacrum for dependent edema. Prevent edema and pruritus-associated skin breakdown by eliminating soaps and using lubricating oils or lotions for bathing. Gently and frequently reposition patient to maintain skin integrity and improve ventilatory function. Teach patient to avoid straining at stool and violent sneezing or nose-blowing, to use a soft toothbrush or sponge-stick for oral care, and, for men, use an electric razor for shaving. No aspirin or aspirin products should be used, the patient should take no over-the-counter drugs without the physician's knowledge and consent, and alcohol may not be ingested. Refer patient and close associates to available alcohol cessation groups such as Alcoholics Anonymous, Al-anon, and Al-ateen. Teach patient about and carry out prescribed therapies, including sodium and fluid restriction, dietary variations, supplemental vitamin therapy, antiemetics, and diuretics, evaluating response and assessing for adverse affects. Administer albumin and assist with paracentesis if prescribed; also prepare patient physically and psychologically for required surgical procedures. Assist patient to adjust to regimen of moderate exercise alternating with periods of rest, and warn against exposure to infections. SEE: *Nursing Diagnoses* in *Appendix*.

   c., **alcoholic.** Cirrhosis occurring in persons who are chronic alcoholics. Approx. 20% of chronic alcoholics develop cirrhosis.

   c., **atrophic.** Cirrhosis in which the liver is decreased in size.

   c., **biliary.** Cirrhosis marked by prolonged jaundice due to chronic retention of bile and inflammation of bile ducts. SEE: *c., obstructive biliary; c., primary biliary*.

   c., **cardiac.** Congestive cirrhosis resulting from passive congestion of the liver due to congestive heart failure.

c., fatty. Cirrhosis with fatty infiltration of the liver cells.

c., hypertrophic. Cirrhosis in which the connective tissue hyperplasia causes the liver to be greatly enlarged.

c., infantile. Cirrhosis occurring in childhood resulting from protein malnutrition. SEE: *kwashiorkor.*

c., macronodular. Cirrhosis characterized by large irregular regenerating nodules and broad bands of fibrous tissue. These areas contain portal spaces and terminal hepatic veins. Seen following viral and idiopathic hepatitis. Formerly termed postnecrotic or posthepatic cirrhosis.

c., metabolic. Cirrhosis due to metabolic disease such as hemochromatosis, glycogen storage disease, or Wilson's disease.

c., micronodular. Cirrhosis characterized by thin bands of fibrotic tissue and small nodules of regeneration. Previously termed portal or Laennec's cirrhosis. SYN: *c., alcoholic.*

c., obstructive biliary. Cirrhosis resulting from obstruction of the common duct by a stone or tumor.

c., primary biliary. A rare, progressive form of cirrhosis characterized by enlargement of the liver, jaundice and pruritus.

c., syphilitic. Cirrhosis occurring in tertiary syphilis, in which gummas form in the liver and, on healing, cause coarse lobulation.

c., toxic. Cirrhosis resulting from toxic substances as in poisoning by carbon tetrachloride or phosphorus.

c., zooparasitic. Cirrhosis resulting from infestation with animal parasites, esp. blood flukes of the genus *Schistosoma,* or liver flukes, *Clonorchis sinensis.*

cirrhotic (sĭ-rŏt'ĭk). Pert. to or affected with cirrhosis.

cirsectomy (sĕr-sĕk'tō-mē) [Gr. *kirsos,* varix, + *ektome,* excision]. Excision of a portion of a varicose vein.

cirsoid (sĕr'soyd) [" + *eidos,* form, shape]. Resembling a varix. SYN: *varicose.*

cirsomphalos (sĕr-sŏm'fä-lŏs) [" + *omphalos,* navel]. Varicose veins around the navel.

cirsotome (sĕr'sō-tōm) [" + *tome,* incision]. Instrument for cutting varicose veins.

cirsotomy (sĕr-sŏt'ō-mē). Treatment of a varicosity by multiple incisions.

C.I.S. *central inhibitory state.*

cis (sĭs) [L., on the same side]. In organic chemistry, a form of isomerism in which similar atoms or radicals are on the same side. In genetics, a prefix meaning the location of two or more genes on the same chro-

mosome of a homologous pair.

cisplatin (sĭs'plă-tĭn). An antineoplastic chemical used in treating testicular tumors and ovarian cancer. The drug's nephrotoxicity may be almost eliminated by ensuring a diuresis of 150 ml/hr. when the drug is administered.

cissa (sĭs'ă) [Gr. *kissa*]. Pica. Abnormal craving to eat inedible materials.

cistern (sĭs'tĕrn). A reservoir for storage of fluid.

cisterna [L.] (pl. *cisternae*). [NA] A reservoir or cavity.

c. chyli. [NA] A dilated sac into which empties the intestinal, two lumbar, and two descending lymphatic trunks; the origin of the thoracic duct. SYN: *receptaculum chyli.*

c. subarachnoidalis. [NA] A wide space in the cranial cavity between the arachnoid and the pia mater. It contains cerebrospinal fluid.

cisternal (sĭs-tĕr'năl). Concerning a cavity filled with fluid.

cisternal puncture. A spinal puncture with a hollow needle between the cervical vertebrae, through the dura mater into the cisterna at the base of the brain.

PURPOSE: To inject a drug or a serum as in cerebral meningitis or cerebral syphilis; to remove spinal fluid for diagnostic purposes, or to reduce intracranial pressure. Should be used as a source of spinal fluid only if fluid cannot be obtained by lumbar puncture. SEE: *cerebrospinal fluid; spinal puncture.*

cisvestitism (sĭs-vĕs'tĭ-tĭzm) [L. *cis,* on the same side, + *vestitus,* dressed, + Gr. *-ismos,* condition]. Wearing of clothes appropriate to one's sex but suitable for a calling or profession other than one's own.

Ex.: A civilian who dresses in a uniform of the armed services.

Citanest. Trade name for prilocaine hydrochloride.

Citelli's syndrome (chē-tĕl'ēz) [Salvatore Citelli, It. laryngologist, 1875–1947]. Insomnia or drowsiness, and lack of concentration associated with intelligence disorders, seen in children with infected adenoids or sphenoid sinusitis.

citrate (sĭt'rāt, sī'trāt). Compound of citric acid and a base.

citrated (sĭt'rāt-ĕd). Combined or mixed with citric acid or a citrate.

citrate solution. Solution used to prevent clotting of the blood. Its use permits whole blood to be stored in a refrigerator until it is needed for transfusion.

citric acid. USP. $C_6H_8O_7$. A tribasic acid present in the juice of many fruits, esp. citrus fruits. SEE: *acid, citric.*

citric acid cycle. A complicated series of reactions in the body involving the oxidative metabolism of pyruvic acid and liberation of energy. It is the main pathway of terminal oxidation in the process of which not only carbohydrates but proteins and fats are utilized. SYN: *Krebs cycle; tricarboxylic acid cycle.* SEE: *Krebs cycle* for illus.

citronella (sĭt″rŏn-ĕl′ă). Volatile oil obtained from *Cymbopogon citratus,* lemongrass. Used in perfumes and as an insect repellent. It contains geraniol and citronellal.

citrovorum factor. Folic acid, q.v.

citrulline (sĭt-rŭl′lĭn). An amino acid, $C_6H_{13}N_3O_3$, formed from ornithine. It is present in watermelons.

citrullinemia (sĭt-rŭl″lĭ-nē′mē-ă). A type of aminoaciduria accompanied by increased amounts of citrulline in the blood, urine, and spinal fluid. Clinically, there will be ammonia intoxication, liver disease, vomiting, mental retardation, convulsions, and failure to thrive.

citrullinuria (sĭt-rŭl″lĭ-nū′rē-ă). Increased amount of citrulline in the urine.

Cl. 1. Chem. symb. for the element chlorine. 2. *chloride; clavicle; Clostridium.*

cladosporiosis (klăd″ō-spō-rē-ō′sĭs) [Gr. *klados,* branch, + *sporos,* seed, + *osis,* condition]. A general term for an infection, usually of the central nervous system, due to the fungus *Cladosporium.*

Cladosporium. A genus of fungi. The condition tinea nigra is caused by either *C. werneckii* or *C. mansonii.*

clairvoyance (klăr-voy′ăns) [Fr.]. Alleged ability to be aware of events that occur at a distance without receiving any sort of sensory information concerning the events.

clamp (klămp) [MD. *klampe,* metal clasp]. Device used in surgery to grasp, join, compress, or support an organ, tissue, or vessel.

    c., rubber-dam. An attachment that fits on the cervical part of the tooth for retention of a rubber-dam. SEE: *rubber-dam.*

clang [L. *clangere,* to peal]. 1. A loud, metallic sound. 2. In psychiatry, clang association is speech directed by the sound of words, as in combining words that rhyme, rather than using appropriate ones.

clap. Colloquial term for gonorrhea.

clapotage, clapotement (klă″pō-tăzh′, klă-pŏt-maw′) [Fr.]. Any splashing sound in succussion of a dilated stomach.

clapping (klăp′ĭng). Percussion of the chest to loosen secretions. The hand is used in a cupped position. Also called cupping or tapping.

Clapton's lines. Green lines on dental margin of gums in copper poisoning.

Clara cells [Max Clara, Austrian anatomist, b. 1899]. Secreting cells in the surface epithelium of the bronchioles. The cells, along with goblet cells, provide secretions for the respiratory tract. The secretion is a mucuspoor protein that coats the epithelium.

clarificant (klăr-ĭf′ĭk-ănt) [L. *clarus,* clear, + *facere,* to make]. Any agent that clears the turbidity of a liquid.

clarification (klăr″ĭ-fĭ-kā′shŭn). 1. Making a solution free of turbidity. 2. In psychiatry, a technique used to help a patient recognize inconsistencies in his or her statements.

Clark's rule. A method of calculating pediatric drug dosages. The weight of the child in pounds is multiplied by the adult dose and the result is divided by 150. SEE: *dosage.*

Clarke, Jacob A. L. British anatomist, 1817–1880.

    C.'s bodies. Alveolar sarcomatous intranuclear bodies of breast.

    C.'s column. The dorsal nucleus of the spinal cord.

Clarke-Hadfield syndrome [Cecil Clarke, 20th century Brit. physician; Geoffrey John Hadfield, Brit. pathologist, 1899–1968]. Infantilism caused by pancreatic insufficiency. A child suffering from this syndrome is underweight and fails to grow.

clasmatodendrosis (klăz-măt″ō-dĕn-drō′sĭs) [Gr. *klasma,* fragment, + *dendron,* tree, + *osis,* condition]. A breaking up of astrocytic protoplasmic expansions.

clasmatosis (klăz″mă-tō′sĭs) [″ + *osis,* condition]. Crumbling into small bits; fragmentation, as of cells.

clasp (klăsp). A device for holding objects or tissues together. In dentistry, a variety of wire or metal retainers or attachments to stabilize dentures or prosthetic devices in the mouth.

clasp-knife phenomenon. Increased resistance in muscle to passive movement of a joint followed by a sudden letting go of the muscle; commonly seen in patients with spasticity.

class [L. *classis,* division]. 1. In biology, a taxonomic group of clearly defined animals or plants classified below a phylum and above an order. 2. In statistics, a group of variables that fall within certain value limits.

classification (klăs″sĭ-fĭ-kā′shŭn). The orderly separation of a group of similar organisms, animals, or individuals into classes according to traits or characteristics that are common to each class or group.

    c., Dukes [Cuthbert E. Dukes, Brit. physician, 1890–1977]. A system of classifying the extent of spread of adenocarcinoma of the colon or rectum.

    c., plant or animal. Plant kingdom is divided as: kingdom, division, class, natural order, and genus. The animal kingdom is divided as: kingdom, subkingdom, phylum, class, order, family (including species), and genus. The names of class categories are Latinized. SEE: *taxonomy.*

clastic (klăs′tĭk) [Gr. *klastos,* broken]. Causing division into parts.

clastogenic (klăs′tō-jĕn″ĭc) [″ + *gennan,* to produce]. Capable of breaking chromosomes, e.g., agents that cause chromosomal abnormalities.

clastothrix (klăs′tō-thrĭks) [″ + *thrix,* hair]. Splitting of the hair. SYN: *trichorrhexis nodosa.*

Claude's syndrome (klawdz) [Henri Claude, Fr. psychiatrist, 1869–1945]. Paralysis of the third cranial nerve, contralateral ataxia and tremor. Caused by a lesion in the red nucleus of the brain.

claudication (klaw-dĭ-kā′shŭn) [L. *claudicare,* to limp]. Lameness; limping.

   c., intermittent. A severe pain in calf muscles occurring during walking but that subsides with rest. It results from inadequate blood supply, which may be due to arterial spasm, atherosclerosis, arteriosclerosis obliterans, or an occlusion of an artery to the limb. This symptom, which occurs more frequently in men than women, is reported to be present in 1.8% of the population under 60 years of age, in 3.7% of those aged 60 to 70, and in 5.2% of those over 70 years of age. Prognosis is favorable in that the condition becomes stable or improves in the majority of patients. Thus, conservative therapy is advisable. Exercise in the form of walking is helpful in increasing the distance that can be walked without experiencing symptoms.

   c., venous. Claudication resulting from inadequate venous drainage.

Claudius' cells (klaw′dē-ŭs) [Friedrich Claudius, Austrian anatomist, 1822–1869]. Large columnar cells external to the organ of Corti.

Claudius' fossa. Small depression in posterior part of pelvis, on either side, in which lies the ovary.

claustrophilia (klaws-trō-fĭl′ē-ă) [L. *claustrum,* a barrier, + Gr. *philein,* to love]. Dread of being in an open space; a morbid desire to be shut in with doors and windows closed.

claustrophobia (klaws-trō-fō′bē-ă) [″ + Gr. *phobos,* fear]. Fear of being confined in any space, as in a locked room; a simple phobia.

claustrum (klŏs′trŭm) [L.]. 1. A barrier. 2. Thin layer of gray matter separating the external capsule of the brain from the island of Reil.

clausura (klaw-sū′ră) [L.]. Atresia of a passage.

clava (klā′vă) [L., club] (pl. *clavae*). An elevation on dorsal surface of the medulla oblon-

gata caused by the underlying nucleus gracilis, the superior extremity of the fasciculus gracilis.

clavate (klā′vāt). Club-shaped.

clavicle (klăv′ĭ-k′l) [L. *clavicula,* little key]. The collarbone; a bone, curved like the letter *f,* that articulates with the sternum and the scapula.

   c., dislocation of. Forward, sternal end: TREAT: Procedure will be done by emergency care physician or orthopedist. Place knee against spine and draw shoulders back; apply clavicle bandage with pad on dislocated end of bone.

   Outer extremity: Bone upon upper surface of acromion or upon anterior part of spine of the scapula.

   SYM: Prominence upon surface of acromion that disappears when arm is raised. Shoulders flattened, arm hanging close to trunk.

   TREAT: Procedure will be done by emergency care physician or orthopedist. Raise shoulder, draw backward; place pad in axilla, bringing elbow close to side; secure arm and forearm to chest with pad in axilla; pressure by pad and gutta percha plate on projecting clavicle strapped in place.

   c., fracture of. SYM: Swelling, pain, protuberance with sharp depression over the injured bone. Patient holds the immobile arm by supporting it at the elbow.

   TREAT: Procedure will be done by emergency care physician or orthopedist. Have assistant draw arms and shoulders backward. Raise shoulders and support in upward, backward, and outward direction. Maintain position by clavicle strap or figure-of-eight wrap between the shoulders and over the back.

   F.A.: Place ball of cloth or one or two handkerchiefs, tightly rolled, under armpit. Apply arm sling; bandage elbow to side, hand and forearm extending across the chest. Or lay patient on back on the floor with rolled-up blanket under shoulders until medical aid arrives. This position keeps shoulders back and prevents broken ends of bone from rubbing.

clavicotomy (klăv″ĭ-kŏt′ō-mē) [″ + Gr. *tome,* incision]. Surgical division of the clavicle.

clavicular (klă-vĭk′ū-lăr). Pert. to the clavicle.

clavus (klā′vŭs) [L., nail]. A corn or callosity.

   c. hystericus. A sharp pain in the head described as feeling like a nail being driven into it.

clawfoot. A deformity of the foot characterized by excessively high longitudinal arch, usually accompanied by dorsal contracture of toes. SYN: *pes cavus.*

clawhand. A hand characterized by hyperextension of the proximal phalanges of the digits and extreme flexion of middle and distal phalanges. Usually the result of injury to ulnar and median nerves. SYN: *main en griffe.*

claw toe. A toe with dorsal flexion of 1st phalanx and plantar flexion of 2nd and 3rd phalanges. SYN: *hammertoe.*

Clayton gas. Sulfur dioxide; used to fumigate ships.

clean-catch method. Procedure for obtaining a urine specimen in order to obtain a sample for culture that will have minimal chance of being contaminated. For females, while the labia are held apart, the periurethral area is cleaned with a mild soap or antibacterial solution, rinsed with copious amounts of plain water, and then, with the labia still held apart, the area is dried, front-to-back, with a dry gauze pad, the urine is passed, and the specimen is collected in a sterile container. It is important that the labia be held apart and that the urine flows directly into the container without touching the skin. It is preferable that the sample be obtained after the urine flow is well established, i.e., a midstream specimen. For males, cleanse the urethral meatus and obtain the midstream specimen in a sterile container. If the male is uncircumcised, be certain that the foreskin is retracted prior to cleansing the penis.

cleaning, ultrasonic. Use of high-frequency vibrations to clean instruments.

clean room. A type of controlled environment facility in which all incoming air passes through a filter capable of removing 99.97% of all particles 0.3 microns and larger. The temperature, pressure, and humidity in the room are controlled. Clean rooms are used in research and in controlling infections, especially for persons who may not have normally functioning immune systems.

Ex.: Individuals who have been treated with drugs that prevent immune response as part of the therapeutic preparation for transplantation of an organ.

In very rare instances a child is born without the ability to develop the immune system. Such children are kept in a clean room while waiting for specific therapy such as bone marrow transplantation. Alternatively, these children may be kept in a suit that completely isolates them from physical contact with the environment but allows them to be mobile. The suit, sometimes called a "space bubble," is attached to filtering devices needed to screen the air supplied to the child.

clearance. The elimination of a substance from the blood plasma by the kidneys. SEE: *renal clearance test.*

clearing agent. Substance that makes tissues prepared for microscopic examination more transparent.

cleavage (klē′vĕj) [AS. *cleofian,* to cleave]. 1. Splitting a complex molecule into two or more simpler ones. 2. Cell division following the fertilization of an egg. SYN: *segmentation.*

cleavage cell. The blastomere.

cleavage lines. Lines indicating the prevailing direction of fibers in the corium of the skin. In a living subject or fresh cadaver, a puncture wound does not remain round but becomes elliptical in the direction of the fibers. Lines in general run obliquely. This is important to the surgeon because an incision parallel to these lines will heal with much less scarring than one across the lines. SYN: *Langer's lines.* SEE: *Langer's lines* for illus.

cleft (klĕft) [ME. *clift,* crevice]. 1. A fissure or elongated opening. 2. Divided or split.

 c., alveolar. An anomaly resulting from lack of fusion between the medial nasal process and the maxillary process. Cleft maxillary alveolar process is usually associated with cleft lip and palate, or both.

 c., branchial. An opening between the branchial arches of an embryo. In lower vertebrates it becomes a gill cleft.

 c., facial. An anomaly resulting from failure of facial processes of embryo to fuse. Common ones are oblique facial cleft, an open nasolacrimal furrow extending from eye to lower portion of nose that is sometimes continuous with a cleft in upper lip, and transverse facial cleft, which extends laterally from the angle of the mouth.

cleft cheek. Transverse facial cleft. SYN: *macrostomia.*

cleft foot. A bipartite foot resulting from failure of a digit and its corresponding metatarsal to develop.

cleft hand. A bipartite hand resulting from failure of a digit and its corresponding metacarpal to develop.

cleft lip. Harelip. A congenital cleft or separation of the upper lip. May be associated with cleft palate.

cleft palate. A congenital fissure in the roof of the mouth forming a communicating passageway between mouth and nasal cavities. May be unilateral or bilateral and complete or incomplete.

cleft sternum. A congenital fissure of the breastbone.

cleft tongue. A bifid tongue; one with a separated tip.

cleido- (klī′dō) [L. *clavis,* key]. Prefix pert. to the clavicle.

cleidocostal (klī″dō-kŏs′tăl) [″ + *costa,* rib]. Concerning the clavicle and ribs.

cleidorrhexis (klī″dō-rĕk′sĭs) [″ + Gr. *rhexis,* rupture]. Fracture or bending of the clavicles of the fetus for delivery.

cleidotomy (klī-dŏt′ō-mē) [″ + Gr. *tome,* incision]. Dividing a fetal clavicle to facilitate delivery.

clemastine fumarate (klĕm′ăs-tēn). USP. An antihistamine drug. Trade name is Tavist.

clenching (klĕnch′ĭng). With the teeth in contact, forcible, repeated contraction of the jaw muscles. This causes pulsating and bilateral contractions of the temporalis and pterygomasseteric muscles. This may be done consciously, subconsciously while awake, or during sleep. SEE: *bruxism.*

cleptomania (klĕp″tō-mā′nē-ă). Kleptomania. Impulsive stealing in which the motive is not related to the intrinsic value of the stolen article. There is often deep regret following the act.

click (klĭk). 1. An abrupt and brief sound heard in listening to the heart sounds. 2. Any brief sound but esp. one heard during a joint movement.

clidinium bromide (klī-dĭn′ē-ŭm). USP. A drug used in treating peptic ulcers and other conditions wherein it is desirable to inhibit the action of the parasympathetic nervous system. Trade name is Quarzan.

client. The patient of a health care professional.

climacteric (klī-măk′tĕr-ĭk, klī-măk-tĕr′ĭk) [Gr. *klimakter,* a rung of a ladder]. The period that marks the cessation of a woman's reproductive ability (female climacteric or menopause); a corresponding period of lessening of sexual activity in the male (male climacteric).

climatology, medical [Gr. *klima,* sloping surface of the earth, + *logos,* word, reason]. Branch of meteorology that includes the study of climate and its relationship to disease. SEE: *bioclimatology.*

climatotherapy (klī″măt-ō-thĕr′ăp-ē) [″ + *therapeia,* treatment]. Treatment of disease by having patient move to a more favorable climate.

climax (klī′măks) [Gr. *klimax,* ladder]. 1. Period of greatest intensity. 2. The sexual orgasm, q.v.

clindamycin hydrochloride (klĭn″dă-mī′sĭn). USP. An antibiotic effective against gram-positive cocci. At one time it was thought to have the side effect of causing colitis. It is now believed that the colitis that may develop during therapy with clindamycin is due to resistant strains of *Clostridium difficile.* Trade name is Cleocin HCl.

clinic (klĭn′ĭk) [Gr. *klinikos,* pert. to a bed]. 1. Medical and dental instruction in which patients are observed directly, symptoms noted, and treatments discussed. 2. A center for physical examination and treatment of ambulant patients who are not hospitalized. 3. A place where preliminary diagnosis is made and treatment given, as in an x-ray clinic, a dental clinic, or child-guidance clinic.

clinical. 1. Founded on actual observation and treatment of patients as distinguished from data or facts obtained by experimentation or pathology. 2. Pert. to a clinic.

clinical analysis. The chemical analysis and study of body fluids, excreta, and tissues in the diagnosis and treatment of disease.

clinical ecology. A form of medical practice based on two concepts: that a broad range of environmental chemicals and foods can be responsible for an illness in which an unlimited variety of symptoms occur in the absence of objective physical findings, pathological abnormalities, or specific, abnormal results of laboratory tests; and that the immune system is functionally depressed by many environmental chemicals. The disease termed environmental illness or a disease related to the mentioned environmental factors has also been known by other names, such as environmentally induced disease, chemical hypersensitivity syndrome, multiple chemical sensitivities, chemically induced immune dysregulation, twentieth century disease, total allergy syndrome, ecologic illness, and food and chemical sensitivity.

clinical judgment. The exercise of the clinician's experience and knowledge in diagnosing and treating illness and disease. SEE: *decision analysis.*

clinical pathology. Division of pathology that utilizes clinical analysis and other laboratory procedures in the diagnosis and treatment of disease.

clinical thermometer. Glass or electronic instrument that measures body temperature. The glass, nondisposable type may be disinfected by first cleansing with cotton and soap solution, using a rotary motion downward to bulb end. This removes adherent mucus, which coagulates in some disinfectants, thereby retaining organisms. Rinse thoroughly in tepid, not hot, water and submerge in 70% alcohol for 10 minutes. Rinse before use. SEE: *thermometer.*

clinical trial. A carefully designed and executed investigation of the effects of a drug administered to human subjects. The goal is to define the clinical efficacy and pharmacologic effects (toxicity, side effects, incompatibilities, or interactions) of the substance. The U.S. government requires strict testing of all new drugs prior to their approval for use as therapeutic agents. SEE: *double-blind technique; randomization.*

clinician (klĭn-ĭsh'ăn) [Gr. *klinikos,* pert. to a bed]. A health professional or nurse with expertise in clinical practice as distinguished from one specializing in research.

c., nurse. A nurse practitioner or clinician is a registered nurse with preparation in a specialized educational program. At present this preparation may be in the context of a formal continuing education program, a baccalaureate nursing program, or an advanced-degree nursing program. It is envisioned that in the future a nurse practitioner or clinician will be academically prepared at the baccalaureate or higher degree level. This preparation enables the nurse practitioner to provide nursing care as a primary health care provider in a variety of settings. Primary care provides health care to individual patients or groups of patients in order to maintain their health status and to prevent serious illness or disability. In any health care setting, the focus is mainly on the maintenance of wellness, the prevention of illness, and dealing with acute or chronic health problems. (Adapted from definition provided by the American Nurses' Association.)

clinicopathologic (klĭn''ĭ-kō-pă''thō-lŏj'ĭk). Concerning the clinical and pathological manifestations of a disease.

clinicopathological conference. ABBR: CPC. A teaching conference in which clinical findings are presented to a physician previously unfamiliar with a case, who then attempts to diagnose the disease that would explain the clinical findings. The exact diagnosis is then presented by the pathologist, who has either examined the tissue removed at surgery or has performed the autopsy. SEE: *medical grand rounds.*

clinocephaly (klī''nō-sĕf'ă-lē) [Gr. *klinein,* to bend, + *kephale,* head]. Congenital flatness or saddleshape of the top of the head. Caused by bilateral premature closure of the sphenoparietal sutures.

clinodactyly (klī''nō-dăk'tĭ-lē) ['' + *daktylos,* finger]. Permanent medial or lateral deflection of one or more fingers.

clinoid (klī'noyd) [Gr. *kline,* bed, + *eidos,* form, shape]. Resembling a bed in shape.

clinoid processes. Three pairs of prominences on upper surface of sphenoid bone.

clinometer (klī-nŏm'ĕ-tĕr) [Gr. *klinein,* to slope, + *metron,* measure]. Instrument for estimation of torsional deviation of eyes. Used to measure ocular muscle paralysis. SYN: *clinoscope.*

clinoscope (klī'nō-skōp) ['' + *skopein,* to examine]. Instrument for measuring the weakness of ocular muscles.

clinostatism (klī'no-stăt''ĭzm). The recumbent position.

clip. A metallic instrument for holding tissue or other material together.

cliseometer (klĭs''ē-ŏm'ĕt-ĕr) [Gr. *klisis,* inclination, + *metron,* measure]. Device for measuring the inclination that the pelvis makes with the spinal column.

Clistin. Trade name for carbinoxamine maleate.

clithrophobia (klĭth''rō-fō'bē-ä) [Gr. *kleithria,* keyhole, + *phobos,* fear]. Morbid fear of being locked in.

clition (klĭt'ē-ŏn) [Gr. *kleitys,* slope]. A craniometric point in center of highest part of the clivus on the sphenoid bone.

clitoridectomy (klī''tō-rĭd-ĕk'tō-mē) [Gr. *kleitoris,* clitoris, + *ektome,* excision]. Excision of clitoris.

clitoriditis (klī''tō-rĭd-ī'tĭs) ['' + *itis,* inflammation]. Inflammation of the clitoris.

clitoridotomy (klī''tō-rĭd-ŏt'ō-mē) ['' + *tome,* incision]. Incision of the clitoris; female circumcision.

clitoris (klī'tō-rĭs, klĭt'ō-rĭs) [Gr. *kleitoris*]. One of the structures of the female genitalia. It is a small erectile body located beneath the anterior labial commissure and partially hidden by the anterior portion of the labia minora. It is homologous to the penis of the male.

STRUCTURE: It consists of three parts: a body, two crura, and a glans. The body, about an inch (2.5 cm) long, consists of two fused corpora cavernosa. It extends from the pubic arch above to the glans below. The two crura are continuations of the corpora cavernosa and serve to attach them to the inferior rami of the pubic bones. They are covered by the ischiocavernosus muscles. The glans, which forms the free distal end, is a small rounded tubercle composed of erectile tissue. It is highly sensitive. The glans is usually covered by a hoodlike prepuce, and its ventral surface is attached to the frenulum of the labia.

clitoris crises. Involuntary attack of sexual excitement in women with tabes dorsalis.

clitorism (klī'tō-rĭzm). 1. The counterpart of priapism. A long-continued, painful condition in the female with recurring erection of the clitoris. 2. Enlargement of the clitoris.

clitoritis (klī''tō-rī'tĭs). Inflammation of the clitoris. SYN: *clitoriditis.*

clitoromegaly (klī''tō-rō-mĕg'ă-lē) ['' + *megas,* large]. Enlargement of the clitoris. May be caused by an endocrine disease, or by use of anabolic steroids by female athletes.

clivus (klī'vŭs) [L., a slope]. A surface that slopes, as the sphenoid bone.

c. blumenbachii. The slope at the base of the skull.

clo. A unit for thermal insulation of clothing. The amount of insulation necessary to maintain comfort in a sitting-resting subject in a normally ventilated room (air movement at the rate of 10 cm/second) at a temperature of 70°F (21°C) with relative humidity of less than 50%.

cloaca (klō-ā′kǎ) [L. *cloaca*, a sewer]. 1. Cavity lined with endoderm at the posterior end of the body that serves as a common passageway for urinary, digestive, and reproductive ducts. Present in adult birds, reptiles, and amphibia, and in the embryos of all vertebrates. 2. An opening in the sheath covering necrosed bone.

clobetasol propionate. A high-potency topical corticosteroid; used for short-term treatment to cortisone-responsive dermatoses.

clock [LL. *clocca*]. Device for measuring time.

c., biological. An internal system in organisms that regulates behavior in a rhythmic manner. Functions such as growth, feeding, the wake-sleep cycle, the menstrual cycle, and reproduction coincide with certain external events such as day and night, the tides, and the seasons. Biological clocks appear to be set by environmental conditions in some animals, but if they are isolated from their environment they continue to function according to the usual rhythm. A gradual change in environment does produce a gradual change in the timing of the biological clocks. SEE: *night work, maladaptation to.*

clofazimine (klō-fǎ′zǐ-mēn). A drug used in treating patients with leprosy who are resistant to the sulfones.

clofibrate (klō-fī′brāt). USP. Drug used to reduce plasma concentration of lipids. Used in treating hyperlipoproteinemias, q.v., types III, IV, and V. Trade name is Atromid-S.

Clomid. Trade name for clomiphene citrate.

clomiphene citrate (klō′mĭ-fēn). USP. A nonsteroidal agent used to stimulate ovulation in women who have potentially functioning pituitary and ovarian systems. Women treated with this medicine who become pregnant have an increased incidence of multiple births. Trade name is Clomid.

clonal (klōn′ǎl). Concerning a clone, q.v.

clonazepam (klō-nǎz′ē-pǎm). USP. An anticonvulsant drug. Trade name is Klonopin.

clone (klōn) [Gr. *klon*, a cutting used for propagation]. 1. In microbiology, the asexual progeny of a single cell. 2. A group of plants propagated from one seedling or stock. Members of the group are identical in character but do not reproduce from seed. 3. In tissue culture, a group of cells descended from a single cell.

clonic (klŏn′ĭk) [Gr. *klonos*, turmoil]. Pert. to clonus; alternate contraction and relaxation of muscles.

clonicity (klŏn-ĭs′ĭ-tē). Condition of being clonic.

clonicotonic (klŏn″ĭ-kō-tŏn′ĭk) [Gr. *klonos*, turmoil, + *tonikos*, tonic]. Both clonic and tonic, as some forms of muscular spasm.

clonic spasm. Spasm marked by muscular rigidity and then relaxation.

clonidine hydrochloride (klō′nĭ-dēn). USP. An antihypertensive drug. Trade name is Catapres.

clonism, clonismus (klŏn′ĭzm, klō-nĭz′mŭs) [″ + *-ismos*, condition of]. Condition of being affected with clonic spasms, or a succession of them.

clonograph (klŏn′ō-grǎf). Device for recording spasmodic contractions and movements.

clonorchiasis (klō″nor-kī′ǎ-sĭs). A disease of the Orient due to the Chinese liver fluke, *Clonorchis sinensis*, which infects the bile ducts of man. Infection occurs when one eats uncooked freshwater fish containing encysted larvae. Early symptoms are loss of appetite and diarrhea; later there may be signs of cirrhosis of the liver. The disease may be prevented by thoroughly cooking fish, or by freezing it at −10°C (14°F) for a minimum of 5 days. The disease rarely causes death, but it may last for 30 years.
TREAT: Praziquantel is effective.

Clonorchis sinensis (klō-nor′kĭs sī-nĕn′sĭs). The trematode fluke, Chinese liver fluke. An important cause of disease, esp. in the Orient. SEE: *clonorchiasis.*

clonospasm (klŏn′ō-spǎzm) [″ + *spasmos*, spasm]. Rapid alternation of muscular contraction and relaxation. The rate is much slower than a tremor. In upper motor neuron paralysis, sharp flexion of the ankle often produces ankle clonus.

clonus (klō′nŭs). Spasmodic alternation of muscular contractions between antagonistic muscle groups due to a hyperactive stretch reflex from an upper motor neuron lesion. Usually, sustained pressure or stretch of one of the muscles will inhibit the reflex.

Cloquet's canal (klō-kāz′) [Jules Germain Cloquet, Fr. surgeon, 1790–1883]. An irregular passage (hyaloid) through the center of the vitreous body in the fetus.

closed-packed position. The joint position where there is maximum congruency of the articular surfaces and where the ligaments and joint capsule usually are taut. Opposite of maximum loose-packed position.

Clostridium (klō-strĭd′ē-ŭm) [Gr. *kloster*, spindle]. A genus of bacteria belonging to the family Bacillaceae. They are anaerobic, spore-forming rods and are widely distributed in nature; over 250 species are recognized. They are common in the soil and in the intestinal tract of man and animals and are frequently found in wound infections. Several are pathogenic in man, being the primary causative agents for gas gangrene.

C. botulinum. Species that grows in improperly processed food. Produces a powerful toxin, the cause of botulism, q.v.

C. chauvoei. Causative organism for blackleg or symptomatic anthrax in cattle.

C. difficile. Species of bacteria, the toxin from which causes enterocolitis. Several antibiotics were at one time thought to cause a particular type of colitis. It was later demonstrated that *C. difficile* was the true cause.

C. histolyticum. A proteolytic organism found in feces and soil, isolated from necrotic war wounds and found in some cases of gas gangrene.

C. novyi. Species found in many cases of gas gangrene.

C. perfringens. Most common causative agent of gas gangrene. SYN: *gas bacillus.*

C. septicum. Species found in cases of gangrene in man, cattle, hogs, and other domestic animals.

C. sporogenes. Species frequently associated with other organisms in mixed gangrenous infections.

C. tetani. The causative organism of tetanus or lockjaw. Produces a powerful exotoxin, a portion of which affects nerve tissue; another portion is hemolytic.

C. welchii. *C. perfringens.*

closure (klō'shŭr). 1. Shutting or bringing together as in suturing together the edges of a laceration type of wound. 2. In psychotherapy, term used to represent the resolution of an issue that was a topic in therapy and a cause of distress for the patient.

clot (klŏt) [AS. *clott*, lump]. 1. A thrombus; a coagulum, as of blood or lymph. SEE: *blood, clotting of; coagulation factors; thrombosis.* 2. To coagulate.

c., agony. Clot formed in the heart when death ensues from prolonged heart failure.

c., antemortem. Clot formed in the heart or its cavities before death.

c., blood. Coagulum formed of blood.

c., chicken fat. Yellow-colored blood clot appearing to contain no erythrocytes.

c., currant jelly. Clot of fibrin of reddish color and jellylike consistency.

c., distal. Clot formed in a vessel on distal side of a ligature.

c., external. Clot formed outside a blood vessel.

c., heart. Clot within the heart.

c., internal. Clot formed by coagulation of blood within a vessel.

c., laminated. Clot formed in a succession of layers filling an aneurysm.

c., muscle. Clot formed in muscle tissue.

c., passive. Clot formed in the sac of an aneurysm.

c., plastic. Clot formed from the intima of an artery at the point of ligation.

c., postmortem. Clot formed in the heart or blood vessel after death.

c., proximal. Clot formed on the proximal side of a ligature.

c., stratified. Clot consisting of layers of different colors.

clothes louse. A body louse. SYN: *Pediculus humanus corporis.* SEE: *pediculosis corporis.*

clothing [AS. *clath*, cloth]. Wearing apparel. Used both functionally and decoratively. From the medical standpoint, clothes serve to conserve heat or to protect the body.

Ex.: gloves, sunhelmets, and shoes. Air spaces in a fabric conserve heat. It is texture, not the material alone, that conserves heat. Woolen fabrics lose in warmth when the material is matted down and the air spaces are destroyed. Wool and silk absorb more moisture than other fabrics, but silk loses it more readily. Cotton and linen come next, but linen loses moisture more quickly than cotton. Knitted fabrics absorb and dry more readily than woven fabrics of the same material. Temperature inside an individual's hat may vary from 13° to 20°F (7° to 11°C) warmer than the outside temperature. Body heat is increased when moisture from wet garments cannot escape. SEE: *clo.*

clotrimazole (klō-trĭm'ă-zōl). USP. An antifungal drug that is also used in treating vulvovaginal candidiasis. Intravaginal use occasionally causes burning, redness, and itching in either the patient, her sex partner, or both. Trade names are Gyne-Lotrimin, Mycelex G, and Lotrimin.

clotting. The formation of a jellylike substance from blood shed at the site of an injury to a blood vessel. This action usually halts blood flow from the wound. SEE: *coagulation, blood.*

clouding of consciousness. A state of mental confusion characterized by insufficiency of perception and impaired attention and resulting in loss of orientation of time and place, amnesia, and ill-adjusted reactions. Occurs in toxic, febrile, and other deliria as well as in cases where insufficient oxygen is being supplied to the brain. SEE: *consciousness.*

cloudy swelling. Microscopic appearance of tissues that have degenerated and become swollen.

cloven spine. Congenital defect of spinal

canal walls caused by lack of union between laminae of the vertebrae. SYN: *spina bifida*.

clove oil [L. *clavus*, a nail or spike]. A volatile oil distilled from the dried flower buds of the clove tree, *Eugenia caryophyllus*.

ACTION/USES: Antiseptic and aromatic. Also used to relieve pain in teeth. It is applied directly to the area.

clownism (klown'izm). Grotesque actions and attitudes, esp. those in certain hysterical states or in epilepsy.

cloxacillin sodium (klŏks″ă-sĭl'ĭn). USP. A penicillinase-resistant antibiotic. Trade names are Cloxapen and Tegopen.

Cloxapen. Trade name for cloxacillin sodium.

clozapine. A drug approved for use in treating schizophrenic patients who have failed to respond to standard antipsychotic drugs. This drug is less likely to produce restlessness or muscle stiffness than standard drugs. In about 8% of cases, the drug will have to be discontinued because of the development of side effects, such as grand mal seizures, sedation, orthostatic hypotension, leukopenia, or agranulocytosis. Trade name is Clozaril.

clubbing (klŭb'ĭng). A condition that affects the fingers and toes in many diseases of varying etiologies. The most outstanding feature of clubbing is a lateral and longitudinal curvature of the nails accompanied by soft tissue enlargement, presenting a bulbous, shiny appearance. Most commonly found in diseases of the lung, infective endocarditis, steatorrhea, and occasionally as a familial condition not associated with pathology. SEE: illus.

clubfoot. Congenital foot deformity. SEE: *talipes*.

clubhand. Deformity of the hand resembling clubfoot. SYN: *talipomanus*.

clue cells. Vaginal epithelial cells coated with coccobacillary organisms. The cells, which have a granular appearance, are seen in bacterial vaginosis. SEE: *bacterial vaginosis; Gardnerella vaginalis vaginitis*.

clump (klŭmp) [AS. *clympre*, a lump]. 1. A mass of bacteria in solution. May be caused by an agglutination reaction. 2. To gather together.

clumping [AS. *clympre*, a lump]. Thick grouping of microorganisms in a culture when specific immune serum is added. SYN: *agglutination*.

clunes (kloo'nēz) [L. pl. of *clunis*, buttock]. [NA] The buttocks; nates.

cluster. A closely grouped series of events or cases of a disease or other health-related phenomena with well-defined distribution patterns, in relation to time or place or both.

cluster headache. A headache similar to mi-

CLUBBING

CLUBBING

graine, occurring as often as two or three times each night over a period of weeks and usually 2 to 3 hours after falling asleep. After this cluster of headaches, the patient may be free of symptoms for weeks or months. Even though the headache may recur in association with stress, overwork, or emotional trauma, the etiology is unknown. SYN: *headache, histamine*.

SYM: The headaches come on abruptly and are characterized by intense throbbing pain behind the nostril and one eye. The eye and nose water, the skin over the throbbing area becomes red, and the pupil of the eye may become constricted. An attack rarely lasts longer than 2 hours.

TREAT: Ergotamine tartrate is effective in treating acute attacks, as is inhalation of oxygen at the rate of about 7 liters/min. Prevention may be accomplished by use of methysergide, prednisone, or lithium.

cluttering (klŭt'ĕr-ĭng). A speech defect characterized by omission of letters or syllables.

Clutton's joint [Henry Hugh Clutton, Brit. surgeon, 1850–1909]. Hydroarthrosis of the knee joint often associated with interstitial keratitis, seen in congenital syphilis.

clysis (klī'sĭs) [Gr. *klyzein*, to cleanse] (pl. *clyses*). Injection of fluid into the body other than orally. This may be done by injecting the fluid into tissue spaces, the rectum, or the abdominal cavity. Technique is used to inject fluids parenterally in situations where venipuncture is not possible.

clysma (klĭs'mă) [Gr. *klysma*, a drenching]. An enema.

clyster (klĭs'tĕr) [Gr. *klyster*, syringe]. An enema; a clysma.

C.M. *chirurgiae magister*, Master in Surgery.

Cm. Chem. symb. for the element curium.

cm. *centimeter*.

c/m. *counts per minute*.

cm². *square centimeter*.

cm³. *cubic centimeter*.

C.M.A. *Canadian Medical Association*.

CMI. *cell-mediated immunity*.

c/min. *counts per minute*.

c.mm. *cubic millimeter*.

CMRR. *common mode rejection ratio*. A term used to describe the ability of an amplifier to amplify a signal in the presence of electrical noise. The higher the number, the better the amplification.

CMT. *certified medical transcriptionist*. SEE: medical transcriptionist.

CN. *cyanogen*.

C.N.A. *Canadian Nurses' Association*.

cnemial (nē'mē-ăl). Pert. to the leg, esp. the shin.

cnemis (nē'mĭs) [Gr. *knemis*, legging]. Shin, lower leg, tibia.

cnemitis (nē-mī'tĭs) [" + *itis*, inflammation]. Inflammation of the tibia.

cnemoscoliosis (nē"mŏ-skŏ"lē-ō'sĭs) [" + *skoliosis*, curvature]. Lateral bending of the leg.

C.N.M. *certified nurse-midwife*.

CNS. *central nervous system; clinical nurse specialist*.

CO. Chem. formula for carbon monoxide; cardiac output.

CO₂. Chem. formula for carbon dioxide.

CO₂ therapy. 1. Therapeutic application of low temperatures with solid carbon dioxide. SEE: *cryotherapy; hypothermia* (def. 2). 2. Inhalation of carbon dioxide to stimulate breathing.

Co. Chem. symb. for the element cobalt.

CoA. Coenzyme A, q.v.

coacervate (kō-ăs'ĕr-vāt) [L. *coacervatus*, heaped up]. The formation of an aggregate in a solution that is about to emulsify or in an emulsion that is demulsifying.

coadaptation (kō"ăd-ăp-tā'shŭn). Mutual adaptation of two independent organisms, organs, or persons.

coadunation (kō"ăd-ū-nā'shŭn) [L. *co-*, together, + *ad*, to, + *unus*, one]. Union or junction of dissimilar substances in one uniform mass.

coagglutination (kō"ă-gloo"tĭn-ā'shŭn) [L.

coagulare, to curdle]. Clumping by an antigen and the homologous antibody of the corpuscles of another organism.

coagula (kō-ăg'ū-lă) [L.]. Pl. of coagulum.

coagulability (kō-ăg"ū-lă-bĭl'ĭ-tē). The condition of being capable of forming clots, esp. blood clots.

coagulable (kō-ăg'ū-lă-b'l). Capable of clotting; apt to clot.

coagulant (kō-ăg'ū-lănt) [L. *coagulans*, congealing]. 1. That which causes a fluid to coagulate. 2. Causing coagulation.

coagulase (kō-ăg'ū-lāz) [L. *coagulum*, blood clot]. Any enzyme, such as thrombin, that causes coagulation.

coagulate (kō-ăg'ū-lāt) [L. *coagulare*, to congeal]. To solidify or to change from a fluid state to a semisolid mass.

coagulated. Clotted or curdled.

coagulated proteins. Derived (insoluble) proteins, resulting from the action of alcohol on protein, or heat on protein solutions.

coagulation, blood (kō-ăg"ū-lā'shŭn) [L. *coagulatio*, clotting]. Coagulation of blood may occur in two pathways, depending upon the beginning of the process.

Extrinsic: Pathway (in an abbreviated outline form) requires the blood to be exposed to a subendothelial tissue factor originating outside the blood. This factor begins a complex pathway involving thromboplastin, factor VII, calcium, plus binding to factor X, leading to its conversion to factor Xa; and this acts to convert prothrombin to thrombin to fibrinogen and, eventually, fibrin.

Intrinsic: The intrinsic pathway (in abbreviated outline form) occurs when blood is drawn without contamination by tissue factor. This clotting pathway does not require an additive. It is triggered when the blood is exposed to a foreign surface and factor XII is activated. Factor XII may also be activated through limited cleavage by kallikrein. This process is accelerated by high molecular weight kininogen (HMWK). This leads to formation of factor XII, a process that produces more HMWK to accelerate the production of kallikrein. The process continues and factor XI, factor IX, and HMWK, in concert with calcium, generates factor Xa. The clotting cascade then continues, as in the extrinsic pathway, and prothrombin is converted to thrombin, which acts on fibrinogen to produce fibrin.

coagulation factors. A great number of terms have been applied to the various factors involved in the coagulation process. The generally accepted terms for the factors as well as their Roman numeral designation are provided here. In the past, factor VI, called accelerin, was used but is no longer employed.

Factor I, fibrinogen. *Factor II*, prothrombin. *Factor III*, tissue factor. *Factor IV*, calcium ions. *Factor V*, an unstable protein substance, proaccelerin, also called labile factor. *Factor VII*, proconvertin or serum prothrombin conversion accelerator. *Factor VIII*, antihemophilic factor. *Factor IX*, Christmas factor. *Factor X*, Stuart-Prower factor. *Factor XI*, plasma thromboplastin antecedent (PTA). *Factor XII*, Hageman or glass factor. *Factor XIII*, fibrin stabilizing factor (FSF). Prekallikrein, also called Fletcher factor. High molecular weight kininogen (HMWK), also called Fitzgerald, or Falujenc, or Williams factor, or contact activation cofactor.

coagulation time. The time required for a small amount of blood to coagulate. This can be determined by collecting blood in a small test tube and noting elapsed time from moment blood is shed to time it coagulates or by collecting blood in a small capillary tube and breaking off small pieces of the tube at 30-second intervals. Coagulation is indicated by the appearance of fine threads of fibrin between the broken ends of the tube. Normal time, using the capillary tube method, is 6 to 17 minutes.

coagulative (kō-ăg′ū-lā″tĭv). Causing coagulation.

coagulometer (kō-ăg″ū-lŏm′ĕt-ĕr) [L. *coagulare*, to congeal, + Gr. *metron*, measure]. Device for measuring the blood's coagulation time.

coagulopathy (kō-ăg″ū-lŏp′ă-thē) [″ + Gr. *pathos*, disease, suffering]. Defect in the blood clotting mechanisms. SEE: *coagulation, blood.*

c., consumption. Disseminated intravascular clotting.

coagulum (kō-ăg′ū-lŭm) [L.] (pl. *coagula*). 1. A blood clot. 2. A curd.

coalesce (kō-ăl-ĕs′) [L. *coalescere*]. To fuse; run or grow together.

coalescence (kō-ă-lĕs′ĕns). Fusion or growing together of two or more parts of bodies.

coal tar. USP. A tar that is produced in the destructive distillation of bituminous coal. Used as an ingredient of ointments for treating eczema and other skin diseases.

coal worker's pneumoconiosis. Form of pneumoconiosis in which carbon and silica accumulate in the lungs due to breathing coal dust. SYN: *black lung.*

coapt (kō′ăpt) [L. *coaptare*, to fit together]. To bring together, as in suturing a laceration.

coaptation (kō″ăp-tā′shŭn) [L. *coaptare*, to fit together]. The adjustment of separate parts to each other, as the edges of fractures.

coarctate (kō-ărk′tāt) [L. *coarctare*, to tighten]. To press or pressed together.

coarctation (kō″ărk-tā′shŭn). 1. Compression of the walls of a vessel. 2. Shriveling. 3. A stricture.

c. of aorta. Localized malformation resulting in narrowing of the aorta.

coarctotomy (kō″ărk-tŏt′ō-mē) [″ + Gr. *tome*, incision]. Cutting or division of a stricture.

coat [L. *cotta*, a tunic]. A covering or a layer in the wall of a tubular structure, as the inner coat (tunica intima), middle coat (tunica media), and outer coat (tunica adventitia) of an artery.

C.O.A.T.S. *Comprehensive Occupational Assessment and Training System.* A pretreatment test battery used to determine interests and abilities that may be used in the rehabilitation regimen of persons with disabilities.

Coats' disease [George Coats, Brit. ophthalmologist, 1876–1915]. Development of large white masses deep in the blood vessels of the retina. This term is now used to describe at least six separate retinal disorders.

cobalamin (kō-băl′ă-mĭn). Chemical that contains cobalt and is contained in all of the several B_{12} vitamins. SEE: *cyanocobalamin.*

cobalamin concentrate. USP. Medicine containing 500 mg of cobalamin in each gram. Used in treating vitamin B_{12} deficiency.

cobalt (kō′bălt). SYMB: Co. At. wt. 59.933; at. no. 27; sp. gr. 8.9. A gray, hard, ductile metal. Cobalt deficiency causes anemia in ruminants, but it has not been demonstrated in man. Cobalt is an essential element in vitamin B_{12}. Even though cobalt stimulates production of red blood cells, its use as a therapeutic agent is not advised. Overdose of cobalt in children may cause death. In adults it may cause anorexia, nausea, vomiting, deafness, and thyroid hyperplasia with resultant compression of the trachea.

cobalt-57. Radioactive isotope of cobalt with a half-life of 272 days.

cobalt-60. Radioactive isotope of cobalt. Used as a source of beta and gamma rays in treating malignancies. It has a half-life of 5.27 years.

cobra (kō′bră). Any one of a group of poisonous snakes native to parts of Africa and Asia. They all have the ability to expand their neck into a flattened hood.

cobra venom solution. Minute quantities of cobra venom in sterile physiological salt solution.

COBS. *cesarean-obtained barrier-sustained*; in reference to animals delivered sterilely by cesarean section and maintained in a germ-free environment.

coca (kō′kă). Dried leaves of the shrub *Erythroxylum coca*, from which several alkaloids, including cocaine, are obtained.

cocaine babies. Term applied to babies born with birth defects who were exposed to cocaine while in utero as a result of the mother's use of that drug. Scientific proof of this cause and effect relationship has been difficult to establish. Part of the reason is that cocaine-using mothers usually have other conditions that could contribute to the development of birth defects, i.e., poor nutrition, smoking, and abuse of alcohol and other drugs. It is known that cocaine crosses the placenta and enters the fetal circulation. In addition, use of cocaine by the father of the child at the time of conception may have a negative effect on sperm quality.

cocaine hydrochloride (kō-kān′, kō′kān). USP. The hydrochloride of an alkaloid obtained from the shrub *Erythroxylum coca*, native to Bolivia and Peru. The plant is cultivated extensively in South America. Cocaine is classed as a drug of abuse when used for nonmedical purposes. "Street" names for cocaine include snow; coke; crack; lady; flake; gold dust; green gold; blow; and toot.

USE: a topical anesthetic applied to mucous membranes. SEE: *crack; free base; freebasing.*

cocaine hydrochloride poisoning, acute. SYM: Initially it produces stimulation of the nervous system with excitement, incoherent talking, restlessness or hallucinations followed by tachycardia, dilated pupils, chills or fever, abdominal pain, vomiting and muscular spasms, irregular respiration, convulsions, coma, and death from respiratory arrest.

TREAT: Administer diazepam intravenously. Give emetic, then gastric lavage if drug was ingested. Succinyl choline if convulsions interfere with respiration. Treat hyperthermia. The hypermetabolic state along with ventricular arrhythmias has been managed with propranolol I.V. Artificial respiration and oxygen may be needed. If patient survives for three hours, prognosis is good.

SEE: *Nursing Diagnoses* in *Appendix.*

Caution: Do not administer morphine or opium derivatives.

---

cocainism (kō′kān-īzm). The habitual use of cocaine. SEE: *cocaine hydrochloride poisoning, acute.*

cocainization (kō″kān-ī-zā′shŭn). Inducing analgesia by use of cocaine.

cocainomania (kō″kān-ō-mā′nē-ă). Intense desire for cocaine and its effects.

cocarboxylase (kō″kăr-bŏk′sĭ-lās). Thiamine pyrophosphate, q.v.

cocarcinogen (kō-kăr′sĭ-nō-jĕn″). Some-

thing, either a chemical or environmental factor, that enhances the action of a carcinogen, the end result of which is the development of a malignancy.

coccal (kok′ăl). Concerning or caused by cocci.

cocci (kok′sī). Pl. of coccus.

Coccidia (kŏk-sĭd′ē-ă) [Gr. *kokkos*, berry]. An order of protozoa belonging to the class Sporozoa. All are intracellular parasites usually infecting epithelial cells of the intestine and associated glands. They are principally parasites of lower animals and cause great economic loss due to their toxic effect upon domestic and game animals. Only one species, *Isospora hominis,* infects humans. The geographic area of infestation is largely confined to the Far East.

coccidian (kŏk-sĭd′ē-ăn). 1. Concerning Coccidia. 2. Any member of the order Coccidia.

Coccidioides. A genus of fungi with but a single species, *Coccidioides immitis,* that is pathogenic for man. SEE: *coccidioidomycosis.*

coccidioidin (kŏk″sĭd-ē-oy′dĭn). USP. An antigenic substance prepared from *Coccidioides immitis.* Used as a skin test in diagnosing coccidioidomycosis.

coccidioidomycosis (kŏk-sĭd″ĭ-oyd-ō-mī-kō′sĭs) [″ + *eidos,* form, shape, + *mykes,* fungus, + *osis,* condition]. A coccidioidal granuloma. Exists in two forms: primary coccidioidomycosis, which is an acute self-limiting disease involving only the respiratory organs, and progressive coccidioidomycosis, a chronic, diffuse, granulomatous disease that may involve almost any part of the body. SYN: *desert rheumatism; granuloma, coccidioidal; valley fever.* SEE: *Nursing Diagnoses* in *Appendix.*

ETIOL: Caused by a pathogenic fungus, *Coccidioides immitis.*

TREAT: None is needed in the primary form of the disease. Amphotericin B is the only effective drug for the progressive granulomatous form. Ketoconazole is effective in suppressing symptoms and preventing progression of infection in patients with pulmonary or disseminated disease. It should not be used to replace Amphotericin B in patients with meningitis or those who are immunocompromised.

PROG: For the primary type, favorable; for the progressive type, grave, often fatal.

coccidiosis (kŏk-sĭd-ē-ō′sĭs) [″ + *osis,* condition]. Pathogenic condition resulting from infestation with coccidia. SEE: *Coccidia.*

coccobacilli (kŏk″ō-bă-sĭl′ī). Bacilli that are short and thick and somewhat ovoid in form. SEE: *bacteria* for illustration.

coccobacteria (kŏk″ō-băk-tē′rē-ă). 1.

Spherical-shaped bacteria. 2. Any kind of cocci.

coccogenous (kŏk-ŏj'ĕn-ŭs) [Gr. *kokkos*, berry, + *gennan*, to produce]. Produced by cocci.

coccoid (kŏk'oyd) [" + *eidos*, form, shape]. Resembling a micrococcus.

coccus (kŏk'ŭs) [Gr. *kokkos*, berry] (pl. *cocci*). A type of bacteria that is spherical or ovoid in form. When cocci appear singly, they are designated micrococci; in pairs, diplococci; in clusters like bunches of grapes, staphylococci; in chains, streptococci; in cubical packets of eight, sarcinae. Many are pathogenic, causing such diseases as septic sore throat, erysipelas, scarlet fever, rheumatic fever, pneumonia, gonorrhea, meningitis, and puerperal fever. SEE: *bacteria.*

coccyalgia, coccydynia (kŏk″sē-ăl'jē-ă, kŏk″sē-dĭn'ē-ă) [Gr. *kokkyx*, coccyx, + *algos*, pain; " + *odyne*, pain]. Pain in the coccyx.

coccygeal (kŏk-sĭj'ē-ăl). Pert. to or in the region of the coccyx.

coccygeal body. Small arteriovenous anastomosis at the level of the coccyx. It is associated with the median sacral artery.

coccygeal nerves. Lowest of spinal nerves; pair of nerves arising from the coccygeal section of the spinal cord and entering into the pudendal plexus.

coccygectomy (kŏk″sĭ-jĕk'tō-mē) [" + *ektome*, excision]. Excision of the coccyx.

coccygeus (kŏk-sĭj'ē-ŭs). Concerning the coccyx.

coccygodynia (kŏk-sī-gō-dĭn'ē-ă) [" + *odyne*, pain]. Pain in the coccygeal region. SYN: *coccyalgia; coccydynia.*

coccyx (kŏk'sĭks) [Gr. *kokkyx*, coccyx]. Small bone at the base of the spinal column in man, formed by four fused rudimentary vertebrae. Usually ankylosed and articulating with the sacrum above.

cochineal (kŏch'ĭn-ēl) [L. *coccinus*, scarlet]. Dried female insect of *Coccus cacti*, used as a dye in laboratory work.

cochlea (kŏk'lē-ă) [Gr. *kokhlos*, land snail]. A winding cone-shaped tube forming a portion of the inner ear. It contains the organ of Corti, the receptor for hearing.

The cochlea is coiled, resembling a snail shell, winding two and three-quarters turns about a central bony axis, the modiolus. Projecting outward from the modiolus is a thin bony plate, the spinal lamina, that partially divides the cochlear canal into an upper passageway, the scala vestibuli, and a lower one, the scala tympani. Lying between the two scalae is the cochlear duct, in the floor of which lies the spiral organ (of Corti). The base of the cochlea adjoins the vestibule. At the cupola or tip, the two scalae are joined at the helicotrema. SEE: illus.

cochlear (kŏk'lē-ăr). Pert. to the cochlea.

cochleare (kŏk″lē-ā'rē) [L., spoon]. Latin word used in writing prescriptions. Indicates a spoon or spoonful.

cochleariform (kŏk″lē-ăr'ĭ-form) [" + L. *forma*, shape]. Spoon-shaped.

cochlear implant. An experimental electrical device that receives sound and transmits the resulting electric signal to electrodes implanted in the cochlea of the ear. That signal stimulates the cochlea and the subject is able to perceive sound. Eventually the ability to perceive noise and the ability to understand speech should be possible through use of this device. SYN: *cochlear prosthesis.*

cochlear nerve. The division of the vestibulocochlear nerve (8th cranial nerve) that supplies the cochlea. SEE: *vestibulocochlear nerve.*

cochleitis (kŏk″lē-ī'tĭs) [Gr. *kokhlos*, land snail, + *itis*, inflammation]. Inflammation of the cochlea. SYN: *cochlitis.*

cochleo-orbicular reflex (kŏk″lē-ō-or-bĭk'ū-lăr). Contraction of orbicularis palpebrarum muscle resulting from sudden noise being produced near ear. SYN: *cochleopalpebral reflex.*

cochleopalpebral reflex (kŏk″lē-ō-păl'pĕ-brăl). Contraction of orbicularis palpebrarum muscle resulting from sudden noise being produced near ear. SYN: *cochleo-orbicular reflex.*

cochleovestibular (kŏk″lē-ō-vĕs-tĭb'ū-lăr) [" + L. *vestibulum*, vestibule]. Pert. to the cochlea and vestibule of the ear.

cochlitis (kŏk-lī'tĭs) [" + *itis*, inflammation]. Cochleitis; inflammation of the cochlea.

cockroach [Sp. *cucaracha*]. *Blatta orientalis*. A common insect belonging to the order Orthoptera that infests homes, and food handling and food storage places. They are swift-running omnivorous insects averaging about 2 cm in length, but may be winged and much larger. Through their dual contact with filth and food, they may mechanically transmit bacteria, protozoan cysts, and helminth ova. Common genera are *Blatta, Blatella,* and *Periplaneta.*

cocktail (kŏk'tāl). Any beverage containing several ingredients.

    c., lytic. Term that originated in France; a mixture of analgesic and phenothiazine derivatives used in anesthesia as a premedication.

cock-up splint. A static splint designed to maintain the wrist in either wrist extension or dorsal flexion.

cock-up toe. Toe deformity with dorsiflexion of the metatarsophalangeal joint and flex-

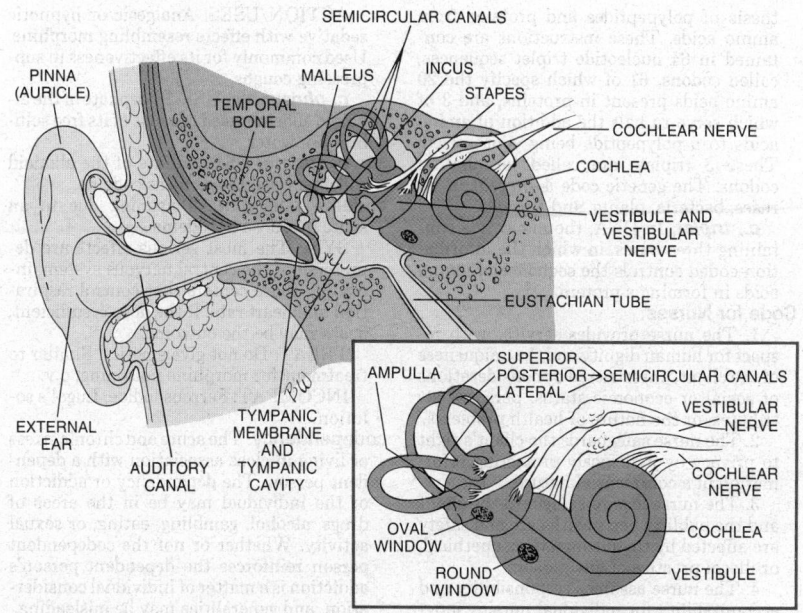

SEMICIRCULAR CANALS
MALLEUS
INCUS
STAPES
PINNA (AURICLE)
TEMPORAL BONE
COCHLEAR NERVE
COCHLEA
VESTIBULE AND VESTIBULAR NERVE
EUSTACHIAN TUBE
EXTERNAL EAR
TYMPANIC MEMBRANE AND TYMPANIC CAVITY
AUDITORY CANAL

AMPULLA
SUPERIOR
POSTERIOR SEMICIRCULAR CANALS
LATERAL
VESTIBULAR NERVE
COCHLEAR NERVE
OVAL WINDOW
COCHLEA
ROUND WINDOW
VESTIBULE

COCHLEA (IN RELATION TO THE INNER EAR AND OUTER AUDITORY APPARATUS)

ion of the interphalangeal and distal interphalangeal joints. SEE: *claw toe; hammertoe.*

cocoa butter. Theobroma oil. The fat obtained from the roasted seed of *Theobroma cacao.*

USES: As a base in suppositories and as a topical skin lubricant.

coconsciousness (kō-kŏn'shŭs-nĕs). Conscious states of which we are unaware because they are not in the focus of attention but are at the fringe of consciousness.

cocontraction (kō"kŏn-trăk'shŭn). Muscular state in which muscles around a joint or the spinal column contract simultaneously to provide stability.

coconut "water" [Sp. and Port. *coco,* coconut, + Eng. *nut*]. The liquid obtained from the unripe coconut. The composition of the "water" varies with the species of coconut, maturation of the fruit, and location where it was grown. Because the fluid is poor in sodium, chloride, and bicarbonate, and rich in potassium, calcium, and magnesium as compared with recommended oral rehydration solution (ORS), it is unsuitable for use in treating acute diarrhea.

Coco-Quinine. Trade name for quinine sul-

fate.

coctolabile (kŏk"tō-lā'bĭl) [L. *coctus,* cooked, + *labilis,* perishable]. Something that is altered or destroyed when heated to the temperature of boiling water.

coctoprecipitin (kŏk"tō-prē-sĭp'ĭt-ĭn) [" + *praecipitare,* to cast down]. A precipitin produced by injecting a serum that has been boiled.

coctostabile (kŏk"tō-stā'bĭl) [" + *stabilis,* resisting]. Incapable of being altered or destroyed by heating to the temperature of boiling water.

code (kōd). 1. A collection of rules and regulations or specifications. 2. A set of symbols for communicating information or for concealing the information from those not familiar with the true meaning of the symbols. 3. A form of coded message used in transmitting information in a hospital, esp. when the information is broadcast over a public address system, e.g., "code blue" or "code 9" could be used to indicate a particular type of emergency to an emergency care team. 4. A system of symbols that represents information contained in a computer data bank.

c., genetic. The instructions present in living cells that specify and control the synthesis of polypeptides and proteins from amino acids. These instructions are contained in 64 nucleotide triplet sequences, called codons, 61 of which specify the 20 amino acids present in proteins, and 3 of which serve to halt the addition of amino acids to a polypeptide being synthesized. These 3 triplets are called termination codons. The genetic code is present in viruses, bacteria, plants, and animals.

c., triplet. In DNA, the nucleotide containing three bases, in which the information coded controls the sequence of amino acids in forming a protein.

Code for Nurses.

1. The nurse provides services with respect for human dignity and the uniqueness of the client, unrestricted by considerations of social or economic status, personal attributes, or the nature of health problems.

2. The nurse safeguards the client's right to privacy by judiciously protecting information of a confidential nature.

3. The nurse acts to safeguard the client and the public when health care and safety are affected by the incompetent, unethical, or illegal practice of any person.

4. The nurse assumes responsibility and accountability for individual nursing judgments and actions.

5. The nurse maintains competence in nursing.

6. The nurse exercises informed judgment and uses individual competence and qualifications as criteria in seeking consultation, accepting responsibilities, and delegating nursing activities to others.

7. The nurse participates in activities that contribute to the ongoing development of the profession's body of knowledge.

8. The nurse participates in the profession's efforts to implement and improve standards of nursing.

9. The nurse participates in the profession's efforts to establish and maintain conditions of employment conducive to high quality nursing care.

10. The nurse participates in the profession's effort to protect the public from misinformation and misrepresentation and to maintain the integrity of nursing.

11. The nurse collaborates with members of the health professions and other citizens in promoting community and national efforts to meet the health needs of the public. [From Code for Nurses with Interpretive Statements, Kansas City, MO, American Nurses' Association, 1976]

codeine (kō'dēn) [Gr. *kodeia*, poppyhead]. USP. An alkaloid obtained from opium, or synthetically from morphine as methylmorphine.

ACTION/USES: Analgesic or hypnotic sedative with effects resembling morphine. Used commonly for its effectiveness in suppressing coughs.

c. phosphate. USP. Phosphate of the alkaloid codeine, used because of its free solubility in water.

c. sulfate. USP. Sulfate of the alkaloid codeine. Used the same as codeine.

codeine poisoning. Poisoning due to an acute overdose of codeine.

SYM: The most serious effects are depression of the central nervous system, including those centers that control respiration and heart rate. If the dose is sufficient, death may be the outcome.

TREAT: Do not give emetics. Similar to treatment for morphine poisoning, q.v.

INCOMPAT: Ferrous iodide, Lugol's solution.

codependency. The acute and chronic stress of living in close association with a dependent person. The dependency or addiction of the individual may be in the areas of drugs, alcohol, gambling, eating, or sexual activity. Whether or not the codependent person reinforces the dependent person's addiction is a matter of individual consideration, and generalities may be misleading.

cod liver oil. A fixed oil obtained from the fresh livers of the codfish. The official oil is standardized for its vitamin A and D content.

ACTION/USES: Formerly widely used in cases of nutritional deficiency to supply vitamins A and D. Esp. used for prophylaxis of rickets in infants. Rarely used now due to the availability of more efficient and more palatable agents.

INCOMPAT: Light and air, both of which cause the oil to become rancid.

codon (kō'dŏn). A sequence of three bases in a strand of DNA that provides the genetic code for a specific amino acid.

Codroxomin. Trade name for hydroxocobalamin.

coefficient (kō"ĕ-fish'ĕnt) [L. *co-*, together, + *efficere*, to produce]. 1. In chemistry, a numerical figure put before a chemical formula or compound to indicate the number of molecules of that substance taking part in the chemical reaction. 2. An expression of a ratio between two different quantities, or the effect produced by varying certain factors.

c., isotonic. Number indicating the amount of salt to be added to distilled water to prevent the destruction of erythrocytes when the salt solution is added to the blood.

c. of absorption. Volume of gas absorbed by a unit volume of a liquid at 0°C and a pressure of 760 mmHg.

Coelenterata (sē-lĕn″tĕr-ā′tă) [Gr. *koilos*, hollow, + *enteron*, intestine]. A phylum of invertebrates that includes corals, hydras, jellyfish, and sea anemones. Contact with some species can result in sting injuries. SEE: *bites or stings*.

coelom (sē′lŏm) [Gr. *koiloma*, a cavity]. The cavity in an embryo between the split layers of lateral mesoderm. In mammals, it develops into the pleural, peritoneal, and pericardial cavities.

c., extraembryonic. In man, the cavity in the developing blastocyst that lies between the mesoderm of the chorion and the mesoderm covering the amniotic cavity and yolk sac.

coenocyte (sē′nō-sīt, sĕn′ō-sīt) [Gr. *koinos*, common, + *kytos*, cell]. A multinucleated mass of protoplasm; a mass of protoplasm in which there are no cell membranes between the nuclei. SEE: *syncytium*.

coenzyme (kō-ĕn′zīm) [L. *co-*, together, + Gr. *en*, in, pl. *zyme*, leaven]. Enzyme activators. A diffusible, heat-stable substance of low molecular weight that, when combined with an inactive protein called apoenzyme, forms an active compound or a complete enzyme called holoenzyme.

Ex.: adenylic acid, riboflavin, and coenzymes I and II.

coenzyme A. An enzyme important to a variety of biological processes. It is a precursor for biosynthesis of fatty acids and sterols and is an acetylating agent. SYN: *acetyl CoA*.

coetaneous (kō″ē-tā′nē-ŭs) [″ + *aetas*, age]. Having the same age or date.

coexcitation (kō-ĕk-sī-tā′shŭn) [″ + *excitare*, to arouse]. Simultaneous excitation of two parts or bodies.

cofactor (kō′făk-tor). A factor acting in conjunction with another. In general, it is necessary that the cofactor be present for the other factor to be active.

coferment (kō-fĕr′mĕnt) [″ + *fermentum*, leaven]. A coenzyme.

coffee. The seed, called coffee beans, of trees of the genus *Coffea*. The roasted beans are pulverized, then brewed with boiling water to prepare the beverage known as coffee. Evidence that drinking coffee is harmful is lacking. SEE: *caffeine* for caffeine content of the beverage.

coffee-ground vomitus. Vomit similar to coffee grounds in pigment and consistency, occurring as a result of the presence of blood in the vomitus.

Cogan's syndrome (kō′găns) [David G. Cogan, U.S. ophthalmologist, b. 1908]. Interstitial keratitis associated with tinnitus, vertigo, and usually deafness.

Cogentin. Trade name for benztropine mesylate.

cognition (kŏg-nĭsh′ŭn) [L. *cognoscere*, to know]. Awareness with perception, reasoning, judgment, intuition, and memory; the mental process by which knowledge is acquired. A patient with normally functioning mental processes would have insight into his or her illness.

cogwheel respiration. Repeated sudden brief interruptions of inspiration and expiration.

cogwheel rigidity. When tremor coexists with rigidity as in Parkinson's syndrome, manual manipulation of body parts may take on the feel of a cogwheel. This can occur as an extrapyramidal side effect of antipsychotic drug therapy.

coherent (kō-hĕr′ĕnt) [L. *cohaerere*, to stick together]. 1. Sticking together, as parts of bodies or fluids. 2. Consistent; making a logical whole.

cohesion (kō-hē′zhŭn). The property of adhering.

cohesive (kō-hē′sĭv). Adhesive; sticky.

Cohnheim's areas (kōn′hīmz) [Julius Friedrich Cohnheim, Ger. pathologist, 1839–1884]. Irregular groups of fibrils seen in a cross section of a striated muscle fiber.

Cohnheim's theory. Theory that tumors result from embryonal cells not utilized for fetal development.

cohort. The component of the population born during a particular period and traced through life as it enters successive time and age periods. SEE: *analysis, cohort*.

cohort study. In epidemiology, a method of investigation is a cohort, q.v.; is followed prospectively or retrospectively.

coil (koyl). 1. A continuous material such as tubing, rope, or a spring arranged in a spiral, loop, or circle. 2. Popular term for a type of intrauterine contraceptive device.

coilonychia (koy″lō-nĭk′ē-ă) [Gr. *koilos*, hollow, + *onyx*, nail]. Koilonychia. Dystrophy of the fingernails in which they are thin and concave with raised edges. Sometimes associated with iron-deficiency anemia.

coin counting. A sliding movement of tips of thumb and index finger over each other in paralysis agitans.

coinfection. The condition of an organism or individual cells being infected simultaneously by two different pathological microorganisms.

coin test. Test for pneumothorax. A coin placed on the chest over the suspected area is struck with another coin. A metallic ringing sound is heard if a cavity containing air is underneath.

coital (kō′ĭ-tăl). Pert. to sexual intercourse.

coition (kō-ĭsh′ŭn) [L. *coire*, to come together]. Coitus; sexual intercourse.

coitophobia (kō″ĭ-tō-fō′bē-ă) [″ + Gr. *phobos*, fear]. Morbid fear of sexual intercourse.

coitus (kō′ĭ-tŭs). Sexual intercourse between man and woman by insertion of the penis into the vagina. SYN: *coition; copulation; sexual intercourse.*

    c. à la vache. Coitus from behind with the female in the knee-chest position.

    c. interruptus. Coitus with withdrawal of the penis from the vagina before seminal emission occurs. This is not an effective method of contraception.

    c. reservatus. Coitus with intentional suppression of ejaculation.

    c. Saxonius. Coitus with manual pressure of the urethra at the underside of the penis or in the perineum to block the emission of semen at the time of ejaculation. This may be done by the female partner to prevent premature ejaculation. SYN: *squeeze technique.*

col (kŏl). The nonkeratinized, depressed gingival tissue that lies between adjacent teeth; it extends labiolingually between the interdental papillae below the interproximal contact of the teeth.

Cola (kō′lă) [W. African *kola*]. A genus of tropical trees that produce the kola nut. An extract of the kola nut is used in pharmaceutical preparations and as a main ingredient in some carbonated beverages.

Colace. Trade name for docusate sodium.

colation (kō-lā′shŭn) [L. *colare*, to strain]. Straining, filtering.

colchicine (kŏl′chĭ-sĭn). USP. Medicine used in treating an acute attack of gout. Because the drug stimulates smooth muscles, diarrhea may be an undesired side effect.

COLD. *chronic obstructive lung disease.* SEE: *COPD.*

cold [AS. *ceald*, cold]. 1. A general term for coryza or inflammation of the respiratory mucous membranes known as the common cold. 2. Lacking heat or warmth; having a low temperature. Opposite of heat.

    c., chest. Cold with inflammation of the bronchial mucous membranes. SYN: *bronchitis.*

    c., common. Acute catarrhal inflammation of any or all parts of the respiratory tract from the nasal mucosa to the nasal sinuses, throat, larynx, trachea, and bronchi. It is highly contagious. Incubation period is from 12 to 72 hours. Lasting immunity does not develop. Even though the common cold does not cause death, its economic importance is vast because it is the greatest cause of absenteeism in industry and schools. SYN: *acute coryza.*

    SYM: Congestion of nasal mucosa with partial or complete occlusion of nostrils; continuous watery discharge with more or less continuous sniffling and blowing of nose. Also sneezing, lacrimation, irritated nasopharynx, chilliness, and malaise. Fever in adults is rare; if fever is present, influenza or other cause of the infection must be suspected. Symptoms are usually resolved within 2 to 10 days. Persons with chronic diseases such as diabetes, or diseases of the heart or lungs, should consult a physician when they have a cold, esp. if it is severe, accompanied by fever, or lasts more than 10 days.

    ETIOL: May be due to any one of a considerable number of viruses including rhinoviruses, coxsackie, and coronaviruses.

    TREAT: Treatment is mainly for the relief of symptoms. Spraying the nasal mucosa with ephedrine hydrochloride, phenylephrine (Neosynephrine), or inhalation of benzedrine or menthol relieves nasal congestion. Analgesics are useful to relieve aching. Preparations containing codeine will usually relieve a cough but should not be used when the cough is productive. An expectorant containing either iodinated glycerol or potassium iodide-saturated solution may relieve cough. Antihistamines in persons with nasal allergy sometimes are effective in controlling the nasal secretions. Bedrest is recommended for febrile patients. There is no evidence that high doses of vitamin C are of benefit in treating the common cold; but some studies have shown a reduced period of disability in persons who took as much as 8 gm of vitamin C on the first day of disease. Analgesics such as aspirin may be of benefit in treating the malaise. There is no effective vaccine. Antibiotics are of use only if there is secondary bacterial infection.

    CONTAGIOUSNESS: The virus may be present in the nasal secretions for a week or longer after the onset of symptoms.

cold agglutinin. A red blood cell agglutinin that acts at only relatively low temperatures (ranging from 0° to 20°C). This agglutinin occurs as part of the disease process in some cases of viral and mycoplasmal infections.

cold agglutinin disease. Term applied to a group of disorders characterized by hemolytic anemia, obstruction of the microcirculation, or both. Due to agglutination of red blood cells by the cold agglutinin. In some this is caused by a transient infectious disease, and in others, the cause is idiopathic. The latter occurs mostly in women over the age of 50.

cold cream. USP. A water-in-oil emulsion ointment base used topically on the skin.

cold pack. Wrapping of a patient or an area in towels dipped in cold water before application. A more effective method is to place crushed ice in a small plastic bag with a small amount of water. Application of cold by this method does not cause frostbite in healthy adults. Cold packs applied to ankle injuries in the first 36 hours reduced recovery time when compared to early heat treatment. Usually used to reduce fever, pain, swelling, or inflammation.

cold pressor test. Test that measures the response of the blood pressure to the immersion of one hand in ice water. An excessive increase in pressure indicates a latent hypertensive state.

cold sore. SEE: *aphthous ulcer.*

coldspray. Aerosol coolant used to quickly lower the temperature and thus harden thermoplastic splinting material during the fitting or molding process.

cold stress. SEE: *hypothermia.*

colectomy (kō-lĕk′tō-mē) [Gr. *kolon,* colon, + *ektome,* excision]. Excision of part or all of the colon.

coleocystitis (kō″lē-ō-sĭs-tī′tĭs) [Gr. *koleos,* sheath, + *kystis,* bladder, + *itis,* inflammation]. Inflammation of the vagina and bladder. SYN: *colpocystitis.*

coleoptosis (kō″lē-ŏp-tō′sĭs) [″ + *ptosis,* a dropping]. Prolapse of the wall of the vagina.

coleotomy (kō″lē-ŏt′ō-mē) [″ + *tome,* incision]. Incision into the pericardium or into the vagina. SYN: *colpotomy.*

colestipol hydrochloride (kō-lĕs′tĭ-pōl). An ion-exchange resin similar in action to cholestyramine, q.v.

colibacillemia (kō″lĭ-băs-ĭl-lē′mē-ă) [Gr. *kolon,* colon, + L. *bacillus,* little rod, + Gr. *haima,* blood]. Colon bacillus in the blood.

colibacillosis (kō″lĭ-băs-ĭ-lō′sĭs) [″ + ″ + Gr. *osis,* condition]. Infection with the colon bacillus.

colibacilluria (kō-lĭ-băs-ĭl-ū′rē-ă) [″ + ″ + Gr. *ouron,* urine]. Presence of *Escherichia coli* in the urine.

colibacillus (kō″lĭ-bă-sĭl′ŭs) [″ + L. *bacillus,* little rod]. The colon bacillus, *Escherichia coli.*

colic (kŏl′ĭk) [Gr. *kolikos,* pert. to the colon]. 1. Spasm in any hollow or tubular soft organ accompanied by pain. 2. Pert. to colon. SEE: *cholecystalgia; tormina.*

   c., biliary. Colic in bile ducts usually associated with a gallstone.

   c., infantile. Colic occurring in infants, principally during the first few months.

   c., intestinal. Colic in which pain may occur throughout the abdomen.

   c., lead. Severe abdominal colic associated with lead poisoning. Lead line may be found on gums and basic stippling in red blood cells.

   c., menstrual. Abdominal pain at the time of menstruation. SYN: *dysmenorrhea.*

   c., renal. Pain in region of one of the kidneys and toward the thigh. Pain radiates from kidney region around and over abdomen into the groin. May be associated with the passage of renal calculi.

   c., uterine. Severe abdominal pain arising in uterus, usually during the menstrual period. SEE: *dysmenorrhea.*

colica (kŏl′ĭ-kă) [L.]. Colic.

colicin (kŏl′ĭ-sĭn). A bacteriocin produced by some strains of *Escherichia coli* that is lethal to other *E. coli.* Since its discovery in 1925, approximately 20 colicins have been described, and some are produced by bacteria other than *E. coli.* All colicins are now called bacteriocins, q.v.

colicky (kŏl′ĭk-ē). Concerning colic or affected by it.

colicolitis (kō″lĭ-kō-lī′tĭs) [Gr. *kolon,* colon, + *kolon,* colon, + *itis,* inflammation]. Colitis due to *Escherichia coli.*

colicoplegia (kō″lĭ-kō-plē′jē-ă) [″ + *plege,* stroke]. Colic and paralysis due to lead poisoning.

colicystitis (kō″lĭ-sĭs-tī′tĭs) [″ + *kystis,* bladder, + *itis,* inflammation]. Inflammation of bladder resulting from infection with *Escherichia coli.*

colicystopyelitis (kō-lĭ-sĭs″tō-pī″ĕ-lī′tĭs) [″ + ″ + *pyelos,* pelvis, + *itis,* inflammation]. Inflammation of bladder and pelvis of kidney caused by *Escherichia coli.*

coliform (kō′lĭ-form) [″ + L. *forma,* form]. 1. Sieve form; cribriform. 2. A general term applied to some species of the family *Enterobacteriaceae,* including *Escherichia coli, Enterobacter,* and *Klebsiella* species. Their presence in water, esp. that of *E. coli,* is presumptive evidence of fecal contamination.

colilysin (kō-lĭl′ĭ-sĭn) [″ + *lysis,* dissolution]. A hemolysin formed by *Escherichia coli.*

colinephritis (kō″lĭ-nē-frī′tĭs) [″ + *nephros,* kidney, + *itis,* inflammation]. Nephritis caused by the colon bacillus, *Escherichia coli.*

coliplication (kō″lĭ-plĭ-kā′shŭn) [″ + L. *plica,* fold]. Operation for correcting a dilated colon.

colipuncture (kō′lĭ-pŭnk″chūr) [″ + L. *punctura,* a piercing]. Puncture of the colon to relieve distention. SYN: *colocentesis.*

colipyuria (kō″lĭ-pī-ū′rē-ă) [″ + *pyon,* pus, + *ouron,* urine]. Pus in urine due to *Escherichia coli.*

colisepsis [″ + *sepsis,* putrefaction]. Infection caused by the colon bacillus.

colistimethate sodium, sterile (kō-lĭs″tĭ-mĕth′āt). USP. A form of colistin, q.v., suitable for use intramuscularly or intravenously. Trade name is Coly-Mycin M Parenteral.

colistin sulfate (kō-lĭs′tĭn). USP. Polymyxin E. An antibiotic effective against some of the gram-negative bacteria, esp. Pseudomonas, that are resistant to other antibiotics. Trade name is Coly-Mycin S.

colitis (kō-lī′tĭs) [″ + *itis*, inflammation]. Inflammation of the colon. SEE: *irritable bowel disease.*

   c., amebic. SEE: *amebiasis.*

   c., mucous. Colon, irritable, q.v.

   c., pseudomembranous. Colitis associated with antibiotic therapy. This is usually due to a toxin produced by *Clostridium difficile*. It is characterized by formation of a pseudomembrane on the mucosa of the colon. The symptoms of diarrhea with gross blood and mucus, abdominal cramps, fever, and leukocytosis usually begin 4 to 10 days after beginning antibiotic therapy.

   TREAT: Discontinue use of the antibiotic and institute therapy with either oral vancomycin or metronidazole.

   c., ulcerative. Ulceration of mucosa of colon. SEE: *Nursing Diagnoses* in *Appendix.*

   SYM: Passage of offensive watery stools with mucus and pus. Abdominal pain, tenderness, or colic. Intermittent or irregular fever. Hemorrhage and perforation may occur. SEE: *irritable bowel disease.*

colitoxemia (kō″lī-tŏk-sē′mē-ă) [Gr. *kolon*, colon, + *toxikon*, poison, + *haima*, blood]. Toxemia caused by the colon bacillus, *Escherichia coli.*

colitoxicosis (kō″lī-tŏk″sĭ-kō′sĭs) [″ + ″ + *osis*, condition]. Systemic poisoning caused by the colon bacillus, *Escherichia coli.*

coliuria (kō″lī-ū′rē-ă) [″ + *ouron*, urine]. Presence of *Escherichia coli* in the urine. SYM: *colibacilluria.*

colla (kŏl′lă). Pl. of collum, q.v.

collagen (kŏl′ă-jĕn) [Gr. *kolla*, glue, + *gennan*, to produce]. A fibrous insoluble protein found in the connective tissue, including skin, bone, ligaments, and cartilage. Collagen represents about 30% of the total body protein. Collagen is the protein typical of dental tissues (except for enamel), forming the matrix of dentin, cementum, and alveolar bone proper. Collagen fibers also form the periodontal ligament which attaches the teeth to their bony sockets.

collagenase (kŏl-lăj′ĕ-nās) [″ + ″ + *-ase*, enzyme]. An enzyme that induces changes in collagen to cause its degradation.

collagenation (kŏl-lăj″ē-nă′shŭn). Presence of collagen in tissue.

collagenic (kŏl″ă-jĕn′ĭk). Producing or containing collagen.

collagenoblast (kŏl-lăj′ĕ-nō-blăst) [″ + ″ + *blastos*, germ]. A fibroblast-derived cell that when mature produces collagen.

collagenolysis (kŏl″ă-jĕn-ŏl′ĭ-sĭs) [″ + ″ + *lysis*, dissolution]. The degradation or destruction of collagen.

collagenosis (kŏl-lăj″ē-nō′sĭs) [″ + ″ + *osis*, condition]. A collagen disease, q.v.

collapse [L. *collapsus*, fallen to pieces]. 1. An abnormal retraction of the walls of an organ. 2. A sudden exhaustion, prostration, or weakness due to decreased circulation of the blood.

   SYM: Similar to those of hemorrhage. The peripheral arteries are depleted of blood, and the veins, esp. in the splanchnic region, are congested; apathy; extreme pallor; cold, clammy perspiration; thin, rapid pulse; fall of blood pressure; unconsciousness.

   NURSING IMPLICATIONS: Lower the head of the bed. Maintain patent airway. Elevate lower extremities slightly to increase venous return. Assess vital signs and level of consciousness for symptoms of shock; administer I.V. fluids as ordered. Keep patient warm but not hot. Remain with the patient and provide reassurance that he or she is being cared for appropriately.

   c., circulatory. Shock, q.v.

   c. of lung. An airless state of all or part of a lung. Normal in fetus. Artificially induced by pneumothorax; thoracoplasty; or avulsion of phrenic nerve. May occur spontaneously due to rupture of a bleb on the pleural surface of the lung.

collapsing. Falling into extreme and sudden prostration resembling shock.

collapsing pulse. Pulse of aortic insufficiency or regurgitation. SYN: *Corrigan's pulse; water-hammer pulse.*

collapsotherapy (kŏ-lăp″sō-thĕr′ă-pē) [L. *collapsus*, fallen to pieces, + Gr. *therapeia*, treatment]. Treatment of pulmonary affections by unilateral pneumothorax and immobilization of affected lung.

collar (kŏl′ăr) [L. *collum*, neck]. 1. A band worn round the neck. 2. Structure or marking formed like a neckband.

   c. of Venus. Mottled appearance of the skin of the neck usually present in late syphilis. SYN: *melanoleukoderma colli; venereal collar.*

collarbone. The clavicle, q.v.

collateral (kō-lăt′ĕr-ăl) [L. *con*, together, + *lateralis*, pert. to a side]. 1. Accompanying, side by side as in a small side branch of a blood vessel or nerve. 2. Subordinate or accessory.

collateral circulation. Circulation of small anastomosing vessels, esp. when a main artery is obstructed.

collateral eminence. An elevation in the floor of the lateral ventricle.

collateral fissure. Fissure on the median surface of the cerebral hemisphere.

collateral ganglia. Ganglia of the sympathetic division of the autonomic nervous system, located near origins of the celiac and mesenteric arteries. These include the celiac and mesenteric ganglia. SYN: *preverte-bral ganglia.*

collateral ligaments. Ligaments which provide medial and lateral stability to joints. These include the medial (ulnar) and lateral (radial) collateral ligaments at the elbow, the medial (tibial) and lateral (fibular) collateral ligaments at the knee, the medial (deltoid) and lateral collateral ligaments at the ankle, and collateral ligaments of the fingers.

collaterals. Pl. of collateral.

collateral trigone. The angle between the diverging inferior and posterior horns of the lateral ventricle.

collecting tubules. Small ducts that receive urine from several renal tubules which join together to provide a passage for the urine to larger straight collecting tubules (papillary ducts of Bellini) that open into the pelvis of the kidney. SEE: illus. at *kidney.*

Colles' fascia (kŏl'ēz) [Abraham Colles, Ir. surgeon, 1773–1843]. Inner layer of superficial fascia of perineum.

Colles' fracture. The transverse fracture of the distal end of the radius (just above wrist) with displacement of hand backward and outward.

NURSING IMPLICATIONS: The emergency room nurse obtains a history of the injury, and assesses the patient for pain, and the distal forearm for swelling, mobility, and any obvious deformity; inspects the extremity above the fracture site; and assesses the area below the fracture site, inspecting for color changes and palpating for temperature change and the presence of pulses and sensation. The affected extremity is temporarily immobilized with a splint. Cold applications may be used to reduce pain and limit swelling. A radiograph is taken.

colliculectomy (kŏl-lĭk″ū-lĕk′tō-mē) [L. *colliculus,* mound, + Gr. *ektome,* excision]. Removal of the colliculus seminalis.

colliculitis (kŏl-lĭk″ū-lī′tĭs) [″ + Gr. *itis,* inflammation]. Inflammation of the colliculus seminalis.

colliculus (kŏl-lĭk′ū-lŭs) [L.] (pl. *colliculi*). A little eminence.

  c. bulbi; c. bulbi intermedius. Erectile tissue encircling the male urethra at the entrance to the bulb.

  c. cervicalis. The crest on the posterior wall of the female urethra.

  c. inferior. [NA] One of two elevations forming the lower portion of the corpora quadrigemina of the midbrain.

  c. seminalis. [NA] An oval enlargement on the crista urethralis, an elevation in the floor of the prostatic portion of the urethra. On its sides are the openings of the ejaculatory ducts and numerous ducts of the prostate gland. SYN: *c. urethralis.*

  c. superior. [NA] One of two elevations forming the upper portion of the corpora quadrigemina of the midbrain.

  c. urethralis. C. seminalis.

collimation (kŏl″ĭ-mā′shŭn) [L. *collineare,* to align]. The process of making parallel. In radiography, the process of limiting the scatter and extent of the x-ray beam to the part being radiographed.

collimator (kŏl′ĭ-mā″tur) [L. *collineare,* to align, direct, aim]. Radiographic device used to limit the scatter and extent of the x-ray beam.

colliquation (kŏl″ĭ-kwā′shŭn) [L. *con,* together, + *liquare,* to melt]. 1. Abnormal discharge of a body fluid. 2. Softening of tissues to liquefaction. 3. A wasting.

colliquative (kŏ-lĭk′wă-tĭv). Pert. to a liquid and excessive discharge, as a colliquative diarrhea.

collodion (kŏ-lō′dē-ŏn) [Gr. *kollodes,* resembling glue]. USP. A preparation containing pyroxylin, a preparation of cellulose nitrate, dissolved thoroughly in ether and alcohol. It is a viscous liquid having an odor of ether and is highly flammable. When applied, it dries to form a strong, thin, transparent film and is useful in sealing the edge of a dressing, esp. on the scalp.

  c., flexible. A preparation of collodion containing camphor and castor oil. It is more elastic than collodion in ether and alcohol.

  c., salicylic acid. Flexible collodion with salicylic acid. Used as a keratolytic agent.

colloid (kŏl′oyd) [Gr. *kollodes,* glutinous]. 1. A type of solution. A gluelike substance such as a protein or starch whose particles (molecules or aggregates of molecules) when dispersed in a solvent to the greatest possible degree remain uniformly distributed and fail to form a true solution. 2. The size of a microscopic colloid; particles ranging from 10^{-9} to 10^{-11} meters (1 to 100 nanometers). 3. A homogenous gelatinous substance found within the follicles of the thyroid gland and containing the thyroid hormones.

  c., thyroid. Semifluid, jellylike substance filling the follicles of the thyroid gland. It contains the thyroid hormones.

colloidal (kŏl-loyd′ăl). Pert. to a colloid.

colloidal dispersion. A mixture containing colloid particles that fail to settle out and are held in suspension. They are common in animal and plant tissues, the protoplasm of cells being a colloidal mixture. Particles of colloidal dispersions are too large to pass through cell membranes and such dispersions usually appear cloudy.

colloid chemistry. The application of chemistry to systems and substances, and the problems of emulsions, mists, foams, and suspensions.

colloid cyst. A sac containing a jellylike liquid.

colloid degeneration. Mucoid degeneration seen in the protoplasm of epithelial cells.

colloidin (kŏl-loy'dĭn). A jellylike substance seen in colloid degeneration.

colloidoclasia (kŏl-oyd″ō-klā'sē-ă) [″ + *klasis*, fracture]. An alteration in the equilibrium of body colloids producing anaphylactic shock. Resulting from entrance into the bloodstream of unaltered colloids such as proteins.

colloidopexy (kŏl-oyd'ō-pĕk″sē) [″ + *pexis*, fixation]. Fixation of colloids during metabolism.

colloid suspension. A mixture holding particles in suspension, the forms of which change with the forces acting upon them, such as milk, or fat.

colloma (kŏ-lō'mă) [Gr. *kolla*, glue, + *oma*, tumor]. A colloid degeneration of a cancer.

collopexia (kŏl″ō-pĕk'sē-ă) [L. *collum*, neck, + Gr. *pexis*, fixation]. Fixation of the cervix uteri.

collum (kŏl'lŭm) [L.] (pl. *colla*). 1. The necklike part of an organ. 2. The neck.

collyrium (kŏ-lĭr'ē-ŭm) [Gr. *kollyrion*, eye salve]. An eyewash or lotion for the eye.

coloboma (kŏl″ō-bō'mă) [Gr. *koloboma*, a mutilation]. A lesion or defect of the eye, usually a fissure or cleft of the iris, ciliary body, or choroid. May be congenital, pathological, or surgical. Sometimes the eyelid is involved.

colocecostomy (kŏ″lō-sē-kŏs'tō-mē) [Gr. *kolon*, colon, + L. *caecum*, blindness, + Gr. *stoma*, mouth]. Surgical joining of the colon to the cecum of the small intestine.

colocentesis (kŏ″lō-sĕn-tē'sĭs) [″ + *kentesis*, puncture]. Surgical puncture of the colon to relieve distention.

colocholecystostomy (kŏ″lō-kō″lē-sĭs-tŏs'tō-mē) [″ + *chole*, bile, + *kystis*, bladder, + *stoma*, mouth]. Surgical formation of a communication between the colon and gallbladder. SYN: *cholecystocolostomy.*

coloclysis, colochlyster (kŏ-lŏk'lĭ-sĭs, kŏ″lō-klĭs'tĕr) [″ + *klysis*, washing]. A colonic enema.

colocolostomy (kō″lō-kō-lŏs'tō-mē) [″ + *kolon*, colon, + *stoma*, mouth]. Formation of a connection between two portions of the colon.

colocutaneous (kō″lō-kū-tā'nē-ŭs) [″ + L. *cutis*, skin]. 1. Concerning the colon and the skin. 2. A pathological or surgically made connection between the colon and the skin. SEE: *colostomy.*

colocynth (kŏl'ō-sĭnth) [Gr. *kolokynthe*, fruit of *Citrullus colocynthis*]. Dried pulp of unripe colocynth fruit.

ACTION/USES: A type of cathartic that has such drastic action that it should not be used.

coloenteritis (kō″lō-ĕn″tĕr-ī'tĭs) [Gr. *kolon*, colon, + *enteron*, intestine, + *itis*, inflammation]. Inflammation of mucous membrane of small and large intestines.

colofixation (kō″lō-fĭk-sā'shŭn). Suspension of the colon in the treatment of ptosis.

Cologel. Trade name for methylcellulose.

colon [L.; Gr. *kolon*]. [NA] The large intestine from the end of the ileum to the rectum, about 59 inches (1.5 meters) long. Divided into the ascending, transverse, descending, and the sigmoid or pelvic colon. Beginning at the cecum, the first part of the large intestine, the ascending colon, passes upward to the right colic or hepatic flexure, where it turns as the transverse colon passing ventral to the liver and stomach. On reaching the spleen, it turns downward (left colic or splenic flexure) and continues as the descending colon to the brim of the pelvis, where it is continuous with the sigmoid colon, and extends to the rectum. SEE: illus.

FUNCT: *Mechanical:* Mixing the intestinal contents. *Chemical:* No digestive enzymes are secreted in the colon, but an alkaline fluid aids in the completion of digestion begun in the small intestine. Those products of bacterial action that are absorbed into the bloodstream are carried by the portal circulation to the liver before they enter into the general circulation. More water is absorbed in the colon than in the small intestine. The fluids of the body are conserved in this way and, in spite of the large volumes of secretions added to the food during its progress through the alimentary canal, the contents of the colon are gradually dehydrated until they assume the consistency of normal feces or even become quite hard. SEE: *absorption; defecation; irritable bowel syndrome.*

c., bacteria of. *Escherichia coli* is the most important but not the most common bacterium that normally inhabits the colon. It is outnumbered by the gram-negative anaerobic *Bacteroides* bacilli by at least 100 to 1. Whatever digestion takes place in the

COLON AND RECTUM

HEPATIC FLEXURE
SPLENIC FLEXURE
TRANSVERSE COLON
ASCENDING COLON
DESCENDING COLON
ILEUM, DISTAL END OF SMALL INTESTINE
RECTOSIGMOID JUNCTION
OPENING OF ILEUM INTO CECUM
SIGMOID COLON
VERMIFORM APPENDIX
RECTUM
ANUS

colon results from bacterial action. A large number of fermentative bacteria are found in the middle portion of the colon. Putrefying bacteria are found in the lower part of the colon. These may produce toxic products, such as indol, skatol; however, if absorbed, such products undergo detoxification in the liver. SEE: *flatus*.

   c., irritable. The most frequently seen gastrointestinal disease. Women are three times more likely to have this disease than men. Both the small and large intestines are involved in this syndrome of disordered motility that is accompanied by pain, usually in the lower abdominal area, and constipation alternating with diarrhea. The pain is usually relieved by the passage of either small-diameter stools of varying consistency or gas and mucus. The symptoms, which may be chronic or recurring at intervals, are usually triggered by anxiety-producing periods of stress from social, family, or occupational problems. Typically, patients will have little insight into their disease and regard their altered bowel habits and stool size as being the cause of their discomfort. The disease

subsides as the stress situation is relieved. SYN: *colitis, mucous; irritable bowel syndrome; spastic colon.*

   ETIOL: Unknown but related to the patient's reaction to stress that induces changes in the motility pattern of the intestinal tract.

   TREAT: A careful history, physical examination, and special studies of the GI tract are required to assure the patient and physician that no organic disease is present. The patient is then treated for chronic anxiety neurosis. It is essential that the patient be reassured that the disease will not cause chronic colitis or cancer of the colon. The use of laxatives for constipation and antispasmodics such as tincture of belladonna for abdominal cramps may be of assistance, but may prevent the patient from learning to recognize the importance of the gastrointestinal signs and symptoms.

   NOTE: Even though the disease will not cause malignancy of the GI tract, it is important to periodically review the patient for such pathologic changes because presence of this syndrome does not mean the individual is free of the potential of developing malignancies in any body site.

c., polyps of. SEE: *polyps, colonic.*

c., toxic dilatation of. Marked dilatation of the colon, esp. the transverse colon, occurring as a complication of a primary disease of the colon. Clinically there are tachycardia, fever, and leukocytosis. There may or may not be abdominal tenderness, a palpable abdominal mass, mental confusion, cramping, and change in number of bowel movements each day. The condition may occur as a complication of ulcerative colitis, Crohn's disease, or amebic colitis.

colon, words pert. to: anus; appendix; cecum; cholecystocolostomy; colalgia; colic; colitis; "colo-" words; diverticulitis; intestines; jejunum; megacolon; peristalsis; polyps, colonic; rectum.

colonalgia (kō″lŏn-ăl′jē-ă) [Gr. *kolon,* colon, + *algos,* pain]. Pain in the colon.

colonic (kō-lŏn′ĭk). Pert. to the colon.

colonic irrigation. Injection into the colon of a large amount of fluid in order to fill and flush it. Administered to wash the wall of the bowel as high as the fluid can reach. Two primary methods; one tube, involving filling the colon to capacity through a single tube and allowing liquid to run out through the same tube; and two-tube method, employing separate inflow and outflow tubes.

colonitis (kō-lŏn-ī′tĭs) [″ + *itis,* inflammation]. Colitis.

colonization (kŏl″ō-nī-zā′shŭn). 1. The process of a group of organisms living together, esp. bacteria. 2. Innidiation, q.v.

colonopathy (kō″lŏ-nŏp′ă-thē) [Gr. *kolon,* colon, + *pathos,* disease]. Any disease of the colon.

colonopexy (kō-lŏn′ō-pĕk″sē) [″ + *pexis,* fixation]. Process of attaching part of colon to abdominal wall.

colonorrhagia (kō″lŏn-ō-rā′jē-ă) [″ + *rhegnynai,* to burst forth]. Hemorrhage from the colon.

colonorrhea (kō″lŏn-ō-rē′ă) [″ + *rhoia,* flow]. 1. Colitis. 2. Discharge of watery fluid from the colon.

colonoscope (kō-lŏn′ō-skōp) [″ + *skopein,* to examine]. Instrument for examination of the colon. SEE: *sigmoidoscope.*

colonoscopy (kō″lŏn-ŏs′kŏ-pē). Examination of the upper portion of the rectum with an elongated speculum or a colonoscope.

colony (kŏl′ō-nē) [L. *colonia*]. A growth of microorganisms in a culture. Usually considered to have grown from a single organism.

colony counter. Apparatus for counting bacterial colonies in a culture plate.

colony-stimulating factor-1. ABBR: CSF-1. A protein present in human serum that promotes monocyte differentiation.

SEE: *granulocyte-monocyte colony stimulating factor (GM-CSF).*

colopexostomy (kō″lō-pĕks-ŏs′tō-mē) [Gr. *kolon,* colon, + *pexis,* fixation, + *stoma,* mouth]. Resection of the colon and fixation to abdominal wall to establish an artificial anus.

colopexotomy (kō″lō-pĕks-ŏt′ō-mē) [″ + ″ + *tome,* incision]. Incision and fixation of colon.

colopexy, colopexia (kō′lō-pĕk″sē, -pĕks′ē-ă). Fixation of the sigmoid or cecum to the abdominal wall by suture.

coloplication (kō″lō-plĭ-kā′shŭn) [″ + L. *plica,* fold]. Surgical creation of a fold in the colon to reduce its lumen.

coloproctectomy (kō″lō-prŏk-tĕk′tō-mē) [″ + *proktos,* anus, + *ektome,* excision]. Surgical removal of the rectum and colon.

coloproctitis [″ + ″ + *itis,* inflammation]. Colonic and rectal inflammation. SYN: *colorectitis.*

coloproctostomy (kō″lō-prŏk-tŏs′tō-mē) [″ + ″ + *stoma,* mouth]. Making a communication between a segment of colon and the rectum.

coloptosia (kō″lŏp-tō′sē-ă) [″ + *ptosis,* dropping]. Prolapse of the colon, esp. of the transverse colon.

coloptosis (kō-lŏp-tō′sĭs). A downward displacement of the colon.

colopuncture (kō′lō-pŭnk-chūr) [″ + L. *punctura,* piercing]. Surgical puncture of the colon to relieve distention. SYN: *colocentesis.*

color [L.]. A visible quality, distinct from form, and light and shade.

c.'s, primary. The three colors of light, red, green, and violet, that can be mixed to produce all of the colors perceived by the human eye. Pigments that can be so mixed are red, yellow, and blue.

color, words pert. to: achromate; achromoderma; "achro-" words; alba; albedo; albicans; albinism; allochroism; allochromasia; anerythropsia; anisochromatic; aurantiasis; auric; carotene; carotenemia; "chrom-" words; isochromatic; melanin; nigrities; pigmentation; rubefacient; rubiginous; rubor; vermilion border; versicolor; xanthic.

color blindness. Absence of or defect in the perception of colors. Color vision is based on perception of red, green, and blue (termed the 1st, 2nd, and 3rd color factors, respectively). If there is a defect in the perception of one of these colors, a color will be perceived as if it were composed only of the other two colors. Based on the color or colors for which there is defective perception, a person may suffer from red, green, or blue blindness. Color blindness in which all colors are perceived as gray is termed monochromasia.

color deficient. A preferred term for color blindness, inability to identify one or more of the primary colors. Children may become unduly alarmed by hearing the words color blindness; thus, color deficient, which is technically correct, is preferred.

colorectal carcinoma. Malignant neoplasm of the colon or rectum. An estimated 62,000 persons in the U.S. die of this disease annually. It is the second most common cause of death from cancer in the U.S.

SYM: These are nonspecific and include change in the usual pattern of bowel habits, esp. in patients over 40 years of age; recent onset of constipation, diarrhea, or tenesmus in an older patient; passage of bright red or dark blood in the stool; presence of hypochronic microcytic anemia.

DIAG: Digital rectal exam; anoscopy; proctosigmoidoscopy; colonoscopy; barium enema exam; biopsy of suspicious lesions and polyps.

TREAT: Surgical resection. Then a combination of levamisole and fluorouracil if the cancer has metastasized to regional lymph nodes.

colorectitis (kō″lō-rĕk-tī′tĭs) [Gr. *kolon*, colon, + L. *rectum*, straight, + Gr. *itis*, inflammation]. Inflammation of colon and rectum. SYN: *coloproctitis.*

colorectostomy (kō″lō-rĕk-tŏs′tŏ-mē) [″ + ″ + Gr. *stoma*, mouth]. Formation of passage between colon and rectum.

colorectum (kōl″ō-rĕk′tŭm). The colon and rectum.

color gustation. A sense of color aroused by stimulation of taste receptors.

color hearing. A sense of color caused by a sound.

colorimeter (kŭl″or-ĭm′ĕ-tĕr) [L. *color*, color, + Gr. *metron*, measure]. Instrument for measuring intensity of color in a substance or fluid, esp. one for determining the amount of hemoglobin in the blood.

color index. An outmoded method of expressing the amount of hemoglobin present in each red cell.

colorrhaphy (kō-lor′ă-fē) [Gr. *kolon*, colon, + *rhaphe*, seam, ridge]. Suture of the colon.

color sense. One of the three parts of visual function. The others are form sense and light sense. This is tested by determining the ability to distinguish colors. SEE: *form sense; light sense.*

coloscopy (kō-lŏs′kō-pē). Visual examination of the colon by use of a sigmoidoscope.

colosigmoidostomy (kō″lō-sĭg″moy-dŏs′tō-mē) [″ + *sigmoeides*, shaped like Gr. S, + *stoma*, mouth]. Surgical joining of the descending colon to the pelvic colon.

colostomy (kō-lŏs′tō-mē) [Gr. *kolon*, colon, + *stoma*, mouth]. The opening of some portion of the colon through the abdominal wall to its outside surface. Performed when it is impossible for the feces to pass through the colon and out the anus due to a pathological condition, or because the distal bowel has been surgically removed. Temporary colostomies are done to divert the fecal flow from an inflamed area or from an operative area. SEE: illus.; *ostomy* for colostomy care.

NURSING IMPLICATIONS: Cleanse the stoma and surrounding skin area gently with soap and water to remove all fecal material, rinsing and drying thoroughly. Apply a drainage bag, fitting the karaya adhesive ring (or other type appliance) close to the stoma to insure a firm seal and prevent leakage, but not so closely as to constrict the stoma. Hypoallergenic skin barriers are also available. Colostomy irrigations may be ordered. The procedure is similar to administering an enema: a soft rubber catheter is used to instill fluid. The object is to stimulate evacuation of feces, rather than to wash out the colon as in colonic irrigation. Follow established procedure for the irrigation. Support the patient in viewing and caring for the colostomy, offering encouragement while teaching proper care.

Instruct the patient to avoid gas-forming foods, such as cabbage, cauliflower, and broccoli, if they cause a problem; also irritating foods, such as nuts and those with seeds. Recognize the difficult adjustment required by the patient and family, and encourage them to verbalize their fears and concerns. Offer support and refer them to available support groups, such as the local chapter of the Ostomy Association. SEE: *Nursing Diagnoses* in *Appendix.*

c., double barrel. Temporary colostomy in which there are two openings into the colon; one distal and one proximal. Elimination occurs through the proximal stoma, thus allowing the distal length of the colon to rest and heal as in colitis, q.v. When healing is complete, the two ends are rejoined and returned to the peritoneal cavity, and normal function resumes.

c., terminal. Colostomy in which the proximal cut end of the colon is formed into a stoma and the distal colon is either resected or closed.

c., wet. 1. Colostomy in the right side of the colon or in the ileum. The drainage from this type of colostomy is liquid. 2. Colostomy in the left colon distal to the point where the ureters have been anastomosed to it. Thus the urine and fecal material are excreted through the same stoma.

COLOSTOMY SITES

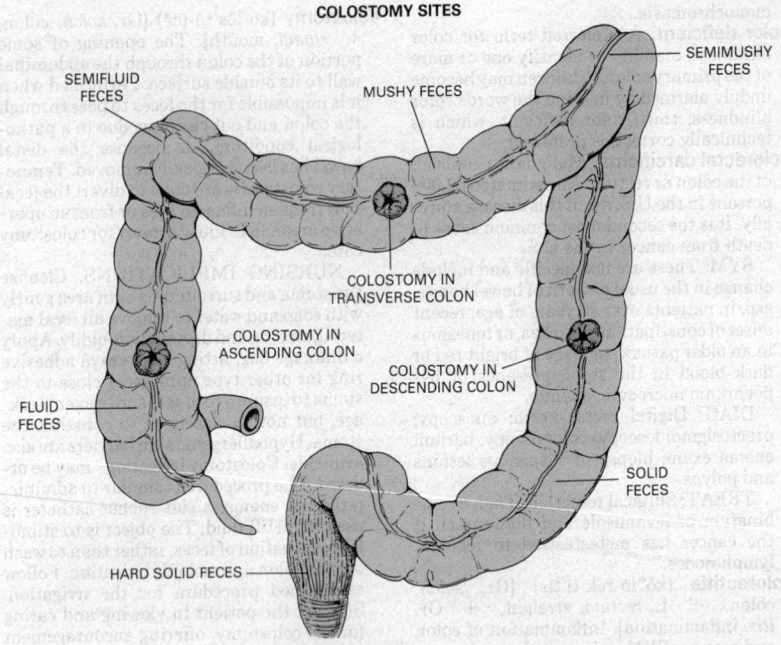

SEMIFLUID FECES

MUSHY FECES

SEMIMUSHY FECES

COLOSTOMY IN TRANSVERSE COLON

COLOSTOMY IN ASCENDING COLON

COLOSTOMY IN DESCENDING COLON

FLUID FECES

SOLID FECES

HARD SOLID FECES

colostrorrhea (kō-lŏs″trō-rē′ă) [L. *colostrum*, colostrum, + Gr. *rhoia*, flow]. Abnormal secretion of colostrum.

colostrum [L.]. Breast fluid that may be secreted from the second trimester of pregnancy onward, but is most evident in the first 2 to 3 days after birth and before the onset of true lactation. This thin yellowish fluid contains a great quantity of proteins and calories in addition to antibodies and lymphocytes.

colotomy (kō-lŏt′ō-mē) [Gr. *kolon*, colon, + *tome*, incision]. Incision of colon.

colovaginal (kō″lō-văj′ĭ-năl). Concerning the colon and vagina or communication between the two.

colovesical (kō″lō-vĕs′ĭ-kăl). Concerning the colon and the urinary bladder or communication between the two.

colpalgia (kŏl-păl′jē-ă) [Gr. *kolpos*, vagina, + *algos*, pain]. Vaginal pain.

colpatresia (kŏl-pă-trē′zē-ă) [″ + *a-*, not, + *tresis*, a perforation]. Occlusion or pathological closure of the vagina; vaginal atresia.

colpectasia (kŏl-pĕk-tā′sē-ă) [″ + *ektasis*, distention]. Dilatation of the vagina.

colpectomy (kŏl-pĕk′tō-mē) [″ + *ektome*, excision]. Surgical removal of the vagina.

colpeurynter (kŏl′pū-rĭn″tĕr) [″ + *eurynein*, to dilate]. A bag for dilatation of the vagina.

colpeurysis (kŏl-pū′rĭs-ĭs). Dilatation of the vagina by surgery.

colpitis (kŏl-pī′tĭs) [″ + *itis*, inflammation]. Inflammation of the vagina. SEE: *vaginitis*.

    c. macularis. Small erythematous lesions present on the squamous epithelium of the upper vagina and cervix. The lesions are seen best by use of colposcopy, q.v., and have the appearance of "strawberry spots." Presence of these spots have a high positive predictive value for women with trichomoniasis. SEE: *trichomonas vaginalis.*

colpocele (kŏl′pō-sēl) [″ + *kele*, tumor, swelling]. Hernia into the vagina.

colpoceliotomy (kŏl″pō-sē″lē-ŏt′ō-mē) [″ + *koilia*, belly, + *tome*, incision]. Entering the abdomen surgically through the vagina. SEE: *culdoscopy.*

colpocleisis (kŏl″pō-klī′sĭs) [″ + *kleisis*, a closure]. Operation of occluding the vagina.

colpocystitis (kŏl″pō-sĭs-tī′tĭs) [″ + *kystis*, bladder, + *itis*, inflammation]. Inflammation of vagina and bladder.

colpocystocele (kŏl″-pō-sĭs′tō-sēl) [″ + kystis, bladder, + kele, tumor, swelling]. Prolapse of the bladder into the vagina.

colpocystoplasty (kŏl″pō-sĭs′tō-plăs″tē) [″ + ″ + plassein, to form]. Surgical treatment of vesicovaginal fistula.

colpocystosyrinx (kŏl″pō-sĭs-tō-sĭr′ĭnks) [″ + ″ + syrinx, fistula]. Fistula between the bladder and vagina.

colpocystotomy (kŏl″pō-sĭs-tŏt′ō-mē) [″ + ″ + tome, incision]. Cutting into the bladder through the vagina.

NURSING IMPLICATIONS: Measure and record intake and output; carefully assess patient for bladder distention. Evaluate retention catheter for patency and character of drainage. If irrigation is required, a three-way catheter should be utilized, allowing continuous or intermittent irrigation as ordered. Irrigation equipment and fluid must be sterile to help prevent nosocomial infection.

colpocytology (kŏl″pō-sī-tŏl′ō-jē) [″ + kytos, cell, + logos, word, reason]. Study of the cells shed by the vaginal mucosa.

colpodynia (kŏl″pō-dĭn′ē-ă) [Gr. kolpos, vagina, + odyne, pain]. Pain in the vagina. SYN: colpalgia.

colpohyperplasia (kŏl″pō-hī-pĕr-plā′zē-ă) [″ + hyper, over, + plasis, a forming]. Excessive growth of mucous membrane of the vagina.

c. cystica. Infectious inflammation of the vaginal walls characterized by the production of small blebs.

colpomicroscope (kŏl″pō-mī′krō-skōp) [″ + mikros, small, + skopein, to view]. Optical device for very high power magnification of the vaginal mucosa and the cervix.

colpomyomectomy (kŏl″pō-mī″ō-mĕk′tō-mē) [″ + mys, muscle, + oma, tumor, + ektome, excision]. Removal of a fibroid tumor of the uterus through the vagina.

colpomyomotomy (kŏl″pō-mī″ō-mŏt′ō-mē) [″ + ″ + ″ + tome, incision]. Incision of the uterus through the vagina for removal of a tumor.

colpoperineoplasty (kŏl″pō-pĕr″ĭn-ē′ō-plăs″tē) [″ + perinaion, perineum, + plassein, to form]. Plastic surgery on vagina and perineum.

colpoperineorrhaphy (kŏl″pō-pĕr″ĭn-ē-or′ră-fē) [″ + ″ + rhaphe, seam, ridge]. Operation for mending perineal tears in the vagina.

colpopexy (kŏl′pō-pĕk″sē) [″ + pexis, fixation]. Suture of a relaxed and prolapsed vagina to the abdominal wall.

colpoplasty (kŏl′pō-plăs″tē) [″ + plassein, to form]. Plastic surgery of the vagina.

colpoptosis (kŏl″pŏp-tō′sĭs) [″ + ptosis, a dropping]. Prolapse of the vagina. SYN:

procidentia.

colporrhagia (kŏl″pō-rā′jē-ă) [″ + rhegnynai, to burst forth]. Excessive vaginal discharge; vaginal hemorrhage.

colporrhaphy (kŏl-por′ă-fē) [″ + rhaphe, seam, ridge]. Suture of the vagina.

colporrhexis (kŏl″pō-rĕk′sĭs) [″ + rhexis, rupture]. Laceration or rupture of the vaginal walls.

colposcope (kŏl′pō-skōp) [″ + skopein, to examine]. An instrument used for examination of the tissues of the vagina and cervix by means of a magnifying lens.

colposcopy (kŏl-pŏs′kō-pē). The examination of vaginal and cervical tissues by using a colposcope. Colposcopy is used in selecting sites of abnormal epithelium for biopsy in patients with abnormal Pap smears. It is helpful in defining tumor extension and for evaluating benign lesions. It has also proved to be valuable in postpubertal vaginal examination of diethylstilbestrol-exposed offspring.

colpospasm, colpospasmus (kŏl″pō-spăzm, kŏl″pō-spăz′mŭs) [Gr. kolpos, vagina, + spasmos, a convulsion]. Spasm of the vagina.

colpostat (kŏl′pō-stăt) [″ + statikos, standing]. Device for holding an instrument, such as a radium applicator, in place in the vagina.

colpostenosis (kŏl″pō-stĕn-ō′sĭs) [″ + stenosis, narrowing]. Stenosis or narrowing of the vagina.

colpostenotomy (kŏl″pō-stĕn-ŏt′ō-mē) [″ + ″ + tome, incision]. A cutting operation for dilating the lumen in stricture of the vagina.

colpotherm (kŏl′pō-thĕrm) [″ + therme, heat]. Electrical heating device introduced into the vagina.

colpotomy (kŏl-pŏt′ō-mē) [″ + tome, incision]. Incision into the wall of the vagina.

colpoureterocystotomy (kŏl″pō-ū-rē″tĕr-ō-sĭs-tŏt′ō-mē) [″ + oureter, ureter, + kystis, bladder, + tome, incision]. Exposure of the ureteral orifices by incision through the walls of the vagina and bladder.

colpoureterotomy (kŏl″pō-ū-rē″tĕr-ŏt′ō-mē) [″ + ″ + tome, incision]. Incision of the ureter through the vagina.

colpoxerosis (kŏl″pō-zē-rō′sĭs) [″ + xerosis, dryness]. Abnormal dryness of the vaginal mucosa.

columbium. Former name for niobium, q.v.

columella (kŏl″ū-mĕl′lă) [L., small column]. 1. A little column. 2. In bacteriology, portion of the sporangiophore upon which are borne the spores.

c. cochleae. The modiolus of the cochlea.

c. nasi. The anterior part of the septum

of the nose.

column (kŏl′ŭm) [L. *columna*, pillar]. A cylindrical supporting structure.

c., anal. Vertical folds in the anal canal.

c., anterior. The anterior portion of the gray matter on each side of the spinal cord. With reference to white matter, the posterior funiculus.

c., Clarke's. A group of large cells in the medial portion of the base of the posterior gray column of the spinal cord.

c., fornix. A column of the fornix, two arched bands of fibers that form the anterior portion of the fornix. Fibers lead to mammillary body.

c., gray. Gray matter in the anterior and posterior horns of the spinal cord.

c., lateral. A column in lateral portion of gray matter of spinal cord. Contains cell bodies of preganglionic neurons of sympathetic nervous system. The lateral funiculus or the white matter between roots of spinal nerves.

c. of Burdach. The fasciculus cuneatus, q.v.

c. of Goll. The fasciculus gracilis, q.v.

c. of Gowers. Tract of ascending fibers anterior to the direct cerebellar column and on the lateral surface of the spinal cord.

c. of Morgagni. One of several vertical ridges in mucous membrane at junction of anus and rectum.

c., posterior. The posterior horn of the gray matter of the spinal cord. It consists of an expanded portion or caput connected by a narrower cervix to the main portion of gray matter. The posterior funiculus of the white matter.

c., rectal. C., anal, q.v.

c., renal. A column of Bertin, cortical material of the kidney that extends centrally, separating the pyramids.

c., spinal. C., vertebral, q.v.

c., vertebral. The portion of the axial skeleton consisting of vertebrae (7 cervical, 12 thoracic, 5 lumbar, the sacrum, and the coccyx) joined together by intervertebral disks. It forms the main supporting axis of the body, encloses and protects the spinal cord, and serves for attachment of the appendicular skeleton and muscles for moving the various body parts. SYN: *spinal column.*

c., vesicular. Line of ganglion cells on inner side of posterior column.

columna (kŏ-lŭm′na) [L.] (pl. *columnae*). [NA] A column or pillar.

c. carnea. A muscular projection within the cardiac ventricles. SYN: *trabecula carnea cordis.*

c. nasi. Nasal septum.

c. rugarum vaginae. Folds of mucous membrane of the vagina that are arranged in a columnar fashion. SYN: *c. vaginalis.*

c. vaginalis. C. rugarum vaginae, q.v.

columnar layer. Retinal rod-and-cone layer.

columning (kŏl′ŭm-ĭng). An outmoded technique using the introduction of tampons in vagina to support the prolapsed uterus. SEE: *pessary.*

Coly-Mycin M. Trade name for colistin sodium.

Coly-Mycin S Oral. Trade name for colistin sulfate.

coma (kō′mă) [Gr. *koma*, a deep sleep]. An abnormal deep stupor occurring in illness, as a result of it, or due to an injury. The patient cannot be aroused by external stimuli. More than 50% of cases are a result of trauma to the head or circulatory accidents in the brain caused by hypertension, arteriosclerosis, thrombosis, tumor, abscess formation, or insufficient flow of blood to the brain. Other frequent causes of coma are acute infections of the brain or meninges; acute infections and bacterial intoxications as in fevers, botulism, and other infectious diseases; effects of drugs (alcohol, atropine, barbiturates, chloral, hyoscine, paraldehyde, and phenols); trauma as in accidents, hemorrhage, and electrocution; gases or fumes such as carbon dioxide or carbon monoxide; extreme temperature; neurosis such as in malingering. SEE: *Glasgow Coma Scale.*

TREAT: Treat symptomatically until there is evidence that definitive therapy is indicated. Institute basic life support measures.

F.A.: Should be cautiously instituted. Patient should not be moved other than to position the head in order to help clear the airway. Sudden movement of the patient by unskilled persons may be dangerous. The shirt collar should be loosened.

Caution: If there is a question of whether the coma is due to an overdose of insulin or diabetic coma, it is safe to give glucose intravenously; administration of insulin might be disastrous.

Urine should be examined for albumin, sugar, narcotics, and acetone. In uremic coma, stimulate diuresis. In coma due to hysteria, the patient requires careful nursing care and observation but no specific therapy, other than maintaining the airway, is indicated.

NURSING IMPLICATIONS: Maintain a patent airway, monitor neurologic status, utilizing Glasgow Coma Scale, and including level of consciousness, pupillary signs, ocular movement, verbal response, sensory and motor function, mental and behavioral status, and vital signs, particularly respiratory patterns, every one to four hours depending on stability. Document findings and report evidence of clinical deterioration. Monitor and maintain fluid and electrolyte balance; maintain GI functions; provide adequate enteral or parenteral nutrition. Assess ventilatory status, auscultating for adventitious lungs sounds, and provide adequate ventilation and oxygenation, repositioning the patient to improve aeration of lung bases and encourage drainage of secretions; also suction oropharynx as necessary. Assess skin and institute plan to prevent or manage decubiti; provide passive range-of-motion exercises to maintain joint mobility; reposition patient frequently to prevent decubiti; and use appropriate supportive devices to prevent external hip rotation and flexion and extension contractures, and use foot board to prevent foot drop. Protect corneas from ulceration. Provide verbal and touch stimulation, consistently orienting patient to person, place, time and activities, as the patient may be aware of surroundings and hear what is said even though unresponsive. SEE: *shock.*

c., alcoholic. Coma due to alcohol.

c., apoplectic. Coma due to intracranial vascular accident; so-called shock or stroke. One side of body and one or more of the extremities may be paralyzed. Initially fever is not present. One pupil may be larger than the other. Coma usually indicates increased intracranial pressure. SEE: *apoplexy; stroke.*

c., barbiturate. Coma caused by ingestion or injection of barbiturates. Used clinically in the treatment of elevated intracranial pressure.

NURSING IMPLICATIONS: Patient is usually intubated and mechanically ventilated. Careful attention to adequate pulmonary toilet and effective operation of mechanical ventilator are necessary. Respiratory status should be monitored frequently.

c., diabetic. Coma occurring in diabetes, due to lack of insulin, which causes metabolic changes with excess production of acetone bodies, q.v., and metabolic acidosis. Paralysis not present. SEE: table. SEE: *Nursing Diagnoses* in *Appendix.*

SYM: Sweet breath. Hyperglycemia is present, and eyeballs may be soft due to dehydration.

TREAT: Correct use of insulin has prevented diabetic coma to a large extent but an overdose may induce hypoglycemic coma. Thus, do not give insulin until the diagnosis of diabetic coma is made. Examine urine hourly for dextrose; if urine is sugar-free,

more dextrose must be given.

c., hepatic. Coma due to liver failure. SEE: *hepatic coma.*

c., hypoglycemic. Unconsciousness due to a decreased level of blood glucose. This may be due to a disease of the pancreas, an overdose of insulin, or starvation. SEE: table.

c., irreversible. Coma from which the patient cannot recover. SYN: *brain death.*

c., Kussmaul's. The coma, acidosis, and deep breathing seen in diabetic coma.

c., nonketotic hyperosmolar. Coma present mostly in diabetic patients with marked hyperglycemia.

c., uremic. The result of disturbed kidney metabolism, causing autointoxication through the retention of metabolic end products that would normally be excreted by the kidneys. Interference with the acid-base balance develops.

SYM: In general, respirations are stertorous, face is livid; skin is dry and may be covered with "uremic frost," which is a collection of urea excreted in the sweat; forceful and rapid pulse; blood pressure elevated; sphincters may be relaxed; urinous odor on breath; urine scanty and containing many casts and albumin. Complete retention may occur.

c., vigil. Coma in which the patient's eyes are open wide, and they are in a vacant stare; face is expressionless; but patient is unconscious. May occur in typhus or typhoid fever, or in organic brain syndrome associated with systemic infection.

coma scale. SEE: *Glasgow Coma Scale.*

comatose (kō'mă-tōs). In a condition of coma.

combustion (kŏm-bŭst'yŭn). 1. Burning. 2. In metabolism, the oxidation of food with production of heat.

comedo (kŏm'ē-dō) [L. *comedere,* to eat up] (pl. *comedones, comedos*). Blackhead. Discolored dried sebum plugging an excretory duct of the skin.

SYM: Commonly affects the face, back, and ears; chronic, frequently associated with seborrheic dermatitis or acne; usually during adolescence.

ETIOL: Either increased activity of sebaceous glands or material secreted is unable to escape through a too-narrow opening.

TREAT: Aside from careful and gentle removal of plugs, treatment is essentially that of acne, q.v.

PROG: Obstinate and persistent, but amenable to treatment.

comes (kō'mēz) [L., companion] (pl. *comites*). A blood vessel that accompanies a nerve or another blood vessel.

Diagnosis of Diabetic and Hypoglycemic Coma

	Diabetic Coma	Hypoglycemic Coma
Onset	Gradual	Often sudden
History	Often of acute infection in a diabetic or insufficient insulin intake. Previous history of diabetes may be absent.	Recent insulin injection, inadequate meal, or excessive exercise after insulin
Skin	Flushed, dry	Pale, sweating
Tongue	Dry or furred	Moist
Breath	Smell of acetone	Acetone odor rare
Thirst	Intense	Absent
Respiration	Deep (air hunger) (Kussmaul)	Shallow
Vomiting	Common	Rare
Pulse	Rapid, feeble	Full and bounding
Eyeball Tension	Low	Normal
Urine	Sugar and acetone present	No sugar or acetone, unless bladder has not been emptied for some hours
Blood Sugar	Raised (over 200 mg/dl)	Subnormal (20–50 mg/dl)
Blood Pressure	Low	Normal
Abdominal Pain	Common and often acute	Absent

Comfolax. Trade name for docusate sodium.

comma tract of Schultze. The fasciculus interfascicularis, a tract of descending fibers located between the fasciculus cuneatus and fasciculus gracilis in the posterior funiculus of the spinal cord.

commensal (kŏ-mĕn'săl) [L. com-, together, + mensa, table]. One of two or more organisms that live in an intimate, nonparasitic relationship. SYN: symbion; symbiont. SEE: symbiosis.

commensalism (kŏ-mĕn'săl-ĭzm″). The symbiotic relationship of two organisms of different species in which neither is harmful to the other and one gains some benefit such as protection or nourishment.
Ex.: nonpathogenic bacteria in human intestine.

comminute (kŏm'ĭ-nūt) [L. com-, together, + minuere, to crumble]. To break into pieces.

comminuted fracture. A fracture in which the bone is splintered or crushed. SEE: compound fracture.

comminution (kŏm″ĭ-nū'shŭn) [L. comminutio, crumbling]. Reducing a solid body to varying sizes by grating, pulverizing, slicing, granulating, and by other processes. SEE: attenuation.

commissura (kŏm″mĭ-sū'ră) [L.] (pl. commissurae). A commissure.

commissural (kŏm-mĭs'ū-răl). Pert. to a commissure.

commissure (kŏm'ĭ-shūr) [L. commissura, a joining together]. 1. A transverse band of nerve fibers passing over the midline in the central nervous system. 2. The coming together across the midline or dividing space of two structures, as the lips, eyelids, or labia.
c., anterior cerebral. Band of white fibers that passes through lamina terminalis, connecting the two cerebral hemispheres.
c., anterior gray. Commissure in spinal cord lying anterior to central canal.
c., anterior white. Commissure in spinal cord lying anterior to central canal and anterior to the anterior gray commissure.
c., of fornix. Band of fibers connecting the two crura.
c., posterior, of brain. Commissure just above the midbrain containing fibers that connect the superior colliculi.
c., posterior, of spinal cord. Gray commissure connecting two halves of spinal cord. It lies posterior to the central canal.

commissurorrhaphy (kŏm″ĭ-shūr-or'ă-fē) [″ + Gr. rhaphe, seam, ridge]. Surgical procedure of joining the parts of a commissure together in order to decrease the size of the opening.

commissurotomy (kŏm″ĭ-shūr-ŏt'ō-mē) [″ + Gr. tome, incision]. Surgical incision of any commissure. May be used in treating mitral stenosis in order to increase the size of the mitral orifice. This is done by incising the adhesions that cause the leaves of the valve to stick together. Commissurotomy may also be used in treating certain psychiatric conditions by incising the anterior commissure of the brain.

commitment (kŏ-mĭt'měnt). The legal procedure for hospitalization of a patient who may not be competent to make that decision or who does not choose to be hospitalized. Usually done in connection with patients with mental illness, but may be used to hospitalize patients with certain contagious diseases. SEE: *certification.*

common bile duct. Duct carrying bile to the duodenum and receiving it from the cystic duct of the gallbladder and the hepatic ducts. SEE: *biliary tract* for illus.

commune (kŏm'yoon). A group of people with common goals and beliefs who live in the same area, usually in one or more small homes or residences. Some communes are committed to the concept of holistic medicine.

communicable disease. 1. A disease that may be transmitted directly or indirectly from one individual to another. 2. Disease due to an infectious agent or toxic products produced by it. SEE: *CDC blood and body fluid precautions;* table.

communicable disease, words pert. to: agent; carrier; CDC blood and body fluid precautions; contagion; endemic; epidemic; host, intermediate; immunity; incidence; incubation; infection; isolation; microbe; microorganism; prevalence; quarantine; transmissible; vector.

communicans (kŏ-mū'ně-kănz) [L. *communicare,* to connect with]. One of a number of communicating nerves or arteries.

communication board. Any of a variety of devices with letters or words that permit communication by patients with impaired physical and verbal ability.

communicator. An electronic device that permits persons with impaired verbal and physical ability to communicate through graphic or symbolic light-emitting diode (LED) displays, printed messages, or synthetic speech.

communis (kŏ-mū'nĭs) [L.]. 1. Common, nonspecific. 2. In anatomy, something such as a vessel that supplies several branches.

community medicine. Health care for all members of a community, with particular emphasis on preventive medicine and public health.

Comolli's sign (kō-mōl'lēz) [Antonio Comolli, It. pathologist, b. 1879]. A triangular swelling corresponding to the outline of the fractured scapula.

comorbid disease. A disease coexisting with the primary disease, e.g., the patient's primary disease could be cancer and the comorbid disease could be emphysema.

compact [L. *compactus,* joined together]. Closely and tightly packed together. Dense; solid.

compact bone. Hard or dense bone, which forms the superficial layer of all bones, in contrast to spongy or cancellous bone found chiefly in the ends of long bones.

compaction (kŏm-păk'shŭn). 1. Simultaneous engagement of the presenting parts of twins in the pelvis so that labor cannot progress. 2. In dentistry, the act or process of joining or packing together powdered gold, mat gold, or gold foil in a prepared cavity in a tooth.

comparative anatomy. Human anatomy compared with that of animals.

comparative negligence. In forensic medicine, negligence of the plaintiff and defendant are measured in terms of percentages. Damages awarded are decreased in proportion to plaintiff's amount of negligence provided it is less than that of defendant.

compartment syndrome. Any condition in which a structure such as a nerve or tendon is being constricted in a space, e.g., *carpal tunnel syndrome.* The sheath or tendon may be enlarged due to disease or inflammation and no longer able to move freely in the compartment. The condition may also be present inside a cast when edema causes increased pressure on the limb immobilized.

NURSING IMPLICATIONS: Evaluate patient at risk for deep, throbbing pain out of proportion to original problem, pain that is not relieved by ordered analgesic drugs, pain occurring in response to passive flexion or extension of digits, decrease in mobility of digits, and paresthesias. Notify physician of findings and elevate the extremity. Remove constricting dressings or casts while supporting injured limb. Prepare for surgical decompression (fasciotomy) if symptoms are not resolved within 30 minutes.

compatibility [L. *compati,* to sympathize with]. 1. State of suitability to be mixed or taken together without unfavorable results, as drugs. 2. Ability of two individuals or groups to live together without undue strife or tension.

compatible. In pharmacology, pertaining to the ability to mix two medicines without interfering with their action.

Compazine. Trade name for prochlorperazine maleate.

compensating. Making up for a deficiency.

compensation [L. *cum,* with, + *pensare,* to weigh]. 1. Making up for a defect, as cardiac circulation competent to meet demands made upon it regardless of valvular

Method of Transmission of Some Common Communicable Diseases

Disease	How Agent Leaves the Bodies of the Sick	How Organisms May Be Transmitted	Method of Entry into the Body
Acquired immuno-deficiency syndrome (AIDS)	Blood, semen, or other body fluids, including breast milk	Inoculation by use of contaminated needles or by direct contact so that infected body fluids can enter the body	Transplacentally to embryo or fetus Nursing at breast
Cholera	Excreta from intestinal tract	As in typhoid fever	As in typhoid fever
Diphtheria	Sputum and discharges from nose and throat Skin lesions	Direct contact Droplet infection from patient coughing Hands of nurse Articles used by and about patient	Through mouth to throat or nose to throat
Gonococcal disease	Lesions Discharges from infected mucous membranes	Direct contact as in sexual intercourse Towels, bathtubs, toilets, etc. Hands of infected persons soiled with their own discharges Hands of attendant	Directly onto mucous membrane Through breaks in membrane
Hepatitis A, viral	Feces	As in typhoid fever	As in typhoid fever, rarely by blood transfusion
Hepatitis B, viral and delta hepatitis	Blood and serum-derived fluids, including semen and vaginal fluids	Contact with blood and body fluids	Transfusion Exposure to body fluids including during hetero- or homosexual intercourse
Hepatitis C	Blood	Transfusion Parenteral drug use Laboratory exposure to blood Health care workers exposed to blood, i.e., dentists and their assistants, and clinical and laboratory staff	Infected blood Contaminated needles
Hookworm	Feces	Direct contact with soil polluted with feces Eggs in feces hatch in sandy soil. Feces may also contaminate food.	Larvae enter through breaks in skin, especially skin of feet, and after devious passage through the body settle in the intestine.

Method of Transmission of Some Common Communicable Diseases
(Continued)

Disease	How Agent Leaves the Bodies of the Sick	How Organisms May Be Transmitted	Method of Entry into the Body
Influenza	As in pneumonia	As in pneumonia	As in pneumonia
Leprosy	Uncertain, may be from lesions Bacilli found in nodules that may break down, forming lesions	Uncertain, probably nasal discharges of untreated patients	Uncertain, probably via upper respiratory tract and broken skin
Measles (rubella)	As in streptococcal sore throat	As in streptococcal sore throat	As in streptococcal sore throat
Meningitis, meningococcal	Discharges from nose and throat	Direct contact Hands of nurse or attendant Articles used by and about patient Flies	Mouth and nose
Mumps	Discharges from infected glands and mouth	Direct contact with persons affected	Mouth and nose
Ophthalmia neonatorum (gonococcal infection of eyes of newborn)	Purulent discharges from the eye	Direct contact with infected areas as vagina of infected mother during birth Other infected babies Hands of doctor or nurse Linens	Directly on the conjunctiva
Pneumonia	Sputum and discharges from nose and throat	Direct contact Hands of nurse Articles used by and about patient	Through mouth and nose to lungs
Poliomyelitis	Discharges from nose and throat, and via feces	Direct contact Hands of nurse or attendant Rarely in milk	Through mouth and nose
Rubeola	Secretions from nose and throat	Droplet spread from nose or throat by direct contact with nasal or throat secretions Airborne spread is possible	Through mouth and nose
Streptococcal sore throat	Discharges from nose and throat skin lesions	Direct contact Hands of nurse Articles used by and about patient	Through mouth and nose

Method of Transmission of Some Common Communicable Diseases
(Continued)

Disease	How Agent Leaves the Bodies of the Sick	How Organisms May Be Transmitted	Method of Entry into the Body
Syphilis	Infected tissues Lesions Blood Transfer through placenta to fetus	Direct contact Kissing or sexual intercourse Contaminated needles and syringes	Directly into blood and tissues through breaks in skin or membrane Contaminated needles and syringes
Tetanus	Excreta from infected herbivorous animals and man	Soil, especially that with manure or feces in it Dust, etc. Articles used about stables	Directly into bloodstream through wounds (organism is an anaerobe and prefers deep, incised wound)
Trachoma	Discharges from infected eyes	Direct contact Hands, towels, handkerchiefs	Directly on conjunctiva
Tuberculosis, bovine		Milk from infected cow	As in tuberculosis, human
Tuberculosis, human	Sputum Lesions Feces	Direct contact such as kissing Droplet infection from person coughing with mouth uncovered Sputum from mouth to fingers, thence to food and other things Soiled dressings	Through mouth to lungs and intestines From intestines via lymph channels to lymph vessels and to tissues
Typhoid fever	Feces and urine	Direct contact with food, water, articles, or insects contaminated with feces, or urine from patients	Through mouth via infected food or water and thence to intestinal tract
Whooping cough	Discharges from respiratory tract	Direct contact with persons affected	Mouth and nose

defect. 2. In psychoanalysis, a psychic mechanism best described by an example. The individual handicapped by a physical deformity or variation or by a character defect may escape the consciousness or revelation of the inferiority by accomplishment resulting from compensatory ambition. More simply, the short man may strut or the incompetent brag. Sublimation, q.v., is

often similar, but varies in that the substitution of a higher social goal gratifies the infrasocial drive by replacement, rather than going to the opposite extreme in a merely camouflaging manner. 3. Restitution by means of payment to a person injured, esp. in the work place.

c., failure of. Inability of heart muscle to cope with cardiac output required. It indicates a diseased heart muscle.

ETIOL: Diseased myocardium; back pressure, due to mitral regurgitation; mitral or aortic stenosis; or aortic regurgitation.

compensatory. To compensate or make up for a loss or lack of some capability or for an injury, e.g., the compensatory increase in strength of the leg opposite to one that has been amputated or paralyzed.

competence (kŏm'pĕ-tĕns). 1. In psychiatry, having the ability to manage one's affairs, and by inference, not to be insane. Usually stated as being mentally competent. 2. To perform in a manner that is satisfactory to the demands of a situation, to interact effectively with the environment.

competition (kŏm"pĕ-tĭsh'ŭn). The simultaneous attempt of similar substances to attach to a receptor site of an enzyme or cell wall.

complaint (kŏm-plānt'). Verbalization or other form of communication of the principal reason the patient is seeking medical assistance.

complement (kŏm'plĕ-mĕnt) [L. *complere*, to complete]. A group of proteins in the blood that influence the inflammatory process and serve as the primary mediator in the antigen-antibody reactions of the B cell mediated immune response, q.v. Components of complement are labeled C1-C9. C3 and C5 are most commonly involved in promoting vasodilation, chemotaxis, q.v., opsonization of antigens, q.v., lysis of cells, and blood clotting. Complement is activated whenever tissue injury occurs, specifically by neutrophil aggregation, antigen-antibody contact, bacterial endotoxins, and the release of blood coagulation proteins. SEE: *antibody; antigen; cytokines, immunity; inflammation; opsonin.*

A deficiency or abnormality in complement, which may be inherited, can increase susceptibility to infection. Specific disorders associated with abnormal complement levels include hypogammaglobulinemia, systemic lupus erythematosus, dermatomyositis, glomerulonephritis, recurrent pyogenic infections, and hereditary angioedema. These diseases associated with specific complement deficiencies illustrate the importance of the complement in maintaining a normal state of health.

complemental, complementary. Supplying something that is lacking in another system or entity.

c. air. Amount of air that can be inspired over and above the tidal air by the deepest inspiration. SEE: *air.*

c. colors. Any two spectral colors that, when blended, produce white light.

complementarity. In individual and group

interactions, the extent of the resolution of the emotional requirements of those involved.

complement fixation. A common blood assay used to determine if antigen-antibody reactions have occurred. Complement that combines with the antigen-antibody complex becomes inactive and is unable to lyse (kill) red blood cells in vitro. The degree of complement fixation is determined by the number of red blood cells that are destroyed, which indicates the amount of free complement not bound to the antigen-antibody complexes. Complement fixation is one way to measure the severity of an infection since it helps indicate the extent and effectiveness of antigen-antibody reactions occurring in the body.

complex [L. *complexus*, woven together]. 1. All the ideas, feelings, and sensations connected with a subject. 2. Intricate. 3. An atrial or ventricular systole as it appears on an electrocardiograph tracing. 4. A subconscious idea (or group of ideas) that has become associated with a repressed wish or emotional experience and that may influence behavior although the person may not have any appreciation of the connection between the repressed thoughts or actions.

In freudian theory, a grouping of ideas with an emotional background. These may be harmless, and the individual may be fully aware of them, e.g., an artist sees every object with a view to a possible picture and is said to have established a complex for art. Often, however, the complex is aroused by some painful emotional reaction such as fright or excessive grief that, instead of being allowed a natural outlet, becomes unconsciously repressed and later manifests itself in some abnormality of mind or behavior. According to Freud, the best method of determining the complex is through the medium of psychoanalysis. SEE: *Electra complex; Jocasta complex; Oedipus complex.*

c., castration. Morbid fear of being castrated.

c., Electra. Excessive love of her father by an adult female. SEE: *Electra complex.*

c., Ghon. The primary lesion in tuberculosis, consisting of the affected area of the lung and a corresponding lymph node. These usually heal and become calcified.

c., Golgi. An organelle present in most cells but larger in secretory cells. Enclosed are vacuoles, sacs, and secretory material. This complex is vital to the cell's function. SEE: *Golgi apparatus; organelle* for illus.

c., inferiority. A state of mind in which one feels inferior to others.

c., Jocasta. SEE: *Jocasta complex.*

c., Oedipus. Excessive love of his mother

by an adult male, usually accompanied by hostility toward father. SEE: *Oedipus complex.*

   c., superiority. Exaggerated conviction of one's own superiority; also pretense of being superior to compensate for a real or imagined inferiority.

complexion (kŏm-plĕk'shŭn). The color and appearance of the facial skin.

complexus (kŏm-plĕk'sŭs) [L.]. Semispinalis capitis muscle.

compliance (kŏm-plī'ăns). 1. The property of altering size and shape in response to application of force, weight, or release from such force. Thus the lung and thoracic cage of a child may have a high degree of compliance as compared to that of an elderly adult. SEE: *elastance.* 2. The extent to which a patient's behavior coincides with medical advice. Compliance may be estimated by carefully questioning the patient and family members, evaluating the degree of clinical response to therapy, presence or absence of side effects of the drug(s) used, serum drug levels or test for excretion of the drug in the urine, and counting remaining pills.

   c., pulmonary. A measure of the force required to distend the lungs.

complication [L. *cum,* with, + *plicare,* to fold]. An added difficulty; a complex state. A disease or accident superimposed upon another without being specifically related, yet affecting or modifying the prognosis of the original disease, e.g., pneumonia is a complication of measles and is the cause of many deaths from that disease.

component. A constituent part.

component blood therapy. SEE: *blood component therapy.*

compos mentis (kŏm"pŭs mĕn'tĭs) [L.]. Of sound mind; sane. SEE: *non compos mentis.*

compound [L. *componere,* to place together]. 1. A substance composed of two or more units or parts combined in definite proportions by weight and having specific properties of its own. Compounds are formed in plants and animals and are of two types, organic and inorganic. 2. Made up of more than one part.

   c., dental. A nonelastic molding or impression material used in dentistry that softens when heated and solidifies without chemical change when cooled, i.e., a thermoplastic material.

   c., inorganic. One of many compounds that, in general, contains no carbon.

   c., organic. Compound containing carbon, such as carbohydrates, proteins, and fats.

compound astigmatism. Myopia of both vertical and horizontal meridians.

compound fracture. Fracture of bone where broken end of bone has penetrated the skin.

compound microscope. A microscope consisting of two or more lenses.

comprehend. To understand something.

compress [L. *compressus,* squeezed together]. 1. (kŏm'prĕs) Cloth, wet or dry, folded and applied firmly to a part. 2. (kŏm-prĕs') To press together into smaller space. 3. To close by squeezing together, as a wound.

   c., chest. Application of two pieces of linen of sufficient size to fit the entire chest from the clavicles down to the umbilicus.

   c., cold. Soft, absorbent cloth, several layers thick, dipped in cold water, slightly wrung out, applied to given part. To maintain constant temperature, compress is frequently renewed or ice bag or rubber coil through which ice water is circulating is placed on it. Duration of application is usually 30 to 60 minutes.

   c., forehead. Soft, moist towel renewed at least every two minutes.

   c., hot. Soft, absorbent cloth folded into several layers, dipped in hot water 107° to 115°F (41.7° to 46.1°C), barely wrung out and placed on part to be treated; covered with a piece of flannel large enough to overlap the linen slightly. Temperature is maintained at constant level by renewing compress or by rubber coil through which hot water 107° to 115°F (41.7° to 46.1°C) is circulated.

   c., wet. Application of two or more folds of soft cloth wrung out of water at prescribed temperatures and covered with flannel.

compression (kŏm-prĕsh'ŭn) [L. *compressio,* a compression]. A squeezing together; state of being pressed together.

   c., cerebral. Pressure on the brain produced by increased intracranial fluids, embolism, thrombosis, tumors, and skull fractures. More serious than concussion, q.v.

   SYM: Deep unconsciousness; full, bounding pulse; deep, stertorous, slow respirations; flushed face; high blood pressure; pupils varying in size. Fever may develop, and there may be retention or incontinence of urine and feces.

   DANGER SIGNALS: Coma; Cheyne-Stokes respiration; fever; quickening of pulse.

   NURSING IMPLICATIONS: Assess patient closely for symptoms of increased intracranial pressure, respiratory distress, convulsions, bleeding from the ears or nose, or drainage of cerebrospinal fluid from the ears or nose (which most probably indicates a fracture). Observe for any alterations in sensory, motor, or mental status. Pupillary size, equality, and ability to react to light are monitored and recorded as frequently as indicated. Maintain seizure precautions. SEE: *coma.*

c., digital. Compression of blood vessels by means of the fingers in order to stop hemorrhage.

c., myelitis. Compression caused by pressure on the spinal cord, often due to a tumor.

compression gloves. Any type of glove made of stretch material so that pressure is maintained against the fingers and hands. This helps to reduce edema.

compressor. 1. An instrument or device that applies a compressive force, as in compaction of gold. 2. A muscle that compresses a part, as the compressor hemispherium bulbi, which compresses the bulb of the urethra.

c., air. A machine that compresses air into storage tanks for use in air syringes, air turbine handpieces, and other air-driven tools.

compromised host. Persons who lack resistance to infection due to a deficiency in any of their host defenses. SEE: *AIDS; host defense mechanisms; immunocompromised.*

compulsion (kŏm-pŭl'shŭn) [L. *compulsio,* compulsion]. Repetitive stereotyped act performed to relieve fear connected with obsession; dictated by the patient's subconscious against the subject's wishes and, if denied, causing uneasiness.

compulsion neurosis. Obsession or psychoneurosis that compels one to perform an absurd act or to say something silly. SYN: *obsessional neurosis.*

compulsive (kŏm-pŭl'sĭv). Pert. to or characterized by compulsion.

compulsive ideas. An idea that continues against one's will to suggest the commitment of an overt act that would normally be against one's better judgment.

compulsory (kŏm-pŭl'sor-ē). Compelling action against one's will.

computer. An electronic device for storing and retrieving numerical or textual information; and, in the case of numerical or mathematical data, for processing and analyzing it. In medicine and in biological sciences in general, the use of computers has made it possible to store on and retrieve from small disks quantities of data that would require an inordinate amount of space if stored in conventional files.

c., digital. A computer that processes information in the form of discrete digits or units.

computer-assisted design. ABBR: CAD. The use of computer systems to assist in designing objects. This may be utilized in plastic surgery to reshape body parts, such as the face; or in orthopedics to design replacement parts, such as an artificial hip.

computer interface. Usually describes a circuit or part required to connect a computer to some external device, such as a printer.

con- [L.]. Prefix meaning together with.

con-A. *concanavalin-A.*

conarium (kō-nā'rē-ŭm) [L.]. The pineal body of the brain.

conation (kō-nā'shŭn) [L. *conatio,* an attempt]. The initiative, impulse, and drive, arising from inside oneself, to act. All of these may be diminished in cerebral diseases, esp. those involving the medial orbital parts of the frontal lobes. SEE: *abulia.*

conative (kŏn'ă-tĭv). Pert. to conation.

concanavalin-A (kŏn"kă-năv'ĭ-lĭn). ABBR: con-A. A mitogen, q.v., protein from the jack bean used in the laboratory to stimulate proliferation of T lymphocytes drawn from multiple sites in the body. SEE: *mitogen.*

concatenation (kŏn-kăt"ĭ-nā'shŭn) [L. *con,* together, + *catena,* chain]. A group of events or effects acting in concert or occurring at the same time.

Concato's disease (kŏn-kŏ'tōs) [Luigi M. Concato, It. physician, 1825–1882]. Polyserositis.

concave (kŏn'kāv, kŏn-kāv') [" + *cavus,* hollow]. Having a spherically depressed or hollow surface.

concavity (kŏn-kăv'ĭ-tē). A surface with curved, bowl-like sides.

concavoconcave (kŏn-kā"vō-kŏn'kāv) [" + *cavus,* hollow, + *con,* with, + *cavus,* hollow]. Concave on opposing sides.

concavoconvex (kŏn-kā"vō-kŏn'vĕks) [" + " + *convexus,* vaulted]. Concave on one side and convex on opposite surface. SEE: *convex.*

conceive (kŏn-sēv') [L. *concipere,* to take to oneself]. 1. To become pregnant. 2. To form a mental image or to bring into mind; to form an idea.

concentration (kŏn-sĕn-trā'shŭn) [L. *con,* together with, + *centrum,* center]. 1. Increase in strength of a fluid by evaporation. 2. Medicine strengthened by removal of part of the liquid in it. 3. Fixation of mind on one subject to exclusion of all other thoughts.

c., hydrogen ion. Concentration of hydrogen ions in a solution; the symbol is pH, q.v.

c., minimum inhibitory. ABBR: MIC. The lowest concentration of an antibiotic in a bacterial culture that prevents the growth of specific bacteria.

concentric (kŏn-sĕn'trĭk) [" + *centrum,* center]. Having a common center.

concentric muscle contraction. SEE: *muscle contraction, concentric.*

concept (kŏn'sĕpt) [L. *conceptum,* something understood]. An idea.

conception (kŏn-sĕp'shŭn). 1. The mental process of forming an idea. 2. The union of the male sperm and the ovum of the female; fertilization. With a cycle of 28 days, menstruation normally lasts 5 days followed by a period of repair and proliferation of the lining of the uterus (endometrium) for about a week. In general, ovulation occurs about 12 to 14 days prior to the beginning of the next menstrual period. Thus, sexual intercourse during the middle of the menstrual cycle is most likely to result in conception. During this period, the ovum is discharged from the follicle and makes its way through the fallopian tube to the uterus. If fertilization does not occur during this time, the ovum disintegrates and for the remaining portion of the menstrual cycle (the 10 days preceding menstruation) conception is less likely to occur.

However, one of the most variable events known in human biology is the menstrual cycle. It is therefore quite difficult, and in many cases impossible, to predict optimum time of conception or the reverse by attempting to calculate ovulation time from the time the last menstrual period occurred. Also, sperm survival time in the female reproductive tract is variable. SEE: *basal temperature chart; contraception.*

conceptual models in nursing. SEE: *Appendix 23.*

conceptus (kŏn-sĕp'tŭs). The products of conception.

concha (kŏng'kă) [Gr. *konche*, shell] (pl. *conchae*). 1. The outer ear or the pinna. 2. One of the three nasal conchae. SEE: *c., nasal.*

   c. auriculae. [NA] A concavity on the median surface of the auricle of the ear, divided by a ridge into the upper cymba conchae and a lower cavum conchae. The latter leads to the external auditory meatus.

   c. bullosa. Distention of turbinate bone due to cyst formation.

   c., nasal. One of the three scroll-like bones that project medially from the lateral wall of the nasal cavity; a turbinate bone. The superior and middle conchae are processes of lateral mass of the ethmoid bone; the inferior concha is a face bone. Each overlies a meatus.

   c. sphenoidalis. [NA] In a fetal skull, one of two curved plates located on anterior portion of body of sphenoid bone. Forms part of roof of nasal cavity.

conchitis (kŏng-kī'tĭs) [" + *itis*, inflammation]. Inflammation of any concha.

conchoidal (kŏng-koy'dăl) [" + *eidos*, form, shape]. Having the shape of a shell.

conchoscope (kŏng'kō-skōp) [" + *skopein*, to examine]. Instrument for examination of the nasal cavity.

conchotome (kŏng'kō-tōm) [" + *tome*, incision]. Device for excision of middle turbinate bone.

conchotomy (kŏng-kŏt'ō-mē). Surgical incision of a nasal concha.

concoction (kŏn-kŏk'shŭn) [L. *con*, with, + *coquere*, to cook]. Mixture of two medicinal substances usually done with the aid of heat.

concomitant (kŏn-kŏm'ĭ-tănt) [" + *comes*, companion]. Accessory; taking place at the same time.

concordance (kŏn-kor'dăns). In twins, the equal representation of a genetic trait in each.

concrement (kŏn'krē-mĕnt) [L. *concrementum*]. A concretion as of protein and other substances. If infiltrated with calcium salts, it is termed a calculus.

concrescence (kŏn-krĕs'ĕns) [L. *con*, with, + *crescere*, to grow]. The union of separate parts; coalescence, esp. the attachment of a tooth to an adjacent one.

concrete (kŏn'krēt, kŏn-krēt') [L. *concretus*, solid]. Condensed, hardened, or solidified.

concretio cordis (kŏn-krē'shē-ō kor'dĭs). Obliteration of the pericardial space due to chronic constrictive pericarditis.

concretion (kŏn-krē'shŭn) [" + *crescere*, to grow]. A calculus.

concussion (kŏn-kŭsh'ŭn) [L. *concussus*, shaken violently]. 1. An injury resulting from impact with an object. 2. Loss of function either partial or complete as that resulting from a blow or fall.

   c. of brain. Cerebral concussion. A common result of a blow to the head or fall on the end of spine with force sufficient to be transmitted upward. This usually causes unconsciousness, either temporary or prolonged. Return of consciousness may be gradual. Patient may suddenly draw up knees and vomit. SEE: *Nursing Diagnoses* in *Appendix.*

   SYM: Vary with location and extent of injury from transient dizziness to various paralyses, or unconsciousness; unequal pupils, shock. If uncomplicated, patient regains consciousness in a short period of time. Period of reaction, accompanied by vomiting, temperature 99° to 100°F (37.2 to 37.8 C), rapid pulse, flushed face, restlessness, headache, cerebral irritation, lasts for 12 to 24 hours.

   F.A.: Keep patient quietly lying down with head and shoulders slightly elevated. Do not give stimulants. Transportation should be delayed if possible. Sedatives are generally contraindicated. Cool applications to head and neck are soothing. Reassure patient if conscious. Maintain suitable temperature. Report any adverse symptoms, such as bleeding, or alteration in pupil size or reaction, at once. SEE: *coma; contusion; transportation of the injured.*

Caution: Do not give morphine.

---

c. of labyrinth. Deafness resulting from a blow to the head or ear.

c., spinal. Loss of function in spinal cord resulting from a blow or severe jarring.

condensation (kŏn"dĕn-sā'shŭn) [" + *densare,* to make thick]. 1. Making more dense or compact. 2. Changing a liquid to a solid or a gas to a liquid. 3. In psychoanalysis, the union of ideas to form a new mental pattern. 4. In chemistry, a type of reaction in which two or more molecules of the same substance react with each other and form a new and heavier substance with different chemical properties. 5. A mechanical process used in dentistry to remove excess mercury from amalgam or to form a dense gold foil restoration; it improves the physical properties of the material used and forces it to adapt more nearly perfectly to the cavity preparation.

condenser (kŏn-dĕn'sĕr). 1. Device for solidifying vapors and liquids. SEE: *capacitance.* 2. An instrument or tool used to compact and condense restorative materials in dental cavity preparations; also called a plugger.

c., electrical. Device for storing of electricity by using two conducting surfaces and a nonconductor.

c., substage. The part of the lens system of a microscope necessary to supply the illumination critical to the resolving power of the instrument. Also called Abbé condenser.

condiment (kŏn'dĭ-mĕnt) [L. *condire,* to pickle]. Appetizing ingredient added to food.

CLASSIFICATION: *Aromatic:* vanilla; cinnamon; cloves; chervil; parsley; bay leaf. *Acrid or peppery:* pepper; ginger; tabasco; all-spice. *Alliaceous or allylic:* onion, mustard; horseradish. *Acid:* vinegar; capers; gherkins; citron. *Animal origin:* caviar; anchovies. *Miscellaneous:* salt; sugar; truffles.

In general, with the exception of sugar, condiments have little nutritional value. They are extremely useful in making food more appetizing.

ACTION: They are appetizers and stimulate the secretion of saliva and intestinal juices.

condition. 1. The state of being a person. 2. State of health; or physical, esp. athletic, fitness. 3. To train a person or animal to respond in a predictable way to a stimulus.

conditioned reflex. Reflex acquired as a result of training and repetition.

conditioning (kŏn-dĭsh'ŭn-ĭng). 1. Improv-

ing the physical capability of a person by an exercise program. 2. In psychology, the use of a special and different stimulus in conjunction with a familiar stimulus. After a sufficient period of time in which the two stimuli have been simultaneously presented, the special stimulus alone will cause the response that could originally be produced only by the familiar stimulus. The late Russian physiologist, Ivan Pavlov, used dogs to demonstrate that the strange stimulus, ringing of a bell, could cause the animal to salivate if the test was done after a period of *conditioning* during which the bell and the familiar stimulus, food, were presented simultaneously. SYN: *classical conditioning.*

c., aversive. SEE: *aversion therapy.*

c., operant. The learning of a particular action or type of behavior that is followed by a reward. This technique was publicized by the contemporary Harvard psychologist, B.F. Skinner, who trained animals to activate (by pecking, in the case of a pigeon, or pressing a bar, in the case of a rat) an apparatus that released a pellet of food.

condom (kŏn'dŭm) [L. *condus,* a receptacle]. A thin, flexible sheath worn over the penis. It is made of rubber (latex) or the cecum of a sheep. A condom is used during sexual intercourse to prevent sperm from entering the vagina and to help prevent venereal disease. SEE: *AIDS; contraception; sexually transmitted diseases.*

c., instructions for use. Keep a supply of condoms at hand, ideally in a cool, dry place, so that one is easily available for use at every intercourse. Do not reuse a condom. Do not test a condom by inflating or stretching it. Handle it gently and keep it away from sharp objects. For maximum effectiveness, put the condom on before genital contact. Either the man or the woman may put the condom in place, but long fingernails may damage it. A man who is reluctant to use a condom may be more receptive to the idea if his partner puts it on for him. Unroll the condom on the erect penis, leaving a space at the end to accommodate the ejaculate. The condom must be placed with the rolled portion out so that it will unroll properly. If desired, lubricate the outside of the condom, using contraceptive jelly or another water-soluble lubricant. Use of oil-based lubricants may damage condom. After ejaculation, be sure that the condom does not become dislodged from the penis. Hold the rim of the condom firmly against the base of the penis during withdrawal. Check the condom for tears before throwing it away. If it has torn, insert a contraceptive suppository, jelly, or foam into the vagina immediately.

conductance (kŏn-dŭk'tăns) [L. *conducere,* to lead]. The conducting ability of a body or a circuit for electricity. The best conductor is one which offers the least resistance, such as gold, silver, and copper. When expressed as a numerical value, conductance is the reciprocal of resistance. The unit is the ohm.

conduction (kŏn-dŭk'shŭn). 1. The process whereby a state of excitation affects successive portions of a tissue or cell, so that the disturbance is transmitted to remote points. Conduction occurs not only in the fibers of the nervous system but also in muscle fibers. 2. The transfer of electrons, ions, heat, or sound waves through a conductor or conducting medium.

   c., bone. Sound conduction through cranial bones.

conduction system, cardiac. SEE: *heart, conduction system of.*

conductivity (kŏn"dŭk-tiv'ĭ-tē). The specific electric conducting ability of a substance. Conductivity is the reciprocal of unit resistance or resistivity. The unit is the ohm/cm. Specific conductivity is sometimes expressed as a percentage. In such cases, the conductivity is given as a percentage of the conductivity of pure copper under certain standard conditions.

conductor (kŏn-dŭk'tor). 1. Medium transmitting a force, a signal, or electricity. 2. A guide directing a surgical knife or probe.

conduit (kŏn'doo-ĭt). A channel or aqueduct, esp. an artificial one surgically constructed.

   c., ileal. Attachment of one or both ureters to one end of an isolated loop of ileum; the other end is attached to an opening in the abdominal wall.

condylar (kŏn'dĭ-lăr) [Gr. *kondylos,* knuckle]. Pert. to a condyle.

condylarthrosis (kŏn"dĭl-ăr-thrō'sĭs) [" + *arthrosis,* a joint]. A form of diarthrosis, q.v.; an ovoid head in an elliptical cavity.

condyle (kŏn'dĭl) [Gr. *kondylos,* knuckle] (pl. *condyles*). A rounded protuberance at the end of a bone forming an articulation.

condylectomy (kŏn"dĭ-lĕk'tō-mē) [" + *ektome,* excision]. Excision of a condyle.

condylion (kŏn-dĭl'ē-ŏn) [Gr. *kondylion,* knob]. A point on either the lateral or medial surface of the mandibular condyle.

condyloid (kŏn'dĭ-loyd) [Gr. *kondylos,* knuckle, + *eidos,* form, shape]. Pert. to or resembling a condyle.

condyloid process. Articular process on ramus of mandible consisting of a capitulum and neck. Articulates with mandibular fossa of temporal bone.

condyloid tubercle. A tubercle on capitulum of condyloid process of the mandible for attachment of temporomandibular ligament.

condyloma (kŏn"dĭ-lō'mă) [Gr. *kondyloma,* wart]. A wartlike growth of the skin, usually seen on the external genitalia or near the anus.

   c. acuminatum. An ordinary wart in the genital and perianal areas. It is caused by a virus and may be spread by one area containing a wart inoculating an area that it contacts. The spread of a wart from one labium to the other by auto-inoculation is possible. The virus that causes the wart is usually sexually transmitted. SYN: *wart, genital.*

   ETIOL: Various types of human papilloma virus.

   TREAT: Podophyllum applied locally; cryosurgery; electrocautery; laser surgery. Also, intralesional injection of interferon alfa is effective in treating some patients in whom other forms of therapy failed.

   c. latum. A mucous patch on the vulva or anus, coated with gray exudate, flattened in form, with delimited area, characteristic of syphilis.

condylomatous (kŏn"dĭ-lō'mă-tŭs). Pert. to a condyloma.

condylotomy (kŏn"dĭ-lŏt'ō-mē) [Gr. *kondylos,* knuckle, + *tome,* incision]. Division without removal of a condyle.

condylus (kŏn'dĭ-lŭs) (pl. *condyli*). Condyle.

cone (kōn) [Gr. *konos,* cone]. 1. A three-dimensional figure with circular base with sides sloping to a point above. May be solid or hollow. 2. In the outer layer of the retina (the layer closest to the front of the eye), the flask-shaped cells that receive visual stimuli. SEE: *rods.* 3. A hollow, tapered, cylindrical device used in upper extremity exercise activities to improve grasp, coordination, and range of motion.

   c., ocular. Cone of light in eye with point on the retina.

   c., retinal. Specialized cone-shaped cells of the retina of the eye. These cells, along with the retinal rods, are light-sensitive. The cones receive color stimuli.

cone of light. Triangular areas of reflected light on the membrana tympani extending downward from the umbo.

cone shell poisoning. The neurotoxin delivered into the wound by pointed hollow teeth of the marine animal contained in the cone shell causes intense local pain, swelling, and numbness that may last several days. In severe poisoning there may be muscular incoordination and weakness that can progress to respiratory paralysis. Even though death can occur, recovery within 24 hours is the usual outcome. There is no specific therapy but supportive measures including artificial respiration and supplemental oxygen may be needed. Use of a tourniquet to slow absorption of the toxin may help.

conexus (kŏ-nĕk′sŭs) [L.]. A connecting structure.

confabulation (kŏn-făb″ū-lā′shŭn) [L. *confabulari*, to talk together]. A behavioral reaction to memory loss in which the patient fills in memory gaps with inappropriate words.

confectio, confection (kŏn-fĕk′shē-ō, -shŭn) [L. *conficere*, to prepare]. Sugarlike soft solids in which one or more medicinal substances are incorporated with the object of affording an agreeable form for their administration and a convenient method for their preservation. Not often prescribed, and not official.

confidentiality. Information the health care team obtains from or about a patient; i.e., laboratory data are considered to be privileged and thus cannot be disclosed to a third party without the patient's consent. In some instances when the information is important to public health, it may be illegal not to disclose those data.

configuration (kŏn-fĭg″ū-rā′shŭn). 1. The shape and appearance of anything. 2. In chemistry, the position of atoms in a molecule.

confinement (kŏn-fīn′mĕnt) [O. Fr. *confiner*, to restrain in a place]. The period of childbirth.

conflict (kŏn′flĭkt) [L. *confligere*, to contend]. 1. Opposing action of incompatibles. 2. In psychiatry, the conscious or unconscious struggle between two opposing desires or courses of action. A technical term applied to a state in which social goals dictate behavior contrary to more primitive (often subconscious) desires.

confluence of sinuses. The union of the sagittal sinus with the transverse sinuses.

confluent (kŏn′floo-ĕnt) [L. *confluere*, to run together]. Running together, as when pustules merge.

conformation (kŏn″for-mā′shŭn). The form or shape of a part, body, material, or molecule.

confrontation (kŏn″frŭn-tā′shŭn) [L. *con*, together with, + *frons*, face]. 1. The examination of two patients together, one with a disease and the other from whom the disease was supposed to be contracted. 2. A method employed in determining extent of visual fields in which that of the patient is compared with that of the examiner. 3. In counseling, a feedback procedure in which a patient's behavior and apparent feelings are presented in an attempt to facilitate better understanding of his or her actions.

confusion (kŏn-fū′zhŭn). Not being aware of or oriented with respect to time, place, or self.

c., mental. An abnormal mental state in which the individual experiences reduction of mental functions, attentiveness, alertness, and the ability to comprehend the immediate situation.

confusional state, acute. This condition is seen frequently in hospitalized patients of any age, but particularly in geriatric patients with dementia. Clinically, there is clouding of consciousness; memory impairment; impaired cognitive function; impaired perception; disturbances of emotion; depression of psychomotor activity, but repetitive, stereotyped activity such as plucking at bed clothes or tossing from side to side may be seen.

ETIOL: Primary neurological disease must be distinguished from confusion due to a systemic disease or toxic causes.

TREAT: Reassurance, attempt to have a relative or friend stay with the patient; in agitated patients sedation with a long-acting tranquilizer or short-term sedation in order to do diagnostic procedures may be required; if present, correct hypoxia, hypoglycemia, hyperthermia, or dehydration; appropriate therapy for the primary disease and provision of an adequate diet.

congelation (kŏn″jĕ-lā′shŭn) [L. *congelare*, to freeze]. Freezing, or a frostbite.

congener (kŏn′jĕn-ĕr) [L. *con*, together, + *genus*, race]. 1. Two or more muscles with the same function. 2. Something that by structure, function, or origin is similar to another. In the production of alcoholic beverages by fermentation, chemical substances termed congeners are also produced. These chemicals, over a hundred of which are known, impart aroma and flavor to the alcoholic compound. The precise role of these congeners in producing toxic effects is unknown.

congenerous (kŏn-jĕn′ĕr-ŭs). Possessing the same function, as synergistic muscles.

congenital (kŏn-jĕn′ĭ-tăl) [L. *congenitus*, born together]. Present at birth.

congenital anomaly. An abnormality present at birth.

congested (kŏn-jĕs′tĕd) [L. *congerere*, to heap together]. Containing an abnormal amount of blood.

congestion. The presence of an excessive amount of blood or tissue fluid in an organ or in tissue. SYN: *hyperemia.*

c., active. Congestion resulting from increased flow of blood to a part or dilatation of blood vessels.

c., passive. Hyperemia resulting from interference with flow of blood from capillaries into venules. May also result from myocardial insufficiency.

c., pulmonary. The accumulation of an abnormal amount of blood in the pulmonary vascular bed. It usually occurs in association with heart failure.

congestive (kŏn-jĕs'tĭv). Pert. to congestion.

conglobate (kŏn'glō-bāt) [L. *con*, together, + *globare*, to make round]. In one mass, as lymph glands.

conglobation (kŏn"glō-bā'shŭn). Aggregation of particles in a rounded mass.

conglomerate (kŏn-glŏm'ĕr-āt) [" + *glomerare*, to heap]. 1. An aggregation in one mass. 2. Clustered; heaped together.

conglutin (kŏn-gloo'tĭn) [L. *conglutinare*, to glue together]. A protein resembling casein found in peas, beans, and almonds.

conglutinant (kŏn-gloo'tĭ-nănt). Promoting adhesion, as of the edges of a wound.

conglutinate (kŏn-gloo'tĭ-nāt). Having the quality of adhesiveness.

conglutination (kŏn-gloo"tĭn-ā'shŭn). 1. Coalescence, adhesion. 2. Reaction, such as agglutination.

congregate housing. Housing for the elderly that provides for individual living units ranging from being independent to those at the institutional level of dependence.

coniasis (kō-nī'ă-sĭs) [Gr. *konis*, dust, + *-iasis*, condition]. Dustlike calculi in gallbladder and bile ducts.

conidia (kō-nĭd'ē-ă) (sing. *conidium*). Asexual spores of fungi.

conidiophore (kŏn-īd'ē-ō-for) [" + *phoros*, bearing]. The stalk supporting conidia.

coniofibrosis (kō"nē-ō-fī-brō'sĭs) [Gr. *konis*, dust, + L. *fibra*, fiber, + Gr. *osis*, condition]. Pneumoconiosis produced by dust such as that from asbestos or silica. This causes fibrosis to develop in the lung.

coniology (kō-nē-ŏl'ō-jē) [" + *logos*, study of]. The study of dust and its effects.

coniosis (kō"nē-ō'sĭs) [" + *osis*, condition]. Any condition caused by inhalation of dust.

coniosporosis (kō"nē-ō-spō-rō'sĭs) [" + *sporos*, seed, + *osis*, condition]. Hypersensitivity reaction consisting of asthma and pneumonitis caused by breathing the spores of *Cryptostroma corticale* or *Coniosporium corticale*. These fungi grow under the bark of some types of trees. Workers who strip the bark from these trees may develop this condition.

coniotomy (kō"nē-ŏt'ō-mē) [Gr. *konos*, cone, + *tome*, incision]. Cricothyrotomy, q.v.

conization (kŏn"ĭ-zā'shŭn) [Gr. *konos*, cone]. Excision of a cone of tissue, as of the mucous membrane of the cervix.

conjugata (kŏn"jū-gā'tă) [L. *conjugatus*, yoked together]. [NA] Diameter of pelvis, measured from center of the promontory of the sacrum to the back of the symphysis pubis. SYN: *conjugate*.

    c. vera. Conjugate, true, q.v.

conjugate (kŏn'jū-gāt). 1. Paired or joined. 2. An important diameter of the pelvis, measured from the center of the promontory of the sacrum to the back of the symphysis pubis. In obstetrics, the diagonal conjugate is measured and the true conjugate is estimated. SYN: *c. diameter*. SEE: *c., diagonal; c., external.*

    c. deviation. Deviation of both eyes to either side.

    c., diagonal. Diameter measured from the lower edge of the symphysis to the promontory of the sacrum, which can be determined during life, whereas the true conjugate cannot be measured. The true conjugate is estimated by deducting 1.5 to 2.0 cm from the length of the diagonal conjugate. It is about ½ to ¾ in. (1.3 to 1.9 cm) longer than the true conjugate, or about 5 in. (12.7 cm).

    c. diameter. Conjugate.

    c., external. Diameter measured from the spine of the last lumbar vertebra to the front of the pubes (this is done by using calipers); it is normally about 8 in. (20.3 cm).

    c., true. In obstetrics, the distance between the midline superior point of the sacrum and the upper margin of the symphysis pubis. It is the anterioposterior diameter of the pelvic inlet. SYN: *conjugata vera.*

conjugation (kŏn"jū-gā'shŭn). A coupling together. In biology, the union of two unicellular organisms accompanied by an interchange of nuclear material as in *Paramecium*.

conjunctiva (kŏn"jŭnk-tī'vă, kŏn-jŭnk'tĭvă) [L. *conjungere*, to join together]. Mucous membrane that lines eyelids and is reflected onto eyeball.

    DIVISIONS: Palpebral conjunctiva covers undersurface of lids; bulbar conjunctiva coats anterior portion of eyeball; fornix conjunctiva is the transition portion forming fold between lid and globe.

    INSPECTION: Palpebral and ocular portions should be examined. Color and degree of moisture and presence of foreign bodies should be observed; also petechial hemorrhages and inflammation.

    PATH: Conditions are trachoma, pannus, and discoloration. Yellowish discoloration is seen in jaundice and pale conjunctivae are observed in anemias.

conjunctival reflex. Closure of eyelids when conjunctiva is touched or threatened.

conjunctivitis (kŏ-jŭnk"tĭ-vī'tĭs) [" + Gr. *itis*, inflammation]. Inflammation of conjunctiva.

    TREAT: Directed against the specific type of infection.

    c., actinic. Conjunctivitis resulting from exposure to ultraviolet (actinic) radiations.

    c., acute contagious. Pinkeye, q.v.

c., angular, of Morax-Axenfeld. Conjunctivitis affecting the inner angle of the conjunctivae.

c., catarrhal. Conjunctivitis due to a variety of causes such as foreign bodies, various bacteria, or irritation from heat, cold, or chemicals.

c., Chlamydial. Conjunctivitis caused by *Chlamydia trachomatis.* In the newborn, conjunctivitis due to *Chlamydia trachomatis* is more frequently encountered than ophthalmia neonatorum, q.v., due to gonococci. Prophylaxis for this is 1% silver nitrate. If the disease develops, tetracycline or sulfonamides are used.

c., epidemic hemorrhagic. Virus infection with sudden pain in the eye. It progresses to swollen eyelids, hyperemia of the conjunctiva, and later subconjunctival hemorrhage. The disease, which is self-limiting and for which there is no specific therapy, usually affects both eyes. Several viral agents can cause this disease. Included are enterovirus 70, echovirus 7, and coxsackievirus A24.

c., follicular. Type of conjunctivitis characterized by pinkish round bodies in retrotarsal fold.

c., gonorrheal. Severe, acute form of purulent conjunctivitis caused by the gonococcus *Neisseria gonorrhea.* SEE: *ophthalmia neonatorum.*

c., granular. Acute contagious inflammatory conjunctivitis with granular elevations on the lids that ulcerate and cicatrize. SYN: *trachoma.*

c., inclusion. Acute purulent inflammation of the conjunctivae caused by *Chlamydia trachomatis.* The neonate is infected as it passes through the mother's genital tract. The adult may be infected while swimming or from a sex partner.

c., membranous. Acute conjunctivitis characterized by a false membrane with or without infiltration.

c. of newborn. Ophthalmia neonatorum, q.v.

c., phlyctenular. Allergenic form of conjunctivitis commonly seen in children. Characterized by nodules that may ulcerate.

c., purulent. Form of conjunctivitis due to organisms producing purulence, esp. gonococci.

c., vernal. Conjunctivitis beginning in the spring. Most probably due to allergy.

conjunctivoma (kŏn-jŭnk″tĭ-vō′mă) [L. *conjungere,* to join together, + Gr. *oma,* tumor]. A tumor of the conjunctiva.

conjunctivoplasty (kŏn″jŭnk-tĭ′vō-plăs″tē) [″ + Gr. *plassein,* to form]. Removal of part of cornea, but replacing with flaps from the conjunctiva.

connective [L. *connectere,* to bind together]. Pert. to that which connects or binds together.

connective tissue. Tissue that supports and connects other tissues and parts. The cells of connective tissue are comparatively few in number, the bulk of the tissue consisting of intercellular substance or matrix, the nature of which gives each type of connective tissue its particular properties. Connective tissues are highly vascular with the exception of cartilage. Connective tissue proper includes the following types: mucous, fibrous (areolar, white fibrous, yellow fibrous, or elastic), reticular, and adipose. Dense connective tissue includes cartilage and bone (osseous tissue).

Conn's syndrome [J. W. Conn, U.S. physician, b. 1907]. Primary hyperaldosteronism; the symptoms and clinical condition include muscle weakness, polyuria, hypertension, hypokalemia, and alkalosis associated with an abnormally high rate of secretion of aldosterone by the adrenal cortex. SEE: *Nursing Diagnoses* in *Appendix.*

conoid (kō′noyd) [Gr. *konos,* cone, + *eidos,* form, shape]. Resembling a cone; conical.

conoid ligament. Lower and inner portion of coracoclavicular ligament.

conoid tubercle. Eminence on inferior surface of clavicle to which is attached the conoid ligament.

consanguinity (kŏn″săn-gwĭn′ĭ-tē) [L. *consanguinitas,* kinship]. Relationship by blood, i.e., being descended from a common ancestor.

conscience (kon′shŭntz). One's inner sense of what is right, wrong, or fair, esp. as this applies to relations with persons or society. This sense can inhibit or reinforce the individual's actions and thoughts. SEE: *superego.*

conscious (kŏn′shŭs) [L. *conscius,* aware]. Being aware and having perception; awake. SEE: *coma.*

consciousness. A state of awareness. It implies an orientation to time, place, and person, i.e., the individual knows approximately the date, the nature of the environment, name, and other pertinent personal data. The content of consciousness is a composite of memories and the comprehension of external reality; the emotional status and the individual's goals also enter. It is, then, a large part of what is described as "personality" in its largest sense.

Consciousness varies its intensity and extent from minute to minute. In crises, vivid ideational association may lead to an exaggerated state of awareness. In states of relaxed contentment, it lessens, to disappear completely in sleep. This differs from the pathological condition of coma, in which the patient cannot be aroused.

In so-called pathological sleep (i.e., encephalitis lethargica) and in stupor, though aroused, the patient is unable to postpone again lapsing into dullness, whereas, up to a point, normal sleep can be adequately combated by the demands of reality. Stupor is produced largely by the factors resulting in coma; the personality is relatively intact but "hazy." However, there are conditions in which a real personality change manifests itself. Clouding of consciousness may simulate the dullness but usually not the other characteristics of stupor. On the contrary, such patients may impress one as being alert.

Alteration of consciousness and attention, and impaired orientation and recent memory, are characteristic of delirium. A quiet delirium may not easily reveal itself, even in certain states of automatism in which one finds evidence of the "real personality"; there may appear on casual examination little to arouse suspicion, yet brutal acts or total absence of memory may indicate major abnormalities.

Again, in somnambulistic (sleepwalking) states, experiences may register but cannot be recalled after return to a normal state. Consciousness, on the other hand, may erroneously appear to be present in so-called "coma vigil" because the eyes are open and expression may be alert. SEE: *c., levels of.*

c., clouding of. A phase of delirium in which the patient's consciousness is cloudy or not clear.

Clouding of consciousness may be diagnosed from the appearance of the patient in catatonic stupor and it may be difficult to realize that the patient is quite lucid and that experiences are being registered accurately and can be later recalled. In true clouding, stimuli usually fail to register.

c., cosmic. The inner reaches of consciousness in which there is recognition of knowledge or facts independent of physical influence.

c., disintegration of. Cause of most mental disorders not resulting from organic conditions. Produced by the contents of the unconscious gradually disrupting the conscious.

c., levels of. The state of consciousness may vary from fully alert to coma. It is important to use a standardized system of describing the state rather than vague terms such as semiconscious, semicomatose, or semistuporous.

Alert wakefulness: Patient clearly appreciates the environment and responds quickly and appropriately to visual, auditory, and other sensory stimuli.

Drowsiness: Patient does not fully appreciate the environment and responds to stimuli appropriately but with delay and slowness. May be roused by verbal stimuli but may ignore some of them. Patient is capable of verbal response unless aphasia, aphonia, or anarthria is present. Lethargy and obtundation are also descriptive of the drowsy state.

Stupor: Patient is aroused by intense stimuli only. Loud noise may elicit a nonspecific reaction. Motor response and reflex reactions are usually preserved unless the patient is paralyzed.

Coma: Patient does not perceive the environment and intense stimuli produce a rudimentary response if any at all. The presence of reflex reactions depends on the location of the lesion(s) in the nervous system.

consensual (kŏn-sĕn'shū-ăl) [L. *consensus,* agreement]. Reflex stimulation of one part or side as the result of excitation of another part or opposite side.

consensual light index. When one eye is exposed to an intensity of light different from that to which the other is exposed, both pupils will react.

consensual light reflex. Pupillary reflex (def. 3), q.v.

consensual reflex. Any reflex occurring on opposite side of body from point of stimulation.

consent. The granting of permission by the patient for an act to be carried out by another person; such as permission for a surgical or therapeutic procedure or experiment to be performed by a physician or dentist.

c., implied. Consent presumed in certain actions by the patient, as when he or she enters the dental office and sits in a dental chair; the consent implying examination, diagnosis, and consultation.

c., informed. Consent that is given by a person after receipt of the following information: the nature and purpose of the proposed procedure or treatment; the expected outcome and the likelihood of success; the risks; the alternatives to the procedure and supporting information regarding those alternatives; and the effect of no treatment or procedure, including the effect on the prognosis and the material risks associated with no treatment. Also included are instructions concerning what should be done if the procedure turns out to be harmful or unsuccessful, and who will pay for additional medical expenses incurred as a result of an unsuccessful procedure.

consenting adult. An adult who consents to participate in social or sexual activity that might be or formerly was regarded as abnormal, e.g., sadomasochistic sexual activity, or homosexual acts.

conservative (kŏn-sĕr'vă-tĭv) [L. *conservare*, to preserve]. Pert. to utilization of a simple rather than a radical method of either medical or surgical therapy.

conservation. Cognitive principle indicating that a certain quantity remains constant in spite of transformation of shape. Children develop conservation ability for number, length, liquid amount, solid amount, space, weight, and volume. First described by Piaget.

conservation model. SEE: *Appendix 23.*

consolidation (kŏn-sŏl-ĭ-dā'shŭn) [L. *consolidare*, to make firm]. The act of becoming solid. Esp. used in connection with the solidification of the lungs due to pathological engorgement of the lung tissues as occurs in acute pneumonia.

constant (kŏn'stănt) [L. *constans*, standing together]. 1. Unchanging. 2. A condition, fact, or situation that does not change.

constellation (kŏn"stĕl-lā'shŭn) [L. *con*, together, + *stella*, star]. A group, set, or configuration of objects, individuals, or conditions.

constipation (kŏn"stĭ-pā'shŭn) [L. *constipare*, to press together]. Difficult defecation; infrequent defecation with passage of unduly hard and dry fecal material; sluggish action of the bowels. SEE: *Nursing Diagnoses* in *Appendix.*

ETIOL: Predisposing factors: No regular bowel habits from childhood; worry, anxiety, fear, sedentary life. Direct factors: Failure to establish definite and regular times for bowel movements; improper diet; intestinal obstruction; tumors; excessive use of laxatives; weakness of intestinal musculature (atony) or excessive tonicity (spasticity); use of certain drugs; presence of anal lesions. It is also a concomitant in some types of insanity.

NOTE: It is virtually impossible to state how frequently the bowels should move in order to be classed as "normal." In healthy individuals, such frequency can vary, ranging from two to three bowel movements per day to two per week.

Caution: A change in frequency of bowel movements may be a sign of serious intestinal or colonic disease, e.g., a malignancy. A change in bowel habits should be discussed with a physician.

TREAT: Plenty of fresh vegetables, fruits, milk, and an abundance of water. Attempt to establish regular bowel habits, exercise, and eating habits.

NURSING IMPLICATIONS: Assess patient's usual bowel habits and patterns. Assess patient's usual intake of fluids and fiber, and daily activity. Encourage patient to increase fluid intake, if free of cardiac or renal diseases, and to consume fruit, vegetable and cereal fiber, including two types at each meal. Encourage increased activity, especially walking. Evaluate patient's response. Request prescription for stool softeners, glycerin or laxative suppositories if necessary to establish regular pattern, but discourage continued use of laxatives.

   c., atonic. Constipation due to weakness of muscles of colon and rectum.

   c., obstructive. Constipation due to an obstruction in the intestines. Surgical aid may be needed. Preoperative diet should contain low-residue and no gas-forming foods.

   c., spastic. Constipation due to excessive tonicity of the intestinal wall, esp. the colon.

constitution [L. *constituere*, to establish]. The physical makeup and functional habits of the body.

constitutional. Pert. to the body as a whole.

constriction [L. *con*, together, + *stringere*, to draw]. 1. A binding or squeezing of a part. 2. The narrowing of a vessel or opening, as constriction of blood vessels or the pupil of the eye.

constrictor. 1. That which binds or restricts a part. 2. A muscle that constricts a vessel, opening, or passageway, as the constrictors of the faucial isthmus and pharynx, the circular fibers of the iris, intestine, and blood vessels.

constructive metabolism. The building-up or anabolic process. SEE: *anabolism; catabolism.*

consultant [L. *consultare*, to counsel]. A consulting health care worker, such as nurse, physician, dentist, pharmacist, or psychologist who acts in an advisory capacity.

consultation. In a specific patient, diagnosis and proposed treatment by two or more health care workers at one time.

consummation. The completion of marriage by the first act of sexual intercourse.

consumption (kŏn-sŭmp'shŭn) [L. *consumere*, to waste away]. 1. Tuberculosis. 2. Wasting. 3. The using up of anything.

consumption-coagulopathy. Clinical condition of altered blood coagulation wherein depletion of the clotting factors I, II, V, VII, and platelets occurs. A pathological state secondary to a variety of diseases. SYN: *disseminated intravascular coagulation.*

consumptive. Pert. to or afflicted with tuberculosis.

contact [L. *con*, with, + *tangere*, to touch].

1. Mutual touching or apposition of two bodies. 2. One who has been recently exposed to a contagious disease.

c., complete. When entire proximal surface of a tooth touches entire surface of an adjoining tooth, proximally.

c., direct. Transmission of a contagious disease by a healthy person coming in contact with a person who is a carrier of or has the disease.

c., indirect. Spread of a contagious disease by some medium other than directly touching an infected person.

c., mediate. C., indirect, q.v.

c., occlusal. The normal contact between teeth when the maxilla and mandible are brought together in habitual or centric occlusion.

c., proximal; c., proximate. Touching of teeth on their adjacent surfaces.

contactant (kŏn-tăk′tănt). A substance that produces an allergic or sensitivity response when in direct contact with the skin.

contact dermatitis. Inflammation of the skin due to coming in contact with an irritating or sensitizing chemical.

contact lens. Device made of various materials, either rigid or flexible, that fit over the cornea or part of the cornea in order to supplement or alter the refractive ability of the lens or cornea of the eye. Contact lenses, no matter what type, require special care with respect to their storage when not being worn, directions for insertion and removal, and the length of time the lenses can be worn. The manufacturer's or dispensing health care worker's instructions should be read and followed. Failure to do this could result in serious eye diseases.

c.l., bifocal. Contact lens that contains two corrections in the same lens.

c.l., extended wear. Lenses made of materials that permit permeation of gas, i.e., oxygen, so that there is less chance for corneal irritation.

c.l., hard. Contact lens made of rigid, translucent materials.

c.l., soft. Contact lens made of flexible, translucent materials. Even though these lenses are more comfortable, can be worn longer, and are harder to displace than hard lenses, there are disadvantages. They may not provide the same degree of visual acuity as hard lenses and they require more cleaning and disinfection. Tear production may be decreased, esp. in older patients. The soft lenses may need to be replaced every 6 to 18 months. Corneal infections can prevent further use of soft lenses, and the infection can cause permanent loss of vision.

contact surface. Proximal surface of a tooth.

contagion (kŏn-tā′jŭn) [L. *contingere*, to touch]. 1. The process of transferring a specific disease by either direct or indirect contact. 2. A contagious disease. 3. Any virus or other microorganism that causes a contagious disease. SEE: *virulent; virus.*

contagious (kŏn-tā′jŭs). Communicable; transmitted readily from one person to another either directly or indirectly, with reference to the organism that causes a disease.

contagious pustular dermatitis. A cutaneous disease of sheep and goats transmitted to man by direct contact. The lesion on man is usually solitary and on the hands, arms, or face. This maculopapular area may progress to a pustule up to 3 cm in diameter and may last 3 to 6 weeks. The etiological agent is *Parapoxvirus,* which is a genus of poxvirus. There is no specific treatment. SYN: *human orf.*

contagium (kŏn-tā′jē-ŭm) [L.]. The agent causing infection or contagion.

containers, care and handling of. Contamination of the container in which a specimen is to be placed may render the results of the examination useless and therefore interfere with the diagnosis. Care must be taken to avoid contamination of any container used for the collection of specimens. Use of sterile disposable containers for collecting specimens is recommended. SEE: *Universal Precautions* in *Appendix.*

Caution: Persons handling specimens should wear rubber gloves in order to protect themselves from accidental exposure to the hepatitis B and AIDS viruses.

Sterilization of glassware: This is accomplished by hot air or dry heat, boiling water, flowing steam, steam under pressure, certain gases, and the use of germicidal chemicals.

Labels: All containers should be labeled with the name of the patient, room number, and the name of the attending physician. Labels should be placed on the container, not on the lid. Request forms, sometimes used as labels, are made up to suit the individual laboratory or hospital. Provision is made for recording necessary data as indicated, including date when specimen was taken, under what circumstances, for what substances the examination is to be done, and any other information desired. SEE: *chain of custody.*

Time: If the required specimen cannot be furnished at once, make a note of what is needed; inform the patient, the supervisor, and any other nurse who may attend the patient in your absence.

Charting: Note on the chart all specimens sent to the laboratory, when sent, and any other data that seem pertinent such as the appearance of the specimen or unusual occurrences while obtaining it.

Care of specimen: Cover immediately after depositing in the container; check label or request form. Make sure that the container is intact and that there is no danger of spilling while in transit. SEE: *Universal Precautions* in *Appendix.*

contaminant (kŏn-tăm′ĭ-nănt). Substance or organism that causes contamination.

contaminate (kŏn-tăm′ĭ-nāt) [L. *contaminare,* to render impure]. 1. To soil, stain, or pollute. 2. To render unfit for use through introduction of a substance that is harmful or injurious. 3. To make impure or unclean. 4. To deposit a radioactive substance in any place where it is not supposed to be.

contamination. 1. The act of contaminating, esp. introduction of disease germs or infectious material into or on normally sterile objects. 2. In psychiatry, the fusion and condensation of words so that they run together when spoken.

c., radiation. Radiation in or on a place where it is not wanted.

content. That which is contained in something.

contiguity (kŏn″tĭ-gū′ĭ-tē) [L. *contiguus,* touching]. Contact or closely associated.

c., amputation in. Amputation through a joint.

c., law of. If two ideas occur in association, they are apt to be repeated.

c., solution of. Dislocation or displacement of two normally contiguous parts.

continence (kŏn′tĭ-nĕns) [L. *continere,* to hold together]. Self-restraint, used esp. in connection with refraining from sexual intercourse. Also used in reference to the ability to control urination and defecation. SEE: *incontinence.*

continent (kŏn′tĭ-nĕnt). 1. Capable of controlling urination and defecation. 2. Not engaging in sexual intercourse. SEE: *continence.*

continued (kŏn-tĭn′ūd). Uninterrupted.

continuing care community. A type of combined health housing and social care insurance for older persons. Elderly persons sign a contract, paying an entrance fee and a monthly service charge. The contract remains in effect as long as the person lives.

continuity (kŏn″tĭ-nū′ĭ-tē) [L. *continuus,* continued]. The state of being continuous or intimately united.

c., amputation in. Amputation through a long bone.

c., solution of. Division of normally continuous parts by fracture, rupture, laceration, incision.

continuous (kŏn-tĭn′ū-ŭs) [L. *continere,* to

hold together]. Without break, cessation, or interruption.

continuous ambulatory peritoneal dialysis. SEE: *dialysis, continuous ambulatory peritoneal.*

continuous passive motion. ABBR: CPM. The use of a mechanical apparatus to provide continuous movement through specific ranges of motion at selected joints. This is used following surgery to reduce complications and promote recovery.

continuous spectrum. An unbroken series of wavelengths, either visible or invisible. Also an unbroken range of radiations of different wavelengths in any portion of the invisible spectrum.

continuous subcutaneous insulin infusion. ABBR: CSII. SEE: *insulin pump.*

contortion (kŏn-tor′shŭn) [L. *contorquere,* to twist together]. A twisting into an unusual shape.

contour (kŏn′toor) [It. *contornare,* to go around]. Outline or surface configuration of a part. To shape or form a surface, as in carving dental restorations to approximate the conditions of the original tooth surface.

c., gingival. The normal festooning of the gingiva along the cervical part of the teeth and rounding off toward the attached gingiva.

c., gingival denture. The form of the denture base or other materials around the cervical parts of artificial teeth.

contoured (kŏn′toord). Having an irregular, undulating surface resembling a relief map, said of bacterial colonies.

contra- [L.]. Prefix indicating opposite or against, as in contraindication.

contra-aperture [L. *contra,* against, + *apertura,* opening]. A second opening made in an abscess.

contraception (kŏn″tră-sĕp′shŭn) [″ + *conceptio,* a conceiving]. The prevention of conception, q.v. SEE: *contraceptive.*

c., postcoital. ABBR: PCC. There are several means of preventing pregnancy in the immediate postcoital period. These include diethylstilbesterol, RU486 (not available in the U.S.), or insertion of an intrauterine device.

contraceptive (kŏn″tră-sĕp′tĭv). Any process, device, or method that prevents conception. Categories of contraceptives include steroids; chemical; physical or barrier; combinations of physical or barrier and chemical; "natural"; abstinence; and permanent surgical procedures. SEE: tables; *abortion; RU486.*

STEROIDS: Oral contraceptives, colloquially termed "the pill," consist of chemicals that are quite similar to natural hormones (estrogen or progesterone). They act

Contraceptive Use of U.S. Women 15 to 44 Years Old Exposed to the Risk of Unwanted Pregnancy, 1987

Exposure and Contraceptive Method*	No. (Millions)†	Percentage of Exposed Women†	Percentage of All Women Aged 15–44†
Exposed users	38.0	92	66
Sterilization	13.8	33	24
Female	8.1	20	14
Male	5.7	14	10
Oral contraceptive	13.2	32	23
Condom	6.9	17	12
Spermicide	2.3	6	4
Withdrawal	2.3	6	4
Diaphragm	1.7	4	3
Periodic abstinence	1.7	4	3
IUD	1.1	3	2
Douche	0.6	1	1
Exposed nonusers	3.3	8	6

Source: Reprinted with permission from *The New England Journal of Medicine*, 320:778, 1989.

* "Users" are women who use some method of contraception; "nonusers" use no contraceptive method. IUD denotes intrauterine device.

† Numbers and percentages do not add up because some women used more than one method.

by preventing ovulation. When taken according to the instructions, these pills are almost 100% effective. Long-acting injectable or implanted steroid contraceptives are available. Diethylstilbestrol is used as a "morning after" contraceptive, esp. in cases of rape or incest. SEE: *Norplant*.

CHEMICAL: Spermicides in the form of foam, cream, jelly, spermicide-impregnated sponge, or suppositories are placed in the vagina prior to intercourse. They may be used alone or in combination with a barrier contraceptive. They act by killing the sperm. Douching after intercourse is not effective enough to be thought of as a method of contraception.

PHYSICAL OR BARRIER: IUDs, or intrauterine contraceptive devices, are plastic or metal objects placed inside the uterus. They are thought to act by preventing the fertilized egg from attaching itself to the lining of the uterus. Their effectiveness is only slightly lower than that of oral contraceptives. Diaphragms are made of a dome-shaped piece of rubber with a flexible spring circling the edge. They are available in various sizes and are inserted into the vagina so as to cover the cervix. A diaphragm must be used in conjunction with a chemical spermicide, which is used prior to positioning the diaphragm. A specially fitted cervical cap is also available as a barrier-type contraceptive. A sponge impregnated with a contraceptive cream or jelly is available. It is placed in the vagina up to several hours prior to intercourse. The male partner can use a condom, a flexible tube-shaped barrier placed over the erect penis so that the ejaculate is contained in the tube and is not deposited in the vagina. Condoms are made of rubber or animal membranes. They are available in dry as well as wet-lubricated forms, and are manufactured in various colors. Used properly, the condom is a reliable means of contraception. It is more effective as a means of contraception if combined with a chemical spermicide. Condoms also help prevent spread of diseases transmitted by sexual intercourse by providing a physical barrier. SEE: *condom, instructions for use.*

NATURAL: Methods involve abstaining from intercourse for a specified number of days before, during, and after ovulation. Rhythm is based on calculating the fertile period by the calendar. In practice, this method has a high rate of failure. Other methods include determining ovulation by charting the woman's basal temperature (SEE: *basal temperature chart*) as well as judging the time of ovulation by observing cyclical changes in the cervical mucus. Sophisticated home-diagnostic tests for the hormonal changes present at time of ovulation are available. Withdrawal, the removal of the penis from the vagina just prior to ejaculation, is a method subject to a high failure rate because sperm may be contained

Rates of Contraceptive Failure According to Method

Method	Failure Rate (per 100 Woman-Years)
Sterilization	
Male	0.02
Female	0.13
Oral contraceptive	
<50 µg of estrogen	0.27
50 µg of estrogen	0.16
>50 µg of estrogen	0.32
Progestin only	1.2
IUD*	
Copper 7	1.5
Loop D	1.3
Diaphragm	1.9
Condom	3.6
Withdrawal	6.7
Spermicide	11.9
Rhythm	15.5

Source: Reprinted with permission from *The New England Journal of Medicine*, 320:778, 1989.
* IUD denotes intrauterine device.

in the pre-ejaculatory fluid from the penis.

PERMANENT: For women: Tubal ligation involves surgical division of the fallopian tubes and ligating the cut ends. This procedure does not interfere with the subsequent enjoyment of sexual intercourse. This form of sterilization is effective but virtually irreversible. For men: Vasectomy consists of cutting the vas deferens and tying each end so that the sperm can no longer travel from the testicle to the urethra. The procedure has to be done bilaterally and the ejaculate tested for several months postoperatively to be certain sperm are not present. Until two successive tests reveal absence of sperm, the method should not be regarded as having been successful. Attempts to reverse this surgical procedure have been successful only in a small percentage of cases. Vasectomy does not interfere with the normal enjoyment of sexual intercourse.

contract (kŏn-trăkt') [L. *contrahere*, to draw together]. 1. To draw together, reduce in size, or shorten. 2. To acquire through infection, as to contract a disease.

contractile (kŏn-trăk'tĭl). Able to contract or shorten.

contractility (kŏn-trăk-tĭl'ĭ-tē). 1. Having the ability to contract or shorten. 2. In cardiac physiology, the force with which left ventricular ejection occurs. It is independent of effects of preload, q.v., or afterload, q.v.

contraction (kŏn-trăk'shŭn). A shortening or tightening, as that of a muscle, or a reduction in size; a shrinking.

  c., Braxton Hicks. SEE: *Braxton Hicks* sign.

  c., carpopedal. Contraction of the flexor muscles of the hands and feet due to tetany hypocalcemia, or hyperventilation.

  c., concentric muscle. SEE: *muscle contraction, concentric.*

  c., eccentric muscle. SEE: *muscle contraction, eccentric.*

  c., isometric. Muscular contraction in which the muscle develops tension but does not change its length. SYN: *static muscle contraction.*

  c., isotonic. Muscular contraction in which the muscle maintains constant tension by changing its length during the action.

  c., tetanic. Continuous contraction of muscles.

  c., tonic. Spasmodic contraction of a muscle for an extended period of time.

contraction stress test. ABBR: CST. A method of testing the condition of the fetus by stimulating the uterus to contract. This can be done by administering oxytocin or by manual stimulation of the nipple. The latter process stimulates the hypothalamus, which in turn causes the posterior lobe of the pituitary to release oxytocin. SEE: *oxytocin challenge test.*

contracture (kŏn-trăk'chŭr) [L. *contractura*]. Fibrosis of connective tissue in skin, fascia, muscle, or joint capsule that prevents normal mobility of the related tissue or joint.

  c., Dupuytren's [Baron Guillaume Dupuytren, Fr. surgeon, 1777–1835]. Contracture of palmar fascia, causing the ring and little fingers to bend into the palm so that they cannot be extended. SEE: illus.

  c., fibrotic. Contraction of a muscle in which the muscle tissue has been replaced by fibrous tissue due to injury.

  c., functional. Decrease of a contracture during anesthesia or sleep.

  c., myostatic. Adaptive shortening of muscle, usually due to immobilization and without the presence of tissue pathology.

  c., physiological. A temporary condition in which tension and shortening of a muscle are maintained for a considerable time although there is no tetanus. May be induced by heat, action of drugs, or acids.

  c., pseudomyostatic. Apparent perma-

CONTRACTION OF THE FLEXOR TENDON OF THE RING FINGER

DUPUYTREN'S CONTRACTURE

nent contraction of a muscle due to a central nervous system lesion, resulting in loss of range of motion and resistance of the muscle to stretch.

    c., Volkmann's. Pronation and flexion of the hand, with atrophy of the muscles of the forearm. Results from circulatory impairment due to pressure from a cast, constricting dressings, or injury to the radial artery. This can be prevented by being alert to signs of coldness, pallor, cyanosis, pain, and swelling of the part below the injury or constriction and removal of the cause.

contrafissura (kŏn″trǎ-fĭ-shū′rǎ) [L. *contra,* against, + *fissura,* fissure]. A skull fracture at a point opposite from where the blow was received. SEE: *contrecoup injury.*

contraindication (kŏn″trǎ-ĭn-dĭ-kā′shŭn) [″ + *indicare,* to point out]. Any symptom or circumstance indicating the inappropriateness of a form of treatment otherwise advisable.

contralateral (kŏn″trǎ-lăt′ĕr-ǎl) [″ + *latus,* side]. Originating in, or affecting, the opposite side of the body. Opposed to homolateral and ipsilateral.

contralateral reflexes. 1. Passive flexion of one part following flexion of another. 2.

Passive flexion of one leg, causing similar movement of opposite leg.

contrast (kŏn′trăst). In radiography, the difference between adjacent densities on a radiograph resulting from the part radiographed and film characteristics.

contrast medium. In radiology, use of radiopaque substance to provide a contrast in density between the tissue or organ being filmed and the medium. Thus barium sulfate will, when swallowed, help to demonstrate the outline of the intestinal tract as x-ray films are taken during the passage of the medium.

    c.m., low-osmolarity. ABBR: LOCM. Contrast media with low osmolarity. These agents produce fewer undesired effects after intravascular administration than do high-osmolarity contrast media.

contrast sprays. Spray administered by having patient sit on side of bathtub, spraying the feet and legs with warm water for one minute and cold water for one minute. Do this for 10 minutes twice daily. This is done to stimulate blood circulation.

contravolitional (kŏn″trǎ-vō-lĭ′shŭn-ǎl) [L. *contra,* against, + *velle,* to wish]. In opposition to or without the will; involuntary.

contrecoup (kŏn-tr-koo′) [Fr., counterblow]. Occurring on the opposite side.

contrecoup injury. An injury to parts of the brain located on the side opposite that of the primary injury, as when the frontal and temporal lobes of the brain are forced against the irregular bones of the anterior portion of the cranial vault as a result of a blow on the back of the head.

contrectation (kŏn″trĕk-tā′shŭn) [L. *contrectare*, to handle]. 1. Touch with the hands. 2. Caressing or sexually fondling one of the opposite sex.

contributory negligence. In forensic medicine, the plaintiff's negligence in combination with defendant's negligence are the causes of plaintiff's injuries or damages.

control (kŏn-trōl′) [L. *contra*, against, + *rotulus*, little wheel]. 1. To regulate or maintain. 2. A standard against which observations or conclusions may be checked in order to establish their validity, as a control animal, one that has not been exposed to the treatment or condition being studied in the other animals. 3. In clinical investigations, the matching of cases and controls with as many major variables as appear to be important in the particular study. This leaves the suspected factor open for study in the two groups.

controlled substance act. The Comprehensive Drug Abuse Prevention and Control Act. A law enacted in 1971 designed to control the distribution and use of all depressant and stimulant drugs and other drugs of abuse or potential abuse as may be designated by the Drug Enforcement Administration of the Department of Justice.

Labels of drugs included in this list include a large "C" followed by a Roman numeral designation. Alternatively the Roman numeral is within the large "C."

The act specifies record-keeping by the pharmacist, the format for prescription writing, and limits the amount of a drug that can be legally dispensed. This and whether refills are allowed varies with the nature of the drug. Centrally acting drugs such as narcotics, stimulants, and certain sedatives are divided into five classes called Schedules I through V. Schedule I drugs are experimental. Prescriptions for Schedule II drugs may not be refilled. Prescriptions for Schedule III and IV drugs may be refilled up to 5 times within 6 months of the time the initial prescription was written. Schedule V drugs are restricted only to the extent that all nonscheduled prescription drugs are regulated.

contrude (kŏn-trood′) [L. *con*, with, + *trudere*, to thrust]. 1. Abnormal lingual curve or line of dental arch. 2. To crowd together, as the teeth.

contrusion (kŏn-troo′zhŭn). Having the teeth crowded.

contuse (kŏn-tooz′) [L. *contundere*, to bruise]. To bruise.

contusion (kŏn-too′zhŭn). An injury in which the skin is not broken; a bruise.

SYM: Pain, swelling, and discoloration.

F.A.: Apply cold applications. Follow with firm bandage to prevent swelling. Twenty-four to 48 hours later, application of heat is desirable, followed by gentle massage. SEE: *concussion*.

conus (kō′nŭs) [Gr. *konos*]. 1. A cone. 2. Posterior staphyloma of myopic eye.

c. arteriosus. [NA] Right cardiac ventricle's upper rounded anterior angle, where pulmonary artery arises.

c. medullaris. [NA] Conical portion of lower spinal cord.

convalescence (kŏn″văl-ĕs′ĕns) [L. *convalescere*, to become strong]. The period of recovery after the termination of a disease or an operation.

convalescent. 1. Getting well. 2. One who is recovering from a disease or operation.

convalescent diet. A diet suitable for the condition from which the patient is recovering. SEE: *soft diet.*

convection (kŏn-vĕk′shŭn) [L. *convehere*, to convey]. The transference of heat by means of currents in liquids or gases.

convergence (kŏn-vĕr′jĕns) [L. *con*, with, + *vergere*, to incline]. 1. The moving of two or more objects toward the same point. 2. In reflex activity, the coming together of several axons or afferent fibers upon one or a few motor neurons; the condition whereby impulses from several sensory receptors converge upon the same motor center, resulting in a limited and specific response. 3. Visual lines directed to a nearby point.

convergent (kŏn-vĕr′jĕnt). Tending toward a common point.

conversion (kŏn-vĕr′zhŭn) [L. *convertere*, to turn round]. 1. Change from one state to another. In obstetrics, the change in position of a fetus in the uterus in order to facilitate delivery. SEE: *version.*

conversion disorder. SEE: *hysteria, conversion.*

conversion reaction. A conversion type of hysterical neurosis in which there is loss of or alteration in physical functioning suggesting a physical disorder but instead representing the expression of a psychological conflict or need. The disturbance is not under voluntary control and cannot be explained by a disease process; it is not limited to pain or sexual dysfunction. SEE: *somatoform disorders.*

conversion symptom. The unconscious change of an anxiety-producing state to a somatic symptom; thus in hysteria the manifestation may be imagined pain, or disability. SEE: *somatoform disorders.*

convex (kŏn'vĕks, kŏn-vĕks') [L. *convexus,* vaulted, arched]. Curved evenly; resembling the segment of a sphere.

convexoconcave (kŏn-vĕk"sō-kŏn'kāv, -kŏn-kāv') [" + *concavus,* vaulted hollow]. Concave on one side and convex on opposite surface. SYN: *concavoconvex.*

convexoconvex [" + *convexus,* arched]. Convex on two opposite faces.

convolute (kŏn'vō-loot) [L. *convolvere,* to roll together]. Rolled, as a scroll.

convoluted. Convolute, rolled.

convoluted tubule. In the kidney, the proximal convoluted tubule, which lies between Bowman's capsule and the loop of Henle; the distal convoluted tubule, which lies between the loop of Henle and the collecting duct. SEE: illus. at *kidney.*

convolution (kŏn'vō-loo'shŭn) [L. *convolvere,* to roll together]. 1. A turn, fold, or coil of anything that is convoluted. 2. In anatomy, a gyrus, one of the many folds on the surface of the cerebral hemispheres. They are separated by grooves (sulci or fissures). SEE: *gyrus.*

  c., angular. A gyrus forming posterior portion of inferior parietal lobule.

  c.'s, annectant. The four gyri connecting the convolutions on upper surface of occipital lobe with parietal and temporosphenoidal lobes.

  c., anterior choroid. Gyrus choroides.

  c., anterior orbital. Convolution that lies in front of the orbital sulcus.

  c., Arnold's. Gyri posteriores inferiores.

  c., ascending frontal. Convolution forming anterior boundary of fissure of Rolando.

  c., ascending parietal. Convolution parallel to ascending frontal convolution, separated from it by fissure of Rolando, except at extremities, where they are generally united.

  c., Broca's. The inferior, or third, frontal convolution.

  c., callosal. Gyrus cinguli.

  c.'s, cerebral. Convolutions of the cerebrum.

  c., cuneate. Gyral isthmus.

  c., dentate. A small, notched gyrus, rudimentary in man, situated in dentate fissure.

  c.'s, exterior olfactory. Small projections forming outer boundary of the olfactory grooves.

  c., hippocampal. Uncinate gyrus.

  c., inferior frontal. The lower and outer part of frontal lobe.

  c., inferior occipital. A small convolu-

tion lying between middle and inferior occipital fissures.

  c., insular. One of a group of small convolutions forming the island of Reil, entirely concealed by the operculum.

  c.'s, intestinal. The coils of the intestines.

  c., marginal. Convolution beginning in front of locus perforatus anterior and bounding longitudinal fissure on mesial aspect of the hemisphere.

  c., middle frontal. Convolution continuous posterior with ascending frontal convolution and extending forward over anterior end of hemisphere to its orbital surface.

  c., middle occipital. Convolution between the first and third occipital convolutions.

  c., middle temporosphenoidal. A small gyrus continuous with the middle occipital or angular gyrus.

  c.'s, occipitotemporal. Two small convolutions on lower surface of temporosphenoidal lobe.

  c. of the corpus callosum. Gyrus fornicatus, q.v.

  c. of the sylvian fissure. Convolution that bounds the fissure of Sylvius.

  c., olfactory. Olfactory lobe.

  c.'s, orbital. Small gyri on orbital surface of frontal lobe.

  c.'s, parietal. Ascending parietal convolution and superior parietal convolution.

  c., posterior orbital. A small convolution on posterior and outer side of orbital sulcus, and continuous with inferior frontal convolution.

  c., second frontal. Convolution on the frontal lobes, lying posteriorly between the superior and inferior frontal sulci. SYN: *c., middle frontal.*

  c., superior frontal. Convolution that bounds great longitudinal fissure, arising posterior from upper end of ascending frontal convolution.

  c., superior occipital. Uppermost of the three convolutions on superior surface of occipital lobe.

  c., superior parietal. Portion of parietal lobe limited anteriorly by upper part of the fissure of Rolando, posteriorly by exterior parieto-occipital fissure, and inferiorly by intraparietal sulcus.

  c., superior temporosphenoidal. Uppermost of three convolutions forming temporosphenoidal lobe. It lies just below and is parallel with sylvian fissure.

  c., supramarginal. The anterior portion of interior parietal lobule behind inferior extremity of intraparietal fissure (sulcus), below which it joins the ascending parietal convolution.

c., transverse orbital. The gyrus occupying posterior portion of inferior surface of frontal lobe, at anterior extremity of fissure of Sylvius.

c., uncinate. Convolution extending from near the posterior extremity of the occipital lobe to apex of the temporosphenoidal.

convulsant (kŏn-vŭl'sănt) [L. *convellere*, to pull together]. 1. An agent that produces a convulsion. 2. Causing onset of a convulsion.

convulsant poisons. Toxic substances that cause the person affected to experience convulsions. The common ones are strychnine and other drugs of the nux vomica group, and various infrequently used drugs, such as picrotoxin.

SYM: These produce a sense of suffocation, dyspnea, and then muscular rigidity; there are powerful tetanic contractions that may be very painful. These spasms may be brought on by trivial stimuli, such as touching the patient, or they may come on spontaneously and involuntarily at varying intervals of from 3 to 30 minutes and may last from 1 to 5 minutes. Trismus, cyanosis, and tachycardia are frequent accompaniments. Death results from asphyxia or exhaustion.

TREAT: Appropriate therapy will depend upon substance that caused the convulsion. General measures for emptying the stomach or attempting to neutralize the drug may be indicated. Sedatives may be ordered by the physician. Oxygen and artificial respiration may be indicated.

convulsion (kŏn-vŭl'shŭn). Paroxysms of involuntary muscular contractions and relaxations.

NOTE: It is important for the person who observes the convulsion to record on the chart the following: time of onset; duration; whether or not convulsion started in a certain area of the body or became generalized from the start; type of contractions; whether or not the patient became incontinent; was there an abnormal odor to the patient's breath; did the convulsion cause the patient to be injured or strike head during the convulsion. This information, in addition to its medicolegal importance, will be quite valuable in diagnosis and in caring for the patient.

ETIOL: General: epilepsy; eclampsia; meningitis; tetanus; uremia; poisoning from camphor, cyanides, strychnine. In children, the cause is often fever. Other causes include rickets; syphilis; malnutrition; malaria; acute infectious disease; or toxemia of pregnancy. In adults, convulsions may be caused by epilepsy; heat cramps; strychnine; brain lesions.

TREAT: Febrile convulsions in children are usually controlled by phenobarbital with or without aspirin as an antipyretic. In adults, the cause must first be found. Keep patient from injuring self. Firm pad between teeth to avoid biting tongue or cheeks. If fever is present, tepid or cool bath. Sedatives or anesthesia may be ordered by physician. Aftercare: rest in bed; absolute quiet; careful diagnosis without unduly disturbing patient. SEE: *febrile convulsions.*

c., clonic. Convulsions having intermittent contractions, muscles being alternately contracted and relaxed.

c., febrile. SEE: *febrile convulsions.*

c., hysterical. Convulsion caused by hysteria.

c., mimetic. A spasm of facial muscles.

c., oscillating. Convulsion involving separate bundles of muscle fibers that contract alternately.

c., puerperal. Eclamptic convulsion in pregnant or puerperal woman.

c., salaam. Nodding spasm.

c., tonic. Convulsion in which the contractions are maintained for a time, as in tetany.

c., toxic. Convulsion caused by action of a toxin on nervous system.

c., uremic. Convulsion caused by uremic condition.

convulsion, words pert. to: anticonvulsive; apoplexy; athetosis; chill; chorea; coma; consciousness; electroconvulsive therapy; epilepsy; hysteria; ictus; mimetic; paroxysm; rabies; strychnine; tetanus; tic; tremor.

convulsive (kŏn-vŭl'sĭv). Pert. to convulsions.

convulsive reflex. Incoordinate contraction of muscles in a convulsive manner.

convulsive tic. Spasm of face.

"cookbook" medicine. The erroneous concept that medical practice may be regulated and supervised by use of a set of guidelines and rules rather than by a comprehensive, holistic approach to the medical needs of a patient.

cooking [L. *coquere*, to cook]. The process of heating foods in order to prepare them for eating. Cooking makes most foods more palatable, easier to masticate, improves their digestibility, and destroys or inactivates harmful organisms or toxins that may be present. Cooking releases the aromatic substances and extractives that contribute odors and taste to foods. These odors help to stimulate the appetite. SEE: *trichinosis.*

Caution: Not all toxic substances are inactivated by heat. Most microorganisms and parasites are destroyed in the ordinary process of cooking, but some require a higher degree of heat and longer cooking to effect this result. Pork has to be cooked completely throughout in order to kill the encysted larvae of *Trichinella*.

ACTION: *Protein:* Soluble proteins become coagulated. *Soluble substances:* These, including heat-labile vitamins, are often inactivated by boiling, and even mineral substances and starches, though insoluble to a certain extent, may be altered in this process. *Starch:* The starch granules now swell and are changed from insoluble (raw) starch to soluble starch capable of being converted into sugar in the process of digestion and of being assimilated in the system.

Cooley's anemia [Thomas Cooley, U.S. pediatrician, 1871–1945]. Anemia resulting from inheritance of a recessive trait responsible for interference with the rate of hemoglobin synthesis. SYN: *thalassemia major*.

Coombs' test [R. R. A. Coombs, Brit. immunologist, b. 1921]. A test for antiglobulins in the red cell; used in diagnosing various hemolytic anemias.

coordination (kō-or″dĭn-ā′shŭn) [L. *co-*, same, + *ordinare*, to arrange]. The working together of various muscles for the production of a certain movement. More generally, the working together of different systems of the body in a given process, as the coordination between the system of glands and involuntary muscles in digestion.

COPD. *chronic obstructive pulmonary disease.* SEE: *COLD.*

cope (kōp) [ME. *caupen*, to contend with]. 1. The ability to deal effectively with and handle the stresses to which one is subjected. 2. The upper half of a flask used in the casting art. 3. In dentistry, the cavity side of a denture flask.

coping. A measure of the individual's resourcefulness and ability to deal with the stress of daily life and unusual challenges posed by chronic disease, disability, and pain.

copodyskinesia (kō″pō-dĭs″kĭn-ē′sē-ă) [Gr. *kopos*, fatigue, + *dys*, difficult, + *kinesis*, motion]. Fatigue of or difficulty in moving a group of muscles used in working. May be out of proportion to that which would be expected from the amount of work done, in which case it is called occupational neurosis. SEE: *chronic fatigue syndrome; writer's cramp*.

copolymer (kō-pŏl′ĭ-mĕr). A polymer composed of two different kinds of monomers.

copper [L. *cuprum*]. SYMB: Cu. At. wt. 63.54; at. no. 29; sp. gr. 8.96. A metal, small quantities of which are utilized by the body. Its salts are irritant poisons. SEE: *Poisons and Poisoning* in *Appendix; Wilson's disease*.

FUNCT: The total body content of copper is 100 to 150 mg; the amount normally ingested each day is less than 2 mg. An essential component of several enzyme systems, it is present in the liver and is excreted by the kidneys and in the bile.

DEFICIENCY SYM: Anemia; weakness; impaired respiration and growth; and poor utilization of iron.

SOURCES: Found in many vegetable and animal tissues.

copperas (kŏp′ĕr-ăs). $FeSO_4 \cdot 7H_2O$. Pale blue-green crystals of ferrous sulfate. Used as disinfectant and deodorizer. SYN: *ferrous sulfate; green vitriol*.

copperhead. A poisonous snake, *Agkistrodon contortrix*, common in the southern United States. SEE: *snakebite; snake, poisonous*.

copper sulfate. $CuSO_4 \cdot 5H_2O$. Blue vitriol. Deep-blue shiny crystals or granular powder. Astringent when used in proper dilution. Also used as an algicide.

copper sulfate poisoning. SYM: A disagreeable coppery metallic taste with tightness in the throat, nausea and vomiting, thirst, abdominal pains, cramps, and suppression of urine.

F.A.: Emesis; wash out stomach. Administer penicillamine or BAL, q.v. Monitor vital signs, treat shock, administer oxygen if needed, control convulsions, and maintain electrolyte balance. Be aware of possible renal and hepatic failure. SEE: *Poisons and Poisoning* in *Appendix*.

copremesis (kŏp-rĕm′ē-sĭs) [Gr. *kopros*, dung, + *emesis*, vomiting]. The vomiting of fecal material.

coproantibody (kŏp″rō-ăn′tĭ-bŏd″ē). Any one of a group of antibodies in the feces to various enteric bacteria. They are of the IgA type. Their ability to protect the host has not been shown.

coprolagnia (kŏp″rō-lăg′nē-ă) [″ + *lagneia*, lust]. An erotic satisfaction at the sight or odor of excreta.

coprolalia (kŏp″rō-lā′lē-ă) [″ + *lalia*, babble]. The use of vulgar, obscene, or sacrilegious language. Seen in schizophrenia, and Gilles de la Tourette's syndrome.

coprolith (kŏp′rō-lĭth) [″ + *lithos*, stone]. Hard, inspissated feces.

coprology (kŏp-rŏl′ō-jē) [″ + *logos*, word, reason]. Study of the feces. SYN: *scatology*.

coprophagy (kŏp-rŏf′ă-jē) [″ + *phagein*, to eat]. The eating of excrement. SYN: *scatophagy*.

coprophilia (kŏp″rō-fĭl′ē-ă) [″ + *philein*, to love]. Abnormal interest in feces; a perversion in adults.

coprophilic. Term applies to organisms that normally live in fecal material.

coprophobia (kŏp″rō-fō′bē-ă) [″ +

phobos, fear]. Abnormal fear of defecation and feces.

coproporphyria (kŏp″rō-por-fĭr′ē-ă) [″ + *porphyra*, purple]. An inherited form of porphyria in which an excess amount of coproporphyrin is excreted in the feces.

coproporphyrin (kŏp″rō-por′fĭr-ĭn). A porphyrin present in urine and feces. Coproporphyrins I and II are normally present in minute and equal amounts, but quantities are altered in certain diseases as poliomyelitis, infectious hepatitis, and in lead poisoning.

coproporphyrinuria (kŏp″rō-por″fĭr-ĭn-ū′ē-ă). Excess coproporphyrin in the urine.

coprozoa (kŏp″rō-zō′ă) [″ + *zoon*, animal]. Protozoa in fecal matter outside of the intestine.

copula (kŏp′ū-lă) [L., link]. 1. Any connecting part. 2. A median elevation on floor of embryonic pharynx representing future root of the tongue; copula linguae.

copulation (kŏp″ū-lā′shŭn) [L. *copulatio*]. Sexual intercourse. SYN: *coition; coitus.*

cor (kor) [L.]. [NA] The heart.

   c. pulmonale. SEE: *cor pulmonale.*

coracoacromial (kor″ă-kō-ă-krō′mē-ăl) [Gr. *korax*, raven, + *akron*, point, + *omos*, shoulder]. Pert. to acromial and coracoid processes.

coracoid (kor′ă-koyd) [″ + *eidos*, form, shape]. Resembling, in shape, a crow's beak.

coracoid process. Process on upper anterior surface of scapula.

cord [Gr. *khorde*]. 1. A stringlike structure. 2. The umbilical cord. 3. A firm elongated structure consistent with a thrombosed vein, esp. one in the extremities, where it may be detected by palpation.

   c., spermatic. Cord by which the testis is connected to the abdominal inguinal ring. It surrounds the ductus deferens, blood vessels, lymphatics, and nerves supplying the testis and epididymis. These are enclosed in the cremasteric fascia, which forms an investing sheath.

   c., spinal. That portion of the central nervous system contained in the spinal canal. The center of the cord consists of gray matter, which is composed of nerve cells, dendrites, and their processes. The white matter is arranged in tracts outside the gray matter. It consists of medullated nerve fibers that are going to and from the brain, connecting various layers of gray matter in the cord, and leaving and entering the spinal column. The cord serves as a conducting pathway for sensory impulses to the brain and motor impulses from the brain. It also serves as a reflex center for many reflex acts. SYN: *medulla spinalis* [NA].

   c., umbilical. Cord that connects the circulatory system of the fetus to the placenta.

   c., vocal. Two thin, reedlike folds of tissue within the larynx that vibrate with the passage of air between them, producing sounds that are the basis of speech.

cordal (kor′dăl). Concerning a cord, e.g., spinal or vocal cord.

cordate (kor′dāt) [L. *cor*, heart]. Shaped like a heart.

cord bladder. Distention of the bladder without discomfort.

   SYM: Tending to void frequently and dribbling after urination.

   ETIOL: Lesion affecting the posterior roots of the spinal column at the level of bladder innervation above the sacral level.

cordectomy (kor-dĕk′tō-mē) [Gr. *khorde*, cord, + *ektome*, excision]. Surgical removal of a cord.

cordiform (kor′dĭ-form) [L. *cor*, heart, + *forma*, shape]. Shaped like a heart.

corditis (kor-dī′tĭs) [Gr. *khorde*, cord, + *itis*, inflammation]. Inflammation of the spermatic cord. SYN: *funiculitis.*

cordocentesis. Technique of obtaining a sample of blood from the umbilical cord while the fetus is in utero.

cordopexy (kor′dō-pĕk″sē) [″ + *pexis*, fixation]. Operative fixation of an anatomical cord, esp. the vocal cords.

cordotomy (kor-dŏt′ō-mē) [″ + *tome*, incision]. Spinal cord section of lateral pathways to relieve pain. SYN: *chordotomy.*

Cordran. Trade name for flurandrenolide.

core (kor). The center of a structure.

coreclisis (kor″ē-klī′sĭs) [Gr. *kore*, pupil of the eye, + *kleisis*, closure]. Occlusion of the pupil. SYN: *iridencleisis.*

corectasia, corectasis (kor-ĕk-tā′zē-ă, -ĕk′tă-sĭs) [″ + *ektasis*, dilatation]. Dilatation of the pupil of the eye resulting from disease.

corectome (kō-rĕk′tōm) [″ + *ektome*, excision]. Instrument used for cutting or removing the iris. SYN: *iridectome.*

corectomy (kō-rĕk′tō-mē). Surgical removal of the iris. SYN: *iridectomy.*

corectopia (kor-ĕk-tō′pē-ă) [″ + *ek*, out of, + *topos*, place]. Having the pupil to one side of the center of the iris.

corediallysis (kō″rē-dī-ăl′ī-sĭs) [″ + *dia*, through, + *lysis*, dissolution]. Separation of outer border of iris from its ciliary attachment.

corediastasis (kor″ē-dī-ăs′tă-sĭs) [″ + *diastasis*, a standing apart]. Dilatation of pupil.

corelysis (kor-ĕl′ī-sĭs) [″ + *lysis*, dissolution]. Obliteration of pupil because of adhesions of iris to cornea.

coremorphosis (kor″ē-mor-fō′sĭs) [″ + *morphe*, form, + *osis*, condition]. Establishment of an artificial pupil.

coreometer (kŏ″rē-ŏm′ĕ-tĕr) [″ + *metron*, measure]. Instrument for measurement of the pupil.

coreometry (kŏ″rē-ŏm′ĕ-trē). Measurement of the pupil of the eye.

coreoplasty (kŏ′rē-ō-plăs″tē) [″ + *plassein*, to form]. Any operation for forming an artificial pupil.

corepressor (kŏ″rē-prĕs′sor). The substance capable of activating the repressor produced by a regulator gene.

corestenoma (kor″ē-stĕn-ō′mă) [″ + *stenoma*, contraction]. Narrowing of pupil.

    c. congenitum. Partial congenital obliteration of pupil by outgrowths from the iris that form a partial gridlike covering over the pupil.

core temperature. The body's temperature in deep structures such as the liver or heart, as opposed to the peripheral areas, such as the mouth or axilla.

coretomedialysis (kor″ĕt-ō-mē-dē-ăl′ĭ-sĭs) [″ + *tome*, incision, + *dialysis, dia*, through, + *lysis*, dissolution]. Making of an artificial pupil through the iris. SYN: *iridodialysis*.

coretomy (kō-rĕt′ō-mē) [″ + *tome*, incision]. Any incision of the iris. SYN: *iridotomy*.

Cori cycle (kō′rē) [Carl Ferdinand Cori, Czech.-born U.S. physician and biochemist, 1896–1984; Gerty T. Cori, Czech.-born U.S. biochemist, 1896–1957]. In carbohydrate metabolism, the breakdown of muscle glycogen, with formation of lactic acid, which enters the bloodstream, is converted to liver glycogen, which in turn breaks down into glucose, which is carried to muscles where it is reconverted to muscle glycogen.

corium (kō′rē-ŭm) [L., skin] (pl. *coria*). [NA] The layer of the skin lying immediately under the epidermis; the true skin. Consists of two layers, papillary and reticular. It is composed of loose connective tissue containing numerous capillaries, lymphatics, and nerve endings. In it lie hair follicles, sebaceous glands, sweat glands and their ducts, and smooth muscle fibers. SYN: *cutis vera; dermis*.

corm (korm) [Gr. *kormos*, a trimmed tree trunk]. A short bulb-shaped, underground stem of a plant such as the colchicum.

corn [L. *cornu*, horn]. Horny induration and thickening of the skin, hard or soft, according to location. SYN: *clavus*.

    SYM: Hard corns on exposed surfaces have a horny core of conical shape extending down into the derma, causing pain and irritation. Soft corns that occur between the toes are kept soft by moisture and maceration. This may lead to inflammation beneath the corn. Infection with pyogenic organisms results in suppuration.

    ETIOL: Pressure or friction or both from ill-fitting shoes.

    TREAT: Remove cause by use of properly fitting shoes of soft leather and proper shape. Materials made from spongelike substances for absorbing energy and thus preventing friction are available for lining shoes or bandaging the area of the foot being abraded. Local application of a keratolytic agent for removal of corn. Corn pads to relieve pressure. Services of a podiatrist may be necessary. Patients with diabetes or a circulatory condition who have corns need special care to prevent infections of the feet.

cornea (kor′nē-ă) [L. *corneus*, horny]. [NA] The clear, transparent anterior portion of the fibrous coat of the eye composing about one-sixth of its surface. Its curvature being greater than that of the remainder of the bulb enables it to function as an important refractive medium. It is continuous at its periphery with the sclera. It is composed of five layers: layer of epithelium; Bowman's membrane (anterior limiting membrane); substantia propria corneae [NA]; Descemets' membrane; and a layer of endothelium. SEE: *geographic ulceration of cornea*.

cornea, words pert. to: abrasio corneae; anterior chamber; arcus senilis; "cera-" words; chemosis; circumcorneal; "kerat-" words; macula cornea; megalocornea; microcornea; nebula; pannus; phlyctenula; pterygium; rhytidosis; staphyloma; synechia.

corneal. Pert. to the cornea.

corneal contact lens. SEE: *lens, corneal contact*.

corneal impression test. In diagnosing rabies, q.v., the staining of material obtained from the corneas of patients suspected of having rabies. The rabies virus may be seen in the stained material.

corneal reflex. Closure of eyelids resulting from direct corneal irritation.

corneal transplant. Transplantation of a cornea from a healthy donor eye. This is the most common organ transplantation procedure in the U.S. There are two major types of procedures: split-thickness technique, in which a portion of the anterior host cornea is removed, and a partial thickness of the donor cornea is attached. This is also called lamellar keratoplasty. The penetrating keratoplasty, or full thickness transplantation, involves complete removal of the patient's cornea and replacement with the donor cornea.

    Transmission of donor disease to the recipient is a rare event but rabies, Creutzfeldt-Jakob disease, and hepatitis B have been acquired by the graft recipient. The technique is more likely to be successful when histocompatibility matching of donor and recipient is as close as possible. The success rate is more than 90% at one year. SEE: *keratoplasty*.

NURSING IMPLICATIONS: Explain surgery to patient and the need to protect the graft from external pressure as well as prevention of increased intraocular pressure by avoiding bending below the waist, etc. Safety precautions should be taken to avoid falls. Ensure that the environment is as calm and restful as possible, and discourage coughing, straining at stool, and quick movements of the eye, esp. in the early postoperative period. Emphasize the importance of compliance with medical regimen, particularly the careful insertion of eye medications at the correct intervals and the reporting of untoward symtoms such as pain. Include patient's family in teaching so that support and assistance can be provided in the recovery period at home.

corneitis (kor″nē-ī′tĭs) [L. *corneus*, horny, + Gr. *itis*, inflammation]. Inflammation of the cornea. SYN: *keratitis*.

Cornell Medical Index. A lengthy, all-inclusive, self-administered history form developed at Cornell University Medical School.

corneoblepharon (kor″nē-ō-blĕf′ă-rŏn) [″ + Gr. *blepharon*, eyelid]. Adhesion of the eyelid to the cornea.

corneoiritis (kor″nē-ō-ī-rī′tĭs) [L. *corneus*, horny, + Gr. *iris*, iris, + *itis*, inflammation]. Inflammation of iris and cornea.

corneomandibular reflex (kor″nē-ō-măn-dĭb′ū-lär). Deflexion of mandible toward opposite side when cornea is irritated while mouth is open and relaxed.

corneosclera (kor″nē-ō-sklē′rǎ) [L. *corneus*, horny, + *skleros*, hard]. The cornea and sclera considered together constituting the tunica fibrosa [NA] or fibrous coat of the eye.

corneous (kor′nē-ŭs) [L. *corneus*]. Horny; hornlike.

corneum (kor′nē-ŭm) [L., horny]. Horny layer of the skin. SYN: *stratum corneum*.

corniculate (kor-nĭk′ū-lāt). Containing small horn-shaped projections.

corniculum (kor-nĭk′ū-lŭm) [L., little horn]. A small, hornlike process.

cornification (kor″nĭ-fĭ-kā′shŭn) [″ + *facere*, to make]. The process by which squamous epithelial cells are converted into hard horny material as in the corneum of the skin or in structures such as nails, horns, hair, and feathers that are derived from epithelium. SYN: *keratinization*.

cornified (kor′nĭ-fīd). Changed into horny tissue.

cornu (kor′nū) [L., horn] (pl. *cornua*). [NA]

Any projection like a horn.

c. ammonis. Hippocampus major of brain.

c. anterius. [NA] Anterior horn of the lateral ventricle.

c. coccygeum. [NA] Two upward projecting processes that articulate with the sacrum.

c. cutaneum. Hornlike excrescence on skin.

c. inferius. [NA] Inferior horn of the lateral ventricle.

c. of the hyoid. Greater and lesser horns of the hyoid bones, q.v.

c. of the sacrum. Two small processes projecting inferiorly on either side of the sacral hiatus leading into the sacral canal.

c. posterius. [NA] Posterior horn of the lateral ventricle.

cornua (kor′nū-ă). Pl. of cornu.

cornual (kor′nū-ăl). Pert. to a cornu.

corona (kŏ-rō′nă) [Gr. *korone*, crown]. [NA] Any structure resembling a crown.

c. capitis. Crown of head.

c. ciliaris. [NA] Circular figure on inner surface of ciliary body.

c. dentis. [NA] Crown of a tooth.

c. glandis. [NA] Posterior border of glans penis.

c. radiata. 1. [NA] Ascending and descending fibers of the internal capsule that, above the corpus callosum, extend in all directions to the cerebral cortex. Many of the fibers arise in the thalamus. 2. A thin mass of follicle cells that adhere firmly to the zona pellucida of the human ovum following ovulation.

c. veneris. Syphilitic blotches on forehead that parallel the hairline.

coronal (kō-rō′năl). Pert. to a corona.

coronal plane. Plane dividing the body into front and back portions.

coronal suture. Suture that joins the parietal and frontal bones of the cranium.

coronary (kor′ō-nă-rē) [L. *coronarius*, pert. to a crown or circle]. Encircling, as the blood vessels that supply blood directly to the heart muscle. Loosely used to refer to the heart and to coronary heart disease. Coronary pain is usually dull and heavy and may radiate to the arm, jaw, or back. Typically, the patient describes the pain as being viselike or producing a feeling of compression or squeezing of the chest.

coronary angiography. Radiographic examination of the coronary arteries after injection of a contrast agent.

coronary arteries. 1. One of a pair of arteries that supply blood to the myocardium of the heart. They arise within the right and left aortic sinuses at base of the aorta. Decreased flow of blood through these arteries

NORMAL AND DISEASED CORONARY ARTERIES

LUMEN

NORMAL

LUMEN

NARROWING DUE TO ATHEROSCLEROSIS

CALCIUM DEPOSIT

LUMEN

VIRTUALLY COMPLETE OCCLUSION BY ATHEROSCLEROSIS OF INTIMAL LINING

LUMEN

ATHEROMA

HEMORRHAGE INTO ATHEROMA LEAVING VERY LITTLE LUMEN

THROMBUS

ATHEROMA

COMPLETE OCCLUSION DUE TO THROMBUS AND ATHEROMA

EARLY ORGANIZATION OF THROMBUS

SMALL LUMEN

RECANALIZATION THROUGH ORGANIZING THROMBUS

induces attacks of angina pectoris, q.v. 2. The cervical branch of the uterine artery.

coronary artery disease. ABBR: CAD. Narrowing of the coronary arteries sufficiently to prevent adequate blood supply to the myocardium. The narrowing is usually caused by atherosclerosis; and it may progress to the point where the heart muscle is damaged due to lack of blood supply. SEE: *angina pectoris; coronary artery bypass surgery; cholesterol; heart disease, ischemic; heart disease, risk factor; lipoprotein; thrombosis, coronary;* illus.

coronary artery spasm. Intermittent constriction of the large coronary arteries. This may lead to angina pectoris in a variety of conditions and is not necessarily associated with exertion; e.g., Prinzmetal's angina, q.v.

coronary artherectomy. Technique of removing obstructions in the coronary artery. This is done by use of a cutting instrument inserted through a cardiac catheter. This same approach has been used experimentally to introduce a laser device into the coronary arteries for removal of plaques.

coronary blood flow. Quantitation of the amount of blood flowing to the coronary arteries of the heart. This may be done by one of several techniques including indicator dilution or use of radioisotopes.

coronary artery bypass surgery. A shunt, established surgically, that permits blood to travel from the aorta to a branch of the coronary artery at a point past an obstruction. Used in treating coronary artery disease. SEE: *Nursing Diagnoses in Appendix.*

coronary care unit. A specially equipped area of a hospital providing intensive nursing and medical care for patients who have acute coronary thrombosis.

coronary heart disease. ABBR: CHD. Decreased flow of blood to the heart muscle to the extent that either basal needs for oxygen are unmet, or the oxygen supply is insufficient when an increased demand for oxygen is made, as in work. The cause is usually due to atherosclerosis of the coronary arteries; any other factor that limits flow of blood through these arteries may be involved. SEE: *angina pectoris; angina, variant; behavior patterns, types A and B; cholesterol; heart disease, risk factors; lipoprotein; percutaneous transluminal coronary angioplasty.*

coronary occlusion. Closing off of a coronary artery. SYN: *coronary thrombosis.*

coronary plexus. A network of autonomic

nerve fibers that lies close to base of heart.

coronary sinus. The vessel cavity or passage that receives the cardiac veins from the heart. It opens into right atrium.

coronary thrombosis. Occlusion of one or more of the coronary arteries of the heart.

coronaviruses (kor″ō-nă-vī′rŭs-ēs) [L. *corona*, crown, + *virus*, poison]. A group of viruses morphologically similar, ether-sensitive, and probably composed of RNA, that are responsible for some but not all common colds. So named because their microscopic appearance is that of a virus particle surrounded by a crown.

coroner (kor′ō-nĕr) [L. *corona*, crown]. An official (originally, English crown officer) who investigates and holds inquests concerning those dead from unknown or violent causes. The coroner may or may not be a physician, depending upon the law in each state.

coronoid (kor′ō-noyd) [Gr. *korone*, something curved, kind of crown, + *eidos*, form, shape]. Shaped like a crown.

coronoidectomy (kor″ō-noy-dĕk′tō-mē) [″ + ″ + *ektome*, excision]. Excision of the coronoid process of the mandible of the jaw.

coronoid fossa. An oval depression on anterior surface of distal end of humerus. Receives coronoid process of ulna.

coronoid process. 1. Process on proximal end of ulna. Forms anterior portion of semilunar notch. 2. Process on the anterior upper end of the ramus of the mandible that serves for attachment of the temporalis muscle.

coroparelcysis (kor″ō-păr-ĕl′sī-sĭs) [Gr. *kore*, pupil, + *parelkein*, to draw aside]. Surgically bringing the pupil to one side so that it no longer is under a scar but lies under a transparent area.

coroscopy (kō-rŏs′kō-pē) [″ + *skopein*, to examine]. Shadow test to determine refractive error of an eye. SYN: *skiascopy*.

corotomy (kō-rŏt′ō-mē) [″ + *tome*, incision]. Surgical incision of the iris. Iridotomy, q.v.

corpora (kor′pō-ră). Pl. of corpus, q.v.

c. arantii. Tubercle found in center of semilunar valves of heart.

c. arenacea. Psammoma bodies found in the pineal body. SYN: *brain sand.*

c. olivaria. Two oval masses behind pyramids of the oblongata.

c. paraaortica. Organs of Zuckerkandl, q.v.

c. quadrigemina. The superior portion of the midbrain consisting of two pairs of rounded bodies, the superior and inferior colliculi.

corporeal (kor-pō′rē-ăl). Consisting of a physical body.

corpse (korps) [L. *corpus*, body]. The dead

human body.

corpsman (kor′măn) (pl. *corpsmen*). An enlisted member of a military medical service, esp. the U.S. Navy. During duty in the armed forces he receives training and experience in one or more health-related fields. In wartime, a corpsman may be assigned as the only medically trained person to a field unit or a small ship.

corpulence (kor′pū-lĕns) [L. *corpulentia*]. Fatness of the body. SYN: *obesity.*

corpulent (kor′pū-lĕnt). Fat; obese.

cor pulmonale. Hypertrophy or failure of right ventricle resulting from disorders of the lungs, pulmonary vessels, or chest wall. Living for an extended period at high altitude also may cause this condition.

corpus (kor′pŭs) [L., body] (pl. *corpora*). [NA] The principal part of any organ; any mass or body.

c. albicans. [NA] A mass of fibrous tissue that replaces the regressing corpus luteum following rupture of the graafian follicle. It forms a white scar that gradually decreases in size and eventually disappears.

c. amygdaloideum. Almond-shaped gray matter in the lateral wall and roof of the third ventricle of the brain.

c. amylaceum. A mass having an irregular laminated structure like a starch grain. Found in the prostate, meninges, lungs, and other organs in various pathological conditions.

c. annulare. Pons varolii.

c. callosum. [NA] The great commissure of the brain between the cerebral hemispheres.

c. cavernosum. Any erectile tissue, esp. the erectile bodies of the penis, clitoris, male or female urethra, bulb of the vestibule, or the nasal conchae.

c. cavernosum penis. [NA] Two columns of erectile tissue on dorsum of the penis.

c. cerebellum. The two lateral portions of the cerebellum exclusive of the central flocculonodular node.

c. ciliare. [NA] Ciliary body.

c. dentale. Gray layer in white substance of the cerebellum. SYN: *c. rhomboidale.*

c. fimbriatum. White layer edging the lower cornu of the lateral ventricle.

c. flavum. Waxy body seen in the central nervous system.

c. fornicis. [NA] Body of the fornix.

c. geniculatum. Medial or lateral geniculate body, q.v.; a mass of gray matter lying in the thalamus.

c. hemorrhagicum. Blood clot formed in the cavity left by rupture of the graafian follicle.

c. highmorianum. Mediastinum testis.

c. interpedunculare. Gray matter between peduncles before the pons varolii.

c. luteum. [NA] Small yellow body that develops within a ruptured ovarian follicle. It is an endocrine structure secreting progesterone. SEE: *ovary* for illus.

c. Luysii. The subthalamic nucleus lying in the ventral thalamus.

c. mammillare. [NA] Mamillary body; a rounded body in the anterior part of the interpeduncular fossa of the brain.

c. restiforme. The restiform body or inferior cerebellar peduncle. A band of fibers, principally ascending, in the medulla oblongata that connects the spinal cord below with the cerebellum.

c. rhomboidale. Gray layer in white substances of the cerebellum. SYN: *c. dentale.*

c. spongiosum. Erectile tissue surrounding the urethra.

c. striatum. [NA] Structure in the cerebral hemispheres consisting of two basal ganglia (the caudate and lentiform nuclei), and the fibers of the internal capsule that separate them.

c. subthalamicum. The subthalamic nucleus (corpus Luysii), lying in the ventral thalamus.

c. trapezoideum. [NA] The trapezoid body q.v.

c. vitreum. [NA] Vitreous portion of eye.

c. wolffianum. Wolffian body.

corpuscle (kor′pŭs-ĕl) [L. *corpusculum*, little body]. 1. Any small rounded body. 2. An encapsulated sensory nerve ending. 3. Old term for a blood cell. SEE: *erythrocyte; leukocyte.*

c., axile; c., axis. The center of a tactile corpuscle.

c., blood. An erythrocyte or leukocyte.

c., bone. A bone cell.

c., cancroid. Characteristic nodule in cutaneous epithelioma.

c., cartilage. A cell characteristic of cartilage.

c., chromophil. Tiny body found in cytoplasm of a nerve cell. SYN: *Nissl body.*

c.′s, chyle. Corpuscles seen in chyle.

c., colloid. Corpus amylaceum.

c., colostrum. A cell containing phagocytosed fat globules present in milk secreted the first few days after parturition. SYN: *colostrum body.*

c.′s, corneal. Connective tissue corpuscles found in fibrous tissue of cornea.

c.′s, Drysdale′s. Transparent cells found in the fluid of certain ovarian cysts.

c.′s, genital. Encapsulated sensory nerve endings resembling pacinian corpuscles present in skin of external genitalia and nipple.

c., ghost. A decolorized red blood cell.

SYN: *achromatocyte; phantom corpuscle.*

c.′s, Gierke′s. Particles seen in the thymus gland. SYN: *Hassall's corpuscles.*

c.′s, Golgi-Mazzoni. Tactile corpuscles in the skin of the fingertips.

c.′s, Hassall′s. Corpuscles found in the thymus gland. SYN: *c.′s, Gierke′s.*

c.′s, Krause′s. Sensory encapsulated nerve endings in mucosa of genitalia, mouth, nose, and eyes.

c., lymph. A lymphocyte.

c., malpighian. 1. A renal corpuscle consisting of a glomerulus and Bowman's capsule, which encloses it. 2. A malpighian body of the spleen.

c.′s, Mazzoni′s. Nerve endings resembling Krause's corpuscles.

c., Meissner′s. An encapsulated touch receptor found in connective tissue immediately underlying the epidermis of the skin, esp. on palmar and volar surfaces of hands and feet. SYN: *c., tactile.*

c.′s, milk. Fat-filled globules present in milk. They represent the distal ends of mammary gland cells that are broken off in apocrine secretion.

c., pacinian. A large, ovoid, sensory end organ consisting of concentric layers or lamellae of connective tissue surrounding a nerve ending. They are present in tendons, intermuscular septa, connective tissue membranes, and sometimes internal organs, and function as proprioceptive receptors and as receptors of deep pressure.

c., phantom. A decolorized red blood cell. SYN: *c., ghost.*

c., Purkinje′s. SEE: *Purkinje cells.*

c., red. An erythrocyte.

c., renal. A glomerulus and the capsule (Bowman's capsule) that surrounds it. It is located at the proximal end of a renal tubule. SYN: *c., malpighian.*

c.′s, reticulated. Erythrocytes that when properly stained show filamentous reticulations.

c., splenic. A nodule of lymphatic tissue present in the spleen.

c., tactile. A sensory end organ that responds to touch, as Meissner's corpuscle, q.v.

c., terminal. A nerve ending. SEE: *nerve.*

c.′s, thymic. Corpuscles found in the thymus.

c., white. A leukocyte.

corpuscular (kor-pŭs′kū-lăr). Pert. to corpuscles.

corpusculum (kŏr-pŭs′kū-lŭm) [L., little body] (pl. *corpuscula*). [NA] Corpuscle.

correction. The altering of a condition that is abnormal or malfunctioning.

corrective (kō-rĕk′tiv) [L. *corrigere*, to correct]. 1. A drug that modifies action of another. 2. Pert. to such a drug.

correlation (kor″ĕ-lā′shŭn) [L. *com-*, together, + *relatio*, relation]. 1. The processes by which the various activities of the body, esp. nervous impulses, occur in proper relation to each other. 2. In statistics, the degree to which one variable increases or decreases with respect to another variable. The positive correlation is greatest when the coefficient of correlation is plus 1.0; the negative correlation is maximum when the coefficient is minus one; the correlation is least when the value is zero. A variable can have a positive or negative correlation with another variable.

correspondence. The act or state of corresponding, i.e., occurring in proper relationship to other phenomena.

   c., retinal. Condition occurring in normal vision in which images formed on the maculae or other points of the retinas of the two eyes are mentally blended and seen as a single image.

corresponding. Agreeing with, matching, or fitting.

corresponding points of retina. Identical points; points on the retinas of the two eyes that when stimulated give rise to a single image.

Corrigan's pulse (kor′ĭ-gǎns) [Sir Dominic J. Corrigan, Ir. physician, 1802–1880]. A full bounding pulse that appears to be completely empty between beats. Associated with aortic insufficiency. SYN: *waterhammer pulse.*

corrosion (kǒ-rō′zhŭn) [L *corrodere*, to corrode]. Slow disintegration or wearing away of something by a destructive agent.

corrosive (kǒ-rō′sĭv). Producing corrosion.

corrosive alkalies. Corrosive hydroxides most commonly of sodium, ammonium, and potassium, as well as carbonates. Because of their great combining power with water and their action on the fatty tissues, they cause rapid deep tissue destruction. They have a tendency to gelatinize tissue, turning it a somewhat grayish color and forming a soapy, slippery surface, accompanied by pain and burning.

corrosive poisoning. Poisoning by strong acids, alkalies, strong antiseptics including bichloride of mercury, carbolic acid (phenol), lysol, cresol compounds, tincture of iodine, and arsenic compounds. These are destructive and cause disintegration similar to that caused by burns. If they are swallowed, any part of the alimentary canal may be affected. Tissues involved are altered, easily perforated, or destroyed. Death comes very shortly from shock or swelling of throat and pharynx, which causes choking, or by closure of esophagus, causing slow starvation, if untreated. SEE: individual poisons in *Poisons and Poisoning* in *Appendix.*

SYM: Intense burning about mouth, throat, pharynx, and abdomen; abdominal cramping, retching, nausea, vomiting, and often collapse. There may be bloody vomitus (hematemesis) and diarrhea; the stools are watery, mucoid, bloody, and possibly stained with the poison or its products, resulting from its action on the contents of the alimentary tract. Stains about the lips, cheeks, tongue, mouth, or pharynx are often characteristic brown; stains on mucous membranes may be violet-colored or black. Carbolic acid or phenol leaves a white or gray stain resembling boiled meat; hydrochloric acid stains are grayish; nitric acid leaves a yellow stain; sulfuric acid leaves tan or dark burns.

TREAT: Immediate treatment preferably in a hospital is mandatory. It is also important to attempt to discover the chemical substance ingested; for this reason save all materials such as bottles, food, jars, or containers that may help to answer this question. This is essential when the patient is either comatose or an infant. In treating corrosive poisoning, DO NOT INDUCE VOMITING; DO NOT ATTEMPT GASTRIC LAVAGE; and DO NOT ATTEMPT TO NEUTRALIZE THE CORROSIVE SUBSTANCE. Vomiting will increase the severity of damage to the esophagus by having the corrosive substance again come in contact with it. Attempting gastric lavage may result in perforating either the esophagus or stomach. Immediately dilute the corrosive substance by having patient drink milk or water. If trachea has been damaged, tracheostomy may be needed. Opiates will be needed to control pain. For esophageal burns begin broad-spectrum antibiotics and corticosteroid therapy. Intravenous fluids will be required if esophageal or gastric damage prevents ingestion of liquids. Long-range therapy will be directed toward preventing or treating esophageal scars and strictures.

corrugator (kor′ū-gā″tor) [L. *con*, together, + *rugare*, to wrinkle]. A muscle that lies above the orbit arising medially from frontal bone and having its insertion on skin of medial half of the eyebrows. It draws the brow medially and inferiorly.

Cortef. Trade name for hydrocortisone.

Cortef Acetate. Trade name for hydrocortisone acetate.

Cortenema. Trade name for hydrocortisone retention enema.

cortex (kor′tĕks) [L., rind] (pl. *cortices*). 1. [NA] The outer layer of an organ as distinguished from the inner medulla as in the adrenal gland, kidney, ovary, lymph node, thymus, and cerebrum and cerebellum of the brain. 2. The outer layer of a structure as a hair or the lens of the eye. 3. The outer superficial portion of the stem or root of a plant.

c., adrenal. The outer layer of the adrenal gland; secretes mineralocorticoids, androgens, and glucocorticoids.

c., cerebellar. The surface layer of the cerebellum consisting of three layers: outer or molecular, middle, and inner or granular layer. Purkinje's cells are present in the middle layer.

c., cerebral. The thin, convoluted surface layer of gray matter of the cerebral hemispheres, consisting principally of cell bodies of neurons arranged in five layers. There are also numerous fibers.

c., interpretive. The temporal cortex, where memories of the past may be evoked by electrical stimulation.

c., renal. SEE: *kidney.*

c., temporal. Outer layer of brain behind the temples.

Corti, Alfonso Giacomo Gaspare (kor'tē). Italian anatomist, 1822 – 1876.

C., canal of. A triangular-shaped canal extending the entire length of the organ of Corti. Its walls are formed by the external and internal pillar cells.

C.'s membrane. A delicate film of gelatinous consistency that covers the cochlear duct of the inner ear. SEE: *C., organ of.*

C., organ of. An elongated spiral structure running the entire length of the cochlea in the floor of the cochlear duct and resting on the basilar membrane. It is the end organ of hearing and contains hair cells, supporting cells, and neuroepithelial receptors stimulated by sound waves. SEE: *C.'s membrane.*

cortiadrenal (kor″tē-ăd-rē′năl) [L. *cortex,* rind, + *ad,* toward, + *ren,* kidney]. Pert. to cortex of adrenal gland.

cortical (kor′tĭ-kăl). Pert. to a cortex.

corticate (kor′tĭ-kāt). Possessing a cortex or bark.

corticectomy (kor″tĭ-sĕk′tō-mē) [″ + Gr. *ektome,* excision]. Surgical removal of a portion of the cerebral cortex.

cortices (kor′tĭ-sēz). Pl. of cortex.

corticifugal (kor″tĭ-sĭf′ū-găl) [L. *cortex,* rind, + *fugere,* to flee]. Conducting impulses away from the outer surface or cortex; particularly denoting axons of pyramidal cells of the cerebral cortex. SYN: *corticoefferent.*

corticipetal (kor″tĭ-sĭp′ĕ-tăl) [″ + *petere,* to seek]. Conducting impulses toward the outer surface, or cortex; particularly denot-

ing fibers of the thalamic radiation conveying impulses to sensory areas of cerebral cortex. SYN: *corticoafferent.*

corticoadrenal (kor″tĭ-kō-ăd-rē′năl) [″ + *ad,* toward, + *ren,* kidney]. Pert. to cortex of adrenal gland.

corticoafferent (kor″tĭ-kō-ăf′fĕr-ĕnt) [″ + *adferre,* to bear to]. Conducting impulses toward the outer surface or cortex; conveying impulses to sensory areas of the cerebral cortex. SYN: *corticipetal.*

corticobulbar (kor″tĭ-kō-bŭl′băr) [″ + *bulbus,* bulb]. Pert. to the cerebral cortex and upper portion of the brain stem, as corticobulbar tract.

corticoefferent (kor″tĭ-kō-ĕf′-ĕr-ĕnt) [″ + *effere,* to bring out of]. Conducting impulses away from the outer surface or cortex; particularly denoting axons of pyramidal cells of the cerebral cortex. SYN: *corticifugal.*

corticoid (kor′tĭ-koyd) [″ + Gr. *eidos,* form, shape]. Any of a number of hormonal steroid substances obtained from the cortex of the adrenal gland. SYN: *corticosteroid.*

corticopeduncular (kor″tĭ-kō-pē-dŭng′kū-lăr) [″ + *pedunculus,* little foot]. Pert. to cortex and cerebral peduncles.

corticopleuritis (kor″tĭ-kō-ploo-rī′tĭs) [″ + Gr. *pleura,* rib, + *itis,* inflammation]. Inflammation of the outer parts of the pleura.

corticopontine (kor″tĭ-kō-pŏn′tīn) [″ + *pons,* bridge]. Concerning or connecting the cerebral cortex and the pons of the brain.

corticospinal (kor″tĭ-kō-spī′năl) [″ + *spina,* thorn]. Pert. to cerebral cortex and spinal cord. SYN: *spinocortical.*

corticosteroid (kor″tĭ-kō-stēr′oyd). Any of a number of hormonal steroid substances obtained from the cortex of the adrenal gland. They are classified according to their biological activity as glucocorticoids, mineralocorticoids, and androgen. Adrenal corticosteroids do not initiate cellular and enzymatic activity, but permit many biochemical reactions to proceed at optimal rates.

corticosterone (kor″tĭ-kŏs′tĕ-rōn). A hormone of the adrenal cortex. Corticosterone influences carbohydrate, potassium and sodium metabolism. It is essential for normal absorption of glucose, the formation of glycogen in the liver and tissues, and the normal utilization of carbohydrates by the tissues. SEE: *adrenocorticotropic hormone.*

corticothalamic (kor″tĭ-kō-thă-lăm′ĭk) [″ + Gr. *thalamos,* chamber]. Concerning or connecting the cerebral cortex and the thalamus of the brain.

corticotrophic, corticotropic (kor″tĭ-kō-trŏf′ĭk, -trŏp′ĭk) [″ + Gr. *trophe,* nourishment;" + Gr. *trope*, a turn]. Pert. to corticotrophin.

corticotrophin, corticotropin (kor″tĭ-kō-trō′fĭn, -trō′pin). The adrenocorticotrophic factor or principle in the anterior lobe of the pituitary gland. Stimulates adrenal cortex to secrete steroid hormones. Trade names are Acthar and Corticotrophin Gel ACTH. Trade name for corticotrophin zinc hydroxide is Cortrophin Zinc ACTH. SYN: *ACTH*.

corticotropin-releasing hormone. ABBR: CRH. A hormone released from the hypothalamus that acts on the anterior pituitary to increase secretion of adrenal corticotropin hormone (ACTH). Also, in response to stress, CRH causes hyperglycemia, increased oxygen consumption, increased cardiac output, decreased sexual activity, suppresses release of growth hormone, diminishes gastrointestinal function, stimulates respiration, and causes behavioral changes.

cortin (kor′tĭn) [L. *cortex*, rind]. An extract of the cortex of the adrenal gland; contains a mixture of the active steroid agents such as corticosterone.

cortisol (kor′tĭ-sŏl). An adrenocortical hormone, usually referred to pharmaceutically as hydrocortisone. Closely related to cortisone, q.v., in physiological effects.

cortisone (kor′tĭ-sōn). A hormone isolated from the cortex of the adrenal gland and also prepared synthetically. It is closely related to cortisol, and is largely inactive in man until it is converted to cortisol. It is important for its regulatory action in metabolism of fats, carbohydrates, sodium, potassium, and proteins. Also used as an anti-inflammatory agent. Trade name for cortisone acetate, USP, is Cortone Acetate.

Cortone Acetate. Trade name for cortisone acetate.

Cortril. Trade name for hydrocortisone.

Cortril Acetate-AS. Trade name for hydrocortisone acetate.

Cortrophin. Trade name for corticotropin (injection).

Cortrophin Zinc ACTH. Trade name for corticotropin zinc hydroxide (suspension, sterile).

Cortrosyn. Trade name for cosyntropin.

coruscation (kŏ-rŭs-kā′shŭn) [L. *coruscare*, to glitter]. The subjective sensation of flashes of light before the eyes. SEE: *Moore's lightning streaks*.

corybantism (kor″ĭ-băn′tĭzm) [Gr. *Korybas*, a priest of Cybele who accompanied the goddess, during her travels, with music and wild dancing, + -*ismos*, condition]. Wild delirium, terrifying hallucinations, and muscular spasms, none of which are conducive to sleep.

Corynebacterium (kō-rī″nē-băk-tē′rē-ŭm) [Gr. *coryne*, a club, + *bacterion*, a small rod]. A genus of the family Corynebacteriaceae. The bacteria are rod-shaped, gram-positive, and nonmotile. Though many of the species are pathogens in domestic animals, birds, reptiles, and plants, the most important is the species *C. diphtheriae*, q.v., pathogenic in man.

C. diphtheriae. The causative agent of diphtheria in man. SYN: *Klebs-Loeffler bacillus*. SEE: *diphtheria*.

C. vaginale. An organism that may cause vaginitis. It was also known as *Haemophilus vaginalis*. The currently accepted name is *Gardnerella vaginalis*, q.v.

coryza (kŏ-rī′ză) [Gr. *koryza*, catarrh]. An acute catarrhal inflammation of the nasal mucous membrane accompanied by profuse nasal discharge. SEE: *cold*.

cosensitize (kō-sĕn′sĭ-tīz) [L. *con*, with, + *sensitivus*, sensitive]. To sensitize to more than one infection.

Cosmegen. Trade name for dactinomycin.

cosmesis [G. *kosmesus*, an arranging]. In surgery, the consideration of the effect the procedure will have on the appearance or beauty of the patient.

cosmetic (kŏz-mĕt′ĭk). 1. Preparation such as powder or cream for improving appearance. 2. Serving to preserve or promote appearance.

cosmetic surgery. Surgical procedures, usually plastic surgery, directed toward preserving appearance or correcting ugly scars or burns.

cosmic (kŏz′mĭk) [Gr. *kosmos*, order, the universe]. Pert. to the universe as a whole.

costa (kŏs′tă) [L.] (pl. *costae*). [NA] Rib.

c. fluctuans. A floating rib.

c. spuria. [NA] A false rib.

c. vera. [NA] A true rib.

costal (kŏs′tăl). Pert. to a rib.

costal cartilage. A cartilage that connects the end of a true rib with the sternum or the end of a rib with the costal cartilage above.

costalgia (kŏs-tăl′jē-ă) [L. *costa*, rib, + Gr. *algos*, pain]. Pain in a rib or in the intercostal spaces as in intercostal neuralgia.

costal pit. Cup-shaped depression at distal end of transverse process of a thoracic vertebra for articulation with tubercle of rib.

costectomy (kŏs-tĕk′tō-mē) [" + Gr. *ektome*, excision]. Operation of excising or resecting a rib.

Costen's syndrome [James B. Costen, U.S. otolaryngologist, 1895–1961]. Temporomandibular joint syndrome, q.v.

costive (kŏs′tĭv) [L. *constipare*, to press together]. Constipated.

costiveness (kŏs′tĭv-nĕs). Constipation.

costocervical (kŏs″tō-sĕr′vĭ-kăl). Concerning the ribs and neck.

costochondral (kŏs″tō-kŏn′drăl) [L. *costa*, rib, + Gr. *chondros*, cartilage]. Pert. to a rib and its cartilage.

costoclavicular (kŏs″tō-klă-vĭk′ū-lăr) [″ + *clavicula*, a little key]. Pert. to ribs and clavicle.

costocoracoid (kŏs″tō-kor′ă-koyd) [″ + Gr. *korax*, crow, + *eidos*, form, shape]. Pert. to ribs and coracoid process of scapula.

costophrenic [″ + Gr. *phren*, diaphragm]. Pertaining to the ribs and diaphragm.

costopneumopexy (kŏs″tō-nū′mō-pĕk″sē) [″ + Gr. *pneumon*, lung, + *pexis*, fixation]. Anchoring a lung to a rib.

costosternal (kŏs″tō-stĕr′năl) [″ + Gr. *sternon*, chest]. Pert. to a rib and the sternum.

costosternoplasty (kŏs″tō-stĕr′nō-plăs″tē) [″ + ″ + *plassein*, to form]. Surgical repair of funnel chest. A portion of a rib is used to support the sternum.

costotome (kŏs′tō-tōm) [″ + Gr. *tome*, incision]. Knife or shears for cutting through a rib or cartilage.

costotomy (kŏs-tŏt′ō-mē). 1. Incision or division of a rib or part of one. 2. Excision of a rib. SYN: *costectomy*.

costotransverse (kŏs″tō-trăns-vĕrs′) [″ + *transvertere*, to turn across]. Pert. to the ribs and transverse processes of articulating vertebrae.

costovertebral (kŏs″tō-vĕr′tĕ-brăl) [″ + *vertebra*, joint]. Pert. to a rib and a vertebra.

costoxiphoid (kŏs″tō-zī′foyd) [″ + Gr. *xiphos*, sword, + *eidos*, form, shape]. Concerning or connecting the ribs and the xiphoid process of the sternum.

cosyntropin (kō-sĭn-trō′pĭn). Synthetic corticotropin used to test for adrenal insufficiency. The medicine is given intramuscularly or intravenously, and the plasma cortisol is determined in order to judge the adequacy of response. Trade name is Cortrosyn.

C.O.T.A. *certified occupational therapy assistant.*

Cotazym. Trade name for pancrelipase.

cotinine. The principal metabolite of nicotine. It is excreted in the urine. Its detection indicates that the individual has recently smoked cigarettes.

cotton [ME. *cotoun*, from Arabic *qutn*, cotton]. A soft, white, fibrous material obtained from the fibers enclosing the seeds of various plants of the Malvaceae, esp. those of the genus *Gossypium*.

  c., purified. USP. Cotton fibers from which the oil has been completely removed, enhancing ability to absorb liquids.

  c., styptic. Cotton impregnated with an astringent.

cotton-wool spot. The appearance of the retina in certain conditions, including hypertension and other diseases.

co-twin (kō-twĭn). Either one of twins.

cotyledon (kŏt″ĭ-lē′dŏn) [Gr. *kotyledon*, hollow of a cup]. 1. Mass of villi on chorionic surface of the placenta. 2. Any of rounded portions into which the placenta's uterine surface is divided. 3. Seed leaf of a plant embryo.

cotyloid (kŏt′ĭ-loyd) [Gr. *kotyloeides*, cupshaped]. Shaped like a cup.

cotyloid cavity. The acetabulum or socket receiving the head of the femur.

cough (kawf) [ME. *coughen*]. A forceful and sometimes violent expiratory effort preceded by a preliminary inspiration. The glottis is partially closed, the accessory muscles of expiration are brought into action, and the air is noisily expelled.

A cough may be due to a variety of conditions, as can be seen below. There is no one course of therapy. Each disease is evaluated and treated accordingly. It is usually inadvisable to suppress completely coughs due to inflammation of the respiratory tract. This is particularly true if sputum is produced as a result of coughing. SEE: *expectoration.*

  c., aneurysmal. Cough that is brassy and clanging, heard in patients suffering from aneurysm.

  c., asthmatic. Cough that is more like an attack of dyspnea.

  c., brassy. Cough heard in patients in whom there is pressure on the left recurrent laryngeal nerve, as in aortic aneurysm.

  c., bronchial. Cough heard in patients with bronchiectasis, q.v. May be provoked by change of posture, as getting up in the morning. Sputum has a fetid odor, is copious, and is dirty gray. Cough heard in bronchitis, q.v., in earlier stages is hacking and irritating; in later stages looser and easier. Sputum is thin frothy mucus.

  c., diphtherial. Cough heard in laryngeal diphtheria; noisy and brassy, with stridulous breathing.

  c., dry. Cough unaccompanied by moisture.

  c., ear. A reflex cough induced by irritation in the ear that stimulates Arnold's nerve (ramus auricularis nervi vagi).

  c., effective. Cough in which sputum or any exudate is expectorated. SYN: *c., productive.*

  c., hacking. A series of repeated efforts, as occurs in the early stages of pulmonary tuberculosis.

  c., harsh. A metallic cough occurring in laryngitis.

  c., moist. A loose cough accompanied by production of mucus or exudate.

c., paroxysmal. Cough occurring in whooping cough and bronchiectasis.

c., productive. Cough in which mucus or an exudate is expectorated. SYN: *c., effective.*

c., pulmonary. Cough that is hard and painful, seen in pneumonia. Hacking and irritating in early stages of tuberculosis; in later stages, frequent and paroxysmal. SEE: *sputum.*

c., reflex. Cough due to irritation from the middle ear, pharynx, stomach, or intestine. It may occur singly or coupled, or may be hacking in character. Stimulation of Arnold's nerve, q.v., of the ear can cause this type of cough.

c., uterine. A reflex cough resulting from irritation of female organs, esp. the uterus.

c., whooping. 1. Pertussis. 2. The paroxysmal cough ending in a whooping inspiration that occurs in pertussis.

coulomb (koo'lŏm, -lōm) [Charles A. de Coulomb, Fr. physicist, 1736–1806]. ABBR: C. Unit of electrical quantity. It is the quantity of electricity that flows across a surface when a steady current of one ampere flows for one second.

Coumadin. Trade name for warfarin sodium.

counseling. The providing of advice and guidance to a patient by a health professional.

count. The computation obtained by determining the number of units of the object being counted per unit of volume or, in the case of radiation, counts per unit of time. Types of counts include bacteria count, various blood cell counts, platelet count, reticulocyte count, differential count of white blood cells, emissions from radioactive substances, and parasite count.

counter (kown'tĕr). Device for counting anything.

c., Coulter. Device for automatically counting the blood cells.

c., Geiger. Device for detecting and counting ionizing radiation.

c., scintillation. Device for detecting and counting radiation. Flashes of light are produced when radiation is detected.

counteract (kown"tĕr-äkt'). To act against or in opposition to.

counteraction (kown"tĕr-äk'shŭn). That action of a drug or chemical agent having an action opposing that of another agent.

countercurrent exchanger. The exchange of chemicals between two countercurrent streams separated by a membrane. This permits the fluid leaving one side of the membrane to be similar to the composition of the fluid entering the other end of the other stream.

counterextension (kown"tĕr-ĕks-tĕn'shŭn)

[L. *contra*, against, + *extendere*, to extend]. Back pull or resistance to extension on a limb.

counterimmunoelectrophoresis (kown" tĕr-ĭm"ū-nō-ē-lĕk"trō-fō-rē'sĭs) [" + *immunis*, safe, + Gr. *elektron*, amber, + *phoresis*, bearing]. Process in which antigens and antibodies are placed in separate wells and an electric current is passed through the diffusion medium. Antigens migrate to the anode and antibodies to the cathode. If the antigen and antibody correspond to each other, they will upon meeting in the diffusion medium precipitate and form a precipitin band or line.

counterincision (kown"tĕr-ĭn-sĭzh'ŭn) [" + *incisio*, incision]. A second incision made either to promote drainage or to relieve the stress on a wound as it is sutured.

counterirritant (kown"tĕr-ĭr'ĭ-tänt) [" + *irritare*, to excite]. An agent such as mustard plaster that is applied locally to produce inflammatory reaction for the purpose of affecting some other part, usually adjacent to or underlying the surface irritated. Three degrees of irritation are produced by the following classes of agents: 1. rubefacients, which redden the skin; 2. vesicants, q.v., which produce a blister or vesicle; and 3. escharotics, which form an eschar or slough or cause death of tissue. SEE: *acupuncture; escharotic; moxibustion; plaster, mustard.*

counterirritation (kown"tĕr-ĭr"ĭ-tā'shŭn). Superficial irritation that relieves some other irritation of deeper structures.

counteropening (kown"tĕr-ō'pĕn-ĭng) [L. *contra*, against, + AS. *open*, open]. A second opening, as in an abscess that is not draining satisfactorily from the first incision.

counterpressure instrument. An instrument that provides counter-retraction to offset that exerted by exit of needle.

counterpulsation, intra-aortic balloon. ABBR: IABC. The use of a balloon attached to a catheter inserted through the femoral artery into the descending thoracic aorta for producing alternating inflation and deflation during diastole and systole respectively. This permits lowering resistance to aortic blood flow during systole and increasing resistance during diastole. The result is to decrease the work of the heart and to increase flow of blood to the coronary arteries. The inflation of the balloon is accomplished by using helium. This technique is rarely used.

counterpuncture [" + *punctura*, puncture]. Counteropening. An additional opening made to help drainage, as an abscess.

countershock. The application of an electric current to the heart directly or indirectly in order to alter a disturbance in cardiac rhythm.

counterstain (kown'tĕr-stān). Application of a different stain to tissues that have already been prepared for microscopic examination by having been stained. The added stain helps to contrast the tissues originally stained.

countertraction (kown"tĕr-trăk'shŭn). Application of traction so the force opposes the traction already established. Used in reducing fractures.

countertransference (kown"tĕr-trăns-fĕr'ĕns). In psychoanalytic theory, the development by the analyst of an emotional (i.e., transference) relationship with the patient. The therapist may in this situation lose objectivity.

coup de soleil (kū-dă-sŏ-lā') [Fr.]. Sunstroke.

couple. 1. To join together. 2. To have sexual intercourse.

coupling (kŭp'lĭng). In cardiology, the regular occurrence of premature systole just after a normal systolic beat.

course, courses (kors, kor'sĕs) [L. *cursus,* a flowing]. Colloquial term for menstruation.

Courvoisier's law (koor-vwă'zē-āz) [Ludwig Georg Courvoisier, Swiss surgeon, 1843–1918]. Law pert. to dilatation of gallbladder. Disease processes that cause sudden blockage of the common bile duct, e.g., a stone, do not usually cause dilatation of the gallbladder. When the duct is obstructed slowly, as would be the case in infiltration of tissue around the duct (as in cancer), dilatation of the gallbladder is usually present.

couvade (koo-văd'). The custom in some primitive cultures of the father remaining in bed as if ill during the time the mother is confined for childbirth.

Couvelaire uterus [Alexandre Couvelaire, French obstetrician, 1873–1948]. The condition wherein, in abruptio placentae, q.v., blood is extravasated into the uterine musculature. This acute condition may be associated with disseminated intravascular coagulation, and hysterectomy may be required. SYN: *uteroplacental apoplexy.*

covalence, covalent (kō-văl'ĕns, -ĕnt). The sharing of electrons between two atoms, which bonds the atoms; pert. to such sharing of electrons.

covariance (kō-vā'rē-ăns). In statistics, the expected value of the product of the deviations of corresponding values of two variables from their respective means.

covariant (kō-vā'rē-ănt). In mathematics, pert. to variation of one variable with another so that a specified relationship is unchanged.

cover. To provide protection, esp. in the sense of assisting the body to protect against that which would normally not require such help or cover.

Ex.: The adrenal gland is normally capable of responding to stress by increasing the secretion of adrenal cortical hormones but, if a patient has received adrenocortical hormones for some time and then discontinues them, the adrenal will for a period of time be unable to respond adequately to stress such as a surgical procedure or trauma. In that case, replacement hormone therapy will be needed until the stress is over. Thus the patient would be covered by receiving adrenocortical hormones in the period of stress.

cover glass, cover slip. Thin glass disk to cover a tissue or bacterial specimen to be examined microscopically.

Cowden's disease or syndrome [Cowden, family name of first patient described]. Hamartoma, multiple, q.v.

Cowling's rule. A method for calculation of pediatric drug dosages. The age of the child at the next birthday is divided by 24. However, the most safe and accurate methods of pediatric dosage calculation include the weight and body surface area or both of the patient. SEE: *Clark's rule; Young's rule.*

Cowper's glands [William Cowper, Brit. anatomist, 1666–1709]. A pair of compound tubular glands less than one cm in size beneath the bulb of the male urethra, and emptying a mucous secretion into it. These small round bodies are yellow in color and correspond to the Bartholin glands, q.v., in the female. SYN: *bulbourethral glands.*

cowperitis (kow"pĕr-ī'tĭs) [*Cowper* + Gr. *itis,* inflammation]. Inflammation of Cowper's glands.

cowpox (kow'poks). Vaccinia; pustular eruption on teats and bag of a cow in form of bluish vesicles, similar to smallpox. When given to humans, usually by vaccination, some degree of immunity against smallpox is obtained. SYN: *vaccinia.* SEE: *Jenner, Edward.*

coxa (kŏk'să) [L.] (pl. *coxae*). [NA] Hip or hip joint.

   c. plana. Aseptic necrosis of the upper end of the epiphysis of the head of the femur.

   c. valga. Deformity produced when angle of the head of the femur with the shaft is increased above 120°. Opposed to coxa vara.

   c. vara. A deformity produced by decrease in the angle made by the head of the femur with the shaft. Normally it should be 120°; but in coxa vara it may be 80° to 90°. Coxa vara occurs in rickets or may result from bone injury.

coxalgia (kŏk-săl'jē-ă) [L. *coxa,* hip, + Gr. *algos,* pain]. 1. Pain in the hip. SYN: *coxodynia.* 2. Hip joint disease. SYN: *coxitis.*

coxarthrosis (kŏks"ărth-rō'sĭs) [" + Gr. *arthron,* joint, + *osis,* condition]. Term used in foreign literature to indicate arthritis of the hip.

Coxiella (kŏk"sē-ĕl'lă) [Harold Rae Cox, U.S. bacteriologist, b. 1907]. A genus of bacteria related to rickettsiae.

    C. burnetii [Cox; Sir Frank Macfarlane Burnet, Australian Nobel prize winner, b. 1899]. Causative organism of Q fever, q.v.

coxitis (kŏk-sī'tĭs) [L. *coxa,* hip, + Gr. *itis,* inflammation]. Hip joint disease. SYN: *coxalgia* (def. 2).

coxodynia (kŏk"sō-dĭn'ē-ă) [" + Gr. *odyne,* pain]. Pain in the hip joint. SYN: *coxalgia* (def.1).

coxofemoral (kŏk"sō-fĕm'ŏ-răl) [" + *femur,* thigh]. Pert. to the hip and femur.

coxotuberculosis (kŏk"sō-tū-bĕr"kū-lō'sĭs) [" + *tuberculum,* a little swelling, + *osis,* diseased condition]. Tuberculous condition of the hip joint.

coxsackievirus (kŏk-săk'ē-vī"rŭs) [*Coxsackie,* a city in N.Y., + L. *virus,* poison]. A group of viruses, the first of which was isolated in 1948 from two children in Coxsackie, N.Y. There are 23 group A and 6 group B coxsackieviruses. Most coxsackievirus infections in man are mild, but the viruses do produce a variety of illnesses including aseptic meningitis, herpangina, epidemic pleurodynia, epidemic hemorrhagic conjunctivitis, acute upper respiratory infection, and myocarditis of the newborn. It is also possible that coxsackie infection during the first trimester of pregnancy is causally related to increased incidence of congenital heart lesions in newborns. SEE: *picornaviruses.*

cozymase (kō-zī'mās). Nicotinamide-adenine dinucleotide. ABBR: NAD.

C.P. *candle power; cerebral palsy; chemically pure.*

C.P.A. *Canadian Physiotherapy Association.*

CPAP. *continuous positive air pressure.*

CPK. *creatine phosphokinase.*

c.p.m. *counts per minute* of ionizing emissions from a radioactive material.

CPPV. *continuous positive pressure ventilation.*

CPR. *cardiopulmonary resuscitation.*

C.P.S. *cycles per second.*

CR. *conditioned reflex.*

C.R. 1. *crown-rump;* the axis for measurement of a fetus. 2. *central ray;* the center of a divergent x-ray beam.

Cr. Chem. symb. for the element chromium.

crab louse. *Phthirus inguinalis* and *Phthirus pubis.* Louse that infests the pubic region and other hairy areas of the body. SEE: *pediculosis.*

''crack.'' Street name for an almost pure form of cocaine. It is prepared from an aqueous solution of cocaine hydrochloride to which ammonia (with or without baking soda) has been added. This causes the alkaloidal form of cocaine to be precipitated. Because "crack" is not destroyed by heating, it may be smoked. The effects of "crack" are very brief compared to ingested or injected cocaine. SEE: *cocaine hydrochloride poisoning, acute.*

''crack'' baby. An infant exposed to "crack" in utero due to the mother's use of the drug during the pregnancy. SEE: *cocaine babies.*

cracked pot sound. Percussion sound resembling that heard when striking a cracked pot, indicative of a pulmonary cavity.

''cracking'' joints. The sound produced by forcible movement of a joint by contracting the muscles that contract or extend a joint, esp. the metacarpophalangeal joints. This is probably caused by the sudden creation of negative pressure in the joint space to produce a temporary vacuum. SEE: *crepitation.*

crackles. Discrete, noncontinuous lung sounds. SEE: *rales.*

    c., coarse. Louder, slightly longer, lower-pitched lung sounds. SEE: *rales.*

    c., fine. Soft, very short, high-pitched lung sounds. SEE: *rales.*

cradle [AS. *cradel*]. Frame for keeping bedclothes from pressing on a wound or fractured part. SYN: *arculus.*

cradle cap. Seborrheic dermatitis of the newborn usually appearing on the scalp, face, and head. Thick, yellowish, crusted lesions will develop on the scalp, and scaling, papules, or fissuring will appear behind the ears and on the face. SEE: *seborrhea.*

    TREAT: Mild shampoo daily; corticosteroid cream to the affected area twice daily.

cramp [ME. *crampe*]. 1. A pain, usually sudden and intermittent, of almost any area of the body, esp. abdominal and pelvic viscera. SEE: *dysmenorrhea.* 2. Painful, involuntary skeletal muscle contractions. SEE: *cramp, muscle; heat cramps; systremma; writer's cramp.*

    TREAT: Depends upon cause and location. In muscular cramps try to extend muscle, compress it, and apply heat and massage.

    c., heat. Painful muscle contractions occurring in persons who have performed hard muscular work in high environmental heat, sweated profusely, and replaced their fluid losses with water. The usual muscles affected are those used during work, i.e., the hand, arm, or leg muscles. The cramps may come on during work or up to 18 hours after completing a work shift.

    c., muscle. Painful, involuntary skeletal muscle contraction. This occurs at rest, mostly at night, is asymmetric, and usually affects the gastrocnemius muscle and small muscles of the foot. Persons with cirrhosis, well-developed muscles, or in the last months of pregnancy may experience this type of cramp. Ordinary muscle cramps are not due to fluid or electrolyte abnormality. These cramps begin when a muscle already in its most shortened position involuntarily contracts.

TREAT: Passive stretching of the involved muscle and active contraction of the antagonists will relieve an established cramp. Quinine, methocarbamol, or chloroquine may help to relieve muscle cramps.

c., occupational. A form of focal dystonia in which agonist and antagonist muscles contract at the same time. This can occur in writers, pianists, typists, and almost any occupation. They are not considered to have an emotional basis.

TREAT: Rest from specific task, anticholinergics and benzodiazepine may provide temporary relief. Injection of botulinum toxin into the most active muscle has been of help.

c., writer's. SEE: writer's cramp.

cranial (krā′nē-ăl) [L. cranialis]. Pert. to the cranium.

cranial bones. Bones that constitute the cranium or brain case.

cranial nerves. Twelve pair of nerves that have their origin in the brain. In addition to the 12 pair of cranial nerves, there is a small combined efferent and afferent nerve that goes from the olfactory area of the brain to the nasal septum. This nerve, which is thought by some anatomists to be the first cranial nerve, is called terminal nerve. SEE: illus.

DIAG: Lesions of the cranial nerves give rise to the following alteration(s) (lesions are described as if one of each pair of nerves were diseased): *First* (Olfactory): Loss or disturbance of the sense of smell. *Second* (Optic): Blindness of various types, depending upon the exact location of the lesion. *Third* (Oculomotor): Ptosis (drooping) of eyelid, deviation of the eyeball outward, dilatation of the pupil, double vision. *Fourth* (Trochlear): Rotation of the eyeball upward and outward, double vision. *Fifth* (Trigeminal): Sensory root: Pain or loss of sensation in face, forehead, temple, and eye. Motor root: Deviation of the jaw toward paralyzed side, difficulty in chewing. *Sixth* (Abducens): Deviation of the eye outward, double vision. *Seventh* (Facial): Paralysis of all the muscles on one side of the face; inability to wrinkle the forehead, to close the eye, to whistle; deviation of the mouth toward the sound side. *Eighth* (Vestibulocochlear):

Deafness or ringing in the ears; dizziness; nausea and vomiting; reeling. *Ninth* (Glossopharyngeal): Disturbance of taste; difficulty in swallowing. *Tenth* (Vagus): Disease of the vagus nerve is usually limited to one or more of its divisions. Paralysis of the main trunk on one side causes hoarseness and difficulty in swallowing and talking. The commonest disease of the vagus is of its left recurrent branch, which causes hoarseness as its principal manifestation. *Eleventh* (Spinal Accessory): Drooping of the shoulder; inability to rotate the head away from affected side. *Twelfth* (Hypoglossal): Paralysis of one side of the tongue; deviation of tongue toward paralyzed side; thick speech.

craniectomy (krā-nē-ĕk′tŏ-mē) [Gr. kranion, skull, + ektome, excision]. Opening of skull and removal of a portion of it.

NURSING IMPLICATIONS: Assess neurologic status every 15 to 30 minutes for the first 12 hours postoperatively, then every hour for the next 12 hours, then every 4 hours depending on stability. This assessment should include level of consciousness, pupillary signs, ocular movement, verbal response, sensory and motor function, mental and behavioral status, and vital signs (particularly respiratory patterns). Report patterns indicating deterioration. Serum electrolyte levels should be evaluated as necessary because decreased sodium, chloride, or potassium levels can alter neurologic signs, and treatment of change in condition should be based on etiology.

cranio- [Gr. kranion, L. cranium, skull]. Prefix pert. to the skull or cranium.

cranioacromial (krā″nē-ō-ă-krō′mē-ăl) [Gr. kranion, skull, + akron, extremity]. Rel. to the cranium and the acromion.

craniocaudal (krā″nē-ō-kawd′ăl) [″ + L. cauda, tail]. Direction from head to foot.

craniocele (krā′nē-ō-sēl) [″ + kele, tumor, swelling]. Protrusion of the brain from the skull. SEE: encephalocele.

craniocerebral (krā″nē-ō-sĕr-ē′brăl) [″ + L. cerebrum, brain]. Rel. to the skull and brain.

cranioclasis (krā″nē-ŏk′lă-sĭs) [″ + klasis, fracture]. Crushing of the fetal head to permit delivery.

cranioclast (krā′nē-ō-klăst) [″ + klastos, broken]. Instrument for crushing fetal skull to facilitate delivery, esp. of a dead or deformed fetus.

cranioclasty (krā′nē-ō-klăs″tē). Crushing of fetal head in dystocia.

craniocleidodysostosis (krā″nē-ō-klī″dō-dĭs-ŏs-tō′sĭs) [″ + kleis, clavicle, + dys, bad, + osteon, bone, + osis, condition]. A congenital condition that involves defective ossification of bones of head, face,

CRANIAL NERVES

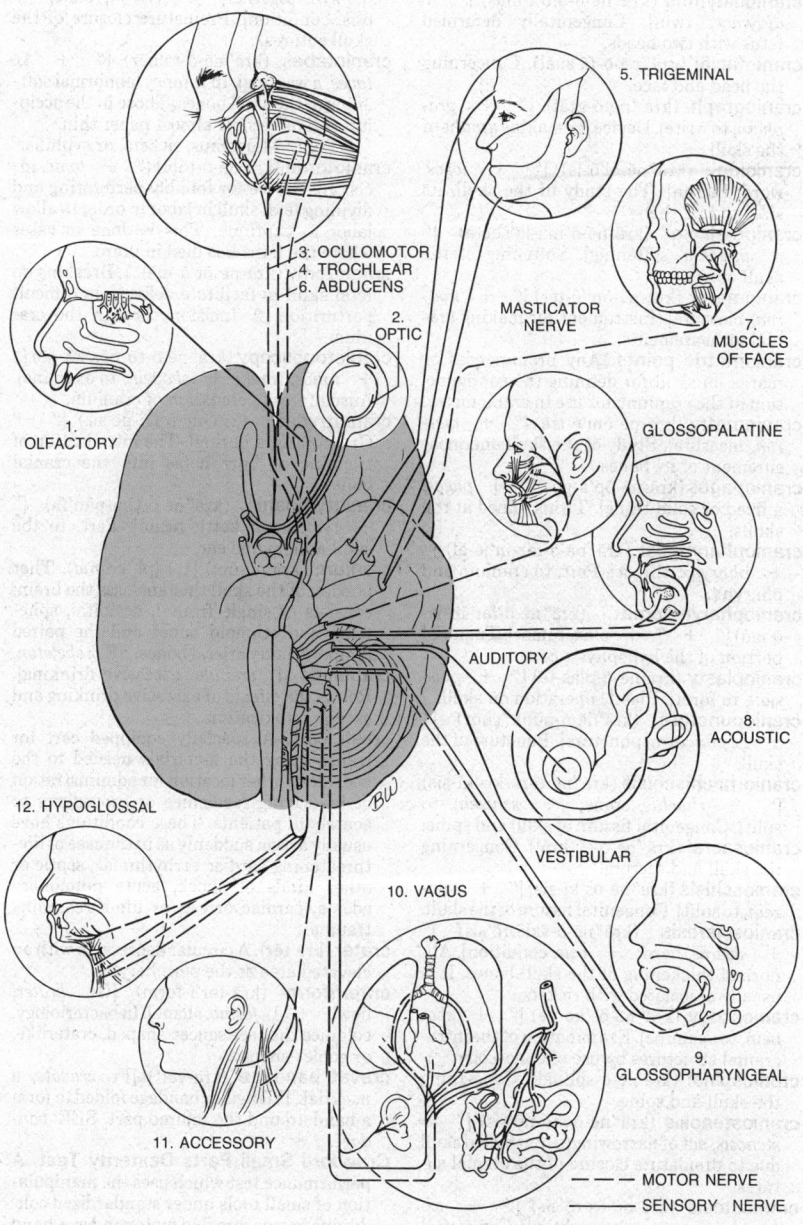

1. OLFACTORY

2. OPTIC

3. OCULOMOTOR
4. TROCHLEAR
6. ABDUCENS

5. TRIGEMINAL

MASTICATOR NERVE

7. MUSCLES OF FACE

GLOSSOPALATINE

AUDITORY

8. ACOUSTIC

VESTIBULAR

12. HYPOGLOSSAL

10. VAGUS

9. GLOSSOPHARYNGEAL

11. ACCESSORY

- - - MOTOR NERVE
—— SENSORY NERVE

and clavicles.

craniodidymus (krā″nē-ō-dĭd′ĭ-mŭs) [″ + *didymos,* twin]. Congenitally deformed fetus with two heads.

craniofacial (krā″nē-ō-fā′shăl). Concerning the head and face.

craniograph (krā′nē-ō-grăf) [″ + *graphein,* to write]. Device for making graphs of the skull.

craniology (krā″nē-ŏl′ō-jē) [″ + *logos,* word, reason]. The study of the skull, its size, and its shape.

craniomalacia (krā-nē-ō-mă-lā′shē-ă) [″ + *malakia,* softening]. Softening of the skull bones.

craniometer (krā-nē-ŏm′ĕ-tĕr) [″ + *metron,* measure]. Instrument for making cranial measurements.

craniometric points. Any prominences or marks on skull for defining the configuration of the cranium; for use in craniometry.

craniometry (krā-nē-ŏm′ĕ-trē) [″ + *metron,* measure]. Study of the skull and measurement of its bones.

craniopagus (krā-nē-ŏp′ă-gŭs) [″ + *pagos,* a fixed or solid thing]. Twins joined at the skulls.

craniopharyngeal (krā″nē-ō-făr-ĭn′jē-ăl) [″ + *pharynx,* throat]. Pert. to cranium and pharynx.

craniopharyngioma (krā″nē-ō-făr-ĭn-jē-ō′mă) [″ + ″ + *oma,* tumor]. Tumor of portion of the hypophysis cerebri.

cranioplasty (krā′nē-ō-plăs-tē) [″ + *plassein,* to form]. Plastic operation on skull.

craniopuncture (krā′nē-ō-pŭnk″chūr) [″ + L. *punctura,* puncture]. Puncture of the skull.

craniorhachischisis (krā″nē-ō-ră-kĭs′kĭ-sĭs) [″ + *rhachis,* spine, + *schizein,* to split]. Congenital fissure of skull and spine.

craniosacral (krā″nē-ō-sā′krăl). Concerning the skull and sacrum.

cranioschisis (krā″nē-ŏs′kĭ-sĭs) [″ + *schizein,* to split]. Congenital fissure of the skull.

cranioclerosis (krā″nē-ō-sklē-rō′sĭs) [″ + *skleros,* hard, + *osis,* condition]. Abnormal thickening of the skull bones. It is usually associated with rickets.

cranioscopy (krā″nē-ŏs′kō-pē) [″ + *skopein,* to examine]. Examination of the intracranial structures by use of endoscopy.

craniospinal (krā′nē-ō-spī′năl). Concerning the skull and spine.

craniostenosis (krā″nē-ō-stē-nō′sĭs) [″ + *stenosis,* act of narrowing]. Contracted skull due to premature closure of the cranial sutures.

craniostosis (krā-nē-ō-ŏs-tō′sĭs) [″ + *osteon,* bone, + *osis,* condition]. Congenital ossification of cranial sutures.

craniosynostosis (krā″nē-ō-sĭn″ŏs-tō′sĭs) [″ + *syn,* together, + *osteon,* bone, + *osis,* condition]. Premature closure of the skull sutures.

craniotabes (krā″nē-ō-tā′bēz) [″ + L. *tabes,* a wasting]. In infancy, abnormal softening of the skull bones. Those in the occipital region become almost paper thin.

ETIOL: Marasmus, rickets, or syphilis.

craniotome (krā′nē-ō-tōm) [″ + *tome,* incision]. Device for forcibly perforating and dividing fetal skull in labor in order to allow labor to continue. This is done in cases where the fetus has died in utero.

craniotomy (krā-nē-ŏt′ō-mē). 1. Breaking up fetal skull to facilitate delivery in difficult parturition. 2. Incision through the cranium.

craniotonoscopy (krā″nē-ō-tō-nŏs′kō-pē) [″ + *tonos,* tone, + *skopein,* to examine]. Auscultatory percussion of cranium.

craniotrypesis (krā″nē-ō-trĭ-pē′sĭs) [″ + Gr. *trypesis,* a boring]. The introduction of trephine or burr holes into the cranial bones.

craniotympanic (krā″nē-ō-tĭm-păn′ĭk) [″ + *tympanon,* kettle-drum]. Pert. to the skull and middle ear.

cranium (krā′nē-ŭm) [L.] (pl. *crania*). That portion of the skull that encloses the brain; consists of single frontal, occipital, sphenoid, and ethmoid bones and the paired temporal and parietal bones. SEE: *skeleton.*

crapulous (L. *crapula,* excessive drinking). Rel. to the effects of excessive drinking and eating; intoxication.

crash cart. A specially equipped cart for transporting the materials needed to the bedside or other location for administration of life-saving medicines or procedures to acutely ill patients. These conditions have usually arisen suddenly as in the case of life-threatening cardiac arrhythmias, septic or other kinds of shock, acute pulmonary edema, cardiac arrest, or life-threatening trauma.

crater (krā′tĕr). A circular depression with an elevated area at the periphery.

crateriform (krā-tĕr′ĭ-form) [Gr. *krater,* bowl, + L. *forma,* shape]. In bacteriology, colonies that are saucer-shaped, craterlike, or goblet-shaped.

cravat bandage (kră-văt′) [Fr. *cravate,* a necktie]. Triangular bandage folded to form a band around the injured part. SEE: *bandage.*

Crawford Small Parts Dexterity Test. A performance test which uses the manipulation of small tools under standardized conditions to measure fine motor and eye-hand coordination.

crazing. Minute fissures on the surface of natural or artificial teeth.

crazy bone. Colloquial term for the medial epicondyle of the humerus; striking it will often cause tingling in the fingers due to the effect on the adjacent ulnar nerve.

C-reactive protein. A globulin that in the presence of calcium ions precipitates the C substance, q.v., of pneumococcal cells. C-reactive protein is an abnormal protein detectable in blood only during the active phase of certain acute illnesses, esp. rheumatic fever.

cream. The fat portion of milk. When untreated milk is allowed to stand undisturbed, the cream rises to the top of the container. The fat content of cream is very high.

cream of tartar. $KHC_4H_4O_6$. Potassium bitartrate.

crease (krēs) [ME. *crest,* crest]. A line produced by a fold.

   c., gluteofemoral. The crease that bounds the inferior border of the buttocks.

creatinase (krē-ăt′in-ās) [Gr. *kreas,* flesh, + *-ase,* enzyme]. An enzyme that decomposes creatinine.

creatine (krē′ă-tĭn) [Gr. *kreas,* flesh]. $NH{:}C(NH_2)N(CH_3) \cdot CH_2COOH + H_2O$. Methylglycocyamine; a colorless, crystalline substance that can be isolated from various animal organs and body fluids. It combines readily with phosphate to form phosphocreatine (creatine phosphate), which serves as a source of high-energy phosphate released in the anaerobic phase of muscle contraction. Found esp. in muscle juice and in blood. Creatine may be present in a greater quantity in the urine of women than men. Creatine excretion is increased in pregnancy and decreased in hypothyroidism.

creatine kinase. Enzyme present in skeletal and cardiac muscle and the brain. Catalyzes the reversible transfer of high-energy phosphate between creatine and phosphocreatine and between adenosine diphosphate (ADP) and adenosine triphosphate (ATP). Serum level is increased 10 to 25 times the normal level in the first few hours following myocardial infarction. The level returns to normal within two to four days. Serum levels are also increased in progressive muscular dystrophy and following trauma to skeletal muscle. It is not elevated in liver disease or pulmonary infarction.

creatinemia (krē″ă-tĭn-ē′mē-ă) [″ + *haima,* blood]. Excess of creatine in circulating blood.

creatinine (krē-ăt′ĭn-ĭn) [Gr. *kreas,* flesh]. $C_4H_7ON_3$. 1-methylglycocyamidine, the end product of creatine metabolism. It also can be isolated as colorless crystals from animal material. Increased quantities of it are found in advanced stages of renal disease. It is a normal, alkaline constituent of urine and blood. About 0.02 gm/kg of body weight is excreted by the kidneys per day.

creatinine phosphokinase. Improper term for creatine kinase.

creatinuria (krē-ă″tĭn-ū′rē-ă) [″ + *ouron,* urine]. Excess concentration of creatinine in urine.

creativity and mental illness. The most important qualities of genius, i.e., persons with high levels of creativity, are high intelligence, a special aptitude, persistence, adventurousness, and intellectual courage. It has long been suggested that persons who are highly creative are more likely to be mentally ill than those who are not creative. Modern studies support this possibility. There is, however, no basis for believing that a person has to be mentally ill in order to be highly creative.

creatorrhea (krē″ă-tō-rē′ă) [″ + *rhoia,* flow]. The presence of undigested muscle fibers in the feces, seen in some cases of pancreatic disease.

Credé's method (krā-dāz′) [Karl S.F. Credé, Ger. gynecologist, 1819–1892]. 1. The means whereby the placenta is expelled by downward pressure on the uterus through the abdominal wall with the thumb on the posterior surface of the fundus uteri and the flat of the hand on the anterior surface, the pressure being applied in the direction of the birth canal. This may cause inversion of the uterus if done improperly. 2. For treatment of the eyes of the newborn, the use of 1% silver nitrate solution instilled into the eyes immediately after birth for the prevention of ophthalmia neonatorum (gonorrheal ophthalmia), q.v. 3. For emptying a flaccid bladder, pressure is placed over the symphysis pubis to expel the urine periodically.

cremains [contraction of cre*mated* re*mains*]. That which remains after the body has been prepared for burial by cremation.

cremaster (krē-măs′tĕr) [L., to suspend]. One of the fascia-like muscles suspending and enveloping the testicles and spermatic cord.

cremasteric (krē-măs′tĕr-ĭk). Pert. to the cremaster muscle.

cremasteric fascia. One of the coverings of the spermatic cord.

cremasteric reflex. Retraction of testis when skin is stroked on front inner side of thigh.

cremate (krē′māt) [L. *crematio,* a burning]. To dispose of the body of a dead person by burning. The ashes may or may not be buried.

crematorium (krē″mă-tō′rē-ŭm) [L.]. A place for the burning of corpses.

crenate (krē′nāt) [L. *crenatus*]. Notched or scalloped, as crenated condition of blood corpuscles.

crenation (krē-nā′shŭn). The conversion of normally round red corpuscles into shrunken, knobbed, starry forms, as when blood is mixed with salt solution of 5% strength. SEE: *plasmolysis.*

crenocyte (krē′nō-sīt). Crenated red blood cell.

creosote (krē′ō-sōt) [Gr. *kreas*, flesh, + *sozein*, to preserve]. A mixture of phenols obtained from the destructive distillation of coal or wood. This toxic substance has been used as a disinfectant and as a preserver of wood.

crepitant (krĕp′ĭ-tănt) [L. *crepitare*]. Crackling; having or making a crackling sound.

crepitation (krĕp-ĭ-tā′shŭn). 1. A crackling sound heard in certain diseases, as the rale heard in pneumonia. 2. A grating sound heard on movement of ends of a broken bone. 3. A clicking or crackling sound often heard in movements of joints, such as the temporomandibular, elbow or patellofemoral joints, due to roughness and irregularities in the articulating surfaces. SEE: *temporomandibular joint syndrome.*

crepitus (krĕp′ĭ-tŭs) [L.]. 1. The noise of gas discharged from the intestines. 2. Crepitation.

    c., joint. Crepitus felt when a joint is moved. May be present when osteoarthritis has caused degeneration of a joint.

    c. redux. Rale indicating approaching recovery in pneumonia.

crepuscular (krē-pŭs′kū-lăr) [L. *crepusculum*, twilight]. Pert. to twilight; used to describe twilight mental state.

crescent (krĕs′ĕnt) [L. *crescens*]. Shaped like a sickle or the new moon.

    c., articular. A crescent-shaped cartilage present in certain joints as the menisci of the knee joint.

    c., myopic. Grayish patch in fundus or eye due to atrophy of choroid.

    c. of Giannuzzi. A crescent-shaped group of serous cells lying at the base of or along the side of a mucous alveolus of a salivary gland.

crescent bodies. Achromocytes, q.v.

crescentic (krĕs-ĕn′tĭk). Sickle-shaped.

Crescormon. Trade name for somatropin.

cresol (krē′sŏl). Yellow-brown liquid obtained from coal tar and containing not more than 5% of phenol.

    USE: A disinfectant in a 1% to 5% solution for articles or areas that do not come in

direct contact with food.

cresomania, croesomania (krē″sō-mā′nē-ă) [Croesus, wealthy king of Lydia, 6th century B.C.]. Hallucination of possessing great wealth.

crest [L. *crista*, crest]. A ridge or an elongated prominence, esp. one on a bone.

    c., alveolar. The most coronal portion of the bone surrounding the tooth; the continuous upper ridge of bone of the alveolar process, which is usually the first bone lost as a result of periodontal disease.

CREST syndrome [Calcinosis, *R*aynaud's (phenomenon), *E*sophageal (dysfunction), *S*clerodactyly, *T*elangiectasia]. Scleroderma, q.v. SYN: *progressive systemic sclerosis.*

cretin (krē′tĭn) [Fr.]. One afflicted with congenital myxedema due to lack of thyroid secretion. Characterized by lack of growth and mental development; the patient rarely if ever exceeds the mental age of 10. The skin is rough and dry, and the hair coarse, dry, and brittle. Teeth erupt slowly and are of poor quality and irregularly placed. The tongue is large and apt to protrude from a mouth that constantly drools saliva. A child with cretinism is characteristically potbellied, swaybacked, and prone to umbilical hernia. SEE: *cretinism.*

cretinism (krē′tĭn-ĭzm) [″ + Gr. *-ismos*, condition]. Congenital condition due to lack of thyroid secretion, characterized by arrested physical and mental development, dystrophy of the bones and soft parts, and lowered basal metabolism. The acquired form of this disease is myxedema, q.v.

    SYM: Myxedema, and impaired mental ability.

    ETIOL: A congenital deficiency in secretion of the thyroid hormones.

    TREAT: Appropriate thyroid preparation.

cretinoid (krē′tĭ-noyd) [″ + Gr. *eidos*, form, shape]. Having the symptoms of cretinism, or resembling a cretin, due to a congenital condition.

cretinous (krē′tĭ-nŭs). Pert. to a cretin or to cretinism.

Creutzfeldt-Jakob disease [Hans Gerhard Creutzfeldt, 1855–1964; Alfons Maria Jakob, 1884–1931. Both were German psychiatrists]. ABBR: CJD. A central nervous system disease that causes presenile dementia, myoclonus, and distinctive EEG changes.

    ETIOL: Unknown, but assumed to be a slow virus. The infectious agent has been isolated but has not been identified. CJD has developed in the recipient of a cornea from a donor with CJD.

    TREAT: None.

COURSE: Fatal.

Caution: The causative agent of CJD is extremely resistant to most sterilization procedures; thus, the same precautions as used for AIDS should be exercised when handling body fluids and tissues from patients with CJD. SEE: *Universal Precautions* in *Appendix.*

crevice (krĕv'ĭs) [Fr. *crever*, to break]. A small fissure or crack.
  c., gingival. The fissure produced by the marginal gingiva with the tooth surface.
crevicular (krĕv-ĭk'ū-lăr). Pert. to the gingival crevice.
CRF. *corticotrophin-releasing factor,* esp. the substance present in extract of the hypothalamus that brings about the release of ACTH from the anterior pituitary.
crib (krĭb) [AS. *cribbe,* manger]. 1. A framework around a denture or a natural tooth to serve as a brace or supporting structure. 2. A small bed with long legs and high sides for an infant or young child.
cribbing (krĭb'ĭng). Aerophagia; swallowing air.
crib death. SEE: *sudden infant death syndrome.*
cribrate (krĭb'rāt) [L. *cribratus*]. Profusely pitted or perforated like a sieve.
cribration (krĭb-rā'shŭn). The state of being perforated.
cribriform (krĭb'rĭ-form) [L. *cribrum,* a sieve, + *forma,* form]. Sievelike.
cribriform fascia. The portion of deep fascia that covers the fossa ovalis of the thigh.
cribriform plate. The thin, perforated, medial portion of the horizontal plate of the ethmoid bone. Also, a synonym for alveolar bone proper, the sievelike layer of bone that makes up the wall of the socket and supports the tooth.
crick. A muscle spasm or cramp, esp. in the neck.
cricoarytenoid (krī"kō-ă-rĭt'ĕn-oyd) [Gr. *krikos,* ring, + *arytaina,* pitcher, + *eidos,* form, shape]. Extending between the cricoid and arytenoid cartilages.
cricoderma (krī-kō-dĕr'mă) [" + *derma,* skin]. Ring-shaped infiltrations in center of indurations on the skin.
cricoid (krī'koyd) [" + *eidos,* form, shape]. Shaped like a signet ring.
cricoid cartilage. The lowermost cartilage of the larynx. It is shaped like a signet ring, the broad portion or lamina being posterior, the anterior portion forming the arch.
cricoidectomy (krī"koyd-ĕk'tō-mē) [" + " + *ektome,* excision]. Excision of cricoid cartilage.
cricoidynia (krī-koy-dĭn'ē-ă) [" + " + *odyne,* pain]. Pain in cricoid cartilage.

cricopharyngeal (krī"kō-făr-ĭn'jē-ăl) [" + *pharynx,* throat]. Pert. to the cricoid cartilage and pharynx.
cricothyroid (krī-kō-thī'royd) [" + *thyreos,* shield, + *eidos,* form, shape]. Pert. to the thyroid and cricoid cartilages.
cricothyrotomy (krī"kō-thī-rŏt'ō-mē) [" + " + *tome,* incision]. Division of the cricoid and thyroid cartilages.
cricotomy (krī-kŏt'ō-mē) [" + *tome,* incision]. Division of the cricoid cartilage.
cricotracheotomy (krī"kō-trā"kē-ŏt'ō-mē) [" + *tracheia,* windpipe, + *tome,* incision]. Division of the cricoid cartilage and upper trachea in closure of the glottis.
cri du chat syndrome (krē-dū-shä). A hereditary congenital anomaly so named because the infant's cry resembles the cry of a cat. Characterized by mental retardation, microcephaly, dwarfism, epicanthal folds, and laryngeal defect. Due to a deletion of the short arm of chromosome 4 or 5 of the B group.
Crigler-Najjar syndrome (krĕg'lĕr-nă'här) [John Fielding Crigler, U.S. physician, b. 1919; Victor A. Najjar, U.S. physician, b. 1914]. A familial form of congenital hyperbilirubinemia associated with brain damage and resembling kernicterus. The syndrome is caused by an enzyme deficiency in the liver and faulty bilirubin conjugation. Transmitted as an autosomal recessive trait; death usually occurs within 15 months after birth.
criminal [L. *crimen,* crime]. 1. Pert. to crime. 2. A person who has committed or been convicted of a crime.
criminology (krĭm"ĭ-nŏl'ō-jē). Scientific study of criminals and their relation to society.
crinogenic (krĭn"ō-jĕn'ĭk) [Gr. *krinein,* to secrete, + *gennan,* to produce]. Producing or stimulating secretion.
cripple. 1. An individual without full use of the body, esp. the arms or legs. 2. One who is physically traumatized with resulting inability to use part of the body.
crisis (krī'sĭs) [Gr. *krisis,* turning point] (pl. *crises*). 1. The turning point of a disease; a very critical period often marked by a long sleep and profuse perspiration. 2. The term used for the sudden descent of a high temperature to normal or below; generally occurs within 24 hours. 3. Sharp paroxysms of pain occurring over the course of a few days in certain diseases. 4. In counseling, an unstable period in a person's life characterized by inability to adapt to a change resulting from a precipitating event.
  c., abdominal. General term for severe abdominal pain due to many possible causes.

c., addisonian. Acute failure of the adrenal gland.

c., celiac. Rapid onset of malnutrition in celiac disease with severe watery diarrhea, vomiting, dehydration, and acidosis. Vigorous antibiotic and nutritional therapy is required.

c., Dietl's. Sudden, severe attack of gastric pain, chills, fever, nausea, and general collapse. In cases of floating kidney, the ureter becomes kinked and urine is obstructed, producing symptoms of renal colic.

c., salt-losing. Acute vomiting, dehydration, hypotension, and sudden death as a result of acute loss of sodium. May be caused by adrenal hyperplasia, salt-losing nephritis, or gastrointestinal disease.

c., sickle cell. Severe abdominal pain due to sickle cell anemia.

c., tabetic. Abdominal pain due to syphilis.

c., thyroid. Sudden increase in severity of symptoms of thyrotoxicosis; marked by fever and extreme tachycardia. Outcome occasionally fatal. SYN: *thyroid storm*, q.v.

c., true. Temperature drop accompanied by a fall in the pulse rate.

crisis intervention. Problem-solving activity intended to correct or prevent the continuation of a crisis, as in poison control centers or suicide prevention services. Usually these activities are mediated through telephone services manned by professional or paraprofessional workers in the medical and social fields. SEE: *Poison Control Centers* in *Appendix*.

crispation (krĭs-pā'shŭn) [L. *crispare*, to curl]. Mild involuntary muscle twitching that causes a sensation of creeping of the skin.

crista (krĭs'tă) [L.] (pl. *cristae*). 1. [NA] A crest or ridge. 2. A projection, sometimes branched, of the inner wall of a mitochondrion into its fluid-filled cavity.

c. ampullaris. [NA] A localized thickening of the membrane lining the ampullae of the semicircular canals; it is covered with neuroepithelium containing auditory cells.

c. galli. [NA] A ridge on the ethmoid bone to which the falx cerebri is attached.

c. lacrimalis posterior. [NA] A vertical ridge on the lateral surface of the lacrimal bone.

c. spiralis. A ridge on the spiral lamina of the cochlea, q.v.

criterion (krī-tē'rē-ŏn) [Gr. *kriterion*, a means for judging] (pl. *criteria*). Standard or attribute for judging a condition or establishing a diagnosis.

critical (krĭt'ĭ-kăl) [Gr. *kritikos*, critical]. 1. Pert. to a crisis. 2. Dangerous.

critical pathway. A statement of nursing and medical processes which must occur in an expected period of time to achieve an appropriate length of stay within an acute care setting. The timing of diagnostic tests, consultations, medications, treatments, and discharge plans are stated as standards of care in order to promote the coordination of continuity of care.

critical period. 1. Phase of life cycle during which cells are responsive to certain regulators. 2. The time during gestation when important organ systems are being formed and during which the fetus is most vulnerable to environmental factors that may cause deformities.

CRNA. *certified registered nurse anesthetist.*

crocodile tears. 1. Excess tear production that occurs when salivary glands are stimulated during eating in patients with incomplete recovery from facial paralysis. 2. Tears produced as an insincere display of grief or concern. So named because crocodiles allegedly weep after eating their victims.

Crohn's disease (krōnz) [Burrill B. Crohn, U.S. gastroenterologist, b. 1884]. Regional ileitis; regional enteritis. SEE: *ileitis, regional*. SEE: *Nursing Diagnoses* in *Appendix*.

cromolyn sodium (krō'mŏ-lĭn). Disodium cromoglycate, a medicine unrelated to steroids or epinephrine that is quite useful in treating airway obstruction associated with asthma. This medicine is used in children and young adults as maintenance therapy. It is of no benefit in treating acute attacks of asthma. Trade name is Intal.

Crookes' dark space [Sir William Crookes, Brit. physicist, 1832–1919]. Nonluminous region enveloping outline of the cathode in a discharge tube. SEE: *cathode.*

Crookes' tube. An early form of vacuum discharge tube used for the study of cathode rays.

Crosby capsule [William Holmes Crosby, Jr., U.S. physician, b. 1914]. A device attached to a flexible tube that is introduced into the gastrointestinal tract per os. It is designed so that a sample of tissue may be obtained from the mucosal surface with which it is in contact. The capsule is then removed and the tissue examined for evidence of pathological changes.

cross [L. *crux*]. 1. Any structure or figure in the shape of a cross. 2. In genetics, the mating or the offspring of the mating of two individuals of different strains, varieties, or species.

crossbirth. Presentation of the fetus where the long axis of the fetus is at right angles to that of the mother and requires version.

cross bite. A form of dental malocclusion in the buccolingual direction.

crossbreeding. Mating of individuals of different breeds or strains.

cross-bridges. In the fine structure of muscles, the thick and thin elements of the A bands of the myofibrils intermix to form dark bands.

cross-dress. To dress in clothing appropriate for one of the opposite sex.

crossed. Passing from one side to the other, as crossed pyramidal tract, in which nerve fibers cross from one side of the medulla to the other.

crossed finger airway technique. Method used to open an unconscious patient's mouth by placing thumb and index finger on opposite rows of teeth and spreading the jaw open.

crossed reflexes. 1. Passive flexion of one part following flexion of another. 2. Passive flexion of one leg causing similar movement of opposite leg.

cross education. Contralateral facilitation or changes resulting from exercise.

cross-eye. Manifest inward deviation of the visual axis of one eye toward that of the other eye when looking at an object. SYN: *esotropia.* SEE: *squint; strabismus.*

cross-fertilization. The fusion of male and female gametes from different individuals.

crossing over. In genetics, the mutual interchange of blocks of genes between two homologous chromosomes. It occurs during synapsis in meiosis.

crossmatching. Test to establish blood compatibility before transfusion. SEE: *blood groups.*

crossover. The result of the reciprocal exchange of genetic material between chromosomes.

cross-training. To train someone in two or more different fields of specialization, e.g., an operating room nurse who is also trained to be an intensive care nurse. This may permit more efficient utilization of the staff.

Crotalus (krŏt′ă-lŭs) [Gr. *krotalon,* rattle]. A genus of snakes that includes most rattlesnakes. All are highly poisonous.

crotamiton (krō″tă-mī′tŏn). USP. An effective scabicide. Eurax is the trade name for a preparation of which crotamiton is a component.

crotaphion (krō-tăf′ē-ŏn) [Gr. *krotaphos,* the temple]. Tip of greater wing of sphenoid bone.

crotonism (krō′tŏn-ĭzm). Poisoning from croton oil.

croton oil (krō′tŏn) [Gr. *kroton,* castor oil plant seed]. Oleum tiglii; a fixed oil expressed from the seed of the croton plant, *Croton tiglium.*

ACTION: Drastic cathartic; externally as a rubefacient. Because this substance is toxic, it is no longer used.

croup (croop). Childhood disease characterized by a resonant barking cough, suffocative and difficult breathing, laryngeal spasm, and sometimes by the formation of a membrane.

NURSING IMPLICATIONS: Evaluate child for respiratory distress: rate and character of respiration, use of accessory muscles, intercostal retractions, substernal retraction, nasal flaring, inspiratory stridor, barking cough. Provide a high humidity atmosphere with cool moisture if fever is present, keeping patient dry to prevent chilling. Approach child and parents in a calm manner to reduce fears and anxiety. Administer prescribed drugs, orally or by nebulization; evaluate response and assess for side effects. SEE: *Nursing Diagnoses* in *Appendix.*

  c., catarrhal. Acute catarrhal laryngitis.

  c., diphtheritic. Diphtheria of the larynx.

  c., membranous. Inflammation of larynx with exudation forming a false membrane. SYN: *laryngitis, croupous.* SEE: *Nursing Diagnoses* in *Appendix.*

SYM: Those of laryngitis; loss of voice; noisy, difficult, and stridulous breathing; weak, rapid pulse; livid skin; moderate fever.

ETIOL: Several viruses may cause this disease. These include parainfluenza, respiratory syncytial, various influenza viruses.

TREAT: Humidification of the air by whatever means is available such as vaporizers or steam. Antibiotics are indicated only if there is secondary bacterial infection. Corticosteroids are of no benefit. If hypoxia is present, inhalation of 40% concentration of well-humidified oxygen is indicated. This is best accomplished by use of a face mask.

PROG: Grave, unless tracheostomy has been performed. The illness usually subsides in three to four days. SEE: *carpopedal spasm; steam tent.*

  c., spasmodic. Recurrent attacks of croup.

croupous (kroo′pŭs). Pert. to croup or having a fibrinous exudation.

Crouzon's disease (kroo-zŏnz′) [Octave Crouzon, Fr. neurologist, 1874–1938]. Congenital disease characterized by hypertelorism (widely spaced eyes), craniofacial dysostosis, exophthalmos, optic atrophy, and divergent squint.

crowing (krō′ĭng). A noisy, harsh sound on inspiration.

crown [L. *corona,* wreath]. The top or highest part of an organ, tooth, or other structure, as the top of the head. Corona [NA].

c., anatomic. The true crown of the tooth formed of enamel.

c., clinical. That portion of the tooth seen above the gingiva; i.e., visible in the mouth.

crowning [L. *corona*, wreath]. Stage in delivery when fetal head presents at the vulva. Crowning occurs when the largest diameter of the infant's head comes through the vulvar opening.

crownwork. Artificial crown for a tooth.

CRP. *C-reactive protein.*

CRT. *cathode-ray tube.*

CRTT. *certified respiratory therapy technician.*

crucial (kroo'shăl) [L. *crucialis*]. 1. Cross-shaped. 2. Decisive; of supreme importance; critical.

cruciate (kroo'shē-āt). Cross-shaped, as in the cruciate ligaments of the knee.

crucible (kroo'sĭ-b'l) [L. *crucibulum*]. A dish or container for substances that are being melted, burned, or dehydrated while exposed to high temperatures.

cruciform (kroo'sĭ-form) [L. *crux*, cross, + *forma*, shape]. Shaped like a cross.

crude (krood) [L. *crudus*, raw]. Raw, unrefined, or in a natural state.

crura (kroo'ră) [L., legs] (sing. *crus*). A pair of elongated masses or diverging bands, resembling legs.

c. cerebelli. Cerebellar peduncles.

c. cerebri. Pair of bands joining cerebrum to medulla and pons.

c. of diaphragm. Two pillars connecting spinal column and diaphragm.

c. of the fornix. Arches made by division of the fornicate extremities.

crural (kroo'răl) [L. *cruralis*] Pert. to the leg or thigh; femoral.

crural arch. Femoral arch.

crural hernia. Femoral hernia.

crural nerve. Femoral nerve. SEE: *Nerves* in *Appendix.*

crural palsies. Palsies of the nerves of the legs (e.g., 12th thoracic, 1st to 5th lumbar, and 1st to 3rd sacral spinal nerves).

crus (krŭs) [L.] (pl. *crura*). [NA] 1. The leg. 2. Any structure resembling the leg.

c. cerebri. [NA] Either of the two peduncles connecting the cerebrum with the pons.

crush syndrome. The result of prolonged, continuous pressure on large muscles, e.g., the legs or arms. As a result of the trauma, the muscle tissue disintegrates. Once the pressure is released and circulation is restored, myoglobin, potassium, and phosphorus leak into the circulation. If left untreated, hypovolemic shock and hyperkalemia are followed by acute renal failure. This condition, also known as traumatic

rhabdomyolysis, is associated with a high rate of morbidity and mortality. SEE: *renal failure, acute; reperfusion; rhabdomyolysis.*

crust [L. *crusta*]. 1. A scab. A secondary lesion; dry serous or seropurulent, brown, yellow, red, or green exudations on a free surface. Seen in eczema, seborrhea, syphilis, impetigo, favus, and ringworm of the scalp. 2. An outer covering or coat.

crusta [L.] (pl. *crustae*). Crust.

crutch [AS. *crycc*]. 1. A device for aiding a paralyzed, weak, or injured person in walking. Usually a long staff with padded crescent-shaped portion at the top for placing under the armpit. A great variety of crutches and devices that serve the same purpose are available; the most common is the axillary; various forms of walkers that provide a mobile stable platform that the patient holds on to while walking; forearm crutch or lofstrand crutch that provides points of contact between the hand and the forearm; the shelf crutch, an adapted forearm crutch that permits a person who can't bear weight on the hands to use a crutch; three- or four-legged cane for the person with poor balance who needs mild support. It is important that the patient be instructed as to the proper use of a crutch, as nerve lesions can result from improper use.

NURSING IMPLICATIONS: Depending on the nature of restrictions, teach patient appropriate gaits for crutch walking. Teach patient how to negotiate stairs and inclines and how to move safely through doorways. Instruct patient not to lean on crutches, to sit rather than stand.

2. In psychoanalysis, the use of some affliction that may be real or imaginary to explain personal inadequacy or failure.

Crutchfield tongs [William Gayle Crutchfield, U.S. surgeon, 1900–1972]. Device for inserting into each side of the skull. Traction is then applied parallel to the long axis of the cervical spine by applying traction to the device.

crutch paralysis. Paralysis or weakness of the muscles of the arm(s) as a result of compression of the nerves of the brachial plexus or radial nerve by the head of the crutch. It is important that crutches be fitted so that the weight of the body is borne by the hands and arms, and not by the head of the crutch as it is forced into the axilla.

Cruveilhier-Baumgarten syndrome (kroo-văl-yă'bŏm'găr-tĕn) [Jean Cruveilhier, Fr. pathologist, 1791–1874; Paul Clemens von Baumgarten, Ger. pathologist, 1848–1928]. Cirrhosis of the liver caused by patency of the umbilical or paraumbilical veins and the resultant collateral circulation. It is associated with prominent periumbilical veins, portal hypertension, liver atrophy, and splenomegaly.

cry (krī). Production of inarticulate sounds, with or without weeping, which may be sudden, loud, or quiet as in a sob. These sounds are made in response to a variety of stimuli: fright, fear, pain, apprehension, sadness, glee, or joy. SEE: *cry reflex.*

   c., cephalic. Sudden shrill cry by an infant. May be indicative of cerebral disease.

   c., epileptic. Sudden, loud cry that may accompany the onset of an epileptic seizure.

   c., hydrocephalic. An involuntary night cry by a child with acute tuberculous meningitis or acute-onset hydrocephalus.

   c., night. Any sudden outcry at night. May be caused by onset of acute joint pain.

cryalgesia (krī-ăl-jē′zē-ă) [Gr. *kryos,* cold, + *algos,* pain]. Pain from the application of cold.

cryanesthesia (krī-ăn-ĕs-thē′zē-ă) [″ + *an-,* not, + *aisthesis,* sensation]. Loss of sense of cold.

cryesthesia (krī-ĕs-thē′zē-ă) [″ + *aisthesis,* sensation]. Sensitiveness to the cold.

cry for help. Actions of individuals who are potentially suicidal or severely depressed to inform others of their distress. This may be done by leaving cryptic messages or making phone calls that are later interpreted to mean that the individual was asking for help more or less covertly.

crymodynia (krī″mō-dĭn′ē-ă) [Gr. *krymos,* frost, + *odyne,* pain]. Pain from cold, esp. rheumatic pain aggravated by cold or damp weather.

crymophilic (krī″mō-fĭl′ĭk) [″ + *philein,* to love]. Showing preference for cold, as in psychrophilic bacteria. SYN: *cryophilic.*

crymophylactic (krī″mō-fī-lăk′tĭk) [″ + *phylaxis,* protection]. Resistant to cold.

crymotherapy (krī″mō-thĕr′ă-pē) [″ + *therapeia,* treatment]. The use of cold in treating disease. SYN: *cryotherapy.*

cryo- [Gr. *krymos,* cold]. Combining form concerning cold.

cryoaerotherapy (krī″ō-ĕr-ō-thĕr′ă-pē) [Gr. *kryos,* cold, + *aer,* air, + *therapeia,* treatment]. Cold air bath in which, by degrees, the patient is accustomed to freezing temperature.

cryoanesthesia. SEE: *anesthesia, refrigeration.*

cryobank (krī′ō-bănk). Storage of biological tissues at very low temperatures.

cryobiology (krī″ō-bī-ŏl′ō-jē) [″ + *bios,* life, + *logos,* word, reason]. Study of effect of cold on biological systems.

cryocautery (krī″ō-kaw′tĕr-ē) [″ + *kauter,* a burner]. Device for application of

cold sufficient to kill tissue.

cryoextraction (krī″ō-ĕks-trăk′shŭn). Use of a cooling probe introduced into the lens of the eye to produce an ice ball limited to the lens. The ice ball, which includes the lens, is then removed. Used in treating cataracts.

cryofibrinogen (krī″ō-fī-brĭn′ō-jĕn). An abnormal fibrinogen that precipitates when cooled and dissolves when reheated to body temperature.

cryogen (krī′ō-jĕn) [″ + *gennan,* to produce]. Substance that produces low temperatures.

cryogenic (krī″ō-jĕn′ĭk). Producing or pert. to low temperatures.

cryoglobulin (krī″ō-glŏb′ū-lĭn) [″ + L. *globulus,* globule]. An abnormal protein, globulin, that precipitates when cooled and dissolves when reheated to body temperature.

cryoglobulinemia (krī″ō-glŏb″ū-lĭn-ē′mē-ă) [″ + ″ + Gr. *haima,* blood]. Presence in the blood of an abnormal protein that forms gels at low temperatures. Found in association with pathological conditions such as multiple myeloma, leukemia, and certain forms of pneumonia.

cryohypophysectomy (krī″ō-hī″pō-fīz-ĕk′tō-mē) [Gr. *kryos,* cold, + *hypo,* under, + *physis,* growth, + *ektome,* excision]. Destruction of the hypophysis by use of cold.

cryolesion. 1. The cooling of an area in order to injure or destroy it. This is done for therapeutic reasons. 2. A lesion produced by exposure to cold, e.g., frostbite.

cryometer (krī-ŏm′ĕ-tĕr) [″ + *metron,* measure]. A thermometer for measuring very low temperatures.

cryophilic (krī″ō-fĭl′ĭk) [″ + *philein,* to love]. Showing preference for cold, as in psychrophilic bacteria. SYN: *crymophilic; psychrophilic.*

cryoprecipitate (krī″ō-prē-sĭp′ĭ-tāt). The precipitate formed when serum from patients with rheumatoid arthritis, glomerulonephritis, systemic lupus erythematosus and other chronic diseases in which immune complexes are pathogenic is stored at 4°C. The joint fluid from rheumatoid arthritis patients will also form a precipitate when so stored.

cryopreservation. Preservation of biological materials, such as tissue, sperm, fluids, blood, or plasma at very low temperatures. This enables the tissue to be used in another individual at a later time, as it remains viable after thawing. The technique is used to preserve human semen for artificial insemination.

cryoprobe (krī′ō-prōb). Device for applying

cold to a tissue. Liquid nitrogen is the coolant frequently used. SEE: *cryoextraction*.

cryoprotectants. Drugs that permit cells to survive freezing and thawing.

cryoprotective (krī″ō-prō-tĕk′tĭv). Pert. to a chemical that protects cells from the effect of cold.

cryoprotein (krī″ō-prō′tē-ĭn). Any protein that precipitates when cooled below body temperature. SEE: *cryofibrinogen; cryoglobulin*.

cryospray (krī′ō-sprā). Spraying of liquid nitrogen on tissues in order to destroy them.

cryostat (krī′ō-stăt). Device for maintaining very low temperatures.

cryosurgery (krī″ō-sĕr′jĕr-ē) [″ + ME. *surgerie*, surgery]. Technique of exposing tissues to extreme cold in order to produce well-demarcated areas of cell injury and destruction. The tissue is usually cooled to below −20°C. Used in treating malignant tumors to control pain, to produce lesions in the brain, and to control bleeding. The cold is usually produced by use of a probe through which liquid nitrogen circulates.

cryothalamotomy (krī″ō-thăl″ă-mŏt′ō-mē) [″ + L. *thalamus*, inner chamber, + Gr. *tome*, incision]. Destruction of a portion of the brain by cooling the end of a slender probe placed in the thalamus. This is usually done by circulating liquid nitrogen through the hollow stylus. Has been used in the treatment of parkinsonism.

cryotherapy (krī-ō-thĕr′ă-pē) [″ + *therapeia*, treatment]. The therapeutic use of cold.

cryotolerant (krī″ō-tŏl′ĕr-ănt) [″ + L. *tolerare*, to bear]. Able to tolerate very low temperatures.

crypt (krĭpt) [Gr. *kryptos*, hidden]. 1. A small sac or cavity extending into an epithelial surface. 2. A tubular gland, esp. one of the intestine.

c., anal. One of a number of small indentations lying immediately behind junction of anal skin and rectal mucosa.

c., bony. A space in the bony jaw occupied by a developing tooth. SYN: *dental crypt*.

c. of iris. An irregular excavation on anterior surface of the iris near pupillary and ciliary margins.

c. of Lieberkühn. A tubular gland of the intestine that secretes intestinal juice. Its wall is composed of columnar epithelium containing argentaffin cells and, at the base of the gland, cells of Paneth. They open between bases of the villi.

c., synoviparous. A saclike extension of the synovial cavity into the capsule of a joint. Sometimes they become blind sacs.

c., tonsillar. A deep invagination of the surface-stratified epithelium into substance of the lingual or palatine tonsils. It is surrounded by lymph nodules and may be branched.

cryptamnesia (krĭpt″ăn-ăm-nē′zē-ă) [″ + *an-*, not, + *amnesia*, forgetfulness]. Subconscious memory. SYN: *cryptomnesia*.

cryptectomy (krĭp-tĕk′tō-mē) [″ + *ektome*, excision]. Excision of a crypt.

cryptesthesia (krĭp-tĕs-thē′zē-ă) [″ + *aisthesis*, sensation]. Subconscious awareness of facts or occurrences other than through the senses or through rational thinking, such as intuition or clairvoyance.

cryptic (krĭp′tĭk) [Gr. *kryptikos*, hidden]. 1. Having a hidden meaning; occult. 2. Tending to hide or disguise.

cryptitis (krĭp-tī′tĭs) [Gr. *kryptos*, hidden, + *itis*, inflammation]. Inflammation of a crypt or follicle, esp. an anal crypt.

cryptocephalus (krĭp″tō-sĕf′ă-lŭs) [″ + *kephale*, head]. Congenital deformity in which the head is inapparent.

cryptococcosis (krĭp″tō-kŏk-ō′sĭs) [″ + *kokkos*, berry, + *osis*, condition]. A systemic fungus infection that may involve any organ of the body, lungs, or skin, but having a marked predilection for the brain and its meninges. SYN: *torulosis*.

SYM: Development of single or multiple abscesses. In the cerebral type there is headache, dizziness, vertigo, stiffness of neck muscles; in final stages, coma and respiratory failure. Often mistaken for brain tumor.

ETIOL: *Cryptococcus neoformans (Torula histolytica)*, a fungus.

TREAT: Amphotericin B is somewhat beneficial in certain cases.

PROG: Poor; cerebral and meningeal forms are usually fatal.

Cryptococcus (krĭp″tō-kŏk′ŭs). A genus of pathogenic yeastlike fungi. The causative agent of cryptococcosis. Former term was *Torula*.

cryptodidymus (krĭp-tō-dĭd′ĭ-mŭs) [″ + *didymos*, twin]. A congenital anomaly in which one fetus is concealed within another.

cryptogenic (krĭp″tō-jĕn′ĭk) [″ + *gennan*, to produce]. Of unknown or indeterminate origin.

cryptogenic infection. The invasion of bacteria without outward evidence of entry into the body. SEE: *infection*.

cryptogenic stroke. SEE: *stroke, cryptogenic*.

cryptolith (krĭp′tō-lĭth) [″ + *lithos*, stone]. A concretion in a glandular follicle.

cryptomenorrhea (krĭp″tō-mĕn″ō-rē′ă) [″ + *men*, month, + *rhoia*, flow]. Monthly subjective symptoms of menses without flow of blood. May be caused by an imperforate hymen.

cryptomerorachischisis (krĭp″tō-mē″rō-rǎ-kĭs′kĭ-sĭs) [″ + *meros*, part, + *rhachis*, spine, + *schisis*, a splitting]. Spina bifida occulta without a tumor but with bony deficiency.

cryptomnesia (krĭp-tŏm-nē′zē-ǎ) [″ + *mnesis*, memory]. Subconscious memory. SYN: *cryptanamnesia.*

cryptophthalmus (krĭp″tŏf-thǎl′mŭs) [″ + *ophthalmos*, eye]. Complete congenital adhesion of eyelids to globe of eye.

cryptoplasmic (krĭp″tō-plǎz′mĭk) [″ + LL. *plasma*, form, mold]. Having existence in a concealed form.

cryptopodia (krĭp″tō-pō′dē-ǎ) [Gr. *kryptos*, hidden, + *pous*, foot]. Fibromata of feet so diffuse as to resemble pads.

cryptopyic (krĭp″tō-pī′ĭk) [″ + *pyon*, pus]. Having concealed suppuration, as a pyemia without apparent etiology.

cryptorchid, cryptorchis (krĭpt-or′kĭd, -or′kĭs) [″ + *orchis*, testis]. An individual with testicles that have not descended into the scrotum.

cryptorchidectomy (krĭpt″or-kĭ-dĕk′tō-mē) [″ + ″ + *ektome*, excision]. Operation for correction of an undescended testicle.

cryptorchidism, cryptorchism (krĭpt-or′kĭd-ĭzm, -kĭzm) [″ + *orchis*, testis, + *-ismos*, condition]. Failure of testicles to descend into scrotum.

cryptorrhea (krĭp-tō-rē′ǎ) [″ + *rhoia*, flow]. Excessive secretion of a ductless gland.

cryptorrhetic, cryptorrheic (krĭp″tō-rĕt′ĭk, -rē′ĭk). Pert. to the internal secretions.

cryptoscope (krĭp″tō-skōp) [″ + *skopein*, to examine]. Fluoroscope.

cryptosporidiosis. A diarrheal disease caused by protozoa of the genus *Cryptosporidium. Cryptosporidium parvum* is the most common species in human infections. The disease was first described in humans in 1976. Travelers to endemic areas have an increased chance of becoming infested with this organism. The typical infection, in immunocompetent individuals, causes explosive diarrhea and abdominal cramps following an incubation period of 4 to 14 days; these usually last for 5 to 11 days but may continue for a month. In immunocompromised patients the disease often causes death. This disease is commonly seen in patients with AIDS and in those cancer and organ transplant patients who are immunocompromised. In the normal patient there is no effective specific therapy, and the disease is self-limiting. In the immunocompro-

mised patient the only effective therapy is reversal of the immunologic defect.

Caution: Stools from these patients are highly infectious. Use standard technique in handling and disposing of them. SEE: *Universal Precautions* in *Appendix.*

Cryptosporidium. A genus of protozoa classed as a coccidian parasite. It is an important cause of diarrhea, esp. in immunocompromised patients. SEE: *cryptosporidiosis.*

cryptotoxic (krĭp″tō-tŏk′sĭk) [″ + *toxikon*, poison]. Having unknown toxic properties.

cryptoxanthin (krĭp″tō-zǎn′thĭn). A substance present in a variety of foods, e.g., eggs and corn, that can be converted to vitamin A in the body.

cry reflex. 1. Normal ability of an infant to cry. Not usually present in premature infants. 2. Spontaneous crying by infants during sleep. Due to some painful disease such as tuberculosis of the joints.

crystal (krĭs′tǎl) [Gr. *krystallos*, ice]. A solid body in which the atoms are arranged in a definite symmetrical pattern and having faces lying at definite angles to each other as crystals formed from salts or water.

c., apatite. In dentistry, refers to the hydroxyapatite crystal typical of calcified tissues. A complex of calcium phosphate and other elements, it is present in bone and in the cementum, dentin, and enamel layers of teeth. The most perfect crystalline pattern (and therefore the most dense) is found in enamel, which is the hardest tissue of the body.

c.'s, Charcot-Leyden. Protein-containing crystals found in diseased tissues wherein eosinophils are being destroyed. Present in sputum from asthma patients, leukemic bloods, and pleural effusions containing large numbers of eosinophils.

c.'s, Charcot-Neumann. Spermin crystals found in semen and some animal tissues.

c.'s, Charcot-Robin. A type of crystal formed in blood in leukemia.

c.'s of hemin. Yellowish or brown crystals that appear when dried blood or hemoglobin is heated after adding a few drops of acetic acid and salt. They are crystals of hemin, the hydrochloride of heme. Their presence constitutes a delicate and reliable test for blood.

c.'s, spermin. Crystals composed of spermine phosphate and seen in prostatic fluid on addition of a drop of ammonium phosphate solution.

crystallin (krĭs′tǎl-ĭn). Globulin of the crystalline lens.

crystalline (kris′tă-lĭn). Resembling crystal.

crystalline deposits. Acid group includes the urates, oxalates, carbonates, and sulfates. The alkaline group includes the phosphates and cholesterin ammonium urate.

crystalline lens. The lens of the eye in the capsule behind the pupil. It separates the aqueous from the vitreous humor. It is transparent and refracts the rays of transmitted light to bring them to focus on the retina.

crystallization (kris″tă-lĭ-zā′shŭn) [Gr. *krystallos,* ice]. The formation of crystals.

crystallography (kris″tă-lŏg′ră-fē) [″ + *graphein,* to write]. Study of crystals. Useful in investigating renal calculi.

crystalloid [″ + *eidos,* form, shape]. 1. Like a crystal. 2. A substance capable of crystallization, which in solution can be diffused through animal membranes. Opposite of colloid.

crystalloiditis (kris″tăl-oyd-ī′tĭs) [″ + ″ + *itis,* inflammation]. Inflammation of crystalline lens.

crystallophobia [Gr. *krystallos,* ice, + *phobos,* fear]. Abnormal fear of glass or objects made of glass.

crystalluria (kris-tă-lū′rē-ă) [″ + *ouron,* urine]. The appearance of crystals in the urine. May occur following the administration of sulfonamides. Their formation can be prevented by administration of adequate amounts of alkali.

Crystodigin. Trade name for digitoxin.

CS. *cesarean section.*

Cs. Chem. symb. for the element cesium.

c-section. *cesarean section,* q.v.

CSF. *cerebrospinal fluid.*

CS gas. A gas, orthochlorobenzalmalonitrile, used in riot control. Named after its two inventors, Corson and Stoughton.

C substance. A complex carbohydrate present in the cell wall of pneumococcal cells. SEE: *C-reactive protein.*

CT. *computerized tomography.*

Ctenocephalides (tĕn-ō-sĕf-ăl′ĭ-dēz) [Gr. *ktenodes,* like a cockle, + *kephale,* head]. A genus of fleas belonging to the order Siphonaptera. Common species are *Ct. canis* and *Ct. felis,* the dog flea and cat flea, respectively. The adults feed on their hosts while larvae live on dried blood and feces of adult fleas. Adults may attack man and other animals. They serve as intermediate host of the dog tapeworm, *Dipylidium caninum,* and may transmit other helminth and protozoan infections.

c-terminal. In chemical nomenclature, the alpha carboxyl group of the last amino acid.

CTZ. *chemoreceptor trigger zone.* A zone in the medulla that is sensitive to certain chemical stimuli. Stimulation of this zone will produce an effect such as nausea.

Cu [L. *cuprum*]. Chem. symb. for the element copper.

cubic measure. A unit or a system of units used to measure volume or capacity as distinguished from liquid measure. SEE: *Cubic Measure* in *Weights and Measures* in *Appendix.*

cubital (kū′bĭ-tăl) [L. *cubitum,* elbow]. Pert. to the ulna or to the forearm.

cubital fossa. Triangular area lying anterior to and below the elbow, bounded medially by the pronator teres and laterally by the brachioradialis muscle. SYN: *antecubital fossa.*

cubitus (kū′bĭ-tŭs) [L]. [NA] Elbow; forearm; ulna.

   c. valgus (pl. *cubitum valgum*). A deformity of the arm in which the forearm deviates laterally. May be congenital or due to injury or disease. In females, slight cubitus valgus is normal and is one of the secondary sex characteristics.

   c. varus. A deformity of the arm in which the forearm deviates medially.

cuboid (kū′boyd) [Gr. *kubos,* cube, + *eidos,* form, shape]. Like a cube.

cuboid bone. Outer bone of the instep bones of the foot that articulates posteriorly with the calcaneus and anteriorly with the 4th and 5th metatarsals.

cu. cm. *cubic centimeter.*

cucurbit (kū-kĕr′bĭt) [L. *cucurbita,* gourd]. Cupping glass. SEE: *cupping.*

cue. In psychology, a stimulus or set of stimuli that results in action or attempted action.

cued speech. A language for the deaf that combines lip reading with cues provided by the hands. The use of this technique permits the deaf person to understand a greater variety of words and the mechanics of language than either sign language or lip reading alone.

cuff (kŭf) [ME. *cuffe,* glove]. Anatomical structure encircling a part.

   c., attached gingival. Attachment or junctional epithelium which is attached to the calcified root of the tooth apical to the gingival sulcus.

   c., gingival. The most coronal portion of the gingiva around the tooth.

cuffed endotracheal tube. An airway catheter used to provide an airway through the trachea and at the same time prevent aspiration of foreign material into the bronchus. This is accomplished by an inflatable cuff that surrounds the tube. The cuff is inflated after the tube is placed in the trachea.

cuff-inflation hypertension. Marked increase in blood pressure in association with inflation of the cuff of the sphygmomanometer. This does not represent true hypertension.

cuffing (kŭf'ĭng). A collection of inflammatory cells in the shape of a ring around small blood vessels.

cuirass (kwē-răs') [Fr. *cuirasse*, breastplate]. A firm bandage around the chest.

cul-de-sac (kŭl"dĭ-săk') [Fr., bottom of the sack]. 1. A blind pouch or cavity. 2. The rectouterine pouch or pouch of Douglas, an extension of the peritoneal cavity, which lies between the rectum and posterior wall of uterus.

culdocentesis (kŭl"dō-sĕn-tē'sĭs) [" + Gr. *kentesis*, puncture]. Obtaining material from the posterior vaginal cul-de-sac by aspiration or surgical incision through the vaginal wall. Procedure is done for therapeutic or diagnostic reasons.

culdoscope (kŭl'dō-skōp). An endoscope used in performing a culdoscopic examination.

culdoscopy (kŭl-dŏs'kō-pē). Examination of the viscera of the pelvic cavity of the female after introduction of an endoscope through the wall of the posterior fornix of the vagina.

-cule, -cle [L.]. Suffix indicating little, as molecule, corpuscle.

Culex (kū'lĕks) [L., gnat]. A genus of small to medium-sized mosquitoes of cosmopolitan distribution. Some species are vectors of disease organisms.

    C. pipiens. The common house mosquito. Serves as a vector of *Wuchereria bancrofti,* the causative agent of filariasis.

    C. quinquefasciatus. Mosquito common in the tropics and subtropics; the most important intermediate host of *Wuchereria bancrofti.*

Culicidae (kū-lĭs'ĭ-dē). A family of insects belonging to the order Diptera. Includes the mosquitoes.

culicide (kū'lĭ-sīd) [L. *culex*, gnat, + *caedere,* to kill]. An agent that destroys gnats and mosquitoes.

culicifuge (kū-lĭs'ĭ-fūj) [L. *culex*, gnat, + *fugere,* to flee]. An agent to repel mosquito attacks.

Cullen's sign (kŭl'ĕnz) [Thomas Stephen Cullen, U.S. gynecologist, 1868–1953]. Bluish discoloration of the periumbilical skin due to intraperitoneal hemorrhage. This may be caused by ruptured ectopic pregnancy or acute pancreatitis.

culling. The process of removal of abnormal or damaged blood cells from the circulation by the spleen. SEE: *pitting, spleen.*

culmen (kŭl'mĕn) [L., summit] (pl. *culmina*). 1. Top or summit of a thing. 2. [NA] Most prominent part of the vermis superior of the cerebellum. Near its anterior extremity.

cult [L. *cultus,* care]. A group of people with an obsessive commitment to an ideal or principle, or to an individual personifying that ideal.

cultivation (kŭl"tĭ-vā'shŭn) [L. *cultivare,* to cultivate]. The propagation of living organisms, esp. growing microorganisms in an artificial medium.

cultural (kŭl'tū-răl) [L. *cultura,* tillage]. Pert. to cultures of microorganisms.

culture (kŭl'tūr). 1. The propagation of microorganisms or of living tissue cells in special media that are conducive to their growth. 2. The manmade part of the environment; man's symbols, ideas, values, traditions, institutions, and technology.

    c., blood. Culture used in the diagnosis of specific infectious diseases. Test consists of withdrawing blood from a vein under sterile precautions, placing it in or upon suitable culture media, and determining whether or not bacteria grow in the media. If organisms do grow, they are identified by bacteriological methods.

    c., cell. An in vitro growth of cells.

    c., contaminated. Culture whereupon bacteria from a foreign source have infiltrated the original bacteria being grown.

    c., continuous flow. Bacterial culture in which a fresh flow of culture media is maintained. This allows the bacteria to maintain their growth rate.

    c., gelatin. Culture of bacteria on a gelatin medium.

    c., hanging block. A thin slice of agar seeded on its surface with bacteria, and then inverted on a cover slip and sealed in the concavity of a hollow glass slide.

    c., hanging drop. Culture accomplished by inoculating the bacterium into a drop on a cover glass and mounting upside down over the depression on a concave slide.

    c., negative. Culture made from suspected matter that fails to reveal the suspected organism.

    c., positive. Culture that reveals the suspected organism.

    c., pure. Culture of a single form of microorganism uncontaminated by other organisms.

    c., slant. Culture in which the medium is placed in a tube that is slanted to allow greater surface for growth of the inoculum of bacteria.

    c., stab. Bacterial culture made by thrusting into the culture medium a point inoculated with the matter under examination.

    c., stock. Permanent culture from which transfers may be made.

    c., streak. Spreading of the bacteria inoculum by drawing a wire containing the inoculum across the surface of the medium.

c., tissue. Growing of tissue cells in artificial nutrient media.

c., type. Standard strains of bacteria that are maintained in a suitable storage area. These permit bacteriologists to compare known strains with unknown or partially identified strains.

cultured keratinocytes. Keratinocytes may be cultured and a small biopsy sample from uninjured skin will grow as a sheet and expand to have a surface area 1000 to 10,000 times the area of the sample. The sheet can be used to cover wounds such as burns. The culture technique requires 2 to 3 weeks and the regeneration of tissue below the sheet may not be complete for 5 to 6 months.

culture medium. A substance on which microorganisms may grow. Those most commonly used are broths, gelatin, and agar, which contain the same basic ingredients.

c.m., defined. SEE: *defined medium.*

culture shock. The emotional trauma of being exposed to the culture, mores, and customs of a culture vastly different from the one to which one has been accustomed.

cu mm. *cubic millimeter.*

cumulative (kū″mū-lă-tĭv) [L. *cumulus*, a heap]. Increasing in effect by successive additions; the total is usually greater than the sum of all the additions.

cumulative drug action. The action of small but repeated doses of drugs that are not immediately eliminated from the body. They tend to accumulate in the system and can produce symptoms of poisoning.

Ex.: lead, silver, and mercurial preparations.

cumulus (kū′mū-lŭs) [L., a little mound]. A small elevation; a heap of cells.

c. oophorus. A solid mass of follicular cells that surrounds the developing ovarian follicle. It projects into the antrum of the graafian follicle. SYN: *discus proligerus.*

cuneate (kū′nē-āt) [L. *cuneus*, wedge]. Wedge-shaped.

cuneate fasciculus. Continuation of postero-external column of cord into the medulla. SYN: *c. funiculus.*

cuneate funiculus. Cuneate fasciculus, q.v.

cuneate nucleus. Gray matter at end of cuneate fasciculus.

cuneiform (kū-nē′ĭ-form) [″ + *forma*, shape]. Wedge-shaped.

cuneiform bones. Bones of the internal, middle, and external tarsus.

cuneiform cartilage. One of two small pieces of yellow elastic cartilage that lie in the aryepiglottic fold of the larynx immediately anterior to the arytenoid cartilage.

cuneo- (kū′nē-ō) [L. *cuneus*, wedge]. Prefix rel. to a wedge.

cuneocuboid (kū″nē-ō-kū′boyd) [″ + Gr. *kubos*, cube, + *eidos*, form, shape]. Pert. to cuboid and cuneiform bones.

cuneohysterectomy (kū″nē-ō-hĭs″tĕr-ĕk′tō-mē) [″ + Gr. *hystera*, womb, + *ektome*, excision]. Excision of a wedge of tissue from the posterior surface of the cervix uteri to correct abnormal anteflexion.

cuneus (kū′nē-ŭs) [L., wedge] (pl. *cunei*). Wedge-shaped lobule of brain on mesial surface of occipital lobe.

cuniculus (kū-nĭk′ū-lŭs) [L., an underground passage] (pl. *cuniculi*). Burrow in epidermis made by the itch mite.

cunnilinguist (kŭn-ĭ-lĭn′gwĭst) [L. *cunnus*, pudenda, + *lingua*, tongue]. One who practices cunnilingus, q.v.

cunnilingus (kŭn-ĭ-lĭn′gŭs). Sexual activity in which the mouth and tongue are used to stimulate the female genitalia. SEE: *fellatio.*

cunnus (kŭn′ŭs) [L.]. The vulva, q.v.; pudenda.

cup [LL. *cuppa*, drinking vessel]. 1. Small drinking vessel. 2. A cupping glass. SEE: *cupping.* 3. An athletic supporter (jockey strap) reinforced with a piece of firm material to cover the male genitalia. Worn to protect the penis and testicles during vigorous and contact sports. 4. Either of the two cup-shaped halves of a brassiere that fits over a breast. 5. A method of producing counterirritation. SEE: *cupping.*

c., favus. A cup-shaped crust that develops in certain fungus infections. SEE: *favus.*

c., glaucomatous. A depression in the optic disk occurring in late stages of glaucoma.

c., optic. In the embryo, a double-layered cuplike structure connected to the diencephalon by a tubular optic stalk. It gives rise to the sensory and pigmented layers of the retina.

c., physiologic. A slight concavity in the center of the optic disk.

cup arthroplasty of hip. Surgical technique for remodeling the femoral head and acetabulum and then covering the head with a metal cup. It is rarely used in treating arthritis of the hip. Total hip replacement, q.v., is usually the procedure of choice in the elderly as well as in young adults on a selective basis.

Cupid's bow. The normal bow-shape of the upper lip of the mouth.

cupola, cupula (kū′pō-lă, -pū-lă) [L. *cupula*, little tub]. 1. The little dome at the apex of the cochlea and spiral canal of the ear. 2. The portion of costal pleura that extends superiorly into the root of the neck. It is dome shaped and accommodates the apex of the lung.

cupping. Application to the skin of a glass vessel, from which air has been exhausted by heat, or of a special suction apparatus in order to draw blood to the surface. This is done to produce counterirritation. SEE: *leech; moxibustion.*

cupric (kū′prĭk). Concerning divalent copper, Cu^{++}, in solution.

cupric sulfate. Copper sulfate, blue vitriol.

cuprous (kū′prŭs). Concerning monovalent copper, Cu^+, in a compound.

cuprum (kū′prŭm) [L.]. Copper, q.v. ABBR: Cu.

cupruresis (kū″proo-rē′sĭs) [L. *cuprum,* copper, + Gr. *ouresis,* to void urine]. Excretion of copper in the urine.

cupulolithiasis (kū″pū-lō-lĭth-ī′ă-sis) [L. dim. of *cupa,* a tub, + Gr. *lithos,* stone, + *iasis,* state or condition of]. Disease of calculi in the cupulo of the posterior semicircular canal of the middle ear. The condition may be associated with positional vertigo.

curare (kū-, koo-rär′ē) [phonetic equivalent of Carib Indian name for extracts of plants used as arrow poisons]. One of several different resinous substances obtained from extracts of South American trees including species of chondrodendron. The pharmacologically active ingredient of curare used medically is the alkaloid D-tubocurarine. This drug is used to facilitate skeletal muscle relaxation during anesthesia. SEE: *tubocurarine chloride.*

curarization (kū″rär-ĭ-zā′shŭn). Condition following introduction of a purified form of curare: eyelids heavy; nystagmus; husky voice; weak jaw and throat muscles; inability to raise head, arms, and legs. Employed to lessen severity of convulsions produced by pentylenetetrazol and electric shock therapy and relaxation of muscles as in tetanus.

curative (kū′ră-tĭv) [L. *curare,* to take care of]. Having healing or remedial properties.

curb cut. An area where a sidewalk has been modified or designed to eliminate the vertical curb. By providing a gradual slope to the street at this point, an environmental obstacle has been removed, thus improving access for persons with wheelchairs, others who have difficulty walking, or those pushing wheeled vehicles.

curd [ME]. Milk coagulum, composed mainly of casein.

cure [L. *cura,* care]. 1. Course of treatment to restore health. 2. Restoration to health.

curet, curette (kū-rĕt′) [Fr. *curette,* a cleanser]. 1. A spoon-shaped scraping instrument for removing foreign matter from a cavity. 2. In dentistry, one of a variety of sharp instruments used to remove calculus and to smooth tooth roots or to remove soft tissues from a periodontal pocket or extrac-

tion site.

curettage (kū″rĕ-tăzh′) [Fr.]. 1. Scraping of a cavity. SYN: *curettement.* 2. The use of a curet in removal of necrotic tissue from around the tooth, dental granulomata, or cysts and tissue fragments or debris from the bony socket after tooth extraction; also called debridement.

   c., periapical. Use of a curet to remove pathological tissues from around the apex of the tooth root.

   c., suction. Vacuum aspiration, q.v.

   c., uterine. Scraping with a curet to remove contents of uterus as is done following inevitable or incomplete abortion; to produce abortion; to obtain specimens for use in diagnosis; and to remove growths, such as polyps.

   NURSING IMPLICATIONS: The procedure should be explained to the patient, and any questions answered. Physical preparation for the procedure should be completed. The patient should be placed in lithotomy position for the procedure. Asepsis should be maintained during the procedure. Postoperatively, a perineal pad count is done to determine the extent of uterine bleeding — excess bleeding should be reported to the physician. Administer analgesics as ordered and needed to keep the patient comfortable.

   Instruct the patient to report any bleeding lasting longer than 10 days, to avoid use of tampons, IUDs, diaphragms, and douches during this time, and to report signs of infection, such as fever or foul-smelling vaginal discharge. Encourage gradual resumption of usual activities as long as they do not cause vaginal bleeding.

curettement (kū-rĕt′mĕnt) [Fr.]. Curettage, q.v.

Curie (kūr′ē, kū-rē′). 1. Marie, Polish-born Fr. chemist, 1867–1934; discovered radioactivity of thorium; discovered polonium and radium, and isolated radium from pitchblende. Awarded Nobel Prize in physics in 1903 with her husband, and in chemistry in 1911. 2. Pierre, Fr. chemist, 1859–1906. He and his wife were awarded the Nobel Prize in 1903.

curie [Marie Curie]. ABBR: Ci. The standard unit of quantity of radon, being the amt. in equilibrium with 1 gm of radium element. This quantity decays at the rate of 3.7×10^{10} disintegrations per second.

curietherapy (kū″rē-thĕr′ă-pē) [″ + Gr. *therapeia,* treatment]. Radium therapy.

curium (kū′rē-ŭm) [Pierre and Marie Curie]. SYMB: Cm. At. wt. of the longest-lived isotope, 247; at. no. 96. A man-made element of the actinide series. The half-life of the most stable isotope is 16 million years.

curled. In bacteriology, said of parallel chains in wavy strands, such as in anthrax colonies.

Curling's ulcer (kŭr'lĭngz) [Thomas Curling, Brit. physician, 1811–1888]. Acute peptic ulcer that sometimes occurs following acute stress, e.g., a severe burn. A form of stress ulcer, q.v.

currant jelly clot. Soft red postmortem blood clot in heart and vessels.

current [L. *currere*, to run]. A flow, as of water or the transference of electrical impulses.

   c., alternating. Current that periodically flows in opposite directions. Alternating current waves may be either sinusoidal or nonsinusoidal. The alternating current wave used most commonly therapeutically is the sinusoidal.

   c., direct. Current that flows in one direction only. When used medically it is called the galvanic current.

curriculum (kŭ-rĭk'ū-lŭm) [L.]. A course of study in a special field or covering a specific time.

Curschmann's spirals (koorsh'mänz) [Heinrich Curschmann, Ger. physician, 1846–1910]. Coiled spirals of mucus occasionally seen in sputum of asthma patients, etc. SEE: *sputum.*

curse (kĕrs). 1. To attempt to inflict injury by appeal to a malevolent supernatural power. 2. Injury assumed to have been inflicted by a malevolent supernatural power.

   c., Ondine's [*Ondine,* character in Greek mythology]. 1. Primary alveolar hypoventilation due to reduced responsiveness of the respiratory center to carbon dioxide. 2. Loss of autonomic respiratory function due to a lesion in the cervical portion of the spinal cord.

curvature. [L. *curvatura,* a slope]. A normal or abnormal bending or sloping away; a curve.

   c., angular. A sharp bending of the vertebral column.

curvature of spine. One of four normal curves or flexures of the vertebral column as seen in profile: cervical, thoracic, lumbar, and sacral. Abnormal curvatures may occur as a result of maldevelopment or disease processes. SEE: *kyphosis; lordosis; scoliosis.*

curve [L. *curvus*]. A bend.

   c., dye-dilution. A graph of the disappearance rate of a known amount of injected dye from the circulation. Used to measure cardiac function.

   c., epidemic. A chart or graph in which the number of new cases is plotted for each time interval selected.

   c., learning. A graph of the effect of learning or practice on the performance of an intellectual or physical task.

   c., normal. In statistics, the theoretical frequency of a set of data. It is usually a bell-shaped curve. SYN: *normal distribution curve; gaussian curve.*

   c. of Carus. An arc corresponding to the pelvic axis.

   c. of Spee. Curve established by viewing the occlusal alignment of teeth, beginning with the tip of the lower canine and extending back along the buccal cusps of the natural premolar and molar teeth to the ramus of the mandible.

curvi- [L. *curvus,* curve]. Combining form meaning curved.

curvilinear. Concerning or pertaining to a curved line.

Cushing, Harvey (koosh'ĭng). U.S. surgeon, 1869–1939.

   C.'s disease. Cushing's syndrome, q.v., in which the hypersecretion of glucocorticoids is secondary to hypersecretion of adrenocorticotrophic hormone from the pituitary.

   C.'s syndrome. Syndrome resulting from hypersecretion of the adrenal cortex in which there is excessive production of glucocorticoids. May be caused by a tumor of the adrenal gland or excess stimulation of that gland as a result of hyperfunction of the anterior pituitary. Prolonged administration of large doses of adrenocortical hormones will also cause this syndrome. Symptoms are protein loss, adiposity, fatigue and weakness, osteoporosis, amenorrhea, impotence, capillary fragility, edema, excess hair growth, diabetes mellitus, skin discoloration and turgidity (plethora), and purplish striae of skin.

   NURSING IMPLICATIONS: When patient requires prolonged administration of therapeutic, as opposed to replacement, doses of adrenocortical hormones, monitor patient for development of potential side effects. Assist patient in adjustment to physical changes in body image and strength. Provide realistic reassurance and emotional support, encouraging verbalization of feelings about losses. Encourage intermittent rest periods, assist patient with mobility, especially in initiating movements requiring arm-shoulder strength, and provide safety measures to prevent falls. Teach patient the importance of employing the smallest possible maintenance dose, usually on an every-other-day regimen, and of gradually decreasing dosage following an increase during an exacerbation. SEE: *Nursing Diagnoses* in *Appendix.*

cushingoid (koosh'ĭng-oyd). Resembling Cushing's syndrome.

cushion. In anatomy, a mass of connective tissue, usually adipose, that acts to prevent undue pressure upon underlying tissues or structures.

cusp (kŭsp) [L. *cuspis*, point]. 1. A rounded or cone-shaped point on the crown of a tooth. 2. One of the leaflike divisions or parts of the valves of the heart. SEE: *bicuspid valve; semilunar cusps; tricuspid valve.*

  c., Carabelli's. An accessory cusp found on the upper molars of most Caucasians and none of the Mongolian race.

cuspid (kŭs'pĭd). The canine teeth. SEE: *dentition* for illus.

cuspidate (kŭs'pĭ-dāt) [L. *cuspidatus*]. Having cusps.

cuspidor (kŭs'pĭ-dor). A rounded glass or metal bowl attached to a dental unit into which a patient may expectorate.

custom. A generally accepted practice or behavior by a particular group of people or a social group.

cut. 1. Separating or dividing tissues by use of a sharp surgical instrument such as a scalpel. 2. To dilute a substance in order to decrease the concentration of the active ingredient.

cutaneous (kū-tā'nē-ŭs) [L. *cutis*, skin]. Pert. to the skin. SYN: *dermal; integumentary.*

cutaneous nerves. Nerves that provide sensory pathways for stimuli to the skin. SEE: *Nerves* in *Appendix.*

cutaneous respiration. The transpiration of gases through the skin.

cutdown (kŭt'down). A surgical procedure for locating a vein or artery to permit intravenous or intra-arterial administration of fluids or drugs. Required in patients with vascular collapse due to shock or other causes.

cuticle (kū'tĭ-k'l) [L. *cuticula*, little skin]. 1. A layer of solid or semisolid substance that covers the free surface of a layer of epithelial cells. It may be of a horny or chitinous consistency; sometimes it is calcified; the enamel cuticle of a tooth, and the capsule of the lens of the eye are considered cuticles. 2. The epidermis of the skin.

  c., acquired. A layer of salivary products, bacteria, and food debris on the surface of the teeth; not a true cuticle. SYN: *pellicle.*

  c., attachment. The glycosaminoglycans layer secreted by junctional or attachment epithelium that attaches the epithelium to the calcified tooth surface. Also called dental cuticle.

  c., dental. The glycosaminoglycans layer produced by attachment epithelium on the cementum of the tooth root. It is continuous with and identical in origin and function to enamel cuticle, which is present on the enamel crown.

  c., enamel. The thin, calcified layer that covers the enamel crown of the tooth prior to eruption. Remnants that persist after de-

calcification of the tooth for microscopy are called Nasmyth's membrane.

cuticula (kū-tĭk'ū-lă) [L.]. Cuticle.

  c. dentis. A skinlike membrane that may cover the teeth after they have erupted and usually is lost in ordinary mastication of food. The membrane is easily removed by a dentist. SYN: *enamel cuticle; Nasmyth's membrane.*

cuticularization (kū-tĭk″ū-lăr-ĭ-zā'shŭn). Growth of skin over a sore or wound.

cutin (kū'tĭn) [L. *cutis*, skin]. A wax that combines with cellulose to form the cuticle of plants.

cutireaction (kū″tĕ-rē-ăk'shŭn). Inflammatory or irritative reaction appearing on the skin; skin reaction.

  c., von Pirquet's. Reaction of skin after inoculation with tuberculosis toxins.

cutis (kū'tĭs) [L.]. [NA] The skin; consisting of the epidermis and the corium (dermis), and resting upon the subcutaneous tissue.

  c. anserina. Gooseflesh caused by erection of skin papillae, as from cold, shock, fright, or fear.

  c. aurantiasis. Yellow discoloration of the skin resulting from ingesting excessive quantities of vegetables, such as carrots, containing carotenoid pigments. SEE: *carotenemia.*

  c. hyperelastica. Congenital or familial condition characterized by excessive elasticity of the skin, loose-jointedness, easy bruisability, and development of pseudotumors at joints. SYN: *Ehlers-Danlos syndrome.*

  c. laxa. Congenital hereditary disorder characterized by dermatolysis or hypertrophy of the skin and subcutaneous tissue.

  c. marmorata. Transitory purplish discoloration of skin on exposure to cold.

  c. pendula. C. laxa, q.v.

  c. testacea. Condition characterized by formation of plates of greasy material on trunk and extremities. SYN: *seborrhea.*

  c. unctosa. Excessive secretion of sebaceous glands. SEE: *seborrhea.*

  c. vera. The corium, q.v.; deep layer of skin, the dermis, q.v.

  c verticis gyrata. Convoluted scalp folds 1 to 2 cm thick. The appearance is that the scalp is too big for the head. The condition may develop any time from birth to adolescence. It is more common in males. The skin cannot be flattened by traction.

cutization (kū-tĭ-zā'shŭn). Skinlike condition of a mucous membrane as a result of continued exposure.

cut throat. Laceration of throat. Seriousness of injury depends upon angle of thrust of cutting object and location, and the amount of tissue damage.

F.A.: Send for physician. Have patient lying down, head and shoulders raised. If trachea is severed, keep open and free from clot. Compress bleeding points with sterile cloths. Reassure such patients, keep their lips moist, do not leave them for an instant. Artificial respiration if necessary.

cuvette (kŭv-ĕt′) [Fr. *cuve,* a tub]. Small transparent glass container, esp. one used to hold liquids that are to be examined photometrically.

CVA. *cerebrovascular accident.*

CVP. *central venous pressure.*

cyanephidrosis (sī″ăn-ĕf″ĭ-drō′sĭs) [″ + *ephidrosis,* sweating]. Bluish sweat.

cyanhemoglobin (sī″ăn-hē″mō-glō′bĭn). Hemoglobin combined with cyanide. The blood containing this is cherry-red.

cyanhidrosis (sī-ăn-hī-drō′sĭs) [″ + *hidrosis,* sweat]. Exuding bluish sweat.

cyanide (sī′ă-nīd″). A compound containing the radical —CN, as potassium cyanide (KCN), sodium cyanide (NaCN).

cyanide poisoning. Cyanides are among the most common and most deadly poisons known. They stop cellular respiration by inhibiting the action of cytochrome oxidase, carbonic anhydrase, and other enzyme systems. The seeds of certain stone fruits, such as apricots, jetberry bush and toyon, and seeds of fruits of some members of the apple family contain chemicals that upon digestion yield cyanide. This occurs only if the seeds are broken. The fatal dose for a small child varies from 5 to 25 seeds. SEE: *Poisons and Poisoning* in Appendix.

SYM: Start within a few seconds, rarely longer than 2 minutes. The patient utters a cry, becomes unconscious, and falls. Respiration is first rapid and convulsive, later slow and gasping. Death usually comes within 5 minutes. When smaller doses are taken, there is an acrid taste, a choking feeling, anxiety, dizziness, confusion, and headache. Convulsions with frothing of the mouth. Often incontinence. Pulse rapid, feeble, and irregular.

F.A.: Must be very prompt. Immediate emesis and gastric lavage, and without delay have victim inhale amyl nitrate immediately for 15 to 30 seconds every 2 to 3 minutes. While this is being done, give I.V. sodium nitrite 0.3 gm in 10 ml of water at rate of 2.5 to 5 ml per minute. As soon as this is completed, administer through the same needle 25 to 50 ml of 50% solution of sodium thiosulfate. Immediate artificial respiration with 100% oxygen is required also. In one hour, repeat half doses of medicines listed above. Hyperbaric oxygen therapy should be used if immediately available. External heat, epinephrine for collapse, and keep the

patient in a recumbent position. An alternative antidote, hydroxocobalamin-thiosulfate mixture, is used outside the U.S. It is given in doses of 4 to 10 grams.

cyanmethemoglobin (sī″ăn-mĕt″hē-mō-glō′bĭn). Combination of cyanide and methemoglobin.

cyano- [Gr. *kyanos,* dark blue]. Combining form meaning dark blue.

cyanoacrylate adhesives. Monomers of *N*-alkyl cyanoacrylate that have been used as a tissue adhesive. This use is limited by the toxicity of the glue. Commercially available versions are called "superglue."

Caution: "Superglue" will cause tissues such as the skin covering fingers to form a firm adhesion. When this happens while using "superglue," the bond may have to be removed surgically.

---

cyanocobalamin (sī″ăn-ō-kō-băl′ă-mĭn). USP. A component of the vitamin B complex. It is essential for blood formation. Used in treating pernicious anemia. Trade names are Berubigen, Betalin 12, Crystallin, Rubramin PC, and Bevatine 12. SYN: *vitamin B₁₂.*

cyanoderma (sī″ă-nō-dĕr′mă) [″ + *derma,* skin]. Blue discoloration of skin. SYN: *cyanosis.*

cyanogen (sī-ăn′ō-jĕn) [″ + *gennan,* to produce]. 1. The radical CN. 2. A poisonous gas, CN—CN.

cyanomycosis (sī″ăn-ō-mī-kō′sĭs) [″ + *mykes,* fungus, + *osis,* condition]. Development of blue pus due to *Micrococcus pyocyaneus.*

cyanopathy (sī″ăn-ŏp′ă-thē) [″ + *pathos,* disease]. Blue discoloration of skin. SYN: *cyanosis.*

cyanophil (sī-ăn′ō-fĭl) [″ + *philein,* to love]. Blue-staining substance of plants and animals.

cyanophilous (sī-ăn-ŏf′ĭl-ŭs). Having an affinity for a blue dye or stain.

cyanopia, cyanopsia (sī-ăn-ō′pē-ă, -ŏp′sē-ă) [″ + *opsis,* vision]. Vision in which all objects appear to be blue.

cyanosed. Affected with cyanosis.

cyanosis (sī-ă-nō′sĭs) [″ + *osis,* condition]. Slightly bluish, grayish, slatelike, or dark purple discoloration of the skin due to presence of abnormal amounts of reduced hemoglobin in the blood. May not appear in patients with severe anemia even though their blood is poorly oxygenated because there is not enough reduced hemoglobin present to cause the blue color to be visible.

ETIOL: Deficiency of oxygen and excess of carbon dioxide in blood caused by gas or any condition interfering with entrance of air into the respiratory tract; overdoses of certain drugs; or any form of asphyxiation.

TREAT: Remove cause. Artificial respiration together with oxygen inhalation or oxygen plus carbon dioxide in patients with chronic lung disease. Stimulants, heat, and massage are valuable adjuncts. SEE: *asphyxia; unconsciousness.*

c., congenital. Cyanosis usually associated with stenosis of the pulmonary orifice, an imperfect ventricular septum, or a patulous foramen ovale or ductus arteriosus. SEE: *tetralogy of Fallot.*

c., delayed. C., tardive.

c., enterogenous. Cyanosis induced by intestinal absorption of toxins or by certain drugs. SEE: *methemoglobinemia.*

c. retinae. Bluish appearance of retina seen in congenital heart disease, polycythemia, and in certain poisonings, such as dinitrobenzol.

c., tardive. Cyanosis resulting from an interatrial or interventricular septal defect.

cyanotic (sī-ăn-ŏt′ĭk). Of the nature of, affected with, or pert. to cyanosis.

cyanuria (sī″ă-nū′rē-ă). The voiding of blue urine.

cybernetics (sī″bĕr-nĕt′ĭks) [Gr. *kybernetes,* helmsman]. The science of control and communication in biological, electronic, and mechanical systems. This includes analysis of feedback mechanisms that serve to govern or modify the actions of various systems.

cyberphilia (sī″bĕr-fĭl′ē-ă) [″ + *philein,* to love]. Fascination with the use of machines, esp. computers, their use, and programming them.

cyberphobia (sī″bĕr-fō′bē-ă) [″ + *phobos,* fear]. Tension, anxiety, and stress in persons required to work with a computer.

cycad (sī′kăd). A variety of plants including *Cycas revoluta* and *C. circinalis,* from which cycasin has been isolated.

cycasin (sī′kă-sĭn). Toxic substance present in cycad plants. The chemical may be important in inducing cancer in some lower animals.

cyclacillin (sī-klă-sĭl′ĭn). USP. An antibacterial drug. Trade name is Cyclapen-W.

cyclamate (sī′klă-māt). A salt of cyclamic acid that is used as a non-nutritive artificial sweetener. It is about 30 times as sweet as sugar. Its general use has been restricted because of the chemical's toxic effect on lower animals.

cyclarthrosis (sī-klăr-thrō′sĭs) [Gr. *kyklos,* circle, + *arthron,* joint, + *osis,* condition]. A lateral ginglymus or pivot joint, which makes rotation possible.

cycle (sī′kl) [Gr. *kyklos,* circle]. A series of movements or events; a sequence usually recurring at regular intervals.

c., cardiac. The series of consecutive movements through which the heart passes in performing one heartbeat; it includes contraction or systole, relaxation or diastole, and a short rest pause called the diastasis cordis. A complete cycle corresponds to one pulse beat, which requires a variable length of time depending upon the heart rate.

c., Cori. A series of reactions that accounts for the disposal of lactate formed during muscular activity, i.e., muscle glycogen to lactic acid to liver glycogen to blood glucose to muscle glycogen.

c., gastric. Progression of peristaltic waves over the stomach wall.

c., genesial. 1. The period from puberty to menopause. 2. The period of sexual maturity.

c., glycolytic. The successive steps by which glucose is broken down in living tissue.

c., Krebs. A series of reactions occurring in muscle cells and possibly all tissues in which pyruvic acid (or two-carbon derivatives of carbohydrate, fat, or protein) formed anaerobically are converted through a series of interrelated oxidation-reduction and other reactions to carbon dioxide and water, with the release of energy principally utilized in the formation of adenosine triphosphate (ATP). It is considered to be the final common pathway for the oxidation of and interconversions between the three primary classes of foods. SYN: *citric acid cycle; tricarboxylic acid cycle (TCA).* SEE: *Krebs cycle* for illus.

c., life. All of the developmental history of an organism whether in a free-living condition or in a host; e.g., as a parasite that experiences part of its cycle inside another organism.

c., menstrual. A series of periodically recurring changes in the hormonal status of women and in the endometrium of the uterus, culminating in menstruation, q.v.

cyclectomy (sī-klĕk′tō-mē) [Gr. *kyklos,* circle, + *ektome,* excision]. 1. Excision of a portion of the ciliary body or muscle. 2. Excision of the ciliary border of the eyelids.

cycles per second. ABBR: cps. SEE: *hertz.*

cyclic (sī′klĭk). Periodic; occurring in cycles.

cyclic AMP. A cyclic nucleotide participating in the activities of many hormones, including catecholamines, ACTH, and vasopressin. SYN: *adenosine 3′,5′-cyclic monophosphate.*

cyclic AMP synthetase. Adenylate cyclase, q.v.

cyclicotomy (sĭk″lĭ-kŏt′ō-mē) [″ + *tome,* incision]. Cutting of the ciliary muscle.

cyclic vomiting. Periodic and recurring attacks of vomiting occurring in persons of a nervous temperament. The condition is usually associated with acidosis. SEE: *nausea; vomiting.*

SYM: Dizziness, loss of appetite, headache, nausea may occur. Patient then vomits about every half hour for 1 to 2 days. Great thirst, slight rise of temperature, rapid pulse, prostration.

NURSING IMPLICATIONS: Monitor vital signs, maintain fluid and electrolyte balance, administer medications as ordered for relief of headache and nausea and vomiting, and provide frequent oral hygiene. A calm, stress-free environment should be provided.

cyclins. A group of proteins important in regulating mitosis.

cyclitis (sĭk-lī′tĭs) [″ + *itis*, inflammation]. Inflammation of the ciliary body of the eye.

SYM: Tenderness in ciliary region, swelling of upper lid, circumcorneal injection, deposits on Descemet's membrane, reduced or hazy vision, increased or decreased tension. Pain in or about the eye, worse at night and on pressure. Its course is rapid, and progressively unfavorable.

COMPLICATIONS: Iritis, choroiditis, scleritis, glaucoma.

TREAT: Local: atropine, heat, protection from light. General: salicylates, induced diaphoresis, rest; treat underlying cause if possible.

c., plastic. Ciliary body inflammation accompanied by that of entire uveal tract, giving rise to a fibrinous exudate in anterior chamber and vitreous.

c., purulent. Suppurative inflammation of ciliary body and iris.

c., serous. Simple inflammation without iritis.

cyclizine hydrochloride. USP. Antihistamine used in treating and preventing motion sickness. Trade name is Marezine hydrochloride.

cyclo- [Gr. *kyklos*, circle]. 1. A combining form meaning circular or pert. to a cycle. 2. A combining form pert. to the ciliary body of the eye.

cyclobenzaprine hydrochloride (sī″klō-bĕn′ză-prēn). USP. A muscle relaxant drug. Trade name is Flexeril.

cycloceratitis (sī″klō-sĕr″ă-tī′tĭs). Inflammation of cornea and ciliary body. SYN: *cyclokeratitis.*

cyclochoroiditis (sī″klō-kō″royd-ī′tĭs) [″ + *chorioeides*, skinlike, + *itis*, inflammation]. Inflammation of ciliary body and choroid coat of eye.

cyclodialysis (sī″klō-dī-ăl′ī-sĭs) [″ + *dialysis*, dissolution]. Operation performed in certain types of glaucoma to produce com-

munication between anterior chamber and suprachoroidal space for the escape of aqueous humor.

cycloid (sī′kloyd) [″ + *eidos*, form, shape]. 1. Resembling a circle. 2. Denoting a ring of atoms. 3. Extreme variations of mood from elation to melancholia. SEE: *cyclothymia.*

cyclokeratitis (sī″klō-kĕr-ă-tī′tĭs) [″ + *keras*, cornea, + *itis*, inflammation]. Inflammation of cornea and ciliary body.

cyclomethycaine sulfate (sī″klō-mĕth′ī-kān). USP. A topical anesthetic. It is relatively effective when used on the mucous membranes of the mouth, nose, eye, and bronchi. Trade name is Surfacaine.

Cyclopar. Trade name for tetracycline hydrochloride.

cyclopentamine hydrochloride (sī″klō-pĕn′tă-mēn). USP. A vasoconstrictor drug.

cyclopentolate hydrochloride (sī″klō-pĕn′tō-lāt). Moderately long-acting drug used as a cycloplegic and mydriatic. Trade name is Cyclogyl.

cyclophoria (sī″klō-fō′rē-ă) [″ + *phoros*, bearing]. Rotation of eyeball due to weakness of oblique muscles. SYN: *periphoria.*

cyclophosphamide (sī″klō-fŏs′fă-mĭd). USP. An effective antineoplastic agent that has also been used as an immunosuppressive agent in organ transplantation. Trade name is Cytoxan.

cyclopia (sī-klō′pē-ă) [Gr. *kyklos*, circle, + *ops*, eye]. Condition of being a cyclops, q.v.

cycloplegia (sī″klō-plē′jē-ă) [″ + *plege*, a stroke]. Paralysis of ciliary muscle can be an anticholinergic side effect of antipsychotic or antidepressant medications.

cycloplegic (sī″klō-plē′jĭk). Producing cycloplegia.

cyclopropane (sī″klō-prō′pān). C_3H_6. A gaseous anesthetic agent, colorless, slightly heavier than air, with a not unpleasant odor. Administered with 70% to 95% oxygen, it produces unconsciousness in 1 to 2 minutes. Fire and explosion must be guarded against.

cyclops (sī′klŏps). A fetal malformation in which there is only one eye.

cycloserine (sī″klō-sĕr′ēn). USP. A broad-spectrum antibiotic that has been used in combination with other drugs in treating tuberculosis. It is contraindicated in patients with epilepsy and in those with depression or anxiety. Trade name is Seromycin.

cyclosis (sī-klō′sĭs) [Gr. *kyklosis*, circulation]. A streaming movement of protoplasm such as is seen in certain plant and animal cells.

cyclosporine (sī′klō-spor-een). An immunosuppressive drug useful in suppressing rejection phenomena in organ transplant recipients. Trade name is Sandimmune.

cyclothiazide (sī″klō-thī′ă-zīd). USP. A diuretic of the benzothiazide group. The drug also acts to lower blood pressure in hypertensive patients. Trade name is Anhydron.

cyclothymia (sī"klō-thī'mē-ă) [" + *thymos*, mind]. In psychiatry, an obsolete term for mild fluctuations of the manic-depressive type.

cyclotomy (sī-klŏt'ō-mē) [" + *tome*, incision]. Surgical incision of the ciliary muscle of the eye.

cyclotron (sī'klō-trŏn). A particle accelerator in which the particle is rotated between magnets, gaining speed with each rotation.

cyclotropia (sī"klō-trō'pē-ă). Permanent cyclophoria, i.e., deviation of the anteriorposterior axis of the eye away from the axis necessary to produce visual fusion.

cycrimine hydrochloride (sī'krĭ-mĭn). USP. Drug used in treating parkinsonism. Trade name is Pagitane Hydrochloride.

cyesis (sī-ē'sĭs) [Gr. *kyesis*]. Pregnancy.

cylicotomy (sĭl"ĭ-kŏt'ō-mē) [Gr. *kylix*, cup, + *tome*, incision]. Cutting of ciliary muscle.

cylinder (sĭl'ĭn-dĕr) [Gr. *kylindros*]. A hollow, tube-shaped body.

   c.'s, crossed. Two cylindrical lenses at right angles to each other. Used in diagnosing astigmatism.

   c.'s, urinary. Cylindrically shaped casts in the urine.

cylindroadenoma (sĭ-lĭn"drō-ăd"ē-nō'mă) [Gr. *kylindros*, cylinder, + *aden*, gland, + *oma*, tumor]. An adenoma containing cylindrical masses of hyaline material.

cylindroid (sĭl-ĭn'droyd) [" + *eidos*, form, shape]. 1. Cylinder-shaped. 2. A mucous, spurious cast in urine. Recognized by their twists and turns, varying markedly in diameter in different places, most frequently pointed at the ends and frequently crossing an entire field. They do not usually have cellular intrusions.

cylindroma (sĭl"ĭn-drō'mă) [" + *oma*, tumor]. Malignant tumor containing a collection of cells forming cylinders.

cylindruria (sĭl"ĭn-drū'rē-ă) [" + *ouron*, urine]. Presence of cylindroids in the urine.

cymbocephalic (sĭm"bō-sĕ-făl'ĭk) [Gr. *kymbe*, boat, + *kephale*, head]. Having a boat-shaped head.

cynanthropy (sĭn-ăn'thrō-pē) [Gr. *kyon*, dog, + *anthropos*, man]. Insanity in which the patient behaves like a dog.

cynic spasm [Gr. *kynikos*, doglike]. Spasm of facial muscles causing a grin or snarl like a dog. SYN: *risus sardonicus*.

cynophobia (sī"nō-fō'bē-ă) [" + *phobos*, fear]. 1. Unreasonable fear of dogs. 2. Morbid fear of rabies. SYN: *lyssophobia* (def. 2).

cypridophobia (sĭp"rĭ-dō-fō'bē-ă) [Gr. *Kypris*, Venus, + *phobos*, fear]. 1. Morbid

fear of venereal disease. 2. Abnormal fear of the sexual act. 3. False belief of having a venereal disease.

cypriphobia (sĭp-rĭ-fō'bē-ă). Morbid aversion to and fear of coitus.

cyproheptadine hydrochloride (sī"prō-hĕp'tă-dēn). USP. An anti-allergy drug that is also used in postgastrectomy dumping syndrome. Trade name is Periactin.

cyrtometer (sĭr-tŏm'ē-tĕr) [Gr. *kyrtos*, bent, + *metron*, measure]. Instrument for measuring circumference of chest and comparison of chest curves. Also used to measure other curved portions of the body.

cyrtosis (sĭr-tō'sĭs) [" + *osis*, condition]. Having any abnormal curvature of the spine. SEE: *kyphosis.*

cyst (sĭst) [Gr. *kystis*, bladder, sac]. 1. A closed sac or pouch, with a definite wall, that contains fluid, semifluid, or solid material. It is usually an abnormal structure resulting from developmental anomalies, obstruction of ducts, or from parasitic infection. 2. In biology, a structure formed by, and enclosing, certain organisms, in which they become inactive, as the cyst of certain protozoans or of the metacercariae of flukes. It may serve as a reproductive structure, as in hydatid cysts.

   c., adventitious. Cyst formed around a foreign body.

   c., alveolar. Dilation and rupture of pulmonary alveoli to form air cysts.

   c., apical. Cyst near the apex of the tooth root.

   c., blood. Bloody tumor. SYN: *hematoma.*

   c., blue dome. Cyst close to the surface of the breast. The blue color is due to bleeding into the cyst.

   c., branchial. C., cervical.

   c., cervical. A closed epithelial sac derived from a branchial groove of its corresponding pharyngeal pouch.

   c., chocolate. Ovarian cyst with darkly pigmented gelatinous content.

   c., colloid. Cyst with gelatinous contents.

   c., congenital. Cyst present at birth resulting from abnormal development, as a dermoid cyst, imperfect closure of a structure as in spina bifida cystica; or nonclosure of embryonic clefts, ducts, or tubules, such as cervical cysts.

   c., daughter. Cyst growing out of the walls of another cyst.

   c., dental. Cyst that forms from any of the odontogenic tissues.

   c., dentigerous. A fluid-filled cyst usually surrounding the crown of an unerupted tooth. Often involves incomplete enamel formation. Also called eruption cyst or follicular cyst. SYN: *odontoma, follicular.* SEE:

c., dermoid.

c., dermoid. Cyst containing elements of hair, teeth, or skin. It occurs commonly in the ovary or testes and contains derivatives of all three germ layers.

c., distention. Cyst formed in a natural enclosed cavity as a follicular cyst of the ovary.

c., echinococcus. C., hydatid, q.v.

c., epidermal. 1. Cyst that forms in skin due to the blockage of a pilosebaceous follicle. 2. Cyst that contains epidermis.

c., extravasation. Cyst arising from hemorrhage into tissues.

c., exudation. Cyst caused by trapping of an exudate in a closed area.

c., follicular. Cyst arising from a follicle, as a follicular cyst of the thyroid gland, ovary, or forming tooth.

c., Gartner's. Cyst developing from a vestigial mesonephric duct (Gartner's duct) in a female.

c., hydatid. Cyst formed by the growth of the larval form of the *Echinococcus granulosus*, usually in the liver.

c., implantation. Cyst resulting from displacement of portions of the epidermis as may occur in injuries.

c., intraligamentary. Cystic formation between the layers of the broad ligament.

c., involutional. Cyst occurring in the normal involution of an organ or structure, as in the mammary gland.

c., keratin. Cyst containing keratin.

c., meibomian. Tumor or cyst produced by inflammation of a meibomian gland of the eyelid. SYN: *chalazion.*

c., mucoid. Cyst containing mucoid material that has formed from degenerating connective tissue. Usually occurs over a distal joint of the finger.

c., mucous. Retention cyst composed of mucus.

c., nabothian. Cystic formation caused by closure of the ducts of the nabothian glands in the cervix uteri as a result of healing of an erosion.

c., odontogenic. Cyst associated with the teeth as a dentigerous or radicular cyst.

c., ovarian. Cystic formation in the ovary. SEE: *ovary.*

c., parasitic. Cyst enclosing the larval form of certain parasites as the cysticercus or hydatid of tapeworms or the larva of certain nematodes, i.e., *Trichinella.*

c., parovarian. Cystic formation of the parovarium.

c., pilar. An epithelial cyst with a wall that resembles follicular epithelium. It is filled with a homogeneous mixture of keratin and lipid. SYN: *trichilemma cyst.*

c., pilonidal. An elongated closed sac lined with stratified epithelium usually containing hair. Occurs in midline over sacral area of back. SYN: *pilonidal sinus.*

c., porencephalic. An anomalous cavity of the brain that communicates with the ventricular system.

c., proliferative. Cyst lined with epithelium that proliferates, forming projections that extend into the cavity of the cyst.

c., radicular. Granulomatous cyst located alongside the root of a tooth.

c., retention. Cyst retaining the secretion of a gland, as in a mucous or sebaceous cyst.

c., sebaceous. Cyst of a sebaceous gland.

c., seminal. Cyst of the epididymis, ductus deferens, or other sperm-carrying ducts that contain semen.

c., suprasellar. Cyst of the hypophyseal stalk just above the floor of the sella turcica. Its wall is frequently calcified or ossified.

c., tubo-ovarian. Ovarian cyst that ruptures into the lumen of an adherent uterine tube.

c., unilocular. Cyst containing only one cavity.

c., vaginal. Cystic formation in the vagina.

c., vitelline. Congenital cyst of the gastrointestinal canal. Lined with ciliated epithelium, it is the remains of the omphalomesenteric duct.

cyst, words pert. to: encysted; endocyst; hydrocyst; hydroma; marsupialization; steatoma.

cystadenocarcinoma (sĭs-tăd″ē-nō-kăr″sĭ-nō′mă) [Gr. *kystis,* bladder, + *aden,* gland, + *karkinos,* crab, + *oma,* tumor]. Glandular malignancy that forms cysts as it grows.

cystadenoma (sĭst″ăd-ĕn-ō′mă) [″ + ″ + *oma,* tumor]. An adenoma containing cysts. Cystoma blended with adenoma.

c., pseudomucinous. Cyst filled with a thick, viscid fluid and lined with tall epithelial cells.

c., serous. Cyst filled with a clear serous fluid and lined with cuboidal epithelial cells.

cystalgia (sĭs-tăl′jē-ă) [″ + *algos,* pain]. Pain in the bladder.

cystathionine (sĭs″tă-thī′ō-nīn). An intermediate compound in the metabolism of methionine to cysteine.

cystathioninuria (sĭs″tă-thī″ō-nī-nū′rē-ă). Hereditary disease caused by a deficiency of the enzyme important in metabolizing cystathionine. Clinically there are mental retardation, thrombocytopenia, and acidosis.

cystauxe (sĭs-tŏk′sē) [″ + *auxe,* increase]. Enlargement or thickening of the urinary bladder.

cystectasy (sĭs-tĕk'tă-sē) [" + *ektasis,* dilatation]. 1. An operation for extracting calculus from the bladder by dividing the membranous portion of the urethra, and then dilating the neck of the bladder. 2. Dilatation of bladder.

cystectomy (sĭs-tĕk'tō-mē) [" + *ektome,* excision]. 1. Removal of a cyst. 2. Excision of the cystic duct and the gallbladder, or just the cystic duct. 3. Excision of the urinary bladder or a part of it.

cysteic acid. Acid produced by the oxidation of cysteine. Further oxidation produces taurine.

cysteine hydrochloride (sĭs'tē-ĭn, sĭs-tē'ĭn). USP. A sulfur-containing amino acid, $C_3H_7NO_2S \cdot HCl \cdot H_2O$, found in many proteins. Valuable as a source of sulfur in metabolism.

cystelcosis (sĭs"tĕl-kō'sĭs) [" + *helkosis,* ulceration]. Ulceration of the urinary bladder.

cystic (sĭs'tĭk) [Gr. *kystis,* bladder]. 1. Of or pert. to a cyst. 2. Pert. to the gallbladder. 3. Pert. to the urinary bladder.

cystic duct. The duct of the gallbladder. It unites with the hepatic duct from the liver to form the common bile duct. SEE: *biliary tract* for illus.

cysticercoid (sĭs"tĭ-sĕr'koyd) [" + *kerkos,* tail, + *eidos,* form, shape]. The larval encysted form of a tapeworm. It differs from a cysticercus in having a much reduced bladder.

cysticercosis (sĭs"tĭ-sĕr-kō'sĭs) [" + " + *osis,* condition]. Infestation with cysticerci.

cysticercus (sĭs"tĭ-sĕr'kŭs) (pl. *cysticerci).* The encysted larval form of a tapeworm, consisting of a rounded cyst or bladder into which the scolex is invaginated. SYN: *bladder worm.*

   c. cellulosae. The bladder worm that is the larva of the pork tapeworm, *Taenia solium.*

cystic fibrosis. ABBR: CF. An inherited disease of exocrine glands affecting the pancreas, respiratory system, and apocrine glands. Usually begins in infancy and is characterized by chronic respiratory infection, pancreatic insufficiency, and increased electrolytes in sweat. CF is the major cause of severe chronic lung disease in children. CF may be associated with nasal polyposis, pansinusitis, rectal prolapse, failure to thrive, and liver disorders. The etiology and primary defect of cystic fibrosis are unknown. CF occurs in 1 in 2000 white and 1 in 17,000 black live births.

   TREAT: Therapy must be individualized, carefully monitored, and continued throughout the life span. Pulmonary disease is controlled with antibiotics. It is essential that secretions be cleaned from the airway. This is accomplished by intermittent aerosol therapy with a mixture of phenylephrine, propylene glycol, and saline. A mucolytic agent such as N-acetycysteine may be helpful; postural drainage; mist inhalation; bronchodilator therapy. Bronchoalveolar lavage has been of use in some patients. SEE: *bronchoalveolar lavage.*

   PROG: Median cumulative survival is approximately 20 years, and males survive much longer than females. The reason for this is not known. SYN: *fibrocystic disease of pancreas; mucoviscidosis.*

   NURSING IMPLICATIONS: Teach patient and family pulmonary chest physiotherapy (positioning, clapping, and vibration) followed by deep breathing and coughing to help mobilize secretions. Encourage fluid intake to thin dry secretions. Administer humidified air with IPPB therapy as prescribed, along with required pancreatic enzyme replacement. Teach patient to avoid respiratory infections, and to initiate prescribed antibiotic prophylaxis promptly. Assist child through developmental stages and tasks, substituting acceptable developmental activities for those the child is forbidden. Involve the child in his or her own care, offering valid choices and encouraging decision-making. Offer realistic reassurance regarding expectations post exacerbations. Provide emotional support to all involved as they work through feelings of anticipatory grief. SEE: *Nursing Diagnoses* in *Appendix.*

cysticotomy (sĭs"tĭ-kŏt'ō-mē) [" + *tome,* incision]. Incision of cystic bile duct. SYN: *choledochotomy.*

cystiform (sĭs"tĭ-form) [" + L. *forma,* form]. Having the form of a cyst.

cystigerous (sĭs-tĭj'ĕr-ŭs) [" + L. *gerere,* to bear]. Containing cysts.

cystine (sĭs'tēn) [Gr. *kystis,* bladder]. $C_6H_{12}N_2S_2O_4$. A sulfur-containing amino acid, which is produced by the action of acids on proteins that contain this compound. It is an important source of sulfur in metabolism.

cystinemia (sĭs"tĭ-nē'mē-ă) [*cystine* + Gr. *haima,* blood]. The presence of cystine in blood.

cystinosis (sĭs'tĭ-nō'sĭs) [" + Gr. *osis,* condition]. An inherited disease of cystine metabolism resulting in abnormal deposition of cystine in body tissues. The cause is disordered proximal renal tubular function. Clinically, failure to grow is accompanied by the development of rickets, corneal opacities, acidosis, and deposition of cystine in tissues. SYN: *cystine storage disease.*

cystinuria (sĭs″tĭ-nū′rē-ă) [″ + *ouron*, urine]. 1. The presence of cystine in urine. 2. A hereditary, metabolic disorder characterized by excretion of large amounts of cystine, lysine, arginine, and ornithine in the urine. Results in the development of recurrent urinary calculi.

cystitis (sĭs-tī′tĭs) [Gr. *kystis*, bladder, + *itis*, inflammation]. Inflammation of the bladder usually occurring secondary to ascending urinary tract infections. Associated organs (kidney, prostate, urethra) may be involved. May be acute or chronic. SEE: *Nursing Diagnoses* in *Appendix.*

   SYM: *Acute:* Frequent and painful urination. *Chronic:* Secondary to some other lesion with possibly pyuria as only symptom.

   TREAT: Antibiotics are useful in treating the infection, but more definitive therapy will be required if the basic cause is a renal calculus or a structural defect in the urinary tract such as obstruction.

   NURSING IMPLICATIONS: Assess patient for pain, urinary frequency, chills or fever. Assess urinary bladder for spasms, distention. Monitor urinary output for volume and frequency. Inspect urine for cloudiness, gross hematuria; send clean-catch specimen to laboratory for urinalysis and culture and sensitivity tests. Encourage fluid intake to dilute urine and decrease pain on voiding. Provide heat to lower abdomen to decrease spasms. Administer and teach patient about prescribed urinary antiseptics, analgesics, and antibiotics, evaluating therapeutic effectiveness and assessing for side effects. Explain that prescribed urinary antiseptics such as phenazopyridine hydrochloride (Pyridium) will color urine reddish-orange and may stain fabric.

   c., interstitial. Inflammation and irritation of the bladder wall. The etiology is unknown, and treatment is not specific.

   SYM: Lower abdominal or vaginal pain, urinary frequency and urgency.

cystitome (sĭs′tĭ-tōm) [″ + *tome*, incision]. Instrument for incision into sac of crystalline lens.

cystitomy (sĭs-tĭt′ō-mē). 1. Surgical incision of a cavity. 2. Incision of capsule of crystalline lens. 3. Incision into the gallbladder. SYN: *cholecystotomy.*

cysto-, cyst- [Gr. *kystis*, bladder]. Prefix pert. to the urinary bladder or a cyst.

cystoadenoma (sĭs″tō-ăd″ĕ-nō′mă) [″ + *aden*, gland, + *oma*, tumor]. Tumor containing cystic and adenomatous elements.

cystocele (sĭs′tō-sēl) [″ + *kele*, tumor, swelling]. A bladder hernia that protrudes into the vagina. Injury to the vesicovaginal fascia during delivery may allow the bladder to pouch into the vagina, causing a cysto-cele. May cause urinary frequency, urgency, and dysuria. SYN: *vesicocele.*

cystocolostomy (sĭs″tō-kō-lŏs′tō-mē) [″ + *kolon*, colon, + *stoma*, mouth]. Formation of communication between the gallbladder and colon.

cystodiaphanoscopy (sĭs″tō-dī″ă-făn-ŏs′kō-pē) [″ + *dia*, through, + *phanein*, to shine, + *skopein*, to examine]. Transillumination of abdomen by an electric light in bladder.

cystodynia (sĭs″tō-dĭn′ē-ă) [″ + *odyne*, pain]. Pain in the urinary bladder. SYN: *cystalgia.*

cystoelytroplasty (sĭs″tō-ē-lĭt′rō-plăs-tē) [″ + *elytron*, sheath, + *plassein*, to form]. Repair of a vesicovaginal fistula.

cystoepiplocele (sĭs″tō-ē-pĭp′lō-sēl) [″ + *epiploon*, omentum, + *kele*, tumor, swelling]. Herniation of a portion of the bladder and the omentum.

cystoepithelioma (sĭs″tō-ĕp″ĭ-thē″lē-ō′mă) [″ + *epi*, upon, + *thele*, nipple, + *oma*, tumor]. Epithelioma in stage of cystic degeneration.

cystofibroma (sĭs″tō-fī-brō′mă) [″ + L. *fibra*, fiber, + Gr. *oma*, tumor]. Fibrous tumor containing cysts.

cystogastrostomy (sĭs″tō-găs-trŏs′tō-mē) [″ + *gaster*, stomach, + *stoma*, mouth]. Joining an adjacent cyst, usually of the pancreas, to the stomach.

cystogram (sĭs′tō-grăm) [″ + *gramma*, something written]. A roentgenogram of the bladder.

cystography (sĭs-tŏg′ră-fē) [″ + *graphein*, to write]. Radiographic study of any cyst into which a radiopaque dye has been instilled, esp. the bladder.

cystoid (sĭs′toyd) [″ + *eidos*, form, shape]. Resembling a cyst.

cystojejunostomy (sĭs″tō-jē-jū-nŏs′tō-mē) [″ + L. *jejunum*, empty, + Gr. *stoma*, mouth]. Joining of an adjacent cyst to jejunum.

cystolith (sĭs′tō-lĭth) [″ + *lithos*, stone]. A vesical calculus.

cystolithectomy (sĭs-tō-lĭ-thĕk′tō-mē) [″ + *lithos*, stone, + *ektome*, excision]. Excision of a stone from the bladder.

cystolithiasis (sĭs-tō-lĭ-thī′ă-sĭs) [Gr. *kystis*, bladder, + *lithos*, stone, + *-iasis*, condition]. Formation of calculi in the bladder.

cystolithic (sĭs″tō-lĭth′ĭk) Pert. to a vesical calculus.

cystolutein (sĭs″tō-loo′tē-ĭn) [″ + L. *luteus*, yellow]. Yellow pigment found in some ovarian cysts.

cystoma (sĭs-tō′mă) [″ + *oma*, tumor] (pl. *cystomata, cystomas*). A cystic tumor; a growth containing cysts.

cystometer (sĭs-tŏm′ĕ-tĕr) [″ + *metron*,

measure]. Device for estimating the capacity of the bladder and pressure changes in it during micturition.

cystometrography (sĭs″tō-mĕ-trŏg′rä-fē) [″ + ″ + *graphein*, to write]. Graphic record of the pressure in the bladder at varying stages of filling.

cystomorphous (sĭs″tō-mor′fŭs) [″ + *morphe*, form]. Cystlike; cystoid.

cystopexy (sĭs′tō-pĕk″sē) [″ + *pexis*, fixation]. Surgical fixation of bladder to wall of abdomen.

cystoplasty (sĭs′tō-plăs″tē) [″ + *plassein*, to form]. Plastic operation upon the bladder.

cystoplegia (sĭs″tō-plē′jē-ă) [″ + *plege*, stroke]. Paralysis of the bladder.

cystoproctostomy (sĭs″tō-prŏk-tŏs′tō-mē) [″ + *proktos*, rectum, + *stoma*, mouth]. Surgical formation of a connection between the urinary bladder and the rectum.

cystoptosia, cystoptosis (sĭs″tŏp-tō′sē-ă, -sĭs) [″ + *ptosis*, a dropping]. Prolapse into the urethra of the vesical mucous membrane.

cystopyelitis (sĭs″tō-pī-ĕ-lī′tĭs) [″ + *pyelos*, pelvis, + *itis*, inflammation]. Inflammation of both the urinary bladder and the renal pelvis.

cystopyelonephritis (sĭs″tō-pī″ĕ-lō-nĕf-rī′tĭs) [″ + ″ + *nephros*, kidney, + *itis*, inflammation]. Cystitis combined with pyelitis.

cystoradiography (sĭs″tō-rā″dē-ŏg′rä-fē) [″ + L. *radius*, ray, + Gr. *graphein*, to write]. Radiography of the gallbladder or urinary bladder.

cystorectostomy (sĭs″tō-rĕk-tŏs′tō-mē) [″ + L. *rectum*, straight, + Gr. *stoma*, mouth]. Establishment of a surgical communication between the bladder and rectum.

cystorrhagia (sĭs″tō-rā′jē-ă) [″ + *rhegnynai*, to burst forth]. Hemorrhage from the urinary bladder.

cystorrhaphy (sĭst-or′ă-fē) [″ + *rhaphe*, seam, ridge]. Surgical suture of the bladder.

cystorrhea (sĭs″tō-rē′ă) [″ + *rhoia*, flow]. A discharge of mucus from the urinary bladder.

cystorrhexis [″ + *rhexis*, rupture]. Rupture of the bladder.

cystosarcoma (sĭs″tō-săr-kō′mă) [″ + *sarx*, flesh, + *oma*, tumor]. Sarcoma containing cysts or cystic formations.

cystoscope (sĭst′ō-skōp) [″ + *skopein*, to examine]. Instrument for interior examination of bladder and ureter. It is introduced through the urethra into the bladder.

cystoscopy (sĭs-tŏs′kō-pē) [″ + *skopein*, to examine]. Examination of the bladder

with the cystoscope.

cystospasm (sĭs′tō-spăzm) [Gr. *kystis*, bladder, + *spasmos*, a convulsion]. Spasmodic contractions of the urinary bladder.

cystostomy (sĭs-tŏs′tō-mē) [″ + *stoma*, mouth]. Surgical incision into the bladder.

cystotome (sĭs′tō-tōm) [″ + *tome*, incision]. Instrument for incision of bladder.

cystotomy (sĭs-tŏt′ō-mē) [″ + *tome*, incision]. Incision of bladder.

c., suprapubic. SEE: *suprapubic cystostomy.*

cystotrachelotomy (sĭs″tō-trā″kē-lŏt′ō-mē) [″ + *trachelos*, neck, + *tome*, incision]. Incision into neck of bladder.

cystoureteritis (sĭs″tō-ū-rē″tĕr-ī′tĭs) [″ + *oureter*, ureter, + *itis*, inflammation]. Inflammation of ureter and urinary bladder.

cystoureterogram (sĭs″tō-ū-rē′tĕr-ō-grăm) [″ + ″ + *gramma*, something written]. Roentgenographic study of the bladder and ureter.

cystourethritis (sĭs″tō-ū″rē-thrī′tĭs) [″ + *ourethra*, urethra, + *itis*, inflammation]. Inflammation of the urinary bladder and the urethra.

cystourethrocele (sĭs″tō-ū-rē′thrō-sēl) [″ + ″ + *kele*, tumor, swelling]. Prolapse of the bladder and urethra of the female.

cystourethrography (sĭs″tō-ū-rē-thrŏg′rä-fē) [″ + ″ + *graphein*, to write]. Roentgenographic examination of the bladder and urethra by use of radiopaque contrast media.

c., chain. Radiological examination in which a sterile beaded radiopaque chain is introduced into the bladder by means of a special catheter so that one end of the chain is in the bladder and the other extends outside via the urethra. This examination is useful in demonstrating anatomical relationships, esp. in female patients with persistent urinary incontinence.

c., voiding. Cystourethrography done prior to, during, and after voiding.

cystourethropexy, retropubic. General term for surgical procedure for correction of stress urinary incontinence.

cystourethroscope (sĭs″tō-ū-rē′thrō-skōp) [″ + *ourethra*, urethra, + *skopein*, to examine]. Device for examining the posterior urethra and urinary bladder.

cystovesiculography (sĭs″tō-vĕ-sĭk-ū-lŏg′rä-fē). Roentgenographic examination of the bladder and seminal vesicles.

cytarabine (sī-tār′ă-bēn). USP. Drug originally developed as an antileukemic agent and now used in treating herpesvirus hominis infections that cause either keratitis or encephalitis. Trade name is Cytosar-U. SYN: *cytosine arabinoside; ara-C.* SEE: *ara-A.*

-cyte (sīt) [Gr. *kytos,* cell]. Suffix denoting cell.

cytidine (sī'tǐ-dǐn). A nucleoside that is one of the four main riboside components of ribonucleic acid. It consists of a cytosine and D-ribose.

cyto-, cyt- [Gr. *kytos,* cell]. Prefix denoting the cell.

cytoanalyzer (sī″tō-ăn″ă-lī′zĕr). Device for detecting malignant cells in microscopic preparations or in fluids. The technique has not been perfected.

cytoarchitectonic (sī″tō-ärk″ĭ-tĕk-tŏn′ĭk) [″ + *architektonike,* architecture]. Pert. to structure and arrangement of cells.

cytobiology (sī″tō-bī-ŏl′ō-jē) [″ + *bios,* life, + *logos,* word, reason]. Biology of cells.

cytobiotaxis (sī″tō-bī-ō-tăk′sĭs) [″ + ″ + *taxis,* arrangement]. The influence of cells upon other living cells. SYN: *cytoclesis.*

cytoblast (sī'tō-blăst) [″ + *blastos,* germ]. A cell nucleus. SEE: *cyton.*

cytocentrum (sī″tō-sĕn′trŭm) [″ + *kentron,* center]. Minute body in cytoplasm of cell close to nucleus. SYN: *centrosome.* SEE: *sphere, attraction.*

cytochalasin B (sī″tō-kăl′ă-sĭn). A substance that destroys the contractile microfilaments in cells. This fragments cells and permits the fragments to be investigated.

cytochemistry (sī″tō-kĕm′ĭs-trē). The chemistry of the living cell.

cytochrome (sī'tō-krōm) [″ + *chroma,* color]. A pigment widely distributed in animals and plants. It plays an important role in cellular respiration. It is a mixture of three hemochromogens, designated cytochromes A, B, and C.

cytochrome oxidase. An enzyme of importance in biological oxidations, functioning in the transfer of electrons from cytochromes to oxygen, thus activating oxygen, which unites with hydrogen to form water.

cytochrome P-450. A protein similar to hemoglobin in the microsomes of liver cells and in organs such as the ovary, adrenal gland, testes, and placenta that produces steroids. Important in catalyzing the metabolism of steroid hormones and fatty acids and in the detoxification of a variety of chemical substances.

cytochylema (sī″tō-kī-lē′mă) [Gr. *kytos,* cell, + *chylos,* juice]. The more fluid constituent of cell protoplasm. SYN: *hyaloplasm.*

cytocidal (sī″tō-sī′dăl) [″ + L. *caedere,* to kill]. Lethal to cells.

cytocide (sī'tō-sīd). An agent that kills cells.

cytoclasis (sī″tŏk′lă-sĭs) [″ + *klasis,* destruction]. Destruction of cells.

cytoclastic [″ + *klasis,* destruction]. De-

structive to cells.

cytoclesis (sī″tō-klē′sĭs) [″ + *klesis,* a call]. The influence of living cells upon other cells. SYN: *cytobiotaxis.*

cytodendrite (sī″tō-dĕn′drīt) [″ + *dendron,* tree]. A dendrite given off from the body of a nerve cell.

cytodiagnosis (sī″tō-dī″ăg-nō′sĭs) [″ + *dia,* through, + *gignoskein,* to know]. Diagnosis of pathogenic conditions by the study of cells present in exudates, fluids, etc.

cytodieresis (sī″tō-dī-ĕr′ē-sĭs) [″ + *diairesis,* division]. Cell division.

cytodistal (sī″tō-dĭs′tăl) [″ + *distare,* to be distant]. Pert. to a neoplasm remote from the cell of origin.

cytogenesis (sī″tō-jĕn′ĕs-ĭs) [″ + *genesis,* generation, birth]. Origin and development of the cell.

cytogenetics (sī″tō-jĕ-nĕt′ĭks). The study of cytology in relation to genetics, esp. the study of chromosomal behavior in mitosis and meiosis. Modern cytogenetics has led to the identification of chromosomes as bearers of the genes and deoxyribonucleic acid (DNA) as the key molecule of the gene. The diagnosis of fetal abnormalities can be made as early as 11 to 14 weeks of gestation by using cytogenetic technique, following obtaining cells from the amniotic fluid or placenta. SEE: *amniocentesis; chorionic villus sampling.*

cytogenic (sī-tō-jĕn′ĭk) [″ + *gennan,* to produce]. Producing cells or promoting the production of cells.

cytogenous (si-tŏj′ĕn-ŭs) [″ + *gennan,* to produce]. Producing cells.

cytogeny (sī-tŏj′ĕ-nē) [″ + *genesis,* generation, birth]. The formation and development of the cell.

cytogerontology. The study of cell aging developed by Leonard Hayflick, M.D.

cytoglycopenia (sī″tō-glī-kō-pē′nē-ă) [″ + *glykys,* sweet, + *penia,* poverty]. Deficient glucose of blood cells. Also called cytoglucopenia.

cytohistogenesis (sī″tō-hĭs″tō-jĕn′ē-sĭs) [″ + *histos,* web, + *genesis,* generation, birth]. The structural development of cells.

cytohyaloplasm (sī″tō-hī′ăl-ō-plăzm) [″ + *hyalos,* glass, + LL. *plasma,* form, mold]. Fibrillary network of protoplasm. SYN: *hyaloplasm.*

cytoid (sī'toyd) [″ + *eidos,* form, shape]. Resembling a cell.

cytoinhibition (sī″tō-ĭn″hī-bĭsh′ŭn) [″ + L. *inhibere,* to restrain]. Phagocytic cell action that prevents the destruction of ingested bacteria by the cell.

cytokalipenia (sī″tō-kăl-ĭ-pē′nē-ă) [″ + L. *kalium,* potassium, + Gr. *penia,* poverty]. A potassium deficiency in body or blood cells.

cytokines. A group of extracellular factors that may be produced by a variety of cells including monocytes, lymphocytes, and other non-lymphoid cells. Cytokines produced by monocytes and lymphocytes are called monokines and lymphokines, respectively. Cytokines include the interleukins, some interferons, and tumor necrosis factor. They act by changing the cells that produce them (autocrine effect), altering other cells close to them (paracrine effect), and by affecting cells systemically (endocrine effect). Cytokines are important in controlling local and systemic inflammatory response. SEE: *acute phase reaction; interleukin-1; lymphokines; monokines; tumor necrosis factor.*

cytokinesis (sī″tō-kī-nē′sĭs) [″ + *kinesis,* movement]. The separation of the cytoplasm into two parts, which occurs in the latter stages of mitosis or cell division. SYN: *cytodieresis.*

cytologist. A person trained in cytology, q.v.

cytology (sī-tŏl′ō-jē) [″ + *logos,* word, reason]. The science that deals with the formation, structure, and function of cells.

cytolymph (sī′tō-lĭmf) [″ + L. *lympha,* lymph]. Matrix of cytoplasm of cells. SYN: *cytochylema; hyaloplasm.*

cytolysin (sī-tŏl′ĭ-sĭn) [″ + *lysis,* dissolution]. An antibody that causes disintegration of cells.

cytolysis (sī-tŏl′ĭ-sĭs). Dissolution or destruction of living cells. Hemolysis is the term used in case of red blood corpuscles, and bacteriolysis for bacteria.

cytomegalic inclusion disease. A disease, esp. of the neonatal period, characterized by variable severity in which an asymptomatic infection may leave no sequelae to a disease with fever, hepatosplenomegaly, microcephaly, and, in neonates, mental or motor retardation and perhaps death. Due to infection with cytomegalovirus, which can occur congenitally, postnatally, or later in life. The virus can produce a latent infection that may be subsequently activated by pregnancy, multiple blood transfusions, or following immunosuppression therapy. SEE: *ganciclovir.* SEE: *Nursing Diagnoses* in *Appendix.*

TREAT: There is no specific therapy.

cytomegalovirus (sī″tō-mĕg″ă-lō-vī′rŭs). One of a group of species-specific herpesviruses. The human cytomegalovirus inhabits the salivary glands and causes cytomegalic inclusion disease, q.v.

Cytomel. Trade name for liothyronine sodium.

cytometaplasia (sī″tō-mĕt″ă-plā′zē-ă) [Gr. *kytos,* cell, + *metaplasis,* change]. Change in form or function of cells.

cytometer (sī-tŏm′ĕ-ter) [″ + *metron,* measure]. Instrument for counting and measuring cells.

   c., flow. Device for measuring thousands of cells as they are forced one at a time through a focused light beam, usually a laser. Cells studied by use of this device need to be in an evenly dispersed suspension.

cytometry (sī-tŏm′ĕ-trē). The counting and measuring of cells.

   c., flow. SEE: *flow cytometry.*

cytomicrosome (sī-tō-mī′krō-sōm) [″ + *mikros,* small, + *soma,* body]. One of the minute granules in the protoplasm (cytoplasm) of the cell.

cytomitome (sī″tō-mī′tōm) [″ + *mitos,* thread]. Any part of the network of the cytoplasm.

cytomorphology (sī″tō-mor-fŏl′ō-jē) [″ + *morphe,* form, + *logos,* word, reason]. The study of the structure of cells.

cytomorphosis (sī″tō-mor-fō′sĭs) [″ + ″ + *osis,* condition]. The cellular transformations that a cell undergoes during its life.

cyton (sī′tŏn) [Gr. *kytos,* cell]. 1. A cell. 2. The body of a nerve cell. SYN: *perikaryon.*

cytopathic (sī″tō-păth′ĭk) [″ + *pathos,* disease]. 1. Concerning pathological changes in a cell. 2. Concerning the ability of an agent, esp. a virus, to injure or destroy a cell.

cytopathogenic effect (sī″tō-păth″ō-jĕn′ĭk) [″ + *pathos,* disease, + *gennan,* to produce]. In tissue culture, the morphologic changes seen in the cultured cells due to the effect of some pathogenic agent such as a virus.

cytopathology (sī″tō-păth-ŏl′ō-jē) [″ + ″ + *logos,* word, reason]. Study of the cellular changes in disease.

cytopenia [″ + *penia,* lack]. Diminution of cellular elements in blood or other tissues.

cytophagocytosis (sī″tō-făg″ō-sī-tō′sĭs) [″ + *phagein,* to eat, + *kytos,* cell, + *osis,* condition]. Destruction of other cells by phagocytes. SYN: *cytophagy.*

cytophagous (sī-tŏf′ă-gŭs). Devouring or destructive of cells.

cytophagy (sī-tŏf′ă-jē). Cell destruction by phagocytes. SYN: *cytophagocytosis.*

cytophilic (sī-tō-fĭl′ĭk) [″ + *philein,* to love]. Having an affinity for or attracted by cells, e.g., antibodies.

cytophotometry (sī″tō-fō-tŏm′ĕ-trē). SEE: *flow cytometry.*

cytophylaxis (sī″tō-fī-lăk′sĭs) [″ + *phylaxis,* protection]. The protection of cells against lysis.

cytophyletic (sī″tō-fī-lĕt′ĭk) [″ + *phyle,* tribe]. Pert. to genealogy of cells.

cytophysics (sī″tō-fĭz′ĭks) [″ + *physike,* (study of) nature]. The physics of cellular activity.

cytophysiology (sī″tō-fĭz-ē-ŏl′ō-jē) [″ + *physis*, nature, + *logos*, word, reason]. Physiology of the cell.

cytopipette (sī″tō-pī′pĕt). A pipette for obtaining specimens of cells, esp. from body fluids or cavities.

cytoplasm (sī′tō-plăzm) [″ + LL. *plasma*, form, mold, from Gr. *plassein*, to mold, spread out]. The protoplasm of a cell outside the nucleus.

cytoplast (sī′tō-plăst). The cytoplasm of a cell body as distinguished from the contents of the nucleus.

cytoproximal (sī″tō-prŏk′sĭ-măl) [″ + L. *proximus*, nearest]. Pert. to the portion of an axon nearest to the cell body from which it originates.

cytoreticulum (sī″tō-rĕ-tĭk′ū-lŭm) [″ + L. *reticulum*, network]. The fibrillar network supporting fluid of protoplasm.

cytorrhyctes (sī″tō-rĭk′tēz) [″ + *oryssein*, to dig]. Inclusion bodies in cells. Composed of virus elementary bodies, they were once thought to be of protozoal origin.

Cytosar-U. Trade name for cytarabine.

cytoscopy (sī-tŏs′kō-pē) [″ + *skopein*, to examine]. Microscopic examination of cells for purposes of diagnosis.

cytosine (sī′tō-sĭn). A pyrimidine base, $C_4H_5N_3O$, which is a component of ribonucleic and deoxyribonucleic acids.

   c. arabinoside. Drug originally developed as an antileukemic agent and now used in treating herpesvirus hominis infections that cause either keratitis or encephalitis. SYN: *cytarabine.*

cytoskeleton (sī″tō-skĕl′ĕ-tŏn). The internal structural framework of a cell consisting of three types of filaments: microfilaments, microtubules, and intermediate filaments. These form a dynamic framework for maintaining cell shape and allowing rapid changes in the three-dimensional structure of the cell.

cytosol (sī′tō-sŏl). The clear fluid portion of a cell. SYN: *hyaloplasm.*

cytosome (sī′tō-sōm) [″ + *soma*, body]. The portion of a cell exclusive of the nucleus.

cytostasis (sī-tŏs′tă-sĭs) [Gr. *kytos*, cell, + *stasis*, standing still]. Stasis of white blood corpuscles, as in the early stage of inflammation.

cytostatic (sī″tō-stăt′ĭk) [″ + *stasis*,

standing still]. Preventing the growth and proliferation of cells.

cytostome (sī′tō-stōm) [″ + *stoma*, mouth]. The mouth opening of one-celled organisms.

cytotactic (sī″tō-tăk′tĭk). Pert. to cytotaxia.

cytotaxia, cytotaxis (sī-tō-tăk′sē-ă, -sĭs) [″ + *taxis*, arrangement]. Attraction or repulsion of cells for each other.

cytotherapy [″ + *therapeia*, treatment]. 1. Treatment by use of glandular extracts; organotherapy. 2. Use of cytotoxic or cytolytic substances or serums in treating disease.

cytothesis (sī-tŏth′ē-sĭs) [″ + *thesis*, a placing]. Restoration or repair of injured cells.

cytotoxic (sī″tō-tŏks′ĭk). Destructive to cells.

cytotoxic agents. Chemicals that destroy cells or prevent their multiplication. They are a group of compounds developed for use in cancer chemotherapy. The ideal agent for such use should destroy the fast-growing cancer cells without injuring the normal cells of the body.

cytotoxin (sī″tō-tŏk′sĭn) [″ + *toxikon*, poison]. An antibody or toxin that attacks the cells of particular organs. SEE: *endotoxin; erythrotoxin; exotoxin; leukocidin; lysis; neurotoxin.*

cytotrophoblast (sī″tō-trō′fō-blăst) [″ + *trophe*, nourishment, + *blastos*, germ]. The thin inner layer of the trophoblast composed of cuboidal cells, the outer layer being the syntrophoblast. SYN: *layer, Langhans'.*

cytotropic (sī″tō-trŏp′ĭk, -trōp′ĭk) [″ + *trope*, a turn]. Having an affinity for cells.

cytotropism (sī-tŏt′rō-pĭzm) [″ + *trope*, a turn, + *-ismos*, condition]. The movement of cells toward or away from a stimulus such as drugs, viruses, bacteria, or physical conditions such as heat or cold.

Cytoxan (sī-tŏk′săn). Trade name for cyclophosphamide, q.v.

cytozoic (sī″tō-zō′ĭk) [″ + *zoon*, animal]. Living within or attached to a cell, as certain protozoa.

cytozoon (sī-tō-zō′ŏn). A protozoon that lives as an intracellular parasite.

cyturia (sī-tū′rē-ă) [Gr. *kytos*, cell, + *ouron*, urine]. Presence of any kind of cells in the urine.

Czermak's spaces (chăr′măks) [Johann Czermak, Ger. physiologist, 1828–1873]. The interglobular spaces in dentin due to failure of calcification.

D

δ, Δ. Lower and upper case delta, q.v., respectively, the fourth letter of the Greek alphabet.

D. 1. L. *da*, give; *date; daughter; deciduous;* L. *detur,* let it be given; *died; diopter; divorced; doctor.* 2. Chem. symb. for deuterium.

D-. In biochemistry, a symbol used as a prefix and written as a small capital letter to indicate the structure of certain organic compounds with asymmetric carbon atoms. If a carbon atom is attached to four different substituent groups that can be arranged in two ways and represent nonsuperimposable mirror images of each other, it is classed as asymmetric. The name of such a compound is preceded by D-. When there are only three dissimilar groups around the carbon atom, only one configuration in space is possible. The carbon atom is classed as symmetrical (or chiral), and the name is preceded by L-.

In other chemical nomenclature, a small letter *d-* or *l-* indicates the direction of rotation of a polarized light shown through a solution of the compound. When the plane of the light is rotated to the right, i.e., dextrorotatory, the compound's name is preceded by *d-*. If the light is rotated to the left, i.e., levorotatory, the name is preceded by *l-*.

If a D-compound that has an asymmetric carbon is also capable of rotating light and does so dextrorotatory, its name is preceded by D(+); if levorotatory, D(−). If the asymmetric carbon is of the L-form and is dextrorotatory, its name is prefixed by L(+); if levorotatory, the name is preceded by L(−).

d. *density;* L. *dexter* or *dextro,* right; L. *dies, day; distal; dorsal; duration.*

2,4-D. Herbicide, 2,4-dichlorophenoxy-acetic acid, that acts by stimulating broad-leaf plants to grow. It is toxic to humans and animals.

D/A. *digital to analog.*

Da. Symbol for dalton.

daboia, daboya (dă-boy′ă). Indian name for Russell's viper, a large poisonous snake of India, Burma, and Thailand. Its venom is used to enhance the action of certain blood coagulation factors.

dacarbazine (dă-kăr′bă-zēn). An alkylating agent used in treating neoplasms including malignant melanoma and Hodgkin's disease. Trade name is DTIC-Dome.

dacnomania (dăk″nō-mā′nē-ă) [Gr. *daknein,* to bite, + *mania,* insanity]. An irrational impulse to kill.

dacryadenalgia (dăk″rē-ăd-ĕn-ăl′jē-ă) [Gr. *dakryon,* tear, + *aden,* gland, + *algos,* pain]. Pain in a lacrimal gland. SYN: *dacryoadenalgia.*

dacryadenitis (dăk″rē-ăd-ĕ-nī′tĭs) [″ + ″ + *itis,* inflammation]. Inflammation of a lacrimal gland.

dacryadenoscirrhus (dăk″rē-ăd″ĕn-ō-skĭr′us) [″ + ″ + *skirrhos,* hardening]. Induration of a lacrimal gland.

dacryagogatresia (dăk″rē-ă-gŏg″ă-trē′sē-ă) [Gr. *dakryon,* tear, + *agogos,* leading, + *a-,* not, + *tresis,* perforate]. Occlusion of a tear duct.

dacryagogue (dăk′rē-ă-gŏg). An agent that stimulates the secretion of tears.

dacrycystalgia (dăk″rē-sĭs-tăl′jē-ă) [″ + *kystis,* cyst, + *algos,* pain]. Pain in a lacrimal sac. SYN: *dacryocystalgia.*

dacryelcosis (dăk″rē-ĕl-kō′sĭs) [″ + *helkosis,* ulceration]. Ulceration of the lacrimal apparatus.

dacryoadenalgia (dăk″rē-ō-ăd″ĕn-ăl′jē-ă) [″ + *aden,* gland, + *algos,* pain]. Pain in a lacrimal gland. SYN: *dacryadenalgia.*

dacryoadenectomy (dăk″rē-ō-ăd″ĕ-nĕk′tō-mē) [″ + ″ + *ektome,* excision]. Surgical removal of the lacrimal gland.

dacryoadenitis (dăk″rē-ō-ăd″ĕn-ī′tĭs) [″ + ″ + *itis,* inflammation]. Inflammation of lacrimal gland. It is rare; seen as complication in epidemic parotitis (mumps involving lacrimal gland); and present in Mikulicz's disease. May be acute or chronic.

dacryoblennorrhea (dăk″rē-ō-blĕn″ō-rē′ă) [″ + *blenna,* mucus, + *rhoia,* flow]. Discharge of mucus from a lacrimal sac, and chronic inflammation of the sac.

dacryocele (dăk′rē-ō-sēl) [″ + *kele,* tumor, swelling]. Protrusion of a lacrimal sac.

dacryocyst (dăk′rē-ō-sĭst) [″ + *kystis,* cyst]. The lacrimal sac.

dacryocystalgia (dăk″rē-ō-sĭs-tăl′jē-ă) [″ + ″ + *algos,* pain]. Pain in a lacrimal sac.

dacryocystectomy (dăk″rē-ō-sĭs-tĕk′tō-mē) [″ + *kystis,* cyst, + *ektome,* excision]. The excision of membranes of the lacrimal sac.

dacryocystitis (dăk″rē-ō-sĭs-tī′tĭs) [″ + ″ + *itis,* inflammation]. Inflammation of the tear sac involving mucous membrane of the lacrimal sac with submucous membrane, which later extends to connective tissue, surrounding it with resulting cellulitis. Usually secondary to prolonged obstruction of the nasolacrimal duct.

SYM: Profuse tearing (epiphora); redness and swelling in area of sac, which may also extend to lids and conjunctiva; pain, esp. on pressure over the lacrimal sac; overflow of tears.

TREAT: Hot compresses applied to area. Appropriate topical and systemic antibiotic therapy depending upon the organisms isolated from the inflamed area. Incision and drainage of inflamed area if fluctuant; attempt to restore permeability of duct with probe when acute symptoms have subsided; in chronic cases extirpate sac or do intranasal operation (dacryocystorhinostomy).

dacryocystoblennorrhea (dăk″rē-ō-sĭs″tō-blĕn-ō-rē′ă) [″ + ″ + *blenna,* mucus, + *rhoia,* flow]. Chronic inflammation of and discharge from the lacrimal sac.

dacryocystocele (dăk″rē-ō-sĭs′tō-sēl) [Gr. *dakryon,* tear, + *kystis,* cyst, + *kele,* tumor, swelling]. Herniated protrusion of lacrimal sac.

dacryocystography (dăk″rē-ō-sĭs-tŏg′ră-fē) [″ + ″ + *graphein,* to write]. Radiographic examination of the nasolacrimal drainage system after introduction of a contrast agent.

dacryocystoptosis (dăk″rē-ō-sĭs-tŏp-tō′sĭs) [″ + ″ + *ptosis,* a dropping]. Prolapse of the lacrimal sac.

dacryocystorhinostenosis (dăk″rē-ō-sĭs″tō-rī-nō-stĕ-nō′sĭs) [″ + ″ + *rhis,* nose, + *stenosis,* act of narrowing]. Narrowing or obliteration of the canal connecting the lacrimal sac with the nasal cavity. Test for patency is done by placing a weak sugar solution in the conjunctival space. If the duct is patent, the patient will report a sweet taste in the mouth.

dacryocystorhinostomy (dăk″rē-ō-sĭs″tō-rī-nŏs′tō-mē) [″ + ″ + ″ + *stoma,* mouth]. Surgical connecting of lumen of tear sac with nasal cavity.

dacryocystorhinotomy (dăk″rē-ō-sĭs″tō-rī-nŏt′ō-mē) [″ + ″ + ″ + *tome,* incision]. Surgical probing of the duct leading from the lacrimal sac into the nose.

dacryocystosyringotomy (dăk″rē-ō-sĭs″tō-sir″ĭn-gŏt′ō-mē) [″ + *kystis,* cyst, + *syrinx,* tube, + *tome,* incision]. Making an opening between the lacrimal sac and the nasal cavity.

dacryocystotome (dăk″rē-ō-sĭs′tō-tōm) [″ + ″ + *tome,* incision]. Device for incision of lacrimal sac.

dacryocystotomy (dăk″rē-ō-sĭs-tŏt′ō-mē). Incision of the lacrimal sac.

dacryocyte. Teardrop or pear-shaped red blood cells. Seen in myelofibrosis and certain anemias. Previously termed poikilocyte. SYN: *teardrop cell.*

dacryogenic. Promoting the shedding of tears.

dacryohelcosis (dăk″rē-ō-hĕl-kŏ′sĭs) [″ + *helcosis,* ulceration]. Ulceration of the lacrimal sac or duct.

dacryohemorrhea (dăk″rē-ō-hĕm″ō-rē′ă) [″ + *haima,* blood, + *rhoia,* flow]. Discharge of bloody tears.

dacryolith, dacryolite [Gr. *dakryon,* tear, + *lithos,* stone]. Concretion in lacrimal passages.

dacryolithiasis (dăk″rē-ō-lĭ-thī′ă-sĭs) [″ + *lithiasis,* formation of stones]. Presence of stones or calculi in the lacrimal apparatus.

dacryoma (dăk″rē-ō′mă) [″ + *oma,* tumor]. 1. A lacrimal tumor. 2. A tumorlike swelling due to obstruction of the lacrimal duct.

dacryon (dăk′rē-ŏn) [Gr. *dakryon*]. The lacrimal point of juncture of the lacrimal, frontal, and upper maxillary bones.

dacryops (dăk′rē-ŏps) [Gr. *dakryon,* tear, + *ops,* eye]. Constant flow of tears; dacryorrhea.

dacryopyorrhea (dăk″rē-ō-pī″ō-rē′ă) [″ + *pyon,* pus, + *rhoia,* discharge]. Discharge of pus from lacrimal duct.

dacryopyosis (″ + *pyosis,* suppuration]. Suppuration in the lacrimal sac or duct.

dacryorrhea (dăk″rē-ō-rē′ă) [″ + *rhoia,* flow]. Excessive flow of tears.

dacryosolenitis (dăk″rē-ō-sō-lĕn-ī′tĭs) [″ + *solen,* duct, + *itis,* inflammation]. Inflammation of a lacrimal or nasal duct.

dacryostenosis (dăk″rē-ō-stĕn-ō′sĭs) [″ + *stenosis,* act of narrowing]. Obstruction of or narrowing of a lacrimal or nasal duct.

dacryosyrinx (dăk″rē-ō-sī′rĭnks) [″ + *syrinx,* tube]. A lacrimal fistula.

DACT. *disposable absorption containment trunk.*

dactinomycin. An antibiotic of the actinomycin complex used as an antineoplastic agent. Trade name is Cosmegen.

dactyl (dăk′tĭl) [Gr. *daktylos,* finger]. A finger or toe; a digit of the hand or foot.

dactyledema (dăk″tĭl-ĕ-dē′mă) [″ + *oidema,* swelling]. Edema of the fingers or toes.

dactylion. Adhesions between or union of fingers or toes.

dactylitis [″ + *itis,* inflammation]. Chronic inflammation of bones of fingers and toes in very young children.

ETIOL: Usually tuberculous or syphilitic.

d., sickle cell. Painful swelling of the feet and hands during the first several years of life of children with sickle cell anemia, q.v.

dactylocampsodynia (dăk″tĭ-lō-kămp″sō-dĭn′ē-ă) [″ + *kampsis,* bend, + *odyne,* pain]. Painful contraction of one or more fingers.

dactylogram [″ + *gramma,* something written]. A fingerprint.

dactylography [″ + *graphein,* to write]. 1.

The study of fingerprints. 2. The act of using a machine for blind deaf-mutes to convey the signs of speech by touch.

dactylogryposis (dăk″tĭ-lō-grĭ-pō′sĭs) [″ + *gryposis*, curve]. Permanent contraction of the fingers.

dactylology (dăk-tĭl-ŏl′ō-jē) [″ + *logos*, word, reason]. Representing words by signs made with the fingers. SEE: *American Sign Language.*

dactylolysis (dăk″tĭ-lŏl′ĭ-sĭs) [″ + *lysis*, dissolution]. Spontaneous dropping off of fingers or toes. Seen in leprosy and ainhum and sometimes produced in utero when a hair firmly wrapped around a digit will cause amputation of the finger or toe.

dactylomegaly (dăk″tĭ-lō-měg′ă-lē) [″ + *megas*, large]. Abnormally large size of fingers and toes. SEE: *acromegaly.*

dactyloscopy (dăk″tĭ-lŏs′kō-pē) [″ + *skopein*, to examine]. Examination of fingerprints for purpose of identification.

dactylospasm (dăk′tĭ-lō-spăzm) [″ + *spasmos*, a convulsion]. Cramp of a finger or toe.

dactylus (dăk′tĭ-lŭs) [Gr. *daktylos*]. A toe or finger.

daily living skills. SEE: *activities of daily living.*

dairy food substitute. Foods resembling existing dairy foods in taste and appearance but differing in composition from the dairy food for which they are substituted.

Dakin's solution (dā′kĭns) [Henry D. Dakin, U.S. chemist, 1880–1952]. A solution for cleansing wounds, developed during World War I. A very dilute neutral solution (0.45% to 0.5%) of sodium hypochlorite and 0.4% boric acid.

Dale reaction [Sir Henry H. Dale, 1875–1968, Brit. scientist and Nobel prize winner in 1936]. A test that demonstrates the ability of muscle tissues from an animal that has been made anaphylactic to contract when re-exposed to the antigen. Either guinea pig uterine muscle or intestines are used. The test is very specific, as unrelated antigens will not cause the sensitized muscle to contract. Werner Schultz demonstrated the same phenomenon independent of Dale's work. SYN: *Schultz reaction.*

Dalmane. Trade name for flurazepam hydrochloride.

dalton (dawl′tŏn). ABBR: Da. An arbitrary unit of mass equal to $\frac{1}{12}$ the mass of carbon 12 or 1.657×10^{-24} gram.

Dalton, John. British chemist, 1766–1844.

D. -Henry law [Joseph Henry, U.S. physicist, 1797–1878]. When a mixture of gases is in equilibrium with a liquid, each gas will dissolve in the liquid in proportion to its partial pressure in the gas.

D.'s law. In a mixture of gases, the total pressure is equal to the sum of the partial pressures of each gas.

dam. A thin sheet of rubber used in dentistry and surgery to isolate a part from the surrounding tissues and fluids. Frequently a rubber dam is used as a surgical drain.

damp. 1. Moist, humid. 2. A noxious gas in a mine.

d., after. A gaseous mixture formed by the explosion of methane and air in a mine; contains large percentage of carbon dioxide, nitrogen, and carbon monoxide.

d., black. An atmosphere formed by the slow absorption of oxygen and the giving off of carbon dioxide by the coal in a mine.

d., cold. Foggy vapor in a mine charged with carbon dioxide.

d., fire. Methane, CH_4, found in coal mines.

d., white. Carbon monoxide formed in a mine following an explosion.

damping. The steady diminution of the amplitude of successive vibrations as of an electric wave or current.

danazol (dă′nă-zōl). USP. Drug that suppresses the action of the anterior pituitary. It is used in treating endometriosis. Trade name is Danocrine.

dance, Saint Vitus'. A disease characterized by involuntary and irregular jerkings and movements in diverse groups of muscles. SEE: *chorea.*

dancing disease. In Europe during the Middle Ages, epidemic dancing mania supposed to have been caused by the bite of the tarantula. SEE: *tarantism.*

dancing mania. Epidemic chorea.

D and C. *dilation* of the cervix and *curettage* of the uterus; a gynecologic procedure.

D and E. *dilation* and *evacuation* of the uterus. SEE: *D and C.*

dander (dăn′dĕr). Small scales from the hair or feathers of animals that may cause allergy in sensitive individuals.

dandruff. Normal exfoliation of the epidermis of the scalp in the form of dry, white scales. Sometimes due to seborrhea, q.v.

dandy fever. Dengue, q.v. An acute, epidemic, febrile disease occurring in tropical areas.

Dandy-Walker syndrome (dăn′dē-wawk′ĕr) [Walter E. Dandy, U.S. neurosurgeon, 1886–1946; Arthur E. Walker, U.S. surgeon, b. 1907]. Congenital hydrocephalus caused by blockage of the foramina of Magendie and Luschka, through which the cerebrospinal fluid passes.

Dane particles [David S. Dane, contemporary Brit. virologist]. The viral particles present in the serum of patients with hepatitis B. They contain DNA and are infectious.

Danocrine. Trade name for danazol, USP.

danthron (dăn'thrŏn). USP. A cathartic that helps to produce soft or semifluid stools. Trade names are Dorbane and Istizin.

Dantrium. Trade name for dantrolene sodium.

dantrolene sodium (dăn'trō-lēn). A muscle relaxant used to relieve spasticity. Trade name is Dantrium.

Danysz phenomenon [Jean Danysz, Polish-born pathologist in France, 1860–1928]. A phenomenon that provides an example of the reversibility of precipitation of complexes of antibodies and antigens. When a specified amount of diphtheria toxin is added all at once to an antitoxin serum, the mixture is nontoxic; but if the same quantity of toxin is added in portions at about 30-minute intervals, the mixture is toxic.

dapsone (dăp'sōn). USP. An antibacterial sulfone that is the drug of choice for treatment of all forms of leprosy. Also used in treatment of dermatitis herpetiformis. Frequent blood studies must be performed on patients receiving this drug for prolonged periods, as hemolysis, leukopenia, and methemoglobinemia can occur. Trade name is Avlosulfon.

Daranide. Trade name for dichlorphenamide.

Daraprim. Trade name for pyrimethamine.

Darbid. Trade name for isopropamide iodide.

Daricon. Trade name for oxyphencyclimine hydrochloride.

Darier's disease (dăr-ē-āz') [Ferdinand Jean Darier, Fr. dermatologist, 1856–1938]. A rare hereditary condition characterized by verrucous papular growths that coalesce into plaques of various sizes on the scalp, face, neck, trunk, and axillae. SYN: *keratosis follicularis.*

Darier's sign [Ferdinand Jean Darier, Fr. dermatologist, 1833–1916]. The skin change produced when the skin lesion in urticaria pigmentosa is briskly rubbed. The area usually begins to itch, becomes raised and surrounded by erythema. SEE: *mastocytosis; urticaria pigmentosa.*

darkroom. A light-tight room for processing photographic and x-ray films; there may be a filtered safe light for visibility according to the types of film used.

Darling's disease (dăr'lĭngz) [Samuel Taylor Darling, U.S. pathologist, 1872–1925]. Histoplasmosis.

dartoid (dăr'toyd) [Gr. *dartos,* skinned, + *eidos,* form, shape]. Resembling the tunica dartos in its slow, involuntary contractions.

dartos [Gr.]. The muscular, contractile tissue beneath the skin of the scrotum. SYN: *tunica dartos* [NA].

dartos muliebris. A veil-like smooth muscle just under the skin of the labia majora.

dartos muscle reflex. Wormlike contraction of dartos muscle following sudden cold application to perineum.

dartrous [Gr. *dartos,* skinned]. Of the nature of herpes; herpetic.

Darvon. Trade name for propoxyphene hydrochloride.

Darvon-N. Trade name for propoxyphene napsylate.

darwinian ear [Charles Robert Darwin, Brit. naturalist, 1809–1882]. An exaggeration of darwinian tubercle, q.v.

darwinian tubercle. A blunt point projecting from upper part of the helix of the ear.

darwinism (dăr'wĭ-nĭzm). The theory of biological evolution, q.v., through natural selection, q.v.

Datril. Trade name for acetaminophen.

Datura (dă-tū'ră). A genus of plants, one member of which, *Datura stramonium,* contains constituents of hyoscyamine and scopolamine, which have anticholinergic properties.

daughter (daw'tĕr). 1. A decay product. 2. A product of cell division, as a daughter cell or daughter nucleus. 3. One's female child.

daunorubicin hydrochloride. USP. An antineoplastic drug used in treating acute leukemia. Trade name is Cerubidine.

Davidsohn's sign [Hermann Davidsohn, Ger. physician, 1842–1911]. The lessening or absence of pupillary light reflex when an electric light is held in the closed mouth. Indicates presence of a tumor or fluid in the maxillary sinus.

DAWN. *Drug Abuse Warning Network.*

dawn phenomenon. In patients with diabetes mellitus of either type and in some normal persons, the insulin requirements between 6 a.m. and 9 a.m. increase markedly as compared to the midnight to 6 a.m. period. The increased dose of insulin required during this period is in contrast to the Somogyi phenomenon, q.v., which is managed by decreasing insulin during the critical period. SEE: *diabetes mellitus.*

day blindness. Inability to see well in a bright light.

day-care center. A place for the care of preschool children both of whose parents are employed or for some other reason are unable to care for their child during normal working hours.

daydream. Mental musing or fantasy while awake.

dazzle. Dimming of the vision due to intense stimulus of very bright light. SEE: *glare.*

dB, db. *decibel.*

D.C. *Doctor of Chiropractic; direct current.*

d/c. *discontinue.*

DDD pacing. SEE: *pacemaker, cardiac, artificial.*

D.D.S. *Doctor of Dental Surgery.* SEE: *D.M.D.*

DDST. *Denver Developmental Screening Test.*

DDT. Dichlorodiphenyltrichloroethane; now called chlorophenothane. A powerful insecticide effective against a wide variety of insects, esp. the flea, fly, louse, mosquito, bedbug, cockroach, Japanese beetle, and European corn borer. However, many species develop resistant populations, and birds and fish that feed on affected insects suffer toxic effects. The United States in 1972 banned DDT except for essential public health use and a few minor uses to protect crops for which there were no effective alternatives.

When ingested orally, it may cause acute poisoning. Symptoms are vomiting, numbness and partial paralysis of limbs, anorexia, tremors, and depression, resulting in death. SEE: *Poisons and Poisoning* in *Appendix.*

de- [L. *de,* from]. Prefix indicating down or from.

deacidification [" + *acidus,* sour, + *facere,* to make]. Neutralization of acidity.

deactivation [" + *activus,* acting]. The process of becoming inactive.

dead [AS. *dead*]. Without life or life processes. SEE: *death.*

dead tooth. A nonvital tooth by clinical standards, having the pulp removed by endodontic treatment; a poor choice of terms for, if the periodontal tissues are healthy, the tooth will continue to function without symptoms.

deaf [AS. *deaf*]. 1. Partially or completely lacking the sense of hearing. 2. Unwillingness to listen; heedless.

deafferentation (dē-ăf″ĕr-ĕn-tā′shŭn). Cutting the afferent nerve supply. SEE: *denervated.*

deaf-mute. A person who is unable to hear or speak.

deaf-mutism. The state of being both deaf and unable to speak.

deafness [AS.]. Complete or partial loss of ability to hear. Some deaf persons will experience the hallucination of hearing music. This is not due to insanity.

ETIOL: May occur from several causes such as injury or disease of that part of the cortex controlling the center for hearing; disease of the middle ear or the eighth cranial nerve; toxic effects of certain drugs; hysteria without any abnormality of the ear or brain; injury of the ear from loud noises such as the firing of a gun at close range, or prolonged and repetitive exposure to loud noise, whether in the workplace or in connection with a hobby that is done in a noisy environment, e.g., loud music or gun shooting; an abnormal mental state producing auditory aphasia or psychic deafness, q.v.; or congenital defects.

Some forms of conduction deafness may be remedied by a fenestration operation or stapes mobilization. SEE: *American Sign Language, otosclerosis.*

NURSING IMPLICATIONS: Teach patient to help prevent damage to hearing by avoiding excessively loud noises by wearing sound muffling ear plugs or muffs if exposed to industrial noise and to recognize that loud music can be as detrimental to hearing as the noise of a jackhammer. Avoid cleaning inside ears or putting sharp objects into ears. Nurses should be aware that many antibiotic and chemotherapeutic drugs are ototoxic, thus hearing should be evaluated continually when suspect drugs are used. When interacting with a person with a hearing deficit, the nurse should make her presence known to the patient by sight or gentle touch before beginning to speak. If possible, decrease background noise or remove patient from noisy area before speaking. Stand so that your face is illuminated to facilitate patient's visualization of lips and expressions; keep hands away from mouth and do not chew gum or food while speaking. Face directly to person's face, or toward ear with best hearing, and do not turn away while speaking. Use short words and simple sentences, speaking clearly and distinctly using a normal tone and speed if the patient is attempting to read your lips. Avoid exaggerated mouthing of words or loud tones. Placing your stethoscope in patient's ears and speaking into the bell may help to cut out extraneous sounds and direct words to the patient's ears, and to take advantage of bony conduction. If the patient is literate use sign language or finger spelling to communicate. If you write information, be clear and use large letters in case the patient has poor visual acuity.

   d., acoustic trauma. Impaired hearing due to repeated exposure to loud noise.

   d., aviator's. A temporary or permanent nerve deafness found in some aviators. It is caused by prolonged exposure to loud noise.

   d., bass. Inability to hear low-frequency tones.

   d., central. Deafness resulting from lesions of auditory tracts of the brain or auditory centers of the cerebral cortex.

   d., cerebral. Deafness due to brain lesion.

   d., ceruminous. Deafness due to plugs of cerumen (ear wax) blocking ear canal.

d., conduction. Deafness resulting from any condition that prevents sound waves from being transmitted to the auditory receptors. May result from wax obstructing the external auditory meatus, inflammation of the middle ear, ankylosis of ear bones, or fixation of footplate of stirrup. SEE: *otosclerosis; Rinne test; Weber test.*

d., cortical. Deafness due to disease of the cortical centers without a lesion.

d., high-frequency. Loss of hearing of high-frequency sounds.

d., hysterical. Deafness that will come and go in a hysterical patient.

d., nerve. Deafness due to a lesion of the auditory nerve or central neural pathways.

d., occupational. Deafness caused by working in places where noise levels are quite high. Persons working in such an environment should wear devices to protect the hearing sense from the noise.

d., ototoxic. Hearing loss due to the toxic effect of certain chemicals or medicines on the eighth nerve.

d., perceptive. Deafness resulting from lesions involving sensory receptors of the cochlea or fibers of the acoustic nerve, or a combination.

d., psychic. Condition in which auditory sensations are perceived but not comprehended.

d., sensineural. Deafness due to defective function of the cochlea or acoustic nerve.

d., tone. Inability to distinguish musical sounds.

d., word. Condition in which sounds are heard but interpretation of the words is impossible. A form of aphasia, q.v.

deamidase (dē-ăm′ĭ-dās). An enzyme that splits amides to form carboxylic acid and ammonia.

deamidization (dē-ăm″ĭ-dĭ-zā′shŭn). The removal of an amide group by hydrolysis.

deaminase. An enzyme that causes the removal of an amino group from organic compounds.

deamination, deaminization. Loss of the NH_2 radical from amino compounds. Alanine can be deaminized to give ammonia and pyruvic acid: $CH_3CH(NH_2)COOH + O = CH_3CO \cdot COOH + NH_3$. Deamination may be simple, oxidative, or hydrolytic. Oxidizing enzymes are called deaminizing enzymes when the oxidation is accompanied by splitting off of amino groups.

dearterialization (dē″ăr′tēr″ē-ăl-ĭ-zā′shŭn) [L. *de*, from, + Gr. *arteria*, artery]. Changing character of arterial into venous blood; deoxygenation.

dearticulation (dē″ăr-tĭk″ū-lā′shŭn). Dislocation of a joint.

death [AS. *death*]. Permanent cessation of all vital functions; the loss of brain stem and spinal reflexes and flat EEGs over at least 24 hours. The following definitions of death have also been considered: (1) Total irreversible cessation of cerebral function, spontaneous function of the respiratory system, and spontaneous function of the circulatory system. (2) The final and irreversible cessation of perceptible heartbeat and respiration. Conversely, as long as any heartbeat or respiration can be perceived, with or without mechanical or electrical aids, and regardless of how the heartbeat and respiration were maintained, death has not occurred.

Conditions such as cardiac standstill or complete lack of renal function meant certain death at one time. But the use of cardiac pacemakers, artificial hearts and kidneys, heart transplants, and kidney transplants has made this definition of death untenable. SEE: *life.*

SIGNS: The principal sign of death is cessation of the heart's action. Other indications are absence of reflexes, cessation of electrical activity in the brain as determined by EEG, manifestations of rigor mortis, q.v., and a mottled discoloration of the body, esp. over all parts where there is pressure. In case of an emergency, the usual symptoms of death often are found to be unreliable. Attempts at resuscitation should continue to be made indefinitely. No harm can be done in attempting to resuscitate one who seems to be deceased; successes are numerous.

Determining time lapse since death occurred: Take the rectal temperature. In general the body loses one degree of Fahrenheit temperature each hour following death. Of course, the rate of heat loss varies with temperature of the surrounding air, water, or snow.

Emotional aspects of dying: Patients and their families rely upon physicians to provide technical expertise when illness occurs. In addition, when the patient is dying, the patient and the family require emotional and physical support. The dying patient who is conscious needs to be touched and assured that, in this final chapter, the physician will be doing what is needed, i.e., to care for the patient. SEE: *advance directive; choosing death; death investigation; death with dignity; do not attempt resuscitation; living will; uniform donor card.*

NURSING IMPLICATIONS: Follow legal procedures concerning requesting organ donation. Be sure appropriate health care professionals are notified of patient and family wishes regarding organ donation so that necessary protocols are followed.

Note the times of cessation of respirations and heartbeat, and notify the physician to certify death. Notify family according to hospital policy and provide emotional support. Document and remove auxiliary equipment (catheters, drainage tubes, venous lines, and all other devices) leaving hospital ID bracelet in place. Place the body in a supine position with the limbs extended and head slightly elevated. Insert dentures and close mouth and eyes. Cleanse the body, applying clean dressings as needed, and pack the rectum with absorbent material to prevent drainage. Cover the body to the chin with a sheet. Collect and record the patient's valuables and belongings. Allow the family to visit as desired, offering comfort and support. Have family member sign for and remove patient belongings according to hospital policy. After family has gone, prepare the body for the morgue, applying chin strap, wrist and ankle protection, and ties and shroud. Identify body with tags tied to wrist or foot and outside of shroud, including name, ID number, room and bed numbers, attending physician, and date and time of death. Transport body to morgue and place in refrigeration unit according to hospital policy.

    d., biologic. Death due directly to natural causes.

    d., black. Former name for bubonic plague.

    d., brain. Brain death, q.v.

    d., crib. Sudden infant death syndrome, q.v.

    d., fetal. Death of a fetus in utero.

    d., functional. Central nervous system death with vital functions being artificially supported.

    d., good. Death in which the rights of the individual concerned have been respected, and during which the dying person was made as comfortable as possible and was in the company of persons he or she knew and loved. SEE: *advance directive; hospice; living will; uniform donor card.*

    d., local. Gangrene or necrosis of a part.

    d., man-made. Death due to something other than natural causes, e.g., murder, war, political violence.

    d., molecular. Death of cell life.

    d., sudden. SEE: *sudden death.*

death, words pert. to: agonal; ante mortem; autopsy; choosing death; death investigation; demise; do not attempt resuscitation; euthanasia; in articulo mortis; in extremis; lethal; "necr-" words; "no code" orders; posthumous; post mortem; putrefaction; rigor mortis; suicide; uniform donor card.

deathbed. 1. The bed on which a person dies. 2. The final hours preceding death.

deathbed statement. A declaration made at the time immediately preceding death. Such a statement, if made with the consciousness and belief that death is impending and in the presence of a witness, may be held in law as equally binding as a statement made under oath. SYN: *antemortem statement.*

death investigation. It is customary that violent, suspicious or unexpected death, and deaths unattended by a physician be investigated. The investigation is, by law, done by an officially appointed person. The investigation system includes medical examiners, coroners, and combined medical examiner and coroner. Which system is used varies from state to state. SEE: *coroner; medical examiner.*

death rate. The number of deaths occurring per 1000 of the population in a given area within a specified time. SYN: *mortality.*

death rattle. A sound heard in the throat of the dying. Caused by the accumulation of mucus in the throat due to absence of the cough reflex. The breath moving through the mucus makes the "rattle" sound.

death sentence. In medicine, discovery or diagnosis of a disease that will almost inevitably lead to the death of the patient.

"death with dignity." A concept resulting from the fact that it is possible to maintain metabolic functions in persons who will or may eventually remain in a coma for the remainder of their lives. In order to prevent this prolongation of life, a patient, or the family if the patient is unconscious, may sign this statement: "I request that I be allowed to die and not be kept alive by artificial means or heroic measures. I ask also that drugs be mercifully administered to me to alleviate terminal suffering even if they may hasten the moment of death." SEE: *advance directive; assisted suicide; do not attempt resuscitation; "no code" orders.*

debilitant [L. *debilis,* weak]. 1. A remedy used to reduce excitement. 2. That which weakens.

debilitate. To produce weakness or debility.

debility. Weakness of tonicity in functions or organs of the body.

débouchement (dā-boosh-mŏn′) [Fr.]. Opening or emptying into another part.

Debove's membrane (dĕ-bōvz′) [Georges Maurice Debove, Fr. physician, 1845–1920]. Layer of connective tissue cells between the epithelium and basement tissue of respiratory and intestinal epithelia.

débride (dā-brēd′) [Fr.]. To perform the action of debridement.

débridement (dā-brēd-mŏn′) [Fr.]. The removal of foreign material and dead or damaged tissue, esp. in a wound.

    d., canal or d., root canal. The removal

of organic and inorganic debris from a dental root canal by mechanical or chemical methods. This procedure is done in preparation for sealing the canal to prevent further decay of the tooth.

   d., enzymatic. Use of proteolytic enzymes to remove dead tissue from a wound. The enzyme does not attack viable tissues.

   d., epithelial. The removal of the entire epithelial lining or attachment epithelium from a periodontal pocket. SEE: *curettage.*

debris (dĕ-brē') [Fr., remains]. The remains of broken down or damaged cells or tissue.

debrisoquin (dĕb-rĭs'ō-kwĭn). An antihypertensive medicine not generally available in the U.S.

debt (dĕt). Deficit.

   d., oxygen. After strenuous, i.e., anaerobic, physical activity, the oxygen required (in addition to that required while resting, in the recovery period) to oxidize the excess lactic acid produced and to replenish the depleted stores of adenosine triphosphate and phosphocreatinase.

deca-, dec- [Gr. *deka*]. Prefix indicating ten.

Decaderm. Trade name for dexamethasone.

Decadron. Trade name for dexamethasone.

Decadron-LA. Trade name for dexamethasone acetate.

Deca-Durabolin. Trade name for nandrolone decanoate.

decagram (dĕk'ă"grăm) [Gr. *deka,* ten, + *gramma,* small weight]. A weight of 10 grams.

decalcification (dē"kăl-sĭ-fĭ-kā'shŭn) [L. *de,* from, + *calx,* lime, + *facere,* to make]. The removal or withdrawal of lime salts from bone or teeth.

decalcify. 1. To soften bone by removal of calcium or its salts by acids. 2. To remove the mineral content from bones or teeth so that sections can be cut and stained for microscopic examination.

decaliter (dĕk'ă-lē"tĕr) [Gr. *deka,* ten, + Fr. *litre,* liter]. A measure of 10 liters, equivalent to 10,000 milliliters, or about 10.57 quarts. SEE: *deciliter.*

decalvant (dē-kăl'vănt) [L. *decalvare,* to make bald]. Destroying hair or making bald.

decameter (dĕk'ă-mē-tĕr) [Gr. *deka,* ten, + *metron,* measure]. A measure of 10 meters; 393.71 in.

decannulation (dē-kăn"nū-lā'shŭn). The removal of a cannula.

decanormal (dĕk"ă-nor'măl) [" + L. *norma,* rule]. Pert. to a solution 10 times as strong as one normal solution. It contains 10 gm equivalent weights of the substance per liter. SEE: *normal.*

decant (dē-kănt') [L. *de,* from, + *canthus,* rim of a vessel]. To pour off liquid so the sediment remains in the bottom of the container.

decantation. The gentle pouring off of a liquid so the sediment remains.

decapitation (dē-kăp"ĭ-tā'shŭn) [" + *caput,* head]. 1. The separation of the head from the body; beheading. 2. Separating the head from the shaft of a bone. SYN: *detruncation.*

decapsulation [" + *capsula,* little box]. Removal of a capsule of an organ.

decarboxylase (dē"kăr-bŏk'sĭ-lās). An enzyme that catalyzes the release of carbon dioxide from compounds such as amino acids.

decarboxylation, decarboxylization (dē" kăr-bŏks-ĭ-lā'shŭn, -ĭl"ĭ-zā'shŭn). A chemical reaction whereby the carboxyl group, —COOH, is removed from an organic compound.

Decaspray. Trade name for dexamethasone.

decavitamin capsules (dĕk"ă-vī'tă-mĭn). USP. A vitamin preparation that contains vitamins A, D, and C; calcium pantothenate; folic acid; niacinamide; pyridoxine hydrochloride (vitamin B_6); riboflavin; thiamine hydrochloride (vitamin B_1); a suitable form of alpha-tocopherol (vitamin E); and cyanocobalamin (vitamin B_{12}).

decay (dē-kā') [" + *cadere,* to fall, die]. 1. Gradual loss of vigor with physical and mental deterioration as in aging. SEE: *senility.* 2. To waste away. 3. Decomposition of organic matter by the action of microorganisms. SEE: *caries; cementoclasia.* 4. Disintegration of radioactive substances.

   d., radioactive. The continual loss of energy by radioactive substances. This disintegration of the nucleus by the emission of alpha, beta, or gamma rays eventually results in the complete loss of radioactivity. The time required for some materials to become stable may be minutes and, for others, thousands of years. SEE: *half-life.*

   d., tooth. Caries, q.v.

deceleration (dē-sĕl"ĕ-rā'shŭn). Decrease in velocity.

deceleration injury. Head injury when the moving head hits a stationary object, such as a dancer hitting a wall.

deception. The deliberate misrepresentation of facts through words or actions in order to make someone else believe that which is not true. In medicine, deception may take the form of not telling a patient the truth or ommitting information that would help the patient make a decision about the medical care providers. Conversely, a patient may decieve the health care team concerning important historical events or present condition.

decerebrate (dē-sĕr'ĕ-brāt) [" + *cerebrum,* brain]. 1. To eliminate cerebral function by decerebration. 2. A person or animal who has been subjected to decerebration.

decerebrate posture. The posture present in an individual with decerebrate rigidity. The extremities are stiff and extended, and the head is retracted.

decerebrate rigidity. SEE: *rigidity, decerebrate.*

decerebration (dē-sĕr-ĕ-brā'shŭn). Removal of the brain or cutting the spinal cord at the level of the brain stem. SEE: *pithing.*

dechlorination, dechloridation [" + Gr. *chloros*, green]. Reduction in the amount of chlorides in the body by reduction of or withdrawal of salt in the diet.

Decholin. Trade name for dehydrocholic acid.

deci- [L. *decimus*, tenth]. Prefix indicating one-tenth.

decibel (dĕs'ĭ-bĕl) [L. *decimus*, tenth, + *bel*, unit of sound]. The unit for expressing logarithmically the pressure or power (and thus degree of intensity or loudness) of sound.

decidophobia [*decide* + Gr. *phobos*, fear]. Fear of making a decision.

decidua (dē-sĭd'ū-ă) [L. *deciduus*, falling off]. The name given to the endometrium or lining of the uterus during pregnancy, and the tissue around the ectopically located fertilized ovum, e.g., in the fallopian tube or peritoneal cavity. The gland structures of the endometrium and the interstitial cells undergo marked hypertrophy. The decidua divides itself into an outer or compact layer and an inner spongy layer.

d. basalis. [NA] That part of the decidua that unites with the chorion to form the placenta. SYN: *d. serotina.*

d. capsularis. [NA] That part of the decidua that surrounds the chorionic sac. SYN: *d. reflexa.*

d. menstrualis. The layer of the uterine endometrium that is shed during menstruation.

d. parietalis. [NA] The endometrium during pregnancy except at the site of the implanted blastocyst. SYN: *d. vera.*

d. reflexa. D. capsularis.

d. serotina. D. basalis.

d. vera. D. parietalis.

decidual (dē-sĭd'ū-ăl). Pert. to or resembling the decidua.

deciduation (dē-sĭd'ū-ā'shŭn). The loss of the decidua during menstruation.

deciduitis (dē-sĭd'ū-ī'tĭs) [" + Gr. *itis*, inflammation]. Inflammation of the decidua.

deciduoma (dē-sĭd'ū-ō'mă) [" + Gr. *oma*, tumor]. A uterine tumor containing decidual tissue. Thought to arise from portions of decidua retained within the uterus following an abortion.

d., benign. During pregnancy, the more or less normal invasion of the uterine musculature by the syncytium, which disappears after the gestation is completed.

d., Loeb's. Decidual tissue produced within the uteruses of experimental animals as a result of mechanical or hormonal stimulation.

d., malignant. Tumor consisting of syncytial and Langhans' cells, which tend to invade the general system by way of the bloodstream. Specific therapy with methotrexate may cause a complete remission. SYN: *choriocarcinoma; chorioepithelioma.*

ETIOL: This tumor may arise following a full-term pregnancy, an ectopic pregnancy, an abortion, a miscarriage, and particularly a vesicular mole.

DIAG: May be made by histological study, aided by the symptoms and the Ascheim-Zondek test, the results of which remain strongly positive during the presence of this type of tumor.

TREAT: Chemotherapy with the folic acid antagonist methotrexate (USP) or dactinomycin.

deciduomatosis (dē-sĭd'ū-ō-mă-tō'sĭs) [" + Gr. *oma*, tumor, + *osis*, condition]. Excessive and irregular formation of decidual tissue in the nonpregnant state.

deciduosarcoma [" + Gr. *sarx*, flesh, + *oma*, tumor]. A tumor of the chorion. SYN: *choriocarcinoma; chorioepithelioma.*

deciduous (dē-sĭd'ū-ŭs) [L. *deciduus*]. Falling off; subject to being shed.

deciduous teeth. An old term for the primary dentition, which begins to appear in the mouth at about 6 months of age and proceeds until the last teeth are replaced by permanent teeth in the 12th or 13th year. SEE: *dentition.*

decigram (dĕs'ĭ-grăm) [L. *decimus*, tenth, + Gr. *gramma*, small weight]. One tenth of a gram.

deciliter (dĕs'ĭ-lē-tĕr) [" + Fr. *litre*]. ABBR: dl. A unit of volume in the SI system of measurement that is equal to 0.1 liter or 100 milliliters.

decimeter (dĕs'ĭ-mē"tĕr) [" + Gr. *metron*, measure]. One tenth of a meter.

decinormal (dĕs"ĭ-nor'măl) [" + *norma*, rule]. Having one-tenth the strength of a normal solution. SEE: *normal.*

decipara (dē-sĭp'ă-ră) [" + *parere*, to bring forth, to bear]. A woman who has given birth for the tenth time to an infant or infants, alive or dead, weighing 500 grams or more. SYN: *para X.*

decision analysis. A logically consistent approach to the common clinical problem of needing to make a decision when its consequences cannot be foretold with certainty.

Definitions of Commonly Used Terms in Epidemiology and Decision Making

Test Result	Disease State	
	Present	Absent
Positive	a (true positive)	b (false positive)
Negative	c (false negative)	d (true negative)

Prevalence (prior probability)	=	$(a + c)/(a + b + c + d)$	= all patients with the disease/all patients tested
Sensitivity	=	$a/(a + c)$	= true-positive test results/all patients with the disease
Specificity	=	$d/(b + d)$	= true-negative test results/all patients without the disease
False-negative rate	=	$c/(a + c)$	= false-negative test results/all patients with the disease
False-positive rate	=	$b/(b + d)$	= false-positive test results/all patients without the disease
Positive predictive value	=	$a/(a + b)$	= true-positive test results/all positive test results
Negative predictive value	=	$d/(c + d)$	= true-negative test results/all patients with negative results
Overall accuracy	=	$(a + d)/(a + b + c + d)$	= true-positive + true-negative test results/all tests

Source: Braunwald, E, et al: Harrison's Principles of Internal Medicine, ed 11. McGraw-Hill, New York, 1987.

The uncertainties in medical practice are due to a great number of factors including biological variation and the inadequacy of the clinical data available for an individual patient. There are three steps in this process: the outcome or consequences of each decision option are described schematically by the use of a decision tree, q.v.; probability is used to quantify the uncertainties inherent in each decision option; each of the possible outcomes of a decision is characterized by a number that serves as a measure of the patient's preference for that outcome as compared with the other outcomes. After the last step is completed, each outcome is assigned a "utility" value in which 1.0 indicates a perfect outcome and 0 is the worst possibility. Use of decision analysis will most probably become increasingly important in helping all members of the professional health care team and the patient make logical choices concerning management of the illness.

decision making. The process of using all of the information available about a patient and arriving at a decision concerning the therapeutic plan. SEE: table.

decision tree. A graphical analysis of the decisions or choices available to the physician in deciding upon a course of action in treating a patient. Included in the graph, i.e. decision tree, will be the probabilities of all of the events that may result from each decision. SEE: decision analysis.

Declaration of Geneva. A statement adopted in 1948 by the Second General Assembly of the World Medical Association. Some medical schools use it at graduation exercises.

"At the time of being admitted as Member of the Medical Profession I solemnly pledge myself to consecrate my life to the service of humanity. I will give to my teachers the respect and gratitude which is their due; I will practice my profession with conscience and dignity; The health of my patient will be my first consideration; I will respect the secrets which are confided in me; I will maintain by all the means in my power, the honor and the noble traditions of the medical profession; my colleagues will be my brothers; I will not permit considerations of religion, nationality, race, party politics or social standing to intervene between my duty and my patient; I will maintain the utmost respect for human life, from the time of conception; even under threat, I will not use my medical knowledge contrary to the laws of humanity. I make these promises solemnly, freely and upon my honor." SEE: Hippocratic oath; Nightingale Pledge; Prayer of Maimonides.

Declaration of Hawaii. The General Assembly of the World Psychiatric Association has laid down the following ethical guidelines for psychiatrists all over the world. These guidelines were unanimously adopted by the association in 1976.

(1) The aim of psychiatry is to promote health and personal autonomy and growth. To the best of his or her ability, consistent with accepted scientific and ethical principles, the psychiatrist shall serve the best interests of the patient and be also concerned for the common good and a just allocation of health resources.

To fulfill these aims requires continuous research and continual education of health care personnel, patients, and the public.

(2) Every patient must be offered the best therapy available and be treated with the solicitude and respect due to the dignity of all human beings and to their autonomy over their own lives and health.

The psychiatrist is responsible for treatment given by the staff members and owes them qualified supervision and education. Whenever there is a need, or whenever a reasonable request is forthcoming from the patient, the psychiatrist should seek the help or the opinion of a more experienced colleague.

(3) A therapeutic relationship between patient and psychiatrist is founded on mutual agreement. It requires trust, confidentiality, openness, cooperation, and mutual responsibility. Such a relationship may not be possible to establish with some severely ill patients. In that case, as in the treatment of children, contact should be established with a person close to the patient and acceptable to him or her.

If and when a relationship is established for purposes other than therapeutic, such as in forensic psychiatry, its nature must be thoroughly explained to the person concerned.

(4) The psychiatrist should inform the patient of the nature of the condition, of the proposed diagnostic and therapeutic procedures, including possible alternatives, and of the prognosis. This information must be offered in a considerate way and the patient be given the opportunity to choose between appropriate and available methods.

(5) No procedure must be performed or treatment given against or independent of a patient's own will, unless the patient lacks capacity to express his or her own wishes or, owing to psychiatric illness, cannot see what is in his or her best interest or, for the same reason, is a severe threat to others.

In these cases compulsory treatment may or should be given, provided that it is done in the patient's best interests and over a reasonable period of time, a retroactive informed consent can be presumed, and, whenever possible, consent has been obtained from someone close to the patient.

(6) As soon as the above conditions for compulsory treatment no longer apply the patient must be released, unless he or she voluntarily consents to further treatment.

Whenever there is compulsory treatment or detention there must be an independent and neutral body of appeal for regular inquiry into these cases. Every patient must be informed of its existence and be permitted to appeal to it, personally or through a representative, without interference by the hospital staff or by anyone else.

(7) The psychiatrist must never use the possibilities of the profession for maltreatment of individuals or groups, and should be concerned never to let inappropriate personal desires, feelings, or prejudices interfere with the treatment.

The psychiatrist must not participate in compulsory psychiatric treatment in the absence of psychiatric illness. If the patient or some third party demands actions contrary to scientific or ethical principles the psychiatrist must refuse to cooperate. When, for any reason, either the wishes or the best interests of the patient cannot be promoted he or she must be so informed.

(8) Whatever the psychiatrist has been told by the patient, or has noted during examination or treatment, must be kept confidential unless the patient releases the psychiatrist from professional secrecy, or else vital common values or the patient's best interest makes disclosure imperative. In these cases, however, the patient must be immediately informed of the breach of secrecy.

(9) To increase and propagate psychiatric knowledge and skill requires participation of the patients. Informed consent must, however, be obtained before presenting a patient to a class and, if possible, also when a case history is published, and all reasonable measures be taken to preserve the anonymity and to safeguard the personal reputation of the subject.

In clinical research, as in therapy, every subject must be offered the best available treatment. His or her participation must be voluntary, after full information has been given of the aims, procedures, risks, and inconveniences of the project, and there must always be a reasonable relationship between calculated risks or inconveniences and the benefit of the study.

For children and other patients who cannot themselves give informed consent this should be obtained from someone close to them.

(10) Every patient or research subject is free to withdraw for any reason at any time from any voluntary treatment and from any teaching or research program in which he or

she participates. This withdrawal, as well as any refusal to enter a program, must never influence the psychiatrist's efforts to help the patient or subject.

The psychiatrist should stop all therapeutic, teaching, or research programs that may evolve contrary to the principles of this Declaration. SEE: *Declaration of Geneva; Hippocratic oath; Nightingale Pledge; Prayer of Maimonides.*

declination (dĕk″lĭ-nā′shŭn). Cyclophoria, q.v.

declinator (dĕk′lĭn-ā″tor) [L. *declinare*, to turn aside]. Instrument used during trephining for holding apart the dura mater.

decline (dē-klīn′). 1. Progressive decrease. 2. Declining period of a disease.

declivis cerebelli (dē-klīv′ĭs sĕr-ĕ-bĕl′ī) [L.]. Sloping posterior portion of the monticulus of the superior vermis of the cerebellum.

decoction (dē-kŏk′shŭn) [L. *de*, down, + *coquere*, to boil]. A liquid medicinal preparation made by boiling vegetable substances with water. When the strength and method of preparation are not otherwise specified, it is made by boiling five parts of the coarsely comminuted drug for 15 minutes with enough water to make 100 parts. There are no official decoctions.

decollation (dē″kŏl-ā′shŭn) [L. *de*, from, + *collum*, neck]. Decapitation, esp. of the fetus during labor. SYN: *decapitation; detruncation.*

décollement (dā-kŏl-mŏn′) [Fr., ungluing]. Separation of two adherent structures.

decoloration (dē-kŭl″or-ā′shŭn). Loss or removal of color or pigment.

decompensation [L. *de*, from, + *compensare*, to make good again]. 1. Failure of heart to maintain adequate circulation. 2. In psychology, failure of defense system mechanism such as occurs in relapses of mental patients.

decomplementize. To remove complement.

decomposition (dē-kŏm-pō-zĭsh′ŭn) [″ + *componere*, to put together]. 1. The putrefactive process; decay. 2. Reducing a compound body to its simpler constituents. SEE: *biodegradation; fermentation; resolution.*

    d., double. Chemical change in which the molecules of two interacting compounds exchange a portion of their constituents.

    d., hydrolytic. Chemical change in substances due to addition of a molecule of water.

    d., simple. Chemical change by which a molecule of a single compound breaks into its simpler constituents or substitutes the entire molecule of another body for one of these constituents.

decompress. 1. To pass from a state of stress to tranquillity. 2. To relieve pressure, esp. that produced by air or gas.

decompression [″ + *compressio*, a squeezing together]. 1. The removal of pressure, as from gas in the intestinal tract. SEE: *Wangensteen tube.* 2. The slow reduction or removal of pressure on deep-sea divers and caisson workers to prevent development of nitrogen bubbles in the tissue spaces. SEE: *caisson disease.*

    d., explosive. In aviators or divers, decompression resulting from an extremely rapid rate of change from one pressure to a much lesser pressure. This may occur if a high-altitude aircraft suddenly loses its cabin pressurization or if a diver ascends quite rapidly. Either of these causes violent expansion of body gases. SEE: *bends.*

decompression illness. A condition that develops in divers subjected to rapid reduction of air pressure after coming to the surface following exposure to compressed air. The cause is nitrogen bubbles in the tissue spaces.

    TREAT: Decompression illness is effectively treated by placing the person in a decompression chamber. The pressure in the chamber is then increased to the level that relieves the patient's symptoms and then decreased very slowly until the pressure inside the chamber is equal to outside pressure. SYN: *caisson disease.* SEE: *bends; hyperbaric chamber.*

decongestant. 1. Reducing congestion or swelling. 2. An agent that reduces congestion, esp. nasal.

decontamination. The process of rendering an object, person, or area free of a contaminating substance such as live bacteria, poison gas, or a radioactive substance.

decorticate posture. Characteristic posture of a patient with a lesion at or above the upper brain stem. The patient is rigidly still with arms flexed, fists clenched, and legs extended.

decortication [″ + *cortex*, bark]. Removal of the surface layer of an organ or structure, as the removal of a portion of the cortex of the brain from the underlying white portion.

    d., pulmonary. Removal of the pleura of the lung or a portion of the surface lung tissue.

    d., renal. Removal of capsule of the kidney.

decrement (dĕk′rĕ-mĕnt) [L. *decrementum*, decrease]. 1. The period in the course of a febrile disease when the fever subsides. 2. The reduction in the response of the nervous system to repeated stimulation. 3. A decrease in the quantity or force of an entity.

decrepitate (dē-krĕp′ĭ-tāt) [L. *decrepitare*, to crackle]. To cause decrepitation or a crackling noise.

decrepitation. A crackling noise.

decrepitude (dē-krĕp'ĭ-tūd). State of general feebleness and decline that sometimes accompanies old age; weak; infirm.

decrudescence (dē-kroo-dĕs'ĕns). Decrease in the severity of the symptoms of disease.

decubation (dē-kū-bā'shŭn) [L. *de*, down, + *cumbere*, to lie]. 1. The act of lying down. 2. The recovery stage of an infectious disease.

decubital. Pert. to a bedsore.

decubitus (dē-kū'bĭ-tŭs) [L., a lying down]. 1. A bedsore. 2. A patient's position in bed.

    d., acute. A severe, sometimes fatal, bedsore that can occur on the affected side in hemiplegia.

    d., Andral's. Position assumed by patient of lying on sound side during early stages of pleurisy.

    d., dorsal. Lying on the back.

    d., lateral. Lying on the side.

    d., ventral. Lying on the stomach.

decubitus projections. Radiographic procedures that use the decubitus positions and the central ray of the x-ray beam placed horizontally; aids in the demonstration of air-fluid levels.

decubitus ulcer. Ulcer, initially of the skin, due to prolonged pressure against areas of skin of a person who is lying down. Nevertheless, pressure ulcers or sores may occur at any site, e.g., on the buttocks of patients confined to wheelchairs. The most common sites are over bony prominences, i.e., the sacrum, heels, trochanter, lateral malleoli, and ischial areas. The pathological process, i.e., the combination of pressure, shearing forces, friction, and moisture, lead to death of tissue due to lack of blood supply. If not treated vigorously, the ulcer will progress from a simple erosion to complete involvement of the deep layers of the skin and may eventually extend to the underlying muscle and bone tissue. SYN: *pressure ulcer or sore.*

    The most important principle is to prevent the continuous pressure that causes the ulcer.

    The size of a pressure sore may be determined by covering the area with a transparent film that is adherent to the ulcer and in contact with the surrounding skin. Sterile isotonic saline is then injected under the film until the film is level with the surrounding skin. The amount of fluid required is recorded. Repetition of this at intervals will provide an index of the healing progress or lack of it.

    NURSING IMPLICATIONS: Try to prevent decubiti through frequent inspection of the skin for redness and signs of skin breakdown. Do not massage areas that are reddened, as this can inflict shearing force and damage to deep layers of tissue, the site of origin of many decubiti. Good skin care, especially over bone prominences; turning and position changes every two hours; passive range-of-motion exercises; early ambulation; and provision of nutritious meals. Special beds and mattresses used in treating or preventing decubiti should be kept in proper working order. Donut cushions should not be used because they decrease blood flow to the area resting in the center of the donut. If decubiti develop, they should be thoroughly cleansed and debrided, and ordered treatments should be carried out. Topical agents that have been used in treating decubiti include absorbable gelatin sponges, granulated sugar, karaya gum patches, antiseptic irrigations, air-permeable clear dressings that allow aspiration of collected fluid, debriding agents, and dextranomer beads. It is questionable whether or not these agents are more effective in treating decubiti than relief of pressure, simple debridement, and appropriate use of antibiotics. Continuity of care is of major importance. Further skin damage should be prevented by avoiding harsh soaps and alcohol-based products.

decurrent (dē-kŭr'ĕnt) [L. *decurrere*, to run down]. Traveling or extending down from above.

decussate (dē-kŭs'āt) [L. *decussare,* to make an X]. 1. To cross, or crossed, as in the form of the letter x. 2. Interlacing or crossing of parts.

decussation. 1. A crossing of structures in form of an x. 2. The place of crossing. SYN: *chiasma.*

    d. of pyramids. Crossing of fibers of pyramids of the medulla oblongata from one pyramid to the other.

    d., optic. Crossing of fibers of the optic nerves; the optic chiasma.

decussorium (dē-kŭs-ō'rē-ŭm). Instrument for depression of the dura following trephining.

dedifferentiation. 1. The return of parts to a homogeneous state. 2. Process by which mature differentiated cells or tissues are sites of origin of immature elements of the same type, as in some cancers.

dedolation (dĕd"ō-lā'shŭn). 1. Removal of a thin shaving of skin using an oblique slicing cut. 2. The feeling that the limbs have been bruised.

deduction (dē-dŭk'shŭn). Reasoning from the general to the particular.

de-efferented state. SYN: *pseudocoma,* q.v. SEE: *locked-in syndrome.*

deep [AS. *deop*]. Below the surface.

deep reflexes. Reflexes within, or fractional

stretch reflexes. Opposed to superficial or skin reflexes.

deer fly. A biting fly, *Chrysops discalis,* that transmits the causative organism of deer fly fever, a form of tularemia.

deer fly fever. Tularemia, q.v.

DEF. *decayed, extracted,* and *filled* teeth.

defamation. In law, an intentional wrong that occurs when a person communicates to a third party information which injures or harms the reputation of another. Oral defamation is slander. Written defamation is libel.

defatted [L. *de,* from, + AS. *faelt,* to fatten]. Freed from or deprived of fat.

defecalgesiophobia (dĕf″ē-kăl″jē-sē-ō-fō′bē-ă) [L. *defaecare,* to remove dregs, + Gr. *algesis,* sense of pain, + *phobos,* fear]. Fear of defecating because of pain.

defecation (dĕf-ē-kā′shŭn) [L. *defaecare,* to remove dregs]. Evacuation of the bowels. The bulk of the feces depends upon the amount and composition of food ingested. One does not, however, have to eat in order to have bowel movements. A large quantity of cellular material is desquamated from the epithelial lining of the intestinal tract each day. The food residues, reaching the rectum, cause the urge to defecate. The sensation is related to periodic increase of pressure within the rectum and contracture of its musculature. The expulsion of a fecal mass is accompanied by coordinated action of the following mechanisms: involuntary contraction of the circular muscle of the rectum behind the bowel mass followed by contraction of the longitudinal muscle; relaxation of the internal (involuntary) and external (voluntary) sphincter ani; voluntary closure of the glottis, fixation of the chest, and contraction of the abdominal muscles, causing an increase in intra-abdominal pressure. SEE: *constipation; feces; stool.*

defecation syncope. Syncope occurring during or immediately after defecation. It may be associated with disease of the gastrointestinal tract, cardiovascular or cerebrovascular systems, or orthostatic hypotension. In many cases the potential cause is not discovered.

defect (dē′fĕkt). A flaw or imperfection.

   d., congenital. Imperfection present at birth.

   d., filling. Interruption of the contour of the inner surface of the stomach or intestine revealed by roentgenography. It may be due to a benign obstruction or a malignancy.

   d., septal. Defect in one or more of the septa between the heart chambers.

defective [L. *defectus,* a failure]. 1. Not perfect. 2. A person deficient in one or more physical, mental, or moral powers.

defeminization (dē-fĕm″ĭ-nĭ-zā′shŭn). The loss of female sexual characteristics.

defendant. In law, the person or party against whom a lawsuit or legal action seeking damages or other legal relief is brought. SEE: *plaintiff.*

defense [L. *defendere,* to repel]. 1. Resistance to disease. 2. Acting to protect oneself from harm or injury.

defense mechanism. 1. Any reaction, whether general or cellular, that serves to protect against something harmful, as in immune reactions. Any defense mechanism occurring in excess can be pathological. 2. In psychoanalysis, a method of unconscious behavior used to resolve or conceal conflicts or anxieties. Ex.: compensation; denial; projection.

defense reflex. Retraction or tension in defense against an action or threatened action.

defensins [term coined by Robert I. Lehrer, U.S. physician, b. 1938]. Antimicrobial peptides present in leukocytes from several species including man. They are active against bacteria, fungi, and enveloped viruses in vitro. They may contribute to host defenses against susceptible organisms.

defensive. Defending; a means of protecting from injury.

defensive medicine. To practice medicine as if each patient is planning a malpractice suit. This is done by ordering an inordinate number of laboratory and test procedures.

deferens (dĕf′ĕr-ĕnz) [L. *deferens,* carrying away]. Deferent.

deferent (dĕf′ĕr-ĕnt). Conveying anything away from or downward. SEE: *afferent; efferent.*

deferentectomy (dĕf-ĕr-ĕn-tĕk′tō-mē) [″ + Gr. *ektome,* excision]. Cutting of a ductus deferens.

deferential (dĕf-ĕr-ĕn′shăl) [L. *deferre,* to bring to]. Pert. to or accompanying the ductus deferens.

deferentitis (dĕf″ĕr-ĕn-tī′tĭs) [″ + Gr. *itis,* inflammation]. Inflammation of the ductus deferens.

deferoxamine mesylate (dē-fĕr-ŏks′ă-mēn). USP. A drug with a very high affinity for iron. It is used parenterally to reduce the iron stored in the body in patients with hemochromatosis, acute iron poisoning, or abnormal storage of iron due to multiple blood transfusions. Trade name is Desferal.

deferred shock. Delayed onset of symptoms of shock.

defervescence [L. *defervescere,* to become calm]. The period that marks the subsidence of fever to normal temperature.

defibrillation. Stopping fibrillation of the heart through the use of drugs or by physical means. SEE: *cardioversion; defibrillation,* *electrical.*

d., electrical. Stopping fibrillation of the heart by using an electrical device that applies countershocks to the heart through electrodes placed on the chest wall. It is hoped that this countershock will allow the heart's normal pacemaker to take over. The electrical "dose" required for defibrillation is less for lightweight individuals than for larger persons. SEE: *cardioversion; cardioverter; pacemaker, cardiac, artificial.*

defibrillator (dē-fĭb″rĭ-lā′tor). Electrical device that produces defibrillation of the heart. It may be used externally or in the form of an automatic implanted cardioverter defibrillator. The latter is implanted in patients who have had a life-threatening ventricular tachyarrhythmia or cardiac arrest, and in whom drug therapy is unsuitable. SEE: *cardioversion.*

d., automatic implanted cardioverter. ABBR: AICD. Device surgically implanted in patients at high risk for sudden cardiac (arrhythmia-induced) death. Machine will automatically function to detect and treat life-threatening arrhythmias.

d., fully automatic. Unit will perform all functions by computer (analyze rhythm, select energy level, charge machine, and shock patient). All operator has to do is apply adhesive paddles and turn machine to "on."

d., manual. Unit requires the operator to assess the need for defibrillation (patient's ECG and condition), select energy level, charge the machine, and deliver shock.

d., semi-automatic. Unit will assess the rhythm and give voice prompts to operator concerning patient's condition, energy level, charging, and shocking patient.

defibrination, defibrinization [L. *de,* from, + *fibra,* fiber]. Process of being deprived of fibrin. SEE: *coagulation, blood.*

deficiency (dē-fĭsh′ĕn-sē) [L. *deficere,* to lack]. A lack; less than the normal amount.

deficiency disease. Condition due to a deficiency of a substance essential in body metabolism. The deficiency may be due to either inadequate intake, digestion, absorption, or utilization of foods, minerals, water, or vitamins. It may also be due to excess loss through excretion or to an intestinal parasite such as hookworm or tapeworm.

Ex.: Night blindness and keratomalacia due to lack of vitamin A; beriberi or polyneuritis due to lack of thiamine; pellagra due to lack of niacin; scurvy due to lack of vitamin C; rickets and osteomalacia due to lack of vitamin D; pernicious anemia due to lack of gastric intrinsic factor and vitamin B_{12}.

deficit (dĕf′ĭ-sĭt). A deficiency or lack, e.g., muscular or mental deficit.

defined medium. In bacteriology, a medium in which the composition is accurately defined and carefully controlled. One use of this culture medium is to investigate the influence of altering ingredients on bacterial cell growth characteristics.

definition [L. *definire,* to limit]. 1. The precise determination of the limits of anything, esp. a disease process. 2. The detail with which images are recorded on radiographic film or screens.

definitive. Clear and final; without question.

deflection (dē-flĕk′shŭn). The turning away from a previous or usual course.

defloration (dĕf″lō-rā′shŭn) [L. *de,* from, + *flos, flor-,* flower]. Rupture of the hymen during coitus, by accident, surgically, or through vaginal examination. Not many females have a hymen that is of such size or consistency as to require its surgical rupture. SEE: *hymen; virginity.*

deflorescence. Disappearance of an eruption of the skin.

defluvium (dē-floo′vē-ŭm) [L.]. Falling out.

d. capillorum. Loss of hair.

defluxio (dē-flŭk′sē-ō) [L.]. A flowing down.

d. capillorum. A falling out of hair.

d. ciliorum. A falling out of eyelashes.

defluxion (dē-flŭk′shŭn). A flowing down; copious discharge or loss of any kind.

deformability (dē-form″ă-bĭl′ĭ-tē). Capable of being deformed.

deformation [L. *de,* from, + *forma,* form]. The act of deforming; a disfiguration.

deformity. An alteration in the natural form of a part or organ. Distortion of any part or general disfigurement of the body. It may be acquired or congenital. If present after injury, deformity usually implies presence of fracture, dislocation, or both. May be due to extensive swelling, extravasation of blood, or rupture of muscles.

d., anterior. Abnormal anterior convexity of the spine. SYN: *lordosis.*

d., gunstock. Deformity in which the forearm, when extended, makes an angle with the arm because of displacement of the axis of the extended arm.

ETIOL: Condylar fracture at the elbow.

d., Madelung's. Distortion of the radius at its lower end with ulnar displacement backward.

d., seal fin. Lateral deviation of the fingers in rheumatoid arthritis.

d., silverfork. The peculiar deformity seen in Colles' fracture of the forearm. SEE: *Colles' fracture.*

d., Sprengel's. Congenital upward displacement of the scapula.

d., Velpeau's. D., silverfork.

d., Volkmann's. Congenital tibiotarsal dislocation.

defundation [" + *fundus,* base]. Excision of the uterine fundus.

defurfuration (dē"fĕr-fū-rā'shŭn) [" + *furfur,* bran]. Shedding of epidermis in scales; branny desquamation. May occur in various skin conditions, including seborrheic dermatitis (dandruff), psoriasis, ichthyosis, and eczema.

deg. *degeneration; degree.*

deganglionate (dē-găn'glē-ŏn-āt") [" + Gr. *ganglion,* knot]. To deprive of ganglia.

degenerate [L. *degenerare,* to fall from one's ancestral quality]. 1. To deteriorate. 2. Characterized by deterioration.

degeneration [L. *degeneratio*]. Deterioration or impairment of an organ or part in structure of cells and the substances of which they are a part. Opposed to regeneration.

　　d., adipose. D., fatty.

　　d., albuminoid. D., amyloid.

　　d., ascending. Nerve fiber degeneration progressing to the center from the periphery.

　　d., calcareous. Infiltration of lime salts into tissues.

　　d., caseous. Cheesy alteration of tissues seen in tuberculosis.

　　d., cloudy swelling. A condition in which protein substances in cells become cloudy, the cells increasing in size with minute droplets of protein substances. It may occur in any inflamed tissue.

　　d., colloid. Jelly-like disorganization of tissues.

　　d., congenital macular. Various forms of congenital degeneration of the macula of the eye.

　　d., cystic. Cyst formation accompanying degeneration.

　　d., descending. Nerve fiber degeneration progressing toward the periphery from the original lesion.

　　d., fatty. Deposition of abnormal amounts of fat in cells, or the replacement or infiltration of tissues by fat cells.

　　d., fibroid. Change of membranous tissue into that of a fibrous nature.

　　d., gray. Degeneration in white nerve tissue due to chronic inflammation, assuming a gray color.

　　d., hepatolenticular. Wilson's disease, q.v.

　　d., hyaline. A form of degeneration in which the tissues assume a homogeneous and glassy appearance. Caused by hyaline deposits replacing musculoelastic elements of blood vessels with a firm, transparent substance that causes loss of elasticity. It is responsible for hardening of the arteries and is often followed by calcification or deposit of lime salts in dead tissue. Calcification also may result in concretions.

　　d., hydropic. Pathological change in cells characterized by the appearance of water droplets in the cytoplasm.

　　d., lipoidal. Deposition of fat droplets in cells.

　　d., macular. SEE: *macular degeneration.*

　　d., mucoid. Deposition of mucus in the connective tissues.

　　d., mucous. Deposition of mucus or mucoid substance in the connective tissue of organs, or epithelial cells.

　　d., myxomatous. D., mucoid.

　　d., Nissl. Nerve cell degeneration after division of the axon.

　　d., pigmentary. Degeneration in which affected cells develop an abnormal color.

　　d., polypoid. Formation of polyp-like growths on mucous membrane.

　　d., secondary. D., wallerian.

　　d., senile. Bodily and mental changes of the aged.

　　d., senile macular. ABBR: SMD. Degeneration of the retina that may come on and increase as a person ages.

　　d., spongy. Familial demyelination of the deep layers of the cerebral cortex. The affected area has a spongy appearance. Symptoms include mental retardation, enlarged head, muscular flaccidity, and blindness. Death usually occurs prior to 18 months of age.

　　d., subacute combined, of spinal cord. Degeneration of the posterior and lateral columns of the spinal column. Clinically, paresthesia, sensory ataxia, and sometimes spastic paraplegia are present. The disease is the result of pernicious anemia.

　　d., vitreous. D., hyaline.

　　d., wallerian. Nerve fiber degeneration after separation from its nutritive center.

　　d., Zenker's. D., hyaline.

degeneration, words pert. to: athetoid; atrophic; cacogenic; caseation; catalysis; colloid; sarcomatosis; steatosis.

degenerative. Pert. to or accompanied by degeneration.

deglutible (dē-gloo'tĭ-bl) [L. *deglutire,* to swallow]. Capable of being swallowed.

deglutition (dē"gloo-tĭsh'ŭn). The act of swallowing.

deglutitive. Pert. to deglutition.

degradation (dĕg"rĕ-dā'shŭn) [LL. *degradare,* to go down a step]. Physical, metabolic, or chemical change to a less complex form. Foods are physically degraded during chewing, and then chemically degraded from complete compounds, such as proteins and starches, to amino acids and sugars, respectively. SEE: *biodegradation.*

degranulation. Loss of granules, esp. in a phagocytic cell.

degree (dē-grē'). 1. A unit of measurement on

a scale. 2. A unit of angular measure. 3. A stage of severity of a disease. 4. Evidence of academic attainment granted by the institution in which the individual studied.

degrees of freedom. ABBR: d.f. In statistics, in defining the properties of the sample, the number of independent observations in a quantity, e.g., if the sample contains a total of 10 children that are being classified by hair color (either brown, black, or white) and it is known that four of the children have blonde hair, then there are two degrees of freedom; if, at the beginning of the investigation, hair color of all subjects was unknown, there would be three degrees of freedom.

degustation (dē″gŭs-tā′shŭn) [L. *degustatio*]. The sense of taste; the function or act of tasting.

dehiscence (dē-hĭs′ĕns) [L. *dehiscere*, to gape]. 1. A bursting open, as of a graafian follicle or a wound, esp. a surgical abdominal wound. 2. In dentistry, an isolated area in which the tooth root is denuded of bone from the margin nearly to the apex. It occurs more often in anterior than posterior teeth; more on the vestibular than the oral surface.

NURSING IMPLICATIONS: Attempt to prevent by providing proper nutrition; preoperative evaluation of risk factors such as obesity, malnourishment; and provide support for the wound during coughing and movements that put strain on the wound.

In surgical dehiscence, notify the surgeon immediately. Cover the wound with a sterile towel or dressing moistened with warm sterile physiological saline solution. Have the patient decrease the tension on abdominal muscles by slightly flexing the knees. Keep the patient calm and quiet, and reassure him or her that the wound will be cared for. Advise the patient that surgery will be required, and prepare for surgery. SEE: *Nursing Diagnoses* in Appendix.

dehumanization (dē-hū″măn-ĭ-zā′shŭn) [L. *de*, from, + *humanus*, human]. Loss of human qualities, as occurs in persons who are psychotic or in previously normal individuals subjected to torture or mental stress imposed by others, as could occur in prisoners.

dehumidifier (dē″hū-mĭd′ĭ-fī″ĕr). Device for removing moisture from the air.

dehydrate [L. *de*, from, + Gr. *hydor*, water]. 1. In chemistry, to deprive of, lose, or become free of water. 2. Loss of or deprivation of water from the body or tissues. To become dry.

dehydration (dē″hī-drā′shŭn). 1. Removal of water from a substance. 2. Condition resulting from excessive loss of body fluid. Occurs when output of fluid exceeds fluid intake.

May result from fluid deprivation, excessive loss of fluid, reduction in total quantity of electrolytes, or injection of hypertonic solutions. SEE: *skin, tenting of.* SEE: *Nursing Diagnoses* in Appendix.

dehydroandrosterone (dē-hī″drō-ăn-drō-stĕr′ōn, -drŏs′tĕr-ōn). Previously used name for dehydroepiandrosterone, q.v.

dehydrocholesterol (dē-hī″drō-kō-lĕs′tĕr-ŏl). A sterol found in the skin and other tissues that after activation by irradiation forms vitamin D.

dehydrocholic acid. USP. A bile salt that stimulates production of bile from the liver. Trade names are Cholan-DH, Decholin, Dilabil, and Ketochol.

dehydrocorticosterone (dē-hī″drō-kor-tĭ-kōs′tĕr-ōn). 11-dehydrocorticosterone (Kendall's compound A). $C_{21}H_{28}O_4$. A physiologically active steroid isolated from the adrenal cortex. It is important in water and salt metabolism. SEE: *adrenal gland.*

dehydroepiandrosterone (dē-hī″drō-ĕp″ē-ăn-drŏs′tĕr-ōn). An androgenic substance, $C_{19}H_{28}O_2$, present in urine. It has about one-fifth the potency of androsterone. The level of this hormone in plasma decreases with age.

dehydrogenase (dē-hī-drŏj′ĕ-nās). An enzyme that catalyzes the oxidation of a specific substance, causing it to give up its hydrogen.

dehydrogenate (dē-hī″drŏj′ĕn-āt). To remove hydrogen from a chemical compound.

dehydroisoandrosterone (dē-hī″drō-ī″sō-ăn-drŏs′tĕr-ōn). A 17-ketosteroid excreted in normal male urine. It possesses androgenic activity.

deinstitutionalization. A planned program for placing hospitalized psychiatric patients in the community by way of halfway houses, residential hotels, group homes, and boarding houses.

deionization (dē-ī″ŏn-ī-zā′shŭn). Removal of ions from a substance, thus producing a substance free of minerals.

Deiters' cells (dī′tĕrz) [Otto F. C. Deiters, Ger. anatomist, 1834–1863]. 1. Supporting cells in organ of Corti. 2. Neuroglia cells.

Deiters' nucleus. Collection of cells behind the acoustic nucleus.

Deiters' process. Axis cylinder process or neuraxon.

déjà entendu (dā′zhä ŏn-tŏn-doo′) [Fr., already heard]. 1. Recognition of something previously understood. 2. The illusion that what one is hearing was heard previously.

déjà vu (dā′zhä voo) [Fr., already seen]. The impression that something seen or some situation being experienced for the first time has been previously seen or experienced.

dejecta (dē-jĕk′tă) [L. *dejectio*, injection].

Feces; intestinal waste.

dejection, dejecture (dē-jĕk′shŭn, -tūr). 1. A cast-down feeling or mental depression. 2. Defecation or act of defecation.

Déjérine, Joseph Jules (dā″zhĕr-ēn′). French neurologist, 1849–1917.

 D.'s disease. Interstitial neuritis of infants.

 D. -Sottas disease [Jules Sottas, Fr. neurologist, 1866–1943]. Progressive and hypertrophic interstitial neuritis of infants. It is slowly progressive, but the life span may be normal.

 D.'s syndrome. Condition in which deep sensation is depressed but tactile sense is normal, caused by lesion of long root fibers of posterior column.

dekaliter. A unit of volume in the SI system of measurement that is equal to 10 liters. SEE: *decaliter; deciliter.*

delacrimation (dē-lăk″rĭ-mā′shŭn) [L. *de,* from, + *lacrima,* tear]. Excessive flow of tears. SEE: *epiphora.*

delactation (dē″lăk-tā′shŭn) [″ + *lactare,* to suckle]. Weaning or cessation of lactation.

Delalutin. Trade name for hydroxyprogesterone caproate.

delamination [″ + *lamina,* plate]. The division into layers, esp. that of a blastoderm into two layers — epiblast and hypoblast.

Delatestryl. Trade name for testosterone enanthate.

de-lead (dē-lĕd). To remove lead from the body or a tissue. SEE: *chelate.*

deleterious (dĕl″ē-tē′rē-ŭs) [Gr. *deleterios*]. Harmful.

deletion (dē-lē′shŭn). In cytogenetics, the loss of a portion of a chromosome.

Delhi boil. Aleppo boil, q.v.

delicate. Having a fine, fragile structure.

deligation (dĕl-ĭ-gā′shŭn) [L. *deligare,* to tie up]. The application of ligatures or binder.

delimitation [L. *de,* from, + *limitare,* to limit]. Determination of limits of an area or organ in diagnosis.

delinquent (dē-lĭn′kwĕnt). One whose behavior is criminal or antisocial.

deliquesce (dĕl″ĭ-kwĕs′) [L. *deliquescere,* to melt away]. To cause liquefaction or moistening.

deliquescence (dĕl″ĭ-kwĕs′ĕns). The process of becoming liquefied or moist as the result of absorption of water from the air. Ordinary table salt has this property.

deliquescent (dĕl″ĭ-kwĕs′ĕnt). Pert. to a substance that absorbs water from the atmosphere.

délire de toucher (dā-lēr′ dŭ too-shā′) [Fr.]. An abnormal desire to touch or feel things.

deliriant, delirifacient (dē-lĭr′ē-ănt, dē-lĭr″ĭ-fā′shĭ-ĕnt) [L. *delirare,* to be deranged]. An

agent that will produce delirium, e.g., atropine or hyoscine.

delirium (dē-lĭr′ē-ŭm) [L.]. A state of mental confusion and excitement characterized by disorientation for time and place, usually with illusions and hallucinations. The mind wanders, speech is incoherent, and the patient is in a state of continual aimless physical activity. There are many forms of delirium, depending on the cause, which may be fever, shock, exhaustion, anxiety, or drug overdose.

 RS: alcoholism; carphologia; dipsomania; restraint.

 d., acute. Delirium developing suddenly and speedily, resulting in recovery or death.

 d., alcoholic. D. tremens.

 d., chronic. Delirium of chronic psychoses without febrile characteristics.

 d. constantium. Delirium of patients with reiteration of fixed idea.

 d. cordis. Atrial fibrillation.

 d. epilepticum. Delirium following an epileptic attack or appearing instead of an attack.

 d., febrile. Delirium occurring with fever.

 d., lingual. Delirium in which meaningless sounds are muttered constantly.

 d. mussitans. Excitement causing lingual delirium.

 d. of negation. Delirium in which patient thinks body parts are missing.

 d. of persecution. Delirium in which patient feels persecuted by surrounding persons.

 d., partial. Delirium reacting on only a portion of the mental faculties, causing only some of the patient's actions to be unreasonable.

 d., post-traumatic. D., traumatic, q.v.

 d., senile. Intermittent or permanent state of disorientation, hallucinations, confusion, and wandering that may come on abruptly in old age or may be associated with senile dementia.

 d., toxic. Delirium produced by a toxin.

 d., traumatic. Delirium following injury or shock.

 d. tremens. ABBR: DTs. A dramatic complication of alcoholism. The onset may follow a period of abstinence following a prolonged drinking spree, or it may occur in the chronic alcoholic who has been admitted to the hospital for an unrelated illness. Its onset is usually sudden and initially may present with any of the following: restlessness, irritability, confusion, tremulousness, insomnia, and, in about 30% of cases, generalized convulsions. This somewhat benign clinical onset progresses to a dramatic condition characterized by visual, auditory, and

delitescence — 509 — delomorphous cells

tactile hallucinations, incessant and incoherent talking, disorientation, tremors, and jerky, restless movements. Signs of overactivity of the autonomic nervous system, with dilated pupils, fever, tachycardia, with profuse sweating are present. Five to 15% of these patients die depending on the presence of pre-existing illness. In the majority of cases, recovery occurs within three to five days. The patient may fall into a deep sleep and awaken with little if any memory of the illness. SEE: *alcoholism; alcohol withdrawal syndrome.* SYN: *acute alcohol withdrawal.*

TREAT: Because the illness is potentially fatal and treatment is controversial, it is important that the patient be hospitalized. This is particularly true for those who have a history of previous attacks.

NURSING IMPLICATIONS: Protect patient and those around him or her, and carry out therapy to relieve withdrawal symptoms. Monitor mental status, cardiopulmonary and hepatic function and vital signs, including body temperature, anticipating complicating hyperthermia or circulatory collapse. Administer ordered drug and fluid therapy, titrating to patient's symptoms and blood pressure response. Evaluate need for and administer prescribed anticonvulsant drugs. Maintain a calm, nonstressful environment, illuminated to reduce visual hallucinations. Call the patient by name, explain procedures, and frequently orient to reality. Observe the patient closely, having someone stay with him or her as much as possible. Physical restraint should be avoided but may be required for combative patients or those who attempt to harm themselves. Be patient, tactful, understanding, and supportive throughout the period of acute withdrawal. Recognize and help the patient to recognize the need for further treatment and supportive counseling. SEE: *Nursing Diagnoses* in Appendix.

Caution: This syndrome is a true medical emergency that should be treated aggressively due to the possibility of death. Also, it is important to be certain there is not a coexisting condition such as head trauma with concussion, or an acute infectious disease; or that the signs and symptoms are not due to some toxic substance other than ethanol.

delitescence (dĕl″ĭ-tĕs′ĕns) [L. *delitescens,* hiding]. 1. An unusually complete and speedy resolution of an inflammation. 2. The latent period prior to development of symptoms following poisoning.

deliver [L. *deliberare,* to free completely]. 1. To aid in childbirth. 2. To remove or extract, as a tumor from a cystic enclosure or a cataract.

delivery. Expulsion of the child with placenta and membranes from the mother at birth. SEE: *labor.*

d., abdominal. Delivery of the child by cesarean section.

d., forceps. Delivery of the child by application of forceps to the fetal head. These may be applied prior to head engagement, and is called high forceps delivery; or applied after the head is visible, this is called low forceps delivery; or, if the forceps are applied after engagement but prior to the head becoming visible, this is called midforceps delivery.

d., postmortem. Delivery of the child either by the abdominal or vaginal route after death of the mother.

d., precipitate. Delivery that occurs under nonsterile conditions and when the physician is not present. In the true sense, it is one that follows a rapid labor, regardless of who is present.

NOTE: Watch the patient carefully. A multipara needs more careful watching than a primipara. Nevertheless, it may occur in a primipara.

When preparing for delivery, do not wait for the head to be visible in a multipara if she is having frequent hard contractions, particularly if she is bearing down. Have a physician see her immediately. In a primipara it is fairly safe to wait in the majority of cases until a small portion of the head is seen at the vaginal orifice during a contraction before putting the patient up for delivery. Remember to watch the primipara or multipara who has received an analgesic, since precipitation can occur with little or no warning. This means watching for bulging of the perineum during the contractions by viewing the vulva and not taking it for granted that because the patient is fairly quiet no progress in labor is being made.

d., premature. Delivery of a fetus before full term.

d., spontaneous. Delivery of an infant without external aid.

d., vaginal. Delivery of an infant through the birth canal.

dellen (dĕl′ĕn). A depression or thinning in the corneal surface of the eye. May be due to swelling of adjacent tissue from wearing contact lenses or degenerative changes.

delomorphous (dĕl″ō-mor′fŭs) [Gr. *delos,* evident, + *morphe,* form]. Having definite form and shape.

delomorphous cells. Granular cells that stain easily. Found next to basement membrane in the stomach and glands in the cardiac region.

delousing (dē-lows'ĭng) [L. *de*, from, + AS. *lus*, louse]. Ridding the body of lice. SEE: *louse*.

delta. 1. Δ or δ, upper and lower case, respectively, of the symbols for the fourth letter of the Greek alphabet. 2. A triangular space. 3. Change in value or amount of something being measured or monitored.

Delta-Cortef. Trade name for prednisolone.

deltacortisone (dĕl″tă-kor′tĭ-sōn). Prednisone, q.v., a steroid hormone with glucocorticoid activity.

delta fornicis (dĕl′tă for′nĭ-sĭs) [L.]. A triangular surface on lower side of fornix.

delta hepatitis virus. ABBR: HDV. SEE: *hepatitis, delta agent*.

Deltasone. Trade name for prednisone.

deltoid [Gr. *delta*, letter d, + *eidos*, form, shape]. Shaped like the capital form of the Greek letter delta (Δ); triangular.

deltoid ligament. Internal lateral ligament of ankle joint.

deltoid muscle. The musculus deltoideus, which covers the shoulder prominence.

deltoid ridge. Ridge on humerus where deltoid muscle is attached.

delusion (dē-loo′zhŭn) [L. *deludere*, to cheat]. A false belief brought about without appropriate external stimulation and inconsistent with the individual's own knowledge and experience. Seen most often in psychoses, in which patients cannot separate delusion from reality. Differs from hallucination, q.v., in that the latter involves the false excitation of one or more of the senses. The most important delusions are those that cause patients to harm others or themselves.

Ex.: fear of being poisoned causing the patient to refuse food; delusions leading to suicide or inflicting injury upon self; false beliefs such as having been guilty of an unpardonable sin; delusions of persecution.

d., depressive. Delusion causing a saddened state.

d., expansive. Unreasonable conviction of one's own power, or importance; seen in manic patients.

d., fixed. Delusion that remains unaltered.

d., fleeting. A type of delusion that comes and goes.

d., nihilistic. Delusion that causes the victim to believe that everything has ceased to exist.

d. of control. Delusion that one's thoughts and actions are under the control of an external force.

d. of grandeur. A false sense of possessing wealth or power. SYN: *megalomania*.

d. of negation. D., nihilistic.

d. of persecution. Delusion in which patients feel everyone around them is against them.

d., reference. Delusion that causes the victim to read a meaning into the acts or words of others that was not intended, often the interpretation is of slight or ridicule.

d., systematized. Logical correlation with false reasoning and deduction.

d., unsystematized. Delusion without any correlation between ideas and surroundings.

delusional. Pert. to a delusion.

demand. Something that is needed.

d., biological oxygen. The amount of oxygen required for a biological reaction, esp. the oxygen required to oxidize materials in natural water supplies, such as rivers or lakes. SEE: *eutrophication*.

demand valve manually cycled resuscitator. Resuscitator utilizing high-low oxygen which is cycled by pushing a button and watching the chest rise. Can be used during CPR efforts, but the high oxygen pressure may result in gastric distention and barotrauma. Trade names are Robershaw valve and Elder valve.

demarcation (dē″măr-kā′shŭn) [L. *demarcare*, to limit]. Setting a limit or boundary.

demasculinization. Loss of male sexual characteristics. This may be caused by lack of the male hormone or due to the action of certain drugs.

demecarium bromide (dĕm″ē-kā′rē-ŭm). USP. An anticholinesterase agent used in treating glaucoma. Trade name is Humorsol.

demeclocycline hydrochloride (dĕm″ē-klō-sī′klēn). USP. A tetracycline-type antibiotic. Trade name is Declomycin.

dement [L. *dementare*, to make insane]. One afflicted with dementia.

demented. Of unsound mind.

dementia (dē-mĕn′shē-ă) [L. *dementare*, to make insane]. A broad (global) impairment of intellectual function (cognition) that usually is progressive and that interferes with normal social and occupational activities. Patients with this condition have little insight into it and care for them is sought by their family or associates.

SYM: Onset of primary dementia may be slow, over a period of months or years; memory deficits; impaired abstract thinking; poor judgment; clouding of consciousness and orientation is not present until the terminal stages; depression, agitation, sleeplessness, and paranoid ideation may be present.

ETIOL: Primary as with Alzheimer's disease; secondary as with brain tumors, fever, or severe medical or surgical diseases.

TREAT: Symptomatic for primary dementia and appropriate specific therapy for the reversible causes of dementia.

d., alcoholic. Dementia in terminal portion of chronic alcoholic state.

d., apoplectic. Dementia following cerebral hemorrhage or tumors.

d., dialysis. SEE: *dialysis dementia.*

d., epileptic. Dementia seen in some cases of long-term epilepsy.

d. paralytica. A form of neurosyphilis characterized by sudden onset with deterioration of memory and concentration and irritability. Behavior deteriorates, and emotional instability develops. Neurasthenia, depression, and delusions of grandeur with lack of insight may be present.

d., postfebrile. Dementia following severe cases of infectious diseases.

d., presenile. Dementia beginning in middle age, usually resulting from cerebral arteriosclerosis. Symptoms are apathy, loss of memory, and disturbances of speech and gait. SEE: *Nursing Diagnoses* in *Appendix.*

d., primary. Dementia associated with Alzheimer's disease, q.v.

d., senile. Dementia occurring in the aged. Characterized by progressive mental deterioration with loss of memory, esp. for recent events, with occasional intercurrent attacks of excitement.

d., syphilitic. Dementia caused by lesion of syphilis.

d., toxic. Dementia due to excessive use of a drug or drugs toxic to the central nervous system.

Demerol (dĕm'ĕr-ōl). Trade name for meperidine hydrochloride, a white, odorless, crystalline compound, soluble in water, having a neutral reaction and an analgesic effect similar to morphine.

Caution: Continued use will lead to addiction.

---

demi- [L. *dimidius*, half]. Prefix indicating half.

demibain (dĕm'ĭ-băn) [Fr., half bath]. Half a bath; sitz bath.

demilune (dĕm'ĭ-loon) [L. *dimidius*, half, + *luna*, moon]. A crescent-shaped group of serous cells that form a caplike structure over a mucous alveolus. They are present in mixed glands, esp. the submandibular gland.

demineralization [L. *de*, from, + *minare*, to mine]. Loss of mineral salts, esp. from the bones. SEE: *decalcification.*

demise (dē-mīz') [L. *dimittere*, to dismiss]. Destruction or death.

demodectic (dĕm-ō-dĕk'tĭk). Concerning or caused by the mite *Demodex.*

Demodex [Gr. *demos*, fat, + *dex*, worm]. Genus of mites and ticks of the class Arach-

nida and order Acarina.

D. folliculorum. The hair follicle or face mite. An almost microscopic elongated wormlike organism that infests hair follicles and sebaceous glands of various mammals, including humans.

demography (dē-mŏg'ră-fē) [Gr. *demos*, people, + *graphein*, to write]. The statistical and quantitative study of characteristics of human populations. Size, growth, density, age and sex distribution, and vital statistics are included in the data collected.

demoniac. Concerning a demon. Frenzied activity, as if possessed by demons or evil spirits.

demorphinization (dē-mor"fĭn-ĭ-zā'shŭn). Gradual decrease in the dose of morphine being used by one addicted to that drug.

demotivate. To cause loss of incentive or motivation.

Demours' membrane (dē-mūr') [Pierre Demours, Fr. ophthalmologist, 1702–1795]. A fine membrane between the endothelial layer of the cornea and the substantia propria. SYN: *Descemet's membrane.*

demucosation (dē"mū-kō-sā'shŭn) [L. *demucosatio*]. Removal of mucosa of any part of body.

demulcent [L. *demulcens*, stroking softly]. An agent that will soothe the part or soften the skin to which applied. The term is usually restricted to agents acting on mucous membrane.

Ex.: glycerin, honey, lanolin, olive oil.

Demulen. Trade name for combination of estrogen with progestogen.

de Musset's sign. SEE: *Musset's sign.*

demyelinate (dē-mī'ĕ-lĭn-āt) [" + Gr. *myelos*, marrow]. Destruction or removal of the myelin sheath of nerve tissue. Seen in Guillain-Barré syndrome, q.v.

demyelinating. An inflammatory process of nerves that destroys normal, healthy myelin.

demyelination (dē-mī"ĕ-lĭ-nā'shŭn). Removal of the myelin sheath of a nerve.

denarcotize (dē-năr'kō-tīz). To withdraw narcotic from an addicted person.

denaturation (dē-nā"chŭr-ā'shŭn). Adding a substance to alcohol that makes it toxic and unfit for human consumption but usually does not interfere with its use for other purposes.

denatured [" + *natura*, nature]. Alteration of the usual nature of a substance, as the addition of methanol to alcohol renders it unfit for consumption.

denatured protein. A protein that has been treated in some manner that caused it to lose some of its physical and chemical properties. Cooking egg white denatures the albumin present.

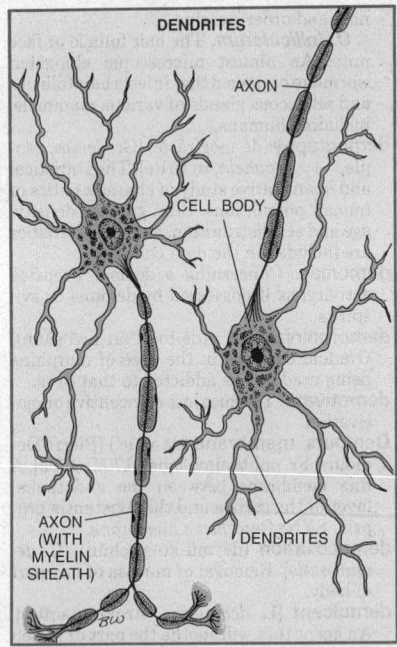

DENDRITES

AXON

CELL BODY

AXON
(WITH
MYELIN
SHEATH)

DENDRITES

dendraxon (dĕn-drăk'sŏn) [Gr. *dendron*, tree, + *axon*, axle]. The terminal filaments of the neuraxon of a nerve cell.

dendric (dĕn'drĭk). Pert. to or possessing a dendron.

Dendrid. Trade name for idoxuridine (IDU).

dendriform (dĕn'drĭ-form) [" + L. *forma*, shape]. Branching, or like a tree in shape.

dendrite (dĕn'drīt) [Gr. *dendrites*, pert. to a tree]. A branched protoplasmic process of a neuron that conducts impulses to the cell body. There are usually several to a cell. They form synaptic connections with other neurons. SYN: *dendron; neurodendrite*. SEE: illus.

    d.'s, extracapsular. Dendrites of neurons of autonomic ganglia that pierce the capsule surrounding the cell and extend for considerable distances from the cell body.

    d.'s, intracapsular. Dendrites of neurons of autonomic ganglia that ramify beneath the capsule, forming a network about the cell body.

dendritic. Treelike in form.

dendritic calculus. A renal stone molded in the form of the pelvis and calyces.

dendroid (dĕn'droyd) [" + *eidos*, form, shape]. 1. Dendriform, pert. to dendrites. 2.

Arborescent, treelike.

dendron (dĕn'drŏn) [Gr., tree]. A dendrite; a protoplasmic branch from a nerve cell. SYN: *neurodendrite*.

dendrophagocytosis (dĕn"drŏ-făg-ō-sī-tō'sĭs) [Gr. *dendron*, tree, + *phagein*, to eat, + *kytos*, cell, + *osis*, condition]. The absorption of portions of astrocytes by microglia cells.

denervated [L. *de*, from, + Gr. *neuron*, nerve]. 1. Excision, incision, or blocking of a nerve supply. 2. A condition in which the afferent and efferent nerves are cut. SEE: *deafferentation*.

dengue (dăng'gă, -gĕ) [Sp.]. An acute febrile disease characterized by sudden onset, with headache, fever, prostration, joint and muscle pain, lymphadenopathy, and a rash that appears simultaneously with a second temperature rise following an afebrile period. SYN: *breakbone fever; dengue fever*.

    SYM: Two fever periods with intermissions; eruptions similar to measles; severe pain in muscles and joints.

    ETIOL: Group B arbovirus transmitted by the mosquito. Incubation period is 3 to 15 days, usually 5 to 6 days.

    TREAT: No specific treatment. Analgesic and sedative agents. Mosquito control for prophylaxis.

denial (dĕ-nī'ăl). 1. Refusal to admit the reality of, or to acknowledge the presence or existence of something; keeping out of conscious awareness anxiety-producing realities. A defense mechanism. 2. In medical care reimbursement context, the decision by the patient's insurer that part or all of the medical care administered was not justified. The result of the denial is that the insurer refuses to pay for all or a portion of the medical costs incurred.

denial and isolation. According to Elisabeth Kübler-Ross, these are the initial emotional reactions to being told of impending death. Individuals refuse to accept the diagnosis and seek additional professional opinions in the hope that the predicted outcome is erroneous. When these efforts are in vain, the patient feels isolated and abandoned. SEE: *acceptance*.

denidation (dĕn"ĭ-dā'shŭn) [L. *de*, from, + *nidus*, nest]. Normal removal of the superficial mucosal surface of the lining of the uterus during menstruation.

denitrify. The removal of nitrogen from something.

denitrogenation. In aerospace medicine, the removal of nitrogen from the body of a person who is preparing to fly in an environment in which the barometric pressure will be much lower than that at sea level. Prior to the flight, the individual will breathe 100% oxygen for a variable length of time, depending upon the degree of reduced barometric pressure to which he or she will be exposed. SYN: *preoxygenation.* SEE: *bends; decompression illness.*

Dennie's line. An extra fold of skin below the lower eyelid. May be present in patients with atopic dermatitis.

dens (dĕnz) [L.] (pl. *dentes*). [NA] 1. A tooth. SEE: *dentition* for illus. 2. The odontoid process of the axis. A process on the body of the axis that serves as a pivot for the rotation of the atlas.

    d. bicuspidus. D. premolaris.

    d. caninus (pl. *dentes canini*). [NA] Canine tooth.

    d. deciduus (pl. *dentes decidui*). [NA] Milk tooth, first tooth.

    d. incisivus (pl. *dentes incisivi*). [NA] Incisor tooth.

    d. molaris (pl. *dentes molares*). [NA] Molar tooth, grinder.

    d. permanens (pl. *dentes permanentes*). [NA] One of the 32 teeth making up the permanent teeth.

    d. premolaris (pl. *dentes premolares*). [NA] One of the premolar teeth.

    d. sapientiae. A wisdom tooth; late tooth; third molar. SYN: *d. serotinus.*

    d. serotinus. [NA] A wisdom tooth; third molar.

densimeter (dĕn-sĭm'ĕ-tĕr) [L. *densus,* thick, + Gr. *metron,* measure]. Instrument for measuring densities.

dens in dente [L., a tooth in a tooth]. A dental anomaly in which the x-ray film of a tooth shows the outline of a second dental structure within the tooth. Outwardly, on inspection, the visible tooth is normal. SYN: *dens invaginatus.*

densitometer (dĕn"sĭ-tŏm'ĕ-tĕr). A special densimeter for measuring bacterial growth and effect of antiseptics and bacteriophages upon it. In radiology, an instrument that measures the optical density of a radiograph.

densitometry (dĕn"sĭ-tŏm'ĕ-trē). 1. Determination of the density of a substance, e.g., bone. 2. Determining the amount of ionizing radiation to which a person has been exposed.

density [L. *densitas,* thickness]. 1. Relative weight of a substance compared with a reference standard. SEE: *specific gravity.* 2. The quality of being dense. 3. The degree of blackness on a radiograph or the relationship between the light given and the light passing through a radiograph.

dental. Pert. to the teeth.

dental arch. The arch formed by the cutting and chewing surfaces of the teeth.

dental assistant. One who assists in the care and treatment of dental patients. The responsibilities vary according to the needs of the dentist, the training and capability of the individual, and the state regulations of duties.

dental caries. Decay of the teeth. SEE: *caries; fluoridation.*

dental chart. A diagrammatic representation of the mouth on which clinical and radiographic findings can be recorded. It often includes the restorations present, decayed surfaces, missing teeth, and periodontal conditions.

dental consonant. A consonant pronounced with the tongue at or near the front upper teeth. Term used in speech therapy.

dental curve. The curve or bow of the line of the teeth in the jaw. The different portions of the curve are described as follows: *alignment curve,* the line passing through the center of the teeth from the middle line through the last molar; *buccal curve,* the curve extending from the cuspid to the 3rd molar; *compensating curve,* the occlusal line of bicuspids and molars; *labial curve,* the curve extending from cuspid to cuspid.

dental disk. A thin circular piece of paper, cloth, or other substance charged with abrasive powder for cutting or polishing teeth and fillings.

dental dysfunction. Malfunctioning of the parts of the dental structure.

dental emergencies. Acute conditions affecting the teeth, such as inflammation of the soft tissues surrounding teeth and post treatment complications of dental surgery, are best treated by dentists. Nevertheless, the primary care physician and other health care professionals need to be familiar with these emergency conditions and their management. SEE: table.

dental engine. A machine operated with foot power or by an electric or a water motor to give a swift rotary motion to drills, burs, and burnishers.

dental engineering. Use of the principles of engineering in dentistry.

dental floss. Waxed or unwaxed thread, or tape used for cleaning and removing plaque between the teeth and testing for defects in the teeth.

dental formula. A brief method of expressing the dentition of mammals in which the numbers of the teeth are given in the form of a fraction, each portion of which represents one quadrant; the numbers of the upper teeth forming the numerator, and those of the lower teeth the denominator.

    The first number listed represents the in-

Signs and Symptoms and Recommended Emergency Management of Odontogenic Problems

Condition	Signs and Symptoms	Recommended Management
Acute periodontal disease		
Acute periodontal abscess	Localized pain Swelling of gingivae Possible sinus tract Lack of response to percussion Periodontal pocketing	Curettage to establish drainage Antibiotics Warm saline rinses Soft diet Referral to dentist
Pericoronitis	Pain and generalized soreness Inflamed operculum over partially erupted tooth	Irrigation Warm saline rinses Gentle massage with toothbrush Antibiotics for fever and lymphadenopathy Referral to dentist for possible tissue excision or tooth removal
Acute necrotizing ulcerative gingivitis	Generalized pain Pain with chewing Bleeding gums Foul breath Generalized gingival inflammation Necrotic tissue Loss of interdental papillae	Brushing, flossing, general debridement Daily saline rinses Hydration Referral to dentist
Acute primary herpetic gingivostomatitis	Gingival ulceration Fever Punctate lesions of gingivae and possibly dorsum of tongue, buccal mucosa, and floor of mouth	Rest Diluted mouthwashes Increased fluid intake Soft diet Topical analgesics Referral to dentist
Pulpitis and periapical problems		
Reversible pulpitis	Sharp, transient pain response to cold stimuli Recent dental restoration	Analgesics Avoidance of thermal stimuli Referral to dentist
Irreversible pulpitis	Spontaneous pain Persistent pain response to thermal stimuli	Referral to dentist for removal of pulp or extraction of tooth
Periapical inflammation	Acute pain on percussion	Examination for lymph node involvement, intraoral and extraoral swelling, and fever Analgesics Referral to dentist

Signs and Symptoms and Recommended Emergency Management of Odontogenic Problems *(Continued)*

Condition	Signs and Symptoms	Recommended Management
Periapical abscess	Tooth sensitive to touch Tooth mobile Fever Swelling	Thorough systemic examination Incision and drainage Antibiotics Analgesics Warm water rinses Referral to dentist
Posttreatment complications		
Alveolar osteitis (dry socket)	Throbbing pain 2–4 days after extraction	Irrigation of extraction site Sedative dressing (eugenol) Analgesics Gauze packs, bone wax, or gelatin sponge to control hemorrhage Referral to dentist
Tooth sensitivity	Thermal sensitivity Pain on closing mouth Imbalance when teeth contact	Referral to dentist

Source: Comer, RW, et al: Dental emergencies. Postgrad Med 85:63, February 15, 1989.

cisors; the second is for the canine; the third, premolar; and the fourth, molar. The dental formula of the upper and lower right half of the mouth of humans is:

$$\frac{2-1-2-3}{2-1-2-3}$$

dental geriatrics. The scientific study and treatment of dental conditions of the aged.

dentalgia (děn-tăl′jē-ă) [L. *dens,* tooth, + Gr. *algos,* pain]. Toothache.

dental handpiece. An instrument designed to hold the rotary instruments used in dentistry to remove tooth structure or to smooth and polish restorative materials; it may be powered by foot pedal, electric motor, air, or water turbines.

dental hygienist. A licensed allied health professional who by training and practice is skilled in performing preventive dental services such as cleaning teeth (i.e., dental prophylaxis), and in promoting dental health by instructing persons how to care for their teeth. A dental hygienist may or may not work under the supervision of a dentist.

dental index. A system of numbers for indicating comparative size of the teeth.

dental instruments. A variety of steel instruments with points or cutting surfaces at either or both ends, which can be sharpened, sterilized, and used in the special procedures of dentistry.

dental materials. The various types of colloids, plastics, resins, and metal alloys used in dentistry to take impressions, restore teeth, or duplicate the dentition; the science or department devoted to research and instruction in the use of restorative materials in dentistry.

dental plaque. A gummy mass of microorganisms that grows on the crowns and spreads along the roots of teeth. It usually is too small to be seen and is both colorless and transparent. Dental plaque is the forerunner of dental caries and periodontal disease. Calcified dental plaque is called calculus. Preventive measures include proper daily self-care of the teeth, careful use of dental floss, and periodic prophylaxis by a dentist or dental hygienist. SEE: *caries; periodontitis; pyorrhea alveolaris.*

dental prosthesis. An artificial part used in the mouth to replace missing structural tissue or teeth. SYN: *denture.*

dental pulp. The embryonic connective tissue that is vascular, well innervated, and occupies the central space within the tooth and its roots.

dental sealants. The application of plastic films to the chewing surfaces of teeth to seal the pits and grooves where food and bacteria can be trapped; used to reduce the occurrence of dental caries. Dental sealants are used in addition to fluorides and other preventive measures.

dental tape. Waxed or unwaxed thin tape used for cleaning and removing plaque between the teeth.

dental trephination. Surgical creation of a drainage tract, with a burr or sharp instrument, in the soft tissue or bone overlying a tooth root apex. This is usually done to permit drainage of an apical abscess. SYN: *apicostomy; apical puncture.*

dentate (děn′tāt) [L. *dentatus,* toothed]. Notched; having short triangular divisions of the margin; toothed.

dentes [L.]. Teeth. Pl. of dens.

denti-, dento-. Combining form concerning teeth.

dentia (děn′shē-ă) [L.]. Process of eruption of teeth.

    d. praecox. Premature eruption of teeth.

    d. tarda. Delayed eruption of teeth.

dentibuccal (děn-tǐ-bŭk′l) [L. *dens,* tooth, + *bucca,* cheek]. Pert. to both the cheek and teeth.

denticle (děn′tǐ-kl) [L. *denticulus,* little tooth]. 1. A small toothlike projection. 2. A calcified structure within the pulp of the tooth. SYN: *pulp stone.*

denticulate [L. *denticulatus,* small-toothed]. Finely toothed or serrated.

denticulate body. Corpus dentatum of the cerebellum.

dentification [L. *dens,* tooth, + *facere,* to make]. Conversion into dental structure.

dentiform [″ + *forma,* shape]. Toothlike.

dentifrice (děn′tǐ-frĭs) [″ + *fricare,* to rub]. A powder or other substance for cleaning teeth.

dentigerous (děn-tĭj′ěr-ŭs) [″ + *gerere,* to bear]. Having or containing teeth.

dentilabial (děn-tǐ-lā′bē-ăl) [″ + *labium,* lip]. Pert. to both the teeth and lips.

dentilingual (děn-tǐ-lǐn′gwăl) [″ + *lingua,* tongue]. Pert. to both the teeth and tongue.

dentimeter (děn-tǐm′ě-těr) [″ + Gr. *metron,* measure]. Device for measuring teeth.

dentin (děn′tǐn) [L. *dens,* tooth]. The calcified part of the tooth surrounding the pulp chamber, covered by enamel in the crown and by cementum in the root area.

dentinal. Pert. to dentin.

dentinitis [″ + Gr. *itis,* inflammation]. Inflammation of dentin.

dentinoblast (děn′tǐn-ō-blăst) [″ + Gr. *blastos,* germ]. An old term meaning a dentin-forming cell. SYN: *odontoblast.*

dentinoclast (děn′tǐn-ō-clăst) [″ + Gr. *clastos,* broken]. A multinucleate cell indistinguishable from an osteoclast. It is involved with resorption of dentin. The same

cells probably resorbed cementum before contacting dentin and would be better called odontoclasts. SEE: *osteoclast.*

dentinogenesis (děn″tǐn-ō-jěn′ě-sǐs) [″ + *genesis,* generation, birth]. Formation of dentin in development of a tooth.

    d. imperfecta. Hereditary aplasia or hypoplasia of the enamel and dentin of a tooth.

dentinoid [″ + Gr. *eidos,* form, shape]. 1. Resembling dentin. 2. The noncalcified matrix of dentin, similar to the noncalcified matrix of bone, which is called osteoid. SYN: *predentin.*

dentinoma [″ + Gr. *oma,* tumor]. A tumor composed of tissues that give origin to the teeth, consisting mainly of dentin.

dentinosteoid (děn″tǐn-ŏs′tē-oyd) [″ + Gr. *osteon,* bone, + *eidos,* form, shape]. A tumor composed of dentin and bone.

dentiparous (děn-tǐp′ă-rŭs) [″ + *parere,* to bring forth, to bear]. Pert. to development and formation of teeth.

dentist [L. *dens,* tooth]. An authorized practitioner of dentistry.

dentistry. 1. That branch of medicine dealing with the care of the teeth and associated structures of the oral cavity. It is concerned with the prevention, diagnosis, and treatment of diseases of the teeth and gums. 2. The art or profession of a dentist. SYN: *dentology; odontology.*

    d., esthetic. Repair and restoration or replacement of carious or broken teeth.

    d. for children. Pedodontics or pedodontology.

    d., forensic. Area of dentistry particularly related to jurisprudence; most often seen as the identification of unknown persons by the details of their dentition and tooth restorations.

    d., four-handed. Concept and practice of extensive utilization of a chairside dental assistant to facilitate and enhance the productivity of the dentist.

    d., geriatric. Area of dentistry devoted to the dental health care of the aged.

    d., hospital. The practice of dentistry in a hospital where the dentist is an integral part of the health team providing comprehensive care.

    d., operative. Branch of dentistry dealing with restorative dental operations on the mouth.

    d., prosthodontic. Replacing defective or missing teeth through the use of artificial appliances such as bridges, crowns, and dentures.

    d., public health. Area of dentistry that seeks to improve the dental health of communities by epidemiological studies, research in preventive methods, and better distribution, management, and utilization

CHILD

ADULT

DENTITION

ERUPTION OF DECIDUOUS (MILK) TEETH

UPPER	ERUPTION
CENTRAL INCISOR	5–7 MO
LATERAL INCISOR	7–10 MO
(CUSPID) CANINE	16–20 MO
FIRST MOLAR	10–16 MO
SECOND MOLAR	20–30 MO

LOWER	
SECOND MOLAR	20–30 MO
FIRST MOLAR	10–16 MO
(CUSPID) CANINE	16–20 MO
LATERAL INCISOR	8–11 MO
CENTRAL INCISOR	6–8 MO

ERUPTION OF PERMANENT TEETH

UPPER	COMPLETED BY
CENTRAL INCISOR	9–10 YR
LATERAL INCISOR	10–11 YR
(CUSPID) CANINE	12–15 YR
FIRST PREMOLAR (BICUSPID)	12–13 YR
SECOND PREMOLAR (BICUSPID)	12–14 YR
FIRST MOLAR	6–7 YR
SECOND MOLAR	14–16 YR
THIRD MOLAR	18–25 YR

LOWER	
THIRD MOLAR	18–25 YR
SECOND MOLAR	13–16 YR
SECOND PREMOLAR (BICUSPID)	13–14 YR
FIRST PREMOLAR (BICUSPID)	12–15 YR
FIRST MOLAR	6–7 YR
(CUSPID) CANINE	10–13 YR
LATERAL INCISOR	9–10 YR
CENTRAL INCISOR	8–9 YR

of dentists.

dentition [L. *dentitio*]. The type, number, and arrangement of teeth in the dental arch. SEE: illus.; *teeth* for illus.

　　d., diphyodont. Condition of having two sets of teeth, i.e., primary and permanent, as in many mammals and humans.

　　d., heterodont. Condition of having teeth of various shapes which may serve different functions; e.g., incisors, canines, and molars.

　　d., homodont. Condition of having morphologically similar teeth, as in the porpoise.

　　d., mixed. Condition of having both primary and permanent teeth, e.g., between the ages of 6 and 13 years in humans. SYN: *transitional dentition.*

　　d., monophyodont. Condition of having a single set of teeth.

　　d., permanent. The eruption of the permanent teeth (32) beginning at about the age of six years in humans. Completed by the 16th year with the exception of wisdom teeth, which appear between the 18th and 25th years. The order of eruption follows: The incisors are followed by the bicuspids (premolars) and the canines; then the second molars are followed by the third molars.

The appearance of the first molars is highly variable, but in some instances they may be the first permanent teeth to appear. SEE: *teeth.*

　　d., polyphyodont. Development of several successive sets of teeth during a lifetime.

　　d., primary. Eruption of 20 primary or deciduous teeth in humans. In general, the order of eruption is two lower central incisors, 6 to 8 months; two upper central incisors, 5 to 7 months; two lower lateral incisors, 8 to 11 months; two upper lateral incisors, 7 to 10 months; four canines (cuspids), lower and upper, 16 to 20 months; four first molars, lower and upper, 10 to 16 months; four second molars, upper and lower, 20 to 30 months.

dentoalveolar (děn″tō-ăl-vē′ō-lăr) [L. *dens,* tooth, + *alveolus,* small hollow]. Pert. to alveolus of a tooth and to the tooth itself.

dentoalveolitis (děn″to-ăl″vē-ō-lī′tĭs) [″ + ″ + Gr. *itis,* inflammation]. A purulent inflammation of the tooth socket linings characterized by looseness of the teeth and shrinkage of the gum. SYN: *pyorrhea alveolaris.*

dentofacial (děn″tō-fā′shăl). Concerning the teeth and face.

dentoid [" + Gr. *eidos,* form, shape]. Dentiform; odontoid; tooth-shaped.

dentoidin. The organic ground substance of dentin. SYN: *predentin.*

dentolegal. Concerning dentistry and legal matters.

dentulous (děn'tū-lŭs). Having one's natural teeth. SEE: *edentulous.*

denture (děn'chūr). A partial or complete set of artificial teeth set in appropriate plastic materials to substitute for the natural dentition and related tissues.

　　NURSING IMPLICATIONS: Dentures should be cleansed after each meal. They should be gently brushed with warm water and scrubbed with moderate pressure. Solutions and mixtures accepted by the American Dental Association are: 1. Ammonia water 28% (2 ml in 30 ml of water); 2. Trisodium phosphate (600 mg in 30 ml water); 3. Sodium hypochlorite (bleach) (2 ml in 120 ml water). Store dentures in an opaque, covered container. They should be stored wet or dry according to their composition. Follow the instructions given to the patient by the dentist. Remove dentures from comatose or moribund patients as well as prior to any surgical procedure.

　　d., full. Denture that replaces all of the teeth in both jaws.

　　d., immediate. A complete set of artificial teeth to be inserted immediately after removal (extraction) of natural teeth.

　　d., partial. A dental appliance replacing less than the full number of teeth in either jaw.

denturism. The movement of dental technicians to be permitted to provide dentures legally to the public independent of supervision of a dentist. SEE: *denturist.*

denturist. A dental technician who fabricates and fits dentures without supervision of a dentist.

denucleated (dē-nū'klē-āt"ĕd) [L. *de,* from, + *nucleus,* kernel]. Deprived of a nucleus.

denudation [L. *denudare,* to lay bare]. Removal of a protecting layer or covering through surgery, pathological change, or trauma.

denutrition (dē"nū-trĭsh'ŭn) [L. *de,* from, + *nutrire,* to nourish]. Malnutrition.

Denver classification. A system for classifying chromosomes based on size and position of the centromere. SEE: *chromosome.*

Denver Developmental Screening Test. ABBR: DDST. Widely used screening test to detect problems in the development of very young children.

deodorant (dē-ō'dor-ănt) [" + *odorare,* to perfume]. An agent that masks or absorbs foul odors. SEE: *odor.*

deodorize (dē-ō'dor-īz) [" + *odor,* odor].

To remove foul odor.

deodorizer (dē-ō'dor-īz-ĕr). That which deodorizes.

deontology (dē"ŏn-tŏl'ō-jē) [Gr. *deonta,* needful, + *logos,* word, reason]. The theory or study of professional obligations and commitments; medical ethics. SEE: *ethics.*

deorsum (dē-or'sŭm) [L.]. Downward.

　　d. vergens. Turning downward.

deorsumduction (dē-or"sŭm-dŭk'shŭn) [L. *deorsum,* downward, + *ducere,* to lead]. Bending downward.

deorsumversion (dē-or"sŭm-vĕr'zhŭn) [" + *vertere,* to turn]. Downward turning or movement of the eyes.

deossification (dē-ŏs"ĭ-fĭ-kā'shŭn) [L. *de,* from, + *os,* bone, + *facere,* to make]. Loss of or removal of mineral matter from bone or osseous tissue.

deoxidate [" + Gr. *oxys,* sharp]. To remove oxygen from a chemical.

deoxidation. Process of depriving a chemical compound of oxygen.

deoxidizer (dē-ŏk'sĭ-dī-zĕr). A deoxidizing agent.

deoxycholic acid (dē-ŏk"sē-kō'lĭk). $C_{24}H_{40}O_4$. A crystalline acid found in bile.

deoxycorticosterone (dē-ŏk"sē-kor"tē-kŏs'tĕr-ōn). A hormone from the adrenal gland. It acts principally on salt and water metabolism.

deoxygenation (dē-ŏk"sĭ-jĕn-ā'shŭn). Removal of oxygen from a chemical compound or tissue.

deoxyribonuclease (dē-ŏk"sē-rī"bō-nū'klē-ās). ABBR: DNase. An enzyme that hydrolyzes and thus depolymerizes deoxyribonucleic acid (DNA).

deoxyribonucleic acid (dē-ŏk"sē-rī"bō-nū-klē'ĭk). ABBR: DNA. A complex nucleic acid of high molecular weight consisting of deoxyribose, phosphoric acid, and four bases (two purines, adenine and guanine, and two pyrimidines, thymine and cytosine). These are arranged as two long chains that twist around each other to form a double helix joined by bonds between the complementary components. Nucleic acid is present in chromosomes of the nuclei of cells and is the chemical basis of heredity and the carrier of genetic information for all organisms except the RNA viruses. Formerly spelled desoxyribonucleic acid. SEE. *chromosome; gene; ribonucleic acid; virus.*

deoxyribonucleoprotein (dē-ŏk"sē-rī"bō-nū"klē-ō-prō'tē-ĭn). Class of conjugated proteins that contain deoxyribonucleic acid.

deoxyribonucleoside (dē-ŏk"sē-rī"bō-nū'klē-ō-sīd). Class of nucleotide in which the pentose is 2-deoxyribose.

deoxyribose (dē-ŏk″sē-rī′bōs). A phosphoric ester of a pentose present in nucleic acid.

depancreatize (dē-păn′krē-ă-tīz). To remove the pancreas surgically.

Department of Health and Human Services. ABBR: HHS. The U.S. Government agency that administers federal health programs. Previous name was Department of Health, Education, and Welfare.

Depen. Trade name for penicillamine.

dependence (dē-pĕn′dĕns) [L. *dependere*, to hang down]. 1. A form of behavior that suggests inability to make decisions. 2. A psychic craving for a drug that may or may not be accompanied by physiological dependency. 3. A state of reliance on another. SEE: *habituation; withdrawal.*

dependent care. Caring for persons who are dependent. Included would be elderly parents and other relatives, as well as children. SEE: *dumping,* def. 2.

depersonalization disorder. The belief that one's own reality is temporarily lost or altered. The patient feels estranged or unreal and may have the sensation that the extremities have changed size. Feeling of being automated or as if in a dream may be present. The onset is usually rapid, and it usually occurs in adolescence or under extreme stress, fatigue, or anxiety.

depersonalize. To make impersonal; to deprive of personality or individuality.

de Pezzer's catheter. Self-retaining urethral catheter that has a bulbous tip.

dephosphorylation (dē-fŏs″for-ī-lā′shŭn) [L. *de,* from, + *phosphorylation*]. Removal of a phosphate group from a compound.

depigmentation (dē″pĭg-mĕn-tā′shŭn). Removal of pigment, esp. from the skin, by use of chemical or physical means.

depilate (dĕp′ĭl-āt) [L. *depilare,* to deprive of hair]. To remove hair.

depilation (dĕp″ĭl-ā′shŭn). The process of hair removal. SEE: *epilation.*

depilatory. An agent used for the removal of hair.

depilatory techniques. Removal of hair from the body may be accomplished by several temporary procedures, including shaving the area; plucking a few unsightly hairs; chemically; or by wax treatment. If chemical depilation is used, care must be taken to avoid skin irritation. The wax treatment involves application of molten wax, allowing it to cool; then, when the wax is pulled away, the hair comes with it. Permanent depilation is accomplished by electrolysis of each hair follicle. This time-consuming process is done by an electrologist trained in the technique. SEE: *electrolysis; hirsutism.*

deplete (dē-plēt′) [L. *depletus,* emptied]. To empty; to produce depletion.

depletion (dē-plē′shŭn). Removal of substances such as blood, fluids, iron, fat, and protein from the body.

deplumation (dē″ploo-mā′shŭn) [L. *de,* from, + *pluma,* feather]. Loss of eyelashes as result of disease.

depolarization (dē-pō″lăr-ĭ-zā′shŭn) [″ + *polus,* pole]. The process of reducing to a nonpolarized condition; neutralization of polarity.

depolymerization (dē-pŏl″ĭ-mĕr-ĭ-zā′shŭn). The breakdown or splitting of polymers into their basic building blocks or monomers.
    Ex.: the glucose monomer may be polymerized to form the large glycogen polymer and then broken down, i.e., depolymerized, to form glucose.

Depo-Medrol. Trade name for methylprednisolone acetate.

Depo-Provera. Trade name for medroxyprogesterone acetate.

deposit (dē-pŏz′ĭt) [L. *depositus,* having put aside]. 1. Sediment; precipitate. 2. Matter collected in any part of an organism.
    d., calcareous. Deposit of calcified material, as in calculus on teeth.
    d., tooth. Soft or hard materials deposited on the surface of a tooth. Also known as plaque or calculus.

deposition. In law, an oral interrogation about the subject at issue. The party or witness is under oath and the interrogation is recorded word for word by a judicial officer such as a court reporter.

depot (dē′pō, dĕp′ō) [Fr. *depot,* fr. L. *depositum*]. A place of storage, esp. in the body, such as fat depot.

depravation (dĕp″ră-vā′shŭn) [L. *depravare,* completely destroyed]. Pathological deterioration of function or secretion.

depressant [L. *depressus,* pressed down]. An agent that will depress a body function or nerve activity, such as sedative medicines.
    d., cardiac. Depressant that decreases heart rate and contractility.
    d., cerebral. Depressant that lessens brain activity, making the patient dull and less active. Large doses may produce sleep.
    d., motor. Depressant that lessens contractions of involuntary muscles.
    d., respiratory. Drug that lessens frequency and depth of breathing.
    d., secretory. Agent causing decreased glandular secretions.

depressed (dē-prĕst′). 1. Below the normal level, as when fragments of bone are forced below their normal level and that of surrounding portions of bone. 2. Low in spirits; dejected. 3. Decreased level of function. SEE: *depression.*

depression (dē-prĕsh′ŭn) [L. *depressio,* a

pressing down]. 1. A hollow or lowered region. 2. The lowering of a part, such as the mandible. 3. The decrease of a vital function such as respiration. 4. Mental depression characterized by altered mood. An estimated 3% to 5% of the world's population experiences depression on any given date. There is loss of interest in all usually pleasurable outlets such as food, sex, work, friends, hobbies, or entertainment. Diagnostic criteria include presence of depressed mood nearly every day, markedly diminished interest or pleasure in most or all activities, and 3 or more of the following: (1) Poor appetite or significant weight loss; or increased weight gain. (2) Insomnia or hypersomnia. (3) Psychomotor agitation or retardation. (4) Feeling of hopelessness. (5) Loss of energy, or fatigue. (6) Feelings of worthlessness, self-reproach, or excessive or inappropriate guilt. (7) Complaints of or evidence of diminished ability to think or concentrate. (8) Recurrent thoughts of death, suicidal ideation, wish to be dead, or attempted suicide.

TREAT: Therapy must be individualized because the various types of depression have different underlying causes. Thus, to attempt to treat all persons suffering depression with the same medication would be ill-advised. SEE: *depression, situational or reactive; electroconvulsive therapy; grief reaction; suicide.*

NURSING IMPLICATIONS: Evaluate the patient's level of physical activity and socialization, feelings of worthlessness, self-esteem versus self-reproach, inappropriate guilt, concern with death, and attempts at self-injury. Provide adequate nutrition and fluids and assistance with grooming and other activities of daily living. Consistently demonstrate warmth and interest in the patient. Guard against use of excessive cheerfulness while maintaining an optimistic attitude. Using positive reinforcement techniques, reduce support gradually as patient demonstrates ability to resume self-care.

d., anaclitic. Depression in infants separated from their mothers between the first months and 1 year of age. These infants have been cared for in a suitable physical situation, but without the love, affection, and nurturing usually present in the mother-child relationship. These infants may have severe disturbances in health, motor, language, and social development. They may die. Symptoms include crying, panic behavior, and increased motor activity at first. Later, there is depression, apathy, staring into space, and silent crying.

d., bipolar. Depression in which disor-

ders of both mood and elation are alternately present.

d., endogenous. D., melancholic, q.v.

d., melancholic. This form of depression is defined by meeting the criteria in def. 4 of depression, q.v., plus the presence of at least 5 of the following: lack of reaction to usually pleasurable stimuli; depression regularly worse in the morning; early morning awakening; psychomotor retardation or agitation; marked anorexia or weight loss; no marked personality disturbance before major depressive episode; one or more previous major depressive episodes followed by complete or near complete recovery; previous good response to specific and adequate somatic antidepressant therapy.

d., postpartum. The signs and symptoms of depression that do not dissipate within several weeks following delivery, or strong feelings of depression and anger that begin 1 to 2 months after childbirth. SEE: *postpartum blues.*

d., situational or reactive. Mental depression usually self-limiting, following severe life disappointments such as a death in the family, loss of a job, or a personal financial catastrophe.

d., unipolar. Mental depression characterized by mind shifts from a normal baseline to a depressed state.

depressomotor (dē-prĕs′ō-mō″tor) [″ + *motor*, mover]. Drug that diminishes muscular movements by lessening the impulses for motion sent from the brain or spinal cord.

depressor [L.]. Instrument for depressing a part.

d., tongue. Device used to depress and displace the tongue in order to facilitate visual examination of the throat.

depressor fibers. Muscles that depress or draw down a part.

depressor nerve. A nerve, the stimulation of which lessens or inhibits the activity of an organ or tissue.

depressor reflex. More or less transient stimulation of depressor fibers.

deprivation (dĕp″rĭ-vā′shŭn) [L. *de,* from, + *privare,* to remove]. Loss or absence of necessary parts or functions.

d., emotional. Isolation of an individual, esp. an infant, from normal emotional stimuli. In infants, this produces impairment of mental and physical development.

d., sensory. A situation or environment wherein the usual sensory stimuli, such as noise and light, as well as human contact are absent or, in the case of noise, masked by a continuous dull noise. Persons exposed partially or completely to such an environment include astronauts, patients in artificial respirators, and patients with temporary loss of a sense (as in bandaging of both eyes). Prolonged exposure to lack of sensory stimuli may cause hallucinations and other signs and symptoms of mental disorder.

d., sleep, effects of. SEE: *sleep deprivation, effects of.*

deprogram. The freeing of an individual from some mentally harmful cult, religion, or political brainwashing program.

depth [ME. *depthe*]. Richness; intensity; quality of being deep.

depth dose. Actual amount of radiation exposure at a specific point below the surface of the body.

depth perception. Perception of spatial relationships; three-dimensional perception.

depth psychology. Psychology of unconscious behavior. Opposed to psychology of conscious behavior.

depulization (dĕ-pūl″ĭ-zā′shŭn) [L. *de,* from, + *pulex,* flea]. Destruction of fleas, including those that carry the plague bacillus.

depurant (dĕp′ū-rănt) [L. *depurare,* to purify]. 1. A medicine that helps to purify by promoting the removal of waste material from the body. 2. Removal of waste material.

depuration. Process of freeing from impurities.

depurative. Having cleansing properties.

depurator. An agent that purifies.

de Quervain's disease. Tenosynovitis due to relative narrowness of the tendon sheath of the abductor pollicis longus and the extensor pollicis brevis.

deradelphus (dĕr-ă-dĕl′fŭs) [Gr. *dere,* neck, + *adelphos,* brother]. Malformed twins, fused above the thorax and having one head, but separated below the chest as two bodies.

deradenitis (dĕr″ăd-ĕn-ī′tĭs) [″ + *aden,* gland, + *itis,* inflammation]. Inflammation of a lymph gland of the neck.

deradenoncus (dĕr″ăd-ĕn-ŏnk′ŭs) [″ + *onkos,* bulk, mass]. Swelling or tumor of a neck gland.

derangement (dĕ-rānj′mĕnt) [Fr. *deranger,* unbalance]. 1. Lack of order or organization, esp. as compared to the previous condition; confusion. 2. A defect in the annulus fibrosus of the intervertebral disk allowing the nucleus pulposus to herniate.

Dercum's disease (dĕr′kŭms) [Francis X. Dercum, U.S. neurologist, 1856–1931]. Scattered areas of painful cutaneous nodules or fat accumulations in menopausal women. SYN: *adiposis dolorosa.*

derealization. The sense that reality has changed; a sense of detachment from one's surroundings.

dereism (dē′rē-ĭzm) [L. *de,* from, + *res,* thing]. In psychiatry, activity and thought based on fantasy and wishes rather than logic or reason.

dereistic (dē″rē-ĭs′tĭk) [″ + *res,* thing]. Pert. to overexercise of the imagination to the extent of ignoring reality, as seen in daydreaming. SEE: *autism.*

derencephalus (dĕr″ĕn-sĕf′ă-lŭs) [Gr. *dere,* neck, + *enkephalos,* brain]. Congenitally deformed fetus with a rudimentary skull and bifid cervical vertebrae.

derivation (dĕr″ĭ-vā′shŭn) [L. *derivare,* to draw off]. The source or origin of a substance.

derivative (dĕ-rĭv′ă-tĭv). 1. That which is not original or fundamental. 2. Anything derived from another body or substance. 3. That which produces derivation. 4. In embryology, that which develops from a preceding structure, as the derivatives of the germ layers.

derm, derma [Gr. *derma,* skin]. The cutis vera, or true skin.

dermabrasion (dĕrm″ă-brā″zhŭn) [″ + L. *abrasio,* wearing away]. A surgical procedure for removal of acne scars, nevi, tattoos, or fine wrinkles on the skin by using sandpaper or mechanical methods on the frozen epidermis. Procedure is dangerous and should not be used indiscriminately. SEE: *chemical peel of skin; planing.*

Dermacentor (dĕr″mă-sĕn′tor). A genus of ticks belonging to the order Acarina, family Ixodidae.

   D. andersoni. The wood tick, a species of ticks that is parasitic on man or other mammals during some part of its life cycle. May transmit causative agents of Rocky Mountain spotted fever, scrub typhus, tularemia, anaplasmosis, brucellosis, Q fever, and several forms of virus encephalomyelitis. Also causes tick paralysis.

   D. variabilis. A species of ticks similar to *D. andersoni.* In central and eastern United States, it is the main vector for Rocky Mountain spotted fever. Parasitic to dogs, horses, cattle, rabbits, and humans.

Dermacort. Trade name for hydrocortisone.

dermad [Gr. *derma,* skin, + L. *ad,* toward]. Toward the skin; externally.

dermadrome (dĕr′mă-drōm). Skin manifestation of a systemic disease.

dermal. Rel. to the skin or derma. SYN: *cutaneous; integumentary.*

dermalaxia (dĕr″mă-lăk′sē-ă) [″ + *malaxis,* softening]. Morbid relaxation or softness of the skin.

dermalgia (dĕr-măl′jē-ă) [″ + *algos,* pain]. Pain localized in the skin.

dermamyiasis (dĕr-mă-mī-ī′ă-sĭs) [″ + *myia,* fly, + *-iasis,* condition]. Skin disease caused by invasion of larvae of dipterous insects.

dermapostasis (dĕr″mă-pŏs′tă-sĭs) [″ + *apostasis*, a falling away]. Abscess formation accompanying a skin disease.

dermat-, dermato- [Gr. *dermatos*]. Prefixes indicating relationship to skin.

dermatalgia (dĕr″mă-tăl′jē-ă) [Gr. *dermatos*, skin, + *algos*, pain]. Paresthesia with localized pain in the skin. SYN: *dermalgia.*

dermatatrophia (dĕrm″ăt-ă-trō′fē-ă) [″ + *atrophia*, atrophy]. Atrophy of the skin.

dermatides. Plural of dermatitis.

dermatitis (dĕr″mă-tī′tĭs) [Gr. *dermatos*, skin, + *itis*, inflammation]. Inflammation of skin evidenced by itching, redness, and various skin lesions.

ETIOL: May be due to one of several causes: systemic disease, skin irritants such as poison ivy, corrosives, acids, and alkalies or hypersusceptibility on part of patient to conditions that would not cause skin irritation in persons who were not hypersusceptible.

TREAT: Remove primary cause if due to systemic effect. If caused by local agent, remove irritant by washing with soap and water.

NURSING IMPLICATIONS: Assist patient to avoid harsh soaps, known irritants, temperature extremes, emotional stress, and other potential precipitants. Use local measures (tepid sponge baths, cool compresses) to relieve pruritus and inflammation. Administer prescribed drug therapy and assess response. Teach patient how to apply topical medicines if they are prescribed; warn about drowsiness related to systemic antihistamine drugs; and instruct about the serious side effects of systemic corticosteroid therapy. Encourage patient to express feelings about condition, and avoid showing distaste when caring for patient's lesions.

    d., actinic. Reaction of skin to sunlight or other sources of photochemical activity such as x-rays or ultraviolet light.

    d., allergic. Inflammation believed to be due to an allergy. SEE: *allergen; allergy.*

    d., atopic. Dermatitis of unknown etiology characterized by itching and scratching in an individual with inherently irritable skin. There may be allergic, hereditary, or psychological components. The disease rarely occurs prior to two months of age and may occur initially quite late in life. In about 70% of all cases there is a family history of the disease. About 3% of all infants have atopic dermatitis. The symptoms are made worse by contact with wool, climatic changes, and excessive exposure to soap, water, and oils. The skin lesion in infants consists of swollen papules that are itchy and become exudative and crusty from scratching. Secondary infection and lymphadenopathy are common. About half of the infantile cases clear up by 18 months of age. The lesions in children and adults are similar to those of infancy but lichenification is present.

TREAT: Avoidance of soaps and ointments. Bathing should be kept to a minimum, but bath oils may help to prevent drying of the skin. Use soft-textured clothing that does not contain wool. Fingernails should be kept short to decrease damage from scratching. Antihistamines may help to reduce itching at night. Avoid heavy exercise because of its induction of perspiration. Use a nonlipid softening lotion followed by a cortisone or hydrocortisone lotion in a propylene glycol base twice daily. Oral antibiotics may be needed for a brief period to control secondary infection.

    d., berlock or d., berloque. A type of phytophotodermatitis with postinflammatory hyperpigmentation at the site of application of perfumes or colognes containing oil of bergamot.

    d. calorica. Inflammation due to heat or cold, as in sunburn.

    d., cercarial. Dermatitis resulting from infestation with the cercaria of blood flukes belonging to the genus *Schistosoma*. SYN: *schistosome dermatitis; swimmer's itch.*

    d., contact. Inflammation and irritation of the skin due to contact with an irritating substance. Usually due to a combination of reduced ability of the skin to resist injury and exposure to a material in strong concentration such as soap or chemical. Some individuals are sensitive to such apparently innocuous compounds as perfumes and deodorants.

TREAT: Remove patient from offending material and treat skin as indicated. SYN: *d. venenata.*

    d., cosmetic. Dermatitis caused by an ingredient in a cosmetic preparation. A form of contact dermatitis.

    d., diaper. Irritation of the skin in contact with a diaper. Possible etiological agents include soap, powder, urine, ammonia, feces, any one of which may be aggravated by the prolonged contact of the skin with moisture.

    d., exfoliative. SEE: *exfoliative dermatitis.*

    d. herpetiformis. Chronic inflammatory disease characterized by erythematous, papular, vesicular, bullous, or pustular lesions with tendency to grouping and with intense itching and burning.

SYM: Lesions develop suddenly and spread peripherally. Disease is variable and erratic, and attack may be prolonged for weeks or months. Secondary infection may follow trauma to the inflamed areas.

ETIOL: Direct cause unknown. Occurs mostly in adult males though no age is exempt. Some patients have associated asymptomatic gluten-sensitive enteropathy. In those persons the HLA-B8 antigen may be present.

TREAT: Oral dapsone will provide substantial relief of symptoms in a few days. Also sulfapyridine may be used.

d. hiemalis. Dermatitis occurring in cold weather.

d. infectiosa eczematoides. Pustular eruption during or following a pyogenic disease.

d. medicamentosa. Drug eruption.

SYM: With exception of bromine and iodine, the eruption is not characteristic and may resemble almost any condition or disease of the skin.

ETIOL: Idiosyncrasy or sensitization to the drug in question. Cosmetics, arsenic, iodides, bromides, phenobarbital, and antibiotics are some of the offending agents.

TREAT: Removal of cause.

d. multiformis. Form of dermatitis with lesions of a pustular nature.

d. papillaris capillitii. Formation on scalp and neck of surface elevations interspersed with pustules and ending in scarlike elevations resembling keloids.

d., poison ivy. Dermatitis resulting from ivy poisoning. SYN: *d., rhus.* SEE: *poison ivy dermatitis.*

d., primary. Skin eruption that is a direct, rather than an allergic, response.

d., radiation. Dermatitis due to radiation exposure.

d., rhus. A contact dermatitis caused by substances present in certain plants. SEE: *poison ivy dermatitis; Toxicodendron.*

d. seborrheica. Acute or subacute inflammatory skin disease of unknown etiology beginning on the scalp, characterized by rounded, irregular, or circinate lesions covered with yellow or brown-gray greasy scales. SYN: *alopecia furfuracea; pityriasis capitis; seborrhea corporis; seborrhea sicca.* SEE: *Nursing Diagnoses* in *Appendix.*

SYM: On the scalp, it may be dry with abundant grayish branny scales, or oozing and crusted, constituting eczema capitis, and may spread to forehead and postauricular regions. On the forehead, it shows scaly and infiltrated lesions with dark red bases, some itching, localized loss of hair. On eyebrows and eyelashes, dry, dirty white scales with itching. On nasolabial folds or vermilion border of lips, inflammation with itching. On sternal region, greasy and unctuous to the touch. May appear in interscapular,

axillary, and genitocrural regions also.

TREAT: When limited to scalp, frequent shampooing and use of mild keratolytic agents. Selenium-containing shampoos have been helpful. Generalized seborrheic dermatitis requires careful attention including scrupulous skin hygiene, keeping skin as dry as possible, dusting powders. Topical and systemic cortisone preparations may be required.

d., stasis. Eczema of the legs with edema, pigmentation, and sometimes chronic inflammation. Usually due to impaired circulation.

d. venenata. Any inflammation caused by local action of various animal, vegetable, or mineral substances contacting the surface of the skin.

SYM: Vary from simple hyperemia to gangrene and sloughing. Majority are erythematous, limited to part touched by irritant, becoming papular, vesicular, or pustular with burning or itching.

ETIOL: Drugs, acids, alkalies, plants (poison ivy, oak, or sumac). Runs an acute course with recurrence on re-exposure to the sensitizing agent.

TREAT: Apply local drying solutions such as aluminum acetate. Calamine lotion is helpful in drying the lesions and for control of itching. In severe cases, the use of topical and systemic cortisone may be needed.

d. verrucosa. Chronic fungal infection of the skin characterized by the formation of wartlike nodules. These may enlarge and form papillomatous structures that sometimes ulcerate. SYN: *chromoblastomycosis,* q.v.

ETIOL: May be due to one of several fungi including *Hormodendrum pedrosoi* or *Phialophora verrucosa.*

d., x-ray. Skin inflammation due to effects of x-rays.

dermatoautoplasty (dĕr″mă-tō-aw′tō-plăs″tē) [Gr. *dermatos,* skin, + *autos,* self, + *plassein,* to form]. Grafting of skin taken from some portion of the patient's own body.

Dermatobia (dĕr″mă-tō′bē-ă) [″ + *bios,* life]. A genus of botflies belonging to the order Diptera of the family Oestridae.

D. hominis. A species of botflies, found in parts of tropical America, whose larvae infest man and cattle. The eggs are transported by mosquitoes.

dermatobiasis (dĕr″mă-tō-bī′ă-sĭs). Infestation by the larvae of *Dermatobia hominis,* the eggs of which are carried to the skin by mosquitoes. The larvae then hatch and bore into the skin while the mosquito feeds. Marblelike boils form at the site of infestation.

dermatocele (dĕr'mă-tō-sēl") [" + *kele*, tumor, swelling]. Tendency of hypertrophied skin and subcutaneous tissue to hang loosely in folds. SYN: *dermatolysis*.

   d. lipomatosa. A pedunculated lipoma with cystic degeneration.

dermatocelidosis (dĕr"mă-tō-sĕl"ĭ-dō'sĭs) [" + *kelis*, spot, + *osis*, condition]. Freckles; a macular eruption. SYN: *dermatokelidosis*.

dermatocellulitis (dĕr"mă-tō-sĕl"ū-lī'tĭs) [" + L. *cellula*, little cell, + Gr. *itis*, inflammation]. Inflammation of subcutaneous connective tissue.

dermatoconiosis (dĕr"mă-tō-kō"nē-ō'sĭs) [" + *konia*, dust]. Any irritation of the skin caused by dust, esp. one due to occupational exposure.

dermatocyst (dĕr'mă-tō-sĭst) [" + *kystis*, cyst]. A skin cyst.

dermatofibroma [" + L. *fibra*, fiber, + Gr. *oma*, tumor]. A nonmalignant skin fibroma. SEE: *dimple sign*.

dermatofibrosarcoma (dĕr"mă-tō-fī"brō-sär-kō'mă) [" + " + Gr. *sarx*, flesh, + *oma*, tumor]. Fibrosarcoma of the skin.

dermatogen (dĕr-măt'ō-jĕn) [" + *gennan*, to produce]. Antigen from a skin disease.

dermatogenous (dĕr"mă-tŏj'ĕn-ŭs). Producing skin or disease of skin.

dermatoglyphics (dĕr"mă-tō-glĭf'ĭks) [" + *glyphe*, a carving]. Study of surface markings of the skin, esp. those of hands and feet. Useful in identification and genetic studies. SEE: *fingerprint* for illus.

dermatographia, dermatography. A form of urticaria due to physical allergy.

dermatoheliosis. Sun-induced degenerative changes in the skin. Included are wrinkling, atrophy, hyper- and hypomelanotic macules, telangiectasia, yellow papules and plaques, keratoses, and degeneration of elastic tissue. This condition can be prevented by avoiding exposure to the sun or by using topically applied effective sunscreens.

dermatoheteroplasty (dĕr"mă-tō-hĕt'ĕr-ō-plăs"tē) [" + *heteros*, other, + *plassein*, to mold]. Skin grafting from a member of a different species.

dermatokelidosis (dĕr"mă-tō-kĕl"ĭ-dō'sĭs) [" + *kelidoun*, to stain]. A macular eruption; freckle.

dermatologist (dĕr"mă-tŏl'ō-jĭst) [Gr. *dermatos*, skin, + *logos*, word, reason]. A physician who specializes in treating diseases of the skin.

dermatology (dĕr"mă-tŏl'ō-jē). The science of the skin and its diseases.

dermatolysis (dĕr"mă-tŏl'ĭ-sĭs) [" + *lysis*, dissolution]. Tendency of hypertrophied skin and subcutaneous tissue to hang in folds. Loose skin. SYN: *cutis laxa; cutis pendula; pachydermatocele* (def. 1).

dermatoma (dĕr"mă-tō'mă) [" + *oma*, tumor]. Circumscribed thickening of skin.

dermatome (dĕr'mă-tōm) [Gr. *derma*, skin, + *tome*, incision]. 1. Instrument for incising the skin or for cutting thin slices for transplantation of skin. 2. A delineated area of skin innervated by a spinal cord segment. Each cord segment has a representative skin area. SEE: illus. 3. The lateral portion of the somite of an embryo, which gives rise to the dermis of the skin; the cutis plate.

dermatomere (dĕr'mă-tō-mēr) [Gr. *dermatos*, skin, + *meros*, part]. A segment of embryonic integument.

dermatomucosomyositis (dĕr"mă-tō-mū-kō"sō-mī-ō-sī'tĭs) [" + L. *mucosa*, mucous membrane, + Gr. *mys*, muscle, + *itis*, inflammation]. Inflammation involving mucosa and muscles.

dermatomycosis (dĕr"mă-tō-mī-kō'sĭs) [" + *mykes*, fungus, + *osis*, condition] (pl. *dermatomycoses*). A skin infection caused by certain fungi of the genera *Trichophyton*, *Epidermophyton*, and *Microsporum*. SYN: *tinea*.

dermatomyoma [" + *mys*, muscle, + *oma*, tumor]. Myoma of the skin.

dermatomyositis (dĕr"mă-tō-mī"ō-sī'tĭs) [" + " + *itis*, inflammation]. A disease of connective tissue. An acute, subacute, or chronic disease of unknown etiology. Characterized by edema, dermatitis, and inflammation of the muscles.

SYM: Fever, malaise, general weakness, weakness of the pelvic and shoulder girdle muscles; skin and mucosal lesions often present. About one third of patients will have dysphagia.

TREAT: Symptomatic: bedrest, physical therapy, salicylates. Adrenocortical steroids are helpful in most cases. Cytotoxic drugs such as azathioprine, cyclophosphamide, or methotrexate may be of benefit in patients who do not respond to adrenocortical steroids.

NURSING IMPLICATIONS: Assess and record level of discomfort, muscle weakness, and range of motion on a daily basis. Careful turning is needed along with frequent position changes. Maintenance of correct body alignment, massage, graduated exercises, and resistance exercises are beneficial in preventing or treating muscle atrophy and contractures. Warm baths and moist heat applications are helpful in relief of stiffness. Mouth lesions may be irrigated with warm saline solution as needed.

Encourage self-help activities to maintain patient independence. Assist patient to avoid scratching. Apply tepid sponge baths

or compresses as needed. Teach patient and family about disease process and possible therapeutic, undesired effects of corticosteroids and cytotoxic drugs. Encourage patient to express fears and concerns; provide realistic support and encouragement.

dermatoneurosis [" + *neuron*, nerve, + *osis*, condition]. Skin disease of nervous origin. SEE: *neurodermatitis*.

dermatopathia [" + *pathos*, disease, suffering]. Any disease of the skin.

dermatopathology [" + " + *logos*, word, reason]. Study of diseases of the skin.

dermatopathy. Any skin disease. SYN: *dermatopathia*.

dermatophiliasis (dĕr"mă-tō-fĭ-lī'ă-sĭs). 1. Infestation with *Tunga penetrans*, a pathogenic actinomycete. 2. Dermatophilosis.

dermatophilosis (dĕr"mă-tō-fĭ-lō'sĭs). An actinomycotic infection that occurs in certain hooved animals and rarely in humans.

dermatophobia [" + *phobos*, fear]. Abnormal fear of having a skin disease.

dermatophylaxis (dĕr'mă-tō-fĭ-lăk'sĭs) [" + *phylaxis*, protection]. Protecting the skin from infection.

dermatophyte (dĕr'mă-tō-fīt) [" + *phyton*, plant]. A fungal parasite that grows in or on the skin. Dermatophytes rarely penetrate deeper than the epidermis or its appendages — hair and nails. They cause such skin diseases as favus, tinea, ringworm, and eczema. Important dermatophytes include the genera *Microsporum*, *Trichophyton*, and *Epidermophyton*.

dermatophytid (dĕr"mă-tŏf'ĭ-tĭd). A toxic rash or eruption occurring in dermatomycosis.

dermatophytosis (dĕr"mă-tō-fĭ-tō'sĭs) [" + *phyton*, plant, + *osis*, condition]. A fungus infection of the skin of the hands and feet, esp. between the toes. SYN: *athlete's foot; ringworm of feet; tinea pedis.*

dermatoplastic [" + *plassein*, to form]. Pert. to skin grafting.

dermatoplasty (dĕr'mă-tō-plăs"tē). Transplanting living skin to cover cutaneous defects caused by injury, operation, or disease.

NURSING IMPLICATIONS: Nursing measures are directed toward protection of the graft site from dislodgement, from trauma or infection; and promotion of healing of the donor site. Monitor signs of infection such as fever and pain and assist patient to cope with altered mobility. Provide pain relief as indicated. As with any patient who has skin grafting, good nutrition is essential.

dermatorrhagia (dĕr"mă-tō-rā'jē-ă) [Gr. *dermatos*, skin, + *rhegnynai*, to burst forth]. Hemorrhage into or from the skin.

dermatorrhea (dĕr"mă-tō-rē'ă) [" +

rhoia, flow]. Excessive secretion of sebaceous glands.

dermatorrhexis [" + *rhexis*, rupture]. Rupture of the skin and capillaries in the skin.

dermatosclerosis (dĕr"mă-tō-sklĕr-ō'sĭs) [" + *sklerosis*, hardening]. Infiltration of the skin with fibrous material.

dermatosis (dĕr"mă-tō'sĭs) [" + *osis*, condition] (pl. *dermatoses*). Any disease of the skin in which inflammation is not necessarily a feature. Not a synonym for dermatitis.

   d. papulosa nigra. Eruption consisting of many tiny tumors or milia on skin of face. Greatest incidence is among blacks.

   d., progressive pigmentary. Reddish papules principally on legs; eruption is slowly progressive.

dermatosome (dĕr'mă-tō-sōm) [" + *soma*, body]. Section of equatorial plate in mitosis.

dermatotherapy [" + *therapeia*, treatment]. Treatment of skin diseases.

dermatotome (dĕr'mă-tō-tōm") [" + *tome*, incision]. 1. One of the fetal skin segments. 2. A knife for incising the skin or small lesions. SYN: *dermatome* (def. 1).

dermatotropic (dĕr"mă-tō-trŏp'ĭk) [" + *trope*, a turning]. Acting preferentially on the skin.

dermatoxerasia (dĕr"mă-tō-zē-rā'zē-ă) [" + *xerasia*, dryness]. Roughening of skin. SYN: *xeroderma*.

dermatozoon [" + *zoon*, animal]. An animal parasite of the skin.

dermatozoonosis (dĕr"mă-tō-zō"ō-nō'sĭs) [" + " + *nosos*, disease]. Any skin disease caused by an animal parasite.

dermatrophia (dĕr-ă-trō'fē-ă) [" + *atrophia*, atrophy]. Atrophy of the skin.

dermic (dĕr'mĭk) [Gr. *derma*, skin]. Pert. to the skin.

dermis (dĕr'mĭs) [L.]. The skin; cutis vera or true skin. SYN: *corium* [NA].

dermoblast [Gr. *derma*, skin, + *blastos*, germ]. Part of mesoblastic layer, developing into the corium.

dermographia, dermography (dĕr-mō-grăf'ē-ă, -ŏg'ră-fē) [" + *graphein*, to write]. A form of urticaria due to allergy.

dermoid (dĕr'moyd) [" + *eidos*, form, shape]. 1. Resembling the skin. 2. A dermoid cyst.

dermoid cyst. An ovarian teratoma. A nonmalignant cystic tumor in which are found elements derived from the ectoderm, such as hair, teeth, or skin. These tumors occur frequently in the ovary but may develop in other organs such as the lungs.

dermoidectomy (dĕr"moyd-ĕk'tō-mē) [" + " + *ektome*, excision]. Excision of a dermoid cyst.

dermolipoma (dĕr″mō-lĭ-pō′mă). 1. Growth of yellow fatty tissue beneath the bulbar conjunctiva. 2. Lipoma of the skin.

dermomycosis (dĕr″mō-mī-kō′sĭs) [″ + *mykes*, fungus, + *osis*, condition]. A skin disease produced by a fungus. SYN: *tinea*.

dermonosology (dĕr″mō-nō-sŏl′ō-jē) [″ + *nosos*, disease, + *logos*, word, reason]. The science of classification of skin diseases.

dermophlebitis (dĕr″mō-flĕ-bī′tĭs) [″ + *phleps*, vein, + *itis*, inflammation]. Inflammation of superficial veins and surrounding skin.

dermoskeleton [″ + *skeleton*]. Apparent external covering of the body; the hair, nails, and teeth in humans. SYN: *exoskeleton*.

dermosynovitis (dĕr″mō-sĭn-ō-vī′tĭs) [″ + L. *synovia*, joint fluid, + Gr. *itis*, inflammation]. Inflammation of the skin overlying an inflamed bursa or tendon.

dermotropic (dĕr″mō-trŏp′ĭk) [″ + *trope*, a turning]. Acting esp. on the skin.

dermovascular (dĕr″mō-văs′kū-lăr) [″ + *vas*, vessel]. Concerning the skin and its blood vessels.

derodidymus (dĕr″ō-dĭd′ĭ-mŭs) [Gr. *dere*, neck, + *didymos*, double]. A malformed fetus with two necks and heads but a single body and normal limbs. SYN: *dicephalus*.

DES. *diethylstilbestrol*, q.v.

desalination. Partial or complete removal of salts from a substance, as from seawater or brackish water, so that it is suitable for agricultural or household purposes.

desaturation [L. *de*, from, + *saturare*, to fill]. A process whereby a saturated organic compound is converted into an unsaturated one, as when stearic acid, $C_{18}H_{36}O_2$, is changed into oleic acid, $C_{18}H_{34}O_2$. The product has different physical and chemical properties after this transformation. SEE: *saturated hydrocarbon.*

Desault's apparatus (dĕ-sōz′) [Pierre J. Desault, Fr. surgeon, 1744–1795]. Bandage used for fracture of clavicle. SEE: *bandage.*

descemetitis (dĕs″ĕ-mĕ-tī′tĭs). Inflammation of Descemet's membrane on the corneal posterior surface. SYN: *cyclitis, serous.*

Descemet's membrane (dĕs-ĕ-māz′) [Jean Descemet, Fr. anatomist, 1732–1810]. A fine membrane between the endothelial layer of the cornea and the substantia propria.

descemetocele (dĕs″ĕ-mĕt′ō-sēl). Protrusion of Descemet's membrane.

descendens (dē-sĕn′dĕns) [L. *de*, from, + *scendere*, to climb]. Descending; a descending structure.

d. hypoglossi. A branch of the hypoglossal nerve given off at the point at which it curves around the occipital artery, which

passes down obliquely across the sheath of the carotid vessels (sometimes within it) to form a loop just below the middle of the neck with branches of the 2nd and 3rd cervical nerves.

descensus (dē-sĕn′sŭs) [L.]. Process of falling, descent.

d. testis. Normal passage of the testicle from the abdominal cavity down into the scrotum. Occurs during last few months of fetal life. SYN: *migration of testicle.*

d. uteri. SEE: *uterus, prolapse of.*

d. ventriculi. Downward displacement of the stomach. SYN: *gastroptosis.*

DES daughters. Daughters of mothers who received diethylstilbestrol (DES) during pregnancy. SEE: *DES syndrome; diethylstilbestrol.*

desensitization. 1. Treatment of allergies by repeated injections of dilute solutions containing the allergen. The concentration of the solution is too weak to cause symptoms, but slowly promotes tolerance of the antigen by the immune system. It increases the levels of IgG, q.v., which block IgE from binding to mast cells and initiating the release of the chemical mediators of inflammation. Although not always successful, densensitization is still commonly used, particularly for patients whose allergic response to an antigen is systemic anaphylaxis, q.v. SEE: *allergy; anaphylaxis.* 2. In psychiatry, the alleviation of an emotionally upsetting life situation.

NURSING IMPLICATIONS: Patients receiving desensitization must be monitored closely for signs of anaphylaxis each time they receive an injection of dilute antigen.

d., systematic. A form of behavior therapy, used particularly for phobias, in which the patient is gradually exposed to anxiety-producing stimuli until they no longer produce anxiety. SEE: *flooding.*

desensitize [L. *de*, from, + *sentire*, to perceive]. 1. To deprive of or lessen sensitivity by nerve section or blocking. 2. To abate anaphylactic sensitiveness by administration of the specific antigen in low dosage.

desert fever, desert rheumatism. Coccidioidomycosis, q.v.

desexualize (dē-sĕks′ū-ăl-īz) [″ + *sexus*, sex]. To castrate; to remove sexual traits.

Desferal. Trade name for deferoxamine mesylate.

desferrioxamine (dĕs-fĕr′ē-ŏks′ă-mēn). Deferoxamine, q.v.

desiccant (dĕs′ĭ-kănt). Causing desiccation or dryness.

desiccate (dĕs′ĭ-kāt) [L. *desiccare*, to dry up]. To dry.

desiccation (dĕs″ĭ-kā′shŭn). The process of

drying up. SEE: *electrodesiccation.*

"designer drug" [Term coined by Gary Henderson, contemporary pharmacologist]. The use of chemical technology to illicitly produce drugs of abuse such as methamphetamine; fentanyl and its analogues; and phencyclidine hydrochloride (PCP). In a number of attempts to produce these drugs, toxic chemicals have been made. Also, the compounds are not standardized with respect to potency, so deaths from overdose may occur.

desipramine hydrochloride (dĕs-ĭp'rä-mēn). USP. An antidepressant. Trade names are Norpramin and Pertofrane.

deslanoside (dĕs-lăn'ō-sīd). USP. A cardiac glycoside, obtained from digitalis leaf, that has the same action as lanatoside C. Trade name is Cedilanid-D.

desmalgia (dĕs-măl'jē-ă) [Gr. *desmos*, band, + *algos*, pain]. Pain in a ligament.

desmectasia, desmectasis (dĕs-mĕk-tă'zē-ă, -ĕk'tă-sĭs) [" + *ektasis*, dilatation]. Stretching of a ligament.

desmepithelium (dĕs-mĕp-ĭ-thē'lē-ŭm) [" + *epi*, upon, + *thele*, nipple]. The epithelial lining of vessels and synovial cavities.

desmitis (dĕs-mī'tĭs) [" + *itis*, inflammation]. Inflammation of a ligament.

desmo- [Gr. *desmos*, band]. Prefix indicating a band, a ligament.

desmocranium (dĕs"mō-krā'nē-ŭm) [" + L. *cranium*]. In the embryo, the earliest form of the skull.

desmocyte (dĕs'mō-sīt) [" + *kytos*, cell]. A supporting tissue cell. SYN: *fibroblast; fibrocyte.*

desmocytoma (dĕs"mō-sī-tō'mă) [" + *oma*, tumor]. A tumor formed of desmocytes; a sarcoma.

desmodynia [" + *odyne*, pain]. Pain in a ligament.

desmoenzyme. An intracellular enzyme.

desmogenous (dĕs-mŏj'ĕ-nŭs) [" + *gennan*, to produce]. Of connective tissue origin.

desmography (dĕs-mŏg'ră-fē) [" + *graphein*, to write]. A description of or treatise on ligaments.

desmoid (dĕs'moyd) [" + *eidos*, form, shape]. 1. Tendonlike; fibroid. 2. A very tough and firm fibroma.

desmology (dĕs-mŏl'ō-jē) [" + *logos*, word, reason]. Science of tendons and ligaments.

desmoma [" + *oma*, tumor]. A tumor of the connective tissue.

desmoneoplasm (dĕs"mō-nē'ō-plăzm) [" + *neos*, new, + LL. *plasma*, form, mold]. A connective tissue tumor.

desmopathy (dĕs-mŏp'ă-thē) [" + *pathos*, disease, suffering]. Any disease affecting ligaments.

desmoplasia (dĕs-mō-plā'zē-ă) [" + Gr. *plassein*, to form]. An abnormal tendency to form fibrous tissue or adhesive bands.

desmoplastic [" + *plassein*, to form]. Causing or forming adhesions.

desmopressin acetate. A synthetic antidiuretic, a vasopressin analogue, with greater antidiuretic activity but less pressor activity than vasopressin. Trade names are DDAVP and Stimate Injection.

desmopyknosis (dĕs"mō-pĭk-nō'sĭs) [" + *pyknosis*, condensation]. Surgical procedure for shortening of round ligaments by attaching them by loops to the anterior uterine wall.

desmorrhexis (dĕs-mō-rĕk'sĭs) [" + *rhexis*, rupture]. Rupture of a ligament.

desmosis (dĕs-mō'sĭs) [" + *osis*, condition]. Any disease of the connective tissue.

desmosome (dĕs'mō-sōm) [" + *soma*, body]. Structure binding adjacent epithelial cells.

desmotomy (dĕs-mŏt'ō-mē) [" + *tome*, incision]. Dissection of ligament.

desoximetasone (dĕs-ŏk"sē-mĕt'ă-sōn). USP. A corticosteroid used topically. Trade name is Topicort.

desoxy-. Prefix meaning deoxidized or a reduced form of. SEE: words beginning with *deoxy-.*

desoxycorticosterone (dĕs-ŏk"sē-kor-tĭ-kŏs'tĕr-ōn). An active steroid hormone produced by the adrenal cortex. It plays an important role in the regulation of water and salt metabolism.

   d. acetate. USP. An acetate ester of desoxycorticosterone and the form in which the hormone is usually administered in its therapeutic use. It may be injected intramuscularly or used buccally. Trade names are Doca Acetate and Percorten Acetate.

desoxyribonucleic acid (dĕs"ŏk-sē-rī"bō-nū'klē-ĭk). Former spelling for deoxyribonucleic acid, q.v.

despair. The eighth stage in Erikson's developmental theory; the opposite of ego integrity. The individual experiences despair over past life events and dismay over a foreshortened life.

despumation (dĕs"pū-mā'shŭn) [L. *de*, from, + *spuma*, froth]. Separation of froth or scum from a liquid.

desquamate (dĕs'kwă-māt) [L. *desquamare*, to remove scales]. To shed or scale off the surface epithelium.

desquamation (dĕs"kwă-mā'shŭn). Shedding of the epidermis.

   d., furfuraceous. Shedding of branlike scales.

desquamative (dĕs-kwŏm'ă-tĭv). Of the nature of desquamation, or pert. to or causing it. SYN: *keratolytic.*

DES syndrome. The occurrence of neoplasms of the vagina in young women whose mothers received diethylstilbestrol, q.v., early in their pregnancy.

destructive [L. *destructus,* destroyed]. Causing ruin or destruction. Opposite of constructive.

destructive lesion. A pathological change such as an infection, tumor, or injury that causes the death of tissue or an organ.

desudation (dē-sū-dā′shŭn) [L. *de,* from, + *sudare,* to perspire]. Excessive sweating often followed by slight pustular eruption.

desulfhydrase (dē″sŭlf-hī′drās). An enzyme that cleaves cysteine into hydrogen sulfide, ammonia, and pyruvic acid.

desynchronosis (dē-sĭn″krŏ-nō′sĭs) [″ + Gr. *synkhronos,* same time]. The time difference between that of a person's present location and that to which the person is accustomed, causing an upset of the individual's internal biological clock. Occurs in persons traveling across a number of time zones in a short period of time. Lay term for this condition is "jet lag."

DET. *diethyltryptamine.*

det. L. *detur,* let it be given.

detachment [O. Fr. *destachier,* to unfasten]. Becoming separate.

   d., retinal. The pathological condition in which the retina or a part of it becomes separated from the choroid.

detail. In radiology, the sharpness with which an image is presented on a radiograph.

detector [L. *detectus,* uncovered]. Device for determining the presence of something.

   d., lie. A polygraph, an instrument for determining minor physical changes assumed to occur under the stress of lying or any other emotion. Variations in respiratory rhythm, pulse rate, blood pressure, and sweating of hands are measured. Increased perspiration lessens resistance to passage of electric current. The test has popular appeal among law enforcement departments, but results obtained are presumptive and not absolute.

   d., optical. The sensor in a typical colorimeter or photometer that senses the light transmitted by the sample.

   d., radiation. Instrument used to detect the presence of radiation.

detergent [L. *detergere,* to cleanse]. 1. Something that purges or cleanses; cleansing. 2. A cleaning or wetting agent prepared synthetically from a variety of chemicals. These are classed as anionic if they have a negative electrical charge or cationic if they have a positive charge. SYN: *wetting agent.* SEE: *soap.*

deterioration [L. *deteriorare,* to deteriorate].

Retrogression; said of impairment of mental or physical functions.

determinant (dē-tĕr′mĭ-nänt) [L. *determinare,* to limit]. That which determines the character of anything.

determination [L. *determinatus,* limiting]. Establishing the nature or precise identity of a substance, organism, or event.

determinism (dē-tĕr′mĭn-ĭzm) [″ + Gr. *-ismos,* condition]. The theory that all human action is the result of predetermined and inevitable physical, psychological, or environmental conditions that are uninfluenced by the will of the individual.

detersive [L. *detergere,* to cleanse]. Detergent; cleansing or purging.

det. in dup. [L. *detur in duplo*]. Let twice as much be given.

detortion, detorsion (dē-tor′shŭn). 1. Surgical therapy for torsion of a testicle, ureter, or volvulus of the bowel. 2. Correction of any bodily curvature or deformity.

detoxicate (dē-tŏk′sĭ-kāt) [L. *de,* from, + Gr. *toxikon,* poison]. To remove the toxic principle of a substance. SYN: *detoxify.*

detoxification [″ + ″ + L. *facere,* to make]. 1. Reduction of the toxic properties of a poisonous substance. SEE: *biotransformation.* 2. Process of removing the physiological effects of a drug or substance from an addicted individual.

detoxify (dē-tŏk′sĭ-fī). 1. To remove the toxic quality of a substance. 2. To treat a toxic overdose of any medicine, but esp. of the toxic state produced by drugs of abuse or acute alcoholism.

detrition (dē-trĭsh′ŭn) [L. *detritus,* to rub away]. The wearing away of a part, esp. through friction, as that of the teeth. SEE: *bruxism.*

detritus (dĭ-trī′tŭs) [L., to rub away]. Any broken down, degenerative, or carious matter produced by disintegration.

detruncation (dē″trŭn-kā′shŭn) [L. *de,* from, + *truncus,* trunk]. Decapitation, esp. of a fetus. SYN: *decollation.*

detrusor urinae (dē-trū′sor ū-rī′nē) [L.]. External longitudinal layer of muscular coat of bladder.

detumescence (dē″tū-mĕs′ĕns) [L. *de,* down, + *tumescere,* to swell]. 1. Subsidence of a swelling. 2. Subsidence of erectile tissue of genital organs (penis or clitoris) following erection.

deutencephalon (dūt-ĕn-sĕf′ă-lŏn) [Gr. *deuteros,* second, + *enkephalos,* brain]. The interbrain. SYN: *diencephalon; thalamencephalon.*

deuteranomalopia (doo″tĕr-ă-nŏm″ă-lō′pē-ă) [″ + *anomalos,* irregular, + *ops,* eye]. Partial color blindness in which the primary colors are perceived but green is poorly appreciated.

deuteranopia, deuteranopsia (dū″tĕr-ăn-ō′pē-ă, -ŏp′sē-ă) [″ + *anopia*, blindness]. Green blindness; color blindness in which there is a defect in the perception of green. SEE: *color blindness.*

deuterate (dū′tĕr-āt). To combine with deuterium.

deuterium (dū-tē′rē-ŭm) [Gr. *deuteros*, second]. SYMB: ^{2}H or D. Heavy hydrogen; the mass two isotope of hydrogen.

   d. oxide. An isotope of water in which hydrogen has been displaced by its isotope, deuterium. Its properties differ from ordinary water in that it has a higher freezing and boiling point and is incapable of supporting life. SYN: *heavy water.*

deutero-, deuter-, deuto- [Gr. *deuteros*, second]. Prefix indicating second or secondary.

deuteron (dū′tĕr-ŏn). SYMB: d. The nucleus of deuterium or heavy hydrogen.

deuteropathia, deuteropathy [Gr. *deuteros*, second, + *pathos*, disease]. A disease associated with or secondary to another disease.

deuteroplasm [″ + LL. *plasma*, form, mold]. The reserve food supply in the yolk or ovum.

deutoscolex (dū″tō-skō′lĕks) [″ + *skolex*, worm]. Secondary daughter cysts that develop on the inner wall of a hydatid cyst.

devasation (dē″văs-ā′shŭn) [L. *de*, from, + *vasa*, vessel]. Destruction of blood vessels.

devascularization (dē-văs″kū-lăr-ĭ-zā′shŭn) [″ + *vascularis*, pert. to a vessel]. 1. Loss or draining of blood from a part. 2. Decrease in the blood supply to a part of the body.

developer. In radiology and photography, the solution used to make the latent image visible on the radiographic film.

development [O. Fr. *desveloper*, to unwrap]. Growth to full size or maturity, as in the progress of an egg to the adult state. SEE: *growth and development.*

   RS: aplasia; apposition; chorista; dysplasia.

   d., cognitive. The sequential acquisition of the ability to learn, reason, and analyze that begins in infancy and progresses as the individual matures.

   d., psychomotor and physical, of infant. SEE: *psychomotor and physical development of infant.*

developmental. Pert. to development.

developmental milestones. Those skills regarded as having special importance in the development of infants and toddlers and usually associated with a particular age range; e.g., sitting, crawling, walking.

deviance [L. *deviare*, to turn aside]. Away

from the accepted norm.

deviant. Something (or someone) that is variant when compared with the norm or an accepted standard.

   d., sex. One whose sexual behavior is considered to be abnormal or socially unacceptable. SEE: *paraphilia.*

deviant behavior. Actions considered to be abnormal.

deviate (dē′vē-āt″) [L. *deviare*, to turn aside]. 1. To move steadily away from a designated norm. 2. An individual whose behavior, esp. sexual behavior, is so far removed from societal norms that it is classed as socially, morally, or legally unacceptable.

deviation (dē-vē-ā′shŭn). Going out of the way; departure from normal.

   d., axis. A change in the direction of the major electrical axis of the heart as determined by the electrocardiogram.

   d., conjugate. Deviation of face and eyes to the same side.

   d., minimum. The smallest deviation that a prism can produce.

   d., standard. ABBR: SD. In statistics, the measure of variability from the central tendency of any frequency curve. It is the square root of the variance.

device (dĭ-vīs′) [O. Fr. *devis*, contrivance]. An apparatus, machine, or shaped object constructed to perform a specific function.

   d., adaptive. An object or tool that has been designed or modified for use by persons with disability. SYN: *assistive device.*

   d., intrauterine contraceptive. Device made in a variety of shapes and from several different materials, including plastic or copper, and placed in the uterus to prevent conception. ABBR: IUCD or IUD.

devil's grip. Epidemic pleurodynia.

deviometer (dē″vē-ŏm′ĕ-tĕr) [L. *de*, from, + *via*, way, + Gr. *metron*, measure]. Device for estimating degree of strabismus.

devisceration (dē-vĭs″ĕr-ā′shŭn) [″ + *viscus*, internal organ]. Removal of viscera. SYN: *evisceration.*

devitalization [″ + *vita*, life]. 1. Destruction or loss of vitality. 2. Anesthetizing sensitive pulp of a tooth; known as killing the nerve.

devolution (dĕv″ō-loo′shŭn) [L. *devolvere*, to roll down]. Any destructive process in which organic substances are broken down into simple compounds; degradation. SYN: *catabolism.*

dew cure. Walking with bare feet in grass wet with dew. A form of hydrotherapy that is of questionable therapeutic value. SYN: *kneippism.*

dew point. Temperature at which dew begins to form as the moisture in the air condenses.

dexamethasone (dĕk″să-mĕth′ă-sōn). USP.

A synthetic glucocorticoid drug. Trade names are Decadron and SK-Dexamethasone.

dexbrompheniramine maleate (děks" brŏm-fĕn-ĭr'ă-mēn). USP. An antihistamine.

dexchlorpheniramine maleate (děks"klor-fĕn-ĭr'ă-mēn). USP. An antihistamine. Trade name is Polaramine.

dexter (děks'tĕr) [L.]. On the right side. SEE: *sinistral.*

dexterity. Skill in using the hands, usually requiring both fine and gross motor coordination.

dextrad (děks'trăd) [L. *dexter,* right, + *ad,* toward]. 1. Toward the right side. 2. A right-handed person.

dextral (děks'trăl). Pert. to the right side.

dextrality (děks-trăl'ĭ-tē). Right-handedness. SEE: *sinistrality.*

dextran (děks'trăn) [L. *dexter,* right]. A polysaccharide produced by the action of *Leuconostoc mesenteroides* on sucrose. It is available in various molecular weights and is used as a plasma volume expander.

dextranomer beads. Cross-linked network of dextran prepared in the form of beads. Because this compound has great ability to absorb moisture, it has been used in helping to debride wounds. Trade name is Debrisan. SEE: *decubitus ulcers.*

dextrase (děks'trās). An enzyme that splits dextrose and converts it into lactic acid.

dextraural (děks-traw'răl) [L. *dexter,* right, + *auris,* ear]. Hearing better with the right ear.

dextriferron (děks"trĭ-fĕr'ŏn). Ferric hydroxide, used in treating iron-deficiency anemia.

dextrin (děks'trĭn) [L. *dexter,* right]. A yellow-white powder that forms mucilaginous solutions in water and can be prepared by the action of heat or acid on starch. It is a carbohydrate of the formula $(C_6H_{10}O_5)_{11}$. In digestion, it is a soluble or gummy matter into which starch is converted by diastase; it is the result of the first chemical change in the digestion of starch.

dextrinuria (děks"trĭn-ū'rē-ă) [" + Gr. *ouron,* urine]. Dextrin in the urine.

dextro- [L. *dexter,* right]. Prefix indicating to the right.

dextroamphetamine sulfate (děks"trō-ăm-fĕt'ă-mēn sŭl'fāt). USP. A compound related to amphetamine sulfate (i.e., an isomer of amphetamine). Sometimes written *d*-amphetamine sulfate or dextro-amphetamine sulfate. Used as a central nervous system stimulant in treatment of mild depression. The drug is of benefit in treating abnormally hyperactive children, but concomitant psychotherapy and parent coun-

seling are essential. Continued use of this drug in children depresses their growth; thus growth should be carefully monitored. The drug has no place in the long-term treatment of obesity. Prolonged use can cause psychological dependence. Trade name is Dexedrine. The "street" name is "speed."

dextrocardia (děks"trō-kăr'dē-ă) [" + Gr. *kardia,* heart]. Having the heart on the right side of the body.

dextrocardiogram [" + " + *gramma,* something written]. A cardiogram representing action of the right ventricle.

dextrocular (děks-trŏk'ū-lăr) [" + *oculus,* eye]. Having a stronger right eye than left.

dextrocularity (děks"trŏk-ū-lăr'ĭ-tē). The condition of having the right eye stronger than the left.

dextroduction [" + *ducere,* to lead]. The movement of visual axis to the right.

dextrogastria [" + Gr. *gaster,* belly]. Having the stomach on the right side of the body.

dextromanual [" + *manus,* hand]. Right-handed.

dextromethorphan (děk"strō-mĕth'or-făn). USP. A cough suppressant. A great number of cough medicines include this drug in their formula.

dextropedal (děks-trŏp'ĕ-dăl) [" + *pes, ped-,* foot]. Having greater dexterity in using the right leg than the left one.

dextrophobia [" + Gr. *phobos,* fear]. Abnormal aversion to objects on right side of body.

dextroposition (děks"trō-pō-zĭsh'ŭn). Displaced to the right.

dextropropoxyphene (děk"strō-prō-pŏk'sē-fēn). Propoxyphene, q.v., an analgesic that can cause addiction.

dextrorotatory (děks"trō-rō'tă-tor-ē) [" + *rotare,* to turn]. Turning rays of light to the right.

dextrose (děks'trōs). USP. $C_6H_{12}O_6$. A simple sugar of the monosaccharose group; a crystalline solid that can be made by the action of acids on starches. It is very soluble in water, is an important constituent of corn syrup and honey, and is an example of one kind of carbohydrate, q.v. The most important of the monosaccharide group. Its presence in the urine in large amounts is most probably a result of diabetes. However, its presence may be associated with brain injuries, cirrhosis of the liver, normal pregnancies, and as a result of the administration of epinephrine or thyroxine. It is formed in the digestive tract by the action of enzymes on carbohydrates. It occurs naturally in plants and in the body fluids of animals.

RS: diabetes; glycosuria; hyperglycemia; hypoglycemia; monosaccharoses.

dextrose and sodium chloride injection. A sterile solution of dextrose, salt, and water for use intravenously. It contains no antimicrobial agents.

dextrosinistral (dĕks″trō-sĭn′ĭs-trăl) [L. *dexter*, right, + *sinister*, left]. From right to left.

dextrosuria (dĕks-trō-sū′rē-ă). Dextrose in the urine.

dextrothyroxine sodium (dĕks″trō-thī-rŏk′sĭn). USP. A thyroxine-like drug used in treating type II hyperlipoproteinemia. Trade name is Choloxin.

dextrotropic, dextrotropous (dĕks″trō-trŏp′ĭk,-trō′pŭs) [″ + Gr. *tropos*, a turning]. Turning to the right.

dextroversion [″ + *vertere*, to turn]. Turned or located toward the right.

DF-2. A gram-negative rod present in the oral cavity of about 8% of dogs. It is an important cause of septicemia and meningitis that occurs within 4 to 8 days following dog or cat bites or scratches. SEE: *dog bite.*

DFP. *diisopropyl fluorophosphate.* SEE: *isoflurophate.*

dg. *decigram.*

DHE-45. Trade name for dihydroergotamine mesylate.

dhobie itch (dō′bē) [Hindi, laundryboy]. Tropical name for form of tinea cruris more intense than that observed in temperate zones.

di- [Gr. *dis*, twice]. Prefix indicating twice, double, or two.

diabetes (dī″ă-bē′tēz) [Gr. *diabetes*, passing through]. A general term for diseases characterized by excessive urination. Usually refers to diabetes mellitus, q.v.

  d., bronze. A disease of iron metabolism characterized by enlargement of the liver, pigmentation of the skin so that it takes a bronzed hue, diabetes mellitus, and frequently cardiac failure. It is a rare condition seen ten times as frequently in males as in females. The majority of cases develop after the fourth decade. SYN: *hemochromatosis.*

  d. insipidus. Polyuria and polydipsia caused by inadequate secretion of vasopressin, the antidiuretic hormone, by the neurohypophysis (main portion of the posterior lobe of the pituitary gland). More common in the young.

    SYM: Urine output of 5 to 10 liters/24 hours is common. Sp. gr. is usually 1.001 to 1.005, and urine is free of sugar and albumin. Thirst, weakness, dry skin.

    ETIOL: In almost half of all cases, the cause is unknown. Trauma to the head that causes damage to the pituitary or a tumor in that area causes the remainder of cases.

    TREAT: Eradication of causative factor if determined. When not due to specific in-

jury of the pituitary, the disease is easily controlled by use of vasopressin replacement therapy. This may be given by injection or nasal spray.

  PROG: Essentially chronic.

  NURSING IMPLICATIONS: Monitor fluid intake and output; evaluate for dehydration and hypovolemic hypotension; monitor urine specific gravity and weight; teach patient procedure for nasal insufflation of vasopressin. Instruct patient to wear or carry medical identification at all times.

  d. mellitus. A chronic disorder of carbohydrate metabolism, characterized by hyperglycemia and glycosuria and resulting from inadequate production or utilization of insulin. Persons fulfilling these conditions are not a homogeneous group. Diabetes mellitus is classified according to two syndromes: Type I, or insulin-dependent diabetes mellitus (IDDM) and Type II, or non-insulin-dependent diabetes mellitus (NIDDM). In Type I, the patients secrete little or no insulin. In the past, this form of diabetes was called juvenile-onset, ketotic, or brittle diabetes. In Type II, insulin is produced, but exogenous insulin is needed to control hyperglycemia. Older terms for this form of diabetes were maturity-onset, nonketotic, or stable diabetes. Type II diabetes occurs much more frequently than Type I. SEE: *dawn phenomenon; d.m., insulin-dependent; d.m., non-insulin-dependent; insulin; insulin pump; insulin resistance; polyneuropathy, diabetic; Somogyi phenomenon.*

  SYM: Principal symptoms are elevated blood sugar (hyperglycemia), sugar in urine (glycosuria), excessive urine production (polyuria), excessive thirst (polydipsia), and increase in food intake (polyphagia); itching, frequently about the genitals. Urine sp. gr. 1.020 to 1.040; sugar excessive; urine contains diacetic acid, beta-hydroxybutyric acid, acetone when disease process is in advanced stage. More common in women and after the age of 40. Fasting blood sugar raised above normal range of 90 to 120 mg/dl of blood; boils and carbuncles; vascular changes may be present. Loss of weight; emaciation; weakness; and debility. When severe diabetes is allowed to progress without proper treatment, coma ensues with weakness and sweet (acetone) odor of breath; nausea, headache, vomiting, dyspnea, sense of intoxication, delirium, and deep coma resulting in death.

  ETIOL: Basic cause is still unknown but the pathological defect is failure of beta cells of the pancreas to secrete an adequate amount of insulin. In most instances diabetes mellitus is the result of a genetic disorder, but it may also result from a deficiency of beta cells caused by inflammation, malignant invasion of the pancreas, or surgery. In the absence of insulin, glycogenesis and glycolysis are adversely affected. After insulin is secreted by the beta cells of the pancreas, it is transported to the cells of the body where it binds to specific insulin receptors. The insulin then acts to promote glucose metabolism in the cell and to inhibit glucose production by the liver.

COMPLICATIONS: Diabetic acidosis due to excessive production of ketone bodies; low resistance to infections, esp. those involving extremities; ulceration of lower extremities; increase in incidence of toxemia in pregnancy; cardiovascular and renal disorders; disturbances in electrolyte balance.

Diabetics are prone to develop retinopathy, glaucoma, and various type of neuropathy. Eye involvement is common, and 0.2% of diabetics become blind each year. This complication is much less frequent in the insulin-dependent type than the non-insulin-dependent type. The retinal changes may be of the nonproliferative type with retinal ischemia and areas of infarction. In the proliferative type, new vessels are formed in the retina and these may lead to retinal detachment. These new vessels are destroyed by use of photocoagulation; this helps to prevent further deterioration of vision.

Diabetic neuropathy is estimated to occur in 40% of patients in whom diabetes has been present 25 years. A single peripheral nerve may be involved, the autonomic nervous sytem may be involved, or cranial nerves may be affected.

Cardiovascular disease is the major cause of death in diabetics. In addition, peripheral vascular disease may lead to ischemia and gangrene of the lower limbs. Amputation(s) may be required.

TREAT: Consists of diet, insulin, exercise, and hygienic measures. At first the patient should be placed on a well-balanced diet adequate in all basic essentials: carbohydrates, proteins, fats, vitamins, minerals, and fluids. In many patients this may be all that is required. Obese persons with this disease should be placed on a diet that will enable them to lose weight. Control of diabetes is much more difficult in an obese person. Blood sugar determinations may need to be made at frequent intervals. Glucose levels in the urine may be monitored by the patient or family as often as necessary. In addition, the availability of kits for use at home make it possible to obtain a blood sample for monitoring the blood glucose level at home. Long-term blood glucose reg-

ulation may be objectively assessed by determining the glycosylated hemoglobin (hemoglobin A_{1c}) in blood. SEE: *hemoglobin* A_{1c}.

NOTE: Blood sugar and glucose are considered to be the same.

When a patient is given an adequate diet and glucose still appears in the urine, use of insulin may be necessary. Its use is not required in every case and may be dangerous if not properly given. Drugs have been given by mouth for the control of mild cases of diabetes. These have been used with success mostly in middle-aged and older patients who still have some beta cell function.

Diet: A balanced diet of approximately 1000 to 1200 Calories may be prescribed. The diet is modified according to the weight of the patient. This should be increased promptly if levels of glucose in the blood are brought within normal limits. The age, weight, and type of work or physical activity in which the patient is engaged are important in planning a diet. Standardized diets have been worked out in which the necessary proportions of carbohydrates, proteins, and fats are outlined. The diets vary from 1200 to 3000 Calories. Frequent feedings (5 to 6 each day) rather than the standard three meals are preferred. The older the patient, as a rule, the smaller the proportion of fat in the diet. SEE: *exchange list.*

Exercise: Physical exercise is important in helping to improve glucose utilization. Thus, a regular exercise program should be encouraged. The individual with diabetes should not be excluded from any athletic endeavor at any level. Initially, high-level physical activity will necessitate careful management of insulin intake and monitoring of glucose levels in the blood.

PROG: Diabetes is a chronic, incurable disease, but symptoms can be ameliorated and life prolonged by proper therapy. The isolation and eventual production of insulin in 1922 by Canadian physicians Banting and Best made it possible to allow persons with the disease to lead a normal life.

NURSING IMPLICATIONS: Carefully assess the patient for symptoms indicative of insulin shock, diabetic acidosis or hyperglycemic, hyperosmolar, nonketotic coma. Do urine analysis for glucose and ketones daily or more often if indicated. Administer insulin, q.v., or oral hypoglycemic agents as ordered; know the action, peak, onset, and duration of action for each specific type of insulin administered. Explain dietary restrictions to the patient, in addition to the need for a steady, consistent level of exercise on a daily basis.

Patients with diabetes must understand

their disease, its possible complications, and treatment. Be certain that the patient understands the need for good hygiene, proper care of the feet, dosage and administration of insulin or oral agent, technique for urine analysis for glucose and ketones, the signs of insulin shock and diabetic acidosis, and what to do if either of these conditions should develop.

Diagnostic aids are available for diabetic patients to use to test their own urine and blood for glucose. Supervision is advisable while patients are learning to use those techniques. Encourage patient, particularly those who are insulin-dependent, to seek regular medical monitoring of condition. Persons with diabetes mellitus should wear a Medic Alert bracelet. SEE: *Nursing Diagnoses in Appendix.*

d.m., brittle. SEE: *d.m., insulin-dependent.*

d.m., chemical. A stage of diabetes mellitus in which the various tests for altered glucose metabolism other than the fasting blood glucose level are abnormal but there are no obvious clinical signs or symptoms of diabetes.

d.m., endocrine. Diabetes mellitus associated with certain diseases of the pituitary, thyroid, or adrenal glands.

d.m., iatrogenic. Diabetes mellitus brought on by administration of drugs such as corticosteroids, certain diuretics, or birth control pills.

d.m., insulin-dependent, Type I. ABBR: IDDM. Diabetes mellitus that usually has its onset prior to the age of 25 years, in which the essential abnormality is related to absolute insulin deficiency. This form usually is quite difficult to regulate. SYN: *brittle diabetes; juvenile-onset diabetes.* SEE: table.

d.m., latent. Diabetes mellitus that manifests itself during times of stress such as pregnancy, infectious disease, obesity, or trauma. Previous to the stress, no clinical or laboratory findings of diabetes are present. There is a very strong chance that such individuals will eventually develop overt diabetes mellitus.

d.m., non-insulin-dependent, Type II. ABBR: NIDDM. A group of forms of diabetes mellitus that occur predominantly in adults. The insulin produced is sufficient to prevent ketoacidosis but insufficient to meet the total needs of the body. This form of diabetes in nonobese patients can usually be controlled by diet and oral hypoglycemic agents. Occasionally insulin therapy is required. Obese patients can be controlled by avoidance of overfeeding. SYN: *maturity-onset diabetes mellitus.* SEE: table.

d., pancreatic. Diabetes associated with disease of the pancreas.

d., phlorhizin. Glycosuria caused by administration of phlorhizin.

d., renal. Renal glycosuria; condition characterized by a low renal threshold for sugar. Glucose tolerance is normal and diabetic symptoms are lacking.

d., true. D. mellitus.

diabetic (dī-ă-bĕt′ĭk). Pert. to diabetes.

diabetic acidosis. SEE: *acidosis, diabetic.*

diabetic center. Area in the floor of the fourth ventricle of the brain.

diabetic coma. Loss of consciousness due to severe diabetes mellitus that has not been treated or to treatment that has not been adequately regulated. SEE: *coma, diabetic.*

diabetic ear. Otitis media diabetica.

diabetic polyneuropathy. SEE: *polyneuropathy, diabetic.*

diabetic tabes. Diabetes with neuritic pains in leg and loss of patellar tendon reflex.

diabetogenic (dī″ă-bĕt″ō-jĕn′ĭk) [″ + *gennan,* to produce]. Causing diabetes.

diabetogenous (dī″ă-bē-tŏj′ĕn-ŭs). Caused by diabetes.

Diabinese. Trade name for chlorpropamide.

diabrosis (dī″ă-brō′sĭs) [Gr., eating through]. A corrosion causing perforation of a vessel or organ.

diabrotic (dī-ă-brŏt′ĭk). 1. Corrosive. 2. An escharotic or corrosive.

diacele (dī′ă-sēl) [Gr. *dia,* between, + *koilia,* a hollow]. The third ventricle of the brain.

diacetate (dī-ăs′ĕ-tāt). A salt of diacetic acid.

diacetemia (dī-ăs″ĕ-tē′mē-ă). Presence of diacetic acid in the blood.

diacetic acid (dī″ă-sĕt′ĭk). Acetoacetic acid, found in acidosis and in the urine of the diabetic. Similar to acetone, it is found in serious diabetes and in any condition that produces starvation and excessive fat metabolism, such as persistent vomiting.

diacetonuria, diaceturia (dī-ăs″ĕ-tō-nū′rē-ă, dī-ăs″ĕ-tū′rē-ă). Diacetic acid in urine.

diacetylmorphine (dī″ă-sē″tĭl-mor′fēn). Heroin.

diacid (dī-ăs′ĭd) [Gr. *dis,* twice, + L. *acidus,* soured]. A chemical compound having two replaceable atoms of hydrogen.

diaclasis (dī-ă-klā′sĭs) [Gr. *dia,* through, + *klan,* to break]. A surgical procedure in which a bone is intentionally fractured. SYN: *osteoclasis.*

diaclast (dī′ă-klăst) [″ + *klan,* to break]. Device for perforating the fetal skull.

diacrinous (dī-ăk′rĭn-ŭs) [Gr. *diakrinein,* to separate]. Pert. to cells that secrete outwardly rather than into circulation. SYN: *exocrine.*

diacrisis (dī-ăk′rĭ-sĭs) [Gr. *diakrisis,* separa-

Comparison of Type I Insulin-Dependent Diabetes Mellitus and Type II Non-Insulin-Dependent Diabetes Mellitus

	Type I	Type II
Age at onset	Usually under 30	Usually over 40
Type of onset	Abrupt	Gradual
Body weight	Normal	Obese — 80%
HLA association	Positive	Negative
Insulin in blood	Little to none	Some usually present
Islet cell antibodies	Present at onset	Absent
Prevalence	0.2%–0.3%	2%–4%
Symptoms	Polyuria, polydipsia, polyphagia, weight loss, ketoacidosis	Polyuria, polydipsia, pruritus, peripheral neuropathy
Control	Insulin and diet	Diet (sometimes only diet control), hypoglycemic agents, sometimes insulin
Vascular and neural changes	Eventually develop	Will usually develop
Stability of condition	Fluctuates, difficult to control	Fairly stable, usually easy to control

tion]. 1. A change in the character of a secretion. 2. Any disease involving an altered secretion. 3. A critical discharge or excretion in a disease.

diacritic, diacritical [Gr. *dia*, through, + *krinein*, to judge]. Diagnostic; said of symptoms.

diaderm [Gr. *dia*, through, + *derma*, skin]. Blastoderm composed of ectoderm and entoderm, and containing between them the segmentation cavity.

diadochokinesia (dī-ăd″ō-kō-kǐn-ē′zē-ă) [Gr. *diadokos*, succeeding, + *kinesis*, movement]. Ability to make antagonistic movements, as pronation and supination of the hands in quick succession. SEE: *disdiadochokinesia*.

diagnose (dī′ăg-nōs) [Gr. *diagignoskein*, to discern]. To determine the cause and nature of a pathological condition; to recognize a disease.

diagnosis (dī″ăg-nō′sĭs) (pl. *diagnoses*). 1. The term denoting name of the disease or syndrome a person has or is believed to have. 2. The use of scientific and skillful methods to establish the cause and nature of a person's illness. This is done by evaluating the history of the disease process; the signs and symptoms present; laboratory data; special tests such as x-ray pictures and electrocardiograms. The value of establishing a diagnosis is to provide a logical basis for treatment and prognosis.

d., antenatal. Diagnostic procedures to determine the health status of the fetus include amniocentesis, cell culture, biochemical methods, amnioscopy, nonstress test, oxytocin challenge test, biophysical profile, amniography, ultrasound, and chorionic villus biopsy.

d. by exclusion. Establishing a diagnosis by eliminating other possibilities.

d., clinical. Diagnosis determined by history, laboratory studies, and symptoms. Most diseases have a symptom or symptoms in common with other diseases.

d., cytological. Diagnosis based on cells present in body tissues or exudates.

d., differential. Comparison of symptoms of two similar diseases to determine the cause of the illness.

d., medical. The entire process of determining the cause of the patient's illness or discomfort. The method of arriving at the diagnosis will depend upon a number of factors including the type of illness or injury present. Indeed, making the diagnosis of a simple and superficial laceration of the skin of the lower leg will be much less involved than would making the diagnosis of a laceration of the scalp. In the latter, the depth of the wound will be of utmost importance in determining the number of layers of the scalp to be sutured. Also the diagnosis of an obscure infectious disease or of an unexplained fever will involve clinical skills as well as sophisticated laboratory investigations that would not be required to diagnose a simple cold or influenza. *Medical diagnosis* is to be differentiated from *nursing diagnosis,* q.v.

 d., nursing. SEE: *nursing diagnosis.*

 d., oral. SEE: *oral diagnosis.*

 d., pathological. Diagnosis based on structural lesions present.

 d., physical. Diagnosis by external examination only.

 d., radiographic. Diagnosis arrived at by the interpretation of radiographic findings. SYN: *roentgenographic d.*

 d., serological. Diagnosis made by using a serological test such as that for syphilis or typhoid.

diagnosis, words pert. to: abdomen; auscultation; blood; breathing; chest; colic; coma; constipation; convulsion; cough; examination; eye; face; fatigue; feces; fever; gait; gums; headache; infection; inflammation; inspection; nail; nausea; oral mucosa; pain; pallor; palpation; palpitation; percussion; perspiration; position; pulse; pus; radiographs; reflexes; respiration; skin; sputum; syncope; teeth; temperature; tongue; unconsciousness; urine; vertigo; vomiting.

diagnosis related group. ABBR: DRG. A system designed to attempt to standardize prospective payment for medical care. The reimbursement for treating all individuals within the same DRG is the same, regardless of actual cost to the health care facility. The facility may earn a profit if the patient's hospitalization is shorter than the specified average length of stay of that category of illness.

diagnostic. Pert to a diagnosis.

Diagnostic and Statistical Manual of Mental Disorders (Third Edition—Revised). ABBR: DSM-III-R. Standard nomenclature of emotional illness used by all health care practitioners. DSM-III-R, introduced in 1987, is the one in current use; it updates and classifies mental illness as well as presents guidelines and diagnostic criteria for various mental disorders. It is published by the American Psychiatric Association.

diagnostician (dī″ăg-nŏs-tĭsh′ŭn) [Gr. *diagignoskein,* to discern]. One skilled in diagnosis.

diakinesis (dī″ă-kĭ-nē′sĭs) [Gr. *dia,* through, + *kinesis,* motion]. In cell division, the final stage in prophase of meiosis. At this time the homologous chromosomes shorten and thicken.

dial (dī′ăl) [L. *dialis,* daily, fr. *dies,* day]. A graduated circular face, similar to a clock

face, upon which some measurement is indicated by a pointer that moves as the entity (pressure, temperature, or heat) being measured changes.

 d., astigmatic. Black lines of uniform width drawn across a circular dial as if they were connecting opposing numbers on the face of a clock. Used in testing for astigmatism.

dialy- [Gr. *dia,* through, + *lysis,* dissolution]. Prefix meaning to separate.

dialysance (dī″ă-lī′săns). In kidney dialysis, the minute rate of net exchange of a substance between blood and dialysis fluid per unit blood-bath concentration gradient.

dialysate (dī-ăl′ĭ-sāt). A liquid that has been dialyzed. In renal failure, dialysate refers to the fluid used to remove or deliver compounds or electrolytes that the failing kidney cannot excrete or retain in the proper concentrations.

dialysis (dī-ăl′ĭ-sĭs) [Gr. *dia,* through, + *lysis,* dissolution]. 1. The passage of a solute through a membrane. 2. Process of diffusing blood across a semipermeable membrane to remove toxic materials and to maintain fluid, electrolyte, and acid-base balance in cases of impaired kidney function or absence of the kidneys. SEE: *hemodialysis.*

 d., continuous ambulatory peritoneal. ABBR: CAPD. A type of maintenance dialysis that utilizes an implanted peritoneal catheter. Fluid is drained into and from the peritoneal cavity by gravity. CAPD is an alternative to chronic hemodialysis and is considerably less expensive.

 d., continuous cyclic peritoneal. ABBR: CCPD. Treatments are performed every night with fluid remaining in the peritoneal cavity until the next night.

 d., intermittent peritoneal. ABBR: IPD. Dialysis using automated equipment. Often performed overnight, the fluid is drained at the end of the treatment from the peritoneal cavity.

 d., peritoneal. Dialysis in which the lining of the peritoneal cavity is used as the dialysis membrane. Dialyzing fluid introduced into the peritoneal cavity is allowed to remain there for one or two hours and is then removed. The procedure may be repeated as often as indicated. Care must be taken to prevent the development of peritonitis. This is done by using strict sterile technique. SEE: *Nursing Diagnoses* in *Appendix.*

 d., renal. Dialysis of blood in order to remove liquid and chemicals that the kidneys would normally remove if they were present and functioning.

dialysis acidosis. Metabolic acidosis due to prolonged hemodialysis in which the pH of the dialysis bath has been inadvertently reduced by the action of contaminating bacteria.

dialysis dementia. A neurologic disturbance seen in patients who have been on dialysis for a number of years. There are speech difficulties, myoclonus, dementia, seizures, and eventually death. The pathologic mechanism is unknown, but may be related to an increased concentration of aluminum in the brain.

dialysis disequilibrium. The symptoms of nausea, vomiting, drowsiness, headache, and seizures that occur shortly after beginning hemodialysis or peritoneal dialysis. The cause is related to the rapid pH changes in the blood and decrease in the osmolarity of the extracellular fluid. The urea in the brain is higher than in the serum.

dialytic. Belonging to or resembling the process of dialysis.

dialyzable (dī-ă-līz′ă-b'l). Capable of dialysis.

dialyze (dī′ă-līz). To make a dialysis or to have made one.

dialyzer (dī′ă-līz″ĕr) [Gr. *dia*, through, + *lysis*, dissolution]. Apparatus used in performing dialysis.

diameter (dī-ăm′ĕ-tĕr) [″ + *metron*, a measure]. Distance from any point on the periphery of a surface, body, or space to the opposite point.

d., anteroposterior, of pelvic cavity. Distance between the middle of the symphysis pubis and the upper border of the 3rd sacral vertebra. It is usually 13.5 cm in the adult female.

d., anteroposterior, of pelvic inlet. Distance from the posterior surface of the symphysis pubis to the promontory of the sacrum (about 11 cm in the adult female). SYN: *true conjugate d. of pelvic inlet.*

d., anteroposterior, of pelvic outlet. Distance between the tip of the coccyx and the lower edge of the symphysis pubis.

d., bigonial. Distance between the two gonia. Gonion is the anthropometric point at the most inferior, posterior, and lateral point on the angle of the mandible.

d., biparietal. Transverse distance between parietal eminences on each side (about 9.25 cm).

d., bitemporal. Distance between the temporal bones (about 8 cm).

d., bitrochanteric. Distance between the highest points of the greater trochanters.

d., bizygomatic. Greatest transverse distance between most prominent points of the zygomatic arches.

d., buccolingual. Measurement of a tooth from the buccal to the lingual surface.

d., cervicobregmatic. Distance between anterior fontanel and junction of the neck with floor of the mouth.

d., diagonal conjugate, of pelvis. Distance from the upper part of the symphysis pubis to the most distant part of the brim of the pelvis.

d., external conjugate. Anteroposterior diameter of the pelvic inlet measured externally; distance from the skin over the upper part of symphysis pubis to the skin over a point corresponding to the sacral promontory.

d., frontomental. Distance from the top of the forehead to point of the chin.

d., interspinous. Distance between the two anterior superior spines of the ilia.

d., labiolingual. Measurement of an anterior tooth from the labial to the lingual surface.

d., mentobregmatic. Distance from the chin to middle of anterior fontanel.

d., mesiodistal. Measurement of a tooth from the ventral or mesial surface to the distal or dorsal surface.

d., obstetric, of pelvic inlet. Shortest distance between the sacrum and symphysis. This diameter is shorter than the true conjugate.

d., occipitofrontal. Distance from the posterior fontanel to the root of the nose.

d., occipitomental. Greatest distance between the most prominent portion of the occiput and point of chin (about 13.5 cm).

d.'s of fetal skull. Important diameters at full term are suboccipitobregmatic, 3.75 in. (9.5 cm); cervicobregmatic, 3.75 in. (9.5 cm); frontomental, 3.2 in. (8.1 cm); occipitomental, 5 in. (12.7 cm); supraoccipitomental, 5.5 in. (14 cm); occipitofrontal, 4.5 in. (11.4 cm); suboccipitofrontal, 4 in. (10.2 cm); biparietal, 3.75 in. (9.5 cm); bitemporal, 3.2 in. (8.1 cm).

d. of pelvis. *Anteroposterior:* the distance between the sacrovertebral angle and the symphysis pubis. *Bi-ischial:* between the ischial spines. *Conjugata diagonalis:* between the sacrovertebral angle and the symphysis pubis. *Conjugata vera:* the true conjugate between the sacrovertebral angle and the middle of the posterior aspect of the symphysis pubis (about 1.5 cm less than the diagonal conjugate). *Intercristal:* between the crests of the ilium. *Interspinous:* between the spines of the ilium. *Intertrochanteric:* between the greater trochanters when the hips are extended and the legs are held together. *Internal conjugate:* between the promontory of the sacrum and the upper edge of the symphysis pubis. *Pelvic:* any diameter of the pelvis found by measuring a straight line between any two points. SEE: *pelvis.*

diamid(e) (dī-ăm'ĭd, -īd) [L. *di*, two, + *amide*]. A compound that contains two amine groups. Sometimes used incorrectly to indicate a diamine or hydrazine.

diamidine (dī-ăm'ĭ-dēn). Any chemical compound that contains two amidine, $C(NH)NH_2$, groups.

diamine (dī-ăm'ĭn, -ēn). A chemical compound with two amino, $-NH_2$, groups.

diaminuria (dī-ăm''ĭ-nū'rē-ă). Presence of diamines in the urine.

Diamox. Trade name for acetazolamide, a carbonic anhydrase inhibitor.

diapause (dī'ă-pawz) [Gr. *dia*, through, + *pausis*, pause]. The state of metabolic inactivity that some plants, seeds, eggs, and insect forms assume in order to survive adverse conditions such as winter.

diapedesis (dī''ă-pěd-ē'sĭs) [" + *pedan*, to leap]. Passage of blood cells, esp. leukocytes, by ameboid movements through the unruptured wall of a capillary vessel.

diaper rash or dermatitis. SEE: *rash, diaper.*

diaphane (dī'ă-fān) [Gr. *dia*, through, + *phainein*, to appear]. A very small electric light utilized in transillumination.

diaphanography. Transillumination of the breast.

diaphanometer (dī''ă-făn-ŏm'ě-těr) [" + " + *metron*, measure]. A device for estimating the amount of solids in a fluid by its transparency.

diaphanometry (dī''ă-făn-ŏm'ě-trē). Determination of translucency of a fluid, as the urine.

diaphanoscope (dī-ă-făn'ō-skōp) [" + *phainein*, to appear, + *skopein*, to examine]. Device for transillumination of body cavities.

diaphanoscopy (dī''ă-făn-ŏs'kō-pē). Examination by the diaphanoscope; transillumination.

diaphemetric (dī''ă-fě-mět'rĭk) [" + *haphe*, touch, + *metron*, measure]. Pert. to degree of tactile sensibility.

diaphorase (dī-ăf'ō-rās). The flavoprotein catalyst of the reoxidation of nicotinamide-adenine dinucleotide (NAD) or nicotinamide-adenine dinucleotide phosphate (NADP) by mitochondrial electron transport chain.

diaphoresis (dī''ă-fō-rē'sĭs) [" + *pherein*, to carry]. Profuse sweating.

diaphoretic (dī''ă-fō-rět'ĭk) [" + *pherein*, to carry]. 1. A sudorific or an agent that increases perspiration. The term sudorific is usually confined to those active agents that cause drops of perspiration to collect on the skin, such as opium or pilocarpine. Heat may also be included as such an agent. 2. A patient who is sweating profusely.

diaphragm (dī'ă-frăm) [Gr. *diaphragma*, a

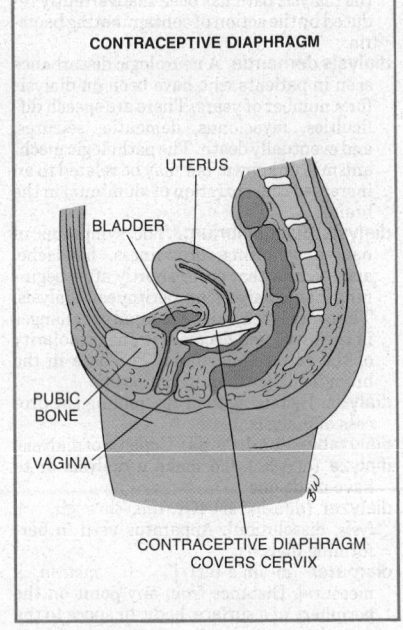

CONTRACEPTIVE DIAPHRAGM

UTERUS

BLADDER

PUBIC BONE

VAGINA

CONTRACEPTIVE DIAPHRAGM COVERS CERVIX

partition]. 1. Thin membrane such as one used for dialysis. 2. In microscopy, an apparatus located beneath the opening in the stage by means of which the amount of light passing through the object can be regulated. 3. A rubber or plastic cup that fits over the cervix uteri and is used for contraceptive purposes. SEE: illus. 4. A musculomembranous wall separating the abdomen from the thoracic cavity with its convexity upward. It contracts with each inspiration, flattening out downward, permitting the descent of the bases of the lungs. It relaxes with each expiration, elevating itself and restoring the inverted basin shape. The deeper the inspiration, the lower the descent of the diaphragm; the greater the expiration, the higher it rises.

Its origin is at a level with the 6th ribs or intercostal spaces anteriorly and the 11th or 12th ribs posteriorly. The right half rises higher than the left. The lower surface is in relation to the suprarenal bodies of the kidney, liver, spleen, and cardiac end of the stomach. It aids in defecation and parturition by its ability to cause an increase in intra-abdominal pressure while the person attempts to exhale with the glottis closed. It becomes spasmodic in hiccoughs and sneez-

MOVEMENT OF RIB CAGE AND DIAPHRAGM DURING RESPIRATION

INHALATION

THE DIAPHRAGM HAS DESCENDED, AND THE RIB CAGE HAS MOVED UP AND OUT TO ALLOW THE LUNGS TO EXPAND

EXHALATION

THE DIAPHRAGM HAS ASCENDED, AND THE RIB CAGE HAS MOVED DOWN AND IN AS THE LUNGS CONTRACT

ing. SEE: illus.; *Boerhaave syndrome; phrenic; "phren-" words; Valsalva's maneuver.*

d., Bucky. A grid suspended immediately beneath the x-ray table and above the film tray, so constructed that the effects of backscatter and secondary radiation are eliminated when radiographs of dense structures are taken.

d., hernia of. Congenital or traumatic protrusion of abdominal contents through the diaphragm.

d., pelvic. The musculofascial layer forming the lower boundary of the abdominopelvic cavity. It is funnel-shaped and is pierced in the midline by the urethra, vagina, and rectum. Consists of a muscular layer made up of the paired levator ani and coccygeus muscles. The fascial layer consists of two portions, the parietal and visceral layers, the former being made up of the peritoneum continuous with the connective tissue sheaths of the psoas and iliac muscles; the visceral layer is split from the parietal layer at the white line passing downward and inward to form the upper sheath of the levator ani muscles; the anterior part of this layer unites the bladder with the posterior wall of the pubes. The middle portion splits

into three parts: the vesical layer, investing bladder and urethra; the rectovaginal layer, forming the rectovaginal septum; the rectal layer, investing the rectum. The posterior part is the base of the broad ligament, where it sheaths the uterine arteries and supports the cervix.

d., urogenital. Urogenital trigone, or triangular ligament. A musculofascial sheath that lies between the ischiopubic rami. It lies superficial to the pelvic diaphragm and in the male surrounds the membranous urethra; in the female, it surrounds the vagina.

diaphragmalgia (dī″ă-frăg-măl′jē-ă) [Gr. *diaphragma*, a partition, + *algos*, pain]. Pain in the diaphragm.

diaphragmatic. Pert. to the diaphragm.

diaphragmatocele (dī″ă-frăg-măt′ō-sēl) [″ + *kele*, tumor, swelling]. Hernia of the diaphragm.

diaphragmitis (dī″ă-frăg-mī′tĭs) [″ + *itis*, inflammation]. Inflammation of the diaphragm.

diaphragmodynia [″ + *odyne*, pain]. Pain in the diaphragm.

diaphyseal (dī″ă-fĭz′ē-ăl). Part of or affecting the shaft of a long bone.

diaphysectomy [Gr. *diaphysis*, a growing through, + *ektome*, excision]. Removal of part of the shaft of a long bone.

diaphysis (dī-ăf'ĭ-sĭs). [NA] The shaft or middle part of a long cylindrical bone. SEE: *apophysis; epiphysis.*

diaphysitis (dī"ă-fĭ-zī'tĭs) [Gr. *diaphysis,* a growing through, + *itis,* inflammation]. Inflammation of shaft of a long bone.

Diapid. Trade name for lypressin.

diaplexus [Gr. *dia,* through, + L. *plexus,* braid]. Choroid plexus of the third ventricle.

diapophysis (dī-ă-pŏf'ĭ-sĭs) [" + *apophysis,* outgrowth]. An upper articular surface of transverse process of a vertebra.

diarrhea (dī-ă-rē'ă) [" + *rhein,* to flow]. Frequent passage of unformed watery bowel movements. It is a frequent symptom of gastrointestinal disturbances. SEE: *cholera; epidemic viral gastroenteropathy; oral rehydration therapy.*

ETIOL: Diet; inflammation or irritation of the mucosa of the intestines; gastrointestinal infections; certain drugs; psychogenic factors.

NURSING IMPLICATIONS: Assess patient for symptoms of dehydration, such as dry mucous membranes, poor skin turgor, soft eyeballs, and, in infants, depressed fontanels; and for indications of metabolic acidosis, such as headache, lethargy, decreasing level of consciousness, and compensatory hyperventilation. Monitor fluid balance, documenting intake and output and daily weight, and administer oral or I.V. fluids, electrolytes, and nutrients as prescribed, evaluating patient response. Prevent spread of infectious diarrhea by practicing and teaching thorough handwashing and hygiene measures, correct care and refrigeration of foods at risk for bacterial contamination, and by reporting unusual numbers of diarrhea cases to appropriate public health authorities. Assess anal area for skin excoriation. Wash gently and rinse thoroughly after each movement, and apply a protective ointment. Administer antidiarrheal medications as prescribed. SEE: *Nursing Diagnoses* in *Appendix.*

d., acute. Diarrhea characterized by sudden onset.

TREAT: Strong tea; whey; rice milk; arrowroot; and blackberry brandy. Adsorbents, such as aluminum hydroxide and bismuth subsalicylate (Pepto-Bismol), are useful. Gradual return to ordinary diet. Basically, these are home remedies that act as demulcents or astringents for the irritated intestinal mucosa. They are often effective, but severe cases of diarrhea may require additional therapy. Specific therapy depends upon the cause of the diarrhea. Also in severe cases fluid- and electrolyte-replacement therapy may be needed. Agents that reduce intestinal activity, such as antispasmodics and paregoric, may provide distinct symptomatic relief.

d., dysenteric. Diarrhea due to dysentery, q.v., characterized by mucous or bloody stools.

d., emotional. Diarrhea caused by emotional stress.

d., epidemic, in newborn. Contagious diarrhea in newborn caused by pathogenic strains of *Escherichia coli,* occurring in epidemics in hospitals.

d., fatty. Diarrhea with stools containing undigested fat particles.

d., infantile. Diarrhea in children under two years. Dysentery, q.v.

SYM: Dry skin, high temperature, thirst, pains, increase in frequency and amount of stools with change of color and consistency.

TREAT: Each year the deaths of thousands of children with diarrhea are prevented by the use of oral rehydration solutions consisting of clean (i.e., potable) water, salt, potassium, bicarbonate, and glucose. SEE: *oral rehydration solution.*

d., lienteric. Watery stools with undigested food particles.

d., membranous. Diarrhea with passage of pieces of intestinal mucosa.

d., mucous. Diarrhea with mucus in stools.

d., purulent. Presence of pus in stools, a result of intestinal ulceration.

d., simple. Variety of diarrhea in which stools contain only normal excreta.

d., summer. Diarrhea occurring in children during summer heat.

d., travelers'. ABBR: TD. Diarrhea experienced by travelers. The cause of some cases is enteropathogenic strains of *E. coli.* There is no completely effective method of prophylaxis. Nevertheless, attempt to avoid eating uncooked food or drinking beverages that could be contaminated. In general, the disease is self-limiting and usually lasts for 3 to 4 days. Symptomatic therapy for tenesmus, fluid loss, vomiting, and malaise is indicated. If diarrhea persists without signs of severe systemic disease such as blood in the stools, the use of paregoric, loperamide (trade name: Imodium), or diphenoxylate will be of benefit. The latter two are the drugs of choice for symptomatic treatment of TD. Diphenoxylate with atropine (trade name: Lomotil) is contraindicated in children under 2 years of age. Bismuth subsalicylate taken as tablets or liquid form of Pepto-Bismol helps to decrease severity of symptoms.

PREVENTION: Avoid ingestion of contaminated water, including ice, and food; do not eat uncooked vegetables or fresh salads.

Pepto-Bismol can be effective in preventing TD. Persons taking Pepto-Bismol should not take other salicylates at the same time. Two antimicrobials, doxycycline or trimethoprim-sulfamethoxazole, may be taken prophylactically and will greatly reduce the attack rate of TD, but like all drugs, their benefit must be weighed against the development of potentially serious side effects from the medicines.

diarthric (dī-ăr′thrĭk) [Gr. *dis*, two, + *arthron*, joint]. Pert. to two or more joints.

diarthrosis [Gr., a movable articulation]. An articulation in which opposing bones move freely; a hinge joint.

diarticular [Gr. *dis*, two, + L. *articulus*, joint]. Pert. to two joints. Specifically, pert. to the temporomandibular joints, where the mandible articulates in two places with the skull.

diascope (dī′ă-skōp) [Gr. *dia*, through, + *skopein*, to examine]. A glass plate held against the skin for examining superficial lesions. Erythematous lesions will show the compressed capillary bed, but a hemorrhagic area will not blanch when the glass is pressed against the skin.

Diasone Sodium Enterab. Trade name for sulfoxone sodium.

diastalsis (dī-ă-stăl′sĭs) [″ + *stalsis*, contraction]. A wave of inhibition before a downward contraction in the intestine. Similar to peristalsis.

diastaltic. 1. Pert. to diastalsis. 2. Denoting reflex action.

diastase (dī′ăs-tās) [Gr. *diastasis*, a separation]. A specific enzyme or ferment in plant cells, such as in sprouting grains and malt and in the digestive juice that converts starch into sugar.

diastasis (dī-ăs′tă-sĭs) [Gr.]. 1. In surgery, injury to a bone involving separation of an epiphysis. 2. In cardiac physiology, the last part of diastole. It follows the period of most rapid diastolic filling of the ventricles, consists of a period of retarded inflow of blood from atria into ventricles, lasts (in humans under average conditions) about 0.2 second, and is immediately followed by atrial systole.

    d. recti. A separation of the two halves of the rectus abdominis muscles in the midline at the linea alba. A benign condition when it occurs in pregnant women.

diastema (dī″ă-stē′mă) [Gr. *diastema*, an interval or space] (pl. *diastemata*). 1. A fissure. 2. A space between two adjacent teeth.

diastematocrania (dī″ă-stĕm″ă-tō-krā′nē-ă) [″ + *kranion*, cranium]. Congenital sagittal fissure of the skull.

diastematomyelia (dī″ă-stĕm″ă-tō-mī-ē′lē-ă) [″ + *myelos*, marrow]. Congenital fissure of the spinal cord, frequently associated with spina bifida cystica, q.v.

diastematopyelia (dī″ă-stĕm″ă-tō-pī-ē′lē-ă) [″ + *pyelos*, pelvis]. Congenital median slit of the pelvis.

diaster [Gr. *dis*, two, + *aster*, star]. Double star figure formed during mitosis, q.v. SYN: *amphiaster*.

diastole (dī-ăs′tō-lē) [Gr. *diastellein*, to expand]. The normal period in the heart cycle during which the muscle fibers lengthen, the heart dilates, and the cavities fill with blood; diastole of the atria occurs before that of the ventricles. Roughly, the period of relaxation alternating with systole or contraction. SEE: *blood pressure; heart; murmur; pulse; systole.*

diastolic (dī-ăs-tŏl′ĭk). Pert. to diastole.

diastolic pressure. ABBR: DP. The period of least pressure in the arterial vascular system.

    d.p., augmented. Increasing the diastolic pressure, usually by an artificial device, such as an intra-aortic balloon pump. SEE: *counterpulsation, intra-aortic balloon.*

diataxia [Gr. *dis*, two, + *ataxia*, lack of order]. Bilateral ataxia.

diatela, diatele (dī-ă-tē′lă, -tēl′) [Gr. *dia*, between, + L. *tela*, web]. Membranous roof of third ventricle.

diaterma [″ + *terma*, end]. Portion of the floor of the third ventricle.

diathermal (dī″ă-thĕr′măl) [Gr. *dia*, through, + *therme*, heat]. Ability to absorb heat rays.

diathermanous. Diathermal.

diathermia [Gr. *dia*, through, + *therme*, heat]. Diathermy.

diathermic. Of the nature of diathermy or of its results.

diathermy (dī′ă-thĕr′mē) [Gr. *dia*, through, + *therme*, heat]. The therapeutic use of a high-frequency current to generate heat within some part of the body. The frequency is greater than the maximum frequency for neuromuscular response and ranges from several hundred thousand to millions of cycles per second. Used to increase blood flow to specific areas. Should not be used in acute stage of recovery from trauma.

    d., medical. Generation of heat within the body by the application of high-frequency oscillatory current for warming, but not damaging, tissues.

    d., short-wave. Treatment by use of wavelengths of 3 to 30 meters.

    d., surgical. Diathermy of high frequency for electrocoagulation or cauterization.

diathesis (dī-ăth′ĕ-sĭs) [Gr. *diatithenai*, to dispose]. Constitutional predisposition to certain disease conditions.

diathetic. Pert. to diathesis.

diatom (dī'ă-tŏm) [Gr. *diatemnein*, to cut through]. One of a group of unicellular microscopic algae. They possess a siliceous or calcium-containing cell wall.

diatomaceous earth (dī"ă-tŏ-mā'shŭs). Substance composed of diatoms. SEE: *diatom.*

diatomic. 1. Containing two atoms; said of molecules. 2. Bivalent.

diatrizoate meglumine (dī"ă-trī-zō'āt). USP. A radiopaque substance used intra-arterially to visualize the arteries and veins of the heart and brain, and great vessels such as the aorta. Also used to visualize the kidneys and bladder. Trade names include Gastrografin, Hypaque Meglumine, and Reno-M.

diatrizoate sodium. USP. A radiopaque substance used to visualize various hollow body organs such as the kidney, bladder, uterus, and fallopian tubes.

diaxon, diaxone [Gr. *dis*, two, + *axon*, axis]. A neuron having two axons.

diazepam (dī-ăz'ĕ-păm). USP. An anti-anxiety and sedative drug used extensively in the United States. It is effective in treating status epilepticus, acute cocaine poisoning, and a variety of anxiety disorders. Trade name is Valium.

diazo-. Prefix used in chemistry to note that a compound contains the —N=N— group.

diazo reaction. A deep red color in urine, produced by the action of p-diazobenzene-sulfonic acid and ammonia on aromatic substances found in the urine in certain conditions.

diazotize (dī-ăz'ō-tīz). In chemistry, conversion of NH_2 groups into diazo, —N=N—, groups.

diazoxide (dī-ăz-ŏk'sīd). USP. Drug used in treating acute hypertension emergencies to produce lowering of the blood pressure; and in treating hypoglycemia due to hyperinsulinism. Trade names are Hyperstat (I.V. only) and Proglycem (oral).

dibasic (dī-bā'sĭk) [" + *basis*, base]. Containing in each molecule two atoms of hydrogen replaceable by a base; said of acid.

Dibenzyline. Trade name for phenoxybenzamine hydrochloride.

diblastula (dī-blăs'tū-lă) [" + *blastos*, sprout]. A blastula containing the ectoderm and entoderm.

Dibothriocephalus (dī-bŏth"rē-ō-sĕf'ăl-ŭs). Former name for the genus *Diphyllobothrium.*

dibucaine hydrochloride. USP. A local anesthetic similar to cocaine in action when applied topically and similar to procaine and cocaine when injected. Trade name is Nupercaine Hydrochloride.

DIC. *disseminated intravascular coagulation.*

dicalcic, dicalcium (dī-kăl'sĭk) [" + L. *calx*, lime]. Containing two atoms of calcium.

dicalcium phosphate (dī-kăl'sē-ŭm fŏs'făt). Dibasic calcium phosphate. Used as a source of calcium to supplement the diet.

dicentric (dī-sĕn'trĭk). Having two centers or two centromeres.

dicephalus (dī-sĕf'ă-lŭs) [" + *kephale*, head]. Congenitally deformed fetus with two heads.

dichloramine-T (dī-klor'ă-mēn). White powder containing about 28% chlorine.
  ACTION/USES: Germicide and disinfectant.

2,4-dichlorophenoxyacetic acid. ABBR: 2,4-D. A toxic substance previously used as a weed killer. SEE: *Poisons and Poisoning* in *Appendix.*

dichlorphenamide (dī"klor-fĕn'ă-mīd). USP. A carbonic anhydrase inhibitor used in treating glaucoma. Trade names are Daranide and Oratrol.

dichorionic (dī"kō-rē-ŏn'ĭk). Having two chorions. This may occur in two-egg (dizygotic) twins.

dichotomy, dichotomization (dī-kŏt'ō-mē, dī-kŏt"ō-mī-zā'shŭn) [Gr. *dicha*, twofold, + *tome*, incision]. 1. Bifurcation of a vein. 2. Cutting or dividing into two parts.

dichroic (dī-krō'ĭk). Pert. to dichroism.

dichroic mirror. An optical device used in some spectrophotometers to split a beam of light into reference and sample beams.

dichroism (dī'krō-ĭzm) [Gr. *dis*, two, + *chroa*, color]. Property of a substance appearing to be one color by direct light and another by transmitted light.

dichromate (dī-krō'māt). A chemical that contains the Cr_2O_7 group.

dichromatic. Being able to see only two colors.

dichromatism (dī-krō'mă-tĭzm). Ability to distinguish only two primary colors.

dichromatopsia (dī"krō-mă-tŏp'sē-ă) [" + *chroma*, color, + *opsis*, sight]. Ability to distinguish only two primary colors.

dichromic. 1. Containing two atoms of chromium. 2. Seeing only two colors.

dichromophil [" + *chroma*, color, + *philein*, to love]. Double staining with both acid and basic dyes.

dichromophilism (dī"krō-mŏf'ĭl-ĭzm) [" + " + " + *-ismos*, condition]. Having the capacity for double staining.

Dick method [George F. Dick, 1881–1967, and Gladys H. Dick, 1881–1963, U.S. bacteriologists]. A toxin-antitoxin injection for the prevention of scarlet fever.

Dick test. A test for susceptibility or immunity to scarlet fever. The erythrogenic toxin from *Streptococcus* is injected intracutaneously. In a negative reaction, some slight inflammatory changes may occur due to irritation by proteins in fluid administered. In a manner somewhat similar to the Schick testing for diphtheria, a person's susceptibility to scarlet fever may be ascertained by the injection of a standardized toxin of the β-hemolytic streptococcus. A positive (susceptible) reaction in the form of erythema appears in about 12 to 24 hours. Patients convalescing from scarlet fever invariably give a negative reaction. SEE: *Schick test*.

dicloxacillin sodium (dī-klŏks″ă-sĭl'ĭn). USP. A semisynthetic penicillin useful in treating penicillinase-resistant staphylococci. Trade names are Dycill and Dynapen.

Dicodid. Trade name for hydrocodone bitartrate.

dicoelous (dī-sē'lŭs) [″ + *koilos*, hollow]. 1. Concave or hollowed out on two sides. 2. Containing two cavities.

dicophane (dī'kō-fān). A powerful insecticide now rarely used because of its toxicity. SYN: *chlorophenothane; DDT*.

dicoria (dī-kō'rē-ă) [″ + *kore*, pupil]. Double pupil in each eye.

dicoumarol (dī-koo'mă-rŏl). Dicumarol, q.v.

dicrotic (dī-krŏt'ĭk) [Gr. *dikrotos*, beating double]. Having one heartbeat for two arterial pulsations; rel. to a double pulse.

dicrotic notch. In a pulse tracing, a notch on the descending limb.

dicrotic wave. A positive wave following the dicrotic notch.

dicrotism (dī'krŏt-ĭzm) [″ + *-ismos*, condition]. The state of being dicrotic.

dictyoma (dĭk″tē-ō'mă) [Gr. *diktyon*, net, + *oma*, tumor]. A tumor of the ciliary epithelium. Also spelled diktyoma.

dictyosome (dĭk'tē-ō-sōm) [″ + *soma*, body]. Cytoplasmic body similar to the Golgi apparatus. It is thought to be a dispersed element of the Golgi apparatus.

dicumarol (dī-koo'mă-rŏl). USP. An anticoagulant that decreases activity of prothrombin in the blood plasma and hence increases prothrombin time. Used in prophylaxis and treatment of intravascular clotting, in postoperative thrombophlebitis, pulmonary embolism, acute peripheral embolism and thrombosis, and recurrent idiopathic thrombophlebitis. Used also in management of acute coronary thrombosis. Frequently an adjunct to heparin, q.v. The dose is determined by periodically testing the prothrombin time. If heparin is being given, it is important that three to four hours elapse between the last dose of heparin and the time the blood is drawn for the prothrombin test.

CONTRA: Subacute bacterial endocar-

ditis, recent brain, spinal, or eye surgery, purpura and blood dyscrasias, in vitamin K deficiency, and in absence of prothrombin determination. The drug is excreted in the mother's milk. Thus, breast-fed infants whose mothers are receiving Dicumarol should be carefully observed for bleeding tendency. In cases of hemorrhage due to this drug, stop the drug immediately and give vitamin K intravenously; whole fresh blood may be needed. SEE: *anticoagulant; heparin; tissue plasminogen activator; vitamin K*.

dicyclic (dī-sī'klĭk). 1. Having or concerning two cycles. 2. In chemistry, containing two cyclic ring structures.

dicyclomine hydrochloride (dī-sī'klō-mēn). USP. An anticholinergic drug used as an antispasmodic. Trade name is Bentyl.

didactic (dī-dăk'tĭk) [Gr. *didaktikos*]. Concerning instruction by lectures and by use of texts as opposed to clinical or bedside teaching of medicine.

didactylism (dī-dăk'tĭ-lĭzm) [Gr. *dis*, two, + *daktylos*, finger]. The congenital condition of having only two digits on a hand or foot.

didanosine. ABBR: DDI. Drug used in treating AIDS. Trade name is Videx.

didelphic (dī-dĕl'fĭk) [″ + *delphys*, uterus]. Having or pert. to a double uterus.

didymalgia, didymodynia (dĭd-ĭ-măl'jē-ă, dĭd″ĭ-mō-dĭn'ē-ă) [Gr. *didymos*, twin, + *algos*, pain]. Pain in a testicle.

didymitis (dĭd-ĭ-mī'tĭs) [″ + *itis*, inflammation]. Inflammation of a testicle. SYN: *orchitis*.

didymus (dĭd'ĭ-mŭs) [Gr. *didymos*, twin]. 1. A twin. 2. A congenital abnormality involving joined twins. 3. A testicle.

die. 1. To cease living. 2. In dentistry, a positive duplicate made from an impression of a tooth.

diechoscope (dī-ĕk'ō-skōp) [Gr. *dis*, two, + *echo*, echo, + *skopein*, to examine]. A stethoscope for simultaneous auscultation from two different sites.

diecious (dī-ē'shŭs) [″ + *oikos*, house]. Having sexually distinct males and females, esp. in botany.

dieldrin (dī-ĕl'drĭn). A chlorinated hydrocarbon used as an insecticide. It is toxic to humans and marine and terrestrial animals. SEE: *Poisons and Poisoning* in *Appendix*.

dielectric [Gr. *dia*, through, + *elektron*, amber]. An insulating substance offering great resistance to passage of electricity by conduction.

diembryony (dī-ĕm'brē-ŏn″ē). The development of two embryos in a single egg.

diencephalon (dī″ĕn-sĕf'ă-lŏn) [Gr. *dis*, two, + *enkephalos*, brain]. Second portion of the brain or that lying between the telencephalon and mesencephalon. It includes the epithalamus, thalamus, metathalamus, and hypothalamus. SYN: *thalamencephalon.*

dienestrol (dī″ĕn-ĕs′trŏl). USP. A nonsteroid, synthetic estrogen used for estrogen therapy.

Dientamoeba (dī″ĕn-tă-mē′bă). A genus of parasitic protozoa characterized by possession of two similar nuclei.

D. fragilis. A species of parasitic amebae inhabiting the intestine of humans. Persons infected may have diarrhea with blood or mucus, abdominal pain, and anal pruritus. This organism has been found inside the eggs of pinworms. Thus, it is thought that these eggs serve as the vector.

dieresis (dī-ĕr′ĕ-sĭs) [Gr. *diairesis,* a division]. 1. Breaking up or dispersion of things normally joined, as by an ulcer. 2. Mechanical separation of parts by surgical means.

dieretic. Pert. to dieresis; dissolvable or separable.

diet [Gr. *diaita,* way of living]. 1. Liquid and solid food substances regularly consumed in the course of normal living. 2. A prescribed allowance of food adapted for a particular state of health or disease, as a diet prescribed for use by a diabetic. 3. To cause to eat or drink sparingly in accordance with prescribed rules. SEE: *energy expenditure, basal.*

d., balanced. Diet adequate in energy-providing substances (carbohydrates and fats), tissue-building compounds (proteins), inorganic chemicals (water and mineral salts), agents that regulate or catalyze metabolic processes (vitamins), and substances for certain physiological processes, such as bulk for promoting peristaltic movements of the digestive tract.

d., macrobiotic. SEE: *macrobiotic diet.*

d., minimum residue. Diet used for short periods of time to insure a minimum of solid material in the intestinal tract. Foods allowed include one glass of milk per day; clear fluids and juices; lean meat; noodles; and refined cereals.

d., reduction. Diet that reduces the caloric content sufficiently to cause weight loss. Normal metabolism must be preserved, as must bulk, mineral, protein, vitamin, and water requirements. During weight loss intake should be 600 to 1500 Cal below maintenance levels for the individual's weight. SEE: *obesity.*

d., very low calorie. Commercially available diet in which caloric intake may be from 400 to 800 Calories per day. The very low calorie diet is usually in the form of a powdered supplement that is taken 3 to 5 times a day with large amounts of water.

This type of diet can be effective, but the long-range efficacy in maintaining the weight loss may be discouraging.

diet, words pert. to: bland diet; calcium (high and low) diet; elimination diet; energy expenditure, basal; fat (low) diet; feeding; fluid diet; liquid diet; roughage diet; salt-free diet; soft diet; weight, set point.

dietary (dī′ĕ-tā″rē). 1. Pert. to diet. 2. A system of dieting. 3. A regulated food allowance.

dietary fiber. SEE: *fiber, dietary.*

dietetic (dī-ĕ-tĕt′ĭk). 1. Pert. to diet or its regulation. 2. Food specially prepared for restrictive diets.

dietetics [Gr. *diaitetikos*]. The science of applying nutritional data to the regulation of the diet of healthy and sick individuals. Some fundamental principles and facts of this science will be summarized here. SEE: *energy expenditure, basal; Appendix.*

CONSERVATION OF ENERGY: In order to obtain metabolic balance, the number of calories consumed must equal the energy required for basic metabolic needs plus additional energy output resulting from muscular work and added heat losses. Thus a person whose basal rate is 1000 Calories (kilogram calories) per 24 hours may during the day do work and lose heat, adding about 075 Calories to the energy output; he or she must, therefore, obtain 2500 Calories.

One gm of fat yields approx. 9 Cal. One gm of carbohydrate or protein yields about 4 Cal.

NOTE: To convert Calories to kilojoules, multiply Calories (kilocalories) by 4.1855.

CONSERVATION OF MATTER: Everything that leaves the body, whether exhaled as carbon dioxide and water or excreted as urea and minerals, must be replaced in the food. Thus, a person excreting 10 gm of nitrogen daily must receive 10 gm of it in his or her diet, for the element can neither be created nor destroyed. This metabolic balance may be monitored by the use of careful chemical analysis of all that is eaten and excreted.

diethazine hydrochloride (dī-ĕth′ă-zēn). An anticholinergic used in treating parkinsonism.

diethylcarbamazine citrate (dī-ĕth″ĭl-kăr-băm′ă-zēn). USP. Medicine used in treating filarial infections.

diethylpropion hydrochloride (dī-ĕth″ĭl-prō′pē-ŏn). USP. An adrenergic drug with actions similar to those of the amphetamines. Trade names are Tenuate and Tepanil.

diethylstilbestrol (dī-ĕth″ĭl-stĭl″bĕs′trŏl). USP. ABBR: DES. A synthetic preparation possessing estrogenic properties. It is several times more potent than natural estrogens and may be given orally. It is used therapeutically in the treatment of menopausal disturbances and other disorders due to estrogen deficiencies. SEE: *DES daughters; DES syndrome.*

Caution: Should not be administered during pregnancy. Such use has been found to be related to subsequent vaginal malignancies in the daughters of mothers who were so treated.

ORIGINAL MIXTURE   MIXTURE AFTER DIFFUSION ACTION

diethyltoluamide (dī-ĕth″ĭl-tŏl-ū′ă-mīd). USP. ABBR: DET. An effective insect repellant, esp. for repelling arthropods.

diethyltryptamine (dī-ĕth″ĭl-trĭp′tă-mĭn). A hallucinogenic agent that at low dose levels has effects similar to those of LSD.

dietitian (dī-ĕ-tĭsh′ăn) [Gr. *diaita*, way of living]. An individual whose training and experience is in the area of nutrition, and who has the ability to apply that information to the dietary needs of the healthy and sick.

Dietl's crisis (dē′tls) [Joseph Dietl, Pol. physician, 1804–1878]. Renal colic resulting from kinking and partial obstruction of the ureter, accompanied by scanty bloodstained urine.

dietotherapy (dī″ĕ-tō-thĕr′ă-pē). Use of the sciences of dietetics and nutrition in treating disease.

Dieulafoy's triad (dyŭ-lă-fwăhz′) [Georges Dieulafoy, Fr. physician, 1839–1911]. Tenderness, muscular contraction, and skin hyperesthesia at McBurney's point in acute appendicitis.

differential (dif″ĕr-ĕn′shăl) [L. *differre*, to carry apart]. Marked by differences.

differential amplifier. An amplifier used to increase the difference between two signals, one of which is usually a reference.

differential blood count. Determination of the number of each variety of leukocytes in one microliter (μl) of blood. SEE: *blood count, differential.*

differential diagnosis. Diagnosis based on comparison of symptoms of two or more similar diseases to determine which the patient is suffering from. SEE: *diagnosis.*

differentiation. 1. Acquisition of functions different from those of the original type. 2. The distinguishing of one disease from another. 3. In psychiatry, the integration of emotional and intellectual functions in an individual.

   d., lymphocyte. The process by which immature lymphocytes are stimulated to become functional T and B cells able to recognize and respond to antigens.

diffraction (dĭ-frăk′shŭn) [L. *diffringere*, to break to pieces]. The change that occurs in light when it passes through crystals,

prisms, or parallel bars in a grating, in which the rays are deflected and thus appear to be turned aside. This produces dark or colored bands or lines or other phenomena. Term is also applied to similar phenomena in sound.

diffraction grating. The device in a spectrophotometer that disperses white light into the colors of the spectrum. This is done to isolate wavelengths.

diffusate (dĭf′ū-sāt) [L. *dis*, apart, + *fundere*, to pour]. In the process of dialysis, that portion of a liquid that passes through a membrane and that contains crystalloid matter in solution. SYN: *dialysate.*

diffuse (dĭ-fūs′). Spreading, scattered, spread.

diffusible (dĭ-fūz′ĭ-bl). Capable of being diffused.

diffusion (dĭ-fū′zhŭn) [″ + *fundere*, to pour]. 1. Absorption of a liquid such as the absorption by cells of water from lymph when the percentage of salt is less in lymph than in the cells. When the percentage is greater in the lymph than in the cells, water is withdrawn from the latter. SEE: *osmosis.* 2. A process whereby various gases interpenetrate and become mixed as a result of the incessant motion of their molecules. Similarly, if aqueous solutions of different materials stand in contact, mixing occurs on standing even if the solutions are separated by thin membranes. SEE: illus. 3. The tendency of molecules of a substance (gaseous, liquid, or solid) to move from a region of high concentration to one of lower concentration.

digastric (dī-găs′trĭk) [Gr. *dis*, twice, + *gaster*, belly]. Having two bellies; said of certain muscles.

digenesis [″ + *genesis*, generation, birth]. Reproduction in which alternate generations are asexual.

Digenetica (dī-jĕ-nĕt′ĭ-kă). An order of parasitic flatworms belonging to the class Trematoda. It is characterized by having an asexual generation, living usually in molluscs, alternating with a sexual generation living in vertebrates as their final host. It includes all four groups of flukes parasitic in man. SEE: *fluke.*

digest [L. *dis*, apart, + *gerere*, to carry]. 1. To undergo digestion, as in the process involved in changing food from a solid physical form to a soft, moisturized mass acted upon in the intestinal tract by chemicals, bacteria, and enzymes. SEE: *metabolism.* 2. To make a condensation of a subject.

digestant. 1. An agent that will digest food or aid in digestion, such as pepsin or pancreatin. 2. A preparation made from the digestive glands or lining membrane of the stomach, classified according to the foods it digests, such as carbohydrate or protein.

digestible. That which is capable of being digested.

digestion [L. *digestio*, a taking apart]. The process by which food is broken down mechanically and chemically in the gastrointestinal tract and converted into absorbable forms. Salt, the simplest sugars (such as glucose), cystalloids in general, and water can be absorbed unchanged, but starches, fats, and proteins for the most part are not absorbable until split into smaller molecules by the process of digestion. Even the sugar sucrose (a disaccharide) must first be split into two simple hexoses, glucose and fructose, in order to be absorbed. The chemical actions are chiefly hydrolytic; they are brought about by a variety of enzymes, each of which acts in an acid or alkaline or neutral juice according to its peculiar properties.

The higher molecular weight carbohydrates are converted into monosaccharides, q.v. A very small proportion of ingested starch is digested in the mouth. Starch is partially digested in the stomach. The remaining starch and other carbohydrates are digested in the stomach and small intestine. Proteins, through successive stages, are ultimately converted into amino acids and fats into fatty acids and glycerine. Almost all of the digestion of fats occurs in the small intestine. A small amount of a fat derived from butter can be digested by an enzyme, tributyrase, in the stomach. In the stomach the soluble casein of milk is converted into insoluble paracasein, resulting in its coagulation or clotting. This is brought about by the enzyme pepsin. This digestive process will not occur in the absence of gastric acid. Proteins are also digested by the action of enzymes secreted into the small intestine from the pancreas, and from enzymes present in the epithelial cells of the small intestine. The enzyme lipase is able to act on emulsified fats. It liberates, for instance, butyric acid from the fats in milk. This chemical causes the characteristic odor of vomitus. The chemical actions are facilitated by the churning wavelike motions, i.e., peristalsis, of the stomach walls. When the chyme is ready to leave the stomach, the pylorus opens from time to time and the chyme is quickly propelled into the duodenum. SEE: table.

    d., artificial. Digestion outside the living organism by a ferment.

    d., duodenal. The chyme, which is usually acid as it comes from the stomach, is made alkaline and the fats it contains are emulsified by the action of bile. Enzymes adapted to these new conditions are supplied by the pancreatic juice, which enters by two ducts, and by the intestinal juice, which comes from small glands in the wall of the intestine itself. The hydrolysis of starches, fats, and proteins is carried to its physiological completion here and in the remainder of the small intestine.

    d., extracellular. Digestion occurring outside the body of the cell.

    d., gastric. Portion of the digestive process taking place in the stomach.

    d., intestinal. Hydrolytic processes continue in the intestines, and absorption of the products is active. From the ileum, the food residues pass in a nearly liquid state through a small opening into the ascending colon. A sphincter muscle prevents backflow. True digestive processes in the colon are slight, but there are normally bacterial action (the products of which are mostly absorbed) and reabsorption of water. The remaining substances, now colored by pigments that entered with bile and changed to a firm consistency by the loss of water, pass on through the transverse colon, the descending colon, and the sigmoid flexure into the rectum. They are retained in the rectum by the action of sphincters until defecation occurs. SEE: *absorption.*

    d., intracellular. Metabolic processes within cells.

    d., oral. Portion of digestive process taking place in the mouth. It includes the physical process of chewing food and the chemical process of starch-splitting by the enzyme ptyalin, present in the saliva.

    d., pancreatic. Portion of digestive process influenced by pancreatic juice.

    d., salivary. Digestive action by the saliva. SEE: *salivary digestion.*

    d., secondary. Cellular assimilation of nutritive material.

digestive (dī-jĕs′tĭv). Pert. to digestion.

digestive juice. One of several secretions that aid in processes of digestion.

digestive system. All the organs and glands associated with ingestion and digestion of food; the tract from the mouth to the anus.

Action of Digestive Enzymes on Foods

Food Component	Enzyme	Secretion	Site of Action
Proteins	Pepsin	Gastric juice, acid	Stomach
	Trypsin	Pancreatic juice, alkaline	Small intestine
Fats	Lipase	Gastric juice	Stomach
	Lipase	Pancreatic juice	Small intestine
	Salivary amylase	Saliva, alkaline	Mouth and, to some small extent, in stomach
Carbohydrates	Ptyalin	Saliva	Mouth
	Pancreatic amylase	Pancreatic juice, alkaline	Small intestine
	Invertase	Succus entericus	Small intestine

Action of Digestive Secretions on Proteins, Fats, and Carbohydrates

Secretion	Proteins	Fats	Carbohydrates
Saliva			Cooked starch into maltose
Gastric Juice	Curdles milk Proteins into peptones		
Pancreatic Juice	Peptones to simpler substances	Fats to fatty acids and glycerol	Raw and cooked starch into maltose Sugars into simpler forms
Bile		Emulsifies fats	
Intestinal Juice	Completes the change of peptones into amino acids		Completes the change of all sugars into the simplest form. NOTE: Disaccharides are hydrolyzed to monosaccharides in the mucosal cells lining the small intestine.

SEE: illus.

digit (dĭj′ĭt) [L. *digitus*, finger] (pl. *digits*). A finger or toe.

digital (dĭj′ĭ-tăl). Pert. to or resembling a finger or toe.

digital amniotome. A small apparatus that fits over the tip of the index finger. A small knifelike projection at the end of the device is used to puncture the bag of waters prior to delivery of the fetus. This usually expedites progression of labor.

digitalis (dĭj″ĭ-tăl′ĭs) [L. *digitus*, finger]. USP. Foxglove. The dried leaves of *Digitalis purpurea* used in powdered form in tablets or capsules. Cardiotonic glycosides, esp. digitoxin and digoxin, are obtained from various species of the digitalis plant. SEE: *Poisons and Poisoning* in *Appendix*.

ACTION/USES: Digitalis glycosides increase the force of myocardial contraction, increase the refractory period of the atrioventricular (A-V) node, and to a lesser degree affect the sinoatrial (S-A) node. Digitalis acts to increase cardiac output by increasing the contractility of cardiac muscle. Digitalis is indicated in congestive heart failure, and its use causes diuresis and general amelioration of this condition. It is usually necessary to continue the drug after the heart failure is controlled. Digitalis is also used in atrial fibrillation and flutter and in paroxysmal atrial tachycardia.

CONTRA: Digitalis is not indicated in sinus tachycardia or premature systoles in

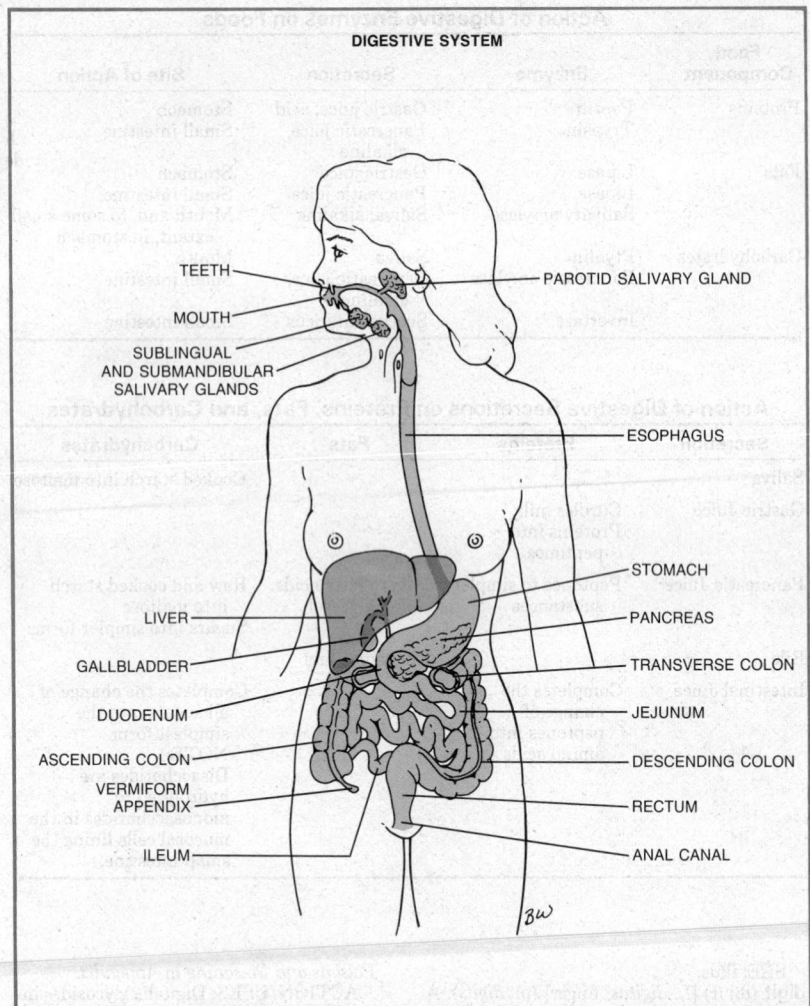

DIGESTIVE SYSTEM

TEETH

MOUTH

SUBLINGUAL
AND SUBMANDIBULAR
SALIVARY GLANDS

PAROTID SALIVARY GLAND

ESOPHAGUS

LIVER

GALLBLADDER

DUODENUM

ASCENDING COLON

VERMIFORM
APPENDIX

ILEUM

STOMACH

PANCREAS

TRANSVERSE COLON

JEJUNUM

DESCENDING COLON

RECTUM

ANAL CANAL

the absence of heart failure. Its use in shock caused by infections is of no benefit and may be harmful. It should not be used in ventricular fibrillation or if the patient is allergic to digitalis.

PRECAUTIONS: Potassium depletion, which may accompany diuresis, sensitizes the myocardium to digitalis and may permit toxicity to develop with what would otherwise be the usual dose. Patients with acute myocardial infarction, severe pulmonary disease, or far-advanced heart failure may be more sensitive to digitalis and thus prone to develop arrhythmia. Calcium affects the heart in a manner similar to digitalis; its use in a digitalized patient may produce serious arrhythmias. In myxedema, digitalis requirements are decreased because excretion rate of the drug is decreased. Patients with incomplete A-V block, esp. those with Stokes-Adams attacks, may develop complete heart block if given digitalis. Because renal insufficiency delays the excretion of digitalis, the dose must be adjusted accordingly in those patients.

digitalis poisoning. Toxicity that may develop acutely or chronically from the cumulative effect of digitalis. Patients on digitalis therapy must know how to take their pulse and be aware of the signs and symptoms of heart block or other adverse effects. They should also include potassium-containing foods in their daily diet. SEE: *Nursing Diagnoses* in *Appendix.*

SYM: Digestive disturbances such as nausea and vomiting, irregular pulse, diarrhea, and yellow vision. Frequently distressing headache. Cardiac irregularities are common, esp. slowing of heart, ventricular extrasystoles, or partial heart block.

F.A.: Evacuate stomach and discontinue digitalis and diuretics. Because these patients are usually chronically ill, special care is necessary in their management. Serious cases of poisoning should be treated with digoxin immune Fab (ovine). Trade name is Digibind.

digitalization (dĭj″ĭ-tăl-ĭ-zā′shŭn). Subjection of an organism to the action of digitalis.

digital radiography. Radiography using computerized imaging instead of the conventional film or screen imaging.

digital reflex. Sudden flexion of terminal phalanx of a finger or thumb when nail is suddenly tapped.

digital subtraction angiography. SEE: *angiography, digital subtraction.*

digitate [L. *digitus*, finger]. Having finger-like impressions or processes.

digitation (dĭj-ĭ-tā′shŭn). A finger-like process.

digiti (dĭj′ĭ-tī). Pl. of digitus.

digitiform (dĭj′ĭ-tĭ-form). Similar to a finger.

digitoxin (dĭj-ĭ-tŏk′sĭn). USP. A cardiotoxic glycoside obtained from various species of the digitalis plant. A heart stimulant, administered orally or parenterally. Trade names are Crystodigin and Purodigin. SEE: *digitalis.*

digit span test. A test of the temporal-sequential organization of a child. The youngster is asked to recall a sequence of numbers immediately after they have been spoken. SEE: *object span test; temporal-sequential organization.*

digitus [L]. (pl. *digiti*) A finger or toe.

diglossia (dī-glŏs′ē-ă) [Gr. *dis*, double, + *glossa*, tongue]. Having a double tongue.

diglyceride (dī-glĭs′ĕr-īd). Glyceride combined with two fatty acid molecules. SEE: *triglyceride.*

dignathus (dĭg-nā′thŭs) [″ + *gnathos*, jaw]. A congenital deformity in which there are two jaws.

digoxin (dī-jŏk′sĭn). USP. A cardiotonic glycoside obtained from *Digitalis lanata*. A heart stimulant administered orally or parenterally. Trade name is Lanoxin.

digoxin immune Fab (ovine) for injection. A biological substance for use in treating severe overdose of digoxin or digitoxin. This fragment antigen binding (Fab) combines with molecules of digoxin or digitoxin which are then excreted by the kidneys. Trade name is Digibind).

dihydric (dī-hī′drĭk). A compound containing two hydrogen atoms.

dihydrocodeinone bitartrate (dī-hī″drō-kō′dē-ĭ-nōn). An opioid analgesic that is used in combination with a number of other drugs.

dihydroergotamine mesylate (dī-hī″drō-ĕr-gŏt′ă-mēn). USP. A vasoconstrictor used in treating migraine. Trade name is DHE-45.

dihydrosphingosine. $CH_3—[CH_2]_{14}—CHOH—CH(NH_2)—CH_2OH$. A long-chain amino alcohol present in sphingolipids. Also known as sphinganine. SEE: *sphingolipids; sphingosine.*

dihydrotachysterol (dī-hī″drō-tăk-ĭs′tĕr-ŏl). USP. A hydrogenated tachysterol; a steroid, obtained by irradiation of ergosterol. Aids absorption of calcium from digestive tract in hypoparathyroidism. Trade name is Hytakerol.

dihydroxyaluminum aminoacetate (dī″hī-drŏk″sē-ă-lū′mĭ-nŭm). An antacid used in treating gastric hyperacidity. Trade name is Robalate.

dihydroxyaluminum sodium carbonate. USP. A gastric antacid preparation. Trade name is Rolaids.

dihydroxycholecalciferol (dī″hī-drŏk″sē-kō″lē-kăl-sĭf′ĕ-rŏl). A group of compounds considered to be hormones because of their ability to influence absorption and metabolism of calcium. One of these, calcitriol, is thought to be the active form of vitamin D, q.v.

3,4-dihydroxyphenylalanine (dī-hī-drŏk″sē-fĕn″ĭl-ăl′ă-nēn). Dopa, q.v.

dihysteria (dī″hĭs-tēr′ē-ă) [Gr. *dis*, double, + *hystera*, womb]. State of having a double uterus.

diiodohydroxyquin (dī″ī-ō″dō-hī-drŏk′sē-kwĭn). Previously used name for iodoquinol, USP.

diktyoma (dĭk-tē-ō′mă) [Gr. *diktyon*, net, + *oma*, tumor]. A tumor of the ciliary epithelium. SYN: *dictyoma.*

dilaceration (dī″lăs-ĕr-ā′shŭn) [L. *dilacerare*, to tear apart]. 1. A tearing apart, as of a cataract. SEE: *discission.* 2. Bending of the root of a tooth due to injury during development.

Dilantin (dī-lăn′tĭn). Trade name for phenytoin sodium, USP. Previously termed diphenylhydantoin sodium. A derivative of glyceryl urea. An anticonvulsant used esp. in the treatment of epilepsy.

dilatant (dī-lā′tănt) [L. *dilatare*, to enlarge]. Anything that causes dilation.

dilatation (dĭl-ă-tā′shŭn). 1. Expansion of an organ or vessel. 2. Expansion of an orifice with a dilator.

d., digital. Dilatation of an opening or a cavity by use of the fingers.

d., heart. Abnormal increase in the size of the cavities of the heart, a common result of valvular disease or hypertension.

d., stomach. Condition in which the stomach is extremely dilated. Acute dilatation of the stomach or acute gastromesenteric ileus may occur as a postoperative or postpartum condition and usually results from obstruction of the duodenum.

dilation. 1. Expansion of an orifice with a dilator. 2. Expansion of an organ, orifice, or vessel. SYN: *dilatation*.

dilation and curettage. ABBR: D and C. A surgical procedure that expands the cervical canal of the uterus (dilation) so that the surface lining of the uterine wall can be scraped (curettage). SEE: *Nursing Diagnoses* in *Appendix.*

dilation and evacuation. ABBR: D and E. During the second trimester, removal of the products of conception by suction curettage and use of forceps.

dilator (dī-lā′tor) [L. *dilatare*, to expand]. Instrument for dilating muscles or for stretching cavities or openings.

d., Barnes′. Rubber bag that is filled with fluid for dilation of the cervix uteri.

d., Bossi′s. Multiple-pronged instrument that dilates by separation of the prongs. Used for dilation of the cervix uteri.

d., Goodell′s. Similar to the Bossi except that it has three prongs.

d., gynecologic. Instrument for dilating the cervix uteri.

d., Hegar′s. Graduated metal sounds that are inserted into the cervical canal and cause a graded dilation.

d., tent. Small cone made of seaweed, sponge, or tree roots that is inserted into the uterine canal dry and, on absorbing moisture, expands to cause a slow dilation. SEE: *Laminaria digitata.*

d., vaginal. Glass, plastic, or metal device for dilating the vagina.

Dilaudid. Trade name for hydromorphone hydrochloride.

dildo, dildoe. An artificial penis-shaped device used intravaginally to produce sexual pleasure.

diluent (dĭl′ū-ĕnt) [L. *diluere*, to wash away]. An agent that dilutes the substance or solution to which it is added.

dilution (dī-loo′shŭn). 1. Process of rendering a substance attenuated or diluted. 2. A diluted substance. SEE: *adulteration.*

dim. Reduced light or action of decreasing light present.

dimenhydrinate (dī″mĕn-hī′drĭn-āt). USP. A drug used to prevent or treat motion sickness and to control nausea, vomiting, and dizziness in other conditions. Trade names are Dommanate and Dramamine.

dimension (dī-mĕn′shŭn). The measure of anything. It is expressed in commonly recognized and accepted units.

dimer (dī′mĕr). 1. In chemistry, esp. polymer chemistry, the combination of two identical molecules to form a single compound. 2. In virology, a capsomer containing two subunits.

dimercaprol (dī-mĕr-kăp′rŏl). USP. $C_3H_8OS_2$. A compound, 2,3-dimercaptopropanol, used as an antidote in poisoning from heavy metals such as arsenic, gold, and mercury. It occurs as a colorless liquid with a disagreeable odor. Mixed with benzyl benzoate and oil, it is administered intramuscularly. Trade name is BAL in Oil.

Dimetane. Trade name for brompheniramine maleate.

dimethicone (dī-mĕth′ĭ-kōn). A silicone oil used to protect the skin against water-soluble irritants.

dimethindene maleate (dī″mĕth-ĭn′dēn). USP. An antihistamine. Trade names are Forhistal Maleate and Triten.

dimethisterone (dī″mĕth-ĭs′tĕr-ōn). A progestational agent.

dimethylamine (dī-mĕth″ĭl-ăm′ĭn). A malodorous product of decaying materials that contain proteins.

p-dimethylaminoazobenzene (dī-mĕth″ĭl-ăm″ĭ-nō-ăz″ō-bĕn′zēn). A carcinogenic dye, butter yellow.

dimethyl phthalate (dī-mĕth″ĭl-thăl′āt). An insect repellant.

dimethyl sulfoxide (dī-mĕth″ĭl sŭlf-ŏks′ĭd). USP. ABBR: DMSO. A solvent used to facilitate absorption of medicines through the skin. It is a colorless liquid with little odor, but when it is applied to the skin and absorbed, the patient will notice a garlic-like taste sensation.

dimethyltryptamine (dī-mĕth″ĭl-trĭp′tă-mēn). An agent that in low doses has hallucinogenic action similar to LSD.

dimetria (dī-mē′trē-ă) [Gr. *dis*, double, + *metra*, uterus]. A double uterus.

dimorphous (dī-mor′fŭs) [″ + *morphe*, form]. Occurring in two different forms.

dimple. A small depression in the skin, esp. of the cheek or chin.

dimple sign. Sign used to differentiate a benign lesion, dermatofibroma, from a nodular melanoma, which it may mimic. Upon application of lateral pressure with the thumb and index finger, the dermatofibroma will dimple or become indented; melanomas, melanocytic nevi, and normal skin protrude above the initial plane.

dimpling. The formation of slight depressions in the flesh due to retraction of the subcutaneous tissue. Occurs in certain carcinomas, such as cancer of the breast. SEE: *peau d'orange.*

2,4-dinitrophenol (dī-nī″trō-fē′nŏl). An isomeric compound formerly used in making dyes. It is very toxic, and is used only as a reagent. SEE: *Poisons and Poisoning* in *Appendix.*

Dinoflagellata (dī″nō-flăj″ē-lā′tă) [″ + *flagellum,* whip]. An order of minute marine protozoa that have been associated with a red discoloration of seawater known as "red tide." They are toxic to fish.

dinoprost tromethamine (dī′nō-prŏst). A drug that causes uterine contractions and may be used to induce abortion during the very early stage of pregnancy. SYN: *prostaglandin F*$_{2a}$.

dinucleotide (dī-nū′klē-ō-tīd). The product of cleaving a polynucleotide.

Dioctophyma (dī-ŏk″tō-fī′mă). A genus of roundworm found in dogs but rarely in man.

dioctyl calcium sulfosuccinate (dī-ŏk′tĭl). A stool softener. Previously used name for docusate calcium.

dioctyl sodium sulfosuccinate. Previously used name for docusate sodium, q.v.

Diodrast (dī′ō-drăst). Trade name for iodopyracet, a radiopaque medium used in x-ray studies, esp. of the urinary tract.

Diogenes syndrome [Diogenes, Gr. philosopher, 4th century B.C.]. Condition found among elderly persons, most of whom live alone, have no interest in personal cleanliness, and are uninterested in the cleanliness of their homes. They are usually undernourished, but this is not necessarily due to poverty. Persons from all walks of life may have this condition.

diopter, dioptre [Gr. *dia,* through, + *optos,* visible]. Refractive power of lens. It is the reciprocal of the focal length expressed in meters. Used as unit of measurement in refraction.

dioptometer (dī″ŏp-tŏm′ē-tĕr) [″ + ″ + *metron,* measure]. Device for measuring ocular refraction.

dioptometry (dī″ŏp-tŏm′ē-trē). The determination of refraction and accommodation of the eye.

dioptral (dī-ŏp′trăl). Pert. to a diopter.

dioptric (dī-ŏp′trĭk). Pert. to refraction of light.

dioptrics. The science of refraction of light.

diovulatory (dī-ŏv′ū-lā-tō″rē). Production of two ova in the same ovarian cycle.

dioxide (dī-ŏk′sīd) [Gr. *dis,* two, + *oxys,* sharp]. A compound having two oxygen atoms per molecule.

dioxin. 2,3,7,8-tetrachlorodibenzo-*p*-dioxin (TCDD). A chemical important because of its being an unwanted and undesirable contaminant in widely used herbicides and preservatives. There are more than 75 different isomers of dioxin. Exposure to dioxin can produce chloracne, liver injury, peripheral neuropathy, central nervous system changes, and psychiatric difficulty. The possibility that dioxin causes cancer in man is being investigated. At low concentrations, dioxin, which is carcinogenic in animals, is one of the most toxic substances to which workers in the industrial and agricultural environment can be exposed. SEE: *Agent Orange; pentachlorophenol; 2,4,5-trichlorophenoxyacetic acid.*

dioxybenzone (dī-ŏks″ī-bĕn′zōn). USP. Chemical for protecting skin from the sun. Trade name is Spectra-Sorb UV 24.

dipeptid(e) (dī-pĕp′tĭd, -tīd) [″ + *peptein,* to digest]. A derived protein obtained by hydrolysis of proteins or condensation of amino acids.

dipeptidase (dī-pĕp′tĭ-dās). An enzyme that catalyzes the hydrolysis of dipeptides to amino acids.

diperodon (dī-pĕr′ō-dŏn). USP. A topical anesthetic.

Dipetalonema perstans (dī-pĕt″ă-lō-nē′mă). A species of filaria that infests wild or domestic animals and occasionally humans. In humans, the adult worm migrates to the subcutaneous tissue and produces a nodule. The adult worm may, rarely, be seen beneath the conjunctiva.

diphallus (dī-făl′ŭs) [″ + *phallos,* penis]. A condition in which there is either a complete or incomplete doubling of the penis or clitoris.

diphasic (dī-fā′zĭk) [″ + *phasis,* a phase]. Having two phases.

diphemanil methylsulfate (dī-fē′mă-nĭl). USP. An anticholinergic drug used in treating gastric hyperacidity. Trade name is Prantal.

diphenhydramine hydrochloride (dī″fĕn-hī′dră-mēn hī-drō-klō′rĭd). USP. An antihistaminic agent. Trade name is Benadryl.

diphenoxylate hydrochloride (dī″fĕn-ŏk′sī-lāt). USP. A smooth muscle relaxant used in combination with atropine in treating diarrhea.

diphenylhydantoin sodium (dī-fĕn″ĭl-hī-dăn′tō-ĭn). A white odorless powder, freely soluble in water. An anticonvulsant used esp. in the treatment of epilepsy. The official name is phenytoin. Trade name is Dilantin.

diphenylpyraline hydrochloride (dī-fēn″ĭl-pī′rǎ-lēn). USP. An antihistamine. Trade name is Hispril.

diphonia (dī-fō′nē-ǎ) [Gr. *dis*, two, + *phone*, voice]. Simultaneous production of two different voice tones.

diphosphatidylglycerol. An extract of beef hearts that contains phosphorylated polysaccharide esters of fatty acids. It is used in certain tests for syphilis.

2,3-diphosphoglycerate. ABBR: 2,3-DPG. An organic phosphate in red blood cells that alters the affinity of hemoglobin for oxygen. Blood cells stored in a blood bank lose 2,3-diphosphoglycerate but once they are infused, the substance is resynthesized or reactivated. SYN: *2,3-bisphosphoglycerate.*

diphtheria (dĭf-thē′rē-ǎ) [Gr. *diphthera*, membrane]. An acute infectious disease characterized by the formation of a false membrane on any mucous surface and occasionally on the skin. Usually accompanied by great prostration. SEE: *antitoxin; Klebs-Loeffler bacillus; Schick test; toxin-antitoxin.*

SYM: Onset gradual. Usually slight headache and malaise. Temperature 100° to 101°F (37.8° to 38.3°C) and sore throat with presence of yellow-white or gray pseudomembrane adherent to tonsils or pharyngeal walls. Cervical adenitis may develop early in severe types. In nasal diphtheria, fever is a much more evident symptom. Adenitis often is severe, with serous discharge from nostrils, which may be blood tinged. Strong fetid odor of breath common. Myocarditis and late neuritis are commonly present.

ETIOL: Causative organism *Corynebacterium diphtheriae*, a gram-positive nonmotile, non-spore-forming, club-shaped bacillus. In stained smears, the bacilli are usually arranged at sharp angles with each other. This gives the characteristic Chinese-letter appearance. The disease is rare under one year of age. The vast majority of cases occur before the age of 10, but older children and adults are not exempt. Both sexes are equally susceptible. Esp. prevalent in fall and winter months. Transmission through direct contact with a human carrier, or as a result of exposure through contact with articles that have been contaminated by the diphtheria patient.

INCUB: Two to five days, occasionally longer.

DIFF. DIAG: Tonsillitis; scarlet fever; acute pharyngitis; streptococcus sore throat; peritonsillar abscess; infectious mononucleosis; Vincent's angina; acute moniliasis; and staphylococcus infections in the respiratory tract following chemo-

therapy. Examination of a smear from infected area is advisable, but cultures should be obtained in every instance for the purpose of confirming the diagnosis. In the laryngeal type, edema of the glottis, foreign bodies, and retropharyngeal abscess need to be considered.

ACTIVE IMMUNIZATION: Not all individuals are susceptible to diphtheria, and this factor may be determined by means of the Schick test, q.v. Therefore, it is advisable to use this test in adults before administering either toxin-antitoxin or toxoid. Routine immunization should begin at age three months, diphtheria toxoid being administered in combination with pertussis vaccine and tetanus toxoid; this is then followed by booster doses. Diphtheria toxoid, following a subcutaneous test for hypersensitivity, is used for immunization of adults.

GENERAL MEASURES: Strict bedrest during acute and convalescent stages of disease. In cases with myocardial involvement, prolonged rest in bed is extremely important.

TREAT: Hospitalize patients in an intensive care unit without delay and administer diphtheria antitoxin I.V. even before culture results are known.

Caution: Skin test for sensitivity to the toxin must precede administration of the antitoxin.

The dose of antitoxin given will be governed by the location and duration of the disease. If the patient is sensitive to antitoxin, desensitization will be required. Specific antimicrobial therapy is needed to eradicate the organisms, but it cannot serve as a substitute for the antitoxin. Erythromycin, penicillin G procaine, or ampicillin are effective. To determine that the organism has been eliminated, 3 consecutive negative cultures must be obtained after completion of antibiotic therapy.

Surgical interference is sometimes a necessity in laryngeal diphtheria. Intubation is always to be preferred to tracheotomy, provided an experienced operator is available, and hospitalization, which will make possible any attention required within a moment's notice, is provided.

Symptomatic patients should be kept in isolation until two cultures are negative for the organism. These should be taken 24 and 48 hours after discontinuing antibiotics.

PROG: Favorable when antitoxin in sufficient amounts is administered within three days from time of onset. If it is given on the first day, death hardly ever occurs. In laryngeal diphtheria, intubation or rarely tracheotomy may be necessary as well as an adequate dose of diphtheria antitoxin. Age is an important factor, with death more frequent in very young or very old patients than in intermediate age group. When therapy is not given promptly, the incidence of nerve damage is quite high. If the patient survives, the myocarditis and neuritis will completely resolve.

    d., cutaneous. Diphtheritic lesions of the skin, usually limited to the site of infection.

    d., laryngeal. Considered to be a complication of diphtheria. Results from extension of the membrane from the pharynx with gradual occlusion of the airway. Signs are restlessness, use of accessory respiration muscles, and development of cyanosis. If this condition is not remedied effectively, death results.

    d., surgical. Diphtheric membrane formation on wounds.

diphtheria antitoxin. USP. The antitoxin used in treating diphtheria.

diphtherial. Pert. to diphtheria.

diphtheria toxin for Schick test. USP. The toxin used for determining immunity to diphtheria. SEE: *Schick test.*

diphtheria toxoid. USP. Immunizing agent for diphtheria.

diphtheric, diphtheritic (dĭf-thē′rĭk, dĭf-thĕr-ĭt′ĭk). Pert. to diphtheria.

diphtherin (dĭf′thē-rĭn). The toxin of diphtheria, from *Corynebacterium diphtheriae.*

diphtheroid (dĭf′thē-royd) [″ + *eidos,* form, shape]. 1. Resembling diphtheria or the bacteria that cause diphtheria. 2. The formation of a false or pseudomembrane not due to the diphtheria bacillus.

diphtherotoxin (dĭf′thĕr-ō-tŏk′sĭn) [″ + *toxikon,* poison]. The specific toxin of the diphtheria bacillus.

diphthongia (dĭf-thŏn′jē-ă) [Gr. *dis,* two, + *phtongos,* voice]. The simultaneous utterance of two vocal sounds of different pitch in pathological conditions of the larynx.

Diphyllobothrium (dī-fĭl″ō-bŏth′rē-ŭm) [″ + *phyllon,* leaf, + *bothrion,* pit]. A genus of tapeworms belonging to the order Pseudophyllidea and characterized by possession of a scolex with two slitlike grooves or bothria. Formerly called *Dibothriocephalus.*

    D. cordatum. The heart-shaped tapeworm, a small species infesting dogs and seals in Greenland, formerly known as *D. mansoni.* The plerocercoids are occasionally found in humans.

    D. erinacei. A species infesting dogs, cats, and other carnivores. Larval stages are occasionally found in humans.

    D. latum. The broad or fish tapeworm.

The adult lives in the intestine of fish-eating mammals, including humans. The largest tapeworm infesting humans, it may reach a length of 50 to 60 feet or 15.2 to 18.3 meters (average 20 feet or 6.1 meters). The eggs develop into ciliated larvae called coracidia. These are eaten by certain species of copepods, in which each becomes an oncosphere, which develops into a procercoid. Further development occurs in a fish, where it develops into a wormlike plerocercoid or sparganum larva. Infection of the final host occurs after eating raw or improperly cooked fish. Infection can be prevented by thoroughly cooking all freshwater fish, or by keeping the fish frozen at $-10°C$ ($14°F$) for 48 hours prior to eating.

    SYM: Pathological effects are abdominal pain, loss of weight, digestive disorders, progressive weakness, and a severe type of anemia that is clinically identical with pernicious anemia.

    TREAT: Niclosamide or paromomycin. The therapy may need to be repeated if examination of the stools indicates presence of infection after three months of treatment.

diphyodont (dĭf′ē-ō-dŏnt) [″ + *phyein,* to produce, + *odous,* tooth]. Having two sets of teeth, a primary and permanent set, as in humans.

diplacusis (dĭp″lă-kū′sĭs) [″ + *akousis,* hearing]. Variety of disturbed perception of pitch characterized by hearing two tones for every sound produced.

diplegia (dī-plē′jē-ă) [Gr. *dis,* twice, + *plege,* a stroke]. 1. Paralysis of similar parts on both sides of the body. 2. In cerebral palsy, usually refers to excessive stiffness in all limbs, but with greater stiffness in the legs than in the arms.

    d., infantile. Birth palsy.

    d., spastic. Congenital spastic stiffness of the limbs.

diplegic (dī-plē′jĭk). Pert. to diplegia.

diplo-. Combining form meaning double or twin.

diploalbuminuria (dĭp″lō-ăl-bū″mĭn-ū′rē-ă) [Gr. *diplous,* double, + L. *albumen,* white of egg, + Gr. *ouron,* urine]. Coexistence of physiologic and pathologic albuminuria.

diplobacillus [″ + L. *bacillus,* a little stick]. A double bacillus, two being linked end to end.

diplobacterium [″ + *bakterion,* little rod]. An organism made up of two adherent bacteria.

diploblastic (dĭp″lō-blăs′tĭk) [″ + *blastos,* germ]. The ectoderm and endoderm having two germ layers.

diplocardia [″ + *kardia,* heart]. Having the two lateral halves of the heart partially separated by a groove.

diplocephaly (dĭp″lō-sĕf′ă-lē) [″ + *ke-phale*, head]. Having two heads.

diplococcemia (dĭp″lō-kŏk-sē′mē-ă) [″ + *kokkos*, berry, + *haima*, blood]. Diplococci in the blood.

diplococci (dĭp″lō-kŏk′sē, -kŏk′ī). Pl. of diplococcus. SEE: *bacteria* for illus.

Diplococcus (dĭp-lō-kŏk′ŭs) [″ + *kokkus*, berry]. A genus of bacteria belonging to the family Lactobacillaceae. They are grampositive organisms occurring in pairs.

    D. pneumoniae. SEE: *Streptococcus pneumoniae.*

diplococcus (dĭp″lō-kŏk′ŭs) (pl. *diplococci*). Any of various spherical bacteria appearing in pairs, esp. of the genus *Diplococcus*. SEE: *bacteria* for illus.

diplocoria (dĭp″lō-kō′rē-ă) [″ + *kore*, pupil]. Double pupil in the eye.

diploë (dĭp′lō-ē) [Gr. *diploē*, fold]. Spongy tissue between the two layers of compact bone of the skull.

diploetic, diploic. Pert. to the diploë.

diplogenesis [Gr. *diplous*, double, + *genesis*, generation, birth]. Having two parts or producing two substances; production of double fetus or the doubling of some fetal parts.

diploid (dĭp′loyd) [″ + *eidos*, form, shape]. Having two sets of chromosomes. Said of somatic cells, which contain twice the number of chromosomes present in the egg or sperm. SEE: *chromosome; meiosis; mitosis.*

diplokaryon (dĭp″lō-kăr′ē-ŏn) [″ + *karyon*, nucleus]. A nucleus containing twice the diploid number of chromosomes.

diplomellituria (dĭp″lō-mĕl″ī-tūr′ē-ă) [″ + *meli*, honey, + *ouron*, urine]. Condition in which diabetic and nondiabetic glycosuria occur either simultaneously or alternately in the same individual.

diplomyelia (dĭp″lō-mī-ē′lē-ă) [″ + *myelos*, marrow]. Condition in certain types of spina bifida in which the spinal cord appears to be doubled due to a lengthwise fissure.

diploneural [″ + *neuron*, nerve]. Having two nerves from different origins, as certain muscles.

diplopagus (dĭp-lŏp′ă-gŭs) [″ + *pagos*, a thing fixed]. Conjoined twins that share some organs.

diplophonia (dĭp-lō-fō′nē-ă) [″ + *phone*, voice]. Having two different voice tones at the same time. SYN: *diphonia.*

diplopia (dĭp-lō′pē-ă) [″ + *ope*, sight]. Double vision. May be monocular.

    d., binocular. Double vision occurring when both eyes are used but not in focus. Seen in disease of the eyeballs, cranial nerve affections, and disease of the cerebellum, cerebrum, and meninges.

    d., crossed. Binocular vision in which the images are on the side opposite to the eye that sees the image.

    d., direct. D., uncrossed.

    d., heteronymous. D., crossed.

    d., monocular. Double vision with one eye.

    d., uncrossed. Double vision in which each image appears on the same side as the eye that sees the image. SYN: *diplopia, homonymous.* SEE: *diplopia, crossed.*

    d., uniocular. D., monocular.

    d., vertical. Diplopia with one of two images higher than the other.

diplopiometer (dĭp-lō″pē-ŏm′ē-tĕr) [Gr. *diplous*, double, + *ope*, sight, + *metron*, measure]. Device for estimating double vision.

diploscope [″ + *skopein*, to examine]. Device for study of binocular vision.

diplosomatia, diplosomia (dĭp″lō-sō-mā′shē-ă, dĭp″lō-sō′mē-ă) [″ + *soma*, body]. Condition in which twins are joined at one or more points.

diplotene (dĭp′lō-tēn). In cell division, the stage of the first meiotic prophase. The homologous pairs of chromatids begin to separate.

dipole (dī′pōl). 1. Two equal and opposite charges separated by a distance. 2. In chemistry, one portion of the molecule has a certain charge and the other portion has an equal and opposite charge.

dipping. 1. Palpation of the liver by a quick depressive movement of the fingers while the hand is held flat on the abdomen. 2. The act of immersing an object in a solution, esp. applied to the dipping of cattle or dogs for the control of ticks.

Diprosone. Trade name for betamethasone dipropionate.

diprosopus (dĭp-rō-sōp′ŭs) [Gr. *dis*, twice, + *prosopon*, face]. A malformed fetus characterized by a double face.

dipsesis (dĭp-sē′sĭs) [Gr., a thirst]. Thirst.

dipsogen (dĭp′sō-jĕn). An agent that induces thirst.

dipsomania (dĭp″sō-mā′nē-ă) [Gr. *dipsa*, thirst, + *mania*, madness]. A morbid and uncontrollable craving for alcoholic beverages. SEE: *alcoholism.*

dipsophobia (dĭp-sō-fō′bē-ă) [″ + *phobos*, fear]. Morbid fear of drinking.

dipsosis (dĭp-sō′sĭs) [″ + *osis*, condition]. Abnormal thirst.

dipsotherapy (dĭp″sō-thĕr′ă-pē) [″ + *therapeia*, treatment]. Limitation of water intake as a means of treatment.

dipstick (dĭp′stĭk). A chemical-impregnated paper strip used for analysis of body fluids, but principally urine.

Diptera (dĭp′tĕr-ă) [Gr. *dipteros*, having two

wings]. An order of insects characterized by having sucking or piercing mouth parts, one pair of wings, and complete metamorphosis. It includes the flies, gnats, midges, and mosquitoes. It contains many species involved in the transmission of pathogenic organisms, as in malaria.

dipterous (dĭp'tĕr-ŭs). Having two wings; characteristic of the order Diptera.

dipygus (dī-pī'gŭs) [Gr. *dis*, two, + *pyge*, rump]. A congenitally deformed fetus with a double pelvis.

dipylidiasis (dĭp"ĭ-lī-dī'ă-sĭs). Infestation with the tapeworm *Dipylidium caninum*.

Dipylidium (dĭp"ĭ-lĭd'ē-ŭm) [Gr. *dipylos*, having two entrances]. A genus of tapeworms belonging to the family Dipyliidae that infests dogs and cats.

   D. caninum. A common parasite of dogs and cats. Occasionally, human infestation may occur through the accidental ingestion of lice or fleas, which serve as the intermediate host.

direct [L. *diregere*, to direct]. Immediate; uninterrupted; straight.

direct current. ABBR: DC or dc. An electric current flowing continuously in one direction only. SEE: *electric shock.*

directionality. Ability to perceive one's position in relationship with the environment; sense of direction. Problems with directionality are frequently found in children with learning disabilities or suspected minimal brain dysfunction.

direct light reflex. Prompt contraction of sphincter of iris when light entering through pupil strikes retina of eye.

director. Grooved device for guiding a knife in surgery.

direct reflex. Reflex in which response occurs on same side as the stimulus.

dirigomotor (dĭr"ĭ-gō-mō'tor) [L. *dirigere*, to direct, + *motor*, mover]. Controlling or directing muscular activity.

Dirofilaria (dī"rō-fĭ-lā'rē-ă). A genus of filaria.

   D. immitis. Heartworm, a species of filaria that occurs in dogs, but may infest humans.

dis- 1. [L. *dis*, apart] Prefix indicating free of, to undo. 2. [Gr. *dis*, twice] Prefix meaning double or twice.

disability (dĭs"ă-bĭl'ĭ-tē). Any restriction or lack of ability to perform an activity in the manner considered normal for a human being. SEE: *handicap.*

   d., developmental. Term used for conditions due to congenital abnormality, trauma, deprivation, or diseases that interrupt or delay the sequence and rate of normal growth, development, and maturation.

disaccharidase (dī-săk'ă-rĭ-dās). A group of enzymes that split disaccharides into monosaccharides.

disaccharide (dī-săk'ĭ-rĭd) [Gr. *dis*, twice, + *sakkharon*, sugar]. A carbohydrate composed of two monosaccharides. SEE: *carbohydrate.*

disarticulation [L. *dis*, apart, + *articulus*, joint]. Amputation through a joint.

disassimilation [" + *ad*, to, + *similare*, to make like]. Changing assimilated material into less complex compounds for the production of energy.

disaster [" + L. *astrum*, star, ill-starred]. A natural or man-made occurrence such as a flood, tornado, earthquake, forest fire, bridge or building collapse, nuclear reactor accident, war, explosion, or train wreck. The need for emergency evacuation and medical services is increased during and following a disaster. It is essential that hospitals and community services have a plan for the expeditious mobilization and use of their services during and following a disaster.

disaster planning. A comprehensive plan of action to cope with a sudden, unexpected event such as a flood, fire, famine, nuclear bomb attack, oil spill, earthquake, explosion, electrical power failure, poison gas attack, aircraft accident, or contamination of the water supply. The plan may be for a community, state, or nation. Involved will be a plan for mobilizing all available emergency sources and to do this in a minimum of time. Frequent disaster planning drills are essential to being adequately prepared for an actual disaster.

disc [Gr. *diskos*, quoit]. A flat, round, platelike structure. SEE: *disk.*

discharge (dĭs-chărj', dĭs'chărj) [ME. *dischargen*, to discharge]. 1. To release from care by a physician, other medical care worker, or a medical care facility. 2. The escape (esp. by violence) of pent up or accumulated energy or of explosive material. 3. The flowing away of a secretion or excretion of pus, feces, urine, etc. 4. The material thus ejected.

   d., cerebrocortical. The violent action of an injured or malfunctioning portion of the cerebral cortex that gives rise to an epileptic paroxysm.

   d., convective. Discharge from a high potential source in the form of electrical energy passing through the air to the patient.

   d., disruptive. Passage of current through an insulating medium due to the breakdown of the medium under electrostatic stress.

   d., lochial. Uterine excretion following childbirth. SEE: *lochia.*

discharge abstract. A summary of the record of hospitalization of a patient. It is prepared at the time the patient leaves the hospital.

discharge summary. A summary of the hospital or clinic record of a patient. Prepared after time of discharge.

discharging. The emission of or the flowing out of material, as the discharge of pus from a lesion. Excreting.

discharging lesion. A lesion of a nerve center in the brain suddenly discharging motor impulses.

dischronation [L. *dis*, apart, + Gr. *chronos*, time]. Lack of a sense of relativity in the consciousness of time.

discission (dĭs-sĭzh′ŭn) [″ + *scindere*, to cut]. Rupture of the capsule of the crystalline lens in operation for cataract.

discitis (dĭs-kī′tĭs) [Gr. *diskos*, quoit, + *itis*, inflammation]. Diskitis.

disclosing agent. A diagnostic aid used in dentistry to reveal areas of the teeth that are not being cleaned adequately. The dye is erythrosine sodium, USP, and is applied to the teeth in a 2% solution or by a tablet that is chewed by the patient.

discoblastic [″ + *blastos*, germ]. Pert. to discoid segmentation of yolk in an impregnated ovum.

discoblastula (dĭs″kō-blăs′tū-lă). A modified blastula found in highly telolecithal eggs, as in birds in which the blastomeres form a cellular cap (germinal disk or blastoderm) that is separated from the yolk by a space, the blastocoele.

discogenic (dĭs″kō-jĕn′ĭk) [″ + *gennan*, to produce]. Caused by an intervertebral disk.

discography (dĭs-kŏg′ră-fē). Use of a contrast medium injected into the intervertebral disk in order to examine it by x-ray.

discoid. Like a disk.

disconnection syndromes. Disturbances of the visual and language functions of the central nervous system due to interruption of the connections between two cerebral hemispheres in the corpus callosum; occlusion of the anterior cerebral artery; or interruption of the connections between different parts of one hemisphere. These syndromes also may be produced by tumors or hypoxia. The syndromes can manifest in a variety of ways including inability, when blindfolded, to match an object held in one hand with that in the other; inability to execute a command with the right hand but not the left; if blindfolded, objects in the right hand are named correctly but not those in the left; being able to speak normally but unable to understand spoken language.

discoplacenta [Gr. *diskos*, quoit, + *plakous*, a flat cake]. A disklike placenta.

discordance (dĭs-kor′dăns). In genetics, the expression of a trait in only one of a twin pair. SEE: *concordance*.

discrete (dĭs-krēt′) [L. *discretus*, separated]. Separate; said of certain eruptions on the skin. SEE: *confluent*.

discrimination [L. *discriminare*, to divide]. The process of distinguishing or differentiating.

d., one-point. Ability to locate specifically a point of pressure on the surface of the skin.

d., tonal. Ability to distinguish one tone from another. This is dependent upon the integrity of the transverse fibers of the basilar membrane of the organ of Corti.

d., two-point. Ability to localize two points of pressure on the surface of the skin and to identify them as discrete sensations. SYN: *tactile discrimination*. SEE: *two-point discrimination test*.

discus [Gr. *diskos*, quoit] (pl. *discuses* or *disci*). [NA] A disk.

d. articularis. [NA] An interarticular fibrocartilage; an articular disk.

d. proligerus. The cumulus oophorus.

disdiaclast (dĭs-dī′ă-klăst) [Gr. *dis*, twice, + *diaklan*, to break through]. A doubly refracting element in the tissues of striated muscles.

disdiadochokinesia (dĭs-dī″ă-dō″kō-kĭ-nē′zē-ă) [L. *dis*, apart, + Gr. *diadochos*, succeeding, + *kinesis*, movement]. Inability to make finely coordinated movements of a part in opposite directions, as when quickly supinating and pronating the hand. SEE: *diadochokinesia*.

disease (dĭ-zēz′) [Fr. *des*, from, + *aise*, ease]. Literally the lack of ease; a pathological condition of the body that presents a group of clinical signs and symptoms and laboratory findings peculiar to it and that sets the condition apart as an abnormal entity differing from other normal or pathological body states.

The concept of disease may include the condition of illness or suffering not necessarily arising from pathological changes in the body. There is a major distinction between disease and illness in that the former is usually tangible and may even be measured, whereas illness is highly individual and personal, as with pain, suffering, and distress. A person may have a serious disease such as hypertension but no feeling of pain or suffering, and thus no illness. Conversely, a person may be extremely ill, as with hysteria or mental illness, but have no evidence of disease as measured by pathological changes in the body. SYN: *dyscrasia*. SEE: *health; syndrome*.

d., acute. Disease having a rapid onset

and of relatively short duration.

d., anticipated. Disease that may be predicted to occur in individuals with a certain genetic, physical, or environmental predisposition.

d., autoimmune. Disease in which the body produces disordered immunological response against itself. Normally the body's immune mechanisms are able to distinguish clearly between a normal and a foreign substance. In autoimmune diseases, this system becomes defective and produces antibodies against normal parts of the body to such an extent as to cause tissue injury. Certain diseases such as hemolytic anemia, some forms of glomerulonephritis, rheumatoid arthritis, myasthenia gravis, and scleroderma are considered to be autoimmune diseases.

d., chronic. Disease having a slow onset and lasting for a long period of time.

d., chronic granulomatous. ABBR: CGD. A genetically determined group of disorders characterized by defects in the ability of polymorphonuclear leukocytes to kill certain bacteria. Clinically, suppurative lymphadenitis, dermatitis, diarrhea, stomatitis, osteomyelitis, brain abscess, pulmonary disease, and hepatosplenomegaly are present. A rare disease that occurs mostly in male infants and children.

DIAG: Use of nitroblue tetrazolium test (NBT). Normal neutrophils have the ability to reduce the yellow dye to blue formazan. The NBT is negative in CGD.

TREAT: Continuous or intermittent antibiotic therapy and bone marrow transplantation have been effective.

d., collagen. SEE: *collagen disease.*

d., communicable. A disease, the causative organism of which is transmissible from one person to another either directly or indirectly through a carrier or vector.

d., complicating. Disease that occurs during the course of another disease.

d., congenital. Disease that is present at birth. May be due to hereditary factors, prenatal infection, injury, or the effect of a drug the mother took during pregnancy.

d., constitutional. Disease due to an individual's hereditary makeup. SEE: *diathesis.*

d., contagious. An infectious disease readily transmitted from one person to another.

d., cystine storage. An inherited disease of cystine metabolism resulting in abnormal deposition of cystine in body tissues. The cause is disordered proximal renal tubular function. Clinically, the child fails to grow, and develops rickets, corneal opacities, and acidosis. SYN: *cystinosis.*

d., deficiency. Disease resulting from inadequate intake or absorption of essential dietary factors such as vitamins or minerals.

d., degenerative. Disease resulting from degenerative changes that occur in tissues and organs, characteristic of old age.

d., degenerative joint. Osteoarthritis, q.v.

d., demyelinating. Disturbance of nerve cells due to destruction of their myelin sheaths.

d., endemic. Disease that is present more or less continuously, or frequently recurs, in a community.

d., epidemic. Disease that attacks a large number of individuals in a community at the same time.

d., epizootic. An epidemic that affects animals of a particular area, usually in a short period of time.

d., extrapyramidal. Any one of several degenerative diseases of the nervous system that involve the extrapyramidal system and the basal ganglion of the brain. Symptoms include tremors, chorea, athetosis, and dystonia. Parkinsonism, q.v., is a form of extrapyramidal disease.

d., familial. Disease that occurs in several members of the same family.

d., focal. Disease located at a specific and distinct area such as the tonsils or adenoids, or in a boil.

d., functional. Disease in which no anatomical changes can be observed to account for the symptoms present.

d., glycogen storage. SEE: *glycogen storage disease.*

d., heavy chain. A group of diseases involving serum immunoglobulins. The globulins contain heavy chain subunits. If the immunoglobulin A (IgA) is affected, abdominal lymphoma and malabsorption occur. When immunoglobulin D (IgD) is involved, a clinical picture similar to multiple myeloma is present. When immunoglobulin G (IgG) is affected, there are lymphadenopathy, weakness, weight loss, and repeated bacterial infections. If immunoglobulin M (IgM) is involved, the lymphadenopathy affects the abdominal lymph nodes, the liver, and the spleen. Bence Jones proteinuria occurs.

d., hemolytic, of the newborn. Erythroblastosis fetalis, q.v.

d., hemorrhagic, of the newborn. Bleeding tendency in the newborn characterized by melena, purpura, and prothrombin deficiency. The disease is self-limiting.

d., hereditary. Disease due to hereditary factors transmitted from parent to offspring.

d., hookworm. SEE: *ancylostomiasis;*

Necator americanus.

d., hypokinetic. Physical and mental illness produced by lack of or insufficient exercise.

d., iatrogenic. Disease caused by medical or surgical intervention. The implication is that the disease would not have occurred if the individual had not sought medical care.

d., idiopathic. Disease for which no causative factor can be recognized.

d., infectious. Disease resulting from the presence of a pathogenic organism in the body.

d., intercurrent. Disease occurring during the course of another unrelated disease.

d., iron storage. Hemochromatosis, q.v.

d., malignant. 1. Cancer. 2. Disease, including but not limited to cancer, in which the progress is extremely rapid and generally threatening or resulting in death within a short time.

d., Mediterranean. SEE: *thalassemia.*

d., metabolic. Disease due to abnormality of the body chemistry. The abnormality may be due to underproduction of a needed substance, such as insulin in diabetes, or overproduction, such as thyroid hormone in thyrotoxicosis.

d., motor neuron. One of several types of diseases of the motor neurons: progressive muscular atrophy, progressive bulbar palsy, and amyotrophic lateral sclerosis. These diseases are characterized by degeneration of anterior horn cells of the spinal cord, the motor cranial nerve nuclei, and the pyramidal tracts. They occur principally in males. In the U.S., amyotrophic lateral sclerosis is commonly known as Lou Gehrig's disease. He was a well-known athlete whose baseball career and life were prematurely ended as a result of this disease.

d., occupational. Disease resulting from factors associated with the occupation in which the patient is engaged.

d., organic. Disease resulting from recognizable anatomical changes in an organ or tissue of the body.

d., pandemic. An extremely widespread epidemic disease involving the entire world.

d., parasitic. Disease resulting from the growth and development of parasitic organisms (plants or animals) in or upon the body.

d., periodontal. SEE: *periodontitis.*

d., psychosomatic. Psychological factors contribute to the initiation or exacerbation of a physical illness. Conditions in the general category of psychosomatic disorders are obesity, tension headache, some types of asthma, neurodermatitis, peptic ulcer, some attacks of angina pectoris, and frequency of urination.

NOTE: It is not possible for a human being to be consciously sick without some interplay between the emotions and the bodily functions.

d., pulmonary veno-occlusive. A rare condition characterized by extensive occlusion of the small and medium-sized veins of the lung by loose, sparsely cellular, fibrous tissue. Some larger veins may be involved. This disease produces severe pulmonary venous hypertension.

d., secondary. Disease occurring as the result of another disease, e.g., obesity may cause secondary diseases of the joints and muscles of the lower extremities due to the increased trauma incident to transporting and supporting the added weight.

d., self-limited. Disease that even if untreated eventually goes away.

d., sporadic. Disease in which only occasional cases occur; not epidemic or endemic.

d., storage. Disorder involving abnormal deposition of a substance in body tissues. SEE: *glycogen storage disease; Wilson's disease.*

d., subacute. Disease in which symptoms are less pronounced but more prolonged than in an acute disease; intermediate between acute and chronic disease.

d., systemic. A generalized disease rather than a localized or focal one.

d., thyrotoxic heart. Disease due to increased activity of the thyroid gland, characterized by cardiac enlargement, atrial fibrillation, and heart failure. SEE: *thyrotoxicosis.*

d., venereal. ABBR: VD. Disease usually acquired through sexual relations. Includes syphilis, gonorrhea, granuloma inguinale, herpes genitalis, *Chlamydia trachomatis* infections, trichomoniasis, anogenital warts, scabies, pediculosis pubis, enteric infections due to anal-oral contacts, lymphogranuloma venereum, and chancroid. SEE: *sexually transmitted diseases.*

disengagement [Fr.]. 1. The emergence of the fetal head from within the maternal pelvis. 2. Any withdrawal from participation in customary social activity. 3. In psychiatry, autonomous functioning with little or no emotional attachment and a distorted sense of independence.

disentanglement. Rescue technique used to free a trapped victim that involves removing the wreckage from around the patient (rather than removing the patient from the wreckage). For example, freeing a person trapped in a crushed car often requires the car to be pried apart with heavy rescue tools capable of cutting through metal.

disequilibrium (dĭs-ē″kwĭ-lĭb′rē-ŭm) [L. *dis,*

apart, + *aequus,* equal, + *libra,* balance]. An unequal and unstable equilibrium.

dish. An open container, usually convex, made of glass, ceramic, plastic, or wood.

d., Petri. SEE: *Petri dish.*

disharmony. Lacking harmony, discordant.

disinfect (dĭs-ĭn-fĕkt') [" + *inficere,* to corrupt]. To free from infection by physical or chemical means.

disinfectant. A substance that prevents infection by killing bacteria. Most disinfectants are used on equipment or surfaces rather than in or upon the body. Common disinfectants are the halogens: chlorine, fluorine, iodine; salts of heavy metals: mercuric chloride (bichloride of mercury), silver nitrate; boric acid; chloride of lime; organic compounds: formaldehyde, alcohol 70%, iodoform, organic acids, phenol (carbolic acid), cresols, benzoic and salicylic acids and their sodium salts; miscellaneous substances: thymol, hydrogen peroxide, potassium permanganate, ethylene oxide. Term is usually applied to a chemical or physical agent that kills vegetative forms of microorganisms.

disinfection. The application of disinfectants. It is not possible to ensure 100% disinfection of a room unless the entire room and its contents are treated with a gaseous agent such as ethylene oxide. Disinfestation, or the killing of vermin by chemicals and their vapors, however, is possible. SEE: table.

d., concurrent. Prompt disinfection and suitable disposal of infected excreta during the entire course of a disease.

d. of blankets and woolens. May be steam-disinfected or soaked for two hours in 5% carbolic acid solution and then washed and rinsed thoroughly. Cotton goods may also be so treated or boiled before washing. Materials that might be harmed by conventional methods of disinfection may be treated in a chamber with ethylene oxide gas.

d. of excreta. Should be soaked in 5% carbolic acid solution for one hour before disposal. All infected excreta should be burned. Sputum may be treated as excreta if impossible to burn.

d. of field of operation. A safe rule is to make the disinfection too extensive. Thus, in operations upon large wounds of the scalp and in all operations on the skull and its contents, the entire scalp must be shaved and disinfected.

In operations upon the breast, the axilla and half of the chest must be prepared. If glands of the neck are involved, the entire neck must be included in field of operation.

In amputation of foot and lower third of the leg, the disinfection must extend as far as the knee, and in all higher amputations it should include the whole limb and corresponding side of pelvis.

In all abdominal operations below the umbilicus, the pubic area must be shaved and the surface disinfection must include the whole anterior surface and both sides as far as the breasts.

In operations on the stomach, liver, and bile ducts, the field extends from the pubic area to the breasts. A general warm bath with liberal use of tincture of green soap should precede disinfection of the field of operation in all abdominal and pelvic operations, including hernia and varicocele.

In operations upon parts of the body difficult to disinfect as scalp, palm of hand, and sole of foot, it is advisable to scrub with warm water and tincture of green soap and then rinse. Use either 70% solution of alcohol; povidone-iodine, USP; benzalkonium chloride; or other suitable disinfectant. Seventy percent ethyl alcohol is useful in hand and surface disinfection.

Caution: The mucous membranes are active, absorbing surfaces so that the use of solutions of carbolic acid, mercuric bichloride, and other potent antiseptics is prohibited in these areas. The use of any of these agents in the vagina, uterus, or rectum frequently has resulted in serious poisoning and in some instances death.

In operations in the oral cavity, such as excision of superior or inferior maxilla, and amputation of tongue, the employment of a disinfecting solution is preceded by thorough cleansing of the teeth and swabbing the mucous membrane with hydrogen peroxide.

In operations upon the rectum, the procedure in common use consists of shaving perianal area and giving cleansing enemas.

Vaginal disinfection is preceded by shaving and disinfection of the external genitals. After a thorough cleansing with warm water and tincture of green soap, a douche of warm water with a suitable disinfectant is recommended.

Catheterization should always be preceded by disinfection of the meatus with green soap and rinsing the area thoroughly with sterile water.

The external ear canal should be mechanically cleansed of wax, dirt, or blood clots, and then carefully disinfected by a low-pressure stream of warm hydrogen peroxide, until it is absolutely clean. This should not be done if the eardrum has been rup-

Methods of Disinfection

Method	Concentration or Intensity	Use	Limitations
Moist heat			
Autoclaving	250°–270°F (121°–132°C)	Sterilize instruments not harmed by heat and water pressure	Moisture will not permeate some materials. Cannot be used for heat-sensitive items
Boiling water	212°F (100°C)	Kill non-spore-forming pathogenic organisms	Does not kill spores. Probably not effective against hepatitis virus
Radiation			
Ultraviolet light		Air and surface disinfection	Penetrates poorly. Harmful to unprotected skin and eyes
Ionizing		Sterilize medicines, some plastics, sutures, and biologicals	Expensive. May alter the medicine or material
Filtration			
Membrane		Water purification	Slow and expensive
Fiberglass filters		Air disinfection	Only cleans incoming air; does not prevent recontamination
Physical cleaning			
Ultrasonic		Disinfect instruments	Aids in cleaning but not effective alone
Washing		Disinfect hands and surfaces	Does not remove all organisms
Chemicals			
Alcohols	70%–90%	Skin degerming	Sometimes irritating. Does not kill spores
Chlorines	100–200 parts per million	Water disinfection. Food surface sanitization	Inactivated by inorganic matter. Does not kill spores. Ineffective at certain pH values
Iodines, tincture	2%	Skin degerming	Not sporicidal. Sometimes irritating
Iodines, iodophors	74–450 parts per million	General disinfectant	Not sporicidal
Phenols	1%–4%	General disinfectant	Ineffective against some bacteria. May be irritating or corrosive
Quaternary ammonia compounds, tincture	0.1%	Skin degerming	Neutralized by soap. Not sporicidal
Quaternary ammonia compounds, aqueous	Diluted one part to 750 parts	General disinfectant	May be incompatible with some water. Ineffective against some bacteria
Mercurials	0.1%	Skin degerming	Slow acting. May be irritating
Formaldehyde (formalin)	5%	Drastic disinfection	Irritating, corrosive
Glutaraldehyde	2%	Instrument sterilization	Irritates mucous membranes. Unstable

Methods of Disinfection *(Continued)*

Method	Concentration or Intensity	Use	Limitations
Germicidal soaps (hexachlorophene)	2%–3%	Skin degerming	Bacteriostatic rather than bactericidal
Gaseous			
Ethylene oxide	450 mg/liter of air	Sterilization of heat-sensitive materials or those that must be kept dry	Temperature, time, humidity critical Treated materials need to air for varying periods of time (depending on composition) following treatment
Formaldehyde gas		Fumigation Sterilization of heat-sensitive materials	Irritating, corrosive, toxic

Source: Adapted from Benarde, MA (ed): Disinfection: A Treatise. Marcel Dekker, New York, 1970.

tured or if there is doubt of its integrity.

d., terminal. Disinfection of the room and infected materials at the end of the infectious stage of a disease.

disinfestation (dĭs″ĭn-fĕs-tā′shŭn) [L. *dis,* apart, + *infestare,* to strike at]. The process of killing infesting insects or parasites.

disinhibition (dĭs″ĭn-hĭ-bĭsh′ŭn). 1. Abolition of or countering inhibition. 2. In psychiatry, freedom to act in accordance with one's drives with a decrease in social or cultural constraint.

disinsected. Freed of insects.

disinsertion. Detachment of the retina at its periphery.

disintegration [″ + *integer,* entire]. 1. The product of catabolism; the falling apart of the constituents of a substance. 2. Disorganization of the psyche.

disjoint. To disarticulate or to separate bones from their natural positions in a joint.

disjunction (dĭs-jŭnk′shŭn). Chromosome separation at the anaphase of the first meiotic division.

disk [Gr. *diskos,* a disk]. A flat, round, platelike structure.

d., anisotropic. A dark, shining, highly refractile disk forming a part of the striation of the myofibril of a striated muscle fiber. SYN: *Q disk.*

d., articular. The biconcave oval disk of fibrous connective tissue that separates the two joint cavities of the temporomandibular joint on each side.

d., Bowman's. Disklike segment of a striated muscle fiber.

d., choked. A swollen optic disk due to inflammation or edema. SYN: *papilledema.*

d., dental. A thin circular paper or other material carrying polishing or cutting materials; it is driven by a dental engine and utilized in a variety of procedures with natural or artificial teeth.

d., embryonic. An oval disk of cells in the blastocyst of a mammal from which the embryo proper develops. Its lower layer, the endoderm, forms the roof of the yolk sac. Its upper layer, the ectoderm, forms the floor of the amniotic cavity. The primitive streak develops on the upper surface of the disk.

d., epiphyseal. Disklike epiphysis at ends of vertebral centrum.

d., germinal. Disk of cells on the surface of the yolk of a teloblastic egg from which the embryo develops. SYN: *blastoderm.*

d., herniated intervertebral. SEE: *herniated disk.*

d., intervertebral. The fibrocartilaginous tissue uniting the vertebral bodies; the outer portion is the anulus fibrosus, the inner portion is the nucleus pulposus.

d., M. A thin line lying in the center of Hensen's disk.

d., Merkel's. Tiny expanded end of a sensory nerve fiber found in epidermis and in epithelial root sheath of a hair. SYN: *tactile disk.*

d., optic. Area of the retina where optic nerve enters it. SEE: *blind spot.*

d., proligerous. D., germinal.

d., Q. D., anisotropic.

d., slipped. Lay term for herniated intervertebral disk.

d., tactile. D., Merkel's.

d., Z. The intermediate disk of a striated muscle fiber. SEE: *striated muscle.*

diskectomy (dĭs-kĕk'tō-mē). Surgical removal of a herniated intervertebral disk.

diskiform (dĭs'kĭ-form). Shaped like a dish or disk.

diskitis (dĭsk-ī'tĭs) [Gr. *diskos,* disk, + *itis,* inflammation]. Inflammation of a disk, esp. an interarticular cartilage. SYN: *meniscitis.*

dislocation [L. *dis,* apart, + *locare,* to place]. The displacement of any part, esp. the temporary displacement of a bone from its normal position in a joint.

   d., closed. D., simple.

   d., complete. Dislocation that completely separates the surfaces of a joint.

   d., complicated. Dislocation associated with other major injuries.

   d., compound. Dislocation in which the joint communicates with the external air.

   d., congenital. Dislocation existing from or before birth.

   d., consecutive. Dislocation in which the luxated bone has changed its position since its first displacement.

   d., divergent. Dislocation in which the ulna and radius are dislocated separately.

   d., habitual. Dislocation that often recurs after replacement.

   d., incomplete. A subluxation; a slight displacement.

   d., mandibular. SEE: *subluxation.*

   d., metacarpophalangeal joint. Dislocation of finger. It is usually complicated by an interposition of tendons or other structures. When reduced, it tends to slip out immediately. In many instances, manipulation of this region only tends to make it more difficult for a subsequent reduction; therefore, immobilize the disturbed area with well-placed and padded splints of hand and wrist. Send patient to physician promptly.

   d., Monteggia's. Dislocation of hip joint in which head of femur is near anterosuperior spine of the ilium.

   d., Nélaton's. Dislocation of the ankle in which the talus is forced up between the end of the tibia and the fibula.

   d., old. Dislocation in which no reduction has been accomplished even after many days, weeks, or months.

   d., partial. D., incomplete.

   d., pathologic. Dislocation resulting from paralysis or disease of joint or supporting tissues.

   d., primitive. Dislocation in which the bones remain as originally displaced.

   d., recent. Dislocation seen shortly after it occurred.

   d., simple. Dislocation in which the joint is not penetrated by a wound.

   d., slipped. SEE: *herniated disk.*

   d., subastragalar. Separation of the calcaneum and the scaphoid from the talus.

   d., traumatic. Dislocation due to injury or violence.

dismember. To remove an extremity or a portion of it.

dismutase (dĭs-mū'tās). An enzyme that acts on two molecules of the same substance. One of these is oxidized and the other reduced, thereby producing two new compounds.

   d., superoxide. An enzyme present in aerobic but not in strictly anaerobic bacteria. It functions to destroy the poisonous highly reactive free-radical form of O_2, superoxide (O_2^-), formed by flavoenzymes. Thus, aerobic bacteria are protected from the lethal effect of superoxide by the action of this enzyme.

disocclude. Loss of contact between opposing teeth.

disomus (dī-sō'mŭs) [Gr. *dis,* twice, + *soma,* body]. A malformed fetus with a double trunk.

disopyramide phosphate (dī-sō-pēr'ă-mĭd). USP. Drug used in treating cardiac arrhythmias. Trade name is Norpace.

disorder. Pathological condition of the mind or body. SEE: *disease.*

   d., character. A personality disorder manifested by a chronic, habitual, maladaptive pattern of reaction that is relatively inflexible, limits the optimal use of potentialities, and often provokes the responses from the environment that the subject wants to avoid.

   d., functional. SEE: *illness, functional.*

disorganization [L. *dis,* apart, + Gr. *organon,* a unified organ]. Alteration in an organic part, causing it to lose most or all of its distinctive characteristics.

disorientation (dĭs"ō-rē-ĕn-tā'shŭn) [" + *oriens,* arising]. Inability to estimate direction or location, or to be cognizant of time or of persons.

disparate [L. *disparitas,* unequal]. Dissimilar, not equally paired.

disparate points (dĭs'păr-ăt, dĭs-păr'ăt) [L. *disparare,* to separate]. Points on the two retinas that are not corresponding or identical, causing objects to appear double.

dispensary [L. *dispensare,* to give out]. Place or clinic for obtaining medical care.

dispensatory (dĭs-pĕn'să-tō-rē) [L. *dispensatorium*]. Publication, in book form, of the description and composition of medicines.

dispense (dĭs-pĕns'). To prepare or deliver medicines.

dispersate (dĭs'pŭr-sāt). Suspension of finely divided particles in a liquid.

disperse (dĭs-pĕrs') [L. *dis,* apart, + *spargere,* to scatter]. 1. To scatter, esp. applied to the scattering of light rays. 2. To dissipate or effect the disappearance of, as of a tumor or the particles of a colloidal system.

dispersion (dĭs-pĕr′zhŭn). 1. Act of dispersing. 2. That which is dispersed.

d., coarse. Mechanical suspension.

d., colloidal. Colloid solution.

d., medium. Liquid in which a colloid is dispersed.

d., molecular. A true solution.

dispersoid. A colloid in which the dispersed phase is great.

dispersonalization (dĭs-pĕr″sŏn-ăl-ĭ-zā′shŭn). Mental state in which the individual denies the existence of his or her personality or parts of the body.

displacement [Fr. deplacer, to lay aside]. 1. Removal from the normal or usual position or place. 2. Adding to a fluid one of greater density, causing the first fluid to be dispersed. 3. Transference of emotion from the original idea with which it was associated to a different idea, thus allowing the patient to avoid acknowledging the original source.

disposable absorption containment trunk. ABBR: DACT. An externally worn device used experimentally to absorb urine and menstrual flow. Designed for use by female astronauts and pilots confined for prolonged periods in surveillance aircraft, e.g., U-2 type "spy" planes.

disposition [L. disponere, to arrange]. 1. A natural tendency or aptitude exhibited by an individual or group. It may be manifested toward acquiring a certain disease, presumably due to hereditary factors. 2. The sum total of a person's behavior as determined by his or her mood. SEE: diathesis.

disproportion (dĭs″prō-por′shŭn). One entity being of a size different from that considered to be normal.

d., cephalopelvic. In obstetrics, the head of the fetus is larger than the pelvic outlet.

dissect (dĭ-sĕkt′, dī-sĕkt′) [L. dissecare, to cut up]. To separate tissues and parts of a cadaver for anatomical study.

dissection (dĭ-, dī-sĕk′shŭn). The cutting of parts for purpose of separation and studying of the same.

dissemble. To mislead, to give a false impression, or to conceal the truth.

disseminated [L. dis, apart, + seminare, to sow]. Scattered or distributed over a considerable area, esp. applied to disease organisms; scattered throughout an organ or the body.

disseminated intravascular coagulation. 075.ABBR: DIC. A pathological form of coagulation that is diffuse rather than localized, as would be the case in normal coagulation. The process damages rather than protects the area involved, and several clotting factors are consumed to such extent

that generalized bleeding may occur. A variety of conditions have been associated with DIC including septic shock; acute intravascular hemolysis; acute viral, rickettsial, and protozoal infections; abruptio placentae; septic abortion; surgical procedures; heat stroke; certain poisonous snake bites; severe head injury; malignancies; retained dead fetus; liver disease; and systemic lupus erythematosis. SEE: *Nursing Diagnoses* in *Appendix.*

TREAT: Treat the primary illness; administer heparin; in adults, administer fibrinolytic inhibitors. This may be dangerous if thrombotic process not previously treated with heparin. Transfusion to reestablish normal hemostatic potential if thrombosis is blocked by heparin.

dissipation (dĭs-ĭ-pā′shŭn) [L. dissipare, to scatter]. 1. Dispersion of matter. 2. Act of being wasteful and living a dissolute life, esp. drinking alcoholic beverages to excess.

dissociation (dĭs-sō″sē-ā′shŭn) [L. dis, apart, + sociatio, union]. 1. Separation, as the separation by heat of a complex compound into simpler molecules. 2. The ability to move one body segment independently of another. 3. In psychiatry, the breaking off of normal thought processes from consciousness, as can occur in amnesia, conversion reaction, or as a result of the action of psychoactive drugs. SEE: hysteria.

d., atrioventricular. Dissociation that occurs when independent pacemakers of the atria and ventricles of the heart are not in harmony.

d., microbic. Change in the morphology of a cultured microbial colony due to mutation or selection.

d. of personality. Split in consciousness resulting in two different phases of personality, neither being aware of the words, acts, and feelings of the other. SEE: dual personality; multiple personality; vigilambulism.

d., psychological. Disunion of mind of which the person is not aware.

Ex.: dual personalities, fugues, somnambulism, selective amnesia.

dissolution [L. dissolvere, to dissolve]. 1. Death. 2. Pathological resolution or breaking up of the integrity of an anatomical entity.

dissolve (dĭ-zŏlv′) [L. dissolvere, to dissolve]. To cause absorption of a solid in and by a liquid.

dissolvent (dĭ-zŏl′vĕnt). 1. Having the power to dissolve. 2. That which is capable of being dissolved.

dissolving. To cause to enter into a solution.

dissonance (dĭs′ō-năns). 1. Discord or disagreement. 2. Unpleasant sounds, particularly musical ones.

d., cognitive. Incongruity of thought, philosophy, or actions.

distad (dĭs'tăd) [L. *distare*, to be distant]. Away from the center.

distal (dĭs'tăl) [L. *distare*, to be distant]. Farthest from the center, from a medial line, or from the trunk. Opposed to proximal. In dental usage, distal refers to teeth farther from the middle of the given arch.

distance. Space between two objects.

d., focal. Distance from the optical center of a lens to the focal point.

d., focal-film. Distance between the focal target of the x-ray and film.

d., interocclusal. Distance between the occlusal surfaces of opposed teeth when the mandible is at rest.

d., interocular. Distance between two eyes. SEE: *hypertelorism.*

d., object-film. ABBR: OFD. In radiography, the distance between the anatomical structure to be imaged and the radiographic film.

d., source-skin. Distance from a radioactive source to the surface of the patient.

d., source-to-image receptor. Distance from the source of radiation to the imaging device.

d., target-skin. Distance between the source of radiation and the skin.

distemper (dĭs-tĕm'pĕr). In veterinary medicine, one of several virus infections of animals.

distend [L. *distendere*, to stretch out]. 1. To stretch out. 2. To become inflated.

distensibility (dĭs-tĕn″sĭ-bĭl′ĭ-tē). The property of being distensible.

distention. The state of being distended.

distichiasis (dĭs″tĭ-kī′ă-sĭs) [Gr. *distichia*, a double row]. Two rows of eyelashes, one or both of which are directed inward toward the eye.

distill (dĭs-tĭl′) [L. *destillare*, to drop from]. Vaporizing by heat and condensing and collecting the volatilized products.

distillate (dĭs'tĭl-āt, dĭs-tĭl′āt). That which has been derived from the distillation process.

distillation. Condensation of a vapor that has been obtained from a liquid heated to the volatilization point, as the condensation of steam from boiling water. Distillation is used for the purification of water and for other purposes. Distilled water should be stored in covered containers because it readily takes up impurities from the atmosphere.

d., destructive. The process of decomposing complex organic compounds by heat in the absence of air and condensing the vapor of the liquid products.

d., dry. Distillation of solids without adding liquids.

d., fractional. Separation of liquids based upon the difference in their boiling points.

distobuccal (dĭs″tō-bŭk′ăl) [L. *distare*, to be distant, + *bucca*, cheek]. Pert. to the distal and buccal walls of bicuspid and molar teeth; also pert. to the distal or buccal walls of a cavity preparation.

distoclusion (dĭs″tō-kloo′zhŭn). Condition in which the lower teeth meet the upper teeth behind the normal position.

distogingival (dĭs″tō-jĭn′jĭ-văl) [″ + *gingiva*, gum]. Pertaining to the distal and gingival walls of a cavity being prepared for restoration.

distolabial (dĭs″tō-lā′bē-ăl) [″ + *labialis*, lips]. Pertaining to the distal and labial surfaces of a tooth.

distolingual (dĭs″tō-lĭng′gwăl) [″ + *lingua*, tongue]. Pertaining to the distal and lingual surfaces of a tooth.

distome. A fluke with two suckers, an oral and a ventral sucker or acetabulum.

distomia (dī-stō′mē-ă) [Gr. *dis*, two, + *stoma*, mouth]. Congenitally deformed fetus with two mouths.

disto-occlusal (dĭs″tō-ŏ-kloo′zăl). Concerning the distal and occlusal surfaces of a tooth or the distal and occlusal walls of a cavity preparation.

distortion [L. *distortio*, twist, writhe]. 1. A twisting or bending out of regular shape. 2. A writhing or twisting movement as of the muscles of the face. 3. A deformity in which the part or structure is altered in shape. 4. In ophthalmology, visual perception of an image that does not provide a true picture. This is due to astigmatism or to retinal abnormalities. 5. In psychiatry, the process of modifying unconscious mental elements so that they can enter consciousness without being censored. 6. In radiology, the difference in size and shape of a radiographic image as compared to the actual part examined. 7. Variations in the amplitude or frequency of a signal. They may be caused by overdriving the amplifier in the circuit.

distractibility. A condition of mental wandering in which the thoughts are attracted by extraneous conditions or influenced by a dissociation of consciousness. Inability to focus one's attention.

distraction (dĭs-trăk′shŭn) [L. *dis*, apart, + *tractio*, a drawing]. 1. State of mental confusion or derangement. 2. Separation of the surfaces of a joint by extension without injury or dislocation of the parts.

distraught (dĭs-trawt′) [L. *distrahere*, to perplex]. The mental state of being in doubt, deeply troubled, and having conflicting thoughts. Patient may be frantic and have need to be continuously occupied.

distress (dǐs-trĕs') [L. *distringere*, to draw apart]. Physical or mental pain or suffering.

    d., fetal. SEE: *fetal distress.*

distribution [L. *dis*, apart, + *tribuere*, to allot]. 1. The dividing and spreading of anything, esp. blood vessels and nerves, to tissues. 2. The presence of entities, such as hair, fat, or nutrients, at various sites or in particular patterns throughout the body. 3. In demography or statistics, the pattern of location of particular individuals who are ill, or of events.

    d., frequency. SEE: *frequency distribution.*

    d., gaussian. Normal distribution, q.v.

    d., normal. SEE: *normal distribution.*

districhiasis (dǐs-trǐk-ǐ'ǎ-sǐs) [Gr. *dis*, double, + *thrix*, hair]. Two hairs growing from the same hair follicle.

distrix (dǐs'trǐks). The splitting of ends of the hairs.

disturbance. 1. Interruption of the normal sequence of continuity. 2. A departure from the considered norm.

    d., emotional. Mental disorder.

disulfate (dī-sŭl'fāt). A compound containing two sulfate radicals. SEE: *bisulfate.*

disulfiram (dī-sŭl'fǐ-răm). USP. A drug administered orally to treat alcoholism. Alcohol is acted on by alcohol dehydrogenase to produce acetaldehyde. The toxic effect of disulfiram is due to the prevention of the further degradation of the toxic substance acetaldehyde. Trade name is Antabuse.

Caution: The reaction to use of alcohol while this drug is being administered may cause severe reactions such as respiratory depression, shock, acute congestive heart failure, myocardial infarction, unconsciousness, convulsions, and sudden death.

---

disulfiram poisoning. SEE: *Antabuse* in *Poisons and Poisoning* in *Appendix.*

dithiazanine iodide (dī"thī-ăz'ǎ-nēn). An anthelmintic.

Dittrich's plugs (dĭt'rĭks) [Franz Dittrich, Ger. pathologist, 1815–1859]. Small particles in fetid sputum composed of pus, detritus, bacteria, and fat globules.

diurese (dī"ū-rēs'). To cause diuresis.

diuresis (dī"ū-rē'sǐs) [Gr. *diourein*, to urinate]. Secretion and passage of large amounts of urine. This condition occurs in diabetes mellitus. It can be an early sign of chronic interstitial nephritis. May also be due to hysteria, result of fear and anxiety, ingestion of large quantities of liquids, diabetes insipidus, or the action of drugs that have the ability to cause diuresis. Cold applications have a diuretic action by con-

tracting superficial vessels and raising blood pressure. SEE: *diuretic.*

diuretic (dī"ū-rĕt'ĭk). Increasing or an agent that increases the secretion of urine. Diuretics act in two ways: by increasing glomerular filtration or by decreasing reabsorption from the tubules. An increase in blood flow in the renal vessels increases urine formation by increasing glomerular filtration-pressure and by increasing the number of glomeruli functioning. SEE: *diuresis.*

Diuril (dī'ū-rĭl). Trade name for chlorothiazide, a diuretic agent.

diurnal [L. *dies*, day]. 1. Daily. 2. Happening in the daytime or pert. to it. SEE: *circadian; clock, biological; desynchronosis; nocturnal.*

divagation (dī-vă-gā'shŭn) [L. *divagatus*, to wander off]. 1. To wander astray. 2. Rambling or incoherent speech.

divalent (dī-vā'lĕnt). A molecule with an electric charge of two; bivalent.

divergence (dī-vĕr'jĕns) [L. *divergere*, to turn aside]. Separation from a common center, esp. that of the eyes.

divergent. Radiating in different directions.

diver's paralysis. Occupational disease due to returning too suddenly to normal atmosphere after working under high air pressure. SYN: *bends; caisson disease.*

diverticula (dī"vĕr-tĭk'ū-lǎ) [L. *devertere*, to turn aside]. Pl. of diverticulum.

diverticulectomy (dī"vĕr-tĭk"ū-lĕk'tō-mē) [" + Gr. *ektome*, excision]. Surgical removal of a diverticulum.

diverticulitis (dī"vĕr-tĭk"ū-lī'tĭs) [" + Gr. *itis*, inflammation]. Inflammation of a diverticulum or of diverticula in the intestinal tract, esp. in the colon, causing stagnation of feces in little distended sacs of the colon (diverticula) and pain.

    NURSING IMPLICATIONS: In acute episode, monitor results of treatment with fluid and electrolyte replacement, antibiotic therapy and nasogastric suction. Observe the patient for symptoms of increasing or decreasing distress. Provide support and reassurance. For chronic form of the disease, teach patient about the disease process and symptoms to watch for. Encourage a well-balanced diet which is non-irritating to the bowel, and medical supervision. SEE: *Nursing Diagnoses* in *Appendix.*

    d., acute. SYM: Similar to appendicitis: inflammation of peritoneum, formation of an abscess, and, finally, gangrene accompanied by perforation may ensue.

    d., chronic. SYM: Constipation growing worse, mucus in stools, griping abdominal pains at intervals. Wall of bowels may thicken, which may produce chronic intestinal obstruction.

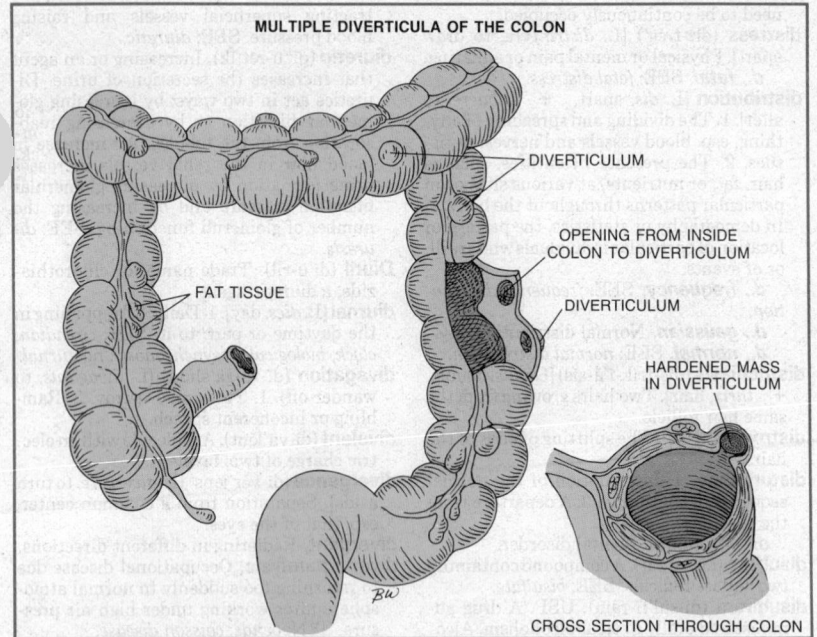

MULTIPLE DIVERTICULA OF THE COLON

DIVERTICULUM

OPENING FROM INSIDE
COLON TO DIVERTICULUM

DIVERTICULUM

FAT TISSUE

HARDENED MASS
IN DIVERTICULUM

CROSS SECTION THROUGH COLON

diverticulosis (dĭ″vĕr-tĭk″ū-lō′sĭs) [″ +
Gr. *osis*, condition]. Diverticula in the colon
without inflammation or symptoms. Only a
small percentage of persons with diverticulosis develop diverticulitis.

diverticulum (dĭ″vĕr-tĭk′ū-lŭm) [L. *devertere*, to turn aside] (pl. *diverticula*). A sac or
pouch in the walls of a canal or organ. SEE:
illus.

    d., false. Diverticulum without muscu-
lar coats in wall or pouch. This type of diverticulum is acquired.

    d., gastric. Pulsion-type diverticula usu-
ally on the lesser curvature of the esophago-
gastric junction.

    d., Meckel's. Diverticulum caused by
continued existence of the omphalomesenteric duct. Its occurrence is fairly common.
Usually located on ileum close to ileocecal
valve.

    d. of colon. Outpocketing of the colon.
These are asymptomatic and cause difficulty when they become inflamed.

    d. of duodenum. Diverticulum com-
monly located near entrance of common bile
and pancreatic ducts.

    d. of jejunum. Diverticulum usually
marked by severe pain in upper abdomen,
followed occasionally by massive hemorrhage from intestine.

    d. of stomach. Diverticulum of wall of
stomach.

    d., true. Diverticula involving all the
coats of muscle in the pouch wall. Usually
congenital.

    d., Zenker's. SEE: *Zenker's diverticu-
lum.*

diving reflex. Submersion of the face and
nose of animals, including humans, in water
produces a complex cardiovascular reflex
that constricts blood flow except to the
brain; decreases cardiac output and rate;
and produces stable or slightly increased arterial blood pressure. The reflex enables
aquatic animals to remain submerged for
long periods because it reduces their oxygen
requirements. In humans, the reflex has
been used to treat paroxysmal atrial tachycardia.

division (dĭ-vĭzh′ŭn) [L. *dividere*, to divide]. 1.
A separation into parts. 2. That which separates, as anatomical boundary, partition, or
wall.

divulge [L. *divulgare*, to make common]. To
reveal something that was not previously
common knowledge.

divulsion (dĭ-vŭl′shŭn) [L. *dis*, apart, +
vellere, to pluck]. Forcibly pulling apart.

divulsor (dĭ-vŭl′sor) [L. *dis*, apart, + *vellere*, to pluck]. Device for dilatation of a part,
esp. the urethra.

    d., pterygium. Instrument for separating corneal portion of the pterygium.

d., tendon. Device for separating tendon from surrounding tissue.

Dix, Dorothea Lynde. A Massachusetts schoolteacher (1802–1887) who crusaded for prison reform and for care of the mentally ill. She was responsible for founding many hospitals in the U.S., Canada, and several other countries. During the Civil War, she organized the nursing service of the Union armies.

dizygotic twins (dī″zī-gŏt′ĭk) [Gr. *dis*, two, + *zygon*, yoke]. Twins who are the product of two ova. SYN: *fraternal twins*. SEE: *monozygotic twins.*

dizziness [AS. *dysig,* foolish]. A sensation of whirling or feeling a tendency to fall. SYN: *giddiness.* SEE: *vertigo.*

DKA. *diabetic ketoacidosis.*

dl. *deciliter.*

DM. *diabetes mellitus.*

D.M.D. *Doctor of Dental Medicine.*

DMF index. The total number of decayed, missing, and filled teeth.

DMSO. *dimethyl sulfoxide,* q.v.

DMT. *dimethyltryptamine,* q.v.

DNA. *deoxyribonucleic acid.*

DNA fingerprinting. A method of using fragments of deoxyribonucleic acid to establish an autoradiograph of that particular DNA sample. Use of the same procedure on a sample suspected of coming from the same person can then be compared. The technique has been used in criminal investigations.

DNA probe. A method of detecting and identifying microorganisms. The use of recombinant DNA technique to isolate, reproduce, and label a portion of the genetic material, DNA, from the nucleus of a microorganism that is specific for it. This fragment can be added to a specimen containing the organisms. The specimen and known DNA are treated so that the DNA strands from the organisms in the specimen are separated into single strands. The DNA from the specimen rejoins (is annealed to) the known labeled DNA and is thereby labeled. This permits the identification of a single pathogenic organism in a specimen that contains many different microorganisms.

DNAR. *do not attempt resuscitation.*

DNR. *do not resuscitate.*

D.O. *Doctor of Osteopathy.*

DOA. *dead on arrival* (at a hospital).

Dobell's solution (dō′bĕlz) [Horace B. Dobell, Brit. physician, 1828–1917]. Carbolic acid, borax, sodium bicarbonate, glycerine, and water in solution.

Dobie's globule (dō′bēz) [William M. Dobie, Brit. physician, 1828–1915]. A very tiny spherical body in the light band of a striated muscle fiber.

dobutamine hydrochloride. A synthetic beta-agonist whose primary effect is to increase cardiac contractility, with little effect on systemic vascular resistance. It produces less tachycardia than dopamine, and has no effect on renal blood flow. It is of use in congestive heart failure and cardiogenic shock.

Doca Acetate. Trade name for desoxycorticosterone acetate.

doctor [L. *docere,* to teach]. 1. The recipient of an advanced degree, such as doctor of medicine (M.D.); doctor of osteopathy (D.O.); doctor of philosophy (Ph.D.); doctor of science (D.Sc.); doctor of science in nursing (D.S.N.); doctor of dental medicine (D.M.D.); doctor of education (Ed.D.); or doctor of divinity (D.D.). 2. One who, after graduating from a medical, veterinary, or dental school, successfully passes an examination and is licensed by a state government to practice medicine, veterinary medicine, or dentistry.

Because of the great variety of doctoral degrees, the use of the word doctor is sometimes confusing. This may be remedied by using the word physician when writing or speaking of those who possess an M.D. or D.O. (doctor of osteopathy) degree. SEE: *optometry; osteopathy.*

d., barefoot. A practitioner of traditional or native medicine in the People's Republic of China. These individuals have not attended a medical school.

doctrine (dŏk′trĭn). The system of principles taught or advocated.

docusate calcium (dŏk′ū-sāt). USP. A stool softener. Trade name is Surfak.

docusate sodium. USP. A stool softener. Trade names are Colace, Modane Soft, and Doxinate.

dog bite. Lacerated or punctured wound by a dog. The dog should be observed for 10 days to determine the presence of rabies.

Caution: The physically handicapped and infants should not be left alone with dogs, esp. large ones. Dogs known to be gentle pets have killed infants living in the same household.

TREAT: Thoroughly cleanse the wound, washing vigorously with soap and water for at least 10 minutes to remove saliva. Flush with a viricidal agent and follow with a clear rinse. Do not stop bleeding (unless massive) because blood flow helps to cleanse the wound. Provide routine tetanus prophylaxis. Obtain information about animal, its location, and owner. Include these data in report to public health authorities. Appropriate antirabies therapy if the animal is known to have rabies. SEE: *DF-2; rabies.*

dogmatic. Pert. to expression of an opinion in an uncompromising, arrogant manner.

Döhle bodies (dě'lē) [Paul Döhle, Ger. pathologist, 1855–1928]. Leukocyte inclusions in the periphery of neutrophils. The bodies are composed of liquefied endoplasmic reticulum. Toxic granulations in the neutrophils frequently accompany Döhle bodies. They are present in association with burns, severe or systemic infections, trauma, and neoplastic diseases.

dol. Symb. for degree of pain intensity registered on the dolorimeter.

Dolene. Trade name for propoxyphene hydrochloride.

dolichocephalic (dŏl″ĭ-kō-sĭ-făl′ĭk) [Gr. *dolichos,* long, + *kephale,* head]. Having a skull with a long anteroposterior diameter.

dolichocolon (dŏl″ĭ-kō-kō′lŏn) [″ + *kolon,* colon]. Abnormally long colon.

dolichofacial (dŏl″ĭ-kō-fā′shăl). Pertaining to a long face.

dolichohieric (dŏl″ĭ-kō-hī-ĕr′ĭk) [″ + *hieron,* sacred]. Having a long, slender sacrum.

dolichomorphic (dŏl″ĭ-kō-mor′fĭk) [″ + *morphe,* form]. Pertaining to a body type that is long and slender. SEE: *ectomorph.*

dolichopellic, dolichopelvic (dŏl″ĭ-kō-pĕl′ĭk,-pĕl′vĭk) [″ + *pyelos,* an oblong trough]. Having an abnormally long or narrow pelvis.

dolichosigmoid (dŏl″ĭ-kō-sĭg′moyd) [″ + *sigmoeides,* sigmoid]. Having an abnormally long sigmoid flexure of the colon.

dolichuranic (dŏl″ĭk-ū-răn′ĭk) [″ + *ouranos,* palate]. Concerning a long alveolar arch of the maxilla.

doll's eye movements. Oculocephalic reflex. SYN: *doll's eye reflex.*

doll's head maneuver. A test of eye movement in comatose patients. The head is quickly rotated from one side to the other. Normally, the eyes deviate together to the side opposite the direction of head rotation. If this response is absent, there may be damage to the brain stem or oculomotor nerves. SEE: *coma.*

Dolophine Hydrochloride. Trade name for methadone hydrochloride.

dolor (dō′lor) [L.] (pl. *dolores*). Pain. One of the principal indications of inflammation. The others are rubor (redness), tumor (swelling), and calor (heat).

dolorific (dō″lor-ĭf′ĭk) [L. *dolor,* pain]. Causing pain.

dolorimeter (dō″lor-ĭm′ĭ-tĕr) [″ + Gr. *metron,* measure]. Device for measuring degree of pain.

dolorogenic [″ + Gr. *gennan,* to produce]. Causing pain.

domain. In immunology, the portion of a pro-

tein, such as an immunoglobulin, that has a functional role independent of the remainder of the protein.

domatophobia (dō-măt-ō-fō′bē-ă) [Gr. *doma,* house, + *phobos,* fear]. Abnormal aversion to being in a house; a form of claustrophobia.

domiciliary (dŏm″ĭ-sĭl′ē-ār″ē) [L. *domus,* house]. Pert. to or carried on in a house.

domiciliary care facilities. Home providing mainly custodial and personal care for persons who do not require medical or nursing supervision, but may need assistance with activities of daily living because of a physical or mental disability. These may also be referred to as board and care homes, personal care homes, or sheltered living environments. SEE: *adult foster care.*

dominance [L. *dominans,* ruling]. 1. Genetic quality through which one of an allelic pair of hereditary factors has the capacity to suppress the expression of the other so that the first prevails in the heterozygote. 2. Often used to refer to the preferred hand or side of the body, as in right-hand dominance. 3. In psychiatry, the tendency to be commanding or controlling of others.

   d., ocular. The use of one eye by choice for particular tasks such as aiming a gun. This may or may not be related to right- or left-hand dominance.

dominant. In genetics, a trait or characteristic that will be expressed in the offspring even though it is carried on only one of the homologous chromosomes. SEE: *recessive.*

domoic acid. An excitotoxin reported to have contaminated mussels.

Donath-Landsteiner phenomenon (dō′năth-lănd′stī-nĕr) [Julius Donath, Austrian physician, 1870–1950; Karl L. Landsteiner, Austrian-born U.S. biologist, 1868–1943]. A test for paroxysmal hemoglobinuria. Blood from the patient is cooled to 5°C, and a cold hemolysin in the plasma combines with the red blood cells if the patient has the illness. Upon warming, the sensitized red cells are hemolyzed by the complement normally present.

donee (dō-nē′) [L. *donare,* to give]. One who receives something, such as a blood transfusion, from a donor.

Don Juan [After the legendary, promiscuous, Spanish nobleman, Don Juan de Tenerio]. A male whose sexual promiscuity arises from insecurity concerning his masculinity or latent and unconscious homosexual preference.

Donnan's equilibrium (dŏn′ănz) [Frederick G. Donnan, Brit. chemist, 1870–1956]. Condition in which an equilibrium is established between two solutions separated by a semipermeable membrane so that the sum of the anions and cations on one side is equal to that on the other side.

donor. 1. One who furnishes blood, tissue, or an organ to be used in another person. 2. In chemistry, a compound that frees part of itself to unite with another compound called an acceptor, q.v.

    d., universal. One whose blood is of group O and is therefore usually compatible with most other blood types. In actual practice this compatibility rarely occurs because of the many factors other than the major blood antigens (A, B, AB) that determine blood compatibility.

donor card. A document used by a person who wishes to make an anatomical gift, at the time of his or her death, of an organ or other body part needed for transplantation. SEE: illus; *transplantation.*

do not attempt resuscitation. ABBR: DNAR. An order somewhat more precise than "do not resuscitate" (DNR). DNR implies that, had resuscitation attempt been made, the patient could have been revived. DNAR indicates resuscitation efforts should not be attempted regardless of expected outcome of those efforts.

Donovan body [Charles Donovan, Ir. physician, 1863–1951]. The common name for the causative organism, *Calymmatobacterium granulomatis,* of granuloma inguinale.

donovanosis. SEE: *granuloma inguinale.*

dopa. A chemical substance, 3,4-dihydroxyphenylalanine, produced by the oxidation of tyrosine to tyrosinase. It is a precursor of catecholamines and melanin.

dopamine hydrochloride (dō′pă-mēn). 1. A catecholamine synthesized by the adrenal gland. It is the immediate precursor in the synthesis of norepinephrine. Dopamine is used to treat hypotension unrelated to hypovolemia (which should be treated with transfusions, IV fluids, and surgery). It has different actions at various doses. Low doses (2-5 mcg/kg/min) cause renal (dopaminergic effects) and mesenteric dilation. Intermediate doses (5-15 mcg/kg/min) increase cardiac contractility, which increases cardiac output, blood pressure, and perfusion pressure. High doses (above 15 mcg/kg/min) cause generalized vasoconstriction by activating alpha-adrenergic receptors. It is also used in the treatment of shock. Trade names are Intropin and Dopastat. 2. A catecholamine neurotransmitter, or brain messenger, implicated in some forms of psychosis and abnormal movement disorders.

Caution: Do not administer by I.V. push. Monitor I.V. line frequently to be certain there is no extravasation. Do not administer with other drugs in the same I.V. line. Discontinue use gradually. When dopamine is used in life-threatening states of shock, blood pressure and renal function must be monitored carefully.

dopaminergic (dō″pă-mēn-ĕr′jĭk). 1. Caused by dopamine. 2. Concerning tissues that are influenced by dopamine.

dopa-oxidase (dō″pă-ŏk′sĭ-dās). Enzyme in some epithelial cells that converts dopa to melanin.

Dopar. Trade name for levodopa.

dope. An imprecise slang term used to describe almost any drug of abuse. SEE: *doping; doping, blood.*

doping. In athletic medicine, use of a drug or blood product that the athlete hopes will improve performance. The existence of a drug that safely accomplishes this has not been demonstrated. The administration of anabolic hormones to females causes signs of masculinization, including facial hair growth, deepening of the voice, and clitoromegaly.

    d., blood. The practice of athletes to store several units of their own blood, and to have it transfused to themselves a day or two prior to competition. The safety and effectiveness of this practice is questionable, and it is unapproved by sports governing bodies.

Doppler echocardiography. A sensitive, noninvasive technique for determining the blood flow velocity in different locations in the heart. It is an adaptation of ultrasound technology. This same method can be used in determining the uterine artery blood flow velocity during pregnancy. SEE: *echocardiography.*

Doppler effect (dŏp′lĕr) [Johann Christian Doppler, Austrian scientist, 1803–1853]. The apparent frequency of waves, such as those of sound, varies with change in distance between the source and the receiver. The frequency seems to increase as the distance decreases and to decrease as the distance increases.

Doppler measurement of blood pressure and fetal heart rate. Use of Doppler sound waves to determine systolic blood pressure, as well as to determine the fetal heart rate.

doraphobia (dō″ră-fō′bē-ă) [Gr. *dora,* hide, + *phobos,* fear]. Abnormal aversion to touching the hair or fur of animals.

Dorello's canal [Primo Dorello, It. anatomist, 1872–1963]. A bony canal in tip of temporal bone enclosing the abducens nerve.

Dorendorf's sign [Hans Dorendorf, Ger. physician, b. 1866]. A filling up or fullness of the supraclavicular groove in aneurysm of the aortic arch.

dornase (dor′nās). Short for deoxyribonu-

UNIFORM DONOR CARD

OF_____

Print or type name of donor

In the hope that I may help others, I hereby make this anatomical gift, if medically acceptable, to take effect upon my death. The words and marks below indicate my desires.

I give: (a) _____ any needed organs or parts

             (b) _____ only the following organs or parts

_____

Specify the organ(s) or part(s)

for the purposes of transplantation, therapy, medical research or education;

             (c) _____ my body for anatomical study if needed.

Limitations or
special wishes, if any : _____

Signed by the donor and the following two witnesses in the presence of each other:

_____   _____
Signature of Donor   Date of Birth of Donor

_____   _____
Date Signed   City & State

_____   _____
Witness   Witness

This is a legal document under the Uniform Anatomical Gift Act or similar laws.

clease.

    d., pancreatic. Dornase prepared from beef pancreas. Used to loosen thick pulmonary secretions.

dorsa [L.]. Pl. of dorsum.

dorsabdominal [L. *dorsum,* back, + *abdomen,* belly]. Pert. to the back and abdomen.

dorsad [″ + *ad,* toward]. Toward the back.

dorsal [L. *dorsum,* back]. 1. Pert. to the back. 2. Indicating a position toward a rear part. Opposed to ventral.

dorsal cord stimulation. Procedure for relieving pain by electric stimulation of the spinal cord through electrodes sutured to the posterior spinal cord.

dorsal elevated position. Position in which patient is on his or her back with head and shoulders elevated at an angle of 30° or more.

dorsalgia (dŏr-săl′jē-ă) [″ + Gr. *algos,* pain]. Pain in the back. SYN: *notalgia; rachialgia.*

dorsalis (dor-sā′lĭs) [L.]. Dorsal, i.e., pertaining to the back.

dorsal nerves. Branches of spinal nerves that pass dorsally to innervate structures or areas near the vertebral column. Also called dorsal rami.

dorsal recumbent position. Similar to dorsal elevated position except the extremities are moderately flexed and rotated outward, the soles of the feet rest upon the bed or table, or the legs may be extended. With legs not flexed, this position is used for examination of chest, abdomen, and lower limbs. With legs flexed, it is used in giving douches, for bathing, for catheterizing, and for applying abdominal compresses. The patient may be placed in this position for bimanual palpation or for vaginal examinations and repair of perineal lesions following parturition.

dorsal reflex. Irritation of the skin over the erector spinal muscles, causing contraction of muscles of the back.

dorsal rigid posture. Position in which both legs (or the right one only) are drawn up. Observed in peritonitis, meningitis, ascites, and tympanites. The right leg is drawn up in appendicitis, pelvic inflammation, renal calculus in right ureter, psoas abscess, and peritonitis on the right side.

dorsal slit. A surgical method of making the foreskin of the penis easily retractable. The foreskin is cut in the dorsal midline but not far enough to extend into the mucous membrane next to the glans.

dorsi-, dorso-, dors- [L.]. Combining form indicating back.

dorsiduct [L. *dorsum*, back, + *ducere*, to lead]. To draw toward the back or backward.

dorsiduction. Drawing toward the back.

dorsiflect (dor′sĭ-flĕkt) [″ + *flectere*, to bend]. To bend backward.

dorsiflexion. Movement of a part at a joint so as to bend the part toward the dorsum or posterior aspect of the body. Thus, dorsiflexion of the foot indicates movement of the foot in a backward direction, in which the foot moves toward the top or dorsum of the foot, the opposite of plantar flexion. Dorsiflexion of the toes indicates moving the toes away from the sole of the foot. When the hand is extended, or bent backward at the wrist, it is dorsiflexed; this is the opposite of palmar flexion or volar flexion of the wrist.

dorsimesal (dor″sĭ-mĕs′ăl). In the direction of the dorsimeson.

dorsimeson (dor-sĭ-mĕs′ŏn) [″ + Gr. *meson*, middle]. The median plane of the back.

dorsispinal (dor″sĭ-spī′năl) [″ + *spina*, thorn]. Pert. to the back and spine.

dorsocephalad (dor″sō-sĕf′ă-lăd) [″ + Gr. *kephale*, head, + L. *ad*, toward]. Situated toward the back of the head.

dorsodynia (dor″sō-dĭn′ē-ă) [″ + Gr. *odyne*, pain]. Pain in the muscles of upper part of the back.

dorsolateral (dor″sō-lăt′ĕr-ăl). Concerning the back and side.

dorsolumbar. Concerning the lower thoracic and upper lumbar (loin) area of the back.

dorsoplantar (dor″sō-plăn′tăr) [″ + *planta*, sole of the foot]. Direction from the top to the bottom of the foot.

dorsosacral [″ + *sacrum*, sacred bone]. Pert. to the lower back.

dorsosacral position. Position in which patient is upon the back as in the dorsal recumbent position, q.v., except that thighs are flexed upon abdomen and legs upon thighs, which are abducted. Leg holders are used to support legs in position. Used for gynecological examinations and treatments, in plastic operations of genital tract, in vaginal hysterectomy, and in diagnosis and treatment of diseases of urethra and bladder. SYN: *lithotomy position.* SEE: *position* for illus.

dorsoventral (dor″sō-vĕn′trăl). Concerning the back and frontal surfaces of the body.

dorsum [L.] (pl. *dorsa*). The back or posterior surface of a part. In the foot, the dorsum is the top of the foot.

dosage [Gr. *dosis*, a giving]. Determination of the amount, frequency, and number of doses of medication or radiation for a patient.

   d. calculation for children. There is no absolutely reliable formula for calculating the dose of a medicine an infant or child should receive. Several rules for calculating a child's dose have been used in the past, but those that use body surface area are most accurate. SEE: *body surface area.*

dose (dōs) [Gr. *dosis*, a giving]. Amount of a medicinal preparation or of radiation to be administered at one time.

   d., absorbed. Dose of ionizing radiation imparted to a tissue or target.

   d., air. The intensity of radiation measured in air at the target.

   d., bolus. A medicine given intravenously at a controlled but rapid rate.

   d., booster. SEE: *booster.*

   d., cumulative. 1. Total dose of radiation resulting from repeated exposures. 2. The summation of dose of a drug present in the body after repeated medication. It takes into account the medicine excreted or biotransformed that is therefore no longer effective.

   d., curative. Dose required to cure an illness or disease.

   d., divided. Fractional portions administered at short intervals.

   d., equianalgesic. A dose of one form of

analgesic drug equivalent in pain-relieving potential to another analgesic. Knowing this equivalence will permit substitution of analgesics in order to attempt to prevent undesired side effects of a medicine for control of pain.

d., erythema. Smallest amount of x-rays that will produce erythema within two weeks following treatment.

d., fatal. Dose that kills. SEE: LD_{50}.

d., infective. The amount of infectious organisms, esp. bacteria and viruses, that will cause disease.

d., maintenance. Dose required to maintain the desired effect.

d., maximum. Largest dose that is safe to administer.

d., maximum permissible. In accordance with radiation protection guidelines, the amount of radiation exposure permitted to persons whose occupation requires working with radioactive sources. These values also apply to the general population and are different for pregnant females.

d., median curative. Dose that cures the disease in half of the persons treated.

d., median infective. Infective dose that causes disease in half of the susceptibles given that dose.

d., median lethal. ABBR: LD_{50}, q.v. The amount of a substance, bacteria, or toxin that will kill 50% of the animals exposed to the material. SEE: *dose, minimum lethal.*

d., minimum. Smallest dose that will be effective.

d., minimum lethal. The smallest amount of a substance that will kill an animal. SEE: LD_{50}.

d., primary. The initial and large dose given to provide a high blood level without delay.

d., skin. Radiation dose to the skin including secondary radiation from backscatter, i.e., radiation reflected from the surroundings.

d., therapeutic. Dose required to produce the desired effect.

d., threshold. SEE: *erythema dose.*

d., tissue tolerance. Largest dose, esp. of radiation, that will not harm tissues.

d., toxic. Dose that causes signs and symptoms of drug toxicity.

dose response curve. A graph in which the degree of the effect of a drug or chemical is charted at specific doses. Connecting these points as the dose is increased produces the curve of response with respect to the dose administered.

dosimeter (dō-sĭm′ĭ-tĕr) [″ + *metron*, measure]. Device for measuring x-ray output.

dosimetric (dō″sĭ-mĕt′rĭk). Pert. to dosimetry.

dosimetry (dō-sĭm′ĕ-trē) [″ + *metron*, measure]. Measurement of doses.

dot. A small speck.

d., Trantas. [Alexios Trantas, Gr. ophthalmologist, 1867–1960] Chalky concretions in the conjunctiva around the limbus of the eye. Seen in vernal conjunctivitis.

dotage [ME. *doten*, to be silly]. Senility; feeblemind-ness of very old age.

double (dŭb′l) [L. *duplus*, twofold]. Combining two things or qualities.

double blind technique. A method of scientific investigation in which neither the subject nor the investigator working with the subject or analyzing data knows what treatment, if any, the subject is receiving. At the completion of the experiment, the "code" is broken and data are analyzed with respect to the various treatments used. This method attempts to eliminate observer and subject bias. SEE: *open-label study.*

double-contrast examination. Radiographic examination in which both a radiopaque and a radiolucent contrast medium are used simultaneously to visualize internal anatomy.

double personality. A split in consciousness, neither personality being aware of acts and words of other. SEE: *dual personality; multiple personality.*

double touch. Exploration with a finger in one cavity and thumb in another.

double uterus. Dihysteria, q.v. SYN: *uterus didelphys.*

double vision. Seeing two images of an object at the same time. SYN: *diplopia.*

double-voided urine. Urine sample voided 30 minutes after the patient has emptied the bladder. SYN: *second-voided urine.*

doubling time. The time required to double in size, as in the growth of a malignant tumor.

douche (doosh) [Fr.]. A current of vapor or stream of hot or cold water directed against a part. A douche may be made of plain water or medicated. It may be for the purpose of personal hygiene or treatment of a local condition.

d., air. Air current directed on body for therapeutic purposes. Usually directed to the tympanum for opening the eustachian tube.

d., alternating. D., Scotch.

d., astringent. Douche containing substances such as alum or zinc sulfate for shrinking the mucous membrane.

d., circular. Needle spray or application of water to body through horizontal jets the size of a needle from a number of small rows of sprays so placed that the water is projected against the skin of bather from four directions simultaneously.

d., cleansing. An external or perineal douche for cleansing genitalia following defecation or following operations such as hemorrhoidectomy, curettage, rectal surgery, circumcision, or perineorrhaphy. Mild antiseptic or disinfectant solution, 98° to 104°F (36.7° to 40°C), poured or sprayed over the parts, followed by gentle drying and inspection for cleanliness.

d., deodorizing. Douche used to deodorize the vagina and vaginal secretions when they have an offensive odor.

d., high. Douche in which the bag is at least 4 feet (1.2 meters) above the hips of the patient.

d., jet. Douche applied to the body in a solid stream from the douche hose.

d., low. Douche in which the bag is 1 to 1½ ft (31 to 46 cm) above the hips of the patient.

d., medicated. Douche containing a medicinal substance for the treatment of local conditions.

d., neutral. Douche given at average surface temperature of body, i.e., 90° to 97°F (32.2° to 36.1°C).

d., perineal. Spray projected upward from a bidet, q.v., placed just above the floor; patient sits on the seat of the bidet and receives douche upon perineum.

d., Scotch. Douche consisting of alternating hot and cold jets of water against local area of skin.

d., vaginal. Douche of vagina used for deodorant, antiseptic, stimulating, or hemostatic purposes. Temperature of solutions: antiseptic or deodorant douche, 105° to 112°F (40.6° to 44.4°C); stimulating or hemostatic douche, 118° to 120°F (47.8° to 48.9°C). Solution should flow slowly with little pressure, the douche solution container being elevated up to 2 feet (61 cm) above patient's pelvis. Quantity generally 2 to 3 qt. (2 or 3 liters) of solution unless otherwise ordered.

NOTE: The vagina, like many other areas of the body, has the ability to cleanse itself. Thus there is very little reason for a normal, healthy woman to use a vaginal douche. Douching can upset the balance of the vaginal flora and change vaginal pH, thus predisposing the woman to vaginitis. There is no evidence that a postcoital vaginal douche is effective as a contraceptive.

In at least one investigation, it has been shown that vaginal douching is a risk factor for pelvic inflammatory disease (PID). The more frequently the subjects douched, the more likely they were to have PID.

Douglas bag [Claude G. Douglas, Brit. physiologist, 1882–1963]. A container, usually a bag made of flexible material, for collecting expired air. It is used in investigating respiratory function and physiology.

Douglas' cul-de-sac, pouch, space [James Douglas, Scot. anatomist, 1675–1742]. Peritoneal space or pouch that lies behind uterus and in front of rectum.

Douglas' fold. The arcuate line of the sheath of the rectus abdominalis muscle.

douglasitis (dŭg-lăs-ī'tĭs). Inflammation of the cul-de-sac of Douglas.

dowager's hump. Cervical lordosis with dorsal kyphosis due to the slow, painless loss of bone, i.e., osteoporosis. This may occur at any age but is seen most commonly in elderly females.

dowel [ME. *dowle*, peg]. Metal pin for fastening an artificial crown to a tooth root.

down. 1. Lanugo, the fine hairs of the skin of the newborn. 2. The fine soft feathers of the young of some birds; and the small feathers underneath the large feathers of adult birds, particularly waterfowl. Used in clothing to protect from the cold.

down regulate. To inhibit or suppress the normal response of an organ or system, e.g., the immune system or the central nervous system. SEE: *immunocompromised.*

Down syndrome [J. Langdon Down, Brit. physician, 1828–1896]. A variety of congenital moderate-to-severe mental retardation. Marked by sloping forehead, small ear canals, gray or very light yellow spots at periphery of iris (Brushfield's spots), short broad hand with a single palmar crease (simian crease), a flat nose or absent bridge, low-set ears, and generally dwarfed physique. SYN: *trisomy 21.*

Women at high risk of giving birth to a child with Down syndrome are those over 40; those who have had a previous child with the syndrome; and those who themselves have Down syndrome (pregnancy is rare in this condition). In addition, there is a high risk of having a child with Down syndrome when there is parental mosaicism with a 21 trisomic cell population.

Down syndrome may be diagnosed antenatally by use of several techniques. SEE: *amniocentesis.* SEE: *Nursing Diagnoses in Appendix.*

ETIOL: Patients with Down syndrome have an extra chromosome, usually number 21 or 22.

doxapram hydrochloride (dŏk'să-prăm). USP. A respiratory stimulant. Trade name is Dopram.

Doxinate. Trade name for docusate sodium.

doxorubicin hydrochloride (dŏk″sō-rū'bĭ-sĭn). USP. An antineoplastic antibiotic agent. Trade name is Adriamycin.

doxycycline (dŏk″sē-sī'klēn). USP. A broadspectrum antibiotic of the tetracycline group. Trade name is Vibramycin.

doxylamine succinate (dŏk-sǐl'ă-mēn). USP. An antihistamine. Trade names are Decapryn Succinate and Unisom.

Doyère's eminence (dwă-yārz') [Louis Doyère, Fr. physiologist, 1811–1863]. Elevation where a nerve filament enters a muscle.

D.P. *Doctor of Pharmacy.*

2,3-D.P.G. *2,3-diphosphoglycerate.*

D.P.H. *Diploma in Public Health.*

D.P.M. *Doctor of Podiatric Medicine.*

D.P.T. Vaccine for diphtheria, pertussis, and tetanus. Used in the immunization program for infants and children.

DR. *reaction of degeneration.*

Dr. *Doctor.*

dr. *drachm; dram.*

drachm (drăm) [Gr. *drachme*, a Gr. unit of weight]. ABBR: dr. SYMB: 3. A unit of weight in apothecaries' system. Also spelled dram.

dracontiasis (drăk″ŏn-tī′ă-sĭs) [Gr. *drakontion*, little dragon]. Dracunculiasis.

dracunculiasis (dră-kŭng″kū-lī′ă-sĭs). Infestation with the nematode *Dracunculus medinensis.*

dracunculosis (dră-kŭng″kū-lō′sĭs). Dracunculiasis.

Dracunculus (dră-kŭng′kū-lŭs). A genus of parasitic nematodes.

D. medinensis. The guinea worm or "fiery serpent." A species of nematode that is a common human parasite, esp. in Africa and India. Infection of the human occurs when water containing infected crustacea of the genus *Cyclops* is swallowed. The larvae are liberated in the stomach or duodenum, then migrate through the viscera and become adults. The adult female, after mating, burrows under the skin of the leg. Larvae are discharged into environment through the ulcer caused by the worm, esp. when legs are in water. The infection may be prevented by boiling suspect water, by treating it with chlorine, or by filtering it to remove the infected *Cyclops.*

TREAT: The head of the adult worm can be seen in the ulcer. Slow traction on the worm will remove it. This is done by making a small incision, grasping the front end of the worm, and winding it around a small object. The winding is increased each day until the worm is removed. Be careful not to break worm. Use of thiabendazole or niridazole may be effective.

draft, draught. A dose of liquid medicine intended to be taken in a single dose.

drag. Street language for clothing of one sex worn by a person, often a homosexual, of the opposite sex.

drain (drān) [AS. *dreahnian*, to draw off]. 1. Exit or tube for discharge of a morbid matter. 2. To draw off a fluid.

d., capillary. Drawing off by capillary attraction.

d., cigarette. Drain made by covering a small strip of gauze with rubber.

d., Mikulicz's. Single layer of gauze pushed into the wound cavity, to which is added thick gauze wicks that project from the cavity.

d., nonabsorbable. Drain made from horsehair, gauze, rubber, glass, or metal. Types are abdominal, antrum, perineal, and suprapubic.

d., Penrose. A cigarette drain made with a piece of small rubber tubing through which gauze has been pulled.

drainage (drān′ĭj). The free flow or withdrawal of fluids from a wound or cavity, as pus from a cavity or wound. SEE: *autodrainage; drain.*

d., capillary. Drainage by method of capillary attraction.

d., closed. Drainage of a wound or body space so that the air is excluded.

d., closed sterile. A sterile tube draining a body site such as the abdominal cavity or pleural space that is designed to prevent the entry of air and bacteria into the tubing or the area being drained.

d., funnel. Drainage with glass funnels.

d., negative pressure. Drainage in which negative pressure is maintained in the tube. Used in treating pneumothorax and in certain types of drains or catheters in the intestinal tract.

d., open. Drainage of a wound or body cavity so that air is not excluded from the area of the cavity.

d., postural. Drainage for the nasal area, bronchi, and sinuses. The patient is placed in a position in which gravity will allow drainage. SEE: *postural drainage* for illus.

d., suction. SEE: *d., negative pressure.*

d., tidal. A method, controlled mechanically, of filling the bladder with solution by gravity and periodically emptying the bladder by siphonage. Usually used when the patient lacks control of the bladder as in injuries or lesions of the spinal cord.

d., Wangensteen. SEE: *Wangensteen tube.*

drainage tube. Device for allowing escape of pus, serum, blood, or other fluids from a wound or abscess.

drained weight. The actual weight of food that has been allowed to drain in order to remove the liquids in which it has been prepared.

dram [Gr. *drachme*]. ABBR: dr. SYMB: 3. A

unit of weight in apothecaries' system. SYN: *drachm*.

d., fluid. A teaspoonful or ⅛ of a fluid ounce or 57.1 gr of distilled water, the equivalent of 3.7 ml. In Great Britain, 54.8 gr of distilled water or 3.5 ml.

Dramamine (drăm′ă-mēn) Trade name for dimenhydrinate, the chlorotheophylline salt of the antihistaminic agent diphenhydramine. Dramamine has a depressant effect on hyperstimulated labyrinthine function and is used to treat or prevent nausea, vomiting, vertigo, and motion sickness.

dramatism [Gr. *drama*, acting, + *-ismos*, condition]. Dramatic behavior and lofty speech seen in psychological disturbances.

drapetomania (drăp″ĕt-ō-mā′nē-ă) [Gr. *drapetes*, runaway, + *mania*, madness]. Insane impulse to wander from home.

drastic [Gr. *drastikos*, effective]. 1. Acting strongly. 2. A very active cathartic, usually producing many explosive bowel movements accompanied by pain and tenesmus. The use of this type of cathartic is not advisable.

draught (drăft) [ME. *draught*, a pulling]. 1. A drink. 2. Drawing liquid into the mouth. 3. Breeze produced by wind or fan. 4. A liquid medicinal dose to be taken all at once.

Draw-a-Person test. A widely used projective assessment that is assumed to reveal information about a patient's body image or self-concept. SYN: *Machover test*.

drawer sign or test. Sign diagnostic of rupture of the cruciate ligament(s) of the knee. The knee is flexed to 90 degrees with the foot stabilized on the examination table. The examiner applies an anterior then posterior force against the upper tibia, perpendicular to the long axis of the leg. There will be an increased glide, anterior or posterior of the tibia, if rupture is present of the anterior or posterior cruciate ligament respectively. This is sometimes called "draw sign."

draw sheet. Historically, the term draw sheet was given to a long roll or bolt of muslin that was stretched across the width of the bed with the free end initially placed under the patient's buttocks. When this became soiled, it was drawn from under the patient and rolled up on the opposite side of the cot or bed, allowing the patient to lie on a clean section of the roll of muslin.

The draw sheet is used to protect the bottom sheet and mattress from drainage and soilage, and it is easier to change, for both the patient and nurse, than the entire bed. When a draw sheet is folded and placed under a patient to use for lifting and turning, it is called a lift sheet. In many hospitals, draw sheets have been replaced by paper

and plastic pads that resemble disposable diapers.

dream [AS. *dream*, joy]. Occurrence of ideas, emotions, and sensations during sleep. Some dreams may be recalled upon awakening; others may not be.

Interpretation of the meaning of dreams has been of interest to the laity as well as psychoanalysts, not to mention the person who recalls having the dream. The idea that a dream conceals a meaning buried deep in the subconscious is questionable. A dream may reveal more than it conceals. Any idea, emotion, or wish may be the subject of a dream. Less controversial is the research results correlating changes in the electroencephalogram and rapid eye movements (REM) during sleep with dream activity. Under experimental conditions, it has been possible to communicate with the person who is dreaming. Some lower animals, i.e., cats and dogs, dream. There is no evidence that two people asleep together have the same dream simultaneously. SEE: *REM; sleep; sleep, disorders of; wet dream.*

drench. A dose of medicine that is administered to an animal by pouring into its mouth.

drepanocyte (drĕp′ă-nō-sīt) [Gr. *drepane*, sickle, + *kytos*, cell]. Sickle or crescent cell.

drepanocytemia (drĕp″ă-nō-sī-tē′mē-ă) [″ + ″ + *haima*, blood]. Sickle cell anemia.

drepanocytic (drĕp″ă-nō-sĭt′ĭk). Pert. to or resembling a sickle cell.

dressing [O. Fr. *dresser*, to prepare]. Covering, protective or supportive, for diseased or injured parts.

NURSING IMPLICATIONS: Explain procedure and ensure patient privacy. Assemble needed equipment and wash hands thoroughly. Follow strict aseptic technique during dressing changes. Dispose of discarded dressings properly. Wash hands following the procedure. Carefully note the presence and character of any drainage on the dressing or around the incision. Also note the condition of the wound or suture line for presence of any erythema or edema.

RS: bandage; compress.

d., absorbent. Gauze, sterilized gauze, or absorbent cotton.

d., antiseptic. Dressing consisting of gauze permeated with an antiseptic solution.

d., clear transparent covering. SEE: *d., transparent synthetic.*

d., dry. Dressing consisting of dry gauze, absorbent cotton, or other dry material.

d., fixed. Dressing permeated with

starch, silicate of soda, or plaster of paris. When this dressing dries, it provides fixation of the part so treated.

d., hot moist. The most common form is a hot normal saline solution, as hot as can be borne by the bare forearm of the nurse. The sterile towel is unfolded, and the gauze dressing is dropped into it. Then immerse the center of the towel in solution and wring out by turning the dry ends in opposite directions. The dressing is applied with sterile forceps directly to the wound. Sometimes a dry sterile towel is used over it to keep the dressing in place. Heat is best maintained by infrared lamp.

Caution: Do not burn the patient.

---

d., nonadherent. Dressing that has little or no tendency to adhere to dried secretions from the wound.

d., occlusive. Dressing that seals a wound completely to prevent infection from without and to prevent moisture from within from escaping through the dressing.

d., pressure. Dressing that is used to apply pressure to the wound. May be used following skin grafting.

d., protective. Dressing applied for the purpose of preventing injury or infection to the part so treated.

d., self-adhering roller. Rolled gauze strip made of a material which adheres to one side of the gauze. Comes in various widths.

d., transparent synthetic. Dressing usually made of a plastic material with the skin-contact side coated with a hypoallergenic adhesive.

d., universal. A large flat bandage that may be folded several times to make a relatively large dressing or folded several more times to make a smaller and thicker bandage. This process can be continued until the unit is suitable for use as a cervical collar. The bandage is easily made and stored. SEE: illus.

d., water. Dressing consisting of gauze, cotton, or similar dressing material that is kept wet by the application of sterilized water.

d., wet-to-dry. Dressing consisting of gauze moistened by sterile saline applied directly to wound and covered with dry gauze pads and a bandage. Used to prevent adherence of gauze to wound.

dressing stick. An adaptive device designed to permit independent dressing by persons with limited motion.

Dressler's syndrome [William Dressler, U.S. physician, 1890-1960]. A syndrome characterized by pericarditis, pericardial and pleural effusion, and fever. Occurs several weeks to many months post myocardial infarction. Etiology is unknown. Symptoms respond to aspirin or indomethacin therapy. SYN: *postmyocardial infarction syndrome.*

DRG. *diagnosis related group,* q.v.

drift. Movement due to an external force, often in an aimless fashion.

d., genetic. The chance variation of genetic frequency, seen most often in a small population.

d., mesial. Movement of teeth in the arch in a mesial or ventral direction due to occlusal forces and interproximal wear of teeth.

drill. Device for rotating a sharp and shaped cutting instrument. Used for preparing teeth for restoration and in orthopedics. SEE: *bur.*

Drinker respirator [Philip Drinker, U.S. engineer in industrial hygiene, 1894–1972]. Apparatus in which alternating positive and negative air pressure upon the patient's thoracic area, by allowing the air in the otherwise immobile lung to be alternately filled with air and emptied, acts to produce artificial respiration. Commonly called the iron lung.

drip [ME. *drippen*, to drip]. 1. To fall in drops. 2. To instill a liquid slowly, drop by drop.

d., intravenous. Slow injection of a suitable solution a drop at a time, intravenously.

d., Murphy. Slow rectal instillation of a fluid drop by drop.

d., nasal. Method of administering fluid slowly to dehydrated babies by means of a catheter with one end placed through the nose into the esophagus.

d., postnasal. A condition due to chronic sinusitis in which a discharge flows from the postnasal region into the pharynx.

drive (drīv) [AS. *drifan*]. The force or impulse to act.

drive controls. A variety of devices and adapted equipment, including hand or foot controls, for modifying a motor vehicle for use by persons with physical disability.

Drolban. Trade name for dromostanolone propionate.

dromomania (drŏ″mō-mā′nē-ă) [Gr. *dromos*, a running, + *mania*, madness]. Insane impulse to wander.

dromostanolone propionate (drŏ″mō-stăn′ō-lōn). USP. An antineoplastic drug. Trade name is Drolban.

dromotropic [″ + *tropikos*, a turning]. Pert. to supposed fibers in cardiac nerves that influence conductivity of muscles.

dronabinol. USP. Synthetic tetrahydrocannabinol, the psychoactive substance in mar-

UNIVERSAL DRESSING

ijuana. It is used as an antiemetic. Trade names are Deltanyne and Marinol.

drop [AS. *dropa*]. 1. A minute spherical mass of liquid. 2. Failure of a part to maintain its normal position. Usually due to paralysis or injury.

d., culture. A bacterial culture in a drop of culture medium.

d.'s, ear-. Medication administered by drops placed in the external canal of the ear.

d.'s, eye-. Medication placed in conjunctival sac.

d., foot. Condition in which toes drag and foot hangs, caused by paralysis of the anterior tibial muscles.

d., hanging. Application of a drop of solution to a small glass coverslip. This is then inverted over a glass slide with a depression in it. The contents of the suspended solution can be examined microscopically.

d.'s, knock-out. The myth that a nonlethal dose, i.e., a few drops, of a substance such as chloral hydrate can cause immediate unconsciousness if given orally or mixed with an alcoholic beverage. Movies have perpetrated and perpetuated this myth.

d.'s, nose. Medication instilled in or sprayed into the nasal cavity.

d., wrist. Paralysis of extensor muscles causing hand to hang down from forearm.

drop attack. A pattern of falling in the elderly due to motor abnormalities and fragility of bones. SEE: *stroke; transient ischemic attack.*

droperidol (drō-pĕr′ĭ-dŏl). USP. A drug used for premedication for surgery. It is neuroleptic, sedative, and tranquilizing. Trade name is Inapsine.

droplet. Very small drop.

droplet infection. Infection conveyed by means of infective particles, as when carried in a spray from the nose or mouth. Usual mode of infection for common cold.

dropper. A tube, usually narrowed at one end for dispensing drops of liquid. If water is so dispensed, about 20 drops will equal one milliliter. SEE: *d., medicine.*

d., medicine. According to *USP XXII,* a medicine dropper consists of a tube made of glass or other suitable transparent material that generally is fitted with a collapsible bulb and, while varying in capacity, is constricted at the delivery end to a round opening having an external diameter of 3 mm. The dropper, when held vertically, delivers water in drops, each of which weighs between 45 mg and 55 mg.

In using a medicine dropper, one should keep in mind that few medicinal liquids have the same surface and flow characteristics as water, and therefore the size of drops may vary considerably from one preparation to another.

When accuracy of dosage is important, a dropper that has been calibrated esp. for the preparation with which it is supplied should be employed. The volume error incurred in measuring any liquid by means of a calibrated dropper should not exceed 15% under normal use conditions.

dropsy (drŏp'sē) [Gr. *hydor*, water]. Obsolete term for generalized edema.

Drosophila (drō-sŏf'ĭ-lă). A genus of flies belonging to the order Diptera. Includes the common fruit flies.

   D. melanogaster. A genus of fruit flies used extensively in the study of genetics. The development of the chromosome theory of heredity was largely the outcome of research on this species.

drowning [ME. *dr(o)unen*, to drown]. Asphyxiation due to immersion in liquid. It may also result from a spasm of the glottis, which allows neither air nor water to pass into the lungs (dry drowning). An acute asphyxial reaction to ingested water or liquid followed by laryngeal relaxation and flooding of the respiratory tract with water is another mechanism of drowning (wet drowning). Drowning can occasionally result from vagally induced cardiac arrest after immersion in extremely cold water.

   NOTE: Delayed death due to hypoxia can occur 15 min to 3 days after immersion. It is imperative that resuscitated patients be kept in the hospital for observation until this possibility can be excluded.

   SYM: Unconsciousness, cessation of respiration, cyanosis, depending upon duration of submersion. Due to action of the epiglottis, there is very little, if any, water in the lung.

   F.A.: It is essential that immediate efforts to aerate the victim's lungs be made, but this will be futile if the airway is not clear. In addition, attempt to remove water that has been aspirated by use of the Heimlich maneuver. Air may be administered artificially by any means available including mouth-to-mouth resuscitation. Cardiac resuscitation may be required.

   It is important to examine for head or neck injuries, esp. if the patient had been diving into water where it was possible to strike a submerged object. If there is damage to the head, neck, or vertebral column, it is important to keep the neck in a neutral position. SEE: *cardiopulmonary resuscitation; diving reflex; drownproofing.*

   NOTE: Prolonged immersion does not necessarily mean that resuscitation will result in a brain-damaged individual. This is esp. true if the individual has been immersed in very cold water. SEE: *diving reflex.*

   RS: artificial respiration; asphyxia; shock; syncope; unconsciousness.

drownproofing. A method of staying afloat by using a minimum amount of energy. May be kept up for hours even by nonswimmers, whereas only the most fit and expert of swimmers could stay afloat for more than 30 minutes. Details of the drownproofing technique may be obtained from local chapters of the American Red Cross. SEE: illus.

   TECHNIQUE: 1. *Rest:* Take a deep breath and sink vertically beneath the surface, relax your arms and legs, keep chin down and allow fingertips to brush against knees. Keep neck relaxed and back of head above the surface. 2. *Get set:* Gently raise arms to a crossed position with back of wrists touching forehead. At the same time step forward with one leg and backward with the other. 3. *Lift head, exhale:* Without moving your arms and legs from the previous position, raise your head quickly but smoothly to the vertical and exhale through your nose. 4. *Stroke and kick, inhale:* To support your head above the surface while you inhale through your mouth, gently sweep the arms outward and downward and step downward with both feet. 5. *Head down, press:* As you drop beneath the surface, put your head down and press downward with your arms and hands to arrest your descent. 6. *Rest:* Important to relax completely as in the first step for six to ten seconds.

drowsiness. The state of almost falling asleep.

   d., day-time. Drowsiness occurring during the day rather than just prior to normal bedtime. The cause may be inadequate sleep the preceding night; however, it may also be associated with anxiety, ill health, or side effects of either prescribed drugs or drugs of abuse. The condition is not equivalent to narcolepsy, q.v.

Dr.P.H. *Doctor of Public Health.*

drug [O. Fr. *drogue,* chemical material]. Any substance that, when taken into the living organism, may modify one or more of its functions.

   d., designer. SEE: *"designer drug."*

   d.'s, generic. SEE: *generic drugs.*

   d.'s, look-alike. A group of solid dosage forms of drugs that mimic by size, shape, color, and markings various prescription drugs. Included may be controlled drugs.

   d., recreational. The abusive use of a drug for enjoyment rather than for a medical purpose.

   d., scheduled. SEE: *controlled substance act.*

drug abuse. The use or overuse, usually by self-administration, of any drug in a manner that deviates from the prescribed pattern.

Drug Abuse Warning Network. ABBR: DAWN. A system for obtaining statistical

DROWNPROOFING TECHNIQUE

1. Rest; 2. Get set; 3. Lift head, exhale; 4. Stroke and kick, inhale; 5. Head down, press; 6. Rest.

data concerning admissions to a sample of emergency treatment facilities for drug abuse.

drug action. Function of a drug in various body systems.

Local: When the drug is applied locally or directly to a tissue or organ, it may combine with the cells' albumin to form an albuminate. This action may be (1) astringent when the drug cannot act because the albuminate does not dissolve, (2) corrosive when the drug is strong enough to destroy cells, or (3) irritating when too much of the drug combines with cells to impair them.

General or systemic action: This occurs when the drug enters the bloodstream by absorption or direct injection, affecting tissues and organs not near the site of entry. Systemic action may be (1) specific when specific in the cure of a certain disease; (2) substitutive or replenishing when it supplies substances deficient in the body; (3) physical when some of the constituents of a cell are dissolved by the action of the drug in the bloodstream; (4) chemical when the drug or some of its principles combine with the constituents of cells or organs to form a new chemical combination; (5) salt action by osmosis, q.v., caused by dilution of salt (also acids, sugars, and alkalies) in the stomach or intestines by fluid withdrawn from the blood and tissues, or by diffusion, q.v., when water is absorbed by cells from the lymph; (6) selective, action produced by drugs that affect only certain tissues or organs; (7) synergistic, the increase in the action of one drug by another drug; (8) antagonistic, counteraction of one drug by another; (9) physiological, the potentially beneficial effect of a drug similar to that which the body normally produces; (10) therapeutic, the effect upon diseased organs or tissues; (11) side action, creating an effect not primarily desired; (12) empiric, an effect produced but not proved by clinical or laboratory tests to be effective; (13) toxicological, a toxic or undesired effect, generally the result of an overdose or long-term usage.

Cumulative: The effect of drugs that are slowly excreted or absorbed so that with repeated doses an accumulation of the drug in the body produces a toxic effect. Such drugs should not be administered continuously.

Incompatible: Production of undesired side effects when some drugs are administered together. This may be due to the antagonistic action of one drug to other drugs or to a physical interaction of the drugs to cause inactivation of one of the drugs, e.g., some drugs mixed in I.V. fluids will precipitate.

RS: active principle; adulteration; antidote; bioequivalence; biotransformation; dosage; dose response curve; double-blind test; names of individual drugs; names of poisons; prescription writing.

drug addiction. A condition caused by excessive or continued use of habit-forming drugs. Illicit drugs may or may not contain the kind and amount of drug the user thought was purchased. For this reason, a user may have a serious reaction (even death) to the unknown substance present in the material.

SYM: The symptom pattern may be changed according to the drug used. In general there may be a change in personality, loss of appetite, dulled appetite, disturbance in normal sleep-rhythm, generally a weight loss. The addict may be dull, sleepy, and uncoordinated in movement, having the appearance of intoxication. The eyes are often tearing and bloodshot; a watery fluid at times dripping from the nose. When intramuscular or intravenous injection is used, there may be scars and hardening and swelling of the arm tissues. Hepatitis or AIDS or both may occur when narcotic addicts use dirty needles and syringes for administering drugs to themselves or fellow addicts. SEE: *AIDS; hepatitis.*

drug administration. *Acids:* When administered orally, acids should be given well diluted through a glass tube or by stomach tube because they are corrosive to the enamel and dentin of the teeth. They should be given with much water, and the drinking tube should be placed well back in the mouth to prevent the fluid coming in contact with the teeth before passing into the throat. Diluted hydrochloric acid is one preparation that should always be given using this technique.

Habit-forming drugs: These should be given as ordered by the physician.

Horse serum: When injections containing it are administered, information should be obtained as to whether the patient has ever received horse serum and what reaction there was at that time. If the patient is allergic to horse serum, a test for sensitivity should always be done by injecting a few drops of the greatly diluted material containing horse serum hypodermically. Within a short time a reaction will occur. A small spot appears at the site of the injection if the patient has a tendency toward an unfavorable reaction. The physician will provide instructions for desensitizing a person allergic to horse serum.

Insulin: When this is administered, it should be given hypodermically or intravenously according to the instructions of the attending physician. The type of insulin, dosage, and frequency of dosage vary greatly with each patient. SEE: *insulin pump.*

Laxatives: These are best given in the evening because it usually takes 6 to 8 hours for them to produce an effect. Saline purgatives are usually given well diluted on an empty stomach in the morning. Other purgatives usually are given as ordered and needed.

Mouthwash: Stock solutions used for mouthwash should be diluted by one half or more before being given to the patient. Only enough for the immediate mouth washing should be given to the patient at a particular time.

Oxygen: The most commonly used method for administration of oxygen consists of inserting a catheter into a nostril or into each nostril. Oxygen may also be given from a tank by means of a mask over the patient's nose and mouth, or the patient may be placed in an oxygen tent, an oxygen chamber, or room. The last two methods are not only expensive and less effective than use of a mask or nasal catheters but are also extremely dangerous and must be used cautiously, as the danger from fire hazard is

very great. Oxygen given by catheter should be hydrated by bubbling through water prior to passage into the nose. Dry oxygen in high concentration for a prolonged period will cause severe irritation of the nasal and respiratory mucosa.

Saline purgatives: Should always be given to the patient when the stomach is empty, preferably in the morning.

Sleeping pills: All such preparations should be given from one-half to one hour before sleep is desired. All procedures should be taken care of before the medicament is given in order that nothing disturbs the patient after the drug is administered.

Vaccines: If the vaccines are alum-precipitated or alumina-absorbed, the preferred route of administration is intramuscular. Typhoid booster injections are given intracutaneously, and all other fluid preparations are given subcutaneously.

drug delivery, new methods of. A variety of methods of drug delivery has been used experimentally. Included are chemical modification of a drug to enable it to penetrate membranes such as the blood-brain barrier; incorporation of microparticles in colloidal carriers made of proteins, carbohydrates, lipids, or synthetic polymers; controlled release systems that permit a drug to be delivered for very long periods; transdermal controlled-release systems, e.g., those currently in use for administration of scopolamine or nitroglycerin. In addition to the use of various carriers for drugs, cell transplantation could be used to provide therapeutic agents, and the possibility of inserting genes into cells to produce desired effects is being explored. SEE: *liposomes.*

drug dependence. A psychic (and sometimes physical) state resulting from interaction of a living organism and a drug. Characterized by behavioral and other responses that include a compulsion to take the drug on a continuous or periodic basis in order to experience its psychic effects or to avoid the discomfort of its absence. Tolerance may or may not be present, and a person may be dependent on more than one drug.

drug eruption. Dermatitis medicamentosa.

drug-fast. Resistance, as of bacteria, to action of a drug or drugs.

drug fever. Fever caused by the administration of a drug or drugs. Almost any drug has the ability to produce in some individuals this undesired side effect.

druggist (drŭg′ĭst). Pharmacist.

drug handling. Carefully read the label or other printed instruction issued with medicine. Measure the ordered doses (quantities) accurately and never guess. A measuring glass or spoon should be used, marked in milliliters, ounces, or both. When giving a dose of medicine, be sure to whom it has to be given, what has to be given, when it has to be given, and the amount to be given. Do not leave the bedside until the patient actually swallows medicines intended to be taken orally.

NOTE: The cover must never be left off the container because a necessary property may evaporate, the drug may become dangerously concentrated, or it may absorb moisture from the air and become difficult to handle or dilute. The drug storage compartment must be kept locked.

drug interaction. The pharmacological interaction of drugs taken concurrently. The result may be antagonism, synergism, and consequently may be lethal in some cases. It is important for the patient, physician, and nurse to be aware of the potential interaction of drugs that are prescribed as well as those that the patient may be self-administering.

Many patients, especially the elderly, may take a variety of medicines each day. The chances of developing an undesired drug interaction increases rapidly as the number of drugs used increases. It is estimated that if 8 or more medications are being used, there is a 100% chance of interaction.

drug overdose. Literally, any excess dose of a drug, but in our present culture, the self-administration of a potentially lethal dose of a drug of abuse. The individual's action may be inadvertent in that the dose was an accustomed one but the potency of the "street drug" was much greater than expected. When such a dose results in coma or death, the person is said to have OD'd, i.e., overdosed. SEE: *Nursing Diagnoses* in *Appendix.*

drug product problem reporting program. A program managed by the United States Pharmacopeial Convention, Inc. The purpose is to inform the product manufacturer, the labeler, and the Food and Drug Administration (FDA) of potential health hazards and defective drug products. The reports may be submitted by any health professional.

drug rashes. Rashes produced in some patients by application or ingestion of drugs. In general, drug rashes are not specific for certain drugs. Therefore, the following should be used only as a rough guide.

Antibiotics: erythema. *Antipyrine:* papular, erythematous rash, sometimes accompanied by edema and much irritation. *Arsenic:* papular or erythematous rash, sometimes urticarial. Prolonged use may produce pigmentation of skin. *Belladonna:*

erythematous rash, usually accompanied by intense itching. *Bromides:* usually like acne vulgaris; sometimes erythema. *Chloral:* papular erythema. *Iodides:* usually papular erythema, sometimes with acnelike pustules. *Phenolphthalein:* macular rash, sometimes purpuric. *Quinine:* very irritable erythema or urticaria. *Salicylate:* erythematous rash, possibly morbilliform.

drug reaction. Adverse and undesired reaction to a substance taken for its pharmacological effects. An estimated 15% of hospitalized patients will develop toxic or allergic drug reactions. SEE: table.

drug receptors. The part or parts of a cell that interact with a drug or drugs. The proteins in cells in the form of enzymes are the most important class of drug receptors. Chemotherapeutic agents used in treating malignancies react with nucleic acid receptors. Some anesthetic agents react with lipid receptors on the cell membrane.

drugs, words pert. to: adulteration; ampule; analeptic; analgesic; anesthetic; antacid; anthelmintic; antiarthritic; antidiuretic; antiemetic; antipyretic; antiseptic; antispasmodic; bioequivalence; carminative; cathartic; convulsant; decoction; demulcent; depressant; diaphoretic; digestant; diuretic; ecbolic; elixir; emetic; expectorant; ferment; glucoside; half-life; hematinic; hemostatic; hormone; hypnotics; insulin pump; laxative; Medic Alert; medicine; oil; ointment; oxytocic; pharmacology; pharmacopeia; pill; purgative; rubefacient; sedative; solution; stimulant; synergism; tablet; tincture; tonic; troche; vaccine; vasoconstrictor; vasodilator; vermicide.

drum. The eardrum of tympanic cavity; the tympanum or cavity of the middle ear.

drunkenness [AS. *drinean,* to drink]. Alcoholic intoxication. In legal medicine, intoxication or being "under the influence" of alcohol is defined according to the concentration of alcohol in the blood or exhaled air. The precise concentration used to define legal intoxication varies between states. Clinically, a blood level of 0.3% to 0.4% of ethyl alcohol is classed as marked intoxication. A level of 0.4% to 0.5% is consistent with alcoholic stupor, and a level over 0.5% is sufficient to cause alcoholic coma.

drusen (droo'zĕn) [Ger. *Druse,* weathered ore]. Small, hyaline, globular pathological growths formed on optic papilla or on Descemet's membrane.

dry eye. In certain conditions there is insufficient lubrication in the eye and the conjunctiva becomes much less moist than normal. This produces pain and discomfort in the eyes. This may occur in any condition that

Comparison of Toxic and Allergic Drug Reactions*

	Toxic	Allergic
Incidence	May occur with any drug	Occurs infrequently
Dosage	Usually high	Therapeutic
Reaction time	May occur with first dose, or may be due to cumulative effect	Usually only upon re-exposure, but some drugs cross-react with chemicals of similar structure
Symptoms	May be similar to pharmacological action of drug	Not related to pharmacological action of drug
Associated disorders	None	Asthma, hay fever

* Differences may be indistinct. Shock from drug overdose may be no different from allergic shock.

causes scars of the cornea, such as erythema multiforme, trachoma, or corneal burns; Sjögren's syndrome; lagophthalmos; Riley-Day syndrome; absence of lacrimal gland; paralysis of the facial or trigeminal nerves; medication with atropine; deep anesthesia; and debilitating diseases. Suitably prepared water-soluble polymers are effective in treating this condition.

dry ice. Solidified carbon dioxide used for commercial refrigeration. Also used in the form of a pencil-shaped block for treating certain skin lesions, such as warts, by freezing. The temperature of solid carbon dioxide is −78.5°C. For this reason it is extremely important to use thick cloth gloves when handling it. Momentary skin contact with dry ice can cause severe frostbite and blisters.

dry measure. A measure of volume for dry commodities. SEE: *Weights and Measures* in *Appendix*.

dry mouth. Decrease or lack of saliva. This condition may be due to the action of drugs such as anorectics, anticholinergics, antidepressants, antihistamines, diuretics, nicotine, caffeine, hypnotics, or sedatives. Radiation therapy in the area of the salivary glands may destroy those glands. SYN: *xerostomia*. SEE: *Sjögren's syndrome; saliva, artificial*.

TREAT: Pilocarpine may help. If saliva is completely absent, saliva substitutes are beneficial. Dry mouth due to dehydration is ameliorated by fluid intake.

Drysdale's corpuscles (drīz'dālz) [Thomas M. Drysdale, U.S. gynecologist, 1831–1904]. Non-nucleated granular cells present in the fluid of certain ovarian cysts.

DSA. *digital subtraction angiography.* SEE: *angiography, digital subtraction.*

DTIC-Dome. Trade name for dacarbazine.

DT's. *delirium tremens.*

dualism (dū'ă-lĭzm) [L. *duo*, two, + Gr.

-ismos, condition]. 1. The condition of being double or twofold. 2. The theory that the human individual consists of two entities, mind and matter, that are independent of each other. 3. The theory that various blood cells arise from two types of stem cells; myeloblasts giving rise to the myeloid elements, and lymphoblasts giving rise to the lymphoid elements.

dual personality. A form of multiple personality seen in hysteria and schizophrenia that results in the expression of two different phases of personality at various intervals, neither personality as a rule being aware of the words, acts, and feelings of the other. When this occurs in schizophrenia, the individual psychic function is split off from the personality as a whole and becomes autonomous. This may be unrelated to and contradictory of the main personality. SEE: *dissociation of personality; multiple personality; vigilambulism.*

duazomycin (dū-ăz"ō-mī'sĭn). An antineoplastic agent.

Dubini's disease (dū-bē'nēz) [Angelo Dubini, It. physician, 1813–1902]. Rapid rhythmic contractions of a group or groups of muscles. SYN: *chorea, electric; spasmus Dubini.*

Dubin-Johnson syndrome [Isadore Nathan Dubin, U.S. pathologist, 1913-1980; Frank B. Johnson, U.S. pathologist, b. 1919]. Inherited defect of bile metabolism that causes retention of conjugated bilirubin in hepatic cells. The patient is mildly jaundiced.

duboisine (dū-bŏy'sēn). Alkaloid derivative of plant *Duboisia myoporoides*. It is a form of hyoscyamine used as a mydriatic.

Dubowitz tool or score [Lilly and Victor Dubowitz, contemporary South African physicians]. A method of estimating the gestational age of an infant based on 21 strictly defined physical and neurological signs.

This method provides the correct gestational age ± 2 weeks in 95% of infants.

Duchenne, Guillaume B. A. (dū-shěn'). French neurologist, 1806–1875.

D.'s disease. Degeneration of the posterior roots and column of the spinal cord and of the brain stem. Characterized by attacks of pain, progressive ataxia, loss of reflexes, functional disorders of the bladder, larynx, and gastrointestinal system, and impotence. Develops in conjunction with syphilis and most frequently affects middle-aged males. SYN: *tabes dorsalis.*

D.'s muscular dystrophy. Pseudohypertrophic muscular dystrophy characterized by weakness and pseudohypertrophy of the affected muscles. The disease begins in childhood, is progressive, and affects the shoulder and pelvic girdle muscles. The disease, mostly of males, is transmitted as a sex-linked recessive trait. Death usually occurs at an early age. SEE: *Nursing Diagnoses* in *Appendix.*

D.'s paralysis. Bulbar paralysis.

Duchenne-Aran disease (dū-shěn'är-än') [Duchenne; Francois Amilcar Aran, Fr. physician, 1817–1861]. Progressive spinal muscular atrophy, characterized by chronic progressive wasting of muscles with subsequent weakness and paralysis. The upper extremity is most commonly involved. Caused by degeneration of the anterior horn cells of the spinal cord. Occasionally the bulbar nuclei of the brain are involved. A variety of conditions may lead to the development of this disease: infections, avitaminosis, or toxins.

Duchenne-Erb paralysis (dū-shěn'ayrb) [Duchenne; Wilhelm Heinrich Erb, Ger. neurologist, 1840–1921]. Paralysis of muscles supplied by nerves from the upper brachial plexus.

Ducrey's bacillus (dū-krāz') [Augusto Ducrey, It. dermatologist, 1860–1940]. Small, rod-shaped organism found in pairs, the cause of chancroid or soft chancre. SYN: *Haemophilus ducreyi.*

duct [L. *ducere,* to lead]. 1. A narrow tubular vessel or channel, esp. one serving to convey secretions from a gland. 2. A narrow enclosed channel containing a fluid, as the semicircular duct of the ear.

d., accessory pancreatic. Duct of the pancreas leading into the pancreatic duct or the duodenum near the mouth of the common bile duct.

d., alveolar. A branch of a respiratory bronchiole that leads to the alveolar sacs of the lungs.

d., Bartholin's. The major duct of the sublingual gland.

d.'s, biliary. Canals that carry bile. The intrahepatic ducts include the bile canaliculi and interlobular ducts; the extrahepatic ducts include the hepatic, cystic, and common bile ducts. SYN: *bile ducts.*

d., cochlear. Canal of the cochlea.

d., common bile. Duct formed by the confluence of the hepatic and cystic ducts. Conveys bile to the duodenum opening at the papilla of Vater. SYN: *ductus choledochus* [NA].

d., cystic. Excretory duct of the gallbladder.

d., efferent. One of a group of 12 to 14 small tubes that constitute the efferent ducts of the testis. They lie within the epididymis and connect the rete testis with the ductus epididymidis. Their coiled portions constitute the lobuli epididymidis.

d., ejaculatory. Duct that conveys semen into uretha.

d., endolymphatic. In the embryo, a tubular projection of the otocyst ending in a blind extremity, the endolymphatic sac. In the adult, it connects the endolymphatic sac with the utricle and saccule.

d., excretory. Any duct that conveys a product from an organ as the excretory duct of a salivary gland.

d., Gartner's. A remnant of the wolffian duct extending from the parovarium through the broad ligament into the vagina.

d.'s, hepatic. Ducts that receive bile from right and left lobes of liver and carry it to the common bile duct. SYN: *ductus hepaticus dexter* [NA]; *ductus hepaticus sinister* [NA].

d., interlobular. Duct passing between lobules within a gland, e.g., one of the ducts carrying bile.

d., lacrimal. One of two short ducts, inferior and superior, that convey tears from the lacrimal lake to the lacrimal sac. Their openings are on the margins of the upper and lower eyelids. SYN: *canal, lacrimal.*

d.'s, lactiferous. A group of 15 to 20 ducts that drain the lobes of the mammary gland. Each opens in a slight depression in the tip of the nipple.

d., Leydig's. D., mesonephric.

d., lymphatic. One of two main ducts conveying lymph to the bloodstream; the left lymphatic duct (thoracic duct) and the right lymphatic duct. SEE: *lymphatic system* for illus.

d., lymphatic, left. D., thoracic.

d., lymphatic, right. Duct that drains lymph from the right side of the body above the diaphragm. Discharges into the right innominate vein. Smaller than the left lymphatic duct.

d.'s, mammary. D.'s, lactiferous.

d., mesonephric. Duct that, in the embryo, connects the mesonephros with the cloaca. In the male, it develops into the reproductive ducts (duct of epididymis, deferent duct, seminal vesicle, and ejaculatory duct). In the female, it gives rise to the duct of the epoophoron, a rudimentary structure. SYN: *wolffian duct.*

d., metanephric. Ureter.

d.'s, milk. D.'s, lactiferous.

d.'s, müllerian. Bilateral ducts in the embryo that form the uterus, vagina, and fallopian tubes. SYN: *Müller's ducts.*

d., nasolacrimal. Duct that conveys tears from the lacrimal sac to the nasal cavity. It opens beneath the inferior nasal concha.

d.'s of Rivinus. Five to 15 ducts (the minor sublingual ducts) that drain the posterior portion of the sublingual gland.

d. of Santorini. Accessory pancreatic duct.

d. of the epoophoron. Gartner's duct, q.v.

d. of Wirsung. D., pancreatic.

d., omphalomesenteric. D., vitelline.

d., pancreatic. Duct that conveys pancreatic juice to the duodenum. SYN: *d. of Wirsung.*

d.'s, papillary. Any of the large collecting tubules of the kidney.

d., paramesonephric. The genital canal in the embryo. In the female, it develops into the oviducts, uterus, and vagina; in the male, it degenerates to form the appendix testis.

d.'s, paraurethral. D.'s, Skene's.

d., parotid. Duct through which secretions from the parotid gland enter into mouth. SYN: *d., Stensen's.*

d.'s, prostatic. About 20 ducts that discharge prostatic secretion into the urethra. SYN: *ductus prostatici* [NA].

d.'s, salivary. Any of the ducts that drain a salivary gland.

d.'s, secretory. The smaller canals of a gland.

d., segmental. A pair of embryonic tubes located between visceral and parietal layers of mesoblast on each side of the body.

d.'s, semicircular. Three membranous tubes forming a part of the membranous labyrinth of the inner ear. They lie within the semicircular canals and bear corresponding names: anterior, posterior, and lateral.

d.,'s seminal. Any of the ducts that convey semen, specifically the ductus deferens and the ejaculatory duct.

d.'s, Skene's. Two slender ducts of Skene's glands that open on either side of the urethral orifice in the female. SYN: *d.'s, paraurethral.*

d., spermatic. Excretory duct of the testicle that later joins the duct of the seminal vesicle to become the ejaculatory duct. SYN: *ductus deferens* [NA]; *vas deferens.*

d., Stensen's. D., parotid.

d., striated. A class of ducts contained within the lobules of glands, esp. salivary glands, that contain radially appearing striations within the cells, denoting the presence of mitochondria.

d.'s, sublingual. Excretory ducts of the sublingual gland. SEE: *d., Bartholin's.*

d., submandibular. Duct of the submandibular gland. It opens on a papilla at the side of the frenulum of the tongue.

d.'s, tear. Ducts that convey tears. Include excretory ducts of lacrimal glands, and lacrimal and nasolacrimal ducts.

d., testicular. D., spermatic.

d., thoracic. The left lymphatic duct. Drains the left side of the body above the diaphragm and all of the body below the diaphragm. Discharges into the left innominate vein.

d., umbilical. D., vitelline.

d., utriculosaccular. A narrow tube emanating from the utricle and opening into the endolymphatic duct.

d., vitelline. The narrow duct that, in the embryo, connects the yolk sac (umbilical vesicle) with the intestine. SYN: *d., umbilical; yolk stalk.*

d., Wharton's. Duct of the submandibular gland. SYN: *d., submandibular.*

d., wolffian. D., mesonephric.

duct ectasia. An inflammatory condition of the lactiferous ducts of the breast. There is nipple discharge, nipple inversion, breast mass, and periareolar sepsis. This occurs at all ages following menarche. The condition resembles carcinoma of the breast. SYN: *nonpuerperal mastitis.*

ETIOL: Unknown, but in some cases may be associated with hyperprolactinemia due to a pituitary tumor.

TREAT: Surgical drainage of abscess and antibiotics.

ductile (dŭk′tĭl) [L. *ductilis*, fr. *ducere*, to lead]. Capable of being elongated without breaking.

duction. In ophthalmology, the rotation of an eye about an axis. This movement is made by the action of the extraocular muscles.

ductless [L. *ducere*, to lead, + AS. *loessa*, less]. Having no duct, secreting only internally.

ductless glands. Glands without ducts; they secrete internally one or more hormones that have a specific action upon the body. SEE: *endocrine gland; exocrine.*

ductule (dŭk′tūl). A very small duct.

d., aberrant. One of a group of small tubules associated with the epididymis. They end blindly, representing the vestigial remains of the caudal group of mesonephric tubules.

ductulus (dŭk′tū-lŭs). Ductule, or small duct.

ductus (dŭk′tŭs) (pl. *ductus*). [NA] Duct, q.v.

d. arteriosus. [NA] A channel of communication between the main pulmonary artery and the aorta of the fetus.

d. arteriosus, patent. SEE: *patent ductus arteriosus.*

d. choledochus. [NA] The common bile duct.

d. cochlearis. [NA] The cochlear duct. SYN: *scala media.*

d. deferens. [NA] Excretory duct of the testicle. Conveys sperm from the epididymis to the ejaculatory duct. SYN: *vas deferens.*

d. epoophori longitudinalis. The caudal part of the mesonephric duct. It normally degenerates but may persist in the female. SYN: *duct of the epoophoron.*

d. hemithoracicus. [NA] Ascending branch of the thoracic duct, opening either into the right lymphatic duct or close to the angle of union of the right subclavian and right internal jugular veins.

d. hepaticus. A duct about 3 in. (7.6 cm) long, formed by union of the cystic and hepatic ducts. Carries the bile to the intestine.

d. hepaticus dexter. [NA] Duct issuing from the right lobe of the liver and uniting with the ductus hepaticus sinister to form the hepatic duct. Drains the right and caudate lobes.

d. hepaticus sinister. [NA] Duct that unites with the ductus hepaticus dexter to form the hepatic duct. Drains the left and caudate lobes.

d. prostatici. [NA] Ducts for carrying secretions from the prostate into the urethra.

d. reuniens. The endolymph-containing canal of the inner ear that connects the saccule with the cochlear duct. SYN: *Hensen's canal.*

d., utriculosaccularis. [NA] Small tube connecting the saccule of the internal ear with the utricle.

d. venosus. [NA] The smaller, shorter, and posterior of two branches into which the umbilical vein divides after entering the abdomen. Empties into the inferior vena cava.

Duffy system. A blood group consisting of two antigens determined by allelic genes. SEE: *blood groups.*

Duke Longitudinal Study. Three studies that focused on the normal aging process in middle-aged and older persons. Subjects were given periodic physical, mental, and social examinations at the Duke University Medical Center.

Duke method. SEE: *bleeding time.*

Dulcolax. Trade name for bisacodyl.

dull [ME. *dul*]. 1. Not resonant on percussion. 2. Not mentally alert. 3. Having a boring personality.

dullness. 1. Lack of normal resonance on percussion. 2. State of being dull.

d., shifting. Upon percussing the abdominal cavity, an area of dullness is found to shift as body position is changed. This indicates that the dullness is related to a collection of peritoneal fluid in the cavity.

dumb [AS.]. Lacking the power or faculty to speak. SYN: *mute.*

dumbness. Muteness.

dumping. 1. In medical care, the practice of transferring a patient who is unable to pay for care to a hospital that accepts such patients. 2. The abandoning of elderly individuals in hospital emergency departments.

dumping syndrome. Syndrome characterized by sweating and weakness after eating. Occurs in patients who have had gastric resections. Exact cause is unknown but rapid emptying (i.e., dumping of the stomach contents) into the small intestine is associated with the symptoms. It is often ameliorated by a regimen of small meals at frequent intervals.

duodenal (dū-ō-dē′năl, dū-ŏd′ĕ-năl) [L. *duodeni*, twelve]. Pert. to the duodenum.

duodenal bulb. Area of duodenum just beyond the pylorus.

duodenal delay. Delay in the movement of food through the duodenum due to conditions such as inflammation of lower portion of the intestine, which reflexly inhibits duodenal movements.

duodenal ulcer. Damaged mucous membrane, usually accompanied by suppuration. Sometimes a sore that bleeds is present. This creates danger of perforation. A duodenal ulcer heals slowly due to constant passage of irritating fluids, enzymes, and food over it. SEE: *peptic ulcer.*

duodenectasis (dū″ō-děn-ěk′tă-sĭs) [″ + Gr. *ektasis*, expansion]. Chronic dilatation of the duodenum.

duodenectomy (dū″ō-děn-ěk′tō-mē) [″ + Gr. *ektome*, excision]. Excision of part or all of the duodenum.

duodenitis (dū″ŏd-ě-nī′tĭs) [″ + Gr. *itis*, inflammation]. Inflammation of the duodenum.

duodenocholecystostomy (dū″ō-dē″nō-kō-lĭ-sĭs-tŏs′tō-mē) [″ + Gr. *chole*, bile, + *kystis*, bladder, + *stoma*, mouth]. Formation by surgical means of a fistula between the duodenum and gallbladder. SYN: *duodenocystostomy.*

duodenocholedochotomy (dū″ō-dē″nō-kō-lěd-ō-kŏt′ō-mē) [″ + Gr. *choledochos,* bile duct, + *tome,* incision]. Surgical incision of the duodenum to reach the gallbladder.

duodenocystostomy (dū″ō-dē″nō-sĭs-tŏs′tō-mē). Duodenocholecystostomy.

duodenoenterostomy (dū″ō-dē″nō-ĕn″tĕr-ŏs′tō-mē) [″ + Gr. *enteron,* intestine, + *stoma,* mouth]. Formation of passage between the duodenum and intestine.

duodenogram (dū-ŏd′ĕ-nō-grăm) [″ + Gr. *gramma,* something written]. A roentgenogram of the duodenum.

duodenography (dū″ō-dē-nŏg′-ră-fē) [″ + Gr. *graphein,* to write]. Radiographic examination of the duodenum.

   d., hypotonic. Radiographic examination of the duodenum after medication has been administered to halt the peristaltic action of the gastrointestinal tract.

duodenohepatic (dū-ŏd″ē-nō″hĕ-păt′ĭk) [″ + Gr. *hepatos,* liver]. Pert. to duodenum and liver.

duodenoileostomy (dū″ō-dē″nō-ĭl″ē-ŏs′tō-mē). Surgical establishment of a communication between the duodenum and ileum.

duodenojejunostomy (dū″ō-dē″nō-jē-joo-nŏs′tō-mē) [″ + *jejunum,* empty, + Gr. *stoma,* mouth]. Making a passage between the duodenum and jejunum.

duodenorrhaphy (dū″ō-dē-nor′ă-fē) [″ + Gr. *rhaphe,* seam, ridge]. Suturing the duodenum.

duodenoscopy (dū″ŏd-ē-nŏs′kō-pē) [″ + Gr. *skopein,* to examine]. Inspection of the duodenum with an endoscope.

duodenostomy (dū″ŏd-ē-nŏs′tō-mē) [″ + Gr. *stoma,* mouth]. Surgical formation of a permanent opening into the duodenum through the wall of the abdomen.

duodenotomy (dū″ŏd-ē-nŏt′ō-mē) [″ + Gr. *tome,* incision]. An incision into the duodenum.

duodenum (dū″ō-dē′nŭm, dū-ŏd′ĕ-nŭm) [L. *duodeni,* twelve]. [NA] The first part of the small intestine, connecting with the pylorus of the stomach and extending to the jejunum. The duodenum receives hepatic and pancreatic secretions through the same duct (duct of Wirsung). It is 8 to 11 in. (20 to 28 cm) long, the average length being 10 in. (25 cm). Brunner's glands and Lieberkühn's glands are found in the duodenum. Chyle is formed there. It is a crucial section of the alimentary canal. In it occurs the mixing of acid chyme from the stomach, bile from the liver and gallbladder, pancreatic juice, and intestinal juices secreted by the glands of Brunner and Lieberkühn. The nerve supply comes from the celiac plexus. Pancreaticoduodenal branches of the hepatic and superior mesenteric arteries and the right gastric artery supply blood. SEE: *abdominal quad-*

rants and *digestive system* for illus.

ACTION: The entry of acid chyme into the duodenum brings about discharge of bile from the gallbladder and the secretion of pancreatic juice by the pancreas. These enter through the duct of Wirsung. Bile salts alkalinize the chyme and emulsify the fats. Through the action of pancreatic enzymes, the following changes occur: steapsin (pancreatic lipase) hydrolyzes neutral fats to fatty acids and glycerol; amylopsin (pancreatic amylase) hydrolyzes starch to maltose; maltase hydrolyzes maltose to glucose. Three proteolytic enzymes (trypsin, chymotrypsin, and peptidase) act on proteins, hydrolyzing them to proteoses, peptones, and amino acids.

Secretory phenomena: At least two substances are secreted by the duodenum. One of these, secretin, q.v., stimulates the pancreas to increase production of its juice. The other, cholecystokinin-pancreozymin, causes the gallbladder to contract and force its contents through the bile duct, to the duct of Wirsung, and then into the duodenum. In addition, nervous mechanisms contribute to the coordination that exists here, regulating the rate of discharge of chyme from the stomach, varying both quality and quantity of the various secretions, and determining the rate of passage through the duodenum.

Motor phenomena: The first part of the duodenum (pars superior, duodenal cap, duodenal bulb) is the small portion immediately following the pylorus of the stomach. It is regularly full of material and consequently visible in roentgenograms as a spade-shaped shadow. The next part (pars descendens) is that into which the common bile duct (ductus choledochus) and pancreatic ducts open. Movement through it and through the pars inferior and the pars ascendens is so rapid that they are normally inconspicuous on x-ray film. Throughout the duodenum the mucosa is thrown into folds (plicae circulares). The folds are permanent and inactive. The villi, which stud the surface of the folds as well as the spaces between them, exhibit waving and thrusting movements.

RS: bile; Brunner's glands; choledochoduodenostomy; digestion; duodenal ulcer; enzyme; gallbladder; gastric juice; intestine; Lieberkühn crypts; liver; pancreas; pancreatic juice; succus entericus.

duplication, duplicature [L. *duplicare,* to double]. A doubling or folding of a part or of an organ, or state of being folded.

duplicitas (dū-plĭs′ĭ-tăs). Fetal abnormality in which an organ or a part is doubled or apparently doubled.

dupp (dŭp). In cardiac auscultation, the expression for the second heart sound heard over the apex. This sound is shorter and of higher pitch than *lubb*, the first heart sound. SEE: *auscultation; heart.*

Dupuytren, Baron Guillaume (dū-pwē-trän'). French surgeon, 1777–1835.
　　D.'s contracture. Contracture of palmar fascia usually causing the ring and little fingers to bend into the palm so that they cannot be extended. This condition tends to occur in families, after middle age, and more frequently in men. There is no correlation between occupation and development of this condition. It is associated with liver disease and long-term use of phenytoin.
　　ETIOL: Unknown.
　　TREAT: Surgical removal of the tissue causing the contracture. SEE: *contracture, Dupuytren's,* for illus.
　　D.'s fracture. Fracture dislocation of the ankle. The talus is displaced upward.

dura (dū'ră) [L. *durus,* hard]. Dura mater.

Durabolin. Trade name for nandrolone phenpropionate.

Duracillin. Trade name for penicillin G procaine.

dural (dū'răl) [L. *durus,* hard]. Pert. to the dura.

dura mater [L., hard mother]. The outer membrane covering the spinal cord (dura mater spinalis [NA]) and brain (dura mater cerebri [NA] or dura mater encephali [NA]). SEE: *pia mater; tentorium cerebelli.*

duramatral. Pert. to the dura. SYN: *dural.*

Durand-Nicolas-Favre disease. Lymphogranuloma venereum, q.v.

duraplasty [" + Gr. *plassein,* to form]. Plastic repair of the dura mater.

Duraquin. Trade name for quinidine gluconate.

duration. The average length of time a disorder is present in a patient.

durematoma (dū"rĕm-ă-tō'mă) [" + Gr. *haima,* blood, + *oma,* tumor]. Accumulation of blood between arachnoid and dura.

duritis (dū-rī'tĭs) [" + Gr. *itis,* inflammation]. Inflammation of the dura. SYN: *pachymeningitis.*

duroarachnitis (dū"rō-ăr"ăk-nī'tĭs) [" + Gr. *arachne,* spider, + *itis,* inflammation]. Inflammation of dura and arachnoid membrane.

Duroziez' murmur (dū-rō"zē-āz') [Paul Louis Duroziez, Fr. physician, 1826–1897]. The systolic and diastolic murmur heard over a large artery when pressure is applied to the area just distal to the stethoscope.

dust. Minute, fine particles of earth; any powder, esp. something that has settled from the air.
　　d., blood. Hemoconia, q.v.

d., ear. Fine calcareous bodies found in the gelatinous substance of the otolithic membrane of the ear; otoconium or otoliths.
　　d., house. The total of particles present in the air in a house. Materials included are mites, hairs, fibers, pollens, and smoke particles.

dust cells. Reticuloendothelial cells in the walls of the alveoli of the lungs that ingest or destroy dust particles.

dusting powder. Any fine powder for dusting on skin.
　　d.p., absorbable. USP. Powder prepared from cornstarch. It is used as a lubricant for surgical gloves.

Duverney's fracture (dū-věr-nāz') [Joseph G. Duverney, Fr. anatomist, 1648–1730]. Fracture of the ilium.

Duverney's gland. The vulvovaginal gland.

Duvoid. Trade name for bethanechol chloride.

D.V.M. *Doctor of Veterinary Medicine.*

dwarf [AS. *dweorg,* dwarf]. An abnormally short or undersized person.
　　d., achondroplastic. Type of dwarfism characterized by normal trunk but shortened extremities, a large head, and prominent buttocks.
　　d., asexual. Dwarf with deficient sexual development.
　　d., hypophyseal. Dwarf whose condition resulted from hypofunction of the anterior lobe of the hypophysis.
　　d., infantile. Dwarf with marked physical, mental, and sexual underdevelopment.
　　d., micromelic. Dwarf with very small limbs.
　　d., ovarian. An undersized female due to absence or underdevelopment of the ovaries.
　　d., phocomelic. Dwarf with abnormally short diaphyses of either pair of extremities or of all four.
　　d., physiologic. A person normally developed except for stature.
　　d., pituitary. D., hypophyseal.
　　d., primordial. Dwarf in whom there is a selective deficiency of growth hormone but with otherwise normal endocrine function.
　　d., rachitic. Dwarf whose condition is due to rickets.
　　d., renal. Dwarf whose condition is due to renal osteodystrophy.
　　d., thanatophoric. Type of dwarfism caused by generalized failure of endochondral bone formation. Characterized by large head, prominent forehead, hypertelorism, saddle nose, and short limbs extending straight out from trunk. Most of these infants die soon after birth.

dwarfism. Condition of being abnormally small. May be hereditary or a result of endocrine dysfunction, deficiency diseases, renal insufficiency, diseases of the skeleton, or other causes.

Dwyer instrumentation. Surgical procedure for stabilization of scoliosis. The spine is approached from the front and bolts are inserted transversely through each vertebral body. A cable attached to the bolts is applied to the convexity of the curve and the vertebrae are pulled together.

Dy. Chem. symb. for the element dysprosium.

dyad [Gr. *duas*, pair]. 1. A pair. 2. A pair of chromosomes formed by the division of a tetrad in meiosis. A dyad represents a single chromosome split precociously for a subsequent division. 3. In chemistry, a bivalent element or radical. 4. In psychiatry, two people in an interactional situation.

dyadic. Pertaining to the social interaction between two people.

Dycem. Registered trademark name for nonslip material often used by persons with use of only one arm to stabilize objects (such as plates) on tables and work surfaces.

Dycill. Trade name for dicloxacillin sodium.

Dyclone. Trade name for dyclonine hydrochloride.

dyclonine hydrochloride (dī'klō-nēn). USP. A topical anesthetic used in otolaryngology. Trade name is Dyclone.

dye. Any substance that is of itself colored or that is used to impart color to another material such as a thin slice of tissue prepared for microscopic examination. Dyes may also be employed in manufacturing test reagents used in medical laboratories.

dying. The condition in which death seems imminent.

Even though death is inevitable, persons in the medical care field receive almost no guidance or instruction in how to deal with the patient who asks, "Am I dying?", or with those related to the patient. The dying person may find it less difficult to discuss death with the physician than with family members or close associates. Another aspect of death, esp. in patients with incurable disease, is how does society and the physician deal with persons who ask for assistance in committing suicide. This problem has not been resolved in the U.S. In some countries, assisted suicide is legal.

Considering all of this, the physician and all concerned health care workers must be prepared to provide emotional, physical, and spiritual support to the dying patient. This is, of course, done in a compassionate, open, and dignified way. Dying patients should not be isolated from their family. The family will need to be reassured that all that can be done is being done for the dying person. SEE: *acceptance; advance directive;*

assisted suicide; death; death with dignity; denial and isolation; do not attempt resuscitation; living will; tender loving care; United Network for Organ Sharing (UNOS).

dynamia (dī-năm'ē-ă) [Gr. *dynamis*, power]. Vital energy or ability to combat disease.

dynamic (dī-năm'ĭk). Pert. to vital force or inherent power. Opposed to static.

dynamics. The science of bodies in motion and their forces.

> **d., group.** SEE: *group dynamics.*
> **d., population.** SEE: *population dynamics.*

dynamic splint. 1. A splint fabricated with moving parts to allow mobility by providing forces that substitute for weak or absent muscle strength. 2. A spring-loaded splint designed to apply a constant low intensity stretch force to a stiff joint or an adaptively shortened musculotendinous unit.

dynamogenesis (dī"nă-mō-jĕn'ē-sĭs) [" + *genesis,* generation, birth]. The capacity to call forth increased energy.

dynamogenic [" + *gennan,* to produce]. Pert. to, or caused by, an increase of energy.

dynamograph (dī-năm'ō-grăf) [" + *graphein,* to write]. Device for recording muscular strength.

dynamometer (dī"nă-mŏm'ē-tĕr) [" + *metron,* measure]. 1. Device for measuring muscular strength. 2. Device for determining the magnifying power of a lens.

dynamoneure (dī-năm'ō-nūr) [" + *neuron,* nerve]. A motor spinal nerve cell.

dynamoscope (dī-năm'ō-skōp) [" + *skopein,* to examine]. Instrument for auscultation of muscles.

dynamoscopy (dī-năm-ŏs'kō-pē). 1. Auscultation of muscles. 2. Visual evaluation of the function of an organ or system.

Dynapen. Trade name for dicloxacillin sodium.

dyne (dīn) [Gr. *dynamis,* power]. Force needed for imparting an acceleration of 1 cm per second to a 1-gm mass.

dynein. A very large protein that has a molecular configuration that resembles arms. Contraction of these dynein arms facilitates the movement of cilia and flagella of bacteria. SEE: *immotile cilia syndrome; Kartagener's syndrome.*

Dyrenium. Trade name for triamterene.

dys- [Gr.]. Prefix meaning bad, difficult, painful, disordered.

dysacousia, dysacusis, dysacousma (dĭs"ă-koo'zē-ă, -koo'sĭs, -kooz'mă) [Gr. *dys,* bad, + *akousis,* hearing]. 1. Discomfort caused by loud noises. 2. Difficulty in hearing.

dysadrenalism (dĭs"ăd-rē'năl-ĭzm). Disordered function or disease of the adrenal gland.

dysantigraphia (dĭs″än-tĭ-grăf′ē-ă) [″ + *anti*, against, + *graphein*, to write]. Inability to copy writing or printed letters.

dysaphia (dĭs-ă′fē-ă) [″ + *haphe*, touch]. Dullness of the sense of touch.

dysaptation, dysadaptation. Impaired ability of the iris of the eye to accommodate to varying intensities of light.

dysarthria (dĭs-ăr′thrē-ă) [″ + *arthroun*, to utter distinctly]. 1. Difficult and defective speech due to impairment of the tongue or other muscles essential to speech. Mental function is intact. 2. Inability to speak in which there is no defect in the ability to understand and, if literate, to read or write. The cause may be due to lower motor neuron disease, certain nervous system diseases, or cerebellar lesions.

dysarthrosis [″ + *arthrosis*, joint]. Joint malformation or deformity.

dysautonomia (dĭs″aw-tō-nō′mē-ă) [″ + *autonomia*, freedom to use own laws]. A rare hereditary disease involving the autonomic nervous system characterized by mental retardation, motor incoordination, vomiting, frequent infections, and convulsions. It is seen almost exclusively in Ashkenazi Jews. SEE: *Mecholyl test.*

dysbarism (dĭs′băr-ĭzm) [″ + *barys*, heavy, + *-ismos*, condition]. Symptom complex following exposure of body to less-than-atmospheric pressure in air flight or altitude chamber. When occurring in severe form, sometimes called decompression sickness or bends, q.v.

dysbasia (dĭs-bā′zē-ă) [″ + *basis*, a step]. Difficulty in walking, esp. when due to disease of the brain or spinal cord.

dysboulia (dĭs-bū′lē-ă) [″ + *boulē*, will]. 1. Inability to fix the attention; difficulty experienced in thinking; mind weariness. 2. Weak and uncertain willpower.

dyscalculia (dĭs″kăl-kū′lē-ă) [″ + L. *calculare*, to compute]. Disability with respect to using mathematics. Although this disorder is common, it is poorly understood.

dyscephaly (dĭs-sĕf′ă-lē). Malformation of the head and facial bones.

dyschezia (dĭs-kē′zē-ă) [″ + *chezein*, to defecate]. Painful or difficult bowel movements.

dyschiria (dĭs-kī′rē-ă) [″ + *cheir*, hand]. Inability to tell which side of the body has been touched. If referred to the wrong side it is called allochiria, q.v., or allesthesia, q.v. If referred to both sides it is called synchiria, q.v. SYN: *achiria.*

dyschondroplasia (dĭs″kŏn-drō-plā′zē-ă) [″ + *chondros*, cartilage, + *plassein*, to form]. Disease, usually hereditary, resulting in disordered growth. Characterized by multiple exostoses of growth of the epiphyses, esp. of the long bones, metacarpals, and phalanges. SYN: *chondrodysplasia; Ollier's disease.*

dyschroa, dyschroia (dĭs-krō′ă, dis-kroy′ă) [″ + *chroia*, complexion]. Discolored skin, esp. of the face; poor or bad complexion.

dyschromatopsia (dĭs″krō-mă-tŏp′sē-ă) [″ + *chroma*, color, + *opsis*, vision]. Imperfect color vision.

dyschromia. Discoloration, as of the skin.

d., nail. Discoloration of fingernails and toenails. Pigmented bands in the nails may be related to Addison's disease, Peutz-Jeghers syndrome, pregnancy, use of minocycline, radiotherapy, cytotoxic drugs, antimalarials, and zidovudine therapy in AIDS patients.

dyschronism (dĭs-krō′nĭzm) [″ + *chronos*, time]. 1. Disturbed time relation, esp. that which occurs when one is transported from one time zone to one that is 5 to 10 hours ahead of or behind the original. This leads to disturbances of biological rhythms. SYN: *jet lag.* 2. Separate as to time.

dyscinesia (dĭs-sĭ-nē′zē-ă). Impairment in ability to perform voluntary movement. SYN: *dyskinesia.*

dyscoria (dĭs-kō′rē-ă) [″ + *kore*, pupil]. Abnormal form or shape of the pupil.

dyscrasia (dĭs-krā′zē-ă) [Gr. *dyskrasia*, bad temperament]. An old term meaning abnormal mixture of the four humors. The word is now used as a synonym for disease.

dyscrasic (dĭs-krā′sĭk). Pert. to dyscrasia.

dyscrinism (dĭs-krī′nĭzm) [Gr. *dys*, bad, + *krinein*, to secrete, + *-ismos*, condition of]. Any disorder of secretions, esp. of an endocrine gland.

dysdiadochokinesia (dĭs″dī-ăd″ō-kō-kĭ-nē′sē-ă) [″ + *diadochos*, succeeding, + *kinesis*, movement]. Inability to quickly substitute antagonistic motor impulses to produce antagonistic muscular movements.

dysembryoplasia (dĭs-ĕm″brē-ō-plā′sē-ă) [″ + *embryon*, embryo, + *plassein*, to form]. Fetal malformation occurring during growth of the embryo.

dysemia [″ + *haima*, blood]. Any blood disease.

dysenteric (dĭs″ĕn-tĕr′ĭk). Pert. to dysentery.

dysentery (dĭs′ĕn-tĕr″ē) [″ + *enteron*, intestine]. A term applied to a number of intestinal disorders, esp. of the colon, characterized by inflammation of the mucous membrane.

SYM: Abdominal pain, tenesmus, diarrhea with passage of mucus or blood.

ETIOL: Bacterial or viral infection; infestation by protozoa or parasitic worms; chemical irritants.

d., amebic. Dysentery due to amebas.

d., bacillary. An acute infectious disease caused by bacteria of the genus *Shigella*, esp. *S. dysenteriae, S. boydii, S. flexneri,* and *S. sonnei.* It may occur sporadically or in epidemics. In addition to intestinal symptoms, a severe toxemia may occur due to exo- and endotoxins produced by the organisms.

d., balantidial. Dysentery caused by the ciliate protozoan *Balantidium coli.*

d., malignant. A form of dysentery in which symptoms are very pronounced and progress rapidly, usually terminating fatally.

d., viral. Dysentery caused by virus.

dysergia (dĭs-ĕr′jē-ă) [Gr. *dys,* bad, + *ergon,* work]. Lack of coordination in muscular voluntary movements.

dysesthesia (dĭs″ĕs-thē′zē-ă) [″ + *esthesia,* sensation]. Abnormal sensations on the skin, such as experiencing a feeling of numbness, tingling, prickling, burning, or cutting pain. SEE: *paresthesia.*

d., auditory. Abnormal discomfort from loud noises. SYN: *dysacusia.*

d. pedis. Severe itching and burning of the plantar surface of the feet and toes. May occur as a reaction to heparin therapy.

dysfunction (dĭs-fŭnk′shŭn) [″ + L. *functio,* a performance]. Abnormal, inadequate, or impaired function of an organ or part.

dysgalactia [″ + *gala,* milk]. Defective milk secretion.

dysgammaglobulinemia. Disproportion in the concentration of immunoglobulins in the blood. May be congenital or acquired.

dysgenesis (dĭs-jĕn′ĕ-sĭs) [″ + *genesis,* generation, birth]. Defective or abnormal development, particularly in the embryo.

d., gonadal. Congenital endocrine disorder caused by failure of the ovaries to respond to pituitary hormone (gonadotropin) stimulation. Clinically there is amenorrhea, failure of sexual maturation, and usually short stature. About one third of these patients have webbing of the neck and may have cubitus valgus. Intelligence may be impaired. SYN: *Turner's syndrome.*

ETIOL: Due to a defect in or absence of the second sex chromosome.

dysgenic [″ + *gennan,* to produce]. Pert. to dysgenesis.

dysgenitalism [″ + L. *genitalia,* organs of reproduction, + Gr. *-ismos,* condition]. Condition caused by abnormal genital development.

dysgerminoma (dĭs″jĕr-mĭn-ō′mă) [″ + L. *germen,* a sprout, + Gr. *oma,* tumor]. A malignant neoplasm of the ovary.

dysgeusia (dĭs-gū′zē-ă) [″ + *geusis,* taste]. Impairment or perversion of the gustatory sense such that normal tastes are inter-

preted as being unpleasant or completely different from the characteristic taste of a particular food or chemical compound. SEE: *hypogeusia, idiopathic; cacogeusia; heterogeusia; phantogeusia.*

dysglandular [″ + L. *glans,* acorn]. Abnormal functioning of glands, esp. those of internal secretion.

dysglobulinemia (dĭs-glŏb″ū-lĭn-ē′mē-ă) [″ + L. *globulus,* globule, + Gr. *haima,* blood]. Abnormality of the amount or quality of blood globulins.

dysgnathia (dĭs-nā′thē-ă) [″ + *gnathos,* jaw]. Abnormality of the mandible and maxilla.

dysgnosia (dĭs-nŏ′sē-ă) [Gr. *dysgnosia,* difficulty of knowing]. Any anomaly of intellect.

dysgonesis (dĭs″gō-nē′sĭs) [Gr. *dys,* bad, + *gone,* seed]. 1. Functional disorder of the genital organs. 2. Poor growth of bacterial culture.

dysgonic. Bacterial cultures of sparse growth.

dysgraphia (dĭs-grăf′ē-ă) [″ + *graphein,* to write]. 1. Inability to write properly. Usually the result of a brain lesion. 2. Writer's cramp.

dyshematopoiesia (dĭs-hĕm″ă-tō-poy-ē′sē-ă) [″ + *haima,* blood, + *poiein,* to make]. Imperfect blood formation.

dyshidria (dĭs-hĭd′rē-ă) [″ + *hidros,* sweat]. Dyshidrosis.

dyshidrosis (dĭs-hī-drō′sĭs) [″ + ″ + *osis,* condition]. 1. Disorder of the sweating apparatus. 2. A recurrent vesicular eruption on skin of hands and feet marked by intense itching. SEE: *pompholyx.*

TREAT: The control of sweating or proper absorption of perspiration will be of benefit. For the feet, wearing absorbent socks, well-ventilated shoes, and application of substances that reduce sweating will help to control symptoms. Individuals who do not wear shoes are rarely found to have this disorder. Acute attacks will respond to treatment with a corticosteroid in an ointment combined with iodoquinol. This is applied at night with an occlusive dressing.

dysidrosis (dĭs-ī-drō′sĭs). Dyshidrosis, q.v.

dyskaryosis (dĭs-kăr″ē-ō′sĭs). Abnormality of the nucleus of a cell.

dyskeratosis (dĭs″kĕr-ă-tō′sĭs) [″ + *keras,* horn, + *osis,* condition]. 1. Epithelial alterations in which a certain number of isolated malpighian cells become differentiated. 2. Any alteration in the keratinization of the epithelial cells of the epidermis. Characteristic of many skin disorders.

dyskinesia (dĭs″kĭ-nē′sē-ă) [″ + *kinesis,* movement]. Defect in voluntary movement.

d. algera. Hysterical condition in which

quick active movement is painful.

d., biliary. Failure of the sphincter of Oddi to relax normally. This prevents the flow of bile from the gallbladder to the intestinal tract.

d. intermittens. Limb disability occurring intermittently.

d., tardive. Condition of slow, rhythmical, automatic stereotyped movements, either generalized or in single muscle groups. These occur as an undesired effect of therapy with certain psychotropic drugs, esp. the phenothiazines.

d., uterine. Pain in the uterus on movement.

dyskinetic. Concerning dyskinesia.

dyslalia (dĭs-lā'lē-ă) [" + lalein, to talk]. Impairment of speech due to defect of speech organs.

dyslexia (dĭs-lĕk'sē-ă) [" + lexis, diction]. An imprecise term concerning a condition in which an individual with normal vision is unable to interpret written language. The condition is more common in males and is usually noticed in the child with reading difficulty in the first grade. These individuals can see and recognize letters but are unable to spell and write words. They have no difficulty recognizing the meaning of objects and pictures. Dyslexia is unrelated to intelligence. Some great intellects, including Thomas Edison, Albert Einstein, Woodrow Wilson, and Winston Churchill, are thought to have been dyslexic.

Exact cause is unknown. Recent evidence indicates that function of the left hemisphere of the brain of dyslexics is different from that of normals. The results of other studies propose that, in dyslexics, there is an error in timing of reception of visual stimuli so that one of two major visual stimuli pathways is not received in the right line sequence. SEE: alexia.

dyslogia (dĭs-lō'jē-ă) [" + logos, word, reason]. Difficulty in expressing ideas.

dysmasesis (dĭs"mă-sē'sĭs) [" + masesis, mastication]. Difficulty in masticating.

dysmaturity. Condition in which infants weigh less than would be expected for the known length of the gestational period. These infants are sometimes referred to as being small-for-date. SYN: intrauterine growth retardation.

dysmegalopsia [" + megas, big, + opsis, vision]. Inability to visualize correctly the size of objects; they appear larger than they really are.

dysmelia (dĭs-mē'lē-ă) [" + melos, limb]. Congenital deformity or absence of a portion of one or more limbs.

dysmenorrhea (dĭs"mĕn-ō-rē'ă) [" + men, month, + rhein, to flow]. Pain in association with menstruation. One of the most frequent gynecologic disorders, it is classified into primary, q.v., and secondary, q.v. An estimated 50% of menstruating women experience this disorder, and about 10% of these are incapacitated for several days each period. This disorder is the greatest single cause of absence from school and work among menstrual-age women. In the U.S., this illness causes the loss of an estimated 140,000,000 work hours each year. SEE: premenstrual tension syndrome.

NURSING IMPLICATIONS: In young women experiencing discomfort or pain during menstruation, encourage medical evaluation to rule out underlying causative disorders. Support and assist the individual to cope with this problem. Encourage well-balanced diet and moderate exercise. Use of mild heat to abdomen may be helpful. Patient may find assistance by using strategies such as biofeedback, and referral to a support or self-help group may be warranted. SEE: Nursing Diagnoses in Appendix.

d., congestive. Condition caused by pelvic congestion.

d., inflammatory. Condition caused by pelvic inflammation.

d., membranous. A severe spasmodic dysmenorrhea that is accompanied by the passage of a cast or partial cast of the uterine cavity.

d., primary. SYM: The pain usually begins just before or at the onset of menstruation. The pain is spasmodic and located in the lower abdomen, but it may also radiate to the back and thighs. Also included in some individuals are nausea, vomiting, diarrhea, low back pain, headache, dizziness, and in severe cases, syncope and collapse. These symptoms may last from a few hours to several days but seldom persist for more than 3 days. These symptoms tend to decrease or disappear after the individual has experienced childbirth the first time, and to decrease with age. It is much more common than secondary dysmenorrhea.

ETIOL: The exact cause is unknown, but uterine ischemia due to increased production of prostaglandins with increased contractility of the muscles of the uterus (i.e., the myometrium) is felt to be the principal mechanism. As in any disease or symptom, the individual's reaction to and tolerance of pain will influence the extent of the disability experienced. Primary dysmenorrhea is not a behavioral or psychologic disorder.

One study revealed that prevalence and severity of dysmenorrhea may be reduced in those who use oral contraceptives, and that severity was increased in those with long duration of menstrual flow, in those who smoked, and in those who had early menarche. Exercise did not influence the prevalence or severity of dysmenorrhea.

DIAG: A cramping, labor-like pain that starts just prior to or at the onset of menstruation. The first attack occurs with or shortly after menarche and occurs subsequently only if preceded by ovulation; pelvic examination is normal. It is essential that secondary dysmenorrhea be ruled out.

TREAT: Oral contraceptives and nonsteroidal, anti-inflammatory drugs including aspirin; mefenamic acid (trade name is Ponstel) or ibuprofen (trade name is Motrin); or naproxen (trade name is Naprosyn). These medicines should be taken in the appropriate dose 3 to 4 times a day and with milk to lessen the chance of gastric irritation.

d., secondary. This condition frequently causes pain quite similar to that of the primary form of dysmenorrhea, but it usually begins some years after menarche. A history of the occurrence of pain in association with pelvic inflammatory disease, or use of an IUD, or endometriosis, or fertility problems suggests the diagnosis of secondary dysmenorrhea.

TREAT: Therapy for the underlying disease and in the meantime use of nonsteroidal, anti-inflammatory drugs.

d., spasmodic. Dysmenorrhea caused by uterine contractions of spasmodic form.

dysmetria (dĭs-mē′trē-ă) [Gr. *dys*, bad, + *metron*, measure]. Inability to fix the range of a movement in muscular activity. Rapid and brusque movements are made with more force than necessary. Seen in cerebellar affections.

RS: adiadochokinesis; asynergia; gait.

dysmetropsia [″ + ″ + *opsis*, vision]. Inability to visualize correctly the size and shape of things.

dysmimia (dĭs-mĭm′ē-ă) [″ + *mimos*, imitation]. 1. Inability to express oneself by gestures or signs. 2. Inability to imitate.

dysmnesia (dĭs-nē′zē-ă) [″ + *mneme*, memory]. Any impairment of memory.

dysmorphophobia (dĭs″mor-fō-fō′bē-ă) [″ + *morphe*, formed, + *phobos*, fear]. Irrational fear of being deformed or the illusion that one is deformed.

dysmorphosis (dĭs″mor-fō′sĭs) [″ + ″ + *osis*, condition]. Not normal in form.

dysmyotonia (dĭs″mī-ō-tō′nē-ă) [″ + *mys*, muscle, + *tonos*, tone]. Muscle atony; abnormal muscle tonicity.

dysnomia. Forgetting words or having difficulty finding words for written or oral expression.

dysodontiasis (dĭs″ō-dŏn-tī′ă-sĭs) [″ + *odous*, tooth, + *-iasis*, process]. Painful or difficult dentition.

dysomnias (dĭs-ōm′nē-ăz) [″ + L. *somnus*, sleep]. Any disturbance involving the amount, quality, or timing of sleep. SEE: *sleep.*

dysontogenesis (dĭs″ŏn-tō-jĕn′ĕ-sĭs) [″ + *ontos*, being, + *gennan*, to produce]. Defective development of an organism, esp. of an embryo.

dysontogenetic. Pert. to dysontogenesis.

dysopia, dysopsia (dĭs-ō′pē-ă, ŏp′sē-ă) [″ + *opsis*, vision]. Defective vision.

dysorexia (dĭs″ō-rĕk′sē-ă) [″ + *orexis*, appetite]. Perverted or lessened appetite.

dysosmia (dĭs-ŏz′mē-ă) [″ + *osme*, smell]. Distortion of normal smell perception.

dysostosis (dĭs″ŏs-tō′sĭs) [″ + *osteon*, bone, + *osis*, condition]. Defective ossification.

d., cleidocranial. A congenital ossification of the skull with partial atrophy of clavicles.

d., craniocerebral. A hereditary disease characterized by ocular hypertelorism, exophthalmos, strabismus, widening of the skull, high forehead, beaked nose, and hypoplasia of the maxilla.

d., mandibulofacial. Hypoplasia of the facial bones; downward sloping of the palpebral tissues; defects of the ear; macrostomia; and a fish-face appearance. It occurs in two forms that are thought to be autosomal dominants.

dysoxidizable [″ + L. *oxidum*, oxide]. Not easy to oxidize.

dyspancreatism [″ + *pankreas*, pancreas, + *-ismos*, condition]. Impaired pancreatic function.

dyspareunia (dĭs″pă-rū′nē-ă) [″ + *pareunos*, lying beside]. Occurrence of pain in the labial, vaginal, or pelvic areas during or after sexual intercourse. This common condition has been difficult to investigate because most women do not discuss it with health care providers.

ETIOL: Infections in the reproductive tract; inadequate vaginal lubrication; uterine myomata; endometriosis; atrophy of vaginal mucosa; psychosomatic causes; and vaginal foreign bodies.

TREAT: Specific therapy for primary disease; counseling with respect to appropriate vaginal and vulval lubrication (Vaseline is of no benefit).

dyspepsia (dĭs-pĕp′sē-ă) [″ + *peptein*, to digest]. Imperfect or painful digestion. Not a disease in itself but symptomatic of other diseases or disorders. Characterized by vague abdominal discomfort, a sense of fullness after eating, eructation, heartburn, nausea and vomiting, and loss of appetite. These symptoms may occur irregularly and in different patterns from time to time. The symptoms are increased in times of stress. SYN: *indigestion*.

d., acid. Dyspepsia due to excessive acidity of the stomach.

d., alcoholic. Dyspepsia caused by excessive use of alcoholic beverages.

d., biliary. Form of dyspepsia in which there is insufficient quantity or quality of bile secretion.

d., cardiac. Form of dyspepsia occurring during heart disease.

d., gastric. Dyspepsia caused by faulty stomach function.

d., gastrointestinal. Dyspepsia caused by faulty function of stomach and intestines.

d., hepatic. Dyspepsia caused by liver disease.

d., hysterical. Dyspepsia present during hysterical attacks.

dyspeptic (dĭs-pĕp′tĭk). 1. Affected with or pert. to dyspepsia. 2. One afflicted with dyspepsia.

dyspermasia [″ + *sperma*, seed]. Dyspermia.

dyspermatism. Dyspermia.

dyspermia. Difficult or painful emission of sperm during coitus.

dysphagia (dĭs-fā′jē-ă) [″ + *phagein*, to eat]. Inability to swallow or difficulty in swallowing. SEE: *achalasia; cardiospasm.*

d. constricta. Dysphagia due to narrowing of the pharynx or esophagus.

d. lusoria. Dysphagia caused by pressure exerted on the esophagus by an anomaly of the right subclavian artery.

d., oropharyngeal. Difficulty in propelling food or liquid from the oral cavity into the esophagus.

d. paralytica. Dysphagia due to paralysis of muscles of deglutition and esophagus.

d., spastica. Dysphagia resulting from a spasm of pharyngeal or esophageal muscles.

dysphagy (dĭs′fă-jē). Dysphagia.

dysphasia (dĭs-fā′zē-ă) [″ + *phasis*, speech]. Impairment of speech resulting from a brain lesion.

dysphonia (dĭs-fō′nē-ă) [″ + *phone*, voice]. Difficulty in speaking; hoarseness.

d. clericorum. Hoarseness due to public speaking.

d. puberum. Change or breaking in voice in boys at time of puberty.

d., spasmodic. Dysphonia due to spasmodic contraction of all of the muscles involved with speech production. Actions involving many of the same muscles, i.e., swallowing and singing, are usually unaffected. The condition is usually nonprogressive and is not thought to be due to psychological factors.

TREAT: In general, therapy has been ineffective. Injection of botulinum toxin into one or both thyroarytenoid muscles of the larynx has been used experimentally. The injections must be repeated several times a year.

dysphoria (dĭs-fō′rē-ă) [″ + *pherein*, to bear]. Exaggerated feeling of depression and unrest without apparent cause; a mood of general dissatisfaction, unpleasantness, restlessness, anxiety, discomfort, unhappiness.

dysphrasia (dĭs-frā′zē-ă) [Gr. *dys*, bad, + *phrasis*, speech]. Impairment of speech due to a brain lesion. SYN: *dysphasia.*

dysphylaxia (dĭs-fĭ-lăk′sē-ă) [″ + *phylaxis*, protection]. Waking too early from sleep.

dyspigmentation (dĭs″pĭg-mĕn-tā′shŭn). Abnormality of the skin or hair pigment.

dyspituitarism (dĭs″pĭ-tū′ĭ-tăr-ĭzm) [″ + L. *pituita*, mucus, + Gr. *-ismos*, condition]. Condition due to disorder of the pituitary body.

dysplasia [″ + *plassein*, to form]. Abnormal development of tissue. SYN: *alloplasia; heteroplasia.*

d., anhidrotic. Congenital condition marked by absent or deficient sweat glands, intolerance of heat, and abnormal development of teeth and nails.

d., cervical. Abnormal changes in the tissues covering the cervix uteri.

d., chondroectodermal. Condition marked by defective development of bones, nails, teeth, and hair and by congenital heart disease. SYN: *Ellis-van Creveld syndrome.*

d., hereditary ectodermal. Hereditary defect marked by few or absent sweat glands and hair follicles, smooth shiny skin, abnormal or absent teeth, nail deformities, cataracts or alterations of cornea, absence of mammary glands, concave face, prominent eyebrows, conjunctivitis, deficient hair growth, and mental retardation.

d., monostotic fibrous. Replacement of bone by fibrous tissue. Marked by pain usually in tibia or femur. Cause is unknown.

d., polyostotic fibrous. Replacement of bone by a vascular fibrous tissue. Marked by difficulty in walking and multiple bone deformities and fractures. Usually commences in childhood. Cause is unknown.

dyspnea (dĭsp-nē′ă, dĭsp′nē-ă) [″ + *pnoē*, breathing]. Air hunger resulting in labored or difficult breathing, sometimes accompanied by pain. Normal when due to vigorous work or athletic activity.

SYM: Audible labored breathing, distressed anxious expression, dilated nostrils, protrusion of abdomen and expanded chest, gasping, marked cyanosis.

ETIOL: Insufficient oxygenation of the blood resulting from disturbances in the lungs, low oxygen pressure of air, circulatory disturbances, hemoglobin deficiency. Other causes may be acidosis, excessive CO_2 content of blood, lesions of the respiratory center, emotional excitation, hyperexcitability of Hering-Breuer reflex, cardiac asthma, and orthopnea. It may be a subjective feeling.

NURSING IMPLICATIONS: Assess for alleviating and aggravating factors. Do a complete respiratory assessment to identify additional symptoms of respiratory distress. Obtain arterial blood gas values. Make sure airway is patent. Place patient in a high Fowler's position, orthopneic position, or position of comfort. Administer oxygen and medications as ordered. Remain with the patient until breathing becomes less labored and anxiety has decreased. When patient is more comfortable, conduct a more thorough interview and examination to obtain data about patient's cardiopulmonary status and previous dyspneic episodes.

_d._, cardiac. Dyspnea due to cardiac insufficiency, as in acute myocardial infarction.

_d._, expiratory. Dyspnea as in asthma and bronchitis; wheezing and painful expiration. Secretions in respiratory tract cause the sound.

_d._, inspiratory. Dyspnea due to interference in passage of air to the lungs.

_d._, paroxysmal nocturnal. Attacks of shortness of breath which usually occur at night and awaken the patient. This is due to advanced forms of heart failure associated with elevations of pulmonary venous and capillary pressures. Previously, incorrectly termed cardiac asthma.

dyspneic (dĭsp-nē'ĭk). Affected with or due to dyspnea.

dyspraxia (dĭs-prăk'sē-ă) [" + _prassein,_ achieve]. A disturbance in the programming, control, and execution of volitional movements. It cannot be explained by absence of comprehension, inadequate attention, or lack of cooperation; usually associated with a stroke, head injury, or any condition affecting the cerebral hemispheres.

dysprosium (dĭs-prō'sē-ŭm). SYMB: Dy. At. wt. 162.50; at. no. 66. A metallic element of the yttrium group of rare earths.

dysprosody (dĭs-prŏs'ō-dē). Lack of the normal rhythm, melody, and articulation of speech. This condition may be present in patients with parkinsonism.

dysraphia, dysraphism (dĭs-rā'fē-ă, -fĭzm)

[" + _rhaphe,_ seam, ridge]. In the embryo, failure of raphe formation or failure of fusion of parts that normally fuse.

_d._, spinal. A general term applied to failure of fusion of parts along the dorsal midline. May involve any of the following structures: skin, vertebrae, skull, meninges, brain, and spinal cord.

dysreflexia. Uncontrollable increase in sympathetic activity that cannot be inhibited in children with spinal cord injury.

dysrhythmia (dĭs-rĭth'mē-ă) [" + _rhythmos,_ rhythm]. Abnormal, disordered, or disturbed rhythm.

dysstasia [" + _stasis,_ standing]. Difficulty in standing.

dysstatic. Exhibiting difficulty in standing.

dyssynergia [" + _synergia,_ cooperation]. Failure of muscular coordination. SYN: _ataxia._

dystaxia (dĭs-tăk'sē-ă) [" + _taxis,_ arrangement]. Partial ataxia.

dystectia (dĭs-tĕk'shē-ă) [" + L. _tectum,_ roof]. In the embryo, failure of closure of the neural tube. Thus, deformities such as spina bifida cystica or meningocele are produced.

dysteleology (dĭs"tē-lē-ŏl'ō-jē) [" + _telos,_ end, + _logos,_ word, reason]. Study of rudimentary organs that have no apparent useful purpose.

dysthymia (dĭs-thī'mē-ă) [" + _thymos,_ mind]. A chronic, mild form of depression that has been present for at least two years. It occurs twice as frequently in women as in men.

dysthyreosis (dĭs"thī-rē-ō'sĭs) [" + _thyreos,_ shield, + _osis,_ condition]. Impaired functional activity of thyroid gland. SYN: _dysthyroidism._

dysthyroidism (dĭs-thī'roy-dĭzm) [" + " + _eidos,_ form, shape, + _-ismos,_ condition]. Imperfect development and function of the thyroid gland.

dystocia (dĭs-tō'sē-ă) [" + _tokos,_ birth]. Difficult labor. May be produced by either the size of the passenger (the fetus) or the small size of the pelvic outlet.

FETAL CAUSES: Usually large babies. Other factors are malpositions of the fetus (transverse, face, brow, breech, or compound presentation); abnormalities of the fetus (hydrocephalus, tumors of the neck or abdomen, hydrops); multiple pregnancy (interlocked twins).

MATERNAL CAUSES: _Uterus:_ Primary and secondary uterine inertia; congenital anomalies of the uterus (bicornuate uterus); tumors of the uterus (fibroids, carcinoma of the cervix); abnormal fixation of the uterus by previous operation. _Bony pelvis:_ Contracted pelvis; generally contracted pelvis; flat and generally contracted pelvis; funnel pelvis; exostoses of the pelvic bones; tumors of the pelvic bones. *Cervix uteri:* Bandl's contraction ring; rigid cervix that will not dilate; stenosis and stricture preventing dilatation. *Ovary:* Ovarian cysts that block the pelvis. *Vagina and vulva:* Cysts; tumors; atresias and stenoses. *Pelvic soft tissues:* Distended bladder or colon.

DIAG: Can generally be made by vaginal examination, ultrasound, and external pelvimetry before the patient goes into labor.

TREAT: Varies according to the condition present that causes the dystocia. The goal is correction of the abnormality in order to allow the fetus to pass. If this is not possible, operative delivery is necessary. SEE: *cesarean section.*

dystonia (dĭs-tō′nē-ă) [″ + *tonos*, tone]. Prolonged muscle contractions that may cause twisting and repetitive movements or abnormal posture. These movements may be in the form of rhythmic jerks. The condition may progress in childhood, but progression is rare in adults. In children the legs are usually affected first.

ETIOL: In most cases no cause can be discovered. The syndrome may be associated with a great variety of metabolic or neurologic diseases and other conditions such as head trauma, viral encephalitis, stroke, brain tumor, toxic levels of manganese or carbon disulfide, wasp stings, and undesired side effects of drugs used in treating parkinsonism and antipsychotic medicines.

TREAT: Discontinue medicines if they are implicated; treat specific diseases associated with the condition. Anticholinergic drugs; levodopa; and injection of botulinum toxin in focal dystonias such as blepharospasm or torticollis; physiotherapy; psychotherapy.

d. musculum deformans. A rare progressive syndrome that usually begins in childhood and in most patients is invariably progressive. Characterized by distorted twisting or movement of a part or all of the body. The posture may be bizarre and the position is sustained. The inherited pattern is seen in families from northern Europe. The patient remains mentally normal. The bizarre posture is abolished in sleep, but eventually it may persist even then.

ETIOL: Unknown.

TREAT: It is important that the patient not be treated as if the disease were due to hysteria or mental illness. There is no specific therapy but anticholinergics and reserpine may be of benefit. The most effective therapy has involved use of cryothalamec-

tomy to destroy a portion of the ventrolateral nucleus of the thalamus. SYN: *torsion dystonia of childhood.*

dystonic. Pert. to dystonia or hyper- or hypotonicity of tissues.

dystopia (dĭs-tō′pē-ă) [″ + *topos,* place]. Malposition; displacement of any organ.

d. canthorum. Lateral displacement of the inner canthi of the eyes.

dystopic (dĭs-tŏp′ĭk). Not in place.

dystopy (dĭs′tō-pē) [″ + *topos,* place]. Dystopia.

dystrophia (dĭs-trō′fē-ă) [″ + *trephein,* to nourish]. Disorder caused by defective nutrition or metabolism. SYN: *dystrophy.*

dystrophic (dĭs-trŏf′ĭk). Pert. to dystrophia.

dystrophoneurosis (dĭs-trŏf″ō-nū-rō′sĭs) [″ + *trephein,* to nourish, + *neuron,* nerve, + *osis,* condition]. Defective nutrition caused by disease of the nervous system.

dystrophy (dĭs′trō-fē). Disorder caused by defective nutrition or metabolism. SYN: *dystrophia.*

d., adiposogenital. A condition characterized by a peculiar type of obesity and hypogenitalism due to a disturbance in the hypothalamus, which controls food intake, and of the pituitary, which controls gonadal development. SYN: *Fröhlich's syndrome.*

d., Landouzy-Déjérine. A hereditary form of progressive muscular dystrophy with onset in childhood or adolescence. Characterized by atrophic changes in muscles of shoulder girdle and face, inability to raise arms above the head, myopathic facies, eyelids that remain partly open in sleep, and inability to whistle or purse lips. SYN: *atrophy, Landouzy-Déjérine.*

d., progressive muscular. A familial disease characterized by progressive atrophy and wasting of muscles. Onset is usually at an early age, and it occurs more frequently in males than females. Its cause is thought to be a genetic defect in muscle metabolism.

d., pseudohypertrophic muscular. A hereditary disease usually beginning in childhood in which muscular ability is lost. At first there is muscular pseudohypertrophy, followed by atrophy.

dysuria (dĭs-ū′rē-ă) [″ + *ouron,* urine]. Painful or difficult urination, symptomatic of numerous conditions. Dysuria may be indicative of cystitis; urethritis; infection anywhere in the urinary tract; urethral stricture; hypertrophied, cancerous, or ulcerated prostate in the male; prolapse of uterus in the female; pelvic peritonitis and abscess; metritis; cancer of the cervix; dysmenorrhea; or psychological abnormalities.

May also be caused by certain medications, esp. opiates and medicines used to prevent motion sickness. Pain and burning may also be caused by concentrated acid urine. SEE: *urinary tract infection.*

dysuriac. One affected with dysuria.

dyszooamylia (dĭs-zō″ō-ăm-ĭl′ē-ă) [″ + *zoon*, animal, + *amylon*, starch]. Failure of liver to transform dextrose into glycogen.

dyszoospermia (dĭs″zō-ō-spĕrm′ē-ă) [″ + ″ + *sperma*, seed]. Imperfect formation of spermatozoa.

E

E. *emmetropia; energy; Escherichia; eye.*
E$_1$. *estrone.*
E$_2$. *estradiol.*
E$_3$. *estriol.*
e. *electric charge; electron;* L. *ex,* from.
ea. *each.*
EACA. *epsilon-aminocaproic acid.*
ead. L. *eadem,* the same.
Eales' disease (ēlz) [Henry Eales, Brit. physician, 1852–1913]. Recurrent hemorrhages into the retina and vitreous, most commonly seen in males in the second and third decades of life. The cause is unknown.
ear [AS. *ear*]. Organ of hearing. Consisting of external, middle, and internal ear. SEE: illus.; *Baranay's caloric test; hearing, functional test for; labyrinth* for additional illus.

EXAM: Hearing ability may be estimated by asking the patient to repeat phrases or answer questions that the examiner states while facing away from the patient. For accuracy, however, the hearing should be tested by using an accurately calibrated audiometer. This is esp. true if the test of hearing acuity is done on an individual who works in a noisy environment. Comparing subsequent tests of hearing with the original or baseline record will permit determining the effect, if any, of the noisy work environment on the individual's hearing.

Also examine for color, size, and shape of ear; discharge from middle or inner ear; tenderness upon pressure in front or back of ear; inflammation or bulging of drum; perforations or scars of drum. Deafness may indicate wax in the external ear canals, blocked eustachian tubes, disorders of the 8th (vestibulocochlear) nerve, disease of the middle ear, or the toxic effect of drugs. Pallor of ears, tongue, and gums indicates shock or anemia. Ringing in ears may be noted in cerebral hyperemia and anemia, in disease of ear, Ménière's disease, and after use of certain drugs such as quinine or those containing salicylic acid, e.g., aspirin; also occurs without any discernible cause. SEE: *hearing, sensorineural.*

NURSING IMPLICATIONS: Teach patients to keep ears clean and protect from trauma and infection by never inserting any object into the ear canal or beyond. Avoid forceful nose blowing that can push secretions into the middle ear via the eustachian tube. Teach patients that over-amplified music, power tools, and hobbies involving exposure to the noise of firearms or any loud noise can cause hearing loss. Protect from prolonged exposure to environmental noise by wearing ear plugs or protectors. Evaluate hearing ability in patients receiving potentially ototoxic drugs. Teach patients correct methods for instillation of ear medications.

e., Blainville's. Congenital asymmetry of the ears.

e., Cagot. An ear without a lower lobe.

e., cauliflower. A deformity consisting of a thickening of the external ear resulting from trauma that caused a hematoma. Commonly seen in boxers.

e., external. Portion of the ear consisting of the auricle and external auditory canal, and separated from the middle ear by the tympanic membrane or eardrum.

e., foreign bodies in. These are usually insects, pebbles, beans, or peas.

SYM: Pain, ringing, or buzzing in the ear. If due to a live insect, there is usually a great noise.

TREAT: Do not attempt to lure insects from the ear canal with a bright light; they may be stimulated to crawl deeper. Drop in bland oil and float insect out. In case of a solid foreign body, oil or water should not be used because they might either push the object further in the ear or cause it to swell and become firmly embedded. Such foreign bodies in the ear do not constitute an emergency and should be left untreated until seen by a physician.

Water sometimes enters the ears of swimmers and will not flow out spontaneously. Usually it can be dislodged by a sudden tap on the side of the head above the ear, or by introducing a long wisp of cotton, which will draw it out by capillary action. Also a few drops of 70% alcohol instilled in the canal will hasten evaporation of the so-called trapped water. Occasionally this sensation of water in the ear is not due to water but to swelling of the cerumen, q.v. In such instances a physician should be consulted.

e., internal. Portion of the ear consisting of the cochlea, containing the sensory receptors for hearing, and the vestibule and semicircular canals, which include the receptors for equilibrium and the sense of position. Innervated by the vestibulocochlear nerve.

e., middle. The tympanic cavity, an irregular air-filled space in the temporal bone. Anteriorly it communicates with the eustachian tube, which forms an open channel between the middle ear and the cavity of the nasopharynx. Posteriorly, the middle ear

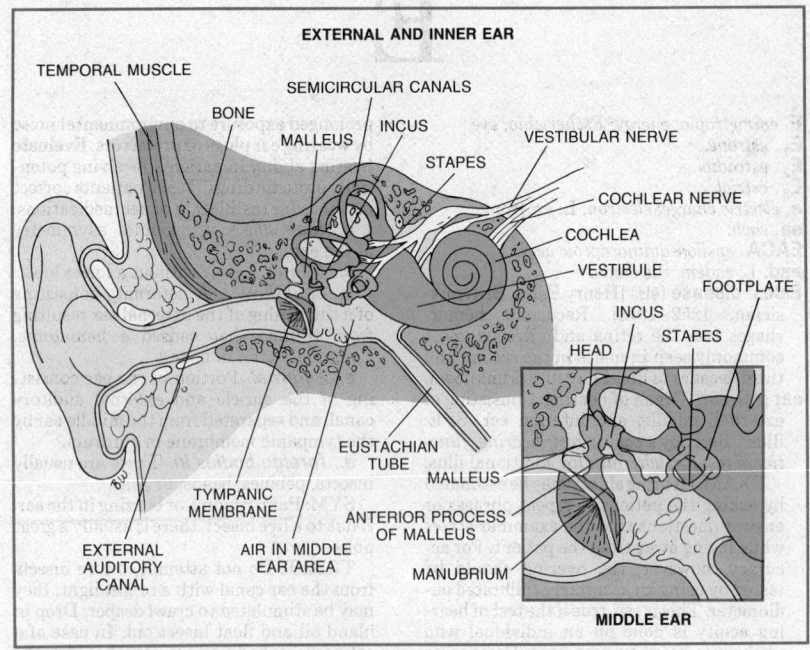

EXTERNAL AND INNER EAR

TEMPORAL MUSCLE
BONE
MALLEUS
SEMICIRCULAR CANALS
INCUS
STAPES
VESTIBULAR NERVE
COCHLEAR NERVE
COCHLEA
VESTIBULE
FOOTPLATE
INCUS
STAPES
HEAD
EUSTACHIAN TUBE
MALLEUS
ANTERIOR PROCESS OF MALLEUS
MANUBRIUM
TYMPANIC MEMBRANE
EXTERNAL AUDITORY CANAL
AIR IN MIDDLE EAR AREA
MIDDLE EAR

opens into the mastoid antrum and this in turn communicates with the mastoid cells. Of the three potential openings into the middle ear, two — the tympanic membrane and the round window — are covered. The third one is for the eustachian tube. Three ossicles (small bones) joined together extend from the tympanic membrane to the fenestra vestibuli; these are the malleus, incus, and stapes. SEE: *eardrum; tympanum.*

   e., Mozart. SEE: *Mozart ear.*

   e., nerve supply of. *External:* branches of facial, vagus, and mandibular nerves and from cervical plexus. *Middle:* tympanic plexus and branches of mandibular, vagus, and facial nerves. *Internal:* vestibulocochlear nerve.

   e., pierced. Ear lobe that has been pierced with a needle so that a permanent channel will remain, thus permitting the wearing of an earring attached to the ear by use of a connector through the channel.

   e., surfer's. SEE: *surfer's ear.*

ear, words pert. to: acoustic meatus; acoustic nerve; aditus ad antrum; angiotitis; annulus tympanicus; antihelix; antitragus; antrotympanitis; audiogram; auditory; auricula; "auris-" words; binaural; cavum

tympani; cerumen; cochlea; cochlear implant; concha; crista ampullaris; cupola; deafness; ear wax; endolymph; epitympanum; eustachian; foreign bodies; hearing; hearing aid; helix; hydrotis; incus; labyrinth; labyrinthitis; malleus; ossicle; "ot-" or "oto-" words; pinna; Rinne's test; scala; socioacusis; tinnitus aurium; tympanum; "utri-" words; vestibule of ear; Weber test.

earache. Pain in the ear. SYN: *otalgia; otodynia.*

ear bones. The ossicles of the tympanic cavity: malleus, incus, and stapes. SEE: *ear* for illus.

eardrops. A medication in liquid form for instillation into the external ear canal.

Caution: Do not use if tympanic membrane is damaged or broken.

eardrum (ēr'drŭm). The cavity in the middle ear. SYN: *tympanum.*

ear dust. Calcareous concretions in the membranous labyrinth. SYN: *otoconia; otolith.*

ear oximeter. Device that determines the oxygen content of the blood flowing through the ear.

ear plug. Device for preventing sound from entering the ear by occluding the external auditory canal.

Caution: Should not be used while swimming because it may interfere with pressure equalization.

earth. 1. The planet on which we live. The diameter of the earth at the equator is 7926 miles (12,755 km). It is 92.9 million miles (149.6 million km) from the sun, and it makes one revolution around the sun every 365.26 days. Its only natural satellite is the moon. 2. The soil on the surface of the world.

e., alkaline. General term for the oxides of calcium, strontium, magnesium, and barium.

e., diatomaceous. Silica containing fossilized shells of diatoms. Used in insulating material, filters, and as an absorbent.

e., fuller's. Clay that is similar to kaolin. Used as an absorbent, as a filler in textiles, and in cosmetics.

earth, age of. At one time, the earth was calculated to have been formed in 4004 B.C. at 9 a.m. Mesopotamian local time, according to the Julian calendar. Now the age of the earth is estimated to be 4.5 billion years.

earth eating. Eating of clay or dirt, sometimes by children as a form of pica, q.v.

ear thermometry. Determining the temperature of the tympanic membrane by use of a device for rapidly sensing infrared radiation from the membrane. Commercially available devices do this in 3 seconds. SEE: *temperature.*

earwax (ēr′wăks). Substance secreted by glands at the outer one-third of the ear canal. In Caucasians and blacks, the wax is a pale honey color, may be moist and sticky or dry; in Mongolians it is usually gray, dry, and brittle. Usually earwax does not accumulate in the ear canal, but it may clog the channel in some persons; in this case, the wax may become impacted and will need to be physically removed, not by irrigation of the canal but by use of a curette. Soft wax is easily removed by gentle syringe instillation of plain water in the canal. SYN: *cerumen.*

eat [AS. *etan*]. 1. To devour as food. 2. To take solid food. 3. To corrode.

eat, words pert. to: acoria; anorexia nervosa; apastia; appetite; bradyphagia; bulimia; dysphagia; fastidium; fasting; geophagia; hunger; hyperorexia; mastication; parorexia; pica; polyphagia; taste.

eating disorders. A subclass of disorders which include any one of multiple disturbances of eating behavior. Anorexia nervosa, bulimia, pica, and rumination disorder of infancy are included in the subclass.

Eaton agent. *Mycoplasma pneumoniae,* one of the several causes of primary atypical pneumonia.

Eaton-Lambert syndrome [Lee McKendree Eaton, U.S. physician, 1905–1958; Edward Howard Lambert, U.S. physiologist, b. 1915]. A type of myasthenia associated with muscle weakness, hyporeflexia, and autonomic dysfunction. About half of the cases are associated with oat cell carcinoma of the lung.

TREAT: 3,4-diaminopyridine alone or with pyridostigmine.

Eberthella (ā″bĕr-tĕl′ă) [Karl Joseph Eberth, Ger. pathologist, 1835–1926]. Formerly a genus of bacteria. Now classified under *Salmonella.*

Ebner's glands [A. G. Victor von Ebner, Austrian histologist, 1842–1925]. Serous glands of the tongue usually found in the vicinity of the circumvallate papillae.

Ebola virus disease [Ebola, Zaire, Africa]. Disease caused by a virus classed as a member of the family *Filoviridae.* Characterized by sudden onset of a high fever, prostration, vomiting, diarrhea, followed by uremia, rash, hemorrhages and central nervous system changes. The disease can be transmitted by handling tissues and cells from African green monkeys, but in some cases the source of the infection is unknown. Clinically, this disease is almost identical to that caused by Marburg virus, but the two viruses are not antigenically related.

DIAG: Isolation of the virus by inoculation into guinea pigs or cell cultures.

TREAT: There is no specific therapy.

PROG: Where excellent medical care was available for supportive therapy, the case-fatality rate was 22%; in rural conditions, 90%.

ebonation (ē″bō-nā′shŭn) [L. *e,* out, + AS. *ban,* bone]. Removal of bony fragments from a wound.

Ebstein's anomaly (ĕb′stīnz) [Wilhelm Ebstein, Ger. physician, 1836–1912]. A congenital condition of the heart, symptoms of which are fatigue, palpitations, and dyspnea, resulting from downward displacement of the tricuspid valve from the annulus fibrosus.

ebullism (ĕb′ū-lizm) [L. *ebullire,* to boil over]. Formation of water vapor in body tissue, which occurs when the body is exposed to extreme reduction in barometric pressure. SEE: *bends; decompression illness.*

eburnation (ĕb″ŭr-nā′shŭn) [L. *eburnus,* made of ivory]. Changes in bone causing it to become dense and hard like ivory.

eburneous (ē-bŭr′nē-ŭs). Resembling ivory; ivory-colored.

EBV. *Epstein-Barr virus.* SEE: *mononucleosis, infectious.*

EC. *Enzyme Commission.*

ecaudate (ē-kaw'dāt) [L. *e*, without, + *cauda*, tail]. Without a tail.

ecbolic (ĕk-bŏl'ĭk) [Gr. *ekbolikos*, throwing out]. 1. Hastening uterine evacuation by causing contractions of the uterine muscles. 2. Any agent producing or hastening labor or abortion. SYN: *oxytocic*.

ECC. *emergency cardiac care; external cardiac compression.* SEE: *cardiopulmonary resuscitation.*

eccentric (ĕk-sĕn'trĭk) [Gr. *ek*, out, + *kentron*, center]. 1. Proceeding away from a center. 2. Peripheral.

eccentric muscle contraction. SEE: *muscle contraction, eccentric.*

eccentro-osteochondrodysplasia (ĕk-sĕn"trō-ŏs"tē-ō-kŏn"drō-dĭs-plā'zhē-ă) [Gr. *ekkentros*, from the center, + *osteon*, bone, + *chondros*, cartilage, + *dys*, bad, + *plassein*, to form]. A pathological condition of bones caused by imperfect bone formation. Ossification occurs in eccentric centers instead of in one common center.

eccentropiesis (ĕk-sĕn"trō-pī-ē'sĭs) [" + *piesis*, pressure]. Pressure from within exerted outward.

ecchondroma (ĕk-ŏn-drō'mă) [Gr. *ek*, out, + *chondros*, cartilage, + *oma*, tumor]. A chondroma or cartilaginous tumor.

ecchondrotome (ĕk-ŏn'drō-tōm) [" + " + *tome*, incision]. Knife for excision of cartilage.

ecchymoma (ĕk-ĭ-mō'mă) [" + *chymos*, juice, + *oma*, tumor]. A swelling resulting from the accumulation of blood in subcutaneous tissues such as occurs following a bruise.

ecchymosis (ĕk-ĭ-mō'sĭs) [" + " + *osis*, condition] (pl. *ecchymoses*). A skin discoloration consisting of large, irregularly formed hemorrhagic areas. The color is blue-black, changing in time to greenish brown or yellow.
ETIOL: Extravasation of blood into skin or mucous membrane.

ecchymotic (ĕk-ĭ-mŏt'ĭk) [" + *chymos*, juice]. Resembling or rel. to an ecchymosis.

eccrine (ĕk'rĭn) [Gr. *ekkrinein*, to secrete]. Pert. to secretion, esp. of sweat. SEE: *apocrine; endocrine; exocrine.*

eccrine sweat glands. Glands distributed over the entire skin surface that, because they secrete sweat, are important in regulating body heat. The total number of glands is from two to five million. There are over 400 per sq. cm on the palms and about 80 per sq. cm on the thighs. SEE: *sweat glands* for illus; *apocrine sweat glands; sweat glands.*

eccritic (ĕk-krĭt'ĭk) [Gr. *ekkritikos*]. Promoting or that which promotes excretion.

eccyclomastopathy (ĕk-sī"klō-măs-tŏp'ă-thē) [Gr. *ek*, out, + *kyklos*, circle, + *mastos*, breast, + *pathos*, disease, suffering]. A mass of lesions of the breast made up of connective tissue and epithelial cells.

ecdysis (ĕk'dĭ-sĭs) [Gr. *ekdysis*, getting out] (pl. *ecdyses*). 1. The shedding or sloughing off of the epidermis of the skin. SYN: *desquamation*. 2. The shedding of the outer covering of the body as occurs in certain animals such as insects, crustaceans, and snakes. SYN: *molt*.

ECG, ecg. *electrocardiogram.*

echidnase (ē-kĭd'nās) [Gr. *echidna*, viper]. An enzyme present in the venom of viper snakes. It produces inflammation.

echidnin (ē-kĭd'nĭn). 1. The venom of poisonous snakes. 2. The active principle present in snake venom.

Echidnophaga (ĕk"ĭd-nŏf'ă-gă). A genus of fleas belonging to the family Pulicidae.
E. gallinacea. The sticktight flea, an important flea pest of poultry. It collects in clusters on the heads of poultry and in the ears of mammals. It may infest humans, esp. children.

echinate (ĕk'ĭ-nāt) [Gr. *echinos*, hedgehog]. 1. Spiny. 2. In agar streak, a growth with pitted or toothed margins along the inoculation line; in stab cultures, coiled growth with pointed outgrowths. SYN: *echinulate*.

echinococcosis (ē-kī"nō-kŏk-ō'sĭs, ĕk"ĭ-nō-kŏk-ō'sĭs) [" + *kokkos*, berry, + *osis*, condition]. Infestation with *Echinococcus*.

echinococcotomy (ē-kī"nō-kŏk-ŏt'ō-mē) [" + " + *tome*, incision]. Operation for evacuation of an echinococcal cyst.

Echinococcus (ē-kī"nō-kŏk'ŭs) (pl. *Echinococci*). A genus of tapeworms. They are minute forms consisting of a scolex and three or four proglottids.
E. granulosus. A species of tapeworms that infests dogs and other carnivores. Its larva, called a hydatid, develops in other mammals, including humans, and causes the formation of hydatid cysts in the liver or lungs. SEE: *hydatid.*
E. hydatidosus. Variety of *Echinococcus* characterized by development of daughter cysts from the mother cyst. SEE: *hydatid.*

echinocyte. Abnormal erythrocytes with multiple, regular, spiny projections from the surface.

echinosis (ĕk"ĭ-nō'sĭs) [Gr. *echinos*, hedgehog, + *osis*, condition]. Crenated red blood cells that are irregular in shape.

Echinostoma (ĕk"ĭ-nŏs'tō-mă) [" + *stoma*, mouth]. A genus of flukes characterized by a spiny body and the presence of a collar of spines near the anterior end. They are found in the intestines of many vertebrates, esp. aquatic birds. They occasionally occur as accidental parasites in humans.

echinulate (ē-kĭn'ū-lāt). A bacterial growth

having pointed processes or spines. SYN: *echinate.*

echo (ĕk′ō) [Gr. *ekho*]. A reverberating sound produced when sound waves are reflected back to their source.

   e., amphoric. Amphoric sound sometimes heard in auscultation of chest. SEE: *chest.*

echoacousia. Subjective echoes of sounds just normally heard.

echocardiogram (ĕk″ō-kăr′dē-ō-grăm″). The graphic record produced by echocardiography, q.v.

echocardiography (ĕk″ō-kăr″dē-ŏg′rä-fē). A noninvasive diagnostic method that uses ultrasound, q.v., to visualize internal cardiac structures. All cardiac valves can be visualized, and the dimensions of each ventricle and the left atrium can be measured.

   e., Doppler. SEE: *Doppler echocardiography.*

echoencephalogram (ĕk″ō-ĕn-sĕf′ă-lō-grăm″). Recording of the ultrasonic echoes of the brain. Esp. useful in diagnosing conditions that cause a shift in the midline structures of the brain.

echogram (ĕk′ō-grăm). The record made by echography.

echography (ĕk-ŏg′rä-fē) [″ + *graphein,* to write]. The use of ultrasonic technique to produce a photograph of the echo produced when sound waves are reflected from tissues of different density. SEE: *ultrasonography.*

echokinesia (ĕk″ō-kĭn-ē′sē-ă) [″ + *kinesis,* movement]. Involuntary repetition of another's gestures.

echolalia (ĕk-ō-lā′lē-ă) [″ + *lalia,* talk, babble]. Involuntary parrotlike repetition of words spoken by others, often accompanied by twitching of muscles. Frequently seen in catatonic schizophrenia.

echolocation. The location of an object by use of the sense of hearing to detect an echo. Used by animals and blind persons to assist in identifying the position of obstructions.

echomimia (ĕk″ō-mĭm′ē-ă) [″ + *mimesis,* imitation]. Imitation of the actions of others as seen in schizophrenia. SYN: *echopraxia.*

echomotism (ĕk″ō-mō′tĭzm) [″ + L. *motus,* moving]. Imitation of movements.

echopathy (ĕ-kŏp′ă-thē) [″ + *pathos,* disease, suffering]. A neurosis in which there is pathological repetition of another's actions and words.

echophotony (ĕk″ō-fŏt′ō-nē) [″ + *phos,* light, + *tonos,* tone]. Mental association of certain sounds with particular colors.

echophrasia (ĕk″ō-frā′sē-ă) [″ + *phrasis,* speech]. Echolalia.

echopraxia (ĕk″ō-prăk′sē-ă) [″ + *prassein,* to perform]. Imitation without meaning of motions made by others. SYN: *echo-*

mimia; echomotism.

echo sign. Repetition of closing word of a sentence, a sign of epilepsy or other brain conditions.

echothiophate iodide (ĕk″ō-thī′ō-fāt). USP. A cholinergic drug used topically in the eye for treatment of glaucoma. Trade name is Phospholine Iodide.

ECHO virus. Virus belonging to the group originally known as *E*nteric *C*ytopathogenic *H*uman *O*rphan group. They are associated with nonbacterial viral meningitis, enteritis, pleurodynia, acute respiratory infection, and myocarditis. More than 34 viruses were assigned to this group initially. Later, some were reclassified. Types 10 and 28 were removed from the ECHO group and classed as reovirus 1 and rhinovirus 1, respectively.

Eck's fistula (ĕks) [N. V. Eck, Russian physiologist, 1847–1908]. Artificial communication between the portal vein and the inferior vena cava; used in experimental surgery in animals.

eclabium (ĕk-lā′bē-ŭm) [Gr. *ek,* out, + L. *labium,* lip]. Eversion of a lip.

eclampsia (ĕ-klămp′sē-ă) [″ + *lampein,* to shine]. Coma and convulsive seizures between the 20th week of pregnancy and the end of the first week postpartum. Develops in 1 out of 200 patients with pre-eclampsia, q.v., and is usually fatal if untreated.

   SYM: Edema of the legs and feet, puffiness of the face, hypertension and albuminuria. Severe headaches, dizziness, spots before the eyes, epigastric pain and nausea, convulsions (beginning with fixation of the eyeballs, rolling of the eyes, twitchings of the face, arms, and hands; the paroxysms then involve the entire body), and coma. There may be one or many convulsions. The pulse is rapid and bounding, the temperature usually rises to 103° or 104° F (39.4 or 40° C) and the blood pressure may be quite elevated. The patient may remain in coma until death.

   ETIOL: Unknown. Occurs more often in primigravidae. Pre-existing hypertension and glomerulonephritis contribute to cause.

   PATH: Seen most frequently in the kidney, liver, brain, and placenta. The kidney shows degenerated tubal nephritis; the tubal epithelium shows cloudy swelling, fatty degeneration, and coagulation necrosis. The liver is enlarged and mottled. There are portal vein thrombosis and degeneration of the periphery of the lobules with subcapsular hemorrhages. Edema, hyperemia, thrombosis, and hemorrhages are present in the brain. In the placenta, there are infarcts, thromboses, and hemorrhages. There is also retinal edema.

TREAT: Prophylaxis is of primary importance. Good prenatal care with careful and frequent observation and recording of the patient's blood pressure, urine output, and weight. Institute appropriate therapy as soon as there are any abnormal findings, and terminate pregnancy if unsuccessful in reducing the signs of danger.

Caution: The routine use of diuretics in pregnancy is contraindicated because diuretics are of no benefit and may do considerable harm by masking signs and symptoms that would alert the patient and the physician to the onset of eclampsia.

Convulsions: Prevent the patient from doing herself bodily harm (restrain her in bed, protect the tongue by keeping the teeth separated). Give magnesium sulfate (MgSO₄) intravenously, by use of an I.V. pump, 4 gm in 10 min and then 1 gm each hour if urinary output is maintained. If the hypertension is not controlled by the MgSO₄, I.V. may be needed. The dose is adjusted to control the blood pressure; but do not lower B.P. less than 130/80 because the uterus could be inadequately perfused below that level, thus risking fetal damage. If MgSO₄ causes an excess fall in B.P., then calcium gluconate I.V. may be used as an antidote. Constant monitoring of blood pressure, pulse, respirations, reflexes, and urinary output.

Delivery: Delivery is not indicated until the patient has reached a stable condition; usually within 4 to 6 hours. If the patient is in active labor, the most conservative methods should be followed. Cesarean section should not be done unless there is some other obstetrical reason. If medical management effects no improvement, labor must be instituted by administration of an oxytocic agent. Cesarean section may be required.

NURSING IMPLICATIONS: Prevent by educating pregnant women about preeclampsia and eclampsia, maternal and fetal nutritional needs, and the importance of prenatal care in early diagnosis and treatment of pre-eclampsia. Monitor protein intake to insure adequate protein levels, normal oncotic pressure, and to limit edema formation. Teach the patient that excessive salt restriction, fluid restriction, and diuretics may be harmful. Encourage bedrest in a left side-lying position to prevent vena caval and aortic compression and to increase renal and uterine perfusion. Provide a non-stimulating environment, call bell, full seizure precautions, and readily available emergency medications and delivery equip-

ment. Continually evaluate the clinical state of the patient and fetus by obtaining maternal vital signs and use of fetal monitor. Observe for impending labor and evaluate response to labor contractions if these occur. Notify the obstetrician of any change in patient or fetus. Provide emergency care of convulsions, administer medication as directed, and monitor patient response. Provide psychological support to patient and family, and prepare them for possible termination of pregnancy. Continue assessment every four hours for 48 hours post delivery; patient is at risk throughout this period.

eclamptic. Rel. to, or of the nature of, eclampsia.

eclamptogenic (ĕk-lămp″tō-jĕn′ĭk) [Gr. *ek*, out, + *lampein*, to shine, + *gennan*, to produce]. Causing convulsions.

eclectic (ĕk-lĕk′tĭk) [Gr. *eklektikos*, selecting]. Selecting from various sources what seems to be the best.

eclecticism (ĕk-lĕk′tĭ-sĭzm) [″ + -*ismos*, state of]. A former system of medicine treating disease through specific remedies for individual signs or symptoms rather than for distinct diseases. Remedies principally botanical.

ecmnesia (ĕk-nē′zē-ä) [Gr. *ek*, out, + *mnesis*, memory]. Inability to remember recent events, as seen in senility. The long-term memory is not affected.

ECMO. *extracorporeal membrane oxygenator.*

ecocide (ĕk″ō-sīd′) [Gr. *oikos*, house, + L. *caedere*, to kill]. Willful destruction of some portion of the environment.

E. coli. *Escherichia coli*, q.v.

ecological terrorism. The threat to use violent acts that would harm the quality of the environment in order to blackmail a group or society. SYN: *environmental terrorism.*

ecologic fallacy. In epidemiology, the erroneous attempt from population studies to determine the risk of a particular individual developing a disease.

ecology (ē-kŏl′ō-jē) [Gr. *oikos*, house, + *logos*, word, reason]. Science of the relations and interactions of the totality of organisms to their environment, including the relations and interactions of organisms to each other in that environment. SYN: *bionomics.*

Economo's disease [Constantin von Economo, Austrian neurologist, 1876–1931]. SEE: *encephalitis lethargica.*

economy of movement [Gr. *oikos,* house + *nomos,* law]. The efficient, energy-sparing motion or activity of the system or body.

écorché (ā″kor-shā′) [Fr.]. A representation of an animal or human form without skin so that the muscles are clearly seen.

ecosphere (ĕk′ō-sfēr″) [Gr. *oikos*, house,

+ L. *sphera*, ball]. Portions of the universe habitable by living organisms and plant life.

ecostate (ē-kŏs'tāt) [L. *e*, without, + *costa*, rib]. Without ribs.

ecosystem (ĕk'ō-sĭs"tĕm). The smallest ecology unit. The living organisms and plants and their environment in a defined area.

Ecotrin. Trade name for aspirin.

écouvillonage (ā-koo"vē-yŏ-nŏzh') [Fr. *ecouvillon*, a stiff brush or swab]. The cleansing and application of remedies to a cavity by means of a brush or swab.

écrasement (ā-krăz-mŏn') [Fr.]. Excision by means of an écraseur.

écraseur (ā-krā-zēr') [Fr., crusher]. A wire loop used for excisions.

EC space. *extracellular space.*

ecstasy (ĕk'stā-sē) [Gr. *ekstasis*, a standing out]. An exhilarated, trancelike condition or state of exalted delight.

ecstrophy (ĕk'strō-fē) [Gr. *ekstrophe*, a turning out]. Turning an organ inside out. SYN: *exstrophy.*

ECT. *electroconvulsive therapy.*

ectad [Gr. *ektos*, outside, + L. *ad*, toward]. Toward the surface; outward; externally.

ectal. External, outer, on the surface.

ectasia, ectasis (ĕk-tā'sē-ă, ĕk'tă-sĭs) [Gr. *ek*, out, + *teinein*, to stretch]. Dilatation of any tubular vessel.

    e., hypostatic. Dilatation of a blood vessel from the pooling of blood in dependent parts, esp. the legs.

    e. iridis. Smallness of the pupil of the eye caused by displacement of the iris.

    e. ventriculi paradoxa. Hourglass stomach.

ectatic. Distensible or capable of being stretched.

ectental [Gr. *ektos*, without, + *entos*, within]. Pert. to entoderm and ectoderm.

ectental line. Point of entodermal and ectodermal junction in the gastrula.

ectethmoid (ĕk-tĕth'moyd) [" + *ethmos*, sieve, + *eidos*, form, shape]. Lateral mass of the ethmoid bone.

ecthyma (ĕk-thī'mă) [Gr. *ek*, out, + *thyein*, to rush]. An infection of the skin. Usually a result of neglected treatment of impetigo, q.v. It is marked by shallow lesions with adherent crusts or scabs. May be followed by pigmentation and scarring. Treatment is the same as that for impetigo, q.v.

ectiris (ĕk-tī-rĭs) [Gr. *ektos*, outside, + *iris*, iris]. The external portion of the iris.

ecto- [Gr. *ektos*, outside]. Prefix meaning outside.

ectoantigen (ĕk"tō-ăn'tĭ-gĕn) [" + *anti*, against, + *gennan*, to produce]. An antigen assumed to have its origin in ectoplasm

of bacterial cells or one loosely attached to the surface of bacteria and capable of being separated from the bacterial cell.

ectoblast (ĕk'tō-blăst) [" + *blastos*, germ]. 1. Ectoderm. 2. Any outer membrane; as a cell wall.

ectocardia (ĕk'tō-kăr'dē-ă) [" + *kardia*, heart]. Displacement of the heart.

ectocervical (ĕk"tō-sĕr'vĭ-kăl). Concerning the ectocervix.

ectocervix (ĕk"tō-sĕr'vĭks). The portion of the canal of uterine cervix that is lined with squamous epithelium.

ectochoroidea (ĕk"tō-kō-roy'dē-ă) [" + *khorioeides*, choroid]. Outer layer of choroid coat of the eye.

ectocolostomy (ĕk"tō-kŏ-lŏs'tō-mē) [" *kolon*, colon, + *stoma*, mouth]. Formation through the abdominal wall of an opening into the colon.

ectocondyle (ĕk"tō-kŏn'dĭl) [" + *kondylos*, knuckle]. The outer condyle of the bone.

ectocornea (ĕk-tō-kor'nē-ă) [" + L. *corneus*, horny]. External layer of the cornea.

ectocuneiform (ĕk-tō-kū'nē-ĭ-form) [" + L. *cuneus*, wedge, + *forma*, form]. External cuneiform bone.

ectocytic (ĕk"tō-sī'tĭk) [" + *kytos*, cell]. Outside of the cell.

ectodactylism (ĕk"tō-dăk'tĭl-ĭzm) [Gr. *ektrosis*, miscarriage, + *daktylos*, finger, + *ismos*, state of]. Lack of a digit or digits.

ectoderm (ĕk'tō-dĕrm) [Gr. *ektos*, outside, + *derma*, skin]. The outer layer of cells in the developing embryo. From it are developed skin structures, teeth and glands of mouth, the nervous system, organs of special sense, part of the pituitary gland, and the pineal and suprarenal glands. SYN: *epiblast.* SEE: *entoderm; mesoderm.*

ectodermal. Rel. to the ectoderm.

ectodermatosis, ectodermosis (ĕk"tō-dĕr"mă-tō'sĭs, -dĕr-mō'sĭs) [" + *derma*, skin, + *osis*, diseased condition]. Illness resulting from congenital maldevelopment of ectodermal structures.

    e. erosiva pluriorificialis. A rare form of erythema multiforme characterized by fever, chills, profuse salivation, small blisters on tongue, lips, and cheeks, and erythematous lesions on the hands. It occurs in children and young persons.

ectodermic. Pert. to the ectoderm. SYN: *ectodermal.*

ectodermoidal (ĕk"tō-dĕr-moyd'ăl) [Gr. *ektos*, outside, + *derma*, skin, + *eidos*, form, shape]. Pert. to or resembling the ectoderm.

ectoentad (ĕk"tō-ĕn'tăd) [" + *entos*, within]. From without inward.

ectoenzyme (ĕk"tō-ĕn'zīm) [" + *en-*, in, + *zyme*, leaven]. An extracellular enzyme, or one that acts outside of the cell that secretes it.

ectogenous (ĕk-tŏj'ĕ-nŭs) [" + *gennan*, to produce]. 1. Having its origin outside of a body or structure, as infection. 2. Ability to grow outside of the body, as a parasite.

ectoglia (ĕk-tŏg'lē-ă) [" + *glia*, glue]. Superficial embryonic layer in beginning of stratification of the medullary tube of the embryo.

ectoglobular (ĕk"tō-glŏb'ū-lăr) [" + L. *globulus*, globule]. Not within blood cells.

ectogony (ĕk-tŏg'ō-nē) [" + *gone*, seed]. Influence of the embryo on the mother.

ectolecithal (ĕk"tō-lĕs'ĭ-thăl) [" + *lekithos*, yolk]. Pert. to ovum having food yolk placed near the surface.

ectomere (ĕk'tō-mēr) [" + *meros*, part]. One of the blastomeres forming the ectoderm.

ectomesoblast (ĕk"tō-mĕs'ō-blăst) [" + *mesos*, middle, + *blastos*, germ]. Cells from which the ectoblast and mesoblast will develop.

ectomorph (ĕk'tō-morf) [" + *morphe*, form]. Body build characterized by predominance of tissues derived from the ectoderm. Characterized by linearity of body build with sparse muscular development. SEE: *endomorph; mesomorph; somatotype.*

-ectomy (ĕk'tō-mē) [Gr. *ektome*]. Suffix denoting excision of any organ or gland.

ectonuclear (ĕk-tō-nū'klē-ăr) [Gr. *ektos*, outside, + L. *nucleus*, kernel]. Occurring outside a cell nucleus.

ectopagus (ĕk-tŏp'ă-gŭs) [" + *pagos*, something fixed]. An abnormal fetus consisting of twins fused at the thorax.

ectoparasite (ĕk"tō-păr'ă-sīt") [" + Gr. *parasitos*, parasite]. A parasite that lives on the outer surface of the body, as fleas, lice, or ticks.

ectoperitonitis (ĕk"tō-pĕr"ĭ-tō-nī'tĭs) [" + *peritonaion*, peritoneum, + *itis*, inflammation]. Inflammation of the parietal layer of peritoneum (layer lining the abdominal wall).

ectophyte (ĕk'tō-fīt) [" + *phyton*, plant]. A parasite of vegetable origin growing on the skin.

ectopia (ĕk-tō'pē-ă) [Gr. *ektopos*, displaced]. Malposition or displacement, esp. congenital, of an organ or structure.

    e. cordis. Malposition of the heart in which it lies outside the thoracic cavity.

    e. lentis. Displacement of the crystalline lens of the eye.

    e. pupillae congenita. Congenital displacement of the pupil.

    e. renis. Displacement of the kidney.

    e. testis. Displacement of the testis.

    e. vesicae. Displacement of the bladder, esp. exstrophy of the bladder.

    e., visceral. An umbilical hernia.

ectopic (ĕk-tŏp'ik). In an abnormal position. Opposite of entopic.

ectopic beat, complex. Electrical stimulation of cardiac contraction beginning at a point other than the sinoatrial node.

ectopic pregnancy. Implantation of the fertilized ovum outside of the uterine cavity. There is usually a poorly developed decidual reaction in the uterus. SEE: *pregnancy, ectopic,* for illus.

    SYM: Amenorrhea; tenderness, soreness, pain on affected side; pallor, weak pulse, signs of shock or hemorrhage; pain may be reflected to shoulder; perhaps bluish discoloration of umbilicus.

    Unruptured: Amenorrhea may or may not be present; vague pains in the abdomen usually on one side; irregular hemorrhage. The diagnosis at this stage can be made by the usual biological tests for pregnancy.

    Ruptured: Without a severe hemorrhage: there is severe pain in the lower abdomen with repeated fainting spells. Diagnosis is made by transvaginal needle puncture into the peritoneal cavity. This will reveal free blood. If bleeding is severe and surgical therapy is not instituted without delay, death may result.

    LOCATIONS: *Abdominal:* In the free abdominal cavity and attached to one of the abdominal viscera. *Interstitial:* In the interstitial portion of the tube. *Ovarian:* In the ovary. The ovarian and primary abdominal types are very rare. *Tubal:* In the fallopian tube, the type most frequently encountered. The pregnancy may be situated in the interstitial, ampullar, or isthmic portion of the tube, the isthmic type being the most common.

    ETIOL: Most commonly associated with inflammatory conditions of the tube and other conditions that mechanically interfere with the downward passage of the ovum, such as diverticula, polypi in the tubal lumen, and peritoneal adhesions. Any variety of pregnancy or any combination of varieties may occur (uterine plus ectopic, bilateral ectopic).

    DIFF. DIAG: Ectopic pregnancy must be differentiated from appendicitis, uterine pregnancy, acute salpingitis, twisting of the pedicle of an ovarian cyst or pedunculated fibroid tumor, and hemorrhage from a ruptured graafian follicle or corpus luteum cyst.

    TREAT: Once the diagnosis of ectopic pregnancy is made, operative treatment is indicated. In those cases in which there is profound shock from hemorrhage, the patient should be supported by blood transfusion and saline infusions before major surgery is attempted. If the pregnancy is tubal, the preservation of the tube is important in order to facilitate a future pregnancy. Ectopic pregnancies of 3.5 cm or less that have not ruptured have been treated experimentally with a single dose of methotrexate. The results were favorable, and side effects were minimal.

NURSING IMPLICATIONS: Gather pertinent historical data, evaluate for pain and shock, monitor vital signs, and have Rh compatible blood cross matched for possible transfusion, if prescribed. Initiate intravenous fluid infusion via wide bore cannula, administer prescribed oxygen and medications. Determine wishes of patient and family regarding religious rites for products of conception; support and reassure patient preoperatively, clarifying information and correcting misconceptions. Postoperatively, assess vital signs, bleeding, and physical and emotional reactions to treatment. Administer prescribed medical therapies. Anticipate grieving process and refer for further counseling as needed. SEE: *Nursing Diagnoses* in *Appendix*.

ectopic rhythm. Any abnormal or irregular cardiac rhythm.

NURSING IMPLICATIONS: Monitor rhythm and report and take action for life-threatening dysrhythmias.

ectopic secretion (ĕk-tŏp′ĭk). The secretion of hormones by tumors arising from tissues that do not normally secrete the hormone or hormones.

ectoplasm [Gr. *ektos*, outside, + LL. *plasma*, form, mold]. The outermost layer of cell protoplasm.

ectoplasmic. Pert. to ectoplasm. SYN: *ectoplastic*.

ectoplast (ĕk′tō-plăst) [″ + *plastikos*, formed]. Cell membrane.

ectoplastic. Formed at the periphery. SYN: *ectoplasmic*.

ectopotomy (ĕk-tō-pŏt′ō-mē) [Gr. *ektopos*, displaced, + *tome*, incision]. Removal of the fetus in ectopic pregnancy.

ectopterygoid (ĕk″tō-tĕr′ĭ-goyd) [Gr. *ektos*, outside, + *pteryx*, wing, + *eidos*, form, shape]. External or lateral pterygoid muscle. Acts to bring jaw forward.

ectopy (ĕk′tō-pē) [Gr. *ektopos*, displaced]. Displacement. SYN: *ectopia*.

ectoretina (ĕk″tō-rĕt′ĭ-nă) [Gr. *ektos*, outside, + L. *rete*, net]. Outer layer of retina.

ectostosis (ĕk-tŏs-tō′sĭs) [″ + *osteon*, bone, + *osis*, condition]. Formation of bone beneath the periosteum.

ectothrix (ĕk′tō-thrĭks) [″ + *thrix*, hair]. Any fungus that produces arthrospores on the hair shafts.

Ectotrichophyton (ĕk″ō-trī-kŏf′ĭ-tŏn) [″

+ *thrix*, hair, + *phyton*, plant]. Former name for *Trichophyton megalosporon ectothrix*, a genus of parasitic fungi causing tinea or ringworm of the hair.

ectozoon (ĕk-tō-zō′ŏn) [″ + *zoon*, animal]. Parasitic animal that lives on the outside of another animal.

ectro- [Gr. *ektrosis*, miscarriage]. Combining form meaning congenital absence of a part.

ectrodactylism (ĕk″trō-dăk′tĭl-ĭzm) [″ + *daktylos*, finger, + *-ismos*, state of]. Congenital absence of all or part of a digit.

ectromelia (ĕk″trō-mē′lē-ă) [″ + *melos*, limb]. Hypoplasia of the long bones of the limbs.

ectromelus (ĕk-trŏm′ē-lŭs) [″ + *melos*, limb]. Individual with ectromelia.

ectropic (ĕk-trō′pĭk) [Gr. *ek*, out, + *trope*, turning]. Pert. to complete or partial eversion of a part, generally the eyelid.

ectropion (ĕk-trō′pē-ŏn). Eversion of an edge or margin, as the edge of an eyelid.

ETIOL: Old age; relaxation of skin; cicatrix following trauma; infection; palsy of facial nerve.

ectropionize. To evert or cause an eversion.

ectrosyndactyly (ĕk″trō-sĭn-dăk′tĭ-lē) [″ + *syn*, together, + *dactylos*, finger]. Congenital absence of one or more fingers; the remaining fingers are fused together.

eczema (ĕk′zĕ-mă) [Gr. *ekzein*, to boil out]. Acute or chronic cutaneous inflammatory condition with erythema, papules, vesicles, pustules, scales, crusts, or scabs alone or in combination. They may be dry or with watery discharge, with thickening, infiltration, and more or less itching or burning. Eczema is more the description of a symptom than of a disease. This word has become synonymous with dermatitis caused by a number of external and internal factors acting singly or in combination. It has therefore no specific connotation, particularly with respect to etiology. SEE: *allergy.* SYN: *dermatitis.*

SYM: Primary type characterized by erythematous, papular, vesicular, or pustular lesions. In secondary type, the lesions evolve from primary variety. Invasion by pathogenic organisms may cause suppuration.

ETIOL: No class, age, or sex is exempt, but those with thin, dry skins are more susceptible. The lesions are not infectious. Two classes of causes: external or exciting (irritation, allergic contact, reaction to exposure to certain microorganisms, occupational and nonoccupational, chemical); and constitutional or predisposing. The latter includes eczema caused by genetic and psychological factors.

TREAT: Depends upon the etiology and will therefore be highly individualized according to the causative agent, organism, or condition.

PROG: Chronic, amenable to treatment but prone to relapse and recurrence.

NURSING IMPLICATIONS: Assist the patient in eliminating allergens from diet and environment and in avoiding precipitating or exacerbating factors, such as irritants (wool, detergents, perfumes), extreme temperature changes, and emotional stress. Teach patient about use and side effects of ordered topical and systemic measures to relieve pruritus and inflammation. Institute measures to decrease excoriation from scratching, such as hand mittens and short, smooth nails. Have patient bathe using tepid water and special nonfat, nonperfumed soap, avoiding soap altogether during acute exacerbations. Do not show anxiety or revulsion when touching lesions during assessment or application of topical medications. Nevertheless, universal precautions, q.v. in *Appendix*, must be observed. Encourage patient to verbalize and examine feelings about altered body image and arrange for further counseling as necessary to assist patient in dealing with associated emotional distress. SEE: *Nursing Diagnoses* in *Appendix*.

e., erythematous. Dry, pinkish, ill-defined patches with itching and burning; slight swelling with tendency to spread and coalesce; branny scaling; roughness and dryness of skin. May become generalized.

e. fissum. Form of eczema with painful fissures.

e. herpeticum. Massive crops of vesicles that become pustular, occurring when infection with herpes simplex virus takes place in a person, usually an infant, with pre-existing eczema. SYN: *Kaposi's varicelliform eruption*. SEE: *AIDS*.

e. hypertrophicum. Eczema with a permanent enlargement of papillae of the skin or with skin growths.

e., lichenoid. Eczema with a thickened condition of the skin.

e. marginatum. Eczema caused by ringworm. SYN: *tinea cruris*.

e., nummular. Lesions are coin- or oval-shaped.

e., pustular. Includes many forms: follicular, impetiginous, or consecutive types including eczema rubrum (red, glazed surface with little oozing), eczema madidans (raw, red, and covered with moisture), eczema fissum (thick, dry, inelastic skin with cracks and fissures), squamous eczema (chronic on soles, legs, scalp; multiple circumscribed, infiltrated patches with thin, dry scales).

e., seborrheic. Eczema marked by ex-

cessive secretion from the sebaceous glands. SYN: *seborrhea*.

e. vaccinatum. Generalized vaccinial lesions or local lesions elsewhere than at vaccination site in persons who have eczema and have been vaccinated. Also may occur as result of accidental contact with a recently vaccinated parent or sibling. SYN: *Kaposi's varicelliform eruption*. SEE: *AIDS*.

eczematous (ĕk-zĕm'ă-tŭs). Marked by or resembling eczema.

ED. *effective dose; erythema dose.*

E.D. *Emergency Department.*

ED₅₀. The median effective dose; produces the desired effect in 50% of subjects tested.

EDC. *expected date of confinement.*

Edecrin. Trade name for ethacrynic acid.

edema (ĕ-dē'mă) [Gr. *oidema*, swelling] (pl. *edemas* or *edemata*). A local or generalized condition in which the body tissues contain an excessive amount of tissue fluid. Generalized edema is sometimes called dropsy, q.v., or anasarca, q.v. Spelled *oedema* in Great Britain.

ETIOL: May result from increased permeability of the capillary walls; increased capillary pressure due to venous obstruction or heart failure; lymphatic obstruction; disturbances in renal functioning; reduction of plasma proteins; inflammatory conditions; fluid and electrolyte disturbances, particularly those causing sodium retention; malnutrition; starvation; chemical substances such as bacterial toxins, venoms, caustic substances, and histamine. May occur by diffusion, q.v., osmosis, q.v., or dialysis, q.v.

TREAT: Bedrest desirable. Salt intake restricted; may be moderate or severe restriction depending upon degree of edema. Fluid intake restricted; may be as low as 600 ml in 24 hours. This prescription may be relaxed when free diuresis has been attained. Diuretics are effective when renal function is good and edema mild and when underlying abnormality of cardiac function, capillary pressure, or salt retention is being corrected simultaneously. One of a variety of effective diuretics may be used. Diuretics are contraindicated in pre-eclampsia, and in the true nephritic edema of acute diffuse glomerulonephritis. They are often useless in cardiac edema associated with advanced renal insufficiency. The diet in edema should be adequate in protein, high in calories, rich in vitamins, and low in salt. When diuresis appears, the patient may resume a normal diet. SEE: *decubitus ulcer*.

NURSING IMPLICATIONS: Assess and document edema according to type (pitting or non-pitting), extent and location, symmetry, and degree of pitting. Palpate for edema against bony prominences, pressing with fingertip for 5 seconds before releasing. The tissue should rebound to original contour immediately. Measure and record depth of indentation. Question patient about increased tightness of rings, shoes, garment waistlines and belts, etc. Also assess for periorbital edema, measure abdominal girth and ankle circumference, monitor patient's weight and fluid intake and output. Protect fragile, edematous tissue from damage by careful handling and positioning and by skin care. Mobilize and elevate edematous extremities to promote venous return, assessing for increasing lung congestion. Administer and teach patient about prescribed therapies, including sodium restriction, diuretics, protein replacement, and elastic stockings.

e., acute circumscribed. Form of edema with localized swelling, usually on the face.

e., angioneurotic. Large areas of swelling of subcutaneous tissues, mucous membranes, and occasionally viscera. May be due to allergic sensitivity to drugs, food, or physical agents such as cold or wind, but in many cases the cause is unknown. SYN: *angioedema.*

e., blue. Hysteric paralysis inducing a swollen, bluish condition of a limb.

e., brain. Swelling of brain tissue due to accumulation of fluid. May be caused by a tumor, toxic chemicals, or infections.

e. bullosum vesicae. Form of edema affecting the bladder.

e., cardiac. Accumulation of fluid in body tissues due to congestive heart failure. It is most apparent in the dependent portion of the body.

e., cerebral. Brain edema, q.v.

e., dependent. Edema or swelling of that part of the body lower than the heart. Thus, the legs are more edematous than are the upper arms.

e., high-altitude. Pulmonary edema that may occur in aviators, mountain climbers, or anyone exposed to decreased atmospheric pressure. SEE: *hypoxia.*

e., inflammatory. Edema due to inflammation.

e., laryngeal. Edema of the larynx, usually resulting from allergic reaction, and causing airway obstruction unless treated. Treat with intravenous or intratracheal epinephrine and emergency tracheostomy or both.

e., malignant. Edema characterized by a rapid course and speedy destruction of tissue.

e. neonatorum. Edema in newborn, esp. premature infants. Condition is usually transitory, involving hands, face, feet, and genitalia, and it rarely becomes generalized.

e. of glottis. Infiltration of the submucosa of the larynx with cough, loss of voice, and feeling of suffocation.

e., pitting. Edema, usually of the skin of the extremities, that when pressed firmly with a finger will maintain the depression produced by the finger.

e., pulmonary. Accumulation of fluid in the lungs due to left-sided failure of the heart, i.e., more blood is supplied to the pulmonary circulation than is removed. May also occur in right-sided heart failure. SEE: *Nursing Diagnoses* in *Appendix.*

e., purulent. Edema caused by purulent infiltration.

e., salt. Form of edema caused by increase of salt in the diet.

edema, words pert. to: angioneurotic edema; cephaledema; chemosis; nephritis; phlegmasia alba dolens; urticaria bullosa.

edematogenic (ĕ-dĕm″ă-tō-jĕn′ĭk). Causing edema.

edematous (ĕ-dĕm′ăt-ŭs) [Gr. *oidema,* swelling]. Pert. to, or affected with, edema.

edentia (ē-dĕn′shē-ă) [L. *e,* without, + *dens,* tooth]. Absence of teeth.

edentulous (ē-dĕnt′ū-lŭs). Without teeth.

edetate calcium disodium (ĕd′ĕ-tāt). USP. The disodium salt of ethylenediaminetetraacetic acid. A chelating agent used in diagnosing and treating lead poisoning. Trade names are Calcium Disodium Versenate and Versene CA.

edetate disodium (ĕd′ĕ-tāt dī-sō′dē-ŭm). A chelating agent, disodium, dihydrogen, ethylenediaminetetraacetate dihydrate. It is used in treating hypercalcemia.

edge. A margin or border.

e., bevel. A tooth edge produced by beveling.

e., chamber. A blunt edge with an obtuse angle.

e., cutting. An angled or sharpened edge for cutting, as an incisor tooth or blade of a knife.

e., denture. A margin or border of a denture.

e., incisal. The sharpened edge of a tooth produced by occlusal wear, the labiolingual margin.

edible (ĕd′ĭ-bl) [L. *edere,* to eat]. Suitable for food; fit to eat, nonpoisonous.

edrophonium chloride (ĕd″rō-fō′nē-ŭm). USP. A cholinergic drug. Trade name is Tensilon. SEE: *edrophonium test.*

edrophonium test. Use of edrophonium chloride to test for the presence of myasthenia gravis. The appropriate dose is injected intravenously; if there is no effect, a larger dose is given within 45 seconds. A positive test demonstrates brief improvement in strength unaccompanied by lingual fasciculation. The test may also be used to determine an overdose of a cholinergic drug. An excessive dose of cholinergic drug produces weakness that closely resembles myasthenia. A very small dose of edrophonium chloride given intravenously will make the weakness worse if it is due to cholinergic drug overdose and will improve the weakness if it is due to myasthenia gravis.

Caution: The test should not be performed unless facilities and staff for respiratory resuscitation are immediately available.

EDTA. *ethylenediaminetetraacetic acid.*

eduction (ē-dŭk'shŭn) [L. *e*, out, + *ducere*, to lead]. Emergence from a particular state or condition; thus, coming out of the effects of general anesthesia is an example of eduction. SEE: *induction* (def. 4).

EEE. *eastern equine encephalitis.*

EEG. *electroencephalogram.*

EENT. *eyes, ears, nose, and throat.*

EFA. *essential fatty acids.*

effacement (ĕ-fās'mĕnt). In obstetrics, during the normal progress of delivery, the dilation of the cervix, enlarging the cross-sectional area of the canal to permit passage of the fetus.

effect (ĕ-fĕkt') [L. *effectus*, to accomplish]. Result of an action or force.

e., additive. Therapeutic effect of a combination of two or more drugs that is equal to the sum of the individual drug effects.

e., Bainbridge. SEE: *reflex, Bainbridge.*

e., cumulative. Drug effect that is apparent only after a number of doses have been given. Caused by excretion or metabolic degradation of only a fraction of each dose given. Sometimes it is therapeutically desirable although this type of effect is usually avoided.

e., piezoelectric. In ultrasound, changing the mechanical action of the ceramic crystals into an electrical impulse. SEE: *triboluminescence.*

effectiveness (ĕ-fĕk'tĭv-nĕs). The ability to cause the expected or intended effect or result.

effector. One of the nerve endings having the efferent process end in a gland or muscle cell. The terminal arborizations of efferent or motor nerves. Also applied to effector organs (muscles and glands).

effector cells. Term used to refer to the active cells of the immune system responsible for destroying or controlling foreign antigens. SEE: *leukocyte.*

effector organ. A structure, specifically muscles and glands, that when stimulated produces an effect.

effeminate. Pert. to the state or condition of a male having the physical characteristics or mannerisms of a female.

effemination (ĕ-fĕm″ĭ-nā'shŭn) [L. *effeminare*, to make feminine]. The production of female physical characteristics in a male. SYN: *feminization.*

efferent [L. *efferens*, to bring out]. Carrying away from a central organ or section, as efferent nerves, which conduct impulses from the brain or spinal cord to the periphery; efferent lymph vessels, which convey lymph from lymph nodes; and efferent arterioles, which carry blood from glomeruli of the kidney. Opposite of afferent, q.v.

efferent nerves. Nerves that carry impulses having the following effects: motor, causing contraction of muscles; secretory, causing glands to secrete; and inhibitory, causing some organs to become quiescent. SYN: *motor nerves.*

effervesce (ĕf″ĕr-vĕs') [L. *effervescere*, to boil up]. To boil or form bubbles on the surface of a liquid.

effervescence (ĕf-ĕr-vĕs'ĕns). Formation of bubbles of gas rising to surface of fluid.

effervescent. Bubbling. Rising in little bubbles of gas.

efficiency. The accomplishing of a task with no undue expenditure of energy or effort.

effleurage (ĕf-loor-äzh') [Fr. *effleurer*, to touch lightly]. Deep or gentle stroking in massage.

efflorescence (ĕf-flor-ĕs'ĕns) [L. *efflorescere*, to bloom]. A rash; a redness of the skin. SYN: *exanthem.*

efflorescent. Becoming powdery or drying from loss of water of crystallization.

effluent (ĕf'loo-ĕnt) [L. *effluere*, to flow out]. 1. A flowing out. 2. Fluid material discharged from a sewage treatment or industrial plant.

effluvium (ĕf-loo-vē-ŭm) (pl. *effluvia*). A malodorous outflow of vapor or gas, particularly one that is toxic.

effort. Expenditure of physical or mental energy.

effort syndrome. A form of anxiety neurosis, q.v., in which fatigue is the presenting symptom. The fatigue is increased by mild exertion, and may be more pronounced in the morning.

effuse (ĕ-fūs') [L. *effusio*, pour out]. Thin, widely spreading. Applied to a bacterial growth that forms a very delicate film over a surface.

effusion (ĕ-fū'zhŭn). Escape of fluid into a part, as the pleural cavity, such as pyothorax (pus), hydrothorax (serum), hemothorax (blood), chylothorax (lymph), pneumothorax (air), hydropneumothorax (serum and air), and pyopneumothorax (pus and air).

e., joint. Increased fluid within a joint cavity. There may be increased production of synovial fluid following trauma or with some arthritic disease processes, or blood accumulating in the joint following trauma, surgery, or due to hemophilia.

e., pericardial. Fluid in the pericardial cavity, between the visceral and parietal pericardium. May produce symptoms of cardiac tamponade.

e., pleural. Fluid in the thoracic cavity between the visceral and parietal pleura. May be seen on chest x-ray if greater than 300 ml.

eflornithine. An antineoplastic and antiprotozoal drug. It has been used to treat African sleeping sickness (African trypanosomiasis). Trade name is Ornidyl.

Efudex. Trade name for fluorouracil.

egesta (ē-jĕs'tă) [L. *egere*, to cast forth]. Waste matter eliminated from the body, esp. excrement.

egg [AS. *aeg*]. 1. The female sex cell or ovum, applied esp. to a fertilized ovum that is passed from the body and develops outside, as in fowls. 2. The mammalian ovum.

eggs, raw. Eggs in their fresh, uncooked state, esp. eggs intended for food. Human consumption of raw or inadequately cooked eggs has caused Salmonella, q.v., infections. To kill Salmonella in eggs, if present, boil for 7 minutes, fry for 3 minutes per side, or poach for 5 minutes. Do not use sauces or dressings made with raw eggs. Fresh eggs should be stored in the cold; cracked eggs should be discarded.

eglandulous (ē-glănd'ū-lŭs) [L. *e*, out, + *glandula*, glandule]. Without glands.

ego (ē'gō, ĕg'ō) [L. *ego*, I]. In psychoanalysis, one of the three major divisions in the model of the psychic apparatus. The others are id and superego. The ego possesses consciousness and memory and serves to mediate between the primitive instinctual or animal drives (the id), internal social prohibitions (the superego), and reality. Thus, the ego allows one to adapt to what might otherwise be a very unpleasant situation. The psychiatric use of the term should not be confused with its common usage in the sense of self-love or selfishness. SEE: *id; superego.*

egocentric (ē"gō-sĕn'trĭk) [L. *ego*, I, + Gr. *kentron*, center]. Pert. to a withdrawal from the external world with concentration upon inner self.

egocentricity. Stage of cognitive development in which the child perceives almost exclusively from his own viewpoint and in his own way. Characteristic of the toddler and early preschool child.

ego-dystonic (ē"gō-dĭs-tŏn'ĭk) [" + Gr. *dys*, bad, + *tonos*, tension]. Pert. to

something repulsive to the individual's self-image.

ego-integrity. The eighth stage in Erikson's developmental theory. The opposite of despair. The individual accepts his or her past life and whatever life has in store in the future.

egoism (ē'gō-ĭzm). An inflated estimate of one's value or effectiveness.

egomania (ē"gō-mā'nē-ă) [" + Gr. *mania*, madness]. Abnormal self-esteem and self-interest.

egophony (ē-gŏf'ō-nē) [Gr. *aix*, goat, + *phone*, voice]. A nasal sound, somewhat like the bleat of a goat, heard in auscultation of the chest when the subject speaks in a normal tone. Present in persons with pleural effusion.

ego strength. The ability of the ego to maintain its various functions, the prime one of which is to perceive reality and adapt to it.

ego-syntonic (ē"gō-sĭn-tŏn'ĭk) [" + Gr. *syn*, together, + *tonos*, tension]. Pert. to something that is consistent with the individual's self-image.

egotism (ē'gō-tĭzm). 1. The tendency to regard oneself more highly than is warranted by the facts, and to boast of one's abilities or achievements. 2. An inflated sense of self-importance; conceit. SEE: *egoism.*

egotropic (ē"gō-trŏp'ĭk) [L. *ego*, I, + Gr. *tropos*, a turning]. Interested chiefly in one's self; self-centered.

Ehlers-Danlos syndrome (ā'lĕrz-dăn'lŏs) [Edvard Ehlers, Danish dermatologist, 1863–1937; H. A. Danlos, Fr. dermatologist, 1844–1912]. An inherited disorder of the elastic connective tissue. The characteristic soft velvety skin is fragile, hyperelastic, and bruises easily. Hyperextensibility of joints, visceral malformations, atrophic scars, pseudotumors, and calcified subcutaneous cysts are present.

ETIOL: Unknown.

TREAT: No specific therapy.

PROG: Patients may be uncomfortable and inconvenienced by their disease, but the prognosis is good.

Ehrenritter's ganglion (ār'ĕn-rĭt"ĕrs) [Johann Ehrenritter, Austrian anatomist, d. 1790]. The superior ganglion of the glossopharyngeal nerve.

Ehrlich's side-chain theory (ār'lĭks) [Paul Ehrlich, Ger. physician, 1854–1915. Awarded Nobel Prize in medicine in 1908]. A theory proposed to explain immune reactions wherein the antigen-antibody reaction is compared to a chemical structure with side chains or chemical receptors. Through these chemical receptors the body cells combine with antigens that eventually are released as circulating antibodies.

Ehrlichiosis, human [P. Ehrlich]. Infection with species of the genus *Ehrlichia*, usually *Ehrlichia canis*. This member of the Rickettsia family causes an illness similar to Rocky Mountain spotted fever except for the absence of a skin rash. The disease may be transmitted by ticks.

TREAT: Tetracycline.

eicosa-. SEE: *icosa.*

eicosanoids. All of the products of the metabolism of arachidonic acid. Prostaglandins, q.v., thromboxanes, q.v., and leukotrienes, q.v., are some of the compounds formed.

eidetic (ī-dĕt′ĭk) [Gr. *eidos,* form, shape]. Rel. to or having the ability of total visual recall of anything previously seen.

eidoptometry (ī-dŏp-tŏm′ĕ-trē) [Gr. *eidos,* form, shape, + *optein,* to see, + *metron,* measure]. Determination of ability to perceive form visually.

eighth cranial nerve. The acoustic nerve. SYN: *vestibulocochlear nerve.*

Eikenella corrodens (ī″kĕn-ĕl′ă). A gram-negative rod normally present in the mouth.

eikonometry (ī″kō-nŏm′ĕ-trē) [Gr. *eikon,* image, + *metron,* measure]. 1. Determination of distance of an object by measuring the image produced by a lens of known focus. 2. Optical instrument used in detecting presence of aniseikonia.

eiloid (ī′loyd) [Gr. *eilein,* to coil, + *eidos,* form, shape]. Having a coil-like structure.

Eimeria (ī-mē′rē-ă). A genus of sporozoan parasites belonging to the class Telosporidia, subclass Coccidia. They are intracellular parasites living in the epithelial cells of vertebrates and invertebrates. They rarely are parasitic to humans.

E. hominis. A species that has been found in empyema in humans.

einsteinium (īn-stīn′ē-ŭm) [Albert Einstein, German-born U.S. physicist, 1879–1955]. SYMB: Es. At. wt. 254.0881; at. no. 99. A radioactive element.

Eisenmenger′s complex [Victor Eisenmenger, Ger. physician, 1864–1932]. Congenital cyanotic heart defect consisting of ventricular septal defect, dextroposition of the aorta, pulmonary hypertension with pulmonary artery enlargement and hypertrophy of the right ventricle.

eisodic (ī-sŏd′ĭk) [Gr. *eis,* into, + *hodos,* way]. Centripetal or afferent, as nerve fibers of a reflex arc.

ejaculate. The semen released during ejaculation.

ejaculatio (ē-jăk″ū-lā′shē-ō) [L.]. Sudden expelling; ejaculation.

e. praecox. Premature ejaculation. Inability to prevent ejaculation of semen at the beginning of copulation or prior to it.

ejaculation (ē-jăk″ū-lā′shŭn) [L. *ejaculari,* to throw out]. Ejection of the seminal fluid from the male urethra.

PHYS: Ejaculation consists of two phases: (1) the passage of semen and the secretions of the accessory organs (bulbourethral and prostate glands and seminal vesicles) into the urethra and (2) the expulsion of the seminal fluid from the urethra. The former is brought about by contraction of the smooth muscle of the ductus deferens and the increased secretory activity of the glands; the latter by the rhythmical contractions of the bulbocavernosus and ischiocavernosus muscles and the levator ani. The prostate discharges its secretions before those of the seminal vesicle. The sensations associated with ejaculation constitute the male orgasm.

Ejaculation is a reflex phenomenon. Afferent impulses arising principally from stimulation of the glans penis pass to the spinal cord by way of the internal pudendal nerves. Efferent impulses arising from a reflex center located in the upper lumbar region of the cord pass through sympathetic fibers in the hypogastric nerves and plexus to the ductus deferens and seminal vesicles. Other impulses arising from the 3rd and 4th sacral segments pass through the internal pudendal nerves to the ischiocavernosus and bulbocavernosus muscles. Erection of the penis usually precedes ejaculation. Ejaculation occurs normally during copulation, masturbation, or as a nocturnal emission. The seminal fluid normally contains 60 to 150 million sperm/ml. The volume of the ejaculation is from 2 to 5 ml. SEE: *electroejaculation; orgasm; semen.*

RS: coitus; excitation; orgasm.

e., premature. SEE: *premature ejaculation.*

e., retrograde. Ejaculation in which the seminal fluid is discharged into the bladder rather than to the outside through the urethra. A condition usually present after prostatectomy. It is possible to retrieve the sperm and then use them for artificial insemination.

ejaculatory. Pert. to ejaculation.

ejaculatory duct. The terminal portion of the seminal duct formed by the union of the ductus deferens and the excretory duct of the seminal vesicle.

ejecta (ē-jĕk′tă) [L. *ejectus,* thrown out, ejected]. Material, esp. waste material, excreted by the body. SYN: *dejecta; egesta.*

ejection (ē-jĕk′shŭn). Removal of something, esp. a sudden removal.

e., ventricular. Forceful expulsion of blood from the ventricles of the heart.

ejection fraction. In cardiac physiology, the percentage of the blood emptied from the ventricle during contraction.

Ekbom's syndrome [K. A. Ekbom, Swedish neurologist, b. 1907]. SEE: *restless legs syndrome.*

EKG. Abbr. for Ger. *elektrokardiogramm.* SEE: *ECG.*

ekphorize (ĕk'fō-rīz) [Gr. *ek*, out, + *phorein*, to bear]. In psychiatry, to bring back the effect of a psychic experience in an attempt to experience it again in memory. SEE: *engram.*

elaboration (ē-lăb″ō-rā'shŭn). The process of metabolizing food so that it may be utilized by the body.

elastance. The character or quality of a material to return to its original form after having been deformed. SEE: *compliance,* def. 1.

elastase (ē-lăs'tās). A pancreatic enzyme that in the presence of trypsin cleaves amino acids from proteins.

elastic (ē-lăs'tĭk) [Gr. *elastikos,* drive on, set in motion]. Capable of being stretched and returning to its original state; having elasticity.

e., intermaxillary. Elastic band between maxillary and mandibular teeth used in orthodontic therapy; also called a maxillomandibular elastic.

e., intramaxillary. Elastic band used in horizontal space closure by attachments within the same arch.

e., vertical. Elastic applied to arch brackets in a manner perpendicular to the occlusal plane for approximating teeth.

elastic bandage. Bandage that can be stretched to exert continuous pressure.

elastic cartilage. Yellow cartilage such as is found in the epiglottis, pharynx, external ears, and auditory tube.

elasticity (ē″lăs-tĭs'ĭ-tē). The quality of returning to original size and shape after compression or stretching.

elastic skin. Rare condition in which there is unusual elastic state of the skin.

elastic stocking. Stocking worn to apply pressure to the extremity, aiding the return of blood from the extremity to the heart through the deep veins.

elastic tissue. Connective tissue supplied with elastic fibers as found in the middle coat of arteries.

elastin (ē-lăs'tĭn). An extracellular connective tissue protein that is the principal component of elastic fibers.

elastinase (ē-lăs'tĭn-ās). An enzyme that dissolves elastin.

elastofibroma (ē-lăs″tō-fĭ-brō'mă) [″ + L. *fibra,* fiber, + Gr. *oma,* tumor]. A benign soft tissue tumor that contains elastic and fibrous elements.

elastoid (ē-lăs'toyd) [″ + *eidos,* form, shape]. Pert. to a substance formed by hyaline degeneration.

elastoma (ē″lăs-tō'mă) [″ + *oma,* tumor]. A chronic disease of the skin; pseudoxanthoma.

elastomer (ē-lăs'tō-mĕr) [″ + *meros,* a part]. A polymeric substance that has elastic properties similar to rubber.

elastometer (ē″lăs-tŏm'ĕ-tĕr) [″ + Gr. *metron,* measure]. Device for measuring elasticity.

elastometry. The measurement of elasticity of tissues.

elastorrhexis (ē-lăs″tō-rĕk'sĭs) [″ + *rhexis,* rupture]. Rupture of elastic tissue.

elastose (ē-lăs'tōs). A peptone resulting from gastric digestion of elastin.

elastosis (ē″lăs-tō'sĭs) [″ + *osis,* condition]. Any disease of elastic tissues.

e., nodular. SEE: *nodular elastosis.*

elation (ē-lā'shŭn) [L. *elatus,* exalted]. Joyful emotion. It is of pathological origin when out of accord with patient's actual circumstances.

Elavil. Trade name for amitriptyline hydrochloride.

elbow (ĕl'bō) [AS. *eln,* forearm, + *boga,* bend]. Joint between arm and forearm. SEE: illus.

e., golfer's. A strain of the medial forearm muscles near their origin on the medial epicondyle of the humerus. SYN: *medial epicondylitis.* SEE: *tennis elbow.*

e., little league. SEE: *little league elbow.*

e., tennis. A strain of the lateral forearm muscles near their origin on the lateral epicondyle of the humerus. SEE: *tennis elbow;* SYN: *epicondylitis, lateral humeral.*

elbow conformer. A splint applied to prevent flexion contractures following burns to the upper extremity. The device is fabricated to conform to the anterior arm. Pressure is applied to the olecranon process by a soft, cupped pad.

elbow jerk. Involuntary bending of elbow caused by striking tendon of biceps or triceps muscle.

elbow joint. Joint between arm and the forearm. Includes the humeroulnar, humeroradial, and proximal radioulnar articulations.

elbow reflexes. Reflexes in the elbow region are the biceps reflex and triceps reflex. SEE: *biceps reflex; triceps reflex.*

elbow unit. A component of the upper extremity prosthesis that permits the arm to bend at the elbow.

Eldecort. Trade name for hydrocortisone.

elderly primigravida. A woman who is 35 years of age or older and pregnant for the first time. In the past, women were informed that delaying childbearing until age 35 or

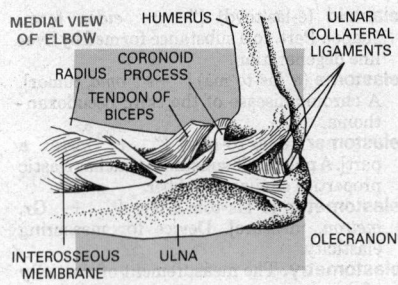

MEDIAL VIEW OF ELBOW
HUMERUS
ULNAR COLLATERAL LIGAMENTS
CORONOID PROCESS
RADIUS
TENDON OF BICEPS
OLECRANON
INTEROSSEOUS MEMBRANE
ULNA

CROSS-SECTION THROUGH ELBOW
HUMERUS

RADIUS
SYNOVIAL SPACE
ULNA

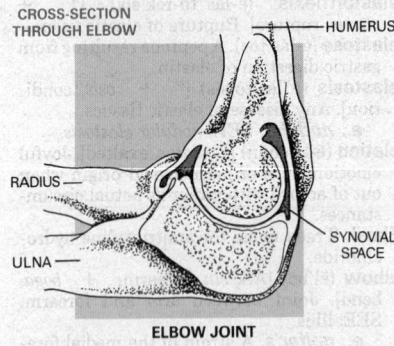

ELBOW JOINT

more would greatly increase the chance of an adverse outcome of pregnancy. A well-controlled study of the outcome of first pregnancy in this age group indicates little, if any, increased risk of adverse fetal outcome. These women did have significantly more antepartum and intrapartum complications than younger women. The patients studied were private patients who were predominantly white, college educated, married, nonsmoking, and had had excellent prenatal care.

elective therapy. A treatment or surgical procedure not requiring immediate attention and therefore planned for the patient's convenience.

Electra complex [Gr. Elektra, Agamemnon's daughter, who helped assassinate her mother because of love for her father, whom the former had slain]. In psychoanalysis, a group of symptoms due to suppressed sexual love of daughter for father. SEE: *Jocasta complex; Oedipus complex.*

electric, -al [Gr. *elektron*, amber]. Pert. to, caused by, or resembling electricity.

electricity. A form of energy that exhibits magnetic, chemical, mechanical, and thermal effects. Electricity is formed from the interactions of positive and negative charges. SEE: *electromotive force.*

    e., frictional. Generation of static electricity by rubbing two articles together.

    e., galvanic. Electricity generated by chemical action.

    e., induced. Electricity generated in a body from another body close by without contact.

    e., magnetic. Electricity induced by means of a magnetic device.

    e., negative. Electrical charge caused by an excess of electrons negatively charged.

    e., positive. Electrical charge caused by loss of negative electrons.

    e., static. Electricity generated by friction of certain materials.

electric light baker. Device for warming a part, as in arthritis. SEE: *baker.*

electric shock. Injury from electricity, which varies according to type and strength of current and length and location of contact. Electric shocks vary from trivial burns to complete charring and destruction of skin; or unconsciousness from paralysis of the respiratory center, fibrillation of the heart, or both. Approximately 1000 persons are electrocuted accidentally each year in the U.S., and 4000 persons are injured. Five percent of admissions to burn centers are related to electrical injury.

    Whether or not an electric shock will cause death is influenced by the pathway the current takes through the body, the amount of current, and the skin resistance. Thus, a very small amount of electric energy applied directly to the heart may be enough to cause the heart to cease activity. As little as one milliampere of 60 cycle current applied directly to the ventricle can cause fibrillation. Conversely, a very large amount of electric energy may be unable to penetrate the dry calloused skin of the fingers and hands and thus be harmless.

    An effective current greater than 15 milliamperes for alternating current and 75 milliamperes for direct current causes muscle tissue to contract. The hand exposed to a sufficient electric current is unable to release its grip. Chest muscles will be paralyzed and respiration will cease if sufficient current passes across the thorax.

    Emergency insulation: Protection against such currents may be made with dry nonconductors such as folded newspapers, magazines, cardboard, wood, rubber, or clothing. These may be used to move patient from the contact or to remove wire from patient. It is always preferable to turn off the current if possible. If patient is in water, remember that it is electrically charged and special precautions must be taken. On a humid or rainy day, ordinary insulators may contain sufficient moisture to conduct electricity. Make sure insulators are dry.

High-tension currents, such as those used about x-ray equipment or in conducting currents for long distances or for special industrial locations, cannot be insulated by such means. Such currents may penetrate or pass through rubber, paper, or strips of wood. A safe procedure is to ascertain the source of current and have it shut off; otherwise, multiple tragedies could result.

SYM: Burns, loss of consciousness.

F.A.: Carefully free victim from source of current with nonconductors or shut off current. Prolonged artificial respiration may be necessary. SEE: *cardiopulmonary resuscitation; lightning safety rules; resuscitation; shock.*

electrify [Gr. *elektron,* amber, + L. *facere,* to make]. To charge a body with electricity.

electrization. The act of charging or treating by use of electricity.

electro-, electr- [Gr. *elektron,* amber]. Prefix indicating relationship to electricity.

electroaffinity (ē-lĕk″trō-ă-fĭn′ĭ-tē). Measure of the capability of ions to retain their charge.

electroanalgesia (ē-lĕk″trō-ăn″ăl-jē′zē-ă) [″ + *analgesia,* want of feeling]. Producing relief from pain by using low-intensity electric currents applied locally or through implanted electrodes.

electroanesthesia (ē-lĕk″trō-ăn″ĕs-thē′ zē-ă) [″ + *an-,* not, + *aisthesis,* sensation]. General anesthesia produced by a device that passes electricity of a certain frequency, amplitude, and wave form through the brain.

electrobiology (ē-lĕk″trō-bī-ŏl′ō-jē) [″ + *bios,* life, + *logos,* word, reason]. Science of electric phenomena in the living body.

electrocardiogram (ē-lĕk″trō-kăr′dē-ō-grăm″) [″ + *kardia,* heart, + *gramma,* something written]. ABBR: ECG. A record of the electrical activity of the heart; shows certain waves called P, Q, R, S, and T waves. Sometimes a U wave is seen. The first or P wave is caused by the depolarization of the atrial muscle tissues, whose electrical changes in turn caused atrial contraction. The Q, R, and S waves (QRS complex) correspond to depolarization of ventricular muscle. The T wave corresponds to ventricular repolarization. The electrocardiogram gives important information concerning the spread of excitation to the different parts of the heart, and it is of value in the diagnosis of cases of abnormal cardiac rhythm and myocardial damage. SEE: illus.

electrocardiograph (ē-lĕk″trō-kăr′dē-ō-grăf) [″ + ″ + *graphein,* to write]. Device for recording electrical variations in action of heart muscles.

electrocardiography. The making and study of graphic records (electrocardiograms) produced by electric currents originating in the heart.

electrocardiophonograph (ē-lĕk″trō-kăr″dē-ō-fō′nō-grăf) [Gr. *elektron,* amber, + *kardia,* heart, + *phone,* sound, + *graphein,* to write]. Device for recording heart sounds.

electrocatalysis (ē-lĕk″trō-kă-tăl′ĭ-sĭs) [″ + *kata,* down, + *lysis,* dissolution]. Chemical decomposition produced by electricity.

electrocautery (ē-lĕk″trō-kaw′tĕr-ē) [″ + *kauterion,* branding iron]. Cauterization by means of an apparatus consisting of a holder containing a wire, which may be heated to a red or white heat by an electric current, either direct or alternating.

electrochemistry [″ + *chemeia,* chemistry]. Science of chemical changes produced by electricity.

electrocision (ē-lĕk′trō-sĭzh′ŭn) [″ + L. *caedare,* to cut]. Excision by electric current.

electrocoagulation (ē-lĕk″trō-kō-ăg″ū-lā′ shŭn) [″ + L. *coagulare,* to thicken]. Coagulation of tissue by means of a high-frequency electric current. The heat producing the coagulation is generated within the tissue to be destroyed.

electrocochleography (ē-lĕk″trō-kŏk-lē-ŏg′ ră-fē). Measurement of electrical activity produced when the cochlea is stimulated. Technique involves placing a needle electrode on the cochlea by passing it through the eardrum. The electrical activity is then recorded.

electrocontractility (ē-lĕk″trō-kŏn-trăk-tĭl′ ĭ-tē) [″ + L. *contrahere,* to contract]. Contraction of muscular tissue by electrical stimulation.

electroconvulsive therapy (ē-lĕk″trō-kŏn-vŭl′sĭv). ABBR: ECT. The use of an electric shock to produce convulsions. At one time, this form of therapy was used so indiscriminately that it fell into disfavor. There is, nevertheless, a place for this type of treatment in specific types of mental illness, esp. in people with acute depression and suicidal intentions.

electrocorticography (ē-lĕk″trō-kor″tĭ-kŏg′ ră-fē). Recording the electrical impulses from the brain by placing electrodes directly on the cerebral cortex.

electrocryptectomy (ē-lĕk″trō-krĭp-tĕk′tō-mē) [″ + *kryptos,* concealed, + *ektome,* excision]. Destruction of tonsillar crypts by diathermy.

electrocution (ē-lĕk″trō-kū′shŭn) [″ + L. *acutus,* sharpened]. The destruction of life by means of electric current. SEE: *electric*

QRST COMPLEX OF ELECTROCARDIOGRAM

ELECTROCARDIOGRAM LEADS

LIMB LEADS

LEAD I   LEAD II   LEAD III

AUGMENTED LIMB LEADS

LEAD aV$_R$ LEAD aV$_L$ LEAD aV$_F$

shock; lightning safety rules.

electrode (ē-lĕk′trōd) [″ + *hodos,* a way]. A medium intervening between an electric conductor and the object to which the current is to be applied. In electrotherapy an electrode is an instrument with a point or a surface from which to discharge current to the body of a patient.

    e., active. Electrode that is smaller in size than a dispersive electrode and produces stimulation in a concentrated area.

    e., calomel. Electrode that develops a standard electrical potential. It is used as a standard in determining the pH of fluids.

    e., depolarizing. Electrode with greater resistance than the part of the body in the circuit.

    e., dispersive. Electrode larger in size than an active electrode. It produces electrical stimulation over a large area.

    e., gas-sending. A chemical sensor that responds to the partial pressure of a gas in solution. Used routinely to measure blood gases.

    e., glass. In chemistry, used to describe the chemical sensors that employ a glass membrane as opposed to those that use organic or solid state membranes as the sensing surface.

    e., hydrogen. Electrode that absorbs hydrogen gas.

    e., immobilized enzyme. A chemical sensor that is highly selective due to a specific enzyme incorporated into its structure.

    e., indifferent. E., dispersive.

    e., internal reference. In chemistry, the metal electrode inside all chemical sensing potentiometric electrodes.

    e., ion-selective. A chemical transducer that yields a response to variations in the concentration of a given ion in solution.

    e., multiple point. Several sets of terminals providing for the use of several electrodes. SEE: *multiterminal.*

    e., negative. Cathode.

    e., point. Electrode with an insulating handle at one end and a metallic point at the other for use in applying static sparks. SYN: *e., spark ball.*

    e., positive. Anode.

    e., reference. A chemical electrode whose cell potential remains fixed and against which an indicator electrode is compared. The most common reference electrode is the (Ag/AgCl) silver/silver chloride electrode.

    e., spark-ball. E., point, q.v.

    e., subcutaneous. Electrode placed beneath the skin.

    e., surface. Electrode placed on the surface of the skin or exposed organ.

    e., therapeutic. Electrode for introduc-

tion of medicines through the skin by ionization. SEE: *iontophoresis.*

electrodermal (ē-lĕk″trō-dĕr′măl). Concerning the electrical properties of skin.

electrodesiccation (ē-lĕk″trō-dĕs″ĭ-kā′shŭn) [Gr. *elektron,* amber, + L. *desiccare,* to dry up]. The destructive drying of cells and tissue by means of short high-frequency electric sparks, in contradistinction to fulguration, which is the destruction of tissue by means of long high-frequency electric sparks. Electrodesiccation is used for hemostasis of very small capillaries or veins that have been severed during surgery.

electrodiagnosis. Use of electrical and electronic devices for diagnostic purposes. Their use is helpful in almost all branches of medicine, but particularly in investigating function of the heart, nerves, and muscles.

electrodialysis (ē-lĕk″trō-dī-ăl′ĭ-sĭs) [″ + *dia-,* apart, + *lysis,* dissolution] (pl. *electrodialyses*). A method of separating electrolytes from colloids by passing a current through a solution containing both.

electrodynamometer (ē-lĕk″trō-dī″nă-mŏm′ĕ-tĕr) [″ + *dynamis,* power, + *metron,* measure]. An instrument to measure the strength of an electric current.

electroejaculation. Production of ejaculation by electrical stimulation from a probe placed in the rectum. This method has been used to produce a semen sample from paraplegic patients. The semen was then used successfully for artificial insemination.

electroencephalogram (ē-lĕk″trō-ĕn-sĕf′ă-lō-grăm) [″ + *enkephalos,* brain, + *gramma,* something written]. ABBR: EEG. A tracing on an electroencephalograph. SEE: illus.; *electroencephalography.*

electroencephalograph (ē-lĕk-trō-ĕn-sĕf′ă-lō-grăf) [″ + ″ + *graphein,* to write]. An instrument for recording electrical activity of the brain. SEE: *electroencephalography.*

electroencephalography. Amplification, recording, and analysis of the electrical activity of the brain. The record obtained is called an electroencephalogram (EEG).

    Electrodes are placed on the scalp in various locations. The difference between the electrical potential of two sites is recorded. The potential between a pair at a time or between many pairs can be obtained simultaneously. The most frequently seen pattern in the normal adult under resting conditions is the alpha rhythm of 8½ to 12 per second. A characteristic change in the wave occurs during sleep, upon opening the eyes, and during mental attention. Some persons who have intracranial disease will have a normal EEG and others with no otherwise demonstrable disease will have an

NORMAL AND ABNORMAL
ELECTROENCEPHALOGRAM WAVE PATTERNS

NORMAL ADULT
10/sec. activity in occipital area

PETIT MAL SEIZURE
Synchronous 3/sec. spikes and waves

GRAND MAL SEIZURE
High-voltage spikes, generalized

TEMPORAL LOBE EPILEPSY
Right temporal spike focus

BRAIN TUMOR
Left frontal slow wave focus

ENCEPHALITIS
Diffuse slowing

Source: Reprinted with permission from The Merck Manual, 13th ed., Merck & Co., Inc., 1977, pp. 1408–1409.

abnormal EEG. Nevertheless, the use of this diagnostic technique has proved to be very helpful in studying epilepsy and convulsive disorders and in localizing lesions in the cerebrum. SEE: *rhythm, alpha; rhythm, beta; wave, theta.*

electrogoniometer (ē-lĕk″trō-gō″nē-ŏm′ē-tĕr). Electrical device for measuring angles of joints and their range of motion.

electrograph. A record usually graphically displayed or recorded of the electrical activity produced by biological tissues. Thus an electrocardiogram is a form of electrograph.

electrohemostasis (ē-lĕk″trō-hē-mŏs′tā-sĭs) [Gr. *elektron,* amber, + *haima,* blood, + *stasis,* standing still]. The arrest of bleeding by means of a high-frequency current. SEE: *cautery.*

electrohysterography (ē-lĕk″trō-hĭs″tĕr-ŏg′ră-fē) [″ + *hystera,* womb, + *graphein,* to write]. Recording the electrical activity of muscle tissue, myometrium, of the uterus.

electrology [″ + *logos,* word, reason]. The branch of science that deals with the phenomena and properties of electricity.

electrolysis (ē″lĕk-trŏl′ĭ-sĭs) [″ + *lysis,* dissolution]. The decomposition of a substance by passage of an electric current through it. Hair follicles may be destroyed by use of this method. SEE: *depilatory techniques.*

electrolyte (ē-lĕk′trō-līt) [″ + *lytos,* soluble]. 1. A solution that is a conductor of electricity. 2. A substance that, in solution, conducts an electric current and is decomposed by the passage of an electric current. Acids, bases, and salts are common electrolytes. 3. Ionized salts in blood, tissue fluids and cells including salts of sodium, potassium, and chlorine. SEE: table.

    e., amphoteric. A solution that produces both hydrogen (H^+) and hydroxyl (OH^-) ions.

electrolytes, direct measurement of. Measurement of serum ions, such as sodium, chloride, potassium, etc., without prior dilution of the sample. The direct measurement of electrolytes is considered to be more nearly accurate than measurement by indirect methods, as it is not prone to error in cases of hyperlipidemia.

electrolytes, indirect measurement of. Measurement of serum ions, such as sodium, chloride, potassium, etc., that employs dilution of the sample prior to analysis. The method is prone to error in cases of hyperlipidemia.

electrolytic (ē-lĕk″trō-lĭt′ĭk). Caused by or rel. to electrolysis.

electrolytic conduction. In metals, the electrical charges are carried by the electrons of inappreciable mass. In solutions, the electrical charges are carried by electrolytic ions, each one of a mass several thousand times as great as the electron. When a direct current passes through an electrolytic solution between metallic electrodes immersed in it, the positive ions move to the cathode, the negative ions to the anode.

electromagnet [″ + *magnes,* magnet]. A magnet consisting of a length of insulated wire wound around soft iron core.

electromagnetic. Pert. to an electromagnet.

electromagnetic induction. Generation of an electromotive force, q.v., in an insulated conductor moving in an electromagnetic field or in a fixed conductor in a moving magnetic field.

electromagnetic radiation. All forms of energy emanating from an electrical source and transmitted through the air. Included are the electromagnetic fields produced by light, radio, x-rays, and gamma rays. The higher the frequency of the fields produced, the more energy contained. Thus, the radiated energy from the 60 cycle frequency of an ordinary household electrical line is quite small. Nevertheless, the long-range effects of exposure to even these low-level fields is being investigated to determine whether or not this type of exposure represents a health hazard.

electromagnetic spectrum. SEE: *spectrum, electromagnetic;* table.

electromagnetism. Magnetism produced by an electric current.

electromassage [″ + Fr. *masser,* to massage]. Massage combined with electrical treatment.

electrometer (ē-lĕk-trŏm′ē-tĕr) [″ + *metron,* measure]. An instrument for measuring differences in electric potential.

electromotive [″ + L. *motor,* mover]. Pert. to passage of electricity in a current or motion produced by it.

electromotive force. ABBR: EMF. The effect of differences of potential that, on the closing of a circuit, causes a flow of electricity from one place to another, giving rise to an electric current. The strength of an electric current is directly proportional to the impressed electromotive force and inversely proportional to the resistance in the case of direct current and to the impedance in the case of alternating current. Electromotive force is measured in volts or in some convenient multiple or fraction of a volt. Microvolt, millivolt, and kilovolt are, respectively, one-millionth volt, one-thousandth volt, and 1000 volts.

    In order to understand the terms used to define electricity, a somewhat simple analogy can be made between water flowing

Electrolytes (Cations and Anions) in Plasma, Interstitial Water (ISW), and Intercellular Water (ICW)

	Plasma mEq/L average	ISW mEq/kg H_2O* average	ICW mEq/kg H_2O average
Cations			
Na^+	140	144	5–10
K^+	4	4	155
Ca^{2+}	5	3	3
Mg^{2+}	2	2	30
Total	151	153	193–198
Anions			
Cl^-	103	114	5–10
HCO_3^-	26	28	10
Protein	16	2	
HPO_4^{2-}; $H_2PO_4^-$	2	1	180†
SO_4^{2-}	1	4	
Organic Acids	4	4	
Total	151	153	195–200

Source: Adapted from Krupp, MA and Chatton, MJ (eds): Current Medical Diagnosis and Treatment 1982. Appleton & Lange, East Norwalk, CT, 1982.
* Concentrations derived by converting plasma concentrations to mEq/L of plasma water, accounting for nonwater volume of plasma and applying Donnan factors of 0.96 for monovalent ions and 0.92 for divalent ions.
† Protein, organic phosphates, other organic compounds.

through a pipe and electricity flowing through a wire. The *amount* of electricity, measured in *amperes*, can be compared to the *amount* of water flowing; the *pressure* of electricity, measured in *volts* and called *electromotive force*, can be compared to the *pressure* forcing the water through the pipe; the *resistance* to the flow of electricity, measured in *ohms*, can be compared to the *resistance* to the flow of water through a pipe. Obviously, as the size of the pipe increases, the resistance decreases.

The relationship of the strength of electric current to electromotive force (volts) and the resistance (ohms) to the flow of electricity in a circuit is expressed by the formula:

$$I = \frac{E}{R}$$

I (current expressed in amperes); E (volts); and R (resistance expressed in ohms). This formula expresses Ohm's law, q.v.

electromyogram (ē-lĕk″trō-mī′ō-grăm) [Gr. *elektron*, amber, + *mys*, muscle, + *gramma*, something written]. A graphic record of the contraction of a muscle as a result of electrical stimulation.

electromyography (ē-lĕk″trō-mī-ŏg′ră-fē)

[″ + ″ + *graphein*, to write]. The preparation, study of, and interpretation of electromyograms.

electron [Gr. *elektron*, amber]. An extremely minute particle with a negative electrical charge that revolves about the central core or nucleus of an atom. Its mass is about ⅟₁₈₄₀ that of a hydrogen atom, or 9.11×10^{-28} grams. The negative electrical charge is 1.602×10^{-19} coulombs. When emitted from radioactive substances, electrons are known as negative beta particles or rays.

electronarcosis (ē-lĕk″trō-năr-kō′sĭs). The induction of narcosis or unconsciousness by the application of electricity to the brain.

electron-dense. In electron microscopy, pert. to tissue of a density that prevents penetration by electrons.

electronegative [″ + L. *negare*, to deny]. Condition of being charged with negative electricity, which results in the attraction of bodies positively charged and the repulsion of bodies negatively charged.

electroneurolysis (ē-lĕk″trō-nū-rŏl′ĭ-sĭs). Destruction of a nerve by use of an electric needle.

electronic. Pert. to electrons.

electronic dental anesthesia. ABBR: EDA. In dentistry, low levels of electric current are used to block pain signals en route to the

Electromagnetic Spectrum

Frequency Hz (cycles per second)	Character of Radiation	Wavelength Cm	
10^{23}		10^{-12}	
	Cosmic Rays		
10^{22}		10^{-11}	
10^{21}			
	Gamma Rays	10^{-10}	
10^{20}		10^{-9}	
10^{19}			
	X-Rays	10^{-8}	
10^{18}		10^{-7}	
10^{17}			
		10^{-6}	
10^{16}	Ultraviolet Radiation		
		10^{-5}	
10^{15}	Visible Light		
		10^{-4}	
10^{14}	Infrared Radiation		
		10^{-3}	
10^{13}			
		10^{-2}	
10^{12}	Submillimeter Waves		
		10^{-1}	
10^{11}			
		1.0	
10^{10}	Microwaves (Radar)		
		10	
10^{9}			UHF (ultra high frequency)
		10^{2}	
10^{8}	Television and FM Radio		VHF (very high frequency)
		10^{3}	
10^{7}	Short Wave Radio		HF (high frequency)
		10^{4}	
10^{6}	AM Radio		MF (medium frequency)
		10^{5}	
10^{5}			LF (low frequency)
	Maritime Communications	10^{6}	
10^{4}			VLF (very low frequency)

Source: Adapted from Van Nostrand's Scientific Encyclopedia, ed 5. Van Nostrand Reinhold Co., New York, 1976.

brain. The patient controls the current through a hand-held box. The current creates no discomfort and, unlike local anesthesia, there is no numbness to wear off once the dental work is completed. SEE: *patient-controlled analgesia.*

electronic fetal monitoring. ABBR: EFM. The use of an electronic device to monitor fetal vital signs.

electronic infusion device. ABBR: EID. A

device for monitoring I.V. infusions. The device may have an alarm in case the flow is restricted because of an occlusion of the line. In that case, the alarm will sound when a preset pressure limit is sensed. The device can also signal that an I.V. is close to completion. The pressure is regulated by the height at which the I.V. container is positioned above the level of the heart when the patient is flat. A height of 36 in. (91 cm) will provide a pressure of 1.3 lb/sq in. (70 mmHg). SEE: *infusion pump.*

electronics. The science of all systems involving the use of electric devices used for communication, information processing, and control.

electronic voice. SEE: *speech synthesizer.*

electronization [Gr. *elektron,* amber]. The use of radiation to restore electrical equilibrium to diseased cells.

electron microscope. SEE: *microscope, electron; microscope, scanning electron.*

electron volt. SYMB: eV. The energy acquired by an electron as it passes through a potential of 1 volt.

electronystagmography (ē-lĕk″trō-nĭs″tăg-mŏg′ră-fē) [″ + *nystagmos,* drowsiness, + *graphein,* to write]. A method of recording nystagmus activity by detecting the electrical activity of the extraocular muscles. SEE: *nystagmus.*

electro-oculogram (ē-lĕk″trō-ŏk′ū-lō-grăm″). Recording of the electric currents produced by eye movements. SEE: *electroretinogram.*

electropathology (ē-lĕk″trō-pă-thŏl′ō-jē) [″ + *pathos,* disease, suffering, + *logos,* word, reason]. Determining electrical reaction of muscles and nerves as means of diagnosis.

electrophobia. Irrational fear of electricity.

electrophoresis (ē-lĕk″trō-for-ē′sĭs) [″ + *phoresis,* bearing]. The movement of charged colloidal particles through the medium in which they are dispersed as a result of changes in electrical potential. Electrophoretic methods are useful in the analysis of protein mixtures as protein particles move with different velocities dependent principally on the number of charges carried by the particle. SEE: *diathermy; iontophoresis; phoresis.*

electrophorus (ē-lĕk″trŏf′ō-rŭs) [″ + *phorein,* to bear]. An instrument for obtaining static electricity by means of induction.

electrophrenic (ē-lĕk″trō-frĕn′ĭk). Pert. to stimulation of the phrenic nerve by electricity.

electrophrenic respiration. Application of intermittent electrical stimuli to cutaneous electrodes over the phrenic nerves in the neck to rhythmically stimulate respiration.

Used in the patient whose respiratory center has been damaged.

electrophysiology (ē-lĕk″trō-fĭz″ē-ŏl′ō-gē) [″ + *physis,* nature, + *logos,* word, reason]. A branch of physiology that deals with the relationships of body functions to electrical phenomena such as the effects of electrical stimulation upon the tissues, the production of electric currents by organs and tissues, and the therapeutic use of electric currents.

electropositive [″ + L. *positivus,* to put, place]. Condition of being subject to repulsion by bodies positively electrified and to attraction by bodies negatively electrified.

electropuncture [″ + L. *punctura,* to prick]. Piercing tissues with an electrically heated needle.

electroradiometer (ē-lĕk″trō-rā-dē-ŏm′ē-tĕr) [″ + L. *radius,* ray, + Gr. *metron,* measure]. An electroscope for differentiation of radiant energy.

electroresection (ē-lĕk″trō-rē-sĕk′shŭn). Removal of tissue by use of an electrical device such as a cautery.

electroretinogram (ē-lĕk″trō-rĕt′ĭ-nō-grăm). ABBR: ERG. A record of the action currents of the retina produced by visual or light stimuli.

electroscission (ē-lĕk″trō-sĭ′zhŭn) [″ + L. *scindere,* to cut]. Division of tissues by electrocautery.

electroscope (ē-lĕk′trō-skōp) [″ + *skopein,* to examine]. An instrument that detects intensity of radiation.

electroshock. Shock produced by an electric current.

electroshock therapy. The induction of convulsive seizures by the passing of an electric current through the brain. Used in the treatment of acute depression. SEE: *electroconvulsive therapy.*

electrosleep. Sleep production as a result of the passage of mild electrical impulses through parts of the brain. Has been used experimentally in treating insomnia and mental illness.

electrostatic [Gr. *elektron,* amber, + *statikos,* causing to stand]. Pert. to static electricity.

electrostatic generator. Device that generates static electricity.

electrostatic unit. Any unit of electrical measurement based on the attraction or repulsion of a static charge as distinguished from an electromagnetic unit, which is defined in terms of the attraction or repulsion of magnetic poles.

electrostimulation (ē-lĕk″trō-stĭm″ū-lā′shŭn). Use of electric current to stimulate a tissue, such as muscle or bone. In the latter case, the stimulation is used experimentally to facilitate and hasten healing of fractures.

electrosurgery (ē-lĕk″trō-sŭr′jĕ-rē) [″ + L. *chirurgia*, surgery]. Surgical procedures in which electricity is required either in the actual surgical apparatus or in the application of electrical cautery.

electrosynthesis (ē-lĕk″trō-sĭn′thĕ-sĭs). Use of electricity to synthesize chemical compounds.

electrotaxis (ē-lĕk″trō-tăk′sĭs) [″ + *taxis*, arrangement]. The movement of a cell or an organism toward or away from an electrical stimulus.

electrothanasia (ē-lĕk″trō-thă-nā′zē-ă) [″ + *thanatos*, death]. Death resulting from electric shock; electrocution.

electrotherapeutics (ē-lĕk″trō-thĕr-ă-pū′tĭks) [″ + *therapeutike*, treatment]. Use of electricity in the treatment of musculoskeletal dysfunction, pain and disease. SYN: *electrotherapy.*

electrotherapist (ē-lĕk″trō-thĕr′ă-pĭst) [″ + *therapeia*, treatment]. An individual who has had special training and has acquired skill in the therapeutic use of electricity. The term is sometimes used incorrectly to designate anyone who administers electrical treatments.

electrotherapy. Use of electricity in treating musculoskeletal dysfunction, pain, or disease. SYN: *electrotherapeutics.*

electrothermotherapy (ē-lĕk″trō-thĕr″mō-thĕr′ă-pē) [″ + ″ + *therapeia*, treatment]. The production of heat within the living tissues for therapeutic purposes by means of bodily resistance to the passing of an electric current.

electrotome (ē-lĕk′trō-tōm) [″ + *tome*, incision]. An electrocautery device used for surgical procedures.

electrotonic (ē-lĕk″trō-tŏn′ĭk) [″ + *tonos*, tension]. Of or pert. to electrotonus.

electrotonus (ē-lĕk-trŏt′ō-nŭs). The change in the irritability of a nerve or muscle during the passage of an electric current.

electrotropism (ē-lĕk-trŏt′rō-pĭzm) [″ + *trope*, a turning, + *-ismos*, condition of]. Reaction of cells to an electric current.

electrovalence (ē-lĕk″trō-vā′lĕns). The ionic linkage between atoms in which each accepts or donates electrons so that each atom ends up with a completed electron shell.

electroversion (ē-lĕk″trō-vĕr′zhŭn). SEE: *cardioversion.*

electuary (ē-lĕk′tū-ă-rē) [Gr. *ekleikhein*, to lick up]. Medicinal substance mixed with honey or sugar to form a paste suitable for oral consumption.

eleidin (ē-lē′ĭ-dĭn) [Gr. *elaion*, oil]. An acidophil substance present in the stratum lucidum of the epidermis.

element [L. *elementum*, a rudiment]. In modern chemistry, a substance that cannot be separated into substances different from itself by ordinary chemical processes. Elements exist in a free and in a combined state. More than 100 have been identified. SEE: *Elements* in *Appendix.*

Elements found in the human body include oxygen, aluminum, carbon, cobalt, hydrogen, nitrogen, calcium, phosphorus, potassium, sulfur, sodium, chlorine, magnesium, iron, fluorine, iodine, copper, manganese, and zinc.

   e.´s, trace. Chemical elements present in the body or in the diet in extremely small amounts. Some are absolutely necessary for metabolism.

element, words pert. to: atom; atomic; chemical change; chemical compound; electron; mineral compounds; neutron; nucleus; oxidation; oxide; radical; radioactive; valence.

eleoma (ĕl″ē-ō′mă) [Gr. *elaion*, oil, + *oma*, tumor]. Swelling in tissue produced by the injection of oil.

eleosaccharum (ĕl″ē-ō-săk′ă-rŭm) [″ + *sakcharon*, sugar]. A mixture of powdered sugar with a volatile oil.

elephantiasis (ĕl″ē-făn-tī′ă-sĭs) [Gr. *elephas*, elephant, + *-iasis*, condition]. A chronic infectious condition characterized by pronounced hypertrophy of the skin and subcutaneous tissues resulting from obstruction of the lymphatic vessels. The lower extremities and the scrotum are parts most frequently involved. SYN: *pachydermatosis.*

ETIOL: Elephantiasis may be congenital (Milroy's disease) or the result of metastatic invasion of the lymph nodes by tumor cells. Inflammatory elephantiasis results from filariasis or local infection of the lymph nodes. Elephantiasis is caused by infection of the lymphatics by one of the three filiarial parasites of man, *Wuchereria bancrofti, Brugia malayi,* or *Brugia timori.* It is common in tropical countries.

TREAT: There is no completely effective therapy, but diethylcarbamazine reduces the number of organisms in the peripheral blood. Surgery to treat hydrocele is indicated. Surgery is not effective in treating lymphedema of the legs.

   e., scrotal. Elephantiasis that is mainly located in the scrotum. SYN: *chyloderma.*

elephant man disease. Colloquial name for Recklinghausen's disease, q.v.

elevation (ĕl″ē-vā′shŭn). A raised area that protrudes above the surrounding area.

   e.´s, tactile. Small raised areas of palms and soles that contain a cluster of nerve endings.

elevator [L. *elevare*, to lift up]. 1. Curved retractor for holding lid away from the globe of the eye. 2. Retractor for raising depressed bones by levers or screws. 3. Instruments of various designs for extracting teeth or removing root or bone fragments.

    e., periosteal. Surgical instrument for separating the periosteum from the bone.

eleventh cranial nerve. Motor nerve made up of a cranial and a spinal part that supplies the trapezius and sternomastoid muscles and pharynx. Accessory portion joins the vagus, to which it supplies motor and some of its cardioinhibitory fibers. SYN: *accessory nerve; spinal accessory nerve.*

eliminant (ē-lĭm'ĭ-nănt) [L. *e,* out, + *limen,* threshold]. 1. Effecting evacuation. 2. Agent aiding in elimination.

eliminate (ē-lĭm'ĭ-nāt). To expel; to rid the body of waste material.

elimination. 1. Excretion of waste products by the skin, kidneys, and intestines. 2. Leaving out, omitting, removing.

elimination, words pert. to: absorption; constipation; defecation; dejecta; egesta; ejecta; enema; evacuate; feces; flatus; stool.

elimination diet. A diet used to determine which foods cause an allergic response. The patient starts with a very few foods and if none of these causes sensitivity, one food is added to the diet. If that causes no reactions, another food is added, etc. Offending foods discovered by this technique are then eliminated from the diet.

elinguation (ē"lĭn-gwā'shŭn) [" + *lingua,* tongue]. The operation of removing the tongue from the oral cavity.

ELISA. *enzyme-linked immunoabsorbent assay.*

elixir (ē-lĭk'sĕr) [L. from Arabic *al-iksir*]. A sweetened, aromatic, hydro-alcoholic liquid used in the compounding of oral medicines. Elixirs constitute one of the most commonly used types of medicinal preparation taken orally in liquid form.

Elixophyllin. Trade name for theophylline.

ellipsis (ē-lĭp'sĭs) [L. *ellipsis* fr. Gr., a falling short, defective]. In psychiatric therapy, the patient's omitting important words or ideas during treatment.

ellipsoid (ē-lĭp'soyd). Spindle-shaped.

elliptocyte (ē-lĭp'tō-sīt). Oval-shaped red cells. About 15% of red cells are normally oval shaped, but in anemia and hereditary elliptocytosis, the percentage is increased. In birds, reptiles, and some other animals, the red cells are normally elliptocytes.

elliptocytosis (ē-lĭp"tō-sī-tō'sĭs). Condition of increased number of elliptocytes. It occurs in some forms of anemia.

    e., hereditary. A benign inherited condition in which the red cells are oval or elliptically shaped. This inherited curiosity occurs

in about one in each 2000 births.

Ellis-van Creveld syndrome. A congenital syndrome consisting of polydactyly, chondrodysplasia with acromelic dwarfism, hydrotic ectodermal dysplasia, and congenital heart defects. It is thought to be transmitted as an autosomal trait. SYN: *dysplasia, chondroectodermal.*

elongation (ē"lŏng-gā'shŭn). The condition of being extended or lengthened, or the process of extending.

elope. Pert. to a patient who leaves a hospital, esp. a psychiatric hospital, without permission.

eluate (ĕl'ū-āt). The material washed out by elution.

eluent (ē-lū'ĕnt). The solvent or dissolving substance used in elution.

elution (ē-lū'shŭn) [L. *e,* out, + *luere,* to wash]. In chemistry, separation of one material from another by washing. If a material contains water-soluble and water-insoluble materials, the passage of water, the eluent, through the mixture will remove that portion of the material that is water soluble, the eluate, and leave the water-insoluble residue.

elutriation (ē-lū-trē-ā'shŭn) [L. *elutriare,* to cleanse]. The separation of insoluble particles from finer ones by decanting the fluid.

emaciate (ē-mā'sē-āt) [L. *emaciare,* to make thin]. To cause to become excessively lean.

emaciated. Excessively thin or lacking in normal amount of tissue. SYN: *wasted.*

emaciation. State of being extremely lean.

    ETIOL: Malnutrition; diseases of gastrointestinal canal. If rapid: marasmus, Addison's disease, tuberculosis, anorexia nervosa, cancer, diabetes, suppuration, hyperthyroidism, chronic diarrhea, stricture of esophagus, pyloric obstruction, parasites, loss of sleep, exophthalmic goiter, starvation. SEE: *anorexia; marasmus; tabes; wasting.*

emaculation (ĕm-ăk"ū-lā'shŭn) [L. *emaculare,* to remove spots]. Removal of spots from the skin.

emailloid (ā-mī'loyd) [Fr. *email,* enamel, + Gr. *eidos,* form, shape]. Tumor having its origin in tooth enamel.

emanation [L. *e,* out, + *manare,* to flow]. 1. Something given off; radiation; emission. 2. A gaseous product of radioactive disintegration.

    e., actinium. Emanation given off by actinium. SYN: *actinon.*

    e., radium. Radioactive gas given off by radium. SYN: *radon.*

    e., thorium. Radioactive gas given off by thorium. SYN: *thoron.*

emancipated minor. Person legally under age but recognized by the state as having the legal capacity to consent for him- or herself. Criteria for being so categorized vary among the states.

emasculation (ē-măs″kū-lā′shŭn) [L. *emasculare,* to castrate]. 1. Castration. 2. Excision of the entire male genitalia. 3. Figuratively, making powerless or ineffective.

embalming (ĕm-bäm′ĭng) [L. *im-,* on, + *balsamum,* balsam]. Use of antiseptics and preservatives in and on the dead body in order to prepare it for burial. This prevents premature biodegradation of the body.

embarrass (ĕm-bǎr′ǎs). To interfere with or compromise function.

Embden-Meyerhof pathway [Gustab G. Embden, Ger. biochemist, 1874–1933; Otto Fritz Meyerhof, Ger. biochemist, 1884–1951]. A series of metabolic and enzymatic changes that occur in many plants and animals when glucose, glycogen, or starch is metabolized anaerobically to produce lactic acid. In the process, energy in the form of adenosine triphosphate (ATP) is produced. This is the principal means of producing energy in mammals, including man.

embedding [″ + AS. *bedd,* to bed]. In histology, the process by which a piece of tissue is placed in a firm medium such as paraffin in order to support it and keep it intact during the subsequent cutting into thin sections for microscopic examination.

embolalia, embololalia (ĕm″bō-lā′lē-ă, ĕm″bō-lō-lā′lē-ă) [Gr. *embolos,* thrown in, + *lalia,* babble]. Meaningless language of the insane. SYN: *embolophrasia.*

embole (ĕm′bō-lē) [Gr. *emballein,* to throw in]. 1. Reduction of a dislocation. 2. Formation of the gastrula by invagination. SYN: *emboly.*

embolectomy (ĕm″bō-lĕk′tō-mē) [″ + *ektome,* excision]. Removal of an embolus from a vessel. It may be done surgically or by use of enzymes that dissolve the clot. The latter method is used in treating acute myocardial infarction and other areas where blood flow is obstructed by a blood clot. SEE: *tissue plasminogen inactivator.*

embolic. Pert. to or caused by embolism.

emboliform [″ + L. *forma,* form]. 1. Resembling a nucleus. 2. Wedge-shaped, as the nucleus emboliformis.

embolism (ĕm′bō-lĭzm) [″ + -*ismos,* condition]. Obstruction of a blood vessel by foreign substances or a blood clot. Diagnosis depends upon predisposing factors. Arteriosclerosis favors a diagnosis of thrombosis while atrial fibrillation, bacterial endocarditis, or thrombophlebitis points to embolism. Embolism is usually due to blood clots. SEE: *tissue plasminogen inactivator.*

    RS: embolus, thrombosis, thrombus.

    e., air. Embolism caused by air bubble.

SEE: *air.*

    NURSING IMPLICATIONS: Prevent by scrupulous flushing of I.V. lines, especially centrally placed lines, and by insuring that connections are intact. Have patient use Valsalva maneuver when changing central line connections. Assess for sudden onset of dyspnea, hypotension, chest pain, hemoptysis, cyanosis, decreasing level of consciousness. Position patient on left side with head down to trap air in right heart. Clamp I.V. tubing, administer oxygen, and notify physician.

    e., crossed. SEE: *e., paradoxical.*

    e., fat. Embolism caused by globules of fat obstructing blood vessels. Frequently occurs after fracture of long and pelvic bones.

    NURSING IMPLICATIONS: Evaluate patients at risk, i.e., those with fracture of long bones or multiple injuries, for agitation, restlessness, and delirium, tachycardia, tachypnea, dyspnea, wheezing, and copious production of thick white sputum. Petechiae often appear on buccal membranes, in conjunctival sacs, and across chest and axillae. Monitor blood gas values for hypoxemia. Support respiratory efforts with positioning and oxygen in high concentrations, and with endotracheal intubation and mechanical ventilation as necessary. Administer prescribed pharmacologic agents. Provide emotional support throughout crisis.

    e., paradoxical. An embolus arising from the venous circulation that enters the arterial circulation by crossing from the right side of the heart to the left side through a patent foramen ovale or septal defect.

    e., pulmonary. Obstruction of the pulmonary artery or one of its branches. Usually caused by an embolus from thrombosis in lower extremities. The risk of developing pulmonary embolism as a result of venous thrombosis in the lower extremity can be reduced by use of subcutaneously administered low doses of heparin prior to and following surgery. In addition, the use of dextran and graduated compression elastic stockings is beneficial. SEE: *thrombosis, deep vein;* illus.

    NURSING IMPLICATIONS: Prevent occurrence of venous stasis, thrombus formation, and thrombophlebitis by using elastic stockings, venous return exercises, and early ambulation. Evaluate patients at risk for chest pain, acute dyspnea, apprehension, and cough. Auscultate for adventitious lung sounds, tachypnea, tachycardia, and cardiac gallop or murmur. Assist with diagnostic studies and medical treatment, support ventilatory function with

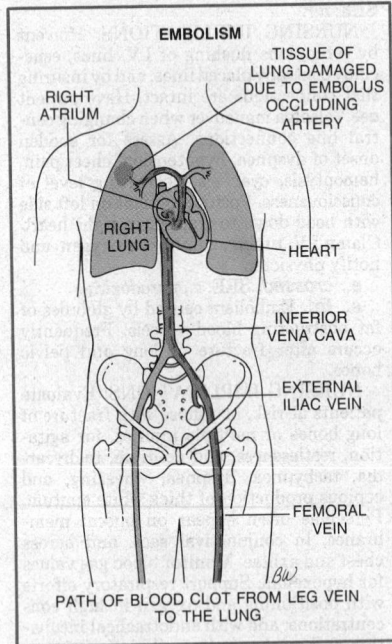

EMBOLISM

TISSUE OF
LUNG DAMAGED
DUE TO EMBOLUS
OCCLUDING
ARTERY

RIGHT
ATRIUM

RIGHT
LUNG

HEART

INFERIOR
VENA CAVA

EXTERNAL
ILIAC VEIN

FEMORAL
VEIN

BW

PATH OF BLOOD CLOT FROM LEG VEIN
TO THE LUNG

head-of-bed elevation, supplemental oxygen as ordered, endotracheal intubation, and mechanical ventilation as necessary. Monitor arterial blood gas values every two to four hours; vital signs, cardiac rhythm, urine output, and level of consciousness every one to two hours. Report deterioration of patient. Instruct women with a history of emboli to avoid use of oral contraceptive drugs.

    e., pyemic. Embolism caused by purulent matter.

embolophrasia (ĕm″bŏ-lō-frā′zē-ă) [″ + *phrasis*, utterance]. Meaningless speech. SYN: *embolalia.*

embolus (ĕm′bō-lŭs) [Gr. *embolos*, stopper] (pl. *emboli*). A mass of undissolved matter present in a blood or lymphatic vessel brought there by the blood or lymph current. Emboli may be solid, liquid, or gaseous. Other emboli may consist of bits of tissue, tumor cells, globules of fat, air bubbles, clumps of bacteria, and foreign bodies. Emboli may arise within the body, or they may gain entrance from without. Occlusion of vessels from emboli usually results in the development of infarcts, q.v. SEE: *thrombosis; thrombus.*

    e., air. An air bubble in the veins, right

atrium or ventricle, or capillaries.

    e., amniotic fluid. Can occur naturally after a difficult labor or from oxytocin-induced hypertonic uterine contractions. A small tear in the amnion or chorion high in the uterus may allow fluid to leak into the chorionic plate and enter the maternal circulation through the venous system. Fluid can also enter at areas of placental separation or cervical tears. Occurs more often in multiparas. Even though it has been thought that the cause of the signs and symptoms is the leak of amniotic fluid into the maternal circulation, the validity of this explanation is in doubt.

    SYM: Respiratory distress, circulatory collapse, acute hemorrhage, and cor pulmonale.

    e., coronary. Embolus in one of the coronary arteries, which may be a complication of arteriosclerosis and cause angina pectoris.

    e., pulmonary. Embolus in pulmonary artery or one of its branches.

emboly (ĕm′bō-lē) [Gr. *emballein*, to throw in]. Formation of the gastrula by invagination. SYN: *embole.*

embolysis (ĕm-bŏl′ĭ-sĭs). The dissolution of an embolus, esp. one due to a blood clot.

embosum. To embrace, envelop, or enclose; to hold to the bosom.

embrace reflex. A defensive reflex consisting of the infant's drawing of its arms across its chest in an embracing manner in response to stimuli produced by striking the surface on which the infant rests. SYN: *Moro reflex; startle reflex.*

embrasure (ĕm-brā′zhŭr) [Fr., window opening from within]. The space formed by the contour and position of adjacent teeth.

    e., buccal. Embrasure spreading toward the cheek between molar and premolar teeth.

    e., labial. Embrasure opening toward the lips between canine and incisor teeth.

    e., lingual. Embrasure opening to the lingual sides of the teeth.

    e., occlusal. Space marked by the marginal ridge on the distal side of one tooth and that on the mesial side of the adjacent tooth, and the contact points.

embryectomy (ĕm″brē-ĕk′tō-mē) [Gr. *embryon*, something that swells in the body, + *ektome*, excision]. Removal of an extrauterine embryo.

embryo (ĕm′brē-ō) [Gr. *embryon*, something that swells in the body]. 1. The young of any organism in an early stage of development. 2. Stage in prenatal development of a mammal between the ovum and the fetus. In humans, stage of development between the 2nd and 8th weeks inclusive. SEE: illus.

STAGES OF DEVELOPMENT OF HUMAN EMBRYO INCLUDING MATURE FETUS

YOLK SAC

4MM

28 DAYS

8MM

35 DAYS

3CM

60 DAYS

UMBILICAL CORD

18.5CM

20-WEEK FETUS

BW

PLACENTA

UMBILICAL CORD

UTERINE WALL

AMNION

CHORION

VAGINA

NINE MONTHS

DEVELOP: *Zygote* (1st week): Following fertilization, cells multiply (cleavage), which results in formation of a morula, which in turn develops into a blastocyst consisting of a trophoblast and inner cell mass. The trophoblast gives rise to the fetal membranes and placenta, after the oosperm enters the uterus and begins implantation. (2nd week): Two cavities (amniotic cavity and yolk sac) arise within the inner cell mass. These are separated by the embryonic disk, which in the second week consists of an ectoderm and an endoderm layer. (3rd week): A mesoderm layer forms between the ectoderm and endoderm layers and these three germ layers develop into the embryo proper.

Embryo (4th through 8th weeks): The embryo increases in length from about 1.5 mm to 23 mm. The germ layers of the embryonic disk give rise to the principal organ systems, and the embryo begins to show the human form. During this period of organogenesis, the embryo is particularly sensitive to the effect of toxic chemicals, including alcohol and tobacco smoke, and is sensitive to hypoxemia.

Fetus (3rd to 9th months): The epithelium of the alimentary canal, liver, pancreas, and lungs develop from endoderm. Muscle, all connective tissues, blood, lymphatic tissue and the epithelium of blood vessels, body cavities, kidneys, gonads, and suprarenal cortex develop from mesoderm. The epidermis, nervous tissue, hypophysis, and the epithelium of the nasal cavity, mouth, salivary glands, bladder, and urethra develop from ectoderm.

embryocardia (ĕm″brē-ō-kăr′dē-ă) [″ + *kardia*, heart]. Heart action in which first and second sounds are equal and resemble the fetal heart sounds. A sign of cardiac distress.

embryocidal (ĕm′brē-ō-sī′dal) [Gr. *embryon*, something that swells in the body, + L. *cida*, killer]. Pert. to anything that kills an embryo.

embryoctony (ĕm″brē-ŏk′tŏ-nē) [″ + *kteinein*, to kill]. Destroying the fetus in utero, as in cases where delivery is impossible, or during abortion. SEE: *craniotomy.*

embryogenetic, embryogenic [″ + *gennan*, to produce]. Pert. to or giving rise to an embryo.

embryogeny (ĕm″brē-ŏj′ĕ-nē). The growth and development of an embryo.

embryography [″ + *graphein*, to write]. A treatise on the embryo.

embryology [″ + *logos*, word, reason]. The science that deals with the origin and development of an individual organism.

embryoma (ĕm-brē-ō′mă) [″ + *oma*, tumor]. A tumor consisting of derivatives of the embryonic germ layers but lacking in organization.

embryonal (ĕm′brē-ō-năl). Pert. to or resembling an embryo.

embryonic (ĕm″brē-ŏn′ĭk) [Gr. *embryon*, something that swells in the body]. Pert. to or in condition of an embryo.

embryonization. Reversion of a cell or tissue to an embryonic structure.

embryonoid (ĕm′brē-ō-noyd) [″ + *eidos*, form, shape]. Having the appearance of an embryo.

embryopathy (ĕm″brē-ŏp′ă-thē) [″ + *pathos*, disease, suffering]. Any pathological condition in the embryo.

embryoplastic [″ + *plassein*, to form]. Having a part in the formation of an embryo; said of cells.

embryoscopy. Direct visualization of the fetus or embryo in the uterus by inserting the light source and image-detecting portion of a fetoscope into the amniotic cavity through a small incision in the abdominal wall. Use of this technique permits visualization of the fetus, photography of the fetus, surgical correction of certain types of congenital defects, as well as obtaining specimens of amniotic fluid for analysis of chemical and cellular materials. SEE: illus.

embryotome (ĕm′brē-ō-tōm″) [″ + *tome*, incision]. Instrument used in dismemberment of fetus in utero.

embryotomy (ĕm″brē-ŏt′ō-mē). The dissection of a fetus to aid delivery.

embryotoxon (ĕm″brē-ō-tŏks′ŏn) [″ + *toxon*, bow]. Congenital marginal opacity of the cornea. SYN: *arcus juvenilis.*

embryo transfer. The technique of implanting a fertilized ovum into the uterus. Fertilization is usually done by placing the sperm and ovum in a special culture tube. SEE: *fertilization, in vitro; GIFT; surrogate mother.*

embryotroph (ĕm′brē-ō-trōf) [″ + *trophe*, nourishment]. A fluid resulting from the enzyme action of the trophoblasts upon the neighboring maternal tissue that nourishes the embryo from the time of implantation into the uterus.

embryotrophy (ĕm″brē-ŏt′rō-fē). Nutrition of the fetus.

embryulcia (ĕm″brē-ŭl′sē-ă) [″ + *elkein*, to draw]. Forcible removal of the fetus by instruments, as in embryotomy.

embryulcus (ĕm″brē-ŭl′kŭs) [Gr. *embryoulkos*, forceps]. Instrument for extracting a dead fetus from the uterus.

emedullate (ē-mĕd′ū-lāt) [L. *e*, out, + *medulla*, marrow]. To remove the marrow from a bone.

emergency [L. *emergere*, to raise up]. 1. Any urgent condition perceived by the patient as

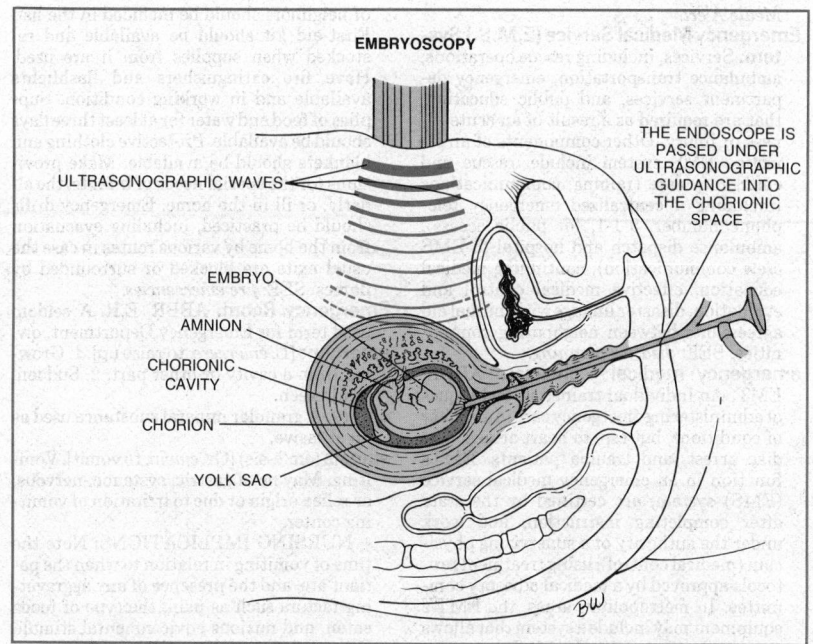

EMBRYOSCOPY

ULTRASONOGRAPHIC WAVES

THE ENDOSCOPE IS PASSED UNDER ULTRASONOGRAPHIC GUIDANCE INTO THE CHORIONIC SPACE

EMBRYO

AMNION

CHORIONIC CAVITY

CHORION

YOLK SAC

requiring immediate medical or surgical evaluation or treatment. 2. An unexpected serious occurrence that may cause a great number of injuries. They usually require immediate attention. SEE: *disaster planning; radiation accidents; Medical Emergencies* in *Appendix*.

emergency, words pert. to: artificial respiration; asphyxia; basic life support; bites or stings; burn; cardiopulmonary resuscitation; choking; convulsion; disaster planning; drowning; fainting; foreign bodies; poison control center; poisoning; radiation accidents, emergency handling of; shock.

emergency cardiac care. ABBR: ECC. All care necessary to deal with sudden and often life-threatening events affecting cardiovascular and pulmonary systems. The most frequent problem requiring ECC is heart disease. For those acute conditions, ECC includes recognizing early warning signs of heart attack; efforts to prevent complications; reassurance of the victim; prompt availability of monitoring and treatment; providing basic life support (BLS) at the scene, when needed; providing advanced cardiac life support (ACLS) at the scene as quickly as possible to stabilize the victim before transporting to a medical care facil-

ity; transferring the stabilized victim to an appropriate hospital where definitive continued cardiac care can be provided. SEE: *advanced cardiac life support; basic life support; cardiopulmonary resuscitation.*

Emergency Department. ABBR: E.D. That portion of a hospital which treats patients experiencing an emergency.

emergency kit. A kit containing the basic equipment and drugs needed to provide initial emergency care to individuals experiencing life-threatening conditions. Included would be a stethoscope; bag-valve-mask; oral airways, adult and pediatric; infusion needle; large-bore I.V. needle, 12-gauge for tracheal obstruction; appropriate sterile syringes and needles; tape; epinephrine 1:1000, 1 ml ampule; diazepam, 10 mg ampule; diphenhydramine hydrochloride, 50 mg ampule; 50% dextrose/water, 50 ml ampule; and blood pressure cuff. Optional items are suction equipment; small oxygen tank; laryngoscopes, adult and pediatric; endotracheal tubes of several sizes; number 18 and number 20 I.V. catheters; normal saline, 250 ml bag; albuterol; atropine, 0.6 mg/ml ampule; nitroglycerin tablets; and morphine sulfate, 10 mg ampule.

emergency medical identification. SEE:

Medic Alert.

Emergency Medical Service (E.M.S.) System. Services, including rescue operations, ambulance transportation, emergency department services, and public education, that are required as a result of an acute illness or injury. Other components of an effective EMS system include: rescue and emergency care training, communications (including a centralized emergency telephone number, 9-1-1, for public access), ambulance dispatch and hospital-to-EMS crew communication), continuing medical education, effective medical control and evaluation, disaster linkage with mutual aid agreements between neighboring communities. SEE: *disaster planning.*

emergency medical technician. ABBR: EMT. An individual trained in techniques of administering emergency care in a variety of conditions, but esp. to heart attack, cardiac arrest, and trauma patients. EMTs function in an emergency medical service (EMS) system, are certified by the state after completing instruction, and work under the authority of a supervising physician (medical control), using treatment protocols approved by a medical advisory committee. In metropolitan areas, the EMT's equipment may include a system that allows communication with a hospital; some can transmit electrocardiograms for analysis by a physician. SEE: *Emergency Medical Service (E.M.S.) System; EMS medical control; EMS treatment protocols; paramedic.*

emergency medicine. The branch of medicine specializing in emergency care of the acutely ill and injured. Board-certified physicians who successfully complete a residency and qualifying examination may use the abbreviation F.A.C.E.P. (Fellow of the American College of Emergency Physicians). SEE: *certified emergency nurse; Emergency Nurses Association; F.A.C.E.P.*

Emergency Nurses Association. Professional organization representing and certifying nurses who are proficient in emergency care.

emergency readiness. Planning in advance for an unexpected crisis, esp. a natural disaster such as a flood or hurricane. Inspect the home for potential hazards and correct those discovered. Isolate flammable materials such as paints, oils, and fuels. Locate utility shut-off valves and point them out to all members of the household. Know location of nearest public shelter and the time required to go there by walking as well as by car. Family members should be trained in basic life support techniques. Emergency phone numbers should be posted and easily accessible. The names and phone numbers of neighbors should be included in the list. First-aid kit should be available and restocked when supplies from it are used. Have fire extinguishers and flashlights available and in working condition. Supplies of food and water for at least three days should be available. Protective clothing and blankets should be available. Make provisions for the special needs of infants, the elderly, or ill in the home. Emergency drills should be practiced, including evacuation from the home by various routes in case the usual exits are blocked or surrounded by flames. SEE: *fire emergencies.*

Emergency Room. ABBR: E.R. A seldom used term for Emergency Department, q.v.

emergent [L. *emergere,* to raise up]. 1. Growing from a cavity or other part. 2. Sudden, unforeseen.

emery. A granular mineral substance used as an abrasive.

emesis (ĕm′ĕ-sĭs) [Gr. *emein,* to vomit]. Vomiting. May be of gastric, systemic, nervous, or reflex origin or due to irritation of vomiting center.

NURSING IMPLICATIONS: Note the time of vomiting in relation to when the patient ate, and the presence of any aggravating factors such as pain, the type of foods eaten, and noxious environmental stimuli. Record the type of vomiting and amount, color, and characteristics of the emesis. The patient should receive good oral hygiene; administer medications as ordered to control vomiting. If the patient who vomits is weak or comatose, take care to prevent aspiration of vomitus into the lungs. The foot of the bed may be elevated, and the patient should be in a side-lying position or with the head turned to the side. Have suction equipment readily available for the comatose patient. SEE: *antemetic; aspiration; emetic; vomit; vomitus.*

e., gastric. Vomiting present in gastric ulcer, gastric carcinoma, acute gastritis, chronic gastritis, hyperacidity and hypersecretion, and pressure upon stomach.

e. gravidarum. Vomiting of pregnancy.

e., irritation. Vomiting caused by drugs, uremia, nephritis, some brain tumors, chloroform, or ether.

e., nervous. Emesis resulting from tumor or abscess of brain, seasickness, acute myelitis, meningitis, anemia and hyperemia of brain, concussion and contusion of brain, fracture of skull, Ménière's disease, or migraine.

e., reflex. Emesis caused by irritation of fauces and pharynx, coughing, removal of viscous secretion from nasopharynx, unpleasant odors and sights, shock, nervousness, anticipation, anxiety, hysteria, morning sickness, gastric crisis of tabes, or hiccoughs.

emesis basin. SEE: *basin, emesis.*

emetic (ĕ-mĕt′ĭk) [Gr. *emein,* to vomit]. An agent that produces vomiting. Emetics may induce vomiting by their local effect, as copper sulfate, zinc sulfate, mustard, and ipecac in small doses diluted in water; or by their effect on the central nervous system, such as is produced by apomorphine hydrochloride given parenterally. SEE: *vomiting; vomitus.*

ADM: Dilute contents of stomach before giving an emetic. Emesis is much more likely to take place when the stomach is distended. Vomiting may be induced by drinking generous amounts of warm water, preferably warm soapy water, and by stimulating the uvula or posterior pharynx. Gastric lavage is preferable to emetics in treating patients who have swallowed poison because the poison may reinjure the esophagus and mouth as it is expelled from the stomach. Emetics may be dangerous because of their own toxic effect as in severe cardiovascular diseases, tuberculosis, advanced pregnancy, hernia, ulcers of the stomach, or corrosive poisoning. For these reasons, the indiscriminate use of chemical emetics is contraindicated.

Caution: Do not administer salt solutions orally to induce vomiting. The absorbed salt can be lethal.

---

    e., direct. Emetic that acts by its presence in the stomach, as mustard.

    e., indirect. Emetic that acts on the vomiting center of brain, as apomorphine.

emetine (ĕm′ĕ-tēn) [Gr. *emein,* to vomit]. Powdered, white alkaloid emetic obtained from ipecac, q.v.

    e. bismuth iodide. A combination of emetine and bismuth containing about 20% emetine and 20% bismuth. Action and uses same as emetine.

    e. hydrochloride. USP. The hydrated hydrochloride of an alkaloid obtained from ipecac. It is used for the treatment of both intestinal and extra-intestinal amebiasis. It should be used cautiously in elderly or debilitated patients. Children, pregnant women, and patients with serious organic disease should not receive emetine.

emetism [″ + *-ismos,* condition of]. Poisoning from overdose of ipecac.

SYM: Acute inflammation of pylorus, hyperemesis, diarrhea, and sometimes coughing and suffocation.

emetocathartic (ĕm″ĕ-tō-kă-thăr′tĭk) [″ + *katharsis,* a purging]. Producing both emesis and catharsis.

emetology (ĕm″ĕ-tŏl′ō-jē) [″ + *logos,*

word, reason]. Study of anatomy and physiology of vomiting.

E.M.F. *electromotive force; erythrocyte maturation factor.*

EMG. *electromyogram,* q.v.

emic. In anthropology and transcultural nursing, emic refers to a type of analysis of disease which focuses on the culture of the patient. The emic perspective emphasizes the subjective experience and cultural beliefs pertinent to the illness experience. For example, in psychiatric settings in the southeastern United States, many patients believe that their illness is caused by a spell or curse from evil spirits. In these cases, a health care worker using an emic perspective would ask an indigenous health care person to consult with the patient in addition to providing care within the traditional health care system. SEE: *etic.*

EMIC. *emergency maternal and infant care.*

emigration [L. *e,* out, + *migrare,* to move]. Passage of white blood corpuscles through the walls of capillaries and veins during inflammation.

eminence [″ + *minere,* to hang on]. A prominence or projection, esp. of a bone.

    e., arcuate. A rounded eminence on upper surface of petrous portion of temporal bone. SYN: *jugum petrosum.*

    e., articular, of the temporal bone. A rounded eminence forming the anterior boundary of the glenoid fossa.

    e., auditory. A collection of gray matter on the floor of 4th ventricle of the brain at its lower part, forming the deep origin of the auditory nerve.

    e., bicipital. A tuberosity for insertion of biceps muscle on radius.

    e., blastodermic. An elevated mass of cells of a developing ovum forming the blastoderm.

    e., canine. A vertical ridge on the external surface of the maxilla.

    e., collateral. Eminence between middle and posterior horns in lateral ventricle of brain.

    e., frontal. A rounded prominence on either side of the median line and a little below center of the frontal bone.

    e., germinal. Mass of follicle cells that surround the ovum. SYN: *cumulus oophorus.*

    e., hypothenar. Eminence on ulnar side of palm, formed by muscles of little finger.

    e., iliopectineal. Eminence on upper aspect of pubic bone above the acetabulum, marking the junction of bone with the ilium.

    e., intercondyloid. Process on the head of the tibia lying between the two condyles.

    e., mamillary. Projection of inner pillars of fornix. SYN: *corpus mamillare* [NA].

e., median. Anterior bodies of medulla oblongata separated by anterior median fissure.

e., nasal. Prominence on vertical portion of frontal bone above the nasal notch and between the two superciliary ridges.

e., occipital. Protuberance on occipital bone.

e. of Doyère. Slight elevation of muscular fiber corresponding to entrance of a nerve fiber into the muscle.

e., olivary. Oval projection at upper part of medulla oblongata above extremity of lateral column. SYN: *oliva* [NA]; *olivary body.*

e., parietal. The marked convexity on outer surface of parietal bone.

e.'s, portal. The small median lobes on the lower surface of the liver.

e., pyramidal. Elevation on the mastoid wall of the tympanic cavity. It contains a cavity in which lies the stapedius muscle. SYN: *pyramid of tympanum.*

e., thenar. Eminence formed by muscles below the thumb on the palm of the hand.

eminentia (ĕm″ĭn-ĕn′shē-ă) [L.] (pl. *eminentiae*). An eminence.

emiocytosis (ē″mē-ō-sī-tō′sĭs) [L. *emitto*, to send forth, + Gr. *kytos*, cell, + *osis*, condition]. The process of movement of intracellular material to the outside. Granules join the cell membrane, which ruptures to allow the substance to be free in the intercellular fluid. SYN: *exocytosis.* SEE: *endocytosis; pinocytosis.*

emissary (ĕm′ĭ-să-rē) [L. *e*, out, + *mittere*, to send]. 1. Providing an outlet. 2. An outlet.

emissary veins. Small veins that pierce the skull and carry blood from the sinuses within the skull to the veins without.

emissio (ē-mĭs′sē-ō) [L.]. A discharge; emission.

emission (ē-mĭsh′ŭn) [L. *e*, out, + *mittere*, to send]. An issuance or discharge; the sending forth or discharge, such as of an atomic particle, exhalation, or of a light or heat wave.

e., nocturnal. Involuntary discharge of semen during sleep. SYN: *wet dream.*

e., thermionic. The process by which electrons are released from the x-ray filament after a current has been passed through it.

emissivity. The ability of a substance or surface to emit radiant energy.

emit. To produce or release something, e.g., light, heat, or sound waves.

emmenagogue (ĕm-ĕn′ă-gŏg) [Gr. *emmena*, menses, + *agogos*, leading]. A substance that promotes or assists the flow of menstrual fluid. SEE: *ecbolic.*

e., direct. That which has a direct effect

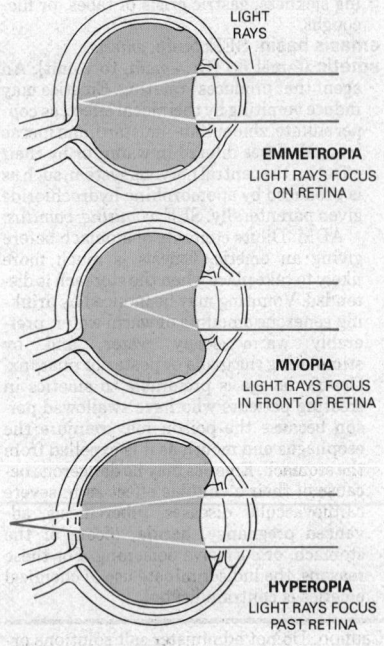

LIGHT
RAYS

EMMETROPIA
LIGHT RAYS FOCUS
ON RETINA

MYOPIA
LIGHT RAYS FOCUS
IN FRONT OF RETINA

HYPEROPIA
LIGHT RAYS FOCUS
PAST RETINA

on the reproductive tract, such as a hormone.

e., indirect. An agent that alters the menstrual function by treatment of a primary illness.

emmenia (ĕ-mē′nē-ă) [Gr. *emmena*]. The menstrual flow.

emmenic. Pert. to the menses.

emmeniopathy (ĕ-mē″nē-ŏp′ă-thē) [Gr. *emmena*, menses, + *pathos*, disease, suffering]. Any disorder of menstruation.

emmenology (ĕm″ĕn-ŏl′ō-jē) [″ + *logos*, word, reason]. Science of menstruation.

emmetrope (ĕm′ĕ-trōp) [Gr. *emmetros*, in measure, + *opsis*, sight]. One endowed with normal vision.

emmetropia (ĕm″ĕ-trō′pē-ă). Normal condition of the eye in refraction in which, when the eye is at rest, parallel rays focus exactly on the retina. SEE: illus.; *astigmatism; myopia.*

emmetropic. Normal vision. SEE: *hypermetropic; myopic.*

Emmet's operation [Thomas A. Emmet, U.S. gynecologist, 1828–1919]. 1. Uterine trachelorrhaphy, i.e., suture of torn uterine cervix. 2. Suturing of a lacerated perineum. 3. Converting a sessile submucous tumor of the uterus into a pedunculated one. 4. Operation for prolapse of uterus.

emollient (ē-mŏl′yĕnt) [L. *e*, out, + *mollire*, to soften]. An agent that will soften and soothe the part when applied locally. The term is usually confined to agents affecting the surface of the body. SEE: *demulcent*.

Ex.: ointment of rose water; olive oil; petrolatum.

emotion (ē-mō′shŭn) [L. *emovere*, to stir up]. 1. Passions or sensibilities characterized by physical changes in the body such as alteration in heart rate and respiratory activity, vasomotor reactions, and changes in muscle tone. 2. A mental state or feeling such as fear, hate, love, anger, grief, or joy arising as a subjective experience rather than as a conscious mental effort. These feelings constitute the drive that brings about the emotional or mental adjustment necessary to satisfy instinctive needs. Physiological changes invariably accompany alteration in the emotions, but such change may not be apparent to either the person experiencing the emotion or an observer.

Frustration is normally associated with displeasure and intensification of perception of personal need; the process of gratification is accompanied by pleasurable feeling that persists for a variable period in less intense form.

Anxiety or fear arises when one doubts one's ability to meet a situation adequately. Neutralization consists of flight from danger or a struggle (fight) to remove the threat. Civilized people may find a goal unattainable because their conditioned (moral) reactions regard the goal as socially objectionable or they may even deny the goal entirely. Thus, conflicts arise and the stage is set for the onset of psychogenic disease.

DISORDERS: Emotions are not felt in the same way by healthy persons as by those suffering from mental disease. In schizophrenia there is a decrease of pleasure, hate, love, and other emotions. There is loss of ability to feel and express emotions such as love or hate. The patients are said to be blunted. The emotions they do show are not in harmony with their ideas. For example, they may smile while describing tortures and terrors.

Unhappiness is marked in manic depressive psychosis. It varies in degree and may lead to suicide. In the excited stage undue happiness is marked. SEE: *anhedonia*.

emotion, words pert. to: anhedonia; anxiety; catharsis; conflict; depression; empathy; disease, psychosomatic; exaltation; fear; frustration; love; mania; manic-depressive; phobia; sympathy.

emotional [L. *emovere*, to stir up]. Rel. to any of the emotions.

emotional need. An individual has inner needs with respect to the emotions of love, fear, anxiety, sadness, loneliness, and anger. These needs may be understood and handled by the healthy individual, but are especially difficult to cope with during illness or mental stress. The medical care team should be alert to the possibility that a patient's needs in these areas must be managed and treated. This is best done by demonstrating empathy for the patient and being close by when needed. In times of stress and anxiety, the therapy of holding an aged patient's hand has remarkable therapeutic effects. SEE: *TLC*.

emotivity (ē″mō-tĭv′ĭ-tē). One's capability for emotional response.

empathic [Gr. *en*, in, + *pathos*, disease, suffering]. Pert. to, or characterized by, empathy.

empathy (ĕm′pă-thē). Objective awareness of and insight into the feelings, emotions, and behavior of another person and their meaning and significance. Not the same as sympathy, which is usually nonobjective and noncritical.

emperipolesis (ĕm-pĕr″ĭ-pō-lē′sĭs) [Gr. *en*, into, + *peripolesis*, a going about]. Penetration by lymphocytes of another cell.

emperor of pruritus. The itching that accompanies poison ivy dermatitis involving the anal area. It is so intense that it is called "the emperor of pruritus."

emphraxis (ĕm-frăk′sĭs) [Gr., an obstruction]. A stoppage or obstruction; an infarction.

emphysema (ĕm″fĭ-sē′mă) [Gr. *emphysan*, to inflate]. 1. Pathological distention of tissues by gas or air in the interstices. 2. A chronic pulmonary disease characterized by increase beyond the normal in the size of air spaces distal to the terminal bronchiole with destructive changes in their walls. SYN: *chronic obstructive pulmonary disease; pulmonary emphysema.*

DIAG: Precise diagnosis of emphysema is difficult to establish. Clinically the patient may have breathlessness that may be present only during exertion. Cough with production of sputum usually indicates the presence of chronic bronchitis.

TREAT: Patient should avoid contact with atmospheric pollution, esp. that caused by cigarette smoke. Bronchodilators, mucolytic agents, weight reduction if patient is obese, antibiotics for infections, and the use of oxygen therapy only if clearly needed to prevent hypoxia.

NURSING IMPLICATIONS: Assist in maintaining a patent airway, eliminating all bronchial irritants such as smoke from the environment. Assist and encourage the patient to increase oral fluid intake as permitted to help liquify inspissated secretions. Administer prescribed medications (bronchodilators, anti-inflammatory agents, expectorants) and teach patient about the desired actions as well as side effects to be reported. Administer prescribed inhalation therapy and chest physiotherapy, including postural drainage, clapping and vibration. Provide pulmonary toilet after therapy, and encourage patient to rest before proceeding with other activities. Teach patient to prevent respiratory infections by avoiding contact with persons with respiratory infections, and by using correct pulmonary hygiene procedures. Assist patient to improve nutritional status by encouraging frequent, small meals and food supplements that are high in protein rather than carbohydrates, which increase carbon dioxide load. Explain that smaller meals reduce intra-abdominal pressure on the diaphragm, thus easing ventilatory effort. Teach the patient breathing exercises such as diaphragmatic breathing to increase ventilatory efficiency and floppy-lipped breathing to keep small airways open, and expiration exercises to improve functional capacity. Teach patient about the dangers of increased oxygen intake to a patient dependent on hypoxic drive for ventilation. Provide emotional support to all throughout frequent exacerbations and remissions, and encourage participation in support groups and services to aid in dealing with decreasing functional abilities. SEE: *Nursing Diagnoses* in *Appendix.*

   e., subcutaneous. Presence of air in subcutaneous tissue.

emphysematous (ĕm″fĭ-sĕm′ă-tŭs). Affected with or pert. to emphysema.

empiric (ĕm-pĭr′ĭk) [Gr. *empeirikos,* skilled, experienced]. 1. Based on experience. SEE: *empirical.* 2. A practitioner whose skill or art is based upon what has been learned through experience.

empirical (ĕm-pĭr′ĭk-ăl). Based on experience rather than on scientific principles.

empiricism (ĕm-pĭr′ĭs-ĭzm) [Gr. *empeirikos,* skilled, experienced, + *-ismos,* condition of]. 1. Experience, not theory, as basis of medical science. 2. Quackery.

emprosthotonos (ĕm″prŏs-thŏt′ŏ-nŏs) [Gr. *emprosthen,* forward, + *tonos,* tension]. A form of spasm in which the body is flexed forward. Sometimes seen in tetanus and strychnine poisoning. Opposite of opisthotonos.

empty follicle syndrome. In in vitro fertilization investigations, the absence of oocytes in the stimulated follicle of the ovary.

This may be a cause of infertility in some individuals.

empty-sella syndrome. On lateral x-ray of the skull, the sella turcica, which normally contains the pituitary gland, is found to be empty. Clinically, the patients may show no endocrine abnormality or may have signs of decreased pituitary function. The only treatment needed is to provide hormonal replacement in those who demonstrate hypopituitarism. In autopsy studies, empty-sella has been found in about 5% of presumably normal persons. SEE: *pituitary gland.*

emptysis (ĕmp′tĭ-sĭs) [Gr., a spitting]. Expectoration of blood or blood-stained mucus. SYN: *hemoptysis.*

empyema (ĕm″pī-ē′mă) [Gr.]. Pus in a body cavity, esp. in the pleural cavity (pyothorax). Usually the result of a primary infection in the lungs.

   SYM: Chills, fever, and sweating. Skin is gray, malar flushed, appetite poor with marked malaise, pain in chest, cough, and emaciation. Dyspnea may ensue.

   TREAT: Antibiotic therapy, aspiration of pleural fluid. Treatment of primary condition. Surgical drainage may be necessary.

   NURSING IMPLICATIONS: In acute condition, evaluate for unilateral chest pain, cough, high fever, and malaise, and in chronic condition evaluate for weight loss, general malaise, and low-grade fever. Depending on amount of fluid present, pulmonary assessment may show unequal chest expansion, dullness to percussion, and decreased or absent breath sounds over the involved area. Assist with drainage by thoracentesis or water-seal chest drainage with suction and with local and systemic administration of antibiotics. Maintain the drainage system and record drainage amounts and characteristics. Protect the patient from accidental disruption of the water seal or dislodgement of the drainage tube. Provide increased fluid and protein intake, and encourage breathing exercises to promote lung expansion.

   e., interlobular. Form of empyema with pus between lobes of lung.

   e. necessitatis. Form of empyema in which pus can escape spontaneously.

   e., pulsating. Form of empyema with cardiac beats causing pulsation of chest wall.

empyesis (ĕm″pī-ē′sĭs) [Gr., suppuration]. 1. Any skin eruption characterized by pustules. 2. Any accumulation of pus. 3. Hypopyon, accumulation of pus in the anterior chamber of the eye.

empyocele (ĕm′pī-ō-sēl) [Gr. *empyein,* to suppurate, + *kele,* tumor, swelling]. A collection of pus in a sacculated cavity, esp.

in the scrotum; a suppurating hydrocele.

empyreuma (ĕm″pī-roo′mă) [Gr., a live coal]. The characteristic odor of animal or vegetable material being burned in a closed container.

EMS. *emergency medical service.*

EMS communication. Communication system which serves to coordinate emergency medical care among ambulances, (telephone) 911 dispatch center, and hospital emergency departments. It includes citizen-to-EMS, dispatcher-to-EMS crew, paramedic-to-doctor, and EMS crew-to-emergency department, as well as EMS-to-other public safety organizations, i.e., police, fire, rescue. SEE: *disaster planning; EMS medical control.*

Components of the EMS communication system include:

EMS base-station. A dispatch and coordination area that transmits and receives radio communications.

EMS mobile transmitters/receivers. Radios located in emergency vehicles.

EMS portable transmitters/receivers. Hand-held portable radios used at emergency scenes.

EMS repeaters. Base stations that receive radio transmissions from mobile and portable transceivers and amplify the signal, extending the range of communication.

EMS biotelemetry. Transmitting electrocardiographic and other patient data via radio or telephone to a distant receiving station from which consultation may be obtained.

EMS medical advisory committee. Representatives of medical groups that provide medical direction to an EMS and emergency department's system.

EMS medical control. Physician direction of life support procedures performed by EMTs and paramedics in pre-hospital care, including on-line and off-line supervision. *On-line* medical control is the instruction a physician provides via radio or telephone to an EMS crew. *Off-line* medical control is the direction and supervision given to EMS crews via treatment protocols, case review, in-service training, and standing orders for treatment.

Medical control is also divided into prospective, immediate, and retrospective forms. *Prospective form* involves development of treatment protocols which EMTs perform under a license of the medical director or medical advisory committee. *Immediate form* involves giving direct medical orders or consultation by radio or telephone (defined above as on-line control). *Retrospective form* involves review of call reports to see if protocols have been followed.

EMS medical director. Physician responsible for insuring the appropriate level of quality of care throughout an EMS system.

EMS standing orders. Instructions preapproved by the medical advisory committee directing EMS crews to perform specific advanced life support measures *before* contacting a medical control physician. These orders are implemented in cases where a delay in treatment could harm the patient (e.g., cardiac arrest).

EMS treatment protocols. Written procedures for diagnosis, triage, treatment, patient transportation or patient transfer between hospitals. These procedures are part of the official policy of the system and approved by representatives of the medical advisory committee.

EMS treatment protocols may either be implemented as standing orders or require prior approval of a medical control physician.

EMT. *emergency medical technician.*

EMT-A. *emergency medical technician-ambulance.* Basic level technician. The "A" and "ambulance" terms are usually omitted.

EMT-D. *emergency medical technician* who is trained in *defibrillation.*

EMT-I. *emergency medical technician-intermediate.* Technician trained to an intermediate level and able to perform some advanced life support skills, such as intravenous fluid administration or endotracheal intubation.

EMT-P. *emergency medical technician-paramedic.* Technician trained to the highest level for delivery of pre-hospital care.

emulsification (ē-mŭl″sĭ-fĭ-kā′shŭn) [L. *emulsio,* emulsion, + *facere,* to make]. 1. Process of making an emulsion. 2. Breaking down of large fat globules in the intestine to smaller, uniformly distributed particles, accomplished largely through the action of bile acids, which lower surface tension.

emulsifier. Anything used to make an emulsion.

emulsify (ē-mŭl′sĭ-fī). To form into an emulsion.

emulsion [L. *emulsio*]. 1. A mixture of two liquids not mutually soluble. If they are thoroughly shaken, one will divide into globules in what is called the discontinuous or dispersed phase; the other is then the continuous phase. Milk is an emulsion in which butterfat is the discontinuous phase. 2. In radiology, that part of the radiographic film sensitive to radiation and containing the image after development.

emulsoid (ē-mŭl′soyd) [″ + Gr. *eidos,* form, shape]. A colloid in an aqueous solution in which the colloid has a marked attraction for water to the extent that the dispersoid, q.v., contains large quantities of water. SYN: *hydrophilic lyophilic colloid.*

Ex.: protoplasm, starch, soap, gelatin, and egg white.

emunctory (ē-mŭnk'tō-rē) [L. *emungere,* to cleanse]. 1. Pert. to organ or duct having an excretory function. 2. An excretory duct, as the pores of skin.

E.N.A. *extractable nuclear antigen.*

enamel (ĕn-ăm'ĕl) [O. Fr. *esmail,* enamel]. The hard, white, dense substance forming a covering for the crown of the teeth. It is the hardest substance in the body. SYN: *enamelum* [NA].

   e., aprismatic. A thin surface layer of the tooth thought to be solid without individual enamel rods or prisms.

   e., cervical. Enamel at the neck of the tooth characterized by shorter enamel rods with more prominent incremental lines and perikymata.

   e., gnarled. Enamel under the cusp of a tooth characterized by twisting, intertwining groups of enamel rods, thought to resist shearing forces.

   e. hypoplasia. Incomplete development of the tooth enamel. Usually due to faulty calcium and phosphate metabolism.

   e., mottled. Condition in which the enamel acquires a mottled appearance as a result of the ingestion of excessive amounts of fluorides in water or foods.

enamel organ. A cup-shaped structure that forms on the dental lamina of an embryo. It produces the enamel and serves as a mold for the remainder of the tooth.

enamel pearls. SEE: *pearls, enamel.*

enamelum. [NA] Enamel.

enanthem, enanthema (ĕn-ăn'thĕm, -ăn-thē'mă) [Gr. *en,* in, + *anthema,* blossoming]. Eruption of mucous membrane. SEE: *exanthem; Koplik's spots; rash.*

enanthematous (ĕn″ăn-thĕm'ă-tŭs). Of the nature of an enanthema.

enanthesis (ĕn″ăn-thē'sĭs) [Gr. *en,* in, + *anthein,* to bloom]. A skin eruption caused by systemic disease such as typhoid fever or syphilis.

enanthrope (ĕn-ăn'thrōp) [″ + *anthropos,* man]. 1. Any disease originating in the body. 2. An autoinfection.

enantio-. Combining form meaning opposite.

enantiobiosis (ĕn-ăn″tē-ō-bī-ō'sĭs) [Gr. *enantios,* opposite, + *bios,* life]. The condition in which associated organisms are antagonistic to each other. SEE: *symbiosis.*

enantiomorph (ĕn-ăn'tē-ō-morf″). One of a pair of isomers, each of which is a mirror image of the other. They may be identical in chemical characteristics, but in solution one rotates a beam of polarized light in the opposite direction of the other. The isomers are called dextro if they rotate light to the right, and levo if they rotate light to the left.

enantiopathy (ĕn-ăn″tē-ŏp'ă-thē) [″ + *pathos,* disease, suffering]. Treatment of one disease by using another disease that produces changes or symptoms antagonistic to it.

enarthrosis (ĕn″ăr-thrō'sĭs) [Gr. *en,* in, + *arthron,* joint, + *osis,* condition] (pl. *enarthroses*). A ball-and-socket joint such as the hip joint. A form of diarthrosis.

en bloc (ĕn blŏk) [Fr., as a whole]. In surgery, to remove as a whole or as a lump.

encanthis (ĕn-kăn'thĭs) [Gr. *en,* in, + *kanthos,* angle of the eye]. An excrescence or new growth at the inner angle of the eye.

encapsulation [″ + *capsula,* a little box]. 1. Enclosure in a sheath not normal to the part. 2. The process of the formation of a capsule or a sheath about a structure.

encatarrhaphy (ĕn″kăt-ăr'ă-fē) [Gr. *enkatarrhaptein,* to sew in]. Insertion of an organ or tissue into a part where it is not normally found.

enceinte (ŏn-sănt') [Fr.]. Pregnant.

encephalalgia (ĕn-sĕf″ăl-ăl'jē-ă) [Gr. *enkephalos,* brain, + *algos,* pain]. Deep-seated head pain. SYN: *cephalalgia.*

encephalatrophy (ĕn-sĕf″ă-lăt'rō-fē) [″ + *a-,* not, + *trophe,* nourishment]. Cerebral atrophy.

encephalic (ĕn″sĕf-ăl'ĭk) [Gr. *enkephalos,* brain]. Pert. to the brain or its cavity.

encephalitis (ĕn-sĕf″ă-lī'tĭs) [″ + *itis,* inflammation]. Inflammation of the brain.

ETIOL: It may be due to a specific disease entity such as rabies or be caused by an arthropod-borne (arbor) virus, or it may occur as a sequela of influenza, measles, German measles, chickenpox, herpesvirus infection, smallpox, vaccinia, or other diseases.

TREAT: Support; therapy for specific cause. SEE: *rabies.*

NURSING IMPLICATIONS: Evaluate for signs of meningeal irritation, such as nuchal rigidity and opisthotonos, changes in level of consciousness, and signs of increased intracranial pressure, such as increased restlessness, projectile vomiting, convulsions, pupil irregularities, and motor function and vital sign changes, and for signs of cranial nerve involvement, such as ptosis, diplopia, or strabismus. Also evaluate for behavioral changes and abnormal sleep patterns. Monitor intake and output to prevent dehydration and avoid overload. Provide frequent oral hygiene. Reposition the patient frequently to prevent neck discomfort and joint pain; and assist with range-of-motion exercises. Assure the patient's family that behavioral changes usually disappear, and refer the patient to a rehabilitation program for treatment of any residual effects once the acute phase is over. SEE: *Nursing Diagnoses* in *Appendix.*

 e., acute disseminated. E., postinfection, q.v.

 e., cortical. Encephalitis of brain cortex only.

 e., epidemic. Any form of encephalitis that occurs as an epidemic.

 e., equine. A mosquito-borne type of viral encephalitis originally isolated as an encephalitis affecting horses.

 e., equine, eastern. Primarily a viral disease of birds and wild animals, transmitted to horses and man by mosquitoes. More severe than other types of encephalitis. Outbreaks have occurred in the eastern and Gulf Coast states.

 e., equine, western. A mild type of viral encephalitis that has occurred in western United States and Canada.

 e., hemorrhagic. Herpes encephalitis in which there is hemorrhage along with brain inflammation.

 e., herpes. Encephalitis due to infection with herpes simplex virus. Though rare, it is frequently fatal. It has been successfully treated with an antiviral agent.

 e. hyperplastica. Acute encephalitis without suppuration.

 e., infantile. Brain inflammation in the young that may cause cerebral palsy.

 e., Japanese (B type). Similar to St. Louis encephalitis, it is caused by a different strain of mosquito-borne virus. Occurs in summer and fall.

 e., lead. Encephalitis due to lead poisoning.

 e. lethargica. A disease of the nervous system thought to be caused by a virus. Characterized by lethargy, oculomotor paralysis, clonic and choreiform movements, rigidity, delirium, stupor, coma, and reversal of sleep rhythm. The disease first appeared pandemically in 1916 to 1917, and is now considered extinct. SYN: *Economo's disease.*

 e., meningo-. Encephalitis combined with meningitis.

 e. neonatorum. A form of encephalitis occurring within the first several weeks of life.

 e. periaxialis. Inflammation of the white matter of the cerebrum, occurring mainly in the young.

 e., postinfection. Encephalitis occurring following a smallpox vaccination or one of the common communicable diseases, as chickenpox.

 e., postvaccinal. Acute encephalitis following vaccination.

 e., purulent. Encephalitis characterized by abscesses in the brain.

 e., Russian spring-summer. Encephalitis due to a tick-borne virus. It may also be transmitted to man by drinking goat milk.

 e., St. Louis. A mosquito-borne virus disease that first occurred epidemically in the summer of 1933 in and around St. Louis, a city in the U.S. Now endemic in the U.S., Trinidad, Jamaica, Panama, and Brazil. Occurs most frequently during summer and early fall.

 e., toxic. Encephalitis resulting from metal poisonings, as lead poisoning.

encephalocele (ĕn-sĕf'ă-lō-sēl) [Gr. *enkephalos*, brain, + *kele*, hernia]. Protrusion of the brain through a cranial fissure. SYN: *hydrencephalocele.*

encephalocystocele (ĕn-sĕf''ă-lō-sĭs'tō-sēl) [" + *kystis*, sac, + *kele*, tumor, swelling]. Hernia of the brain. The hernia sac is filled with cerebrospinal fluid.

encephalogram (ĕn-sĕf'ă-lō-grăm) [" + *gramma*, something written]. Roentgenogram of the brain. Usually done with air injected into the ventricles in order to provide contrast in the picture.

encephalography (ĕn-sĕf''ă-lŏg'ră-fē) [" + *graphein*, to write]. X-ray examination of the head, esp. examination following the introduction of air into the ventricles through a lumbar or cisternal puncture.

encephaloid (ĕn-sĕf'ă-loyd) [" + *eidos*, form, shape]. 1. Resembling the cerebral substance. 2. A malignant neoplasm of brainlike texture.

encephalolith (ĕn-sĕf'ă-lō-lĭth) [" + *lithos*, stone]. A calculus of the brain.

encephaloma (ĕn-sĕf''ă-lō-mă) [" + *oma*, tumor]. Tumor of the brain.

encephalomalacia (ĕn-sĕf''ă-lō-mă-lā'sē-ă) [" + *malakia*, softening]. Cerebral softening.

encephalomeningitis (ĕn-sĕf''ă-lō-mĕn''ĭn-jī'tĭs) [" + *meninx*, membrane, + *itis*, inflammation]. Inflammation of the brain and its membranes.

encephalomeningocele (ĕn-sĕf''ă-lō-mĕ-nĭng'gŏ-sēl) [" + " + *kele*, tumor, swelling]. Protrusion of membranes and brain substance through the cranium.

encephalomere (ĕn-sĕf'ă-lō-mēr'') [" + *meros*, part]. A primitive segment of the embryonic brain. SYN: *neuromere.*

encephlometer (ĕn-sĕf''ă-lŏm'ĕ-tĕr) [" + *metron*, measure]. An instrument for measuring the cranium and locating brain regions.

encephalomyelitis (ĕn-sĕf''ă-lō-mī-ĕl-ī-'tĭs) [" + *myelos*, marrow, + *itis*, inflammation]. Acute inflammation of the brain and spinal cord.

e., acute disseminated. Acute disorder of the brain and spinal cord due to causes such as vaccination or acute exanthema. SYN: *e., postinfectious.*

e., benign myalgic. Epidemic disease of unknown etiology. It usually occurs in young institutionalized persons. There are the usual symptoms of encephalitis but few physical signs. It may be confused with poliomyelitis. SYN: *Icelandic disease.*

e., equine. Virus disease of horses that may be communicated to man. Includes eastern and western equine encephalitis.

e., postinfectious. E., acute disseminated, q.v.

e., postvaccinal. Encephalomyelitis following smallpox vaccination.

encephalomyeloneuropathy (ĕn-sĕf″ă-lō-mī″ĕ-lō-nū-rŏp′ă-thē). Any disease involving the brain, spinal cord, and nerves.

encephalomyelopathy (ĕn-sĕf″ă-lō-mī″ĕl-ŏp′ă-thē) [″ + ″ + *pathos,* disease, suffering]. Any disease of the brain and spinal cord.

encephalomyeloradiculitis (ĕn-sĕf″ă-lō-mī″ĕ-lō-ră-dĭk″ū-lī′tĭs). Inflammation of the brain, spinal cord, and nerve roots.

encephalomyocarditis (ĕn-sĕf″ă-lō-mī″ō-kăr-dī′tĭs). Any disease involving the brain and cardiac muscle.

encephalon (ĕn-sĕf′ă-lŏn) [Gr. *enkephalos,* brain]. [NA] The brain, including the cerebrum, cerebellum, medulla oblongata, pons, diencephalon, and midbrain.

encephalopathy (ĕn-sĕf″ă-lŏp′ă-thē) [″ + *pathos,* disease, suffering]. Any dysfunction of the brain.

e., hepatic. SEE: *hepatic coma.*

encephalopuncture (ĕn-sĕf″ă-lō-punk′tūr) [″ + L. *punctura,* a piercing]. Puncture into the brain substance.

encephalopyosis (ĕn-sĕf″ă-lō-pī-ō′sĭs) [″ + *pyosis,* suppuration]. Abscess of the brain.

encephalorrhagia (ĕn-sĕf″ă-lō-rā′jē-ă) [″ + *rhegnynai,* to burst forth]. Cerebral hemorrhage. SEE: *hemorrhage, cerebral.*

encephalosclerosis (ĕn-sĕf″ă-lō-sklē-rō′sĭs) [″ + *sklerosis,* hardening]. Hardening of the brain.

encephalospinal [″ + L. *spina,* thorn, spine]. Pert. to the brain and spinal cord.

encephalotome (ĕn-sĕf′ă-lō-tŏm) [Gr. *enkephalos,* brain, + *tome,* incision]. Instrument for incising brain tissue.

encephalotomy (ĕn-sĕf″ă-lŏt′ō-mē). 1. Brain dissection. 2. Surgical destruction of the brain of a fetus to facilitate delivery.

enchondroma (ĕn″kŏn-drō′mă) [Gr. *en,* in, + *chondros,* cartilage, + *oma,* tumor]. A benign cartilaginous tumor occurring generally where cartilage is absent or within

a bone where it expands the diaphysis. SYN: *enchondrosis.*

enchondrosarcoma (ĕn-kŏn″drō-săr-kō′mă) [″ + ″ + *sarx,* flesh, + *oma,* tumor]. Sarcoma made up of cartilaginous tissue.

enchondrosis (ĕn-kŏn-drō′sĭs) [″ + ″ + *osis,* condition]. A benign cartilaginous outgrowth from bone or cartilaginous tissue. SYN: *enchondroma.*

enclave (ĕn′klāv) [Fr. *enclaver,* to enclose]. A mass of tissue that becomes enclosed by tissue of another kind.

enclitic (ĕn-klĭt′ĭk) [Gr. *enklinein,* to lean on]. Having the planes of the fetal head inclined to those of the maternal pelvis.

enclosure. Any anatomically enclosed space or area.

encode. To convert something such as a message to a coded form in order to make translation back to the original difficult for someone unfamiliar with the code.

encolpitis (ĕn-kŏl-pī′tĭs) [Gr. *en,* in, + *kolpos,* vagina, + *itis,* inflammation]. Inflamed condition of the vaginal mucosa. SYN: *endocolpitis.*

encopresis (ĕn-kō-prē′sĭs) [″ + *kopros,* excrement]. Condition associated with constipation and fecal retention. Watery colonic contents bypass the hard fecal masses and pass through the rectum. Often confused with diarrhea.

encranial [″ + *kranion,* cranium]. Intracranial or within the cranium.

enculturation. Process of transmitting to the members of the community the values, beliefs, and customs of the family, the cultural group, and the larger society.

encyesis (ĕn″sī-ē′sĭs) [″ + *kyesis,* pregnancy]. Normal uterine pregnancy.

encysted (ĕn-sĭst′ĕd) [″ + *kystis,* bladder, pouch]. Surrounded by membrane; encapsulated. SYN: *saccate.*

end-, endo-. Combining form meaning within.

end [AS. *ende*]. A termination; extremity.

endadelphos (ĕnd″ă-dĕl′fŏs) [Gr. *endon,* within, + *adelphos,* brother]. A congenitally deformed fetus, the twin of which is enclosed in the body or in a cyst on the fetus.

Endamoeba (ĕn″dă-mē′bă). *Entamoeba.*

endangeitis, endangiitis (ĕnd″ăn-jē-ī′tĭs) [Gr. *endon,* within, + *angeion,* vessel, + *itis,* inflammation]. Inflammation of the endangium or inner coat of blood vessels.

endangium (ĕn-dăn′jē-ŭm) [″ + *angeion,* vessel]. Innermost coat or intima of blood vessels.

endaortitis (ĕnd″ā-or-tī′tĭs) [″ + *aorte,* aorta, + *itis,* inflammation]. Inflammation of inner coat of the aorta.

endarterectomy (ĕnd″ăr-tĕr-ĕk′tō-mē). Surgical removal of the lining of an artery. It is performed on almost any major artery that is diseased or blocked, such as carotid, femoral, or popliteal arteries.

e., carotid. SEE: *carotid endarterectomy.*

endarterial (ĕnd″ăr-tē′rē-ăl) [″ + *arteria,* artery]. 1. Pert. to the inner portion of an artery. 2. Within an artery.

endarteritis, endoarteritis (ĕnd-ăr-tĕr-ī′tĭs) [″ + ″ + *itis,* inflammation]. Inflammation of innermost coat (intima) of an artery, resulting from syphilis, trauma, pyogenic bacteria, or infective thrombi.

e., acute. Rare inflammation of large arteries.

e., chronic. Degeneration of arterial coats in the aging. SYN: *atheroma.*

e. deformans. Thickening of intima or replacement with atheromatous or calcareous deposits.

e. obliterans. Chronic progressive thickening of intima leading to stenosis or obstruction of lumen.

e., syphilitic. Endarteritis caused by syphilis.

end artery. An artery that does not communicate with other arteries.

endbrain. Telencephalon.

end-bud. The terminal of a sensory nerve. SYN: *end-bulb.*

end-bulb. The terminal portion of a sensory nerve. SYN: *end-bud.*

e. of Krause. An encapsulated nerve ending found in the skin and mucous membranes.

endemic [Gr. *en,* in, + *demos,* people]. Pert. to a disease that occurs continuously in a particular population, but has low mortality, such as measles. Used in contrast to *epidemic.*

endemoepidemic (ĕn-dĕm″ō-ĕp-ĭ-dĕm′ĭk) [″ + ″ + *epi,* on, among, + *demos,* people]. Endemic, but becoming epidemic periodically.

endergonic (ĕnd″ĕr-gŏn′ĭk) [Gr. *endon,* within, + *ergon,* work]. Pert. to chemical reactions that require energy in order to occur.

endermatic, endermic [Gr. *endon,* within, + *derma,* skin]. Administration of medicine by absorption through the skin.

endermosis [″ + ″ + *osis,* condition]. 1. Administration of medicines through the skin. 2. Herpetic affection of any mucous membrane.

end feel. In physical therapy and rehabilitation, the feel experienced by an evaluator when overpressure is applied to tissue at the end of the available range of motion. It is interpreted as abnormal when the quality of the feel is different from normal response at that joint. The feel may be soft as when two muscle groups are compressed or soft tissues are stretched, firm as when a normal joint or ligament is stretched, or hard as when two bones block motion. Abnormal end feels may include a springy sensation when cartilage is torn within a joint, muscle guarding when a muscle involuntarily responds to acute pain, or muscle spasticity when there is increased tone due to an upper motor neuron lesion or when the feel is different from that normally experienced for the joint being tested.

end-feet. Terminal buttons; the enlarged ends of nerve fibers that terminate adjacent to the dendrite of another nerve cell.

ending. The finish or final portion of a tissue or cell.

endoaneurysmorrhaphy (ĕn″dō-ăn″ū-rĭs-mor′ăf-ē) [Gr. *endon,* within, + *aneurysma,* aneurysm, + *rhaphe,* seam, ridge]. Opening an aneurysmal sac and suturing its orifice.

endoangiitis (ĕn″dō-ăn-jē-ī′tĭs) [″ + *angeion,* vessel, + *itis,* inflammation]. Inflammation of the inner coat of blood vessels. SYN: *endangiitis; endoarteritis; endophlebitis.*

endoantitoxin (ĕn″dō-ăn-tē-tŏk′sĭn) [″ + *anti,* against, + *toxikon,* poison]. An antitoxin within a cell.

endoappendicitis (ĕn″dō-ă-pĕn″dĭ-sī′tĭs) [″ + L. *appendere,* to hang, + Gr. *itis,* inflammation]. Inflammation of mucosa of the vermiform appendix.

endoauscultation (ĕn″dō-ăws″kŭl-tā′shŭn) [″ + L. *auscultare,* to listen to]. Auscultation by esophageal tube passed into the stomach or by a tube passed into the heart.

endobiotic (ĕn″dō-bī-ŏt′ĭk) [″ + *bios,* life]. Pert. to an organism living parasitically in the host.

endoblast (ĕn′dō-blăst) [″ + *blastos,* germ]. The immature cell that is the precursor of an endodermal cell.

endobronchitis (ĕn″dō-brŏng-kī′tĭs). Inflammation of the smaller bronchi.

endocardiac, endocardial [″ + *kardia,* heart]. Within the heart or arising from the endocardium.

endocarditis (ĕn″dō-kăr-dī′tĭs) [″ + ″ + *itis,* inflammation]. Inflammation of the lining membrane of the heart. It is usually confined to the external lining of the valve, sometimes to the lining membrane of its chambers. May be due to invasion of microorganisms or an abnormal immunological reaction.

TREAT: If due to bacterial invasion, use appropriate antibiotic therapy for as long as a month or, in the case of some organisms, up to two months.

NURSING IMPLICATIONS: During the acute phase, it is essential to maintain the patient on bedrest and provide a calm, quiet environment. Take vital signs, including apical pulse rate, every 2 to 4 hours (or more frequently if ordered). You may place the patient in Fowler's position with arms supported on pillows at sides to help relieve dyspnea. Administer antibiotics as ordered. When patient begins activity or ambulation, take pulse before and after the activity to determine the effects of the stress on the heart muscle. Teach the patient the importance of taking prescribed prophylactic antibiotics. SEE: *Nursing Diagnoses* in *Appendix.*

*e., **acute bacterial.*** Endocarditis that begins abruptly and progresses rapidly. Usually caused by virulent organisms such as staphylococci or pneumococci.

*e., **atypical verrucous.*** Nonbacterial endocarditis in which the accumulation of debris on the endocardium is associated with various wasting diseases.

*e., **bacterial.*** SEE: *e., acute bacterial.*

*e., **chronic.*** E., ulcerative.

*e., **infective.*** Endocarditis due to microorganisms.

*e., **Libman-Sacks.*** Nonbacterial endocarditis. SEE: *e., atypical verrucous.*

*e., **malignant.*** A fatal type of endocarditis that is usually secondary to suppurative inflammation elsewhere. SEE: *e., ulcerative.*

*e., **mural.*** Endocarditis of the lining of the heart chambers but not including the heart valve.

*e., **rheumatic.*** Endocarditis that occurs following rheumatic fever.

*e., **subacute bacterial.*** A condition usually caused by colonization of the *Streptococcus viridans* group (mainly *S. salivarius, S. mitis, S. bovis, S. fecalis, S. sanguis*) in an abnormal heart or in valves damaged previously by rheumatic fever.

*e., **syphilitic.*** Endocarditis due to syphilis having extended from aortic involvement to the aortic valves.

*e., **tuberculous.*** Endocarditis involving the heart valves; caused by the tubercle bacillus.

*e., **ulcerative.*** A rapidly destructive form of acute bacterial endocarditis characterized by necrosis or ulceration of the valves and the deposition of colonies of micrococci. Usually fatal.

*e., **valvular.*** Endocarditis affecting only the covering of the valves and not the lining of the heart chambers.

*e., **vegetative.*** Endocarditis associated with fibrinous clots on ulcerated valvular surfaces.

*e., **verrucous.*** Nonbacterial endocarditis occurring frequently in lupus erythematosus.

*e. **viridans.*** E., subacute bacterial.

endocardium [Gr. *endon*, within, + *kardia*, heart]. [NA] Serous lining membrane of inner surface and cavities of the heart. It is continuous with the intima or interior coat of arteries.

endocervical (ĕn″dō-sĕr′vĭ-kăl) [″ + L. *cervix*, neck]. Pert. to the endocervix.

endocervicitis (ĕn″dō-sĕr″vĭ-sī′tĭs) [″ + ″ + Gr. *itis*, inflammation]. Inflammation of mucous lining of the cervix uteri. Usually chronic, due to infection, and accompanied by cervical erosion.

SYM: White or yellow mucoid discharge.

TREAT: Electrocauterization of cervical lesion. An antibiotic for local application may be prescribed. SEE: *carcinoma in situ.*

endocervix (ĕn″dō-sĕr′vĭks) [″ + L. *cervix*, neck]. The lining of the canal of the cervix uteri.

endochondral (ĕn″dō-kŏn′drăl) [″ + *chondros*, cartilage]. Within a cartilage.

endochondral bone formation. One of the two types of bone formation in skeletal development. Each long bone is formed as a cartilage model before bone is laid down, replacing the cartilage.

endochorion (ĕn″dō-kō′rē-ŏn) [″ + *chorion*, chorion]. The inner chorion; vascular layer of allantois.

endocolitis (ĕn″dō-kō-lī′tĭs) [″ + *kolon*, colon, + *itis*, inflammation]. Inflammation of the mucosa of colon. SEE: *colitis.*

endocolpitis (ĕn″dō-kŏl-pī′tĭs) [″ + *kolpos*, vagina, + *itis*, inflammation]. Inflammation of the vaginal mucosa. SYN: *encolpitis.*

endocorpuscular (ĕn″dō-kor-pŭs′kū-lăr) [″ + L. *corpusculum*, small body (corpuscle)]. Within a corpuscle.

endocranial (ĕn″dō-krā′nē-ăl) [″ + *kranion*, cranium]. 1. Intracranial or within the cranium. 2. Pert. to the endocranium.

endocranitis (ĕn″dō-krā-nī′tĭs) [″ + ″ + *itis*, inflammation]. Inflammation of endocranium.

endocranium (ĕn″dō-krā′nē-ŭm). The dura mater of the brain, which forms the lining membrane of the cranium.

endocrinasthenia (ĕn″dō-krĭn″ăs-thē′nē-ă) [Gr. *endon*, within, + *krinein*, to secrete, + *astheneia*, weakness]. Neurasthenia due to dysfunction of the endocrine system.

endocrine (ĕn′dō-krīn, -krĭn, -krēn) [″ + *krinein*, to secrete]. 1. An internal secretion. 2. Pert. to a gland that secretes directly into the bloodstream.

endocrine gland. A ductless gland that produces an internal secretion discharged into the blood or lymph and circulated to all parts of the body. Hormones, the active principles of the glands, produce effects on tissues more or less remote from their place of origin. In addition to their endocrine function, some glands produce an external secretion.

The endocrine glands include hypophysis (pituitary gland), thyroid gland, parathyroid glands, adrenal (suprarenal) glands, islands of Langerhans of the pancreas, and the gonads (ovaries and testes). In addition, the hypothalamus produces releasing hormones that exert an effect on the production of some hormones. Other structures such as the gastrointestinal mucosa and the placenta have an endocrine function.

The hormones secreted by the ductless glands may have a specific effect on an organ or tissue or a general effect on the entire body, as in the case of the thyroid hormone, which affects the rate of metabolism. Among the physiological processes affected by hormones are rate of metabolism and the metabolism of specific substances, growth and developmental processes, the secretory activity of other endocrine glands, the development and functioning of the reproductive organs, sexual characteristics and libido, the development of personality and higher nervous functions, the ability of the body to meet conditions of stress, and resistance to disease.

Endocrine dysfunction may result from hyposecretion, in which an inadequate amount of the hormone(s) is secreted, or from hypersecretion, in which excessive amounts of hormones are produced. Secretion of endocrine glands may be under nervous control, under control of chemical substances in the blood, or, in some cases, under control of other hormones. Many pathological conditions are the result of or are associated with the malfunctioning of the endocrine glands. SEE: illus.; table.

endocrine neoplasm, multiple. SEE: *multiple endocrine neoplasm.*

endocrino- [Gr. *endon,* within, + *krinein,* to secrete]. Combining form for endocrine.

endocrinologist. A medical scientist skilled in endocrinology.

endocrinology (ĕn″dō-krĭn-ŏl′ō-jē) [″ + ″ + *logos,* word, reason]. The science of the endocrine, or ductless, glands and their functions.

endocrinopathic. Of the nature of endocrinopathy.

endocrinopathy (ĕn″dō-krĭn-ŏp′ă-thē) [″ + ″ + *pathos,* disease, suffering]. Any disease resulting from disorder of an endocrine gland or glands.

endocrinotherapy (ĕn″dō-krĭn″ō-thĕr′ă-pē) [″ + ″ + *therapeia,* treatment]. Treatment with endocrine preparations.

endocyst (ĕn′dō-sĭst) [″ + *kystis,* bladder, pouch]. The innermost layer of any hydatid cyst.

endocystitis (ĕn″dō-sĭs-tī′tĭs) [″ + ″ + *itis,* inflammation]. Inflammation of mucous membrane of bladder. SEE: *cystitis.*

endocytosis. A method of ingestion of a foreign substance by a cell. The cell wall invaginates to form a space for the material and then the opening closes to trap the material inside the cell. SEE: *phagocytosis; pinocytosis; exocytosis; emiocytosis.*

endoderm (ĕn′dō-dĕrm) [″ + *derma,* skin]. Inner layer of cells of an embryo. SYN: *entoderm; hypoblast.*

endodermal. Pert. to the entoderm. SYN: *entodermal.*

Endodermophyton (ĕn″dō-dĕr-mŏf′ĭ-tŏn) [″ + *derma,* skin, + *phyton,* a growth]. Former name of a genus of parasitic fungi growing in the epidermis of the skin. Now included in the genus *Trichophyton.*

endodiascope (ĕn″dō-dī′ă-skōp) [″ + *dia,* through, + *skopein,* to examine]. X-ray tube that may be placed within a cavity of the body for radiological examination and radiation therapy.

endodiascopy (ĕn″dō-dī-ăs′kō-pē). X-ray examination of a body cavity with an endodiascope.

endodontia (ĕn″dō-dŏn′shē-ă) [″ + *odous,* tooth]. Endodontics.

endodontics (ĕn″dō-dŏn′tĭks). A branch of dentistry concerned with diagnosis, treatment, and prevention of diseases of the dental pulp and its surrounding tissues.

endodontist. A specialist in the practice of endodontics.

endodontitis (ĕn″dō-dŏn-tī′tĭs) [″ + *odous,* tooth, + *itis,* inflammation]. Inflammation of the dental pulp. SYN: *pulpitis.*

endodontologist. An endodontist.

endodontology. Endodontics.

endoectothrix (ĕn″dō-ĕk′tō-thrĭks) [″ + *ektos,* outside, + *thrix,* hair]. Any fungus growth on and in the hair.

endoenteritis (ĕn″dō-ĕn″tĕr-ī′tĭs) [″ + *enteron,* intestine, + *itis,* inflammation]. Inflammation of mucous membrane of intestines.

endoenzyme (ĕn″dō-ĕn′zīm) [″ + *en,* in, + *zyme,* leaven]. An intracellular enzyme.

endogamy (ĕn-dŏg′ă-mē) [″ + *gamos,* marriage]. 1. The custom or tribal restriction of marriage within a tribe or group. 2. In biology, reproduction by joining together gametes descended from the same ancestral cell.

endogastric (ĕn″dō-găs′trĭk) [″ + *gaster,* belly]. Pert. to the stomach's interior.

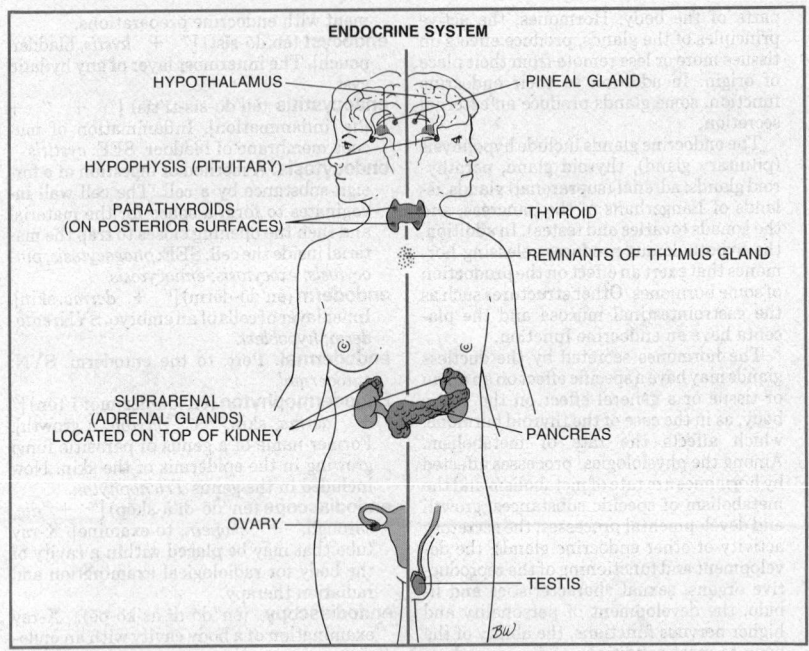

ENDOCRINE SYSTEM

HYPOTHALAMUS

PINEAL GLAND

HYPOPHYSIS (PITUITARY)

PARATHYROIDS
(ON POSTERIOR SURFACES)

THYROID

REMNANTS OF THYMUS GLAND

SUPRARENAL
(ADRENAL GLANDS)
LOCATED ON TOP OF KIDNEY

PANCREAS

OVARY

TESTIS

endogastritis (ĕn″dō-găs-trī′tĭs) [″ + ″ + *itis,* inflammation]. Inflammation of the lining membrane of the stomach.

endogenic (ĕn″dō-jĕn′ĭk) [″ + *gennan,* to produce]. Having origin within the organism. SYN: *endogenous.*

endogenous (ĕn-dŏj′ĕ-nŭs). 1. Produced or arising from within a cell or organism. 2. Concerning spore formation within the bacterial cell. SYN: *endogenic.*

endogenous opiate-like substance. SEE: *endorphins; enkephalins; opiate receptor.*

endogeny (ĕn-dŏj′ĕ-nē). Growth within the cell.

endoglobar, endoglobular (ĕn″dō-glŏb′ăr, ĕn″dō-glŏb′ū-lăr) [Gr. *endon,* within, + L. *globulus,* a globule]. Within the blood corpuscles.

endognathion (ĕn″dō-năth′ē-ŏn) [Gr. *endon,* within, + *gnathos,* jaw]. A point in the inner segment of the intermaxillary bone or premaxilla.

endointoxication (ĕn″dō-ĭn-tŏk″sĭ-kā′shŭn) [″ + L. *in,* into, + Gr. *toxikon,* poison]. Poisoning due to an endogenous toxin.

endolabyrinthitis (ĕn″dō-lăb″ĭ-rĭn-thī′tĭs) [″ + *labyrinthos,* labyrinth, + *itis,* inflammation]. Inflamed condition of the membranous labyrinth.

endolaryngeal (ĕn″dō-lă-rĭn′jē-ăl) [″ + *larynx,* larynx]. Within the larynx.

Endolimax nana (ĕn″dō-lī′măks nă′nă) [″ + *leimax,* meadow]. A species of ameba inhabiting the intestines of humans, monkeys, and other mammals. It is usually nonpathogenic in humans and is found in the intestines of healthy persons.

endolumbar [″ + L. *lumbus,* loin]. In the lumbar portion of the spinal cord.

endolymph (ĕn′dō-lĭmf) [″ + L. *lympha,* clear fluid]. Pale transparent fluid within the labyrinth of the ear.

endolymphatic. Rel. to the endolymph.

endolymphatic duct. A slender duct extending from posterior surface of the saccule of the inner ear. It ends blindly in the petrous portion of the temporal bone as a dilated pouch, the endolymphatic sac.

endolysin (ĕn-dŏl′ĭ-sĭn) [″ + *lysis,* dissolution]. Bacterial substance within a leukocyte that destroys bacteria.

endomastoiditis (ĕn″dō-măs″toy-dī′tĭs) [″ + *mastos,* breast, + *eidos,* form, shape, + *itis,* inflammation]. Inflammation of mucosa lining the mastoid cavity and cells.

endometer (ĕn-dŏm′ē-tĕr). Electronic device used to determine the length of a tooth's root canal.

Principal Endocrine Glands

Name	Position	Function	Endocrine Disorders
Thyroid	Two lobes in anterior portion of neck	Influences basal metabolic rate; indirectly influences growth and nutrition	Hypofunction— Cretinism in young; myxedema in adult; goiter Hyperfunction— Goiter; thyrotoxicosis
Parathyroid	Four or more small glands near thyroid	Calcium and phosphorus metabolism; indirectly affects muscular irritability	Hypofunction— Tetany Hyperfunction— Resorption of bone; renal calculi
Adrenal Cortex	One above each kidney	Steroid hormones regulating carbohydrate metabolism and salt and water balance; some effects on sexual characteristics	Hypofunction— Addison's disease Hyperfunction— Adrenogenital syndrome; Cushing's syndrome
Adrenal Medulla	The inner portion of the adrenal gland. It is surrounded by the adrenal cortex.	Effects on sympathetic nervous system and carbohydrate metabolism	Hypofunction— Almost unknown Hyperfunction— Pheochromocytoma
Anterior Pituitary	Small gland at base of brain	Influences growth, sexual development, skin pigmentation, thyroid function, adrenocortical function through effects on other endocrine glands (except for growth factor, which acts directly on cells)	Hypofunction— Dwarfism in child; decrease in all other endocrine gland functions except parathyroids Hyperfunction— Acromegaly in adult; diabetes, gigantism in child
Posterior Pituitary	Attached to anterior pituitary	Oxytocic factor influencing some aspects of uterine contraction Antidiuretic factor influencing absorption of water by kidney tubule	Unknown Hypofunction— Diabetes insipidus
Testes and Ovaries	Testes—in the scrotum Ovaries—in the pelvic cavity	Development of secondary sex characteristics; some effect on metabolism	Hypofunction—Lack of sex development or regression in adult Hyperfunction— Abnormal sex development

Principal Endocrine Glands (Continued)

Name	Position	Function	Endocrine Disorders
Pancreas (endocrine portion)	Abdominal cavity; head adjacent to duodenum; tail close to spleen and kidney	Secretes insulin and glucagon, which regulate carbohydrate metabolism	Hypofunction — Diabetes mellitus Hyperfunction — If a tumor produces excess insulin, hypoglycemia; if excess glucagon, diabetes mellitus

endometrectomy (ĕn″dō-mē-trĕk′tō-mē) [″ + metra, uterus, + ektome, excision]. Excision of uterine mucosa. SEE: curettage.

endometrial (ĕn″dō-mē′trē-ăl) [″ + metra, uterus]. Pert. to the lining of the uterus.

endometrial cyst. An ovarian cyst or tumor lined with endometrial tissue. Usually seen in ovarian endometriosis.

endometrial dating. Microscopic examination of a suitable, stained specimen from the endometrium of the uterus in order to establish the number of days to the next menstrual period. The dating is on the basis of an ideal 28-day cycle. Thus, day 8 indicates menstruation is 20 days away and day 23 that it is 5 days away. This system was devised by the late Dr. John Rock, a physician at Harvard University, to enable gynecologists to visualize endometria being discussed without having to provide detailed descriptions of the material studied.

endometrial jet washing. Collection of fluid that has been used to irrigate the uterine cavity. Cells present in the fluid are examined for evidence of malignancy. Method is used as a screening test for endometrial carcinoma.

endometrioma (ĕn″dō-mē″trē-ō′mă) [Gr. endon, within, + metra, uterus, + oma, tumor]. A tumor containing shreds of ectopic endometrium; found most frequently in the ovary, cul-de-sac, rectovaginal septum, and the peritoneal surface of the posterior portion of the uterus.

endometriosis (ĕn″dō-mē″trē-ō′sĭs) [″ + ″ + osis, condition]. Ectopic endometrium located in various sites throughout the pelvis or in the abdominal wall. It is estimated this occurs in 1% to 7% of women in the U.S.

SYM: Pelvic pain, adnexal mass, infertility. SEE: illus. SEE: Nursing Diagnoses in Appendix.

e., direct. Invasion of the myometrium by the mucous membrane lining the uterus.

e., implantation. E., peritoneal.

e., internal. E., direct.

e., metastatic. Extraperitoneal lesions in circumstances resembling metastatic pelvic carcinoma.

e., peritoneal. Endometrial tissue found throughout the pelvis.

e., primary. E., direct.

e., transplantation. Endometriosis occurring within an abdominal incision scar following pelvic surgery.

endometritis (ĕn″dō-mē-trī′tĭs) [″ + ″ + itis, inflammation]. Inflammation of the endometrium.

ETIOL: Produced by bacterial invasion. May be acute, subacute, or chronic, the acute cases most commonly resulting from infection by staphylococci, E. coli bacilli, or gonococci; trauma; septic abortion. The subacute and chronic types are the result of repeated acute attacks. Occasionally the chronic type may be due to infection with the tubercle bacillus. Many other conditions are labeled as endometritis but are of either vascular or endocrine origin. Some of these conditions are senile endometritis, hyperplastic endometritis, and hypertrophic endometritis.

SYM: In acute cases the symptoms are usually low back and low abdominal pain, dysmenorrhea, menorrhagia, sterility, and constipation. In chronic endometritis, there is scant serosanguineous vaginal discharge. A positive diagnosis cannot be made without a curettage and a histological study of the recovered material. SEE: cervix uteri; endometrium; uterus.

e., cervical. Inflammation of the inner portion of the cervix uteri.

e., decidual. Inflammation of the mucous membrane of a gravid uterus.

e. dissecans. Endometritis accompanied by development of ulcers and shedding of the mucous membrane.

e., puerperal. Acute endometritis following childbirth.

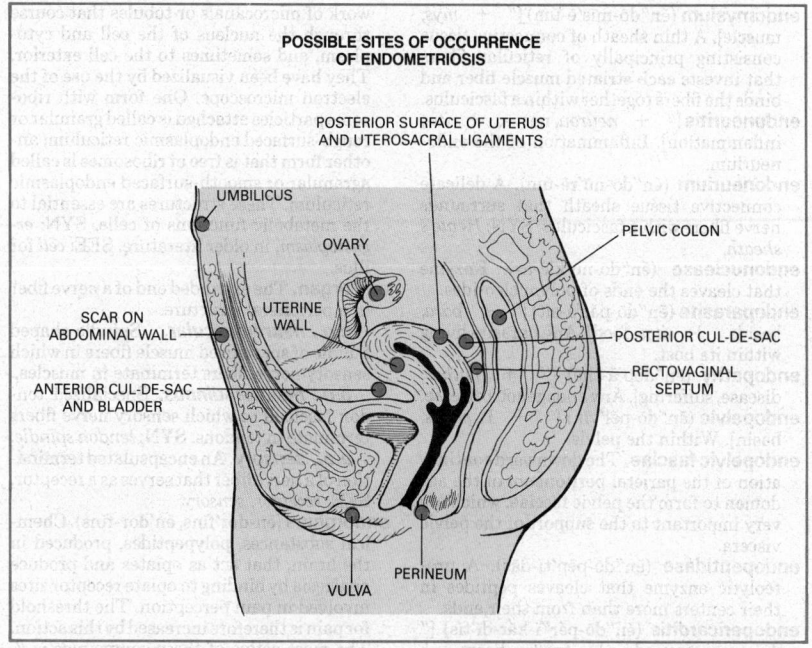

POSSIBLE SITES OF OCCURRENCE
OF ENDOMETRIOSIS

POSTERIOR SURFACE OF UTERUS
AND UTEROSACRAL LIGAMENTS

UMBILICUS

OVARY

PELVIC COLON

SCAR ON
ABDOMINAL WALL

UTERINE
WALL

POSTERIOR CUL-DE-SAC

RECTOVAGINAL
SEPTUM

ANTERIOR CUL-DE-SAC
AND BLADDER

PERINEUM

VULVA

endometrium (ĕn-dō-mē'trē-ŭm) [Gr.
endon, within, + *metra,* uterus]. [NA]
The mucous membrane lining the inner surface of the uterus. Histologically it consists
of a surface epithelium made up of a single
layer of columnar cells, a few of which bear
cilia. Invaginations of the epithelium form
simple, branched tubular glands that extend
to the myometrium. The glands are separated by connective tissue resembling mesenchyme, which forms the stroma. There is
no submucosa, the mucosa lying closely attached to the myometrium.

The endometrium is supplied by two
types of arteries: straight arteries, supplying
the deeper third or basal layer of the endometrium, and spiral arteries, supplying the
spongy and compact layers. They penetrate
between the glands and form a subepithelial
capillary plexus. These arteries show
marked changes in response to hormonal
stimulation during the menstrual cycle. Beginning with menarche and ending at
menopause, the uterine endometrium
passes through cyclic changes that constitute the menstrual cycle, q.v. These changes
are related to the development and maturation of the graafian follicle in the ovary, the
discharge of the ovum, and the subsequent

development of the corpus luteum in the
ovary.

Following fertilization of the ovum, the
endometrium serves as nesting place and
implantation occurs. The endometrium
fuses with the developing chorion of the embryo and at birth there is a splitting off and
shedding of the uterine lining or decidua.
During pregnancy, the decidua basalis, the
endometrium lying between the chorionic
vesicle and myometrium, develops into the
maternal portion of the placenta, q.v.

The endometrial lining is shed if the
ovum is not fertilized or if the fertilized
ovum does not implant. When this is completed, the cycle begins again. SEE: *ovary*
for illus.

endometry (ĕn-dŏm'ĕ-trē) [Gr. *endon,*
within, + *metron,* measure]. Measurement of the interior of a cavity or organ.

endomorph (ĕn″dō-morf′) [″ + *morphe,*
form]. Body build characterized by predominance of tissues derived from the endoderm. SEE: *ectomorph; mesomorph; somatotype.*

endomyocarditis (ĕn″dō-mī-ō-kăr-dī′tis) [″
+ *mys,* muscle, + *kardia,* heart, +
itis, inflammation]. Inflammation of the endocardium and myocardium.

endomysium (ĕn″dō-mīs′ē-ŭm) [″ + *mys,* muscle]. A thin sheath of connective tissue consisting principally of reticular fibers that invests each striated muscle fiber and binds the fibers together within a fasciculus.

endoneuritis [″ + *neuron,* nerve, + *itis,* inflammation]. Inflammation of the endoneurium.

endoneurium (ĕn″dō-nū′rē-ŭm). A delicate connective tissue sheath that surrounds nerve fibers with a fasciculus. SYN: *Henle's sheath.*

endonuclease (ĕn″dō-nū′klē-ās). Enzyme that cleaves the ends of polynucleotides.

endoparasite (ĕn″dō-păr′ă-sīt) [″ + *para,* beside, + *sitos,* food]. Any parasite living within its host.

endopathy (ĕn″dŏp′ă-thē) [″ + *pathos,* disease, suffering]. Any endogenous disease.

endopelvic (ĕn″dō-pĕl′vĭk) [″ + L. *pelvis,* basin]. Within the pelvis.

endopelvic fasciae. The downward continuation of the parietal peritoneum of the abdomen to form the pelvic fasciae, which are very important to the support of the pelvic viscera.

endopeptidase (ĕn″dō-pĕp′tĭ-dās). A proteolytic enzyme that cleaves peptides in their centers more than from their ends.

endopericarditis (ĕn″dō-pĕr″ĭ-kăr-dī′tĭs) [″ + *peri,* around, + *kardia,* heart, + *itis,* inflammation]. Endocarditis complicated by pericarditis.

endoperimyocarditis (ĕn″dō-pĕr″ĭ-mī″ō-kăr-dī′tĭs) [″ + ″ + *mys,* muscle, + *kardia,* heart, + *itis,* inflammation]. Inflammation of the pericardium, myocardium, and endocardium.

endoperitonitis (ĕn″dō-pĕr″ĭ-tō-nī′tĭs) [″ + *peritonaion,* peritoneum, + *itis,* inflammation]. Inflammation of the peritoneum.

endophasia (ĕn″dō-fā′zē-ă) [″ + *phasis,* utterance]. Formation of words by the lips without producing sound.

endophlebitis (ĕn″dō-flē-bī′tĭs) [″ + *phleps,* vein, + *itis,* inflammation]. Inflammation of the inner coat or membrane of a vein.

    e. obliterans. Endophlebitis causing obliteration of a vein.

    e. portalis. Inflammation of the portal vein.

endophthalmitis (ĕn″dŏf-thăl-mī′tĭs) [″ + *ophthalmos,* eye, + *itis,* inflammation]. Inflammation of the inside of the eye that may or may not be limited to a particular chamber, i.e., anterior or posterior.

endoplasm [″ + LL. *plasma,* form, mold]. The central, more fluid portion of the cytoplasm of a cell. Opposed to ectoplasm.

endoplasmic reticulum. A connecting net-

work of microcanals or tubules that course through the nucleus of the cell and cytoplasm, and sometimes to the cell exterior. They have been visualized by the use of the electron microscope. One form with ribosome particles attached is called granular or rough-surfaced endoplasmic reticulum; another form that is free of ribosomes is called agranular or smooth-surfaced endoplasmic reticulum. These structures are essential to the metabolic functions of cells. SYN: *ergastoplasm,* in older literature. SEE: *cell* for illus.

end organ. The expanded end of a nerve fiber in a peripheral structure.

    e.o., neuromuscular. Spindle-shaped bundle of specialized muscle fibers in which sensory nerve fibers terminate in muscles.

    e.o., neurotendinous. Specialized tendon fasciculi in which sensory nerve fibers terminate in tendons. SYN: *tendon spindle.*

    e.o., sensory. An encapsulated termination of a nerve fiber that serves as a receptor. SEE: *receptor, sensory.*

endorphins (ĕn-dor′fĭns, ĕn′dor-fĭns). Chemical substances, polypeptides, produced in the brain, that act as opiates and produce analgesia by binding to opiate receptor sites involved in pain perception. The threshold for pain is therefore increased by this action. The most active of these compounds is β-endorphin. SYN: *endogenous opiate-like substance.* SEE: *enkephalins; opiate receptor; substance P.*

endorrhachis (ĕn″dō-rā′kĭs) [Gr. *endon,* within, + *rhachis,* spine]. Membrane lining of the spinal canal.

endosalpingitis (ĕn″dō-săl″pĭn-jī′tĭs) [″ + *salpinx,* tube, + *itis,* inflammation]. Inflammation of lining of fallopian tubes.

endosalpingoma (ĕn″dō-săl″pĭn-gō′mă). Adenomyoma of the uterine tube.

endosalpinx (ĕn″dō-săl′pĭnks) [″ + *salpinx,* tube]. The mucous membrane lining the uterine tube.

endoscope (ĕn′dō-skōp) [″ + *skopein,* to examine]. A device consisting of a tube and optical system for observing the inside of a hollow organ or cavity. This observation may be done through a natural body opening or through a small incision.

endoscopic laser cholecystectomy. SEE: *laparoscopic laser cholecystectomy.*

endoscopic retrograde cholangiopancreatography. ABBR: ERCP. Injection of a radiopaque material into the papilla of Vater. This is done by use of a fiberoptic endoscope guided by use of fluoroscopy. The procedure is helpful in determining the cause of jaundice. SEE: *jaundice; percutaneous transhepatic cholangiography.*

endoscopy (ĕn-dŏs′kō-pē). Inspection of

body organs or cavities by use of the endoscope.

endosepsis (ĕn″dō-sĕp′sĭs) [″ + *sepsis*, decay]. Septicemia having its origin within the body.

endoskeleton [″ + *skeleton*, skeleton]. Internal bony framework of the body. Opposite of exoskeleton.

endosmometer (ĕn″dŏs-mŏm′ĕ-tĕr) [″ + *osmos*, a thrusting, + *metron*, measure]. Device for estimating passage by osmosis of a substance through a membrane or tissue.

endosmosis (ĕn″dŏs-mō′sĭs) [″ + ″ + *osis*, condition]. Osmosis in which flow of water is from the outside liquid to the solution within a membranous cell.

endosome (ĕn′dō-sōm) [″ + L. *soma*, body]. The vacuole formed when material is absorbed in the cell by the process of endocytosis, q.v. The vacuole fuses with lysosomes. SYN: *receptosome*.

endospore [″ + *sporos*, a seed]. A thick-walled spore within a bacterium.

endosteitis (ĕn″dŏs-tē-ī′tĭs) [″ + *osteon*, bone, + *itis*, inflammation]. Inflammation of the endosteum or of medullary cavity of a bone. SYN: *endostitis*.

endosteoma (ĕn-dŏs″tē-ō′mă) [″ + ″ + *oma*, tumor]. A tumor in the medullary cavity of a bone.

endosteum (ĕn-dŏs′tē-ŭm) [″ + *osteon*, bone]. Membrane lining the medullary cavity of a bone.

endostitis (ĕn″dŏs-tī′tĭs) [″ + ″ + *itis*, inflammation]. Inflammation of the endosteum or the medullary cavity of a bone. SYN: *endosteitis*.

endostoma (ĕn-dŏs-tō′mă) [″ + ″ + *oma*, tumor]. Osseous tumor within a bone.

endostosis (ĕn″dŏs-tō′sĭs) [″ + ″ + *osis*, condition]. The development of an endostoma.

endotendineum (ĕn″dō-tĕn-dĭn′ē-ŭm) [″ + L. *tendo*, tendon]. The connective tissue in tendons between the bundles of fibers.

endothelial (ĕn″dŏ-thē′lē-ăl) [Gr. *endon*, within, + *thele*, nipple]. Pert. to or consisting of endothelium.

endothelin. An endothelium-derived vasoactive peptide that acts to cause blood vessels to constrict.

endotheliocyte (ĕn″dŏ-thē′lē-ō-sīt″) [″ + ″ + *kytos*, cell]. An endothelial cell.

endotheliocytosis (ĕn″dŏ-thē″lē-ō-sī-tō′sĭs) [″ + ″ + ″ + *osis*, condition]. Abnormal increase in endothelial cells.

endotheliolysin (ĕn″dŏ-thē-lē-ŏl′ĭ-sĭn) [″ + *thele*, nipple, + *lysis*, dissolution]. An antibody found in snake venom that dissolves endothelial cells.

endotheliolytic (ĕn″dŏ-thē-lē-ō-lĭt′ĭk). Capable of destroying endothelial tissue.

endothelioma (ĕn″dŏ-thē-lē-ō′mă) [″ + *thele*, nipple, + *oma*, tumor]. Malignant growth of lining cells of the blood vessels.

endotheliomyoma (ĕn″dŏ-thē″lē-ō-mī-ō′mă) [″ + ″ + *mys*, muscle, + *oma*, tumor]. Muscular tumor with elements of endothelium.

endotheliomyxoma (ĕn″dŏ-thē″lē-ō-mĭks-ō′mă) [″ + ″ + *myxa*, mucus, + *oma*, tumor]. Myxoma with element from endothelium.

endotheliosis (ĕn″dŏ-thē″lē-ō′sĭs). Increased growth of endothelium.

endotheliotoxin (ĕn″dŏ-thē-lē-ō-tŏks′ĭn) [″ + ″ + *toxikon*, poison]. A specific toxin that acts on endothelial capillary cells and causes hemorrhages.

endothelium (ĕn″dŏ-thē′lē-ŭm) [″ + *thele*, nipple]. [NA] A form of squamous epithelium consisting of flat cells that line the blood and lymphatic vessels, the heart, and various other body cavities. It is derived from mesoderm.

endothelium-derived relaxing factor. ABBR: EDRF. A potent vasodilator released by normal vascular endothelium. It also acts synergistically with prostacyclin to inhibit platelet aggregation.

endothermal, endothermic [Gr. *endon*, within, + *therme*, heat]. 1. Storing up potential energy or heat. 2. Absorbing heat. 3. Absorption of heat during chemical reactions.

endothermy (ĕn′dō-thĕr″mē). Elevation of temperature of deep body tissue in response to high-frequency current.

endothrix (ĕn′dō-thrĭks) [″ + *thrix*, hair]. Any fungus growing inside the hair shaft.

endothyropexy (ĕn″dō-thī′rō-pĕks″ē) [″ + *thyreos*, shield, + *pexis*, fixation]. Surgery involving displacement of the thyroid gland and fixing it to the side of the neck.

endotoscope (ĕn-dō′tō-skōp) [″ + *ous*, ear, + *skopein*, to examine]. An ear speculum. SYN: *otoscope*.

endotoxemia (ĕn″dō-tŏks-ē′mē-ă). Toxemia due to the presence of endotoxins in the blood.

endotoxicosis (ĕn″dŏ-tŏk″sĭ-kō′sĭs) [Gr. *endon*, within, + *toxikon*, poison, + *osis*, condition]. Poisoning due to an endotoxin.

endotoxin. Bacterial toxin confined within the body of a bacterium, freed only when the bacterium is broken down. SEE: *cytotoxin; enterotoxin; erythrotoxin; exotoxin; neurotoxin.*

endotoxin shock. Shock due to release of endotoxins from bacteria. Endotoxins are present in the lipopolysaccharide (LPS) component of the cell wall of gram-negative bacteria. LPS stimulates host responses that are beneficial but, at the same time, initiate a number of toxic reactions that may lead to disseminated intravascular coagulation (DIC), widespread capillary damage, hypotension, adult respiratory distress syndrome (ARDS), and fever. Unless these toxic reactions are treated vigorously, death may be the outcome.

TREAT: Supportive therapy for the shock; identify source of gram-negative bacteria and eradicate or remove it. To be effective, these therapeutic measures must be instituted immediately, literally within minutes of when the patient is seen. Therapy with corticosteroids or nonsteroidal anti-inflammatory agents may be of help. The use of tissue necrosis antibodies is experimental. SEE: *shock; tissue necrosis factor; toxic shock syndrome.*

endotracheal tube, cuffed. Tube used inside the trachea to provide an airway through the trachea while preventing aspiration of foreign material into the bronchus. This is accomplished by an inflatable cuff that surrounds the tube. It is inflated after the tube is placed in the trachea.

endotracheitis (ĕn″dō-trā-kē-ī′tĭs) [″ + *tracheia,* trachea, + *itis,* inflammation]. Inflammation of the tracheal mucosa.

endotrachelitis (ĕn″dō-trā-kĕl-ī′tĭs) [″ + *trachelos,* neck, + *itis,* inflammation]. Inflammation of the endocervical tissues of the uterine cervix. SYN: *endocervicitis.*

endovasculitis (ĕn″dō-văs″kū-lī′tĭs) [″ + L. *vasculum,* vessel, + Gr. *itis,* inflammation]. Inflammation of the endangium or inner coat of a blood vessel. SYN: *endangeitis.*

endovenous (ĕn″dō-vē′nŭs) [″ + L. *vena,* vein]. Within a vein. SYN: *intravenous.*

endplate. The terminal mass of a nerve fiber ending on a muscle cell.

   e., motor. An ending in a striated muscle fiber. SYN: *myoneural junction.*

end product. The final material or substance left at the completion of a series of reactions, either chemical or physical.

end result. The ultimate or final result.

end-stage. The final phase of a disease process.

Enduron. Trade name for methyclothiazide.

endyma (ĕn′dĭm-ă) [Gr., a garment]. Membranous lining of cerebral ventricles and central canal of spinal cord. SYN: *ependyma.*

enema (ĕn′ĕ-mă) [Gr.]. 1. Introduction of solutions into the rectum and colon in order to stimulate bowel activity and to cause emptying of the lower intestine; to introduce food or medicine for therapeutic purposes; to give anesthesia; or to aid in roentgenogra-

phy. 2. Solution introduced into the rectum.

   e., barium. Administration of barium sulfate in solution as a diagnostic aid in x-ray examination of colon.

   e., cleansing. Enema to empty the lower intestine or the colon. Use 15 to 60 ml for an infant, 240 to 360 ml for a child, and 500 to 1000 ml (approx. 1 to 2 L) for an adult.

NURSING IMPLICATIONS: Explain procedure to the patient and ensure privacy. Assemble all needed equipment, position the patient properly, and drape to ensure privacy. Follow hospital procedure for administration of enema. Be sure that during enema, the container is no more than 18 inches above the rectum, and that the solution is at the correct temperature. Clear tubing of air. Lubricate tip of rectal tube and insert into rectum. Fluid should flow into the rectum slowly. Coach the patient to breathe slowly and deeply during the procedure to help relax abdominal muscles. When the procedure is completed, position patient on a bedpan or assist to the bathroom. Chart the amount, type, and consistency of return from enema.

   e., double-contrast. Enema of barium or other radiopaque material that is injected and evacuated. This is followed by injection of air. Roentgenograms of the lower intestinal tract are then taken.

   e., emollient. Enema given to soothe and protect the intestinal mucosa by making a coating over membranes, to allay local pain and irritation, and to act as a vehicle for the rectal administration of drugs. It should be given at a temperature of about 105°F (40.6°C). The record must show if the patient felt relieved and to what extent and if the solution was retained.

   e., high. Enema designed to reach most of the colon. Rubber tube is inserted into rectum to carry water as far as possible.

   e., lubricating. Enema administered after an operation for hemorrhoids in order to soften the feces and lubricate the anal canal. When there is an impaction of feces, a lubricating enema may be given, followed in two hours by a cleansing enema. Warmed olive or mineral oil, 4 to 6 oz (120 to 180 ml), may be given. The patient should remain in a prone position with hips elevated for one-half hour following the enema in order to help retain the oil, thus aiding it in passing higher into the colon.

   e., medicinal. An enema to which some drug or medication has been added on order of the attending physician. It may be given to medicate diseased conditions of the rectum, sigmoid, or colon or to aid in absorption of a medicine for its systemic effects. It is necessary that this enema be retained and absorbed.

e., nutrient. Enema containing predigested foods for the purpose of giving sustenance to a patient unable to be fed otherwise. SYN: *nutritive enema.*

e., one-two-three. Mixture of 1 oz (30 ml) magnesium sulfate, 2 oz (60 ml) glycerine, and 3 oz (90 ml) hot water. This mixture must be given with a small tube because of the small quantity and the action desired. The results following the injection are more satisfactory if given very carefully with assistance to help the patient retain it.

e., physiological salt solution. A normal salt solution is five grams or one teaspoon of salt to a pint (473 ml) of water. The distention made by this enema excites peristalsis and evacuation. There is no harm in retaining this enema. Often ordered to be retained in treating dehydration.

e., retention. Enema that may be used to provide nourishment or medication. This enema must be formulated from constituents that will not stimulate the nerve endings and reflexly promote peristalsis. It necessarily must consist of a small amt. of solution, usually 100 to 240 ml.

NURSING IMPLICATIONS: Inform the patient of the purpose of this procedure so that full cooperation can be attained. Place patient on left side with knees flexed. Insert the rectal tube high (6 in. or 15 cm or more). Expel air from the tubing before it is inserted. Once inserted, the tube should not be moved — unless absolutely necessary — until the procedure is completed. The fluid should run in slowly, stopping at intervals, to aid retention. If the patient experiences the least desire to expel the solution, fluid should be stopped until the desire to evacuate is passed. Withdraw the tube quickly, and place pressure on the buttocks (compressing them together) for a minute or two to prevent evacuation.

e., saline. Enema consisting of normal saline solution or magnesium sulfate in warm water.

e., soapsuds. Use prepared soapsuds or, if liquid soap is used, 30 to 1000 ml of water is the right proportion. Strong soapsuds should not be used because of the danger of injuring intestinal mucosa. Mild white soaps, such as castile, are best.

enema, words pert. to: clysis; coloclyster; colonic irrigation; enteroclysis; medication routes, rectal; rectal feeding; rectum.

energetics (ĕn″ĕr-jĕt′ĭks). Science of study of energy esp. in relation to human use of energy in the form of food and the expenditure of energy in doing work or athletic exercise.

energy (ĕn′ĕr-jē) [Gr. *energeia*]. The capacity of a system for doing work or its equivalent

in the strict physical sense. Energy is manifested in various forms: motion (kinetic energy), position (potential energy), light, heat, ionizing radiation, or sound.

Changes in energy may be physical or chemical or both. Movement of a part of the body shortens and thickens the muscles involved and changes the position and size of cells temporarily, but the intake of oxygen in the blood combined with sugar and fat creates a chemical change and produces heat (energy) and waste products within the cells, which in turn produce fatigue. SEE: *calorie; energy expenditure, basal.*

e., conservation of. The theory that energy cannot be created or destroyed, but is transformed into other forms.

e., kinetic. Energy of motion.

e., latent. Energy that exists but is not being used.

e., potential. Stored energy.

e., radiant. Form of energy that is transmitted through space without the support of a sensible medium. Radio waves, infrared waves, visible rays, ultraviolet waves, x-rays, gamma rays and cosmic rays are energy in this form. SEE: *electromagnetic spectrum* for table.

energy, words pert. to: kinetic; metabolism; radiant; unit.

energy expenditure, basal. ABBR: BEE. In calculating the daily energy requirements for an individual, a fundamental datum needed is the amount of energy the individual needs if no work were done at all. The BEE (expressed as Calories) may be calculated for any individual by using the Harris-Benedict equations. These account for sex, age, height, and weight. If the individual is sedentary, moderately active, or engaged in strenuous activity, add 30%, 50%, or 100%, respectively, to the BEE.

The Harris-Benedict equation involves W (weight in kg), H (height in cm), and A (age in years). The formulae are:

$$\text{For women: BEE} = 6.55 + (9.6 \times W) + (1.8 \times H) - (4.7 \times A)$$

$$\text{For men: BEE} = 66 + (13.7 \times W) + (5 \times H) - (6.8 \times A)$$

Hospitalized patients who are nonstressed will require 20% more calories than for basal needs.

Energy expended is increased by about 13% over basal needs for each °C of fever; burn and trauma patients will require 40% to 100% more calories than for basal requirements. SEE: *diet; dietetics; food.*

enervation [L. *enervatio*]. 1. Deficient in nervous strength; weakness. 2. Resection or removal of a nerve.

enflagellation (ĕn″flăj-ĕl-lā′shŭn). Production and development of flagella.

enflurane (ĕn′floo-rān). USP. An anesthetic agent. Trade name is Ethrane.

ENG. *electronystagmography*.

engagement. 1. In obstetrics, the entrance of the fetal head or the part being presented into the superior pelvic strait. SYN: *lightening*. SEE: *labor*. 2. In the behavioral sciences, a term often used to convey the active involvement of an individual in everyday activities which have personal meaning.

Engelmann's disk [Theodor W. Engelmann, Ger. physiologist, 1843–1909]. A narrow zone of transparent material lying on each side of the intermediate disk in the isotropic or I disk of a striated muscle fiber.

engine. Device for converting energy into mechanical motion.

    e., dental. A machine that rotates dental instruments.

    e., high-speed. In dentistry, a machine that rotates a dental instrument in excess of 12,000 rpm.

    e., ultraspeed. A machine that rotates a dental instrument at speeds from 100,000 to 300,000 rpm.

engineering. In medical science, the practical application of principles of pure sciences such as physics or chemistry in attempting to provide solutions to medical problems. Branches of this science include human, dental, genetic, and biomechanical factors.

engorged (ĕn-gorjd′) [O. Fr. *engorgier*, to obstruct, to devour]. Distended, as with blood or fluids.

engorgement. Vascular congestion; distention.

engram (ĕn′grăm) [Gr. *engramm*]. A durable mark or trace. The protoplasmic change left by a stimulus in neural tissue.

enhancement (ĕn-hăns′mĕnt). Increasing the effect of ionizing radiation on tissues by use of oxygen or other chemicals.

enissophobia (ĕn-ĭs″ō-fō′bē-ă) [Gr. *enissein*, to reproach, + *phobos*, fear]. Fear of criticism, esp. for having committed a sin.

enkatarrhaphy (ĕn″kă-tăr′ăf-ē) [Gr. *enkatarrhaptein*, to sew in]. Burying of structure by suturing adjacent tissue over it.

enkephalins (ĕn-kĕf′ă-lĭns). Chemical substances, polypeptides, produced in the brain. They act as opiates and produce analgesia by binding to opiate receptor sites involved in pain perception. The threshold for pain is therefore increased by this action. It is possible that enkephalins have a role in explaining the withdrawal signs of narcotic addiction. SYN: *endogenous opiate-like substance*. SEE: *endorphins; opiate receptor*.

enlargement (ĕn-lărj′mĕnt). An increase in size of anything, esp. of an organ or tissue.

enol (ē′nŏl). A form that a ketone may take by a method known as tautomerism. A substance changes from the enol form to the ketone form by the oscillation of a hydrogen atom from the enol form to the ketone form.

enolase (ē′nō-lās). An enzyme present in muscle tissue that converts phosphoglyceric acid to phosphopyruvic acid.

enology (ē-nŏl′ō-jē) [Gr. *oinos*, wine, + *logos*, word, reason]. The science of production and evaluation of wine. Also spelled oenology.

enomania (ē″nō-mā′nē-ă) [″ + *mania*, madness]. Craving for alcoholic beverages.

enophthalmos (ĕn″ŏf-thăl′mŭs) [Gr. *en*, in, + *ophthalmos*, eye]. Recession of eyeball into orbit. Opposite of exophthalmos.

enosimania (ĕn″ŏs-ĭ-mā′nē-ă) [Gr. *enosis*, a quaking, + *mania*, madness]. A mental state characterized by excessive and irrational terror.

enostosis (ĕn″ŏs-tō′sĭs) [Gr. *en*, in, + *osteon*, bone, + *osis*, condition]. An osseous tumor within the cavity of a bone.

enriched. The addition of something extra. For example, the addition of vitamins or minerals to a food in order to *enrich* it.

ensiform (ĕn′sĭ-form) [L. *ensis*, sword, + *forma*, form]. Swordlike structure.

ensisternum (ĕn″sĭs-tĕr′nŭm) [″ + Gr. *sternon*, sternum]. The lowest portion of the sternum. SYN: *xiphoid process*.

enstrophe (ĕn′strō-fē) [Gr. *en*, in, + *strephein*, to turn]. Inversion; a turning inward, esp. of eyelids.

ENT. *ear, nose, and throat*.

entad (ĕn′tăd) [″ + L. *ad*, toward]. Toward the inside; inwardly.

ental (ĕn′tăl) [Gr. *entos*, within]. Pert. to the interior; inside, central.

entamebiasis (ĕn″tă-mē-bī′ă-sĭs) [″ + *amoibe*, change]. Infestation with *Entamoeba*.

Entamoeba (ĕn″tă-mē′bă). A genus of parasitic ameba, several of which are found in the human digestive tract.

    E. buccalis. E. gingivalis.

    E. coli. Species normally found in the human intestinal tract. Nonpathogenic to man.

    E. gingivalis. Nonpathogenic species that inhabits the mouth.

    E. histolytica. Pathogenic species of ameba, the cause of amebic dysentery and tropical liver abscess. SEE: *amebiasis*.

    E. kartulisi. Species found in the pus of necrotic bone abscesses.

    E. tetragena. Species now considered identical with *E. histolytica*.

    E. undulans. Species found in the intestine.

enteradenitis (ĕn″tĕr-ăd″ĕ-nī′tĭs) [Gr. *enteron*, intestine, + *aden*, gland, + *itis*, inflammation]. Inflammation of intestinal glands.

enteral (ĕn′tĕr-ăl) [Gr. *enteron*, intestine]. Within or by way of the intestine.

enteral tube feeding. Feeding of the appropriate formula to a patient by means of a tube passed into the stomach from the nasal passage. It is used for patients who for some reason are unwilling or unable to masticate or swallow food.

enteralgia (ĕn″tĕr-ăl′jē-ă) [″ + *algos*, pain]. Neuralgia or pain in the intestines. Intestinal cramps or colic.

enterectasia (ĕn″tĕr-ĕk-tā′sē-ă) [″ + *ektasis*, dilatation]. Dilatation of the small intestines.

enterectomy (ĕn″tĕr-ĕk′tō-mē) [″ + *ektome*, excision]. Excision of a portion of the intestines.

enterelcosis (ĕn″tĕr-ĕl-kō′sĭs) [″ + *helkosis*, ulceration]. Intestinal ulceration.

enteric (ĕn-tĕr′ĭk) [Gr. *enteron*, intestine]. Pert. to the small intestine.

enteric-coated. A type of drug formulation in which tablets or capsules are coated with a special compound that will not dissolve until the pill or tablet is exposed to the fluids in the small intestine.

enteric fever. Typhoid fever, q.v.

enteritis (ĕn″tĕr-ī′tĭs) [″ + *itis*, inflammation]. Inflammation of the intestines, more particularly of the mucous and submucous tissues of the small intestines. SEE: *Nursing Diagnoses in Appendix.*

   e., regional. SEE: *ileitis, regional.*

entero-, enter- [Gr. *enteron*, intestine]. Prefix denoting some relationship to the intestines.

enteroanastomosis (ĕn″tĕr-ō-ăn-ăs″tō-mō′sĭs) [″ + *anastomosis*, opening]. Intestinal anastomosis.

enteroantigen (ĕn″tĕr-ō-ăn′tĭ-jĕn) [″ + *anti*, against, + *gennan*, to produce]. An antigen derived from the intestines.

enteroapokleisis (ĕn″tĕr-ō-ăp″ō-klī′sĭs) [″ + *apokleisis*, a shutting out]. Operation for exclusion of a part of the intestine.

Enterobacter. A group of enteric gram-negative rods of the family Enterobacteriaceae that occur in soil, dairy products, water, sewage, and the intestinal tracts of man and animals; often secondary pathogens, or opportunistic infections. In man, many of these infections are hospital acquired.

   E. aerogenes. A species of *Enterobacter*. It occurs normally in the intestine of man and other animals and is found in decayed matter, on grains and plants. The organism is important in causing urinary tract infections and intestinal disease when antibiotic therapy causes elimination of other organisms. Formerly called *Aerobacter aerogenes.*

   E. agglomerans. An organism formerly called *Erwinia*. Has been associated with serious systemic infections, particularly septicemia from contaminated I.V. fluids.

Enterobacteriaceae (ĕn″tĕr-ō-băk-tē″rē-ā′sē-ē). A family of gram-negative, nonspore-forming rods. Some of the genera are intestinal pathogens. Included in the family are *Shigella, Salmonella, Escherichia, Klebsiella, Proteus,* and *Yersinia.*

enterobacteriotherapy (ĕn″tĕr-ō-băk-tē″rē-ō-thĕr′ă-pē) [″ + *bakterion*, little rod, + *therapeia*, treatment]. Use of vaccines containing intestinal bacteria.

enterobiasis (ĕn″tĕr-ō-bī′ă-sĭs) [Gr. *enteron*, intestine, + *bios*, life]. Infestation with pinworms *(Enterobius vermicularis).* SYN: *oxyuriasis.*

enterobiliary (ĕn″tĕr-ō-bĭl′ē-ār-ē) [″ + L. *bilis*, bile]. Pert. to the intestines and the bile passages.

Enterobius (ĕn″tĕr-ō′bē-ŭs) [″ + *bios*, life]. A genus of parasitic nematode worms, formerly *Oxyuris vermicularis.*

   E. vermicularis. A species of nematode worms, the adult form of which inhabits the large intestine in humans. The genital organs and bladder may become infected in females, causing cystitis due to the bacteria that the female worm carries. Infestations are characterized by irritation of the anal region and allergic reaction of the neighboring skin accompanied by intense itching, which may result in loss of sleep, excessive irritability, and a secondary infection of the area around the anus as a result of the scratching. Distribution is worldwide. It is estimated that in temperate climates 20% of children have this condition. Female worms average 8 to 13 mm in length and males 2 to 5 mm. SYN: *pinworm.*

   DIAG: Finding adult worms in feces or on the anus; or by applying transparent, pressure-sensitive tape to the perianal area and then examining the tape microscopically for eggs. This latter test is more likely to be positive in the morning prior to bathing.

   TREAT: Pyrantel pamoate or mebendazole is effective. Family recurrences may be prevented if the entire family is treated.

enterocele (ĕn′tĕr-ō-sēl) [″ + *keke*, hernia]. 1. A hernia of the intestine through the vagina. 2. Posterior vaginal hernia.

enterocentesis (ĕn″tĕr-ō-sĕn-tē′sĭs) [″ + *kentesis*, puncture]. Puncture of intestine to withdraw gas or fluids.

enterocholecystostomy (ĕn″tĕr-ō-kō″lē-sĭs-tŏs′tō-mē) [″ + *chole*, bile, +

kystis, bladder, + *stoma,* mouth]. Making an opening between the gallbladder and small intestine. SYN: *cholecystenterostomy.*

enterocholecystotomy (ĕn″tĕr-ō-kō″lē-sĭs-tŏt′ō-mē) [″ + ″ + ″ + *tome,* incision]. Incision of both gallbladder and intestine.

enterocinesia (ĕn″tĕr-ō-sĭn-ē′sē-ă) [″ + *kinesis,* movement]. Intestinal movement. SYN: *peristalsis.*

enterocinetic (ĕn″tĕr-ō-sĭn-ĕt′ĭk). Pert. to or promoting peristalsis.

enteroclysis (ĕn″tĕr-ŏk′lĭ-sĭs) [″ + *klysis,* a washing out]. 1. Injection of a nutrient or medicinal liquid into bowel. 2. Irrigation of colon with large amt. of fluid intended to fill the colon completely and flush it. SEE: *enema.*

enterococcus (ĕn″tĕr-ō-kŏk′ŭs). Any species of streptococcus inhabiting the human intestine.

enterocoele (ĕn′tĕr-ō-sēl) [″ + *koilia,* hollow]. The abdominal cavity.

enterocolectomy (ĕn″tĕr-ō-kō-lĕk′tō-mē) [″ + *kolon,* colon, + *ektome,* excision]. Surgical removal of the terminal ileum, cecum, and ascending colon.

enterocolitis (ĕn″tĕr-ō-kō-lī′tĭs) [″ + ″ + *itis,* inflammation]. Inflammation of intestines and colon. This serious condition may be so acute as to require immediate treatment of shock, regulation of electrolyte balance, and antibiotics if ordered by physician.

    e., neonatal necrotizing. A severe disease of the GI tract of the newborn, esp. the premature. Etiology is unknown and treatment is vigorous and symptomatic. The death rate may be as high as 50%.

enterocolostomy (ĕn″tĕr-ō-kō-lŏs′tō-mē) [″ + ″ + *stoma,* mouth]. Surgical joining of the small intestine to the colon.

enterocutaneous (ĕn″tĕr-ō-kū-tā′nē-ŭs). Communication between the skin and intestine.

enterocyst (ĕn′tĕr-ō-sĭst) [Gr. *enteron,* intestine, + *kystis,* bladder]. A benign cyst of the intestinal wall.

enterocystocele (ĕn″tĕr-ō-sĭs′tō-sēl) [″ + *kele,* tumor, swelling]. Hernia of the bladder wall and intestine.

enterocystoma (ĕn″tĕr-ō-sĭs-tō′mă) [″ + ″ + *oma,* tumor]. Cystic tumor of the intestinal wall.

enterocystoplasty (ĕn″tĕr-ō-sĭs′tō-plăs″tē) [″ + ″ + *plastos,* formed]. A plastic surgical procedure involving the use of a portion of intestine to enlarge the bladder.

enterodynia (ĕn″tĕr-ō-dĭn′ē-ă) [″ + *odyne,* pain]. Pain in the intestine. SYN: *enteralgia.*

enteroenterostomy (ĕn″tĕr-ō-ĕn″tĕr-ŏs′tō-mē) [″ + *enteron,* intestine, + *stoma,* mouth]. Formation of a communication between two intestinal segments that are not continuous.

enteroepiplocele (ĕn″tĕr-ō-ē-pĭp′lō-sēl) [″ + *epiploon,* omentum, + *kele,* tumor, swelling]. Hernia of small intestine and omentum.

enterogastritis (ĕn″tĕr-ō-găs-trī′tĭs) [″ + *gaster,* belly, + *itis,* inflammation]. Inflammation of stomach (gastritis) and intestines (enteritis).

enterogastrone (ĕn″tĕr-ō-găs′trōn). A hormone secreted by the intestinal mucosa that, by depressing gastric motility and secretion, controls the release of food from the stomach into the duodenum. A meal high in fat content will cause greater secretion of this hormone than will a normal feeding.

enterogenous (ĕn″tĕr-ŏj′ĕ-nŭs) [″ + *gennan,* to produce]. Originating in the small intestines.

enterogram [″ + *gramma,* something written]. Tracing or graph of intestinal movements.

enterography [″ + *graphein,* to write]. 1. A description of the intestines. 2. Making of an enterogram.

enterohemorrhagic E. coli. SEE: *Escherichia coli.*

enterohepatic (ĕn″tĕr-ō-hĕ-păt′ĭk) [″ + *hepar,* liver]. Pert. to the intestines and liver.

enterohepatitis (ĕn″tĕr-ō-hĕp-ă-tī′tĭs) [″ + ″ + *itis,* inflammation]. Inflamed condition of the intestine and liver.

enterohydrocele (ĕn″tĕr-ō-hī′drō-sēl) [″ + *hydor,* water, + *kele,* tumor, swelling]. Hydrocele with loop of intestine in the sac.

enteroidea (ĕn″tĕr-oy′dē-ă) [″ + *eidos,* form, shape]. The intestinal fevers; those caused by intestinal bacilli, including typhoid fever.

enteroinvasive E. coli. SEE: *Escherichia coli.*

enterokinase (ĕn″tĕr-ō-kī′nās) [″ + *kinesis,* movement]. Previous term for enteropeptidase, q.v.

enterokinesia. Peristalsis, q.v.

enterolith (ĕn″tĕr-ō-lĭth) [″ + *lithos,* stone]. An intestinal concretion.

enterolithiasis (ĕn″tĕr-ō-lĭ-thī′ă-sĭs). The formation or existence of intestinal calculi.

enterology [″ + *logos,* word, reason]. The study of the intestinal tract.

enterolysis (ĕn″tĕr-ŏl′ĭ-sĭs) [″ + *lysis,* dissolution]. Surgical therapy of intestinal adhesions.

enteromegalia, enteromegaly (ĕn″tĕr-ō-mĕ-gā′lē-ă, ĕn″tĕr-ō-mĕg′ă-lē) [″ + *megas,* large]. Abnormal enlargement of the intestines. SYN: *megacolon*.

Enteromonas hominis (ĕn"tĕr-ŏm'ō-năs hŏm'ĭn-ĭs). A minute, flagellated, protozoan parasite that lives in the intestine of humans. It is rare and considered nonpathogenic.

enteromycosis (ĕn"tĕr-ō-mī-kō'sĭs) [" + *mykes*, fungus, + *osis*, diseased condition]. Disease of intestine resulting from bacteria or fungi.

enteromyiasis (ĕn"tĕr-ō-mī-ī'ă-sĭs) [" + *myia*, fly]. Disease caused by the presence of maggots (the larvae of flies) in the intestines.

enteron (ĕn'tĕr-ŏn) [Gr.]. The alimentary canal.

enteroneuritis (ĕn"tĕr-ō-nū-rī'tĭs) [" + *neuron*, nerve, + *itis*, inflammation]. Inflammation of nerves of the intestines.

enteroparesis (ĕn"tĕr-ō-păr'ē-sĭs) [" + *paresis*, relaxation]. Reduced peristalsis of the intestines followed by dilation of the walls.

enteropathogen (ĕn"tĕr-ō-păth'ō-jĕn) [" + *pathos*, disease, suffering, + *gennan*, to produce]. Any microorganism that causes intestinal disease.

enteropathogenic E. coli. SEE: *Escherichia coli.*

enteropathy (ĕn"tĕr-ŏp'ă-thē) [" + *pathos*, disease, suffering]. Any intestinal disease.

enteropeptidase (ĕn"tĕr-ō-pĕp'tĭ-dās). An enzyme occurring in the mucosa of the duodenum, necessary for the activation of the trypsinogen of the pancreatic juice that is converted into trypsin.

RS: enzyme; trypsin; trypsinogen.

enteropexy (ĕn'tĕr-ō-pĕks"ē) [" + *pexis*, fixation]. Fixation of the intestine to the abdominal wall or to another portion of the intestine.

enteroplasty (ĕn'tĕr-ō-plăs"tē) [" + *plassein*, to form]. Plastic operation on intestines. SEE: *laparotomy.*

enteroplegia (ĕn"tĕr-ō-plē'jē-ă) [" + *plege*, stroke]. Paralysis of intestines. SEE: *paralytic ileus.*

enteroplex (ĕn'tĕr-ō-plĕks) [" + *plexis*, a weaving]. Instrument for joining cut edges of intestines.

enteroplexy. Union of divided parts of the intestine. SYN: *enteroanastomosis.*

enteroproctia (ĕn"tĕr-ō-prŏk'shē-ă) [" + *proktos*, anus]. The condition of having an artificial anus.

enteroptosis (ĕn"tĕr-ŏp-tō'sĭs) [" + *ptosis*, a dropping]. Prolapse of the intestine or abdominal organs.

enterorrhaphy (ĕn"tĕr-or'ă-fē) [" + *rhaphe*, seam, ridge]. The stitching of an intestinal wound or of the intestines to some other structure.

enterorrhexis (ĕn"tĕr-ō-rĕks'ĭs) [" + *rhexis*, rupture]. Rupture of the intestine.

enteroscope (ĕn"tĕr-ō-skōp") [" + *skopein*, to examine]. Device for visually examining the inside of the intestines.

enterosepsis (ĕn"tĕr-ō-sĕp'sĭs) [" + *sepsis*, decay]. Intestinal toxemia; sepsis developed from the intestinal contents. SYN: *enterotoxism.*

enterospasm (ĕn'tĕr-ō-spăzm) [Gr. *enteron*, intestine, + *spasmos*, spasm]. Intermittent painful contractions of the intestines.

enterostasis (ĕn"tĕr-ō-stā'sĭs) [" + *stasis*, a standing]. Cessation of or delay in the passage of food through the intestine.

enterostenosis (ĕn"tĕr-ō-stĕ-nō'sĭs) [" + *stenosis*, a narrowing]. Narrowing or stricture of the intestine.

enterostomal therapist. Individual trained to assist patients who have had an ostomy in learning the proper methods of caring for their ostomy sites.

enterostomy (ĕn"tĕr-ŏs'tō-mē) [" + *stoma*, mouth]. Surgical formation of a permanent opening into the intestine through the abdominal wall.

enterotome (ĕn'tĕr-ō-tōm) [" + *tome*, incision]. Instrument for incision of intestines.

enterotomy (ĕn-tĕr-ŏt'ō-mē). Incision or dissection of the intestines.

enterotoxemia (ĕn"tĕr-ō-tŏk-sē'mē-ă). Condition in which toxins are absorbed from the intestine and are circulating in the blood.

enterotoxigenic (ĕn"tĕr-ō-tŏk"sī-jĕn'ĭk). Producing enterotoxins, as in enterotoxigenic strains of the bacillus *E. coli.* These bacilli are important in causing "travelers' diarrhea."

enterotoxigenic E. coli. SEE: *Escherichia coli.*

enterotoxin (ĕn"tĕr-ō-tŏk'sĭn) [" + *toxikon*, poison]. 1. Toxin produced in or originating in the intestinal contents. 2. Exotoxin specific for the cells of the mucosa. 3. Exotoxin produced by certain species of bacteria that cause various diseases, including food poisoning and toxic shock syndrome.

enterotoxism. Absorption of toxins from the intestinal contents.

enterotropic [" + *trope*, a turning]. Affecting or attracted by the intestines.

Enterovirus. A group of viruses that originally included the viruses of polio, coxsackie, and ECHO, which infected the human gastrointestinal tract. Enteroviruses are now classed as a genus of picornaviruses. SEE: *picornaviruses.*

enterozoic (ĕn"tĕr-ō-zō'ĭk) [" + *zoon*, animal]. Pert. to parasites inhabiting the intestines.

enterozoon (ĕn″tĕr-ō-zō′ŏn) (pl. *enterozoa*). Any intestinal animal parasite.

enthesis (ĕn′thĕ-sĭs) [Gr., a putting in]. 1. The use of metallic or other inert substances to substitute for or replace lost tissue. 2. Site of attachment of bone to a tendon, ligament, or joint capsule.

enthesitis. Tenderness to palpation at the site of attachment of bone to a tendon, ligament, or joint capsule. It is usually caused by trauma to the area.

enthetic (ĕn-thĕt′ĭk). 1. Pert. to enthesis, q.v. 2. Introduced from outside. SYN: *exogenous*.

enthlasis (ĕn′thlă-sĭs) [Gr., dent caused by pressure]. Depressed fracture of the skull containing bone fragments, i.e., comminuted.

entire. In bacteriology, the smooth, regular border of a bacterial colony.

entity (ĕn′tĭ-tē) [L. *ens*, being]. 1. A thing existing independently, containing in itself all the conditions necessary to individuality. 2. That which forms a complete whole, denoting a distinct condition or disease.

ento- [Gr. *entos*, within]. Prefix indicating within, inside.

entoblast (ĕn′tō-blăst) [″ + *blastos*, germ]. Endoblast, q.v.

entocele (ĕn′tō-sēl) [″ + *kele*, tumor, swelling]. 1. Internal hernia. 2. Displacement of a part inwardly.

entochondrostosis (ĕn″tō-kŏn″drŏs-tō′sĭs) [″ + *chondros*, cartilage, + *osis*, condition]. The development of bone within cartilage.

entochoroidea (ĕn″tō-kō-roy′dē-ă) [″ + *chorioeides*, choroid]. The inner layer of the choroid; coat of the eye.

entocineria (ĕn″tō-sĭn-ē′rē-ă) [″ + L. *cinereus*, ashen]. The internal gray matter of nerve centers, esp. of the brain.

entocone (ĕn′tō-kōn) [″ + *konos*, cone]. The inner posterior cusp of an upper molar tooth.

entocornea (ĕn″tō-kor′nē-ă) [″ + L. *corneus*, horny]. Posterior or inner lining membrane of cornea. SYN: *Descemet's membrane*.

entocyte (ĕn′tō-sīt) [″ + *kytos*, cell]. Material inside the cell wall.

entoderm (ĕn′tō-dĕrm) [″ + *derma*, skin]. Inner layer of cells in the blastoderm, q.v. Innermost of the three primary germ layers of a developing embryo. It gives rise to the epithelium of the digestive tract and its associated glands, the respiratory organs, bladder, vagina, and urethra. SYN: *endoderm*.

entoectad (ĕn″tō-ĕk′tăd) [″ + *ektos*, without, + L. *ad*, toward]. Proceeding from within outward.

entome (ĕn′tōm) [Gr. *en*, in, + *tome*, incision]. Knife for division of urethral stricture.

entomion (ĕn-tō′mē-ŏn) [Gr. *entome*, notch]. The tip of mastoid angle of the parietal bone.

entomology (ĕn″tō-mŏl′ō-jē) [Gr. *entomon*, insect, + *logos*, word, reason]. The study of insects.

  e., medical. That branch of entomology that deals with insects and their relationship to disease, esp. to disease of humans.

entophyte (ĕn′tō-fīt) [Gr. *entos*, within, + *phyton*, plant]. Any vegetable parasite living within the body.

entopic [Gr. *en*, in, + *topos*, place]. Normally situated; in a normal place. Opposite of ectopic.

entoptic (ĕn-tŏp′tĭk) [Gr. *entos*, within, + *optikos*, seeing]. Pert. to the interior of the eye.

entoptic phenomena. Visual phenomena arising from within the eye, characterized by seeing floating bodies, circles of light, black spots, and transient flashes of light. May be due to individuals seeing their own blood cells move through the retinal vessels, or floaters, which are small specks of tissue floating in the vitreous fluid. SEE: *photopsia; Moore's lightning streaks; muscae volitantes.*

entoretina (ĕn″tō-rĕt′ĭ-nă) [″ + L. *rete*, a net]. Internal layer of the retina.

entotic (ĕn-tō′tĭk, ĕn-tŏt′ĭk) [″ + *ous*, ear]. Pert. to interior of ear or to perception of sound as a result of condition of the auditory apparatus.

entozoon (ĕn″tō-zō′ŏn) [″ + *zoon*, animal] (pl. *entozoa*). Any animal parasite living within the body of another animal.

entrails. The intestines of an animal.

entrain. To alter the biological rhythm of an organism so that it assumes a cycle different from a 24-hour one.

entropion (ĕn-trō′pē-ŏn) [Gr. *en*, in, + *trepein*, to turn]. Inversion or turning inward of an edge, esp. the margin of the lower eyelid.

  e., cicatricial. An inversion resulting from scar tissue on the inner surface of the lid.

  e., spastic. An inversion resulting from a spasm of the orbicularis oculi muscles.

entropionize (ĕn-trō′pē-ō-nīz). To invert or correct by turning in.

entropy (ĕn′trŏ-pē) [Gr. *en*, in, + *trope*, a turning]. 1. That portion of energy within a system that cannot be utilized for mechanical work but is available for internal use. 2.

The quantity or degree of randomness, disorder, or chaos in a system.

enucleate (ē-nū′klē-āt) [L. *enucleare,* to remove the kernel of]. 1. To remove a part or a mass in its entirety. 2. To destroy or take out the nucleus of a cell. 3. To remove the eyeball surgically. 4. To remove a cataract surgically.

enucleation (ē-nū″klē-ā′shŭn). Removal of an entire mass or part without rupture, esp. pert. to a tumor or the eyeball.

enucleator (ē-nū′klē-ā-tor). Instrument for separating a tumor mass, as a myoma.

enuresis (ĕn″ū-rē′sĭs) [Gr. *enourein,* to void urine]. Involuntary discharge of urine after the age by which bladder control should have been established. In children, voluntary control of urination is usually present by the age of five. Nevertheless, nocturnal enuresis is present in about 10% of otherwise healthy five-year-old children and 1% of normal children at age 15. Enuresis is slightly more common in boys than in girls and occurs more frequently in the first-born child. This condition has a distinct family tendency. SEE: *bladder drill; Sioux alarm.*

ETIOL: In the great majority of cases, there is no organic basis for persistent enuresis. In these cases, the cause is most probably due to inadequate or misguided attempts at toilet training. Also, emotional stress, such as the birth of a sibling, death in the family, or separation from the family, may be associated with the onset of enuresis in a previously continent child. Conditions that may cause enuresis include urinary tract infection, increased fluid intake due to diabetes mellitus, any disease that interferes with the formation of concentrated urine, trauma to or disease of the spinal cord, and epilepsy.

TREAT: When no organic disease is present, the use of imipramine as a temporary adjunct may be helpful. This is usually given in a dose of 10 to 50 mg orally at bedtime, but the effectiveness may decrease with continued administration. The bladder may be trained to hold larger amounts of urine. This procedure has decreased the rate of occurrence of enuresis. No matter what the cause, the child should not be made to feel guilty or ashamed, and enuresis should be considered by the family and the child as any other condition that lends itself to appropriate therapy. If the child tries too hard to control the condition, it may worsen. Conditioning devices that sound an alarm when bedwetting occurs should not be used unless prescribed by a health care professional familiar with the treatment of enuresis.

Caution: Imipramine is not recommended for children under six years of age. Blood counts should be taken at least monthly during therapy to detect the possible side effect of granulocytosis.

e., diurnal. Urinary incontinence during the day. Its etiology is usually of a pathological nature. It may be caused by muscular contractions brought about by laughing, coughing, or crying. Often persists for long periods of time, esp. after protracted illness. It occurs more commonly in females.

e., nocturnal. Urinary incontinence during the night. It is irregular and unaccompanied by urgency or frequency. Incontinence may cease for several weeks only to return. This type is more common in boys than in girls.

Fluid should be restricted late in day and diurnal voidings should be spaced at more than ordinary intervals. The child may be awakened once or twice in the night and, when fully awake, robed and walked to the bathroom. As improvement is noticed, the number of awakenings may be lessened. The foot of the bed may also be elevated. Electronic devices that awaken the child the moment the bed is wet are available.

e., primary. Enuresis in which a child has never been dependably dry.

e., secondary. Occurrence of enuresis in a child in whom there had been no history of incontinence for a year or more.

envelope (ĕn′vĕ-lōp). A covering, or container.

e., nuclear. A double-membrane layer of lipids and proteins surrounding the nucleus of a cell.

envenomation (ĕn-vĕn″ō-mā′shŭn). The introduction of poisonous venoms into the body by means of a bite or sting.

environment [O. Fr. *en-,* in, + *viron,* circle]. The surroundings, conditions, or influences that affect an organism or the cells within an organism.

environmental control unit. ABBR: ECU. An electronic device operated by persons with severe disabilities that permits remote control of various home functions, such as heating, lighting, telephone, television, doorlocks, drapes, and air conditioning.

environmental illness. SEE: *chemical ecology.*

envy. To be unhappy about or to wish to possess the qualities or physical belongings of someone else.

e., penis. SEE: *penis envy.*

enzootic (ĕn″zō-ŏt′ĭk) [Gr. *en,* in, + *zoon,* animal]. An endemic disease limited to a

Summary of the Main Enzymatic Processes in Digestion

Site	Secretion	Enzyme	Substrate	Degree of Digestion	Products of Digestion
Mouth	Saliva	Amylases	Starch and glycogen	Slight	Dextrins, maltose
		Ptyalin	Raw starch	Slight	Dextrins, maltose
Stomach	Gastric juice	Pepsins	Protein	Incomplete	Proteoses, peptones
		Lipase	Triglycerides	Very slight	Fatty acids, glycerol
Intestine	Pancreatic juice	Trypsin Chymotrypsin Carboxypeptidase	Proteins Proteoses Peptones Peptides	Nearly complete	Amino acids
		Amylases	Starch and glycogen	Nearly complete	Dextrins, maltose
	Intestinal juice and intestinal mucosa	Enteropeptidase	Trypsinogen	Complete	Trypsin
		Maltase	Maltose	Complete	Glucose
		Lactase	Lactose	Complete	Glucose, galactose
		Sucrase	Sucrose	Usually complete	Glucose, fructose
		Nucleosidases (in mucosa)	Nucleosides	Usually complete	Purine bases, ribose

small number of animals.

enzygotic (ĕn″zī-gŏt′ĭk) [Gr. *en*, in, + *zygon*, yoke]. Developed from the same ovum.

enzygotic twins. Twins developed from one ovum. SYN: *monozygotic twins.* SEE: *dizygotic twins.*

enzyme (ĕn′zīm) [″ + *zyme*, leaven]. An organic catalyst produced by living cells but capable of acting independently. Enzymes are complex proteins that are capable of inducing chemical changes in other substances without being changed themselves. This aspect of enzymes allows a given amount of an enzyme to produce virtually unlimited quantities of the end product of the reaction. Enzymes are reaction-specific and act in just one way to produce the end result; this means that the entire reaction is exceptionally pure. They are present in digestive juices, where they act upon food substances, causing them to break down into simpler compounds. They are capable of accelerating the speed of chemical reactions. SEE: table.

ACTION: The reactions effected by the digestive enzymes are chiefly decompositions of a hydrolytic nature, but enzymes are equally important in the synthetic reactions of assimilation.

Each hydrolytic enzyme has been given a name indicating the substance upon which it acts with the addition of the suffix *-ase.* Lipases indicate fat-splitting enzymes; amylases, starch-splitting ones; and proteases, protein-splitting enzymes. Some of them take a qualifying adjective, as salivary or pancreatic enzymes. Some of the best-known enzymes such as rennin, pepsin, trypsin, and thrombin do not end in *-ase* because they were named before this method of nomenclature was instituted.

The substance acted upon by an enzyme is called the substrate. Proenzyme or zymogen is the name given to precursors of an enzyme. The more common groups of digestive tract enzymes are hydrolytic; fat, protein-, starch-, and sugar-splitting enzymes; coagulating enzymes or those that cause clotting, such as thrombin; oxidases or oxidizing enzymes; deamidizing enzymes, those that are important in removing amines or amino groups during oxidation; reductases or reducing enzymes; splitting enzymes; and joining enzymes.

Enzymes are specific in their action; they will act only upon a certain substance or a group of closely related chemical substances and no other. Each enzyme has an optimum temperature at which it acts with greatest efficiency; each is influenced by the reaction of the medium in which it acts, there being an optimum degree of acidity or alkalinity.

Enzyme activity can be retarded or inhibited by temperature extremes, presence of salts of heavy metals (copper, mercury), dehydration, and ultraviolet radiation.

Enzymes sometimes require the presence of additional substances to make them active. Nonspecific substances that activate enzymes are called activators (Ex.: HCl for pepsin). Specific substances that act selectively with certain enzymes only are called coenzymes (Ex.: enteropeptidase for trypsinogen). Several hundred enzymes have been identified, but as many as a thousand are thought to be present in mammals.

e., activating. Enzyme that catalyzes the attaching of an amino acid to the appropriate transfer ribonucleic acid.

e.'s, allosteric. Enzymes that can have their activity modified by binding certain types of effectors, called allosteric effectors, to a non-active site on the enzyme.

e., amylolytic. Enzyme that catalyzes the conversion of starch to sugar.

e., autolytic. Enzyme that produces autolysis or cell digestion.

e., bacterial. Enzyme developed by bacteria.

e.'s, branching. Enzymes, glycosyltransferases, that transfer a carbohydrate unit from one molecule to another.

e., coagulating. Enzyme that catalyzes the conversion of soluble proteins into insoluble ones. SYN: *coagulase.*

e., deamidizing. Enzyme that splits amine off amino acid compounds.

e., debranching. Enzyme, dextrin-1-6-glucosidase, that removes a carbohydrate unit from molecules that contain short carbohydrate units attached as side chains.

e., decarboxylating. Enzyme, such as carboxylase, that separates CO_2 from organic acids.

e., digestive. Any enzyme involved in digestive processes in the alimentary canal.

e., extracellular. Enzyme that produces its effects outside the cell that produces it.

e., fermenting. Enzyme produced by bacteria or yeasts that brings about the fermentation of substances, esp. carbohydrates.

e., glycolytic. Enzyme that catalyzes the oxidation of sugar.

e., hydrolytic. Enzyme that catalyzes hydrolysis.

e., inhibitory. Enzyme that blocks a chemical reaction.

e., inorganic. A metallic colloidal solution, acting somewhat like an enzyme.

e., intracellular. Enzyme that acts within the cell that produces it.

e., inverting. Enzyme that catalyzes the hydrolysis of sucrose.

e., lipolytic. Enzyme that catalyzes the hydrolysis of fats. SYN: *lipase.*

e., mucolytic. Enzyme that depolymerizes mucus by splitting mucoproteins. They are called mucinases. Examples are lysozyme and hyluronidase.

e., oxidizing. Enzyme that catalyzes oxidative reactions. SYN: *oxidase.*

e., proteolytic. Enzyme that catalyzes conversion of proteins into peptides.

e., redox. Any enzyme that catalyzes oxidation-reduction reactions.

e., reducing. Enzyme that removes oxygen. SYN: *reductase.*

e., respiratory. Enzyme that acts within tissue cells catalyzing oxidative reactions with the release of energy, such as cytochromes, and flavoproteins.

e., splitting. Any enzyme that acts to facilitate removal of part of a molecule.

e., steatolytic. E., lipolytic, q.v.

e., transferring. Any enzyme that facilitates the moving of one molecule to another compound. SYN: *transferase.*

e., uricolytic. Enzyme that catalyzes conversion of uric acid into urea.

e., yellow. One of a group of flavoproteins involved in cellular oxidations.

Enzyme Commission. ABBR: EC. A commission created in 1956 by the International Union of Biochemistry to standardize enzyme nomenclature.

enzyme induction. The adaptive increase in the number of molecules of a specific enzyme secondary either to an increase in its rate of synthesis or a decrease in its rate of degradation.

enzyme-linked immunoabsorbent assay. ABBR: ELISA. A rapid enzyme immunoassay method in which either an antibody or an antigen can be coupled to an enzyme. The resulting complex will retain both immunological and enzymatic activity. Use of this method provides for detection of either an antigen or an antibody. Certain bacterial antigens and antibodies as well as hormones can be detected by use of the ELISA method. The sensitivity is enhanced by the addition of an antibody to an enzyme such as alkaline phosphatase. In reacting with the substance, an intense color reaction is produced. These assays are quite sensitive and specific as compared with the radioimmune assay (RIA) tests, and have the advantage of not requiring radioisotopes and the expensive counting apparatus.

enzymology (ĕn″zī-mŏl′ō-jē). The study of

enzymes and their actions.

enzymolysis (ĕn-zī-mŏl′ĭ-sĭs) [Gr. *en,* in, + *zyme,* leaven, + *lysis,* dissolution]. Chemical change or disintegration due to an enzyme.

enzymopathy (ĕn″zī-mŏp′ă-thē). Any disease in which an enzyme deficiency is involved.

enzymopenia (ĕn-zī″mō-pē′nē-ă). Deficiency of an enzyme.

enzymuria (ĕn″zī-mū′rē-ă) [″ + ″ + *ouron,* urine]. Presence of enzymes in the urine.

EOA. *esophageal obturator airway.*

EOM. *extraocular muscles.*

EOP. *external occipital protuberance.*

eosin (ē′ō-sĭn) [Gr. *eos,* dawn (rose-colored)]. Several synthetic dyes, including bluish and yellow ones. They are used in staining tissues for microscopic examination.

eosinoblast (ē″ō-sĭn′ō-blăst) [″ + *blastos,* germ]. A bone marrow cell that develops into a myelocyte. SYN: *myeloblast.*

eosinopenia (ē″ō-sĭn-ō-pē′nē-ă) [″ + *penia,* poverty]. Abnormally small number of eosinophilic cells in the peripheral blood.

eosinophil (ē″ō-sĭn′ō-fĭl) [″ + *philein,* to love]. One type of granulocytic white blood cell characterized by a polymorphic nucleaus cytoplasmic granules that stain with eosin or other acid stains. Although their activity is not entirely clear, eosinophils are known to destroy parasitic organisms and to play a major role in allergic reactions. Some of the major chemical mediators that cause bronchoconstriction in asthma are released by eosinophils. Eosinophils make up 1% to 3% of the white cell count. SEE: *leukocyte.*

eosinophilia (ē″ō-sĭn-ō-fĭl′ē-ă) [Gr. *eos,* dawn, + *philein,* to love]. 1. Presence of unusual number of eosinophils in the blood. 2. Condition of staining readily with eosin.

    e., urinary. Presence of increased amount of eosinophils in urine.

eosinophilia-myalgia syndrome, tryptophan-induced. Eosinophilia and severe myalgia seen in patients with a history of taking oral preparations of the amino acid L-tryptophan.

    SYM: Abrupt onset, within a week or so, of pain, edema, and induration of the extremities, esp. the lower. Skin involvement includes alopecia, transient rash, and subjective weakness. The disease is disabling and chronic. Eosinophilia is greater than 1×10^9 cells per liter. In order to establish the diagnosis, other diseases that could cause these findings, e.g., infections or neoplasia, must be excluded.

    ETIOL: The outbreak that occurred in 1989 was most probably due to a chemical constituent associated with specific manufacturing conditions at one company.

    TREAT: Supportive; discontinue taking tryptophan.

eosinophilic (ē″ō-sĭn-ō-fĭl′ĭk). Readily stainable with eosin.

eosinophilous (ē″ō-sĭn-ŏf′ĭ-lŭs) [″ + *philein,* to love]. 1. Easily stainable with eosin. 2. Having eosinophilia.

eosinotactic (ē″ō-sĭn-ō-tăk′tĭk) [″ + *taktikos,* arranged]. Attraction or repulsion of eosinophil cells.

epactal (ē-păk′tăl) [Gr. *epaktos,* added to]. Supernumerary.

eparterial (ĕp″ăr-tē′rē-ăl) [Gr. *epi,* over, upon, + *arteria,* artery]. Located over or above an artery.

epaxial (ĕp-ăk′sē-ăl) [″ + L. *axis,* axis]. Situated above or behind any axis.

epencephalon (ĕp″ĕn-sĕf′ă-lŏn) [″ + *enkephalos,* brain]. The anterior portion of the embryonic hindbrain (rhombencephalon) from which arise the pons and cerebellum. SYN: *metencephalon.*

ependyma (ĕp-ĕn′dĭ-mă) [Gr. *ependyma,* an upper garment, wrap]. [NA] Membrane lining the cerebral ventricles and central canal of spinal cord.

ependymal (ĕp-ĕn′dĭ-măl). Pert. to the ependyma.

ependymal cells. Cells of the developing neural tube that give rise to the ependyma. They arise from spongioblasts derived from the neural epithelium.

ependymal layer. The innermost of three layers that form the neural tube of an embryo.

ependymitis (ĕp″ĕn-dĭ-mī′tĭs) [″ + *itis,* inflammation]. Inflammation of the ependyma.

ependymoblast (ĕp-ĕn′dĭ-mō-blăst) [″ + *blastos,* germ]. An embryonic ependymal cell or ependymocyte.

ependymocyte (ĕp-ĕn′dĭ-mō-sīt) [″ + *kytos,* cell]. An ependymal cell.

ependymoma (ĕp-ĕn″dĭ-mō′mă) [″ + *oma,* tumor]. A tumor arising from fetal inclusion of ependymal elements.

ephebiatrics (ĕ-fē-bē-ăt′rĭks) [Gr. *epi,* at, + *hebe,* youth, + *iatrikos,* medical]. A branch of medicine dealing with adolescents. SYN: *adolescent medicine.*

ephebic (ĕ-fē′bĭk) [Gr. *ephebikos*]. Pert. to adolescence.

ephebology (ĕf-ē-bŏl′ō-jē) [″ + ″ + *logos,* word, reason]. The study of puberty and its changes.

ephedrine (ĕ-fĕd′rĭn, ĕf′ĕ-drēn). An alkaloid originally obtained from species of *Ephedra;* first isolated by Nagai in 1887. In ancient Chinese medicine it was used as a diaphoretic and antipyretic. It was not until much later, however, that its action was studied and its valuable therapeutic properties made known. It is a sympathomimetic drug usually produced synthetically. Action is similar to that of epinephrine. Its effects, although less powerful, are more prolonged, and it exerts an action when given orally, whereas epinephrine is effective only by injection. Ephedrine orally (or by injection) dilates the bronchial muscles, contracts the nasal mucosa, and raises the blood pressure. Chiefly used for its bronchodilator effect in asthma, and for its constricting effects on the nasal mucosa in hay fever.

INCOMPAT: Calcium chloride; iodine; tannic acid.

e. hydrochloride. A more soluble salt of the alkaloid, having the same action and uses as ephedrine.

e. sulfate. USP. The sulfate of ephedrine. It occurs as fine white crystals or as a powder. Its action and uses are the same as those of ephedrine. Trade name is Isofedrol.

ephelis (ĕf-ē'lĭs) [Gr. *ephelis,* freckle] (pl. *ephelides*). Freckle.

ephemeral (ē-fĕm'ĕr-ăl) [Gr. *epi,* on, + *hemera,* day]. Of brief duration.

ephidrosis (ĕf″ĭ-drō'sĭs) [Gr., a sweating]. Abnormal amt. of sweating.

e. cruenta. Sweat containing blood.

e. tincta. Colored sweat. SYN: *chromidrosis.*

epi-, ep- [Gr.]. Prefix meaning upon, over, at, in addition to, after.

epiandrosterone (ĕp″ē-ăn-drŏs'tĕr-ōn). An androgenic hormone normally present in the urine.

epiblast (ĕp'ĭ-blăst) [Gr. *epi,* upon, + *blastos,* germ]. Outer layer of cells of the blastoderm. SYN: *ectoderm.*

epiblastic (ĕp-ĭ-blăs'tĭk). Pert. to the epiblast.

epiblepharon (ĕp″ĭ-blĕf'ă-rŏn) [″ + Gr. *blepharon,* eyelid]. A fold of skin passes across the margin of either the upper or lower eyelid so that the eyelashes are pressed against the eye.

epibole, epiboly (ē-pĭb'ŏ-lē) [Gr. *epibole,* cover]. Inclusion of the hypoblast within the epiblast, due to swifter growth of the latter. SEE: *emboly.*

epibulbar (ĕp″ĭ-bŭl'băr). Lying upon the bulb of any structure; more specifically, located upon the eyeball.

epicanthus [Gr. *epi,* upon, + *kanthos,* canthus]. A vertical fold of skin extending from the root of the nose to the median end of the eyebrow, covering the inner canthus and caruncle. It is a characteristic of certain ethnic groups and may occur as a congenital anomaly in others.

epicardia (ĕp″ĭ-kărd'ē-ă) [″ + *kardia,*

heart]. The abdominal portion of the esophagus extending from the diaphragm to the stomach, about 2 cm in length.

epicardium. [NA] The inner or visceral layer of the pericardium, q.v., which forms a serous membrane forming the outermost layer of the wall of the heart.

epichordal (ĕp″ĭ-kord'ăl) [″ + *khorde,* cord]. Located dorsad to the notochord.

epichorion (ĕp″ĭ-kō'rē-ŏn) [″ + *chorion*]. The portion of the decidua of the placenta that covers the ovum.

epicomus (ē-pĭk'ō-mŭs) [″ + *kome,* hair]. A congenital malformation consisting of a parasitic twin or head attached to the summit or vertex of the skull.

epicondylalgia (ĕp″ĭ-kŏn-dĭ-lăl'jē-ă) [″ + *kondylos,* condyle, + *algos,* pain]. Pain in the elbow joint in the region of the epicondyles.

epicondyle (ĕp-ĭ-kŏn'dīl) [″ + *kondylos,* condyle]. The eminence at the articular end of a bone above a condyle.

epicondylitis (ĕp″ĭ-kŏn″dĭ-lī'tĭs) [″ + ″ + *itis,* inflammation]. Inflammation of the epicondyle of the humerus and surrounding tissues.

e., lateral humeral. Tennis elbow, q.v.

e., medial humeral. Golfer's elbow, q.v.

epicranium [″ + *kranion,* cranium]. Soft parts covering the cranium.

epicranius (ĕp″ĭ-krā'nē-ŭs). Occipitofrontal muscle and scalp.

epicrisis (ĕp″ĭ-krī″sĭs) [″ + *krisis,* crisis]. A secondary crisis following the initial critical stage of a disease.

epicritic (ĕp-ĭ-krĭt'ĭk) [Gr. *epikritikos,* judging]. 1. Pert. to acute sensibility, such as that of the skin when it discriminates between degrees of sensation caused by touch or temperature. 2. Pert. to an epicrisis. 3. Something such as pain or itching that is well localized.

epicystitis [Gr. *epi,* upon, + *kystis,* bladder, + *itis,* inflammation]. Inflammation of cellular tissue above the bladder.

epicystotomy (ĕp″ĭ-sĭs-tŏt'ō-mē) [″ + ″ + *tome,* incision]. Opening above the symphysis pubis into the bladder.

epicyte (ĕp'ĭ-sīt) [″ + *kytos,* cell]. 1. An epithelial cell. 2. A cell membrane.

epidemic (ĕp″ĭ-dĕm'ĭk) [″ + *demos,* people]. Appearance of an infectious disease or condition that attacks many people at the same time in the same geographical area. SEE: *endemic; epizootic; pandemic.*

epidemic viral gastroenteropathy. A disease that occurs in outbreaks affecting groups of adults and children. The disease usually is self-limiting, but may cause severe dehydration and death. Symptoms include nausea, vomiting, diarrhea, mild fever, and abdominal pain.

ETIOL: Norwalk virus group and Rotavirus.

TREAT: Vigorous fluid replacement therapy, esp. in infections due to Rotavirus. This may be lifesaving in infected children. Oral rehydration solutions (ORS) are of distinct benefit and may be the only effective therapy available for infants and children in developing countries. SYN: *acute infectious nonbacterial gastroenteritis; winter vomiting disease.* SEE: *oral rehydration solutions; oral rehydration therapy.*

epidemiologic (ĕp″ĭ-dē-mē-ŏ-lŏj′ĭk) [″ + *demos*, people, + *logos*, study]. Pert. to the study of epidemics.

epidemiologist (ĕp″ĭ-dē-mē-ŏl′ō-jĭst). A specialist in the field of epidemiology.

epidemiology (ĕp″ĭ-dē-mē-ŏl′ō-jē). Study of the distribution and determinants of health-related states and events in populations, and the application of this study to the control of health problems.

Thus, epidemiology is concerned with the traditional study of epidemic diseases caused by infectious agents and with such health-related events as accidents, suicide, climate, toxic agents such as lead, air pollution, and catastrophes due to ionizing radiation. SEE: *pharmacoepidemiology.*

epidermal, epidermic [″ + *derma*, skin]. Pert. to the epidermis.

epidermal growth factor. ABBR: EGF. An amino acid polypeptide that stimulates growth of a number of different cells, including keratinocytes. It has been used experimentally to promote wound healing.

epidermatoplasty (ĕp″ĭ-dĕr-măt′ō-plăs-tē) [″ + ″ + *plassein*, to mold]. Grafting with pieces of epidermis with the underlying layer of the corium.

epidermis (ĕp″ĭ-dĕr′mĭs) [″ + *derma*, skin]. Skin, q.v.

epidermitis (ĕp″ĭ-dĕr-mī′tĭs) [″ + ″ + *itis*, inflammation]. Inflammation of the superficial layers of the skin.

epidermization (ĕp″ĭ-dĕr″mĭ-zā′shŭn). 1. Skin grafting. 2. Conversion of deeper germinative layer of cells into outer layer of epidermis.

epidermodysplasia verruciformis (ĕp″ĭ-dĕr″mō-dĭs-plā′sē-ă). Generalized warts of the skin.

epidermoid (ĕp″ĭ-dĕr′moyd) [Gr. *epi*, upon, + *derma*, skin, + *eidos*, form, shape]. 1. Resembling or pert. to the epidermis. 2. A tumor arising from aberrant epidermal cells. SYN: *cholesteatoma.*

epidermolysis (ĕp″ĭ-dĕr-mŏl′ĭ-sĭs) [″ + ″ + *lysis*, dissolution]. Loosening of the epidermis.

e. bullosa. A genetically transmitted

form characterized by formation of deep-seated bullae appearing after irritation or rubbing of a part.

epidermoma (ĕp″ĭ-dĕr-mō′mă) [″ + ″ + *oma*, tumor]. An excrescence on the skin.

epidermomycosis (ĕp-ĭ-dĕr″mō-mī-kō′sĭs) [″ + ″ + *mykes*, fungus, + *osis*, condition]. Skin disease caused by a fungus.

Epidermophyton (ĕp″ĭ-dĕr-mŏf′ĭ-tŏn) [″ + ″ + *phyton*, plant]. A genus of fungi, similar to *Trichophyton* but affecting the skin and nails instead of the hair.

E. floccosum. The causative agent of certain types of tinea, esp. tinea pedis (athlete's foot), tinea cruris, tinea unguium, and tinea corporis.

epidermophytosis (ĕp″ĭ-dĕr-mō-fī-tō′sĭs) [″ + ″ + ″ + *osis*, condition]. Infection by a species of *Epidermophyton.*

epididymectomy (ĕp″ĭ-dĭd″ĭ-mĕk′tō-mē) [″ + *didymos*, testis, + *ektome*, excision]. Removal of the epididymis.

epididymis (ĕp″ĭ-dĭd′ĭ-mĭs) (pl. *epididymides*). A small oblong body resting upon and beside the posterior surface of the testes, consisting of a convoluted tube 13 to 20 ft (3.97 to 6.1 meters) long, enveloped in the tunica vaginalis, ending in the ductus deferens. It consists of the head (caput or globus major), which contains 12 to 14 efferent ducts of the testis, the body, and the tail (cauda or globus minor). It constitutes the first part of the excretory duct of each testis. The epididymis is supplied by the internal spermatic, deferential, and external spermatic arteries; it is drained by corresponding veins. SEE: illus.

epididymitis (ĕp″ĭ-dĭd″ĭ-mī′tĭs) [″ + *didymos*, testis, + *itis*, inflammation]. Inflammation of the epididymis. SEE: *Nursing Diagnoses* in *Appendix.*

SYM: Fever and chills, pain in inguinal region, swollen epididymis.

ETIOL: May be complication of gonorrhea, syphilis, tuberculosis, mumps, prostatitis, urethritis, prostatectomy, or following prolonged use of indwelling catheter.

TREAT: Bedrest, support of scrotum, and appropriate antibiotic.

epididymodeferentectomy (ĕp″ĭ-dĭd″ĭ-mō-dĕf″ĕr-ĕn-tĕk′tō-mē) [″ + ″ + L. *deferens*, carrying away, + Gr. *ektome*, excision]. Excision of epididymis and ductus deferens.

epididymodeferential (ĕp″ĭ-dĭd″ĭ-mō-dĕf″ĕr-ĕn′shăl). Concerning both the epididymis and ductus deferens.

epididymography (ĕp″ĭ-dĭd″ĭ-mŏg′ră-fē) [″ + ″ + *graphein*, to write]. Radiographic examination of the epididymus after the introduction of a contrast agent.

epididymoorchitis (ĕp″ĭ-dĭd″ĭm-ō-or-kī′tĭs)

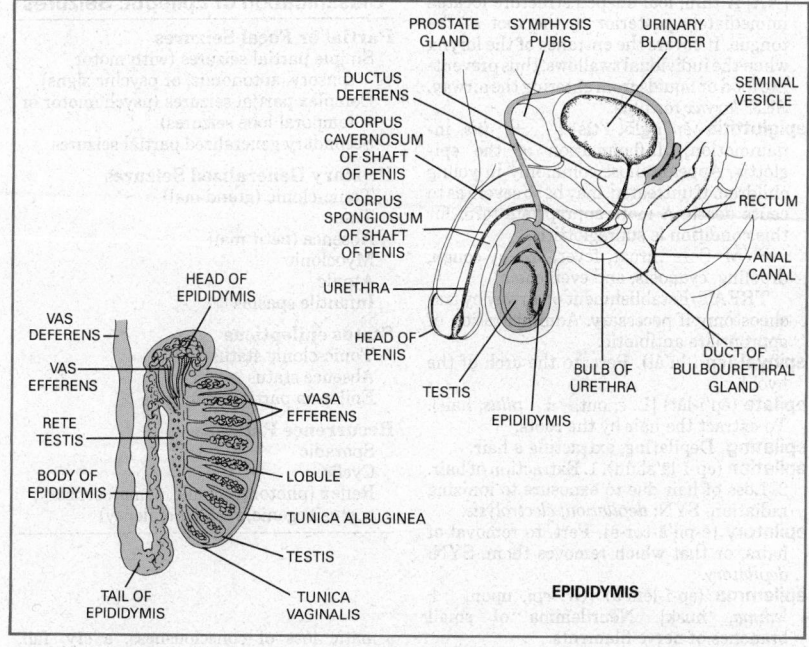

EPIDIDYMIS

[" + *didymos*, testis, + *orchis*, testis, + *itis*, inflammation]. Epididymitis with orchitis, q.v.

epididymotomy (ĕp″ĭ-dĭd″ĭ-mŏt′ō-mē) [" + " + *tome*, incision]. Incision into the epididymis.

epididymovasostomy (ĕp-ĭ-dĭd″ĭ-mō-văs-ŏs′tō-mē) [" + " + L. *vas*, vessel, + Gr. *stoma*, mouth]. Anastomosing between the epididymis and the vas.

epididymovesiculography (ĕp″ĭ-dĭd″ĭ-mō-vĕ-sĭk″ū-lŏg′ră-fē). Radiographic examination of the epididymus and seminal vesicle after introduction of a contrast agent.

epidural [Gr. *epi*, upon, + L. *durus*, hard]. Located over or upon the dura.

epidural space. Space outside of dura mater of the brain and spinal cord.

epifascial (ĕp″ĭ-făsh′ē-ăl). On or upon a fascia.

epifolliculitis (ĕp″ĭ-fŏl-lĭk″ū-lī′tĭs) [" + L. *folliculus*, follicle, + Gr. *itis*, inflammation]. Inflammation of hair follicles of the scalp.

epigaster [" + *gaster*, belly]. Embryonic structure that develops into the large intestine. SYN: *hindgut*.

epigastralgia (ĕp″ĭ-găs-trăl′jē-ă) [" + " + *algos*, pain]. Pain in the epigastrium.

epigastric. Pert. to the epigastrium. SEE: *precordium.*

epigastric reflex. Contraction of the upper portion of the rectus abdominis muscle when skin of the epigastric region is scratched.

epigastrium (ĕp″ĭ-găs′trē-ŭm) [" + *gaster*, belly]. Region over the pit of the stomach. SEE: *Auenbrugger's sign.*

epigastrocele (ĕp″ĭ-găs′trō-sēl) [" + *kele*, hernia]. Hernia in the epigastrium.

epigastrorrhaphy (ĕp″ĭ-găs-tror′ă-fē) [" + " + *rhaphe*, seam, ridge]. Suture of an abdominal wound in the epigastric area.

epigenesis (ĕp″ĭ-jĕn′ĕ-sĭs) [" + *genesis*, generation, birth]. In embryology, the theory that parts of an organism arise by a process of progressive development from simple to complex structures through the utilization of cells as building units.

epiglottidean (ĕp″ĭ-glŏ-tĭd′ē-ăn) [" + *glottis*, glottis]. Pert. to the epiglottis.

epiglottidectomy (ĕp″ĭ-glŏt″ĭd-ĕk′tō-mē) [" + " + *ektome*, excision]. Excision of the epiglottis.

epiglottiditis (ĕp″ĭ-glŏt″tĭd-ī′tĭs) [" + " + *itis*, inflammation]. Inflammation of the epiglottis. SYN: *epiglottitis.*

epiglottis (ĕp″ĭ-glŏt′ĭs) [Gr.] (pl. *epiglottides*).

[NA] A thin, leaf-shaped structure located immediately posterior to the root of the tongue. It covers the entrance of the larynx when the individual swallows, thus preventing food or liquids from entering the airway. SEE: *larynx* for illus.

epiglottitis (ĕp″ĭ-glŏt-ī′tĭs) [″ + *itis*, inflammation]. Inflammation of the epiglottis. Appears most commonly in young children. If untreated, may be so severe as to cause death. A more appropriate term for this condition is supraglottitis.

SYM: Sore throat, fever, croupy cough, drooling, cyanosis, and even coma.

TREAT: Establishment of airway by tracheostomy if necessary. Administration of appropriate antibiotic.

epihyal (ĕp-ĭ-hī′ăl). Pert. to the arch of the hyoid.

epilate (ĕp′ĭ-lāt) [L. *e*, out, + *pilus*, hair]. To extract the hair by the roots.

epilating. Depilating; extracting a hair.

epilation (ĕp-ĭ-lā′shŭn). 1. Extraction of hair. 2. Loss of hair due to exposure to ionizing radiation. SYN: *depilation; electrolysis.*

epilatory (ĕ-pĭl′ă-tor-ē). Pert. to removal of hairs, or that which removes them. SYN: *depilatory.*

epilemma (ĕp-ĭ-lĕm′ă) [Gr. *epi*, upon, + *lemma*, husk]. Neurilemma of small branches of nerve filaments.

epilepsy (ĕp′ĭ-lĕp″sē) [Gr. *epilepsia*, to seize]. A recurrent paroxysmal disorder of cerebral function characterized by sudden, brief attacks of altered consciousness, motor activity, or sensory phenomena. Convulsive seizures are the most common form of attacks. Some but not all recurrent seizure patterns are due to epilepsy.

OCCURRENCE: Over 1 million persons in the U.S. are estimated to be subject to recurrent seizures. The estimated prevalence is 6.42 cases per 100,000 population.

ETIOL: Attempts to find a cause for the sudden abnormal discharge of cerebral neurons is not possible in all types of epilepsy. In some cases a brain tumor, scar tissue remaining from trauma to the brain, or a progressive neurological disease may be responsible. In the great majority of cases, however, no pathologic basis for the seizures is evident, either during life or at autopsy. The latter type of seizure has been classed as "idiopathic." In certain circumstances, e.g., fever, convulsant drugs, hypoxia, or hypoglycemia in normal persons, the response may include seizure(s). If these events are isolated and do not recur, these patients are not classed as having epilepsy.

SYM: These may vary from the almost imperceptible alteration in consciousness, as in absence seizures (petit mal) to the dra-

Classification of Epileptic Seizures

Partial or Focal Seizures
 Simple partial seizures (with motor, sensory, autonomic, or psychic signs)
 Complex partial seizures (psychomotor or temporal lobe seizures)
 Secondary generalized partial seizures

Primary Generalized Seizures
 Tonic-clonic (grand mal)
 Tonic
 Absence (petit mal)
 Myoclonic
 Atonic
 Infantile spasms

Status epilepticus
 Tonic-clonic status
 Absence status
 Epilepsia partialis continua

Recurrence Patterns
 Sporadic
 Cyclic
 Reflex (photomyoclonic, somatosensory, musicogenic, reading epilepsy)

---

matic loss of consciousness, a cry, fall, tonic-clonic convulsions of all extremities, urinary and fecal incontinence, and amnesia for the event. Some attacks are preceded by an aura; others provide no warning. Other forms are limited to muscular contractions of a localized area or only one side of the body. SEE: Classification of Epileptic Seizures table; *postictal confusion.*

TREAT: A thorough investigation of the patient is made to identify any remedial cause of the seizures. These would include metabolic diseases, endocrine system disturbances, cerebral tumors, abscess of the brain, meningioma.

The patient needs to understand the illness and realize that he or she does not have to live as an invalid. Persons whose convulsions are controlled by medications can participate in sports; and most countries will permit a person to drive an automobile if he or she has experienced no seizures for six months to one year. The family, physician, and associates should encourage the patient to work and live a normal life. If, however, seizures are uncontrolled, automobile driving, swimming, operation of unguarded machinery, and ladder climbing should not be allowed. Epileptics should not drink alcoholic beverages.

Medical therapy for prevention and control of seizures is available and each type of epilepsy may require a specific therapeutic regimen. Antiepileptic drugs available include phenytoin, carbamazepine, phenobarbital, primidone, ethosuximide, methsuximide, clonazepam, valproate sodium, and trimethadione. In addition, if the seizures are related to a lesion in the brain, neurosurgical treatment is indicated.

Surgical therapy is estimated to be indicated in 40% of cases of partial epilepsy. About one-third of patients treated at a center dedicated to this type of surgery were seizure free; another one-third had marked reduction of seizure attacks.

PROG: Grand mal seizures can be controlled completely in about 50% of cases, and greatly reduced in frequency in another 35%. Petit mal can be controlled in 40% of cases, and frequency reduced in 35%. Psychomotor attacks can be controlled in 35% of cases, and frequency reduced in 50%. Virtually all epilepsy patients are normal between attacks.

The seizure disorders (epilepsy) were classified in 1970 and revised in 1981 according to the clinical form of the seizure and the EEG changes. SEE: table. The term *epilepsy* has a negative aspect to it, and for that reason, it is advisable to use the term *seizure* when talking with the patient.

Simple partial seizures: These are limited to a portion of the body, and there is no loss of consciousness. The area involved may spread until the entire side is involved. This type of seizure, with motor, sensory, or autonomic signs, was originally called jacksonian epilepsy. *Complex partial seizures:* Episodic changes in behavior accompanied by loss of consciousness. The seizure is preceded by an aura with complex hallucinations or sensory illusions. While unconscious, the patient may drive a car or continue to read a book, but will not respond to questions or commands. There is amnesia for the seizure, and recovery may take as long as one hour. *Secondary generalized partial seizures:* The progression of a seizure from simple or complex to a generalized seizure.

Primary generalized seizures: Tonic-clonic (grand mal). A common seizure pattern with sudden onset of unconsciousness, tonic contraction of muscles, loss of postural control, and a cry caused by contraction of respiratory muscles forcing exhalation. This is followed by generalized contraction of the muscles of the four extremities. After 2 to 5 minutes of unconsciousness and subsidence of clonic contractions, the patient gradually regains consciousness. Fecal and urinary incontinence, as well as biting of the tongue, may occur. The patient is amnestic for the event and may not be completely functional for several days.

Tonic seizures: Quite similar to the generalized seizures but the muscular activity is tonic rather than clonic, and it may last for a shorter time. *Absence seizures (petit mal):* Seizures in which there is sudden cessation of activity for a few seconds to several minutes. No fall or convulsive muscular contractions occur. The seizures begin in childhood and in many cases patients outgrow the condition. The patients are normal except for the seizures that may occur as frequently as 100 times a day. *Atypical absence seizures:* Seizures similar to absence seizures in patients who have other forms of generalized seizures. *Myoclonic seizures:* Sudden and brief contractions of a single group of muscles or of the entire body. The patients fall but do not lose consciousness. *Atonic seizures:* Brief loss of consciousness and a fall but without muscular contractions. *Infantile spasms:* Generalized seizures occurring in the first year of life. These are synchronous contractions of the muscles of the neck, trunk, and arms. About 90% of these children are mentally deficient. *Status epilepticus:* A series of grand mal seizures that may occur when the patient is awake and active or during sleep, but consciousness is not completely regained between attacks. This serious condition requires therapy without delay. *Epilepsia partialis continua:* A special type of focal motor status epilepticus in which there is clonic twitching of one group of muscles, and this is repeated at regular intervals of a few seconds and may persist for hours or indefinitely.

NURSING IMPLICATIONS: During seizure, protect patient from injury and prevent aspiration. Cradle head if on hard surface, but do not attempt to restrain movement. Loosen tight clothing. Turn patient to side to allow tongue to fall away from airway and permit drainage of saliva. If present at onset of seizure (before tonic phase begins), insert oral airway, padded tongue blade, or other soft object between teeth. DO NOT force objects between closed jaws as teeth or object may shatter and fragments be aspirated. Remain with the patient throughout the seizure, noting time of onset and duration, patient activity at time of onset, sequence of events, sensory phenomena, motor activity, postural tone, laterality of movements, incontinence, tongue biting, pupillary, skin or respiratory changes, and patient response following seizure. Offer comfort and reassurance following seizure activity. Evaluate patient's knowledge of epilepsy and its treatment, and correct misconceptions. Assist patient to express and deal with fear, anxiety, and grief, and refer for further counseling regarding altered self-concept and role disturbance as necessary. Teach patient and family importance of compliance with prescribed pharmacologic regimen, concerns for side effects, and need for follow-up care. Persons with epilepsy should wear a Medic Alert bracelet. SEE: *Nursing Diagnoses* in *Appendix.*

e., sleep. Spasmodic uncontrollable desire to sleep. SYN: *narcolepsy.*

e., television. Epileptic attacks that occur while the patient is viewing television. The pattern of the horizontal and vertical lines of a black and white TV picture may be the cause of the seizure rather than the stroboscopic or "flicker" effect.

e., traumatic. Epilepsy caused by trauma to the brain.

epileptic (ĕp″ĭ-lĕp′tĭk) [Gr. *epileptikos*]. 1. Concerning epilepsy. 2. Individual suffering from attacks of epilepsy.

epileptiform (ĕp″ĭ-lĕp′tĭ-form) [Gr. *epilepsia*, to seize, + L. *forma*, form]. Having the form of epilepsy.

epileptogenic, epileptogenous (ĕp″ĭ-lĕp-tō-jĕn′ĭk, -tŏj′ĕ-nŭs) [″ + *gennan*, to produce]. Giving rise to epileptoid convulsions.

epileptoid [″ + *eidos*, form, shape]. Resembling epilepsy. SYN: *epileptiform.*

epileptology [″ + *logos*, word, reason]. Study of epilepsy.

epiloia (ĕp″ĭ-lŏy′ă). Tuberous sclerosis, q.v.

epimandibular (ĕp″ĭ-măn-dĭb′ū-lăr) [Gr. *epi*, upon, above, + L. *mandibulum*, jaw]. Located upon the lower jaw.

epimer (ĕp′ĭ-mĕr). One of a pair of isomers that differ only in the position of the hydrogen atom and the hydroxyl group attached to one asymmetric carbon atom.

epimere (ĕp′ĭ-mēr) [Gr. *epi*, upon, + *meros*, apart]. In embryology, the dorsal muscle-forming portion of the somite.

epimerite (ĕp″ĭ-mĕr′īt) [″ + *meros*, part]. An organelle of certain protozoa by which they attach themselves to epithelial cells.

epimorphosis (ĕp″ĭ-mor′fō-sĭs) [″ + *morphoun*, to give shape, + *osis*, condition]. Regeneration of a part of an organism by growth at the cut surface.

epimysium (ĕp″ĭ-mĭz′ē-ŭm) [″ + *mys*, muscle]. Outermost sheath of connective tissue that surrounds a skeletal muscle. Consists of irregularly distributed collagenous, reticular, and elastic fibers, connective tissue cells, and fat cells. SYN: *perimysium externum.*

epinephrine (ĕp″ĭ-nĕf′rĭn) [″ + *nephros*, kidney]. USP. $C_9H_{13}NO_3$. A hormone secreted by the adrenal medulla in response to

stimulation of the sympathetic nervous system. This substance and norepinephrine are the two active hormones produced by the adrenal medulla. It causes some of the physiological expressions of fear and anxiety and has been found to be in excess in some anxiety disorders. Epinephrine, which has been synthesized, is also produced by tissues other than the adrenal. It is employed therapeutically as a vasoconstrictor, to treat cardiac dysrhythmias, and to relax bronchioles. Its effects are similar to those brought about by stimulation of the sympathetic division of the autonomic nervous system. Used to check local hemorrhage and to relieve asthmatic attacks. Also used to prolong action of local anesthetics by constricting blood vessels to prevent rapid absorption. Trade names are Adrenalin, Bronkaid Mist, Primatene Mist, and Sus-Phrine. SYN: *adrenaline.*

INCOMPAT: Light; heat; air; iron salts; and alkalies.

e. bitartrate. USP. $C_9H_{13}NO_3C_4H_6O_6$. A white or grayish-white crystalline powder. It is a sympathomimetic agent used for topical application to the eye. Trade names are Asmatane Mist, Lyophrin, Medihaler-Epi, and Suprarenin.

epinephrinemia (ĕp″ĭ-nĕf″rĭ-nē′mē-ă) [″ + ″ + *haima*, blood]. Epinephrine in the blood.

epinephritis (ĕp″ĭ-nĕf-rī′tĭs) [″ + *nephros*, kidney, + *itis*, inflammation]. Inflammation of an adrenal gland.

epinephroma (ĕp-ĭ-nĕ-frō′mă) [″ + ″ + *oma*, tumor]. A lipomatoid tumor of the kidney. SYN: *hypernephroma.*

epineural (ĕp″ĭ-nū′răl) [″ + *neuron*, nerve]. Located upon a neural arch.

epineurium (ĕp″ĭ-nū′rē-ŭm). The general connective tissue sheath of a nerve. SEE: *nerve.*

epiotic (ĕp″ē-ŏt′ĭk) [″ + *ous*, ear]. Located above the ear.

epiotic center. Ossification center of temporal bone forming upper and posterior part of the auditory capsule.

epipastic (ĕp″ĭ-păs′tĭk) [″ + *passein*, to sprinkle]. Resembling a dusting powder.

epipharynx (ĕp″ĭ-făr′ĭnks) [″ + *pharynx*, throat]. Nasal portion of pharynx. SYN: *rhinopharynx.*

epiphenomenon (ĕp″ĭ-fĕ-nŏm′ĕ-nŏn) [″ + *phainomenon*, phenomenon]. An exceptional symptom or occurrence in a disease that is not related to the usual course of the disease.

epiphora (ĕ-pĭf′ō-ră) [Gr., downpour]. Abnormal overflow of tears down the cheek due to excess secretion of tears or to obstruction of the lacrimal duct.

epiphyseal (ĕp″ĭ-fĭz′ē-ăl) [″ + *physis*, growth]. Pert. to or of the nature of an epiphysis. Also spelled *epiphysial*.

epiphyseolysis (ĕp″ĭ-fĭz″ē-ŏl′ĭ-sĭs) [″ + ″ + *lysis*, dissolution]. Separation of an epiphysis. Also spelled *epiphysiolysis*.

epiphyseopathy (ĕp″ĭ-fĭz-ē-ŏp′ă-thē) [″ + ″ + *pathos*, disease, suffering]. Any disease of an epiphysis or of the pineal gland. Also spelled *epiphysiopathy*.

epiphysial (ĕp″ĭ-fĭz′ē-ăl). SEE: *epiphyseal*.

epiphysis (ē-pĭf′ĭ-sĭs) [Gr., a growing upon] (pl. *epiphyses*). [NA] 1. In the developing infant and child, a secondary bone-forming (ossification) center separated from a parent bone in early life by cartilage. As growth proceeds and at a different time for each epiphysis, it becomes a part of the larger (or parent) bone. It is possible to judge the biological age of a child from the development of these ossification centers as shown radiographically. 2. A center for ossification at each extremity of long bones. SEE: *diaphysis*.

epiphysitis (ē-pĭf″ĭ-sī′tĭs) [″ + *itis*, inflammation]. Inflammation of an epiphysis, esp. that at the hip, knee, and shoulder in infants.

epipial (ĕp″ĭ-pī′ăl) [″ + L. *pia*, tender]. Situated above or upon the pia mater.

epiplocele (ē-pĭp′lō-sēl) [Gr. *epiploon*, omentum, + *kele*, tumor, swelling]. Hernia containing omentum.

epiploenterocele (ē-pĭp″lō-ĕn′tĕr-ō-sēl) [″ + *enteron*, intestine, + *kele*, tumor, swelling]. Hernia consisting of omentum and intestine.

epiploic (ĕp″ĭ-plō′ĭk) [Gr. *epiploon*, omentum]. Pert. to the omentum.

epiploic foramen. The opening between the greater and lesser peritoneal cavities.

epiploitis (ē-pĭp″lō-ī′tĭs) [″ + *itis*, inflammation]. Inflammation of the omentum.

epiplomerocele (ē-pĭp″lō-mē′rō-sēl) [″ + *meros*, thigh, + *kele*, tumor, swelling]. Femoral hernia containing omentum.

epiplomphalocele (ē-pĭp″lŏm-făl′ō-sēl) [″ + *omphalos*, navel, + *kele*, hernia]. Umbilical hernia with omentum protruding.

epiploon (ē-pĭp′lō-ŏn) [Gr., omentum]. The omentum, esp. the greater omentum. SYN: *omentum*.

epiplopexy (ē-pĭp′lō-pĕks″ē) [″ + *pexis*, fixation]. Suturing of omentum to the anterior abdominal wall.

epiplosarcomphalocele (ē-pĭp″lō-săr″kŏm-făl′ō-sēl) [″ + *sarx*, flesh, + *omphalos*, navel, + *kele*, tumor, swelling]. An umbilical hernia with protruding omentum. SYN: *epiplomphalocele*.

epiploscheocele (ē-pĭp″lŏs-kē′ō-sēl) [″ +

oscheon, scrotum, + *kele*, tumor, swelling]. Omental hernia into the scrotum.

epipygus (ĕp″ĭ-pī′gŭs) [Gr. *epi*, upon, + *pyge*, buttocks]. A developmental anomaly in which an accessory limb is attached to the buttocks. SEE: *pygomelus*.

episclera (ĕp″ĭ-sklē′ră) [″ + *skleros*, hard]. Outermost superficial layer of the sclera of the eye.

episcleral (ĕp″ĭ-sklē′răl). 1. Pert. to the episclera. 2. Overlying the sclera of the eye.

episcleritis (ĕp″ĭ-sklē-rī′tĭs) [″ + *skleros*, hard, + *itis*, inflammation]. Inflammation of the subconjunctival layers of the sclera.

episioelytrorrhaphy (ē-pĭs″ē-ō-ĕl″ĭ-tror′ă-fē) [Gr. *epision*, pubic region, + *elytron*, vagina, + *rhaphe*, seam, ridge]. Surgical narrowing of vagina and vulva in order to support a prolapsed uterus.

episioperineoplasty (ē-pĭs″ē-ō-pĕr″ĭ-nē′ō-plăs″tē) [″ + *perinaion*, perineum, + Gr. *plassein*, to form]. Plastic surgery of the perineum and vulva.

episioperineorrhaphy (ē-pĭs″ē-ō-pĕr″ĭ-nē-or′ă-fē) [″ + ″ + *rhaphe*, seam, ridge]. Suturing the vulva and perineum for the support of a prolapse of the uterus.

NURSING IMPLICATIONS: Give perineal care as needed, and teach the patient the correct perineal hygiene of wiping from front to back. Anesthetic sprays or creams may be ordered, and local heat applications through use of a heat lamp, warm soaks, or sitz baths may be ordered and should be administered for pain relief. Inspect the perineum at intervals to assess for symptoms of infection or hematoma formation.

episioplasty (ē-pĭs″ē-ō-plăs′tē) [″ + *plassein*, to form]. Plastic surgery on the vulva.

episiorrhaphy (ē-pĭs″ē-or′ă-fē) [″ + *rhaphe*, seam, ridge]. Suture of a lacerated perineum.

episiostenosis (ē-pĭs″ē-ō-stĕ-nō′sĭs) [″ + *stenosis*, narrowing]. Narrowing of the vulvar slit.

episiotomy (ē-pĭs″ē-ŏt′ō-mē) [″ + *tome*, incision]. Incision of perineum at end of second stage of labor to avoid spontaneous laceration of perineum and to facilitate delivery.

episome (ĕp′ĭ-sōm). Bacterial elements that can replicate either autonomously or in association with the chromosome. SEE: *plasmid*.

epispadias (ĕp″ĭ-spā′dē-ăs) [Gr. *epi*, upon, + *spadon*, a rent]. Congenital opening of urethra on dorsum of penis.

episplenitis (ĕp″ĭ-splē-nī′tĭs) [″ + *splen*, spleen, + *itis*, inflammation]. Inflammation of the splenic capsule.

epistasis (ē-pĭs′tă-sĭs) [Gr., stoppage]. 1. A

film that forms on urine that has been allowed to stand. 2. The suppression of any discharge. SEE: *hypostasis.*

epistaxis (ĕp″ĭ-stăk′sĭs) [Gr.]. Hemorrhage from nose; nosebleed. SEE: *Kiesselbach's area.*

ETIOL: May occur secondary to local infections (vestibulitis, rhinitis, sinusitis); systemic infections (scarlet fever, typhoid); drying of nasal mucous membrane; trauma (including picking the nose); arteriosclerosis; hypertension; and bleeding tendencies associated with anemias.

TREAT: Lie quietly propped up in bed, cold compresses, epinephrine locally, and if necessary, followed by cautery of bleeding vessel. Posterior packing of the nasal cavity may be needed, or use of balloon tamponade. This is done by inserting a Foley-like catheter into the nose and inflating the balloon after it is placed posteriorly. Traction is then placed on the catheter so that the vessels in the area are compressed. SEE: *nosebleed* for illus.

NURSING IMPLICATIONS: Evaluate patient's airway clearance, discomfort and anxiety, and history of previous nosebleeds. Sit patient upright and assist to lean forward to expectorate blood and to prevent aspiration, and limit nausea and vomiting due to swallowed blood. Attempt to stop bleeding by pinching the nostrils against the nasal septum for 5 to 10 minutes while patient mouth-breathes. Pressure across or under upper lip and cold applications over the nose or nape of neck may help to stop bleeding. If posterior packing or balloon tamponade is ordered, evaluate patient for hypoxemia and administer supplemental oxygen by face mask as necessary. Evaluate nares for evidence of pressure necrosis. Teach patient to avoid blowing or picking at nose. Patient may benefit from increased humidity if dryness is a factor. Teach patient simple measures to stop a nosebleed.

episternal (ĕp″ĭ-stĕr′năl) [Gr. *epi,* upon, + *sternon,* chest]. Situated above the sternum.

episternum. Upper portion of the sternum. SYN: *manubrium sterni.*

epistropheus (ĕp″ĭ-strŏ′fē-ŭs) (pl. *epistrophei*). Former term for axis of the second cervical vertebra.

epitaxy (ĕp″ĭ-tăk′sē) [Gr. *epi-,* upon, + *taxis,* arrangement]. The oriented growth of one crystal on the surface of a different crystal.

epitendineum (ĕp″ĭ-tĕn-dĭn′ē-ŭm) [″ + L. *tendere,* to stretch]. The fibrous sheath enveloping a tendon.

epitenon (ĕp-ĭ-tĕn′ŏn) [″ + *tenon,* tendon]. The connective tissue holding a tendon within its sheaths. SYN: *epitendineum.*

epithalamus (ĕp″ĭ-thăl′ă-mŭs) [″ + *thalamos,* chamber]. [NA] The uppermost portion of the diencephalon of the brain. It includes the pineal body, trigonum habenulae, habenula, and the habenular commissure.

epithelia [″ + *thele,* nipple] (pl. of *epithelium*). Epithelial layer of cells. SEE: *epithelium.*

epithelial (ĕp″ĭ-thē′lē-ăl). Pert. to or composed of epithelium.

epithelial attachment. The area of soft tissue attached to the tooth. SYN: *gingival cuff; junctional epithelium.*

epithelial cancer. Carcinoma composed of epithelial cells. SYN: *epithelioma.*

epithelial casts. Aggregations of renal epithelium with cells filled with granules or fat droplets. They often preserve their original form in the epithelial tubes.

epithelial cells. Cells that are irregular in shape, having a single nucleus. Frequently two or three are joined together.

epithelial diaphragm. The epithelial extension of Hertwig's root sheath that determines the number and size of tooth roots. It induces dentin formation locally as the root elongates. SEE: *Hertwig's root sheath.*

epithelialization (ĕp″ĭ-thē″lē-ăl-ĭ-zā′shŭn). The growth of skin over a wound.

epithelial tissue. Those cells that form the outer surface of the body and line the body cavities and the principal tubes and passageways leading to the exterior. These cells form the secreting portions of glands and their ducts and are important parts of certain sense organs. The cells of epithelial tissues lie closely approximated to each other and contain very little intercellular substance. They are arranged in one or a few layers and are devoid of blood vessels. SEE: illus.; *tissue.*

epitheliitis (ĕp″ĭ-thē″lē-ĭ′tĭs). Overgrowth and inflammation of the mucosal epithelium following injury such as could be caused by ionizing radiation.

epithelioblastoma (ĕp″ĭ-thē″lē-ō-blăs-tō′mă) [″ + *thele,* nipple, + *blastos,* germ, + *oma,* tumor]. Epithelial cell tumor.

epitheliogenic, epitheliogenetic (ĕp″ĭ-thē″lē-ō-jĕn′ĭk, -jĕ-nĕt′ĭk) [″ + ″ + *gennan,* to produce]. Caused by epithelial proliferation.

epithelioglandular (ĕp″ĭ-thē″lē-ō-glăn′dū-lăr). Concerning the epithelial cells of a gland.

epithelioid (ĕp″ĭ-thē′lē-oyd) [″ + ″ + *eidos,* form, shape]. Resembling epithelium.

epitheliolysin (ĕp″ĭ-thē-lē-ŏl′ĭ-sĭn) [″ + ″ + *lysis,* dissolution]. A specific lysin formed in blood serum of an animal in which epithelial cells of an animal of a different species were injected. Epitheliolysin de-

EPITHELIAL TISSUES

UNILAMINAR (SIMPLE)

SQUAMOUS

CUBOIDAL

WITHOUT SURFACE SPECIALIZATION

WITH MICROVILLI (BRUSH/STRIATED BORDER)

CILIATED

GLANDULAR

PSEUDO-STRATIFIED

COLUMNAR

GUSTATORY

OLFACTORY

STATO-ACOUSTIC

SENSORY

MYOEPITHELIOCYTE

MUTILAMINAR

NON-KERATINIZING

KERATINIZING

STRATIFIED SQUAMOUS

MAY INCLUDE PIGMENTED COMPONENTS

STRATIFIED CUBOIDAL/COLUMNAR

(RELAXED)

(STRETCHED)

UROTHELIUM (TRANSITIONAL)

COMPLEX DERIVED STRUCTURES

EXOCRINE

ENDOCRINE

MULTICELLULAR GLANDS

TOOTH GERM

NERVOUS TISSUE (OFTEN CLASSIFIED AS A SEPARATE TISSUE, BUT RETAINS MANY CHARACTERISTICS OF ITS EPITHELIAL ORIGINS)

SEMINIFEROUS EPITHELIUM

stroys the cells of an animal of the same species as that from which the epithelial cells were derived.

epitheliolysis (ĕp″ĭ-thē-lē-ŏl′ĭ-sĭs). Death of epithelial tissue. The destruction or dissolving of epithelial cells by an epitheliolysin.

epithelioma (ĕp″ĭ-thē-lē-ō′mă) [″ + *thele*, nipple, + *oma*, tumor]. A malignant tumor consisting principally of epithelial cells; a carcinoma. A tumor originating in the epidermis of the skin or in a mucous membrane.

   e. adamantinum. Tumor of the jaw arising from the enamel organ. Of low-grade malignancy; may be solid or partly cystic. SYN: *adamantinoma.*

   e. adenoides cysticum. Basal cell carcinoma of low malignancy occurring on the surface of the body, esp. the face. Characterized by formation of cysts. SYN: *acanthoma.*

   e., basal cell. Epithelioma derived from cells in the basal layer of the epidermis (stratum germinativum).

   e., deep-seated. Epithelioma that involves lymphatic glands with irregular rounded ulcers occurring after several months.

epitheliomatous (ĕp″ĭ-thē-lē-ō′mă-tŭs). Pert. to epithelioma.

epitheliosis (ĕp″ĭ-thē″lē-ō′sĭs) [″ + *thele*, nipple, + *osis*, condition]. Trachomatous proliferation of the conjunctival epithelium.

epithelium (ĕp″ĭ-thē′lē-ŭm) [″ + *thele*, nipple] (pl. *epithelia*). [NA] The layer of cells forming the epidermis of the skin and the surface layer of mucous and serous membranes. The cells rest on a basement membrane and lie closely approximated to each other with little intercellular material between them. The epithelium may be simple, consisting of a single layer, or stratified, consisting of several layers. Cells making up the epithelium may be flat (squamous), cube-shaped (cuboidal), or cylindrical (columnar). Modified forms of epithelium include ciliated, pseudostratified, glandular, and neuroepithelium. The epithelium may include goblet cells, which secrete mucus. Stratified squamous epithelium may be keratinized for a protective function or abnormally in pathologic response. Squamous epithelium is classified as endothelium, which lines the blood vessels and the heart, and mesothelium, which lines the serous cavities. Epithelium serves the general functions of protection, absorption, and secretion, and specialized functions such as movement of substances through ducts, production of germ cells, and reception of stimuli. Its ability to regenerate is excellent; and it may replace itself as frequently as every 24 hours. SEE: *skin.*

   e., ciliated. Epithelial cells with fine hairlike protuberances, called cilia, on their free border. These cells are able to sweep particles in a certain direction.

   e., columnar. Epithelium composed of cells shaped like pillars.

   e., cuboidal. Epithelium consisting of cube-shaped or prismatic cells with height approx. equal to width.

   e., germinal. Epithelium that covers the surface of the genital ridge of the urogenital folds of an embryo. It gives rise to seminiferous tubules of the testes and the surface layer of the ovary. It was once thought to give rise to the germ cells (spermatozoa and ova).

   e., glandular. Epithelium consisting of cells that secrete.

   e., laminated. E., stratified.

   e., mesenchymal. Epithelium of the squamous type that lines the subarachnoid and subdural cavities, the chambers of the eye, and the perilymphatic spaces of the ear.

   e., pavement. Epithelium of flat, platelike cells in a single layer.

   e., pigmented. Epithelium containing pigment granules.

   e., pseudostratified. Epithelium in which the bases of cells rest on the basement membrane but the distal ends of some do not reach the surface. Nuclei of the cells lie at different levels, giving the appearance of stratification.

   e., reduced enamel. Combined epithelial layers of the enamel organ, which form a protective layer over the enamel crown as it erupts, and then become the primary attachment epithelium surrounding the tooth.

   e., squamous. E., pavement.

   e., stratified. Epithelium with the cells in layers.

   e., sulcular. The nonkeratinized epithelium that lines the gingival sulcus.

   e., transitional. A form of stratified epithelium in which the cells have the ability to adjust themselves to mechanical changes such as stretching and contracting. Found only in the urinary system (pelvis and kidney, ureter, bladder, and a part of the urethra).

epitope (ĕp′ĭ-tōp). Any component of an antigen molecule that functions as an antigenic determinant by permitting the attachment of certain antibodies. SEE: *paratope.* SYN: *antigenic determinant.*

epitrichial layer. Periderm, q.v.

epitrichium (ĕp″ĭ-trĭk′ē-ŭm) [Gr. *epi*, upon, + *trichion*, hair]. Superficial layers of the epidermis of the fetus. SYN: *periderm.*

epitrochlea (ĕp″ĭ-trŏk′lē-ă) [″ + *trochalia*,

pulley]. The inner condyle of the humerus.

epitrochlear (ĕp″ĭ-trŏk′lē-ăr). Pert. to the inner condyle of the humerus.

epiturbinate (ĕp″ĭ-tĕr′bĭn-āt) [″ + L. *turbo*, top]. The tissue upon or covering the turbinate bone.

epitympanum (ĕp″ĭ-tĭm′pă-nŭm) [″ + *tympanon*, drum]. Attic of the middle ear; area above the drum membrane.

epizoic (ĕp″ĭ-zō′ĭk) [″ + *zoon*, animal]. Living as a parasite on the exterior of an animal.

epizoicide (ĕp″ĭ-zō′ĭ-sīd) [″ + ″ + L. *caedere*, to kill]. That which destroys epizoa.

epizoon (ĕp″ĭ-zō′ŏn) [″ + *zoon*, animal] (pl. *epizoa*). An animal organism living as a parasite on the exterior of the host animal.

epizootic. Any disease of animals that attacks many animals in the same area.

epoetin alfa. Synthetic human erythropoietin. Trade name is Epogen. SEE: *erythropoietin.*

eponychium (ĕp″ō-nĭk′ē-ŭm) [″ + *onyx*, nail]. 1. The horny embryonic structure from which the nail develops. 2. Perionychium [NA].

eponym (ĕp′ō-nĭm) [Gr. *eponymos*, named after]. A name for anything (diseases, organs, functions, places) adapted from the name of a particular person.

epoophorectomy (ĕp″ō-ō-fō-rĕk′tō-mē) [Gr. *epi*, upon, + *oophoron*, ovary, + *ektome*, excision]. Removal of the parovarium.

epoophoron (ĕp″ō-ŏf′ō-rŏn). A rudimentary structure located in the mesosalpinx. Consisting of a longitudinal duct (duct of Gartner) and ten to fifteen transverse ducts, it is the remains of the upper portion of the mesonephros and is the homologue of the head of the epididymis in the male. SYN: *Rosenmüller's body; parovarium.*

epoxide. Any chemical compound that contains two carbon atoms joined to a single oxygen atom.

epoxy (ē-pŏk′sē). General term for polymers that contain molecules wherein oxygen is attached to two different carbon atoms. They are widely used as adhesives.

epsilon-aminocaproic acid. A synthetic substance used to correct an overdose of certain fibrinolytic agents. Also useful in treating excessive bleeding due to increased fibrinolytic activity in the blood.

epsom salt (ĕp′sŭm). Magnesium sulfate.

EPSP. *excitatory postsynaptic potential.*

Epstein-Barr virus [M. A. Epstein, Brit. physician, b. 1921; Y. M. Barr, contemporary Canadian physician]. ABBR: EBV. A virus, discovered in 1964, believed to be the causative agent in infectious mononucleosis. In South African children, it is associated with Burkitt's lymphoma; in Asian populations, with nasopharyngeal carcinoma. Why the virus has these different and varied associations in different geographical areas is unknown.

Epstein's pearls [Alois Epstein, Czech. pediatrician, 1849–1918]. In newborn infants, whitish-yellow accumulation of epithelial cells, or retention cysts on the hard palate. They are harmless and disappear within a few weeks.

epulis (ĕp-ū′lĭs) [Gr. *epoulis*, a gumboil] (pl. *epulides*). A fibrous sarcomatous tumor having its origin in the periosteum of the lower jaw.

epuloid (ĕp′ū-loyd) [″ + *eidos*, form, shape]. 1. Like an epulis. 2. Tumor of the jaw or gum resembling an epulis.

epulosis (ĕp″ū-lō′sĭs) [Gr. *epoulosis*]. Cicatrization; a cicatrix.

epulotic (ĕp″ū-lŏt′ĭk) [Gr. *epoulotikos*]. Promoting cicatrization.

Equal Rights Amendment. ABBR: ERA. In the U.S., a proposed amendment to the Constitution to prohibit discrimination on the basis of sex.

Equanil. Trade name for meprobamate.

equation [L. *aequare*, to make equal]. 1. State of being equal. 2. In chemistry, a symbolic representation of a chemical reaction.

    e., personal. SEE: *personal equation.*

equator [L. *aequator*]. Line encircling a round body and equidistant from both poles.

    e. oculi. An imaginary line encircling the bulb of the eye midway between anterior and posterior poles.

    e. of cell. The boundary of a plane through which the division of a cell occurs.

    e. of crystalline lens; e. lentis. Line that marks the junction of the anterior and posterior surfaces. To it are attached the fibers of the suspensory ligament.

equatorial. Pert. to an equator.

equatorial plate. Mass of chromosomes at equator of the nuclear spindle during karyokinesis.

equi- [L. *aequus*, equal]. Prefix meaning equal.

equianalgesic. A dose of one form of analgesic drug equivalent in pain-relieving potential to another analgesic. Knowing this equivalence will permit substitution of analgesics in order to attempt to prevent undesired side effects of a medicine for control of pain.

equilibrating (ē-kwĭl′ĭ-brāt-ĭng) [L. *aequilibris*, in perfect balance]. Maintaining equilibrium.

equilibration. The process of modifying the masticatory forces or occlusal surfaces of teeth to produce simultaneous occlusal contacts between upper and lower teeth, and to equalize the stress of occlusal forces of the supporting tissues of the teeth.

equilibrium [L. *aequus*, equal, + *libra*, balance]. State of balance. Condition in which contending forces are equal.

e., nitrogenous. Condition in which the nitrogen excreted equals the nitrogen intake.

e., physiological. Having egesta equal to the ingesta.

equilin (ĕk'wĭl-ĭn) [L. *equus*, horse]. Crystalline estrogenic hormone derived from pregnant mares' urine.

equimolar. In comparing chemical substances quantitatively, having the same molar concentration.

equine (ē'kwīn) [L. *equus*, horse]. Concerning or originating from a horse.

equinovarus (ē-kwī″nō-vā'rŭs) [L. *equinus*, equine, + *varus*, bent inward]. A form of clubfoot with a combination pes equinus and pes varus, i.e., walking without touching the heel to the ground and with the sole turned inward.

equipotential (ē″kwĭ-pō-tēn'shăl) [L. *aequus*, equal, + *potentia*, ability]. Having the same electrical charge or physical strength.

equivalence (ē-kwĭv'ă-lĕns) [″ + *valere*, to be worth]. Quality of being equivalent.

equivalent (ē-kwĭv'a-lĕnt). 1. Equal in power, force, or value. 2. Amount of weight of any element needed to replace a fixed weight of another body.

equivalent weight. The weight of a chemical element that is equivalent to and will replace a hydrogen atom (1.008 grams) in a chemical reaction.

E.R. *external resistance; Emergency Room.*

Er. Chem. symb. for the element erbium.

eradication. Complete elimination of a disease, esp. one that is epidemic or endemic.

Erben's reflex (ĕrb'ĕnz) [Siegmund Erben, Austrian physician, b. 1863]. Retardation of pulse when head and trunk are forcibly bent forward.

erbium (ĕr'bē-ŭm). SYMB: Er. At. wt. 167.26; at. no. 68; sp. gr. 9.051. A rare metallic element.

Erb's paralysis [Wilhelm Heinrich Erb, Ger. neurologist, 1840–1921]. Paralysis of group of muscles of shoulder and upper arm involving cervical roots of 5th and 6th spinal nerves. The arm hangs limp, the hand rotates inward, and normal movements are lost. SYN: *Erb's palsy.*

Erb's point. The point on the side of the neck 2 to 3 cm above the clavicle and in front of the transverse process of the sixth cervical vertebra. Electrical stimulation over this area causes various arm muscles to contract.

ERCP. *endoscopic retrograde cholangiopancreatography.*

erectile (ĕ-rĕk'tīl) [L. *erigere*, to erect]. Able to become erect.

erectile tissue. Vascular tissue that, when filled with blood, becomes erect or rigid, as the clitoris, penis, or nipples.

erection. The state of swelling, hardness, and stiffness observed in the penis and to a lesser extent in the clitoris of the female, generally due to sexual excitement. Caused by engorgement with blood of the corpora cavernosa and the corpus spongiosum of the penis and the corpus cavernosa clitoridis of the female.

Erection is necessary in the male for the natural intromission of the penis into the vagina of the female but not for the emission of semen. The blood withdraws from the penis after ejaculation and the erection is reduced. Erection of the penis may occur as the result of sexual excitement, during sleep, or due to physical stimulation of the penis. Abnormal persistent erection of the penis due not to sexual excitement but to certain disease states is called priapism, q.v. SEE: *nocturnal emission; penile prosthesis.*

erector [L. *erigere*, to erect]. A muscle that raises a part.

erector spinae reflex. Irritation of the skin over the erector spinae muscles causing contraction of muscles of the back. SYN: *dorsal reflex; lumbar reflex.*

eremophobia (ĕr″ĕm-ō-fō'bē-ă) [Gr. *eremos*, solitary, + *phobos*, fear]. Dread of being alone.

erethism (ĕr'ĕ-thĭzm) [Gr. *erethismos*, irritation]. Excessive excitement or response to irritating stimuli. Opposite of apathism.

e. mercurialis. Mental illness occurring as a result of chronic mercury poisoning.

erethismic (ĕr″ĕ-thĭz'mĭk). Pert. to or causing erethism. SYN: *erethitic.*

erethisophrenia (ĕr″ĕ-thĭ-zō-frē'nē-ă) [″ + *phren*, mind]. Unusual mental excitability.

erethistic (ĕr″ĕ-thĭs'tĭk) [Gr. *erethismos*, irritation]. Erethismic, exciting.

erethitic (ĕr″ĕ-thĭt'ĭk). Causing erethism; irritable, excited.

ereuthrophobia (ĕr″ū-thrō-fō'bē-ă) [Gr. *erythros*, red, + *phobos*, fear]. Pathological fear of blushing. SYN: *erythrophobia.*

ERG. *electroretinogram.*

erg [Gr. *ergon*, work]. In physics, the amount of work done when a force of 1 dyne acts through a distance of 1 cm. One erg is roughly ⅟₉₈₀ gram-centimeter. That is, to raise a load of 1 gm against gravity the distance of 1 cm requires that a force of 980 dynes operate through a distance of 1 cm and hence that 980 ergs of work be done.

ergasiomania (ĕr-gā″sē-ō-mā'nē-ă) [Gr. *ergasia*, work, + *mania*, madness]. An abnormal desire to be busy at work.

ergasiophobia (ĕr-gā″sē-ō-fō′bē-ă) [″ + *phobos*, fear]. Abnormal dislike for work of any kind or for assuming responsibility.

ergasthenia (ĕr″găs-thē′nē-ă) [Gr. *ergon*, work, + *astheneia*, weakness]. A symptom, condition, or weakness due to overwork.

ergastic (ĕr-găs′tĭk) [Gr. *ergastikos*]. Possessing potential energy.

ergastoplasm. SEE: *endoplasmic reticulum.*

ergocalciferol (ĕr-gō-kăl-sĭf′ĕr-ōl). USP. Vitamin D_2, an activated product of ergosterol. Primarily used in prophylaxis and treatment of vitamin D deficiency. Trade names are Deltalin and Drisdol.

ergogenic (ĕr″gō-jĕn′ĭk) [Gr. *ergon*, work, + *gennan*, to produce]. To increase work, esp. to increase potential for work output.

ergograph (ĕr′gō-grăf) [″ + *graphein*, to write]. An apparatus for recording the contractions of muscles and measuring the amount of work done.

Ergomar. Trade name for ergotamine tartrate.

ergometer (ĕr-gŏm′ĕ-tĕr) [″ + *metron*, measure]. An apparatus for measuring the amount of work done by a human or animal subject.

  e., bicycle. Stationary bicycle used in determining the amount of work performed by the rider.

ergonomic aids. In athletic medicine, the questionable and in many cases harmful use of various substances in an attempt to enhance performance. Some of these materials — such as blood transfusions, anabolic steroids, amphetamines, amino acids, and human growth hormone — are standard medicines approved for uses other than those intended by the athlete. Others are not only not indicated for any illness but may be harmful, esp. when the amount of the active ingredient in the product is unknown. Included in this latter group are cyproheptadine, taken to increase appetite, strength and, allegedly, testosterone production; ginseng, q.v.; pangamic acid, q.v.; octacosanol, a 28 carbon straight-chain alcohol obtained from wheat germ oil, the biological effects of which are unknown; guarana, prepared from the seeds of the *Paulliania cupana* tree, used for its alleged ability to increase energy; gamma-oryzanol, an isomer of oryzanol extracted from rice bran oil, allegedly of assistance in decreasing recovery time after exercise; proteolytic enzymes, e.g., chymotrypsin, trypsin-chymotrypsin, and papain, the safety and efficacy of which have not been established, esp. when used with oral anticoagulants or by pregnant or lactating women; and bee

pollen, which is taken to improve athletic performance, although there is no evidence that it is effective. SEE: *anabolic agents; blood doping.*

ergonomics (ĕr″gō-nŏm′ĭks) [″ + *nomikos*, law]. The science concerned with how to fit a job to man's anatomical, physiological, and psychological characteristics in a way that will enhance human efficiency and well-being.

ergonovine maleate (ĕr″gō-nō′vĭn). USP. An ergot derivative used in treating migraine, and in obstetrics to stimulate contractions of the uterus. Trade name is Ergotrate Maleate.

ergophobia (ĕr″gō-fō′bē-ă) [″ + *phobos*, fear]. Morbid dread of working.

Ergostat. Trade name for ergotamine tartrate.

ergosterol (ĕr-gŏs′tĕr-ōl). A sterol found in plant and animal tissues. It is converted to vitamin D_2 by irradiation.

ergot (ĕr′gŏt). A drug obtained from *Claviceps purpurea*, a fungus that grows parasitically on rye. Several valuable alkaloids, as ergotamine, q.v., are obtained from ergot.

ergotamine (ĕr-gŏt′ă-mēn). $C_{33}H_{35}O_5N_5$. A crystalline alkaloid derived from ergot.

  e. tartrate. USP. A white crystalline substance that stimulates smooth muscle of blood vessels and the uterus, inducing vasoconstriction and uterine contractions. Used in the treatment of migraine. Trade names are Ergomar, Ergostat, and Gynergen.

ergotherapy (ĕr″gō-thĕr′ă-pē) [″ + *therapeia*, treatment]. Work used as a treatment of disease.

ergotism (ĕr′gō-tĭzm). Poisoning resulting from excessive use of ergot or from eating food made from rye or wheat infected with the fungus *Claviceps purpurea.* May be acute or chronic. SEE: *ergot poisoning.*

ergot poisoning. May result from eating bread made with grain contaminated with the *Claviceps purpurea* fungus; or by taking overdoses of the drug.

  SYM: Appear several hours after ingestion. Vomiting, burning, and cramping in abdomen; great thirst; profound weakness; diarrhea; slow weak pulse; anesthesia, tingling, and twitching in extremities; dilated pupils; occasionally convulsions; anuria. If patient survives, generalized gangrene, particularly of the extremities, may develop.

  F.A.: Slurry of activated charcoal by mouth followed by emesis or gastric lavage and instillation of a saline cathartic, external heat. Amyl nitrite by inhalation to counteract arterial spasms; anticonvulsants if needed. SEE: *Poisons and Poisoning* in *Appendix.*

ergotrate (ĕr′gō-trāt). An active principle

isolated from ergot.

Ergotrate Maleate. Trade name for ergonovine maleate.

Eristalis (ĕr-ĭs′tă-lĭs). A genus of flies belonging to the family Syrphidae. The larva, called rat-tailed maggot *(E. tenax),* may cause intestinal myiasis in humans.

erode (ē-rōd′) [L. *erodere*]. 1. To wear away. 2. To eat away by ulceration.

erogenous (ĕr-ŏj′ĕ-nŭs) [Gr. *eros,* love, + *gennan,* to produce]. Causing sexual excitement. SYN: *erotogenic.*

erogenous zone. Any part of the body, touching or stroking of which can cause sexual excitement. SEE: *zone, erogenous.*

eros. 1. In psychoanalysis, the collective instincts for self-preservation. 2. Eros, the Greek god of love.

E rosette. A laboratory test performed to identify human T lymphocytes. When T lymphocytes combine with sheep red blood cells (SRBC) in a culture, a cluster of cells forms called a rosette. This test is often replaced by the use of monoclonal antibodies, q.v., that identify the CD4 receptor specific for T cells.

erosion (ē-rō′shŭn) [L. *erodere,* to gnaw away]. An eating away of tissue. External or internal destruction of a surface layer by physical or inflammatory processes.

e., dental. The wearing away of the surface layer (enamel) of a tooth. SEE: *abrasion, attrition; bruxism.*

e. of cervix uteri. The alteration of the epithelium on a portion of the cervix as a result of irritation by infection.

SYM: In the early stages, the epithelium shows necrosis; in healing, there is a downgrowth of epithelium from the endocervical canal. If this is accomplished by a single layer of tissue having a grossly granular appearance, it is called a simple granular erosion. If the growth is excessive and shows papillary tufts, it is called a papillary erosion. Histologically, the papillary erosion shows many glands of the branching racemose type whose epithelium is the mucus-bearing cell with the nucleus at the base. In the healing process, squamous epithelium grows over the eroded area with the following results: the squamous cells take the place of the tissue beneath it completely, giving a complete healing, or the glands fill with squamous plugs and remain in that state, or the mouths of the glands are occluded by the squamous cells and cysts are formed (nabothian cysts). In the congenital type of erosion, the portio is covered by high columnar epithelium. SEE: *carcinoma-insitu; Papanicolaou test.*

TREAT: Prophylaxis, proper care of the cervix following delivery. Cauterization of the early erosion with electrocautery is usually curative. Cryotherapy may be used.

erosive (ē-rō′sĭv). 1. Able to produce erosion. 2. An agent that erodes tissues or structures.

erotic (ē-rŏt′ĭk) [Gr. *erotikos*]. 1. Stimulating sexual desire. 2. Concerning sexual love. 3. A person who stimulates sexual desire.

eroticism (ĕ-rŏt′ĭ-sĭzm) [″ + *-ismos,* condition]. Sexual desire.

e., allo-. Eroticism directed to an external object rather than to self.

e., anal. Sensations of pleasure experienced through defecation during a stage in the development of children. In psychiatry, fixation of the libido at the anal-erotic developmental stage.

e., auto-. 1. Self-gratification of the sexual instinct. Usually by manual stimulation of erogenous areas, esp. the penis or clitoris. SEE: *asphyxia, sexual; masturbation; urolagnia.* 2. Self-admiration combined with sexual emotion, such as that obtained from viewing one's naked body or one's genitals.

e., oral. 1. In psychiatry, fixation of the libido to the oral phase of development. 2. Sexual pleasure derived from use of the mouth.

erotism (ĕr′ō-tĭzm). Eroticism.

erotogenic (ĕ-rō″tō-jĕn′ĭk) [Gr. *eros,* love, + *gennan,* to produce]. Producing sexual excitement. SEE: *zone, erogenous.*

erotology (ĕr″ŏ-tŏl′ō-jē) [″ + *logos,* word, reason]. The study of love and its manifestations.

erotomania (ĕ-rō″tō-, ĕ-rŏt″ō-mā′nē-ă) [″ + *mania,* madness]. Pathological exaggeration of sexual behavior.

erotopathia (ĕ-rō″tō-, ĕ-rŏt″ō-păth′ē-ă) [″ + *pathos,* disease, suffering]. Any abnormal sex impulse.

erotophobia (ĕ-rō″tō-, ĕ-rŏt″ō-fō′bē-ă) [″ + *phobos,* fear]. Aversion to sexual love or its manifestations.

erratic [L. *errare,* to wander]. Wandering, having an unpredictable or fluctuating course or pattern. SYN: *eccentric.*

errhine (ĕr′īn) [Gr. *en,* in, + *rhis,* nose]. 1. Causing increased nasal discharge. 2. An agent that increases nasal secretion or discharge.

error. A mistake or miscalculation.

e., type I. In statistics, experimental medicine and epidemiology, erroneously rejecting a hypothesis.

e., type II. In statistics, experimental medicine and epidemiology, erroneously accepting a hypothesis.

erubescence [L. *erubescere,* to grow red]. Reddening of the skin; a blush.

eructation (ē-rŭk-tā′shŭn) [L. *eructare*]. Producing gas from the stomach, usually with a characteristic sound; belching.

eruption (ē-rŭp'shŭn) [L. *eruptio,* a breaking out]. 1. Breaking out and becoming visible, esp. applied to the appearance of a skin lesion or rash accompanying a disease such as measles or scarlet fever. 2. The appearance of a lesion such as redness or spotting on the skin or mucous membrane. 3. The breaking through of a tooth through the gum; the cutting of a tooth.

    e., active. Movement of the tooth toward the occlusal plane.

    e., creeping. A skin lesion characterized by a tortuous elevated red line that progresses at one end while fading out at the other. It is caused by the migration into the skin of the larvae of certain nematodes, esp. *Ancylostoma braziliense* and *A. canis,* which are present in ground exposed to dog or cat feces. SYN: *larva migrans.*

    e., delayed. The most common variation in the tooth eruption pattern; may be due to crowding or a variety of genetic, endocrine, or physiological factors.

    e., drug. Skin reaction resulting from the ingestion of certain drugs such as iodides. SYN: *dermatitis medicamentosa.*

    e., passive. Increased size of the clinical crown of a tooth by apical migration of the attachment epithelium and periodontium.

    e., serum. Eruption that occurs following the injection of a serum. May be accompanied by chills and fever.

eruptive. Pert. to breaking out.

eruptive stage. The stage of tooth eruption when the tooth is moving towards the occlusal plane prior to function. Root formation is coincident with eruption but is only one of several factors related to the mechanism of tooth eruption.

erysipelas (ĕr″ĭ-sĭp'ĕ-lăs) [Gr. *erythros,* red, + *pella,* skin]. Acute febrile disease with localized inflammation and redness of skin and subcutaneous tissue accompanied by systemic signs and symptoms.

    SYM: Fever; chills; nausea; vomiting; painful and warm skin; face and head lesions that are hot and red usually seen within 24 to 48 hours. Bullae may develop.

    ETIOL: Almost always group A streptococci.

    TREAT: Penicillin or erythromycin. Cool magnesium sulfate solution compresses for skin. May be fatal if untreated.

    PROG: Excellent with treatment. If untreated, nephritis, abscesses, and septicemia may develop.

    NURSING IMPLICATIONS: The patient is not usually hospitalized, thus provide support and encourage compliance with medical regimen. Emphasize the importance of taking prescribed antibiotics. During acute phase, encourage rest and elevation of the body part affected. Application of mild heat to affected part may be helpful. If symptoms do not subside, urge medical follow-up in order to detect early signs of complications and to institute prescribed therapy. Encourage hygienic measures to prevent the spread of the infection to other members of the household.

erysipelatous (ĕr″ĭ-sĭ-pĕl'ă-tŭs). Of the nature of or pert. to erysipelas.

erysipeloid (ĕr-ĭ-sĭp'ĕ-loyd) [″ + ″ + *eidos,* form, shape]. An infective dermatitis resembling erysipelas usually limited to the hands and characterized by hyperemia, edema, and occasionally systemic complications.

    ETIOL: Caused by *Erysipelothrix rhusiopathiae,* usually acquired by handling shellfish, poultry, or meat.

    TREAT: Penicillin or erythromycin.

Erysipelothrix rhusiopathiae (ĕr″ĭ-sĭ-pĕl'ŏ-thrĭks) [″ + ″ + *thrix,* hair]. A species of gram-positive branching filamentous, rod-shaped, nonmotile bacteria. They cause erysipeloid, q.v.

erysipelotoxin (ĕr″ĭ-sĭp″ĕ-lō-tŏk'sĭn). The toxin produced by *Streptococcus pyogenes,* the causative agent of erysipelas.

erysiphake (ĕr-ĭs'ĭ-fāk). A small spoon-shaped device used in cataract surgery to remove the lens by suction.

erythema (ĕr″ĭ-thē'mă) [Gr., redness]. A form of macula showing diffused redness over the skin.

    ETIOL: Caused by capillary congestion, usually due to dilatation of the superficial capillaries as a result of some nervous mechanism within the body, inflammation, or some external influence such as heat, exposure to ionizing radiation, sunlight, or cold.

    e. ab igne. Localized erythema due to exposure to heat.

    e. annulare. Erythema that is ring-shaped.

    e. chronicum migrans. ABBR: ECM. An annular erythema following an insect bite, esp. that of the tick infected with the spirochete which causes Lyme disease, q.v. The erythema develops following the bite, and the annular inflamed border moves away from the site and becomes a large, bluish-red area with a firm border. In time, multiple rings without a central bite may develop and produce intersecting patterns. This form of erythema is a marker for Lyme disease.

    e. congestivum. Erythema with congestive state of skin.

    e., diffuse. Erythema that is widely spread over body.

    e. induratum. Chronic vasculitis of the skin occurring in young adult females.

Characterized by hard cutaneous nodules that break down to form necrotic ulcers and leave atrophic scars. SYN: *Bazin's disease*.

e. infectiosum. A mild, moderately contagious disease, seen mostly in children. Characteristic of the clinical presentation is a marked erythema of the face as if the child has been slapped. The reddening of the skin fades and recurs. It is caused by the parvovirus B-19 agent. Usually, there are mild constitutional symptoms, but B-19 infection may be associated with transient aplastic crisis in patients with hereditary hemolytic anemias, and other hematologic changes in immunocompromised patients with bone marrow suppression and non-immune hydrops fetalis. The rash will last from 2 to 34 days. No treatment or isolation is indicated for this nonfatal disease, but it is important to distinguish it from rubella, a disease that can mimic it. SYN: *Fifth disease*. SEE: *parvovirus B-19*.

e. intertrigo. Chafing of opposing surfaces with erythema and often with maceration and abrasion. SYN: *chafing*.

e. marginatum. A form of erythema multiforme in which the center of the area fades, leaving elevated edges.

e. multiforme. A macular eruption with dark red papules or tubercles. Usually on extremities appearing in successive eruptions of short duration. No itching, burning, or rheumatic pains. May appear in separate rings, concentric rings, disk-shaped patches, distributed elevations, and figured arrangements.

e. neonatorum. Erythema toxicum neonatorum, q.v.

e. nodosum. Red and painful nodules on legs, associated with rheumatism. Also caused by certain drugs and food poisoning.

e., punctate. Erythema occurring in minute points, as scarlet fever rash.

e. toxicum neonatorum. A benign, self-limited occurrence of firm, yellow-white papules or pustules from 1 to 2 mm in size present in about 50% of full-term infants. The cause is unknown, and the lesions disappear without need for treatment.

e. venenatum. Form of erythema caused by contact with a toxic substance.

erythematic, erythematous (ĕr″ĭ-thĕ-măt′ĭk, ĕr″ĭ-thĕm′ă-tŭs) [Gr. *erythema*, redness]. Pert. to or marked by erythema.

erythemogenic (ĕr″ĭ-thē″mō-jĕn′ĭk) [″ + *gennan*, to produce]. Pert. to erythema.

erythralgia (ĕr″ĭ-thrăl′jē-ă) [″ + *algos*, pain]. A condition of painful redness of the skin. SYN: *erythromelalgia*.

erythrasma (ĕr″ĭ-thrăz′mă). Red-brown eruption in patches in the axillae and groin

caused by *Corynebacterium minitissimum*.

erythredema (ĕ-rĭth″rĕ-dē′mă) [″ + *oidema*, swelling]. An infantile disease characterized by lesions of the skin on the hands and feet, swelling of the extremities, digestive disturbances, and itching. It is frequently followed by arthritis involving multiple joints and with muscle weakness. Its cause is unknown, but mercury may be an etiological agent. SYN: *acrodynia*.

erythremia (ĕr″ĭ-thrē′mē-ă) [″ + *haima*, blood]. Polycythemia vera, q.v.

erythrism (ĕ-rĭth′rĭzm) [″ + *-ismos*, condition of]. Redness of the hair and beard with ruddy complexion.

erythristic (ĕr″ĭ-thrĭs′tĭk). Having a ruddy complexion and red hair.

erythrityl tetranitrate (ĕ-rĭth′rĭ-tĭl). USP. Drug used to dilate the coronary arteries. Used in treating angina pectoris. Trade name is Cardilate.

erythro- [Gr. *erythros*]. Prefix meaning red.

erythroblast (ĕ-rĭth′rō-blăst) [″ + *blastos*, germ]. Any form of nucleated red corpuscles. The earliest stages in the development are pronormoblast, basophilic normoblast, polychromatic normoblast, and orthochromatic normoblast. Nucleated red cells are not normally seen in the circulating blood. Erythroblasts contain hemoglobin. In the embryo they are found in blood islands of the yolk sac, body mesenchyma, liver, spleen, and lymph nodes; after the third month they are restricted to the bone marrow.

erythroblastemia (ĕ-rĭth″rō-blăs-tē′mē-ă) [″ + ″ + *haima*, blood]. An excessive number of erythroblasts in the blood.

erythroblastic. Pert. to erythroblasts.

erythroblastoma (ĕ-rĭth″rō-blăs-tō′mă) [″ + *blastos*, germ, + *oma*, tumor]. A tumor (myeloma) with cells resembling megaloblasts.

erythroblastosis (ĕ-rĭth″rō-blăs-tō′sĭs) [″ + ″ + *osis*, condition]. A condition marked by the presence of erythroblasts in the blood.

e. fetalis. A hemolytic disease of the newborn characterized by anemia, jaundice, enlargement of the liver and spleen, and generalized edema (hydrops fetalis). SEE: *hemolytic disease of the newborn*.

erythrochloropia (ĕ-rĭth″rō-klor-ō′pē-ă) [Gr. *erythros*, red, + *chloros*, green, + *ops*, eye]. Partial color blindness with ability to see red and green, but not blue and yellow.

erythrochromia (ĕ-rĭth″rō-krō′mē-ă) [″ + *chroma*, color]. Hemorrhagic red pigmentation of the spinal fluid.

Erythrocin Lactobionate-I.V. Trade name for erythromycin lactobionate for injection.

erythroclasis (ĕr″ĕ-thrŏk′lă-sĭs). The splitting up of red blood cells.

erythroclastic (ĕ-rĭth-rō-klăs′tĭk) [″ + *klasis*, a breaking]. Destructive to red blood cells.

erythrocyanosis (ĕ-rĭth-rō-sī″ă-nō′sĭs) [″ + *kyanos*, blue, + *osis*, condition]. Red or bluish discoloration on the skin with swelling, itching, and burning.

erythrocyte (ĕ-rĭth′rō-sīt) [″ + *kytos*, cell]. A mature red blood cell or corpuscle. Each is a non-nucleated, biconcave disk averaging 7.7 microns in diameter. The body of the cell consists of a spongelike stroma containing a respiratory pigment, hemoglobin, enclosed in a cell membrane of proteins in combination with lipoid substances. Hemoglobin is a conjugated protein consisting of a colored iron-containing portion (hematin) and a simple protein (globin). It combines readily with oxygen to form an unstable compound (oxyhemoglobin). The total surface area of the red cells of an average adult is 3820 square meters or about 2000 times greater than the total body surface area. SEE: *blood cell* for illus.

NUMBER: In a normal person, the number of erythrocytes averages about 5,000,000 per cu. mm (5,500,000 for males, 4,500,000 for females). The total number in an average-sized person is about 35 trillion. The number per cu. mm varies with age (being higher in infants), time of day (being lower during sleep), activity and environmental temperature (increasing in both conditions), and altitude. Persons living at altitudes of 10,000 ft (3048 m) or more may have a red cell count of 8,000,000 per cu. mm or more.

If an individual has a normal blood volume of 5 L (70 ml per kg of body weight), 5,000,000 red blood cells per cu. mm of blood, and the erythrocytes have an average life span of 120 days, then the body needs to produce 2,400,000 red blood cells per second in order to maintain this concentration of blood.

PHYS: The primary function of the red blood cells is to carry oxygen and carbon dioxide. They also play a role in the regulation of the acid-base balance of the blood and in the formation of bile pigments, which are derived from decomposition products of hemoglobin.

DEVELOP: Red cell formation (erythropoiesis) in the adult takes place in the red bone marrow, principally in the vertebrae, ribs, sternum, diploë of cranial bones, and proximal ends of the humerus and femur. They arise from large nucleated stem-cells (promegaloblasts), which give rise to pro-

normoblasts, in which hemoglobin appears. These give rise to normoblasts, which extrude their nuclei. Red cells at this stage possess a fine reticular network and are known as reticulocytes. This reticular structure is lost before the cells enter circulation as mature erythrocytes. The proper formation of erythrocytes depends upon several factors, among them healthy condition of the bone marrow, dietary substances such as iron, cobalt, and copper, all essential for the formation of hemoglobin, plus essential amino acids and certain vitamins, esp. B_{12} and folic acid (pteroylglutamic acid).

The average length of life of a red blood cell is 120 days. Cells are continuously dying, disintegrating, and being replaced. The cellular debris is picked up by the cells of the reticuloendothelial system, esp. those of the spleen, liver, and bone marrow. Hemoglobin is broken down, and proteins and iron are stored and utilized in the formation of new erythrocytes. The iron-containing portion (hematin) gives rise to bilirubin, which is excreted in the bile as one of the bile pigments.

VARIETIES: On microscopic examination erythrocytes may reveal variations in the following respects: size (anisocytosis); shape (poikilocytosis); staining reaction (achromia, hypochromia, hyperchromia, polychromatophilia); structure (possession of bodies such as Cabot's rings, Howell-Jolly bodies, Heinz bodies; parasites such as malaria; a reticular network; or nuclei); and number (anemia, polycythemia). SEE: *blood, synthetic.*

   e., achromatic. Erythrocyte from which the hemoglobin has been dissolved; a colorless corpuscle.

   e., basophilic. Erythrocyte in which cytoplasm stains blue, indicating the presence of basophilic material. May be diffuse (basophilic material uniformly distributed) or punctate (material appearing as pinpoint dots).

   e., crenated. Erythrocyte with a serrated or indented edge, usually the result of withdrawal of water from the cell as occurs when cells are placed in hypertonic solutions.

   e., immature. An erythroblast; any immature erythrocyte.

   e., orthochromatic. Erythrocyte that stains with acid stains only, cytoplasm appearing pink.

   e., polychromatic. Erythrocyte that does not stain uniformly.

erythrocyte reinfusion. The infusion of blood obtained from a donor into the donor.

This is usually done by obtaining the unit or two of blood, freeze-preserving the erythrocytes, and then reinfusing them at a later date. This is also done in healthy persons who wish to attempt to enhance their athletic performance. SYN: *doping, blood.*

erythrocyte sedimentation rate. SEE: *sedimentation rate.*

erythrocythemia (ĕ-rĭth″rō-sī-thē′mē-ă) [Gr. *erythros,* red, + *kytos,* cell, + *haima,* blood]. Enormous increase in circulating red blood cells. SEE: *erythremia; polycythemia vera.*

erythrocytolysin (ĕ-rĭth″rō-sī-tŏl′ĭ-sĭn). Anything that hemolyzes red blood cells.

erythrocytolysis (ĕ-rĭth″rō-sī-tŏl′ĭ-sĭs) [″ + ″ + *lysis,* dissolution]. Dissolution of red blood corpuscles with the escape of hemoglobin.

erythrocytometer (ĕ-rĭth″rō-sī-tŏm′ĕ-tĕr) [″ + ″ + *metron,* measure]. Instrument for counting red blood cells.

erythrocytoopsonin (ĕ-rĭth″rō-sī″tō-ŏp-sō′nĭn) [″ + ″ + *opsonein,* to buy food]. A substance opsonic for red corpuscles.

erythrocytopenia (ĕ-rĭth″rō-sī″tō-pē′nē-ă) [″ + ″ + *penia,* poverty]. Decreased number of red blood cells in the body. SYN: *erythropenia.*

erythrocytopoiesis (ĕ-rĭth″rō-sī″tō-poy-ē′sĭs) [″ + ″ + *poiesis,* making]. Formation of red blood cells; erythropoiesis.

erythrocytorrhexis (ĕ-rĭth″rō-sī″tō-rĕk′sĭs) [″ + ″ + *rhexis,* rupture]. The breaking up of red blood cells with particles or fragments of the cell escaping into the plasma. SYN: *plasmorrhexis.*

erythrocytoschisis (ĕ-rĭth″rō-sī-tŏs′kĭ-sĭs) [″ + ″ + *schisis,* division]. The breaking up of red blood cells into small disk-like particles resembling blood platelets.

erythrocytosis (ĕ-rĭth″rō-sī-tō′sĭs) [″ + ″ + *osis,* increasing condition]. Abnormal increase in the number of red blood cells in circulation, secondary to many disorders.

erythroderma (ĕ-rĭth″rō-dĕr′mă) [″ + *derma,* skin]. Abnormal redness of skin, usually pert. to widespread areas of erythema. SYN: *erythrodermia.*

    e. desquamativum. A disease, resembling seborrhea, of breast-fed infants. Characterized by redness of skin and development of scales.

    e. ichthyosiforme congenitum. A congenital condition characterized by thickening and redness of the skin; may resemble ichthyosis or lichen.

erythrodermia (ĕ-rĭth″rō-dĕr′mē-ă). Erythroderma.

erythrodextrin (ĕ-rĭth″rō-dĕx′trĭn) [″ + L. *dexter,* right]. Dextrin formed by hydrolysis of starch. When iodine is mixed with it, a red color is produced. SEE: *achroodextrin.*

erythrodontia (ĕ-rĭth″rō-dŏn′shē-ă) [″ + *odous,* tooth]. Reddish-brown or yellow discoloration of the dentin of the teeth. May be present in patients with congenital erythropoietic porphyria.

erythrogenesis (ĕ-rĭth″rō-jĕn′ĕ-sĭs) [″ + *genesis,* generation, birth]. The development of red blood cells.

erythroid (ĕr′ĭ-throyd) [″ + *eidos,* form, shape]. 1. Of a reddish color. 2. Concerning the red blood cells.

erythrokeratodermia (ĕ-rĭth″rō-kĕr″ă-tō-dĕr′mē-ă) [″ + *keras,* horn, + *derma,* skin]. Reddening and hardening of the skin.

erythrokinetics (ĕ-rĭth″rō-kī-nĕt′īks) [″ + *kinesis,* movement]. The quantitative description of the rate of production of red blood cells and their life span.

erythroleukemia (ĕ-rĭth″rō-loo-kē′mē-ă) [Gr. *erythros,* red, + *leukos,* white, + *haima,* blood]. A variant of acute myelogenous leukemia with anemia, bizarre red cell morphology, erythroid hyperplasia in the bone marrow, and hepatosplenomegaly in a few cases. The leukocyte count may be extremely high or quite low.

erythroleukosis (ĕ-rĭth″rō-loo-kō′sĭs) [″ + ″ + *osis,* condition]. Abnormal increase of red cells and granulocytes.

erythrolysin (ĕr″ĭ-thrōl′ĭ-sĭn) [″ + *lysis,* dissolution]. An agent causing erythrolysis. SYN: *erythrocytolysin; hemolysin.* SEE: *lysin.*

erythrolysis. Dissolution of red blood corpuscles. SYN: *erythrocytolysis.*

erythromania (ĕ-rĭth″rō-mā′nē-ă) [″ + *mania,* madness]. Uncontrolled blushing.

erythromelalgia (ĕ-rĭth″rō-mĕl-ăl′jē-ă) [″ + *melos,* limb, + *algos,* pain]. A condition affecting the extremities, esp. the feet, characterized by burning and throbbing sensations, which come and go. SYN: *acromelalgia.*

erythromelia (ĕ-rĭth″rō-mē′lē-ă) [″ + *melos,* limb]. Painless erythema of extensor surfaces of extremities.

erythromycin (ĕ-rĭth″rō-mī′sĭn) [″ + *mykes,* fungus]. USP. An antibiotic from *Streptomyces erythreus.* It is effective orally against many gram-positive and some gram-negative organisms. Trade name is Erythrocin.

erythron (ĕr′ĭ-thrŏn) [Gr. *erythros,* red]. The concept of blood as a body system including the circulating red cells and the organ from which they arise.

erythroneocytosis (ĕ-rĭth″rō-nē″ō-sī-tō′sĭs) [″ + *neos,* new, + kytos, cell, + *osis,* condition]. Presence of immature red blood cells in the peripheral blood.

erythronoclastic (ĕ-rĭth″rō-nō-klăs′tĭk) [″ + *klan*, to break]. Destructive to the erythron.

erythroparasite (ĕ-rĭth″rō-păr′ă-sīt) [″ + *parasitos*, parasite]. A red blood cell parasite.

erythropathy (ĕr″ĭ-thrŏp′ă-thē) [″ + *pathos*, disease, suffering]. Disease of the red blood cells.

erythropenia (ĕ-rĭth″rō-pē′nē-ă) [″ + *penia*, poverty]. Deficiency in number of red blood cells. SYN: *erythrocytopenia.*

erythrophage (ĕ-rĭth′rō-fāj) [″ + *phagein*, to eat]. A phagocyte that destroys red blood cells.

erythrophagia. Destruction of red blood cells by phagocytes.

erythrophile, erythrophilous (ĕ-rĭth′rō-fĭl, ĕr″ĭ-thrŏf′ĭ-lŭs) [″ + *philein*, to love]. Readily staining red.

erythrophobia (ĕ-rĭth″rō-fō′bē-ă) [″ + *phobos*, fear]. 1. Abnormal dread of blushing or fear of being diffident or of being embarrassed. 2. A morbid fear of, or aversion to, anything colored red.

erythrophose (ĕ-rĭth′rō-fōz) [″ + *phos*, light]. Any red subjective perception of a bright spot. SEE: *phose.*

erythrophthisis (ĕ-rĭth″rō-thī′sĭs) [″ + *phthisis*, wasting]. Serious damage to the restorative power of red corpuscles. SEE: *anemia, hypoplastic.*

erythropia, erythropsia (ĕr″ĭ-thrō′pē-ă, -thrŏp′sē-ă) [″ + *opsis*, vision]. Condition in which objects appear to be red.

erythroplasia (ĕ-rĭth″rō-plā′zē-ă) [″ + *plasis*, molding, forming]. Condition characterized by the appearance of erythematous lesions of the mucous membranes.

   e. of Queyrat. A rare precancerous dermatosis of the genital mucosa that occurs predominantly in uncircumcised men. Treatment with fluorouracil is usually effective.

erythropoiesis (ĕ-rĭth″rō-poy-ē′sĭs) [″ + *poiesis*, making]. The formation of red blood cells.

erythropoietic (ĕ-rĭth″rō-poy-ĕt′ĭk). Pert. to red blood cells.

erythropoietin (ĕ-rĭth″rō-poy′ĕ-tĭn). A hormone that stimulates red blood cell production. It is an alpha-globulin produced primarily by the kidneys in response to hypoxia. It has been synthesized and is commercially available. Trade name is Epogen. SEE: *epoetin alfa.*

Caution: Erythropoietin has been used by athletes in an attempt to enhance performance. When the hormone is used without medical supervision and in large doses, it may cause an abnormal increase in red cell mass and can lead to a fatal outcome. SEE: *blood doping.*

erythroprosopalgia (e-rĭth″rō-prō-sō-păl′jē-ă) [″ + *prosopon*, face, + *algos*, pain]. A neuropathy characterized by redness and pain in the face.

erythropsia (ĕr-ĭ-thrŏp′sē-ă) [″ + *opsis*, vision]. Perversion of color vision in which all objects look red.

erythropsin (ĕ-rĭth-rŏp′sĭn) [″ + *opsis*, vision]. Pigment in the external portion of the rods of the retina. SYN: *rhodopsin.*

erythrorrhexis (ĕ-rĭth″rō-rĕks′ĭs) [″ + *rhexis*, rupture]. Rupture of a red cell and escape of its plasma. SYN: *erythrocytorrhexis; plasmorrhexis.*

erythrosine sodium. USP. A dye used as a dental disclosing agent. Applied to the teeth in a 2% solution or in soluble tablets, which are chewed. SEE: *disclosing agent.*

erythrosis (ĕr-ĭ-thrō′sĭs) [″ + *osis*, condition]. A reddish-purple discoloration of the skin and mucous membranes in polycythemia.

erythrostasis (ĕ-rĭth″rō-stā′sĭs) [″ + *stasis*, standing still]. Accumulation of red blood cells in vessels due to blood flow having ceased. SEE: *sludged blood.*

erythrotoxin (ĕ-rĭth″rō-tŏk′sĭn) [″ + *toxikon*, poison]. An exotoxin that attacks red blood cells.

erythruria (ĕr-ĭ-thrū′rē-ă) [″ + *ouron*, urine]. Red color of the urine.

Es. Chem. symb. for the element einsteinium.

escape [O. Fr. *escaper*]. 1. To break out of confinement; leak or seep out. 2. The act of attaining freedom.

   e., vagal. Occurrence of a ventricular contraction when the normal rhythmical beat of the heart has been stopped or inhibited by stimulation of the vagus nerve.

   e., ventricular. Occurrence of single or repeated ventricular contractions from impulses arising in the atrioventricular node rather than the sinoauricular node. SYN: *extrasystole, nodal.*

escape beat. SEE: *beat, escape.*

escape phenomenon. The development of resistance to the effects of a continuously present stimulus.

eschar (ĕs′kăr) [Gr. *eschara*, scab]. A slough, esp. one following a cauterization or burn. SEE: *escharotic.*

escharotic (ĕs-kăr-ŏt′ĭk) [Gr. *escharotikos*]. Agent used to destroy tissue and to cause sloughing, which produces what is known as an eschar. Escharotics may be acids, alkalies, metallic salts, phenol or carbolic acid, carbon dioxide, or electric cautery.

escharotomy (ĕs-kăr-ŏt′ō-mē) [Gr. *eschara*, scab, + *tome*, incision]. Removal of the eschar formed on the skin and underlying tissue of severely burned areas. Procedure is particularly helpful in restoring circulation to the extremities of patients in which the eschar forms a tight swollen band around the circumference of the limb.

Escherichia (ĕsh-ĕr-ĭk′ē-ă). A genus of bacteria belonging to the family Enterobacteriaceae, tribe Eschericheae. They are common inhabitants of the alimentary canal of humans and other animals.

Escherichia coli (E. coli). The colon bacillus. Short, plump, gram-negative, non-spore-forming motile bacilli almost constantly present in the alimentary canal of humans and other animals. They are normally non-pathogenic in the intestinal tract. Outside the body and under certain conditions, particularly in the urinary tract, *E. coli* is responsible for infections in other systems and for enteritis in infants and adults. Certain enterotoxigenic strains are a principal cause of travelers' diarrhea. The presence of the bacilli in milk or water is an indicator of fecal contamination.

   E.c., enterohemorrhagic. ABBR: EHEC. The strain of *E. coli* that causes a diarrheal syndrome in which the bloody discharges are copious and there is no fever.
   TREAT: Maintain fluid and electrolyte balance; appropriate antibiotic.

   E.c., enteroinvasive. ABBR: EIEC. A type of *E. coli* that invades and multiplies in the epithelial cells of the distal ileum and colon. The clinical syndrome is the same as for Shigella, q.v., infections.
   TREAT: Maintain fluid balance and use of appropriate antibiotic, usually trimethoprim-sulfamethoxazole.

   E.c., enteropathogenic. ABBR: EPEC. A type of *E. coli* infection that produces infantile diarrhea.
   TREAT: Maintain fluid and electrolyte balance, and oral nonabsorbable antibiotics. SEE: *oral rehydration therapy.*

   E.c., enterotoxigenic. ABBR: ETEC. A type of *E. coli* infection that can cause diarrhea in infants and travelers. Fluid loss may be as severe as in cholera.
   TREAT: Maintain fluid and electrolyte balance, antidiarrheal medicines, and trimethoprim-sulfamethoxazole or doxycycline. SEE: *oral rehydration therapy; travelers' diarrhea.*

Escherich's reflex (ĕsh′ĕr-ĭks) [Theodor Escherich, Ger. physician, 1857–1911]. Pursing or muscular contraction of lips resulting from irritation of mucosa of lips.

eschrolalia (ĕs-krō-lā′lē-ă) [Gr. *aischros*, indecent, + *lalia*, babble]. Meaningless utterance of obscene words. SYN: *coprolalia.*

escorcin (ĕs-kor′sĭn). A stain derived from escalin. It is used to stain and identify de-

fects or injury of the cornea of the eye.

esculent (ĕs′kū-lĕnt). Suitable for use as food.

escutcheon (ĕs-kŭch′ăn) [L. *scutum*, a shield]. The pattern of pubic hair growth. It is different in the male and female.

eserine (ĕs′ĕr-ĭn) [*esere*, African name for the Calabar bean]. Physostigmine, q.v.

ESF. *erythropoietic stimulating factor.* SEE: *erythropoietin.*

Esidrix. Trade name for hydrochlorothiazide.

-esis. A Greek suffix used to form nouns of action or process, e.g., hematopoiesis, paracentesis.

Eskabarb. Trade name for phenobarbital.

Eskalith. Trade name for lithium carbonate.

Esmarch's bandage (ĕs′märks) [Johannes F. A. von Esmarch, Ger. surgeon, 1823–1908]. 1. A triangular bandage. 2. A rubber bandage used to control bleeding. Before surgery is begun, the bandage is applied tightly to the limb, commencing at the distal end and reaching above the site of operation, where a rubber tourniquet is firmly applied. The bandage is then removed, rendering the surgical area virtually bloodless. SEE: *bandage.*

Caution: Tourniquet must not be applied so tightly as to cause nerve damage and it must be removed in time to prevent injury caused by lack of blood flow to the distal tissues.

esodic (ē-sŏd′ĭk) [Gr. *es*, toward, + *hodos*, way]. Pert. to sensory nerves conducting impulses toward the brain and spinal cord. SYN: *afferent; centripetal.*

esoethmoiditis (ĕs″ō-ĕth″moy-dī′tĭs) [Gr. *eso*, inward, + *ethmos*, sieve, + *eidos*, form, shape, + *itis*, inflammation]. Inflammation of membrane of ethmoid cells.

esogastritis (ĕs″ō-găs-trī′tĭs) [″ + *gaster*, belly, + *itis*, inflammation]. Inflammation of the gastric mucous membrane.

esophagalgia (ē-sŏf-ă-găl′jē-ă) [Gr. *oisophagos*, esophagus, + *algos*, pain]. Pain in the esophagus.

esophageal (ē-sŏf″ă-jē′ăl). Pert. to the esophagus.

esophageal apoplexy. Intramural hematoma of esophagus.

esophageal obturator airway. ABBR: EOA. Airway device (primarily used in EMS systems) in which the tube is blindly inserted into the esophagus, thereby blocking vomitus and permitting lung ventilation.

esophageal varices. Varices of the esophagus, esp. the distal portion. These may be associated with any condition that causes chronic obstruction of venous drainage from the esophageal veins into the portal vein of the liver. Cirrhosis of the liver, q.v., is frequently associated with this condition. SEE: *Mallory-Weiss syndrome; Muller maneuver.*

esophageal web. Thin membranous structures that include mucosal and submucosal coats across the esophagus. They may be congenital or may follow trauma, inflammation, or ulceration of the esophagus. SEE: *Plummer-Vinson syndrome.*

esophagectasia, esophagectasis (ē-sŏf″ă-jĕk-tā′sē-ă, -jĕk′tă-sĭs) [″ + *ektasis,* distention]. Dilatation of the esophagus.

esophagectomy (ē-sŏf″ă-jĕk′tō-mē) [″ + *ektome,* excision]. Excision of a part of the esophagus.

esophagismus (ē-sŏf-ă-jĭs′mŭs) [″ + *-ismos,* condition]. Esophageal spasm.

esophagitis (ē-sŏf-ă-jī′tĭs) [″ + *itis,* inflammation]. Inflammation of the esophagus. SEE: *acid reflux test.*

esophagobronchial (ē-sŏf″ă-gō-brŏng′kē-ăl) [″ + *bronchos,* windpipe]. Concerning the esophagus and bronchus.

esophagocele (ē-sŏf′ă-gō-sēl) [″ + *kele,* tumor, swelling]. Hernia of the esophagus.

esophagodynia (ē-sŏf″ă-gō-dĭn′ē-ă) [Gr. *oisophagos,* esophagus, + *odyne,* pain]. Pain in the esophagus.

esophagoenterostomy (ē-sŏf″ă-gō-ĕn-tĕr-ŏs′tō-mē) [″ + *enteron,* intestine, + *stoma,* mouth]. Formation of communication between the esophagus and intestine following excision of stomach.

esophagogastrectomy (ē-sŏf″ă-gō-găs-trĕk′tō-mē) [″ + *gaster,* belly, + *ektome,* excision]. Surgical removal of all or part of the stomach and esophagus.

esophagogastroanastomosis (ē-sŏf″ă-gō-găs″trō-ă-năs″tō-mō′sĭs) [″ + ″ + *anastomosis,* opening]. Joining the esophagus to the stomach.

esophagogastroplasty (ē-sŏf″ă-gō-găs′trō-plăs″tē) [″ + ″ + *plassein,* to form]. Plastic repair of the esophagus and stomach.

esophagogastroscopy (ē-sŏf″ă-gō-găs-trŏs′kō-pē) [″ + ″ + *skopein,* to examine]. Inspection of the esophagus and stomach by using a type of endoscope.

esophagogastrostomy (ē-sŏf″ă-gō-găs-trŏs′tō-mē) [″ + ″ + *stoma,* mouth]. Formation of a communication between the esophagus and stomach.

esophagojejunostomy (ē-sŏf″ă-gō-jĕ-jū-nŏs′tō-mē) [″ + L. *jejunum,* empty, + Gr. *stoma,* mouth]. Surgical anastomosis of a free end of the jejunum to the esophagus. It provides a bypass for food in cases of esophageal stricture.

esophagomalacia (ē-sŏf″ă-gō-mă-lā′sē-ă) [Gr. *oisophagos,* esophagus, + *malakia,* softness]. Softening of the esophageal walls.

esophagomycosis (ē-sŏf″ă-gō-mī-kō′sĭs) [″ + *mykes,* fungus, + *osis,* condition]. Bacterial or fungus disease of esophagus.

esophagomyotomy (ē-sŏf″ă-gō-mī-ŏt′ō-mē) [″ + *mys,* muscle, + *tome,* incision]. Cutting of the muscular coat of the esophagus. May be used in treating stenosis of the lower esophagus. SEE: *Schatzki ring.*

esophagoplasty (ē-sŏf′ă-gō-plăs″tē) [″ + *plassein,* to form]. Repair of the esophagus by a plastic operation.

esophagoplication (ē-sŏf″ă-gō-plĭ-kā′shŭn) [″ + L. *abplicare,* to fold]. The surgical procedure of reducing dilation of the esophagus by taking tucks in its walls.

esophagoptosia, esophagoptosis (ē-sŏf″ă-gŏp-tō′sē-ă, -sĭs) [″ + *ptosis,* a dropping]. Relaxation and prolapse of the esophagus.

esophagoscope (ē-sŏf′ă-gō-skōp) [″ + *skopein,* to examine]. A type of endoscope for examination of the esophagus.

esophagospasm (ē-sŏf′ă-gō-spăzm″) [″ + *spasmos,* a convulsion]. Spasm of the esophagus.

esophagostenosis (ē-sŏf″ă-gō-stĕn-ō′sĭs) [″ + *stenosis,* act of narrowing]. Stricture or narrowing of the esophagus.

esophagostomy (ē-sŏf-ă-gŏs′tō-mē) [″ + *stoma,* mouth]. Surgical formation of an opening into the esophagus.

esophagotome (ē-sŏf′ă-gō-tōm) [″ + *tome,* incision]. Instrument for forming an esophageal fistula.

esophagotomy (ē-sŏf-ă-gŏt′ō-mē). Surgical incision into the esophagus. SEE: *achalasia; cardiospasm; dysphagia.*

esophagotracheal (ē-sŏf″ă-gō-trā′kē-ăl). Concerning the esophagus and the trachea, or a communication between the two.

esophagus (ē-sŏf′ă-gŭs) [Gr. *oisophagos*] (pl. *esophagi*). [NA] A muscular canal extending from the pharynx to the stomach. This vital structure is essential for carrying swallowed foods and liquids from the mouth to the stomach. Length about 9 to 9.75 in. (23 to 25 cm).

e., foreign bodies in. The patient may complain of pain or an uncomfortable feeling deep in the chest.

Foreign bodies are ordinarily not dangerous and usually pass through the alimentary tract in a few days without danger. However, it may be dangerous to give cathartics or enemas. These patients should always be under the care of a physician. SEE: *Heimlich maneuver.*

F.A.: The article often can be dislodged by making the patient vomit by using the finger to stimulate the oral pharynx or back part of the throat.

esophoria (ĕs-ō-fō′rē-ă) [Gr. *eso,* inward, + *phorein,* to bear]. Tendency of visual lines to converge. Inward turning or amount of inward turning of the eye. Opposite of exophoria. SYN: *esotropia*. SEE: *heterotropia*.

esosphenoiditis (ĕs″ō-sfē-noyd-ī′tĭs) [″ + *sphen*, wedge, + *eidos*, form, shape, + *itis*, inflammation]. Osteomyelitis of the sphenoid bone.

esotropia (ĕs-ō-trō′pē-ă) [″ + *tropos*, turning]. Marked turning inward of eye; crossed eyes. SYN: *esophoria*.

ESP. *extrasensory perception.*

ESR. *electron spin resonance.* A technique used in medical imaging that identifies atoms by their electron spin characteristics; *erythrocyte sedimentation rate.*

ESRD. *end stage renal disease.*

-ess [O. Fr.-*esse*]. Suffix noting female sex.

essence [L. *essentia*, being or quality]. 1. The spirit or principle of anything. 2. An alcoholic solution of volatile oil.

essential [L. *essentialis*]. 1. Pert. to an essence. 2. Indispensable. 3. Independent of a local abnormal condition, having no obvious external cause. SEE: *idiopathic.*

essential oils. SEE: *oils, essential.*

essential tremor. SEE: *tremor, essential.*

EST. *electroshock therapy.* SEE: *electroconvulsive therapy.*

ester [L. *aether*, ether]. In organic chemistry, a compound formed by the combination of an organic acid with an alcohol. Water is eliminated in this reaction.

Ex.: Ethyl acetate is an ester formed by combining acetic acid with ethyl alcohol. Esters are commonly liquids with characteristic fruity or flowery odors.

esterase (ĕs′tĕr-ās). Generic term for an enzyme that catalyzes the hydrolysis of esters.

esterification (ĕs-tĕr″ĭ-fĭ-kā′shŭn). Combination of an organic acid with an alcohol to form an ester.

esterize. To convert into an ester.

esthematology (ĕs″thĕm-ă-tŏl′ō-jē) [Gr. *aisthema*, sensation, + *logos*, word, reason]. Science of the sense organs and their function.

esthesia (ĕs-thē′zē-ă) [Gr. *aisthesis*, sensation]. 1. Perception, feeling, sensation. 2. Any disease that affects sensation or perception.

esthesiology (ĕs-thē″zē-ŏl′ō-jē) [″ + *logos*, word, reason]. Science of sensory phenomena. SYN: *esthematology.*

esthesiometer, aesthesiometer (ĕs-thē-zē-ŏm′ĕ-tĕr) [″ + *metron*, measure]. Device for measuring tactile sensibility.

esthesioneurosis (ĕs-thē″zē-ō-nū-rō′sĭs) [″ + *neuron*, nerve, + *osis*, condition]. Any sensory impairment.

esthesiophysiology (ĕs-thē″sē-ō-fĭs-ē-ŏl′ō-jē) [″ + *physis*, nature, + *logos*, study]. Physiology of the sense organs.

esthesioscopy (ĕs-thē″zē-ŏs′kō-pē) [″ + *skopein*, to examine]. Testing tactile and other forms of sensibility.

estheticokinetic (ĕs-thĕt″ĭ-kō-kĭn-ĕt′ĭk) [″ + *kinesis*, movement]. Being both sensory and motor.

esthetics (ĕs-thĕt′ĭks). Aesthetics, q.v.

Estinyl. Trade name for ethinyl estradiol.

estival (ĕs′tĭ-văl) [L. *aestivus*]. Rel. to or occurring in summer.

estivoautumnal [″ + *autumnalis*, pert. to autumn]. Pert. to summer and autumn, formerly applied to a type of malaria.

Estrace. Trade name for estradiol.

estradiol (ĕs-tră-dī′ŏl). USP. $C_{18}H_{24}O_2$, a steroid produced by the ovary and possessing estrogenic properties. Large quantities are found in the urine of pregnant women and mares and in the urine of stallions, the latter two serving as sources of the commercial product. Estradiol is effective when given subcutaneously or intramuscularly but not when administered orally. It is converted to estrone in the body. Trade names are Estrace and Progynon. SEE: *diethylstilbestrol; estrogen.*

e. dipropionate. An ester of estradiol.

estrin (ĕs′trĭn). Estrogen.

estrinization (ĕs″trĭn-ĭ-zā′shŭn). Production of vaginal epithelial changes characteristic of estrogen stimulation.

estriol (ĕs′trē-ŏl). USP. $C_{18}H_{24}O_3$ Estrogenic hormone considered to be the metabolic product of estrone and estradiol. It is found in the urine of the female.

estrogen (ĕs′trō-jĕn) [Gr. *oistros*, mad desire, + *gennan*, to produce]. Any natural or artificial substance that induces estrogenic activity; more specifically the estrogenic hormones, estradiol and estrone, produced by the ovary; the female sex hormones. Estrogens are responsible for the development of secondary sexual characteristics and for cyclic changes in the vaginal epithelium and endothelium of the uterus. Natural estrogens include estradiol, estrone, and their metabolic product, estriol. When used therapeutically, estrogens are usually given in the form of a conjugate such as ethinyl estradiol, conjugated estrogens, USP, q.v., or the synthetic estrogenic substance, diethylstilbestrol. These preparations are effective when given by mouth.

Estrogens provide a satisfactory replacement hormone for the treatment of menopause. It is important to observe closely patients treated this way for any malignant changes in the breast or endometrium. Estrogen should be administered intermittently and in the lowest effective dose.

e.'s, conjugated. USP. Estrogenic substances, principally estrone and equilin, excreted in the urine of pregnant mares. Trade name is Premarin.

estrogenic (ĕs-trō-jĕn'ĭk). Causing estrus; acting to produce the effects of an estrogen.

estrone (ĕs'trōn). USP. $C_{18}H_{22}O_2$. An estrogenic hormone found in the urine of pregnant women and mares. It is also prepared synthetically. Used in the treatment of estrogen deficiencies. It is less active than estradiol but more active than estriol. Trade name is Theelin.

estropipate. USP. Estrogen. Previously used name was piperazine estrone citrate. Trade name is Ogen.

estrual (ĕs'troo-ăl) [Gr. *oistros*, mad desire]. Pert. to estrus of animals.

estruation. The sexually fertile period in animals; the so-called period of heat.

estrus, oestrus [Gr. *oistros*, mad desire]. The cyclic period of sexual activity in nonhuman female mammals, characterized by congestion of and secretion by the uterine mucosa, proliferation of vaginal epithelium, swelling of the vulva, ovulation, and acceptance of the male by the female. During estrus the animal is said to be "in heat."

estrus cycle. The cycle from the beginning of one estrus period to the beginning of the next. Includes proestrus, estrus, and metestrus followed by a short period of quiescence called diestrus.

estuarium (ĕs''tū-ā'rē-ŭm) [L.]. Vapor bath.

état criblé (ā-tā' krĕb-lā') [Fr., sievelike state]. Multiple irregular perforations of Peyer's patches of the intestines. These patches are characteristic of typhoid fever.

état mamelonné (ā-tā' mă-mĕl-ŏn-ā') [Fr., knobby state]. Condition of gastric mucosa in chronic inflammation with nodular projections.

etching (ĕch'ĭng) [Ger. *ätzen*, to feed]. Application of a corrosive or abrasive material to a glass or metal surface to create a pattern or design.

  e., acid. A dental procedure used to produce a roughened surface on tooth enamel for better mechanical retention in bonding resin to tooth structure.

ethacrynic acid. USP. A diuretic drug. Trade name is Edecrin.

ethambutol hydrochloride (ĕ-thăm'bū-tōl). USP. A drug used in treating tuberculosis. It is used in combination with isoniazid. Trade name is Myambutol.

Ethamide. Trade name for ethoxzolamide.

ethanol (ĕth'ă-nŏl). Ethyl alcohol. SEE: *alcohol.*

ethaverine hydrochloride (ĕth''ă-vĕr'ēn). Drug used to produce coronary artery relaxation. Its use is of questionable value.

ethchlorvynol (ĕth-klor'vĭ-nŏl). USP. A sedative hypnotic drug that may produce ad-

diction. Trade name is Placidyl.

ethene (ĕth-ēn'). Ethylene, $CH_2{=}CH_2$.

ether [Gr. *aither*, air]. Any organic compound in which an oxygen atom links together with carbon chains. The ether used for anesthesia is diethyl ether, $C_4H_{10}O$. As an anesthetic it causes postoperative nausea and profuse salivation.

ether anesthesia. $C_4H_{10}O$. Diethyl ether, the common ether previously used in anesthesia. It is rarely used now.

Caution: Ether is highly flammable and should be handled with great care. Also, it should not be stored once its container has been opened because toxic products form when ether is exposed to light.

NURSING IMPLICATIONS: Observe the patient's level of consciousness, take vital signs, and observe for nausea and vomiting as the patient recovers from the effects of the anesthesia. Position the patient on side or with head turned to the side to decrease chance of aspiration if vomiting occurs. Cold compresses may be placed on the head. Rectal irrigations or insertion of a rectal tube may be ordered to relieve gas pressure.

ether asphyxia. Suffocation during ether anesthetization. SEE: *resuscitation.*

ether bed. Bed prepared to receive patient immediately following an operative procedure requiring anesthesia.

ethereal (ĕ-thē'rē-ăl) [Gr. *aither*, air]. Pert. to or made with ether.

etherization (ē''thĕr-ĭ-zā'shŭn). Administration of ether to induce anesthesia.

etherize (ē'thĕr-īz). To anesthetize by use of ether.

etheromania (ē''thĕr-ō-mā'nē-ă) [" + *mania*, madness]. Addiction to use of ether.

ethics [Gr. *ethos*, moral custom]. A system of moral principles or standards governing conduct. SEE: *Declaration of Geneva; Declaration of Hawaii; Hippocratic oath; Nightingale Pledge; Prayer of Maimonides.*

  e., dental. A system of principles governing dental practice; a moral obligation to render the best possible quality of dental service to the patient and to maintain an honest relationship with other members of the profession and people in general.

  e., medical. A system of principles governing medical conduct. It deals with the relationship of a physician to the patient, the patient's family, fellow physicians, and society at large. SEE: *Hippocratic oath.*

  e., nursing. A system of principles governing conduct of a nurse. It deals with the relationship of a nurse to the patient, the patient's family, associates and fellow nurses, and society at large. SEE: *Nightingale Pledge.*

ethinamate (ĕ-thĭn′ă-māt). USP. A mild sedative and hypnotic drug. Trade name is Valmid.

ethinyl estradiol (ĕth′ĭ-nĭl). USP. Trade names are Estinyl and Feminone. SEE: *estradiol.*

ethionamide (ĕ-thī″ŏn-ăm′ĭd). USP. A drug used in treating tuberculosis. It is used in combination with other drugs. Trade name is Trecator-SC.

ethionine (ĕ-thī′ō-nĭn). A progestational agent used in some oral contraceptives.

ethmocarditis (ĕth″mō-kăr-dī′tĭs) [Gr. *ethmos*, sieve, + *kardia*, heart, + *itis*, inflammation]. Inflammation of cardiac connective tissue.

ethmoid (ĕth′moyd) [″ + *eidos*, form, shape]. Sievelike; cribriform.

ethmoidal. Pert. to the ethmoid bone or sinuses.

ethmoid bone. Sievelike spongy bone that forms a roof for the nasal fossae and part of the floor of the anterior fossa of the skull. It contains a number of thin-walled cellular cavities, the ethmoidal cells, which are arranged in three groups. They open into the nasal cavity.

ethmoidectomy (ĕth-moy-dĕk′tō-mē) [″ + *eidos*, form, shape, + *ektome*, excision]. Excision of ethmoid cells that open into nasal cavity.

ethmoiditis (ĕth″moy-dī′tĭs) [″ + ″ + *itis*, inflammation]. Inflammation of ethmoidal cells. May be acute or chronic.
    SYM: Headache, acute pain between eyes, nasal discharge.

ethmoid sinus. Air cells or space inside the ethmoid bone, opening into nasal cavity.

ethnic (ĕth′nĭk) [Gr. *ethnikos*, of a nation]. Concerning groups of people within a cultural system who desire or are given special status based on traits such as religion, culture, language, or appearance.

ethnobiology (ĕth″nō-bī-ŏl′ō-jē) [Gr. *ethnos*, race, + *bios*, life, + *logos*, word, reason]. Study of the biological characteristics of various races.

ethnocentric. Refers to a belief that one's own way of viewing and experiencing the world is superior to others' perspectives. In health care, an ethnocentric perspective would support the worldview of the caretaker, rather than consider the patient's perspective of health and illness.

ethnocentrism. Mindset that causes one to judge the actions and beliefs of others according to one's own cultural background rules.

ethnography (ĕth-nŏg′ră-fē) [″ + *graphein*, to write]. The study of the culture of a single society. Data are gathered during a period of residence with the group by direct observation. SEE: *anthropology.*

ethnology (ĕth-nŏl′ō-jē) [″ + *logos*, word, reason]. The comparative study of cultures using ethnographic data. SEE: *anthropology.*

ethology (ĕ-, ē-thŏl′ō-jē) [Gr. *ethos*, manners, habits, + *logos*, word, reason]. Scientific study of customs and behavior of animals in their natural habitat, as well as in captivity.

ethopropazine hydrochloride (ĕth″ō-prō′pă-zēn). USP. An autonomic nervous system blocking agent used in treating parkinsonism. Trade name is Parsidol.

ethosuximide (ĕth″ō-sŭk′sĭ-mĭd). USP. An anticonvulsant drug. Trade name is Zarontin.

ethotoin (ĕ-thō′tō-ĭn). An anticonvulsant that, because of its moderate effectiveness, is little used. Trade name is Peganone.

ethoxzolamide (ĕth″ŏks-zōl′mĭd). USP. A carbonic anhydrase inhibitor used in treating glaucoma.

ethyl (ĕth′ĭl) [Gr. *aither*, air, + *hyle*, matter]. In organic chemistry, the radical C_2H_5, which is contained in a great number of compounds, including ethyl ether, ethyl alcohol, and ethyl acetate.

    e. acetate. $C_4H_8O_2$. A colorless flammable liquid used as a solvent.

    e. alcohol. C_2H_6O. Grain alcohol. SEE: *alcohol; Poisons and Poisoning* in *Appendix.*

    e. aminobenzoate. Benzocaine, a topical anesthetic.

    e. biscoumacetate. An anticoagulant drug.

    e. chaulmoograte. The ethyl esters of the fatty acids of chaulmoogra oil. Used in the treatment of leprosy.

    e. chloride. USP. C_2H_5Cl. A very volatile liquid with a pleasant odor. When sprayed on the skin, it evaporates so quickly that the tissue is cooled immediately. Because of this property, the skin is anesthetized.
    USES: Local anesthetic in minor surgery. It is a topical anesthetic and is used only for very short periods of anesthesia.

    e., vanillin. A flavoring agent.

ethylamine (ĕth″ĭl-ăm′ĭn). $CH_3CH_2NH_2$. An amine formed in the decomposition of certain proteins.

ethylcellulose (ĕth″ĭl-sĕl′ū-lōs). An ether of cellulose. It is used in preparing drugs.

ethylene (ĕth′ĭl-ēn). CH_2CH_2. A flammable and explosive, colorless gas prepared from alcohol by dehydration. Present in illuminating gas. It is colorless and has a sweetish taste but a pungent, foul odor. It is lighter than air and diffusible when liberated.

    e. glycol. $C_2H_6O_2$. The simplest glycol; a colorless alcohol used as an antifreeze. SEE:

Poisons and Poisoning in *Appendix.*

e. oxide. A chemical, C_2H_4O, that in its gaseous state is used to sterilize materials that cannot withstand heat or steam. Also used as a fumigant.

ethylene anesthesia. Because ethylene is a rather weak anesthetic, it usually is given as a combination of oxygen 20%, cyclopropane 10%, and ethylene 70%.

PHYS. EFFECTS: Ethylene causes less alteration in the blood gases than nitrous oxide. Ethylene alone causes very little muscular relaxation; the blood pressure may rise and respiration is not depressed. Analgesia results before loss of hearing or before complete unconsciousness. Nausea and vomiting seldom persist as long as 24 hr, but generally disappear before consciousness has returned.

ADVAN: Slightly stimulating to cardiac and respiratory systems. It is not irritating to mucous glands and kidneys. It has a short period of induction and makes possible a very rapid recovery. There is an absence of cyanosis and a minimum of emesis.

DISADVAN: It has an objectionable smell; it is highly flammable and explosive; lives have been lost because someone was careless and a spark was produced from some immediate source.

PRECAUTIONS: Ethylene should be stored where there is adequate ventilation. It should be administered away from fire, electrical appliances, or x-ray apparatus. To prevent sparks, all lights should be turned on before bringing the tanks into the room. Furniture should never be dragged or rolled into the room while the anesthetic is being given. The humidity of the room should be controlled during the administration of this anesthetic. Nylon clothing or undergarments should not be worn by anyone in the room; friction from the material may generate static electricity.

Ethylene does not combine as readily with air as do other anesthetics but floats around as clouds. The vapor rises in a cloudlike form and any gust of air may carry it out of the room; a devastating explosion will result if someone on the outside is smoking or if the fumes contact an electrical spark.

Ethylene always is stored in red tanks; oxygen in green tanks; nitrous oxide in blue tanks; carbon dioxide in gray tanks.

ethylenediamine (ĕth″ĭ-lēn-dī′ă-mēn). USP. Drug used as a solvent for theophylline; it is therefore present in aminophylline injection.

ethylenediaminetetraacetic acid. ABBR: EDTA. A chelating agent used in treating exposure to toxic chemicals.

ethylmorphine (ĕth″ĭl-mor′fēn). A drug sim-

ilar to codeine, used as an anti-cough preparation.

ethylnorepinephrine hydrochloride (ĕth″ĭl-nor-ĕp″ĭ-nĕf″rĭn). USP. An adrenergic drug used in treating asthma. Trade name is Bronkephrine.

ethynodiol diacetate (ĕ-thī″nō-dī′ŏl). USP. A progestational drug.

ethynyl (ĕth′ĭ-nĭl). An organic radical, $HC\equiv C{-}$.

etic. In anthropology and transcultural nursing, etic refers to a kind of analysis that emphasizes the universal or culture-free aspects of disease. The categories of Western biomedicine may be viewed as an etic classification because diagnostic objective measures are used to formulate a diagnosis irrespective of the patient's cultural and subjective perspectives. For example, hallucinations are classified as an "illness" from an etic perspective when, in fact, hallucinations may be a component of normal grieving in some cultures. SEE: *emic.*

etio-. Combining form indicating causation.

etiocholanolone (ē″tē-ō-kō-lăn′ō-lōn). A steroid produced by testosterone catabolism. It is excreted in the urine.

etiologic, etiological (ē″tē-ō-lŏj′ĭk, -ĭ-kăl) [Gr. *aitia,* cause, + *logos,* word, reason]. Pert. to the cause or causes of disease.

etiology (ē″tē-ŏl′ō-jē). 1. The study of the causes of disease. 2. The cause of a disease.

etiotropic (ē″tē-ō-trŏp′ĭk) [Gr. *aita,* cause, + *tropos,* turning]. Directed against the cause of a disease; said of a drug or treatment that destroys or inactivates the causal agent of a disease. Opposite of nosotropic.

etodolac. A nonsteroidal anti-inflammatory agent. Trade name is Lodine.

etretinate. Drug used in the treatment of severe recalcitrant psoriasis. Trade name is Tegison.

Caution: Must not be used by women who are pregnant or who intend to become pregnant; should be prescribed only by physicians knowledgeable in the systemic use of retinoids.

---

etymology (ĕt″ĭ-mŏl′ō-jē) [L. *etymon,* origin of a word, + *logos,* word, reason]. The science of the origin and development of words. Most medical words are derived from Latin and Greek, but many of those from the Greek have reached us through the Latin, being modified by that language. Generally when two Greek words are used to form one word, they are connected by the letter "o." Many medical words have been formed from one or more roots, forms used or adapted from the Latin or Greek, and many of them are modified by either a prefix or a suffix, or by both. A knowledge of important Latin or Greek roots and prefixes will reveal the meanings of a great many other words. SEE: *Abbreviations, Prefixes, and Suffixes* in *Appendix*.

Eu. Chem. symb. for the element europium.

eu- [Gr. *eus*, good]. Prefix meaning healthy, normal, good, well.

Eubacteriales (ū″băk-tē-rē-ā′lēz) [Gr. *eus*, good, + *bakterion*, little rod]. An order of bacteria that includes many of the microorganisms pathogenic to man.

Eubacterium (ū″băk-tē′rē-ŭm). Genus of bacteria that is a member of the order Eubacteriales.

eubiotics (ū″bī-ŏt′ĭks) [″ + *bios*, life]. The science of healthy and hygienic living.

eubolism (ū′bŏl-ĭzm). Normal metabolism.

eucalyptol (ū″kă-lĭp′tōl) [″ + *kalyptein*, to cover]. A substance obtained from oil of eucalyptus. Has an aromatic odor and has been used in expectorants.

eucalyptus oil (ū-kă-lĭp′tŭs). Oil distilled from fresh leaves of the plant. Used as an expectorant.

eucapnia (ū-kăp′nē-ă) [″ + *kapnos*, smoke]. Presence of normal amounts of carbon dioxide in the blood.

eucatropine hydrochloride (ū-kăt′rō-pēn). USP. An anticholinergic used as a mydriatic. It is applied topically to the eye.

euchlorhydria (ū″klor-hī′drē-ă). Presence of the normal amount of free hydrochloric acid in the gastric juice.

eucholia (ū-kō′lē-ă) [″ + *chole*, bile]. Normal condition of bile regarding its constituents and amount secreted.

euchromatin (ū-krō′mă-tĭn) [″ + *chroma*, color]. Chromatin that is rich in nucleic acid and is genetically active. SEE: *heterochromatin*.

euchylia (ū-kī′lē-ă) [″ + *chylos*, juice]. Normal condition of the chyle.

eucrasia (ū-krā′sē-ă) [″ + *krasis*, mixture]. Condition of normal health; state of the body in which all activities are in normal balance.

eudiaphoresis (ū″dī-ă-fō-rē′sĭs) [″ + *dia*, through, + *pherein*, to carry]. Normal secretion of perspiration.

eudiometer (ū″dē-ŏm′ē-tĕr) [Gr. *eudia*, good weather, + *metron*, measure]. An instrument for testing purity of air and making analysis of gases.

euesthesia (ū-ĕs-thē′sē-ă) [Gr. *eus*, good, + *aisthesis*, sensation]. Having normal senses.

eugenics (ū-jĕn′ĭks) [″ + *gennan*, to produce]. The science that deals with the genetic and prenatal influences that affect the expression of certain characteristics in offspring.

eugenol (ū′jĕn-ŏl). USP. A material obtained from clove oil and other sources. A topical analgesic used in dentistry. It is also mixed with zinc oxide to form a material that will harden sufficiently to be used as a temporary dental filling.

euglobulin (ū-glŏb′ū-lĭn). A true globulin, or one that is insoluble in distilled water and soluble in dilute salt solution. SEE: *pseudoglobulin*.

euglycemic. Normal concentration of glucose in the blood.

eugonic (ū-gŏn′ĭk) [Gr. *eus*, good, + *gone*, seed]. Pert. to a luxuriant growth of bacteria.

euhydration. Normal amount of water in the body.

eukaryon (ū-kăr′ē-ŏn) [″ + *karyon*, nucleus]. The nucleus of a eukaryote cell.

eukaryote (ū-kăr′ē-ōt). An organism in which the cell nucleus is surrounded by a membrane. SEE: *prokaryote*.

eukinesia (ū-kĭn-ē′sē-ă) [″ + *kinesis*, movement]. Normal power of movement.

Eulenburg's disease (oyl′ĕn-bŭrgz) [Albert Eulenburg, Ger. neurologist, 1840–1917]. Myotonia congenita. SYN: *Thomsen's disease; paramyotonia congenita*.

Eumycetes (ū″mī-sē′tēz) [″ + *mykes*, fungus]. A class of Thallophyta including all the true fungi.

eunuch (ū′nŭk) [Gr. *eune*, bed, + *echein*, to guard]. Castrated male; one who has had his testicles removed, esp. before puberty so that secondary sexual characteristics do not develop. Absence of the male hormone produces certain symptoms, such as a female type of voice and loss of hair on the face. In Middle Eastern and some Asian countries, eunuchs were employed to guard the women of a harem.

eunuchism (ū′nŭk-ĭzm) [″ + ″ + *-ismos*, condition]. Condition resulting from complete lack of male hormone. It may be due to atrophy or removal of testicles.

e., pituitary. Condition produced by failure of the anterior lobe of the pituitary to secrete gonadotrophic hormones; secondary hypogonadism.

eunuchoid (ū′nŭ-koyd) [″ + ″ + *eidos*, form, shape]. Having the characteristics of a eunuch such as retarded development of sex organs, absence of beard and bodily hair, high-pitched voice, and striking lack of muscular development.

eunuchoidism (ū-′nŭk-oyd-ĭzm) [″ + ″ + ″ + *-ismos*, condition]. Deficient production of the male hormone androgen by the testes.

eupancreatism (ū-păn′krē-ă-tĭzm) [Gr. *eus*, good, + *pankreas*, pancreas, + *-ismos*, condition]. Normal condition of the pancreas.

eupepsia [" + *pepsis,* digestion]. Normal digestion as distinguished from dyspepsia.

eupeptic. Pert. to good digestion.

euphonia (ū-fōn'ē-ă) [" + *phone,* voice]. Having a normal clear voice.

euphoria (ū-for'ē-ă) [" + *phoros,* bearing]. 1. A condition of good health. 2. In psychiatry, an exaggerated feeling of well-being; mild elation.

euphoriant. Something that induces euphoria.

euplastic (ū-plăs'tĭk) [" + *plastikos,* formed]. Healing quickly and well.

euploidy (ū-ploy'dē) [" + *ploos,* fold, + *eidos,* form, shape]. In genetics, the state of having complete sets of chromosomes.

eupnea (ŭp-nē'ă) [" + *pnein,* to breathe]. Normal breathing as distinguished from dyspnea and apnea.

eupraxia (ū-prăks'ē-ă) [" + *prassein,* to do]. Normal capacity to execute a motor pattern. SEE: *paralysis.*

eupraxic (ū-prăks'ĭk). Contributing to proper functioning.

europium (ū-rō'pē-ŭm). SYMB: Eu. At. no. 63; at. wt. 151.96. A rare element of the lanthanide series.

Eurotium (ū-rō'shē-ŭm) [Gr. *euros,* mold]. A genus of molds.

eury- (ū'rē) [Gr. *eurys,* wide]. A prefix indicating broad.

eurycephalic (ū"rē-sĕ-făl'ĭk) [" + *kephale,* head]. Having a broad or wide head.

eustachian (ū-stā'kē-ăn, -shĕn) [Bartolomeo Eustachio (Eustachi), It. anatomist, 1520–1574]. Pert. to the auditory tube. SEE: *ear; eustachian tube.*

eustachian catheter. Instrument for insertion into eustachian tube.

eustachianography. Radiologic examination of the eustachian tube and middle ear after the introduction of a contrast agent.

eustachian tube. The auditory tube, extending from the middle ear to the pharynx, 3 to 4 cm long and lined with mucous membrane. Occlusion of the tube leads to the development of otitis media. SEE: *politzerization.* SYN: *otopharyngeal tube.*

eustachian valve. Valve at the entrance of the inferior vena cava.

eustachitis (ū"stā-kī'tĭs). Inflammation of the eustachian tube.

eusystole (ū-sĭs'tō-lē) [Gr. *eus,* good, + *systellein,* to draw together]. A state of the systole of the heart that is normal in time and force.

eutectic (ū-tĕk'tĭk) [Gr. *eutektos*]. Easily melted.

eutectic mixture. A mixture of two or more substances that has a melting point lower than that of any of its constituents.

euthanasia (ū-thă-nā'zē-ă) [Gr. *eus,* good, + *thanatos,* death]. 1. Dying easily, quietly, and painlessly. 2. The act of willfully ending life in individuals with an incurable disease. Ethical considerations of this act are being actively debated. One difficulty is how will the physician or society determine that the time for acting to kill the patient has come. SEE: *advance directive; assisted suicide; death; death with dignity; dying; hopelessly ill patients; living will.*

euthenics (ū-thĕn'ĭks) [Gr. *euthenia,* well- + being]. The science of improvement of a population through modification of the environment.

Eutheria. Mammals with a true placenta.

Euthroid. Trade name for liotrix.

euthyroid (ū-thī'royd). Normal thyroid gland function.

Eutonyl. Trade name for pargyline hydrochloride.

Eutrombicula (ū"trŏm-bĭk'ū-lă). A genus of mites.

eutrophication (ū-trŏf"ĭ-kă'shŭn) [Gr. *eutrophein,* to thrive]. Alteration of the environment by increasing the nutrients required by one species to the disadvantage of other species in the ecosystem, esp. in an aquatic environment.

ev, eV, EV. *electron volt.*

evacuant (ē-văk'ū-ănt) [L. *evacuans,* making empty]. Drug that stimulates the bowels to move.

evacuate [L. *evacuatio,* emptying]. 1. To discharge, esp. from the bowels; to empty the uterus. 2. To move patients from place or site of accident or catastrophe to a hospital or shelter.

evacuation (ē-văk"ū-ā'shŭn). 1. Act of emptying, esp. the bowels. 2. The material discharged from the bowels; stool. 3. Removal of air from a closed container; the production of a vacuum. 4. Act of moving people to a safe place, esp. from a disaster or a wartorn area.

evacuator (ē-văk'ū-ā-tor). Device for emptying, as of the bowels, or for irrigating the bladder and removing calculi.

evaginate (ē-văj'ĭ-nāt) [L. *evaginare,* to unsheath]. Pert. to protrusion of some part or organ from its normal place.

evagination (ē-văj-ĭ-nā'shŭn). 1. Emergence from a sheath. 2. Protrusion of an organ or part. SEE: *invagination.*

evaluation. 1. The judgment of anything. 2. In medicine, consideration of the health and physical and mental capability and potential of a patient or of one considered to be healthy. 3. The final step of the nursing process, q.v. It is essential in assuring the quality and effectiveness of the nursing process. Included in this step will be providing answers concerning the accuracy of the nursing diagnoses, the effectiveness of the nursing plan in meeting the needs of the patient, the usefulness of the nursing interventions in attaining the goals of the planning process, and the need for changing any aspects of the nursing process in order to improve the quality of nursing care. SEE: *nursing assessment; nursing intervention; nursing process; planning; problem-oriented medical record.* 4. In physical therapy, the procedures used to determine the state of the patient prior to initiation of therapeutic intervention, and change in status to determine the continued appropriateness or need for adaptation of the therapeutic program.

evanescent (ĕv″ă-nĕs′ĕnt) [L. *evanescere*, to vanish]. Not permanent; of brief duration; passing gradually.

Evans blue [Herbert M. Evans, U.S. anatomist, 1882–1971]. USP. A diazo dye occurring as a blue-green powder, very soluble in water. It is used intravenously as a diagnostic agent.

Evans syndrome [Robert S. Evans, U.S. physician, b. 1912]. An autoimmune disease characterized by thrombocytopenia and hemolytic anemia.

evaporation [L. *e*, out, + *vaporare*, to steam]. 1. Change from liquid form to vapor. 2. Loss in volume due to conversion of a liquid into a vapor.

evenomation (ē-vĕn″ō-mā′shŭn) [L. *ex*, from, + *venenum*, poison]. Removal of venom from the biting insect or reptile; or removal of venom from the victim of a bite.

eventration (ē″vĕn-trā′shŭn) [L. *e*, out, + *venter*, belly]. 1. Partial protrusion of the abdominal contents through an opening in the abdominal wall. 2. Removal of contents of the abdominal cavity.

eversion (ē-vĕr′zhŭn) [″ + *vertere*, to turn]. Turning outward. SEE: *chilectropion.*

evidement (ā-vēd-mŏn′) [Fr., a scooping out]. Scraping away diseased tissue.

evidence. In forensic medicine, all of the tangible items and record materials pertinent to the legal considerations.

evil [AS. *yfel*]. Disease or illness.

eviration (ē″vī-rā′shŭn) [L. *e*, out, + *vir*, man]. 1. Castration. 2. In psychiatry, delusion in a male who thinks he has become a woman.

evisceration (ē-vĭs″ĕr-ā′shŭn) [″ + *viscera*, viscera]. 1. Removal of the viscera or of the contents of a cavity. 2. Spilling out of abdominal contents resulting from wound dehiscence.

NURSING IMPLICATIONS: Contact physician immediately. Cover the wound with a sterile towel moistened with sterile physiological saline (warm). Tension on the abdomen may be decreased by having the patient flex knees slightly and by placing patient in Fowler's position. Reassure the patient and inform him or her that surgery will be required. Prepare patient for surgery.

evisceroneurotomy (ē-vĭs″ĕr-ō-nū-rŏt′ō-mē) [″ + ″ + Gr. *neuron*, nerve, + *tome*, incision]. Scleral evisceration of the eye with division of optic nerve.

evocation (ĕv″ō-kā′shŭn) [″ + *vocare*, to call]. Creating anew by memory recall or by imagination.

evoked responses. The record of electrical activity produced at various levels in the central nervous system in response to stimulation of an area of the sensory nerve system. The record is obtained by using the electroencephalogram. Analysis of the response can provide important information concerning the function of the peripheral and central nervous systems. SEE: *brain stem auditory evoked responses; somatosensory evoked responses; visual evoked responses.*

evolution (ĕv″ō-lū′shŭn) [L. *e*, out, + *volvere*, to roll]. A process of orderly and gradual change or development. More generally, any orderly and gradual process of modification whereby a system, whether physical, chemical, social, or intellectual, becomes more highly organized.

    e., theory of. The theory that all species of plants and animals, including humans, have come into existence by gradual continuous change from earlier forms. SEE: *natural selection.*

evulsion (ē-vŭl′shŭn) [″ + *vellere*, to pluck]. 1. Tearing away of a part or new growth. 2. Forcible extraction as of teeth.

Ewing's tumor or sarcoma (ū′ĭngz) [James Ewing, U.S. pathologist, 1866–1943]. A diffuse endothelioma or endothelial myeloma forming a fusiform swelling on a long bone.

ex- [L., Gr. *ex*, out]. Prefix indicating out, away from, completely.

exa-. In the SI system, a combining form indicating 10^{18}.

exacerbation (ĕks-ăs″ĕr-bā′shŭn) [″ + *acerbus*, harsh]. Aggravation of symptoms or increase in the severity of a disease.

exaltation [L. *exaltare*, to lift up]. A mental state characterized by feelings of grandeur, excessive joy, elation, and optimism; an abnormal feeling of personal well-being or self-importance.

examination [L. *examinare*, to examine]. The act or process of inspection of the body and its systems to determine the presence or absence of disease. Terms employed indicate type of examination: physical, bimanual, digital, oral, rectal, OB (obstetrical), roentgenological, cystoscopic.

Local physical examination includes specific parts and organs. Four procedures utilized are inspection, palpation, percussion, and auscultation. Laboratory examination includes urinalysis, blood tests, cultures, and various special means of visualizing body spaces and organs and their functions. SEE: *abdominal examination.*

e., bimanual. SEE: *pelvic examination.*

e., dental. Careful consideration of the surfaces of teeth and dental fillings, usually with a sharp-pointed explorer to detect areas of demineralization or caries or failing margins of restorations. The depth of the gingival sulcus is also probed and measured around each tooth to assess the state of health of the periodontium.

e., oral. A careful and thorough inspection and palpation of the mouth, tongue, cheek, and tissues of the neck to assess the state of health of the tissues. SEE: *oral diagnosis.*

examinations, National Board. Examinations administered to test the qualifications of medical, dental, and other professional students. Successful completion of the basic science and clinical parts of the examinations is required for licensure in most states.

exanthem (ĕks-ăn'thĕm) [Gr. *exanthema*, eruption] (pl. *exanthems*). Any eruption of the skin accompanied by inflammation, such as measles, scarlatina, erysipelas.

e. subitum. An acute disease of infants. Probably due to a virus. Marked by high fever for three or four days and sometimes convulsions at the onset. A diffuse maculopapular rash usually appears just at the time the fever suddenly subsides. Treatment is symptomatic. SYN: *roseola infantum.* SEE: *convulsion.*

exanthema (ĕks-ăn-thē'mă) [Gr.] (pl. *exanthemas, -mata*). Exanthem.

exanthematous (ĕks″ăn-thĕm'ă-tŭs). Pert. to an eruption or rash.

exanthrope (ĕks'ăn-thrōp) [Gr. *ex*, out, + *anthropos*, man]. A cause or source of a disease originating outside the body.

exarticulation (ĕks″är-tĭk-ū-lā'shŭn) [L. *ex*, out, + *articulus*, joint]. 1. Amputation of a limb through a joint. 2. Excision of a part of a joint.

excavation (ĕks″kă-vā'shŭn) [″ + *cavus*, hollow]. 1. A hollow or depression. 2. Formation of a cavity.

e., atrophic. A hollow or cupped appearance of the optic nerve head as seen by use of the ophthalmoscope.

e., dental. The preparation of a cavity in a tooth prior to filling.

e. of optic nerve. A slight depression in the center of the optic papilla or disk from which retinal vessels emerge. Depression is

total in glaucoma as a result of high intraocular pressure.

e., rectouterine. The rectouterine pouch or pouch of Douglas.

excavator (ĕks'kă-vā″tor). Instrument for removing tissue or bone. It may be spoonshaped if used on soft tissue and spoonshaped with sharp edges if used in dentistry.

excerebration (ĕk″sĕr-ĕ-brā'shŭn) [″ + *cerebrum*, brain]. Removal of the brain, esp. that of the dead fetus in order to facilitate delivery.

exchange. To give up or substitute something for something else. In dietetics, the exchange of an equal amount of one food substance for another so that the caloric intake remains the same.

exchange list. A grouping of foods to assist people on special diets. In each group, foods are listed in serving sizes that are interchangeable with respect to carbohydrates, fats, protein, and calories. The groups are starch/bread, meat, vegetables, fruit, milk, and fats. This approach is esp. useful in managing diabetics.

exchange, sister chromatid. The exchange of DNA segments between sister chromatids.

exchange transfusion. Transfusion and withdrawal of small amounts of blood repeated until blood volume is almost entirely exchanged. Used in infants born with hemolytic disease and dangerously high levels of serum bilirubin, in patients with uremia, and in treating some types of poisoning. SEE: *hemolytic disease of the newborn; kernicterus.*

excipient (ĕk-sĭp'ē-ĕnt) [L. *excipiens*, excepting]. Any substance added to a medicine to permit it to be formed into the proper shape and consistency; the vehicle for the drug.

excise (ĕk-sīz') [L. *ex*, out, + *caedere*, to cut]. To cut out or remove surgically.

excision (ĕk-sĭ'zhŭn) [L. *excisio*]. An act of cutting away or taking out.

excitability [L. *excitare*, to arouse]. Sensitiveness to being stimulated.

e., independent. Power of a muscle to respond to a stimulus without intervention of motor nerves.

e., muscle. The property of a muscle fiber to be excited to contract. This is a function of the chemical state of the nerve membrane and the time since a previous stimulus was applied.

e., nerve. The property of a nerve to produce an action potential. This is a function of the permeability of the nerve membrane. The membrane is influenced by physical, chemical, and electrical forces. Also, the intensity of electrical stimuli will influence the ability of the nerve to be excited.

e., reflex. Sensitiveness to reflex irritation.

excitant (ĕk-sīt'änt). An agent that will excite a special function of the body; subdivided, according to action, as motor, cerebral, etc. Amphetamine, cocaine, and strychnine are examples of medical excitants.

excitation [L. *excitatio*]. 1. The act of exciting. 2. Condition of being stimulated or excited.

e., direct. Stimulation of a muscle by placing an electrode in it or physically stimulating it.

e., indirect. Stimulation of a muscle via its nerve.

excitation wave. The wave of irritability originating in the sinoatrial node that sweeps over the conducting tissue of the heart and induces contraction of the atria and ventricles.

exciting. Causing excitement.

excitoglandular (ĕk-sīt"ō-glăn'dū-lăr) [L. *excitare*, to arouse, + *glans*, kernel]. Increasing glandular function.

excitometabolic (ĕk-sīt"ō-mĕt"ă-bŏl'ĭk) [" + Gr. *metabole*, change]. Inducing metabolic changes.

excitomotor (ĕk-sīt"ō-mō'tor) [" + *motor*, moving]. Increasing rapidity of muscular activity.

excitomuscular (ĕk-sīt"ō-mŭs'kū-lăr) [" + Gr. *mys*, muscle]. Causing muscular activity.

excitor (ĕk-sī'tor) [L. *excitare*, to arouse]. That which incites to greater activity. SYN: *stimulant*.

excitosecretory (ĕk-sīt"ō-sē'krē-tor-ē) [" + *secretio*, a hiding]. Tending to bring about secretion.

excitotoxin. Neurotransmitters, e.g., glutamate and aspartate, that can cause cell death if their action is prolonged. These chemicals are thought to be important in damaging cells of the brain during ischemia.

excitovascular (ĕk-sī"tō-văs'kū-lăr) [" + *vascularis*, pert. to a vessel]. Increasing circulation activity.

exclave (ĕks'klāv) [Gr. *ex*, out, + L. *clavis*, key]. A detached portion of an organ, an accessory gland such as a spleen or pancreas.

exclusion (ĕks-kloo'zhŭn) [L. *exclusio*, fr. *ex*, out, + *claudere*, to shut]. Shutting off or removing from the main part.

excochleation (ĕks-kŏk-lē-ā'shŭn) [L. *ex*, out, + *cochlea*, spoon]. Scraping out or curetting the contents of a cavity.

excoriation (ĕks-kō-rē-ā'shŭn) [" + *corium*, skin]. Abrasion of the epidermis or of the coating of any organ of the body by trauma, chemicals, burns, or other causes.

excrement (ĕks'krē-mĕnt) [L. *excrementum*]. Waste material passed out of the body, esp. feces. SEE: *excretion*.

excrementitious (ĕks"krē-mĕn-tĭsh'ŭs). Of the nature of excrement.

excrescence (ĕks-krĕs'ĕns) [L. *ex*, out, + *crescere*, to grow]. Any abnormal growth from the surface of a part.

excreta (ĕks-krē'tă) [L.]. Waste matter excreted from the body, including feces, urine, and perspiration. In some diseases, the excreta of the patient contains infectious material. This must be disinfected and handled carefully by hospital personnel. SEE: *AIDS*.

Pads made of absorbent materials should be placed under the patient who has involuntary discharges. When disposed of, the pads should be placed in sturdy plastic bags. In handling all infected discharges, the nurse should wear rubber gloves and a face mask.

Caution: When using the following disinfecting materials, be certain they do not come in contact with skin or eyes.

Phenol: A 5% solution to be used in quantity at least equal to the amount of the material to be disinfected.

Chlorinated lime: Dissolve in the proportion of 4 oz (120 ml) to 1 gal (3.8 L) of water. One qt (946 ml) of this solution for disinfection of each liquid discharge. For solid fecal matter a stronger solution or a larger quantity of this solution will be required.

excrete (ĕks-krēt') [L. *excretus*, sifted out]. To expel or eliminate waste material from the body, blood, or organs.

excretion (ĕks-krē'shŭn) [L. *excretio*]. 1. Waste matter, excreta. 2. The elimination of waste products from the body.

ORGANS: *Intestines:* indigestible residue, water, and bacteria. *Kidneys:* water, nitrogenous substances (urea, uric acid, creatine, creatinine), mineral salts. *Respiratory system:* carbon dioxide, water vapor, and other gases. *Skin:* small amt. through perspiration of water, salts, minute quantities of urea. Its excretory function is stimulated by kidney inactivity. In renal failure, diaphoretics, hot packs, and warm blankets stimulate skin, thus helping to avoid uremic coma.

excretion, words pert. to: defecation; dejecta; diarrhea; elimination; enema; excrement; excreta; expectoration; feces; hydragogue; incontinence; lung; perspiration; pore; respiration; skin; sputum; stool; sweat; urine; void; vomit; vomiting; vomitus.

excretory (ĕks'krē-tō-rē) [L. *excretus*, sifted out]. Pert. to or bringing about excretion.

excursion (ĕks-kŭr'zhŭn) [L. *excursio*]. 1. Wandering from the usual course. 2. Extent of movement of a part such as the extremities or eyes.

Exercise: Energy Required*

Calories Required per Hour of Exercise	Activity†
80	Sitting quietly, reading
200	Golf with use of powered cart
250	Walking 3 miles/hr (4.83 km/hr); housework; light industry; cycling 6 miles/hr (9.7 km/hr)
330	Heavy housework; walking 3.5 miles/hr (5.6 km/hr); cycling 6 miles/hr (9.7 km/hr); golf, carrying own bag; tennis, doubles; ballet exercises
400	Walking 5 miles/hr (8 km/hr); cycling 10 miles/hr (16.1 km/hr); tennis, singles; water skiing
500	Manual labor; gardening; shoveling
660	Running 5.5 miles/hr (8.9 km/hr); cycling 13 miles/hr (20.9 km/hr); climbing stairs; heavy manual work
1020	Running 8 miles/hr (12.9 km/hr); climbing stairs with 30-pound (13.61 kg) load

* These estimates are approximate and can serve only as a general guide. They are based on an average person who weighs 160 pounds (72.58 kg).
† Energy requirements for swimming are not provided because of the variables such as temperature of the water, whether the water is fresh or salt, buoyancy of the individual, and whether the water is calm or not.

---

excurvation (ĕks″kŭr-vā′shŭn) [Gr. *ex*, out, + L. *curvus*, bend]. A curvature outward.

excystation (ĕk″sĭs-tā′shŭn) [″ + *kystis*, cyst]. Pert. esp. to the escape of certain organisms (parasitic worms or protozoa) from an enclosing cyst wall or envelope. Process that occurs in the life cycle of an intestinal parasite after encysted form is ingested.

exencephalia (ĕks″ĕn-sĕf-ā′lē-ă) [″ + *enkephalos*, brain]. A congenital anomaly in which the brain is located outside the skull. A term for encephalocele, hydrencephalocele, and meningocele.

exenteration (ĕks-ĕn″tĕr-ā′shŭn) [″ + *enteron*, intestine]. Evisceration.

exercise [L. *exercitus*, having drilled]. Performed activity of the muscles, voluntary or otherwise, esp. to maintain fitness. SEE: table.

 e., active. Form of bodily movement that the patient performs by voluntary contraction and relaxation of muscles.

 e., assistive. Form of bodily movement that the patient performs by voluntary contraction and relaxation of muscles with the aid of a therapist.

 e., blowing. Exercise in which the patient blows into a tube connected to a bottle containing water. That bottle is attached to another bottle so that the air pressure produced forces water from the one into the other. This increases intrabronchial pressure, which tends to aid in expansion of the lung. Research has indicated that emphysema cavities are irreversible. Thus, blowing exercise is used only to lessen the formation of these cavities. SEE: *atelectasis; empyema; pneumonia.*

 e., Buerger's postural. Exercise used for circulatory disturbances of the extremities.

 e., Codman's. A type of gentle active motion of the upper extremity following immobilization with the purpose of re-establishing range of motion and function following fracture. SYN: *Codman's movements; pendulum exercises.*

 e., concentric. Exercise in which the muscle action overcomes resistance or the muscle contracts. SEE: *muscle contraction, concentric; muscle contraction, eccentric.*

 e., corrective. Use of specific exercises to correct deficiencies caused by trauma or inactivity.

 e., eccentric. Exercises where there is overall lengthening of the muscle in response to an external resistance. SEE: *muscle contraction, concentric; muscle contraction, eccentric.*

 e.'s, flexibility. Exercises designed to increase range of motion and extensibility of muscle.

 e., free. Bodily movement that is carried through by patient with no external assistance.

 e., isokinetic. An exercise, usually using a specially designed machine, which controls the velocity of muscle shortening or lengthening, so that the force generated by the muscle is maximum through the full range of motion.

e., isometric. Active contraction where the force generated by the muscle is equal to the resistance. There is no change in muscle length, and no movement results.

e., isotonic. Active muscle contraction where the force exerted remains constant and muscle length changes.

e.'s, Kegel. SEE: *Kegel exercises.*

e., muscle-setting. Contracting and relaxing a skeletal muscle or group of muscles without moving the part or changing the muscle length. Setting is a non-stressful form of isometric exercise where no external resistance is used. SYN: *e., isometric; e., static.*

e., passive. Form of bodily movement that is carried through by the therapist without the assistance or resistance of the patient.

e., range of motion. Movements of joints through their available range of motion. Can be used to prevent loss of motion. SEE: illus.

e., resistive. Form of supervised bodily movement, with or without apparatus, that offers resistance to muscle action.

e., static. Alternate contraction and relaxation of a skeletal muscle or group of muscles without movement of the joint. SYN: *e., isometric; e., muscle-setting.*

e., stretching. Therapeutic exercise maneuvers, utilizing physiologic principles, designed to increase range of motion of joints or increase extensibility of pathologically shortened connective tissue structures.

e., therapeutic. Scientific supervision of bodily movement, with or without apparatus, for purpose of restoring normal function to diseased or injured tissues.

exercise during pregnancy. During pregnancy in which both the mother and the fetus are normal, exercise may and should be continued. The amount and type of exercise is an individual matter. The woman who, prior to her pregnancy, has exercised regularly should experience no difficulty with continuing; on the other hand, a previously sedentary woman should not attempt to institute a vigorous exercise program such as long distance running or jogging during her pregnancy. No matter what type of exercise is undertaken it is important to remember that, with the progress of pregnancy, the center of gravity will change and most probably prevent participation at the same level and skill as when she was not pregnant. Sports that should be avoided include water skiing, horseback riding, and scuba diving. In high speed falls, water skiing could cause miscarriage due to an inad-

vertent, forceful vaginal douche. In horseback riding, in addition to the possibility of falling from the horse, the repeated bouncing may lead to inflammation of the symphysis pubis. Scuba diving may lead to decompression sickness and bends, q.v., and intravascular air embolism in the fetus. Women who breast feed their children can continue exercising provided they maintain hydration and adequate breast support.

exercise electrocardiogram. Electrocardiogram taken during graded increases in rate of exercise. SEE: *stress test.*

exercise-induced asthma. Asthmatic attacks that occur during exercise. They can usually be prevented by breathing air at body temperature fully saturated with water vapor.

exercise prescription. An exercise schedule usually for the purpose of increasing the state of physical fitness of a previously sedentary individual who has recently had a serious illness such as myocardial infarction, or who is physically fit and wants to know the amount, frequency, and kind of exercise to take in order to develop and maintain a state of fitness. The actual prescription is individualized, taking into account the person's age and health status and the availability of facilities and of adequate supervision, particularly in the case of persons who have or have had evidence of chronic disease of any kind, but esp. of the heart and lungs. SEE: *physical activity and exercise.*

exercise tolerance test. A test to determine the efficiency of the cardiorespiratory system. It may be performed on healthy individuals or those thought to have cardiac disease. The subject is placed on a treadmill and is monitored with an ECG and a device that measures the amount of oxygen utilized. The rate of the treadmill is increased during the test until the subject reaches the point of exhaustion, or until the first signs of distress in a patient with cardiac disease. Analysis of the data reveals the state of cardiorespiratory fitness. SYN: *exercise stress test.*

Caution: It is essential that emergency medical equipment be available during the testing.

---

exeresis (ĕks-ĕr′ĕ-sĭs) [Gr. *exairesis,* taking out]. Excision of any part.

exergonic (ĕk″sĕr-gŏn′ĭk) [Gr. *ex,* out, + *ergon,* work]. Pert. to chemical reactions that produce energy when they occur.

exfetation (ĕks-fē-tā′shŭn) [Gr. *ex,* out, + L. *fetus,* fetus]. Ectopic gestation.

exflagellation (ĕks″flăj-ĕ-lā′shŭn) [″ + L. *flagellum,* whip]. The formation of microgametes (flagellated bodies) from the micro-

RANGE-OF-MOTION EXERCISES

EXTENSION AND FLEXION OF THE WRIST

FLEXION OF ELBOW WHILE HANDS ARE IN PRONATION

FLEXION OF ELBOW WHILE HANDS ARE IN SUPINATION

FLEXION AGAINST GRAVITY OF ARM WITH HANDS PRONATED

FLEXION AGAINST GRAVITY OF ARM WITH HANDS IN SUPINATION

FLEXION OF SHOULDER AGAINST GRAVITY WHEN ELBOW IS IMMOBILIZED

ABDUCTION AND EXTERNAL ROTATION OF ARM AGAINST GRAVITY WHEN ELBOW IS IMMOBILIZED gametocytes. Occurs in the malarial organism *(Plasmodium)* in the stomach of a mosquito.

exfoliatin. Toxin produced by *Staphylococcus aureus*; responsible for the "scalded skin" syndrome.

exfoliation (ĕks″fō-lē-ā′shŭn) [″ + L. *folium,* leaf]. The shedding of something, such as leaves off a tree, human skin, or the primary set of human teeth.

exfoliative dermatitis. An erythematous condition in which scaling occurs following the erythema. In addition to the increased loss of exfoliated skin there is systemic involvement with lymphadenopathy in 60% of cases, and hepatomegaly in about a third of the cases; fever without other signs of infection; anemia in 65% of the cases; eosinophilia in 30% of the cases; and hypothermia in some cases. Even though the cause of idiopathic exfoliative dermatitis is unknown, the condition is secondary to or associated with a large number of other disease processes of the skin (atopic dermatitis, contact dermatitis, mycosis fungoides, psoriasis), systemic diseases (Hodgkin's disease, lymphomas, leukemias, certain cancers), and toxic chemicals and drugs (antibiotics, arsenic, mercury, aspirin, codeine, BAL, gold, iodine, quinidine).

When the skin involvement is extensive the patient may become depressed because of the cosmetic changes.

TREAT: If cause can be determined, remove or treat appropriately. For the idiopathic type, treatment is with corticosteroids, emollients, and antihistamines for pruritis.

Caution: Do not use corticosteroids if this condition is a manifestation of psoriasis.

---

exhalation (ĕks″hă-lā′shŭn) [″ + L. *halare,* to breathe]. The process of breathing out; emanation of a gas or vapor. Opposite of inhalation.

exhaustion [″ + L. *haurire,* to drain]. 1. State of being exhausted, extreme fatigue, or weariness; loss of vital powers; inability to respond to stimuli. 2. Process of removing the contents of or using up a supply of anything. 3. The act of drawing or letting out.

e., heat. A condition resulting from exposure to high temperatures. Characterized by drowsy state of mind, rapid breathing, paleness, cold and sweaty skin, and normal or below normal temperature. May be due to salt deficiency, failure of the sweating mechanism, deficient water intake, or a combination of these factors. SYN: *prostration, heat.*

exhibit (ĕgs-hĭb′ĭt) [L. *exhibere,* to display]. 1. To show. 2. Collection of objects for public inspection.

exhibitionism [″ + Gr. *-ismos,* condition]. 1. Tendency to attract attention to oneself by any means. 2. A psychoneurosis manifesting itself in an abnormal impulse that causes one to expose the genitals to one of the opposite sex.

exhibitionist. 1. One with an abnormal desire to attract attention. 2. One who yields to an impulse to expose the genitals to the view of one of the opposite sex.

exhilarant (ĕg-zĭl′ăr-ănt) [L. *exhilarare,* to gladden]. That which is mentally stimulating.

exhumation (ĕks″hū-mā′shŭn) [L. *ex,* out, + *humus,* earth]. Removal of a dead body from the grave after it has been buried. SYN: *disinterment.*

exitus (ĕk′sĭ-tŭs) [L., going out]. Death.

Ex-Lax. Trade name for a laxative containing phenolphthalein.

Exna. Trade name for benzthiazide.

Exner's nerve (ĕks′nĕrz) [Siegmund Exner, Austrian physiologist, 1846–1926]. Nerve from the pharyngeal plexus to the cricothyroid membranes.

Exner's plexus. A plexus of nerve fibers forming a layer near the surface of the cerebral cortex.

exo- [Gr. *exo,* outside]. Prefix indicating without; outside of.

exobiology (ĕk″sō-bī-ŏl′ō-jē). The biological science of the universe, exclusive of our planet.

exocardia (ĕk″sō-kăr′dē-ă) [″ + *kardia,* heart]. Congenitally abnormal position of the heart.

exocardial. Occurring outside of the heart.

exocataphoria (ĕks″ō-kăt-ă-for′ē-ă) [″ + *kata,* down, + *phoros,* bearing]. Condition in which there is a downward and outward turning of the visual axes.

exocolitis (ĕks″ō-kō-lī′tĭs) [″ + *kolon,* colon, + *itis,* inflammation]. Inflammation of the peritoneum of the colon.

exocrine (ĕks′ō-krĭn) [″ + *krinein,* to separate]. 1. The external secretion of a gland. Opposed to endocrine. 2. Term applied to glands whose secretion reaches an epithelial surface either directly or through a duct.

exocytosis (ĕks″ō-sī-tō′sĭs) [″ + *kytos,* cell, + *osis,* condition]. The discharge of particles from a cell. They are too large to pass through the cell membrane by diffusion or osmosis. SEE: *pinocytosis.*

exodeviation (ĕk″sō-dē″vē-ā′shŭn). Turning outward. When this condition occurs in eyes, it is termed exotropia.

exodontia (ĕks-ō-dŏn′shē-ă) [″ + *odous,* tooth]. The subdivision of dentistry that specializes in the extraction of teeth. Exodontia is often included with other procedures in a department or division of oral and maxillofacial surgery.

exodontology (ĕks″ō-dŏn-tŏl′ō-jē) [″ + ″ + *logos*, word, reason]. Branch of dentistry concerned with extraction of teeth.

exoenzyme (ĕk-sō-ĕn′zīm) [″ + *en*, in, + *zyme*, leaven]. Enzyme that does not function within the cells from which it is secreted.

exoerythrocytic (ĕk″sō-ē-rĭth″rō-sī′tĭk) [″ + *erythros*, red, + *kytos*, cell]. Occurring outside the red cells. Part of the life cycle of the malaria parasite in the human host is inside the red cell; the rest is outside, i.e., exoerythrocytic.

exogamy (ĕks-ŏg′ă-mē) [″ + *gamos*, marriage]. 1. Marriage outside of a particular group. 2. In biology, conjugation between protozoan gametes of different ancestry.

exogastritis (ĕks″ō-găs-trī′tĭs) [″ + *gaster*, belly, + *itis*, inflammation]. Inflammation of the peritoneal coat of stomach.

exogenous (ĕks-ŏj′ĕ-nŭs) [″ + *gennan*, to produce]. Originating outside an organ or part.

exohysteropexy (ĕks″ō-hĭs′tĕr-ō-pĕks″ē) [″ + *hystera*, womb, + *pexis*, fixation]. Fixation of the uterus by implanting the fundus into the abdominal wall.

exometritis (ĕks-ō-mē-trī′tĭs) [″ + *metra*, womb, + *itis*, inflammation]. Inflammation of the peritoneal coat of the uterus.

exomphalos (ĕks-ŏm′fă-lŭs) [Gr. *ex*, out, + *omphalos*, navel]. 1. Umbilical protrusion. 2. Umbilical hernia.

exons. The coding regions of the DNA of genes. SEE: *introns.*

exopathic (ĕk″sō-păth′ĭk) [Gr. *exo*, outside, + *pathos*, disease, suffering]. Pert. to a disease or pathogen originating outside of the body.

exophoria (ĕks″ō-fō′rē-ă) [″ + *phoros*, bearing]. Tendency of visual axes to diverge outward. Opposite of esophoria.

exophthalmia (ĕks″ŏf-thăl′mē-ă) [″ + *ophthalmos*, eye]. Abnormal protrusion of the eyeball. SYN: *exophthalmos.*

    e. cachectica. Exophthalmic goiter.

    e. fungosa. Late state of glioma retinae.

exophthalmic (ĕks″ŏf-thăl′mĭk). Pert. to protrusion of the eyeball.

exophthalmic goiter. A condition marked by protrusion of the eyeballs, increased heart action, enlargement of the thyroid gland, weight loss, nervousness. SYN: *thyrotoxicosis.* SEE: *hyperthyroidism.*

exophthalmometer (ĕk″sŏf-thăl-mŏm′ē-tĕr). Device for measuring the degree of protrusion of the eyeballs.

exophthalmos, exophthalmus (ĕks″ŏf-thăl′mōs, -mŭs). Abnormal protrusion of eyeball. May be due to thyrotoxicosis, tumor of the orbit, orbital cellulitis, leukemia, or aneurysm.

    e., pulsating. Exophthalmos accompanied by pulsation and bruit due to an aneurysm behind the eye.

exoplasm (ĕk′sō-plăzm) [″ + LL. *plasma*, form, mold]. Outer protoplasm of a cell. SYN: *ectoplasm.*

exoserosis (ĕks″ō-sĕr-ō′sĭs) [″ + *serum*, whey, + Gr. *osis*, condition]. An oozing of serum or discharging of an exudate.

exoskeleton (ĕk″sō-skĕl′ĕ-tŏn) [″ + *skeleton*, a dried-up body]. 1. The hard outer covering of certain invertebrates such as the molluscs and arthropods. Composed of chitin, calcareous material, or both. 2. In vertebrates, the hard outer covering such as the shell of a turtle or, more specifically, the hard parts of the body surface derived principally from the ectoderm. These include such structures as hair, hooves, horns, nails, feathers, and scales.

exosmosis (ĕks″ŏs-mō′sĭs) [″ + *osmos*, a thrusting, + *osis*, condition]. Diffusion of a fluid from within outward, as from a blood vessel.

exosplenopexy (ĕks″ō-splēn′ō-pĕks-ē) [″ + *splen*, spleen, + *pexis*, fixation]. Suturing the spleen to opening in the abdominal wall.

exostosis (ĕks″ŏs-tō′sĭs) [″ + *osteon*, bone] (pl. *exostoses*). A bony growth that arises from the surface of a bone, often involving the ossification of muscular attachments. SYN: *hyperostosis; osteoma; osteoncus.*

    e. bursata. Exostosis arising from the epiphysis of a bone and covered with cartilage and a synovial sac.

    e. cartilaginea. Exostosis consisting of cartilage underlying the periosteum.

    e., dental. Exostosis on the root of a tooth.

    e., multiple osteocartilaginous. A hereditary disorder of growth characterized by the development of multiple exostoses, usually located on the diaphyses of long bones near the epiphyseal lines. Results in irregularities of growth of the epiphyses and often secondary deformities.

exoteric (ĕks″ō-tĕr′ĭk) [Gr. *exoterikos*, outer]. Pert. to causes developing outside the body. SYN: *exopathic.*

exothermal, exothermic [Gr. *exo*, outside, + *therme*, heat]. Chemical reaction with production of heat.

exothymopexy (ĕks″ō-thī′mō-pĕks″ē) [″ + *thymos*, thymus, + *pexis*, fixation]. Suturing of an enlarged thymus gland to the sternum.

exothyropexy (ĕks″ō-thī′rō-pĕks″ē). Suture of the thyroid and external fixation to induce atrophy.

exotic (ĕg-zŏt′ĭk) [Gr. *exotikos*]. Not native; originating in another part of the world.

exotoxin (ĕks″ō-tŏks′ĭn) [Gr. *exo*, outside, + *toxikon*, poison]. A toxin produced by a microorganism and excreted into its surrounding medium. It can usually be recovered from the liquid medium in which the toxin-producing organisms have developed. Exotoxins usually are unstable, being sensitive to the effects of chemicals, light, and heat. They are produced by certain bacteria, including diphtheria and tetanus organisms. Exotoxins differ with regard to the particular tissues of the host that may be affected.
RS: cytotoxin; endotoxin; erythrotoxin; leukocidin; leukotoxic; neurotoxin.

exotropia (ĕks″ō-trō′pē-ă) [″ + *tropos*, turning]. Divergent strabismus; abnormal turning of one or both eyes outward.

expander (ĕk-spăn′dĕr) [L. *expandere*, to spread out]. That which increases the size, volume, or amount of something. SEE: *plasma volume expander.*

expansion (ĕks-păn′shŭn) [L. *expandere*, to spread out]. Increase of volume; spreading out.

expansive delusion. Overvaluation of one's power and wealth, accompanied by a feeling of well-being. These beliefs are not consistent with reality. SEE: *megalomania.*

expectant [Gr. *ex*, out, + L. *spectare*, to watch]. Waiting.

expectation. Hoping, anticipation.

expected date of confinement. ABBR: EDC. The predicted date of childbirth. SEE: *pregnancy* for table.

expectorant (ĕk-spĕk′tō-rănt) [Gr. *ex*, out, + L. *pectus*, breast]. An agent that facilitates the removal of the secretions of the bronchopulmonary mucous membrane. Expectorants are classed as sedative or stimulating. Ammonium carbonate, ammonium chloride, and ipecac are considered expectorants.

expectoration (ĕk-spĕk″tō-rā′shŭn). The act or process of spitting out saliva or coughing up materials from the air passageways leading to the lungs. Expulsion of mucus or phlegm from the throat or lungs. It may be mucous, mucopurulent, serous, or frothy. In pneumonia, it is viscid and tenacious, sticks to anything, and is rusty in appearance. In bronchitis, it is frothy, often streaked with blood, and greenish-yellow because of pus. In advanced tuberculosis, it varies from small amount of frothy fluid to abundant offensive greenish-yellow sputum often streaked with blood. SEE: *sputum.*

expel (ĕks-pĕl′) [L. *expellere*]. To drive out.

experience. 1. Personally encountering or having undergone an event. 2. The obtaining of knowledge or wisdom from one's own observations.

experiment [L. *experimentum*, to test]. The scientific procedure used to test the validity of a hypothesis, to gain further evidence or knowledge, or to test the usefulness of a drug or type of therapy that has not been tried previously.

expiration (ĕks″pĭ-rā′shŭn) [Gr. *ex*, out, + L. *spirare*, to breathe]. 1. The expulsion of air from the lungs in breathing. Normally the duration of expiration is shorter than that of inspiration. In general, if the duration of expiration is longer than inspiration, a pathological condition such as emphysema or asthma is present. Muscles used in expiration are the internal intercostal muscles, musculus rectus abdominis [NA], musculus transversus abdominis [NA], the triangularis sterni, and possibly the iliocostalis, serratus posterior inferior, and quadratus lumborum. SEE: *diaphragm* for illus.; *inspiration; respiration.* 2. Death.

e., active. Expiration accomplished as a result of muscular activity, as in forced respiration. The muscles used in respiration are the muscles of the abdominal wall (external and internal oblique, rectus, and transversus abdominis); the internal intercostals, serratus posterior inferior, platysma, and quadratus lumborum.

e., passive. Expiration during quiet respiration in which no muscular effort is required. It is brought about by the elasticity of the lung, recoil of the elastic tissues of the chest such as the costal cartilages, and the weight of the thoracic wall.

expiratory (ĕks-pī′ră-tor″ē). Pert. to expiration.

expiratory center. The part of the respiratory center in the medulla controlling expiratory movements.

expire. 1. To breathe out or exhale. 2. To die.

explant (ĕks-plănt′) [″ + L. *planta*, sprout]. To remove a piece of living tissue from the body and transfer to an artificial culture medium for growth as in tissue culture. Opposite of implant.

explode (ĕks-plōd′) [L. *explodere*, fr. *ex*, out, + *plaudere*, to clap the hands]. To burst or to have rapid onset such as an epidemic; or sudden decompression of a cavity. Explosive decompression occurs when the pressure in the cabin of an airplane flying at high altitude is suddenly decreased.

exploration [L. *explorare*, to search out]. Examination of an organ or part by various means.

exploratory. Pert. to an exploration.

explorer. An instrument used in exploration,

esp. a device used to locate foreign bodies or to define passageways in body sinuses or cavities.

e., dental. A sharp-pointed instrument used to detect unsound enamel, carious lesions, or imperfect margins of restorations in teeth.

explosive decompression. SEE: *decompression, explosive.*

explosive speech. Sudden and explosive utterance. SEE: *speech.*

exponent (ĕks'pō-nĕnt). The mathematical method of indicating the power to which the entity symbolized is to be raised. It is placed as a superscript; e.g., 10^2 or x^2 indicates that 10 and x are to be squared or multiplied by themselves. The exponent can have any numerical value and may be positive or negative; it does not have to be a whole number. SEE: *Scientific Notation* in *Appendix.*

expose. 1. To open up as in surgically opening the abdominal cavity. 2. To be without heat or shelter. 3. To have been in contact with an infected person or agent. 4. To display one's genitalia publicly, esp. when members of the opposite sex are present. Colloquially, this is termed "flashing." 5. To deliver an amount of radiation.

exposure. The amount of radiation being delivered or received over a given area or to the entire body.

express [L. *expressare*]. To squeeze out.

expression. 1. Expelling anything by pressure. 2. Facial disclosure of feeling or a physical state. SYN: *facies.* SEE: *face.*

expressivity. The extent to which a heritable trait is manifest in the individual carrying the gene.

expulsion rate. In gynecology, the rate of spontaneous expulsion of an intrauterine contraceptive device (IUD) in the group of women who use them. Usually expressed with respect to the time elapsed following implantation.

expulsive [L. *expellere*, to drive out]. Having a tendency to expel.

exquisite [L. *exquirere*, sought after]. Unusually intense with respect to pain, pleasure, beauty, or excellence.

exsanguinate (ĕks-săn'gwĭn-āt) [Gr. *ex*, out, + *sanguis*, blood]. Loss of blood to the point at which life can no longer be sustained.

exsanguination (ĕk-săn"gwĭn-ā'shŭn). The process of expressing blood from a part.

exsanguine (ĕks-săn'gwĭn). Anemic; bloodless.

exsection (ĕk-sĕk'shŭn) [L. *exsectus*, having cut]. Excision.

Exsel. Trade name for selenium sulfide.

exsiccant (ĕk-sĭk'ănt) [L. *exsiccare*, to dry out]. 1. Absorbing or drying up a discharge.

2. An agent that absorbs moisture. 3. A dusting or drying powder.

exsiccation (ĕk"sī-kā'shŭn). 1. A drying up. 2. In chemistry, removing the water from compounds or solutions. SYN: *desiccation.*

exsiccative (ĕk-sĭk'ă-tĭv). Causing to dry up or that which dries. SYN: *desiccative.*

exsomatize (ĕk-sŏ'mă-tīz) [Gr. *ex*, out, + *soma*, body]. To remove from the body.

exsorption (ĕk-sorp'shŭn). Movement of material including cells and electrolytes from the blood to the lumen of the intestines. In pathological conditions such as intestinal obstruction, this process may cause a great increase in pressure inside the area of the intestinal tract affected.

exstrophy (ĕks'trō-fē) [" + *strephein*, to turn]. A congenital turning inside out of an organ. SYN: *eversion.*

e. of bladder. A congenital malformation in which the lower portion of the abdominal wall and anterior wall of the bladder are missing and the bladder is everted through the opening. SYN: *ectopia vesicae.*

exsufflation (ĕk"sŭ-flā'shŭn) [" + *sufflatio*, blown up]. Forceful expulsion of air from a cavity by artificial means, such as use of a mechanical exsufflator.

ext. L. *extractum*, extract.

extemporaneous [LL. *extemporaneus*]. Not prepared according to formula but devised for the occasion.

extend (ĕk-stĕnd') [Gr. *ex*, out, + L. *tendere*, to stretch]. 1. To straighten a leg or arm. 2. To move forward.

extended care facility. A medical care institution for patients who require long-term custodial or medical care, esp. for a chronic disease or one requiring prolonged rehabilitation therapy.

extended family. Members of the immediate family plus grandparents and other relatives.

extender (ĕk-stĕn'dĕr) That which causes an increase in the time something lasts or has an effect. The time required for absorption of some medicines given intramuscularly may be increased by injecting them with a substance such as an oil, which slows absorption.

e., leg. A device added to the legs of furniture (e.g., beds, tables) to increase their height to accommodate the needs of persons in wheelchairs.

extension (ĕks-tĕn'shŭn) [L. *extensio*]. 1. The movement by which both ends of any part are pulled apart. A movement that brings the members of a limb into or toward a straight condition. Opposite of flexion. 2. The application of a pull (traction) to a fractured or dislocated limb. 3. To increase the angle between the bones forming a joint.

e., Buck's. A method of producing traction by applying adhesive tape or flannel-backed adhesive tape to the skin and keeping it in smooth close contact by means of circular bandaging of the part to which it is applied.The adhesive strips are placed along the long axis of the arm or leg, the superior ends being about 1 in. (2.5 cm) from the fracture site. Weights sufficient to produce the required extension are fastened to the inferior end of the adhesive strips by means of a rope that is run over a pulley to permit free motion.

extensor [L.]. A muscle that extends a part.

exterior [L.]. Outside of; external.

exteriorize. 1. To expose a part temporarily in surgery. SEE: *marsupialization.* 2. In psychiatry, to turn one's interests outward.

extern (ĕks'tĕrn) [L. *externus,* outside]. A medical student, living outside of a hospital, who assists in the medical and surgical care of patients. SEE: *intern.*

external. Exterior; lateral; opposite of medial or internal.

external fixator. Device(s) for holding fractured bones in place by use of external rather than internal fixation.

externalia (ĕks"tĕr-nā'lē-ă) [L. *exter,* outside, + *genitalis,* genital]. External genitals.

externalize (ĕks-tĕr'nă-līz). 1. In surgery, to provide exposure to the outside. 2. In psychiatry, to direct one's inner conflicts to the outside rather than keeping them hidden inside.

exteroceptive (ĕks"tĕr-ō-sĕp'tĭv) [L. *externus,* outside, + *receptus,* having received]. Pert. to end organs receiving impressions from without.

exteroceptor (ĕks"tĕr-ō-sĕp'tor). A sense organ, as found in the eye, ear, or skin, adapted for the reception of stimuli from outside the body.

extima (ĕks'tĭ-mă) [L., outermost]. The outer layer. SEE: *intima.*

extinction [L. *exstinctus,* having extinguished]. 1. The process of extinguishing or putting out. 2. The complete inhibition of a conditioned reflex as a result of failure to reinforce it.

extinguish (ĕks-tĭng'gwĭsh) [L. *extinguere,* to render extinct]. To abolish, esp. to remove a reflex, by surgical, psychological, or pharmacologic means depending upon the type of reflex involved.

extirpation (ĕks-tĭr-pā'shŭn) [L. *extirpare,* to root out]. Excision of a part; taking out by the roots.

extorsion (ĕks-tor'shŭn) [Gr. *ex,* out, + L. *torsio,* twisting]. Rotation of an organ or limb outward.

extra- [L. *extra,* outside]. Prefix meaning outside of, in addition to, beyond.

extra-articular [" + *articulus,* joint]. Outside a joint.

extra beat. Extrasystole.

extracapsular (ĕks"tră-kăp'sū-lăr). Outside a capsule, e.g., a joint capsule or the capsule of the lens of the eye.

extracapsular extraction. Basic surgical technique for cataract removal. The nucleus, cortex, and anterior capsule are removed; the posterior capsule is left intact. Often done by phacoemulsification, q.v., under local anesthesia using a microscope.

extracellular (ĕks"tră-sĕl'ū-lăr). Outside the cell.

extracellular space. SEE: *space, extracellular.*

extrachromosomal. Not connected to the chromosomes; as in exerting an effect other than through the action of chromosomes.

extracorporeal (ĕks"tră-kor-por'ē-ăl) [" + *corpus,* body]. Outside the body.

extracorporeal membrane oxygenator. ABBR: ECMO. A device external to the body that oxygenates blood delivered to it from the body and then returns it to the patient. It has been used experimentally in patients with acute respiratory failure.

extracorporeal shock-wave lithotriptor. A technique for breaking up kidney stones. The shock waves are focused on the stones. This disintegrates them and permits their passage in the urine. Technique is also used to treat gallstones. SEE: *calculus, renal; percutaneous ultrasonic lithotriptor.*

extracorticospinal (ĕks"tră-kor"tĭ-kō-spī'năl). Outside the corticospinal tract of the central nervous system.

extracranial (ĕks"tră-krā'nē-ăl). Outside the skull.

extract (ĕks-trăkt', ĕks'trăkt) [L. *extractum*]. 1. To pull out or remove forcibly, as to extract a tooth. 2. A solid or semisolid preparation made by extracting the soluble portion of a compound by using water or alcohol and evaporating the solution. 3. Active principle of a drug obtained by distillation or chemical processes.

e., alcoholic. Extract in which alcohol acts as the solvent.

e., aqueous. Extract in which water is the solvent.

e., aromatic fluid. Extract made from an aromatic powder.

e., compound. Extract prepared from more than one drug or substance.

e., ethereal. Extract using ether as the vehicle.

e., fluid. Extract made into a solution from a vegetable drug that contains medicinal components.

e., powdered. A dried crushed extract.

e., soft. Extract of the consistency of

honey.

e., solid. Extract made by evaporating the fluid part of a solution.

extraction [L. *extractum*, drawing out]. 1. Pulling out, as a tooth. 2. The removing of the active portion of a drug from its vehicle.

extractive (ĕks-trăk′tĭv). That which has been extracted or removed.

extractor. Instrument for removing foreign bodies. Varieties include esophageal, throat, bronchial, and tissue.

e., vacuum. SEE: *vacuum extractor*.

extractum (ĕks-trăk′tŭm) [L., a drawing out] (pl. *extracta*). An extract. SEE: *fluidextract*.

extracystic (ĕks″tră-sĭs′tĭk) [L. *extra*, outside, + Gr. *kystis*, bladder]. Outside or unrelated to a bladder or cystic tumor.

extradural (ĕks-tră-dū′răl) [″ + *durus*, hard]. 1. On outer side of the dura mater. 2. Unconnected with the dura mater.

extraembryonic (ĕks″tră-ĕm″brē-ŏn′ĭk) [″ + Gr. *embryon*, something that swells in the body]. Apart from and outside the embryo, e.g., the amnion.

extragenital (ĕks″tră-jĕn′ĭ-tăl) [″ + *genitalis*, genital]. Outside or unrelated to the genital organs.

extrahepatic (ĕks″tră-hĕ-păt′ĭk) [L. *extra*, outside, + Gr. *hepatos*, liver]. Outside or unrelated to the liver.

extraligamentous [″ + *ligare*, to bind]. Outside or unrelated to a ligament.

extramalleolus (ĕks″tră-măl-lē′ō-lŭs) [″ + *malleolus*, little hammer]. The external or lateral malleolus of the ankle.

extramarginal (ĕks″tră-măr′jĭ-năl) [″ + *margo*, margin]. Pert. to subliminal consciousness.

extramarital. Outside of marriage; e.g., extramarital sexual intercourse.

extramastoiditis (ĕks″tră-măs″toyd-ī′tĭs) [″ + Gr. *mastos*, breast, + *eidos*, form, shape, + *itis*, inflammation]. Inflammation of outside tissues contiguous to the mastoid process.

extramedullary (ĕks″tră-mĕd′ū-lă-rē) [″ + *medulla*, marrow]. Outside or unrelated to any medulla, esp. the medulla oblongata.

extramural (ĕks″tră-mū′răl) [″ + *murus*, wall]. Outside the wall of the organ or vessel.

extraneous (ĕks-tră′nē-ŭs) [L. *extraneus*, external]. Outside and unrelated to an organism.

extranuclear [L. *extra*, outside, + *nucleus*, kernel]. Outside a nucleus.

extraocular (ĕks″tră-ŏk′ū-lăr) [″ + *oculus*, eye]. Outside the eye, as in extraocular eye muscles.

extraocular eye muscles. ABBR: EOM. Muscles attached to the eyeball that control eye movement and coordination.SEE: illus.

extrapolar [″ + *polus*, pole]. Outside instead of between poles, as the electrodes of a battery.

extrapyramidal (ĕks″tră-pĭ-răm′ĭ-dăl). Outside the pyramidal tracts of the central nervous system.

extrapyramidal syndrome. Any one of several degenerative diseases of the nervous system that involve the extrapyramidal system and the basal ganglion of the brain. The symptoms include tremors, chorea, athetosis, and dystonia. Parkinsonism, q.v., is an extrapyramidal syndrome.

extrapyramidal system. SEE: *system, extrapyramidal*.

extrasensory. Pert. to forms of perception not dependent upon the five primary senses, such as thought transference.

extrasensory perception. ABBR: ESP. Perception of external events by other than the five senses.

extrasystole (ĕks″tră-sĭs′tō-lē) [″ + Gr. *systole*, contraction]. Premature contraction of the heart. In humans, it is the result of some factor that initiates a stimulus in the impulse-conducting system. It may occur in either the presence or absence of organic heart disease. It may be of reflex origin, being initiated by stimuli from almost any part of the body, or it may be of central origin. It may be induced experimentally by stimulating the heart at any time except during the absolute refractory period.

e., atrial. Premature contraction of the atrium at some point outside the S-A node.

e., junctional. Extrasystole, nodal, q.v.

e., nodal. Extrasystole occurring as a result of the origin of an impulse in the A-V node.

e., ventricular. Extrasystole occurring after the normal contraction of the ventricle has ceased. Usually followed by a long compensatory pause. Originates in either the ventricular muscle tissue or Purkinje fibers or both.

extratubal (ĕks″tră-tū′băl). Outside a tube, esp. the uterine tube.

extrauterine (ĕks″tră-ū′tĕr-ĭn) [″ + *uterus*, womb]. Outside the uterus.

extravaginal (ĕks″tră-văj′ĭ-năl) [″ + *vagina*, sheath]. Outside the vagina.

extravasate (ĕks-trăv′ă-sāt) [″ + *vas*, vessel]. 1. To escape from a vessel into the tissues, said of serum, blood, or lymph. 2. Fluids escaping from vessels into surrounding tissue.

extravasation (ĕks-trăv″ă-sā′shŭn). The escape of fluids into the surrounding tissue. SYN: *suffusion*.

extravascular (ĕks″tră-văs′kū-lăr) [″ + *vasculum*, vessel]. Outside a vessel.

extraventricular [″ + *ventriculus*, little belly]. Outside any ventricle, esp. one of the

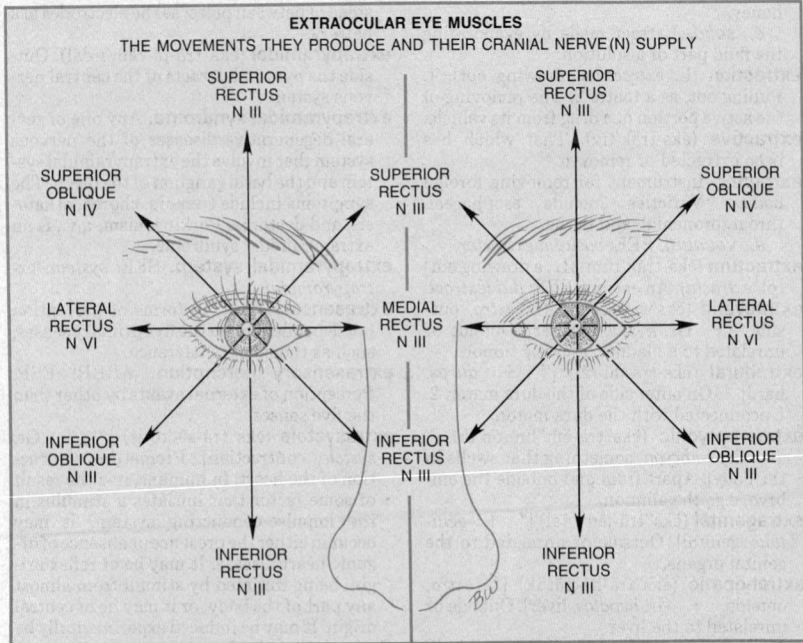

EXTRAOCULAR EYE MUSCLES
THE MOVEMENTS THEY PRODUCE AND THEIR CRANIAL NERVE (N) SUPPLY

SUPERIOR
RECTUS
N III

SUPERIOR
RECTUS
N III

SUPERIOR
OBLIQUE
N IV

SUPERIOR
RECTUS
N III

SUPERIOR
OBLIQUE
N IV

LATERAL
RECTUS
N VI

MEDIAL
RECTUS
N III

LATERAL
RECTUS
N VI

INFERIOR
OBLIQUE
N III

INFERIOR
RECTUS
N III

INFERIOR
OBLIQUE
N III

INFERIOR
RECTUS
N III

INFERIOR
RECTUS
N III

heart.

extremital (ĕks-trĕm'ĭ-tăl) [L. *extremus*, outermost]. Pert. to an extremity. SYN: *distal*.

extremity. 1. The terminal part of anything. 2. An arm or leg.

    e., lower. The lower limb, including the hip, thigh, leg, ankle, and foot.

    e., upper. The upper limb, including the shoulder, arm, forearm, wrist, and hand.

extrinsic (ĕks-trĭn'sĭk) [LL. *extrinsecus*, outer]. From, or coming from, without.

extrinsic muscles. ABBR: e.m. Those muscles attached partly to the trunk and partly to a limb, such as the muscles that attach in the forearm and cross the wrist and hand to move the fingers, or attach in the leg and cross the ankle to move the toes. Those muscles outside an organ that control the position of that organ, such as e.m. of eye or e.m. of tongue.

extrospection (ĕks″trō-spĕk'shŭn) [L. *extra*, outside, + *spectare*, to look]. Continual inspection by the patient of his or her skin for evidence of dirt. Associated with mysophobia, compulsive fear of dirt.

extroversion (ĕks″trō-vĕr'zhŭn) [″ + *vertere*, to turn]. 1. Eversion; turning inside out. 2. The direction of attention and energy outward from the self. SEE: *introversion*.

extrovert. A personality-reaction type; one who is interested mainly in external objects and actions. The extreme pathological extrovert reaction is seen in manic-depressive psychosis. Opposite of introvert.

extrude (ĕks-trūd') [L. *extrudere*, to squeeze out]. To push or force out.

extrusion (ĕks-troo'zhŭn). 1. Something occupying an abnormal external position. 2. In dentistry, position of a tooth when pushed forward from line of occlusion. 3. Describing a herniated nucleus pulposus where the nuclear material ruptures through the outer fibers of the annulus fibrosis and is present in the spinal canal but is still partially within the disk and still attached to it.

extrusion reflex. Infantile reflex in which the tongue moves outward after it has been touched. Present from birth to 4 months.

extubation (ĕks″tū-bā'shŭn) [Gr. *ex*, out, + L. *tuba*, tube]. Removal of a tube, as a laryngeal tube.

exuberant (ĕg-zū'bĕr-ănt) [L. *exuberare*, to be very fruitful]. 1. Excessive as in the increased and excessive growth of granulation tissue or bacterial culture. 2. Joyful, happy.

exudate (ĕks'ū-dāt) [L. *exsudare*, to sweat out]. Accumulation of a fluid in a cavity, or matter that penetrates through vessel walls into adjoining tissue, or the production of pus or serum.

In comparison with a transudate, there are more cells, protein, lactic dehydrogenase, and solid material in an exudate. Exudates may be classified as catarrhal, fibrinous, hemorrhagic, diphtheritic, purulent, and serous, the fluids being different in various affections. A fibrinous exudate may wall off a cavity, resulting in adhesions following surgery, as in empyema and appendicitis. Inflammatory processes tend to wall off the injured area to localize the inflammation and to prevent its spread. SEE: *empyema; exudation; infection; inflammation; pus; resorption; transudate.*

exudation (ĕks″ū-dā′shŭn). Pathological oozing of fluids, usually the result of inflammatory conditions. SEE: *exudate.*

exudative (ĕks′ū-dā″tĭv). Having the property of exudation.

exude (ĕg-zūd′, ĕk-sūd′) [L. *exsudare,* to sweat out]. To pass off slowly through the tissues; said of a semisolid or fluid.

exumbilication (ĕks″ŭm-bĭl″ĭ-kā′shŭn) [Gr. *ex,* out, + L. *umbilicus,* navel]. Protrusion of navel. SYN: *exomphalos.*

exuviae (ĕks-ū′vē-ē) [L.]. Material cast off or shed.

eye [AS. *eage*]. Organ of vision. SEE: illus.

ANAT: Composed of three coats. From inside the eye out they are retina, sensory for light; uvea (choroid, ciliary body, and iris); sclera and cornea, serving as protection for the delicate retina. These layers enclose two cavities, the more anterior or ocular chamber being the space lying in front of the lens. It is divided by the iris into an anterior chamber and a posterior chamber, both of which are filled with a watery aqueous humor. The cavity behind the lens is much larger and filled with a jellylike vitreous body. The lens is suspended behind the iris by the ciliary zonule. Anteriorly, the cornea is covered by the conjunctiva, which continues and forms the inner layer of the eyelids. Movements of the eyeball are brought about by six muscles: the superior, inferior, medial, and external rectus muscles, and the superior and inferior oblique muscles.

Nerve supply: 2nd or optic nerve. *Eye muscles:* 3rd or oculomotor, 4th or trochlear, and 6th or abducens. *Lid muscles:* facial nerve to orbicularis oculi and oculomotor nerve to levator palpebrae. Sensory fibers to the orbit are furnished by ophthalmic and maxillary fibers of the 5th or trigeminal nerve. Sympathetic postganglionic fibers are derived from the carotid plexus, their cell bodies lying in the superior cervical ganglion. They supply the dilator muscle of the iris, lacrimal gland, and smooth muscle fibers in the eyelid; parasympathetic fibers from the ciliary ganglion pass to the ciliary muscle and constrictor muscles of the iris.

PHYS: Light entering the eye passes through the cornea, then through the pupil, an opening in the iris, and on through the crystalline lens and the vitreous body to the retina. The aqueous humor, lens, and vitreous body constitute the refracting media of the eye. Through changes in the curvature of the lens brought about by its elasticity and contraction of the ciliary muscles, light rays are focused on the retina, where they stimulate the rods and cones, the sensory receptors. The cones are concerned with color vision and the rods with vision in dim light. Sensory impulses are conveyed over the optic nerve to the brain where, in the visual area of the cerebral cortex located in the occipital lobe, they register as visual sensations. The amount of light entering the eye is regulated by the pupil, its size being controlled by the dilator and constrictor muscles of the iris. The eye can distinguish nearly 8 million differences in color. As the eye ages, objects appear to have a greater degree of greenness. The principal functions of the eye are color sense, light sense, movement, and form sense, q.v.

DIAG: Following trauma to the head and in certain disease states, the size, shape, motion, and reactions of the pupils provide extremely important diagnostic information.

Contracted pupils: May denote irritative lesions of the 3rd nerve in early stages of some types of anesthesia or during alcoholic excitement, or may result from therapeutic dose of an opiate such as morphine. Contraction of one pupil indicates irritative lesion of the opposite side of the brain, situated at the 3rd nerve nuclei, or a paralysis of the sympathetic nerve fibers due to a lesion somewhere in their course.

Dilated pupils: May result from taking the medicines belladonna or atropine, or from irritation of the sympathetic nerve fibers. May occur during attacks of dyspnea in the last stages of anesthesia. Dilation of one pupil indicates a paralysis of the 3rd nerve from some brain lesion or an irritation of the cervical sympathetic nerve fibers.

Floating specks: Most individuals see little specks of material, which are small pieces of tissue, floating in the vitreous humor. These are called *muscae volitantes,* which is Latin for "flying flies." These specks are the remainder of intraocular embryonic tissue that did not completely disappear. This is not an abnormal condition. *Squint:* This is an unfavorable symptom in the course of a brain disease.

ANATOMY OF EYE

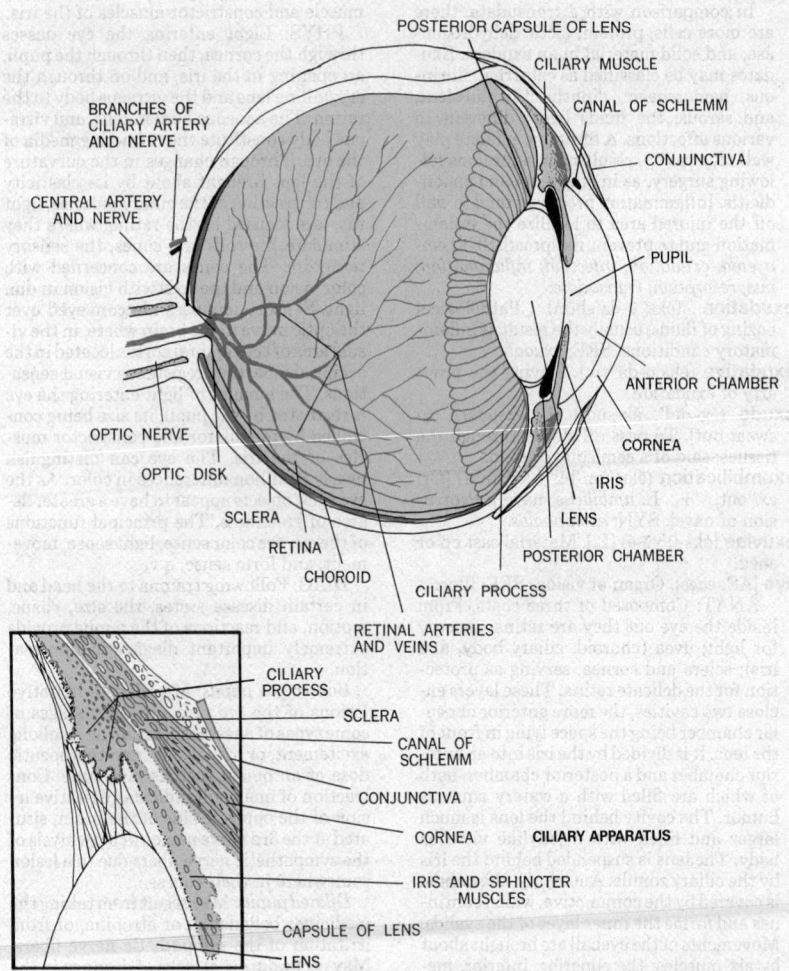

POSTERIOR CAPSULE OF LENS

CILIARY MUSCLE

CANAL OF SCHLEMM

CONJUNCTIVA

BRANCHES OF
CILIARY ARTERY
AND NERVE

PUPIL

CENTRAL ARTERY
AND NERVE

ANTERIOR CHAMBER

CORNEA

IRIS

OPTIC NERVE

LENS

OPTIC DISK

POSTERIOR CHAMBER

SCLERA

RETINA

CHOROID

CILIARY PROCESS

RETINAL ARTERIES
AND VEINS

CILIARY
PROCESS

SCLERA

CANAL OF
SCHLEMM

CONJUNCTIVA

CORNEA

CILIARY APPARATUS

IRIS AND SPHINCTER
MUSCLES

CAPSULE OF LENS

LENS

EYE COMPRESSES: *Cold compresses:* Used to relieve congestion of eyelids; to control intraocular hemorrhage; occasionally for conjunctivitis and early lid injuries to prevent hemorrhage into tissues. Use the following procedure: scrub hands, wring out compresses moistened by isotonic saline solution with forceps and place on ice to chill; place compresses over lids and extend over cheek; change every two or three minutes. Each compress may be used over and over if there is no pus. When pus is present, each compress may be used only once.

Hot compresses: Used to increase the blood supply to the eyelids and eyeballs, and to relieve pain. Scrub hands, apply petroleum jelly with clean swab to area to which compresses are to be applied; wring compresses dry with forceps, test on wrist, and apply as hot as patient can tolerate. To increase blood supply to eyelids, place compresses over lids and extend over cheek; to increase blood supply to eyeballs, place compresses over lids and extend over brow.

TECHNIQUE FOR EXAMINATION OF CONJUNCTIVA

FINGER IS PLACED OVER LASHES AND GENTLY MOVED DOWN TO EXPOSE CONJUNCTIVA. AT THE SAME TIME, THE PATIENT IS ASKED TO LOOK UP.

FINGER IS PLACED OVER LASHES AND GENTLY MOVED UP. AT THE SAME TIME, THE PATIENT IS ASKED TO LOOK DOWN.

PULL UPPER LID DOWN AND PLACE SMOOTH STICK OVER UPPER LID.

WITH THE STICK IN PLACE, THE UPPER LID IS PULLED UP AND OVER THE STICK SO THE UPPER CONJUNCTIVA IS NOW COMPLETELY VISIBLE.

Use new compresses for each application if pus is present; dry the eyelid when last compress is removed. SEE: *lacrimal apparatus; Universal Precautions* in *Appendix.*

NURSING IMPLICATIONS: The patient with an eye injury, either minor or major, will fear blindness. Reassurance is therefore essential. Visual acuity should be tested at once. If the globe has been penetrated, do not apply a patch to the eye but use a suitable shield. Do not attempt to remove a penetrating foreign body. Withhold all medicines, esp. corticosteroids, until the patient has been seen by a physician.

During convalescence, teach patients about the need for periodic eye examinations and to protect the eye from trauma by wearing safety goggles when working with or near tools that could throw off potentially penetrating materials; and protect from excessive exposure to bright light by using tinted lenses. Teach patients to avoid rubbing the eyes and correct methods for instillation of prescribed medications. SEE: *eyedrops; tears, artificial.*

Caution: Do not administer corticosteroids topically or systemically until the patient has been seen by a physician, preferably an ophthalmologist. *Remember: A red eye due to herpes simplex plus use of corticosteroids can cause blindness in that eye.*

---

   e., aphakic. Eye from which the crystalline lens has been removed.

   e., artificial. A prosthesis for placement in the orbit of an individual whose eye has been removed. SEE: *ocularist.*

   e., black. Ecchymosis of the tissues surrounding the eye.

   e., crossed. Strabismus with deviation of the visual axis of one eye toward that of the other eye.

   e., dark-adapted. Eye that has become adjusted for viewing objects in dim light; one adapted for scotopic or rod vision. Depends upon the regeneration of a light-sensitive substance, visual purple.

   e. deviation. In eye muscle imbalance and "crossed eyes," the eye that is not aligned.

   e., dominant. Eye to which a person unconsciously gives preference as a source of stimuli for visual sensations. The dominant eye is usually used in sighting a gun or in using a monocular microscope.

   e., dry. Dry eye, q.v.

   e., exciting. In sympathetic ophthalmia, the damaged eye, which is the source of sympathogenic influences.

   e., fixating. In strabismus, the eye that is directed toward the object of vision.

e., foreign body in. Manifested by pain, lacrimation, spasm of the eye; later redness, swelling, and occasionally headache occur. Infection may be carried into the eye, resulting in an ulcer of the cornea. Metal produces a chemical effect as it disintegrates, an action that affects the eyeball. The roentgenogram is sometimes used to detect any tiny particles of metal, and the electromagnet to assist in removing them. Sympathetic ophthalmia, q.v., the transference of inflammation from an injury of one eye to the normal eye, may be produced by wounds that pierce the eyeball. Loss of vision in both eyes may result if the affected eye is not removed.

F.A.: Tearing often washes dust from the eye; or bringing the upper lid over the lower and directing the patient to roll the eye often deposits the dust on the margin of the lower lid.

Great care is necessary in removing larger particles. This should be done in a quiet, well-lighted place with clean, preferably sterile, materials. Follow by instillation of 1 or 2 drops of a bland oil into the eye. If the eye is inflamed, use repeated hot compresses.

If the patient cannot be taken care of at once, the eye should be bandaged to keep it closed and thus avoid scratching the conjunctiva. There should be no delay in having the speck removed, as serious injury to the eyeball or to the vision may result. In general, the longer the foreign body remains in the eye, the deeper it becomes embedded.

e., light-adapted. Eye that has become adjusted to viewing objects in bright light; one adapted for phototic or cone vision; one in which visual purple has been bleached.

e., pink-. Acute contagious conjunctivitis. SEE: *pink-eye.*

e., squinting. Eye that deviates from the object of fixation in strabismus.

e., sympathizing. In sympathetic ophthalmia, the uninjured eye, which reacts to the pathologic process in the injured eye.

e., trophic ulceration of. A noninfectious ulceration of the corneal epithelium of the eye due to repeated trauma.

eyeball. The globe of the eye. Tension and position of the globe in relation to orbit should be noted.

PATH: *Exophthalmos:* If the protrusion is bilateral, the condition may be due to goiter. The eye may appear to protrude in fright, asthma, and spasmodic croup. It is noted in thrombosis of superior longitudinal sinus, cardiac atrophy, laryngeal stenosis, and paralysis of ocular movements. One or both may be affected by hemorrhage in orbit, aneurysm, exostosis, or tumor of orbit, or enlarged lacrimal glands. *Enophthalmos:* Bilateral or unilateral recession of eyeball.

eyeball, voluntary propulsion of. The ability to voluntarily cause the globe of the eye to protrude by as much as 10 mm (0.4 inch). This is not harmful to the eye or visual acuity.

eye bank. An organization that collects and stores corneas for transplantation.

eyebrow. The arch over the eye; also its covering, esp. the hairs.

eye contact. The meeting of the gaze of the eyes of two persons; looking directly into the eyes of another.

eyecup. 1. The optic vesicle, evagination of the embryonic brain from which the retina develops. 2. A small cup that fits over the eye, used for bathing the surface of the eye.

eyedrops. Any medicinal substance intended to be dropped in liquid form onto the conjunctiva.

In applying eyedrops, the head should be held back; the drops will not pass from under the upper lid to under the lower lid or vice versa. The smaller the eyedrops, the better. Too much liquid in the eye causes the patient to blink, and the medication is then washed away by the increased lacrimal secretion.

Caution: Many medicines are not absorbed from the conjunctiva; they may be readily absorbed from the nasolacrimal duct. For this reason, esp. in children, it is advisable to close off the duct by applying pressure to the inner canthus of the eye for a few minutes after each instillation. This is of particular importance when using drugs such as belladonna to which young children are especially sensitive.

eye-gaze communicator. An electronic device that allows a person to control a computer by looking at words or commands on a video screen. A very low intensity light shines into one of the user's eyes. Reflections from the cornea and retina are picked up by a TV camera. As the direction of gaze moves, the relative position of the two reflections changes, and this information is used by the computer to determine the area at which the user is looking. The computer then executes the command.

eyeglass. A glass lens used to aid the defective eye in seeing.

eyeground. Fundus of eye, seen with ophthalmoscope.

eyelash. A stiff hair on the margin of the eyelid. SYN: *cilium.*

eyelid. One of two movable protective folds that when closed cover the anterior surface of the eyeball. They are separated by the palpebral fissure. The upper (palpebrae superior) is the larger and more movable. It is raised by contraction of the levator palpebrae superioris muscle. Angles formed by the lids at inner and outer ends are known as the canthi. The cilia, or eyelashes, arise from the edges of the eyelids. The posterior surface is lined by the conjunctiva, a mucous membrane.

   e., drooping. Ptosis of the eyelid.

   e., fused. A congenital anomaly resulting from failure of the fetal eyelids to separate.

eyelid closure reflex. Contraction of orbicularis palpebrarum with closure of lids resulting from percussion above supraorbital nerve. SYN: *McCarthy's reflex; supraorbital reflex.*

eye muscle imbalance. Pathological condition of the extraocular muscles of one or both eyes. It causes the eyes to be misaligned in one or more axes. SEE: *eye, crossed; esophoria; exophoria.*

eyepiece (ī'pēs). The portion of an optical device such as a microscope closest to the viewer's eye.

eye protection. Use of goggles, plastic or glass face masks, or protective glasses to prevent injury to the eye when working or playing in situations that could cause severe damage to the eye, e.g., working with a grinding machine, sports involving use of a small ball, fishing, or hiking in an area where tree branches must be dodged.

eye stones. Very small stones placed in the conjunctival sac to remove a mobile foreign body from the eye.

eyestrain. Tiredness of the eye due to overuse.

eyewash. Any suitable liquid material used to wash the eye. Ex.: sterile physiological saline or sterile water.

F

F. 1. *Fahrenheit; femto-; field of vision; folic acid; formula; function; Fusiformis.* 2. Chem. symb. for the element fluorine.

F₁. In genetics, the first filial generation, the offspring of a cross between two unrelated individuals.

F₂. The second filial generation or the offspring of a cross between two individuals of the F₁ generation.

FA., F.A. *fatty acid; filterable agent; first aid; fluorescent antibody.*

F.A.A.N. *Fellow of the American Academy of Nursing.*

Fab. *fragment antigen binding.*

fabella (fă-bĕl′lă) [L., little bean] (pl. *fabellae*). Fibrocartilage or bones that sometimes develop in the head of the gastrocnemius muscle.

fabism (fā′bĭzm) [L. *faba*, bean, + Gr. *-ismos*, condition]. Favism, q.v.

fabrication (făb″rĭ-kā′shŭn) [L. *fabricatus*, having built]. A deliberately false statement told as if it were true. Present in Korsakoff's syndrome, q.v.

Fabry's disease (fā′brēz) [J. Fabry, Ger. physician, 1860–1930]. An inherited metabolic disease in which a glycolipid, ceramide trihexoside, accumulates in the organs and tissues. The excessive amounts present in the kidneys and other organs impair their function. Renal transplantation may be of benefit.

F.A.C.C.P. *Fellow of the American College of Chest Physicians.*

F.A.C.D. *Fellow of the American College of Dentists.*

face [L. *facies*]. Anterior part of the head from forehead to chin, extending laterally to but not including the ears; the visage or countenance. SEE: illus.; *facial expression.*

ANAT: There are 14 bones in the face. The blood supply is bilateral from the facial, maxillary, and superficial temporal branches of the external carotid artery and the ophthalmic branch of the internal carotid artery. The veins include exterior and interior jugular.

DIAG: The following conditions affect the features: mouth breathing, chronic alcoholism, narcotic drug use, abdominal diseases, pain, fear, mental depression, fatigue, facial hemiplegia, cretinism, myxedema, congenital syphilis, exophthalmic goiter, paralysis agitans, encephalitis lethargica, locomotor ataxia, acromegaly, Down syndrome, acute diffuse peritonitis, dyspnea, hysteria, late stages of pulmonary tuberculosis, lobar pneumonia, renal diseases, typhoid fever, hippocratic facies.

Brownish-yellow spots: Commonly called liver spots. Seen in pregnancy, malignancies of liver or uterus, and in exophthalmic goiter. Cosmetics and facial irritants, sunburn, and exposure to weather are also factors. Occur in many diseases including Addison's disease, diabetes, hemochromatosis, pellagra, acanthosis nigricans. Also occur in arsenic poisoning.

Depigmentation: Vitiligo or scars.

Yellowish discoloration: Jaundice due to presence of excess of bile pigments in the blood. Carotenemia may cause a yellowish discoloration.

Cyanosis: Deficient oxygenation of the blood, which may be due to acquired or congenital malformations of the heart, to asthma, whooping cough, pulmonary tuberculosis, croup, obstruction of trachea, aneurysm, tumor, asphyxia, drug poisoning, emphysema, or dilation of right side of the heart.

Flushing (hyperemia): May be permanent or evanescent. If due to emotions or sunburn, it will be temporary. Chronic flushing may be due to febrile diseases, pulmonary tuberculosis, convulsions, alcoholism, ovarian tumors, goiter, plethora, or hypertension.

Pallor: Absence of color may be due to use of cosmetics, excessive confinement indoors, malnourishment, anemia, hemorrhage, shock, fright.

Quiver chin: Quivering of the chin most often seen in children who are emotionally stressed and close to tears.

Redness alternating with pallor: Emotion such as anger, cerebrospinal meningitis, typhoid, menopause, and general vasomotor disturbances.

Sallowness: Cachexia, cancer, lead poisoning, some anemias, Addison's disease, and diseases of the liver.

Edema: Swelling of the face from edema is noted in cardiac, renal, and blood diseases, pneumothorax, mediastinal tumors, and aneurysm. It may be localized and evanescent due to urticaria, angioneurotic edema, or anaphylaxis. Seen in thrombosis of superior longitudinal sinus.

Absence of expression from half the face, with face drawn and distorted: Indicates facial paralysis of opposite side.

Anxious or pinched look: Anxiety, fear, or apprehension.

Risus sardonicus: A sardonic smile caused by contraction or spasm of mouth muscles.

MUSCLES OF FACE AND SCALP

FRONTAL BELLY OF OCCIPITOFRONTALIS
ORBICULARIS OCULI
DEPRESSOR SUPERCILII
LEVATOR LABII SUPERIORIS ALAEQUE NASI
NASALIS
LEVATOR LABII SUPERIORIS
ZYGOMATICUS MINOR
ZYGOMATICUS MAJOR
ORBICULARIS ORIS
DEPRESSOR LABII INFERIORIS
MENTALIS
DEPRESSOR ANGULI ORIS
RISORIUS
PLATYSMA

AURICULARIS SUPERIOR
AURICULARIS ANTERIOR
OCCIPITAL BELLY OF OCCIPITOFRONTALIS
AURICULARIS POSTERIOR
SEMISPINALIS CAPITIS
STERNOCLEIDOMASTOID
SPLENIUS CAPITIS
TRAPEZIUS

Spasms: May be intermittent, continuous, bilateral, or unilateral. May be due to dental disorders or diseases of skin, nose, or eyes. May be mimic or habit spasms; choreic, winking spasms; convulsive tic; blepharospasm. Closure of eyelids caused by spasm of orbicular muscles due to affection of the nerve supply, the eye muscles, or to eye diseases. Spasm of eyelids, chin, upper lips, or muscles of face seen in early stages of meningitis. Tonic spasms due to tetanus, spasms following paralysis, hysteria, and tic douloureux.

RS: anemia; argyria; Bell's palsy; chloasma; cranial nerves; cyanosis; edema; exophthalmic goiter; expression; eye; eyelid; facial; facies; flush; forehead; hyperemia; jaundice; jaw; lip; mouth; nose; poisoning; risus sardonicus; sallow; skeleton; skin; skull; spasm; tic; vitiligo.

f., moon. Full, round face seen in Cushing's syndrome, q.v. May also be an undesired side effect of corticosteroid therapy.

face-lift. Nonscientific term for plastic surgery of the face. SEE: *rhitidectomy.*

facet, facette (făs'ĕt) [Fr. *facette,* small face]. A small, smooth area on a bone or other hard surface.

facetectomy (făs″ĕ-tĕk'tō-mē) [″ + Gr.

ektome, excision]. Surgical removal of the auricular facet of a vertebra.

facet joints. The zygapophyseal joints of the vertebral column between the articulating facets of each pair of vertebrae.

facial [L. *facialis*]. Pert. to the face.

facial bones. The 14 bones that make up the face: maxillae (2); nasal (2); palatine (2); inferior nasal conchae (2); mandible (1); zygoma (2); lacrimal (2); vomer (1).

facial center. Brain center causing facial movements.

facial expression. The human face has a great store and variety of expressions. Normally, these can convey almost any human emotion or reaction. Expressions may convey different meanings in different cultures. Also, certain disease states, i.e., schizophrenia, may limit the ability to interpret facial expression, and parkinsonism is associated with facial rigidity. In certain cultures, a smile is to be expected and in other societies a smile may be an infrequent facial expression.

facial nerve. Seventh cranial nerve, a mixed nerve consisting of efferent fibers supplying the facial muscles, the platysma muscle, the submandibular and sublingual glands; afferent fibers from taste buds of the anterior

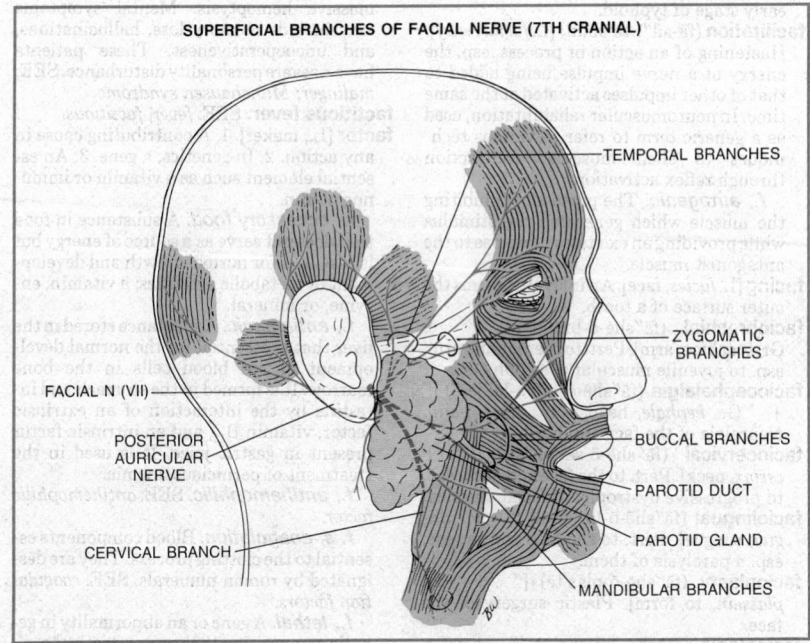

SUPERFICIAL BRANCHES OF FACIAL NERVE (7TH CRANIAL)

TEMPORAL BRANCHES

ZYGOMATIC BRANCHES

FACIAL N (VII)

POSTERIOR AURICULAR NERVE

BUCCAL BRANCHES

PAROTID DUCT

PAROTID GLAND

CERVICAL BRANCH

MANDIBULAR BRANCHES

two-thirds of the tongue and from the muscles. Afferent fibers originate from geniculate ganglion; motor and secretory fibers from nuclei in the pons. They are distributed throughout the ear, face, palate, and tongue. Branches are tympanic, chorda tympani, posterior auricular, digastric, stylohyoid, temporal, zygomatic, malar, buccal, mandibular, and cervical. SEE: *cranial nerves; illus.*

facial paralysis. Paralysis affecting the muscles of the face. The 7th cranial nerve is involved.

facial reflex. Contraction of facial muscles following pressure on eyeball.

facial spasm. An involuntary contraction of muscles supplied by the facial nerve, involving one side of the face or the region around the eye. SEE: *cranial nerves; tic.*

-facient. Suffix indicating to make happen, or to cause.

facies (fā′shē-ēz) [L] (pl. *facies*). [NA] 1. The face or the surface of any structure. 2. The expression or appearance of the face.

    f. abdominalis. Pinched, anxious, shrunken, and drawn expression seen in abdominal problems.

    f., adenoid. Dull, lethargic appearance with open mouth. May be due to hyper-

trophy of adenoids, or chronic mouth breathing.

    f. aortica. Expression seen in aortic valve insufficiency with bluish sclerae, sunken cheeks, and sallow face.

    f. hepatica. Facies seen in liver disease. Skin is sallow, conjunctivae yellow, and eyeballs sunken.

    f. hippocratica. Facies seen in those dying from long-continued illness or from cholera. Cheeks and temples hollow, eyes sunken, complexion leaden, and lips relaxed.

    f. leontina. Lion-like face seen in certain forms of leprosy.

    f., masklike. Expressionless face with little or no animation; seen in parkinsonism.

    f. mitralis. Facies seen in mitral insufficiency. Capillaries more or less visible, cheeks pink, more or less cyanotic.

    f., myopathic. Facies due to muscular relaxation. Lids drop and lips protrude.

    f., parkinsonian. Mask-like face with infrequent eye blinking. The individual can move the face, but in repose, it is expressionless. Characteristic of parkinsonism.

    f., typhoid. Dusky complexion, injected conjunctivae, and dull expression seen in early stage of typhoid.

facilitation (fă-sĭl"ĭ-tā'shŭn) [L. *facilis*, easy]. Hastening of an action or process, esp. the energy of a nerve impulse being added to that of other impulses activated at the same time. In neuromuscular rehabilitation, used as a generic term to refer to various techniques to elicit muscular contraction through reflex activation.

f., autogenic. The process of inhibiting the muscle which generated the stimulus while providing an excitatory impulse to the antagonist muscle.

facing [L. *facies*, face]. An inlay that forms the outer surface of a tooth.

faciobrachial (fā"shē-ō-brā'kē-ăl) [" + Gr. *brachion*, arm]. Pert. to the face and arm, esp. to juvenile muscular dystrophy.

faciocephalalgia (fā"shē-ō-sĕf"ă-lăl'jē-ă) [" + Gr. *kephale*, head, + *algos*, pain]. Neuralgia of the face and head.

faciocervical (fā"shē-ō-sĕr'vĭ-kăl) [" + *cervix*, neck]. Pert. to the face and neck, esp. to progressive dystrophy of facial muscles.

faciolingual (fā"shē-ō-lĭn'gwăl) [" + *lingua*, tongue]. Pert. to the face and tongue, esp. a paralysis of them.

facioplasty (fā"shē-ō-plăs'tē) [" + Gr. *plassein*, to form]. Plastic surgery of the face.

facioplegia (fā"shē-ō-plē'jē-ă) [" + Gr. *plege*, stroke]. Facial paralysis. SYN: *prosopoplegia.*

facioscapulohumeral (fā"shē-ō-skăp"ū-lō-hū'mĕr-ăl) [" + *scapula*, shoulder blade, + *humerus*, shoulder]. Pert. to the face, scapula, and upper arm.

facioscapulohumeral muscular dystrophy. Landouzy-Déjérine dystrophy.

F.A.C.O.G. *Fellow of the American College of Obstetricians and Gynecologists.*

F.A.C.P. *Fellow of the American College of Physicians.*

F.A.C.S. *Fellow of the American College of Surgeons.*

F.A.C.S.M. *Fellow of the American College of Sports Medicine.*

factitious (făk-tĭsh'ŭs) [L. *facticius*, made by art]. Something produced artificially; not natural.

factitious disorders. Disorders that are not real, genuine, or natural. The symptoms, physical and psychological, are produced by the individual and are under voluntary control. These symptoms and the behavior are used to pursue goals that are involuntarily adopted. The goal is to assume the role of patient and to stay in a hospital. This is attained by a variety of means such as taking anticoagulants, feigning right lower quadrant pain with nausea and vomiting, dizziness, fainting, fever of unknown origin, and

massive hemoptysis. Mental symptoms may include memory loss, hallucinations, and uncooperativeness. These patients have a severe personality disturbance. SEE: *malinger; Munchausen syndrome.*

factitious fever. SEE: *fever, factitious.*

factor [L., maker]. 1. A contributing cause in any action. 2. In genetics, a gene. 3. An essential element such as a vitamin or immunoglobulin.

f., accessory food. A substance in food that does not serve as a source of energy but is essential for normal growth and development or metabolic activities; a vitamin, enzyme, or mineral.

f., antianemic. A substance stored in the liver that is essential for the normal development of red blood cells in the bone marrow. It is formed in the stomach and intestine by the interaction of an extrinsic factor, vitamin B_{12}, and an intrinsic factor present in gastric juice. It is used in the treatment of pernicious anemia.

f., antihemophilic. SEE: *antihemophilic factor.*

f.'s, coagulation. Blood components essential to the clotting process. They are designated by roman numerals. SEE: *coagulation factors.*

f., lethal. A gene or an abnormality in genetic composition that causes death of a zygote or of an individual before the reproductive age.

f., milk. A substance present in certain strains of mammary cancer prone mice that is transferred to offspring through milk from the mammary glands. It is capable of inducing the development of mammary cancer in suckling mice exposed to the factor.

f., proliferation inhibiting. A lymphokine that inhibits cell division in tissue culture.

f., Rh. An antigen present on the surface of erythrocytes. SEE: *Rh blood group.*

Factorate. Trade name for antihemophilic factor (AHF).

facultative (făk'ŭl-tā"tĭv) [L. *facultas*, capability]. 1. Having the capacity to do something that is not compulsory. 2. In biology and particularly bacteriology, having the ability to live under certain conditions. Thus, a microorganism may be facultative with respect to oxygen and be able to live with or without oxygen.

faculty. 1. A normal mental attribute or sense; ability to function. 2. Persons employed as teachers at a college or university.

FAD. *flavin adenine dinucleotide.*

Faget's sign [Jean C. Faget, Fr. physician, 1818–1884]. Pulse slower than would be expected with the elevated temperature

Fahrenheit and Celsius Scales

F	C	F	C	F	C
500°	260°	203°	95°	98°	36.67°
401	205	194	90	97	36.11
392	200	176	80	96	35.56
383	195	167	75	95	35
374	190	140	60	86	30
356	180	122	50	77	25
347	175	113	45	68	20
338	170	110	43.33	50	10
329	165	109	42.78	41	5
320	160	108	42.22	32	0
311	155	107	41.67	23	− 5
302	150	106	41.11	14	−10
284	140	105	40.56	+ 5	−15
275	135	104	40.00	− 4	−20
266	130	103	39.44	−13	−25
248	120	102	38.89	−22	−30
239	115	101	38.33	−40	−40
230	110	100	37.78	−76	−60
212	100	99	37.22		

$$1.0°F = 0.54°C$$
$$1.8°F = 1.0 \ °C$$
$$3.6°F = 2.0 \ °C$$
$$4.5°F = 2.5 \ °C$$
$$5.4°F = 3.0 \ °C$$

present. May be seen in some viral infections.

faggot. 1. Slang for a male homosexual. 2. In Britain, a demeaning term for a woman.

Fahrenheit scale (făr'ĕn-hīt″) [Daniel Gabriel Fahrenheit, Ger.-Dutch physicist, 1686–1736]. A temperature scale with the freezing point of water at 32° and the boiling point at 212°. Indicated by F. SEE: table; *Celsius scale; Kelvin scale; thermometer; Miscellaneous Units of Measurement* in *Appendix.*

fail safe. The idea that a device, system, or program can be manufactured, planned, or conceived in such a manner as to prevent failure or malfunction, and to be problemfree or to be infallible.

failure (fāl'yĕr). Inability to function, esp. loss of that which was once present, as in failing eyesight or hearing.

    f., heart. Condition in which the heart is not able to perform adequately its function of pumping blood. It may be temporary or chronic.

    f., kidney or renal. Condition in which the kidneys are not able to perform their functions adequately. It may be partial, temporary, chronic, acute, or complete.

    f., multisystem organ. SEE: *multiple system organ failure.*

    f., respiratory. Condition in which the lungs are unable to perform adequately their function of moving air into and carbon dioxide out of the lungs. It may be due to disease of the lung tissue, or paralysis or weakness of the respiratory muscles.

failure to thrive. ABBR: FTT. Condition in which infants and children not only fail to gain weight but also may lose it. It is seen more often in institutionalized and retarded children. The organic causes include almost any severe chronic condition. The causes of non-organic failure to thrive (NOFTT) include starvation, emotional deprivation, and social disruption. SEE: *Nursing Diagnoses* in *Appendix.*

faint [O. Fr. *faindre,* to feign]. 1. To feel weak as though about to lose consciousness. 2. Weak. 3. Syncope: loss of consciousness due to cerebral anemia or insufficient blood to the brain.

    SYM: Prior to onset patient may be pale, weak, dizzy, have cold perspiration and uncomfortable abdominal sensation. Patient may fall to the ground unconscious. Pulse is usually weak, rapid, and often irregular.

    F.A.: It is important that the individual be placed in a horizontal position, preferably with the head low in order to facilitate blood flow to the brain. At the same time, be certain that there is a clear airway and that the clothing is loose, esp. if a tight collar was being worn. It is important to ascertain that respiratory and cardiac functions are within normal limits. Fainting usually is of short duration and is counteracted by the individual's being in a supine position. Nevertheless it is important to attempt to establish the cause of the faint prior to dismissing the episode as being of no consequence. If recovery from fainting is not prompt, the patient should be moved to a hospital.

RS: apoplexy; asphyxia; coma; shock; swoon; syncope; unconsciousness.

faintness. 1. A sensation of impending loss of consciousness. 2. A sensation due to lack of food.

faith healing. Healing accomplished by supplication to a divine being or power to the exclusion of medical or surgical therapy. Although this area is open to dangerous and fraudulent practice, the medical community cannot completely ignore the psychosomatic aspects of illness that may be affected positively in this manner.

falcate (făl′kāt) [L. *falx*, sickle]. Sickle-shaped.

falces (făl′sēz) [L.]. Pl. of falx.

falcial (făl′shăl). Pert. to the falx.

falciform (făl′sĭ-form) [L. *falx*, sickle, + *forma*, form]. Sickle-shaped.

falciform ligament. The triangular ligament attached to sides of the sacrum and coccyx by its base.

falciform ligament of liver. A wide, sickle-shaped reflection of the peritoneum that serves as a principal attachment of the liver to the diaphragm, and serves to separate the right from the left lobes of the liver. Its broad attachment extends from the posterior, superior portion of the liver to the anterior convex portion connected to the internal surface of the right rectus abdominis muscle.

falciform process. That portion of the falciform ligament along the inner margin of the ramus of the ischium.

falcular. 1. Sickle-shaped. 2. Pert. to the falx cerebelli.

fallectomy (făl-ĕk′tō-mē). Cutting away part of a fallopian tube.

falling drop. 1. In physical diagnosis, a metallic tinkle heard over the normal stomach and bowel when inflated. 2. The same sound heard over large cavities containing fluid and air, as in hydropneumothorax.

fallopian canal (fă-lō′pē-ăn) [Gabriele Fallopio, It. anatomist, 1523–1562]. Canal in petrous bone. The facial nerve passes through this canal.

fallopian ligament. Round ligament of the uterus.

fallopian tube. The tube or duct that extends laterally from the lateral angle of the fundal end of the uterus and terminates near the ovary. It serves to convey the ovum from the ovary to the uterus and spermatozoa from the uterus toward the ovary. Medially each tube opens into the uterus; distally each opens into the peritoneal cavity. Each lies in the superior border of the broad ligament.

ANAT: The narrow region near the uterus, the isthmus, continues laterally as a wider ampulla. The latter expands to form the terminal funnel-shaped infundibulum, at the bottom of which lies a small opening, the ostium, through which the ovum enters the oviduct. Surrounding each ostium are a number of finger-like processes called fimbria extending toward the ovary. Each tube averages about 4½ in. (11.4 cm) in length and ¼ in. (6 mm) in diameter. Its wall consists of three layers: mucosa, muscular layer, and serosa. The epithelium of the mucosa consists of ciliated and nonciliated cells. Ciliary action aids in the movement of the ovum toward the uterus. The muscular layer consists of an inner circular and outer longitudinal layer of smooth muscle. The serosa consists of connective tissue underlying the outermost layer of peritoneum. The blood supply is derived from branches of the uterine and ovarian arteries. The nerve supply is from the pelvic, ovarian, and uterine nerve plexuses, sending fibers to the tubes. SYN: *oviduct; uterine tube*. SEE: *uterus; genitalia, female*, for illus.

Fallot, tetralogy of (făl-ō′). [Etienne L. A. Fallot, Fr. physician, 1850–1911] A congenital condition characterized by defect in the interventricular septum, stenosis of the pulmonary artery, dextroposition of the aorta, and hypertrophy of the right ventricle. Modern surgical therapy has made it possible to treat this condition effectively.

fallotomy (făl-ŏt′ō-mē). Division of the fallopian tubes. SYN: *salpingotomy*.

fallout. Settling of radioactive fission products from the atmosphere after release of such materials into the air after explosion of an atomic bomb or device; or from a radiation accident such as could occur at any installation using radioactive materials.

falls. In the elderly, falls are the leading cause of death. It is important for those providing medical care to search for the cause(s) of the fall. Risk factors for falling include reduced visual acuity and hearing, vestibular dysfunction, peripheral neuropathy, musculoskeletal disorders, postural hypotension, and use of medicines such as antidepressants, sedatives, or vasodilators. By careful clinical investigation, the cause of falls can be determined and appropriate steps taken to prevent them in the future.

Hazards in the home which increase the chances of being involved in a fall are scatter rugs that are not secure or slip-resistant, out-of-the-way light switches, cluttered access to paths through a room or entrance, poorly lighted steps and stairways, lack of handrails on the entire length of a stairway, and tubs and showers that are not fitted with sturdy grab bars and which have slippery surfaces upon which to stand.

false [L. *falsus*]. That which is untrue or incorrect.

false imprisonment. In law, an intentional error that occurs when a person is unlawfully detained without consent by either force or constraint without confinement.

false-negative (făwls′nĕg′ă-tĭv). A test or procedure that indicates that the abnormality or disease being investigated is not present when in fact it is. SEE: *false-positive*.

false-positive (făwls′pŏs′ĭ-tĭv). A test or procedure that indicates that the abnormality or disease being investigated is present when in fact it is not. SEE: *false-negative*.

false ribs. The lower five pairs of ribs that do not unite directly with the sternum. SEE: *rib; vertebrae.*

falsification (făwl″sĭ-fĭ-kā′shŭn). The act of writing or stating that which is not true.

f., retrospective. Deliberate or unconscious alteration of memory for past events or situations. A mental mechanism for ego preservation.

falx [L.] (pl. *falces*). [NA] Any sickle-shaped structure.

f. cerebelli. [NA] A fold of the dura mater that forms a vertical partition between the hemispheres of the cerebellum.

f. cerebri. [NA] A fold of the dura mater that lies in the longitudinal fissure and separates the two cerebral hemispheres.

f. inguinalis. [NA] The conjoined or conjoint tendon that forms the origin of the transversus abdominis and internal oblique muscles.

f. ligmentosa. The broad ligament of the liver. SYN: *falciform ligament of liver.*

fames (fā′mēz) [L.]. Hunger.

familial [L. *familia*, family]. Pert. to or common to the same family; e.g., a disease occurring more frequently in a family than would be expected by chance.

familial Mediterranean fever. An inherited autosomal recessive disorder seen most commonly in Middle Eastern ethnic groups but has appeared in family clusters in persons of Irish or Italian descent. The attacks, which almost always include fever, first appear between the ages of 5 and 15. Included in the syndrome are some of the following:

abdominal pain resembling peritonitis, chest pain of pleural or pericardial origin, erysipelas-like redness near the ankle, and joint involvement. Duration and frequency of attacks are unpredictable. Some of the patients develop amyloidosis. Otherwise, the prognosis is favorable even though there is no specific therapy.

familial periodic paralysis. A rare familial disease in which attacks of flaccid paralysis, often at time of awakening, occur. This condition is usually associated with hypokalemia, but is sometimes present even though the blood potassium level is normal or elevated. In affected individuals, the condition may be precipitated by administration of glucose in patients who are hypokalemic; and by administering potassium chloride in those with hyperkalemia.

Caution: These tests may cause cardiac or respiratory changes and should not be done by inexperienced physicians.

TREAT: Acetazolamide is used to prevent either hypokalemia or hyperkalemia. Oral potassium chloride is given in attacks accompanied by hypokalemia.

family. 1. A group of individuals who have descended from a common ancestor. 2. In biological classification, the division between an order and a genus. 3. A group of people living in a household who share common attachments, such as mutual caring, emotional bonds, regular interactions, and common goals, which include the health of the individuals in the family.

family care leave. Being permitted to be absent from work in order to care for a family member who is pregnant, ill, disabled, or incapacitated.

family planning. The planning and spacing of conception of children according to the wishes of the couple rather than to chance. It is accomplished by practicing some form of birth control.

family practice. Comprehensive medical care with particular emphasis on the family unit, in which the physician's continuing responsibility for health care is not limited by the patient's age or sex nor by a particular organ system or disease entity.

Family practice is the specialty that builds upon a core of knowledge derived from other disciplines, drawing most heavily on Internal Medicine, Pediatrics, Obstetrics and Gynecology, Surgery and Psychiatry, and establishes a cohesive unit, combining the behavioral sciences with the traditional biological and clinical sciences. The core of knowledge encompassed by the discipline of Family Practice prepares the family physician for a unique role in patient management, problem solving, counseling and as a personal physician who coordinates total health care delivery. (Definition supplied by The American Academy of Family Physicians.)

family therapy. Treatment of the members of a family together, rather than an individual "patient"; the family unit is viewed as a social system important to all of its members.

famine. Pronounced scarcity of food, causing hunger and starvation.

Fanconi's syndrome [Guido Fanconi, Swiss pediatrician, 1892–1979]. 1. Congenital hypoplastic anemia. 2. Aminoaciduria associated with rickets, q.v., due to failure of the proximal renal tubules or to dysfunction of the deamination process. Symptoms include rickets, polyuria, and growth failure. Dietary therapy is of some help but the patients usually die prior to puberty.

fang [AS., to plunder]. 1. A sharp-pointed tooth. 2. The root of a tooth.

fango (făn'gō) [Italian, mud]. Mud obtained from thermal springs in Battaglia, Italy. Used in treating rheumatism and gout.

Fannia (făn'ē-ă). A genus of small houseflies.

fantast (făn'tăst) [Gr. *phantasia,* imagination]. A daydreamer.

fantasy (făn'tă-sē) [Gr. *phantasia,* imagination]. The mechanism of creating in one's mind that which is unreal and may be disordered and weird; may also be creative.

F.A.O.T.A. *Fellow of the American Occupational Therapy Association.*

FAPTA. *Fellow of the American Physical Therapy Association.*

farad (făr'ăd) [Michael Faraday, Brit. physicist, 1791–1867]. A unit of electrical capacity. The capacity of a condenser that, charged with 1 coulomb, gives a difference of potential of 1 volt. This unit is so large that one-millionth part of it has been adopted as a practical unit called a microfarad.

faraday (făr'ă-dā). The amount of electrical charge associated with one gram equivalent of an electrochemical reaction. Equal to approx. 96,000 coulombs. SEE: *coulomb; farad.*

faradic. Pert. to induced electricity.

faradism. The therapeutic use of an interrupted current to stimulate muscles and nerves. Such a current is derived from the secondary or induction coil.

faradization. 1. The treatment of nerves or muscles with faradic current. 2. The condition of nerves or muscles so treated.

faradotherapy. Treatment of disease by faradic current.

farcy (făr'sē) [L. *farcire,* to stuff]. A chronic form of glanders, q.v.

    f., button. Farcy marked by dermal tubercular nodules.

farina (fă-rē'nă) [L.]. Finely ground meal commonly made from wheat or other grain. Used as cereal and flour.

farinaceous (făr″ĭ-nā'shŭs). 1. Starchy. 2. Pert. to flour.

farmer's lung. A form of hypersensitivity alveolitis caused by exposure to moldy hay that has fermented. *Actinomyces micropolyspora faeni* and *Thermoactinomyces vulgaris* are the causative microorganisms. SEE: *alveolitis; bagassosis; hypersensitivity.*

farpoint. The farthest point of vision at which objects can be seen distinctly with eyes in complete relaxation.

Farre's tubercles (fărz) [John R. Farre, Brit. physician, 1775–1862]. Carcinomatous masses on surface of the liver.

farsighted. Pert. to farsightedness.

farsightedness. An error of refraction in which, with accommodation completely relaxed, parallel rays come to a focus behind the retina. Individuals affected can see distant objects clearly, but cannot see near objects in proper focus. SYN: *hyperopia.*

fart [Old High Ger. *fezan,* to break wind]. Term for passage of intestinal gas via the anus. SEE: *flatus.*

fascia (făsh'ē-ă) [L., a band] (pl. *fasciae*). [NA] A fibrous membrane covering, supporting, and separating muscles. It also unites the skin with underlying tissue. Fascia may be superficial, a nearly subcutaneous covering permitting free movement of the skin, or it may be deep, enveloping and binding muscles.

    f., Abernethy's. A layer of areolar tissue separating the external iliac artery from the iliac fascia over the psoas muscle.

    f., anal. Fascia of connective tissue covering levator ani muscle from the perineal aspect.

    f., aponeurotic. Thick fascia that provides attachment for a muscle.

    f., Buck's. Fascial covering of the penis, derived from Colles' fascia.

    f., cervical, deep. Fascia of the neck covering the muscles, vessels, and nerves.

    f., cervical, superficial. Fascia of the neck just inside the skin.

    f., Cloquet's. Femoral fascia.

    f., Colles'. Inner layer of the perineal fascia.

    f., cremasteric. Fascia covering the cremaster muscle of the spermatic cord.

    f., cribriform. Fascia of the thigh covering the saphenous opening.

    f., crural. Deep fascia of the leg.

    f., deep. The connective tissue covering for all of the body. It is just below the superficial fascia and adipose tissue.

    f., dentate. Gray matter in the cerebral dentate convolution. SYN: *gyrus, dentate.*

f., endothoracic. Fascia that separates the pleura of the lung from the inside of the thoracic cavity and the diaphragm.

f., extrapleural. Endothoracic fascia.

f., intercolumnar. Fascia derived from the external abdominal ring sheathing the spermatic cord and testis.

f. lata femoris. [NA] Wide fascia encasing the hips and the thigh muscles.

f., lumbodorsal. Deep investing membrane covering deep muscles of the trunk and back.

f., pectineal. Pubic section of fascia lata.

f., pelvic. Fascial tissues of extreme importance in the maintenance of normal strength in the pelvic floor. SEE: *diaphragm, pelvic.*

f., pharyngobasilar. Sheet of connective tissue lying between the mucosal and muscular layers of the pharyngeal wall. SYN: *aponeurosis, pharyngeal.*

f., plantar. Sheet of connective tissue investing the muscles of the sole of the foot. SYN: *aponeurosis, plantar.*

f., Scarpa's. The deep layer of the superficial fascia of the abdomen.

f., superficial. The connective tissue layer just below the skin.

f., thyrolaryngeal. Fascia covering the thyroid gland.

f. transversalis. Fascia located between the perineum and transversalis muscle. It lines the abdominal cavity.

fasciae (făsh′ē-ē). Pl. of fascia.

fascial (făsh′ē-ăl) [L. *fascia,* a band]. Pert. to or of the nature of fascia.

fascial reflex. Muscular contraction resulting from percussing facial fascia.

fasciaplasty (făsh′ē-ă-plăs″tē) [″ + Gr. *plassein,* to form]. Plastic surgery of fascia.

fascicle (făs′ĭ-kl) [L. *fasciculus,* little bundle]. A fasciculus.

fascicular (fă-sĭk′ū-lăr). 1. Arranged like a bundle of rods. 2. Pert. to a fasciculus.

fasciculation (fă-sĭk″ū-lă′shŭn). 1. Formation of fascicles. 2. Involuntary contraction or twitching of muscle fibers. These can be seen under the skin. 3. Spontaneous contractions of muscle fibers that do not cause movement at a joint. A bioelectric potential caused by deterioration of anterior horn cells.

fasciculus (fă-sĭk′ū-lŭs) (pl. *fasciculi*). [NA] A small bundle, esp. of nerve or muscle fibers. More specifically, a division of a funiculus of the spinal cord consisting of fibers of one or more tracts. Sometimes the term is used as a synonym for tract. SYN: *fasciola.*

f. cuneatus. A triangular-shaped bundle of nerve fibers lying in the dorsal funiculus of the spinal cord. Its fibers enter the cord through the dorsal roots of spinal nerves

and terminate in the medulla. SYN: *column of Burdach.*

f., dorsolateral. Tract, dorsolateral, q.v.

f., fundamental. Portion of anterior column of the spinal cord continuing into the medulla oblongata.

f. gracilis. A bundle of nerve fibers lying in the dorsal funiculus of the spinal cord medial to the fasciculus cuneatus. Conducts sensory impulses from the periphery to the medulla. SYN: *column of Goll.*

f., longitudinal, dorsal. A bundle of association fibers connecting the frontal lobe with the occipital and temporal lobes.

f., longitudinal, inferior. A bundle of association fibers connecting the occipital and temporal lobes of the brain.

f., longitudinal, medial. A bundle of fibers running from the spinal cord to the upper portion of the midbrain.

f., longitudinal, posterior. Nerve fiber bundle running between corpora quadrigemina and nuclei of 4th and 6th nerves.

f., unciform. Fibers within sylvian fissure connecting frontal and temporosphenoid lobes. SYN: *uncinate fasciculus.*

fasciectomy (făsh″ē-ĕk′tō-mē) [L. *fascia,* band, + Gr. *ektome,* excision]. Excision of strips of fascia.

fasciitis (făs″ē-ī′tĭs). Inflammation of any fascia.

fasciodesis (făsh″ē-ŏd′ē-sĭs) [″ + Gr. *desis,* binding]. Operation of attaching a fascia to a tendon or another fascia.

Fasciola (fă-sī′ō-lă) [L. *fasciola,* a band]. A genus of flukes belonging to the class Trematoda.

F. hepatica. A species of flukes infesting the liver and bile ducts of cattle, sheep, and other herbivores; the common liver fluke. An occasional parasite of man. Intermediate hosts are snails belonging to the genus *Lymnaea.*

fasciola (fă-sī′ō-lă, fă-sē′ō-lă) [L., a band] (pl. *fasciolae*). A bundle of nerve or muscle fibers.

f. cinerea. Upper portion of dentate fascia.

fasciolar (fă-sē′ō-lăr). Pert. to the fasciola cinerea.

fasciolopsiasis (făs″ē-ō-lŏp-sī′ă-sĭs). Infection of the body with a genus of trematode worms, *Fasciolopsis buski.* It is contracted by ingesting plants grown in water infested by the intermediate host, snails. SYN: *distomiasis.*

SYM: Diarrhea, abdominal pain, anasarca, and eosinophilia.

TREAT: Praziquantel.

Fasciolopsis buski (făs″ē-ō-lŏp′sĭs). A fluke that infests the intestinal tract of certain mammals including man. Symptoms include vomiting, anorexia, and diarrhea alternating with constipation. The number of flukes present may be sufficient to cause intestinal obstruction. The disease occurs in Asia, including central and southern China. SEE: *fasciolopsiasis.*

fascioplasty (făsh′ē-ō-plăs″tē) [L. *fasciola,* a band, + Gr. *plassein,* to form]. Plastic operation on a fascia.

fasciorrhaphy (făsh-ē-or′ă-fē) [″ + Gr. *rhaphe,* seam, ridge]. Suturing a fascia.

fasciotomy (făsh-ē-ŏt′ō-mē) [″ + Gr. *tome,* incision]. Surgical incision and division of a fascia.

fascitis (fă-sī′tĭs) [″ + Gr. *itis,* inflammation]. Inflamed condition of a fascia.

FASRT. *Fellow of the American Society of Radiologic Technologists.*

fast. 1. [AS. *faest,* fixed] Resistant to the effects or action of a chemical substance. 2. [AS. *faestan,* to hold fast] Abstention from food, usually voluntary.

f., acid-. Term applied to bacteria, esp. the Mycobacteria, that after staining are not decolorized when treated with acid.

fast food. A nonspecific term for food served in commercial establishments that can serve prepared food with minimal delay.

fastidious. In microbiology, an organism that has precise nutritional and environmental requirements for growth and survival.

fastidium (făs-tĭd′ē-ŭm) [L., aversion]. Aversion to food or to eating. Sometimes seen in hysteria, but not as the result of delusions.

fastigium (făs-tĭj′ē-ŭm) [L., ridge]. 1. The highest point. The full period of development of acute, infectious diseases when the temperature reaches the maximum. 2. The most posterior portion of the 4th ventricle formed by the junction of the anterior and posterior medullary vela projecting into the medullary substance of the cerebellum.

fasting [AS. *faestan,* to hold fast]. Going without food. Energy requirements of body metabolism during fasting are supplied by the oxidization of fats, which, if glucose is not supplied, results in the products of incomplete fat metabolism such as fatty acids, diacetic acid, and acetone, producing ketosis and a mild acidosis. This condition occurs quickly in children as they have little glycogen reserve.

Caution: Unsupervised fasting in order to lose weight can cause death.

fastness [AS. *faest,* fixed]. Ability of bacteria to resist stains or destructive agents.

fat [AS. *faett*]. 1. Adipose tissue of the body, which serves as an energy reserve. SEE: *obesity.* 2. Grease, oil. 3. In chemistry, triglyceride ester of fatty acids; one of a group of organic compounds closely associated in nature with the phosphatides, cerebrosides, and sterols. The term lipid, q.v., is applied in general to a fat or fatlike substance. Fats are insoluble in water but soluble in ether, chloroform, benzene, and other fat solvents. Upon hydrolysis, fats break down into fatty acids and glycerol (an alcohol). Fats are hydrolyzed by the action of acids, alkalies, lipases (fat-splitting enzymes) and superheated steam.

CHEM. STRUCTURE: In the fat molecule, one molecule of glycerol is combined with three of fatty acids. Three fatty acids, oleic acid ($C_{18}H_{34}O_2$), stearic acid ($C_{18}H_{36}O_2$), and palmitic acid ($C_{16}H_{32}O_2$), constitute the bulk of fatty acids present in neutral fats found in body tissues. According to the fatty acid with which the glycerol is combined, corresponding fats are triolein, tristearin, and tripalmitin. These three fats are the principal fats present in foods.

PHYS.: Fats serve as a source of energy. Subcutaneous fat also provides an insulating layer that inhibits heat loss. Fat acts to support and protect certain organs such as the eye and kidney; provides a concentrated reserve of food; provides essential fatty acids necessary for normal growth and development; and in foods is a vehicle for natural fat-soluble vitamins. In conjunction with carbohydrates, fats serve as protein sparers. They are an important constituent of cell structure, forming an integral part of the cell membrane. When properly distributed, fat gives a pleasing contour to the body.

Because certain fatty acids (linoleic, *d*-linolenic, and arachidonic) are necessary for formation of other products in the body and because they are not themselves synthesized in the body, they are classed *essential fatty acids.* Linolenic acid can, however, be converted into other fatty acids including arachidonic acid. Arachidonic acid is of particular importance because it is essential to the formation of prostaglandins, thromboxanes, prostacyclins, and leukotrienes. These three essential fatty acids are obtainable in the diet from plant sources.

Animals fed a fat-free diet develop dermatitis, fail to grow; the liver becomes fatty, and there are neurological disturbances. These changes can be prevented or reversed by adding linoleic and linolenic acids to the diet. The human diet should consist of about 4% of the calories from linoleic and 1% from linolenic acids.

The importance of fats as a stored source of energy in the body is apparent when the fact that only enough carbohydrate in the form of glycogen can be stored to supply bodily energy needs for about 12 hours; but in the 70-kg man of average build, 12 kg of stored fat (in the form of triacylglycerols) is enough to supply the energy needs for as long as 8 weeks.

DIGESTION AND ABSORPTION: In the stomach, emulsified fats such as cream or egg yolk are acted on by gastric lipase; however, most fats undergo digestion in the intestine, where they are acted on by a pancreatic lipase, steapsin, which hydrolyzes them to fatty acids and glycerol. Although containing no lipolytic enzymes, bile is essential for the digestion of fats. It aids in the emulsification of fats and has a hydrotropic action, i.e., renders substances such as fatty acids, which are normally insoluble in water, readily soluble in the intestinal juices. Bile salts also act as specific activators of the pancreatic lipase. Bile salts react with fatty acids, forming water-soluble, diffusible soaps that facilitate the emulsification of fats. Glycerol and fatty acids enter the epithelial cells, where they recombine to form neutral fats, most of which enter the lacteals. The fats are carried in the lymph through lymph vessels to the thoracic duct, from which they enter the bloodstream. After a meal rich in fats, the mesenteric lymph vessels are filled with a milklike fluid, the chyle, containing finely emulsified fat particles called chylomicrons.

METABOLISM: Absorbed fats are utilized in the following ways: oxidized with the release of energy; deposited in adipose tissue as storage fat; incorporated in the cells of tissues as an integral part of the protoplasm; desaturated and stored in the liver; excreted in the secretions of the mammary and sweat glands and in the feces.

Intermediary metabolism: In the oxidation of fat to carbon dioxide and water, several intermediary substances (ketones) are formed. The principal ones are acetoacetic acid, betahydroxybutyric acid, and acetone. Excessive production of ketone bodies, which occurs when fats are incompletely oxidized, is called ketosis. This especially occurs when there is an interference in carbohydrate metabolism, as in diabetes. Ketosis also occurs in starvation, in certain fevers, toxemias of pregnancy, and hyperthyroidism. Ketosis results in acidosis.

SOURCES: In addition to fat being absorbed from the intestine, body fat may arise from the conversion of carbohydrates (glucose) or proteins into fat. Fatty acids cannot be converted directly to glucose in the body, but a portion of the molecule of fatty acids of certain length can be utilized as carbohydrate.

NUTRITION: Fats have a high caloric value, yielding about 9 Cal per gm as compared with about 4 Cal for carbohydrates and proteins. The average diet of 3000 Cal may derive 40% of the caloric value from fats. Nutritionists and epidemiologists feel that decreasing fat in the diet to 30% would decrease the risk of developing cancer, esp. of the colon, breast, and prostate. In addition to their nutritive values, fats improve the taste and odor of foods, provide a feeling of satiety, and because of their high caloric content are of special importance in high-caloric diets.

CONTRA: Fat intake should be reduced in certain diseases such as hepatitis and in low-caloric diets.

RS: bile; fatty acid; gallbladder; glycerin; ketone; ketosis; lipase; liver.

f., neutral. Compounds of the higher fatty acids (palmitic, stearic, and oleic) with glycerol. They are the common fats of animal and plant tissues.

fat, words pert. to: absorption; acid; "adip-" words; anorexia nervosa; body composition; caloric excess; calorie; cholesterol; chondrolipoma; diet; digestion; energy; fasting; fatty acid; food; food requirements; fuel value; glucose; hydrogenation; ketogenic diet; ketone; ketosis; "lip-" words; obesity; palmitic acid; palmitin; reduction diet; steapsin; stearin; stearrhea; triacylglycerols.

fatal (fāt′l) [L. *fatalis*]. 1. Inevitable. 2. Causing death.

fatality. A death, especially from an accident or a disaster.

fat emulsion. Combination for liquid, lipid, and an emulsifying system suitable for I.V. use. This isotonic solution should not be mixed with other materials given I.V.

fatigability (făt″ĭ-gă-bĭl′ĭ-tē). Condition of becoming easily tired or exhausted.

fatigue (fă-tēg′) [L. *fatigare*, to tire]. 1. A feeling of tiredness or weariness resulting from continued activity or as a side effect from some psychotropic drug. 2. The state or condition of an organ or tissue in which its response to stimulation is reduced or lost as a result of overactivity. 3. To bring about a condition of fatigue.

Fatigue may be the result of excessive activity, which results in the accumulation of metabolic waste products such as lactic acid; malnutrition (deficiency of carbohydrates, proteins, minerals, or vitamins); circulatory disturbances such as heart disease or anemia, which interfere with the supply of oxygen and energy materials to tissues; respiratory disturbances, which interfere with the supply of oxygen to tissues; infectious diseases, in which toxic products are produced or body metabolism altered; endocrine disturbances such as occur in diabetes, hyperinsulinism, and menopause; psychogenic factors such as emotional conflicts, frustration, anxiety, neurosis, boredom; physical factor such as being crippled. Environmental noise and vibration contribute to the development of fatigue. SEE: *chronic fatigue syndrome.*

   f., acute. Fatigue with sudden onset such as occurs following excessive exertion; relieved by rest.

   f., chronic. Long-continued fatigue not relieved by rest. Indicative of disease such as tuberculosis or diabetes or other conditions of altered body metabolism.

   f., muscular. The reduced capacity of a muscle to perform work as a result of repeated contractions. Fatigue may be partial or complete.

fat overload syndrome. A rare complication of intravenous administration of fat emulsion. Symptoms include sudden elevation of serum triglyceride level, fever, hepatosplenomegaly, coagulopathy, and dysfunction of other organs. Specific therapy is not available, but plasma exchange has been used experimentally.

fat replacements. Substances developed to provide all of the characteristics of fats but have either relatively few calories or none at all. Simplesse is the trade name for a fat substitute made of milk and egg white. It provides 1 to 2 calories per gram. A calorie-free fat replacement may be available, as the product Olestra. It performs the same functions as fat but it is not digested by the body and is not absorbed from the gastrointestinal tract.

fatty (făt′ē). Of, or pert. to, fats or fatty substances; adipose. SEE: *fat; heart; obesity.*

fatty acid. A hydrocarbon in which one of the hydrogen atoms has been replaced by a carboxyl (COOH) group; a monobasic aliphatic acid made up of an alkyl radical attached to a carboxyl group.

   Saturated fatty acids have single bonds in their carbon chain with the general formula $C_nH_{2n}O_2$. They include acetic, butyric, caproic, caprylic, capric, lauric, formic, myristic, palmitic, and stearic acids. Unsaturated fatty acids have one or more double or triple bonds in the carbon chain. They include those of the oleic series (oleic, tiglic, hypogeic, and palmitoleic) and the linoleic or linolic series (linoleic, linolenic, clupanodonic, arachidonic, hydrocarpic, and chaulmoogric acids). Fatty acids are insoluble in water. This would prevent their being absorbed from the intestines were it not for the action of bile salts on the fatty acids to enable them to be absorbed. SEE: *fat.*

   f.a., essential. The unsaturated fatty acids (linoleic, linolenic, and arachidonic)

cannot be synthesized in the body and have been considered to be essential to maintain health. SEE: *digestion.*

   f.a., free. ABBR: FFA. The form of fatty acids as they leave the cell to be transported for use in another part of the body. These acids are not esterified. In the plasma they immediately combine with albumin.

fatty acids, omega-3 (ω3). SEE: *acids, omega-3 fatty.*

fatty casts. Casts seen in the urine sediments. They are usually abnormal and consist of a mass of fat globules.

fatty change. Any abnormal accumulation of fat within parenchymal cells. This may occur in the heart or other organs. It is seen in the liver, usually resulting from the effect of excessive and prolonged alcohol intake.

fatty degeneration. A change involving the deposition of fat in the cytoplasm of cells.

fauces (fŏ′sēz) [L.]. [NA] The constricted opening leading from the mouth and the oral pharynx. It is bounded by the soft palate, base of the tongue, and the palatine arches. The anterior pillars of the fauces are known as the glossopalatine arch, and the posterior pillars as the pharyngopalatine arch. SEE: *fossa.*

faucial (fŏ′shăl) [L. *fauces,* throat]. Pert. to the fauces.

faucial reflex. Gagging or vomiting resulting from irritation of the fauces.

faucitis (fŏ-sī′tĭs) [″ + Gr. *itis,* inflammation]. Inflammation of the fauces.

fauna (faw′nă) [L. *Faunus,* mythical deity of herdsmen]. All of the animals, including microscopic forms, in the area considered. SEE: *flora.*

faveolate (fă-vē′ō-lăt) [L. *faveolus,* little honeycomb]. Honeycombed. SYN: *alveolate.*

faveolus (fă-vē′ō-lŭs) [L., little honeycomb]. A depression or small pit, esp. on the skin. SYN: *foveola.*

favism (fā′vĭzm) [It. *fava,* bean, + Gr. *-ismos,* condition]. A hereditary condition common in Sicily and Sardinia resulting from sensitivity to a species of bean, *Vicia faba.* It is characterized by fever, acute hemolytic anemia, vomiting, diarrhea, and may lead to prostration and coma. It is caused by ingestion of the beans or inhalation of the pollen of the plant by persons who have an inherited deficiency of the enzyme glucose-6-phosphate dehydrogenase.

favus (fā′vŭs) [L., honeycomb]. Skin disease caused by the fungus *Trichophyton schoenleinii.* It is characterized by pinhead to pea-sized, saucer-shaped, yellowish crust (scutulum) over hair follicles of the scalp and is accompanied by musty odor and itching. It may spread all over the body. SEE: *scutulum.*

F.C.A.P. *Fellow of the College of American Pathologists.*

Fc fragments. Small pieces, i.e., fragments, of immunoglobulins (antibodies) used by macrophages in their processing and presenting of foreign antigens to T lymphocytes. SEE: *macrophage processing; specific immune response.*

Fc receptors. Receptors on monocytes and macrophages that bind Fc fragments, q.v., of immunoglobulins G and E, q.v. SEE: *immunoglobulin; macrophage processing; phagocytosis.*

F.D. *fatal dose; focal distance.*

F.D.A. *Food and Drug Administration.*

FDP. *fibrin degradation products.*

Fe [L. *ferrum*]. Chemical symbol for the element iron.

fear [AS. *faer*]. Fright, dread. Primitively, the emotional reaction to an environmental threat; it now also presents itself frequently as an indicator of inner problems. Fear is present in anxiety disorders and depression. At the somatic level, hyperthyroidism and hyperadrenalism may strongly simulate the fear state. SEE: *emotion; Phobias* in *Appendix.*

features. Any part of the face.

febricide (fĕb'rĭ-sīd) [L. *febris*, fever, + *cidus*, killing]. Destructive to fever. SYN: *antipyretic.*

febrifacient (fĕb-rĭ-fā'sē-ĕnt) [" + *facere*, to make]. Producing fever.

febrifugal (fĕb-rĭf'ū-găl) [" + *fugare*, to put to flight]. Reducing fever.

febrifuge (fĕb'rĭ-fūj). That which reduces fever. SYN: *antipyretic.*

febrile (fē'brĭl, fē'brĭl, fĕb'rĭl) [L. *febris*, fever]. Feverish; pert. to a fever. SEE: *fever.*

febrile convulsions. About three to five percent of children will experience a convulsion associated with fever. Most will have this in the period between six months and two to three years of age. Febrile convulsions are rare after age six to eight. Boys are more susceptible than girls to this type of convulsion. It is important to do a complete history and physical examination including neurological appraisal for the possibility of another cause, such as tetany, epilepsy, acute lead encephalopathy, cerebral concussion or hemorrhage or tumor, hypoglycemia, or poisoning with a convulsant drug. SEE: *epilepsy.*

TREAT: Appropriate therapy for reduction of the elevated body temperature, and a sedative dose of phenobarbital, 3 mg/kg/day of body weight. It is important that the measures to reduce the temperature not be so vigorous as to cause hypothermia. The application of cool compresses with gentle flow of air over the body will suffice. A hypo-

thermia blanket is also suitable for use. Ice water baths and vigorous fanning of the child as alcohol is applied will most probably produce hypothermia and should not be used. In the past, the recommendation has been made that a child who has experienced a single febrile convulsion should have daily anticonvulsant therapy for a two- to four-year period. The efficacy and advisability of this have not been proved.

Caution: 1. If the fever is due to influenza or varicella, do not administer salicylates; their use could increase the risk of developing Reye's syndrome. 2. Prolonged treatment with phenobarbital depresses cognitive function in children.

---

febrile state. A term used to describe constitutional symptoms that accompany a rise in temperature. Pulse and respiration usually rise with headache, pains, malaise, loss of appetite, concentrated and diminished urine, constipation, restlessness, insomnia, and irritability.

febriphobia (fĕb"rĭ-fō'bē-ă) [" + Gr. *phobos*, fear]. Anxiety or fear induced by a rise in body temperature.

febris (fē'brĭs) [L.]. Fever.

    f. enterica. Typhoid fever.

    f. flava. Yellow fever.

    f. undulans. Brucellosis.

fecal (fē'kăl) [L. *faeces*, refuse]. Pert. to, or of the nature of, feces.

fecal impaction. The formation of a firm mass of feces in the distal colon or rectum. The size and firmness of the mass prevents its passage.

    ETIOL: Congenital megacolon in children; psychiatric disorders; painful anal conditions that inhibit the patient's desire to defecate; intestinal obstruction; dehydration; immobility in elderly debilitated patients; spinal cord injury; rectal neoplasms; and use of narcotics.

    TREAT: Manual extraction is the indicated and usual initial treatment. This may require local anesthesia. The impaction is fragmented by using a scissoring action of the fingers. After the impaction is fragmented, use of mild laxatives, such as mineral oil instilled into the rectum, will provide lubrication and assist in passage of the fragments. Rarely will surgery be required.

fecalith (fē'kă-lĭth) [" + Gr. *lithos*, stone]. A fecal concretion. SYN: *coprolith.*

fecaloid (fē'kă-loyd) [" + Gr. *eidos*, form, shape]. Resembling feces.

fecaloma (fē"kăl-ō'mă) [" + Gr. *oma*, tumor]. A large mass of accumulated feces in the rectum resembling a tumor. SYN: *scatoma; stercoroma.*

fecaluria (fē″kăl-ū′rē-ă) [″ + Gr. *ouron*, urine]. Fecal matter in the urine.

fecal vomit. Feces in vomitus. Occurs in strangulated hernia or intestinal obstruction preventing normal bowel movements.

feces (fē′sēz) [L. *faeces*]. Stools; excreta; dejecta; excrement. Body waste such as food residue, bacteria, epithelium, and mucus, discharged from the bowels by way of the anus. SYN: *stool.*

COMP: The total weight of the stool in a healthy adult male on a normal diet will be 100 to 200 gm daily. Of this, 65% will be water and the remainder dry matter. Excreted nitrogen will be less than 1.7 gm daily. The stool is composed of residue of food including undigested cellulose; water; secretions from intestinal glands, stomach, and liver; indole; skatole; cholesterol; mucus and epithelial cells; purine bases; pigment; microorganisms; inorganic salts; and sometimes foreign substances. The normal reaction is neutral or slightly alkaline. The stools of infants usually are acid.

DIAG: Inspection should include color, form, odor, and the presence of any observable foreign substances.

Color: May be indicative of various disorders. *Black* or *tarry* stools can indicate bleeding or hemorrhage into the gastrointestinal tract. Tarry is used to describe stools containing digested blood. May also follow the use of drugs such as bismuth, iron, tannin, manganese, or charcoal. *Bloody:* May indicate hemorrhoids, cancer of the rectum, ulcers, fissures, abraded rectal membrane from dry feces, eroded rectal polypus, acute proctitis, foreign bodies, colitis, intussusception or strangulated hernia in children, cancer of the colon, typhoid fever, or phosphorus poisoning. *Clay-colored:* May denote impaired bile formation or obstruction, phosphorus poisoning, or yellow atrophy of the liver. *Green:* In general, this indicates in children and infants that the bowel contents have passed quickly through the intestinal tract.

Form and Consistency: Normally soft and formed. Hard, nodular, or scybalous in constipation. Fluid or mushy in diarrhea. Consistently flattened or ribbonlike in rectal obstruction or spastic colitis. Greasy in jaundice.

Mucus: Amount should be noted. Present in abnormal as well as normal circumstances. May occur as superficial gelatinous streaks or blobs; mixed with the stool and only apparent after making a thin paste with water; mixed with blood as in dysentery of the stool. Mucus may be the principal component.

Odor: This varies with disease and dietary differences. Variations such as sour, pungent, or putrid occur in different diseases. SEE: *flatus. Offensive odor:* In jaundice, acute indigestion, enteritis, typhoid fever, and occasionally constipation. *Putrid odor:* May be the result of syphilitic or carcinomatous ulceration of the rectum or gangrenous dysentery. *Sour odor:* Normal stools of infants.

Parasites: The presence of various intestinal parasites can be determined by examination of the feces. Gross examination may reveal the presence of nematodes (roundworms) or tapeworms; however, microscopic examination is necessary to determine the presence of protozoa, helminth ova, or larvae. In examination of feces, stools are collected in clean dry containers. For microscopic examination, representative bits of feces or mucus are emulsified in saline solution on a clean slide, then spread evenly, and covered with a coverglass. Diagnosis of pinworms is done by examination of scrapings or contact slides from the anal and perianal regions.

feces, words pert. to: anus; colon; constipation; defecation; diarrhea; elimination; enema; excreta; excretion; impaction; intestine; meconium; melanorrhea; melena; rectum; scatology; sigmoid; steatorrhea; stool.

Fechner's law (fĕk′nĕrz) [Gustav Theodor Fechner, Ger. psychologist, 1801–1887]. A theory stating that the magnitudes of sensation produced by given stimuli form an arithmetical progression, the stimuli forming a geometrical progression.

Fe(C₃H₅O₃)₂. Ferrous lactate; lactate of iron.

FeCl₂. Ferrous chloride.

FeCl₃. Ferric chloride.

FeCO₃. Ferrous carbonate.

fecula (fĕk′ū-lă) [L. *faecula*, dregs]. 1. Sediment. 2. Starch.

feculent (fĕk′ū-lĕnt) [L. *faeculentus*]. Having sediment.

fecund. Fertile.

fecundate (fē′kŭn-dāt) [L. *fecundare*, to bear fruit]. To fertilize or impregnate or render fertile.

fecundation (fē″kŭn-dā′shŭn). Impregnation; fertilization.

 f., artificial. Impregnation by injecting the seminal fluid into the uterus by mechanical means. SYN: *artificial insemination.*

fecundity (fē-kŭn′dĭ-tē). Ability to produce offspring; fertility.

feedback. 1. The return of some output to the place of origin by the system that receives it.

 To a certain degree, blood pressure and blood sugar are regulated by feedback mechanisms. Feedback may be negative or positive. Thus, a positive feedback signal indicates that more blood glucose needs to be made available when blood sugar level falls. Conversely, a negative feedback signal occurs when the blood sugar level rises to normal, indicating that production of blood sugar should be reduced or stopped. 2. In psychiatry, the expressed verbal reaction or physical reaction, i.e., body language, of one person to another person's actions or behaviors.

feeder. A device permitting independent eating by persons with severe motor control problems.

feeding [AS. *fedan*, to give food to]. Taking or giving nourishment.

f., artificial. 1. Providing a liquid food preparation through a tube passed into the stomach or the rectum. Also through gastrostomy or duodenostomy. SEE: *hyperalimentation.* 2. Feeding of a baby with food other than mother's milk.

f., breast. Feeding of an infant at the breast.

f., forced. Tube feeding to an individual who doesn't want to eat or to be fed by this means.

f., intravenous. Administration of fluids and nutrients through a vein.

f., rectal. Type rarely used, because little nourishment can be absorbed through colon. Normal saline often used with glucose, making a 5% to 10% solution by adding 15 to 30 gm of sugar to 10 oz (300 ml) of normal saline.

f., tube. Feeding through a tube that extends through the mouth or nostril and into the stomach. Indicated for patients who cannot swallow or masticate food, but who have functioning GI tracts. The nasal method is most often used, and requires a much smaller tube and a little more dexterity but is less likely to be successfully resisted. A tube lubricated with glycerin is gently passed into pharynx and, avoiding the larynx, is passed into the stomach. Entry into the larynx may produce struggling and cyanosis.

Caution: Prior to feedings be certain that tube is in stomach and not in the bronchus. This can be determined by aspirating the tube and observing for gastric contents or by listening to the end of the tube. If air comes out of the tube with each expiration, the tube is not in the stomach. If the position of the tube is in doubt, inject a small amount of air into it and at the same time auscultate the stomach area. If the tube is present in the stomach, a gurgling should be heard as the air is injected. Foods or nutritional substances as ordered by the phy-

sician are fed slowly.

feeding center. An area in the hypothalamus that may act to control food intake. SEE: *satiety center; weight, set point.*

feeling [AS. *felan*, to feel]. The conscious phase of nervous activity. The emotions are centrally stimulated feelings and those sensations peripherally produced by excitation of peripheral nerves, including those of the special senses.

Feen-A-Mint. Trade name of phenolphthalein.

Feer's disease (fārz) [Emil Feer, Swiss pediatrician, 1864–1955]. Acrodynia, q.v.

feet [AS. *fet*] (sing. *foot*). The pedal extremities of the legs. SEE: *foot.*

Fehling's solution (fā′lĭngz) [Hermann von Fehling, Ger. chemist, 1812–1885]. A solution used for detecting the presence of sugar in urine. It consists of equal parts of solutions A and B prepared as follows: Solution A (copper solution): dissolve 34.66 gm of copper sulfate crystals in an amount of water to make 500 ml. Solution B (alkaline tartrate solution): dissolve 173 gm of crystallized potassium sodium tartrate and 50 gm of sodium hydroxide in an amount of water to make 500 ml. Mix equal portions of solutions A and B just before using. This mixture is then added to the urine sample and the liquid is boiled. If sugar is present, a red precipitate of cuprous oxide is formed.

Feingold diet. (fīn′gōld) [Benjamin Feingold, U.S. pediatrician, 1900–1982]. A diet in which all foods containing artificial coloring, flavoring, and preserving materials are excluded. Used in treating hyperactive children.

fel (fĕl) [L.]. Bile.

feline (fē′lĭn) [L. *feles*, cat]. Concerning cats.

fellatio (fĕl-ā′shē-ō) [L. *fellare*, to suck]. Oral (not vocal) stimulation of the penis. SEE: *cunnilingus.*

fellatrix, fellatrice. A female who performs fellatio.

felon (fĕl′ŏn) [ME. *feloun*, malignant]. Infection or abscess of soft tissue of terminal joint of a finger. SYN: *whitlow.*

feltwork. 1. Fibrous network. 2. A plexus of nerve fibrils.

Felty's syndrome (fĕl′tēz) [Augustus Roi Felty, U.S. physician, b. 1895]. Chronic rheumatoid arthritis associated with splenomegaly, neutropenia, and in some cases anemia and thrombocytopenia. Occurs most commonly in patients with long-standing disease.

female [L. *femella*, little woman]. 1. An individual of the sex that produces ova or bears young. 2. Characteristics of this sex. SEE:

genitalia, female.

feminine (fĕm′ĭ-nĭn). Concerning or being of the female sex.

feminism [L. *femininus*]. The development of female secondary sexual characteristics in the male. SEE: *gynecomastia.*

feminization. The normal development of female secondary sexual characteristics, or the pathologic development of these in the male. SEE: *sex determination.*

    f., testicular. An apparent female in whom genetic sex is male. Caused by the inability of the tissues to respond to the male hormone produced by the testicles. External genitalia are rudimentary, and the testicles may be in the abdomen.

Feminone. Trade name for ethinyl estradiol.

femoral (fĕm′or-ăl) [L. *femoralis*]. Pert. to the thigh bone or femur.

femoral artery. Artery that begins at the external iliac artery and terminates behind the knee as the popliteal artery on the inner side of the femur. SYN: *arteria femoralis* [NA].

femoral reflex. Extension of knee and flexion of foot resulting from irritation of skin over upper anterior third of thigh.

femoral vein. Continuation of the popliteal vein upward toward the external iliac vein. SYN: *vena femoralis* [NA].

femorocele (fĕm′ō-rō-sēl′) [L. *femur*, thigh, + Gr. *kele*, tumor, swelling]. Femoral hernia.

femorotibial (fĕm″ō-rō-tĭb′ē-ăl) [″ + *tibia*, pipe]. Rel. to the femur and tibia.

femto- [Danish *femten*, fifteen]. In metric system nomenclature, a prefix indicating that the entity following is to be multiplied by 10^{-15}. Thus a femtogram is 10^{-15} gram. SEE: *Metric System* in *Appendix.*

femur (fē′mŭr) [L.] (pl. *femora*). [NA] The thigh bone. It extends from the hip to the knee and is the longest and strongest bone in the skeleton. SEE: illus.

    RS: calcar femorale; cavalry bone; femoral; trochanter.

fenestra (fĕn-ĕs′tră) [L., window] (pl. *fenestrae*). 1. An aperture frequently closed by a membrane. 2. An open area, as in the blade of a forceps.

    f. cochleae. [NA] The opening leading into the cochlea. It is closed by a membrane, the secondary tympanic membrane.

    f. rotunda. Window, cochlear, q.v.; window, round, q.v.

    f. vestibuli. [NA] An oval opening on the inner wall of the middle ear or tympanum leading to the vestibule, into which the base of the stapes fits.

fenestrated (fĕn′ĕs-trāt″ĕd) [L. *fenestra*, window]. Having openings.

fenestration. 1. Condition of having a fenestra. 2. An operation in which an artificial

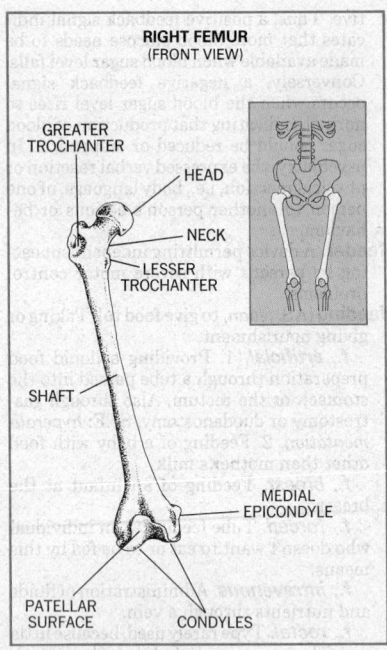

RIGHT FEMUR
(FRONT VIEW)

GREATER
TROCHANTER

HEAD

NECK

LESSER
TROCHANTER

SHAFT

MEDIAL
EPICONDYLE

PATELLAR
SURFACE

CONDYLES

opening is made into the labyrinth of the ear. Performed in cases of otosclerosis, to treat the associated deafness.

fenfluramine hydrochloride (fĕn-floor′ă-mēn). An adrenergic agent. Trade name is Pondimin.

fenoprofen calcium (fĕn-ō-prō′fĕn). USP. A nonsteroidal anti-inflammatory agent. Trade name is Nalfon.

fentanyl citrate (fĕn′tă-nĭl). USP. A potent synthetic analgesic. Trade name is Sublimaze. SEE: *"designer drug."*

Feosol. Trade name for ferrous sulfate.

Feostat. Trade name for ferrous fumarate.

feral (fĕr′ŭl) [L. *fera*, wild animal]. Existing in a wild, untamed, and undomesticated state.

Fergon. Trade name for ferrous gluconate.

ferment (fĕr-mĕnt′, fĕr′mĕnt) [L. *fermentum*]. 1. To decompose. 2. A substance capable of producing fermentation in other substances. 3. A catalytic agent that is capable of inducing fermentation in substances with which it comes in contact.

    RS: enzyme; pancreatin; papain; steapsin; trypsin; trypsinogen; tyrosinase; yeast.

fermentation. The oxidative decomposition of complex substances through the action of enzymes or ferments, produced by microorganisms. Bacteria, molds, and yeasts are the principal groups of organisms involved in fermentation. Fermentations of economic importance are those involved in the production of alcohol, alcoholic beverages, lactic and butyric acids, and the baking of bread.

f., acetic. Production of acetic acid by the bacterial oxidation of ethyl alcohol under aerobic conditions.

f., alcoholic. Production of ethyl alcohol from carbohydrates, usually through the action of yeasts.

f., amylolytic. Process of hydrolysis of starch with the formation of sugar.

f., autolytic. Disintegration of tissues after death due to enzymes present in the tissues.

f., butyric. Formation of butyric acid from bacterial action on carbohydrates under anaerobic conditions.

f., citric acid. Formation of citric acid from action of molds on carbohydrates.

f., invertin. Fermentation that converts cane sugar into dextrose and levulose.

f., lactic. Formation of lactic acid from carbohydrates by action of bacteria. The genera *Streptococcus* and *Lactobacillus* are the forms usually involved. Bacterial action is responsible for the souring of milk.

f., oxalic acid. Formation of oxalic acid from carbohydrates from the action of certain molds, esp. *Aspergillus.*

f., propionic acid. Formation of propionic acid from carbohydrates from action of certain bacteria.

f., viscous. Production of gelatinous material by different forms of bacilli.

fermentum (fĕr-mĕn'tŭm) [L.]. Yeast; a ferment.

fermium (fĕr'mē-ŭm) [Enrico Fermi, It.-U.S. physicist and Nobel Prize winner, 1901–1954]. SYMB: Fm. At. wt. 257; at. no. 100. Radioactive element.

fern [AS. *fearn*]. A flowerless plant belonging to the class Filicinae of the division Tracheophyta. At one time a substance derived from male ferns was used in treating certain kinds of intestinal parasites.

fern pattern, ferning. The palm leaf (arborization) pattern that cervical mucus assumes when placed in a thin layer on a glass slide and allowed to dry. This is seen on microscopic examination of the slide. It occurs only during certain stages of the menstrual cycle. The pattern, caused by crystallization of the mucus as it dries, is dependent upon the concentration of electrolytes present, esp. sodium chloride. The salt concentration is determined by the amount of estrogen in the mucus. Usually seen at midcycle in normal menstruating women; therefore it may be helpful in determining time of ovu-

lation in women who have difficulty becoming pregnant. The mucus has a beaded, i.e., nonferning, pattern at other times in the cycle and during pregnancy. SYN: *cervical mucus arborization.*

Fero-Gradumet. Trade name for ferrous sulfate.

-ferous [L. *ferre*, to bear]. Suffix meaning producing.

ferrated (fĕr-āt'ĕd) [L. *ferrum*, iron]. Combined with iron or containing iron.

ferri-, ferro- [L. *ferrum*, iron]. Prefix used to indicate presence of iron.

ferric. 1. Pert. to or containing iron. SYN: *ferruginous.* 2. Denoting a compound containing iron in its trivalent form.

f. chloride. FeCl₃. Used principally in form of tincture as an astringent applied to the throat.

ferrin. An iron-containing compound isolated from liver tissue.

ferritin (fĕr'ĭ-tĭn). An iron-phosphorus-protein complex containing about 23% iron. It is formed in the intestinal mucosa by the union of ferric iron with a protein, apoferritin. Ferritin is the form in which iron is stored in the tissues, principally in the reticuloendothelial cells of the liver, spleen, and bone marrow.

ferrokinetics (fĕr″rō-kĭ-nĕt'ĭks) [″ + Gr. *kinesis*, movement]. Consideration of the absorption, utilization, storage, and excretion of iron.

ferropexia (fĕr-ō-pĕks'ē-ă). Iron fixation.

ferroprotein (fĕr″ō-prō'tē-ĭn). A protein combined with an iron-containing radical. Ferroproteins are important oxygen-transferring enzymes (e.g., Warburg's enzyme, cytochrome, oxidase).

ferrotherapy (fĕr″ō-thĕr'ă-pē) [″ + Gr. *therapeia*, treatment]. Use of iron in treating anemia.

ferrous (fĕr'ŭs) [L. *ferrum*, iron]. 1. Pert. to iron. SYN: *ferruginous.* 2. Denoting a compound containing bivalent iron.

f. fumarate. USP. C₄H₂FeO₄. An iron preparation used to treat anemias. Trade name is Feostat.

f. gluconate. USP. C₁₂H₂₂FeO₁₄. Occurs as a yellowish powder or granules. Used as a hematinic. Trade name is Fergon.

f. sulfate. USP. FeSO₄. Iron sulfate. Pale, bluish-green crystals that are taken orally as a hematinic. Incompatible with alkalies, chlorides, tannic acid, and oxidizing agents. Trade names are Feosol, Fero-Gradumet, and Mol-Iron.

ferruginous (fĕr-ū'jĭ-nŭs) [L. *ferrugo*, iron rust]. 1. Pert. to or containing iron. 2. Of the color of iron rust.

ferrule (fĕr'ūl) [L. *viriola*, little bracelet]. A band or ring of metal applied to the end of

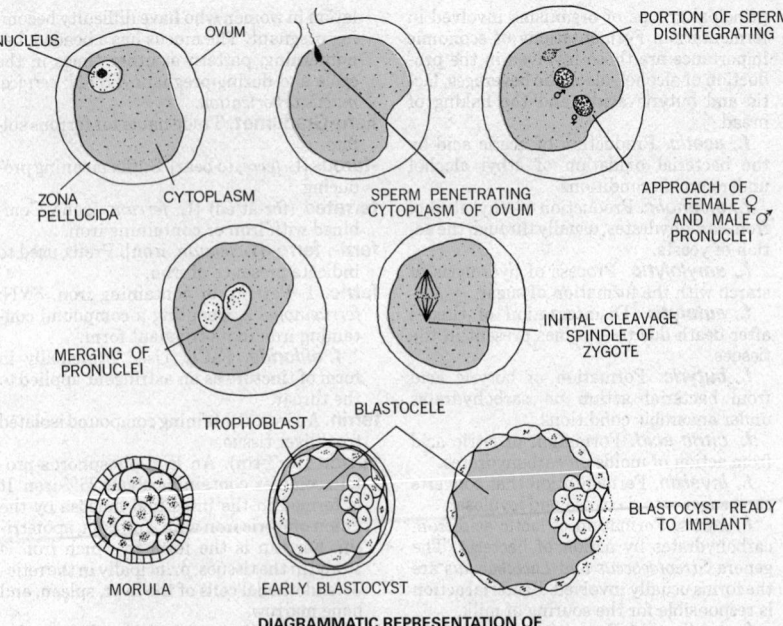

NUCLEUS   OVUM   PORTION OF SPERM DISINTEGRATING

ZONA PELLUCIDA   CYTOPLASM   SPERM PENETRATING CYTOPLASM OF OVUM   APPROACH OF FEMALE ♀ AND MALE ♂ PRONUCLEI

MERGING OF PRONUCLEI   INITIAL CLEAVAGE SPINDLE OF ZYGOTE

BLASTOCELE

TROPHOBLAST   BLASTOCYST READY TO IMPLANT

MORULA   EARLY BLASTOCYST

DIAGRAMMATIC REPRESENTATION OF OVUM AND EVENTS OF FERTILIZATION

the root or crown of a tooth in order to strengthen it.

ferrum (fĕr′ŭm) [L., iron]. SYMB: Fe. Iron.

fertile (fĕr′tĭl) [L. *fertilis*]. Capable of reproduction.

fertility (fĕr-tĭl′ĭ-tē). Quality of being productive or fertile.

fertilization [L. *fertilis,* reproductive]. 1. Fecundation; union of an ovum with the spermatozoon of the male, the male sex cell being carried in the seminal discharge. This usually takes place in the fallopian tube. Viable spermatozoa have been found in the tube 48 hours after the last coitus. After the ovum is fertilized, cell division begins. The fertilized ovum then enters the uterus, where it may implant for continued nurture and development. 2. In botany, the union of the male and female gametes. In higher plants, when the pollen tube enters the ovule, two gametes emerge, one uniting with the egg to form the zygote, from which the embryo develops; the other uniting with two endosperm nuclei to form a primary endosperm cell, from which the endosperm (reserve food) develops. SEE: illus.

RS: coitus; conception; contraceptive; embryo transfer; GIFT; impregnation; in vitro fertilization; ovum; spermatozoa; sterile; sterility.

f., heterologous. SEE: *heterologous fertilization.*

f., homologous. SEE: *homologous fertilization.*

f., in vitro. Exposure of mature oocytes to sperm in vitro. After fertilization the ova are then placed in the uterus. SEE: *embryo transfer; GIFT.*

fertilizin (fĕr″tĭ-lī′zĭn). A substance, possibly a glycoprotein, extracted from starfish or sea urchin eggs that causes agglutination of the sperm of the same species. It probably aids in fertilization by fixing sperm to the egg membrane. It is complementary to antifertilizin, a substance extracted from sperm that agglutinates eggs.

fervescence (fĕr-vĕs′ĕns) [L. *fervescere,* to grow hot]. Increase of fever.

fester (fĕs′tĕr) [L. *fistula,* ulcer]. To become inflamed and suppurate.

festinant (fĕs′tĭ-nănt). Increasing in speed, accelerating.

festination (fĕs″tĭ-nā′shŭn) [L. *festinatio*]. Abnormal and involuntary increase in speed of walking in an attempt to catch up with the displaced center of gravity due to the patient's leaning forward. Seen in certain neurological diseases.

festoon (fĕs-toon′) [L. *festus,* festal]. A carving in the base material of a denture that simulates the natural indentations of the gums.

FET. *forced expiratory time.*

fetal (fē′tăl) [L. *fetus,* fetus]. Pert. to fetus.

fetal alcohol syndrome. ABBR: FAS. Birth defects in infants born to mothers whose chronic alcoholism persisted during the gestation period. Shortly after birth these infants may exhibit signs of alcohol withdrawal. In addition, some of the infants will have physical abnormalities, e.g., deficiency in growth and mental deficiency.

fetal circulation. The course of the flow of blood in a fetus. Blood, oxygenated in the placenta, passes through the umbilical vein and ductus venosus to the inferior vena cava and thence to the right atrium, from which it may follow one of two courses: 1) through the foramen ovale to the left atrium and thence through the aorta to the tissues or 2) through the right ventricle, pulmonary artery, and ductus arteriosus to the aorta, and thence to the tissues. In either case the blood bypasses the lungs, which are not functioning before birth. Blood is returned to the placenta through the umbilical arteries, which are continuations of the hypogastric arteries. At birth or shortly after, the ductus arteriosus and the foramen ovale close, establishing normal circulation. Failure of either to close may cause the baby to be blue. SEE: illus; *ductus arteriosus, patent.*

fetal distress. A clinical diagnosis indicating a pathological condition in the fetus. Usually the distress is due to anoxia and is judged by fetal heart rate or biochemical changes in the amniotic fluid or fetal blood.

fetal heart rate monitoring. Obtaining the heart rate of the fetus. This may be done by auscultation, use of an electronic device, or by Doppler ultrasound. SEE: *Doppler echocardiography; fetal monitoring in utero.*

fetalism (fē′tăl-ĭzm) [″ + Gr. *-ismos,* condition]. Retention of fetal structures after birth.

fetal membranes. The membranous structures that serve to protect and support the embryo or fetus and provide its nutrition, respiration, and excretion. The structures are the yolk sac, allantois, amnion, chorion, decidua, and placenta.

fetal monitoring in utero. Technique of obtaining information on the physical condition of the fetus. This includes recording the fetal EKG, respiratory rate and, by invasive techniques, fetal blood gas and pH data. SEE: *amniocentesis; chorionic villus sampling; Doppler echocardiography; fetal heart rate monitoring.*

feticide (fē′tĭ-sīd) [″ + *cidus,* kill]. Killing the fetus. SEE: *infanticide.*

fetid (fē′tĭd) [L. *fetidus,* stink]. Rank or foul in odor.

fetish (fē′tĭsh) [Portug. *feitico,* charm, sorcery]. 1. An object, such as an idol or charm, that is thought to have mysterious, magical, and supernatural power. 2. In psychiatry, the love object of a person who suffers from fetishism, q.v.

fetishism (fē′tĭsh-, fĕt′ĭsh-ĭzm) [″ + Gr. *-ismos,* condition]. 1. Belief in some object as possessing power or capable of being a stimulus. SEE: *voodoo.* 2. Erotic stimulation or sexually arousing fantasies involving contact with nonliving objects, such as articles of dress or a braid of hair.

fetochorionic (fē″tō-kor-ē-ŏn′ĭk) [L. *fetus,* fetus, + Gr. *chorion,* membrane]. Pert. to the fetus and the chorion or chorionic membrane of the placenta.

fetoglobulin (fē″tō-glŏb′ū-lĭn). Fetoprotein, q.v.

fetography (fē-tŏg′ră-fē). Roentgenography of the fetus in utero.

fetology (fē-tŏl′ō-jē) [″ + Gr. *logos,* word, reason]. Study of the fetus.

fetometry (fē-tŏm′ĕ-trē) [L. *fetus,* fetus, + Gr. *metron,* measure]. Estimation of size of the fetus or its head before delivery.

fetoplacental (fē″tō-plă-sĕn′tăl) [″ + *placenta,* a flat cake]. Pert. to the fetus and its placenta.

fetoprotein (fē″tō-prō′tēn). An antigen present in the human fetus and in certain pathological conditions in the adult. The amniotic fluid level can be used to evaluate fetal development. Elevated serum levels are found in adults with certain kinds of liver diseases. SEE: *alpha-fetoprotein.*

fetor (fē′tor) [L.]. Stench; an offensive odor.

f. ex ore. Offensive breath, halitosis.

f. hepaticus. A mousy odor in the breath of persons with severe liver impairment. SEE: *hepatic coma.*

f. oris. Halitosis.

fetoscope. An optical device, usually flexible and made of fiberoptic materials, used for direct visualization of the fetus in the uterus. SEE: *fetoscopy; embryoscopy.*

fetoscopy. Direct visualization of the fetus in the uterus by using a fetoscope. SEE: *embryoscopy.*

fetotoxic (fē″tō-tŏk′sĭk) [L. *fetus,* fetus, + Gr. *toxikon,* poison]. Anything that is toxic to the fetus. Materials that have been found to be potentially fetotoxic are alcohol, morphine, salicylates, coumarin anticoagulants, sedatives, tetracyclines, thiazides, tobacco smoke, and large doses of vitamin K. SEE: *teratogenic; thalidomide.*

fetus (fē′tŭs) [L.]. 1. The latter stages of the developing young of an animal within the

FETAL CIRCULATION

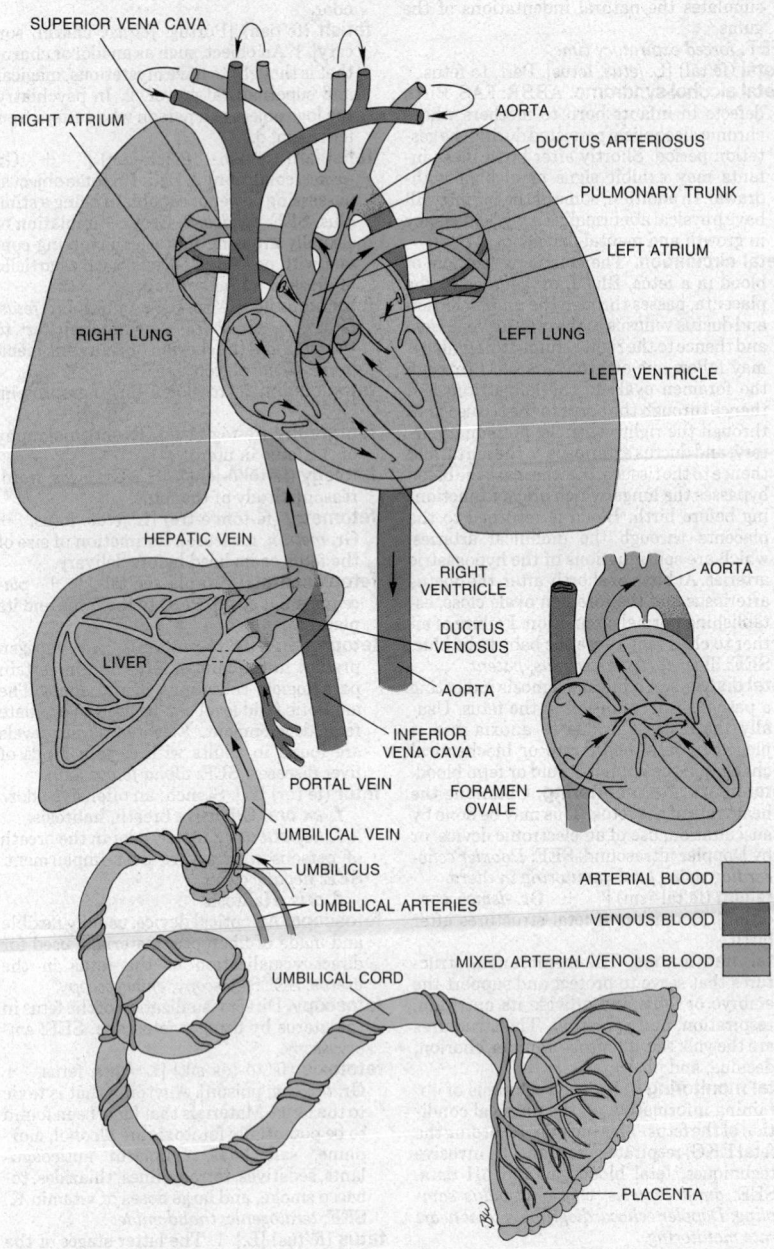

SUPERIOR VENA CAVA

RIGHT ATRIUM

RIGHT LUNG

HEPATIC VEIN

LIVER

PORTAL VEIN

UMBILICUS

UMBILICAL VEIN

UMBILICAL ARTERIES

UMBILICAL CORD

AORTA

DUCTUS ARTERIOSUS

PULMONARY TRUNK

LEFT ATRIUM

LEFT LUNG

LEFT VENTRICLE

RIGHT VENTRICLE

DUCTUS VENOSUS

AORTA

INFERIOR VENA CAVA

AORTA

FORAMEN OVALE

ARTERIAL BLOOD

VENOUS BLOOD

MIXED ARTERIAL/VENOUS BLOOD

PLACENTA

Development of Fetal Tissue

Ectoderm

Epidermis
Epithelium of:
  External and internal ear
  Nasal cavity
  Mouth
  Anus
  Amnion and chorion
  Distal portion of male urethra
Nervous tissue

Mesoderm

Connective tissues
  Skeleton
Male and female reproductive tracts
Blood vessels, lymphatics
Kidneys, ureters, trigone of bladder
Pleura, peritoneum, pericardium
Muscles

Entoderm

Respiratory tract except nose
Digestive tract except mouth and anus
Bladder except trigone
Proximal portion of male urethra
Female urethra

uterus or within an egg. 2. In humans, the child in utero from the third month to birth. Prior to that time it is called an embryo. SEE: table.

f. amorphus. A shapeless fetal anomaly, one scarcely recognizable as a fetus.

f., calcified. Fetus that has died in utero and become calcified. SYN: *lithopedion.*

f. in fetu. F., parasitic.

f., mummified. A dead fetus that has assumed a mummified form upon failure of resorption to occur.

f. papyraceus. In twin pregnancy, the dead fetus pressed flat by the development of the living twin.

f., parasitic. Condition in which a small imperfect fetus, called parasite, is contained within the body of another fetus, the autosite. SYN: *fetus in fetu.* SEE: *dermoid cyst.*

FEV$_1$. Forced expiratory volume in 1 second. A form of timed vital capacity test. After full inspiration the person exhales as hard and fast as possible into a lightweight spirometer. The amount of air exhaled during the first second is recorded. The test results provide an excellent index of pulmonary function.

fever [L. *febris*]. 1. Elevation of temperature

above the normal. The normal temperature taken orally is 98.6°F (37°C). However, it may be within the range of normal if it is 1° above or 2° below this value. On the other hand, if a person whose normal temperature is 97.8°F (36.5°C) has become ill, 98.6°F (37°C) could represent fever in that individual. Thus it is not practical to attempt to designate a precise level of normal body temperature. Rectal temperature will be 0.5° to 1.0°F higher than oral temperature. The basal energy expenditure is estimated to be increased about 12% for each °C of fever. SYN: *pyrexia.* SEE: *energy expenditure, basal; temperature.* 2. A disease characterized by an elevation of body temperature, such as typhoid fever, yellow fever.

SYM: Face flushed; hot, dry skin; anorexia; headache; nausea and sometimes vomiting; constipation and sometimes diarrhea; aching all over; scant, highly colored urine. Delirium is possible if temperature is over 105°F (40.5°C) or in some cases with less fever. Convulsions may follow, esp. in children; coma. SEE: *convulsion.*

ETIOL: Moderate increase in body temperature in the young may result from minor causes and is of less significance than in the adult. After childhood, fevers may be caused by a hot environment; generation of body heat by physical means such as exercise; neurogenic factors such as injury to the hypothalamus; dehydration such as occurs after excessive diuresis; many therapeutic drugs, which have the ability to cause fever as an undesired side effect of their use; chemical substances such as caffeine or cocaine when injected into the bloodstream; injection of proteins or their products, or the breakdown of necrotic tissue (these are the aseptic fevers such as follow surgery or coronary occlusion); infectious diseases or inflammation (fever is the result of the breakdown of bacterial proteins or toxins liberated by the disease organisms that affect the heat-regulating centers); severe hemorrhage.

TREAT: Traditionally, the onset of fever elicited a response from caregivers to take steps to lower the temperature. This was done by using antipyretic drugs such as aspirin or acetaminophen, cool baths, cooling blankets, or combinations of these. At the present time the rationale for such therapy is not clear, and the benefit to the patient's comfort is questionable. Except when due to causes such as dehydration, heat stroke, or heat exhaustion, fever may be of benefit to the patient. To automatically assume that antipyretic therapy is indicated may be invalid.

CLASSIF: *Intermittent:* A temperature

curve that returns to normal during the day and reaches its peak in the evening. *Remittent:* A fever that fluctuates but does not return to normal. *Sustained:* A temperature that remains elevated with little fluctuation. *Relapsing:* Periods of fever interspersed with periods of normal temperature.

PERIODS: *Invasion or onset of fever:* While temperature is rising and until maximum is reached. Gradual as in typhoid or sudden as in scarlet fever. *Fastigium or stadium:* When the fever is more or less stationary with variations often reaching the maximum observed in that illness. This highest point in the fever is known as the fastigium. *Defervescence:* During which the fever declines until temperature is normal. When sudden, it is known as crisis, as in lobar pneumonia; when gradual, lysis, as in measles.

Caution: When evaluating a patient's temperature, you must consider that the thermometer may be inaccurate or that the patient may heat the thermometer to feign fever.

f., childbed. An infection of the birth canal following trauma from childbirth. SYN: *puerperal sepsis.*

f., continuous. A sustained fever, as in scarlet fever, typhus, or pneumonia, in which there is slight diurnal variation.

f., drug. Fever caused by the administration of a drug. Almost any drug has the ability to produce this undesired side effect in some individuals.

f., factitious. The artificial production of fever by the patient. This is done by artificially heating the thermometer or by self-administered pyrogenic substances. The possibility of the fever being artificial may be suspected when it is noted that the pulse rate is much less than would be expected for the degree of fever noted. This diagnosis should be considered in all patients wherein there is no other plausible explanation for the fever. Patients with this condition may have serious psychiatric problems. SYN: *psychogenic fever.* SEE: *factitious disorders; malinger; Munchausen syndrome.*

f., induced. Fever artificially produced to treat certain diseases such as central nervous system syphilis. Sustained fever of 105°F (40.5°C), or even higher, maintained for 6 to 8 or 10 hours may be induced by the use of medical diathermy or injection of malarial parasites.

f., intermittent. Fever that comes and goes.

f. of unknown origin. ABBR: FUO. An illness of at least three weeks' duration with

fever exceeding 38.3°C on several occasions and diagnosis not established after one week of hospital investigation. The main causes are systemic and localized infections, neoplasms, or collagen-vascular diseases such as rheumatoid arthritis, disseminated lupus erythematosus, and polyarteritis nodosa. Less common causes are granulomatous disease, inflammatory disease of the bowel, pulmonary embolization, drug fever, cirrhosis of the liver, and rare disease such as Whipple's disease. Some cases remain undiagnosed. SEE: *fever, factitious.*

f., periodic. Familial Mediterranean fever. An inherited disease of unknown etiology of Sephardic Jews, Armenians, and Arabs. Symptoms are intermittent attacks of fever, abdominal pain, and pleurisy. Joint changes are similar to those of rheumatoid arthritis. Renal failure due to amyloidosis sometimes occurs. There is no known therapy.

f., relapsing. Any one of a group of acute infectious diseases caused by a variety of *Borrelia.* There are alternating periods of fever and normal temperature, the typical temperature curve being a characteristic of the disease. SEE: *relapsing fever.*

f., remittent. Fever that never falls to a normal temperature but shows some diurnal variation.

f., septic. Fever due to septic matter in the body. SEE: *septicemia.*

fever, words pert. to: ague; antifebrile; apyrexia; calor; chill; crisis; dengue; factitious; fastigium; febrifacient; febrifuge; febrile convulsions; fever, factitious; FUO; heat; infection; inflammation; influenza; lysis; malaria; Munchausen syndrome; pulse; "pyr-" words; quartan; quintan; quotidian; respiration; sepsis; suppuration; temperature.

fever blister. Area of inflammation of the lips or mucous membrane of the mouth. Caused by herpes simplex virus, usually type I. SYN: *fever sore.*

F.F.D. *focal film distance.* Distance from the focal spot of the x-ray tube to the film.

FH₄. *5,6,7,8-tetrahydrofolic acid,* folacin, the active form of folic acid.

fiat (fi′ăt) [L.]. Let there be made, a term used in writing prescriptions.

fiber [L. *fibra*]. 1. Threadlike or filmlike element, as a nerve fiber. A neuron or the axonal portion of a neuron. 2. An elongated threadlike structure. A fiber may be cellular in composition, as nerve fiber or muscle fiber, or may be a cellular product, as collagen fiber, elastic fiber, oxytalan fiber, or reticular fiber. 3. A slender cellulosic fiber derived from plants such as cotton. SEE: *rayon, purified.*

RS: chondrofibroma; cilia; cimbia; cingulum; "fibr-" words; filament; filum.

f., accelerator. Fiber nerve pathway causing increased heart rate upon stimulation.

f., afferent. Fiber carrying incoming impulses to nerve cells.

f., dietary. Components of food that are resistant to chemical digestion. Includes foods made up of cellulose, hemicellulose, lignin, gums, mucilages, and pectin. These substances add bulk to the diet to produce a large bulky bowel movement.

Dietary fibers are classified according to their solubility in water. Fibers that are water-insoluble include cellulose, lignin, and some hemicelluloses. Natural gel-forming fibers such as gums, mucilages, and some hemicelluloses are water-soluble. Most foods of plant origin contain both soluble and insoluble dietary fiber. A great number of disease processes such as hypertension, diabetes, hypercholesterolemia, polyps of the colon, colon cancer, gallstones, and irritable bowel syndrome have been investigated with respect to their relation to dietary fiber intake. These studies have not provided clear-cut evidence of the benefit. It is clear, though, that dietary fiber, particularly those derived from wheat, oats, and other insoluble fiber sources are useful in the prevention and treatment of constipation.

Foods rich in fiber include whole-grain foods, bran flakes, beans, fruits, leafy vegetables, nuts, root vegetables and their skins, and prunes, which also contain the laxative substance diphenylisatin.

f., efferent. Fiber carrying outgoing impulses.

f., inhibitory. Fiber nerve pathway causing slower heart action upon stimulation.

f., man-made. Synthetic fiber made from chemicals, e.g., rayon, polyester (Dacron).

f., medullated. Nerve fiber in which axis cylinder is sheathed in myelin.

f., nerve. Part of a nerve cell that carries impulses. SEE: *nerve.*

f., nonmedullated. Nerve fiber in which there is no myelin sheath between axis cylinder and neurilemma. SYN: *f., unmyelinated.*

f.'s, Purkinje. Atypical muscle fibers lying beneath the endocardium that form the impulse-conducting system of the heart.

f., synthetic. F., man-made.

f., unmyelinated. F., nonmedullated, q.v.

fibercolonoscope (fī″bĕr-kō-lŏn′ō-skōp). Fiberoptic endoscope for examining the colon.

fibergastroscope (fī″bĕr-găs′trō-skōp). Fiberoptic endoscope for examining the stomach.

fiberglass. Glass spun into fine fibers. It is used in the building industry for insulation. The fibers are irritating to the skin.

fiber-illuminated (fī′bĕr-ĭl-loo″mĭn-ā″tĕd). Transmission of light to an object by use of fiberoptic bundles.

fiberoptic. Flexible material of glass or plastic that transmits light along its course by reflecting it from the side or wall of the fiber. Use of this principle permits transmission of light and therefore visual images around sharp curves and corners. Devices utilizing fiberoptic materials are quite useful in endoscopic examinations.

fiberscope (fī′bĕr-skōp). A flexible endoscope that uses fiberoptic, q.v., materials for visualization.

fibra (fī′brǎ) [L.] (pl. *fibrae*). [NA] A fiber.

fibralbumin (fī″brăl-bū′mĭn) [L. *fibra,* fiber, + *albumen,* white of egg]. Globulin.

fibremia (fī-brē′mē-ǎ) [" + Gr. *haima,* blood]. Fibrin formed in the blood, causing embolism or thrombosis. SYN: *inosemia.*

fibril (fī′brĭl) [L. *fibrilla*]. A small fiber. A very small filamentous structure, often the component of a cell or a fiber.

f., muscle. An extremely minute fibril found within the cytoplasm of smooth muscle cells and in the sarcoplasm of striated and cardiac muscle fibers. SYN: *myofibril.*

f., nerve. Delicate fibril found in the cell body and processes of a neuron. SYN: *neurofibril.*

fibrilla (fī-brĭl′ǎ) [L.] (pl. *fibrillae*). A fibril or small fiber.

fibrillar, fibrillary. Pert. to, or consisting of, fibrils.

fibrillated (fī′brĭ-lāt′d) [L. *fibrilla,* little fiber]. Composed of minute fibers. SYN: *fibrillar; fibrous.*

fibrillation (fī″brĭl-ā′shŭn). 1. The formation of fibrils. 2. Quivering or spontaneous contraction of individual muscle fibers. 3. An abnormal bioelectric potential occurring in neuropathies and myopathies.

f., atrial. Extremely rapid, incomplete contractions of the atria resulting in fine, rapid, irregular, and uncoordinated movements.

f., ventricular. The primary mechanism and arrhythmia seen in sudden cardiac arrest. Organized electrical activity and synchronized mechanical pumping activity is absent. The ECG shows a chaotic, wavy baseline. If not terminated rapidly with defibrillation, brain damage will occur due to lack of blood flow to that organ. Untreated ventricular fibrillation will lead to death. SEE: *defibrillation; pacemaker, cardiac, arti-*

ficial.

fibrillogenesis (fĭ-brĭl″ō-jĕn′ĕ-sĭs). Formation of fibrils.

fibrillolysis (fĭ″brĭl-ŏl′ĭ-sĭs) [″ + Gr. *lysis,* dissolution]. Dissolution of fibrils.

fibrillolytic (fĭ″brĭl-ō-lĭt′ĭk). Dissolving fibrils.

fibrin (fī′brĭn) [L. *fibra,* fiber]. A whitish, filamentous protein formed by the action of thrombin on fibrinogen. The conversion of fibrinogen, a hydrosol, into fibrin, a hydrogel, is the basis for the clotting of the blood. The fibrin is deposited as fine interlacing filaments in which are entangled red and white blood cells and platelets, the whole forming a coagulum or clot. SEE: *coagulation, blood.*

    RS: blood clot; coagulation; fibrinogen; prothrombin; thrombin.

fibrinocellular (fī″brĭ-nō-sĕl′ū-lăr). Composed of fibrin and cells, as in certain exudates.

fibrinogen (fī-brĭn′ō-jĕn) [″ + Gr. *gennan,* to produce]. A protein present in the blood plasma that through the action of thrombin and in the presence of calcium ions is converted into fibrin; this is essential for clotting of blood. Also called factor I. SEE: *blood, clotting of; coagulation factors.*

fibrinogenic, fibrinogenous. Producing fibrin.

fibrinogenolysis (fī″brĭ-nō-jĕ-nŏl′ĭ-sĭs) [″ + ″ + *lysis,* dissolution]. Decomposition or dissolution of fibrin.

fibrinogenopenia (fī-brĭn″ō-jĕn″ō-pē′nē-ă) [″ + Gr. *gennan,* to produce, + *penia,* poverty]. Reduction in the amount of fibrinogen in the blood, usually the result of a liver disorder.

fibrinoid (fī′brĭ-noyd) [″ + Gr. *eidos,* form, shape]. Resembling fibrin.

fibrinoid change. Alteration in connective tissues in response to immune reactions. The tissue becomes swollen, homogenous, and bandlike in appearance.

fibrinoid material. A fibrinous substance that develops in the placenta, increasing in quantity as the placenta develops. Its origin is attributed to the degenerating decidua and trophoblast. It forms an incomplete layer in the chorion and decidua basalis and also occurs in the form of small irregular patches on the surface of the chorionic villi. In late pregnancy, the material may have a striated or canalized appearance, to which the term canalized fibrinoid is applied.

fibrinolysis (fī″brĭn-ŏl′ĭ-sĭs). Dissolution of fibrin by fibrinolysin. Caused by the action of a proteolytic enzyme system. This system is continually active in the body, but its action is greatly increased by various stress stimuli such as intense exercise, anoxia, hy-

poglycemia, or bacterial infections.

fibrinolytic (fī″brĭn-ō-lĭt′ĭk). Pert. to the splitting up of fibrin.

fibrinopenia (fī″brĭn-ō-pē′nē-ă) [″ + Gr. *penia,* poverty]. Fibrin and fibrinogen deficiency in the blood.

fibrinopeptide (fī″brĭ-nō-pĕp′tīd). The substance removed by thrombin from fibrinogen during blood coagulation.

fibrinoplastic (fī″brĭn-ō-plăs′tĭk) [″ + Gr. *plassein,* to form]. Concerning fibroplastin.

fibrinopurulent (fī″brĭ-nō-pū′roo-lĕnt) [″ + *purulentus,* festering]. Consisting of pus and fibrin.

fibrinosis (fī-brĭ-nō′sĭs) [″ + Gr. *osis,* condition]. Excess of fibrin in the blood.

fibrinous (fī′brĭn-ŭs) [L. *fibra,* fiber]. Pert. to, of the nature of, or containing fibrin.

fibrin split products. The materials produced when the crosslinked fibrin in a blood clot is digested by plasmin, q.v. SYN: *fibrin degradation products.*

fibrinuria (fī-brĭn-ū′rē-ă) [″ + Gr. *ouron,* urine]. Passage of fibrin in the urine.

fibro- [L. *fibra*]. Prefix indicating relationship to fibers or fibrous tissues.

fibroadenia (fī″brō-ă-dē′nē-ă) [L. *fibra,* fiber, + Gr. *aden,* gland]. Fibrous degeneration of glandular tissue.

fibroadenoma (fī″brō-ăd″ĕ-nō′mă) [″ + ″ + *oma,* tumor]. Adenoma with fibrous tissue forming a dense stroma.

fibroadipose [″ + *adeps,* fat]. Being fibrous and fatty.

fibroangioma [″ + Gr. *angeion,* vessel, + *oma,* tumor]. A fibrous tissue angioma.

fibroareolar (fī″brō-ă-rē′ō-lăr) [″ + *areola,* little space]. With fibrous and areolar tissue.

fibroblast (fī′brō-blăst) [″ + Gr. *blastos,* germ]. Any cell or corpuscle from which connective tissue is developed. SYN: *desmocyte; fibrocyte.*

fibroblast growth factors. A group of proteins usually present intracellularly that have important angiogenic function and are important in enhancing wound healing and tissue repair. Overactivity of these factors has been associated with neoplasia.

fibroblastoma (fī″brō-blăs-tō′mă) [″ + ″ + *oma,* tumor]. Tumor of connective tissue or fibroplastic cells.

fibrocalcific (fī″brō-kăl-sĭf′ĭk). Partially calcified fibrous material.

fibrocarcinoma (fī″brō-kăr″sĭ-nō′mă) [″ + Gr. *karkinos,* cancer, + *oma,* tumor]. A carcinoma in which the trabeculae are resistant and thickened with granular degeneration of the cells.

fibrocartilage (fī″brō-kăr′tĭ-lĭj) [″ + *cartilago,* gristle]. A type of cartilage in which the matrix contains thick bundles of white or collagenous fibers. Found in the intervertebral disks.

fibrocellular (fĭ″brō-sĕl′ū-lăr) [″ + *cellula*, little cell]. Both fibrous and cellular. SYN: *fibroareolar*.

fibrochondritis (fĭ″brō-kŏn-drī′tĭs) [″ + Gr. *chondros*, cartilage, + *itis*, inflammation]. Inflammation of fibrocartilage.

fibrochondroma (fĭ″brō-kŏn-drō′mă) [″ + ″ + *oma*, tumor]. Tumor of fibrous tissue and cartilage.

fibrocyst (fĭ′brō-sĭst) [″ + Gr. *kystis*, cyst]. A fibrous tumor that has undergone cystic degeneration or one that has accumulated fluid in the interspaces.

fibrocystic (fĭ″brō-sĭs′tĭk). 1. Consisting of fibrocysts. 2. Fibrous with cystic degeneration.

fibrocystic disease of the breast. A nonspecific diagnosis for a condition in which there are palpable lumps in the breasts, usually associated with pain and tenderness, that fluctuate with the menstrual cycle and become progressively worse until menopause. At least 50% of women of reproductive age have palpably irregular breasts caused by this condition.

Women with fibrocystic disease of the breast have a 2 to 5 times greater risk of developing breast cancer. Some women with this disease have atypical hyperplasm of the lesion. If these patients also have a family history of breast cancer, then their risk of developing cancer of the breast is greatly increased. They should have a breast examination every six months and mammography once a year. SYN: *chronic cystic mastitis*. SEE: *breast, self-examination of.*

NURSING IMPLICATIONS: Teach patient importance of monthly breast self-examination, mapping known lumps (round, movable and well-delineated), also examination by a health professional and mammography every six months. Teach the patient that knowing the contours (feel, texture) of her breasts will make it possible for her to detect any changes, often sooner or more accurately than the health care provider who examines her infrequently. Discuss use of fine-needle aspiration as diagnostic and treatment modality, encouraging patient to verbalize feelings and concerns. Wearing a well-fitted, supportive brassiere both day and night can help reduce discomfort, as can application of ice packs intermittently to tender areas and ingestion of aspirin or nonsteroidal anti-inflammatory drugs available over the counter. In severe cases, hormone therapy may be prescribed. Nurse should caution patient that relief may not be noted for 4 to 6 months, and should assess for annoying and upsetting side effects such as weight gain, amenor-

rhea, and masculinization. Provide emotional support for patient, who may have a heightened awareness of and fear about developing breast cancer.

fibrocystic disease of pancreas. Cystic fibrosis, q.v.

fibrocystoma (fĭ″brō-sĭs-tō′mă) [″ + Gr. *kystis*, cyst, + *oma*, tumor]. Fibroma combined with cystoma.

fibrocyte (fĭ′brō-sīt) [″ + Gr. *kytos*, cell]. A mature, older, fiber-forming cell or fibroblast.

fibrodysplasia (fĭ″brō-dĭs-plā′sē-ă) [″ + Gr. *dys*, bad, + *plassein*, to form]. Fibrous dysplasia.

fibroelastic (fĭ″brō-ē-lăs′tĭk) [″ + Gr. *elastikos*, elastic]. Pert. to connective tissue containing both white nonelastic collagenous fibers and yellow elastic fibers.

fibroelastosis (fĭ″brō-ē″lăs-tō′sĭs). Overgrowth of fibroelastic tissue.

  f., endocardial. Fibroelastosis of the endocardium, leading to cardiac failure.

fibroenchondroma (fĭ″brō-ĕn″kŏn-drō′mă) [″ + Gr. *en*, in, + *chondros*, cartilage, + *oma*, tumor]. Enchondroma containing fibrous elements.

fibroepithelial polyp. SEE: *polyp, fibroepithelial.*

fibroepithelioma (fĭ″brō-ĕp″ĭ-thē″lē-ō′mă) [″ + Gr. *epi*, upon, + *thele*, nipple, + *oma*, tumor]. A new growth containing fibrous and epithelial elements.

fibroglia (fĭ-brŏg′lē-ă) [″ + Gr. *glia*, glue]. Supporting tissue of fibroblasts.

fibroid (fĭ′broyd) [″ + Gr. *eidos*, form, shape]. 1. Containing or resembling fibers. SEE: *degeneration*. 2. A colloquial term for fibroma, esp. fibroma of the uterus.

  f., interstitial. Tumor in muscular wall of uterus that may grow inward and form a polypoid fibroid, or outward and become a subperitoneal fibroid.

  f., uterine. Fibroid in uterus. SEE: *fibroma, uterine.*

fibroidectomy (fĭ-broyd-ĕk′tō-mē) [″ + ″ + *ektome*, excision]. Surgical removal of a fibroid tumor.

fibrolipoma (fĭ″brō-lĭ-pō′mă) [″ + Gr. *lipos*, fat, + *oma*, tumor]. A lipoma having excessive fibrous tissue.

fibroma (fĭ-brō′mă) [″ + Gr. *oma*, tumor] (pl. *fibromata*). A fibrous, encapsulated, connective tissue tumor. It is irregular in shape, slow in growth, and has a firm consistency. Pressure or cystic degeneration may cause pain. May be found in the periosteum. May affect the jaws, the occiput, pelvis, vertebrae, ribs, long bones, and sternum.

  f., intramural. Tumor located in muscle tissue of the uterus between the peritoneal coat and endometrium.

f. of breast. A benign, nonulcerative, and painless tumor of the breast.

f., submucous. Fibroma encroaching upon endometrial cavity; sessile or pedunculated.

f., subserous. Fibroma lying beneath peritoneal coat of uterus, often pedunculated.

f., uterine. A fibroid tumor of the uterus. It is the most common tumor found in women.

SYM: Fibromata rarely cause symptoms before the age of 30. Although their cardinal symptoms are supposed to be dysmenorrhea, menorrhagia, and leukorrhea, these are found infrequently, and the symptomatology is directly related to the location of the tumors in the uterus. Thus, tumors that encroach upon the bladder region cause frequency and dysuria; those pressing on the rectum cause rectal tenesmus; those that encroach upon the endometrium may cause menorrhagia and dysmenorrhea, and very large subserous growths may be symptomless.

Use of oral contraceptive pills reduces the risk of fibroma of the uterus, as does cigarette smoking; obesity increases the risk. Fibroids may, because of their size or location, cause infertility. Whether or not fibroids enlarge during pregnancy is unclear. SYN: *fibroids.* SEE: *dysmenorrhea; dysuria; menorrhagia; tenesmus.*

PATH: A benign tumor varying in size from a few millimeters in diameter to a size large enough to fill the entire abdominal cavity. May be single or multiple. The tumors usually increase in size during the reproductive years and may regress after the menopause. They are completely encapsulated by a fibrous connective tissue capsule in which the blood vessels that supply the tumor are found. They are subjected to numerous benign degenerations such as necrobiotic changes (red and gray degeneration), hyaline changes, telangiectatic and lymphangiectatic changes, calcareous degeneration, fatty degeneration, and infection. Occasionally, a fibroid will show sarcomatous degeneration.

TREAT: Fibromata producing no symptoms should be left in place and the patient kept under observation. Medical treatment involving luteinizing hormone-releasing hormone (LHRH) analogues will cause fibroids to shrink; but the growth returns when LHRH is discontinued. If unusually rapid growth is evidenced, they should be removed. Small submucous tumors may be removed during hysteroscopy by using electrocautery. Laser technique has been used to remove these tumors. If pregnancy is a possibility, tumors of such size as to interfere with childbearing should be removed.

fibromatosis (fi″brō-mă-tō′sĭs) [L. *fibra*, fiber, + Gr. *oma*, tumor, + *osis*, condition]. The simultaneous development of many fibromas. SYN: *fibrosis.*

f. gingivae. An inherited condition in which there is hypertrophy of the gums prior to the time of eruption of the teeth. Hypertrichosis is usually present.

f., palmar. Dupuytren's contracture, q.v.

fibromatous (fī-brō′mă-tŭs). Pert. to, or of the nature of, a fibroma.

fibromectomy (fī″brō-mĕk′tō-mē) [″ + Gr. *oma*, tumor, + *ektome*, excision]. Removal of a fibroid tumor.

fibromembranous (fī″brō-mĕm′bră-nŭs) [″ + *membrana*, web]. Having both fibrous and membranous tissue.

fibromuscular (fī″brō-mŭs′kū-lăr) [″ + *musculus*, muscle]. Consisting of muscle and connective tissue.

fibromyalgia [″ + Gr. *mys*, muscle, + *algos*, pain]. Chronic pain in muscles and soft tissues surrounding joints. Efforts to classify this condition have resulted in the American College of Rheumatology criteria for classification of fibromyalgia, published in 1990. SEE: table.

TREAT: A variety of therapeutic approaches have been tried. Essential to the management of this condition are reassurance, elimination of contributing factors, physical therapy with the objective of restoration of normal neuromuscular function, institution of a cardiovascular fitness program, and appropriate medications for sleep disturbances. Anti-inflammatory agents, including corticosteroids, have not been useful in the experience of some investigators. SYN: *tension myalgia.* SEE: *trigger point or zone.*

fibromyitis (fī″brō-mī-ī′tĭs) [″ + Gr. *mys*, muscle, + *itis*, inflammation]. SEE: *fibromyalgia.*

fibromyoma (fī″brō-mī-ō′mă) [″ + ″ + *oma*, tumor]. 1. Fibrous tissue myoma. 2. A fibroid tumor of the uterus that contains more fibrous than muscle tissue.

fibromyomectomy (fī″brō-mī″ō-mĕk′tō-mē) [″ + ″ + *ektome*, excision]. Removal of a fibromyoma from the uterus, leaving that organ in place.

fibromyositis (fī″brō-mī″ō-sī′tĭs) [″ + Gr. *mys*, muscle, + *itis*, inflammation]. SEE: *fibromyalgia.*

fibromyotomy (fī″brō-mī-ŏt′ō-mē) [″ + ″ + *tome*, incision]. Opening of a fibroid tumor.

fibromyxoma (fī″brō-mĭk-sō′mă) [″ + Gr. *myxa*, mucus, + *oma*, tumor]. A fibroma

The American College of Rheumatology 1990 Criteria for Classification of Fibromyalgia*

1. History of widespread pain

   Definition: Pain is considered widespread when all the following are present — pain in the left side of the body, pain in the right side of the body, pain above the waist, and pain below the waist. In addition, axial skeletal pain (cervical spine, anterior chest, thoracic spine, or low back) must be present. In this definition, shoulder and buttock pain is considered as pain for each involved side. "Low back" pain is considered lower segment pain.

2. Pain in 11 of 18 tender point sites on digital palpation

   Definition: On digital palpation, pain must be present in at least 11 of the following 18 tender point sites:
   - *Occiput* — bilateral, at the suboccipital muscle insertions
   - *Low cervical* — bilateral, at the anterior aspects of the intertransverse spaces at C5-7
   - *Trapezius* — bilateral, at the midpoint of the upper border
   - *Supraspinatus* — bilateral, at origins, above the scapular spine near the medial border
   - *Second rib* — bilateral, at the second costochondral junctions, just lateral to the junctions on upper surfaces
   - *Lateral epicondyle* — bilateral, 2 cm distal to the epicondyles
   - *Gluteal* — bilateral, in upper outer quadrants of buttocks in anterior fold of muscle
   - *Greater trochanter* — bilateral, posterior to the trochanteric prominence
   - *Knee* — bilateral, at the medial fat pad proximal to the joint line

   Digital palpation should be performed with an approximate force of 4 kg.
   For a tender point to be considered "positive," the subject must state that the palpation was painful. "Tender" is not to be considered "painful."

Source: American College of Rheumatology, Multicenter Criteria Committee. By permission.
* For classification purposes, patients will be said to have fibromyalgia if both criteria are satisfied. Widespread pain must have been present for at least 3 months. The presence of a second clinical disorder does not exclude the diagnosis of fibromyalgia.

that has undergone partial myxomatous degeneration.

fibromyxosarcoma (fī″brō-mĭk″sō-săr-kō′mä) [″ + ″ + *sarkos,* flesh, + *oma,* tumor]. 1. A sarcoma containing fibrous and myxoid tissue. 2. A sarcoma that has undergone mucoid degeneration.

fibronectin. Any one of a group of proteins present in blood plasma and extracellular matrix. The presence of fetal fibronectin in the cervical and vaginal secretions may be a marker by which subsequent development of preterm labor may be predicted.

fibroneuroma (fī″brō-nū-rō′mä) [″ + Gr. *neuron,* nerve, + *oma,* tumor]. A mixed neuroma and fibroma. SYN: *neurofibroma.*

fibro-osteoma (fī″brō-ŏs-tē-ō′mä) [″ + Gr. *osteon,* bone, + *oma,* tumor]. Tumor containing bony and fibrous elements. SYN: *osteofibroma.*

fibropapilloma (fī″brō-păp-ĭ-lō′mä) [″ + *papilla,* nipple, + Gr. *oma,* tumor]. A mixed fibroma and papilloma sometimes occurring in the bladder.

fibroplasia (fī″brō-plā′sē-ă) [″ + Gr. *plasis,* a molding]. The development of fibrous tissue, as in wound healing.

f., retrolental. Rentrolental fibroplasia, q.v.

fibroplastic (fī″brō-plăs′tĭk) [″ + Gr. *plassein,* to form]. Giving formation to fibrous tissue.

fibropurulent (fī″brō-pūr′ū-lĕnt) [″ + *purulentus,* festering]. Pus containing flakes of fibrous tissue.

fibrosarcoma (fī″brō-săr-kō′mä) [L. *fibra,* fiber, + Gr. *sarkos,* flesh, + *oma,* tumor]. A spindle-celled sarcoma containing much connective tissue.

fibrose (fī′brōs). To form or produce fibrous tissue, e.g., a scar.

fibroserous (fī″brō-sē′rŭs) [″ + *serosus,* serous]. Containing fibrous and serosal elements. The pericardium is such a tissue.

fibrosis (fī-brō′sĭs) [″ + Gr. *osis,* condition]. Abnormal formation of fibrous tissue.

f., arteriocapillary. Arteriolar and capillary fibroid degeneration.

f., diffuse interstitial pulmonary. Hamman-Rich syndrome, q.v.

f. of lungs. Formation of scar tissue in connective tissue framework of lungs following inflammation or pneumonia and in pulmonary tuberculosis.

f., postfibrinosis. Development of fibrosis in a tissue in which fibrin has been deposited.

f., proliferative. Formation of new fibrous tissue from connective tissue cells.

f., pulmonary. Fibrosis of the lung following any pulmonary disease.

f., retroperitoneal. Fibrosis, of unknown etiology, of the retroperitoneal area. It may progress to cause obstruction of the great blood vessels and ureters.

f. uteri. Diffuse growth of fibrous tissue throughout the uterus.

fibrositis (fĭ-brō-sī'tĭs) [" + Gr. *itis,* inflammation]. Fibromyositis, q.v. SYN: *fibromyalgia; fibromyositis.*

fibrothorax (fĭ"brō-thō'răks) [" + Gr. *thorax,* chest]. Fibrosis that causes the two pleural surfaces of the lung to adhere to each other.

fibrotic (fĭ-brŏt'ĭk). Marked by or pert. to fibrosis.

fibrous (fī'brŭs) [L. *fibra,* fiber]. Composed of or containing fibers.

fibula (fĭb'ū-lă) [L., pin]. [NA] The outer and smaller bone of the leg from the ankle to the knee, articulating above with the tibia and below with the tibia and talus. One of longest and thinnest bones of the body.

fibular. Pert. to the fibula.

fibulocalcaneal (fĭb"ū-lō-kăl-kā'nē-ăl) [L. *fibula,* pin, + *calcaneus,* pert. to the heel]. Pert. to the fibula and calcaneus or os calcis.

ficin (fī'sĭn) [L. *ficus,* fig]. Sap from the fig tree. It contains an enzyme that is capable of hydrolyzing proteins.

Fick method [Adolf Eugen Fick, Ger. physician, 1829–1901]. A method of determining cardiac output.

F.I.C.S. *Fellow of the International College of Surgeons.*

FID. *flame ionization detector.* A detector employed in gas chromatography in which a sample burned in a flame changes the conductivity between two electrodes.

fidget [Norwegian *fiskjat,* to be eager]. To move about nervously or impatiently.

field [AS. *feld*]. A specific area in relationship to an object.

f., auditory. The space or distance within the limit of hearing.

f., high-power. The portion of the object seen when the high magnification lenses of the microscope are used.

f., low-power. The portion of the object seen when the low magnification lenses of the microscope are used.

f. of vision. That portion of space that the fixed eye can see. SEE: *perimetry.*

fifth cranial nerve. A large mixed nerve arising superficially from the side of the pons near its superior border. It is connected to

the brain stem by two roots: a large sensory root and a small motor root. SYN: *trigeminal nerve.*

Fifth disease. So called because it was the fifth disease described with a similar rash. SEE: *erythema infectiosum.*

fifth ventricle. Space separating the two layers of the septum pellucidum of the brain.

fight-or-flight reaction of Cannon [Walter B. Cannon, U.S. physiologist, 1871–1954]. The generalized response to an emergency situation. This includes intense stimulation of the sympathetic nervous system and the adrenal gland. The heart and respiratory rates, blood pressure, and blood flow to muscles are increased. This is the body's response to an emergency in order to be prepared to either flee or fight.

FIGLU, FIGlu. *formiminoglutamic acid.*

FIGLU excretion test. Test for folic acid deficiency. When histidine is administered to a patient with folic acid deficiency, formiminoglutamic (FIGLU) acid in the urine will increase.

FIGO staging system. The staging system for cancer of the cervix uteri developed by the International Federation of Gynecology and Obstetrics.

figurate (fĭg'ū-rāt) [L. *figuratum,* figured]. Skin lesions that have a certain form, such as geographic, annular, or circular.

figure [L. *figura*]. 1. A body, form, shape, or outline. 2. A number.

figure-ground discrimination. The ability to perceive visually the outline of an object from visually competing background stimuli. This ability is often impaired following central nervous system damage.

fila (fī'lă) [L. *filum,* thread]. Pl. of filum.

filaceous (fĭ-lā'shŭs). Composed of filaments.

filament [L. *filamentum*]. 1. A fine thread. 2. A threadlike coil of tungsten found in the x-ray tube that is the source of electrons.

f., axial. A fine filament forming the central axis of the tail of a spermatozoon.

filamentous. Made up of long, interwoven or irregularly placed threadlike structures.

filar (fī'lăr) [L. *filum,* thread]. Filamentous.

Filaria (fĭl-ā'rē-ă) [L. *filum,* thread]. Term formerly applied to a genus of nematodes belonging to the superfamily Filarioidea.

F. bancrofti. Wuchereria bancrofti.

F. loa. Loa loa.

F. medinensis. Dracunculus medinensis.

F. sanguinis hominis. Wuchereria bancrofti.

filaria (fĭl-ā'rē-ă) [L. *filum,* thread]. A long filiform nematode belonging to the superfamily Filarioidea. The adults live in vertebrates. In humans, they may be found in the lymphatic vessels and lymphatic organs, circulatory system, connective tissues, subcutaneous tissues, and serous cavities. Typically, the female produces larvae called microfilariae, which may be sheathed or sheathless. They reach the peripheral blood or lymphatic vessels, where they may be ingested by a blood-sucking arthropod (mosquitoes, gnats, flies). In the intermediate host, they transform into rhabditoid larvae that metamorphose into infective filariform larvae. These migrate to the proboscis and are deposited in or on the skin of the vertebrate host. SEE: *elephantiasis.*

filarial (fĭ-lā′rē-ăl). Pert. to or caused by filariae.

filariasis (fĭl-ă-rī′ă-sĭs) [″ + Gr. *-iasis,* condition]. A chronic disease due to one of the filariae species. SEE: *elephantiasis.*

filaricidal (fĭ-lăr″ĭ-sīd′ăl) [″ + *caedere,* to kill]. Pert. to that which is destructive to *Filaria.*

Filarioidea (fĭ-lăr″ē-oy′dē-ă). A superfamily of filarial nematodes that parasitize many animal species, including man. SEE: *filariasis.*

file (fīl). 1. A metal device with a roughened surface. It is used for shaping bones and teeth. 2. In computers, a term used to describe data stored in a specifically designated area of the computer's memory system.

filial generation. In genetics, the first offspring of a specific mating or crossmating. This is abbreviated F_1. Descendants resulting from F_1 matings are known as the F_2 or second filial generation.

filiform (fĭl′ĭ-form) [″ + *forma,* form]. 1. In biology, pert. to a growth that is uniform along the inoculation line in stab or streak cultures. 2. Hairlike, filamentous.

fillet (fĭl′ĕt) [Fr. *filet,* a band]. 1. A loop of thread, cord, or tape used for providing traction or suspension of tissue during surgery. 2. Bundles of sensory fibers in the medulla, pons, and brain.

filling (fĭl′ĭng) [AS. *fyllan,* to fill]. 1. The material for insertion in a prepared tooth cavity, usually amalgam. 2. The operation of filling tooth cavities.

film. 1. A thin skin, membrane, or covering. 2. A thin sheet of material, usually cellulose, coated with a light-sensitive emulsion used in taking photographs. 3. In microscopy, a thin layer of blood or other material spread on a slide or coverslip.

   f., bite-wing. Roentgenogram taken with a part of the film holder held between the teeth and the film parallel to the teeth. This technique permits films to be taken of several upper and lower teeth at the same time.

   f., spot. An x-ray film of a small anatom-

ical area.

   f., x-ray. A special photographic film that is sensitive to x-rays.

film badge. A badge containing film that is sensitive to x-rays. Used to determine the cumulative exposure to x-rays of persons who work in radiology.

filopressure (fĭ′lō-prĕ″shŭr) [L. *filum,* thread, + *pressura,* pressure]. Pressure on a blood vessel caused by a ligature.

filovaricosis (fī″lō-văr-ĭ-kō′sĭs) [″ + *varix,* a dilated vein, + Gr. *osis,* condition]. Dilatation or thickening of the axis cylinder of a nerve fiber.

filter [L. *filtrare,* to strain through]. 1. To pass a liquid through any porous substance that prevents particles larger than a certain size to pass through. 2. Device for filtering liquids, light rays, or radiations. SEE: *absorption; osmosis.*

   f. bed. Large-scale filter to purify the water supply.

   f., Berkefeld. A diatomaceous earth filter designed to remove bacteria from solutions passed through it, but allow virus-sized particles to pass through into the filtrate.

   f., infrared. Filter that permits passage of only infrared waves of certain wavelength.

   f., Kitasato's. Suction variety of filter using porcelain dilator.

   f., membrane. Filter made from biologically inert cellulose esters, polyethylene, or other porous materials.

   f., Millipore. Trademark name of a filter with controlled pore size that separates particles above specific sizes from the solutions that flow through.

   f., optical. Device that passes only a portion of the visible light spectrum. Absorption filters function by absorbing the unwanted wavelengths. Interference filters employ the wave effects of constructive and destructive superposition to pass or inhibit appropriate wavelengths.

   f., Pasteur-Chamberland. Filter of unglazed porcelain capable of retaining bacteria and some viruses. Either pressure or suction is required to force or draw the liquid through the filter.

   f., umbrella. Filter placed in a blood vessel in order to prevent emboli from passing that point. Has been used in the vena cava to prevent emboli in the veins from reaching the lungs.

   f., wedge. A filter used in radiography and radiation therapy to vary the intensity of the x-ray beam in order to compensate for a difference in the thickness of the part being exposed to radiation.

   f., Wood's. A glass screen allowing passage of ultraviolet radiation and absorbing rays of visual light. Used in diagnosing certain dermatological conditions, esp. tinea capitis.

filterable [L. *filtrare*, to strain through]. Capable of passing through the pores of a porcelain filter, through which bacteria cannot pass.

filtrate (fĭl′trāt). The fluid that has been passed through a filter. The residue is the precipitate.

    f., glomerular. The fluid that passes from the blood through the capillary walls of the glomeruli of the kidney. It is a protein-free plasma from which urine is formed.

filtration (fĭl-trā′shŭn). The process of removing particles from a solution by allowing the liquid portion to pass through a membrane or other partial barrier. This barrier contains holes or spaces through which the liquid may pass but which are too small to permit the solid particles to pass. SEE: *filter.*

filtration of roentgen rays. The absorption of some of the relatively longer wavelengths of roentgen radiation by placing some absorbing medium in the path of the rays such as aluminum, copper, or zinc.

filtrum [L.]. A filter.

filum (fī′lŭm) [L.] (pl. *fila*). [NA] A threadlike structure.

    f. coronaria. A fibrous band extending from the base of the medial cusp of the tricuspid valve to the aortic annulus.

    f. terminale. [NA] A long, slender filament at the end of the spinal cord.

fimbria (fĭm′brē-ă) [L., fringe] (pl. *fimbriae*). Any structure resembling fringe or border.

    f. ovarica. The longest fringelike extremity of the fallopian tubes; extending from the infundibulum close to the ovary.

    f. tubae. Fringelike portion at abdominal end of the fallopian tubes.

fimbriate (fĭm′brē-āt″). 1. Having finger-like projections. 2. Fringed.

fimbriated [L. *fimbria*, fringe]. Fringed.

fimbriocele (fĭm′brē-ō-sēl″) [″ + Gr. *kele*, tumor, swelling]. Hernia including the fimbriated portion of the oviduct.

fine motor skills. Skills pertaining to the synergy of small muscles, primarily in the hand, and related to manual dexterity and coordination.

finger [AS.]. One of the five digits of the hand.

    f., baseball. Condition resulting from violent backward dislocation of the terminal phalanx onto the dorsum of the middle phalanx, as when a finger is struck on its tip when extended. SEE: *f., hammer.*

    f., clubbed. Enlarged terminal phalanx of the finger. May be present in chronic obstructive pulmonary disease, cyanotic con-

genital heart disease; carcinoma of the lung; bacterial endocarditis; and carcinoma of the thyroid.

    f., dislocation of. Dislocations of a finger occur only at a joint. If there has been a crushing injury, assume that a fracture is present until an x-ray examination has been performed. Dislocations of a finger usually are easily diagnosed and quite easily reduced. They may be caused by blows, falls, and similar accidents.

First, be certain that there is no fracture. Then treat the dislocation by asking the patient to steady and support his wrist (or have somebody else do so) for countertraction. Take hold of the finger beyond the dislocated muscles and tendons and, with the free hand, slip the dislocated bone into place. Apply a splint from the tip of the finger well into the palm of the hand. The splint may be made of plastic, of tongue depressors, or temporarily of heavy cardboard.

Caution: Do not under any circumstances attempt to reduce a dislocation of the thumb joint nearest to the palm of the hand until x-ray examination has ruled out the possibility of fracture.

---

    f., hammer. Permanent flexion of the terminal phalanx of the finger; due to damage of the extensor tendon.

    f., hippocratic. F., clubbed, q.v.

    f., mallet. F., hammer, q.v.

    f., seal. SEE: *seal finger.*

    f., webbed. Condition in which some or all of the fingers are congenitally fused. Syndactylism.

finger, words pert. to: acroataxia; acrodynia; arachnodactyly; camptodactylia; dactyl; dactylus; digit; nail; phalanx.

finger cot. A protective covering for a finger. Usually made of plastic, rubber, or metal so that an injured finger may be protected from trauma during the healing process.

finger ladder. A device attached to a wall and in which notches are cut along an inclined line. The patient "walks" up this notched ladder by placing the fingertips in the notches. This activity assists with shoulder flexion or abduction to maintain range of motion, and may be used as a self-stretching technique to stretch the extensors or adductors of the shoulder to increase shoulder flexibility.

fingernail. SEE: *nail.*

fingerprint. An imprint made by the cutaneous ridges of the fleshy portion of the distal end of a finger. Fingerprints are used for purposes of identification, as they are individually unique. SEE: illus.

finger spelling. A method of communication

FINGERPRINTS

SIMPLE ARCH   ULNAR LOOP   SIMPLE WHORL

DERMATOGLYPHIC AREAS OF THE HAND

ULNAR LOOP
ARCH
RADIAL LOOP
TRIRADII
WHORL
FLEXION CREASES

used by persons with hearing or visual impairment in which words are spelled out letter by letter rather than depicted with single signs as in American Sign Language (ASL). Finger spelling can be done visually as well as tactually.

finger splint. A padded strip of malleable metal used to immobilize a fractured finger. As an alternative, the injured finger is often "buddy-taped" to an adjoining finger for support.

finger spreader. An orthotic device for the hand, usually made of foam rubber, used to hold the thumb and fingers in an extended position while maintaining the normal arches of the hand.

finger spring. Device for assisting extension or flexion of joints of fingers.

finger-stall. A protective covering for the finger. It may be made of rubber, plastic, metal, or leather. SYN: *finger cot.*

finger-to-nose test. A clinical test of cerebellar function. The individual stands with eyes closed and arms at the side and is asked to touch their nose with the tip of their finger.

finite. Having limits or boundaries.

fire [AS. *fyr*]. 1. Flame producing heat. 2. Fever.

f., St. Anthony's. Former term for erysipelas.

fire ant stings. The bite of fire ants, *Solenopsis,* cause local redness and tenderness; and the allergic response may be life-threatening.

TREAT: Wash area, which may contain multiple bites, with soap and water. Give epinephrine 0.3 to 0.5 ml of a 1:1000 aqueous solution subcutaneously, repeated every 20 to 30 minutes. This may be lifesaving. Use of a tourniquet will slow absorption of the venom. Application of ice packs to the area will relieve pain. Oxygen, endotracheal intubation, and vasopressors may be needed. Corticosteroids and antibiotics may be required.

firearm injuries. In 1985, 31,566 persons in the U.S. died as a result of firearm injuries. This important public health problem is the subject of research, but very little progress has been made.

fire emergencies. If a person's clothing catches fire, he or she should be rolled in a rug or blanket to smother flames. Running only fans the flames. It may be necessary to trip a burning person in order to prevent his or her running about. If an individual is outdoors, rolling in the dirt will smother flames.

If the victim is trapped in a burning building, the occupied room should have doors and windows closed to prevent cross breezes from increasing the fire. The window should be opened only if the victim is to be rescued through it. Do not open any door more than a few inches to ascertain possibility of escape. A burst of flame or hot air may push door in and asphyxiate anyone in the room. Wet cloths or towels should be held over mouth and nostrils to keep out smoke and gases. SEE: *burn; flames; gases; transportation.*

Caution: In attempting to escape from an area filled with smoke or fire it is important to crawl rather than run. The heat several feet above floor level may be lethal but, at floor level, cool enough to tolerate.

Even with crawling, it is important to proceed as quickly as possible because the toxic gas carbon monoxide will be present in higher concentration at floor level because it is heavier than air.

---

first aid. The administration of emergency assistance to individuals who have been injured or otherwise disabled, prior to the arrival of a physician or transportation to a hospital or physician's office. First aid should never be the substitution for definitive medical care. SEE: *basic life support; burn; cardiopulmonary resuscitation; Medi-*

cal Emergencies in *Appendix*.

RS: artificial respiration; bites or stings; burn; choking; coma; convulsion; dislocation; drowning; electric shock; fainting; fish poisoning; flames, inhalation of; food poisoning; foreign bodies; fracture; freezing; frostbite; fumes; insect bites and stings; laceration; poison; poison control center; poisoning; radiation accidents, emergency handling of; radioactive patient; shock; snakebite; unconsciousness.

first cranial nerves. Nerves supplying the nasal olfactory mucosa. Consist of delicate bundles of unmyelinated fibers, the fila olfactoria, which pass through the cribriform plate and terminate in the olfactory glomeruli of the olfactory bulb. The fila are the central processes of bipolar receptor neurons of olfactory mucous membrane. SYN: *olfactory nerves*.

first-degree A-V block. Cardiac dysrhythmia caused by delayed conduction through or from the atrioventricular node and characterized by a prolonged P-R interval. Usually requires no treatment.

first intention healing. Healing that takes place when wound edges are held or sutured together without granulation tissue having been formed. SEE: *healing*.

Fishberg concentration test (fish'bĕrg) [A. M. Fishberg, U.S. physician, b. 1898]. A test of the ability of the kidneys to concentrate, i.e., produce a urine of high specific gravity.

fish poisoning. A form of food poisoning caused by eating certain fish. Some fish are inherently poisonous; others become poisonous through decomposition, through infestation with certain parasites, or by poisonous metabolic substances produced during the spawning season.

Ciguatera poisoning: Poisoning produced when certain types of bottom-dwelling shore fish are ingested. This includes grouper, red snapper, and barracuda. The toxin, ciguatoxin, is present in fish that feed on protozoa. The toxin acts within 5 hours of ingestion, and symptoms may persist for 8 days or longer. SYM: Abdominal cramps, nausea, vomiting, diarrhea, paresthesia, hypotension, and respiratory paralysis. TREAT: Supportive.

Scromboid fish poisoning: Poisoning due to eating fish that have spoiled and are infested with bacteria, usually *Proteus morganii*, that degrade the protein in fish to produce scrombotoxin. SYM: About 30 minutes to 2 hours after eating the fish, a peppery sensation of the tongue develops, then a rash, pruritus, headache, dizziness, periorbital edema, thirst, nausea, vomiting, diarrhea, and abdominal cramps develop. These last about 12 to 24 hours. TREAT:

Symptomatic, but antihistamines may be of benefit. If stomach hasn't been emptied by vomiting, use gastric lavage. SEE: *anisakiasis; shellfish, paralytic poisoning from; sushi.*

fishskin disease. A disease of the skin characterized by increase of the horny layer and deficiency of the skin secretions. SYN: *ichthyosis*.

fission (fĭsh'ŭn) [L. *fissio*]. 1. Splitting into two or more parts. 2. A method of asexual reproduction in bacteria, protozoa, and other lower forms of life. The cell or the body divides into two or more parts, each of which develops into a complete individual. 3. Bombarding or splitting the nucleus of a heavy atom to release energy and neutrons.

fissiparous (fĭ-sĭp'ă-rŭs) [L. *fissus*, cleft, + *parere*, to bring forth]. Reproducing by fission.

fissura (fĭs-ū'ră) [L.] (pl. *fissurae*). [NA] Fissure. SYN: *cleft; sulcus*.

fissural (fĭsh'ū-răl). Pert. to a fissure.

fissure (fĭsh'ūr) [L. *fissura*]. 1. A groove or natural division, cleft or slit, deep furrow in the brain, liver, spinal cord, and other organs. 2. Ulcer or cracklike sore. 3. A break in the enamel of a tooth.

f., anal. A linear ulcer on the margin of the anus.

f., auricular. Fissure of petrous portion of the temporal bone.

f., branchial. SEE: *branchial clefts*.

f., Broca's. Fissure encircling the third left frontal convolution of the brain.

f., Burdach's. Fissure connecting lateral surface of insula and inner surface of operculum of the brain.

f., calcarine. Fissure extending from the cerebrum's occipital end to the occipital fissure.

f., callosomarginal. A conspicuous sulcus in mesial surface of cerebral hemisphere running above and concentric with the curved upper surface of the corpus callosum.

f., central. F., Rolando's.

f., Clevenger's. Inferior temporal sulcus of the brain.

f., collateral. Fissure on the inferior surface of cerebral hemisphere separating subcalcarine and subcollateral gyri.

f.'s, Henle's. Connective tissue areas between the muscular fibers of heart.

f., hippocampal. Fissure of brain extending from posterior part of corpus callosum to the tip of temporal lobe.

f., inferior orbital. Fissure at the apex of the orbit through which pass the infraorbital blood vessels and maxillary branch of the trigeminal nerve.

f., interparietal. Intraparietal sulcus.

f., longitudinal. Fissure on the lower surface of the liver.

f., occipitoparietal. Fissure between the occipital and parietal lobes of the brain.

f. of Bichat. Fissure below the corpus callosum in the cerebellum.

f. of Sylvius. Fissure separating the frontal and parietal lobes from the temporal lobe of the brain.

f., palpebral. Opening separating the upper and lower eyelids.

f., portal. Opening into the liver on its undersurface; continues into the liver as the portal canal.

f., Rolando's. Fissure separating frontal and parietal lobes of the brain.

f., sphenoidal. Fissure separating the wings and body of the sphenoid.

f., transverse. 1. Fissure between the cerebellum and cerebrum of the brain. 2. Fissure on lower surface of the liver that serves as the hilum transmitting vessels and ducts to the liver.

f., umbilical. Anterior portion of liver's longitudinal fissure, which contains the round ligament, the obliterated umbilical vein.

f., Wernicke's. Fissure dividing the temporal and parietal lobes from the occipital lobe of the brain.

f., zygal. A transverse cerebral sulcus that connects two parallel sulci. The three sulci are in the form of an H.

fisting. Slang term for the sadomasochistic practice of using the fist to penetrate the rectal area via the anal canal. This practice may cause severe or fatal rectal trauma. SYN: *fist fornication.* SEE: *Universal Precautions* in *Appendix.*

fistula (fĭs′tū-lă) [L., *fistula*, pipe]. An abnormal tubelike passage from a normal cavity or tube to a free surface or to another cavity. May be due to congenital incomplete closure of parts or may result from abscesses, injuries, or inflammatory processes.

f., anal. Fistula near the anus.

f., arteriovenous. Direct communication between an artery and vein.

f., biliary. Fistula through which bile is discharged after a biliary operation.

f., blind. Fistula open at only one end.

f., branchial. An open branchial cleft.

f., cervical. 1. An abnormal opening into the cervix uteri. 2. An opening in the neck leading to the pharynx, resulting from incomplete closure of the branchial clefts.

f., complete. Fistula with both external and internal openings.

f., craniosinus. Communication between the intracranial space and a paranasal sinus.

f., enterovaginal. Fistula between the bowel and vagina.

f., fecal. Fistula in which there is a discharge of feces through the opening.

f., gastric. Direct communication between the stomach and the skin over the abdomen.

f., horseshoe. Perianal fistula in which the tract goes around the rectum and communicates with the skin at one or more points.

f., incomplete. Fistula that has only one opening and that is to the skin, i.e., it does not communicate with an internal cavity or organ.

f., metroperitoneal. Fistula between uterine and peritoneal cavities.

f., parotid. Fistula from the parotid gland to the skin surface.

f., perineovaginal. Opening from the vagina through the perineum.

f., pulmonary arteriovenous, congenital. Direct communication within the lung of a pulmonary artery with a pulmonary vein. This congenital condition allows blood to bypass the oxygenation process in the lungs.

f., rectovaginal. Opening between the rectum and vagina.

f., thyroglossal. A midline fistula just above the thyroid that connects the openings in the skin to a persistent embryonic thyroglossal duct.

f., umbilical. Direct communication between the umbilicus and the gut. Usually due to the failure of closure of the urachal duct.

f., ureterovaginal. Opening between the ureter and vagina.

f., vesicouterine. Opening between the uterus and bladder.

f., vesicovaginal. Opening from the bladder into the vagina.

fistulatome (fĭs′tū-lă-tōm″) [″ + Gr. *tome*, incision]. Instrument for incising a fistula.

fistulectomy (fĭs″tū-lĕk′tō-mē) [″ + Gr. *ektome*, excision]. Excision of a fistula.

fistulization (fĭs″tū-lĭ-zā′shŭn) [L. *fistula*, pipe]. Becoming fistulous.

fistuloenterostomy (fĭs″tū-lō-ĕn-tĕr-ŏs′tō-mē) [″ + Gr. *enteron*, intestine, + *stoma*, mouth]. Operative closure of a biliary fistula and formation of new passage of bile into the intestine.

fistulous (fĭs′tū-lŭs). Pert. to, or containing, a fistula.

fit (fĭt) [AS. *fitt*]. 1. A sudden attack, convulsion, or paroxysm. SEE: *convulsion.* 2. Modification of one structure to that of another, as in dental restoration.

fitness, biologic. The ability of an individual with a disease to produce or father children who survive to adult life and are themselves able to reproduce.

fitness, physical. SEE: *physical fitness.*

fix. 1. To stain microscopic specimens for examination. 2. Slang for receiving a dose of a drug of abuse. 3. During the development of film, the process that stops the development action and makes the recorded image permanent.

fixation [L. *fixatio*]. 1. The act of holding or fastening in a fixed position. Immobilizing, making rigid. 2. The condition of being fixed. 3. A phase of Freudian psychosexual development in which the libido is arrested at an early or presexual level. 4. SEE: *fix* (def. 1). 5. The process of making an image recorded on film permanent.

 f., binocular. Focusing of both eyes on the target.

 f., complement. The action of a complement, a constituent of fresh blood serum, on an antigen, which in turn has been acted on by its antibody. During the uniting of antigen, antibody, and complement, the complement is rendered inactive or destroyed. This process is known as fixation of complement and is the basis of the Wassermann and Kolmer tests for syphilis. SEE: *complement.*

 f., external. Use of external devices, such as pins, in the fractured bone segments in order to keep them in place.

 f., field of. The widest limits of vision in all directions within which the eyes can fixate.

 f., internal. Use of internal wires, screws, or pins applied directly to the fractured bone segments in order to keep them in place.

 f. of eyes. The movement of the eyes for the most acute vision in which they are directed toward an object so that the visual axes meet and the image of the object falls on corresponding points of each retina.

fixation point. The fovea or the point on the retina where the visual axes (lines) meet the point of clearest vision.

fixative (fĭk′să-tĭv) [L. *fixus*, fastened]. 1. A substance that serves to make firm or fixed. 2. A substance used to harden and preserve pathological specimens.

fixed eruption. Skin lesions that appear in response to exposure to a drug. The eruption reappears at approx. the same site when the drug is again administered. Discontinuation of the medication is indicated.

fixed partial denture. A dental restoration of one or more missing teeth which is cemented to prepared natural teeth. SEE: *denture.*

fixing. In histology, rapid killing of tissue elements so that their normal living form is preserved. It is done to permit accurate and undistorted microscopic visualization of the tissues.

Fl. *fluid.*

flaccid (flăk′sĭd) [L. *flaccidus*, flabby]. Relaxed, flabby, having defective or absent muscular tone.

flaccid paralysis. Paralysis in which there is loss of muscle tone, loss of or reduction of tendon reflexes, atrophy and degeneration of muscles, and reaction of degeneration. Due to lesions of lower motor neurons of spinal cord.

flagella (flă-jĕl′ă) [L.]. Pl. of flagellum.

flagellant (flăj′ĕ-lănt) [L. *flagellum*, whip]. 1. Pert. to flagellum. 2. Pert. to stroking in massage. 3. One who practices flagellation.

flagellate (flăj′ĕ-lāt). 1. With one or more flagella. 2. A protozoon with one or more flagella.

flagellation (flăj″ĕ-lā′shŭn). 1. Whipping. 2. Massage by strokes. 3. A form of sexual aberration in which the libido is stimulated by whipping oneself, being whipped, or whipping someone else.

flagelliform (flă-jĕl′ĭ-form) [″ + *forma*, shape]. Shaped like a flagellum.

flagellum (flă-jĕl′ŭm) [L., whip] (pl. *flagella*). A hairlike, motile process on the extremity of a bacterium or protozoon.

flag sign. A peculiar change in hair color in which there is depigmentation of the hair in a band perpendicular to the long axis of the hair. This is seen in kwashiorkor, q.v., and indicates a period of severe malnutrition.

Flagyl. Trade name for metronidazole.

flail arm splint. ABBR: FAS. An upper extremity orthotic device used to provide support and limited function, consisting of a shoulder-operated harness, a volar supporting structure fabricated from low temperature thermoplastic material, and a terminal device which allows the arm to grasp or stabilize objects.

flail chest. A condition of the chest wall due to two or more fractures on each affected rib resulting in a segment of rib(s) which is not attached on either end; the flail segment moves paradoxically in with inspiration and out during expiration.

flail joint. A joint with excessive mobility usually due to paralysis of the muscles that control it.

flames, inhalation of. SYM: Intense irritation of nose, throat, pharynx, windpipe, and lungs with choking, coughing, interference with respiration, and intense swelling of the throat. Breathing is markedly limited. Shock is a common result, and should be suspected in any persons exposed to flames or smoke. Patient may also have facial burns, singed nose hairs, and elevated carboxyhemoglobin. The condition may cause adult respiratory distress syndrome (ARDS) and, later on, pulmonary complications including pneumonia, atelectasis, and thromboembolism. The immediate threat to life is carbon monoxide (CO) poisoning, q.v., and upper airway obstruction.

TREAT: Be prepared to treat CO poisoning and to promptly intubate or do a tracheostomy and provide supplemental oxygen if the airway is significantly obstructed. Corticosteroids may be used for edema; however, be aware that infection, which is a major complication, could be facilitated by such therapy. Prophylactic antibiotics are not useful and may promote infection with resistant organisms. Bronchoscopy is indicated to remove mucous plugs. SEE: *burn; fire; gases.*

flammable. Burning easily. SYN: *inflammable.*

flange (flănj). A border that projects above the main structure. In dentistry, the part of an artificial denture that extends from the imbedded teeth to the border of the denture.

flank [O. Fr. *flanc*]. The part of the body between ribs and upper border of ilium. Also loosely used to refer to the outer side of the thigh, hip, and buttock. SEE: *latus.*

flannelmouth. A person whose speech is thick.

flap [Dutch *flappen,* to strike]. 1. A mass of partially detached tissue used in plastic surgery of an adjacent area or in covering the end of a bone after resection. 2. An uncontrolled movement seen in some diseases. SEE: *asterixis.*

    f., amputation. Flap of skin used to cover the end of a part left after an amputation.

    f., extraction. Removal of cataract so as to make a flap in the cornea.

    f., island. Skin flap in which the edges are free but the center is attached and contains the vascular supply.

    f., jump. Skin flap moved from place to place by successively cutting one end and attaching it to a new site.

    f., mucoperiosteal. A flap of mucosal tissue, including the underlying periosteum, reflected from the bone during oral surgery.

    f., pedicle. Flap made by suturing the edges to form a tube. Then one end of the tube is cut and sutured to another site. By use of the jump flap technique, such a flap may be moved, in several stages, a great distance.

    f., periodontal. A section of soft tissue surgically separated from underlying bone and removed or repositioned to eliminate periodontal pockets or to correct mucogingival defects.

    f., skin. Flap containing only skin.

    f., sliding. Horizontal movement of a flap to cover a nearby raw area.

    f., tube. A long pedicle flap. SEE: *f., pedi-*

cle.

flare. A flush or spreading area of redness that surrounds a line made by drawing a pointed instrument across the skin. It is the second reaction in the triple response, q.v., of skin to injury and is due to dilatation of the arterioles.

flash. 1. Hot flash. SEE: *hot flashes.* 2. Excess material from a mold.

flashbacks. The return of imagery and hallucinations after the immediate effects of hallucinogens have worn off. They may occur for an extended period. They may be of a frightening or threatening form but may consist only of perceptual distortion.

flash method. Means of pasteurizing milk by rapidly raising its temperature to 178°F (80.1°C), maintaining it there for a few minutes, and rapidly chilling it until the temperature is 40°F (4.4°C).

flash point. The temperature at which a substance will burst into flame spontaneously.

flask [LL. *flasco*]. A small bottle with a narrow neck.

flatfoot. Abnormal flatness of sole and arch of foot. This condition may exist without causing symptoms or interfering with normal function of the foot. The inner longitudinal and anterior transverse metatarsal arches are those that may be depressed. It may be acute, subacute, or chronic. SYN: *pes planus; splayfoot.*

    f., spasmodic. Flatfoot in which the foot is held everted by spasmodic contraction of the peroneal muscle.

flatness. Resonance heard on percussion over solid organs or when there is fluid in the thoracic cavity.

flatplate. Term used to describe a radiographic examination requiring a frontal projection of the abdomen or other body part with the patient in a supine position.

flatulence (flăt'ū-lĕns) [L. *flatulentus*]. Excessive gas in the stomach and intestines. SEE: *distention; gastrointestinal decompression; paralytic ileus; Wangensteen tube.*

NURSING IMPLICATIONS: Auscultate bowel sounds. Evaluate for abdominal distention, the presence and location of pain and cramping, and the passage of flatus rectally. Encourage active ambulation to increase peristalsis. If the patient cannot ambulate or if ambulation is ineffective, insert a lubricated rectal tube 15 cm (6 in.) into the rectum and allow to remain in place for no more than 30 minutes. Unless contraindicated, local heat may be applied to the abdomen. If bowel sounds decrease or abdominal distention increases and flatus is not passed, notify the physician, as the patient may be developing paralytic ileus.

flatulent (flăt'ū-lĕnt). Affected with or caused

by gas in the alimentary tract.

flatus (flā′tŭs) [L., a blowing]. 1. Gas in the digestive tract. 2. Expelling of gas from a body orifice; esp. the anus. The average person excretes 400 to 1200 cc of gas each day. The gas passages may average a dozen a day in some persons and up to a hundred in some persons. Flatus from the lower intestinal tract contains hydrogen, methane, skatoles, indoles, carbon dioxide, and small amounts of oxygen and nitrogen. SEE: *borborygmus; eructation.*

Foods that are known for their ability to cause excess intestinal gas include beans, peas, lentils, cabbage, onions, Brussels sprouts, bananas, apples, raisins, apricots, high-fiber cereals, whole wheat products, milk and milk products, and sorbitol present in some dietetic foods.

TREAT: In some persons with excess intestinal gas this can be controlled by avoiding foods they have found to be flatulogenic. In others in whom there is no distinct relationship to the type of food eaten, they should be reassured that flatulence, though sometimes socially awkward or embarrassing, is not detrimental to health.

    f., vaginal. Expulsion of air from the vagina.

flatus tube. A rectal tube to facilitate expulsion of flatus. It is used in cases of severe distention and before a saline enema.

NURSING IMPLICATIONS: Gas in the lower bowel may be relieved by a rectal tube. The tube is lubricated and inserted for 20 minutes. The tube may be reinserted every four hours. Hot water bottle or heating pad applied to the abdomen may also be ordered.

flatworm. A worm belonging to the phylum Platyhelminthes.

flavedo (flă-vē′dō) [L.]. Yellowness, as of the skin; sallowness; jaundice.

flavescent (flă-vĕs′ĕnt). Yellowish.

flavin (flā′vĭn). One of a group of natural water-soluble pigments occurring in milk, yeasts, bacteria, and some plants. All contain the flavin or isoalloxazine nucleus and are yellow in color. Present in riboflavin and in Warburg's yellow enzyme.

flavism (flā′vĭzm) [L. *flavus,* yellow, + Gr. *-ismos,* condition]. Having a yellow tinge.

flavivirus (flā″vē-vī′rŭs). A genus of Togaviridae. They were previously called group B arboviruses. Viruses that cause yellow fever, certain types of encephalitis, and dengue are species in this genus.

flavo- [L. *flavus,* yellow]. Prefix indicating yellow.

Flavobacterium. A genus of rod-shaped bacteria belonging to the Achromobacteraceae. They are found in soil and water and produce an orange-yellow pigment in cultures.

Flavobacterium meningosepticum is especially virulent for the premature infant, in whom it causes meningitis. The fatality rate is quite high.

flavone (flā′vōn). The chemical from which the natural colors of many vegetables are derived.

flavoprotein. One of a group of conjugated proteins that constitute the yellow enzymes essential in cellular respiration.

flavor (flā′vor). 1. The quality of a substance that affects the sense of taste. It may also stimulate the sense of smell. 2. A material added to a food or medicine to improve its taste.

Flaxedil. Trade name for gallamine triethiodide.

flaxseed. Seed of *Linum usitatissimum.* SYN: *linseed.*

fl. dr. *fluidram.*

flea (flē) [AS. *flea*]. Any insect of the order Siphonaptera. Fleas are wingless, suck blood, and have legs adapted for jumping. Usually they are parasitic on warm-blooded animals including man. Fleas of the genus *Xenopsylla* transmit the bacillus of plague *(Pasteurella pestis)* from rats to humans. Fleas may transmit other diseases such as tularemia, endemic typhus, and brucellosis. They serve as intermediate hosts for the cat and dog tapeworms.

    f., cat. Ctenocephalides felis.

    f., chigger. Tunga penetrans. SYN: *chigger; jigger; sand flea.*

    f., dog. Ctenocephalides canis.

    f., human. Pulex irritans.

    f., rat. Xenopsylla cheopis.

flea bites. Hemorrhagic puncta surrounded by erythematous and urticarial patches as the result of the injection of flea saliva.

TREAT: Ice applied to the site will decrease the pain. Application of a corticosteroid cream may decrease the inflammatory response.

PREVENTION: Treat the skin with an insect repellent available in form of a powder, spray, or oil for topical use.

flea infestation. A home with dogs or cats may become infested with fleas. It is possible to kill the flea population by treating the house for 24 hr by using naphthalene. This substance is available in flake form for use as a moth repellent. The flakes are spread on newspapers in the middle of each room, and the house is closed for 24 hr.

Caution: It is essential to disconnect all electrical equipment in the house prior to this procedure because an electrical spark could cause the fumes to explode. Any plants, pets, or humans could suffer adverse effects if they remain in the house during the treatment period.

The house should be thoroughly ventilated after the treatment period in order to remove the fumes.

Another possibility is to drown the fleas by allowing them to jump into a shallow pan containing water and a detergent. The pan is left in the flea-infested area at night in a dark room except for a light over the pan. The fleas are attracted to the light and, when they jump, land in the water, where they sink and drown because of the detergent in the water.

fleam (flēm) [Fr. *flieme*]. Lancet used in venesection.

flecainide acetate. Antiarrhythmic drug. Trade name is Tambocor.

Flechsig's areas (flĕk'zĭgz) [Paul E. Flechsig, Ger. neurologist, 1847–1929]. Anterior, lateral, and posterior areas of each lateral half of the medulla.

fleece of Stilling. Meshwork of white fibers that surrounds the dentate nucleus of the cerebellum.

Fleet Bisacodyl. Trade name for bisacodyl.

Fleet Enema. Trade name for sodium biphosphate.

Fleet Mineral Oil Enema. Trade name for mineral oil.

Fleming, Sir Alexander (flĕm'ĭng). Scottish physician, 1881–1955, who in 1945, along with Ernst B. Chain and Sir Howard W. Florey, was awarded the Nobel Prize in medicine and physiology for the discovery of penicillin.

flesh [AS. *flaesc*]. The soft tissues of the animal body, esp. the muscles. SEE: *carnivorous; meat.*

   f., examination of animal. Examine for color, consistency, proportion of fat, odor, and, after cooking, its taste. In general, it should be neither very pale nor dark purple; it should be marbled and of firm and elastic consistency; it should be free from odor; touching the flesh should not moisten the finger.

   NOTE: *Yellow:* May be produced by food eaten by animal. In disease, due to animals having been jaundiced. *Brown:* Rare except in old meat undergoing decomposition. *Dark Purple:* May indicate animal died a natural death or suffered from acute fever, tuberculosis, or rinderpest. Avoid. *Dark Reddish-Brown:* May indicate animal was hunted or overdriven; poisoned, drowned, or suffocated. Such meat is to be avoided. *Scarlet:* Rare. Indicates arsenic or carbon monoxide poisoning. *Redness:* Indicates that animal may have been poisoned or the meat frozen. *Green or Violet:* Indicates the beginning of dangerous putrefaction. *Saffron:* Indicates artificial coloring. *Brilliant Red:* Due

to poisonous bacteria. *Gray:* Usually in sausages. Due to bacteria. *Phosphorescent:* Not due to putrefaction. Usually found in fish and shellfish. Increased by heat. Sometimes in meat, esp. veal, caused by bacteria, and generally transmitted from fish kept in the same place with meat. *White:* Rare except in veal. Found in certain diseases. Avoid.

   f., goose. Cutis anserina.

   f., proud. Excessive granular tissue in a wound or ulcer.

Fletcher factor. A blood clotting factor, prekallikrein.

fletcherism [Horace Fletcher, U.S. dietitian, 1849–1919]. Taking small amounts of food at a time. These small bites are chewed for a prolonged period prior to swallowing. SEE: *psomophagia.*

flex [L. *flexus*, bent]. To bend upon itself, as a muscle.

flexibilitas cerea (flĕks"ĭ-bĭl'ĭ-tăs sē'rē-ă) [L.]. A cataleptic state in which limbs retain any position in which they are placed. Characteristic of catatonic patients. SEE: *catalepsy.*

flexibility [L. *flexus*, bent]. Quality of being bent without breaking; adaptability. SYN: *pliability.*

flexible. Capable of being bent without breaking.

flexile (flĕks'īl) [L. *flexus*, bent]. Pliant, flexible.

flexion (flĕk'shŭn) [L. *flexio*]. 1. The act of bending or condition of being bent in contrast to extension. SEE: *antecurvature.* 2. To decrease the angle between the bones forming a joint.

flexor (flĕks'or) [L.]. A muscle that brings two bones closer together, causing flexion of the part or a decreased angle of the joint. Opposite to extensor.

flexura (flĕk-shoo'ră) [L.]. Flexure.

flexure (flĕk'shĕr) [L. *flexura*]. A bend.

   f., colic, left. Bend in the colon at which point the transverse colon becomes the descending colon.

   f., colic, right. Bend at the transition point where the ascending colon becomes the transverse colon.

   f., dorsal. Convex curve in the thoracic area of the spine.

   f., duodenojejunal. Curve at meeting point of jejunum and duodenum.

   f., hepatic. Right flexure of the colon. The bend in the large intestine forming the junction of the ascending with the transverse colon.

   f., sigmoid. S-like loop (in left iliac fossa) of the descending colon as it joins the rectum. SEE: *colon.*

   f., splenic. Left flexure of the colon. The bend at junction of transverse with descending colon.

flicker. The visual sensation of alternating intervals of brightness caused by rhythmically interrupting light stimuli.

flicker phenomenon. When an intermittent light stimulus is seen, there is a rate that will produce the sensation that the light is continuous.

flight into disease. Readily assuming the status of being sick in order to escape reality.

flight into health. Voluntary and temporary suppression of symptoms in order to prevent further psychoanalytic probing into the patient's psyche.

flight of ideas. Continuous but fragmentary stream of talk. The general train of thought can be followed but direction is frequently changed, often by chance stimuli from the environment. May be seen in acute manic states.

flint disease. Pneumonoconiosis associated with the inhalation of dust produced by stone cutting. SYN: *chalicosis.*

flip-flop. In computers, a circuit that yields as an output one of two possible conditions: high (1) or low (0). Used in memory circuits and counters.

floaters (flō′tĕrs) [AS. *flotian,* float]. Translucent specks of various sizes and shapes that float across the visual field. They are due to small bits of protein or cells floating in the vitreous. The great majority of people have these benign materials in their eyes. SEE: *muscae volitantes.*

floating [AS. *flota,* a raft]. Moving about; out of normal location.

floating kidney. Kidney movable from its normal bed of fat.

floating ribs. The 11th and 12th ribs, which do not articulate with the sternum.

floats. Glass capsules containing labels to float in an exposed liquid to designate its nature.

floccillation, floccitation (flŏk″sĭ-lā′shŭn, -tā′shŭn) [L. *floccilatio*]. Semiconscious picking at bedclothes in association with fever, stupor, and delirium. SYN: *carphologia; carphology.*

floccose (flŏk′ōs) [L. *floccosus,* full of wool tufts]. In biology, pert. to a growth made up of short and densely but irregularly interwoven filaments.

floccular (flŏk′ū-lär) [L. *flocculus,* little tuft]. Pert. to the flocculus of the cerebellum.

flocculation (flŏk″ū-lā′shŭn). The gathering together of the fine dispersed particles in a solution into larger, usually visible particles.

flocculation reaction. Flocculation of a serum reaction.

flocculence (flŏk′ū-lĕns″). State of being flocculent or resembling shreds or tufts of cotton.

flocculent (flŏk′ū-lĕnt). Resembling the white portion of floating island or a fluid or culture containing whitish shreds of mucus.

flocculus (flŏk′ū-lŭs) [L., little tuft] (pl. *flocculi*). 1. A small tuft of woollike fibers. 2. [NA] A lobe below and behind the middle peduncle of the cerebrum on each side of the median fissure.

flood. 1. Pathological uterine hemorrhage. 2. Excessive menstrual bleeding.

flooding (flŭd′ĭng). 1. Colloquial term for excessive amount of menstrual flow. 2. In treating phobias, repeated exposure to the disturbing ideas, situations, or conditions until these conditions no longer produce anxiety.

Flood's ligament [Valentine Flood, Ir. surgeon, 1800–1847]. A band of ligaments attached to the lower part of the lesser tuberosity of the humerus.

floor [AS. *flor*]. The surface that forms the lower limit of a cavity or space, as the floor of the cranial cavity, fourth ventricle, mouth, nasal fossa, pelvis, or a cavity preparation in a tooth.

floppy-valve syndrome. SYN: *mitral valve prolapse,* q.v.

flora [L. *flos,* flower]. 1. Plant life as distinguished from animal life. 2. Plant life occurring or adapted for living in a specific environment. Thus one speaks of the intestinal, vaginal, or skin flora. SEE: *fauna.*

florid [L. *floridus,* blossoming]. Having a bright deep-red color. Used to describe skin coloration.

Florinef Acetate. Trade name for fludrocortisone acetate.

Floropryl. Trade name for isoflurophate.

floss. To use dental floss or tape to remove plaque and calculus from the otherwise inaccessible dental surfaces between teeth.

   f., dental. A waxed or unwaxed tape or thread used to clean and remove plaque between teeth and below the gumline.

flour [L. *flos,* flower]. Finely ground meal obtained from wheat or other grain; any soft fine powder. SEE: *Foods* in Appendix.

flow [AS. *flowan,* to flow]. 1. Action of flowing with respect to time. 2. The act of moving or running freely.

flow cell. A flow-through optical cell employed in photometers and cell counters through which the sample and any standards are passed for detection. SEE: *flow cytometry.*

flow cytometry. A sophisticated technique for analyzing individual cells as they flow in single file through a detector system. The cells, which have been tagged with a monoclonal antibody with a fluorescent label, pass through the detector at about 10,000 cells per second. Flow cytometry has a great number of clinical and research applications, e.g., analysis of cell size, structure, and viability; examination of DNA and RNA in the cells; determination of pH in the cells; chromosome analysis; determination of the percentage of cells in a population that are in various stages of development, thus providing means of estimating the extent or control of a malignant tumor. Monitoring the number of populations of T cells, B cells, and T helper and suppressor cells, and using that information to calculate the helper: suppressor ratio is of assistance in determining the patient's immune status. Flow cytometry has been used in monitoring survival of transplants of organs and tissues such as bone marrow. SEE: *cell sorting.*

flower [L. *flos,* flower]. That part of a plant that comprises the organs of reproduction such as the anthemis, arnica, and matricaria. A complete flower includes a calyx, corolla, stamens, which produce pollen, and a pistil, which produces the ovule.

flow, laminar. SEE: *laminar air flow.*

flowmeter. Device for measuring the flow of a gas or liquid. Used esp. in monitoring flow of anesthetic gases.

flow state. An altered state of consciousness in which the mind functions at its peak, time may seem to be distorted, and a sense of happiness seems to pervade that period. In such a state the individual feels alive and fully attentive to what is being done. This state is distinguished from strained attention in which the person forces himself or herself to perform a task in which he or she has little interest.

floxuridine (flŏks-ŭr′ĭ-dēn). USP. An antimetabolite used in treating certain forms of cancer.

fl. oz. *fluidounce,* 29.57 milliliters.

flu (floo). Influenza.

flucticuli (flŭk-tĭk′ū-lī) [L., little waves] (sing. *flucticulus*). Wavelike markings on lateral wall of third ventricle.

fluctuant (flŭk′chū-ănt). Varying, or unstable. SEE: *fluctuation.*

fluctuation [L. *fluctuatio*]. 1. A variation from one course to another. 2. A wavy impulse felt in palpation and produced by vibration of body fluid.

DIAG: If fluctuation is felt over the lower abdomen, ascites usually is present. May be caused by peritoneal hemorrhage. If it is confined to limited portion of abdomen, tuberculous peritonitis may be implicated; over central portion, bladder distention; in lower abdomen in women, an ovarian cyst or pregnancy; in right hypochondrium, a hydatid cyst, abscess of liver, distended gallbladder; over left hypochondrium, cysts or abscess; above umbilicus, dilated colon or stomach partly filled with fluid and gas.

flucytosine (flū-sī′tō-sēn″). An antifungal drug. It is usually used with amphotericin B in order to decrease the emergence of resistant strains of yeasts and fungi. Trade name is Ancobon.

fludrocortisone (floo″drō-kor′tĭ-sōn). A synthetic corticosteroid.

f. acetate. A corticosteroid drug. Trade name is Florinef Acetate.

fluid [L. *fluidus*]. A nonsolid, liquid, or gaseous substance. SEE: *secretion.*

f., allantoic. Fluid present in the allantoic sac.

f., amniotic. A clear yellowish fluid that fills the fetal membranes in pregnancy Spec. grav. approx. 1.006. It is composed of albumin, salts (chiefly urea), and water, and suspended in it are lanugo, epidermal cells, vernix caseosa, and meconium. It is derived from the amnion. Its chief function is to provide protection for the fetus. SEE: *amnion; meconium.*

f., cerebrospinal. Fluid found in central canal of spinal cord, in the ventricles of the brain, and in the subarachnoid space about the brain and spinal cord. It is formed by the choroid plexuses of the ventricles.

f., extracellular. Tissue fluid or fluid occupying spaces between the tissue cells.

f., extravascular. All the body fluids outside the blood vessels. Includes tissue fluid, fluids within the serous and synovial cavities, the cerebrospinal fluid, and lymph.

f., interstitial. F., extracellular.

f., intracellular. Fluid contained within cells and constituting about 50% of body weight.

f., intraocular. Fluid within the anterior and posterior chambers of the eye.

f., repair. Solution in water of electrolytes and usually glucose, given intravenously to correct or repair fluid and electrolyte imbalance. SEE: *fluid replacement.*

f., seminal. Semen.

f., serous. Fluid in the serous cavities.

f., spinal. Cerebrospinal fluid present in the spinal canal of the spinal cord.

f., synovial. Fluid contained within synovial cavities, bursae, and tendon sheaths. SYN: *synovia.*

fluid balance. Regulation of amount of water in the body. The balance is upset when fluids are lost by vomiting, diarrhea, bleeding, or when dehydration occurs. Treatment of fluid imbalance depends upon the cause, the kind and quantity of fluids lost, and the state of renal function. SEE: *fluid replacement.*

fluid diet. Diet for those unable to tolerate solid food or for patients whose gastrointestinal tract needs to be free of solid matter.

fluidextract, fluidextractum [L. *fluidus,* fluid, + *extractum,* extract]. Solution of the soluble constituents of vegetable drugs of such strength that each cc or ml represents 1 gm of the drug. Fluidextracts contain alcohol as a solvent or preservative, and many of these form precipitates when water is added.

   f., aromatic cascara. USP. Liquid preparation of cascara sagrada, magnesium oxide, glycyrrhiza extract, saccharin, anise oil, coriander oil, methyl salicylate, alcohol, and water. Used as a laxative.

   f., glycyrrhiza. A liquid preparation of glycyrrhiza.

   f., ipecac. A fluid preparation of the powdered rhizome and roots of *Cephaelis ipecacuanha* or *C. acuminata.* It is used as an emetic and expectorant.

fluidotherapy. A dry heat modality consisting of cellulose particles held in a container and moved in air. The turbulence of the gassolid mixture generates a thermal effect when objects are immersed in the medium. Treatment temperature ranges from 43–50°C.

fluidounce. SYMB: f℥. Measure of apothecaries' fluid volume, equal to eight fluidrams or 29.57 ml.

fluidram. SYMB: f℈. Apothecaries' measure of fluid volume, equal to 3.697 ml.

fluid replacement. Administering fluids by any route to attempt to correct a fluid deficit. The deficit may be "physiologic" as in dehydration due to perspiring in a hot, dry climate while doing hard physical labor or sports, or due to inadequate intake of fluids; or "pathological" as in traumatic or septic shock, adult respiratory distress syndrome, fluid loss due to severe vomiting or diarrhea or both, metabolic and endocrine conditions such as diabetic ketosis, chronic renal failure, adrenal insufficiency.

   The goal of fluid replacement is to correct both the fluid imbalance as well as the electrolyte (acid base) imbalance(s). The oral route of replacement is used if possible. The intravenous, intraperitoneal, or subcutaneous routes are also used, with the intravenous route being used most frequently. Fluid composition may be isotonic, hypotonic, hypertonic; certain crystalloids such as sodium, potassium, chloride or calcium; or osmotically active substances including glucose, protein, starch, and the synthetic plasma volume expanders, dextran or hetastarch. The composition, rate of administration, and route will depend upon the clinical condition being treated. SEE: *catheter, central venous; central line; intravenous infusion pump; oral rehydration therapy; solution;* illus. for intravenous infusion techniques.

Caution: During fluid replacement in the critically ill, monitor patient frequently to be certain that fluid overload is prevented and to be sure the solution is flowing and that it isn't extravasating. This is especially important when treating infants and small children.

---

fluid retention. Failure to eliminate fluid from the body because of renal, cardiac, or metabolic disease, or combinations of these disorders. Retention of salt is another cause of fluid retention. Excess salt in the body requires retention of water to maintain the proper chemical and physical properties of body fluids. A low-sodium diet is indicated in fluid retention. The advisability of using diuretics will depend upon the functional state of the kidneys.

fluke (flook) [AS. *floc,* flatfish]. A parasitic worm belonging to the class Trematoda, phylum Platyhelminthes. Those parasitic in man belong to the order Digenea. Most flukes have complex life cycles that include asexual generations that live in a mollusc (snail or bivalve). Stages of a typical fluke include adult, egg, miracidium, sporocyst, redia, cercaria, and metacercaria.

   f., blood. A schistosome; flukes of the genus *Schistosoma, S. haematobium, S. mansoni,* and *S. japonicum.* Adults live principally in the mesenteric and pelvic veins. They cause schistosomiasis and schistosome dermatitis (swimmer's itch).

   f., intestinal. Species of intestinal flukes infesting man include *Gastrodiscoides hominis, Fasciolopsis buski, Heterophyes heterophyes,* and *Metagonimus yokogawai.*

   f., liver. Species living in the liver and bile ducts. Those infesting man include *Clonorchis sinensis, Fasciola hepatica, Dicrocoelium dendriticum,* and *Opisthorchis felineus.*

   f., lung. Fluke that infests lung tissue. Only one species is common in man, namely *Paragonimus westermani.*

flumethasone pivalate (floo-měth′ă-sōn). USP. A synthetic corticosteroid. Trade name is Locorten.

flumina pilorum (floo′mĭ-nă pī-lō′rŭm) [L., rivers of hair]. [NA] The curved lines along which the hairs of the body are arranged, esp. in the fetus; hairs lying in same direction.

fluo-. Prefix indicating flow.

fluocinolone acetonide (floo-ō-sĭn′ō-lōn). USP. A synthetic corticosteroid. Trade names are Fluonid and Synalar.

Fluogen. Trade name for influenza virus vaccine, trivalent.

Fluonid. Trade name for fluocinolone acetonide.

fluor albus (floo′or ăl′bŭs) [L., white flow]. White discharge from the uterus or vagina. SYN: *leukorrhea.*

fluorescein sodium (floo″ō-rĕs′ē-ĭn). USP. A red crystalline powder. Used chiefly for diagnostic purposes and for detecting foreign bodies in or lesions of the cornea of the eye. Trade names are Fluor-I-Strip A.T., Fluorescite, Ful-Glo, and Funduscein.

fluorescence (floo″ō-rĕs′ĕnts). Property of certain substances to emit light when exposed to certain types of light radiation, usually ultraviolet. This was first noted in fluorspar. The mechanism is absorption of certain wavelengths and simultaneous emission of a longer wavelength that terminates simultaneously with the cessation of the incident exciting radiation.

fluorescent (floo-ō-rĕs′ĕnt). 1. In biology, having one color by transmitted light and another by reflected light. 2. Luminous when exposed to other light rays.

fluorescent antibody. ABBR: FA. An antibody that has been stained or marked by a fluorescent material. Use of the fluorescent antibody technique permits rapid diagnosis of various kinds of infections.

fluorescent polarization immunoassay. ABBR: FPIA. An antigen-antibody analysis utilizing the measurement of both fluorescence and polarization of light by fluorescent tagged molecules. Small molecules rotate rapidly and lose polarization while large molecules rotate slowly and retain their polarization.

fluorescent screen. 1. A sheet of cardboard, paper, or glass coated with a material that fluoresces visibly, such as calcium tungstate. It is used in fluoroscopy when roentgen rays, radium rays, or electrons impinge upon it. 2. A sheet of cardboard, paper, or glass, coated with anthracene or other fluorescing materials to observe ultraviolet radiations. SYN: *intensifying screen.*

fluorescent treponemal antibody-absorption test. ABBR: FTA-ABS. Test for syphilis using fluorescent antibody, q.v., technique.

Fluorescite. Trade name for fluorescein sodium, USP.

fluoridation (floo″or-ĭ-dā′shŭn). The addition of fluorides to a water supply as a means of helping to prevent dental caries.

The development of dental caries in the deciduous and permanent teeth can be decreased by providing fluoride either as a supplement in the drinking water, by topical application to the teeth, or by daily medication with fluoride. There are several important considerations: fluoride in excess daily dose will cause discoloration of the teeth if the fluoride is ingested while the teeth are developing, i.e., from birth to 8 or 10 years. If fluoridated water is consumed during pregnancy, the deciduous teeth, which begin to mineralize during the 4th or 5th month in utero, will incorporate that compound and be more resistant to caries. In the adult tooth, when enamel has lost mineral (white spot lesion), the remineralization is greatly enhanced by the presence of fluoride, which leads to the precipitation of calcium phosphate.

The rate of loss of teeth in individuals receiving fluoride from infancy will be only one-quarter that of persons who received no fluoride. The most certain and effective method of administering fluoride is by providing drinking water that contains one part per million, 1 mg/1000 ml, of fluoride. This will assure a daily dose of fluoride of 0.25 to 0.50 mg per day.

Caution: Children drinking water that is fluoridated should not be given supplemental fluoride medication.

fluoride (floo′ō-rīd). A compound of fluorine with a radical; a salt of hydrofluoric acid.

   f., stannous. A compound applied topically to the teeth to prevent dental caries.

fluoride dental treatment. The application of a fluoride solution or gel to the teeth as a means of controlling or preventing caries. SEE: *dental sealants.*

fluoride poisoning. SEE: *Poisons and Poisoning* in *Appendix.*

fluorine (floo′ō-rēn, floor′ēn). SYMB: F. At. wt. 18.9984; at. no. 9. Gaseous chemical element found in the soil in combination with calcium. SEE: *fluoridation.*

Fluor-I-Strip A.T. Trade name for fluorescein sodium, USP.

fluoroacetate (floo″or-ō-ăs′ē-tāt). A salt of fluoroacetic acid. SEE: *Poisons and Poisoning* in *Appendix.*

fluoroapatite. A compound formed when the enamel of teeth is treated with appropriate concentrations of the fluoride ion. The modified hydroxyapatite is less acid-soluble and therefore resistant to caries. Fluoroapatite is also formed in bone, as well as in enamel and dentin of teeth, when fluoride is taken systemically.

fluorocarbon. General term for hydrocarbons in which some of the hydrogen atoms have been replaced with fluorine. Their use in aerosol sprays was discontinued because of an adverse effect on the atmosphere. SYN: *fluorinated hydrocarbons.*

fluorometer (floo-or-ŏm′ĕ-tĕr). 1. Device for determining the amount of radiation produced by x-rays. 2. Device for adjusting a fluoroscope in order to establish better the location of the target and to produce an undistorted image or shadow.

fluorometholone (floor"ō-mĕth'ō-lōn). USP. A synthetic corticosteroid. Trade names are Oxylone and FML Liquifilm.

Fluoroplex. Trade name for fluorouracil.

fluoroscope (floo'or-ō-skōp). A device consisting of a fluorescent screen suitably mounted, either separately or in conjunction with a roentgen tube, by means of which the shadows of objects interposed between the tube and the screen are made visible.

fluoroscopy. The use of a fluoroscope for medical diagnosis or for testing various materials by roentgen rays.

fluorosis (floo-or-ō'sĭs). Chronic fluorine poisoning, sometimes marked by mottling of tooth enamel. Often results from too much fluoride in drinking water.

fluorouracil (floor"ō-ŭr'ă-sĭl). USP. An antimetabolite used in treating certain forms of cancer. Trade names are Adrucil, 5-FU, Efudex, and Fluoroplex.

fluoxetine hydrochloride. An antidepressant. Trade name is Prozac.

fluoxymesterone (floo-ŏk"sē-mĕs'tĕr-ōn). USP. An anabolic and androgenic hormone. Trade names are Ora-Testryl and Halotestin.

fluphenazine enanthate (floo-fĕn'ă-zēn). USP. A phenothiazine-type tranquilizer. Trade name is Prolixin Enanthate.

fluprednisolone (floo"prĕd-nĭs'ō-lōn). A corticosteroid drug. Trade name is Alphadrol.

flurandrenolide (floor"ăn-drĕn'ō-līd). USP. A corticosteroid drug. Trade name is Cordran.

flurazepam hydrochloride (floor-ăz'ĕ-păm). A sedative-hypnotic drug. Trade name is Dalmane.

flurogestone acetate (floor"ō-jĕs'tōn). A progestational drug.

flurothyl (floor'ō-thĭl). USP. A central nervous system stimulant.

fluroxene (floor-ŏks'ēn). An anesthetic agent administered by inhalation.

Caution: It may be flammable and explosive.

---

flush [ME. *flusshen*, to fly up]. 1. Sudden redness of the skin. 2. Irrigation of a cavity with water.

f., hectic. Redness of the cheeks seen in some chronic febrile diseases such as pulmonary tuberculosis.

f., hot. Flush accompanied with sensation of heat; common in neuroses, psychoneuroses, and during menopause.

f., malar. A bright-colored flush over the malar area and cheekbones. May be associated with any febrile disease.

flutter [AS. *floterian*, to fly about]. A tremulous movement, esp. of the heart, as in atrial and ventricular flutter.

f., atrial. Condition in which contractions of the atrium become extremely rapid (200 to 400 per min). In pure flutter, a regular rhythm is maintained; in impure flutter, the rhythm is irregular.

f., diaphragmatic. Rapid contractions of the diaphragm. They may occur intermittently or be present for an extended period. The cause is unknown.

f., mediastinal. Abnormal side-to-side motion of the mediastinum during respiration.

f., ventricular. Ventricular contractions of the heart at a rate of 250 or more.

flutter-fibrillation. Cardiac dysrhythmia alternating between atrial fibrillation and atrial flutter, or one that could be either when seen on a cardiac monitor.

flux [L. *fluxus,* a flow]. An excessive flow or discharge from an organ or cavity of the body.

fly [AS. *fleoge*]. An insect belonging to the order Diptera, characterized by possessing sucking mouth parts, one pair of wings, and incomplete metamorphosis, such as the May fly, house fly, or dragonfly. Term is sometimes applied to insects belonging to other orders. SEE: *Diptera.*

f., black. A fly of the genus *Simulium.*

f., blow. Flies of the family Calliphoridae. They breed in dung or the flesh of dead animals. SYN: *bluebottle flies.* SEE: *Calliphora vomitoria.*

f., bot-. SEE: *botfly.*

f., flesh. The Sarcophagidae.

f., house. Musca domestica.

f., sand-. Phlebotomus.

f., screwworm. A fly belonging to the families Calliphoridae and Sarcophagidae.

f., Spanish. Cantharides.

f., tsetse. *Glossina palpalis;* fly that transmits African sleeping sickness or trypanosomiasis.

f., warble. Dermatobia.

Fm. Chem. symb. for the element fermium.

f.m. L. *fiat mistura*, make a mixture. An abbreviation used in prescription writing.

foam (fōm) [AS. *fam*]. A mixture of finely divided gas bubbles interspersed in a liquid.

focal [L. *focus*, hearth]. Pert. to a focus.

focal infection. Infection occurring near a focus, such as the cavity of a tooth.

focal lesion. A limited central lesion.

focal spot. Area on the x-ray tube target that is bombarded with electrons to produce x radiation.

foci (fō'sī) [L.]. Pl. of focus.

focus [L., hearth] (pl. *foci*). 1. The point of

convergence of light rays or waves of sound.
2. The starting point of a disease process.

f., real. Point at which convergent rays intersect.

f., virtual. Point at which divergent rays would intersect if prolonged backward.

FOD. *focus-object distance.* The distance from the target of the x-ray tube to the surface being radiographed.

fog. Droplets suspended in a gas, as water droplets in air.

fogging. 1. A method of testing vision, used particularly in testing astigmatism and in postcycloplegic examination. 2. Method of intense application of an insecticide. The solution is nebulized and appears in the air as a fog. 3. Unwanted density on the radiographic film resulting from exposure to secondary radiation, light, chemicals, or heat.

foil. A thin, pliable sheet of metal. In dentistry, various types of gold foil are used for restorations or the preparation of appliances.

folacin. Folic acid, q.v.

fold [AS. *fealdan,* to fold]. A ridge; a doubling back. SYN: *plica.*

f., amniotic. Folded edge of the amniotic membrane where it rises over and finally encloses the embryo of birds, reptiles, and some mammals.

f., aryepiglottic. The ridgelike lateral walls of the entrance to the larynx.

f., circular. A large fold that extends into the lumen of the small intestine.

f., costocolic. Ligament arising from the peritoneum that attaches the splenic flexure of the colon to the diaphragm.

f., Douglas'. Fold of peritoneum extending on each side to the base of the broad ligament. This forms the rectouterine space, called Douglas' pouch.

f.'s, gastric. Folds of mucosa, mostly longitudinal, in the empty stomach.

f., genital. Fold of skin in the embryo on each side of the genital tubercle that develops into the labia minora in the female.

f., gluteal. The linear crease in the skin that separates the buttocks from the thighs.

f., lacrimal. A valvelike fold in the lower part of the nasolacrimal duct.

f., mesouterine. Fold of peritoneum supporting the uterus.

f., mucosal. Fold of mucosal tissue.

f., nail. The folded-in epidermal tissue surrounding the sides and base of nails.

f., palmate. The ridges on the cervical canal of the uterus.

f., semilunar, of conjunctiva. Fold of conjunctiva at the inner angle of the eye.

f., transverse, of rectum. Transverse mucosal folds of the rectum. SYN: *valves of Houston.*

f., ventricular; f., vestibular. The false vocal cord.

f., vestigial. Ligament of the left superior vena cava. SYN: *Marshall's fold.*

f., vocal. F., ventricular, q.v.

folia (fō'lē-ä) [L.]. Pl. of folium.

foliaceous (fō-lē-ā'shē-ŭs) [L. *folia,* leaves]. Resembling or pert. to a leaf.

folic acid (fō'lĭk). USP. $C_{19}H_{19}N_7O_6$. A member of the vitamin B complex. Used in treatment of sprue. Found naturally in green plant tissue, liver, and yeast. Also called pteroylglutamic acid. Trade name is Folvite.

Caution: Folic acid should not be used in treatment of pernicious anemia because it does not protect patients against the development of changes in the central nervous system that accompany this type of anemia.

---

folie (fō-lē') [Fr.]. Mania; psychosis.

f. à deux. Occurrence of psychosis, usually of the paranoid type, at the same time in two closely associated persons. Rarely more than two persons are involved.

f. du doute. Abnormal doubts about ordinary acts and beliefs; inability to decide upon definite course of action or conduct.

f. du pourquoi. Unreasonable and unrelenting questioning.

f. gémellaire. Psychosis occurring in both twins.

folinic acid. The active form of folic acid. Used in counteracting the effects of folic acid antagonists, and in treating anemia due to folic acid deficiency. Trade name is Calcium Folinate.

folium (fō'lē-ŭm) [L., leaf] (pl. *folia*). Thin, broad, leaflike structure.

f. vermis. [NA] Fold on the posterior part of the upper surface of the vermis of the cerebellum.

follicle [L. *folliculus,* little bag]. A small secretory sac or cavity.

f.'s aggregated. An aggregation of solitary nodules or groups of lymph nodules found chiefly in the ileum near its junction with the colon. They are circular or oval, about 1 cm wide and 2 to 3 cm long. They lie in the mucosa and submucosa and always occur on the side of the intestine opposite to the attachment of mesentery. In typhoid fever, they undergo hyperplasia and often become ulcerated. SYN: *Peyer's patch.*

f., atretic. An ovarian follicle that has undergone degeneration or involution.

f., dental. The connective tissue structure that encloses the developing tooth within the substance of the jaw prior to tooth eruption. The dental sac and its contents.

f., gastric. The glands in the gastric mucosa of the stomach.

f., graafian. The complete development of the primary oocyte in the cortex of the ovary to the stage where the ovum is fully developed. SEE: *graafian follicle; ovary; ovum* for illus.

f., growing. A developing follicle of the ovary.

f., hair. An invagination of the epidermis from which a hair develops.

f., lymphatic. The densely packed collection of lymphocytes and lymphoblasts that make up the cortex of lymph glands.

f., nabothian. Dilated cyst of the glands of the cervix uteri.

f., ovarian. A spherical structure in the cortex of the ovary consisting of an oogonium or an oocyte and its surrounding epithelial (follicular) cells. Follicles are of three types: primary, consisting of an oogonium and a single layer of follicular cells; growing, in which the follicle cells proliferate, forming several layers, and the first maturation division occurs; vesicular, or graafian follicle, which possesses a cavity (antrum) containing the follicular fluid (liquor folliculi). The oocyte lies in the cumulus oophorus, a mass of cells on the inner surface. The cells lining the follicle constitute the stratum granulosum. The follicle is a secretory structure producing estrogen and progesterone. SEE: *corpus luteum.*

f., primordial. Follicle of the ovary, which consists of the ovum enclosed in a single layer of cells.

f., sebaceous. Oil gland of the skin.

f., solitary. A single lymph nodule of the intestine.

f., thyroid. Spherical or ovoid structure found in the thyroid gland lined with a single layer of cuboidal epithelial cells, which secrete the thyroid hormone. The follicles are filled with colloid, a viscid substance rich in iodine.

f., vesicular. Follicle containing a cavity; a mature ovarian or graafian follicle.

follicle-stimulating hormone. ABBR: FSH. Hormone produced by the anterior pituitary. It stimulates growth of the follicle in the ovary and spermatogenesis in the testis.

follicular. Pert. to a follicle or follicles.

follicular tonsillitis. Inflammation of follicles on surface of the tonsil, which become filled with pus.

follicular tumor. A sebaceous cyst.

folliculitis (fŏ-lĭk″ū-lī′tĭs) [L. *folliculus,* little bag, + Gr. *itis,* inflammation]. Inflammation of a follicle or follicles.

f. barbae. Ringworm of the beard.

f. decalvans. Purulent follicular inflammation of the scalp resulting in irregular

alopecia and scarring.

SYM: Initial inflammatory papule or pustule at mouth of follicle pierced by a hair is followed by crusting and desiccation, when it drops off along with loosened hair. Bald patches with slight depressed whitish center surrounded by inflamed margin. Extends peripherally.

ETIOL: Cause unknown. Believed to be caused by staphylococci. Affects mostly males between 2nd and 4th decades.

PATH: Sebaceous gland atrophy and flattened papillae.

TREAT: Externally, topical antibiotics or corticosteroids and frequent shampoos.

PROG: Loss of hair in affected areas is permanent, although extension may be arrested.

f., keloidal. Chronic dermatitis with production of hard papules that join together to form keloid tissue.

folliculogenesis, induction of. The stimulation of follicle development in the ovary by the use of drugs or hormones, e.g., clomiphene, or human menopausal gonadotropin. SEE: *fertilization in vitro; gamete intrafallopian transfer.*

folliculoma (fŏ-lĭk″ū-lŏ′mă) [″ + Gr. *oma,* tumor]. A tumor of the ovary originating in a graafian follicle in which the cells resemble the cells of the stratum granulosum.

folliculose (fŏ-lĭk′ū-lōs). Composed of follicles.

folliculosis (fŏ-lĭk″ū-lŏ′sĭs) [″ + Gr. *osis,* condition]. Presence of an abnormal quantity of lymph follicles.

folliculus (fŏ-lĭk′ū-lŭs) [L.] (pl. *folliculi*). [NA] A follicle.

follow-up. The continued care or monitoring of a patient after the initial visit or examination.

Follutein. Trade name for chorionic gonadotropin.

Folvite. Trade name for folic acid.

fomentation (fō″mĕn-tā′shŭn) [L. *fomentatio*]. A hot, wet application for the relief of pain or inflammation. SEE: *dressing, hot moist; stupe.*

fomes (fō′mēz) [L., tinder] (pl. *fomites*). Any substance that adheres to and transmits infectious material.

fomites (fō′mĭ-tēz). Pl. of fomes.

Fontana's spaces (fŏn-tă′năz) [Felice Fontana, It. scientist, 1730–1805]. Spaces between the processes of ligamentum pectinatum of the iris. These convey the aqueous humor.

fontanel, fontanelle (fŏn″tă-nĕl′) [Fr. *fontanelle,* little fountain]. An unossified space or soft spot lying between the cranial bones of the skull of a fetus. SEE: illus.

f., anterior. Fontanel at the junction of

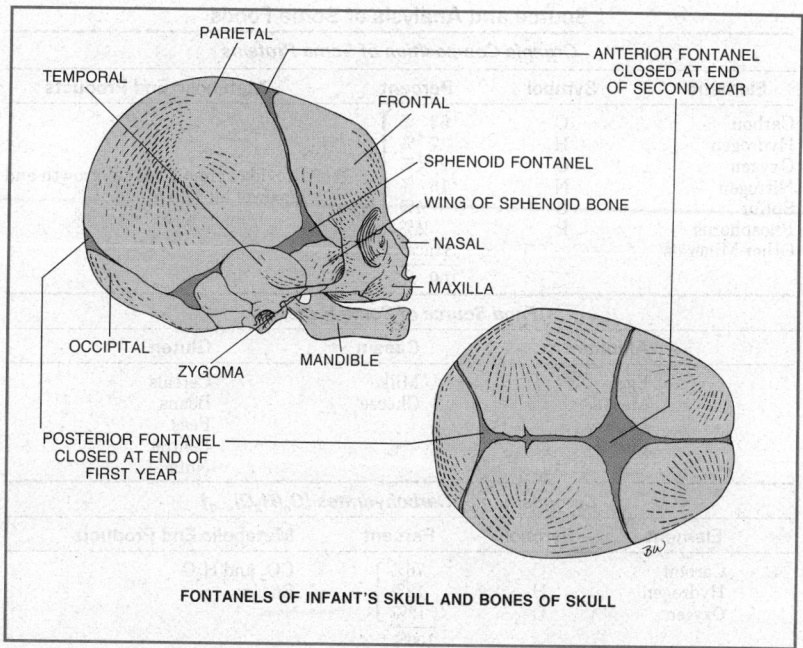

FONTANELS OF INFANT'S SKULL AND BONES OF SKULL

TEMPORAL

PARIETAL

FRONTAL

ANTERIOR FONTANEL
CLOSED AT END
OF SECOND YEAR

SPHENOID FONTANEL

WING OF SPHENOID BONE

NASAL

MAXILLA

OCCIPITAL

ZYGOMA

MANDIBLE

POSTERIOR FONTANEL
CLOSED AT END OF
FIRST YEAR

the coronal, frontal, and sagittal sutures.

    f., posterior. Fontanel at the junction of the sagittal and lambdoid sutures.

fonticulus (fŏn-tĭk'ū-lŭs) [L., little fountain]. [NA] Fontanel.

food [AS. *foda*] (pl. *foods*). Any material that provides the nutritive requirements of an organism to maintain growth and physical well-being. SEE: table; *Foods, Nutritive Value of* in *Appendix; Recommended Daily Dietary Allowances* in *Appendix.*

    COURSE: *Alimentary canal:* Foods enter the mouth and in the buccal area are reduced to a pulp or semifluid mass through the processes of mastication and insalivation (the mixing of food with saliva). Swallowing or deglutition then occurs. In swallowing, the food mass or bolus passes into the pharynx and then through the esophagus to the stomach, the entrance to which is controlled by the cardiac sphincter.

    Stomach: In the stomach the food is stored and mixed with gastric juice. This action combined with the gastric acidity kills many of the microorganisms present in food. After it attains a certain fluid consistency, it passes through the pyloric sphincter into the small intestine.

    Small intestine: In the first portion or du-

odenum, the intestinal contents (now called chyme) are mixed with bile secreted by the liver and with pancreatic juice, both of which enter through the opening of the common bile duct. In the next two portions, the jejunum and ileum, the chyme is mixed with the intestinal juice secreted by the intestinal glands or crypts of Lieberkühn. In the small intestine, digestion is completed and the end products of digestion (simple sugars, amino acids, fatty acids, and glycerol) are absorbed into the capillaries and lacteals of the intestinal mucosa.

    Large intestine: Remaining material passes from the small intestine into the large intestine (colon) through the ileocecal valve located at the junction of the ascending colon and the cecum, a blind pouch that terminates in the vermiform appendix. The material continues through the colon (ascending, transverse, descending, and sigmoid) to the rectum, from which it is discharged as feces through the anal canal at the anus, or anal orifice. In the large intestine, the major portion of the water of the intestinal contents is absorbed. Digestive changes are limited to the action of bacteria, which brings about putrefaction and fermentation of incompletely digested foods.

748

Source and Analysis of Some Foods

Organic Composition of Some Proteins

Element	Symbol	Percent	Metabolic End Products
Carbon	C	53 %	
Hydrogen	H	7 %	
Oxygen	O	22 %	Provide amino acids for growth and repair of all cells
Nitrogen	N	16 %	
Sulfur	S	½%	
Phosphorus	P	½%	
Other Minerals		trace	
		100 %	

Food Source of Some Proteins

Albumen	Casein	Gluten
Eggs	Milk	Cereals
Meat	Cheese	Beans
Poultry		Peas
Fish		Lentils
		Nuts

Composition of Carbohydrates [$C_n(H_2O)_{n-1}$]

Element	Symbol	Percent	Metabolic End Products
Carbon	C	76%	CO_2 and H_2O
Hydrogen	H	12%	Energy
Oxygen	O	12%	
		100%	

Examples of Carbohydrates in Food

Glucose	Sucrose	Cellulose, Glycogen, and Starch
$C_6H_{12}O_6$	$C_{12}H_{22}O_{11}$	$(C_6H_{10}O_5)_n$

Carbohydrates and fats are sources of heat and energy, but neither can take the place of proteins, the only food source of nitrogen. Carbohydrates consist principally of sugars, starch, glycogen, and cellulose.

Composition of Some Fats

Element	Symbol	Percent	Metabolic End Products
Carbon	C	45%	CO_2 and H_2O
Hydrogen	H	6%	Produce heat and energy but do not build tissues or cells
Oxygen	O	49%	
		100%	

Examples of Origin of Fats

Animal	Oils	Nuts	Fruits
Butter, Oleomargarine, Eggs, Lard, Cooking Oils, Meat, Dairy Products	Cottonseed, Corn, Sunflower, Safflower	Peanuts	Palm, Olive

Additional Dietary Requirements

Water, Minerals (Iodine, Iron, Magnesium, Calcium, Copper, Chromium, Cobalt, Zinc, Selenium, Manganese, and Molybdenum), Vitamins

f., contamination of. Food may be the cause of illness because it may act as the carrier of pathogenic organisms such as those that cause enteritis *(Salmonella)* or tuberculosis, parasites such as those that cause trichinosis, or certain types of worms (roundworms, tapeworms).

f., convenience. Food in which one or more steps in preparation have been completed before the product is offered for retail sale. Examples include frozen vegetables, bake mixes, and heat-and-serve types of food.

f., dietetic. Food that has been modified in nutrient content in some way in order to be used in special diets, esp. for diabetics.

f., enriched. Food in which the vitamin and mineral content has been increased either by addition or by irradiation.

f., fast. SEE: *fast food.*

f., nutrient substances of. Substances that in the body serve as a source of energy or provide material for the growth and repair of tissue. Foods are organic substances (proteins, carbohydrates, fats) present in animal and plant tissues. The term "food" is commonly used to refer to any substance taken into the body that serves a nutrient function. Thus, any discussion of food would include vitamins, minerals, water, and trace elements (zinc, chromium, cobalt, magnesium, manganese, molybdenum, selenium).

f., textured. Food products manufactured from a variety of nutritional components. In texture they may resemble conventional protein-source foods such as meat, seafood, or poultry.

food additives. Substances or a mixture of substances other than basic foodstuff that are present in a food as a result of any aspect of production, processing, storage, or packaging. Accidental contaminants are not considered to be food additives.

food adulterant. A substance that makes food impure or inferior, such as toxic organisms, filth, pesticide residues, radioactive fallout, any poisonous or deleterious substance, or any substance added to increase bulk or weight in a food product.

food allergies. Allergic, i.e., immunologic, reactions resulting from ingestion of foods to which a person has become sensitized. One may become sensitive to almost any food; however, certain foods such as milk, eggs, wheat, shellfish, chocolate, and oranges are frequent offenders.

SYM: Urticaria (hives), certain eczemas, nausea, vomiting, diarrhea, and intestinal cramps. A syndrome (angioneurotic edema) characterized by a transient swelling of various parts of the body and spasm of the intestine may result.

Food and Drug Administration. ABBR: FDA. In the U.S., an official regulatory body for foods, drugs, cosmetics, and medical devices. It is a part of the U.S. Department of Health and Human Services.

food and drug interactions. Drugs may interfere with absorption or utilization of food, particularly certain vitamins. Excess intake of food high in vitamin K may interfere with the action of anticoagulants. Prolonged use of antacids may cause phosphate depletion. SEE: *monoamine oxidase inhibitors.*

food ball. Gastric stone made up of fruit and vegetable skins, seeds, and fibers. SYN: *phytobezoar.*

food chain. The sequential transfer of food energy from green plants to animals that eat plants, then to animals that eat the plant-eating animals; e.g., cows eat plants, other animals including man eat the meat of cows. Interruption of the chain at any point may produce an ecological disaster.

food exchange. Commonly used foods grouped according to similarities in composition so that such foods may be used interchangeably in diet planning.

food hypersensitivity reactions. SEE: *food allergies.*

food intolerance. An abnormal, nonimmunologic response to ingested food. The basis for the intolerance may be pharmacologic, toxic, or metabolic. Pharmacologic intolerance is the body's reaction to a component of the food that produces effects like a drug; metabolic intolerance is due to the effect of the food on the person's metabolism; and food toxicity is caused by toxins in the food or released by microorganisms contaminating the food.

food labels. The information provided on food packages and labels indicating the various nutrients, calories, and food additives present in the food. Unfortunately, the labels may not be as informative as the consumer would like. The problem may be due to the esoteric chemical names listed or the tendency of the supplier to use meaningless terms such as "fresh," "light," "lite," "natural," or "organic," or providing the names of oils and fats without being specific about the percent of saturated and unsaturated fat. Food and Drug Administration regulations are aimed at correcting some of these inadequacies, but until this program is complete the consumer must be aware of the fact that a food label may be inaccurate or misleading.

food poisoning. An imprecise term indicating an illness resulting from the ingestion of foods containing poisonous substances.

True food poisoning includes mushroom poisoning, shellfish poisoning, poisoning resulting from foods contaminated with poisonous insecticides or toxic substances such as lead or mercury, and milk sickness (due to milk from cows that have fed on certain poisonous plants). Also, occasionally poisoning resulting from eating foods that have undergone putrefaction or decomposition or poisoning from bacteria. SEE: *anisakiasis; fish poisoning; sushi.*

food requirements. It is assumed that an average healthy man (154 lb or 70 kg) performing light to moderate muscular work requires 2700 Cal/day and that an average healthy woman (128 lb or 58 kg) requires 2000 Cal/day. This would be supplied in part by protein, but mostly by fat and carbohydrates. Persons in sedentary occupations require fewer calories. In general, adults require 1 gm of protein per day for each kilogram of their ideal weight.

A diet made up of ordinary foods and supplying the necessary amounts of protein and energy undoubtedly supplies an abundance of mineral matter. The assumption is usually made that, provided a woman is engaged in some moderately active occupation, she requires fewer calories each day because of her comparatively smaller build. Calculated on the basis of food energy required per kilogram of body weight, children and pregnant women require more food than other adults. In patients with fever, basal energy expenditure is increased about 12% for each °C of fever.

The criteria for an adequate diet are difficult to define because food habits vary from one area to another as well as from individual to individual. No single diet or individual food is essential for life or health. Also, it is not possible to state that the ideal diet, with respect to assuring maximum growth and development, would be the one that would assure maximum longevity. SEE: *energy expenditure, basal; Foods, Nutritive Value of* in *Appendix; Recommended Daily Dietary Allowances* in *Appendix.*

food trap. SEE: *trap, food.*

foot [AS. *fot*]. 1. The terminal portion of the lower extremity. The bones of the foot include the tarsus, metatarsus, and phalanges. SEE: illus.; *skeleton.* 2. A unit of measurement containing 12 in. (30.48 cm). ABBR: ft.

    f., arches of. Four arches: internal or medial longitudinal, outer or lateral longitudinal, and two transverse arches.

    f., athlete's. Fungus infection of the foot.

    f., cleft. Condition in which a cleft extends between the digits to the metatarsal

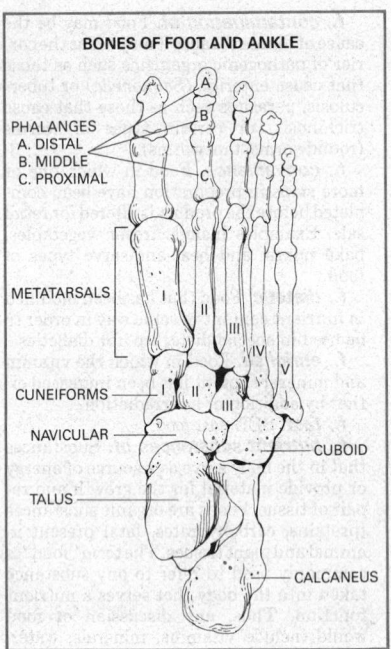

BONES OF FOOT AND ANKLE

PHALANGES
A. DISTAL
B. MIDDLE
C. PROXIMAL

METATARSALS

CUNEIFORMS

NAVICULAR

TALUS

CUBOID

CALCANEUS

region, usually due to a missing digit.

    f., flat-. Abnormal flatness of sole and arch of foot. This condition may exist without causing symptoms or interfering with normal function of the foot. The inner longitudinal and anterior transverse metatarsal arches are those that may be depressed. It may be acute, subacute, or chronic. SYN: *pes planus.*

    f., immersion. Condition of foot resulting from prolonged immersion of the feet in water.

    f., Madura. SEE: *Madura foot.*

    f., march. Spontaneous fracture of one of the metatarsal bones of the foot.

    f., splay-. Flatfoot accompanied by extreme width of the foot.

    f., trench. Degeneration of the skin of the feet due to prolonged exposure to moisture. The condition may be prevented by being certain that clean, dry socks are worn at all times. The feet do not have to be exposed to cold to develop this condition.

foot and mouth disease. A viral disease of cattle and horses that is rarely transmitted to humans.

    SYM: In humans, fever, headache, malaise with dryness and burning sensation of the mouth. Vesicles develop on the lips, tongue, mouth, palms, and soles.

TREAT: Symptomatic. Full recovery occurs in 2 to 3 weeks.

foot board. A board or similar material placed at the foot end of the patient's bed. It is angled slightly away from the patient and extends up above the mattress. When used properly, it will help to prevent footdrop. The patient should be positioned in bed so that when the legs are fully extended, the soles of the feet just touch the board.

foot-candle. An amount of light equivalent to 1 lumen, q.v., per square foot.

footdrop. Plantar flexion of the foot due to weakness or paralysis of the anterior muscles of the lower leg. It may occur in any patient who is in bed continuously, esp. if comatose. For bedridden patients, a foot board, q.v., should be used to prevent footdrop.

footling presentation. Presentation of feet foremost in labor.

footplate. The flat part of the stapes, a bone in the middle ear.

foot pound. The amount of energy required to lift one pound of mass a vertical distance of one foot.

footprint. An impression of the foot, esp. an ink impression used for identification of infants.

forage (fō-rŏzh') [Fr., boring]. Creating a channel through an enlarged prostate by use of an electric cautery. This technique may be used in other tissues.

foramen (for-ā'mĕn) [L.] (pl. *foramina*). [NA] A passage or opening; an orifice, a communication between two cavities of an organ, or a hole in a bone for passage of vessels or nerves.

f., apical. Opening in the end of the root of the tooth through which the blood, lymphatic, and nerve supply to the dental pulp passes.

f., condyloid, anterior. Opening above the condyle of the occipital bone. The twelfth cranial nerve passes through it.

f., condyloid, posterior. Opening behind the condyle of the occipital bone. A small vein passes through it.

f., epiploic. Opening connecting the peritoneal cavity to its lesser sac.

f., ethmoidal. One of the openings in the medial wall of the orbit. The ethmoidal nerve and artery pass through these openings.

f., external auditory. The external auditory meatus through which sound waves travel in order to reach the tympanic membrane and the inner ear.

f., incisive. One of the small openings sometimes present in the incisive fossa of the hard palate.

f., infraorbital. Opening in the maxilla for the infraorbital branch of the maxillary nerve.

f., internal auditory. The opening in the petrous portion of the sphenoid bone through which the seventh and eighth cranial nerves pass.

f., interventricular. The opening between the lateral ventricle and the third ventricle of the brain. SYN: *foramen of Monro.*

f., intervertebral. Opening between adjacent articulated vertebrae for passage of nerves to and from spinal cord.

f., jugular. Opening in the base of the skull through which pass the sigmoid and inferior petrosal sinus, and the ninth, tenth, and eleventh cranial nerves.

f., Magendie's. SEE: *Magendie's foramen.*

f. magnum. Opening in the occipital bone through which passes the spinal cord from the brain.

f., mandibular. Opening on the medial surface of the mandibular ramus through which the inferior alveolar vessels and nerve enter the mandibular canal.

f., mastoid. Opening in the mastoid part of the temporal bone. A small vein passes through it.

f., mental. Opening on the ventral surface of the body of the mandible. The mental nerve and artery exit through it for superficial distribution.

f., obturator. Large oval foramen below acetabulum bounded by the pubis and ischium. SEE: *Magendie's foramen.*

f. of Bochdalek. Opening through the left diaphragm between the abdomen and thorax. Most common site for a diaphragmatic hernia, q.v.

f. of Monro. Opening between the third and lateral ventricles of the brain.

f. of Vesalius. Opening sometimes present in the sphenoid bone, medial to the foramen ovale. A vein from the cavernous sinus passes through it.

f. of Winslow. F., epiploic, q.v.

f., olfactory. Opening in the ethmoid bone for passage of the olfactory nerves.

f., optic. Opening in the lesser wing of the sphenoid bone. The optic nerve and ophthalmic artery pass through it.

f. ovale. 1. Opening between the two atria of the heart in the fetus. It closes shortly before or after birth in most cases. If it remains open, the defect can be repaired surgically. 2. Oval opening in posterior margin of great sphenoidal wing for mandibular branch of the trigeminal nerve and small meningeal artery.

f., palatine. F., incisive, q.v.

f., palatine (greater and lesser). Openings of the palatine canals through which nerves pass to the mucosa of the hard and soft palate.

f. rotundum. Opening in the great wing of the sphenoid bone through which the maxillary branch of the trigeminal nerve passes.

f., sacral, anterior. One of the openings on the anterior aspect of the sacrum through which pass the anterior primary branches of the sacral nerve.

f., sacral, posterior. One of the openings on the posterior aspect of the sacrum through which pass the posterior primary branches of the sacral nerve.

f., Scarpa's. Opening behind the upper medial incisor tooth through which passes the nasopalatine nerve. This opening is not always present.

f., sciatic, greater. Opening bounded by the hip bone, sacrum, and the sacrotuberous ligament.

f., sciatic, lesser. Opening bounded by the hip bone, sacrum, and sacrospinous ligament.

f., sphenopalatine. Opening between the palatine and sphenoid bones. It provides a passage from the pterygopalatine fossa to the nasal cavity for the sphenopalatine artery and nasal nerves.

f., spinous. Opening in the spine of the sphenoid bone through which passes the middle meningeal artery.

f., supraorbital. Opening that is sometimes present above the superior border of the orbit. The supraorbital nerve and vessels pass through it.

f., thebesian. One of the openings leading directly into the atria and ventricles of the heart. Very small thebesian veins empty into these openings.

f., transverse. Opening in the transverse process of a cervical vertebra.

f., vena caval. Opening in the diaphragm through which pass the vena cava and branches of the right vagus nerve.

f., vertebral. The large opening between the neural arch and the body of the vertebra.

f., Weitbrecht's. Opening in the articular capsule of the shoulder joint.

f., zygomatico-orbital. One or more small openings on the outer surface of the zygomatic bone. The zygomatic nerve passes through it.

Forbes' disease [Gilbert B. Forbes, U.S. pediatrician, b. 1915]. Glycogen storage disease, type III, q.v.

force. An external influence, a push or a pull exerted on an object. The metric unit for force is the newton. One newton equals 0.225 pound force.

f., catabolic. Energy produced by metabolism of food.

f., electromotive. ABBR: EMF. Energy that causes flow of electricity in a conductor. The energy is measured in volts.

f., G. The gravitational constant. In aerospace medicine, the term is used to indicate the forces on the human body during the accelerative forces encountered in certain flight maneuvers. Thus, a force of two positive G's means that the aviator is being subjected to a force twice that of gravity with a doubling of his weight in that condition; i.e., the force against the seat would be two G's. G force may be in any axis and may be negative or positive.

f., reserve. The energy available above that required for normal functioning of the heart.

f., unit of. Arbitrary definition of a certain amount of force. For example, a dyne is the amount of force acting continuously on a mass of one gram that will accelerate the mass one cm per second per second.

forced expiratory time. ABBR: FET. The time required to forcibly exhale a specified volume of air from the lung.

forceps (for'sĕps) [L.]. Pincers for holding, seizing, or extracting. There are many distinct types of forceps, varying according to the operation for which they are intended. In obstetrics, forceps application is classified according to the position of the fetal head when the forceps are applied, i.e., outlet forceps, low forceps, and midforceps. SEE: *station.*

f., alligator. Sturdy toothed forceps with a double clamp.

f., Allis. Forceps with curved, serrated edges. Used to firmly grasp tissue.

f., artery. Forceps for holding ends of an artery in order to perform ligation.

f., axis-traction. Obstetrical forceps fitted with a handle that makes it possible to provide traction in line with the way the head needs to be moved.

f., bone. Forceps used for cutting bone and for removal of bone fragments.

f., capsule. Forceps for removal of the lens of the eye in membranous cataract.

f., Chamberlen. The original obstetric forceps named after the inventor Peter Chamberlen (1560–1631) or his son Peter (1601–1683). They kept their development secret until Hugh Chamberlen (1664–1726) disclosed it.

f., clamp. Any forceps with an automatic lock.

f., dental. Forceps of varying shapes for grasping teeth during extraction procedures.

f., dressing. Forceps for general use in

dressing wounds and for removal of dead tissue and drainage tubes.

f., Halsted's. F., mosquito, q.v.

f., mosquito. A very small, delicately pointed hemostat. SYN: *f., Halsted's.*

f., needle. Forceps for grasping and holding a needle.

f., obstetric. Forceps used to extract the fetal head from the pelvis during delivery. They serve the dual purpose of allowing withdrawal force to be applied to the fetal head and protecting the head during the passage.

f., rongeur. Forceps used for cutting bone.

f., tissue. Forceps with tiny teeth for grasping delicate tissues.

f., towel. Forceps for clipping towels to the site of the operative wound.

forcipate (for'si-pāt) [L. *forceps,* tongs]. Shaped like forceps.

forcipressure [" + *pressura,* pressure]. Arresting hemorrhage by pressure on an artery with forceps.

Fordyce's disease (for'dī-sēs) [John Fordyce, U.S. dermatologist, 1858–1925]. Enlarged ectopic sebaceous glands in the mucosa of the mouth and genitals. They appear as small yellow spots, called Fordyce's spots. They are asymptomatic and present in the majority of people.

Fordyce-Fox disease (for'dīs-fŏks') [John Fordyce; George Henry Fox, U.S. dermatologist, 1846–1937]. A chronic pruritic papular eruption of areas of the skin that contain apocrine sweat glands. The intra-epidermal ducts of the apocrine glands are obstructed and, because of that, they rupture. Disease occurs mostly in those 13 to 35 years of age and is seen about 10 times more frequently in women than men. It does not occur prior to puberty.

TREAT: A number of agents, including estrogens, corticosteroids, and topical tretinoin cream have been used, but with little benefit. SYN: *Fox-Fordyce disease; miliaria, apocrine.*

Fordyce's spots. SEE: *Fordyce's disease.*

fore- [AS.]. Prefix meaning before or in front of.

forearm [AS. *fore,* in front, + *arm,* arm]. The portion of the arm between the elbow and wrist.

forebrain [" + *bregen,* brain]. Anterior portion of the brain of the embryo. SYN: *prosencephalon.*

forefinger. The first or index finger.

forefoot. The part of the foot in front of the tarsometatarsal joint.

foregut [" + *gut,* a pouring]. First part of the embryonic digestive tube from which pharynx, esophagus, stomach, and duode-

num are formed. SYN: *protogaster.*

forehead [AS. *forheafod*]. Anterior part of the head below the hairline and above the eyes. SYN: *frons.*

foreign bodies. Slivers, cinders, dirt, or small objects that lodge in the skin, ears, eyes, or nose, or internally. They frequently lead to infection. If not removed, they may lead to unsightly marks or tattooing of the skin and inflammation of the tissue involved.

F.A.: *In skin:* Carefully clean the areas involved. Foreign material can be removed carefully piece by piece or by vigorous swabbing with gauze or brush and a soapy solution. Follow with a sterile dressing.

In attempting to remove a small foreign body, first cleanse the area with mild soap and warm water. Sterilize a clean needle by heating it to a dull or bright red color in a flame; this can be done with a single match. Inasmuch as both ends of the needle get hot, it is wise to hold the far end in a nonconductor of heat such as folds of paper or stick it in a cork or in the edge of a small book. Allow it to cool, and disregard black deposit on the needle; it is sterile carbon and will not interfere with the procedure. Introduce the needle at right angles to the direction of sliver and lift it out. Most persons attempt to stick the needle in direction of the foreign body and consequently have to thrust many times before they manage to lift the sliver out. When it is removed, apply an antiseptic and cover wound with a sterile dressing. Tetanus antitoxin or a tetanus booster may be required, depending on the history of immunization.

In the ear: Water should not be introduced if any vegetable matter is in the ear because it may cause the foreign body to be pushed further into the ear or cause it to swell and become firmly embedded. Place a globule of ordinary glue on the end of a match stick or an applicator; gently introduce it until it touches the foreign body and then remove gently.

If an insect is in the ear, the patient may experience loud buzzing, pain, and dizziness. Flood ear with warm oil or water, letting insect float out.

In the vagina: A great variety of foreign body objects may be present in the vagina, esp. in children and in the insane. Also, it is possible to forget to remove a vaginal tampon, pessary, or contraceptive diaphragm. The treatment is to remove the foreign body. Antibiotic therapy is not usually necessary.

In wounds: Foreign bodies are often present in wounds. Generally these should be left undisturbed if a surgeon is available within a short time. If the foreign body is large, it might be embedded in large blood vessels, or muscles. Removing it might result in much loss of blood or might cause breaking off of splinters, particles of rust, or dirt. Within a few moments, blood and the natural reaction of swelling would tend to fill in the wound and cover this foreign material, making it exceedingly difficult for the physician to care for the patient. Therefore it is much wiser to leave a large foreign body in position and obtain the services of a physician promptly.

forelock. A lock of hair that grows on the forehead.

    f., white. A white tuft of hair that grows on the forehead. It is associated with Waardenburg syndrome, q.v.

forensic (for-ĕn'sĭk) [L. *forensis,* public]. Pert. to the law; legal.

forensic dentistry. The branch of dentistry that deals with the application of the art and science of dentistry to the purposes of law.

    Whereas forensic medicine will often be utilized to establish the time and cause of death, forensic dentistry may be called upon to establish the identity of an individual based on dental records only.

forensic medicine. Medicine in relation to the law; as in autopsy proceedings, or the determination of time or cause of death, or in the determination of sanity. Also, the legal aspects of medical ethics and standards.

foreplay. Fondling of the sex partner in order to produce mutual sexual arousal and pleasure prior to intercourse.

forepleasure [AS. *fore,* in front, + L. *placere,* to please]. Sexual pleasure preceding orgasm.

foreskin [" + O. Norse *skinn,* skin]. Prepuce, q.v., or loose skin at and covering the end of the penis or clitoris, like a hood. Excision of the prepuce constitutes circumcision. Smegma praeputii, q.v., is secreted by Tyson's glands and collects under foreskin. SEE: *circumcision.*

    NURSING IMPLICATIONS: In infants, see that the prepuce is not adherent or interfering with urination. Retract foreskin daily to prevent interference with urination, and formation of adhesions. Teach parents to clean area properly with mild soap and water daily and whenever diaper is changed. Report abnormalities to the physician.

forewaters (for'wăt-ērz). The thin mucus secretion discharged from the vagina during pregnancy. It is produced by the uterine glands and is considered to be normal.

forgetting. Being unable to remember something previously known or learned.

fork. An elongated instrument that splits at the end to form two or more prongs.

    f., tuning. Device that when struck at the forked end vibrates and thus can be heard and felt. It is used in testing the sensations of hearing, including bone conductions and vibration. A fork that vibrates at 256 cycles per second is suitable for use in these tests.

form. The distinctive size, shape, and external appearance of anything.

-form [L. *forma*]. Suffix meaning having the form of.

formaldehyde (for-măl'dĕ-hīd). HCOH. A colorless, pungent, irritant gas commonly made by oxidation of methyl alcohol; the simplest member of the group of aldehydes. It is used as a preservative as an aqueous solution of 37% formaldehyde. This chemical has been shown to be carcinogenic in certain animals and is possibly a carcinogen in man.

    ACTION/USES: A disinfectant, preservative, or fumigant. A 10% solution is useful as an astringent. A 1% or 2% solution is used for cleansing dishes, instruments, or fabrics. Formaldehyde is a powerful disinfectant, esp. in the form of gas, because of its penetrating power, but it is active only in the presence of an abundance of moisture. The solution is germicidal in the strength of 1% to 2%, but the action may require 20 to 30 minutes. It hardens tissues and is often used in histology for tissue preservation. It has a similar hardening effect on the living skin; it is very irritating to mucous membranes and produces reddening, inflammation, and necrosis if applied repeatedly or continuously. It is sometimes used in soap for disinfection of the hands. A 10% solution is used for sterilizing feces, urine, and sputum; 5% to 10% for clothing and towels. SEE: *aldehyde; fumigation.*

formaldehyde poisoning. SYM: Local irritation of eyes, nose, mouth, throat, respiratory and gastrointestinal tracts, and central nervous system, causing vertigo, stupor, abdominal pain, convulsions, unconsciousness, renal damage. SEE: *Poisons and Poisoning* in *Appendix.*

    F.A.: Administration of 0.2% ammonia water changes formaldehyde into methenamine. This should be given with large amounts of milk, water, and egg white. Then use gastric lavage or induce vomiting. After that, leave milk in stomach. Morphine may be needed for pain. Treat acidosis with sodium bicarbonate. Shock and respiratory distress should be treated as needed.

formalin (for'mă-lĭn). Aqueous solution of 37% formaldehyde. SEE: *aldehyde.*

formate (for'māt). A salt of formic acid.

formatio (for-mā'shē-ō) [L.] (pl. *formationes*). [NA] A structure with definite arrangement and shape.

    f. reticularis. Dorsal part of the medulla

oblongata.

formation. 1. A structure, shape, or figure. 2. The giving of form or shape to, or the development of, a structure.

f., reticular. A reticular structure formed of gray matter and interlacing fibers of white matter found in the medulla oblongata between the pyramids and the floor of the 4th ventricle. It is also present in the spinal cord, midbrain, and pons. Fibers from this structure are believed to be able to activate the cortex of the brain independently of specific sensory or other neural systems. Thus reticular formation is part of the reticular activating or alerting system.

forme fruste (form froost) [Fr., defaced] (pl. *formes frustes*). An aborted or incomplete form of disease arrested before running its course. Thus the disease appears in an atypical and indefinite form.

formic [L. *formica*, ant]. Pert. to ants, or to formic acid.

formic acid. HCOOH. A clear, pungent liquid obtained from the oxidation of formaldehyde or wood alcohol. Originally it was obtained from the distillation of the bodies of red ants. It is the cause of the pain and swelling resulting from the bites or stings of certain insects.

formic aldehyde. Formaldehyde.

formication. A sensation as of insects creeping upon the body; a form of paresthesia. One of the more common side effects of cocaine withdrawal.

formic ether. Volatile anesthetic liquid ethyl formate.

formiciasis (for″mĭs-ī′ă-sĭs) [L. *formica*, ant, + Gr. *-iasis*, condition]. Irritation caused by ant bites.

formilase (for′mĭ-lās). An enzyme that catalyzes conversion of acetic acid to formic acid.

formiminoglutamic acid. ABBR: FIGLU. A chemical intermediate in the metabolism of histidine to glutamic acid. Folacin, FH_4, is an essential coenzyme for this reaction. If there is a deficiency of folic acid, excess amounts of formiminoglutamic acid will appear in the urine.

formol (for′mŏl). Formaldehyde solution. SEE: *formalin.*

form sense. An element of visual function, q.v. It is tested by determining visual acuity. The other elements of visual function are color sense and light sense. SEE: *color sense; light sense.*

formula [L., a little form] (pl. *formulas, -lae*). 1. A rule prescribing ingredients and proportions for the preparation of a compound. 2. In chemistry, an expression by symbols of the constitution of a molecule consisting of letters, each denoting one atom of one elementary substance, with figures written as subscripts denoting the number of atoms present.

Ex.: water consists of two molecules of the element hydrogen and one of oxygen. The formula is H_2O. It may also be written HOH or H—O—H.

Collections of atoms that constitute a group by themselves (radical) are often separated by periods or parentheses, and in this case, figures prefixed or appended to the parentheses or placed before an expression contained within periods apply to all the symbols embraced by the parentheses or periods. In all other cases, a figure prefixed to a symbolical expression for a molecule, like a coefficient in an algebraic formula, is understood to be a multiplier of all the symbols following.

f., Arneth's. Method of estimating number of immature leukocytes by means of an elaborate differential blood count, based upon their shape and number of lobes in the nucleus. It is seldom used.

f., chemical. SEE: *formula* (def. 2).

f., dental. Formula showing the number and arrangement of the teeth. For human permanent teeth:

$$\frac{2-1-2-3}{2-1-2-3} \text{ (right upper jaw)}$$
(right lower jaw)

In this formula the numerators indicate the number in the maxilla and the denominators those in the mandible; the incisor, canine, premolar, and molar are listed in order, respectively. Using the formula, if one upper incisor were missing, that portion of the formula would be written one over two. If a lower molar were missing, the notation would be three over two.

f., empirical. The formula of a compound that shows the atoms and their numbers in a molecule, as H_2O.

f., molecular. The chemical formula indicating the elements and number of each present but providing no information concerning the two- or three-dimensional arrangement of the chemical elements in the formula. SEE: *f., spatial or stereochemical.*

f., official. Formula in a pharmacopeia.

f., spatial or stereochemical. A method of depicting chemical formulas so that the elements and their number are known as well as the position of the elements in space in relation to each other.

f., structural. Formula of a compound that shows the relationship of the atoms to each other in a molecule. The atoms are shown joined by valence bonds, e.g., H—O—H.

formulary [L. *formula*, a little form]. A book of formulas.

F., National. ABBR: NF. A book that provides standards and specifications for drugs. Previously issued by the American Pharmaceutical Association, it is now published by the U.S. Pharmacopeial Convention, Inc.

formyl. The radical of formic acid, HCO.

fornicate 1. [L. *fornicatus*] Arched or vaultlike. 2. [L. *fornicari*] To have sexual intercourse with a partner to whom one is not married.

fornication. Sexual intercourse between unmarried partners.

fornices (for'nĭ-sēz) [L.]. Pl. of fornix.

fornicolumn [L. *fornix*, arch, + *columna*, column]. The anterior pillar of the fornix.

fornicommissure (for-nĭ-kŏm'ĭ-sūr) [" + *commissura*, a joining together]. The commissure or body of the fornix uteri.

fornix [L., arch] (pl. *fornices*). [NA] 1. A fibrous vaulted band connecting the cerebral lobes. 2. Any body with vaultlike or arched shape.

 f. conjunctivae. [NA] Loose folds connecting palpebral and bulbar conjunctivae.

 f. uteri. Anterior and posterior spaces into which the upper vagina is divided. These recesses are formed by protrusion of the cervix uteri into the vagina.

 f. vaginae. [NA] F. uteri.

Fort Bragg fever [Fort Bragg, North Carolina, a U.S. military base]. Pretibial fever, q.v.

fortification spectrum. Appearance of dark patch with zigzag outline in visual field, causing a temporary blindness in that portion of the eye. SYN: *teichopsia.*

Foscarnet. A drug used for treatment of cytomegalovirus (CMV) retinitis. CMV retinitis is present in about 20% of people with AIDS, q.v.

Foshay's test [Lee Foshay, U.S. physician, 1896–1961]. The intradermal injection of a suspension of killed *Francisella tularensis*, the causative agent of tularemia. The appearance of an area of erythema at the injection site is considered a positive reaction.

fossa (fŏs'ä) [L.] (pl. *fossae*). [NA] A furrow or shallow depression.

 f., amygdaloid. Depression containing the tonsil.

 f., articular, of mandible. Depression on the inferior surface of the temporal bone that accepts the condyle of the mandible. SYN: *f., glenoid; f., mandibular; f., articular, of temporal bone.*

 f., articular, of temporal bone. F., articular, of mandible, q.v.

 f., axillary. The armpit; axilla.

 f., canine. The wide, shallow depression on the external surface of the maxilla superolateral to the canine tooth. It serves as the origin of the levator anguli oris muscle.

 f., cerebral. Any one of several depressions on the inside floor of the cranium.

 f., Claudius'. Triangular area harboring the ovary.

 f., condylar. Depression behind the occipital epicondyle.

 f., coronoid. Depression on the anterior surface of the lower end of the humerus. During full flexion of the forearm, the coronoid process of the ulna fits into the depression.

 f., cranial. F., cerebral, q.v.

 f., digastric. Depression behind the lower margin of the mandible at the side of the symphysis menti. The anterior belly of the digastric muscle attaches here.

 f., epigastric. Pit of the inside of the stomach.

 f., ethmoid. The groove in the cribriform plate of the ethmoid bone. The olfactory bulb of the brain occupies the depression. SYN: *olfactory groove.*

 f., glenoid. Depression on the scapula that provides space for articulation with the head of the humerus; also glenoid fossa of the temporal bone which articulates with the condyle of the mandible.

 f., hyaloid. Depression on the anterior surface of the vitreous body of the eye. The lens is located there.

 f., hypophyseal. The deep depression in the sphenoid bone in which the pituitary gland rests. SYN: *sella turcica.*

 f., iliac. One of the concavities of the iliac bones of the pelvis.

 f., incisive. Depression on the anterior surface of the body of the maxilla medial to the root of the canine incisor tooth.

 f., infratemporal. Shallow depression under and medial to the zygomatic arch. It contains the muscles of mastication, the first two parts of the maxillary artery, pterygoid venous plexus, and branches of the mandibular nerve, the third division of the trigeminal nerve.

 f., intercondyloid. Depression on the inferior surface of the femur between the femoral condyles; for passage of the cruciate ligaments.

 f., interpeduncular. The deep groove in the anterior surface of the midbrain, between the cerebral peduncles. The third cranial nerve emerges here.

 f., ischiorectal. Space on either side of the lower end of the rectum and anal canal. It is bounded laterally by the obturator internus muscle and the tuberosity of the ischium, medially by the levator ani and coccygeus muscles, and posteriorly by the gluteus maximus muscle.

 f., lacrimal. Hollow of frontal bone holding the lacrimal gland.

f., mandibular. Depression in the temporal bone. The condyle of the mandible fits into this fossa. SYN: *mandibular fossa of temporal bone.*

f., mastoid. Small triangular area between the posterior wall of the acoustic meatus and the posterior root of the zygomatic process of the temporal bone.

f., nasal. Cavity between the anterior opening to the nose and the nasopharynx.

f., navicular. Fossa between the vulva and fourchette.

f., olecranon. Depression on the posterior surface of the lower end of the humerus. During full extension of the forearm, the olecranon process of the ulna fits into this depression.

f. ovalis. Opening in thigh through which the large saphenous vein passes.

f. ovalis cordis. [NA] Remnant of embryonic foramen ovale in right cardiac atrium.

f., ovarian. Depression in the parietal peritoneum of the pelvis in which rests the ovary.

f., pituitary. F., hypophyseal, q.v.

f., popliteal. The soft tissue depression posterior to the knee.

f., Rosenmüller's. Depression in the pharynx posterior to opening of eustachian tube.

f., sphenomaxillary. SYN: *pterygopalatine fossa.*

f., sublingual. A shallow depression on the inner surface of the body of the mandible above the anterior part of the mylohyoid ridge. It is occupied by the major salivary gland in the area, the sublingual gland.

f., submandibular. An oblong depression between the mylohyoid ridge and the inferior border of the medial surface of the body of the mandible. It is occupied by the submandibular gland. Previously referred to as the submaxillary gland and submaxillary fossa.

f., subpyramidal. Depression in the inferior wall of the middle ear. It is inferior to the round window and posterior to the pyramid.

f., supraspinous. The concave triangular area above the spinous process of the posterior surface of the clavicle.

f. supratonsillaris. [NA] Space between anterior and posterior pillars of the fauces above the tonsil.

f., temporal. Depression on the side of the skull below the temporal lines. It is deep to the zygomatic arch and continuous with the infratemporal fossa.

fossae (fŏs'ē) [L.]. Pl. of fossa.

fossette (fŏ-sĕt') [Fr.]. 1. A small depression or fossa. 2. A small, but deep, corneal ulcer.

fossula (fŏs'ū-lä). Small fossa.

foster care. The care of particular individuals in a group or private home. These are usually abandoned, orphaned, or delinquent children who are the responsibility of a governmental agency which provides the funds for their care.

f.c., adult. SEE: *adult foster care.*

Fothergill's disease (fŏth'ĕr-gĭlz) [John Fothergill, Brit. physician, 1712–1780]. 1. Scarlatina anginosa, an ulcerative sore throat present in severe scarlet fever. 2. Trigeminal neuralgia.

foulage (foo-lŏzh') [Fr.]. Massage by kneading with pressure on the muscles.

foundation, denture. The area upon which a denture rests.

fourchet, fourchette (foor-shĕt') [Fr. *fourchette,* a fork]. A tense band or transverse fold of mucous membrane at the posterior commissure of the vagina, connecting the posterior ends of the labia minora. The fossa navicularis, a more or less deep cul-de-sac anterior to the fourchette, separates it from the hymen. It disappears after defloration or parturition, leaving a more open vulva below and behind. SYN: *frenulum labiorum pudendi* [NA]. SEE: *vestibule of vagina.*

fourth cranial nerve. A small mixed nerve making its exit from the dorsal surface of the midbrain. It contains efferent motor fibers to the superior oblique muscle of the eye and afferent sensory fibers conveying proprioceptive impulses from the same muscle. SYN: *trochlear nerve.*

fovea (fō'vē-ä) [L.] (pl. *foveae*). [NA] A pit or cuplike depression. SEE: *fossa.*

f. capitis. The depression on the head of the femur for attachment of the ligamentum teres.

f. centralis retinae. [NA] Pit in the middle of macula lutea.

foveate (fō'vē-āt) [L. *foveatus*]. Pitted; having depressions.

foveation (fō"vē-ā'shŭn). Pitting, as in smallpox.

foveola (fō-vē'ō-lä) [L., little pit] (pl. *foveolae*). A minute pit or depression.

Fowler's position [George R. Fowler, U.S. surgeon, 1848–1906]. A semi-sitting position. The head of an adjustable bed can be elevated to the desired height to produce angulation of the body, usually 45° to 60°. Knees may or may not be bent. A wedge support can be used to elevate the head and back of the patient if an adjustable bed is not available. The position is used to facilitate breathing and drainage and for the comfort of the bedridden patient while eating or talking.

NOTE: Hips (knees) may or may not be

flexed in this position which has three variations: high, sitting upright in bed; regular, head or torso elevated 45° or more; and low or semi-, head and torso elevated to 30°.

Fowler's solution [Thomas Fowler, Brit. physician, 1736–1801]. An arsenical solution containing 0.95 to 1.5 gm of arsenic trioxide for each 100 ml of solution. SYN: *potassium arsenite solution.*

Fox-Fordyce disease (fŏks-for'dĭs). SEE: *Fordyce-Fox disease.*

foxglove (fŏks'glŏv). Common name for the plant *Digitalis purpurea,* from which the drug digitalis is obtained. Foxglove was mentioned in the writings of Welsh physicians in 1250 and by William Withering in a book published in 1785.

Fr. Chem. symb. for the element francium.

fraction [L. *fractio,* act of breaking]. In biological chemistry, the separable part of a substance such as blood or plasma.

   f. of inspired oxygen. ABBR: FiO_2. The concentration of oxygen in the inspired air, esp. that supplied as supplemental oxygen by mask or catheter. Concentrations of oxygen greater than 50% are toxic if administered for other than brief periods.

fractional. Pert. to a fraction or a portion of a whole.

fractional test meal. Fractional examination of stomach contents. The method for collection and examination of stomach contents follows: First the residual contents are removed and then the test meal given; after the meal, samples are removed every 15 min. for 2 hours, examined, and submitted for chemical tests. Free hydrochloric acid, bile, blood, starch, mucus, and the total of acids are analyzed. Free hydrochloric and total acids are normally present in small amounts. In peptic ulcers there is a high acid curve. There is a low curve in carcinoma, and an absence of acid in pernicious anemia.

fractionation. In radiation therapy, the process of spreading the total required treatment dose over an extended time.

fracture [L. *fractura,* break]. 1. A sudden breaking of a bone. 2. A broken bone. SEE: illus.

   CAUSES: In certain diseases and conditions such as osteomalacia, syphilis, and osteomyelitis, bones break spontaneously without trauma.

   Direct violence: The bone is broken directly at the spot where the force was applied, as in fracture of the tibia by being run over. *Indirect violence:* The bone is fractured by a force applied at a distance from the site of fracture and transmitted to the fractured bone, as fracture of the clavicle by falling on the outstretched hand. *Muscular contraction:* The bone is broken by a sudden violent

contraction of the muscles.

   SIGNS: Loss of power of movement; pain with acute tenderness over the site of fracture; swelling and bruising; deformity and possible shortening; unnatural mobility; crepitus or grating that is heard when the ends of the bone rub together. Do not try to obtain these last two signs. Use roentgenography to find the type of fracture and the exact position of the bone fragments.

   F.A.: In simple fractures, the limb or part must be kept immovable by means of splints. If proper wooden, plastic, or metal splints are unavailable, they may be improvised by using magazines or folded newspapers. The clothing should not be removed unless there is dangerous hemorrhage. If it is necessary to remove clothing, do so by cutting the cloth away so as to disturb the area as little as possible.

   If it is an upper extremity, it should be supported in a sling, and the patient may then walk. If a lower limb is injured, the patient should remain supine and make no attempt to walk.

   TREAT: The physician will reduce the fracture, that is, place the fragments in proper position. Keep the bone in position by means of a cast until union has taken place. Then restore the limb to complete function by physical therapy and exercise.

   In compound fractures, any bleeding must be arrested before treating the fracture. Open reduction may be required. The wound is then washed and cleaned with sterile saline. If the area is grossly contaminated, mild soap solution may be used provided it is thoroughly washed away by using generous amounts of sterile saline. When the wound is quite clean, a sterile dressing is secured by a bandage. A cast is then applied as in simple fractures.

   A weak electric current applied to fractured bones has been found to promote healing.

Caution: First aid for fractures of the spine requires extreme care with respect to moving the patient. Unnecessary or improper movement may injure or even transect the spinal cord.

   NURSING IMPLICATIONS: Evaluate the patient for pain and point tenderness, nerve and vascular impairment distal to the fracture site, swelling, crepitus, discoloration and open wounds near the fracture site. Immobilize the fracture by splinting the site and the joints above and below the site. Cover an open fracture with a sterile or clean dressing. Elevate the injured extremity to minimize edema. Control bleeding with direct pressure. Monitor the patient's

FRAGMENTS
UNDISPLACED

FRAGMENTS SEPARATED
DUE TO BREAK FROM
WITHIN
(COMPOUND FRACTURE)

FRAGMENTS SEPARATED
BY EXTERNAL FORCE
SUCH AS BULLET
(COMPOUND FRACTURE)

PROXIMAL
PORTION OF
BONE

MIDDLE
PORTION OF
BONE

DISTAL
PORTION
OF BONE

UNDISPLACED

DISPLACED

INCOMPLETE

COMPLETE

COMMINUTED

SEGMENTAL

BUTTERFLY

SPIRAL

HAIR-
LINE

TYPES OF FRACTURES AND TERMINOLOGY

overall condition for shock and other complicating factors. Assessment of vascular and neurologic status of limb distal to fracture is essential following immobilization therapy with traction, casting, or fixation device. Also evaluate patients for infection, fat embolism, and delayed union or nonunion. SEE: *Nursing Diagnoses* in *Appendix*.

RS: buttonhole fracture; cerclage; extension; greenstick fracture; malunion; splint.

f., avulsion. Tearing of a piece of bone away from the main bone by the force of muscular contraction.

f., bimalleolar. Fracture of the medial and lateral malleoli of the ankle joint.

f., blow-out. Fracture of the floor of the orbit where fragments are displaced downward due to a blow to the eye.

f., boxer's. A fracture of the distal end of the fifth metacarpal with posterior displacement of the proximal structures.

f., clay shoveler's. Fracture of the base of the spinous process of the lower cervical spine associated with sudden flexion of the neck. May also be caused by direct trauma.

f., closed. Fracture of the bone, but with no skin wound.

f., Colles'. SEE: *Colles' fracture.*

f., comminuted. Fracture in which the bone is broken or splintered into pieces.

f., complete. Fracture in which the bone is completely broken, i.e., neither fragment is connected to the other.

f., complicated. Fracture in which the bone is broken and has injured some internal organ, such as a broken rib piercing a lung.

f., compound. Fracture in which the bone is broken, an external wound leads down to the site of fracture, or fragments of bone protrude through the skin.

f., compression. Fracture of a vertebra by pressure along the long axis of the vertebral column.

f., depressed. Fracture in which a piece of the skull is broken and driven inward.

f., diastatic. Fracture that follows a cranial suture and causes separation of that suture.

f., direct. Fracture at the site where force was applied.

f., dislocation. Fracture near a joint that is dislocated.

f., double. Two fractures of the same bone.

f., Duverney's. Fracture of ilium just below the anterior superior spine.

f., epiphyseal. Separation of the epiphysis from the bone. Takes place between the shaft of a bone and its growing end. Occurs only in young patients.

f., fatigue. SEE: *stress fracture.*

f., fissured. A narrow split in the bone. The split does not go through to the other side of the bone.

f., greenstick. Fracture in which the bone is partially bent and partially broken, as when a green stick breaks. It occurs in children, esp. in those with rickets.

f., hairline. A minor fracture in which all the portions of the bone are in perfect alignment. The fracture is seen on roentgenogram as a very thin hair line between the two segments, but not extending entirely through the bone. SEE: *stress fracture.*

f., hangman's. SEE: *hangman's fracture.*

f., impacted. Fracture in which the bone is broken, and one end is wedged into the interior of the other.

f., incomplete. Fracture in which the line of fracture does not include the whole bone. SEE: *stress fracture.*

f., indirect. Fracture distant to the place where the force was applied.

f., intrauterine. Fracture of a bone in the fetus while it is in utero.

f., lead pipe. Fracture in which the bone is compressed and bent so that one side of the fracture bulges and on the other side there is a slight crack.

f., LeFort. Fracture of one or more of the bones of the face: maxillary, nasal, orbital, or zygomatic.

f., march. Stress fracture, q.v.

f., nonunion of. SEE: *nonunion.*

f., open. Fracture in which an open wound is present at the fracture site. SYN: *f., compound.*

f., overriding. Fracture in which the ends of the fractured bones slide past each other.

f., pathologic. Fracture of a diseased or weakened bone produced by a force that would not have fractured a healthy bone. The underlying disease may be metastases from the primary cancer, cancer of the bone, or osteoporosis.

NURSING IMPLICATIONS: Support limbs and joints of patient gently and carefully when repositioning, exercising, or mobilizing. Consider fracture a potential cause or result if such a patient falls or is otherwise injured. Support community efforts to obtain "kneeling camel" type step-access for public transportation vehicles, since high step can be the cause of pathologic hip fracture in an osteoporotic individual.

f., ping-pong. A depressed fracture of the skull that resembles the indentation that can be made by pressing firmly on a ping-pong ball.

f., Pott's. Fracture of the lower end of the fibula with outward displacement of the ankle and foot. The medial malleolus of the fibula may or may not be fractured.

f., pretrochanteric. Fracture that passes through the greater trochanter of the femur.

f., Smith's. Colles' fracture, q.v.

f., spiral. An oblique fracture.

f., spontaneous. F., pathologic, q.v.

f., stellate. Fracture in which cracks emerge from the central point.

f., stress. SEE: *stress fracture.*

f., torus. Fracture in which the bony cortex is not broken but is buckled.

f., transcervical. Fracture through the neck of the femur.

f., transverse. Fracture in which the fracture line is at right angles to the long axis of the bone.

f., trimalleolar. Fracture of the lateral and medial malleoli of the ankle joint with an additional fracture of the posterior edge of the distal tibia.

f., tripod. Fracture in which the zygoma is separated from attachment to the maxilla, the temporal, and the frontal bones.

fracture dislocation. Fracture near a joint that is dislocated.

fragile X syndrome. Condition of an X-linked mutation associated with a fragile site near the tip of the long arm of the X chromosome. Most males and 30% of females with this syndrome are mentally deficient. The males also develop greatly enlarged testicles (macro-orchidism), usually after puberty; but this change has been reported as early as age 5 months.

fragilitas (fră-jĭl′ĭ-tăs) [L.]. Fragility.

f. crinium. Brittleness, as of the hair, showing splitting and breaking of the shaft. Cause unknown.

f. ossium. Brittleness of bones.

f. unguium. Abnormal brittleness of nails.

fragility. State of brittleness.

f., capillary. Breaking down of capillaries with hemorrhage into almost any site but most noticeably in the skin.

f., erythrocyte. Increased tendency of the red blood cells to rupture when the salt content of the blood is decreased.

f. of blood. Tendency of red blood cells to rupture. This is determined by subjecting the cells in laboratory tests to different concentrations of saline.

If red blood cells are placed in distilled water, they swell rapidly and burst because they normally are suspended in a solution of much greater osmotic pressure. This phenomenon is called hemolysis. If they are suspended in a solution of normal saline, the cells retain their normal shape and do not burst. If they are placed in successively weaker solutions of saline, a point is reached at which some of the cells burst and liberate their hemoglobin within a given length of time, while others do not (partial hemolysis). Finally, at a given dilution, all of the cells have burst within the allotted time, which is usually two hours. The cells of normal blood begin to hemolyze in about 0.44%, and complete hemolysis occurs in about 0.35% saline solution.

fragment (frăg′mĕnt). A part broken off a larger entity.

fragment antigen binding. ABBR: Fab. A part of the antibody molecule that contains the antigen-binding site. It is obtained by enzymatic hydrolysis of the antibody.

fragmentation [L. *fragmentum,* detached part]. Breaking up into fragments.

frail elderly. Older individuals experiencing physical, mental, and emotional disability, any one of which could limit their independence and promote dependency on and require assistance from another. Seen more commonly in those 75 years of age or older.

frambesia (frăm-bē′zē-ă) [Fr. *framboise,* raspberry]. An infectious tropical disease caused by a spirochete, *Treponema pertenue.* SYN: *yaws.*

frambesioma (frăm-bē-zē-ō′mă) [″ + Gr. *oma,* tumor]. Primary lesion of yaws in the form of a protruding nodule. This mother yaw appears at the site of inoculation of the causative agent, *Treponema pertenue.*

frame. A supporting structure.

f., Balkan. A framework that fits over the bed. Suspended from the frame and connected through ropes and pulleys are weights used to produce desired continuous traction while permitting freedom of motion, thus maintaining desired immobilization of the part being treated.

f., Bradford [Edward H. Bradford, U.S. orthopedic surgeon, 1848–1926]. An oblong frame, about 7 × 3 feet (2.13 × 0.91 meters), made of 1 in. (2.5 cm) pipe covered with movable canvas strips that run from one side of the frame to the other. Used for patients with fractures or disease of the hip or spine, thus permitting them to urinate and defecate without moving the spine or changing position.

f., quadriplegic standing. Device for supporting a patient with all four extremities paralyzed.

f., Stryker. SEE: *Stryker frame.*

f., trial. An eyeglass frame for holding trial lenses while a person is being fitted for glasses.

framework. The basic system or design of anything.

Franceschetti's syndrome (frăn″chĕs-kĕt′ēz) [Adolphe Franceschetti, Swiss ophthalmologist, 1896–1968]. Mandibulofacial dysostosis with hypoplasia of the facial bones, downward angulation of the palpebral fissures, macrostomia, ear defects, and defectively formed extremities. SYN: *Treacher-Collins syndrome.*

Franciscella tularensis (frän″sĭ-sĕl′ă too″lă-rĕn′sĭs) [Edward Francis, Tulare County, California]. A short, nonmotile, encapsulated, non-spore-forming, gram-negative organism that causes tularemia, q.v., in man. Formerly classed as *Pasteurella tularensis.*

francium (frăn′sē-ŭm) [Named for France, the country in which it was discovered]. SYMB: Fr. At. no. 87. The at. wt. of the most stable isotope is 233. A radioactive metallic element occurring as a natural isotope.

frank. Obvious, esp. in reference to a clinical sign or condition such as blood in the urine, sputum, or feces.

Frankenhäuser's ganglion (fräng′kĕn-hoy″zĕrs) [Ferdinand Frankenhäuser, Ger. gynecologist, 1832–1894]. A nerve ganglion sometimes found in lateral walls of the cervix uteri.

Frankfort horizontal plane. A cephalometric plane joining the anthropometric landmarks of porion and orbitale; the reproducible position of the head when the upper margin of the ear openings and lower margin of the orbit of eye are horizontal.

Franklin glasses [Benjamin Franklin, U.S. statesman and inventor, 1706–1790]. Bifocal spectacles.

fraternal twins. Two offspring that have developed in the uterus at the same time, but are the result of independent fertilization of two ova. SYN: *dizygotic twins.* SEE: *monozygotic twins.*

fratricide (frăt′rĭ-sīd″) [L. *fratricidium*]. Murder of one's brother or sister.

Fraunhofer's lines (frown′hōf-ĕrz) [Joseph von Fraunhofer, Ger. optician, 1787–1826]. Absorption bands or lines seen in a spectrum, caused by the absorption of groups of light rays in their passage through solids, liquids, or gases.

F.R.C.P. *Fellow of the Royal College of Physicians.*

F.R.C.P.(C.). *Fellow of the Royal College of Physicians of Canada.*

F.R.C.S. *Fellow of the Royal College of Surgeons.*

F.R.C.S.(C.). *Fellow of the Royal College of Surgeons of Canada.*

freckle (frĕk′l) [O. Norse *freknur*]. Small local brownish or yellowish pigmentation of the skin due to an accumulation of melanin. SYN: *ephelis; lentigo.*

ETIOL: Exposure to sun usually stimulates melanin production.

f., Hutchinson's. A noninvasive malig-

nant melanoma.

free association. 1. Trend of thoughts when not under mental restraint or direction. 2. The procedure in psychoanalysis that requires the patient to speak aloud his thought flow, word for word, without censorship.

free base. A form of cocaine used by addicts. It is prepared by alkalinizing the hydrochloride salt, extracting it with an organic solvent such as ether, and then heating the extract to 90°C. The inhaled material is rapidly absorbed from the lung. SEE: *cocaine hydrochloride; crack; freebasing.*

freebasing. The inhalation of a form of cocaine called free base, q.v. SEE: *cocaine hydrochloride; crack.*

free medical clinics. Clinics that are established by the community rather than a hospital and provide free medical care. They are unusual in that their purpose is to deal with illnesses and conditions that are both medical and social.

free radical. SEE: *radical, free.*

freeze-drying. Preservation of tissue by rapidly freezing the specimen and then dehydrating it in a high vacuum. SYN: *lyophilization.*

freezing [AS. *freosan*]. 1. Passing from liquid to solid state because of loss of heat. 2. Becoming stiff, rigid, and inflexible from cold. Frigidity of a limb can result from exposure to cold. Most common in the debilitated, the exhausted, and those alcoholics who fall asleep in a location exposed to extreme cold. SEE: *frostbite; windchill factor.*

SYM: Paleness, cyanosis, coldness. Unconsciousness usually develops.

F.A.: Protect part with a cradle and apply dry heat at room temperature. Alternatively, the patient may be placed in tepid bath water. Sudden applications of intense heat are contraindicated; however, rapid rewarming in warm water at a temperature of 40–42°C (104–108°F) is mandatory. This is done until thawing is complete. After rewarming is accomplished, treat with analgesics for pain, tetanus prophylaxis, nonsteroidal anti-inflammatory agents, and intravenous penicillin for 48 to 72 hours.

freezing mixtures. For ice bags, 5 oz (150 ml) each of ammonium chloride and potassium nitrate, and one part water.

freezing point. Temperature at which liquids freeze.

Freiberg's infraction (frī′bĕrgz) [Albert Henry Freiberg, U.S. surgeon, 1868–1940]. Osteochondritis of the head of the second metatarsal bone of the foot.

fremitus (frĕm′ĭ-tŭs) [L.]. Vibratory tremors, esp. those felt through the chest wall by palpation. Varieties are vocal or tactile, friction, hydatid, rhonchal or bronchial, cavernous on succussion, pleural, pericardial, tussive, thrills. SEE: *palpation; thrill.*

f., tactile. The vibration or thrill felt while the patient is speaking and the hand is held against the chest.

f., tussive. Vibrations felt when the hand is held against the chest when the patient coughs.

f., vocal. Vibrations of the voice transmitted to the ear on auscultation of the chest of a person speaking. In determining the vocal fremitus, observe the following precautions: Palpate symmetrical parts of the chest, making firm pressure. When comparing, use the same pressure on both sides. Apply hands as nearly parallel to ribs as possible; remember that the fremitus normally increases over the right apex. It is decreased in pleural effusions (air, pus, blood, serum, or lymph); emphysema; pulmonary collapse from an obstructed bronchus; pulmonary edema; and morbid growths of the lung.

frenal (frē′năl) [L. *fraenum,* bridle]. Pert. to the frenum.

French scale. A system used to indicate the outer diameter of catheters and sounds. Each unit on the scale is approx. equivalent to ⅓ mm; thus a 21 French sound is 7 mm in diameter.

frenectomy (frē-něk′tō-mē) [″ + Gr. *ektome,* excision]. Surgically cutting of any frenum, usually the frenum of the tongue.

frenotomy (frē-nŏt′ō-mē) [″ + Gr. *tome,* incision]. Division of any frenum, esp. for tongue-tie.

frenuloplasty (frěn′ū-lō-plăs″tē) [″ + Gr. *plassein,* to form]. Surgical correction of an abnormally attached frenulum.

frenulum (frěn′ū-lŭm) [L., a little bridle] (pl. *frenula*). 1. [NA] A small frenum. SYN: *vinculum.* 2. A small fold of white matter on the upper surface of the anterior medullary velum extending to corpora quadrigemina.

f. clitoridis. [NA] The union of inner parts of the labia minora on undersurface of the clitoris, q.v.

f. labiorum pudendi. [NA] Fold of membrane connecting the posterior ends of the labia minora.

f. linguae. [NA] Fold of mucous membrane that extends from the floor of the mouth to the inferior surface of the tongue along its midline.

f. of ileocecal valve. Prolongation of the two lips of the ileocolic valve around the inner wall of the colon.

f. of the lips, labialis oris. Fold of mucous membrane extending from the middle of the inner surface of the lip to the alveolar mucosa; seen in both upper and lower jaws.

f. of tongue. Frenulum that attaches the lower side of the tongue to the floor of the buccal cavity. At birth this may be tight, in which case it is called tongue-tie, q.v.

f. preputii. [NA] Frenulum that unites the foreskin (prepuce) to the glans penis.

frenum (frē′nŭm) [L. *fraenum,* bridle] (pl. *frena*). A fold of mucous membrane that connects two parts, one more or less movable, and serves to check the movement of this part. SEE: *frenulum.*

frenzy (frěn′zē) [ME. *frenesie*]. A state of violent mental agitation; maniacal excitement. SEE: *panic.*

frequency [L. *frequens,* often]. 1. The number of repetitions of a phenomenon in a certain period of time or within a distinct population, as the frequency of heartbeat, frequency of sound vibrations, or frequency of a disease entity. SEE: *incidence.* 2. The rate of oscillation or alternation in an alternating current circuit, in contradistinction to periodicity in the interruptions or regular variations of current in a direct current circuit. Frequency is computed on the basis of a complete cycle, a complete cycle being one in which the current rises from zero to a positive maximum, returns to zero, and descends to an opposite negative minimum and returns to zero.

frequency distribution. In statistics, the grouping of data by frequency of occurrence at arbitrarily determined values even though the variable may be continuously variable, e.g., disease occurrences could be grouped by weeks, months, or years rather than the precise day of occurrence. SEE: *normal distribution.*

fresh frozen plasma. ABBR: FFP. Fluid portion of one unit of human blood that has been centrifuged, separated, and frozen solid within six hours of collection. SEE: *blood component.*

F response. In electrodiagnostic study of spinal reflexes, the time required for a stimulus applied to a motor nerve to travel in the opposite direction up the nerve to the spinal cord and return.

fretum (frē′tŭm) [L.]. A constriction.

Freud, Sigmund (froyd). A famous Austrian neurologist and psychoanalyst (1856–1939) whose teachings involved a procedure for investigating mental function by use of free-association dream interpretation; and analysis of resistance and transference. Freud did not consider psychoanalysis to be scientific. The real purpose of psychoanalysis was to elucidate the darkest recesses of the mind and soul and to enable the individual to integrate the emotional and intellectual sides of his nature, i.e., the forces of love and death, to develop better knowledge of

freudian (froy'dē-ăn). Pert. to Sigmund Freud's theories of unconscious or repressed libido or past sex experiences or desires as the cause of various neuroses, the cure for which is the restoration of such conditions to consciousness through psychoanalysis. SEE: *Freud, Sigmund.*

freudian slip [From Freudian psychology]. A mistake in speaking or writing that is felt to provide insight into the individual's unconscious thoughts, motives, or wishes.

Freund's adjuvant (froynds) [Jules Thomas Freund, Hungarian-born U.S. immunologist, 1890 – 1960]. Mixture of killed microorganisms, usually mycobacteria, in an oil and water emulsion. The material is administered to induce antibody formation. Because the oil retards absorption of the mixture, the antibody response is much greater than if the killed microorganisms were administered alone.

friable (frī'ă-b'l) [L. *friabilis*]. Easily broken or pulverized.

friction [L. *frictio*]. Rubbing. In massage, strong circular manipulations always followed by centripetal stroking. In hydrotherapy, friction is used in drying patients after tonic baths, and in shampoos and drip sheet rubs.

f., deep transverse. Also called cross fiber. A massage technique where stroking is applied across the longitudinal direction of the tissues of muscles, tendons, ligaments or fascia in order to prevent adhesions, increase mobility of the tissue, and align new fibers along the lines of stress.

f., dry. Friction using no liquid.

f., moist. Friction using a liquid or oil.

frictional electricity. Electricity produced by friction. SEE: *electricity, static.*

friction rub. The distinct sound heard when two dry surfaces are rubbed together. If the sound is loud enough, the condition producing the sound can also be felt.

f.r., pericardial. Friction rub that may be present in pericarditis, particularly when the disease process first starts.

f.r., pleural. Creaking, grating sounds made when inflamed pleural surfaces move during respiration. Often heard only during the first day or two of a pleurisy. SEE: *pericardial friction rub.*

Friedländer's bacillus (frēd'lĕn-dĕrz) [Carl F. Friedländer, Ger. physician, 1847 – 1887]. *Klebsiella pneumoniae*, a species of bacteria that causes pneumonia and is a secondary invader in bronchitis or sinusitis.

Friedländer's disease. Endarteritis obliterans, inflammation of an artery sufficient to cause complete closure of the lumen.

Friedman's test (frēd'mănz) [Maurice H. Friedman, U.S. physiologist, b. 1903]. Pregnancy test. The injection of the urine of a woman suspected of pregnancy into an unmated female rabbit will cause the formation of corpora lutea and corpora hemorrhagica in the rabbit at the end of two days if the woman is pregnant. Tests that are less difficult to perform are available.

Friedreich's ataxia (frēd'rīks) [Nikolaus Friedreich, Ger. neurologist, 1825 – 1882]. An inherited degenerative disease with sclerosis of the dorsal and lateral columns of the spinal cord. Accompanied by ataxia, speech impairment, lateral curvature of the spinal column, and peculiar swaying and irregular movements, with paralysis of the muscles, esp. of the lower extremities. Onset occurs in childhood or early adolescence. SYN: *ataxia, hereditary spinal.*

Friedreich's sign. 1. Sudden collapse of the cervical veins that were previously distended at each diastole. Caused by an adherent pericardium. 2. Lowering of the pitch of the percussion note that occurs over an area of cavitation during inspiration.

fright [AS. *fryhto*]. Extreme sudden fear.

f., precordial. Nausea and fear felt before the onset of manic-depressive illness.

fright neuroses. Traumatic hysteria.

frigid (frĭj'ĭd) [L. *frigidus*]. 1. Cold. 2. Irresponsive to emotion, applied esp. to the inability on the part of a woman to feel sexual desire. SEE: *impotence.*

frigidity (frĭ-jĭd'ĭ-tē). Inhibited sexual excitement during sexual activity. In males, it manifests as partial or complete failure to attain or maintain erection until completion of the sex act.

In females, there is partial or complete failure to attain or maintain the vaginal lubrication-swelling response of sexual excitement until completion of the sex act.

frigolabile (frĭg"ō-lā'bĭl) [L. *frigor*, cold, + *labilis*, unstable]. Capable of being destroyed by low temperature.

frigorific (frĭg"ō-rĭf'ĭk) [L. *frigorificus*]. Generating cold.

frigorism [L. *frigor*, cold, + Gr. *-ismos*, condition]. Very poor blood circulation caused by long exposure to cold.

frigostabile (frĭg"ō-stā'b'l) [" + *stabilis*, firm]. Incapable of being destroyed by low temperature.

frigotherapy (frĭg"ō-thĕr'ă-pē) [" + Gr. *therapeia*, treatment]. The use of cold in treatment of disease. SYN: *cryotherapy.*

frit (frĭt) [It. *fritta*, fry]. 1. The material from which glass or the glazed portion of pottery is made. 2. A similar material for making the glaze of artificial teeth.

frog belly. Flaccid abdomen in children afflicted by rickets, and atony of abdominal cells resulting from dyspepsia, accompanied by flatulence.

frog face. Flatness of face resulting from intranasal disease.

Fröhlich's syndrome (frā'lĭks) [Alfred Fröhlich, Austrian neurologist, 1871–1953]. Condition characterized by obesity and sexual infantilism, atrophy or hypoplasia of the gonads, and altered secondary sex characteristics. Due to disturbance of the hypothalamus and hypophysis, usually secondary to a neoplasm. SYN: *adiposogenital dystrophy.*

Froin's syndrome (frō-änz') [Georges Froin, Fr. physician, b. 1874]. Yellow cerebrospinal fluid that rapidly coagulates. It contains an excess of lymphocytes and protein, particularly globulin.

frolement (frōl-mŏn') [Fr.]. 1. Very light friction with the hand in massage. SEE: *massage*. 2. A sound resembling rustling heard in auscultation.

Froment's sign (frō-mäz') [Jules Froment, Fr. physician, 1878–1946]. Flexion of the distal phalanx of the thumb when a sheet of paper is held between the thumb and index finger. An indication of ulnar nerve palsy.

Frommann's lines (frŏm'änz) [Carl Frommann, Ger. anatomist, 1831–1892]. Transverse lines in the axis cylinder of medullated nerve fibers. Demonstrated by staining with silver nitrate.

frons (frŏnz) [L.]. [NA] The forehead.

frontad [L. *frons, front-*, brow, + *ad*, toward]. Toward the frontal aspect.

frontal [L. *frontalis*]. 1. Anterior. 2. Pert. to the forehead bone.

frontal bone. Forehead bone.

frontal lobe. Four main convolutions in front of the central sulcus of the cerebrum.

frontal plane. A plane parallel with the long axis of the body and at right angles to the median sagittal plane.

frontal sinuses. A pair of hollow spaces in the frontal bone lying above the orbits. They are lined with mucous membrane, contain air, and communicate with the middle nasal meatus by means of the nasofrontal duct.

fronto- [L. *frons*, brow]. Prefix indicating anterior position or relationship with the forehead.

frontomalar (frŏn"tō-mā'lăr) [" + *mala*, cheek]. Rel. to the frontal and malar bones.

frontomaxillary (frŏn"tō-măx'ĭ-lār"ē) [" + *maxilla*, jawbone]. Rel. to the frontal and maxillary bones.

frontoparietal (frŏn"tō-pă-rī'ĕ-tăl) [" + *parietalis*, pert. to a wall]. Pert. to the frontal and parietal bones.

frontotemporal [" + *tempora*, the tem-

ples]. Pert. to the frontal and temporal bones.

front-tap reflex. Contraction of gastrocnemius muscles when stretched muscles of the extended leg are percussed.

frost [AS.]. Frozen vapor deposit.

    f., uremic. Deposit of urea crystals on the skin from evaporation of sweat in a patient whose kidneys are severely impaired, such as in uremia.

frostbite. Freezing or effect of freezing of a part of the body. Exposed areas such as ears, cheeks, nose, fingers, and toes are usually affected. SEE: *freezing; frostnip.* SEE: *Nursing Diagnoses* in *Appendix.*

    SYM: Tingling, redness followed by paleness and numbness of affected area. It is of three degrees: transitory hyperemia following numbness; formation of vesicles; and gangrene.

    F.A.: Do not rub part with snow. Rapid rewarming in water at 40–42°C (104–108°F). Give tetanus prophylaxis, analgesics, nonsteroidal anti-inflammatory agents, and antibiotics if blistered. Stimulate with orally administered hot fluids such as tea, coffee, or beef bouillon. Patient should not be allowed to smoke. Administer artificial respiration if indicated. Patients have been known to recover without loss of fingers or toes even though amputation seemed inevitable. If sloughing of tissue occurs, treat as for a burn. SEE: *freezing* for treatment of frozen parts.

frost-itch. Itching of skin provoked by cold temperatures. SYN: *pruritus hiemalis.*

frostnip. A mild form of cold injury. The reversible changes in areas farthest removed from the core of the body, such as earlobes, cheeks, nose, fingers, and toes, consist of blanching of the skin and numbness. SEE: *frostbite.*

frottage (frō-tŏzh') [Fr., rubbing]. Massage technique using rubbing. SEE: *frotteurism.*

frotteurism. Recurrent intense sexual urges and fantasies involving touching and rubbing against a nonconsenting person. These acts are usually done in crowded places where arrest is unlikely. Persons who commit this type of behavior are usually young males. The individual who has acted on these urges is usually distressed about them.

frozen section. The cutting of a thin piece of tissue from a frozen specimen to permit rapid examination under the microscope. A technique used while the patient is still anesthetized. The surgeon's further action will be influenced by the results of this rapid test.

"frozen watchfulness." The hopeless reproachful stare of battered children. SEE: *abused person.*

F.R.S. *Fellow of the Royal Society.*

F.R.S.C. *Fellow of the Royal Society (Canada).*

fructofuranose (frŭk″tō-fū′ră-nōs). The furanose form of fructose.

fructokinase (frŭk″tō-kī′nās). Enzyme that catalyzes transfer of high-energy phosphate from a donor to fructose.

fructose (frŭk′tōs) [L. *fructus,* fruit]. USP. Levulose; fruit sugar. A monosaccharide and a hexose, having the same empirical formula as glucose, $C_6H_{12}O_6$, and found in corn syrup, honey, fruit juices, and in the syrup resulting from the inversion of sucrose, an invert sugar. It is metabolized to provide a source of energy or may be stored in the body after being converted to glycogen. SEE: *disaccharide.*

fructose intolerance. Inability to metabolize the carbohydrate fructose due to a hereditary absence or deficiency of the enzyme 1-phosphofructaldolase. Clinical signs develop early in life. They include hypoglycemia, jaundice, hepatomegaly, vomiting, lethargy, irritability, and convulsions. Fructose can be identified in the urine. Do not use fructose tolerance test, because to do so may induce irreversible coma.

    TREAT: Acute attacks are treated by administering glucose. For long-term therapy, all foods containing fructose, which is present in sweet fruits and sugar cane, and sucrose and sorbitol, the latter used as a sweetening agent in foods and drugs, must be eliminated from the diet.

fructosemia (frŭk″tō-sē′mē-ă) [″ + Gr. *haima,* blood]. Presence of fructose in the blood.

fructoside (frŭk′tō-sīd). A carbohydrate that upon hydrolysis yields fructose.

fructosuria (frŭk″tō-sū′rē-ă) [″ + Gr. *ouron,* urine]. Fructose in the urine.

fruit [L. *fructus,* fruit]. A ripened ovary of seed-bearing plants and the surrounding tissue as the pod of a bean, nut, grain, or berry. The edible product of a plant consisting of ripened seeds and the enveloping tissue. Fruits in general tend to add bulk to the diet. This quality, as well as their containing specific laxative substances in some cases, makes fruits quite helpful in treating constipation.

    COMP: Carbohydrates in the form of fruit sugars are the chief nutritive value of fruits. Seventy-five percent of it is a mixture of dextrose and levulose. Good source of vitamins, minerals, and iodine.

    Pectose bodies: The principle in fruits that causes them to jell. Pectose is found in unripe fruit; pectin is found in ripe fruit or fruit that has been cooked in a weak acid solution.

    Principal acids: Acetic in wine and vinegar. Citric in lemons, oranges, limes, and citron. Malic in apples, pears, apricots, peaches, currants, and gooseberries. Oxalic in rhubarb, sorrel, and cranberries. Tartaric in grapes, pineapples, and tamarinds. Salicylic in currants, cranberries, cherries, plums, grapes, and crabapples.

    Combined acids: Citric and malic in raspberries, strawberries, gooseberries, and cherries. Citric, malic, and oxalic in cranberries.

frumentaceous (froo-mĕn-tā′shŭs) [L. *frumentum,* grain]. Resembling or belonging to grain.

frustration [L. *frustratus,* disappointed].1. The failure of libido to find adequate outlet. 2. The condition that results from the thwarting or prevention of acts that if performed would bring satisfaction or gratification of physical or personality needs.

Fryns syndrome. A pattern of lethal, multiple congenital malformations first described in 1979 by J.P. Fryns et al.

FSH. *follicle-stimulating hormone.* Secreted by the anterior lobe of the hypophysis.

FSH-RF. *follicle-stimulating hormone releasing factor.*

ft. L. *fiat* or *fiant,* let there be made; *florentium,* former name for promethium; *foot.*

FTA-ABS. *fluorescent treponemal antibody-absorption test for syphilis.*

FTT. *failure to thrive.*

5-FU. Trade name for fluorouracil.

fuchsin (fook′sĭn). A red dye that can be prepared in an acid or basic form.

fucose (fū′kōs). A mucopolysaccharide present in blood group substances and in human milk.

fucosidosis (fū″kō-sī-dō′sĭs). Hereditary disease resulting from absence of the enzyme required to metabolize fucosidase. Clinically, neurological deterioration begins shortly after a period of normal early development. Heart disease, thick skin, and hyperhidrosis develop and are followed by death at an early age.

-fuge [L. *fugare,* to put to flight]. Suffix meaning to expel or drive away.

fugitive (fū′jĭ-tĭv) [L. *fugitivus*]. 1. Temporary, transient. 2. Wandering; pert. to inconstant symptoms.

fugue (fūg) [L. *fuga,* flight]. A dissociative disorder in which the person acts in a normal manner but has almost complete amnesia for what happened when recovery occurs.

    f., psychogenic. Sudden, unexpected travel away from one's home or place of work with inability to recall one's past. The individual may partially or completely assume a new identity. The condition is not due to organic brain disease. The condition may follow severe mental stress such as marital quarrels or a natural disaster. It is usually of short duration but can last for months. Recovery is the usual outcome without recurrences.

fulcrum. The object or point upon which a lever moves.

fulgurant (fŭl'gū-rănt) [L. *fulgurans*]. Severe and sudden coming and going like a flash of light, as a shooting pain.

fulgurating [L. *fulgurare*, to lighten]. Pert. to fulguration.

fulguration (fŭl-gū-rā'shŭn). Destruction of tissue by means of high-frequency electric sparks. SEE: *electrodesiccation*.

fulling [O. Fr. *fauler*, to fill]. A movement in massage; kneading with the limb held between the hands, rolling it backward and forward.

full term. In obstetrics, an infant born during the time between completion of 38 to 41 weeks of gestation. SYN: *infant, term*.

fulminant (fool'-, fŭl'mĭ-nănt) [L. *fulminans*]. Sudden, severe onset; coming in lightning-like flashes of pain, as in tabes dorsalis. SYN: *fulgurant*.

fulminating. Occurring with very great rapidity, said of certain pains and diseases. SYN: *fulgurant*.

Fulvicin-P/G. Trade name for griseofulvin ultramicrosize.

Fulvicin-U/F. Trade name for griseofulvin microsize.

fumarase (fū'mă-rās). An enzyme present in many plants and animals. It catalyzes the production of L-malic acid from fumaric acid.

fumaric acid. One of the organic acids in the citric acid cycle for the metabolism of the acetate produced from fats, carbohydrates, and proteins.

fumes [L. *fumus*, smoke]. Vapors, esp. those having irritating qualities.

    f., nitric acid. Used in various chemical processes. Poisoning is produced by the action of the corrosive fumes on the respiratory tract.

    SYM: Choking, gasping, swelling of mucous membranes, tightness in chest, pulmonary edema, cough, and shock. Symptoms may last for one week or more.

    TREAT: Immediately remove the patient from the fumes, then maintain good ventilation of lungs. Administer therapy for shock and pulmonary edema. Administration of oxygen under pressure using a mask may be required along with analgesics for anxiety. Remove clothes if they are contaminated. Cortisone may be helpful in diminishing inflammatory response in lungs.

fumigant (fū'mĭ-gănt) [L. *fumigare*, to make smoke]. An agent used in disinfecting a room. The substance used produces fumes that are lethal to insects and rodents. Chemicals used include hydrogen cyanide gas, acrylonitrile, carbon tetrachloride, ethylene oxide, and methyl bromide.

Caution: All of these chemicals are highly toxic, potentially lethal, and, in some cases, explosive. They should be used only by persons skilled in their application.

---

fumigation (fū'mĭ-gā'shŭn). 1. The use of poisonous fumes or gases to destroy living organisms, esp. rats, mice, insects, and other vermin. Fumigants are relatively ineffective against bacteria and viruses; consequently terminal disinfection of the sick room, formerly a common practice, has been discontinued. 2. The disinfection of rooms by gases.

fuming [L. *fumus*, smoke]. Having a visible vapor.

function (fŭng'shŭn) [L. *functio*, performance]. 1. The action performed by any structure. In a living organism this may pertain to a cell or a part of a cell, tissue, organ, or system of organs. 2. The act of carrying on or performing a special activity. Normal function is the normal action of an organ. Abnormal activity or the failure of an organ to perform its activity is the basis of disease or disease processes. Structural changes in an organ constitute pathological changes and are common causes of malfunctioning, although an organ may act abnormally in the absence of observable structural changes. In humans, function can pertain to the manner in which the individual is able to successfully perform the tasks and roles required for everyday living.

function, words pert. to: absorption; anabolism; assimilation; catabolism; digestion; excretion; malfunction; metabolism; secretion.

functional. 1. Pert. to function. 2. A word applied to disturbances of function in a variety of ways, such as the disturbance of function in which there is no organic disease to account for the altered function.

functional disease. General term for inorganic disease or one in which changes of an organ are not in evidence; a disturbance of any organ's functions.

functional independence measure. An objectively scored measure of functional independence used by rehabilitation practitioners. Includes items related to self-care, sphincter control, mobility, locomotion, communication, and social cognition.

functional overlay. The emotional response to physical illness. It may take the form of a conversion or hysterical response, affective overreaction, prolonged symptoms of physical illness after signs of the illness have subsided, or combinations of these reactions. Functional overlay may appear to be the primary disease and require skillful diagnosis to determine the actual cause of illness.

functional psychosis. Disorder exhibited in psychosis in which there is no apparent pathology of the central nervous system.

functional residual capacity. The amount of air remaining in the lungs after a normal, resting expiration.

functioning tumor. A tumor that is capable of synthesizing the same product as the normal tissues from which it arises, esp. endocrine or nonendocrine tumors that produce hormones.

funda (fŭn'dă) [L., sling]. A four-tailed bandage.

fundal (fŭn'dăl) [L. *fundus*, base]. Pert. to a fundus.

fundament (fŭn'dă-měnt) [L. *fundamentum*]. 1. A foundation. 2. The anus.

fundectomy (fŭn-děk'tō-mē) [L. *fundus*, base, + Gr. *ektome*, excision]. Removal of the fundus of any organ.

fundic (fŭn'dĭk). Pert. to a fundus.

fundiform (fŭn'dĭ-form) [L. *funda*, sling, + *forma*, shape]. Sling-shaped or looped.

fundoplication (fŭn"dō-plĭ-kā'shŭn). Surgical reduction of the size of the opening into the fundus of the stomach and suturing the previously removed end of the esophagus to it. Used in treating reflux of gastric contents into the esophagus.

fundoscopy (fŭn-dŏs'kō-pē) [L. *fundus*, base, + Gr. *skopein*, to examine]. Literally, the examination, esp. visual, of the fundus of any organ. In ophthalmology, visual examination of the fundus of the eye. SYN: *ophthalmoscopy.*

fundus [L., base] (pl. *fundi*). [NA] 1. The larger part, base or body of a hollow organ. 2. The portion of an organ most remote from its opening.

   f. oculi. Posterior inner part of eye as seen with ophthalmoscope.

   f. of bladder. Base of the urinary bladder, the portion closest to the rectum.

   f. of gallbladder. Lower dilated portion of the gallbladder.

   f. of stomach. Uppermost portion of the stomach, posterior and lateral to the entrance of the esophagus.

   f. tympani. Floor of the tympanic cavity close to the jugular fossa. It contains the bulb of the internal jugular vein.

   f. uteri. Body of the uterus above the openings of the fallopian tubes.

funduscope (fŭn'dŭs-skōp) [L. *fundus*, base, + Gr. *skopein*, to examine]. Device, an ophthalmoscope, for examining the fundus

of the eye.

fundusectomy (fŭn"dŭs-ĕk'tō-mē) [" + Gr. *ektome*, excision]. Excision of the fundus of the stomach. SYN: *cardiectomy.*

fungal (fŭn'găl). Caused by fungus or pert. to fungus.

fungal septicemia. Presence of pathogenic fungi in the blood. May be seen as a complication of parenteral hyperalimentation. SYN: *fungemia.*

fungate (fŭn'gāt) [L. *fungus*, mushroom]. To grow like a fungus.

fungating (fŭn'gāt-ĭng). Growing rapidly like a fungus, applied to certain tumors.

fungemia (fŭn-jē'mē-ă) [" + Gr. *haima*, blood]. Presence of fungi in the blood. SYN: *fungal septicemia.*

Fungi (fŭn'jī) [L. *fungus*, mushroom]. A division of plant-like organisms that includes molds and yeasts. Fungi grow as single cells as in yeast or as multicellular filamentous colonies as in molds and mushrooms. They do not contain chlorophyll and thus are dependent upon a saprophytic or parasitic existence. True fungi have a plant body composed of hyphae. Included are the algal fungi (Phycomycetes), sac fungi (Ascomycetes), club fungi (Basidiomycetes), and imperfect fungi (Fungi Imperfecti or Deuteromycetes). Many forms are pathogenic to plants and animals.

fungi. Pl. of fungus.

fungicide (fŭn'jĭ-sīd) [L. *fungi*, mushrooms, + *cidus*, killing]. An agent that kills fungi and their spores.

fungiform (fŭn'jĭ-form) [" + *forma*, shape]. Fungus-shaped.

fungiform papillae. Small rounded eminences on middle and anterior parts of dorsum and esp. along sides of tongue.

fungistasis (fŭn-jĭ-stā'sĭs) [" + Gr. *stasis*, a halting]. A condition in which the growth of fungi is inhibited.

fungistat (fŭn'jĭ-stăt) [" + Gr. *statikos*, standing]. An agent that inhibits the growth of fungi.

fungistatic. Inhibiting the growth of fungi.

fungitoxic (fŭn"jĭ-tŏk'sĭk). A toxic effect on fungi.

fungoid (fŭn'goyd) [" + Gr. *eidos*, form, shape]. Having the appearance of a fungus.

fungosity (fŭn-gŏs'ĭ-tē). A soft, spongy fungus-like growth.

fungous (fŭn'gŭs). Pert. to a fungus.

fungus (fŭn'gŭs) [L., mushroom] (pl. *fungi*). 1. A vegetable cellular organism that subsists on organic matter. 2. A plantlike organism belonging to the division Fungi. 3. A sponge-like morbid growth on the body that resembles fungi. SEE: *actinomycosis.*

funic (fū'nĭk) [L. *funis*, cord]. Pert. to the umbilical cord.

funicle (fū′nĭ-k'l) [L. *funiculus*, little cord]. A small, threadlike structure. SYN: *funiculus*.

funic souffle. The purring sound heard over the pregnant uterus and having the same rate as the fetal heartbeat. The sound is from blood flowing through vessels in the umbilical cord.

funicular (fū-nĭk′ū-lăr). Pert. to the spermatic or umbilical cord.

funicular process. That part of the tunica vaginalis that covers the spermatic cord.

funiculitis (fū-nĭk″ū-lī′tĭs) [″ + Gr. *itis*, inflammation]. Inflammation of the spermatic cord.

funiculopexy (fū-nĭk′ū-lō-pĕks″ē) [″ + Gr. *pexis*, fixation]. Suturing the spermatic cord to the tissues in cases of undescended testicle.

funiculus (fū-nĭk′ū-lŭs) [L., little cord] (pl. *funiculi*). 1. [NA] Any small structure resembling a cord. 2. A division of the white matter of the spinal cord consisting of fasciculi or fiber tracts lying peripherally to the gray matter. Differentiated into dorsal, lateral, and ventral funiculi.

funiform (fū′nĭ-form) [L. *funis*, cord, + forma, shape]. Cordlike.

funipuncture [L. *funis*, a cord, + *punctura*, to prick]. Puncture of the vein of the umbilical cord in order to obtain a fetal blood sample. This is done in utero by using ultrasound technique to direct the needle.

funis (fū′nĭs) [L., cord]. A cordlike structure, such as the spermatic cord or the umbilical cord.

funisitis. Infection of the umbilical cord.

funnel [L. *fundere*, to pour]. Conical, wide-open-mouthed device for pouring through its open tube at end into another vessel.

funnel breast, funnel chest. Congenital anomaly consisting of sternal depression of chest walls so that the chest is funnel-shaped.

funny bone. The medial epicondyle of the humerus. So termed because pressure applied over this area stimulates the ulnar nerve and produces a distinct sensation.

F.U.O. *fever of unknown origin.*

Furacin. Trade name for nitrofurazone.

Furadantin. Trade name for nitrofurantoin.

furcal [L. *furca*, fork]. Forked.

furcation (fŭr-kā′shŭn). The anatomical area of a multirooted tooth where the roots divide. SYN: *furca*.

furcula (fŭr′kū-lă) [L., little fork]. The hypobranchial eminence, an elevation in the floor of the embryonic pharynx at the level of the 3rd and 4th branchial arches. It gives rise to the epiglottis and the aryepiglottic folds.

furfur [L., bran] (pl. *furfures*). Dandruff scales.

furfuraceous (fŭr-fū-rā′shŭs). Scaly or resembling scales.

furor [L., rage]. Extremely violent outbursts of anger, often without provocation.

   f. femininus. Nymphomania, q.v.

furosemide (fū-rō′sĕ-mīd). USP. A diuretic. Trade name is Lasix.

furred [O. Fr. *forre*, lining]. Said of the tongue on which a dustlike deposit has formed.

furrow [AS. *furh*]. A groove.

   f., atrioventricular. Groove demarcating the atria of the heart from the ventricles.

   f., digital. Any one of several transverse lines on the palmar surface of the fingers across the joints.

   f., gluteal. Vertical groove on the skin between the buttocks.

furuncle (fū′rŭng-k'l) [L. *furunculus*]. A boil. SYN: *furunculus*.

furuncular (fū-rŭng′kū-lăr). Pert. to a boil.

furunculoid (fū-rŭng′kū-loyd) [L. *furunculus*, a boil, + Gr. *eidos*, form, shape]. Resembling a furuncle or boil. SYN: *furunculus*.

furunculosis (fū-rŭng″kū-lō′sĭs) [″ + Gr. *osis*, condition]. A condition resulting from boils.

furunculous. Pert. to or of the nature of a boil or boils.

furunculus (fū-rŭng′kū-lŭs) [L., a boil] (pl. *furunculi*). Boil, furuncle. Acute, deep-seated phlegmonous inflammation formed in the skin, usually ending in suppuration and necrosis.

SYM: Neck, axillae, face, buttocks, and breasts are common sites of predilection. Begins in hair follicle or sudoriparous gland as a subcutaneous swelling or acuminate pustule around a hair shaft. The skin is smooth and shining with pain and tenderness. The lesion may come to a head or become boggy and fluctuant, or regression may take place before suppuration, resulting in disappearance by absorption. Lesion ruptures spontaneously or following incision, discharging necrotic tissue and pus. Healing follows.

ETIOL: Staphylococcal infection of follicular or sebaceous glands.

TREAT: Moist heat, incision at the time the lesion points (comes to a head), and appropriate systemic antibiotic.

NURSING IMPLICATIONS: Teach patient the importance of scrupulous personal and family hygiene. Urge the patient not to share towels or washcloths and to boil these before reuse. Caution the patient against squeezing a boil as it may rupture into the surrounding area and spread. Teach patient aseptic technique in caring for boil and disposing of dressings. Encourage compliance with medical treatment.

Fusarium (fū-zā′rē-ŭm) [L. *fusus*, spindle]. A

genus of fungi.

fuscin (fŭs′ĭn) [L. *fuscus*, dark brown]. A brown pigment, a melanin, present in the outermost layer (pigmented epithelium) of the retina.

fuse (fūz) [L. *fusus*, poured]. 1. A safety device consisting of a strip of wire of easily fusible (meltable) metal, the conductance of which is predetermined. The metal fuses and breaks circuit when excess of current passes through. 2. To unite or blend together as the coherence of adjacent body structures.

fusible (fū′zĭ-b′l). Capable of being melted.

fusiform (fū′zĭ-form) [L. *fusus*, spindle, + *forma*, shape]. Tapering at both ends; spindle-shaped.

fusimotor (fū″sĭ-mō′tor). Concerning the motor innervation of the intrafusal muscle fibers arising from the gamma efferent neurons of the anterior gray matter of the spinal cord.

fusion (fū′shŭn) [L. *fusio*]. 1. Meeting and joining together through liquefaction by heat. The process of fusing or uniting. 2. Union of adjacent tooth germs to form an oversize tooth of abnormal configuration or two teeth partially fused at the crown or root.

f., diaphyseal-epiphyseal. Surgical obliteration of the epiphyseal line of a bone so that epiphysis and diaphysis are joined.

f., nuclear. Joining of the nucleus of two atoms to form a larger nucleus. It occurs when temperatures reach millions of degrees.

f., spinal. Surgical fusion of two or more vertebrae. SYN: *spondylosyndesis.*

Fusobacterium. A genus of non-spore-forming, nonencapsulated, nonmotile, gram-negative bacteria usually found in necrotic lesions of the mouth and bowel. Their role in causing acute ulcerating gingivitis (trench mouth) has not been established.

fusocellular [L. *fusus*, spindle, + *cellulus*, little cell]. Spindle-celled.

fusospirochetal (fū″sō-spī-rō-kē′tăl) [″ + Gr. *speira*, coil, + *chaite*, hair]. Pert. to fusiform bacilli and spirochetes.

fusospirochetosis (fū″sō-spī″rō-kē-tō′sĭs) [″ + ″ + ″ + *osis*, condition]. Infection with fusiform bacilli and spirochetes.

fustigation (fŭs″tĭ-gā′shŭn) [L. *fustigatio*]. In massage, beating with light rods.

futility. In medical practice, the realization that a potential action will not be in the best interest of the patient, esp. if the patient has, prior to the illness, directed that resuscitation efforts should not be used in the event of the development of a terminal illness. SEE: *advance directive.*

fututrix (fū-tū′trĭks). A female who practices tribadism, q.v.

F wave. Flutter waves in atrial fibrillation. Detectable on the ECG at 250 to 350 per minute.

FWB. *full weight bearing.*

G

γ. Third letter of Greek alphabet; gamma is the anglicized equivalent. Symbol for microgram and immunoglobulin.

G. 1. The newtonian constant of gravitation. 2. Symbol for giga, 10^9, in SI units.

g. 1. Symbol for the standard force of attraction of gravity, 980.665 meters/second^2; or about 32.17 ft./second^2. 2. *gingival*. 3. *gram*. 4. *gender*.

Ga. Chem. symb. for the element gallium.

GABA. *gamma-aminobutyric acid.*

gadfly. A fly belonging to the family Tabanidae, q.v., that lays eggs under the skin of its victim, causing swelling simulating a boil. Multiple furuncles appear with hatching of larvae. SEE: *botfly.*

gadolinium (găd″ō-lĭn′ē-ŭm). SYMB: Gd. At. wt. 157.25; at. no. 64. A very rare element.

GAF. *Global Assessment of Functioning.*

gag. 1. Device for keeping the jaws open during surgery. 2. To retch or cause to retch.

gage (gāj). Gauge.

gag reflex. Gagging and vomiting resulting from irritation of throat or pharynx.

gain. 1. To increase something such as weight, strength, or health. 2. In electronics, the term used to describe the amplification factor for a given circuit or device.

    g., primary. In psychiatry, the relief of symptoms upon converting emotional anxiety to what the patient perceives as an organic illness, e.g., hysterical paralysis or blindness. SEE: *hysteria, conversion.*

    g., secondary. The obvious advantage that a person gains from his illness, such as being taken care of, release from responsibility, attention from others. SEE: *hysteria, conversion.*

Gaisböck's syndrome (gīs′bĕks) [Felix Gaisböck, Ger. physician, 1869–1955]. Abnormal number of red corpuscles in blood without other signs and symptoms characteristic of polycythemia vera.

gait (gāt) [ME. *gait*, passage]. Manner of walking.

    g., antalgic. Gait pattern in which the patient experiences pain during the stance phase and thus remains on the painful leg for as short a time as possible.

    g., ataxic. Gait characterized by staggering and unsteadiness.

    g., cerebellar. A staggering movement seen in cerebellar disease.

    g., double step. Gait in which alternate steps are of a different length or at a different rate.

    g., drag-to. Gait in which the feet are dragged to the crutches rather than lifted.

    g., equine. Gait characterized by high steps; characteristic of tibialis anterior paralysis. In a rigid equinus posture of the ankle, the person walks on his toes. This is also seen in spastic gait patterns.

    g., festinating. Gait in which patient walks on toes as though pushed. Starts slowly, increases, and may continue until the patient grasps some object in order to stop. Characteristic of parkinsonism.

    g., four-point. Gait in which the right crutch and then the left foot are advanced consecutively; then the left crutch and the right foot are moved forward.

    g., gluteus maximus. Leaning of the trunk backward to keep the hip extended during the stance phase. Caused by weakness of the gluteus maximus.

    g., gluteus medius. Leaning of the trunk to the affected side during the stance phase. Caused by paralysis of the gluteus medius muscle.

    g., helicopod. Gait in which the feet or foot describes a half circle with each step. Sometimes seen in hysteria.

    g., hemiplegic. Gait in which patient abducts the paralyzed limb, swings it around, and brings it forward so that the foot comes to the ground in front. During stance phase the patient bears very little weight on the involved leg.

    g., quadriceps. Leaning of the trunk forward at the beginning of the stance phase of gait in order to lock the knee when there is weakness or paralysis of the quadriceps femoris muscle.

    g., scissor. Gait in which legs cross in walking. Seen in upper motor neuron lesion accompanied by spasticity.

    g., spastic. A stiff movement, toes seeming to catch and drag, legs held together, hips and knee joints slightly flexed. Seen in spastic paraplegia, sclerosis of lateral pyramidal columns of cord, tumor of spinal cord, and arachnoiditis.

    g., steppage. Gait in which the foot is lifted high to clear the toes; there is no heel strike, the toes hit the ground first. Seen with anterior tibialis paralysis, peripheral neuritis, late stages of diabetic neuropathy, alcoholism, and chronic arsenic poisoning.

    g., swing-through. Gait in which the crutches are advanced and the legs are swung between and past them.

    g., swing-to. Gait in which the crutches are advanced and the legs are advanced to the crutches.

g., tabetic. The high-stepping ataxic walk in which the feet slap the ground. It is caused by tabes dorsalis.

g., three-point. Gait in which the crutches and the affected leg are advanced, then the other leg is advanced.

g., two-point. Gait in which the right foot and left crutch are advanced simultaneously, then the left foot and right crutch are moved forward.

g., waddling. Gait in which feet are wide apart and walk resembles that of a duck. Seen in coxa vara and double congenital displacement of hip when lordosis is present.

galact-, galacto- [Gr. *gala*, milk]. Combining forms pert. to milk.

galactacrasia (gă-lăk″tă-krā′zē-ă) [″ + *akrasia*, bad mixture]. An abnormal composition of milk from the breast.

galactagogue (gă-lăk′tă-gŏg) [″ + *agogos*, leading]. Agent that promotes the flow of milk.

galactan (gă-lăk′tăn). A complex carbohydrate that forms galactose upon hydrolysis.

galactase. An enzyme or proteolytic ferment of milk.

galactemia (gă-lăk-tē′mē-ă) [″ + *haima*, blood]. Milky condition of the blood.

galactic (gă-lăk′tĭk). Pert. to flow of milk.

galactischia (găl″ăk-tisk′ē-ă) [″ + *ischein*, to suppress]. Suppression of the secretion and flow of milk.

galactoblast (gă-lăk′tō-blăst) [″ + *blastos*, germ]. Body found in mammary acini; contains fat globules.

galactocele (gă-lăk′tō-sēl) [″ + *kele*, tumor, swelling]. 1. A tumor caused by occlusion of a milk duct. 2. Hydrocele containing a milk-like liquid.

galactoid. Resembling milk.

galactokinase (gă-lăk″tō-kī′nās). Enzyme that catalyzes transfer of high-energy phosphate groups from a donor to D-galactose. D-galactose-1-phosphate is produced by this reaction.

galactolipin [″ + *lipos*, fat]. A phosphorus-free lipid combined with galactose; a cerebroside.

galactoma (găl-ăk-tō′mă) [″ + *oma*, tumor]. Cystic tumor of female breast. SYN: *galactocele* (def. 1).

galactometer [″ + *metron*, measure]. Device for measuring the specific gravity of milk. SYN: *lactometer.*

galactopexic (găl-ăk-tō-pĕk′sĭk) [″ + *pexis*, fixation]. Holding galactose.

galactopexy (gă-lăk′tō-pĕk″sē). The fixation of galactose by the liver.

galactophagous (găl″ăk-tŏf′ă-gŭs) [″ + *phagein*, to eat]. Feeding upon milk.

galactophore (găl-ăk′tō-for) [″ + *pherein*, to bear]. A milk duct.

galactophoritis (găl-ăk″tō-for-ī′tĭs) [″ + ″ + *itis*, inflammation]. Inflammation of a milk duct.

galactophygous (găl-ăk-tŏf′ĭ-gŭs) [″ + *phyge*, flight]. Arresting flow of milk.

galactoplania (gă-lăk″tō-plā′nē-ă) [″ + *plane*, wandering]. Secretion of milk in some part of the body other than the mammary gland.

galactopoietic (gă-lăk″tō-poy-ĕt′ĭk) [″ + *poiein*, to make]. 1. Having to do with the production of milk. 2. A substance that promotes the secretion of milk.

galactorrhea (gă-lăk″tō-rē′ă) [″ + *rhoia*, flow]. 1. Continuation of lactation or flow of milk at intervals after cessation of nursing. 2. Excessive flow of milk.

galactosamine (gă-lăk″tō-săm′ĭn). Galactose containing an amine group on the second carbon.

galactose (gă-lăk′tōs). $C_6H_{12}O_6$. A dextrorotatory monosaccharide or simple hexose sugar. Galactose is an isomer of glucose and is formed, along with glucose, in the hydrolysis of lactose. It is a component of cerebrosides. Galactose is readily absorbed in the digestive tract; in the liver it is converted into glycogen.

galactosemia (gă-lăk″tō-sē′mē-ă). An inborn error of metabolism inherited as an autosomal recessive trait characterized by inability to convert galactose to glucose. It is due to congenital absence of the enzyme that is required for conversion of galactose to glucose and its derivatives. This enzyme is galactose-1-phosphate uridyl transferase. Diagnosis is confirmed by testing the newborn's urine for noncarbohydrate reducing substances. The infant with galactosemia will fail to thrive within a week after birth due to anorexia, vomiting, and diarrhea unless galactose and lactose are removed from the diet. If untreated, the disease may progress to starvation and death. Untreated children who do survive usually fail to grow, are mentally retarded, and have cataracts. If galactose is excluded from the diet early in life, the prognosis is good.

Galactosemia can be diagnosed in utero by amniocentesis. If a pregnant woman is a known carrier, it is advisable that she exclude lactose and galactose from her diet.

galactosidase (gă-lăk″tō-sī′dās). Enzyme that catalyzes the metabolism of galactosides.

galactosides (gă-lăk′tō-sīds). Carbohydrates that contain galactose.

galactostasis (găl″ăk-tŏs′tă-sĭs) [″ + *stasis*, a stopping]. Cessation or checking of milk secretion.

galactosuria (găl-ăk″tō-sū′rē-ă) [″ +

ouron, urine]. Galactose in the urine.

galactotherapy (gă-lăk″tō-thĕr′ă-pē) [″ + *therapeia,* treatment]. 1. Treatment of a nursing infant by drugs administered to the mother. 2. Therapeutic use of milk, as a milk diet. SYN: *lactotherapy.*

galactotoxin (gă-lăk″tō-tŏks′ĭn) [″ + *toxikon,* poison]. A toxic substance in milk produced by bacteria.

galactotoxism (gă-lăk″tō-tŏk′sĭzm). Poisoning due to drinking milk that contains toxic substances.

galactotrophy (găl″ăk-tŏt′rō-fē) [″ + *trophe,* nourishment]. Feeding with nothing but milk.

galactozymase (gă-lăk″tō-zī′mās) [″ + *zyme,* leaven]. A starch-hydrolyzing enzyme in milk.

galacturia (găl-ăk-tū′rē-ă) [″ + *ouron,* urine]. The passing of milky urine. SYN: *chyluria.*

galea (gā′lē-ă) [L. *galea,* helmet]. 1. [NA] A helmet-like structure. 2. A type of head bandage.

    g. aponeurotica. The aponeurosis of the scalp. It connects the anterior and posterior bellies of the occipitofrontalis muscle.

galeanthropy (gā″lē-ăn′thrō-pē) [Gr. *gale,* cat, + *anthropos,* man]. A delusion that one has become transformed into a cat.

Galeazzi's sign [Riccardo Galeazzi, It. orthopedic surgeon, 1866–1952]. A clinical test for determining the presence of congenital hip dislocation in infants and toddlers. With the child lying in a supine position and the knees flexed and hips flexed at 90°, dislocation is evidenced if one knee is higher than the other.

Galen, Claudius. A noted Greek physician and medical writer, circa A.D. 130–200, residing in Rome, where he was physician to Marcus Aurelius. Recognized as the authority on medicine through the Middle Ages. Called the father of experimental physiology.

    G.'s veins. The veins running through the tela choroidea formed by the joining of the terminal and choroid veins and forming the vena cerebri magna, which empties into the straight sinus of the brain.

galena (gă-lē′nă). Lead sulfide ore.

galenic (gă-lĕn′ĭk). Pert. to Galen, q.v., or his teachings.

galenicals, galenics (gă-lĕn′ĭ-kăls, -ĭks). 1. Herb and vegetable medicines. 2. Crude drugs and medicinals as distinguished from pure active principles contained in them. 3. A medicine prepared according to an official formula.

galeophilia (găl″ē-ō-fĭl′ē-ă) [Gr. *gale,* cat, + *philein,* to love]. Fondness for cats.

galeophobia (găl″ē-ō-fō′bē-ă) [″ +

phobos, fear]. Abnormal aversion to cats.

galeropia, galeropsia (găl-ĕr-ō′pē-ă, -ŏp′sē-ă) [Gr. *galeros,* cheerful, + *opsis,* vision]. Unusual clearness of vision.

gall [AS. *gealla,* sore place]. 1. An excoriation. 2. The bitter secretion of the liver stored in the gallbladder; bile. It has no enzymes, but it assists in the emulsifying of fats. It also stimulates the intestines and multiplies the action of the pancreatic juice threefold. It is discharged through the cystic duct into the duodenum.

    RS: bile ducts; calculus; "chol-" words; colic, biliary; cystic duct.

gallamine triethiodide (găl′ă-mīn trī″ē-thī′ō-dīd). USP. A drug that inhibits transmission of nerve impulses across the myoneural junction of voluntary muscles. Trade name is Flaxedil.

Gallant reflex. Infantile reflex in which the trunk curves toward the side of stimulation in a prone infant. Present from birth to 2 months.

gallate (găl′lāt). A salt of gallic acid.

gallbladder [AS. *gealla,* sore place, + *blaedre,* bladder]. Pear-shaped sac on undersurface of right lobe of liver holding bile from the liver. The bile is stored and while in the gallbladder is concentrated by removing water. About 500 to 600 ml of bile is secreted each day, and it is approximately 82% water. The bile is then discharged through the cystic duct, which is 3 to 4 in. (7.6 to 10.2 cm) long, 1 in. (2.54 cm) greatest diameter. The cystic duct leads into the common bile duct which empties into the small intestine.

gall duct [″ + L. *ductus,* a passage]. Tube carrying bile from the liver and gallbladder. SYN: *bile duct.*

gallium (găl′ē-ŭm) [L. *Gallia,* Gaul]. SYMB: Ga. At. wt. 69.72; at. no. 31. A rare metal, small amounts of which are found in bauxite and zinc blends.

    Gallium-68 (^{68}Ga) is used in studies involving use of radioactive materials. It has a half-life of 68 minutes.

gallon [Med. L. *galleta,* jug]. Four liquid measure quarts; 231 cubic inches or 3.79 liters. In England the Imperial liquid gallon is 277.4 cubic inches or 4.55 liters.

gallop rhythm. The third and fourth heart sounds coincide with the two stages of diastolic filling during the cardiac cycle. One occurs at mid-diastole passively, and the other is due to active filling of the ventricle by atrial contraction and occurs in presystole. These two sounds may be normal or abnormal, but in either case they may resemble a gallop rhythm.

gallstone [AS. *gealla,* sore place, + *stan,* stone]. Concretion formed in the gallbladder or bile ducts. The most common type is the cholesterol-containing stone. Gallstones form when the bile contains more cholesterol than can be kept in solution. The cholesterol precipitates out to form gallstones. The incidence of gallstones in women is approximately twice that in men. Obesity increases the risk of developing gallstones. SEE: *Nursing Diagnoses in Appendix.*

SYM: Stone may remain dormant and give little distress unless inflammation and distention of the gallbladder take place or unless it enters and is unable to pass through the biliary ducts, thus producing colic. The pain may radiate to the back and right shoulder, usually several hours after eating and when the stomach is empty. Flatulence is a common symptom. Jaundice is usually absent.

TREAT: Analgesics, meperidine being the drug of choice. Morphine is thought to increase spasm of the sphincter of Oddi and thus is not used for pain relief. Persistent pain or enlargement of the gallbladder due to its distention with gallstones may require surgery. Percutaneous instillation of methyl *tert*-butyl ether into the gallbladder will dissolve gallstones. The use of lithotripsy, i.e., extracorporeal shock-wave therapy, has been used to disintegrate stones.

RS: bilifuscin; calculus; cholelithiasis.

GALT. *gut-associated lymphoid tissue.*

Galton's whistle [Sir Francis Galton, Brit. scientist, 1822–1911]. A whistle used to test hearing.

galvanic [Luigi Galvani, It. physiologist, 1737–1798]. Pert. to galvanism.

galvanic battery. A series of cells, giving a combined effect of all the units, and generating electricity by chemical reaction.

galvanic cell. One of a series of cells generating electricity through chemical reaction.

galvanic current. Direct electric current, usually from a battery.

galvanism. Therapeutic use of direct current of electricity.

galvanization (găl″văn-ĭ-zā′shŭn). Employment of a galvanic current as a therapeutic measure.

galvanocautery (găl″vă-nō-kaw′tĕr-ē) [*galvanism* + Gr. *kauterion*, cautery]. Cauterization of tissue by means of an electric current. SEE: *electrocautery.*

galvanocontractility (găl″vă-nō-kŏn″trăk-tĭl′ĭ-tē) [″ + L. *contractus*, drawn together]. Capability of a muscle to contract under a galvanic stimulation.

galvanofaradization (găl″vă-nō-făr″ă-dĭ-zā′shŭn). Combined use of continuous and interrupted electric current in treating a nerve or a muscle.

galvanometer (găl″vă-nŏm′ĕ-tĕr) [″ +

Gr. *metron*, measure]. An instrument that measures current by electromagnetic action. SYN: *rheometer* (def. 1).

galvanopalpation (găl″vă-nō-păl-pā′shŭn) [″ + L. *palpare*, to touch]. A method of measuring tactile sensibility of the nerves of the skin by use of electric current.

galvanopuncture (găl″vă-nō-pŭng′chŭr) [″ + L. *punctura*, puncture]. Introduction of needles to complete a galvanic current.

galvanoscope (găl-văn′ō-skōp) [″ + Gr. *skopein*, to examine]. Instrument that shows the presence and direction of a galvanic current.

galvanosurgery (găl″vă-nō-sĕr′jĕr-ē) [″ + Gr. *cheir*, hand, + *ergon*, work]. Use of galvanism in surgery.

galvanotaxis (găl″vă-nō-tăk′sĭs) [″ + Gr. *taxis*, arrangement]. The tendency of a living organism to arrange itself in a medium so that its axis bears a certain relationship to the direction of the electric current in the medium.

galvanotherapeutics, galvanotherapy (găl″vă-nō-thĕr″ă-pū′tĭks, -thĕr′ă-pē) [″ + Gr. *therapeia*, treatment]. Treatment by means of electricity. SYN: *electrotherapy.*

galvanothermy (găl″văn-ō-thĕrm′ē) [″ + Gr. *therme*, heat]. Treatment by the heat from a galvanic battery.

galvanotonus (găl-văn-ŏt′ō-nŭs) [″ + Gr. *tonos*, tension]. Tonic contractions caused by a galvanic current.

galvanotropism (găl″văn-ŏt′rō-pĭzm) [″ + Gr. *tropos*, a turn]. The tendency of an organism to grow, turn, or move in relationship with an electric current.

gamete (găm′ēt) [Gr. *gamein*, to marry]. A mature male or female reproductive cell; the spermatozoon or ovum. SEE: *chromosome; meiosis.*

RS: conception; fertilization; gene; ovum; spermatozoon.

gamete intrafallopian transfer. ABBR: GIFT. A procedure developed by Ricardo Asch, a contemporary U.S. physician, to assist couples who have an infertility problem. Through use of a laparoscope, ova are obtained from a mature follicle and then analyzed in a Petri dish. Sperm are placed in a separate Petri dish. If the two specimens are judged to be suitable for use, first an ovum is aspirated into a special catheter followed by sperm; then another egg is drawn into the catheter. The ova and sperm are then placed in the fallopian tube where fertilization will have an opportunity to take place naturally. SEE: *embryo transfer; fertilization, in vitro.*

gametic (găm-ĕt′ĭk). Pert. to gametes.

gametocide (găm′ĕ-tō-sīd″) [″ + L. *caedere*, to kill]. An agent destructive to gametes or gametocytes, particularly those of malaria.

gametocyte (gă-mē'tō-sīt) [" + *kytos*, cell]. A stage of the malarial protozoon that reproduces in the blood of the Anopheles mosquito.

gametogenesis (găm"ĕt-ō-jĕn'ĕ-sĭs) [" + *genesis*, generation, birth]. Development of gametes: oogenesis or spermatogenesis.

gametogony (găm"ē-tŏg'ō-nē). The phase in the life cycle of the malarial parasite (Plasmodium) in which male and female gametocytes, which infect the mosquito, are formed.

gametophyte (găm'ē-tō-fīt) [" + *phyton*, plant]. In plants, the sexual or gamete-producing generation that alternates with the asexual or spore-producing generation.

gamic (găm'ĭk) [Gr. *gamein*, to marry]. Sexual, esp. as applied to eggs that develop only after fertilization in contrast to those that develop without fertilization. SEE: *parthenogenesis.*

gamma. 1. Third letter of the Gr. alphabet, γ. 2. In chemistry it is used to designate the third of a series, as the third carbon atom in an aliphatic chain. 3. One microgram; or one thousandth of a milligram (0.001 mg); one millionth of a gram.

gamma-aminobutyric acid. ABBR: GABA. An amino-acid-inhibiting transmitter in the central nervous system.

gamma benzene hexachloride (găm'ă bĕn' zēn hĕk"să-klor'īd). An insecticide used in treating scabies. Trade name is Kwell. SYN: *lindane.*

gammacism. Inability to pronounce correctly g and k sounds.

Gammagee. Trade name for immune globulin.

gamma globulin. A protein formed in the blood. Ability to resist infection is related to concentration of such proteins. SEE: *immunoglobulin.*

gamma knife stereotaxic radiosurgery. A method for delivering a high dose of radiation to a specific site in the brain.

Gammar. Trade name for immune globulin.

gamma rays. Electromagnetic waves of extremely short wavelength emitted by radioactive substances. They are thought to be of the same nature as x-rays and have greater penetrating power than alpha or beta rays. SEE: *ray.*

gammopathy (găm-ŏp'ă-thē). A disease in which there is an increase in serum immunoglobulin, as in myeloma, but Bence Jones protein is not present in the urine.

gamo- [Gr. *gamos*, marriage]. Combining form indicating relationship to marriage or sexual union.

gamogenesis (găm"ō-jĕn'ĕ-sĭs) [" + *gen-*

esis, generation, birth]. Sexual reproduction.

gamont (găm'ŏnt) [" + *on*, being]. A sexual form of certain protozoa. SEE: *gametocyte.*

gamophobia (găm"ō-fō'bē-ă) [" + *phobos*, fear]. Neurotic fear of marriage.

gampsodactylia (gămp"sō-dăk-tĭl'ē-ă) [Gr. *gampsos*, curved, + *daktylos*, digit]. Deformity of the toes causing them to resemble claws. SYN: *clawfoot.*

ganciclovir. A synthetic antiviral drug. It has been used intravenously in treating cytomegalovirus (CMV) retinitis in immunocompromised patients. Trade name is Cytovene. SEE: *cytomegalic inclusion disease.*

ganglia (găng'glē-ă). Plural form of ganglion.

ganglial (găng'lē-ăl) [Gr. *ganglion*, knot]. Pert. to a ganglion. SYN: *ganglionic.*

gangliated (găng'lē-ā-tĕd). 1. Having ganglia. 2. Intermixed.

gangliectomy (găng"glē-ĕk'tō-mē) [" + *ektome*, excision]. Excision of a ganglion.

gangliform (găng'li-form) [" + L. *forma*, shape]. Formed like a ganglion.

gangliitis (găng"glē-ī'tĭs) [" + *itis*, inflammation]. Inflammation of a ganglion.

ganglioblast (găng'glē-ō-blăst") [" + *blastos*, germ]. An embryonic ganglion cell.

gangliocyte (găng'glē-ō-sīt") [" + *kytos*, cell]. A ganglion cell.

gangliocytoma (găng"glē-ō-sī-tō'mă) [" + " + *oma*, tumor]. Ganglioneuroma.

ganglioglioma (găng"glē-ō-glī-ō'mă) [" + *glia*, glue, + *oma*, tumor]. A ganglion-cell glioma.

ganglioglioneuroma (găng"glē-ō-glī"ō-nū-rō'mă) [" + " + *neuron*, nerve, + *oma*, tumor]. Ganglion cells, glia cells, and nerve fibers in a nerve tumor.

ganglioma (găng-lē-ō'mă) [" + *oma*, tumor]. 1. Tumor of a lymphatic gland. 2. A swelling of lymphoid tissue.

ganglion (găng'lē-ŏn) [Gr.] (pl. *ganglia* or *ganglions*). 1. A mass of nervous tissue composed principally of nerve-cell bodies and lying outside the brain or spinal cord. Ex.: the chains of ganglia that form the main sympathetic trunks; the dorsal root ganglion of a spinal nerve. 2. Cystic tumor developing on a tendon or aponeurosis; sometimes occurs on the back of the wrist.

 g., abdominal. Any one of the abdominal ganglia.

 g., anterior cerebral. Corpus striatum. Corpus striatum and corpus lenticulare considered together.

 g., aorticorenal. Ganglion lying near the lower border of the celiac ganglion. It is located near the origin of the renal artery.

 g., Arnold's auricular. Tiny ganglion located beneath the foramen ovale of the ear. SYN: *g., otic.*

g., auricular. G., Arnold's auricular.

g., autonomic. Ganglion of the autonomic division of the nervous system.

g., basal. Mass of gray matter beneath the 3rd ventricle. Consisting of the caudate, lentiform, and amygdaloid nuclei and the claustrum.

g., basal optic. Mass of gray matter beneath the 3rd ventricle.

g., cardiac. Tiny ganglion toward which converge the fibers of superficial cardiac plexus. It lies on the right side of the ligamentum arteriosus. SYN: *Wrisberg's ganglion.*

g., carotid. Ganglion formed by filamentous threads from the carotid plexus beneath the carotid artery.

g., celiac. One of a pair of prevertebral or collateral ganglia located near the origin of the celiac artery. They form a part of the celiac plexus.

g., cephalic. One of the parasympathetic ganglia in the head: otic, pterygopalatine, and submandibular ganglia.

g., cerebral. Main cerebral nerve centers.

g., cervical. One of the three pairs of ganglia (superior, middle, inferior) located in the neck region. They are the ganglia of the cervical portion of the sympathetic trunk.

g., cervicothoracic. G., stellate, q.v.

g., cervicouterine. Ganglion near the uterine cervix. SYN: *g., Frankenhäuser's.*

g., ciliary. Tiny ganglion located in the rear portion of the orbit. SYN: *g., lenticular; g., ophthalmic.*

g., coccygeal. Ganglion located in the coccygeal plexus and forming the lower termination of the two sympathetic trunks; sometimes absent.

g., collateral. One of several ganglia of the sympathetic nervous system. They are in the mesenteric nervous plexuses near the abdominal aorta.

g., Corti's. Ganglion on the cochlear nerve.

g., dorsal root. Ganglion located on the dorsal root of a spinal nerve. Contains the cell bodies of sensory neurons. SYN: *g., spinal.*

g., false. An enlargement on a nerve that does not contain a ganglion.

g., Frankenhäuser's. Cervical ganglion of the uterus.

g., gasserian. G., trigeminal, q.v.

g., geniculate. Ganglion on the pars intermedia, the sensory root of the facial nerve. It lies in the anterior border of the anterior geniculum of the facial nerve.

g., inferior mesenteric. A prevertebral sympathetic ganglion located in the inferior

mesenteric plexus near the origin of the inferior mesenteric artery.

g., intervertebral. G., spinal.

g., jugular. Ganglion located on the root of the vagus nerve and lying in upper portion of jugular foramen.

g., lateral. One of a chain of ganglia forming the main sympathetic trunk.

g., lenticular. G., ciliary.

g., lumbar. One of the ganglia usually occurring in fours in the lumbar portion of the sympathetic trunk.

g., lymphatic. Lymph nodes.

g., nodose. Ganglion of the trunk of the vagus nerve. Located immediately below the jugular ganglion. It makes connections with the spinal accessory nerve, hypoglossal nerve, and the superior cervical ganglion of the sympathetic trunk.

g., ophthalmic. G., ciliary.

g., otic. A small ganglion located deep in the zygomatic fossa immediately below the foramen ovale. It lies medial to the mandibular nerve. It supplies postganglionic parasympathetic fibers to the parotid gland. SYN: *g., Arnold's auricular.*

g., parasympathetic. One of the ganglia on the cholinergic nerves of the sympathetic nervous system.

g., petrous. Ganglion located on lower margin of temporal bone's petrous portion.

g., pharyngeal. Ganglion in contact with the glossopharyngeal nerve.

g., phrenic. One of a group of ganglia joining the phrenic plexus.

g., pterygopalatine. G., sphenopalatine, q.v.

g., renal. One of a group of ganglia joining the renal plexus.

g., sacral. One of the four small ganglia located in the sacral portion of the sympathetic trunk. They lie on the anterior surface of the sacrum and are connected to the spinal nerves by gray rami.

g., Scarpa's. G., vestibular, q.v.

g., semilunar. G., trigeminal, q.v.

g., sensory. One of the ganglia of the peripheral nervous system that transmits sensory stimuli.

g., simple. Cystic tumor in a tendon sheath.

g., sphenopalatine. Ganglion associated with the great superficial petrosal nerve (branch of facial nerve) and the maxillary nerve. It transmits both sympathetic and parasympathetic fibers to the nasal mucosa, palate, pharynx, and orbit.

g., spinal. Ganglionic enlargement of spinal nerves' dorsal roots. SYN: *g., dorsal root.*

g., spiral. A long, coiled ganglion in the cochlea of the ear. It contains bipolar cells, the peripheral processes of which terminate in the organ of Corti. The central processes form the cochlear portion of the acoustic nerve and terminate in the cochlear nuclei of the medulla.

g., stellate. Ganglion formed by joining of the inferior cervical ganglion with the first thoracic sympathetic ganglion.

g., submandibular. Ganglion lying between the mylohyoideus and hyoglossus muscles and suspended from the lingual nerve by two small branches. Peripheral fibers pass to the submandibular, sublingual, lingual, and adjacent salivary glands.

g., superior mesenteric. A prevertebral ganglion of the sympathetic nervous system. It lies close to the celiac ganglion and with it forms a part of the celiac plexus. It lies close to the base of the superior mesenteric artery.

g., suprarenal. Ganglion situated in the suprarenal plexus.

g., sympathetic. One of the ganglia of the thoracolumbar (sympathetic) division of the autonomic nervous system. Includes vertebral or lateral ganglia (those forming the sympathetic trunk) and prevertebral or collateral ganglia, more peripherally located.

g., temporal. Tiny ganglion joining the anterior branches of the superior cervical ganglion.

g., terminal. Ganglion of the autonomic division of the nervous system that lies close to or within the organ innervated.

g., thoracic. One of 11 or 12 ganglia of the thoracic area of the sympathetic trunk.

g., trigeminal. Ganglion on the sensory portion of the fifth cranial nerve.

g., tympanic. An enlargement on the tympanic portion of the glossopharyngeal nerve.

g., vestibular. A bilobed ganglion located on the vestibular branch of the acoustic nerve at the base of the internal acoustic meatus. Its peripheral fibers arise in the maculae of the sacculus and utriculus and the cristae of the ampullae of the semicircular ducts.

g., Wrisberg's. Collection of autonomic nerve cells in the superficial cardiac plexus.

g., wrist. G., simple.

ganglionated. Having or consisting of ganglia.

ganglionectomy (găng″lē-ō-nĕk′tō-mē) [Gr. ganglion, knot, + ektome, excision]. Excision of a ganglion.

ganglioneuroma (găng″lē-ō-nū-rō′mă) [″ + neuron, nerve, + oma, tumor]. A neuroma containing ganglion cells.

ganglionic (găng-lē-ŏn′ĭk). Pert. to or of the nature of a ganglion.

ganglionic blockade. Blocking the transmission of stimuli in autonomic ganglia. Pharmacologically, this is done by using drugs that occupy receptor sites for acetylcholine, and by stabilizing the postsynaptic membranes against the actions of acetylcholine liberated from presynaptic nerve endings. The usual effects of drugs that cause ganglionic blockade are vasodilatation of arterioles with increased peripheral blood flow; hypotension; dilation of veins with pooling of blood in tissues, decreased venous return, and decreased cardiac output; tachycardia; mydriasis; cycloplegia; reduced tone and motility of the gastrointestinal tract with consequent constipation; urinary retention; dry mouth; and decreased sweating. Ganglionic blocking drugs are little used in treating hypertension, but are used in treating autonomic hyperreflexia, and to produce controlled hypotension during certain types of surgery. Two drugs used for ganglionic blocking are mecamylamine hydrochloride, USP; and trimethaphan camsylate, USP.

ganglionitis (găng″lē-ŏn-ī′tĭs) [″ + itis, inflammation]. Inflamed condition of a ganglion.

ganglionostomy (găng″glē-ō-nŏs′tō-mē) [″ + stoma, mouth]. Surgical incision of a simple ganglion. SEE: ganglion, simple.

ganglioplegia (găng″glē-ō-plē′jē-ă) [″ + plege, stroke]. Failure of nervous stimuli to be transmitted by a ganglion. SEE: ganglionic blockade.

ganglioplegic. Any medicine that prevents transmission of nervous impulses through sympathetic or parasympathetic ganglia. Drugs that have this action have limited therapeutic applicability because of undesired side effects. They are useful in treating hypertensive crises and to decrease blood pressure and thus limit bleeding during certain surgical procedures.

ganglioside (găng′glē-ō-sīd). A particular class of glycosphingolipid present in nerve tissue and in the spleen.

gangliosidosis (găng″glē-ō-sī-dō′sĭs) (pl. gangliosidoses). Accumulation of abnormal amounts of specific gangliosides in the nervous system. SEE: sphingolipidosis.

gangosa (găng-gō′să) [Sp. gangosa, muffled voice]. Ulceration of the nose and hard palate, regarded as a late stage of yaws.

gang rape. SEE: rape, gang.

gangrene (găng′grēn) [Gr. gangraina, an eating sore]. A necrosis, or death, of tissue, usually due to deficient or absent blood supply. SEE: necrosis.

ETIOL: Usually results from obstruction of the blood supply to an organ or tissue. May result from inflammatory processes, injury, or degenerative changes such as arteriosclerosis. It is commonly a sequela of boils, frostbite, crushing injuries, or diseases such as diabetes mellitus and Raynaud's disease. Emboli in large arteries in almost any part of the body will cause gangrene of the area distal to that point. The part that dies is known as a slough if the soft tissues are involved or a sequestrum if it is a bone that dies. The dead matter must be removed before healing can take place.

g., angioneurotic. State resulting from thrombotic arteries and veins.

g., diabetic. Condition arising in some diabetics as a result of vascular pathology.

g., dry. Condition that results when the part that dies has little blood and remains aseptic. The arteries but not the veins are obstructed. The tissues dry and drop off, the process continuing for weeks or months. SEE: *Nursing Diagnoses* in *Appendix.*

SYM: Pain in early stages. The part is cold and black and begins to atrophy. The most distal parts are generally affected first, the necrosis then spreading upward. Usually seen in arteriosclerosis associated with diabetes.

g., embolic. Gangrenous condition arising subsequent to an embolic obstruction.

g., gas. Gangrene in a wound infected by a gas bacillus, the most common etiologic agent being *Clostridium perfringens.*

TREAT: Antibiotics, clostridial antitoxin. In some cases, surgical intervention may be necessary.

g., humid. G., moist.

g., idiopathic. Gangrene of unknown etiology.

g., inflammatory. Gangrene associated with acute infections and inflammation.

g., moist. Gangrene that is wet as a result of tissue necrosis and bacterial infection.

SYM: The part is hot and red; later it is cold and bluish, commencing to slough. It spreads rapidly, and there is an offensive odor. Death may result in a few days.

g., primary. Gangrene developing in a part without previous inflammation.

g., secondary. Gangrene developing subsequent to local inflammation.

g., symmetric. Gangrene on opposite sides of the body in corresponding parts. Usually the result of vasomotor disturbances. Characteristic of Raynaud's and Buerger's disease.

g., traumatic. Gangrene resulting from extensive injuries.

gangrenous. Of the nature of gangrene.

ganoblast (găn'ō-blăst) [Gr. *ganos,* brightness, + *blastos,* cell]. The cell that forms

enamel of a tooth. SYN: *ameloblast.*

Ganser's syndrome (găn'zĕrz) [Sigbert J. M. Ganser, Ger. psychiatrist, 1853–1931]. A factitious disorder, q.v., characterized by the individual mimicking behavior he or she thinks is typical of a psychosis; e.g., provides nonsense answers and does things incorrectly. The person is not psychotic.

Gantanol. Trade name for sulfamethoxazole.

Gantrisin. Trade name for sulfisoxazole.

gantry (găn'trē) [Gr. *kanthēlios,* pack ass]. Housing for the imaging source and detectors into which the patient is placed for computerized tomography and magnetic resonance imaging.

gap [Old Norse *gap,* chasm]. An opening or a break; an interruption in continuity.

g., auscultatory. A period of silence that sometimes occurs in the determination of blood pressure by the auscultatory method. The exact cause is unknown, but it may occur in patients with hypertension or aortic stenosis. SEE: *blood pressure.*

Garamycin. Trade name for gentamicin sulfate.

Gardnerella vaginalis [Herman Gardner, U.S. physician, d. 1947]. A bacterium that may cause vaginitis in otherwise healthy women. Formerly called *Haemophilus vaginalis* or *Corynebacterium vaginale.*

Gardnerella vaginalis vaginitis. Vaginitis due to the bacterium *Gardnerella vaginalis* (formerly termed *Haemophilus vaginalis*). The bacilli are usually gram-negative but may be gram-variable in old cultures. The disease is most probably sexually transmitted. Diagnosis is best made clinically rather than microbiologically in that *Gardnerella* bacteria are often found in healthy, asymptomatic individuals. Clinically, there is a characteristic malodorous discharge, elevated vaginal pH, and wet preparation of vaginal epithelial cells that are heavily stippled with bacteria. These are called "clue cells." Mixing a 10% solution of potassium hydroxide with the vaginal secretion produces a fishy odor. SYN: *bacterial vaginosis.* SEE: *clue cells.*

TREAT: Metronidazole.

Gardner's syndrome [Eldon J. Gardner, U.S. geneticist, b. 1909]. Familial polyposis of the colon associated with a high risk of developing carcinoma of the colon. Also present are multiple osteomas and soft-tissue tumors of the skin. The condition is inherited as an autosomal dominant trait.

gargarism (găr'găr-ĭzm) [Gr. *gargarisma*]. A gargle or throat wash.

gargle [Fr. *gargouille,* throat; but may be onomatopoeia for gargle]. 1. A wash for the throat. 2. To wash out the mouth and throat by tipping the head back, allowing the fluid to accumulate in the back of the throat while agitating it by the forceful expiration of air.

gargoylism (găr′goyl-ĭsm). A condition, usually congenital, characterized by dwarfism, kyphosis, and other skeletal abnormalities, disturbances in lipoid metabolism, and usually mental deficiency. SYN: *Hurler's syndrome; lipochondrodystrophy*.

garlic [AS. *gar*, spear, + *leac*, the leek]. An edible, strongly flavored bulb of *Allium sativum* used mainly for seasoning. The chemical allicin, responsible for the smell of garlic, is not evident until the clove is cut or crushed. At that time, the precursors of allicin act to produce allicin. Garlic has antibiotic and antithrombotic actions and may reduce cardiovascular risk factors. The active ingredient in natural garlic may vary. Extracts of garlic contain very little allicin.

garment, front-opening. Any female garment that has been chosen or modified to open from the front rather than the rear to improve dressing convenience for persons with limited function.

Garré's disease (găr-āz′) [Carl Garré, Swiss surgeon, 1858–1928]. Chronic sclerosing osteitis or osteomyelitis due to pyogenic cocci.

Garren gastric bubble [Lloyd and Mary Garren, contemporary U.S. gastroenterologists]. A deflated bladder is placed in the stomach and then inflated; used to assist in treating morbid obesity by reducing the effective volume of the stomach and reducing hunger.

Gartner's duct [Hermann T. Gartner, Danish surgeon and anatomist, 1785–1827]. A small duct lying parallel to the uterine tube. It is a vestigial structure representing the persistent mesonephric duct. SYN: *duct of the epoophoron; ductus epoophori longitudinalis* [NA].

G.A.S. *general adaptation syndrome*. SEE: *stress*.

gas. One of the basic forms of matter. The molecules are free and move swiftly in all directions. Thus, a gas not only takes the shape of the containing vessel but expands and fills the vessel no matter what its volume. Among the common important gases are oxygen; nitrogen; hydrogen; helium; sewer gas, which contains carbon monoxide; carbon dioxide; the anesthetic gases; ammonia; and the poisonous war gases. Liquids and solids when heated may give off toxic fumes. SEE: *anesthesia; g.'s, war*.

 g., binary. Toxic nerve gas formed when two relatively harmless components are mixed. Devised for use in chemical warfare. SEE: *g.'s, war*.

 g.'s, blood. The principal gases found in the blood are oxygen, nitrogen, and carbon dioxide. They may be dissolved in the plasma or they may exist in loose chemical combination with other compounds, as oxygen combined with hemoglobin.

 g., Clayton. SEE: *Clayton gas*.

 g., coal. A flammable, explosive, and toxic gas produced from the distillation of coal; it is used for heating and lighting. The principal constituents are methane, carbon monoxide, and hydrogen.

 g.'s, digestive tract. Among the gases in the digestive tract are oxygen, nitrogen, hydrogen, carbon dioxide, methane; and those produced by bacterial decomposition of proteins, such as hydrogen sulfide, indole, and skatole.

 g., illuminating. A mixture of various combustible gases including hydrogen and carbon monoxide. Its poisonous effects are largely due to carbon monoxide, q.v.

 g., inert. Gas such as helium, argon, neon, or krypton, which reacts little if at all with other substances.

 g., intestinal. SEE: *flatus*.

 g., laughing. Nitrous oxide, N_2O, which has analgesic and anesthetic properties and is commonly used for minor operations and some dental procedures.

 g., lewisite. A poisonous gas that contains arsenic and has the odor of geraniums.

 SYM: Similar to those of vesicant gas but come on at once and as a rule are not so severe. Arsenic can be recovered from the serum of the blisters, and symptoms of arsenic poisoning may occur.

 TREAT: Similar to that for vesicant gas. SEE: *g., vesicant; g.'s, war*.

 g., lung irritant. Gas causing irritation of lungs, such as chlorine or phosgene. SEE: *Nursing Diagnoses in Appendix*.

 SYM: Burning sensation of the eyes, nose, and throat; bronchitis and pneumonia. Sometimes followed by pulmonary edema and probably death.

 TREAT: Remove patient from exposure and apply respirator. If the patient was exposed to phosgene (which has the odor of musty hay), symptoms may be delayed and the patient may collapse later. It is important, therefore, to provide complete rest, remove patient on a stretcher, and provide warmth. Supplemental oxygen may be required over a fairly long period. SEE: *g.'s, war*.

 g., marsh. Methane.

 g., mustard. Dichlorethyl sulfide. Poisonous gas used in warfare. SEE: *g., vesicant; g.'s, war*.

 g., nerve. Gas that acts by interfering

with or preventing transmission of nerve impulses. SEE: *g.'s, war.*

g., nose irritant. Diphenylchloroarsine, an irritant smoke.

SYM: Intense pain in the nose, throat, and air passages; sneezing followed by headache and aching in teeth and jaws; acute mental depression; and sometimes vomiting.

TREAT: The patient must be reassured that no permanent harm is done and should be warned against removing respirator in spite of the fact that the symptoms may get worse after donning it. Nasal douching with warm sodium bicarbonate solution is helpful. SEE: *g.'s, war.*

g., sewer. Gas produced by decaying matter in sewage. It is toxic, usually flammable, and explosive.

g., suffocating. Any of several war gases, such as phosgene, or diphosgene, made from chlorine compounds. It causes irritation of bronchi and lungs, resulting in pulmonary edema. SEE: *g., lung irritant; g.'s, war.*

g., tear. Gas such as bromoacetone that irritates the conjunctiva and produces a flow of tears.

TREAT: As a rule, none is necessary. When the victim is removed from the contaminated area, the symptoms tend to subside gradually. Irrigating the eyes with large amounts of clear water or physiological saline will hasten recovery.

g., toxic. Any harmful gas.

g., vesicant. A type of gas that attacks the skin in every part of the body, causing blisters. Clothing and boots become contaminated and a source of danger. Mustard and lewisite gas are examples.

SYM: Symptoms do not appear at once; may be six hours or longer before the patient is aware of anything being wrong. Pain in the eyes, lacrimation, and discharge may be the first evidence. The eyelids swell and the patient is unable to see. A diffuse redness of the skin is followed by blistering and ulceration.

TREAT: Decontamination is essential and must be thorough. Bathe eyes freely with normal saline or plain water; a drop or two of castor oil will prevent lids from sticking; no bandage should be worn. The patient should be scrubbed, if possible, under a hot or warm shower for 10 minutes. If, in spite of these precautionary measures, blisters arise, they should be treated with a mild antiseptic and a protective dressing.

PROG: Healing is very slow, but generally complete if correct treatment is promptly begun.

g., vomiting. Gas that induces emesis, specifically chloropicrin.

g.'s, war. Any chemical substances, whether solid, liquid, or vapor, used to produce poisonous gases with irritant effects. They can be classified as lacrimators, sternutators (sneeze-causing), lung irritants, vesicants, and those that act as a systemic poison such as nerve gas. Some gases have multiple effects.

Gases are known as persistent or nonpersistent, i.e., those that diffuse and are dispersed fairly rapidly and those that linger and evaporate slowly.

NURSING IMPLICATIONS: Persons rendering first aid should avoid becoming casualties by taking appropriate precautions. Be certain all of the gas masks are in working order and in good condition. Rescuers should first put on own mask, then fit masks to patients. Skin should be covered, and any exposed skin flooded with water to flush off chemical contaminant if suspected. Maintain strict discipline during gas raids to avoid panic. Thorough gas training and well-organized efforts to follow established protocols and to ascertain that everyone follows instructions for equipment use and survival techniques will prevent hysteria and panic as well as lessening the effects of the gas.

Decontamination centers are essential. Nurses must understand the vital importance of decontamination, and participate in the thorough decontamination of patients, clothing, boots, and equipment, even the ambulances used. Such decontamination should precede admitting the patient to emergency care areas, in order to prevent unaffected persons in the area from becoming casualties.

gas bacillus. Term for *Clostridium perfringens.*

gas distention. Distention resulting from abnormal gaseous accumulation in the abdominal cavity. It may be acute, chronic, local, or general, and may involve the abdominal wall, or intra-abdominal viscera in addition to the cavity. A preoperative enema may prevent gas formation. Gas can develop postoperatively as a complication of surgery. It is usually limited to the lower part of the small intestine and all of the large intestine.

TREAT: No cold fluids. Change of posture, insertion of a rectal tube. Enema only as advised by surgeon.

gaseous. Of the nature or form of gas.

gas gangrene. Gangrene, q.v., caused by *Clostridium perfringens.*

gasoline. A product of the destructive distillation of petroleum. Commercial gasolines may contain toxic additives such as tetraethyl lead or tricresyl phosphate.

Caution: The practice of using one's mouth to produce suction on a tube in order to siphon gasoline from a gas tank is dangerous because of the possibility of inhaling or swallowing this toxic substance.

---

gasoline poisoning. SYM: Giddiness; headache; intoxication; nervous disturbance; muscular tremors; difficulty in respiration; paralyses; convulsions; cyanosis; unconsciousness; pulmonary hemorrhage. Usually no local disturbance of stomach unless the gasoline has been swallowed.

F.A.: Fresh air, inhalation of oxygen and carbon dioxide; artificial respiration when necessary. Otherwise, treat symptoms. If clothing and skin have been grossly contaminated, all precautions to prevent sparks and open flames must be taken. Gasoline is highly flammable and when mixed with air is also explosive.

gasometric (găs″ō-mĕt′rĭk). Pert. to measurement of gases.

gasometry (găs-ŏm′ĕ-trē). Estimation of amount of gas present in a mixture.

gasp [Old Norse *geispa*]. To catch the breath; to inhale and exhale with quick, difficult breaths; the act of gasping.

gas pains. Abdominal pain produced by distention by gas of all or part of the intestinal tract. May be a sign of postsurgical paralytic ileus. SEE: *flatulence.*

gasserectomy (găs″ĕr-ĕk′tō-mē). Excision of the gasserian ganglion. SEE: *ganglion, gasserian.*

gaster-, gastero-, gastro- [Gr. *gaster*, belly]. Combining forms indicating stomach or the region of the stomach.

gasteralgia (găs-tĕr-ăl′jē-ă) [″ + *algos*, pain]. Gastralgia.

Gasterophilus (găs″tĕr-ŏf′ĭ-lŭs). A genus of botflies belonging to the family Oestridae, order of Diptera. The larvae infest horses.

   G. hemorrhoidalis. A species that infests horses.

   G. intestinalis. Botflies that infest the stomachs of horses.

   G. nasalis. The chin fly. Eggs are laid on shafts of hair on the lower lip and jaw of horses.

gastorrhagia (găs-tor-ā′jē-ă) [″ + *rhegnynai*, to burst forth]. Gastrorrhagia.

gastralgia (găs-trăl′jē-ă) [″ + *algos*, pain]. Pain in the stomach from any cause.

gastratrophia (găs″tră-trō′fē-ă) [″ + *atrophia*, atrophy]. Atrophy of the stomach.

gastrectasia, gastrectasis [″ + *ektasis*, dilatation]. Dilatation of the stomach. May be acute or chronic.

SYM: *Acute:* Severe, sudden pain accompanied by collapse. Small rapid pulse, temperature subnormal, upper abdominal pain resembling angina pectoris. Distended and tympanic abdomen. Vomiting of fluids and eructation of gas. *Chronic:* Vomiting of food taken several days before. Vomitus is sour and contains fatty acids, mucus, and bacteria.

ETIOL: Obstruction of pylorus; atony, overeating, omental hernia, periduodenal adhesions.

gastrectomy (găs-trĕk′tō-mē) [″ + *ektome*, excision]. Surgical removal of a part of or the whole of the stomach.

gastric (găs′trĭk) [Gr. *gaster*, stomach]. Pert. to the stomach. SEE: *digestion; stomach.*

gastric analysis. Analysis of gastric contents of the stomach to determine quality of secretion, amount of free and combined hydrochloric acid, absence or presence of blood, bile, bacteria, fatty acids. The test is particularly helpful in suspected cases of gastric bleeding, gastric carcinoma, or pernicious anemia.

gastric digestion. The phase of digestion that occurs in the stomach while food is being temporarily stored and mixed in it. The semisolid mass of food known as chyme is mixed with the salivary juices, and certain other substances are added from the stomach, including hydrochloric acid, mucus, pepsin, and some lipase.

CHEM. ASPECTS: During the meal, stimuli from the brain are carried to the stomach by way of the vagi; they result from the sensations of sight, smell, and taste. In addition, the stretching of the stomach wall stimulates the gastric glands. This causes the hormone gastrin to be discharged from the pyloric region into the blood. The circulating gastrin reaches the gastric glands and causes them to secrete.

The following changes occur in the food while in the stomach. Pepsin acts on proteins of high molecular weight, hydrolyzing them to peptones. Pepsin also coagulates milk. Hydrochloric acid is essential for the activity of pepsin. It is responsible for the antiseptic action of the gastric juice. SEE: *digestion.*

MOTOR ASPECTS: When food enters the stomach initially, there is relaxation, then the stomach increases its pressure upon the contents. The cardiac sphincter closes firmly to prevent regurgitation into the esophagus. The pyloric part of the stomach begins to exhibit wavelets of contraction that travel toward the pylorus. They become deeper, and their focus of origin shifts in the direction of the cardia. At first the pylorus, like the cardia, remains firmly closed, and the wavelets result only in physically mixing the food. Now the pylorus begins to open occasionally, allowing the acid chyme to spurt at intervals into the duodenum. The further course of the chyme is described under *digestion, duodenal.* How quickly the chyme leaves the stomach is influenced by the amount of the feeding, its osmotic character, and the amount of fat present. In general, a high-fat-content meal will leave the stomach at a slower rate than a low-fat meal.

gastric glands. Cardiac, fundic or oxyntic, and pyloric excretory glands of the stomach. These are tubular glands in the mucosa of the wall. The general result of gastric digestion is the reduction of the ingested mass to a mushy, gray mixture called acid chyme. Gastric glands contain zymogenic or peptic cells, which secrete pepsinogen, the inactive form of pepsin; parietal border or oxyntic cells, which secrete hydrochloric acid; and mucous cells found in the neck of the gland, which secrete mucin.

gastric inhibitory polypeptide. ABBR: GIP. A polypeptide in cells of the duodenum and jejunum which acts to inhibit secretion of gastric acid. SEE: *enterogastrone.*

gastric juice. The digestive juice of the gastric glands of the stomach. It is a thin colorless fluid containing pepsin, hydrochloric acid, mucin, small quantities of inorganic salts, and the intrinsic factor of the antianemic principle. It is strongly acid, having a pH of 0.9 to 1.5, its total acidity being equivalent to 10 to 50 ml of tenth-normal (10%) hydrochloric acid; free HCl is from 0 to 30 ml of tenth-normal HCl. The amount secreted in 24 hours varies greatly. The mixture of acid and pepsin has effects that neither substance has alone, and acts upon some proteins with remarkable speed. There is also a lipase present.

   DIAG: *Achlorhydria:* Pernicious anemia is the most common cause of this finding in persons who do not have gastric cancer. *Carcinoma:* Bacteria, blood, and sometimes tumor cells are present; frequently no hydrochloric acid is found. *Hyperacidity:* May indicate gastric ulcer. *Pus cells:* Indicate severe inflammation of the stomach. *Red cells:* Same significance as pus cells plus evidence of hemorrhage.

   RS: digestion; gastric analysis; hydrochloric acid; hyperchlorhydria; hypochlorhydria; stomach.

gastric lavage. Washing out of the stomach. Used to empty stomach when contents are irritating, as in prolonged postanesthetic vomiting and in some cases of regurgitant vomiting in acute intestinal obstruction. Also to clean cavity before an operation is performed upon it; to remove poison in cases in which this method of treatment is indicated; and to remove a test meal.

   NURSING IMPLICATIONS: Assess level of consciousness, and ability and willingness of patient to cooperate with therapy. Explain need for lavage, what patient may expect (procedure and sensations), and what you will expect of patient. Gather and prepare equipment: plastic or rubber large-lumen gastric tube, ice in bowl if rubber tube is used, water-soluble lubricant, disposable irrigation set with bulb syringe, and adhesive tape to secure tube after insertion, clamp, safety pin and rubber band, gloves, stethoscope, tissues, glass of water with straw, emesis basin, container for aspirant, at least 500 to 1000 ml of irrigating solution as prescribed (usually physiological saline solution), and antidote specified by Poison Control Center. Restraints may also be required, especially for child or irrational individual. Place patient in high Fowler's position if conscious and cooperative, and cover chest with bib. If patient is unconscious, position to prevent aspiration of stomach contents, and have suction available. Measure distance for tube insertion by placing tip of tube at tip of nose, extending tube to ear lobe and then to xiphoid process. Mark this location on tube, or note length of tubing that will remain outside the patient after insertion. Test for patency of nostril by having patient sniff through one nostril, then the other. Use nostril that is free of obstruction. Give patient emesis basin to hold. Lubricate tip of tubing, hyperextend patient's neck, and pass tube into nasopharynx rather than through mouth. This produces less gag reflex. Pass tube downward to enter nasopharynx. Having patient dry-swallow during this phase of passage helps prevent gagging. Do not force tube. If obstruction is met, remove tube, let patient rest, relubricate tube, and attempt again. Notify physician if tube cannot be passed without traumatizing mucosa. When tube is in nasopharynx, have patient flex neck slightly to bring head forward, closing airway and positioning throat for safe and effective swallowing. Give patient glass of water with straw (if permitted), and encourage patient to swallow tube with small sips of water (or dry-swallow if water not permitted). Rotating tube toward opposite nostril as this phase of passage begins often helps direct it toward esophagus and away from trachea. Use hand on nose to secure tube, while dominant hand steadily but gently moves tube forward and patient swallows in response to repeated commands to do so. Provide positive reinforcement and encouragement to patient throughout procedure. When tube has been passed to predetermined depth, verify placement by aspirating stomach contents with bulb syringe, or by injecting small volume (10 to 15 cc) of air while auscultating over the epigastrium for whooshing sound. Inspect back of throat for any evidence of coiled tubing, especially if patient is gagging or uncomfortable and restless. Secure tubing to nares.

Caution: Prior to attempting to instill liquids into the stomach via the tube, be certain that end of tube is in stomach and not in bronchus. If proper placement of the tube is in doubt, careful instillation of a very small amount of sterile water will help to demonstrate its location. If the tube is in the bronchus, the air will cause the water to return during expiration.

Instill desired volume of irrigation fluid as prescribed, being careful to prevent entrance of air. Instillation of a large volume of solution, 500 ml or more, may be required to distend stomach. This will expose all areas to solution. Large volume also dilutes harmful liquids and thins or liquefies other materials, decreasing their absorption rate. Monitor patient for signs of retching. If this occurs, apply suction to remove some of instilled fluid. Repeat process as necessary to cleanse and empty stomach. Instill antidote or activated charcoal slurry if appropriate and prescribed. Document procedure, including volume of irrigant instilled, and volume and character of aspirant. Send aspirant specimen to laboratory for analysis as directed. Tube may remain in place, attached to intermittent low suction as required, or be removed immediately following procedure. For removal, tube should be clamped securely, thus preventing aspiration of its contents when distal opening reaches pharynx. Untape tube and rotate tube gently to be certain it is free of mucus, then gently but steadily pull tube outward, folding it into gloved hand. Pull glove off over tube, then second glove over fist to effectively "double-bag" tube. Provide patient with tissues to wipe eyes and blow nose, and assist with oral hygiene. Provide fresh linens as necessary. Document response to procedure.

gastric ulcer. An ulcer of the stomach. SYN: *peptic ulcer.*

gastrin. A hormone secreted by the mucosa of the pyloric area of the stomach and duodenum in various species of animals, including man. The hormone is released into gastric venous blood, from which it flows into the liver and into the general circulation. When the hormone reaches the glands of the stomach, gastric acid secretion is stimulated.

Gastrin causes the lower esophageal sphincter to contract and relaxes the ileocecal sphincter. Also, it has a mild effect on small intestine motility and gallbladder motility. Gastrin is released in response to meat extracts, ethyl alcohol in about 10% concentration, and by distention of the antrum of the stomach. SEE: *Zollinger-Ellison syndrome.*

gastrinoma (găs"trĭn-ō'mă). The tumor associated with Zollinger-Ellison syndrome, q.v.

gastritis (găs-trī'tĭs) [Gr. *gaster,* stomach, + *itis,* inflammation]. Inflammation of the stomach. Characterized by epigastric pain or tenderness, nausea, vomiting, and systemic electrolyte changes if vomiting persists. The mucosa may be atrophic or hypertrophic.

ETIOL: Generally unknown. May result from infection, excessive indulgence in alcoholic beverages, or dietary indiscretions. Pain in the region of the stomach may be due to causes other than gastritis, such as cancer. Gastritis may be due to an excess or a deficiency of hydrochloric acid.

g., acute. SYM: Moderate fever; anorexia, coated tongue; intense pain in epigastrium; persistent vomiting; thirst; prostration.

TREAT: Medical therapy, including antisecretory drugs. For severe prolonged bleeding, surgery may be required. SEE: *Nursing Diagnoses* in *Appendix.*

g., atrophic. Chronic gastritis with atrophied mucosa and glands.

g., chronic. SYM: Usually asymptomatic, but one or more of the following may be present: mild nausea and anorexia; sense of distention or fullness after eating a small meal; bad taste in mouth; pain over epigastrium may be mild or acute.

TREAT: Antispasmodics, antacids, reassurance and sedatives. SEE: *Nursing Diagnoses* in *Appendix.*

g., giant hypertrophic. Gastritis with excessive proliferation of the folds of mucosa of the stomach. SYN: *Ménétrier's disease,* q.v.

g., toxic. Gastritis due to any toxic agent, including poisons, or corrosive chemicals.

gastro- [Gr. *gaster,* stomach]. Used as a combining form to denote the stomach.

gastroanastomosis (găs"trō-ăn-ăs"tō-mō'sĭs) [" + *anastomosis,* outlet]. Formation of passage between the pyloric and cardiac ends of the stomach for relief of hourglass contraction.

gastrocamera (găs"trō-kăm'ĕ-ră). A camera, small enough to be swallowed, that is used to photograph the inside of the stomach.

gastrocardiac (găs″trō-kăr′dē-ăk) [″ + *kardia*, heart]. Concerning the stomach and heart.

gastrocele (găs′trō-sēl) [″ + *kele*, hernia]. Hernia of the stomach.

gastrocnemius (găs″trŏk-nē′mē-ŭs) [″ + *kneme*, leg]. The large muscle of the posterior portion of the lower leg. It is the most superficial of the calf muscles. Plantar flexes the foot and helps to flex the knee upon the thigh.

gastrocolic (găs″trō-kŏl′ĭk) [″ + *kolon*, colon]. Pert. to the stomach and colon.

gastrocolic omentum. The greater omentum. SYN: *epiploon.*

gastrocolic reflex. Peristaltic wave in colon induced by entrance of food into fasting stomach.

gastrocolitis (găs″trō-kō-lī′tĭs) [″ + ″ + *itis*, inflammation]. Inflammation of the stomach and colon.

gastrocoloptosis (găs″trō-kŏl″ŏp-tō′sĭs) [″ + ″ + *ptosis*, dropping]. Downward prolapse of the stomach and colon.

gastrocolostomy (găs″trō-kŏl-ŏs′tō-mē) [″ + ″ + *stoma*, mouth]. Establishment of a permanent passage between the stomach and colon.

gastrocolotomy (găs″trō-kō-lŏt′ō-mē) [″ + ″ + *tome*, incision]. Incision into the stomach and colon.

gastrocolpotomy (găs″trō-kŏl-pŏt′ō-mē) [″ + *kolpos*, vagina, + *tome*, incision]. An incision through the abdominal wall into upper part of the vagina.

gastrocutaneous (găs″trō-kū-tā′nē-ŭs) [″ + L. *cutis*, skin]. Concerning the stomach and skin, or a communication between the two.

gastrodialysis (găs″trō-dī-ăl′ĭ-sĭs) [″ + *dia*, through, + *lysis*, dissolution]. Dialysis, i.e., washing out, of the stomach in order to help clear both the stomach and the blood of toxic materials that are secreted into the stomach.

gastrodidymus (găs″trō-dĭd′ĭ-mŭs) [″ + *didymos*, twin]. Congenitally deformed twins united by a common abdominal cavity.

gastrodisciasis (găs″trō-dĭs-kī′ă-sĭs). Infestation by a fluke, *Gastrodiscoides hominis.*

Gastrodiscoides (găs″trō-dĭs-koy′dēz). A genus of flukes belonging to family Gastrodiscidae, suborder Amphistomata.

   G. hominis. A species of flukes commonly infesting hogs but occasionally found in humans.

gastroduodenal (găs″trō-dū″ō-dēn′ăl) [Gr. *gaster*, stomach, + L. *duodeni*, twelve]. Rel. to the stomach and duodenum.

gastroduodenitis (găs″trō-dū-ŏd″ĕn-ī′tĭs) [″ + ″ + Gr. *itis*, inflammation]. Inflam-

mation of the stomach and duodenum.

gastroduodenoscopy (găs″trō-dū″ō-dē-nŏs′kō-pē) [″ + ″ + *skopein*, to examine]. Use of an endoscope for visual examination of the stomach and duodenum.

gastroduodenostomy (găs″trō-dū″ō-dĕn-ŏs′tō-mē) [″ + ″ + Gr. *stoma*, mouth]. Formation of an artificial opening between the stomach and duodenum.

gastrodynia (găs″trō-dĭn′ē-ă) [″ + *odyne*, pain]. Pain in the stomach. SYN: *gastralgia.*

gastroenteralgia (găs″trō-ĕn″tĕr-ăl′jē-ă) [″ + *enteron*, intestine, + *algos*, pain]. Pain in the stomach and intestines.

gastroenteric (găs″trō-ĕn-tĕr′ĭk). Pert. to the stomach and intestines or to a condition involving both.

gastroenteritis (găs″trō-ĕn-tĕr-ī′tĭs) [″ + *enteron*, intestine, + *itis*, inflammation]. Inflammation of the stomach and intestinal tract. SEE: *Nursing Diagnoses in Appendix.*

gastroenteroanastomosis (găs″trō-ĕn″tĕr-ō-ă-năs″tō-mō′sĭs). Surgically joining the stomach to the small intestine.

gastroenterocolitis (găs″trō-ĕn″tĕr-ō-kŏl-ī′tĭs) [″ + ″ + *kolon*, colon, + *itis*, inflammation]. Inflammation of the stomach, small intestine, and colon.

gastroenterocolostomy (găs″trō-ĕn″tĕr-ō-kō-lŏs′tō-mē) [″ + ″ + ″ + *stoma*, mouth]. Creation of a passage between the stomach, small intestine, and colon.

gastroenterology (găs″trō-ĕn″tĕr-ŏl′ō-jē) [″ + ″ + *logos*, word, reason]. The branch of medical science concerned with study of the physiology and pathology of the stomach, intestines, and related structures, such as the esophagus, liver, gallbladder, and pancreas.

gastroenteropathy (găs″trō-ĕn″tĕr-ŏp′ă-thē). Any disease of the gastrointestinal tract.

gastroenteroptosis (găs″trō-ĕn″tĕr-ŏp-tō′sĭs) [″ + ″ + *ptosis*, a dropping]. Prolapse of the stomach and intestines.

gastroenterostomy (găs″trō-ĕn-tĕr-ŏs′tō-mē) [″ + *enteron*, intestine, + *stoma*, mouth]. Surgical anastomosis between the stomach and small bowel. This operation is required for patients suffering from carcinoma or cicatricial stricture of the pyloric orifice of the stomach.

gastroenterotomy (găs″trō-ĕn″tĕr-ŏt′ō-mē) [″ + ″ + *tome*, incision]. Incision of the stomach and intestine through abdominal wall.

gastroepiploic (găs″trō-ĕp″ĭ-plō′ĭk) [″ + *epiploon*, omentum]. Pert. to the stomach and greater omentum.

gastroesophageal (găs″trō-ĕ-sŏf″ă-jē′ăl) [″ + *oisophagos*, esophagus]. Concerning the stomach and esophagus.

gastroesophageal reflux. Reflux of gastric contents into the esophagus. This may occur at any time when the pressure in the stomach is greater than that in the esophagus. Reflux may occur in association with obesity, pregnancy, or incompetence of the lower esophageal sphincter. This condition may cause esophagitis. The principal symptom is heartburn.

Gastroesophageal reflux occurs in runners, in whom it is usually associated with belching.

TREAT: Neutralize acid with use of antacids and H_2 antagonists. Also weight reduction if patient is obese; sleep with head of bed elevated. Avoid foods that produce symptoms and do not use anticholinergics. Surgery is rarely indicated.

g.r., chronic. Persistent reflux of the acid contents of the stomach into the lower esophageal area. The principal symptom is heartburn.

TREAT: Neutralize acid with use of antacids and H_2 antagonists. Also weight reduction if patient is obese; sleep with head of bed elevated. Avoid foods that produce symptoms and do not use anticholinergics. Surgery is rarely indicated.

gastroesophagitis (găs″trō-ē-sŏf″ă-jī′tĭs) [″ + ″ + itis, inflammation]. Inflammation of the stomach and esophagus.

gastroesophagostomy (găs″trō-ē-sŏf″ă-gŏs′tō-mē) [″ + ″ + stoma, mouth]. Formation of passage from the esophagus into the stomach.

gastrofiberscope (găs″trō-fī′bĕr-skōp). A flexible endoscope utilizing fiber optics for visual examination of the stomach.

gastrogastrostomy (găs″trō-găs-trŏs′tō-mē) [″ + gaster, stomach, + stoma, mouth]. Surgical formation of passage in persistent hourglass contraction of the stomach between the two gastric pouches. SYN: gastroanastomosis.

gastrogavage (găs″trō-gă-văzh′) [″ + Fr. gavage, cramming]. Artificial feeding through an opening into the stomach or a tube passed into the stomach.

gastrogenic (găs″trō-jĕn′ĭk) [″ + gennan, to produce]. Having its origin in the stomach.

Gastrografin. Trade name for oral diatrizoate meglumine used as contrast medium in radiographic examinations of the alimentary tract.

gastrohepatic [″ + hepar, liver]. Pert. to the stomach and liver.

gastrohepatitis (găs″trō-hĕp-ă-tī′tĭs) [″ + ″ + itis, inflammation]. Combination of gastritis and hepatitis.

gastroileac (găs-trō-ĭl′ē-ăk) [″ + L. ileum, groin]. Pert. to the stomach and ileum.

gastroileal reflex. Physiologic relaxation of ileocecal valve resulting from food in stomach.

gastroileitis (găs″trō-ĭl-ē-ī′tĭs). Inflammation of the stomach and ileum.

gastroileostomy (găs″trō-ĭl-ē-ŏs′tō-mē). Surgical anastomosis between the stomach and ileum.

gastrointestinal [″ + L. intestinalis, intestine]. Pert. to the stomach and intestine.

gastrointestinal bleeding. Bleeding from the gastrointestinal tract. It is an important sign that requires prompt therapy, and its cause must be determined.

gastrointestinal decompression. Removal of gases from the intestinal tract by use of suction through a tube inserted through the nostrils and into the digestive tract. SEE: Wangensteen tube.

gastrojejunostomy (găs-trō-jĕ-jū-nŏs′tō-mē) [″ + L. jejunum, empty, + Gr. stoma, mouth]. Surgical anastomosis between the stomach and jejunum.

gastrolienal (găs″trō-lī′ĕn-ăl) [″ + L. lien, spleen]. Concerning the stomach and spleen.

gastrolith (găs′trō-lĭth) [″ + lithos, stone]. A calculus in the stomach.

gastrolithiasis (găs″trō-lĭth-ī′ă-sĭs). Formation of calculi in the stomach.

gastrology (găs-trŏl′ō-jē) [″ + logos, word, reason]. Study of function and diseases of the stomach.

gastrolysis (găs-trŏl′ĭ-sĭs) [″ + lysis, dissolution]. Surgical breaking of adhesions between the stomach and adjoining structures.

gastromalacia (găs-trō-mă-lā′shē-ă) [″ + malakia, softening]. Softening of the stomach walls.

gastromegaly (găs″trō-mĕg′ă-lē) [″ + megas, large]. Enlargement of the stomach.

gastromycosis (găs″trō-mī-kō′sĭs) [″ + mykes, fungus, + osis, condition]. Disease of the stomach due to fungi.

gastromyotomy (găs″trō-mī-ŏt′ō-mē) [″ + mys, muscle, + tome, incision]. Incision of circular muscle fibers of the stomach.

gastromyxorrhea (găs″trō-mĭks″ō-rē′ă) [″ + myxa, mucus, + rhoia, flow]. Excessive secretion of gastric mucus.

gastropancreatitis (găs″trō-păn″krē-ă-tī′tĭs) [″ + pan, all, + kreas, flesh, + itis, inflammation]. Inflammation of the stomach and pancreas at same time.

gastroparalysis (găs″trō-păr-ăl′ĭ-sĭs) [″ + para, beyond, + lyein, to loosen]. Paralysis of the stomach.

gastropathy (găs-trŏp′ă-thē) [″ + pathos, disease, suffering]. Any disorder of the stomach.

gastropexy, gastropexis (găs′trō-pĕk″sē,

-sĭs) [" + *pexis*, fixation]. Suturing of the stomach to the abdominal walls for correction of displacement.

gastrophrenic (găs"trō-frĕn'ĭk) [" + *phren*, diaphragm]. Rel. to the stomach and diaphragm.

gastroplasty (găs'trō-plăs"tē) [" + *plassein*, to form]. Plastic surgery of the stomach. This procedure has been used in several ways to decrease the size of the stomach in order to treat morbid obesity. The success of these techniques is questionable.

gastroplegia (găs"trō-plē'jē-ă) [" + *plege*, stroke]. Paralysis of the stomach.

gastroplication (găs"trō-plĭ-kā'shŭn) [" + L. *plicare*, to fold]. Stitching the walls of the stomach to reduce dilatation.

gastroptosis (găs"trō-tō'sĭs) [" + *ptosis*, falling]. Downward displacement of the stomach. It rarely if ever causes symptoms or illness.

gastropulmonary (găs"trō-pŭl'mō-năr-ē) [" + L. *pulmo*, lung]. Concerning the stomach and lungs.

gastropylorectomy (găs"trō-pī"lor-ĕk'tō-mē) [" + *pyloros*, pylorus, + *ektome*, excision]. Excision of the stomach at pyloric end.

gastropyloric. Rel. to the stomach and pylorus.

gastroradiculitis (găs"trō-ră-dĭk"ū-lī'tĭs) [" + L. *radix*, root, + Gr. *itis*, inflammation]. Inflammation of the posterior spinal nerve roots, the sensory fibers of which supply the stomach.

gastrorrhagia (găs"trō-rā'jē-ă) [" + *rhegnynai*, to burst forth]. Hemorrhage from the stomach.

gastrorrhaphy (găs-tror'ă-fē) [" + *rhaphe*, seam, ridge]. 1. Suture of an injured stomach wall. 2. Gastroplication.

gastrorrhea (găs-trō-rē'ă) [" + *rhoia*, flow]. An excessive secretion of gastric juice.

gastrorrhexis. Rupture or tearing of the stomach.

gastroschisis (găs-trŏs'kĭ-sĭs) [" + *schisis*, a splitting]. A congenital fissure that remains open in the wall of the abdomen.

gastroscope (găs'trō-skōp) [" + *skopein*, to examine]. An endoscope for inspecting the stomach's interior.

gastroscopy (găs-trŏs'kō-pē). Examination of the stomach and abdominal cavity by use of a gastroscope.

gastrospasm (găs'trō-spăzm) [" + *spasmos*, spasm]. A spasm of the stomach.

gastrosplenic (găs"trō-splĕn'ĭk) [" + *splen*, spleen]. Of or pert. to the stomach and spleen.

gastrostaxis (găs"trō-stăk'sĭs) [" + *staxis*, trickling]. Oozing of blood from the mucosa of the stomach.

gastrostenosis (găs"trō-stĕn-ō'sĭs) [" + *stenosis*, narrowing]. Contracted state of the stomach.

   g. cardiaca. Stenosis of cardiac orifice of the stomach.

   g. pylorica. Stenosis of pylorus of the stomach.

gastrostogavage (găs-trŏs"tō-gă-văzh') [" + *stoma*, mouth, + Fr. *gaver*, to stuff]. Feeding by means of a tube leading from outside the body into the stomach through a gastric fistula. SEE: *gavage.*

gastrostolavage (găs-trŏs"tō-lă-văzh') [" + Fr. *lavage*, fr. L. *lavare*, to wash]. Irrigation of the stomach through a gastric fistula, or surgically constructed gastrostomy.

gastrostoma (găs-trŏs'tō-mă) [" + *stoma*, mouth]. A fistula of the stomach.

gastrostomy (găs-trŏs'tō-mē). Surgical creation of a gastric fistula through the abdominal wall. It is necessary in some cases of cicatricial stricture of the esophagus for the purpose of introducing food into the stomach.

   NURSING IMPLICATIONS: Keep the skin around the gastrostomy tube clean and dry, and protect the skin from excoriating gastric secretions. Prevent pulling on the tube because the incision may widen and allow spillage of gastric secretions on skin or into tissues. Before feeding, assess tube position and stomach contents. After feedings, flush the tube with water to prevent clogging. Teach the patient and family correct technique for care and feeding through the gastrostomy tube. Perform oral hygiene at least once a day. SEE: *gastrostomy feeding button.*

gastrostomy feeding button. A device inserted in the stoma of a gastrostomy. The device allows feeding to be injected into the stomach with a minimum of difficulty and stomal care. It is equipped with a one-way valve to prevent reflux of gastric contents. Patients can be instructed to clean these devices.

gastrosuccorrhea (găs"trō-sŭk"or-ē'ă) [" + L. *succus*, juice, + Gr. *rhoia*, flow]. An excessive secretion of gastric juice with increased acidity. SYN: *hypersecretion.*

gastrotherapy (găs"trō-thĕr'ă-pē) [" + *therapeia*, treatment]. Treatment of gastric diseases.

gastrothoracopagus (găs"trō-thō"ră-kŏp'ă-gŭs) [" + *thorax*, chest, + *pagos*, thing fixed]. Congenitally deformed twins joined at the stomach and thorax.

gastrotome (găs'trō-tōm) [" + *tome*, incision]. Instrument for incising stomach or abdomen.

gastrotomy (găs-trŏt'ō-mē) [" + *tome*, incision]. Gastric or abdominal incision.

gastrotonometer (găs″trō-tō-nŏm′ĕ-tĕr) [″ + *tonos*, tension, + *metron*, measure]. Instrument for measuring intragastric pressure.

gastrotropic (găs″trō-trŏp′ĭk) [″ + *tropos*, turning]. Attracted to or affecting the stomach.

gastrotympanites (găs″trō-tĭm″pă-nī′tēz) [″ + *tympanites*, distention]. Distention of the stomach by gas or air.

gastrula (găs′troo-lă) [L., little belly]. Stage in embryonic development following the blastula in which the embryo assumes a two-layered condition. The outer layer is the ectoderm or epiblast; the inner layer, the endoderm or hypoblast. The latter lines a cavity, the gastrocoele or archenteron, that opens to the outside through an opening, the blastopore.

gastrulation (găs″troo-lā′shŭn). Development of the gastrula in the embryo.

Gatch bed [Willis Dew Gatch, U.S. surgeon, 1878–1962]. A bed in which the patient can be raised and held in a half-sitting position.

gate. In computers, a term used to describe the smallest decision-making circuit (logic circuit) possible.

gate theory. The hypothesis that painful stimuli may be prevented from reaching higher levels of the central nervous system by stimulation of larger sensory nerves. This is one of the proposed explanations of the action of acupuncture.

gating. In radiology, procedure used to reduce image artifacts caused by involuntary motion.

   g., cardiac. Medical image information consistently collected during a specific phase of the cardiac cycle.

   g., respiratory. Medical image information consistently collected during a specific phase of respiration.

gatism (gă′tĭzm) [Fr. *gâter*, to spoil]. Urinary or rectal incontinence.

Gaucher, Philippe C. E. (gō-shā′). French physician, 1854–1918.

   G.'s cells. Large reticuloendothelial cells seen in Gaucher's disease, q.v. They contain a small, eccentrically placed nucleus and kerasin.

   G.'s disease. A chronic congenital disorder of lipid metabolism caused by a deficiency of the enzyme beta-glucocerebrosidase. The severe form is rare, but milder forms frequently occur, esp. in people of Jewish extraction. Fatty substances called glycosphingolipids accumulate in the reticuloendothelial cells.

   There are three clinical subtypes of the disease. Type 1 includes 99% of the cases. It is associated with enlarged liver and spleen, increased skin pigmentation, and painful bone lesions. Type 2 is characterized by neurologic symptoms including oculomotor apraxia, strabismus, and hypertonicity. These occur, usually in the first year of life, with death following within the first 18 months of life. Type 3 is similar to Type 2 but onset of symptoms is much later and the course is longer. SYN: *lipoidosis, cerebroside.*

   TREAT: Until recently, therapy was entirely symptomatic. Alglucerase, an altered form of the enzyme beta-glucocerebrosidase, may be curative. However, the annual cost of therapy with this enzyme, trade name Ceredase, may be as much as $100,000.

gauge (gāj). 1. Device for measuring size, capacity, amount, or power of an object or substance. 2. A standard of measurement.

Gaultheria Oil. Trade name for a compound that contains methyl salicylate.

Gault's reflex (gawlts). Contraction of orbicularis palpebrarum muscle to produce a blinking of the eye following a loud noise close to the ear. The reflex is tested in cases of suspected malingering to feign deafness. SEE: *malingerer.*

gauntlet (gawnt′lĕt) [Fr. *gant*, glove]. A glovelike bandage that fits the hand and fingers.

gauss (gows) [Johann Carl F. Gauss, Ger. physicist, 1777–1855]. The unit of intensity of a magnetic flux.

gaussian distribution [J. C. F. Gauss]. Normal distribution, q.v.

Gauss' sign (gows) [Carl J. Gauss, Ger. gynecologist, 1875–1957]. Unusual mobility of the uterus in the early weeks of pregnancy.

gauze (gawz) [O. Fr. *gaze*, gauze]. Thin, loosely woven muslin or similar material used for bandages and surgical sponges.

   g., absorbent. USP. Gauze made of absorbent material.

   g., antiseptic. Gauze containing an antiseptic substance.

   g., aseptic. Gauze that is sterilized. Often packaged in an aseptic container, usually paper, and ready for use.

   g., petrolatum. USP. Absorbent gauze saturated with petrolatum. It has been sterilized.

gavage (gă-văzh′) [Fr. *gaver*, to stuff]. Feeding with a stomach tube or with a tube passed through the nares, pharynx, and esophagus into the stomach. The food is in liquid or semiliquid form at room temperature. SEE: *gastrostogavage.*

Gavard's muscle (gă-vărz′) [Hyacinthe Gavard, Fr. anatomist, 1753–1802]. The oblique muscular fibers of the stomach's coat.

gay. Homosexual.

Gay's glands [Alexander H. Gay, Russian

anatomist, 1842–1907]. Large sebaceous circumanal glands.

Gay-Lussac's law (gā″lū-săks′) [Joseph L. Gay-Lussac, Fr. chemist and physicist, 1778–1850]. Law stating that if pressure remains constant, the volume of a gas will vary directly with change in the absolute temperature. SYN: *Charles' law*. SEE: *Boyle's law*.

gaze (gāz). To look or stare intently in one direction.

GB. *gallbladder.*

Gd. Chem. symb. for the element gadolinium.

Ge. Chem. symb. for the element germanium.

Gee, Samuel J. (gē). Brit. physician, 1839–1911.

 G.'s disease. Infantile nontropical sprue. Also called *Gee-Herter disease; Gee-Herter-Heubner disease.*

 G.- Thaysen disease. Adult form of nontropical sprue.

geezer. Slang term for an odd or eccentric man. Describes individuals who are usually old, have survived hardships, and are fiercely independent. Such persons may be difficult to manage when they are confronted with an illness that jeopardizes their being self-sufficient.

gegenhalten (gā″gĕn-hält′ĕn) [Ger.]. In cerebrocortical disease, involuntary resistance to passive movement.

Geigel's reflex (gī′gĕlz) [Richard Geigel, Ger. physician, 1859–1930]. Reflex in females involving a contraction of muscular fibers, adjacent to the superior portion of Poupart's ligaments, when the inner anterior aspect of the upper thigh is stroked. Corresponds to the cremasteric reflex, q.v., in males.

Geiger counter (gī′gĕr) [Hans Geiger, Ger. physicist in England, 1882–1945]. An instrument for detecting ionizing radiation.

gel (jĕl) [L. *gelare,* to congeal]. A semisolid condition of a precipitated or coagulated colloid; jelly; a jellylike colloid. It contains a large amount of water.

 g., aluminum hydroxide. USP. A white, viscous suspension of aluminum hydroxide used as an antacid.

gelasmus (jĕ-lăs′mŭs) [Gr. *gelasma,* a laugh]. 1. Spasmodic laughter of the insane. 2. Hysterical laughter.

gelate (jĕl′āt). To cause formation of a gel.

gelatin (jĕl′ă-tĭn) [L. *gelatina,* gelatin]. 1. A derived protein obtained by the hydrolysis of collagen present in the connective tissues of the skin, bones, and joints of animals.

 USES: As a food, in preparation of pharmaceuticals, and as a medium for culture of bacteria.

 2. The substance on an x-ray film in which the silver halide crystals are suspended in the radiographic emulsion.

 g., nutrient. Bacterial culture medium composed of broth and gelatin.

gelatin culture. Gelatinous base used for bacterial growth.

gelatiniferous (jĕl″ăt-ĭn-ĭf′ĕr-ŭs) [″ + *ferre,* to bear]. Producing gelatin.

gelatinize (jĕl-ăt′ĭn-īz) [L. *gelatina,* gelatin]. To convert into gelatin.

gelatinoid (jĕl-ăt′ĭn-oyd) [″ + Gr. *eidos,* form, shape]. Resembling gelatin.

gelatinolytic (jĕl-ăt″ĭn-ō-lĭt′ĭk) [″ + Gr. *lysis,* dissolution]. Dissolution or splitting up of gelatin.

gelatinous (jĕl-ăt′ĭn-ŭs). Containing or of the consistency of gelatin.

gelatin sponge, absorbable. USP. Gelatin in the form of a sterile absorbable sponge. Used as a hemostat to control oozing of blood from minute vessels. Trade name is Gelfoam.

Caution: This material may seem effective if used when blood pressure is decreased, as could be the condition during surgery, but may fail as the patient becomes normotensive.

---

gelation (jĕl-ā′shŭn). The transformation of a colloid from a sol into a gel.

Gelfoam. Trade name for absorbable gelatin sponge, which acts as a hemostat. SEE: *gelatin sponge, absorbable.*

Gellé's test (zhĕl-āz′). [Marie Ernst Gellé, Fr. physician, 1834–1923] A tuning fork is connected with a rubber tube inserted in the ear. Pressure or suction in the tube is produced by an attached bulb. If ear is normal, vibrations are felt.

gelose (jĕ′lōs) [L. *gelare,* to congeal]. 1. Gelatinous element of agar, $(C_6H_{10}O_5)_n$. 2. Bacterial culture medium.

gelosis (jĕl-ō′sĭs). A hard lump that is so firm as to appear frozen. Occurs esp. in muscle tissue.

gelotherapy (jĕl″ō-thĕr′ă-pē) [Gr. *gelos,* laughter, + *therapeia,* treatment]. Inducing hilarity in treatment of certain forms of mental illness.

gelotripsy (jĕl′ō-trĭp″sē) [L. *gelare,* to congeal, + Gr. *tripsis,* a rubbing]. The massaging away of indurated swellings.

-gels. Suffix indicating colloids in a solid state.

gemellipara (jĕm″ĕl-lĭp′ă-ră) [L. *gemelli,* twins, + *parere,* to produce]. One who has borne twins.

gemellology (gĕm″ĕl-ŏl′ō-jē) [L. *gemellus,* twin, + Gr. *logos,* study]. Study of twins.

gemellus (jĕm-ĕl′ŭs) [L., twin] (pl. *gemelli*). Either of two muscles inserted in the obturator internus tendon.

gemfibrozil (jĕm-fĭ′brō-zĭl). Drug used to alter the blood lipids in order to delay the progress or development of atherosclerosis. Trade name is Lopid.

geminate (jĕm'ĭ-nāt) [L. *geminatus,* paired]. In pairs.

gemination (jĕm-ĭ-nā'shŭn). 1. Development of two teeth or two crowns within a single root. 2. A doubling.

gemistocyte (jĕm-ĭs'tō-sīt) [Gr. *gemistos,* laden, full, + *kytos,* cell]. In the central nervous system, an astrocyte that is swollen and has an eccentric nucleus. Seen adjacent to areas of edema or infarct.

gemma (jĕm'mă) [L., bud]. 1. A small budlike reproductive structure produced by lower forms of life. 2. Any small budlike structure such as a taste bud or end-bulb.

gemmation (jĕm-mā'shŭn) [L. *gemmare,* to bud]. Cell reproduction by budding. Budlike processes or daughter cells, each containing chromatin, separate from the mother cell from which the bud is projected.

gemmule (jĕm'ūl) [L. *gemmula,* little bud]. 1. A gemma. 2. One of numerous minute processes present on the dendrites of a neuron.

-gen [Gr. *genes,* born or producing]. Combining form meaning that which produces.

gena (jē'nă) [L.]. The side of the face; cheek.

genal (jē'năl). Pert. to the cheek. SYN: *buccal.*

gender [L. *genus,* kind]. The sex of an individual, i.e., male or female.

gender identity. The sex classification of an individual. An inner sense of maleness or femaleness; influenced by culture, as opposed to sexual identity, which is biological.

g.i., mistaken. Assignment of incorrect sex to a newborn. This may lead to the individual's having a gender role opposite of the chromosomal sex.

gender role. The characteristic lifestyle and behavior pattern of a person with respect to sexual and social conditions associated with being of a particular sex. Usually this behavior represents how the individual feels about his or her own sexual preference; it may not coincide with the true chromosomal and anatomic sexual differentiation of the person.

gender testing. A test to verify the gender of persons competing as females in athletic competition. This test is done by examining the sex chromatin of the athletes.

gene (jēn) [Gr. *gennan,* to produce] (pl. *genes*). The basic unit of heredity. Each gene occupies a certain location on a chromosome. They are self-producing, ultramicroscopic structures capable under certain circumstances of giving rise to a new character, such a change being called a mutation. Hereditary traits are controlled by pairs of genes in the same position on a pair of chromosomes. These gene pairs, or alleles, may both be dominant or both be recessive in their expression of that trait. In either of those cases the individual is said to be homozygous for the trait controlled by that gene pair. If the gene pair (alleles) consists of one dominant and one recessive gene, the individual is heterozygous for the trait controlled by that gene pair. SEE: *chromosome; DNA; RNA.*

g.'s, allelic. Pairs of genes located at the same site on chromosome pairs.

g.'s, complementary. Nonallelic, independent genes neither of which will express its effect without the presence of the other.

g., dominant. Gene that will express its effect without assistance from its allele.

g., histocompatibility. Gene that controls the specificity of the antigenic response of tissues.

g., holandric. Gene located in the nonhomologous portion of the Y chromosome of males.

g., inhibiting. Gene that prevents the expression of another gene.

g., lethal. Gene that, when in a homozygous condition, brings about an effect that results in the death of an individual, usually in utero.

g., modifying. Gene that influences or alters the effect of another gene.

g., mutant. An altered gene that permanently functions in a different manner than it did prior to the alteration.

g., operator. One of certain genes believed to have a role in controlling the actions of other genes. SYN: *operon.*

g., pleiotropic. A gene that has multiple effects.

g., recessive. Gene that expresses its effect only when present in both chromosomes. Simplistically, a "double dose" is required.

g., regulator. Gene that can control some specific activity of another gene.

g., sex-linked. Gene contained within the X or Y chromosome.

g., structural. Gene that determines the structure of polypeptide chains by controlling the sequence of amino acids.

g., X-linked. Gene located on the X chromosome. The X and Y chromosomes determine sex.

genealogy. Study of the ancestry of an individual or of a group. Such investigations are of particular importance in tracing the inheritance of genetically transmitted conditions or traits. One of the most important collections of geneological information is that in the archives of the Church of Latter Day Saints, i.e., the Mormon Church, in Salt Lake City, Utah.

gene amplification. The duplication of regions of DNA to form multiple copies of a specific portion of the original region. This method of gene enhancement is important in increasing a tumor cell's resistance to cytotoxic drugs, and in allowing multiple drug resistance to a wide range of unrelated drugs after resistance to a single agent has developed.

gene map. A map of the human genome, i.e., a map of each chromosome. A project for mapping all of the genes in human chromosomes has begun. The goal is to eventually identify all of the functions of each part of the normal human chromosome. It is estimated that humans have 100,000 genes that determine the amino acid structure of proteins. Only about 1% have been mapped. SEE: *genome*.

gene probe. In molecular biology, the technique of matching a short segment of DNA or RNA with the matching sequence of bases on a chromosome. Use of this method permits identification of the precise area on a chromosome responsible for the genetic abnormality being investigated. SEE: *gene splicing*.

genera. Pl. of genus.

general adaptation syndrome. ABBR: G.A.S. Syndrome described by Hans Selye [Austrian-Canadian endocrinologist, 1907 –1982] as the total organism's nonspecific response to stress. The response occurs in the following three stages: (1) Alarm reaction, in which the body recognizes the stressor and the pituitary-adrenocortical system responds by producing the hormones essential to either flight or fight. In this stage heart rate increases, blood sugar is elevated, pupils dilate, and digestion slows. (2) Resistance or adaptive stage, in which the body begins to repair the effect of the arousal. The acute stress symptoms diminish or disappear. If, however, the stress continues, adaptation fails in its attempts to maintain the defense. (3) Exhaustion stage occurs when the body can no longer respond to the stress. As a consequence, one or several of a great variety of diseases such as emotional disturbances, cardiovascular and renal diseases, and certain types of asthma may develop. SEE: *stress*.

generalize [L. *generalis*]. 1. To become or render nonspecific. 2. To become systemic, as a local disease.

generation (jĕn″ĕr-ā′shŭn) [L. *generare*, to beget]. 1. An act of forming a new organism. 2. A group of animals or plants the same distance removed from an ancestor, as the first filial (F_1) generation. SEE: *filial generation*. 3. The average period of time between the birth of parents and the birth of their children. This could be 16 to 20 years in some cultures and 20 to 25 years in others. Also

the time would be different if only female parents were considered in computing this average unless all marriages occurred between persons of the same age. 4. The production of an electric current.

   g., alternate. A mode of reproduction in which sexual generation alternates with an asexual generation, characteristic of all plants above the division Thallophyta. It also occurs in some of the lower animals.

   g., asexual. Reproduction that occurs without the union of sexual elements or gametes, such as reproduction by fission or spore production.

   g., filial. The offspring of a given mating or cross; F_1.

   g., parental. In genetics, the generation in which a specific study is begun.

   g., sexual. Reproduction by the union of male and female cells.

generative (jĕn′ĕr-ă-tĭv). Concerned in reproduction of, or affecting, the species.

generator (gĕn′ĕr-ā″tor). That which produces something, esp. a device that produces heat, electricity, or impulses.

   g., aerosol. A device that produces minute particles from liquid materials such as medicines in solution. These may be used in inhalation therapy.

   g., electric. Device that changes mechanical energy into electrical energy.

   g., pulse. Device that produces stimuli intermittently; thus, a cardiac pacemaker requires this type of generator.

   g., x-ray. The portion of the x-ray unit which includes the high voltage transformer, the filament transformer, and the rectifiers. Used to create an electrical current appropriate for producing x-rays.

generic (jĕn-ĕr′ĭk) [L. *genus*, kind]. 1. General. 2. Pert. to a genus. 3. Distinctive.

generic drugs. Nonproprietary drugs, i.e., not protected by a trademark. In the U.S., generic drugs are required to meet the same bioequivalency test as the original brand name drugs. Manufacturers of brand name drugs produce the majority of generic drugs and allow them to be sold without the original brand name. Generic and brand name drugs may experience manufacturing defects. More than 8000 generic drugs are available in the U.S. SYN: *nonproprietary drugs*.

genesiology (jĕn-ē-zē-ŏl′ō-jē) [Gr. *genesis*, generation, birth, + *logos*, word, reason]. The science of reproduction.

genesis (jĕn′ē-sĭs). 1. Act of reproducing; generation. 2. The origin of anything.

gene splicing. In molecular biology, a portion of DNA from one gene is spliced into the DNA of another gene.

gene therapy. The replacement in the

human of a defective or malfunctioning gene by introducing a gene that does function adequately and properly. This was first done in September 1990 by use of molecular biology techniques by doctors R. Michael Blaese, W. French Anderson, and Kenneth W. Culver at the U.S. National Institutes of Health. The patient was a 4-year-old girl who lacked the ability to produce an enzyme essential to keeping immune cells alive. Deficiency of the specific enzyme adenosine deaminase (ADA) was the cause of her immunodeficiency.

Gene therapy may eventually be used to treat a variety of medical conditions caused by defective or inadequate genes.

g.t., somatic. An experimental method of cloning genes and reintroducing them into cells for the purpose of correcting inherited disease.

genetic (jĕn-ĕt'ĭk). Pert. to reproduction.

genetic burden. The impact of pathological changes, i.e., diseases and deaths, due to inherited traits or diseases.

genetic code. The information system in living cells that determines the amino acid sequence in polypeptides. By this action all of the genetic information transmitted to an offspring is specified. The code is universal in that it applies to all living things.

genetic counseling. The application of what is known about human genetics in providing advice to those concerned about the possibility of their offspring being free of hereditary abnormality.

genetic engineering. The synthesis, alteration, replacement, or repair of genetic material by synthetic means.

geneticist (jĕn-ĕt'ĭ-sĭst) [Gr. *gennan,* to produce]. One who specializes in genetics.

genetics. The study of heredity and its variation.

g., biochemical. Science of the biochemistry of genes and chemical influences on the gene.

g., clinical. Clinical investigation of the importance of genetics in health and disease.

g., molecular. Study of genetics at the molecular level, in contrast with the study of entire genes or chromosomes. SEE: *gene splicing.*

genetotrophic (jĕ-nĕt"ō-trŏf'ĭk). Concerning genetics and nutrition.

genetous (jĕ-nĕt'ŭs). Congenital.

gene transfer. Transfer of a gene from one person to another to repair an inherited defect in the recipient. This has not been done in human beings.

Geneva Convention. In 1864 the major military powers met in Geneva, Switzerland, to establish regulations concerning the status of those wounded in military action on land. The sick and wounded and all those involved in their care, including physicians, nurses, corpsmen, ambulance drivers, and chaplains, were declared to be neutral and, therefore, would not be the target of military action. These provisions were expanded in 1868 to include naval military action. Much evidence indicates that warring nations have not always abided by the provisions of the Convention.

genial (jē'nē-ăl) [Gr. *geneion,* chin]. Rel. to the chin.

genic (jĕn'ĭk) [Gr. *gennan,* to produce]. Rel. to or caused by genes.

-genic. Suffix indicating generation or production.

genicular (jĕ-nĭk'ū-lăr). Concerning the knee.

geniculate (jĕ-nĭk'ū-lāt) [L. *geniculare,* to bend the knee]. 1. Bent, like a knee. 2. Pert. to the ganglion or geniculum of the facial nerve.

geniculate otalgia. Pain transmitted from the facial nerve to the ear.

geniculocalcarine tract. Radiation, optic, q.v.

geniculum (jĕn-ĭk'ū-lŭm) [L. *geniculum,* little knee]. A structure resembling a knot, or a knee. Indicates an abrupt bend or angle in a small structure.

genion (jē'nē-ŏn) [Gr. *geneion,* chin]. Apex of the mental spine of the mandible.

genioplasty (jē'nē-ō-plăs"tē) [" + *plassein,* to form]. Plastic surgery of the chin or cheek.

genital (jĕn'ĭ-tăl) [L. *genitalis,* belonging to birth]. Pert. to the genitals.

genital herpes. SEE: *herpes genitalis.*

genitalia, genitals (jĕn-ĭ-tāl'ē-ă, jĕn'ĭ-tăls). Organs of generation; reproductive organs.

g., ambiguous. The external genitalia are not clearly distinguishable as being of either sexual form.

g., female. Organs concerned with reproduction in the female sex. The external genitalia collectively are termed the vulva or pudendum and include the mons veneris, labia majora, labia minora, clitoris, fourchet, fossa navicularis, vestibule, vestibular bulb, Skene's glands, glands of Bartholin, hymen and vaginal introitus, and perineum. The internal genitalia are the two ovaries, two fallopian tubes, uterus, and vagina. SEE: illus.

g., male. Reproductive organs of the male sex. Two bulbourethral (Cowper's) glands, two ejaculatory ducts, two glandular organs producing spermatozoa (the testes or gonads), penis with urethra, two seminal ducts (vasa deferentes or ductus deferentes), two seminal vesicles, two spermatic

FEMALE GENITAL ORGANS

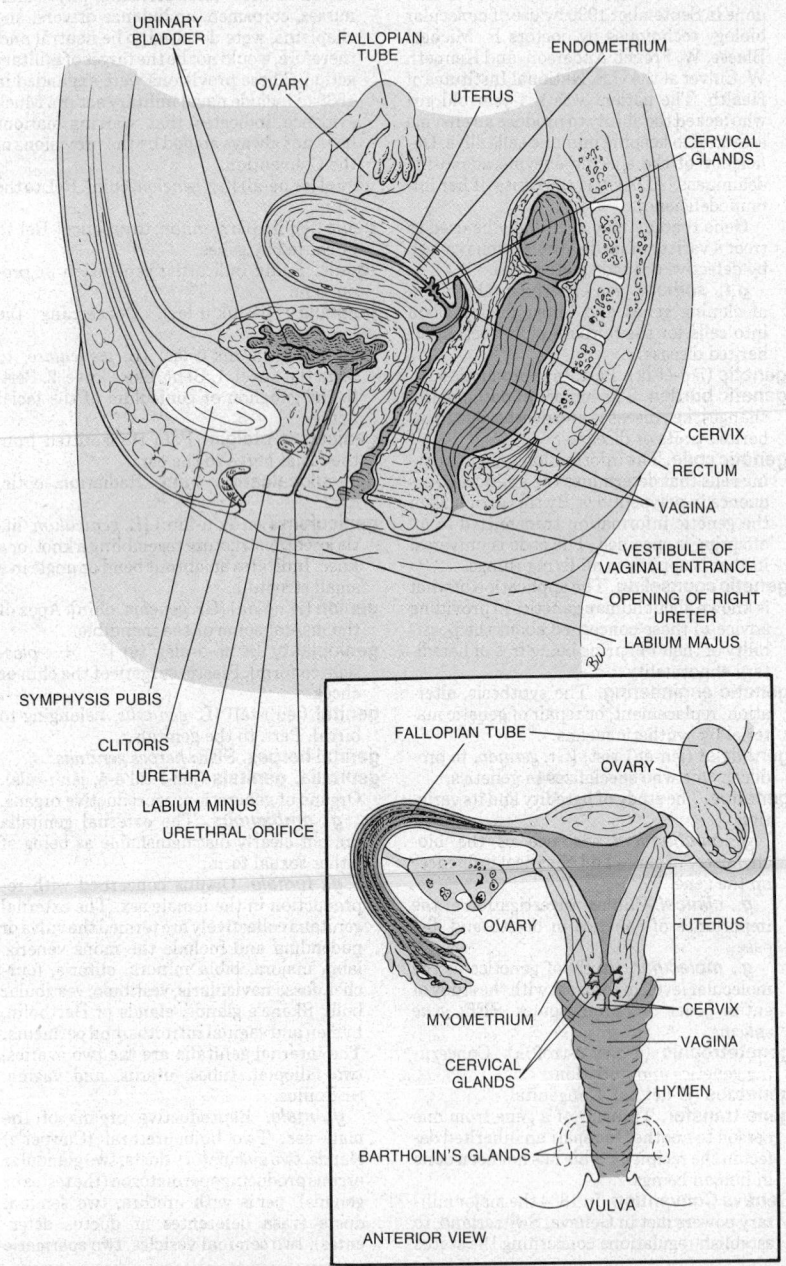

URINARY BLADDER

FALLOPIAN TUBE

OVARY

UTERUS

ENDOMETRIUM

CERVICAL GLANDS

CERVIX

RECTUM

VAGINA

VESTIBULE OF VAGINAL ENTRANCE

OPENING OF RIGHT URETER

LABIUM MAJUS

SYMPHYSIS PUBIS

CLITORIS

URETHRA

LABIUM MINUS

URETHRAL ORIFICE

FALLOPIAN TUBE

OVARY

OVARY

UTERUS

MYOMETRIUM

CERVICAL GLANDS

CERVIX

VAGINA

HYMEN

BARTHOLIN'S GLANDS

VULVA

ANTERIOR VIEW

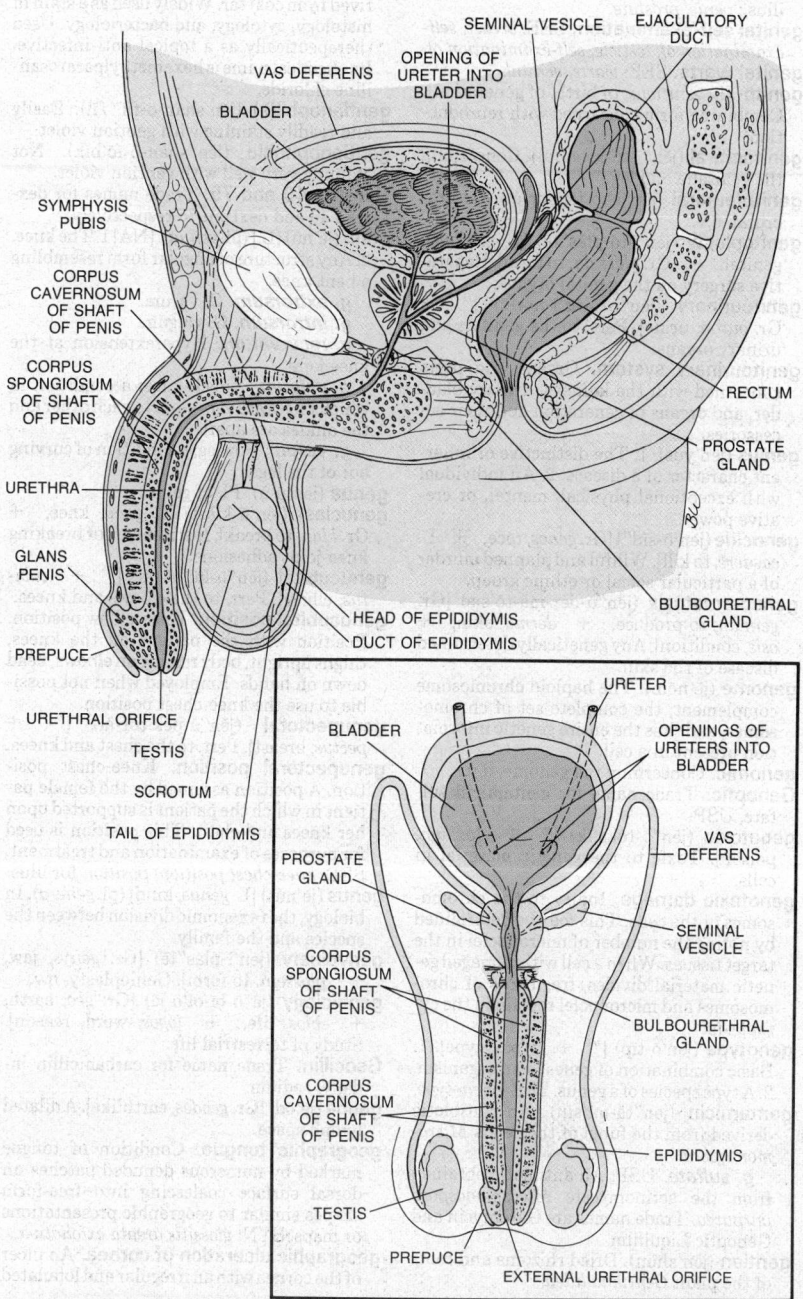

MALE GENITAL ORGANS

SEMINAL VESICLE

EJACULATORY DUCT

OPENING OF URETER INTO BLADDER

VAS DEFERENS

BLADDER

SYMPHYSIS PUBIS

CORPUS CAVERNOSUM OF SHAFT OF PENIS

CORPUS SPONGIOSUM OF SHAFT OF PENIS

URETHRA

GLANS PENIS

PREPUCE

URETHRAL ORIFICE

TESTIS

SCROTUM

TAIL OF EPIDIDYMIS

HEAD OF EPIDIDYMIS

DUCT OF EPIDIDYMIS

RECTUM

PROSTATE GLAND

BULBOURETHRAL GLAND

URETER

BLADDER

OPENINGS OF URETERS INTO BLADDER

VAS DEFERENS

SEMINAL VESICLE

PROSTATE GLAND

CORPUS SPONGIOSUM OF SHAFT OF PENIS

BULBOURETHRAL GLAND

CORPUS CAVERNOSUM OF SHAFT OF PENIS

EPIDIDYMIS

TESTIS

PREPUCE

EXTERNAL URETHRAL ORIFICE

cords, scrotum, and prostate gland. SEE: illus.; *penis; prostate.*

genital self-examination. SEE: *breast, self-examination of; testicle, self-examination of.*

genital warts. SEE: *warts, genital.*

genito- [L. *genitivus*, of birth, of generation]. Combining form concerned with reproduction.

genitocrural (jĕn″ĭ-tō-kroo′răl). Concerning the genitalia and leg.

genitofemoral (jĕn″ĭ-tō-fĕm′or-ăl). Genitocrural, q.v.

genitoplasty (jĕn″ĭ-tō-plăs″tē) [L. *genitalis*, genital, + Gr. *plassein*, to form]. Reparative surgery on the genital organs.

genitourinary (jĕn″ĭ-tō-ūr′ĭ-nār-ē) [″ + Gr. *ouron*, urine]. Pert. to the genitals and urinary organs.

genitourinary system. Organs and parts concerned with the kidneys, urinary bladder, and organs of generation and their accessories.

genius (jĕn′yŭs). 1. The distinctive or inherent character of a disease. 2. An individual with exceptional physical, mental, or creative power.

genocide (jĕn′ō-sīd″) [Gr. *genos*, race, + L. *caedere*, to kill]. Willful and planned murder of a particular social or ethnic group.

genodermatosis (jĕn″ō-dĕr-mă-tō′sĭs) [Gr. *gennan*, to produce, + *derma*, skin, + *osis*, condition]. Any genetically determined disease of the skin.

genome (jĕ′nōm). The haploid chromosome complement; the complete set of chromosomes, and thus the entire genetic information present in a cell.

genomic. Concerning the genome, q.v.

Genoptic. Trade name for gentamicin sulfate, USP.

genotoxic (jĕn″ō-tŏks′ĭk) [″ + *toxikon*, poison]. Toxic to the genetic material in cells.

genotoxic damage. Injury to the chromosomes of the cells. This may be determined by noting the number of micronuclei in the target tissues. When a cell with damaged genetic material divides, fragments of chromosomes and micronuclei remain in the cytoplasm.

genotype (jĕn′ō-tīp) [″ + *typos*, type]. 1. Basic combination of genes of an organism. 2. The species of a genus. SEE: *phenotype.*

gentamicin (jĕn″tă-mī′sĭn). An antibiotic derived from the fungi of the genus *Micromonospora.*

g. sulfate. USP. An antibiotic obtained from the actinomycete *Micromonospora purpurea.* Trade names are Garamycin and Genoptic Liquifilm.

gentian (jĕn′shŭn). Dried rhizome and roots of the plant *Gentiana lutea.*

g. violet. USP. $C_{25}H_{30}ClN_3$. A dye derived from coal tar. Widely used as a stain in histology, cytology, and bacteriology. Used therapeutically as a topical anti-infective. Its chemical name is hexamethylpararosaniline chloride.

gentianophil(e) (jĕn′shăn-ō-fĭl, fīl). Easily and readily staining with gentian violet.

gentianophobic (jĕn″shăn-ō-fō′bĭk). Not staining very well with gentian violet.

Gentran 40 and 75. Trade names for dextran 40 and dextran 75 respectively.

genu (jē′nū) [L.] (pl. *genua*). [NA] 1. The knee. 2. Any structure of angular form resembling a bent knee.

g. extrorsum. G. varum.

g. introrsum. G. valgum.

g. recurvatum. Hyperextension at the knee joint.

g. valgum. Knock-knee; a condition in which knees are very close to each other and the ankles are apart.

g. varum. Bowleg; a condition of curving out of the legs.

genua (jĕn′ū-ă). Pl. of genu.

genuclast (jĕn′ū-klăst) [L. *genu*, knee, + Gr. *klan*, to break]. Instrument for breaking knee-joint adhesions.

genucubital (jĕn″ū-kū′bĭ-tăl) [″ + *cubitus*, elbow]. Pert. to the elbows and knees.

genucubital position. Knee-elbow position. Position with the patient on the knees, thighs upright, body resting on elbows, head down on hands. Employed when not possible to use the knee-chest position.

genupectoral (jĕn″ū-pĕk′tor-ăl) [″ + *pectus*, breast]. Pert. to the chest and knees.

genupectoral position. Knee-chest position. A position assumed by the female patient in which the patient is supported upon her knees and chest. This position is used for purposes of examination and treatment. SEE: *knee-chest position; position* for illus.

genus (jē′nŭs) [L. *genus*, kind] (pl. *genera*). In biology, the taxonomic division between the species and the family.

genyplasty (jĕn′ĭ-plăs″tē) [Gr. *genys*, jaw, + *plassein*, to form]. Genioplasty, q.v.

geobiology (jē″ō-bī-ŏl′ō-jē) [Gr. *geo*, earth, + *bios*, life, + *logos*, word, reason]. Study of terrestrial life.

Geocillin. Trade name for carbenicillin indanyl sodium.

geode (jē′ōd) [Gr. *geodes*, earthlike]. A dilated lymph space.

geographic tongue. Condition of tongue marked by numerous denuded patches on dorsal surface coalescing into free-form shapes similar to geographic presentations or maps. SYN: *glossitis areata exfoliativa.*

geographic ulceration of cornea. An ulcer of the cornea with an irregular and lobulated border.

geomedicine (jē″ō-mĕd′ĭ-sĭn) [Gr. *geo*, earth, + L. *medicina*, medicine]. Study of the influence of geography and thus climate on health. SYN: *medical geography*.

Geopen. Trade name for carbenicillin disodium, USP.

geophagia, geophagism, geophagy (jē-ō-fā′jē-ă, -ŏf′ă-jĭzm, -ŏf′ă-jē) [″ + *phagein*, to eat]. A condition in which the patient eats inedible substances, as chalk, clay, or earth. SYN: *geotragia*. SEE: *pica*.

geotaxis (jē″ō-tăk′sĭs) [″ + *taxis*, arrangement]. Geotropism, q.v.

geotragia (jē″ō-trā′jē-ă) [″ + *trogein*, to chew]. Earth eating. SYN: *geophagia*.

geotrichosis (jē″ō-trĭ-kō′sĭs). Infection by the fungus *Geotrichum*, which usually attacks the lungs. Symptoms resemble those of chronic bronchitis or tuberculosis. May also infect the mouth or intestine.

Geotrichum (jē-ŏt′rĭ-kŭm). A genus of fungi belonging to the family Eremascaceae; the causative agent of geotrichosis.

geotropism (jē″ŏt′rō-pĭzm) [″ + *tropos*, a turning]. The influence of gravity on living organisms.

gephyrophobia (jē-fĭ″rō-fō′bē-ă) [Gr. *gephyra*, bridge, + *phobos*, fear]. Aversion to bodies of water, to crossing on bridges over water, or to traveling on boats.

Gerdy's fibers (zhĕr′dēz) [Pierre N. Gerdy, Fr. physician, 1797–1856]. The superficial transverse ligament of the palm.

geriatric day hospital. A form of adult day care providing rehabilitative, medical, and personal care services as well as social and recreational services for the elderly. The concept was originally developed in England. SEE: *care, respite*.

geriatrics (jĕr″ē-ăt′rĭks) [Gr. *geras*, old age, + *iatrike*, medical treatment]. Branch of medicine concerned with the problems of aging. Included are all aspects of aging, including physiological, pathological, psychological, economic, and sociological problems. The importance of geriatrics is emphasized by the fact that the expected lifespan is increasing. It is estimated that 25,000 persons in the U.S. are 100 years old or older and that by the year 2080 this number will increase to over 1,000,000. SYN: *geriatric medicine*. SEE: *age is not a diagnosis; gerontology*.

   g., dental. The special area of dentistry dealing with the problems of aging as it relates to dental treatment. Also called gerodontics, gerodontology.

Gerlach's valve (gĕr′lăks) [Joseph von Gerlach, Ger. anatomist, 1820–1896]. An inconstant valve present at the opening of the vermiform process (appendix) into the cecum.

germ [L. *germen*, sprout, fetus]. 1. A microorganism, esp. one that causes disease. 2. The first rudiment of an organism.

   g., dental. The embryonic structure that gives rise to the tooth; it consists of the enamel organ, dental papilla, and dental sac. SYN: *tooth bud*.

   g., hair. The rudimentary structure from which a hair develops. Consists of an ingrowth of epidermal cells called hair peg, which pushes into the corium.

   g., wheat. The vitamin-rich embryo of the wheat seed or kernel. It contains vitamin E, thiamine, riboflavin, and other vitamins.

germanium (jĕr-mā′nē-ŭm) [L. *Germania*, Germany]. SYMB: Ge. At. wt. 72.59; at. no. 32; sp. gr. 5.323 (25°C). A grayish-white metallic element of the silicon group.

German measles. SEE: *rubella*.

germ cell. An ovum or spermatozoon.

germ epithelium. Ridge of epithelium in the embryo from which the sexual portions of the body are derived.

germicidal (jĕrm″ĭ-sī′dăl) [L. *germen*, sprout, + *caedere*, to kill]. 1. Destructive to germs. 2. Pert. to an agent destructive to germs.

germicide (jĕr′mĭ-sīd). A substance that destroys microorganisms. Bacteria and their spores may be killed by boiling for 30 minutes, by dry heat at 160° to 170°C for one hour, and by steam at 121°C for 20 minutes. SEE: *antiseptics; disinfectant*.

germinal [L. *germen*, sprout]. Pert. to a germ or reproductive cells (egg or sperm), or to germination.

germinal center. A light area of lymphocytopoietic cells that occupies the center of lymphatic nodules of the spleen, tonsils, and lymph nodes.

germinal disk. A disk of cells on the surface of the yolk of a teloblastic egg from which the embryo develops. SYN: *blastoderm*.

germinal epithelium. 1. The epithelium that covers the surface of the genital ridge of an embryo. 2. The epithelium that covers the surface of a mature mammalian ovary.

germinal vesicle. Purkinje vesicle, q.v.

germination [L. *germinare*, to sprout]. 1. Development of an impregnated ovum into an embryo. 2. The sprouting of the spore or seed of a plant.

germinoma (jĕr″mĭ-nō′mă). Neoplasm arising from germ cells in the testis or ovary.

germ layers. Three primary cell layers in the embryo from which the organs and tissues develop. They are the ectoderm, mesoderm, and endoderm.

germ plasm. The reproductive tissues.

germ theory. Theory that certain diseases are the result of the presence of pathologic microorganisms in the body.

gero- [Gr. *geras*, old age]. Combining form relating to old age.

geroderma, gerodermia (jĕr-ō-dĕr′mă, -mē-ă) [″ + *derma*, skin]. Appearance of senility brought about by premature loss of hair, wrinkling of the skin, and general atrophy.

gerodontology (jĕr″ō-dŏn-tŏl′ō-jē). Branch of dentistry that deals with dental problems of the aged.

geromarasmus (jĕr″ō-măr-ăs′mŭs) [″ + *marasmos*, a wasting]. Emaciation that accompanies extreme old age.

geromorphism (jĕr″ō-mor′fizm) [″ + *morphe*, form, + *-ismos*, state of]. Appearance of age in youth.

Gerontological Society of America. ABBR: GSA. An organization established in 1945 for the main purpose of promoting scientific study of aging. Researchers, practitioners and educators are members. The society publishes *The Journal of Gerontology* and *The Gerontologist.*

gerontology (jĕ-rŏn-tŏl′ō-jē) [″ + *logos*, word, reason]. Scientific study of the effects of aging and of age-related diseases on the human. SEE: *geriatrics.*

gerontophilia (jĕr″ŏn-tō-fil′ē-ă) [″ + *philein*, to love]. Fondness or love for old people.

gerontophobia. Fear of aging.

gerontotherapeutics (jĕr-ŏn″tō-thĕr″ă-pū′tĭks) [″ + *therapeia*, treatment]. Therapy of the aged, the goal of which is to prevent or slow the onset of senescence.

gerontoxon (jĕ-rŏn-tŏks′ŏn) [″ + *toxon*, bow]. Degenerative circle about corneal exterior surface seen in the aged. SYN: *arcus senilis.*

Gerota's capsule (gā-rō′tăz) [Dimitru Gerota, Rumanian anatomist, 1867–1939]. The perirenal fascia.

gestagen (jĕs′tă-jĕn). That which produces progestational effects. This general term is usually applied to natural or synthetic steroid hormones used to alter reproductive physiology.

gestalt (gĕs-tawlt′) [Ger. *Gestalt*, form]. The concept that the configuration of objects and experience is present as a whole formation that cannot be analyzed by breaking it into its component parts.

   g. therapy. A form of therapy that emphasizes the treatment of the person as a whole, with a focus on the reality of the present time and place and with an emphasis on personal growth and enhanced self-awareness.

gestation (jĕs-tā′shŭn) [L. *gestare*, to bear]. In mammals, the length of time from conception to birth. The average gestation time is a species-specific trait. In humans, the average length, as calculated from the first day of the last normal menstrual period, is 280 days, with a normal range of 259 days (37 weeks) to 287 days (41 weeks). Infants born prior to the 37th week are classed as premature, and those born after the 41st week are postmature. SEE: *gestational assessment; pregnancy.*

   g., abdominal. Ectopic gestation in which the product of conception develops in the peritoneal cavity.

   g., cornual. Gestation in an ill-developed cornu of a bicornuate uterus.

   g., ectopic. Gestation in which the fetus develops outside the uterus.

   g., interstitial. Tubal gestation in which the ovum is developed in a portion of the fallopian tube that traverses the wall of the uterus.

   g., multiple. The presence of two or more embryos in the uterus. The incidence of this in the U.S. is about 1.5% of all births. Up to 40% of twin gestations are undiagnosed prior to labor and delivery. When twins are diagnosed by use of ultrasound early in the first trimester, in about half of these cases one twin will silently abort, and this may or may not be accompanied by bleeding. This has been termed the vanishing twin. The incidence of birth defects in each fetus of a twin pregnancy is twice that in singular pregnancies.

   g., ovarian. A form of ectopic gestation in the ovary.

   g., plural. Gestation in which there is more than one embryo.

   g., prolonged. Gestation prolonged beyond the usual period.

   g., secondary. Gestation in which the ovum becomes dislodged from the original seat of implantation and continues to develop in a new situation.

   g., secondary abdominal. Extrauterine gestation in which the fetus, originally situated in the oviduct or elsewhere, has developed in the abdominal cavity.

   g., tubal. Ectopic gestation in which the product of conception grows in the fallopian tube.

   g., tuboabdominal. Extrauterine gestation in which the fetal sac is formed partly of the abdominal extremity of the oviduct and partly of plastic exudation in the area.

   g., tubo-ovarian. Extrauterine gestation in which the fetal sac is made up of the ovary and the abdominal end of the fallopian tube.

   g., uterotubal. Gestation in which the ovum develops partially in the uterine end of the fallopian tube and partially within the cavity of the uterus.

gestational assessment. Determining the

prenatal age of the fetus. This information is essential for obstetric care because the decision to intervene or not and at what time will be influenced by the estimated age of the fetus. The age has been estimated by evaluating the menstrual history, time of initial detection of fetal heart tones, and date the level of the fundus reaches the umbilicus. These methods are not precise, especially if the date of the last menstrual period is either vaguely remembered or unknown.

Use of ultrasound to obtain measurements of the crown-rump length in the first trimester and biparietal diameter in the second trimester, and other measurements, have enabled obstetricians to have a more nearly precise estimate of gestational age. Even so, these techniques, because of biological variation of fetal size and early intrauterine growth failure, may not be consistently accurate. SEE: *Dubowitz tool or score.*

gestation sac. The amnion and its contents.

gestation time. The duration of a normal pregnancy for a particular species. SEE: *pregnancy* for table.

gestosis (jĕs-tō′sĭs) [L. *gestare*, to bear, + Gr. *osis*, condition]. Any disorder of pregnancy.

gesture. 1. A body movement that assists in the expression of thoughts or when emphasizing speech. SEE: *body language.* 2. An act, written or spoken, to indicate a feeling.

geumaphobia (gū″mă-fō′bē-ă) [Gr. *geuma*, taste, + *phobos*, fear]. Abnormal dislike or fear of tastes.

GFR. *glomerular filtration rate.*

GH. *growth hormone.*

Ghon's primary lesion, tubercle (gănz) [Anton Ghon, Czech. pathologist, 1866–1936]. A small, sharply defined shadow in roentgenographic film of the lung seen in certain cases of pulmonary tuberculosis in children. It is usually the primary lesion of tuberculosis in children.

ghost corpuscle. Depigmented red blood corpuscle. SYN: *phantom corpuscle.*

GH-RH. *growth hormone-releasing hormones.*

GI. *gastrointestinal.*

Giannuzzi's cells (jăn-noot′sēz) [Guiseppe Giannuzzi, It. anatomist, 1839–1876]. Crescent-shaped groups of serous cells found in the mixed salivary glands. They appear as darkly staining cells forming a caplike structure on the alveoli.

giant [Gr. *gigas*, giant]. An individual or structure much larger than normal.

giant cell. A large cell with several nuclei, appearing to be made up of many cells, but not clearly outlined. Found in both kinds of marrow, esp. in red marrow and spleen. Also found in tissues that are healing, around foreign bodies, and in the inflammatory reaction to tuberculosis. SYN: *megakaryocyte.*

giant cell tumor. 1. A tumor of bone that probably arises from connective tissue of the bone marrow. Histologically, it contains a vascular reticulum of stromal cells and multinucleated giant cells. It may or may not be malignant. 2. A yellow giant cell tumor of a tendon sheath. 3. Epulis. 4. Chondroblastoma.

giantism (jī′ăn-tĭzm). Excessive development of the size of a body or its parts. SYN: *gigantism.*

Giardia (jē-ăr′dē-ă) [Alfred Giard, Fr. biologist, 1846–1908]. A genus of protozoa possessing flagella. They inhabit the small intestine of humans and other animals, are pear-shaped, and have two nuclei and four pairs of flagella. They attach themselves to the cells of the intestinal mucosa, from which they absorb nourishment. The concentration of chlorine routinely used in treating domestic water supplies does not kill *Giardia* cysts. Boiling water inactivates *Giardia* cysts.

    G. lamblia. Species of *Giardia* found in man, to whom they are transmitted by ingestion of cysts in fecally contaminated water or food. *Giardia* are found worldwide. Formerly considered nonpathogenic, evidence indicates that they interfere with the absorption of fats. The most frequently observed symptoms of infection with *G. lamblia* are diarrhea, fever, cramps, anorexia, nausea, weakness, weight loss, abdominal distention, flatulence, greasy stools, belching, and vomiting. Onset of the symptoms begins about two weeks after exposure, and the disease may persist for up to two to three months.

    There is no known chemoprophylaxis for giardiasis, but treatment with metronidazole, tinidazole, or quinacrine is highly effective. SEE: *water, emergency preparation of safe drinking.*

    DIAG: Identification of cysts or trophozoites in feces. This is done three times before being considered negative. Duodenal contents can be examined by aspiration or string test.

giardiasis (jī″ăr-dī′ă-sĭs). Infection with the flagellate protozoan *Giardia lamblia.* SYN: *lambliasis.*

Gibbon's hydrocele (gĭb′ŏns) [Quinton V. Gibbon, U.S. surgeon, 1813–1894]. A hydrocele and large hernia combined.

gibbosity (gĭ-bŏs′ĭ-tē) [LL. *gebbosus*, humped]. 1. Condition of having a humpback. 2. A hump or gibbus, as the deformity of Pott's disease.

gibbous (gĭb′bŭs). Humped; protuberant or humpbacked.

gibbus (gĭb′ŭs) [L. *gibbosus*]. Hunchback, gibbous.

Gibney's boot, bandage (gĭb′nēz) [Virgil P. Gibney, U.S. surgeon, 1847–1927]. A basket-weave bandage made of adhesive tape, used to treat ankle sprain, or to support the ankle.

Gibson's murmur (gĭb′sŭnz) [George A. Gibson, Scot. physician, 1854–1913]. A continuous cardiac murmur that increases in systole. It is heard best at the left of the sternum in the first and second intercostal spaces. It occurs in patients with patent ductus arteriosus.

giddiness [AS. *gydig,* insane]. A lightheaded sensation. SYN: *dizziness.* SEE: *vertigo.*

Giemsa's stain (gēm′zăs) [Gustav Giemsa, Ger. chemist, 1867–1948]. A stain for blood smears. Used for differential leukocyte counts and for the detection of parasitic microorganisms.

Gifford's reflex (gĭf′fordz) [Harold Gifford, U.S. ophthalmologist, 1858–1929]. Pupillary contraction resulting from endeavoring forcibly to close eyelids that are held apart.

GIFT. *gamete intrafallopian transfer,* q.v.

giga (jĭg′ă, jī′gă). In SI units, a prefix indicating that the entity following is to be multiplied by 10^9. SEE: *Metric System* in *Appendix.*

gigantism (jī′găn-tĭzm) [Gr. *gigas,* giant, + *-ismos,* state of]. Excessive development of the body or of a part. SYN: *giantism.*

  g., acromegalic. Gigantism in which overgrowth of the bones of the hands, feet, and face is present. Due to excessive production of the pituitary growth hormone after full skeletal growth has been attained.

  g., eunuchoid. Gigantism accompanied by eunuchoid features and sexual insufficiency.

  g., normal. Gigantism in which the bodily proportions and sexual development are normal. Usually the result of hypersecretion of growth hormone.

gigantoblast (jī-găn′tō-blăst) [″ + *blastos,* germ]. A very large nucleated red corpuscle.

gigantocyte (jī-găn′tō-sīt) [″ + *kytos,* cell]. 1. A giant cell. 2. A very large erythrocyte.

gigantosoma (jī-găn″tō-sō′mă) [″ + *soma,* body]. Abnormal size of the body. SYN: *giantism; gigantism.*

Gigli's saw (jēl′yēz) [Leonardo Gigli, It. gynecologist, 1863–1908]. A wire saw originally used to cut the symphysis pubis to facilitate delivery of a fetus. Now used in removing part of the skull in craniotomy.

Gilbert's syndrome (zhēl-bārz′) [Nicolas A. Gilbert, Fr. physician, 1858–1927]. A hereditary disease due to a deficiency of the enzyme glucuronyl transferase, to excess bilirubin production, or to a hemolytic dis-

order. This benign condition causes no symptoms, but an excess of unconjugated serum bilirubin is present. The presence of jaundice may not be noticed by the patient until it is detected by a laboratory test for bilirubin. Persons with this syndrome will have an increase in serum bilirubin following two days of fasting.

Gilchrist's disease (gĭl′krĭsts) [Thomas Caspar Gilchrist, U.S. dermatologist, 1862–1927]. Blastomycosis, q.v.

Gilles de la Tourette's syndrome [Georges Gilles de la Tourette, Fr. neurologist, 1857–1904]. A rare disease of unknown etiology that begins in childhood and may continue throughout life. It is now thought to be a neurological rather than a psychiatric disease. The disease, which affects boys three times more frequently than girls, is estimated to affect 0.1 to 0.5 per thousand in the U.S. Symptoms include lack of muscle coordination, involuntary purposeless movements, tics, and incoherent grunts and barks that may represent stifled obscenities. Some victims at the time of puberty will begin to experience attacks of coprolalia and involuntary swearing. This aspect of the disease complicates social adjustment.

  TREAT: Certain drugs including haloperidol or clonidine have allowed dramatic improvement in some patients. SYN: *Tourette's syndrome.* SEE: *tic.*

Gimbernat's ligament (hĭm-bĕr-năts′) [Antonio de Gimbernat, Sp. surgeon, 1734–1790]. Pectineal portion of the inguinal ligament. Its lateral free edge forms the medial portion of the femoral ring.

ginger. A pungent, spicy material obtained from the root (rhizome) of the plant *Zingiber officinale.* It is used as a flavoring agent in medicines and in cooking.

gingiva (jĭn-jī′vă, jĭn′jī-vă) [L.]. The gum; the tissue that surrounds the necks of the teeth and covers the alveolar processes of the maxilla and mandible.

  g., alveolar. The part of the gums that covers the alveolar process of the teeth.

  g., attached. Gingiva lying between the free gingival groove and the mucogingival line. It is firmly attached by lamina propria to underlying periosteum, bone, and tooth.

  g., free. The unattached portion of the gingiva. It forms part of the wall of the fissure surrounding the anatomic crown of a tooth.

  g., labial. Gingiva covering labial surfaces of the teeth.

  g., lingual. Gingiva covering lingual surface of the teeth.

  g., marginal. The crest of the free gingiva surrounding the tooth like a collar. It is about 1 mm wide and forms the soft tissue portion of the gingival sulcus.

gingival (jĭn′jĭ-văl) [L. *gingiva*, gum]. Rel. to the gums.

gingivalgia (jĭn″jĭ-văl′jē-ă) [″ + Gr. *algos*, pain]. Pain in the gums.

gingival hypertrophy. Excess growth of gingival tissue. May be associated with prolonged therapy with phenytoin.

gingivally (jĭn′jĭ-văl″lē). Toward the gums.

gingivectomy (jĭn″jĭ-věk′tō-mē) [″ + Gr. *ektome*, excision]. Excision of diseased gum tissue in periodontal pathologies. SYN: *ulectomy.*

gingivitis (jĭn-jĭ-vī′tĭs) [″ + Gr. *itis*, inflammation]. Inflammation of the gums characterized by redness, swelling, and tendency to bleed. SYN: *ulitis.*

ETIOL: May be local due to improper dental hygiene, poorly fitting dentures or appliances, or poor occlusion. It may accompany generalized stomatitis associated with mouth and upper respiratory infections. May also occur in deficiency diseases such as scurvy, blood dyscrasias, or metallic poisoning.

 g., acute necrotizing. An ulcerative necrotizing inflammation.

TREAT: Debridement of ulceration, proper dental hygiene, rinsing of mouth with saline or suitable hydrogen peroxide solution. Avoid chemical or physical trauma to mucosa. Force fluids and provide proper nutrition. Systemic antibiotics are usually not required. SYN: *trench mouth.*

 g., expulsive. Osteoperiostitis of a tooth in which the tooth is expelled from its socket.

 g., gravidum. Gingivitis of pregnancy. Characterized by generalized hypertrophy of the gums that may progress to the state of tumor formation.

 g., hyperplastic. Gingivitis associated with overgrowth of the gingiva. May be caused by dental plaque or due to prolonged use of phenytoin.

 g., interstitial. Inflammation of the gums and alveolar processes that precedes pyorrhea.

 g., necrotizing ulcerative. ABBR: NUG. An acute gingivitis characterized by ulceration and necrosis of the gingival margin and interdental papillae. SYN: *Vincent's angina; trench mouth.*

 g., phagedenic. A rapidly spreading ulceration of the gums accompanied by extensive ulceration and sloughing of tissue.

 g., Vincent's. G., acute necrotizing, q.v.

gingivoglossitis (jĭn″jĭ-vō-glŏs-sī′tĭs) [″ + Gr. *glossa*, tongue, + *itis*, inflammation]. Inflammation of the gums and tongue. SYN: *stomatitis.*

gingivolabial (jĭn″jĭ-vō-lā′bē-ăl). Concerning the gums and lips.

gingivoplasty (jĭn′jĭ-vō-plăs″tē) [″ + Gr. *plassein*, to form]. Surgical correction of the gingival margin.

gingivostomatitis (jĭn″jĭ-vō-stō″mă-tī′tĭs) [″ + Gr. *stoma*, mouth, + *itis*, inflammation]. Inflammation of the gingival tissue and the mucosa of the mouth.

 g., acute necrotizing ulcerative. ABBR: ANUG. Severe stomatitis with ulceration and necrosis of the oral mucosa and the gingival tissue. SYN: *trench mouth.*

 g., herpetic. Inflammation of the gingival tissue and oral mucosa due to infection with herpes simplex virus.

ginglyform (jĭng′lĭ-form) [Gr. *ginglymos*, hinge, + L. *forma*, shape]. In the form of a hinged joint. SYN: *ginglymoid.*

ginglymoarthrodial (jĭng″lĭ-mō-ăr-thrō′dē-ăl) [″ + *arthrodia*, gliding joint]. Pert. to a joint that is both hinged and arthrodial. SEE: *arthrodia.*

ginglymoid (jĭng′lĭ-moyd) [″ + *eidos*, form, shape]. Pert. to or shaped like a hinged joint.

ginglymus (jĭng′lĭ-mŭs) [Gr. *ginglymos*, hinge]. A hinge joint; diarthrosis. SEE: *joint.*

ginseng (jĭn′sĕng) [Chinese *jen-shen*, man, man image]. The root of the Chinese or American ginseng. Species of Asiatic ginseng are different from those in North America. It is used therapeutically by some cultures as an aphrodisiac or stimulant. The medical evidence to support such use is controversial.

Giraldés′ organ (hĭr-ăl-dās′) [Joachim A. C. C. Giraldés, Portuguese surgeon in Paris, 1808–1875]. A vestige of the wolffian body at posterior side of the testicle. SYN: *paradidymis.*

girdle (AS. *gyrdel*, girdle]. 1. A zone or belt; cingulum, the waist. 2. A structure that resembles a circular belt or band.

 g., pelvic. The portion of the lower extremities to which the lower limbs are attached. Composed of the two innominate or hip bones.

 g., shoulder. The portion of the upper extremities to which the upper limbs are attached. Composed of the two clavicles and two scapulae.

girdle pain. Zonesthesia, q.v.

girdle symptom. A symptom in tabes as of a tight girdle, such as a feeling of constriction about the chest; also found in compression of the cord due to collapse of the vertebrae as in Pott's disease.

Gitaligin. Trade name for gitalin.

gitalin (jĭt′ă-lĭn). A cardiac glycoside extracted from digitalis. Trade name is Gitaligin.

gitter cell. A honeycombed cell packed with a number of lipoid granules. SYN: *microglia*, q.v.

giving-up. The state, in either a patient or those providing care, of feeling the situation, condition, or illness is one in which the course and prognosis are inevitably dismal. It leads to the feeling of complete hopelessness and despair. Obviously the act of giving up is inappropriate in any situation but particularly when the diagnosis may be incorrect. SEE: *grief reaction; helplessness; hopelessness.*

gizzard (gĭz′ărd). The very strong muscular stomach of certain birds. Food is mixed with gastric juice and macerated with the aid of small stones, called grit, that are ingested and remain in the gizzard.

glabella [L. *glaber*, smooth]. The smooth surface of the frontal bone lying between the superciliary arches; the portion directly above the root of the nose.

glabrate, glabrous [L. *glaber*, smooth]. 1. Bald. 2. Smooth.

glacial (glā′shăl) [L. *glacialis*, icy]. Glassy; resembling ice.

gladiate (glā′dē-āt) [L. *gladius*, sword]. Sword-shaped. SYN: *ensiform; xiphoid.*

glairy. Viscous; albuminous; mucoid.

gland [L. *glans*, acorn]. 1. A secretory organ or structure. 2. A cell or a group of cells that can manufacture a secretion discharged and used in some other part of the body.

On the basis of complexity of structure, glands may be simple (consisting of one or a few secreting units) or compound (consisting of many secreting units whose secretions leave the gland by a common duct). Simple tubular glands may be straight, coiled, or branched. Glands consisting of one cell are called unicellular; those of more than one cell, multicellular.

On the basis of their secretion, glands are mucous (those producing a viscous slimy secretion); serous (those producing a clear watery secretion); or mixed (those producing both).

On the basis of the presence or absence of ducts, glands are exocrine (those that possess ducts that carry the secretions to an epithelial surface) and endocrine (those without ducts and whose secretions enter the blood or lymph). The latter are gonads or sex glands and pineal, pituitary, thyroid, parathyroid, thymus, and adrenal glands.

On the basis of the shape of the secreting units, glands are tubular (secreting portion elongated with a narrow lumen) or saccular (secreting portion in the form of a sac or flask). If the lumen of the secreting portion is wide, it is termed an alveolus; if narrow, an acinus. Glands composed of these types of units are termed alveolar and acinar respectively.

On the basis of the manner by which secretion is accomplished, glands are merocrine (secretion forms within cells and is passed through cell membranes into excretory ducts); apocrine (secretion forms in apical ends of cells, which break off and form a part of the secretion) such as the mammary gland; and holocrine (entire cell with its contents is extruded as the secretion) such as sebaceous glands. SEE: *cell* for illus.

g., accessory. A small gland functioning as an accessory to another gland of similar structure some distance removed.

g., acinotubular. Gland structurally midway between an acinous and a tubular gland.

g., acinous. Gland whose secreting units are composed of saclike structures, each possessing a narrow lumen.

g., adrenal. An endocrine gland lying above each kidney.

g.'s, aggregate. Lymphatic glands in patch formation found mainly in ileum. SYN: *Peyer's patches.*

g.'s, albuminous. Digestive tract glands secreting a fluid containing albumin.

g.'s, anal. Glands in the region of the anus.

g., apocrine. Gland whose cells lose some of their cytoplasmic contents in the formation of secretion. Examples include the mammary glands and some sweat glands. SEE: *eccrine sweat glands.*

g.'s, areolar. Large sebaceous and rudimentary milk glands present in the areola surrounding the nipple of the female breast. SYN: *Montgomery's glands.*

g.'s, auricular. External otic lymph nodes.

g.'s, axillary. Axillary lymph nodes.

g.'s, Bartholin's. Numerous glands that open into the vestibule of the vagina. Homologous to bulbourethral glands of the male.

g.'s, Blandin's. Tiny racemose glands that secrete mucus and saliva. Located near the tip of the undersurface of the tongue.

g.'s, Bowman's. Simple branched tubular glands present in the olfactory mucosa of the nasal cavity.

g.'s, brachial. Lymph glands in the arm and forearm.

g.'s, bronchial. Mixed glands lying in the submucosa of the bronchi and bronchial tubes.

g.'s, Bruch's. Conjunctival lymph nodes in lower lids.

g.'s, Brunner's. Glands in the duodenal submucosa secreting intestinal juice.

g.'s, buccal. Acinous glands in the cheek tissue.

g., bulbourethral. One of two small glands above the bulb of corpus spongiosum, whose secretion forms part of seminal fluid. SYN: *Cowper's glands.*

g.'s, cardiac. Glands of the stomach near the cardiac orifice of the esophagus.

g., carotid. Tiny gland at bifurcation of the common carotid artery. SYN: *carotid body.*

g.'s, celiac. Several lymph nodes anterior to the abdominal aorta.

g.'s, ceruminous. Glands in the external auditory canal that excrete cerumen.

g.'s, cervical. Lymph glands situated in the neck.

g.'s, ciliary. G.'s, Moll's.

g.'s, circumanal. G.'s, anal.

g.'s, Cobelli's. Glands in the esophageal mucosa.

g., coccygeal. G., Luschka's.

g., compound. Gland consisting of a number of branching duct systems that open into the main excretory duct.

g., compound tubular. Gland composed of numerous minute tubules leading to a lone duct.

g., conglobate. G., lymph.

g., Cowper's. G., bulbourethral.

g.'s, cutaneous. Glands of the skin, esp. the sebaceous and sudoriferous glands. Includes modified forms such as the ciliary, ceruminous, anal, preputial, areolar, and meibomian glands.

g., cytogenic. A gland that produces living cells, such as the testis or ovary.

g., ductless. A gland that lacks an excretory duct. SEE: *endocrine gland.*

g.'s, duodenal. G.'s, Brunner's.

g.'s, Ebner's. Serous glands of the tongue located in the region of the vallate papillae, their ducts opening into the furrows surrounding the papillae.

g., eccrine. A simple sweat gland of the skin. SEE: *eccrine sweat glands; g., apocrine.*

g., endocrine. An organ or structure that secretes a hormone that is absorbed into the blood or lymph; a ductless gland. Principal endocrine glands are the pituitary, ovary, adrenals, pancreas, placenta, thyroid, and testes, q.v. SEE: *endocrine gland.*

g.'s, female. Bartholin's, nabothian, Skene's, uterine, and mammary glands; the ovaries and glans clitoridis.

g.'s, Fraenkel's. Tiny glands located below the margin of the vocal cords.

g.'s, fundic. Glands of the body and fundus of the stomach; gastric glands, which secrete gastric juice.

g., gastric. Any one of three different types of glands in the mucosa of the stom-

ach: cardiac in the superior area; oxyntic in the fundus; and pyloric in the distal portion.

g.'s, Gay's. Multiple sweat glands developed to a great extent in the perianal area.

g., genal. Gland in buccal submucosa.

g.'s, genital. Ovaries in female and testes in male.

g.'s, hair. Sebaceous glands opening into each hair follicle.

g.'s, haversian. Glands that secrete synovial fluid.

g.'s, hematopoietic. Glands that participate in blood production.

g.'s, hemolymph. Modified glands that contain blood and lymph sinuses and probably participate in the formation of leukocytes and the destruction of red blood corpuscles.

g.'s, hepatic. Lymph nodes located in front of the portal vein.

g., holocrine. SEE: *holocrine.*

g.'s, inguinal. Lymph nodes in the inguinal region.

g., interscapular. Embryonic lymphatic tissue.

g., interstitial. Gland in connective tissue of seminiferous tubules of testes that produces internal secretions. SYN: *Leydig's cells.*

g.'s, intestinal. Simple or branched tubular glands of the intestine that secrete the succus entericus. Include Brunner's glands and crypts of Lieberkühn.

g.'s, jugular. G.'s, cervical.

g.'s, Krause's. Small glands in the conjunctiva of the eyelids.

g.'s, labial. Multiple acinous glands between the mucosa of the lips and the opening on the inner lip.

g., lacrimal. A compound tubuloalveolar gland, located in the roof of the orbit, that secretes tears.

g.'s, lactiferous. G., mammary.

g.'s, Lieberkühn's. Tiny tubular glands on the intestinal mucosa.

g.'s, lingual. Glands of the tongue; includes the anterior lingual glands (glands of Nuhn), posterior lingual glands (glands of von Ebner), and mucous glands at the root of the tongue.

g.'s, Littré's. Tiny mucous glands in the urethral mucosa in the cavernous portion.

g.'s, lumbar. Lymphatics located behind the peritoneal region and the lower section of the diaphragmatic posterior part.

g., Luschka's. Gland located near the coccygeal tip.

g., lymph; g., lymphatic. Nodule of lymphatic tissue, found along the path of a lymphatic vessel.

g., mammary. A compound alveolar gland that secretes milk. In the human female, these glands are made up of lobes and lobules bound together by areolar tissue. The main ducts number 15 to 20 and are known as lactiferous ducts, each one discharging through a separate orifice on the surface of the nipple. The dilatations of the ducts form reservoirs for the milk during lactation, q.v. The pink or dark-colored skin around the nipple is called the areola, q.v.

g.'s, meibomian. G.'s, tarsal.

g., merocrine. Gland in which the cells remain intact in the process of the elaboration and discharge of their secretion. SEE: *eccrine sweat glands.*

g., Méry's. G., bulbourethral.

g., mixed. 1. Gland that has both endocrine and exocrine function. An example is the pancreas. 2. Salivary glands that secrete both mucous and serous secretion, often with both cell types in the same acinus. SEE: *submandibular gland.*

g.'s, Moll's. Modified sweat glands in the eyelid.

g.'s, Montgomery's. G.'s, areolar.

g.'s, Morgagni's. G.'s, Littré's.

g.'s, muciparous. Glands that secrete mucus.

g.'s, nabothian. Dilated mucous glands in the uterine cervix.

g.'s, odoriferous. Glands exuding odoriferous materials, as those around the prepuce or anus.

g.'s of Zeis. Large sebaceous glands found in the eyelids associated with the follicles of the eyelashes.

g.'s, olfactory. Glands in the olfactory mucous membranes.

g.'s, oxyntic. Gastric glands usually found in the abdominal cardiac region.

g.'s, palatine. Mucous glands in the tissue of the palate.

g.'s, palpebral. G.'s, tarsal.

g.'s, parathyroid. One of the several small endocrine glands about 6 mm long by 3 to 4 mm broad on the back of, and at lower edge of the thyroid gland, or embedded within its substance. These glands secrete parathyroid hormone, which regulates calcium and phosphorus metabolism.

g.'s, paraurethral. Small rudimentary glands that open on either side of the posterior portion of the urethral orifice in the female. SYN: *g.'s, Skene's.*

g., parotid. Largest salivary gland, located in front of the ear. It is a compound tubuloacinous serous gland.

g., peptic. G., gastric, q.v.

g.'s, Peyer's. G.'s, aggregate.

g., pineal. Tiny glandular body of conical shape located between two superior quadrigeminal bodies. Connected with the thalamus but not a part of the brain.

g., pituitary. A small, gray, rounded body attached to the base of the brain by the infundibular stalk, a downward extension of the floor of the third ventricle. It averages $1.3 \times 1.0 \times 0.5$ cm in size and about 0.6 gm in weight. SYN: *hypophysis.*

g.'s, preputial. G.'s, Tyson's.

g., prostate. In the male, a gland that surrounds the neck of the bladder and the urethra. It is partly glandular, with ducts opening into the prostatic portion of the urethra, and partly muscular. It secretes a thin, opalescent, slightly alkaline fluid that forms part of semen. Consists of a median lobe and two lateral lobes. About $2 \times 4 \times 3$ cm and weighing about 20 gm, it is enclosed in a fibrous capsule containing smooth muscle fiber in its inner layer. Muscular fibers separate glandular tissue and encircle the urethra.

g.'s, pyloric. Gastric glands near the pylorus that secrete gastric juice.

g., racemose. G., acinous.

g., Rivinus. G., sublingual.

g., saccular. G., acinous.

g., salivary. One of the three salivary glands of the mouth: parotid, sublingual, and submandibular.

g., sebaceous. A simple or branched alveolar gland that secretes sebum. They are found in the skin. Their ducts usually open into hair follicles.

g., sentinel. An enlarged lymph gland due to a pathological process in the area drained by the lymph channels leading to that gland.

g., seromucous. A mixed serous and mucous gland.

g.'s, serous. G.'s, albuminous.

g., sex. The ovary or testis.

g.'s, Skene's. Glands lying just inside of and on the posterior aspect of the urethra in the female. When the margins of the urethra are drawn apart and the mucous membrane is gently everted, the two small openings of Skene's glands, one on each side of the floor of the urethra, become visible. Trauma frequently causes a gaping of the urethra, exposing the glands; and in acute gonorrhea, they are almost always infected.

g.'s, solitary. G.'s, intestinal.

g., sublingual. The smallest of the salivary glands of the mouth. SYN: *Rivinus gland.*

g., submandibular. The mixed serous-mucous salivary glands that lie below the mandible.

g.'s, sudoriferous. Glands, situated in the skin, that secrete perspiration. SYN: *sweat glands.*

g., suprarenal. G., adrenal.

g.'s, sweat. G.'s, sudoriferous. SEE:

sweat glands for illus.

g.'s, synovial. Glands that secrete synovial fluid. SYN: *g.'s, haversian.*

g., target. Any gland affected by the action or secretion of another gland, e.g., the thyroid is a target gland of the pituitary.

g.'s, tarsal. Glands situated in the eyelid. They secrete sebaceous substance that keeps the lids from adhering to each other. SYN: *meibomian gland.*

g., thymus. The thymus body or thymus, q.v.

g., thyroid. A ductless gland located in the base of the neck on both sides of the lower part of the larynx and upper part of the trachea. It consists of two lateral lobes connected by an isthmus. Sometimes a third medial or pyramidal lobe extends upward from the isthmus. Histologically it consists of a large number of closed vesicles, called follicles, that contain the thyroglobulin, which in turn contains various active substances such as thyroxine. The thyroid gland is enlarged in goiter, and it may appear to pulsate due to the increased blood supply.

g.'s, tracheal. Acinous glands of the tracheal mucosa.

g., tubular. Gland whose terminal secreting portions are narrow tubes.

g.'s, Tyson's. Tiny sebaceous glands found on the inner surface of the prepuce and on the glans of the penis.

g., unicellular. Mucus-secreting cells present in columnar or pseudostratified columnar epithelial tissue layers. Also called goblet cells.

g.'s, urethral. G.'s, Littré's.

g.'s, vaginal. Acinous glands in the vaginal mucosa. They are found only in the uppermost portion near the cervix. The major portion of the vaginal mucosa is devoid of glands.

g.'s, vestibular. Glands of the vaginal vestibule. They include the minor vestibular glands and the major vestibular glands (Bartholin's gland).

g.'s, vulvovaginal. G.'s, Bartholin's.

g.'s, Waldeyer's. Glands in the eyelid.

g.'s, Weber's. Glands in the tongue mucosa.

g., Zuckerkandl's. Tiny yellowish lobe occasionally seen between geniohyoid muscles. An accessory thyroid gland.

gland, words pert. to: "aden-" words; "adreno-" words; endocrine; holocrine; name of each gland; seborrhea; "sial-" words.

glanders (glăn′dĕrz). Contagious infection caused by *Pseudomonas mallei* in horses, donkeys, and mules. It is communicable to humans, but no cases have occured in the Western Hemisphere since 1938.

SYM: Fever, inflammation of the skin and mucous membranes, esp. those of the nasal cavity, with formation of ulcers and abscesses. Small subcutaneous nodules develop, which break down, giving rise to ulcers. Beginning as small areas, these tend to spread and coalesce and finally involve large areas that exude a viscid, mucopurulent discharge with a foul odor. May occur in acute or chronic form. In the acute septicemic form, prognosis is grave. It is almost ˙ variably fatal.

TREAT: Experience with the disea limited but sulfadiazine is the reco mended therapy.

glandilemma (glăn″dĭ-lĕm′ă) [L. *glans,* acorn, + Gr. *lemma,* sheath]. The outer covering or capsule of a gland.

glandula (glăn′dū-lă) (pl. *glandulae*). A small gland. SYN: *glandule.*

glandular [L. *glandula,* little acorn]. Pert. to or of the nature of a gland.

glandular therapy. Treatment of disease with endocrine glands or their extracts. SYN: *organotherapy.*

glandule (glăn′dūl). A small gland. SYN: *glandula.*

glans [L. *glans,* acorn] (pl. *glandes*). A gland.

g. clitoridis. [NA] The head of the clitoris. SEE: *clitoris.*

g. penis. [NA] Bulbous end of the penis. SEE: *penis.*

Glanzmann's thrombasthenia (glänz′mänz) [Edward Glanzmann, Swiss pediatrician, 1887–1959]. A rare congenital abnormality of blood platelets, characterized by easy bruising and epistaxis that sometimes requires blood transfusions. Bleeding is prolonged, clot retraction is diminished, and platelets do not aggregate during blood coagulation or after addition of ADP (adenosine diphosphate). The only therapy is platelet transfusions.

glare [ME. *glaren,* to gleam]. A condition causing temporary blurring of vision with possible permanent injury to retina. Caused by intense light (visible radiation) emanating from highly reflecting objects such as sunlight reflected from water or snow or projected by automobile headlight or by a therapeutic light. SEE: *dazzle.*

glaserian artery (glā-sē′rē-ăn) [Johann Heinrich Glaser, Swiss anatomist, 1629–1679]. A branch of the internal maxillary artery, it supplies the tympanum. SYN: *tympanic artery.*

glaserian fissure. A narrow slit posterior to the mandibular fossa of the temporal bone. The chorda tympani nerve passes through it. SYN: *petrotympanic fissure.*

Glasgow Coma Scale. A scale for evaluating

and quantitating the degree of coma by determining the best motor, verbal, and eye-opening response to standardized stimuli. Coma is diagnosed by absence of motor and verbal response and eye opening. A score of 7 or less is classed as coma when this scale is used. A score of 9 or greater excludes the diagnosis of coma. SEE: *coma; Trauma Score.*

glass [AS. *glaes*]. A hard, brittle, amorphous, transparent material composed of silica and various bases.

    g., leaded. Safety glass that contains lead. Used in radiology to help protect technicians from x-rays.

    g., photochromic. Glass that is manufactured clear and uncolored until light strikes it. When used in sunglasses, the lens becomes dark and reduces the amount of light transmitted, becoming clear again when no longer exposed to bright light.

    g., polarized. A medium that permits the exiting light waves to vibrate in only one direction.

    g., safety. A type of laminated glass that meets specific requirements concerning the force necessary to break it and is so designed that it breaks without shattering. Its use in automobiles reduces the risk of injury involving broken glass.

    g., tempered. Glass that has been treated with heat so that the force required to break it is increased in comparison with ordinary glass.

    g., ultraviolet transmitting. Glass designed to admit ultraviolet radiation through it. The glass is designed to transmit about half of the solar radiation, between the wavelengths of 290 and 320 nanometers.

    g., watch. Shallow, saucer-like glass dish, resembling the glass cover widely used to cover the face of a large pocket watch.

glasses [AS. *glaes*, glass]. 1. Transparent refractive device worn to correct refraction errors in the patient's eyes. 2. Device worn to protect eyes from glare or particles in the air.

    g., bifocal. Glasses in which the refracting power of the lower portion differs from that in the upper portion, the lower portion being used for viewing near objects or reading, the upper portion for distant objects. SYN: *Franklin glasses.*

    g., safety. Glasses using heat-treated glass or impact-resistant plastic lenses. Their use serves to protect the eyes from dangerous slivers of glass that are produced when ordinary lenses are broken in an accident. Use of glass of this kind in manufacturing lenses for eyeglasses is mandatory in the U.S.

    g., sun-. Glasses with tinted lenses for decreasing the intensity of light seen through them. SEE: *sunglasses.*

    g., trifocal. Glasses with three different corrections in each lens: one each for near, intermediate, and far vision.

glassy. Hyaline; vitreous. Descriptive term to indicate a tissue that looks like glass and is smooth and shiny.

Glauber's salt (glō′bĕrz) [Johann Rudolf Glauber, Dutch physician, 1604–1668]. Sodium sulfate.

glaucoma (glaw-kō′mă) [L., cataract]. A group of eye diseases characterized by increase in intraocular pressure, which results in atrophy of the optic nerve and may result in blindness. There are three major categories of glaucoma: angle closure glaucoma, that comes on in persons whose eyes are anatomically predisposed to develop the condition; open angle glaucoma in which the angle that permits the drainage of aqueous humor from the eye appears to be normal but does not function adequately; and congenital, in which the intraocular pressure is increased, but why this occurs is not known. The increased pressure causes the globe of the eye to be enlarged; a condition known as buphthalmia, q.v. The acute type of glaucoma is attended by acute pain. The chronic type has an insidious onset. Normal tonometer reading is 13 to 22. An early sign of glaucoma is subjective complaint that lights appear to have halos around them.

    ETIOL: Failure of removal, i.e., drainage, of aqueous humor from the eye at a rate to keep up with its production in the anterior chamber. Thus, narrowing or closure of the filtration angle that interferes with drainage of aqueous through the canal of Schlemm will cause an accumulation of intraocular fluid followed by increased intraocular pressure. Glaucoma may develop, however, even though the filtration angle is normal and the canal of Schlemm appears to be functioning; the cause of this form of glaucoma is not known.

    DIAG: Glaucoma may not cause symptoms, but is detected by measuring the intraocular pressure. In other cases, the frequent need to change eyeglass prescriptions, vague visual disturbances, mild headache, seeing a halo around lights, and impaired dark adaptation may be present.

    TREAT: *Nonoperative:* Miotics (eserine, pilocarpine); timolol maleate; I.V. mannitol; parenteral acetazolamide. Experimental studies indicate that marijuana, q.v., alleviates the symptoms of severe glaucoma. Control of associated disorders such as diabetes. *Operative:* Paracentesis of cornea; iridectomy (broad peripheral); cyclodialysis;

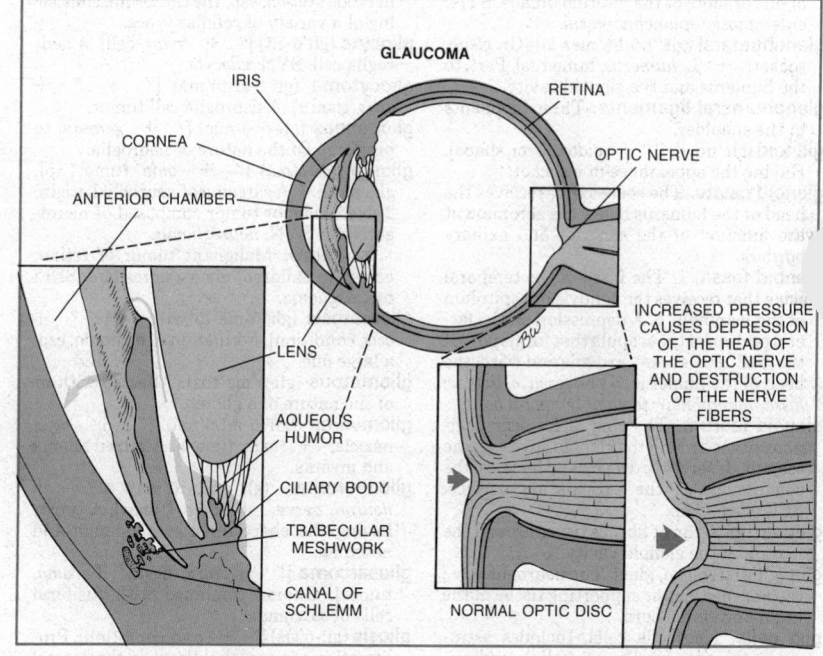

GLAUCOMA

IRIS

CORNEA

ANTERIOR CHAMBER

RETINA

OPTIC NERVE

INCREASED PRESSURE CAUSES DEPRESSION OF THE HEAD OF THE OPTIC NERVE AND DESTRUCTION OF THE NERVE FIBERS

LENS

AQUEOUS HUMOR

CILIARY BODY

TRABECULAR MESHWORK

CANAL OF SCHLEMM

NORMAL OPTIC DISC

anterior sclerotomy; sclerotomy with inclusion of iris, as iridotasis or iridencleisis; sclerectomy. SEE: illus.; *ciliarotomy; trabeculoplasty.*

Caution: Acute glaucoma may be precipitated in patients with angle closure glaucoma by dilating the pupils.

NURSING IMPLICATIONS: Patients with glaucoma need to know and understand that the disease can be controlled, but not cured. Teach them that fatigue, emotional upsets, excess fluid intake, and use of antihistamines may increase intraocular pressure. Patients should wear a Medic Alert bracelet or tag. Instruct patient about medications, including technique for eyedrop administration. Encourage strict adherence to regimen of prescribed drugs.

Public education is important to encourage early detection of the disease before vision is seriously and permanently impaired; investigation of such symptoms as seeing rings around lights, diplopia, and clumsiness due to reduced peripheral field of vision should be investigated.

    g., absolute. Glaucoma in which the eye is completely blind; cornea is insensitive; anterior chamber shallow; excavated optic disk; eye is as hard as stone; extremely painful.

    g., chronic. Glaucoma in which the tonometer indicates intraocular pressure reading of up to 45 or 50; enlargement of anterior ciliary veins; cornea is clear; dilated pupil; pain; poor vision during attacks; visual field may be normal; cupping of the optic disk is not present in the early stages.

    g., narrow angle. Glaucoma caused by a shallow anterior chamber and thus a narrow filtration angle through which the aqueous humor normally passes. Because the rate of movement of the aqueous is impaired, increased intraocular tension develops. SYN: *g., closed angle.*

    g., open angle. Any form of glaucoma in which the filtration angle is normal.

glaucomatous (glaw-kō'mă-tŭs). Pert. to glaucoma.

GLC. *gas-liquid chromatography.* SEE: *chromatography, gas-liquid.*

gleet (glēt). A mucous discharge from the urethra in chronic gonorrhea.

Glénard's disease (glā-nărz') [Frantz Glénard, Fr. physician, 1848–1920]. Prolapse of one or more of the internal organs. SYN: *enteroptosis; splanchnoptosia.*

glenohumeral (glē″nō-hū′mĕr-ăl) [Gr. *glene,* socket, + L. *humerus,* humerus]. Pert. to the humerus and the glenoid cavity.

glenohumeral ligaments. Three ligaments in the shoulder.

glenoid (glē′noyd) [″ + *eidos,* form, shape]. Having the appearance of a socket.

glenoid cavity. The socket that receives the head of the humerus below the acromion at the junction of the superior and axillary borders.

ᴇnoid fossa. 1. The fossa of the temporal bone that receives the condyle or capitulum of the mandible. 2. A depression on the lateral portion of the scapula that forms part of the ball and socket articulation with the head of the humerus. SYN: *fossa, articular; fossa, mandibular; fossa of temporal bone.*

glenoid labrum. The ring of fibrocartilaginous tissue around the glenoid cavity on the scapula. It serves to deepen and increase the congruency of the articulating surface. SEE: *glenoid lip.*

glenoid lip. A rim of fibrous tissue around the margin of the glenoid cavity.

glia (glī′ă) [Gr. *glia,* glue]. The neuroglia, q.v.; the non-nervous or supporting tissue of the brain and spinal cord.

glia cells. Neuroglia cells. Includes astrocytes, oligodendroglia (oligoglia), and microglia. SEE: *cell; neuroglia.*

gliacyte (glī′ă-sīt) [″ + *kytos,* cell]. A neuroglia cell.

gliadin (glī′ă-dĭn). A water-insoluble protein present in the gluten of wheat. It is deficient in the essential amino acid lysine. The sticky mass that results when wheat flour and water are mixed is due to gliadin. In some individuals the intestinal mucosa lacks the ability to digest this substance, thus damaging the lining and causing gluten-induced enteropathy, q.v.

glial (glī′ăl). Concerning glia or neuroglia.

gliarase (glī′ă-rās) [Gr. *glia,* glue]. Astrocytic mass with incomplete fission of cytoplasm.

glide. 1. To move in a smooth, virtually frictionless manner. 2. Movement in a smooth, virtually frictionless manner. 3. A joint mobilization technique where the therapist applies a translatoric force or glide against one of the bones of a joint causing it to move parallel to a defined treatment plane in the joint. Use to maintain or increase joint play.

g., mandibular. The movement of the mandible in any direction as the teeth come into contact.

glioblastoma (glī″ō-blăs-tō′mă) [″ + *blastos,* germ, + *oma,* tumor]. A neuroglia cell tumor. SYN: *glioma.*

g. multiforme. A neoplasm of the central

nervous system, esp. the cerebrum, consisting of a variety of cellular types.

gliocyte (glī′ō-sīt) [″ + *kytos,* cell]. A neuroglia cell. SYN: *gliacyte.*

gliocytoma (glī-ō-sī-tō′mă) [″ + ″ + *oma,* tumor]. A neuroglia cell tumor.

gliogenous (glī-ŏj′ĕ-nŭs) [″ + *gennan,* to produce]. Of the nature of neuroglia.

glioma (glī-ō′mă) [″ + *oma,* tumor] (pl. *gliomata*). 1. A sarcoma of neuroglial origin. 2. Neoplasm or tumor composed of neuroglia cells. SYN: *neuroglioma.*

g. retinae. Malignant tumor of retina; occurs in children; metastasizes late. SEE: *pseudoglioma.*

gliomatosis (glī″ō-mă-tō′sĭs) [″ + ″ + *osis,* condition]. Formation of a glioma, esp. a large one.

gliomatous (glī-ō′mă-tŭs). Affected with or of the nature of a glioma.

gliomyoma (glī″ō-mī-ō′mă) [″ + *mys,* muscle, + *oma,* tumor]. A mixed glioma and myoma.

glioneuroma (glī″ō-nū-rō′mă) [″ + *neuron,* nerve, + *oma,* tumor]. A tumor having the characteristics of glioma and neuroma.

gliosarcoma [″ + *sarx,* flesh, + *oma,* tumor]. Glioma combined with fusiform cells of sarcoma.

gliosis (glī-ō′sĭs) [″ + *osis,* condition]. Proliferation of neuroglial tissue in the central nervous system.

gliosome (glī′ō-sōm) [″ + *soma,* body]. One of the rounded bodies seen in neuroglia cells.

gliotoxin (glī″ō-tŏk′sĭn). An antibiotic obtained from several different fungi.

Glisson, Francis (glĭs′ŭn). British physician and anatomist, 1597–1677.

G.'s capsule. The outer capsule of fibrous tissue investing the liver.

G.'s disease. Rickets, q.v.

glissonian cirrhosis. Inflammation of peritoneal coat of the liver. SYN: *perihepatitis.*

glissonitis. Inflammation of Glisson's capsule.

globi (glō′bī) [L.]. Plural of globus.

globin (glō′bĭn) [L. *globus,* globe]. 1. A protein constituent of hemoglobin. 2. One of a particular group of proteins.

globoid (glō′boyd) [″ + Gr. *eidos,* form, shape]. Resembling a globe. SYN: *spheroid.*

globular (glŏb′ū-lăr) [L. *globus,* a globe]. Resembling a globe or globule; spherical.

globule (glŏb′ūl) [L. *globulus,* globule]. Any small, rounded body.

globulin (glŏb′ū-lĭn) [L. *globulus,* globule]. One of a group of simple proteins insoluble in pure water but soluble in neutral solutions of salts of strong acids. Examples include serum globulin; fibrinogen; myosinogen; lactoglobulin.

g., Ac. Accelerator globulin; a globulin present in blood serum that speeds up the conversion of prothrombin to thrombin in the presence of thromboplastin and calcium ions.

g., antihemophilic. A clotting component present in the plasma that is essential for the normal agglutination and disintegration of blood platelets. It is deficient in the blood of hemophiliacs. SEE: *hemophilia.*

g., antilymphocyte. Globulin from a person who has become immunized to lymphocytes. Used as an immunosuppressant.

g., gamma. That fraction of serum globulin with which most of the immune antibodies are associated. Most of the antibodies to viruses, bacterial agglutinogens, exotoxins, and injected foreign proteins are contained in the gamma globulin fraction. SEE: *immunoglobulin.*

g., immune. USP. A sterile, nonpyrogenic solution of globulins normally present in human blood. It is used in passive immunization of nonimmune persons exposed to infectious hepatitis, poliomyelitis, mumps, rubella, rubeola, and varicella. Previously used name: immune serum globulin, human. Trade names are Gamastan, Gamimune, Gammagee, Gammar, Immu-G, and Immuglobulin.

g., Rh$_o$(D) immune. A sterile nonpyrogenic solution of globulins derived from human blood plasma that contains antibodies to the erythrocyte factor Rh$_o$(D). It is used to prevent development of Rh$_o$(D) antibodies in Rh$_o$(D)-negative mothers following a miscarriage, therapeutic abortion, or delivery of an Rh$_o$(D)-positive fetus or child. This is of benefit in preventing the development of erythroblastosis fetalis, q.v., in the next pregnancy.

g., serum. Globulins present in blood plasma or serum; the fraction of the blood serum with which antibodies are associated. By electrophoresis, they can be separated into alpha, beta, and gamma globulins, which differ in their isoelectric points.

g., varicella-zoster immune. SEE: *varicella-zoster immune globulin.*

globulinuria (glŏb″ū-lĭn-ū′rē-ă) [L. *globulus,* globule, + Gr. *ouron,* urine]. Globulin in the urine.

globulose (glŏb′ū-lōs) [L. *globulus,* globule]. Albumose or protein produced by the digestion of globulins.

globus [L.]. A globe or sphere.

g. hystericus. A lump in the throat in hysteria and other neuroses. SYN: *spheresthesia.*

g. major. Head of epididymis.

g. minor. Lower end of epididymis.

g. pallidus. [NA] Pale section within the lenticular nucleus of the brain. SEE: *paleostriatum.*

glomangioma (glō-măn″jē-ō′mă) [L. *glomus,* a ball, + Gr. *angeion,* vessel, + *oma,* tumor]. A benign tumor that develops from an arteriovenous glomus (cluster of blood cells) of the skin.

glomectomy (glō-měk′tō-mē). Surgical removal of any glomus.

glomerate (glŏm′ĕr-āt) [L. *glomerare,* t wind into a ball]. Conglomerate, clustere grouped.

glomerular (glō-měr′ū-lăr) [L. *glomerulu* little ball]. Pert. to a glomerulus; clustered.

glomerular disease. A large group of diseases that have basic pathological involvement of the glomerulus. They may be classified by clinical severity, by histologic changes in the kidney, or by etiology. Etiologic factors include *primary glomerular disease;* disease secondary to *systemic disease* such as lupus erythematosus or polyarteritis; *infectious disease* such as streptococcal infection, malaria, syphilis, or schistosomiasis; *metabolic disease* such as diabetes or amyloidosis; *toxins* such as mercury, gold, or snake venom; or *serum sickness;* and *hypersensitivity* to drugs.

Glomerular disease may also be associated with hereditary disorders, e.g., Alport's syndrome, q.v., and Fabry's disease, q.v. SEE: *glomerulonephritis; kidney; nephritis; nephrotic syndrome.*

Clinical findings are those associated with the primary dysfunction and pathological changes in the glomerulus, which include proteinuria and hypertension. If protein loss exceeds 5 grams a day, the nephrotic syndrome, q.v., will develop.

glomeruli (glō-měr′ū-lī) [L. *glomerulus,* little ball] (sing. *glomerulus*). 1. Small structures in the malpighian body of the kidney made up of capillary blood vessels in a cluster and enveloped in a thin wall. 2. A group of twisted capillaries or nerve fibers.

glomerulitis (glō-měr″ū-lī′tĭs) [″ + Gr. *itis,* inflammation]. Inflammation of glomeruli, esp. of the renal glomeruli.

glomerulonephritis (glō-měr″ū-lō-nĕ-frī′tĭs) [″ + Gr. *nephros,* kidney, + *itis,* inflammation]. A form of nephritis in which the lesions involve primarily the glomeruli. May be acute, subacute, or chronic. Acute glomerulonephritis and acute nephritic syndrome are synonymous. This condition frequently follows infections, esp. those of the upper respiratory tract due to particular strains of streptococci. It may also be caused by systemic lupus erythematosus, subacute bacterial endocarditis, cryoglobulinemia, various forms of vasculitis including polyarteritis nodosa, Henoch-Schönlein purpura, and visceral abscess. Characterized by hematuria, proteinuria, red-cell casts, oliguria, edema, and hypertension. Investigation of serum complement and renal biopsy will facilitate diagnosis and help to establish the prognosis. SEE: *glomerulonephritis, rapidly progressive; glomerular disease.*

NURSING IMPLICATIONS: Assess the patient for symptoms of glomerulonephritis such as hematuria, edema, nausea, irritability, flank pain, constipation, decreased urine output, increased urine specific gravity, headache, and hypertension.

Overall nursing care for the patient includes observations for changes in amount of edema, daily weighing, measuring and recording intake and output, taking vital signs every two to four hours, and searching for signs of skin breakdown. The patient will need proper skin care and turning, as well as instruction in dietary and fluid restriction. In addition, the patient will need diversional activities, encouragement, and emotional support. Limit activity to reduce energy expenditure during period of acute hematuria, azotemia, and gross edema, and while blood pressure is elevated. Encourage self-care as possible based on fatigue and changes in blood pressure as activity is increased. SEE: *Nursing Diagnoses in Appendix.*

g., rapidly progressive. ABBR: RPGN. Any glomerular disease in which there is rapid loss of renal function in which usually over 50% of the glomeruli are damaged.

glomerulopathy (glō-měr″ū-lŏp′ă-thē). Any disease of the glomerulus of the kidney.

glomerulosclerosis (glō-měr″ū-lō-sklē-rō′sĭs). Fibrosis of the renal glomeruli.

g., diabetic. A type of glomerulosclerosis seen in some cases of diabetes mellitus. Eosinophilic material is present in various parts of the glomerulus. SYN: *g., intercapillary.*

g., intercapillary. G., diabetic, q.v.

glomerulus (glō-měr′ū-lŭs) [L.] (pl. *glomeruli*). 1. A group of twisted capillaries or nerve fibers. 2. One of the small structures in the malpighian body of the kidney made up of capillary blood vessels in a cluster and enveloped in a thin wall. SEE: *kidney* for illus.

g., olfactory. A rounded body found in the olfactory bulb, formed by the numerous terminal branches of the dendrites of a mitral cell intertwining with the terminal fibers of several olfactory receptor cells.

glomoid (glō′moyd). Similar in appearance to a glomus.

glomus (glō′mŭs) [L., a ball]. A small, round

swelling made up of tiny blood vessels and found in stroma containing many nerve fibers.

g. caroticum. [NA] A flat structure at the bifurcation of the common carotid body. Contains cells that respond to changes in concentration of oxygen in the blood and to changes in blood pressure.

g. choroideum. [NA] An enlargement of the choroid plexus at its entrance into the lateral ventricle.

g. coccygeum. [NA] The coccygeal body.

glossa [Gr. *glossa*, tongue]. The tongue.

glossal. Rel. to the tongue.

glossalgia (glŏs-săl′jē-ă) [″ + *algos*, pain]. Pain in the tongue. SYN: *glossodynia.*

glossectomy (glŏs-ĕk′tō-mē) [″ + *ektome*, excision]. Partial or complete excision of the tongue. SYN: *elinguation.*

Glossina (glŏs-sī′nă). A genus of flies called tsetse flies. Includes about 20 species of bloodsucking flies that are confined principally to central and southern Africa. They transmit the trypanosomes *(Trypanosoma gambiense, T. rhodesiense)*, the causative agents of sleeping sickness in man, and other trypanosomes that infect wild and domestic animals. Important species are *Glossina palpalis, G. morsitans, G. tachinoides,* and *G. swynnertoni.* SEE: *sleeping sickness; Trypanosoma.*

glossitis (glŏs-sī′tĭs) [″ + *itis*, inflammation]. Inflammation of the tongue.

g., acute. Glossitis associated with stomatitis, q.v. The tongue is covered with ulcers and is tender and painful. Another form affects the parenchyma of tongue and is characterized by edema, which may spread to surrounding structures, producing asphyxia and necessitating tracheostomy.

SYM: Tongue is painful; saliva thick and viscid, rendering swallowing difficult. Marked malaise, and often a rise in temperature.

TREAT: Oral cleanliness with frequent antiseptic mouthwashes. Anesthetic oral solution for pain. Bland or liquid diet.

g. areata exfoliativa. Condition of tongue marked by numerous denuded patches on the dorsal surface coalescing into free-form shapes similar to geographic areas on a map. SYN: *geographic tongue.*

g. desiccans. A painful, raw, and fissured tongue.

g., median rhomboid. An inflammatory area, somewhat diamond-shaped, found on the dorsum of the tongue anterior to the vallate papillae.

g., Moeller's. A chronic superficial inflammation of the tongue characterized by burning or pain and increased sensitivity to hot and spicy foods.

g. parasitica. Black or hairy tongue, characterized by the appearance on the dorsum of the tongue of a dark, furlike patch consisting of hypertrophied filiform papillae, pigment, and shed epithelial cells. SYN: *glossophytia.*

glosso- [Gr. *glossa,* tongue]. Prefix pert. to the tongue.

glossocele (glŏs′sō-sēl) [″ + *kele,* swelling]. Swelling and protrusion of the tongue as a result of disease or malformation.

glossodynamometer (glŏs″sō-dī″nă-mŏm′ĕ-tĕr) [″ + *dynamis,* power, + *metron,* measure]. Device for measuring contractile power of the tongue muscles.

glossodynia (glŏs″ō-dĭn′ē-ă) [″ + *odyne,* pain]. Pain in the tongue. SYN: *glossalgia.* SEE: *burning mouth syndrome.*

g. exfoliativa. A chronic superficial inflammation of the tongue characterized by burning or pain and increased sensitivity to hot and spicy foods.

glossoepiglottic (glŏs″ō-ĕp-ĭ-glŏt′ĭk) [″ + *epi,* upon, + *glottis,* back of tongue]. Pert. to the ligament between the base of the tongue and epiglottis.

glossoepiglottidean (glŏs″ō-ĕp-ĭ-glŏ-tĭd′ē-ăn). Rel. to the tongue and epiglottis.

glossoepiglottidean folds. Three mucous membrane folds from base of the tongue to the epiglottis. SYN: *plicae epiglotticae.*

glossoepiglottidean ligament. Elastic band from base of the tongue to the epiglottis in middle glossoepiglottidean fold.

glossograph (glŏs′ō-grăf) [″ + *graphein,* to write]. An instrument for recording the tongue's movements in speaking.

glossohyal (glŏs″ō-hī′ăl) [″ + *hyoeides,* U-shaped]. Rel. to the tongue and hyoid bone. SYN: *hyoglossal.*

glossokinesthetic (glŏs″ō-kĭn″ĕs-thĕt′ĭk) [″ + *kinesis,* movement, + *aisthetikos,* perceptive]. Pert. to movements of the tongue, esp. those in speech.

glossolabial (glŏs″ō-lā′bē-ăl) [″ + L. *labium,* lip]. Pert. to the tongue and lips.

glossolalia (glŏs″ō-lā′lē-ă) [″ + *lalia,* babble]. Repetition of senseless remarks not related to the subject or situation involved.

glossology (glŏ-sŏl′ō-jē) [″ + *logos,* word, reason]. Study of the tongue and its diseases. SYN: *glottology.*

glossopalatine (glŏs″ō-păl′ă-tīn). Pert. to the tongue and palate.

glossopathy (glŏs-sŏp′ă-thē) [″ + *pathos,* disease, suffering]. Disease of the tongue.

glossopharyngeal (glŏs″ō-fă-rĭn′jē-ăl) [″ + *pharynx,* throat]. Rel. to the tongue and pharynx.

glossopharyngeal breathing. A technique of breathing whereby the patient with in-spiratory muscle weakness increases the volume of air breathed in by taking several "gulps" of air, closing the mouth, and forcing air into the lungs.

glossopharyngeal nerve. Ninth cranial nerve. Function: Special sensory (taste), visceral sensory, and motor. Origin: By several roots from the medulla oblongata. Distribution: Pharynx, ear, meninges, posterior third of tongue, parotid gland. Branches: Carotid, tympanic, pharyngeal, lingual, tonsillar, and sinus nerve of Hering. SEE:s.

glossoplasty (glŏs′ō-plăs″tē) [″ + *plassein,* to form]. Reparative surgery of the tongue.

glossoplegia (glŏs″ō-plē′jē-ă) [″ + *plege,* stroke]. Paralysis of the tongue, usually unilateral. SYN: *glossolysis.*

ETIOL: Cerebral hemorrhage, disease, or injury that involves the hypoglossal nerve.

glossoptosis (glŏs″ŏp-tō′sĭs) [″ + *ptosis,* a dropping]. Dropping of the tongue downward out of normal position.

glossopyrosis (glŏs″ō-pī-rō′sĭs) [″ + *pyrosis,* a burning]. A burning sensation of the tongue. SEE: *burning mouth syndrome.*

glossorrhaphy (glŏ-sor′ă-fē) [″ + *rhaphe,* seam, ridge]. Suture of wound of the tongue.

glossospasm (glŏs′ō-spăzm) [″ + *spasmos,* spasm]. Spasmodic contraction of muscles of the tongue.

glossotomy (glŏ-sŏt′ō-mē) [″ + *tome,* incision]. Incision of the tongue.

glossotrichia (glŏs″ō-trĭk′ē-ă) [″ + *thrix,* hair]. Hairy tongue due to greatly elongated filiform papillae that give the tongue a hairy appearance; may be associated with antibiotic therapy.

glossy. Smooth and shining.

glossy skin. Shiny appearance of the skin due to atrophy or injury to nerves.

glottic [Gr. *glottis,* back of tongue]. Of or pert. to the tongue or glottis.

glottis (glŏt′ĭs) [Gr. *glottis,* back of tongue] (pl. *glottises* or *glottides*). [NA] The sound-producing apparatus of the larynx consisting of the two vocal folds and the intervening space, the rima glottidis. A leaf-shaped lid of fibrocartilage (the epiglottis) protects this opening.

g., edema of. The accumulation of fluid in the tissues lining the larynx. It may result from irritation of the larynx from improper use of the voice, excessive use of tobacco or alcohol, chemical fumes, acute infections, or more serious conditions such as tuberculous or syphilitic laryngitis.

SYM: Hoarseness, and later complete aphonia; extreme dyspnea at first on inspiration but later on expiration also. Stridulous respiration; barking cough when epi-

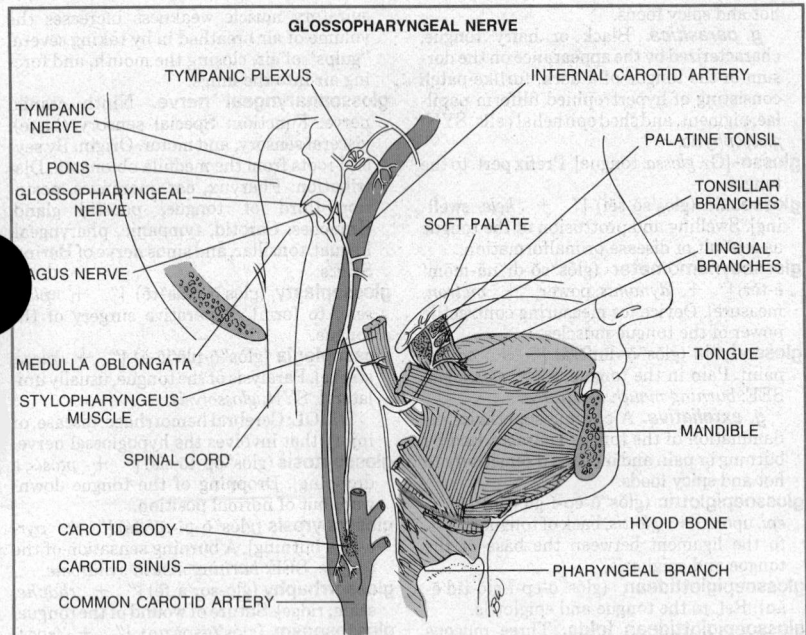

GLOSSOPHARYNGEAL NERVE

TYMPANIC PLEXUS
INTERNAL CAROTID ARTERY
TYMPANIC NERVE
PONS
GLOSSOPHARYNGEAL NERVE
PALATINE TONSIL
TONSILLAR BRANCHES
SOFT PALATE
LINGUAL BRANCHES
VAGUS NERVE
MEDULLA OBLONGATA
TONGUE
STYLOPHARYNGEUS MUSCLE
SPINAL CORD
MANDIBLE
CAROTID BODY
HYOID BONE
CAROTID SINUS
PHARYNGEAL BRANCH
COMMON CAROTID ARTERY

glottis is involved.

glottology (glŏ-tŏl′ō-jē) [″ + *logos*, word, reason]. The study of the tongue and its diseases. SYN: *glossology*.

glove. A protective covering for the hand. In medical care the glove is made of a flexible impervious material that will permit full movement of the hand and fingers. Gloves are used to prevent the contamination of the operative site with organisms from the person wearing the glove and to prevent pathogens from the patient contaminating the hands of the health care worker. These factors are particularly important when the patient has a disease such as hepatitis B or AIDS. SEE: *Universal Precautions* in *Appendix*.

Caution: It is not advisable to wash gloves and to wear them while treating another patient.

glucagon (gloo′kǎ-gŏn). USP. A polypeptide hormone that has the property of increasing the concentration of glucose in the blood. It is obtained from pork and beef pancreas glands. Glucagon is secreted by the alpha cells of the human pancreas. Parenteral administration of glucagon produces relaxation of the smooth muscle of the stomach, duodenum, small bowel, and colon.

glucagonoma (glū″kǎ-gŏn-ō′mǎ). A malignant tumor of the alpha cells of the islets of Langerhans of the pancreas. Principal signs and symptoms include weight loss, diabetes mellitus, skin rash, glossitis, elevated serum glucagon levels, and anemia. Treatment is surgical.

gluciphore (gloo′sĭ-for). Glucophore.

glucocerebroside (gloo″kō-sĕr′ĕ-brō-sīd″). Cerebroside with the carbohydrate glucose contained in the molecule. Present in tissues in Gaucher's disease.

glucocorticoid (gloo″kō-kort′ĭ-koyd) [Gr. *gleukos*, sweet (new wine), + L. *cortex*, cortex, + Gr. *eidos*, form, shape]. A general classification of adrenal cortical hormones that are primarily active in protecting against stress and in affecting protein and carbohydrate metabolism. SEE: *mineralocorticoid*.

glucofuranose (gloo″kō-fū′rǎ-nōs). The form of glucose containing the furanose ring.

glucogenesis (gloo″kō-jĕn′ĕ-sĭs). Formation of glucose from glycogen.

glucohemia (gloo″kō-hē′mē-ǎ) [″ + *haima*, blood]. Sugar in the blood. SYN: *glycosemia*.

glucokinase (gloo″kō-kī′nās). An enzyme in the liver and pancreas. In the presence of ATP, it catalyzes the conversion of glucose to glucose 6-phosphate.

glucokinetic (gloo″kō-kī-nĕt′ĭk). Acting to maintain the blood glucose level.

Glucometer. A battery-operated device used to measure blood glucose by using a few drops of blood obtained from the finger.

gluconeogenesis (gloo″kō-nē″ō-jĕn′ē-sĭs) [″ + *neos,* new, + *genesis,* generation, birth]. The formation of glycogen from non-carbohydrate sources such as amino or fatty acids. It occurs in the liver under such conditions as low carbohydrate intake or starvation. SYN: *glyconeogenesis.*

glucopenia (gloo″kō-pē′nē-ă) [″ + Gr. *penia,* lack]. Abnormally low concentration of blood glucose.

glucophore (gloo′kō-for) [″ + *phorein,* to carry]. The portion of a chemical compound that imparts a sweet taste to the substance.

glucoprotein (gloo″kō-prō′tē-ĭn). Glycoprotein.

glucopyranose (gloo″kō-pī′ră-nōs). The form of glucose containing the six-carbon pyran ring.

glucuronyl transferase. Enzyme that converts unconjugated or indirect bilirubin to conjugated or direct bilirubin.

glucosamine (gloo″kō-săm′ēn). An aminosaccharide present in chitin and mucus.

glucose (gloo′kōs) [Gr. *gleukos,* sweet (new wine)]. 1. A sugar. In medicine, the word is used to indicate the sugar dextrose. This is also called D-glucose. 2. An intermediate in metabolism of carbohydrates in the body.

Glucose is the most important carbohydrate in body metabolism. It is formed during digestion from the hydrolysis of di- and polysaccharides, esp. starch. It is absorbed from the intestines into the blood of the portal vein. In its passage through the liver, excess glucose is converted into glycogen (glycogenesis). The concentration of sugar in the blood is approximately 0.1% (100 mg/dl), the amount being maintained at a fairly constant level (80 to 120 mg/dl) through the action of insulin produced by the islets of Langerhans of the pancreas. Failure of the pancreas to produce adequate insulin results in hyperglycemia, in which the blood sugar (glucose) level may rise to 200 mg/dl or higher. When above the renal threshold (about 160 to 180 mg/dl), glucose appears in the urine (glycosuria). This is a symptom of diabetes. Overproduction of insulin or injection of insulin as in insulin shock treatment reduces the blood sugar below normal, a condition known as hypoglycemia, q.v.

In the tissue, glucose may be converted into glycogen, utilized to form fat, or oxidized to carbon dioxide and water. Free glucose is not used in the tissues until phosphorylated by ATP (adenosine triphosphate). This occurs through the action of an enzyme, hexokinase, with the resultant production of glucose-6-phosphate. Through a complex series of reactions involving several enzymes, the action of certain hormones, and the formation of several intermediate products including lactic and pyruvic acids, oxidation to carbon and water is brought about. Hormones of the anterior lobe of the hypophysis, the adrenal gland (cortex and medulla), thyroid, and the gonads play a role in carbohydrate metabolism.

When the blood sugar is below normal, fat stores are metabolized. Incomplete metabolism of fats leads to the formation of ketone bodies, also a symptom of diabetes. Blood sugar acts as a protein sparer, q.v. Nervous tissue is esp. dependent upon glucose as its source of energy, the brain being able to oxidize glucose directly. SEE: *carbohydrate.*

g., blood level of. The glucose found in the bloodstream has a dual origin. First, glucose is present normally in both the whole blood and plasma; secondly, the greater percentage of the normal glucose concentration has an exogenous origin — that is, from the food intake. The normal glucose concentration in the blood is 80 to 120 mg/dl. Increased concentration is associated with acromegaly; adrenal tumors; increased intracranial pressure; diabetes mellitus; hemochromatosis; hyperthyroidism; hyperpituitarism; hyperadrenalism. Decreased concentration is associated with Addison's disease; adenoma or carcinoma of islets of Langerhans; cretinism; hyperinsulinism; hypopituitarism; hypothyroidism; insulin shock; muscular dystrophy; myxedema.

g., liquid. A liquid obtained from the incomplete hydrolysis of starch. It is a thick syrupy liquid, sweet in taste, containing D-glucose (dextrose), dextrins, and other carbohydrates. It is used for nutritive purposes and in various pharmaceutical and food preparations.

glucose-6-phosphate dehydrogenase. ABBR: G-6-PD. An enzyme that dehydrogenates glucose-6-phosphate to form 6-phosphoglucon. This is the initial step in the pentose phosphate pathway of glucose catabolism.

glucose polymer. A glucose saccharide mixture of 3% glucose, 7% maltose, 5% maltotriose, 85% polysaccharides of 4 to 15 glucose units. Because it is virtually tasteless, its use as the source of glucose in the carbohydrate tolerance test has been helpful in making the test better accepted by patients.

Trade name is Polycose. SEE: *glucose tolerance test.*

glucose tolerance test. A test performed by giving a certain amount of glucose to a patient orally or intravenously. Blood samples are drawn at specified intervals and the blood glucose determined in each sample. By this means, the ability of the patient to metabolize glucose can be determined. In suspected cases of hyperinsulinism, the test is prolonged to six hours with samples of blood being drawn hourly and analyzed for sugar content. If the blood-sugar level continues to drop after three hours, falling below 80 mg/dl, hyperinsulinism is indicated, although other conditions may produce a deficiency in blood sugar (hypoglycemia).

A dose of oral cortisone 8½ hours and 2½ hours prior to giving the glucose is sometimes administered. This is called the oral cortisone glucose tolerance test. The cortisone increases the demand for insulin and thus reveals deficiency in insulin response. SEE: *glucose polymer.*

glucosidase (gloo-kō'sĭ-dās). An enzyme that catalyzes the hydrolysis of a glucoside.

glucoside (gloo'kō-sĭd). A glycoside that upon hydrolysis yields a sugar, glucose, and one or two additional products. Glucosides are numerous and widely distributed in plants. Many glucosides have medicinal properties; for example, digitalin and strophanthin, present in digitalis and strophanthus respectively, have a specific effect upon the heart. SEE: *glycoside.*

glucosin (gloo'kō-sĭn). Any one of a series of bases derived by action of ammonia on glucose.

glucosulfone sodium (gloo"kō-sŭl'fōn). A derivative of dapsone used in treating leprosy.

glucosuria (gloo"kō-sū'rē-ă) [" + *ouron,* urine]. Abnormal amount of sugar in the urine. SYN: *glycosuria.*

glucuronic acid. An important acid, $CHO(CHOH)_4COOH$, in human metabolism by virtue of its detoxifying action. It combines with certain toxic substances and renders them harmless.

β-glucuronidase (gloo"kū-rŏn'ĭ-dās). An enzyme that splits glycosidic linkages in glucuronides. It is involved in cell division.

glucuronide (gloo-kū'rŏn-īd). The combination of glucuronic acid with phenol, alcohol, or any acid containing the carboxyl, COOH, group.

glue ear. A descriptive term for chronic accumulation of a high-viscosity fluid in the middle ear. Occurs principally in children 5 to 8 years old. It causes deafness, which can be treated by removal of the exudate.

glue-sniffing. Inhaling the vapor from types of glue or solvents that contain toxic chemicals such as benzene, toluene, or xylene. This produces an altered state of consciousness and has occasionally caused death.

Gluge's corpuscles (gloo'gēz) [Gottlieb Gluge, Ger. pathologist, 1812–1898]. Granular cells containing fat droplets, usually found in degenerating nervous tissue.

glutamate (gloo'tă-māt). Salt of glutamic acid.

glutamic acid (gloo-tăm'ĭk) [L. *gluten,* glue, + *ammonium*]. $COOH \cdot (CH_2)_2 \cdot CH(NH_2) \cdot COOH$. An amino acid formed in the hydrolysis of proteins. It is the only amino acid metabolized by the brain.

glutamic-oxaloacetic transaminase. ABBR: GOT, or SGOT for serum glutamic-oxaloacetic transaminase. Enzyme that is involved in the transfer of the amino group of glutamic acid to oxaloacetic acid to form α-ketoglutaric acid and aspartic acid. When cells of either the liver or heart are injured, this enzyme's blood level is increased, thus providing a chemical indicator of hepatitis or myocardial tissue damage. SYN: *aspartate aminotransferase.*

glutamic-pyruvic transaminase. ABBR: GPT, or SGPT for serum glutamic-pyruvic transaminase. Enzyme that is involved in the transfer of the amino group of glutamic acid to pyruvic acid to form α-ketoglutaric acid and L-alanine. When cells of either the liver or heart are injured, this enzyme's blood level is increased, thus providing a chemical indicator of hepatitis or myocardial tissue damage. SYN: *alanine aminotransferase.*

glutaminase (gloo-tăm'ĭ-nās). An enzyme that catalyzes the breakdown of glutamine into glutamic acid and ammonia.

glutamine (gloo'tă-mĭn, -mēn"). The monoamide of aminoglutaric acid. It is present in the juices of many plants and is essential in the hydrolysis of proteins.

γ-glutamyl transpeptidase. A tissue enzyme that is elevated in many conditions involving hepatic damage including alcohol-induced hepatic injury; in patients with renal disease, pancreatitis, diabetes mellitus, coronary artery disease, and carcinoma of the prostate; and in individuals taking phenytoin and barbiturates.

glutaral (gloo'tă-răl). USP. A solution of glutaraldehyde in sterile water.

glutaraldehyde (gloo"tă-răl'dĕ-hīd). 1. A sterilizing agent effective against all microorganisms including viruses and spores. 2. An excellent primary fixative agent for electron microscopy, usually followed by osmium in the preparation of material for transmission electron microscopy.

glutathione (gloo-tă-thī'ŏn) [" + Gr. *theion*, sulfur]. A tripeptide of glutamic acid, cysteine, and glycine. Found in small quantities in active animal tissues; takes up and gives off hydrogen; fundamentally important in cellular respiration.

    g., reduced. The form of glutaraldehyde present in red blood cells. It detoxifies hydrogen peroxide that forms either spontaneously or after drug administration, thus protecting red cells from injury due to hydrogen peroxide.

gluteal (gloo'tē-ăl) [Gr. *gloutos*, buttock]. Pert. to the buttocks.

gluteal fold. Crease between the thigh and the buttocks. SEE: *rump.*

gluteal reflex. Contraction of gluteal muscles from stimulation of overlying skin.

glutelin (gloo'tĕ-lĭn) [L. *gluten*, glue]. A simple protein found in grain seeds, soluble in alkalies and dilute acids but not in neutral solutions. SEE: *protein.*

gluten [L., glue]. Vegetable albumin, a protein that can be prepared from wheat and other grain.

gluten-free diet. Elimination of gluten from the diet by avoiding all products containing wheat, rye, oats, or barley. Gluten is present in a large number of foods where thickening sauces are used; thus it is essential that the diet be discussed with a dietitian.

gluten-induced enteropathy. Adult celiac disease due to gluten intolerance which leads to malabsorption of essential nutrients. Signs and symptoms include steatorrhea, bloating, and malnutrition. SYN: *celiac disease.* SEE: *gluten-free diet; sprue.*

    TREAT: Eliminate gluten from the diet.

glutethimide (gloo-tĕth'ĭ-mĭd). USP. A hypnotic drug. Trade name is Doriden.

glutin. The viscid portion of wheat gluten. SYN: *gliadin.*

glutinous (gloo'tĭn-ŭs) [L. *glutinosus*, glue]. Adhesive; sticky.

glutitis [Gr. *gloutos*, buttock, + *itis*, inflammation]. Inflammation of the muscles of the buttocks.

glycase (glī'kās) [Gr. *glykys*, sweet]. The enzyme that converts maltose into dextrose. SEE: *enzyme.*

glycemia (glī-sē'mē-ă) [" + *haima*, blood]. Sugar or glucose in the blood. SYN: *glycosemia.*

DL-glyceraldehyde (glĭs"ĕr-ăl'dĕ-hīd). An aldose, CHOCH(OH)CH$_2$OH, produced by the metabolism of fructose in the liver.

glyceride (glĭs'ĕr-īd) [Gr. *glykys*, sweet]. An ester of glycerin compounded with an acid.

glycerin (glĭs'ĕr-ĭn). USP. C$_3$H$_8$O$_3$. A trihydric alcohol, trihydroxy-propane, present in chemical combination in all fats. It is a syrupy colorless liquid, soluble in all propor-

tions in water and alcohol. It is made commercially by the hydrolysis of fats, esp. during the manufacture of soap. Used extensively as a solvent, as a preservative, and as an emollient in various skin diseases. Given orally, it is effective in reducing intracranial pressure; and preoperatively in reducing intraocular pressure in glaucoma. Trade names are Glyrol, Ophthalgan, and Osmoglyn.

glycerite (glĭs'ĕr-īt) [L. *glyceritum*]. A medicine mixed in a glycerin solution.

glycerol (glĭs'ĕr-ŏl) [Gr. *glykys*, sweet]. Glycerin.

glyceryl (glĭs'ĕr-ĭl). The trivalent radical C$_3$H$_5$ of glycerol.

    g. monostearate. An emulsifying agent used in preparing creams and ointments.

    g. triacetate. Previously used name for triacetin, q.v.

    g. trinitrate. Nitroglycerin, USP. A valuable medicine used in treating angina pectoris or in preventing an attack if given prior to exercise.

    NOTE: Tablets should be stored in tightly sealed, dark containers to prevent loss of potency.

glycine (glī'sēn, -sĭn) [Gr. *glykys*, sweet]. USP. C$_2$H$_5$NO$_2$. A nonessential amino acid, q.v. SYN: *glycocin; aminoacetic acid.*

glyco-, glyc- (glī-kō) [Gr. *glykys*, sweet]. Prefix used in chemical compounds to indicate relationship to sugar or the presence of glycerol or similar substance.

glycobiarsol (glī"kō-bī-ăr'sŏl). USP. An amebicide.

glycocalyx (glī"kō-kăl'ĭks). A thin layer of glycoprotein and polysaccharide that covers the surface of some cells, such as muscle cells, fibroblasts, pericytes, and epithelial cells, and contributes to the basal lamina.

glycocholate (glī"kō-kŏl'āt). A salt of glycocholic acid.

glycocholic acid. A substance present in bile. It is a conjugate of cholic acid and glycine. SEE: *acid, glycocholic.*

glycocin. Glycine.

glycoclastic (glī"kō-klăs'tĭk) [" + *klan*, to break]. Pert. to the hydrolysis and digestion of sugars.

glycocoll (glī'kō-kŏl) [" + *kolla*, glue]. Glycine.

glycogen (glī'kō-jĕn) [" + *gennan*, to produce]. C$_6$H$_{10}$O$_{5x}$. A polysaccharide commonly called animal starch, a whitish powder that can be prepared from mammalian liver and muscle and other animal tissues. Formation of glycogen from carbohydrate sources is called glycogenesis; from noncarbohydrate sources, glyconeogenesis. The conversion of glycogen to glucose is called glycogenolysis. Glycogen is the form in which carbohydrate is stored in the animal body for future conversion into sugar and for subsequent use in performing muscular work or for liberating heat. SEE: *glycogen storage disease; glyconeogenesis.*

Glycogen usually is formed from sugar. It is converted when needed by the tissues into glucose. It is utilized by muscles and, with their contraction, breaks down into lactic acid. Oxygen is then needed to convert lactic acid back into glycogen, at which time some of the lactic acid is metabolized, producing carbonic acid and heat.

glycogenase (glī-kō'jĕn-ās). An enzyme in the liver that hydrolyzes glycogen. Its end product is dextrose.

glycogenesis (glī"kō-jĕn'ĕ-sĭs) [" + *genesis*, generation, birth]. The formation of glycogen from glucose.

glycogenetic. Pert. to the formation of glycogen.

glycogenic. Rel. to glycogen.

glycogenolysis (glī"kō-jĕn-ŏl'ĭ-sĭs) [" + *gennan*, to produce, + *lysis*, dissolution]. Conversion of glycogen into glucose in body tissues.

glycogenolytic (glī"kō-jĕn"ō-lĭt'ĭk) [" + " + *lysis*, dissolution]. Pert. to the hydrolysis of glycogen.

glycogenosis (glī"kō-jĕn-ō'sĭs) [" + " + *osis*, condition]. Abnormal accumulation of normal or abnormal forms of glycogen in tissue. The so-called glycogen storage diseases are grouped into various types according to the enzyme deficiency responsible.

glycogen storage disease. Any one of several heritable diseases characterized by abnormal storage and accumulation of glycogen in tissues, esp. the liver.

    g.s.d., phosphorylase b kinase deficiency. This storage disease was previously called type VIa, VIII, or IX.

    g.s.d. type Ia. This storage disease usually has its onset in the first year of life. It is an autosomal recessive genetic disorder and is due to a glucose-6-phosphatase deficiency. Also called von Gierke disease.

    g.s.d. type Ib. Storage disease similar to type Ia but occurring at only $\frac{1}{10}$ the frequency of Ia. The defect is due to a deficiency of glucose-6-phosphatase microsomal translocase.

    g.s.d. type II. Storage disease due to a deficiency of lysosomal α-glucosidase.

    g.s.d. type III. Deficiency of two debranching enzymes in liver and muscle tissues.

    g.s.d. type IV. Branching enzyme deficiency. Present are liver and spleen enlargement and hepatic failure, followed by death. SYN: *Andersen's disease.*

    g.s.d. type V. Muscle phosphorylase deficiency. SYN: *McArdle's disease.*

    g.s.d. type VI. Deficiency of liver phosphorylase, characterized by growth retardation, hepatomegaly, hypoglycemia, and acidosis. SYN: *Hers disease.*

    g.s.d. type VII. Deficiency of muscle phosphofructokinase, characterized by weakness and cramping of muscles following exercise.

glycogeusia (glī"kō-jū'sē-ă) [Gr. *glykys*, sweet, + *geusis*, taste]. A sweet taste.

glycohemia (glī"kō-hē'mē-ă) [" + *haima*, blood]. Abnormal amount of sugar in the blood. SYN: *glycosemia.*

glycol (glī'kōl, -kŏl) [" + *alcohol*]. Any one of the dihydric alcohols related to ethylene glycol, $C_2H_6O_2$.

glycolipid(e) (glī"kō-lĭp'ĭd) [" + *lipos*, fat]. Compound of fatty acids with a carbohydrate, containing nitrogen, but no phosphoric acid. Found in myelin sheath of nerves.

glycolysis (glī-kŏl'ĭ-sĭs) [" + *lysis*, dissolution]. Hydrolysis of sugar by an enzyme in the body.

glycolytic. Pert. to hydrolyzing sugar.

glycolytic enzyme. An enzyme that catalyzes the hydrolysis of sugars.

glycometabolic (glī"kō-mĕt-ă-bŏl'ĭk) [" + *metabole*, change]. Rel. to metabolism of sugar.

glycometabolism (glī"kō-mĕ-tăb'ŏ-lĭzm). Utilization of sugar, q.v., by the body. SEE: *metabolism.*

glyconeogenesis (glī"kō-nē"ō-jĕn'ĕ-sĭs) [" + *neos*, new, + *genesis*, generation, birth]. The formation of glycogen from noncarbohydrates, such as fat or amino acids from protein. SYN: *gluconeogenesis.*

glyconucleoprotein (glī"kō-nū"klē-ō-prō'tē-ĭn) [" + L. *nucleus*, kernel, + Gr. *protos*, first]. A nucleoprotein so named to emphasize the presence of sugar units in the substance.

glycopenia (glī-kō-pē'nē-ă) [" + *penia*, poverty]. Abnormally low level of blood glucose; hypoglycemia.

glycopexic (glī"kō-pĕks'ĭk) [" + *pexis*, fixation]. Pert. to the fixing or storing of sugar.

glycopexis (glī"kō-pĕk'sĭs). The storing of glycogen in the liver.

glycophorin (glī"kō-fō'rĭn). Glycoprotein that spans the bilipid layer of the erythrocyte membrane. The outside end of this complex substance contains blood group antigens and sites to which some viruses attach. This protein also functions as the channel for the passage of anions in and out of the red cell.

glycopolyuria (glī"kō-pŏl"ē-ū'rē-ă) [" + *polys*, much, + *ouron*, urine]. Diabetes mellitus with moderately increased sugar in the urine but greatly increased uric acid.

glycoprival, glycoprivous (glī″kō-prī′văl, -vŭs) [″ + L. *privus,* deprived of]. Lacking in or without carbohydrates.

glycoprotein (glī″kō-prō′tē-ĭn) [″ + *protos,* first]. A compound consisting of a carbohydrate and protein.

glycoptyalism (glī″kō-tī′ăl-ĭzm) [″ + *ptyalon,* saliva, + *-ismos,* condition]. Excretion of glucose in the saliva. SYN: *melitoptyalism.*

glycopyrrolate (glī″kō-pĭr′rō-lāt). USP. An anticholinergic drug. Trade name is Robinul.

glycorrhachia (glī-kō-rā′kē-ă) [″ + *rhachis,* spine]. Sugar in the cerebrospinal fluid.

glycorrhea (glī″kō-rē′ă) [″ + *rhoia,* flow]. Discharge of sugar from the body as in urine.

glycosecretory (glī″kō-sē-krē′tō-rē) [″ + L. *secretus,* separate]. Pert. to or determining the formation of glycogen.

glycosemia (glī-kō-sē′mē-ă) [″ + *haima,* blood]. Abnormal amount of sugar in the blood.

glycosialia (glī″kō-sī-ăl′ē-ă) [″ + *sialon,* saliva]. Glucose in the saliva.

glycosialorrhea (glī″kō-sī″ăl-ō-rē′ă) [″ + ″ + *rhoia,* flow]. Excessive secretion of saliva containing glucose.

glycoside. A substance derived from plants that upon hydrolysis yields a sugar and one or more additional products. Depending on the sugar formed, glycosides are designated glucosides or galactosides. SEE: *glucoside.*

glycosphingolipids (glī″kō-sfĭng″ō-lĭp′ĭds). A group of carbohydrate-containing fatty acid derivatives of ceramide, q.v. Three classes of these lipids are cerebrosides, gangliosides, and ceramide oligosaccharides. When the enzymes essential to the metabolism of these compounds are absent, the glycosphingolipids accumulate, particularly in the nervous system. Death is the usual outcome.

glycostatic (glī″kō-stăt′ĭk) [Gr. *glykys,* sweet, + *statikos,* standing]. Acting to maintain the level of sugar in the body.

glycosuria (glī″kō-sū′rē-ă) [″ + *ouron,* urine]. The presence of glucose in the urine. Traces of sugar, particularly glucose, may occur in normal urine but are not detected by ordinary qualitative methods. In routine urinalyses the presence of a reducing sugar is suspicious of diabetes mellitus. It is found when the blood sugar level exceeds the renal threshold (about 170 mg/dl of blood). Fasting level of blood glucose is usually between 80 and 120 mg/dl of blood.

Glycosuria may result from pancreatic (insulin) insufficiency; disorders of the endocrine glands, esp. the hypophysis, adrenals, thyroid, or ovaries; excessive carbohy-

drate intake; excessive glycogenolysis; or reduction of renal threshold. SYN: *glycuresis.*

g., alimentary. Glycosuria following ingestion of large amounts of starches or sugars.

g., diabetic. Glycosuria resulting from hyposecretion of insulin.

g., emotional. Glycosuria resulting from emotional states such as worry or anxiety.

g., phloridzin. Glycosuria resulting from the injection of phloridzin, which reduces the renal threshold for glucose.

g., pituitary. Glycosuria resulting from dysfunction of the anterior pituitary.

g., renal. Glycosuria occurring when glucose is persistent and not accompanied by hyperglycemia. It occurs when the renal threshold for glucose is decreased.

glycosyl (glī′kō-sĭl). The radical obtained when a certain OH group is detached from a saccharide.

glycosylated hemoglobin. SEE: *hemoglobin A_{1c};* TREAT under *diabetes mellitus.*

glycotropic (glī″kō-trŏp′ĭk) [″ + *tropos,* a turning]. Acting to antagonize insulin or to increase the blood sugar level.

glycuresis (glī″kū-rē′sĭs) [″ + *ouresis,* urination]. Presence of glucose in the urine. SYN: *glycosuria.*

glycuronuria (glī-kū″rō-nū′rē-ă). Glycuronic acid in the urine.

glycylglycine (glīs″ĭl-glīs′ĭn). The simplest form of a polypeptide.

glycyltryptophan (glīs″ĭl-trĭp′tō-făn). A dipeptide of glycine and tryptophan.

glycyrrhiza (glīs-ĭ-rī′ză) [″ + *rhiza,* root]. NF. The dried root of *Glycyrrhiza glabra,* known commercially as Spanish licorice. Used as an ingredient of glycyrrhiza fluidextract and glycyrrhiza syrup, both of which are used as flavoring agents in compounding medicine. This substance has a weak cortisone-like action. SEE: *licorice.*

glyoxalase (glē-ōk′să-lās). An enzyme that catalyzes the conversion of methylglyoxal to lactic acid by the addition of water.

glyoxylic acid. An acid produced by the action of glycine oxidase on glycine or sarcosine.

Glysennid. Trade name for sennosides A and B.

gm. *gram.*

GML. *glabellomeatal line.* Imaginary line through the glabella and the external auditory meatus.

gnashing. Grinding the teeth. SEE: *bruxism.*

gnat (năt). Any of a number of small insects belonging to the order Diptera, suborder Orthorrhapha. Term applied generally to insects smaller than mosquitoes. Includes black flies, midges, and sandflies.

g., buffalo. A small dipterous insect belonging to the genus *Simulium,* q.v.

gnathalgia (năth-ăl'jē-ă) [Gr. *gnathos,* jaw, + *algos,* pain]. Pain in the jaw. SYN: *gnathodynia.*

gnathic (năth'ĭk) [Gr. *gnathos,* jaw]. Pert. to an alveolar process or to the jaw.

gnathion (năth'ē-ŏn). Lowest point of middle line of lower jaw; a craniometric point.

gnathitis (năth-ī'tĭs) [" + *itis,* inflammation]. Inflammation of the jaw or adjacent soft parts.

gnatho- (năth'ō) [Gr. *gnathos,* jaw]. Prefix pert. to jaw or cheek.

gnathocephalus (năth"ō-sĕf'ă-lŭs) [" + *kephale,* head]. A malformed fetus in which the head consists principally of the jaws.

gnathodynamometer (năth"ō-dī"nă-mŏm'ĕ-tĕr) [" + *dynamis,* power, + *metron,* measure]. Device for measuring biting force.

gnathodynia (năth"ō-dĭn'ē-ă) [" + *odyne,* pain]. Pain in the jaw. SYN: *gnathalgia.*

gnathoplasty (năth'ō-plăs"tē) [" + *plassein,* to form]. Reparative surgery of jaws or cheek.

gnathoschisis (năth-ŏs'kĭ-sĭs) [" + *schizein,* to split]. Congenital jaw cleft.

Gnathostoma (năth-ŏs'tō-mă) [" + *stoma,* mouth]. A genus of nematode worms that infest the stomach walls of domestic and wild animals. They occasionally accidentally infest man.

gnathostomiasis (năth"ō-stō-mī'ă-sĭs). Infestation with *Gnathostoma.*

gnosia (nō'sē-ă) [Gr. *gnosis,* knowledge]. The perceptive faculty of recognizing persons, things, and forms.

gnotobiotics (nō"tō-bī-ŏt'ĭks) [Gr. *gnotos,* known, + *bios,* life]. Study of animals that have been raised in germ-controlled or germ-free surroundings.

GnRH. *gonadotropin-releasing hormone.*

goat's milk. Milk obtained from goats and used in infants who are unable to tolerate cow's milk. It should be pasteurized prior to use.

goblet cell. A type of secretory cell found in the epithelium of the intestinal and respiratory tracts: a unicellular gland that secretes mucus. Mucin droplets accumulate in the distal end of the cell, forming a large ovoid mass that causes the cell to become swollen and distorted in shape. The free surface of the cell finally ruptures and liberates the mucus. SYN: *cell, mucous; chalice cell.* SEE: *cell; gland; mucus; secretion.*

goggle-eyed. Having abnormally protruding eyes. SYN: *exophthalmic.*

goiter (goy'tĕr) [L. *guttur,* throat]. An enlargement of the thyroid gland. SYN: *struma.*

ETIOL: May be due to lack of iodine in diet, thyroiditis, inflammation from infection, tumors, or hyperfunction or hypofunction of the thyroid gland.

g., aberrant. Supernumerary thyroid enlargement.

g., acute. Goiter that grows rapidly.

g., adenomatous. Thyroid enlargement due to growth of encapsulated adenomata.

g., colloid. Goiter in which there is a great increase of follicular contents.

g., congenital. Goiter present at birth.

g., cystic. Goiter in which a cyst or cysts are formed. May result from the degeneration of tissue or liquefaction within an adenoma.

g., diffuse. Goiter in which the thyroid tissue is diffuse in contrast to its nodular form as in adenomatous goiter.

g., diving. A movable goiter, located either below or above the sternal notch.

g., endemic. Goiter development in certain geographic localities, esp. those in which iodine is deficient in food and water.

g., exophthalmic. Goiter with exophthalmos. SYN: *Graves' disease; hyperthyroidism: thyrotoxicosis.*

SYM: Bulging eyeballs, i.e., exophthalmos, generally present; enlarged thyroid, tremor of fingers and muscles of hands, tachycardia, increased metabolism, vomiting and diarrhea, profuse perspiration, nervous irritability, skin eruptions, emaciation, anemia, hyperglycemia. Goiters are more prevalent in fresh water and lake areas and less so on the sea coast, due to the lack of iodine in fresh water. Iodine, iodized salt, and antithyroid drugs are used in treating the disease. SEE: *thyroid storm.*

ETIOL: Unknown, but may be related to malfunction of the immune system. Incidence is higher in females.

DIAG: The disease is diagnosed by using laboratory tests that measure the levels of various thyroid hormones in the serum, or the ability of the thyroid gland to take up radioactive iodine. SEE: *Graves' ophthalmopathy.*

NURSING IMPLICATIONS: Evaluate for blood pressure elevation, cardiac dysrhythmias, and emotional stress. Help the patient cope with related anxiety. Promote high-protein, high-calorie nutrition to counteract increased protein catabolism. Teach the patient comfort measures to deal with elevated body temperature and GI complaints (abdominal cramps, frequent bowel movements). Protect the patient from eye injuries. Follow special instructions related to therapeutic use of radioactive iodide.

g., fibrous. Goiter with hyperplastic capsule and struma of the thyroid gland.

g., follicular. G., parenchymatous.

g., hyperplastic. G., parenchymatous.

g., intrathoracic. Goiter in which a portion of the thyroid tissue lies within the thoracic cavity.

g., lingual. Hypertrophied mass forming a tumor at the posterior portion of the dorsum of the tongue.

g., nodular. Enlarged thyroid that contains nodules.

g., parenchymatous. Goiter characterized by multiplication of cells lining the follicles or alveoli. There is usually a reduction in colloid, and the follicular cavities assume various sizes and are often obliterated by infoldings of their walls. Fibrous tissue may increase markedly. Iodine content of gland is low. Goiter usually of a diffuse nature.

g., perivascular. Goiter surrounding a large blood vessel.

g., retrovascular. Goiter development behind a large blood vessel.

g., simple. Thyroid gland hyperplasia unaccompanied by constitutional symptoms.

g., substernal. Enlargement of lower part of thyroid isthmus.

g., suffocative. Goiter that causes shortness of breath due to pressure.

g., toxic. Exophthalmic goiter or goiter in which there is an excessive production of the thyroid hormone. SEE: *goiter, exophthalmic.*

g., vascular. Goiter due to distention of blood vessels of thyroid gland.

goitrogens (goy'trō-jĕns) [L. *guttur*, throat, + *gennan*, to produce]. Substances that cause goiters. They occur in nature in certain foods, including turnips, rutabaga, and cabbage.

gold. SYMB: Au (from L. *aurum*, gold). At. wt. 196.967; at. no. 79; sp. gr. 19.32. A metallic element, yellow in color. Its salts have been used in early rheumatoid arthritis and in nondisseminated lupus erythematosus. Radioactive gold, Au 198 injection, is used in treatment of certain types of cancer and as an aid in outlining certain organs, as in liver scanning. SEE: *scanning.*

g. alloy. An alloy of gold with copper, silver, platinum, or others added for strength or hardness. Pure gold is rated 24 carats. Gold that contains other metals in the alloy are less than 24 carats. Thus, 18 parts of gold mixed with 6 parts of another metal would be rated as 18 carat gold.

g. alloy, dental casting. A hard or extrahard alloy used principally for crowns, inlays, clasps, splints, and orthodontic and prosthetic appliances.

G. Au 198 Injection. USP. A sterile colloidal solution of radioactive gold (^{198}Au).

g. sodium thiomalate. USP. A water-soluble gold preparation. Has been used in treating rheumatoid arthritis when there was active inflammation of joints. Trade name is Myochrysine.

goldbeater's skin. A strong, thin membrane prepared from the cecum of the ox. It has been used as a surgical dressing.

Goldblatt kidney [Harry Goldblatt, U.S. physician, 1891–1977]. Kidney of a dog that has been deprived of part of its blood supply in order to induce hypertension experimentally. This condition may occur in humans due to vascular disease.

gold standard. In medical care and experimental medicine, a therapeutic action, drug, or procedure that is the best that is currently available and to which other therapeutic actions, drugs, or procedures are compared in order to determine if they are as effective or better than the "gold standard."

Golgi apparatus (gŏl'jē) [Camillo Golgi, It. pathologist, 1843–1926]. A lamellar membranous structure near the nucleus of almost all cells. It contains curved parallel series of flattened saccules that are often expanded at their ends. The structure is best seen by electron microscopy. In secretory cells the apparatus functions to concentrate and package the secretory product. Its function in other cells, though apparently important, is poorly understood.

Golgi's cells or neurons. Multipolar nerve cells in the cerebral cortex and posterior horns of spinal cord. Type I possesses long axons, and Type II possesses short axons.

Golgi's tendon organ. ABBR: GTO. This structure is thought to function as a feedback system which works to sense muscle tension through tendon stretch, inhibit muscle contraction of the agonist and facilitate contraction of the antagonist muscle. The purpose of this mechanism, known as autogenic facilitation, is to prevent overuse and damage to the muscle and corresponding joint.

Goll's tract (gölz) [Friedrich Goll, Swiss anatomist, 1829–1903]. Tract in the posterior white column of the spinal cord. SYN: *fasciculus gracilis* [NA].

Golytely. Trade name for polyethylene glycol electrolyte for gastrointestinal lavage solution.

gomphosis (gŏm-fō'sĭs) [Gr., bolting together]. [NA] A conical process fitting into a socket in an immovable joint.

Ex.: a tooth in its bony socket in the alveolus.

gonad (gō'năd, gŏn'ăd) [Gr. *gone*, seed]. 1. The embryonic sex gland before differentiation into definitive testis or ovary. 2. A generic term referring to both the female sex glands, or ovaries, and the male sex glands, or testes. Each forms the cells necessary for human reproduction, spermatozoa from the testes, ova from the ovaries.

INTERNAL SECRETIONS: *Female:* The vesicular follicles of the ovaries secrete estrogen, which is important in regulating and controlling female reproductive function including the development of secondary sex characteristics. The corpus luteum produces progesterone, which helps to prepare the lining of the uterus (endometrium) to receive and assist in the implantation of the fertilized ovum. *Male:* The interstitial cells of the testes secrete the androgen testosterone, which stimulates metabolism, increases muscular strength, and influences the development of secondary sex characteristics.

Hormones from both sexes have been isolated and standardized and are used in the treatment of conditions arising from an insufficiency of these hormones. SEE: *estrogen; ovary; testicle; testosterone.*

gonadal (gō′năd-ăl). Pert. to a gonad. SYN: *gonadial.*

gonadal dysgenesis. Congenital endocrine disorder caused by failure of the ovaries to respond to pituitary hormone (gonadotropin) stimulation. Clinically there are amenorrhea, failure of sexual maturation, and usually short stature. About one third of these patients have webbing of the neck, and many have marked cubitus valgus, q.v. Intelligence may be impaired. These patients usually have only 45 chromosomes, the second X chromosome being absent. SYN: *Turner's syndrome.*

gonadectomy (gŏn-ă-dĕk′tō-mē) [Gr. *gonos,* genitals, + *ektome,* excision]. Excision of a testis or ovary.

gonadial (gō-năd′ē-ăl). Pert. to a reproductive gland. SYN: *gonadal.*

gonadopathy (gŏn″ă-dŏp′ă-thē) [″ + *pathos,* disease, suffering]. Any disease of the sexual glands.

gonadotherapy (gŏn″ă-dō-thĕr′ă-pē) [″ + *therapeia,* treatment]. Treatment by injection of extracts containing testicular or ovarian hormones.

gonadotrope (gŏ-năd′ō-trōp) [″ + *trope,* turning]. A gonadotrophic hormone.

gonadotrophic (gŏn″ă-dō-trŏf′ĭk) [″ + *trophe,* nourishment]. Rel. to stimulation of the gonads.

gonadotrophic hormones. Gonadotropins, q.v., or gonad-stimulating hormones.

gonadotropin (gŏn″ă-dō-trō′pĭn). A gonad-stimulating hormone.

  g.'s, anterior pituitary. Hormones produced by the anterior lobe of the hypophysis. Include the follicle-stimulating hor-

mone (FSH) and luteinizing hormone (LH). In the male this is called the interstitial cell-stimulating hormone (ICSH).

  g., chorionic. Gonadotropins produced by the chorionic villi of the placenta. They are present in the blood and urine of pregnant women and in the blood of pregnant mares. Detection of their presence in urine is the basis of the pregnancy tests. SYN: *hormone, anterior pituitary.*

gonadotropin-releasing hormone. The releasing hormone produced in the hypothalamus. It acts on the pituitary to cause release of the gonadotrophic substances luteinizing hormone and follicle-stimulating hormone. This hormone is approved for use in treating endometriosis.

gonaduct (gŏn′ă-dŭkt) [″ + L. *ductus,* canal]. The seminal duct or the oviduct.

gonalgia (gō-năl′jē-ă) [Gr. *gony,* knee, + *algos,* pain]. Pain in the knee.

gonangiectomy (gŏn″ăn-jē-ĕk′tō-mē) [Gr. *gone,* seed, + *angeion,* vessel, + *ektome,* excision]. Excision of the vas deferens or a part of it. SYN: *vasectomy.*

gonarthritis (gŏn″ăr-thrī′tĭs) [Gr. *gony,* knee, + *arthron,* joint, + *itis,* inflammation]. Inflammation of knee joint.

gonarthromeningitis (gŏn-ăr″thrō-měn-ĭn-jī′tĭs) [″ + ″ + *meninx,* membrane, + *itis,* inflammation]. Synovitis of the knee joint.

gonarthrotomy (gŏn″ăr-thrŏt′ō-mē) [″ + ″ + *tome,* incision]. Incision of knee joint.

gonatocele (gŏn-ăt′ō-sēl) [″ + *kele,* tumor, swelling]. White swelling; tumor of the knee.

gonecyst, gonecystis (gŏn′ē-sĭst, gŏn-ē-sĭs′tĭs) [Gr. *gone,* seed, + *kystis,* a bladder]. A seminal vesicle.

gonecystitis (gŏn″ē-sĭs-tī′tĭs) [″ + ″ + *itis,* inflammation]. Inflammation of seminal vesicles.

gonecystolith (gŏn″ē-sĭs′tō-lĭth) [″ + ″ + *lithos,* stone]. A concretion or calculus in a seminal vesicle.

Gongylonema (gŏn″jĭ-lō-nē′mă) [Gr. *gongylos,* round, + *nema,* thread]. A genus of nematode worms belonging to the suborder Spirurata. They are parasitic in the wall of the esophagus and stomach of domestic animals. Occasionally, they are accidental parasites in man. *G. pulchrum* is the species most frequently involved.

goniometer (gō″nē-ŏm′ē-ter) [Gr. *gonia,* angle, + *metron,* measure]. Apparatus to measure joint movements and angles. Various sizes and types of goniometers are available, including finger goniometers, bubble goniometers, gravity goniometers, and recording electrogoniometers.

gonion (gō′nē-ŏn) [Gr. *gonia,* angle]. Point of

angle of the mandible or lower jaw.

goniopuncture (gō″nē-ō-pŭnk′tūr). Surgical procedure for allowing aqueous humor to drain from the eye. Used in treating glaucoma.

gonioscope (gō′nē-ō-skōp) [″ + *skopein*, to examine]. An instrument for inspecting the angle of the anterior chamber of the eye and for determining ocular motility and rotation.

goniosynechia (gō″nē-ō-sĭ-nĕk′ē-ă). Adhesion of the iris to the cornea of the eye.

goniotomy (gō″nē-ŏt′ō-mē) [″ + *tome*, incision]. Surgical procedure for removing obstructions to the free flow of aqueous humor into the canal of Schlemm of the eye.

gono-, gon- (gŏn′ō) [Gr. *gonos*, genitals]. Prefix meaning generation, genitals, offspring, semen.

gonocide (gŏn′ō-sīd) [″ + L. *caedere*, to kill]. Destructive to the gonococcus.

gonococcal (gŏn″ō-kŏk′ăl) [″ + *kokkos*, berry]. Rel. to or caused by gonococci.

gonococcal conjunctivitis. SEE: *conjunctivitis, gonorrheal.*

gonococcemia (gŏn″ō-kŏk-sē′mē-ă) [″ + ″ + *haima*, blood]. Gonococci in the blood. SYN: *gonohemia.*

gonococci (gŏn″ō-kŏk′ sī). Pl. of gonococcus.

gonococcic (gŏn″ō-kŏk′sĭk) [″ + *kokkos*, berry]. Pert. to the gonococcus.

gonococcic smears. Stains used are Gram's method and methylene blue. Gonococci appear in pairs and tetrads. They are gram-negative and intracellular.

gonococcide (gŏn″ō-kŏk′sīd) [″ + ″ + L. *caedere*, to kill]. An agent that kills gonococci.

gonococcocide (gŏn″ō-kŏk′ō-sīd). Gonococcide.

gonococcus (gŏn″ō-kŏk′ŭs) [Gr. *gonos*, genitals, + *kokkos*, berry] (pl. *gonococci*). The organism causing gonorrhea, a member of the species *Neisseria gonorrhoeae.* It is an intracellular diplococcus and tends to occur in pairs. It is classified as a gram-negative bacterium and may be found in or on the genitals, in the blood, the joints, the heart, the eye, urine, feces, and in boils. SEE: *gonorrhea.*

gonocyte (gŏn′ō-sīt) [″ + *kytos*, cell]. The primitive reproductive cell.

gonohemia (gŏn″ō-hē′mē-ă) [″ + *haima*, blood]. Gonococcal septicemia. SYN: *gonococcemia.*

gonorrhea (gŏn″ō-rē′ă) [″ + *rhoia*, flow]. A specific, contagious, catarrhal inflammation of the genital mucous membrane of either sex. The disease also may affect other structures of the body such as the heart, conjunctiva, oral mucosa, rectum, or joints. In the female the parts involved may be the urethra, vulva, vulvovaginal glands, vagina, endocervix, Skene's glands, Bartholin's glands, or fallopian tubes. SEE: *safe sex; Universal Precautions* in *Appendix.*

SYM: *Male:* Yellow mucopurulent discharge from the penis resulting from inflammation of the urethra. May become deep-seated and affect the prostate. Slow, difficult, and painful urination, and sometimes painful induration of the penis.

Caution: It was previously thought that gonorrhea in the male was always symptomatic. This is not true, and suspected cases should always have cultures for the gonococcus. To be certain the patient is cured, the infected sites should be cultured one and two weeks after completion of treatment.

NOTE: In either sex, it is important to obtain a serological test for syphilis prior to starting antibiotic therapy. Penicillin therapy may mask a case of syphilis. Also, it is important to test all sexual contacts of the patient for presence of gonorrhea and syphilis.

Female: Gonorrhea in the female may be asymptomatic, and even when symptoms are present, they may not cause enough discomfort for the patient to seek medical care. Symptoms include one or more of the following: urethral or vaginal discharge; painful or frequent urination; lower abdominal pain; tenderness in the area of Bartholin's and Skene's glands; acute pelvic inflammatory disease.

ETIOL: Infection by the gonococcus, *Neisseria gonorrhoeae.*

DIAG: Gram's stain of the urethral discharge is almost 100% accurate in diagnosing gonorrhea in the male. This is not true for the female. The material for diagnosis in the female should be obtained from multiple sites including the cervix, vaginal vault, and urethra, and by milking of Bartholin's and Skene's glands. The material should be inoculated without delay on Thayer-Martin medium. It is important to evaluate the patient for presence of other sexually transmitted diseases, including syphilis and Chlamydia.

PROPH: Use of condoms during sexual activity or avoidance of contact with infected persons; immediate penicillin as a preventive following contact. In newborn, instillation of one drop of 1% silver nitrate in conjunctival sac of each eye. If the mother has gonorrhea, both she and the infant should be treated with parenteral penicillin. SEE: *ophthalmia neonatorum.*

TREAT: Amoxocillin plus probenicid, except in cases due to penicillinase-producing strains of *Neisseria gonorrhoeae* (PPNG). In those individuals, the drug of choice is spectinomycin I.M. or cefoxitin I.M. with oral probenecid. Give doxycycline or tetracycline in addition to the other drug to cure a concurrent Chlamydial infection. Neither of these drugs alone is considered to be adequate therapy for gonorrhea. Also, spectinomycin is not effective for pharyngeal gonococcal infection. Local therapy may be required for eradication of foci of infection in the female, involving such structures as Skene's duct, Bartholin's glands, and the cervix.

PROG: The inflammation may clear up without serious results, or it may become chronic (involving deeper tissues and producing urethral stricture) or produce complications (prostatitis, epididymitis, orchitis, cystitis, arthritis, and endocarditis). No case of acute gonorrhea in the female should be considered cured until three successive negative smears from the cervix and Bartholin's and Skene's glands are obtained, at least two of which should be examined immediately after a menstrual period.

NURSING IMPLICATIONS: Instruct the patient to take antibiotics as prescribed, to have moist heat applied or sitz baths done as ordered, and to refrain from sexual intercourse until the disease has been properly treated. The patient should also know that his or her sexual contacts should receive treatment. Discuss prevention of future infections. Wear gloves and eye protection when obtaining cultures or specimens from persons suspected of having gonorrhea.

Assess patient for allergies, especially antibiotic sensitivity, and observe for drug reactions. Warn patient that infection will continue and can be transmitted until cultures become negative. Double bag contaminated instruments and soiled dressings. Report case and known sexual contacts to local public health department. SEE: *Nursing Diagnoses* in *Appendix*.

gonorrheal. Of the nature of or pert. to gonorrhea.

gonorrheal arthritis. Arthritis or rheumatism resulting from gonorrheal infection.

Gonyaulax catanella (gŏn″ē-aw′lăks). A species of plankton that causes certain shellfish that eat them to become toxic. It is also one of the causes of "red tide" when present in massive numbers in the ocean, a condition that has occurred on certain beaches of North America. Shellfish present in such water contain the toxin present in the plankton.

gonycampsis (gŏn″ĭ-kămp′sĭs) [Gr. *gony*, knee, + *kampsis*, bending]. Abnormal curvature of the knee.

gonycrotesis (gŏn″ĭ-krō-tē′sĭs) [″ + *krotesis*, knocking]. Knock-knee, genu valgum.

gonyectyposis (gŏn″ē-ĕk-tĭ-pō′sĭs) [″ + *ektyposis*, modeling in relief]. Bowlegs. SYN: *genu varum*.

gonyocele (gŏn′ē-ō-sēl) [″ + *kele*, swelling]. Tuberculous synovitis of the knee.

gonyoncus (gŏn″ē-ŏn′kŭs) [″ + *onkos*, tumor]. Tumor of the knee.

Goodell's sign [William Goodell, U.S. gynecologist, 1829–1894]. Softening of the cervix in pregnancy.

Goodpasture's syndrome [Ernest William Goodpasture, U.S. pathologist, 1886–1960]. Progressive glomerulonephritis, hemoptysis, and hemosiderosis. It is a rare disease. Death is usually due to renal failure.

Good Samaritan Law. Legal stipulation for protection of those who give first aid in an emergency situation. The necessity for such legislation arose when physicians who assisted in giving emergency care were later accused of malpractice by the victim.

goose flesh. A skin reaction caused by erection of skin papillae from cold or shock due to contraction of the arrector pili muscles. This causes transient roughness of the skin. SYN: *cutis anserina; piloerection.*

Gordon's reflex [Alfred Gordon, U.S. neurologist, 1874–1953]. Extension of great toe when sudden pressure is made on deep flexor muscles of calf of leg. It is present in pyramidal tract disease. SEE: *Babinski's reflex.*

Gore-Tex. Trade name for a synthetic fabric that has the properties of being waterproof and yet allowing moisture in the form of water vapor to escape through it. SEE: *polytetrafluoroethylene; Teflon.*

gorget (gor′jĕt) [Fr. *gorge*, throat, because of shape of instrument]. An instrument grooved to protect soft tissues from injury as a pointed instrument is inserted in a body cavity.

Gossypium (gŏ-sĭp′ē-ŭm) [L.]. A genus of perennial shrub of the Malvaceae family. Widely grown because of cotton fiber derived from the covering of seeds. Bark of some species is diuretic, emmenagogic, and oxytocic. SEE: *cotton; gossypol.*

gossypol. A toxic chemical present in cottonseed. It has been used experimentally as an infertility agent in the male.

GOT. *glutamic-oxaloacetic transaminase.* SYN: *aspartate aminotransferase.*

gouge (gowj). Instrument for cutting away hard tissue of bone.

goundou (goon′doo) [African]. Condition of periostitis of the nasal processes of the maxillae due to prior infection with yaws or syphilis. The nasal bones become quite enlarged, and the orbit may be involved. The appearance of the nose has been characterized colloquially as "big nose" or "dog nose." SEE: *anakré*.

gout (gowt) [L. *gutta*, drop]. Hereditary metabolic disease that is a form of acute arthritis and is marked by inflammation of the joints. Joints affected may be at any location, but gout usually begins in the knee or foot.

SYM: Most persons with hyperuricemia are asymptomatic. When an attack of acute gouty arthritis does develop, it usually begins at night with moderate pain that increases in intensity to the point where no body position provides relief.

ETIOL: Excessive uric acid in blood and deposits of urates of sodium in and around joints. Several different metabolic abnormalities may cause hyperuricemia.

TREAT: Acute gout responds to colchicine. Nonsteroidal anti-inflammatory agents are also useful in acute attacks. Long-term therapy is directed to preventing hyperuricemia by giving uricosuric drugs such as probenecid or allopurinol. Patients with gout have a tendency to form uric acid kidney stones. To help prevent this, fluids should be forced at the rate of 3 liters each day. Because salicylates interact to interfere with the uricosuric action of either probenecid or allopurinol, they should be avoided.

DIET: Should be well balanced and devoid of purine-rich foods.

NURSING IMPLICATIONS: Assess patient for hypertension, back pain, albuminuria or other indicators of nephrolithiasis or renal dysfunction, low-grade fever, and inflamed joints (hot, tender, dusky-red or cyanotic). During the acute phase the patient is usually placed on bedrest for the initial 24 hours, and with the affected joints elevated and immobilized and protected by a bed-cradle. Administer analgesics and apply compresses (hot or cold) as prescribed for pain relief. Administer colchicine, allopurinol, probenecid, or other prescribed drugs, teaching patient about and assessing for side effects while evaluating for desired therapeutic effect. Encourage oral fluid intake to 3000 ml per day to promote uric acid excretion and prevent kidney stone formation, monitoring serum uric acid levels and alkalinizing urine with sodium bicarbonate if prescribed. Instruct patient concerning low-purine diet and explain the importance of gradual weight reduction if obesity is a factor. If soft-tissue tophi are present, teach patient to wear soft clothing to cover these areas, thus preventing irritation and rupture, and to use meticulous skin care and sterile dressings to prevent infection of open lesions. Explain that surgery may be required to excise or drain infected or ulcerated tophi or to correct joint deformities or improve joint function. However, be aware of and teach patients that even minor surgery may precipitate gout attacks (usually within 24 to 96 hours after surgery). SEE: *Nursing Diagnoses* in *Appendix*.

   g., abarticular. Gout that involves structures other than the joints.

   g., chronic. Persistent form of gout.

   g., lead. Gout-like symptoms associated with lead poisoning. SYN: *saturnine gout*.

   g., saturnine. G., lead.

   g., tophaceous. Gout marked by the development of tophi (deposits of sodium urate) in the joints, the external ear, and about the fingernails.

gouty. Of the nature of or rel. to gout.

gouty diathesis. Predisposition to gout.

Gowers' sign or maneuver [Sir William R. Gowers, Brit. neurologist, 1845–1915]. A clinical sign of muscular dystrophy in childhood, evidenced through observation of children's use of their arms to push themselves erect by moving their hands up their thighs. This permits assuming the standing position from one of kneeling. It is indicative of weakness of the hip and knee extensors.

Gowers' tract (gow'ĕrz). Tract formed of fibers from posterior roots of lateral tract of the spinal cord reaching the cerebellum by way of the superior peduncle.

G.P. *general practitioner.*

G-6-PD. *glucose-6-phosphate dehydrogenase.*

GPT. *glutamic-pyruvic transaminase.* SYN: *alanine aminotransferase.*

gr. *grain.*

graafian follicle (grăf'ē-ăn) [Regnier de Graaf, Dutch physician and anatomist, 1641–1673]. A mature vesicular follicle of the ovary. Beginning with puberty and continuing until the menopause, except during pregnancy, a graafian follicle develops at approx. monthly intervals. Each follicle contains a nearly mature ovum (an oocyte) that, upon rupture of the follicle, is discharged from the ovary, a process called ovulation. Ovulation occurs usually about the 13th day of the menstrual cycle, dated from the first day of the menstrual period. Within the ruptured graafian follicle, the corpus luteum develops. Both the follicle and the corpus luteum are glands of internal secretion, the former secreting estrogens, and the latter, estrogen and progesterone. SEE: *ovum* for illus.

gracile (grăs'īl) [L. *gracilis*, slender]. Slender; slight.

gracile nucleus. Mass of medullary gray matter terminating the funiculus gracilis.

gracilis (grăs'ĭ-lĭs) [L., slender]. A long

slender muscle on the medial aspect of the thigh.

gradatim (gră-dă'tĭm) [L.]. Gradually or by degrees.

Gradenigo's syndrome (gră-dĕn-ē'gōz) [Giuseppe Gradenigo, It. physician, 1859–1926]. Suppurative otitis media with abducens nerve paralysis and pain in temporal region.

gradient (grā'dē-ĕnt). A slope or grade; an increase or decrease of varying degrees or the curve that represents such.

　g., axial. A gradient of physiological or metabolic activity exhibited by embryos and many adult animals, the principal one of which follows the main axis of the body, being highest at the anterior end and lowest at the posterior end.

graduate (grăd'ū-āt, -ăt) [L. gradus, a step]. 1. A vessel marked by lines for measuring liquids. 2. One who has been awarded an academic or professional degree from a college or university.

graduated. Marked by a series of lines indicating degrees of measurement, weight, or volume.

graduated tenotomy. Partial surgical division of tendon of an eye muscle.

Graefe's sign (grā'fēz) [Albrecht von Graefe, Ger. ophthalmologist, 1828–1870]. Failure of the upper lid to follow a downward movement of the eyeball when the patient changes his or her vision from looking up to looking down. Seen in Graves' disease (hyperthyroidism) with exophthalmos.

graft (grăft) [L. graphium, grafting knife]. 1. Tissue that is transplanted or implanted in a part of the body to repair a defect. Homograft involves grafting material from another individual of the same species. Heterograft indicates that the grafted tissue or organ was obtained from a species different from the recipient. 2. The process of placing tissue at a different site than from where it was derived to repair a defect.
　RS: autograft; transplantation; zoografting.

　g., allogeneic. Graft from a genetically nonidentical donor of the same species as the recipient. SYN: allograft.

　g., autodermic. G., autogenous.

　g., autogenous. Graft taken from another part of the patient's body.

　g., autologous. G., autogenous.

　g., avascular. Graft in which vascular infiltration does not occur.

　g., bone. A piece of bone generally taken from the tibia and inserted elsewhere in the body to replace another osseous structure. Banks for storage of bone have been established.

　g., cable. Nerve graft made up of bundles of segments from an unimportant nerve.

　g., cadaver. Grafting tissue, including skin, cornea, or bone, obtained from a body immediately after death.

　g., delayed. A skin graft that is partially elevated and then replaced so that it may be moved later to another site.

　g., dermal. A split-skin or full-thickness skin graft. The graft will grow hair and have active sweat and sebum glands.

　g., fascia. Use of fascia usually removed from the fascia lata for repairing defects in other tissues.

　g., fascicular. Nerve graft with each bundle of nerves being separately sutured.

　g., free. Graft that is completely separated from its original site and then transferred.

　g., full-thickness. Graft of the entire layer of skin without the subcutaneous fat.

　g., gingival. A sliding graft employing the gingival papilla as the graft material.

　g., heterodermic. Graft in which the donor is of another species.

　g., heteroplastic. Graft taken from another person.

　g., heterotopic. SEE: transplant, heterotopic.

　g., homologous. Graft in which the donor is of the same species as the recipient.

　g., isologous. Graft in which the donor and recipient are genetically identical, i.e., are usually identical twins. SYN: isograft.

　g., lamellar. Very thin corneal graft used to replace surface layer of opaque corneal tissue.

　g., mesh. Split-skin graft which contains multiple perforations or slits. These slits allow the graft to be expanded so that a much larger area is covered. The holes in the graft are covered by new tissue as the graft spreads.

　g., nerve. Transplantation of a healthy nerve to replace a segment of a damaged nerve.

　g., Ollier-Thiersch. Wide, thin strips of skin used to cover a wound.

　g., omental. Use of a portion of the omentum to cover or repair a defect in a hollow viscus, or to cover a suture line in an abdominal organ.

　g., ovarian. Implantation of a section of an ovary into the muscles of the abdominal wall.

　g., pedicle. A skin graft that is left attached at one end until the free end has begun to receive nourishment from the new site.

　g., periosteum. Application of a piece of bone and its periosteum to another site.

　g., pinch. Graft consisting of small bits of skin.

g., postmortem. Tissue taken from a body after death and stored under proper conditions to be used later on a patient requiring a graft of such tissue.

g., punch. Full-thickness graft, usually circular, for transplanting skin containing hair follicles to a bald area.

g., rope. G., cable.

g., sieve. Graft in which a section of skin is removed except for small, regularly spaced areas that remain. The removed portion is used at the new site. The small remaining areas will grow to cover the entire area at the donor site. Similar to mesh graft.

g., skin. Removal of small sections of skin to a clean, raw surface, such as a large superficial burn.

g.'s, split-skin. Grafts of a part of the skin thickness.

g., sponge. Small piece of sponge placed over an ulcerating part to stimulate epidermal growth.

g., thick-split. Grafts of about half or more of the thickness of the skin.

g., Thiersch's. Graft in which only epidermis and small amount of dermis are used.

g.'s, Wolfe's. Graft in which the whole thickness of the skin is used.

g., zooplastic. Graft taken from an animal.

grafting. Implantation of skin or tissue from a healthy site to an injured site.

graft-versus-host reaction. The pathological reaction between the host and tissue grafted. Occurs when the host's immune response is deficient because of immunosuppressive therapy.

Graham's law (grā'ămz) [Thomas Graham, Brit. chemist, 1805–1869]. The rate of diffusion of a gas is inversely proportional to the square root of its density.

grain [L. *granum*]. 1. The seed or seedlike fruit of many members of the grass family, esp. corn, wheat, oats, and other cereals. 2. A weight; 0.065 of a gram. ABBR: gr. 3. Direction of fibers or layers.

gram. ABBR: gm; g. A unit of weight (mass) of the metric system. It equals approx. the weight of a cubic centimeter or a milliliter of water. It is equal to 15.432 grains or 0.03527 ounce (avoirdupois). One thousand grams equal one kilogram. SEE: table.

gram-equivalent. In chemistry, the weight in grams of a substance that will react with one gram of hydrogen.

gramicidin (grăm"ĭ-sī'dĭn). USP. One of the antibiotics produced by *Bacillus brevis.*

grammeter. A unit of work energy equivalent to that expended in raising a weight of one gram vertically one meter.

Gram's method [Hans C. J. Gram, Danish physician, 1853–1938]. A method for stain-

ing bacteria. It is of importance in the identification of bacteria.

PROCEDURE: Prepare a film on a slide, dry, and fix with heat. Stain with aniline gentian violet of ammonium oxalate crystal violet one minute. Rinse in water, then immerse in Gram's iodine solution for one minute. Rinse off iodine solution and decolorize in 95% ethyl alcohol or acetone. Counterstain with dilute carbolfuchsin or safranine for 30 seconds. Rinse with water, blot dry, and examine. Gram-positive bacteria will retain the violet stain and gram-negative bacteria will adopt the red counterstain.

NOTE: In order to provide a simple means of checking on the accuracy of the staining materials, a small amount of material from between one's teeth can be placed on the slide at the opposite end from that of the specimen being examined. Gram-negative and gram-positive organisms are always present in the mouth. Thus, that end of the slide is examined first. If both types of organisms are seen, proceed to examine the specimen.

gram molecule. The weight in grams of a substance equal to its molecular weight. SYN: *mole.*

gram-negative. Losing the stain and taking the color of the red counterstain in Gram's method of staining. A primary characteristic of certain microorganisms. SEE: *Gram's method;* table.

gram-positive. Retaining the color of the gentian violet stain in Gram's method of staining. SEE: *Gram's method;* table.

Grancher's disease (grän-shăz') [Jacques J. Grancher, Fr. physician, 1843–1907]. Pneumonia with splenization, q.v., of the lung. SYN: *splenopneumonia.*

Grancher's sign. Raised pitch of expiratory murmur in pulmonary consolidation.

grandiose (grän'dē-ōs). In psychiatry, concerning one's unrealistic and exaggerated concept of self-worth, importance, wealth, and ability.

grandiosity. An exaggerated sense of self-importance, power, or status.

grand mal (grän măl) [Fr., great evil]. SEE: *epilepsy.*

grand rounds, medical. SEE: *medical grand rounds.*

granular [L. *granulum*, little grain]. Of the nature of granules. Roughened by prominences like those of seeds.

granular cast. Coarse or fine granule, short and plump, sometimes yellowish, similar to hyaline cast. Soluble in acetic acid. Seen in inflammatory and degenerative nephropathies. SEE: *cast.*

granulatio (grăn"ū-lā'shē-ō) [L.]. A granule.

Gram Conversion into Ounces (Avoirdupois)*

Gm	Oz	Gm	Oz	Gm	Oz	Gm	Oz
1	0.03	30	1.06	59	2.08	88	3.10
2	0.07	31	1.09	60	2.12	89	3.14
3	0.11	32	1.13	61	2.15	90	3.17
4	0.14	33	1.16	62	2.18	91	3.21
5	0.18	34	1.20	63	2.22	92	3.24
6	0.21	35	1.23	64	2.26	93	3.28
7	0.25	36	1.27	65	2.29	94	3.31
8	0.28	37	1.30	66	2.33	95	3.35
9	0.32	38	1.34	67	2.36	96	3.38
10	0.35	39	1.37	68	2.40	97	3.42
11	0.39	40	1.41	69	2.43	98	3.46
12	0.42	41	1.44	70	2.47	99	3.49
13	0.45	42	1.48	71	2.50	100	3.53
14	0.49	43	1.51	72	2.54	125	4.41
15	0.53	44	1.55	73	2.57	150	5.30
16	0.56	45	1.59	74	2.61	175	6.18
17	0.60	46	1.62	75	2.64	200	7.05
18	0.63	47	1.65	76	2.68	250	8.82
19	0.67	48	1.69	77	2.71	300	10.58
20	0.70	49	1.73	78	2.75	350	12.34
21	0.74	50	1.76	79	2.79	400	14.11
22	0.77	51	1.80	80	2.82	450	15.87
23	0.81	52	1.83	81	2.85	454	16.00
24	0.84	53	1.87	82	2.89	500	17.64
25	0.88	54	1.90	83	2.93	600	21.16
26	0.91	55	1.94	84	2.96	700	24.69
27	0.95	56	1.97	85	3.00	800	28.22
28	0.99	57	2.01	86	3.03	900	30.75
29	1.02	58	2.04	87	3.07	1000	35.27

* One gram is equal to 0.03527 ounce (avoirdupois).

granulation. 1. Formation of granules or state or condition of being granular. 2. Fleshy projections formed on the surface of a gaping wound that is not healing by first intention or indirect union. Each granulation represents the outgrowth of new capillaries by budding from the existing capillaries and then joining up into capillary loops supported by cells that will later become fibrous scar tissue. Granulations bring a rich blood supply to the healing surface.

g., arachnoidal. Villuslike projections of the subarachnoid layer of the meninges that project into the superior sagittal sinus and other venous sinuses of the brain. Through them, cerebrospinal fluid re-enters the bloodstream. SYN: *pacchionian bodies.*

g., exuberant. An excessive mass of granulation tissue formed in the healing of a wound or ulcer; proud flesh.

granule (grăn′ūl) [L. *granulum*, little grain]. 1. A small, grainlike body. 2. In histology, a minute mass in a cell that has an outline but no apparent structure.

g.'s, acidophil. Granules that stain readily with acid dyes.

g., albuminous. Cytoplasmic granule in many normal cells. Not affected by ether or chloroform, but disappears from view when acetic acid is added.

g., Altmann's. Mitochondria.

g., amphophil. Granule that stains with both acid and basic dyes. SYN: *g., beta.*

g., azurophil. Granule that takes a stain with azure dyes easily. Found in lymphocytes and monocytes; small and red or reddish-purple in color. They are inconstant in number, being present in about 30% of the cells.

g., basal. A small, deeply staining granule, found in certain protozoa, from which the flagellum arises. SYN: *blepharoplast.*

g.'s, basophil. Cellular granules that stain with a basic dye.

g., beta. An azurophil granule found in beta cells of the hypophysis or islets of Langerhans of the pancreas. SYN: *g., amphophil.*

g., chromophil. Granule of chromophil substance present in the cytoplasm of neu-

Some of the Gram-Negative Bacteria

Genus	Species	Colloquial or Old Names	Disease Caused in Man
Bordetella	B. pertussis	Bordet-Gengou bacillus	Whooping cough
Brucella	B. melitensis	Micrococcus melitensis	Brucellosis
	B. abortus	Bang's bacillus	
	B. suis		
Escherichia	E. coli	Bacillus coli	Occasionally suppuration, cystitis, pyelitis
Hemophilus	H. influenzae	Pfeiffer's bacillus	Meningitis and conjunctivitis
Klebsiella	K. pneumoniae	Pneumobacillus or Bacillus mucosus capsulatus	Occasionally pneumonia
Legionella	L. pneumophila		Pneumonia
Neisseria	N. meningitidis	Meningococcus	Cerebrospinal meningitis
	N. gonorrhoeae	Gonococcus	Gonorrhea
	N. catarrhalis	Micrococcus catarrhalis	Nasopharyngeal catarrh
Proteus	P. vulgaris	Bacillus proteus	Suppuration
Pseudomonas	P. mallei	Bacillus mallei or the glanders bacillus	Glanders
	P. aeruginosa	Bacillus pyocyaneus	Suppuration ("blue pus")
Salmonella	S. typhosa	Typhoid bacillus	Typhoid fever
	S. paratyphi (A&B)	Bacillus paratyphosus, etc.	Paratyphoid fever, gastroenteritis (food poisoning)
	S. enteritidis	(Salmonella group)	
	S. typhimurium		
Shigella	S. dysenteriae	Dysentery bacilli	Bacillary dysentery
Vibrio	V. cholera	Comma bacillus	Cholera
Yersinia	Y. pestis	Pasturella pestis; plague bacillus	Plague

rons. SYN: *g., Nissl.*

g.'s, cone. The nuclei of the cones, sensory cells of the retina. They form the outer zone of the outer nuclear layer of the retina.

g.'s, delta. Small granules in the delta cells of the pancreas.

g., eosinophil. One of various granules that react with acid dyes. They are present in the eosinophils of the leukocytes.

g., glycogen. Minute particles of glycogen seen in liver cells following fixation.

g.'s, juxtaglomerular. Secretory granules in the juxtaglomerular cells of the glomerulus of the kidney.

g., Kölliker's interstitial. Granule in the sarcoplasm of a striated muscle fiber.

g.'s, metachromatic. Granules found in protoplasm of numerous bacteria; irregular in size. Stain deeply.

g.'s, Much's. Granules sometimes seen in sputum from patients with tuberculosis. They do not stain with acid-fast stain but do take Gram's stain. These particles are probably degenerated tubercle bacilli.

g.'s, neutrophil. Granules such as those found in neutrophil leukocytes, which stain with both basic and acid dyes, assuming a neutral tint.

g., Nissl. A chromophil granule found in the cell bodies of neurons. SYN: *Nissl bodies.*

g.'s, pigment. Granules of coloring matter seen in pigment cells.

g., Plehn's. Basophilic granule seen in the conjugating form of *Plasmodium vivax.*

g., protein. Protein particles of minute size in cells.

g., rod. Nucleus of the rod visual cell found in the external nuclear layer of the retina connected with the rods.

g., Schüffner's. Polychrome methylene blue-staining granule found in parasitized erythrocytes of tertian malaria; coarse and red.

The Chief Gram-Positive Bacteria

Genus	Species	Colloquial or Old Names	Disease Caused in Man
Bacillus	B. anthracis	Anthrax bacillus	Anthrax
	B. subtilis	Hay bacillus	Eye infections (rarely)
Clostridium	C. tetani	Tetanus bacillus	Tetanus
	C. botulinum	Bacillus botulinus	Botulism
	C. perfringens	C. welchii	Gas gangrene
Corynebacterium	C. diphtheriae	Diphtheria bacillus Klebs-Loeffler bacillus	Diphtheria
Diplococcus	D. pneumoniae	Streptococcus pneumoniae	Lobar and bronchopneumonia; other infections
Gardnerella	G. vaginalis	Haemophilus vaginalis Corynebacterium vaginale	Bacterial vaginosis
Sarcina	S. lutea		Rarely suppuration
Staphylococcus	S. aureus	S. albus	Suppuration, pyemia, gastroenteritis, pneumonia, osteomyelitis, toxic shock syndrome, scalded skin syndrome
	S. epidermidis		Endocarditis
Streptococcus	S. pyogenes		Suppuration, scarlet fever, septicemia, toxic shock-like syndrome
	S. viridans	S. mitis	Subacute bacterial endocarditis

g.'s, secretory. G.'s, zymogen.

g., seminal. Minute particles in semen, supposed to derive from disintegrated nuclei in nutritive cells from seminiferous tubules.

g.'s, zymogen. Granules present in gland cells, esp. the secretory cells of the pancreas, the chief cells of the gastric glands, and serous cells of the salivary glands. They are the precursors of the enzymes secreted. SYN: *g.'s, secretory.*

granulitis (grăn-ū-lī'tĭs) [L. *granulum*, little grain, + Gr. *itis*, inflammation]. Acute miliary tuberculosis.

granuloadipose (grăn″ū-lō-ăd′ĭ-pōs). Fatty degeneration with the presence of fatty granules.

granuloblast (grăn′ū-lō-blăst) [″ + Gr. *blastos*, germ]. Mother cell of a granulocyte. A myeloblast found in bone marrow.

granulocyte (grăn′ū-lō-sīt″) [″ + Gr. *kytos*, cell]. A granular leukocyte; a polymorphonuclear leukocyte (neutrophil, eosinophil, or basophil).

granulocyte colony-stimulating factor.

ABBR: G-CSF. Naturally occurring cytokine glycoprotein which stimulates proliferation and functional activity of neutrophils. Effective in treating bone marrow deficiency following cancer chemotherapy or bone marrow transplantation. G-CSF's generic name is filgrastim. Trade name is Neupogen. SEE: *colony-stimulating factor-1 (CSF-1).*

granulocyte-macrophage colony-stimulating factor. ABBR: GM-CSF. Naturally occurring cytokine glycoprotein which stimulates production of neutrophils, monocytes, and macrophages. Effective in treating bone marrow deficiency following cancer chemotherapy or bone marrow transplantation. GM-CSF's generic name is sargramostim. Trade names are Leukine and Prokine. SEE: *colony-stimulating factor-1 (CSF-1).*

granulocytopenia (grăn″ū-lō-sī″tō-pē′nē-ă) [″ + ″ + *penia*, poverty]. Abnormal reduction of granulocytes in the blood. SYN: *granulopenia.*

granulocytopoiesis (grăn″ū-lō-sī″tō-poy-ē′

sĭs) [" + " + *poiein*, to form]. The formation of granulocytes.

granulocytosis (grăn"ū-lō-sī-tō'sĭs) [" + " + *osis*, condition]. Abnormal increase in the number of granulocytes in the blood.

granuloma [" + Gr. *oma*, tumor]. A granular tumor or growth, usually of lymphoid and epithelioid cells. It occurs in various infectious diseases such as leprosy, cutaneous leishmaniasis, yaws, and syphilis.

   g. annulare. A condition of the skin characterized by development of reddish nodules arranged in the form of a circle.

   g., apical. G., dental.

   g., benign, of thyroid. A lymphadenoma of the thyroid.

   g., coccidioidal. A chronic, generalized granulomatous disease caused by the fungus *Coccidioides immitis.* SEE: *coccidioidomycosis.*

   g., dental. Granuloma developing at the tip of tooth root, usually the result of pulpitis. It consists of a proliferating mass of chronic inflammatory tissue and possibly epithelial nests or colonies of bacteria. It may be encapsulated by fibrous tissue of the periodontal ligament. SYN: *chronic apical periodontitis; g., apical; g., periapical.*

   g., eosinophilic. A form of xanthomatosis, q.v., accompanied by eosinophilia and formation of cysts on bone.

   g. fissuratum. A circumscribed, firm, fissured, fibrotic tumor caused by chronic irritation. It may occur where hard objects such as dentures or the ear pieces of glasses rub against the labioalveolar fold or the retroauricular fold, respectively. The tumor is not malignant and disappears when the irritating object is removed.

   g., foreign body. Chronic inflammation around foreign bodies such as sutures, talc, splinters, or gravel.

   g. fungoides. Mycosis fungoides.

   g., infectious. Any infectious disease in which granulomas are formed, such as tuberculosis or syphilis. Granulomas are also formed mycoses, protozoan infections, and certain metazoal diseases.

   g. inguinale. A granulomatous ulcerative disease in which the initial lesion commonly appears in the genital area as a painless nodule.

   ETIOL: A short, gram-negative bacillus, *Calymmatobacterium granulomatis.* These microorganisms are commonly called Donovan bodies, q.v.

   TREAT: Streptomycin, chloramphenicol, trimethoprim/sulfamethoxazole, or tetracyclines. Streptomycin will not prevent the development of incubating syphilis. When treatment is completed, the pa-

tient should be followed for six months to determine if syphilis was contracted along with the granuloma.

   g. iridis. Granuloma that develops on the iris.

   g., lipoid. Granuloma that contains fatty tissue or cholesterol.

   g., lipophagic. Granuloma in which the macrophages have phagocytosed the surrounding fat cells.

   g., Majocchi's. G., trichophytic.

   g., malignant. Lymphogranulomatosis; Hodgkin's disease.

   g., paracoccidioidal. Paracoccidioidomycosis.

   g. pyogenicum. Granuloma containing pyogenic organisms that develop at the site of a wound. They may also occur at the tip of the fingers along the sides of the nails or beneath the free edge of the nail. They bleed easily and are usually painful to touch. SYN: *septic granuloma.*

   g., swimming pool. Chronic skin infection with *Mycobacterium balnei.* This organism may be present in unchlorinated swimming pools.

   g., telangiectaticum. A very vascular granuloma at any site, but esp. in the nasal mucosa or pharynx.

   g.'s, trichophytic. Granulomas of the skin of the follicles and follicular areas of the legs. Caused by fungi, usually *Trichophyton rubrum.*

granulomatosis (grăn"ū-lō"mă-tō'sĭs) [L. *granulum*, little grain, + Gr. *oma*, tumor, + *osis*, condition]. The development of multiple granulomas.

   g., Wegener's. Rare disease of unknown etiology characterized by widespread granulomatous lesions of the bronchi, necrotizing arteriolitis, and glomerulonephritis.

granulomatous (grăn"ū-lŏm'ă-tŭs). Containing granulomas.

granulopenia (grăn"ū-lō-pē'nē-ă) [" + Gr. *penia*, poverty]. Abnormal decrease of granulocytes in the blood. SYN: *granulocytopenia.*

granuloplasm (grăn'ū-lō-plăzm). Granular cytoplasm.

granuloplastic (grăn"ū-lō-plăs'tĭk) [" + Gr. *plassein*, to form]. Developing granules.

granulopoiesis (grăn"ū-lō-poy-ē'sĭs) [" + Gr. *poiein*, to make]. The formation of granulocytes.

granulopotent (grăn"ū-lō-pō'tĕnt) [" + *potentia*, power]. Potentially capable of forming granules.

granulosa (grăn"ū-lō'să). Layer of cells in the theca of the graafian follicle.

granulosa cell tumor. Tumor of the ovary. The cells resemble those of the primordial follicle. The neoplasm is associated with development of feminization.

granulosa-theca cell tumor. Tumor of the ovary in which the cells are derived from the graafian follicle. The tumor is associated with signs of feminization.

granulose (grăn'ū-lōs). The soluble portion of starch. It is converted into sugar by hydrolysis.

granulosis (grăn"ū-lō'sĭs) [" + Gr. *osis*, condition]. A mass of minute granules.

  g. rubra nasi. Disease of the skin of the nose.

  SYM: Moist erythematous patch on numerous macules.

  ETIOL: Inflammatory infiltration about the nose with slightly elevated papules and dilated sweat glands.

granum (grā'nŭm) [L.]. Grain.

grape. 1. The fruit of the genus *Vitis*. Contains acid potassium tartrate. Acidity decreases with the age of the grape and sugar increases. The sugar is nearly all glucose and is more abundant than in any other fruit. Raisins (sweet dried grapes) contain more sugar and less water. 2. Structure or growth resembling a grape or bunch of grapes.

grape sugar. Dextrose.

graph (grăf). 1. A visual presentation of statistical, clinical, or experimental data represented by a relationship between two sets of numbers or variables on an abscissa (y) (vertical) axis and the ordinate (x) (horizontal) axis. 2. Any visual representation of a numerical relationship.

-graph [Gr. *graphos*, drawn or written; one who draws]. Combining form indicating something written; or an instrument used to make a drawing or record.

graphesthesia (grăf"ĕs-thē'zē-ă) [" + *aisthesis*, sensation]. The ability by which outlines, numbers, words, or symbols traced or written upon the skin are recognized.

graphite (grăf'īt) [Gr. *graphein*, to write]. A soft form of carbon.

grapho- [Gr. *graphein*, to write]. Prefix meaning to write.

graphology (grăf-ŏl'ō-jē) [" + *logos*, word, reason]. Examination of handwriting in diseases of the nerves as a means of diagnosis or as a means of analyzing personality.

graphomotor (grăf"ō-mō'tor) [" + L. *motor*, mover]. Pert. to movements involved in writing.

graphophobia (grăf"ō-fō'bē-ă) [" + *phobos*, fear]. Abnormal fear of writing.

graphorrhea (grăf"ō-rē'ă) [" + *rhoia*, flow]. Writing of many meaningless words and phrases.

graphospasm (grăf'ō-spăzm) [" + *spas-*

mos, spasm]. Writer's cramp.

-graphy [Gr. *grapho*, to write]. Combining form concerning drawing, writing, recording, or the method for that process.

GRAS List. Indicates food additives *generally recognized as safe* by the U.S. Food and Drug Administration. SEE: *food additives*.

grasp. Specific types of prehension involving the fingers or the palmar surface or both. Types of grasp include: cylindrical, as in holding a cylinder, where the fingers and palmar surface are in opposition, and ball grasp, as in holding a spherical object, where the fingers, thumb, and palmar surface surround an object. Related terms: prehension, pinch, hook.

grass. Artifact seen on oscilloscope tracings, especially in hemodynamic monitoring, resembling the random addition of vertical lines to the pattern. In hemodynamic monitoring, caused by rapid movement of the end of the catheter, usually because of malplacement.

gratification. Being gratified.

gratify. To give satisfaction or to be satisfied, esp. with regard to personal needs.

grating. In spectrophotometry, describes the element used in a monochromator that disperses white light into the visible spectrum.

grattage (gră-tăzh') [Fr., a scraping]. Removal of morbid growths by rubbing with a brush or harsh sponge.

grave [L. *gravis*, heavy]. Serious; dangerous; severe.

gravel [Fr. *gravelle*, coarse sand]. Crystalline dust or concretions of crystals from the kidneys. Generally made up of phosphates, calcium, oxalate, and uric acid.

Graves' disease [Robert James Graves, Irish physician, 1796–1853]. Exophthalmic goiter. SEE: *goiter, exophthalmic*.

Graves' ophthalmopathy. Ophthalmopathy associated with hyperthyroidism. Clinically, there is exophthalmos, periorbital edema, periorbital and conjunctival inflammation, decreased extra-ocular muscle mobility, corneal injury. Accompanying these may be lacrimation, eye pain, blurring of vision, photophobia, diplopia, and loss of vision.

  TREAT: Therapy for the hyperthyroidism, sleep with head of bed elevated, methylcellulose eyedrops, and diuretics will help to relieve eye discomfort. If the condition is severe and progressive, surgical decompression of the orbit will be required to treat impaired retinal function and exposure keratopathy. SEE: *goiter, exophthalmic*.

gravid (grăv'ĭd) [L. *gravida*, pregnant]. Pregnant; heavy with child.

gravida (grăv'ĭ-dă) [L.]. A pregnant woman.

gravida macromastia. Rapid enlargement of the breasts during pregnancy. This may progress to cause severe distention with sloughing of breast tissue with bleeding and infection. Surgical therapy may be required.

gravidism [L. *gravida,* pregnant, + Gr. -*ismos,* state of]. State of being pregnant.

graviditas (gră-vĭd'ĭ-tăs). Pregnancy.

gravidity (gră-vĭd'ĭ-tē) [L. *gravida,* pregnant]. Pregnancy.

gravidocardiac (grăv"ĭd-ō-kăr'dē-ăk) [" + Gr. *kardia,* heart]. Pert. to cardiac disorders resulting from pregnancy.

gravimetric (grăv"ĭ-mĕt'rĭk) [L. *gravis,* heavy, + Gr. *metron,* measure]. Determined by weight.

gravistatic (grăv"ĭ-stăt'ĭk) [" + Gr. *statikos,* causing to stand]. Resulting from gravitation, as in a form of gravistatic pulmonary congestion.

gravitation [L. *gravitas,* weight]. Force and movement tending to draw every particle of matter together, esp. the attraction of the earth for bodies at a distance from its center.

gravity. Property of possessing weight. The force of the earth's gravitational attraction.

    g., specific. ABBR: sp. gr. Weight of a substance compared with an equal volume of water. Water is used as a standard and considered to have a specific gravity of 1 (1.000).

Gravlee jet washer [Leland Clark Gravlee, Jr., U.S. obstetrician and gynecologist, 1928–1984]. Proprietary device for irrigating the endometrial cavity with sterile isotonic saline and then removing the solution and the dislodged cells. The cells are stained and examined for evidence of malignancy.

gray. 1. Color without hue between extremes of black and white. 2. A unit of absorbed radiation energy in the SI system. One gray equals 100 rads. ABBR: Gy.

gray matter. Nervous tissue of a grayish color in which myelinated nerve fibers do not predominate. It contains large numbers of cell bodies of neurons. The term is generally applied to the gray portions of the central nervous system, which include the cerebral cortex, basal ganglia, and nuclei of the brain, and the gray columns of the spinal cord, which form an H-shaped region surrounded by white matter. Sympathetic ganglia and nerves may also be gray. SYN: *substantia grisea* [NA].

gray syndrome of the newborn. The appearance of vomiting, lack of sucking response, irregular and rapid respiration, abdominal distention, and cyanosis in newborn infants treated at birth with chloramphenicol. Flaccidity and an ashen-gray color are present within 24 hours. Death occurs in about 40% of the patients, most frequently on the fifth day of life.

Caution: Children less than one month of age being treated with chloramphenicol should receive no more than 25 mg/kg of body weight each day.

green. A color intermediate between blue and yellow, afforded by rays of wavelength between 492 and 575 nanometers. SEE: words beginning with *chloro-*.

    g., brilliant. A derivative of malachite green. Used in staining bacteria.

    g., indocyanine. A dye used intravenously to determine blood volume.

    g., malachite. A dye used as a stain and antiseptic.

green blindness. A type of color blindness in which green colors cannot be distinguished. SYN: *aglaucopsia.*

Greenfield's disease [J. Godwin Greenfield, Brit. neuropathologist, 1884–1958]. Metachromatic leukodystrophy, q.v.

green soap. USP. A potassium soap made by the saponification of suitable vegetable oils without the removal of glycerin.

green soap tincture. Green soap to which lavender oil and alcohol have been added.

greenstick fracture. Fracture involving only part of the thickness of a bone. SEE: *fracture.*

green vitriol. Ferrous sulfate. SYN: *copperas.*

greffotome (grĕf'ō-tōm) [Fr. *greffe,* graft, + Gr. *tome,* incision]. Instrument for making tissue grafts.

grenz rays [Ger. *Grenze,* boundary]. Roentgen rays with an average wavelength of two angstroms. SEE: *ray.*

grid. 1. A chart with an abscissa (y) (vertical) axis and an ordinate (x) (horizontal) axis upon which to plot graphs. 2. A device made of parallel lead pieces used to screen scattered radiation when taking radiographs.

    g., Fixott-Everett. A plastic-embedded screen placed over dental radiographic film prior to exposure to x-rays. It facilitates measurement of bone loss and other tissue changes.

grief reaction. The emotional reaction that follows the loss of a love object. Somatic symptoms include easy fatigability, hollow or empty feelings in the chest and abdomen, sighing, hyperventilation, anorexia, insomnia, and the feeling of having a lump in the throat. Psychological symptoms begin with an initial stage of shock and disbelief accompanied by an inner awareness of mental discomfort, sorrow, and regret. These may be followed by tears, sobbing, and cries of pain. The duration of the reaction is variable but may last for over a year.

griffe des orteils (grĕf dāz or-tă´) [Fr.]. Muscular atrophy of foot with contraction. SYN: *clawfoot.*

Grifulvin V. Trade name for griseofulvin microsize.

grinder (grīn´dĕr) [AS. *grindan,* to gnash]. A molar tooth. SYN: *dens molaris* [NA].

grinders' disease. Chronic lung disease due to dust inhalation. SYN: *pneumoconiosis; siderosis.*

grinding. Forceful rubbing together as in chewing. SEE: *bruxism.*

    g., selective. Altering and correcting the occlusion of teeth by grinding in accordance with what is required.

grip, grippe (grĭp) [Fr. *gripper,* to seize]. Acute infectious disease marked by fever, prostration, pains in head and back, and upper respiratory tract symptoms such as cough and nasal congestion. SYN: *influenza.*

gripes (grīps) [AS. *gripan,* to grasp]. Intermittent severe pains in bowels. SYN: *colic.*

griping. An acute intermittent cramplike pain, esp. in the abdomen.

Grisactin. Trade name for griseofulvin microsize.

griseofulvin. An antifungal antibiotic for oral administration. Especially effective in ringworm. Trade names for griseofulvin are Fulvicin-U/F, Gris-PEG, and Grifulvin V.

Gris-PEG. Trade name for griseofulvin.

gristle (grĭs´ĕl) [AS.]. Cartilage.

grits. Coarsely ground corn. It may be prepared as a thick mush, or it can be poured into a mold, allowed to set and solidify, and then sliced and fried.

grocers' itch. Eczema of the hands due to irritation from handling flour and sugar. SEE: *eczema.*

groin [AS. *grynde,* abyss]. The depression between the thigh and trunk. The inguinal region.

grommet (grŏm´ĭt). A device, also known as a ventilation tube, placed in an artificial opening in the tympanic membrane in order to permit air to flow freely between the inner ear and the external auditory canal. The prosthesis is used as a treatment adjunct in managing chronic otitis media with effusion.

groove [MD. *groeve,* ditch]. Long narrow channel, depression, or furrow. SYN: *sulcus.*

    g., bicipital. Groove for the long tendon of the biceps brachii located on the anterior surface of the humerus. SYN: *g., intertubercular.*

    g., branchial. Groove in the embryo that is lined with ectoderm and lies between two branchial arches. SEE: *branchial arches; branchial grooves.*

    g., carotid. A broad groove on the inner surface of the sphenoid bone lateral to the body. It lodges the carotid artery and the cavernous sinus.

    g., costal. Groove on the lower internal border of a rib. It lodges the intercostal vessels and nerve. SYN: *g., subcostal.*

    g., costovertebral. A broad groove that extends along each side of the vertebrae. It lodges the sacrospinalis muscle and its subdivisions. SYN: *g., vertebral.*

    g., Harrison's. Groove or line extending laterally from the xiphoid process of the sternum. It marks the attachment of the diaphragm to the costal margins. Seen in severe rickets in children.

    g., infraorbital. Groove on the orbital surface of the maxilla that transmits the infraorbital vessels and nerve.

    g., intertubercular. G., bicipital.

    g., labial. Groove that develops in each of the primitive jaws. It gives rise to the vestibule separating the lips from the gums.

    g., lacrimal. 1. Groove on the posterior surface of the frontal process of the maxilla. 2. Groove on the anterior surface of the posterior lacrimal crest of the lacrimal bone. The two grooves lodge the lacrimal sac.

    g., laryngotracheal. Groove along the ventral surface of the anterior portion of the embryonic gut that gives rise to the respiratory organs.

    g., malleolar. Groove on the anterior surface of the distal end of the tibia that lodges tendons of the tibialis posterior and flexor digitorum longus musculi.

    g., medullary. G., neural.

    g.'s, meningeal. Depressions on the internal surface of the cranial bones where blood vessels follow the meningeal and osseous structures of the skull.

    g., musculospiral. G., radial.

    g., mylohyoid. Groove on the inner surface of the mandible that runs obliquely forward and downward and lodges the mylohyoid nerve and artery. In the embryo it lodges Meckel's cartilage.

    g., nasolacrimal. Groove extending from the inner angle of the eye to the primitive olfactory sac in the embryo. It separates the maxillary and lateral nasal processes; its epithelial lining gives rise to the nasolacrimal duct.

    g., nasopalatine. Groove on the vomer that lodges the nasopalatine nerve and vessels.

    g., neural. A longitudinal groove on the dorsal surface of the embryo lying between the neural folds. Upon closure of the folds to form the neural tube, the groove becomes the cavity of the neural tube, eventually giving rise to the ventricles of the brain and the central canal of the spinal cord.

g., obturator. Groove at the superior and posterior angle of the obturator foramen through which pass the obturator vessels and nerve.

g., olfactory. A shallow groove on the superior surface of the cribriform plate of the ethmoid on each side of the crista galli. It lodges the olfactory bulb.

g., palatine. One of a number of grooves on the inferior surface on the palatine process of the maxilla. They lodge the palatine vessels and nerves.

g., peroneal. 1. A shallow groove on the lateral aspect of the calcaneus. 2. A deep groove on the inferior surface of the cuboid bone. Each transmits the tendon of the peroneus longus muscle.

g., pharyngeal. G., branchial.

g., primitive. In the embryo, a shallow groove in the primitive streak of the blastoderm, bordered by the primitive folds.

g., pterygopalatine. Groove on the maxillary surface of the perpendicular portion of the palatine bone that, with corresponding grooves on the maxilla and pterygoid process of the sphenoid, transmits the palatine nerve and descending palatine artery.

g., radial. A broad, shallow groove running in a spiral direction on the posterior surface of the humerus. It transmits the radial nerve and the profunda branchi artery. SYN: *g., musculospiral.*

g., rhombic. One of seven transverse grooves in the floor of the developing rhombencephalon. They separate the neuromeres.

g., sagittal. A shallow groove on the inner surface of the parietal bones that lodges the superior sagittal sinus. SYN: *sagittal sulcus.*

g., sigmoid. Groove on the inner surface of the mastoid portion of the temporal bone. It transmits the transverse sinus.

g., subcostal. G., costal.

g., tympanic. Groove at the bottom of the exterior auditory meatus that receives the inferior portion of the tympanic membrane.

g., urethral. Groove on the caudal surface of the genital tubercle or phallus bordered by the urethral folds. The latter close, transforming the groove into the cavernous urethra.

g., vertebral. G., costovertebral.

g., visceral. G., branchial.

gross (grōs) [L. *grossus*, thick]. 1. Visible to the naked eye. 2. Consisting of large particles or components; coarse or large. 3. Having an insensitiveness or lack of social refinement.

gross anatomy. Study of organs and parts seen without the aid of a microscope.

gross lesion. Lesion visible to the eye without the aid of a microscope.

gross motor skills. Skills pertaining to the synergy of large muscle groups, as in balancing, running, and throwing.

ground. 1. Basic substance or foundation; reduced to a powder; pulverized. 2. In electronics, the negative or earth pole that has zero electrical potential.

ground bundle. A bundle of nerve fibers that immediately surrounds the gray matter of the spinal cord. It is divided into three regions, the anterior, lateral, and posterior bundles, which lie in the corresponding funiculi. These consist principally of short descending fibers.

ground itch. Inflammation of the skin resulting from the invasion of the larvae of hookworms (*Ancylostoma* or *Necator*). SYN: *ancylostomiasis.* SEE: *larva migrans.*

ground substance. The fluid, semifluid, or solid material that occupies the intercellular spaces in fibrous connective tissue, cartilage, or bone. SYN: *matrix.*

group [It. *gruppo*, knot]. A number of similar objects or structures taken or considered together; thus, bacteria with similar metabolic characteristics are considered together as a group. Atomic molecules and compounds with similar structures or properties are classified with certain groups.

g., alcohol. The hydroxyl, —OH, group, which imparts alcoholic characteristics to organic compounds. These may be in three forms: primary, —CH₂OH; secondary, =CHOH; and tertiary, ≡COH.

g., azo. In chemistry, the group —N=N—.

g., coli-aerogenes. Coliform bacteria.

g., colon-typhoid-dysentery. Collective term for *Escherichia, Salmonella,* and *Shigella* bacteria.

g., peptide. The —CONH— radical.

g., prosthetic. 1. In a conjugated protein, the nonprotein portion of the molecule. 2. The nonprotein component of a coenzyme.

g., saccharide. The monosaccharide unit, C₆H₁₀O₅, which is a component of higher polysaccharides.

group dynamics. In politics, sociology, and psychology, a study of the forces and conditions that influence the actions of the entire group as well as the relations of the individuals to each other in the group.

grouping. Classification of individual traits according to a shared characteristic.

g., blood. Classification of blood of different individuals according to agglutinating and hemolyzing qualities before making a blood transfusion. SEE: *blood groups;*

blood transfusion.

grouping serum. A serum used for determining the blood group to which unknown cells belong. The grouping serums commonly used are human serums secured from donors and rabbit antiserums prepared commercially.

group therapy. A form of simultaneous psychotherapy involving two or more patients and one or more psychotherapists for the purpose of treating each patient's mental illness or improving health.

group transfer. An oxidation-reduction chemical reaction involving the exchange of chemical groups. A transferase enzyme is required.

Grover's disease [R. W. Grover, contemporary U.S. dermatologist]. A common itchy (pruritic) condition with sudden onset characterized by a few or numerous smooth or warty papules, vesicles, eczematous plaques, or shiny translucent nodules. The pruritus may be mild or severe, and it is aggravated by heat. Even though the condition is self-limiting, it may last months or years. SYN: *transient acantholytic dermatosis.*

    TREAT: Symptomatic. Avoid heat and sweat-inducing activities. Retinoic acid may be helpful.

growing pains. An imprecise term indicating ill-defined pain in the musculoskeletal system of young persons. Typically, the pain comes on after bedtime. There is no evidence that the pain is related to rapid growth.

    TREAT: Reassurance, aspirin, application of local heat, and massage. Quinine sulfate given prior to bedtime may help.

growth [AS. *growan,* to grow]. The progressive development or increase in size of a living thing. This may be normal, as in growth of an embryo or child, or pathological, as in a cyst or benign or malignant tumor.

    METHOD: By the synthesis of new protoplasm and multiplication of cells.

    TYPES: (1) General body growth is seen in the increase in the physical size of the body and increase in the total weight of the muscles and various internal organs. Growth is usually slow and steady but has a marked acceleration just after birth and at the time of puberty (the growth spurt).

    (2) Organs of the lymphoid type, such as the thymus and the lymph nodes, grow fastest early in life, reach their peak of development at about the age of 12 years, and then stop growing or regress.

    (3) The neural type of organ, such as the brain, cord, eye, and meninges, grows in childhood but is close to its adult size by the age of 8 years. This size is maintained without regression.

    (4) The genital type of growth is seen in the testes, ovaries, and other genitourinary structures. Their growth is the slowest of these four types in infancy, but at puberty they grow faster and cause the striking changes in appearance that make up the secondary sex characteristics.

    Not all of the organs of the body are included in the above four types. Some structures, such as the mammary glands, have several cycles of growth and regression in a lifetime.

growth hormone, human. Hormone that is liberated by the anterior pituitary and is important in regulating growth. SYN: *somatotropin.*

    The aging process usually includes loss of lean body mass, thinning of the skin, and expansion of the adipose tissue mass. These changes are probably related to the decline in secretion of growth hormone by the pituitary. This begins after age 30 and continues. The possibility that these age-related changes may be altered by administration of human growth hormone is being investigated.

growth hormone, human synthetic. SEE: *human growth hormone, synthetic.*

gruel [L. *grutum,* meal]. Any cereal boiled in water.

grumose, grumous (groo'mōs,-mŭs) [L. *grumus,* heap]. 1. Made up of coarse granular bodies in the center. 2. Lumpy, clotted.

Grünfelder's reflex (groon'fĕld-ĕrs). Fanlike spreading of toes with upward flexion of great toe resulting from pressure over posterior fontanel.

gryposis (grĭ-pō'sĭs) [G. *grypōsis,* a crooking]. Abnormal curvature of any part of the body, esp. the nails.

GSA. *Gerontological Society of America.*

GSR. *galvanic skin response.*

G-suit. A coverall-type garment designed for use by aviators. It contains compartments that inflate and bring pressure on the legs and abdomen to prevent blood from pooling there. In aviators this helps to prevent unconsciousness caused by positive acceleration with resulting pooling of blood in the lower extremities. The suit has been used in medicine to treat postural hypotension. SEE: *MAST.*

gt. L. *gutta,* a drop.

gtt. L. *guttae,* drops.

GU. *genitourinary.*

guaiac (gwī'ăk) [NL. *Guaiacum*]. A resin obtained from trees of the genus *Guaiacum;* either *G. officinale* or *G. sanctum.* An alcoholic solution of guaiac is used in testing for occult blood in feces.

guaiacol (gwī'ă-kōl). *o*-Methoxyphenol. A

substance similar to phenol obtained by fractional distillation of creosote or by synthetic means. Used as antiseptic and germicide, intestinal antiseptic, and expectorant.

guaifenesin (gwī-fĕn'ĕ-sĭn). USP. An expectorant. Trade name is Robitussin.

guanase (gwăn'ās) [Sp. *guano*, from Quechua *huanu*, dung]. An enzyme in a number of glands; it converts guanine into xanthine.

guanethidine (gwăn-ĕth'ĭ-dēn). A drug that depresses the function of postganglionic adrenergic nerves. Thus sympathetic nerve activity is inhibited. Guanethidine is used in treating hypertension.

  g. sulfate. USP. An adrenergic blocking agent used in treating hypertension.

guanidine (gwăn'ĭ-dēn). A crystalline organic compound, $(NH_2)_2C=NH$, found among the decomposition products of proteins.

guanidinemia (gwăn″ĭd-ĕn-ē'mē-ă) [*guanidine* + Gr. *haima*, blood]. Guanidine in the blood.

guanidoacetic acid. A chemical formed in the liver, kidney, and other tissues. It is then metabolized to form creatine.

guanine (gwă'nēn). $C_5H_5N_5O$. An organic compound that occurs as a natural constituent of animal and vegetable nucleic acids. It is abundant in liver, muscle, glandular tissue such as pancreas, and seeds. Uric acid is its metabolic end point.

guanosine (gwăn'ō-sĭn). The nucleoside formed from guanine and ribosome. It is a major constituent of RNA and DNA.

guard. A device for protecting something, e.g., a mouth guard or a face guard.

guardian ad litem [L.]. In cases of child abuse, a guardian for the child appointed by the court to protect the best interests of the child.

guardianship. Legal arrangement whereby one person or institution assumes responsibility for an adult individual. When a guardian is appointed, it is assumed that the individual receiving the care is incompetent and unable to care for himself.

guarding. A body defense method to prevent movement of an injured part, esp. spasm of abdominal muscles when an examiner attempts to palpate inflamed areas or organs in the abdominal cavity.

gubernaculum (gū″bĕr-năk'ū-lŭm) [L., helm]. 1. A structure that guides. 2. A cordlike structure uniting two structures.

  g. dentis. A connective tissue band that connects the tooth sac of an unerupted tooth with the overlying gum.

  g. testis. [NA] A fibrous cord in the fetus that extends from the caudal end of the testis through the inguinal canal to the scrotal swelling. It plays a role in the descent of the testis into the scrotum.

Gubler's line (goob'lĕrz) [Adolphe Gubler, Fr. physician, 1821–1879]. The level of superficial origin of the trigeminus or fifth nerve.

Gubler's paralysis. Hemiplegia affecting parts on opposite sides of the body. SYN: *hemiplegia, alternate.*

Gubler's tumor. A fusiform swelling on the wrist in lead palsy.

Gudden's inferior commissure (gŭd'ĕnz) [Bernard A. von Gudden, Ger. neurologist, 1824–1886]. Fibers of optic tract.

Gudden's law. In the division of a nerve, degeneration in the proximal portion is toward the nerve cell.

guidance. The act of guiding or counseling a patient.

guide. A mechanical aid or device that assists in setting a course or directing the motion either of one's hand or of an instrument one holds.

guide dog. A dog specifically trained to assist blind or partially sighted persons with mobility. SYN: *seeing eye dog.*

guideline. An instructional guide or reference to indicate a course of action in a specified situation, e.g., critical care guideline.

guidewire. Device used to assist in positioning and moving an intravenous catheter.

guile. Use of deception or cunning in accomplishing something.

Guillain-Barré syndrome [Georges Guillain, Fr. neurologist, 1876–1961; J. A. Barré, Fr. neurologist, b. 1880]. ABBR: GBS. Acute febrile polyneuritis. A disease of unknown etiology but thought to have an autoimmune basis. Onset is usually preceded by a history of nonspecific febrile illness. From one to three weeks later, signs and symptoms of multiple nerve involvement develop. Characterized by pain; and weakness that is symmetrical and begins in the extremities, ascends to involve the entire limb, and may involve the trunk and abdominal and thoracic muscles. The muscles of the head and face may be paralyzed bilaterally. Almost all of the patients have some sensory nerve symptoms but these are usually mild. Recovery after a period varying from several weeks or months is the usual outcome.

This disease has been described by various terms: acute polyneuritis with facial diplegia, acute infectious polyneuritis, and Landry-Guillain-Barré syndrome. All are believed to be the same disease.

TREAT: Respiratory assistance as needed and careful nursing care. Where plasmapheresis is instituted within 2 weeks of onset, recovery is hastened. Tracheostomy may be needed.

NURSING IMPLICATIONS: Assess patient for extent of involvement and paralysis. Note and document swallowing difficulty and signs of respiratory distress. Take appropriate measures if either or both occur. Administer prescribed analgesic. Place emergency tracheostomy tray at bedside. Provide passive range of motion exercises three to four times a day to prevent formation of contractures. Maintain fluid and electrolyte balance if swallowing reflex is impaired. SEE: *Nursing Diagnoses* in *Appendix.*

guillotine (gĭl'ŏ-tēn) [Fr., instrument for beheading]. Instrument for excising tonsils and laryngeal growths.

guilt (gĭlt). Emotion resulting from doing what is thought to be wrong, associated with self-reproach, the need for punishment; excesses or absence of guilt characterize a variety of psychiatric disorders.

guinea pig (gĭn'ē pĭg). 1. A small rodent used in laboratory research. 2. A colloquial term for persons being used in medical experiments.

guinea worm. *Dracunculus medinensis.*

Gull's disease [Sir William W. Gull, Brit. physician, 1816–1890]. Atrophy of the thyroid gland, which causes myxedema, q.v.

gullet [L. *gula,* throat]. The esophagus.

Gullstrand's slit lamp (gŭl'strändz) [Allvar Gullstrand, Swedish ophthalmologist, 1862–1930]. A device for illuminating the eye so that its anterior portion can be examined by use of a microscope.

gum. 1. A substance given out by or extracted from certain plants. It is sticky when moist but hardens upon drying. Roughly, any resinlike substance given out by plants. 2. The fleshy substance or tissue covering the alveolar processes of the jaws. SYN: *gingiva.*

DIAG: *Bleeding easily:* Indicates scurvy or inflammation as in trench mouth or pyorrhea. *Blue:* Silver poisoning. *Bluish red:* Indicates mercurial stomatitis or lead poisoning if bluish line is at edge of teeth. *Greenish line:* At edge of teeth may indicate copper poisoning. *Purplish line or color:* Scurvy. *Red line:* In youth, indicates gingivitis, pyorrhea, scurvy. *Spongy gum and ulceration:* Gingivitis; scurvy; stomatitis; leukemia; tuberculosis; and diabetes.

RS: diagnosis; gingiva; uletic.

gumboil. Abscess of the gum. SYN: *parulis.*

SYM: Gum is red, swollen, tender, and very painful. A fluctuating swelling containing pus may appear. It may point and break or require incision.

ETIOL: Subperiosteal infection associated with a carious tooth. May be caused by irritation or injury by a denture.

TREAT: Hot mouthwashes and applications over gum or externally. Warn patient not to swallow pus. Frequent mouthwashes after lesion is evacuated.

gumma (gŭm'mă) [L. *gummi,* gum]. A soft tumor of the tissues characteristic of the tertiary stage of syphilis. It is a granuloma varying in size from a millimeter to a centimeter or more in diameter. May be single or multiple, and tends to be encapsulated. Each consists of a central necrotic mass surrounded by an inflammatory zone and fibrosis. The necrotic portion may be firm or elastic, gelatinous or hyalinized. Infectious organisms may be present. The tumor occurs most frequently in the liver but may occur in other organs, such as the brain, testis, heart, skin, and in bone. SEE: *syphilis.*

SYM: Depend upon location. Bursting of a gumma leads to a gummatous ulcer that is painless but slow to heal. The base is formed by a "wash-leather" slough but surrounding tissues are healthy.

gummatous (gŭm'ă-tŭs). Having the character of a gumma.

gummose (gŭm'ōs). $C_6H_{12}O_6$. A sugar from animal gum.

gummy [L. *gummi,* gum]. Sticky, swollen, puffy.

Gunn's dots (gŭnz) [Robert Marcus Gunn, Brit. ophthalmologist, 1850–1909]. White spots on the retina of the eye, close to the macula.

Gunn's syndrome. SEE: *Marcus Gunn syndrome.*

gunshot wound. Penetrating or perforating wound that may contain a foreign body, as a bullet. SEE: *wound, bullet.*

gunstock deformity. Deformity in which the long axis of the extended forearm turns outwardly from the arm, caused by fracture at the elbow.

Günther's disease [Hans Günther, Ger. physician, 1884–1956]. Congenital erythropoietic porphyria.

gurney (gĕr'nē). A litter, equipped with wheels, used in hospitals for transporting patients.

gustation (gŭs-tā'shŭn) [L. *gustare,* to taste]. Sense of taste.

gustatory (gŭs'tă-tō-rē). Pert. to sense of taste.

gustatory sweating. Sweating and flushing over the distribution of the auriculotemporal nerve in response to chewing.

gustometry (gŭs-tŏm'ĕ-trē) [" + Gr. *metron,* measure]. Measurement of acuteness of the sense of taste.

gut [AS.]. 1. The bowel or intestine. 2. The primitive gut or embryonic digestive tube, which includes the foregut, midgut, and hindgut. 3. Short term for catgut.

gut-associated lymphoid tissue. ABBR: GALT. Term used for all lymphoid tissue associated with the gastrointestinal tract, including the tonsils, appendix, and Peyer's patches. GALT contains lymphocytes, primarily B cells, and is responsible for controlling organisms entering the body via the digestive system.

Guthrie test. Diagnostic test to detect phenylketonuria (PKU). Required by law in most states. SEE: *phenylketonuria.*

gutta [L., a drop] (pl. *guttae*). ABBR: gt. (pl. *gtt.*). A drop. The amount in a drop varies with the nature of the liquid and its temperature. It is therefore not advisable to use the number of drops per minute of a solution as anything more than a general guide to the amount of material being administered intravenously.

gutta-percha (gŭt″ă-pĕr′chă). USP. Purified dried latex of certain trees. Used in dentistry as a temporary filling.

guttate [L. *gutta*, drop]. Resembling a drop, said of certain cutaneous lesions.

guttatim (gŭt-tā′tĭm) [L.]. Drop by drop.

guttering (gŭt′ĕr-ĭng). Cutting a channel or groove in a bone.

guttur (gŭt′ŭr) [L. *gutter*, throat]. The throat.

guttural (gŭt′ŭ-răl). Pert. to the throat.

gutturotetany (gŭt″ŭr-ō-tĕt′ă-nē) [″ + Gr. *tetanos*, tension]. Laryngeal spasm of throat with temporary stutter.

Guyon's sign (gē-yŏnz′) [Felix J. C. Guyon, Fr. surgeon, 1831–1920]. Ballottement of kidney.

Gwathmey's method (gwăth′mēz) [James T. Gwathmey, U.S. surgeon, 1863–1944]. Use of anesthetic consisting of ether and olive oil solution. This is placed in the rectum and colon, where it is absorbed.

Gy. *gray*, q.v., in the SI system, the unit of absorbed radiation energy.

gymnastics [Gr. *gymnastikos*, pert. to nakedness]. Systematic body exercise with or without special apparatus.

g., ocular. Systematic exercise of the eye muscles to improve muscular coordination and efficiency.

g., Swedish. A system of movements made by a patient against a resistance provided by the attendant. This system was, at one time, used throughout the world. It influenced the development of modern gymnastics.

gymnophobia (jĭm-nō-fō′bē-ă) [Gr. *gymnos*, naked, + *phobos*, fear]. Abnormal aversion to viewing a naked body.

gynander (jĭ-năn′dĕr, jī-, gī-) [Gr. *gyne*, woman, + *aner, andros*, man]. An individual possessing both male and female characteristics. SYN: *gynandromorph; pseudohermaphrodite.*

gynandrism (jĭ-năn′drĭzm). 1. Male hermaphroditism. 2. Partial female pseudohermaphroditism.

gynandroid (jĭ-năn′droyd, jī-, gī-) [″ + ″ + *eidos*, form, shape]. An individual having sufficient hermaphroditic sexual characteristics to be mistaken for a person of the opposite sex.

gynatresia (jī-nă-trē′zē-ă , jī-, gī-) [″ + *a-*, not, + *tresis*, perforation]. Atresia, q.v., of the vagina.

gynecic (jĭ-nē′sĭk, jī, gī-) [Gr. *gyne*, woman]. Pert. to women.

gyneco-, gyno- [Gr.]. Prefix meaning woman, female.

gynecogenic (jĭn″ē-kō-jĕn′ĭk) [Gr. *gyne*, woman, + *gennan*, to produce]. Producing female characteristics.

gynecoid (jĭn′ē-koyd) [″ + *eidos*, form, shape]. Resembling the female of the species.

gynecologic, gynecological (gī″nē-kŏ-lŏj′ĭk, jī″-, jĭn″ē-; -ĭ-kăl) [″ + *logos*, word, reason]. Pert. to gynecology or study of diseases peculiar to women.

gynecologic operative procedures. NURSING IMPLICATIONS: *Post-operative:* Count and chart pulse every 15 minutes for first few hours. Report immediately any change in rate or volume. Watch for shock or internal hemorrhage. Keep warm and quiet; no visitors. Fluids when tolerated, tap water being best.

Care must be taken to prevent retention of urine. Sterile, closed, continuous drainage of the bladder may be preferable to repeated catheterization. Patient catheterized as ordered every 12 hours after operation, then every 8 hours until able to void. Thrombophlebitis with embolism is a serious complication. Have the patient exercise her legs frequently. Elastic stockings up to the knees, not circular elastic bandages, should be worn continuously while the patient is bedridden.

gynecologist (gī″nē-kŏl′ō-jĭst, jī″-, jĭn″ē-). Physician who specializes in gynecology.

gynecology (gī″nē-kŏl′ō-jē, jī″-, jĭn″ē-) [″ + *logos*, word, reason]. The study of the diseases of the female reproductive organs, including the breasts.

gynecomania (jī″nē-kō-mā′nē-ă, gī″-, jĭn″ē-) [″ + *mania*, madness]. Abnormal sex desire in the male. SYN: *satyriasis.*

gynecomastia (jī″nē-kō-măs′tē-ă, gī″-, jĭn″ē-) [″ + *mastos*, breast]. Development of abnormally large mammary gland in the male; sometimes may secrete milk.

gynecopathy (jī-nē-kŏp′ă-thē, gī″-, jĭn″ē-) [″ *pathos*, disease, suffering]. Diseases peculiar to women.

gynecophonus (jī″nē-kŏf′ŏn-ŭs, gī″-, jĭn″ē-) [″ + *phone*, voice]. Having an effeminate voice.

Gyne-Lotrimin. Trade name for clotrimazole.

gynephobia (jĭ″nĕ-fō′bē-ă, gī″-, jĭn″ē-) [″ + *phobos*, fear]. Abnormal aversion to the company of women, or fear of them.

Gynergen. Trade name for ergotamine tartrate.

gynesic (gĭ-nē′sĭk, jĭ-, jĭn-ē′-) [Gr. *gyne*, woman]. Pert. to the diseases of women.

gyniatrics (jĭ″nē-ăt′rĭks , gī″-, jĭn″ē-) [″ + *iatrikos*, medical treatment]. Treatment of diseases of women.

gynopathic [″ + *pathos*, disease, suffering]. Pert. to diseases of women.

gynoplastics [″ + *plassein*, to form]. Reparative surgery of female genitalia.

gynoplasty. Gynoplastics.

gypsies. A tightly knit cultural group whose origins were in India more than 500 years ago. They have migrated to Europe and the U.S. Many gypsies are nomadic. Medically they are prone to develop hypertension, diabetes, and occlusive vascular disease, some part of which may be related to their practice of inbreeding.

gypsum (jĭp′sŭm) [L.; G. *gypsos*, chalk]. 1. A natural form of hydrated calcium sulfate. When heated to 130°C, it loses its water and becomes plaster of paris. 2. When heated, gypsum is allowed to dehydrate in the presence of sodium succinate or calcium hydrochloride; the result is a hemihydrate of gypsum, used as dental stone in preparing investments for dental casting.

gyrate (jī′rāt) [Gr. *gyros*, circle]. 1. Ring-shaped, convoluted. 2. To revolve.

gyration (jī-rā′shŭn). A rotary movement.

gyre (jīr) [Gr. *gyros*, circle]. Convolution. SYN: *gyrus.*

gyrectomy (jī-rĕk′tō-mē) [″ + *ektome*, excision]. Surgical removal of a cerebral gyrus.

gyrencephalic (jī-rĕn-sĕ-făl′ĭk) [″ + *enkephale*, head]. Having a brain marked by numerous convolutions.

gyri (jī′rī). Pl. of gyrus.

gyri breves insulae. [NA] Preinsular gyri.

gyro- [Gr.]. Combining form meaning a circle, spiral, ring.

gyroma (jī-rō′mă) [Gr. *gyros*, circle, + *oma*, tumor]. Ovarian tumor consisting of a convoluted mass.

gyrometer (jī-rŏm′ĕ-ter) [″ + *metron*, measure]. A device for measuring the cerebral gyri.

gyrose (jī′rōs). In bacteriology, marked by wavy lines or circles. Applied to bacterial colonies.

gyrospasm (jī′rō-spăzm) [″ + *spasmos*, a convulsion]. Spasmodic rotary head movement.

gyrous (jī′rŭs) [Gr. *gyros*, circle]. Marked by circular lines. SYN: *gyrose.*

gyrus (jī′rŭs) (pl. *gyri*). [NA] One of the convolutions of the cerebral hemispheres of the brain. The gyri are separated by shallow grooves (sulci) or deeper grooves (fissures). SEE: *convolution.*

   g., angular. Gyrus of the parietal lobe that embraces the posterior end of the superior temporal sulcus.

   g., annectent. Any of many short folds of gray matter formed as a result of short branches or twigs of sulci extending into adjacent gyri. They are not always present.

   g., anterior central. Gyrus of the frontal lobe extending vertically between the precentral and central sulci.

   g., Broca´s. G., frontal, inferior.

   g., callosal. A large gyrus on the medial surface of the cerebral hemisphere that lies directly above the corpus callosum and arches over its anterior end.

   g. cerebelli. Layer of the cerebellum.

   g., cingulate. Arch-shaped convolution of the cingulum, curved over the surface of the corpus callosum, from which it is separated by the callosal sulcus.

   g., dentate. Gyrus marked by indentations that lie on the upper surface of the hippocampal gyrus.

   g. fornicatus. Gyrus on the medial surface of the cerebrum, which includes the gyrus cinguli, the isthmus, the hippocampus, the hippocampal gyrus, and the uncus.

   g., frontal, inferior. A convolution on the external surface of the frontal lobe of the cerebrum located between the sylvian fissure and the inferior frontal sulcus.

   g., frontal, middle. Gyrus between the superior and inferior frontal sulci.

   g., frontal, superior. Convolution of the cerebral frontal lobe situated above the superfrontal fissure.

   g., fusiform. Gyrus beneath the collateral fissure joining the occipital and temporal lobes.

   g., Heschl´s. Transverse temporal gyrus.

   g., hippocampal. Gyrus situated between the hippocampal and collateral fissures.

   g., infracalcarine. G., lingual.

   g., lingual. Gyrus between the calcarine and collateral fissures.

   g. longus insulae. [NA] Lengthy gyrus composing the postinsula.

   g., marginal. G., frontal, superior.

   g., middle temporal. Gyrus located between the middle temporal sulcus and superior temporal sulcus.

   g., occipital. Any of the gyri on the lateral surface of the occipital lobe. They are not always present. Classified roughly into two groups, the inferior or lateral occipital gyri and the superior occipital gyri.

g., occipitotemporal. G., fusiform.

g., orbital. One of four gyri (anterior, posterior, lateral, and medial) forming the inferior surface of the frontal lobe.

g., paracentral. Area on mesial aspect of the cerebrum; the paracentral lobule. Lies above cingulate sulcus.

g., parahippocampal. Gyrus on the lower surface of each cerebral hemisphere between the hippocampal and collateral sulci.

g., paraterminal. A small area of the cerebral cortex anterior to the lamina terminalis and below the rostrum of the corpus callosum.

g., parietal. Gyrus on lateral aspect of parietal lobe. Includes posterior central gyrus, superior and inferior parietal gyri.

g., postcentral. Gyrus immediately posterior to the central sulcus of the cerebrum. It contains most of the general sensory area of the brain. SYN: *posterior central gyrus.*

g., precentral. Gyrus immediately anterior to the central sulcus of the cerebrum. It contains the pyramidal area.

g., profundi cerebri. One of the very deep gyri of the cerebrum.

g. rectus. [NA] Gyrus on the orbital aspect of the frontal lobe, located between the mesial margin and the olfactory sulcus.

g., Retzius. The supra- and subcallosal gyri.

g., subcallosal. A narrow band of gray matter on the medial surface of the hemisphere below the rostrum of the corpus callosum.

g., subcollateral. G., fusiform.

g., supracallosal. A rudimentary gyrus on the upper surface of the corpus callosum.

g., supracallosus. Gray matter layer covering the corpus callosum.

g., supramarginal. Gyrus in the inferior parietal lobule twisting about the upper terminus of the sylvian fissure.

g., temporal. One of the three gyri (superior, middle, inferior) on lateral surface of the temporal lobe.

g. transitivus. G., annectent.

g., uncinate. Anterior hooked portion of the hippocampal gyrus.

H

H. Chem. symb. for the element hydrogen.

H., h. *haustus,* a draft of medicine; *height; henry; hora* or *hour; horizontal; hypermetropia.*

h. Symbol for hecto, a term used in SI units.

h. Symbol for Planck's constant.

H⁺. Chem. symb. for hydrogen ion.

[H⁺]. Symbol for hydrogen ion concentration.

¹H. Chem. symb. for protium.

²H. Chem. symb. for deuterium, an isotope of hydrogen.

Ha. Chem. symb. for hahnium.

HAA. *hepatitis-associated antigen.*

Haab's reflex (hŏbz) [Otto Haab, Swiss ophthalmologist, 1850–1931]. Contraction of pupils without alteration of accommodation or convergence when gazing at a bright object. May indicate a cortical lesion.

HaAg. *hepatitis A antigen.*

habena (hă-bē'nă) [L., rein] (pl. *habenae*). 1. A frenum. 2. Bandage for a wound. 3. Pineal gland peduncle. SYN: *habenula* [NA].

habenal, habenar [L. *habena,* rein]. Pert. to the habena or habenula.

habenula (hă-bĕn'ū-lă) [L., little rein, strap]. 1. A frenum or any rein- or whiplike structure. 2. [NA] A peduncle or stalk attached to the pineal body of the brain. Fibers that travel posteriorly along the dorsomedial border of the thalamus to the habenular ganglia (epithalamus) resemble reins. 3. A narrow bandlike stricture.

   h. **urethralis.** One of two whitish bands between the clitoris and meatus urethra in young females.

habenular. Pert. to the habenula, esp. the stalk of the pineal body.

habenular commissure. A band of transverse fibers connecting the two habenular areas.

habenular trigone. A depressed triangular area located on the lateral aspect of the posterior portion of the third ventricle. Each contains a medial and lateral habenular nucleus.

habilitation (hă-bĭl″ĭ-tā'shŭn). The process of educating or training persons with disadvantage or disability to improve their ability to function in society.

habit [L. *habere, habitus,* to have, hold]. 1. A motor pattern executed with facility following constant or frequent repetition; an act performed in a voluntary manner but that after sufficient repetition is performed as a reflex action. Habits result from the passing of impulses through a particular set of neurons and synapses many times. 2. A particular type of dress or garb. 3. Mental or moral constitution or disposition. 4. Bodily appearance or constitution, esp. as related to a disease or predisposition to a disease, as the apoplectic habit. SYN: *habitus.* 5. Addiction to the use of drug or beverage as the drug habit or alcoholic habit.

   h., **chorea.** H., spasm.

   h., **masticatory.** The sequence and pattern of jaw movement in chewing by an individual. It is influenced by the type of food, occlusal problems or missing teeth, personal habits, or state of mind and may be unilateral or bilateral. Under some conditions it would be recognized as clenching or bruxing habit. SEE: *bruxism.*

   h., **spasm.** A spasmodic voluntary movement that has become involuntary. Often due to something irritating; sometimes from mimicry. SYN: *tic.*

habit disorders. Initially, usually in childhood, a tension-discharging phenomenon such as head banging, body rocking, thumb sucking, nail biting, hair pulling, tics, and teeth grinding. How important these are depends upon their etiology and their persistence. Almost all children will demonstrate some of these disorders during their development, but if they do not interfere with function they should not be of concern.

habit training. Development by young children of specific behavior patterns concerning basic activities such as eating, dressing, using the toilet, and sleeping.

habituation. Act of becoming accustomed to anything from frequent use or exposure. In drug addiction, the mental equivalent of physical tolerance and dependence on drugs.

habitus [L., habit] (pl. *habitus*). 1. A physical appearance, body build, or attitude. 2. A physical appearance that indicates a tendency for a person to develop a specific disease.

hachement (hăsh-mŏn') [Fr., chopping]. In massage, a chopping stroke with the edge of the hand.

hacking cough. Recurrent, nonproductive cough. SYN: *cough, dry.*

haem. Heme.

haem-. SEE: words beginning with *hem-.*

Haemadipsa (hē″mă-dĭp'să) [Gr. *haima,* blood + *dipsa,* thirst]. A genus of terrestrial leeches found in Asia that attach to humans and animals.

   H. **ceylonica.** Species of leech found in certain humid, tropical areas.

Haemagogus (hē″mă-gŏg′ŭs) [″ + *agogos*, leading]. A genus of mosquitoes. Includes species that serve as vectors of jungle yellow fever. Similar to *Aedes* species.

Haemaphysalis (hĕm″ă-fĭs′ă-lĭs) [″ + *physallis*, bubble]. A genus of ticks. Various species serve as vectors for diseases including tick-borne typhus and Rocky Mountain spotted fever. Some species are reservoirs for rickettsiae but do not bite man.

Haemophilus (hē-mŏf′ĭl-ŭs) [″ + *philein*, to love]. A genus of bacteria that require either the growth factor X or V, or both, provided by blood. The small, nonmotile, gram-negative bacilli are aerobic and do not form spores. The V factor is destroyed by enzymes present in unheated red blood cells. Thus chocolate agar is the preferred culture medium.

H. aegyptius. Koch-Weeks bacillus; the cause of one form of contagious conjunctivitis.

H. ducreyi. The causative organism of chancroid or soft chancre. SEE: *chancroid.*

H. influenzae. An organism found in respiratory infections and formerly thought to be the cause of influenza but now considered to be a primary and a secondary invader. It is the causative organism of influenzal meningitis, conjunctivitis, septicemia, and respiratory infections. SEE: *Pfeiffer's bacillus.*

H. vaginalis. Bacteria that cause vaginitis in otherwise healthy women. This organism is now called *Gardnerella vaginalis.*

Haemophilus influenza type b infections. An important cause of meningitis in children between the ages of 1 month and 4 years. In children, this organism also causes acute epiglottitis, pneumonia, septic arthritis, and cellulitis.

TREAT: Use ampicillin unless the organism is beta-lactamase resistant, in which case use chloramphenicol. If organism is not susceptible to either of these drugs, use cefotaxime or ceftriaxone.

PREVENTION: Administer Haemophilus influenza type b vaccine when child is 2 years of age or older. SEE: *vaccine* for table.

Haemosporidia (hē″mō-spō-rĭd′ē-ă). An order of sporozoa that live in the blood cells of vertebrates and reproduce sexually in invertebrates; includes the genus *Plasmodium*, which causes malaria in man.

hafnium (hăf′nē-ŭm) [L. *Hafnia*, Copenhagen]. SYMB: Hf. At wt. 178.49; at no. 72; sp. gr. 13.31. A rare chemical element.

Hagedorn needle (hă′gĕ-dorn) [Werner Hagedorn, Ger. surgeon, 1831–1894]. A curved surgical needle with flattened sides.

hahnium (hähn′ē-ŭm) [Named after Otto Hahn, Ger. scientist, 1879–1968]. SYMB: Ha. Name proposed for the artificially made element 105.

Hailey-Hailey disease [W. H. Hailey, 1898–1967; H. E. Hailey, b. 1909, U.S. dermatologists]. Benign familial pemphigus.

hair [AS. *haer*]. 1. A keratinized, threadlike outgrowth from the skin of mammals. 2. Collectively, the threadlike outgrowths that form the fur of animals or that grow on the human body.

A hair is a thin, flexible shaft of cornified cells that develops from a cylindrical invagination of the epidermis, the hair follicle. Each consists of a free portion or shaft (scapus pili) and a root (radix pili) embedded within the follicle. The shaft consists of three layers of cells: the cuticle or outermost layer; the cortex, forming the main horny portion of the hair; and the medulla, the central axis. SEE: illus. Hair color is due to pigment in the cortex.

Hair in each part of the body has a definite period of growth, after which it is shed. In the adult human there is a constant gradual loss and replacement of hair. Hair of the eyebrows lasts only three to five months; that of the scalp two to five years. Baldness or alopecia results when replacement fails to keep up with hair loss. It may be due to hereditary factors or pathological conditions such as infections or injury from irradiation. Also cytotoxic agents used in cancer chemotherapy may cause temporary loss of hair. SEE: *alopecia.*

h., auditory. An epithelial cell to which are attached delicate hairlike processes. These are present in the ear in the spiral organ of Corti, concerned with hearing; and in the crista ampullaris, macula utriculi, and macula sacculi, concerned with equilibrium.

h., bamboo. Sparse, brittle hair with bamboolike nodes. These apparent nodes are actually partial fractures of the hair shaft. This is caused by an atrophic condition of the hair. SYN: *trichorrhexis nodosa.*

h., beaded. Swellings and constrictions in the hair shaft due to a developmental defect known as monilethrix, q.v.

h., burrowing. Hair that grows horizontally under the skin, causing a foreign body reaction.

h., gustatory. One of several fine hairlike processes extending from the ends of gustatory cells in a taste bud. They project through the inner pore of a taste bud.

h., ingrown. Hair that reenters the skin and causes a foreign body reaction.

h., kinky. Short, sparse, kinky hair that may be poorly pigmented. Associated with kinky hair disease, q.v.

h., lanugo. SEE: *lanugo.*

HAIR AND ADJACENT STRUCTURES OF CROSS-SECTION OF SKIN

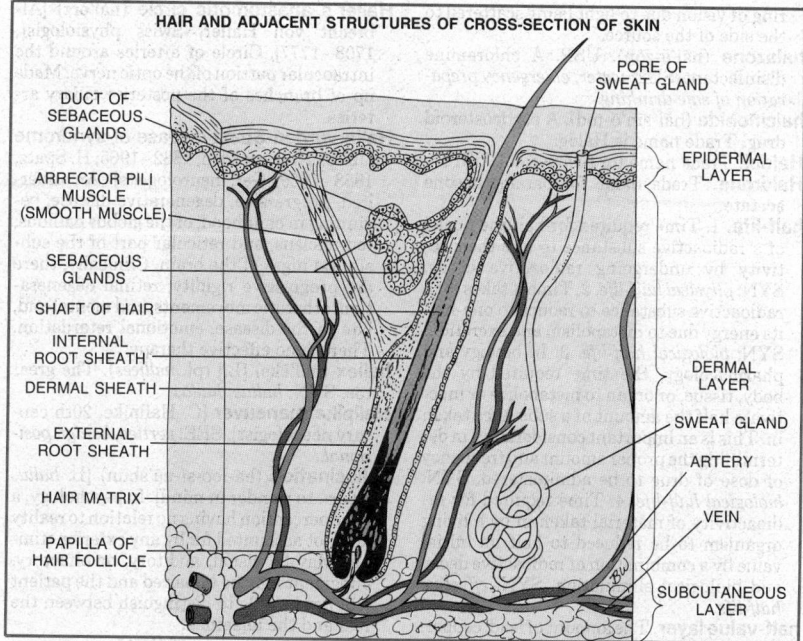

DUCT OF SEBACEOUS GLANDS

ARRECTOR PILI MUSCLE (SMOOTH MUSCLE)

SEBACEOUS GLANDS

SHAFT OF HAIR

INTERNAL ROOT SHEATH

DERMAL SHEATH

EXTERNAL ROOT SHEATH

HAIR MATRIX

PAPILLA OF HAIR FOLLICLE

PORE OF SWEAT GLAND

EPIDERMAL LAYER

DERMAL LAYER

SWEAT GLAND

ARTERY

VEIN

SUBCUTANEOUS LAYER

h., moniliform. Monilethrix, q.v.

h., pubic. Hair that appears over the pubes at the onset of sexual maturity.

h., sensory. Specialized epithelial cells with hairlike processes.

h., tactile. Hair that is capable of receiving tactile or touching stimuli.

h., taste. Hairlike projections from the ends of the taste cells in the taste buds.

h., terminal. Long, coarse, pigmented hair of the adult.

h., twisted. Congenitally deformed hair that is short, brittle, and twisted.

hair analysis. Investigation of the chemical composition of hair. It is used in studying exposure to toxic chemicals in the environment, in poisoning investigations, in nutritional studies; and in monitoring the course of certain diseases. The sample should be obtained from new-growth hair within 5 cm of the scalp to reduce the chance of contamination of the hair by air pollutants.

hairball. A mass of hair in the stomach. SYN: *trichobezoar.*

hair bulb. The lower expanded portion of a hair root. Growth of a hair results from the proliferation of cells of the hair bulb.

hair cell. An epithelial cell possessing fine nonmotile cilia found in the maculae and the organ of Corti of the membranous labyrinth of the inner ear. They are receptors for the senses of position and hearing.

hair follicle. An invagination of the epidermis that forms a cylindrical depression, penetrating the corium into the connective tissue that holds the hair root. Sebaceous glands, which secrete an oily fluid, and tiny muscles (arrectores pili) that cause the hair to stand are attached to these follicles.

hair papilla. A projection of the corium that extends into the hair bulb at the bottom of a hair follicle. It contains capillaries through which a hair receives nourishment.

hair transplantation. A surgical procedure for placing plugs of skin containing hair follicles from one body site to another. This technique is very time consuming, but has some success in treatment of alopecia of the scalp.

hairy tongue. Tongue covered with hairlike papillae entangled with threads produced by the fungus *Aspergillus niger* or *Candida albicans.* Usually seen as the result of antibiotic therapy that inhibits growth of bacteria normally present in the mouth. This permits overgrowth of fungi. SYN: *tongue, black hairy.*

halation (hăl-ā'shŭn) [Gr. *alos*, a halo]. Blur-

halazone (hăl'ă-zōn). USP. A chloramine disinfectant. SEE: *water, emergency preparation of safe drinking.*

halcinonide (hăl-sĭn'ō-nīd). A corticosteroid drug. Trade name is Halog.

Haldol. Trade name for haloperidol, USP.

Haldrone. Trade name for paramethasone acetate.

half-life. 1. Time required for half the nuclei of a radioactive substance to lose their activity by undergoing radioactive decay. SYN: *physical half-life.* 2. Time it takes for a radioactive substance to reduce to one-half its energy due to metabolism and excretion. SYN: *biological half-life.* 3. In biology and pharmacology, the time required by the body, tissue, or organ to metabolize or inactivate half the amount of a substance taken in. This is an important consideration in determining the proper amount and frequency of dose of drug to be administered. SYN: *biological half-life.* 4. Time required for radioactivity of material taken in by a living organism to be reduced to half its initial value by a combination of radioactive decay and biological elimination. SYN: *effective half-life.*

half-value layer. The amount of lead, copper, cement, or material that would dissipate the beam of radiation by 50%. The number of half-value layers required for safety in blocking the area on a patient is five, because that represents 50% of 50% and 50% of that, etc. For example, $50\% + 25\% + 12.5\% + 6.23\% + 3.12\% = 96.9\%$. Thus the patient would be shielded from all but about 3% of the radiation. (Examples of the amount of material required to protect from radiation are 2 inches [5 cm] of lead and 2 feet [61 cm] of cement.)

half-value thickness. The thickness of a substance that, when placed in the path of a given beam of rays, will lower its intensity to one-half of the initial value.

halfway house. A facility to house mental patients who do not need hospitalization but who are not ready for independent living.

halibut liver oil. An oil obtained from the liver of the halibut fish. It is rich in vitamins A and D.

halide (hăl'īd). Compound containing a halogen, i.e., bromine, chlorine, fluorine, or iodine, combined with a metal or some other radical.

halitosis (hăl-ĭ-tō'sĭs) [L. *halitus,* breath, + Gr. *osis,* condition]. Offensive breath. SEE: *bad breath.*

halitus (hăl'ĭ-tŭs). 1. The breath. 2. Warm vapor.

Haller's anastomotic circle (hăl'ĕrz) [Albrecht von Haller, Swiss physiologist, 1708–1777]. Circle of arteries around the intraocular portion of the optic nerve. Made up of branches of the posterior ciliary arteries.

Hallervorden-Spatz disease or syndrome [Julius Hallervorden, 1882–1965; H. Spatz, 1888–1969, Ger. neurologists]. An inherited, progressive, degenerative disease, beginning in childhood, of the globus pallidus, red nucleus, and reticular part of the substantia nigra of the brain. Clinically, there are progressive rigidity, retinal degeneration, athetotic movements, and mental and, late in the disease, emotional retardation. There is no effective therapy.

hallex (hăl'ĕks) [L.] (pl. *hallices*). The great toe. SYN: *hallus; hallux.*

Hallpike maneuver [C. Hallpike, 20th century neurologist]. SEE: *vertigo, benign positional.*

hallucination (hă-loo-sĭ-nā'shŭn) [L. *hallucinari,* to wander in mind]. In psychology, a false perception having no relation to reality and not accounted for by any exterior stimuli. May be visual, auditory, or olfactory. Judgment may be impaired and the patient will not be able to distinguish between the real and the imagined.

Structural disease of the sensory organ and conducting mechanism may contribute to the formation of hallucinations, e.g., deafness following otitis media often is associated with tinnitus. An irritative lesion of the visual cortex may produce hallucination.

RS: acousma; delusion; hallucinosis; hypnagogic; illusion.

    h., auditory. Imaginary perception of sounds, usually voices.

    h., extracampine. Hallucination that arises from outside the normal sensory field or range, as people having the sensation of seeing something behind them.

    h., gustatory. Sense of tasting something that is not present.

    h., haptic. Hallucination pert. to touching the skin, or to sensations of temperature or pain.

    h., hypnagogic. Pre-sleep phenomenon having the same practical significance as a dream but experienced while consciousness persists. Includes sense of falling, sinking, or of the ceiling moving.

    h., kinetic. Sensation of flying or moving the body or a part of it.

    h., microptic. Hallucination in which things seem reduced in size.

    h., motor. Imaginary perceptions of movement.

    h., olfactory. Hallucination involving

smell.

h., somatic. Sensation of pain attributed to visceral injury.

h., stump. Phantom limb, q.v.

h., tactile. False sense of touching something.

h., visual. Sensation of seeing objects that are not real.

hallucinogen (hă-loo'sĭ-nō-jĕn) [″ + Gr. *gennan,* to produce]. Drug that produces hallucinations. LSD, peyote, mescaline, PCP, and sometimes ethyl alcohol are hallucinogens.

hallucinogenesis (hă-lū″sĭ-nō-jĕn'ĕ-sĭs). Production of or causing hallucinations.

hallucinosis (hă-loo″sin-ō'sĭs) [″ + Gr. *osis,* condition]. The state of having hallucinations more or less persistently. SEE: *hallucination.*

h., acute alcoholic. Alcoholic psychosis marked by fear or anxiety and auditory hallucinations.

hallus. Hallux.

hallux (hăl'ŭks) [L.] (pl. *halluces*). [NA] The great toe.

h. dolorosus. Pain in the metatarsophalangeal joint of the great toe due to flatfoot.

h. flexus. Hammertoe.

h. malleus. Hammertoe of the great toe.

h. rigidus. Restriction or loss of motion of the joint connecting the great toe to the metatarsal. It is painful upon walking.

h. valgus. Displacement of great toe toward other toes.

h. varus. Displacement of great toe away from other toes.

halmatogenesis (hăl″mă-tō-jĕn'ĕ-sĭs) [Gr. *halma,* jump, + *genesis,* generation, birth]. A sudden deviation of type from one generation to the other. SEE: *mutation.*

halo [Gr. *halos,* a halo]. 1. The areola, esp. of the nipple. 2. A ring surrounding the macula lutea in ophthalmoscopic images. 3. A circle of light surrounding a shining body.

h., Fick's. A colored halo around light; this is observed by some persons due to the wearing of contact lenses.

h., glaucomatous. Visual perception of rainbowlike colors seen around lights. This is due to glaucoma-induced edema of the cornea.

h., senile peripapillary. A ring of choriodoretinal atrophy around the head of the optic nerve. This may occur in the aged.

halodermia (hăl″ō-dĕr'mē-ă). Skin eruption caused by exposure to a halogen.

Halog. Trade name for halcinonide.

halogen (hăl'ō-jĕn) [Gr. *hals,* salt, + *gennan,* to produce]. A salt former; one of a group of elements (chlorine, Cl; bromine, Br; iodine, I; and fluorine, F) having very similar chemical properties. They combine

with hydrogen to form acids and with metals to form salts.

haloid (hăl'oyd) [″ + *eidos,* form, shape]. Resembling salt or a halogen.

haloid salt. A salt made up of a base and a halogen.

halometer (hă-lŏm'ĕ-tĕr) [Gr. *halos,* a halo, + *metron,* measure]. 1. Device for measuring diffraction halo of a red blood cell. 2. Device for measuring the halo around the optic disk.

haloperidol (hă″lō-pĕr'ĭ-dŏl). USP. An antipsychotic drug. Uses include the treatment of psychotic disorders, such as schizophrenia, and the treatment of Gilles de la Tourette's syndrome.

halophilic (hăl″ō-fĭl'ĭk) [″ + *philein,* to love]. Concerning or having an affinity for salt or any halogen.

halosteresis (hă-lŏs″tĕr-ē'sĭs) [Gr. *hals,* salt, + *steresis,* privation]. Deficiency of lime salts in the bones. SYN: *halisteresis.* SEE: *osteomalacia; osteoporosis.*

halo symptom. Colored circle or circles around lights. These are seen by patients with glaucoma or with punctate lens opacities.

Halotestin. Trade name for fluoxymesterone, USP.

halothane (hăl'ō-thān). USP. A fluorinated hydrocarbon used as a general anesthetic.

Halsted's operation (hăl'stĕdz) [William Stewart Halsted, U.S. surgeon, 1852–1922]. 1. Operation for inguinal hernia. 2. Radical mastectomy for cancer of the breast.

Halsted's suture. An interrupted suture for intestinal wounds.

ham [AS. *haum,* haunch]. 1. The popliteal space or region behind the knee. 2. Common name for the thigh, hip, and buttock.

hamartoma (hăm-ăr-tō'mă) [Gr. *hamartia,* defect, + *oma,* tumor]. A tumor resulting from new growth of normal tissues. The cells grow spontaneously, reach maturity, and then do not reproduce. Thus the growth is self-limiting and benign.

h., multiple. Congenital malformations that present a slowly growing mass of abnormal tissue in multiple sites. The tissues are appropriate to the organ in which the hamartomas are located, but they are not normally organized. They may appear in blood vessels as hemangiomata, and in the lung and kidney. They are not malignant but cause symptoms because of the space they occupy.

hamartomatosis (hăm″ăr-tō-mă-tō'sĭs) [″ + ″ + *osis,* condition]. Existence of multiple hamartomas.

hamate (hăm'ăt). Hooked.

hamate bone. The medial bone in the distal row of carpal bones of the wrist. Also called *unciform.*

hamatum (hă-mā'tŭm) [L. *hamatus*, hooked]. The hamate bone of the wrist. SYN: *os hamatum.*

hamaxophobia [Gr. *amaxa*, a carriage, + *phobos*, fear]. Fear of riding in a vehicle.

Hamman, Louis (hăm'ăn). U.S. physician, 1877–1946.

    H.'s disease. Spontaneous mediastinal emphysema.

    H.-Rich syndrome [Arnold Rich, U.S. pathologist, 1893–1968]. Previously used term for idiopathic pulmonary fibrosis, q.v.

hammer. 1. An instrument with a head attached crosswise to the handle for striking blows. 2. Common name for the malleus, the hammer-shaped bone of the middle ear.

    h., dental. A mallet or motor-driven hammer used for condensing direct filling gold or silver amalgam during the placement of fillings in teeth.

    h., percussion. Hammer with a rubber head used for tapping surfaces of the body in order to produce sounds for diagnostic purposes. SEE: *plexor.*

    h., reflex. Hammer used for tapping parts of the body such as a muscle, tendon, or nerve in order to initiate certain reflex responses.

hammer finger. Flexion deformity of the distal joint of a finger. It is caused by avulsion of the extensor tendon. SYN: *mallet finger.*

hammertoe. A toe with dorsal flexion of 1st phalanx and plantar flexion of 2nd and 3rd phalanges. SYN: *claw toe.*

hamster. A rodent, *Cricetus cricetus*, belonging to the family Cricetidae, common in Europe and western Asia. It is extensively used as a research animal.

hamstring [AS. *haum*, haunch]. One of the tendons that form the medial and lateral boundaries of the popliteal space.

    h.'s, inner. Tendons of the semimembranosus, semitendinosus, and gracilis muscles.

    h., outer. Tendon of the biceps femoris.

hamstrings. Three muscles on the posterior aspect of the thigh, the semitendinosus, semimembranosus, and biceps femoris. They flex the leg and adduct and extend the thigh.

Ham test. Test for diagnosing paroxysmal nocturnal hemoglobinuria. The red cells are tested for resistance to lysis during incubation with acidified serum.

hamular (hăm'ū-lăr) [L. *hamulus*, a small hook]. Unciform; hook-shaped.

hamulus (hăm'ū-lŭs) [L., a small hook] (pl. *hamuli*). 1. Any hook-shaped structure. 2. Hooklike process on the hamate bone.

    h. cochleae. Hooklike process at the tip of the osseous spiral lamina of the cochlea.

    h. lacrimalis. [NA] Hooklike process on the lacrimal bone.

    h. pterygoideus. [NA] Hooklike process at the tip of the medial pterygoid process of the sphenoid bone.

hand [AS.]. That part of the body attached to the forearm at the wrist. It includes the wrist (carpus) with its 8 bones, the metacarpus or body of the hand (ossa metacarpalia) having 5 bones, and the phalanges (fingers) with their 14 bones. In some occupations and recreational endeavors, workers use their hands as hammers. This may cause damage to the ulnar nerve and artery with consequent signs of ischemia and neuropathy. SYN: *manus* [NA]. SEE: illus.

    h., accoucheur's. Obstetrician's hand, q.v.

    h., ape. Deformity of the hand in which the thumb is permanently extended. Usually due to a median nerve injury. The result will be paralysis and atrophy of the thenar muscles.

    h., claw. SEE: *clawhand.*

    h., cleft. Deformity of the hand in which the division between the fingers, particularly between the third and fourth, extends into the carpus.

    h., drop. Wrist drop.

    h., functional position of. Principle used in splint fabrication whereby wrist is dorsiflexed 20° to 35°, there is a normal transverse arch, and the thumb is in abduction and opposition and aligned with the pads of the four fingers. Proximal interphalangeal joints are flexed 45° to 60°.

    h., lobster-claw. Cleft hand.

    h., obstetrician's. Hand in tetany with extension at the metacarpophalangeal and the interphalangeal joints, and adduction of the thumb. SYN: *accoucheur's hand.*

    h., opera-glass. Deformity of the hand caused by chronic arthritis. The phalanges appear to be telescoped into one another like an opera glass.

    h., resting position of. Principle used in splint fabrication whereby the forearm is midway between pronation and supination, wrist is at 12° to 20° dorsiflexion, and phalanges are slightly flexed. Thumb is in partial opposition and forward.

    h., writing. The tips of the thumb and first finger are touching and the other fingers are flexed as if writing. Seen in paralysis agitans.

H. and E. *hematoxylin* and *eosin*, a staining method used in histology.

handedness. The tendency to use one hand in preference to the other. Preferential use of the left hand is called sinistrality and of the right hand dextrality.

    Over 90 percent of people are right-

BONES OF THE RIGHT HAND AND WRIST

RADIUS
ULNA
SCAPHOID
LUNATE
PISIFORM
CAPITATE
TRIQUETRUM
TRAPEZIUM
HAMATE
TRAPEZOID
METACARPAL
PROXIMAL PHALANX
MIDDLE PHALANX
DISTAL PHALANX

VIEW FROM PALMAR SIDE

ULNA
RADIUS
LUNATE
SCAPHOID
PISIFORM
TRAPEZIUM
TRIQUETRUM
TRAPEZOID
HAMATE
CAPITATE
METACARPAL
PROXIMAL PHALANX
MIDDLE PHALANX
DISTAL PHALANX

VIEW FROM BACK OF THE HAND

handed. Being left-handed may be hereditary or due to disease of the left cerebral hemisphere in early life. Left hemisphere dominance for language occurs in 95 percent of right-handed people and in 50 percent of those who are left-handed. A disturbance in language is produced in almost all right-handed persons by unilateral brain damage that affects the left hemisphere.

hand-foot-and-mouth disease. Painful ulcerative and vesicular lesions of the oral mucosa and tongue with vesicular lesions of the hands and feet. It is highly infectious. Various types of coxsackievirus group A, esp. type 16, and enterovirus 71 are the usual etiologic agents.

handicap. Disadvantage for a given individual, resulting from an impairment or a disability, that limits or prevents the fulfillment of a role that is normal, depending on age, sex, and social and cultural factors for that individual. SEE: *disability.*

handpiece (hănd′pēs). Hand instrument used in dentistry. It contains a chuck for holding tools used in preparing teeth for restoration, polishing, and condensing. The tool may rotate or vibrate.

   h., air-bearing turbine. Handpiece driven by compressed air, having a turbine and air bearings and capable of rotary speeds up to 400,000 r.p.m.

   h., contra-angle. Handpiece with one or more bends so that the shaft of the rotary instrument is at an angle to the handpiece to facilitate reaching less accessible areas of the mouth for dental work.

   h., high-speed. Handpiece that operates at speeds about 12,000 r.p.m.

Hand-Schüller-Christian disease (hănd-shĭl′ĕr-krĭs′chăn) [Alfred Hand, Jr., U.S. pediatrician, 1868–1949; Artur Schüller, Austrian neurologist, b. 1874; Henry A. Christian, U.S. physician, 1876–1951]. A rare disease of unknown cause in which lipids accumulate in the body and manifest as histiocytic granulomas in bone (particularly the skull), the skin, and viscera. Exophthalmos and diabetes insipidus may be present. The disease is seen in children and young adults. Adrenal cortical hormones have been of some help in treating the illness. SYN: *xanthoma disseminatum.*

handsock. A type of glove that covers the hand but, because it has no individual spaces for the fingers, makes grasping objects difficult. Use of handsocks during infancy may inhibit the rate of development of hand skills.

hand syringe. A hollow rubber bulb which is fitted to a nozzle and delivers air when squeezed.

hanging drop culture. A method of culturing

microorganisms by placing a drop of the culture medium containing organisms on a coverslip, then inverting the coverslip over a concavity of a hanging drop slide.

hangman's fracture. The fracture produced when judicial hanging is done properly. At the time the dropped victim fully extends the rope, the hangman knot causes fracture dislocation of the upper cervical spine and transection of the spinal cord or medulla. If the knot is not made or applied properly, death is usually due to asphyxia.

hangnail [AS. *ang-*, tight, painful, + *naegel*, nail]. Partly detached piece of skin at root or lateral edge of finger or toenail.

hangover. A nontechnical term for describing the malaise that may be present following the ingestion of a considerable amount of an alcoholic beverage or other central nervous system depressant. Usually present upon awakening after stuporous sleep. Characterized by some if not all of the following: mental depression, headache, thirst, nausea, irritability, fatigue. Symptoms and severity will vary with the individual.

The presence of congeners, q.v., in alcoholic beverages is felt to be related to the development of a hangover. Therapy of hangover is not specific. SEE: *alcoholism, acute; delirium tremens.*

Hanot's disease (ä-nōz') [Victor C. Hanot, Fr. physician, 1844–1896]. Hypertrophic cirrhosis of liver with jaundice.

Hansen's bacillus [Gerhard H. A. Hansen, Norwegian physician, 1841–1912]. *Mycobacterium leprae*, the cause of leprosy, which Hansen discovered in 1871.

Hansen's disease. Leprosy.

hapalonychia (hăp″ăl-ō-nĭk′ē-ă) [Gr. *hapalos*, soft, + *onyx*, nail]. Lack of rigidity of the nails. SYN: *onychomalacia.*

haphalgesia (hăf″ăl-jē′zē-ă) [Gr. *haphe*, touch, + *algesis*, sense of pain]. A sensation of pain upon touching the skin lightly or with an object that is not an irritant.

haphephobia (hăf″ē-fō′bē-ă) [″ + *phobos*, fear]. Aversion to being touched by another person.

haplodont (hăp′lō-dŏnt) [″ + *odous*, tooth]. Having teeth without ridges or tubercles on the crown.

haploid [Gr. *haploos*, simple, + *eidos*, form, shape]. Possessing half the diploid or normal number of chromosomes found in somatic or body cells. Such is the case of the germ cells — ova or sperm — following the reduction divisions in gametogenesis, the haploid number being 23 in man. SEE: *chromosome; diploid.*

haploidy (hăp′loy-dē). The state of haploids.

haplopia (hăp-lō′pē-ă) [″ + *ops*, vision]. Single vision; condition in which an object

viewed by two eyes appears as a single object, in contrast to diplopia, in which it appears as two objects.

haplotype. The combination of several alleles, q.v., in a gene cluster. SEE: *histocompatibility antigens.*

hapten(e) (hăp′tĕn, -tēn) [Gr. *haptein*, to seize]. A substance that normally does not act as an antigen or stimulate an immune response. However, it can be combined with an antigen and, at a later time, initiate a specific antibody response on its own.

haptic (hăp′tĭk) [Gr. *haptein*, to touch]. Pert. to touch. SYN: *tactile.*

haptics. The science of the touch sense.

haptin (hăp′tĭn). Hapten.

haptoglobin (hăp″tō-glō′bĭn). A mucoprotein to which hemoglobin released from lysed red cells into plasma is bound. It is increased in certain inflammatory conditions and decreased in hemolytic disorders.

haptometer (hăp-tŏm′ĕ-tĕr) [″ + *metron*, measure]. Device for measuring the acuteness of the sense of touch.

hardening [AS. *heardian*, to harden]. 1. Rendering a pathological or histological specimen firm or compact for making thin sections for microscopic study. 2. The development of increased resistance to extremes of environmental temperature. SEE: *acclimation.*

hardening of the arteries. Colloquial expression used for arteriosclerosis.

hardness. 1. Quality of water containing certain substances, esp. soluble salts of calcium and magnesium. These react with soaps, forming insoluble compounds that are precipitated out of solution, thus interfering with their cleansing action. 2. That quality of x-rays determining their penetrating power. Hardness lessens as wavelengths become longer. 3. The quality of firmness or density of a material imparted by the cohesion of the particles that compose it.

   h. of a gas tube. Term used to qualify the condition of a tube according to the degree of rarefaction of the residual gas. The higher the vacuum, the harder the tube and the rays emitted, the higher the voltage required to cause a discharge with a cold cathode, and hence the shorter the wavelength of the resulting roentgen rays.

hardness number. A number on a calibrated scale indicating the relative hardness as determined by a particular system of testing; e.g., Knoop, Mohs, Rockwell, Vickers hardness tests. A steel ball or diamond point is applied with a known variable load for a determined period of time to produce an indent whose depth or diameter can be measured.

harelip [AS. *hara*, hare, + *lippa*, lip]. A vertical cleft or clefts in the upper lip. It is congenital, resulting from the faulty fusion of the median nasal process and the lateral maxillary processes. Nongenetic factors may also be responsible for causing this condition. It is usually unilateral and on the left side, although it may be bilateral. It may involve the lip or the upper jaw alone or both together, and often occurs with cleft palate. The incidence of harelip is from one in 600 to one in 1250 births. SYN: *cleft lip.*

harelip suture. A twisted figure-of-eight suture used in surgical correction of harelip.

harlequin fetus. A newborn infant with abnormal skin that resembles a thick horny armor. The skin is divided into areas by deep red fissures and the infants die within a few days. Also known as ichthyosis foetalis and ichthyosiform erythroderma. These were at one time regarded as separate diseases but are now known to represent different degrees of severity of the same entity.

harlequin sign. Benign transient color change seen in neonates in which one half of the body blanches while the other half becomes redder with a clear line of demarcation.

harmonic. In physics, concerning wave forms, an oscillation or frequency that is a whole number multiple of the basic frequency.

harmony (hăr′mō-nē). The condition of working or living together smoothly.

h., functional occlusal. The ideal occlusion of the teeth so that in all mandibular positions during chewing, the teeth will be functioning efficiently and without trauma to supporting tissues.

h., occlusal. Proper occlusion of the teeth in various mandibular positions.

harness. In rehabilitation that part of an upper extremity prosthesis that fits around the shoulder and back to permit mechanical control of the terminal device and hold the socket firmly around the stump.

harpoon (hăr-poon′) [Gr. *harpazein,* to seize]. Device with a hook on the end for obtaining small pieces of tissue such as muscle for examination.

Harrison's groove [Edwin Harrison, Brit. physician, 1779–1847]. Depression on lower edge of the thorax caused by tug of the diaphragm; seen in rickets and any disease of infants that tends to obstruct inspiration.

Hartmann's solution [Alexis F. Hartmann, U.S. pediatrician, 1849–1931]. Lactated Ringer's injection. A sterile solution of 0.6 gram of sodium chloride, 0.03 gram of potassium chloride, 0.02 gram of calcium chloride, and 0.31 gram of sodium lactate diluted with water for injection to make 100 ml. Used for fluid and electrolyte treatment.

Hartnup disease [*Hartnup,* the family name of the first reported case]. A rare hereditary metabolic disease in which amino acid absorption and excretion are abnormal, esp. that of tryptophan. Resorption of amino acids by the kidney is also defective. Clinical signs resemble pellagra, with a rash that is worsened by exposure to sunlight.

harvest. To obtain samples or remove bacteria or other microorganisms from a culture.

harvest mite. Mite, similar in appearance to scabies, that lives in grain stems, grasses and bushes. It is common in the southern U.S. The larvae attach to the skin and inject a secretion that causes itching.

Harvey, William (hăr′vē). British physician, 1578–1657, who described the circulation of the blood.

Hashimoto's struma [Hakaru Hashimoto, Japanese surgeon, 1881–1934]. Thyroiditis, Hashimoto's, q.v.

hashish (hăsh′ĭsh) [Arabic, hemp, dried grass]. A more or less purified extract prepared from the flowers, stalks, and leaves of the hemp plant *Cannabis sativa.* The gummy substance is smoked or chewed for its euphoric effects. SEE: *cannabis; marijuana.*

Hasner's valve or fold [Joseph R. Hasner, Prague ophthalmologist, 1819–1892]. A fold of the mucous membrane at the opening of the nasolacrimal duct in the inferior meatus of the nasal cavity. SYN: *plica lacrimalis.*

Hassall's corpuscles [Arthur H. Hassall, Brit. chemist and physician, 1817–1894]. Spherical or oval bodies present in the medulla of the thymus. Each consists of central area of degenerated cells surrounded by concentrically arranged flattened or polygonal cells.

Hatchcock's sign. Tenderness just beyond the angle of the jaws when the finger follows on the undersurface of the mandible toward the angle. Found in mumps before any swelling can be detected.

haunch (hawnsh) [Fr. *hanche*]. The hips and buttocks.

haustra (haws′trä) [L. *haurire,* to draw, drink] (sing. *haustrum*). The sacculated pouches of the colon.

h. coli. Sacculations of the colon resembling tucks caused by the fact that the gut is longer than the longitudinal bands or taeniae.

haustral (haw′străl). Pert. to the colonic haustra.

haustration (haws-trä′shŭn). The process of formation of a haustrum.

haustrum (haw′strŭm) [L. *haurire,* to draw, drink] (pl. *haustra*). [NA] One of the sacculations of the colon caused by longitudinal bands that are shorter than the gut. SYN: *haustra coli.*

haustus (haws′tŭs) [L., a drink]. A swallow, or draft, of medicine.

HAV. *hepatitis A virus.*

Haverhill fever (hā′vĕr-ĭl) [Haverhill, Mass., U.S., where the initial epidemic occurred]. A febrile disease transmitted to man by a rat, usually by rat bite. *Streptobacillus moniliformis* is the etiological agent. SYN: *rat bite fever due to Streptobacillus moniliformis.*

haversian canal (hă-vĕr′shăn) [Clopton Havers, Brit. physician and anatomist, 1650–1702]. Minute vascular canals found in osseous tissue.

haversian canaliculi. Delicate canals extending from the lacunae into the matrix of bone. They anastomose with canaliculi of adjacent lacunae, forming a network of fine channels that communicate with haversian and Volkmann's canals. They transmit nutrient materials.

haversian gland. Minute projections from the surface of the synovial tissue into the joint space. SEE: *gland, haversian.*

haversian system. Architectural unit of bone consisting of a central tube (haversian canal) with alternate layers of intercellular material (matrix) surrounding it in concentric cylinders. Alternating layers of matrix and cells are called haversian lamellae. SEE: *bone.*

hay fever. A Type I hypersensitivity reaction or allergic disease of mucous membranes of nose and upper air passages induced by external irritation. SYN: *pollinosis; rhinitis, vasomotor.* SEE: *Nursing Diagnoses* in *Appendix.*

SYM: Inflammation, catarrh, watery discharges from the eyes, coryza, headache, asthmatic symptoms.

ETIOL: Airborne pollens or occasionally fungus spores. Spring type is due to pollens of trees such as oak, elm, hickory, ash. Summer type is due to pollens of plants such as grasses, plantain, and sorrel. Fall type is due principally to the pollen of ragweeds. Nonseasonal hay fever may result from inhalation of irritating substances such as the danders of animals or dust such as hay, straw, or house dust or from ingestion of drugs or foods to which the subject is allergic.

TREAT: Either remove the patient from contact with the allergen or remove the allergen from the patient's environment. Filtration of air by masks and nasal filters may be helpful. Drug therapy in which epinephrine, antihistamines, or other drugs are given orally or used as nose drops, or nasal sprays. Antihistamines that are free of anticholinergic side effects, e.g., astemizole and terfenadine, are available. If nasal obstruction persists, inhaled corticosteroids should be tried. In situations in which it is not possible to avoid contact with the allergen, prophylactic treatment consisting of desensitization by injection of pollen extracts of allergens (other than food) to which the subject is sensitive may be of benefit.

Hayflick limit [Leonard Hayflick, U.S. microbiologist, b. 1928]. The limit of time that cells in culture will live. Using data obtained from investigations of cell cultures, Dr. Hayflick has estimated that the limit of life of human beings could be over 100 years.

Haygarth's deformities [John Haygarth, Brit. physician, 1740–1827]. Exostoses or bony tumors on joints in rheumatoid arthritis.

hazardous material. Any material handled in such a way that people coming into contact with it can suffer personal injury or property damage. The hazard of any material is determined by the chemical, physical, and biological properties of the material and the possibility of exposure to that material. SEE: *health hazard; permissible exposure limits; right to know law; toxic substance.*

hazmat. Contraction for hazardous material.

HB. *hepatitis B.*

Hb. *hemoglobin.*

HB Ag. *hepatitis B antigen.*

Hbg. *hemoglobin.*

H2 blockers. SEE: *H2-receptor antagonists.*

HBV. *hepatitis B virus.*

HC Cream. Trade name for hydrocortisone cream.

HCG. *human chorionic gonadotrophin.*

HCl. *hydrochloric acid.*

HCO$_3$⁻. Chemical formula for bicarbonate ion.

H$_2$CO$_3$. Chemical formula for carbonic acid.

H.D. *hearing distance.*

h.d. L. *hora decubitus,* the hour of going to bed.

HDCV. *human diploid cell vaccine* (for rabies).

H. disease. *Hartnup disease,* q.v.

HDL. *high-density lipoprotein.*

He. Chem. symb. for the element helium.

head [AS. *heafod*]. 1. Caput [NA]. That part of the animal body containing the brain and organs of sight, hearing, smell, and taste. It includes the facial bones. 2. The proximal end of a bone. 3. The larger extremity of any structure or body.

ABNORM: *Abnormal fixation* of the head may be caused by postpharyngeal abscess, arthritis deformans, swollen cervical glands, rheumatism, traumatism of the neck, sprains of cervical muscles, congenital spasmodic torticollis, caries of a molar tooth, burn scars, or eye muscle imbalance (hyperphoria). Inability to move the head may be due to caries of the cervical vertebrae and diseases of articulation between the occiput and atlas or paralysis of neck muscles.

Abnormal movements include habit spasms such as nodding. Rhythmical nodding is seen in aortic regurgitation, chorea, torticollis, q.v. A retracted head is seen in acute meningitis, cerebral abscess, tumor, thrombosis of the superior longitudinal sinus, acute encephalitis, laryngeal obstruction, tetanus, hydrophobia, epilepsy, spasmodic torticollis, strychnine poisoning, hysteria, rachitic conditions, and painful neck lesions at the back.

    h., after-coming. Childbirth with the head delivered last.

    h., articular. A projection on bone that articulates with another bone.

    h., nerve. The optic disk.

head, words pert. to: acromegaly; caput; "ceph-" words; coryza; face; gyrospasm; macrocephalous; nutation; occipital; sinciput; skeleton; temple; vertex.

headache [AS. *heafod,* head, + *acan,* to ache]. A diffuse pain in different portions of the head and not confined to any nerve distribution area. May be acute or chronic. It may be frontal, temporal, or occipital; confined to one side of the head or to the region immediately over one eye. The character of pain may vary. It may be dull and aching or acute and almost unbearable. It may be an intermittent intense pain, a throbbing pain, a pressure pain when the head feels as if it will burst, or a penetrating pain driving through the head. SYN: *cephalgia.* SEE: *migraine.*

    ETIOL: Transient acute headaches may be due to a variety of causes including diseases of the paranasal sinuses, teeth, eye, ear, nose, or throat; acute infections; or trauma to the head. Chronic headaches may be caused by a variety of conditions including physical, emotional, psychosomatic, or psychogenic factors; fevers; metabolic conditions; or exposure to toxic chemicals. The exact cause can be determined by thorough analysis of the data obtained from history, physical examination, tests, and laboratory studies, which may include roentgenography of the skull, electroencephalography, and metabolic studies.

    Toxic factors: (1) Exogenous origin: Foul air from poor ventilation; poisonous gases, including fumes from furnaces or gas fires; drugs (quinine, morphine, atropine, histamine); alcohol; tobacco; wines with high histamine content. (2) Endogenous origin: Any absorption of the toxins of bacterial infection will cause headache. Includes chronic infections (nose and sinuses, teeth, middle ear, pharynx, tonsils, appendix, gallbladder, pelvic viscera); fever; bacteremias

(typhoid fever, malaria, smallpox, tuberculosis, grippe and influenza, puerperal fever).

    Systemic diseases: Nephritis with uremia, biliary tract disease including acute yellow atrophy of the liver, rheumatism, diabetes, anemia, polycythemia, eclampsia, central nervous system syphilis.

    Gastrointestinal disturbances: Dyspepsia, gastric hyper- and hypoacidity, intestinal stasis, and constipation. *Physicochemical disturbances:* Acidosis, alkalosis. *Cardiovascular disturbances:* Myocardial and valvular insufficiency causing congestive heart failure; constriction, dilatation, or edema of intracranial blood vessels.

    Endocrine disorders: Pituitary, thyroid, adrenal, and ovarian tumors; carcinoid tumors. *Gynecological factors:* Functional disturbances of one or more of the endocrine glands, puberty, dysmenorrhea, premenstrual tension, menstruation, pregnancy, menopause. *Psychoneurological factors:* Nervous exhaustion; worry, excitement, anger, or nervous tension; migraine; hysteria; epilepsy; psychoneuroses.

    Diseases of special sense organs: Iritis, glaucoma, conjunctivitis; adenoids, deviated septum; middle ear affections. *Organic disease of brain:* Causing pressure such as tumor, abscess, gumma, cyst, hydrocephaly, intracranial hemorrhage; subdural hematoma; intracranial vascular disease; arteriosclerosis; embolism, thrombosis, or aneurysm; encephalitis; various forms of meningitis; meningismus.

    Miscellaneous causes: Almost any disturbance of body function may cause headache. Other causes are external pressure and constriction of head; trauma to head; sunstroke; any form of motion sickness; irritation of mucous membrane of nose and sinuses by dust, pollen; fatigue (physical or mental); insomnia; travel to an altitude sufficient to produce hypoxia. Spinal puncture or diagnostic examination involving injecting dyes or radioactive substances into cranial arteries or air into the ventricles of the brain may be followed by headache. Orgasm is a rare cause of headache.

    TREAT: Depends entirely upon cause.

    IMPORTANT: A headache that may be the symptom of a serious disease should not be treated symptomatically without attempting to find its cause.

    NURSING IMPLICATIONS: Evaluate character, severity, location, radiation, prodromata or associated symptoms; and any palliative measures the patient uses to provide relief. Note temporal factors and any relationship of recurring headaches to other activities. Provide non-invasive comfort measures and prescribed medical treatment and evaluate patient responses.

h., cluster. SEE: *cluster headache.*

h., coital. Headache that begins suddenly during coitus, or immediately after orgasm. These are uncommon, occur more frequently in men than women, and may last for minutes or hours. There is no significant underlying pathology.

h., exertional. An acute headache of short duration that appears after strenuous physical activity. It is usually benign and is relieved by aspirin. It can be prevented by changing to a less strenuous exercise.

h., histamine. Headache resulting from ingestion of histamine (some wines contain histamine), injection of histamine, or excessive histamine in circulating blood. Due to dilatation of branches of the carotid artery. SEE: *cluster headache.*

h., postlumbar puncture. Of patients having lumbar puncture, 10% to 40% will develop a severe headache. It is thought to be related to the leakage of spinal fluid through the hole that fails to close when the needle is removed from the dura. The use of a small-gauge spinal puncture needle helps to prevent this headache.

TREAT: Bedrest in a completely flat and prone position without use of a pillow, forced oral and intravenous fluids, and cortical steroids are useful in treating the headache. If the headache persists in spite of therapy, it may be possible to stop the leakage of spinal fluid by injection of 10 ml of the patient's blood in the epidural space at the site of the lumbar puncture. The blood may provide a patch for the hole in the dura.

h., tension. 1. Headache associated with chronic contraction of the muscles of the neck and scalp. 2. Headache associated with emotional or physical strain.

h., thundering. Sudden acute headache that may accompany intracranial hemorrhage. Its absence does not rule out intracranial hemorrhage.

head banging. In children, a tension-discharging action in which the head is repeatedly banged against the crib. May be part of a temper tantrum.

headgear. A covering for the head, esp. a protective one; a steel helmet for use by soldiers; a helmet used by participants in certain sports.

headgut. Part of the embryo that develops into the pharynx, lungs, stomach, liver, duodenum, and esophagus. SYN: *foregut.*

head injury. Injury to the head due to trauma.

head trauma. Injury to the head, esp. to the scalp and cranium. The injury may be limited to soft tissue damage or may include the cranial bones and the brain.

heal (hēl) [AS. *hael*, whole]. To cure; to make whole or healthy.

healer. 1. A person who heals. 2. One who heals by use of an alternative method such as spiritual healing. SEE: *holistic medicine.*

healing. The restoration to a normal mental or physical condition, but esp. of an inflammation or a wound.

Healing by first intention: This process closes the edge of a wound with little or no inflammatory reaction and in such a manner that little or no scar is left to reveal the site of the injury. New cells are formed to take the place of dead ones, and the capillary walls stretch across the wound to join themselves to each other in a smooth surface. New connective tissue may form an almost imperceptible scar that proves temporary. In repairing lacerations and surgical wounds, the goal is to produce a repaired area that will heal by first intention.

Healing by second intention: This is healing by granulation or indirect union. Granulation tissue is formed to fill the gap between the edges of the wound with a thin layer of fibrinous exudate. It excludes bacteria and aids in checking bleeding by the coagulation of the blood. Connective tissue cells support the new capillaries. This form of healing is slower than that by first intention, and its gray-red surface may become pale and flabby if the healing is too long delayed. If the granulations show above the surface, they may have to be removed with caustics. If the granulations first form at the top instead of the bottom of the wound, it may have to be kept open by drainage.

Healing by third intention: Healing of an ulcer or cavity by filling with granulation tissue. This type of healing usually leads to the formation of a scar.

COMPLICATIONS: These may result from the formation of a scar that interferes with the functioning of a part and possible deformity; the formation of a keloid, q.v., the result of overgrowth of connective tissue forming a tumor in the surface of a scar; necrosis of the skin and mucous membrane that produces a raw surface, which results in an ulcer; a sinus or fistula, which may be due to bacteria or some foreign substance remaining in the wound; proud flesh, which represents excessive growth of granulation tissue. SEE: illus.

health (hĕlth) [AS. *haelth*, wholeness]. A condition in which all functions of the body and mind are normally active. The World Health Organization defines health as a state of complete physical, mental, or social well-being and not merely the absence of disease or infirmity. This definition is of limited usefulness when evaluating an individual and when one asks who determines

---

WOUND HEALING

HEALING BY FIRST INTENTION

SCAB

MITOSES

NEUTROPHILS PLATELETS CLOT

GRANULATION TISSUE: MACROPHAGES, FIBROBLASTS
3-7 DAYS

FIBROUS UNION, REMODELED TISSUE
WEEKS

HEALING BY SECOND INTENTION

SCAB

PLATELETS CLOT

GRANULATION TISSUE
3-7 DAYS

HEALING BY THIRD INTENTION

WOUND CONTRACTION
WEEKS

---

well-being, the health professional or the individual. Many persons enjoy a state of well-being even though they might be classed as unhealthy by others.

h., bill of. Public health certificate stating that passengers on a public conveyance or ship are free of infectious disease.

h., board of. A public body, appointed or elected, concerned with administering the laws pertaining to the health of the public.

h., department of. Branch of a government (city, county, or nation) for regulation and protection of the people's health.

h., industrial. Health of employees of industrial firms.

h., public. State of health of the population of a particular community, as opposed to individual or personal health.

health care proxy. A legal document that allows individuals to name someone they know and trust to make health care decisions for them if, for any reason and at any time, the individual becomes unable to make or communicate those decisions.

Some states limit the age at which such a proxy may be established and prohibit certain persons, such as an estate administrator or an employee of a health care facility in which the person making the proxy is a resident, from being appointed to make health care decisions unless he or she is related to the person by blood, marriage, or adoption. SEE: *advance directive; do not attempt resuscitation; living will; donor card* for illus.

health certificate. An official statement signed by a physician attesting to the state of health of a particular individual.

health education. Educational process or program designed for improvement and maintenance of health. It is directed to the general public in contrast to a health education program organized for instructing persons who will become health educators.

health examination, periodic. SEE: *periodic health examination.*

healthful. Conducive to good health.

health hazard. Literally, any thing, condition, or circumstance that may be or is harmful to health. With respect to chemicals, a substance is considered to be a health hazard if at least one study, conducted in accordance with established scientific principles, documents that acute or chronic effects may occur in connection with use of or exposure to that chemical. SEE: *hazardous material; permissible exposure limits; right to know law; toxic substance.*

Health Maintenance Organization. ABBR: HMO. A prepaid health care program of group practice with comprehensive medical care being provided and with an emphasis on preventive medicine.

health risk appraisal. Analysis of all that is known about a person's entire life situation including personal and family medical history, occupation, and social environment in order to estimate his or her risk of disability or death as compared to the national averages. The data used for comparison will vary with the age, sex, ethnic background, and income of the patient; and the skill of the evaluator and the sensitivity and specificity of the tests used in the evaluation. SEE: *risk factors.*

healthy. Being in a state of health or enjoying it.

healthy persons, medical evaluation of. Examination of healthy individuals in an attempt to determine their state of health at that time; and to discover asymptomatic and latent indicators of disease(s) that may develop later. In most economies, the benefits obtained weighed against the cost of such an evaluation make such medical evaluation inadvisable.

hearing [AS. *hieran*]. The act or power of perceiving sound.

FUNCT. TESTS: Hearing acuity can be determined by the distance at which a person can hear a certain sound such as a watch tick, the use of audiometers, and bone conduction. In audiometers, electrically produced sounds are conveyed by wires to a receiver applied to the subject's ear. Intensity and pitch of sound can be altered and are indicated on the dials. Results are plotted on a graph known as an audiogram. In bone conduction tests, a device such as a tuning fork or an apparatus that converts an electric current into mechanical vibrations is applied to the skull. This is of value in distinguishing between perceptive and conduction deafness. SEE: *acoustic reflex threshold; audiogram; auditory evoked response; cochlear implant; ear; hearing impaired; Rinne's test; Weber test.*

    h., after-. Perception of sound after the stimulus producing it has ceased to act.

hearing aid. An apparatus used by those with impaired hearing for amplifying sound. The modern electronic hearing aid may simply amplify sound or it may be designed to attenuate certain portions of the sound signal and amplify others. The cost may vary from several hundred dollars to more than a thousand dollars. A variety of hearing aids are available, and it is important that patients use the type most suitable for their needs and comfort. It is also important for patients to have a trial period prior to making the final decision to purchase the device.

hearing distance. Distance at which a given sound can be heard. On the prairies and in Arctic air, a voice may be heard for two miles or more.

hearing hallucinations. Subjective sensations of sound such as hearing voices when none actually exists.

hearing impaired. A term used to describe individuals whose ability to hear has decreased to a degree that is noticeable by others as well as themselves.

hearing loss. Decreased ability to perceive sounds as compared to what the individual or examiner would regard as normal. SEE: *audiogram; audiometry.*

heart (härt) [AS. *heorte*]. A hollow, muscular, contractile organ, the center of the circulatory system. It provides the propulsive force for circulating the blood throughout the vascular system. Its wall possesses three layers: the outer epicardium, a serous layer; the middle myocardium, composed of cardiac muscle; and the inner endocardium, a layer that lines the four chambers of the heart and covers the valves. The heart is enclosed in a fibroserous sac, the pericardium,

ANTERIOR VIEWS OF EXTERIOR AND INTERIOR OF HEART AND VESSELS

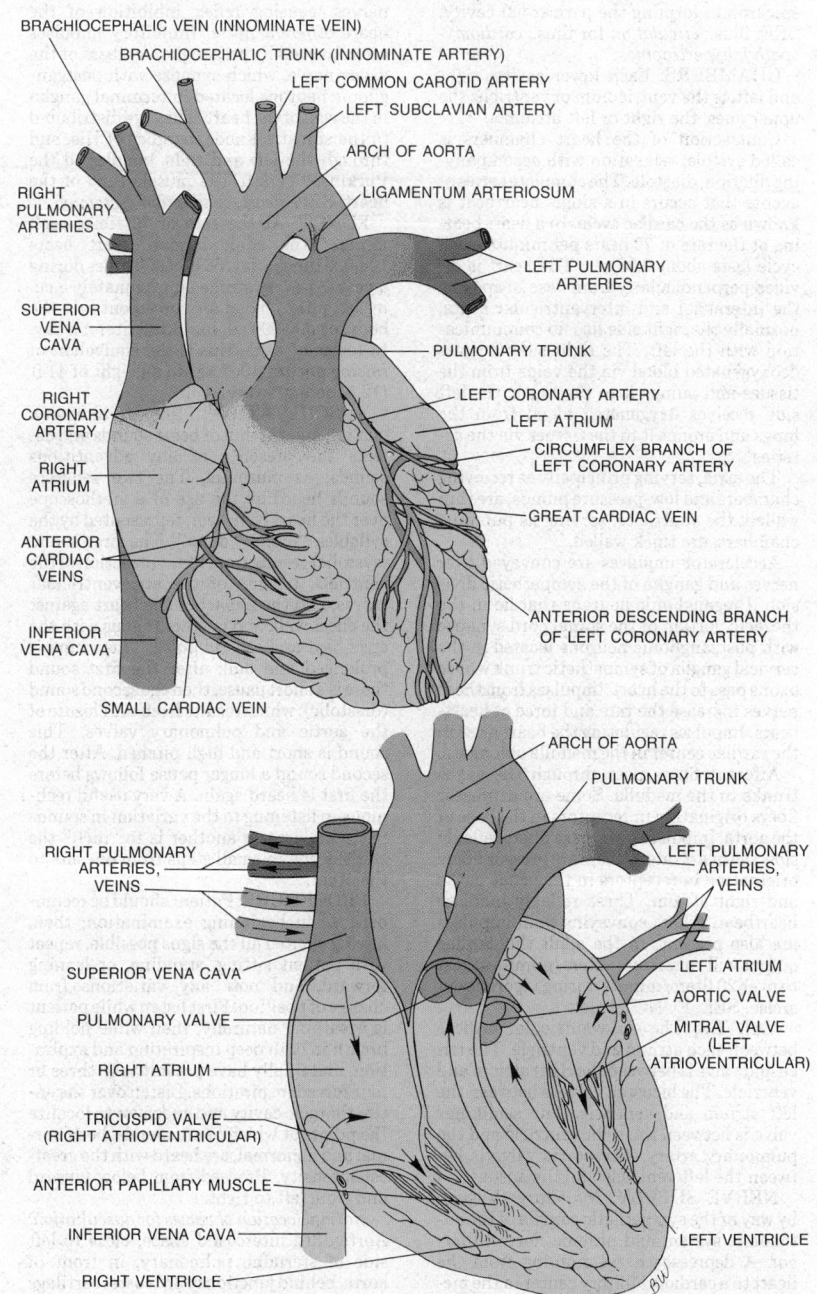

BRACHIOCEPHALIC VEIN (INNOMINATE VEIN)

BRACHIOCEPHALIC TRUNK (INNOMINATE ARTERY)

LEFT COMMON CAROTID ARTERY

LEFT SUBCLAVIAN ARTERY

ARCH OF AORTA

LIGAMENTUM ARTERIOSUM

RIGHT PULMONARY ARTERIES

LEFT PULMONARY ARTERIES

SUPERIOR VENA CAVA

PULMONARY TRUNK

LEFT CORONARY ARTERY

LEFT ATRIUM

CIRCUMFLEX BRANCH OF LEFT CORONARY ARTERY

RIGHT CORONARY ARTERY

RIGHT ATRIUM

GREAT CARDIAC VEIN

ANTERIOR CARDIAC VEINS

INFERIOR VENA CAVA

ANTERIOR DESCENDING BRANCH OF LEFT CORONARY ARTERY

SMALL CARDIAC VEIN

ARCH OF AORTA

PULMONARY TRUNK

RIGHT PULMONARY ARTERIES, VEINS

LEFT PULMONARY ARTERIES, VEINS

SUPERIOR VENA CAVA

LEFT ATRIUM

AORTIC VALVE

PULMONARY VALVE

MITRAL VALVE (LEFT ATRIOVENTRICULAR)

RIGHT ATRIUM

TRICUSPID VALVE (RIGHT ATRIOVENTRICULAR)

ANTERIOR PAPILLARY MUSCLE

INFERIOR VENA CAVA

LEFT VENTRICLE

RIGHT VENTRICLE

the space between the pericardium and the epicardium forming the pericardial cavity. SEE: illus.; *circulation* for illus.; *cardiomyopathy, hypertrophic.*

CHAMBERS: Each lower cavity, right and left, is the ventriculum or ventricle; the upper ones, the right or left atrium.

Contraction of the heart chambers is called systole; relaxation with accompanying dilation, diastole. The complete series of events that occurs in a single heartbeat is known as the cardiac cycle. In a heart beating at the rate of 72 beats per minute, each cycle lasts about 0.85 sec. The heart is divided perpendicularly from base to apex by the interatrial and interventricular septa; normally the right side has no communication with the left. The right side receives deoxygenated blood via the veins from the tissues and pumps it to the lungs; the left side receives oxygenated blood from the lungs and pumps it to the tissues via the arteries.

The atria, serving principally as receiving chambers and low-pressure pumps, are thin walled; the ventricles, serving as pumping chambers, are thick walled.

Accelerator impulses are conveyed over nerves and ganglia of the sympathetic division. Preganglionic neurons that lie in the thoracic portion of the spinal cord synapse with postganglionic neurons located in the cervical ganglia of sympathetic trunk whose axons pass to the heart. Impulses from these nerves increase the rate and force of heartbeats. Impulses regulating the heart arise in the cardiac center in the medulla oblongata. Afferent fibers pass through the vagus trunks to the medulla. Some are depressor fibers originating in receptors in the base of the aorta. Impulses over these fibers reflexly slow the heart rate. Others are pressor fibers originating in receptors in the venae cavae and right atrium. These reflexly increase heartbeat. Fibers conveying pain impulses are also present. In the adult the cardiac output will vary from 5 liters/minute at rest to over 20 liters/minute during vigorous exercise. SEE: FUNCT below.

VALVES: The atrioventricular orifices between each atrium and ventricle. The tricuspid valve is between the right atrium and ventricle. The bicuspid valve is between the left atrium and ventricle. The semilunar valve is between the right ventricle and the pulmonary artery. The aortic valve is between the left ventricle and the aorta.

NERVE SUPPLY: *Inhibitory* (Vagus): by way of the sympathetic ganglia of the autonomic system and phrenic nerve. *Afferent:* A depressor nerve running from the heart to a cardioinhibitory center in the medulla, through the sheath of the vagus nerves, causing reflex inhibition of the heart. *Efferent fibers:* Inhibitory impulses are conveyed by preganglionic fibers of the vagus nerve, which synapse with postganglionic neurons located in terminal ganglia in the wall of the heart. They are distributed to the sinoatrial node, bundles of His, and through the left and right bundles to the Purkinje fibers to the muscle cells of the heart. SEE: *heart, conduction system of.*

FUNCT: At the rate of 72 times each minute, the adult human heart beats 104,000 times a day, 38,000,000 times in a year. At every stroke approximately 5 cu. in. (82 ml) of blood are forced out into the body, or 500,000 cu. in. (8,193 liters) a day. In terms of work, this is the equivalent of raising one ton (907 kg) to a height of 41 ft (12.5 meters) every 24 hr.

AUSCULTATION: Shows intensity, quality, and rhythm of heart sounds and detects the presence of any adventitious sounds, as murmurs. The two separate sounds heard by the use of a stethoscope over the heart have been represented by the syllables "lubb," "dupp." The first sound (systolic) results from the contraction of the ventricle, tension of the atrioventricular valves, and the impact of the heart against the chest wall, and is synchronous with the apex beat and carotid pulse. This sound is prolonged and dull; after the first sound there is a short pause, then the second sound (diastolic), which results from the closure of the aortic and pulmonary valves. This sound is short and high pitched. After the second sound a longer pause follows before the first is heard again. A very useful technique in listening to the variation in sounds from one area to another is to "inch" the stethoscope in small steps from one site to the other.

PROCEDURE: Patient should be recumbent when beginning examination; then, having elicited all the signs possible, repeat with patient sitting, standing, or leaning forward, and note any variations from change of position. First listen while patient is breathing naturally, then while holding breath in both deep inspiration and expiration, and finally have patient take three or four forced inspirations. Listen over the entire thoracic cavity and endeavor to localize the points at which heart sounds, both normal and abnormal, are heard with the greatest intensity. Proceed from below upward and from left to right.

Normal location of valves for auscultation: Aortic, 3rd intercostal space, close to left side of sternum; pulmonary, in front of aorta, behind junction of 3rd costal cartilage

PROJECTION OF HEART AND GREAT VESSELS ON CHEST WALL

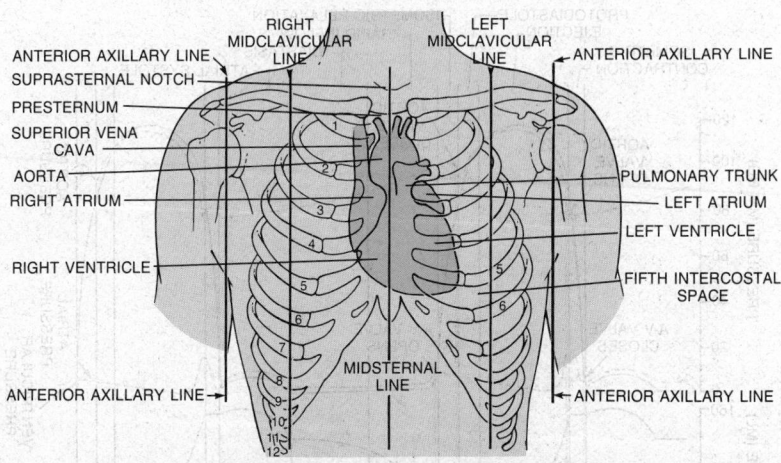

ANTERIOR AXILLARY LINE
SUPRASTERNAL NOTCH
PRESTERNUM
SUPERIOR VENA CAVA
AORTA
RIGHT ATRIUM

RIGHT VENTRICLE

ANTERIOR AXILLARY LINE

RIGHT MIDCLAVICULAR LINE
LEFT MIDCLAVICULAR LINE
MIDSTERNAL LINE

ANTERIOR AXILLARY LINE
PULMONARY TRUNK
LEFT ATRIUM
LEFT VENTRICLE
FIFTH INTERCOSTAL SPACE
ANTERIOR AXILLARY LINE

**PROJECTION OF HEART AND VALVES ON CHEST WALL
HEART SOUNDS FROM EACH VALVE ARE HEARD BEST OVER AREAS SHOWN**

AORTIC
TRICUSPID

PULMONIC
MITRAL

with sternum, left side; tricuspid, behind middle of sternum about level of 4th costal cartilage; mitral, behind 3rd intercostal space about 1 in. (2.5 cm) to the left of sternum. SEE: illus.

Intensity: Both sounds are either heard better or actually accentuated in increased heart action from any cause, normal or abnormal, such as anemia, vigorous exercise, cardiac hypertrophy, subjects with thin chest walls, and consolidation of the lung as in pneumonia. Accentuation of the aortic second sound results from hypertrophy of the left ventricle, increased arterial resist-

ance as in arteriosclerosis with hypertension, or aortic aneurysm. Accentuation of the pulmonary second sound results from pulmonary obstruction as in emphysema, pneumonia, or hypertrophy of the right ventricle. Both heart sounds are poorly heard or actually decreased in intensity in general obesity, general debility, degeneration or dilatation of the heart, pericardial or pleural effusion, and emphysema.

Reduplication of heart sounds: Probably due to a lack of synchronous action in the valves of both sides of the heart. Results from many conditions but notably from in-

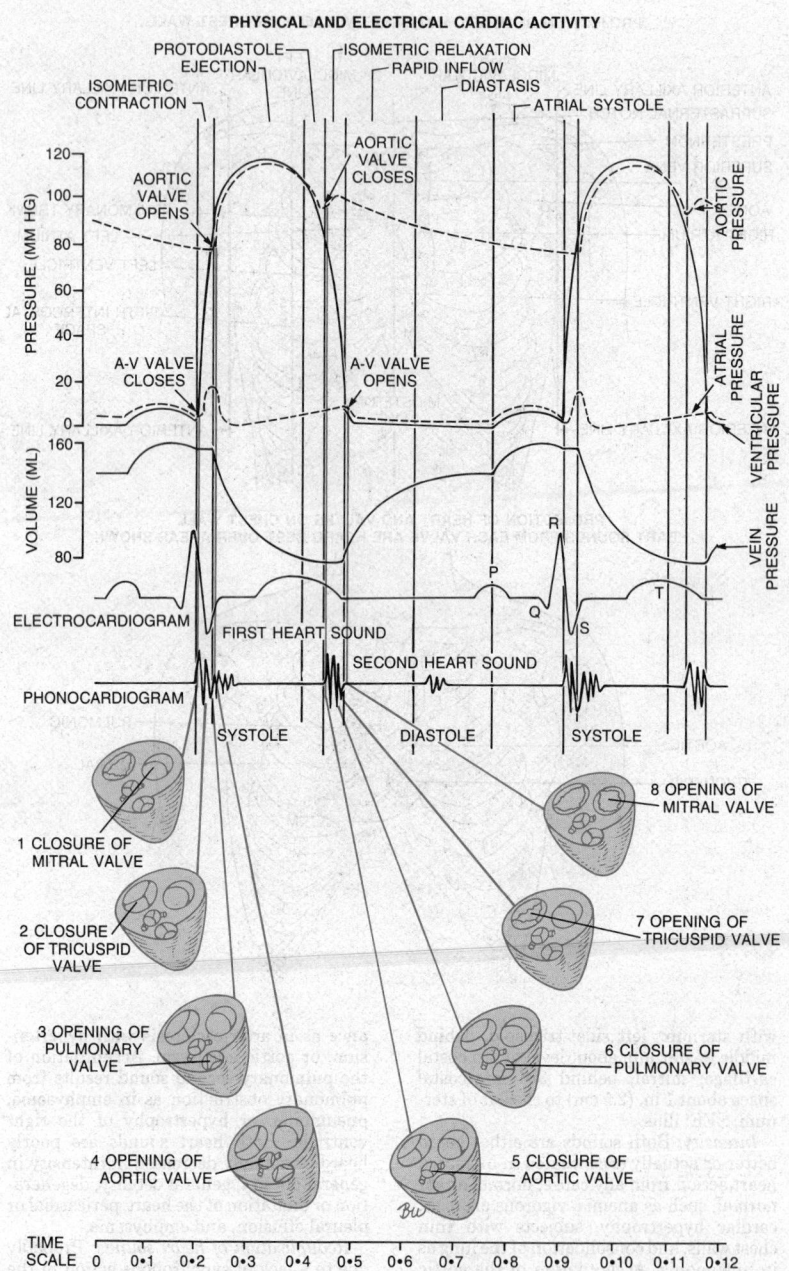

PHYSICAL AND ELECTRICAL CARDIAC ACTIVITY

ISOMETRIC CONTRACTION

PROTODIASTOLE EJECTION

ISOMETRIC RELAXATION
RAPID INFLOW
DIASTASIS

ATRIAL SYSTOLE

AORTIC VALVE OPENS

AORTIC VALVE CLOSES

A-V VALVE CLOSES

A-V VALVE OPENS

AORTIC PRESSURE

ATRIAL PRESSURE

VENTRICULAR PRESSURE

VEIN PRESSURE

PRESSURE (MM HG)

120
100
80
60
40
20
0

VOLUME (ML)

160
120
80

ELECTROCARDIOGRAM

P Q R S T

FIRST HEART SOUND

SECOND HEART SOUND

PHONOCARDIOGRAM

SYSTOLE   DIASTOLE   SYSTOLE

1 CLOSURE OF MITRAL VALVE

2 CLOSURE OF TRICUSPID VALVE

3 OPENING OF PULMONARY VALVE

4 OPENING OF AORTIC VALVE

5 CLOSURE OF AORTIC VALVE

6 CLOSURE OF PULMONARY VALVE

7 OPENING OF TRICUSPID VALVE

8 OPENING OF MITRAL VALVE

TIME SCALE   0   0•1   0•2   0•3   0•4   0•5   0•6   0•7   0•8   0•9   0•10   0•11   0•12 creased resistance in the systemic or the pulmonary circulation, as in arteriosclerosis and emphysema. Frequently noted in mitral stenosis and pericarditis.

Murmurs: A murmur is an abnormal sound heard over the heart or blood vessels and may result from obstruction or regurgitation at the valves following endocarditis; dilatation of the ventricle or relaxation of its walls rendering the valves relatively insufficient; aneurysm; a change in the blood constituents, as in anemia; roughening of the pericardial surfaces, as in pericarditis; irregular action of the heart. Murmurs produced within the heart are termed endocardial; those outside, exocardial; those produced in aneurysms, bruits; those produced by anemia, hemic murmurs.

Hemic murmurs: Soft and blowing in character, usually systolic in time, heard best over pulmonary valves. Associated with symptoms of anemia.

Aneurysmal murmur or bruit: Usually loud, booming in character, systolic in time, heard best over the aorta or base of heart, often associated with an abnormal area of dullness and pulsation, and with symptoms resulting from pressure on neighboring structures.

Pericardial friction sounds: Superficial, rough, and creaking in quality, to and fro in time, not transmitted beyond the precordium and may be modified by pressure of the stethoscope.

PALPATION AND INSPECTION: Not only determines position, force, extent, and rhythm of apex beat, but also detects existence of any fremitus or thrill. A thrill is a vibratory sensation likened to that received when the hand is placed on the back of a purring cat. Thrills at base of heart may result from valvular lesions, atheroma of aorta, aneurysm, and from roughened pericardial surfaces as in pericarditis. A presystolic thrill at apex is almost pathognomonic of mitral stenosis. In children especially, a precordial bulge or substernal thrust or apical heave suggest cardiac enlargement.

PERCUSSION: Determines shape and extent of cardiac dullness. The normal area of superficial or absolute percussion dullness (part uncovered by lung) is detected by light percussion and extends from the 4th left costosternal junction to the apex beat; from the apex beat to the juncture of the xiphoid cartilage, with the sternum, and thence up the left border of the sternum. The normal area of deep percussion dullness (the heart projected on the chest wall) is detected by firm percussion and extends from 3rd left costosternal articulation to the apex beat; from apex beat to junction of the xi-

phoid cartilage with the sternum; and hence up right border of sternum to the 3rd rib. The lower level of the cardiac dullness fuses with the liver dullness and can rarely be determined. The area of cardiac dullness is increased in hypertrophy and dilation of the heart; pericardial effusion. The area of detectable cardiac dullness is diminished in emphysema, pneumothorax, and pneumocardium.

h., abdominal. Heart that is displaced into the abdominal cavity.

h., armored. Condition characterized by deposit of calcareous matter in the pericardium.

h., artificial. Device that will pump the blood the heart would normally pump. It may be located inside or outside the body. SEE: *heart-lung machine.*

h., beriberi. Heart failure due to deficiency of the vitamin thiamine.

h., boatshaped. Heart in which one ventricle is dilated and hypertrophied as a result of aortic regurgitation.

h., bony. Heart with calcareous patches in its walls and pericardium.

h., cervical. Heart that is displaced into the neck region.

h., conduction system of. Specialized nervous tissue in the heart which conducts the electrical impulses throughout the heart. Consists of (in order of normal conduction) the sinoatrial node, the intra-atrial tracts, the atrioventricular node, the bundle of His, the right and left bundle branches, and the Purkinje fibers.

h., dilatation of. Enlargement of heart due to stretching of its walls. Varieties are dilatation with thickening of walls and dilatation with thinning walls.

SYM: As long as the associated hypertrophy keeps pace with the dilatation, no symptoms result. Otherwise there are dyspnea, edema, and cough, the signs of heart failure.

h., fatty degeneration of. Condition in which the myocardium has undergone fatty degeneration.

SYM: All signs of heart failure, i.e., dyspnea; cough; weak, irregular pulse; edema; dyspepsia; attacks of syncope.

PROG: Unfavorable. Death may occur on slight exertion.

h., fatty infiltration of. Abnormal amount of fat deposited in and upon heart.

SYM: Shortness of breath increased by exertion; weak but regular pulse; precordial distress; tendency to pulmonary congestion with resulting bronchitis.

PROG: Depends upon cause. If due to a correctable condition, it is favorable.

h., fibroid. Chronic myocarditis in which

fibrous tissue develops within the muscular tissue of the heart.

SYM: Same as fatty degeneration, condition dependent upon atheroma or sclerosis of coronary arteries.

h., hypertrophy of. Enlargement of heart due to increased size of myocardium.

h., irritable. Neurocirculatory asthenia or effort syndrome. Characterized by breathlessness, palpitation, weakness, and exhaustion.

h., left. The left atrium and ventricle. This portion of the heart receives the aerated blood from the lungs and propels it into the systemic circulation.

h., palpitation of. Heartbeat that is easily noticed by the person. Frequently rapid, irregular, or both. May result from dyspepsia; mental or physical excitement; organic heart disease; hyperthyroidism; anemia; hysteria; an independent neurosis; or endocarditis, myocarditis, and pericarditis due to infection and trauma; circulatory disturbances; disorders of metabolism, nutrition, and growth.

h., right. The right atrium and ventricle. This portion of the heart receives the venous blood and propels it to the lungs.

heart attack. Myocardial infarction, q.v.

heartbeat. The rhythmic contraction of the heart.

heart block. Condition in which the conductile tissue of the heart, the sinoatrial (S-A) and atrioventricular (A-V) nodes, bundle of His, Purkinje fibers, fails to conduct impulses normally from the atrium to the ventricles. This causes altered rhythm of the heartbeat. Known as arrhythmia, the condition may be present in several forms.

ETIOL: Structural changes as from tumor or damage of the myocardium due to coronary artery occlusion. Toxic effects of drugs or the toxins of infections. Nutritional or endocrine factors may also be of importance.

h.b., atrioventricular. A form in which impulses are impeded at the A-V node.

h.b., bundle branch. Condition in which impulses are blocked in one of the branches of the bundle of His, resulting in ventricles beating out of rhythm with each other so that one ventricle is stimulated to beat slightly before the other. SYN: *heart block, interventricular.*

h.b., complete or third-degree. Condition in which there is a complete dissociation between atrial and ventricular systoles. Ventricles may beat at a rate of 30 to 40/min while atria are beating the normal 70 beats/min.

h.b., congenital. Heart block present at birth due to improper development of the impulse-conducting system.

h.b., fasicular. Conduction defect in either or both of the subdivisions of the left bundle branch.

h.b., first-degree. Heart block in which conduction time of impulses is prolonged but all atrial beats are followed by ventricular beats; usually recognized only by electrocardiograph by prolonged P-R interval.

h.b., interventricular. H.b., bundle branch.

h.b., partial or second-degree. Heart block in which one of two or three impulses passes from the atrium to the ventricle. Has two variants, Wenckebach or Mobitz I and Mobitz II. In Wenckebach, the P-R intervals become progressively longer until a QRS complex is dropped, and the cycle repeats. In Mobitz II, a regular absence of QRS complexes occurs, with constant length of P-R intervals.

h.b., sinoatrial. Heart block in which there is interference in the passage of impulses from the sinoatrial node. May be partial or complete. SEE: *sick sinus syndrome.*

heartburn. Burning sensation in the substernal area due to reflux of acid contents of the stomach into the lower esophagus. This condition is known to occur in persons whose exercise program includes running, even if no food is present in the stomach. SEE: *gastroesophageal reflux, chronic.* SYN: *brash; pyrosis.*

heart disease. Term used to describe any pathological condition of the heart.

h.d., ischemic. Lack of oxygen supply to the heart with consequent altered cardiac function. The most common cause of myocardial ischemia is atherosclerosis of the coronary arteries. Depending upon several factors, including oxygen demand of the myocardium, degree of narrowing of the lumen of the arteries, and duration of the ischemia, the end result is temporary or permanent damage to the heart. SEE: *coronary arteries; coronary artery disease; coronary heart disease; heart disease, risk factors.*

h.d., risk factors. From a variety of studies it is known that certain conditions and lifestyle variations are more likely to be present in persons with ischemic heart disease than in the general population. These may be divided into those that are not reversible: aging, male sex, genetic factors; reversible ones: use of tobacco, hypertension, obesity, sedentary lifestyle, stress; and others that may or may not be reversible: hyperlipidemia, hyperglycemia, diabetes mellitus, decreased levels of high-density lipoproteins, and behavior patterns. SEE: *behavior patterns, types A and B.*

heart failure. 1. Cessation of the heartbeat. 2.

A syndrome or clinical condition resulting from failure of the heart to maintain adequate circulation of blood. May result from failure of the right or left ventricle or both.

SYM: Dyspnea, cardiac asthma, stasis in systemic or portal circulation, edema, cyanosis, hypertrophy of heart. Symptoms vary depending on which side of the heart is affected.

ETIOL: Hypertension, infections, pericardial effusion, valvular insufficiency, coronary disease, congenital malformations, arteriosclerosis, constrictive pericarditis, atherosclerosis, hyperthyroidism.

h.f., backward. Heart failure in which venous return to the heart is reduced with resulting venous stasis and congestion. Due principally to failure of the right ventricle.

h.f., congestive. Condition characterized by weakness, breathlessness, abdominal discomfort, edema in lower portions of body resulting from venous stasis and reduced outflow of blood from the left side of the heart. SEE: *dyspnea, paroxysmal nocturnal.*

h.f., forward. Heart failure in which forward flow of blood to the tissues is inadequate due either to inability of left ventricle to pump sufficient blood or to insufficient blood arriving at the ventricle.

h.f., high output. Heart failure even though the cardiac output is high.

h.f., left-sided. Failure of the heart to maintain left ventricular output. SYN: *left ventricular heart failure.*

h.f., left ventricular. H.f., left-sided, q.v.

h.f., low output. Failure of the heart to maintain blood output.

h.f., right-sided. Inadequate output by the right ventricle. SYN: *right ventricular heart failure.*

h.f., right ventricular. H.f., right-sided, q.v.

heart-lung machine. Device for maintaining the functions of the heart and lungs while either or both are unable to continue to function adequately. The device pumps the blood and oxygenates it and removes carbon dioxide. In animal studies and in open-heart surgery, such devices take over the function of the heart and lungs while these organs are being treated or possibly replaced. Also called *heart-lung bypass.*

heart murmur. Sounds from the heart other than those normally present. A murmur is produced by the blood passing over a roughened valve as could be the case in rheumatic heart disease, by flowing through a constricted opening such as a narrowed mitral valve, an interventricular septal defect, or by backflow of blood through an incompetent valve. SEE: AUSCULTATION under *heart.*

heart pump, nuclear-powered. An artificial heart powered by nuclear energy.

heart rate. The number of beats of the heart per unit of time, usually expressed or written as number per minute.

heart reflex. Any reflex in which the stimulation of a sensory nerve brings about an increase or decrease in the heart rate. An example is the Bainbridge reflex, in which stimulation of sensory receptors in the right atrium by increased venous return results in an increase in heart rate.

heart sounds. SEE: AUSCULTATION under *heart.*

heart test. Nonspecific term for any of the various methods of clinically testing the heart.

heart transplantation. Surgical transplantation of the heart from a patient who died of trauma or some other disease that left the heart intact and capable of functioning in the recipient. This procedure became quite frequent in the 1970s, and then very few were done. As techniques for matching the donor and recipient have improved, the procedure is once again being done in special centers.

heart valve, prosthetic. A substitute valve used to replace a diseased valve. Most valves are artificial and not made of biologic tissues.

heat [AS. *haetu*]. 1. Condition of being hot; warmth. Opposed to cold. 2. High temperature; generalized fever or localized heat due to an infection. Calor (fever) and dolor, rubor, and tumor (pain, redness, and swelling) represent the four classic signs of inflammation. SEE: *febrile convulsions; fever.* 3. Sexual excitement in lower animals; period of such excitement. SYN: *estrus.* 4. Form of energy that increases the temperature of surrounding tissues or objects by conduction, convection, or radiation. 5. Sensation of warmth or an increase in temperature.

Heat is constantly being produced within the body as a result of exothermic chemical processes occurring in metabolic processes. Ultimately all heat produced in the body results from oxidative processes. Body temperature (normally 98.6°F or 37°C) is the result of a balance between heat production (thermogenesis) and heat loss (thermolysis). SEE: table. The temperature of the body is not uniform. Oral temperatures range from 96.6° to 100°F (37° to 37.8°C). Axillary temperature is somewhat lower and rectal temperature is somewhat higher. Change in mean body temperature is not easily measured but should not be estimated to be precisely equivalent to changes in rec-

Elimination of Body Heat

The mode of elimination and the percentage of heat lost through each of the following is:

Radiation	55%*
Convection and conduction	15%
Evaporation through skin and lungs	24%
Warming inspired air	2%
Elimination of CO_2 from lungs	3%
Warming ingested food and water, and loss through feces and urine	1%

* Figures are approximate and vary with physiological activity of the body, type of clothing worn, relative humidity, and degree of acclimatization to a particular environment.

tal or oral temperature. SEE: *core temperature*.

Reducing the temperature of the skin reflexly brings about a constriction of the blood vessels, thus reducing heat loss and conserving heat within the body. The application of heat reflexly induces the dilation of blood vessels, thus increasing blood flow to the skin with consequent increase in heat loss.

The application of heat to the skin reflexly produces effects in the deeper portions of the body. It induces muscle relaxation, increases blood supply, and stimulates metabolic activity. Physiological effects resulting are hyperemia and sedation of sensory or motor activity. Application of moderate cold tends to produce the opposite effects.

Relaxation of muscular tissue results in relief of pain, which may be due to rigidity and spasm in tissues. Local hot applications may have some reflex effect on deep organs. This is the basis of treating certain conditions by means of counterirritation such as that produced by liniments or mustard plaster.

h., acclimatization to. Adjustment of an organism to heat in the environment. Exposure to high environmental temperature requires a period of adjustment in order for the body to function efficiently. The amount of time required will depend upon the temperature, humidity, and duration of exposure each day. Significant physiological adjustments will occur in five days and will be completed within two weeks to a month.

h., application of. *General:* May be dry or moist. The effect is first to produce a slight contraction of vessels in skin, thus increasing blood pressure. This makes patients feel that their head is full and bursting. However, this effect is only of very short duration, and discomfort can be avoided by application of a cold compress or ice bag to the head. The true effect follows immediately when the blood vessels in the skin are dilated due to the relaxation of involuntary

muscle contained in their walls. The skin is reddened, increased blood supply to the sweat glands causes them to act freely, and heat loss is accelerated. During a general application of heat it is necessary to watch the patient carefully, noting any apparent discomfort, state of pulse and respiration, and color, and to be certain patient does not become dehydrated or suffer heat exhaustion, q.v.

Caution: Do not apply heat to extremities that have reduced blood supply as could be the case in most forms of arteriosclerosis or advanced diabetes.

Local: May be dry or moist. Dry applications include hot water bottles; bags of hot salt previously heated in an oven; radiant heat; electric pads; and diathermy.

Moist: Considered more penetrating than dry heat but this is due more to the fact that water-soaked materials lose heat slower than dry ones. The application should be approx. 120°F (48.9°C). Compresses may be kept warm by keeping hot water bottles at proper temperature next to them. Do not use electric heating devices next to moist dressings. Devices that force hot water at a selected temperature through soft flexible tubing are available. These may be used to heat wet or dry compresses.

h., conductive. Term applied to heat transferred by conduction from a heat source to an object that is cold when the two materials are in contact with each other.

h., convective. Flow of heat to an object or part of the body by passage of heated particles, gas, or liquid from the heat source to the colder body.

h., conversive. Heat generated in the tissues by a current of electricity or by some form of radiant energy.

h., diathermy. Electrical energy is converted into heat by the use of diathermy and short wave.

h., dry. Heat that has no moisture. May be administered in form of hot, dry pack; hot water bottle; electric light bath; heliotherapy; hot bricks; resistance coil; electric pad or blanket; hot air bath; or therapeutic lamp.

h., initial. Muscular heat produced during contraction when tension is increasing, during maintenance of tension, and during relaxation when tension is diminishing.

h., latent. Heat required to convert a solid into a liquid or a liquid into a gas at a given temperature.

h., latent, of fusion. Heat required to convert 1 gm of a solid into liquid at the same temperature, e.g., when 1 gm of ice at 0°C is converted into water at 0°C; this process requires 80 Cal, and until it is completed there will be no rise of temperature.

h., latent, of vaporization. Heat required to change 1 gm of a liquid at its boiling point to vapor at the same temperature. The latent heat of steam is 540 Cal; therefore, when steam cools to liquid, each gm gives out 540 Cal. This explains why a scald from steam is much more severe than one caused by boiling water.

h., luminous. Heat derived from light. This form may be tolerated better than other forms of radiation. Light may be converted into heat. Short infrared rays penetrate subcutaneous tissues to a greater extent than long, invisible rays.

h., mechanical equivalent of. The value of heat units in terms of work units. One Calorie (kilocalorie) is equal to 4.1855×10^4 joules.

h., moist. Heat that has moisture content. May be applied as hot bath pack, hot wet pack, hot foot bath, fomentations, poultices, or vapor bath. Watch for chill, fainting, dizziness, headache, collapse, faintness, increased pulse, weakness. Cold applications to head should be used during and after treatment. Opinion regarding therapeutic use of heat or cold differs.

h., molecular. Result of multiplying a substance's molecular weight by its specific heat.

h. of evaporation. The heat absorbed per unit of mass when a substance is converted from a liquid to a gas, e.g., the change of water to steam when it is heated sufficiently. For water, the amount of heat required to transform water into steam is 540 calories per gram of water.

h., prickly. Vesicles due to obstruction or acute inflammation of sweat glands. SYN: *miliaria.*

h., radiant. Heat given off from a heated body; it passes through the air in form of waves.

h., sensible. Heat producing a temperature rise when absorbed by a body.

h., specific. Heat needed to raise the temperature of 1 gm of a substance 1°C.

heat cramps. Acute painful spasms of voluntary muscles following hard work in a hot environment without adequate fluid and salt intake.

F.A.: Move the patient to a cool place and give a salt solution (¼ tsp or 1 gm of table salt in a glass of water) by mouth. Repeat at 5- to 30-minute intervals until cramping stops.

PROPH: Ingestion of 1 to 2 grams (65 to 130 mg) of salt taken three or four times a day with at least two glasses (16 ounces or ½ liter) of water with each dose. SEE: *heat exhaustion.*

heat exhaustion. Acute reaction to heat exposure. Not the same as heatstroke, q.v. SEE: table.

SYM: Weakness, dizziness, nausea, headache, and finally collapse. Skin is cold and clammy, pupils dilated. Body temperature is usually normal, but blood pressure may be decreased.

F.A.: Move the patient to a cool place, loosen clothing, place in a head-low position. Intravenous infusion of isotonic saline is rarely needed.

PROG: Favorable if properly treated.

heat gun. Device used in splint fabrication that produces heated air to render thermoplastic splinting materials malleable for fitting.

heat labile. Thermolabile, q.v.

heatstroke. An acute and dangerous reaction to heat exposure. Characterized by high body temperature, usually above 105°F (40.6°C); cessation of sweating; headache; numbness; tingling and confusion prior to sudden delirium or coma; fast pulse; rapid respiratory rate; usually elevated blood pressure. The basic defect is failure of the heat-regulating mechanisms of the body. SYN: *sunstroke.* SEE: table; *peritoneal dialysis.*

TREAT: Effective therapy may save the patient's life. Without delay, the nude patient should be placed in a bathtub filled with cold water. This will not cause pain, shock, or cutaneous vasoconstriction. The patient's temperature will need to be monitored carefully. Remove from bath when temperature falls to 103°F (39.4°C). If cold water and a bathtub are not available, place wet sheets on nude body, fan vigorously, and massage the skin. Do not apply alcohol to the skin. Take temperature every 10 minutes and do not allow it to fall below 101°F (38.5°C) to prevent changing hyperthermia to hypothermia. Careful observation of patient for signs of fluid and electrolyte imbalance, and renal failure will be required for several days.

Comparison of Heatstroke and Heat Exhaustion

Heatstroke	Heat Exhaustion
Definition: A condition or derangement of the heat-control centers due to exposure to the rays of the sun or very high temperatures. Loss of heat is inadequate or absent.	**Definition:** A state of very definite weakness produced by the excess loss of normal fluids and sodium chloride in the form of sweat.
History: Exposure to sun or extreme heat	**History:** Exposure to heat, usually indoors
Differential Symptoms:	**Differential Symptoms:**
Face: Red, dry, and hot	*Face:* Pale, cool, and moist
Skin: Hot, dry, and no sweating	*Skin:* Cool, clammy, with profuse diaphoresis
Temperature: High, 106° to 110°F (41.1° to 43.3°C)	*Temperature:* Subnormal
Pulse: Full, strong, bounding	*Pulse:* Weak, thready, and rapid
Respirations: Dyspneic and sonorous	*Respirations:* Shallow and quiet
Muscles: Tense and possible convulsions	*Muscles:* Tense and contracted
Eyes: Pupils are dilated but equal	*Eyes:* Pupils are normal; eyeballs may be soft
Treatment: Absolute rest with head elevated; keep body cool by any means available until hospitalized, but do not use alcohol applied to skin. Take temperature every 10 minutes, and do not allow it to fall below 38.5°C (101°F).	**Treatment:** Keep patient quiet; head should be lowered; keep body warm to prevent onset of shock.
Drugs: Allow no stimulants; give infusions of normal saline (to force fluids).	*Drugs:* Salty fluids and fruit juices should be given frequently in small amounts. Intravenous isotonic saline will be required if patient is unconscious.

Peritoneal lavage using ice cold, sterile saline has also been used to treat heatstroke. SEE: *peritoneal dialysis*.

NURSING IMPLICATIONS: Participate in efforts to educate the public about heat illnesses. Teach athletes and coaches the signs and symptoms of heat problems and the importance of treatment. Advise patients, particularly the elderly, those with diabetes, and alcoholics, about hot weather precautions to avoid heat illnesses: Clothing should be lightweight and loose fitting, frequent rest breaks should be taken when strenuous activity is undertaken, adequate fluid and electrolyte solutions should be ingested, and hot locations should be avoided if possible. Elderly and obese individuals are at special risk for overheating as are patients taking phenothiazine drugs. SEE: *Nursing Diagnoses* in *Appendix*.

heat unit. Unit of heat produced by exposure to x-rays. It is the product of the milliamperage times the seconds of exposure times the kilovoltage peak.

heaves (hēvs). Vomiting.

heavy chain disease. Any one of several abnormalities of immunoglobulins in which excessive quantities of alpha, gamma, delta, epsilon, or mu chains are produced. The immunoglobulins formed are incomplete, causing, in some cases, distinct clinical signs and symptoms including weakness, recurrent fever, susceptibility to bacterial infections, lymphadenopathy, hepatosplenomegaly, erythema, and edema of the soft palate; anemia, leukopenia, thrombocytopenia, eosinophilia, and abnormal protein electrophoretic patterns are also produced.

Heberden's disease (hē′bĕr-dĕnz) [William Heberden, Brit. physician, 1710–1801]. Arthritis with deformity that begins in the fingers and progresses. The concomitant deformity is caused by ankylosis, exostosis, and atrophy of soft parts. SYN: *arthritis deformans*.

Heberden's nodes. Hard nodules or enlargements of tubercles of last phalanges of fingers; seen in osteoarthritis.

hebetic (hē-bĕt′ĭk) [Gr. *hebetikos*, youthful]. Pert. to or occurring at the time of puberty.

hebetude [L. *hebet*, dull]. Being dull or lethargic.

hebosteotomy (hē-bŏs″tē-ŏt′ō-mē) [Gr. *hebe*, youth, + *osteon*, bone, + *tome*, incision]. Hebotomy, q.v.

hebotomy (hē-bŏt'ō-mē). Section through the pubis to facilitate labor. SYN: *pubiotomy.*

hecateromeric, hecatomeric (hĕk"ă-tĕr"ō-mĕr'ĭk, hĕk"ă-tō-mĕr'ĭk) [Gr. *hekateros,* each of two, + *meros,* part]. Having two processes on a spinal neuron, one supplying each side of the spinal cord.

hecto- [Gr. *hekaton,* hundred]. In the metric system, a prefix indicating 100 times (10^2) the unit named. Thus hectoliter (10^2 liters) is 100 liters.

hectogram [" + *gramma,* small weight]. One hundred grams, or 3.527 avoirdupois ounces.

hectoliter (hĕk'tō-lē"tĕr) [" + *litra,* a pound]. One hundred liters.

hectometer (hĕk-tōm'ĕ-tĕr) [" + *metron,* measure]. One hundred meters.

hedonism (hēd'ŏn-ĭzm) [Gr. *hedone,* pleasure, + *-ismos,* condition]. A theory or standard of conduct in which the principal object of life is pleasure. SEE: *pleasure principle.*

hedrocele (hĕd'rō-sēl) [Gr. *hedra,* anus, + *kele,* tumor, swelling]. Hernia or prolapse through the anus. SYN: *proctocele.*

heel [AS. *huela,* heel]. Rounded posterior portion of the foot under and behind the ankle. SYN: *calx.*

    h., Thomas [Hugh Owen Thomas, Brit. orthopedic surgeon, 1834–1891]. A corrective shoe in which the heel is approximately 12 mm longer and 4 to 6 mm higher on the medial edge. This produces varus of the foot and prevents depression of the head of the talus.

heel bone. Bone at back of tarsus. SYN: *calcaneus; os calcis.*

heel puncture. Method for obtaining a blood sample from a newborn or premature infant.

Caution: The puncture should be made in the lateral or medial areas of the plantar surface of the heel and avoid the posterior curvature of the heel; go no deeper than 2.4 mm. Do not use a previous puncture site.

HEENT. *head, eyes, ears, nose, throat.*

Heerfordt's disease (hār'forts) [C. F. Heerfordt, Danish ophthalmologist, b. 1871]. Uveoparotid fever, a form of sarcoidosis.

Hegar's sign (hā'gărz) [Alfred Hegar, Ger. gynecologist, 1830–1914]. Sign that may be present during second and third months of pregnancy. On bimanual examination, the lower part of the uterus is easily compressed between fingers placed in the vagina and those of the other hand over the pelvic area. This is due to the softening of lower segments of the uterus and to the fact that the fetus does not fill the uterine cavity at this stage, leaving an empty space in the lower part. The sign is not a positive one for pregnancy.

Heidenhain's demilunes (hī'dĕn-hīnz) [Rudolph Peter Heinrich Heidenhain, Ger. physiologist, 1834–1897]. Crescent-shaped groups of serous cells at the base of, or along the sides of, the mucous alveoli of the salivary glands, esp. sublingual and submandibular. SYN: *crescents of Giannuzzi.*

height (hīt) [AS. *hiehthu*]. Vertical distance from the bottom to the top of an organ or structure.

Heimlich maneuver (hīm'lĭk) [H. J. Heimlich, U.S. physician, b. 1920]. Technique for removing a foreign body from the trachea or pharynx, where it is preventing flow of air to the lungs. The obstruction usually is due to a bolus of food.

    The maneuver consists of applying subdiaphragmatic pressure by: (1) wrapping your arms around the victim's waist from behind; (2) making a fist with one hand and placing it against the victim's abdomen between the navel and the rib cage; (3) clasping your fist with your free hand and pressing in with a quick forceful upward thrust. Repeat several times if necessary. If one is alone and experiences airway obstruction due to a foreign body, this technique could be self-applied.

    This treatment is quite effective in dislodging the obstruction by forcing air against the mass much as pressure from a carbonated beverage will forcibly remove a cork or cap from a bottle. The average airflow produced is 225 liters/min. SEE: *choking;* illus.

Heimlich sign. Grasping one's throat with the thumb and index finger to signal that the individual is choking.

Heineke-Mikulicz pyloroplasty (hī'nĕ-kĕ-mĭk'ū-lĭch) [Walter Hermann Heineke, Ger. surgeon, 1834–1901; Johann von Mikulicz-Radecki, Polish surgeon, 1850–1905]. Pyloroplasty of the stomach, done to enlarge the outlet of the stomach.

Heinz bodies [Robert Heinz, Ger. pathologist, 1865–1924]. Granules in red blood cells due to damage of the hemoglobin molecules. Seen in premature infants, in certain forms of drug sensitivity, and in a certain type of hereditary hemolytic anemia. The bodies are best seen when the blood is stained with a special stain.

Heinz body anemia. Hemolytic anemia of infancy associated with the finding of Heinz bodies in the red cells.

Heister, spiral valve of (hī'stĕr) [Lorenz Heister, Ger. anatomist, 1683–1758]. A spiral fold of the mucous membrane lining the cystic duct. It serves to keep the lumen

HEIMLICH MANEUVER
(FOR REMOVAL OF A FOREIGN BODY BLOCKING THE AIR PASSAGE)

1.
CLASPED HANDS PLACED
JUST BELOW MIDDLE OF
RIB CAGE

MANEUVER FOR VICTIM WHO
IS STANDING

2.
HANDS PLACED
JUST BELOW
RIB CAGE
AT DISTAL
END OF
STERNUM

FOR VICTIM WHO IS SUPINE

4.
BACK OF
CHAIR TO
PRESS AGAINST
THE BODY
JUST BELOW
RIB CAGE

3.
POSITION FOR
SELF-ADMINISTERING MANEUVER

open.

HeLa cells (hē'lă). Cell, HeLa, q.v.

helcoid (hĕl'koyd) [Gr. *helkos,* ulcer, + *eidos,* form, shape]. Resembling an ulcer.

helcology (hĕl-kŏl'ō-jē) [" + *logos,* word, reason]. The study of ulcers.

helcoma (hĕl-kō'mă) [" + *oma,* tumor]. Ulcer of the cornea.

helcoplasty (hĕl'kō-plăs-tē) [" + *plassein,* to form]. Grafting healthy skin on ulcers. SEE: *dermatoplasty.*

helcosis (hĕl-kō'sĭs) [" + *osis,* condition]. The development of an ulcer. SYN: *ulceration.*

helianthine (hē-lē-ăn'thĭn). Methyl orange used as an indicator in determining pH.

helical (hĕl'ĭ-kăl). In the shape of a helix.

helicine (hĕl'ĭ-sĭn) [Gr. *helix,* coil]. 1. Spiral. 2. Pert. to a helix or coil.

helicine arteries. Tortuous arteries in cavernous tissue of the penis and clitoris, and in the uterus.

Helicobacter pylori. An organism that has been associated with gastritis. Previously used name was *Campylobacter pylori.*

helicoid (hĕl'ĭ-koyd) [" + *eidos,* form, shape]. Resembling a helix or spiral.

helicopodia (hĕl''ĭ-kō-pō'dē-ă) [" + *pous,* foot]. A peculiar movement in which the foot, when brought forward, drags and describes a partial arc. Results in a gait such as seen in spastic hemiplegia.

helicotrema (hĕl''ĭ-kō-trē'mă) [" + *trema,* a hole]. [NA] The opening at the tip of the cochlear canal where the scala tympani and scala vestibuli unite.

heliophobia (hē''lē-ō-fō'bē-ă) [Gr. *helios,* sun, + *phobos,* fear]. Abnormal fear of the sun's rays, esp. by one who has suffered a sunstroke.

heliosis (hē''lē-ō'sĭs) [" + *osis,* condition]. Sunstroke.

heliotaxis (hē-lē-ō-tăk'sĭs) [" + *taxis,* arrangement]. A reaction in plants that causes them to respond negatively or positively to the sunlight.

    h., negative. Turning away from the sun.

    h., positive. Turning toward the sun.

heliotherapy (hē''lē-ō-thĕr'ă-pē) [" + *therapeia,* treatment]. Exposure to sunlight for therapeutic purposes.

heliotropism (hē''lē-ŏt'rō-pĭzm) [" + *trepein,* to turn, + *-ismos,* condition]. Tendency of living organisms to turn or grow toward the sun.

helium (hē'lē-ŭm) [Gr. *helios,* sun]. USP. SYMB: He. At. wt. 4.0026; at. no. 2. A liter of the gas at sea level pressure and 0°C weighs 0.1785 gram. A gaseous element. It is given off by radium and other radioactive elements as charged helium ions known as

alpha rays. Because of its low density, it being next to the lightest element known, it is mixed with air or oxygen and used in the treatment of various respiratory disorders. Because of its low solubility, it is mixed with air supplied to workers laboring under high atmospheric pressure, as in caissons. When so used, it reduces time required in adjusting to increasing or decreasing air pressure and reduces the danger of bends.

helix (hē'lĭks) [Gr., coil]. 1. A coil or spiral. 2. [NA] Margin of the external ear.

    h., Watson-Crick. A double helix named after the two scientists who established its structure. Each half of the helix contains chemical compounds arranged in a specific sequence. Variation in the sequence of these compounds enables genetic information to be transmitted. The double helix is the structure of DNA or deoxyribonucleic acid, q.v.

Heller's test [Johann F. Heller, Austrian pathologist, 1813–1871]. A test for the presence of albumin in urine. To make the test, pour pure nitric acid into a clean test tube to a depth of ½ in. (13 mm) and carefully overlay it with an equal quantity of urine. The presence of albumin is indicated by the appearance of an opaque white ring at the junction of the fluids. Certain drugs in the urine and urates in highly concentrated specimens may give false-positive test results. SEE: *urine.*

Hellin's law [Dyonizy Hellin, Polish pathologist, 1867–1935]. Law stating that twins occur once in 80 pregnancies, triplets once in 6400 (80²) pregnancies, quadruplets once in 512,000 (80³) pregnancies.

helminth [Gr. *helmins,* worm]. 1. A wormlike animal. 2. Any animal, either free-living or parasitic, belonging to the phyla Platyhelminthes (flatworms), Acanthocephala (spinyheaded worms), Nemathelminthes (threadworms or roundworms), or Annelida (segmented worms).

helminthagogue (hĕl-mĭnth'ă-gŏg) [" + *agogos,* leading]. A medicine or treatment that causes parasitic worms to be expelled from the intestinal tract. SYN: *vermifuge.*

helminthemesis (hĕl-mĭn-thĕm'ĕ-sĭs) [" + *emesis,* vomiting]. The vomiting of intestinal worms.

helminthiasis (hĕl-mĭn-thī'ă-sĭs) [" + *iasis,* condition]. Having intestinal parasites or worms.

helminthic (hĕl-mĭn'thĭk). 1. Pert. to worms. 2. Pert. to that which expels worms. SYN: *anthelmintic; vermifugal.*

helminthicide (hĕl-mĭn'thĭ-sīd) [" + L. *cidus,* to kill]. A medicine that kills worms. SYN: *vermicide.*

helminthoid (hĕl-mĭn'thoyd) [" + *eidos,*

form, shape]. Wormlike or resembling a worm.

helminthology (hĕl″mĭn-thŏl′ō-jē) [″ + *logos,* word, reason]. The study of parasitic intestinal worms.

helminthoma (hĕl″mĭn-thō′mă) [″ + *oma,* tumor]. A tumor caused by parasitic worms.

helminthophobia (hĕl-mĭn″thō-fō′bē-ă) [″ + *phobos,* fear]. Morbid dread of worms or delusion of being infested by them.

heloma (hē-lō′mă) [Gr. *helos,* nail, + *oma,* tumor]. A callosity or corn. SYN: *clavus.*

helotomy (hē-lŏt′ō-mē) [″ + *tome,* incision]. Surgical treatment of corns.

helper T cells. Term used for a subpopulation of T lymphocytes that secrete interleukin-2, q.v., and play a major role in directing the specific immune response, q.v. SYN: *T4 cell.*

helplessness. A state that may arise when a patient has a condition in which he or she is dependent on an outside source for life support. Such patients feel unable to alter their situation and experience anxiety due to inability to relieve their own discomfort. A fear of the necessary dependency on other people or even on mechanical supports may also be present. SEE: *giving-up; hopelessness.*

Helweg's bundle (hĕl′vĕgz) [Hans K. S. Helweg, Danish physician, 1847–1901]. A small tract passing from the olivary body to the anterior horn cells in the cervical region. Part of the extrapyramidal motor system. SYN: *olivospinal tract.*

hema- (hē′mă, hĕm′-ă) [Gr. *haima,* blood]. Combining form indicating blood.

hemachrosis (hē″mă-, hĕm″ă-krō′sĭs) [″ + *chrosis,* coloring]. Abnormal redness of blood. It is present in carbon monoxide poisoning.

hemacytometer (hē″mă-, hĕm″ă-sī-tŏm′ĭ-tĕr) [″ + *kytos,* cell, + *metron,* measure]. Apparatus used in counting blood cells.

hemacytozoon (hē″mă-, hĕm″ă-sī-tō-zō′ŏn) [″ + ″ + *zoon,* animal]. A protozoan parasite infesting red blood corpuscles.

hemad (hē′măd) [Gr. *haima,* blood, + L. *ad,* toward]. 1. Pert. to blood or blood vessels. 2. Toward the ventral or hemal aspect of the body. Opposed to neural or dorsal. SYN: *hemal.*

hemadostenosis (hē″mă-, hĕm″ă-dō-stĕn-ō′sĭs) [″ + *stenosis,* act of narrowing]. Contraction of blood vessels.

hemadsorption (hĕm″ăd-sorp′shŭn). Adherence of red blood cells to other cells or surfaces.

hemadynamometer (hē″mă-, hĕm″ă-dī″nă-mŏm′ĭ-ter) [″ + *dynamis,* power, + *metron,* measure]. Device for determin-

ing blood pressure.

hemafecia (hē″mă-, hĕm-ă-fē′sē-ă) [″ + L. *faeces,* refuse]. Feces containing blood. SEE: *occult blood.*

hemagglutination (hĕm″ă-gloo-tĭ-nā′shŭn) [″ + L. *agglutinare,* to paste to]. The clumping of red blood corpuscles.

hemagglutination inhibition. Prevention of hemagglutination by interaction or blocking of the antibody or virus that would otherwise cause hemagglutination.

hemagglutinin (hĕm″ă-gloo′tĭ-nĭn). An antibody that induces clumping of red blood corpuscles.

h., cold. Agglutination of erythrocytes (usually of sheep) at low temperatures by the serum of patients with certain diseases.

h., warm. An agglutinin effective only at body temperature, 37°C.

hemagogue (hē″mă-, hĕm′ă-gŏg) [″ + *agogos,* leading]. An agent that promotes the flow of blood, esp. menstrual flow. SEE: *emmenagogue.*

hemal (hē′măl). 1. Pert. to the blood or blood vessels. 2. Pert. to side of the body in which the heart is located. SYN: *hemad.*

hemal arch. The ribs, breastbone, and that part of the vertebrae that, together, enclose the heart and viscera.

hemal gland. A hemal or hemolymph node.

hemal node. A body resembling a lymph node in structure but associated with blood vessels instead of lymph vessels. Present in certain ungulates. SYN: *hemal gland.*

hemanalysis (hē″măn-, hĕm″ăn-ăl′ĭ-sĭs) [Gr. *haima,* blood, + *analysis,* a dissolving]. Any type of blood analysis. SEE: *blood.*

hemangiectasis (hē″măn-, hĕm″ăn-jē-ĕk′tă-sĭs) [″ + *angeion,* vessel, + *ektasis,* dilatation]. Dilatation of blood vessels.

hemangioblast (hē-măn′jē-ō-blăst) [″ + ″ + *blastos,* germ]. A mesodermal cell that can form either vascular endothelial cells or hemocytoblasts.

hemangioblastoma (hē-măn″jē-ō-blăs-tō′mă) [″ + ″ + *oma,* tumor]. A hemangioma of the brain, usually located in the cerebellum.

hemangioendothelioblastoma (hē-măn″jē-ō-ĕn″dō-thē″lē-ō-blăs-tō′mă) [″ + ″ + *endon,* within, + *thele,* nipple, + *blastos,* germ, + *oma,* tumor]. A neoplasm of the epithelial cells lining blood vessels.

hemangioendothelioma (hē″măn-jē-ō-ĕn″dō-thē-lē-ō′mă) [″ + ″ + ″ + ″ + *oma,* tumor]. An overgrowth of the endothelium of the minute capillary vessels. They are variable in size and are commonly seen in the capillary net of the cerebral meninges.

hemangiofibroma (hē-măn″jē-ō-fī-brō′mă)

[" + " + L. *fibra*, fiber, + Gr. *oma*, tumor]. A fibrous hemangioma.

hemangioma (hē-măn"jē-ō'mă) [" + *angeion*, vessel, + *oma*, tumor] (pl. *hemangiomata*). A benign tumor of dilated blood vessels.

hemangiomatosis (hē-măn"jē-ō-mă-tō'sĭs) [" + " + " + *osis*, condition]. Multiple angiomata of blood vessels.

hemangiopericytoma (hē-măn"jē-ō-pĕr"ē-sī-tō'mă). A tumor arising in capillaries. It is composed of pericytes.

hemangiosarcoma (hē-măn"jē-ō-săr-kō'mă) [" + " + *sarkos*, flesh, + *oma*, tumor]. A malignant neoplasm originating from blood vessels. SYN: *angiosarcoma*.

hemaphein (hĕm"ă-fē'ĭn) [" + *phaios*, dusky, gray]. Brown coloring material in the blood and urine.

hemapoiesis (hĕm"ă-poy-ē'sĭs) [" + *poiesis*, formation]. Blood formation. SYN: *hematopoiesis*.

hemapoietic (hĕm-ă-poy-ĕt'ĭk) [" + *poiein*, to form]. Pert. to hematopoiesis. SYN: *hematopoietic*.

hemapophysis (hĕm-ă-pŏf'ĭ-sĭs) [" + *apo*, from, + *physis*, growth]. Portion of a developing vertebra that forms a rib and costal cartilage.

hemarthros, hemarthrosis (hĕm-ăr'thrōs, hĕm-ăr-thrō'sĭs) [" + *arthron*, joint]. Bloody effusion into cavity of a joint.

hematapostema (hĕm"ăt-ă-pŏs-tē'mă) [Gr. *haimatos*, blood, + *apostema*, abscess]. An abscess that contains blood.

hematein (hĕm"ă-tē'ĭn). A stain obtained by oxidation of hematoxylin.

hematemesis (hĕm-ăt-ĕm'ē-sĭs) [" + *emesis*, vomiting]. Vomiting of blood. SEE: *hemoptysis* for table; *hemorrhage*.

SYM: Blood often clotted and mixed with food; acid in reaction. Subsequent stools may be tarry. If of gastric origin, the blood is generally dark and acid. If of pharyngeal origin, it is bright red and alkaline in reaction. If loss of blood is severe enough, shock and collapse may occur.

TREAT: Absolute rest, nothing by mouth. Feed intravenously if necessary. No stimulants. Have patient lie down. Surgery may be necessary.

NURSING IMPLICATIONS: Evaluate character and quantity of vomitus, monitor vital signs, and note associated symptoms, including state of alertness. Support patient while vomiting to prevent aspiration. Provide oral hygiene after episodes of vomiting and as needed while the patient is not taking anything by mouth.

hematencephalon (hĕm"ăt-ĕn-sĕf'ă-lŏn) [" + *enkephalos*, brain]. Cerebral hemorrhage.

hematherapy (hĕm"ă-thĕr'ă-pē) [Gr. *haima*, blood, + *therapeia*, treatment]. Administration of fresh blood in treatment of disease.

hemathermal (hĕm"ă-, hē"mă-thĕr'măl) [" + *therme*, heat]. Warm blooded; applied to animals whose blood remains at a fairly constant temperature. SYN: *hemathermous; hematothermal.* SEE: *homotherm; poikilotherm.*

hemathermous (hĕm"ă-thĕr'mŭs). Warm blooded. SYN: *hemathermal; hematothermal.*

hemathidrosis, hematidrosis (hē-măt"hĭ-drō'sĭs) [Gr. *haimatos*, blood, + *hidros*, sweat, + *osis*, condition]. Condition in which sweat contains blood.

hematic (hē-măt'ĭk). 1. Rel. to the blood. 2. A drug used in treating anemia. SYN: *hematinic.*

hematimeter (hĕm-ă-tĭm'ē-tĕr) [" + *metron*, measure]. Apparatus used in counting blood corpuscles in a cu. mm of blood. SYN: *hematometer; hemocytometer.*

hematin (hĕm"ă-tĭn). The nonprotein portion of the hemoglobin molecule wherein the iron is in the ferric (Fe^{+++}) rather than the ferrous (Fe^{++}) state. SEE: *ferritin; heme.*

hematinemia (hē-mă-, hĕm-ă-tĭn-ē'mē-ă). Heme in the circulating blood.

hematinic (hē-mă-, hĕm-ă-tĭn'ĭk) [Gr. *haima*, blood]. 1. Pert. to blood. 2. An agent that increases the amount of hemoglobin in the blood

hematinuria (hē"mă-tĭn-ū'rē-ă). Hematin in the urine. SYN: *hemoglobinuria.*

hemato- (hē'mă-tō, hĕm'ă-tō) [Gr. *haimatos*, blood]. Prefix indicating blood.

hematobilia (hĕm"ă-tō-bĭl'ē-ă) [" + L. *bilis*, bile]. Blood in the bile or bile ducts.

hematobium (hē"mă-, hĕm"ă-tō'bē-ŭm) [" + *bios*, life]. A parasite that lives in the blood.

hematoblast (hē'mă-, hĕm'ă-tō-blăst) [" + *blastos*, germ]. A hemocytoblast.

hematocele (hē'mă-, hĕm'ă-tō-sēl) [" + *kele*, tumor, swelling]. 1. A blood cyst. 2. Effusion of blood into a cavity. 3. Swelling due to effusion of blood into the tunica vaginalis testis.

  h., parametric. Tumor formed by blood effusion in the cul-de-sac of Douglas walled off by adhesions.

  h., pudendal. A blood-filled swollen area of the labium.

hematocelia (hĕm"ă-tō-sē'lē-ă) [" + *koilia*, cavity]. Hemorrhage into the peritoneal cavity.

hematocephalus (hē"mă-, hĕm"ă-tō-sĕf'ă-lŭs) [" + *kephale*, head]. Fetus born with hemorrhage in the head.

hematochezia (hĕm″ă-tō-kē′zē-ă) [″ + chezein, to go to stool]. Passage of stools containing red blood rather than tarry stools.

hematochromatosis (hĕm″ă-tō-krō″mătō′- sĭs) [″ + chroma, color, + osis, condition]. Hemochromatosis, q.v.

hematochyluria (hē″mă-, hĕm″ă-tō-kī-lū′ rē-ă) [″ + chylos, juice, + ouron, urine]. Blood and chyle in the urine.

hematocolpometra (hē″mă-, hĕm″ă-tō-kŏl″pō-mē′tră) [″ + kolpos, vagina, + metra, uterus]. Retention of menstrual blood in the vagina and uterus. May be due to an imperforate hymen.

hematocolpos (hē″mă-, hĕm″ă-tō-kŏl′pŏs). Retained menstrual blood in the vagina caused by an imperforate hymen.

hematocrit (hē-măt′ō-krĭt) [″ + krinein, to separate]. 1. Centrifuge for separating solids from plasma in the blood. 2. The volume of erythrocytes packed by centrifugation in a given volume of blood. The hematocrit is expressed as the percentage of total blood volume that consists of erythrocytes or as the volume in cubic centimeters of erythrocytes packed by centrifugation of blood. Normal values at sea level: men, average 47%, range 40% to 54%; women, average 42%, range 37% to 47%; children, varies with age from 35% to 49%; newborn, 49% to 54%. SEE: blood; buffy coat.

hematocyst (hē′mă-, hĕm′ă-tō-sĭst) [Gr. haimatos, blood, + kystis, a bladder]. 1. Hemorrhage into a cyst or the urinary bladder. 2. A blood-filled cyst.

hematocyte (hē′mă-, hĕm′ă-tō-sīt) [″ + kytos, cell]. 1. A red blood cell. 2. Any blood cell.

hematocytoblast (hĕm″ă-tō-sī′tō-blăst) [″ + ″ + blastos, germ]. Hemocytoblast, q.v.

hematocytometer (hē″mă-, hĕm″ă-tō-sī-tŏm′ĕ-ter) [″ + ″ + metron, measure]. Device for counting number of blood cells in given quantity of blood.

hematocytozoon (hē″mă-, hĕm″ă-tō-sī-tō-zō′ŏn) [″ + ″ + zoon, animal]. A parasite that lives in red blood cells.

hematocyturia (hē″mă-, hĕm″ă-tō-sī-tū′rē-ă) [″ + ″ + ouron, urine]. Red blood cells in urine; hematuria, as differentiated from hemoglobinuria, q.v.

hematogenesis (hē″mă-, hĕm″ă-tō-jĕn′ē-sĭs) [″ + genesis, generation, birth]. The development of blood cells. SYN: hematopoiesis.

hematogenic, hematogenous (hē″mă-, hĕm″ă-tō-jĕn′ĭk, -tŏj′ĕ-nŭs) [″ + gennan, to produce]. 1. Pert. to formation of blood. SYN: hematopoietic. 2. Pert. to or originating in the blood.

hematohidrosis (hē″mă-, hĕm″ă-tō-hī-drō′ sĭs) [″ + hidros, sweat, + osis, condition]. Secretion of sweat containing blood. SYN: hematohidrosis.

hematoid (hē′mă-, hĕm′ă-toyd) [″ + eidos, form, shape]. Resembling blood.

hematoidin (hē″mă-, hĕm-ă-toy′din). The yellow crystalline substance, biliverdin, that remains when red blood cells are destroyed in bruised tissue.

hematokolpos. Hematocolpos.

hematologist (hē″mă-, hĕm″ă-tŏl′ō-jĭst) [″ + logos, word, reason]. One who specializes in the study of the blood and in the diagnosis and treatment of disorders of blood and blood-forming tissues.

hematology (hē″mă-, hĕm″ă-tŏl′ō-jē). The science concerned with blood and the blood-forming tissues.

hematolymphangioma (hē″mă-, hĕm″ă-tō-līmf-ăn″jē-ō′mă) [″ + L. lympha, lymph, + Gr. angeion, vessel, + oma, tumor]. A tumor consisting of dilated blood vessels and lymphatics.

hematolysis (hē″mă-, hĕm-ă-tŏl′ĭ-sĭs) [″ + lysis, dissolution]. Hemolysis.

hematolytic (hĕm-ă-tō-lĭt′ĭk). Pert. to hemolysis.

hematoma (hē″mă-, hĕm-ă-tō′mă) [Gr. haimatos, blood, + oma, tumor]. A swelling or mass of blood (usually clotted) confined to an organ, tissue, or space and caused by a break in a blood vessel.

　h. auris. Hematoma beneath the perichondrium of the ear cartilage.

　h., epidural. Hematoma above the dura mater. Usually arterial, except in posterior fossa.

　h., intracerebral. Hemorrhage localized in one area of the brain.

　h., pelvic. Hematoma present in cellular tissue of the pelvis.

　h., subarachnoid. Hemorrhage between the arachnoid membrane and the pia mater; usually caused by the rupture of a congenital intracranial aneurysm, a berry aneurysm, by hypertension, or by trauma. It usually results from an arterial bleed.

　h., subdural. Hematoma located beneath the dura, usually the result of head injuries.

　h., vulvar. Hematoma occurring on the vulva.

hematomediastinum (hē″mă-, hĕm″ă-tō-mē″dē-ă-stī′nŭm) [″ + L. mediastinus, in the middle]. Blood effusion into the mediastinum.

hematometer (hē-mă-tŏm′ĕ-tĕr) [″ + metron, measure]. Hemoglobinometer.

hematometra (hē″mă-, hĕm″ă-tō-mē′tră) [″ + metra, uterus]. 1. Hemorrhage in the uterus. 2. Accumulation of menstrual blood in the uterus. SEE: *hematocolpos; hydrometra; pyometra.*

hematometry (hĕm″ă-tŏm′ĕ-trē) [″ + *metron*, measure]. Determination of varieties and number of blood cells and amount of hemoglobin in the blood.

hematomphalocele (hē″mă-, hĕm″ăt-ŏm-făl′ō-sēl) [″ + *omphalos*, navel, + *kele*, tumor, swelling]. Effusion of blood into an umbilical hernia.

hematomyelia (hē″mă-, hĕm″ă-tō-mī-ē′lē-ă) [″ + *myelos*, marrow]. Hemorrhage of blood into the spinal cord.

hematomyelitis (hē″mă-, hĕm″ă-tō-mī″ĕl-ī′tĭs) [″ + ″ + *itis*, inflammation]. Inflammation of spinal cord accompanied by bloody effusion.

hematomyelopore (hē″măt-, hĕm″ăt-ō-mī′ĕl-ō-por) [″ + ″ + *poros*, passage]. Formation of cavities and channels in the spinal cord as a result of hemorrhage.

hematonephrosis (hē″mă-, hĕm″ă-tō-nĕ-frō′sĭs) [″ + *nephros*, kidney, + *osis*, condition]. Accumulation of blood in the pelvis of the kidney.

hematopathology [″ + *pathos*, disease, suffering, + *logos*, word, reason]. The study of pathological conditions of the blood.

hematopericardium (hē″mă-, hĕm″ă-tō-pĕr″ĭ-kăr′dē-ŭm) [″ + *peri*, around, + *kardia*, heart]. Bloody effusion into the pericardial sac.

hematoperitoneum (hē″mă-, hĕm″ă-tō-pĕr″ĭ-tō-nē′ŭm) [″ + *peritonaion*, peritoneum]. Bloody effusion into the peritoneal cavity. SYN: *hemoperitoneum.*

hematopexin (hĕm″ă-tō-pĕk′sĭn) [″ + *pexis*, fixation]. Hemopexin, q.v.

hematophage (hĕm′ă-tō-fāj) [″ + *phagein*, to eat]. A phagocytic cell that destroys red blood cells.

hematophagia (hĕm″ă-tō-fā′jē-ă). 1. Subsistence of blood. 2. Destruction of blood cells by phagocytes.

hematophagous (hĕm-ă-tŏf′ă-gŭs). Living on blood. SEE: *hematophagia.*

hematophilia (hĕm″ă-tō-fĭ′ē-ă) [″ + *philein*, to love]. Hemophilia.

hematophobia (hē″mă-, hĕm″ă-tō-fō′bē-ă) [″ + *phobos*, fear]. Hemophobia.

hematophyte (hē″mă-, hĕm″ă-tō-fīt) [″ + *phyton*, plant]. Plant organism or bacteria in the blood.

hematoplastic [″ + *plassein*, to form]. Pert. to formation of blood. SYN: *hematopoietic.*

hematopoiesis (hē″mă-, hĕm″ă-tō-poy-ē′sĭs) [Gr. *haimatos*, blood, + *poiesis*, formation]. Production and development of blood cells, normally in the bone marrow. Tissues that produce blood cells are said to be hematopoietic.

h., extramedullary. Production of blood cells in tissues other than bone marrow. This occurs in severe anemia and other diseases affecting the blood.

hematopoietic (hē″mă-, hĕm″ă-tō-poy-ĕt′ĭk). 1. Pert. to the production and development of blood cells. 2. A substance that assists in or stimulates the production of blood cells. SYN: *hematogenic; hematoplastic.*

hematopoietic growth factors. A group of at least 7 substances involved in the production of blood cells. Included are several interleukins and erythropoietin, q.v.

hematopoietic malignancies. Leukemias and lymphomas are cancers that arise from unregulated clonal proliferation of hematopoietic stem cells. The individual cells, most of which are incompetent and useless, mature slowly and survive longer than normal. The lethal aspect of these conditions, leukemia and lymphoma, is not due to the rapid production of new cells but to the constant generation of defective new cells. SEE: *leukemia; lymphoma.*

hematopoietic system. The blood-forming organs, esp. bone marrow and lymph nodes.

hematoporphyrin (hē″mă-, hĕm″ă-tō-por′fī-rĭn) [″ + *porphyra*, purple]. Iron-free heme, a decomposition product of hemoglobin present in the urine in certain conditions.

hematoporphyrinuria (hē″mă-, hĕm″ă-tō-por″fī-rĭn-ū′rē-ă) [″ + ″ + *ouron*, urine]. Hematoporphyrin in urine.

hematorrhachis (hĕm-ă-tor′ă-kĭs) [″ + *rhachis*, spine]. Hemorrhage into the spinal cord.

hematorrhea (hĕm″ă-tō-rē′ă) [″ + *rhoia*, flow]. Profuse hemorrhage.

hematosalpinx (hē″mă-, hĕm″ă-tō-săl′pĭnks) [″ + *salpinx*, tube]. Retained menstrual fluid in the fallopian tube.

hematoscheocele (hĕm-ă-tŏs′kē-ō-sēl) [″ + *oscheon*, scrotum, + *kele*, tumor, swelling]. Blood accumulated in the scrotum.

hematosepsis (hĕm″ă-tō-sĕp′sĭs) [″ + *sepsis*, putrefaction]. Septicemia.

hematospermatocele (hĕm″ă-tō-spĕr-măt′ō-sēl) [″ + *sperma*, seed, + *kele*, tumor, swelling]. A blood-filled spermatocele.

hematospermia (hĕm″ă-tō-spĕr′mē-ă). Semen that contains blood; hemospermia.

h. spuria. Hematospermia coming from the prostatic urethra.

h. vera. Hematospermia coming from the seminal vesicles.

hematostatic (hĕm″ă-tō-stăt′ĭk) [Gr. *haimatos*, blood, + *stasis*, standing]. 1. Retaining blood in a part. 2. Pert. to the arrest of blood flow in a hemorrhage. SYN: *hemostatic.*

hermatosteon (hĕm-ă-tŏs'tē-ŏn) [" + *osteon*, bone]. Bleeding into the medullary cavity of a bone.

hematothermal (hĕm"ă-tō-thĕr'măl) [" + *therme*, heat]. Warm blooded. SYN: *hemathermal; hemathermous.*

hematothorax (hĕm"ă-tō-thō'răks) [" + *thorax*, chest]. Blood in the pleural space. SYN: *hemothorax.*

hematotoxic (hĕm"ă-tō-tŏk'sīk) [" + *toxikon*, poison]. 1. Pert. to septicemia. 2. Toxic to blood cells.

hematotrachelos (hĕm"ă-tō-tră-kē'lōs) [" + *trachelos*, neck]. Retained menstrual blood in the uterus, usually due to obstruction of the cervical canal.

hematotropic (hĕm"ă-tō-trŏp'ĭk) [" + *tropos*, a turning]. Having special affinity for red blood cells.

hematotympanum (hĕm"ă-tō-tĭm'păn-ŭm) [" + *tympanon*, drum]. Blood in the middle ear.

hematoxylin (hĕm"ă-tŏk'sĭ-lĭn). $C_{16}H_{14}O_6$. A colorless crystalline compound obtained by ether extraction of the wood portion of the tree *Haematoxylon campechianum.* Upon oxidation it is converted into hematein, an oxidation product of hematoxylin, which stains certain structures a deep blue color. It is an excellent nuclear stain and widely used in histological work.

hematozoon (hē"mă-, hĕm"ă-tō-zō'ŏn) [" + *zoon*, animal]. Any living organism in the blood.

hematozymosis (hē"mă-, hĕm"ă-tō-zī-mō'sĭs) [" + *zymosis*, fermentation]. Blood fermentation.

hematuria (hē"mă-, hĕm"ă-tū'rē-ă) [" + *ouron*, urine]. Blood in the urine.

SYM: Urine may be slightly smoky, reddish, or very red.

ETIOL: Lesion of urinary tract; blood dyscrasia; contamination during menstruation or puerperium; prostatic disease; trauma; tumors; poisoning, esp. carbolic acid and cantharides; malaria, toxemias; or calculus in urinary tract.

DIAG: If blood is well mixed with urine, it probably came from the kidneys. If clotted in tubular casts of ureters, it came from the kidneys and ureters. If passed at beginning of urination, from the urethra; if at the end, from the bladder.

NOTE: The occurrence of bright red blood in the urine and its appearance in the toilet bowl are quite frightening to the patient. The patient, physician, and nurse should realize that a very small amount of blood may cause the entire toilet bowl to appear to be full of blood.

h., micro-. The detection of red blood cells in the urine upon microscopic examination of a specimen. Even though this finding in asymptomatic persons may, in 20-25% of cases, represent a pathologic process, the remaining cases may be unexplained. In the normal individual, about 1500 erythrocytes are excreted in the urine each minute.

h., renal. Urine smoky, sometimes bright red.

h., urethral. Always bright red. Precedes urination.

h., vesical. Urine bright red, not uniform.

heme (hēm). An iron-containing nonprotein portion of the hemoglobin molecule wherein the iron is in the ferrous (Fe^{++}) state. SEE: *ferritin; hematin.*

hemeralopia (hĕm"ĕr-ăl-ō'pē-ă) [Gr. *hemera*, day, + *alaos*, blind, + *ops*, eye]. Diminished vision in bright light. Term formerly erroneously applied to night blindness or nyctalopia, q.v. Nyctalopia indicates inability to see in dim light, though otherwise vision is normal.

In hemeralopia, the sight is poor in sunlight and in good illumination; it is good at dusk, at twilight, and in poor illumination. This is noted in albinism, retinitis with central scotoma, toxic amblyopia, coloboma of the iris and choroid, opacity of the crystalline lens or cornea, and in conjunctivitis with photophobia.

hemi- (hĕm'ē) [Gr.]. Prefix meaning half.

hemiacephalus (hĕm"ē-ă-sĕf'ă- lŭs) [" + *a-*, not, + *kephale*, head]. A malformed fetus with a markedly defective head. SEE: *anencephalus.*

hemiachromatopsia (hĕm"ē-ă-krō-mă-tŏp' sē-ă) [" + " + *chroma*, color, + *opsis*, vision]. Color blindness in one-half, or in corresponding halves, of the vision field.

hemiageusia (hĕm"ē-ă-gū'zē-ă) [" + " + *geusis*, taste]. Loss of sense of taste on one side of the tongue.

hemialbumin (hĕm"ē-ăl-bū'mĭn) [" + L. *albumen*, white of egg]. A product resulting from the digestion of albumin.

hemialbumose (hĕm"-ē-ăl'bū-mōs). An albumoid product from the digestion of certain proteins. It is found in bone marrow.

hemialbumosuria (hĕm"ē-ăl-bū"mō-sū'rē-ă) [" + " + Gr. *ouron*, urine]. Hemialbumose in the urine.

hemialgia (hĕm-ē-ăl'jē-ă) [" + *algos*, pain]. Pain in half of the body.

hemiamaurosis (hĕm"ē-ăm"ŏ-rō'sĭs) [" + *amaurosis*, darkness]. Blindness in one-half of the visual field. SYN: *hemiamblyopia; hemianopia.*

hemiamblyopia (hĕm"ē-ăm"blē-ō'pē-ă) ["

+ *amblys,* dim, + *ops,* sight]. Blindness in one-half of the visual field. SYN: *hemiamaurosis; hemianopia.*

hemiamyosthenia (hĕm″ē-ă″mī-ŏs-thē′nē-ă) [Gr. *hemi-,* half, + *a-,* not, + *mys,* muscle, + *sthenos,* strength]. Absence of normal muscular power on one side of the body. SYN: *hemiparesis.*

hemianacusia (hĕm″ē-ăn″ă-kū′zē-ă) [″ + *an-,* not, + *akousis,* hearing]. Deafness in one ear.

hemianalgesia (hĕm″ē-ăn-ăl-jē′zē-ă) [″ + ″ + *algos,* pain]. Lack of sensibility to pain (analgesia) on one side of the body.

hemianencephaly (hĕm″ē-ăn″ĕn-sĕf′ă-lē) [″ + *an-,* not, + *enkephalos,* brain]. Congenital absence of half of the brain.

hemianesthesia (hĕm″ē-ăn-ĕs-thē′zē-ă) [″ + ″ + *aisthesis,* sensation]. Anesthesia of half of the body.

hemianopia, hemianopsia (hĕm″ē-ă-nō′pē-ă, -nŏp′sē-ă) [″ + *an-,* not, + *ops,* eye]. Blindness for half the field of vision in one or both eyes. SYN: *hemiamaurosis; hemiamblyopia.*

   h., altitudinal. Blindness in upper or lower half of the visual field of one or both eyes.

   h., binasal. Affection of nasal half of the visual field in each eye.

   h., bitemporal. Affection of temporal half of visual field in each eye.

   h., complete. Blindness in half the visual field.

   h., crossed. Either bitemporal or binasal hemianopsia.

   h., heteronymous. H., crossed.

   h., homonymous. Blindness of nasal half of the visual field of one eye and temporal half of the other, or right-sided or left-sided hemianopsia of corresponding sides in both eyes.

   h., incomplete. Blindness in less than half of the visual field of each eye.

   h., quadrant. Blindness of symmetrical quadrant of the field of vision in each eye.

   h., unilateral. Hemianopsia affecting only one eye.

hemianosmia (hĕm″ē-ăn-ŏs′mē-ă) [Gr. *hemi-,* half, + *an-,* not, + *osme,* smell]. Loss of smell in one nostril.

hemiapraxia (hĕm″ē-ă-prăks′ē-ă) [″ + *a-,* not, + *prassein,* to do]. Incapacity to exercise purposeful movements on one side of the body.

hemiarthrosis (hĕm″ē-ăr-thrō′sĭs) [″ + *arthron,* joint, + *osis,* condition]. A false articulation between two bones. SYN: *synchondrosis.*

hemiasynergia (hĕm″ē-ă″sĭn-ĕr′jē-ă) [″ + *a-,* not, + *syn,* with, + *ergon,* work]. Lack of coordination of parts affecting one side of the body.

hemiataxia (hĕm″ē-ă-tăks′ē-ă) [″ + *ataxia,* lack of order]. Impaired muscular coordination causing awkward movements of the affected side of the body.

hemiathetosis (hĕm″ē-ăth″ē-tō′sĭs) [″ + *athetos,* without fixed position, + *osis,* condition]. Athetosis of one side of the body.

hemiatrophy (hĕm-ē-ăt′rō-fē) [″ + *atrophia,* atrophy]. Impaired nutrition resulting in atrophy of one side of the body or of an organ or part.

hemiballism (hĕm-ē-băl′ĭzm) [″ + *balismos,* jumping]. Jerking and twitching movements of one side of the body. SYN: *hemichorea.*

hemiblock (hĕm′ī-blŏk). In heart block, failure of conduction in one of the two main divisions of the left branches of the conducting bundle.

hemic (hē′mĭk, hĕm′ĭk) [Gr. *haima,* blood]. Pert. to blood. SYN: *hemal.*

hemicanities (hĕm″ē-kăn-ĭsh′ī-ēz) [Gr. *hemi-,* half, + L. *canities,* gray hair]. Grayness of hair on one side only.

hemicardia (hĕm-ē-kăr′dē-ă) [″ + *kardia,* heart]. Half of a four-chambered heart.

hemicastration (hĕm″ē-kăs-trā′shŭn) [″ + L. *castrare,* to prune]. Removal of one ovary or testicle. At one time, removal of the left testicle was done on the erroneous assumption that sperm from the right testicle produced only sons.

hemicellulose (hĕm-ē-sĕl′ū-lōs). One of a group of polysaccharides that differ from cellulose in that they may be hydrolyzed by dilute mineral acids, and from other polysaccharides in that they are not readily digested by amylases. Includes pentosans, galactosans (agar-agar), and pectins.

hemicentrum (hĕm-ē-sĕn′trŭm) [″ + *kentron,* center]. Either lateral half of the centrum of a vertebra.

hemicephalia (hĕm″ē-sĕ-fā′lē-ă) [″ + *kephale,* head]. Congenital absence of one-half of the skull and brain.

hemicephalus (hĕm-ē-sĕf′ă-lus). A congenitally deformed child with only one cerebral hemisphere.

hemicerebrum (hĕm″ē-sĕr′ē-brŭm) [″ + L. *cerebrum,* brain]. Half of the cerebral hemisphere.

hemichorea (hĕm-ē-kō-rē′ă) [″ + *choreia,* dance]. Convulsive movements of one side of the body. SYN: *hemiballism.*

hemichromatopsia (hĕm″ē-krō-mă-tŏp′sē-ă) [″ + *chroma,* color, + *opsis,* vision]. Blindness to color in one-half of the visual field. SYN: *hemiachromatopsia.*

hemicolectomy (hĕm″ē-kō-lĕk′tō-mē) [″ + *kolon,* colon, + *ektome,* excision]. Surgical removal of half or less of the colon.

hemicorporectomy (hĕm″ē-kor″pō-rĕk′tō-mē) [″ + L. *corpus*, body, + Gr. *ektome*, excision]. Surgical removal of the lower half of the body.

hemicrania (hĕm-ē-krā′nē-ă) [″ + *kranion*, skull]. 1. Unilateral head pain, usually migraine. 2. Malformed fetus having only one-half of the skull development.

hemicraniectomy (hĕm″ē-krā-nē-ĕk′tō-mē) [″ + ″ + *ektome*, excision]. Surgical division of cranial vault from front backward, exposing half of the brain.

hemicraniosis (hĕm″ē-krā-nē-ō′sĭs) [″ + ″ + *osis*, condition]. Enlargement of half of cranium or face.

hemidesmosome. The half of a desmosome produced by epithelial cells for attachment of basal surface of the cell to the underlying basement membrane or the enamel or cementum tooth surface in the case of junctional epithelium.

hemidiaphoresis (hĕm″ē-dī″ă-for-ē′sĭs) [″ + *dia*, through, + *pherein*, to carry]. Sweating on one side of the body. SYN: *hemidrosis; hemihidrosis.*

hemidiaphragm (hĕm″ē-dī′ă-frăm) [″ + ″ + *phragma*, wall]. Half of the diaphragm.

hemidrosis (hĕm″ĭ-drō′sĭs). 1. [″ + *hidrosis*, sweating]. Sweating on one side of the body. SYN: *hemidiaphoresis; hemihidrosis.* 2. [Gr. *haima*, blood, + *hidrosis*, sweating] Secretion of sweat containing blood. SYN: *hemathidrosis.*

hemidysergia (hĕm″ē-dĭs-ĕr′jē-ă) [Gr. *hemi-*, half, + *dys*, bad, + *ergon*, work]. Lack of coordination of muscles on one side of the body.

hemidysesthesia (hĕm″ē-dĭs-ĕs-thē′zē-ă) [″ + ″ + *aisthesis*, sensation]. Impaired sensation of half of the body.

hemidystrophy (hĕm″ē-dĭs′trō-fē) [″ + ″ + *trophe*, nourishment]. Inequality in development of the two sides of the body.

hemiectromelia (hĕm″ē-ĕk-trō-mē′lē-ă) [″ + *ektro*, abortion, + *melos*, limb]. Deformed extremities on one side of the body.

hemiepilepsy (hĕm″ē-ĕp′ĭ-lĕp-sē) [″ + *epilepsia*, seizure]. Epilepsy with convulsions confined to one side of the body.

hemifacial (hĕm″ē-fā′shăl) [″ + L. *facies*, face]. Pert. to one side of the face.

hemigastrectomy (hĕm″ē-găs-trĕk′tō-mē) [″ + *gaster*, belly, + *ektome*, excision]. Excision of half of the stomach.

hemigeusia (hĕm-ē-gū′sē-ă) [″ + *geusis*, taste]. Loss of sense of taste on one side of the tongue.

hemiglossal (hĕm″ē-glŏs′săl) [″ + *glossa*, tongue]. Concerning one side of the tongue.

hemiglossectomy (hĕm″ē-glŏs-sĕk′tō-mē) [″ + ″ + *ektome*, excision]. Surgical removal of half of the tongue.

hemiglossitis [″ + ″ + *itis*, inflammation]. Vesicular eruption on half of the tongue and inner surface of the cheek. Herpetic in character.

hemignathia (hĕm″ē-năth′ē-ă) [″ + *gnathos*, jaw]. Congenital absence of one-half of the lower jaw.

hemihepatectomy (hĕm″ē-hĕp″ă-tĕk′tō-mē) [″ + *hepatos*, liver, + *ektome*, excision]. Surgical removal of half of the liver.

hemihidrosis (hĕm″ē-hī-drō′sĭs) [″ + *hidros*, sweat, + *osis*, condition]. Sweating on only one side of the body. SYN: *hemidiaphoresis; hemidrosis* (def. 1).

hemihypalgesia (hĕm″ē-hī″păl-jē′zē-ă) [″ + *hypo*, under, + *algesis*, sense of pain]. Partial anesthesia on one side of the body.

hemihyperesthesia (hĕm″ē-hī-pĕr-ĕs-thē′zē-ă) [″ + *hyper*, over, + *aisthesis*, sensation]. Abnormal tactile and painful sensitiveness of one side of the body.

hemihyperidrosis (hĕm″ē-hī-pĕr-ĭ-drō′sĭs) [″ + ″ + *hydrosis*, sweating]. Excessive perspiration confined to one side of the body. SYN: *hemihyperhidrosis.*

hemihyperplasia (hĕm″ē-hī″pĕr-plā′zē-ă) [″ + ″ + *plassein*, to form]. Excessive development of one side or one-half of the body or of an organ.

hemihypertonia (hĕm″ē-hī″pĕr-tō′nē-ă) [″ + ″ + *tonos*, tone]. Exaggerated tonicity of muscles on one side of the body.

hemihypertrophy (hĕm″ē-hī-pĕr′trō-fē) [″ + ″ + *trophe*, nourishment]. Hypertrophy of muscles of half of the body or face.

hemihypesthesia, hemihypoesthesia (hĕm″ē-hī″pĕs-thē′zē-ă, -pō-ĕs-thē′zē-a) [Gr. *hemi-*, half, + *hypo*, under, + *aisthesis*, sensation]. Diminished sensibility on one side of the body.

hemihypoplasia (hĕm″ē-hī″pō-plā′zē-ă) [″ + ″ + *plassein*, to form]. Decreased development of half of the body or of an organ.

hemihypotonia (hĕm″ē-hī-pō-tō′nē-ă) [″ + ″ + *tonos*, tone]. Partial loss of tonicity of muscles on one side of the body.

hemikaryon (hĕm″ē-kăr′ē-ŏn) [″ + *karyon*, nucleus]. A cell nucleus with half the diploid number of chromosomes.

hemilaminectomy (hĕm″ē-lăm″ĭ-nĕk′tō-mē) [″ + L. *lamina*, thin plate, + Gr. *ektome*, excision]. Surgical removal of the lamina of the vertebral arch on one side.

hemilaryngectomy (hĕm″ē-lăr″in-jĕk′tō-mē) [″ + *larynx*, larynx, + *ektome*, excision]. Surgical removal of the lateral half of the larynx.

hemilateral [″ + L. *latus*, side]. Rel. to one side only.

hemilesion (hĕm″ē-lē′zhŭn) [″ + L. *laesio*, a wound]. A lesion on one side of the body.

hemilingual (hĕm″ē-lĭng′gwăl) [″ + L. *lin-*

gua, tongue]. Affecting or concerning one lateral half of the tongue.

hemimacroglossia (hĕm″ē-măk″rō-glŏs′ē-ă) [″ + *makros*, large, + *glossa*, tongue]. Enlargement of one lateral half of the tongue.

hemimandibulectomy (hĕm″ē-măn-dĭb-ū-lĕk′tō-mē) [″ + L. *mandibula*, lower jawbone, + Gr. *ektome*, excision]. Surgical removal of half of the mandible.

hemimelus (hĕm″ĭ-mē′lŭs) [″ + *melos*, limb]. A malformed fetus with defective development of the extremities, esp. the distal portion.

hemin (hē′mĭn) [Gr. *haima*, blood]. A brownish-red crystalline salt of heme formed when hemoglobin is heated with glacial acetic acid and sodium chloride. The iron is present in the ferric (Fe^{+++}) state. Used in testing for presence of blood. SEE: *heme*.

heminephrectomy (hĕm″ē-nĕ-frĕk′tō-mē) [Gr. *hemi-*, half, + *nephros*, kidney, + *ektome*, excision]. Excision or removal of a portion of a kidney.

hemineurasthenia (hĕm″ē-nū-răs-thē′nē-ă) [″ + *neuron*, nerve, + *astheneia*, weakness]. Neurasthenia affecting one side of the body only.

hemiopalgia (hĕm″ē-ŏp-ăl′jē-ă) [″ + *ops*, eye, + *algos*, pain]. Pain in one side of the head and the eye on that side.

hemiopia (hĕm-ē-ō′pē-ă) [″ + *ops*, eye]. Blindness in half of the visual field. SYN: *hemianopia*.

hemiopic (hĕm-ē-ŏp′ĭk) [″ + *ops*, eye]. Pert. to hemiopia.

hemipagus (hĕm-ĭp′ă-gŭs) [″ + *pagos*, a thing fixed]. Twins fused at the navel and thorax.

hemiparalysis [″ + *paralyein*, to disable]. Paralysis of one side of the body only.

hemiparaplegia (hĕm″ē-păr-ă-plē′jē-ă) [″ + ″ + *plege*, stroke]. Paralysis of the lower half of one side or of one leg. A confusing term because paraplegia indicates paralysis of both lower extremities.

hemiparesis (hĕm″ē-păr′ē-sĭs, hĕm-ē-păr-ē′sĭs) [″ + *paresis*, paralysis]. Paralysis affecting only one side of the body.

hemiparesthesia (hĕm″ē-păr-ĕs-thē′zē-ă) [″ + *para*, beyond, + *aisthesis*, sensation]. Numbness of one side of the body.

hemipelvectomy (hĕm″ē-pĕl″vĕk′tō-mē) [″ + L. *pelvis*, basin, + Gr. *ektome*, excision]. Surgical removal of half of the pelvis, and the leg.

hemiplegia (hĕm-ē-plē′jē-ă) [″ + *plege*, a stroke]. 1. Paralysis of only one side of the body. SEE: *Benedikt's syndrome; paralysis; thalamic syndrome.*

ETIOL: A brain lesion involving the upper motor neurons and resulting in paral-

ysis of the opposite side of the body. May result from disturbed blood flow to a portion of the brain. This may be due to hemorrhage, cerebral thrombosis, embolism, or a tumor of the cerebrum.

F.A.: Elevate head and shoulders. See that tongue does not obstruct breathing. Avoid stimulants. Do not move patient until arrival of someone competent in emergency medical care.

NURSING IMPLICATIONS: Carefully assess the patient's neurological status. Intervene to prevent contracture formation through range-of-motion exercises at least once a day. Turn the patient frequently and provide good skin care to prevent skin breakdown. Patient should cough and breathe deeply and change position every two hours to prevent hypostatic pneumonia. When able, the patient should be encouraged to assist with his or her activities of daily living. Encourage the use of assistive devices, maintain a positive attitude, and assist patient and family to establish and work toward realistic goals. Before discharge, teach the patient about the use of maintenance drugs, and arrange for home care and referrals for specialized therapies.

h., capsular. Hemiplegia resulting from a lesion of the internal capsule of the brain.

h., cerebral. Hemiplegia caused by brain lesion.

h., facial. Paralysis of muscles of one side of the face.

h., spastic. Hemiplegia accompanied by spasticity, usually occurring in infants.

h., spinal. Hemiplegia resulting from a lesion of the spinal cord. SEE: *Brown-Séquard's paralysis.*

hemiplegic (hĕm-ē-plē′jĭk). 1. Pert. to hemiplegia. 2. Colloquial reference to a patient having hemiplegia.

Hemiptera (hĕm-ĭp′tĕr-ă) [Gr. *hemi-*, half, + *pteron*, wing]. The true bugs; an order of insects characterized by piercing and sucking mouth parts. The first pair of wings is leathery at the base and membranous at the tip; the second pair is membranous. There is incomplete metamorphosis. Includes bedbugs, kissing bugs, and several other species that are pests or transmitters of pathogenic organisms.

hemipyocyanin (hĕm″ē-pī″ō-sī′ă-nĭn). Antibacterial pigment produced by *Pseudomonas pyocyanea.*

hemirachischisis (hĕm″ē-ră-kĭs′kĭ-sĭs) [″ + *rhachis*, spine, + *schisis*, a splitting]. Rachischisis in which protrusion of the spinal meninges does not occur. SYN: *spina bifida occulta.*

hemisacralization (hĕm″ē-să″krăl-ī-zā′shŭn). Abnormal development of one-half of the fifth lumbar vertebra so that it is fused with the sacrum.

hemisection (hĕm″ē-sĕk′shŭn) [″ + L. *sectio,* a cutting]. In surgery or anatomy, cutting an organ or tissue in half. SYN: *bisection.*

hemisomus (hĕm″ē-sō′mŭs) [″ + *soma,* body]. Fetus with lateral half of body missing or malformed.

hemispasm (hĕm′ē-spăzm) [″ + *spasmos,* a convulsion]. Spasm of only one side of the body or face.

hemisphere (hĕm′ĭ-sfēr) [″ + *sphaira,* sphere]. Either half of the cerebrum or cerebellum.

　　h., dominant. The cerebral hemisphere in which the higher cortical functions, esp. those rel. to speech and certain motor activities, are associated; the left one in right-handed individuals. Results in phenomenon known as cerebral dominance.

hemispheric specialization. Referring to the differences in function affected by damage to either the right or left cerebral hemisphere; for example, damage to the right hemisphere may produce difficulties with visual-perceptual abilities while damage to the left hemisphere frequently results in difficulties with language, analytic thought, and abstract concepts.

hemisyndrome (hĕm″ē-sĭn′drōm) [″ + *syndrome,* a running with]. Syndrome indicating a unilateral lesion of the spinal cord.

hemithermoanesthesia (hĕm″ē-thĕr″mō-ăn″ĕs-thē′zē-ă) [Gr. *hemi-,* half, + *therme,* heat, + *an-,* not, + *aisthesis,* sensation]. Unilateral loss of sensitivity to heat and cold.

hemithorax (hĕm″ē-thō′răks) [″ + *thorax,* chest]. One-half of the chest.

hemithyroidectomy (hĕm″ē-thī″royd-ĕk′tō-mē) [″ + *thyreos,* shield, + *eidos,* form, shape, + *ektome,* excision]. Surgical removal of one-half of the thyroid gland tissue.

hemitomias (hĕm″ĭ-tō′mē-ăs) [Gr. *hemitomias,* half a eunuch]. A person with one testicle.

hemitremor (hĕm″ē-trĕm′or). Tremor present in one lateral half of the body.

hemivertebra (hĕm″ē-vĕr′tĕ-bră). Congenital absence or failure to develop of half of a vertebra.

hemizygosity (hĕm″ē-zī-gŏs′ĭ-tē) [″ + *zygotos,* yoked]. Possessing only one of the gene pair that determines a particular genetic trait.

hemlock [AS. *hemleac*]. 1. A species of evergreen plant. 2. Volatile oil extracted from dried, unripe fruit of *Conium maculatum,* poison hemlock.

hemlock poisoning. SYM: Weakness, drowsiness, nausea, vomiting, difficult breathing, paralysis, and death.

　　TREAT: Empty stomach by means of a stomach pump or an emetic. Give cathartic. Treat respiratory failure with artificial respiration and oxygen.

Hemlock Society. An organization that has published information about suicide for terminally ill patients.

hemo-. Prefix meaning blood. SEE: words beginning with *haemo-, haem-, hem-, hema-,* and *hemato-.*

hemoagglutination (hē″mō-ă-gloo″tĭ-nā′shŭn) [Gr. *haima,* blood, + L. *agglutinans,* gluing]. The clumping of red blood corpuscles.

hemoagglutinin (hē″mō-ă-gloo′tĭ-nĭn). An agglutinin that clumps the red blood corpuscles.

hemobilia (hē″mō-bĭl′ē-ă). Blood in the bile or bile ducts.

hemobilinuria (hē″mō-bĭl-ĭn-ū′rē-ă) [″ + L. *bilis,* bile, + Gr. *ouron,* urine]. Urobilin in the blood and urine.

hemochromatosis (hē″mō-krō″mă-tō′sĭs) [″ + *chroma,* color, + *osis,* condition]. A hereditary disease of iron metabolism that causes the body to absorb and store too much iron. The liver becomes enlarged; the skin is pigmented so that it has a bronze hue; and diabetes and cardiac failure may be present. It is a rare disease seen ten times as frequently in males as females. The majority of cases develop after the fourth decade.

　　TREAT: Removal of blood on a weekly basis until iron stores return to a normal level. SYN: *diabetes, bronze.*

　　h., exogenous. Excess deposition of iron in tissues due to multiple transfusions or excess intake of iron.

hemochrome (hē′mō-krōm). Hemoglobin.

hemochromogen (hē″mō-krō′mō-jĕn) [″ + *chroma,* color, + *gennan,* to produce]. General term applied to compounds of heme with nitrogen-containing substances such as a protein.

hemochromoprotein (hē″mō-krō″mō-prō′tē-ĭn). Any protein combined with the blood pigment hemochrome.

hemoclip. A metal clip used to ligate blood vessels.

hemoconcentration. A relative increase in the number of red blood cells resulting from a decrease in the volume of plasma. SYN: *anhydremia.*

hemoconia (hē″mō-kō′nē-ă) [Gr. *haima,* blood, + *konis,* dust]. Minute colorless bodies in blood thought to be the products of disintegration of red blood cells. SYN: *blood dust.*

hemoconiosis (hē″mō-kō″nē-ō′sĭs) [″ + ″ + *osis,* condition]. Having an abnormal amt. of hemoconia in the blood.

hemocuprein (hē″mō-kū′prē-ĭn). A blue copper-containing compound present in red blood cells.

hemocyanin (hē″mō-sī′ă-nĭn) [″ + kyanos, blue]. An oxygen-carrying blue pigment in the plasma of arthropods and molluscs.

hemocyte (hē′mō-sīt) [″ + kytos, cell]. 1. Any blood cell. 2. Red blood cell.

hemocytoblast (hē″mō-sī′tō-blăst) [″ + ″ + blastos, germ]. The primitive reticulo-endothelial stem cell found in bone marrow from which all cells normally present in blood are thought to arise.

hemocytogenesis (hē″mō-sī″tō-jĕn′ĕ-sĭs) [″ + kytos, cell, + genesis, generation, birth]. Hematopoiesis.

hemocytology (hē″mō-sī-tŏl′ō-jē) [″ + ″ + logos, word, reason]. Study of the structure and function of blood cells.

hemocytometer (hē″mō-sī-tŏm′ĕ-tĕr) [″ + ″ + metron, measure]. Device for determining number of cells in a stated volume of blood.

hemocytophagia. Phagocytic ingestion of red blood cells.

hemocytotripsis (hē″mō-sī″tō-trĭp′sĭs) [″ + ″ + tribein, to rub]. Destruction of red blood cells due to extreme pressure.

hemocytozoon (hē″mō-sī″tō-zō′ŏn) [″ + ″ + zoon, animal]. A protozoan parasite of the blood cells. SYN: hematobium.

hemodiagnosis (hē″mō-dī″ăg-nō′sĭs) [″ + dia, through, + gnosis, knowledge]. Examination of the blood for diagnostic purposes.

hemodialysis (hē″mō-, hĕm″ō-dī-ăl′ĭ-sĭs) [″ + ″ + lysis, dissolution]. A method for providing the function of the kidneys by circulating blood through tubes made of semi-permeable membranes. These dialyzing tubes are continually bathed by solutions that selectively remove unwanted material. Use of this technique in patients in whom one or both kidneys are defective or absent is life-saving. SEE: hemoperfusion. SEE: *Nursing Diagnoses* in Appendix.

hemodialyzer (hē″mō-dī′ă-līz″ĕr). Device used in performing hemodialysis.

hemodiastase (hē″mō-dī′ăs-tās) [″ + diastasis, separation]. An amylolytic enzyme in the blood.

hemodilution (hē″mō-dī-lū′shŭn). An increase in the volume of blood plasma resulting in reduced relative concentration of red blood cells.

hemodynamics (hē″mō-dī-năm′ĭks) [Gr. haima, blood, + dynamis, power]. A study of the forces involved in circulating blood through the body.

hemoendothelial (hē″mō-ĕn-dō-thē′lē-ăl).
Pert. to the relationship between blood of the mother and the endothelium of chorionic vessels. SEE: *placenta.*

Hemofil. Trade name for antihemophilic factor (AHF), USP.

hemofiltration (hē″mō-fĭl-trā′shŭn). Use of ultrafiltration technique to remove excess accumulation of normal metabolic products from the blood. The technical aspects are similar to renal dialysis in that the blood flows from the body to the hemofilter and is then returned to the body.

Caution: Depending upon the type of filter membrane used, essential materials will be removed from the blood. It is important to replace the excess crystalloids removed.

---

h., continuous arteriovenous. ABBR: CAVH. Technique using a hemofilter to facilitate removal of water, electrolytes and small to medium molecular weight molecules from the vascular space. Used in patients with renal failure or fluid overload.

hemoflagellate (hē″mō-flăj′ĕ-lāt″) [″ + L. flagellum, whip]. Any flagellate protozoan of the blood. The most important genera are *Trypanosoma* and *Leishmania.*

hemofuscin (hē″mō-fū′sĭn) [″ + L. fuscus, brown]. Brown pigment derived from hemoglobin. In urine, it produces a reddish color.

hemoglobin (hē″mō-, hĕm″ō-glō′bĭn) [″ + L. globus, globe]. ABBR: Hbg; Hgb. The iron-containing pigment of the red blood cells. Its function is to carry oxygen from the lungs to the tissues. The amount of hemoglobin in the blood averages 12–16 gm/100 ml of blood in adult females; 14–18 in males; and somewhat less in children. One gm of hemoglobin can combine with 1.36 cc of oxygen, the resulting compound being oxyhemoglobin. Hemoglobin is a crystallizable, conjugated protein consisting of an iron-containing pigment called heme and a simple protein, globin. In the lungs it combines readily, by a process called oxygenation, with oxygen to form a loose, unstable compound called oxyhemoglobin. In the tissues where oxygen tension is low and carbon dioxide tension is high, oxyhemoglobin liberates its oxygen in exchange for carbon dioxide. A chemical important in these exchanges is 2,3-diphosphoglycerate, q.v. Hemoglobin liberated from disintegrating red blood cells is removed from circulation by the cells of the reticuloendothelial system, esp. those of the liver and spleen. The globin is converted to amino acids and reutilized. Iron from the iron-containing portion is stored in the liver and spleen and reutilized; the non-iron-containing pigment is converted to bilirubin, which is excreted as one of the bile pigments.

Hemoglobin combines with carbon monoxide to form the stable compound carboxyhemoglobin, which is unable to liberate oxygen for use by tissues. Oxidation of the ferrous iron of hemoglobin to the ferric state produces methemoglobin.

Many different types of hemoglobin have been discovered. Study of these has facilitated the investigation of human genetics. Hemoglobin is named according to the way the amino acid components of the globin move when studied by electrophoresis. There are more than a hundred different types of abnormal hemoglobin. SEE: *blood.*

ABNORM: Abnormal forms of hemoglobin are due to mutations. Because of the size of the hemoglobin molecule, the number of possible mutant forms is enormous. Only a few of the diseases caused by these forms are described here:

Hemoglobin S: The first disease discovered to be due to a molecular abnormality of hemoglobin was sickle cell anemia. It is caused by the presence of an abnormal hemoglobin that under proper conditions alters its physical structure to cause red blood cells to assume a sickle shape. In sickle cell trait, the patient is asymptomatic because of being genetically heterozygous for hemoglobin S. In sickle cell disease, individuals are homozygous for hemoglobin S and are symptomatic. SEE: *sickle cell anemia.*

Hemoglobin C disease: A chronic hemolytic anemia with splenomegaly, arthralgias, and abdominal pain.

Hemoglobin E disease: A mild form of hemolytic anemia observed in those native to Southeast Asia.

Hemoglobin SC disease: Present in persons who have inherited two abnormal forms of hemoglobin, S and C. Symptoms include hematuria and pain in bones, joints, abdomen, and chest.

Hemoglobin M disease: An abnormal hemoglobin associated with congenital cyanosis. The iron in the hemoglobin is present in the ferric (Fe^{+++}) state and is unable to combine with oxygen. This type of hemoglobin is called methemoglobin. There is no effective therapy; even so, the course of the disease is benign because of the presence of normal hemoglobin.

h., A₁c. ABBR: Hb A₁c. Hemoglobin A that contains a glucose group linked to the terminal amino acid of the beta chains of the molecule. In diabetes mellitus, when the blood glucose level is optimally and carefully regulated over a long period, five to six weeks, the Hb A₁c level is normal. If the blood glucose level has not been controlled (and has been abnormally elevated) in the preceding five to six weeks, the Hb A₁c blood level is increased. SYN: *glycosylated hemoglobin.*

h., fetal. Hemoglobin found in the erythrocytes of the fetus. It is capable of taking up and giving off oxygen at lower oxygen tensions than that in the erythrocytes of the adult. SYN: *hemoglobin F.*

h., glycosylated. Hemoglobin A₁c, q.v.

hemoglobinemia (hē″mō-glō-bĭn-ē′mē-ă) [Gr. *haima*, blood, + L. *globus*, globe, + Gr. *haima*, blood]. Presence of hemoglobin in the blood plasma.

hemoglobinocholia (hē″mō-glō″bĭn-ō-kō′lē-ă) [″ + ″ + Gr. *chole*, bile]. Hemoglobin in the bile.

hemoglobinolysis (hē″mō-glō-bĭn-ŏl′ĭ-sĭs) [″ + ″ + Gr. *lysis*, dissolution]. Dissolution of hemoglobin.

hemoglobinometer (hē″mō-glō-bĭn-ŏm′ē-ter) [″ + ″ + Gr. *metron*, measure]. Device for determining the amount of hemoglobin in the blood.

hemoglobinopathies (hē″mō-glō″bĭ-nŏp′ă-thēz). The group of diseases caused by or associated with the presence of one of several forms of abnormal hemoglobin in the blood. SEE: *hemoglobin.*

hemoglobinopepsia (hē″mō-glō″bĭn-ō-pěp′sē-ă) [″ + L. *globus*, globe, + Gr. *pepsis*, digestion]. Destruction of hemoglobin. SYN: *hemoglobinolysis.*

hemoglobinophilic (hē″mō-glō-bĭn-ō-fĭl′ĭk) [″ + ″ + Gr. *philein*, to love]. Pert. to organisms that grow better in presence of hemoglobin.

hemoglobinous (hē″mō-glō′bĭ-nŭs). Pert. to or containing hemoglobin.

hemoglobinuria (hē″mō-glō-bĭn-ū′rē-ă) [″ + L. *globus*, globe, + Gr. *ouron*, urine]. Presence of hemoglobin in the urine, but free from red blood cells. Occurs when hemoglobin from disintegrating red blood cells or from rapid hemolysis of red cells exceeds the ability of the blood proteins to combine with the hemoglobin.

ETIOL: Hemolytic anemia; scurvy; purpura; certain chemicals such as arsenic, phosphorus; typhus fever; or septicemia.

h., cold. Hemoglobinuria following local or general exposure to cold. SYN: *h., paroxysmal.*

h., epidemic. Hemoglobinuria of the newborn characterized by jaundice, cyanosis, and fatty degeneration of heart and liver. SYN: *Winckel's disease.*

h., intermittent. Paroxysmal nocturnal hemoglobinuria.

h., malarial. Blackwater fever.

h., march. Hemoglobinuria that occurs following strenuous exercise; e.g., running a marathon.

h., paroxysmal. Intermittent, recurring attacks of hemoglobinuria following exposure to cold (cold hemoglobinuria) or strenuous exercise (march hemoglobinuria). Results from increased fragility of red blood cells or presence of a thermolabile autohemolysin.

h., toxic. Hemoglobinuria resulting from toxic substances such as muscarine or snake venom; toxic products of infectious diseases such as yellow fever, typhoid fever, syphilis, and certain forms of hemolytic jaundice; organisms such as *Plasmodium malariae*, which destroy red blood cells; foreign protein in blood as may follow blood transfusion.

hemoglobinuric (hē″mō-glō″bĭ-nū′rĭk). Rel. to or marked by hemoglobinuria.

hemolith (hē′mō-lĭth) [″ + *lithos*, stone]. A calculus in the wall of a blood vessel.

hemolymph (hē′mō-lĭmf″) [″ + L. *lympha*, lymph]. Blood and lymph.

hemolymphangioma (hē″mō-lĭm-făn″jē-ō′mă). Hematolymphangioma, q.v.

hemolysate (hē-mŏl′ĭ-sāt). The product of hemolysis.

hemolysin (hē-mŏl′ĭ-sĭn) [″ + *lysis*, dissolution]. An agent or condition that disrupts red blood cells.

hemolysis (hē-mŏl′ĭ-sĭs) [″ + *lysis*, dissolution]. The destruction of red blood cells with the liberation of hemoglobin, which diffuses into the surrounding fluid. May occur as a result of the effects of bacterial toxins, snake venoms, immune bodies (hemolysins), and hypotonic saline solutions. Their stroma is ruptured or dissolved and the hemoglobin is liberated into the plasma. As a result, the blood, examined grossly, appears to be more transparent and to have a richer, red color; under the microscope, the dissolution of the red corpuscles can be observed.

When hemolysis occurs within the blood vessels, the body is unable to retain the hemoglobin, which is lost through the kidneys and imparts a red color to the urine. This condition is called hemoglobinuria, q.v.

Injection of a hypotonic saline solution or distilled water into the bloodstream induces hemolysis and may result in death. The red blood cells swell and become globular; their membranes rupture and hemoglobin is liberated. All solutions injected intravenously must be isotonic with the blood. Hemolysis may result from infection by certain disease organisms, e.g., certain streptococci, staphylocci and the tetanus bacillus. Hemolysis also occurs in smallpox and diphtheria and following severe burns. SEE: *fragility of blood.*

hemolytic (hē″mō-lĭt′ĭk). Pert. to the breaking down of red blood cells.

hemolytic anemia. Anemia resulting from hemolysis of red blood cells. Is either congenital (familial) or acquired from the effects of toxic agents.

hemolytic disease of the newborn. Disease of the newborn characterized by anemia, jaundice, enlargement of the liver and spleen, and generalized edema (hydrops fetalis).

ETIOL: Due to transplacental transmission of maternal antibody, usually evoked by maternal and fetal blood group incompatibility. Incompatibilities of the ABO system are common but are not severe. Rh compatibility can result in profound anemia in the fetus, causing death in utero.

Rh incompatibility develops when an Rh-negative woman carries an Rh-positive fetus. Fetal red blood cells cross the placenta and enter the maternal circulation, stimulating maternal antibody production against the Rh factor. These antibodies cross the placenta to the fetal circulation and destroy fetal red blood cells.

TREAT: In cases of Rh incompatibility, the condition can be controlled during pregnancy by following the anti-Rh titer of the mother's blood and the bilirubin level of the fetus by amniocentesis. These indices indicate whether the pregnancy should be allowed to go to full term and if intrauterine transfusion is indicated; or if labor should be induced earlier. Delivery should be as free of trauma as possible and the placenta is not manually removed. The infant with erythroblastosis should be immediately seen by a physician who is capable of and has the facilities and blood supplies available for exchange transfusion. The use of $Rh_o(D)$ immune globulin (trade name: RhoGAM) has been of great benefit in preventing sensitization of an Rh negative mother by an Rh positive fetus, thus preventing hemolytic disease of the newborn in that pregnancy. SYN: *erythroblastosis fetalis.* SEE: *Rh blood group.*

hemolytic jaundice. SEE: *jaundice, hemolytic.*

hemolytic uremic syndrome. An acute condition consisting of microangiopathic hemolytic anemia, thrombocytopenia, and acute nephropathy. The etiology is unknown. Children are most often affected. Onset may be with gastroenteritis and diarrhea or with an upper respiratory tract infection. Following, there is acute onset of purpura, irritability, lethargy, and oliguria. The acute phase continues with splenomegaly, mild jaundice, seizures in some patients, hepatomegaly, pulmonary edema, oliguria-anuria, cardiomegaly, and tachycardia.

Urine may be dark yellow or brownish-red. The acute phase may last from 1 to 2 weeks in mild cases and much longer in severe cases.

TREAT: The treatment is for renal failure and the anemia. Transfusions may be needed, but the circulatory system should not be overloaded; thus, hemoglobin should not be increased beyond 7 to 8 gm/dl.

PROG: The usual outcome is complete recovery, but about 10% develop end-stage renal disease.

hemolyze (hē'mō-līz). To produce hemolysis.

hemomediastinum (hē″mō-mē″dē-ă-stī′nŭm) [Gr. *haima*, blood, + L. *mediastinus*, in the middle]. Effusion of blood into mediastinal spaces. SYN: *hematomediastinum*.

hemometra (hē″mō-mē′tră) [″ + *metra*, uterus]. Retention of blood within the uterus. SYN: *hematometra*.

hemonephrosis (hē″mō-nĕ-frō′sĭs) [″ + *nephros*, kidney, + *osis*, condition]. Blood in the pelvis of the kidney. SYN: *hematonephrosis*.

hemopathic (hē″mō-păth′ĭk) [″ + *pathos*, disease, suffering]. Rel. or due to disease of the blood.

hemopathology (hē″mō-pă-thŏl′ō-jē) [″ + ″ + *logos*, word, reason]. The science of blood disorders.

hemopathy (hē-mŏp′ă-thē). A disease of the blood.

hemoperfusion. Perfusion of blood through substances, such as activated charcoal or ion-exchange resins, to remove toxic materials. The blood is then returned to the patient. This technique differs from hemodialysis, q.v., in that the blood is not separated from the chemicals or solutions by a semipermeable dialysis membrane. SEE: *hemodialysis*.

hemopericardium (hē″mō-pĕr″ĭ-kăr′dē-ŭm) [″ + *peri*, around, + *kardia*, heart]. Accumulation of blood in the pericardial sac.

hemoperitoneum (hē″mō-pĕr″ĭ-tō-nē′ŭm) [″ + *peritonaion*, peritoneum]. Effusion of blood into the peritoneal cavity.

hemopexin (hē″mō-pĕks′ĭn) [″ + *pexis*, fixation]. A glycoprotein of the B-globulin class that binds hemin but not hemoglobin.

hemophage (hē′mō-fāj) [″ + *phagein*, to eat]. A cell destroying red blood cells by phagocytosis.

hemophagocyte (hē″mō-făg′ō-sīt) [″ + ″ + *kytos*, cell]. A phagocyte that ingests red blood cells.

hemophagocytosis (hē″mō-făg″ō-sī-tō′sĭs) [″ + ″ + ″ + *osis*, condition]. Ingestion of red blood cells by phagocytes.

hemophil (hē′mō-fĭl) [″ + *philein*, to love].

Bacteria that grow very well on agar that contains blood.

hemophilia (hē″mō-, hĕm″ō-fĭl′ē-ă) [″ + *philein*, to love]. A hereditary blood disease characterized by greatly prolonged coagulation time. The blood fails to clot and abnormal bleeding occurs. It is a sex-linked hereditary trait transmitted by normal heterozygous females who carry the recessive gene. It occurs almost exclusively in males. There are two types: hemophilia A and B. SEE: *blood*.

The term *hemophilia* has been used to designate a variety of coagulation disorders of blood. This has led to confusion that can be prevented by using the word to mean what it originally meant and to designate conditions resembling it by the name of the specific coagulation factor which is lacking.

SYM: Abnormal tendency to bleed. May cause swelling of the joints.

ETIOL: The cause of hemophilia A and B is deficiency of a factor in plasma, factor VIII in hemophilia A and factor IX in hemophilia B, necessary for coagulation of blood.

TREAT: There is no cure for hemophilia. When hemorrhage occurs in patients with hemophilia A, coagulation factor IX is given; factor VIII is given when hemorrhage occurs in patients with hemophilia B. These factors are available from various sources and special care has been taken to be as sure as possible that they are free of the AIDS virus (HIV) and hepatitis viruses. Many hemophiliacs learn to self-administer these factors to control bleeding episodes. Desmopressin (DDVAP) may be used to treat mild cases of hemophilia A. Hemophiliac patients should avoid trauma. They should wear a bracelet indicating that they are hemophiliac. Information concerning hemophilia is available to the lay and medical public from the National Hemophilia Foundation, 110 Greene St., Suite 303, New York, NY 10012; (212) 219-8180.

Caution: It is important that hemophiliac patients not be given aspirin; its use can further complicate the bleeding tendency.

PROG: The development of concentrated clotting factors VIII and IX has improved the prognosis.

NURSING IMPLICATIONS: Provide emergency care to clean the wound and stop bleeding through application of pressure. Safety is a major concern for the patient with hemophilia, and nursing care should be done gently and carefully. Because hemarthrosis is a common complication, assess the patient for development of this condition and provide care as needed. This will include elevating the affected part, applying ice, and immobilizing the joint in a slightly flexed position. Exercise is generally not begun until at least 48 hours after a bleeding episode has subsided.

The patient and family will be anxious. In order to allay this fear, help them identify activities in which the patient may safely participate. They should also be taught ways to manage attacks of bleeding at home. It is possible for the family to administer cryoprecipitate at home to treat a bleeding episode.

Assess the patient's and family's knowledge of the disease and its treatment, and the impact of the illness on the patient, siblings, and parents' marital relationship. Teach the parents about the seriousness of head injuries and the need for immediate observation and treatment. Explain the use of transfusion therapy, and offer all available methods of obtaining such therapy. Encourage regular dental examinations and gentle, careful oral care. SEE: *Nursing Diagnoses* in *Appendix.*

h., vascular. SEE: *von Willebrand's disease.*

hemophilia A. Hemophilia due to a deficiency of blood coagulation factor VIII. SEE: *hemophilia.*

hemophilia B. This term refers to Christmas disease, a hemophilia-like disease caused by a lack of factor IX, plasma thromboplastin component. This condition can be treated with a lyophilized product that contains concentrated factor IX. SEE: *hemophilia.*

hemophiliac (hē″mō-fĭl′ē-ăk). One afflicted with hemophilia.

hemophilic (hē″mō-fĭl′ĭk). 1. Fond of blood, said of bacteria that grow well in culture media containing hemoglobin. 2. Pert. to hemophilia or hemophiliacs.

Hemophilus SEE: *Haemophilus.*

hemophobia (hē″mō-fō′bē-ă) [Gr. *haima,* blood, + *phobos,* fear]. Aversion to seeing blood or to bleeding.

hemophoric (hē″mō-for′ĭk) [″ + *phoros,* bearing]. Conveying blood.

hemophthalmia, hemophthalmus (hē″mŏf-thăl′mē-ă, hē″mŏf-thăl′mŭs) [″ + *ophthalmos,* eye]. Effusion of blood into the eye.

hemopleura (hē″mō-ploo′ră). Blood in the pleural space. SEE: *hemothorax.*

hemopneumopericardium (hē″mō-nū″mō-pĕr″ĭ-kăr′dē-ŭm) [″ + *pneuma,* air, + *peri,* around, + *kardia,* heart]. Blood and air in the pericardial cavity.

hemopneumothorax (hē″mō-nū-mō-thō′răks) [″ + ″ + *thorax,* chest]. Blood and air in the pleural cavity.

hemopoiesis (hē″mō-poy-ē′sĭs) [″ + *poie-*

sis, formation]. Production or formation of blood cells. SYN: *hematopoiesis.*

hemoprecipitin (hē″mō-prē-sĭp′ĭ-tĭn). A precipitin in blood.

hemoprotein (hē″mō-prō′tē-ĭn). Any protein combined with the heme, blood pigment.

hemopsonin (hē″mŏp-sō′nĭn) [″ + *opsonein,* to buy food]. An antibody that makes red blood cells more susceptible to phagocytosis.

hemoptysis (hē-mŏp′tĭ-sĭs) [″ + *ptyein,* to spit]. Expectoration of blood arising from the oral cavity, larynx, trachea, bronchi, or lungs. SEE: table; *bleeding; hematemesis; hemorrhage.*

SYM: Sudden attack of coughing with production of sputum containing frothy bright red blood and having a salty taste.

TREAT: Cold applications over the chest.

NURSING IMPLICATIONS: Keep the patient quiet and in a calm, reassuring environment. Take vital signs every 4 hours. Frequency of obtaining vital signs depends on their stability; every 4 hours if stable, every ½ to 1 hour as necessary if unstable. Provide tepid fluids. Patient should be kept warm, but not hot. If it is known from which side the patient is bleeding, lean patient toward that side. Place patient at bedrest with head slightly elevated, discourage coughing; but if patient must cough, teach him or her to do so with open glottis and without straining. Apply ice packs and administer sedatives as prescribed. Note the amount, consistency, and color of blood to assist in determining the site of the bleeding. (Blood from lungs is red and frothy; blood from GI tract is dark red to black in color.) Save blood for inspection by physician. SEE: *Nursing Diagnoses* in *Appendix.*

h., parasitic. Spitting of blood resulting from infection of the lungs by *Paragonimus westermani,* q.v., a parasitic fluke.

hemorrhage (hĕm′ĕ-rĭj) [″ + *rhegnynai,* to burst forth]. Abnormal, severe internal or external discharge of blood. May be venous, arterial, or capillary from blood vessels into tissues, into or from the body. Venous blood is dark red; flow is continuous. Arterial blood is bright red; flows in spurts. Capillary blood is of a reddish color; exudes from tissue.

SYM: Diagnosis is obvious when hemorrhage is visible. When internal, diagnosis may be made from the general condition. Patient is in shock; pulse weak, rapid, and irregular; face pale; skin cold and moist.

NURSING IMPLICATIONS: Elevate the bleeding part as far above the head as practical, then apply pressure or a pressure dressing directly to the wound. If this is not

Comparison of Hemoptysis and Hematemesis

Hemoptysis	Hematemesis
Probable previous history of tuberculosis.	Probable previous history of gastric or duodenal trouble.
Blood is coughed up.	Blood is vomited.
Blood is frothy, bright red, and alkaline in reaction.	Blood is usually (not always) dark, usually not frothy, and acid in reaction. Often clotted.
Blood may be mixed with sputum.	Blood may be mixed with food.
There is some dyspnea, pain, and a tickling sensation in the chest.	There is often nausea and pain referred to stomach.

effective, apply strong finger pressure to the pressure point, q.v., of the main artery supplying the wound. The use of a tourniquet should be avoided because of concern for producing increased blood loss and an ischemic limb.

Pneumatic splints may be used to delay effects of internal hemorrhage during transportation. Such devices should not be removed until fluid replacement is initiated. Take appropriate measures to prevent or control shock.

Caution: Universal precautions should be used. SEE: *Universal Precautions* in *Appendix.*

h., accidental. In obstetrics and gynecology, a hemorrhage caused by premature rupture of the placenta. SEE: *ablatio placentae.*

h., antepartum. Hemorrhage appearing before the onset of labor.

h., arterial. In arterial bleeding, which is bright red, the blood ordinarily comes through in waves or spurts. However, the flow may be steady if the torn artery is deep or buried.

F.A.: Almost all arterial bleeding can be controlled with direct pressure to the wound with gauze pads and elevation. Pressure should be applied for twenty minutes. If the blood soaks through, add more gauze to the wad, but do not remove the pads and replace with new ones because this will dislodge clots. A tourniquet is almost never needed and should be reserved for the rare conditions when the above measures fail to stop the bleeding and the patient's life is in jeopardy. A tourniquet should be used only when the limb is considered sacrificable in order to save the patient's life. SEE: *bleeding* for table; *pressure points; tourniquet.*

h., capillary. Bleeding from minute

blood vessels, present in all bleeding. When large vessels are not injured, capillary bleeding may be controlled by simple elevation and pressure with a sterile dry compress.

h., carotid artery. Usually accompanied by bleeding from the jugular veins. May be fatal in a short time.

F.A.: Compression with the thumbs transversely across the neck, both above and below the wound, the fingers directed around the back of the neck to aid in compression. It may be more desirable to pack the wound with sterile gauze and compress it with the closed fist. Wounds of the jugular vein are sometimes the cause of air embolism.

h., cerebral. Escape of blood into tissues of the brain. SEE: *stroke.*

SYM: Unconsciousness, slow pulse, stertorous breathing, hemiplegia, death. May be speech disturbance, incontinence of bladder and rectum, or constipation according to area of brain damage.

ETIOL: Hypertension; arteriosclerosis or atherosclerosis; rupture of aneurysm; trauma.

TREAT: Supportive therapy to maintain airway and oxygenation. Be certain patient is positioned properly to prevent nerve compression of arms. Maintain hydration and fluid and electrolyte balance. Long-range therapy includes physical therapy, speech therapy, and counseling.

h., concealed. Hemorrhage into an area where it is not visible. SYN: *h., internal.*

h., fibrinolytic. Hemorrhage due to a defect in the fibrin component in blood coagulation.

h., gastrointestinal. Bleeding into the stomach (gastric) or duodenum.

h., internal. H., concealed, q.v.

h., intracranial. Bleeding into the cranium.

h., lung. Blood bright red and frothy, frequently coughed up.

h. of knee. TREAT: At the knee or below, apply pad with pressure. If behind knee, apply pad at site and bandage leg firmly. Follow same precautions as with tourniquet with respect to loosening at 12- to 15-minute intervals.

h., petechial. Hemorrhage in form of small rounded spots or petechiae occurring in the skin or mucous membranes.

h., postmenopausal. Bleeding from the uterus after menopause has been established. It may be a sign of malignancy of the reproductive tract and should be carefully and thoroughly investigated.

h., postpartum. Abnormal bleeding from the uterus following childbirth.

h., primary. Hemorrhage immediately following any trauma.

h., retroperitoneal. Bleeding into the retroperitoneal space.

h., secondary. Hemorrhage occurring some time after primary hemorrhage. It may occur after 24 hours or at time of separation of ligature, usually between 7th and 10th day. Usually due to sepsis.

h., stomach. Blood dark, perhaps clotted or mixed with stomach contents, usually vomited. May be from rupture of esophageal varices.

TREAT: Histamine-receptor type two blockers (H₂), carafate. Surgery may be required if bleeding continues. If hemorrhage is from esophagus, compression of bleeding site with a special intraesophageal tube balloon may be helpful.

h., thigh. Upper part near groin.

TREAT: Insert pad or gauze into wound and apply pressure or press thumb in center of fold of groin against bone until bleeding stops below groin. Pad or tourniquet with pad under.

h., typhoid. Gross hemorrhage occurs in approx. 10% of cases of typhoid that progress to the stage of ulceration of gastrointestinal tract. Loss may be 1000 ml. It may occur singly or in succession, the latter being more serious than large hemorrhages. Hemorrhages take place at the end of the second week and during the third week of the disease.

h., unavoidable. Ceaseless, painless bleeding from placenta previa, q.v.

h., uterine. Hemorrhage into the cavity of the uterus. There are three types of pathological uterine hemorrhage: essential uterine hemorrhage (metropathia haemorrhagica) occurs in connection with pelvic, uterine, or cervical diseases; intrapartum hemorrhage occurs during labor; and postpartum hemorrhage occurs after third stage of labor. The latter may be caused by rupture, lacerations, relaxation of the uterus, hematoma, or retained products of conception including the placenta or membrane fragments.

ETIOL: Common causes are trauma; congenital abnormalities; pathological processes such as tumors; infections, esp. of alimentary, respiratory, and genitourinary tracts; generalized vascular disorders such as various purpuras; coagulation defects; retained products of conception following criminal or therapeutic abortion.

TREAT: Application of an umbrella pack will apply pressure to uterine arterial supply. A retained placenta, when present and causing hemorrhage, should be removed with uterine forceps. If the uterus is flaccid, it can usually be stimulated to contract by administering oxytocin I.V. The patient may need transfusion and, in some cases, surgery will be required to prevent fatal hemorrhage. SEE: *pack, umbrella.*

h., venous. Characterized by steady, profuse bleeding of rather dark blood.

F.A.: Keep patient quiet and try to relieve anxiety; elevate the bleeding part if possible. Apply a sterile pressure dressing directly over the wound. Elevation and pressure will control most venous bleeding. Observe closely for signs of shock. SEE: *tourniquet.*

h., vicarious. Hemorrhage from a part due to suppression in another part. SEE: *vicarious menstruation.*

hemorrhage, words pert. to: anthemorrhagic; autotransfusion; bleeding; clotting; coagulation, blood; hematorrhea; hemophilia; rhinorrhagia; Werlhof's disease; wound.

hemorrhagenic (hĕm″ō-ră-jĕn′ĭk) [″ + *rhegnynai,* to burst forth, + *gennan,* to form]. Producing hemorrhage.

hemorrhagic (hĕm-ō-răj′ĭk). Pert. to or marked by hemorrhage.

hemorrhagic disease of the newborn. Hemorrhaging due to inadequate supply of prothrombin received from mother or delay in establishment of bacterial flora of intestine that produces vitamin K. Administration of vitamin K corrects the condition.

hemorrhagic fevers. A group of diseases due to arthropod-borne viruses. This includes yellow fever, Omsk hemorrhagic fever, Crimean hemorrhagic fever, Korean hemorrhagic fever, North and South Vietnam hemorrhagic fever, Argentinian hemorrhagic fever, Bolivian hemorrhagic fever, and Kyasanur Forest disease (India).

hemorrhagic nephrosonephritis. An acute infectious disease with abrupt onset of fever that lasts three to eight days, conjunctival injection, prostration, anorexia, and vomiting. Renal involvement may be mild or progress to acute renal failure, and this may last several weeks. The mode of transmission is unknown; the incubation period varies from 9 to 35 days; and it is apparently not transmitted from person to person. SYN: *epidemic hemorrhagic fever; Korean hemorrhagic fever.*

ETIOL: Hantan virus.

TREAT: Treat shock and renal failure. There is no specific therapy.

hemorrhagiparous (hĕm″ō-răj-ĭp′ă-rŭs) [″ + *rhegnynai*, to burst forth, + L. *parere*, to bring forth, to bear]. Producing hemorrhage. SYN: *hemorrhagenic.*

hemorrhoid (hĕm′ō-royd) [Gr. *haimorrhois*]. A mass of dilated, tortuous veins in the anorectum involving the venous plexuses of that area. There are two kinds: external, those involving veins distal to the anorectal line; internal, those involving veins proximal to the anorectal line. SEE: *Nursing Diagnoses* in *Appendix.*

TREAT: Depends upon the severity of the symptoms, not the extent of the hemorrhoids. In many instances, the only therapy required is improvement in anal hygiene and administration of stool softeners to prevent straining to have a bowel movement. The decision concerning the necessity of surgery or ligature with rubber bands should not be made until acute symptoms and inflammation have subsided. This allows tissues to regain their usual shape. SEE: *hemorrhoidectomy; piles.*

h., external. Dilated vein or veins at the junction of anal mucosa with the anal skin. SEE: illus.

h., internal. Dilated veins of the lower rectum at the anorectal junction. SEE: illus.

h., prolapsed. Protrusion of an internal hemorrhoid through the anus.

h., strangulated. Prolapsed hemorrhoid that is trapped by the anal sphincter, thus cutting off blood flow to the vein in the hemorrhoid.

hemorrhoidal (hĕm-ō-roy′dăl). 1. Rel. to hemorrhoids. 2. Pert. to certain anal arteries; arteria hemorrhoidalis.

hemorrhoidectomy (hĕm″ō-royd-ĕk′tō-mē) [Gr. *haimorrhois*, vein liable to bleed, + *ektome*, excision]. Removal of hemorrhoids by one of several techniques including surgery, cryotherapy, infrared photocoagulation, or ligation by use of rubber bands, called surgical banding, applied to the base of the hemorrhoid. The latter method is used mostly for external hemorrhoids.

NURSING IMPLICATIONS: *Preop:* Follow physician's orders for type of bowel preparation (enemas and stool softeners may be ordered, as well as a low-residue diet). Assess hemorrhoids for size, bleeding, or presence of drainage. Sitz baths should be done as ordered.

Postop: Take vital signs each hour and check rectal area for bleeding every hour in the immediate post-op period. Keep the patient comfortable by gentle cleansing of the rectal area as often as needed; sitz baths; apply ointment as ordered. Keep the rectal area clean and dry, and teach the patient proper perineal hygiene. Avoid use of rubber rings for sitting, as they can contribute to local venous stasis and edema formation. Administer ordered analgesics regularly during the first 24 to 48 hours after surgery to control pain; encourage use of sitz baths to relieve discomfort and promote healing. Administer stool softeners and encourage oral fluid intake to facilitate initial defecation. Teach patient that dietary intake should include 2 liters of fluid, fruit, vegetable, and cereal fiber daily and to avoid straining at stool. SEE: *Nursing Diagnoses* in *Appendix.*

hemosalpinx (hē″mō-săl′pĭnks) [Gr. *haima*, blood, + *salpinx*, tube]. Blood accumulated in an oviduct. SYN: *hematosalpinx.*

hemosiderin (hē″mō-sĭd′ĕr-ĭn) [″ + *sideros*, iron]. An iron-containing pigment derived from hemoglobin from disintegration of red blood cells. It is one method whereby iron is stored until it is needed for making hemoglobin.

hemosiderosis (hē″mō-sĭd-ĕr-ō′sĭs) [″ + ″ + *osis*, condition]. Condition characterized by the deposition, esp. in liver and spleen, of hemosiderin. Occurs in diseases in which there is marked red cell destruction such as hemolytic anemias, pernicious anemia, and chronic infection. SEE: *hemochromatosis.*

hemospasia (hē″mō-spā′zē-ă) [″ + *spaein*, to draw]. Withdrawal of blood by cupping or leeching.

hemospermia (hē″mō-spĕr′mē-ă) [″ + *sperma*, seed]. Bloody semen. SYN: *hematospermia.*

Hemosporida (hē″mō-spor-ĭ′dē-ă) [″ + *sporos*, seed]. An order of parasites found in the blood of various animals, including man.

hemostasis, hemostasia (hē-mŏs′tă-sĭs, hē″mō-stā′zē-ă) [″ + *stasis*, standing still]. 1. Arrest of bleeding or of circulation. 2. Stagnation of blood.

hemostat (hē′mō-stăt) [″ + *statikos*, standing]. 1. Device or medicine that arrests the flow of blood. 2. Compressor for controlling hemorrhage of the tonsils.

hemostatic (hē″mō-stăt′ĭk). 1. Checking hemorrhage. 2. Any drug, medicine, or blood component that serves to stop bleeding, such as vasopressin, gamma-aminobutyric acid, vitamin K, whole blood, or epinephrine

HEMORRHOIDS

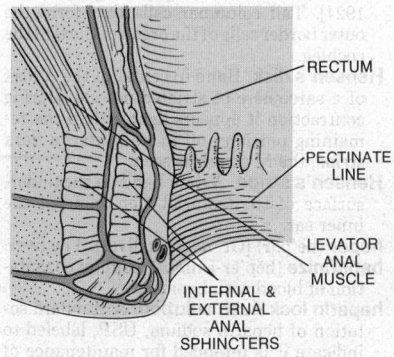

ANATOMY OF RECTUM

ORIGIN OF HEMORRHOIDS ARE
ABOVE PECTINATE LINE
(INTERNAL PLEXUS)

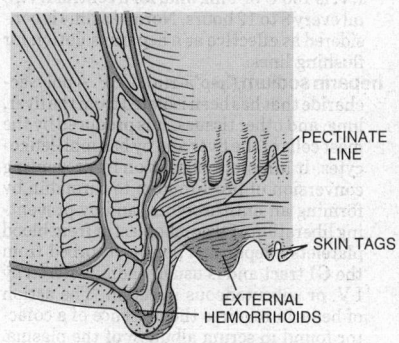

ORIGIN OF HEMORRHOIDS ARE
BELOW PECTINATE LINE
(EXTERNAL PLEXUS)

ORIGIN OF HEMORRHOID IS
ABOVE AND BELOW PECTINATE LINE
(INTERNAL AND EXTERNAL PLEXUS)

applied locally.

hemostyptic (hē-mō-stĭp′tĭk) [″ + *stypti-kos*, astringent]. An astringent that stops bleeding; chemically hemostatic.

hemotherapeutics (hē″mō-thĕr″ă-pū′tĭks) [″ + *therapeutike*, medical practice]. The use of blood, by transfusion, in treatment of disease.

hemotherapy (hē″mō-thĕr′ă-pē) [″ + *therapeia*, treatment]. Blood transfusion as a therapeutic measure.

hemothorax (hē″mō-thō′răks) [″ + *thorax*, chest]. Blood or bloody fluid in the pleural cavity caused by rupture of blood vessels, due to inflammation of the lungs in pneumonia or pulmonary tuberculosis, or

malignant growth or trauma.

hemotoxin (hē″mō-tŏks′ĭn) [″ + *toxikon*, poison]. A toxin destructive of red blood cells. SYN: *hemolysin*.

hemotrophe (hē′mō-trŏf) [″ + *trophe*, nourishment]. Nutrients supplied to the developing embryo by the mother.

hemotrophic (hē-mō-trŏf′ĭk) [″ + *trophe*, nourishment]. Pert. to nutrient substances carried in the blood.

hemotrophic nutrition. Nutrition of the fetus by substances in the maternal blood that pass to the blood of the fetus through vessels within the villi of the placenta. SEE: *histotrophic nutrition*.

hemotropic (hē-mō-trŏp′ĭk) [″ + *tropos*,

turning]. Attracted to or having an affinity for blood or blood cells.

hemotympanum (hē″mō-tĭm′pă-nŭm) [″ + *tympanon*, drum]. Blood in the middle ear.

hemozoin (hē″mō-zō′ĭn). A dark pigment found within malarial organisms *(plasmodia),* derived from the disintegration of hemoglobin.

hemozoon (hē″mō-zō′ŏn). A hematozoon.

Henderson-Hasselbalch equation [Lawrence Joseph Henderson, U.S. biochemist, 1878–1942; K. A. Hasselbalch, Danish physician, 1874–1962]. An equation for stating the expression for the dissociation constant of an acid. In fluid and electrolyte balance, this important equation may be expressed in terms of the bicarbonate (HCO_3^-) system as: pH equals 6.1 + log $HCO_3^-/\alpha(PaCO_2)$ where α equals 0.03 mM/L/mm Hg at 38°C. At the normal pH of the blood, 7.4, the ratio of HCO_3^- to $\alpha(PaCO_2)$ is 20 to 1.

Henle, Friedrich G. J. (hĕn′lē). German anatomist, 1809–1885.

H.'s ampulla. Ductus deferens dilatation just above the ejaculatory duct.

H.'s fissure. Fibrous tissue between the cardiac muscle fibers.

H.'s layer. Outer layer of cells of inner root sheath of hair follicle.

H.'s ligament. Conjoint tendon of the transversus abdominis muscle.

H.'s loop. U-shaped portion of a renal tubule lying between the proximal and distal convoluted portions. Consists of a thin descending limb and a thicker ascending limb.

H.'s membrane. Bruch's layer forming inner boundary of the choroid of the eye.

H.'s sheath. Connective tissue support of individual nerve fibers in a funiculus. SYN: *endoneurium.*

H.'s tubules. Portion of the nephron following the proximal tubule. SEE: *nephron.*

Henoch-Schönlein purpura (hĕn′ŏk-shān′lĭn) [Eduard H. Henoch, Ger. pediatrician, 1820–1910; Johann Lukas Schönlein, Ger. physician, 1793–1864]. A form of allergic purpura with erythema, urticaria, effusions of serum into subcutaneous or submucous tissue or viscera, accompanied by gastrointestinal and joint symptoms. Occurs mostly in children.

henry (hĕn′rē) [Joseph Henry, U.S. physicist, 1797–1878]. Unit designating electrical inductance.

Henry's law (hĕn′rēz) [William Henry, Brit. chemist, 1774–1836]. The weight of a gas dissolved by a given volume of liquid at a constant temperature is directly proportional to the pressure.

Hensen's cells (hĕn′sĕns) [Victor Hensen, Ger. anatomist and physiologist, 1835–1924]. Tall columnar cells that form the outer border cells of the organ of Corti of the cochlea.

Hensen's disk. Band in center of the A disk of a sarcomere of striated muscle. During contraction it appears lighter than the remaining portion and in its center, a dark stripe, the M stripe, is seen.

Hensen's stripe. A dark band on the undersurface of the tectorial membrane of the inner ear.

hepar (hē′păr) [Gr. *hepatos,* liver]. The liver.

heparinize (hĕp′ĕr-ĭ-nīz). To inhibit coagulation of blood with heparin.

heparin lock flush solution. A standard solution of heparin sodium, USP, labeled to indicate it is intended for maintenance of patency of intravenous injection devices only, and is not to be used for anticoagulant therapy. Standard concentration is 100 units/ml. Standard dose for a peripheral I.V. is 100 U or 1 ml; and, for a central I.V., 3 ml every 8 to 12 hours. Normal saline is considered as effective as a heparin solution for flushing lines.

heparin sodium (hĕp′ă-rĭn). USP. A polysaccharide that has been isolated from the liver, lung, and other tissues. It is produced by the mast cells of the liver and by basophil leukocytes. It inhibits coagulation by preventing conversion of prothrombin to thrombin by forming an antithrombin, and by preventing liberation of thromboplastin from blood platelets. Heparin is poorly absorbed from the GI tract and is usually administered by I.V. or subcutaneous injection. The action of heparin requires the presence of a cofactor found in serum albumin of the plasma. Trade names are Hep-Lock, Lipo-Hepin, and Liquaemin Sodium.

USES: An anticoagulant in prevention and treatment of thrombosis and embolism and in treatment of frostbite. Sometimes employed concurrently with dicumarol, q.v. The antagonist for an overdose is protamine sulfate.

heparin sulfate. A chemical, the degradation of which is essential to mucopolysaccharide metabolism. When it is not degraded, it accumulates in connective tissue and causes the clinical manifestation of some of the mucopolysaccharidoses. SEE: *mucopolysaccharidosis.*

hepatalgia (hĕp″ă-tăl′jē-ă) [Gr. *hepatos,* liver, + *algos,* pain]. Pain in the liver. SYN: *hepatodynia.*

hepatalgic (hĕp″ă-tăl′jĭk). Pert. to hepatalgia.

hepatatrophia (hĕp″ăt-ă-trō′fē-ă) [″ + *atrophia,* atrophy]. Atrophied condition of the liver.

hepatauxe (hĕp″ăt-awk′sē) [″ + *auxe*, increase]. Enlargement or hypertrophy of the liver.

hepatectomize (hĕp″ă-tĕk′tō-mīz) [″ + *ektome*, excision]. Surgical removal of the liver.

hepatectomy (hĕp″ă-tĕk′tō-mē) [″ + *ektome*, excision]. Excision of part or all of the liver.

hepatic (hĕ-păt′ĭk) [Gr. *hepatikos*]. Pert. to the liver.

hepatic amebiasis. Infection of the liver by *Entamoeba histolytica* resulting in hepatitis and abscess formation. Usually a sequel to amebic dysentery. SEE: *amebiasis*.

hepatic coma. Impaired central nervous system function due to liver disease. The disease permits venous blood to bypass portal circulation, thus allowing an accumulation of products in the blood that are usually metabolized by the liver (e.g., ammonia). Any condition that is associated with increased ammonia production promotes hepatic coma in patients with severely impaired liver function. Causes include high-protein diet, gastrointestinal bleeding, fluid and electrolyte imbalance, infections, and drugs such as sedatives, tranquilizers, anesthetics, analgesics, diuretics, and alcohol.

SYM: Impaired consciousness, sluggish or impaired speech, drowsiness, confusion, stupor, and coma. The patient will be unable to explain the meaning of simple sayings and may have difficulty in telling the day of the week or month. Attempts to draw simple figures will be unsuccessful. A "mousy" odor of the breath (fetor hepaticus) is usually present. A distinctive type of flapping tremor of the hand called *asterixis*, q.v., will be present in severe cases. Ataxia may be present along with altered deep tendon reflexes. An electroencephalogram will be abnormal, and the blood ammonia level will be elevated.

TREAT: Administer protein-restricted, high-carbohydrate diet. Free the intestinal tract of blood, if present, by enemas or mild cathartics. Oral neomycin will control bacteria that favor ammonia production, and oral lactulose helps to decrease ammonia production in the intestinal tract. Exchange transfusions to remove ammonia from the blood have been used, but they have not been effective.

hepatic duct. Canal that receives bile from the liver. It unites with the cystic duct to form the common bile duct.

hepatic encephalopathy. SEE: *hepatic coma*.

hepatic flexure. The bend of the colon under the liver. The junction of the ascending and transverse colon.

hepatic lobes. Divisions of the liver.

hepaticoduodenostomy (hĕ-păt″ĭ-kō-dū″ō-dĕ-nŏs′tō-mē) [″ + L. *duodeni*, duodenum, + Gr. *stoma*, mouth]. Making an artificial opening between the hepatic duct and duodenum.

hepaticoenterostomy (hĕ-păt″ĭ-kō-ĕn-tĕr-ŏs′tō-mē) [″ + *enteron*, intestine, + *stoma*, mouth]. Operation for artificial opening between the hepatic duct and intestine.

hepaticogastrostomy (hĕ-păt″ĭ-kō-găs-trŏs′tō-mē) [″ + *gaster*, stomach, + *stoma*, mouth]. Operation for a passage between the hepatic duct and the stomach.

hepaticojejunostomy (hĕ-păt′ĭ-kō-jē″jū-nŏs′tō-mē) [″ + L. *jejunum*, empty, + Gr. *stoma*, mouth]. Surgically joining the hepatic duct and the jejunum.

hepaticolithotomy (hĕ-păt″ĭ-kō-lĭ-thŏt′ō-mē). Surgical removal of gallstones from the hepatic duct.

hepaticolithotripsy (hĕ-păt″ĭ-kō-lĭth′ō-trĭp-sē) [″ + *lithos*, stone, + *tripsis*, a crushing]. Crushing of a biliary calculus in the hepatic duct.

hepaticostomy (hĕ-păt″ĭ-kŏs′tō-mē) [″ + *stoma*, mouth]. Establishment of a permanent fistula into the hepatic duct.

hepaticotomy (hĕ-păt″ĭ-kŏt′ō-mē) [″ + *tome*, incision]. Incision into the hepatic duct.

hepatic veins. The three vessels returning blood from the liver and discharging into the inferior vena cava.

hepatic zones. Venous, arterial, and portal regions.

hepatitis (hĕp″ă-tī′tĭs) [″ + *itis*, inflammation]. Inflammation of the liver. It may be caused by a variety of agents, including viral infections, bacterial invasion, and physical or chemical agents. Clinically it is usually accompanied by systemic signs including fever, jaundice, and an enlarged liver.

COMPARISON OF THE TYPES OF HEPATITIS: *Incubation Period:* For hepatitis A, q.v., it is 15 to 50 days with an average of 28 to 30 days. For hepatitis B, q.v., it is 2 weeks to 6 months with an average of 60 to 90 days. For hepatitis C, q.v., it is usually 6 to 8 weeks, but may be as short as 10 days and as long as 11 weeks. The incubation period for delta agent hepatitis (hepatitis D), q.v., is 14 to 70 days, but may be much longer.

Onset: Usually acute for hepatitis A and may be acute for delta agent hepatitis. The onset is usually slow for hepatitis B and C.

Age of Patients: Hepatitis A usually occurs in children or young adults. The other types may occur at any age, but delta agent hepatitis may occur as an epidemic in infants.

Transmission: Hepatitis A and delta agent hepatitis are spread mostly by person to person via the fecal-oral route but may occur by water or food contaminated by the virus. Hepatitis B and hepatitis C are spread by blood and serum-derived fluids; and by direct contact with body fluids.

Severity: Hepatitis A and hepatitis C are usually mild, but the latter may be particularly severe when it occurs in the third trimester of pregnancy. In those cases, the fatality rate may be 10%. Hepatitis B may be quite mild, but some cases progress rapidly to death due to acute necrosis of the liver. All forms of hepatitis except hepatitis A may progress to chronic hepatitis, q.v.

Preventive Measures: For hepatitis A, educate the public about good sanitation and personal hygiene, with emphasis on hygienic disposal of feces. This is particularly important in managing day-care centers. Hands should be washed thoroughly after every diaper change. Travelers to highly endemic areas may be given immunoglobulin (Ig) prior to arrival. For travel in the area for two months or less, the dose for adults is 0.02 to 0.04 ml/kg. If the stay is for longer periods, give adults 0.06 ml/kg. This dose should be repeated every four to six months if the individual remains in the area. If hepatitis A develops in a day-care center, the staff should receive immune serum globulin. For hepatitis B, a vaccine is available. The vaccine is given I.M. in three separate doses. All donated blood should be tested for presence of hepatitis B antigen. Persons who have a history of AIDS exposure or viral hepatitis, q.v., or who have received a blood transfusion or tattoo in the preceding six months or have a history of drug addiction should not be accepted as blood donors. For delta agent hepatitis, the preventive measures are the same as for hepatitis B. For prevention of hepatitis C, the instructions are the same as for hepatitis A. The value of immune serum globulin is not known in this form of hepatitis. Hepatitis E, q.v., is not transmitted by the water route when drinking water is boiled. SEE: *cirrhosis; hepatitis, acute viral; Universal Precautions* in *Appendix.*

h. A. Hepatitis due to hepatitis A virus (HAV). SEE: *hepatitis, acute viral.*

h., acute anicteric. Hepatitis marked by slight fever, gastrointestinal upset, and anorexia, but no jaundice.

h., acute viral. A systemic infection that involves the liver. Four categories of viral agents are known to cause this illness: hepatitis A virus; hepatitis B virus; hepatitis C

virus; and delta agents. Each of these four produces a clinically similar disease. The illness may be so mild as to be inapparent or so severe that the patient may die.

The initial signs and symptoms may include: low-grade fever, anorexia, nausea, vomiting, fatigue, malaise, muscle and joint pain, headache, photophobia, pharyngitis, cough, and coryza. During that phase, which lasts from 2 to 14 days, it is not uncommon to think that the illness is due to influenza. Dark urine and clay-colored stools are present several days prior to appearance of jaundice. After the onset of jaundice, the liver enlarges and becomes tender. Splenomegaly and cervical adenopathy may also be present. Certain liver function tests, including the serum aminotransferases, are abnormal.

The clinical course of acute viral hepatitis is quite variable; after the jaundice (which may last for two weeks) has gone away, the patient begins to feel better. The convalescence period, during which there is some malaise and susceptibility to fatigue, may last from several weeks to months. For comparison of the different aspects of infections with three of these four categories of viral agents, SEE: table at *incubation.*

TREAT: Because there is no specific treatment for acute viral hepatitis, each case is treated symptomatically. Heroic measures, such as massive doses of corticosteroids, exchange transfusion, plasmapheresis, and hemoperfusion, have not been shown to be effective. SEE: *cirrhosis; hepatitis B vaccine; hepatitis, chronic; Universal Precautions* in *Appendix.*

NURSING IMPLICATIONS: Depending on the severity of this phase of the disease, the patient may or may not be hospitalized. For patients at home, instruct about the nature and course of the illness, care and treatment, and signs and symptoms of complications. Encourage the patient to restrict activity and rest, eat a well-balanced diet, drink adequate fluids, and observe character of urine and feces. Emphasize the need for scrupulous attention to linens, dishes, handling of food, etc., to prevent spread to other household members. Instruct to avoid use of alcohol as directed by physician. Urge avoidance of close physical contact with others until tests of enzyme levels are shown to be within normal ranges. Encourage continuing medical follow-up because recovery may require a considerable length of time. Offer emotional support and reassurance, as interference with the patient's habits and lifestyle may be considerable. SEE: *Nursing Diagnoses* in *Appendix.*

h., amebic. The syndrome of a tender,

enlarged liver, pain over the liver, fever, and leukocytosis in a patient with amebic colitis. This name is a misnomer in that the liver changes are not due to an infestation of that organ with amebae but a part of the nonspecific reaction to the infection in the intestinal tract. Nevertheless, occasionally a liver abscess will develop and the walls of the abscess will contain amebae.

TREAT: Metronidazole plus iodoquinol; or chloroquine phosphate plus either emetine or dehydroemetine. These latter two drugs are toxic and should be given only if their course can be carefully observed by using a cardiac monitor. The drugs should not be given to patients with cardiac disease or to a patient who is pregnant.

h. B. Hepatitis caused by hepatitis B virus (HBV).

Caution: Any member of the health care team who comes in contact with blood, body fluids, or body tissues has an increased chance of developing this type of viral hepatitis. This risk can be assessed by testing persons so exposed for presence of HBV antigens. Health care workers who do not have the protection afforded by the HBV antigen should be immunized with hepatitis B vaccine. SEE: *hepatitis B virus vaccine inactivated.*

h. C. Hepatitis caused by hepatitis C virus. Previously, this virus was termed non-A, non-B. It is the most common posttransfusion hepatitis in the U.S. Clinically and epidemiologically, the disease resembles hepatitis B. SEE: *hepatitis, acute viral.*

h., chronic. Symptoms that last for more than several months are considered to represent a chronic state. If these signs and symptoms increase rather than remain mild, cirrhosis may be the outcome. In some hepatitis B cases a persistent carrier state results as evidenced by continued presence of the hepatitis B surface antigen (HBsAg) in the blood. Those individuals are highly likely to be able to transmit hepatitis B.

h., delta agent. This type agent is able to cause hepatitis when it is present in the body along with the hepatitis B surface antigen (HBsAg). The clinical course and epidemiological characteristics of this type of hepatitis are quite similar to those of hepatitis B. Interferon alfa has been used in treating chronic delta hepatitis.

h. E. An important form of hepatitis that is rarely encountered in the U.S. It is caused by a virus that has not been fully characterized but is possibly related to Norwalk agent. It is usually contracted from sewage-contaminated water and can be spread from person to person. Chronic infection probably does not occur, but acute infection in pregnant individuals can be fatal in up to 20% of cases.

h., fulminant. Hepatitis marked by sudden onset of nausea and vomiting, chills, high fever, severe and early jaundice, convulsions, shock, deep coma, and death usually within 10 days.

h., infectious. A previously used term for what is now known as hepatitis A.

h., serum. A previously used term for what is now known to include hepatitis due to either hepatitis B or hepatitis C.

h., toxic or drug-induced. Inflammation of the liver caused by the entry of toxins or drugs into the body. Included in the great number of agents known to be able to cause this type of hepatitis are common drugs and chemicals used in either the treatment of disease or in the workplace.

h., viral. SEE: *hepatitis A; hepatitis B; hepatitis C.*

hepatitis-associated antigen. The original term applied to the Australian antigen. It is now called hepatitis B surface antigen (HBsAg). Its discovery made possible the differentiation of hepatitis B from other forms of viral hepatitis.

hepatitis B immune globulin. USP. Standard solution consisting of globulins derived from blood plasma of human donors who have high titers of antibodies against hepatitis B surface antigen. Trade names are H-Big, Hep-B-Gammagee, and HyperHep.

hepatitis B surface antigen. ABBR: HBsAg. The antigen to hepatitis B virus. It was originally called hepatitis-associated antigen.

hepatitis B virus vaccine inactivated. USP. Vaccine prepared directly from human blood. It is used to vaccinate persons who are at high risk of coming in contact with carriers of hepatitis B, or with blood or fluids from such individuals. Included in the high-risk group are blood bank and dialysis workers, dental hygienists, drug addicts, and some homosexuals. Trade name is Heptavax-B.

hepatization (hĕp″ă-tĭ-zā′shŭn). The second and third stages in consolidation in lobar pneumonia. The surface of the lung has the appearance of liver tissue.

hepato- [Gr. *hepatikos*]. Prefix indicating the liver.

hepatoblastoma (hĕp″ă-tō-blăs-tō′mă) [″ + *blastos*, germ, + *oma*, tumor]. A malignant teratoma of the liver.

hepatocarcinogen. Anything that causes cancer of the liver.

hepatocarcinoma (hĕp″ă-tō-kăr″sin-ō′mă) [″ + *karkinos*, crab, + *oma*, tumor]. Carcinoma of the liver.

hepatocele (hĕp′ă-tō-sĕl) [+ *kele,* tumor, swelling]. Hernia of the liver.

hepatocellular (hĕp″ă-tō-sĕl′ū-lăr). Concerning the cells of the liver.

hepatocholangiocystoduodenostomy (hĕp″ă-tō-kō-lăn″jē-ō-sĭs″tō-dū″ō-dĕ-nŏs′tō-mē) [″ + *chole,* bile, + *angeion,* vessel, + *kystis,* bladder, + L. *duodenum,* duodenum, + Gr. *stoma,* mouth]. Establishment of drainage of bile ducts into the duodenum through the gallbladder.

hepatocholangioduodenostomy (hĕp″ă-tō-kō-lăn″jē-ō-dū-ō-dĕ-nŏs′tō-mē) [″ + ″ + ″ + L. *duodenum,* duodenum, + Gr. *stoma,* mouth]. Establishment of drainage of bile ducts into the duodenum.

hepatocholangioenterostomy (hĕp″ă-tō-kō-lăn″jē-ō-ĕn″tĕr-ŏs′tō-mē) [″ + ″ + ″ + *enteron,* intestine, + *stoma,* mouth]. Establishment of a passage between the liver and intestine.

hepatocholangiogastrostomy (hĕp″ă-tō-kō-lăn″jē-ō-găs-trŏs′tō-mē) [″ + ″ + ″ + *gaster,* belly, + *stoma,* mouth]. Establishment of drainage of bile ducts into the stomach.

hepatocholangiostomy (hĕp″ă-tō-kō-lăn-jē-ŏs′tō-mē) [″ + ″ + ″ + *stoma,* mouth]. Establishment of free drainage by opening into the gall duct.

hepatocholangitis (hĕp″ă-tō-kō-lăn-jī′tis) [″ + ″ + ″ + *itis,* inflammation]. Inflammation of the cells of the liver and bile ducts.

hepatocirrhosis (hĕp″ă-tō-sĭ-rō′sĭs) [″ + *kirrhos,* tawny, + *osis,* condition]. Cirrhosis of the liver.

hepatocolic (hĕp″ă-tō-kŏl′ĭk) [″ + *kolon,* colon]. Rel. to both the liver and colon.

hepatocuprein (hĕp″ă-tō-koo′prĭn). A copper-containing protein in the liver.

hepatocystic (hĕp″ă-tō-sĭs′tĭk) [″ + *kystis,* bladder]. Rel. to the gallbladder or to both the liver and gallbladder.

hepatocyte (hĕp′ă-tō-sīt). A parenchymal liver cell.

hepatoduodenostomy (hĕp″ă-tō-dū″ō-dĕ-nŏs′tō-mē) [″ + L. *duodenum,* duodenum, + Gr. *stoma,* mouth]. Establishment of an opening from the liver into the duodenum. SYN: *hepaticoduodenostomy.*

hepatodynia (hĕp″ă-tō-dĭn′ē-ă) [″ + *odyne,* pain]. Pain in the liver.

hepatoenteric (hĕp″ă-tō-ĕn-tĕr′ĭk) [″ + *enteron,* intestine]. Rel. to the liver and intestines.

hepatogastric (hĕp″ă-tō-găs′trĭk) [Gr. *hepatikos,* liver, + *gaster,* belly]. Rel. to the liver and stomach.

hepatogenic (hĕp″ă-tō-jĕn′ĭk) [″ + *gennan,* to produce]. Having its origin in the liver.

hepatogenous (hĕp″ă-tŏj′ĕ-nŭs). Originating in the liver.

hepatogram (hĕp′ă-tō-grăm″) [″ + *gramma,* something written]. Roentgenographic examination of the liver.

hepatography (hĕp″ă-tŏg′ră-fē) [″ + *graphein,* to write]. Roentgenography of the liver.

hepatohemia (hĕp″ă-tō-hē′mē-ă) [″ + *haima,* blood]. Liver congestion.

hepatoid [″ + *eidos,* form, shape]. Having the structural form of the liver.

hepatojugular (hĕp″ă-tō-jŭg′ū-lăr). Concerning the liver and jugular vein.

hepatojugular reflex. Pressure on the liver causing an increase in the cervical venous pressure in persons with right-sided heart failure.

hepatolenticular (hĕp″ă-tō-lĕn-tĭk′ū-lăr) [″ + L. *lenticula,* lentil, lens]. Rel. to the lenticular nucleus of the eye and liver.

hepatolenticular degeneration. A hereditary syndrome transmitted as an autosomal recessive trait in which a decrease of ceruloplasmin, q.v., permits accumulation of copper in various organs (brain, liver, kidney, and cornea) associated with increased intestinal absorption of copper. A pigmented ring (Kayser-Fleischer ring) at the outer margin of the cornea is pathognomonic. Syndrome is characterized by degenerative changes in the brain, cirrhosis of the liver, splenomegaly, tremor, muscular rigidity, involuntary movements, spastic contractures, psychic disturbances, dysphagia, and progressive weakness and emaciation. SYN: *Wilson's disease.*

TREAT. Prevention of further accumulation of copper by avoiding eating organ meats, shellfish, nuts, dried legumes, chocolate, whole cereals, and all foods and water high in copper. D-penicillamine is given orally to reduce the free plasma copper to normal levels. This therapy in carefully controlled doses will probably be required for the patient's entire lifetime.

hepatolienography (hĕp″ă-tō-lī″ĕ-nŏg′ră-fē) [″ + L. *lien,* spleen, + Gr. *graphein,* to write]. Roentgenographic examination of the liver and spleen. Usually done after intravenous injection of a radiopaque material.

hepatolienomegaly (hĕp″ă-tō-lī″ĕ-nō-mĕg′ă-lē) [″ + ″ + *megas,* large]. Enlargement of the liver and spleen.

hepatolith (hĕp′ă-tō-lĭth) [″ + *lithos,* stone]. A biliary concretion of the liver.

hepatolithectomy (hĕp″ă-tō-lĭ-thĕk′tō-mē) [″ + *lithos,* stone, + *ektome,* excision]. Surgical removal of a calculus from the liver.

hepatolithiasis (hĕp″ă-tō-lĭ-thī′ă-sĭs) [″ + ″ + *-iasis,* disease condition]. Calculi or concretions in the liver.

hepatologist (hĕp″ă-tŏl′ō-jĭst) [″ + *logos*, word, reason]. A specialist in diseases of the liver.

hepatology (hĕp″ă-tŏl′ō-jē) [″ + *logos*, word, reason]. Study of the liver.

hepatolytic (hĕp″ă-tō-lĭt′ĭk). Destructive to tissues of the liver.

hepatoma (hĕp″ă-tō′mă) [″ + *oma*, tumor]. A tumor of the liver.

hepatomalacia (hĕp″ă-tō-mă-lā′sē-ă) [″ + *malakia*, softening]. Softening of the liver.

hepatomegaly (hĕp″ă-tō-mĕg′ă-lē) [″ + *megas*, large]. Enlargement of the liver.

hepatomelanosis (hĕp″ă-tō-mĕl″ă-nō′sĭs) [″ + *melas*, black, + *osis*, condition]. Pigmented deposits or melanosis in the liver.

hepatomphalocele (hĕp″ă-tŏm′fă-lō-sēl″) [Gr. *hepatikos*, liver, + *omphalos*, navel, + *kele*, tumor, swelling]. Protrusion of a part of the liver through the umbilicus. The liver is covered by a membrane.

hepatonecrosis (hĕp″ă-tō-nĕ-krō′sĭs) [″ + *nekrosis*, state of death]. Gangrene of the liver.

hepatonephric (hĕp″ă-tō-nĕf′rĭk) [″ + *nephros*, kidney]. Concerning the liver and kidney.

hepatonephritis (hĕp″ă-tō-nĕ-frī′tĭs) [″ + ″ + *itis*, inflammation]. Inflammation of both liver and kidneys.

hepatonephromegaly (hĕp″ă-tō-nĕf″rō-mĕg′ă-lē) [″ + ″ + *megas*, large]. Hypertrophy of the kidneys or both liver and kidney.

  h. glycogenica. Disease characterized by hypertrophy of liver and excess accumulation of glycogen resulting from failure of glycogenolysis to occur. SYN: *von Gierke's disease.*

hepatopathy (hĕp-ĕ-tŏp′ă-thē) [″ + *pathos*, disease, suffering]. Any disease of the liver.

hepatoperitonitis (hĕp″ă-tō-pĕr″ĭ-tō-nī′tĭs) [″ + *peritonaion*, peritoneum, + *itis*, inflammation]. Inflammation of the peritoneal covering of the liver. SYN: *perihepatitis.*

hepatopexy (hĕp′ă-tō-pĕks″ē) [″ + *pexis*, fixation]. Fixation of a movable liver to the abdominal wall.

hepatophage (hĕp′ă-tō-fāj) [″ + *phagein*, to eat]. A phagocyte that attacks liver cells.

hepatopleural (hĕp′ă-tō-ploo′răl) [″ + *pleura*, side]. Concerning the liver and pleura.

hepatopneumonic (hĕp″ă-tō-nū-mŏn′ĭk) [″ + *pneumonikos*, of the lungs]. Concerning the liver and lungs.

hepatoportogram (hĕp″ă-tō-por′tō-grăm). Roentgenography of the portal vein and its branches in the liver.

hepatoptosia, hepatoptosis (hĕp″ă-tŏp-tō′sē-ă, -tō′sĭs) [″ + *ptosis*, a dropping]. Downward displacement of the liver.

hepatopulmonary (hĕp″ă-tō-pŭl′mō-năr″ē) [″ + L. *pulmo*, lung]. Rel. to both liver and lungs.

hepatorenal (hĕp″ă-tō-rē′năl) [″ + L. *renalis*, kidney]. Pert. to both liver and kidneys.

hepatorrhaphy (hĕp-ă-tor′ă-fē) [″ + *rhaphe*, seam, ridge]. The suturing of a wound of the liver.

hepatorrhexis (hĕp″ă-tō-rĕks′-ĭs) [″ + *rhexis*, rupture]. Rupture of the liver.

hepatoscan (hĕp′ă-tō-skăn). A radioautograph of the liver.

hepatoscopy [″ + *skopein*, to examine]. Inspection of the liver.

hepatosis (hĕp″ă-tō′sĭs) [″ + *osis*, condition]. Any noninflammatory disease of the liver.

hepatosplenitis (hĕp″ă-tō-splē-nī′tĭs) [″ + *splen*, spleen, + *itis*, inflammation]. Inflamed condition of both liver and spleen.

hepatosplenography (hĕp″ă-tō-splē-nŏg′ră-fē) [″ + ″ + *graphein*, to write]. X-ray examination of the liver and spleen.

hepatosplenomegaly (hĕp″ă-tō-splē″nō-mĕg′ă-lē) [″ + ″ + *megas*, large]. Enlargement of both liver and spleen.

hepatosplenopathy (hĕp″ă-tō-splē-nŏp′ă-thē) [″ + ″ + *pathos*, disease, suffering]. Disease that affects the liver and spleen.

hepatostomy (hĕp″ă-tŏs′tō-mē) [″ + *stoma*, mouth]. Surgical incision of the liver with establishment of an opening to the outside of the body.

hepatotherapy (hĕp″ă-tō-thĕr′ă-pē) [″ + *therapeia*, treatment]. 1. Treatment of liver disease. 2. Use of liver or liver extract.

hepatotomy (hĕp″ă-tŏt′ō-mē) [″ + *tome*, incision]. Incision into the liver.

hepatotoxemia (hĕp″ă-tō-tŏks-ē′mē-ă) [″ + *toxikon*, poison, + *haima*, blood]. Autointoxication due to malfunctioning of the liver.

hepatotoxic. Toxic to the liver.

hepatotoxin (hĕp″ă-tō-tŏk′sĭn). A cytotoxin specific for liver cells.

heptachromic (hĕp″tă-krō′mĭk) [Gr. *hepta*, seven, + *chroma*, color]. Possessing normal color vision.

heptapeptide (hĕp″tă-pĕp′tĭd) [″ + *peptein*, to digest]. A polypeptide containing seven amino acids.

heptaploidy (hĕp″tă-ploy′dē) [″ + *ploos*, fold]. Having seven sets of chromosomes.

heptose (hĕp′tōs). Any sugar containing seven carbon atoms in its molecule.

heptosuria (hĕp″tō-sū′rē-ă) [″ + *ouron*, urine]. Heptose in the urine.

herb (ĕrb) [L. *herba*, grass]. A plant with a soft stem containing little wood, esp. one of the aromatic plants used in medicine or as seasoning. The plant usually produces seeds and then dies down at the end of the growing season.

herbalist. One who attempts to promote healing or health through the use of herbs.

herbicide. A substance (such as a chemical) that kills plants or inhibits plant growth.

herbicide poisoning. Poisoning due to the use of a toxic herbicide, such as 2, 4-D, q.v.

herbivorous (hĕr-bĭv′ō-rŭs) [″ + *vorare*, to eat]. Feeding on grasses and herbs. SYN: *vegetarian.*

herd [AS. *heord*]. Any large aggregation of people or animals.

herd immunity. Vaccination of an individual provides immune protection and it may reduce the spread of the infecting agent in the population.

hereditary (hĕ-rĕd′ĭ-tĕr-ē) [L. *hereditarius,* an heir]. Pert. to a genetic characteristic transmitted from parent to offspring. SEE: *chromosome; gene.*

heredity (hĕ-rĕd′ĭ-tē) [L. *hereditas,* heir]. The transmission of genetic characteristics from parent to offspring.

heredo- [L. *hereditas,* heir]. Prefix meaning heredity.

heredoataxia (hĕr″ĕ-dō-ă-tăks′ē-ă) [″ + Gr. *ataxia,* lack of order]. Hereditary spinal ataxia. SYN: *Friedreich's ataxia.*

heredodegeneration (hĕr″ĕ-dō-dē-jĕn″ĕr-ā′shŭn). Inherited degeneration due to defective or diseased hyaloplasm. It is seen in Marie's ataxia.

heredofamilial (hĕr″ĕ-dō-fă-mĭl′ē-ăl). Referring to any disease that occurs in families due to the inherited defect or process to develop the condition.

heredoimmunity (hĕr″ĕ-dō-ĭ-mū′nĭ-tē). Inherited immunity.

Hering, Heinrich Ewald. German physiologist, 1866–1948.

     H.-Breuer reflex [Josef Breuer, Austrian physician, 1842–1925]. Reflex inhibition of inspiration resulting from stimulation of pressoreceptors by inflation of the lungs.

     H.'s nerves. Afferent nerve fibers leading from the carotid sinus by way of the glossopharyngeal nerve to the brain. They are pressoreceptor nerves responding to changes in blood pressure that reflexly control heart rate. An increase in pressure diminishes heart rate.

Hering, Karl Ewald K. (hĕr′ĭng). German physiologist, 1834–1918.

     H.'s theory. Theory of color vision in which it is assumed that the retina possesses three photochemical substances that, depending on their decomposition or resynth-

esis, produce different color sensations by their stimulation of different nerve endings.

heritable. Able to be inherited.

heritage. The genetic and other characteristics transmitted to offspring.

hermaphrodism (hĕr-măf′rō-dĭzm). Hermaphroditism, q.v.

hermaphrodite (hĕr-măf′rō-dīt) [Gr. *Hermaphroditos,* son of Hermes and Aphrodite, who was man and woman combined]. One possessing genital and sexual characteristics of both sexes. The clitoris is usually enlarged, resembling the penis of the male. SYN: *androgyne.*

hermaphroditism (hĕr-măf′rō-dīt-ĭzm). Conditions in which both ovarian and testicular tissue exist in the same individual. Occurs rarely in humans. SYN: *hermaphrodism.* SEE: *intersex.*

     h., bilateral. Condition in which an ovary and testicle are present on both sides.

     h., complex. Having internal and external organs of both sexes.

     h., dimidiate. H., lateral.

     h., false. Possession of the sex glands of one sex (ovary or testis) but accompanied by secondary sexual characteristics and external genitalia of the opposite sex. SYN: *pseudohermaphroditism.*

     h., lateral. Possession of a testis on one side and an ovary on the other.

     h., spurious. H., false.

     h., transverse. Having the outward organs of one sex and the internal organs of the other.

     h., true. Hermaphroditism in which the individual possesses both ovarian and testicular glands.

     h., unilateral. Hermaphroditism in which an ovary and a testis or an ovotestis are present on one side and either an ovary or testis is present on the other side.

hermetic (hĕr-mĕt′ĭk) [L. *hermeticus*]. Airtight.

hernia (hĕr′nē-ă) [L.]. Protrusion or projection of an organ or a part of an organ through the wall of the cavity that normally contains it. SYN: *rupture.* SEE: *herniotomy.*

     ETIOL: Failure of certain normal openings to close during development; weakness resulting from debilitating illness, old age, or injury; prolonged distention as from tumors, pregnancy, or corpulence; increased intra-abdominal pressure resulting from lifting heavy loads or coughing.

     TREAT: Surgery or mechanical reduction. In very large hernias, mechanical devices or trusses may be used on a temporary basis.

     h., abdominal. Hernia through the abdominal wall.

     h., acquired. Hernia that develops any

time after birth in contrast to one present at birth (congenital hernia). Usually the result of excessive strain on the muscular wall. Frequently occurs following injuries or operations.

h., bladder. Protrusion of the bladder or a part of the bladder through a normal or abnormal orifice.

h., cerebral. Hernia of the brain through the cranial wall.

h., Cloquet's. A type of femoral hernia. SEE: *h., femoral.*

h., complete. Hernia in which sac and its contents have passed through the aperture.

h., concealed. Hernia that is imperceptible when palpated.

h., congenital. Hernia existing from birth.

h., crural. Hernia that protrudes behind the femoral sheath.

h., cystic. H., bladder.

h., direct. H., inguinal.

h., diverticular. Protrusion of an intestinal congenital diverticulum.

h., encysted. Scrotal protrusion that, enveloped in its own sac, passes into the tunica vaginalis.

h., epigastric. Hernia of the intestine through an opening in the midline above the umbilicus.

h., fascial. Protrusion of muscular tissue through its fascial covering.

h., fatty. Protrusion of fatty tissue through the abdominal wall.

h., femoral. Descending of intestines through femoral ring.

h., funicular. Hernia into the umbilical or spermatic cord.

h., hiatal. Protrusion of the stomach upward into the mediastinal cavity through the esophageal hiatus of the diaphragm. SEE: illus. SEE: *Nursing Diagnoses in Appendix.*

h., Holthouse's. H., inguinocrural.

h., incarcerated. Hernia causing complete bowel obstruction.

h., incisional. Hernia through a surgical scar.

h., incomplete. Hernia that has not gone completely through the aperture.

h., indirect. H., inguinal.

h., inguinal. Protrusion of the hernial sac containing the intestine at the inguinal opening. In indirect inguinal hernia, the sac protrudes through the internal inguinal ring into the inguinal canal often descending into the scrotum. In direct inguinal hernia, the hernial sac protrudes through the abdominal wall in the region of Hesselbach's triangle, a region bounded by the rectus abdominal muscle, inguinal ligament, and inferior epigastric vessels. Inguinal hernias

account for about 80% of all hernias.

h., inguinocrural. Hernia that is both femoral and inguinal.

h., internal. Hernia that occurs within the abdominal cavity. May be intraperitoneal or retroperitoneal.

h., interstitial. Form of inguinal hernia in which the hernial sac lies between layers of the abdominal muscles.

h., irreducible. Hernia that cannot be returned to its original position out of its sac by manual methods.

h., labial. Protrusion of a loop of bowel into the labium majus.

h., lateral. H., inguinal.

h., lumbar. Hernia in lumbar regions or loins.

h., medial. H., inguinal.

h., mesocolic. Hernia between the layers of the mesocolon.

h., nuckian. Hernia into canal of Nuck.

h., oblique. H., inguinal.

h., obturator. Hernia through the obturator foramen.

h. of diaphragm. There are three types: congenital, acquired or traumatic, and esophageal. In the latter, a portion of the diaphragm is pushed through the esophageal hiatus into the stomach or the hernia protrudes through the diaphragm.

h., omental. Hernia containing a portion of the omentum.

h., ovarian. Presence of an ovary in a hernial sac.

h., phrenic. Hernia projecting through the diaphragm into one of the pleural cavities.

h., posterior vaginal. Hernia of Douglas' sac downward between the rectum and posterior vaginal wall. SYN: *enterocele.*

h., properitoneal. Hernia that protrudes through the peritoneum and into the abdominal wall.

h., reducible. Hernia that can be replaced by manipulation.

h., retroperitoneal. Hernia into the peritoneal sac extending behind the peritoneum into the iliac fossa.

h., Richter's. Hernia in which only a portion of wall of intestine protrudes, the main portion of the intestine being excluded from the hernial sac and the lumen remaining open.

h., scrotal. Hernia that descends into the scrotum.

h., sliding. A form of hernia that may develop and then return to normal by the viscus sliding in and out of the sac of the hernia. This condition may occur with hiatal hernia or in other types of abdominal hernias.

h., strangulated. Hernia so tightly con-

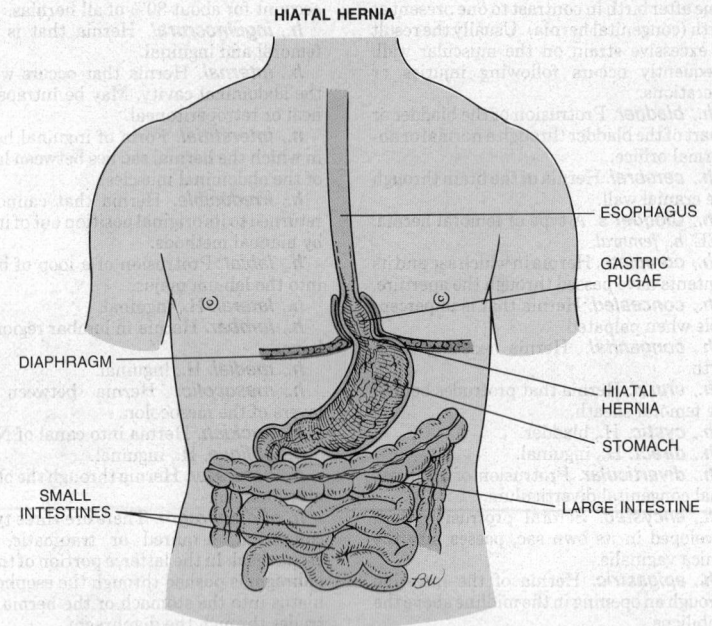

HIATAL HERNIA

ESOPHAGUS

GASTRIC RUGAE

DIAPHRAGM

HIATAL HERNIA

STOMACH

SMALL INTESTINES

LARGE INTESTINE

stricted that gangrene results if surgery does not relieve it. Not reducible by ordinary means.

h., umbilical. Hernia occurring at the navel. Seen mostly in children. Usually it requires no therapy.

h., uterine. Presence of the uterus in the hernial sac.

h., vaginal. Hernial protrusion of the vaginal wall into the surrounding area, usually the pouch of Douglas.

h., vaginolabial. Hernia of a viscus into the posterior end of the labium majus.

h., ventral. Hernia through the abdominal wall. If stretching and thinning of an abdominal scar occur, pressure from the abdomen may cause protrusion of part of the gut. It is then protected only by a layer of thin scar tissue.

hernial (hĕr'nē-ăl) [L. *hernia*, rupture]. Pert. to a hernia.

hernial sac. The pouch of peritoneum pushed before a hernia and into which it descends.

herniated. Having a hernia.

herniated disk. Rupture or herniation of the nucleus pulposus, esp. between lumbar vertebrae. It usually causes pain in the affected side.

herniation (hĕr-nē-ā'shŭn). Development of a hernia.

h. of nucleus pulposus. Prolapse of the nucleus pulposus of the intervertebral disk into the spinal canal. SEE: *Nursing Diagnoses* in *Appendix*.

h., tonsillar. Protrusion of the cerebellar tonsils through the foramen magnum. It causes pressure on the medulla oblongata; and may be fatal.

h., transtentorial. Herniation of the uncus and adjacent structures into the incisure of the tentorium of the brain. It is caused by increased pressure in the cranium. SYN: *uncal herniation*.

hernioenterotomy (hĕr"nē-ō-ĕn"tĕr-ŏt'ō-mē) [" + Gr. *enteron*, intestine, + *tome*, incision]. Herniotomy and enterotomy done during the same surgical procedure.

herniography (hĕr"nē-ŏg'ră-fē) [" + Gr. *graphein*, to write]. Radiographic examination of a hernia after the introduction of a contrast medium.

hernioid (hĕr'nē-oyd) [" + Gr. *eidos*, form, shape]. Resembling a hernia.

herniolaparotomy (hĕr"nē-ō-lăp"ă-rŏt'ō-mē) [" + Gr. *lapara*, loin, + *tome*, incision]. Abdominal surgery for the treatment of hernia.

herniology (hĕr"nē-ŏl'ō-jē) [" + Gr. *logos*, word, reason]. The science of hernias.

hernioplasty (hĕr'nē-ō-plăs"tē) [" + Gr. *plassein*, to form]. Surgical operation for hernia.

herniopuncture (hĕr"nē-ō-pŭnk'chŭr) [" + *punctura*, prick]. Puncture of a hernia with hollow needle for withdrawal of fluid or gas.

herniorrhaphy (hĕr-nē-or'ă-fē) [" + Gr. *rhaphe*, seam, ridge]. Surgical procedure for hernia.

herniotomy (hĕr-nē-ŏt'ō-mē) [" + Gr. *tome*, incision]. Surgery for the relief of hernia; an operation for the correction of irreducible hernia, esp. strangulated hernia.

heroic measures. In medical practice, the undertaking of a procedure or therapy that has an element of daring or boldness to it. Usually, such action is taken to attempt to save a patient's life.

heroin (hĕr'ō-ĭn). A narcotic derived from morphine. Importation, sale, and use of this drug are illegal in the United States. SYN: *diacetylmorphine*. SEE: *drug addiction; endorphins.*

heroin toxicity. Poisoning by heroin.

SYM: Acute poisoning causes euphoria, flushing, itching of the skin, miosis, drowsiness, decreased respiratory rate and depth, bradycardia, hypotension, and a decrease in body temperature. If emergency condition is not treated without delay, cyanosis and death may be the outcome.

TREAT: In acute toxicity, establish and maintain an airway. Remove false teeth, and clean mouth and pharynx of mucus or blood. Give mouth-to-mouth or mouth-to-nose artificial respiration if necessary. Assess and treat any abnormality of cardiac function. Use cardiac massage, defibrillator, or cardiac pacer as needed. Treat pulmonary edema with continuous positive-pressure respiration and oxygen therapy.

Intravenously administer (may have to use femoral or jugular vein) the opiate antagonist nalorphine hydrochloride according to directions in package. Also administer a respiratory stimulant such as 3 to 5 ml of doxapram hydrochloride, USP, intravenously.

Stay with patient until he or she is fully responsive. A long-acting narcotic may continue to act after a short-acting antagonist has worn off. If patient fails to respond to treatment, look for another cause for the coma. SEE: *Universal Precautions* in *Appendix.*

heroinism (hĕr'ō-ĭn-ĭzm) [*heroin* + Gr. *-ismos*, condition]. Addiction to use of heroin. SEE: *drug addiction.*

herpangina (hĕrp-ăn-jī'nă, hĕrp-ăn'jĭ-nă) [Gr. *herpes*, creeping skin disease, + L. *angina*, a choking]. A benign infectious disease of children and, less commonly, of young adults. Occurs in epidemic form throughout the world, most often in summer and early fall.

SYM: Sudden onset of fever, severe sore throat, nausea, vomiting, excess salivation, and malaise. The throat and posterior area of the mouth are covered with vesicles 1 to 2 mm in diameter that rupture and form ulcers.

ETIOL: One of several strains of group A coxsackievirus and rarely other enteroviruses.

TREAT: Symptomatic and supportive. There is no specific therapy, but recovery is prompt.

herpes (hĕr'pēz) [Gr. *herpes*, creeping skin disease]. A word that was used to indicate vesicular eruption caused by a virus, esp. herpes simplex, q.v., or herpes zoster, q.v., and the condition lay people call cold sore or fever blister. When used as a single word, it usually refers to herpes simplex. SEE: *Nursing Diagnoses* in *Appendix.*

h. corneae. Inflammation of the cornea due to herpesvirus.

h. facialis. A form of herpes simplex, q.v., that occurs on the face.

h. febrilis. Herpes simplex of the lips and nasal mucosa.

h. genitalis. Infection of the genital and anorectal skin and mucosa with herpes simplex virus type 2. It is usually spread by sexual contact and is classed as a sexually transmitted disease. This viral infection may be transmitted to the fetus during delivery and may be fatal.

SYM: Itching and soreness are usually present before a small patch of erythema develops. Then a vesicle that erodes appears. These are usually painful and heal in about 10 days. They may occur in any part of the genitalia.

TREAT: Acyclovir has been of considerable benefit in treating the initial infection. SEE: *Universal Precautions* in *Appendix.*

Caution: The lesions are highly contagious, and persons caring for the patient must avoid contact with the exudates.

h. labialis. A form of herpes simplex, q.v., that occurs on the lips. SYN: *cold sore; blister, fever.*

h. menstrualis. Herpetic lesions appearing at the time of the menstrual period.

h., ocular. Herpes of the eye.

h. praeputialis. Herpes simplex of the male genitals.

h. progenitalis. Herpes simplex of the vulva.

h. simplex. An infectious disease caused

by herpes simplex virus type 1. Characterized by thin-walled vesicles that tend to recur in the same area of the skin, usually at a site where the mucous membrane joins the skin; however, they may be limited to the gingiva, oropharynx, or conjunctiva. In newborn infants, meningoencephalitis or a panvisceral infection may occur. In adults 5% to 7% of cases of aseptic meningitis are due to herpes simplex virus. SEE: *Nursing Diagnoses* in *Appendix.*

TREAT: Acyclovir applied locally has been effective. Antibiotics may be helpful in treating secondary infection. Eye lesions should be treated by an ophthalmologist.

h., traumatic. Herpes at the site of a wound.

h. zoster. An acute infectious disease caused by the varicella-zoster virus. It is limited to man and is characterized by inflammation of the posterior root ganglia of only a few segments of the spinal or cranial nerves. A painful vesicular eruption occurs along the course of the nerve and is almost always unilateral. The incubation period is from 7 to 21 days. The total duration of the disease from onset to complete recovery varies from 10 days to 5 weeks. If all the vesicles appear within 24 hours, the total duration is usually short. In general, the disease lasts longer in adults than in children. The virus that causes reactivation of herpes zoster is the same as that which causes chickenpox, i.e., varicella. SYN: *shingles.* SEE: *Nursing Diagnoses* in *Appendix.*

TREAT: Directed toward making the patient comfortable. If the eye is affected, idoxuridine should be used and the treatment supervised by an ophthalmologist.

h. zoster ophthalmicus. Herpes zoster affecting the first division of the 5th cranial nerve. The area of the face, eye, and nose supplied by this nerve is affected. Ocular complications can be quite serious. It is important that the eye be treated early with idoxuridine and that therapy be supervised by an ophthalmologist.

herpesviruses. A family, *Herpesviridae,* of structurally similar viruses. Included in this family are a number of viruses important to man. SEE: *herpes.*

herpesvirus simiae encephalomyelitis. A severe, almost always fatal, encephalomyelitis due to the herpesvirus simiae (also called B virus). It occurs among veterinarians, laboratory workers, and others who have come in contact with infected monkeys.

herpetic (hĕr-pĕt'ĭk) [Gr. *herpes,* creeping skin disease]. Pert. to herpes.

herpetic neuralgia. Neural pain with herpes zoster.

herpetic sore throat. Herpetic tonsillitis.

herpetiform (hĕr-pĕt'ĭ-form) [" + L. *forma,* form]. Resembling herpes.

herpetism (hĕr'pĕ-tĭzm) [" + *-ismos,* condition]. Predisposition of herpetic eruption.

Herplex Liquifilm. Trade name for idoxuridine, USP.

Herring bodies [Percy T. Herring, Brit. physiologist, 1872–1967]. Accumulation of neurosecretory material seen in the pars nervosa of the pituitary in the terminal nerve endings of the hypothalamus, hypophyseal tract. The neurosecretory material is thought to be a protein related to the hormones oxytocin and vasopressin.

Herring track. Equipment item used in rehabilitation of the upper extremity. Designed to exercise an arm in various positions and areas of motion.

hersage (âr-sǎzh') [Fr., a harrowing]. Splitting of a nerve trunk into separate fibers.

Herter's infantilism [Christian Archibald Herter, U.S. physician, 1865–1910]. A form of infantilism resulting from defective fat and calcium absorption. Resembles sprue in adults. SYN: *celiac disease.*

Hertig-Rock embryos [Arthur T. Hertig, U.S. pathologist, b. 1904; John Rock, U.S. gynecologist, 1890–1984]. Very beautifully preserved and dated embryos obtained experimentally in 1952.

Hertig-Rock ovum. Fertilized human ovum 7 to 7½ days old, described in 1945.

Hertwig's root sheath [Wilhelm August Oscar Hertwig, Ger. physiologist, 1849–1922]. A downgrowth of epithelium from the cervical loop of the enamel organ that induces dentin formation of the forming tooth root and determines its shape. The epithelial diaphragm, a horizontal extension of the Hertwig's root sheath, will determine the number and size of the tooth roots.

hertz [Heinrich R. Hertz, Ger. physicist, 1857–1894]. ABBR: Hz. A unit of frequency equal to one cycle/second.

hesitancy. Involuntary delay in initiating urination. This symptom should not be ignored, because it may accompany serious disease of the urinary tract or prostate.

Hespan. Trade name for hetastarch.

hesperidin (hĕs-pĕr'-ĭ-dĭn). A bioflavonoid present in orange and lemon peel.

Hesselbach's hernia (hĕs'ĕl-bŏks) [Franz K. Hesselbach, Ger. surgeon, 1759–1816]. A lobated hernia that passes through the cribriform fascia.

Hesselbach's triangle. The triangular space bounded by Poupart's ligament below, exterior border of rectus muscle internally, and epigastric artery exteriorly.

hetacillin (hĕt"ă-sĭl'ĭn). USP. An antibiotic that is rapidly hydrolyzed in the body to ampicillin and acetone. Trade name is Versapen.

hetastarch. A synthetic polymer plasma volume expander composed of over 90% amylopectin. It has an average molecular weight of 450,000. Trade name is Hespan. SEE: *fluid replacement.*

heteradelphia (hĕt″ĕr-ă-dĕl′fē-ă) [Gr. *heteros*, other, + *adelphos*, brother]. Congenitally joined fetuses in which one twin is more nearly developed than the other.

heteradenia (hĕt″ĕr-ă-dē′nē-ă) [″ + *aden*, gland]. 1. Glandular substance in a part that does not normally contain glands. 2. Abnormal glandular tissue.

heteradenic (hĕt″ĕr-ă-dĕn′ĭk). Pert. to heteradenia.

heteradenoma (hĕt″ĕr-ăd-ē-nō′mă) [″ + *aden*, gland, + *oma*, tumor] (pl. *heteradenomata*). A glandular tumor arising from an area that does not usually contain glands.

heterecious (hĕt″ĕr-ē′shŭs) [″ + *oikos*, house]. Denoting a parasite living on different hosts at different stages of development. SYN: *metoxenous.*

heterecism (hĕt″ĕr-ē′sĭzm). Development of different cycles of existence on different hosts, said of certain parasites.

heteresthesia (hĕt″ĕr-ĕs-thē′zē-ă) [″ + *aisthesis*, sensation]. Variation in degree (plus or minus) of sensory response to cutaneous stimuli.

hetero-, heter- [Gr. *heteros*, other]. Prefix indicating different, or relationship to another.

heteroagglutination (hĕt″ĕr-ō-ă-gloo″tĭ-nă′shŭn). The agglutination by one animal's serum of the red blood cells of an animal of another species.

heteroagglutinin (hĕt″ĕr-ō-ă-glū′tĭ-nĭn). 1. Agglutinin formed as the result of an injection of an antigen from an animal of a different species. 2. Agglutinin capable of agglutinating blood cells of other species of animals.

heteroalbumose (hĕt″ĕr-ō-ăl′bū-mōs) [″ + L. *albumen*, white of egg]. Albumose insoluble in water but soluble in saline solutions or in acid or alkaline solutions. SYN: *hemialbumose.*

heteroantibody (hĕt″ĕr-ō-ăn″tĭ-bŏd′ē). An antibody corresponding to an antigen from another species.

heteroantigen (hĕt″ĕr-ō-ăn′tĭ-jĕn). An antigen in one species that produces a corresponding antibody in another species.

heteroautoplasty (hĕt″ĕr-ō-aw′tō-plăs-tē) [″ + *autos*, self, + *plassein*, to form]. Grafting skin from one person to another.

heteroblastic (hĕt″ĕr-ō-blăs′tĭk) [″ + *blastos*, germ]. Having origin in tissue of another kind. Opposite of homoblastic.

heterocellular (hĕt″ĕr-ō-sĕl′ū-lăr). Composed of different kinds of cells.

heterocephalus (hĕt″ĕr-ō-sĕf′ă-lŭs) [″ + *kephale*, head]. Congenitally deformed fetus with two heads of unequal size.

heterochiral (hĕt″ĕr-ō-kī′răl) [″ + *cheir*, hand]. Reversed as to right and left, but otherwise of the same form and size. Said of images in a plane mirror and of the hands.

heterochromatin (hĕt″ĕr-ō-krō′mă-tĭn) [″ + *chroma*, color]. A type of chromatin that stains less distinctly than the euchromatin, forming clear disks interposed between dark bands on chromosomes. In interphasic nuclei, it constitutes the chromocenters. It is believed to control certain metabolic activities of cells. It is genetically inert. SEE: *euchromatin.*

heterochromatosis (hĕt″ĕr-ō-krō-mă-tō′sĭs) [″ + ″ + *osis*, condition]. 1. Pigmentation of skin from foreign substances. 2. Difference in color. SYN: *heterochromia.*

heterochromia (hĕt″ĕr-ō-krō′mē-ă). A difference in color.

    h. iridis. Different color of iris or sector of iris in the two eyes. It may occur naturally or be due to previous disease in the lighter-colored eye. Rarely it is associated with Waardenberg syndrome, q.v.

heterochromosome (hĕt″ĕr-ō-krō′mō-sōm). 1. The X and Y or sex chromosomes. 2. A chromosome containing material, heterochromatin, that stains differently from the remainder of the chromatin material.

heterochromous (hĕt″ĕr-ō-krō′mŭs) [″ + *chroma*, color]. With abnormal difference in coloration.

heterochronia (hĕt″ĕr-ō-krō′nē-ă) [″ + *chronos*, time]. Denoting an abnormal time for the occurrence of a phenomenon or production of a structure.

heterochronic (hĕt″ĕr-ō-krŏn′ĭk). Occurring at different or at abnormal times.

heterochthonous (hĕt″ĕr-ŏk′thō-nŭs) [Gr. *heteros*, other, + *chthon*, a particular land or country]. Having its origin in a different place from where it was found.

heterocinesia (hĕt″ĕr-ō-sĭ-nē′zē-ă) [″ + *kinesis*, movement]. Movements different from those the patient is instructed to make.

heterocladic (hĕt″ĕr-ō-klăd′ĭk) [″ + *klados*, branch]. Pert. to an anastomosis between branches of two different arteries. Opposite of homocladic.

heterocrisis (hĕt″ĕr-ŏk′rĭ-sĭs) [″ + *krisis*, division]. Irregular or unexpected crisis with abnormal symptoms.

heterocyclic (hĕt″ĕr-ō-sīk′lĭk) [″ + *kyklos*, circle]. Pert. to ring compounds that contain one or more elements other than carbon in the ring.

heterodermic (hĕt″ĕr-ō-dĕr′mĭk) [″ +

derma, skin]. Pert. to a method of skin grafting in which grafts are taken from another person. SYN: *dermatoheteroplasty.*

heterodont (hĕt″ĕr-ō-dŏnt) [″ + *odous,* tooth]. Having teeth of various shapes.

heterodromus (hĕt″ĕr-ŏd′rō-mŭs) [″ + *dromos,* running]. Acting, arranged, or moving in the opposite direction.

heteroerotic. Alloerotism, q.v. SEE: *autoerotism.*

heteroerotism (hĕt″ĕr-ō-ĕr′ō-tĭzm) [″ + *eros,* love, + *-ismos,* condition]. Sexual desire for a person of the opposite sex. SEE: *autoerotic.*

heterogametic (hĕt″ĕr-ō-gă-mĕt′ĭk) [″ + *gamos,* marriage]. Pert. to the production of unlike gametes, applied esp. to a male that produces two types of sperm, one containing the X chromosome, the other the Y chromosome. SEE: *homogametic.*

heterogamy (hĕt″ĕr-ŏg′ă-mē). The union of gametes that are dissimilar in size and structure. Occurs in higher plants and animals. SEE: *isogamy.*

heterogeneity (hĕt″ĕr-ō-jĕ-nē′ĭ-tē). The quality of being heterogeneous.

heterogeneous (hĕt″ĕr-ō-jē′nē-ŭs) [″ + *genos,* type]. Of unlike natures; composed of unlike substances. Opposite of homogeneous.

heterogeneous vaccine. Vaccine made from some source other than patient's own tissues or cells. Opposite of autogenous vaccine.

heterogenesis (hĕt″ĕ-rō-jĕn′ĕ-sĭs) [″ + *genesis,* generation, birth]. Production of offspring that have different characteristics in alternate generations, as in the alternation of an asexual generation with a sexual one. SYN: *metagenesis.* SEE: *homogenesis.*

heterogenetic (hĕt″ĕ-rō-jĕ-nĕt′ĭk). Rel. to heterogenesis.

heterogeusia (hĕt″ĕr-ō-gū′sē-ă) [″ + *geusis,* taste]. Perception of an inappropriate quality of taste when food is present in the mouth or when it is chewed. The taste sensation is unexpected and unusual but not necessarily unpleasant.

heterograft (hĕt″ĕ-rō-grăft) [″ + L. *graphium,* stylus]. Graft taken from another individual or an animal of a different species from the one for whom it is intended. SEE: *autograft; graft; isograft.*

heterography (hĕt″ĕr-ŏg′ră-fē) [″ + *graphein,* to write]. Writing different words from those the writer intended.

heterohemagglutination (hĕt″ĕr-ō-hĕm″ă-gloo″tĭ-nā′shŭn). Agglutination of red blood cells by hemagglutinins from another species.

heterohemagglutinin (hĕt″ĕr-ō-hĕm″ă-gloo′tĭ-nĭn). Hemagglutinin from one species that will agglutinate red blood cells from another species.

heterohemolysin (hĕt″ĕr-ō-hē-mŏl′ĭ-sĭn). A hemolysin present in one animal that will hemolyze the red blood cells of another species.

heteroimmunity (hĕt″ĕr-ō-ĭm-mū′nĭ-tē). Having immunity to an antigen from another species.

heteroinfection (hĕt″ĕr-ō-ĭn-fĕk′shŭn) [Gr. *heteros,* other, + L. *in,* in, + *facere,* to make]. Infection by a microorganism from outside the body.

heteroinoculation (hĕt″ĕr-ō-ĭn-ŏk″ū-lā′shun) [″ + ″ + *oculus,* bud]. Inoculation with a microorganism from a source outside the body.

heterokeratoplasty (hĕt″ĕr-ō-kĕr′ă-tō-plăs″tē) [″ + *keras,* horn, + *plassein,* to form]. Plastic surgery of the cornea utilizing tissue from the cornea from another species.

heterolalia (hĕt″ĕr-ō-lā′lē-ă) [″ + *lalia,* babbling]. The use of meaningless words instead of those intended. SYN: *heterophasia; heterophemia.*

heterolateral (hĕt″ĕr-ō-lăt′ĕr-ăl) [″ + L. *latus,* side]. Situated or occurring on the other side. SEE: *ipsilateral.*

heteroliteral (hĕt″ĕr-ō-lĭt′ĕr-ăl). In speaking, pert. to an incorrect letter being substituted for the correct one.

heterologous (hĕt″ĕr-ŏl′ō-gŭs) [″ + *logos,* word, reason]. 1. Made up of cell tissue not normal to the part. 2. A tissue, cells, or blood obtained from a different individual or species. SEE: *homologous.*

heterologous fertilization. Fertilization of the female egg with sperm from a donor other than the husband. SEE: *homologous fertilization.*

heterology (hĕt″ĕr-ŏl′ō-jē). State of abnormality in structure or method of growth.

heterolysin (hĕt″ĕr-ŏl′ĭ-sĭn) [″ + *lysis,* solution]. Lysins formed from an antigen from an animal of a different species. SEE: *autolysis; hemolysis.*

heterolysis (hĕt″ĕr-ŏl′ĭ-sĭs). Hemolytic action of blood serum of an animal upon corpuscles of another species. SEE: *hemolysis; isolysis.*

heteromeric (hĕt″ĕr-ō-mĕr′ĭk) [″ + *meros,* a part]. 1. Pert. to spinal neurons with processes extending to opposite side of cord. 2. Possessing a different chemical composition.

heterometaplasia (hĕt″ĕr-ō-mĕt″ă-plā′zē-ă) [″ + *meta,* beyond, + *plassein,* to form]. Transformation of tissue into a type foreign to the part where it was produced.

heterometropia (hĕt″ĕr-ō-mĕ-trō′pē-ă). The ability of one eye to refract differently as compared with the other. This produces perceived images of different size. The condition is probably prevalent in many individuals who are completely unaware of it.

heteromorphosis (hĕt″ĕr-ō-mor-fō′sĭs) [″ + morphe, form, + osis, condition]. 1. The regeneration of an organ different from the one that it replaced. 2. Any disease in which malformation or deformity is characteristic. 3. Abnormal position of an organ or tissue.

heteromorphous (hĕt″ĕr-ō-mor′fŭs) [″ + morphe, form]. Deviating from the normal type.

heteronomous (hĕt″ĕr-ŏn′ō-mŭs) [″ + nomos, law]. Abnormal; differing from type.

heteronymous (hĕt″ĕr-ŏn′ĭ-mŭs) [″ + onyma, name]. 1. Having different names that are indicative of a correlation. SEE: hemianopia, crossed. 2. In opposite relation.

hetero-osteoplasty (hĕt″ĕr-ō-ŏs′tē-ō-plăs″tē) [″ + osteon, bone, + plassein, to form]. Grafting of bone, esp. with a graft from an animal.

heteropathy (hĕt″ĕr-ŏp′ă-thē) [″ + pathos, disease, suffering]. 1. Abnormal reaction to irritation or to stimuli. 2. Creation of a pathological condition to neutralize another disorder. SEE: allopathy.

heterophagocytosis. Phagocytosis of materials from the exterior of the cell by the process of endocytosis, q.v. SEE: autophagocytosis; phagocytosis; phagolysosome; phagosome; pinocytosis.

heterophany (hĕt″ĕr-ŏf′ă-nē) [″ + phainein, to appear]. Having different manifestations of the same disorder.

heterophasia (hĕt″ĕr-ō-fā′zē-ă) [″ + phasis, speech]. Expression of meaningless words instead of those intended. SYN: heterolalia; heterophemia.

heterophemia, heterophemy (hĕt″ĕr-ō-fē′mē-ă, hĕt-ĕr-ŏf′ĕ-mē) [″ + pheme, speech]. Expressing one thing when another is intended. SYN: heterolalia; heterophasia.

heterophil(e) (hĕt′ĕr-ō-fĭl, -fĭl) [″ + philein, to love]. 1. In man, the neutrophil leukocyte. 2. Pert. to an antibody reacting with other than the specific antigen. 3. Pert. to a tissue or microorganism that takes a stain other than the ordinary one.

heterophilic (hĕt″ĕr-ō-fĭl′ĭk) [Gr. heteros, other, + philein, to love]. 1. Having affinity for something abnormal. 2. Having antibody response to an antigen other than the specific one.

heterophonia (hĕt″ĕr-ō-fō′nē-ă) [″ + phone, voice]. Change of voice, esp. that which occurs at puberty.

heterophoralgia (hĕt″ĕr-ō-for-ăl′jē-ă) [″ + phoros, bearing, + algos, pain]. Deviation of one eye accompanied by pain.

heterophoria (hĕt″ĕ-rō-for′ē-ă) [″ phoros, bearing]. Tendency of the eyes to deviate from their normal position for visual alignment, esp. when one eye is covered; latent deviation or squint. SEE: -phoria.
ETIOL: Imbalance or insufficiency of ocular muscles.

heterophthalmos (hĕt″ĕr-ŏf-thăl′mŏs) [″ + ophthalmos, eye]. Difference in appearance of the eyes due to the irides differing in color. SEE: heterochromia.

Heterophyes (hĕt″ĕr-ŏf′ĭ-ēz) [″ + phye, stature]. A genus of flukes belonging to the family Heterophyidae.

H. heterophyes. A species of intestinal fluke commonly infesting man. In heavy infestations, it may cause diarrhea, nausea, and abdominal discomfort.

heterophyiasis (hĕt″ĕr-ō-fī-ī′ă-sĭs) [″ + ″ + -iasis, diseased condition]. Infestation by any fluke belonging to the family Heterophyidae.

Heterophyidae. A family of Trematoda (flukes) that infests the intestines of dogs, cats, and other mammals including humans. Infestations are common in Egypt and in the Far East. Includes the genera Heterophyes, Haplorchis, Diorchitrema, and Metagonimus. Intermediate hosts are snails, the cercaria encysting in fish, esp. mullets, or frogs.

heteroplasia (hĕt″ĕr-ō-plā′zē-ă) [″ + plassein, to mold]. Development of tissue at a location where that type of tissue would not normally occur. SYN: alloplasia.

heteroplastic (hĕt″ĕr-ō-plăs′tĭk). Rel. to heteroplasia.

heteroploid (hĕt′ĕr-ō-ployd) [″ + ploos, fold]. Possessing a chromosome number that is not a multiple of the haploid number common for the species.

heteroprosopus (hĕt″ĕr-ō-prō′sō-pŭs) [″ + prosopon, face]. A congenitally deformed fetus having one head and two faces.

heteropsia (hĕt″ĕr-ŏp′sē-ă) [″ + opsis, vision]. Inequality of vision in the two eyes.

heteroptics (hĕt″ĕr-ŏp′tĭks). Perversion of vision such as seeing objects that do not exist or misinterpreting what is seen.

heteropyknosis (hĕt″ĕr-ō-pĭk-nō′sĭs) [″ + pyknos, dense, + osis, condition]. The property whereby various parts of a chromosome stain with varying degrees of intensity. Thought to be due to variations in concentration of nucleic acid.

heteroscopy (hĕt″ĕr-ŏs′kō-pē) [″ + skopein, to examine]. 1. Finding range of vision in strabismus. 2. Unequal vision in the eyes.

heteroserotherapy (hĕt″ĕr-ō-sē″rō-thĕr′ă-pē) [″ + L. serum, whey, + Gr. therapeia, treatment]. Treatment by serum from another person.

heterosexual (hĕt"ĕr-ō-sĕk'shū-ăl) [" + L. *sexus*, sex]. 1. Pertaining to the opposite sex. 2. One whose sexual orientation is to persons of the opposite sex.

heterosexuality (hĕt"ĕr-ō-sĕk"shū-ăl'ĭ-tē). Sexual attraction for one of the opposite sex.

heterosis (hĕt-ĕr-ō'sĭs) [Gr., alteration]. Greater strength, size, vigor, and growth rate seen in the first hybrid generation. SYN: *hybrid vigor.*

heterosmia (hĕt"ĕr-ŏs'mē-ă) [Gr. *heteros*, other, + *osme*, odor]. Consistent perception of an inappropriate smell when an odorant is inhaled. The smell perceived is unusual and unexpected but not unpleasant. SYN: *allotriosmia.*

heterotaxia (hĕt"ĕr-ō-tăk'sē-ă) [" + *taxis*, arrangement]. Abnormal position of organs or parts. SEE: *dextrocardia; situs inversus viscerum.*

heterotherm (hĕt"ĕr-ō-thĕrm"). An animal that is heterothermic. SEE: *heterothermy.*

heterothermy (hĕt'ĕr-ō-thĕr"mē) [" + *therme*, heat]. Condition of animals in which the temperature varies considerably in various situations. It is *not* poikilothermic, q.v.

heterotopia (hĕt"ĕr-ō-tō'pē-ă) [" + *topos*, place]. 1. Development of a normal tissue in an abnormal location. 2. Displacement of an organ or part from its normal location.

heterotopic (hĕt"ĕr-ō-tŏp'ĭk). Misplaced; pert. to heterotopia.

heterotopy (hĕt"ĕr-ŏt'ō-pē) [" + *topos*, place]. Displacement of an organ or a portion of the body.

heterotoxin (hĕt"ĕr-ō-tŏk'sĭn) [" + *toxikon*, poison]. A toxin introduced from without the patient's body.

heterotransplant (hĕt"ĕr-ō-trăns'plănt) [" + L. *trans*, across, + *plantare*, to plant]. An organ, tissue, or structure taken from an animal and grafted into, or on, another animal of a different species. Such transplants usually atrophy.

heterotrichosis (hĕt"ĕr-ō-trī-kō'sĭs) [" + *trichosis*, growth of hair]. Growth of different kinds or color of hairs on the scalp or body.

heterotroph (hĕt'ĕr-ō-trōf) [" + *trophe*, food]. An organism such as man that requires complex organic food in order to grow and develop, in contrast to plants, which can synthesize food from inorganic materials.

heterotropia (hĕt"ĕr-ō-trō'pē-ă) [" + *tropos*, a turning]. Manifest deviation of the eyes due to absence of binocular equilibrium. SEE: *strabismus.*

heterotypic (hĕt"ĕr-ō-tĭp'ĭk). Concerning something of a different type than that which is being discussed or examined, esp. a tissue.

heterovaccine (hĕt"ĕr-ō-văk'sĕn) [" + L. *vaccinus*, pert. to a cow]. A vaccine from a microbial source other than that causing the disease for which it is intended.

heteroxanthine (hĕt"ĕr-ō-zăn'thĭn) [" + *xanthos*, yellow]. Methylxanthine, an alloxuric base found in the urine.

heteroxenous (hĕt"ĕr-ŏk'sē-nŭs) [" + *xenos*, stranger]. Property of a parasite that requires two different hosts in order to complete its life cycle.

heterozygosis (hĕt"ĕr-ō-zī-gō'sĭs) [" + *zygone*, yoke, pair, + *osis*, condition]. The state of having different alleles at a specific locus. SEE: *homozygosis.*

heterozygote (hĕt"ĕr-ō-zī'gōt). An individual with different alleles for a given characteristic. SEE: *allele.*

heterozygous (hĕt"ĕr-ō-zī'gŭs). Possessing different alleles at a given locus. SEE: *homozygous.*

Heubner, Johann Otto L. (hoyb'nĕr). German pediatrician, 1843–1926.

   H.'s disease. Syphilitic endarteritis of the brain.

   H.-Herter disease [Christian Archibald Herter, U.S. physician, 1865–1910]. Nontropical sprue in infants.

heuristic (hū-rĭs'tĭk) [Gr. *heuriskein*, to find out, discover]. Helping to discover or experiment, esp. the encouragement of students to learn through their own investigation.

H.E.W. U.S. Department of *Health, Education,* and *Welfare.* This agency is now the U.S. Department of Health and Human Services.

hex (hĕks) [Ger. *Hexe*, witch, sorceress]. To practice witchcraft on. SEE: *voodoo; zombie.*

hex-, hexa- [Gr. *hex*, six]. Prefix indicating six.

hexabasic [Gr. *hex*, six, + *basis*, base]. An acid that contains six hydrogen atoms (H) that can be replaced by six hydroxyl (OH) radicals.

hexachlorophene (hĕks"ă-klō'rō-fēn). USP. A bactericidal and bacteriostatic compound, used in emulsions and soaps for preoperative cleansing of skin and for scrubbing the nurse's and surgeon's hands prior to surgery.

hexachromic [" + *chroma*, color]. Able to distinguish only six of the seven colors of the spectrum or unable to distinguish violet from indigo.

hexad (hĕk'săd). 1. Six similar things. 2. An element with a valence of six.

hexadactylism (hĕks"ă-dăk'tĭl-ĭzm) [" + *daktylos*, finger, + *-ismos*, condition]. Possession of six fingers or six toes on one limb.

hexadecimal (hĕks"ă-dĕs'ĭ-mŭl) [" + L.

decimus, tenth]. In computers, a number system using the base sixteen rather than base two (binary) or ten (decimal).

hexafluorenium bromide (hĕk″să-flūr-ĕn′ē-ŭm). USP. A neuromuscular blocking agent. Trade name is Mylaxen.

hexamethonium (hĕks″ă-mĕ-thō′nē-ŭm). A compound that acts as a ganglionic blocking agent. Used in the treatment of hypertension.

hexaploidy (hĕk′să-ploy″dē) [″ + *ploos,* fold]. Condition of having six sets of chromosomes.

Hexapoda (hĕks-ăp′ō-dă) [″ + *pous,* foot]. The insects or six-legged arthropods. SYN: *Insecta.*

hexatomic (hĕks″ă-tŏm′ĭk) [″ + *atomos,* indivisible]. Pert. to a compound consisting of six atoms or one with six replaceable hydrogen or univalent atoms.

hexavaccine (hĕks″ă-văk′sēn) [″ + L. *vaccinus,* pert. to a cow]. A vaccine made from six different microorganisms.

hexavalent (hĕks″ă-vā′lĕnt) [″ + L. *valere,* to have power]. Having a chemical valence of six. SYN: *sexivalent.*

hexavitamin capsules or tablets. USP. A standardized vitamin preparation containing vitamins A, D, C, B, riboflavin, and niacinamide.

hexing. Use of witchcraft to cast a spell upon someone, e.g., to will another person's death. SEE: *voodoo.*

hexobarbital (hĕk″sō-bǎr′bĭ-tǎl). USP. A barbiturate sedative. Trade name is Sombulex.

hexokinase (hĕks″ō-kī′nās) [″ + *kinein,* to move, + *-ase,* enzyme]. An enzyme present in muscle tissue that catalyzes the phosphorylation of glucose. It has also been isolated from yeast.

hexosamine (hĕk′sōs-ăm″ĭn). A sugar containing an amino group in place of a hydroxyl group. Glucosamine is one example.

hexose (hĕk′sōs). Any monosaccharide of the general formula $C_6H_{12}O_6$; the group includes particularly dextrose, q.v., and levulose, q.v.

hexosephosphate (hĕks″ōs-fōs′fāt) [Gr. *hex,* six, + *phosphoros,* phosphorus]. A phosphoric acid ester of glucose. One of several esters formed in the muscles and other tissues in the metabolism of carbohydrates.

hexylcaine hydrochloride (hĕk′sĭl-kān). USP. A local anesthetic agent.

hexylresorcinol (hĕks″ĭl-rĕ-sor′sĭ-nŏl). USP. $C_{12}H_{18}O_2$. White needle-shaped crystals used as an anthelmintic.

Hey's ligament (hāz) [William Hey, Brit. surgeon, 1736–1819]. The semilunar lateral margin (falciform margin) of the fossa ovalis, which lies between the iliac and pubic portions of the fascia lata.

HF. 1. *Hageman factor,* blood coagulation factor XII. 2. *high frequency.*

Hf. Chem. symb. for the element hafnium.

Hg [L. *hydrargyrum*]. Chem. symb. for the element mercury.

Hgb. *hemoglobin.*

HgCl₂. Chem. symb. for mercuric chloride; corrosive sublimate.

Hg₂Cl₂. Chem. symb. for mercurous chloride; calomel.

HGF. 1. *human growth factor.* 2. *hyperglycemic-glycogenolytic factor* (glucagon).

HgI₂. Chem. symb. for mercuric iodide.

HgO. Chem. symb. for mercuric oxide.

HgS. Chem. symb. for mercuric sulfide.

HgSO₄. Chem. symb. for mercuric sulfate.

HHS. *Department of Health and Human Services* (of the U.S.).

5-HIAA. 5 *hydroxyindoleacetic acid.*

hiatal hernia. SEE: *hernia, hiatal.*

hiatus (hī-ā′tŭs) [L., an opening]. 1. [NA] An opening, a foramen. 2. An aperture.

   h. aorticus. [NA] Opening in the diaphragm through which pass the aorta and the thoracic duct.

   h. canalis facialis. Hiatus of canal for greater petrosal nerve. SYN: *hiatus fallopii.*

   h. esophageus. [NA] Opening in the diaphragm through which the esophagus passes.

   h. fallopii. H. canalis facialis.

   h. maxillaris. [NA] Opening of maxillary sinus into the nasal cavity, located on the nasal surface of the maxillary bone.

   h., sacral. Opening on the inferior-posterior surface of the sacrum into the sacral canal.

   h. semilunaris. [NA] Groove in the external wall of the middle meatus of the nasal fossa into which the frontal sinus, maxillary sinus, and anterior ethmoid cells drain.

hibernation (hī″bĕr-nā′shŭn) [L. *hiberna,* winter]. Condition of spending the winter asleep and in an almost comatose condition. Some animals adapt to winter by this method.

   h., artificial. State of hibernation produced therapeutically by use of drugs alone or drugs and hypothermia. The rate of metabolism is greatly reduced in this state.

hibernoma (hī″bĕr-nō′mă). A rare multilobular encapsulated tumor that contains fetal fat tissue closely resembling the fat stored in the foot pads of hibernating animals.

Hibiclens. Trade name for chlorhexidine gluconate.

hiccough, hiccup (hĭk′ŭp) [probably of imitative origin]. Spasmodic periodic closure of the glottis following spasmodic lowering of the diaphragm, causing a short, sharp, inspiratory cough. SYN: *singultus.*

ETIOL: It may be caused by indigestion, irritation of diaphragm, alcoholism, new growths of the pleura, certain cerebral lesions, or hysteria. May be due to a disturbance of the phrenic nerve. If prolonged, it has serious significance.

TREAT: Antiemetic drugs, rebreathing in a paper bag, inhalation of carbon dioxide. Stimulation of the nasopharynx with a soft rubber tube; placement of a thin coating of dry granulated sugar in the hypopharynx. If these are not effective, anesthetization of the phrenic nerve may be helpful.

Hicks sign [John Braxton Hicks, Brit. gynecologist, 1823–1897]. Intermittent painless uterine contractions that may occur every 10 to 20 minutes. These contractions may be inapparent to the individual. They appear after the third month of pregnancy. They do not represent true labor pains but are often so interpreted. SYN: *Braxton Hicks sign.*

hidebound disease [AS. *hyd,* a skin, + *bindan,* to tie up]. Hardening and thickening of the skin with loss of elasticity. SYN: *scleroderma.*

hidradenitis (hī-drăd-ĕ-nī′tĭs) [Gr. *hidros,* sweat, + *aden,* gland, + *itis,* inflammation]. Inflammation of sweat glands.

hidradenoma (hī″drăd-ĕ-nō′mă) [″ + ″ + *oma,* tumor]. Adenoma of the sweat glands.

hidrocystoma (hī″drō-sĭs-tō′mă) [″ + *kystis,* cyst, + *oma,* tumor]. A cystic tumor of a sweat gland. SYN: *hydrocystoma.*

hidropoiesis (hī″drō-poy-ē′sĭs) [″ + *poiesis,* formation]. The formation of sweat.

hidropoietic (hī″drō-poy-ĕt′ĭk). Pert. to hidropoiesis. SYN: *sudorific.*

hidrorrhea (hī-drō-rē′ă) [″ + *rhoia,* flow]. Abnormal sweating.

hidrosadenitis (hī″drōs-ăd″ē-nī′tĭs) [″ + *aden,* gland, + *itis,* inflammation]. Inflammation of sweat glands. SYN: *hidradenitis.*

hidrosis (hī-drō′-sĭs) [″ + *osis,* condition]. 1. Formation and excretion of sweat. 2. Excessive sweating.

hidrotic (hī-drŏt′ĭk). 1. Causing the secretion and excretion of sweat. SYN: *diaphoretic; sudorific.* 2. Any drug or medicine that induces sweating.

hieralgia (hī-ĕr-ăl′jē-ă) [Gr. *hieron,* sacrum, + *algos,* pain]. Pain in the region of the sacrum.

hierarchy (hī′răr-kē). The ordering or classification of anything in descending order of importance, or value in the case of numerical data. Thus, one may list the needs of a human being in order of importance, e.g., air, water, food, health, protection from the elements and predators, security, esteem, and love.

hierolisthesis (hī″ĕr-ō-lĭs-thē′sĭs) [″ + *olisthanein,* to slip]. Displacement of the sacrum.

hierophobia (hī″ĕr-ō-fō′bē-ă) [Gr. *hieros,* sacred, + *phobos,* fear]. Abnormal fear of sacred things or persons connected with religion.

high, runners'. SEE: *runners' high.*

high blood pressure. Blood pressure that is above the normal range. A diagnostic judgment or opinion, which must be considered with respect to the person's age, body build, previous blood pressure, and state of mental and physical health at the time the blood pressure is obtained. In general it is not advisable to declare that a person has elevated blood pressure if the opinion is based on one determination of the blood pressure.

RS: blood; blood pressure; hypertension; hypotension; pulse pressure.

high-calorie diet. Diet that includes more calories than normally would be required for a particular individual's metabolic and energy needs. Three meals plus between-meal feedings. Fermentable and bulky foods to be avoided.

IND: Prevention of weight loss in wasting diseases; in high basal metabolism; and after long illness. In deficiency caused by anorexia, poverty, and poor dietary habits. During lactation when 1000 and 1200 extra Cal each day are indicated.

high-cellulose diet. SEE: *high-residue diet.*

high frequency jet ventilation. SEE: *ventilation, high frequency jet.*

Highmore, antrum of (hī′mor) [Nathaniel Highmore, Brit. surgeon, 1613–1685]. The maxillary sinus. SEE: *antrocele.*

Highmore's body. Fibrous tissue mass, a prolongation of albuginea testis, projecting forward along the posterior border of the testis. SYN: *mediastinum testis* [NA].

high-residue diet. Diet that contains considerable amounts of substances such as fiber or cellulose, which the human body is unable to metabolize and absorb. The diet is particularly useful in treating constipation. There is increasing evidence that a diet producing high residue may be beneficial in preventing certain diseases of the gastrointestinal tract. Lay persons refer to high-residue diet as one containing a lot of roughage, q.v. SEE: *fiber.*

high-tech medicine. The recent advances in medical knowledge and technique that have resulted in improved diagnostic, therapeutic, and rehabilitative procedures.

hila (hī′lă) [L.]. Pl. of hilum. SEE: *hilus.*

hilar (hī′lăr). Concerning or belonging to the hilus.

hilitis (hī′lĭ′tĭs) [L. *hilus,* a trifle, + Gr. *itis,* inflammation]. Inflammation of any hilum, esp. the hilum of the lung.

hillock (hĭl'ŏk) [ME. *hilloc*]. A small eminence or projection.

    h., anal. One of two small eminences that lie lateral and posterior to the cloacal membrane and, later, the anal fissure in the embryo.

    h., axon. A small conical elevation on the cell body of a neuron from which the axon arises.

    h., seminal. The colliculus seminalis [NA].

Hill sign [Sir Leonard Erskine Hill, Brit. physiologist, 1866–1952]. When the blood pressure in the leg is 20 to 40 mm of mercury higher than in the arm, this test is classed as positive and indicative of aortic regurgitation.

Hilton's law [John Hilton, Brit. surgeon, 1804–1878]. The trunk of a nerve not only sends branches to a particular muscle, but also sends branches to the joint moved by that muscle and to the skin overlying the insertion of the muscle.

Hilton's line. A white line at the junction of the skin of the perineum and anal mucosa.

Hilton's muscle. The aryepiglottic muscle.

Hilton's sac. A pit along the external portion of the false vocal cords. SYN: *saccule, laryngeal.*

hilum (hī'lŭm) [L.] (pl. *hila*). Hilus.

hilus (hī'lŭs) [L., a trifle] (pl. *hili*). [NA] 1. Depression or recess at exit or entrance of a duct into a gland or of nerves and vessels into an organ. 2. The root of the lungs at level of 4th and 5th dorsal vertebrae.

himantosis (hī″măn-tō'sĭs) [Gr. *himantosis,* a long strap]. Abnormal lengthening of the uvula.

hindbrain (hīnd'brān) [AS. *hindan,* behind, + *bragen,* brain]. The most caudal of the three divisions of the embryonic brain. It differentiates into the metencephalon, which gives rise to the cerebellum and pons, and the myelencephalon, which gives rise to the medulla oblongata. SYN: *rhombencephalon* [NA].

hindfoot (hīnd'foot). Posterior part of the foot consisting of the talus and calcaneus.

hindgut (hīnd'gŭt). The caudal portion of the entodermal tube, which develops into the alimentary canal. It gives rise to the ileum, colon, and rectum.

hind-kidney (hīnd-kĭd'nē). The most caudal of three embryonic kidneys which persists and develops into the permanent kidney. SYN: *metanephros.*

hinge joint. An articulation that permits flexion and extension about a single axis. SYN: *ginglymus.*

Hinton's test [William A. Hinton, U.S. bacteriologist, 1883–1959]. A serological test for syphilis.

hip [AS. *hype*]. 1. Upper part of thigh, formed by the femur and innominate bones. Its three portions are the ilium, ischium, and pubis. SYN: *os coxae.* 2. The region on each side of the pelvis. SEE: *hip joint.*

    h., congenital dislocation of. A congenital defect of the hip joint that is most probably due to multifactorial effects of several abnormal genes.

    h., dislocation of. Dislocation of the hip is very often accompanied by a fracture, and it is extremely difficult even for a well-trained surgeon to distinguish a pure dislocation from a fracture dislocation without roentgenography.

    SYM: Pain, rigidity, loss of function. The dislocation may be obvious by the abnormal position in which the leg is held, or by seeing or feeling the head of the femur in an abnormal position.

    DIAG: Person has great difficulty in straightening the hip following an accident. It is always accompanied by pain. The knee on the injured side resistantly points inwardly toward the other knee, and it is difficult to straighten the leg.

    F.A.: Place the patient on a large splint as for fractured back. In addition, place a large pad, such as a pillow, under the knee of the affected side. Treat for shock if required.

    h., dislocation of, backward. Dislocation of the hip onto the dorsum ilii or sciatic notch.

    SYM: Inward rotation of thigh, with flexion, inversion, adduction, shortening; pain, tenderness; loss of function and immobility.

    TREAT: Patient should be anesthetized. Dorsal position with leg flexed on thigh, and the latter upon the abdomen. Adduct thigh, rotate outward; circumduction outwardly across abdomen, back to straight position. Traction may be required.

    h., dislocation of, downward. This type of hip dislocation is rare.

    TREAT: Traction in flexed position. Outward rotation and extension.

    h., dislocation of, forward. Dislocation of the hip through obturator foramen, on pubis, in perineum, or through fractured acetabulum.

    SYM: Pain, tenderness, and immobility. Shortening in pubic and suprapubic forms; lengthening in obturator and perineal forms.

    TREAT: Hyperextension and direct traction. Flexion, abduction with inward rotations, adduction.

    h., fracture of. A very common occurrence in older persons. It is estimated to occur in one of every three white women older than 85. Osteoporosis, q.v., is the principal condition that predisposes an elderly person to hip fracture.

h., snapping. A slipping around of the hip joint, sometimes producing an audible snapping sound.

h., total replacement of. Orthopedic surgical procedure involving total replacement of the head of the femur and the acetabular portion of the hip joint.

hip joint. Articulation between the femur and the innominate bone. A ball and socket (enarthrosis) formed by the head of the femur fitting into a concavity, the acetabulum.

hip-joint disease. Any disease of the hip joint, esp. tuberculosis.

Hippel's disease, von Hippel-Lindau disease (hĭp′ĕlz, vŏn hĭp′ĕl-lĭn′dow) [Eugen von Hippel, Ger. ophthalmologist, 1867–1939; Arvid Lindau, Swedish pathologist, 1892–1958]. Angiomatosis of the retina and various areas of the body including the central nervous system, spinal cord, and visceral organs.

hippocampal (hĭp″ō-kăm′păl) [Gr. *hippokampos*, seahorse]. Pert. to the hippocampus.

hippocampal commissure. A thin sheet of fibers passing transversely under posterior portion of the corpus callosum. They connect the medial margins of the crura of the fornix. SYN: *commissure of fornix.*

hippocampal fissure. Fissure above the temporal lobe on mesial surface of cerebrum.

hippocampal formation. Olfactory structures lying along the medial margin of the pallium. It includes the hippocampus, dentate gyrus, supracallosal gyrus, longitudinal striae, subcallosal gyrus, diagonal band of Broca, and hippocampal commissure.

hippocampus major. Elevation of floor of the inferior horn of the lateral ventricle of the brain, occupying nearly all of it.

h., digitations of. Three or four shallow grooves on anterior portion of hippocampus.

hippocampus minor. A small elevation on the medial wall of the lateral ventricle formed by end of the calcarine fissure. SYN: *calcar avis* [NA].

Hippocrates (hĭ-pŏk′ră-tēz) [ca. 460–375 B.C.]. Greek physician referred to as the Father of Medicine because he was the first healer to attempt to record medical experiences for future reference. By so doing he established the foundation for the scientific basis of medical practice. SEE: *Hippocratic oath.*

hippocratic facies. The appearance of the face at the time of impending death.

SYM: Dark brown, livid, or lead-colored skin; hollow appearances of eyes; collapse of temples; sharpness of nose; lobes of ears contracting and turning outward.

Hippocratic oath. Oath exacted of his students by Hippocrates: "I swear by Apollo the physician, and Aesculapius, and Hygeia, and Panacea, and all the gods and goddesses, that according to my ability and judgment, I will keep this oath and its stipulation — to reckon him who taught me this art equally dear to me as my parents, to share my substance with him, and to relieve his necessities if required; to look upon his offspring in the same footing as my own brothers, and to teach them this art if they shall wish to learn it, without fee or stipulation, and that by precept, lecture, and every other mode of instruction, I will impart a knowledge of the art to my own sons, and those of my teachers, and to disciples bound by a stipulation and oath according to the law of medicine, but to none other.

"I will follow that system of regimen which, according to my ability and judgment, I consider for the benefit of my patients, and abstain from whatever is deleterious and mischievous. I will give no deadly medicine to anyone if asked, nor suggest any such counsel; and in like manner I will not give to a woman a pessary to produce abortion. With purity and with holiness I will pass my life and practice my art. I will not cut persons laboring under the stone, but will leave this to be done by men who are practitioners of this work. Into whatever houses I enter, I will go into them for the benefit of the sick, and I will abstain from every voluntary act of mischief and corruption; and, further, from the seduction of females or males, of freemen and slaves. Whatever, in connection with my professional practice, or not in connection with it, I see or hear, in the life of men, which ought not to be spoken of abroad, I will not divulge, as reckoning that all such should be kept secret.

"While I continue to keep this Oath unviolated, may it be granted to me to enjoy life and the practice of this art, respected by all men, in all times. But should I trespass and violate this Oath, may the reverse be my lot."

SEE: *Declaration of Geneva; Declaration of Hawaii; Nightingale Pledge; Prayer of Maimonides.*

hippurase (hĭp′ū-rās). Hippuricase, q.v.

hippuria (hĭ-pū′rē-ă) [Gr. *hippos*, horse, + *ouron*, urine]. Large quantities of hippuric acid in the urine.

hippuric acid. Acid formed and excreted by the kidneys. It is formed in the human body from the combination of benzoic acid and glycine, the synthesis taking place in the liver and to a limited extent in the kidney.

hippuricase (hĭ-pūr'ĭ-kās). An enzyme found in the liver, kidney, and other tissues that catalyzes the synthesis of hippuric acid from benzoic acid and glycine. SYN: *hippurase.*

hippus (hĭp'ŭs) [Gr. *hippos,* horse]. Rhythmical and rapid dilatation and contraction of the pupils. Tremor of iris, spasmodic in character.

  h., respiratory. Dilatation during inspiration, and contraction of pupil during expiration.

hirci (hĭr'sī) [L., goats] (sing. *hircus*). Axillary hairs.

hircismus (hĭr-sĭs'mŭs). A malodorous condition of the axillae caused by bacterial action on the sweat.

hircus (hĭr'kŭs) [L., goat]. Sing. of hirci.

Hirschberg's reflex (hĭrsh'bĕrgz) [Leonard Keene Hirschberg, U.S. neurologist, b. 1877]. Adduction of foot when sole at base of great toe is irritated.

Hirschsprung's disease (hĭrsh'sprŭngz) [Harald Hirschsprung, Dan. physician, 1830–1916]. Megacolon due to failure of development of the myenteric plexus of the rectosigmoid area of the large intestine. The colon above the inactive area of the sigmoid dilates and there is chronic constipation, abdominal distention, and fecal impaction.

  TREAT: Surgical excision of affected bowel is the treatment of choice. The remaining normal colon is anastomosed to the anus. SYN: *megacolon.*

hirsute (hŭr'sūt) [L. *hirsutus,* shaggy]. Hairy.

hirsuties (hŭr-sū'shē-ēz). Hirsutism.

hirsutism (hŭr'sūt-ĭzm). Condition characterized by the excessive growth of hair or the presence of hair in unusual places, esp. in women. Hirsutism in women is usually caused by abnormalities of androgen production or metabolism. This may, in patients who do not have an adrenal tumor, be treated symptomatically by shaving, depilatories, or electrolysis. The goal of medical therapy is to decrease androgen production. This may involve use of various agents including hormones or an anti-androgen, cyproterone acetate.

hirudicide (hĭ-rū'dĭ-sīd) [L. *hirudo,* a leech, + *caedere,* to kill]. Any substance that destroys leeches.

hirudin (hĭ-rū'dĭn). A substance present in the secretion of the buccal glands of the leech that prevents coagulation of the blood by inactivating thrombin.

Hirudinea (hĭr"ū-dĭn'ē-ă). A class of Annelida. They are hermaphroditic, lack setae or appendages, and usually possess two suckers. Includes the bloodsucking leeches. A number of species, including *H. medicinalis,* were formerly used extensively for bloodletting.

hirudiniasis (hĭr"ū-dĭn-ī'ă-sĭs). Infestation by leeches. In external hirudiniasis, leeches attach themselves to the skin and suck blood. After the leeches drop off, bleeding may continue as a result of the action of hirudin. Bites may become infected or ulcerate.

  h., internal. Results from accidental ingestion of leeches in drinking water. They may attach themselves to the wall of the pharynx, nasal cavity, or larynx.

Hirudo (hĭ-roo'dō) [L., leech]. A genus of leeches belonging to the family Gnathobdellidae.

His, Jr., Wilhelm (hĭs). German physician, 1863–1934.

  H., bundle of. Atrioventricular bundle (A-V bundle), a group of modified muscle fibers, Purkinje fibers, forming a part of the impulse-conducting system of the heart. It arises in the atrioventricular node and continues in the interventricular septum as a single bundle, the crus commune, which divides into two trunks that pass respectively to the right and left ventricles, fine branches passing to all parts of the ventricles. It conducts impulses from the atria to the ventricles, and this initiates ventricular contraction.

  H.-Werner disease [Heinrich Werner, Ger. physician, 1874–1946]. Trench fever.

Hispanic. An imprecise term that does not indicate a person of a particular ancestry. SEE: *Latino.*

histaffine (hĭs'tă-fēn) [Gr. *histos,* tissue, + L. *affinis,* having affinity for]. Having affinity for tissues.

histaminase (hĭs-tăm'ĭ-nās). An enzyme widely distributed in the body that inactivates histamine.

histamine (hĭs'tă-mĭn, -mēn). A substance, produced from the amino acid histidine, which is normally present in the body. It exerts a pharmacologic action when released from injured cells. The red flush of a burn is due to the local production of histamine. If histamine is injected intradermally and if circulation is normal, a triple response characterized by a small red spot appears within a few seconds, reaches a maximum in about one minute, and then becomes bluish. This is followed by a wheal surrounded by a flare, suggesting a mosquito bite. The final reaction is the development of localized edema at the site of the small red spot. This lasts about 90 seconds. Given intravenously, histamine stimulates gastric secretion, flushing of skin, lowered blood pressure, and headache. Blood pressure returns to normal in a short time because the circulatory system adjusts to the vascular changes and the histamine is inactivated.

Functions of histamine include increasing gastric secretion, dilatation of capillaries, and contraction of bronchial smooth muscle.

h. phosphate. USP. Water-soluble colorless crystals. Sometimes called histamine acid phosphate or histamine diphosphate. Used most frequently as a diagnostic agent in determining the acid-secreting power of the stomach.

histamine blocking agents. Drugs that block the stimulation of cells by histamine. These agents act by interfering with the action of histamine rather than by preventing its secretion. Two classes, the H_1 receptor blocking agents and the H_2 receptor blocking agents, are known and act at different receptor sites. Cimetidine is an example of an H_2 receptor blocking agent.

histamine headache. When histamine is given by injection, an intense headache may appear. Its precise relationship to histaminic cephalalgia is not clear. Some persons will experience headache after drinking types of wine that contain histamine.

histaminemia (hĭs-tăm″ĭ-nē′mē-ă) [histamine + Gr. haima, blood]. Histamine in the blood.

histaminia (hĭs″tă-mĭn′ē-ă). Shock induced by histamine in the body.

histenzyme (hĭst-ĕn′zīm) [Gr. histos, tissue, + en, in, + zyme, leaven]. An enzyme in renal tissues that splits up hippuric acid into benzoic acid and glycocol. SYN: histozyme.

histidase. An enzyme present in the liver that acts on 1-histidine. It splits the imidazole ring with the resultant formation of glutamic and formic acids and ammonia. SYN: histidine ammonia-lyase.

histidine (hĭs′tĭ-dĭn, -dēn). $C_6H_9N_3O_2$. An amino acid obtained by hydrolysis from tissue proteins. Necessary for tissue repair and growth.

histidinemia (hĭs″tĭ-dĭ-nē′mē-ă). A hereditary metabolic disease caused by lack of the enzyme histidase ammonia-lyase, which is normally present in the urine.

histidinuria (hĭs″tĭ-dĭ-nū′rē-ă). Presence of histidine in the urine.

histioblast (hĭs′tē-ō-blăst″). A tissue histiocyte.

histiocyte (hĭs′tē-ō-sīt″) [Gr. histion, little web, + kytos, cell]. A macrophage present in all loose connective tissues. Part of the reticuloendothelial system (RES), q.v., responsible for phagocytosis of foreign antigens. These cells easily ingest trypan blue, colloidal carbon, and other foreign substances of a particulate nature.

histiocytoma (hĭs″tē-ō-sī-tō′mă) [″ + ″ + oma, tumor]. A tumor containing histiocytes.

histiocytosis (hĭs″tē-ō-sī-tō′sĭs) [″ + ″ + osis, condition]. Histocytes in the blood in unusual numbers.

h., lipid. Neimann-Pick disease.

h. X. Letterer-Siwe disease, Hand-Schüller-Christian disease.

histiogenic (hĭs-tē-ō-jĕn′ĭk) [″ + gennan, to form]. Formed by the tissues. SYN: histogenous.

histioid (hĭs′tē-oyd) [″ + eidos, form, shape]. Resembling or composed of one of the body tissues. SYN: histoid.

histioirritative (hĭs″tē-ō-ĭr′ĭ-tā′tĭv) [″ + L. irritare, to excite]. Irritative to connective tissue.

histioma (hĭs″tē-ō′mă) [″ + oma, tumor]. A tissue tumor. SYN: histoma.

histionic (hĭs″tē-ŏn′ĭk). Belonging to or originating in a tissue.

histo- [Gr. histos, web, tissue]. Prefix indicating rel. to tissue.

histoblast (hĭs′tō-blăst) [″ + blastos, germ]. A tissue cell.

histochemistry (hĭs″tō-kĕm′ĭs-trē). Study of chemistry of cells and tissues. It involves use of both light and electron microscopy and special chemical tests and stains.

histochromatosis (hĭs″tō-krō″mă-tō′sĭs) [″ + chroma, color, + osis, condition]. A general term for disorders of the reticuloendothelial system.

histoclastic (hĭs″tō-klăs′tĭk) [″ + klastos, breaking]. Decomposing tissue.

histocompatibility (hĭs″tō-kŏm-păt″ĭ-bĭl′ĭ-tē) A term used to refer to tissues that have antigens of the same HLA complex, q.v., and, therefore, will not cause an immunologic response following transplantation of these tissues from one individual to another.

histocompatibility locus antigens. ABBR: HLA. The multiple antigens, q.v., present on all nucleated cells in the body that identify the cells as "self." These markers determine the compatibility of tissue for transplantation from one individual to another. Creation of histocompatibility antigens is controlled by genes at several sites (loci) on chromosome 6.

By international agreement, the major histocompatibility gene complex (MHC) is called the HLA complex because these antigens were originally found on human lymphocytes, giving them the name human lymphocyte antigens. Antigens from seven sites on chromosome 6, divided into two classes, have been identified in humans. Class I antigens are formed at HLA sites A, B, and C; Class II antigens at HLA sites D, DR, DQ, and DP.

These antigens are important in controlling the presence and magnitude of antibody response. In addition, the HLAs are important in graft-versus-host reactions and autoimmunity.

The presence of specific antigens has been correlated with specific diseases; e.g., HLA-B27 with ankylosing spondylitis; HLA-DR2 with multiple sclerosis; and insulin-dependent (Type I) diabetes mellitus with HLA-DR3, HLA-DR4, and HLA-BfF1. SEE: *major histocompatibility complex.*

histocompatibility genes. The genes comprising the HLA complex that determine the histocompatibility antigenic markers on all nucleated cells. These genes create the antigens by which the immune system recognizes "self" and, therefore, are important in determining the success of transplanted organs and tissues. Many different forms of one particular histocompatibility gene are found at the seven sites on chromosome 6. These different forms are called alleles, q.v. SEE: *histocompatibility locus antigens.*

histocyte (hĭs′tō-sīt) [″ + *kytos,* cell]. A tissue cell. SYN: *histiocyte.*

histodiagnosis (hĭs″tō-dī″ăg-nō′sĭs) [″ + *dia,* through, + *gnosis,* knowledge]. Diagnosis made from examination of the tissues, esp. by use of microscopy.

histodialysis (hĭs″tō-dī-ăl′ĭ-sĭs) [″ + *dialysis,* a loosening]. Disintegration of tissue. SYN: *histolysis.*

histodifferentiation (hĭs″tō-dĭf″ĕr-ĕn″shē-ā′shŭn). The process of cellular maturation in which a primitive cell develops into specific cellular tissue types.

histogenesis (hĭs-tō-jĕn′ĕ-sĭs) [″ + *genesis,* generation, birth]. Development into differentiated tissues of the germ layer; origin and development of tissue.

histogenetic (hĭs″tō-jĕ-nĕt′ĭk). Pert to histogenesis.

histogenous (hĭs-tŏj′ĕ-nŭs). Made by the tissues.

histogram (hĭs′tō-gram) [L. *historia,* observation, + Gr. *gramma,* something written]. A graph showing frequency distributions.

histohematin (hĭs″tō-hĕm′ă-tĭn) [″ + *haima,* blood]. A hemoglobin pigment in various tissues.

histohematogenous (hĭs″tō-hĕm″ă-tŏj′ĕ-nŭs) [″ + ″ + *gennan,* to form]. Arising from both the tissues and the blood.

histoid (hĭs′toyd) [″ + *eidos,* form, shape]. 1. Resembling one of the tissues. 2. Developed from a single tissue, as fibroma.

histoincompatible. Concerning tissues that are sufficiently different from an immunologic standpoint to prevent their use for transplantation. SEE: *histocompatibility antigens.*

histokinesis (hĭs-tō-kĭ-nē′sĭs) [″ + *kine-*

sis, movement]. Movement in the tissues of the body.

histological (hĭs″tō-lŏj′ĭ-kăl) [″ + *logos,* word, reason]. Pert. to histology.

histologist (hĭs-tŏl′ō-jĭst). An individual who specializes in the study of cells and microscopic tissues.

histology (hĭs-tŏl′ō-jē). Study of the microscopic structure of tissue.

    h., normal. Study of healthy tissue.

    h., pathologic. Study of diseased tissue.

histolysis (hĭs-tŏl′ĭ-sĭs) [″ + *lysis,* dissolution]. Disintegration of tissues.

histolytic (hĭs″tō-lĭt′ĭk). Pert. to histolysis.

histoma (hĭs-tō′mă) [″ + *oma,* tumor]. A tumor composed of tissue. SYN: *histioma.*

histone (hĭs′tŏn, -tōn) [Gr. *histos,* web, tissue]. A class of simple proteins present in the chromatin of somatic eukaryote cells. There are at least five classes of histones. Histones combine with the DNA of the cell nucleus.

histonomy (hĭs-tŏn′ō-mē) [″ + *nomos,* law]. The law governing development and structure of tissues.

histonuria (hĭs-tōn-ū′rē-ă) [″ + *ouros,* urine]. Excretion of histones in the urine.

histopathology (hĭs″tō-pă-thŏl′ō-jē) [″ + *pathos,* disease, suffering, + *logos,* word, reason]. Histology of diseased tissues.

histophysiology (hĭs″tō-fĭz″ē-ŏl′ō-jē) [″ + *physis,* nature, + *logos,* word, reason]. Study of functions of cells and tissues.

Histoplasma (hĭs″tō-plăz′mă) [″ + LL. *plasma,* form, mold]. A genus of parasitic fungi.

    H. capsulatum. The causative agent of histoplasmosis, q.v.

histoplasmin (hĭs″tō-plăz′mĭn). USP. An antigen prepared from cultures of *Histoplasma capsulatum* and used as a skin test for the diagnosis of histoplasmosis.

histoplasmosis (hĭs″tō-plăz-mō′sĭs) [″ + ″ + Gr. *osis,* condition]. A systemic, fungal, respiratory disease due to *Histoplasma capsulatum.*

    SYM: The signs and symptoms vary from those of a mild self-limited infection to a severe fatal disease. In the severe form there are fever, anemia, enlargement of spleen and liver, leukopenia, pulmonary involvement, adrenal necrosis, and ulcers of the gastrointestinal tract.

    TREAT: Amphotericin B intravenously.

history (hĭs′tō-rē) [Gr. *historia,* inquiry]. A systematic record of past events as they relate to a person, a period, a country, or a particular group of people.

    h., dental. A record of all aspects of a person's oral health, previous evaluations and treatments, as well as the state of general physical and mental health. SEE: *oral* diagnosis.

h., family. A record of the state of health and medical history of members in the immediate family of the patient that may be of interest to the physician because of genetic or familial tendencies noted.

h., medical. A record of past illnesses and conditions, including prior treatment or medications, that could affect the health of the patient. SEE: *medical history; medical record.*

histotherapy (hĭs″tō-thĕr′ă-pē) [Gr. *histos*, web, tissue, + *therapeia*, treatment]. Administration of animal tissues in the treatment of disease. SYN: *organotherapy.*

histothrombin (hĭs″tō-thrŏm′bĭn) [″ + *thrombos*, a clot]. A thrombin derived from connective tissue.

histotome (hĭs′tō-tōm) [″ + *tome*, incision]. Instrument for cutting tissue into very thin slices for microscopic study of its minute structure. SYN: *microtome.*

histotoxic (hĭs″tō-tŏk′sĭk) [″ + *toxikon*, poison]. Toxic to tissue.

histotribe (hĭs′tō-trīb) [″ + *tribein*, to crush]. Instrument for crushing the tissues to stop bleeding.

histotroph (hĭs′tō-trōf) [″ + *trophe*, nourishment]. Nutritive material, other than the mother's blood, that the embryo utilizes in early development.

histotrophic (hĭs-tō-trŏf′ĭk). 1. Pert. to or favoring the formation of tissue. 2. Pert. to histotroph, q.v.

histotropic (hĭs″tō-trŏp′ĭk) [″ + *trope*, a turning]. Having attraction for tissue cells, as certain parasites, stains, or chemicals.

histozoic (hĭs″tō-zō′ĭk) [″ + *zoe*, life]. Living within or on tissues, said of certain protozoan parasites.

histozyme (hĭs′tō-zīm) [″ + *zyme*, leaven]. A renal enzyme that converts hippuric acid into benzoic acid and glycine, causing fermentation.

histrionic (hĭs″trē-ŏn′ĭk) [L. *histrio*, an actor]. Theatrical, dramatic.

histrionic mania. Dramatic gestures, expressions, and speech in certain psychiatric states.

histrionic personality disorder. Conscious or unconscious overly dramatic behavior for the purpose of drawing attention to one's self.

HIV. *human immunodeficiency virus.* SEE: *AIDS.*

hives (hīvz) [of uncertain origin]. Eruption of very itchy wheals, caused by contact with or ingestion of an allergic substance or food. Sudden sharp changes in climate may produce hives in some persons who are allergic to heat or cold. SYN: *nettle rash; urticaria.*

HL or Hl. latent hyperopia.

hl. hectoliter.

HLA. *histocompatibility locus antigens; human leukocyte antigen.* SEE: *histocompatibility locus antigens.*

HLA complex. The name given to the major histocompatibility complex. It refers to the genes on chromosome 6 that determine the antigenic or "self" markers on all nucleated cells in the body. SEE: *histocompatibility locus antigens.*

Hm. *manifest hyperopia.*

HMD. *hyaline membrane disease.*

HMG. *human menopausal gonadotrophin.*

HMO. *Health Maintenance Organization.*

HMS Liquifilm Ophthalmic. Trade name for medrysone, USP.

HNO₂. Chem. symb. for nitrous acid.

HNO₃. Chem. symb. for nitric acid.

Ho. Chem. symb. for the element holmium.

H₂O. Chem. symb. for water.

H₂O₂. Chem. symb. for hydrogen peroxide.

hoarseness [AS. *has*, harsh]. A rough quality of the voice.
ETIOL: Simple chronic inflammations secondary to chronic nasopharyngitis, chemical irritants, tobacco, or alcohol. Specific causes of chronic laryngitis include: syphilis, tuberculosis, leprosy, neoplasms, papilloma, angioma, fibroma, singer's nodes, carcinoma, paralyses, and prolapse of ventricle of larynx. Virilization of the female usually causes hoarseness. May be caused by overuse of the vocal cords.

hobnail liver. Liver with an irregular surface. SEE: *liver, cirrhosis of; cirrhosis, atrophic.*
ETIOL: Cirrhosis from one of a variety of causes.

Hochsinger's sign (hōk′zĭng-ĕrz) [Karl Hochsinger, Austrian pediatrician, b. 1860]. Closure of fist in tetany when the inner side of the biceps muscle is pressed.

Hodara's disease (hō-dăr′ăz) [Menahem Hodara, Turkish physician, died 1926]. Trichorrhexis nodosa.

Hodgkin's disease (hŏj′kĭns) [Thomas Hodgkin, Brit. physician, 1798–1866]. ABBR: HD. Solid tumor of the lymphoreticular system that can have its origin in any lymphoid tissue, but usually begins in lymph nodes of the supraclavicular, high cervical, or mediastinal area. The malignancy will, if untreated, invade adjacent areas and kill the patient by invading or obstructing vital organs. HD is curable in over 70% of cases. SEE: *Nursing Diagnoses* in *Appendix.*
SYM: Painless enlargement of lymph nodes beginning in the cervical region, then the axillary, inguinal, mediastinal, and mesenteric regions. There are signs due to pressure caused by lymphoid infiltration of blood vessels and organs such as the liver

and spleen. Other symptoms include fever, night sweats, loss of appetite, and weight loss. Some patients experience severe pruritus.

DIAG: Presence of the giant polypoid Reed-Sternberg (RS) cell in tissue obtained for biopsy is diagnostic.

INCIDENCE: The annual crude incidence of HD in the U.S. is 35/million for white males and 26/million for white females. Average age at diagnosis is 32 years, and the mortality rate is about 20%.

TREAT: The goal of therapy is cure, not palliation. This is accomplished in over 70% of patients by use of radiation and combination chemotherapy. Drugs used include nitrogen mustard, vincristine, procarbazine, and prednisone (MOPP), and others. SEE: *lymphoma, non-Hodgkin's.*

Hodgson's disease (hŏj'sŏnz) [Joseph Hodgson, Brit. physician, 1788–1869]. Aneurysmal dilatation of the aorta.

hodoneuromere (hō″dō-nū′rō-mēr) [Gr. *hodos*, path, + *neuron*, nerve, + *meros*, part]. Portion of the primitive trunk including neurons and processes.

hof [Ger., court]. The hollow area of the cell cytoplasm in which the nucleus is imbedded.

Hofbauer cell (hŏf′bow-ĕr) [J. Isfred Isidore Hofbauer, U.S. gynecologist, 1878–1961]. A histiocyte found in the connective tissue of chorionic villi. It is thought to be phagocytic.

Hoffmann's reflex or sign [Johann Hoffmann, Ger. neurologist, 1857–1919]. Flicking or nipping the nail of either the second, third, or fourth finger will, if the reflex is present, cause a flexion of these fingers and maybe the thumb. Its presence indicates tendon reflexes are hyperactive.

hol-, holo- [Gr. *holos*, entire]. Combining form indicating complete, entire, or homogenous.

holandric (hŏl-ăn′drĭk) [″ + *aner*, man]. Transmitted, i.e., inherited only through the males. Thus the genes involved are located on the Y chromosome. SEE: *hologynic.*

holarthritis (hŏl″ăr-thrī′tĭs) [″ + *arthron*, joint, + *itis*, inflammation]. Inflammation of all or many joints.

Holden's line (hōl′dĕnz) [Luther Holden, Brit. anatomist, 1815–1905]. A wrinkle or indistinct furrow in the groin at the junction of the thigh and the abdomen.

holding area. An Emergency Department area in which patients are kept temporarily prior to being transferred to an intensive care unit.

holergastic (hŏl′ĕr-găs′tĭk). Pert. to any psychiatric disorder of major magnitude.

holism (hōl′ĭzm). The philosophy which holds that, in nature, entities such as individuals and other complete organisms function as complete units that cannot be reduced to the sum of their parts. Originally discussed by Jan C. Smuts.

holistic (hō-lĭs′tĭk). Pert. to holism.

holistic medicine. Comprehensive and total care of a patient. In this system, the needs of the patient in all areas, such as physical, emotional, social, spiritual, and economic, are considered and cared for.

Hollenhorst plaques or bodies [R. W. Hollenhorst, U.S. ophthalmologist, b. 1913]. Atheromatous plaques that have lodged in the retinal vessels after having been broken off from the lining of other vessels. They appear as shiny irregular patches in the vessels of the retina.

hollow (hŏl′ō). A depressed area, lower than the surrounding tissue.

 h., Sebileau's [Pierre Sebileau, Fr. anatomist, 1860–1953]. A depression in the floor of the mouth between the tongue and the sublingual glands.

hollow-back. Anterior posterior spinal curvature. SYN: *lordosis.*

Holmgren's test (hōlm′grĕnz) [Alarik F. Holmgren, Swedish physiologist, 1831–1897]. A test in which the patient matches colored skeins of yarn to test for color blindness.

holmium (hŏl′mē-ŭm). SYMB: Ho. At. wt. 164.930; at. no. 67. A rare earth metal.

holoacardius (hŏl″ō-ă-kăr′dē-ŭs) [Gr. *holos*, entire, + *a-*, not, + *kardia*, heart]. A congenitally deformed monozygotic fetus with no heart. The in utero circulation is obtained from the heart of the twin to which the deformed fetus is attached.

holoblastic ova (hŏl″ō-blăs′tĭk) [″ + *blastos*, germ]. Cleavage with segmentation of the entire yolk. Complete division of the egg as opposed to partial or meroblastic cleavage.

holocrine (hŏl′ō-krĭn) [″ + *krinein*, to secrete]. Pert. to a secretory gland or its secretions consisting of altered cells of the same gland. Opposite of merocrine. SEE: *apocrine.*

holodiastolic (hŏl″ō-dī″ă-stŏl′ĭk) [″ + *diastellein*, to expand]. Rel. to the entire diastole, esp. a murmur that occurs during all of diastole.

holoendemic (hŏl″ō-ĕn-dĕm′ĭk) [″ + *en*, in, + *demos*, people]. 1. Term used mostly by those who investigate the epidemiology of malaria. It indicates a spleen rate (spleen enlargement) of 75% or greater in children under age 10. 2. Disease that affects all of the population in the stated area.

holoenzyme (hŏl″ō-ĕn′zīm) [″ + *en*, in, + *zyme*, leaven]. A type of enzyme consisting of a protein portion (apoenzyme) and a non-amino acid part or prosthetic group. SEE: *apoenzyme; prosthetic group.*

holography (hŏl-ŏg′ră-fē) [″ + *graphein,* to write]. A method of producing pictures in which the image appears as a three-dimensional representation of the original object. The picture obtained is called a hologram, i.e., whole message.

hologynic (hŏl″ŏ-jĭn′ĭk) [″ + *gyne,* woman]. Inheritance through females only. SEE: *holandric.*

holomastigote (hŏl″ō-măs′tĭ-gōt) [″ + *mastix,* lash]. Having flagella over the entire surface.

holophrases. Single words, usually verbs, used to convey a variety of meanings. It is common in the development of speech in toddlers.

holophytic (hŏl″ō-fĭt′ĭk) [″ + *phyton,* plant]. Having plantlike characteristics, esp. in reference to protozoa that resemble plants in their metabolic processes.

holoprosencephaly (hŏl″ō-prŏs″ĕn-sĕf′ă-lē) [″ + *proso,* before, + *enkephalos,* brain]. A congenital defect due to an extra chromosome, either trisomy 13-15 or trisomy 18, which causes deficiency in the forebrain.

holorachischisis (hŏl″ō-ră-kĭs′kĭ-sĭs) [″ + *rhachis,* spine, + *schisis,* a splitting]. Complete spina bifida.

holosystolic (hŏl″ō-sĭs-tŏl′ĭk) [″ + *systellein,* to draw together]. Rel. to the entire duration of systole.

holotetanus, holotonia (hŏl-ō-tĕt′ă-nŭs, hŏl″ō-tō′nē-ah) [″ + *tetanos,* tetanus; ″ + *tonos,* tension]. Muscular spasm of the entire body.

holotonic (hŏl″ō-tŏn′ĭk). Pert. to or affected by holotonia.

holotrichous (hŏl-ŏt′rĭ-kŭs) [″ + *thrix,* hair]. Covered entirely with cilia, said of certain protozoa and bacteria.

holozoic (hŏl″ō-zō′ĭk) [″ + *zoion,* animal]. Resembling an animal as to its method of nutrition in which organic materials serve as a source of energy.

Holter monitor. A portable device small enough to be worn by a patient during normal activity. It consists of an electrocardiograph and a recording system capable of storing up to 24 hours of recording of the individual's ECG record. It is particularly useful in obtaining a record of cardiac arrhythmia that would not be discovered by means of an ECG record of only a few minutes' duration.

Holthouse's hernia (hŏlt′howz-ĕs) [Carsten Holthouse, Brit. surgeon, 1810-1901]. Inguinal hernia protruding along the folds of the groin.

homalocephalus (hŏm″ă-lō-sĕf′ă-lŭs) [Gr. *homalos,* level, + *kephale,* head]. A person with a flat skull.

Homans' sign (hō′mănz) [John Homans, U.S. surgeon, 1877-1954]. Pain in the calf when the toe is passively dorsiflexed. An early sign in venous thrombosis of the deep veins of the calf.

homatropine hydrobromide (hō-măt′rō-pēn). USP. An antimuscarinic drug that acts like belladonna. Trade name is Isopto Homatropine.

homatropine methylbromide. USP. An antimuscarinic drug that acts like belladonna. Trade name is Homapin.

homaxial (hō-măk′sē-ăl) [Gr. *homos,* same, + L. *axis,* axis]. Having all axes alike, as a sphere.

home assessment. An evaluation of the home environment of persons with disability, usually by an occupational therapist, for purposes of identifying architectural barriers and safety hazards and recommending modifications or devices for improving mobility, safety, and independent function.

home care. The provision of equipment and services to the patient in the home for the purpose of restoring and maintaining maximal levels of comfort, function, and health of the individual.

homeless person. Literally, a person who, by choice or circumstances, has no place that would be considered a home. The person may sleep in a regular place on the street, in an alley, on a park bench, or in a public place such as a waiting room or subway car, but these locations cannot be classed as homes. Homeless persons are usually, but not necessarily, without financial resources. Generally, these individuals have enormous health care needs.

homeo- [Gr. *homoios,* like, similar]. Prefix indicating likeness or resemblance.

homeodynamics. A principle within the nursing theory of Martha Rogers which suggests that the nature of man is dynamic, everchanging, and holistic. In contrast to homeostasis in which man adapts to his environment, the principle of homeodynamics suggests that man interacts with his environment. Nursing assessment then focuses upon the pattern, rhythm, and source of energy of the patient, rather than coping mechanisms and modes of adaptation.

homeomorphous (hō″mē-ō-mor′fŭs) [″ + *morphe,* form]. Of like shape but not of same composition.

homeo-osteoplasty (hō″mē-ō-ŏs′tē-ō-plăs″tē) [″ + *osteon,* bone, + *plassein,* to form]. Grafting of a piece of bone like the one upon which it is grafted.

homeopathic (hō″mē-ō-păth′ĭk) [″ + *pa-*

thos, disease, suffering]. Pert. to homeopathy.

homeopathist (hō-mē-ŏp'ă-thĭst). One who practices homeopathy.

homeopathy (hō-mē-ŏp'ă-thē) [Gr. *homoios*, like, + *pathos*, disease]. School of medicine, founded by Dr. Samuel Christian Friedrich Hahnemann (1755–1843) in the late 18th century, based on the theory that large doses of drugs that produce symptoms of a disease in healthy people will cure the same symptoms when administered in small amounts. This is loosely based on the theory that "like cures like." SEE: *allopathy*.

homeoplasia (hō"mē-ō-plā'zē-ă) [" + *plassein*, to form]. Formation of new tissue similar to that already existing in a part.

homeoplastic (hō"mē-ō-plăs'tĭk). Rel. to or resembling the structure of adjacent parts.

homeostasis (hō"mē-ō-stā'sĭs) [" + *stasis*, a standing]. State of equilibrium of the internal environment of the body that is maintained by dynamic processes of feedback and regulation. Homeostasis is a dynamic equilibrium.

homeostatic (hō"mē-ō-stăt'ĭk). Pert. to homeostasis.

homeotherapy (hō"mē-ō-thĕr'ă-pē) [" + *therapeia*, treatment]. Treatment or prevention of disease with a substance similar to but not identical with the active causative agent, such as jennerian vaccination.

homeothermal (hō"mē-ō-thĕr'măl) [" + *therme*, heat]. Pert. to a homoiotherm, q.v.

homeotransplant (hō"mē-ō-trăns'plănt) [" + L. *trans*, across, + *plantare*, to plant]. Tissue from one individual transplanted into another of the same species.

homeotransplantation (hō"mē-ō-trăns"plăn-tā'shŭn). Tissue transplantation from one to another of the same species.

homeotypical (hō"mē-ō-tĭp'ĭ-kăl) [" + *typos*, type]. Resembling the typical or normal.

homesickness [AS. *ham*, home, + *seoc*, ill]. Sadness and depression incident to being away from home or loved ones.

homicide (hŏm'ĭ-sīd) [L. *homo*, man, + *caedere*, to kill]. 1. Murder. 2. A murderer.

hominid (hŏm'ĭ-nĭd) [" + *eidos*, form, shape]. A primate of the Hominidae family. Man is the only surviving species.

Homo (hō'mō) [L., man]. A genus of primates of the family Hominidae. The sole living species is man, *Homo sapiens*. Evidence from fossils indicates extinct species, e.g., *Homo habilis, H. erectus, H. australopithecus.*

homo- [Gr. *homos*, same]. Prefix meaning the same or a likeness.

homoblastic (hō"mō-blăs'tĭk) [" + *blastos*, germ]. Developing from a single type of tissue. Opposite of heteroblastic.

homocentric (hō"mō-sĕn'trĭk) [" + *kentron*, center]. Having the same center.

homochronous (hō-mŏk-rō'nŭs) [" + *chronos*, time]. Occurring at the same time or at the same age in each generation.

homocladic (hō"mō-klăd'ĭk) [" + *klados*, branch]. Pert. to an anastomosis between branches of the same artery. Opposite of heterocladic.

homocysteine (hō"mō-sĭs-tē'ĭn). In the catabolism of methionine, the next highest homologue.

homocystine (hō"mō-sĭs'tĭn). A homologue of cystine formed during the catabolism of methionine.

homocystinuria (hō"mō-sĭs-tĭn-ū'rē-ă). An inherited disease caused by the absence of the enzyme essential to the metabolism of homocystine. Clinically the disease is similar to Marfan's syndrome. Patients are mentally retarded and have subluxated lenses, tendency to seizures, liver disease, and failure to grow at a normal rate.

homocytotropic (hō"mō-sī"tō-trŏp'ĭk) [" + *kytos*, cell, + *tropos*, a turning]. Having an affinity for cells of the same species.

homodromous (hō-mŏd'rō-mŭs) [" + *dromos*, running]. Moving in the same direction or toward the same goal.

homoerotic (hō"mō-ĕ-rŏt'ĭk). Homosexual.

homogametic (hō"mō-gă-mĕt'ĭk) [" + *gamos*, marriage]. Pert. to the production of one kind of gamete as regards the sex chromosome. In humans, the XX female is the homogametic sex, as all ova produced contain the X chromosome. SEE: *heterogametic.*

homogenate (hō-mŏj'ĕ-nāt). The material obtained when something is homogenized.

homogeneous (hō"mō-jē'nē-ŭs) [" + *genos*, kind]. Uniform in structure, composition, or nature. Opposite of heterogeneous.

homogenesis (hō-mō-jĕn'ĕ-sĭs) [" + *genesis*, generation, birth]. Reproduction by the same process in succeeding generations. Opposite of heterogenesis.

homogenize (hō-mŏj'ĕ-nīz). To make homogeneous; to produce a uniform emulsion or suspension of two substances normally immiscible.

homogentisic acid. Alkaptone; an acid in the urine due to incomplete oxidation of tyrosine.

homogentisuria (hō"mō-jĕn"tĭ-sū'rē-ă). Alkaptonuria, q.v.

homoglandular (hō"mō-glăn'dū-lăr) [" + L. *glandula*, a little acorn]. Rel. to the same gland.

homograft (hō'mō-grăft). Transplant tissue obtained from the same species. The tissues that survive best are cornea, bone, artery, and cartilage. SYN: *allograft.*

homoiopodal (hō″moy-ŏp′ō-dăl) [Gr. *homoios,* like, + *pous, pod-,* foot]. Having only one kind of process, as nerve cells.

homoiotherm (hō-moy′ō-thĕrm) [″ + *therme,* heat]. A warm-blooded organism. Opposite of poikilotherm.

homokeratoplasty (hō″mō-ker′ă-tō-plăs″tē). A homograft of corneal tissue.

homolateral [Gr. *homos,* same, + L. *latus,* side]. Pert. to or on the same side. Opposite of contralateral. SYN: *ipsilateral.*

homologous (hō-mŏl′ō-gŭs) [″ + *logos,* word, reason]. Similar in fundamental structure and in origin but not necessarily in function. SEE: *heterologous.*
  Ex.: the arm of man, forelimb of a dog, and wing of a bird are homologous structures.

homologous fertilization. Fertilization of the female egg by sperm from the woman's husband. In this context, this is done artificially; i.e., the egg and sperm are united while both are outside the body and then placed intravaginally during the optimum time for fertilization. SEE: *heterologous fertilization.*

homologous organs. Structures that are morphological equivalents, as the arm of man and forelimb of quadrupeds; penis of male and clitoris of female.

homologous series. Compounds with a similar chemical structure and properties, arranged in order of their molecular complexity, such as methane and ethane.

homologous tissues. Tissues identical in structure.

homologous vaccine. Vaccine from the microorganism infecting the patient. SYN: *vaccine, autogenous.*

homologue (hŏm′ō-lŏg). 1. An organ or part common to a number of species. 2. One that corresponds to a part or organ in another structure. 3. In chemistry, any member of a series that resembles the other members in action and general structure but will have a constant compositional difference such as a methyl, CH_3, group.

homology (hō-mŏl′ō-jē) [″ + *logos,* word, reason]. Similarity in structure but not necessarily in function. Opposite of analogy.

homolysin (hō-mŏl′ĭ-sĭn) [″ + *lysis,* dissolution]. An agent in serum destructive to erythrocytes. SYN: *isolysin.*

Homonidae [L. *homo,* man, + Gr. *ideos,* pertaining to]. A family of primates that includes modern and ancient man.

homonomous (hō-mŏn′ō-mŭs) [″ + *nomos,* law]. Pert. to parts arranged in a series that are similar in form and structure, as metameres of a segmented animal or the fingers and toes.

homonymous (hō-mŏn′ĭ-mŭs) [″ + *onyma,* name]. Having the same name.

homonymous diplopia. Diplopia in which the image seen by the right eye is on the right side and vice versa.

homophil (hō-mō-fĭl) [″ + *philein,* to love]. Pert. to an antibody reacting only with a specific antigen.

homophile (hō-mō-fĭl′). Homosexual.

homophobe. One who fears or dislikes homosexuals.

homophobia. Abnormal fear of homosexuals.

homoplastic (hō″mō-plăs′tĭk) [″ + *plassein,* to form]. Having similar form and structure.

homoplasty (hō′mō-plăs″tē). Repair by tissue similar to the one replaced.

Homo sapiens (hō′mō sā′pē-ĕnz) [L. *homo,* man, + *sapiens,* wise, sapient]. The species to which modern man belongs. SEE: *Homo.*

homosexual (hō″mō-sĕks′ū-ăl) [Gr. *homos,* same, + L. *sexus,* sex]. 1. One sexually attracted to another of the same sex. SYN: *homophile.* 2. Pert. to attraction to another of same sex. SEE: *AIDS; asexual; bisexual; gay; heterosexual; homophobe; lesbian.*

homosexuality (hō″mō-sĕks″ū-ăl′ĭ-tē). A condition in which the libido is directed toward one of the same sex.

homostimulant (hŏm″ō-stĭm′ū-lănt) [″ + L. *stimulare,* to arouse]. Stimulating the organ from which an extract is derived.

Homo-Tet. Trade name for tetanus immune globulin.

homothallic (hŏm″ō-thăl′ĭk). In bacteriology, indicating the possibility of mating cells of the same strain.

homotherm (hō′mō-thĕrm) [″ + *therme,* heat]. An animal whose body temperature remains constant regardless of the temperature of the environment. SYN: *animal, warm-blooded.* SEE: *poikilotherm.*

homothermal (hŏm″ō-thĕr′măl). Characterized by maintenance of body temperature at a fairly constant level regardless of the temperature of the environment. SYN: *homoiothermal.*

homotonic (hŏm″ō-tŏn′ĭk) [″ + *tonos,* tension]. Of uniform tension.

homotopic (hŏm″ō-tŏp′ĭk) [″ + *topos,* place]. Occurring at the same site on the body.

homotype (hō′mō-tīp) [″ + *typos,* type]. One organ or part similar in form and function to another, as one of two paired parts or organs.

homotypic (hō′mō-tīp′ĭk). Of the same form and type.

homovanillic acid. ABBR: HVA. Metabolite of catecholamine found in the urine of patients with neuroblastoma. The higher the amount prior to treatment, the better the prognosis of response to treatment.

homozygosis (hōm″ō-zī-gō′sīs) [″ + zygon, yoke, pair, + osis, condition]. Formation of a zygote by the union of gametes that have one or more identical alleles. SEE: heterozygosis.

homozygote (hōm″ō-zī′gōt). A homozygous individual; an individual developing from gametes with similar alleles and thus possessing like pairs of genes for a given hereditary characteristic.

homozygous (hōm″ō-zī-′gŭs). 1. Produced by similar alleles. 2. Said of an organism when germ cells transmit nearly identical alleles resulting from inbreeding.

homunculus (hō-mŭn′kū-lŭs) [L. diminutive of homo, man]. A dwarf in which the parts of the body develop in their normal proportions.

honey [AS. hunig]. A sweet thick liquid substance produced by bees from the nectar gathered from flowers and stored by them for food. The color and flavor are determined by the flowers used. Honey has been used by man as a food since ancient times when it was the principal source of sugar. Allegedly, one of the first fermented sources of alcohol was produced from honey. The alcoholic beverage produced from honey is called mead. About 80% of honey is levulose and dextrose, the remainder mostly water.

Honey is not sterile. Its use in preparing infant's formula has caused botulism. SEE: propolis.

honorific [L. honorificus, honor-making]. To convey honor upon a person, esp. while writing or speaking about an individual. SEE: pejorative.

hook [AS. hok, an angle]. 1. A curved instrument. 2. Term used for the terminal device in an upper extremity orthosis.

hookworm. A parasitic nematode belonging to the superfamily Strongyloidea, esp. Ancylostoma duodenale and Necator americanus, q.v.

hookworm disease. A condition brought about by the presence of the hookworm in the intestinal tract. For complete description and treatment SEE: ancylostomiasis and Necator americanus. SYN: ancylostomiasis; uncinariasis.

Hoover sign [Charles F. Hoover, U.S. physician, 1865-1927]. A test used in suspected unilateral hysterical paralysis. The examiner places a hand under the heel of the paralyzed leg and asks the patient to raise the normal leg against resistance. In hysterical paralysis, the examiner will feel pressure against the hand under the allegedly paralyzed leg. In true paralysis, no pressure will be felt.

hopelessly ill patients. Patients whose illness is such that recovery is not possible and who will die, esp. in the foreseeable future. The question of the physician's ethical responsibility to the patient and close relatives when euthanasia or assisted suicide is requested or discussed is controversial. In 1987 the World Health Association declared: "Euthanasia, that is the act of deliberately ending the life of a patient, even at his own request or at the request of his close relatives, is unethical. This does not prevent the physician from respecting the will of a patient to allow the natural process of death to follow its course in the terminal phase of a sickness." SEE: advance directive; euthanasia; living will; "no code" orders.

hopelessness. The reaction from the feeling that a situation, condition, or illness is without solution or amelioration. This reaction can be seen in either the patient or the health care personnel or both. In certain situations such as grief reaction, q.v., or mourning, there occurs a normal period of feelings of despair, helplessness, and apathy. If this continues for an inordinately long period, hopelessness develops. The alert medical and nursing team will be aware of the development of this reaction and take the appropriate action to prevent its continuation. When those responsible for providing medical care develop the feeling that a patient's condition is hopeless, this leads to the development of their giving up in their efforts to treat the patient effectively. SEE: giving-up; grief reaction; helplessness.

hordeolum (hor-dē′ō-lŭm) [L., barleycorn]. Inflammation of a sebaceous gland of the eyelid. SYN: sty.

h. internum. Suppuration of Zeiss or meibomian glands.

horizontal [L. horizontalis]. 1. Parallel to or in the plane of the horizon. 2. A transverse plane of the body that is at right angles to the vertical axis of the body.

horizontal position. A position in which the patient lies supine and parallel to the floor. Employed in palpitation and auscultation of fetal heartbeat and in operative procedures.

In the abdominal horizontal position the patient lies flat on the abdomen. This position is used in the examination of the back and spinal column.

hormesis (hor-mē′sīs) [Gr. hormesis, rapid motion]. 1. The stimulating effect of a small dose of a substance that is toxic in a larger dose. 2. The controversial hypothetical consideration that very low doses of ionizing radiation may not be harmful, but may even have beneficial effects.

hormion (hor'mē-ŏn) [Gr., little chain]. Junction of the posterior border of the vomer with the sphenoid bone.

hormonagogue (hor-mŏn'ă-gŏg) [Gr. *hormon*, urging on, + *agogos*, leading]. Stimulating or increasing the production of a hormone.

hormonal (hor-mō'năl). Rel. to or acting as a hormone.

hormone (hor'mōn) [Gr. *hormon*, urging on]. 1. A substance that originates in an organ, gland, or part and is conveyed through the blood to another part of the body, stimulating it by chemical action to increase functional activity or to increase secretion of another hormone. 2. The secretion of the ductless glands, e.g., insulin from the pancreas. SEE: *endocrine gland.*

h., adaptive. Hormone produced in response to adapting to stress or some other powerful stimulus.

h., adrenocortical. Hormone secreted by the cortex of the adrenal gland. SEE: *adrenal gland.*

h., adrenocorticotropic. ABBR: ACTH. Hormone secreted by the anterior lobe of the hypophysis (pituitary gland) that stimulates the adrenal cortex. SYN: *corticotropin.*

h.'s, adrenomedullary. Hormones, epinephrine and norepinephrine, produced by the adrenal medulla.

h., androgenic. Hormone that regulates the development and maintenance of the male secondary sexual characteristics; an androgen, q.v. Androgens are secreted by the interstitial tissue of the testis and by the adrenal cortex of both sexes. Includes testosterone, androsterone, and dehydroandrosterone.

h.'s, anterior pituitary. Hormones secreted by the anterior lobe of the hypophysis. They include the growth hormone; thyrotropic (TH); gonadotropic; follicle-stimulating (FSH); interstitial cell-stimulating or luteotropic (ICSH); prolactin; melanocyte-stimulating; and adrenocorticotropic (ACTH) hormones.

h., antidiuretic. Vasopressin. A hormone formed in supraoptic and paraventricular nuclei of hypothalamus and transported to posterior lobe of hypophysis through the hypothalamo-hypophyseal tract. It has an antidiuretic and a pressor effect that elevates blood pressure.

h., calcitonin. Hormone produced in the thyroid gland. Important in regulating calcium and bone metabolism.

h., corpus luteum. Progesterone.

h., cortical. H., adrenocortical, q.v.

h., estrogenic. Hormone, as estrogen, that stimulates the development and main-
tenance of female sexual characteristics. Estrogens are secreted by the ovaries and the placenta in women and by the adrenal cortex in both sexes. Estrogenic hormones include estradiol, estrone, and estriol.

h., follicle. Hormone secreted by the ovarian follicles; an estrogen.

h., follicle-stimulating. ABBR: FSH. Hormone secreted by the anterior lobe of the hypophysis that stimulates maturation of the ovarian follicles in the female. In the male the hormone is important in maintaining spermatogenesis.

h., follicle-stimulating, releasing hormone. ABBR: FSHRH. Hormone from the hypothalamus that regulates release of follicle-stimulating hormone.

h., gastric. Gastrin.

h., gonadotropic. Anterior pituitary hormone affecting the gonads.

h., gonadotropin-releasing. ABBR: GnRH. SEE: *hormone, luteinizing, releasing hormone.*

h., growth, human growth. ABBR: GH. Anterior pituitary hormone promoting normal growth. SYN: *somatotropin.*

h., human placental lactogen. SEE: *human placental lactogen.*

h., immunoregulatory. Hormone that influences components of the immune system, q.v., including the number and activity of the white blood cells. Hormones secreted by almost all of the glands in the body, particularly the hypothalamus and adrenal glands, have been identified as immunoregulatory. They include growth hormone, prolactin, thyroxine, and parathormone, as well as those secreted by and controlling the gonads.

h., inhibitory. Substances that inhibit the release of certain hormones from the pituitary. Somatostatin, which inhibits the release of growth hormone, is included in this group.

h., interstitial cell-stimulating. ABBR: ICSH. H., luteinizing.

h., intestinal. Hormone produced by the mucosa of the intestine. SEE: *cholecystokinin-pancreozymin; secretin.*

h., lactogenic. Prolactin, q.v.

h., lipolytic. Nonspecific term for any hormonal substance that promotes release of free fatty acids from fat tissue, e.g., epinephrine, glucagon, and cortisol.

h., luteal. Hormone produced by the corpus luteum. SYN: *progesterone.*

h., luteinizing. ABBR: LH. Hormone produced by the anterior lobe of the hypophysis that stimulates development of interstitial cells of the testes and the secretion of testosterone by those cells. In the female this hormone, working in conjunction with follicle-stimulating hormone, is responsible for maturation of the follicle of the ovary, and its rupture and transformation into the corpus luteum. SYN: *h., interstitial cell-stimulating (ICSH).*

h., luteinizing, releasing hormone. ABBR: LHRH. Hormone from the hypothalamus that stimulates the synthesis and secretion of follicle-stimulating hormone (FSH) and luteinizing hormone (LH). SYN: *gonadotropin-releasing hormone.*

h., luteotropic. Hormone produced by the anterior lobe of the hypophysis that stimulates the secretion of progesterone by the corpus luteum and secretion of milk by the mammary gland.

h., melanocyte-stimulating. ABBR: MSH. Hormone from the anterior pituitary. It causes pigmentation of the skin.

h., ovarian. Hormone produced by the ovary. SEE: *estradiol; estriol; estrogen; estrone; progesterone.*

h., pancreatic. Hormone produced by the islets of Langerhans of the pancreas. SEE: *insulin.*

h., parathyroid. Hormone secreted by the parathyroid glands that regulates calcium and phosphorus metabolism. Deficiency results in tetany. SEE: *parathormone.*

h.'s, placental. Hormones secreted by the placenta. Include chorionic gonadotropin; a hormone similar to thyroid stimulating hormone (TSH); melanocyte stimulating hormone; and a variety of ACTH.

h., posterior pituitary. Hormone secreted by the posterior lobe of the hypophysis. Includes vasopressin, which produces vasopressor and antidiuretic effects, and oxytocin, which causes contraction of smooth muscle of the uterus.

h., progestational. Progesterone, q.v. SEE: *progestational agent.*

h., progesterone. $C_{21}H_{30}O_2$, a steroid hormone obtained from the corpus luteum or adrenals. It is responsible for changes in uterine endometrium in the second half of the menstrual cycle in preparation for implantation of the blastocyst; development of maternal placenta after implantation; and development of mammary glands.

USES: In treatment of menstrual disorders (amenorrhea, dysmenorrhea) and threatened abortion.

h., prolactin. Hormone of the anterior pituitary that is important in initiating and maintaining lactation.

h., releasing. Substances secreted by the hypothalamus that control or inhibit the release of various hormones. Thyrotropin releasing hormone, gonadotropin releasing hormone, dopamine, growth hormone stim-

ulating hormone, corticotropin hormone-releasing hormone, and somatostatin are included in this group. Dopamine and somatostatin act to inhibit release of the hormones they act upon.

h.'s, sex. Androgenic and estrogenic hormones.

h., somatotrophic. Growth hormone.

h., somatrophin releasing. Growth hormone releasing factor.

h., testicular. Hormone produced by the interstitial tissue of the testis, e.g., testosterone, androsterone, and dehydroandrosterone, q.v.

h., thyroid. Hormone secreted by follicles of the thyroid gland.

h., thyrotropic. Hormone produced by the anterior lobe of the hypophysis that regulates development and functioning of the thyroid gland.

hormonic (hor-mŏn´ĭk) [Gr. *hormon*, urging on]. Rel. to or acting as a hormone. SYN: *hormonal.*

hormonogenesis (hor″mō-nō-jĕn´ĕ-sĭs) [″ + *genesis*, generation, birth]. Production of an internal secretion. SYN: *hormonopoiesis.*

hormonogenic (hor″mō-nō-jĕn´ĭk) [″ + *gennan*, to produce]. Producing hormones. SYN: *hormonopoietic; hormopoietic.*

hormonology (hor″mō-nŏl´ō-jē) [″ + *logos*, word, reason]. The study of hormones. SYN: *clinical endocrinology.*

hormonopoiesis (hor″mō-nō-poy-ē´sĭs) [″ + *poiesis*, formation]. The production of hormones. SYN: *hormonogenesis.*

hormonopoietic (hor″mō-nō-poy-ĕt´ĭk). Rel. to hormones and their formation.

hormonotherapy (hor″mō-nō-thĕr´ă-pē). Therapeutic use of hormones.

hormonotropic (hor″mō-nō-trŏp´ĭk). Stimulation of production of a hormone.

horn. A cutaneous outgrowth composed chiefly of keratin. A hornlike projection. SYN: *cornu.*

h., anterior, of spinal cord. The horn-shaped portion of the gray substance of anterior part of the spinal cord. SEE: *spinal cord.*

h., cicatricial. Cutaneous horn originating in scar tissue.

h., cutaneous. A hard, horny outgrowth from the skin. It is slow-growing, benign, and may be small or large, 10 to 12 cm, in diameter.

h., dorsal. Posterior projection of gray matter of the spinal cord.

h. of Ammon. Hippocampus.

h., posterior. The horn-shaped portion of the gray substance of the posterior part of the spinal cord. SEE: *spinal cord.*

h., sebaceous. A hard protrusion from a

sebaceous gland.

h., ventral. Anterior projection of gray matter of the spinal cord.

h., warty. A hard outgrowth from a wart.

Horner's syndrome (hor'nĕrz) [Johann F. Horner, Swiss ophthalmologist, 1831–1886]. Contraction of the pupil, partial ptosis of the eyelid, enophthalmos, and sometimes loss of sweating over the affected side of the face. Due to paralysis of the cervical sympathetic nerve trunk.

hornet sting. A general urticaria that may result from the sting of this insect.

TREAT: Remove the stinger; apply cold compresses. Household ammonia in 10% solution applied to the area is beneficial, and subsequent soothing lotions such as calamine lotion may be used. If pain is intense, a local anesthetic may be injected. If the systemic reaction is intense, 1 ml of epinephrine of 1:1000 concentration may be given subcutaneously to adults. An injectable antihistamine may be administered subcutaneously or intravenously if given slowly.

horny. 1. Resembling or consisting of horn. 2. Increased sexual drive and interest. The interest may not be accompanied by ability to participate in sexual intercourse.

horopter (hō-rŏp'tĕr) [Gr. *horos*, limit, + *opter*, observer]. Sum of all points in space that have a corresponding point on the retina of the eye.

horripilation (hor''ĭ-pī-lā'shŭn) [L. *horrere*, to bristle, + *pilus*, hair]. Gooseflesh. SYN: *cutis anserina; piloerection.*

horror. A feeling of intense fear, revulsion, or dread caused by seeing or hearing something that is terrifying, shocking, or perceived to be life-threatening to the individual or to others.

horsepower. A unit of power equal to 745.7 watts, or 33,000 foot pounds per minute.

horseshoe fistula. A fistulous tract in a semicircle in front of or behind the anus.

horseshoe kidney. A congenital abnormality in which both kidneys are united at their lower poles, thus forming a horseshoe-shaped mass.

hospice (hŏs'pĭs). An interdisciplinary program of palliative care and supportive services that addresses the physical, spiritual, social, and economic needs of terminally ill patients and their families. This care may be provided in the home or a hospice center.

hospital [L. *hospitalis*, pert. to a guest]. Institution for treatment of the sick and injured.

h., base. A hospital unit within the lines of an army for reception from the front of wounded and sick patients as well as for those within the line.

h., camp. An immobile military unit for care of sick and wounded in camp.

h., evacuation. A mobile advance hospital unit to take the place of field hospitals and to supplement base hospitals.

h., field. A portable military hospital beyond the zone of conflict and beyond the dressing stations.

h., teaching. A hospital concerned with instructing medical students, house officers (residents), and allied health personnel. These endeavors are carried out in conjunction with the hospital's providing medical care. The teaching programs may or may not be part of degree-granting programs, but most are part of a required curriculum for becoming licensed or eligible for certification in a medical or surgical specialty.

hospitalism [L. *hospitalis*, pert. to a guest, + Gr. *-ismos*, condition]. 1. The air of depression and apathy that often surrounds a group of seriously ill patients, esp. if they are in the same and overcrowded ward. 2. A neurotic tendency to seek hospitalization and, once hospitalized, to resist being discharged.

hospitalization. Removal of a patient to, and confinement in, a hospital.

host [L. *hospes*, a stranger]. 1. The organism from which a parasite obtains its nourishment. 2. In embryology, the larger and relatively normal of conjoined twins. 3. In transplantation of tissue, the individual who receives the graft.

h., accidental. Host other than the usual or normal host.

h., alternate. H., intermediate.

h., definitive. 1. The final host or the host in which the parasite reaches sexual maturity. 2. The vertebrate, when the intermediate host is an invertebrate.

h., final. H., definitive.

h., immunocompromised. SEE: *immunocompromised.*

h., intermediate. 1. Host in which a parasite passes through its larval or asexual stages of development. 2. The invertebrate host, when final host is a vertebrate.

h. of predilection. Host preferred by a parasite.

h., primary. H., final.

h., reservoir. Host other than the usual or normal one, one in which a parasite is capable of living and serving as a source of infestation.

h., secondary. H., intermediate.

h., transfer. An interim host that is not essential for the completion of the life cycle of the parasite.

host defense mechanisms. A complex interacting system that protects the host from endogenous and exogenous microorganisms. Included are physical and chemical barriers, inflammatory response, reticuloendothelial system, and immune responses. SEE: *cytokines; interleukin-1; interferon.*

hostility (hŏ-stĭl'ĭ-tē). In psychiatry, the manifestation of anger, animosity, or antagonism in a situation in which such a reaction is unwarranted. Hostility may be directed toward oneself, others, or inanimate objects. It is almost always a symptom of depression.

hot [AS. *hat*, hot].1. Possessing a high temperature. 2. Actively conducting an electric current. 3. Contaminated with dangerous radioactive material.

hot flashes. A symptom complex usually associated with menopause, q.v. Hot flashes, or hot flushes, may start with an aura followed by a feeling of discomfort in the abdominal area, perhaps a chill quickly followed by a feeling of heat moving toward the head. Next the face becomes red, then there is sweating followed by exhaustion. The cause of hot flashes is not completely understood and is controversial. SYN: *hot flushes.* SEE: *menopause.*

hotline. A continuously manned telephone for communicating with persons knowing about or experiencing a crisis, such as suicide contemplation, rape, child abuse, or illicit drug distribution.

Hottentot apron [Hottentot, southern African population]. Excessive elongation of the labia minora seen in Hottentot women. SYN: *velamen vulvae.*

hottentotism (hŏt'ĕn-tŏt-ĭsm) [*Hottentot* + Gr. *-ismos,* condition]. Abnormal form of stuttering.

hot water bag. Rubber or plastic bag of various shapes and sizes for applying dry heat to circumscribed areas and for keeping moist applications warm.

Hounsfield unit. In computerized tomography, a number or value which represents the attenuation of x-rays through a voxel, q.v., in the body, and is assigned to the corresponding pixel, q.v., on the image. This number is relative to the standard which is absorption of x-ray in water.

hourglass contraction. Excessive, irregular contraction of an organ at its center. SEE: *ectasia.*

hourglass stomach. Division of stomach (in form of an hourglass) by a muscular constriction; often associated with gastric ulcer.

housefly. *Musca domestica,* a fly belonging to the order Diptera. Serves as a transmitter of organisms of many infectious diseases.

housemaid's knee. A traumatism resulting from kneeling, which produces a swelling of the bursa anterior to the patella.

house officer. An intern or resident appointed by a hospital to assist in providing medical care. These supervised individuals are receiving medical training in order to meet the requirements for licensure or certification in a medical specialty. SEE: *hospital, teaching.*

house physician. A physician, esp. an intern or resident, who is responsible for caring for patients under the direction of the medical and surgical staff.

house staff. A nonspecific term for interns, residents, and other allied health professionals employed as part of the medical care team for a hospital. Their activities are supervised by the permanent staff of the hospital.

house surgeon. ABBR: H.S. The senior surgical member of the hospital staff who acts for the attending surgeon in his or her absence.

Houston's muscle (hūs'tŏns) [John Houston, Irish surgeon, 1802–1845]. The anterior part of the musculus bulbocavernosus of the penis.

Houston's valves. The normal folds of mucous membrane or valves formed by them in the rectum. They are crescent-shaped. SYN: *plicae transversales recti.*

Howell-Jolly bodies [William H. Howell, U.S. physiologist, 1860–1945; Justin Jolly, Fr. histologist, 1870–1953]. Spherical granules seen in erythrocytes in slides of stained blood. They are thought to be nuclear particles. The bodies are seen in cases of congenital absence of the spleen; following splenectomy; in hemolytic anemia; in pernicious anemia; in thalassemia; and in leukemia.

Howship's lacunae [John Howship, Brit. surgeon, 1781–1841]. Small pits, grooves, or depressions found where resorption of bone is occurring. They are usually occupied by osteoclasts. SEE: *osteoclast.*

Howship's symptom. Paresthesia or pain in the obturator hernia on the inner side of the thigh.

Hp. *haptoglobin.*

H.P. Acthar Gel. Trade name for corticotropin.

HPG. *human pituitary gonadotropin.*

HPL. *human placental lactogen.*

HPLC. *high pressure or high performance liquid chromatography.* Liquid chromatography employing high pressure and short columns to provide separation.

HPO₃. Metaphosphoric acid.

H₃PO₂. Hypophosphorous acid.

H₃PO₃. Phosphorous acid.

H₃PO₄. Orthophosphoric acid.

H₄P₂O₆. Hypophosphoric acid.

hr. *hour.*

H2-receptor antagonists. Chemicals that block the interaction of histamine or acetylcholine with their receptors or parietal cells of the stomach. These agents act as potent inhibitors of gastric acid secretion. Commonly termed H2 blockers. SEE: *hyperchlorhydrosis; peptic ulcer.*

H reflex [after Hoffmann who described it in 1918]. In electrodiagnostic studies of spinal reflexes, the time required for a stimulus applied to a sensory nerve to travel to the spinal cord and return down the motor nerve. SEE: *F response.*

H.S. *house surgeon.*

h.s. *hora somni,* at bedtime.

H₂S. Hydrogen sulfide.

HSA. *human serum albumin.*

H₂SO₃. Sulfurous acid.

H₂SO₄. Sulfuric acid.

H-substance. A substance similar to or identical with histamine.

5-HT. *5-hydroxytryptamine,* serotonin.

Ht. *total hypermetropia.*

ht. *height.*

HTLV-I. *human T-cell lymphotropic virus type I.*

HTLV-II. *human T-cell lymphotropic virus type II.*

HTLV-III. *human T-cell lymphotropic virus type III.*

Hubbard tank. Tank of suitable size and shape for use in active or passive underwater exercises.

hue. A property of color that permits distinguishing one color from another.

Huguier's canal (ū-gē-āz′) [Pierre C. Huguier, Fr. surgeon, 1804–1873]. Canal through which the chorda tympani nerve exits from the cranium.

Huhner test (hoon′ĕr) [Max Huhner, U.S. urologist, 1873–1947]. Test for sterility in the male consisting of aspiration of the vagina within an hour after unprotected coitus to investigate for the presence of motile sperm.

hum. A soft continuous sound.

    h., venous. Sound from large veins in certain anemias.

human [L. *humanus,* human]. Pert. to or characterizing man or mankind.

human bite. Wound caused by human teeth.

    SYM: The aerobic and anaerobic organisms in the mouth cause a severe necrotizing lesion.

    TREAT: Clean the wound thoroughly but do not suture it. Apply a moist dressing and administer tetanus prophylaxis. Both penicillin and a beta-lactamase-resistant penicillin should be given.

human growth hormone, synthetic. Synthetic growth hormone made by using recombinant DNA techniques. Trade name is Humatrope. SEE: *growth hormone, human.*

human immunodeficiency virus. ABBR: HIV. The causative agent of Acquired Immune Deficiency Syndrome (AIDS). SEE: *AIDS.*

human insulin. Insulin prepared by a synthetic process involving use of recombinant DNA technology utilizing strains of *Escherichia coli.* In its effect it is similar to highly purified animal insulins. Trade names are Humulin and Novolin.

humanism. The concept that human interests, values, and dignity are of utmost importance. This concept is integral to the actions and thoughts of those who care for the sick.

human placental lactogen. ABBR: hPL. A hormonal substance produced by the placenta and released to maternal blood. It acts in the last stage of gestation to prepare the breasts for milk production. SYN: *human chorionic somatomammotropin.*

human T-cell lymphotropic virus type I. ABBR: HTLV-I. A virus associated with adult T-cell leukemia.

human T-cell lymphotropic virus type II. ABBR: HTLV-II. A virus associated with hairy cell leukemia.

human T-cell lymphotropic virus type III. ABBR: HTLV-III. A slow-acting virus that causes human immunodeficiency syndrome (AIDS). SYN: *human immunodeficiency virus.*

Humatin. Trade name for paromomycin sulfate.

humectant (hū-mĕk′tănt) [L. *humectus,* moist]. A moistening agent.

humeral (hū′mĕr-ăl) [L. *humerus,* upper arm]. Pert. to the humerus.

humeroradial (hū″mĕr-ō-rā′dē-ăl) [″ + *radius,* wheel spoke, ray]. Pert. to the humerus and radius, esp. in comparison of their length.

humeroscapular (hū″mĕr-ō-skăp′ū-lăr) [″ + *scapula,* shoulder blade]. Concerning the humerus and scapula.

humeroulnar (hū″mĕr-ō-ŭl′năr) [″ + *ulna,* elbow]. Pert. to the humerus and ulna, esp. in comparison of their length.

humerus (hū′mĕr-ŭs) [L., upper arm]. Upper bone of the arm from the elbow (articulating with the ulna and radius) to the shoulder joint, where it articulates with the scapula. SEE: illus.

    h., fracture of. If the fracture is of the upper end, the arm is abducted on a wire splint for about four weeks. Movements of the elbow and wrist are started early, and active movements of the shoulder are begun in about three weeks. SEE: *acromiohumeral; capitellum; cubitus; glenoid cavity.*

    In a fracture of the shaft and lower end of the humerus, the limb is put in plaster in a position midway between pronation and supination with the humerus at right angles to

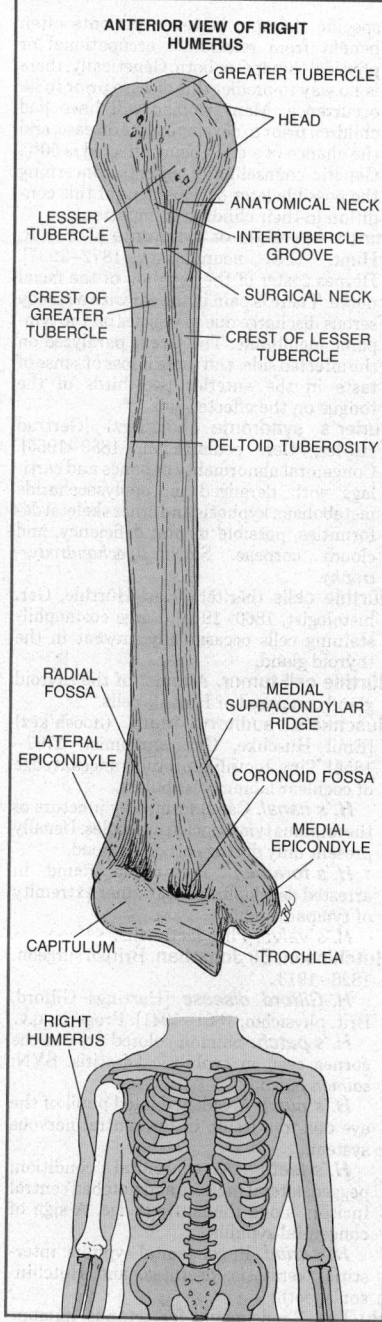

ANTERIOR VIEW OF RIGHT HUMERUS

GREATER TUBERCLE

HEAD

ANATOMICAL NECK

LESSER TUBERCLE

INTERTUBERCLE GROOVE

CREST OF GREATER TUBERCLE

SURGICAL NECK

CREST OF LESSER TUBERCLE

DELTOID TUBEROSITY

RADIAL FOSSA

MEDIAL SUPRACONDYLAR RIDGE

LATERAL EPICONDYLE

CORONOID FOSSA

MEDIAL EPICONDYLE

CAPITULUM

TROCHLEA

RIGHT HUMERUS

Air At Sea Level is Completely Saturated with Water Vapor

At:		If It Contains
F	C	grams
50°	10°	9.6 grams/cubic meter
60°	15.5°	13.3 grams/cubic meter
70°	21°	18.1 grams/cubic meter
90°	32°	32.7 grams/cubic meter

the forearm. Movement of the shoulder, wrist, and finger is allowed at once.

humid [L. *humidus*, moist]. Moist, damp, esp. when pert. to air.

humid gangrene. Gangrene with serous exudation and rapid decomposition. SEE: *gangrene.*

humidifier (hū-mĭd′ĭ-fī″ĕr). Apparatus to increase moisture content of the air in a room.

humidity [L. *humiditas*]. Moisture in the atmosphere.

The moisture content of air usually is expressed as relative humidity. This indicates the amount of water vapor in the air compared to the maximum amount of moisture the air could contain at that temperature and atmospheric pressure. Air that is fully saturated with moisture has 100% relative humidity. When air that is fully saturated is cooled, the excess condenses as in the case of dew or moisture on a cold glass in the summer.

If air was saturated at a temperature of 70°F (21.1°C), water would condense on all objects if the temperature fell to 68°F (20°C). Air can contain at 90°F (32.2°C) almost twice as much water as at 70°F (21.1°C). SEE: table.

Moist air is less dense than completely dry air. This is another reason for humidifying oxygen or air used in inhalation therapy. Also humid air is much less irritating to the respiratory tract mucosa than dry air.

h., relative. Ratio of amount of water vapor present in an air sample to the amount that could be present if the sample were saturated with water vapor. This value is always related to the temperature of the air sample. SEE: table.

humor (hū′mor) [L. *humor*, fluid]. 1. Any fluid or semifluid substance in the body. 2. In ancient medicine, any of the four juices or fluids (blood, phlegm, black bile, yellow bile) of which the body was thought to be composed.

h., aqueous. The clear, watery fluid in the anterior and posterior chambers of the eye. It is produced by the ciliary processes and passes from the posterior to the anterior chamber, and then to the venous system by way of the canal of Schlemm.

h., crystalline. The fluidlike substance of the crystalline lens of the eye.

h., vitreous. The vitreous body. A semifluid, transparent substance occupying the space between the lens and retina.

humoral (hū'mor-ăl) [L. *humor*, fluid]. Pert. to body fluids or substances contained in them.

humpback (hŭmp'băk). 1. Curvature of the spine to such an extent that the back appears to have a lump or protuberance on it. 2. An individual with a humpback. SYN: *gibbous; kyphosis.*

Humulin. Trade name for human insulin.

hunchback (hŭnch'băk). A person with kyphosis such that there is a prominent rounded deformity of the back.

hunger [AS. *hungur*]. 1. A sensation resulting from lack of food, characterized by dull or acute pain referred to the epigastrium or lower part of chest. Usually accompanied by weakness and an overwhelming desire to eat. Hunger pains coincide with powerful contractions of the stomach. Hunger is distinguished from appetite in that the latter is a pleasant sensation based on previous experience that causes one to seek food for the purpose of tasting and enjoying it. 2. To have a strong desire.

h., air. Dyspnea; breathlessness.

hunger contractions. Contractions occurring in the normal empty stomach. They may be painful. A series of such contractions is followed by a period of rest, after which they may return with great intensity unless food is taken.

hunger cure. Restricted diet or fasting for cure of disease.

Hunner's ulcer (hŭn'ĕrz) [Guy LeRoy Hunner, U.S. surgeon, 1868–1957]. SEE: *interstitial cystitis.*

Hunter's canal [John Hunter, Scot. anatomist and surgeon, 1728–1793]. Canalis adductorius. SEE: *canal, adductor.*

Hunter's disease [Charles H. Hunter, Canadian physician, 1873–1955]. Mucopolysaccharidosis II.

hunterian chancre. Indurated, syphilitic chancre. SEE: *chancre.*

Huntington chorea or disease [George Huntington, U.S. physician, 1850–1916]. An inherited disease of the central nervous system that usually has its onset between 30 and 50 years of age. The patient has progressive dementia with bizarre involuntary movements characteristic of chorea. The posture is abnormal. The disease slowly progresses, and death is usually due to an intercurrent infection. There is no effective

specific therapy; however, patients often benefit from referral to occupational or physical therapy, or both. Genetically, there is no way to predict this disease prior to its occurrence. Many women will have had children prior to developing the disease, and the chance of a child being affected is 50%. Genetic counseling of parents concerning the possible later development of this condition in their children is important.

Hunt's neuralgia or syndrome [James R. Hunt, U.S. neurologist, 1872–1937]. Herpes zoster of the ganglion of the facial nerve. There is pain in the ear with a bloody serous discharge due to vesicles on the tympanic membrane. The face is paralyzed on the affected side, and there is loss of sense of taste in the anterior two-thirds of the tongue on the affected side.

Hurler's syndrome (hoor'lĕrz) [Gertrud Hurler, Ger. pediatrician, 1889–1965]. Congenital abnormality of bones and cartilage with deranged mucopolysaccharide metabolism, kyphosis and other skeletal deformities, possible mental deficiency, and cloudy corneae. SYN: *lipochondrodystrophy.*

Hürthle cells (hĕr'tĕl) [Karl Hürthle, Ger. histologist, 1860–1945]. Large eosinophil-staining cells occasionally present in the thyroid gland.

Hürthle cell tumor. A tumor of the thyroid gland composed of Hürthle cells.

Huschke's auditory teeth (hoosh'kēz) [Emil Huschke, Ger. anatomist, 1797–1858]. Tiny, toothlike protuberances at edge of cochlear labium vestibulare.

H.'s canal. Canal formed by juncture of the annulus tympanicus tubercules. Usually present only during early childhood.

H.'s foramen. Perforation found in arrested development near inner extremity of tympanic plate.

H.'s valve. Plica lacrimalis.

Hutchinson, Sir Jonathan. British surgeon, 1828–1913.

H.-Gilford disease [Hastings Gilford, Brit. physician, 1861–1941]. Progeria, q.v.

H.'s patch. Salmon-colored area in the cornea seen in syphilitic keratitis. SYN: *salmon patch.*

H.'s pupil. A widely dilated pupil of the eye due to a lesion in the central nervous system.

H.'s teeth. A congenital condition; pegged, lateral incisors and notched central incisors along the cutting edge. A sign of congenital syphilis.

H.'s triad. In congenital syphilis: interstitial keratosis, deafness, and Hutchinson's teeth.

Hu-Tet. Trade name for tetanus immune

globulin.

Huxley's layer (hŭks'lēz) [Thomas H. Huxley, Brit. physiologist and naturalist, 1825–1895]. Inner layer of nucleated cells forming the inner root sheath of a hair follicle.

HVA. *homovanillic acid.*

hyalin (hī'ă-lĭn) [Gr. *hyalos*, glass]. 1. A clear substance present in tissues that have undergone amyloid degeneration. 2. Material deposited in the glomerulus in certain forms of glomerulonephritis.

hyaline (hī'ă-lĭn). A histologic term rather than a specific indicator of cell injury. It refers to any alteration within cells or in the extracellular space, which gives a homogeneous, glassy, pink appearance in reactive histologic sections stained with hematoxylin and eosin.

hyaline bodies. Homogeneous substance; the result of colloid degeneration; found in degenerated cells. SEE: *degeneration, hyaline.*

hyaline cartilage. The true cartilage. Smooth and pearly, it covers the articular surfaces of bones.

hyaline casts. The most common form of cast found in the urine. They are transparent, pale, and have homogeneous rounded ends. They indicate nephropathy.

hyaline membrane disease. A respiratory disease of the newborn infant. SEE: *respiratory distress syndrome.*

hyalinization (hī'ă-lĭn''ĭ-zā'shŭn). The development of an albuminoid mass in a cell or tissue.

hyalinosis (hī''ă-lĭn-ō'sĭs) [Gr. *hyalos*, glass, + *osis*, condition]. Waxy or hyaline degeneration.

hyalinuria (hī''ă-lĭn-ū'rē-ă) [″ + *ouron*, urine]. Hyalin present in the urine.

hyalitis (hī-ă-lī'tĭs) [″ + *itis*, inflammation]. Inflammation of the vitreous humor. SYN: *hyaloiditis.*

   h., asteroid. One of the spherical or star-shaped bodies in the vitreous of the eye. Due to inflammation.

   h. punctata. A form marked by minute opacities in the vitreous humor.

   h. suppurativa. A purulent inflammation of the vitreous humor.

hyalo- [Gr. *hyalos*, glass]. Prefix indicating resemblance to glass.

hyaloenchondroma (hī''ă-lō-ĕn''kŏn-drō'mă) [″ + *en*, in, + *chondros*, cartilage, + *oma*, tumor]. A chondroma composed of hyaline cartilage.

hyalogen (hī-ăl'ō-jĕn) [″ + *gennan*, to produce]. A protein substance in cartilage and the vitreous humor.

hyaloid (hī'ă-loyd) [″ + *eidos*, form, shape]. Hyaline, glassy.

hyaloid artery. A fetal artery that supplies nutrition to the lens. It disappears in later months of gestation.

hyaloid canal. SEE: *canal, hyaloid.*

hyaloiditis (hī''ă-loyd-ī'tĭs) [″ + *eidos*, form, shape, + *itis*, inflammation]. Inflammation of the hyaloid membrane of the vitreous humor. SYN: *hyalitis.*

hyaloid membrane. Membrane that envelops the vitreous humor.

hyalomere (hī'ă-lō-mēr″) [″ + *meros*, part]. Homogeneous part of a blood platelet, pale in color, as contrasted with the chromomere.

hyalomucoid (hī''ă-lō-mū'koyd) [″ + L. *mucus*, mucus, + Gr. *eidos*, form, shape]. Mucoid in the vitreous body.

hyalonyxis (hī''ă-lō-nĭk'sĭs) [″ + *nyxis*, puncture]. The surgical procedure of puncturing the vitreous body.

hyalophagia, hyalophagy (hī''ă-lō-fā'jē-ă, hī''ă-lŏf'ă-jē) [″ + *phagein*, to eat]. The eating of glass by the demented.

hyalophobia (hī''ă-lō-fō'bē-ă) [″ + *phobos*, fear]. Fear of touching glass.

hyaloplasm (hī'ă-lō-plăzm) [″ + LL. *plasma*, form, mold]. The fluid portion of protoplasm. The basic ground substance; also called basic or fundamental protoplasm. SYN: *hyalotome.*

hyalosis (hī''ă-lō'sĭs) [″ + *osis*, condition]. Pathological changes in the vitreous humor of the eye.

   h., asteroid. Suspended spherical white bodies, made of calcium salts, in the vitreous of the eye.

hyalosome (hī-ăl'ō-sōm) [″ + *soma*, body]. An oval or round structure that resembles the nucleolus of a cell but stains only faintly.

hyalotome (hī-ăl'ō-tōm) [Gr. *hyalos*, glass]. Fluid portion of protoplasm. SYN: *hyaloplasm.*

hyaluronic acid. An acid mucopolysaccharide found in the ground substance of connective tissue that acts as a binding and protective agent. Also found in the synovial fluid and vitreous and aqueous humors.

hyaluronidase (hī''ă-lŭr-ŏn'ĭ-dās). An enzyme found in the testes and present in semen. It depolymerizes hyaluronic acid, thereby increasing the permeability of connective tissues by dissolving the substances that hold body cells together. It acts to disperse the cells of the corona radiata about the newly ovulated ovum, thus facilitating entry of the sperm.

Hyazyme. Trade name for hyaluronidase.

hybrid (hī'brĭd) [L. *hybrida*, mongrel]. The offspring of parents that are different, such as different species.

hybridization (hī'brĭd-ī-zā'shŭn). The production of hybrids by crossbreeding.

hybridoma (hī'''brĭ-dō'mă). The cell produced

by the fusion of an antibody-producing cell and a multiple myeloma cell. This hybrid cell is capable of producing a continuous supply of identical antibodies. SEE: *monoclonal antibodies.*

hydantoin (hī-dăn′tō-ĭn). A colorless base, glycolyl urea, $C_3H_4N_2O_2$, derived from urea or allantoin. SEE: *phenytoin sodium.*

hydatid (hī′dă-tĭd) [Gr. *hydatis*, watery vesicle]. 1. A cyst formed in the tissues, esp. liver, resulting from the development of the larval stage of the dog tapeworm, *Echinococcus granulosus*. The cyst develops slowly, forming a hollow bladder from the inner surface of which hollow brood capsules are formed. These are attached to the mother cyst by slender stalks, or they may fall free into the fluid-filled cavity of the mother cyst. Scolices form on the inner surface of the older brood capsules. In older cysts there is a granular deposit of brood capsules and scolices called hydatid sand. Hydatids may grow for years, sometimes attaining an enormous size. Albendazole, a drug available only from its manufacturer, Smith-Kline Beecham, has been used to treat this disease. It is poorly absorbed and must be used for a prolonged period. It can be toxic to the liver. The cysts should be removed surgically. SYN: *echinococcosis.* 2. A small cystic remnant of an embryonic structure.

    h., sessile. Morgagnian hydatid connected with a testicle.

    h., stalked. Morgagnian hydatid connected with a fallopian tube.

hydatid disease. The disease produced by the cysts of the larval stage of the tapeworm *Echinococcus.* SYN: *echinococcosis.* SEE: *hydatid.*

hydatid fremitus. A tremulous sensation felt on palpating a hydatid tumor.

hydatidiform (hī″dă-tĭd′ĭ-form) [″ + L. *forma*, shape]. Having the form of a hydatid.

hydatid mole. Degenerative process in chorionic villi, which gives rise to multiple benign cysts and rapid growth of uterus with hemorrhage.

    DIAG: Indicated by the hemorrhaging and expulsion of some of the cysts.

hydatidocele (hī″dă-tĭd′ō-sēl) [″ + *kele*, tumor, swelling]. Hydatid cyst of the scrotum or testicle.

hydatid of Morgagni. Cystlike remnant of the mullerian duct that is attached to the fallopian tube.

hydatidoma (hī″dă-tĭd-ō′mă) [″ + *oma*, tumor]. Tumor consisting of hydatids.

hydatidosis (hī″dă-tĭd-ō′sĭs) [Gr. *hydatis*, watery vesicle, + *osis*, condition]. Condition caused by infestation with hydatids.

hydatidostomy (hī″dă-tĭ-dŏs′tō-mē) [″ + *stoma*, mouth]. Evacuation of a hydatid cyst by means of surgery.

hydatidiform (hī-dăt′ĭ-form) [″ + L. *forma*, form]. Hydatidiform.

hydatism (hī′dă-tĭzm) [″ + *-ismos*, condition]. The sound produced by fluid in a cavity.

hydradenitis (hī″drăd-ĕn-ī′tĭs) [Gr. *hydros*, sweat, + *aden*, gland, + *itis*, inflammation]. Inflammation of a sweat gland.

hydradenoma (hī″drăd-ĕ-nō′mă) [″ + ″ + *oma*, tumor]. Tumor of a sweat gland.

hydraeroperitoneum (hī-dră″ĕr-ō-pĕr″ĭ-tō-nē′ŭm) [Gr. *hydor*, water, + *aer*, air, + *peritonaion*, peritoneum]. Collection of fluid and gas in the peritoneal cavity.

hydragogue (hī′dră-gŏg) [″ + *agogos*, leading]. Drug promoting watery evacuation of the bowels, such as magnesium sulfate or sodium phosphate.

hydralazine hydrochloride (hī-drăl′ă-zēn). USP. An antihypertensive drug. Trade name is Apresoline Hydrochloride.

Hydralyn. Trade name for hydralazine hydrochloride, USP.

hydramnion, hydramnios (hī-drăm′nē-ŏn, -ŏs) [″ + *amnion*, a caul on a lamb]. An excess of liquor amnii, which leads to overdistention of the uterus and the possibility of malpresentation. The normal amount is 500 to 1000 ml. It may increase to 2500 ml and not be regarded as abnormal.

    Liquor amnii is secreted by the fetus, and abnormal amounts are probably due to some abnormality of the fetus. Nearly half the cases occur in twin pregnancies. Hydramnion begins about the fifth month and the pressure of the enlarged uterus gives rise to breathlessness, edema, cyanosis, and varicose veins in the mother. The uterus is large for the length of pregnancy. The fetus may be felt bobbing about in the liquor, and the fetal heart is not easily heard.

hydranencephaly (hī″drăn-ĕn-sĕf′ă-lē) [″ + *an-*, not, + *enkephalos*, brain]. Internal hydrocephalus due to congenital absence of the cerebral hemispheres.

hydrargyria (hī″drăr-jĭr′ē-ă) [″ + *argyros*, silver]. Mercury poisoning.

hydrarthrosis (hī″drăr-thrō′sĭs) [″ + *arthron*, joint, + *osis*, condition]. Serous effusion in a joint cavity; white swelling.

    h., intermittent. Intermittent and usually painless swelling of the same joint, a condition that lasts for three to five days. Women are affected more often than men. The period between attacks is commonly two to four weeks, during which time the joints are normal. The knee is the usual joint involved but the elbow, hip, and ankle may be affected. There is no satisfactory treatment.

hydrase (hī′drās). An enzyme that catalyzes

the addition or withdrawal of water from a compound without hydrolysis occurring.

hydrate (hī'drāt). A crystalline substance formed by water combining with various compounds.

hydrated (hī'drā-tĕd) [L. *hydratus*]. Combined chemically with water, forming a hydrate.

hydration (hī-drā'shŭn). 1. The chemical combination of a substance with water. 2. Addition of water to a substance or tissue.

hydraulics (hī-draw'lĭks) [Gr. *hydor*, water, + *aulos*, pipe]. The science of fluids.

hydrazine (hī'drā-zēn). 1. H₄N₂. A colorless gas with a peculiar odor; soluble in water. 2. One of a class derived from hydrazine.

Hydrea. Trade name for hydroxyurea, USP.

hydremia (hī-drē'mē-ă) [Gr. *hydor*, water, + *haima*, blood]. Excess of watery fluid in the blood.

hydrencephalocele (hī"drĕn-sĕf'ă-lō-sēl) [" + *enkephalos*, brain, + *kele*, tumor]. Hernia through a cranial defect of brain substance and meninges, in which fluid occupies the space between the two. SYN: *hydroencephalocele.*

hydrencephalomeningocele (hī"drĕn-sĕf"ă-lō-mĕ-nĭng'gō-sēl) [" + " + *meninx*, membrane, + *kele*, tumor, swelling]. Herniation through a defect in the skull. It contains brain substance and cerebrospinal fluid covered by meningeal tissues.

hydrencephalus (hī"drĕn-sĕf'ă-lŭs). Accumulation of fluid in the cerebral ventricles or outside of the brain. SYN: *hydrocephalus.*

hydrepigastrium (hī"drĕp-ĭ-găs'trē-ŭm) [" + *epi*, upon, + *gaster*, belly]. Accumulation of fluid between the peritoneum and the abdominal muscles.

hydride (hī'drīd). Chemical compound containing hydrogen and an element or radical.

hydrion (hī-drī'ŏn). The hydrogen ion (H⁺).

hydro- [Gr. *hydor*, water]. Prefix pert. to water or to hydrogen.

hydroa (hĭd-rō'ă). Any bullous skin eruption.

hydroappendix (hī"drō-ă-pĕn'dĭks) [" + L. *appendere*, to hang upon]. Watery fluid distending the vermiform appendix.

hydrobilirubin (hī"drō-bĭl"ĭ-roo'bĭn) [" + L. *bilis*, bile, + *ruber*, red]. A brownish-red bile pigment, derived from bilirubin, and thought to be identical with stercobilin and urobilin.

hydrobromate (hī"drō-brō'māt) [" + *bromos*, stench]. A salt of hydrobromic acid.

hydrocalycosis (hī"drō-kăl"ĭ-kō'sĭs) [" + *kalyx*, cup, + *osis*, condition]. Cystic dilation of the renal calix due to obstruction.

hydrocarbon (hī"drō-kăr'bŏn) [" + L. *carbo*, coal]. Compound made up only of hydrogen and carbon.

h., alicyclic. Hydrocarbon that contains cyclic and straight-chain components.

h., aliphatic. A straight-chain hydrocarbon that contains no cyclic component.

h., aromatic. Hydrocarbon in which the carbon atoms are in a ring, or cyclic, configuration.

h., cyclic. Hydrocarbon in which the carbon atoms are in a ring configuration.

h., saturated. Hydrocarbon in which the carbon atoms are linked by a single electron pair and in which all valences are satisfied.

h., unsaturated. Hydrocarbon in which carbon atoms share two or three pairs of electrons.

hydrocele (hī'drō-sēl) [" + *kele*, tumor, swelling]. The accumulation of serous fluid in a saclike cavity, esp. in the tunica vaginalis testis; serous tumors of the testes or associated parts.

h., acute. Most common hydrocele. The majority of cases occur suddenly between the second and fifth years, usually the result of inflammation of the epididymis or testis.

h., cervical. Hydrocele in the neck resulting from accumulation of serous fluid in persistent cervical duct or cleft.

h., chronic. Hydrocele usually seen in men of middle age. May result from filariasis.

h., congenital. Hydrocele present at birth, resulting from failure of closure of the vaginal process.

h., encysted. Hydrocele in the vaginal process in which openings to the scrotal and peritoneal cavities are closed.

h. feminae. Hydrocele in the labium majus or canal of Nuck.

h. hernialis. Condition in which hernia accompanies infantile or congenital hydrocele and there is an accumulation of peritoneal fluid in a hernial sac.

h., infantile. Peritoneal fluid in the tunica vaginalis and vaginal process with the latter closed at the abdominal ring.

h. muliebris. H. feminae.

h., spermatic. Spermatic fluid in the tunica vaginalis of the testes.

h. spinalis. Spina bifida cystica.

hydrocelectomy (hī"drō-sē-lĕk'tō-mē) [" + " + *ektome*, excision]. Surgical removal of a hydrocele.

hydrocephalic [" + *kephale*, head]. Pert. to or affected with hydrocephalus.

hydrocephalocele (hī"drō-sĕf'ă-lō-sēl) [" + " + *kele*, tumor]. Watery hernia of the brain. SYN: *hydrencephalocele.*

hydrocephaloid (hī"drō-sĕf'ă-loyd) [" + " + *eidos*, form, shape]. Resembling or pert. to hydrocephalus.

hydrocephaloid disease. Disease resembling hydrocephalus, but the fontanels of the infant are depressed due to dehydration.

hydrocephalus (hī-drŏ-sĕf'ă-lŭs) [" + *kephale,* head]. The increased accumulation of cerebrospinal fluid within the ventricles of the brain. Results from interference with normal circulation and with absorption of the fluid and esp. from destruction of the foramina of Magendie and Luschka. This may result from developmental anomalies, infection, injury, or brain tumors.

In severe cases in children, the head is usually globular or pyramidal in shape. The face is disproportionately small with eyes hidden in sockets and turned upward. Sutures are separated with bulging fontanels and thin cranial bones. In older individuals, after the skull has formed, there are headache, vomiting, choked disks, atrophy of optic nerve, and mental disturbances. SYN: *hydrencephalus.*

TREAT: If hydrocephalus progresses, the condition is treated by a surgical procedure that utilizes a shunt through which the cerebrospinal fluid flows. The shunt connects the ventricular system with a suitable cavity such as the peritoneum.

PROG: In untreated cases of congenital hydrocephalus, the outcome is fatal in about half of the patients. The prognosis for an uncomplicated course is excellent when hydrocephalus is promptly treated by use of a surgically instituted shunt.

NURSING IMPLICATIONS: *Preop:* Assess for signs of increased intracranial pressure. Particularly in the infant, note bulging of the anterior fontanel and increases in head circumference. Provide adequate nutrition (the infant will need extra head support during feeding). Because the infant's head may be large, head position should be changed frequently, and the head should be assessed for signs of skin breakdown. Lambs' wool may be placed under the infant's head to prevent breakdown of skin in that area.

Postop: Take vital signs every 1 to 2 hours, and do systematic neurological assessment every hour in the immediate postoperative period. In infants, assess the anterior fontanel for bulging or depression. Position the patient as ordered by the physician. Measure and record intake and output, and observe the patient for development of complications such as increased intracranial pressure, dehydration, intracranial infection or septicemia.

The parents will need calm reassurance and emotional support, not only concerning the surgery, but also in terms of the disease process and long-term rehabilitation of their child. SEE: *Nursing Diagnoses* in *Appendix.*

h., communicating. Hydrocephalus in which normal communication between the 4th ventricle and subarachnoid space is maintained.

h., congenital. Chronic type of hydrocephalus occurring in infancy.

h., external. Accumulation of fluid in subdural spaces.

h., internal. Accumulation of fluid within ventricles of the brain.

h., noncommunicating. Hydrocephalus in which a blockage at any location in the ventricular system prevents flow of cerebrospinal fluid to the subarachnoid space.

h., normal pressure. Type of hydrocephalus with enlarged ventricles of the brain with no increase in the spinal fluid pressure or no demonstrable block to the outflow of spinal fluid. Shunting fluids from the dilated ventricles to the peritoneal cavity may be helpful. SEE: *hydrocephalus.*

h., secondary. Hydrocephalus following injury or infections such as meningitis or syphilis.

hydrochlorate (hī''drŏ-klō'rāt) [Gr. *hydor,* water, + *chloros,* green]. Any salt of hydrochloric acid.

hydrochloric acid. An aqueous solution of hydrogen chloride (HCl), containing 35% to 38% HCl by weight. Crude commercial hydrochloric acid is known as muriatic acid.

This normal constituent of gastric juice is produced by the parietal (or oxyntic) cells of gastric glands. The HCl concentration in the stomach is variable, depending upon several factors, including rate of secretion of gastric juice and the type of food eaten. It serves the following functions: converts pepsinogen into pepsin and produces an acid medium favorable for the activity of pepsin; dissolves and disintegrates nucleoproteins and collagen; hydrolyzes sucrose; precipitates caseinogen; inhibits multiplication of bacteria, esp. putrefactive organisms that ferment lactic acid and certain pathogenic forms; stimulates secretion by the duodenum; inhibits the action of ptyalin and thus stops salivary digestion in the stomach.

Average amount found in the food content of stomach is small because of dilution and neutralization by alkaline contents. In pernicious anemia, hydrochloric acid is absent from the stomach (achlorhydria).

hydrochloride (hī''drŏ-klō'rīd). An alkaloid or other base combined with hydrochloric acid.

hydrochlorothiazide (hī''drŏ-klō''rō-thī'ă-zīd). USP. A diuretic. Trade names are Esidrix, HydroDIURIL, Thiuretic, and Zide.

hydrocholecystis (hī''drŏ-kō''li-sĭs'tĭs) [" + *chole,* bile, + *kystis,* bladder]. Dropsy of the gallbladder.

hydrocholeresis (hī″drŏ-kō″lĕr-ē′sĭs) [″ + ″ + *hairesis*, a taking]. Choleresis in which water content of the bile is increased, resulting in production of bile with reduced specific gravity, viscosity, and total solid content.

hydrocholeretic (hī″drŏ-kō″lĕr-rĕt′ĭk). Anything that increases the output of bile without increasing the solids secreted in it.

hydrocirsocele (hī″drŏ-sĭr′sō-sēl) [″ + *kirsos*, varix, + *kele*, tumor, swelling]. Hydrocele combined with varicose veins of spermatic cord.

hydrocodone bitartrate (hī″drŏ-kō′dōn). USP. An analgesic drug. Trade name is Vicodin.

hydrocolloid (hī″drŏ-kŏl′loyd) [″ + *kollodes*, glutinous]. A colloidal suspension in which water is the liquid.

   h. dressing. A flexible dressing made of an adhesive, gumlike (hydrocolloid) material such as karaya or pectin covered with a water-resistant film. The dressing keeps the wound surface moist, but because it excludes air it may promote anaerobic bacterial growth. It should not be used on wounds that are, or are suspected to be, infected. Follow the directions that come with the dressing.

hydrocolpos (hī″drŏ-kŏl′pŏs) [″ + *kolpos*, vagina]. Retention cyst of the vagina containing watery, nonsanguineous fluid or mucus.

hydroconion (hī″drŏ-kō′nē-ŏn) [″ + *konis*, dust]. An atomizer that emits a fine spray.

hydrocortisone (hī′drŏ-kor′tĭ-sōn). The corticosteroid hormone produced by the adrenal cortex. SYN: *cortisol*, q.v.

   h. acetate. Trade names are Cortef Acetate and Cortril Acetate-AS.

hydrocyanic acid. Hydrogen cyanide. SEE: *cyanide poisoning.*

hydrocyst (hī′drŏ-sĭst) [Gr. *hydor*, water, + *kystis*, bladder]. A cyst containing watery fluid.

hydrocystoma [″ + ″ + *oma*, tumor]. Disease marked by small cysts that originate in the sweat gland. Sudamina on the face, esp. in women after middle age. SYN: *hidrocystoma.*

hydrodiascope (hī″drŏ-dī′ă-skōp) [″ + *dia*, through, + *skopein*, to examine]. Device used to treat astigmatism.

hydrodictiotomy (hī″drŏ-dĭk″tē-ŏt′ŏ-mē) [″ + *diktyon*, retina, + *tome*, incision]. A surgical procedure to correct displacement of the retina.

HydroDIURIL. Trade name for hydrochlorothiazide, USP.

hydroencephalocele (hī″drŏ-ĕn-sĕf′ă-lō-sēl) [″ + *enkephalos*, brain, + *kele*, tumor, swelling]. Brain substance expanded into a watery sac protruding through a cleft in the cranium. SYN: *hydrencephalocele.*

hydroflumethiazide (hī″drŏ-floo″mĕ-thī′ă-zīd). USP. A diuretic and antihypertensive drug. Trade names are Diucardin and Saluron.

hydrogel (hī′drŏ-jĕl) [″ + L. *gelare*, to congeal]. A colloid containing water that solidifies in gelatinous form.

hydrogen [″ + *gennan*, to produce]. SYMB: H. At. wt. 1.0079; at. no. 1; sp. gr. 0.069. A liter of the gas at sea level and at 0°C weighs 0.08988 gm. An element existing as a colorless, odorless, and tasteless gas, it possesses one valence electron. Three isotopes of hydrogen (protium, deuterium, and tritium) exist, having atomic weights of approx. 1, 2, and 3, respectively.

   OCCURRENCE: Hydrogen is present in the sun and stars. Even though it is the most abundant element in the known universe, its concentration in the earth's atmosphere is only 0.00005%. Hydrogen occurs in its free state (in natural gases and volcanic eruptions) only in minute quantities. It occurs principally on the earth as hydrogen oxide (water, H_2O) and is a constituent of all hydrocarbons. It is present in all acids and in ionic form is responsible for the properties characteristic of acids. It is present in nearly all organic compounds and is a component of all carbohydrates, proteins, and fats.

   USES: It is highly flammable and used in the oxyhydrogen flame in welding; in hydrogenation of oils for solidifying purposes; as a reducing agent; and in many syntheses.

hydrogen acceptor. In oxidation-reduction reactions, a substance that receives hydrogen atoms from another substance, the donor. SEE: *coenzyme.*

hydrogenase (hī′drŏ-jĕn-ās). An enzyme that catalyzes reduction by molecular hydrogen.

hydrogenate (hī′drŏ-jĕn-āt″). To bring about a combination with hydrogen.

hydrogenation (hī″drŏ-jĕn-ā′shŭn). A process of changing an unsaturated fat to a solid saturated fat by the addition of hydrogen in the presence of a catalyst.

hydrogen cyanide. Hydrocyanic acid, q.v.

hydrogen dioxide. Hydrogen peroxide (H_2O_2).

hydrogen donor. In oxidation-reduction reactions, a substance that gives up hydrogen atoms to another substance, the acceptor.

hydrogen iodide. Acid, hydriodic, q.v.

hydrogen ion. H^+, the positively charged nucleus of a hydrogen atom.

hydrogen ion concentration. [H^+], the relative proportion of hydrogen ions in a solution, the factor responsible for the acidic properties of a solution. SEE: *pH*.

hydrogen ion scale. A scale used to express the degree of acidity or alkalinity of a solution. It extends from 0.00 (total acidity) to 14 (total alkalinity), the numbers running in inverse order of H-ion concentration. The pH value is the negative logarithm of the H-ion concentration of a solution, expressed in gram ions (moles) per liter.

As the hydrogen ion concentration decreases, a change of 1 pH unit means a tenfold decrease in hydrogen ion concentration or true acidity. Thus a solution with a pH of 1.0 is ten times more acid than one with a pH of 2.0 and 100 times more acid than one with a pH of 3.0. A pH of 7.0 indicates neutrality.

As the hydrogen ion concentration varies in a definite reciprocal manner with the hydroxyl ion (OH^-) concentration, a pH reading above 7.0 indicates alkalinity. The arterial blood is slightly alkaline, having a pH of approximately 7.35. SYN: *pH scale*. SEE: *pH*.

hydrogen peroxide. H_2O_2. A colorless syrupy liquid with an irritating odor and acrid taste. It decomposes readily, liberating oxygen. Light is particularly effective in decomposing H_2O_2; therefore it should be stored in tightly sealed glass jars in a dark place.

USES: As a commercial bleaching agent, as an oxidizing and reducing agent. In a 3% aqueous solution, as a mild antiseptic, germicide, and cleansing agent.

h. p., solution of. USP. A standardized aqueous solution of hydrogen peroxide. It has the ability to kill bacteria, and this is its most important use. However, its germicidal activity has been greatly overrated. Organic matter has a tendency to decompose it and as long as there is effervescence when the solution is applied to a wound, there is no great destruction of bacteria.

A solution of hydrogen peroxide has value as a cleansing agent for suppurating wounds and inflamed mucous membranes. It is esp. useful for this purpose because of its development of gas that tends to loosen adherent deposits and detritus, q.v., which might form a breeding place for microorganisms.

Hydrogen peroxide solution is sometimes injected into deep cavities to determine the presence of pus, which will be indicated by effervescence. Because of its lack of toxicity, it is a favored disinfectant for application to various mucous membranes, esp. those of the nose and throat. Diluted with equal parts of water, it is used as a gargle in pharyngitis or mouthwash in stomatitis.

hydrogen sulfide. H_2S. A poisonous, flammable, colorless compound with a characteristic odor of rotten eggs. SEE: *Poisons and Poisoning* in *Appendix*.

hydroglossa (hī″drō-glŏs′ă) [Gr. *hydor*, water, + *glossa*, tongue]. Cystic tumor beneath the tongue. SYN: *ranula*.

hydrogymnasium (hī″drō-jĭm-nā′zē-ŭm) [″ + *gymnazein*, to train naked]. Pool for underwater exercises.

hydrogymnastics (hī″drō-jĭm-năs′tĭks). Underwater exercises.

hydrohematonephrosis (hī″drō-hĕm″ă-tō-nĕf-rō′sĭs) [″ + *haima*, blood, + *nephros*, kidney, + *osis*, condition]. Bloody urine distending the pelvis of the kidney.

hydrohymenitis (hī″drō-hī″mĕn-ī′tĭs) [″ + *hymen*, membrane, + *itis*, inflammation]. Any inflammation of a serous membrane.

hydrokinetics (hī″drō-kī-nĕt′ĭks) [″ + *kinesis*, movement]. Science of fluids in motion.

hydrolabile (hī″drō-lā′bĭl). Having the tendency to lose weight because of loss of fluids, decreased intake of salt or carbohydrate, or excess loss of fluid due to gastrointestinal disease.

hydrolase (hī′drō-lās). An enzyme that causes hydrolysis.

hydrology (hī-drŏl′ō-jē) [″ + *logos*, word, reason]. Science of water in all its aspects.

hydrolysate (hī-drŏl′ĭ-sāt). That produced as a result of hydrolysis.

    h., protein. The amino acids obtained from splitting proteins by hydrolysis. Used as a source of amino acids in certain diets.

hydrolysis (hī-drŏl′ĭ-sĭs) [″ + *lysis*, dissolution]. Any reaction in which water is one of the reactants, more specifically the combination of water with a salt to produce an acid and a base, one of which is more dissociated than the other. Opposed to neutralization. A chemical decomposition in which a substance is split into simpler compounds by the addition or the taking up of the elements of water.

Reactions of this kind are extremely frequent in life processes. The conversion of starch to maltose, of fat to glycerol and fatty acid, and of protein to amino acids are examples of hydrolysis, as are other reactions involved in digestion. A simple example is the reaction in which the hydrolysis of ethyl acetate yields acetic acid and ethyl alcohol: $C_2H_5C_2H_3O_2 + H_2O = CH_3COOH + C_2H_5OH$. Usually such reactions are reversible; the reversed reaction is called neutralization, esterification, or condensation. SEE: *assimilation; enzyme*.

hydrolytic (hī-drō-lĭt′ĭk). Rel. to hydrolysis.

hydrolyze (hī′drō-līz). To cause to undergo hydrolysis.

hydroma (hī-drō′mă) [Gr. *hydor*, water, + *oma*, tumor]. 1. Hygroma. 2. Any cyst containing a watery substance.

hydromassage. Production of massage by use of a stream of water.

hydromeiosis (hī″drō-mī-ō′sĭs) [″ + *meiosis*, diminution]. Swelling of the epidermis after it is exposed to water with consequent blockage of the sweat ducts. This phenomenon limits loss of fluids from sweating when the body is immersed in water.

hydromeningitis (hī″drō-mĕn″ĭn-jī′tĭs) [″ + *meninx*, membrane, + *itis*, inflammation]. 1. Inflammation of membranes of brain with serous effusion. 2. Inflammation of Descemet's membrane.

hydromeningocele (hī″drō-mĕn-ĭn′gō-sēl) [″ + ″ + *kele*, tumor, swelling]. Protrusion of meninges or spinal cord in a sac of fluid.

hydrometer (hī-drŏm′ĕ-tĕr) [″ + *metron*, measure]. An instrument that measures the density of a liquid by the depth to which a graduated scale sinks into the liquid.

hydrometra (hī″drō-mē′tră) [″ + *metra*, uterus]. Collection of watery fluid or mucus in the uterus.

hydrometrocolpos (hī″drō-mē″trō-kŏl′pŏs) [″ + *metra*, uterus, + *kolpos*, vagina]. Distention of the uterus by a collection of watery fluid.

hydromicrocephaly (hī″drō-mī″krō-sĕf′ă-lē) [″ + *mikros*, small, + *kephale*, head]. Condition in which there is a small head that contains an increased amount of cerebrospinal fluid.

hydromorphone hydrochloride (hī″drō-mor′fŏn). USP. An analgesic drug. Trade name is Dilaudid.

Hydromox. Trade name for quinethazone, USP.

hydromphalus (hī-drŏm′fă-lŭs) [″ + *omphalos*, navel]. Watery tumor at the umbilicus.

hydromyelia (hī″drō-mī-ē′lē-ă) [″ + *myelos*, marrow]. Increased fluid in the central canal of the spinal cord. SYN: *hydrorrhachis.*

hydromyelocele (hī″drō-mī-ĕl′ō-sēl) [″ + ″ + *kele*, tumor, swelling]. Protrusion of a sac with cerebrospinal fluid through a spina bifida.

hydromyelomeningocele (hī″drō-mī″ĕ-lō-mĕ-nĭng′gō-sēl) [″ + *myelos*, marrow, + *meninx*, membrane, + *kele*, tumor, swelling]. Deformity of the spine through which a fluid-filled sac containing the spinal cord tissue and membranes protrudes.

hydromyoma (hī″drō-mī-ō′mă) [″ + *mys*, muscle, + *oma*, tumor]. Cystic fibroid, usually uterine, filled with fluid.

hydronephrosis (hī″drō-nĕf-rō′sĭs) [″ +

nephros, kidney, + *osis*, condition]. Collection of urine in the renal pelvis due to obstructed outflow, forming a cyst by production of distention and atrophy of organ. SYN: *nephrohydrosis; nephrydrosis.*

DIAG: Large, fluctuating, soft mass in region of kidney, appearing and disappearing as retained urine passes into the ureters and bladder.

TREAT: Aspiration, nephrectomy, or nephrotomy depending on the severity of the disease. Medical or surgical removal of the cause of the retention is indicated.

hydroparasalpinx (hī″drō-păr′ă-săl′pĭnks) [Gr. *hydor*, water, + *para*, beside, + *salpinx*, tube]. Accumulation of serous fluid in the accessory tubes of the fallopian tube.

hydroparotitis (hī″drō-păr″ō-tī′tĭs) [″ + ″ + *ous*, ear, + *itis*, inflammation]. Accumulation of fluid in the parotid gland.

hydropenia (hī″drō-pē′nē-ă) [″ + *penia*, poverty]. Deficiency in body water.

hydropericarditis [″ + *peri*, around, + *kardia*, heart, + *itis*, inflammation]. Serous effusion accompanying pericarditis.

hydropericardium (hī″drō-pĕr″ĭ-kăr′dē-ŭm). Pericardial dropsy. Accumulation of water in pericardial sac without inflammation.

SYM: Distress in region of heart; diminished cardiac function with signs of heart failure; dysphagia; and dyspnea.

TREAT: Paracentesis. Definitive therapy depends upon cause of disease.

hydroperinephrosis (hī″drō-pĕr″ĭ-nĕ-frō′sĭs) [″ + *peri*, around, + *nephros*, kidney, + *osis*, condition]. Accumulation of serum of connective tissue surrounding the kidney.

hydroperion (hī″drō-pĕr′ē-ŏn) [″ + ″ + *oon*, egg]. Fluid present between decidua capsularis and decidua parietalis; occurs early in pregnancy.

hydroperitoneum (hī″drō-pĕr″ĭ-tō-nē′ŭm) [″ + *peritonaion*, peritoneum]. Accumulation of fluid in peritoneal cavity. SYN: *ascites.*

hydropexis (hī″drō-pĕk′sĭs) [″ + *pexis*, fixation]. The retaining or fixing of water.

hydrophilia (hī-drō-fĭl′ē-ă) [″ + *philein*, to love]. Hydrophilism, q.v.

hydrophilic ointment. USP. A standardized ointment preparation used topically as an emollient. It is an oil-in-water emulsion.

hydrophilism (hī-drŏf′ĭ-lĭzm) [″ + ″ + *-ismos*, condition]. Tendency of tissues to attract and hold water. SYN: *hydrophilia.*

hydrophilous (hī-drŏf′ĭ-lŭs). Taking up moisture. SYN: *bibulous; hygroscopic.*

hydrophobia (hī-drō-fō′bē-ă) [Gr. *hydor*, water, + *phobos*, fear]. 1. Morbid fear of water. 2. Common name for rabies, q.v., resulting from bite of a rabid animal. SYN: *lyssa.*

hydrophobophobia (hī″drō-fō″bō-fō′bē-ă) [″ + ″ + *phobos*, fear]. Morbid fear of contracting hydrophobia (rabies), sometimes resulting in a hysterical condition resembling hydrophobia.

hydrophthalmos (hī″drŏf-thăl′mŏs) [″ + *ophthalmos*, eye]. Distention of the eyeball due to accumulation of fluid within it.

hydrophysometra (hī″drō-fī″sō-mē′tră) [″ + *physa*, air, + *metra*, uterus]. Presence of water and gas in the uterus.

hydropic (hī-drŏp′ĭk) [Gr. *hydropikos*]. Dropsical or pert. to dropsy.

hydropneumatosis (hī″drō-nū″mă-tō′sĭs) [″ + *pneumatosis*, inflation]. Liquid and gas in the tissues producing combined edema and emphysema.

hydropneumopericardium (hī″drō-nū″mō-pĕr-ĭ-kăr′dē-ŭm) [″ + ″ + *peri*, around, + *kardia*, heart]. Serous effusion with gas in the pericardium.

hydropneumoperitoneum (hī″drō-nū″mō-pĕr″ĭ-tō-nē′ŭm) [″ + ″ + *peritonaion*, peritoneum]. Gas and serous fluid in the peritoneal cavity.

hydropneumothorax (hī″drō-nū″mō-thō′răks) [″ + ″ + *thorax*, chest]. Gas and serous effusion in pleural cavity. SYN: *pneumohydrothorax.*

hydrops, hydropsy (hī′drŏps, hī-drŏp′sē) [Gr.]. Dropsy or edema.

    h. abdominis. Edema of the abdominal cavity. SYN: *ascites.*

    h., endolymphatic. H., labyrinthine.

    h. fetalis. The clinical condition in infants of cardiac decompensation with hepatosplenomegaly, respiratory distress, and circulatory distress. This may be caused by erythroblastosis fetalis; infections; tumors; pulmonary, hepatic, or renal disease; diabetes mellitus; Gaucher's disease; or multiple congenital anomalies. SEE: *erythroblastosis fetalis.*

    h. folliculi. Accumulation of fluid in the graafian follicle of the ovary.

    h. gravidarum. Edema accompanying pregnancy.

    h., labyrinthine. Dilatation due to an accumulation of fluid in the endolymphatic space of the ear. A characteristic of Ménière's disease, q.v.

    h. tubae. Collection of fluid in a fallopian tube. SYN: *hydrosalpinx.*

    h. tubae profluens. Edema of the fallopian tube in which the distention becomes so great that the tube is forced to empty itself by the pressure, the emptying taking place via the uterine cavity. SYN: *hydrosalpinx, intermittent.*

hydropyonephrosis (hī″drō-pī″ō-nĕf-rō′sĭs) [Gr. *hydor*, water, + *pyon*, pus, + *nephros*, kidney, + *osis*, condition]. Dilatation of kidney pelvis with pus and urine.

hydroquinone (hī″drō-kwĭn′ōn). USP. A weak but safe depigmenting agent, used topically. Trade names include Black and White Bleaching Cream, Eldoquin, and Eldopaque.

hydrorheostat (hī″drō-rē′ō-stăt) [″ + *rheos*, current, + *histanai*, to place]. A device used to control the flow of electric current by changes in water resistance.

hydrorrhachis (hī-dror′ă-kĭs) [″ + *rhachis*, spine]. Condition of increased cerebrospinal fluid between membranes and the spinal cord or its central canal or cavities. SYN: *hydromyelia.*

hydrorrhachitis (hī-dror-ă-kī′tĭs) [″ + ″ + *itis*, inflammation]. Serous effusion from the spinal cord or its membranes with inflammation of the cord.

hydrorrhea (hī″drō-rē′ă) [″ + *rhoia*, flow]. Copious watery discharge from any part, as from the nose.

    h. gravidarum. Discharge of a watery fluid from the vagina during pregnancy.

hydrosalpinx (hī″drō-săl′pĭnks) [″ + *salpinx*, tube]. Distention of the fallopian tube by clear fluid.

    h., intermittent. A discharge of watery fluid from the fallopian tube. SYN: *hydrops tubae profluens.*

hydrosarcocele (hī″drō-săr′kō-sēl) [″ + *sarx*, flesh, + *kele*, tumor, swelling]. Hydrocele with chronic swelling of the testis.

hydroscheocele (hī-drŏs′kē-ō-sēl″) [″ + *oscheon*, scrotum, + *kele*, tumor, swelling]. Scrotal hernia that contains serous fluid.

hydrosis (hī-drō′sĭs). Hidrosis.

hydrosol (hī′drō-sŏl). The fluid state of a colloidal solution; a sol. State of a colloidal solution in which the colloid particles, separated by water in a continuous phase, are free to move about. SEE: *hydrogel.*

hydrosphygmograph (hī″drō-sfĭg′mō-grăf) [″ + *sphygmos*, pulse, + *graphein*, to write]. Sphygmograph with indicator consisting of a column of water.

hydrostat (hī′drō-stăt) [″ + *statikos*, standing]. Device that maintains the water level in a container at a predetermined level.

hydrostatic (hī″drō-stăt′ĭk) [″ + *statikos*, standing]. Pert. to the pressure of liquids in equilibrium and that exerted on liquids.

hydrostatic densitometry. An underwater weighing technique for the determination of the specific gravity of an individual. The amount of water displaced by the body is corrected for the air contained in the lungs. An accurate determination of body components (e.g., the percentage of fat) can be made. SYN: *hydrostatic weighing.*

hydrostatics (hī″drō-stăt′ĭks). Science of properties of fluids in equilibrium.

hydrostatic test. Putting lungs of a dead infant in water. If they float, the infant has breathed prior to death.

hydrostatic weighing. Hydrostatic densitometry, q.v.

hydrosudotherapy (hī″drō-soo″dō-thĕr′ă-pē) [″ + L. *sudor,* sweat, + Gr. *therapeia,* treatment]. Treatment of disease by sweating and hydrotherapy.

hydrosulfuric acid. Hydrogen sulfide.

hydrosyringomyelia (hī″drō-sĭr-ĭng″ō-mī-ē′lē-ă) [″ + *syrinx,* tube, + *myelos,* marrow]. Distention of the central canal of the spinal cord with effusion of fluid and formation of cavities.

hydrotaxis (hī″drō-tăk′sĭs) [″ + *taxis,* arrangement]. The response of an organism or cell toward or away from moisture. SEE: *hydrotropism.*

hydrotherapeutics (hī″drō-thĕr″ă-pū′tĭks) [Gr. *hydor,* water, + *therapeia,* treatment]. Treatment of disease with water. SYN: *hydrotherapy.*

hydrotherapist (hī″drō-thĕr′ă-pĭst). One who practices hydrotherapy.

hydrotherapy (hī-drō-thĕr′ă-pē) [″ + *therapeia,* treatment]. Scientific application of water in treatment of disease. The therapeutic effects of hydrotherapy are as follows:

Buoyancy: Used to treat conditions such as arthritis or paralysis where the buoyancy effects relieve the stress of weight bearing and allow freer motion.

Brief hot tub and shower baths: Relieve fatigue, produce general relaxation.

Cold baths and applications: Cool the body or body part and stimulate it, esp. if followed by friction and percussion. They contract the small blood vessels when applied locally.

Cold and hot applications: One followed by the other stimulates the cardiovascular system both generally and locally.

Gradually elevated temperature of hot tub and vapor baths: Produces general muscular relaxation.

Hot baths: Relax tissues, including capillaries of skin, drawing blood from deeper tissues; also relieve pain.

Resistance: Viscosity of the water causes resistance to movement and can be used for therapeutic exercise. The faster the movement, the greater the resistance.

Whirlpool: A water bath where the water is agitated by an electric turbine. Besides the value of water temperature, buoyancy, and viscosity, debridement of wounds is assisted.

hydrothermic (hī″drō-thĕr′mĭk). Concern-

ing the effect of heated water.

hydrothionammonemia (hī″drō-thī″ō-năm″ō-nē′mē-ă) [″ + *theion,* sulfur, + *ammoniakos,* of Amen, from near whose temple it came, + *haima,* blood]. Ammonium sulfide in the blood.

hydrothionemia (hī″drō-thī″ō-nē′mē-ă) [″ + ″ + *haima,* blood]. Condition caused by hydrogen sulfide in the blood.

hydrothionuria (hī″drō-thī″ō-nū′rē-ă) [″ + ″ + *ouron,* urine]. Condition caused by hydrogen sulfide in the urine.

hydrothorax (hī″drō-thō′răks) [″ + *thorax,* chest]. A noninflammatory collection of fluid in the pleural cavity.

SYM: Dyspnea; absence of vesicular breath sounds; murmur; flatness over location of fluid.

hydrotis (hī-drō′tĭs) [″ + *ous,* ear]. Serous effusion in the internal ear or tympanum.

hydrotomy (hī-drŏt′ō-mē) [″ + *tome,* incision]. Dissection of tissue by forcible injection of water.

hydrotropism (hī″drō-trō′pĭzm) [″ + *trope,* a turning]. Response of plants toward (positive hydrotropism) or away from (negative hydrotropism) moisture.

hydrotympanum (hī″drō-tĭm′pă-nŭm) [″ + *tympanon,* drum]. Edema fluid in the middle ear.

hydroureter (hī″drō-ū-rē′tĕr) [″ + *oureter,* ureter]. Distention of ureter with fluid due to obstruction.

hydrous (hī′drŭs). Containing water. SEE: *anhydrous.*

hydrovarium (hī″drō-vā′rē-ŭm) [″ + LL. *ovarium,* ovary]. Edema or cyst of the ovary.

hydroxide (hī-drŏk′sīd) [″ + *oxys,* sour]. A compound that contains the hydroxyl (—OH) group, such as NaOH (sodium hydroxide, or caustic soda).

hydroxocobalamin (hī-drŏk″sō-kō-băl′ă-mĭn). USP. A chemical that has the activity of vitamin B_{12}. Its use intramuscularly is contraindicated because it can stimulate the production of antibodies to vitamin B_{12}. Trade names are alphaRedisol and NeoBetalin 12.

hydroxy acids (hī-drŏk′sē). Acids containing one or more hydroxyl (—OH) groups in addition to the carboxyl (C—O—O—H) group, such as lactic acid, $CH_3COHCOOH$.

hydroxyamphetamine hydrobromide (hī-drŏk″sē-ăm-fĕt′ă-mēn hī″drō-brō′mīd). USP. An amphetamine with little ability to stimulate the central nervous system. Used as a solution placed in the eye, where it has ephedrine-like action. Trade name is Paredrine.

hydroxyapatite (hī-drŏk″sē-ăp′ă-tīt). The apatite form of calcium phosphate present with calcium carbonate in the bones and skeleton. In teeth it is soluble in the acids of soft drinks or carbohydrate fermentation, but it becomes decay-resistant fluoroapatite after combining with fluoride ions present in fluoridated water or fluoride supplement.

hydroxybenzene (hī-drŏk″sē-bĕn′zēn). Phenol.

hydroxybutyric acid. An acid present in the urine, esp. in diabetes, when fat is abnormally metabolized in ketosis.

hydroxybutyric dehydrogenase. A serum enzyme that is increased in myocardial infarction.

hydroxychloroquine sulfate (hī-drŏk″sē-klō′rō-kwĭn). USP. An antimalarial drug. Trade name is Plaquenil Sulfate.

25-hydroxycholecalciferol (hī-drŏk″sē-kō″lē-kăl-sĭf′ĕ-rŏl). A vitamin D derivative.

17-hydroxycorticosterone (hī-drŏk″sē-kor″tĭ-kō-stēr′ōn). Hydrocortisone.

hydroxydione sodium succinate (hī-drŏk″sē-dī′ōn). A steroid drug used intravenously as an anesthetic. It has no hormonal action.

hydroxyl. The univalent radical OH, that, when combined with a metallic ion or a radical that acts as a metal (e.g., NH_4), forms a hydroxide. Commonly called a base or alkali.

hydroxylase (hī-drŏk′sĭ-lās). Any enzyme that catalyzes the introduction of hydrogen into a substrate.

hydroxylysine (hī″drŏk-sĭl′ĭ-sĭn). An amino acid found in collagen.

hydroxyprogesterone caproate (hī-drŏk″sē-prō-jĕs′tĕr-ōn). USP. A progestational drug. Trade name is Gesterol LA 250.

hydroxyproline (hī-drŏk″sē-prō′lĭn). An amino acid found in collagen.

hydroxypropyl methycellulose. USP. Cellulose hydroxypropyl methyl ester. A substance used to increase the viscosity of solutions. Trade names are Goniosol, Lubafax, and Tearisol.

hydroxystilbamidine isethionate (hī-drŏk″sē-stĭl-băm′ĭ-dēn). USP. An antiprotozoal drug used in treating North American blastomycosis.

5-hydroxytryptamine (hī-drŏk″sē-trĭp′tă-mēn). Serotonin.

hydroxyurea (hī-drŏk″sē-ū-rē′ă). USP. A cytotoxic drug. Trade name is Hydrea.

hydroxyzine hydrochloride (hī-drŏk′sĭ-zēn). USP. An antihistamine drug. Trade names are Atarax and Vistaril Parenteral.

hygiene (hī′jēn) [Gr. *hygieinos*, healthful]. The study of health and observance of health rules. Study of the methods and means of preserving health.

h., community. That branch of hygiene that deals with the health of a large group of individuals such as in a city, state, or nation,

and esp. with the control of communicable diseases.

h., dental. SEE: *h., oral.*

h., industrial. That branch of hygiene that deals primarily with health of industrial workers, esp. study, treatment, and prevention of occupational diseases.

h., mental. Science of developing and maintaining mental health and preventing mental illness.

h., oral. The personal maintenance of hygiene and cleanliness of the teeth and oral structures by toothbrushing, flossing, and other procedures recommended by a dentist or dental hygienist.

hygienic (hī″jē-ĕn′ĭk). 1. Pert. to health or its preservation. 2. In a healthy condition.

hygienist (hī-jē′nĭst, hī′jē-ĕn-ĭst). A specialist in hygiene.

h., dental. An individual trained in dental prophylaxis who usually works under the supervision of a dentist. The hygienist is essential in patient education as well as in cleaning and polishing teeth. In some states hygienists' expanded duties include dental radiography, application of fluoride solutions, and placing and carving amalgam fillings.

hygienization (hī″jē-ĕn-ī-zā′shŭn). The establishment of sanitary conditions and rules of hygiene.

hygric (hī′grĭk) [Gr. *hygros*, moisture]. Pert. to moisture.

hygro-. Prefix indicating relationship to moisture.

hygroblepharic (hī″grō-blĕ-făr′ĭk) [″ + *blepharon*, eyelid]. Any structure such as the lacrimal gland or agent that moistens the eye.

hygroma (hī-grō′mă) [″ + *oma*, tumor] (pl. *hygromas* or *hygromata).* A sac or bursa containing fluid.

h., cystic. A rapidly growing hygroma of lymphatic origin. Usually located in the neck but may be in the thorax.

hygrometer (hī-grŏm′ē-tĕr) [″ + *metron*, measure]. Instrument for measuring the amount of moisture in the air.

hygroscopic (hī-grō-skŏp′ĭk) [″ + *skopein*, to examine]. 1. Pert. to hygroscopy. 2. Absorbing moisture readily. SYN: *bibulous; hydrophilous.*

hygroscopy (hī-grŏs′kō-pē). Estimation of the quantity of moisture in the atmosphere.

hygrostomia (hī-grō-stō′mē-ă) [″ + *stoma*, mouth]. Excess flow of saliva. SYN: *ptyalism; salivation.*

Hygroton. Trade name for chlorthalidone, USP.

hyl-, hylo- [Gr. *hyle*, matter]. Combining form indicating wood or matter.

hyla (hī′lă). A lateral extension of the aqueductus cerebri.

hyloma (hī-lō′mă) [Gr. *hyle*, matter, + *oma*, tumor]. A tumor composed of or in the hylic tissues, such as hypohyloma and mesohyloma.

hymen (hī′mĕn) [Gr.] [NA] A fold of mucous membrane that partially covers the entrance of the vagina. Contrary to folklore, presence or absence of the hymen cannot be used to prove or disprove virginity or history of sexual intercourse. Its rupture or absence is not evidence of loss of virginity. Conversely, pregnancy has occurred even though the hymen has not been entered.
RS: defloration; hymenorrhaphy; hymenotome.

h., annular. Hymen with a ring-shaped opening in the center.

h. biforis. Hymen with two parallel openings with a thick septum between.

h., cribriform. Hymen with many small perforations.

h. denticulatus. Hymen with an opening with serrated edges.

h., fenestrated. H., cribriform.

h., imperforate. Hymen with no opening in it.

h., lunar. Hymen shaped like the moon.

h., ruptured. Hymen that has been torn by coitus, injury, or surgery.

h., septate. Hymen in which the opening is separated by a thin septum.

h., unruptured. H., imperforate.

hymenal (hī′mĕn-ăl). Pert. to the hymen.

hymenectomy (hī″mĕn-ĕk′tō-mē) [″ + *ektome*, excision]. 1. In surgery and gynecology, incision or removal of the hymen. 2. Excision of a membrane.

hymenitis (hī-mĕn-ī′tĭs) [″ + *itis*, inflammation]. Inflammation of the hymen or a membrane.

Hymenolepis (hī″mĕ-nŏl′ĕ-pĭs) [″ + *lepis*, rind]. A genus of tapeworm. Parasitic in birds and mammals.

H. nana. The dwarf tapeworm, a parasite in the intestine of rats and mice; also commonly found in man. It averages about 1 in. (2.5 cm) in length and differs from other tapeworms in that it is capable of completing its life cycle within a single host. It causes severe toxic symptoms, esp. in children.

hymenology (hī′mĕn-ŏl′ō-jē) [″ + *logos*, word, reason]. Science of the membranes and their diseases.

Hymenoptera (hī″mĕn-ŏp′tur-ă) [Gr. *hymenopteros*, membrane-winged]. An order of insects that includes ants, bees, hornets, and wasps. SEE: *insect bites and stings.*

hymenorrhaphy (hī″mĕn-or′ă-fē) [″ + *rhaphe*, seam, ridge]. Plastic operation on the hymen to restore it to the preruptured state.

hymenotome (hī-mĕn′ō-tōm) [″ + *tome*, incision]. Knife used to divide membranes.

hymenotomy (hī″mĕn-ŏt′ō-mē). 1. Incision of the hymen. 2. Dissection of the membrane.

hyo- [Gr. *hyoeides*, U-shaped]. Prefix indicating connection with the hyoid bone.

hyobasioglossus (hī″ō-bā″sē-ō-glŏs′ŭs) [″ + *basis*, base, + *glossa*, tongue]. The part of hyoglossal muscle attached to the hyoid bone.

hyoepiglottic, hyoepiglottidean (hī″ō-ĕp″ĭ-glŏt′ĭk, hī″ō-ĕp″ĭ-glŏt-ĭd′ē-ăn) [″ + *epiglottis*, epiglottis]. Rel. to the hyoid bone and epiglottis.

hyoglossal (hī″ō-glŏs′ăl) [″ + *glossa*, tongue]. 1. Pert. to the hyoglossus. 2. Extending to the tongue from the hyoid bone.

hyoglossus (hī″ō-glŏs′ŭs). Muscle arising from the body and greater cornu of the hyoid bone and inserted into the dorsum of the tongue. It draws sides down and retracts tongue.

hyoid (hī′oyd) [Gr. *hyoeides*, U-shaped]. 1. Shaped like the Gr. letter upsilon, *v.* 2. Pert. to the hyoid bone, q.v.

hyoid arch. Second branchial arch.

hyoid bone. Horseshoe-shaped bone lying at the base of the tongue. SEE: illus.

hyopharyngeus (hī″ō-făr-ĭn′jē-ŭs) [″ + *pharynx*, throat]. Middle pharyngeal constrictor.

hyoscine hydrobromide. Previously used name for scopolamine hydrobromide.

hyoscyamus (hī″ō-sī′ă-mŭs) [Gr. *hys*, a pig, + *kyamos*, bean]. Dried leaves of the plant *Hyoscyamus niger.* A narcotic that also acts as an antispasmodic. SYN: *henbane.*

hyoscyamus poisoning. Related to atropine. SEE: *atropine* in *Poisons and Poisoning* in *Appendix.*

hypacousia, hypacusia, hypacusis (hī″pă-koo′sē-ă, -kū′sē-ă, -sīs) [Gr. *hypo*, under, + *akousis*, hearing]. Impaired hearing. SEE: *hearing; presbyacusis.*

hypalbuminosis (hī″păl-bū-mĭn-ō′sĭs) [″ + L. *albumen*, white of egg, + Gr. *osis*, condition]. Deficiency in proportion of albumin in blood.

hypalgesia (hī-păl-jĕ′zē-ă) [″ + *algesis*, sense of pain]. Lessened sensitivity to pain. Opposed to hyperalgesia.

hypalgia (hī-păl′jē-ă) [″ + *algos*, pain]. Lessened sensitivity to pain. SYN: *hypalgesia.*

hypamnios (hī-păm′nē-ŏs) [″ + *amnion*, caul of a lamb]. Deficiency in amount of amniotic fluid.

hypaphrodisia (hī-păf″rō-dĭz′ē-ă) [Gr. *hypo*, under, + *aphrodisia*, sexual pleasure]. Decreased or deficient sexual desire.

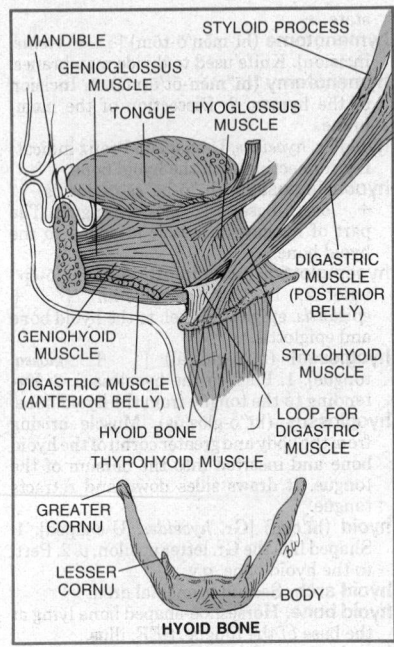

MANDIBLE
STYLOID PROCESS
GENIOGLOSSUS MUSCLE
TONGUE HYOGLOSSUS MUSCLE
DIGASTRIC MUSCLE (POSTERIOR BELLY)
GENIOHYOID MUSCLE
STYLOHYOID MUSCLE
DIGASTRIC MUSCLE (ANTERIOR BELLY)
LOOP FOR DIGASTRIC MUSCLE
HYOID BONE
THYROHYOID MUSCLE
GREATER CORNU
LESSER CORNU
BODY

HYOID BONE

hypaxial (hī-păks′ē-ăl) [″ + *axon*, axle]. Situated beneath the body axis.

hyper- [Gr. *hyper*, over, above, excessive]. Prefix meaning above, excessive, or beyond.

Hyperab. Trade name for rabies immune globulin.

hyperacid (hī″pĕr-ăs′ĭd) [″ + L. *acidus*, sour]. Containing too much acid.

hyperacidaminuria (hī″pĕr-ăs″ĭd-ăm-ĭn-ū′rē-ă) [″ + ″ + *amine* + Gr. *ouron*, urine]. Presence of an excess of amino acids in the urine. SYN: *acidaminuria*.

hyperacidity (hī″pĕr-ă-sĭd′ĭ-tē) [″ + L. *acidus*, sour]. 1. Excess of acid. 2. Excess of acid in the stomach. SEE: *hyperchlorhydria*.

hyperactive child syndrome. SEE: *attention deficit disorder*.

hyperactivity. 1. Increased or excessive activity that may refer to the entire organism (see below) or to a particular entity, e.g., hyperactivity of the heart or thyroid. 2. Excessive muscular activity. The term commonly refers to manifestations of disturbed behavior in children or adolescents characterized by constant overactivity, distractibility, impulsiveness, inability to concentrate, and aggressiveness. This condition is not easily defined because the claim that the child is hyperactive may be based on a low level of

tolerance of the persons caring for the child. Hyperkinetic behavior usually lessens as a child grows older and usually disappears during adolescence.

ETIOL: Emotional disorders; central nervous system dysfunction; mental retardation; or an exaggeration of a normal personality trait.

hyperacuity (hī″pĕr-ă-kū′ĭ-tē) [Gr. *hyper*, over, above, excessive, + L. *acuitas*, sharpness]. Abnormal acuteness of one of the special senses such as hearing or sight.

hyperacusis (hī″pĕr-ă-kū′sĭs) [″ + *akousis*, hearing]. Abnormal sensitivity to sound. Sometimes found in hysteria. SYN: *oxyacusis*.

hyperacute (hī″pĕr-ă-kūt′). The state of any of the senses when they are very acute.

hyperadiposis, hyperadiposity (hī″pĕr-ăd″ĭ-pō′sĭs, -pŏs′ĭ-tē) [″ + L. *adeps*, fat, + Gr. *osis*, condition]. Excessive fatness.

hyperadrenalism (hī″pĕr-ă-drē′năl-ĭzm). Increased secretion from the adrenal gland.

hyperadrenocorticalism (hī″pĕr-ă-drē″nō-kor′tĭ-kăl-ĭzm). Increased secretion from the cortex of the adrenal gland.

hyperalbuminemia (hī″pĕr-ăl-bū″mĭ-nē′mē-ă) [″ + L. *albumen*, white of egg, + Gr. *haima*, blood]. Increased albumin in the blood.

hyperaldosteronism (hī″pĕr-ăl″dō-stĕr′ōn-ĭzm). Excessive production of aldosterone by the adrenal gland. SEE: *aldosteronism*.

hyperalgesia (hī″pĕr-ăl-jē′zē-ă) [″ + *algesis*, sense of pain]. Excessive sensitivity to pain. Opposite of hypalgesia. SYN: *hyperalgia*.

hyperalgia (hī-pĕr-ăl′jē-ă) [″ + *algos*, pain]. Excessive sensitivity to pain. SYN: *hyperalgesia*.

hyperalimentation (hī″pĕr-ăl″ĭ-mĕn-tā′shŭn). The enteral and parenteral infusion of a solution that contains sufficient amino acids, glucose, fatty acids, electrolytes, vitamins, and minerals to sustain life, maintain normal growth and development, and provide for needed tissue repair. The GI tract is the route of choice if it is functional. Intravenous hyperalimentation may be infused via peripheral vessels, but in lesser concentrations because of the increased potential for chemical phlebitis. Infusion through a central line catheter into the superior vena cava provides a sufficient blood volume to rapidly dilute more hypertonic solution, but increases the potential for sepsis.

NURSING IMPLICATIONS: Monitor patient's fluid balance (intake, output, and daily weight), also vital signs and electrolyte values. Monitor for indications of fluid overload. Monitor urine specific gravity and test urine for presence of glucose and acetone every six hours. If hyperalimentation is enteral, know where tube is placed (above or below pyloric sphincter), auscultate bowel sounds, inspect and measure for abdominal distention, and assess for, document, report, and treat nausea, vomiting, or diarrhea. As appropriate, monitor stomach contents for residual volume. If hyperalimentation is via peripheral blood vessels, frequently assess insertion site for evidence of phlebitis; if by a central line, assess insertion site for evidence of infection, and patient for signs and symptoms of sepsis. Redress according to agency protocol. For all intravenous hyperalimentation: Never speed up flow to "catch up" a delayed infusion without specific direction from a physician. Notify physician if line becomes occluded or fluids are stopped or slowed for any reason, and assess for hypoglycemia or fluid deficit. For all hyperalimentation: Mobilize patient as much as possible or permitted to enhance utilization of nutrients. Monitor nutritional status weekly in order to have a record of weight gain. Maintain strict aseptic technique in handling fluids and equipment, being especially vigilant if patient is in an anergic state.

hyperalkalinity (hī″pĕr-ăl-kă-lĭn′ĭ-tē). A condition of excess alkalinity.

hyperaminoacidemia (hī″pĕr-ăm″ĭ-nō-ăs″ĭ-dē′mē-ă). Abnormal amount of amino acids in the blood.

hyperammonemia (hī″pĕr-ăm″mō-nē′mē-ă). Excess of ammonia in the blood. SEE: *ammonia toxicity.*

   h., congenital. Accumulation of an excess of ammonia in the body due to a congenital deficiency of enzymes, either carbamyl phosphate synthetase or ornithine transcarbamylase, essential to the metabolism of ammonia. Clinical signs of ammonia toxicity, q.v., are present. These include vomiting, lethargy, coma, and eventually death.

hyperamylasemia (hī″pĕr-ăm″ĭl-ās-ē′mē-ă). Increased blood amylase.

hyperanacinesia, hyperanacinesis (hī″pĕr-ăn″ă-sĭn-ē′zē-ă, -sĭs). Hyperanakinesis.

hyperanakinesis (hī″pĕr-ăn″ă-kĭ-nē′sĭs) [″ + *anakinesis,* exercise]. Excessive function or movement activity of an organ or part such as of the stomach or intestines.

hyperaphia (hī″pĕr-ā′fē-ă) [″ + *haphe,* touch]. Excessive sensitiveness to touch.

hyperaphic (hī-pĕr-ăf′ĭk). Marked by extreme sensitiveness to touch.

hyperazotemia (hī″pĕr-ăz″ō-tē′mē-ă) [″ + L. *azotum,* nitrogen, + Gr. *haima,* blood]. Increased amount of nitrogenous substances, such as urea, in the blood.

hyperazoturia (hī″pĕr-ăz″ō-tū′rē-ă) [″ + ″ + Gr. *ouron,* urine]. Excessive amount of nitrogenous matter in the urine.

hyperbaric chamber. A chamber large enough to hold a patient and a medical or surgical team. The pressure in the chamber can be increased in order to increase the amount of oxygen in the inspired air or in contact with wounds. SEE: *decompression illness; hyperbaric oxygen.*

hyperbaric oxygen. Oxygen under greater pressure than at normal atmospheric pressure. Pressure chambers in which the oxygen is hyperbaric have been used in treating gas gangrene, decompression sickness (bends), air embolism, smoke inhalation, and carbon monoxide poisoning. Chambers have also been used experimentally in surgery in congenital cyanotic heart disease. It is usually used at 1½ to 3 times absolute atmospheric pressure. SEE: *hyperbaric oxygen therapy.*

hyperbaric oxygen therapy. Use of a hyperbaric chamber containing oxygen to treat carbon monoxide poisoning, gas gangrene, necrotizing fasciitis, crush injuries with acute ischemia of tissues, compromised skin grafts and flaps, mixed soft tissue reactions, burns, smoke inhalation, soft tissue radiation necrosis, chronic refractory osteomyelitis, and conditions requiring recompression, such as bends, q.v., and gas embolism.

   Consultation at any hour concerning treatment of patients in a hyperbaric chamber is available from Divers Alert Network coordinated by Duke University Medical Center, (919) 684-8111.

Caution: Do not use in untreated pneumothorax, premature infants.

---

hyperbarism (hī″pĕr-băr′ĭzm). The condition of being exposed to or having pressure greater than atmospheric. Miners and deep sea divers are exposed to this condition. SEE: *bends; caisson disease.*

hyperbetalipoproteinemia (hī″pĕr-bā″tă-lĭp″ō-prō″tē-ĭn-ē′mē-ă). Excessive amount of β-lipoproteins in the blood. SEE: *hyperlipoproteinemia.*

hyperbilirubinemia (hī″pĕr-bĭl″ĭ-roo-bĭn-ē′mē-ă) [Gr. *hyper,* over, above, excessive, + L. *bilis,* bile, + *ruber,* red, + Gr. *haima,* blood]. Excessive amount of bilirubin in the blood.

hyperbrachycephaly (hī″pĕr-brăk″ē-sĕf′ă-lē) [″ + *brachys,* short, + *kephale,* head]. Excessive degree of brachycephaly; having a cephalic index over 85.

hypercalcemia (hī″pĕr-kăl-sē′mē-ă) [″ + L. *calx,* lime, + Gr. *haima,* blood]. Excessive amount of calcium in the blood. SYN:

calcemia.

h., idiopathic. Type of hypercalcemia seen in infants, caused by vitamin D intoxication. SEE: *bends.*

hypercalciuria (hī″pĕr-kăl″sē-ū′rē-ă) [″ + ″ + Gr. *ouron,* urine]. Excessive quantity of calcium in the urine.

hypercapnia (hī″pĕr-kăp′nē-ă) [″ + *kapnos,* smoke]. Increased amount of carbon dioxide in the blood.

hypercarbia. Hypercapnia, q.v.

hypercatharsis (hī″pĕr-kă-thär′sĭs) [″ + *katharsis,* purge]. Excessive bowel movement in response to administration of cathartics.

hypercellularity (hī″pĕr-sĕl″ū-lār′ĭ-tē). Increased number of cells in any location but esp. in the bone marrow.

hypercementosis (hī″pĕr-sē″mĕn-tō′sĭs) [″ + L. *cementum,* cement, + Gr. *osis,* condition]. Overgrowth of tooth cement (cementum).

hyperchloremia (hī″pĕr-klō-rē′mē-ă) [″ + *chloros,* green, + *haima,* blood]. Increase in chloride content of the blood.

hyperchlorhydria (hī″pĕr-klor-hī′drē-ă) [″ + ″ + *hydor,* water]. An excess of hydrochloric acid in the gastric secretion. It causes a burning sensation in the stomach in the absence of ingested foods. The amount secreted above what is needed to combine with albumoid and basic substances is known as free hydrogen chloride.

The ability of the stomach to produce hydrochloric acid can be evaluated clinically by administering pentagastrin, the chemical that stimulates gastric production, or histamine or betazole. The amount of acid produced is measured by aspirating the stomach four times at 15-minute intervals. SEE: *achlorhydria; gastrin; gastritis; H_2-receptor antagonists; hydrochloric acid; hypochlorhydria; peptic ulcer; Zollinger-Ellison syndrome.*

hyperchloridation (hī″pĕr-klō′rĭ-dā′shŭn). A dosing with large amounts of sodium chloride.

hypercholesterolemia (hī″pĕr-kō-lĕs″tĕr-ōl-ē′mē-ă) [″ + *chole,* bile, + *stereos,* solid, + *haima,* blood]. Excessive amount of cholesterol in the blood.

h., familial. A type of hyperlipoproteinemia, type IIA, in which the low-density lipoproteins are increased and the very low-density lipoproteins are normal. SEE: *hyperlipoproteinemia.*

hypercholesterolia (hī″pĕr-kō-lĕs″tĕr-ō′lē-ă) [″ + ″ + *stereos,* solid]. Excessive cholesterol in the bile.

hypercholia (hī″pĕr-kō′lē-ă) [″ + *chole,* bile]. Abnormal secretion of bile.

hyperchromasia (hī″pĕr-krō-mā′zē-ă) [Gr. *hyper,* over, above, excessive, + *chroma,* color]. Hyperchromatism.

hyperchromatic (hī″pĕr-krō-măt′ĭk) [″ + *chroma,* color]. Overpigmented.

hyperchromatic cell. Cell or a part of a cell that contains more than the normal number of chromosomes and hence stains more densely.

hyperchromatism (hī″pĕr-krō′mă-tĭzm) [″ + ″ + *-ismos,* condition]. 1. Excessive pigmentation. 2. Increased staining capacity of any structure. SYN: *hyperchromatosis.*

hyperchromatopsia (hī″pĕr-krō″mă-tŏp′sē-ă) [″ + ″ + *opsis,* vision]. Defect of vision in which all objects appear colored.

hyperchromatosis (hī″pĕr-krō″mă-tō′sĭs) [″ + *chroma,* color, + *osis,* condition]. 1. Excessive pigmentation, esp. of the skin. 2. Increased staining capacity. SYN: *hyperchromatism.*

hyperchromia (hī″pĕr-krō′mē-ă). Excessive pigmentation. SYN: *hyperchromatism.*

hyperchromic (hī-pĕr-krō′mĭk). 1. Pert. to excessive pigmentation. 2. Intensely colored.

hyperchylia (hī″pĕr-kī′lē-ă) [Gr. *hyper,* over, above, excessive, + *chylos,* juice]. Abnormal secretion of gastric juice.

hyperchylomicronemia (hī″pĕr-kī″lō-mī″krō-nē′mē-ă). Excessive accumulation of fat particles, chylomicrons, in the blood.

hypercoagulability (hīp″ĕr-kō-ăg″ū-lă-bĭl′ĭ-tē). Increased ability of anything to coagulate, but esp. the blood.

hypercorticism (hī″pĕr-kor′tĭ-sĭzm). Excessive production of adrenal cortical hormones in the body.

hypercrinism (hī″pĕr-krī′nĭsm) [″ + *krinein,* to separate, + *-ismos,* condition]. Condition due to excessive activity of any endocrine gland.

hypercryalgesia (hī″pĕr-krī″ăl-jē′zē-ă) [″ + *kryos,* cold, + *algesis,* sense of pain]. Excessive sensitivity to cold. SYN: *hypercryesthesia.*

hypercryesthesia (hī″pĕr-krī″ĕs-thē′zē-ă) [″ + ″ + *aisthesis,* sensation]. Excessive sensitivity to cold. SYN: *hypercryalgesia.*

hypercupremia (hī″pĕr-kū-prē′mē-ă). Increased level of copper in the blood. SEE: *Wilson's disease.*

hypercyanosis (hī″pĕr-sī″ă-nō′sĭs) [″ + *kyanos,* dark blue, + *osis,* condition]. Extreme cyanosis.

hypercyanotic (hī″pĕr-sī″ă-nŏt′ĭk). Denoting extreme cyanosis.

hypercyesis (hī″pĕr-sī-ē′sĭs) [″ + *kyesis,* gestation]. Presence of more than one fetus in a uterus because of fertilization of a second ovum within a short time. The second ovum may be fertilized by a sex partner other than the one who fertilized the first ovum. SYN: *superfetation.*

hypercythemia (hī″pĕr-sī-thē′mē-ă) [″ + *kytos,* cell, + *haima,* blood]. Condition of having an excessive number of red blood corpuscles. SYN: *erythrocytosis.*

hypercytosis (hī″pĕr-sī-tō′sĭs) [″ + ″ + *osis,* condition]. Abnormal increase in leukocytes in the blood. SYN: *leukocytosis.*

hyperdactylia (hī″pĕr-dăk-tĭl′ē-ă) [Gr. *hyper,* over, above, excessive, + *daktylos,* finger]. State of having supernumerary fingers or toes.

hyperdicrotic (hī″pĕr-dī-krŏt′ĭk) [″ + *dikrotos,* beating double]. Abnormally dicrotic. SEE: *dicrotic.*

hyperdistention (hī″pĕr-dĭs-tĕn′shŭn) [″ + L. *distendere,* to stretch out]. Excessive inflation or distention.

hyperdontia (hī″pĕr-dŏn′shē-ă). Presence of more than the normal number of teeth. SYN: *polyodontia.*

hyperdynamia (hī″pĕr-dī-nā′mē-ă) [″ + *dynamis,* force]. Muscular restlessness or extreme violence.

h. uteri. Abnormal uterine contractions in labor.

hypereccrisia, hypereccrisis (hī″pĕr-ĕk-krĭs′ē-ă, -ĕk′krĭ-sĭs) [″ + *ekkrisis,* excretion]. Abnormal amount of excretion.

hypereccritic (hī-pĕr-ĕk-krĭt′ĭk). Pert. to hypereccrisis.

hyperemesis (hī″pĕr-ĕm′ĕ-sĭs) [″ + *emesis,* vomiting]. Excessive vomiting.

h. gravidarum. Nausea and vomiting during pregnancy of such severity and duration that systemic effects such as acidosis, dehydration, and weight loss occur. About two out of each 1000 pregnant women have this disease with such severity as to require hospitalization. If the severe form is untreated, it can be fatal. SEE: *Nursing Diagnoses* in *Appendix.*

SYM: The condition may start as a simple vomiting of early pregnancy, but with combined vomiting, first of gastric contents and later of bile, there develop a chloride depletion, acidosis, and, finally, with severe and continued vomiting, pathological changes in the liver take place.

ETIOL: The cause is unknown.

TREAT: In early cases, rest in bed; small amounts of carbohydrates taken frequently; moderate restriction of fluids; mild sedation and antiemetic drugs are usually effective. In severe cases, the patient is hospitalized, with complete bedrest and no visitors until vomiting ends and eating begins. Treatment includes nothing by mouth for 24 hours; maintain nutritional and electrolyte balance by giving parenteral fluids and pro-

teins as required. Rarely, nasogastric feeding or total parenteral nutrition will be required.

The necessity for emptying the uterus should occur only rarely if the patient is seen early and the proper treatment instituted at once. When the patient improves, food taken by mouth should consist of a light solid diet given in frequent small feedings, with fruit juice or milk between feedings.

Caution: During therapy monitor retina for evidence of hemorrhagic retinitis; and, if it occurs, the pregnancy should be terminated without delay. The death rate in patients with this complication is 50%.

h. lactentium. Vomiting in nursing infants.

hyperemia (hī″pĕr-ē′mē-ă) [″ + *haima,* blood]. 1. Congestion. An unusual amount of blood in a part. 2. A form of macula; red areas on skin that disappear on pressure. 3. In physical therapy, increase in the quantity of blood flowing through any part of the body, shown by redness of the skin caused by the application of heat.

h., active. Hyperemia caused by increased blood inflow. SYN: *h., arterial.*

h., arterial. H., active.

h., Bier's. Passive hyperemia, q.v., produced by application of an elastic bandage and by suction. SYN: *h., constriction.*

h., constriction. H., Bier's.

h., leptomeningeal. Pia-arachnoid congestion.

h., passive. Hyperemia caused by decreased blood outflow. SYN: *h., venous.*

h., reactive. The increased presence of blood in an area after restoration of blood flow following a decreased supply.

h., venous. H., passive.

hyperemization (hī″pĕr-ē″mī-zā′shŭn). Hyperemia produced artificially for therapeutic purposes.

hyperemotivity (hī″pĕr-ē″mō-tĭv′ĭ-tē) [Gr. *hyper,* over, above, excessive, + L. *emovere,* to disturb]. Excessive emotivity or response to stimuli.

hypereosinophilic syndrome, idiopathic. Persistent eosinophilia for which no cause can be found. This rare, world-wide disease is more common in men than in women. Almost any organ can be affected, but most have bone marrow, cardiac and central nervous system involvement.

TREAT: Anticoagulants for patients with thromboembolic complication; corticosteroids. Patients unresponsive to corticosteroids have had marked improvement when given cytotoxic agents such as hydroxyurea.

hypereosinophilia (hī″pĕr-ē″ō-sĭn-ō-fĭl′ē-ă) [″ + *eos*, dawn, + *philein*, to love]. Marked increase in number of eosinophils in the blood.

hyperepinephrinemia (hī″pĕr-ĕp″ĭ-nĕf″rĭ-nē′mē-ă) [″ + ″ + *nephros*, kidney, + *haima*, blood]. Abnormally large amount of epinephrine in the blood.

hyperequilibrium (hī″pĕr-ē″kwĭ-lĭb′rē-ŭm) [″ + L. *aequus*, equal, + *libra*, balance]. Tendency to vertigo when making even slight turning movements.

hypererethism (hī″pĕr-ĕr′ĭ-thĭzm) [″ + *erethisma*, stimulation]. Excessive irritability.

hyperergasia (hī″pĕr-ĕr-gā′sē-ă) [″ + *ergasia*, work]. Unusual functional activity.

hyperergia (hī″pĕr-ĕr′jē-ă). 1. Excessive or increased functional activity. SYN: *hyperergasia.* 2. Abnormal sensitivity to allergens.

hyperergy (hī′pĕr-ĕr″jē) [″ + *ergon*, energy]. Hypersensitivity or condition in which there is an exaggerated response. SEE: *allergy; anaphylaxis.*

hyperesophoria (hī″pĕr-ĕs″ō-fō′rē-ă) [″ + *eso*, inward, + *phorein*, to bear]. Tendency of the visual axis to deviate upward and inward due to muscular imbalance. A form of heterophoria, q.v.

hyperesthesia (hī″pĕr-ĕs-thē′zē-ă) [″ + *aisthesis*, sensation]. Increased sensitivity to sensory stimuli, such as pain or touch. SYN: *algesia; oxyesthesia.*

   h., acoustic. Abnormal sensitivity to sound.

   h., cerebral. Hyperesthesia caused by a cerebral lesion.

   h., gustatory. Oversensitivity of taste.

   h., muscular. Muscular sensitivity to pain and tiredness.

   h., optic. Abnormal sensitivity to light.

   h. sexualis. Abnormal increase in libido.

   h., tactile. Abnormal sensitivity of touch.

hyperesthetic (hī″pĕr-ĕs-thĕt′ĭk). Pert. to hyperesthesia.

hyperexophoria (hī″pĕr-ĕks″ō-fō′rē-ă) [″ + *exo*, outward, + *phorein*, to bear]. Tendency of visual axis to deviate upward and outward due to muscular imbalance. A form of heterophoria, q.v.

hyperexplexia. Excessive reaction to being startled. SEE: *Gilles de la Tourette's syndrome; startle syndromes.*

hyperextension (hī″pĕr-ĕks-tĕn′shŭn) [″ + L. *extendere*, to stretch out]. Extreme or abnormal extension.

hyperferremia (hī″pĕr-fĕr-rē′mē-ă). Excess amount of iron in the blood. SEE: *hemochromatosis.*

hyperfibrinogenemia (hī″pĕr-fī-brĭn″ō-jĕ-nē′mē-ă). Increased amount of fibrinogen in the blood.

hyperflexion (hī″pĕr-flĕk′shŭn). Increased flexion of a joint, usually due to trauma.

hyperfunction [Gr. *hyper*, over, above, excessive, + L. *functio*, performance]. Excessive activity.

hypergalactia (hī-pĕr-găl-ăk′shē-ă) [″ + *gala*, milk]. Excessive milk secretion.

hypergammaglobulinemia (hī″pĕr-găm″ă-glŏb″ū-lĭ-nē′mē-ă). Excessive amount of gamma globulin in the blood.

hypergamy (hī-pĕr′gă-mē) [″ + *gamos*, marriage]. The tendency of females to reproduce with males of equal or higher social standing.

hypergasia (hĭp-ĕr-gā′sē-ă). Hypoergasia, decreased sensitivity to allergens.

hypergenesis (hī″pĕr-jĕn′ĕ-sĭs) [″ + *genesis*, generation, birth]. Redundancy of organs or parts; overproduction. SYN: *hyperplasia.*

hypergenitalism (hī″pĕr-jĕn′ĭt-ăl-ĭzm) [″ + L. *genitalis*, genital]. Excessive development of the genital organs.

   ETIOL: Disturbances in endocrine secretions of the adrenal gland or gonads, or hypothalamic disorders.

hypergeusesthesia, hypergeusia (hī″pĕr-gūs-ĕs-thē′sē-ă, -gū′sē-ă) [″ + *geusis*, taste + *aisthesis*, perception]. Excessive acuteness of sense of taste.

hypergia (hī-pĕr′jē-ă). Decreased sensitivity to allergens.

hyperglandular (hī″pĕr-glăn′dū-lăr) [″ + L. *glandula*, a little acorn]. Having excessive glandular secretions.

hyperglobulinemia (hī″pĕr-glŏb″ū-lĭn-ē′mē-ă) [″ + L. *globulus*, a globule, + Gr. *haima*, blood]. Excessive globulin in the blood.

hyperglycemia (hī″pĕr-glī-sē′mē-ă) [″ + *glykys*, sweet, + *haima*, blood]. Increase of blood sugar as in diabetes. This condition increases susceptibility to infection and it often precedes diabetic coma. SEE: *hypoglycemia.*

hyperglyceridemia (hī″pĕr-glĭs″ĕr-ĭ-dē′mē-ă). Accumulation of glycerides, esp. triglycerides in the blood.

hyperglycinemia (hī″pĕr-glī″sĭ-nē′mē-ă). Accumulation of glycine in the blood. It is caused by a congenital defect in the ability to metabolize the amino acid glycine. There are at least six forms of this disease, all of which are associated with mental and growth retardation.

hyperglycogenolysis (hī″pĕr-glī″kō-jĕn-ŏl′ĭ-sĭs) [″ + ″ + *gennan*, to form, + *lysis*, dissolution]. Excessive conversion of glycogen into glucose by hydrolysis.

hyperglycorrhachia (hī″pĕr-glī″kō-rā′kē-ă)

[" + *glykys,* sweet, + *rhachis,* spine].
Excess of sugar in the cerebrospinal fluid.

hyperglycosemia (hī″pĕr-glī-kō-sē′mē-ă) ["
+ " + *haima,* blood]. Excessive sugar
in the blood. SYN: *hyperglycemia.*

hyperglycosuria (hī″pĕr-glī″kō-sū′rē-ă) ["
+ " + *ouron,* urine]. Excessive sugar in
the urine. SEE: *glycosuria.*

hypergnosia (hī″pĕr-nō′sē-ă) [" + *gnosis,*
knowledge]. Distorted or exaggerated perception influenced by the unconscious projection of emotional subjective experiences.

hypergonadism (hī″pĕr-gō′năd-ĭzm) [" +
gone, seed, + *-ismos,* state of]. Excessive
secretion of the sex glands.

hyperguanidinemia (hī″pĕr-gwăn″ĭ-dĭn-ē′
mē-ă) [" + Sp. *guano,* dung, + *haima,*
blood]. Abnormal amt. of guanidine in
blood.

hyperhedonia, hyperhedonism (hī″pĕr-hē-
dŏ′nē-ă, -hē′dŏn-ĭzm) [Gr. *hyper,* over,
above, excessive, + *hedone,* pleasure,
+ *-ismos,* state of]. 1. Abnormal pleasure
in anything. 2. Abnormal sexual excitement.

Hyper-Hep. Trade name for hepatitis B immune globulin.

hyperhidrosis (hī″pĕr-hī-drō′sĭs) [" +
hidros, sweat, + *osis,* condition]. Sweating greater than would be expected in the
temperature of the environment.

ETIOL: Functional overactivity of sweat
glands caused by debilitating disease or
stimulants. Increased in rheumatic, malarial, relapsing, and septic fever. Occurs in
neuralgia and migraine and follows certain
drugs and hot drinks. Locally it affects
hands and feet in hysteria, fright, nervous
irritability, and hyperthyroidism. May be
associated with hot flashes experienced
during menopause. SEE: *bromidrosis;
sweat.*

TREAT: If due to a systemic disease, appropriate therapy for that condition is indicated. If localized, application of a 20% solution of aluminum chloride hexahydrate in
absolute alcohol at night using occlusive
dressings will be of benefit. The dressed
sites must be dried prior to application, and
the salt is washed away in the morning.
Twice weekly treatment of the areas with
tap water electrophoresis may be of benefit.
In chronic cases that do not respond to therapy, cervical sympathectomy may be required.

hyperhydration (hī″pĕr-hī-drā′shŭn). Excess of water in the body.

hyperimmune (hī″pĕr-ĭm-mūn′). State of
immunity greater than normal.

hyperinflation (hī″pĕr-ĭn-flā′shŭn). Excess
of air in anything, esp. the lungs.

hyperinosemia (hī″pĕr-ī″nō-sē′mē-ă) ["

+ *inos,* fiber, + *haima,* blood]. Abnormal coagulability of the blood; excess of fibrinogen in the blood.

hyperinosis (hī″pĕr-ī-nō′sĭs) [" + *inos,*
fiber, + *osis,* condition]. Excessive fibrinogen in the blood. SYN: *hyperinosemia.*

hyperinsulinism (hī″pĕr-ĭn′sū-lĭn-ĭzm) ["
+ L. *insula,* island, + Gr. *-ismos,* con-
dition]. An excessive amount of insulin in
the blood.

SYM: Those consistent with hypoglycemia, q.v. Hunger; weakness; sweating; staggering; diplopia; rarely convulsions; coma;
and death. Occasionally spontaneous, in
which case symptoms are similar to but last
longer than those in insulin shock.

ETIOL: Tumor on islets of Langerhans or
excessive sensitivity of the islet tissue to an
increase in blood-sugar level. May be caused
by an overdose of insulin. SEE: *insulin; insulin shock; shock.*

hyperinvolution (hī″pĕr-ĭn″vō-lū′shŭn) ["
+ L. *involvere,* to enwrap]. 1. Reduction in
size of uterus below normal after childbirth.
2. Reduction in size below normal of any
organ following hypertrophy. SYN: *superinvolution.*

h. uteri. Extreme atrophy of the uterus
seen following prolonged lactation or severe
puerperal sepsis.

hyperirritability (hī″pĕr-ĭr″ĭ-tă-bĭl′ĭ-tē). Increased response to a stimulus.

hyperisotonic [" + *isos,* equal, + *tonos,*
tension]. Said of one of two solutions that
has the greater osmotic pressure. SYN: *hypertonic.*

hyperkalemia, hyperkaliemia (hī″pĕr-kă-
lē′mē-ă, -kăl″ē-ē′mē-ă) [" + L. *kalium,*
potassium, + Gr. *haima,* blood]. Excessive amount of potassium in the blood.

hyperkeratinization (hī″pĕr-kĕr″ă-tĭn″ĭ-
zā′shŭn) [" + *keras,* horn]. Thickening of
the horny layers of the skin, esp. of the
palms and soles. May be caused by vitamin
A deficiency or chronic arsenic toxicity.

hyperkeratomycosis (hī″pĕr-kĕr″ă-tō-mī-
kō′sĭs) [" + " + *mykes,* fungus, +
osis, condition]. Hypertrophy of horny layer
of the epidermis due to a parasitic fungus.

hyperkeratosis [" + " + *osis,* condi-
tion]. 1. Overgrowth of the cornea. 2. Overgrowth of the horny layer of the epidermis.
SYN: *keratodermia; keratosis.*

h. congenitalis. Hyperkeratosis in the
harlequin fetus.

h., epidermolytic. Congenital disorder
characterized by hyperkeratosis, erythema,
and blisters.

hyperketonemia (hī″pĕr-kē″tō-nē′mē-ă).
Accumulation of an excess of ketone bodies
in the blood.

hyperketonuria (hī″pĕr-kē-tō-nūr′ē-ă). Excessive quantity of ketones in urine.

hyperketosis (hī″pĕr-kē-tō′sĭs). Abnormally high ketone production in the body.

hyperkinesia, hyperkinesis (hī″pĕr-kī-nē′zē-ă, -nē′sĭs) [Gr. *hyper*, over, above, excessive, + *kinesis*, movement]. Increased muscular movement and physical activity. In children it may be due to minimal brain dysfunction, q.v. SEE: *hyperactivity*.

hyperlactation (hī″pĕr-lăk-tā′shŭn) [″ + L. *lactare*, to suckle]. Excessive milk secretion. SYN: *superlactation*.

hyperlipemia (hī″pĕr-lĭp-ē′mē-ă) [″ + *lipos*, fat, + *haima*, blood]. Excessive quantity of fat in the blood.

hyperlipidemia. An increase of lipids in the blood.

hyperlipoproteinemia (hī″pĕr-lĭp″ō-prō″tē-ĭn-ē′mē-ă). Increased lipids in the blood due to either an increased rate of synthesis or decreased rate of breakdown of lipoproteins. The lipoproteins transport triglycerides and cholesterol in the plasma. Clinically, an increased level of lipoproteins may cause atherosclerosis and pancreatitis. Hyperlipoproteinemias can develop as a result of a primary and heritable biochemical defect of either lipoprotein lipase activity or one of the cofactors essential to the function of that enzyme; or they may be secondary to certain endocrine and metabolic disorders, including diabetes mellitus; glycogen storage disease, type I; Cushing's syndrome; acromegaly; hypothyroidism; anorexia; use of drugs such as alcohol, oral contraceptives, and glucocorticoids; renal disease; liver diseases; immunologic disorders; and stress. The hyperlipoproteinemias have been divided into five different lipoprotein patterns describing the changes found in the plasma. These patterns are not descriptive of specific diseases. SEE: *cholesterol; lipoprotein*.

hyperliposis (hī″pĕr-lĭ-pō′sĭs) [″ + *lipos*, fat, + *osis*, condition]. Abnormal amt. of fat in the body.

hyperlithuria (hī″pĕr-lĭth-ū′rē-ă) [″ + *lithos*, stone, + *ouron*, urine]. Excessive excretion of lithic (uric) acid in the urine. SYN: *hyperuricuria*.

hyperlucency. In radiology, increased radiolucency.

hypermastia (hī″pĕr-măs′tē-ă) [″ + *mastos*, breast]. 1. Excessively large mammary glands. May be unilateral. SYN: *gynecomastia*. 2. Presence of abnormal number of mammary glands. SYN: *polymastia; polymazia*.

hypermature (hī″pĕr-mă-tūr′) [″ + L. *maturus*, ripe]. 1. Pert. to anything that has passed the stage of maturity. 2. Overripe, as a cataract or abscess that has gone past the optimum time for incision.

hypermature cataract. An advanced cataract in which the lens has changed shape by contracting.

hypermelanoses. Disorders of melanin pigmentation resulting in increased melanin in either the epidermis (melanoderma) in which the coloration is brown; or in the dermis, in which the color of the skin is blue or slate gray (ceruloderma).

    ETIOL: A number of diseases and conditions, including pregnancy, ACTH- producing tumors, Wilson's diseases, porphyria, biliary cirrhosis, chronic renal failure, certain drugs, suntanning, chronic pruritus. SYN: *melanoderma*. SEE: *ceruloderma; hypomelanoses*.

hypermenorrhea (hī″pĕr-mĕn″ō-rē′ă) [″ + *men*, month, + *rhoia*, flow]. Abnormal increase in the duration or amount of menstrual flow.

hypermetabolic state (hī″pĕr-mĕt″ă-bŏl′ĭk). Condition of abnormally increased rate of metabolism. Seen in fever, and in salicylate poisoning.

hypermetabolism (hī″pĕr-mĕ-tăb′ō-lĭzm). Increased rate of metabolism.

    h., extrathyroidal. Increased rate of metabolism not related to thyroid disease.

hypermetaplasia (hī″pĕr-mĕt″ă-plā′sē-ă) [″ + *meta-*, after, + *plassein*, to form]. Overactivity in tissue replacement or transformation from one type of tissue to another, as cartilage to bone.

hypermetria (hī″pĕr-mē′trē-ă) [Gr. *hyper*, over, above, excessive, + *metron*, measure]. Unusual range of movement; motor incoordination in which muscular movement causes a person to overreach the objective.

hypermetrope (hī″pĕr-mĕt′rōp) [″ + ″ + *ops*, eye]. One who is farsighted. SYN: *hyperope*.

hypermetropia (hī″pĕr-mē-trō′pē-ă). Farsightedness. Opposite of myopia. SYN: *hyperopia*.

hypermetropic (hī″pĕr-mē-trŏp′ĭk). Pert. to farsightedness.

hypermimia (hī″pĕr-mĭm′ē-ă) [″ + *mimesis*, imitation]. Use of a great number of gestures while speaking.

hypermnesia (hī″pĕrm-nē′zē-ă) [″ + *mneme*, memory]. 1. Great ability to remember names, dates, and details. 2. An exaggeration of memory involving minute details of a past experience. It occurs in manic phase of manic-depressive psychosis; in delirium and hypnoses; at the moment of shock and fright in life-threatening situations; with fever; during neurosurgical procedures in which the temporal lobe is stimulated; and following some brain injuries.

hypermobility (hī″pĕr-mō-bĭl′ĭ-tē). Excessive joint play (movement) that permits increased mobility. It is present in certain diseases of children such as Marfan's or Ehlers-Danlos syndromes. SYN: *hypermobile joint syndrome.*

hypermorph (hī′pĕr-morf) [″ + *morphe,* form]. One whose length of limb and consequent standing height is high in proportion to the sitting height. SEE: *hypomorph; somatotype.*

hypermotility (hī″pĕr-mō-tĭl′ĭ-tē) [″ + L. *motio,* motion]. Unusual motility. SYN: *hyperkinesia.*

hypermyatrophy (hī″pĕr-mī-ăt′rō-fē) [″ + *mys,* muscle, + *atrophia,* atrophy]. Unusual wasting of muscle.

hypermyesthesia (hī″pĕr-mī″ĕs-thē′sē-ă) [″ + ″ + *aisthesis,* sensation]. Muscular hyperesthesia.

hypermyotonia (hī″pĕr-mī″ō-tō′nē-ă) [″ + ″ + *tonos,* tone]. Excessive muscular tonus.

hypermyotrophy (hī″pĕr-mī-ŏt′rō-fē) [″ + ″ + *trophe,* nourishment]. Abnormal muscular development.

hypernatremia (hī″pĕr-nă-trē′mē-ă) [″ + L. *natron,* sodium, + Gr. *haima,* blood]. Excess of sodium in the blood.

hypernephroma (hī″pĕr-nĕ-frō′mă) [″ + *nephros,* kidney, + *oma,* tumor]. Renal cell carcinoma.

hyperneurotization (hī″pĕr-nū-rŏt′ĭ-zā′shŭn) [″ + *neuron,* nerve]. Grafting of a motor nerve into a muscle that has an intact nerve supply.

hypernitremia (hī″pĕr-nī-trē′mē-ă) [″ + *nitron,* niter, + *haima,* blood]. Excess of nitrogen in the blood.

hypernormal (hī″pĕr-nor′măl) [″ + L. *norma,* rule]. Abnormal.

hypernormocytosis (hī″pĕr-nor″mō-sī-tō′sis) [″ + ″ + Gr. *kytos,* cell, + *osis,* condition]. An increased proportion of neutrophils in the blood.

hypernutrition (hī″pĕr-nū-trĭsh′ŭn) [″ + L. *nutrire,* to nourish]. Supernutrition; overfeeding.

hyperonychia (hī″pĕr-ō-nĭk′ē-ă) [″ + *onyx,* nail]. Overgrowth (hypertrophy) of the nails.

hyperope (hī′pĕr-ōp) [″ + *ops,* eye]. One who is farsighted. SYN: *hypermetrope.*

hyperopia (hī″pĕr-ō′pē-ă) [″ + *ops,* eye]. Farsightedness. Defect in vision in which parallel rays come to a focus behind the retina due to flattening of the globe of the eye or to error in refraction. SYN: *hypermetropia.* SEE: *emmetropia* for illus.

    SYM: Ocular fatigue and poor vision.

    h., absolute. Hyperopia in which the eye cannot accommodate.

    h., axial. Hyperopia caused by shortness of the eye's anteroposterior axis.

    h., facultative. Hyperopia that can be corrected by accommodation.

    h., latent. Hyperopia in which the error of refraction is overcome and disguised by ciliary muscle action.

    h., manifest. Total amount of hyperopia that can be neutralized by a convex lens without interfering with clarity of vision.

    h., relative. Hyperopia in which vision is clear only when excessive convergence is made.

    h., total. Complete hyperopia combining both latent and manifest types; the amt. of hyperopia present when accommodation is completely suspended by paralyzing the ciliary muscle. This is done by use of a cycloplegic drug.

hyperorchidism (hī″pĕr-or′kĭd-ĭzm) [Gr. *hyper,* over, above, excessive, + *orchis,* testicle, + *-ismos,* state of]. Abnormal activity of testicular secretion.

hyperorexia (hī″pĕr-ō-rĕks′ē-ă) [″ + *orexis,* appetite]. Abnormal hunger. Usually satisfied by frequent small meals, as in gastric diseases, diabetes, hysteria, psychosis, hyperthyroidism and brain tumors. It is found in helminthiasis, diabetes, hysteria, convalescence from acute diseases, psychosis, hyperthyroidism, brain tumors, diseases of the stomach in which hypermotility and hypersecretion are present. SYN: *bulimia.*

hyperorthocytosis (hī″pĕr-or″thō-sī-tō′sis) [″ + *orthos,* straight, + *kytos,* cell, + *osis,* condition]. Increased white blood cells with normal proportion of various forms and without immature forms.

hyperosmia (hī″pĕr-ŏz′mē-ă) [″ + *osme,* smell]. Abnormal sensitivity to odors.

hyperosmolar hyperglycemic nonketotic coma. ABBR: HHNC. Coma caused by increased blood osmolarity and glucose but not associated with ketoacidosis. It usually occurs in diabetes but may be present as a complication of burns, hyperalimentation, and renal dialysis. The blood glucose level may be as high as 1000 mg/dl. The metabolic disorder is treated with insulin, potassium, and sodium until the condition is corrected. The total water deficit may be as much as 10 to 12 liters. When adequate urine flow is established, it is essential to prevent excess administration of potassium.

hyperosmolarity (hī″pĕr-ŏz″mō-lăr′ĭ-tē). Increased osmolarity of the blood.

hyperostosis (hī″pĕr-ŏs-tō′sis) [″ + *osteon,* bone, + *osis,* condition]. Abnormal growth of osseous tissue. SYN: *exostosis; torus.*

    h., frontal internal. Osteoma, usually multiple or arising from the internal area of the frontal bone.

h., infantile cortical. Increased growth of subperiosteal bone occurring most frequently in the mandible and clavicles with fever and other systemic manifestations.

h., Morgagni's. H., frontal internal.

hyperovaria (hī"pĕr-ō-vā'rĭ-ă) [Gr. *hyper*, over, above, excessive, + L. *ovarium*, ovary]. Precocity of sexual development in young girls due to excessive ovarian secretion as the result of unusual and premature development of the ovaries.

hyperovulation. Production of a large number of ova, usually in response to hormonal intervention. This is done in an attempt to improve the chance of pregnancy in a patient who has had difficulty conceiving.

hyperoxaluria (hī"pĕr-ŏk"să-lū'rē-ă). Increased oxalic acid in the urine.

h., enteric. Hyperoxaluria caused by disease of or surgical removal of the ileum.

h., primary. An inherited metabolic disease caused by a defect in glyoxalate metabolism. This causes an increased secretion of oxalate in the urine, renal calculi, renal failure, and generalized deficit of oxalate crystals in tissues.

hyperoxemia (hī"pĕr-ŏk-sē'mē-ă) [" + *oxys*, sharp, + *haima*, blood]. Increased oxygen content in blood.

hyperoxia (hī"pĕr-ŏk'sē-ă). Increased oxygen in the blood.

hyperpancreatism (hī"pĕr-păn'krē-ă-tĭzm) [" + *pankreas*, pancreas, + *-ismos*, condition]. Abnormal amount of secretion from the pancreas.

hyperparasitism (hī"pĕr-păr'ă-sī"tĭzm). Condition in which a parasite lives in or upon another parasite.

hyperparathyroidism (hī"pĕr-păr"ă-thī'roy-dĭzm) [" + *para*, beyond, + *thyreos*, shield, + *eidos*, form, shape, + *-ismos*, condition]. Condition due to increased activity of the parathyroid glands. SYN: *osteitis fibrosa cystica generalisata.*

hyperpathia [" + *pathos*, disease, suffering]. Hypersensitivity to sensory stimuli. Includes hyperesthesia, allodynia, and hyperalgesia.

hyperpepsia (hī"pĕr-pĕp'sē-ă) [" + *pepsis*, digestion]. Indigestion due to hyperchlorhydria.

hyperpepsinia (hī"pĕr-pĕp-sĭn'ē-ă) [" + *pepsis*, digestion]. Excess of pepsin in the gastric secretion.

hyperperistalsis (hī"pĕr-pĕr"ĭ-stăl'sĭs) [" + *peri*, around, + *stalsis*, contraction]. Overactive peristalsis.

hyperphagia [" + Gr. *phagein*, to eat]. Eating more food than required; gluttony. May be due to a lesion in the hypothalamus of the brain.

hyperphalangism (hī"pĕr-făl-ăn'jĭzm) [" + *phalanx*, closely knit row, + *-ismos*, state of]. Having an extra phalanx on a finger or toe. SYN: *polyphalangism.*

hyperphasia (hī"pĕr-fā'zē-ă) [" + *phasis*, speech]. Abnormal desire to talk.

hyperphenylalaninemia (hī"pĕr-fĕn"ĭl-ăl"ă-nĭ-nē'mē-ă). Increased phenylalanine in the blood. SEE: *phenylketonuria.*

hyperphonia (hī"pĕr-fō'nē-ă) [" + *phone*, voice]. 1. Stuttering or stammering due to irritability of the vocal cords. 2. Explosive speech exhibited by those who stammer.

hyperphoria (hī"pĕr-fō'rē-ă) [" + *phorein*, to bear]. Tendency of one eye to turn upward.

hyperphosphatasemia (hī"pĕr-fŏs"fă-tă-sē'mē-ă). Increased alkaline phosphatase in the blood.

hyperphosphatemia (hī"pĕr-fŏs"fă-tē'mē-ă) [" + L. *phosphas*, phosphate, + Gr. *haima*, blood]. Abnormal amount of phosphorus in the blood.

hyperphosphaturia (hī"pĕr-fŏs-fă-tū'rē-ă) [" + " + Gr. *ouron*, urine]. Increased amount of phosphates in the urine.

hyperphospheremia (hī"pĕr-fŏs-fĕr-ē'mē-ă) [" + " + Gr. *haima*, blood]. Abnormal amount of phosphorous compounds in the blood. SYN: *hyperphosphatemia.*

hyperphrenia (hī"pĕr-frē'nē-ă) [Gr. *hyper*, over, above, excessive, + *phren*, mind]. 1. Excessive mental activity. Seen in the manic phase of manic-depressive psychosis. 2. Mental ability and capacity much greater than normal.

hyperpiesia, hyperpiesis (hī"pĕr-pī-ē'zē-ă, -pī'ĕ-sĭs) [" + *piesis*, pressure]. Abnormally high blood pressure.

hyperpietic (hī"pĕr-pī-ĕt'ĭk). Rel. to extremely high blood pressure.

hyperpigmentation (hī"pĕr-pĭg'mĕn-tā'shŭn). Increased pigmentation, esp. of the skin.

hyperpituitarism (hī"pĕr-pĭ-tū'ĭ-tăr-ĭsm) [" + L. *pituita*, mucus, + Gr. *-ismos*, condition]. Condition resulting from overactivity of the anterior lobe of the pituitary. SEE: *acromegaly; gigantism.*

hyperplasia (hī"pĕr-plā'zē-ă) [" + *plassein*, to form]. Excessive proliferation of normal cells in the normal tissue arrangement of an organ. SYN: *hypergenesis.*

h., fibrous. Connective-tissue cell increase following inflammation.

hyperplastic (hī"pĕr-plăs'tĭk). Rel. to hyperplasia.

hyperploidy (hī"pĕr-ploy'dē). Condition of having one extra chromosome and thus not balanced sets of chromosomes. SEE: *Down syndrome; trisomy 21.*

hyperpnea (hī"pĕrp-nē'ă) [" + *pnoia*,

breath]. An increased respiratory rate or breathing that is deeper than that usually experienced during normal activity. A certain degree of hyperpnea is normal after exercise.

ETIOL: Pain, respiratory disease, febrile or cardiac disease, certain drugs, hysteria, or atmospheric conditions experienced at high altitude.

hyperpotassemia (hī″pĕr-pŏt″ă-sē′mē-ă). Increased potassium in the blood. SYN: *hyperkalemia.*

hyperpragic (hī″pĕr-pră′jĭk) [″ + *praxis,* action]. Denoting excessive activity, especially mental activity.

hyperpraxia (hī″pĕr-prăk′sē-ă). Excessive activity and restlessness seen in some mental disorders.

hyperprolactinemia (hī″pĕr-prō-lăk″tĭn-ē′mē-ă). Excess secretion of prolactin thought to be due to hypothalamic-pituitary dysfunction. This is usually associated with amenorrhea with or without galactorrhea.

hyperprolinemia (hī″pĕr-prō″lĭ-nē′mē-ă). An inherited metabolic disease of amino acid metabolism that results in an excess of proline in the body.

hyperproteinemia (hī″pĕr-prō″tĕ-ĭn-ē′mē-ă) [″ + *protos,* first, + *haima,* blood]. Excess of protein in the blood plasma.

hyperproteinuria (hī″pĕr-prō″tē-ĭn-ū′rē-ă) [″ + ″ + *ouron,* urine]. Excess of protein in the urine.

hyperpselaphesia (hī″pĕrp-sĕl″ă-fē′zē-ă) [Gr. *hyper,* over, above, excessive, + *pselaphesis,* touch]. Abnormal sensitivity to touch. SYN: *hyperaphia.*

hyperptyalism (hī″pĕr-tī′ăl-ĭzm) [″ + *ptyalon,* spittle]. Excessive secretion of saliva. SYN: *salivation.* SEE: *xerostomia.*

ETIOL: May be due to pregnancy, stomatitis, rabies, exophthalmic goiter, menstruation, epilepsy, hysteria, nervous conditions, and gastrointestinal disorders. May be induced by mercury, iodides, pilocarpine, and other drugs.

hyperpyretic (hī″pĕr-pī-rĕt′ĭk). Pert. to high body temperature (hyperpyrexia).

hyperpyrexia (hī″pĕr-pī-rĕks′ē-ă) [″ + *pyressein,* to be feverish]. Elevation of body temperature above 106°F (41.1°C). Produced by physical agents such as hot baths, diathermy, hot air, or by reaction to infection caused by microorganisms. SEE: *fever, induced.*

h., malignant. A severe form of pyrexia that occurs during the use of muscle relaxants and general inhalation anesthesia (usually succinylcholine and halothane) in those who have inherited this ability as an autosomal dominant trait. During general anesthesia the temperature rises readily and there are signs of increased muscle metabolism. This condition progresses rapidly and if it is untreated, 70% of patients die. Persons who are susceptible may be diagnosed by elevated CPK levels and histochemical studies on muscle biopsy; and history of exposure to halothane. Persons who are susceptible to this and who need anesthesia should have local anesthesia or neuroleptic anesthesia, q.v. SYN: *hyperthermia, malignant.*

hyperpyrexial (hī″pĕr-pī-rĕk′sē-ăl). Denoting high body temperature.

hyperreactive (hī″pĕr-rē-ăk′tĭv). Pert. to an increased response to stimuli.

hyperreflexia (hī″pĕr-rē-flĕk′sē-ă) [″ + L. *reflexus,* bent back]. Increased action of the reflexes.

hyperresonance (hī″pĕr-rĕz′ō-năns) [″ + L. *resonare,* to resound]. Increased resonance produced when the area is percussed.

hypersalemia (hī″pĕr-săl-ē′mē-ă). Increased salt in the blood.

hypersalivation (hī″pĕr-săl″ĭ-vā′shŭn) [″ + L. *salivatio,* salivation]. Excessive secretion of saliva.

hypersecretion (hī″pĕr-sē-krē′shŭn) [″ + L. *secretio,* separation]. Abnormal amount of secretion.

hypersensibility (hī″pĕr-sĕn″sĭ-bĭl′ĭ-tē) [″ + L. *sensibilitas,* sensibility]. Increased sensitivity in general or to stimuli.

hypersensitiveness (hī″pĕr-sĕn′sĭ-tĭv-nĕs) [″ + L. *sensitivus,* sensitive]. Excessive and abnormal susceptibility to the action of a given agent, as pollen or foreign protein. SEE: *allergy; anaphylaxis; hay fever.*

hypersensitive tooth. Usually a tooth sensitive to temperature changes, sweets, or percussion. Exhibits gingival recession, exposed root dentin, caries, or periodontal disease.

hypersensitivity (hī″pĕr-sĕn″sĭ-tĭv′ĭ-tē). Abnormal sensitivity to a stimulus of any kind.

hypersensitivity reactions. The reaction of the body to antigens. These immunologic responses may be trivial or serious and potentially lethal. They are classed as follows: Type I or immediate, anaphylactic hypersensitivity. This causes formation of immunoglobulin E (IgE) antibodies. An example is the reaction to ragweed pollen. Type II reactions are mediated by the reaction of antigens and antibodies at cell surfaces. Clinical examples include reactions to transfusion with incompatible blood cells and erythroblastosis fetalis. Type III reaction is a reaction between antigens and antibodies that occur in extracellular fluid spaces. It produces toxic complexes which lead to reactions that cause serum sickness and glomerulonephritis. Type IV is a cell-mediated or delayed reaction mediated by the interaction of the antigen with T lymphocytes and subsequent release of lymphokines. Examples include tuberculosis, contact dermatitis, and transplant rejection.

hypersensitization (hī″pĕr-sĕn″sĭ-tĭ-zā′shŭn). 1. Producing or inducing increased sensitivity to an organism or drug. 2. The condition of being highly sensitive to something.

hypersialosis (hī″pĕr-sī″ă-lō′sĭs). Ptyalism, q.v.

hypersomnia (hī″pĕr-sŏm′nē-ă) [″ + L. *somnus*, sleep]. Sleeping for pathological lengths of time. May be associated with psychiatric illness, drug or alcohol use, or narcolepsy, q.v.

hypersplenism (hī″pĕr-splĕn′ĭzm). Increased activity of the spleen in which increased amounts of blood cells of all types are removed from the circulation.

hypersthenia (hī″pĕr-sthē′nē-ă) [Gr. *hyper*, over, above, excessive, + *sthenos*, strength]. Abnormal strength or excessive tension of the entire body or part of it.

hypersthenic (hī″pĕr-sthĕn′ĭk). 1. Denoting excessive strength or tension. 2. Body habitus characterized by a broad, deep thorax, short thoracic cavity, and a large abdominal cavity; a massive build.

hypersthenuria (hī″pĕr-sthĕn-ū′rē-ă) [″ + *sthenos*, strength, + *ouron*, urine]. Passage of abnormally concentrated urine. Usually due to dehydration or excess loss of fluids in sweat.

hypersusceptibility (hī″pĕr-sŭ-sĕp″tĭ-bĭl′ĭtē) [″ + L. *suscipere*, to take up, + *-bilis*, able]. Unusual susceptibility to a disease, pathological conditions, chemicals, or parasites. SEE: *allergy; anaphylaxis.*

hypersystole (hī″pĕr-sĭs′tō-lē) [″ + *systole*, contraction]. Unusual force or duration of the systole, q.v.

hypersystolic (hī″pĕr-sĭs-tŏl′ĭk). Pert. to hypersystole.

hypertelorism (hī″pĕr-tĕl′or-ĭzm) [″ + *telouros*, distant]. Abnormal width between two paired organs, esp. the eyes.

hypertensinogen (hī″pĕr-tĕn-sĭn′ō-jĕn). A globulin present in blood plasma that when acted upon by the enzyme renin forms angiotensin, q.v.

hypertension [″ + L. *tensio*, tension]. 1. Tension or tonus that is greater than normal. 2. A condition in which the patient has a higher blood pressure than that judged to be normal.

ETIOL: The primary factor in hypertension is an increase in peripheral resistance resulting from vasoconstriction or narrowing of peripheral blood vessels. The specific etiology for this condition can be determined in only a small number of patients with hypertension; however, it is important to attempt to define the exact etiology because, if the disease is due to certain pathological states, definitive and curative therapy can be instituted. Causes in this category include coarctation of the aorta; hyperthyroidism with thyrotoxicosis; patent ductus arteriosus; arteriovenous fistula; pheochromocytoma; psychogenic causes; certain forms of renal disease, particularly when limited to one kidney; adrenal tumors; primary aldosteronism; and polycythemia. SEE: *blood pressure, indirect recording of; heart disease, risk factors; infrasonic recorder; pseudohypertension.*

DIAG: There are no precise rules concerning what blood pressure reading is considered to represent hypertension. In general, if on several separate occasions the systolic pressure is above 140 mmHg or the diastolic above 90 mm, the patient is considered to have elevated blood pressure. Normal systolic blood pressure is not 100 plus the individual's age. Coronary artery disease and cerebral vascular disease, the great causes of death and disability, are much more frequent in those who have elevated blood pressure than in those who are normotensive. On the other hand, a patient's blood pressure may register high merely because of being excited when the pressure is taken. For this reason it is advisable to take the pressure on several separate occasions to be certain that the true blood pressure is being obtained. SEE: *human growth hormone, synthetic; hypertensive crisis.*

NURSING IMPLICATIONS: Help prevent or diagnose hypertension by encouraging people to have periodic blood pressure checks, by teaching individuals what their blood pressure reading is and what the numbers mean, and by encouraging lifestyle changes that may prevent hypertension, such as reducing sodium intake and maintaining normal weight and regular exercise patterns. Encourage hypertensive patients to have regular medical examinations, to comply with prescribed medical therapy, to reduce other risk factors for cardiac disease, and to practice stress reduction and management techniques. SEE: *Nursing Diagnoses* in *Appendix.*

RS: blood pressure; blood pressure, indirect recording of; diastolic pressure; heart disease, risk factors; hypotension; infrasonic recorder; pseudohypertension; pulse; pulse pressure; systolic pressure.

h., benign. Hypertension that progresses slowly. The basic disease process may progress to the same endpoint as in malignant hypertension but at a slower rate.

h., essential. Hypertension that develops without apparent cause. SYN: *h., primary.*

h., Goldblatt. Hypertension that resembles renal hypertension produced in experimental animals by decreasing the blood flow to the kidney.

h., malignant. A form of hypertension that progresses rapidly, accompanied by severe vascular damage. It may progress to the point of death.

h., portal. Increased pressure in the portal vein caused by obstruction of flow of blood through the liver.

h., primary. H., essential, q.v.

h., renal. Hypertension accompanied by kidney disease. Hypertension produced experimentally by constriction of renal arteries. It is due to a humoral substance, renin, produced in an ischemic kidney.

hypertensive (hī″pĕr-tĕn′sĭv). Marked by a rise in blood pressure.

hypertensive crisis. Arbitrarily defined as severe elevation in diastolic blood pressure above 120 to 130 mmHg. This is considered to be an emergency if there is evidence of rapid or progressive central nervous system, myocardial, hematologic, or renal deterioration.

TREAT: Reduce blood pressure without delay by use of appropriate therapy, usually sodium nitroprusside, labetalol, and diazoxide. If crisis is due to eclampsia, sodium nitroprusside (SNP) may not be indicated because of risk to fetus.

Caution: Infusion of SNP at the maximum dose rate of 8 µg/kg/min should never last for more than 10 minutes. For treatment of overdose, SEE: *cyanide poisoning.*

Hyper-Tet. Trade name for tetanus immune globulin, human.

hyperthecosis (hī″pĕr-thē-kō′sĭs). Hyperplasia of the theca interna of the ovary. Hirsutism and amenorrhea may be present.

hyperthelia (hī″pĕr-thē′lē-ă) [Gr. *hyper,* over, above, excessive, + *thele,* nipple]. The presence of more than two nipples.

hyperthermalgesia (hī″pĕr-thĕrm″ăl-jē′zē-ă) [″ + *therme,* heat, + *algesis,* sense of pain]. Unusual sensitiveness to heat.

hyperthermia (hī″pĕr-thĕr′mē-ă) [″ + *therme,* heat]. 1. Unusually high fever. SYN: *hyperpyrexia.* 2. Treatment of disease by raising bodily temperature, accomplished by introduction of the malaria organism, injection of foreign proteins, or by physical means. SEE: *fever, induced.*

NURSING IMPLICATIONS: Reduce external covering to encourage heat loss through radiation, but do not induce chilling. Bathe the patient with tepid water, promoting reduction in the surface temperature by convection and evaporation. Increase fluid intake to 3 liters per day if cardiac and renal function are normal to replace fluids lost through sweating, insensible loss, and increased metabolism. Give oral hygiene frequently since dehydration dries oral mucosa. Ensure bed rest and administer supplemental oxygen. Prevent chilling and shivering, which further increases metabolic rate and body temperature. Monitor all vital signs. Administer antipyretics and apply hypothermia blankets only as prescribed by the physician.

h., malignant. Hyperpyrexia, malignant, q.v.

hyperthermoesthesia (hī″pĕr-thĕrm″ō-ĕs-thē′zē-ă) [″ + ″ + *aisthesis,* sensation]. Unusual sensitiveness to heat. SYN: *hyperthermalgesia.*

hyperthrombinemia (hī″pĕr-thrŏm″bĭn-ē′mē-ă) [″ + *thrombos,* clot, + *haima,* blood]. Excess of thrombin in the blood. This tends to promote intravascular clotting.

hyperthymia (hī″pĕr-thī′mē-ă) [″ + *thymos,* mind]. 1. Pathological sensitiveness or excitability. 2. Sudden cruelty or foolhardiness.

hyperthyroidism (hī″pĕr-thī′royd-ĭzm) [″ + *thyreos,* shield, + *eidos,* form, shape, + *-ismos,* state of]. A condition caused by excessive secretion of the thyroid glands, which increases the basal metabolic rate, causing an increased demand for food to support this metabolic activity. SEE: *thyroid function tests.*

SYM: Exophthalmic goiter, fine tremor of the extended fingers and tongue, increased nervousness, weight loss, altered bowel activity, heat intolerance, excessive sweating, increased heart rate.

TREAT: Surgical, by removal of the thyroid gland following proper medical preparation. Medical, by use of antithyroid drugs (as propylthiouracil, methimazole, or carbimazole) or iodide.

NURSING IMPLICATIONS: Monitor vital signs and weight. Promote high-calorie, high-vitamin, high-mineral diet including between-meal snacks and avoidance of caffeinated beverages during treatment. Encourage a cool and restful environment. The nurse can be of great assistance in helping the patient adjust to this disease as it is being treated. Almost invariably there will be emotional and personality changes and problems in the areas of hyperactivity, heat intolerance, and sexual dysfunction. It will be necessary to reassure the patient that these signs and symptoms will be alleviated by therapy. SEE: *Nursing Diagnoses* in *Appendix.*

hyperthyrosis (hī"pĕr-thī-rō'sĭs). Hyperthyroidism.

hyperthyroxinemia (hī"pĕr-thī-rŏk"sĭ-nē'mē-ă). Excess of thyroxine in the blood.

hypertonia (hī"pĕr-tō'nē-ă) [" + *tonos,* tension]. Abnormal tension of arteries or muscles.

hypertonic (hī"pĕr-tŏn'ĭk). 1. Having a higher osmotic pressure than a compared solution. Pert. to a solution of higher osmotic pressure than another. 2. Being in a state of greater than normal tension or of incomplete relaxation. Said of muscles. Opposite of hypotonic.

hypertonicity (hī"pĕr-tŏn-ĭ'sĭ-tē). Excess of muscular tonus or intraocular pressure. SYN: *hypertonia.*

hypertonus (hī"pĕr-tō'nŭs). Increased tension, as muscular tension in spasm.

hypertoxicity (hī"pĕr-tŏk-sĭs'ĭ-tē) [" + *toxikon,* poison]. The state of being excessively poisonous.

hypertrichiasis (hī"pĕr-trĭk-ĭ'ă-sĭs) [" + *thrix,* hair, + *-iasis,* diseased condition]. Hypertrichosis.

hypertrichophobia (hī"pĕr-trĭk"ō-fō'bē-ă) [" + " + *phobos,* fear]. Fear of hair on the body.

hypertrichophrydia (hī"pĕr-trĭk"ŏ-frĭd'ē-ă) [" + " + *ophrys,* eyebrow]. Undue thickness of the eyebrows.

hypertrichosis (hī"pĕr-trĭ-kō'sĭs) [" + " + *osis,* condition]. Growth of hair in excess of normal.
ETIOL: May be due to endocrine disease, esp. of the adrenal gland, and in the female, also the ovary.

hypertriglyceridemia (hī"pĕr-trī-glĭs"ĕr-ĭ-dē'mē-ă). Increased triglycerides in the blood.

hypertrophia (hī"pĕr-trō'fē-ă) [Gr. *hyper,* over, above, excessive, + *trophe,* nourishment]. Increased size of an organ, or of the body, due to growth. SYN: *hypertrophy.*

hypertrophic (hī"pĕr-trŏf'ĭk) [" + *trophe,* nourishment]. Pert. to hypertrophy.

hypertrophy (hī-pĕr'trŏ-fē) [" + *trophe,* nourishment]. Increase in size of an organ or structure that does not involve tumor formation. Term is generally restricted to an increase in size or bulk not resulting from an increase in number of cells or tissue elements, as in the hypertrophy of a muscle. Term sometimes used to apply to any increase in size as a result of functional activity. SYN: *hypertrophia.* SEE: *hyperplasia.*

h., adaptive. Hypertrophy in which an organ increases in size to meet increased functional demands, as hypertrophy of the heart that accompanies valvular disorders.

h., benign prostatic. SEE: *benign prostatic hypertrophy.*

h., cardiac. Increase in size of the heart resulting from hypertrophy of muscle tissue but without increase in size of chambers.

h., compensatory. Hypertrophy resulting from increased function of an organ because of a defect or impaired function of the opposite of a paired organ.

h., concentric. Hypertrophy in which the walls of an organ become thickened without enlargement but with diminished capacity.

h., eccentric. Hypertrophy of an organ with dilatation.

h., false. Hypertrophy with degeneration of one constituent of an organ and its replacement by another.

h., gingival. SEE: *gingival hypertrophy.*

h., Marie's. Chronic periostitis that causes the soft tissues surrounding the joints to enlarge.

h., numerical. Hypertrophy caused by increase in structural elements.

h., physiological. Hypertrophy due to natural rather than pathological factors.

h., pseudomuscular. A disease, usually of childhood, characterized by paralysis, depending upon degeneration of the muscles, which, however, become enlarged from a deposition of fat and connective tissue.
SYM: Weakness of muscles. Patient is awkward and stumbles and seeks support in walking. As paralysis increases, the muscles, particularly those of the calf, thigh, buttocks, and back, enlarge. Upper extremities are less frequently affected. When patient stands erect, the feet are wide apart, the abdomen protrudes, and spinal column shows a marked curvature with convexity forward. Patient rises from recumbent position by grasping the knees or by resting the hands on the floor in front, extending the legs and pushing the body backwards. Gait is waddling. In course of few years paralysis becomes so marked patient is unable to leave bed. This leads to muscular atrophy.
TREAT: Physical therapy helps to prevent contractures, but there is no effective therapy.
PROG: Unfavorable.

h., simple. Hypertrophy due to increase in size of structural parts.

h., true. Hypertrophy caused by increase in size in all the different tissues composing a part.

h., ventricular. Increased size and muscular content of the myocardium of the ventricles.

h., vicarious. Hypertrophy of an organ when another organ of allied function is disabled or destroyed.

hypertropia [Gr. *hyper*, over, above, excessive, + *tropos*, turning]. Vertical strabismus upward.

hyperuricemia (hī″pĕr-ū″rĭs-ē′mē-ă) [″ + *ouron*, urine, + *haima*, blood]. Abnormal amount of uric acid in the blood.

hyperuricuria (hī″pĕr-ū″rĭk-ū′rē-ă) [″ + ″ + *ouron*, urine]. Abnormal amount of uric acid in the urine.

hypervalinemia (hī″pĕr-văl″ĭn-ē′mē-ă). An inherited condition caused by a deficiency of the enzymes essential to the metabolism of valine. Clinically the child is mentally retarded, has nystagmus, vomits, and fails to thrive.

hypervascular (hī″pĕr-văs′kū-lăr) [″ + L. *vasculus*, vessel]. Excessively vascular.

hyperventilation (hī″pĕr-vĕn″tĭ-lā′shŭn) [″ + L. *ventilatio*, ventilation]. Increased minute volume ventilation which results in a lowered carbon dioxide (CO_2) level (hypocapnia). It is a frequent finding in many disease processes such as asthma, metabolic acidosis, pulmonary embolism, pulmonary edema, and also in anxiety-induced states. SEE: *carpopedal spasm*.

TREAT: Treatment is directed at the underlying cause. Immediate therapy consists of decreasing the rate of loss of CO_2. This is best done by having the patient breathe through only one nostril, with the mouth closed. The patient can close one nostril by placing a finger against that side of the nose. This method is simpler than having the patient breathe into a paper bag over the head. After the acute phase of the hyperventilation episode has been treated it will be necessary to determine the underlying cause and provide appropriate therapy.

hyperviscosity (hī″pĕr-vĭs-kŏs′ĭ-tē) [″ + L. *viscosus*, gummy]. Excessive viscosity or exaggeration of adhesive properties. Seen in anemias and inflammatory diseases.

hypervitaminosis (hī″pĕr-vī″tă-mĭn-ō′sĭs) [″ + L. *vita*, life, + *amine* + Gr. *osis*, condition]. A condition caused by an excessive amount of vitamins in the diet; most commonly due to excessive ingestion of vitamin pills.

hypervolemia (hī″per-vŏl-ē′mē-ă) [″ + L. *volumen*, volume, + Gr. *haima*, blood]. Plethora of blood; abnormal increase in the volume of circulating blood.

hypesthesia (hī″pĕs-thē′zē-ă) [Gr. *hypo*, under, beneath, below, + *aisthesis*, sensation]. Lessened sensibility to touch. Variant of hypoesthesia.

hypha (hī′fă) [Gr. *hyphe*, web] (pl. *hyphae*). A filament of mold, or part of a mold mycelium.

hyphedonia (hĭp″hĕ-dō′nē-ă) [Gr. *hypo*, under, beneath, below, + *hedone*, pleasure]. Abnormal diminution of pleasure in acts that should normally give pleasure.

hyphema (hī-fē′mă) [Gr. *hyphaimos*, suffused with blood]. Blood in the anterior chamber of the eye, in front of the iris.

hyphidrosis (hĭp-hĭd-rō′sĭs) [Gr. *hypo*, under, beneath, below, + *hidros*, sweat]. Diminished secretion of sweat.

Hyphomycetes (hī″fŏ-mī-sē′tēz) [Gr. *hyphe*, web, + *mykes*, fungus]. The Fungi Imperfecti. Filamentous fungi with branched or unbranched threads. They do not have sexual spores.

hypnagogic (hĭp-nă-gŏj′ĭk) [Gr. *hypnos*, sleep, + *agogos*, leading]. 1. Inducing sleep or induced by sleep. SYN: *hypnotic*. SEE: *zones, hypnogenic*. 2. In psychology, pert. to hallucinations or dreams just before loss of consciousness.

hypnagogic state. A transitional state between sleeping and awaking and delusions that may result therefrom.

hypnagogue (hĭp′nă-gŏg). Concerning or causing sleep or drowsiness.

hypnalgia (hĭp-năl′jē-ă) [″ + *algos*, pain]. False sense of pain experienced in a dream.

hypnic (hĭp′nĭk) [Gr. *hypnos*, sleep]. Causing sleep. SYN: *somnifacient; somniferous*.

hypno-. Combining form relating to sleep or hypnosis.

hypnoanalysis (hĭp″nō-ă-năl′ĭ-sĭs) [″ + *analysis*, a dissolving]. Combined psychoanalytic therapy and hypnosis.

hypnoanesthesia (hĭp″nō-ăn″ĕs-thē′zē-ă). Use of hypnosis to produce anesthesia.

hypnodontics (hĭp″nō-dŏn′tĭks). The application of controlled suggestion and hypnosis to the practice of dentistry.

hypnogenetic (hĭp″nō-jĕ-nĕt′ĭk) [″ + *gennan*, to produce]. Producing sleep.

hypnoidal (hĭp-noy′dăl) [″ + *eidos*, form, shape]. Pert. to a condition between sleep and waking, resembling sleep.

hypnoidization (hĭp″noy-dī-zā′shŭn) [″ + *eidos*, form, shape]. Induction of hypnosis.

hypnolepsy (hĭp′nō-lĕp″sē) [″ + *lepsis*, seizure]. Irresistible sleepiness. SYN: *narcolepsy*.

hypnology (hĭp-nŏl′ō-jē) [″ + *logos*, word, reason]. Scientific study of sleep.

hypnonarcoanalysis (hĭp″nō-năr″kō-ă-năl′ĭ-sĭs). A psychiatric interview combining hypnosis with drug-induced sedation or narcosis.

hypnonarcosis (hĭp″nō-năr-kō′sĭs). Combination of hypnosis and narcosis.

hypnophobia (hĭp″nō-fō′bē-ă) [″ + *phobos,* fear]. Morbid fear of falling asleep.

hypnopompic (hĭp″nō-pŏm′pĭk) [″ + *pompe,* procession]. Pert. to dreams or visual images persisting after sleep and prior to complete awakening.

hypnosis (hĭp-nō′sĭs) [″ + *osis,* condition]. A subconscious condition in which the objective manifestations of the mind are more or less inactive, accompanied by abnormal sensibility to suggestions made by the hypnotist. Hypnosis has been used in treating phobias and anxiety, and in managing pain. SEE: *autohypnosis; hypnotism; sleepwalking; somnambulism.*

hypnosophy (hĭp-nŏs′ō-fē) [″ + *sophia,* wisdom]. The study of sleep.

hypnotherapy (hĭp″nō-thĕr′ă-pē) [″ + *therapeia,* treatment]. Treatment by hypnotism or by inducing prolonged sleep.

hypnotic (hĭp-nŏt′ĭk) [Gr. *hypnos,* sleep]. 1. Pert. to sleep or hypnosis. 2. An agent that induces sleep or that dulls the senses, such as chloral hydrate.

hypnotics (hĭp-nŏt′ĭks) [Gr. *hypnos,* sleep]. Drugs that cause insensitivity to pain by inhibiting afferent impulses or by inhibiting the receiving of sensory impressions in the cortical centers of the brain, thus causing partial or complete unconsciousness. Hypnotics include sedatives, analgesics, anesthetics, and intoxicants. They are sometimes called somnifacients and soporifics when used to induce sleep.

RS: analgesic; anesthetic; intoxicant; sedative; somnifacient; soporific.

hypnotism (hĭp′nō-tĭzm) [″ + *-ismos,* condition]. An induced sleeplike state during which the patient is peculiarly susceptible to the suggestions of the hypnotist.

hypnotist (hĭp′nō-tĭst) [Gr. *hypnos,* sleep]. One who practices hypnotism.

hypnotize (hĭp′nō-tīz). To put under hypnosis.

hypnotoxin (hĭp″nō-tŏk′sĭn). Theoretically, a toxic substance that accumulates in the blood during wakefulness, the effect of which is to induce sleep.

hypo (hī′pō) [Gr. *hypo,* under, beneath, below]. Popular name for hypodermic syringe or injection.

hypo-, hyp- [Gr. *hypo,* under, beneath, below]. Prefix indicating less than, below, or under. SYN: [L.] *sub.*

hypoacidity (hī″pō-ă-sĭd′ĭ-tē) [″ + L. *acidus,* sour]. A condition of decreased acid in the stomach caused by lowered hydrochloric acid secretion. Secondary to other disorders, such as pernicious anemia.

TREAT: Administer dilute HCl by mouth.

Caution: In order to protect the teeth, it is important to have the patient suck the acid solution through a straw.

---

hypoacusis (hī″pō-ă-kū′sĭs) [″ + *akousis,* hearing]. Decreased sensitivity to sound stimuli.

hypoadrenalism (hī″pō-ăd-rē′năl-ĭzm) [″ + L. *ad,* to, + *renalis,* pert. to kidney, + Gr. *-ismos,* state of]. Adrenal insufficiency.

hypoadrenocorticism (hī″pō-ă-drē″nō-kor′tĭ-sĭzm). Decreased secretion or effect of the adrenal cortical hormone.

hypoaffectivity (hī″pō-ăf′fĕk-tĭv′ĭ-tē). Decreased responsiveness to emotional stimuli. SEE: *obtund.*

hypoalbuminemia (hīpō-ăl-bū″mĭn-ē′mē-ă). Decreased albumin in the blood.

hypoaldosteronism (hī″pō-ăl″dō-stēr′ŏn-ĭzm). Decreased aldosterone in the blood associated with hypotension and increased salt excretion.

hypoalimentation [″ + L. *alimentum,* nourishment]. Insufficient nourishment.

hypoallergenic [″ + *allos,* other, + *ergon,* work]. Diminished potential for causing an allergic reaction.

hypoazoturia (hī″pō-ăz-ō-tū′rē-ă) [″ + L. *azotum,* nitrogen, + Gr. *ouron,* urine]. Diminished urea in the urine.

hypobaric (hī″pō-băr′ĭk) [″ + *baros,* weight]. Decreased atmospheric pressure. SEE: *bends; edema, high altitude.*

hypoblast (hī′pō-blăst) [″ + *blastos,* germ]. The inner cell layer or entoderm, which develops during gastrulation. The external layer is called ectoderm.

hypoblastic (hī-pō-blăs′tĭk). Pert. to the inner layer of the blastoderm.

hypobulia (hī″pō-bū′lē-ă) [″ + *boule,* will]. Impairment of will power. SEE: *abulia.*

hypocalcemia (hī″pō-kăl-sē′mē-ă) [″ + L. *calx,* lime, + Gr. *haima,* blood]. Abnormally low blood calcium.

hypocalciuria (hī″pō-kăl″sē-ū′rē-ă). Decreased calcium in the urine.

hypocapnia (hī″pō-kăp′nē-ă) [Gr. *hypo,* under, beneath, below, + *kapnos,* smoke]. Decreased amount of carbon dioxide in the blood.

hypocarbia (hī″pō-kăr′bē-ă). Decreased carbon dioxide in the blood. Excess rate of respiration will cause this.

hypocellularity (hī″pō-sĕl″ū-lăr′ĭ-tē). Decreased cell content of any tissue.

hypochloremia (hī″pō-klō-rē′mē-ă) [″ + *chloros,* green, + *haima,* blood]. Deficiency of the chloride content of the blood.

hypochlorhydria (hī″pō-klor-hī′drē-ă) [″

+ " + *hydor,* water]. Diminished secretion of hydrochloric acid. Decreased acid may be indicative of carcinoma or anemia. SEE: *achlorhydria; hyperchlorhydria.*

hypochlorite salts. A salt of hypochlorous acid used in household bleach and as an oxidizer, deodorant, and disinfectant.

hypochlorite salts poisoning. SEE: *Poisons and Poisoning* in *Appendix.*

hypochlorization (hī″pō-klō″rī-zā′shŭn). Diminished sodium chloride in the diet. Used in treating hypertension and certain kidney diseases.

hypochlorous acid. An acid, HClO, used as a disinfectant and as a bleaching agent. It is usually used in the form of one of its salts.

hypochloruria (hī″pŏ-klor-ū′rē-ă) [" + *chloros,* green, + *ouron,* urine]. Diminution of chlorides in the urine.

hypocholesteremia (hī″pō-kō-lĕs-tĕr-ē′mē-ă) [" + *chole,* bile, + *stereos,* solid, + *haima,* blood]. Decreased blood cholesterol.

hypochondria (hī″pō-kŏn′drē-ă) [" + *chondros,* cartilage]. Abnormal concern about health with false belief of suffering from some disease. SYN: *hypochondriasis.*

hypochondriac (hī″pō-kŏn′drē-ăk). 1. Pert. to the region of the hypochondrium, q.v., or upper lateral region on each side of the body and below the thorax; beneath the ribs. 2. One having an abnormal and excessive interest in and fear of disease, esp. in persons who are otherwise healthy.

hypochondriac region. Part of abdomen beneath the lower ribs on both sides of the epigastrium. SYN: *hypochondrium.*

hypochondriacal (hī″pō-kŏn-drī′ă-kăl) [" + *chondros,* cartilage]. Affected with a pathological interest in health and disease.

hypochondrial reflex (hī″pō-kŏn′drē-ăl). A sudden inspiratory act resulting from sudden pressure below the costal border.

hypochondriasis (hī″pō-kŏn-drī′ă-sĭs) [" + *chondros,* cartilage, + *-iasis,* diseased condition]. Abnormal anxiety about one's health; a frequent symptom in depressed patients. The patient fears or believes that he or she has a disease that persists despite medical reassurance. SYN: *hypochondria.*

hypochondrium (hī″pō-kŏn′drē-ŭm). Part of the abdomen beneath the lower ribs on each side of the epigastrium.

hypochromasia (hī″pō-krō-mā′sē-ă) [" + *chroma,* color]. Lack of hemoglobin in the red blood cells.

hypochromatism (hī″pō-krō′mă-tĭzm) [" + *chroma,* color]. 1. Lack of or decreased color. 2. A cell, esp. its nucleus, with decreased pigment. 3. Decreased hemoglobin in the red cells.

hypochromatosis (hī″pō-krō-mă-tō′sĭs) [" + " + *osis,* condition]. Disappearance of the chromatin or nucleus in a cell. SYN: *chromatolysis.*

hypochromia (hī″pō-krō′mē-ă). Condition of the blood in which the red blood cells have a reduced hemoglobin content.

hypochromic (hī″pō-krōm′ĭk). Pert. to hypochromia.

hypochylia (hī″pō-kī′lē-ă) [Gr. *hypo,* under, beneath, below, + *chylos,* juice]. Lack of normal secretion of gastric juice.

hypocinesia (hī″pō-sĭn-ē′zē-ă) [" + *kinesis,* movement]. Diminished power of movement. SYN: *hypokinesia.*

hypocomplementemia (hī″pō-kŏm″plĕmĕn-tē′mē-ă). Decreased complement in the blood.

hypocondylar (hī″pō-kŏn′dĭ-lăr) [" + *kondylos,* condyle]. Below a condyle.

hypocone (hī″pō-kōn) [" + *konos,* cone]. The distolingual cusp of an upper molar tooth.

hypoconid (hī″pō-kō′nĭd). The distobuccal cusp of a lower molar tooth.

hypoconulid. The distal, or 5th, cusp of the mandibular first molar tooth. SEE: *hypoconid.*

hypocorticism (hī″pō-kor′tĭ-sĭzm). Decreased adrenal cortical hormone.

hypocrinism (hī″pō-krī′nĭzm) [" + *krinein,* to separate, + *-ismos,* condition]. Deficient secretion of any gland, esp. an endocrine gland.

hypocupremia (hī″pō-kū-prē′mē-ă). Decreased copper in the blood.

hypocyclosis (hī″pō-sī-klō′sĭs) [" + *kyklos,* circle]. Deficient accommodation of the eye.

   h., ciliary. Weakness of ciliary muscle.

   h., lenticular. Lack of elasticity in crystalline lens.

hypocystotomy (hī″pō-sĭs-tŏt′ō-mē) [" + *kystis,* a bladder, + *tome,* incision]. Perineal opening of the bladder.

hypocythemia (hī″pō-sī-thē′mē-ă) [" + *kytos,* cell, + *haima,* blood]. Decrease in the number of blood cells, esp. red blood cells.

hypodactylia (hī″pō-dăk-tĭl′ē-ă) [" + *daktylos,* finger]. Having a decreased number of fingers or toes.

Hypoderma (hī″pō-dĕr′mă) [" + *derma,* skin]. A genus of warble flies of the family Oestridae. The larvae of some species attack cattle and, rarely, man. They cause a subcutaneous channel of inflammation as they burrow under the skin. SEE: *larva migrans, cutaneous.*

hypodermatoclysis (hī″pō-dĕr-mă-tŏk′lĭ-sĭs). Hypodermoclysis.

hypodermatomy (hī″pō-děr-măt′ō-mē) [″ + *derma*, skin, + *tome*, incision]. Subcutaneous incision or section, as of a muscle or tendon.

hypodermiasis (hī″pō-děr-mī′ă-sĭs) [″ + ″ + *-iasis*, condition]. Infection with *Hypoderma*.

hypodermic (hī″pō-děr′mĭk) [″ + *derma*, skin]. Under or inserted under the skin, as a hypodermic injection. It may be given subcutaneously (under the skin), intracutaneously (into the skin), intramuscularly (into a muscle), intraspinally (into the spinal canal), or intravascularly (into a vein or artery). It is given to secure prompt action of a drug when the drug cannot be taken by mouth, when it may not be readily absorbed in the stomach or intestines, when it might be changed by action of the gastric secretions, or to act as an anesthetic about the site of injection. SEE: *anesthesia, local.*

Caution: When injected substance is not intended for intravascular injection, pull back on the syringe plunger after the needle is inserted to determine if the needle is in a vein or artery. If blood is obtained, the needle must be repositioned and the procedure repeated. It may be necessary to use a fresh needle and syringe. Because medicines not intended to be injected intravenously produce serious undesired effects when given intravascularly, do not inject the medicine if the needle is in a vessel.

If medicine is to be injected into an artery or vein, do not administer it unless pulling back on the plunger permits blood to freely enter the syringe.

---

    h., intracutaneous. Injection into the skin.

    h., intramuscular. Injection given in gluteal or lumbar muscular region. Used when a drug is not easily absorbed, when it is irritating, or when large quantity of liquid is to be used.

    h., intraspinal. Injection into the spinal canal.

    h., intravenous. Injection into a vein, the usual site being the median basilic or median cephalic vein of the arm.

    h., subcutaneous. Injection given just under the skin, usually in outer surface of arms and forearm.

hypodermoclysis (hī″pō-děr-mŏk′lĭ-sĭs) [Gr. *hypo*, under, beneath, below, + *derma*, skin, + *klysis*, a washing out]. Injection of fluids into the subcutaneous tissues to supply the body with liquids quickly, as after shock, hemorrhage, or diarrhea; it may be given in any condition in which it is

impossible to give sufficient water by mouth, by rectum, or by vein.

When necessary to maintain a larger amount of water in the tissues in order to keep up proper metabolism, hypodermoclysis may be ordered. The purpose is about the same as that of intravenous infusions. Physiological salt solution (normal salt solution) is generally used because it is compatible with the constituents of the blood. There are other solutions given by this method as preferred by the attending physician. If the solution is not of the correct osmolarity, hemolysis, q.v., may occur. It is essential that the solution be the proper temperature, which should be from 108° to 115°F (42.2° to 46.1°C) in the flask because it cools rapidly while passing through the tubing.

Site of injection may be in the loose tissues at the base of the breasts; in the thighs or buttocks (care being taken to avoid the large blood vessels); in the axillary line (esp. for men); beneath the skin of the abdomen (halfway between the navel and the anterior superior spine); and intraperitoneally in children. The inner aspect of the thighs should be used as site of injection only with great caution because of the closeness of the femoral vessels.

hypodipsia (hī″pō-dĭp′sē-ă) [″ + *dipsa*, thirst]. Decreased intake of fluids due to lack of thirst.

hypodontia (hī″pō-dŏn′shē-ă). Diminished development, or absence, of teeth.

hypodynamia (hī″pō-dī-nā′mē-ă) [″ + *dynamis*, power]. Diminished muscular power or energy. SEE: *adynamia.*

hypoeccrisia (hī″pō-ĕk-krĭs′ē-ă) [″ + *ek*, out, + *krisis*, separation]. Diminished excretion of waste material.

hypoeccritic (hī″pō-ĕk-krĭt′ĭk). 1. Retarding normal excretion. 2. Pert. to insufficient or defective excretion.

hypoendocrisia (hī″pō-ĕn″dō-krĭz′ē-ă). Insufficiency of endocrine secretion. SYN: *hypoendocrinism.*

hypoeosinophilia (hī″pō-ē″ō-sĭn″ō-fĭl′ē-ă) [Gr. *hypo*, under, beneath, below, + *eos*, dawn, + *philein*, to love]. Diminished quantity of eosinophil leukocytes of the blood.

hypoepinephria (hī″pō-ĕp″ĭ-nĕf′rē-ă) [″ + *epi*, upon, + *nephros*, kidney]. Diminished secretion of epinephrine.

hypoergasia (hī″pō-ĕr-gā′sē-ă) [″ + *ergon*, work]. Decreased functional activity.

hypoergia (hī″pō-ĕr′jē-ă). 1. Mild allergy due to decreased response to allergic stimuli. 2. Diminished response to any stimulus.

hypoergic (hī″pō-ĕr′jĭk). 1. Concerning hypoergia. 2. Pert. to decreased energy level.

hypoergy (hī″pō-ĕr′jē) [″ + *ergon*, work]. Hyposensitiveness to allergens.

hypoesophoria (hī″pō-ĕs″ō-fō′rē-ă) [″ + *eso*, inward, + *phorein*, to bear]. Downward and inward deviation of the eye.

hypoesthesia (hī″pō-ĕs-thē′zē-ă) [″ + *aisthesis*, sensation]. Dulled sensitivity to touch.

hypoexophoria (hī″pō-ĕks-ō-fō′rē-ă) [″ + *exo*, outward, + *phorein*, to bear]. Downward and outward deviation of the eye.

hypoferremia (hī″pō-fĕ-rē′mē-ă). Iron deficiency as indicated by diminished iron in the blood.

hypofibrinogenemia (hī″pō-fī-brĭn″ō-jĕ-nē′mē-ă). Decreased fibrinogen in the blood.

hypofunction (hī″pō-fŭnk′shŭn). Decreased function.

hypogalactia (hī″pō-gă-lăk′shē-ă) [″ + *gala*, milk]. Deficient milk production.

hypogammaglobulinemia (hī″pō-găm″ă-glŏb″ū-lĭ-nē′mē-ă). Decreased gamma globulins in the blood, resulting in a state of immunodeficiency.

h., acquired. A form of hypogammaglobulinemia that has its onset in early childhood.

h., congenital. An inherited form of hypogammaglobulinemia in which all of the immunoglobulins are decreased. This usually manifests as immunodeficiency at 6 months of age, by which time the maternal immunoglobulins have disappeared.

hypogastric (hī″pō-găs′trĭk) [″ + *gaster*, belly]. Pert. to lower middle of the abdomen or hypogastrium.

hypogastric artery. Arteria iliaca interna.

hypogastric plexus. Sympathetic nerve plexus in the pelvis.

hypogastric region. The hypogastrium. SEE: *abdominal regions.*

hypogastrium (hī″pō-găs′trē-ŭm). Region below the umbilicus or navel, between the right and left inguinal regions.

hypogenesis (hī″pō-jĕn′ĕ-sĭs) [Gr. *hypo*, under, beneath, below, + *genesis*, generation, birth]. Cessation of growth or development at an early stage, causing defective structure. SEE: *ateliosis.*

hypogenitalism (hī″pō-jĕn′ĭ-tăl-ĭzm) [″ + L. *genitalis*, a genital, + Gr. -*ismos*, condition]. Condition in which the genital organs are underdeveloped. Characterized by reduced size of genital organs, failure of testes to descend in some cases, and incomplete development of secondary sex characteristics. SEE: *hypogonadism.*

hypogeusia (hī″pō-gū′sē-ă) [″ + *geusis*, taste]. Blunting of sense of taste.

h., idiopathic. A syndrome consisting of decreased taste and olfactory acuity, and with or without perverted taste (dysgeusia) and smell. Its cause is unknown. In experimental studies, certain trace elements such as zinc added to the diet appear to correct some of the symptoms.

hypoglossal (hī″pō-glŏs′ăl) [″ + *glossa*, tongue]. Situated under the tongue.

hypoglossal alternating hemiplegia. Medulla lesion paralyzing the tongue by involving the 12th nerve fibers as they course through the uncrossed pyramid. The pathology may extend across the midline or dorsally, involving the medial fillet, causing contralateral anesthesia.

hypoglossal nerve. A mixed cranial nerve, it carries afferent proprioceptive impulses as well as efferent motor impulses. Originates in the medulla oblongata. Distribution: extrinsic and intrinsic muscles of the tongue. SYN: *twelfth cranial nerve.*

hypoglottis (hī″pō-glŏt′ĭs). Undersurface of tongue.

hypoglycemia (hī″pō-glī-sē′mē-ă) [″ + *glykys*, sweet, + *haima*, blood]. Deficiency of sugar in the blood. A condition in which the glucose in the blood is abnormally low. SEE: *Nursing Diagnoses* in *Appendix.*

SYM: Acute fatigue, restlessness, malaise, marked irritability, and weakness. In severe cases, mental disturbances, delirium, coma, and possibly death. SEE: *coma, diabetic* for table.

ETIOL: Hyperfunction of the islets of Langerhans; injection of excessive quantity of insulin, or failure to eat after taking insulin; often precipitated by increased energy need, as in exercise. If the diabetic ingests alcohol, the insulin dose will need to be adjusted. SEE: *coma; hyperglycemia; hyperinsulinism.*

F.A.: If patient is awake with an intact gag reflex and can swallow, give sugar in the form of juice or candy bar. If unresponsive, do not put anything in patient's mouth, as the patient may aspirate it.

hypoglycemic (hī″pō-glī-sē′mĭk). Pert. to or causing hypoglycemia.

hypoglycemic agents, oral. Sulfonylurea compounds that cause a decrease in blood sugar. Acetohexamide, tolbutamide, and chlorpropamide are examples. There is no proof that their use in diabetes mellitus helps prevent the long-term complications of diabetes. Trade names for these are Dimelor, Orinase, and Diabinese, respectively.

Caution: The sulfonylureas should be used only in patients with diabetes of the insulin-independent type who cannot be treated with diet alone and are unwilling or unable to take insulin if weight reduction and dietary control fail.

hypoglycemic shock. Production of shock, q.v., by induction of hypoglycemia by intramuscular administration of insulin in the treatment of schizophrenia.

hypoglycogenolysis (hī″pō-glī′kō-jĕn-ŏl′ĭ-sĭs) [Gr. *hypo*, under, beneath, below, + *glykys*, sweet, + *gennan*, to produce, + *lysis*, dissolution]. Defective hydrolysis of glycogen (glycogenolysis).

hypoglycorrhachia (hī″pō-glī″kō-rā′kē-ă) [″ + ″ + *rhachis*, spine]. Decreased amount of glucose in the cerebrospinal fluid. It usually occurs in meningitis.

hypognathous (hī-pŏg′nă-thŭs) [″ + *gnathos*, jaw]. Having a lower jaw smaller than the upper jaw.

hypogonadism (hī″pō-gō′năd-ĭzm) [″ + *gone*, semen, + *-ismos*, condition]. Defective internal secretion of the gonads.

hypogonadotropic (hī″pō-gŏn″ă-dō-trŏp′ ĭk). Concerning or caused by deficiency of gonadotropin.

hypohepatia (hī″pō-hĕ-pă′tē-ă) [″ + *hepar*, liver]. Deficient liver function.

hypohidrosis (hī″pō-hī-drō′sĭs) [″ + *hidros*, sweat, + *osis*, condition]. Diminished perspiration. SYN: *hyphidrosis*.

hypohyloma (hī″pō-hī-lō′mă) [″ + *hyle*, matter, + *oma*, tumor]. A tumor formed by embryonic tissue. Derived from hypoblastic tissue.

hypoinsulinism [″ + L. *insula*, island, + Gr. *-ismos*, condition]. Insufficient secretion of insulin. SYN: *diabetes mellitus*.

hypoisotonic (hī″pō-ī″sō-tŏn′ĭk) [″ + *isos*, equal, + *tonos*, tension]. Hypotonic.

hypokalemia (hī″pō-kă-lē′mē-ă) [″ + Mod. L. *kalium*, potash, + Gr. *haima*, blood]. Extreme potassium depletion in the circulating blood, commonly manifested by episodes of muscular weakness or paralysis, tetany, and postural hypotension. SYN: *hypopotassemia*.

hypokalemic (hī″pō-kă-lē′mĭk). Concerning hypokalemia.

hypokinesia (hī″pō-kĭ-nē′zē-ă) [″ + *kinesis*, movement]. Decreased motor reaction to stimulus.

hypokinetic (hī″pō-kĭ-nĕt′ĭk). Pert. to hypokinesia.

hypolemmal (hī″pō-lĕm′ăl) [″ + *lemma*, sheath]. Situated below a sheath or membrane.

hypoleydigism (hī″pō-lī′dĭg-ĭzm). Decreased secretion of androgen by the interstitial (Leydig) cells of the testicles.

hypolipidemic (hī″pō-lĭp″ĭ-dē′mĭk). Decreasing the lipid concentration of the blood.

hypoliposis (hī″pō-lĭ-pō′sĭs) [″ + *lipos*, fat, + *osis*, condition]. Deficiency of fat in the tissues.

hypologia (hī-pō-lō′jē-ă) [″ + *logos*, word, reason]. A cerebral symptom marked by inadequate speech.

hypolymphemia (hī″pō-lĭm-fē′mē-ă) [″ + L. *lympha*, lymph, + Gr. *haima*, blood]. Decreased lymphocytes in the blood with normal number of leukocytes.

hypomagnesemia (hī″pō-măg″nĕ-sē′mē-ă). Decreased magnesium in the blood. Clinically, there will be increased neuromuscular irritability.

hypomania (hī″pō-mā′nē-ă) [″ + *mania*, madness]. Mild mania and excitement with moderate change in behavior.

hypomastia (hī-pō-măs′tē-ă) [″ + *mastos*, breast]. Condition of having abnormally small breasts. SYN: *hypomazia*.

hypomazia (hī″pō-mā′zē-ă) [″ + *mazos*, breast]. Hypomastia, q.v.

hypomelanoses. Disorders of melanin pigmentation in which melanin in the epidermis is decreased or absent.

  ETIOL: Albinism, chronic protein deficiency, burns, trauma, vitiligo. SYN: *leukoderma*. SEE: *hypermelanoses*.

hypomenorrhea (hī″pō-mĕn-ō-rē′ă) [″ + *men*, month, + *rhoia*, flow]. Deficient amount of menstrual flow, but periods are regular. SEE: *oligomenorrhea*.

hypomere (hī′pō-mēr) [″ + *meros*, part]. That portion of the mesoderm that later forms the pleuroperitoneal walls. SEE: *epimere; mesomere*.

hypometabolism (hī″pō-mĕ-tăb′ō-lĭzm) [″ + *metabole*, change, + *-ismos*, condition]. Lowered metabolism.

hypometria (hī″pō-mē′trē-ă) [″ + *metron*, measure]. Shortened range of movement.

hypometropia (hī″pō-mĕ-trōp′ē-ă) [″ + ″ + *ops*, eye]. Myopia or shortsightedness.

hypomnesia, hypomnesis (hī″pŏm-nē′zē-ă, -nē′sĭs) [″ + *mnesis*, memory]. Impaired memory.

hypomobility. Restricted joint movement (play) that limits normal range of motion. Opposite of hypermobility.

hypomorph (hī′pō-morf) [″ + *morphe*, form]. An individual with disproportionately short legs with respect to length of trunk. Opposite of hypermorph, q.v. SEE: *somatotype*.

hypomotility (hī″pō-mō-tĭl′ĭ-tē) [″ + L. *motus*, moved]. Hypokinesia.

hypomyotonia (hī″pō-mī″ō-tō′nē-ă) [″ + *mys*, muscle, + *tonos*, tension]. Lacking in muscular tonus.

hypomyxia (hī″pō-mĭks′ē-ă) [″ + *myxa*, mucus]. Diminished secretion of mucus.

hyponanosoma (hī″pō-năn-ō-sō′mă) [″ + *nanos*, dwarf, + *soma*, body]. Extreme dwarfism.

hyponatremia (hī″pō-nă-trē′mē-ă) [″ + L. *natron*, sodium, + Gr. *haima*, blood]. Decreased concentration of sodium in the blood.

hyponeocytosis (hī″pō-nē″ō-sī-tō′sĭs) [″ + *neos*, new, + *kytos*, cell, + *osis*, condition]. Decreased number of leukocytes (leukopenia) with immature cells in the blood.

hyponoia (hī″pō-noy′ă) [″ + *nous*, mind]. Diminished or sluggish mental activity.

hyponychium (hī-pō-nĭk′ē-ŭm) [Gr. *hypo*, under, beneath, below, + *onyx*, nail]. [NA] The nail bed. SYN: *matrix unguis.*

hyponychon (hī-pŏn′ĭ-kŏn) [″ + *onyx*, nail]. Extravasation of blood beneath the nail.

hypo-orthocytosis (hī″pō-or″thō-sī-tō′sĭs) [″ + *orthos*, regular, + *kytos*, cell, + *osis*, condition]. Leukopenia in which the proportions of white blood cells are normal.

hypopallesthesia (hī″pō-păl″ĕs-thē′zē-ă) [″ + *pallein*, to shake, + *aisthesis*, sensation]. Decreased ability to perceive vibratory sense.

hypopancreatism (hī″pō-păn′krē-ă-tĭzm) [″ + *pankreas*, pancreas, + *-ismos*, condition]. Diminished activity of the pancreas.

hypoparathyreosis (hī″pō-păr-ă-thī-rē-ō′sĭs) [″ + *para*, beside, + *thyreos*, shield, + *osis*, condition]. A condition due to lessened or absent secretion of the parathyroids. SYN: *hypoparathyroidism.*

hypoparathyroidism (hī″pō-păr-ă-thī′royd-ĭzm) [″ + ″ + ″ + *eidos*, form, shape, + *-ismos*, condition]. Insufficient secretion of the parathyroid glands. SYN: *hypoparathyreosis.* SEE: *Nursing Diagnoses in Appendix.*

hypopepsia (hī″pō-pĕp′sē-ă) [″ + *pepsis*, digestion]. Impaired digestion due to lack of pepsin.

hypopepsinia (hī″pō-pĕp-sĭn′ē-ă). Deficient pepsin in the gastric juice.

hypoperistalsis (hī″pō-pĕr″ĭ-stăl′sĭs). Diminished peristalsis. SEE: *paralytic ileus.*

hypophalangism (hī″pō-fă-lăn′jĭzm). State of having fewer than the normal number of fingers or toes or both.

hypopharynx (hī″pō-făr′ĭnks) [″ + *pharynx*, throat]. The lowermost portion of the pharynx, which leads to the larynx and esophagus. SYN: *laryngopharynx.*

hypophonesis (hī″pō-fō-nē′sĭs) [″ + *phone*, voice]. A diminished or fainter sound in auscultation or percussion.

hypophonia (hī″pō-fō′nē-ă). Abnormally weak voice due to incoordination of speech muscles, including weakness of muscles of respiration.

hypophoria (hī″pō-fō′rē-ă) [″ + *phorein*, to bear]. Tendency of one visual axis to fall below the other one.

hypophosphatasia (hī″pō-fŏs″fă-tā′zē-ă). An inherited metabolic disease in which there is a deficiency of alkaline phosphatase in the cells. Clinically there are abnormalities of the skeleton such as rickets, osteomalacia, defective tooth development, and phosphoethanolamine in the urine.

hypophosphatemia (hī″pō-fŏs″fă-tē′mē-ă) [″ + L. *phosphas*, phosphate, + Gr. *haima*, blood]. Abnormally decreased amount of phosphates circulating in the blood.

hypophosphaturia (hī″pō-fŏs″fă-tū′rē-ă) [″ + ″ + Gr. *ouron*, urine]. Decreased excretion of phosphate in the urine.

hypophrenia (hī″pō-frē′nē-ă) [″ + *phren*, mind]. Mental deficiency.

hypophrenic (hī″pō-frĕn′ĭk) [″ + *phren*, diaphragm, mind]. 1. Mental deficiency. 2. Below the diaphragm.

hypophyseal (hī″pō-fĭz′ē-ăl) [″ + *physis*, growth]. Pert. to the hypophysis or pituitary.

hypophysectomy (hī-pŏf″ĭ-sĕk′tō-mē) [″ + ″ + *ektome*, excision]. Excision of the hypophysis cerebri.

hypophyseoportal (hī″pō-fĭz″ē-ō-por′tăl). Concerning the portal system of the pituitary gland. SEE: *system, hypophyseoportal.*

hypophyseoprivic (hī″pō-fĭz″ē-ō-prĭv′ĭk). Deficiency of hormone secretion from the pituitary.

hypophysis (hī-pŏf′ĭ-sĭs) [Gr., an undergrowth] (pl. *hypophyses*). 1. An undergrowth. 2. [NA] The pituitary body or gland, q.v. Gland of internal secretion lying in the sella turcica of the sphenoid bone. It consists of two portions, the adenohypophysis (anterior lobe) and the neurohypophysis (posterior lobes), which are attached to the hypothalamus of the brain by the hypophyseal stalk. SEE: *pituitary gland.*

 h. cerebri. The pituitary gland.

hypophysitis (hī-pŏf″ĭ-sī′tĭs) [Gr. *hypo*, under, beneath, below, + *physis*, growth, + *itis*, inflammation]. Inflammation of the pituitary body.

hypopiesis (hī″pō-pī-ē′sĭs) [″ + *piesis*, pressure]. Lower than normal blood pressure.

hypopigmentation (hī″pō-pĭg″mĕn-tā′shŭn). Diminished pigment in a tissue.

hypopinealism (hī″pō-pĭn′ē-ăl-ĭzm) [″ + L. *pineus*, pert. to pine cone, + Gr. *-ismos*, condition]. Diminished secretion of the pineal gland.

hypopituitarism (hī″pō-pī-tū″ĭ-tă-rĭzm) [″ + L. *pituita*, mucus, + Gr. *-ismos*, condition]. A condition resulting from diminished secretion of pituitary hormones, esp. those of the anterior lobe.

hypoplasia (hī″pō-plā′zē-ă) [″ + *plasis*, formation]. Underdevelopment of a tissue organ or body. SEE: *tissue.*

hypopnea (hī″pō-nē′ă) [″ + *pnoia*, breath]. Decreased rate and depth of breathing.

hypoporosis (hī″pō-pō-rō′sĭs) [″ + *poros*, callus, + *osis*, condition]. Deficient development of a callus at site of a bone fracture.

hypoposia (hī″pō-pō′zē-ă) [″ + *posis*, drinking]. Decreased intake of fluids.

hypopotassemia (hī″pō-pō″tăs-sē′mē-ă) [″ + *potassium* + Gr. *haima*, blood]. Hypokalemia.

hypoproteinemia (hī″pō-prō″tē-ĭn-ē′mē-ă) [″ + *protos*, first, + *haima*, blood]. Decrease in the amount of protein in the blood.

hypoproteinosis (hī″pō-prō″tē-ĭ-nō′sĭs). Condition of deficient proteins in the body or diet.

hypoprothrombinemia (hī″pō-prō-thrŏm″bĭn-ē′mē-ă) [″ + L. *pro*, for, + Gr. *thrombos*, clot, + *haima*, blood]. Deficiency of blood clotting factor II (prothrombin) in the blood.

hypopselaphesia (hī″pŏp-sĕl-ă-fē′zē-ă) [″ + *pselaphesis*, touch]. Blunted tactile sense.

hypoptyalism (hī″pō-tī′ăl-ĭzm) [″ + *ptyalon*, saliva, + *-ismos*, condition]. Decreased salivary secretion.

hypopyon (hī-pō′pē-ŏn) [″ + *pyon*, pus]. Pus in anterior chamber of the eye in front of the iris but behind the cornea, seen in corneal ulcer.

hyporeactive (hī″pō-rē-ăk′tĭv). Decreased response to stimuli.

hyporeflexia [″ + L. *reflexus*, bent back]. Diminished function of the reflexes.

hyposalemia (hī″pō-săl-ē′mē-ă) [″ + L. *sal*, salt, + Gr. *haima*, blood]. Decreased amount of sodium chloride in the blood.

hyposalivation (hī″pō-săl″ĭ-vā′shŭn). Abnormal decrease in flow of saliva.

hyposarca (hī″pō-săr′kă) [″ + *sarx*, flesh]. Extreme edema of subcutaneous connective tissue. SYN: *anasarca.*

hyposcleral (hī″pō-sklē′răl). Beneath the sclera of the eye.

hyposecretion (hī″pō-sē-krē′shŭn). Lowered amt. of secretion.

hyposensitive (hī″pō-sĕn′sĭ-tĭv) [″ + L. *sentire*, to feel]. Having reduced ability to respond to stimuli.

hyposensitization (hī″pō-sĕn″sĭ-tī-zā′shŭn). Production of hyposensitiveness.

hyposialadenitis (hī″pō-sī″ăl-ăd-ĕ-nī′tĭs) [Gr. *hypo*, under, beneath, below, + *sia-*

lon, saliva, + *aden*, gland, + *itis*, inflammation]. Inflammation of the submandibular salivary gland.

hyposmia (hī-pŏz′mē-ă) [″ + *osme*, smell]. Defect in sense of smell.

hyposmolarity (hī-pŏz″mō-lăr′ĭ-tē). Decreased osmolar concentration, esp. of the blood or urine.

hyposomnia (hī″pō-sŏm′nē-ă). Decreased ability to sleep. SYN: *insomnia.*

hypospadia, hypospadias (hī″pō-spā′dē-ă, -ăs) [″ + *span*, to draw]. 1. An abnormal congenital opening of the male urethra upon the undersurface of the penis. 2. A urethral opening into the vagina.

hyposphresia (hī″pŏs-frē′sē-ă) [″ + *osphresis*, smell]. Hyposmia.

hypostasis (hī″pŏs′tă-sĭs) [″ + *stasis*, a standing]. 1. Diminished blood flow or circulation. 2. Deposit of sediment due to decreased flow of a body fluid such as blood or urine.

hypostatic (hī″pō-stăt′ĭk) [″ + *statikos*, standing]. 1. Of or pert. to hypostasis. 2. In genetics, hidden or suppressed, said of a gene whose effect is suppressed by the presence of another gene.

hypostatic pneumonia. SEE: *pneumonia, hypostatic.*

hyposteatolysis (hī″pō-stē-ă-tŏl′ĭ-sĭs) [″ + *stear*, fat, + *lysis*, dissolution]. Diminished emulsification of fats during digestion.

hyposthenia (hī″pŏs-thē′nē-ă) [″ + *sthenos*, strength]. Subnormal strength; an enfeebled state; weakness.

hypostheniant (hī″pŏs-thē′nē-ănt). One whose strength and vital forces are reduced; debilitant.

hyposthenic (hī-pŏs-thĕn′ĭk). 1. Debilitant. 2. Body habitus characterized by a long, shallow thorax, a long thoracic cavity, a long, narrow abdominal cavity, and a slender build.

hyposthenuria (hī″pŏs-thĕn-ū′rē-ă) [″ + *sthenos*, strength, + *ouron*, urine]. The secretion of urine of low specific gravity, chiefly in chronic nephritis.

h., tubular. Hyposthenuria resulting from disease of the renal tubule epithelial cells.

hypostomia (hī″pō-stō′mē-ă) [″ + *stoma*, mouth]. Congenital defect in which the mouth is small.

hypostosis (hĭp″ŏs-tō′sĭs) [″ + *osteon*, bone, + *osis*, condition]. Deficient development of bone.

hypostypsis (hī″pō-stĭp′sĭs) [″ + *stypsis*, a contracting]. State of being slightly astringent.

hypostyptic (hī″pō-stĭp′tĭk). Slightly astringent.

hyposynergia (hī″pō-sĭn-ĕr′jē-ă) [″ + *syn*, together, + *ergon*, work]. Poor coordination.

hypotelorism (hī″pō-tĕl′ō-rĭzm) [″ + *telouros*, distant]. Decreased distance between organs, esp. the eyes.

hypotension [″ + L. *tensio*, tension]. 1. Decrease of systolic and diastolic blood pressure below normal. 2. Deficiency in tonus or tension.

Occurs in shock, in hemorrhages, infections, fevers, cancer, anemia, neurasthenia, Addison's disease; in debilitating or wasting diseases; and approaching death. SEE: *blood pressure, chronic low.*

h., orthostatic. Hypotension occurring upon suddenly arising from a recumbent position or from standing still.

hypotensive. Denoting low blood pressure.

hypothalamus (hī″pō-thăl′ă-mŭs) [″ + *thalamos*, chamber]. [NA] The portion of the diencephalon comprising the ventral wall of the third ventricle below the hypothalamic sulcus and including structures forming the ventricular floor, including the optic chiasma, tuber cinereum, infundibulum, and mamillary bodies. It lies beneath the thalamus and laterally is continuous with the subthalamic regions. It contains neurosecretions that are of importance in the control of certain metabolic activities, such as maintenance of water balance, sugar and fat metabolism, regulation of body temperature, and secretion of releasing and inhibiting hormones. It is the chief subcortical region for the integration of sympathetic and parasympathetic activities. SEE: *hormone, releasing; hormone, stimulating.*

hypothenar (hī-pŏth′ĕ-năr) [″ + *thenar*, palm]. The fleshy prominence on the inner side of the palm next to the little finger.

hypothenar eminence. Prominence on the palm below the little finger.

hypothermal (hī″pō-thĕr′măl) [″ + *therme*, heat]. 1. Tepid. 2. Subnormal temperature.

hypothermia (hī″pō-thĕr′mē-ă). 1. Having a body temperature below normal. 2. A technique of lowered body temperature, usually between 78° and 90°F (26° and 32.5°C), to reduce oxygen need during surgery (esp. cardiovascular and neurological procedures) and in hypoxia, to reduce blood pressure, and to alleviate hyperpyrexia. SEE: *hyperthermia.*

h., accidental. Hypothermia due to causes other than as a result of a systemic disorder such as shock, trauma, or carcinoma. This form of hypothermia may be lethal in anyone, but especially in the elderly. It may occur in those exposed to the cold, i.e., skiers, hunters, sailors, climbers, the indigent, homeless persons in winter, and swimmers.

SYM: In the elderly, it is characterized by impaired speech, disorientation and a generalized lethargy. Hypothermia depresses the central nervous system. Initially there is tachycardia followed by bradycardia and atrial and ventricular dysrhythmias. Respirations are increased at first and then depressed, and renal function is depressed after initial diuresis.

TREAT: *Emergency at site:* many persons with hypothermia will not be where comprehensive medical care is available; nevertheless, take immediate steps to prevent further heat loss, then begin rewarming. Immobilize patient; massage of extremities is contraindicated; warm stimulant fluids by mouth are of no help; make plans for transporting patient to a hospital; administration of warm heated air is of benefit, as is heated 5% dextrose in normal saline given I.V. SEE: *frostbite.*

Caution: Oral thermometers are likely to be inaccurate in the cold, outdoors. Remember the treatment slogan "No one is dead until warm and dead."

hypothermia blanket. A specially designed blanket for cooling patients with hyperthermia. It has flexible tubing between the layers of cloth, and cold water is pumped through the tubing.

hypothesis (hī-pŏth′ĕ-sĭs) [″ + *thesis*, a placing) (pl. *hypotheses*). 1. An assumption not proved by experiment or observation. It is assumed for the sake of testing its soundness or to facilitate investigation of a class of phenomena. 2. A conclusion drawn before all the facts are established and tentatively accepted as a basis for further investigation.

hypothrombinemia (hī″pō-thrŏm-bĭn-ē′mē-ă) [″ + *thrombos*, clot, + *haima*, blood]. Deficiency of thrombin in the blood.

hypothymia (hī″pō-thī′mē-ă) [″ + *thymos*, mind]. Decreased emotional response to stimuli.

hypothymism (hī″pō-thī′mĭzm) [″ + ″ + *-ismos*, condition]. Decreased activity of the thymus.

hypothyroid (hī″pō-thī′royd) [″ + *thyreos*, shield, + *eidos*, form, shape]. Marked by insufficiency of thyroid secretion.

hypothyroidism (hī″pō-thī′royd-ĭzm). A condition due to deficiency of the thyroid secretion, resulting in a lowered basal metabolism. A lesser degree of cretinism. SEE: *thyroid function tests.*

SYM: May be obesity; dry skin and hair, both of which become lusterless. Low blood pressure, slow pulse, sluggishness of all functions, depressed muscular activity, intolerance of cold, goiter.

TREAT: Replacement therapy with natural or synthetic thyroid hormone preparations. Increase iodine in diet if iodine is deficient.

NURSING IMPLICATIONS: Assess the patient for indications of decreased metabolic rate, easy fatigability, cool, dry, and scaly skin, hypercarotenemia, hair and eyebrow loss, brittle nails, facial puffiness and periorbital edema, paresthesias, ataxias, cold intolerance, bradycardia, reduced cardiac output, aching muscles and joint stiffness, change in bowel habits, irregular menses, and decreased libido. Assist with and explain diagnostic testing. Carry out medical therapies aimed at restoring a normal metabolic state. Help the patient and family to deal with the psychosocial and psychomotor effects of decreased metabolism. Be alert for GI and cardiac complications. Protect patient from chilling, infection, stress, and trauma. SEE: *Nursing Diagnoses* in *Appendix*.

hypotonia (hī″pō-tō′nē-ă) [″ + *tonos*, tone]. 1. Reduced tension; relaxation of arteries. 2. Loss of tonicity of the muscles or intraocular pressure.

hypotonic (hī-pō-tŏn′ĭk). 1. Pert. to defective muscular tone or tension. 2. A solution of lower osmotic pressure than that of a reference solution or of an isotonic solution.

hypotoxicity (hī″pō-tŏks-ĭs′ĭ-tē) [″ + *toxikon*, poison]. A reduced toxic quality; only slightly poisonous.

hypotrichosis (hī″pō-trĭ-kō′sĭs) [″ + *thrix*, hair, + *osis*, condition]. Abnormal deficiency of hair.

hypotrophy (hī-pŏt′rŏ-fē) [″ + *trophe*, nourishment]. Progressive degeneration and functional loss of cells and tissues. SYN: *abiotrophy; atrophy*.

hypotropia (hī″pō-trō′pē-ă) [″ + *trope*, a turning]. Vertical strabismus downward.

hypotympanotomy (hī″pō-tĭm″pă-nŏt′ō-mē). Surgical incision of the tympanic membrane of the ear.

hypotympanum (hī″pō-tĭm′pă-nŭm). The part of the middle ear beneath the level of the tympanic membrane.

hypouricuria (hī″pō-ū-rĭ-kū′rē-ă) [″ + *ouron*, urine, + *ouron*, urine]. Deficient uric acid in the urine.

hypovenosity (hī″pō-vēn-ōs′ĭ-tē) [″ + L. *venosus*, pert. to a vein]. Incomplete development of the venous system in an area, resulting in atrophy or degeneration.

hypoventilation (hī″pō-vĕn″tĭ-lā′shŭn) [″ + L. *ventilatio*, ventilation]. Reduced rate and depth of breathing.

hypovitaminosis (hī″pō-vī″tă-mĭn-ō′sĭs) [″

+ L. *vita*, life, + *amine* + Gr. *osis*, condition]. A condition due to a lack of vitamins in the diet.

hypovolemia (hī″pō-vō-lē′mē-ă) [″ + L. *volumen*, volume]. Diminished blood volume. SYN: *oligemia; oligohemia*.

hypovolia (hī″pō-vō′lē-ă). Decreased water content.

hypoxanthine (hī″pō-zăn′thĭn, -thēn) [″ + *xanthos*, yellow]. A purine derivative, $C_5H_4N_4O$, in muscles and tissues in a stage of urea and uric acid formation. It is formed during protein decomposition. It is normal in urine in small amounts.

hypoxemia (hī-pŏks-ē′mē-ă) [″ + *oxygen* + *haima*, blood]. Insufficient oxygenation of the blood. SYN: *hypoxia*. SEE: *respiration*.

hypoxia (hī″pŏks′ē-ă). 1. Deficiency of oxygen. 2. Decreased concentration of oxygen in the inspired air. SEE: *anoxia; hypoxemia; posthypoxia syndromes*.

hypoxic lap swimming. A practice by competitive swimmers of holding their breath for a number of laps. The goal of the training is to increase the tolerance to oxygen debt during races. The practice is potentially dangerous and may lead to drowning.

hypsarrhythmia (hĭp″săr-ĭth′mē-ă) [Gr. *hypsi*, high, + *a-*, not, + *rhythmos*, rhythm]. An abnormal electroencephalographic pattern of persistent generalized slow waves and very high voltage. Clinically it is often associated with infantile spasm and progressive mental deterioration. Etiological factors are unknown.

hypsibrachycephalic (hĭp″sē-brăk″e-sĕ-făl′ĭk) [Gr. *hypsi*, high, + *brachys*, broad, + *kephale*, head]. Having a broad and high skull.

hypsicephalic (hĭp″sē-sĕ-făl′ĭk) [″ + *kephale*, head]. Having a skull with a cranial index over 75.1°. SYN: *hypsistenocephalic*.

hypsicephaly (hĭp-sē-sĕf′ă-lē). The condition of having a skull with a cranial index over 75.1°.

hypsiconchous (hĭp″sē-kŏng′kŭs) [″ + *konche*, shell]. Having an orbital index of about 85°.

hypsiloid (hĭp′sĭ-loyd) [Gr. *upsilon*, U or Y, + *eidos*, form]. U- or Y-shaped. SYN: *hyoid*.

hypsiloid ligament. Ligamentum iliofemorale.

hypsistenocephalic (hĭp″sē-stĕn″ō-sē-făl′ĭk) [″ + *stenos*, narrow, + *kephale*, head]. Having a cranial index over 75.1°. SYN: *hypsicephalic*.

hypsocephalous (hĭp″sō-sĕf′ă-lŭs) [Gr. *hypsos*, height, + *kephale*, head]. Having a cranial index over 75.1°. SYN: *hypsicephalic*.

hypsokinesis (hĭp″sō-kĭ-nē′sĭs) [″ + *kinesis*, movement]. Tendency to fall backward when standing; seen in paralysis agitans.

hypsophobia (hĭp″sō-fō′bē-ă) [″ + *phobos*, fear]. Fear of being at great heights. SYN: *acrophobia.*

hypurgia (hī-pŭr′jē-ă) [Gr. *hypourgia,* help]. Any minor factor that changes the course of a disease, esp. for the better.

hysteralgia (hĭs-tĕr-ăl′jē-ă) [Gr. *hystera,* womb, + *algos,* pain]. Uterine pain. SYN: *hysterodynia.*

hysteratresia (hĭs″tĕr-ă-trē′zē-ă) [″ + *a-,* not, + *tresis,* perforation]. Atresia of the uterus.

hysterectomy (hĭs-tĕr-ĕk′tō-mē) [″ + *ektome,* excision]. Surgical removal of the uterus through the abdominal wall or through the vagina. The presence of benign or malignant tumors is the most frequent reason for hysterectomy.

In preparation for abdominal hysterectomy, the patient is placed in dorsal position. The table is ready to be tipped into the Trendelenburg position. As soon as incision is made through the peritoneum, table should be put into Trendelenburg position. This procedure is the same for all abdominopelvic surgery. This position allows the intestines and abdominal organs to fall away from pelvis, so that they may be easily packed off with large pads or with a large roll of packing.

NURSING IMPLICATIONS: *Preop:* Prepare patient using procedural and sensation messages; carry out surgeon's preparatory protocol.

Postop: Monitor vital signs, inspect dressings and vaginal introitus for bleeding or symptoms of hemorrhage. Assess for bladder distention and catheterize as needed, or monitor urinary output from indwelling catheter, then assess bladder emptying and evaluate for urinary retention when catheter is removed. Administer prescribed analgesia or monitor patient-administered analgesia, evaluating response. Prevent respiratory complications by encouraging patient to breathe deeply and cough every 1 to 2 hours and by splinting any incision and turning the patient side to side every 2 hours until patient is able to assume responsibility for mobility. Employ thigh-high elastic stockings or pneumatic leg dressings as prescribed, and encourage leg exercises and early ambulation to prevent venous stasis that may result in phlebitis or deep vein phlebothrombosis. Assess patient for presence of Homans' sign, q.v. Maintain fluid and electrolyte balance via prescribed I.V. replacement therapy, assessing for nausea and vomiting and treating with anti-

emetic as prescribed and required. Maintain nasogastric drainage if present, and assess for bowel sounds as paralytic ileus is a concern. Use rectal tube, ambulation, and analgesia to assist patient to deal with gaseous distention as required. Provide a high-protein, high vitamin C diet to encourage tissue healing when the GI tract is functional. Teach patient about the need to maintain good nutrition and adequate fluid intake, and to report vaginal bleeding, wound infection, or prolonged GI complaints. Explain that tub baths, douching, and coitus usually are restricted until after a postoperative evaluation, and assist patient in scheduling this visit. Explain the rationale for hormone replacement if prescribed following ovary removal, initiating therapy when patient is able to take oral fluids. Teach patient that altered femininity and sexuality following hysterectomy are myths, and assist patient to verbalize and deal with any feelings of loss or grief. Assist patient in dealing with chemotherapy or radiation if these are required. SEE: *Nursing Diagnoses* in *Appendix.*

h., abdominal. Removal of the uterus through an abdominal incision.

h., cesarean. Surgical removal of the uterus at the time of cesarean section.

h., Porro. Subtotal hysterectomy following cesarean section.

h., radical. Surgical removal of the uterus, tubes, ovaries, adjacent lymph nodes, and a part of the vagina. SYN: *Wertheim's hysterectomy.*

h., subtotal. Removal of the uterus, leaving the cervix uteri in place.

h., supracervical. H., subtotal.

h., supravaginal. H., subtotal.

h., total. Removal of both the body of the uterus and the cervix.

h., vaginal. Removal of the uterus through the vagina.

hysteresis (hĭs″tĕr-ē′sĭs) [Gr., a coming too late]. 1. Failure of related phenomena to keep pace with each other. 2. Failure of the manifestation of an effect to keep up with its cause. 3. A transformer loss of power due to the alternating of its magnetic field.

hystereurynter (hĭs″tĕr-ū-rĭn′tĕr) [Gr. *hystera,* uterus, + *eurynein,* to stretch]. An instrument for dilating the os uteri. SYN: *metreurynter.*

hysteria (hĭs-tē′rē-ă) [Gr. *hystera,* uterus]. A mental disorder, usually temporary, presenting somatic symptoms, simulating almost any type of physical disease. The condition occurs in the absence of organic disease to account for the symptoms.

The mental attitude is calm. Easy laughing and crying episodes may be present, possibly without any apparent explanation, and may occur during sleep. Episodic states known as fugues (sleepwalking is similar, occurring in sleep). In these disorders, certain dissociated (repressed) ideas, emotions, and goals develop a reality sufficient to constitute a secondary personality that functions apart from the primary personality.

When the primary consciousness reasserts itself, there is a forgetting (amnesia) of the secondary state. The multiplication or alternation of personalities is quite distinct from schizophrenic splitting in which incongruities and confusion result from the coexistence of each phase of the personality more or less continuously.

NOTE: Currently accepted nomenclature for mental disorders does not include the term *hysteria;* nevertheless, it has been in use for centuries and is included here at least for historical reasons. SEE: *mass psychogenic illness.*

SYM: Emotional instability, various sensory disturbances, and a marked craving for sympathy, which sometimes leads to fraud.

ETIOL: Variable, as in most psychic disturbances. It occurs in both sexes before and after adolescence and at periods of emotional and physical stress.

TREAT: Place patient in a quiet place devoid of spectators. Cold applications to head, face, and neck are helpful. Quiet, firm suggestions are important. Sedatives are to be used under the direction of a physician.

h., anxiety. Hysteria combined with an anxiety neurosis.

h., conversion. Apparent loss of physical function, but there is no organic basis for signs and symptoms such as deafness, blindness, tunnel vision, paralysis, anesthesia, parathesias, or aphonia. SYN: *conversion disorder.* SEE: *gain, primary; gain, secondary.*

h., epidemic. Hysteria in a group of people, usually closely associated in school or work place. The inciting incident might be a rumor; an unaccustomed odor, e.g., paint fumes in a work place; or vomiting after an individual has just eaten. The latter may lead to a hysterical reaction by the group who feel that the food they ate was toxic. SYN: *hysteria, mass.* SEE: *mass psychogenic illness.*

h., major. Very severe hysteria accompanied by epileptiform convulsions.

h., mass. SYN: *hysteria, epidemic.* SEE: *mass psychogenic illness.*

h., minor. Mild form of hysteria without loss of consciousness.

h., rabies. SEE: *rabies.*

hysteriac (hĭs-tĕr′ē-ăk) [Gr. *hystera,* womb].

A hysterical person.

hysteric, hysterical. Pert. to hysteria.

hysterical paralysis. SEE: *paralysis, hysterical.*

hysteric ataxia. Loss of sensation in leg muscles and skin in hysteria.

hysteric chorea. A form of hysteria with choreiform movements.

hystericoneuralgic (hĭs-tĕr″ĭk-o-nū-răl′jĭk) [″ + *neuron,* nerve, + *algos,* pain]. Pert. to pain of hysterical origin, but resembling neuralgia.

hysteritis (hĭs-tĕr-ī′tĭs) [″ + *itis,* inflammation]. Inflammation of the uterus.

hystero-, hyster- [Gr. *hystera,* womb]. Prefix indicating either womb or hysteria.

hysterobubonocele (hĭs″tĕr-ō-bū-bŏn′ō-sēl) [″ + *boubon,* groin, + *kele,* tumor, swelling]. Inguinal hernia surrounding the uterus.

hysterocele (hĭs′tĕr-ō-sēl) [″ + *kele,* tumor, swelling]. Hernia of the uterus, esp. when gravid.

hysterocleisis (hĭs″tĕr-ō-klī′sĭs) [″ + *kleisis,* closure]. Surgical closure of the os uteri.

hysterocystocleisis (hĭs″tĕr-ō-sĭs″tō-klī′sĭs) [″ + *kystis,* a bladder, + *kleisis,* closure]. Operation fastening the cervix uteri in the wall of the bladder.

hysterodynia (hĭs″tĕr-ō-dĭn′ē-ă) [″ + *odyne,* pain]. Uterine pain. SYN: *hysteralgia.*

hysterogastrorrhaphy (hĭs″tĕr-ō-găs-tror′ă-fē) [″ + *gaster,* belly, + *rhaphe,* seam, ridge]. Fixation of uterus to the gastric wall. SYN: *hysteropexy.*

hysterogenic (hĭs″tĕr-ō-jĕn′ĭk) [″ + *gennan,* to produce]. Causing hysteria.

hysterogram (hĭs″tĕr-ō-grăm). Roentgenogram of the uterus.

hysterography (hĭs″tĕ-rŏg′ră-fē) [″ + *graphein,* to write]. Recording of the frequency and intensity of contractions of the uterus.

hysteroid (hĭs′tĕr-oyd) [″ + *eidos,* form, shape]. 1. Resembling hysteria. 2. Pert. to hysteria.

hysterolaparotomy (hĭs″tĕr-ō-lăp″ă-rŏt′ō-mē) [″ + *lapara,* flank, + *tome,* incision]. Uterine incision through abdominal wall; abdominal hysterectomy.

hysterolith (hĭs′tĕr-ō-lĭth) [″ + *lithos,* stone]. A calculus in the uterus.

hysterology (hĭs-tĕr-ŏl′ō-jē) [″ + *logos,* word, reason]. Sum of what is known about the uterus.

hysterolysis (hĭs″tĕr-ŏl′ĭ-sĭs) [″ + *lysis,* dissolution]. Operation of loosening the uterus from its adhesions.

hysteromania (hĭs″tĕr-ō-mā′nē-ă) [″ + *mania,* madness]. 1. Hysterical mania. 2. Nymphomania.

hysterometer (hĭs″tĕ-rŏm′ĕ-tĕr) [″ + *metron*, measure]. Device for measuring the uterus.

hysterometry (hĭs″tĕ-rŏm′ĕ-trē). Measurement of the size of the uterus.

hysteromyoma (hĭs″tĕr-ō-mī-ō′mă) [Gr. *hystera*, womb, + *mys*, muscle, + *oma*, tumor]. Myoma or fibromyoma of the uterus.

hysteromyomectomy (hĭs″tĕr-ō-mī″ō-mĕk′tō-mē) [″ + ″ + *ektome*, excision]. Excision of a uterine fibroid.

hysteromyotomy (hĭs″tĕr-ō-mī-ŏt′ō-mē) [″ + ″ + *tome*, incision]. Uterine incision for removal of a solid tumor.

hystero-oophorectomy (hĭs″tĕr-ō-ō″ō-for-ĕk′tō-mē) [″ + *oon*, egg, + *phoros*, bearing, + *ektome*, excision]. Removal of the uterus and one or both ovaries.

hysteropathy (hĭs″tĕr-ŏp′ă-thē) [″ + *pathos*, disease, suffering]. Any uterine disorder.

hysteropexy (hĭs′tĕr-ō-pĕk″sē) [″ + *pexis*, fixation]. Surgical fixation of the uterus. SYN: *hysterogastrorrhaphy*.

hysteropia (hĭs″tĕr-ō′pē-ă) [″ + *ops*, eye]. A hysterical visual defect.

hysteropsychosis (hĭs″tĕr-ō-sī-kō′sĭs) [″ + *psyche*, mind, + *osis*, condition]. Mental disorder due to uterine disease.

hysteroptosia, hysteroptosis (hĭs″tĕr-ŏp-tō′sē-ă, -sĭs) [″ + *ptosis*, a dropping]. Prolapse of the uterus. SYN: *procidentia*.

hysterorrhaphy (hĭs-tĕr-or′ă-fē) [″ + *rhaphe*, seam, ridge]. Suture of the womb.

hysterorrhexis (hĭs″tĕr-ō-rĕk′sĭs) [″ + *rhexis*, rupture]. Rupture of the uterus, esp. when pregnant.

hysterosalpingectomy (hĭs″tĕr-ō-săl″pĭn-jĕk′tō-mē) [″ + *salpinx*, tube, + *ektome*, excision]. Surgical removal of the uterus and tubes.

hysterosalpingography (hĭs″tĕr-ō-săl″pĭn-gŏg′ră-fē) [″ + ″ + *graphein*, to write]. Roentgenography of the uterus and oviducts after radiopaque material is injected into those organs.

hysterosalpingo-oophorectomy (hĭs″tĕr-ō-săl-pĭng″gō-ō″ō-for-ĕk′tō-mē) [″ + ″ + *oon*, egg, + *phoros*, bearing, + *ektome*, excision]. Surgical removal of the uterus, oviducts, and ovaries.

hysterosalpingostomy (hĭs″tĕr-ō-săl″pĭng-ōs′tō-mē) [″ + ″ + *stoma*, mouth]. Anastomosis of the uterus with the distal end of the fallopian tube after excision of a strictured portion of the tube.

hysteroscope (hĭs′tĕr-ō-skōp) [″ + *skopein*, to examine]. Instrument for examining the uterine cavity. SYN: *metroscope*.

hysteroscopy (hĭs″tĕr-ŏs′kō-pē). Inspection of the uterus by use of a special endoscope. SEE: *hysteroscope*.

hysterospasm (hĭs′tĕr-ō-spăzm″) [Gr. *hystera*, womb, + *spasmos*, a convulsion]. Uterine spasm.

hysterostomatocleisis (hĭs″tĕr-ō-stō″mă-tō-klī′sĭs) [″ + *stoma*, mouth, + *kleisis*, closure]. Operation for vesicovaginal fistula. Consists of closure of the cervix uteri, making the vesical and uterine cavities into a common cavity by means of the opening between them.

hysterostomatomy (hĭs″tĕr-ō-stō-măt′ō-mē) [″ + ″ + *tome*, incision]. Surgical enlargement of the os uteri; incision of the os or cervix uteri.

hysterotome (hĭs′tĕr-ō-tōm) [″ + *tome*, incision]. Instrument for incision of the uterus.

hysterotomy (hĭs-tĕr-ŏt′ō-mē). 1. Incision of the uterus. 2. Cesarean section.

hysterotrachelectomy (hĭs″tĕr-ō-trā″kĕl-ĕk′tō-mē) [″ + *trachelos*, neck, + *ektome*, excision]. Amputation of the uterine cervix.

hysterotracheloplasty (hĭs″tĕr-ō-trā″kĕl-ō-plăs″tē) [″ + ″ + *plassein*, to form]. Plastic surgery or repair of the cervix.

hysterotrachelorrhaphy (hĭs″tĕr-ō-trā″kĕl-or′ă-fē) [″ + ″ + *rhaphe*, seam, ridge]. Plastic surgery of a lacerated cervix by paring the edges and suturing them together.

hysterotrachelotomy (hĭs″tĕr-ō-trā″kĕl-ŏt′ō-mē) [″ + ″ + *tome*, incision]. Surgical incision of the neck of the uterus.

hysterotraumatic (hĭs″tĕr-ō-traw-măt′ĭk) [″ + *trauma*, wound]. Pert. to traumatic hysteria.

hysterotubography (hĭs″tĕr-ō-tū-bŏg′ră-fē). Hysterosalpingography, q.v.

hysterovagino-enterocele (hĭs″tĕr-ō-văj″ĭn-ō-ĕn′tĕr-ō-sēl) [″ + L. *vagina*, sheath, + Gr. *enteron*, intestine, + *kele*, tumor, swelling]. Hernia surrounding the uterus, vagina, and intestines.

Hytakerol. Trade name for dihydrotachysterol, USP.

Hz. *hertz*.

HZV. *herpes zoster virus*.

I

I. 1. Chem. symb. for the element iodine. 2. Symbol for quantity of electricity expressed in amperes.

¹³¹I. Radioactive iodine. At. wt. 131.

¹³²I. Radioactive iodine. At. wt. 132.

i. *optically inactive.*

-ia. Suffix indicating condition, esp. an abnormal state.

IABC. *intra-aortic balloon counterpulsation.*

IABP. *intra-aortic balloon pump.*

I.A.D.R. *International Association for Dental Research.*

I and O. *intake and output.*

ianthinopsia (ī-ăn″thĭ-nŏp′sē-ă) [Gr. *ianthinos,* violet colored, + *opsis,* vision]. Abnormality of vision in which all objects appear to be violet.

-iasis [Gr.]. Suffix, same as or interchangeable with *-osis,* meaning the state or condition of, particularly a pathological condition.

iatraliptics (ī″ă-tră-lĭp′tĭks) [Gr. *iatreia,* cure, + *aleiphein,* to anoint]. Treatment by friction, as when medicated ointment is rubbed into an area.

iatric (ī-ăt′rĭk) [Gr. *iatrikos,* medical]. Combining form referring to medicine, the medical profession, or physicians.

iatro- [Gr. *iatros,* physician]. Combining form indicating relationship to medicine or a physician.

iatrochemistry (ī-ăt″rō-kĕm′ĭs-trē) [″ + *chemeia,* chemistry]. Seventeenth-century opinion that chemistry is the basis of all physiological phenomena.

iatrogenic disorder (ī″ăt-rō-jĕn′ĭk) [″ + *gennan,* to produce]. Any adverse mental or physical condition induced in a patient by effects of treatment by a physician or surgeon. Term implies that such effects could have been avoided by proper and judicious care on the part of the physician, surgeon, or dentist.

iatrogeny (ī″ă-trŏj′ĕ-nē). An adverse state or condition induced by a physician.

iatrology (ī″ă-trŏl′ō-jē) [″ + *logos,* word, reason]. Medical science.

iatrotechniques (ī-ăt″rō-tĕk-nēks′) [″ + *techne,* art]. The art and technique of medicine and surgery.

I band. Isotropic, light band (segment) of a muscle fiber.

IBC. *iron-binding capacity.*

IBD. *inflammatory bowel disease.*

IBS. *irritable bowel syndrome.*

ibuprofen. USP. A nonsteroidal anti-inflammatory agent with antipyretic and analgesic properties. Although its exact mechanism of action is unknown, it does not stimulate the pituitary-adrenal system. Used in treating chronic symptomatic rheumatoid arthritis and osteoarthritis. This drug has antiprostaglandin activity, and is useful in treating primary dysmenorrhea. Trade names are Advil, Motrin, and Nuprin.

IBW. *ideal body weight.*

IC. *inspiratory capacity.*

-ic. A suffix indicating that the word has some characteristic of, e.g., hysteric, hemic, acidic.

ICD. *intrauterine contraceptive device; International Classification of Diseases.*

"ice." Street name for methamphetamine, a drug of abuse. It is usually sold in the form of crystals (from which its name is derived).

ice (īs) [AS. *is*]. A solid form of water. Water becomes ice at a temperature of 32°F (0°C). Ice may be chilled lower than the freezing point. An ice bag, cap, collar, and cravat are devices for holding ice to be applied to a patient to obtain the effect of continuous cold in a circumscribed area. The part so treated should always be covered with several thicknesses of cloth to prevent cold injury to the tissues.

i., dry. Carbon dioxide cooled to the point where it is a solid. This occurs at −110°F (−78.9°C). Used as a commercial refrigerant and for therapeutic refrigeration in the treatment of certain skin conditions, including warts. SEE: *carbon dioxide.*

ice bag. A flexible, watertight bag with a sealable opening large enough to permit ice cubes or chipped ice to be added. Used in any localized condition requiring application of cold. In an emergency any sturdy bag made of flexible plastic can be used. That type of bag can be sealed by tying a knot in the open end.

Caution: Do not place dry ice in an ice bag.

---

iceberg phenomenon. Term for recognition of the gross conditions and diseases and failure to recognize the great majority of conditions that are mild and do not become clinically apparent.

Iceland disease. Epidemic neuromyasthenia.

Iceland moss. An edible lichen containing a form of starch; a slightly tonic demulcent. SYN: *Cetraria.*

ice massage. Application of ice to obtain a therapeutic numbing effect. Paper cups containing water previously frozen are preferable. The cups are rubbed over a localized area in small circles for 5 to 10 minutes in order to numb the part and prepare it for deep pressure or deep transverse friction massage. Ice massage is also used to treat traumatized tissues and joints.

Caution: Direct application of ice may damage the area. The ice should be contained in cloth.

---

ice treatment. Use of ice applied either directly or in a suitable container to cool an injured area. Ice therapy, at least in the first 24 to 48 hours following injury, is believed to be much more beneficial than heat in treating superficial bruises, contusions, and sprains. Application of cold or of ice water in immediate treatment of a burn helps to reduce the extent of inflammation and pain.

ICF. *intracellular fluid.*

ichnogram (ĭk'nō-grăm) [Gr. *ichnos*, footstep, + *gramma*, something written]. A footprint taken while standing.

ichor (ī'kor) [Gr. *ichor*, serum]. Thin, fetid discharge from an ulcer or from a wound.

ichoremia (ī"kor-ē'mē-ă) [" + *haima*, blood]. Septicemia or blood poisoning.

ichorous (ī'kor-ŭs) [Gr. *ichor*, serum]. Resembling ichor or watery pus.

ichthammol (ĭk'thă-mŏl). USP. A reddishbrown viscous fluid obtained by the destructive distillation of certain bituminous shale. The distillate is sulfonated and the final compound contains 10% organic sulfonates. Used as a mild antiseptic and local stimulant in certain skin diseases. Trade name is Ichthyol.

ichthyism, ichthyismus (ĭk'thē-ĭzm, ĭk"thē-ĭz'mŭs) [Gr. *ichthys*, fish, + *-ismos*, condition]. Poisoning from eating decomposed or toxic fish. SEE: *tetrodotoxin*.

ichthyo- [Gr. *ichthys*, fish]. Combining form meaning fish.

ichthyoacanthotoxism (ĭk"thē-ō-ă-kăn"thō-tŏk'sĭzm) [" + *akantha*, thorn, + *toxikon*, poison, + *-ismos*, condition]. Toxin or venom present in the sting, spines, or "teeth" of certain venomous fish.

ichthyohemotoxin (ĭk"thē-ō-hē"mō-tŏk'sĭn) [" + *haima*, blood, + *toxikon*, poison]. Toxin present in the blood of certain poisonous fish.

ichthyoid (ĭk'thē-oyd) [" + *eidos*, form, shape]. Fishlike.

ichthyology (ĭk"thē-ŏl'ō-jē) [" + *logos*, word, reason]. The study of fish.

ichthyootoxin (ĭk"thē-ō"ō-tŏk'sĭn) [" + *oon*, egg, + *toxikon*, poison]. Toxin present in the roe of certain fish.

ichthyophagous (ĭk"thē-ŏf'ă-gŭs) [" + *phagein*, to eat]. Subsisting on fish.

ichthyophobia (ĭk-thē-ō-fō'bē-ă) [" +

phobos, fear]. Aversion to fish.

ichthyosarcotoxin (ĭk"thē-ō-săr"kō-tŏk'sĭn) [" + *sarx*, flesh, + *toxikon*, poison]. Toxin present in the flesh of certain fish.

ichthyosis (ĭk"thē-ō'sĭs) [" + *osis*, condition]. Condition in which the skin is dry and scaly, resembling fish skin. Because ichthyosis is so easily recognized, a variety of diseases have been called by this name.

A mild nonhereditary form is called xeroderma. This is often seen on the legs of older patients, esp. during the winter months. It may be more prevalent in those who bathe frequently, thus causing excessive dryness of the skin.

TREAT: The application of lotions or ointments that soften and soothe the skin provide symptomatic relief for all forms of ichthyosis. Removal of dry scales can be accomplished by applying a combination of 6% salicylic acid in a gel containing propylene glycol, ethyl alcohol, hydroxy propylene cellulose, and water. This is most effective when applied to moistened skin at night, and covered with an occlusive dressing. Soaps should be used sparingly.

i. congenita. Severe form of ichthyosis present at birth. SYN: *harlequin fetus.*

i. fetalis. I. congenita.

i. hystrix. Linear nevus. The skin contains bands or lines of rough, thick, warty, hypertrophic papillary growths.

i., lamellar, of newborn. Rare form of inherited ichthyosis with lamellar desquamation.

i. vulgaris. Hereditary form of ichthyosis that includes two genetically distinct types. Dominant ichthyosis vulgaris is produced by an autosomal dominant gene. Characterized by dry, rough, scaly skin, it is not present at birth and is usually noticed between the ages of one and four. Many cases improve in later life. The second type is sex-linked ichthyosis vulgaris. It is present only in males and is transmitted by the female as a recessive gene. Onset of scattered large brown scales is seen in early infancy. The scalp may be involved, but the face is spared except for the sides and in front of the ear. There is little tendency to improve with age.

ichthyotic (ĭk"thē-ŏt'ĭk) [Gr. *ichthys*, fish]. Rel. to ichthyosis.

ichthyotoxicology (ĭk"thē-ō-tŏk"sĭ-kŏl'ō-jē) [" + *toxikon*, poison, + *logos*, word, reason]. The study of poisons and toxins produced by certain fish.

ichthyotoxin (ĭk"thē-ō-tŏk'sĭn) [" + *toxikon*, poison]. Any toxin present in fish.

ICIDH. *International Classification of Impairment, Disability and Handicap.*

icing. 1. A technique of cutaneous stimulation

using ice (12° to 17°C) to evoke or facilitate reflex muscular responses in patients with central nervous system dysfunction. 2. Application of ice to a recently traumatized area in order to reduce pain and swelling.

ICN. *International Council of Nurses.*

iconolagny (ī-kŏn″ŏ-lăg′nē) [Gr. *eikon*, image, + *lagneia*, lewdness]. Sexual stimulation produced by suggestive pictures, statues, or objects.

icosa- (ī-kō′să) [Gr. *eikosi*, twenty]. Combining form used in chemistry to indicate twenty. Also spelled *eicosa.*

ICP. *intercranial pressure.*

ICS. *intercostal space.*

I.C.S. *International College of Surgeons.*

ICSH. *interstitial cell-stimulating hormone.* In males, this hormone stimulates the production of testosterone by the interstitial cells of the testes. SYN: *luteinizing hormone.*

ictal (ĭk′tăl) [L. *ictus*, a blow or stroke]. Pert. to or caused by a sudden attack or stroke such as acute epilepsy. SEE: *postictal.*

icteric (ĭk-tĕr′ĭk) [Gr. *ikteros*, jaundice]. Pert. to jaundice.

icteritious (ĭk-tĕr-ĭsh′ŭs). Yellowish; resembling jaundice. SYN: *icteroid.*

icteroanemia (ĭk″tĕr-ō-ă-nē′mē-ă) [″ + *an-*, not, + *haima*, blood]. Icterus associated with anemia, hemolysis, and splenic enlargement.

icterogenic, icterogenous (ĭk″tĕr-ō-jĕn′ĭk, -ŏj′ĕn-ŭs) [″ + *gennan*, to produce]. Causing jaundice.

icterohematuric (ĭk″tĕr-ō-hēm″ă-tū′rĭk) [″ + *haima*, blood, + *ouron*, urine]. Concerning icterus and hematuria.

icterohemoglobinuria (ĭk″tĕr-ō-hē″mō-glō″bĭ-nū′rē-ă) [″ + *haima*, blood, + L. *globus*, globe, + Gr. *ouron*, urine]. Concerning icterus and hemoglobinuria.

icterohepatitis (ĭk″tĕr-ō-hĕp-ă-tī′tĭs) [″ + *hepar*, liver, + *itis*, inflammation]. Liver inflammation with jaundice.

icteroid (ĭk′tĕr-oyd) [″ + *eidos*, form, shape]. Resembling jaundice; yellow-hued.

icterus (ĭk′tĕr-ŭs) [Gr. *ikteros*, jaundice]. Pigmentation of the tissues, membranes, and secretions with bile pigments. SYN: *jaundice.*

   i. gravis neonatorum. Hemolytic jaundice of the newborn. It is usually due to isoimmunization with the Rh factor, q.v. SEE: *erythroblastosis fetalis.*

   i., hemolytic. Rare chronic form of icterus, frequently congenital, with periodic attacks of intense hemolysis. SYN: *icterus, nonobstructive.*

   SYM: Much the same as in obstructive icterus, q.v. Sometimes found in acute yellow atrophy, the anemias, and infectious fevers. Enlarged spleen.

   i. neonatorum. Hemolytic jaundice of the newborn. It is usually mild, self-limiting and requires no treatment. If the infant's level of serum bilirubin rises after birth or persists more than a week, an alternative cause must be searched for. SYN: *physiologic jaundice of the newborn.* SEE: *hemolytic disease of the newborn; kernicterus; phototherapy; transfusion, exchange.*

   i., nonobstructive. I., hemolytic.

   i., obstructive. Jaundice caused by obstruction to the flow of bile in the common or hepatic duct.

   SYM: Skin, mucous membrane, sclera, and secretions stained yellow; first noticed in the conjunctivae. Stool light or clay-colored, urine dark, pulse low, temperature slightly subnormal. In extreme cases, delirium, convulsions, coma.

   ETIOL: Cholangitis, carcinoma, gallstones, cirrhosis of liver, cysts, parasites in ducts, pressure by tumors, hepatic abscess.

ictus [L., stroke] (pl. *ictus*). A blow or sudden attack.

   i. cordis. The heartbeat.

   i. epilepticus. Epileptic convulsion.

   i. sanguinis. Apoplexy; cerebrovascular accident.

ICU. *intensive care unit.*

ID. *identification; infective dose; inside diameter; intradermal.*

ID$_{50}$. The infective dose of microorganisms that will produce illness in 50% of the individuals who receive that dose.

id [L. *id*, it; later translators of Freud's writings believed that the word *es* should have been translated to *it* and not to id]. In psychiatry, one of the three divisions of the psyche, the others being the ego, q.v., and superego, q.v. The id is the obscure, inaccessible part of our personality that serves as a repository of instinctual drives continually striving for expression. Expression is manifest as an impulsion to obtain satisfaction for the instinctive needs in accordance with the pleasure-pain principle.

id. L. *idem*, the same.

-id [Gr. *eidos*, form, shape]. Suffix indicating certain secondary skin eruptions that appear some distance from site of primary infection. If etiological agent of primary infection is known, the secondary lesion is designated by adding -id, as in tuberculid and trichophytid.

IDDM. *insulin-dependent diabetes mellitus.*

-ide. Suffix indicating a binary chemical compound, as *sodium chloride.*

idea [Gr., form]. A mental image; a concept.

   i., autochthonous. A thought that comes into the mind independent of train of thoughts, in an unaccountable way.

   i., compulsive. A persistent, obsessional

impulse or thought.

i., dominant. Idea that controls all one's actions and thoughts.

i., fixed. Idea that completely dominates the mind despite evidence to the contrary; a delusion. SYN: *idée fixe.*

i.'s, flight of. Rapid speech, often disconnected and incoherent, in certain mental diseases.

i. of reference. An impression that the conversation or actions of others have reference to oneself.

ideal [L. *idea*, model]. A goal or endeavor regarded as a standard of perfection.

ideation (ī-dē-ā'shŭn). The process of thinking; formation of ideas. It is slow in dementias, depressions, and other organic brain diseases, and in narcotic intoxications, but quickened in early stage of some types of intoxications. It is unduly active in manic-depressive states.

idée fixe (ē-dā' fēks') [Fr.]. An obsession; a fixed idea. SYN: *idea, fixed,* q.v.

identical [L. *identicus,* the same]. Exactly alike.

identification [" + *facere,* to make]. 1. A kind of daydream, as when one identifies oneself with the hero of a book or play. 2. The process of determining the sameness of a thing or person with that described or known to exist. 3. A defense mechanism, operating unconsciously, by which a person patterns himself or herself after some other person. This plays a major role in personality development.

i., dental. The use of the unique characteristics of a person's teeth or dental work as recorded in dental charts, radiographs, and records to establish the person's identity.

identification, palm and sole system of. A system based on prints of the palmar surface of the hand and the plantar surface of the foot. SEE: *dermatoglyphics.*

identity (ī-dĕn'tǐ-tē). 1. The concept that each individual has of his or her body in space and his or her thought processes in relation to the social and intellectual environment. 2. The physical and mental characteristics by which an individual is known and recognized.

i., ego. The sense of self that provides a unity of personality.

i., gender. One's self-concept with respect to being male or female, or confused about one's true sexual identity.

identity testing. SEE: *paternity analysis.*

ideo- [Gr. *idea,* form]. Prefix pert. to mental images.

ideogenous, ideogenetic (ĭd-ē-ŏj'ĕn-ŭs, -ō-jĕ-nĕt'ĭk) [" + *gennan,* to produce]. Stimulated by an idea.

ideology (ī"dē-ŏl'ō-jē) [" + *logos,* word,

reason]. 1. The science of ideas or thought. 2. A system or schema of ideas; a philosophy.

ideomotion (ī"dē-ō-mō'shŭn) [" + L. *motus,* moving]. Muscular automatic movement activated by a dominant idea.

ideomotor (ī"dē-ō-mō'tor). Pert. to ideomotion.

ideomuscular (ī"dē-ō-mŭs'kū-lăr) [" + L. *musculus,* muscle]. 1. Indicating muscular activity produced in connection with a thought. 2. Concerning both ideation and muscular activity.

ideophrenic (ĭd"ē-ō-frĕn'ĭk) [" + *phrenitikos,* insane]. Marked by abnormal ideas of a perverted nature.

ideoplastia (ĭd-ē-ō-plăs'tē-ă) [" + *plassein,* to form]. Condition of the mind of a hypnotized person in which the person is capable of receiving and responding to suggestions of the hypnotist.

ideovascular (ĭd"ē-ō-văs'kū-lăr). Pert. to vascular changes induced by ideas, memories, or emotions; as when a state of mental stress produces an elevation in blood pressure.

idio- [Gr. *idios,* own]. Prefix indicating individual or distinct.

idiochromosome (ĭd"ē-ō-krō'mō-sōm) [" + *chroma,* color, + *soma,* body]. Any sex chromosome.

idiocrasy (ĭd"ē-ŏk'ră-sē) [" + *krasis,* temperament]. Peculiarity that renders one susceptible to certain habits or drugs. SEE: *idiosyncrasy.*

idiocratic (ĭd"ē-ō-krăt'ĭk). Pert. to idiocrasy.

idiocy [Gr. *idiotes,* ignorant person]. Severe mental deficiency, usually due to an arrest in development, or defective development, as opposed to the loss of mental competence. The cause, which occurs either in utero or in the first years after birth, may be genetic, traumatic, or due to severe disease. SEE: *mental retardation.*

i., complete. Idiocy in which primitive instincts are lacking, even that of self-preservation.

i., cretinoid. Endemic idiocy accompanied by goiter. SEE: *cretinism.*

i., epileptic. Idiocy accompanied by epilepsy.

i., genetous. Idiocy of congenital origin.

i., hemiplegic. Hemiplegia accompanied by idiocy in infants.

i., hydrocephalic. Idiocy accompanied by chronic hydrocephalus.

i., intrasocial. Idiocy in which the mentality permits the individual to learn an occupation.

i., microcephalic. Idiocy accompanied by microcephalia.

i., paralytic. Idiocy combined with paralysis.

i., paraplegic. Idiocy combined with paraplegia.

i., sensorial. Mental deficiency caused by loss of one of the special senses.

i., traumatic. Idiocy caused by an injury received in infancy or in early childhood.

idiogamist (ĭd″ē-ŏg′ă-mĭst) [Gr. *idios,* own, + *gamos,* marriage]. An individual who is sexually potent with only one or a few partners.

idiogenesis (ĭd″ē-ō-jĕn′ē-sĭs) [″ + *gennan,* to produce]. Of self-origin or origin without known cause, esp. with reference to disease.

idioglossia (ĭd″ē-ō-glŏs′ē-ă) [″ + *glossa,* tongue]. Inability to articulate properly, so that the sounds emitted are like those of an unknown language.

idiogram (ĭd′ē-ō-grăm″) [″ + *gramma,* something written]. Graphic representation of the karyotype, or chromosome complement of a cell.

idioisolysin (ĭd″ē-ō-ī-sŏl′ĭ-sĭn) [″ + *isos,* equal, + *lysis,* dissolution]. A hemolysin active against the cells of an individual of the same species.

idiolysin (ĭd″ē-ŏl′ĭ-sĭn) [″ + *lysis,* dissolution]. A lysin normally present in blood.

idiometritis (ĭd″ē-ō-mĕ-trī′tĭs) [″ + *metra,* uterus, + *itis,* inflammation]. Inflammation of the uterine parenchyma.

idiomiasma (ĭd″ē-ō-mī-ăz′mă) [″ + *miasma,* stain]. An offensive odor produced by one's own body.

idiomuscular (ĭd″ē-ō-mŭs′kū-lăr) [″ + L. *musculus,* a muscle]. Pert. to the muscles independent of nerve control.

idiomuscular contraction. Motion produced by degenerated muscles without nerve stimulus.

idiopathic (ĭd″ē-ō-păth′ĭk) [″ + *pathos,* disease, suffering]. Pert. to conditions without clear pathogenesis, or disease without recognizable cause, as of spontaneous origin.

idiopathic pulmonary fibrosis. A form of interstitial lung disease with a rapid deterioration in clinical course due to diffuse interstitial pneumonitis or fibrosis. Symptoms vary with the degree but include dyspnea, rapid respirations, anoxia, and weight loss with subsequent weakness and fatigue. At first pulmonary symptoms are not prominent unless there is bronchial involvement with exudate. As the disease progresses, finger clubbing, cyanosis, and heart failure develop. SYN: *Hamman-Rich syndrome.*

ETIOL: Unknown.

DIAG: Based on characteristic clinical signs and symptoms. Definitive diagnosis can be established only by open lung biopsy.

TREAT: Corticosteroids are usually of considerable benefit but are not curative. Supportive therapy consists of supplementary oxygen, antibiotics, and treatment for heart failure. Cyclophosphamide is also used to suppress the neutrophil component of inflammation.

PROG: Usually fatal 4 to 5 years after date of onset.

idiopathy (ĭd-ē-ŏp′ă-thē). A primary disease without apparent cause.

idiophrenic (ĭd″ē-ō-frĕn′ĭk) [″ + *phren,* mind]. Pert. to or originating in the mind alone.

idiopsychologic (ĭd″ē-ō-sī″kō-lŏj′ĭk) [″ + *psyche,* mind, + *logos,* word, reason]. Concerning ideas produced in one's own mind.

idioreflex (ĭd″ē-ō-rē′flĕks) [″ + L. *reflexus,* reflected]. A reflex resulting from a stimulus that arises within the organ in which the reflex takes place.

idiospasm (ĭd′ē-ō-spăzm) [″ + *spasmos,* convulsion]. Spasm confined to one area.

idiosyncrasy (ĭd″ē-ō-sĭn′kră-sē) [″ + *syn,* together, + *krasis,* mixture]. 1. Special characteristics by which persons differ from each other. 2. That which makes one react differently from others. A peculiar or individual reaction to an idea, action, drug, food, or some other substance through unusual susceptibility.

idiosyncrasy of effect. When doses of a drug that would have a known and predictable effect cause a toxic or opposite effect, an unusual effect, or no effect.

idiosyncrasy to a drug. An unusual response to a drug. It can manifest as an accelerated, toxic, or inappropriate response to the usual therapeutic dose of a drug.

idiosyncratic (ĭd″ē-ō-sĭn-krăt′ĭk). Pert. to an idiosyncrasy.

idiot [Gr. *idiotes,* ignorant person]. Former term for a person with severe mental deficiency. SEE: *idiocy; mental retardation.*

idiotic. Like an idiot; said of an idea or action.

idiotrophic (ĭd″ē-ō-trŏf′ĭk) [Gr. *idios,* own, + *trophe,* nourishment]. Capable of securing its own nourishment.

idiotropic (ĭd″ē-ō-trŏp′ĭk) [″ + *trope,* a turning]. Turning inward mentally and emotionally. SYN: *egocentric; introspective.*

idiotropic type. In psychology, an introvert type who is satisfied by his or her own emotions and by inner contemplation and pursuits and who is content to live apart from social contacts.

idiot-savant (ēd-jō′să-vănt) [Fr., learned idiot]. An individual who is generally mentally retarded but has the ability to do complicated tasks such as play instruments, recall dates, or accurately and rapidly perform mathematical calculations. SEE: *autism.*

idiotype. In immunology, the specific region of the antibody-binding (Fab) region of the immunoglobulin molecule to which the specific antigen binds. SEE: *isotypes.*

idiotypic (ĭd″ē-ō-tĭp′ĭk) [Gr. *idios,* own, + *typos,* type]. Rel. to heredity.

idiovariation (ĭd″ē-ō-văr″ē-ā′shŭn) [″ + L. *variare,* to vary]. A mutation that occurs without known cause.

idioventricular (ĭd″ē-ō-vĕn-trĭk′ū-lăr) [″ + L. *ventriculus,* little belly]. Pert. to the cardiac ventricle alone when dissociated from the atrium. A heart rhythm that arises in the ventricle is an example.

idoxuridine (ī-dŏks-ūr′ĭ-dēn). 5-iodo-2′ deoxyuridine. USP. ABBR: IDU. Used to treat herpesvirus infections of the eye. Trade names are Herplex Liquifilm and Stoxil.

IDU. *5-iodo-2′deoxyuridine; idoxuridine.*

Ifosfamide. A cytotoxic agent used in treating metastatic germ-cell testicular cancer. This drug is usually given with mesna to help reduce the toxicity of its metabolites. Trade name is Ifex. SEE: *mesna; testicular cancer, germ-cell.*

IgA. *immunoglobulin gamma A.*

IgD. *immunoglobulin gamma D.*

IgE. *immunoglobulin gamma E.*

IgG. *immunoglobulin gamma G.*

IgM. *immunoglobulin gamma M.*

ignatia (ĭg-nā′shē-ă) [L.]. Seeds of a climbing plant native to the Philippine Islands. The seeds contain about 3% strychnine and brucine.

igniextirpation (ĭg″nē-ĕks″tĭr-pā′shŭn) [L. *ignis,* fire, + *exstirpare,* to root out]. Cautery excision.

ignioperation (ĭg″nē-ŏp″ĕr-ā′shŭn) [″ + *operatio,* a working]. An operation by use of cautery.

ignipuncture (ĭg″nē-pŭnk′chūr) [″ + *punctura,* a piercing]. The use of heated needles in cauterization by puncture.

ignis (ĭg′nĭs) [L., fire]. Fire; cautery. SYN: *moxa.*

   i. infernalis. Ergotism.

I.H. *infectious hepatitis.*

ILD. *interstitial lung disorders.*

ilea. Pl. of ileum.

ileac (ĭl′ē-ăk). 1. Pert. to the ileum. 2. Pert. to ileus.

ileal (ĭl′ē-ăl). Pert. to the ileum.

ileal bypass. Surgical procedure for decreasing absorption of nutrients from the small intestine by anastomosing one portion of the upper small intestine to another portion some distance farther along the intestine. Method is used in treating obesity.

ileal conduit. Method of diverting the urinary flow by transplanting the ureter into a prepared and isolated segment of the ileum, which is sutured closed on one end. The other end is connected to an opening in the abdominal wall. Urine is collected there in a special receptacle.

ileectomy (ĭl″ē-ĕk′tō-mē) [L. *ileum,* ileum, + Gr. *ektome,* excision]. Excision of the ileum.

ileitis (ĭl″ē-ī′tĭs) [″ + Gr. *itis,* inflammation]. Inflammation of the ileum. The membrane becomes inflamed and ulcerates, the affected portion becoming thick, rigid, and edematous, and the lumen progressively narrowed. The lymph glands enlarge and the adjacent mesentery becomes thickened. Most often found in the terminal ileum, but it may spread to other parts of the bowel and to the cecum. Adhesions may be formed. Pain is centered around the umbilicus and right lower quadrant. Abdominal distention is present. Diarrhea may alternate with constipation. Vomiting may occur.

   i., regional. A nonspecific, chronic, inflammatory, granulomatous lesion involving the terminal ileum. It is nontuberculous. The disease may extend over many years with exacerbations and remissions of diarrhea, abdominal pain, anemia, loss of weight, fistula formation, and eventually obstructive intestinal symptoms. Stools are soft and gray or brown in color with abundant fecal particles. Any part of the gastrointestinal tract may be involved, but the ileum is the principal site. The cause is unknown.

   TREAT: Dietary and symptomatic with respect to the anemia and dehydration. Corticosteroids are indicated in acute attacks. Very low daily doses may be of benefit when the acute attack is over. Antibiotics are needed for bacterial complications. If symptoms persist or there is recurrent intestinal obstruction, resection of the inflamed bowel may be palliative but not curative. SYN: *Crohn's disease.*

ileo- (ĭl″ē-ō) [L. *ileum*]. Combining form indicating relationship to the ileum.

ileocecal (ĭl′ē-ō-sē′kăl) [″ + *caecus,* blind]. Rel. to the ileum and cecum.

ileocecal valve. Sphincter muscles that serve to close the ileum at the point where the small intestines open into the ascending colon. It prevents food material from re-entering the small intestine.

ileocecostomy (ĭl″ē-ō-sē-kŏs′tō-mē) [″ + ″ + Gr. *stoma,* opening]. Surgical formation of an opening between the ileum and cecum.

ileocecum (ĭl″ē-ō-sē′kŭm). The ileum and cecum combined.

ileocolic (ĭl″ē-ō-kŏl′ĭk) [″ + Gr. *kolon,* colon]. Pert. to the ileum and colon.

ileocolitis (ĭl″ē-ō-kō-lī′tĭs) [″ + ″ + *itis*, inflammation]. Inflammation of mucous membrane of the ileum and colon. SEE: *Nursing Diagnoses* in *Appendix*.

ileocolostomy (ĭl″ē-ō-kō-lŏs′tō-mē) [″ + ″ + *stoma*, mouth]. Anastomosis between the ileum and colon.

ileocolotomy (ĭl″ē-ō-kō-lŏt′ō-mē) [″ + ″ + *tome*, incision]. Incision of the ileum and colon.

ileocystoplasty (ĭl″ē-ō-sĭst′ō-plăs″tē) [″ + Gr. *kystis*, bladder, + *plassein*, to form]. Use of a portion of the ileum to increase the size of the bladder.

ileocystostomy (ĭl″ē-ō-sĭs-tŏs′tō-mē) [″ + ″ + *stoma*, mouth]. Surgical formation of an opening between the ileum and bladder.

ileoileostomy (ĭl″ē-ō-ĭl″ē-ŏs′tō-mē) [″ + *ileum*, small intestine, + Gr. *stoma*, mouth]. Surgical formation of an opening between two parts of the ileum.

ileoproctostomy (ĭl″ē-ō-prŏk-tŏs′tō-mē) [″ + Gr. *proktos*, rectum, + *stoma*, mouth]. Establishment of opening between the ileum and rectum. SYN: *ileorectostomy*.

ileorectal (ĭl″ē-ō-rĕk′tăl) [″ + *rectum*, rectum]. Concerning the ileum and rectum.

ileorectostomy (ĭl″ē-ō-rĕk-tŏs′tō-mē) [″ + ″ + Gr. *stoma*, mouth]. Formation of a passage between the ileum and rectum. SYN: *ileoproctostomy*.

ileorrhaphy (ĭl″ē-or′ă-fē) [″ + Gr. *rhaphe*, seam, ridge]. Surgical repair of the ileum.

ileosigmoidostomy (ĭl″ē-ō-sĭg″moyd-ŏs′tō-mē) [″ + Gr. *sigma*, letter S, + *eidos*, form, shape, + *stoma*, mouth]. Surgical opening between the ileum and sigmoid flexure.

ileostomy (ĭl″ē-ŏs′tō-mē) [″ + Gr. *stoma*, mouth]. Creation of a surgical passage through the abdominal wall into the ileum. The fecal material drains into a bag worn on the abdomen. SEE: *Nursing Diagnoses* in *Appendix*.

   i., urinary. Surgical formation of an opening between the ileum and the urinary bladder.

ileotomy (ĭl″ē-ŏt′ō-mē) [″ + Gr. *tome*, incision]. Incision into the ileum.

ileotransversostomy (ĭl″ē-ō-trăns″vĕr-sŏs′tō-mē) [″ + *transversus*, crosswise, + Gr. *stoma*, mouth]. Connection of the ileum with the transverse colon.

ileum (ĭl′ē-ŭm) [L., ileum (pl. *ilea*). [NA] Lower three-fifths of the small intestines from the jejunum to the ileocecal valve. Its length varies in the adult male from 31 ft 6 in. (9.6 meters) to 15 ft 6 in. (4.72 meters). SEE: *abdominal regions* and *digestive system* for illus.

   i., duplex. Congenital doubling of the ileum.

ileus (ĭl′ē-ŭs) [Gr. *eileos*, a twisting]. Intestinal obstruction. Originally meant colic due to intestinal obstruction. SEE: *Nursing Diagnoses* in *Appendix*.

   SYM: Acute obstruction; sudden pain, paroxysmal, then continuous; constipation; persistent fecal vomiting; abdominal distention; collapse.

   i., adynamic. Ileus caused by intestinal muscle paralysis.

   i., dynamic. Ileus caused by intestinal muscle contraction.

   i., mechanical. Ileus produced by an obstruction.

   i., meconium. Ileus of the newborn due to obstruction of the bowel with meconium.

   i. paralyticus. I., adynamic.

   i., postoperative. Ileus resulting from handling the bowel during surgery, anesthesia, electrolyte imbalance, or wound infection.

   i., spastic. Ileus due to spasm of a segment of the intestine.

   i. subparta. Ileus due to pressure of the pregnant uterus on the colon.

ilia. Pl. of ilium.

iliac [L. *iliacus*, pert. to ilium]. Rel. to the ilium.

iliac crest. The hip. Upper free margin of the ilium.

iliac fascia. Transversalis fascia over the anterior surface of the iliopsoas muscle.

iliac fossa. One of the concavities of the iliac bones of the pelvis.

iliac region. Inguinal region on either side of the hypogastrium.

iliac roll. Sausage-shaped mass in the left iliac fossa. Caused by induration of the sigmoidal walls.

iliac spine. One of four spines of the ilium, namely the anterior and posterior inferior spines and the anterior and posterior superior spines.

ilio- [L. *ilium*, flank]. Combining form indicating relationship to the ilium or flank.

iliococcygeal (ĭl″ē-ō-kŏk-sĭj′ē-ăl) [″ + Gr. *kokkyx*, coccyx]. Concerning the ilium and coccyx.

iliocolotomy (ĭl″ē-ō-kō-lŏt′ō-mē) [″ + Gr. *kolon*, colon, + *tome*, incision]. Opening into the colon in the iliac or inguinal region.

iliocostal (ĭl″ē-ō-kŏs′tăl) [″ + *costa*, rib]. Joining or concerning the ilium and ribs.

iliofemoral (ĭl″ē-ō-fĕm′or-ăl) [″ + *femoralis*, pert. to femur]. Pert. to the ilium and femur.

iliohypogastric (ĭl″ē-ō-hī″pō-găs′trĭk) [″ + Gr. *hypo*, under, + *gaster*, stomach]. Concerning the ilium and hypogastrium.

ilioinguinal (ĭl″ē-ō-ĭn′gwĭ-năl) [″ + *in-*

guinalis, pert. to groin]. Pert. to the groin and iliac regions.

iliolumbar (ĭl″ē-ō-lŭm′bar) [″ + *lumbus,* loin]. Rel. to the iliac and lumbar regions.

iliopagus (ĭl″ē-ŏp′ă-gŭs) [″ + Gr. *pagos,* thing fixed]. Twins joined in the iliac region.

iliopectineal (ĭl″ē-ō-pĕk-tĭn′ē-ăl) [L. *ilium,* flank, + *pecten,* a comb]. Rel. to the ilium and pubes.

iliopelvic (ĭl″ē-ō-pĕl′vĭk) [″ + *pelvis,* basin]. Concerning the iliac area and pelvis.

iliopsoas (ĭl″ē-ō-sō′ăs) [″ + Gr. *psoa,* loin]. The compound iliacus and psoas magnus muscles.

iliopsoas abscess. An abscess in the psoas and iliacus muscles.

iliosacral (ĭl″ē-ō-sā′krăl) [″ + *sacralis,* pert. to sacrum]. Pert. to the sacrum and ilium.

iliosciatic (ĭl″ē-ō-sī-ăt′ĭk) [″ + *sciaticus,* pert. to the ischium]. Concerning the ilium and ischium.

iliospinal (ĭl″ē-ō-spī′năl) [″ + *spinalis,* pert. to the spine]. Concerning the ilium and spinal column.

iliothoracopagus (ĭl″ē-ō-thō″ră-kōp′ă-gŭs) [″ + Gr. *thorax,* chest, + *pagos,* thing fixed]. Twins joined from pelvis to thorax.

iliotibial (ĭl″ē-ō-tĭb′ē-ăl) [″ + *tibialis,* pert. to tibia]. Pert. to the ilium and tibia.

iliotibial band. A thick, wide fascial layer from the iliac crest along the lateral thigh to the fascia around the lateral aspect of the knee joint. Fibers from the tensor fascia lata and gluteus maximus insert into the proximal band.

ilioxiphopagus (ĭl″ē-ō-zī-fōp′ă-gŭs) [″ + Gr. *xiphos,* sword, + *eidos,* form, shape, + *pagos,* thing fixed]. Twins joined from the pelvis to the xiphoid process.

ilium (ĭl′ē-ŭm) [L., groin, flank] (pl. *ilia*). 1. One of the bones of each half of the pelvis. It is the superior and widest part and serves to support the flank. In the child, prior to fusion with adjacent pelvic bones, it is a separate bone. SYN: *os ilium* [NA]. 2. The flank. SEE: *sacroiliac.*

ill (ĭl) [Old Norse *illr,* bad]. Sick; not healthy; diseased.

illaqueation (ĭl″ăk-wē-ā′shŭn) [L. *illaqueare,* to ensnare]. Turning an inverted eyelash by drawing a loop of thread behind it.

illegitimate. 1. Illegal; against the law. 2. Born out of wedlock.

illinition (ĭl-ĭ-nĭsh′ŭn) [L. *illinire,* to smear]. Inunction, q.v.

illiterate. Being unable to read and write or to use written language as in understanding graphs, charts, tables, maps, symbols, and formulae.

illiterate, functionally. Being unable to read materials considered to be essential for the usual forms of employment.

illness (ĭl′nĭs) [Old Norse *illr,* bad, + AS. *-ness,* state of]. 1. State of being sick. 2. Ailment.

    i., catastrophic. An unusually prolonged or complex illness, esp. one that requires a large expenditure of money for the medical care involved.

    i., functional. An illness for which no organic explanation is present. SYN: *functional disorder.* SEE: *organic disease.*

    i., terminal. An illness which, because of its nature or because of the specific circumstances of the patient, is destined to cause the death of the patient, esp. cancers for which there is little hope that therapeutic interventions will be helpful.

illuminating gas. A mixture of various combustible gases, including hydrogen and carbon monoxide. Its poisonous effects are largely due to carbon monoxide, q.v. Treat by resuscitation, q.v.

illumination (ĭl-lū-mĭn-ā′shŭn) [L. *illuminare,* to light up]. 1. The lighting up of a part for examination or of an object under a microscope. 2. Amount of light thrown upon anything.

    i., axial. Light transmitted along the axis of a microscope.

    i., central. I., axial.

    i., dark-field. Illumination of an object under a microscope in which the central or axial light rays are stopped and the object is illuminated by light rays coming from the sides, the object then appearing light against a dark background. Used to observe extremely small objects such as spirochetes or colloid particles.

    i., direct. Illumination of an object under a microscope by directing light rays upon its upper surface.

    i., focal. Concentration of light upon an object by means of a mirror or a system of lenses.

    i., oblique. Illumination of an object from one side.

    i., through. SEE: *transillumination.*

    i., transmitted light. Illumination in which the light is directed through the object. Light may come directly from a light source or be reflected by a mirror.

illuminism. Condition in certain psychotic states in which the patient has delusions of talking or communing with supernatural or exalted beings.

illusion [L. *illusio*]. Inaccurate perception; misinterpretation of sensory impressions, as opposed to a hallucination, which has no source in fact. Vague stimuli are conducive to the production of illusions, but essentially it is a disorder of ideation. If an illusion becomes fixed, it is said to be a delusion.

i., optical. A visual impression that is inaccurate with respect to what was available to be seen.

illusional. Pert. to, or of the nature of, an illusion.

Ilosone. Trade name for erythromycin estolate.

Ilotycin. Trade name for erythromycin, USP.

Ilozyme. Trade name for pancrelipase.

I.M. *intramuscular(ly).*

im-. Prefix that is used in place of *in-* before words beginning with *b, m,* or *p.*

I.M.A. *Industrial Medical Association.*

ima (i′mă) [L.]. Lowest.

image (ĭm′ĭj) [L. *imago,* likeness]. 1. A mental picture representing a real object. 2. A more or less accurate likeness of a thing or person. 3. The picture of an object such as that produced by a lens or mirror.

i., body. The concept an individual has of his or her physical self. Many individuals have inappropriate self-images. For example, some obese individuals have the body image of a much less obese person.

i., direct. Picture from rays not yet focused.

i., double. Condition occurring in strabismus when the visual axes of the eyes are not directed toward the same object. SEE: *diplopia.*

i., false. I., double.

i., inverted. Image that is turned upside down.

i., latent. In radiology, the image on an exposed radiograph that is invisible because it has not been developed.

i., mirror. Image of an object reflected in a mirror. Right and left are reversed in that image. The term is also used to indicate the similarity of chemical substances, or persons with quite similar personalities and looks. Identical twins are also often described as being mirror images of each other.

i., radiographic. An image created on a fluorescent screen or photographic film by x-rays passed through a structure or tissue. Also called *x-ray image.*

i., real. Image formed by convergence of rays of light from an object.

i., true. I., double.

i., virtual. I., direct.

image intensifier. Device used in radiology to increase the brightness of an image produced in x-ray and x-ray fluoroscopy studies. The technique permits discrimination of much smaller objects in the image and greatly decreases the patient's and the examiner's exposure to the radiation.

imagery (ĭm′ĭj-rē) [L. *imago,* likeness]. Imagination; the calling up of events or mental pictures. Mental imagery may be of various types.

i., auditory. Mental image of sounds that can be recalled, as thunder or wind.

i., smell. Mental concept of odor sensations previously experienced. Often very weak.

i., tactile. Mental image of the feeling of an object.

i., taste. Mental concept of taste sensations previously experienced. Often very weak.

i., visual. Mental concept of an object seen previously. This is probably the commonest type of imagery. SEE: *afterimage.*

imagination [L. *imago,* likeness]. Formation of mental images of things, persons, or situations that are wholly or partially different from those previously known or experienced.

imaging. Production of a picture, image, or shadow that represents the object being investigated. In diagnostic medicine the classic technique for imaging is x-ray. Techniques that involve the use of computer-generated images produced by x-ray, ultrasound, magnetic resonance, or infrared are available.

imago (ĭ-mā′gō) [L., likeness]. 1. An image or shadow. 2. A memory, esp. of a loved one, developed during childhood that has become clouded by idealism and imagination, and is not always correct. 3. The adult, sexually mature form of an insect.

Imavate. Trade name for imipramine hydrochloride, USP.

imbalance [L. *in-,* not, + *bilanx,* two scales]. Out of balance. Without equality in power between opposing forces.

i., autonomic. Imbalance between sympathetic and parasympathetic divisions of the autonomic nervous system, esp. as pertains to vasomotor reactions.

i., sympathetic. Increased excitability of the vagus nerve. SYN: *vagotonia.*

i., vasomotor. Excessive vasoconstriction or vasodilation resulting from impulses to blood vessels.

imbecile (ĭm′bĕ-sĭl) [L. *imbecillus,* feeble]. Former term for severe mental deficiency. SEE: *mental retardation.*

imbecility. A state of severe mental deficiency.

imbed [L. *in,* in, (put) into, + AS. *bedd,* bed]. In histology, to surround with a firm substance, such as paraffin, preparatory to cutting sections. SEE: *embedding.*

imbibition (ĭm″bĭ-bĭsh′ŭn) [″ + *bibere,* to drink]. The absorption of fluid by a solid body or gel.

imbricate, imbricated (ĭm′brĭ-kāt, -ĕd) [L. *imbricare,* to tile]. Overlapping, as tiles or fish scales; overlapping aponeurotic layers.

imbrication (ĭm″brĭ-kā′shŭn) [L. *imbricare,*

to tile]. 1. Overlapping, as tiles. 2. The overlapping of aponeurotic layers in abdominal surgery.

Imferon. Trade name for iron dextran.

imidazole (ĭm″ĭd-ăz′ōl″). An organic compound, $C_3H_4N_2$, characterized structurally by the presence of the heterocyclic ring

$$R-C=C-H$$

which occurs in histidine and histamine.

imide (ĭm′ĭd). A compound with the bivalent atom group (NH).

imipramine hydrochloride (ĭ-mĭp′ră-mēn). USP. An antidepressant drug of the tricyclic class. This drug is also used in treating enuresis in children over 6 years of age. Trade names are Imavate, Janimine, Presamine, SK-Pramine, and Tofranil.

immature (ĭm″mă-tūr′) [L. *in-*, not, + *maturus*, ripe]. Not fully developed or ripened.

immediate [″ + *mediare*, to be in middle]. Direct; without intervening steps.

immedicable (ĭ-mĕd′ĭ-kă-b′l) [L. *immedicabilis*]. Incurable; pert. to that which cannot be healed.

immersion (ĭm-ĕr′shŭn) [L. *in*, into, + *mergere*, to dip]. 1. Placing a body under water or other fluid. 2. In microscopy, the act of immersing the objective (then called an immersion lens) in water or oil, preventing total reflection of rays falling obliquely upon peripheral portions of the objective.

   i., homogeneous. Immersion in which the stratum of air between objective and cover glass is replaced by a medium that deflects as little as possible the rays of light passing through the cover glass.

immersion foot. Damage to the entire foot due to continued exposure to water or to moisture. It can occur in a hot or cold climate in a situation in which it is not possible to maintain proper foot hygiene. From military experience, it was found that the condition could be prevented by changing to dry socks as frequently as required. SEE: *trench foot.*

immersion lens, oil. A special lens with oil placed between the lens and the object being visualized. This produces a higher magnification than would be the case if the oil were not used.

immiscible (ĭ-mĭs′ĭ-bl) [L. *in-*, not, + *miscere*, to mix]. Pert. to that which cannot be mixed, as oil and water.

immobilization [″ + *mobilis*, movable]. The making of a part or limb immovable.

NURSING IMPLICATIONS: Assess the patient for development of any of the complications of immobilization, such as pneumonia, thrombophlebitis, fat emboli, renal calculi, urinary tract infections, decubitus ulcers, muscle atrophy, and contracture formation.

   Institute nursing interventions to prevent complications of immobilization by having the patient cough and breathe deeply every two hours, change position every two hours, wear elastic stockings, do quadriceps-setting, gluteal-setting, and range-of-motion exercises at least daily, ensure good body hygiene, and maintain an increased oral fluid intake. Good skin care is essential; inspect the skin daily for redness and signs of breakdown, and massage the skin; provide a suitable diet. If the patient has a casted or splinted extremity, make sure that the cast is not too tight and thereby constricting blood supply. Always evaluate the neurovascular status of the extremity distal to the site of the cast, splint, or traction by assessing for good color, presence of a pulse, extremity warmth, movement, and sensation.

immotile cilia syndrome. An inherited condition in which the motion of the cilia, normally 1000 cycles per minute, is defective. The cilia have deficient dynein arms that are essential to their movement. Clinically, these patients have the illness described by Kartagener. SEE: *dynein; Kartagener's syndrome.*

immune (ĭm-ūn′) [L. *immunis*, safe]. Protected from or resistant to a disease or infection by a pathogenic organism due to the development of antibodies, q.v., or T cell mediated immunity.

immune body. Antibody, q.v.

immune complex. Substance formed when antibodies attach to antigens to destroy them. These complexes circulate in the blood and may eventually attach to the walls of blood vessels, producing a local inflammatory response. Immune complexes form in Type III hypersensitivity reactions and are involved in the development of glomerulonephritis, serum sickness, arthritis, and vasculitis.

immune globulin, intravenous. ABBR: IVIG. An immune globulin preparation used intravenously in patients with immunodeficiency syndromes and in immunosuppressed recipients of bone marrow transplants. In conjunction with aspirin, it is the standard of care for children during the first 10 days of Kawasaki disease to prevent the development of coronary aneurysms. The risks of using IVIG are minimal.

immune reaction. 1. Demonstrated antigenic response to a specific antibody. 2. The specific reaction of host cells to antigenic stimulation. SEE: *immune response*.

immune response. The reaction of the body to foreign antigens so that they are neutralized or eliminated, preventing damage. It requires that the body recognize the antigen as "nonself" or foreign. SEE: *antigen*.

Cell-mediated immune response: involves the production of lymphocytes by the thymus (T cells) in response to exposure to an antigen. This reaction is important in delayed hypersensitivity; rejection of tissue transplants; response to malignant growths; and in some infections. SEE: *B cells; T cells*.

Humoral immune response: involves production of plasma lymphocytes (B cells) in response to antigen exposure with subsequent antibody formation. This response can produce immunity or hypersensitivity. SEE: *B cells; T cells*.

Nonspecific immune response: the response of the body's tissues and cells to injury from any source, e.g., trauma, organisms, chemicals, ischemia. The initial response of the immune system to any threat, it involves vascular, chemical, and white blood cell activities. SYN: *acute phase response; inflammation*. SEE: *inflammation*.

Specific immune response: required when inflammation is inadequate to cope with injury or invasion of an organism. It is directed and controlled by T and B lymphocytes. Cellular immunity is used to refer to the T lymphocyte response. Humoral immunity is the term previously used to refer to B lymphocyte response. SEE: *B cell mediated immunity; T cell mediated immunity*.

immune response genes. Genes that control the ability of lymphocytes to respond to specific antigens. SEE: *antigen; B cell; HLA complex; T cell*.

immune system. The tissues, organs and physiological processes used by the body to identify a protein as abnormal or foreign and prevent it from harming the organism.

immunifacient (ĭ-mū″nĭ-fā′shĕnt) [″ + *facere*, to make]. Making immune.

immunity [L. *immunitas*]. State of being immune to or protected from a disease, esp. an infectious disease. Usually induced by having been exposed to the antigenic marker on an organism that invades the body; or by having been immunized with a vaccine that has the capability of stimulating production of specific antibodies. SEE: *autoimmune disease; immune response; immunoglobulin; vaccine*.

i., acquired. Immunity resulting from the development of active or passive immu-

nity, as opposed to natural or innate immunity.

i., active. Immunity resulting from the development within the body of antibodies or sensitized T lymphocytes that neutralize or destroy the infective agent. This may result from the immune response to an invading organism or from inoculation with a vaccine containing antibodies. SEE: *immune response; vaccination*.

i., cell-mediated. Immunity resulting from activation of sensitized T lymphocytes. SYN: *cellular immunity*. SEE: *T cell mediated immunity*.

i., congenital. Immunity present at birth. It may be natural or acquired, the latter being dependent upon antibodies received from the blood of the mother.

i., herd. Vaccination of an individual provides immune protection and it may reduce the spread of the infecting agent in the population.

i., humeral. Immunity mediated by antibodies in body fluids such as plasma or lymph. These antibodies are synthesized and secreted by B lymphocytes, q.v. SEE: *B cell immunity; immunity, cell-mediated; lymphocytes; T cells*.

i., local. Immunity limited to a given area or tissue of the body.

i., natural. A more or less permanent immunity to disease with which an individual is born, the result of natural inherent factors. It may be the heritage of an individual, a race, or a species. It may be due to the natural presence of immune bodies, but other factors such as diet, differences in metabolism or temperature, or adaptive features of infective organisms may be involved.

i., passive. Immunity acquired by the introduction of preformed antibodies into an unprotected individual. This can occur through injection or in utero from antibodies that pass from the mother to the fetus through the placenta, or acquired by the newborn by ingesting the mother's milk.

immunization [L. *immunitas*, immunity]. The process of creating immunity to a specific disease in an individual. SEE: *vaccination; vaccine*.

immunoassay (ĭm″ū-nō-ăs′sā) [L. *immunis*, safe, + O. Fr. *assai*, trial]. Measuring the protein and protein-bound molecules that are concerned with the reaction of an antigen with its specific antibody. SEE: *immunoelectrophoresis; immunofluorescence; radioimmunoassay*.

immunobiologics. A general term for antigenic substances such as vaccines and toxoids, and antibody-containing preparations including globulins and antitoxins from human or animal donors. These products are used to produce active or passive immunization or therapy. Examples are vaccines; toxoids; immune globulins; specific immune globulins, e.g., hepatitis immune globulin (HBIG), rabies immune globulin, varicella-zoster immune globulin, and tetanus immune globulin; and antitoxins.

immunobiology (ĭm″ū-nō-bī-ŏl′ō-jē) [″ + Gr. *bios*, life, + *logos*, word, reason]. Study of immune phenomena in biological systems, including the immune response to infectious diseases, transplantation of organs, allergy, autoimmunity, and cancer.

immunochemistry (ĭm″ū-nō-kĕm′ĭs-trē) [″ + Gr. *chemeia*, chemistry]. The chemistry of immunization. The chemistry of antigens, antibodies, and their relation to each other.

immunochemotherapy (ĭm″ū-nō-kē′mō-thĕr″ă-pē) [″ + ″ + *therapeia*, treatment]. Alteration of the immune response or mechanisms by use of drugs. The goal of such therapy is to enhance or depress the immune response. May be used as part of the therapeutic regimen in treating certain types of malignancies.

immunocompetence (ĭm″ū-nō-kŏm′pĕ-tĕns). The ability of the body's immune system to respond to pathogenic organisms and tissue damage. This ability may be diminished by drugs specifically developed to inhibit immune cell function (e.g., chemotherapeutic agents used to treat leukemia and drugs used to prevent organ transplant rejections), by diseases that attack elements of the immune system, or by overwhelming infections. SEE: *immunocompromised.*

immunocompromised. Having an immune system incapable of reacting to pathogens or tissue damage. This may be due to a genetic disorder, disease process, or drugs such as corticosteroids or immunosuppressive agents given to treat a disorder that inhibits immune function. SYN: *immunodeficient.* SEE: *AIDS; compromised host; immunocompetence.*

immunoconglutinin (ĭm″ū-nō-kŏn-gloo′tĭ-nĭn) [″ + *conglutinare*, to glue together]. Autoantibody against certain fixed complement components of an antigen-antibody complex.

immunocytoadherence. A laboratory test used to identify antibody-bearing cells by the formation of rosettes composed of red blood cells and those cells bearing antibodies.

immunodeficiency (ĭm″ū-nō-dĕ-fĭsh′ĕn-sē). Decreased or compromised ability to respond to antigenic stimuli by appropriate cellular immunity reaction. This state may be secondary to loss of immunoglobulins or an abnormality of B or T cell lymphocytes.

SEE: *AIDS; immunocompetence.*

immunodeficiency disease, severe combined. ABBR: SCID. A rare genetic disorder in which there is partial or complete dysfunction of the immune system. To prevent lethal infectious diseases from developing in the children afflicted with SCID, they are kept in a protected environment. Thus, they have been called "bubble babies." In about one third of the cases, a deficiency of the enzyme adenosine deaminase is the cause. Those patients may be treated parenterally with enzyme replacement therapy provided by the drug pegademase bovine. The treatment must be continued for life. SEE: *adenosine deaminase conjugated with polyethylene glycol.*

immunodeficient. The lack of an adequate immune system capable of controlling invading pathogenic organisms. SYN: *immunocompromised.* SEE: *immunocompetence.*

immunodiagnosis (ĭm″ū-nō-dī″ăg-nō′sĭs). Use of specific immune responses in diagnosing medical conditions.

immunodiffusion (ĭm″ū-nō-dĭ-fū′zhŭn). A test method in which an antigen and antibody are placed in a gel where they diffuse toward each other. When they meet, a precipitate is formed.

immunoelectrophoresis (ĭ-mū″nō-ē-lĕk″trō-fō-rē′sĭs). A method of investigating the amount and character of proteins and antibodies in body fluids by using electrophoresis.

immunofluorescence (ĭm″ū-nō-floo″ō-rĕs′ĕns). The use of fluorescein-stained or fluorescein-labeled antibodies to locate antigen in tissues. The antibodies combine with the specific antigen for that antibody. Evidence of the presence of the antigen then can be determined by examining the preparation with a microscope equipped with a fluorescent light. The typical fluorescent light reaction will be present if the antigen is in the preparation.

immunofluorescent method. Detection of antibodies by using special proteins labeled with fluorescein. If the specific organism or antibody that is being searched for is present, it is observed as a fluorescent material when examined microscopically while illuminated with a fluorescent light source.

immunogen (ĭ-mū-nō-jĕn) [″ + Gr. *gennan*, to produce]. A substance capable of producing an immune response. Proteins and polysaccharides may be strong immunogens, but lipids and nucleic acids may also be immunogenic. SEE: *antigen.*

immunogenetics (ĭm″ū-nō-jĕ-nĕt′ĭks) [″ + Gr. *gennan*, to produce]. The study of genetics by use of immune responses. Included would be investigations of immunoglobulins and histocompatibility antigens.

immunogenic (ĭm″ū-nō-jĕn′ĭk). Capable of inducing an immune response. This response depends on the properties of both the immunogen and the host. It is essential that the host recognize that the immunogen is foreign, i.e., nonself.

immunogenicity (ĭm″ū-nō-jĕ-nĭs′ĭ-tē). The capacity to induce a detectable immune response.

immunoglobulin (ĭm″ū-nō-glŏb′ū-lĭn). ABBR: Ig. One of a family of closely related though not identical proteins capable of acting as antibodies. All antibodies are immunoglobulins, but researchers have not yet determined if all immunoglobulins have antibody functions.

i. A. ABBR: IgA. The principal immunoglobulin in exocrine secretions such as milk, respiratory and intestinal mucin, saliva, and tears. This is probably important in protecting mucosal surfaces from invasion by pathogenic bacteria and viruses. Its presence in colostrum, q.v., helps to protect the suckling newborn from infection.

i. D. ABBR: IgD. USP. Previously used name: Rh₀(D) immune globulin. Immune globulin prepared from the plasma of persons with a high concentration of Rh antibodies. Administration of the gamma globulin to an Rh-negative mother within 72 hours after delivery of an Rh-positive infant usually prevents isoimmunization and thus prevents hemolytic disease of the newborn in subsequent pregnancies. The dose must be repeated after each delivery. It is also given on the same schedule after an Rh-negative mother has an abortion and the fetus is Rh positive. Trade names are Gamulin Rh, Hydro-D, and RhoGAM. SEE: *erythroblastosis fetalis.*

i. E. ABBR: IgE. An immunoglobulin which attaches to mast cells in the respiratory and intestinal tracts and plays a major role in allergic reactions. About 50% of patients with allergic diseases have increased IgE levels. IgE is also important in the formation of reagin, a type of immunoglobulin gamma E (IgGE), found in the blood of individuals with an atopic hypersensitivity.

i. G. ABBR: IgG. The principal immunoglobulin in human serum. Because it moves across the placental barrier, IgG is important in producing immunity in the infant prior to birth. It is the major antibody for antitoxins, viruses, and bacteria. It also activates complement and serves as an opsonin, q.v. As gamma globulin, IgG may be given to provide temporary resistance to hepatitis or other diseases.

i. M. ABBR: IgM. A globulin formed in almost every immune response during the early period of the reaction. IgM controls the A, B, O blood group antibody responses and is the most efficient antibody in stimulating complement activity, q.v. Its size prevents its moving across the placenta to the fetus.

immunohematology (ĭ-mū-nō-hēm″ă-tŏl′ō-jē) [L. *immunis,* safe, + Gr. *haima,* blood, + *logos,* word, reason]. Study of blood diseases including certain autoimmune diseases by use of immunological techniques.

immunoincompetent. Inability to produce an immune response. SEE: *immunodeficiency.*

immunologic (ĭm″ū-nō-lŏj′ĭk) [″ + Gr. *logos,* word, reason]. Pert. to immunology.

immunologic diseases. Those diseases caused by the action of antibodies, as in allergic hypersensitiveness to antigens or to specific reactivity of the tissues. SEE: *anaphylaxis; serum sickness.*

immunologist (ĭm″ū-nŏl′ō-jĭst). An individual whose special training and experience is in immunology.

immunology (ĭm″ū-nŏl′ō-jē) [″ + Gr. *logos,* word, reason]. Study of immunity to diseases. SEE: *serology; serum; toxin; vaccination.*

immunomagnetic technique. Use of magnetic microspheres, q.v., in treating bone marrow in order to purge malignant cells. This technique is experimental. SEE: *bone marrow transplant, autologous.*

immunomodulation. Term used for the effects of various chemical mediators, hormones, and drugs on the immune system. SYN: *immunoregulation.*

immunopathology (ĭm″ū-nō-pă-thŏl′ō-jē). Study of tissue alterations that result from immune or allergic reactions.

immunoprecipitation (ĭm″ū-nō-prē-sĭp″ĭ-tā′shŭn). Formation of a precipitate when an antigen and antibody interact.

immunoproliferative (ĭm″ū-nō-prō-lĭf′ĕr-ă-tĭv). Proliferation of cells and tissues involved in producing antigens.

immunoprotein (ĭm″ū-nō-prō′tē-ĭn) [″ + Gr. *protos,* first]. Any protein or substance that confers immunity.

immunoreactant (ĭ-mū″nō-rē-ăk′tănt). Any one of the substances involved in immunologic reactions. Included are immunoglobulins, complement components, and specific antigens.

immunoreaction (ĭ-mū″nō-rē-āk′shŭn). Reaction of an antibody to an antigen.

immunoselection (ĭm″ū-nō-sē-lĕk′shŭn). Selective survival of cell lives due to their having the least amount of cell surface antigenicity. This aspect allows those cells to escape the destructive activity of either antibodies or immune lymphoid cells.

immunostimulant (ĭm″ū-nō-stĭm′ū-lănt). An agent that will cause antibody formation.

immunosuppression (ĭm″ū-nō-sŭ-prĕsh′ŭn). Prevention of formation of immune response.

immunosuppressive (ĭm″ū-nō-sŭ-prĕs′ĭv). Acting to suppress the body's natural immune response to an antigen.

immunosuppressive agent. A substance that suppresses or interferes with normal immune response. These are used in controlling autoimmune diseases and in enhancing the chances for survival of foreign tissue grafts and transplants. A wide variety of drugs are used as immunosuppressive agents.

immunosurgery (ĭ-mū″nō-sĕr′jĕr-ē). The use of specific antigenic substances in surgical therapy.

immunosurveillance (ĭm″ū-nō-sĕr-vā′lĕns). The immune system's recognition and destruction of newly developed abnormal cells that arise from mutations of cell lines. This would occur in cancer cells that contained new antigens.

immunotherapy (ĭm″ū-nō-thĕr′ă-pē) [″ + Gr. *therapeia*, treatment]. The production or enhancement of immunity.

immunotoxin (ĭm″ū-nō-tŏk′sĭn) [″ + Gr. *toxikon*, poison]. Toxic agents can be attached to antibody molecules and they may be used because of this enhanced toxicity to combat tumor cells. This technique has been used to eliminate malignant tumors in the bone marrow.

immunotransfusion (ĭ-mū″nō-trăns-fū′zhŭn) [″ + *trans*, across, + *fusus*, poured]. Transfusion of blood that contains known antibodies.

Imodium. Trade name for loperamide hydrochloride. An antiperistaltic drug used in treating diarrhea. SEE: *diarrhea, travelers'*.

impacted [L. *impactus*, pressed on]. Pressed firmly together so as to be immovable. Term may be applied to any of the following: a fracture in which ends of bones are wedged together; a tooth so placed in the jaw bone that eruption is impossible; a fetus wedged in the birth canal; cerumen; calculi; or accumulation of feces in the rectum.

impaction (ĭm-păk′shŭn) [L. *impactio*, a pressing together]. Condition of being tightly wedged into a part, as eruption of a tooth blocked by other teeth; overloading of an organ, as the feces in the bowels.

impairment. Any loss or abnormality of psychological, physiological, or anatomical structure or function.

impaled object. A foreign body that penetrates the skin and remains imbedded in body tissue. Such objects should not be removed outside of the operating room because hemorrhage may occur from vessels that were damaged in such a way that the foreign body, while in place, prevents hemorrhage. Instead, impaled objects should be stabilized to prevent movement, and allowed to remain in place while the patient is transported to the hospital.

impalpable (ĭm-păl′pă-bl) [L. *in-*, not, + *palpare*, to touch]. Felt with difficulty if at all; hardly perceptible to the touch.

impar (ĭm′păr) [L., unequal]. Unpaired. SYN: *azygous*.

imparidigitate (ĭm-păr″ĭ-dĭj′ĭ-tāt) [″ + *digitus*, finger]. Having an uneven number of fingers or toes.

impatent (ĭm-pă′tĕnt) [″ + *patere*, to be open]. Closed; not patent.

impedance (ĭm-pē′dăns) [L. *impedire*, to hinder]. Resistance met by alternating currents in passing through a conductor; consists of resistance, reactance, inductance, or capacitance. The resistance due to the inductive and condenser characteristics of a circuit is called reactance.

  i., acoustic. Resistance to the transmission of sound waves.

imperative [L. *imperativus*, commanding]. Obligatory; not controlled by the will; involuntary.

imperception [L. *in-*, not, + *percipere*, to perceive]. Inability to form a mental picture; lack of perception.

imperforate (ĭm-pĕr′fō-rāt) [″ + *per*, through, + *forare*, to bore]. Without an opening.

imperforate hymen. A hymen without an opening. Menstruation occurs, but the blood cannot escape from the vagina because of the obstruction of the hymen. The treatment is surgical incision of the hymen. SEE: *hymen*.

imperforation [L. *imperforatus*, not open]. State of being closed or occluded. SYN: *atresia*.

imperious acts. Tics and motions not under control of the will. SEE: *impulsion*.

impermeable [L. *in-*, not, + *permeare*, to pass through]. Not allowing passage, as of fluids; impenetrable.

impervious [L. *impervius*]. Unable to be penetrated.

impetiginous (ĭm″pĕ-tĭj′ĭ-nŭs) [L. *impetiginosus*]. Rel. to impetigo.

impetigo (ĭm-pĕ-tī′gō, -tē′gō) [L.]. Inflammatory skin disease marked by isolated pustules, which become crusted and rupture. Occurs principally around the mouth and nostrils. Usually caused by either staphylococcal, streptococcal, or a combined infection. SEE: *Nursing Diagnoses* in *Appendix*.

i. **contagiosa.** A contagious form of impetigo. Children are esp. susceptible.

SYM: Discrete, thin-walled vesicles and bullae, which become pustular and thin-crusted appearing in crops. They may be flat and umbilicated with no tendency to rupture, and they are filled with a straw-colored fluid. They dry up as thin yellow crusts.

ETIOL: Streptococci or staphylococci.

TREAT: Appropriate systemic antibiotic. Either cephalexin or a β-lactamase resistant penicillin is the drug of choice. Crusts can be removed by applying room-temperature aqueous soaks.

NURSING IMPLICATIONS: Care is given by the nurse in a hospital or by a parent at home. Note the appearance and location of the lesions. The patient is placed in a single room, and isolation procedures are followed. If the patient is a child, apply mittens or cut the fingernails short to prevent the child from injuring the area by scratching. The child is held, comforted, and encouraged to play and to become involved in diversional activities. Administer medications as prescribed to relieve itching. Keep lesions clean and dry. The child will be allowed to return to school when all lesions have healed. Teach parents about good hygiene and wound care, importance of early diagnosis, and treatment for any purulent eruption to limit spread to others.

i. **herpetiformis.** A rare pustular eruption of unknown etiology that occurs esp. during pregnancy and in association with hypocalcemia.

implant [L. *in-*, into, + *plantare*, to plant]. 1. (im-plănt′) To transfer a part, to graft, to insert. Opposite of explant. 2. (ĭm′plănt) That which is implanted, such as a piece of tissue, a tooth, a pellet of medicine, or a tube or needle containing a radioactive substance. Also included are liquid and solid plastic materials used to augment tissues or to fill in areas traumatically or surgically removed. Artificial joints are another example of an implant. SEE: *mammaplasty, augmentation.*

i., **brain.** SEE: *brain implant.*

i., **dental.** A prosthetic device placed in the jaw to which a tooth or denture may be anchored. Endosseous, subperiosteal, or mucosal or endodontic implants are those most frequently used.

i., **radioactive.** A radioactive source that is placed in a body part to increase the radiation effect on a tumor. SEE: *brachytherapy.*

i., **tooth.** Placement of artificial teeth directly into the jawbone or into a frame attached to the jawbone. In some cases, an implant is used to stabilize a loose tooth. This is done by placing an implant through the natural tooth into the jaw. Subperiosteal implants rest on the jawbone, and the gingival tissue grows over the framework; and artificial teeth are attached to the framework. SEE: *implantation; reimplantation.*

implantation (ĭm″plăn-tā′shŭn) [″ + *plantare*, to plant]. 1. Grafting of tissue or insertion of an organ such as tooth, skin or tendon into a new location in the body. 2. Artificial placement of a substance or material into the blood or the uterine canal. 3. Embedding of the developing blastocyst in the uterine mucosa six or seven days following fertilization.

i., **hypodermic.** Introduction of an implant under the skin. Usually a solid substance placed by forcing a small amount out of a hypodermic needle.

i., **teratic.** Union of an abnormal fetus with a nearly normal fetus.

implosion. A violent collapse inward.

implosion flooding. A method of treating fear due to a phobia by exposing the person to the worst possible phobic situation. The fear is experienced at maximum intensity for up to an hour until the patient is no longer capable of experiencing further fear. The phobic situation is imagined in the first sessions and later produced in reality. SEE: *phobic desensitization.*

imponderable [L. *in-*, not, + *pondus*, weight]. Incapable of being weighed or measured.

impostors, medical. Persons who practice medicine without a license and who have not previously been graduated from an accredited medical school.

impotence, impotency [″ + *potentia*, power]. Weakness, esp. inability of the male to achieve or maintain erection. Having attained a certain age in the adult has no etiologic influence on sexual potency. The etiology of impotence with respect to attributing the cause to physical conditions or psychiatric disorders may be tested in the male by measuring nocturnal penile tumescence (NPT). This involves monitoring frequency and intensity of erections that normally accompany rapid eye movement sleep. There is no appreciable decline in those with psychogenic impotence. SYN: *erectile impotence.*

TREAT: Specific therapy for those conditions that can be treated. Particularly useful in patients with vascular insufficiency, neurologic impairment, and possible in patients with psychogenic impotence is intracavernosal injection of vasoactive drugs such as papaverine, phentolamine, or prostaglandin E. These drugs may be injected by the patient. Self-injection is not appropriate in patients with poor manual dexterity, poor visual acuity, or morbid obesity. SEE: *penile prosthesis; sexual dysfunction.*

i., anatomic. Impotence caused by a defect in the genitalia.

i., atonic. Impotence resulting from paralysis of nervi erigentes.

i., functional. Impotence not due to an organic or anatomical defect; usually of psychogenic origin. The individual may experience impotence with one or more sexual partners, but not others.

i., neurogenic. Impotence due to central nervous system lesions, paraplegia, or diabetic neuropathy.

i., pharmacologic. Impotence due to the side effects of certain drugs and medications, e.g., alcohol, cytotoxic agents, barbiturates, beta blockers, marijuana, cimetidine, clonidine, guanethidine, immunosuppressives, lithium, opiates, phenothiazine, some antihypertensive agents, some diuretics, antidepressants, and anticholinergics.

i., psychic. Impotence due to mental disturbance.

i., vasculogenic. Impotence due to inadequate supply of arterial blood to the corpora cavernosa.

impotent (im'pō-tĕnt). 1. Unable to copulate. 2. Sterile; barren.

impotentia (im"pō-tĕn'shē-ā) [L.]. Impotence, q.v.

impregnate (im-prĕg'nāt) [L. *impregnare*, to make pregnant]. 1. To render pregnant. To fertilize an ovum. 2. To saturate.

impregnated. 1. Rendered pregnant 2. Saturated.

impregnated carbon. Electrode having a carbon shell with core of various metals or salts of metals for use in a carbon arc lamp.

impregnation (im"prĕg-nā'shŭn) [L. *impregnare*, to make pregnant]. 1. Fertilization of an ovum. SYN: *fecundation.* 2. Saturation.

i., artificial. Artificial implantation of semen in the female reproductive tract. SYN: *artificial insemination.*

impressio (im-prĕs'sē-ō) [L. impression] (pl. *impressiones*). [NA] A mark, as of one part upon another.

i. cardiaca hepatis. [NA] Impression on surface of the liver corresponding to the position of the heart.

i. colica. [NA] Depression the undersurface of the right lobe of the liver where it contacts the colon.

i. duodenalis. [NA] Depression on the undersurface of the liver beside the gallbladder indicating position of the duodenum.

i. gastrica. [NA] Hollow under the left

lobe of the liver indicating position of the stomach.

i. renalis. [NA] Hollow on the undersurface of the right lobe of the liver adjacent to the right kidney.

impression [L. *impressio*]. 1. A hollow or depression in a surface. 2. Effect produced upon the mind by external stimuli. 3. The imprint of all or part of the dental arch, individual teeth, or cavity preparations, using appropriate dental materials, for the purpose of records or restorative procedures.

i., complete dental. A negative impression of the entire edentulous area, e.g., the area that originally provided the base for the normal teeth.

i., digitate. Impression on inner surface of frontal bone for convolutions of the cerebrum.

i., final. Impression that is used for making the master cast for a dental prosthesis.

i., partial dental. A negative impression of part of the area that previously provided the base for the missing teeth.

impressiones digitatae. [NA] Depressions on the inner cranial surface.

impression materials. A variety of materials appropriate for different dental procedures, including special waxes, plaster of paris modeling compounds, rubber, zinc oxide paste, reversible colloids, and alginate materials.

impression tray. A receptacle or device used to carry the impression material to the mouth and to hold it in apposition to the tissues being recorded.

imprinting. A special type of learned response that occurs in some animals at a critical period in their development.

Ex.: goslings mothered by a hen may adopt the hen as if she were their mother.

impulse (im'pŭls) [L. *impulsus*]. 1. Act of driving onward with sudden force. SEE: *conation.* 2. An incitement of the mind, prompting an unpremeditated act. 3. In physiology, a change transmitted through certain tissues, esp. nerve fibers and muscles, resulting in physiological activity or inhibition.

i., cardiac. 1. The heartbeat felt at the left side of the chest over the apex of the heart. This is a physical impulse. 2. Impulse transmitted over conducting pathway of the heart and responsible for the contraction of the muscular tissue of the heart. This is an electrical impulse. SEE: *heart.*

i., ectopic. A cardiac impulse arising in some part of the heart other than the sinoatrial node.

i., enteroceptive. An afferent nerve impulse arising from stimuli originating in receptors located in internal organs.

i., excitatory. Impulse that stimulates activity.

i., exteroceptive. An afferent nerve impulse arising from stimuli originating in sense organs located on the body surface.

i., inhibitory. Impulse that lessens activity.

i., nervous. A self-propagated excitatory state transmitted along a nerve fiber. It is the result of physicochemical changes occurring in the membrane of the nerve fiber. The impulse on reaching the termination of the fiber may induce an impulse in another nerve cell, induce activity in a tissue such as in muscles (contraction) or in glands (secretion), or give rise to a sensation in the higher nervous centers.

i., proprioceptive. An afferent nerve impulse arising from stimuli originating in joints, muscles, or tendons, or other sensory endings that respond to pressure or stretch.

impulsion. Idea to do something or commit some act or crime suddenly imposed upon the subject that tortures him or her until the act is accomplished. Clear consciousness of the proposed act followed by an agonizing struggle, defeat, and sense of relief following the act are characteristics of impulsions, obsessions, and inhibitions. Impulsions may include folie du doute or doubting mania (e.g., repeatedly checking to determine whether something has been done); obsessive fears of contact or delirium of touch; agoraphobia; dipsomania; pyromania; kleptomania; homicidal or suicidal impulsion; onomatomania; arithmomania; exhibitionism.

IMV. *intermittent mandatory ventilation; intermittent mechanical ventilation.*

In. Chem. symb. for the element indium.

in-. 1. [L. *in*, into]. Prefix indicating in, inside, within; and also intensive action. 2. [L. *in-*, not]. Negative prefix.

inaction (ĭn-ăk'shŭn) [L. *in-*, not, + *actio*, act]. Failure of or decreased response to a stimulus.

inactivate [″ + *activus*, acting]. To make inactive, esp. the alteration or destruction of an enzyme system or a biologically active agent such as a microorganism or antigen.

inactivation. Rendering anything inert by using heat or other means.

inactivation of complement. Loss of activity caused by heating serum to about 55°C (131°F) for one-half hour.

inadequacy (ĭn-ăd'ē-kwă-sē) [″ + *adaequare*, to be equal]. Insufficiency; incompetence.

inane. Insignificant or silly.

inanimate [″ + *animatus*, alive]. 1. Not alive; not animate. 2. Dull, lifeless.

inanition (ĭn″ă-nĭsh'ŭn) [L. *inanis*, empty]. A debilitated condition due to lack of sufficient food material essential to the body, such as in starvation or malabsorption syndrome.

ETIOL: May be due to causes other than the food supply, such as malabsorption, or other disease of the gastrointestinal system that prevents absorption of food.

inapparent. Not noticeable, esp. a disease process that does not alert the patient or the physician to the presence of a disease.

inappetence (ĭn-ăp'ē-tĕns) [″ + *appetere*, to long for]. Lack of craving or desire, esp. for food.

Inapsine. Trade name for droperidol.

inarticulate [″ + *articulus*, joined]. 1. Not jointed; without joints. 2. Unable to pronounce distinct syllables or express oneself intelligibly. 3. Not given to expressing oneself verbally.

in articulo mortis (ĭn ăr-tĭk'ū-lō mor'tĭs) [L.]. At the very moment of death.

inassimilable (ĭn″ă-sĭm'ĭ-lă-bl) [″ + *assimilis*, to make similar]. Not capable of being utilized by the body for nutrition.

inattention. Not paying attention; negligence.

inborn. 1. Innate or inherent, said of characteristics both structural and functional that are inherited or developed during intrauterine development. 2. Inherited, as in inborn error of metabolism.

inbreeding [″ + AS. *bredan*, to cherish]. Mating of individuals that are closely related.

incandescent [L. *incandescere*, to glow]. Glowing with light; white hot.

incapacitate. Being made incapable of some function, act or strength. This may be purely physical or intellectual or both.

incaparina. A mixture of cereal grains and oilseed meals of a given range of protein and quality fortified with vitamins and minerals. Developed at INCAP (Institute of Nutrition of Central America and Panama). Distributed in Latin American countries for feeding young children in order to prevent kwashiorkor, q.v., and other forms of malnutrition.

incarcerated [L. *incarcerare*]. Imprisoned, confined, constricted, as an irreducible hernia.

incarceration. 1. Legal confinement. 2. Imprisonment of a part; constriction as in a hernia.

incarial bone (ĭn-kā'rē-ăl). Os incae; interparietal bone.

incarnatio (ĭn″kăr-nā'shē-ō). 1. To grow in. 2. The process of being converted to flesh.

i. unguis. The ingrowing of a toenail or fingernail.

incasement. Becoming surrounded by a

structure or wall.

incentive spirometry. Spirometry, q.v., in which visual and vocal stimuli are given to the subject in an attempt to stimulate the maximum effort in performing the test.

inception [L. *inceptio*, taking in, beginning]. 1. The beginning of anything. 2. Ingestion. 3. Intussusception.

incest (ĭn′sĕst) [L. *incestus*, unchaste, incest]. Coitus between close blood relatives.

incidence [L. *incidens*, falling upon]. 1. The frequency of occurrence of any event or condition over a period of time and in relation to the population in which it occurs, as incidence of a disease. SEE: *prevalence*. 2. The falling or impinging upon, touching, or affecting in some way.

incident. 1. A happening, event, or occurrence. 2. Falling or striking, as a ray of light.

incineration (ĭn-sĭn″ĕr-ā′shŭn) [L. *in*, into, + *cineres*, ashes]. Destruction by fire. SYN: *cremation*.

incipient (ĭn-sĭp′ē-ĕnt) [L. *incipere*, to begin]. Beginning; coming into existence.

incisal (ĭn-sī′zăl). Cutting.

incise (ĭn-sīz′) [L. *incisus*]. To cut, as with a sharp instrument.

incised (ĭn-sīzd′). Cut with a knife.

incision (ĭn-sĭzh′ŭn) [L. *incisio*]. A cut made with a knife, esp. for surgical purposes.

incisive (ĭn-sī′sĭv) [L. *incisivus*]. 1. Cutting; having the power of cutting. 2. Rel. to the incisor teeth.

incisive bone. An obsolete term for the part of the maxilla that supports the incisor teeth and was derived from the median nasal process embryologically; commonly called the premaxilla.

incisor (ĭn-sī′zor) [L., a cutter]. 1. That which cuts. 2. That which applies to the incisor teeth. 3. One of the cutting teeth. The four front teeth in each jaw of the adult. SEE: *dentition*.

   i.'s, central. The two upper and lower incisors adjacent to the midsagittal plane.

   i., prostatic. Surgical knife for incision of an enlarged prostate.

incisura (ĭn-sī-sū′ră) [L.](pl. *incisurae*). 1. An incision. 2. [NA] Incisure; notch; emargination; indentation at the edge of any structure.

   i. angularis gastrica. A fold or notch on the distal end of the lesser curvature of the stomach.

incisure (ĭn-sīz′ūr) [L. *incisura*, a cutting into]. A notch or slit.

   i. of Rivinus. Tympanic incisure.

   i.'s of Schmidt-Lanterman. Oblique lines on medullated nerve fiber sheaths.

incitant (ĭn-sīt′ănt) [L. *incitare*, to set in motion]. The stimulus that sets off a reaction, disease, or incident.

inclination [L. *inclinere*, to slope]. Leaning from the normal, or from the vertical, as a tooth, or the pelvis.

inclinometer (ĭn″klĭ-nŏm′ĕ-ter) [″ + Gr. *metron*, measure]. Device for measuring ocular diameter from vertical and horizontal lines.

inclusion [L. *inclusus*, enclosed]. Being enclosed or included.

   i., cell. Lifeless, temporary constituent of the protoplasm of a cell. SEE: *cell.*

   i., dental. A tooth unable to erupt because of excessive surrounding tissue. SEE: *impacted tooth.*

   i., fetal. Malformed twins in which one, the parasite, is completely enclosed within its host, the autosite. SEE: *teratoma.*

inclusion blennorrhea. Inclusion conjunctivitis, q.v., of the newborn.

inclusion bodies. Bodies present in the nucleus of cytoplasm of certain cells in cases of infection by filtrable viruses. SEE: *Negri bodies.*

inclusion conjunctivitis. Inflammation of the conjunctiva of the eye due to the organism *Chlamydia trachomatis.* SEE: *ophthalmia neonatorum.*

incoagulability (ĭn″kō-ăg″ū-lă-bĭl′ĭ-tē) [L. *in-*, not, + *coagulare*, to congeal]. Not coagulable.

incoercible (ĭn″kō-ĕr′sĭ-bl) [L. *in-*, not, + *coercere*, to restrain]. Uncontrollable; not able to be held in check.

incoherence (ĭn″kō-hēr′ĕns) [″ + *cohairens*, adhering]. Inability to express oneself coherently or to present ideas in a related order.

incoherent (ĭn″kō-hē′rĕnt). Not coherent or understandable.

incombustible [″ + *combustus*, burned]. Incapable of being burned.

incompatibility [L. *incompatibilis*]. 1. The quality of not being suitable for mixture. Can be applied to a state that renders admixture of medicines unsuitable through chemical action or interaction, insolubility, formation of poisonous or explosive compounds, difference in solubility, or antagonistic action. The quality of not being mixed without chemical changes, or without countering the action of other ingredients in a compound. 2. Condition of not being in harmony with one's surroundings or associates, esp. a spouse or friend.

   i., physiological. A condition in which one or more substances in a mixture have a physiological action antagonistic to that of one of the other compounds.

incompatible. 1. Not capable of uniting. 2. Antagonistic in action, said of some drugs. 3. Not being in harmony with one's environment, situation, or associates, esp. a spouse or friend.

incompetence, incompetency [L. *in-*, not, + *competere*, to be suitable]. Inadequate ability to perform the function or action normal to an organ or part.

  i., aortic. Regurgitation of blood through the aortic valves.

  i., ileocecal. Inability of ileocecal valve to stop the return of the material from the colon to the ileum.

  i., mental. Mental inability to retain charge of one's self or possessions.

  i., muscular. Imperfect closure of the cardiac valve due to weak action of papillary muscles.

  i., pyloric. Weakness of pylorus, which permits undigested food to leave the stomach and enter the duodenum.

  i., relative. Excessive dilatation of a cardiac cavity, which makes perfect closure of the cardiac valves leading in and out of the chamber impossible.

  i., valvular. Leaky condition of one or more cardiac valves permitting regurgitation of blood at the time the valves should be completely closed.

incompetent. 1. One legally unable to execute a contract, such as a brain-damaged individual, or one with marked mental retardation or insanity. 2. The inability to perform necessary activities and tasks expected of one's life roles.

incompetent palatal syndrome. Incomplete or ineffective separation by the soft palate of the nasopharynx from the oropharynx, characterized by hypernasality and distortion of speech called whinolalia.

  ETIOL: May be due to congenital or acquired defects of the palate or to psychiatric disorders.

incompressible [" + *compressus*, pressed together]. Compact; not compressible.

incontinence [" + *continere*, to stop]. 1. Inability to retain urine, semen, or feces, through loss of sphincter control or because of cerebral or spinal lesions. 2. Absence of restraint with respect to sexual activity. SEE: *bladder drill; continence.*

  TREAT: The specific therapy needed for urinary incontinence will depend upon the cause. Symptomatic management of urinary incontinence is facilitated by use of one of several different types of leakproof underpants, panty liners, or a variety of collection devices.

  i., active. Discharge of feces and urine in the normal way at regulated intervals but involuntarily.

  i., anal. Failure of the anal sphincter to prevent involuntary expulsion of gas, liquid, or solids from the lower bowel.

  i., giggle. The occurrence of involuntary uncontrollable passage of urine induced by laughter. Laughter triggers full-scale micturition that cannot be stopped, often until the bladder is empty, even if the laughter stops. It starts at about five to seven years and tends to improve or disappear with increasing age. This condition, which may be due to a central nervous system disease, is distinct from urinary stress incontinence. SEE: *i., urinary stress.*

  i., intermittent. Loss of control of the bladder upon sudden pressure or movement, because of interruption of the voluntary path above the lumbar center.

  i. of milk. Excessive milk flow. SYN: *galactorrhea.*

  i. of urine. Absence of voluntary control of urination. Sphincter muscle always relaxed. SEE: *enuresis.*

  i., overflow. Incontinence characterized by small frequent voidings due to overfilling of the bladder or a bladder with pathologically decreased volume.

  i., paralytic. Constant voiding of small amount of urine and feces due to defective nervous control of sphincters.

  i., passive. Urinary incontinence of a form in which there is a full bladder that doesn't empty normally but urine drips away upon pressure.

  i., urinary stress. Inability to prevent escape of small amounts of urine during stress such as laughing, coughing, sneezing, lifting, or sudden movement. Occurs frequently enough in young women to be classed as normal. Nevertheless, it should be investigated to be certain that it is not caused by a structural abnormality. The urine should be cultured to rule out urinary tract infection. SEE: *bladder drill; i., giggle.*

  NURSING IMPLICATIONS: Teach patient Kegel exercises, q.v., to strengthen pubococcygeal muscles. Encourage patient to practice during urination (stopping and starting urinary stream intermittently) as well as at frequent intervals throughout the day. Instruct patient about importance of keeping vulva clean, dry, and odor free, and about use of commercial barrier products to protect clothing. Encourage patient to continue or resume usual activities while using protective barriers, avoiding social isolation. Evaluate patient's response to exercise regimen periodically.

incoordinate [L. *in-*, not, + *coordinare*, to arrange]. 1. Not able to make coordinated muscular movements. 2. Unable to adjust one's work harmoniously with others.

incoordination (ĭn″kō-or″dĭ-nā′shŭn). Inability to produce harmonious, rhythmic, muscular action that is not due to weakness.

  ETIOL: The condition may be sensory,

due to failure of afferent impulses to be transmitted from muscles, bones, and joints to coordination centers, or it may be motor, due to disturbance in tone or harmony between simultaneously acting muscle groups. SYN: *asynergy*. SEE: *disdiadochokinesia*.

incorporation [L. *in*, into, + *corporare*, to form into a body]. Combining two ingredients to form a homogenous mass.

increase. To grow larger, or to enhance strength.

increment (ĭn′krĕ-mĕnt) [L. *incrementum*]. 1. An increase or addition in number, size, or extent; an enlargement. 2. Something added or gained.

incrustation [L. *in*, on, + *crusta*, crust]. Formation of crusts or scabs.

incubation (ĭn″kū-bā′shŭn) [L. *incubare*, to lie on]. 1. The interval between exposure to infection and the appearance of the first symptom. SYN: *latent period* (def. 2). SEE: table. 2. In bacteriology, the period of culture development. 3. The development of an impregnated ovum. 4. The care of a premature infant in an incubator.

incubator. 1. Enclosed crib, in which the temperature and humidity may be regulated, for care of premature babies. 2. Apparatus for providing suitable atmospheric conditions for culturing bacteria or for maintaining eggs until they hatch.

incubus (ĭn′kū-bŭs) [L. *incubare*, to lie upon]. A nightmare.

incudal (ĭng′kū-dăl) [L. *incus*, anvil]. Rel. to the incus.

incudectomy (ĭng″kū-dĕk′tō-mē) [″ + Gr. *ektome*, excision]. Surgical removal of all or part of the incus of the middle ear.

incudiform (ĭn-kū′dĭ-form) [″ + *forma*, shape]. Like an anvil in shape.

incudomalleal (ĭng″kū-dō-măl′ē-ăl) [″ + *malleus*, a hammer]. Pert. to the incus and malleus and articulation of the anvil and hammer in the tympanum; in the middle ear.

incudostapedial (ĭn″kū-dō-stă-pē′dē-ăl) [″ + *stapes*, a stirrup]. Pert. to the incus and stapes and the articulation between the anvil and stirrup in the tympanum; in the middle ear.

incurable [L. *in-*, not, + *curare*, to care for]. Not capable of being cured.

incurvation (ĭn″kŭr-vā′shŭn) [L. *incurvare*, to bend in]. State of being bent or curved in.

incus (ĭng′kŭs) [L., anvil] (pl. *incudes*). [NA] In the middle ear, the middle of the three ossicles in the tympanum; the anvil. SEE: *ear* for illus.

  *i., **lenticular process of.*** The long process of the incus, a middle ear ossicle. It articulates with the head of the stapes. SYN: *orbiculare*.

incyclophoria (ĭn-sī″klō-for′ē-ă) [L. *in-*, not, + Gr. *kyklos*, circle, + *phoros*, bearing]. Median or negative cyclophoria; the affected eye, when covered, turns inward about its anteroposterior axis.

incyclotropia (ĭn-sī″klō-trō′pē-ă) [″ + ″ + *tropos*, turning]. Cyclotropia in which the eye turns inward toward the nose even when both eyes are open.

in d. L. *in dies*, daily.

indagation (ĭn″dă-gā′shŭn) [L. *indagatus*, searching]. A careful, searching investigation, esp. examination of the genitalia at termination of puerperium.

indecision. Inability to make up one's mind.

indentation [L. *in*, in, + *dens*, tooth]. A depression or hollow.

independent living. Term used by many disabled persons and professionals that emphasizes the rehabilitation goals of active community involvement and assuming responsibility for directing one's own life.

independent living skills. Activities of daily living, q.v.

independent practice associations. ABBR: IPA. A method of arranging for medical care wherein the individual(s) have contracts with office-based practitioners who agree to see patients on a prenegotiated fee schedule.

index (ĭn′dĕks) [L., an indicator] (pl. *indexes* or *indices*). 1. The forefinger. 2. The ratio of the measurement of a given substance with that of a fixed standard.

  *i., **alveolar.*** I., gnathic.

  *i., **cardiac.*** The cardiac output of blood expressed as liters per minute divided by the body surface area expressed in square meters.

  *i., **cephalic.*** Skull breadth multiplied by 100 and divided by its length.

  *i., **cerebral.*** Ratio of greatest transverse to the greatest anteroposterior diameter of the cranium.

  *i., **DMF.*** Index of dental health and caries experience based on the number of DMF teeth or tooth surfaces. D is the number of decayed teeth, M is missing teeth, and F is filled or restored teeth.

  *i., **leukopenic.*** In allergic individuals, a test of sensitivity to foods. A precipitous decrease in white blood cell count in 90 minutes following ingestion of the test food indicates that the food is incompatible with that individual.

  *i., **opsonic.*** Ratio of number of bacteria that are ingested by leukocytes contained in normal serum, compared with the number ingested by leukocytes in the patient's own blood serum.

  *i., **oral hygiene.*** Index based on the presence and amount of debris and calculus on

Incubation and Isolation Periods in Common Infections*

Infection	Incubation Period	Isolation of Patient
AIDS	Serological evidence in several months. Clinical development of signs and symptoms may require years. Approx. half of infected patients will have developed clinical signs and symptoms by 11 years post infection.	Blood and body fluid precautions. Private room if personal hygiene habits are poor.
Brucellosis	Highly variable, usually 5–21 days; may be months	None
Chickenpox	2–3 weeks	1 week after appearance of vesicles
Cholera	A few hours–5 days	Enteric precautions
Common cold	12 hr–3 days	None
Diphtheria	Usually 2–5 days	Until two cultures from nose and throat, taken at least 24 hr apart, are negative; cultures to be taken after cessation of antibiotic therapy
Dysentery, amebic	From a few days to several months, commonly 2–4 weeks	None
Dysentery, bacillary (shigellosis)	1–7 days	As long as stools remain positive
Encephalitis, mosquito-borne	5–15 days	None
Giardiasis	Variable; median 7–10 days	Enteric precautions
Gonorrhea	2–7 days; may be longer	No sexual contact until cured
Hepatitis A	Variable, 15–50 days; mean about 30 days	Enteric precautions until 1 week after onset of jaundice.
Hepatitis B	Variable, usually 45–180 days; mean 60–90 days	Blood and body fluid precautions until antibodies to virus disappear
Hepatitis C	15–64 days	As for hepatitis A
Influenza	1–3 days	As practical
Legionella	2–10 days	None
Malaria	12 days for *Plasmodium falciparum*; 14 days for *P. vivax, P. ovale*; 30 days for *P. malariae*	Protect from mosquitoes
Measles (rubeola)	8–13 days from exposure to onset of fever; 14 days until rash appears	From diagnosis to 7 days after appearance of rash; strict isolation from children under 3 years

* SEE: *Universal Precautions* in *Appendix.*

Incubation and Isolation Periods in Common Infections* (Continued)

Infection	Incubation Period	Isolation of Patient
Meningitis, meningococcal	2–10 days	Until 24 hr after start of chemotherapy
Mononucleosis, infectious	4–6 weeks	None; disinfect articles soiled with nose and throat discharges
Mumps	2–3 weeks	Until the glands recede
Paratyphoid fevers	1–3 weeks for fever; 1–10 days for gastroenteritis	Until 3 stools are negative
Pneumonia, pneumococcal	Believed to be 1–3 days	Until 24 hr after administration of antibiotics
Poliomyelitis	3–35 days	1 week from onset
Puerperal fever, streptococcal	1–3 days	Transfer from maternity ward
Rabies	Usually 2–8 weeks; occasionally only 10 days	Strict for duration of illness; danger to attendants
Rubella (German measles)	16–18 days with range of 23 days	None, but avoid contact with nonimmune pregnant women
Salmonellosis	6–72 hr; usually 12–36 hr	Until stool cultures are salmonella-free on two consecutive specimens collected not less than 24 hr apart
Scabies	2–6 weeks before onset of itching in patients without previous infections; 1–4 days after re-exposed	Excuse patient from school or work until day after treatment
Scarlet fever	1–3 days	7 days; may be terminated in 24 hr
Smallpox	8–17 days	Strict; in screened hospital wards until all scabs have disappeared
Syphilis	10 days–10 weeks; usually 3 weeks	In noncooperative patients, it should be enforced until surface lesions are healed
Tetanus	4 days–3 weeks	None
Toxic shock syndrome	Unknown but may be as brief as several hours	None
Trachoma	5–12 days	Until lesions disappear, but usually not practical
Tuberculosis	4–12 weeks to demonstrable primary lesion or significant tuberculin reactions	Variable, depending on conversion of sputum to negative after specific therapy and on ability of patient to understand and carry out personal hygiene methods

* SEE: Universal Precautions in Appendix.

Incubation and Isolation Periods in Common Infections* *(Continued)*

Infection	Incubation Period	Isolation of Patient
Tularemia	2–10 days	None
Typhoid fever	Usually 1–3 weeks	Until 3 cultures of feces and urine are negative. These should be taken not earlier than 1 month after onset.
Typhus fever	7–14 days	None
Whooping cough	Usually 1 week	For 3 weeks after onset of spasmodic cough

* SEE: *Universal Precautions* in *Appendix.*

six preselected tooth surfaces.

i., pelvic. Ratio of pelvic conjugate and transverse diameters.

i., periodontal (Ramfjord). An extensive consideration of the periodontal status of six teeth by evaluating gingival condition, depth of gingival sulcus or pocket, plaque or calculus, attrition, tooth mobility, and extent of tooth contact.

i., phagocytic. Average of bacteria ingested per leukocyte of blood.

i., refractive. Refraction coefficient.

i., therapeutic. The maximum tolerated dose of a drug divided by the minimum curative dose.

i., thoracic. Ratio of thoracic anteroposterior diameter to transverse diameter.

i., vital. Ratio of the number of births to the number of deaths in a population over a stated period of time.

index case. The initial individual whose condition led to investigation of a hereditary disorder. SEE: *cohort.*

indican (ĭn′dĭ-kăn). 1. Potassium salt of indoxylsulfate, found in sweat and urine, and formed when intestinal bacteria convert tryptophan to indole. 2. In plants, a yellow glycoside, the precursor of the dye indigo.

indicanemia (ĭn″dĭ-kăn-ē′mē-ă) [*indican* + Gr. *haima,* blood]. Indican in the blood.

indicant (ĭn′dĭ-kănt). 1. Something such as a sign or symptom that points to the presence of a disease. 2. Something such as loss of a symptom or sign that indicates that the treatment of the disease is proper and effective.

indicanuria (ĭn″dĭ-kăn-ū′rē-ă) [″ + Gr. *ouron,* urine]. Excess of indoxylsulfate of potassium, a derivative of indole, in urine. It is found in small quantities in normal urine. SYN: *urocyanosis.*

indication [L. *indicare,* to show]. A sign or circumstance that indicates the proper treatment of a disease.

i., causal. Treatment shown by a knowl-

edge of the cause of a disease.

i., symptomatic. Treatment provided because of the symptoms of a disease rather than because of precise knowledge of the actual disease process; e.g., a patient may be given aspirin or antibiotics without knowing the cause of the symptoms of headache or fever.

indicator [L. *indicare,* to show]. In chemical analysis, a substance that can be used to determine pH. In a more general sense, any substance that can be used to determine the completeness of a chemical reaction, as in volumetric analysis. SEE: table.

USES: 1. In titration of ammonia and other weak bases. 2. Topfer's reagent, for determining free acid in gastric juice. 3. In titrating weak acids and for determining combined acid in gastric juice.

indifferent [L. *in-,* not, + *differre,* to differ]. 1. Neutral; tending in no specific direction. 2. Not responsive to normal stimuli; apathetic. 3. Pert. to cells that have not differentiated.

indigenous (ĭn-dĭj′ĕn-ŭs) [L. *indigenus,* born in]. Native to a country or region.

indigestible (ĭn″dĭ-jĕs′tĭ-bl) [L. *in-,* not, + *digerere,* to separate]. Not digestible.

indigestion [″ + *digerere,* to separate]. Incomplete or imperfect digestion, usually accompanied by one or more of the following symptoms: pain, nausea and vomiting, heartburn and acid regurgitation, accumulation of gas and belching. SYN: *dyspepsia.*

indigitation (ĭn-dĭj″ĭ-tā′shŭn) [L. *in,* in, + *digitus,* finger]. Displacement of intestines by intussusception, q.v. SYN: *invagination.*

indigo. A blue dye obtained from plants or made synthetically.

Indigo Carmine. Trade name for indigotindisulfonate, USP.

indigotindisulfonate sodium (ĭn″dĭ-gō″tĭn-dī-sŭl′fō-nāt). USP. A dye used in testing renal function. Trade name is Indigo Carmine.

Colors of Indicators of pH

	Color		
	Toward Acid	Toward Alkali	Range of pH
Methyl yellow	Red	Yellow	2.9–4.0
Congo red	Blue	Red	3.0–5.2
Methyl orange	Red	Yellow	3.1–4.4
Methyl red	Red	Yellow	4.2–6.2
Litmus	Red	Blue	4.5–8.3
Bromcresol purple	Yellow	Purple	5.2–6.8
Bromothymol blue	Yellow	Blue	6.0–7.6
Phenol red	Yellow	Red	6.8–8.4
Phenolphthalein	Colorless	Pink	8.2–10.0

indigouria (ĭn″dĭ-gō-ū′rē-ă) [Gr. *indikon*, Indian dye, + *ouron*, urine]. Indigo in the urine.

indisposition [L. *in-*, not, + *dispositus*, arranged]. Disorder; any slight or temporary illness.

indium (ĭn′dē-ŭm) [L. *indicum*, indigo]. SYMB: In. At. wt. 114.82; at. no. 49; sp. gr. 7.31. A rare metallic element.

indium-111 (¹¹¹In). An isotope of indium which has a half-life of 2.8 days. Used in radioactive tracer studies.

individuation (ĭn″dĭ-vĭd″ū-ā′shŭn). 1. During development, the emergence of specific and individual structures and functions. 2. Process by which a healthy, integrated personality is developed.

Indocin. Trade name for indomethacin.

indocyanine green. USP. A dye used in testing hepatic and renal function. Trade name is Cardio-Green.

indolaceturia (ĭn″dō-lăs″ē-tū′rē-ă) [*indole* + L. *acetum*, vinegar, + Gr. *ouron*, urine]. Excretion of an increased amount of indoleacetic acid in the urine. This occurs in patients with phenylketonuria and may also be increased by eating serotonin-containing foods, e.g., bananas.

indole (ĭn′dōl). C_8H_7N. A solid, crystalline substance found in feces. It is the product of bacterial decomposition of tryptophan and is largely responsible for the odor of feces. In intestinal obstruction it is absorbed and eliminated in the urine in the form of indican, q.v.

indolent (ĭn′dō-lĕnt) [LL. *indolens*, painless]. 1. Indisposed to action. 2. Inactive; not developing; sluggish.

indolent ulcer. Ulcer that is slow to heal but not painful.

indologenous (ĭn″dō-lŏj′ĕn-ŭs) [*indole* + Gr. *gennan*, to produce]. Causing the production of indole.

indoluria (ĭn″dŏl-ū′rē-ă) [″ + Gr. *ouron*, urine]. The presence of indole in urine.

indomethacin (ĭn″dō-mĕth′ă-sĭn). USP. Drug that has anti-inflammatory, analgesic, and antipyretic properties. Primary use is in rheumatoid arthritis, ankylosing spondylitis, and degenerative joint disease when salicylates are ineffective or cannot be tolerated. Because of the high incidence and severity of side effects associated with prolonged administration, its use as a mild antipyretic or analgesic is not recommended. Has also been used in treating attacks of arthritis due to gout and as an antipyretic in Hodgkin's disease when fever fails to respond to other therapy. Indomethacin is also useful in stimulating the closure of patent ductus arteriosus in premature infants who are otherwise healthy. Trade name is Indocin.

indoxyl (ĭn-dŏk′sĭl) [Gr. *indikon*, indigo, + *oxys*, sharp]. C_8H_7NO. An oily substance sometimes found in urine of the apparently healthy, formed from the decomposition of tryptophan by intestinal bacteria.

indoxylemia (ĭn-dŏk″sĭl-ē′mē-ă) [″ + ″ + *haima*, blood]. Indoxyl in the blood.

indoxyluria (ĭn″dŏk-sĭl-ū′rē-ă) [″ + ″ + *ouron*, urine]. Excretion of indoxyl in urine.

induced (ĭn-dūsd′) [L. *inducere*, to lead in]. Produced; caused.

inducer (ĭn-dūs′ĕr). In chemistry, a compound that increases the concentration of another molecule or, in molecular biology, something that facilitates the development of a gene. SEE: *catalyst*.

inductance. That property of an electric circuit by virtue of which a varying current induces an electromotive force in that circuit or a neighboring circuit. The unit of inductance, or self-induction, is the henry.

induction (ĭn-dŭk′shŭn) [L. *inductio*, leading in]. 1. The process of causing or producing, as induction of labor with oxytocic drugs in cases of uterine dysfunction. 2. The generation of electric current in a body by electricity in another body near it. 3. In embryology, the production of a specific morphogenic effect by a chemical substance from one part of the embryo to another. SYN: *evocation*. 4. In anesthesia, the period from the initial inhalation or injection of an anesthetic gas or drug until optimum level of anesthesia is reached.

inductor (ĭn-dŭk'tĕr). 1. Any substance that will cause cells exposed to it to differentiate into an organized tissue. 2. In electronics, a component that employs the principles of electromagnetic induction. It is used in filter circuits and transformers.

inductorium (ĭn″dŭk-tō'rē-ŭm). Device used to produce high-voltage electrical discharges. It is used in physiological investigations.

inductotherm (ĭn-dŭk'tō-thĕrm) [L. *inducere*, to lead in, + Gr. *therme*, heat]. Device for producing pyrexia by electricity.

inductothermy. Treatment of disease by artificial production of fever by electromagnetic induction.

indulin (ĭn'dū-lĭn). Any one of a group of dyes used in histology.

indulinophil(e) (ĭn″dū-lĭn'ō-fĭl, -fīl). The state of being readily stained with indulin.

indurate (ĭn'dū-rāt) [L. *in*, in, + *durus*, hard]. 1. To harden. 2. Hardened.

indurated. Hardened.

induration. 1. The act of hardening. 2. An area of hardened tissue. SEE: *sclerosis; skin*.

i., black. Anthracosis of the lung.

i., brown. Pigmentation and fibrosis of the lung due to chronic venous congestion of the lung.

i., cyanotic. Induration from long continued venous hyperemia, pressure on vessels causing transudation of blood and serum, and formation of a dark, hard mass. In the liver or spleen it leads to absorption of the parenchyma with formation of scar tissue.

i., granular. Fibrosis of an organ such as the liver or kidney in which small fibrotic granules are present.

i., gray. Pneumonia with fibrosis and no pigmentation.

i., red. Chronic interstitial pneumonia with severe congestion.

indurative (ĭn'dŭr-ā″tĭv). Pert. to induration.

indusium (ĭn-dū'zē-ŭm) [L., tunic]. 1. A membranous covering. 2. The amnion.

i. griseum. [NA] A rudimentary gyrus located on the upper surface of the corpus callosum. SYN: *gyrus, supracallosal*.

inebriant (ĭn-ē'brē-ănt) [L. *inebrius*, drunken]. 1. Any intoxicant. 2. Making drunk.

inebriate. To make drunk or to become intoxicated.

inebriation (ĭn-ē″brē-ā'shŭn). State of intoxication. SYN: *drunkenness; intoxication*.

inelastic [L. *in-*, not, + Gr. *elastikos*, elastic]. Not elastic.

inert (ĭn-ērt′) [L. *iners*, unskilled, idle]. 1. Not active; sluggish. 2. In chemistry, having little or no tendency or ability to react with other chemicals.

inertia (ĭn-ēr'shē-ă) [L., inactivity]. 1. In physics, tendency of a body to remain in its state (at rest or in motion) until acted upon by an outside force. 2. Sluggishness; lack of activity.

i., uterine. Absence or weakness of uterine contractions in labor.

in extremis (ĭn ĕks-trē'mĭs) [L.]. At the point of death.

infancy. The very early period of life in which the child is still unable to walk or to feed itself. SEE: *infant*.

infant [L. *infans*]. A liveborn fetus from time of birth through the completion of one year of age. SEE: *neonate*.

i., development of. For three days after birth a baby loses weight; in the next four days, however, a baby should regain the loss and weigh as much as at birth.

Average weekly weight gain in the first three months is 210 gm for boys and 195 gm for girls; from three to six months it is 150 gm for both girls and boys; from six to nine months, 90 gm for boys and 105 gm for girls; from 9 to 18 months 60 gm for both sexes; and from 18 to 24 months 45 gm, both sexes.

The newborn is aware of shadow, movement, and voice. By the fourth week the infant lifts the head momentarily; by the 16th week, holds the head erect, coos, or laughs; walks with hands held by 52nd week; by 15th month, toddles alone and may have a vocabulary of a few words. SEE: *psychomotor and physical development of infant*.

i., post-term. Infant born after beginning of the 42nd week of gestation (longer than 288 days).

i., preterm. Infant born prior to the completion of 37 weeks (259 days) of gestation. SEE: *prematurity*.

i., respiration of. At birth, 40 to 50 per min; first year, 20 to 40; fifth year, 20 to 25; 15th year, 15 to 20. SEE: *pulse; respiration; temperature*.

i., temperature of. Normal (rectal) temperature may have a daily variation of 1° to 1.5°C (1.8° to 2.7°F). It is usually highest between 5 and 8 p.m. and lowest between 3 and 6 a.m. There is therefore no specific normal temperature, but the values given should be regarded as ranging around the value of 37.6°C (99.7°F) when the temperature is taken rectally.

Infants have poorly developed temperature-regulating mechanisms, and need to be protected from chilling and overheating.

i., term. Infant born between the beginning of the 38th week through the 41st week of gestation (260 to 287 days).

infanticide (ĭn-făn′tĭ-sīd) [LL. *infanticidium*]. The killing of an infant.

infantile (ĭn′făn-tīl) [Fr. *infantilis*]. Pert. to infancy or an infant.

infantilism (in-făn′tĭl-ĭzm, ĭn′făn-tĭl-ĭzm″) [″ + Gr. *-ismos*, condition]. 1. Condition in which the mind and body make slow development and the individual fails to attain adult characteristics. Characterized by mental retardation, stunted growth, and sexual immaturity. 2. Childishness.

i., angioplastic. Infantilism due to defective development of vascular system.

i., Brissaud's. Cretinism.

i., cachectic. Infantilism caused by chronic infection or poisoning.

i., celiac. Infantilism caused by intestinal malabsorption due to intolerance to gluten in the diet.

i., dysthyroidal. Infantilism caused by a defective thyroid.

i., hepatic. Infantilism combined with cirrhosis of the liver.

i., hypophyseal. Dwarfism resulting from inadequate secretion of growth hormone from the hypophysis. SYN: *hypophyseal dwarfism.*

i., idiopathic. Variety of arrested physical development of unknown cause.

i., intestinal. Infantilism associated with chronic intestinal disorder, causing poor growth.

i., myxedematous. Cretinism.

i., pituitary. I., hypophyseal.

i., renal. Infantilism caused by a defect in renal function.

i., sex. Continuation of childish traits, esp. sex characteristics, beyond the age of puberty.

i., symptomatic. Infantilism caused by poor tissue development.

i., universal. Infantilism marked by dwarfed stature and absence of secondary sexual characteristics.

infant mortality rate. SEE: *rate, infant mortality.*

infant stimulation. The use of various techniques to provide multisystems input to neonates and infants identified or at risk of delay in development. The purpose is to provide an environment that provides the stimulation necessary for normal development.

infarct [L. *infarctus*]. An area of tissue in an organ or part that undergoes necrosis following cessation of blood supply. May result from occlusion or stenosis of the supplying artery or more rarely from occlusion of the vein that drains the tissue.

i., anemic. Infarct in which blood pigment is lacking or decoloration has occurred. SYN: *i., pale; i., white.*

i., bland. Infarct in which infection is absent.

i., calcareous. Infarct in connective tissue in which calcareous salts have been deposited.

i., cicatrized. Infarct that has been replaced or encapsulated by fibrous tissue.

i., hemorrhagic. I., red.

i., infected. Infarcted tissue that has been invaded by pathogenic organisms.

i., pale. I., anemic.

i., red. Infarct that is swollen and red as a result of hemorrhage. SYN: *i., hemorrhagic.*

i., septic. I., infected, q.v.

i., uric acid. Infarct in kidney due to obstruction of renal tubules by uric acid crystals.

i., white. I., anemic.

infarction. 1. Formation of an infarct. 2. An infarct.

i., cardiac. Myocardial infarction.

i., cerebral. Infarction in the brain due to failure of blood supply to the area.

i., evolution of. Normal healing process after myocardial infarction. Seen on ECG as progressive changes in the S-T segment.

i., extension of. An increase in the size of a myocardial infarction, occurring after the initial infarction and usually accompanied by a return of acute symptoms, such as angina unrelieved by appropriate medicines.

i., myocardial. Infarction in cardiac muscle, usually resulting from formation of a thrombus in the coronary arterial system.

The immediate therapeutic need involves assuring the patient that comprehensive care will be given and at the same time instituting whatever needs to be done to put the patient at rest and to arrange for immediate transport to a hospital, doctor's office, or any place where appropriate therapy may be provided. Because the majority of deaths occur in the first several hours following infarction, it is essential that treatment not be delayed. SEE: *tissue plasminogen inactivator.*

i., pulmonary. Infarction in the lung usually resulting from pulmonary embolism.

Immediate therapy includes control of pain, oxygen administered continuously by mask, and treatment of circulatory collapse (shock) if present.

i., silent myocardial. Actual infarction

Common Protozoal Infections

Disease	Primary Site of Infection	Parasite	Mode of Transmission
Malaria			
Benign tertian		*Plasmodium vivax*	
Benign quartan	Erythrocytes	*P. malariae*	Mosquito (female *Anopheles*)
Malignant tertian		*P. falciparum*	
Sleeping sickness	Blood plasma	*Trypanosoma gambiense*	Tsetse fly (*Glossina palpalis*)
Rhodesian sleeping sickness	Blood plasma	*T. rhodesiense*	Tsetse fly (*Glossina morsitans*)
Leishmaniasis, visceral (kala-azar)	Reticuloendothelial cells and plasma	*Leishmania donovani*	Sandfly (*Phlebotomus argentipes*)
Amebic dysentery	Wall of large intestine	*Entamoeba histolytica*	Fecal (cyst) contamination of food and water

of the myocardium, but the patient has none of the signs or symptoms of this illness.

infect [ME. *infecten*]. To cause pathogenic organisms to be present in or upon, as to infect a wound.

infection (in-fĕk′shŭn). The state or condition in which the body or a part of it is invaded by a pathogenic agent (microorganism or virus) that, under favorable conditions, multiplies and produces injurious effects. Localized infection is usually accompanied by inflammation, but inflammation may occur without infection. SEE: tables.

SYM: The symptoms of infection are those of inflammation. The five classical symptoms listed by early medical writers are dolor (pain), calor (heat), rubor (redness), tumor (swelling), and functio laesa (disordered function).

Pain: This is esp. prominent when the infection is confined within closed cavities, causing pressure. The pain is in proportion to the virulence and extent of the infection. Pain associated with intra-abdominal infection is often due to contact of infected organs with peritoneum. *Redness and swelling:* Not evident when infection is within some rigid tissue or deep within some cavity; more apparent when superficial structures are involved. Discoloration would be a better term than redness, as the color is more blue or purple in advanced bacterial infections, while tuberculosis infections have long been called white swellings. *Heat:* May not be evident on the surface, but there may be considerable elevation of body temperature even with minor infections.

Disordered function: This depends upon the part affected as well as the virulence. With almost all acute bacterial infections there is an increase of polymorphonuclear leukocytes, either absolute or relative. The degree of prostration may be out of proportion to the extent of the injury or apparent infection. There have been many deaths from infection following pricks of needles, small splinters of bone, a trifling cut, or an infection from the bristle of a brush, in which streptococci were the inciting cause. In this type of infection, a red streak may be seen extending up the extremity from the site of injury and following the superficial lymphatics. The lay term for this is "blood poisoning." This red line is absent in staphylococcal infections of the lymphatic vessels.

ETIOL: The principal causes of infection are agents belonging to the following groups of microorganisms: viruses, bacteria, rickettsiae, fungi, and animal parasites.

SITE: Infection may be local or general. Local infections may be at the portal of entry or remote if transferred by the blood or lymph. Microorganisms may gain entry to the tissues through the gastrointestinal tract as in typhoid fever, through the respiratory tract as in tuberculosis and common colds, through wounds as in rabies, from contaminated objects as in tetanus, or from bites of insects as in malaria and yellow fever.

Some medicines, but esp. prolonged therapy with adrenocortical hormones and certain antibiotics, upset either the immune mechanism or the bacterial interrelations

Fungus Infections

Disease	Causative Organisms	Structures Infected	Microscopic Appearances
Ringworm (tinea, otomycosis)	*Microsporum* (*audouinii*, etc.)	Horny layer of epidermis and hairs, chiefly of scalp	Fine septate mycelium inside hairs and scales; spores in rows and mosaic plaques on hair surface
	Trichophyton (*tonsurans*, etc.)	Hairs of scalp, beard, and other parts; nails	Mycelium of chained cubical elements and threads in and on hairs; often pigmented
Favus (tinea favosa)	*Trichophyton schönleini*	Yellow disks in epidermis around a hair; all parts of body; nails	Vertical hyphae and spores in epidermis; sinuous branching mycelium and chains in hairs
Epidermophytosis (dhobie itch, etc.)	*Epidermophyton* (*floccosum*, etc.)	Inflamed patches in inguinal, axillary, and interdigital folds; hairs not affected	Long, wavy, branched and segmented hyphae and spindle-shaped cells in stratum corneum

Systemic Infections

Disease	Causative Organisms	Structures Infected	Microscopic Appearances
Thrush and other forms of candidiasis	*Candida albicans*	White patches on tongue, mouth, throat; also may cause lesions of vagina and skin	Yeastlike budding cells and oval thick-walled bodies in lesion
Actinomycosis	*Actinomyces bovis, A. israelii*	Usually in neck	Branched filaments on radiating rods, forming colonies
Nocardiosis	*Nocardia asteroides*	Lower extremities or lung	Closely resemble bacteria; found in pus
Blastomycosis	*Blastomyces brasiliensis, B. dermatitidis*	Skin and lungs	Yeastlike cells demonstrated in lesion
Coccidioidomycosis	*Coccidioides immitis*	Respiratory tract	Nonbudding spores containing many endospores, in sputum
Cryptococcosis	*Cryptococcus neoformans*	Meninges; sometimes lungs	Yeastlike fungus having gelatinous capsule; demonstrated in spinal fluid

so that the growth of certain microorganisms is encouraged. The resultant superinfection may be quite difficult to control and may be so severe as to cause death. Cortisone therapy encourages the recurrence or resurgence of previous lesions of tuberculosis. SEE: *opportunistic infections.*

METHODS: *Airborne:* Pathogenic organisms in the respiratory tract discharged from the mouth or nose may be borne on the air and settle on food, clothing, walls, and floors. If they are of the type that resists drying for a long period, as would be the case with infections due to spore-forming organisms, they may remain virulent until transmitted to another person. Coughing, sneezing, and expectorating may be responsible for droplet infection because bacteria are expelled into the air.

Animal carriers: Some microorganisms

may be carried from an animal to man by direct contact, indirect transfer, or by intermediary hosts.

Contact: The result of transmission from person to person as in kissing, coming into contact with those afflicted with communicable diseases, or with utensils handled by one with an infection.

Food-borne: Bacteria may be contained in food. Root and salad vegetables may contain bacteria from the soil or from manure used as fertilizer. Cooking safeguards by destroying microorganisms on food, but improperly prepared canned foods may contain the *Clostridium botulinum* toxin, which causes botulism.

Human carriers: Some parasites may live in or upon the bodies of persons who themselves do not suffer from them, but the parasites may be carried by them to others. Carriers may be contact carriers, or those who never show symptoms; incubationary carriers, or those in whom the infection is starting but has not completed the incubation period; and convalescent carriers, or those who have recovered but who still harbor the organism causing their disease.

Insect vectors: An insect, as the housefly, may act as a physical carrier, which may transmit the typhoid bacillus from one point to another, or as an active intermediate host, such as the female *Anopheles* mosquito, which transmits malaria organisms present in her saliva by injecting them into the host while biting that person or animal.

Prenatal: The result of the fetus being infected transplacentally or from contiguity with the maternal membranes.

Soil-borne: Soil-borne, spore-forming organisms commonly enter the body through wounds, as in tetanus and gas gangrene.

Water-borne: Organisms producing typhoid, dysentery, cholera, and amebic infections may be carried through a water supply or through water in public pools used for bathing. These organisms may pass into the water from the feces of an infected person and be communicated to others.

i., acute. Infection that appears suddenly and may be of brief or prolonged duration.

i., airborne. Infectious organisms that have been transported through the air.

i., apical. Infection located at the tip of the root of a tooth.

i., chronic. Infection having a protracted course.

i., concurrent. Existence of two or more infections at the same time. SEE: *superinfection.*

i., contagious. Infectious disease communicable by contact with an infected individual.

i., cross. Transfer of an infectious organism or disease from one patient in a hospital to another.

i., droplet. Infection acquired by inhalation of a microorganism in the air, esp. one added to the air by someone's breath or cough.

i., dustborne. Airborne infection in which the infectious organism is carried by dust.

i., endogenous. Infection caused by bacteria, normally nonpathogenic and inhabiting the digestive tract.

i., exogenous. Infection caused by organisms not present in the body.

i., fungus. Infection with a fungus.

i., local. Infection caused by germs lodging and multiplying at one point in a tissue and remaining there, as a boil.

i., low-grade. Loosely used term for a subacute or chronic infection with only mild inflammation and without pus formation.

i., metastatic. Local infection caused by microorganisms circulated from a focus of infection.

i., mixed. Infection caused by two or more organisms.

i., nosocomial. Infection that is acquired during hospitalization.

i., opportunistic. SEE: *opportunistic infections.*

i., protozoal. Infection with a protozoon, e.g., malaria.

i., pyogenic. Infection resulting from pus-forming organisms.

i., secondary. Infection caused by a different organism than the one causing the primary infection.

i., simple. Infection due to a single species of organism.

i., subacute. Infection intermediate between acute and chronic.

i., subclinical. Infection that is immunologically confirmed but does not show clinical symptoms in the individual.

i., systemic. Infection in which the infecting agent or organisms are throughout the body rather than restricted to a local area as in an abscess.

i., terminal. Infection occurring in the late stage of a disease. Generally acute and septic, usually causing death.

i., waterborne. Infection caused by organisms present in water.

infectious (in-fĕk'shŭs) [ME. *infecten*, infect]. 1. Capable of being transmitted with or without contact. 2. Pert. to a disease due to a microorganism. 3. Producing infection.

infectious disease. Any disease caused by growth of pathogenic microorganisms in the body. May or may not be contagious. SEE: *quarantine; incubation* for Incubation and Isolation Periods in Common Infections table.

infectious mononucleosis. SEE: *mononucleosis, infectious.*

infecundity (ĭn-fē-kŭn′dĭ-tē) [L. *infecunditas,* sterility]. Barrenness; inability to conceive.

inferior (ĭn-fē′rē-or) [L. *inferus,* below]. 1. Beneath; lower. 2. [NA] Used medically in reference to the undersurface of an organ or indicating a structure below another structure.

inferiority complex. In psychology, a repressed state of mind in which one feels inferior to others. Such ideas may be manifested by the assumption of superiority, often resulting in overcompensation. Opposite of superiority complex. SEE: *complex.*

infertility. Inability or diminished ability to produce offspring; unproductivity. Condition may be present in either or both sexual partners and is usually reversible. Diagnostic investigation includes special tests of both partners as well as a complete physical examination. Some factors responsible for infertility are immature or abnormal reproductive systems, anomalies of other organs in that vicinity, infections, endocrine dysfunction, and emotional problems. SEE: *tuboplasty, transcervical balloon.*

* i., secondary.* Infertility in which one or more pregnancies have occurred prior to the present condition of infertility.

infest [L. *infestare,* to attack]. To overrun to a harmful extent. Said esp. of parasites.

infestation. The harboring of animal parasites, esp. macroscopic forms such as ectoparasites and arthropod endoparasites.

infibulation (ĭn-fĭb-ū-lā′shŭn) [L. *in,* in, + *fibula,* clasp]. The process of fastening, as in joining the lips of wounds by clasps. Also suturing together of the labia of females or the foreskin of males to prevent sexual intercourse.

infiltrate (ĭn-fĭl′trāt, ĭn′fĭl-trāt) [″ + *filtrare,* to strain through]. 1. To pass into or through a substance or a space. 2. The material that has infiltrated.

infiltration (ĭn″fĭl-trā′shŭn). The process of a substance passing into and being deposited within the substance of a cell, tissue, or organ.

  Ex.: infiltration of a tissue or organ with blood corpuscles, or of a cell by fatty particles. Infiltration must not be confused with degeneration; in the latter condition the foreign substances are from changes within the cell.

* i., adipose.* I., fatty, q.v.

* i., amyloid.* Infiltration of tissue or viscera with a glycoprotein.

* i., anesthesia.* Injection of an anesthetic solution directly into the tissue. SEE: *anesthesia.*

* i., calcareous.* Deposits of calcium or magnesium salts within a tissue.

* i., cellular.* Infiltration of cells, esp. blood cells, into tissues; invasion by cells of malignant tumors into adjacent tissue.

* i., fatty.* Deposit of fat in the tissues, or oil or fat globules in the cells.

* i., glycogenic.* Glycogen deposit in cells.

* i., lymphocytic.* Infiltration of tissue by lymphocytes.

* i., pigmentary.* Infiltration of pigments.

* i., purulent.* Pus cells in a tissue.

* i., serous.* Infiltration with diluted lymph.

* i., urinous.* Infiltration with urine.

* i., waxy.* Amyloid degeneration.

infinite distance. 1. A distance without limits. 2. In vision, light rays coming from a point of any distance beyond 20 feet (6.1 meters) are practically parallel and accommodation is unnecessary.

infinity. 1. Condition of being infinite. 2. Space, time, or quantity without limits.

infirm [L. *infirmis*]. Weak or feeble, esp. from old age or disease.

infirmary [L. *infirmarium*]. A small hospital; a place for the care of sick or infirm persons.

infirmity. 1. Weakness. 2. A sickness or illness.

Inflamase. Trade name for prednisolone sodium phosphate, USP.

inflammation [L. *inflammare,* to flame within]. The non-specific immune response that occurs in response to any type of bodily injury. It is a stereotyped response that is identical whether the injurious agent is a pathogenic organism, foreign body, ischemia, physical trauma, ionizing radiation, electrical energy, or extreme temperature. Inflammation is a conservative process modified by whatever produces the reaction, but it should not be confused with infection; the two are relatively different conditions, although one may arise from the other. The reactions produced during inflammation and repair may be harmful, e.g., hypersensitivity reactions, the processes that lead to rheumatoid arthritis, excess scar formation. SEE: *infection.*

  SYM: The cardinal signs include rubor (redness), calor (heat), tumor (swelling), and dolor (pain). In addition, fever commonly occurs with extensive inflammation.

  Process: The first step in inflammation is local vasodilation that increases blood flow (causing redness and heat), followed by increased vascular permeability that enables plasma to move out of the capillaries and into the tissues, producing local edema and pain secondary to pressure on nerve endings. Neutrophils, and later monocytes, move out of the blood stream and into the injured tissues. Chemical mediators are released by the leukocytes and tissues to continue the inflammatory response. The arrival of additional neutrophils and macrophages (chemotaxis, q.v.) is also stimulated by the release of mediators. Following destruction of the organism or control of the damage, tissue repair can begin. If the inflammatory response is inadequate to deal with the invading organisms, the specific immune response, q.v., is required.

Chemical mediators in inflammation include histamine, kinins, complement, and arachidonic acid metabolites. These promote continued vasodilation, capillary permeability, and the emigration of neutrophils. Other chemicals released during inflammation are interleukin-1 (IL-1) by macrophages which stimulates the activity of other white blood cells and produces fever. Interferons, q.v., may be released by the leukocytes if the invading organism is a virus.

Inflammation is the basis of all disease processes with "itis" in their names (e.g., appendicitis, bronchitis, cholecystitis), as well as other pathologic disorders (e.g., adult respiratory distress syndrome, which occurs as the result of massive neutrophil aggregation, and emphysema, which occurs following chronic inflammation of the alveoli). However, most inflammation occurs as a normal part of the immune response, not a pathologic response. It is only when inflammation occurs inappropriately, as in autoimmune disorders, or when it is prolonged or overwhelming that inflammation is considered pathologic.

i., acute. Inflammation of rapid onset and rapid resolution. The majority of the response is usually over within 12 hours.

i., chronic. Inflammation that is usually less intense and of prolonged duration. May be characterized by chronically elevated white blood cell count, low grade fever, and pain.

i., exudative. Inflammatory process in which the fluid leaving the capillaries is rich in plasma proteins.

i., fibrinous. Inflammation in which the exudate is rich in fibrin.

i., granulomatous. Inflammation with considerable production of granular tissue. Seen esp. in tuberculosis, syphilis, and in some fungal infections.

i., hyperplastic. Inflammation characterized by excess production of young fibrous tissue.

i., interstitial. Inflammation involving principally the noncellular or supporting elements of an organ.

i., proliferative. I., hyperplastic, q.v.

i., pseudomembranous. Inflammation in which a pseudomembrane is formed. It is due to a toxin that necrotizes the tissues, and is seen in the oral, nasal, and respiratory tract tissues in diphtheria.

i., purulent. Inflammation in which pus is formed. SYN: *i., suppurative.*

i., serous. Inflammation in which the exudate is composed principally of serum.

i., subacute. Mild inflammatory process with minimal signs and symptoms. May progress to a chronic process and, over time, do serious damage.

i., suppurative. I., purulent.

i., ulcerative. Formation of an ulcer over an area of inflammation.

inflammatory [L. *inflammare,* to flame within]. Rel. to or marked by inflammation.

inflammatory response. The tissue and cellular changes that occur with inflammation; the hemodynamic and permeability changes and migration of leukocytes to an area of tissue injury that attempt to produce a localized protective action.

inflation (in-flā′shŭn) [L. *in,* into, + *flare,* to blow]. Distention of a part by air, gas, or liquid.

inflator (in-flā′tor). Device for forcing air into an organ. This may be done for diagnostic or therapeutic purposes.

inflection (in″flĕk′shŭn) [″ + *flectere,* to bend]. 1. An inward bending. 2. Change of tone or pitch of the voice; nuance.

influenza (in″flū-ĕn′ză) [It., influence]. An acute, contagious respiratory infection characterized by sudden onset, fever, chills, headache, myalgia, and sometimes prostration. Coryza, cough, and sore throat are common. It is usually a self-limited disease that lasts from 2 to 7 days. SYN: *flu.* SEE: *cold.*

SYM: Begins abruptly with lassitude, malaise, chilliness, severe pain in head and back, fever from 101° to 103°F (38.3° to 39.4°C). Prostration out of proportion to the fever. Eyes injected, sneezing, hoarseness, and hard paroxysmal cough. Coryza is moderate to severe. Less frequently, gastrointestinal symptoms including anorexia, nausea, vomiting, and diarrhea are present.

ETIOL: The causative agent is a virus of which several genera, A, B, and C, and subtypes, such as H_0N_1 (A_0 human); H_1N_1 (A_1); H_2N_2 (A_2); H_3N_2 (A_{HK}, A_3); $H_{SW}N_1$ (swine); $H_{eq}N$ (2 equine); and $N_{av}N$ (8 avian), have been identified. The influenza virus has shown great genetic variation. This ability provides the basis for development of epidemics in populations that have previously been exposed to influenza caused by other subtypes.

EPIDEMIOLOGY: Usually more prevalent in winter and spring. Young adults, in robust health, appear to be particularly susceptible. The disease is contagious and is spread by discharges from the mouth and nose of infected persons. It may occur sporadically, epidemically, or pandemically. The incidence is highest in ages 5 to 9. The very young and the very old are most at risk of dying. Even during an epidemic, the number of people infected who remain asymptomatic is high as compared to those who are symptomatic. The influenza virus is the only organism that still causes acute nationwide epidemics.

INCUBATION: One to three days.

DIFF. DIAG: Typhoid fever, smallpox in the prodromal stage, cerebrospinal meningitis, and rarely, pulmonary tuberculosis.

COURSE: Ordinarily lasts from four to five days, and may terminate by crisis or speedy lysis. Pulse rate is usually not increased in proportion to fever; may be 90 to 100. Blood pressure low; nosebleed not uncommon. Examination of blood demonstrates a leukopenia. Urinalysis generally demonstrates presence of albumin and casts. Even though fairly rapid recovery is the rule, some patients will experience lassitude for weeks or even months after the acute phase disappears.

The principal complications are secondary bacterial infections of the nasal sinuses, middle ear, and lungs.

PREVENTION: Vaccines are available and are effective in reducing the incidence rate if the vaccine contains the inactivated virus of the strain causing the disease. The vaccine should be given to the elderly and to persons who have chronic diseases, esp. of the heart or lungs. The vaccine does not produce permanent immunity. Amantadine and rimantadine are effective in preventing influenza A.

TREAT: Symptomatic, force fluids, bedrest, antipyretics, analgesics, nasal decongestants. Antibiotics are not indicated unless there is a secondary bacterial infection. Amantadine or rimantadine, if given early in the course of the disease, are helpful in treating influenza A.

PROG: As a rule, outcome is favorable in absence of pulmonary complications. In patients with cyanosis, severe nerve disturbances, or bloody expectoration, prognosis is extremely guarded.

Death may occur but mostly in infants under one year and in those over 60 or in persons who have a chronic disease. SEE: *Reye's syndrome.*

NURSING IMPLICATIONS: Advise evaluation for hypersensitivity to chicken feathers or eggs before administering the vaccine. Explain the possible side effects (local site discomfort, fever, and malaise). SEE: *Nursing Diagnoses* in *Appendix.*

i., Asian. Influenza caused by a variant strain of influenza virus type A.

influenzal (ĭn″flū-ĕn′zăl) [It. *influenza*, influence]. Relating to influenza.

influenza virus vaccine. USP. A sterile aqueous suspension of suitably inactivated influenza virus types A and B either individually or combined. Trade names for influenza virus vaccine are Fluax and Fluogen.

infolding. Process of enclosing within a fold; an operation employed in the treatment of stomach ulcer in which the walls on either side of the lesion are sutured together.

informed consent. Competent and voluntary permission for a medical procedure, test, or medication. The consent is given based on understanding the nature, risks, and alternatives of the procedure or test. The purpose is to promote individual autonomy, protect patients, avoid duress, encourage introspection by health care professionals, and involve the public in promoting autonomy and controlling biomedical research.

infra- [L. *infra*, below, underneath]. Prefix meaning below; under; beneath; inferior to; after.

infra-axillary (ĭn″fră-ăks′ĭl-ă-rē) [″ + *axilla*, little axis]. Below the axilla.

infrabulge (ĭn′fră-bŭlj). The surfaces of the tooth gingival to the height of contour.

infraclavicular (ĭn″fră-klă-vĭk′ū-lăr) [″ + *clavicula*, little key]. Below the clavicle.

infracortical (ĭn″fră-kor′tĭ-kăl) [″ + *cortex*, rind]. Beneath the cortex of any organ.

infracostal (ĭn″fră-kŏs′tăl) [″ + *costa*, rib]. Below the rib.

infracotyloid (ĭn″fră-kŏt′ĭ-loyd) [″ + Gr. *kotyloeides*, cup shaped]. Beneath the cotyloid cavity of the acetabulum of the hip.

infraction (ĭn-frăk′shŭn) [L. *infractus*, to destroy]. An incomplete fracture of a bone in which parts do not become displaced.

infradentale. A craniometric landmark; it is the bony point between the mandibular central incisors. SEE: *cephalometry.*

infradiaphragmatic (ĭn″fră-dī″ă-frăg-măt′ĭk). Below the diaphragm. SYN: *subdiaphragmatic.*

infraglenoid (ĭn″fră-glē′noyd) [L. *infra*, below, underneath, + Gr. *glene*, cavity, + *eidos*, form, shape]. Beneath the glenoid fossa. SYN: *subglenoid.*

infraglottic (ĭn″fră-glŏt′ĭk) [″ + Gr. *glottis*, back of tongue]. Below the glottis.

infrahyoid (ĭn″frā-hī′oyd) [″ + Gr. *hyoeides*, U-shaped]. Below the hyoid bone.

inframammary [″ + *mamma*, breast]. Below the mammary gland.

inframandibular (ĭn″frā-măn-dĭb′ū-lăr) [″ + *mandibula*, lower jawbone]. Below the mandible.

inframarginal [″ + *margo*, a margin]. Below any edge or margin.

inframaxillary [″ + *maxilla*, jawbone]. Below the upper jaw (maxilla).

infranuclear (ĭn″frā-nū′klē-ăr) [″ + *nucleus*, kernel]. In the nervous system, peripheral to a nucleus.

infraocclusion [″ + *occlusio*, a shutting up]. Location of a tooth below the line of occlusion.

infraorbital (ĭn-frā-or′bĭ-tăl) [″ + *orbita*, track]. Beneath the orbit.

infrapatellar (ĭn″frā-pă-tĕl′ăr) [″ + *patella*, a small plate]. Below the patella.

infrapsychic (ĭn″frā-sī′kĭk) [″ + Gr. *psyche*, mind]. Below the level of consciousness; automatic.

infrapubic [″ + *pubes*, hair on genitals]. Below the pubis.

infrared rays. Invisible heat rays beyond the red end of the spectrum.

Their wavelength ranges from 7700 angstrom units (A.U.) to 1 mm. Long-wave infrared rays (15,000 to 150,000 A.U.) are emitted by all heated bodies and exclusively by bodies of low temperature such as hotwater bottles and electrical heating pads; short-wave infrared rays (7200 to 15,000 A.U.) are those emitted by all incandescent heaters.

SOURCES: The sun, electric arc, incandescent globe, and so-called infrared burners.

USES: Their energy is transformed into heat in a superficial layer of the tissues. They are used therapeutically to stimulate local and general circulation and for relief of pain. The infrared thermograph, a device for detecting and photographing infrared rays, has been useful in studying the heat of tissues. This device has many applications such as in investigation of the rate of blood flow through a part. SEE: *radiation; ray*.

infrascapular [″ + *scapula*, shoulder blade]. Beneath the shoulder blade.

infrasonic (ĭn″frā-sŏn′ĭk) [L. *infra*, below, underneath, + *sonus*, sound]. Sound wave frequency lower than those normally heard.

infrasonic recorder. A device that can be used to determine blood pressure. It detects and records the subaudible oscillations of the arterial wall under an occluding cuff. The results are comparable to the values determined by use of an intra-arterial catheter. SEE: *blood pressure, indirect measurement of; pseudohypertension*.

infraspinous [″ + *spina*, thorn]. Beneath the scapular spine.

infrasternal [″ + Gr. *sternon*, chest]. Beneath the sternum.

infratemporal (ĭn″frā-tĕm′pō-răl) [″ + *temporalis*, pert. to the temple]. Below the temporal fossa of the skull.

infratonsillar (ĭn″frā-tŏn′sĭ-lăr) [″ + *tonsilla*, almond]. In the pharynx below the tonsils.

infratrochlear (ĭn″frā-trŏk′lē-ăr) [″ + *trochlea*, pulley]. Beneath the trochlea.

infraumbilical (ĭn″frā-ŭm-bĭl′ĭ-kăl) [″ + *umbilicus*, a pit]. Below the umbilicus.

infraversion (ĭn″frā-vĕr′zhŭn) [″ + *versio*, a turning]. Downward deviation of the eye.

infriction [L. *in*, into, + *frictio*, rubbing]. Rubbing of ointments into the skin. SYN: *inunction*.

infundibulectomy (ĭn″fŭn-dĭb″ū-lĕk′tō-mē) [L. *infundibulum*, funnel, + Gr. *ektome*, excision]. Surgical excision of the infundibulum of any structure or organ, esp. the heart.

infundibuliform (ĭn″fŭn-dĭb′ū-lĭ-form) [″ + *forma*, form]. Funnel-shaped.

i. fascia. The membranous layer investing the spermatic cord.

infundibulopelvic (ĭn″fŭn-dĭb″ū-lō-pĕl′vĭk) [″ + *pelvis*, basin]. Concerning the infundibulum and pelvis of an organ, esp. the kidney.

infundibulum (ĭn″fŭn-dĭb′ū-lŭm) [L.]. 1. [NA] Funnel-shaped passage or structure. 2. Tube connecting the frontal sinus with the middle nasal meatus. 3. Stalk of the pituitary gland. 4. Any renal pelvis division. 5. Cavity formed by fallopian fimbriae. 6. Terminus of a bronchiole. 7. Terminus at upper end of cochlear canal. 8. [NA] Conelike upper anterior angle at right cardiac ventricle from which the pulmonary artery arises. SYN: *conus arteriosus*.

i., ethmoidal. The area in the middle meatus of the nose. The anterior ethmoidal air cells and the frontal nasal duct from the frontal sinus open into this area.

i. of hypothalamus. Infundibulum of the hypothalamus. It extends from the stalk of the hypothalamus to the posterior lobe of the hypothalamus.

i. of the uterine tube. The funnel-shaped opening at the lateral end of the uterine tube.

infusible. 1. [L. *in-*, not, + *fusio*, fusion] Not capable of being fused or melted. 2. [L. *in*, into, + *fundere*, to pour] Capable of being made into an infusion.

infusion (ĭn-fū′zhŭn) [L. *infusio*]. 1. A liquid substance introduced into the body via a vein for therapeutic purposes. 2. Steeping a substance in hot or cold water in order to obtain its active principle. 3. Product obtained from process described in def. 2.

i., bone marrow. A method of obtaining immediate vascular access, esp. in children. Access is obtained by percutaneous insertion of a bone marrow aspiration needle into the marrow cavity of a long bone, usually into the proximal tibia. Once access is gained, substances may be injected into the bone marrow where they are absorbed almost immediately into the general circulation. This avenue of access does not collapse in the presence of shock or peripheral circulatory collapse.

i., continuous. A controlled method of prolonged drug administration that includes the ability to control the delivery rate. This system permits the drug to be available to the body at a constant level. It has proved to be more effective than other regimens in the treatment of certain neoplastic diseases, including acute leukemia.

i., intravenous. Injection of a solution directly into a vein, usually the cephalic or median basilic vein of the arm. SEE: *intravenous infusion.*

i., subcutaneous. Infusion of solutions into the subcutaneous space.

infusion pump. Use of a pump to infuse material into an artery or vein. These are useful in overcoming arterial resistance or when administering thick solutions. Also, the rate of administering the solution may be controlled. SEE: *electronic infusion device.*

infusodecoction (ĭn-fū″sō-dē-kŏk′shŭn) [″ + *de,* down, + *coquere,* to boil]. 1. Infusion followed by decoction. 2. A medicine made from a crude drug steeped in cold water and then in boiling water.

Infusoria (ĭn-fū-sō′rē-ă). Name formerly applied to a class of Protozoa, now called Ciliata, q.v.

infusum (ĭn-fū′sŭm) [L., infusion]. Product obtained from steeping a substance in hot or cold water. SYN: *infusion* (def. 3).

ingesta (ĭn-jĕs′tă) [L. *in,* into, + *gerere,* to carry]. Food and drink received into the body through the mouth.

ingestant (ĭn-jĕs′tănt) [″ + *gerere,* to carry]. Any substance such as food and drink taken orally.

ingestion. The process of taking material (particularly food) into the gastrointestinal tract or the process by which a cell takes in foreign particles.

Ingrassia's apophyses (ĭn-grä′sē-ăs) [Giovanni Filippo Ingrassia, It. anatomist, 1510–1580]. The lesser wings of the sphenoid.

ingravescent (ĭn″grăv-ĕs′ĕnt) [″ + *grave-*

sci, to grow heavy]. Becoming more severe.

ingredient (ĭn-grē′dē-ĕnt) [L. *ingredi,* to enter]. Any part of a compound or a mixture; a unit of a more complex substance.

ingrowing [L. *in,* into, + AS. *growan,* to grow]. Growing inward so that a portion that is normally free becomes covered.

ingrown nail. Growth of the nail edge into the soft tissue, thus causing inflammation and pain. May be due to improper paring of the nail or pressure on the nail edge from improperly fitted shoes.

inguen (ĭn′gwĕn) [L.] (pl. *inguina*). [NA] The groin.

inguinal (ĭng′gwĭ-năl) [L. *inguinalis,* pert. to the groin]. Pert. to the region of the groin.
RS: bubo; groin; hernia; venereal bubo.

inguinal canal. The canal carrying the spermatic cord in the male and the round ligament in the female. It is 1½ in. (3.8 cm) long. A potential source of weakness, it may be the site of a hernia or an undescended testicle.

inguinal glands. Lymph nodes of the groin.

inguinal hernia. Hernia in inguinal region. SEE: *hernia, inguinal.*

inguinal ligament. A fibrous band extending from the anterior superior iliac spine to the pubic tubercle. SYN: *Poupart's ligament.*

inguinal reflex. Reflex in females resembling cremasteric reflex, q.v., in males.

inguinal region. The iliac region on either side of the pubes. SYN: *groin.*

inguinal ring. Interior opening of the inguinal canal (abdominal inguinal ring) and the end of the inguinal canal (subcutaneous inguinal ring).

inguinocrural (ĭng″gwĭ-nō-kroo′răl) [L. *inguen,* groin, + *cruralis,* pert. to the leg]. Concerning the inguinal and thigh areas.

inguinodynia (ĭn″gwĭ-nō-dĭn′ē-ă) [″ + Gr. *odyne,* pain]. Pain in the groin or inguinal region.

inguinolabial (ĭng″gwĭ-nō-lā′bē-ăl) [″ + *labialis,* pert. to the lips]. Concerning the inguinal and labial areas.

inguinoscrotal (ĭng″gwĭ-nō-skrō′tăl) [″ + *scrotum,* a bag]. Concerning the inguinal and scrotal areas.

INH. isoniazid.

inhalant [L. *inhalare,* to inhale]. Medication or compound suitable for inhaling.

inhalation (ĭn″hă-lā′shŭn) [L. *inhalatio*]. 1. Act of drawing breath, vapor, or gas into the lungs; inspiration. 2. Introduction of dry or moist air or vapor into the lungs for therapeutic purposes, such as aromatic spirits of ammonia used to overcome fainting.

　　SUBSTANCES: Mixture of oxygen and carbon dioxide to relieve depressed breathing. Steam inhalations are given to reduce dryness of mucous membranes and to provide heat and moisture to the membranes of the lungs.

inhalation therapy. Administration of medicines, water vapors, gases (such as oxygen, carbon dioxide, or helium), or anesthetics by inhalation. The medicines usually are nebulized by using an aerosol or spray apparatus. SEE: *intermittent positive-pressure breathing.*

inhale (ĭn-hāl′) [L. *inhalare*]. To draw in the breath; to inspire.

inhaler. 1. Device for administering medicines by inhalation. 2. One who inhales.

inherent (ĭn-hĕr′ĕnt) [L. *inhaerens,* to inhere]. Belonging to anything naturally, not as a result of circumstances, and existing as an essential character of something. SYN: *innate; intrinsic.*

inherent cauterization. Deep cauterization.

inheritance (ĭn-hĕr′ĭ-tăns) [L. *inhereditare,* to inherit]. The sum total of all that is inherited; that which is the result of hereditary factors contained within the egg and sperm.

    i., alternative. Inheritance of a trait from one parent.

    i., extrachromosomal. Inherited traits governed by mechanisms other than by chromosomes.

    i., holandric. Inherited traits carried only by males; thus, the operative gene is on the Y chromosome.

    i., hologynic. Transmission of traits from mothers only to daughters.

    i., multifactorial. Inheritance of traits influenced by a number of genetic and nongenetic factors; but none of these has a major effect.

    i., sex-influenced. Inherited traits influenced by the sex chromosomes, i.e., autosomal, but of variable importance in each sex.

    i., sex-limited. A trait that can be expressed in only one sex.

    i., sex-linked. Inheritance of traits regulated by either of the autosomal, i.e., X or Y, chromosomes.

inherited. Body traits and genetic make-up received due to genetic transmission rather than acquired.

inhibin (ĭn-hĭb′ĭn). A testicular hormone that acts to inhibit luteinizing hormone secretion by the anterior pituitary gland.

inhibited sexual excitement. SEE: *frigidity.*

inhibition (ĭn″hĭ-bĭsh′ŭn) [L. *inhibere,* to restrain]. 1. Repression or restraint of a function. 2. In physiology, a stopping of an action or function of an organ, as in the slowing or stopping of the heart produced by electrical stimulation of the vagus. 3. In psychiatry, restraint of one mental process almost simultaneously by another opposed mental process; an inner impediment to free activity.

    i., competitive. Inhibiting the function of an active material by competing for the cell receptor site.

    i., contact. Inhibition of cell division due to the close contact of similar cells.

    i., noncompetitive. Inhibition of enzyme activity due only to the concentration of the inhibitor.

    i., psychic. Arrest of an impulse, thought, action, or speech. The term is commonly applied to the denial of the sex instinct. SYN: *suppression.*

    i., selective. I., competitive, q.v.

inhibitor. That which inhibits.

    Ex.: a chemical substance that stops enzyme activity or a nerve that suppresses activity of an organ innervated by it.

inhibitory (ĭn-hĭb′ĭ-tō-rē). Restraining, preventing.

inhibitory nerve. Nerve that carries impulses that act to slow down or inhibit action in the organ or tissue supplied by its fibers.

inhibitrope (ĭn-hĭb′ĭ-trōp) [″ + Gr. *tropos,* a turning]. Person in whom certain stimuli cause partial arrest of function.

inhomogeneity (ĭn-hō″mŏ-jĕ-nē′ĭ-tē) [L. *in-,* not, + Gr. *homos,* same, + *genos,* kind]. Lack of uniform quality or consistency.

iniac, inial (ĭn″ē-ăk, -ăl) [Gr. *inion,* back of the head]. Pert. to the inion.

iniencephalus (ĭn″ē-ĕn-sĕf′ă-lŭs) [″ + *enkephalos,* brain]. Congenitally deformed fetus in which brain substance protrudes through a fissure in the occiput, so that the brain and spinal cord occupy a single cavity.

inion (ĭn′ē-ŏn) [Gr.]. External occipital protuberance. SEE: *antinion.*

iniopagus (ĭn″ē-ŏp′ă-gŭs) [″ + *pagos,* thing fixed]. Twins fused at the occiput.

iniops (ĭn′ē-ŏps) [″ + *ops,* eye]. A double deformity in which there is joining of the two fetuses from the posterior thorax up, so that one complete face is anterior, with the suggestion of a face posteriorly.

initial (ĭn-ĭsh′ăl) [L. *initium,* beginning]. Rel. to the beginning or commencement of a thing or process. SYN: *incipient.*

initial scene survey. The appearance of the accident scene that yields information about which occult injuries a patient may have sustained. Information obtained can include how the accident occurred, number of patients, need for additional services (police, fire, rescue), and danger to patient or rescuers (threat of fire, explosions from the vehicle or an oil/gas spill, downed power wires, etc.).

initis (ĭn-ī′tĭs) [Gr. *inos,* fiber, + *itis,* inflammation]. 1. Inflammation of fibrous tissue. SYN: *fibrositis.* 2. Inflammation of a tendon. SYN: *tendinitis.* 3. Inflamed condition of a muscle. SYN: *myositis.*

inject [L. *injicere,* to throw in]. To introduce fluid into the body or its parts artificially.

injectable. Capable of being injected.

injected [L. *injectus,* thrown in]. 1. Filled by injection of fluid. 2. Congested.

injection (ĭn-jĕk′shŭn). 1. Forcing of a fluid into a vessel or cavity intramuscularly or under the skin. 2. Substance introduced in this manner. 3. State of being injected; congestion.

Caution: Wear gloves when handling blood or blood products or in situations in which it is possible to be contaminated with the patient's blood. SEE: *AIDS; Universal Precautions* in *Appendix.*

NURSING IMPLICATIONS: All equipment used in preparing and administering an injection should be sterile. Choose appropriate needle length for administration route and site. Wash hands prior to and following procedure; wear gloves if preparing a chemotherapeutic agent. Measure dose accurately. Choose appropriate site by identifying anatomical landmarks, and cleanse area with alcohol swab. Insert needle at appropriate angle for route. After insertion in muscle, aspirate to ensure that there is no blood return. This will help to prevent accidental injection into a blood vessel. Slowly inject the prescribed medication. Remove the needle, applying pressure to the site if appropriate. If the intended injection is in a vein, the chance of bleeding into the soft tissue after removal of the needle may be decreased if the injection area, e.g., the arm, is elevated above the level of the heart. Do this for several minutes. Do not recap used needle, but destroy and dispose of needle and syringe according to prescribed method. Document injection time and site.

i., epidural. Injection of anesthetic solution or other medicine into the epidural space of the spinal cord.

i., fractional. Process of injecting small amounts at a time until the total injection is complete.

i., hypodermic. Term originally indicating injection of a substance beneath the skin. It is preferable to state the specific route of administration, as in intramuscular. SEE: *anesthesia, local.*

i., intra-alveolar. Infiltration method of anesthesia where the anesthetic is introduced into the soft tissues adjacent to the tooth.

i., intracardial. Injection into the heart.

i., intracutaneous. Injection into the skin, a method employed in giving of serums

and vaccines when a local reaction is desired.

i., intralingual. Injection of medicines into the tongue. Usually done as an emergency measure when a vein suitable for use is not available because of circulatory collapse.

i., intramuscular. Injection into intramuscular tissue usually in the anterior thigh, deltoid, or in one of the buttocks. SEE: illus.

i., intraosseous. Injection of anesthetic solution directly into the cancellous bone of the alveolar process adjacent to the tooth to produce a localized effect.

i., intraperitoneal. Injection into the peritoneal cavity.

i., intravenous. Injection into a vein.

i., jet. Technique of injecting medicines and vaccines through the skin without puncturing it. A nozzle ejects a fine spray of liquid at such speed as to penetrate the skin. The skin is not harmed and the procedure is harmless. Esp. useful in immunizing a great number of persons quickly and economically. Hypospray is the trade name for a device used in this procedure.

i., rectal. Instillation, i.e., not an injection, into the rectum; an enema.

i., sclerosing. Injection into a vessel or into a tissue of a substance that will bring about obliteration of the vessel or hardening of the tissues.

i., spinal. Injection into the spinal canal.

i., subcutaneous. Injection beneath the skin. The usual sites are the skin over the deltoid, upper outer arm.

i., vaginal. Instillation, i.e., not an injection, into the vagina. A douche.

i., Z-track. An injection technique in which the surface (skin and subcutaneous) tissues are pulled and held to one side prior to insertion of the needle deep into the muscle in the identified site. The medication is injected slowly, followed by a 10-second delay, then the needle is removed and the tissues quickly permitted to resume their normal position. This provides a Z-shaped track which makes it difficult for the injected irritating drug to seep back into subcutaneous tissues.

injector. Device for making injections.

i., jet. SEE: *injection, jet.*

i., pressure. Device that delivers a substance to be injected over a specified time or at a specified pressure.

injury [L. *injurius,* unjust]. Trauma or damage to some part of the body. SEE: *transportation of the injured.*

SYM: These will depend on the nature, extent, and severity of the damage. If the injuries are severe, there may be signs of shock

INTRAMUSCULAR INJECTION

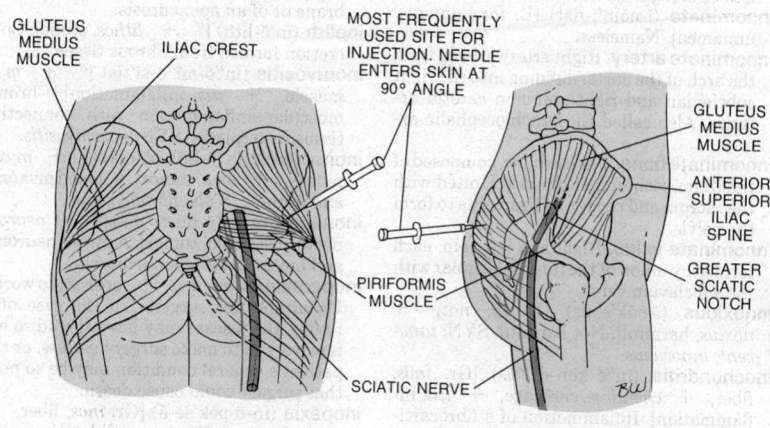

GLUTEUS MEDIUS MUSCLE

ILIAC CREST

MOST FREQUENTLY USED SITE FOR INJECTION. NEEDLE ENTERS SKIN AT 90° ANGLE

GLUTEUS MEDIUS MUSCLE

ANTERIOR SUPERIOR ILIAC SPINE

GREATER SCIATIC NOTCH

PIRIFORMIS MUSCLE

SCIATIC NERVE

POSTERIOR VIEW

LATERAL VIEW

with progressive fall in blood pressure; subnormal temperature; shallow, rapid breathing; cold, clammy, pale skin.

i., egg-white. Injury resulting from biotin deficiency. It is produced in experimental animals by feeding raw egg white or its antibiotin component, avidin. SEE: *biotin.*

i., internal. SEE: *internal injury.*

i., steering wheel. Injury following an automobile accident in which the driver is thrown forward against the steering wheel. This may cause contusion of the heart and trauma to the ribcage.

ink poisoning. Many of the poisonings ascribed to ink are forms of dermatitis. Several types of materials may be responsible. Ordinary ink may cause irritation because of its composition or because of the sensitivity of particular individuals to certain ingredients. Sometimes cleaning materials used in removing ink stains have been found to be toxic.

SYM: Redness, occasionally small pustules and cracking.

F.A.: Wash with alcohol, soap, and water. Rinse carefully and apply a bland dressing such as cold cream.

inlay (ĭn′lā) [L. *in,* in, + AS. *lecgan,* to lay]. A solid filling made to the precise shape of a cavity of a tooth and cemented into it; usually the inlay is made of casting alloy, but it may be porcelain.

inlet. Passage leading to a cavity.

i. of pelvis. SEE: *pelvic inlet.*

INN. *International Nonproprietary Names,* a list of pharmaceuticals published periodically by the World Health Organization.

innate (ĭn-nāt′) [″ + *natus,* born]. 1. Belonging to the essential nature of something. SYN: *inherent; intrinsic.* 2. Existing in or belonging at birth.

innervate (ĭn-nĕr′vāt, ĭn′ĕr-vāt) [″ + *nervus,* nerve]. To stimulate a part, as the nerve supply of an organ.

innervation (ĭn″ĕr-vā′shŭn). 1. Stimulation of a part through the action of nerves. 2. The distribution and function of the nervous system. 3. The nerve supply of a part.

i., collateral. Development of the nerve supply in a nerve tract adjacent to the original nerve supply that has been injured or destroyed.

i., double. Innervation of an organ with both sympathetic and parasympathetic fibers.

i., reciprocal. Innervation of antagonistic muscles of a limb by which impulses of central origin that induce an action such as flexion bring about inhibition of the opposing extensors.

innidiation (ĭ-nĭd″ē-ā′shŭn) [″ + *nidus,* nest]. Multiplication of cells in a part to which they have been carried by metastasis.

innocent (ĭn′ō-sĕnt) [L. *innocens*]. Harmless or benign; clinically unimportant; not malignant (a heart murmur may be called innocent in this sense). SYN: *innocuous; innoxious.*

innocuous (ĭ-nŏk'ū-ŭs) [L. *innocuus*]. Harmless or benign. SYN: *innocent; innoxious.*

innominate (ĭ-nŏm'ĭ-nāt) [L. *innominatus,* unnamed]. Nameless.

innominate artery. Right artery arising from the arch of the aorta, dividing into the right subclavian and right common carotid arteries. Also called the brachiocephalic artery.

innominate bone. The hip bone, composed of the ilium, ischium, and pubis. United with the sacrum and coccyx by ligaments to form the pelvis.

innominate veins. Right and left vein, each formed by union of the internal jugular with the subclavian vein.

innoxious (ĭ-nŏk'shŭs) [L. *in,* not, + *noxius,* harmful]. Not harmful. SYN: *innocent; innocuous.*

inochondritis (ĭn″ō-kŏn-drī'tĭs) [Gr. *inos,* fiber, + *chondros,* cartilage, + *itis,* inflammation]. Inflammation of a fibrocartilage.

inochondroma (ĭn″ō-kŏn-drō'mă) [″ + ″ + *oma,* tumor]. Chondroma or tumor with much fibrous tissue. SYN: *fibrochondroma.*

inoculability (ĭn-ŏk″ū-lă-bĭl'ĭ-tē) [″ + *oculus,* bud]. State of being inoculable.

inoculable. 1. Transmissible by inoculation. 2. Susceptible to a transmissible disease. 3. Capable of being inoculated.

inoculate. To inject an antigen, antiserum, or antitoxin into an individual to produce immunity to a specific disease.

inoculation (ĭn-ŏk″ū-lā'shŭn). The process of being inoculated. This can be accomplished by using a needle and syringe, by scarification of the skin, or by some special technique such as a very high-speed jet of air capable of a force sufficient to carry a liquid solution into the skin. SEE: *injection, jet.*

    i., animal. The injection of serums, microorganisms, or viral organisms into laboratory animals for the purpose of immunizing them or for the purpose of investigating the effects of the inoculated material upon the animals.

inoculum (ĭn-ŏk'ū-lŭm) [L.]. Substance introduced by inoculation.

inocyst (ĭn'ō-sĭst) [Gr. *inos,* fiber, + *kystis,* a bladder]. A fibrous capsule.

inocyte (ĭn'ō-sīt) [″ + *kytos,* cell]. Fibroblast.

inogenesis (ĭn″ō-jĕn'ĕ-sĭs) [″ + *genesis,* generation, birth]. Formation of fibrous tissue.

inogenous (ĭn-ŏj'ĭ-nŭs) [″ + *gennan,* to produce]. Forming tissue or produced from it.

inoglia (ĭn-ŏg'lē-ă) [″ + *glia,* glue]. The supporting tissue of fibroblasts.

inohymenitis (ĭn″ō-hī″mĕn-ī'tĭs) [″ + *hymen,* membrane, + *itis,* inflammation]. Inflammation of any fibrous membrane or of an aponeurosis.

inolith (ĭn'ō-lĭth) [″ + *lithos,* stone]. Concretion formed from fibrous tissue.

inomyositis (ĭn″ō-mī″ō-sī'tĭs) [″ + *mys,* muscle, + *itis,* inflammation]. Chronic muscular inflammation with connective tissue hyperplasia. SYN: *fibromyositis.*

inomyxoma (ĭn″ō-mĭk-sō'mă) [″ + *myxa,* mucus, + *oma,* tumor]. A mixed myxoma and fibroma. SYN: *fibromyxoma.*

inoneuroma (ĭn″ō-nū-rō'mă) [″ + *neuron,* nerve, + *oma,* tumor]. A mixed neuroma and inoma. SYN: *fibroneuroma.*

inoperable [L. *in-,* not, + *operari,* to work]. Unsuitable for surgery. In the case of a tumor, the disease may have spread so extensively as to make surgery useless, or the patient's general condition may be so poor that surgery could cause death.

inopexia (ĭn-ō-pĕk'sē-ă) [Gr. *inos,* fiber, + *pexis,* fixation]. Tendency of blood to coagulate spontaneously in the vessels.

inorganic [L. *in-,* not, + Gr. *organon,* an organ]. 1. In chemistry, occurring in nature independently of living things. Sometimes considered to indicate chemical compounds that do not contain carbon. 2. Not pert. to living organisms.

inorganic acid. An acid composed of inorganic constituents. SYN: *mineral acid.*

inorganic chemistry. Chemistry dealing only with inorganic compounds.

inorganic compound. A chemical compound without carbon.

inosclerosis (ĭn″ō-sklē-rō'sĭs) [Gr. *inos,* fiber, + *skleros,* hard]. Increased fibroustissue density.

inoscopy [″ + *skopein,* to examine]. Diagnosis by examining fibrinous deposits in body fluids.

inosculating [L. *in,* in, + *osculum,* little mouth]. Directly communicating. SYN: *anastomosing.*

inosculation (ĭn-ŏs″kū-lā'shŭn). Union of two vessels. SYN: *anastomosis.*

inose (ĭn'ōs). Inositol.

inosemia (ĭn-ō-sē'mē-ă) [Gr. *inos,* fiber, + *haima,* blood]. 1. An excessive amount of fibrin in the blood. 2. The presence of inositol in the blood.

inosinic acid [″ + L. *acidus,* sour]. A mononucleotide that is present in muscular tissue and also is a product of nucleic acid. Upon hydrolysis, it yields hypoxanthine and D-ribose-5-phosphoric acid.

inosite (ĭn'ō-sīt). Inositol.

inositis (ĭn″ō-sī'tĭs) [″ + *itis,* inflammation]. Inflammation of fibrous tissue.

inositol (ĭn-ŏs'ĭ-tŏl). $C_6H_6(OH)_6$. Hexahydroxycyclohexane, a sugarlike crystalline substance found in the liver, kidney, skeletal and heart muscle, and also present in the leaves and seeds of most plants. It is part of the vitamin B complex. Deficiency of inositol in experimental animals results in loss of hair, eye defects, and growth retardation. Its significance in human nutrition has not been established.

inosituria (ĭn"ō-sĭ-tū'rē-ă) [*inositol* + Gr. *ouron*, urine]. Inositol in the urine.

inosuria (ĭn-ō-sū'rē-ă). 1. [Gr. *inos*, fiber, + *ouron*, urine] Fibrinous excess in urine. 2. [*inositol* + Gr. *ouron*, urine] Inositol in the urine. SYN: *inosituria.*

inotropic (ĭn"ō-trŏp'ĭk) [Gr. *inos*, fiber, + *trepein*, to influence]. Influencing the force of muscular contractility.

inpatient. Patient who is hospitalized. SEE: *outpatient.*

inquest [L. *in*, into, + *quaerere*, to seek]. 1. In legal medicine, official examination and investigation into the cause, circumstance and manner of sudden, unexpected violent, or unexplained death. 2. The act of inquiring.

insalivation [" + *saliva*, spittle]. The process of mixing saliva with food, as in chewing.

insalubrious (ĭn-săl-ū'brē-ŭs) [L. *in*, not, + *salus*, health]. Not healthy; not contributing to health.

insane (ĭn-sān') [" + *sanus*, sound]. Mentally deranged; pert. to insanity.

insanitary. Not conducive to health; unhealthful; esp. pert. to filth.

insanity [L. *insanitas*, insanity]. A severe mental disorder such as a psychosis. An imprecise term for mental disorder or psychosis; now obsolete except as a legal term. In legal medicine, the state or mental condition characterized by inability to distinguish between right and wrong, possession of delusions or hallucinations that prevent individuals from looking after their own affairs with ordinary prudence or that render them a menace to others, or actions resulting from impulses of such intensity that they cannot be resisted.

During lucid intervals, an insane person may enter into a legal contract, marriage, business, or buying and selling, providing at the time he or she is capable of entering into such matters with an understanding of all that is implied. The mental capacity at the time determines the validity of such acts and not the condition before or after. SEE: *neurosis; psychosis.*

insatiable (ĭn-sā'shē-ă-bl) [L. *insatiabilis*]. Incapable of being satisfied or appeased.

inscriptio (ĭn-skrĭp'shē-ō) [L.]. Inscription.

i. tendinea. Tendinous band traversing a muscle.

inscription (ĭn-skrĭp'shŭn) [L. *in*, upon, + *scribere*, to write]. Body of a prescription, which gives the names of the drug(s) prescribed and dosage.

insect [L. *insectum*]. Common name for any of the class Insecta of the phylum Arthropoda. Insects of medical importance are flies, mosquitoes, lice, fleas, ticks, spiders, scorpions, bees, hornets, and wasps.

Insecta. A class of the phylum Arthropoda characterized by three distinct body divisions (head, thorax, abdomen), three pairs of jointed legs, trachea, and usually two pairs of wings. Insects are of medical significance in that some are parasitic; some serve as carriers or vectors of pathogenic organisms; and some are annoying pests causing injury by their bites or stings. SYN: *Hexapoda.*

insect bites and stings. In some cases the venom of a stinging insect may be more toxic than that of a poisonous snake. Fortunately the insect injects a very small amount of venom into the body.

Obviously the reaction of a previously sensitized person is a potentially life-threatening medical emergency that requires prompt, effective therapy. Insect stings and bites cause more deaths than do snake bites. An estimated four persons in 1000 are severely sensitive to insect stings.

F.A.: Remove the stinger if it is present, and cool the area as quickly and efficiently as possible to prevent the venom from gaining access to the general circulation. To prevent injecting further venom, gently tease the stinger out by grasping the stinger with fingernails or forceps. If a specific therapy or antiserum is available, it should be administered.

An antivenin for *black widow spiders (Latrodectus mactans)* is available. One ampule is given I.V. in 10 to 50 ml of saline after the appropriate skin test has been done. For acute pain and muscle contraction, give 10 ml of calcium gluconate I.V. or I.M., and repeat as necessary. SEE: *spider, black widow.*

There is no antiserum for the bite of the *brown recluse spider (Loxosceles reclusus),* but hydrocortisone and supportive measures will help.

For *bees, wasps, and hornets* 0.2 to 0.5 ml of epinephrine subcutaneously and an antihistamine suitable for intravenous injection should be given slowly. If shock and collapse appear to be imminent, hydrocortisone should be given. Apply an ice pack to the sting. If muscle spasms occur, intravenous infusion of calcium lactate or calcium gluconate should be given. In some cases curare (dimethyl tubocurarine chloride) will be required to relieve muscle spasms. SEE: *fire ant stings.*

insecticide (ĭn-sĕk'tĭ-sīd) [L. *insectum*, insect, + *caedere*, to kill]. 1. An agent used to exterminate insects. 2. Destructive to insects.

insectifuge (ĭn-sĕk'tĭ-fūj) [" + *fugare*, to put to flight]. Insect repellant.

Insectivora (ĭn"sĕk-tĭv'ō-ră) [" + *vorare*, to devour]. An order of small mammals including moles and shrews.

insectivore (ĭn-sĕk'tĭ-vor). A member of the order Insectivora.

insect repellents. Solutions, creams, sprays, or lotions containing chemicals that repel insects. Users should be aware that these chemicals can cause allergic or toxic effects.

insecurity. Feelings of helplessness, apprehension, vulnerability, and inability to cope with situations or people.

insemination (ĭn-sĕm"ĭn-ā'shŭn) [L. *in*, into, + *semen*, seed]. 1. Discharge of semen from the penis into the vagina during coitus. 2. Fertilization of an ovum.

  i., artificial. ABBR: AI. Introduction of viable sperm into the vagina, cervical canal, or uterus by artificial means. SEE: *impregnation.*

  i., heterologous artificial. Artificial insemination in which the semen is obtained from a donor other than the husband.

  i., homologous artificial. Artificial insemination in which the semen is obtained from the husband.

insenescence (ĭn"sĕ-nĕs'ĕns) [" + *senescens*, growing old]. 1. Process of growing old or the approaching of old age. 2. Old age in which infirmity and senility would normally be expected to be present but they are not.

insensible [L. *in-*, not, + *sensibilis*, appreciable]. 1. Unconscious; without feeling or consciousness. 2. Not perceptible.

insertion [L. *in*, into, + *serere*, to join]. 1. The movable attachment of the distal end of a muscle, which produces shape changes or skeletal movement when the muscle contracts. 2. Placement or implanting of something into something else, e.g., in dentistry, the process of placing a filling or inlay in a cavity preparation or placing dentures or other prostheses in the mouth.

  i., velamentous. Attachment of the umbilical cord to the edge of the placenta.

insheathed (ĭn-shēthd') [" + AS. *sceath*, sheath]. Enclosed, as by a sheath or capsule. SYN: *encysted.*

insidious (ĭn-sĭd'ē-ŭs) [L. *insidiosus*, cunning]. Used to indicate a disease that comes on in such a manner (lacking symptoms) as to make the patient unaware of its onset.

insight. 1. Self-understanding. 2. In psychia-try, the patients' comprehension that they are ill in mind; and awareness of the character of the illness or of the unconscious factors responsible for the emotional conflict involved.

  In dealing with psychiatric patients with insight into their illness, it is important to determine whether or not the condition into which the patient has insight is, in reality, a fact. For example, one of Jung's patients complained of birds attacking her. At first Jung treated this as a delusion, but later found out the birds did indeed attack his patient. Also, even though the patient may have gained insight into the illness, this does not indicate a cure; the patient is still ill.

insipid (ĭn-sĭp'ĭd) [LL. *insipidus*]. Without taste; lacking in spirit or animation.

in situ (ĭn sī'tū, sĭt'ū) [L.]. 1. In position, localized. 2. In the normal place without disturbing or invading the surrounding tissue.

insolation (ĭn"sō-lā'shŭn) [L. *insolare*, to expose to the sun]. 1. Any exposure to the rays of the sun. 2. Heatstroke or sunstroke.

  In the past it was felt that exposure to the sunlight was a powerful therapeutic measure. It is now known that exposure to excess sunlight on either an acute or a chronic basis may be unwise. Acute overexposure leads to severe sunburn of the skin. People with light skin who experience chronic exposure to the sun have an increased chance of developing malignant neoplasms of the skin. SEE: *heat; heat exhaustion; hyperpyrexia.*

insoluble (ĭn-sŏl'ū-bl) [L. *insolubilis*]. Incapable of solution or of being dissolved.

insomnia (ĭn-sŏm'nē-ă) [L. *insomnis*]. SEE: *sleep, disorders of.*

insomniac (ĭn-sŏm'nē-ăk). One who has insomnia.

insorption (ĭn-sorp'shŭn) [L. *in*, into, + *sorbere*, to suck in]. The passage of material into the blood as in the case when substances move from the gastrointestinal tract into the bloodstream.

inspect [L. *inspectare*, to examine]. To examine visually.

inspection. Visual examination of the external surface of the body as well as of its movements and posture. SEE: *abdomen; chest; circulatory system.*

inspectionism (ĭn-spĕk'shŭn-ĭzm). Voyeurism.

inspersion (ĭn-spĕr'zhŭn) [L. *in*, upon, + *spargere*, to sprinkle]. Sprinkling with powder or a fluid.

inspiration (ĭn"spĭr-ā'shŭn) [L. *in*, in, + *spirare*, to breathe]. Inhalation; drawing air into the lungs. Opposite of expiration. The average rate is 12 to 18 respirations per minute in a normal adult at rest. SEE: *diaphragm* for illus.; *respiration.*

Inspiration may be costal or abdominal, the latter being deeper. The breaking point for breath holding is quite variable. Some professional divers and others are able to prolong it for more than two minutes.

MUSCLES: External intercostals; diaphragm; levatores costarum; pectoralis minor; scaleni; serratus posterior; and superior sternocleidomastoid.

RS: air; apnea; asphyxia; breathing; chest; Cheyne-Stokes respiration; dyspnea; hyperpnea; inhalation therapy; lung; respiration; ventilation.

i., crowing. Peculiar noise in laryngismus stridulus, q.v., or spasmodic croup. SEE: *croup, spasmodic.*

i., external. Interchange of gases in the lungs.

i., forcible. Inspiration in which the muscles of inspiration are assisted by inspiration auxiliaries (i.e., muscles attached to the chest that by contraction increase the volume of the thoracic cavity directly or indirectly by furnishing fixed support whereby other muscles may act more advantageously). If movements become excessively labored, there is brought into coordinate action every muscle in the body that can either directly or indirectly increase the capacity of the thorax.

i., full. Inspiration in which lungs are filled as completely as possible (voluntarily, as in determining the amount of complemental air, or involuntarily, as in cardiac dyspnea).

i., internal. Interchange of gases in the tissues. SEE: *respiration, cell.*

inspirator (ĭn′spĭ-rā″tor). A type of respirator or inhaler.

inspiratory (ĭn-spīr′ă-tor″e). Pert. to inspiration.

inspiratory capacity. The maximum amount of air a person can breathe in after a resting expiration.

inspirometer (ĭn″spĭ-rŏm′ĕ-tĕr) [″ + ″ + Gr. *metron,* measure]. Device for determining the amount of air inspired.

inspissate (ĭn-spĭs′āt) [L. *inspissatus,* thickened]. To thicken by evaporation or absorption of fluid.

inspissated (ĭn-spĭs′ă-tĕd). Thickened by absorption, evaporation, or dehydration.

inspissation (ĭn-spĭ-sā′shŭn). 1. Thickening by evaporation or absorption of fluid. 2. Diminished fluidity or increased thickness.

instar. Any one of the various stages of insect development during successive molts.

instep. The arched medial portion of the foot.

instillation (ĭn″stĭl-ā′shŭn) [L. *in,* into, + *stillare,* to drop]. Slowly pouring or dropping a liquid into a cavity or onto a surface.

instillator. An apparatus for introducing, drop by drop, liquids into a cavity.

instinct (ĭn′stĭngkt) [L. *instinctus,* instigation]. The inherited tendency for the members of specific species to react to certain environmental conditions and stimuli in a particular way. The nature of the reaction is that which has through many generations enabled the individuals and species involved to adapt and survive. Instincts are best understood when considered against the evolutionary background of the individuals and species being observed. Freud spoke of instinct, but present-day psychoanalytic terminology would refer to the forces Freud described as being drive instead of instinct.

i., death. In psychoanalytic theory, the unconscious will to destroy oneself. The counterinstinct for the instinct to live.

i., herd. The basic drive to be associated with a group.

instinctive. Determined by instinct.

institutionalization. A process where individuals live together and gradually develop patterns of behavior; e.g., behaviors frequently associated with nursing home institutionalization are sick role and depression apathy. The movement in medicine and nursing is to move away from this and attempt to create a normalized home environment.

institutional review board. ABBR: IRB. A board whose members are independent of the hospital or medical institution involved. It is established to oversee the plans for conducting medical investigations involving human subjects. The purpose of the board is to protect the rights of those subjects. SEE: *informed consent.*

instruction. 1. Directions or commands. 2. The act of teaching or furnishing information.

i., dental hygiene. A program in which patients are taught the methods of oral hygiene and the importance of plaque control by proper toothbrushing, flossing, and appropriate nutrition.

instrument (ĭn′stroo-mĕnt) [L. *instrumentum,* tool]. 1. A mechanical device. 2. A special tool for accomplishing specific tasks. Thus a reflex hammer, microscope, stethoscope, cystoscope, and surgeon's scalpel are all examples of instruments. SEE: *instruments, care and sharpening of.*

i., dental. Any instrument used in the practice of dentistry including a variety of hand or machine-driven cutting instruments for soft and calcified tissues, forceps, elevators, clamps, reamers, wire pliers, pluggers, carvers, explorers, and other instruments unique to the dental specialties: oral surgery, endodontics, orthodontics, periodontics, prosthodontics, restorative dentistry, etc.

instrumental. 1. Pert. to instruments. 2. An important factor in achieving a result or goal.

instrumental activities of daily living. Those daily living skills, such as shopping, cooking, cleaning, and child care, that are necessary for maintaining the home environment.

instrumentarium (ĭn'stroo-mĕn-tā'rē-ŭm). Instruments required for a surgical or other procedure.

instrumentation 1. The use of instruments and their care. 2. Accomplishment of a task by use of instruments.

Ex.: removal of a foreign body from the bronchus by means of a bronchoscope.

instruments, care and sharpening of. *Cleansing.* Following surgery, collect, count, and unlock the instruments. First rinse with warm water to remove blood, and next, wash with hot water and soap. Then place under the hot water faucet and run boiling water on and through them. Dry at once with gauze. To remove rust, use cleanser sparingly; otherwise, the surface of the instrument will be damaged in the course of time.

Reliable bacterial sterilization of instruments before an operation can always be assured by boiling in a 1% solution of sodium bicarbonate for 15 minutes. This helps to prevent rusting of the instruments. The dipping of an instrument into alcohol or even pure carbolic acid cannot be relied upon to sterilize it.

Caution: Boiling water does not kill the hepatitis viruses. To be certain that this virus is destroyed, either autoclaving or the use of some chemical method of sterilization such as ethylene oxide gas is required.

Sharpening. Washita stone is best for sharpening dull instruments because it cuts away the metal faster. Arkansas stone is better for finishing. Glycerin is a suitable lubricant. The entire edge of the knife should be covered in one sweep. Hold knife so that the edge of the blade is at an angle of 30°. Blunt instruments should be kept highly polished. Rub with fine emery paper and polish with rouge and chamois skin or gauze. Do not use emery paper on saws. Silver instruments should not come in contact with rubber or be exposed to atmosphere. Wrap in dry gauze.

insufficiency (ĭn″sŭ-fĭsh′ĕn-sē) [L. *in-*, not, + *sufficiens*, sufficient]. The condition of being inadequate for a given purpose.

i., adrenal. Decreased or abnormally low production of adrenal cortical hormone by the adrenal gland. The result is Addison's disease.

i., aortic. An imperfect closure of the aortic valve.

i., cardiac. Inability of the heart to function normally.

i., coronary. Diminished blood flow through the coronary arteries of the heart.

i., gastric. Inability of the stomach to empty itself.

i., hepatic. Inability of the liver to function properly.

i., ileocecal. Failure of the ileocecal valve to prevent the back flow of intestinal contents from the cecum to the ileum.

i., mitral. Condition in which the mitral valve closes inefficiently with rhythmic action of the heart.

i., muscular. Condition in which a muscle is unable to exert its normal force and bring about normal movement of the part to which it is attached. Term applied esp. to eye muscles.

i. of ocular muscles. Absence of dynamic equilibrium of ocular muscles.

i., pulmonary valvular. Failure of the pulmonary valve between the right atrium and right ventricle of the heart to close completely.

i., renal. Inability of the kidney to remove waste products from the blood at the normal rate.

i., respiratory. Inadequate functional capacity of the respiratory system.

i., thyroid. Hypothyroidism.

i., valvular. Imperfect cardiac valve closure, permitting leakage of blood.

i., venous. Failure of the valves of the veins to function. This interferes with venous return to the heart.

insufflate [L. *insufflare*, to blow into]. 1. To blow into, as in the lungs of a newborn infant. 2. To blow a medicated powder or medicinal vapor into a cavity.

insufflation. The act of blowing a vapor or powder into a cavity, as the lungs.

i., perirenal. Instillation of air into the perirenal space in order to visualize the adrenal gland better on x-ray studies.

i., tubal. Transuterine insufflation with carbon dioxide to test patency of fallopian tubes. SYN: *Rubin's test.*

insufflator (ĭn'sŭ-flā″tor). Device for blowing powders into a cavity.

insula (ĭn'sū-lă) [L.]. 1. [NA] The central lobe of the cerebral hemisphere. It is a triangular area of the cerebral cortex lying in the floor of the lateral fissure. SYN: *island of Reil.* 2. Any round cutaneous body or patch.

insular (ĭn'sū-lăr) [L. *insula*, island]. Rel. to

any insula, as in pancreatic islets.

insulation [L. *insulare*, to make into an island]. 1. The protection of a body or substance with a nonconducting medium to prevent the transfer of electricity, heat, or sound. 2. The material or substance that insulates.

insulator. That which insulates. Specifically, a substance or body that interrupts the transmission of electricity to surrounding objects by conduction; anything that exerts great resistance to the passage of an electric current by conduction. The electrical resistance of an insulator is expressed in ohms. SEE: *nonconductor*.

insulin [L. *insula*, island]. 1. A hormone secreted by the beta cells of the islets of Langerhans of the pancreas. It can be readily crystallized as a zinc salt, although nickel, calcium, and cobalt also are effective. It is a protein with a molecular weight of approx. 5700. Insulin is essential for the proper metabolism of blood sugar (glucose) and for maintenance of the proper blood sugar level. Inadequate secretion of insulin results in improper metabolism of carbohydrates and fats and brings on diabetes characterized by hyperglycemia and glycosuria. The secretion of insulin is primarily dependent upon the concentration of blood glucose, an increase of blood sugar bringing about an increase in the secretion of insulin. SEE: *diabetes mellitus*, at ETIOL.

2. USP. A protein, obtained from the pancreas of healthy bovine and porcine animals used for food by man, that affects the metabolism of glucose.

3. A preparation used in medical treatment of diabetes. Prepared synthetically or from animal pancreas, usually pork or beef. First discovered and used successfully in diabetes by Sir F. G. Banting. Insulin is not a cure, and it is not necessary in every case of diabetes. Insulin, when injected (it is not active orally) into an individual with diabetes, produces the following effects: normal storage of glycogen in the liver and muscle tissue; reduction in blood sugar level by facilitating metabolism of glucose; disappearance of ketosis and hyperlipemia; prevention of excessive breakdown of protein; and increase in respiratory quotient.

DOSAGE: Should always be expressed in units rather than in milliliters or minims. There is no average dose of insulin for diabetics; each case must be cared for individually.

ADMIN: Insulin preparations are divided into three categories according to how quickly they act and their potency and duration following subcutaneous administration. The types include fast-, intermediate-, and long-acting. Examples of these are given in the subentries. SEE: table.

Syringes for use by blind patients with diabetes are available.

Caution: Persons taking insulin should wear an easily seen bracelet or necklace indicating that they have diabetes and take insulin. This will facilitate diagnosis and treatment in case of coma due to insulin. SEE: *Medic Alert*.

STORAGE: The FDA requires that all preparations of insulin contain instructions *to keep in a cold place and to avoid freezing*. Studies have shown that Prompt Insulin Zinc Suspension, Insulin Zinc Suspension, and Extended Insulin Zinc Suspension retain their potency for 24 months when stored at a temperature of 75°F (24°C). Under the same conditions, Protamine Zinc Insulin Suspension and Isophane Insulin Suspension retain their potency for 36 months. However, Insulin Injection, USP, does lose potency when stored at this temperature. It is advisable to store all types of insulin in the coolest possible area if refrigeration is not available.

i., human. USP. Insulin prepared by a synthetic process involving use of recombinant DNA technology utilizing strains of *Escherichia coli*. In its effect it is similar to highly purified animal insulins. Trade name is Humulin.

i., NPH. SEE: *insulin suspension, isophane*.

i., single component or monocomponent. Highly purified insulin that contains less than 10 parts per million of proinsulin, a substance that is capable of inducing formation of anti-insulin antibodies.

i. suspension, isophane. USP. Intermediate-acting insulin with onset in one-half to 1 hour and duration of 18 to 28 hours. SYN: *insulin, NPH*.

i. suspension, protamine zinc. USP. Long-acting insulin with onset in 6 to 8 hours and duration of 30 to 36 hours.

i., synthetic. Insulin made by the use of recombinant DNA methodology.

i. zinc suspension, extended. USP. Long-acting insulin with onset in 5 to 8 hours and duration of over 36 hours.

i. zinc suspension, prompt. USP. Fast-acting insulin with onset under 1 hour and duration of 12 to 16 hours.

insulinase (ĭn'sū-lĭn-ās). An enzyme that inactivates insulin.

insulinemia (ĭn-sū-lĭn-ē'mē-ă) [L. *insula*, island, + Gr. *haima*, blood]. An excess amount of insulin in the blood.

insulin injection sites. Because insulin is administered at least daily, it is important to

Duration of Effect of Various Insulins When Given by Subcutaneous Injection*

Type of Insulin	Synonym or Trade Name	Onset	Maximum	Duration
		(Given in Hours)		
Insulin, USP	Insulin. May be derived from one of several animals, e.g., pork, beef, ox.	0.5–1.0	2–3	5–7
Insulin Human, USP	Humulin; Novolin	0.5–1.0	2–3	5–7
Insulin Isophane Suspension, USP	NPH Iletin	0.5–1.0	6–10	18–28
Insulin Protamine Zinc Suspension, USP	Insulin Protamine Zinc	6–8	14–20	30–36
Insulin Zinc Extended Suspension, USP	Ultralente Insulin	5–8	16–18	over 36
Insulin Zinc Prompt Suspension, USP	Semilente Iletin	0.5–0.75	3–6	12–16
Insulin Zinc Suspension, USP	Lente Insulin	1.0–1.5	8–12	18–24

* These times are "average" and may be quite different in an individual patient.

have a plan for selecting the site. Rather than shift from one arm to the other, then to the leg, it is advisable to map out a number of injection sites in one area, use those and then use other sites.

insulin lipodystrophy. A complication of insulin administration characterized by changes in the subcutaneous fat at the site of injection. The changes may take the form of atrophy or hypertrophy; rarely are both types present in the same patient. Atrophy develops in as many as one-third of children and adult females who use insulin regularly, but rarely in adult males. The subcutaneous fat appears to have melted away and leaves a saucerlike depression. Hypertrophy at the injection site occurs in the form of a spongy localized area. This complication is slightly more common in males than in females. It is usually associated with a history of prolonged use of the same injection site.

insulinogenesis (ĭn″sū-lĭn-ō-jĕn′ĕ-sĭs) [″ + Gr. *genesis,* generation]. Production of insulin by the pancreas.

insulinogenic (ĭn″sū-lĭn″ō-jĕn′ĭk) [″ + Gr. *gennan,* to produce]. 1. Caused by insulin whether administered or produced by the pancreas. 2. Pert. to production of insulin.

insulinoid (ĭn′sū-lĭn-oyd) [″ + Gr. *eidos,* form, shape]. Resembling or having the properties of insulin.

insulinoma (ĭn″sū-lĭn-ō′mă) [″ + Gr. *oma,* tumor]. Insuloma, q.v.

insulin pump. A small battery-driven pump that delivers insulin subcutaneously into the abdominal wall. The pump can be programmed to deliver varying doses of insulin in accordance with changes in need for insu-

lin during different conditions; e.g., prior to eating.

insulin resistance. A cellular level phenomenon that prevents insulin from exerting its effect on glucose metabolism.

insulin shock. A condition resulting from an overdose of insulin resulting in reduction of the blood sugar level below normal (hypoglycemia). SEE: *Nursing Diagnoses* in *Appendix.*

SYM: Rapid bounding pulse, pale moist skin, weakness, coma. Acetone odor on breath is not present.

TREAT: Eating sugar or candy, orange juice, glucose, other carbohydrates and injections of strong glucose solution intravenously. Epinephrine is of great but transient value.

Caution: Persons taking insulin should wear an easily seen bracelet or necklace indicating that they have diabetes and take insulin. This will facilitate diagnosis and treatment in case of coma due to insulin. SEE: *Medic Alert.*

insulitis (ĭn″sū-lī′tĭs) [″ + Gr. *itis,* inflammation]. Inflammation of the islets of Langerhans of the pancreas.

insuloma (ĭn″sū-lō′mă) [″ + Gr. *oma,* tumor]. Tumor of the islets of Langerhans of the pancreas.

insulopathic (ĭn″sū-lō-păth′ĭk) [″ + Gr. *pathos,* disease, suffering]. Rel. to or caused by abnormal insulin secretion.

insult. In medicine, an injury or trauma.

insultus (ĭn-sŭl′tŭs) [L.]. An attack.

insusceptibility (ĭn″sŭ-sĕp″tĭ-bĭl′ĭ-tē) [L. *in,* not, + *suscipere,* to take up]. Immunity or lack of susceptibility to infection or disease.

intake (ĭn-tāk'). That which is taken in, esp. food and liquids.

  i. and output. ABBR: I and O. A record of the oral and parenteral intake of foods and fluids; and all of the output including urine, feces, vomitus, and if required, an estimate of loss of fluid due to perspiration.

Intal. Trade name for cromolyn sodium.

integration (ĭn″tĕ-grā'shŭn) [L. *integrare*, to make whole]. The bringing together of various parts or functions so that they function as a harmonious whole.

  i., primary. Early recognition of the body and its psyche as apart from one's environment.

  i., secondary. The process involved in developing the adult personality so that the individual coordinates the components into unified and socialized action.

integrator (ĭn′tĕ-grā″tor). Device for measuring body surfaces.

integrity. To be in undiminished or unimpaired state.

integument (ĭn-tĕg″ū-mĕnt) [L. *integumentum*, a covering]. A covering; the skin, consisting of the corium or dermis, and epidermis.

integumentary (ĭn-tĕg-ū-mĕn′tă-rē). Rel. to the integument. SYN: *cutaneous; dermal.*

integumentary system. The skin and its appendages, including the hair and nails.

intellect [L. *intelligere*, to understand]. The mind, or understanding; conscious brain function.

intellectual. 1. Pert to the mind. 2. Possessing intellect.

intellectualization (ĭn″tĕ-lĕk″chū-ăl-ĭ-zā′shŭn). The analysis of personal or social problems on an intellectual basis despite the individual's personal and emotional reactions to those problems.

intelligence [L. *intelligere*, to understand]. The capacity to comprehend relationships. The ability to think; to solve problems and to adjust to new situations. It is doubtful that using a single test to estimate the intelligence of persons from different social, racial, cultural, or economic backgrounds is reliable.

  i., artificial. SEE: *artificial intelligence.*

intelligence quotient. ABBR: IQ. An index of relative intelligence determined through the subject's answers to arbitrarily chosen questions. Intelligence quotient is merely a standard score that places an individual in reference to the scores of others within the age group. The test utilized may be relevant when administered to persons of one culture but not to another. Also, the IQ test may not be an accurate indicator of an individual's

Classification of IQ

IQ	Classification
Above 140	Near genius or genius
120–140	Very superior intelligence
110–119	Superior intelligence
90–109	Normal or average intelligence
80–89	Dull normal
70–79	Borderline deficiency
55–69	Educable mentally retarded
40–54	Trainable
20–39	Severe mentally retarded
Below 20	Profoundly mentally retarded

skills or potential in creative, artistic, or motor skills areas. SEE: table; *intelligence; intelligence test.*

intelligence test. A test designed to determine the intelligence of an individual. Tests are used as a basis for determining intelligence quotient (IQ), q.v. It is now believed that some of the standardized tests of intelligence were more nearly achievement tests. SEE: *intelligence.*

intemperance [L. *in,* not, + *temperare,* to moderate]. Excess in the use of anything; lack of moderation.

intensifying [L. *intensus,* intense, + *facere,* to make]. Making intense; magnifying.

intensifying screen. A thin sheet of celluloid or other substance coated with a finely divided substance that fluoresces under the influence of roentgen rays and is intended to be used in close contact with the emulsion of a photographic plate or film for the purpose of reinforcing the image. SYN: *fluorescent screen.*

intensimeter (ĭn″tĕn-sĭm′ĭ-tĕr) [″ + Gr. *metron,* measure]. An instrument, often a selenium cell or ionization chamber, designed to measure the intensity of roentgen rays.

intensity (ĭn-tĕn′sĭ-tē). 1. The degree or extent of activity, strength, force, electric current, etc. 2. The state of being intense.

intensive (ĭn-tĕn′sĭv). Rel. to or marked by intensity.

intention (ĭn-tĕn′shŭn) [″ + *tendere,* to stretch]. 1. A natural process of healing, q.v. 2. Goal or purpose.

  i., first. Healing without granulation or suppuration.

  i., second. Healing by adhesion of two granulated surfaces.

  i., third. Healing of an ulcer, wound, or cavity by filling with granulation tissue and by cicatrization. SEE: *granulation; resolution.*

intention tremor. Tremor exhibited or intensified when attempting coordinated movements.

inter- [L.]. Prefix meaning in the midst, between.

interacinar (ĭn″tĕr-ăs′ĭ-năr) [L. *inter*, between, + *acinus*, grape]. Located between acini of a gland.

interalveolar (ĭn″tĕr-ăl-vē′ō-lăr) [″ + *alveolus*, little tub]. Between the alveoli, esp. the alveoli of the lungs.

interarticular [″ + *articulus*, joint]. 1. Between two joints. 2. Situated between two articulating surfaces.

interarytenoid (ĭn″tĕr-ăr″ē-tē′noyd) [″ + Gr. *arytaina*, ladle, + *eidos*, form, shape]. Between the arytenoid cartilages of the larynx.

interatrial (ĭn″tĕr-ā′trē-ăl) [″ + *atrium*, hall]. Located between the atria of the heart.

interauricular (ĭn″tĕr-aw-rĭk′ū-lăr) [″ + *auricula*, little ear]. Situated between the auricles of the heart. The preferred term for auricle is atrium.

interbrain [″ + AS. *braegen*, brain]. The hind original part of the forebrain including the thalamus, pineal body (epithalamus), and geniculate bodies (metathalamus). SYN: *diencephalon; thalamencephalon.*

intercadence (ĭn″tĕr-kā′dĕns) [″ + *cadere*, to fall, die]. A supernumerary pulse wave between two regular beats.

intercalary (ĭn-tĕr′kă-lĕr″ē) [″ + *calare*, to call]. 1. Inserted or interposed between. SYN: *extraneous; interposed.* 2. Pert. to an upstroke on a pulse tracing that comes between two pulse beats. SYN: *intercalated.*

intercalated (ĭn-tĕr′kăl-āt-ĕd) 1. Inserted between as something interposed. SYN: *extraneous.* 2. Pert. to an upstroke on a pulse tracing that comes between two pulse beats. SYN: *intercalary.*

intercalated ducts. Short, narrow ducts that lie between secretory ducts and the terminal alveoli in the parotid and submandibular glands and in the pancreas.

intercanalicular (ĭn″tĕr-kăn″ă-lĭk′ū-lăr) [″ + *canalicularis*, pert. to a canaliculus]. Between the canaliculi of a tissue.

intercapillary (ĭn″tĕr-kăp′ĭ-lăr-ē) [″ + *capillaris*, hairlike]. Between the capillaries.

intercarotic (ĭn″tĕr-kă-rŏt′ĭk) [L. *inter*, between, + Gr. *karos*, deep sleep]. Between the external and internal carotid arteries.

intercarpal (ĭn″tĕr-kăr′păl) [″ + Gr. *karpalis*, pert. to the carpus]. Between the carpal bones.

intercartilaginous (ĭn″tĕr-kăr″tĭ-lăj′ĭ-nŭs) [″ + *cartilago*, cartilage]. Connecting or between cartilages.

intercavernous (ĭn″tĕr-kăv′ĕr-nŭs) [″ + L. *caverna*, a hollow]. Between the cavernous sinuses.

intercellular (ĭn″tĕr-sĕl′ū-lăr) [″ + *cella*, compartment]. Between the cells of a structure.

intercellular junctions. The microscopic space between cells. The spaces are important in assisting the transfer of small molecules across capillary walls. These junctions may be widened by chemical or physical factors, and are acted upon by chemical mediators of inflammation to increase vascular permeability.

intercerebral (ĭn″tĕr-sĕr′ē-brăl) [″ + *cerebrum*, brain]. Between the two cerebral hemispheres.

interchange. In dispensing drugs, the use of a generic form of the drug in place of the proprietary form. Some states mandate that prescriptions be filled with use of generic drugs unless the instructions specifically indicate "interchange not permitted."

interchondral (ĭn″tĕr-kŏn′drăl) [″ + Gr. *chondros*, cartilage]. Between cartilages. SYN: *intercartilaginous.*

intercilium (ĭn″tĕr-sĭl′ē-ŭm) [″ + *cilium*, eyelash]. The space between the eyebrows. SYN: *glabella.*

interclavicular (ĭn″tĕr-klă-vĭk′ū-lăr) [″ + *clavicula*, clavicle]. Between the clavicles.

intercoccygeal (ĭn″tĕr-kŏk-sĭj′ē-ăl) [″ + Gr. *kokkyx*, coccyx]. Between the segments of the coccyx.

intercolumnar (ĭn″tĕr-kō-lŭm′năr) [″ + *columna*, column]. Between columns.

intercolumnar fascia. A membrane between pillars of the abdominal ring, enclosing the spermatic cord.

intercolumnar fibers. Intercrural fibers.

intercondylar, intercondyloid, intercondylous [″ + Gr. *kondylos*, knuckle]. Between two condyles.

intercostal [″ + *costa*, rib]. Between the ribs.

intercostal muscles, external. Outer layer of muscles between the ribs, originating on the lower margin of each rib and inserted on the upper margin of the next rib. They draw adjacent ribs together and act to increase the volume of the thorax.

intercostal muscles, internal. Muscles between the ribs, lying beneath the external intercostals. Their function is the same as the external intercostal muscles.

intercostobrachial (ĭn″tĕr-kŏs″tō-brā′kē-ăl) [″ + ″ + *brachium*, arm]. Pert. to the intercostal space and the arm, as the posterior lateral branch of the second intercostal nerve supplying the skin of the arm, or a similar branch of the third intercostal nerve. Formerly called intercostohumeralis.

intercostohumeral (ĭn″tĕr-kŏs-tō-hū′mĕr-ăl) [″ + ″ + *humerus*, upper arm]. Concerning or connecting an intercostal space and the humerus.

intercourse [L. *intercursus*, running between]. Social interaction between individuals or groups. Communication.

   i., sexual. Coitus, q.v.

intercricothyrotomy (ĭn″tĕr-krī″kō-thī-rŏt′ō-mē) [L. *inter*, between, + Gr. *krikos*, ring, + *thyreos*, shield, + *tome*, incision]. Surgical separation of the cricothyroid membrane in order to incise the larynx.

intercristal (ĭn″tĕr-krĭs′tăl) [″ + *crista*, crest]. Between two crests of a bone, organ, or process.

intercrural (ĭn″tĕr-krū′răl) [″ + *crus*, limb]. Between two crura.

intercurrent [″ + *currere*, to run]. 1. Intervening. 2. Pert. to a disease attacking a patient with another malady.

intercusping [″ + *cuspis*, point]. The natural fitting together of the surfaces of opposing teeth. SEE: *occlusion*.

interdent. A specially designed knife used for removing interdental tissue.

interdental [″ + *dens*, tooth]. Between adjacent teeth in the same arch. SYN: *interproximal*. SEE: *interocclusal*.

interdentium (ĭn″tĕr-dĕn′shē-ŭm). The space between any two contiguous teeth.

interdigitation [″ + *digitus*, digit]. 1. Interlocking of toothed or fingerlike processes. 2. Processes so interlocked.

interdisciplinary. Involving or overlapping of two or more fields of medical science.

interest checklist. An assessment approach used by occupational therapists to determine the unique play and leisure interests of an individual.

interface. In computers, a device that enables two normally noncompatible circuits or parts to function together.

interfascicular (ĭn″tĕr-făs-ĭk′ū-lăr) [″ + *fasciculus*, bundle]. Between fasciculi.

interfemoral [″ + *femoralis*, pert. to the thigh]. Between the thighs.

interference [″ + *ferire*, to strike]. Clashing or colliding.

interference of impulses. Condition in which two excitation waves, upon approaching each other and meeting in any part of the heart, are mutually extinguished.

interferometer (ĭn″tĕr-fĕr-ŏm′ĕ-tĕr). Optical device that acts on the interference of two beams of light. This permits examination of the structure of spectral lines. Also used in examining prisms of lenses for faults.

interferon (ĭn-tĕr-fēr′ŏn). ABBR: INF. A group of proteins released by white blood cells and fibroblasts when the invading organism is a virus. They inhibit production of the virus within infected cells, prevent the spread of the virus to other cells, enhance the activity of macrophages, natural killer cells, and cytotoxic T cells, and may inhibit the growth of certain tumor cells.

   i., alpha. A Type I INF released by all leukocytes when stimulated by a virus.

   i., beta. A Type I INF released by fibroblasts stimulated by invasion of a virus.

   i., gamma. A Type II (immune) INF released by T lymphocytes in response to stimulation by multiple antigens or mitogens. Macrophages stimulated by gamma INF are called "angry macrophages" because of their heightened phagocytic ability.

interferon Alfa-n3. An antiviral medicine. Previously used name: leukocyte interferon. Trade name is Wellferon.

interfibrillar, interfibrillary (ĭn″tĕr-fĭb′rĭ-lăr, -rĭ-lăr″ē) [″ + *fibrilla*, a small fiber]. Between fibrils.

interfilamentous (ĭn″tĕr-fĭl″ă-mĕn′tŭs) [″ + *filamentum*, filament]. Between filaments.

interfilar (ĭn-tĕr-fī′lăr) [″ + *filum*, thread]. Between the fibrils of a reticulum.

interfilar mass. The fluid portion of the protoplasm.

interganglionic [″ + *ganglion*, a swelling]. Between ganglia.

intergemmal (ĭn″tĕr-jĕm′ăl) [″ + *gemma*, bud]. Between taste buds.

interglobular [″ + *globulus*, globule]. Between globules.

interglobular dentin. Dentin of the tooth that contains spaces or hypomineralized areas between mineralized globules or calcospherites.

interglobular spaces. Gaps in dentin due to failure of calcification. SYN: *Czermak's spaces*.

intergluteal (ĭn″tĕr-gloo′tē-ăl) [″ + Gr. *gloutos*, buttock]. Between the buttocks.

intergonial. Anthropometric line between the tips of the two angles of the mandible.

intergyral (ĭn″tĕr-jī′răl) [″ + Gr. *gyros*, circle]. Between the cerebral gyri.

interhemicerebral (ĭn″tĕr-hĕm″ĭ-sĕr′ē-brăl) [″ + Gr. *hemi*, half, + L. *cerebrum*, brain]. Intercerebral.

interictal (ĭn″tĕr-ĭk′tăl) [″ + *ictus*, a blow]. Between seizures.

interior [L. *internus*, within]. The internal portion or area of something; situated within.

interischiadic (ĭn″tĕr-ĭs″kē-ăd′ĭk) [L. *inter*, between, + Gr. *ischion*, hip]. Between the ischia of the pelvis.

interkinesis (ĭn″tĕr-kĭ-nē′sĭs) [″ + Gr. *kinesis*, movement]. Interval between first and second meiotic division of cells.

interlabial. Between the lips or any two labia.

interlamellar (ĭn″tĕr-lă-mĕl′ăr) [″ + *lamella*, layer]. Between lamellae.

interleukin-1. ABBR: IL-1. A monokine, q.v., or chemical mediator that permits the cells of the immune system to "talk" to one another, coordinating the immune response. IL-1 is released by macrophages, q.v., and activates other cells by binding at specific receptor sites. It helps regulate the activities of T lymphocytes, particularly helper/T4 cells, q.v. IL-1 is also responsible for the systemic effects of inflammation: fever, increased production and release of leukocytes, especially lymphocytes, and decreased levels of iron and other metals in the blood. It also acts as an OAF, q.v. The factor called endogenous pyrogen is actually IL-1. All of the specific activities of IL-1 under different conditions are still being investigated. SYN: *lymphocyte activating factor.*

interleukin-2. ABBR: IL-2. A lymphokine released primarily by T4 lymphocytes as the result of stimulation by IL-1 and a foreign antigen. IL-2 stimulates the production of IL-2 receptors on the surface of other immune effector cells, increasing the growth and activity of macrophages, B lymphocytes, natural killer cells and other white blood cells as part of the immune response. In vitro incubation of IL-2 with peripheral T lymphocytes produces lymphokine-activated killer (LAK) cells that have been used in the treatment of cancer to kill tumor cells. IL-2 therapy has increased the survival time in patients with renal cell carcinoma and metastatic melanoma. The toxic side effects are less if the drug is given by continuous infusion.

interleukin-3. ABBR: IL-3. A lymphokine, q.v., produced by T cells whose activities have not yet been completely identified. It is known to stimulate proliferation and differentiation of monocytes and lymphocytes and, possibly, some precursors of blood cells in the bone marrow.

interleukin-6. ABBR: IL-6. A lymphokine, q.v., that works with IL-2 to stimulate the growth and maturation of T lymphocytes.

interlobar (ĭn″tĕr-lō′băr) [″ + *lobus*, lobe]. Between lobes.

interlobitis (ĭn″tĕr-lō-bī′tĭs) [″ + ″ + Gr. *itis*, inflammation]. Inflammation of the pleura separating the pulmonary lobes.

interlobular (ĭn″tĕr-lŏb′ū-lăr) [″ + *lobulus*, lobule]. Between lobules of an organ.

interlobular emphysema. Air between the lobes of the lung.

intermalleolar (ĭn″tĕr-mă-lē′ō-lăr) [″ + *malleolus*, little hammer]. Between the malleoli.

intermammary (ĭn″tĕr-măm′ă-rē) [″ + *mamma*, breast]. Between the breasts.

intermamillary (ĭn″tĕr-măm′ĭ-lăr″ē) [″ +

mammilla, nipple]. Between the nipples of the breasts.

intermarriage [″ + *maritare*, to marry]. 1. Marriage between persons of two distinct populations. SEE: *miscegenation.* 2. Marriage between related individuals.

intermaxillary [″ + *maxilla*, jawbone]. 1. Between the two maxillae, as in intermaxillary suture. 2. Formerly meaning between the two jaws.

intermediary (ĭn″tĕr-mē′dē-ăr-ē) [″ + *medius*, middle]. 1. Situated between two bodies. 2. Occurring between two periods of time.

intermediary metabolism. The series of intermediate compounds formed during digestion before the final excretion or oxidation products are formed or eliminated from the body.

intermediate (ĭn″tĕr-mē′dē-ĭt) [″ + *medius*, middle]. Between the two extremes; after the beginning and before the end.

intermedin (ĭn″tĕr-mē′dĭn). A substance secreted by the pars intermedia of the pituitary. It is important in controlling pigment cells of the skin of some reptiles, fish, and amphibians.

intermediolateral [″ + ″ + *latus*, side]. Intermediate but not central.

intermedius (ĭn″tĕr-mē′dē-ŭs) [″ + *medius*, middle]. The middle of three structures.

intermembranous (ĭn″tĕr-mĕm′brā-nŭs) [″ + *membrana*, membrane]. Between membranes.

intermeningeal (ĭn″tĕr-mĕn-ĭn′jē-ăl) [″ + *meninx*, membrane]. Between the meninges.

intermenstrual (ĭn″tĕr-mĕn′stroo-ăl) [″ + Gr. *men*, month]. Between the menses or menstrual periods.

intermetacarpal (ĭn″tĕr-mĕt″ă-kăr′păl) [″ + Gr. *meta*, beyond, + *karpos*, wrist]. Between the carpal bones.

intermission [″ + *mittere*, to send]. 1. Interval between two paroxysms of a disease. 2. Temporary cessation of symptoms.

intermittence [″ + *mittere*, to send]. 1. Condition marked by intermissions in the course of a disease or of a process. 2. A loss of one or more pulse beats.

intermittent (ĭn″tĕr-mĭt′ĕnt). Suspending activity at intervals. Coming and going.

intermittent fever. Fever in which there is complete absence of symptoms between paroxysms. SEE: *malaria; undulant fever.*

intermittent positive-pressure breathing. ABBR: IPPB. Method used to assist breathing. The patient breathes through a mask connected to a device that produces intermittent positive air pressure. When the pressure is increased, the lungs are inflated; then the pressure is released and the patient exhales.

intermittent pulse. Pulse in which a beat is dropped at intervals.

intermural (ĭn″tĕr-mū′răl) [L. *inter,* between, + *murus,* wall]. Between the walls or sides of an organ.

intermuscular [″ + *musculus,* muscle]. Between muscles.

intern (ĭn′tĕrn) [L. *internus,* within]. Physician or surgeon on a hospital staff, usually a recent graduate receiving a year of postgraduate training prior to being eligible to be licensed to practice medicine. SEE: *extern.*

internal [L. *internus,* within]. Within the body. Within or on the inside; enclosed; inward. Opposite of external.

internal bleeding. Hemorrhage from an internal organ or site, esp. the gastrointestinal tract.

internal ear. The vestibule, semicircular canals, and cochlea of the ear.

internal injury. Any injury not visible from the outside, as injury to the organs occupying the thoracic, abdominal, or cranial cavities.

SYM: Vary with structures involved. Ordinarily, profound shock. Patient is pale, cold, perspiring freely, has an anxious expression, may be semicomatose. Pain is usually intense at first, and may continue or gradually diminish as patient grows worse. In severe injuries, pain may not be manifested. Pulse is very feeble, fast, often irregular. Patient may be very restless, breathless, and usually has shallow respiration.

F.A.: Above all, patient should be kept very quiet and comfortably warm but not hot. Do not give anything by mouth. Do not give stimulants because they may exaggerate bleeding. The patient's vital signs are monitored carefully and frequently for evidence of shock and altered cerebral function. If patient is in shock, shoulders should be lowered and the lower extremities elevated at least 45°.

internalization (ĭn-tĕr″năl-ĭ-zā′shŭn). The unconscious mental mechanism in which the values and standards of society and one's parents are taken as one's own.

internal medicine. That branch of medicine that treats diseases of the internal organs by other than surgical means. In effect, internal medicine is based on experimental work in physiology and physiochemistry and the implication that investigators and practitioners in the specialty have special training, knowledge, and skills.

internal secretion. Secretion of the ductless glands, which, entering the bloodstream, activates other glands and organs. SYN:

INTERNATIONAL SYMBOL OF ACCESS

hormones. SEE: *ductless glands; endocrine; hormone; secretion.*

internarial (ĭn″tĕr-nā′rē-ăl) [L. *inter,* between, + *nares,* nostrils]. Between the nares.

internasal (ĭn″tĕr-nā′zăl) [″ + *nasus,* nose]. Between the nasal bones.

internatal (ĭn″tĕr-nā′tăl) [″ + *nates,* buttocks]. Between the buttocks.

International Association for Dental Research. ABBR: I.A.D.R. An association founded in 1920 to provide research in dental science and application of research to develop better treatment and oral health.

International Classification of Diseases. ABBR: ICD. A multivolume codification of diseases, injuries, causes of death, and procedures including operations and diagnostic and nonsurgical procedures. ICD's principal use is to standardize reporting of illness, death, and procedures. The publication is essential to the compilation of statistical information about diseases in a format that allows international comparison of those data.

International Classification of Impairment, Disability and Handicap. ABBR: ICIDH. A standard originated by the World Health Organization for classifying and coding conditions requiring rehabilitation.

International Symbol of Access. A symbol used to identify buildings and facilities that are barrier-free and therefore accessible to disabled persons with restricted mobility, including wheelchair users. SEE: illus.

International System of Units. ABBR: SI. An internationally standardized system of units. The basic quantity measured and the names of the units are meter (length), kilogram (mass), second (time), ampere (electric current), kelvin (temperature), candela (luminous intensity), and mole (amount of a substance). All other units of measurement are derived from these seven basic units.

SEE: *Units of Measurement* in *Appendix.*

international unit. ABBR: I.U. An internationally accepted amount of a substance. Usually this form of expressing quantity is used for fat-soluble vitamins and some hormones, enzymes, and biologicals such as vaccines. These units are defined by the International Conference for Unification of Formulae.

interneuron (ĭn″tĕr-nū′rŏn) [L. *inter*, between, + Gr. *neuron*, nerve]. A neuron located between neurons in a chain of neurons.

internist. A physician who specializes in internal medicine.

internode [″ + *nodus*, knot]. Space between adjacent nodes.

internship (ĭn′tĕrn-shĭp). The period an intern spends in training, usually in a hospital.

internuclear (ĭn″tĕr-nū′klē-ăr) [″ + *nucleus*, a kernel]. 1. Between nuclei. 2. Between outer and inner nuclear layers of the retina.

internuncial (ĭn″tĕr-nŭn′shē-ăl) [″ + *nuncius*, messenger]. Acting as a connecting medium.

internuncial neuron. Neuron situated between two other neurons in a neural pathway.

internus (ĭn-tĕr′nŭs) [L., within]. Internal.

interocclusal (ĭn″tĕr-ŏ-kloo′zăl) [L. *inter*, between, + *occlusio*, a shutting up]. Between the occlusal surfaces or cusps of opposing teeth of the maxillary and mandibular arches. SEE: *interdental; interproximal.*

interoceptive [L. *internus*, within, + *capere*, to take]. In nerve physiology, concerned with sensations arising within the body itself, as distinguished from those arising outside the body.

interoceptor (ĭn″tĕr-ō-sĕp′tor). A receptor activated by stimuli within the body.

   i., general. An end-organ carrying sensations of hunger, thirst, visceral pain, nausea, sexual and circulatory sensations.

   i., special. A receptor for smell and taste.

interofective (ĭn″tĕr-ō-fĕk′tĭv) [″ + *afficere*, to influence]. Pert. to that which concerns the interior of an organism.

interoinferior (ĭn″tĕr-ō-ĭn-fē′rē-or) [″ + *inferus*, below]. Pert. to an inward and downward position.

interolivary [L. *inter*, between, + *oliva*, olive]. Between the olivary bodies.

interorbital [″ + *orbita*, orbit]. Between the orbits.

interosseous [″ + *os*, bone] (pl. *interossei*). Situated or occurring between bones, as muscles, ligaments, or vessels; specific muscles of the hands and feet.

interpalpebral (ĭn″tĕr-păl′pĕ-brăl) [″ + *palpebra*, eyelid]. Between the eyelids.

interparietal (ĭn″tĕr-pă-rī′ĕ-tăl) [″ + *paries*, wall]. 1. Between walls. 2. Between the parietal bones. 3. Between the parietal lobes of the cerebrum.

interparietal bone. Squamous portion of the occipital bone.

interparietal suture. Sagittal suture.

interparoxysmal (ĭn″tĕr-păr″ŏk-sĭz′măl) [″ + Gr. *paroxysmos*, spasm]. Between paroxysms.

interpeduncular (ĭn″tĕr-pĕ-dŭnk′ū-lăr) [L. *inter*, between, + *pedunculus*, peduncle]. Between peduncles.

interpersonal. Concerning the relations and interactions between persons.

interphalangeal (ĭn″tĕr-fă-lăn′jē-ăl) [″ + Gr. *phalanx*, closely knit row]. In a joint between two phalanges.

interphase. 1. The resting stage of a cell between divisions. 2. The area or zone where two phases of a substance, such as a gas and a liquid, contact each other.

interpolar (ĭn″tĕr-pō′lăr) [″ + *polus*, pole]. Between two poles.

interpolar path. Path of galvanic current through tissues between poles.

interpolation (ĭn-tĕr″pō-lā′shŭn). 1. In surgery, the transfer of tissues from one site to another. 2. In statistics, the calculation of an intermediate value from the observed values larger and smaller than the unknown intermediate.

interposed (ĭn′tĕr-pōzd). Inserted between parts.

interposition (ĭn″tĕr-pō-zĭsh′ŭn). The state of being interposed.

interpretation. In psychotherapy, the deeper analysis of the meaning and significance of what the patient says or does. It is explained to the patient in order to help provide insight.

interproximal [″ + *proximus*, next]. Between two adjoining surfaces.

interproximal radiograph. An intraoral radiograph taken, using bitewing film, to show the interproximal surfaces of teeth and the supporting interdental bone.

interproximal space. Triangular space between two adjacent teeth.

interpubic (ĭn-tĕr-pū′bĭk) [″ + *pubes*, pubes]. Between the pubic bones.

interpupillary [″ + *pupilla*, pupil]. Between the pupils.

interpupillary distance. Distance between centers of the pupils of the eyes.

interradicular. Between the roots of teeth; the furcation area.

interradicular bone. The alveolar bone between the roots of multirooted teeth.

interradicular fibers. The collagen fibers of the periodontal ligament in the interradicular area, attaching the tooth to alveolar bone.

interrenal (ĭn″tĕr-rē′năl) [L. *inter,* between, + *ren,* kidney]. Between the kidneys.

interrogatory. In law, a written question sent by plaintiff or defendant to discover additional information about a person, party, event, or subject at issue in a lawsuit.

interscapilium (ĭn″tĕr-skă-pĭl′ē-ŭm) [″ + *scapula,* shoulder blade]. Area between the shoulders or scapulae. SYN: *interscapular.*

interscapular. Between the scapulae.

interscapular reflex. Scapular muscular contraction following percussion or stimulus between the scapulae.

interscapulum (ĭn-tĕr-skăp′ū-lŭm). Section of back between the shoulder blades. SYN: *interscapilium.*

intersection. The site where one structure crosses another or joins a similar structure.

intersegmental (ĭn″tĕr-sĕg-mĕn′tăl) [″ + *segmentum,* a portion]. Between segments.

interseptal (ĭn″tĕr-sĕp′tăl) [″ + *saeptum,* a partition]. Between two septa.

intersex (ĭn′tĕr-sĕks). An individual having both male and female characteristics. The term has some descriptive but little or no diagnostic value. Determination of sex in individuals who appear to have both male and female characteristics is a complex task. The diagnosis should be made after careful study of the chromosomes and of the gross and microscopic anatomical findings. SEE: *hermaphrodite; hermaphroditism.*

   i., female. A genetic female with external sexual characteristics of both sexes.

   i., male. A genetic male with external sexual characteristics of both sexes.

   i., true. The genetic sex of the individual may be either male or female and the sexual characteristics are of both sexes.

intersexuality (ĭn″tĕr-sĕks″ū-ăl′ĭ-tē). Varying expression of male and female physical and sexual characteristics in the same individual. SEE: *intersex.*

interspace. Space between two similar parts, as between two ribs.

interspinal (ĭn-tĕr-spī′năl) [″ + *spinalis,* pert. to the spine]. Between two spinous processes of the spine.

interstice (ĭn-tĕr′stĭs) [L. *interstitium*]. Space or gap in a tissue or structure of an organ. SYN: *interstitium.*

interstitial (ĭn″tĕr-stĭsh′ăl). 1. Placed or lying between. 2. Pert. to interstices or spaces within an organ or tissue.

interstitial cells of testes. Cells of Leydig located in groups between the seminiferous tubules. They produce the hormone (testosterone) of the testes.

interstitial cell-stimulating hormone. ABBR: ICSH. Luteinizing hormone. SEE: *hormone, luteinizing.*

interstitial cystitis. Inflammation and irritation of the bladder. This disease of unknown etiology is most commonly seen in middle-aged women.

   SYM: Frequent urination due to scar tissue causing contraction of the bladder; dysuria, and hematuria. NOTE: Hunner's ulcer of the bladder is thought to have the same pathological basis as this disease.

   TREAT: Dilation of bladder under anesthesia; anticholinergic drugs; and instillation of dimethyl sulfoxide in the bladder.

interstitial fluid. Fluid that surrounds cells.

interstitial lung disorders. ABBR: ILD. A large group of diseases with different causes but with the same or similar clinical and pathological changes. These are due to chronic, nonmalignant, noninfectious diseases of the lower respiratory tract characterized by inflammation and disruption of the walls of the alveoli. This manifests clinically as a limitation in the ability of the lungs to transfer oxygen from the alveoli to the pulmonary capillary bed. Patients with these disorders are dyspneic first in connection with exercise and, as the disease condition progresses, even at rest.

   There are almost 200 different types of ILD, not all of which have a known cause. Known causes include inhalation of irritating or toxic environmental agents such as organic dusts, fumes, vapors, aerosols, and inorganic dusts; drugs; radiation; poisons; and following recovery from adult respiratory distress syndrome. SEE: *idiopathic pulmonary fibrosis.*

interstitial tissue. Intercellular connective tissue.

interstitium (ĭn″tĕr-stĭsh′ē-ŭm) [L.]. The very small space between body parts, tissues, or cells.

intersystole (ĭn″tĕr-sĭs′tō-lē) [L. *inter,* between, + Gr. *systole,* contraction]. Period between the end of the atrial systole and the commencement of the ventricular systole.

intertarsal (ĭn″tĕr-tăr′săl) [″ + Gr. *tarsos,* a broad, flat surface]. Between the tarsal bones of the foot.

intertransverse (ĭn″tĕr-trăns-vĕrs′) [″ + *transversus,* turned across]. Between vertebrae or joining the transverse processes of a vertebra.

intertriginous (ĭn″tĕr-trĭj′ĭ-nŭs). Having the character of intertrigo or having intertrigo.

intertrigo (ĭn″tĕr-trī′gō) [″ + *terere,* to rub]. A superficial dermatitis in the folds of the skin. SEE: *erythema intertrigo.*

intertrochanteric (ĭn″tĕr-trō″kăn-tĕr′ĭk) [″ + Gr. *trochanter,* trochanter]. Situated between the greater and lesser trochanters of the femur.

intertrochanteric line. Ridge between the greater and lesser trochanters of the femur on the posterior aspect of the bone.

intertubular (ĭn″tĕr-tū′bū-lăr) [″ + *tubulus*, tubule]. Between or among tubules.

interureteral, interureteric (ĭn″tĕr-ū-rē′tĕr-ăl, ĭn″tĕr-ū″rĕ-tĕr′ĭk) [″ + Gr. *oureter*, ureter]. Between the two ureters.

intervaginal (ĭn″tĕr-văj′ĭ-năl) [″ + *vagina*, sheath]. Between sheaths.

interval [″ + *vallum*, a breastwork]. 1. Space or time between two objects or periods. 2. Break in the course of disease or between paroxysms.

    i., atriocarotid. In a venous pulse tracing, the interval between onset of the presystolic wave (a) and the systolic (c) wave. It indicates the time required for impulses to travel from the S-A node to the ventricle, normally about 0.2 sec.

    i., A-V. Interval between the beginning of atrial systole and ventricular systole, measured in man from an electrocardiogram.

    i., cardioarterial. Time between the apex beat and radial pulsation.

    i., focal. Distance between the anterior and posterior focal points of the eyes.

    i., isometric. Distance between onset of ventricular systole and opening of the semilunar valves. SYN: *i., presphygmic.*

    i., lucid. Brief remission of symptoms in a psychosis.

    i., passive. The rest period of the heart.

    i., postsphygmic. Interval between closure of the semilunar valves and opening of semilunar valves and opening of atrioventricular valves.

    i., P-R. In the electrocardiogram, period between the onset of the P wave and the beginning of the QRS complex.

    i., presphygmic. Brief period between the ventricular systole and opening of the semilunar valves. SYN: *i., isometric.*

    i., Q-R. In the electrocardiogram, period between the onset of the QRS complex and the peak of the R wave.

    i., QRS. On ECG, interval between the beginning of the Q wave and the end of the S wave. Normal is less than 0.12 sec.

    i., QRST. The ventricular complex of the electrocardiogram. SEE: *electrocardiogram* for illus.

    i., Q-T. On ECG, interval between the beginning of the Q wave and the end of the T wave.

intervalvular (ĭn″tĕr-văl′vū-lăr) [L. *inter*, between, + *valva*, leaf of a folding door]. Between valves, esp. the heart valves.

intervascular [″ + *vasculum*, a vessel]. Situated between blood vessels.

intervention (ĭn″tĕr-vĕn′shŭn). Taking actions so as to modify an effect.

    i., crisis. In psychiatry, the immediate institution of all appropriate forms of therapy for an individual experiencing a personal crisis.

    i., nursing. SEE: *nursing intervention.*

interventricular [″ + *ventriculum*, a small cavity]. Between the ventricles.

intervertebral [″ + *vertebra*, joint]. Situated between two adjacent vertebrae.

intervertebral disk. Broad and flattened disk of fibrocartilage between the bodies of vertebrae. SEE: *herniated disk.*

intervillous (ĭn″tĕr-vĭl′ŭs) [″ + *villus*, tuft]. Between villi.

intestinal [L. *intestinum*, intestine]. Pert. to the intestines. SEE: *digestion; intestine.*

intestinal bypass surgery. Production of controlled intestinal malabsorption by surgically short-circuiting the small intestine. It is done by anastomosing the jejunum to the ileum and removing the small intestine between the anastomotic sites. This procedure is used in treatment of massive obesity.

intestinal flora. Bacteria present in the intestines. The chemical nature of the contents of the intestines varies considerably with respect to the portion of the tract being considered. There are no bacteria in the intestines at birth, but they are present very shortly thereafter. Favorable bacteria may protect the body from invasion by unfavorable ones that cannot thrive in an acid condition. Also, certain medicines, particularly antibiotics, may cause drastic alterations in the number and kinds of bacteria present.

intestinal gases. Gaseous compounds, such as carbon dioxide, hydrogen, methane, methylmercaptan, and hydrogen sulfide, present in the intestinal tract. They are produced by digestive processes. SEE: *digestion; flatus.*

intestinal juice. An imprecise term used to denote the liquid substances secreted into the intestine, esp. the small intestine. It contains a number of enzymes, peptidases, lipase, maltase, and sucrase. Each is important in digesting food.

intestinal obstruction. Blockage of the lumen of the intestine.

    Acute: Small intestine usually involved. Due to intussusception, strangulation, volvulus (twists), foreign bodies, adhesions, tumors, stricture, and gallstones in intestines. Auscultation of the abdomen may reveal a high-pitched tinkle or no sound at all.

    SYM: Pain localized and intense. Temperature subnormal or normal; vomiting, constipation, and distention of abdomen.

    TREAT: Relief of intestinal and gastric distention by use of gastric and intestinal suction tubes. Fluid balance must be maintained. Surgical exploration may be necessary to determine the cause. Parenteral antibodies are indicated for peritonitis.

Chronic: Involves large intestine. Due to stricture, inflammation, abscesses, tumors, fecal matter or chronic peritonitis; gallstones may obstruct feces. Gradual constipation, pain becoming more severe in a few days followed by acute symptoms. SEE: *Nursing Diagnoses in Appendix.*

intestinal perforation. Abdominal crisis due to escape of contents of perforated intestines into the peritoneal cavity. SEE: *perforation of stomach or intestine.*

intestinal putrefaction. The chemical changes by bacteria in the intestine, forming the following: indole, skatole, paracresol, phenol, phenylpropionic acid, phenylacetic acid, paraoxyphenylacetic acid, hydroparacumaric acid, fatty acids, carbon dioxide, hydrogen, methane, methylmercaptan, and sulfurated hydrogen.

intestinal reflex. Intestinal contraction and relaxation above a portion of bowel that is stimulated.

intestinal tubes. Flexible tubes, usually made of plastic or rubber, placed in the intestinal tract for the purpose of sucking gas, fluid, or solids from the stomach or intestines; or for administering fluids, electrolytes, or nutrients to the patient. The tubes may be passed through the nose, mouth, or anus, or through a colostomy opening.

NURSING IMPLICATIONS: When an intestinal tube is inserted, the nurse must aid its movement into the intestinal tract. The patient is usually placed on the right side for one-half hour, then the left side for one-half hour, and then on the back. These position changes, as well as ambulation, will facilitate movement of the tube into the intestinal tract.

Because the tube may drain feces, drainage should be kept from the patient's view. Frequent oral hygiene is needed to prevent oral ulceration because the patient will not be taking fluids by mouth. When the tube is removed, the patient's emotional reaction must be considered. Immediate oral hygiene is performed, particularly since drainage from the tube can easily cause the patient to become nauseated.

While the tube is in, teach the patient not to mouth breathe or swallow air. This enhances entry of air into the gastrointestinal tract and works counter to the principle of intestinal tubes and drainage.

intestine (ĭn-tĕs′tĭn) [L. *intestinum*]. The alimentary canal extending from the pylorus to the anus. It is divided into the small intestine and large intestine or colon. The length of the intestine given is based on measurements made at autopsy. During life the small intestine is approx. 7 meters (23 feet) long. The total surface of the inside of the small intestine is estimated to be 800 square meters (8611 square feet or 956.8 square yards).

PALPATION: Fecal accumulations feel similar to tumors but are hard and resistant; however, if one finger is pressed steadily upon them for one or two minutes, they will indent. They most frequently collect in descending colon.

PERCUSSION: In normal conditions, the large intestine furnishes a more amphoric percussion sound than the stomach. When the large intestine is filled with liquid or solid accumulations, the situation of these accumulations can be marked out on the surface by dullness on percussion. Because these accumulations most frequently occur in the descending colon, the percussion sound over this portion is usually less resonant than over the ascending or transverse colon.

i., large. The large intestine extends from the ileum to the anus and consists of the cecum with vermiform appendix, colon, and rectum. The mucous coat resembles that of small intestine, although glands are smaller. The large intestine resorbs fluid from the intestinal contents. If the bowel is hyperactive, diarrhea is likely to occur.

The beginning of the large intestine is the cecum, a pouch situated on the right side, adjoining the ascending colon. Attached to the cecum is the vermiform appendix, about 7.5 to 10.4 cm (3 to 4 in.) long. The colon is approx. 1.5 meters (5 ft) in length. The first portion of ascending colon extends from the cecum to the undersurface of the liver, where it turns to the left as the transverse colon. Its bend is the right colic or hepatic flexure. The transverse colon passes horizontally to the left to the region of the spleen, where it turns downward as the descending colon. This turn is the splenic flexure. The descending colon continues downward on the left side of the abdomen until it reaches the pelvic brim and curves like the letter S and is placed in front of the sacrum to become the rectum. This S-shaped section is known as the sigmoid colon. The rectum, about 10.2 to 12.7 cm (4 to 5 in.) long, passes downward to terminate in the lower opening of the tract, the anus or anal opening.

i., small. The small intestine begins with the duodenum, approx. 20.3 to 25.4 cm (8 to 10 in.) long, which receives the food mass from the stomach through the pylorus, the bile from the liver and gallbladder, and the pancreatic juice from the pancreas. It connects with the jejunum, about 2.8 meters (9 feet) long. The jejunum, in turn, joins the ileum or twisted intestine, about 4.2 meters (13.7 ft) long, which is attached to the large intestine by the ileocecal or colic valve, which controls passage of food into the large intestine.

In the wall of the small intestine are the Brunner's glands, intestinal glands (crypts of Lieberkühn), blood and lymph vessels (lacteals), and lymphatic tissue in the form of solitary nodules or aggregated nodules (Peyer's patches). The inner surface is thrown into folds (circular folds). Lining the entire surface are minute fingerlike villi through which the products of digestion (simple sugars, amino acids, and fatty acids and carbohydrates) are absorbed. The villi are from 0.5 to 1.5 mm long and there are from 10 to 40 per sq. mm of intestinal mucosa. SEE: *digestive system* for illus.

intestinum (ĭn″tĕs-tī′nŭm) [L.] (pl. *intestina*). Intestine.

  i. crassum. [NA] The large intestine.

  i. rectum. The rectum.

  i. tenue. [NA] The small intestine.

intima (ĭn′tĭ-mă) [L.]. [NA] Innermost coat of a structure, as a blood vessel. SYN: *tunica intima.*

intimal (ĭn′tĭ-măl). Pert. to the inner coat of a blood vessel, the intima.

intimitis (ĭn″tĭ-mī′tĭs) [L. *intima*, innermost, + Gr. *itis*, inflammation]. Inflammation of an intima.

intolerance [L. *in-*, not, + *tolerare*, to bear]. Inability to endure or incapacity for bearing pain or the effects of a drug or other substance.

intorsion (ĭn-tor′shŭn) [L. *in*, toward, + *torsio*, twisting]. Rotation of the eye inward toward the nose on the anterior-posterior axis of the eye. In this condition, twelve o'clock on the corneal margin would be closer to the nose than normal.

intoxicant (ĭn-tŏks′ĭ-kănt). An agent that produces intoxication.

intoxication [L. *in*, in, + Gr. *toxikon*, poison]. 1. State of being intoxicated, esp. of being poisoned by a drug or toxic substance. 2. Intoxicated from overindulgence in alcoholic beverages.

The determination of alcohol content of the blood (i.e., ethyl alcohol, the alcohol present in commercial beverages such as beer, wine, and whiskey) is frequently of value in the diagnosis of intoxication from alcohol, esp. in differentiating other disorders. Normally the alcohol content of body tissues and fluids is negligible. Upon ingestion, alcoholic fluids are absorbed slowly or quickly depending upon the amount swallowed, presence of food in the stomach, and rate of gastric emptying. The amount of al-

cohol found in each ml of blood will also depend upon body size. Thus if 70-kg (154-lb) and 90-kg (198-lb) individuals drink the same amount of alcohol in the same time and under similar conditions, the concentration of alcohol in each ml of blood will be least in the person who weighs the most.

The amount of alcohol present in expired air will also provide an estimate of the alcohol content of the blood. The amount of alcohol present in the blood does not provide completely valid information about the degree of intoxication because of the ability of the central nervous system to adapt to alcohol. SEE: *alcoholism; Breathalyzer.*

  i., water. Intoxication resulting from excessive intake or undue retention of water.

intra- [L.]. Prefix meaning within.

intra-abdominal [L. *intra*, within, + *abdomen*, belly]. Within the abdomen.

intra-acinous (ĭn-tră-ăs′ĭ-nŭs) [″ + *acinus*, grape]. Within an acinus.

intra-aortic balloon counterpulsation. ABBR: IABC. The use of a balloon attached to a catheter inserted through the femoral artery into the descending thoracic aorta to produce alternating inflation and deflation during diastole and systole respectively. This permits lowering resistance to aortic blood flow during systole and increasing resistance during diastole. The result is to decrease the work of the heart and increase flow of blood to the coronary arteries. Inflation of the balloon is accomplished with helium. This method is useful in treating shock. SEE: *Nursing Diagnoses* in Appendix.

intra-arterial [″ + Gr. *arteria*, artery]. Within the artery(ies).

intra-articular (ĭn″tră-ăr-tĭk′ū-lăr) [″ + *articulus*, little joint]. Within a joint.

intra-atrial (ĭn″tră-ā′trē-ăl) [″ + Gr. *atrion*, hall]. Within the atrium or atria of the heart.

intrabronchial (ĭn″tră-brŏng′kē-ăl) [″ + Gr. *bronchos*, windpipe]. Within a bronchus.

intrabuccal (ĭn″tră-bŭk′ăl) [″ + *bucca*, cheek]. Within the tissue of the cheek or within the mouth.

intracanalicular (ĭn″tră-kăn″ă-lĭk′ū-lăr) [″ + *canalicularis*, pert. to a canaliculus]. Within a canaliculus.

intracapsular [″ + *capsula*, little box]. Within a capsule.

intracapsular extraction. Basic surgical technique for cataract removal. Nucleus, cortex, and capsule are removed as one unit. SEE: *cataract.*

intracapsular fracture. Fracture occurring within the capsule of a joint.

intracardiac. Within the heart.

intracarpal (ĭn″tră-kăr′păl) [″ + Gr. *kar-*

palis, pert. to the carpus]. Within the wrist.

intracartilaginous (ĭn″tră-kär″tĭ-lăj′ĭn-ŭs) [″ + *cartilago*, gristle]. Within a cartilage or cartilaginous tissue.

intracellular (ĭn″tră-sĕl′ū-lăr) [″ + *cellula*, cell]. Within cells.

intracellular fluid. SEE: *fluid, intracellular.*

intracerebellar (ĭn″tră-sĕr″ĕ-bĕl′ăr) [″ + *cerebellum*, little brain]. Within the cerebellum of the brain.

intracerebral (ĭn″tră-sĕr′ĕ-brăl) [″ + *cerebrum*, brain]. Within the main portion of the brain.

intracervical (ĭn″tră-sĕr′vĭ-kăl) [″ + *cervicalis*, pert. to the neck]. In the cervical canal of the uterus.

intracisternal (ĭn″tră-sĭs-tĕr′năl) [″ + *cisterna*, cavity]. Within a cistern of the brain.

intracostal (ĭn″tră-kŏs′tăl) [″ + *costa*, rib]. On the inner surface of a rib.

intracranial [″ + Gr. *kranion*, skull]. Within the cranium or skull.

intractable (ĭn-trăk′tă-b'l). Incurable or resistant to therapy.

intracutaneous [″ + *cutis*, skin]. Within the substance of the skin. SYN: *intradermal.*

intracutaneous injection. Hypodermic injection into the skin.

intracutaneous reaction. Reaction following injection of a substance into the skin. SYN: *intradermal reaction.*

intracystic [″ + Gr. *kystis*, bladder]. Inside a bladder or cyst.

intrad (ĭn′trăd). Inwardly; toward the inner part.

intradermal [″ + Gr. *derma*, skin]. ABBR: ID. Within the substance of the skin. SYN: *intracutaneous.*

intradermal reaction (ĭn″tră-dĕr′măl rē-ăk′shŭn) [″ + ″ + L. *re*, back, + *agere*, to do]. Reaction resulting from the injection of a reagent into substance of the skin. SYN: *intracutaneous reaction.*

intraduct (ĭn′tră-dŭkt) [″ + *ductus*, a canal]. Inside a duct.

intraduodenal (ĭn″tră-dū″ō-dē′năl) [″ + *duodeni*, twelve]. Within the duodenum.

intradural (ĭn-tră-dū′răl) [″ + *durus*, hard]. Within or enclosed by the dura mater.

intraepidermal (ĭn″tră-ĕp′ĭ-dĕr′măl) [L. *intra*, within, + Gr. *epi*, upon, + *derma*, skin]. Within the epidermis.

intraepithelial (ĭn″tră-ĕp″ĭ-thē′lē-ăl) [″ + ″ + *thele*, nipple]. Within the epithelium or located between its cells.

intrafebrile [″ + *febris*, fever]. During the febrile stage. SYN: *intrapyretic.*

intrafilar (ĭn-tră-fī′lăr) [″ + *filum*, thread]. Within a network or reticulum.

intragastric [″ + Gr. *gaster*, belly]. Within the stomach.

intragastric balloon. An inflatable device placed in the stomach in an uninflated state. In place, it is inflated. This method of treating obesity has not been effective on a long-term basis.

intragemmal (ĭn″tră-jĕm′ăl) [″ + *gemma*, bud]. Within a bud or the expanded ending of a nerve, as a taste bud.

intraglandular [″ + *glans*, acorn]. Within a gland.

intragyral (ĭn″tră-jī′răl) [″ + Gr. *gyros*, circle]. Within a gyrus of the brain.

intrahepatic (ĭn″tră-hĕ-păt′ĭk) [″ + Gr. *hepatikos*, pert. to the liver]. Within the liver.

intraintestinal [″ + *intestinum*, intestine]. Within the intestine.

intralaryngeal (ĭn″tră-lă-rĭn′jē-ăl) [″ + Gr. *larynx*, larynx]. Within the larynx.

intralesional (ĭn″tră-lē′zhŭn-ăl) [″ + *laesio*, a wound]. Within a lesion.

intraligamentary [″ + *ligamentum*, a binding]. Within the leaves of a ligament. Usually used in referring to fibroid tumors or cysts of the ovary that have grown within the broad ligament.

intraligamentous. Within a ligament.

intralingual. Within the tongue.

intralobar (ĭn″tră-lō′băr) [″ + *lobus*, a lobe]. Within a lobe.

intralobular (ĭn″tră-lŏb′ū-lăr) [″ + *lobulus*, a lobule]. Within a lobule.

intralocular (ĭn″tră-lŏk′ū-lăr) [″ + *loculus*, a cavity]. Within the cavity of any structure.

intralumbar [″ + *lumbus*, loin]. Within the lumbar region or portion of the spinal cord.

intraluminal (ĭn″tră-lū′mĭ-năl) [″ + *lumen*, light]. Within any tubular structure. SYN: *intratubal.*

intramastoiditis (ĭn″tră-măs″tŏyd-ī′tĭs) [″ + Gr. *mastos*, breast, + *eidos*, form, shape, + *itis*, inflammation]. Inflammation of the antrum and mastoid process. SYN: *endomastoiditis.*

intramedullary (ĭn″tră-mĕd′ū-lăr″ē) [″ + *medullaris*, marrow]. 1. Within the medulla oblongata of the brain. 2. Within the spinal cord. 3. Within the marrow cavity of a bone.

intramembraneous bone. Bone formed directly from a condensation of mesenchyme which differentiates into osteoblasts. It forms layers of bone without any cartilage model; includes bones of the face and cranium.

intramural [″ + *murus*, a wall]. Within the walls of a hollow organ or cavity.

intramuscular [″ + *musculus*, a muscle]. ABBR: I.M. Within a muscle.

intramuscular injection. Injection of drugs into a muscle.

intranasal [″ + *nasus*, nose]. Within the

nasal cavity.

intranatal ["   +   *natalis*, birth]. Occurring during birth.

intraocular ["   +   *oculus*, eye]. Within the eyeball.

intraoperative (ĭn"tră-ŏp'ĕr-ā"tĭv) [L. *intra*, within,   +   *operativus*, working]. Occurring during surgery.

intraoral ["   +   *oralis*, pert. to the mouth]. Within the mouth.

intraorbital ["   +   *orbita*, mark of a wheel]. Within the orbit.

intraosseous (ĭn"tră-ŏs'ē-ŭs) ["   +   *os*, bone]. Within the bone substance.

intraosseous infusion. Infusion of fluids, blood, or medications in an emergency situation in which intravenous access is not available, into the tibia in young children. SEE: illus.

intraovarian (ĭn"tră-ō-vā'rē-ăn) ["   +   *ovarium*, ovary]. Within the ovary.

intraparietal (ĭn"tră-pă-rī'ĕ-tăl) ["   +   *paries*, wall]. 1. Within the parietal lobe of the cerebrum. 2. Intramural.

intrapartal. The period from the onset of labor to its termination, marked by delivery of the placenta.

intrapartum (ĭn"tră-păr'tŭm) ["   +   *partus*, birth]. Happening during childbirth.

intrapelvic (ĭn"tră-pĕl'vĭk) ["   +   *pelvis*, basin]. Within the pelvis.

intraperitoneal ["   +   Gr. *peritonaion*, peritoneum]. Within the peritoneal cavity.

intraplacental (ĭn"tră-plă-sĕn'tăl) ["   +   *placenta*, a flat cake]. Within the placenta.

intrapleural ["   +   Gr. *pleura*, rib]. Within the pleural cavity.

intrapontine (ĭn"tră-pŏn'tīn) ["   +   *pons*, bridge]. Within the pons varolii.

intrapsychic, intrapsychical (ĭn"tră-sī'kĭk, -kĭ-kăl) ["   +   Gr. *psyche*, mind]. Having a mental origin or basis, such as conflicts and complexes.

intrapulmonary ["   +   *pulmo*, lung]. Within the lung substance.

intrapyretic (ĭn"tră-pī-rĕt'ĭk) ["   +   Gr. *pyretos*, fever]. During the period of fever. SYN: *intrafebrile.*

intrarectal (ĭn"tră-rĕk'tăl) ["   +   *rectum*, straight]. Within the rectum.

intrarenal (ĭn"tră-rē'năl) ["   +   *renalis*, pert. to the kidney]. Within the kidney.

intraretinal (ĭn"tră-rĕt'ĭ-năl) ["   +   *retina*, retina]. Within the retina of the eye.

intrascrotal (ĭn"tră-skrō'tăl) ["   +   *scrotum*, a bag]. Within the scrotum.

intraspinal [L. *intra*, within,   +   *spina*, thorn]. 1. Ensheathed, within a sheath. 2. Within the spinal canal.

intrathecal (ĭn"tră-thē'kăl) ["   +   Gr. *theke*, sheath]. 1. Within the spinal canal. 2. Within a sheath.

intrathoracic (ĭn"tră-thō-răs'ĭk) ["   +   Gr. *thorax*, chest]. Within the thorax.

intratracheal (ĭn"tră-trăk'ē-ăl) ["   +   Gr. *tracheia*, trachea]. Introduced into, or inside, the trachea.

intratracheal anesthesia. Anesthesia administered through a catheter passed to the level of the trachea.

intratubal ["   +   *tubus*, hollow tube]. Within a tube, esp. the fallopian tube. SYN: *intraluminal.*

intratympanic (ĭn"tră-tĭm-păn'ĭk) ["   +   Gr. *tympanon*, drum]. Within the tympanic cavity.

intrauterine (ĭn"tră-ū'tĕr-ĭn) ["   +   *uterus*, womb]. Within the uterus.

intrauterine contraceptive device. ABBR: IUCD or IUD. Device made in a variety of shapes and from several different materials, including plastic and copper, and placed in the uterus for a prolonged period of time to prevent conception. Because of undesired side effects, the use of IUDs in the U.S. declined. Two IUDs are available for sale in the U.S. One is made of copper, the other contains slowly released progesterone.

intrauterine growth retardation. ABBR: IUGR. Decreased rate of growth of the fetus. This may be the result of any condition that interferes with the blood supply to or state of health of the placenta or the general health and nutrition of the mother. SEE: *prematurity.*

intravasation (ĭn-trăv"ă-zā'shŭn) ["   +   *vas*, vessel]. Passage into the blood vessels of matter formed outside of them through traumatic or pathological lesions.

intravascular. Within blood vessels.

intravenous (ĭn-tră-vē'nŭs) ["   +   *vena*, vein]. ABBR: I.V. Within or into a vein.

intravenous feeding. Providing total nutritional requirements intravenously; essential in treating some diseases. It is accomplished by carefully controlling the composition of fluid given with respect to total calories derived from protein hydrolysate and dextrose, and the electrolytes, minerals, and vitamins. Patients have been maintained for months on nothing but the nutrients and fluids given intravenously, usually through a major vein, such as the subclavian or the jugular. SEE: *parenteral hyperalimentation.*

intravenous infusion. Injection into a vein of a solution to secure an immediate result as in hemorrhage, shock, or collapse. SEE: illus.

    SOLUTIONS: Many liquid preparations are given by intravenous infusion. Those commonly used include isotonic saline, Ringer's lactated, dextrose 5% in water, and potassium chloride 0.2% in 5% dextrose.

INTRAOSSEOUS INFUSION

TIBIAL TUBEROSITY

TIBIAL TUBEROSITY

FIBULA

AVOID GROWTH PLATE (EPIPHYSIS)

TIP NEEDS TO PENETRATE CORTEX AND ENTER MARROW

FEMUR

PATELLA

ANTERIOR TIBIAL TUBEROSITY

20 GAUGE NEEDLE

EPIPHYSEAL PLATE

TIBIA

MEDULLARY CAVITY OF BONE MARROW

The quantity depends on the needs of the patient. May be given continuously at the rate of from 1 to 2 or more liters per day. In severe shock up to 4 liters may be necessary.

SITE: Usually, in the arm, the median basilic or median cephalic vein, but veins at various areas may be used. Preparation is the same as for intravenous injection, but a needle or cannula is used. The vein must be exposed if cannula is used. Introduction of solution should be at the rate required to deliver the amount of fluid and contained electrolytes, medicines, or nutrients in a prescribed time.

intravenous infusion pump. A special pump designed to provide constant but adjustable rate of flow of solutions given intravenously. The pump may work by applying intermittent pressure on the tubing carrying the solution so that the fluid is not actually in contact with the pump itself.

intravenous injection. Insertion of a needle requires a degree of skill which is easily obtained if proper instruction is available. The vein may be distended by applying a tourniquet with sufficient pressure to stop venous return but not arterial flow. The tourniquet is applied several inches above the injection site. If the patient does not have vascular collapse, the arterial pulse can be palpated; if not, the tourniquet is too tight. Application of heat to the extremity for 15 minutes

INTRAVENOUS INFUSION TECHNIQUE

TOURNIQUET

BASILIC VEIN

CEPHALIC VEIN

MEDIAN CUBITAL VEIN

CEPHALIC VEIN

NEEDLE

ACCESSORY CEPHALIC VEIN

ONE OF SEVERAL SITES FOR ENTERING VEIN

PUNCTURING LEFT ARM (ANTERIOR SURFACE)

45°

TECHNIQUE IN PUNCTURING VEIN: 1 PIERCE SKIN AT A 45° ANGLE

NEEDLE PIERCING VEIN

SKIN

VEIN   FAT

2 DECREASE ANGLE TO 15° TO PUNCTURE VEIN

PUNCTURING VEIN OF HAND

prior to starting will also help distend the vessels. Use of a needle attached to a 5- or 10-ml syringe will greatly facilitate controlling the course of the needle. It is best to insert the needle into the vein with the bevel side face out and then, after the needle is in the vein, to rotate it so that the bevel is face in. There will be resistance as the needle goes through one side of the vein wall. The vein should be entered with the needle making only a narrow angle with the long axis of the vein. This will help to prevent pushing the needle clear through the vein.

NOTE: In patients with collapsed veins it may be possible to make the veins apparent by placing a tourniquet around the arm or leg and then inserting a 23 or 25 gauge catheter into a tiny superficial vein. Instillation of sterile I.V. fluid into the vein while the catheter is in place will distend the entire larger vein proximal to the small vein. A larger needle or catheter can then be inserted into the larger vein. SEE: *cutdown; infusion, interosseous; Universal Precautions* in *Appendix.*

intravenous medication. The injection of a sterile solution of a drug or an infusion into a vein.

intravenous treatment. Intravenous injection or intravenous infusion. *Injection* is use of a hypodermic syringe to instill a single dose of medicine. An *infusion* is the introduction of a solution in a larger quantity — 250 to 500 ml by means of a bottle connected to the needle by a plastic or rubber tubing. The rate of infusion may be regulated by adjusting the number of drops per minute. Flow is usually by gravity but can be given under pressure.

Caution: I.V. infusions should be discontinued or infusion fluid replenished when the bottle being administered is depleted. If this is not done, it is possible for air to be introduced into the bloodstream. Clotting of blood in needle occurs when infusion is not continuous.

NURSING IMPLICATIONS: Insure that the correct fluid is infusing; observe the I.V. infusion site every half hour for symptoms of infiltration; calculate and maintain the correct flow rate; insure needle security and that the patient is restrained as needed to maintain the I.V. Change the dressing on the infusion site daily, according to hospital policy. Also assess the patient for complications of I.V. therapy such as circulatory or electrolyte overload, thrombophlebitis, and air embolism.

intraventricular [L. *intra,* within, + *ventriculus,* ventricle]. Within a ventricle.

intravesical (ĭn″tră-vĕs′ĭ-kăl) [″ + *vesica,*

bladder]. Within the urinary bladder.

intravital [″ + *vita*, life]. During period of life.

intravital stain. One that when introduced into a living organism is taken up by living cells.

intra vitam (ĭn″tră vī′tăm) [L.]. During life.

intravitelline (ĭn″tră-vī-tĕl′ĭn) [″ + *vitellus*, yoke]. Within the vitelline or yolk.

intravitreous (ĭn″tră-vĭt′rē-ŭs) [″ + *vitreus*, glassy]. Within the vitreous of the eye.

intrinsic [L. *intrinsicus*, on the inside]. 1. Belonging to the essential nature of a thing. It is both essential and natural, not merely apparent or accidental. SYN: *inherent; innate.* 2. In anatomy, structures belonging solely to a certain body part, as intrinsic nerves or muscles. 3. Due to causes or elements within the body, an organ, or a part.

intrinsic factor. A substance normally present in the gastric juice of humans that makes absorption of vitamin B_{12} possible. Absence of this factor leads to vitamin B_{12} deficiency and pernicious anemia.

intrinsic muscles. Muscles having their origin and insertion entirely within a structure, as the intrinsic muscles of the tongue, larynx, eye, hand or foot.

intro- [L.]. Prefix meaning in or into.

introducer [L. *intro*, into, + *ducere*, to lead]. Device for controlling, directing, and placing an intubation tube within the trachea, a blood vessel, or the heart (as in Swan-Ganz catheter placement). SYN: *intubator.*

introflexion (ĭn″trō-flĕk′shŭn) [″ + *flexus*, bent]. A bending inward.

introitus (ĭn-trō′ĭ-tŭs) [L.]. [NA] An opening or entrance into a canal or cavity, as the vagina.

i. canalis sacralis. Terminal opening of the spinal canal at the end of the sacrum.

i. laryngis. Upper opening of larynx.

i. vaginae. Exterior orifice of vagina.

introjection [″ + *jacere*, to throw]. In psychoanalysis, identification of the self with another or with some object, the victim assuming the supposed feelings of the other personality.

intromission (ĭn″trō-mĭsh′ŭn) [″ + *mittere*, to send]. An insertion or placing of one part into another, esp. insertion of the penis into the vagina.

intromittent (ĭn-trō-mĭt′ĕnt). Conveying or injecting into a cavity or body.

introns. The noncoding space between the discrete coding regions (exons) of the DNA of the gene.

Intropin. Trade name for dopamine hydrochloride.

introspection [″ + *spicere*, to look]. Looking within, esp. examination of one's own mind.

introsusception (ĭn″trō-sŭ-sĕp′shŭn) [″ + *suscipere*, to receive]. Intussusception.

introversion (ĭn″trō-vĕr′shŭn) [″ + *versio*, a turning]. 1. Turning inside out of a part or organ. 2. Condition of an introvert, q.v. Preoccupation with one's self.

introvert. 1. A personality-reaction type characterized by withdrawal from reality; fantasy formation, and stress on the subjective side of life adjustments, seen pathologically in extreme form in schizophrenia. 2. To turn one's psychic energy inward upon oneself.

intubate (ĭn′tū-bāt) [L. *in*, into, + *tuba*, a tube]. To insert a tube in a part, esp. the larynx. SEE: *catheterization.*

intubation (ĭn″tū-bā′shŭn). Insertion of a tube into any hollow organ, as into the larynx or trachea through the glottis for entrance of air, or to dilate a stricture.

POSITION: Patient, who is usually anesthetized, so held that body, neck, and head are kept in a straight line. Neck hyperextension may aid in endotracheal intubation.

i., endotracheal. Insertion of a tube through the nose or mouth into the trachea for the purpose of maintaining the airway, or in order to administer an anesthetic gas or oxygen, or to aspirate secretions.

i., nasotracheal. Insertion of a tube through the nose into the trachea. SEE: *intubation, endotracheal.*

intubator. Device used in inserting a tube into the larynx. SYN: *introducer.*

intuition. Knowing something without going through a rational process of thinking.

intumesce (ĭn-tū-mĕs′) [L. *intumescere*]. To enlarge or swell.

intumescence. 1. A swelling. 2. The process of enlarging. SYN: *tumefaction.*

intumescent (ĭn-tū-mĕs′ĕnt). Swelling or becoming enlarged.

intussusception (ĭn″tŭs-sŭ-sĕp′shŭn) [L. *intus*, within, + *suscipere*, to receive]. Invagination. The slipping of one part of an intestine into another part just below it. Noted chiefly in children, usually in the ileocecal region. SYN: *indigitation; introsusception; invagination.*

PROG: Good if surgery is performed immediately. High mortality if untreated within 24 hours. SEE: *ileus.*

intussusceptum (ĭn″tŭs-sŭ-sĕp′tŭm) [L.]. The inner segment of intestine that has been pushed into another segment.

intussuscipiens (ĭn″tŭs-sŭ-sĭp′ē-ĕns). [L.]. That portion of intestine that receives the intussusceptum.

Inuit [Eskimo people]. People native to Arctic America.

inulase (ĭn′ū-lās). An enzyme that converts

inulin into levulose.

inulin. A polysaccharide found in plants. Yields levulose when hydrolyzed. It is used to study renal function.

inunction (ĭn-ŭngk′shŭn) [L. *in*, into, + *unguere*, to anoint]. Ointment or medicated substance rubbed into the skin to secure a local or a more general systemic effect. SYN: *enepidermic.*

inustion (ĭn-ŭs′chŭn) [″ + *urere*, to burn]. 1. To apply cautery. 2. Deep cauterization.

in utero (ĭn ū′tĕr-ō) [L.]. Within the uterus.

in vacuo (ĭn văk′ū-ō) [L.]. Within a cavity or a space from which air has been exhausted.

invaginate (ĭn-văj′ĭn-āt) [L. *invaginatio*]. 1. To ensheath. 2. To insert one part of a structure within a part of the same structure. 3. In embryology, to grow in or from an ingrowth or inpocketing, esp. the ingrowth of the wall of the blastula, which results in the formation of the gastrula.

invaginated. Enclosed in a sheath; ensheathed.

invagination. The process of becoming ensheathed. SYN: *intussusception.* SEE: *evagination.*

invalid [L. *in-*, not, + *validus*, strong]. 1. Not well; weak. 2. A sickly person, particularly one confined to a bed or wheelchair.

invasion [L. *in*, into, + *vadere*, to go]. 1. That period of a disease following entrance of infective organisms and preceding the appearance of symptoms. 2. The entrance of bacteria or other infectious organisms into the body and their distribution to the tissues.

invasive. Tending to spread, esp. the tendency of a malignant process or growth to spread into healthy tissue.

invasive procedure. Procedure in which the body cavity is entered — e.g., by use of a tube, needle, device, or even by ionizing radiation — or any other invasion that could interfere with bodily function.

inventory. Any list of items, esp. items to describe an individual's personality.

invermination [″ + *vermis*, worm]. Infestation by intestinal worms.

inverse-square law. Law stating that the intensity of radiation or light at any distance is inversely proportional to the square of the distance between the irradiated surface and a point source. Thus a light with a certain intensity at a 4-foot distance will have only one-fourth that intensity at 8 feet and would be four times as intense at a 2-foot distance.

Inversine. Trade name for mecamylamine hydrochloride.

inversion (ĭn-vĕr′zhŭn) [L. *inversio*, to turn inward]. 1. Reversal of normal relationship. 2. Turning inside out of an organ, e.g., the uterus. 3. In chemistry, the process of converting sucrose (which rotates the plane of polarized light to the right) into a mixture of dextrose and levulose, which mixture rotates the plane to the left. The resulting mixture is called invert sugar, and the enzyme that catalyzes this conversion is called invertase. SEE: *enzyme.*

i., uterine. A condition in which the uterus is turned inside out so that the internal surface protrudes into the vagina or beyond it.

invert (ĭn-vĕrt′). To turn inside out or upside down.

invertase (ĭn-vĕr′tās). A sugar-splitting enzyme found in the intestinal juice. It causes the inversion of sugar. SYN: *invertin.*

invertebrate [L. *in-*, not, + *vertebratus*, vertebrate]. Without a backbone; species of animals that do not have a backbone.

invertin (ĭn-vĕr′tĭn). An intestinal ferment that converts cane sugar into invert sugar. SYN: *invertase; zymose.*

invertor (ĭn-vĕr′tor). Muscle that rotates a part inward.

invert sugar. A term usually applied to a mixture of levulose and dextrose, formed by inversion of sucrose by the enzyme invertase. SEE: *carbohydrates; inversion; sugar.*

investing [L. *in*, into, + *vestire*, to clothe]. Ensheathing, encircling with a sheath or coating, as tissue; surrounding.

investment. A covering or sheath.

inveterate [″ + *vetus*, old]. Chronic; firmly seated, as a disease or a habit.

inviscation (ĭn″vĭs-kā′shŭn) [L. *in*, among, + *viscum*, slime]. The mixing of saliva with food during chewing.

in vitro (ĭn vē′trō) [L., in glass]. In glass, as in a test tube. An in vitro test is one done in the laboratory, usually involving isolated tissue, organ, or cell preparations. SEE: *in vivo.*

in vivo (ĭn vē′vō) [L., in the living body]. In the living body or organism. A test performed on a living organism. SEE: *in vitro.*

involucre, involucrum (ĭn′vō-lū″kĕr, ĭn″vō-lū′krŭm) [″ + *volvere*, to wrap]. 1. A sheath or covering. 2. The covering of newly formed bone enveloping the sequestrum in infection of the bone.

involuntary [L. *in-*, not, + *voluntas*, will]. Independent of or even contrary to volition.

involution (ĭn″vō-lū′shŭn) [″ + *volvere*, to roll]. 1. A turning or rolling inward. 2. The reduction in size of the uterus following delivery. 3. The retrogressive change in vital processes after their functions have been fulfilled, such as the change that follows the menopause. 4. A backward change. 5. Diminishing of an organ in vital power or in size. 6. In bacteriology, digression from the usual morphological type such as occurs in certain bacteria, esp. when grown under unfavorable conditions; degeneration.

i. of uterus. Return of uterus to normal size after childbirth.

i., senile. Atrophy of an organ or part from old age.

i., sexual. Cessation of menstrual function. SYN: *climacteric; menopause.*

involutional (ĭn-vō-lū'shŭn-ăl). Concerning involution or a turning inward.

involutional melancholia. Depressive psychosis that occurs during the involutional period (40 to 55 years of age in women; 50 to 65 in men). There is usually no previous history of mental illness. Characteristic symptoms include depression; delusions of sin, guilt, or poverty; an obsession with death; imagined gastrointestinal tract disease; and sometimes delusions of being persecuted. The patient manifests agitation and dejection. The condition may be successfully treated with antidepressant drugs or electroconvulsive therapy.

Io. Chem. symb. for ionium.

iocetamic acid. USP. A radiopaque agent used in certain x-ray studies. Trade name is Cholebrine.

Iodamoeba (ī"ō-dă-mē'bă). A genus of amebas found in the intestinal tract. Their cysts are peculiar in that they are irregular in shape, the nucleus usually is single, and they possess a vacuole filled with glycogen that stains brown in iodine.

I. bütschlii. A small, sluggish ameba found in the large intestine of man. Also found in monkeys and pigs. It is usually nonpathogenic. Also: *I. williamsi.*

iodide (ī'ō-dīd). A compound of iodine containing another radical or element, as potassium iodide.

i., cesium. A phosphor used in radiographic image intensifiers that emits light when struck by radiation.

iodide I 125 solution, sodium. USP. Na^{131}. A standardized solution of radioactive iodide, ^{125}I.

iodinate (ī-ō'dĭ-nāt). To combine with iodine.

iodinated I 131 albumin injection. USP. A standardized preparation of albumin iodinated with the use of radioactive iodine, ^{131}I.

iodine (ī'ō-dīn, ī'ō-dēn) [Gr. *ioeides,* violet colored]. USP. SYMB: I. At. wt. 126.904; at. no. 53; sp. gr. (solid, 20°C) 4.93. A nonmetallic element belonging to the halogen group. It is a black crystalline substance having a melting point of 113.5°C; it boils at 184.4°C, giving off a characteristic violet vapor.

FUNCT: Iodine aids in the development and functioning of the thyroid gland, formation of thyroxine and prevention of goiter. The amount of iodine in the entire body averages 50 mg, of which one-third to one-fifth (10 to 15 mg) is found in the thyroid. Adult daily requirement for iodine is from 100 to 150 μg. A growing child or a pregnant woman needs more than this amount. Those under emotional strain, and adolescents, also need more iodine.

DEFICIENCY SYM: Iodine deficiency in diet may lead to simple goiter characterized by thyroid enlargement and hypothyroidism. This may result in retardation of physical, sexual, and mental development in the young, a condition called cretinism.

SOURCES: In vegetables, esp. those growing near the seacoast, in iodized salt, and in seafoods, esp. in liver of halibut and cod, or the fish liver oils.

USES: Tincture of iodine contains 2% iodine and 2.4% sodium iodide diluted in 50% ethyl alcohol. It is used as a disinfectant for the skin, and as a germicide. It may be used to make contaminated water safe for drinking. Adding three drops of tincture of iodine to a quart of water will kill amebas and bacteria within 30 minutes, and the water will still be palatable. If water to be treated by this method is cloudy or turbid, it should be allowed to settle. Then the clear portion should be decanted and treated with iodine.

i., protein-bound. Iodine that is attached to serum protein.

i., radioactive. ^{131}I. An isotope of iodine with an at. wt. of 131. Used in diagnosis of thyroid disorders and in the treatment of toxic goiter and thyroid carcinoma.

i., tincture of. A 2% solution of iodine and sodium iodide in dilute alcohol.

iodine poisoning. Iodism. SEE: *Poisons and Poisoning* in *Appendix.*

SYM: Brown stains on lips and mouth; burning pain in mouth, throat, and stomach; vomiting (blue vomitus if stomach contained starches, otherwise yellow vomitus); bloody diarrhea.

F.A.: Give immediately by mouth a cornstarch or flour solution, 15 gm in 500 ml (2 cups) of water. Lavage with starch solution or 2% sodium thiosulfate solution. Morphine for pain; and mild stimulants as indicated. Following this therapy, promote catharsis with 30 gm of sodium sulfate and 15 gm of starch in 250 ml (one cup) of water. INCOMPAT: Alkaloids.

iodine tincture. USP. A standardized preparation of iodine in alcohol and water.

iodinophilous (ī"ō-dĭn-ŏf'ĭ-lŭs) [Gr. *ioeides,* violet colored, + *philos,* love]. Easily stained with iodine.

iodipamide meglumine injection. USP. A combination of iodipamide and meglumine used to aid in x-ray examination of the gallbladder. Trade name is Cholografin Meglumine.

iodipamide sodium I 131. USP. Radioactive chemical used in examining body organs and cavities. Trade name is Radio-Cholografin.

iodism (ī'ō-dĭzm). Condition induced by prolonged and excessive use of iodine or its compounds. SEE: *iodine poisoning.*

iodize. To administer or impregnate with iodine.

iodized. Impregnated with iodine.

iodized salt. In the U.S., salt containing about 100 μg of sodium or potassium iodide in each grain of salt. SEE: *salt.*

5-iodo-2'-deoxyuridine. ABBR: IDU. A substance used to treat herpesvirus infections of the eye. SEE: *Mace.* SYN: *idoxuridine.*

iododerma (ī-ō"dō-dĕr'mă) [" + *derma*, skin]. Dermatitis due to iodine.

iodoform (ī-ō'dō-form) [Gr. *ioeides*, violet colored, + L. *forma*, form]. CHI_3. Yellow crystals having a disagreeable odor. Produced by the action of iodine on acetone in the presence of an alkali. Used topically it has mild antibacterial action.

iodoformism (ī'ō-dō-form"ĭzm) [" + " + Gr. *-ismos*, state of]. Poisoning caused by iodoform.

iodoglobulin (ī"ō-dō-glŏb'ū-lĭn) [" + L. *globus*, globe]. A globulin protein that contains iodine.

iodohippurate sodium I 131 injection (ī-ō"dō-hĭp'ū-rāt). USP. A radioactive dye used in testing renal function. Trade name is Hippuran I 131.

iodophilia (ī"ō-dō-fĭl'ē-ă) [" + *philein*, to love]. Condition in which certain cells, when stained, esp. polymorphonuclear leukocytes, show a pronounced affinity for iodine, the cells acquiring a brownish-red color. Seen in pathologic conditions such as acute infections and anemia.

    i., extracellular. Iodophilia in which substances in the plasma outside the cells are colored.

    i., intracellular. Iodophilia in which color changes occur within the cells.

iodophor (ī-ō'dō-for). A combination of iodine and a solubilizing agent or carrier that liberates free iodine in solution. Some forms are used as general antiseptics; they are less irritating than elemental forms of iodine. SEE: *povidone-iodine.*

iodopyracet (ī-ō"dō-pī'ră-sĕt). A radiopaque medium used in intravenous pyelography and urography. Trade name is Diodrast.

iodoquinol (ī-ō"dō-kwĭn'ŏl). USP. $C_9H_5I_2NO$. An antiamebic agent used in the treatment of amebiasis and *Trichomonas hominis* infection of intestines. Previously used name was diiodohydroxyquin. Trade name is Yodoxin. Outside the U.S. this drug is sold under a great number of names.

Caution: Use of this drug has been associated with production of a severe disease of the central nervous system called subacute myelo-optic neuropathy, q.v.
---

iodotherapy [Gr. *ioeides*, violet colored, + *therapeia*, treatment]. Use of iodine medication.

iodum (ī-ō'dŭm) [L.]. Iodine.

IOML. *infraorbitomeatal line;* line through the infraorbital margin and the external auditory meatus.

ion [Gr. *ion*, going]. A particle carrying an electric charge, consisting of an atom or group of atoms into which the molecules of an electrolyte are divided or one of the electrified particles into which the molecules of a gas are divided by ultraviolet rays, gamma rays, or x-rays, or by other ionizing agents.

    Ions occur in gases, esp. at low pressures, under the influence of strong electrical discharges, x-rays, and radium; in solutions of acids, bases, and salts. Such moving particles render the gas or solution capable of conducting the electric current and, on reaching the electrodes, they are discharged.

    Ions that carry positive charges and that consequently discharge at the negative electrode (cathode) are called cations.

    Ex.: hydrogen in aqueous solutions of acids and sodium in aqueous solutions of sodium chloride.

    Ions that carry negative charges will appear at the positive electrode (anode) and are, therefore, called anions.

    Ex.: chlorine in aqueous solutions of hydrochloric acid or of sodium chloride. Thus the reaction in ionization of hydrogen chloride (hydrochloric acid) when dissolved in water is represented as

$$HCl \rightarrow H^+ + Cl^-$$

It means that when the electric current is passed through the solution, hydrogen gas will appear as bubbles at the cathode while chlorine will appear at the anode.

    i., dipolar. Ion that contains both positive and negative charges.

    i., hydrogen. A hydrogen atom that has lost an electron. It has a positive charge, and its symbol is H^+.

    i., hydroxyl. The negatively charged ion of hydrogen and oxygen. The symbol for it is OH^-.

Ionamin. Trade name for phentermine.

ion-exchange resins. Synthetic organic substances of high molecular weight. They replace certain negative or positive ions that they encounter in solutions.

ionic

ionic [Gr. *ion*, going]. Pert. to ions.

ionic medication. Ionotophoresis, def. 2, q.v.

ionium (ī-ō'nē-ŭm). A natural radioactive isotope of thorium. It has a mass number of 230.

ionization. The dissociation of compounds (acids, bases, salts) into their constituent ions.

ionization chamber. Device for determining the number of ions produced by a radioactive source.

ionize. To separate into ions; ionization.

ionogen (ī-ŏn'ō-jĕn) [Gr. *ion*, going, + *gennan*, to produce]. Anything that can be ionized.

ionometer [" + *metron*, measure]. An instrument consisting of an ionization chamber, an electroscope, and an electric charging current designed to measure the amount of radiation used by roentgen rays or radium and to measure the intensity of the rays themselves. SYN: *iontoquantimeter; iontoradiometer.*

ionophose (ī'ō-nō-fōz) [" + *phos*, light]. Production of a violet color.

ionotherapy (ī"ŏn-ō-thĕr'ă-pē) [" + *therapeia*, treatment]. Introduction of ions into the body. SYN: *iontophoresis.*

iontophoresis (ī-ŏn"tō-fō-rē'sĭs) [" + *phorein*, to carry]. 1. Process of electrical current traveling through salt solution causing migration of metal (positive) ion to negative pole and radical (negative) ion to positive pole. 2. Introduction of various ions into tissues through the skin by means of electricity. SYN: *ionic medication.*

iontoquantimeter (ī-ŏn"tō-kwŏn-tĭm'ĕ-ter) [" + L. *quantus*, how much, + Gr. *metron*, measure]. Instrument used to measure the amount of radiation used by, and the intensity of, roentgen rays. SYN: *ionometer; iontoradiometer.*

iontoradiometer (ī-ŏn"tō-rā"dē-ŏm'ĭ-tĕr) [" + L. *radius*, ray, + Gr. *metron*, measure]. Instrument for measuring the amount and intensity of roentgen rays. SYN: *ionometer; iontoquantimeter.*

iontotherapy (ī-ŏn"tō-thĕr'ă-pē) [" + *therapeia*, treatment]. Treatment by introducing ions into the body electrically.

IOP. *intraocular pressure.*

iopanoic acid. USP. A radiopaque dye used in radiographic studies of the gallbladder. Trade name is Telepaque.

iophendylate (ī"ō-fĕn'dĭ-lāt). USP. A radiopaque material used in myelography. Trade name is Pantopaque.

iophobia (ī"ō-fō'bē-ă) [Gr. *ios*, poison, + *phobos*, fear]. 1. Fear of being poisoned. SYN: *toxicophobia.* 2. Fear of touching any rusty object.

iotacism (ī-ō'tă-sĭzm) [Gr. *iota*, letter i]. Defective utterance marked by constant substitution of an ē sound (Greek iota) for other vowels.

iothalamate meglumine injection (ī-ō-thăl'ă-māt). USP. A radiopaque material used in investigation of arteries of the brain as well as in the rest of the body, and in studying kidney function. Trade names are Conray, Cysto-Conray.

I.P. intraperitoneal; isoelectric point.

ipecac (ĭp'ē-kăk). USP. Dried root of the plant ipecacuanha grown in Brazil. It is the source of emetine, q.v. SEE: *Poisons and Poisoning* in Appendix.
  ACTION/USES: Emetic.

I.P.L. *interpupillary line;* line between the center of both pupils.

ipodate calcium (ī'pō-dāt). USP. A radiopaque material used in x-ray studies of the gallbladder. Trade name is Oragrafin Calcium.

ipodate sodium. USP. A radiopaque material used in x-ray studies of the gallbladder. Trade name is Oragrafin Sodium.

IPPB. *intermittent positive-pressure breathing.*

IPPV. *intermittent positive-pressure ventilation.*

ipratropium bromide. An anticholinergic administered by inhalation. Used in treating asthma. Trade name is Atrovent.

iproniazid (ī"prō-nī'ă-zĭd). An antitubercular drug.

ipsi- [L. *ipse*, same]. Combining form indicating the same.

ipsilateral (ĭp"sĭ-lăt'ĕr-ăl) [" + *latus*, side]. On the same side; affecting the same side of the body. Thus, when the right patellar tendon is tapped, a knee-jerk is observed on the same side. Said of findings (paralysis) appearing on same side of body as brain or spinal cord lesion producing them. Opposite of crossed, contralateral. SYN: *homolateral.*

IPSP. *inhibitory postsynaptic potential.*

IQ. *intelligence quotient.*

IR. *infrared.*

I.R. *internal resistance.*

Ir. Chem. symb. for the element iridium.

iralgia (ĭr-ăl'jē-ă) [Gr. *iris*, colored circle, + *algos*, pain]. Pain felt in the iris. SYN: *iridalgia.*

irascible (ĭ-răs'ĭ-bl) [LL. *irascibilis*]. Marked by outbursts of temper or irritability. Easily angered.

IRB. *institutional review board.*

irid- [Gr. *iridos*, colored circle]. Combining form indicating relationship to the iris of the eye.

iridadenosis (ĭr"ĭd-ăd-ĭn-ō'sĭs) [L. *iris*, colored circle, + Gr. *aden*, gland, + *osis*, condition]. A glandular affection of the iris.

iridal (ī'rĭd-ăl). Rel. to the iris. SYN: *iridic; iri-*

tic.

iridalgia (ĭr″rĭd-ăl′jē-ă) [″ + *algos*, pain]. Pain felt in the iris. SYN: *iralgia.*

iridauxesis (ĭr″ĭd-ŏk-sē′sĭs) [″ + *auxesis*, increase]. Increase in thickness of the iris.

iridectome (ĭr″ĭ-dĕk′tōm) [″ + *tome*, incision]. Instrument for cutting the iris in iridectomy.

iridectomesodialysis (ĭr″ĭ-dĕk″tō-mēs″ō-dī-ăl′ĭ-sĭs) [″ + *ektome*, excision, + *mesos*, middle, + *dialysis*, loosening]. Formation of an artificial pupil, by separating adhesions on inner margin of iris.

iridectomize (ĭr″ĭd-ĕk′tō-mīz) [″ + *ektome*, excision]. To excise a portion of the iris.

iridectomy. Surgical removal of a portion of the iris.

   i., optical. Iridectomy done for purpose of making an artificial pupil.

iridectropium (ĭr-ĭ-dĕk-trō′pē-ŭm) [″ + *ektrope*, a turning aside]. Partial eversion of the iris.

iridemia (ĭr-ĭ-dē′mē-ă) [″ + *haima*, blood]. Bleeding from the iris.

iridencleisis (ĭr″ĭ-dĕn-klī′sĭs) [″ + *enklein*, to lock in]. An operation for relieving increased intraocular pressure, as in glaucoma, in which the iris and a portion of the limbus are excised to allow increased volume of the aqueous humor under the conjunctiva.

iridentropium (ĭr″ĭ-dĕn-trō′pē-ŭm) [″ + *en*, in, + *tropein*, to turn]. Partial inversion of the iris.

irideremia (ĭr″ĭd-ĕr-ē′mē-ă) [″ + *eremia*, lack]. Partial or total congenital absence of the iris. SYN: *aniridia.*

irides (ĭr′ĭ-dēz) [Gr.]. Plural of iris.

iridescence (ĭr″ĭ-dĕs′ĕns) [L. *iridescere*, to gleam like a rainbow]. Having the capability to disperse light into the colors of the spectrum.

iridesis (ĭ-rĭd′ĕ-sĭs) [″ + *desis*, a binding]. Formation of an iris artificially, by ligation. SYN: *iridodesis.*

iridic (ĭ-rĭd′ĭk) [Gr. *iris*, colored circle]. Rel. to the iris. SYN: *iridal; iritic.*

iridis, rubeosis. SEE: *rubeosis iridis.*

iridium (ĭ-rĭd′ē-ŭm) [Gr. *iris*, colored circle]. SYMB: Ir. At. wt. 192.2; at. no. 77. A white, hard metallic element.

irido- [Gr. *iridos*, colored circle]. Combining form pert. to the iris.

iridoavulsion (ĭr″ĭ-dō-ăv-ŭl′shŭn) [″ + L. *avulsio*, a pulling away from]. Tearing away (avulsion) of the iris.

iridocapsulitis (ĭr″ĭd-ō-kăp-sū-lī′tĭs) [″ + L. *capsula*, little box, + Gr. *itis*, inflammation]. Iritis with inflammation of the capsule of the lens.

iridocele (ĭ-rĭd′ō-sēl) [″ + *kele*, tumor,

swelling]. Protrusion of a portion of the iris through a defect in the cornea.

iridochorioiditis, iridochoroiditis (ĭr″ĭ-dō-kō″rē-oy-dī′tĭs, ĭr″ĭ-dō-kō-roy-dī′tĭs) [″ + *chorioeides*, skinlike, + *itis*, inflammation]. Inflamed condition of both iris and choroid.

iridocoloboma (ĭr″ĭd-ō-kŏl″ō-bō′mă) [″ + *koloboma*, mutilation]. Congenital defect or fissure of the iris.

iridoconstrictor (ĭr″ĭ-dō-kŏn-strĭk′tor). A muscle or drug that acts to constrict the pupil of the eye.

iridocyclectomy (ĭr″ĭ-dō-sī-klĕk′tō-mē) [″ + *kyklos*, circle, + *ektome*, excision]. Surgical removal of iris and ciliary body.

iridocyclitis (ĭr″ĭd-ō-sī-klī′tĭs) [″ + ″ + *itis*, inflammation]. Inflammation of the iris and ciliary body.

   i., heterochromic. Inflammation of the iris that leads to depigmentation.

iridocyclochoroiditis (ĭr″ĭ-dō-sī″klō-kō″roy-dī′tĭs) [″ + ″ + *chorioeides*, skinlike, + *itis*, inflammation]. Inflammation of the iris, ciliary body, and choroid of the eye.

iridocystectomy (ĭr″ĭ-dō-sĭs-tĕk′tō-mē) [″ + *kystis*, bladder, + *ektome*, excision]. Operation for removal of a cyst from the iris.

iridodesis (ĭr-ĭ-dŏd′ĕ-sĭs) [″ + *desis*, a binding]. Ligature of part of the iris to form an artificial one. SYN: *iridesis.*

iridodiagnosis [″ + *dia*, through, + *gnosis*, knowledge]. Diagnosis of disease by examination of the iris.

iridodialysis (ĭr″ĭd-ō-dī-ăl′ĭ-sĭs) [″ + *dialysis*, loosening]. Separation of the outer margin of the iris from its ciliary attachment.

iridodilator [″ + L. *dilatare*, to dilate]. Substance causing dilatation of the pupil.

iridodonesis (ĭr″ĭd-ō-dō-nē′sĭs) [″ + *donesis*, tremor]. Tremulousness of iris, seen in an aphakic eye or one with subluxated lens. SYN: *hippus.*

iridokeratitis (ĭr″ĭ-dō-kĕr″ă-tī′tĭs) [″ + *keras*, horn, + *itis*, inflammation]. Inflammation of the iris and cornea.

iridokinesis (ĭr″ĭd-ō-kĭn-ē′sĭs) [Gr. *iridos*, colored circle, + *kinesis*, movement]. The contracting and expanding movements of the iris.

iridoleptynsis (ĭr″ĭ-dō-lĕp-tĭn′sĭs) [″ + *leptynsis*, attenuation]. Thinning or atrophy of the iris.

iridology (ĭr″ĭ-dŏl′ō-jē) [″ + *logos*, word, reason]. The study of changes in the iris during the course of a disease.

iridomalacia (ĭr″ĭd-ō-mă-lā′shē-ă) [″ + *malakia*, softness]. Softening of the iris.

iridomedialysis (ĭr″ĭd-ō-mē-dē-ăl′ĭ-sĭs) [″ + L. *medius*, in middle, + Gr. *dialysis*, loosening]. Separation of inner marginal adhesions of the iris. SYN: *iridomesodialysis.*

iridomesodialysis (ĭr″ĭd-ō-mĕs″ō-dī-ăl′ĭ-sĭs) [″ + *mesos,* middle, + *dialysis,* loosening]. Separation of adhesions around the inner border of iris. SYN: *iridomedialysis.*

iridomotor [″ + L. *motor,* that which moves]. Rel. to movements of the iris.

iridoncus (ĭr-ĭ-dong′kŭs) [″ + *onkos,* bulk]. Tumefaction of the iris or development of a tumor.

iridoparalysis [″ + *paralyein,* to disable]. Paralysis of the iris. SYN: *iridoplegia.*

iridoparelkysis (ĭr″ĭ-dō-păr-ĕl′kĭ-sĭs) [″ + *parelkysis,* protraction]. Surgically induced prolapse of the iris in order to displace the pupil artificially.

iridopathy (ĭr″ĭ-dŏp′ă-thē) [″ + *pathos,* disease, suffering]. Disease of the iris.

iridoperiphacitis, iridoperiphakitis (ĭr″ĭdō-pĕr″ĭ-fă-sī′tĭs, -pĕr″ĭ-fă-kī′tĭs) [″ + *peri,* around, + *phakos,* lens, + *itis,* inflammation]. Inflammation of the iris and anterior portion of the capsule of the lens.

iridoplegia (ĭr″ĭ-dō-plē′jē-ă) [″ + *plege,* stroke]. Paralysis of the sphincter of the iris. SYN: *iridoparalysis.*

  i., accommodative. Inability of iris to contract when stimulated by accommodation.

  i., complete. Iridoplegia in which the iris fails to respond to any stimulation. Seen in Adie's pupil, q.v.

  i., reflex. Absence of light reflex with retention of accommodation reflex (Argyll Robertson pupil).

iridoptosis (ĭr″ĭ-dŏp-tō′sĭs) [″ + *ptosis,* a falling]. Prolapse of the iris.

iridopupillary (ĭr″ĭ-dō-pū′pĭ-lĕr″ē) [″ + L. *pupilla,* pupil]. Concerning the iris and the pupil of the eye.

iridorrhexis (ĭr″ĭd-ō-rĕk′sĭs) [″ + *rhexis,* rupture]. Rupture of or a tearing of the iris away from its attachment.

iridoschisis (ĭr″ĭ-dŏs′kĭ-sĭs) [″ + *schisis,* a splitting]. Separation of the stroma of the iris into two layers with disintegration of the anterior layer.

iridosclerotomy (ĭr″ĭd-ō-sklē-rŏt′ō-mē) [″ + *skleros,* hard, + *tome,* incision]. Piercing of the sclera and the border of the iris.

iridosteresis (ĭr″ĭ-dō-stē-rē′sĭs) [″ + *steresis,* loss]. Removal of the iris or a portion of it.

iridotasis (ĭr-ĭ-dŏt′ă-sĭs) [″ + *tasis,* a stretching]. Stretching the iris in treatment of glaucoma.

iridotomy (ĭr-ĭ-dŏt′ō-mē) [″ + *tome,* incision]. Incision of the iris without excising a portion, done for the purpose of making a new aperture in the iris when the pupil is closed. Indicated in eyes that had been operated on for cataract but that have lost their sight through subsequent iridocyclitis. SYN: *iritomy; irotomy.*

iris [Gr.] (pl. *irides*). The colored contractile membrane suspended between the lens and the cornea in the aqueous humor of the eye, separating the anterior and posterior chambers of the eyeball and perforated in the center by the pupil. By contraction and dilatation it regulates the entrance of light.

  ANAT: The free inner edge rests on the lens when the pupil is contracted or partially dilated. The iris contains two muscles, the sphincter pupillae (circular fibers), about one millimeter wide, and the dilator pupillae (meridionally arranged fibers), extending from the sphincter pupillae to the root of the iris. The former is supplied through the oculomotor nerve with parasympathetic fibers derived from the ciliary ganglion; the latter by sympathetic fibers from the superior cervical ganglion. The color of the iris depends on the pigment in the stroma cells and in the cells of the retinal layers. SEE: *aniridia; choroidoiritis; heterochromia iridis; iris, chromatic asymmetry of; rubeosis iridis;* "irid-" words.

  i. bombé. Condition seen in annular posterior synechia. The iris is bulged forward by the pressure of the aqueous humor, which cannot reach the anterior chamber.

  i., chromatic asymmetry of. Difference in color of the two irides (heterochromia). One may be blue or gray and the other brown. May occur in early iritis or cyclitis, or may be present without an associated pathological process.

  i., piebald. Dark discoloration in irregularly shaped area. May be in one or both eyes.

Irish moss. A genus of seaweeds, *Chondrus crispus;* source of a demulcent used in pharmacologic preparations. SYN: *carrageen.*

irisopsia (ī″rĭs-ŏp′sē-ă) [Gr. *iris,* colored circle, + *opsis,* vision]. Visual defect in which colored circles are seen around lights.

iritic (ĭ-rĭt′ĭk) [Gr. *iris,* colored circle]. Rel. to the iris. SYN: *iridal; iridic.*

iritis [″ + *itis,* inflammation]. Inflammation of the iris.

  SYM: Pain, photophobia, lacrimation, diminution of vision. The iris appears swollen, dull, and muddy, and the pupil is contracted, irregular, and sluggish in reaction.

  TREAT: One percent atropine is used, as an ointment or in drop form, frequently enough to keep the pupil dilated. Cortisone or hydrocortisone is used systemically as well as topically. If the primary disease causing the iritis is known it should be treated. However, the etiological factor is usually not known.

i., plastic. Iritis in which the fibrinous exudate forms new tissue.

i., primary. Condition in which the process develops in the iris itself. Seen in general diseases as syphilis, tuberculosis; metastatic in infectious diseases, gonorrhea, and focal infections; also occurs in trauma and sympathetic ophthalmia.

i., purulent. Iritis with a purulent exudate.

i., secondary. Iritis in which the inflammation has spread from neighboring parts as diseases of cornea and sclera.

i., serous. Serum forming the exudate.

iritoectomy (ĭ″rĭ-tō-ĕk′tō-mē) [″ + *ektome,* excision]. In cataract treatment, excision of the part of the iris that is inflamed and occluding the pupil.

iritomy (ĭ-rĭt′ō-mē) [″ + *tome,* incision]. Formation of an artificial pupil, or incision into the iris. SYN: *iridotomy; iromoty.*

iron (ĭ′ẽrn) [AS. *iren;* L. *ferrum*]. SYMB: Fe. At. wt. 55.847; at. no. 26. A metallic element widely distributed in nature. Compounds (oxides, hydroxides, salts) exist in two forms: ferrous, in which iron has a valence of two (Fe^{++}), and ferric, in which it has a valence of three (Fe^{+++}). It is widely used in the treatment of certain forms of anemia. Iron is essential for the formation of chlorophyll in plants, although it is not a constituent of chlorophyll. It is part of the hemoglobin and myoglobin molecules. SEE: *ferritin.*

FUNCT: Because it is essential to hemoglobin formation, iron is essential to life. Iron is also present in enzymes that permit cellular respiration to occur. It plays a role in the nutrition of epithelial tissues. There are approximately 3.45 gm of iron in the adult male body and approximately 2.45 gm in the female, distributed as follows: 60% to 70% in hemoglobin; 10% to 12% in myoglobin and enzymes; and, as ferritin, 29% in females and 10% in males, stored in the liver, spleen, and bone marrow. Iron is stored in the tissues principally as ferritin. Iron is absorbed from the food in the small intestine; it passes, in the blood, to the bone marrow; here it is used in making hemoglobin, which is incorporated into the red corpuscles. A corpuscle, after circulating in the blood for approx. 120 days, is destroyed, and its iron is used over again. The adult male requires from 0.5 to 1.0 mg of iron a day. A female of menstrual age will require about double this amount. During pregnancy and lactation from 2 to 4 mg of iron per day will be required. Prior to puberty and after menopause the female requires no more iron than the male.

Because only a fraction of the iron present in food is absorbed, it is necessary to provide from 15 to 30 mg of iron in the diet to be certain that 1 to 4 mg will be absorbed.

Copper in the food is necessary for the utilization of iron. It is stored in the body and reused repeatedly.

In the first few months of life, the infant will use up most of its iron stores, and the typical diet or formula may not have sufficient iron to replenish those stores. It is therefore important to add iron-containing foods to the diet of an infant by age six months.

Manganese and cobalt, in addition to copper, are necessary for proper utilization of iron.

Iron, as a component of hemoglobin, is essential in the transportation of oxygen. It is needed for tissue respiration and the development of blood cells.

DEFICIENCY SYM: Anemia, lowered vitality, pale complexion, conjunctival pallor, retarded development, decreased amount of hemoglobin in each red cell.

NOTE: Sometimes a disturbance in iron metabolism occurs in which an iron-containing pigment, hemosiderin, and hemofuscin are deposited in the tissues. This gives rise to hemochromatosis. Excessive deposition of hemosiderin in the tissues, such as may occur as a result of excessive breakdown of red cells, is called hemosiderosis.

SOURCES: Almonds; asparagus; bran; beans; cauliflower; celery; chard; dandelions; Boston brown bread; graham bread; egg yolk; kidney; lettuce; liver; oatmeal; oysters; soybeans; whole wheat. Other good sources are apricots; greens; beets; beef; cabbage; cucumbers; currants; dates; duck; goose; lamb; molasses; oranges; parsnips; peppers; peas; potatoes; prunes; radishes; raisins; rhubarb; pineapple; tomatoes; peanuts; turnips; cornmeal; mushrooms. Only 50% of the iron in spinach and similar vegetables is assimilable by the body.

iron dextran injection. USP. A preparation of iron suitable for parenteral use. Trade name is Imferon.

Caution: At time of intravenous use, one or two drops are administered over a period of five minutes to determine whether any signs of anaphylaxis appear.

---

iron lung. Device for automatically providing artificial respiration for patients whose respiratory muscles are paralyzed.

iron poisoning. Acute poisoning usually caused by the accidental ingestion by infants or small children of iron-containing medications intended for the use of adults.

SYM: Vomiting, usually within an hour of taking the iron. Vomiting of blood and melena may occur. If untreated, restlessness, hypotension, rapid respirations, and cyanosis may be followed within a few hours by coma and death.

F.A.: Prompt emptying of the stomach. By digital stimulation of the pharynx if done in the home or by gastric lavage if done in the emergency room. Administration of warm solution of baking soda may help to induce vomiting and the bicarbonate helps to prevent absorption of the iron. Gastric lavage with a solution containing 4 gm of sodium bicarbonate per 100 ml is done and then either 60 ml of the bicarbonate solution or 5 to 10 gm of deferoxamine, q.v., in solution is left in the stomach. The deferoxamine may be administered intramuscularly in an initial dose of 1 gm. This dose may be repeated intramuscularly in four to eight hours and then at 12-hour intervals if needed. If the patient is in shock, treat by the usual methods.

iron sorbitex injection. USP. A preparation of iron suitable for parenteral use.

iron storage disease. Hemochromatosis, q.v.

irotomy (ī-rŏt′ō-mē) [Gr. *iris*, colored circle, + *tome*, incision]. Formation of an artificial pupil. SYN: *iridotomy; iritomy.*

irradiate (ĭ-rā′dē-āt) [L. *in*, into, + *radiare*, to emit rays]. 1. To expose to radiation. 2. To treat with roentgen rays or other forms of radiation. SEE: *irradiation.*

irradiating. Diverging or spreading out from a common center.

irradiation. 1. Therapeutic application of roentgen rays, radium rays, ultraviolet rays or other radiation to a patient. 2. Application of form of radiation to an object or substance to give it therapeutic value, or increase that which it already has. 3. Phenomenon in which a bright object on a dark background appears larger than a dark object of the same size on a bright background. 4. The spreading in all directions from a common center, as nerve impulses, the sensation of pain.

RS: heliotherapy; lamp; light therapy; radiotherapy; radiothermy; radium therapy; radium; radon; ray, roentgen; roentgenotherapy; ultraviolet.

i., interstitial. Therapeutic irradiation by the insertion into the tissues of capillary tubes containing radon.

i. of reflexes. The spread of a reflex to an increasing number of motor units upon increasing the strength of the stimulus.

irrational. Contrary to what is reasonable or logical; i.e., irrational behavior is conduct that cannot be explained by normal reasoning.

irreducible (ĭr″rē-dū′sĭ-bl) [L. *in-*, not, + *re*, back, + *ducere*, to lead]. Not capable of being reduced or made smaller, as a fracture or dislocation.

irrelevance [″ + *relevans*, raising]. Inappropriate to or unrelated to that which was asked or being discussed.

irrespirable (ĭr″rĕ-spī′ră-bl) [″ + *respirare*, to breathe again]. Unfit for breathing, as a gas, or incapable of being breathed.

irresponsible. Not capable of or willing to take responsibility for one's actions.

irreversible. Not being possible to reverse.

irrigate [L. *in*, into, + *rigare*, to carry water]. To wash out with a fluid.

irrigation. The cleansing of a canal by flushing with water or other fluids; the washing of a wound. SYN: *lavage.* SEE: *lavage, gastric.*

Solutions should be sterile and have an approx. temperature slightly warmer than body temperature (100° to 115°F or 37.8° to 46.1°C).

i., bladder. Washing out of the bladder for treatment of inflammation. Can be accomplished by forcing oral fluids.

NURSING IMPLICATIONS: Assemble necessary sterile equipment and the ordered irrigation solution. Follow hospital procedure for catheterization. Insert catheter. Instill irrigation solution in the specified amount using a bulb syringe; clamp the catheter and allow the solution to remain in the bladder for the specified amount of time. Unclamp the catheter and allow the irrigation solution to flow into a basin. Repeat the irrigation as often as ordered. Carefully observe the return from the irrigation, and particularly note the presence of any drainage. The catheter should be removed when the irrigations have been completed. Record treatment done, amount and type of solution used, return from irrigation, and response of patient to procedure. Intermittent and continuous bladder irrigation can be accomplished using a three-lumen indwelling catheter in which one channel leads to the inflation balloon, one channel is for instillation of irrigation fluid, and one channel provides drainage.

i., colonic. Flushing of the colon with water. This procedure is done to wash out material in the colon and to cleanse the bowel as high as possible.

irrigator. Device with hose attachment used to flush or wash a part or cavity with fluids.

irritability [L. *irritabilis*, irritable]. 1. Excitability. 2. Ability to respond in a specific way to a change in environment, a property of all living tissue. 3. Condition in which a person, organ, or a part responds excessively to a stimulus. 4. Quick response to annoyance; impatience.

    i., muscular. Normal response of muscle to a stimulus.

    i., nervous. Response of nerve to stimulus.

irritable. 1. Capable of reacting to a stimulus. 2. Sensitive to stimuli.

irritable bowel syndrome. A disturbance of intestinal function of unknown cause. Clinically, the patient has intermittent symptoms of abdominal discomfort, including cramping and altered bowel activity. The syndrome does not produce fever or weight loss. Symptoms are often initiated or exacerbated by mental or social stress. It is the most frequent gastrointestinal disorder.

    TREAT: Supportive therapy. Reassure patient that the illness is not life-threatening. Antispasmodics may be necessary, as will non-narcotic analgesics. Constipation may be treated with hydrophilic colloids (Metamucil). Use as few drugs as possible.

irritant. An agent that, when used locally, produces more or less local inflammatory reaction. Anything that induces or gives rise to irritation, such as iodine.

irritant poisons. These include a large number of poisons of great variety, not including the corrosive acids or alkalies. They cause pain in the mouth, esophagus, and stomach; nausea; vomiting; great thirst; abdominal cramping; bloody diarrhea; diminished urine.

    TREAT: SEE: individual poisons in *Poisons and Poisoning* in *Appendix.*

irritation [L. *irritatio*]. 1. Reaction to that which is irritating. It is important to distinguish between irritation and sensitization. For example, a substance contacting the skin may cause no irritation when initially applied but can cause a sensitization reaction that will not become obvious until the material is applied the second time. SEE: *allergen; sensitization.* 2. Extreme reaction to pain or pathological conditions. 3. Normal response to stimulus of a nerve or muscle.

    i., spinal. A neurasthenic condition characterized by tenderness along the spinal column, numbness and tingling in the limbs, and susceptibility to fatigue.

    i., sympathetic. The response of an organ to irritation in another organ.

irritative. Pert. to that which causes irritation.

ischemia (ĭs-kē′mē-ă) [Gr. *ischein*, to hold back, + *haima*, blood]. Local and temporary deficiency of blood supply due to obstruction of the circulation to a part.

    i., intestinal. SEE: *angina, intestinal.*

    i., myocardial. Insufficient blood supply to the heart muscle. SEE: *myocardial ischemia.*

ischesis (ĭs-kē′sĭs). Suppression of a discharge, esp. a normal one.

ischia (ĭs′kē-ă) [L.]. Pl. of ischium.

ischiac, ischiadic (ĭs′kē-ăk, ĭs-kē-ăd′ĭk). Ischiatic; sciatic.

ischial (ĭs′kē-ăl) [Gr. *ischion*, hip]. Pert. to the ischium.

ischialgia (ĭs″kē-ăl′jē-ă) [″ + *algos*, pain]. Neuralgic pain in the hip. SYN: *sciatica.*

ischiatic (ĭs″kē-ăt′ĭk) [Gr. *ischion*, hip]. Pert. to the ischium or hip bone. SYN: *ischiac; ischiadic; sciatic.*

ischiatitis (ĭs″kē-ă-tī′tĭs) [″ + *itis*, inflammation]. Sciatic nerve inflammation.

ischidrosis (ĭs″kĭ-drō′sĭs) [Gr. *ischein*, to hold back, + *hidrosis*, sweat]. Suppression of perspiration.

ischio- [Gr. *ischion*, hip]. Prefix pert. to the ischium.

ischioanal (ĭs″kē-ō-ā′năl) [″ + L. *anus*, anus]. Concerning the ischium and anus.

ischiobulbar (ĭs″kē-ō-bŭl′băr) [″ + L. *bulbus*, bulb]. Rel. to the ischium and urethral bulb.

ischiocapsular (ĭs″kē-ō-kăp′sū-lăr) [″ + L. *capsula*, capsule]. Concerning the ischium and capsule of the hip.

ischiocavernosus (ĭs″kē-ō-kă″vĕr-nō′sŭs) [″ + L. *cavernosus*, cavernous]. A muscle extending from the ischium to the penis or clitoris and assisting in their erection.

ischiocele (ĭs′kē-ō-sēl) [″ + *kele*, tumor, swelling]. Hernia through the sciatic notch.

ischiococcygeus (ĭs″kē-ō-kŏk-sĭj′ē-ŭs) [″ + *kokkyx*, coccyx]. 1. Coccygeus muscle. 2. Posterior portion of the levator ani.

ischiodynia (ĭs″kē-ō-dĭn′ē-ă) [″ + *odyne*, pain]. Pain in the ischium.

ischiofemoral (ĭs″kē-ō-fĕm′or-ăl) [″ + L. *femur*, thigh]. Rel. to the ischium and femur.

ischiofibular (ĭs″kē-ō-fĭb′ū-lăr) [″ + L. *fibula*, pin]. Rel. to the ischium and fibula.

ischiohebotomy (ĭs″kē-ō-hē-bŏt′ō-mē) [″ + *hebe*, pubes, + *tome*, incision]. Surgical division of the ascending ramus of the pubes and the ischiopubic ramus. SYN: *ischiopubiotomy.*

ischioneuralgia (ĭs″kē-ō-nū-răl′jē-ă) [″ + *neuron*, nerve, + *algos*, pain]. Neuralgic pain in the hip. SYN: *sciatica.*

ischionitis (ĭs″kē-ō-nī′tĭs) [″ + *itis*, inflammation]. Inflammation of the tuberosity of the ischium.

ischiopubic (ĭs″kē-ō-pū′bĭk) [″ + L. *pubes*, the pubes]. Rel. to the ischium and pubes.

ischiopubiotomy (ĭs″kē-ō-pū″bē-ŏt′ō-mē). Ischiohebotomy.

ischiorectal (ĭs″kē-ō-rĕk′tăl) [″ + L. *rectus*, straight]. Pert. to the ischium and rectum.

ischiorectal abscess. Collection of pus in fatty tissue on either side of the rectum.

ischiosacral (ĭs″kē-ō-sā′krăl) [″ + L. *sacralis*, pert. to the sacrum]. Concerning the ischium and sacrum.

ischiovaginal (ĭs″kē-ō-văj′ĭ-năl) [″ + L. *vagina*, sheath]. Concerning the ischium and vagina.

ischium (ĭs′kē-ŭm) [Gr. *ischion*, hip] (pl. *ischia*). Lower portion of the innominate or hip bone.

ischo- (ĭs′kō) [Gr. *ischein*, to hold back]. Prefix meaning to suppress or restrain.

ischogalactic (ĭs″kō-gă-lăk′tĭk) [″ + *gala*, milk]. 1. Causing suppression of breast milk. 2. Agent that checks milk secretion. SYN: *antigalactic.*

ischuretic (ĭs″kū-rĕt′ĭk) [″ + *ouron*, urine]. 1. Relieving or pert. to ischuria. 2. That which relieves urinary retention or suppression.

ischuria (ĭs-kū′rē-ă) [″ + *ouron*, urine]. Suppression or retention of the urine.

I.S.C.L.T. *International Society of Clinical Laboratory Technologists.*

iseikonia (ĭs″ī-kō′nē-ă) [Gr. *isos*, equal, + *eikon*, image]. Condition in which the image in both eyes is the same. SYN: *isoiconia.*

isinglass (ī′sĭn-glăs). A transparent gelatin prepared from the bladder of certain fish.

island [AS. *igland*, island]. A structure detached from surrounding tissues or characterized by difference in structure; an islet.

i., blood. A small area of blood accumulation present in the yolk sac of the early embryo.

i.'s of Calleja. Groups of densely packed, small cells in the cortex of the gyrus hippocampi.

i.'s of Langerhans. Islets of Langerhans, q.v.

i. of Reil. The insula, a lobe of the cerebral cortex comprising a triangular area lying in the floor of the lateral or sylvian fissure. It is overlapped and hidden by the gyri of the fissure, which constitute the operculum of the insula.

i., pancreatic. I.'s of Langerhans.

islet (ī′lĕt). A tiny isolated mass of one kind of tissue within another type.

i.'s of Calleja. Islands of Calleja.

i.'s of Langerhans [Paul Langerhans, Ger. pathologist, 1847–1888]. Clusters of cells in the pancreas. They are of three types: alpha, beta, and delta cells. The beta cells are found in greatest abundance and produce insulin. Destruction or impairment of function of the islets of Langerhans may result in diabetes or hypoglycemia.

i.'s, Walthard's [Max Walthard, Swiss gynecologist, 1867–1933]. Embryological nests of epithelial-like cells in the superfi-

cial part of the ovaries, tubes, and uterine ligaments. They may also appear as minute cysts. Brenner's tumor is thought to arise from these islets.

-ism [Gr. *-ismos*]. Suffix meaning condition or theory of; principle or method.

Ismelin. Trade name for guanethidine sulfate, USP.

I.S.O. *International Standards Organization.*

iso- [Gr. *isos*, equal]. Combining form meaning equal.

isoagglutination (ī″sō-ă-gloo″tĭ-nā′shŭn) [″ + L. *agglutinare*, to glue to]. Agglutination of red blood cells by agglutinins from the blood of another member of the same species.

isoagglutinin (ī″sō-ă-glū′tĭn-ĭn) [″ + L. *agglutinare*, to glue to]. Antibody in a serum that agglutinates the blood cells of those of the same species from which it is derived. SEE: *agglutinin; blood groups; isohemagglutinin.*

isoagglutinogen (ī″sō-ă-glū-tĭn′ō-jĕn). One of two substances designated A and B that may be present on the surface of red blood cells. Cells containing these substances become agglutinated when mixed with serum containing corresponding isoagglutinins (anti-A or anti-B). SEE: *blood groups.*

isoanaphylaxis (ī″sō-ăn″ă-fĭ-lăk′sĭs) [″ + *ana*, against, + *phylaxis*, protection]. Anaphylaxis produced by serum from another member of the same species.

isoantibody (ī″sō-ăn′tĭ-bŏd″ē). An antibody produced by an isoantigen, q.v.

isoantigen (ī″sō-ăn′tĭ-jĕn) [″ + L. *anti*, against, + *gennan*, to produce]. A substance present in certain individuals that stimulates production of antibodies in other members of the same species but not in the donor. SYN: *alloantigen.*

Ex.: blood group isoantigens that are harmless to the donor but may produce severe antibody response in a recipient of a different blood group or type.

isobar (ī′sō-băr) [″ + *baros*, weight]. In chemistry, one of two or more chemical bodies having same atomic weight, but with different atomic numbers.

isobaric (ī″sō-băr′ĭk). Specific gravity equal to that with which it is being compared. Thus an anesthetic solution used in spinal anesthesia, if isobaric, would be of the same specific gravity as the spinal fluid.

isobucaine hydrochloride (ī″sō-bū′kăn). USP. A local anesthetic agent.

isocaloric (ī″sō-kă-lō′rĭk) [″ + L. *calor*, heat]. Containing the same number of calories as the food or diet with which it is being compared.

isocarboxazid (ī″sō-kăr-bŏk′să-zĭd). USP. An antidepressant drug. Trade name is

Marplan.

isocellular [" + L. *cellula*, cell]. Composed of equal and similar cells.

isochromatic (ī″sō-krō-măt′ĭk) [" + *chroma*, color]. 1. Having the same color. 2. Of uniform color. SYN: *isochroous*.

isochromatophil(e) (ī″sō-krō-măt′ō-fĭl, -fīl) [" + " + *philein*, to love]. Having the same affinity for a dye.

isochromosome (ī″sō-krō′mō-sōm) [" + " + *soma*, body]. A chromosome with arms that are morphologically identical and contain the same genetic loci. This is the result of the transverse rather than the longitudinal splitting of a chromosome.

isochronal (ī-sŏk′rō-năl) [" + *chronos*, time]. Acting in uniform time, or taking place at regular intervals. SYN: *isochronous*.

isochronia (ī″sō-krō′nē-ă) [Gr. *isos*, equal, + *chronos*, time]. The correspondence of events with respect to time, rate, or frequency.

isochronous (ī-sŏk′rō-nŭs). Isochronal, q.v.

isochroous (ī-sŏk′rō-ŭs) [" + *chroa*, color]. Of uniform color. SYN: *isochromatic*.

isocitrate dehydrogenase (ī″sō-cĭt′rāt dē″hī-drŏj′ĕn-ās). An enzyme present in tissues. It catalyzes the conversion of isocitric acid to α-ketoglutaric acid.

isocolloid (ī-sō-kŏl′oyd) [" + *kollodes*, glutinous]. A colloid having the same composition in every transformation.

isocomplement [" + L. *complere*, to complete]. Complement from an individual of the same species.

isocoria (ī″sō-kō′rē-ă) [" + *kore*, pupil]. Equality of size of both pupils. SEE: *anisocoria*.

isocortex (ī″sō-kor′tĕks) [" + L. *cortex*, bark]. The neopallium or nonolfactory portion of the cerebral cortex. It is composed of six layers of fibrous and cellular tissue having a similar distribution pattern. SYN: *neocortex; neopallium*.

isocytosis (ī″sō-sī-tō′sĭs) [" + *kytos*, cell, + *osis*, condition]. Cells of equal size.

isocytotoxin (ī″sō-sī″tō-tŏk′sĭn) [" + " + *toxikon*, poison]. Cytotoxin destructive to homologous cells of the same species.

isodactylism (ī-sō-dăk′tĭl-ĭzm) [" + *daktylos*, finger]. Condition of having fingers or toes of equal length.

isodiametric (ī″sō-dī-ă-mĕt′rĭk) [" + *dia*, across, + *metron*, measure]. Having equal diameters.

isodontic (ī″sō-dŏn′tĭk) [" + *odous*, tooth]. Having teeth of equal size.

isodose (ī′sō-dōs). In radiology, to have equal doses of radiation to different areas.

isodose curve. In radiation therapy, a graph on which the points plot areas or levels of equal radiation dose.

isodynamic (ī″sō-dī-năm′ĭk) [" + *dynamis*, power]. Having equal power.

isoelectric (ī″sō-ē-lĕk′trĭk) [" + *elektron*, amber]. Having equal electric potentials.

isoelectric period. In an occurrence that normally produces an electric force, such as a muscle contraction, the time or point when no electric energy is produced. In an electrocardiogram, the period when the electrical tracing is at zero and is neither positive or negative.

isoenergetic [Gr. *isos*, equal, + *energeia*, energy]. Showing equal force or activity.

isoenzyme (ī″sō-ĕn′zīm) [" + *en*, in, + *zyme*, leaven]. One of several forms in which an enzyme may exist in various tissues. Although the isoenzymes are similar in catalytic qualities, they may be separated from each other by special chemical tests. SYN: *isozyme*. SEE: *lactic dehydrogenase*.

isoetharine hydrochloride (ī-sō-ĕth′ā-rēn). USP. A sympathomimetic drug used as a bronchodilator. Trade name is Bronkosol.

Isofedrol. Trade name for ephedrine sulfate, USP.

isoflurophate (ī-sō-floo′rō-fāt). USP. An anticholinesterase drug used in treating glaucoma as well as atony of the smooth muscle of the intestinal tract and urinary bladder. Trade name is Floropryl.

isogamete (ī″sō-găm′ĕt) [" + *gamete*, wife, *gametes*, husband]. 1. A cell that, through conjugation or fusion with a similar cell, reproduces. 2. A gamete of the same size as the one with which it fuses or unites.

isogamy (ī-sŏg′ă-mē) [" + *gamos*, marriage]. Reproduction resulting from conjugation of isogametes or identical cells.

isogeneic (ī″sō-jĕn-ē′ĭk). Syngeneic, q.v.

isogeneric (ī″sō-jĕ-nĕr′ĭk) [" + L. *genus*, kind]. Of the same kind; concerning or obtained from members of the same genus.

isogenesis (ī″sō-jĕn′ĕ-sĭs) [" + *genesis*, generation, birth]. Similarity in morphological development.

isogenic (ī″sō-jĕn′ĭk). Isologous, q.v.

isograft [" + L. *graphium*, grafting shoot]. Graft taken from another individual or animal of the same genotype as the recipient. SEE: *autograft*.

isohemagglutination (ī″sō-hĕm″ă-gloo″tĭ-nā′shŭn) [" + *haima*, blood, + L. *agglutinare*, to glue to]. Isoagglutination, q.v.

isohemagglutinin (ī″sō-hĕm″ă-glū′tĭn-ĭn) [" + *haima*, blood, + L. *agglutinare*, to glue to]. Substance normally present in most human blood serum; responsible for the clumping of corpuscles observed when incompatible bloods are mixed. The clumping is ascribed to the interaction of an agglutinogen in the corpuscles with a specific agglutinin in the foreign serum. In transfusions, the corpuscles of the donor are exposed to an overwhelming quantity of the recipient's plasma; therefore the agglutinogen content of the donor's corpuscles and the agglutinin content of the recipient's serum are the factors that determine compatibility.

Assuming that there are but two possible agglutinogens, red corpuscles from a given donor may contain both, either, or neither. If the agglutinin, alpha, can react only with agglutinogen A, one can construct a table to illustrate which blood types will be compatible or incompatible with other types. SEE: *agglutinin; agglutinogen.*

isohemolysin (ī″sō-hē-mŏl′ĭ-sĭn) [″ + ″ + *lysis,* dissolution]. Substance that destroys red blood corpuscles of animals of the same species from which it is obtained. SYN: *isolysin.* SEE: *hemolysin.*

isohemolysis (ī″sō-hē-mŏl′ĭ-sĭs). Action of an isohemolysin. SYN: *isolysis.* SEE: *hemolysis.*

isohypercytosis (ī″sō-hī″pĕr-sī-tō′sĭs) [″ + *hyper,* over, above, excessive + *kytos,* cell, + *osis,* condition]. Condition in which the total number of white blood cells is increased but the proportions of the polymorphonuclear leukocytes remain stable.

isohypocytosis (ī″sō-hī″pō-sī-tō′sĭs) [″ + *hypo,* under, beneath, below, + *kytos,* cell, + *osis,* condition]. Condition in which the total number of white blood cells is decreased but the proportions of polymorphonuclear leukocytes remain stable.

isoiconia (ī″sō-ī-kŏ′nē-ă) [Gr. *isos,* equal, + *eikon,* image]. Equality of both retinal images.

isoiconic (ī″sō-ī-kŏn′ĭk). Having equal retinal images.

isoimmunization [″ + L. *immunis,* safe]. Immunization of an individual against the blood of an individual of the same species, esp. the development of Rh-negative agglutinins in an Rh-negative mother in response to agglutinogens present in transfused Rh-positive blood or developed in an Rh-positive fetus.

isokinetic exercise. Contraction of a muscle where the speed is controlled and maximum exertion occurs through its full range of motion, whether eccentric or concentric. Usually, a machine is used to control the velocity and record the torque output. SEE: *isotonic exercise.*

isolate [It. *isolato,* isolated]. 1. To separate or detach from other persons, as during an infectious disease. 2. In chemistry, to obtain a substance in pure form from the mixture or solution that contains it.

isolation. 1. The fear of interrelating with another individual. 2. Limitation of movement and social contacts of patient suffering from, or a known carrier of, communicable disease, in contradistinction to quarantine, which limits the movements of exposed or contact persons. SEE: *incubation* for table; *quarantine.*

NURSING IMPLICATIONS: A patient is placed in isolation to prevent the spread of disease-causing agents from the patient to others or from others to the patient at risk. The rules to be followed are based on the mode of transmission of the organism, e.g., if the organism is spread by droplet, then all items that come in contact with the upper respiratory tract of the patient are isolated and destroyed or disinfected. Most institutions use readily disposable paper plates, cups, and plastic utensils for patients who are isolated. The hands of the personnel caring for the patient, the doctor, nurse, allied health personnel, and family are the commonest means of transmitting infection. Handwashing and keeping the hands away from the face, esp. the nose and mouth, are the best ways to control the spread of disease. Upon leaving the patient, remove gowns, masks, and caps used in the sickroom and place them in an appropriate container. Contaminated items are double bagged for safe disposal. Follow hospital procedure for the specific type of isolation that is in effect. The purpose for isolation precautions should be explained to the patient and family to decrease their fears and increase compliance. SEE: *i., infectious; i., protective; Universal Precautions* in *Appendix.*

i., infectious. Isolation technique that protects health care personnel from a patient who has or is suspected of having an infectious disease.

i., protective. Protective isolation, q.v.

i., reverse. Protective isolation, q.v.

isolation ward. Hospital ward where patients suffering from communicable disease may be kept apart from the rest of the patients.

isoleucine (ī″sō-lū′sēn). USP. An amino acid formed during hydrolysis of fibrin and other proteins. It is essential in the diet.

isologous (ī-sŏl′ō-gŭs). Genetically identical. In transplantations, being isologous (or isogenic) indicates the absence of any tissue incompatibility between the recipient of tissue and the tissue or organ itself. SYN: *isogenic; syngeneic.*

isolophobia (ī″sō-lō-fō′bē-ă) [It. *isolato,* isolated, + Gr. *phobos,* fear]. Fear of being alone. SEE: *agoraphobia.*

isolysin (ī-sŏl′ĭ-sĭn) [Gr. *isos,* equal, + *lysis,*

dissolution]. Substance that dissolves red corpuscles of animals of the same species from which it is obtained. SYN: *isohemolysin.*

isolysis (ī-sŏl'ĭ-sĭs). Destruction of red blood corpuscles produced by an isolysin. SYN: *isohemolysis.* SEE: *hemolysis.*

isolytic (ī-sō-lĭt'ĭk). Rel. to isolysis.

isomer (ī'sō-mĕr) [Gr. *isos*, equal, + *meros*, part]. One of two or more chemical substances that have the same molecular formula but different chemical and physical properties due to different arrangement of the atoms in the molecule. Dextrose is an isomer of levulose. SEE: *polymer.*

isomerase (ī-sŏm'ĕr-ās). Any enzyme that catalyzes the isomerization of its substrate. For example, phosphoglucose isomerase interconverts glucose and fructose-6-phosphate. SEE: *isomerism.*

isomeric (ī'sō-mĕr'ĭk). Pert. to isomerism.

isomerism (ī-sŏm'ĕr-ĭzm). State of being composed of compounds of the same number of atoms but having different atomic arrangement in the molecule. SEE: *metamerism; polymerism.*

isomerization (ī-sŏm''ĕr-ī-zā'shŭn). The conversion of one chemical substance to an isomer. SEE: *isomer; isomerism.*

isometric [" + *metron*, measure]. Having equal dimensions. SEE: *isotonic.*

isometric contraction. SEE: *contraction, isometric.*

isometric contraction phase. The first phase in contraction of the ventricle of the heart in which ventricular pressure increases but there is no decrease in volume of contents because semilunar valves are closed.

isometric exercise. SEE: *exercise, isometric.*

isometropia (ī'sō-mĕ-trō'pē-ā) [" + " + *ops*, eye]. Same refraction of the two eyes.

isomorphism (ī-sō-mor'fĭzm) [" + *morphe*, form, + *-ismos*, state of]. Condition marked by possession of the same form.

isomorphous (ī'sō-mor'fŭs). Possessing the same shape.

isoniazid (ī'sō-nī'ă-zĭd). USP. ABBR: INH. $C_6H_7N_3O$. An odorless compound occurring as colorless or white crystals or as a white crystalline powder. An antibacterial, used principally in treating tuberculosis. Trade names are Cotinazin, Dinacrin, and Nydrazid. Treatment for isoniazid overdose is pyridoxine.

isonicotinoylhydrazine (ī'sō-nĭk''ō-tĭn''ō-il-hī'dră-zēn). Isoniazid.

isonormocytosis (ī'sō-nor''mō-sī-tō'sĭs) [" + L. *norma*, rule, + Gr. *kytos*, cell, + *osis*, condition]. State of having leukocytes normal in number and proportion of

varieties.

isopathy (ī-sŏp'ă-thē) [Gr. *isos*, equal, + *pathos*, disease, suffering]. Therapeutic administration of the causative agent of the disease or its products. SYN: *isotherapy.*

isophoria (ī''sō-fō'rē-ă) [" + *phorein*, to carry]. Equal tension of vertical muscles of each eye with visual lines in the same horizontal plane. Absence of hyperphoria, q.v., and hypophoria, q.v.

isopia (ī-sō'pē-ă) [" + *ops*, vision]. Equal vision in the eyes.

isoplastic (ī''sō-plăs'tĭk) [" + *plastos*, formed]. Term applied to a graft taken from one individual and transplanted to another of the same species. SEE: *isograft.*

isoprecipitin (ī''sō-prē-sĭp'ĭ-tĭn) [" + L. *praecipitare*, to cast down]. A precipitin that reacts with antigens from other members of the same species, but they are genetically dissimilar.

isopropamide iodide (ī''sō-prō'pă-mīd). USP. A synthetic antimuscarinic drug that acts similarly to belladonna. Trade name is Darbid.

isopropanol (ī''sō-prō'pă-nŏl). Isopropyl alcohol.

isopropyl alcohol. C_3H_8O. A clear flammable liquid similar to ethyl alcohol and propyl alcohol. Used in medical preparations for external use, antifreeze, cosmetics, and as a solvent.

Caution: Toxic when taken internally. SEE: *Poisons and Poisoning* in *Appendix.*

isoproterenol hydrochloride (ī''sō-prō''tĕ-rē'nŏl). USP. A sympathomimetic amine used to relieve bronchoconstriction in asthma. It is also used as a cardiac stimulant in heart block. Trade names are Isuprel Hydrochloride, Norisodrine Aerotrol and Vapo-Iso.

Caution: Overdosage administered by inhalation can be fatal.

isopters (ī-sŏp'tĕrz) [" + *opter*, observer]. Lines on a chart of the field of vision that connect points of equal visual acuity.

Isopto Atropine. Trade name for atropine sulfate.

Isopto Carbachol. Trade name for carbachol.

Isopto Carpine. Trade name for pilocarpine hydrochloride, USP.

Isopto Cetamide. Trade name for sulfacetamide sodium, USP.

Isopto Eserine. Trade name for physostigmine salicylate, USP.

Isopto Frin. Trade name for phenylephrine hydrochloride, USP.

Isopto Homatropine. Trade name for homatropine hydrobromide.

Isopto Hyoscine. Trade name for scopolamine hydrobromide.

isopyknosis (ī″sō-pĭk-nō′sĭs) [″ + *pyknosis*, condensation]. Having uniform density, esp. being in a state of equal condensation as in comparing different chromosomes.

Isordil. Trade name for isosorbide dinitrate.

isoserotherapy (ī″sō-sē″rō-thĕr′ă-pē) [″ + L. *serum*, whey, + Gr. *therapeia*, treatment]. Treatment with serum from one having had the same disease as the patient.

isoserum (ī″sō-sē′rŭm). A serum from one having had the disease for which a patient is to receive treatment.

isosexual (ī″sō-sĕks′ū-ăl). Concerning or characteristic of the same sex.

isosmotic (ī″sŏs-mŏt′ĭk) [″ + *osmos*, impulsion]. Having the same total concentration of osmotically active molecules or ions in solution as the solution or body fluid to which it is being compared. SEE: *isotonic*.

isosorbide dinitrate tablets (ī″sō-sor′bĭd). USP. An antianginal drug used sublingually. Trade names are Isordil and Sorbitrate.

Isospora (ī-sŏs′pō-ră) [″ + *sporos*, spore]. A genus of Sporozoa belonging to the order Coccidia.

   I. hominis. A parasitic, nonpathogenic protozoon inhabiting the small intestine of man.

isospore (ī′sō-spor) [Gr. *isos*, equal, + *sporos*, spore]. A nonsexual spore from plants with only one kind of spore. It grows to maturity without conjugating.

isosthenuria (ī″sŏs-thĕn-ū′rē-ă) [″ + *sthenos*, strength, + *ouron*, urine]. Condition of the urine being of a uniform specific gravity and osmolarity despite variations in fluid intake. A sign of marked impairment of renal function.

isostimulation [″ + L. *stimulare*, to goad]. Stimulation of an animal by the use of antigenic material derived from another animal of the same species.

isotherapy (ī″sō-thĕr′ă-pē) [″ + *therapeia*, treatment]. Treatment of disease by active causative agent of the same disease. SYN: *isopathy*.

isothermal [″ + *therme*, heat]. Having equal temperature.

isothermognosis (ī″sō-thĕrm″ŏg-nō′sĭs) [″ + ″ + *gnosis*, knowledge]. Abnormal perception in which stimulations by pain, heat, and cold are all felt as heat.

isotherms (ī′sō-thĕrmz). Lines on a chart or map connecting points that have the same temperature.

isotones (ī′sō-tōnz). Nuclides with the same number of neutrons but a different number of protons in their nuclei.

isotonia (ī″sō-tō′nē-ă) [″ + *tonos*, tone]. The state of equal osmotic pressure of two or more solutions or substances.

isotonic (ī″sō-tŏn′ĭk). An isotonic muscle contraction occurs when tension is developed in a muscle, usually with a constant resistance force, and the muscle length decreases or is lengthened during the performance of work or exercise.

isotonic exercise. SEE: *exercise, isotonic.*

isotonicity (ī″sō-tō-nĭs′ĭ-tē). The state or condition of being isotonic.

isotonic solution. A solution that has a concentration of electrolytes, nonelectrolytes, or a combination of the two that will exert equivalent osmotic pressure as that solution with which it is being compared.

   Ex.: Either 0.16 molar sodium chloride solution (approx. 0.95% salt in water) or 0.3 molar nonelectrolyte solution is approx. isotonic with human red blood cells.

isotope (ī′sō-tōp) [″ + *topos*, place]. One of a series of chemical elements that have nearly identical chemical properties but differ in their atomic weights and electric charge. Many isotopes are radioactive.

   i., radioactive. Radioisotope. An isotope in which the nuclear composition is unstable.

isotope cisternography. Use of a radioactive tracer to investigate the circulation of cerebrospinal fluid. A tracer such as ^{131}I serum albumin is injected in the lumbar subarachnoid space. Flow of the tracer toward the head and into areas of the brain can be recorded by means of serial scintillation scanning. This technique is useful in studying hydrocephalus.

isotretinoin. A keratolytic agent used in treating acne. Trade name is Accutane.

Caution: This medicine should not be used by pregnant women or those who are sexually active and at risk of becoming pregnant.

---

isotropic (ī″sō-trŏp′ĭk) [″ + *tropos*, a turning]. 1. Possessing similar qualities in every direction. 2. Having equal refraction.

isotropy (ī-sŏt′rō-pē). State of being isotropic, q.v.

isotypes. In immunology the determinants on the immunoglobulin molecule that distinguish among the main classes of antibodies of a given species. They are the same for all normal individuals of that species. SEE: *idiotype.*

isotypical (ī-sō-tĭp′ĭ-kăl) [″ + *typos*, mark]. Belonging to the same variety or classification.

isovalericacidemia (ī″sō-vă-lĕr″ĭk-ăs″ĭ-dē′mē-ă). An inherited metabolic disease in which leucine metabolism is affected. Iso-valeric acid accumulates in the blood during periods of increased amino acid metabolism, i.e., during infections or following ingestion of proteins. Coma and death may occur.

isoxsuprine hydrochloride (ĭ-sŏk'sŭ-prēn). USP. A vasodilator drug. Its therapeutic usefulness has not been established. Trade name is Vasodilan.

isozyme (ī'sō-zīm). Isoenzyme, q.v.

issue (ĭsh'ū) [ME.]. 1. Offspring. 2. A suppurating sore maintained by a foreign body in the tissue to act as a counterirritant. 3. A discharge of pus or blood.

isthmectomy (ĭs-mĕk'tō-mē) [Gr. *isthmos*, isthmus, + *ektome*, excision]. Excision of an enlarged isthmus, esp. of the thyroid gland.

isthmian (ĭs'mē-ăn). Rel. to an isthmus.

isthmitis (ĭs-mī'tĭs) [" + *itis*, inflammation]. Inflammation of the throat or fauces.

isthmoparalysis (ĭs″mō-pă-răl'ĭ-sĭs) [" + *para*, beyond, + *lyein*, to loosen]. Paralysis of the muscles of the fauces. SYN: *isthmoplegia*.

isthmoplegia (ĭs″mō-plē'jē-ă) [" + *plege*, a stroke]. Faucial paralysis. SYN: *isthmoparalysis*.

isthmospasm (ĭs'mō-spăzm″) [" + *spasmos*, a convulsion]. Isthmian spasm, as of the fauces or of the fallopian tubes.

isthmus (ĭs'mŭs) [L.; Gr. *isthmos*, isthmus] (pl. *isthmuses* or *isthmi*). 1. A narrow passage connecting two cavities. 2. A narrow structure connecting two larger parts. 3. A constriction between two larger parts of an organ or anatomical structure.

   i., aortic. Constriction in the fetal aorta between the ductus arteriosus and left subclavian artery. Sometimes persists in adults.

   i. faucium. [NA] Constriction connecting the posterior mouth cavity proper with the pharynx.

   i. glandulae thyroideae. [NA] A narrow portion of the thyroid gland connecting the left and right lobes. SYN: *i. of thyroid.*

   i. of eustachian tube. I. tubae auditivae.

   i. of thyroid. I. glandulae thyroideae.

   i. of uterine tube. I. tubae uterinae.

   i. of uterus. I. uteri.

   i., pharyngeal. I. pharyngonasalis.

   i. pharyngonasalis. [NA] Opening between the nasopharynx and oral pharynx.

   i. tubae auditivae. [NA] Narrowest portion of the eustachian tube.

   i. tubae uterinae. [NA] The constricted portion (the medial third) of the uterine (fallopian) tube nearest the uterus.

   i. uteri. [NA] A slight constriction on the surface of the uterus midway between the uterine body and the cervix.

Isuprel Hydrochloride. Trade name for isoproterenol hydrochloride, USP.

isuria (ī-sū'rē-ă) [Gr. *isos*, equal, + *ouron*, urine]. Excretion of urine at a uniform rate.

itch [ME. *icchen*]. 1. Irritation of skin, inducing desire to scratch. Itching is caused by the skin being stimulated by a bite or scratching to release histamine. Scratching has the immediate effect of soothing the superficial nerves of the skin, but this may increase the itching by stimulating the release of histamine. SYN: *pruritus*. 2. Scabies.

   i., baker's. Rash that occurs on the hands and forearms of bakers. It may be due to mechanical or chemical factors.

   i., barber's. A fungus infection of the bearded portion of the face and neck. SYN: *tinea barbae.*

   i., dhobie. A fungus infection of the groin and perineum. SYN: *jock itch; tinea cruris.*

   i., grain. Dermatitis caused by mites.

   i., grocer's. Dermatitis caused by mites in grain or cheese; dermatitis caused by sugar.

   i., ground. Local irritation produced by penetration of the skin of the foot by hookworm larvae, especially *Necator americanus.*

   i., jock. A fungus infection of the groin and perineum. SYN: *dhobie itch; tinea cruris.*

   i., seven-year. Scabies.

   i., swimmer's. Dermatitis that develops after swimming in water containing the larval form of schistosomes.

   i., water. Itch, swimmer's, q.v.

   i., winter. Dermatitis that occurs in the winter. SYN: *pruritus hiemalis.*

itching. Pruritus; irritation of the skin, causing desire to rub or scratch the part.

itch mite. *Sarcoptes scabiei.* SEE: *scabies.*

-ite [Gr.]. 1. Suffix meaning of the nature of. 2. In chemistry, a salt of an acid having the termination *-ous.*

iter (ī'tĕr) [L.]. Passageway between two anatomical parts.

iteral (ī'tĕr-ăl). Pert. to an iter.

iteroparity (ĭt″ĕr-ō-păr'ĭ-tē) [L. *iterare*, to repeat, + *parere*, to bear]. Condition of reproducing more than once in a lifetime.

ithycyphosis, ithyokyphosis (ĭth″ĭ-sĭ-fō'sĭs, ĭth″ē-ō-kī-fō'sĭs) [Gr. *ithys*, straight, + *kyphos*, humped]. Kyphosis with backward projection of the spine.

ithylordosis (ĭth″ĭ-lor-dō'sĭs) [" + *lordosis*, a bending forward]. Lordosis without lateral curvature of the spine.

-itis (ī'tĭs) [Gr.]. Suffix meaning inflammation of.

ITP. *idiopathic thrombocytopenic purpura.*

I.U. *immunizing unit; international unit.*

IUCD. *intrauterine contraceptive device.*

IUD. *intrauterine device.*

IUGR. *intrauterine growth retardation.*

I.V. *intravenous(ly).*

Ivadantin. Trade name for nitrofurantoin sodium, USP.

IVC. *intravenous cholangiography.*

IVCD. *intraventricular conduction defect.* Used in electrocardiography to refer to abnormal conduction in ventricular muscle. SEE: *bundle branch block.*

ivermectin. An antiparasitic drug used in veterinary medicine. Its use in treating human onchocerciasis (river blindness) is being investigated. The drug is also being used experimentally as part of the therapeutic protocol for colorectal carcinoma. Trade names are Eqvalan and Ivomec.

IVF. *in vitro fertilization.*

I.V.P. *intravenous pyelography;* radiographic examination of the kidneys, ureters, and bladder after introduction of a contrast medium.

I.V. push. Administration of medicine intravenously by quick and forcible injection.

I.V.T. *intravenous transfusion.*

I.V.U. *intravenous urography.*

Ivy method (ī′vē) [Andrew C. Ivy, U.S. physiologist, 1893–1978]. SEE: *bleeding time.*

ivy poisoning. Dermatitis caused by contact with poison ivy. SEE: *poison ivy dermatitis.*

Ixodes (īks-ō′dēz) [Gr. *ixodes,* like birdlime]. A genus of ticks of the family Ixodidae, q.v., many of which are parasitic on man and animals.

ixodiasis (īks″ō-dī′ă-sĭs). 1. Lesions of the skin caused by tick bites. 2. Any disease caused by ticks, as Rocky Mountain spotted fever.

ixodic (īks-ŏd′ĭk). Pert. to or caused by ticks.

Ixodidae (īks-ŏd′ĭ-dē). A family of ticks belonging to the order Acarina, class Arachnida. Comprises the hard-bodied ticks including the genera *Amblyomma, Boophilus, Dermacentor, Haemaphysalis, Hyalomma, Ixodes,* and *Rhipicephalus.* All are parasitic and of importance as pests or in the transmission of disease in domestic animals and man. Among diseases transmitted are Rocky Mountain spotted fever, relapsing fever, and tularemia.

Ixodides (īks-ŏd′ĭ-dēz). Ticks.

Ixodoidea (īks″ō-doy′dē-ă). A superfamily of Acarina, the ticks, in which the adults have a thick cuticle.

ixomyelitis (īks″ō-mī-ĕ-lī′tĭs) [Gr. *ixodes,* like birdlime, + *myelos,* marrow, + *itis,* inflammation]. Inflammation of the spinal cord in the lumbar region.

J

J. Symb. for joule.

Jaboulay's amputation (zhă″boo-lāz′) [Mathieu Jaboulay, Fr. surgeon, 1860–1913]. Amputation of the thigh and removal of the hip bone.

Jaboulay's button. Two cylinders that may be screwed together for lateral intestinal anastomosis without the use of sutures.

jacket [O. Fr. *jacquet*, jacket]. A bandage usually applied to the trunk to immobilize the spine or correct deformities.

　　j., porcelain. A jacket crown tooth restoration made of porcelain.

　　j., Sayre's. Plaster-of-paris jacket used as a support for deformity of the spinal column.

　　j., strait-. Device for restraining a patient or criminal who is violent. It has sleeves that extend beyond the hands, the ends of which may be secured, thereby preventing movement of the arms and trunk. SYN: *camisole*.

jackknife position. Position in which the patient lies on the back with shoulders elevated, lower legs flexed on thighs, and the thighs at right angles to the trunk. May be employed when passing a urethral sound. SYN: *position, reclining*.

jackscrew. A threaded screw used for expanding the dental arch or for positioning bone fragments after a fracture.

jacksonian epilepsy [John Hughlings Jackson, Brit. neurologist, 1835–1911]. A localized form of epilepsy with spasms confined to one part or one group of muscles. SEE: *epilepsy*.

Jacob, Arthur. Irish ophthalmologist, 1790–1874.

　　J.'s membrane. Retinal layer of rods and cones.

　　J.'s ulcer. Epithelioma, usually of the face, that slowly destroys soft tissue and bones. SYN: *rodent ulcer*.

Jacobson, Ludwig. Danish anatomist, 1783–1843.

　　J.'s cartilage. One of two narrow longitudinal cartilages lying along the anterior inferior border of the nasal septum. They are rudimentary in man.

　　J.'s nerve. Tympanic nerve.

　　J.'s organ. Rudimentary sac in nasal septum. SYN: *vomeronasal organ*. SEE: *organ of Jacobson*.

　　J.'s sulcus. Portion of the middle ear containing branches of the tympanic plexus.

Jacquemier's sign (zhăk-mē-āz′) [Jean Jac-

quemier, Fr. obstetrician, 1806–1879]. Blue or purple color of the vaginal mucosa. A presumptive sign of pregnancy.

jactatio (jăk-tā′shē-ō) [L.]. Restless tossing of the head and body. Seen in acute illness.

jactatio capitis nocturna [L. *jactatio*, tossing, + *caput*, head, + *nocturnus*, night]. A form of sleep disturbance characterized by nocturnal head banging.

jactitation (jăk″tĭ-tā′shŭn) [L. *jactitatio*, tossing]. In acute disease, the restless to-and-fro movement of the body.

Jaeger's test types (yā′gĕrz) [Jaeger, Eduard, Ritter von Jaxtthal, Austrian ophthalmologist, 1818–1884]. Lines of type of various sizes, printed on a card for testing near vision. The smallest type read at the closest distance is recorded.

jamais vu (zhăm′ā voo) [Fr., never seen]. Subjective mental reaction of being in a completely strange environment when in familiar surroundings. May be associated with temporal lobe lesions. SEE: *déjà vu*.

James fibers [T. N. James, U.S. cardiologist and physiologist, b. 1925]. Pathway for conduction of cardiac impulses so they bypass the atrioventricular node. This alternate fiber pathway permits pre-excitation of the ventricle with resultant tachycardia.

Janeway lesions [Edward Gamaliel Janeway, U.S. physician, 1841–1911]. Small, painless, red-blue macular lesions a few millimeters in diameter; found on the palms and soles in acute bacterial endocarditis. SEE: *Roth's spots*.

janiceps (jăn′ĭ-sĕps) [L. *Janus*, a two-faced god, + *caput*, head]. Deformed embryo with a face on the anterior and posterior aspects of the single head.

Janimine. Trade name for imipramine hydrochloride.

Jansky-Bielschowsky syndrome (jăn′skē-bē-ăl-show′skē) [Jan Jansky, Czech physician, 1873–1921; Max Bielschowsky, Ger. neuropathologist, 1869–1940]. Early juvenile cerebral sphingolipidosis. SEE: *sphingolipidosis*.

jar. 1. A container made of glass, plastic, or other sturdy materials. It is usually taller than wide and may be cylindrical, square, or another shape. 2. A sudden movement, as a jolt or shock.

　　j., bell. A glass vessel with an opening at only one end.

　　j., heel. Production of pain by having the patient stand on tiptoes and suddenly bring the heels to the floor. This may be diagnostic of tuberculosis of the spine, pelvic inflammatory disease in the female, or renal calculus.

jargon (jăr′gŭn) [O. Fr., a chattering]. 1. Unintelligible speech. SYN: *paraphasia*. 2. The technical language or specialized terminology of those in a specific profession or group.

Jarvis′ snare [William C. Jarvis, U.S. laryngologist, 1855–1895]. A snare for removing growths in the nasal cavities.

jaundice (jawn′dĭs) [Fr. *jaune,* yellow]. Condition characterized by yellowness of skin, whites of eyes, mucous membranes, and body fluids due to deposition of bile pigment resulting from excess bilirubin in the blood (hyperbilirubinemia). It may be caused by obstruction of bile passageways, excess destruction of red blood cells (hemolysis), or disturbances in functioning of liver cells.

Jaundice is a symptom that may be the indicator of a benign and curable disease, such as a gallstone blocking the common duct. It may be due to carcinoma of the head of the pancreas involving the opening of the bile duct into the duodenum. It is therefore important to make the correct diagnosis.

The diagnostic studies to determine the cause of jaundice include noninvasive procedures such as ultrasonography and computed tomography, in addition to clinical laboratory studies and expert clinical evaluation. Invasive studies include cholangiography, endoscopic retrograde cholangiopancreatography (ERCP), or percutaneous transhepatic cholangiography (PTC).

In the newborn, severe jaundice may damage the cells of the basal ganglia and the brain stem; also, the bilirubin level may be sufficiently high to cause deafness, cerebral palsy, or death. The cause may be red cell (Rh) incompatibility or septicemia. Depending on the cause, jaundice in the newborn may be treated with exchange transfusion or phototherapy, or both. SYN: *icterus.* SEE: *hemolytic disease of the newborn; kernicterus; phototherapy; transfusion, exchange.*

    j., acholuric. Jaundice without bile pigment in the urine.

    j., cholestatic. Jaundice due to failure of bile to reach the duodenum, whether due to blockage of the flow of bile or to liver cell changes.

    j., congenital. Jaundice occurring at or shortly after birth due to maldevelopment of biliary apparatus.

    j., hematogenous. J., hemolytic.

    j., hemolytic. A rare chronic form of jaundice that results from increased destruction of red blood cells. The serum bilirubin may be only slightly elevated even though bile pigment production may be increased to as much as six times normal. The bilirubin, which is mostly unconjugated and therefore insoluble in water, does not appear in the urine. The spleen is usually enlarged. SYN: *icterus, hemolytic.*

    j., hemorrhagic. Jaundice present with leptospirosis.

    j., hepatocanalicular. Jaundice resulting from changes in the bile canaliculi, with the liver cells remaining relatively normal.

    j., hepatocellular. Jaundice resulting from disease of liver cells.

    j., hepatogenous. Jaundice due to disease of the liver.

    j., infectious. Infectious hepatitis.

    j., leptospiral. Jaundice present with leptospirosis.

    j., nonhemolytic. Jaundice due to abnormal metabolism of bilirubin. By implication, the jaundice is not due to excessive destruction of red blood cells.

    j., obstructive. Jaundice due to a mechanical impediment in the flow of bile from the liver to the duodenum. SYN: *icterus, obstructive.*

    j. of newborn. Jaundice affecting newborn infants. SYN: *icterus neonatorum.*

    j., parenchymatous. J., hepatocellular.

    j., physiologic. Simple jaundice in the newborn lasting only a few days and not requiring therapy.

    j., posthepatic. Jaundice resulting from obstruction of flow of bile ducts. May be incomplete or complete.

    j., regurgitation. Jaundice due to bile entering lymph channels of the liver and thence being conveyed to the blood. May result from biliary obstruction or lesions involving bile capillaries.

    j., retention. Jaundice resulting from inability of liver cells to remove bile pigment from circulation.

    j., spirochetal. An acute infectious disease due to a spirochete, *Leptospira interrogans icterohaemorrhagiae.* SYN: *Weil's disease.*

    j., toxic. Jaundice resulting from bacterial toxins or poisons such as phosphorus, arsphenamine, carbon tetrachloride.

Javelle water (zhŭ-vĕl′) [Javel, a city now part of Paris]. An aqueous solution of potassium or sodium hypochlorite used as a bleach and disinfectant.

jaw [ME. *iawe*]. Either or both of the maxillary and mandibular bones, bearing the teeth and forming the mouth framework. SEE: illus.

    j., cleft. Early embryonic malformation resulting in lack of fusion of the right and left mandible into a single bone.

    j., crackling. Noise in the normal or diseased temporomandibular joint during

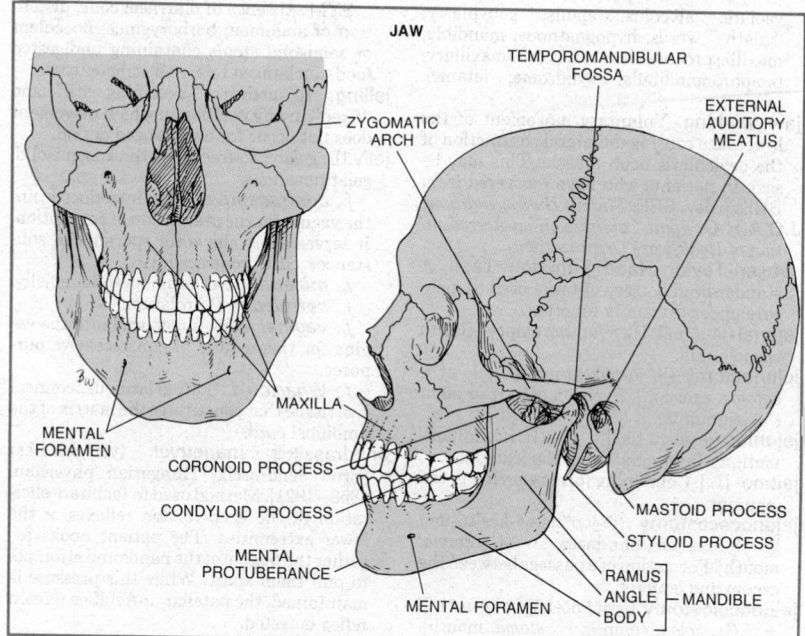

JAW

TEMPOROMANDIBULAR FOSSA

EXTERNAL AUDITORY MEATUS

ZYGOMATIC ARCH

MENTAL FORAMEN

MAXILLA

CORONOID PROCESS

CONDYLOID PROCESS

MENTAL PROTUBERANCE

MENTAL FORAMEN

MASTOID PROCESS

STYLOID PROCESS

RAMUS
ANGLE — MANDIBLE
BODY

movement of the jaw. SYN: *crepitation*.

j., dislocation of. Jaw dislocations are uncomfortable and extremely embarrassing to the patient. They may occur on either side, in which instance the tip of the jaw is pointed away from the dislocation. On the unaffected side, just in front of the ear, may be felt a little hollow or depression that is often tender. If both sides of the jaw are dislocated, the jaw is pushed downward and backward. In either event, there is pain and difficulty in speech and the condition is often accompanied by shock. Backward dislocation of jaw is rare.

CAUSES: Most often caused by a blow to the face or by keeping the mouth open for long periods as in dental treatment, but occasionally caused by chewing large chunks of food, by yawning, or by hearty laughing. A fall or blow on the chin could cause dislocation, but backward dislocation seldom occurs without fracture or extreme trauma.

REDUCTION: These dislocations are reduced by placing well-padded thumbs inside of the mouth on the lower molar (back) teeth with the fingers running along the outside of the jaw as a lever. The thumbs should press the jaw downward and backward. The jaw will glide posteriorly over the ridge of bone (articular eminence), which can be felt, and just as this occurs the jaw usually snaps into place. When this motion is noted, the thumbs should be moved laterally toward the cheeks to keep them from being crushed between the molars.

This snapping into place is due to an involuntary spasm of the muscles, which pulls the jaw as though an overstretched rubber band were attached to it. Following the reduction, an immobilizing bandage or double cravat should be applied.

Caution: It is important that the hands be protected by a heavy glove to prevent trauma by the teeth. SEE: *Universal Precautions* in *Appendix.*

j., lumpy. Fungal disease affecting the jaw, brain, lungs, and gastrointestinal tract. Common in cattle and sometimes affects humans. SYN: *actinomycosis.*

j., swelling of. *Lower:* May be due to alveolar abscess, a cyst, gumma, sarcoma, or actinomycosis. *Upper:* Occurs in alveolar abscess, parotid tumor, parotitis, carcinoma, sarcoma, necrosis of bone, or disease of antrum.

jaw, words pert. to: agnathia; alveolar; alveolate; alveolus; epulis; genyplasty; "gnath-" words; hypognathous; mandible; maxilla; prognathism; ramus; submaxillary; temporomandibular syndrome; tetanus; trismus.

jaw winking. Voluntary movement of the lower face causing unilateral contraction of the orbicularis oculi muscle. This may be seen in patients who have recovered from Bell's palsy. SEE: *Marcus Gunn syndrome.*

J.C.A.H.O. *Joint Commission on Accreditation of Healthcare Organizations.*

Jebsen-Taylor Hand Function Test. A standardized battery of tasks used to measure upper extremity function.

jejunal (jĕ-jū′năl) [L. *jejunum,* empty]. Rel. to the jejunum.

jejunectomy (jĕ″jū-nĕk′tō-mē) [″ + Gr. *ektome,* excision]. Excision of part or all of the jejunum.

jejunitis (jĕ″jū-nī′tĭs) [″ + Gr. *itis,* inflammation]. Inflammation of the jejunum.

jejuno- [L.]. Combining form referring to the jejunum.

jejunocecostomy (jĕ-joo″nō-sē-kŏs′tō-mē) [″ + *caecum,* blindness, + Gr. *stoma,* mouth]. Formation of a passage between the cecum and jejunum.

jejunocolostomy (jē-jū″nō-kōl-ŏs′tō-mē) [″ + Gr. *kolon,* colon, + *stoma,* mouth]. Formation of an artificial passage between the jejunum and colon.

jejunoileal (jē-joo″nō-ĭl′ē-ăl) [″ + *ileum,* small intestine]. Concerning the jejunum and ileum.

jejunoileitis (jē-jū″nō-ĭl″ē-ī′tĭs) [″ + ″ + Gr. *itis,* inflammation]. Inflamed condition of the jejunum and ileum.

jejunoileostomy (jē-jū″nō-ĭl″ē-ŏs′tō-mē) [″ + ″ + Gr. *stoma,* mouth]. Formation of a passage between the jejunum and ileum.

jejunojejunostomy (jē-jū″nō-jē″jū-nŏs′tō-mē) [″ + *jejunum,* empty, + Gr. *stoma,* mouth]. Formation of a passage between two parts of the jejunum.

jejunorrhaphy (jē″joo-nor′ă-fē) [″ + Gr. *rhaphe,* seam, ridge]. Surgical repair of the jejunum.

jejunostomy (jĕ″jū-nŏs′tō-mē) [″ + Gr. *stoma,* mouth]. Surgical creation of a permanent opening into the jejunum.

jejunotomy (jĕ″jū-nŏt′ō-mē) [″ + Gr. *tome,* incision]. Surgical incision into the jejunum.

jejunum (jē-jū′nŭm) [L., empty]. [NA] The second portion of the small intestine extending from the duodenum to the ileum. It is about 8 ft (2.4 meters) in length, making up about two-fifths of the small intestine.

   j., inflammation of. May be present in bacterial infections of the intestinal tract or in regional enteritis.

SYM: Absence of diarrhea; colic; distention of abdomen; borborygmus; flocculent or semisolid stools containing undigested food, unchanged bile, and some mucus.

jelling. In arthritis, becoming stiff and "fixed" in any position in which movement does not occur for a prolonged period.

jelly [L. *gelare,* to freeze]. A thick, semisolid, gelatinous mass.

   j., contraceptive. Jelly introduced into the vagina for the prevention of conception. It serves as a vehicle for spermicidal substances. SEE: *contraceptive.*

   j., mineral. Petrolatum; petroleum jelly.

   j., petroleum. Petrolatum.

   j., vaginal. Jelly introduced into the vagina for therapeutic or contraceptive purposes.

   j., Wharton's. Soft, gelatinous, connective tissue that constitutes the matrix of the umbilical cord.

Jendrassik's maneuver (yĕn-drä′sĭks) [Ernö Jendrassik, Hungarian physician, 1858–1921]. Method used to facilitate elicitation of the deep tendon reflexes of the lower extremities. The patient hooks together the fingers of the hands and attempts to pull them apart. While this pressure is maintained, the patellar or Achilles tendon reflex is tested.

Jenner, Edward. [British physician 1749–1823]. Inventor of the vaccination for smallpox. Prior to Jenner's work, it was known that individuals exposed to a mild case of the disease for the first time would suffer a mild case and then be immune to smallpox. Jenner observed that individuals exposed to cowpox, such as those who milked cows, would develop a minor lesion and then be immune to smallpox. From this observation he developed a vaccine from cowpox lesions, now known to be the vaccinia virus, which gives immunity to smallpox.

Jenner's stain [Louis Jenner, Brit. physician, 1866–1904]. Eosin methylene blue stain.

jerk (jĕrk). 1. A sudden muscular movement. 2. Certain reflex actions resulting from striking or tapping a muscle or tendon. SEE: *reflex.*

   j., Achilles; j., ankle. Contraction of the calf muscles produced by tapping the stretched Achilles tendon.

   j., biceps. Reflex contraction of the biceps brachii produced by tapping over the insertion of the tendon at the head of the radius. Usually, the evaluator places a thumb against the tendon and taps the nail of the thumb to elicit the reflex.

   j., elbow. Involuntary extension of forearm produced by external stimulation of the stretched triceps tendon.

j., jaw. Movement that is a result of tapping the mandible when the jaw is half open. It may be increased when there are bilateral supranuclear cerebral lesions.

j., knee. Forward jerk of lower leg upon striking patellar tendon when knee is flexed at right angles. Absent in locomotor ataxia, infantile paralysis, meningitis, destructive lesions of lower part of spinal cord, and certain forms of paralysis. Increased in lesions of pyramidal areas, brain tumors, spinal irritability, and cerebrospinal sclerosis. SYN: *patellar-tendon reflex.* SEE: *reflex, knee-jerk.*

j., tendon. The contraction of a muscle after tapping its tendon.

j., triceps surae. J., Achilles, q.v.

jet injector. A device that uses a high-speed air jet to deliver medicines, esp. vaccines, intradermally without puncturing the skin.

jet lag. SEE: *desynchronosis; dyschronism.*

jigger. Common name for parasitic fleas called *Tunga penetrans,* q.v. SEE: *chiggers.*

jimson weed. Stramonium, q.v.

jitters (jit′ĕrz). Shakes, q.v.

Jobst pressure garment. Elastic garment fabricated to apply varying pressure gradients to an area. It may be worn over severely burned areas for the purpose of reducing hypertrophic scarring as wounds heal or may be used to prevent or control lymphedema in the arm or legs.

Job's syndrome [Job, Biblical person]. Recurrent infections of the skin related to impaired defenses, the precise nature of which are unclear. SYN: *hyperimmunoglobulin E recurrent infection syndrome.*

Jocasta complex (jō-kăs′tă) [Jocasta, mother in the Oedipus complex, who was the wife and mother of Oedipus]. A term implying psychological or emotional fixation of a mother to her son. SEE: *Oedipus complex.*

Joffroy's reflex (zhŏf-rwhăz′) [Alexis Joffroy, Fr. physician, 1844–1908]. Twitching of gluteal muscles when pressure is made against buttocks.

Joffroy's sign. 1. Absence of facial muscle contraction when eyes turn upward in exophthalmic goiter. 2. Inability to do simple sums in arithmetic. An early sign of general paralysis of the insane caused by central nervous system syphilis.

jogger's heel. Irritation of the fibrous and fatty tissue covering the heel. Due to the type of running characteristic of jogging, in which the heel strikes the surface first, rather than that of sprinting, in which the toes strike first. Persons prone to develop this may diminish the risk by wearing pads

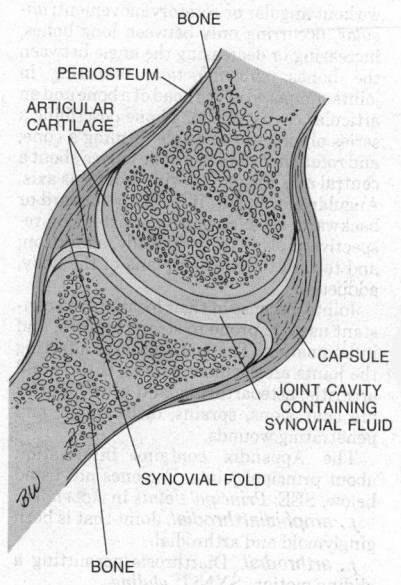

TYPICAL SYNOVIAL JOINT

on their heels and by running on surfaces softer than wood, concrete, or asphalt.

jogging. Running for enjoyment or to maintain physical fitness. In contrast to running, jogging is not a competitive exercise.

joint [L. *junctio,* a joining]. An articulation. The point of juncture between two bones. A joint is usually formed of fibrous connective tissue and cartilage. It is classified as being immovable (synarthrosis), slightly movable (amphiarthrosis), and freely movable (diarthrosis). *Synarthrosis* is a joint in which the two bones are separated only by an intervening membrane, such as the cranial sutures. *Amphiarthrosis* is a joint having a fibrocartilaginous disk between the bony surfaces (symphysis), such as the symphysis pubis, or a joint with a ligament uniting the two bones (syndesmosis), such as the tibiofibular articulation. *Diarthrosis* is a joint in which the adjoining bone ends are covered with a thin cartilaginous sheet and joined by ligament lined by a synovial membrane, which secretes a lubricant. SEE: illus.

Joints are grouped according to motion: ball and socket (enarthrosis); hinge (ginglymus); condyloid; pivot (trochoid); gliding (arthrodia); and saddle joint.

Joints can move in four ways: *gliding*, in which one bony surface glides on another without angular or rotatory movement; *angular*, occurring only between long bones, increasing or decreasing the angle between the bones; *circumduction*, occurring in joints composed of the head of a bone and an articular cavity, the long bone describing a series of circles, the whole forming a cone; and *rotation*, in which a bone moves about a central axis without moving from this axis. Angular movement, if it occurs forward or backward, is called flexion or extension respectively; away from the body, abduction; and toward the median plane of the body, adduction.

Joints, because of their location and constant use, are prone to stress, injuries, and inflammation. The main diseases affecting the joints are rheumatic fever, rheumatoid arthritis, osteoarthritis, and gout. Injuries are contusions, sprains, dislocations, and penetrating wounds.

The Appendix contains information about principal joints. For ones not listed below, SEE: *Principal Joints in Appendix.*

j., amphidiarthrodial. Joint that is both ginglymoid and arthrodial.

j., arthrodial. Diarthrosis permitting a gliding motion. SYN: *j., gliding.*

j., ball-and-socket. Joint in which the round end of one bone fits into the cavity of another bone. SYN: *enarthrosis; j., multiaxial; j., polyaxial.*

j., biaxial. Joint possessing two chief movement axes at right angles to each other.

j., bilocular. Joint separated into two sections by interarticular cartilage.

j., bleeders'. Hemorrhage into joint space in hemophiliacs.

j., Brodie's. Arthrodial neuralgia due to hysteria.

j., Budin's. Congenital cartilaginous band between squamous and condylar parts of the occipital bone.

j., cartilaginous. Joint in which there is cartilage connecting the bones.

j., Charcot's. A disease in tabes dorsalis or syringomyelia. Joint enlargement due to wasting away of muscles below the joint.

j., Chopart's. Union of remainder of tarsal bones with os calcis and astragalus.

j., cochlear. Hinge joint permitting lateral motion. SYN: *j., spiral.*

j., compound. Joint made up of several bones.

j., condyloid. Joint permitting all forms of angular movements except axial rotation.

j.'s, craniomandibular. The encapsulated, double synovial joints between the heads of the mandible and the temporal bones of the cranium. The double synovial joints are separated by an articular disk and function as an upper gliding joint and a lower modified hinge or ginglymoid joint. SYN: *j.'s, temporomandibular.*

j., diarthrodial. Joint characterized by the presence of a cavity within the capsule separating the bony elements, thus permitting considerable freedom of movement.

j., dry. Arthritis of chronic villous type.

j., ellipsoid. Joint having two axes of motion through the same bone.

j., enarthrodial. J., ball-and-socket. SYN: *j., multiaxial.*

j., false. False joint formation subsequent to a fracture.

j.'s, fibrous. Joints connected by fibrous tissue.

j., flail. Joint that is extremely relaxed, the distal portion of the limb being almost beyond the control of the will.

j., ginglymoid. A synovial joint having only forward and backward motion, as a hinge. SYN: *ginglymus; j., hinge.*

j., gliding. Diarthrosis permitting a gliding motion. SYN: *j., arthrodial.*

j., hemophilic. J., bleeders'.

j., hinge. Joint having only a forward and backward motion, as a hinge. SYN: *j., ginglymoid.*

j., hip. A stable ball-and-socket type of joint in which the head of the femur fits into the acetabulum of the hip bone.

j., immovable. Joint in which a cavity is lacking between the bones. SYN: *synarthrosis.*

j.'s, intercarpal. Articulations the carpal bones form in relation to one another.

j., irritable. Recurrent inflamed condition of joint of unknown cause.

j., knee. Joint between the femur, patella, and tibia.

j., midcarpal. Joint separating the navicular, lunate, and triangular bones from the distal row of carpal bones.

j., mixed. Joint with surfaces joined by fibrocartilaginous disks.

j., movable. Slightly movable or freely movable joint, amphiarthrosis and diarthrosis, respectively.

j., multiaxial. J., ball-and-socket. SYN: *j., enarthrodial; j., polyaxial.*

j., pivot. Joint that permits rotation of a bone, the joint being formed by a pivotlike process that turns within a ring, or by a ringlike structure that turns on a pivot. SYN: *j., rotary; j., trochoid.*

j., plane. Synovial joint between bone surfaces. Only gliding movements are possible.

j., polyaxial. J., ball-and-socket. SYN: *j., enarthrodial; j., polyaxial.*

j., receptive. J., saddle.

j., rotary. J., pivot. SYN: *j., trochoid.*

j., saddle. Joint in which the opposing surfaces are reciprocally concavoconvex. SYN: *j., receptive.*

j., simple. Joint composed of two bones.

j., spheroid. Multiaxial joint with spheroid surfaces.

j., spiral. J., cochlear.

j., sternoclavicular. The joint space between the sternum and the medial extremity of the clavicle.

j.'s, subtalar. The three articular surfaces on the inferior surface of the talus.

j., synarthrodial. J., immovable.

j., synovial. Joint separated by space containing synovial fluid. SEE: illus.

j.'s, tarsometatarsal. Joint made up of three arthrodial joints, the bones of which articulate with the bases of the metatarsal bones.

j.'s, temporomandibular. J.'s, craniomandibular.

j., trochoid. J., pivot. SYN: *j., rotary.*

j., uniaxial. Joint moving on a single axis.

j., unilocular. Joint with a single cavity.

joint approximation. A rehabilitation technique whereby joint surfaces are compressed together while the patient is in a weight-bearing posture for the purpose of facilitating co-contraction of muscles around a joint.

joint capsule. The saclike structure that encloses the ends of bones in a diarthrodial joint. Consists of an outer fibrous layer and an inner synovial layer and contains synovial fluid.

joint cavity. The articular cavity or space enclosed by the synovial membrane and articular cartilages. It contains synovial fluid.

joint manipulation. Passive therapeutic techniques used to stretch restricted joints or reposition a subluxation. The techniques are sometimes applied with rapid thrust movements, or are applied with the patient under anesthesia to assure maximum relaxation. SEE: *joint mobilization.*

joint mice. Free bits of cartilage or bone present in the joint space, esp. the knee joint. These are usually the result of previous trauma. They may or may not be symptomatic. SYN: *loose bodies.*

joint mobilization. Passive therapeutic techniques that are applied specifically to joint structures and utilize principles of arthrokinematics, q.v., to increase joint play and range of motion or to treat pain.

joint play. 1. The motions of sliding, rolling, spinning, compressing or distracting which

occur between bony surfaces within a joint when the bones move through ranges of motion. 2. The distensibility or "give" of the joint capsule and ligaments that allows motion to occur between bony partners within a joint.

joint protection. Techniques for minimizing stress on joints, including proper body mechanics and the avoidance of continuous weight-bearing or deforming postures. SYN: *joint preservation.*

Jones criteria [T.D. Jones, U.S. physician, 1899–1954]. The criteria for diagnosis of acute rheumatic fever. SEE: *rheumatic fever.*

joule (jūl) [James Prescott Joule, Brit. physicist, 1818–1889]. ABBR: **J**. Work done in one second by current of one ampere against a resistance of one ohm. One kilogram calorie (kcal or Calorie) is equal to 4185.5 joules. One calorie (small calorie) is equal to 4.1855 joules.

JRA. *juvenile rheumatoid arthritis.*

JRCEDMS. *Joint Review Committee on Education in Diagnostic Medical Sonography.*

JRCERT. *Joint Review Committee on Education in Radiologic Technology.*

jugal [L. *jugalis,* of a yoke]. 1. Connected or united as by a yoke. 2. Pert. to the malar or zygomatic bone.

jugal bone. Malar or zygomatic bone.

jugale (jū-gā'lē). The point at the margin of the zygomatic process.

jugal process. Temporal bone process forming the zygomatic arch. SYN: *zygomatic process.*

jugate (jū'gāt) [L. *jugatus,* joined]. 1. Coupled, yoked. 2. Having ridges.

jugomaxillary (joo″gō-măk'sĭ-lăr″ē). Concerning the maxilla and the zygomatic bone.

jugular (jŭg'ū-lăr) [L. *jugularis*]. Pert. to the throat.

jugular foramen. Opening formed by jugular notches of the occipital and temporal bones.

jugular fossa. Depression in the petrosal portion of the temporal bone for the jugular vein.

jugular ganglion. Nodes of vagus root and glossopharyngeal nerve in jugular foramen.

jugular process. Projection from occipital bone toward the temporal bone.

jugular veins. *External,* receives the blood from the exterior of the cranium and the deep parts of the face. It lies superficial to the sternocleidomastoid muscle as it passes down the neck to join the subclavian vein. *Internal,* receives blood from the brain and superficial parts of the face and neck. It is directly continuous with the transverse sinus, accompanying the internal carotid as it passes down the neck, and joins with the subclavian vein to form the innominate vein. The jugular veins are more prominent during expiration than during inspiration and are also prominent during cardiac decompensation.

When the patient is sitting or in a semirecumbent position, the height of the jugular veins and their pulsations can provide an accurate estimation of central venous pressure and give important information about cardiac compensation.

jugulate (jŭg′ū-lāt) [L. *jugulare*, to cut the throat]. To quickly arrest a process or disease by therapeutic measures.

jugulation (jŭg″ū-lā′shŭn). Sudden arrest of a disease by therapeutic means.

jugulum (jŭg′ū-lŭm) [L.]. Neck or throat.

jugum (jū′gŭm) [L., a yoke] (pl. *juga*). 1. [NA] Ridge or furrow connecting two points. 2. A type of forceps.

    j. penis. Forceps for temporarily compressing the penis.

    j. petrosum. Eminence on petrous section of the temporal bone showing the position of the superior semicircular canal. SYN: *arcuate eminence.*

juice [L. *jus*, broth]. Liquid excreted, secreted, or expressed from any part of an organism.

    j., alimentary. The digestive juices.

    j., gastric. Secretions of the stomach, consisting of water, salts, pepsin, and free hydrochloric acid.

    j., intestinal. A clear, yellow, viscid fluid secreted by Lieberkühn's crypts. It is alkaline in reaction. SYN: *succus entericus.*

    j., pancreatic. A clear, viscid, alkaline digestive juice of the pancreas poured into the duodenum. It contains the enzymes trypsin, amylase, and lipase or steapsin.

jujitsu, jiujitsu (jū-jĭt′sū) [Japanese]. A system of physical training for developing the art of self-defense without weapons. The opponent's weight and strength are used to his or her disadvantage.

jumentous (jū-mĕn′tŭs) [L. *jumentum*, beast of burden]. Like that of a horse, said of odor of urine in certain diseased conditions.

Jumping Frenchmen of Maine. A condition, characterized by a sudden, single, sometimes violent movement or cry that occurs in response to a sharp unexpected sound or touch. The individual may also blurt out whatever was being thought of at the time of the stimulus. The condition may begin in childhood and be lifelong. It has been most frequently described in persons of French descent living in Maine, but may occur in a person of almost any nationality or geographic location. The cause is unknown and there is no effective therapy. SEE: *Gilles de la Tourette's syndrome; mir-*

yachit; startle syndromes.

jump sign. During physical examination, an involuntary reaction to stimulation of a tender area or trigger point, q.v. This may take the form of wincing or sudden jerking of the part being examined, of adjacent areas, or even of the entire body. This sign should not be confused with the startle reaction seen in Jumping Frenchmen of Maine, q.v.

junction (jŭnk′shŭn) [L. *junctio*, a joining]. The place of union or coming together of two parts or tissue layers.

    j., amelodentinal. SEE: *j., dentinoenamel.*

    j., atrioventricular (A-V). Area of cardiac conduction pathway composed of the A-V node and bundle of His.

    j., cementodentinal. Interface of dentin and cementum of the tooth. SYN: *dentinocemental junction.*

    j., cementoenamel. The line around the tooth that marks the boundary between the crown and root of the tooth; the interface between enamel and cementum.

    j., dentinocemental. SEE: *j., cementodentinal.*

    j., dentinoenamel. The plane or interface between the dentin of the tooth and the enamel crown; histological sections show it to be a scalloped boundary at the site of the basement membrane which separated the cell layers that formed the calcified enamel and dentin. SYN: *amelodentinal junction.*

    j., dentogingival. The interface and zone of attachment between the gingiva and enamel or cementum of the tooth. It holds in place the junctional or attachment epithelium.

    j., interneuronal. Junction of adjacent neurons consisting of the terminal ending of one neuron and the dendrite or body of the second neuron. SYN: *synapse.*

    j., mucocutaneous. Junction between the skin and a mucous membrane.

    j., mucogingival. A scalloped, indistinct boundary between the gingiva and the oral mucosa on the alveolar process. The coral color of gingiva may be contrasted with the more vascular oral mucosa. Also called the mucogingival line.

    j., myoneural. Meeting point of a nerve with the muscle to which it is distributed. SYN: *motor endplate.*

    j., sclerocorneal. Meeting point between the sclera and the cornea marked on the external surface of the eyeball by the outer scleral sulcus.

    j., squamocolumnar. Point in the cervical canal at which the squamous and columnar epithelia meet. Most cervical cancers begin in this area; therefore, it is important to obtain cells from this location for the Pap test.

j., tight. A part of the junctional complex at the lateral interface between epithelial cells. Also called zonula occludens.

junctional epithelium. The zone of soft tissue attached to the tooth. SYN: *attachment epithelium; gingival cuff.*

junctional rhythm. An ECG rhythm arising in the A-V junction. Appears as a narrow QRS complex that lacks an upright P wave preceding it.

junctura (jŭnk-tū'ră) [L., a joining] (pl. *juncturae*). Suture of bones; articulation.

juniper tar (joo'nĭ-pĕr). USP. A volatile oil obtained from the wood of *Juniperus oxycedrus.* It is used in shampoos and bath emulsions.

junket [L. *juncus*]. 1. Curds and whey; a type of cream cheese. 2. Commonly, a flavored and sweetened custard set by rennet.

jurisprudence (joor"ĭs-proo'dĕns) [L. *juris prudentia*, knowledge of law]. The scientific study or application of the principles of law and justice.

j., dental. The application of the principles of law as they relate to the practice of dentistry, to the obligations of the practitioners to their patients, and to the relations of dentists to each other and to society in general. This term and forensic dentistry are sometimes used as synonyms, but some authorities consider the first as a branch of law and the second as a branch of dentistry.

j., medical. The application of the principles of law as they relate to the practice of medicine, to the obligations of the practitioners to their patients, and to the relations of physicians to each other and to society in general.

jury-mast (jūr'ē-măst) [L. *jurare*, to be right, + AS. *masc*, a stick]. Apparatus for support of head in disease of the spine.

jusculum (jŭs'kū-lŭm) [L.]. Broth or soup.

Juster's reflex [Emile Juster, 20th century Fr. neurologist]. Finger extension instead of flexion when palm of hand is irritated.

justo major (jŭs'tō mā'jor) [L.]. Bigger than normal, as a pelvis.

justo minor (jŭs'tō mī'nor) [L.]. Smaller than normal, as a pelvis.

jute (jūt) [Sanskrit *juta*, matted hair]. Fiber obtained from tropical shrubs. Once used in making dressings.

juvenile (jū'vĕ-nīl") [L. *juvenis*, young]. 1. Pert. to youth or childhood. 2. Young; immature.

juvenile cell. The early developmental form of white blood cells.

juvenile rheumatoid arthritis. SEE: *arthritis, juvenile rheumatoid.*

juxta- [L., near]. Prefix indicating close proximity.

juxta-articular (jŭks"tă-ăr-tĭk'ū-lăr) [" + *articulus*, joint]. Situated close to a joint.

juxtaglomerular (jŭks"tă-glō-mĕr'ū-lăr) [" + *glomus*, ball]. Near or adjacent to a glomerulus.

juxtaglomerular apparatus. A structure consisting of myoepithelioid cells forming a cuff surrounding the arteriole leading to a glomerulus of the kidney. It is concerned with the production of renin and is involved in sodium metabolism.

juxtaglomerular cells. Myoepithelioid cells resembling those of the carotid body present in the juxtaglomerular apparatus.

juxtangina (jŭks"tăn-jī'nă) [" + *angina*, a choking]. Inflamed condition of pharyngeal muscles.

juxtaposition (jŭks"tă-pō-zĭ'shŭn) [" + *positio*, place]. Position that is adjacent or side by side. SYN: *apposition; contiguity.*

juxtapyloric (jŭks"tă-pī-lor'ĭk) [" + Gr. *pyloros*, pylorus]. Near the pylorus or pyloric orifice.

juxtaspinal (jŭks"tă-spī'năl) [" + *spina*, thorn]. Near the spinal column.

K

K [L. *kalium*]. Chem. symb. for the element potassium.

K, k. 1. Symb. for Gr. letter *kappa*. 2. Used in some formulae in chemistry and physics to indicate a constant or value that does not change. 3. Kelvin temperature scale. 4. Symb. for kilo.

Ka. *cathode;* also Ca.

Kabikinase. Trade name for streptokinase.

Kader's operation [Bronislaw Kader, Polish surgeon, 1863–1937]. Surgical formation of a gastric fistula with the feeding tube inserted through a valvelike flap.

kaif (kīf) [Arabic, quiescence]. A dreamy, tranquil state induced by drugs.

kainophobia (kī-nō-fō'bē-ă) [Gr. *kainos*, new, + *phobos*, fear]. Abnormal aversion to new situations and things. SYN: *neophobia.*

kaiserling (kī'zĕr-lĭng) [Karl Kaiserling, Ger. pathologist, 1869–1942]. Liquid used in preserving pathological specimens.

kakidrosis (kăk-ĭ-drō'sĭs) [Gr. *kakos*, bad, + *hidrosis*, sweat]. Unpleasant odor of the sweat. SYN: *bromidrosis.*

kakke (kŏk'kă) [Japanese]. Endemic form of polyneuritis. SYN: *beriberi.*

kakosmia (kăk-ŏz'mē-ă) [Gr. *kakos*, bad, + *osme*, smell]. Perception of bad odors that do not exist. SYN: *cacosmia.* SEE:*parosmia.*

kakotrophy (kăk-ŏt'rō-fē) [" + *trophe*, nourishment]. Malnutrition. SYN: *cacotrophy.*

kala-azar (kä'lă ă-zăr') [Hindi, black fever]. An infectious disease, common in the rural parts of tropical and subtropical areas of the world. There are several types, which differ as to preference for children or adults, incidence in domestic animals, and transmitting agent. The disease is characterized by lesions of the reticuloendothelial system, esp. the liver and spleen. It is often fatal. SYN: *leishmaniasis, visceral.*

ETIOL: *Leishmania donovani,* a flagellated protozoon. The organism is transmitted by the bite of infected sandflies of the genus *Phlebotomus.*

PROPHYLAXIS: Control of the sandflies that transmit the organisms can be accomplished by use of insecticides that have residual action. In addition, elimination of breeding grounds of the flies is helpful, as is avoidance of animals that are known reservoirs. If exposure to flies is inevitable, then protective clothing should be worn.

TREAT: Sodium stibogluconate (Pentostam) or meglumine antimonate (Glucan-time).

kaliemia (kă-lē-ē'mē-ă) [Arabic, *gali*, potash, + Gr. *haima*, blood]. Potassium in the blood.

kaligenous (kă-lĭj'ĕ-nŭs) [" + Gr. *gennan*, to produce]. Forming potash.

kalimeter (kă-lĭm'ĕ-ter) [" + Gr. *metron*, measure]. Device for determining degree of alkalinity of a substance. SYN: *alkalimeter.*

kaliopenia (kă''lē-ō-pē'nē-ă) [L. *kalium*, potassium, + Gr. *penia*, poverty]. Hypokalemia, i.e., decreased potassium in the blood.

kalium (kā'lē-ŭm) [L.]. SYMB: K. A mineral element necessary to the growth of cells esp. those of the muscles and blood. SYN *potassium.*

kaliuresis (kă''lē-ū-rē'sĭs) [L. *kalium*, potassium, + Gr. *ouresis*, urination]. Excretion of potassium in the urine.

kallidin (kăl'ĭ-dĭn). A plasma kinin. SEE: *kinin.*

kallikrein (kăl-ĭ-krē'ĭn) [Gr. *kallikreas*, pancreas]. An enzyme normally present in blood plasma, urine, and body tissue in an inactive state. When activated, kallikrein is one of the most potent vasodilators. It forms kinin, q.v.

kallikreinogen (kăl''ĭ-krī'nō-jĕn) [" + *gennan*, to produce]. The precursor of kallikrein, q.v., in blood plasma.

kanamycin sulfate (kăn''ă-mī'sĭn). USP. An antibiotic. Trade names are Kantrex and Kantrim.

Kanner syndrome [Leo Kanner, Austrian psychiatrist in the U.S., b. 1894]. Infantile autism. SEE: *autism; autistic child.*

Kantrex. Trade name for kanamycin sulfate, USP.

Kaochlor. Trade name for potassium chloride, USP.

kaolin (kā'ō-lĭn) [Fr., from Mandarin Chinese *kao*, high, + *ling*, mountain]. A yellowwhite or gray clay powder occurring in a natural state as a form of hydrated aluminum silicate. Used internally as an absorbent, externally as a protective by absorbing moisture. SYN: *China clay.*

kaolinosis (kă''ō-lĭn-ō'sĭs). Pneumonoconiosis caused by inhaling kaolin particles.

Kaon. Trade name for potassium gluconate.

Kaon-Cl. Trade name for potassium chloride, USP.

Kaopectate. Trade name for a combination product containing kaolin, USP.

Kaposi, Moritz K. (kăp'ō-sē''). Austrian physician, 1837–1902. Originally his name was Moritz Kohn.

K.'s disease. Xeroderma pigmentosum, q.v. SYN: *xanthelasmoidea*.

K.'s sarcoma. Multiple areas of cell proliferation initially in the skin and eventually in other body sites. These lesions may eventually become sarcomatous. This condition is felt to be related to the immunocompromised state that accompanies AIDS. SEE: *AIDS*.

K.'s varicelliform eruption. Skin disease resulting from infection with herpes simplex or vaccinia virus in the presence of another skin disease such as eczema.

Kappadione. Trade name for menadiol sodium diphosphate.

karaya gum (kăr′ă-ă). Dried gum from *Sterculia* plants. It becomes gelatinous when moist. Used as an adhesive and as a bulk laxative.

Karman catheter [Harvey Karman, U.S. psychologist, b. 1924]. Catheter used in performing suction curettage of the uterus.

Karnofsky Index (or Scale) [D.A. Karnofsky, 20th century physician]. Clinical estimate of a patient's physical state, performance, and prognosis. The scale is from 100, perfectly well, to 0, dead. It has been used in studying cancer and chronic illness.

Kartagener's syndrome (kăr′tă-gā″nĕrz) [Manes Kartagener, Swiss physician, 1897–1975]. Hereditary syndrome consisting of bronchiectasis, maldevelopment of the sinuses, and transposition of the viscera. SEE: *cilia, immotile, syndrome*.

karyo- [Gr. *karyon*, kernel]. Prefix referring to a cell's nucleus.

karyochromatophil (kăr″ē-ō-krō-măt′ō-fĭl) [″ + *chroma*, color, + *philein*, to love]. Having a nucleus that stains.

karyochrome (kăr′ē-ō-krōm″). The cell of a nerve with an easily staining nucleus.

karyoclasis (kăr-ē-ŏk′lă-sĭs) [Gr. *karyon*, kernel, + *klasis*, a breaking]. The fragmentation of a cell nucleus. SYN: *karyorrhexis*.

karyocyte (kăr′ē-ō-sīt) [″ + *kytos*, cell]. Normoblast, the nucleated red blood cell.

karyogamy (kăr-ē-ŏg′ă-mē) [″ + *gamos*, marriage]. Union of nuclei in cell conjugation.

karyogenesis (kăr″ē-ō-jĕn′ē-sĭs) [″ + *genesis*, generation, birth]. Formation and development of a cell nucleus.

karyokinesis (kăr″ē-ō-kĭn-ē′sĭs) [″ + *kinesis*, movement]. The equal division of nuclear material that occurs in cell division. SEE: *cytokinesis; mitosis*.

karyokinetic (kăr″ē-ō-kĭ-nĕt′ĭk). 1. Pert. to karyokinesis. 2. Ameboid.

karyoklasis (kăr″ē-ŏk′lă-sĭs) [″ + *klasis*, a breaking]. Disintegration of the cell nucleus.

karyolobism (kăr″ē-ō-lō′bĭzm) [″ + L. *lobus*, lobe, + Gr. -*ismos*, state of]. Condition in which the nucleus of a cell is lobed, as in polymorphonuclear leukocytes.

karyolymph [″ + L. *lympha*, lymph]. Fluid in meshes of the nucleus; now known to contain active submicroscopic components of the nucleoplasm. Thus the terms karyolymph and nuclear sap do not describe clearly definable entities and should not be used. SEE: *cell; organelle*.

karyolysis (kăr-ē-ŏl′ĭ-sĭs) [″ + *lysis*, dissolution]. Destruction of a nucleus or loss of affinity for basic dyes. SYN: *chromatolysis*.

karyolytic (kăr-ē-ō-lĭt′ĭk). Producing or rel. to karyolysis.

karyomegaly (kăr″ē-ō-mĕg′ă-lē) [″ + *megas*, large]. Abnormal enlargement of the cell nucleus.

karyomere (kăr′ē-ō-mēr″) [″ + *meros*, part]. 1. Chromomere (def. 1), q.v. 2. A vesicle containing only a small portion of the nucleus.

karyomicrosome (kăr″ē-ō-mī′krō-sōm) [″ + *mikros*, small, + *soma*, body]. 1. Any one of the small particles in the karyoplasm. 2. Any one of the small tangible bodies or segments of chromatin fiber.

karyomitome (kăr″ē-ŏm′ĭ-tōm) [″ + *mitos*, thread]. The nuclear network.

karyomitosis (kăr″ē-ō-mī-tō′sĭs) [″ + *mitos*, thread, + *osis*, condition]. Nuclear changes in mitosis or cell division. SYN: *karyokinesis*.

karyomorphism (kăr-ē-ō-mor′fĭzm) [″ + *morphe*, form, + -*ismos*, state of]. The form of a cell nucleus.

karyon (kăr′ē-ŏn) [Gr.]. The nucleus of a cell.

karyophage (kăr′ē-ō-fāj) [Gr. *karyon*, kernel, + *phagein*, to eat]. An intracellular protozoan parasite that destroys the nucleus of a cell.

karyopyknosis (kăr″ē-ō-pĭk-nō′sĭs) [″ + *pyknos*, thick, + *osis*, condition]. Shrinkage of the nucleus of the cell with condensation of the chromatin.

karyorrhexis (kăr″ē-ō-rĕk′sĭs) [″ + *rhexis*, rupture]. Fragmentation of the chromatin in nuclear disintegration. SYN: *karyoclasis*.

karyosome (kăr′ē-ō-sōm) [″ + *soma*, body]. Irregular clumps of nondividing chromatin material seen in the nuclei of cells. SYN: *chromocenter; prochromosome*.

karyostasis (kăr″ē-ŏs′tă-sĭs) [″ + *stasis*, standing]. Stage of resting of a cell nucleus.

karyotheca (kăr″ē-ō-thē′kă) [″ + *theke*, sheath]. The enveloping membrane of a cell nucleus.

karyotype (kăr′ē-ō-tīp) [″ + *typos*, mark]. A photomicrograph of a single cell in the metaphase, q.v., stage of division that is arranged to show the chromosomes in descending order of size. SEE: *chromosome* for illus.

karyozoic (kăr″ē-ō-zō′ĭk) [″ + *zoon*, animal]. Living in the cell nucleus, as would occur with a protozoal parasite.

Kasabach-Merritt syndrome [Haig H. Kasabach, U.S. pediatrician, 1898–1943; K. K. Merritt, U.S. physician, b. 1886]. Capillary hemangioma associated with thrombocytopenic purpura. SYN: *hemangioma-thrombocytopenia syndrome*.

Kashin-Beck disease [N. I. Kashin, Russian physician, 1825–1872; E. V. Beck (Bek)]. Endemic polyarthritis limited to certain areas of Asia. It is believed to be a form of mycotoxicosis caused by eating grain contaminated with the fungus *Fusarium sporotrichiella*.

kata- [Gr. *kata*, down]. Prefix meaning down, reversing process, wrongly, back, against. SEE: words beginning with *cata-*.

katabolism (kă-tăb′ō-lĭzm) [″ + *ballein*, to throw, + *-ismos*, state of]. Catabolism.

kataplasia (kăt-ă-plā′sē-ă). Cataplasia.

katathermometer (kăt″ă-thĕr-mŏm′ĕ-ter) [″ + *therme*, heat, + *metron*, measure]. Two thermometers, one a dry bulb and the other a wet bulb. Both are heated to 110°F (43.3°C) and the time required for each thermometer to fall from 100° to 90°F (37.8° to 32.2°C) is noted. The dry bulb gives the cooling power by radiation and convection. The wet bulb gives the cooling power by radiation, convection, and evaporation. Attempts to use this type of thermometer to measure wind velocity were in vain.

katatonia (kăt-ă-tō′nē-ă) [″ + *tonos*, tension]. Catatonia.

kathisophobia (kăth″ĭ-sō-fō′bē-ă) [Gr. *kathizein*, to sit down, + *phobos*, fear]. Fear of sitting down, and subsequent inability to sit still.

kation (kăt′ē-ŏn) [Gr., descending]. Cation.

katophoria (kăt″ō-fō′rē-ă). Katotropia, q.v.

katotropia (kăt″ō-trō′pē-ă) [Gr. *kata*, down, + *tropos*, a turning]. Tendency of the eyeball to deviate downward. SYN: *katophoria*.

katzenjammer (kăts′ĕn-yăm′ĕr) [Ger. *katzen*, cats, + *jammer*, distress, misery]. German for hangover.

kava [Tongan, bitter]. 1. Root of *Piper methysticum*, a tropical shrub. 2. A Polynesian beverage made from the root of *Piper methysticum*. It has the effect of a tranquilizer and muscle relaxant with caffeinelike properties. Continued use may cause a scaly skin disease.

Kawasaki disease [Tomsaku Kawasaki, contemporary Japanese pediatrician]. An acute febrile disease of children that resembles scarlet fever. The fever is present on the first day of the illness and may last from 1 to 3 weeks. The child is irritable, lethargic, and has bilateral congestion of the conjunctivae. The oral mucosa is deep red, and strawberry tongue is prominent. Lips are dry, cracked, and red. On the third to fifth day, the palms and soles are distinctly red, and edema of the hands and feet is present. The skin on the tips of the fingers and toes peels in layers. A macular erythematous rash free of crusts and vesicles spreads from the extremities to the trunk. Cervical lymphadenopathy is present in the first 3 days and lasts more than 3 weeks. The disease is rarely fatal in the acute phase, but children may die suddenly from coronary artery disease some years later. This disease was previously called *mucocutaneous lymph node syndrome*. SEE: *toxic shock syndrome*.

TREAT: Supportive. If given within 10 days of onset of fever, immune gamma globulin I.V. in high doses and aspirin will decrease the risk of coronary artery dilation and aneurysms. Antibiotics and corticosteroids are not beneficial. Frequent follow-up care in the first 2 months to detect heart disease is important, as is prolonged low-dose aspirin therapy to help prevent platelet aggregation.

Kay Ciel. Trade name for potassium chloride, USP.

Kayser-Fleischer ring (kī′zĕr-flī′shĕr) [Bernard Kayser, 1869–1954; Bruno Fleischer, 1848–1904, Ger. physicians]. SEE: *Wilson's disease.*

KBr. Potassium bromide.

kc. *kilocycle.*

K cells. A type of T lymphocyte activated by an antigen-antibody reaction that directly lyses (kills) infected cells.

KC₂H₃O₂. Potassium acetate.

KCl. Potassium chloride.

KClO. Potassium hypochlorite.

KClO₃. Potassium chlorate.

K₂CO₃. Potassium carbonate.

kc.p.s. *kilocycles per second.*

keep vein open. ABBR: KVO. An order indicating that a vein be kept open so that I.V. solutions or medicines can be administered. The implication is that even though I.V. medication is not needed at the moment, the line carrying I.V. solutions should remain functional. This is done using the lowest possible infusion rate.

kefir, kefyr (kĕf′ĕr) [Caucasus region of Russia]. A preparation of curdled milk made originally in the Caucasus by adding kefir grains to milk.

Keflex. Trade name for cephalexin, USP.

Keflin. Trade name for cephalothin sodium, USP.

Kegel exercises [A. H. Kegel, contemporary

U.S. physician]. An exercise for strengthening the pubococcygeal and levator ani muscles. Basically, the patient tightens those muscles that could be used in attempting to prevent defecation or urination. Dr. Kegel placed a bulb in the vagina and attached it to a manometer. While doing the exercises, the patient could observe the pressure increase and decrease as the muscles were contracted and relaxed. For this technique to be effective, it is imperative that the patient receive detailed instruction. Increase in the strength of the muscles helps to control urinary and fecal incontinence, aids in the childbirth process, and may enhance the pleasure derived from sexual intercourse. SEE: *incontinence, urinary.*

Keith's bundle, node (kēths) [Sir Arthur Keith, Brit. anatomist, 1866–1955]. Sinoatrial node of the heart.

Keith-Flack node [Sir Arthur Keith; Martin William Flack, Brit. physiologist, 1882–1931]. Sinoatrial node of the heart.

Keith-Wagener-Barker classification. Classification of the funduscopic findings in hypertensive patients. Grades 1 to 4 indicate progressive pathological changes. Grade 1 is moderate narrowing of the retinal arterioles; Grade 2 indicates retinal hemorrhages in addition to arteriolar narrowing; in Grade 3 there are cotton-wool exudates; Grade 4 shows papilledema.

kelis (kē'lis) [Gr., blemish]. Keloid.

Kell blood group. One of the human blood groups. It is composed of three forms of antigens present on the surface of the red blood cells. SEE: *blood groups.*

Kelly's pad [Howard A. Kelly, U.S. surgeon, 1858–1943]. A drainage pad for the operating table or bed made by wrapping one end of a rubber sheet over a rolled small blanket, forming a bolster. The bolster is twisted round like a horseshoe to form the pad, the free part of the sheet forming the apron. A commercial inflatable rubber pad of horseshoe shape may be used in same way.

keloid (kē'loyd) [Gr. *kele*, tumor, + *eidos*, form, shape]. Scar formation in the skin following trauma or surgical incision. Tissue response is out of proportion to the amount of scar tissue required for normal repair and healing. The result is a raised, firm, thickened red scar that may grow for a prolonged period of time. The increase in scar size is due to deposition of an abnormal amount of collagen into the tissue. Blacks are esp. prone to developing keloids.

    TREAT: Injection of a corticosteroid into the scar has been effective in some patients. Laser therapy has been tried, as have pharmacologic agents that interfere with collagen synthesis.

k., acne. Keloid that develops at site of acne pustule.

keloidosis (kē″loy-dō′sĭs) [″ + ″ + *osis*, condition]. The formation of keloids.

kelotomy (kē-lŏt′ō-mē) [″ + *tome*, incision]. Operation for strangulated hernia through tissues of the constricting neck.

kelp. 1. Any member of the brown seaweeds of the order Laminariales. 2. The ash of seaweed from which potassium and iodine salts are prepared.

Kelvin scale [Lord (William Thompson) Kelvin, Brit. physicist, 1824–1907]. ABBR: K. Temperature scale in which absolute zero is equal to minus 273° on the Celsius scale. On the Kelvin scale the freezing point of water is 273°K; and the boiling point of water is 373°K.

Kemadrin. Trade name for procyclidine hydrochloride.

Kempner rice-fruit diet (kĕmp′nĕr) [Walter Kempner, U.S. physician, b. 1903]. Rigid salt restriction diet used in treating hypertension. It consists of rice, fruit, and sugar for no more than 2000 Calories per day and 7 mEq of sodium per day.

Kenacort. Trade name for triamcinolone.

Kenalog. Trade name for triamcinolone acetonide.

Kenny treatment [Sister Elizabeth Kenny, Australian nurse, 1886–1952]. Physical therapy used in treating poliomyelitis. Consists of application of hot, moist packs to affected muscles and early re-education of muscles, first through passive exercise and then by active movements as soon as possible. Rigid fixation of paralyzed limbs is discouraged.

kenophobia (kĕn″ō-fō′bē-ă) [Gr. *kenos,* empty, + *phobos,* fear]. Fear of empty spaces.

Kent's bundles [Albert Frank Stanley Kent, Brit. physiologist, 1863–1958]. Accessory conduction fiber bundles in the heart which rapidly convey atrial impulses across the atrioventricular tissue. They are usually present in the Wolff-Parkinson-White syndrome, q.v.

kerasin (kĕr′ă-sĭn). A cerebroside isolated from brain tissue.

keratalgia (kĕr″ă-tăl′jē-ă) [Gr. *keras,* horn, + *algos,* pain]. Neuralgia of the cornea.

keratectasia (kĕr″ă-tĕk-tā′sē-ă) [″ + *ektasis,* extension]. Conical protrusion of the cornea.

keratectomy (kĕr-ă-tĕk′tō-mē) [″ + *ektome,* excision]. Excision of a portion of the cornea.

keratiasis (kĕr-ă-tī′ă-sĭs) [″ + *-iasis,* condition]. Horny wart formations on the skin.

keratic (kĕr-ăt′ĭk). 1. Rel. to keratin. SYN: *horny.* 2. Rel. to the cornea.

keratic precipitates. Inflammatory cells of the anterior chamber of the eye that adhere to the endothelial surface of the cornea. These may be large, heavy, fat precipitates or small and punctate.

keratin (kĕr'ă-tĭn). An extremely tough protein substance in hair, nails, and horny tissue, insoluble in water, weak acids, or alkalis, and unaffected by most proteolytic enzymes. The fibrous protein is produced by keratinocytes and is found in two forms, hard or soft.

   k., hard. Found in hair and nails.

   k., soft. Found in the epidermis of skin as the flexible, tough stratum corneum in the form of flattened non-nucleated scales which slough continually.

keratinase (kĕr'ă-tĭ-nās). Enzyme that hydrolyzes the protein keratin.

keratinization. 1. The process of keratin formation that takes place within the keratinocytes as they progress upward through the layers of the epidermis of skin to the surface stratum corneum. 2. Keratinization may occur normally on moist oral mucosa due to the abrasion of masticatory forces, pathological changes (keratoses) due to an autosomal dominant gene, or environmental trauma, e.g., the heat or toxins of tobacco or other carcinogens.

keratinize (kĕr'ă-tĭn-īz) [Gr. *keras,* horn]. To become hard or horny. Usually said of tissue.

keratinocyte (kĕ-răt'ĭ-nō-sīt) [" + *kytos,* cell]. Any one of the cells in the skin that synthesize keratin.

   k., cultured. SEE: *cultured keratinocytes.*

keratinous (kĕr-ăt'ĭ-nŭs). Pert. to or composed of keratin.

keratitis (kĕr-ă-tī'tĭs) [" + *itis,* inflammation]. Inflammation of the cornea, which is usually associated with decreased visual acuity. Pain is the most common symptom.

   ETIOL: May be caused by microorganisms, trauma, or immune-mediated reactions.

   TREAT: Therapy depends upon the causative organism or other causes, e.g., removal of a foreign body from the cornea.

   NURSING IMPLICATIONS: Due to the seriousness of this condition, the patient should be urged to seek immediate medical attention for signs of inflammation and pain. Instruct the patient to refrain from rubbing the eye as this can result in complications. Encourage him or her to follow medical regimen carefully. In particular, the instillation of prescribed eye medications and follow-up examinations should be emphasized. Encourage the patient to follow a well-balanced diet, as nutritional deficiencies can increase susceptibility to this condition. Provide emotional support and reassurance as this disease can be very distressing to the patient.

   k., band-shaped. White or gray band extending across the cornea.

   k. bullosa. The formation of large, quite resistant blebs with increased tension in the cornea of blind trachomatous eyes.

   k., deep. K., interstitial.

   k., dendritic. Superficial branching corneal ulcers.

   k. disciformis. Gray, disk-shaped opacity in the middle of the cornea.

   k., fascicular. Corneal ulcer resulting from phlyctenules that spread from limbus to center of cornea accompanied by fascicle of blood vessels.

   k., herpetic. Vesicular keratitis in herpes zoster.

   k., hypopyon. Serpentlike ulcer with pus in the anterior chamber of the eye.

   k., interstitial. Deep form of nonsuppurative keratitis with vascularization, occurring usually in syphilis and rarely in tuberculosis. Commonly found between fifth and fifteenth years. SYN: *k., deep; k., parenchymatous.*

   SYM: Pain, photophobia, lacrimation, and loss in vision.

   k., lagophthalmic. Drying due to air exposure of cornea due to defective closure of lids.

   k., mycotic. Keratitis produced by fungi.

   k., neuroparalytic. Dull and slightly cloudy insensitive cornea seen in lesions of the fifth nerve.

   k., parenchymatous. K., interstitial, q.v.

   k., phlyctenular. Circumscribed inflammation of conjunctiva and cornea accompanied by formation of small projections called phlyctenules, which consist of accumulations of lymphoid cells. The phlyctenules soften at the apices, forming ulcers.

   k., punctate. Cellular deposits on the posterior surface of the cornea seen in diseases of uveal tract.

   k., purulent. Keratitis with formation of pus.

   k., sclerosing. Triangular opacity in deeper layers of cornea, associated with scleritis.

   k., superficial punctate. Small gray spots in superficial layers of cornea beneath Bowman's membrane. Occurs in young persons.

   k., trachomatous. Keratitis with abnormal membrane on cornea. SYN: *pannus.*

   k., traumatic. Keratitis caused by a wound of the cornea.

   k., xerotic. Softening, desiccation, and

ulceration of cornea due to dryness of the conjunctiva.

kerato-, kerat- [Gr. *keras*, horn]. Combining form indicating relation to horny substances or to the cornea.

keratoacanthoma (kĕr″ă-tō-ăk″ăn-thō′mä) [″ + *akantha*, thorn, + *oma*, tumor]. A papular lesion filled with a keratin plug that can resemble squamous cell carcinoma. It is benign and usually subsides spontaneously within 6 months.

keratocele (kĕr-ăt′ō-sēl) [″ + *kele*, tumor, swelling]. Protrusion or herniation of Descemet's membrane through a weakened or absent corneal stroma as a result of injury or ulcer.

keratoconjunctivitis (kĕr″ă-tō-kŏn-jŭnk″tĭ-vī′tĭs). Inflammation of the cornea and the conjunctiva.

   k., epidemic. An acute, self-limited keratoconjunctivitis due to a highly infectious virus. SYN: *k., virus.*

   k., flash. Painful keratoconjunctivitis resulting from exposure of the eyes to intense ultraviolet irradiation. Arc welders whose eyes are not properly protected will develop this acute condition.

   k., phlyctenular. Acute inflammation of areas of the conjunctiva due to an allergic response of a portion of the cornea or conjunctiva to an unknown allergen. The inflamed area is called a phlyctenule, q.v. SYN: *eczematous conjunctivitis.*

   SYM: Photophobia, pain, lacrimation, conjunctival injection, and diminished visual acuity.

   k. sicca. Dryness with hyperemia of the conjunctiva due to decreased lacrimal function. The corneal epithelium may be thickened and visual acuity may be impaired. SYN: *dry eyes; keratitis sicca; xerophthalmia.* SEE: *Schirmer's test; Sjögren's syndrome.*

   TREAT: Artificial tears solutions.

   k., virus. K., epidemic.

keratoconus (kĕr-ă-tō-kō′nŭs) [″ + *konos*, cone]. Conical protrusion of the center of the cornea without inflammation. Occurs most often in pubescent females.

keratocyte (kĕr′ă-tō-sīt). A red blood cell of normal cell volume that is deformed with two or more horn-shaped points. SYN: *horn cell.*

keratoderma (kĕr″ă-tō-dĕr′mä) [″ + *derma*, skin]. A localized or disseminated disease of the horny layer of the skin.

   k. blennorrhagica. Prominent hyperkeratotic scaling lesions of the palms, soles, penis, around the nails, and occasionally other areas.

   ETIOL: Associated with Reiter's syndrome, q.v.

   k. climactericum. Hyperkeratosis of the palms and soles of women. This may occur during menopause.

keratodermatitis (kĕr″ă-tō-dĕr″mă-tī′tĭs) [″ + ″ + *itis*, inflammation]. Inflammation of the horny layer of the skin with proliferation.

keratodermia. Hypertrophy of the stratum corneum or horny layer of the epidermis, esp. on the palms of hands and soles of feet, producing a horny condition of the skin.

keratogenous (kĕr-ă-tŏj′ĕ-nŭs) [″ + *gennan*, to produce]. Causing horny tissue development.

keratoglobus (kĕr″ă-tō-glō′bŭs) [″ + L. *globus*, circle]. Globular protrusion and enlargement of cornea seen in congenital glaucoma.

keratohelcosis (kĕr″ă-tō-hĕl-kō′sĭs) [″ + *helkosis*, ulceration]. Corneal ulceration.

keratohemia (kĕr″ă-tō-hē′mē-ă) [″ + *haima*, blood]. Presence of blood in the cornea of the eye.

keratohyalin. A substance present in the form of granules in the cytoplasm of cells in the stratum granulosum of keratinized mucosa or epidermis of the skin.

keratoid (kĕr′ă-toyd) [″ + *eidos*, form, shape]. Horny; resembling corneal tissue.

keratoiditis (kĕr″ă-toyd-ī′tĭs) [″ + ″ + *itis*, inflammation]. Inflammation of the cornea.

keratoiritis (kĕr″ă-tō-ī-rī′tĭs) [″ + *iris*, iris, + *itis*, inflammation]. Inflammation of the cornea and iris.

keratoleptynsis (kĕr″ă-tō-lĕp-tĭn′sĭs) [″ + *leptynein*, to make thin]. A cosmetic operation performed on a sightless eye. The procedure involves removing the corneal surface and covering the area with bulbar conjunctiva.

keratoleukoma (kĕr″ă-tō-lū-kō′mä) [″ + *leukos*, white, + *oma*, tumor]. White corneal opacity.

keratolysis (kĕr-ă-tŏl′ĭ-sĭs) [″ + *lysis*, dissolution]. 1. Loosening of horny layer of the skin. 2. Shedding of the skin at regular intervals.

   k., pitted. Hyperkeratotic areas of the soles and palms with erosion and pitting. Etiology is unknown but may involve infection with *Corynebacterium* or *Actinomyces.* It occurs mostly in barefooted adults in the tropics.

keratolytic (kĕr″ă-tō-lĭt′ĭk). 1. Rel. to or causing keratolysis. SYN: *desquamative.* 2. An agent that causes or promotes keratolysis.

keratoma (kĕr″ă-tō′mä) [″ + *oma*, tumor]. 1. A callosity. 2. A horny growth. SYN: *keratosis.*

keratomalacia (kĕr″ă-tō-mă-lā′shē-ă) [″

+ *malakia*, softness]. Softening of the cornea seen in early childhood due to deficiencies of vitamin A. SYN: *xerotic keratitis*.

keratome (kĕr′ă-tōm) [″ + *tome*, incision]. Knife for incising the cornea.

keratometer (kĕr-ă-tŏm′ĕ-ter) [″ + *metron*, measure]. An instrument for measuring the curves of the cornea.

keratometry (kĕr″ă-tŏm′ĕ-trē) [″ + *metron*, measure]. Measurement of the cornea.

keratomileusis (kĕr″ă-tō-mī-loo′sĭs) [″ + *smileusis*, carving]. Plastic surgery of the cornea in which a portion is removed and frozen, its curvature is reshaped, and then it is reattached to the cornea.

keratomycosis (kĕr″ă-tō-mī-kō′sĭs) [″ + *mykes*, fungus, + *osis*, condition]. Fungus growth on the cornea.

keratonosis (kĕr″ă-tō-nō′sĭs) [″ + *nosos*, disease]. Any noninflammatory disease or deformity of the horny layer of the skin.

keratonyxis (kĕr″ă-tō-nĭks′ĭs) [″ + *nyssein*, to puncture]. Corneal puncture, esp. surgical puncture.

keratopathy, band (kĕr″ă-tŏp′ă-thē) [″ + *pathos*, disease]. Calcium deposits in the superficial layer of the cornea and Bowman's membrane. Occurs with chronic intraocular inflammation and with systemic diseases in which there is hypercalcemia.

keratoplasty (kĕr′ă-tō-plăs″tē) [″ + *plassein*, to form]. Plastic operation on the cornea. SEE: *lens, corneal contact*.

   k., optic. Removal of a corneal scar and replacement with corneal tissue.

   k., refractive. Treatment of myopia or hyperopia by removing a portion of the cornea, freezing it in order to reshape it surgically to correct refractive error, and then replacing it after it has thawed. SEE: *keratomileusis*.

   k., tectonic. Use of corneal tissue to replace that lost due to trauma or disease.

keratoprotein (kĕr″ă-tō-prō′tē-ĭn) [″ + *protos*, first]. The protein of the hair, nails, and epidermis.

keratorrhexis (kĕr″ă-tō-rĕks′ĭs) [″ + *rhexis*, rupture]. Corneal rupture.

keratoscleritis (kĕr″ă-tō-sklĕr-ī′tĭs) [″ + *skleros*, hard, + *itis*, inflammation]. Inflammation of both cornea and sclera.

keratoscope (kĕr′ăt-ō-skōp) [″ + *skopein*, to examine]. Instrument for examination of the cornea.

keratoscopy. Examination of the cornea and its reflection of light.

keratose (kĕr′ă-tōs) [Gr. *keras*, horn]. Horny.

keratosis (kĕr-ă-tō′sĭs) [″ + *osis*, condition] (pl. *keratoses*). 1. Horny growth. 2. Any condition of the skin characterized by the formation of horny growths or excessive development of the horny growth.

   k., actinic. A horny, keratotic, premalignant lesion of the skin caused by excess exposure to sunlight. SYN: *keratosis, solar*. SEE: *sunscreen*.

   k. climactericum. A skin disease occurring in women during menopause, characterized by a circumscribed hyperkeratosis of the palms and soles.

   k. follicularis. A rare hereditary condition characterized by verrucous papular growths that coalesce into plaques of various sizes on the scalp, face, neck, trunk, and axillae. SYN: *Darier's disease*.

   k. nigricans. Acanthosis nigricans.

   k., oral. Keratinization of the mucosa of the mouth to an unusual extent, or in locations normally not keratinized, due to an inherited autosomal dominant gene or the more common effect of tobacco and other carcinogens.

   k. palmaris et plantaris. Congenital abnormality of the palms and soles, characterized by dense thickening of the keratin layer of the palms and soles.

   k. pharyngis. Horny projections from the pharyngeal tonsils and adjacent lymphoid tissue.

   k. pilaris. Chronic inflammatory disorder of area surrounding the hair follicles. Etiology is unknown.

   SYM: Accumulation of horny material at follicular orifices of persons with rough, dry skin. Most pronounced in winter on lateral aspects of thighs and upper arms with possible extension to legs, forearms, and scalp.

   TREAT: There is no specific therapy. Keratolytic lotions may be of some value.

   k. punctata. Discrete horny projections from the sweat pores of the palms and soles.

   k., seborrheic. A benign skin tumor that may be pigmented. Quite common in the elderly. It is composed of immature epithelial cells. SYN: *wart, seborrheic*.

   SYM: Keratoid, nevoid, acanthoid, or verrucose types occurring in elderly and in those with long-standing dry seborrhea, on face, scalp, interscapular or sternal regions, and backs of hands. Yellow, gray, brown, sharply circumscribed lesions covered with a firmly adherent scale, greasy or velvety on trunk or scalp but harsh, rough, and dry on face or hands. The tendency as time passes is for the lesions to increase in number. It is doubtful that they ever become malignant.

   ETIOL: Unknown.

   TREAT: Thorough curettage is quite effective. This leaves a flat surface that becomes covered with normal skin within about one week. Pedunculated lesions can be removed surgically. Cautery may produce scarring; therefore, it should not be used.

   k. senilis. Dry, harsh skin of the aged.

keratotome (kĕr-ăt'ō-tōm) [" + *tome,* incision]. A knife for incising the cornea. SYN: *keratome.*

keratotomy (kĕr-ă-tŏt'ō-mē). Incision of cornea.

 k., radial. Surgical therapy for nearsightedness. Very shallow, bloodless, hairline, radial incisions are made in the outer portion of the cornea where they will not interfere with vision. This allows the cornea to flatten and to help correct the nearsightedness. About two-thirds of patients undergoing this procedure will be able to eliminate the use of glasses or contact lenses.

keraunoneurosis (kĕ-raw"nō-nū-rō'sĭs) [Gr. *keraunos,* lightning, + *neuron,* nerve, + *osis,* condition]. A neurosis caused by fear of a thunderstorm or stroke of lightning.

keraunophobia (kĕ-raw"nō-fō'bē-ă) [" + *phobos,* fear]. Dread of thunder and lightning.

Kerckring's folds (kĕrk'rĭngz) [Theodorus Kerckring, Dutch anatomist, 1640–1693]. Transverse folds of the mucous membrane of the small intestine. SYN: *plicae circulares; valvulae conniventes.*

kerectomy (kē-rĕk'tō-mē) [Gr. *keras,* horn, + *ektome,* excision]. Excision of a portion of the cornea.

kerion (kē'rē-ŏn) [Gr., honeycomb]. In tinea capitis, q.v., an inflammatory, boggy mass containing broken hairs and oozing purulent material from follicular orifices. This is an unusual occurrence.

Kerley lines [P. J. Kerley, Brit. radiologist, b. 1900]. Thickening of the interlobular septa, seen on chest roentgenography. May be due to cellular infiltration or edema associated with pulmonary vein hypertension.

kernicterus (kĕr-nĭk'tĕr-ŭs) [Ger.]. A form of icterus neonatorum occurring in infants. The basal ganglia and other areas of the brain and spinal cord are infiltrated with bilirubin, a yellow pigmented substance produced by the breakdown of hemoglobin. Develops during the second to eighth day of life. Prognosis is quite poor if untreated. For prevention and treatment, SEE: *erythroblastosis fetalis; hemolytic disease of the newborn; phototherapy.*

Kernig's sign (kĕr'nĭgz) [Vladimir Kernig, Russ. physician, 1840–1917]. A symptom of meningitis evidenced by reflex contraction and pain in the hamstring muscles when attempting to extend the leg after flexing the thigh upon the body.

kerosene (kĕr'ō-sēn). A flammable liquid fuel distilled from petroleum. It is used as a solvent as well as a fuel source. SEE: *Poisons and Poisoning* in *Appendix.*

Ketaject. Trade name for ketamine hydrochloride, USP.

Ketalar. Trade name for ketamine hydrochloride, USP.

ketamine hydrochloride. USP. A nonbarbiturate substance, $C_{13}H_{16}ClNO \cdot HCl$, that is used intravenously or intramuscularly to produce anesthesia. The patient becomes cataleptic and may appear to be awake, but is unaware of the environment and unresponsive to pain. Laryngeal reflexes are depressed, and for this reason an endotracheal tube is used to prevent aspiration. Most frequently used for diagnostic procedures and minor operations in which muscle relaxation is not required. Trade names are Ketaject, Ketaset, and Ketalar. SEE: *anesthesia, dissociative.*

 NURSING IMPLICATIONS: Administer on an empty stomach to prevent vomiting and possible aspiration, and following administration of a prescribed anticholinergic to reduce stimulated saliva flow. Permit patient to reawaken in a quiet area with minimal stimulation to reduce severity of hallucinations and delirium. Premedication with prescribed diazepam or a narcotic also may reduce severity of recovery period symptoms. Warn patient about possibility of flashback-type hallucinations within 24 hours of having received ketamine anesthesia. Monitor blood pressure for hypertension, and respiratory status for airway patency, depressed laryngeal and pharyngeal reflexes, respiratory depression, and apnea. Have resuscitative equipment available. Do not discharge patient following anesthesia recovery unless accompanied by responsible adult. Caution patient against driving or operating other motorized equipment for 24 hours after anesthesia.

keto acid (kē'tō-ăs'ĭd). Any organic acid containing the ketone CO (carbonyl radical).

ketoacidosis (kē"tō-ă"sĭ-dō'sĭs) [Ger. *keton,* alter. of *azeton,* acetone, + L. *acidus,* sour, + Gr. *osis,* condition]. Acidosis due to an excess of ketone bodies.

ketoaciduria (kē"tō-ăs"ĭ-dū'rē-ă) [" + " + Gr. *ouron,* urine]. Presence of keto acids in the urine.

ketogenesis (kē-tō-jĕn'ĕ-sĭs) [" + Gr. *genesis,* generation, birth]. Production of ketones or acetone substances.

ketogenic diet (kē-tō-jĕn'ĭk) [" + Gr. *gennan,* to produce]. Diet that produces acetone or ketone bodies, or mild acidosis.

ketohexose (kē"tō-hĕks'ōs) [" + *hex,* six, + *-ose*]. A nonsaccharide consisting of a six-carbon chain and containing a ketone group in addition to alcohol groups. Fructose is an example.

ketolysis (kē-tŏl'ĭ-sĭs) [" + Gr. *lysis,* dissolution]. The dissolution of acetone or ketone bodies.

ketolytic. Pert. to ketolysis.

ketone (kē′tōn). A substance containing the carbonyl group ($C=O$) attached to two carbon atoms. Oxidation product of a secondary alcohol. Organic chemical substance of the general formula:

$$R$$
$$|$$
$$C = O$$
$$|$$
$$R$$

Acetone, C_3H_6O, is an example of a simple ketone. The ketone acids in the body are the end products of fat metabolism.

ketone bodies. A group of compounds produced during the oxidation of fatty acids, including acetoacetic acid, β-hydroxybutyric acid, and acetone. SEE: *acetone; ketosis.*

ketonemia (kē″tō-nē′mē-ă) [″ + Gr. *haima,* blood]. Acetone bodies in the blood. Their presence causes the characteristic fruity breath odor in ketoacidosis. SYN: *acidosis.*

ketone threshold. Level of ketone in the blood above which ketone bodies appear in the urine.

ketonuria (kē-tō-nū′rē-ă) [″ + Gr. *ouron,* urine]. Acetone bodies in the urine.

ketoplasia (kē-tō-plā′sē-ă) [″ + Gr. *plassein,* to form]. The formation or excretion of ketones.

ketoplastic [″ + Gr. *plastikos,* formed]. Pert. to ketoplasia or formation of ketones.

ketose. A carbohydrate containing the ketones.

ketosis (kē-tō′sĭs) [″ + Gr. *osis,* condition]. The accumulation in the body of the ketone bodies: acetone, beta-hydroxybutyric acid, and acetoacetic acid. It is frequently associated with acidosis and is often miscalled acidosis. Ketosis results from the incomplete metabolism of fatty acids, generally from carbohydrate deficiency or inadequate utilization, and is commonly observed in starvation, high-fat diet, pregnancy, following ether anesthesia, and most significantly in inadequately controlled diabetes mellitus. Large quantities of these ketone bodies may be eliminated in the urine (ketonuria). The presence of ketosis is easily determined by testing for the presence of acetone or diacetic acid in the urine. Ketonuria is an early sign of acidosis in patients with diabetes mellitus.

17-ketosteroid. One of a group of neutral steroids having a ketone group in carbon position 17. They are produced by the adrenal cortex and gonads and appear normally in the urine. Among them are androsterone, dehydroisoandrosterone, corticosterone, compound E, and 11-hydroxyisoandrosterone. A greater than normal or less than normal excretion in the urine is indicative of certain endocrine disorders. SEE: *perhydrocyclopentanophenanthrene.*

ketosuria (kē″tō-sū′rē-ă). Presence of ketone bodies in the urine. SEE: *ketosis.*

ketotic. Pertaining to ketosis.

keV. *kiloelectron volts.*

Key-Retzius foramina (kē′rĕt′zē-ŭs) [Ernst A. H. Key, Swedish physician, 1832–1901; Gustav Magnus Retzius, Swedish anatomist, 1842–1919]. Passages in the pia mater carrying the choroid plexus to the fourth ventricle. SYN: *Luschka's foramen.*

kg. *kilogram.*

kg-m. *kilogram-meter.*

KHCO₃. Potassium bicarbonate.

KHSO₄. Potassium bisulfate.

kHz. *kilohertz.*

KI. Potassium iodide.

kibbutz childrearing. Communal form of childrearing pioneered in Israel in which care is provided by the group but parents retain parental relationships with children.

kidney [ME. *kidenei*]. Paired organs, purple-brown in color, situated at the back (retroperitoneal area) of the abdominal cavity, one on each side of the spinal column. Their function is to excrete urine and to help regulate the water, electrolyte, and acid-base content of the blood.

The upper level of the kidneys is opposite the 12th thoracic (dorsal) vertebra; the lower level is opposite the 3rd lumbar vertebra. The right kidney is slightly lower than the left one.

Weight: 113 to 170 gm (4 to 6 oz). Size: about 11.4 cm (4½ in.) long, 5 to 7.5 cm (2 to 3 in.) broad, and 2.5 cm (1 in.) thick. The kidneys in the newborn are about three times as large in proportion to body weight as in the adult.

ANAT: Each kidney is surrounded by fatty tissue and by the renal fascia, a sheath of fibrous tissue, which helps to hold the kidney in place. The concave border of the kidney faces the median line, the center of the concave border opening into a fissure called the hilum or hilus.

Each ureter conducts urine from the pelvis of the kidney to the bladder. The outer portion of the kidney is the cortex, a mass of cortical substance; the inner portion (medullary substance) is the medulla. Within the cortical substance are found the arteries, veins, convoluted tubules, and glomerular capsules, while the medulla contains the renal pyramids, conical masses with papillae projecting into the cuplike cavities (calyces) of the pelvis. Each kidney contains 8 to 18 pyramids made up of collecting tubules, lymphatics, and blood vessels, the pyramids being penetrated by the cortical substance and supporting them. These extensions are known as the renal columns, or columns of Bertin.

The cortical and medullary substance is composed of renal tubules, connective tissue, blood vessels, nerves, and lymphatics. The renal tubule or nephron constitutes the structural and functional unit of the kidney. Each consists of a capsule, proximal convoluted portion, loop of Henle, and distal convoluted portion, which leads to a collecting duct. The capsule, called the glomerular or Bowman's capsule, encloses a globular mass of capillaries, the glomerulus. The capsule and the enclosed glomerulus compose the malpighian or renal corpuscle. The renal corpuscles are located principally in the cortex. SEE: illus.

FORMATION OF URINE: Urine consists of water (95%) and solids (5%), the latter being in solution. The solids include organic constituents (urea, hippuric acid, uric acid, creatinine) and inorganic constituents, principally salts of sodium and potassium. The kidneys remove these substances from the blood, thus acting to maintain homeostasis of the blood and body fluids. Urine is formed by the processes of filtration and reabsorption. As blood passes through the glomerulus, water and dissolved substances are filtered through the capillary walls and the inner or visceral layer of Bowman's capsule, resulting in formation of the glomerular filtrate. Blood cells and colloidal substances such as proteins are retained within the capillaries. The glomerular filtrate passes through the renal tubules to the collecting ducts, during the course of which all of the sugar and some of the salts and other substances are selectively reabsorbed into the capillaries surrounding the tubule. Substances such as uric acid and hydrogen ions may be added to the urine by the cells of the tubules through the process of secretion. The final product, now known as urine, passes through straight collecting ducts into larger collecting ducts (papillary ducts) that open on the tips of the renal papillae. There urine is discharged into the minor calyces of the renal pelvis, and then passes via the ureters to the bladder. Periodically the bladder is voluntarily emptied and its contents are discharged to the outside through the urethra. This is called micturition, urination, or voiding. If a normally hydrated individual ingests a large volume of aqueous fluids, in about 42 min. a sufficient quantity will have been excreted into the bladder to cause the urge to urinate.

Substances that are entirely or almost entirely reabsorbed during passage through the tubule are known as high-threshold substances. These include glucose and chlorides of sodium, potassium, calcium, and magnesium. These are important blood constituents and excreted only when their concentrations in the blood are above normal. Low or nonthreshold substances are those that are reabsorbed only in limited quantities or not at all. These are usually end products of metabolism such as urea, uric acid, and creatine, which appear in considerable quantities in the urine.

The formation of urine is a continuous process, the rate of filtration being dependent primarily upon the blood pressure within the glomeruli and the daily fluid intake.

The volume of urine excreted daily varies from 1000 to 2000 ml (averaging 1500 ml). The amount varies with water intake, nature of diet, degree of body activity, environmental and body temperature, age, blood pressure, and many other factors. Pathological conditions may affect the volume and nature of the urine excreted. However, patients with only one kidney have been found to have normal renal function even after half of that kidney was removed because of cancer. There is no evidence that forcing fluids is detrimental to the kidneys.

NERVE SUPPLY: From renal plexuses forming rich networks about renal vessels. Includes both sympathetic and parasympathetic (vagal) fibers.

SYM. OF KIDNEY DISORDER: Lumbar pain, renal colic, fever, disturbances in micturition (anuria, oliguria, or pain on micturition), presence of blood or pus in the urine, tenderness or swelling in costovertebral region, enlargement or diminution in size of kidney, edema.

EXAM: By palpation, intravenous pyelography, CAT scan, cystoscopy, retrograde cystoscopy, or panendoscopy. SEE: *dialysis; glomerulonephritis; nephropathy; nephritis; renal failure.*

k., amyloid. Kidney infiltrated with amyloid. SYN: *k., lardaceous; k., waxy.*

k., artificial. Device that receives blood from the patient, treats it by dialysis in order to remove wastes just as the kidney does, and returns the blood to the patient. Used in treating patients with renal failure or absent kidneys.

k., cake. Congenitally fused kidneys.

k., contracted. The small kidney characteristic of chronic interstitial or diffuse nephritis.

k., cystic. Kidney that has undergone

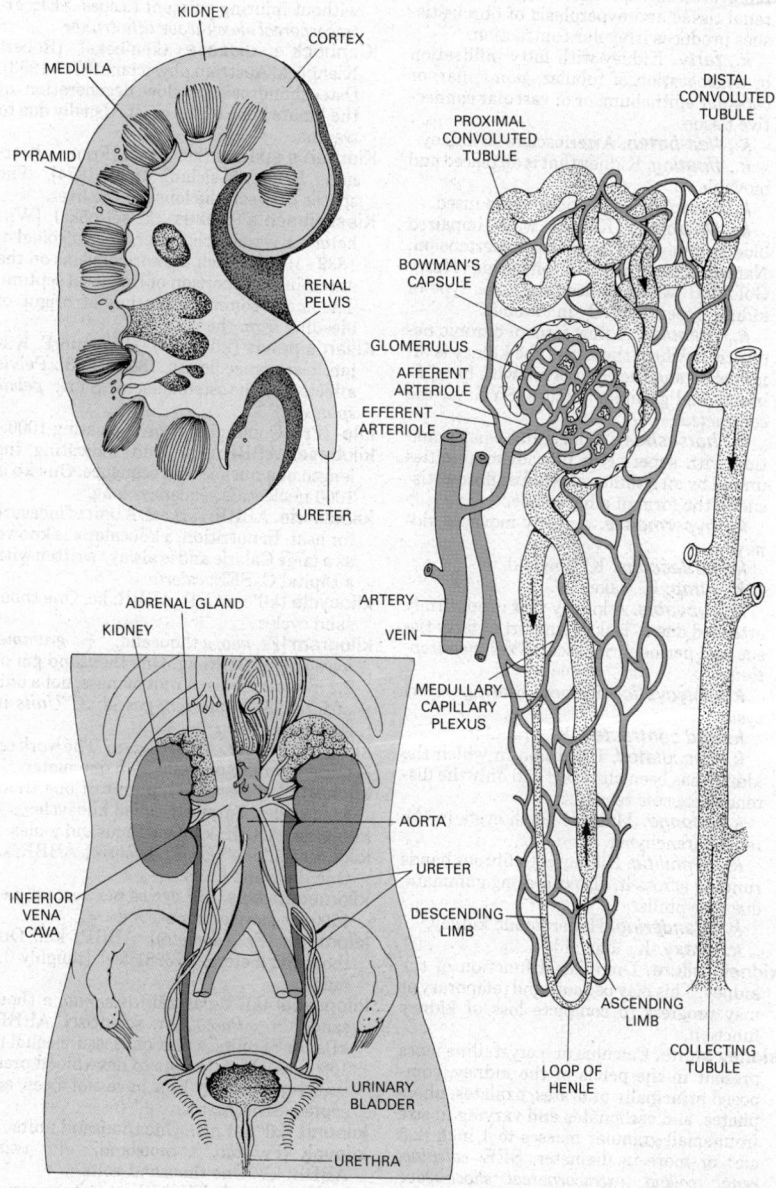

KIDNEY

KIDNEY

CORTEX

MEDULLA

PYRAMID

RENAL PELVIS

URETER

PROXIMAL CONVOLUTED TUBULE

DISTAL CONVOLUTED TUBULE

BOWMAN'S CAPSULE

GLOMERULUS

AFFERENT ARTERIOLE

EFFERENT ARTERIOLE

ARTERY

VEIN

MEDULLARY CAPILLARY PLEXUS

DESCENDING LIMB

ASCENDING LIMB

COLLECTING TUBULE

LOOP OF HENLE

ADRENAL GLAND

KIDNEY

AORTA

URETER

INFERIOR VENA CAVA

URINARY BLADDER

URETHRA

cystic degeneration.

k., embolic contracted. A contracted kidney in which embolic infarction of the renal arterioles produces degeneration of renal tissue and hyperplasia of fibrous tissues produces irregular contraction.

k., fatty. Kidney with fatty infiltration or degeneration of tubular, glomerular, or capsular epithelium, or of vascular connective tissue.

k., flea-bitten. Arteriosclerotic kidney.

k., floating. Kidney that is displaced and movable.

k., fused. The two kidneys are fused.

k., Goldblatt. Kidney with impaired blood supply and resulting hypertension. Named after the U.S. physician Harry Goldblatt, who produced the same type of kidney experimentally in animals.

k., granular. A slow form of chronic nephritis in which the size of the kidney is diminished and the color is red with hard, fibrous, and granular texture. SYN: *k., red contracted.*

k., horseshoe. Congenital malformation with superior or inferior extremities united by an isthmus of renal or fibrous tissue in the form of a horseshoe.

k., hypermobile. A freely movable kidney.

k., lardaceous. K., amyloid.

k., lump. K., cake, q.v.

k., movable. A kidney that is not firmly attached due to lack of support of fatty tissue and perinephric fascia. SYN: *nephroptosis.*

k., polycystic. Kidney bearing many cysts.

k., red contracted. K., granular.

k., sacculated. Condition in which the kidney has been absorbed and only the distended capsule remains.

k., sponge. Multiple small cysts in the renal parenchyma.

k., syphilitic. Kidney with fibrous bands running across it, also caseating gummata, due to syphilis.

k., wandering. Hypermobile kidney.

k., waxy. K., amyloid.

kidney failure. Diminished function of the kidney. This may be acute and temporary or may progress to complete loss of kidney function.

kidney stone. Calculus or a crystalline mass present in the pelvis of the kidney, composed principally of urates, oxalates, phosphates, and carbonates and varying in size from small granular masses to 1 inch (2.5 cm) or more in diameter. SEE: *calculus, renal; colloid; extracorporeal shock-wave lithotriptor.*

kidney stone removal, laser treatment for.
Use of a laser to disintegrate renal calculi. A fiberoptic device is inserted via the urethra, bladder, and ureter to the calculus. The laser is activated and this destroys the stone without injuring adjacent tissues. SEE: *extracorporeal shock-wave lithotriptor.*

Kienböck's disease (kēn'bĕks) [Robert Kienböck, Austrian physician, 1871–1953]. Osteochondrosis or slow degeneration of the lunate bone of the wrist. Usually due to trauma.

Kiernan's spaces (kēr'nănz) [Francis Kiernan, Brit. physician, 1800–1874]. The spaces between the lobes of the liver.

Kiesselbach's plexus (kē'sĕl-bŏks) [Wilhelm Kiesselbach, Ger. laryngologist, 1839–1902]. A rich network of veins on the anteroinferior portion of the nasal septum. The most common location of origin of bleeding from the nose.

Kilian's pelvis (kĭl'ē-ănz) [Hermann F. Kilian, Ger. gynecologist, 1800–1863]. Pelvis affected with osteomalacia. SYN: *pelvis spinosa.*

kilo- [Fr.]. Combining form indicating 1000.

kilobase. ABBR: kb. Unit indicating the length of a nucleic acid sequence. One kb is 1000 nucleotide sequences long.

kilocalorie. ABBR: C.; kcal. A unit of measure for heat. In nutrition, a kilocalorie is known as a large Calorie and is always written with a capital C. SEE: *calorie.*

kilocycle (kĭl'ō-sī"k'l). ABBR: kc. One thousand cycles.

kilogram [Fr. *kilo*, a thousand, + *gramme*, a weight]. ABBR: kg. One thousand gm or 2.2 lb avoirdupois. A unit of mass, not a unit of force. SEE: *newton; pascal; SI Units* in Appendix.

kilogram-meter. ABBR: kg.-m. The work required to raise one kilogram one meter.

kilohertz. In electricity, a unit of one thousand cycles. Formerly called kilocycle.

kilojoule. ABBR: kJ. One thousand joules.

kiloliter (kĭl'ō-lē"tĕr) [Fr. *kilolitre*]. ABBR: kl. One thousand liters.

kilomegacycles. 10^9 cycles per second; i.e., 1000 megacycles per second.

kilometer [Fr. *kilometre*]. ABBR: km. One thousand meters, or 3281 feet (roughly 0.6 mile).

kilopascal (kĭl"ō-păs-kăl') [Fr. *kilo*, a thousand, + *Pascal*, Fr. scientist]. ABBR: kPa. In SI units, a unit of pressure equal to 1000 pascals. Attempts to have blood pressure expressed in kPa have not been accepted. SEE: *pascal.*

kilounit (kĭl'ō-ū'nĭt). One thousand units.

kilovolt [Fr. *kilo*, a thousand, + *volt*]. ABBR: kV. One thousand volts.

kilovoltage peak. The highest voltage occurring during an electrical cycle.

ANATOMY OF THE SUPPORTING STRUCTURES OF THE KNEE

USP.

Klumpke's paralysis (kloomp'kĕz) [Madame Augusta Déjérine-Klumpke, Fr. neurologist, 1859–1927]. Atrophic paralysis of forearm.

Klüver-Bucy syndrome [Heinrich Klüver, Ger.-born U.S. neurologist, 1897–1979; Paul C. Bucy, U.S. neurologist, b. 1904]. Behavioral syndrome usually following bilateral temporal lobe removal. It is characterized by loss of recognition of people, loss of fear, rage reactions, hypersexuality, excessive oral behavior, memory deficit, and overreaction to certain stimuli.

K-Lyte. Trade name for potassium bicarbonate; trade name for a combination product containing citric acid and potassium bicarbonate.

km. *kilometer.*

kMc. *kilomegacycle.*

KMnO₄. Potassium permanganate.

Knapp's forceps (năps) [Herman J. Knapp, U.S. ophthalmologist, 1832–1911]. A forceps with rollerlike blades for expressing trachomatous granulations on the palpebral conjunctiva.

kneading (nēd'ĭng) [AS. *cnedan*]. A form of massage consisting of grasping, wringing, lifting, rolling, or pressing part of a muscle or group of muscles. SYN: *pétrissage.*

knee [AS. *cneo*]. 1. The anterior aspect of the leg at the articulation of the femur and tibia and the articulation itself, covered anteriorly with the patella or kneecap. Formed by the femur, tibia, and patella. SEE: illus. 2. Any structure shaped like a semiflexed knee. SYN: *geniculum.*

RS: geniculate; geniculum; "genu-" words; "gon-" words; patella; popliteal.

k., Brodie's. A chronic fungoid synovitis of the knee joint in which the affected parts become soft and pulpy.

k., dislocation of. Displacement of the knee. Dislocations in themselves are un-

usual. The so-called dislocation of the knee is usually due to various injuries of the joint and of the complicating structures of the knee, such as the tearing of the crushed tendons or ligaments, or the slipping of cartilages. Dislocations should be treated either by a straight splint, as in a fracture of the kneecap, or by two splints, one on either side of the knee, as in a fracture involving the knee joint. The patient should be transported to a hospital as quickly as possible.

k., game. A lay term for internal derangement of the knee joint.

SYM: Pain or instability, locking, and weakness.

PATH: Usually a torn internal cartilage, a fracture of the tibial spine, or an injury to the collateral or cruciate ligaments.

F.A.: Immobilize with a posterior splint. Surgical exploratory arthrotomy or arthroscopy may be necessary.

k., housemaid's. Inflamed condition of the bursa anterior to the patella with accumulation of fluid therein. May be seen in those who have to kneel frequently or continually while working.

k., knock-. Condition in which the knees come together while the ankles are far apart, caused by an outward distortion of the leg that throws the knee inside the normal line. SYN: *genu valgum.* SEE: *bowleg; genu varum.*

k., locked. Condition in which the leg cannot be extended. Usually due to displacement of semilunar cartilage.

k., replacement of. Replacement of the knee joint. Particularly useful in treating patients with severe disabling arthritis of the knee. When done by those skilled in the technique, total knee replacement relieves pain in more than 95% of patients and improves function in more than 90%.

kneecap. The patella.

knee-chest position. Position in which the

patient is on knees with thighs straight, head and upper part of chest resting on table, and arms crossed and on the surface in front of the head. Employed in displacement of prolapsed fundus, dislodgement of impacted head of fetus, management of transverse presentation, replacement of retroverted uterus or displaced ovary, or endoscopic examination of the rectum and colon. SYN: *genupectoral position*. SEE: *position* for illus.

knee-jerk reflex. The reflex contraction or clonic spasm of the quadriceps muscle, produced by sharply striking the ligamentum patellae when the leg hangs loosely flexed at right angles. It is seen in healthy individuals but is usually absent in locomotor ataxia, multiple neuritis, lesions of the lower portion of the spinal cord, lesions of the anterior gray horns of the cord, meningitis, infantile paralysis, pseudohypertrophic paralysis, and atrophic paralysis. It is increased in lesions of the pyramidal tract, cerebral tumors, and sclerosis of the brain and cord. SYN: *patellar reflex*. SEE: *Jendrassik's maneuver; jerk.*

knee joint. The articulation of the femur and tibia.

knee of internal capsule. The curve at the meeting place of the anterior and posterior limbs of the internal capsule of the brain.

Kneipp cure (nīp) [Rev. Father Sebastian Kneipp, Ger. priest, 1821–1897]. Application of water in various forms and degrees of temperature in the cure of disease, esp. wading in cold, dewy grass. SEE: *hydrotherapy.*

kneippism (nīp'ĭzm). Walking barefoot in dewy grass or bathing in cold water as a form of hydrotherapy.

knemometry (nē-mŏm'ĕt-rē) [Gr. *kneme*, shinbone, + *metron*, measure]. A precise method of determining the length of a limb, esp. the lower leg. It has been used to record the effect of administering growth hormone to children with deficiency of the hormone.

knife (nīf) [AS. *cnif*]. A cutting instrument.

 k., electric. A knife that functions by use of a high-frequency cutting current.

 k., gold. A special contra-angle knife used to trim direct filling gold.

 k., interdental. A double-ended knife used in periodontal surgery for removing tissue between teeth.

 k., periodontal. A surgical knife with a scaler-shaped blade whose entire perimeter is a cutting edge. It is used in gingivectomy and other periodontal surgery.

 k., plaster. A stout knife used for cutting and trimming plaster study models in dental practice.

knismogenic (nĭs"mō-jĕn'ĭk) [Gr. *knismos*, tickling, + *gennan*, to produce]. Producing a tickling sensation.

knitting [AS. *cnyttan*, to make knots]. The process of healing by union of pieces of a fractured bone.

KNO₃. Potassium nitrate, niter, q.v., saltpeter.

knob (nŏb) [ME. *knobbe*]. A protuberance on a surface or extremity; a mass, q.v., or nodule, q.v.

knock-knee. Knee, knock-, q.v.

knock-out drops. SEE: *drops, knock-out.*

knot [AS. *cnotta*]. 1. An intertwining of a cord or cordlike structure to form a lump or knob. 2. In surgery, the intertwining of the ends of a suture, ligature, bandage, or sling so that the ends will not slip or become separated. SEE: *square knot;* illus. 3. In anatomy, an enlargement forming a knoblike structure.

 k., false. An external bulging of the umbilical cord resulting from the coiling of the umbilical blood vessels.

 k., granny. A double knot in which the ends of the cord do not lie parallel, but alternate being over and under each other.

 k., Hensen's. A knoblike structure at the anterior end of the primitive streak. SEE: *primitive streak.*

 k., primitive. K., Hensen's.

 k., square. A double knot in which the ends of the second knot are in the same place as the ends of the first knot. SEE: *square knot;* illus.

 k., surgical. A double knot in which the cord is passed through the first loop twice.

 k., syncytial. A protuberance formed by many nuclei of the syntrophoblast and found on the surface of a chorionic villus.

 k., true. A knot formed by the fetus slipping through a loop of the umbilical cord.

knuckle (nŭk'ĕl) [Middle Low Ger. *knokel*]. Prominence of the dorsal aspect of any of the phalangeal joints, esp. of the distal heads of the metacarpals when the fist is clenched.

knuckle pads. Discrete fibromatous pads appearing over the finger joints. Usually appear between ages of 15 and 30. Etiology is unknown but trauma is not a significant factor.

K.O.C. *cathodal opening contraction.* SYN: *COC.*

Koch, Heinrich Herman Robert (kōk). German bacteriologist, 1843–1910.

 K.'s bacillus. The bacillus causing tuberculosis in mammals. SYN: *Mycobacterium tuberculosis.*

 K.'s law. Criterion used in proving an organism is the cause of a disease or lesion: the microorganism in question is regularly found in the lesions of the disease; pure cultures can be obtained from it. When inoculated into susceptible animals, pure cultures

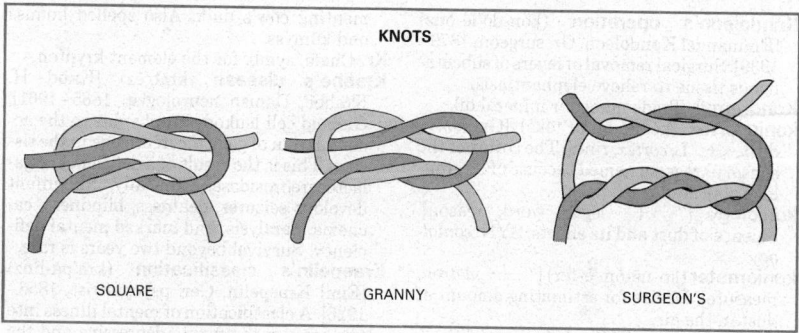

KNOTS

SQUARE   GRANNY   SURGEON'S

can reproduce the disease or pathological condition; and the organism can be obtained again in pure culture from the inoculated animal.

K.'s phenomenon. Local inflammatory reaction resulting from injection of tuberculin into the skin of a person who has been previously exposed to the tubercle bacillus.

K.'s postulates. K.'s law, q.v.

Koch, Walter (kōk). German surgeon, b. 1880.

K.'s node. The atrioventricular node.

kocherization (kōk″ĕr-ī-zā′shŭn). Operative technique in opening the duodenum to expose the ampulla of the common bile duct.

Kocher's reflex (kō′kĕrz) [Theodor Kocher, Swiss surgeon, 1841–1917]. Contraction of abdominal muscles following moderate compression of the testicle.

Koebner phenomenon [Heinrich Koebner, Ger. dermatologist, 1838–1904]. The appearance of a skin lesion as a result of nonspecific trauma (e.g., sunlight, burn, operative wound). It will appear at the trauma site and may be of a type found elsewhere on the skin. May be seen in lichen planus or eczema but is particularly characteristic of psoriasis. The lesion must be sufficient to act on the papillary and epidermal layers of the skin and will appear in 3 to 18 days following the trauma. SYN: *isomorphic phenomenon.*

KOH. Potassium hydroxide.

Köhler's disease (kā′lĕrz) [Alban Köhler, Ger. physician, 1874–1947]. 1. Aseptic necrosis of the navicular bone of the wrist. 2. Osteochondrosis of the head of the second metatarsal bone of the foot.

Kohlrausch's fold (kōl′rowsh-ĕs) [Otto L. B. Kohlrausch, Ger. physician, 1811–1854]. The rectal valve; horizontal folds of the mucosa of the rectum. SYN: *Houston's valves; plicae transversales recti* [NA].

Kohnstamm's phenomenon (kōn′stămz) [Oscar Kohnstamm, Ger. physician, 1871–

1917]. Persistent and spontaneous contraction of a muscle after a strong contraction against resistance has ceased. This is easily demonstrated by standing and forcibly pushing the arm against a wall while standing with the frontal plane perpendicular to the wall. When this is stopped and you have moved away from the wall, the arm will involuntarily adduct and be elevated. SYN: *aftermovement.*

koilocyte (koy′lō-sīt) [Gr. *koilos,* hollow, + *kytos,* cell]. An abnormal cell of the squamous epithelium of the cervix. It is associated with infection with human papillomavirus and eventual development of cervical intraepithelial neoplasia.

koilocytotic atypia (koy″lō-sī-tŏt′ĭk ā-tĭp′ē-ă) [″ + ″ + *osis,* condition, + *a-,* not, + *typicalis,* typical]. Abnormality of the top layers of the epithelium of the uterine cervix wherein the cells undergo vacuolization and enlargement. SEE: *koilocyte.*

koilonychia (koy-lō-nĭk′ē-ă) [″ + *onyx,* nail]. Dystrophy of the fingernails in which they are thin and concave with raised edges. Sometimes associated with iron-deficiency anemia.

koilorrhachic (koy″lō-răk′ĭk) [″ + *rhachis,* spine]. Pert. to a spinal column that has an excessive anterior curve.

koilosternia (koy″lō-stĕr′nē-ă) [″ + Gr. *sternon,* sternum]. Condition in which the chest has a funnel-like depression in the middle of the thoracic wall.

kolp- [Gr. *kolpos,* vagina]. Prefix indicating vagina. SEE: words beginning with *colp-.*

kolpitis (kōl-pī′tĭs) [″ + *itis,* inflammation]. Inflammation of vaginal mucous membrane. SYN: *colpitis.*

kolypeptic (kō″lē-pĕp′tĭk) [Gr. *kolyein,* to hinder, + *pepsis,* digestion]. Retarding digestion.

Konakion. Trade name for phytonadione, USP.

Kondoleon's operation (kŏn-dō'lē-ŏnz) [Emmanuel Kondoleon, Gr. surgeon, 1879–1939]. Surgical removal of layers of subcutaneous tissue to relieve elephantiasis.

Kondremul. Trade name for mineral oil.

koniocortex (kō"nē-ō-kor'tĕks) [Gr. *konis*, dust, + L. *cortex*, rind]. The cortex of the sensory areas, so named because of its granular appearance.

koniology [" + *logos*, word, reason]. Science of dust and its effects. SYN: *coniology*.

koniometer (kō-nē-ŏm'ĕ-ter) [" + *metron*, measure]. Device for estimating amount of dust in the air.

koniosis (kō-nē-ō'sĭs) [" + *osis*, condition]. Any disease condition caused by dust. SYN: *coniosis*. SEE: *pneumonoconiosis*.

Konyne HT. Trade name for factor IX complex.

kophemia (kō-fē'mē-ă) [Gr. *kophan*, to become stupid, + *pheme*, speech]. Word deafness.

Koplik's spots [Henry Koplik, U.S. pediatrician, 1858–1927]. Small red spots with blue-white centers on the oral mucosa, particularly in the region opposite the molars. A diagnostic sign in measles before the rash appears. Not infrequently, the spots disappear as the eruption develops.

kopophobia (kŏp"ō-fō'bē-ă) [Gr. *kopos*, fatigue, + *phobos*, fear]. Abnormal fear of fatigue or exhaustion.

Korányi's sign (kō-răn'yēz) [Friedrich von Korányi, Hung. physician, 1828–1913]. Increased resonance on percussion of the dorsal spine, a sign of pleural effusion.

koro (kō'rō). In China and Southeast Asia, a hysterical phobia that the penis will retract into the abdomen.

koronion (kō-rō'nē-ŏn) [Gr. *korone*, crest]. Apex of coronoid process of the mandible.

Korotkoff's sounds (kō-rŏt'kŏfs) [Nikolai S. Korotkoff, Russ. physician, 1874–1920]. Sounds heard in auscultation of blood pressure. SEE: *blood pressure*.

Korsakoff's syndrome (kor'să-kŏfs) [Sergei S. Korsakoff, Russ. neurologist, 1854–1900]. Personality characterized by a psychosis with polyneuritis, disorientation, muttering delirium, insomnia, illusions, and hallucinations. Painful extremities, rarely a bilateral wrist drop, more frequently bilateral foot drop with pain or pressure over the long nerves. May occur as a sequel to chronic alcoholism. SYN: *polyneuritic psychosis*.

kosher (kō'shĕr) [Hebrew *kasher*, proper]. Pert. to food prepared and served according to Jewish dietary laws.

koumiss (koo'mĭs) [Tartar *kumyz*]. Fermented cow's milk or substance used for fermenting cow's milk. Also spelled kumiss and kumyss.

Kr. Chem. symb. for the element krypton.

Krabbe's disease (krăb'ēz) [Knud H. Krabbe, Danish neurologist, 1885–1961]. Globoid cell leukodystrophy due to the accumulation of galactocerebroside in the tissues. This is the result of a deficiency of galactocerebrosidase. Clinically, the infant develops seizures, deafness, blindness, cachexia, paralysis, and marked mental deficiency. Survival beyond two years is rare.

Kraepelin's classification (krā'pā-lĭnz) [Emil Kraepelin, Ger. psychiatrist, 1856–1926]. A classification of mental illness into two groups: the manic-depressive and the schizophrenic.

krait (krāt). Small venomous snake of the genus *Bungarus* indigenous to India.

kraurosis (krŏ-rō'sĭs) [Gr. *krauros*, dry]. Atrophy and dryness of skin and any mucous membrane, esp. of the vulva. The subcutaneous fat of the mons pubis and labia disappears, clitoris and prepuce atrophy, and stenosis of the vaginal orifice is common. Fissures may develop.

k. penis. Kraurosis in which the glans penis atrophies and becomes shriveled.

k. vulvae. Atrophic disease affecting the female external genitalia seen most often in older women. Characterized by severe itching and a white marble-like appearance of the skin, frequently with excoriations. If untreated, the skin may undergo malignant degeneration. SYN: *Breisky's disease; leukoplakia vulvae.*

Krause, Karl (krowz). German anatomist, 1797–1868.

K.'s glands. Small mucous acinous glands located beneath the fornix conjunctiva. They are accessory lacrimal glands that open into the fornix.

K.'s valve. Fold of mucous membrane of the lacrimal sac at the junction of the lacrimal duct. SYN: *Beraud's valve.*

Krause, Wilhelm (krowz). German anatomist, 1833–1910.

K.'s bulbs; K.'s end bulbs. Widely distributed encapsulated nerve endings present superficially in the skin, cornea, and organs such as the testicles.

K.'s membrane. A thin, dark disk that transversely crosses through and bisects the clear zone of a striated muscle and bisects the clear zone (isotropic disk) of a striated muscle fiber. The portion between two disks constitutes a sarcomere. SYN: *Z disk.*

Krebs cycle [Sir Hans Krebs, Ger. biochemist, 1900–1981, co-winner of a Nobel prize in 1953. He lived and worked in Britain.]. A complicated series of reactions in the body involving the oxidative metabolism of pyruvic acid and liberation of energy. It is the main pathway of terminal oxidation in the process of which not only carbohydrates but proteins and fats are utilized. SYN: *citric acid cycle; tricarboxylic acid cycle.* SEE: illus.

Krönig's area (krä′nĭgz) [Georg Krönig, Ger. physician, 1856–1911]. Resonant region in the thorax over the apices of the lungs.

Krukenberg's chopsticks [Hermann Krukenberg, Ger. surgeon, 1863–1935]. Condition occurring after surgical separation of the remaining ulna and radius of a forearm stump after traumatic removal of a lower arm. This allows the ulna and radius to act as crude pincers, i.e., chopsticks.

Krukenberg's tumor (kroo′kĕn-bĕrgz) [Frederick Krukenberg, Ger. pathologist, 1871–1946]. A malignant tumor of the ovary, usually bilateral and frequently secondary to malignancy of the gastrointestinal tract. Histologically, these tumors consist of myxomatous connective tissue and cells having a signet ring arrangement of their nuclei. The epithelial tissue resembles malignancy of the original site.

krypton (krĭp′tŏn) [Gr. *kryptos,* hidden]. SYMB: Kr. At. wt. 83.80; at. no. 36. A gaseous element found in small amounts in the atmosphere.

K₂SO₄. Potassium sulfate.

KUB. *kidneys, ureters, bladder.* Used in reference to roentgen-ray study of the abdomen.

kubisagari (koo-bĭs″ă-gä′rē) [Japanese, hang-head]. Ptosis and bulbar weakness in nutritionally deficient children; endemic in Japan. A similar disorder was observed in prisoners of war in Japan. Parenteral administration of thiamine has been beneficial.

Kufs′ disease [H. Kufs, Ger. psychiatrist, 1871–1955]. Adult form of cerebral sphingolipidosis, q.v. Onset of symptoms is between 21 and 26 years of age. Diagnosed by the development of dementia, myoclonic jerks, blindness, and retinitis pigmentosa.

Kugelberg-Welander disease [Eric Klaus Henrik Kugelberg, Swedish neurologist, 1913–1983; L. Welander, b. 1909; Swedish neurologists]. Juvenile spinal muscular atrophy.

kumiss, kumyss (koo′mĭs) [Tartar *kumyz*]. Koumiss, q.v.

Kümmell's disease or spondylitis (kĭm′ĕlz) [Hermann Kümmell, Ger. surgeon, 1852–1937]. Spondylitis following compression fracture of the vertebrae.

Kupffer's cells (koop′fĕrz) [Karl W. von Kupffer, Ger. anatomist, 1829–1902]. The name given to macrophages lining the sinusoids of the liver. Over 50% of all macrophages are found in the liver to remove old or damaged cells, pathogens, or abnormal cells

from the blood by phagocytosis. SEE: *macrophage; reticuloendothelial system.*

kuru (koo′roo). A rapidly progressive neurological disease that is invariably fatal. The disease affects mostly adult women and children of both sexes of members of the Fore tribe of New Guinea. Probably due to a transmissible slow infection (rather than a slow virus). The disease is transmitted by the practice of ingesting tissue from a victim who has died (ritual cannibalism) and rubbing infected tissues over the body of women and children kin to the victim. With the decline of this practice, the incidence of kuru has decreased.

Kussmaul, Adolph (koos′mowl). German physician, 1822–1902.

    K.′s breathing. Very deep gasping type of respiration associated with severe diabetic acidosis and coma.

    K.′s disease. Periarteritis nodosa.

kv. *kilovolt.*

KVO. *keep vein open.*

kvp. *kilovoltage peak.*

kwashiorkor (kwăsh-ē-or′kor) [Ghana, Africa, deposed child, i.e., child that is no longer suckled]. A severe protein-deficiency type of malnutrition of children. It occurs after the child is weaned. The clinical signs are, at first, a vague type of lethargy, apathy, or irritability and, later, failure to grow, mental deficiency, inanition, increased susceptibility to infections, edema, dermatitis, and liver enlargement.

    TREAT: In addition to dietary therapy, the acute problems of infections, diarrhea, poor renal function, and shock need immediate attention. At first the diet must be carefully supervised to prevent overloading the system with calories or protein. In the first weeks of therapy, the child may lose weight due to the loss of edema. If the disease has been severe and longstanding, the child may never attain full growth and mental development.

Kwell. Trade name of a shampoo and lotion for treatment of scabies and lice.

Kyasanur Forest disease. One of the Russian tick-borne encephalitides.

kyestein, kiestein (kī-ĕs′tē-ĭn) [Gr. *kyesis,* pregnancy]. A scum or film on stale urine; formerly thought to be a sign of pregnancy.

kymatism [Gr. *kyma,* wave, + *-ismos,* state of]. Twitching of isolated segments of muscle. SYN: *myokymia.*

kymogram (kī′mō-grăm). A tracing or recording made by a kymograph.

kymograph (kī′mō-grăf) [Gr. *kyma,* wave, + *graphein,* to write]. 1. An apparatus for recording movements of a writing pen; designed so that the pen moves in response to force applied to it. Widely used in physiol-

KREBS CYCLE
(TRICARBOXYLIC ACID CYCLE)

GLYCOLYSIS

$$CH_3-\overset{\overset{\displaystyle O}{\|}}{C}-\overset{\overset{\displaystyle O}{\|}}{C}-OH$$
PYRUVIC ACID

$-CO_2$

(O)

FATTY ACID CYCLE

$$CH_3-\overset{\overset{\displaystyle O}{\|}}{C}-S-CoA$$
ACETYL COENZYME A

$$\begin{array}{c} O \\ \| \\ C-OH \\ | \\ C-OH \\ | \\ CH_2-C-OH \\ \| \\ O \end{array}$$
OXALOACETIC ACID

TO RESPIRATORY CHAIN $-(H:^- + H^+)$

$$\begin{array}{c} O \\ \| \\ HO-C-H \\ | \\ CH_2-C-OH \\ \| \\ O \end{array}$$
MALIC ACID

KREBS CYCLE

$+H_2O$

$$\begin{array}{c} H \quad O \\ | \quad \| \\ HO-C-C \quad CH \\ \| \\ \end{array}$$
FUMARIC ACID

TO RESPIRATORY CHAIN $-(H:^- + H^+)$

$$\begin{array}{c} CH_2-C-OH \\ | \quad \| \\ CH_2 \quad O \\ | \\ \end{array}$$
SUCCINIC ACID

$$\begin{array}{c} CH_2 \\ | \\ CH_2 \\ | \\ O=C \\ \end{array}$$
α-KETOGLUTARIC ACID

$+H_2O$
$-CO_2$

TO RESPIRATORY CHAIN $-(H:^- + H^+)$

$$\begin{array}{c} CH_2-C-OH \\ | \\ HO-C-C-OH \\ | \\ CH_2-C-OH \\ \| \\ O \end{array}$$
CITRIC ACID

$-H_2O$

$$\begin{array}{c} CH_2-C-OH \\ | \\ C-C-OH \\ \| \\ CH-C-OH \\ \end{array}$$
cis-ACONITIC ACID

$+H_2O$

$$\begin{array}{c} CH_2-C-OH \\ | \\ CH-C-OH \\ | \\ HO-C-C-OH \\ \end{array}$$
ISOCITRIC ACID

$-(H:^- + H^+)$ TO RESPIRATORY CHAIN

$$\begin{array}{c} CH_2-C-OH \\ | \\ CH-C-OH \\ \| \\ O=C-C-OH \\ \end{array}$$
OXALOSUCCINIC ACID

$-CO_2$

ogy to record activities such as blood pressure changes, muscle contractions, respiratory movements, etc. Consists of a drum rotated by a spring or electric motor. Drum is covered by a paper upon which the record is made by the stylus of a pen. 2. A radiographic device for recording the range of motion of involuntary movements of the heart or diaphragm.

kymography. Radiographic examination in which the range of involuntary movements such as those of the heart or diaphragm is recorded.

kynocephalus (kī″nō-sĕf′ă-lŭs) [Gr. *kyon*, dog, + *kephale*, head]. Deformed fetus in which the head resembles that of a dog.

kynurenine (kī″nū-rĕn′ĭn) [″ + L. *ren*, kidney]. An intermediate compound in tryptophan metabolism.

kypho- [Gr. *kyphos*, a hump]. Prefix indicating humped.

kyphorachitis (kī″fō-răk-ī′tĭs) [″ + *rhachis*, spine, + *itis*, inflammation]. Rachitic deformity involving the thorax and spinal column. Results in development of anteroposterior hump.

kyphos (kī′fŏs) [Gr., hump]. Convex prominence of the spine.

kyphoscoliosis (kī″fō-skō″lē-ō′sĭs) [″ + *skoliosis*, curvation]. Lateral curvature of the spine accompanying anteroposterior hump.

kyphosis (kī-fō′sĭs) [Gr., humpback]. Exaggeration or angulation of normal posterior curve of spine. Gives rise to condition commonly known as humpback, hunchback, or Pott's curvature. Also refers to excessive curvature of the spine with convexity backward. The former may be due to congenital anomaly, disease (tuberculosis, syphilis), malignancy, or compression fracture. The latter may result from faulty posture, osteoarthritis or rheumatoid arthritis, rickets, or other conditions. SYN: *humpback; spinal curvature.*

kyphotic (kī-fŏt′ĭk). Affected by or pert. to kyphosis.

kyrtorrhachic (kĭr″tō-răk′ĭk) [Gr. *kyrtos*, curved, + *rhachis*, spine]. Spinal curvature with posterior concavity.

kyto- [Gr. *kytos*, cell]. Prefix denoting a cell. SEE: words beginning with *cyto-*.

L

Λ, λ. In the Greek alphabet, symbol for lambda.

L., l. *Lactobacillus; Latin; left; left eye; length; lethal; light sense; liter.*

L₊. Symb. for limes tod.

L₀. Symb. for limes nul.

L-. In biochemistry a symbol used as a prefix to indicate the carbon atom is symmetrical (or achiral) and that only three dissimilar groups attach to it. The names of such compounds would be preceded by L-. SEE: D-.

LA. *left atrium.*

La. Chem. symb. for the element lanthanum.

lab. 1. German for the enzyme rennin. 2. Colloquial for laboratory.

Labbé's vein (lăb-āz′) [Léon Labbé, Fr. surgeon, 1832–1916]. Vein that connects the superficial middle cerebral vein and the transverse sinus of the brain. SYN: *inferior anastomotic vein.*

label. The attachment of a radioactive marker or other chemical to a biologically active substance such as a drug or body chemical (such as glucose, protein, or fat). The metabolic fate of the labeled material may be investigated by detecting the presence of the label in various body sites or in excretions. The label material itself is chosen so that it does not alter the metabolism or action of the substance being investigated. SEE: *tracer.*

labeling. SEE: *tag, radioactive; tagging.*

la belle indifférence [Fr., beautiful indifference]. An unrealistic degree of indifference to, or complacency about, startling and gross symptoms of hysterical anesthesia or paralysis. Seen in conversion reaction.

labetalol hydrochloride. An alpha and beta adrenergic blocking agent used in treating hypertension. Trade names are Normodyne and Trandate. SEE: *hypertensive crisis.*

labia (lā′bē-ă) [L.]. Plural of labium.

   l. majora. The two folds of cellular adipose tissue lying on either side of the vaginal opening and forming the lateral borders of the vulva. Their medial surfaces unite anteriorly above the clitoris to form the anterior commissure; posteriorly they are connected by a poorly defined posterior commissure. They are separated by a cleft, the rima pudendi, into which the urethra and vagina open. In young girls, their medial surfaces are in contact with each other, concealing the labia minora and vestibule. In older women, the labia minora may protrude between them.

   l. minora. Two thin folds of integument that lie just inside the vestibule of the vagina and between the labia majora and the hymen. They enclose the vestibule. Anteriorly each divides into two smaller folds that unite with similar folds from the other side and enclose the clitoris, the more anterior one forming the prepuce (preputium clitoridis) of the clitoris, the posterior one forming the frenulum clitoridis. In younger children, they are hidden entirely by the labia majora.

   RS: clitoris; Hottentot apron; mons veneris; nympha; nymphoncus; nymphotomy; smegma; vagina.

labial (lā′bē-ăl) [L. *labialis*]. Pert. to the lips.

labial glands. Many racemose glands between the labial mucosa and orbicularis muscle opening on the lip's inner surface.

labialism (lā′bē-ăl-ĭzm) [L. *labium*, lip, + Gr. *-ismos*, state of]. Defective speech in which labial sounds are stressed.

LaBID. Trade name for theophylline, USP.

labile (lā′bĭl) [L. *labi*, to slip]. Not fixed; unsteady; easily disarranged; rapidly shifting and changing emotions.

   l., heat. Easily altered or decomposed by heat. SYN: *thermolabile.*

lability (lă-bĭl′ĭ-tē). State of being unstable or changeable.

   l., emotional. Excessive emotional reactivity associated with frequent changes or swings in emotions and mood.

labioalveolar (lā″bē-ō-ăl-vē′ō-lăr) [L. *labium*, lip, + *alveolus*, little hollow]. Pert. to lips and tooth sockets.

labiocervical (lā″bē-ō-sĕr′vĭ-kl) [″ + *cervix*, neck]. Pert. to the buccal surface of the lips and the neck of a tooth.

labiochorea (lā″bē-ō-kō-rē′ă) [″ + Gr. *choreia*, dance]. Spasm of the lips in chorea. It causes stammering.

labioclination (lā″bē-ō-klī-nā′shŭn) [″ + Gr. *klinein*, to slope]. In dentistry, deviation of a tooth from the normal vertical toward the labial side.

labiodental (lā″bē-ō-dĕn′tăl) [″ + *dens*, tooth]. 1. Concerning the lips and teeth, esp. the labial surface of a tooth. 2. Referring to the pronunciation of certain letters that require interaction of the teeth and lips.

labiogingival (lā″bē-ō-jĭn′jĭ-văl) [″ + *gingiva*, gum]. Concerning the lips and gums or referring to the labial and gingival surfaces of a tooth.

labioglossolaryngeal (lā″bē-ō-glŏs″ō-lăr-ĭn′jē-ăl) [″ + Gr. *glossa*, tongue, + *larynx*, larynx]. Pert. to the lips, tongue, and larynx.

labioglossopharyngeal (lā″bē-ō-glŏs″ō-făr-ĭn′jē-ăl) [″ + ″ + *pharynx*, throat]. Pert. to the lips, tongue, and pharynx.

labiograph (lā′bē-ō-grăf) [″ + Gr. *graphein*, to write]. Device for registering lip movements in speaking.

labiomental (lā″bē-ō-mĕn′tăl) [″ + *mentum*, chin]. Pert. to the lower lip and chin.

labiomycosis (lā″bē-ō-mī-kō′sĭs) [″ + Gr. *mykes*, fungus, + *osis*, condition]. Any disease of the lips due to presence of a fungus.

labionasal (lā″bē-ō-nā′zăl) [″ + *nasus*, nose]. Concerning the nose and lips.

labiopalatine (lā″bē-ō-păl′ă-tīn) [″ + *palatum*, palate]. Rel. to the lips and palate.

labioplasty (lā′bē-ō-plăs″tē) [″ + Gr. *plassein*, to form]. Plastic surgery of the lips. SYN: *cheiloplasty*.

labiotenaculum (lā″bē-ō-tĕn-ăk′ū-lŭm) [″ + *tenaculum*, a hook]. Instrument for holding lips during an operation.

labioversion (lā″bē-ō-vĕr′zhŭn) [″ + *versio*, a turning]. State of being twisted in a labial direction, esp. a tooth.

labium (lā′bē-ŭm) [L.] (pl. *labia*). [NA] A lip or a structure like one; an edge or fleshy border.

   l. cerebri. Margin of the cerebral hemispheres overlapping the corpus callosum.

   l. inferius oris. [NA] Lower lip.

   l. majus. SEE: *labia majora*.

   l. minus. SEE: *labia minora*.

   l. minus pudendi. SEE: *labia minora*.

   l. oris. [NA] The skin and muscular tissue surrounding the mouth; lips of the mouth.

   l. superius oris. [NA] The upper lip.

   l. tympanicum. Outer edge of organ of Corti.

   l. urethrae. Lateral margin of meatus urinarius externus.

   l. uteri. Thickened margin of the cervix uteri.

   l. vestibulare. Vestibular or inner edge of organ of Corti.

labor [L., work]. The physiological process by which the fetus is expelled from the uterus into the vagina and then to the outside of the body. SYN: *childbirth; parturition.* SEE: illus.

Approx. 95% of normal full-term babies are born 265 to 300 days from the first day of the last menstrual period. Average duration of normal pregnancy is 282 days.

Traditionally labor is divided into three stages, but *lightening* most often occurs up to four weeks prior to onset of labor in primigravid women. It may occur during labor in a woman who has borne a previous child or children. The shape of the abdomen changes, with the lower portion becoming more pendulous and the costal area looking flatter. This change is due to the presenting part having descended into the pelvis to the level of the ischial spines.

FIRST STAGE (stage of dilatation): Period from the onset of regular contractions of the uterus until the cervix is fully dilated and effaced. Averages 12 hours in primigravidas and eight in multiparas.

Identification of this stage is particularly important to the woman who is having her first baby. Diagnosis is complicated by the fact that many persons experience false labor pains. These may begin as early as three to four weeks before onset of true labor. False labor pains are quite irregular, usually confined to the lower part of the abdomen and groin, and do not extend from the back around the abdomen as in true labor. False labor pains do not increase with time and are not made more intense by walking. The conclusive distinction is made by determining the effect of the pains on the cervix. False labor pains do not cause effacement and dilatation of the cervix as do true labor pains. SEE: *Braxton Hicks sign*.

A reliable sign of impending labor is *show*. The appearance of a slight amount of vaginal blood-tinged mucus is a good indication that labor will begin within the next 24 hours. Loss of more than a few milliliters of blood at this time must be regarded as being due to a pathological process. SEE: *placenta previa*.

SECOND STAGE (stage of expulsion): Period from complete dilatation of the cervix through the birth of the fetus. Averages 50 minutes in primigravidas and 20 minutes in multigravidas. Labor pains are severe, occur at two- or three-minute intervals, and last from a little less than one minute to a little more than one and one-half minutes.

Rupture of the membranes (bag of waters) usually occurs during the early part of this stage, accompanied by a gush of amniotic fluid from the vagina. The muscles of the abdomen contract involuntarily during this portion of labor. The patient directs all her strength to bearing down during the pains. She may be quite flushed during the pains and perspire. As labor continues the perineum bulges and, in a head presentation, the scalp of the fetus appears through the vulvar opening. With cessation of each pain the fetus recedes from its position and then advances a little more when the pains return. This continues until more of the head is visible and the vulvar ring encircles the head. This is called *crowning*.

At this time the decision is made concerning an incision in the perineum, i.e., episiotomy, to facilitate delivery. If done, it is most commonly a midline posterior episiotomy.

SEQUENCE OF LABOR AND CHILDBIRTH

1. LABOR BEGINS, MEMBRANES INTACT.

2. EFFACEMENT OF CERVIX, WHICH IS NOW PARTIALLY DILATED.

3. HEAD IS ROTATED, PARTIALLY EXTENDED, AND NOW PRESENTS. MEMBRANES ARE RUPTURED.

4. HEAD IS ALMOST DELIVERED.

5. DELIVERY OF HEAD.

6. DELIVERY OF SHOULDERS.

7. DELIVERY OF INFANT IS COMPLETE. UTERUS BEGINS TO CONTRACT.

8. UMBILICAL CORD HAS BEEN TIED AND CUT. PLACENTA HAS BEGUN TO SEPARATE FROM UTERUS.

When the head is completely removed from the vagina it falls posteriorly; later the head rotates as the shoulders turn to come through the pelvis. There is usually a gush of amniotic fluid as the shoulders are delivered.

THIRD STAGE (placental stage): Period following birth of the fetus through expulsion of the placenta and membranes. As soon as the fetus is delivered, the remainder of the amniotic fluid escapes. It will contain a small amount of blood. Uterine contractions and pains begin, and usually within eight to ten minutes the placenta and membranes are delivered. Following this, there is a certain amount of bleeding from the uterus. The amount may vary from 100 to 500 ml or more, but the average is 200 ml.

Amount of blood loss will vary directly with the size of the fetus. The probability that blood loss will exceed 500 ml is less than 5% if the fetus weighs 5 lb (2268 gm) or less. The chances that blood loss will exceed 500 ml is 25% if the fetus weighs more than 9 lb (4082 gm). Other factors such as episiotomy or perineal laceration will also affect the amount of blood loss. SEE: *birthing chair; Credé's method* for assisting the expulsion of the placenta.

NURSING IMPLICATIONS: Preparation for labor, delivery, and care of the newborn is most frequently carried out in classes taught by obstetric nurses. Expectant couples attend classes together, and are taught exercises, breathing techniques, and supportive care measures for labor, delivery, and the postpartum period, and also are taught neonatal care and feeding techniques. The goals of expectant parent education are the birth of a healthy infant and a positive experience for the couple.

Labor and delivery may take place in a hospital, birthing center, or at home. Hospitals offer care in traditional labor and delivery rooms and, in some facilities, in birthing rooms which attempt to simulate the home environment. Prenatal records are made available in order to review medical, surgical, and gynecologic history, blood type and Rh, and especially any prenatal problems in this pregnancy. If the mother is Rh-negative, and the Rh status of the fetus is unknown or Rh-positive, the mother will receive Rh immune globulin within 72 hours after delivery.

Admission work-up of the patient in labor includes assessing vital signs, height and weight, fetal heart tones and activity, and labor status, i.e., condition of membranes, show, onset time of regular contractions, contraction frequency and duration, and patient response (anxiety, pain or discomfort). Initial laboratory studies are carried out based on agency protocol. The patient is prepared for examination, which may be carried out by her obstetrician, resident physician or other house staff, or by a midwife or obstetrical nurse, depending on the site and the hospital policy. The abdomen is examined to help determine fetal position and presentation (Leopold's maneuvers), and a sterile vaginal examination determines cervical dilatation and effacement, fetal station and position of presenting part. An electronic monitor (applied externally, or internally if membranes have ruptured and head is low) may be used to monitor fetal heart rate and response to contractions, as well as contraction frequency and duration on a continuous or intermittent basis, or this ongoing assessment may be carried out intermittently by the attending nurse, using hands and fetoscope. The frequency of assessment and repetition of vaginal examination are determined by the patient's labor activity, stage, and fetal response. In the past, admission to a labor suite usually included a perineal shave-prep and enema, preparatory for delivery, but these procedures have largely been discontinued and are currently done only if prescribed for the particular patient. The patient is asked to urinate and to have a bowel movement, if possible. Bladder distension is to be avoided, but catheterization is carried out only if all other efforts to encourage voiding fail. The perineum is cleansed (protecting the vaginal introitus from entry of cleansing solutions) and kept as clean as possible throughout the patient's labor, with special cleansing prior to examination and delivery and following any expulsion of feces or urine.

First stage: Patient may be up and walking about depending on activity, membrane status, and fetal position. Electrolyte-rich oral liquids may be prescribed, or I.V. fluid therapy initiated. The nurse functions to support the patient's husband or support person and the patient herself, and monitors the progress of the labor and the response of the fetus, notifying the physician or midwife of any abnormal findings. When membranes rupture spontaneously or are ruptured artificially by the midwife or obstetrician, the nurse immediately observes and documents the color and volume of the fluid, especially noting the presence of meconium staining or unusual odor. The fluid may be tested for pH using nitrazine paper in order to distinguish it from a sudden spurt of urine. The nurse also immediately notes the fetal heart rate, an indicator of fetal response to the occurrence. The nurse provides prescribed analgesia as desired and required by the individual patient, and assists with and monitors regional anesthetic use.

Second stage: Patient may deliver in any position previously agreed upon, including lithotomy or modified lithotomy, sitting or side-lying, in a birthing chair, birthing bed, or on a delivery table. The nurse continues to monitor patient and fetus, prepares the patient for delivery (draping and cleansing), sets up the delivery equipment, and supports the father or support person (positioned near patient's head), and positions the mirror or TV monitor to permit viewing of delivery by couple. The nurse also notes the time of delivery and provides initial infant care following delivery, including further suctioning of the naso- and oropharynx as necessary (initial suctioning is done by deliverer before delivering shoulders), drying and warming infant (head covering, blanket wrap, or thermal warmer), application of cord clamp (after double-clamping and cutting between clamps by deliverer), and positive identification (footprint of infant and fingerprint of mother, application of number band to ankle of infant and wrist of mother), and eye prophylaxis for gonococcal ophthalmia. An Apgar score, q.v., of the infant's overall condition is conducted at 1 and 5 minutes after birth. The infant in good condition is placed on the mother's chest or abdomen or put to breast, and the couple is encouraged to inspect and interact with the infant. An infant in distress is hurried to the nursery, usually with the father attending, so that specialized care can be provided.

Third stage: The nurse continues to monitor the status of the patient's fundus through delivery of the placenta and membranes, examination of vagina and uterus for trauma or retained products, and repair of any laceration or surgical episiotomy. The placenta is examined to ascertain that no fragments remain in the uterus. Perineal area is cleansed.

Fourth stage: The nurse continues to observe the patient and be alert to hemorrhage or other complications by frequent assessment, including: monitoring vital signs, palpating the fundus for firmness and position in relation to the umbilicus at intervals determined by hospital policy or patient condition, and massaging the fundus or administering prescribed oxytocic drugs to maintain uterine contractions and limit bleeding. The nurse also intermittently assesses vaginal bleeding for character and volume, and bladder for distension, encouraging the patient to void and catheterizing only if necessary. The obstetrician or mid-

wife is notified if any problems occur or persist. This period also is used for parent-infant bonding. The nurse encourages the couple to examine the infant and supports the couple's responses to the newborn and to the labor and delivery experience.

l., active. Regular uterine contractions with increasing dilatation of the cervix and descent of the presenting part.

l., arrested. Failure of labor to proceed through the normal stages. May be due to uterine inertia, obstruction of the pelvis, or systemic disease.

l., artificial. L., induction of.

l., complicated. Labor occurring with an accompanying abnormal condition, i.e., hemorrhage or inertia.

l., dry. Labor after most of the amniotic fluid has been drained away. Usually associated with premature rupture of the membranes.

l., false. Uterine contractions occurring before the onset of actual labor. These contractions eventually subside.

l., induction of. Use of oxytocics or other methods to stimulate uterine contractions prior to the time they normally would occur. Contraction of the uterus may be stimulated by gently squeezing the nipples.

Caution: Oxytocin should be used only intravenously, using a device that permits precise control of flow rate. While oxytocin is being administered, the fetal heart rate and uterine contractions should be monitored electronically.

---

l., instrumental. Labor completed by mechanical means, such as the use of forceps.

l., missed. 1. Labor, false, q.v. 2. True labor pains begin but subside. This may be a sign of a dead fetus or extrauterine pregnancy.

l., normal. Progressive dilatation and effacement of the cervix with descent of the presenting part.

l., precipitate. Labor that lasts less than 2 to 3 hours from onset to delivery.

l., premature. Labor that begins prior to the completion of 36 weeks' gestation. SYN: *preterm labor.* SEE: *gestation; prematurity.*

l., spontaneous. Labor that is completed without mechanical or operative interference.

l., trial of. Permitting labor to continue long enough to determine if normal birth appears to be possible.

labor, words pert. to: abortion; "amni-" words; afterbirth; afterpains; ante partum; axis traction; bag of waters; ballottement; bipara; biparous; birthing chair; bradytocia;

breech presentation; bruit, placental; caput succedaneum; caul; cephalhematoma; cephalic version; cephalotomy; cesarean section; cesarotomy; cleidotomy; conception; conjugate; Credé's method; cross birth; delivery; disengagement; dystocia; ecbolic; eclampsia; embryectomy; embryo; embryoctony; embryotocia; eutocia; fetus; gestation; Hegar's sign; herpes; hourglass contraction; hydramnion; impetigo herpetiformis; Lamaze technique or method; Leboyer method; maneuver; midwife; multipara; nullipara; nurse-midwife; obstetrician; obstetrics; ophthalmia neonatorum; oxytocic principle; oxytocin; parturient; parturifacient; partus; placenta; placenta previa; postpartum; presentation, brow; primipara; psychoprophylactic childbirth; puerpera; puerperal; puerperium; quintuplet; restitution; Rh; show; twins; uterus.

laboratory (lăb′ră-tor″ē) [L. *laboratorium*]. A room or building equipped for scientific experimentation, research, testing, or clinical studies of materials, fluids, or tissues obtained from patients.

Laborde's method (lă-bordz′) [Jean B. V. Laborde, Fr. physician, 1830–1903]. Stimulation of the respiratory center in asphyxiation by a series of rhythmical traction movements upon the tongue.

labret (lā′brĕt) [L. *labrum*, lip]. A distinctive plug of ivory, bone, stone, or bottle top worn by some primitive people in a hole artificially produced in the lips of adolescent boys.

labrocyte (lăb′rō-sīt) [Gr. *labros*, greedy, + *kytos*, cell]. A mast cell.

labrum (lā′brŭm) [L., lip] (pl. *labra*). 1. Lip or liplike structure. 2. The upper lip of an insect.

labyrinth (lăb′ĭ-rĭnth) [Gr. *labyrinthos*, maze]. 1. Intricate communicating passages. 2. The internal ear consisting of osseous and membranous labyrinths. These structures are essential to maintaining physical equilibrium of the body. SEE: illus.

   l., bony. L., osseous.

   l., ethmoidal. The lateral mass of the ethmoid bone. Includes the superior and middle conchae and encloses the ethmoidal air cells. SYN: *l., olfactory*.

   l., membranous. Structure in osseous labyrinth consisting of utricle and saccule of vestibule, three semicircular ducts, and the cochlear duct. All are filled with endolymph.

   l., olfactory. L., ethmoidal.

   l., osseous. Consists of vestibule, three semicircular canals, and cochlea. SYN: *l., bony*.

labyrinthectomy (lăb-ĭ-rĭn-thĕk′tō-mē) [″ + *ektome*, excision]. Excision of the laby-

LABYRINTH OF INNER EAR

SUPERIOR

POSTERIOR

LATERAL

SEMICIRCULAR CANALS

ROUND WINDOW

COCHLEA

VESTIBULAR NERVE

COCHLEAR NERVE

rinth.

labyrinthine (lăb-ĭ-rĭn′thīn). 1. Pert. to a labyrinth. 2. Intricate or involved, as a labyrinth. 3. Often used to describe speech that wanders aimlessly from subject to unconnected subject, as seen in schizophrenia.

labyrinthitis (lăb″ĭ-rĭn-thī′tĭs) [″ + *itis*, inflammation]. Inflammation (acute or chronic) of labyrinth; otitis externa. SEE: *Ménière's disease*.

   SYM: Vertigo, vomiting, nystagmus.

   ETIOL: Primary infection; trauma; complication of influenza, otitis media, or meningitis.

labyrinthotomy (lăb″ĭ-rĭn-thŏt′ō-mē) [″ + *tome*, incision]. Surgical incision into labyrinth.

labyrinthus (lăb″ĭ-rĭn′thŭs) [L., Gr. *labyrinthos*, maze]. A labyrinth.

lac (lăk) [L.]. 1. Milk. 2. Milky medicinal substance.

lacerable (lăs′ĕr-ă-b′l) [L. *lacerare*, to tear]. Having the capability of being lacerated.

lacerate (lăs′ĕr-āt) [L. *lacerare*, to tear]. To tear, as into irregular segments.

lacerated. Torn; broken.

laceration. A wound or irregular tear of the flesh.

laceration of cervix. Bilateral, stellate, or unilateral tear of the cervix uteri caused by childbirth.

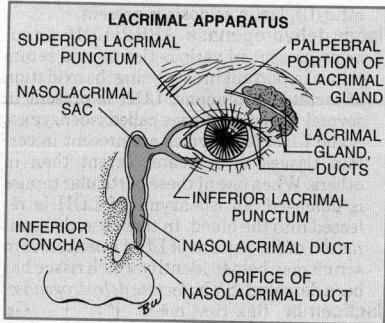

LACRIMAL APPARATUS

SUPERIOR LACRIMAL PUNCTUM
PALPEBRAL PORTION OF LACRIMAL GLAND
NASOLACRIMAL SAC
LACRIMAL GLAND, DUCTS
INFERIOR LACRIMAL PUNCTUM
INFERIOR CONCHA
NASOLACRIMAL DUCT
ORIFICE OF NASOLACRIMAL DUCT

laceration of perineum. Injury of perineum caused by childbirth. If it extends through the sphincter ani muscle, it is complete or fourth degree. SEE: *episiotomy.*

lacertus (lă-sĕr′tŭs) [L., lizard]. 1. Muscular part of the arm. 2. A muscular or fibrous band.

   l. cordis. A muscular tissue band on the inner cardiac surface. SYN: *trabeculae carneae cordis* [NA].

   l. fibrosus. Aponeurotic band from the biceps tendon to the bicipital or semilunar fascia of forearm.

laciniate (lă-sĭn′ē-āt) [L. *lacinia,* fringe]. Being jagged or fringed.

lacrima (lăk′rĭ-mă) [L.]. Tear fluid from eye.

lacrimal (lăk′rĭm-ăl) [L. *lacrima,* tear]. Pert. to the tears.

lacrimal apparatus. Structures concerned with secretion and conduction of tears. Includes lacrimal gland and its excretory ducts, lacrimal canaliculi, lacrimal sac, and nasolacrimal duct, which empties into the nasal cavity. SEE: illus.

   Patency of the lacrimal duct may be tested by placing a dilute solution of sugar in the conjunctival sac; if the duct is patent, the individual will report the sensation of sweetness in the mouth; if not, the sugar will not be perceived.

lacrimal bone. Bone at inner side of the orbital cavity.

lacrimal duct. One of two ducts (superior and inferior) that convey tears from the lacrimal lake to the lacrimal sac.

lacrimal gland. Gland that secretes tears. A tubuloalveolar gland located in orbit, superior and lateral to the eyeball. Consists of a large superior portion (pars orbitalis) and a smaller inferior portion (pars palpebralis).

lacrimal lake. The small pouch formed by the junction of the conjunctiva at the internal canthus of the eye.

lacrimal reflex. Secretion of fluid resulting from irritation of corneal conjunctiva.

lacrimal sac. Upper dilated portion of nasolacrimal duct situated in groove of lacrimal bone. The upper part is behind the internal tarsal ligament. Measures 12 to 15 mm in length.

lacrimation [L. *lacrima,* tear]. Secretion and discharge of tears.

   l., test for. A strip of filter paper, 35 × 5 mm, is sharply bent 5 mm from one end, and is then hooked into the lower conjunctival sac without applying anesthesia. The measured length of saturation of the strip provides a measure of the functional ability to lacrimate and the nerve supply to the lacrimal apparatus. SYN: *Schirmer's test.*

lacrimator. Substance that increases the flow of tears.

lacrimatory (lăk′rĭ-mă-tō″rē). Causing the production of tears.

lacrimonasal (lăk″rĭ-mō-nā′zăl) [″ + *nasus,* nose]. Concerning the nose and lacrimal apparatus.

lacrimotome (lăk′rĭ-mō-tōm) [″ + Gr. *tome,* incision]. A cutting instrument used for incising the lacrimal sac or duct.

lacrimotomy (lăk″rĭm-ŏt′ō-mē) [″ + Gr. *tome,* incision]. Incision of lacrimal duct.

lactacid. Lactic acid.

lactacidemia (lăk-tăs″ĭ-dē′mē-ă) [″ + ″ + Gr. *haima,* blood]. Accumulation of an excess of lactic acid in the blood. It occurs normally following strenuous and prolonged exercise.

lactaciduria (lăkt-ă-sĭd-ū′rē-ă) [″ + ″ + Gr. *ouron,* urine]. Lactic acid excreted in the urine.

lactagogue (lăk′tă-gŏg) [″ + Gr. *agogos,* leading]. Agent that induces secretion of milk. SYN: *galactagogue.*

lactalbumin [″ + *albumen,* coagulated white of egg]. The albumin of milk and cheese; a soluble simple protein. Lactalbumin is present in higher concentration in human milk than in cow's milk. When milk is heated, the lactalbumin coagulates and appears as a film on the surface of the milk.

lactam (lăk′tăm). An organic chemical that contains the —NH—CO group in a ring form. It is formed by the removal of a molecule of water from certain amino acids.

β-lactamase-resistant antibiotics. Antibiotics that are resistant to the action of β-lactamase. This property makes them effective against microbial organisms that produce β-lactamase.

β-lactamases (bā″tă-lăk′tă-mās). A group of enzymes that act on certain antibodies to inactivate them.

lactase [″ + *-ase,* enzyme]. An intestinal sugar-splitting enzyme converting lactose into dextrose and galactose; found in intestinal juice. SEE: *enzyme; maltase; sucrase; sugar.*

lactase deficiency syndrome. Absence of the lactase enzyme in intestinal mucosa leads to symptoms in persons who ingest lactase; those are abdominal cramps, bloating, and diarrhea. This enzyme deficiency may be hereditary but can be present in almost any digestive tract disease that damages the intestinal mucosa.

    TREAT: Avoidance of milk. SEE: *breath test for lactase deficiency; yogurt.*

lactate (lăk′tāt). 1. Any salt derived from lactic acid. 2. To secrete milk.

lactate dehydrogenase. Lactic dehydrogenase, q.v.

lactation (lăk-tā′shŭn) [L. *lactatio*, a sucking]. 1. The period of suckling in mammals. 2. The function of secreting milk.

    DIET: During this period the mother needs additional calcium to offset her loss of milk; and adequate intake of calories, fluids, and protein. Fruits, vegetables, and wholegrain cereal should also be included.

lactation amenorrhea method. ABBR: LAM. The method of causing decreased fertility in a woman by nursing a newborn for a lengthy period, i.e., several years or more. In general, the longer a woman breast-feeds, the longer she prevents ovulation.

lacteal (lăk′tē-ăl) [L. *lacteus*, of milk]. 1. Pert. to milk. 2. An intestinal lymphatic that takes up chyle and passes it to the lymph circulation and, by way of the thoracic duct, to the blood vascular system. SEE: *lymph.*

lactescence (lăk-tĕs′ĕns) [L. *lactescere*, to become milky]. Condition of becoming or resembling milk.

lactic (lăk′tĭk) [L. *lac*, milk]. Pert. to milk.

lactic acid. USP. A mixture of lactic acid, $C_3H_6O_3$, and lactic acid lactate, $C_6H_{10}O_5$, equivalent to a total of not less than 85% and not more than 90%, by weight, of $C_3H_6O_3$. A colorless syrupy liquid formed in milk, sauerkraut, and in certain types of pickles by the fermentation of the sugars by microorganisms. It is also formed during muscular activity by the breakdown of glycogen (glycolysis).

lactic acid fermentation. The production of lactic acid from carbohydrates by the action of various bacteria. Occurs commonly in milk and milk products.

lactic acidosis. ABBR: LA. Accumulation of lactic acid in the blood without respect to the etiology. Lactic acid is produced at a faster rate than normal when there is inadequate oxygenation of skeletal muscle and other tissues. Thus, any disease that leads to tissue hypoxia may cause this condition. In general, when blood pH is less than 7.35 and lactate is greater than 5 to 6 mmol/L (5 to 6

mEq/L), lactic acidosis is present.

lactic dehydrogenase. ABBR: LDH. An enzyme present in various tissues and serum that is important in catalyzing the oxidation of lactate. In humans, LDH is present in several molecular forms called isoenzymes. Some LDH isoenzymes are present in certain tissues to a greater extent than in others. When one of these particular tissues is damaged, an isoenzyme of LDH is released into the blood. In that case, determination of the pattern of LDH isoenzymes in serum may help to identify which tissue has been damaged. SYN: *lactate dehydrogenase.*

lacticemia (lăk-tĭ-sē′mē-ă) [″ + Gr. *haima*, blood]. Lactic acid in the blood. SYN: *lactacidemia.*

lactiferous (lăk-tĭf′ĕr-ŭs) [″ + *ferre*, to bear]. Secreting and conveying milk.

lactiferous ducts. Ducts of the mammary gland.

lactiferous glands. 1. The mammary glands. 2. Montgomery's glands, consisting of 20 to 24 glands in the areola of the nipples.

lactification (lăk″tĭ-fĭ-kā′shŭn) [″ + *facere*, to make]. Lactic acid production.

lactifuge (lăk′tĭ-fūj) [″ + *fugare*, to expel]. 1. Stopping milk secretion. 2. Agent stopping milk secretion.

lactigenous (lăk-tĭj′ĕn-ŭs) [″ + Gr. *gennan*, to produce]. Producing milk.

lactigerous (lăk-tĭj′ĕr-ŭs) [″ + *gerere*, to carry]. Secreting or conveying milk.

lactinated (lăk′tĭ-nāt″ĕd). Containing or prepared with lactose, milk sugar.

lactivorous (lăk-tĭv′or-ŭs) [″ + *vorare*, to devour]. Living upon milk.

Lactobacillus (lăk-tō-bă-sĭl′ŭs) [″ + *bacillus*, little rod]. A genus of bacteria belonging to the family Lactobacillaceae. They are gram-positive, nonmotile, rod-shaped organisms that do not produce spores and are acid resistant. They produce lactic acid from carbohydrates. They are responsible for the souring of milk.

    L. acidophilus. Organism that produces lactic acid by fermenting the sugars in milk. Found in milk, feces of infants fed by bottle, and adults. Also present in carious teeth, saliva, and the human vagina.

    L. bulgaricus. Bacillus found in fermented milk. Milk fermented with this organism is known as Bulgarian milk.

    L. casei. Bacillus found in milk and cheese.

    L. helveticus. Bacillus found in Swiss cheese.

lactobutyrometer (lăk″tō-bū-tĭ-rŏm′ĕ-tĕr) [″ + Gr. *boutyron*, butter, + *metron*, measure]. Instrument for estimating the cream content of milk.

lactocele (lăk′tō-sēl) [″ + Gr. *kele*, tumor,

swelling]. Cystic tumor of the breast due to occlusion of a milk duct. SYN: *galactocele.*

lactoferrin. An enzyme released in phagocytosis by neutrophils and macrophages that combines with iron in the blood. As a result, the iron is unavailable to invading pathogens for their reproduction.

lactogen (lăk'tō-jĕn) [L. *lac,* milk, + Gr. *gennan,* to produce]. Any substance that stimulates the production of milk. SEE: *prolactin.*

   l., human placental. ABBR: HPL. A hormone formed by the placenta. It is not present in the maternal circulation 2 days after delivery.

lactogenic [" + Gr. *gennan,* to produce]. Inducing the secretion of milk.

lactogenic hormone. Prolactin.

lactoglobulin (lăk"tō-glŏb'ū-lĭn) [" + *globulus,* globule]. A protein found in milk. Casein and lactoglobulin are the most common proteins in cow's milk.

   l.'s, immune. Antibodies present in the colostrum.

lactometer (lăk-tŏm'ĕ-tĕr) [" + Gr. *metron,* measure]. Device for determining the specific gravity of milk.

lacto-ovo-vegetarian (lăk"tō-ō"vō-vĕj"ĕ-tā'rē-ăn). A person who is a vegetarian but also utilizes eggs and dairy products in his or her diet.

lactophosphate (lăk"tō-fŏs'fāt) [" + *phosphas,* phosphate]. A salt derived jointly from lactic and phosphoric acid.

lactoprotein (lăk"tō-prō'tē-ĭn) [" + Gr. *protos,* first]. Any protein present in milk.

lactorrhea (lăk-tō-rē'ă) [" + Gr. *rhoia,* flow]. Discharge of milk between nursings and after weaning of offspring. SYN: *galactorrhea.*

lactose. 1. A disaccharide that on hydrolysis yields glucose and galactose. Bacteria can convert it into lactic and butyric acids, as in the souring of milk. The milk of mammals contains 4% to 7% lactose. Its presence in the urine may be indicative of obstruction to flow of milk after cessation of nursing. Commercially, a fine-powdered, white substance that will not dissolve in cold water. 2. A sugar, $C_{11}H_{22}O_{11}$, obtained from evaporation of cow's milk. Used in manufacturing tablets, as a diluent, and in making capsules.

lactose intolerance. Intolerance to milk and some dairy products. It is characterized by gastrointestinal symptoms associated with malabsorption of food. The intolerance may be congenital or have a late onset beginning at several years of age.

   ETIOL: Deficiency of the enzyme lactase, which is essential to the absorption of lactose from the intestinal tract. The deficiency may be present in the newborn or it may be acquired as an adult.

   TREAT: Limit milk consumption to one glass or less each day. The frequency of that "dose" can be determined by the patient's reaction. Yogurts may be consumed instead of milk. Enzyme tablets containing lactose to predigest milk are helpful.

lactoserum (lăk-tō-sēr'ŭm) [" + *serum,* whey]. Blood serum of an animal inoculated with milk; used to precipitate specific caseins from milk.

lactosuria (lăk-tō-sū'rē-ă) [" + Gr. *ouron,* urine]. Occurrence of milk sugar (lactose) in the urine. Frequent during pregnancy and lactation.

lactotherapy (lăk-tō-thĕr'ă-pē) [" + Gr. *therapeia,* treatment]. 1. Treatment with milk diet. 2. Medicinal treatment of nursing infant with drugs given to mother to be excreted in milk. SYN: *galactotherapy.*

lactotoxin (lăk"tō-tŏks'ĭn) [" + Gr. *toxikon,* poison]. Any toxic substance occurring in milk that has decomposed.

lactovegetarian. 1. Pert. to milk and vegetables. 2. One who lives on a diet of milk, other dairy products, and vegetables.

lactulose. A synthetic disaccharide, 4-*O*-β-D-galactopyranosyl-D-fructofuranose, that is not hydrolyzed or absorbed in humans. It is metabolized by bacteria in the colon with the production of organic acids. Used in treating the encephalopathy that develops in patients with advanced cirrhosis of the liver. The unabsorbed sugar produces diarrhea and the acid pH helps to contain ammonia in the feces. Trade names are Cephulac and Chronulac.

lacuna (lă-kū'nă) [L., a pit] (pl. *lacunae*). [NA] A small pit, space, or cavity.

   l., absorption. Howship's lacunae, q.v.

   l., Howship's. A pit or groove in bone where resorption or dissolution of bone is occurring. Usually contains osteoclasts.

   l., intervillous. A space in the placenta occupied by maternal blood and into which fetal placenta villi project.

   l. laterales. Irregular diverticula on either side of the superior sagittal sinus of the brain into which the arachnoidal granulations project.

   l. magna. The largest pitlike recess in the fossa navicularis of the distal end of the male urethra.

   l. of the urethra. One of several recesses in the mucous membrane of the urethra, esp. along the floor and in the bulb. They compose the openings of the urethral glands.

   l. pharyngis. Pit at pharyngeal end of the eustachian tube.

   l., trophoblastic. Irregular cavities in the syntrophoblast that develop into intervillous spaces or lacunae. SYN: *l., blood.* SEE: *l., intervillous.*

l. vasorum. [NA] Space for passage of femoral vessels to the thigh.

lacunae (lă-kū′nē) [L.]. Pl. of lacuna.

lacunar (lă-kū′năr) [L. *lacuna*, pit]. Pert. to lacunae.

lacunula (lă-kū′nū-lă) [L., little pit]. Small or minute lacuna.

lacunule (lă-kū′nŭl) [L. *lacunula*]. Lacunula, q.v.

lacus (lā′kŭs) [L., lake]. Collection of fluid in small hollow or cavity.

l. lacrimalis. [NA] Space at the inner canthus of the eye where tears collect.

LAD. *left anterior descending* (branch of the left coronary artery).

Laënnec's cirrhosis (lā″ĕ-nĕks′) [René T. H. Laënnec, Fr. physician and the inventor of the stethoscope, 1781–1826]. Cirrhosis of the liver associated with chronic excessive alcohol ingestion. SYN: *hobnail liver.* SEE: *liver, cirrhosis of.*

Laënnec's pearls. Round gelatinous masses seen in asthmatic sputum.

Laënnec's thrombus. Globular thrombus in the heart.

Laetrile. Amygdalin; a glycoside derived from pits or other seed parts of plants, including apricots and almonds. Amygdalin contains sufficient cyanide to be fatal when taken in large doses. Laetrile, also known as vitamin B$_{17}$, has no known therapeutic or nutritional value. SYN: *amygdalin.*

There is no evidence that Laetrile is effective in treating cancer.

Caution: Those who administer Laetrile should be prepared to treat acute cyanide poisoning, q.v. Signs of chronic cyanide poisoning (weakness of arms and legs and disorders of the central nervous system) should also be kept in mind.

Lafora, Gonzalo R. (lă-fō′ră). Spanish physician, 1887–1971.

L.'s bodies. Cytoplasmic inclusion bodies that are made of acid mucopolysaccharides and are present in neuronal tissue of the brain in familial myoclonus epilepsy.

L.'s disease. Familial progressive epilepsy.

lag. 1. Period of time between application of stimulus and resulting reaction. 2. Early period following bacterial inoculation into culture medium. Growth is slow during this time. SYN: *lag phase; latent period.*

lageniform (lă-jĕn′ĭ-form) [L. *lagena*, flask, + *forma*, shape]. Flask-shaped.

lagophthalmos, lagophthalmus (lăg″ŏf-thăl′mōs, -mŭs) [Gr. *lagos*, hare, + *ophthalmos*, eye]. Incomplete closure of pal-

pebral fissure when an attempt is made to shut the eyelids. This results in exposure and injury to bulbar conjunctiva and cornea.

ETIOL: Contraction of a scar of the eyelid, facial nerve injury, atony of orbicularis palpebrarum, exophthalmos. Incomplete closure of the lids during sleep is seen in hysteria, in exhausted adults, and often in healthy children.

l., nocturnal. Failure of the eyelids to remain closed during sleep. This may be an etiologic factor in chronic keratitis.

lag phase. Latent period (def. 2), q.v.; lag (def. 2), q.v.

la grippe (lă grĭp′) [Fr.]. Influenza.

laity (lā′ĭ-tē) [Gr. *laos*, the people]. 1. The collective of individuals not in the clergy. 2. Individuals who are not members of a particular profession such as law, dentistry, medicine, or the ministry.

LAK cells. *Lymphokine-activated killer* cells, which are cytotoxic lymphoid cells activated by interleukin-2 (IL-2) that act against malignant tumor cells. The LAK cells can be produced outside the body and administered or produced inside the body by injection of IL-2. SEE: *interleukin-2.*

lake [L. *lacus*]. A small cavity of fluid. SEE: *lacus.*

l., venous. Small subcutaneous blebs filled with blood. May be present on the lips, mouth or ears.

laked. Said of the blood in hemolysis, q.v., or disintegration of the red blood corpuscles, freeing the hemoglobin into the blood plasma.

laking. Freeing of hemoglobin from red blood corpuscles.

LAL. *limulus amebocyte lysate.*

La Leche League. An organization whose purpose is to promote breast feeding. The address is Franklin Park, Illinois 60131, U.S.A.

laliatry (lăl-ī′ă-trē) [Gr. *lalia*, talk, + *iatria*, therapy]. Study and treatment of speech disorders and defects.

lallation (lă-lā′shŭn) [L. *lallatio*]. A babbling form of stammering. Infantile form of speech.

lalognosis (lăl-ŏg-nō′sĭs) [Gr. *lalia*, talk, + *gnosis*, understanding]. Science of understanding speech, particularly lallation, q.v.

lalopathology (lăl″ō-pă-thŏl′ō-jē) [″ + *pathos*, disease, + *logos*, word, reason]. The medical area concerned with speech pathology.

lalopathy (lă-lŏp′ă-thē) [″ + *pathos*, disease]. Any disorder of the speech.

lalophobia (lăl″ō-fō′bē-ă) [″ + *phobos*, fear]. Morbid reluctance to speak due to fear of stammering or committing errors.

laloplegia (lăl-ō-plē′jē-ă) [″ + *plege*, a

stroke]. A paralysis of speech muscles without affecting action of tongue.

lalorrhea (lăl″ō-rē′ă) [″ + *rhoia*, flow]. Abnormal flow of speech.

Lamarck's theory (lă-mărks′) [Jean Baptiste P. A. Lamarck, Fr. naturalist, 1744–1829]. Theory, popular in the 19th century, that evolutionary changes are the result of environmental changes, and that acquired characteristics are inherited and passed on to descendants. This theory has been rejected. SEE: *natural selection.*

Lamaze technique or method (lă-măz′) [Fernand Lamaze, Fr. obstetrician, 1890–1957]. A method of psychoprophylaxis for childbirth in which the mother is instructed in breathing techniques that permit her to facilitate delivery by relaxing at the proper time with respect to the involuntary contractions of abdominal and uterine musculature. Those who are able to use the method require little if any anesthesia during delivery. SEE: *labor.*

lambda (lăm′dă) [Gr.]. 1. Letter in Gr. alphabet (Λ, λ). Also signified by letter L or l. 2. Point or angle of junction of lambdoid and sagittal sutures.

lambdacism (lăm′dă-sĭzm) [Gr. *lambdakismos*]. 1. Stammering of "l" sound. 2. Inability to pronounce "l" sound properly. 3. Substitute of "l" for "r" in speaking.

lambdoid, lambdoidal (lăm′doyd, lăm-doyd′ăl) [Gr. *lambda*, + *eidos*, form, shape]. Shaped like Gr. letter Λ.

lambdoid suture. Suture between the occipital and two parietal bones.

lambert [Johann H. Lambert, Ger. physicist, 1728–1777]. A unit of brightness equal to that seen when a perfectly diffusing surface radiates or reflects one lumen of light per square centimeter. SEE: *lumen* (def. 2).

Lambert-Eaton myasthenia syndrome. SEE: *Eaton-Lambert syndrome.*

lame [AS. *lama*]. Disabled in one or more limbs, esp. in a leg or foot, so that ability for normal locomotion is impaired. Also applied to a weak or painful condition, such as a lame back.

lamella (lă-měl′ă) [L., a little plate] (pl. *lamellae*). 1. A thin plate or scale. 2. A medicated disk of gelatin inserted under lower eyelid and against the eyeball; used as a local application to eye.

l., bone. Thin layer of ground substance of osseous tissue.

l., circumferential. Layer of bone that underlies the periosteum.

l., concentric. Plate of bone surrounding a haversian canal.

l., enamel. Microscopic cracks or calcification imperfections in the enamel surface of a tooth. They may be shallow or extend into the underlying dentin and occur as a developmental defect or a microfracture due to temperature change or shearing forces.

l., ground. L., interstitial, q.v.

l., haversian. L., concentric, q.v.

l., interstitial. Bone lamella filling irregular spaces within the haversian system.

l., medullary. Osseous lamella surrounding and forming the wall of the medullary cavity of tubular bones.

l., periosteal. Bone lamella next to and parallel with the periosteum, forming the external portion of bone.

l., triangular. Small fibrous lamina between the choroid plexuses of the third ventricle of the brain.

l., vitreous. Innermost layer of the choroid next to the retina. SYN: *Bruch's membrane; lamina basalis of choroid.*

lamellar (lă-měl′ăr). 1. Arranged in thin plates or scales. 2. Pert. to lamella.

lameness. Limping, abnormal gait, or hobbling resulting from partial loss of function in a leg. May be due to maldevelopment, injury, or disease.

lamina (lăm′ĭ-nă) [L.] (pl. *laminae*). [NA] 1. A thin flat layer or membrane. 2. The flattened part of either side of the arch of a vertebra.

l., alar. Alar plate of the spinal cord in the human embryo; later becomes the sensory portion.

l., anterior elastic. Thin, tough membrane just below the corneal epithelium. SYN: *Bowman's membrane; l., Bowman's.*

l., basal. 1. Basal plate of spinal cord in the human embryo; later becomes the motor portion. 2. A mucopolysaccharide layer on the basal surface of epithelial cells which separates them functionally from the underlying connective tissue of the body.

l. basalis choroideae. The membrane covering the inner surface of the choroid. SYN: *Bruch's membrane.*

l. basilaris ductus cochlearis. The membranous portion of the spiral lamina of the cochlea of the inner ear.

l., Bowman's. Basement membrane beneath the epithelium of the cornea. SYN: *l, anterior elastic; Bowman's membrane.*

l. cartilaginis cricoideae. [NA] The posterior portion of the cricoid cartilage.

l. choriocapillaris. [NA] Middle layer of the choroid, containing close mesh of capillaries.

l. cribrosa. [NA] Cribriform plate of the ethmoid bone.

l. cribrosa sclerae. Portion of sclera forming a sievelike plate through which pass fibers of the optic nerve to the retina.

l., dental. A U-shaped downgrowth of oral epithelium in both the maxillary and mandibular regions that forms into enamel organs which produce the teeth. SEE: *enamel organ*.

l. dura. A radiographic term describing the compact bone (alveolar bone proper) that surrounds the roots of teeth; in a state of health, it appears on a radiograph as a dense radiopaque line.

l., epithelial. The epithelial layer covering the choroid plexus of the eye.

l. fusca sclerae. Layer of thin pigmented connective tissue on the inner surface of the sclera of the eye.

l., interpubic fibrocartilaginous. Part of the articulation of the pubic bones; it connects the opposing surfaces of these bones.

l., labial. A thickened band of epithelium that grows from the ectodermal covering of the primitive jaw. The ectodermal plate splits and separates lip from gum. SYN: *vestibular*.

l., medullary, internal. Layer of white substance that divides the gray substance of the thalamus into three parts: anterior, medial, and lateral.

l. multiformis. Polymorphic layer of the isocortex of the cerebral cortex.

l. of vertebral arch. Laminae extending from the pedicles of the vertebral arches and fusing together to form the dorsal portion of the arch. The spinous process extends from the center of these laminae.

l. papyracea. Thin, smooth plate of bone on the lateral surface of the ethmoid bone; it forms part of the orbital plate.

l., perpendicular. Thin sheet of bone forming the perpendicular plate of the ethmoid bone. Supports the upper portion of the nasal septum.

l. propria mucosae. Thin layer of fibrous connective tissue that lies immediately beneath the surface epithelium of mucous membranes. SYN: *tunica propria*.

l., pterygoid. Internal and external laminae make up the pterygoid process of the sphenoid bone and are areas of attachment for muscles of mastication.

l., rostral. Continuation of the rostrum of the corpus callosum and the lamina terminalis of the third ventricle.

l. suprachoroidea. [NA] The outermost layer of the choroid.

l., terminal. Thin sheet of tissue forming the anterior border of the third ventricle.

l., vestibular. SEE: *l., labial*.

l. vitrea. L. basalis of choroid.

l. zonalis. Outer or plexiform layer of the isocortex.

laminae (lăm′ĭ-nē). Pl. of lamina.

laminagram (lăm′ĭ-nă-grăm) [L. *lamina*, thin plate, + Gr. *gramma*, something written]. A roentgenogram taken of a section of the body so that the area being investigated appears as if only a slice through the tissue is depicted. SEE: *tomogram*.

laminagraph (lăm′ĭ-nă-grăf) [″ + Gr. *graphein*, to write]. An x-ray technique for producing a laminagram, q.v.

laminagraphy (lăm″ĭ-năg′ră-fē) [″ + Gr. *graphein*, to write]. Study of body tissues by use of laminagrams. SEE: *tomography*.

laminar air flow. Filtered air moving along separate parallel flow planes to surgical theaters, nurseries, bacteriology work areas, or food preparation areas. This method of air flow helps to prevent bacterial contamination and collection of hazardous chemical fumes in areas where they would pollute the work environment.

Laminaria digitata (lăm-ĭ-nār′ē-ă dĭj-ĭ-tä′tä). Genus of kelp or seaweed that when dried has the ability to absorb water and expand with considerable force. Has been used to dilate the uterine cervical canal in induced abortion.

laminarin (lăm″ĭ-nă′rĭn). A polysaccharide obtained from *Laminaria* species of seaweed. It consists principally of glucose residues.

laminated (lăm′ĭn-āt″ĕd) [L. *lamina*, thin plate]. Arranged in layers or laminae.

lamination (lăm″ĭn-ā′shŭn). 1. Layerlike arrangement. 2. In embryotomy, the slicing of the skull.

laminectomy (lăm″ĭ-nĕk′tō-mē) [″ + Gr. *ektome*, excision]. Excision of a vertebral posterior arch.

NURSING IMPLICATIONS: *In the immediate postoperative period:* Patient should be kept flat for 1 to 2 hours, after which change of position from side to side by log rolling every 2 hours is indicated. Ensure that proper assistance is available for proper support and safety during dangling, standing and ambulation as ordered in the early postoperative period. Ensure that patient has voided in first 8 to 12 hours and use nursing measures to promote voiding before resorting to catheterization. Observe dressing for bleeding or cerebrospinal fluid leakage. Administer ordered pain medications as needed by the patient. Apply antiembolic stockings if ordered.

Rehabilitation: Encourage gradual increase in level of activity. Instruct patient to reduce strain on back by avoiding lifting of heavy or moderately heavy objects for at least 8 weeks, by using nonstressful body movements and by good posture. Counsel against long periods of sitting. Encourage involvement in an exercise program after 6 weeks, beginning very gradually in order to strengthen abdominal muscles. Reinforce importance of follow-up visit to physician in

6 weeks' time. SEE: *Nursing Diagnoses* in *Appendix*.

laminitis (lăm-ĭn-ī'tĭs) [" + Gr. *itis*, inflammation]. Inflammation of a lamina.

laminotomy (lăm"ĭ-nŏt'ō-mē) [" + Gr. *tome*, incision]. Division of one of the vertebral laminae.

lamp [Gr. *lampein*, to shine]. Device for producing and applying light, heat, radiation, and various forms of radiant energy for the treatment of disease.

   l., Gullstrand's. L., slit, q.v.

   l., infrared. Heat lamp; a lamp that develops a high temperature, emitting infrared rays. Rays penetrate only a short distance (5 to 10 mm) into the skin. Principal effect is to cause heating of the skin.

   l., slit. Lamp constructed so that an intense light is emitted through a slit; used for examination of the eye.

   l., sun. Lamp that produces ultraviolet light.

   l., ultraviolet. L., sun, q.v.

lamprophonia (lăm"prō-fō'nē-ă) [Gr. *lampros*, clear, + *phone*, voice]. Marked distinctness or clearness of voice.

lamprophonic (lăm"prō-fŏn'ĭk). Possessing a clear voice.

lana (lăn'ă) [L.]. Wool.

lanatoside C (lăn-ăt'ō-sĭd). Glycoside of *Digitalis lanata;* an agent used for digitalization.

lance (lăns) [L. *lancea*]. 1. Two-edged surgical knife. 2. To incise with a lancet.

Lancefield classification (lăns'fēld) [Rebecca Craighill Lancefield, U.S. bacteriologist, 1895 - 1981]. A classification of hemolytic streptococci into various groups according to antigenic structure.

lancet (lăn'sĕt) [L. *lancea*, lance]. Pointed surgical knife with two edges.

lancinating (lăn'sĭ-nāt"ĭng) [L. *lancinare*, to tear]. Sharp or cutting, as pain.

L and A. Abbreviation for the reaction of the pupils of the eye to *light* and *accommodation.*

Landau reflex. Infantile reflex in which the body flexes when the head is passively flexed forward in a prone position. Appears at three months and is absent in children with cerebral palsy and gross motor retardation.

landmark. A recognizable skeletal or soft tissue structure used as a reference point in measurements or in describing the location of other anatomical structures. SEE: *cephalometry; craniometry.*

   l., bony. A structure or spot on a bone that serves as a reference for measurement.

   l., cephalometric. A bony point that serves in living persons or radiographs for measurements of the head or face or orientation of the head in certain positions.

   l., craniometric. A bony point or area on the skull used for measurements or orientation of the skull.

   l., orbital. A cephalometric point located at the lowest point of the orbital margin.

   l., radiographic. A cephalometric, craniometric, or soft tissue landmark used for orientation or measurements.

   l., soft tissue. An area or point on a soft tissue which serves as a point of reference for measurements of the body or its parts.

Landouzy-Déjérine dystrophy (lăn-dū-zē' dĕ"zhē-rēn') [Louis T. J. Landouzy, Fr. physician, 1845 - 1917; Joseph Jules Déjérine, Fr. neurologist, 1849 - 1917]. A slowly progressive dystrophy involving principally the musculature of the face and shoulders. SYN: *facioscapulohumeral dystrophy.*

   TREAT: Supportive; no specific therapy is known. Encourage patient to maintain as full and normal a life as possible and to avoid prolonged bed rest.

Landry-Guillain-Barré syndrome. Guillain-Barré syndrome, q.v.

Landsteiner's classification (lănd'stī-nĕrz) [Karl L. Landsteiner, Austrian-born U.S. biologist, 1868 - 1943; Nobel prize winner in medicine in 1930]. A classification of blood types designating O, A, B, and AB based on the presence of antigens on the erythrocytes.

Lane's kinks [Sir William Arbuthnot Lane, Brit. surgeon, 1856 - 1943]. Bending or twisting of the last few centimeters of the ileum with external adhesions between the folded loops of intestines. This may cause intestinal obstruction.

Langerhans' islands (läng'ĕr-hänz) [Paul Langerhans, Ger. pathologist, 1847 - 1888]. SEE: *islets of Langerhans.*

Langer's lines (läng'ĕrz) [Carl (Ritter von Edenberg) Langer, Austrian anatomist, 1819 - 1887]. The structural orientation of the fibrous tissue of the skin. They form the natural cleavage lines that, though present in all body areas, are visible only in certain sites such as the creases of the palm. These lines are of particular importance in surgery. Incisions made parallel to them make a much smaller scar upon healing than those made at right angles to the lines. SEE: illus.

Langer's muscle. Muscular fibers from insertion of pectoralis major muscle, over the bicipital groove to the insertion of the latissimus dorsi.

Lange's test (läng'ĕz) [Carl Lange, Ger. physician, b. 1883]. Diagnosis of cerebrospinal syphilis by degree of gold precipitation in varying concentrations of colloidal gold solution and spinal fluid.

Langhans' layer (läng'häns) [Theodor Langhans, Ger. pathologist, 1839 - 1915]. A

LANGER'S LINES

cellular layer present in chorionic villi of the placenta. SYN: *cytotrophoblast.*

language. A group of words written or spoken used in accordance with a system common to people of the same community or country and of the same cultural background. Use of language, spoken or written, permits a person to attempt to influence the behavior of another and to express the result of thought processes termed thinking.

languor (lăng′gĕr) [L. *languere,* to languish]. Feeling of weariness or exhaustion as from illness; lack of vigor or animation; lassitude.

laniary (lăn′ē-ā′rē) [L. *laniare,* to tear to pieces]. Adapted or designed for tearing, as are the canine teeth.

lanolin (lăn′ō-lĭn) [L. *lana,* wool]. USP. The purified, fatlike substance obtained from the wool of sheep. Used as an ointment base.
l., anhydrous. USP. Wool fat containing not more than 0.25% water. Used as an ointment base that has the ability to absorb water.

Lanoxin. Trade name for digoxin, USP.

lanthanum (lăn′thă-nŭm). SYMB: La. At. wt. 138.906; at. no. 57. A metallic element. One of a group of elements called lanthanides.

lanuginous (lă-nū′jĭn-ŭs). Covered with lanugo.

lanugo (lă-nū′gō) [L. *lana,* wool]. 1. Downy hair covering the body. 2. Fine downy hairs that cover the body of the fetus, esp. when premature.

LAO. *left anterior oblique* position.

laparectomy (lăp″ă-rĕk′tō-mē) [Gr. *lapara,* flank, + *ektome,* excision]. Excision of strips or gores in abdominal wall to relieve extreme weakness of abdominal muscles.

laparo- [Gr. *lapara,* flank]. Combining form pert. to the flank and to operations through the abdominal wall.

laparocele (lăp′ă-rō-sēl) [″ + *kele,* tumor, swelling]. An abdominal hernia.

laparocholecystotomy (lăp″ăr-ō-kōl″ē-sĭs-tŏt′ō-mē) [″ + *chole,* bile, + *kystis,* bladder, + *tome,* incision]. Incision into the gallbladder through the abdominal wall.

laparocolectomy (lăp″ă-rō-kō-lĕk′tō-mē) [″ + *kolon,* colon, + *ektome,* excision]. Colectomy.

laparocolostomy, laparocolotomy (lăp″ăr-ō-kō-lŏs′tō-mē, lăp″ăr-ō-kō-lŏt′ō-mē) [″ + ″ + *stoma,* mouth]. Formation of a permanent opening into the colon through the abdominal wall.

laparocystectomy (lă″pă-rō-sĭs-tĕk′tō-mē) [″ + *kystis,* bladder, + *ektome,* excision]. Removal of extrauterine fetus or a cyst through an abdominal incision. SYN: *laparocystotomy.*

laparocystidotomy (lăp″ăr-ō-sĭst-ĭ-dŏt′ō-mē) [″ + ″ + *tome,* incision]. Incision of bladder through the abdominal wall.

laparocystotomy (lăp″ăr-ō-sĭs-tŏt′ō-mē). Incision of abdomen to remove contents of a cyst or an extrauterine fetus. SYN: *laparocystectomy.*

laparoenterostomy (lăp″ăr-ō-ĕn″tĕr-ŏs′tō-mē) [″ + *enteron,* intestine, + *stoma,* mouth]. Formation of an artificial opening into the intestine through the abdominal wall.

laparoenterotomy (lăp″ăr-ō-ĕn″tĕr-ŏt′ō-mē) [″ + ″ + *tome,* incision]. Opening into the intestinal cavity by incision through the loins.

laparogastroscopy (lăp″ă-rō-găs-trŏs′kō-pē) [″ + *gaster,* belly, + *skopein,* to examine]. Inspection of the inside of the stomach after gastrotomy.

laparogastrostomy (lăp″ăr-ō-găs-trŏs′tō-mē) [″ + ″ + *stoma,* mouth]. Formation of a permanent gastric fistula through the abdominal wall. SYN: *celiogastrostomy.*

laparogastrotomy (lăp″ă-rō-găs-trŏt′ō-mē) [″ + ″ + *tome,* incision]. Abdominal incision into the stomach.

laparohepatotomy (lăp″ăr-ō-hĕp″ă-tŏt′ō-mē) [″ + *hepar,* liver, + *tome,* incision]. Incision of the liver through the abdominal wall.

laparohysterectomy (lăp″ăr-ō-hĭs″tĕr-ĕk′tō-mē) [″ + *hystera,* womb, + *ektome,* excision]. Removal of the uterus through an incision in the abdominal wall.

laparohystero-oophorectomy (lăp″ăr-ō-hĭs″tĕr-ō-ō″ō-for-ĕk′tō-mē) [″ + ″ + *oon,* ovum, + *phoros,* bearer, + *ektome,* excision]. Removal of uterus and ovaries through an abdominal incision.

laparohysteropexy (lăp″ăr-ō-hĭs′tĕr-ō-pĕks-ē) [″ + ″ + *pexis,* fixation]. Abdominal fixation of the uterus.

laparohysterosalpingo-oophorectomy (lăp″ăr-ō-hĭs″tĕr-ō-săl-pĭn″gō-ō″ō-fō-rĕk′tō-mē) [″ + *hystera,* womb, + *salpinx,* tube, + *oon,* ovum, + *phoros,* bearer, + *ektome,* excision]. Removal of uterus, fallopian tubes, and ovaries through abdominal incision.

laparohysterotomy (lăp″ăr-ō-hĭs″tĕr-ŏt′ō-mē) [″ + ″ + *tome,* incision]. Surgery of the uterus through an abdominal incision. SEE: *cesarean section.*

laparoileotomy (lăp″ăr-ō-ĭl-ē-ŏt′ō-mē) [″ + L. *ileum,* ileum, + Gr. *tome,* incision]. Abdominal incision into the ileum.

laparomyitis (lăp″ăr-ō-mī-ī′tĭs) [″ + *mys,* muscle, + *itis,* inflammation]. Inflammation of the muscular portion of the abdominal wall.

laparomyomectomy (lăp″ăr-ō-mī′ō-mĕk′tō-mē) [″ + ″ + *oma,* tumor, + *ek-*

tome, excision]. Abdominal excision of a muscular tumor.

laparonephrectomy (lăp″ăr-ō-nĕ-frĕk′tō-mē) [″ + *nephros*, kidney, + *ektome*, excision]. Renal excision through the loin.

laparorrhaphy (lăp-ă-ror′ă-fē) [″ + *rhaphe*, seam, ridge]. Suture of wound in the abdominal wall. SYN: *celiorrhaphy*.

laparosalpingectomy (lăp″ăr-ō-săl-pĭn-jek′tō-mē) [″ + *salpinx*, tube, + *ektome*, excision]. Excision of a fallopian tube through an abdominal incision.

laparosalpingo-oophorectomy (lăp″ăr-ō-săl-pĭn″gō-ō″ŏf-ō-rĕk′tō-mē) [″ + ″ + *oon*, ovum, + *phoros*, bearer, + *ektome*, excision]. Removal of fallopian tubes and ovaries through an abdominal incision.

laparosalpingotomy (lăp″ăr-ō-săl-pĭn-gŏt′ō-mē) [″ + ″ + *tome*, incision]. Incision of a fallopian tube through an abdominal incision. SYN: *celiosalpingotomy*.

laparoscope (lăp′ă-rō-skōp″) [″ + *sko-pein*, to examine]. An endoscope designed to permit visual examination of the peritoneal cavity.

laparoscopic cholecystectomy. SEE: *cholecystectomy, laparoscopic.*

laparoscopic laser cholecystectomy. Removal of gallbladder with laser technique. This procedure is not attempted for patient who has severe acute cholecystitis, a palpable gallbladder, or evidence of a stone in the common bile duct. Previously called endoscopic laser cholecystectomy.

laparoscopy (lăp-ăr-ŏs′kō-pē) [″ + *sko-pein*, to examine]. Abdominal exploration employing a type of endoscope called a laparoscope.

laparosplenectomy (lăp″ăr-ō-splēn-ĕk′tō-mē) [″ + *splen*, spleen, + *ektome*, excision]. Abdominal excision of the spleen.

laparosplenotomy (lăp″ăr-ō-splēn-ŏt′ō-mē) [″ + ″ + *tome*, incision]. Incision of the spleen through the abdominal wall.

laparotomy (lăp-ăr-ŏt′ō-mē) [″ + *tome*, incision]. The surgical opening of the abdomen; an abdominal operation.

PREOPERATIVE PREPARATION: Follow the physician's orders regarding diet, shaving of abdomen and pubic area, enemas, douches, and collecting of urine specimens.

NURSING IMPLICATIONS: *Preop:* As the patient may be fearful about the findings, allow time for discussion and expression of feelings. Perform and document preoperative teaching, using procedural and sensation messages. Prepare the patient physically in accordance with hospital or surgeon protocol. Apply thigh-high antiembolic dressings as prescribed.

Postop: Monitor vital signs, dressing status, and bowel sounds. Monitor fluid balance and provide prescribed fluid and electrolyte replacement therapy, initiating high-protein, high-vitamin C diet when GI activity is established. Provide analgesia for pain relief, or monitor patient-controlled analgesia, evaluating effectiveness. Assess ventilatory status and provide respiratory toilet (deep breathing, coughing, oral hygiene, and repositioning) as required by patient response. Encourage urinary output, assessing for bladder distention, and encourage leg mobilization and early ambulation to promote flatus and to prevent venous stasis. Initiate early discharge planning and follow through on any referrals and patient teaching.

laparotrachelotomy (lăp″ăr-ō-trā-kēl-ŏt′ō-mē) [″ + *trachelos*, neck, + *tome*, incision]. Cesarean section with the incision through the lower segment of the uterus.

laparotyphlotomy (lăp″ăr-ō-tī-flŏt′ō-mē) [″ + *typhlon*, cecum, + *tome*, incision]. Incision of cecum through lateral abdominal incision.

lap board. A wheelchair attachment serving as a tray or platform over the lap to support hands and arms or to permit manual activities.

lapinization (lăp″ĭn-ī-zā′shŭn) [Fr. *lapin*, rabbit]. In virology, serial passage of a virus through rabbits in order to modify the virus.

lapis (lă′pĭs) [L.]. Stone.

lard [L. *lardum*, fat]. Purified fat from the hog. The sole nutrient is fat; a 100-gm portion contains 902 Cal.

   l., benzoinated. Lard containing 1% benzoin. It is used as a vehicle for certain types of topically applied medicines.

lardaceous (lăr-dā′shŭs) [L. *lardum*, fat]. Resembling lard; waxy, fatty.

Largon. Trade name for propiomazine hydrochloride.

Larodopa. Trade name for levodopa, USP.

larva [L., mask] (pl. *larvae*). General term applied to the developing form of an insect after it has emerged from the egg and before it transforms into a pupa, from which it emerges as an adult.

   l. currens. A type of larva migrans. The organism, *Strongyloides stercoralis*, travels subcutaneously at the rate of about 10 cm an hour rather than at the slow rate of larva migrans.

   l. migrans, cutaneous. A skin lesion characterized by a tortuous elevated red line that progresses at one end while fading out at the other. It is caused by the subcutaneous migration of the larvae of certain nematodes, esp. *Ancylostoma braziliense* and *A. caninum*, that occur as accidental invaders of humans.

l. migrans, visceral. Infestation of viscera by larvae of animal nematodes such as *Toxocara canis.* These migrate and cause eosinophilia, hepatomegaly, fever and hyperglobulinemia. Occurs mostly in children who play in soil or sand contaminated with dog and cat feces. SEE: *toxocariasis.*

Caution: The ocular symptoms may lead to the erroneous clinical diagnosis of retinoblastoma. There is no specific therapy but cortisone may be useful in controlling hypersensitivity reaction.

---

larval (lär′văl) [L. *larva,* mask]. Concerning larva.

larvate [L. *larva,* mask]. Hidden, concealed. Term applied to an atypical or hidden symptom.

larvicide [″ + *caedere,* to kill]. An agent that destroys insect larvae.

larviphagic (lär″vĭ-fā′jĭk) [″ + Gr. *phagein,* to eat]. Consuming larva, as is done by certain fish.

laryngalgia (lăr-ĭn-găl′jē-ă) [Gr. *larynx,* larynx, + *algos,* pain]. Neuralgia of the larynx.

laryngeal (lăr-ĭn′jē-ăl) [Gr. *larynx,* larynx]. Pert. to the larynx.

laryngeal reflex. Cough as result of irritation of larynx or fauces.

laryngeal vertigo. Vertigo and fainting during a coughing spell in patients with chronic bronchitis. SYN: *tussive syncope.*

laryngectomee (lăr″ĭn-jĕk′tō-mē) [″ + *ektome,* excision]. An individual whose larynx has been removed.

laryngectomy (lăr″ĭn-jĕk′tō-mē) [″ + *ektome,* excision]. Excision of larynx.
NURSING IMPLICATIONS: *Preop:* Prepare patient for changes that will occur in voice and airway following surgery; to aid explanation, use diagrams and actual equipment patient will require. Prepare patient for postsurgical communication changes, and establish communication methods that are most appropriate for and agreeable to the particular patient (e.g., simple sign language, flash cards, magic slate). Explain postoperative setting and care to the patient, validating assessment measures, therapies and equipment. Explain what nutritional modalities (parenteral, enteral, tube feeding) may be used. Support the patient through anticipatory grieving, and refer as necessary for further psychologic or religious support.
Postop: Monitor vital signs, especially respiratory rate and effort, also level of consciousness, arterial blood gas values, and status of dressings and drains. Assess airway patency, care for and suction laryngos-

tomy tube as needed (prevent crust formation with increased humidity and fluid intake), and provide frequent oral care and assistance in managing saliva. Monitor fluid and electrolyte balance, and maintain prescribed replacement therapy. Be attentive to and predictive of patient needs, allowing time for communication and reassuring patient that verbal communication ability will be regained through surgically implanted assistive devices, speech therapy, or external mechanical aids. Support the patient through grief over real losses (usual voice, smell, nose-blowing, laughing and crying sounds, and sucking, plus activites such as swimming), and assist with problems related to body image changes and self-esteem. Assess for early complications such as respiratory distress related to edema, hemorrhage (check posterior aspect of neck as well as dressings and vital signs), and for later ones such as fistula formation, tracheal stenosis, and carotid artery rupture. Encourage patient and significant other to participate in local self-help groups and services (e.g., Lost Chord, Laryngectomee Club), and encourage rapid return to employment, with assistance of social service agencies if employment changes are required.

laryngemphraxis (lăr″ĭn-jĕm-frăk′sĭs) [″ + *emphraxis,* an obstruction]. Obstruction of the larynx.

laryngismal (lăr″ĭn-jĭs′măl) [″ + *-ismos,* condition]. Concerning or resembling affection with laryngeal spasm.

laryngismus (lăr″ĭn-jĭs′mŭs) [″ + *-ismos,* condition]. Spasm of the larynx.

laryngitic (lăr-ĭn-jĭt′ĭk) [Gr. *larynx,* larynx]. 1. Resulting from laryngitis. 2. Rel. to laryngitis.

laryngitis (lăr-ĭn-jī′tĭs) [″ + *itis,* inflammation]. Inflammation of larynx. SEE: *croup.* SEE: *Nursing Diagnoses* in Appendix.

l., acute catarrhal. Acute congestive laryngitis; catarrhal inflammation of laryngeal mucosa and the vocal cords.
SYM: Hoarseness and aphonia and occasionally pain on phonation and deglutition.
ETIOL: Improper use or overuse of voice; exposure to cold and wet; extension from infections in nose and throat; inhalation of irritating vapors and dust; associated with systemic diseases such as whooping cough or measles.
TREAT: Complete rest of voice; promotion of diaphoresis; liquid or soft diet; steam inhalations; codeine or non-narcotic cough suppressants for cough and pain. If due to a virus, there is no specific therapy; if bacterial, use appropriate antibiotics. If acute or

chronic bronchitis is present, treatment of that condition will help control laryngitis.

l., atrophic. Laryngitis leading to diminished secretion and atrophy of the mucous membrane.

SYM: Tickling sensation in throat, hoarseness, cough, dyspnea when crusts are thick and accumulate on vocal cords so as to narrow the breathing aperture.

TREAT: Inhalants and medicated sprays to loosen the crusts; strict attention to associated nose and throat pathology.

l., chronic. A type of laryngitis due to a recurrent irritation, or following the acute form. Often secondary to sinus or nasal pathology, improper use of voice, excessive smoking, drinking, or neoplasms.

SYM: Tickling in throat, huskiness of voice, dysphonia.

TREAT: Correction of preexisting nose and throat pathology, discontinuance of alcohol and tobacco, avoidance of excessive use of voice and proper vocal placement.

l., croupous. Laryngitis occurring mainly in infants and young children and characterized by a barky cough, hoarseness, and stridor.

l., diphtheritic. Invasion of larynx by diphtheria bacilli, usually with formation of membrane.

l., membranous. Laryngitis characterized by inflammation of larynx with the formation of a false membrane of nondiphtheritic origin.

l., syphilitic. A chronic form of laryngitis due to syphilis.

SYM: Hoarseness, cough, simple catarrh, formation of broad condylomata, follicular hyperplasia, syphiloma, syphilitic perichondritis.

Secondary stage in form of mucous patches or tertiary in form of gumma. Secondary syphilis is a diffuse infection, and one sees luetic patches spread over large areas of larynx. In tertiary syphilis, the gummatous lesion can occur in any part of larynx. There is marked redness over the infiltrated area as well as in the surrounding mucous membrane. When breakdown occurs, the resultant ulceration is deep with sharp edges. Pain is usually absent and fixation of the cord is late. Cicatrization and deformity follow healing of gumma.

TREAT: Appropriate antibiotic therapy for syphilis.

l., tuberculous. Laryngitis secondary to pulmonary tuberculosis.

SYM: Hoarseness, aphonia, pain in swallowing, cough. Lesion located in interarytenoid area, vocal cords, epiglottis, or false cords. Lesions are relatively pale; ulceration occurs early.

laryngo- [Gr. *larynx,* larynx]. Prefix pert. to the larynx.

laryngocele (lăr-ĭn″gō-sēl) [″ + *kele,* tumor, swelling]. A congenital air sac connected to the larynx. Its presence is normal in some animals but abnormal in man.

laryngocentesis (lăr-ĭn″gō-sĕn-tē′sĭs) [″ + *kentesis,* puncture]. Incision or puncture of the larynx.

laryngoedema. Swelling of the larynx. It is due to an allergic reaction. Requires immediate endotracheal intubation or tracheostomy.

laryngofissure (lăr-ĭng″gō-fĭsh′ūr) [″ + L. *fissura,* a cleft]. The operation of opening the larynx by a median line incision through the thyroid cartilage.

laryngogram (lă-rĭng′gō-grăm) [″ + *gramma,* something written]. Roentgenogram of the larynx.

laryngograph (lăr-ĭng′ō-grăf) [″ + *graphein,* to write]. Device for making a record of laryngeal movements.

laryngography (lăr″ĭn-gŏg′ră-fē). 1. Description of the larynx. 2. Roentgenography of the larynx after application of a radiopaque dye.

laryngologist (lăr″ĭn-gŏl′ō-jĭst) [″ + *logos,* word, reason]. Specialist in laryngology.

laryngology. The specialty of medicine concerned with the pharynx, throat, larynx, nasopharynx, and tracheobronchial tree.

laryngomalacia (lăr-ĭng″gō-mă-lā′shē-ă) [″ + *malakia,* softness]. Softening of the tissues of the larynx.

laryngometry (lăr″ĭn-gŏm′ĕ-trē) [″ + *metron,* measure]. Systematic measurement of the larynx.

laryngoparalysis (lăr-ĭn″gō-păr-ăl′ĭ-sĭs) [″ + *paralyein,* to disable at one side]. Paralysis of muscles of the larynx.

laryngopathy (lăr″ĭn-gŏp′ă-thē) [″ + *pathos,* disease]. Any disease of the larynx.

laryngopharyngeal (lăr-ĭn″gō-făr-ĭn′jē-ăl) [″ + *pharynx,* throat]. Rel. jointly to the larynx and pharynx.

laryngopharyngectomy (lăr-ĭn″gō-făr-ĭn-jĕk′tō-mē) [″ + ″ + *ektome,* excision]. Removal of the larynx and pharynx.

laryngopharyngeus (lă-rĭng″gō-fă-rĭn′jē-ŭs). The muscle that constricts the inferior pharynx.

laryngopharyngitis (lăr-ĭn″gō-făr-ĭn-jī′tĭs) [″ + ″ + *itis,* inflammation]. Inflammation of the larynx and pharynx. SYN: *pharyngolaryngitis.*

laryngopharyngography (lă-rĭng″gō-fă-rĭn-jŏg′ră-fē) [″ + ″ + *graphein,* to write]. Radiographic examination of the larynx and pharynx when filled with air.

laryngopharynx (lăr-ĭn″gō-făr′ĭnks) [Gr. *larynx,* larynx, + *pharynx,* throat]. Lower portion of the pharynx that extends from the cornua of the hyoid bone or vestibule of the larynx to the lower border of the cricoid cartilage.

laryngophony (lăr″ĭn-gŏf′ō-nē) [″ + *phone*, voice]. Voice sounds heard in auscultating the pharynx.

laryngophthisis (lăr″ĭng-gŏf′thĭ-sĭs) [″ + *phthisis*, a wasting]. Tuberculosis of the larynx.

laryngoplasty (lăr-ĭn′gō-plăs″tē) [″ + *plassein*, to form]. Plastic reparative surgery of the larynx.

laryngoplegia (lă-rĭng″gō-plē′jē-ă) [″ + *plege*, stroke]. Paralysis of laryngeal muscles.

laryngoptosis (lă-rĭng″gō-tō′sĭs) [″ + *ptosis*, a dropping]. Condition in which the larynx is positioned somewhat lower than usual at birth. It may also occur in old age.

laryngorhinology (lăr-ĭn″gō-rīn-ŏl′ō-jē) [″ + *rhis*, nose, + *logos*, word, reason]. The branch of medical science concerned with diseases of the larynx and nose.

laryngorrhagia (lăr″ĭn-gō-rā′jē-ă) [″ + *rhegnynai*, to flow forth]. Laryngeal hemorrhage.

laryngorrhea (lăr″ĭn-gō-rē′ă) [″ + *rhoia*, flow]. Excessive discharge of laryngeal mucus.

laryngoscleroma (lăr-ĭn″gō-sklĕ-rō′mă) [″ + *skleros*, hard, + *oma*, tumor]. Scleroma affecting the larynx.

laryngoscope (lăr-ĭn′gō-skōp) [″ + *skopein*, to examine]. Instrument for examining the larynx.

laryngoscopic (lăr″ĭn-gō-skŏp′ĭk) [″ + *skopein*, to examine]. Pert. to observation of the interior of the larynx with the aid of a small long-handled mirror. SEE: *laryngoscopy*.

laryngoscopist (lăr″ĭng-gŏs′kō-pĭst) [″ + *skopein*, to examine]. An individual trained in laryngoscopy.

laryngoscopy (lăr″ĭn-gŏs′kō-pē). Examination of the interior of the larynx.

NURSING IMPLICATIONS: Explain procedure to patient. Assist physician as necessary. Reassure patient during the procedure. After procedure, place the patient in semi-Fowler's position and check vital signs frequently. Omit oral intake until swallowing reflex returns, usually in 2 to 8 hours. Instruct patient to spit saliva into emesis basin and observe sputum for blood, reporting excessive bleeding. Apply an ice collar to help minimize edema. Immediately report subcutaneous crepitus around face or neck, as this may indicate tracheal perforation. Instruct the patient not to cough, clear throat, or smoke for at least 24 hours to prevent irritation.

l., direct. Laryngoscopy with laryngeal speculum or laryngoscope.

l., indirect. Laryngoscopy with a mirror.

laryngospasm (lăr-ĭn′gō-spăzm) [″ + *spasmos*, a convulsion]. Spasm of laryngeal muscles.

laryngostenosis (lăr-ĭng″gō-stĕ-nō′sĭs) [″ + *stenosis*, a narrowing]. Stricture of the larynx.

l., compression. Stricture of the larynx due to outside causes such as abscess, tumor, or goiter.

l., occlusion. Stricture of the larynx due to congenital bands or membranes, foreign bodies, tumors, cicatricial contraction following ulceration as in diphtheria and tertiary syphilis, penetrating wounds, or corrosive fluid.

SYM: Dyspnea, esp. on inspiration and exertion. Loud breathing that becomes a stridulous choking respiration; pulse weak and fast; face anxious and cyanotic.

TREAT: Depends on cause. Tracheotomy is often necessary.

laryngostomy (lăr-ĭn-gŏs′tō-mē) [″ + *stoma*, mouth]. Establishing a permanent opening through the neck into the larynx.

laryngostroboscope (lăr″ĭn-gō-strō′bō-skōp) [″ + *strobos*, whirl, + *skopein*, to view]. Instrument for inspection of vibration of vocal cords.

laryngotomy (lăr-ĭn-gŏt′ō-mē) [″ + *tome*, incision]. Incision of the larynx.

l., inferior. Surgical incision of the larynx through the cricoid cartilage.

l., median. Surgical incision of the larynx through the thyroid cartilage.

l., subhyoid or superior. Surgical incision of the larynx through the thyroid membrane.

laryngotracheal (lă-rĭng″gō-trā′kē-ăl) [″ + *tracheia*, trachea]. Concerning the larynx and trachea.

laryngotracheitis (lăr-ĭn″gō-trā-kē-ī′tĭs) [″ + ″ + *itis*, inflammation]. Inflamed condition of the larynx and trachea.

laryngotracheobronchitis (lă-rĭng″gō-trā″kē-ō-brŏng-kī′tĭs) [″ + ″ + *bronchos*, windpipe, + *itis*, inflammation]. Inflammation of the larynx, trachea, and bronchi.

laryngotracheotomy (lăr-ĭn″gō-trā-kē-ŏt′ō-mē) [″ + ″ + *tome*, incision]. Incision of the larynx with section of upper tracheal rings.

laryngoxerosis (lăr-ĭn″gō-zĕr-ō′sĭs) [″ + *xeros*, dry, + *osis*, condition]. Abnormal dryness of the larynx.

larynx (lăr′ĭnks) [Gr.] (pl. *larynges*). The enlarged upper end of the trachea below the root of the tongue; a musculocartilaginous structure lined with mucous membrane; the organ of voice. SEE: illus.

EPIGLOTTIS

HYOID BONE
THYROID CARTILAGE
CRICOID CARTILAGE
TRACHEA

ARYTENOID CARTILAGE

FRONT   LATERAL   POSTERIOR   INTERIOR

VOCAL FOLD

RIMA GLOTTIDIS

RIMA GLOTTIDIS ALMOST CLOSED   RIMA GLOTTIDIS OPEN

LARYNX

STRUCTURE: Consists of nine cartilages bound together by an elastic membrane and moved by muscles. Cartilages include three single (cricoid, thyroid, and epiglottic) and three paired (arytenoid, corniculate, and cuneiform). The extrinsic muscles include the omohyoid, sternohyoid, sternothyroid, and several others; intrinsic muscles include the cricothyroid, external and internal thyroarytenoid, transverse and oblique arytenoid, and external and internal thyroarytenoid. The cavity of the larynx contains two pairs of folds, the ventricular folds (false vocal cords) and vocal folds (true vocal cords), and is divided into three regions (vestibule, ventricle, and inferior entrance to the glottis). An opening between the true vocal folds forms a narrow slit, the rima glottidis or glottis.

NERVES: From interior and external branches of superior laryngeal.

BLOOD SUPPLY: Inferior thyroid, branch of thyroid axis and superior thyroid, branch of external carotid.

RS: cricoarytenoid; epiglottis; glottis; "laryng-" words; prominentia laryngea; vestibule; vocal cord.

l., foreign bodies in. SYM: Violent spasmodic cough and dyspnea; fixed pain at par-

ticular spot; loss of voice.

NURSING IMPLICATIONS: American Heart Association current recommendations for aspiration of foreign body include recognition of foreign body obstruction. If patient is able to speak or cough, do not interfere with patient's attempts to expel the object. If patient is unable to speak, cough, or breathe, apply Heimlich maneuver, squeezing abdomen 6 to 10 times rapidly in succession. Use inward and upward thrusts with fist made by wrapping arms around victim from behind, making fist with one hand and covering with other, and placing against abdomen, slightly above umbilicus and well below xiphoid process. Sudden expulsion of air should dislodge obstructing foreign body. If patient loses consciousness, lower carefully to floor, protecting head and neck, and continue efforts, applying abdominal thrusts 6 to 10 times from a position kneeling astride victim's thighs. Also initiate CPR for unconscious victim, as required based on assessment of airway, breathing and circulation. Following abdominal thrusts, open airway and attempt to remove visible obstruction. For an obese or pregnant victim or a child, administer chest thrusts applied to the middle of the sternum rather than abdominal thrusts. Back blows should be utilized on infant prior to chest thrusts. Emergency tracheotomy or cricothyrotomy may be required.

Lasan. Trade name for anthralin, USP.

lascivia (lă-siv′ē-ă) [L. *lascivire*, to be wanton]. Abnormal sexual desire. SEE: *nymphomania; satyriasis.*

Lasègue's sign (lă-sĕgz′) [Ernest C. Lasègue, Fr. physician, 1816–1883]. Pain and discomfort in the back when the fully extended leg of the supine patient is gently raised.

laser (lā′zĕr). Acronym for *l*ight *a*mplification by *s*timulated *e*mission of *r*adiation. A device that emits intense heat and power at close range. The instrument converts various frequencies of light into one small and extremely intense unified beam of one wavelength radiation. The laser can be focused on a very small target. Lasers have multiple treatment applications. In ophthalmology, they are used in treating glaucoma, retinal detachment, and diabetic retinopathy; in cardiology, lasers are used experimentally to vaporize arterial blockage; in dermatology, to remove port-wine nevus, tattoos, and warts; in gynecology, to remove vulval lesions, including genital warts; in gastroenterology, for control of bleeding in the gastrointestinal tract; in surgery and dentistry to remove tumors.

l., excimer. A type of laser used experimentally to remove corneal tissue. It is used in treating myopia and corneal scars.

laser angioplasty. Experimental technique for removing occlusions of arteries caused by atherosclerosis.

laser cane. An experimental cane that helps a blind person detect objects ahead of, above, and below his or her path.

Lasix. Trade name for furosemide, USP.

Lassa fever [Lassa, city in Africa]. A disease caused by arenavirus, first reported in Nigeria in 1969. A reservoir for the virus is a rat, *Mastomys natalensis,* indigenous to Africa.

SYM: Abrupt onset of high fever that is continuous or intermittent spiking with generalized myalgia, chest and abdominal pain, headache, sore throat, cough, dizziness with flushing of the face, conjunctival injection, and nausea, diarrhea, and vomiting. Hemorrhagic areas of the skin and mucous membranes may appear on the fourth day. Mortality in Africa varies from 16% to 45%.

TREAT: Ribavirin given in the first week of illness and continued for 10 days has been very effective in reducing the death rate. This medicine should also be given orally for 10 days prophylactically to those who have been percutaneously exposed to the virus.

Convalescent plasma that has been tested and found to be free of arenavirus and to contain neutralizing antibodies to the virus has been of benefit in treating the disease, but of less benefit than ribavirin. Patients are isolated in special isolation units that filter the air leaving the room and maintain negative pressure. All sputum, blood, excreta, and objects that the patient has contacted are disinfected. SEE: *Universal Precautions* in *Appendix.*

lassitude (lăs′ĭ-tūd) [L. *lassitudo*, weariness]. Weariness; exhaustion.

last sacraments. A religious rite performed by a clergyman to the individual just prior to death.

latah (lă′tă). A type of mental disorder that occurs in people of Southeast Asia, esp. in women. It is characterized by imitative behavior, coprolalia, echolalia, and automatic obedience. It may be provoked by startling, tickling, or frightening the patient. SEE: *Jumping Frenchmen of Maine; miryachit.*

latchkey children. Children who have a key to their home. This is needed when they return home at a time when there is no adult present to supervise them. These children are at a higher risk of accidents, abusing drugs, and smoking cigarettes.

latency (lā′tĕn-sē) [L. *latens*, lying hidden]. State of being concealed, hidden, inactive, or inapparent. SYN: *latent period.*

latency period. The time between the initiation of a stimulus, or contracting of a disease, and the response or clinical manifestation of the disease, respectively.

latent. 1. Lying hidden. 2. Quiet; not active.

latent content. In psychology, that part of a dream or unconscious mental content that cannot be brought into the objective consciousness through any effort of will to remember.

latent heat. Caloric or heat energy absorbed by matter changing from solid to liquid or liquid to vapor without a change in temperature.

latent image. Invisible image formed on the radiographic film because of exposure to x-rays, made visible by the development process.

latent period. 1. Time between a stimulus and its response. SYN: *lag phase.* 2. Time during which a disease is supposed to be existent without manifesting itself; period of incubation. 3. Time from exposure to ionizing radiation to the first visible sign of the effects.

laterad (lăt′ĕr-ăd) [L. *latus*, side, + *ad*, toward]. Toward a side or lateral aspect.

lateral (lăt′ĕr-ăl) [L. *lateralis*]. Pert. to the side.

lateralis (lăt″ĕr-ā′lĭs) [L.]. Indicating that the

laterality (lăt″ĕr-ăl′ĭ-tē). Condition of being on one side or toward the side. Term is used to specify which side of the body or brain is dominant.

l., crossed. Mixed dominance of certain body parts so that the left arm and right leg would be dominant.

l., dominant. Preferential dominance and use of the parts of one side of the body such as the eye, arm, leg, or hand.

lateral sinus. Transverse and sigmoid portion of two cranial venous sinuses. Extends from occipital protuberance to jugular bulb.

latericeous, lateritious (lăt″ĕr-ĭsh′ŭs) [L. *later*, brick]. Resembling brick dust.

lateroabdominal (lăt″ĕr-ō-ăb-dŏm′ĭ-năl) [L. *lateralis*, pert. to side, + *abdomen*, belly]. Concerning the side of the body and the abdominal area.

laterodeviation (lăt″ĕr-ō-dē″vē-ā′shŭn) [″ + *deviare*, to turn aside]. Deviation or displacement to one side.

lateroduction (lăt″ĕr-ō-dŭk′shŭn) [″ + *ducere*, to lead]. Movement to one side, esp. of the eye.

lateroflexion (lăt″ĕr-ō-flĕk′shŭn) [″ + *flexis*, bending]. Bending or curvature toward one side.

laterognathism. Asymmetry of the mandible due to retarded growth, fractures, tumors, or soft tissue atrophy or hypertrophy.

lateroposition (lăt″ĕr-ō-pō-zĭsh′ŭn) [″ + *positio*, position]. Displacement to one side.

lateropulsion (lăt″ĕr-ō-pŭl′shŭn) [L. *lateralis*, pert. to side, + *pulsus*, driving]. Involuntary tendency in cerebellar and labyrinthine disease to fall to one side.

laterosemiprone position (lăt″ĕr-ō-sĕm″ē-prōn′). Position in which patient is on left side leaning forward on chest, with right knee and thigh drawn up, and left arm along back. SYN: *Sims' position.*

laterotorsion (lăt″ĕr-ō-tor′shŭn) [″ + *torsio*, a twisting]. Twisting to one side.

lateroversion (lăt″ĕr-ō-vĕr′shŭn) [″ + *versio*, a turning]. Tendency or a turning toward one side.

latex (lā′tĕks) [L., fluid]. The fluid or sap produced by some plants. Natural rubber is produced from the latex of certain tropical trees.

lathyrism (lăth′ĭ-rĭzm) [Gr. *lathyros*, vetch]. Disease presumably caused by eating certain plants of the genus *Lathyrus*. Characterized by muscular weakness and paraplegia that are irreversible.

lathyrogen (lăth′ĭ-rō-jĕn) [″ + *gennan*, to produce]. Something that produces lathyrism.

Latino. Person residing in the U.S. whose nationality group, or the country in which the person or person's parents or ancestors were born, is a Latin American country in the Western Hemisphere. SEE: *Hispanic.*

latissimus (lă-tĭs′ĭ-mŭs) [L., widest]. Denoting a broad anatomical structure such as a muscle.

latitude. In radiology, a range of exposure that would produce a technically correct radiograph.

latrine (lă-trēn′) [L. *latrina*]. A toilet, particularly one in a military camp.

l., pit. Type of latrine installed outdoors and used where it is impractical to provide a standard, flushing-type toilet. The structure may be manufactured and installed so that odors and flies are not problematical.

latrodectism (lăt″rō-dĕk′tĭzm) [*Latrodectus* + Gr. *-ismos*, condition]. The toxic reaction to the bite of spiders of the genus *Latrodectus*. SEE: *spider, black widow.*

Latrodectus (lăt″rō-dĕk′tŭs) [L. *latro*, robber, + Gr. *daknein*, biting]. A genus of small black spiders belonging to the family Theridiidae.

L. mactans. The black widow or hourglass spider, a species widely distributed in the United States. The bite of the female produces serious symptoms and may result in death. SEE: *spider, black widow.*

LATS. *long-acting thyroid stimulator.*

lattice (lăt′ĭs). 1. A network or framework formed by structures intertwined usually at right angles with each other. 2. In physics, the arrangement of atoms in a crystal.

latus (lā′tŭs) [L., broad] (pl. *latera*). [NA] The side; the flank.

latus, lata, latum (lā′tŭs, lā′tă, lăt′ŭm) [L., broad]. Broad, as the uterine broad ligament.

laudable [L. *laudabilis*, praiseworthy]. Commendable; healthy; normal; formerly said erroneously of pus.

laudanum (lăw′dăn-ŭm). Tincture of opium. SEE: *morphine.*

laugh (lăf) [ME. *laughen*, to laugh]. 1. Sound produced by laughing. SYN: *risus.* 2. To express emotion, usually happiness or mirth, by a series of inarticulate sounds. Typically the mouth is open and a wide smile is present.

l., sardonic. Spasm of facial muscles producing a grinning effect that is inappropriate to the situation. SYN: *risus sardonicus.*

laughing gas (lăf′ĭng). Nitrous oxide gas.

laughter. The role of humor and laughter in promoting a positive attitude and health and in preventing the progress of some diseases has been documented. This does not mean that laughter and a positive attitude can substitute for proven medical therapy.

laughter, compulsive. Laughter without cause, occurring in certain psychoses, esp. schizophrenia.

laughter reflex (lăf'tĕr). Uncontrollable laughter resulting from tickling or pretense of tickling.

Laurence-Moon-Biedl syndrome (law'rĕns-moon'bē'dĕl) [John Zachariah Laurence, Brit. ophthalmologist, 1829–1870; Robert C. Moon, U.S. ophthalmologist, 1844–1914; Arthur Biedl, Prague endocrinologist, 1869–1933]. The combination of girdle-type obesity, sexual underdevelopment, mental retardation, retinal degeneration, polydactyly, and deformity of the skull. The condition is inherited as an autosomal recessive trait.

lavage (lă-văzh') [Fr., from L. *lavare*, to wash]. Washing out of a cavity. SYN: *irrigation*.

l., gastric. Washing out of the stomach. A stomach tube or catheter is used. Solutions such as sterile water, normal saline, 1% to 5% sodium bicarbonate, or activated charcoal may be used. The latter is particularly helpful in certain types of poisoning in which intubation will not damage the esophagus or stomach.

Quantity of solution: Not more than 10 oz at a time, repeated until fluid runs clear.

Temperature and time: 105°F (40.6°C). Preferably before breakfast.

Position: Semirecumbent or low enough to prevent inhalation of returning fluid. In poisoning, save siphoned fluid for examination. If patient is unconscious, use a mouth gag.

Purpose: To remove and dilute irritants or poisons; to cleanse the stomach preoperatively or postoperatively. SEE: *colonic irrigation; irrigation, bladder.*

law [AS. *laga*, law]. 1. Scientifically, a statement that is found to hold true uniformly for a whole class of natural occurrences. 2. A body of rules, regulations, and legal opinions of conduct and action that are made by controlling authority and are legally binding.

l., all-or-none. The weakest stimulus capable of producing a response produces the maximum response contraction in cardiac and skeletal muscles and nerves.

l., Avogadro's. If temperature and external pressure are the same, all gases contain the same number of molecules in equal volumes.

l., Bell's. Anterior spinal nerve roots are motor, and posterior spinal nerve roots are sensory. SYN: *l. of Magendie.*

l., biogenetic. Ontogeny recapitulates phylogeny, i.e., an individual in its development recapitulates stages in its evolutionary development. SYN: *l., Haeckel's.*

l., Boyle's. The volume occupied by a fixed quantity of every gas is inversely proportional, and density directly proportional, to pressure applied to the gas. SYN: *l., Mariotte's.*

l., Charles'. When pressure is constant, volume of a gas varies as the absolute temperature.

l., Courvoisier's. When the common bile duct is obstructed by a calculus, dilatation of the gallbladder is rare; when otherwise obstructed, dilatation is common.

l., Fechner's. The intensity of sensation is proportional to the logarithm of the strength of the stimulus.

l., Gay-Lussac's. L., Charles', q.v.

l., Graham's. The rate at which a gas diffuses through a porous membrane is inversely proportional to the square root of the density of the gas.

l., Haeckel's. L., biogenetic.

l., Hilton's. A nerve trunk supplying any joint supplies the muscles that move the joint and skin over insertion of such muscles.

l., Hooke's. The stress used to stretch or compress a body is proportional to the strain as long as the elastic limits of the body have not been exceeded.

l., Koch's. To prove an organism to be the cause of a given disease or lesion: the microorganism in question is regularly found in the lesions of the disease; pure cultures can be obtained from it; pure cultures when introduced into susceptible animals reproduce the disease or pathological condition; the organism can be obtained again in pure culture from the inoculated animal. SYN: *Koch's postulates.*

l., Marey's. Heart rate varies inversely with arterial blood pressure; that is, a rise or fall in arterial blood pressure brings about, respectively, a slowing or speeding up of heart rate.

l., Mariotte's. L., Boyle's.

l.'s, Mendel's. A number of principles of heredity established by Mendel (1822–1884) that laid the foundation for the modern science of genetics. Includes the principles of unit characters, dominance, segregation, and independent assortment. SEE: *Mendel's laws.*

l., Murphy's. If something can go wrong, it will.

l., Nysten's. Rigor mortis travels progressively from muscles of mastication, through the face, neck, trunk, and arms, reaching the legs and feet last.

l. of definite proportions. Two or more elements when united to form a new substance do so in a constant and fixed proportion by weight.

l. of the heart. Other things being equal, the stroke volume of the heart varies as the extent of diastolic filling or the energy of contraction is a function of the initial length of the muscle fibers.

l. of the intestine. Moderate distention of the intestine at a point causes relaxation below (aborally to the point) and contraction above.

l. of Magendie. L., Bell's.

l. of mass action. In chemical reactions, the amount of change taking place is proportional to the action mass of the reacting substance.

l. of multiple proportions. When two substances unite to form a series of chemical compounds, the proportions in which they unite are simple multiples of one another or of one common proportion.

l. of reciprocal proportions. In chemistry, the proportions in which two elementary bodies unite with a third one are simple multiples or simple fractions of the proportions in which these two bodies unite with each other.

l. of specificity of nervous energy. Law that states that excitation of a receptor always gives rise to the same sensation regardless of the nature of the stimulus.

l., periodic. The physical and chemical properties of chemical elements are periodic functions of their atomic weight. A natural classification of elements is made according to their atomic weight. When arranged in order of their atomic weight or atomic number, elements show regular variations in most of their physical and chemical properties.

l.'s, Rubner's. 1. Law of constant energy consumption: Rapidity of growth is proportional to intensity of the metabolic process. 2. Law of constant growth quotient: The same proportional part, or growth quotient, of total energy is utilized for growth.

l., Sutton's. SEE: *Sutton's law.*

l., Waller's, of degeneration. If a spinal nerve is completely divided, the distal portion undergoes fatty degeneration.

l., Weber's. The increase in stimulus necessary to produce the smallest perceptible increase in sensation bears a constant ratio to the strength of the stimulus already acting.

l., Wolff's. Changes in form and function of bones result in definite changes in their internal structure.

lawrencium (lă-rĕn′sē-ŭm) [Ernest O. Lawrence, U.S. physicist, 1901–1958]. SYMB: Lr. At. wt. of most stable isotopes is 260; at no. 103. A synthetic transuranic chemical element.

lax (lăks) [L. *laxus,* slack]. 1. Without tension. 2. Loose and not easily controlled. Said of bowel movements.

laxative (lăk′să-tĭv) [L. *laxare,* to loosen]. A food or chemical substance that acts to loosen the bowels (i.e., facilitate passage of bowel contents at time of defecation), and, therefore, to prevent or treat constipation. Laxatives may act by increasing peristalsis by irritating the intestinal mucosa, lubricating the intestinal walls, softening the bowel contents by increasing the amount of water in the intestines, and increasing the bulk of the bowel contents. Many individuals feel that it is essential to have one or more bowel movements a day, and if they do not, they may develop the habit of taking some form of laxative daily. They should be instructed that missing a bowel movement is not harmful and bowel movements do not necessarily occur at regular intervals. SYN: *aperient; cathartic; purgative.* SEE: *constipation; enema.*

Caution: A sudden change in bowel habits may be the first sign of a malignancy of the intestinal tract. When this happens, the individual should consult a physician without delay.

---

laxative regimen. The diet may be modified to avoid chronic constipation by maintaining adequate volume of food; eating high-bulk foods that contain high fiber content; eating foods that tend to stimulate bowel activity such as stewed fruits and vegetables; maintaining adequate fluid intake; and participating in regular exercise. In addition, foods that the individual has found to cause constipation should be avoided. Some persons are esp. liable to be constipated by certain cheeses.

laxator (lăk-să′tor) [L. *laxare,* to loosen]. That which has a relaxing effect.

l. tympani. One of two muscles or ligaments of the malleus of the inner ear.

layer (lā′ĕr) [ME. *leyer*]. A stratum; a thin sheetlike structure of more or less uniform thickness.

l., ameloblastic. Enamel layer of the tooth.

l., bacillary. Rod and cone layer of the retina of the eye.

l., basal. Outermost layer of the uterine endometrium lying next to the myometrium.

l., blastodermic. L., germ, q.v.

l., choriocapillary. Lamina choriocapillaris.

l., claustral. Layer of gray matter between the external capsule and insula.

l., clear. Stratum lucidum of the skin.

l., columnar. 1. A layer of tall, narrow

cells forming a covering or lining. 2. The rod and cone layer of the retina of the eye.

l., compact. The compact surface layer of the uterine endometrium.

l., cuticular, of epithelium. A striated layer secreted by and covering the free surface of an epithelial sheet, esp. that on the surface of columnar epithelium of the intestine.

l., enamel. L., ameloblastic, q.v.

l., ependymal. Inner layer of cells of the embryonic neural tube.

l., ganglionic. 1. Fifth layer of cerebral cortex. 2. Inner layer of ganglion cells in the retina whose axons form the fibers of the optic nerve.

l., germ. One of the three primary layers of the developing embryo from which the various organ systems develop. SEE: *ectoderm; endoderm; mesoderm.*

l., germinative. Innermost layer of the epidermis, consisting of a basal layer of cells and a layer of prickle cells (stratum spinosum). SYN: *malpighian layer; stratum germinativum.*

l., granular exterior. Second layer of cerebellar cortex, lying within the molecular layer and separated from it by a single row of Purkinje cells. Consists principally of granule cells.

l., granular interior. Fourth layer of the cerebral cortex, consisting principally of closely packed stellate cells.

l., half-value. In radiology, the thickness of an absorber that will reduce by one half the intensity of a beam of radiation.

l., Henle's. Layer of clear cells forming the outermost layer of the inner epithelial root sheath of a hair.

l., horny. Outermost layer of the skin, consisting of clear, dead, scalelike cells, those of the surface layer being constantly desquamated. SYN: *stratum corneum.*

l., Huxley's. Middle layer of the inner epithelial root sheath of a hair.

l., Langhans'. Cytotrophoblast of a chorionic villus of the placenta.

l., malpighian. L., germinative.

l., mantle. Middle layer of the neural tube of the developing embryo.

l., molecular. 1. Outermost layer of the cerebral or cerebellar cortex. 2. Inner or outer plexiform layer of the retina.

l., nervous. The nerve-containing portion of the retina of the eye.

l., odontoblastic. Layer of connective tissue cells at the outer edge of the pulp where they produce the dentin of the tooth.

l. of pyramidal cells. The exterior pyramidal layer; the third layer of the cerebral cortex.

l. of rods and cones. Layer of the retina

of the eye next to the pigment layer. It contains the rods and cones.

l., osteogenic; l., Ollier's. Innermost or bone-forming layer of the periosteum.

l., outer nuclear. Layer of the retina containing the nuclei of the visual cells (rods and cones).

l., papillary. Superficial layer of the corium lying immediately under the epidermis into which it extends, forming dermal papillae.

l., pigment. Outermost layer of the retina. Cells contain a pigment called fuscin.

l., prickle cell. Stratum spinosum epidermidis; the layer between the granular and basal layers of the skin. Prickle cells are present in this layer.

l., Purkinje. A single row of large flask-shaped cells (Purkinje cells, q.v.) lying between molecular and granular layers of the cerebellar cortex.

l., reticular. Inner layer of the corium lying beneath the papillary layer.

l., somatic. In the embryo, a layer of extra-embryonic mesoderm that forms a part of the somatopleure, the outer wall of the coelom.

l., spinous. L., prickle cell, q.v.

l., splanchnic. Layer of extra-embryonic mesoderm that with the endoderm forms the splanchnopleure.

l., spongy. Middle layer of the uterine endometrium. Contains dilated portions of uterine glands. SYN: *stratum spongiosum.*

l., subendocardial. Layer of loose connective tissue immediately under the endocardium that binds it to the myocardium. Contains fibers of the conducting system of the heart.

l., subendothelial. Layer of fine fibers and fibroblasts lying immediately under the endothelium of the tunica intima of larger arteries and veins.

l., Tomes' granular. Layer of interglobular dentin beneath the dentinocemental junction in the root of a tooth.

l., Weil's basal. A relatively cell-free zone just below the odontoblastic layer in the dental pulp. Also called subodontoblastic layer; cell-free zone of Weil; cell-poor zone.

l., zonal, of hypothalamus. Layer of myelinated fibers covering the thalamus of the brain.

lazaretto (lăz″ă-rĕt′ō) [It. *lazzaro*, a leper]. 1. A quarantine station. 2. Hospital for treatment of contagious diseases.

lb. *pound.*

LBBB. *left bundle branch block.*

LD. *lethal dose.*

LD$_{50}$. *median lethal dose* of a substance, which will kill 50% of the animals receiving that dose. Dose is usually calculated on amount of material given per gram or kilogram of body weight or amount per unit of body surface area.

LDH. *lactic dehydrogenase.*

LDL. *low-density lipoprotein.*

L-dopa. L-3,4-dihydroxyphenylalanine. A drug used in the treatment of Parkinson's disease. SYN: *levodopa.*

L.E. *lupus erythematosus.*

leachate. Water that has passed through a material and in doing so becomes contaminated with substances dissolved in the water. These substances are the leachates, a term used esp. in describing water that has passed through waste disposal sites.

leaching (lēch′ĭng) [AS. *leccan,* to wet]. Extraction of a substance from a mixture by washing the mixture with a solvent in which only the desired substance is soluble. SYN: *lixiviation.*

lead (lēd) [AS. *laedan,* to guide]. A conductor attached to an electrocardiograph. The three common leads are lead I, right arm to left arm; lead II, right arm to left leg; lead III, left arm to left leg. These are known as standard leads, bipolar limb leads, or indirect leads. SEE: *electrocardiogram* for illus.

   l., bipolar. In electrocardiography, any lead that consists of an electrode at one site and another at a different body site. A standard limb lead, I, II, or III, is a bipolar lead.

   l., esophageal. One lead is placed in the esophagus.

   l., limb. Any lead, unipolar or bipolar, in which a limb is the location of one of the electrodes.

   l., precordial. Record taken when one electrode is placed over the precordium, the other over an indifferent region.

   l., unipolar. Record made when one electrode is placed on chest wall overlying the heart, where potential changes are of considerable magnitude, and the other (distant or indifferent electrode) is placed where potential changes are of small magnitude.

lead (lĕd) [L. *plumbum*]. SYMB: Pb. At. wt. 207.2; at. no. 82; sp. gr. 11.35. A metallic element. Its compounds are poisonous. Accumulation and toxicity occur if more than 0.5 mg per day is absorbed. Any level of lead in the blood is abnormal.

   Most cases of lead poisoning occur in children who live in homes where lead was used in the paint. Children eat the paint and thus develop signs of lead toxicity. SEE: *lead encephalopathy, acute; lead poisoning, acute; lead poisoning, chronic; pica.*

   l. acetate. A lead compound that is used in solution as an astringent.

   l. monoxide. A reddish-brown compound used to prepare lead subacetate.

lead apron. An apron that contains lead but is sufficiently pliable to allow it to be worn as protection from ionizing radiation. Used by fluoroscopists, radiologic technologists, and dental technicians as well as patients to protect the gonads during x-ray studies of other parts of the body.

lead colic. Colic due to lead poisoning.

lead encephalopathy, acute. A syndrome seen mostly in children that follows rapid absorption of a large amount of lead. Initially there is clumsiness, vertigo, ataxia, falling, headache, insomnia, restlessness, and irritability. With progression of the syndrome, there will be forceful vomiting, excitement, confusion, convulsions, and coma. There is also a sudden and marked increase in intracranial pressure. In the past, the mortality rate was as high as 25%, and about half of the survivors show evidence of permanent damage to the central nervous system, including mental retardation, EEG abnormalities, cerebral palsy, and optic atrophy.

   TREAT: Discontinue exposure to lead. Corticosteroids and intravenous mannitol, 20% solution, will relieve increased intracranial pressure. Lead can be removed from the body by giving dimercaprol (BAL) and calcium disodium edetate, USP, in a carefully administered dose schedule. Control convulsions with phenobarbital, hydantoin, or diazepam. Maintain hydration with I.V. administration of fluids, but avoid sodium-containing materials. Do not give oral fluids or food for at least 3 days.

lead line. Bluish line on gums in lead poisoning.

lead pipe contraction. Cataleptic condition during which limbs remain in any position in which placed.

lead poisoning, acute. Ingestion or inhalation of a large amount of lead causes abdominal pain, metallic taste in mouth, anorexia, vomiting, diarrhea, headache, stupor, convulsions, and coma. SEE: *Nursing Diagnoses* in *Appendix.*

   TREAT: Establish adequate urine flow; control convulsions with diazepam. Calcium disodium edetate and dimercaprol are administered to promote removal of lead from the body. After acute therapy is completed, penicillamine is given orally for three to six months for children and up to two months for adults. Reduce or eliminate exposure to lead.

Caution: Patients receiving penicillamine therapy must be monitored weekly for adverse reactions including diffuse erythematous rashes, angioneurotic edema, proteinuria, and neutropenia. Penicillamine is contraindicated in patients with a history of penicillin sensitivity, or renal disease, or both.

lead poisoning, chronic. Chronic ingestion or inhalation of lead causes damage to the central and peripheral nervous systems, the blood-forming organs, and the gastrointestinal tract. Early symptoms include loss of appetite, weight loss, anemia, vomiting, fatigue, weakness, headache, lead line on gums, apathy or irritability, and a metallic taste in mouth. Later symptoms of paralysis, sensory loss, incoordination and vague pains develop.

LABORATORY DIAGNOSIS: Anemia; blood lead level above 5 μg/dl; free erythrocyte protoporphyrin (FEP) elevated; increased excretion of lead in urine; characteristic x-ray changes in the ends of growing bones.

TREAT: Eliminate exposure to lead. Provide adequate diet with added vitamins. If hematologic disorders are present, give penicillamine as if poisoning were acute.

NURSING IMPLICATIONS: Identify causative factors and remove. Administer antiemetic as prescribed for nausea and vomiting, hemopoietic for anemia, antispasmodic for abdominal cramps, and analgesic and muscle relaxant for muscle and joint pain. Administer ordered chelating agent(s) to eliminate lead from the body, rotating sites of painful injections and providing physical and emotional comfort measures to relieve distress from injections. Maintain hydration, and assess for signs of toxicity from chelating agents. Educate and support parents to prevent recurrence, and educate the public about the dangers of lead ingestion and the signs and symptoms indicating toxicity and the need for treatment.

Provide tissues and disposal containers for salivation. Establish an active or passive range of motion exercise schedule to prevent muscle atrophy. SEE: *Nursing Diagnoses* in *Appendix.*

leads (lēdz). Insulated wires connecting a monitoring device to a patient.

leaf (lēf) [AS.]. A plant organ usually shooting out from the side of a stem or branch; somewhat flattened and oval in shape, and green in color. SEE: *belladonna; digitalis; hyoscyamus.*

lean (lēn) [AS. *hlaene*, without flesh]. Without flesh, emaciated.

lean body mass. The weight of the body minus the fat content.

learned helplessness. A passive, rather fatalistic behavior based on the feeling that one is helpless. Lack of control in the elderly experiencing chronic illness and environmental and familial losses lead to a sense of passivity and acceptance.

learning. A change in behavior or skill level that follows gaining experience and practice.

l., latent. Learning that is inapparent to the individual at the time it occurs but later becomes evident when the learning is facilitated beyond what would be expected in the area of the original learning.

l., programmed. A system of education in which information is presented in small increments and one does not progress to the next step until a correct answer is provided. This may be done by use of a machine or it may be self-administered by use of a workbook. SEE: *Skinner box.*

learning curve. SEE: *curve, learning.*

learning disability. Inability or defect in ability to learn. Occurs in children and is manifested by difficulty in learning basic skills such as writing, reading, and mathematics.

learning theory. An approach to understanding how learning comes about by applying certain laws of learning; learning represents a change in behavior that has come about due to practice, education, and experience.

Leber's disease (lā'bĕrz) [Theodor Leber, Ger. ophthalmologist, 1840–1917]. Hereditary form of atrophy of the optic nerve that usually affects young males.

Leber's plexus. Plexus of venules in the eye between Schlemm's canal and Fontana's spaces.

Leboyer method (lĕ-boy-yā') [Frederick Leboyer, Fr. obstetrician, b. 1918]. A procedure for childbirth that emphasizes the provision of a gentle and peaceful environment for the birth process. Basic to this is the physical contact between the mother and the child immediately after delivery. Caressing and massaging the infant begins immediately and is continued daily for several months. The method is believed to facilitate mental and physical development of the child.

Lecat's gulf (lā-käz') [Claude Nicholas Lecat, Fr. surgeon, 1700–1768]. The hollow of the bulbous portion of the urethra.

L.E. cell. Abbrev. for *lupus erythematosus,* q.v., cell. A mature neutrophilic polymorphonuclear leukocyte containing the phagocytosed nucleus of another cell. It is characteristic of lupus erythematosus.

This distinctive cell may form when the blood of patients with systemic lupus erythematosus is incubated and further processed according to a specified method. The plasma of some patients contains an antibody to the nucleoprotein of leukocyte nuclei. These altered nuclei, which are swollen, pink, and homogenous, are ingested by phagocytes. These are the L.E. cells. The ingested material, when stained properly, is lavender in color and displaces the nucleus of the phagocyte to the edge of the cell wall. The L.E. cell phenomenon can be demonstrated in most patients with systemic lupus erythematosus, but it is not essential for the diagnosis. SEE: *lupus erythematosus, systemic.*

lechery (lĕtch′ĕr-ē) [Fr. *lecher*, to lick]. Lewdness; sensualism.

lecithal (lĕs′ĭ-thăl) [Gr. *lekithos*, egg yolk]. Concerning the yolk of an egg.

lecithin (lĕs′ĭth-ĭn) [Gr. *lekithos*, egg yolk]. A fatty substance of the group called phospholipids (phosphoglycerides), found in blood, bile, brain, egg yolk, nerves, and other animal tissues, and yielding stearic acid, glycerol, phosphoric acid, and choline on hydrolysis.

lecithinase (lĕs′ĭ-thĭn-ās). An enzyme that catalyzes the decomposition of lecithin.

   l., cobra. An enzyme present in certain snake venoms.

lecithin/sphingomyelin ratio. ABBR: L/S ratio. The ratio of lecithin to sphingomyelin in the amniotic fluid. It is used to assess maturity of the fetal lung. Until about the 34th week of gestation the lungs produce less lecithin than sphingomyelin. As the fetal lung begins to mature, more lecithin than sphingomyelin is produced. Delivery prior to the reversal of the ratio is associated with an increased risk of hyaline membrane disease in the infant. Use of the test enables the obstetrician to determine the optimum time for elective termination of pregnancy.

lecithoblast (lĕs′ĭ-thō-blăst″) [″ + *blastos*, germ]. One of the cells that proliferates to form the yolk-sac.

lecithoprotein (lĕs″ĭ-thō-prō′tē-ĭn) [″ + *protos*, first]. A protein in which lecithin is part of the conjugate.

lectin (lĕk′tĭn) [L. *legere*, to pick and choose]. One of several plant proteins that stimulate lymphocytes to proliferate. Phytohemagglutinin, q.v. and concanavalin A, q.v., are lectins. SEE: *mitogen.*

lectual (lĕkt′ū-ăl) [L. *lectus*, bed]. Pert. to a bed or couch.

LED. *light-emitting diode.*

leech (lētch) [AS. *laece*]. A bloodsucking water worm, belonging to the phylum Annelida, class Hirudinea. It is parasitic on humans and other animals, producing a condition known as hirudiniasis, q.v. Leeches were used as a means of bloodletting, a practice common up to the middle of the 19th century but now almost completely abandoned. They are a source of hirudin, an anticoagulating principle secreted by their buccal glands. In modern times leeches have been used to evacuate periorbital hemorrhage (black eye) and to remove congested

venous blood from the suture lines of reimplanted fingers.

   Leeches may be purchased from Leeches U.S.A. Ltd., 300 Shanes Drive, Westbury, NY 11590. Tel. (516) 333-2570.

   l., artificial. Cup and suction pump or syringe for drawing blood.

Lee's ganglion (lēz) [Robert Lee, Brit. gynecologist and obstetrician, 1793–1877]. Cervical uterine ganglion formed from 3rd and 4th sacral nerves and hypogastric and ovarian plexuses.

lees. Sediment obtained by allowing a solution to settle, esp. the dregs at the bottom of a wine bottle.

Leeuwenhoek's disease (lū′ĕn-hōks) [Antoni van Leeuwenhoek, Dutch microscopist, 1632–1723]. Repetitive involuntary contractions of the diaphragm and accessory muscles of respiration. The patient complains of shortness of breath and epigastric pulsations. SYN: *respiratory myoclonus.*

   ETIOL: Abnormality of the respiratory control system of the brain stem.

   TREAT: Diphenylhydantoin may be effective. If not, section of the phrenic nerve may be necessary.

left. The opposite of right. SYN: *sinistral.*

left-handedness. Condition of being more adept in use of left hand. SYN: *sinistrality.*

left lateral recumbent position. Position in which the patient is reclining on the left side.

leg (lĕg) [ME.]. One of the two lower extremities, including the femur, tibia, fibula, and patella; specifically the part between the knee and ankle. SEE: illus.

   RS: Buerger's disease; calf; crural; crus; saphena; saphenous; sura; systremma; thrombophlebitis; tibia.

   l., badger. Inequality in the length of the legs.

   l., baker. Genu valgum; knock-knee.

   l., bandy. L., bow-.

   l., Barbados. Elephantiasis of the legs.

   l., bayonet. Uncorrected backward displacement of the knee bones, followed by ankylosis at the joint.

   l., bird. Reduction in size of the leg as a result of atrophy of the muscles.

   l., boomerang. A disease of the leg bones occurring among Australian natives, causing a curvature of the leg resembling a boomerang.

   l., bow-. An outward curving of the legs at the knees. SYN: *bandy leg; genu varum.*

   l., milk. Phlebitis of the femoral vein occasionally following parturition and typhoid fever. It is characterized by swelling of the leg, usually without redness. SYN: *phlegmasia alba dolens; white leg.*

MUSCLES OF LEG

ANTERIOR VIEW

POSTERIOR VIEW

l., restless. A sense of uneasiness and uncomfortableness of the legs that comes on at bedtime. Moving the legs tends to relieve the condition. This syndrome is sometimes present at the onset of renal colic due to renal calculi.

l., scissor. Crossed-leg deformity, a result of double hip disease, in which the patient walks with the legs swinging across the midline with each step.

l., white. L. milk. SEE: *phlegmasia alba dolens.*

Legg-Calvé-Perthes disease (lĕg′kăl-vā′pĕr′tĕz) [Arthur T. Legg, U.S. surgeon, 1874–1939; Jacques Calvé, Fr. orthopedist, 1875–1954; Georg C. Perthes, Ger. surgeon, 1869–1927]. Legg's disease, q.v.

Legg's disease (lĕgz) [Arthur T. Legg]. Osteochondritis of the upper femoral epiphysis. SYN: *Legg-Calvé-Perthes disease.*

leggings (lĕg′gĭngs) [ME. *leg*, leg]. Sterile leg coverings used on patient in operating room.

Legionella pneumophila. The gram-negative, rod-shaped bacterium that causes Legionnaires' disease. SEE: *Legionnaires' disease.*

Legionnaires' disease [after individuals stricken while attending an American Legion convention in Philadelphia, PA, in 1976]. A severe, often fatal disease characterized by pneumonia, dry cough, myalgia, and sometimes gastrointestinal symptoms. As the disease progresses, there is evidence of dysfunction of other major organs, and in fatal cases, there is eventual cardiovascular collapse. SYN: *legionellosis.*

ETIOL: A gram-negative bacillus not previously recognized as an agent of human disease. The organism has been termed *Legionella pneumophila.* The organism causes disease by being inhaled from aerosols produced by water cooling towers, air conditioning units, water faucets, shower heads, humidifiers, and contaminated respiratory therapy equipment. Person-to-person transmission does not occur.

TREAT: Erythromycin given early in the course of the disease and for a prolonged period is the drug of choice. Rifampin is also of benefit.

legitimacy (lĕ-jĭt′ĭ-mă-sē) [L. *legitimus*, lawful]. 1. Condition of being legal. 2. Condition of being born in wedlock.

legume (lĕ′gūm) [L. *legumen*, pulse, bean]. Fruit or pod of beans, peas, or lentils.

COMP: Nitrogen: almost equal to that in meat. Legumin, a globulin, is present.

VITAMINS: Sprouted beans are a good source of vitamin B complex. Vitamin A and ascorbic acid are present in small amounts.

CARBOHYDRATES: Generally in the form of starch in about the same proportion

as the cereals but with more cellulose.

legumelin (lĕg-ū′mĕl-ĭn) [L. *legumen*, pulse, bean]. An albumin present in many leguminous seeds, as in peas. SEE: *legume; legumin.*

legumin (lĕ-gū′mĭn). A globulin present in legumes such as peas and beans.

Leiner's disease (lī′nĕrz) [Karl Leiner, Austrian pediatrician, 1871–1930]. Exfoliative dermatitis.

-leio [L. *leios*, smooth]. Combining form meaning smooth.

leiodermia (lī″ō-dĕr′mē-ă) [Gr. *leios*, smooth, + *derma*, skin]. Dermatitis characterized by abnormal glossiness and smoothness of the skin.

leiomyofibroma (lī″ō-mī″ō-fī-brō′mă) [″ + *mys*, muscle, + L. *fibra*, fiber, + Gr. *oma*, tumor]. A benign tumor composed principally of smooth muscle and fibrous connective tissue.

leiomyoma (lī″ō-mī-ō′mă) [″ + ″ + *oma*, tumor]. Myoma consisting principally of smooth muscle tissue.

l., epithelioid. Smooth muscle tumor usually of the stomach.

l. uteri. Fibroma, uterine, q.v.

leiomyosarcoma (lī″ō-mī″ō-săr-kō′mă) [″ + ″ + *sarx*, flesh, + *oma*, tumor]. Combined leiomyoma and sarcoma.

leiotrichous (lī-ŏt′rĭ-kŭs) [″ + *thrix*, hair]. Possessing smooth or straight hair.

Leishman-Donovan bodies. SEE: *body, Leishman-Donovan.*

Leishmania (lēsh-mā′nē-ă) [Sir William B. Leishman, Brit. medical officer, 1865–1926]. A genus of parasitic flagellate protozoa that occur as typical leishmanian forms in vertebrate hosts but as leptomonad forms in invertebrate hosts or in cultures. They are transmitted by the bite of the female phlebotomines (sandflies).

L. braziliensis. Causative agent of American leishmaniasis.

L. donovani. Causative agent of kala-azar (visceral leishmaniasis).

L. tropica. Causative agent of Oriental sore (cutaneous leishmaniasis).

leishmaniasis (lēsh″mă-nī′ă-sĭs). Infection with a species of *Leishmania*, affecting the skin, nasal cavities, and pharynx. One form causes Oriental sore and another kala-azar.

l., American. Leishmaniasis caused by *L. braziliensis*, involving principally nasopharyngeal and mucocutaneous membranes. Common in Central and South America.

l., cutaneous. Leishmaniasis due to infection with *L. tropica.* SYN: *Aleppo boil; Oriental sore.*

l., mucocutaneous. A form of cutaneous leishmaniasis found in parts of Central and

South America. The causative organism is *Leishmania braziliensis* transmitted by sandflies usually of the genus *Lutzomyia*. SYN: *American leishmaniasis*.

  l., visceral. Leishmaniasis caused by *L. donovani*. SYN: *kala-azar*.

lema (lē'mă) [Gr. *leme*]. The dried secretion of the tarsal glands that collects in the inner canthus of the eye. SYN: *sebum palpebrale*.

lemmocyte (lĕm'ō-sīt) [Gr. *lemma*, husk, + *kytos*, cell]. A cell that becomes a neurilemma cell. SEE: *nerve fiber*.

lemniscus (lĕm-nĭs'kŭs) [Gr. *lemniskos*, a ribbon] (pl. *lemnisci*). [NA] A bundle of sensory fibers (lateral or exterior and median or interior) in the medulla and pons.

lemon [Persian *limun*, lemon]. Fruit of the tree *Citrus limon*, containing citric acid. Lemons contain enough ascorbic acid to prevent or treat scurvy.

  May be used in place of vinegar, spices, and aromatic substances by those who cannot use such items. Diabetics may use.

Caution: Food faddists who drink large quantities of lemon juice by sucking directly from the raw fruit may develop erosion of the enamel of their teeth.

---

lemoparalysis (lē"mō-pă-răl'ĭ-sĭs) [Gr. *laimos*, gullet, + *para*, beside, + *lyein*, to loosen]. Paralysis of the esophagus.

lemostenosis [" + *stenosis*, act of narrowing]. Stricture of the esophagus.

length. Measurement of the distance between two points.

  l., basialveolar. Distance from the basion of the foramen magnum of the skull to the intermaxillary suture of the jaw.

  l., basinasal. Distance from the basion of the foramen magnum of the skull to the center of the suture between the frontal and nasal bones.

  l., crown-heel. In the embryo, fetus, or newborn, the distance from the crown of the head to the heel.

  l., crown-rump. In the embryo, fetus, or newborn, the distance from the crown of the head to the apex of the buttocks.

  l., focal. In optics, the distance from the lens to the point of focus of light rays passing through the lens.

  l., wave. In the line of progression of a wave, the distance from one point on the wave to the same point on the next wave. The length of a wave determines whether or not the wave is a visible light, x-ray, gamma, or radio wave.

lenitive (lĕn'ĭ-tĭv) [L. *lenire*, to soothe]. 1. Demulcent, soothing, slightly laxative. 2. A palliative.

lens (lĕnz) [L. *lens*, lentil]. 1. A transparent refracting medium; usually made of glass. 2. [NA] The crystalline lens of the eye.

  RS: capsulociliary; circle of diffusion; vitreous chamber.

  l., achromatic. Lens that corrects chromatic aberration.

  l., aplanatic. Lens that corrects spherical aberrations.

  l., apochromatic. Lens that corrects both spherical and chromatic aberrations.

  l., biconcave. Lens that has a concave surface on each side. SEE: *biconcave* for illus.

  l., biconvex. Lens that has a convex surface on each side. SEE: *biconvex* for illus.

  l., bifocal. Corrective lens containing in either its upper or lower segment a lens of different power. The main lens is for distant vision; the secondary lens is for near vision.

  l., concave spherical. Lens formed of prisms with their apices together and, therefore, thin at the center and thick at the edge. Used in myopia.

  l., contact. A custom-fitted curved lens of glass or synthetic material that is applied to the eye for correction of refractive errors.

  l., convexoconcave. Lens that has a convex surface on one side and a concave surface on the opposite side.

  l., convex spherical. Lens formed of prisms with their bases together and, therefore, thick at the center and thin at the edge. Used in hyperopia.

  l., corneal contact. A type of contact lens that adheres to and covers only the cornea.

  l., crystalline. Transparent colorless structure in the eye, biconvex in shape, enclosed in a capsule, and held in place just behind the pupil by the suspensory ligament. Consists principally of lens fibers that at the periphery are soft, forming the cortex lentis, and in the center of harder consistency, forming the nucleus lentis. Beneath the capsule on the anterior surface is a thin layer of cells, the lens epithelium. Function is to focus rays so that they form a perfect image on the retina.

  l., cylindrical. Segment of a cylinder parallel to its axis, used in correcting astigmatism.

  l., implanted. Artificial lens implanted at the time a cataract is removed. This procedure may also be used in correcting other lens defects.

  l., omnifocal. Lens used in making eyeglasses. Its power to alter light rays varies from the top to the bottom of the lens. This permits a smooth transition from one power lens to the other as one moves the eyes. This is in contrast to an eyeglass lens with the usual two-component bifocal lens.

l., orthoscopic. Lens that produces no distortion of the periphery of the image.

l., soft contact. Contact lens for correcting refractive errors. They are of soft plastic material and cause less discomfort than conventional contact lenses.

l., spherical. Lens in which all surfaces are spherical.

l., trial. Any lens used in testing the vision.

l., trifocal. Corrective lens containing three segments — for near, intermediate, and distant vision.

lentectomy (lĕn-tĕk'tō-mē) [L. *lens,* lentil, + Gr. *ektome,* excision]. Surgical removal of the lens of the eye.

lenticonus (lĕn"tĭ-kō'nŭs) [" + *conus,* cone]. Conical protrusion of the anterior or posterior surface of the lens.

lenticular [L. *lenticularis,* lentil]. 1. Lens shaped. SYN: *lentiform.* 2. Pert. to a lens.

lenticular fossa. Depression in the anterior surface of the vitreous for reception of the crystalline lens.

lenticular glands. Small masses of lymphatic tissue in the lamina propria of the pyloric region of the stomach.

lenticular nucleus. Mass of gray matter forming part of the corpus striatum. Consists of the putamen and globus pallidus.

lenticulostriate (lĕn-tĭk"ū-lō-strī'āt) [" + *striatus,* streaked]. Rel. to the lenticular nucleus and corpus striatum.

lenticulothalamic. Pert. to the lenticular nucleus and the thalamus.

lentiform (lĕnt'ĭ-form) [L. *lens,* lentil, + *forma,* shape]. Lentil or lens shaped. SYN: *lenticular.*

lentigines. Flat, brown spots appearing on aged exposed skin, frequently on the back of the hands due to the accumulation of lipofuscin in tissues as one ages. Lay term frequently used is "liver spots." However, there is no physiological relationship to the liver.

lentiginosis (lĕn-tĭj"ĭ-nō'sĭs) [L. *lentigo,* freckle, + Gr. *osis,* condition]. Presence of multiple lentigines. SEE: *lentigo.*

lentiginous (lĕn-tĭj'ĭn-ŭs) [L. *lentigo,* freckle]. 1. Affected by lentigo. 2. Covered with very small dots.

lentiglobus (lĕn"tĭ-glō'bŭs) [L. *lens,* lentil, + *globus,* sphere]. A lens of the eye that has extreme anterior spherical bulging.

lentigo (lĕn-tī'gō) [L., freckle] (pl. *lentigines*). Small brown macules or yellow-brown pigmented areas on skin sometimes caused by exposure to sun and weather. SYN: *ephelis; freckle.*

l. maligna. A noninvasive malignant melanotic freckle. SYN: *freckle, Hutchinson's.*

lentitis (lĕn-tī'tĭs) [L. *lens,* lentil, + Gr. *itis,* inflammation]. Inflammation of the crystalline lens. SYN: *phakitis.*

lentivirus [L. *lentus,* slow]. A group of retroviruses that cause slowly developing diseases. The virus that causes acquired immunodeficiency syndrome (AIDS), human immunodeficiency virus (HIV), is included in this group of viruses.

leontiasis (lē"ŏn-tī'ă-sĭs) [Gr. *leon,* lion, + *-iasis,* condition]. Lionlike appearance of the face seen in certain diseases, esp. lepromatous leprosy. SYN: *facies leontina.*

l. ossea. Enlargement and distortion of facial bones, giving one the appearance of a lion. The condition is rare and not fatal.

Leopold's maneuver [Christian Gerhard Leopold, Ger. physician, 1846 – 1911]. In obstetrics, the use of four steps in palpating the uterus in order to determine the position and presentation of the fetus.

leotropic (lē-ō-trŏp'ĭk) [Gr. *laios,* left, + *tropos,* a turning]. Wound in a spiral form going from right to left.

leper (lĕp'ĕr) [Gr. *lepros,* scaly]. Person afflicted with leprosy.

lepidic (lĕ-pĭd'ĭk) [Gr. *lepis,* scale]. Concerning scales, or a scaly covering.

lepido- [Gr. *lepis,* scale]. Combining form referring to flakes or scales.

Lepidoptera (lĕp"ĭ-dŏp'tĕr-ă) [" + *pteron,* feather, wing]. An order of the class Insecta that includes the butterflies, moths, and skippers. Characterized by scaly wings, sucking mouth parts, and complete metamorphosis.

lepidosis (lĕp"ĭ-dō'sĭs) [" + *osis,* condition]. Any scaly or desquamating eruption such as pityriasis.

lepothrix (lĕp'ō-thrĭks) [" + *thrix,* hair]. Condition in which the shaft of the hair is encased in hardened, scaly, sebaceous matter.

lepra (lĕp'ră) [Gr. *lepra,* leprosy]. A term formerly used for leprosy. Now used to indicate a reaction that occurs in leprosy patients consisting of aggravation of lesions accompanied by fever and malaise. It can occur in any form of leprosy and may be prolonged.

l. alba. Skin is anesthetic and white, and different forms of paralysis follow.

l. Arabum. True or nodular leprosy.

l. maculosa. Form of lepra with pigmented cutaneous areas.

leprechaunism (lĕp'rĕ-kŏn"ĭzm). Hereditary disease in which the elfin features of the face are accompanied by retardation of physical and mental development, a variety of endocrine disorders, emaciation, and susceptibility to infections. SYN: *Donohue's syndrome.*

leprid (lĕp'rĭd) [Gr. *lepra,* leprosy, + *eidos,*

form, shape]. Leprous cutaneous lesion.

leprology (lĕp-rŏl′ō-jē) [″ + *logos*, word, reason]. The study of leprosy and methods of treating it.

leproma (lĕp-rō′mă) [″ + *oma*, tumor]. A cutaneous nodule or tubercle characteristic of leprosy.

lepromatous (lĕp-rō′mă-tŭs). Concerning lepromas. SEE: *leprosy.*

leprosarium. An institution for the care of lepers.

leprostatic (lĕp″rō-stăt′ĭk) [″ + *statikos,* standing]. Either inhibiting the growth of *Mycobacterium leprae,* or an agent that inhibits that organism's growth.

leprosy (lĕp′rō-sē) [Gr. *lepros,* scaly]. A chronic communicable disease caused by the acid-fast *Mycobacterium leprae.* It may occur in various clinical forms. The two principal forms are lepromatous and tuberculoid. SYN: *Hansen's disease.*

The *lepromatous* (LL) form is characterized by skin lesions and symmetrical involvement of peripheral nerves with anesthesia, muscle weakness, and paralysis. In this form, the lesions are limited to the cooler portions of the body such as skin, upper respiratory tract, and testes. In *tuberculoid* (TT) leprosy, which is usually benign, the nerve lesions are asymmetrical and skin anesthesia is an early occurrence. Visceral involvement is not seen. Because of the anesthesia, rats have been able to remove digits while the patient sleeps. For some time this loss of digits was thought, erroneously, to be due to spontaneous amputation as a part of the disease process.

Lepromatous leprosy is much more contagious than the tuberculoid form. In the latter, *Mycobacterium leprae* are found in lesions only rarely except during reactions.

Between the two major forms are *borderline* (BB) and *indeterminate* leprosy. In the borderline group, the clinical and bacteriological features represent a combination of the two principal types. In the indeterminate group, there are fewer skin lesions and bacteria are much less abundant in the lesions. In many respects, this infection resembles tuberculosis and for many years was regarded as incurable; this is no longer considered to be valid.

SYM: Onset very gradual. The first signs of infection are usually skin changes, but they may be so nonspecific and so slow to progress as to go unrecognized for years.

ETIOL: Caused by *Mycobacterium leprae.* May occur at practically any age.

DIAG: Biopsy of a suspected skin lesion. The bacilli may not be present in tuberculoid lesions. In vitro tests of the immunologic response can be accomplished by the lymphocyte transformation test and the leukocyte migration inhibition test.

INCUB: May be 1 to 30 years, but usually 3 to 5 years.

COMPLICATIONS: Bacterial infections of skin, ulcers, traumatic amputation of fingers due to anesthesia. Tuberculosis is a much more common complication in untreated cases of lepromatous leprosy than in the tuberculoid form. Amyloidosis may be the cause of death in advanced cases.

TREAT: Dapsone (4,4′-diamino-diphenyl sulfone, DDS) is the form of sulfone used, but widespread development of sulfone resistance necessitates combined chemotherapy treatment with dapsone, rifampin, and clofazimine.

Treatment may be complicated by an acute reversal reaction in tuberculoid or indeterminate forms of leprosy in which the lesions become erythematous and edematous and may become necrotic and ulcerated. Also, the erythema nodosum leprosum (ENL) reaction may develop. This occurs most commonly during the end of the first year of therapy. In this reaction, multiple painful red nodules develop and then may become ulcerated and necrotic; they may last a short time, but new lesions appear. The ENL reaction may be of short or long duration. Thalidomide is the drug of choice for treatment of the ENL reaction. Severe reactions may also require corticosteroid therapy. Thalidomide does not alter the primary disease. This drug is available in the U.S. from Gillis W. Long Hansen's Disease Center, Carville, LA 70721, (800) 642-2477. Thalidomide is contraindicated in women of childbearing age.

The management of patients with leprosy is complex and may require expert consultation. Such assistance may be obtained by contacting physicians at Carville.

Segregation of patients in colonies or hospitals until bacterial tests have been negative for six months is not the preferred or effective method of isolating patients. Ambulatory treatment of patients at general clinics has been found to be much more effective. Patients are usually not infectious after three months of therapy with dapsone or clofazimine; and after three days of rifampin. Thus, children need not be removed from the household in which an adequately treated person with leprosy resides.

PROG: With proper therapy, the outlook for recovery is good.

leprotic (lĕp-rŏt′ĭk) [Gr. *lepra,* leprosy]. 1. Rel. to leprosy. 2. Affected with leprosy. SYN: *leprous.*

leprous (lĕp′rŭs). 1. Pert. to leprosy. 2. Affected by leprosy. SYN: *leprotic.*

lepto- [Gr. *leptos*, thin, fine, slim]. Combining form indicating thin, fine, slight, delicate.

leptocephalia (lĕp″tō-sĕ-fā′lē-ă) [Gr. *leptos*, slender, + *kephale*, head]. Having an abnormally vertically elongated, narrow skull.

leptocephalus. An individual possessing an abnormally vertically elongated, narrow skull.

leptochromatic (lĕp″tō-krō-măt′ĭk) [″ + *chromatin*]. Having a fine chromatin network.

leptocyte (lĕp′tō-sīt) [″ + *kytos*, cell]. Target cell, q.v.

leptocytosis (lĕp″tō-sī-tō′sĭs) [″ + ″ + *osis*, condition]. Presence of leptocytes in the blood. SEE: *target cell.*

leptodactyly (lĕp″tō-dăk′tĭ-lē) [″ + *daktylos*, finger]. Abnormally slim fingers.

leptomeninges (lĕp″tō-mĕn-ĭn′jēs) [″ + *meninx*, membrane] (sing. *leptomeninx*). The pia mater and arachnoid as distinct from the dura mater, because of their thinner and more delicate structure.

leptomeningitis (lĕp″tō-mĕn-ĭn-jī′tĭs) [″ + ″ + *itis*, inflammation]. Inflammation of the pia and arachnoid membranes. SYN: *piarachnitis.* SEE: *meningitis.*

SYM: Acute headache, pain in back, rigidity of spine, irritability, drowsiness ending in coma. Clinically, it cannot be distinguished from pachymeningitis, q.v.

ETIOL: Tubercle bacillus, spirochete of syphilis, and other organisms.

leptomeningopathy (lĕp″tō-mĕn″ĭn-gŏp′ă-thē) [″ + ″ + *pathos*, disease]. Disease of the leptomeninges of the brain.

leptomeninx. Sing. of leptomeninges.

leptonema (lĕp″tō-nē′mă) [″ + *nema*, thread]. Early stage of prophase in meiosis. At this stage the chromatin contracts into long, thin filaments. SEE: *cell division.*

leptopellic (lĕp″tō-pĕl′ĭk) [″ + *pellis*, basin]. Having an abnormally narrow pelvis.

leptophonia (lĕp″tō-fō′nē-ă) [″ + *phone*, voice]. Weakness or feebleness of voice.

leptoprosopia (lĕp″tō-prō-sō′pē-ă) [″ + *prosopon*, face]. Narrowness of the face.

leptorhine, leptorrhine (lĕp′tor-rīn) [″ + *rhis*, nose]. Having a very thin or slender nose.

leptoscope (lĕp′tō-skōp) [″ + *skopein*, to examine]. Optical device for measuring the thickness of cell membranes.

leptosome (lĕp′tō-sōm) [″ + *soma*, body]. Person of thin, slight stature.

Leptospira (lĕp-tō-spī′ră) [″ + *speira*, coil]. Genus of thin, spiral, and hook-ended spirochetes.

L. interrogans icterohaemorrhagiae. Serotype causing infectious, hemorrhagic, spirochetal jaundice (Weil's disease, q.v.).

leptospire (lĕp′tō-spīr). Any organism belonging to the genus *Leptospira.*

leptospirosis (lĕp″tō-spī-rō′sĭs) [″ + ″ + *osis*, condition]. Condition resulting from *Leptospira* infection.

leptospiruria (lĕp″tō-spĭr-ū′rē-ă) [″ + ″ + *ouron*, urine]. Presence of *Leptospira* organisms in the urine.

leptotene (lĕp′tō-tēn) [″ + *tainia*, ribbon]. The initial stage of the prophase of cell division. The chromosomes become visible as separate entities but are not yet paired.

leptothricosis (lĕp″tō-thrī-kō′sĭs) [″ + *thrix*, hair]. Disease from *Leptothrix* infection.

Leptus autumnalis. Parasitic mite larvae causing itch and sometimes wheals. SEE: *chiggers.*

leresis (lē-rē′sĭs) [Gr.]. Loquacity in old age; garrulousness.

Leriche's syndrome (lĕ-rēsh′ĕz) [René Leriche, Fr. surgeon, 1879–1955]. Occlusion of the abdominal aorta by a thrombus at its bifurcation. This causes intermittent ischemic pain, i.e., claudication, in the lower extremities and buttocks, impotence, and absent or diminished femoral pulses.

Leri's pleonosteosis (lā′rēz) [André Leri, Fr. physician, 1875–1930]. A form of hereditary physical malformation characterized by upward slanting palpebral fissures, broad thumbs, short stature, and flexion contractures of the fingers.

lesbian (lĕs′bē-ăn) [Gr. *lesbios*, pert. to island of Lesbos]. 1. Pert. to lesbianism, q.v., or sexual orientation in women for those of their own sex. SEE: *bisexual; homosexual.* 2. One who practices lesbianism.

lesbianism. Sexual desire of women for one of their own sex. SYN: *sapphism.*

Named from the Island of Lesbos, where the practice of lesbianism was reputed to have been general in ancient days.

Lesch-Nyhan disease [M. Lesch, b. 1939, William Leo Nyhan, b. 1926, U.S. pediatricians]. An inherited metabolic disease that affects only males. Clinically there is mental retardation, aggressive behavior, self-mutilation, and renal failure. Biochemically there is excess uric acid production due to a virtual absence of an enzyme essential for purine metabolism.

lesion (lē′zhŭn) [L. *laesio*, a wound]. 1. A circumscribed area of pathologically altered tissue. 2. An injury or wound. 3. Single infected patch in a skin disease.

Primary or initial lesions include macules, vesicles, blebs or bullae, chancres, pustules, papules, tubercles, wheals, and tumors, q.v. Secondary lesions are the result of primary lesions. They may be crusts, excoriations, fissures, pigmentations, scales, scars, and ulcers, q.v.

RS: abscess; boil; cancer; carbuncle; cerebropsychosis; chancre; chancroid; felon; gumma; mole; neoplasm; pimple; pus; rash; sebaceous cyst; tumefaction; verruca; wound.

l., degenerative. Lesion caused by or showing degeneration.

l., diffuse. Lesion spreading over a large area.

l., discharging. 1. Brain lesion that discharges nervous impulses. 2. Lesion that discharges an exudate.

l., focal. Lesion of a small definite area.

l., indiscriminate. Lesion affecting separate systems of the body.

l., initial, of syphilis. Hard chancre. SEE: *chancre; syphilis.*

l., irritative. Lesion that stimulates or excites activity in the part of the body where it is situated.

l., local. Lesion of nervous system origin giving rise to local symptoms.

l., peripheral. Lesion of the nerve endings.

l., primary. First lesion of a disease, esp. used in referring to chancre of syphilis, q.v.

l., structural. Lesion that causes change in tissue.

l., systemic. Lesion confined to organs of common function.

l., toxic. Lesion resulting from poisons or toxins from microorganisms.

l., vascular. Lesion of a blood vessel.

LET. *linear energy transfer.* A measure of the rate of energy transfer from ionizing radiation to soft tissue.

lethal [Gr. *lethe*, oblivion]. Pert. to or that which causes death.

lethargic (lĕ-thär′jĭk) [Gr. *lethargos*, drowsiness]. 1. Affected with lethargy. 2. Rel. to lethargy. 3. Sluggish.

lethargy (lĕth′ăr-jē) [Gr. *lethargos*, drowsiness]. A condition of functional torpor or sluggishness; stupor.

l., African. Sleeping sickness. SEE: *encephalitis lethargica.*

l., hysteric. The sleep of hypnotic lethargy, the state in which many cases of apparent death and resurrection are found.

l., induced. Hypnotic trance.

l., lucid. Retention of intellect but loss of willpower with a consequent total lack of muscular response. The subject knows what is going on, may resent it, but is unable to exercise sufficient will to bring about muscular defense.

lethe (lē′thē) [Gr., oblivion]. Amnesia.

letholologica (lĕth-ō-lŏj′ĭ-kă) [Gr. *lethe*, forgetfulness, + *logos*, word, reason]. Temporary inability to remember a word or name, or an intended action.

Letterer-Siwe disease (lĕt′ĕr-ĕr-sī′wĕ) [Erich Letterer, Ger. physician, b. 1895; S. August Siwe, Ger. physician, b. 1897]. A histiocytosis syndrome characterized by proliferation of histiocytes in the viscera and bones. It begins before age 3 and is fatal if untreated. The spleen and liver are enlarged, and there is widespread pulmonary infiltration. There is bone marrow failure accompanied by fever and severe infections. The skin is involved and a variety of lesions are present, including papulovesicular eruption and inflamed pruritic lesions around the anal and vaginal areas. The cause is unknown and there is no specific treatment, but cortisone is used to control lung pathology. It is felt that this disease, eosinophilic granuloma of bone, Hand-Schüller-Christian syndrome, histiocytosis X, and reticuloendotheliosis share a common pattern of the development of granulomatous lesions with histiocytic proliferation.

Leu. *leucine.*

leuc-. SEE: words beginning with *leuk-.*

leucine (loo′sĭn) [Gr. *leukos*, white]. $C_6H_{13}NO_2$. An amino acid found among the products of digestion of proteins. It is present in body tissues and is essential for normal growth and metabolism.

leucine aminopeptidase. ABBR: LAP. A proteolytic enzyme present in the pancreas, liver, and small intestine. Its serum level is elevated in disease of the pancreas, esp. acute pancreatitis, and in obstruction of the common bile duct.

leucinosis (loo″sĭn-ō′sĭs) [″ + *osis*, condition]. Excess of leucine in the body, thus producing leucine in the urine.

leucinuria (loo″sĭn-ū′rē-ă) [″ + *ouron*, urine]. Presence of leucine in urine.

leucism (loo′sĭzm) [″ + *-ismos*, condition]. A form of incomplete albinism.

leucismus (loo-sĭz′mŭs) [″ + *-ismos*, condition]. Condition of being white.

leucitis (loo-sī′tĭs) [″ + *itis*, inflammation]. Inflammation of the sclera. SYN: *scleritis.*

leucovorin calcium (loo″kō-vō′rĭn). USP. The calcium salt of folic acid. It is used in the treatment of megaloblastic anemias. It is also used to antagonize the effect of methotrexate on normal cells when methotrexate is being used to treat malignancies. When so used, large doses of leucovorin are required and the optimum timing and dosage are difficult to establish. This use is called leucovorin "rescue."

leukapheresis (loo″kă-fĕ-rē′sĭs) [″ + *aphairesis*, removal]. Separation of leukocytes from blood that is then transfused back into the patient.

leukemia (loo-kē'mē-ă) [Gr. *leukos,* white, + *haima,* blood]. A chronic or acute disease of unregulated clonal proliferation of the stem cells of the blood-forming tissues. These cells are unable to mature normally and eventually, even though slow-growing, replace the resident cells by tumor cells. This overgrowth is the result of a chromosomal abnormality that prevents maturation of the blood cell precursors. Classification of leukemia is controversial, but there is general agreement that they can be grouped into the broad categories of acute or chronic. Further classification includes those affecting precursors of the granulocytes or the lymphocytes. Leukemias may be caused by a genetic aberration or by exposure to environmental factors such as ionizing radiation or certain toxic chemicals.

INCIDENCE: Leukemias cause about 3% of all malignancies. About 60% of leukemias are myelogenous and 80% of these are the acute myelogenous (AML) type. In adults AML represents about 90% of all leukemias. SEE: *hematopoietic malignancies.* SEE: *Nursing Diagnoses* in *Appendix.*

l., acute myelogenous. ABBR: AML. Malignant disease of hemopoietic stem cells. The clinical features are anemia, pallor, fatigue, easy bruising, bone pain, splenomegaly, and predisposition to infections. There are several subclasses of AML, including acute promyelocytic (APL); acute myelomonocytic (AMML); acute monoblastic (AMoL); acute erythroleukemia (AEL); acute megakaryoblastic leukemia (AMegL); acute lymphatic (ALL); and acute mast cell. SYN: *acute nonlymphocytic leukemia (ANLL).*

TREAT: Cytotoxic chemotherapy and bone marrow transplant after the patient's bone marrow has been treated with radiation.

PROG: The goal of therapy is to produce a remission and to have this continue indefinitely. Remissions are much less likely to occur in patients over 50 years of age.

l., chronic myelogenous. ABBR: CML. A neoplastic disease in which over 90% of cases are associated with a unique chromosome abnormality called the Philadelphia chromosome (Ph¹). CML includes those that are Ph¹ positive and Ph¹ negative. Also included are chronic myelomonocytic (CMML); chronic lymphatic (CLL); prolymphocytic (PLL); Sezary syndrome; and hairy cell (HCL). Chronic lymphatic leukemia (CLL) is further divided into chronic B cell leukemia (B cell CLL) and chronic T cell leukemia (T cell CLL).

CML is a slowly progressive disorder with few symptoms initially. The abnormality of the blood may be discovered as an incidental finding in a person having a routine blood count. Onset of the disease is seldom seen prior to age 50.

SYM: Malaise, fatigue, low exercise tolerance, anemia, night sweats, weight loss, bone pain, splenomegaly, and recurrent infections.

TREAT: Cytotoxic chemotherapy and bone marrow transplant.

PROG: Median survival for patients receiving chemotherapy is 47 months.

l., hairy cell. A malignant, lymphoproliferative disease characterized by pancytopenia, splenomegaly, and abnormal mononuclear cells with irregular cytoplasmic projections. These so-called hairy cells are especially evident in the spleen. This chronic disease has a median age of onset of about 50 years, and 80% of cases are in men.

TREAT: Splenectomy may produce a long-term remission. Use of interferon has been useful in preliminary studies.

PROG: Most patients live 5 years after diagnosis and some live for more than 10 years.

leukemic (loo-kēm'ĭk) [" + *haima,* blood]. 1. Rel. to leukemia. 2. Affected with leukemia.

leukemid (loo-kē'mĭd). Any nonspecific skin lesion associated with leukemia. The lesions may or may not contain leukemia cells.

leukemogenesis (loo-kē"mō-jĕn'ĕ-sĭs) [" + " + *genesis,* generation, birth]. The induction of leukemia.

leukemoid (loo-kē'moyd) [" + " + *eidos,* form, shape]. Having symptoms of leukemia that are actually due to other conditions.

Leukeran. Trade name for chlorambucil, USP.

leukin (loo'kĭn). A thermostable bactericidal substance present in leukocytes.

leuko-, leuk- [Gr. *leukos,* white]. Combining forms signifying white, colorless, or rel. to leukocyte.

leukoagglutinin (loo"kō-ă-gloo'tĭ-nĭn) [" + L. *agglutinans,* gluing]. An antibody that agglutinates white blood cells.

leukocidin (loo-kō-sī'dĭn) [" + L. *caedere,* to kill]. A bacterial toxin that destroys leukocytes.

leukocoria, leukokoria. White or abnormal pupillary reflex. This reflex may be present in infants and children who have retinoblastoma, cataract, retinal detachment, and intraocular infections. Patients with this reflex should be referred to an ophthalmologist without delay.

leukocyte (loo'kō-sīt) [" + *kytos,* cell]. White blood corpuscle. There are two types: granulocytes (those possessing, in their cytoplasm, large granules that stain different colors under a microscope) and agranulocytes (those lacking granules). Granulocytes include basophils, q.v., eosinophils, q.v., and neutrophils, q.v. Agranulocytes include monocytes, q.v., and lymphocytes, q.v. Clinically, granulocytes are often referred to as "polys" because they are all polymorphonuclear (multi-lobed nuclei), while agranulocytes are called mononuclear (one nucleus).

Neutrophils, which make up approximately 60% of all white blood cells (WBCs), are the most active phagocytic cells in the body, and serve as the primary effector cell in inflammation. Eosinophils, 1 to 4% of total WBCs, destroy parasites and are a major component of allergic reactions. The role of basophils, which make up less than 1% of all WBCs, is unclear although it is known that they release many of the chemicals involved in the inflammatory process. Monocytes, 3 to 8% of all WBCs, are extremely phagocytic. Those that have left the blood stream and settled in the tissues are called macrophages, q.v. Next to neutrophils, macrophages are the most important phagocytic WBCs.

Leukocytes are formed from two stem cells, q.v., in the bone marrow. The myeloid stem cell line produces granulocytes and monocytes, and the lymphoid stem cell produces lymphocytes. Lymphoid cells travel to the thymus, spleen and lymph nodes, where they mature and differentiate into active, antigen-specific, q.v., lymphocytes.

FUNCT: Leukocytes are the primary effector cells against infection and tissue damage. They not only neutralize or destroy organisms, but also act as scavengers, cleaning up damaged cells by phagocytosis, q.v., to initiate the repair process. Leukocytes travel by ameboid movement and are able to penetrate tissue and then return to the blood stream. Their movement is directed by chemicals released by injured cells, a process called chemotaxis, q.v. After coming in contact with and recognizing an antigen, they engulf it (phagocytosis) and then destroy it through the release of lysosomes, q.v., from granules in their cytoplasm. When leukocytes are killed along with the pathogenic organisms they have destroyed, the resulting material is called pus, commonly found at the site of localized infections. Pus that collects because of inadequate blood or lymph drainage is called an abscess.

Microscopic examination: Leukocytes can be measured in any bodily secretion. They are normally present in blood and, in small amounts, in spinal fluid and mucus. The presence of WBCs in urine, sputum, or fluid drawn from the abdomen is an indication of infection or trauma. The type of WBC present is identified by the shape of the cell or by the staining of granules. Granules in eosinophils stain red, those in basophils stain blue, and those in neutrophils are purple.

Clinically, serum WBC counts are important in detecting infection or immune system dysfunction. The normal WBC level is 5000 to 10,000/mm^3. An elevated (greater than 10,000) leukocyte count (leukocytosis) indicates an acute infection or disease process (such as certain types of leukemia), while a decrease in the number of leukocytes (less than 5000) indicates either immunodeficiency, q.v., or an overwhelming infection which has depleted WBC stores. In addition to the total WBC count, the differential count is also frequently important. A differential count measures the number of each type of cell, e.g., neutrophil, monocyte, lymphocyte. The differential also measures the number of immature cells of each cell type as an indication of production by the bone marrow. Immature cells are called "blasts" (Ex: lymphoblasts, myeloblasts). During an infection, the number of blasts is increased as large numbers of immature cells are released. SEE: *inflammation.*

   l., acidophilic. L., eosinophilic.

   l., agranular. L., nongranular, q.v.

   l., basophil. Leukocyte with cytoplasmic granules that stain with basic dyes. Stain a deep purple with Wright's stain. Constitute 0% to 0.75% of white cell count.

   l., eosinophilic. A granular leukocyte with cytoplasmic granules that stain with acid dyes. Appear reddish when stained with Wright's stain. Constitute 1% to 3% of white cell count. SYN: *l., acidophil.*

   l., granular. Leukocyte containing granules in cytoplasm.

   l., heterophilic. Neutrophilic leukocyte of certain animals whose granules stain with an acid stain.

   l., lymphoid. L., nongranular, q.v.

   l., neutrophilic. Leukocyte with fine cytoplasmic granules that do not stain with acid or basic stains but have an affinity for neutral stains.

   l., nongranular. An agranulocyte; a lymphocyte or monocyte.

   l., polymorphonuclear. Leukocyte with a nucleus consisting of several lobes. One of the granulocytes (neutrophil, eosinophil, basophil).

leukocyte migration inhibition factor. ABBR: LMIF. A lymphokine, q.v., that inhibits movement of neutrophils.

leukocytic (loo″kō-sĭt′ĭk) [″ + *kytos,* cell].

Pert. to leukocytes.

leukocytoblast (loo″kō-sī′tō-blast) [″ + ″ + *blastos,* germ]. Cell from which leukocytes arise.

leukocytogenesis (loo″kō-sī″tō-jĕn′ĕ-sĭs) [″ + *kytos,* cell, + *genesis,* generation, birth]. Leukocyte formation. SYN: *leukopoiesis.*

leukocytoid (loo′kō-sī″toyd) [″ + ″ + *eidos,* form, shape]. Resembling a leukocyte.

leukocytolysin. A lysin that destroys leukocytes. SEE: *leukocidin.*

leukocytolysis (loo″kō-sī-tŏl′ĭ-sĭs) [″ + *kytos,* cell, + *lysis,* dissolution]. Destruction of leukocytes.

leukocytoma (loo″kō-sī-tō′mă) [″ + ″ + *oma,* tumor]. 1. Tumor composed of cells resembling leukocytes. 2. Tumorlike mass of leukocytes.

leukocytopenia (loo″kō-sī″tō-pē′nē-ă) [″ + ″ + *penia,* want]. An abnormal decrease in leukocytes, usually below 5000 per cu. mm. SYN: *leukopenia.*

leukocytoplania (loo″kō-sī″tō-plā′nē-ă) [″ + ″ + *plane,* wandering]. The passage of leukocytes from blood vessels into the tissues, or through membranes.

leukocytopoiesis (loo″kō-sī″tō-poy-ē′sĭs) [″ + ″ + *poiein,* to make]. Formation of white blood cells.

leukocytosis (loo″kō-sī-tō′sĭs) [″ + *kytos,* cell, + *osis,* condition]. Increase in number of leukocytes (above 10,000 per cu. mm) in the blood, generally caused by presence of infection and usually transient. It also may accompany or occur after the following conditions: hemorrhage, extensive operations, coronary occlusion, malignant growth, pregnancy, certain intoxications, and toxemias. Eosinophilic leukocytosis occurs in some allergies, animal parasite infestation, and Hodgkin's disease.

Leukemias, however, are associated with production of immature leukocytes due to abnormal condition of blood-forming organs. Leukocytosis is present in most infections but not usually in those due to a virus.

In leukocytosis the numbers of white cells may vary from a 50% increase to many times more than normal. In leukemia there may be as many as one million white cells per cu. mm. Leukocytosis is early and marked in severe infections when the patient's resistance is good; if infection and resistance are less marked it appears later to a lesser degree and disappears more quickly. Leukocytosis may occur in unusually virulent infections, such as diphtheria, pneumonia, and sepsis. SEE: *leukopenia.*

   l., basophilic. An increase in the basophils in the blood.

   l., mononuclear. An increase in the monocytes in the blood.

   l., pathologic. Leukocytosis due to a disease such as an infection.

leukocytotaxis (loo″kō-sī″tō-tăk′sĭs) [Gr. *leukos,* white, + *kytos,* cell, + *taxis,* arrangement]. The movement of leukocytes either toward or away from an area such as a traumatized or infected site.

leukocytotoxin (loo″kō-sī″tō-tŏk′sĭn) [″ + ″ + *toxikon,* poison]. A toxin that destroys leukocytes.

leukocyturia (loo″kō-sī-tū′rē-ă) [″ + ″ + *ouron,* urine]. Leukocytes in the urine.

leukoderma (loo-kō-dĕr′mă) [″ + *derma,* skin]. Deficiency of pigmentation of the skin, esp. in patches. SEE: *vitiligo.*

   l., syphilitic. Macular depigmentation esp. of the skin of the neck and shoulders. Seen in late syphilis.

leukodiagnosis (loo″kō-dī″ăg-nō′sĭs) [″ + *dia,* through, + *gnosis,* knowledge]. Diagnosis by observance of number, variety, or reaction of leukocytes.

leukodystrophy (loo″kō-dĭs′trō-fē). Disease of the central nervous system in which the formation of the myelin is abnormal. This may be due to a specific biochemical defect. This is an incurable disease.

   l., metachromatic. A type of hereditary leukodystrophy caused by a deficiency of the enzyme cerebroside sulfatase, an enzyme that is essential for the degradation of sulfatide. Deficiency of the enzyme allows excess deposition of sulfatide in nerve tissues. Clinical signs of this disease usually appear at about one year of age. They include gait disturbance, inability to learn to walk, spasticity of limbs, hyperreflexia, dementia, and eventually death. The disease, for which there is no specific therapy, is usually fatal by age 10.

leukoedema (loo″kō-ĕ-dē′mă) [″ + *oidema,* swelling]. A benign leukophakia-like abnormality of the mucosa of the mouth or tongue. The affected areas are opalescent or white, and wrinkled.

leukoencephalitis (loo″kō-ĕn-sĕf-ă-lī′tĭs) [″ + *enkephalos,* brain + *itis,* inflammation]. Inflammation of the white matter of the brain.

leukoencephalopathy, progressive multifocal. ABBR: PML. Widespread demyelinating lesions of the brain, brain stem, and cerebellum. It is usually associated with chronic neoplastic diseases including Hodgkin's disease, chronic lymphocytic leukemia, and lymphosarcoma. It also occurs as a complication of AIDS, and in immunocompromised patients. Clinically there is paralysis, blindness, aphasia, ataxia, dysarthria, dementia, confusional states, and coma. Death occurs in 3 to 6 months of onset of neurological symptoms.

    ETIOL: JC virus (the initials of the first patient from whom the virus was isolated). TREAT: There is none.

leukoerythroblastosis (loo″kō-ĕ-rĭth″rō-blăs-tō′sĭs) [″ + *erythros,* red, + *blastos,* germ, + *osis,* condition]. Anemia due to any condition that causes the bone marrow to be infiltrated and thus inactivated.

leukokeratosis (loo″kō-kĕr-ă-tō′sĭs) [″ + *keras,* horn, + *osis,* condition]. White patch formation on the surface of the mucosa of the tongue, cheek, and gums. SYN: *leukoplakia.*

leukokoria (loo″kō-kō′rē-ă) [″ + *kore,* pupil]. Leukocoria, q.v.

leukokraurosis (loo″kō-kraw-rō′sĭs) [″ + *krauros,* dry, + *osis,* condition]. Kraurosis vulvae, q.v.

leukolymphosarcoma (loo″kō-lĭm″fō-săr-kō′mă) [″ + L. *lympha,* lymph, + Gr. *sarx,* flesh, + *oma,* tumor]. Lymphosarcoma cell leukemia.

leukolysis (loo-kŏl′ĭ-sĭs) [″ + *lysis,* dissolution]. Destruction of leukocytes. SYN: *leukocytolysis.*

leukoma (loo-kō′mă) [″ + *oma,* tumor]. A white, opaque corneal opacity.

    l. adherens. Corneal scar with incarcerated iris tissue.

leukomaine (loo′kō-mān) [Gr. *leukoma,* whiteness]. A group of substances normally present in living tissues. They resemble alkaloids, some are toxic, and some are physiologically active.

leukomainemia (loo″kō-mā-nē′mē-ă) [″ + *haima,* blood]. Excess of leukomaines in the blood.

leukomatous (loo-kō′mă-tŭs) [Gr. *leukos,* white, + *oma,* tumor]. 1. Pert. to leukoma. 2. Suffering from leukoma.

leukomyelitis (loo″kō-mī-ĕ-lī′tĭs) [″ + *myelos,* marrow, + *itis,* inflammation]. Inflammation of the white matter of the spinal cord.

leukomyelopathy (loo″kō-mī-ĕl-ŏp′ă-thē) [″ + ″ + *pathos,* disease]. Disease involving the white matter of the spinal cord.

leukonecrosis (loo″kō-nĕ-krō′sĭs) [″ + *nekrosis,* state of death]. Dry, light-colored, or white gangrene.

leukonychia (loo″kō-nĭk′ē-ă) [″ + *onyx,* nail]. White spots or streaks on the nails. SYN: *canities unguium.*

leukopathia (loo″kō-păth′ē-ă) [″ + *pathos,* disease]. 1. Absence of pigment in the skin. SEE: *leukoderma.* 2. Disease involving leukocytes.

    l. unguium. Leukonychia, q.v.

leukopedesis (loo″kō-pĕ-dē′sĭs) [″ + *pedan,* to leap]. Passage of leukocytes through walls of blood vessels.

leukopenia (loo″kō-pē′nē-ă) [″ + *penia,* lack]. Abnormal decrease of white blood corpuscles usually below 5000 per cu. mm. A great number of drugs may cause leukopenia, as can failure of the bone marrow. SYN: *granulocytopenia; leukocytopenia.*

leukoplakia (loo″kō-plā′kē-ă) [″ + *plax,* plate]. Formation of white spots or patches on the mucous membrane of the tongue or cheek. The spots are smooth, irregular in size and shape, hard, and occasionally fissured. The lesions may become malignant.

    l. buccalis. Leukoplakia of the mucosa of the cheek.

    l. lingualis. Leukoplakia of the tongue.

    l. vulvae. Atrophic disease affecting the female external genitalia seen most often in older women. Characterized by severe itching and a white marblelike appearance of the skin, frequently with excoriations. Without medical intervention, the skin may undergo malignant degeneration. SYN: *kraurosis vulvae.*

leukoplasia (loo-kō-plā′zē-ă). White patch formation on buccal mucosa. SYN: *leukoplakia.*

leukopoiesis (loo″kō-poy-ē′sĭs) [″ + *poiesis,* formation]. Leukocyte production. SYN: *leukocytogenesis.*

leukopoietic (loo″kō-poy-ĕt′ĭk) [″ + *poiein,* to make]. Forming leukocytes.

leukopsin. A substance formed in the rods of the retina from rhodopsin under the influence of light.

leukorrhagia (loo″kō-rā′jē-ă) [″ + *rhegnynai,* to burst forth]. Profuse white vaginal discharge. SYN: *leukorrhea.*

leukorrhea (loo″kō-rē′ă) [″ + *rhoia,* flow]. Usually white or yellow mucous discharge from the cervical canal or the vagina. There is frequently a so-called physiological leukorrhea that may be constantly present but somewhat increased preceding and following menstruation, and during sexual excitement. It may be of considerable concern to the young girl at the time of menarche because she has not been told that this white fluid would tend to collect on the vulvae. Leukorrhea may be abnormal if it is increased in amount; has a change in color; is malodorous; or contains blood.

    SYM: Usually indications of acute inflammation—pain, heat, redness of parts involved. Pain in groin, hypogastrium, sacral regions, and small of back. Urethra often implicated, causing painful micturition. Symptoms that may occur in connection with chronic leukorrhea are innumerable. Discharge may be of any consistency: thin and watery or viscid and tenacious; and it may or may not have a foul odor.

ETIOL: Pathological states of the endocervix and vagina. Infection by *Trichomonas vaginalis, Candida albicans,* and other pathogens.

TREAT: If due to a specific microorganism, treat with appropriate antibiotic. In general, douches are ineffective in curing the cause of this symptom. If due to senile changes in the vagina, estrogen-containing cream or ointment applied locally is quite effective.

leukosarcoma (loo″kō-sǎr-kō′mǎ) [Gr. *leukos,* white, + *sarx,* flesh, + *oma,* tumor]. A variation of malignant lymphoma in which the blood cells become leukemic.

leukosis (loo-kō′sĭs) [″ + *osis,* condition]. Abnormal proliferation of leukocyte-forming tissues.

leukotactic (loo″kō-tǎk′tĭk) [″ + *taxis,* arrangement]. Possessing the power of attracting leukocytes.

leukotaxine (loo″kō-tǎk′sĭn). A noncellular nitrogenous substance present in injured tissue.

leukotaxis (loo″kō-tǎks′ĭs). Possessing the power of attracting (positive leukotaxis) or repelling (negative leukotaxis) leukocytes.

leukotomy (loo-kŏt′ō-mē) [″ + *tome,* incision]. Lobotomy, q.v.

leukotoxic (loo″kō-tŏks′ĭk) [″ + *toxikon,* poison]. Destructive to leukocytes.

leukotoxin (loo″kō-tŏk′sĭn) [″ + *toxikon,* poison]. Leukocytotoxin, q.v.

leukotrichia (loo″kō-trĭk′ē-ǎ) [″ + *thrix,* hair]. Whiteness of the hair. SYN: *canities.*

leukotrienes. A group of arachidonic acid metabolites that function as chemical mediators of inflammation. Leukotrienes C4, D4 and E4, which constitute what was formerly known as the slow-releasing substance of anaphylaxis (SRS-A), are released by the mast cells after an IgE-antigen reaction. They are extremely powerful bronchial constrictors and vasodilators and mediate the adverse vascular and bronchial effects of systemic anaphylaxis. Leukotriene B4 also promotes chemotaxis, q.v.

leukous (loo′kŭs) [Gr. *leukos,* white]. White, esp. rel. to the skin.

levallorphan tartrate (lěv″ǎl-lor′fǎn). USP. A narcotic antagonist used to counteract morphine or opioid-induced respiratory depression. Trade name is Lorfan.

levamisole hydrochloride. An antihelminthic drug used originally in veterinary medicine. It is now used as adjuvant therapy in treating metastatic colorectal cancer. Trade name is Tramisol.

levarterenol bitartrate (lěv″ǎr-tě-rē′nŏl bī-tǎr′trāt). Previously used name for norepinephrine bitartrate, q.v. A sympathomimetic agent that, due to its vasopressor effect, may be useful in treating hypotension that accompanies shock. It is usually administered intravenously because it is rapidly inactivated. Trade name is Levophed.

levator (lē-vā′tor) [L., lifter] (pl. *levatores*). 1. [NA] A muscle that raises or elevates a part. Opposite of depressor. 2. An instrument that lifts depressed portions.

l. ani. A broad muscle that helps to form the floor of the pelvis.

l. palpebrae superioris. A muscle that elevates the upper eyelid.

LeVeen shunt [Harry LeVeen, U.S. surgeon, b. 1917]. Shunt from the peritoneal cavity to the venous circulation. Used to help control ascites by allowing ascitic fluid to enter the venous circulation.

level of activities. In the nervous system, connector neurons are grouped into levels corresponding to different stages of development: spinal cord level; medullary level; midbrain level; basal ganglial level; cortical level. Each level is responsible for certain activities but controlled by the one above it.

lever (lěv′ěr, lē′věr) [L. *levare,* to raise]. Rigid bar used to modify direction, force, and motion. A type of simple machine that provides the user with a mechanical advantage. Levers are used to facilitate the moving and lifting of objects too heavy or awkward for one to move unassisted.

levigation (lěv″ĭ-gā′shŭn) [L. *levigare,* to render smooth]. The grinding of a substance into a fine state, usually in water, and then letting the material settle in order to separate the coarser particles from the fine.

Levin's tube (lē-vĭnz′) [Abraham L. Levin, U.S. physician, 1880–1940]. A catheter that is usually introduced through the nose and extends through the stomach into the duodenum. It is used to help prevent accumulation of intestinal liquids and gas during and following intestinal surgery.

levitation [L. *levitas,* lightness]. The subjective sensation of rising in the air or moving through the air unsupported. Occurs in dreams, altered states of consciousness, and certain mental disorders.

levocardia (lē″vō-kǎr′dē-ǎ) [L. *laevus,* left, + Gr. *kardia,* heart]. Term describing the normal position of the heart when other viscera are inverted. SEE: *dextrocardia.*

levocarnitine. An amino acid-derived drug used in treating primary carnitine deficiency. Trade names are Carnitor, Vitacarn. SEE: *carnitine.*

levoclination (lē″vō-klī-nā′shŭn) [″ + *clinatus,* leaning]. Torsion or twisting of the upper meridians of the eyes to the left.

levocycloduction (lē″vō-sī″klō-dŭk′shŭn) [″ + Gr. *kyklos,* circle, + L. *ducere,* to lead]. Levoduction, q.v.

levodopa. USP. L-3,4-dihydroxyphenylalanine. Drug used in the treatment of Parkinson's disease. Trade names are Bendopa, Dopar, and Levopa. SYN: L-*dopa.*

Levo-Dromoran. Trade name for levorphanol tartrate, USP.

levoduction (lē″vō-dŭk′shŭn) [L. *laevus,* left, + *ducere,* to lead]. Movement or drawing toward the left, esp. of an eye.

levonordefrin (lē″vō-nor′dĕ-frĭn). USP. A vasoconstrictor drug used to prolong the action of local anesthetic agents. Trade name is Neo-Cobefrin.

Levopa. Trade name for levodopa, USP.

Levophed. Trade name for norepinephrine bitartrate.

levophobia (lĕv″ō-fō′bē-ă) [″ + Gr. *phobos,* fear]. Morbid dread of objects on the left side of the body.

Levoprome. Trade name for methotrimeprazine.

levopropoxyphene napsylate (lē″vō-prō-pŏk′sĕ-fēn). USP. An anticough drug used orally.

levorotation (lē″vō-rō-tā′shŭn) [″ + *rotare,* to turn]. Twisting or turning to the left. SYN: *levotorsion.*

levorotatory (lē″vō-rō′tă-tor-ē). Causing to turn toward the left, applied esp. to substances that turn polarized light rays to the left. SYN: *levogyrous.*

levorphanol tartrate (lĕv-or′fă-nōl). USP. A synthetic analgesic that acts similarly to morphine. Trade name is Levo-Dromoran.

levothyroxine sodium (lē″vō-thī-rŏk′sēn). USP. The sodium salt of the natural isomer of thyroxine used in treating thyroid deficiency. Trade name is Synthroid.

levotorsion, levoversion (lē″vō-tor′shŭn, lē″vō-vĕr′shŭn) [″ + *torsio,* a twisting]. 1. A twisting to the left. SYN: *levorotation.* 2. Levoclination, q.v.

levulinic acid. An acid formed when certain simple sugars are acted on by dilute hydrochloric acid.

levulose (lĕv′ū-lōs) [L. *laevus,* left]. SEE: *fructose.*

levulosemia (lĕv″ū-lō-sē′mē-ă) [″ + Gr. *haima,* blood]. Presence of fructose in the blood.

levulosuria (lĕv″ū-lō-sū′rē-ă) [″ + Gr. *ouron,* urine]. Presence of fructose in the urine.

lewisite (lū′ĭ-sīt) [Warren Lee Lewis, U.S. chemist, 1878–1943]. A toxic gas similar in action to mustard gas used in warfare to disable and kill. It acts as a vesicant in the lungs.

   TREAT: Dimercaprol, q.v.

Lewy bodies [Frederic H. Lewy, Ger. neurologist, 1885–1950]. Neuronal cells with pigmented inclusion bodies. They are found in the brain in the substantia nigra and locus ceruleus, esp. in Parkinson's disease.

Leyden jar (lī′dĕn) [Ernest V. von Leyden, Ger. physician, 1832–1910]. A glass jar coated partially inside and out with metal; it is used as a capacitor or collector of electricity.

Leydig cells (lī′dĭg) [Franz von Leydig, Ger. anatomist, 1821–1908]. Interstitial tissue cells in the testicles that produce testosterone.

L.F.A. *left frontoanterior* fetal position.

L-forms [named for *Lister* Institute]. Spontaneous variants of bacteria that replicate as spherically structured, filterable elements with defective or absent cell walls. They are filterable because of their flexibility rather than their size. Stable forms may grow for an indefinite time in a wall-less state. Organisms of the unstable form are capable of regenerating their cell walls and reverting to their antecedent bacterial form. The ability of L-forms to cause disease is doubtful. SYN: *L-phase variants.*

L.F.P. *left frontoposterior* fetal position.

L.F.T. *left frontotransverse* fetal position.

LGA. *large for gestational age.*

LH. *luteinizing hormone.*

Lhermitte's sign (lār′mĭts) [Jacques Jean Lhermitte, Fr. neurologist, 1877–1959]. The symptom (rather than a sign) of a pain resembling a sudden electric shock throughout the body produced by flexing the neck.

   ETIOL: Trauma to the cervical portion of the spinal cord, multiple sclerosis, cervical cord tumor, or cervical spondylosis.

LHRH. *luteinizing hormone releasing hormone.*

Li. Chem. symb. for the element lithium.

libidinous (lĭ-bĭd′ĭ-nŭs) [L. *libidinosus,* pert. to desire]. Characterized by sexual desires.

libido (lĭ-bī′dō, -bē′dō) [L., desire]. 1. The sexual drive, conscious or unconscious. 2. In psychoanalysis, the energy or force that is the driving force of human behavior. Variously identified as the sex urge, desire to live, desire for pleasure or satisfaction.

Libman-Sacks disease (lĭb′măn-săks′) [Emanuel Libman, U.S. physician, 1872–1946; Benjamin Sacks, U.S. physician 1896–1939]. Verrucous, nonbacterial endocarditis.

Libritabs. Trade name for chlordiazepoxide.

Librium. Trade name for chlordiazepoxide hydrochloride, USP.

lice. Pl. of louse.

licensure. In the health care profession, the granting of permission — official or legal, or both — to perform medical actions that are legally forbidden to be done by persons who are not so licensed. Whether or not one is qualified for such a license is usually determined by some official body representing the federal or state government.

l., individual. In the health care profession, licensure of an individual to perform certain medical actions.

l., institutional. In the health care business, the licensing of institutions such as hospitals, clinics, or corporations to perform certain medical care functions.

licentiate (lī-sĕn′shē-ăt). 1. An individual who practices a profession by the authority granted by a license. 2. In some countries, a medical practitioner who has no medical degree.

lichen (lī′kĕn) [Gr. *leichen*, lichen]. 1. Any form of papular skin disease; usually noting lichen planus. 2. In botany, any one of numerous plants consisting of a fungus growing symbiotically with certain algae. They form characteristic scaly or branching growths on rocks or barks of trees.

l., myxedematous. Generalized eruption of asymptomatic nodules due to mucinous deposits in the upper layers of the skin and in vessels and organs.

l. nitidus. A rare skin condition characterized by small, chronic, asymptomatic papules that are usually pink and are usually located only on the penis, abdomen, and flexor surfaces of the elbows and palms.

l. pilaris. L. spinulosus, q.v.

l. planopilaris. A form of lichen planus in which white shiny follicular papules are present along with the usual plane papules.

l. planus. Inflammatory pruritic lesions of the skin.

SYM: Begins with pinhead-sized papules, reddish or violaceous, glistening, then coalescing, forming rough, scaly patches; acute, subacute, or chronic itching, usually symmetrical lesions on the flexor surface of the arms, trunk, and genitalia, and on the oral and vaginal mucosa. According to type of lesion the disease may be lichen planus atrophicus, erythematosus, hypertrophicus, linearis or ruber moniliformis.

ETIOL: Unknown, but exposure to some chemicals may cause similar lesions on the skin.

TREAT: The disease, for which there is no specific therapy, is self-limiting but may last years, or recur. If exposure to a chemical is related to the onset of the disease, discontinue exposure to it. Local symptomatic therapy for itching and occlusive dressing with corticosteroid cream will be helpful. If mucosal lesions are severe, systemic corticosteroids are indicated.

PROG: Prolonged but favorable.

l. ruber moniliformis. Large verrucous

lesions of lichen planus arranged as the beads in a necklace.

l. ruber planus. L. planus, q.v.

l. sclerosus et atrophicus. Chronic skin eruption consisting of discrete or confluent flat-topped ivory-white papules, each of which contains a black keratotic plug. The lesions may be associated with intractable itching, esp. when they are in the anal and genital areas. Kraurosis vulvae, q.v., is frequently associated with this disease.

l. scrofulosus. An eruption of tiny punctate reddish-brown papules arranged in circles or groups in young persons with tuberculosis. The lesions are caused by the spread of the tubercle bacilli through the blood to the skin.

l. simplex chronicus. An itching papular eruption that is circumscribed and located on skin that has become thickened and pigmented due to the rubbing of it. SYN: *Vidal's disease.*

l. spinulosus. Form of lichen with a spine developing in each follicle. SYN: *keratosis pilaris.*

l. striatus. A papular eruption usually seen on one extremity of a child. It is arranged in linear groups and consists of pink papules. The disease, though self-limiting, may last for a year or longer.

l. tropicus. Form of lichen with redness and inflammatory reaction of the skin. SYN: *miliaria rubra; prickly heat.*

lichenification (lī-kĕn″ĭ-fĭ-kā′shŭn) [Gr. *leichen,* lichen, + L. *facere,* to make]. 1. Cutaneous thickening and hardening from continued irritation. 2. Changing of an eruption into one resembling a lichen.

lichenin (lī′kĕ-nĭn). A starch obtained from Icelandic moss. SYN: *moss starch.*

lichenoid (lī′kĕn-oyd) [″ + *eidos,* form, shape]. Resembling lichen.

Lichtheim's syndrome (lĭkt′hīmz) [Ludwig Lichtheim, Ger. physician, 1845–1928]. Subacute combined degeneration of the spinal cord associated with pernicious anemia.

licorice (lĭk′ĕr-ĭs, -ĕr-ĭsh) [ME.]. A dried root of *Glycyrrhiza glabra* used as a flavoring agent, demulcent, and mild expectorant. Glycyrrhiza is prepared from licorice. Ingestion of large amounts of licorice can cause salt retention, excess potassium loss in the urine, and elevated blood pressure. SYN: *glycyrrhiza.*

lid [ME.]. An eyelid.

Lida-Mantle. Trade name for lidocaine, USP.

lidocaine (lī′dō-kān). USP. A local anesthetic drug. Trade name is Xylocaine.

l. hydrochloride. USP. A local anesthetic that is also used intravenously to treat certain cardiac arrhythmias, esp. ventricular dysrhythmias. Trade names are

Lida-Mantle and Xylocaine.

lid reflex. Closure of eyelids resulting from direct corneal stimulation. SYN: *corneal reflex.*

lie, transverse. A position of the fetus in utero in which the long axis of the fetus is across the long axis of the mother. SEE: *presentation* for illus.

Lieberkühn crypts (lē′bĕr-kēn) [Johann N. Lieberkühn, Ger. anatomist, 1711–1756]. Simple tubular glands present in the intestinal mucosa. In their epithelium are found goblet cells, cells of Paneth, and argentaffin cells. The glands form minute invaginations opening between the bases of the villi. They lie in the lamina propria, their blind ends extending to the muscularis mucosa. In the large intestine they are longer and contain few if any Paneth cells and more goblet cells. They are arranged vertically with much regularity. SYN: *glands, Lieberkühn's.*

lie detector. A polygraph; an instrument for determining minor physiological changes assumed to occur under the stress of lying (or any other emotion). Variations in respiratory rhythm, pulse rate, blood pressure, and sweating of the hands are among the functions that are monitored. Increased perspiration lessens resistance to passage of electrical current. The test has popular appeal among law enforcement departments but results obtained are presumptive and not absolute; nevertheless, interpretations of polygraph data have been admitted as evidence in some legal proceedings. The advisability of accepting the results of polygraph tests is controversial.

lien (lī′ĕn) [L.]. [NA] The spleen.

  l. accessorius. [NA] Accessory spleen.

  l. mobilis. Floating spleen.

lienal (lī-ē′năl) [L. *lien,* spleen]. Rel. to the spleen. SYN: *splenic.*

lienitis (lī″ĕ-nī′tĭs) [″ + Gr. *itis,* inflammation]. Inflammation of the spleen. SYN: *splenitis.*

lienocele (lī-ē′nō-sēl) [″ + Gr. *kele,* tumor, swelling]. Splenic hernia. SYN: *splenocele.*

lienography (lī″ē-nŏg′ră-fē) [″ + Gr. *graphein,* to write]. Radiographic examination of the spleen after introduction of a contrast medium.

lienomalacia (lī-ē″nō-mă-lā′shē-ă) [″ + Gr. *malakia,* softening]. Softening of the spleen. SYN: *splenomalacia.*

lienomedullary (lī-ē″nō-mĕd′ū-lăr-ē) [″ + *medulla,* marrow]. Rel. to both the spleen and bone marrow.

lienomyelogenous (lī-ē″nō-mī-ĕl-ŏj′ĕ-nŭs) [″ + Gr. *myelos,* marrow, + *gennan,* to produce]. Derived from both the spleen and bone marrow.

lienomyelomalacia (lī-ē″nō-mī″ĕl-ō-mă-lā′ shē-ă) [″ + ″ + *malakia,* softening]. Softening of the spleen and bone marrow.

lienopancreatic (lī-ē″nō-păn″krē-ăt′ĭk) [″ + Gr. *pankreas,* pancreas]. Rel. to the spleen and pancreas.

lienorenal (lī-ē″nō-rē′năl) [″ + *renalis,* pert. to kidney]. Rel. to the spleen and kidney.

lienotoxin (lī-ē″nō-tŏk′sĭn) [″ + Gr. *toxikon,* poison]. Splenotoxin, q.v.

lientery (lī′ĕn-tĕr″ē) [Gr. *leios,* smooth, + *enteron,* intestine]. Diarrhea in which the stool contains undigested food.

lienunculus (lī″ĕn-ŭng′kū-lŭs). Accessory spleen.

life (līf) [AS.]. 1. State of being alive; quality manifested by metabolism, growth, reproduction, and adaptation to environment; state in which the organs of an animal or plant are capable of performing all or any of their functions. 2. Time between birth or inception and death of an organism. Biologically, the life of a system begins at the moment of conception and ends at death; however, for legal and other reasons the definition of when life begins and death occurs has been subject to a variety of interpretations. SEE: *death.* 3. The sum total of those properties that distinguish living things (animals or plants) from nonliving inorganic chemical matter or dead organic matter.

  RS: antibiotic; "bio-" words; death; vital; vitality.

life, beginning of. There is considerable controversy over the question of when life begins. This is so because some of those who favor abortion feel that life begins some considerable time after conception; others feel that life begins at the moment of conception.

life expectancy. The number of years that an average person of a given age may be expected to live as determined by mortality tables. The data from which such tables are constructed may be obtained as much as two decades or more prior to their date of publication. This is particularly true for data used for insurance purposes. SEE: table.

life extension. The concept that certain types of intervention may allow a person to live longer than would have been the case if those interventions had not been used. Examples would be in the areas of nutrition, exercise, abstinence from cigarettes, and not driving while intoxicated.

life lost, years of. SEE: *years of life lost.*

life review therapy. A type of insight-oriented therapy which was first described by Robert Butler in 1964. Life review therapy has a psychoanalytic theoretical base and is focused on conflict resolution. Life review

Life Expectancy (In Years)

Age	National Center for Health Statistics		
	1979–1981	1983	1984*
Total Population			
0	73.9	74.6	74.7
15	60.2	60.8	60.8
25	50.8	51.3	51.4
35	41.4	41.9	42.0
45	32.3	32.7	32.7
55	23.9	24.1	24.2
65	16.5	16.7	16.8
75	10.5	10.7	10.7
Male			
0	70.1	71.0	71.1
15	56.5	57.3	57.3
25	47.4	48.0	48.1
35	38.2	38.8	38.8
45	29.2	29.7	29.8
55	21.1	21.4	21.5
65	14.2	14.5	14.5
75	8.9	9.0	9.0
Female			
0	77.6	78.1	78.3
15	63.8	64.2	64.3
25	54.2	54.5	54.6
35	44.5	44.9	44.9
45	35.2	35.4	35.5
55	26.4	26.6	26.7
65	18.4	18.6	18.7
75	11.6	11.8	11.9

* Provisional
Source: Adapted from Statistical Bulletin, Jul–Sep 1986, p. 26.

therapy is generally conducted with persons who are near the end of their life cycle. The therapeutic process allows the patients to review their lives, come to terms with conflict, gain meaning from their lives, and die peacefully.

life satisfaction. Attitudes possessed by individuals concerning their present life situation and the extent to which they are either content or discontent. Sometimes used simultaneously with morale, successful aging, well-being.

life satisfaction index. ABBR: LSI. A self-reporting instrument measuring life satisfaction in the elderly. A total of five rating scales are used.

life sciences. All of the scientific disciplines concerned with living organisms and forces that affect living things; included are biology, zoology, medicine, dentistry, surgery, nursing, and psychology.

life span. The maximal obtainable age by a member of a species.

lifestyle. The pattern of living and behavior

of an individual, society, or culture, esp. as it distinguishes individuals concerned or included in the groups from other individuals or groups.

life support. Use of any technique, therapy, or device to assist in sustaining life. SEE: *basic life support.*

life support, withholding. Removal of or not giving medical interventions with the expectation that the patient will die as a result.

life-sustaining therapy. Therapy of a critically ill patient that if discontinued would cause the patient to die.

ligament (lĭg′ă-mĕnt) [L. *ligamentum*, a band]. 1. A band or sheet of strong fibrous connective tissue connecting the articular ends of bones serving to bind them together and to facilitate or limit motion. 2. A thickened portion or fold of peritoneum or mesentery that supports a visceral organ or connects it to another viscus. 3. A band of fibrous connective tissue connecting bones, cartilages, and other structures and serving for support or for attachment of fascia or muscles. 4. A cordlike structure representing the vestigial remains of a fetal blood vessel.

l., accessory. Ligament that supplements another, esp. one on the lateral surface of a joint. One outside of and independent of the capsule of a joint.

l., acromioclavicular. Ligament extending from the clavicle to the acromial process of the scapula.

l., alar. Ligament connecting the odontoid process of the atlas to the occipital bone. SYN: *l., apical.*

l., annular. A circular ligament, esp. one enclosing a head or radius or one holding the footplate of the stapes in the fenestra vestibuli.

l., apical. A single median ligament extending from the odontoid process to the occipital bone. SYN: *l., alar.*

l.'s, arcuate. The lateral, medial, and exterior ligaments that extend from the 12th rib to the transverse process of the 1st lumbar vertebra, to which the diaphragm is attached.

l., arterial. A fibrous cord extending from the pulmonary artery to the arch of the aorta, the remains of the ductus arteriosus of the fetus.

l.'s, auricular. The anterior, posterior, and superior auricular ligaments uniting the external ear to the temporal bone.

l., broad, of liver. A wide, sickle-shaped fold of peritoneum, attached to the lower surface of the diaphragm, the internal surface of the right rectus abdominis muscle, and the convex surface of the liver.

l., broad, of uterus. Folds of peritoneum attached to lateral borders of the uterus from insertion of the fallopian tube above to the pelvic wall. It consists of two leaves between which are found the remnants of the wolffian ducts, cellular tissues, and the major blood vessels of the pelvis.

l.'s, capsular. Heavy fibrous structures, lined with synovial membrane and surrounding articulations.

l.'s, carpal. Ligaments uniting the carpal bones.

l., caudal. Bundles of fibrous tissue uniting dorsal surfaces of the two lower coccygeal vertebrae and superjacent skin.

l., check. Ligament that restrains motion of a joint, esp. the lateral odontoid ligaments.

l., collateral. SEE: *collateral ligaments.*

l., conoid. Posterior portion of the coracoclavicular ligament.

l., coracoacromial. Broad triangular ligament attached to the outer edge of the coracoid process of the scapula and the tip of the acromion.

l., coracoclavicular. Ligament uniting the clavicle and coracoid process of the scapula.

l., coracohumeral. Broad ligament connecting the coracoid process of the scapula to the greater tubercle of the humerus.

l., coronary, of liver. A fold of peritoneum extending from the posterior edge of the liver to diaphragm.

l., costocolic. Ligament attaching the splenic flexure of the colon to the diaphragm.

l., costocoracoid. Ligament joining the first rib and coracoid process of the scapula.

l.'s, costotransverse. Ligaments uniting ribs with transverse processes of vertebrae.

l., costotransverse, middle. Ligament consisting of parallel fibers extending between a vertebra and its adjacent rib.

l.'s, costovertebral. Ligaments uniting the ribs and vertebrae.

l., cricopharyngeal. A ligamentous bundle between the upper and posterior border of the cricoid cartilage and the anterior wall of the pharynx.

l., cricothyroid. Ligament uniting cricoid and thyroid cartilages and the location for the horizontal incision (called coniotomy) to prevent choking.

l., cricotracheal. The ligamentous structure uniting the upper ring of the trachea and the cricoid cartilage.

l., cruciate. 1. Ligament of the ankle passing transversely across the dorsum of the foot that holds tendons of the anterior muscle group in place. 2. A cross-shaped ligament of the atlas consisting of the transverse ligament and superior and inferior bands, the former passing upwards and attaching to the margin of the foramen magnum, the latter passing downwards and attaching to the body of the atlas. 3. Two ligaments of the knee, the anterior passing from tibia to medial aspect of the lateral condyle of the femur, the posterior passing from the tibia to the lateral aspect of the medial condyle.

l., cruciform. A structure consisting of one ligament crossing another.

l., crural. L., inguinal.

l., deltoid. Interior lateral ligament of the ankle.

l., dentate. A fibrous band of pia mater extending the length of the spinal cord on each side between the spinal nerves. It has a scalloped appearance as it pierces the arachnoid to attach to the dura mater at regular intervals.

l., dentoalveolar. SYN: *periodontal ligament.*

l., falciform, of liver. A wide, sickle-shaped fold of peritoneum attached to the lower surface of the diaphragm, internal surface of the right rectus abdominis muscle, and convex surface of the liver.

l., fundiform, of penis. Ligament extending from lower portion of the linea alba and Scarpa's fascia to dorsum of the penis.

l., gastrophrenic. A fold of peritoneum between the esophageal end of the stomach and the diaphragm.

l., Gimbernat's. Triangular flat expansion of aponeurosis of abdominal external oblique muscle. Forming medial boundary of femoral ring. SYN: *l., lacunar.*

l., gingivodental. That part of the periodontal ligament that extends into the gingiva and blends with the connective tissue lamina propria.

l.'s, glenohumeral. Fibers of the coracohumeral ligament passing into the joint and inserted into the inner and upper part of the bicipital groove.

l., glenoid. Ligament that extends between palmar surfaces of phalanges and corresponding metacarpal bone.

l., Henle's. The lateral extension of the tendinous insertion of the rectus abdominis muscle. It is posterior to the falx inguinalis.

l., hepaticoduodenal. A fold of peritoneum from transverse fissure of liver to vicinity of the duodenum and right flexure of colon, forming anterior boundary of foramen of Winslow.

l., iliofemoral. Bundle of fibers forming the upper and anterior portion of the capsular ligament of the hip joint. Ligament that extends from ilium to intertrochanteric line. SYN: *Y ligament.*

l., iliolumbar. Ligament extending from 4th and 5th lumbar vertebrae to iliac crest.

l., iliopectineal. A portion of the pelvic fascia attached to the iliopectineal line and to the capsular ligament of the hip joint.

l., infundibulopelvic. The upper free edge of the broad ligament in which the ovarian artery is found. SYN: *l., suspensory, of ovary.*

l., inguinal. Ligament extending from anterior superior iliac spine to pubic tubercle. Forms lower margin of aponeurosis of exterior oblique muscle. SYN: *l., crural; l., Poupart's.*

l., interclavicular. Bundle of fibers between sternal ends of the clavicles, attached to interclavicular notch of sternum.

l., interspinal. Ligament extending from the superior margin of a spinous process of one vertebra to lower margin of one above.

l., ischiocapsular. Ligament extending from ischium to ischial border of acetabulum.

l., lacunar. L., Gimbernat's, q.v.

l., lateral occipitoatlantal. Ligament on each side between transverse processes of atlas and jugular process of the occipital bone.

l.'s, lateral odontoid. Strong ligaments extending between sides of odontoid process of the axis and inner sides of condyles of the occipital bone.

l.'s, lateral, of liver. Folds of peritoneum extending from lower surface of diaphragm to adjacent borders of right and left lobes of the liver. SYN: *triangular ligaments.*

l.'s, Lisfranc's. Cuneometatarsal interosseous ligaments. Ligaments that join the cuneiform bone to the metatarsal bone.

l., Lockwood's. Suspensory ligament of the eye.

l., medial. A broad ligament that connects the medial malleolus of the tibia to the tarsal bones.

l.'s, meniscofemoral. Two small ligaments of the knee, one anterior and one posterior. The anterior one attaches to the posterior area of the lateral meniscus and the anterior cruciate ligament. The posterior one attaches to the posterior area of the lateral meniscus and the medial condyle of the femur.

l.'s, nephrocolic. Fibrous strands that connect the kidneys with the ascending and descending colon.

l., nuchal. The upward continuation of the supraspinous ligament, extending from the 7th cervical vertebra to the occipital bone.

l.'s, palpebral. Two ligaments, medial and lateral, extending from tarsal plates of the eyelids to the frontal process of maxilla and the zygomatic bone respectively.

l., patellar. A strong, flat band securing the patella to the tibia. It is a continuation of the tendon of the quadriceps femoris muscle.

l., pectineal. A triangular-shaped ligament that extends from the medial end of the inguinal ligament and the pectineal line of the pubis.

l., periodontal. The connective tissue that surrounds the roots of teeth and holds them in the sockets of the teeth.

l., Petit's. A thickened portion of the pelvic fascia between the cervix and vagina. It passes posteriorly in the rectouterine fold to attach to the anterior surface of the sacrum.

l., phrenocolic. A fold of peritoneum joining the left colic flexure of the colon to the adjacent costal portion of the diaphragm.

l., popliteal arcuate. Ligament on the posterolateral side of the knee, extending from the head of the fibula to the joint capsule.

l., Poupart's. L., inguinal.

l., pterygomandibular. Band of fiber extending between apex of internal pterygoid plate of sphenoid bone and the posterior extremity of internal oblique line of mandible.

l.'s, pubic arcuate. Ligaments connecting the pubic bones at the symphysis pubis. Include anterior and superior pubic ligaments and the arcuate (inferior) ligament.

l., pulmonary. A fold of pleura that extends from the hilus of the lung to the base of the medial surface of the lung.

l., rhomboid, of clavicle. A strong structure extending from the tuberosity of the clavicle to outer surface of the cartilage of the first rib.

l., round, of femur. Ligament of the head of the femur that is attached to the anterior superior part of the fovea of the head of the femur and to the sides of the acetabular notch.

l., round, of liver. Fibrous cord extending upward from the umbilicus and enclosed in lower margin of the falciform ligament. Represents obliterated left umbilical vein of the fetus.

l., round, of uterus. Ligament attached to uterus immediately below and in front of the entrance of the fallopian tube. Each extends laterally in the broad ligament to the pelvic wall, where it passes through inguinal ring, terminating in the labium majus.

l.'s, sacroiliac. Two ligaments, the anterior and posterior, that connect sacrum and ilium.

l., sacrospinous. Ligament extending from the spine of the ischium to sacrum and coccyx in front of the sacrotuberous ligament.

l., sacrotuberous. Ligament extending from tuberosity of the ischium to posterior superior and inferior iliac spines and to lower part of sacrum and coccyx.

l., sphenomandibular. Ligament attached superiorly to spine of sphenoid and inferiorly to lingula of mandible.

l., spiral, of cochlea. The thickened periosteum of the peripheral wall of the osseous cochlear canal. The basilar membrane is attached to its inner surface.

l., stylohyoid. A thin fibroelastic cord between lesser cornu of hyoid bone and apex of styloid process of the temporal bone.

l., stylomandibular. A thin fibrous band of tissue extending between styloid process of temporal bone and lower part of posterior border of ramus of the mandible. SYN: *stylomaxillary ligament.*

l., suprascapular. A thin fibrous band of tissue extending from base of coracoid process of scapula to inner margin of suprascapular notch.

l., supraspinal. Ligament uniting apices of spinous processes of vertebrae.

l., suspensory. Ligament suspending an organ.

l., suspensory, of axilla. The continuation of the clavipectoral fascia down to attach to the axillary fascia.

l., suspensory, of lens. The zonula ciliaris (ciliary zonule); the fibers holding the crystalline lens in position.

l., suspensory, of ovary. Ligament extending from tubal end of ovary laterally to pelvic wall. It lies in layers of the broad ligament. SYN: *l., infundibulopelvic.*

l., suspensory, of penis. A triangular bundle of fibrous tissue extending from anterior surface of the symphysis pubis and adjacent structures to the dorsum of the root of the penis.

l.'s, suspensory, of uterus. The broad ligaments, the round ligaments, and the rectouterine folds of the uterus.

l.'s, sutural. Thin, fibrous layers interposed between articulating surfaces of bones united by suture.

l., temporomandibular. The thickened portion of the joint capsule that passes from the articular tubercle at the root of the zygomatic arch to attach to the subcondylar neck of the mandible.

l., tendinotrochanteric. Ligament that forms a part of the capsule of the hip joint.

l., transverse crural. Ligament lying on anterior surface of leg just above ankle.

l., transverse humeral. A fibrous band that bridges the bicipital groove of the humerus in connecting the lesser and greater tuberosities.

l., transverse, of atlas. A strong ligament passing over the odontoid process of the axis.

l., transverse, of hip joint. A ligamentous band extending across cotyloid notch of the acetabulum.

l., transverse, of knee joint. A fibrous band extending from anterior margin of external semilunar fibrocartilage of knee to extremity of the internal semilunar fibrocartilage.

l., trapezoid. Anterior exterior portion of the coracoclavicular ligament.

l.'s, triangular, of liver. Two ligaments, right and left, that connect posterior aspects of right and left lobes with corresponding portions of the diaphragm.

l., umbilical, lateral. Fibrous cord extending from bladder to umbilicus. Represents obliterated interior iliac artery of fetus.

l., umbilical, median. Fibrous cord extending from apex of bladder to umbilicus. Represents the remains of the urachus of fetus.

l., uterorectosacral. Ligament that arises from the sides of the cervix and passes upwards and backwards, passing around the rectum, to the second sacral vertebra. They are enclosed within the rectouterine folds, which demarcate borders of the rectouterine pouch.

l., uterosacral. L., Petit's, q.v.

l., venous, of liver. A solid fibrous cord representing obliterated ductus venosus of the fetus. It lies between the caudate and left lobes of the liver and connects the left branch of the portal vein to the interior vena cava.

l., ventricular, of larynx. The lateral free margin of the quadrangular membrane. It is enclosed within and supports the ventricular fold.

l., vesicouterine. Ligament that attaches the anterior aspect of the uterus to the bladder.

l., vestibular. A thin fibrous band attached anteriorly to the lamina of the thyroid cartilage and posteriorly to the anterior portion of the arytenoid cartilage.

l., vocal. The thickened free edges of the elastic cone extending from thyroid angle to vocal processes of arytenoid cartilages. They support the vocal folds, q.v.

l., Weitbrecht's. The oblique band connecting the ulna and radius.

l.'s, yellow. Ligaments connecting laminae of adjacent vertebrae.

ligamenta. Pl. of ligamentum.

ligamentopexis (lĭg″ă-měn″tō-pěks′ĭs) [L. *ligamentum*, band, + Gr. *pexis*, fixation]. Suspension of uterus on the round ligament.

ligamentous (lĭg″ă-měn′tŭs) [L. *ligamentum*, band]. 1. Rel. to a ligament. 2. Like a ligament.

ligamentum (lĭg″ă-měn′tŭm) [L., a band] (pl. *ligamenta*). [NA] Ligament.

ligand (lī′gănd, lĭg′ănd) [L. *ligare*, to bind]. 1. In chemistry, an organic molecule attached to a central metal ion by multiple bonds. 2. In immunology, a small molecule bound to another chemical group or molecule.

ligase (lī′gās, lĭg′ās). General term for a class of enzymes that catalyze the joining of the ends of two chains of DNA.

ligate (lī′gāt). To apply a ligature.

ligation (lī-gā′shŭn). The application of a ligature.

ligature (lĭg′ă-chūr) [L. *ligatura*, a binding]. 1. Process of binding or tying. 2. A band or bandage. 3. A thread or wire for tying a blood vessel or other structure in order to constrict or fasten it. Cord or material used may be catgut, q.v., synthetic suture materials such as nylon or Dacron, kangaroo gut, polyglycolic acid, and natural fibers such as

silk or cotton. Sometimes strips of fascia obtained from the patient are used as a ligature. SEE: *suture*.

light (līt) [AS. *leohte*, not heavy]. 1. Not heavy. 2. Pale.

light (līt) [AS. *lihtan*, to shine]. The sensation produced by electromagnetic radiation that falls on the retina. Radiant energy producing a sensation of luminosity on the retina is limited to a wavelength of about 400 nanometers (extreme violet) to 770 nanometers (extreme red). SEE: *laser; ray; seasonal affective disorder.*

l., axial. Light with rays parallel to each other and to optic axis.

l., cold. Any form of light that is not perceptibly warm. The heat of ordinary light rays is dissipated when they are passed through some medium such as quartz.

l., diffused. Rays broken by refraction.

l., idioretinal; l., intrinsic. The sensation of light when there are no retinal stimuli to produce that sensation.

l., oblique. Light that strikes a surface obliquely.

l., polarized. Light in which waves vibrate in one direction only.

l., reflected. Light rays that are thrown back by an illuminated object such as a mirror.

l., refracted. Rays bent from original course.

l., transmitted. Light that passes through an object.

l., white. Light that contains all of the visible wavelengths of light.

l., Wood's. Ultraviolet light of approximately 365 nanometers wavelength, used in diagnosing fungus infections of the scalp and in detecting materials that fluoresce.

light, words pert. to: "actin-" words; Fraunhofer's lines; heliotherapy; lambert; lumen; lux; "phot-" words; "radi-" words; ray; reflection; reflector; refraction; spectrum.

light adaptation. Changes that occur in a dark-adapted eye in order for vision to occur in moderate or bright light. Principal changes are contraction of pupil and bleaching of visual purple in the rods. Bright sunlight is 30,000 times the intensity of bright moonlight, but the eye adapts so that visual function is possible under both conditions. SEE: *night vision; vision.*

light cast. A cast used in orthopedics. It is made of a lightweight material that is usually applied and then hardened by treating with the heat from a light.

light diet. Diet consisting of all foods allowed in soft diet, q.v., plus whole-grained cereals, easily digested raw fruits and vegetables. Foods not pureed or ground. Used as an intermediate regimen for patients who do not require a soft diet but are not yet able to resume a full diet.

light difference. The difference with respect to sensitiveness to intensity of light between the two eyes.

lightening [AS. *leohte,* not heavy]. Descent of presenting part of fetus into the pelvis. This often occurs two to three weeks prior to the beginning of the first stage of labor. It may not occur in multiparas until active labor begins. SEE: *labor.* SYN: *engagement.*

light-headed. Feeling of dizziness or of being about to faint. May be a sign of postural hypotension. SEE: *vertigo, benign positional.*

lightning. The discharge of atmospheric electricity from cloud to cloud or cloud to earth. About 100 lightning strokes hit the earth every second. Thirty percent of persons struck by lightning will die. SEE: *lightning safety rules.*

lightning safety rules. The estimated 100 deaths that occur annually in the U.S. from electrocution due to lightning could be reduced by observing these rules: During a lightning storm remain indoors; do not stay near open doors, fireplaces, radiators, appliances; do not use plug-in electric equipment such as hair dryers, electric toothbrushes, or electric razors; do not take laundry off clotheslines; do not work on fences, computers or word processors, a telephone or telephone line, power lines, pipelines, or structural steel construction, or metal objects such as fishing rods or golf clubs; if working on a tractor, get off it and either seek shelter or, if none is available, drop to the ground away from tractor, avoid hilltops; in a forest, seek shelter in a low area under a thick growth of small trees; avoid open spaces, wire fences, metal clotheslines, exposed sheds, and all electrically conductive elevated objects; get out of water and off small boats; stay in the automobile if traveling; if an electrical charge is evidenced by hair standing on end or tingling of skin, drop to the ground immediately because of immediate danger of being struck by lightning.

lightning streaks, Moore's. SEE: *Moore's lightning streaks.*

light reflex. Constriction of the pupil when light is flashed into the eye.

light sense. One of the three parts of visual function. The others are color sense and form sense. It is tested by visual field examination. SEE: *color sense; form sense.*

light therapy. The use of light rays in the treatment of disease. Includes use of ultraviolet and infrared radiations. Light intensity, esp. in winter, may have an important influence on seasonal depression. SYN: *phototherapy.*

light unit. A foot-candle. This is the amount

of light measured one foot from a standard candle. The ideal amount of light required for work varies with the specific type of work being done. The term foot-candle took the place of candle power, but light intensity in the International System of Units is indicated by lumen.

lignin (lĭg′nĭn). A polysaccharide present in plants that combines with cellulose to form the cell walls.

lignocaine (lĭg′nō-kān). A local anesthetic. SEE: *lidocaine hydrochloride.*

lignoceric acid. A saturated, naturally occurring fatty acid, $C_{24}H_{48}O_2$, present in certain foods, including peanuts.

limb (lĭm) [AS. *lim*]. 1. An arm or leg. 2. An extremity. 3. A limblike extension of a structure.

RS: anisomelia; appendicular; extremity; member.

   l., anacrotic. The ascending portion of the pulse wave.

   l., anterior, of internal capsule. The lenticulocaudate portion that lies between lenticular and caudate nuclei.

   l., ascending, of renal tubule. Portion of tubule between the bend in Henle's loop and the distal convoluted section.

   l., catacrotic. The descending portion of the pulse wave.

   l., descending, of renal tubule. Portion of tubule between proximal convoluted section and the bend in Henle's loop.

   l., pectoral. The arm.

   l., pelvic. The lower extremity.

   l., phantom. The perception and sensation that an amputated limb is still present. It may be associated with painful paresthesias, pain, and itching.

   l., thoracic. The upper extremity.

limbic (lĭm′bĭk) [L. *limbus,* border]. Pert. to a limbus or border. SYN: *marginal.*

limbic system. A group of brain structures, including the hippocampus, amygdala, dentate gyrus, cingulate gyrus, gyrus fornicatus, the archicortex, and their interconnections and connections with the hypothalamus, septal area, and a medial area of the mesencephalic tegmentum. The system is activated by motivated behavior and arousal, and it influences the endocrine and autonomic motor systems.

limbus (lĭm′bŭs) [L., border] (pl. *limbi*). [NA] The edge or border of a part.

   l. alveolaris. 1. The upper free edge of the alveolar process of the mandible. 2. The lower free edge of the alveolar process of the maxilla. SYN: *arcus alveolaris maxillae.*

   l. conjunctivae. The edge of the conjunctiva overlapping the cornea.

   l. corneae. [NA] The edge of the cornea where it unites with the sclera.

l., corneoscleral. In the eye, a transitional dome 1 or 2 mm wide where the cornea joins the sclera and conjunctiva.

l. fossae ovalis. [NA] The thickened margin of the fossae ovalis, esp. the rim of the septum secundum bounding the fossa.

l. laminae spiralis osseae. Thickening of the periosteum of the osseous spiral lamina of the cochlea to which the tectorial membrane is attached.

limbi palpebrales, anteriores. The anterior margin of the free edge of the eyelids from which the cilia or eyelashes grow.

limbi palpebrales, posteriores. The posterior margin of the free edge of the eyelids; the region of transition of skin to conjunctival mucous membrane.

l. sphenoidalis. Ridge on anterior portion of upper surface of sphenoid bone.

lime (līm) [AS. *lim*, glue]. USP. Calcium oxide, CaO. A substance obtained from limestone. Calcium oxide is prepared from limestone, $CaCO_3$, by heating it sufficiently to drive off the carbon dioxide. When lime is mixed with water, heat is produced. Lime is an ingredient of cement and mortar. SYN: *calcium oxide; quicklime.* SEE: *calcium.*

Caution: Avoid contact with eyes when working with lime.

---

l., chlorinated. Substance resulting from chlorination of slaked lime, consisting chiefly of calcium chloride and calcium hypochlorite. Used principally as a disinfectant and in aqueous solution as a bleaching agent.

l., slaked. The substance produced when lime is allowed free access to water and carbon dioxide from the atmosphere. It is a mixture of calcium hydroxide, $Ca(OH)_2$, and calcium carbonate, $CaCO_3$.

l., soda. A combination of calcium oxide and sodium hydroxide.

l., sulfurated. USP. Solution of lime, sublimated sulfur, and water. Used as a topical solution in treating skin disease.

l. water. Alkaline solution of calcium hydroxide, $Ca(OH)_2$, in water; a weak base used as an antacid.

lime [Fr.]. Fruit of *Citrus aurantifolia.* Its juice is antiscorbutic.

limen (lī'měn) [L.] (pl. *limina*). [NA] Entrance, threshold.

l. nasi. The boundary line between the bony and cartilaginous portion of the nasal cavity. It is also at this point that the nasal cavity proper and the vestibule of the nose meet.

l. of insula. The portion of the cortex of the brain that provides a threshold to the insula. The middle cerebral artery passes over

this threshold to extend to the insula.

limes nul. The greatest amount of toxin that when mixed with one unit of antitoxin and injected into a guinea pig weighing 250 gm will cause no local reaction. SYMB: L_0.

limes tod. The least amount of toxin that when mixed with one unit of antitoxin and injected into a guinea pig weighing 250 gm will kill it within 96 hours. SYMB: L_+.

limestone. Rock formed of organic fossil remains of shells. It contains mostly calcium carbonate. SEE: *lime.*

liminal (lĭm'ĭ-năl) [L. *limen*, threshold]. Hardly perceptible; rel. to a threshold as of consciousness or vision. SEE: *subliminal.*

limit (lĭm'ĭt). 1. A boundary. 2. A point or line beyond which something cannot or may not progress.

l., assimilation. The amount of carbohydrate that can be absorbed or ingested without causing glycosuria.

l., audibility. The limits of sound frequencies at both the low and high ends of the sound scale beyond which sound cannot be heard. The lower limit is approximately 8 to 16 Hz (cycles per second) and the upper limit between 12,000 and 20,000 Hz, depending upon various factors, including age. In general, the upper limit of audible sound decreases with age.

l., elastic. The extent to which something may be stretched or bent and still have the ability to return to its original shape.

l., Hayflick's. The number of cell divisions that will take place in human cell cultures prior to dying out. This is estimated to be about 50 cell divisions.

l. of flocculation. The amount of a toxin or toxoid that causes the most rapid flocculation when combined with its antitoxin.

l. of perception. The smallest object that can be detected by the eye. Such an object usually subtends a visual image of one minute. This produces a retinal image slightly larger than the diameter of a retinal cone, i.e., about 0.004 mm. SYN: *normal limit of visual acuity.*

l., quantum. The minimum wavelength present in the spectrum produced by x-rays.

limitans (lĭm'ĭ-tăns) [L. *limitare*, to limit]. 1. Used in conjunction with other words to denote limiting. 2. Used synonymously to indicate membrane limitans.

limitation (lĭm"ĭ-tā'shŭn). Condition of being limited.

limitation of motion. The restriction of movement or range of motion of a part or joint, esp. that imposed by disease or trauma to joints and soft tissues.

limnology [Gr. *limne*, pool, + *logos,* study]. Scientific study of all of the features of a body of fresh water such as a pond, lake, or river that are important ecologically, i.e., potability, pH, degree of pollution, mineral content, and variation with seasonal and climatic changes.

limosis (lĭ-mō′sĭs) [Gr. *limos*, hunger]. Abnormal hunger; perverted appetite.

limotherapy (lĭ″mō-thĕr′ă-pē) [″ + *therapeia*, treatment]. Treatment of obesity by restriction of diet or by fasting.

limp. To walk with abnormal, jerky movements.

limulus amebocyte lysate test. ABBR: LAL test. Limulus amebocyte lysate is formed from the lysed circulating amebocytes of the horseshoe crab *(Limulus polyphemus)*. The lysate is used to detect minute quantities of bacterial endotoxins, and has been used to test for pyrogens in various materials. It is also used to detect septicemia due to gram-negative bacteria.

Lincocin. Trade name for lincomycin hydrochloride.

lincomycin hydrochloride (lĭn″kō-mī′sĭn). USP. An antibiotic obtained from *Streptomyces lincolnensis*. Trade name is Lincocin.

lincture, linctus (lĭnk′tŭr, -tŭs) [L. *linctus*, a licking]. A thick, sweet, syrupy medicinal preparation given for its effect on the throat. Usually taken in sips or may be licked or sucked as with a throat lozenge.

lindane (lĭn′dān). USP. A miticide used in treating scabies. Trade names are Scabene and Kwell, whose formulations include lindane.

Lindau's disease (lĭn′dowz) [Arvid Lindau, Swedish pathologist, 1892–1958]. Lindau-von Hippel disease, q.v.

Lindau-von Hippel disease (lĭn′dow-vŏn hĭp′ĕl) [Arvid Lindau; Eugen von Hippel, Ger. ophthalmologist, 1867–1939]. Angiomata of the retina and cysts and angiomata of the brain and certain visceral organs.

line (lĭn) [L. *linea*]. 1. Any long, relatively narrow mark. 2. A boundary or an outline. 3. A wrinkle. 4. In anthropometry or cephalometry, an imaginary line connecting two anatomical points. This is necessary to establish a plane or an axis. 5. A catheter or a wire attached to a patient, as an I.V. line or arterial line.

l., abdominal. Line indicating abdominal muscle boundaries.

l., absorption. A black line in the continuous spectrum of light passing through an absorbing medium.

l., alveolobasilar. Line from basion to alveolar point.

l., alveolonasal. Line from alveolar point to nasion.

l., auriculobregmatic. Line from auricular point to bregma.

l.'s, axillary. Anterior, posterior, and midaxillary lines that extend downward from the axilla.

l., base. Line from the infraorbital ridge through the middle of the external auditory meatus to midline of occiput.

l., basiobregmatic. Line from basion to bregma.

l., Baudelocque's. Exterior conjugate diameter of pelvis.

l.'s, Beau's. Transverse lines on the fingernails formed at the base of the nail, usually in response to local trauma, malnutrition, or systemic disease. They become visible as the nail grows. Their distance from the base of the nail can provide a rough estimate of the time of occurrence of the cause.

l., biauricular. Line from one auditory meatus over vertex to the other.

l., blue. Line seen on gums in chronic lead poisoning.

l., canthomeatal. Imaginary line extending from the canthus of the eye to the center of the external auditory meatus. SYN: *orbitomeatal line.*

l., cement. The refractile boundary of an osteon or the haversian system of a bone.

l., cervical. 1. Line of junction of cementum and enamel of a tooth. 2. Line on neck of tooth where gum is attached.

l.'s, cleavage. Langer's lines, q.v.

l., costoarticular. Line from sternoclavicular joint to point on 11th rib.

l., costoclavicular. Line midway between nipple and sternum border.

l., Douglas'. A crescent-shaped line at the lower limit of the posterior sheath of the rectus abdominis muscle. It is sometimes indistinct.

l., epiphyseal. Line at the junction of the epiphysis and diaphysis of a long bone. It is at this junction that bone growth occurs.

l., gingival. Line determined by the extent of coverage of the tooth by gingiva; the shape of the gingival line is similar to the curvature of the cervical line but they rarely coincide. Also called free gingival margin.

l., glabelloalveolar. An imaginary line through the glabella on the frontal bone and the alveolar process of the maxilla.

l., glabellomeatal. Imaginary line that extends from the glabella to the center of the external auditory meatus and is used for radiographic positioning of the skull.

l.'s, gluteal. Three lines, anterior, posterior, and inferior, on exterior surface of ilium.

l., gum. Line formed by the gingival margin of the neck of the tooth. SYN: *gingival line.*

l., iliopectineal. Bony ridge marking the brim of the pelvis.

l., incremental One of the lines seen in a microscopic section of the enamel of a tooth. They resemble growth lines in a tree.

l., incremental, of Retzius. Periodic dark lines seen in the enamel of a tooth that represent occasional metabolic disturbances of mineralization.

l., incremental, of von Ebner. Very light lines in the dentin of a tooth that represent the boundary between the layers of dentin produced daily.

l., infraorbitomeatal. Imaginary line from the inferior orbital margin to the external auditory meatus, which is used for radiographic positioning of the skull.

l., interauricular. Line joining the two auricular points.

l., intercondylar. Transverse ridge joining condyles of femur above the intercondyloid fossa.

l., interpupillary. Imaginary line between the centers of the eyes, which is used for radiographic positioning of the skull.

l., intertrochanteric. Ridge upon posterior surface of femur exterior between the greater and lesser trochanters.

l., intertuberal. Line joining inner borders of the ischial tuberosities below the small sciatic notch.

l.'s, Kerley's. Lines present on roentgenograms of the chest of patients with any disease that causes thickening or infiltration of the interlobular septa. Those in the costophrenic angle area are called Kerley B lines, and those extending peripherally from the hilum are termed Kerley A lines. Kerley C lines are fine lines in the middle of pulmonary tissue.

l., lead. An irregular dark line in the gingival margin. The line is present in chronic lead poisoning and is caused by the deposition of lead in that portion of the gum.

l., lip. The highest or lowest point the lips reach on the teeth or gums during a broad smile.

l., mamillary. Vertical line through the center of the nipple.

l., mammary. Horizontal line from one nipple to the other.

l., median. Line joining any two points in the periphery of the median plane of the body or one of its parts.

l., mentomeatal. Imaginary line from the mental point of the mandible to the external auditory meatus used in radiography of the skull.

l., milk. The mammary ridge, an ectodermal thickening in the embryo exterior between bases of limb buds.

l., mucogingival. SEE: *junction, mucogingival.*

l., mylohyoid. Ridge on the inner surface of the mandible. It extends from a point beneath the mental spine upward and back to the ramus past the last molar. The mylohyoid muscle and the superior constrictor muscle of the pharynx attach to this ridge.

l., nasobasilar. Line through basion and nasion.

l., nuchal, superior and inferior. Two curved ridges on occipital bone extending laterally from exterior occipital crest.

l., oblique, of fibula. The medial crest of posteromedial border; a line extending from the medial side of the head and terminating distally at the interosseous crest.

l., oblique, of radius. Faint ridge on anterior surface passing downward and laterally from radial tuberosity.

l. of demarcation. Line of division between healthy and diseased tissue.

l. of fibula, oblique. Prominent ridge on the interior surface of the shaft of the fibula.

l. of fixation. Imaginary line drawn from subject viewed to the fovea centralis.

l. of ilium, intermediate. Ridge upon crest of ilium between inner and outer lip.

l. of mandible, oblique. Ridge on outer surface of lower jaw.

l.'s of Owen [Sir Richard Owen, Brit. anatomist, 1804–1892]. Occasional prominent growth lines or bands in the dentin of a tooth. They provide a record of the growth of the coronal or radicular dentin. SYN: *contour lines.*

l., parasternal. Line midway between nipple and border of sternum.

l., pectineal. Line on posterior surface of femur extending downward from lesser trochanter. That portion of the iliopectineal line formed by the os pubis.

l., popliteal, of femur. Oblique line on posterior surface of tibia.

l., popliteal, of tibia. Line of posterior surface of tibia, extending obliquely downward from the fibular facet on lateral condyle to the medial border of bone.

l., resting. Smooth cement line seen in microscopic sections that separates old bone from newly formed bone.

l., reversal. Cement line seen in microscopic sections of bone that shows scallops and irregularites representing earlier bone resorption. Resorption to that point occurred before the process reversed and new bone was formed by apposition. SEE: *Howship's lacunae.*

l., scapular. Line extending downward from the lower angle of the scapula.

l., semilunar. The curved groove in the external abdominal wall. This is over the lateral border of the sheath of the rectus abdominis muscle. SYN: *spigelian line.*

l., Shenton's. In a roentgenogram of the

hip joint, a curved line extending from the upper limit of the obturator foramen to the middle of the neck of the femur.

l., sight. Line from center of pupil to viewed object.

l., sternal. Medial line of the sternum.

l., sternomastoid. Line from between heads of sternomastoid muscle to mastoid process.

l.'s, supracondylar, medial and lateral. Two ridges on posterior surface of distal end of femur, formed by diverging lips of the linea aspera.

l., supraorbital. Line across forehead above root of exterior angular process of frontal bone.

l., temporal, of frontal bone. Two curved lines on lateral surface of skull, passing upwards and backwards from zygomatic process of frontal bone and terminating posteriorly at supramastoid crest.

l., umbilicopubic. That portion of median line extending from umbilicus to symphysis pubis.

l., visual. Line that extends from object to macula lutea passing through the nodal point. SYN: *visual axis.*

l.'s, Zöllner's. Parallel lines, usually three long ones, with a series of short lines drawn at regular intervals across one of the lines at approximately 60°. Similar lines are drawn across the second line at the angle of approximately 120°. Short lines are drawn across the third at the same angle as on the first lines. These lines produce the optical illusion that the long lines are converging or diverging.

linea (lĭn'ē-ă) [L.,line](pl. *lineae*). [NA] An anatomical line.

l. alba. [NA] The white line of connective tissue in middle of abdomen from sternum to pubis.

lineae albicantes. Lines seen on the abdomen, buttocks, and breasts. Frequently due to pregnancy, obesity, or prolonged adrenal cortical hormone therapy, but may occur as the result of abdominal distention due to any cause. SYN: *striae atrophicae.*

l. aspera. [NA] A longitudinal ridge on posterior surface of middle third of the femur.

l. costoarticularis. Line between the sternoclavicular articulation and point of the 11th rib.

l. nigra. Black line or discoloration of the abdomen that may be seen in pregnant women during latter part of term. It runs from above the umbilicus to the pubes.

l. semilunaris. Spigelian line, q.v.

l. splendens. A thickening of the pia mater extending along the anterior median surface of the spinal cord. It ensheaths the anterior spinal artery.

l. sternalis. Median line of the sternum.

lineae striae atrophicae. Lines, or striae, of atrophic skin. Seen esp. in Cushing's syndrome.

l. terminalis. [NA] Bony ridge on inner surface of ilium continued on to pubis that divides true and false pelvis.

lineae transversae ossis sacri. Ridges formed by lines of union of the 5th sacral vertebrae.

linear (lĭn'ē-ăr) [L. *linea*, line]. Pert. to or resembling a line.

linear energy transfer. A measure of the rate of energy transfer from ionizing radiation to soft tissue.

liner (lĭn'ĕr). Anything applied to the inside of a hollow body or structure.

l., cavity. A layer of material applied to a cavity preparation to protect the pulp of the tooth. It is usually a suspension of zinc phosphate or calcium hydroxide and is used to neutralize the acidity of the base or cement material.

l., soft. Material applied to the underside of a denture to provide a soft surface contact with the oral tissues. Some acrylic or silicone resins have been made resilient and are used as liners. Also called cushion liner; resilient liner.

lingua (lĭng'gwă) [L.] (pl. *linguae*). [NA] Tongue or tonguelike structure.

l. frenata. Tongue with a very short frenum, resulting in tongue-tie. SYN: *ankyloglossia.*

l. geographica. Geographic tongue.

l. nigra. Condition in which the tongue has a brown furlike area on its dorsum. The area is composed of hypertrophied filiform papillae pigment and possibly microorganisms. Sometimes results from excessive use of oxygen-liberating mouthwashes or antibiotic therapy. SYN: *tongue, black hairy.*

l. plicata. A fissured tongue.

lingual (lĭng'gwăl) [L. *lingua*, tongue]. 1. Pert. to the tongue. 2. Tongue-shaped.

linguiform (lĭng'gwĭ-form) [" + *forma*, shape]. Tongue-shaped.

lingula (lĭng'gū-lă) [L., little tongue]. [NA] Tongue-shaped process, esp. lingula cerebelli.

l. cerebelli. [NA] Tonguelike process of cerebellum prolonged forward on upper surface of superior medullary velum.

l. of lung. Projection of lung that separates cardiac notch from inferior margin of left lung.

l. of mandible. Projection of bone that forms the medial boundary of the mandibular foramen and gives attachment to the sphenomandibular ligament.

l. of sphenoid. Ridge between the body and ala magna of the sphenoid.

lingulectomy (lǐng″gū-lěk′tō-mē) [L. *lingula,* little tongue, + Gr. *ektome,* excision]. Surgical removal of the lingula of the upper lobe of the left lung.

linguo- [L. *lingua,* tongue]. Combining form indicating the tongue.

linguoclasia (lǐng′gwō-klā′zē-ă) [L. *lingua,* tongue, + Gr. *klasis,* destruction]. Displacement of a tooth toward the tongue.

linguoclination (lǐng′gwō-klī-nā′shŭn) [″ + *clinatus,* leaning]. Angulation of a tooth in its vertical axis toward the tongue.

linguodental. Relating to the tongue and teeth, such as the speech sound "th," which is produced with the aid of the tongue and teeth.

linguodistal (lǐng″gwō-dǐs′tăl) [″ + *distare,* to be distant]. Concerning the distal part of a tooth and the tongue.

linguogingival (lǐng″gwō-jǐn′jǐ-văl) [″ + *gingiva,* gum]. Concerning the tongue and the gingiva, or pertaining to the lingual and gingival walls of a cavity preparation.

linguomesial. Pertaining to the lingual and mesial surfaces of a tooth or the lingual and mesial walls of a cavity preparation.

linguo-occlusal (lǐng″gwō-ō-kloo′zăl) [″ + *occludere,* to shut up]. Concerning or bounded by the lingual and occlusal surfaces of a tooth.

linguopapillitis (lǐng″gwō-păp″ǐ-lī′tǐs) [″ + *papilla,* nipple, + Gr. *itis,* inflammation]. Small ulcers of the papillae of the edge of the tongue.

linguopulpal. Pertaining to the lingual and pulpal surfaces of a cavity preparation.

linguoversion (lǐng″gwō-vĕr′zhŭn) [″ + *versio,* a turning]. Displacement of a tooth toward the tongue.

liniment [L. *linimentum,* smearing substance]. A liquid containing a medicament and oil, alcohol, or water for use externally. Applied by friction method or on a bandage.

l., camphor. A preparation of camphor and a suitable vehicle, such as an oil, that is used topically as an irritant.

l., medicinal soft soap. Tincture of green soap.

linimentum (lǐn-ǐ-měn′tŭm) [L.]. Liquid preparation for external use and usually applied by rubbing. SYN: *liniment.*

linitis (lǐn-ī′tǐs) [Gr. *linon,* flax, + *itis,* inflammation]. Inflammation of the lining of the stomach.

l. plastica. Linitis with thickening of the wall of the stomach usually due to neoplastic tissue. SYN: *stomach, leather-bottle.*

linkage. In genetics, the association between distinct genes that occupy closely situated loci on the same chromosome. This results in an association in the inheritance of these genes.

l., sex. A genetic characteristic that is located on the X or Y chromosome.

linseed [AS. *linsaed*]. Seeds of the common flax, *Linum usitatissimum.* It is the source of linseed oil. Linseed is used as a demulcent and emollient. SYN: *flaxseed.*

lint (lǐnt) [L. *linteum,* made of linen]. 1. Linen scraped until soft and wooly for dressing wounds. 2. Cotton fiber. 3. Household dust.

lintin (lǐn′tǐn). Prepared absorbent cotton; fabric used in dressings.

liothyronine sodium (lī″ō-thī′rō-nēn). USP. Sodium salt of triiodothyronine. Used in treating hypothyroidism. Trade name is Cytomel. SEE: *thyroid function tests.*

liotrix tablets (lī′ō-trǐks). USP. A combination of levothyroxine sodium and liothyronine sodium. Used in treating thyroid deficiency. Trade names are Euthroid and Thyrolar.

lip [AS. *lippa*]. 1. Soft external structure that forms the boundary of the mouth or opening to the oral cavity. SYN: *labium* (or *labia*) *oris.* 2. One of the lips of the pudendum (labium majus or minus). 3. A liplike structure forming the border of an opening or groove.

PATH: *Chancre:* It is not unusual to have the initial lesion of syphilis appear upon the lip of the mouth as an indurated base with a thin secretion and accompanied by enlargement of the submaxillary glands. *Condyloma latum:* This appears as a mucous patch, flattened, coated with gray exudate, with strictly delimited area, usually at the angle of the mouth. *Eczema:* Dry fissures, often covered with a crust, bleeding easily, and occurring on both lips. *Epithelioma:* May be confused with chancre. Seldom appears before the age of 40, but there are exceptions. It may appear as a common cold sore, a painless fissure, or other break of the lower lip. A crust or scab covers the lesion, leaving a raw surface if removed. Pain does not appear until the lesion is well advanced. Much more common on lower lip than upper. *Herpes:* Appears on the lips in pneumonia, typhoid, common cold, other febrile diseases, and idiopathically. *Tuberculous ulcer:* At inner portion of lip close to angle of mouth. Pathological examination necessary for verification.

DIAG: Examination is considered to be incomplete unless lips are everted to expose buccal surfaces. *Bluish or purplish:* May appear in the aged, in those exposed to great cold, and in carbon monoxide poisoning. *Dry:* May be seen in fevers or be caused by drugs such as atropine, by thirst, or by mouth breathing. *Fissured:* May occur after exposure to cold, in avitaminosis, and in children with congenital syphilis. The dribbling of saliva and a toothless condition may cause fissures in the corners of the mouth. *Pale:* May be seen in anemia and wasting diseases, in prolonged fever, and after a hemorrhage. *Rashes:* May be manifestations of typhoid fever, meningitis, or pneumonia. Mucous patches may appear in secondary syphilis, chancre, cancer, and epithelioma.

RS: buccal; cheilitis; cheilosis; "chil-" words; labia; labium; labrum.

l., cleft. Harelip.

l., double. A redundant fold of mucous membrane in the mouth on either side of the midline of the lip.

l., glenoid. Thickened fibrocartilaginous structure surmounting margin of acetabulum.

l., Hapsburg. A thick, overdeveloped lower lip.

l.'s, oral. Upper and lower lips that surround mouth opening and form anterior wall of buccal cavity.

l., tympanic. Lower border of the sulcus spiralis internus of the cochlea.

l., vestibular. Upper border of the sulcus spiralis internus of the cochlea.

lipacidemia (lĭp″ăs-ĭ-dē′mē-ă) [Gr. *lipos,* fat, + L. *acidus,* acid, + Gr. *haima,* blood]. Excess fatty acids in the blood.

lipaciduria (lĭp″ăs-ĭ-dū′rē-ă) [″ + ″ + Gr. *ouron,* urine]. Fatty acids in the urine.

liparocele (lĭp′ă-rō-sēl) [″ + *kele,* tumor, swelling]. 1. Scrotal hernia containing fat. 2. A fatty tumor.

liparous (lĭp′ă-rŭs) [Gr. *lipos,* fat]. Obese; fat.

lipase (lĭ′pās, lī′pās) [″ + *-ase,* enzyme]. A lipolytic or fat-splitting enzyme found in the blood, pancreatic secretion, and tissues. Emulsified fats of cream and egg yolk are changed in the stomach to fatty acids and glycerol by gastric lipase. SEE: *digestion; enzyme.*

l., pancreatic. Steapsin, q.v.

lipasuria (lĭp″ăs-ū′rē-ă) [″ + ″ + Gr. *ouron,* urine]. Lipase in the urine.

lipectomy (lĭ-pĕk′tō-mē) [″ + *ektome,* excision]. Excision of fatty tissues.

l., suction. Removal of subcutaneous fat tissue by use of a blunt-tipped cannula introduced into the fatty area through a small incision. Suction is then applied and fat tissue is removed. SYN: *lipoplasty.*

lipedema (lĭp″ĕ-dē′mă) [″ + *oidema,* swelling]. Swelling of the skin, esp. of the lower extremity, due to accumulation of fat and fluid subcutaneously.

lipemia (lĭ-pē′mē-ă) [″ + *haima,* blood]. Abnormal amount of fat in the blood.

l., alimentary. Accumulation of fat in the blood after eating.

l. retinalis. Condition in which retinal vessels appear reddish white or milk. Found in cases of hyperlipidemia. SEE: *hyperlipoproteinemia.*

lipid(e) (lĭp′ĭd, -īd) [Gr. *lipos,* fat]. Any one of a group of fats or fatlike substances, characterized by their insolubility in water and solubility in fat solvents such as alcohol, ether, and chloroform. The term is descriptive rather than a chemical name such as protein or carbohydrate. Includes true fats (esters of fatty acids and glycerol); lipoids (phospholipids, cerebrosides, waxes); and sterols (cholesterol, ergosterol). SEE: *fat; lipoprotein.*

lipid histiocytosis. Niemann-Pick disease.

lipidosis. Any disorder of fat metabolism. SYN: *lipoidosis.*

lipiduria (lĭp″ĭ-dū′rē-ă) [″ + Gr. *ouron,* urine]. Lipids in the urine.

lipin (lĭp′ĭn) [Gr. *lipos,* fat]. SEE: *lipid(e).*

Lipiodol (lĭp-ī′ō-dŏl) [″ + L. *oleum,* oil]. Trade name for an iodized oil used as a contrast medium in x-ray studies.

lipo-, lip- (Gr. *lipos,* fat]. Combining forms pert. to fat.

lipoarthritis (lĭp″ō-ărth-rī′tĭs) [″ + *arthron,* joint, + *itis,* inflammation]. Inflammation of fatty tissues of joints.

lipoatrophia, lipoatrophy (lĭ″pō-ă-trō′fē-ă, lĭ″pō-ăt′rō-fē) [″ + *a-,* not, + *trophe,* nourishment]. Atrophy of fat tissue. May occur at the site of insulin injection. SEE: *lipodystrophy.*

lipoblast (lĭp′ō-blăst) [″ + *blastos,* germ]. An immature fat cell.

lipoblastoma (lĭp″ō-blăs-tō′mă) [″ + ″ + *oma,* tumor]. A benign tumor of fatty tissue. SYN: *adipoma; lipoma.*

lipocardiac (lĭp″ō-kăr′dē-ăk) [″ + *kardia,* heart]. 1. Pert. to fatty heart degeneration. 2. One who suffers from fatty degeneration of heart.

lipocatabolic (lĭp″ō-kăt″ă-bŏl′ĭk) [″ + *katabole,* a casting down]. Concerning the breaking down of fat tissue during metabolism.

lipocele (lĭp′ō-sēl) [″ + *kele,* tumor, swelling]. Presence of fatty tissue in a hernia sac. SYN: *adipocele; liparocele.*

lipoceratous (lĭp″ō-sĕr′ă-tŭs) [″ + L. *cera,* wax]. Concerning the waxy substance formed when a body decomposes in a moist area, as when buried in wet soil. SYN: *adipoceratous.*

lipocere (lĭp′ō-sēr) [″ + L. *cera,* wax]. Waxy substance resulting from exposure of fleshy tissue to moisture with the exclusion of air. SYN: *adipocere.*

lipochondrodystrophy (lĭp″ō-kŏn″drō-dĭs′trō-fē) [″ + *chondros,* cartilage, + *dys,* bad, + *trephein,* to nourish]. Congenital abnormality in the skeletal bones and cartilage with deranged mucopolysaccharide metabolism, kyphosis and other deformity, possible mental deficiency, and cloudy corneae. SYN: *Hurler's syndrome; mucopolysaccharidosis I.*

lipochondroma (lĭp″ō-kŏn-drō′mă) [″ + ″ + *oma,* tumor]. Tumor that is both fatty and cartilaginous.

lipochrome (lĭp′ō-krōm) [″ + *chroma,* color]. A group of fat-soluble pigments. SEE: *carotene.*

    Ex.: carotene, the fat-soluble yellow pigment found in carrots, sweet potatoes, egg yolk, butter, body fat and corpus luteum.

lipocyte (lĭp′ō-sīt) [″ + *kytos,* cell]. Fat cell.

lipodystrophy (lĭp″ō-dĭs′trō-fē) [″ + *dys,* bad, + *trophe,* nourishment]. Disturbance or defectiveness of fat metabolism.

    l., insulin. A complication of insulin administration characterized by changes in the subcutaneous fat at the site of injection. The changes may take the form of atrophy or hypertrophy; rarely are both types present in the same patient. Atrophy develops in as many as one-third of children and adult females who use insulin regularly, but rarely in adult males. The subcutaneous fat appears to have melted away and leaves a saucerlike depression. Hypertrophy at the injection site occurs in the form of a spongy localized area. This type of complication of insulin administration is slightly more common in males than in females. It is usually associated with a history of prolonged use of the same injection site.

    l., intestinal. Disease characterized principally by fat deposits in intestinal and mesenteric lymphatic tissue, fatty diarrhea, loss of weight and strength, and arthritis.

    l., progressive. A pathological condition in which there is progressive, symmetrical loss of subcutaneous fat from the upper part of the trunk, face, neck, and arms.

    l., trochanteric. Excess accumulation of fatty tissue over the thighs. This condition is called saddlebag thighs.

lipofibroma (lĭp″ō-fī-brō′mă) [″ + L. *fibra,* fiber, + Gr. *oma,* tumor]. A lipoma having much fibrous tissue. SYN: *fibrolipoma.*

lipofuscin (lĭp″ō-fūs′sĭn) [″ + L. *fuscus,* brown]. One of a class of insoluble lipid pigments present in cardiac and smooth muscle cells. It is known as aging pigment. It is the indigestible residue of portions of the cell that have been injured and phagocytosed. This is frequently seen in cells undergoing atrophy. Its presence is not injurious to the cell. SEE: *atrophy, brown; radical, free.*

lipofuscinosis (lĭp″ō-fū″sĭn-ō′sĭs) [″ + Gr. *osis,* condition]. Abnormal deposition of lipofuscin in tissues.

Lipo Gantrisin. Trade name for sulfisoxazole acetyl, USP.

lipogenesis (lĭp″ō-jĕn′ĕ-sĭs) [Gr. *lipos,* fat, + *genesis,* generation, birth]. Fat formation.

lipogenetic, lipogenic (lĭp″ō-jĕ-nĕt′ĭk, lĭp″ō-jĕn′ĭk). Producing fat. SYN: *lipogenous.*

lipogenous (lĭp-ŏj′ĕ-nŭs). Producing fat. SYN: *lipogenetic.*

lipogranuloma (lĭp″ō-grăn-ū-lō′mă) [″ + L. *granulum,* granule, + Gr. *oma,* tumor]. Inflammation of fatty tissue with granulation and development of oily cysts.

lipogranulomatosis (lĭp″ō-grăn″ū-lō-mă-tō′sĭs) [″ + ″ + ″ + *osis,* condition]. A disorder of fat metabolism in which a nodule of fat undergoes central necrosis and the surrounding tissue becomes granulomatous.

Lipo-Hepin. Trade name for heparin sodium, USP.

lipoid (lĭp′oyd) [″ + *eidos,* form, shape]. 1. Similar to fat. 2. Substance resembling fats in appearance and solubility, but containing groups other than the glycerol and fatty acids that make up the true fats. SYN: *lipid.*

    Ex.: cholesterol; kephalin; lecithin.

lipoidemia (lĭp″oy-dē′mē-ă) [″ + ″ + *haima,* blood]. Excess of lipoids in the blood.

lipoidosis (lĭp-oy-dō′sĭs) [″ + ″ + *osis,* condition]. Condition in which lipids accumulate in excessive quantities in body tissue. SYN: *lipidosis.* SEE: *xanthomatosis.*

    l., arterial. Arteriosclerosis.

    l., cerebroside. A familial disease characterized by deposition of glucocerebroside in cells of the reticuloendothelial system. SYN: *Gaucher's disease.*

lipoiduria (lĭp″oy-dū′rē-ă) [″ + ″ + *ouron,* urine]. Lipoids in the urine.

lipolipoidosis (lĭp″ō-lĭp″oy-dō′sĭs) [″ + *lipos,* fat, + *eidos,* form, shape, + *osis,* condition]. Infiltration of fats and lipoids into a tissue.

lipolysis (lĭp-ŏl′ĭ-sĭs) [″ + *lysis,* dissolution]. The decomposition of fat.

lipolytic (lĭp-ō-lĭt′ĭk). Rel. to lipolysis.

lipolytic digestion. The conversion of neutral fats by hydrolysis into fatty acids and glycerol; fat splitting.

lipolytic enzyme. Fat-splitting enzyme. SYN: *lipase.* SEE: *enzyme.*

lipoma (lĭ-pō′mă) [Gr. *lipos,* fat, + *oma,* tumor]. A fatty tumor. It is frequently found in multiple but is not metastatic. SYN: *adipoma.* SEE: *chondrolipoma.*

    l. arborescens. An abnormal treelike accumulation of fatty tissue in a joint.

    l., cystic. Lipoma containing cysts.

    l., diffuse. Lipoma not definitely circumscribed.

    l. diffusum renis. Condition in which fat

displaces parenchyma of the kidney.

l. durum. Lipoma in which there is marked hypertrophy of the fibrous stroma and capsule.

l., hernial. Lipocele.

l., nasal. A fibrous growth of the subcutaneous tissue of the nostrils.

l., osseous. Lipoma in which the connective tissue has undergone calcareous degeneration.

l. telangiectodes. A rare form of lipoma containing a large number of blood vessels.

lipomatoid (lĭ-pō′mă-toyd) [″ + ″ + eidos, form, shape]. Similar to a lipoma.

lipomatosis (lĭp″ō-mă-tō′sĭs) [″ + oma, tumor + osis, condition]. Condition marked by excessive deposit of fat in a localized area. SYN: *liposis; obesity.*

l. renis. Fatty infiltration of renal parenchyma. SYN: *lipoma diffusum renis.*

lipomatous (lĭp-ō′mă-tŭs). 1. Of the nature of lipoma. 2. Affected with lipoma.

lipomeningocele (lĭp″ō-mĕ-nĭng′gō-sēl) [″ + meninx, membrane, + kele, tumor, swelling]. A meningocele associated with lobules of fat tissue.

lipomeria (lĭ″pō-mē′rē-ă) [Gr. leipein, to leave, + meros, a part]. In a deformed fetus, congenital absence of a limb.

lipometabolic (lĭp″ō-mĕt″ă-bŏl′ĭk) [Gr. lipos, fat, + metabole, change]. Rel. to metabolism of fat.

lipometabolism (lĭp-ō-mĕ-tăb′ŏl-ĭzm) [″ + ″ + -ismos, condition]. Fat metabolism.

lipomyoma (lĭp″ō-mī-ō′mă) [″ + mys, muscle, + oma, tumor]. A myoma containing fatty tissue.

lipomyxoma (lĭp″ō-mĭks-ō′mă) [″ + myxa, mucus, + oma, tumor]. A mixed lipoma and myxoma. SYN: *myxolipoma.*

lipopectic (lĭp-ō-pĕk′tĭk) [″ + pexis, fixation]. Characterized by lipopexia.

lipopenia (lĭp″ō-pē′nē-ă) [″ + penia, poverty]. Deficiency of lipids.

lipopenic (lĭp″ō-pē′nĭk). Concerning lipopenia.

lipopeptid, lipopeptide (lĭp″ō-pĕp′tĭd, -tīd). A complex of lipids and amino acids.

lipopexia (lĭp″ō-pĕk′sē-ă). Accumulation of fat in the body.

lipophage (lĭp′ō-fāj) [″ + phagein, to eat]. Fat-absorbing cell.

lipophagia, granulomatous (lĭp″ō-fā′jē-ă). Lipodystrophy, intestinal, q.v.

lipophagic (lĭp-ō-fā′jĭk). Consuming, destroying, or absorbing fat.

lipophagy (lĭ-pŏf′ă-jē). The ingestion of fat cells by phagocytes.

lipophanerosis (lĭp″ō-făn″ē-rō′sĭs) [″ + phaneros, visible, + osis, condition]. The alteration of fat in a cell so that it becomes visible as droplets.

lipophil (lĭp′ō-fĭl) [″ + philein, to love]. 1. Having an affinity for fat. 2. Absorbing fat.

lipophilia (lĭp″ō-fĭl′ē-ă) [″ + philos, love]. Affinity for fat.

lipopolysaccharide (lĭp″ō-pŏl″ē-săk′ă-rīd). The linkage of molecules of lipids with polysaccharides.

lipoprotein. Conjugated proteins consisting of simple proteins combined with lipid components: cholesterol, phospholipid, and triglyceride. Most plasma lipids do not circulate in an unbound state, but are chemically linked with proteins. These large molecules are categorized with respect to their chemical properties and densities as determined by ultracentrifugation. Analysis of their concentrations and proportions in the blood can provide important clues as to their role in certain diseases, particularly cardiovascular abnormalities, hypertension, atherosclerosis, and coronary artery disease. Lipoproteins are classified as very low density (VLDL), low-density (LDL), and high-density (HDL). It is thought that individuals with high blood levels of HDL are less predisposed to coronary heart disease as compared with those with high blood levels of VLDL or LDL. SEE: *hyperlipoproteinemia.*

l., high-density. ABBR: HDL. Plasma lipids bound to albumin, consisting of lipoproteins. They contain more protein than either very low density lipoproteins or low-density lipoproteins.

l., low-density. ABBR: LDL. Plasma lipids bound to albumin, consisting of lipoproteins that contain more protein than the very low density lipoproteins.

l., very low density. ABBR: VLDL. Plasma lipids bound to albumin and consisting of chylomicrons and pre-lipoproteins. This class of plasma lipoproteins contains a greater ratio of lipid than the low-density lipoproteins and is the least dense.

lipoprotein lipase. ABBR: Lp(a). An enzyme produced by many tissues. It is present on capillary walls where it is activated to hydrolyze fat (chylomicrons) and very low density lipoprotein (VLDL) to monoglycerides to free fatty acids and intermediate-density lipoprotein (IDL). This enzyme, similar to plasminogen, is an important regulator of lipid and lipoprotein metabolism. Even though the physiological functions of Lp(a) and apo(a) are not fully understood, there is a positive association of plasma Lp(a) and premature myocardial infarction. Deficiency of this enzyme leads to an increase in chylomicrons, VLDLs, and low levels of HDL. Diseases associated with acquired causes of decreased lipoprotein lipase include acute ethanol ingestion, diabetes mellitus, hypothyroidism, chronic renal failure, and nephrotic syndrome.

liposarcoma (lĭp″ō-săr-kō′mă) [Gr. *lipos*, fat, + *sarx*, flesh, + *oma*, tumor]. A malignant tumor derived from embryonal lipoblastic cells.

liposis (lĭ-pō′sĭs) [″ + *osis*, condition]. Abnormal accumulation of fat in the body. SYN: *adiposis*.

liposoluble (lĭp″ō-sŏl′ū-b'l) [″ + L. *solubilis*, soluble]. Soluble in fats.

liposome (lĭp′ō-sōm) [″ + *soma*, body]. The sealed concentric shells formed when certain lipid substances are in an aqueous solution. As it forms, the liposome entraps a portion of the solution in the shell. Liposomes may be manufactured and filled with a variety of medications. These have been used to deliver substances to particular organs. These drug forms may be more effective and less toxic than drugs given by other means.

lipostomy (lĭ-pŏs′tō-mē) [Gr. *leipein*, to fail, + *stoma*, mouth]. Congenital absence or extreme smallness of the mouth.

lipothymia (lī″pō-thī′mē-ă) [″ + *thymos*, mind]. Faintness; syncope.

lipotrophy (lĭ-pŏt′rō-fē) [Gr. *lipos*, fat, + *trophe*, nourishment]. Increase in body fat.

lipotropic (lĭp-ō-trŏp′ĭk) [″ + *trope*, a turning]. Having an affinity for lipids.

Ex.: certain dyes such as Sudan III, which stains fat readily.

lipotropic factors. Compounds that promote the transportation and utilization of fats and help to prevent accumulation of fat in the liver.

lipotropism, lipotropy (lĭ-pŏt′rō-pĭzm, -pē) [″ + *trope*, a turn, + *-ismos*, condition]. 1. Having the action of removing fat deposits in the liver. 2. An agent that acts to remove fat from the liver.

lipovaccine (lĭp″ō-văk′sēn). A vaccine suspended in vegetable oil.

lipoxeny (lĭ-pŏks′ĕ-nē) [Gr. *leipein*, to fail, + *xenos*, host]. Desertion of host by parasitic organism after completion of its development.

lipoxidase (lĭ-pŏk′sĭ-dās). An enzyme that catalyzes the oxidation of the double bonds of an unsaturated fatty acid.

lipoxygenase (lĭ-pŏks′ĭ-jĕ-nās). Lipoxidase, q.v.

Lippes loop (lĭ′pēz) [Jacob Lippes, U.S. obstetrician, b. 1924]. A type of intrauterine contraceptive device.

lipping (lĭp′ĭng). A growth of bony tissue beyond the joint margin in degenerative joint disease.

lippitude (lĭp′ĭ-tūd) [L. *lippitudo*, fr. *lippus*, blear-eyed]. Ulcerations of the margins of the eyelids. SYN: *blepharitis*.

lip reading. Interpreting what is being said by watching the speaker's lip and facial movements and expression. This method is used very effectively by deaf people.

lip reflex. Reflex movement of lips when angle of mouth is suddenly and lightly tapped during sleep.

lipsis (lĭp′sĭs) [Gr. *leipein*, to fail]. Ending or cessation.

   l. animi. Fainting.

lipuria (lĭ-pū′rē-ă) [Gr. *lipos*, fat, + *ouron*, urine]. Fat in the urine.

Liquaemin Sodium. Trade name for heparin sodium, USP.

liquefacient (lĭk″wē-fā′shĕnt) [L. *liquere*, to flow, + *facere*, to make]. 1. Agent that converts a solid substance into liquid. 2. Converting a solid into liquid.

liquefaction (lĭk″wē-făk′shŭn). 1. Conversion of a solid into a liquid. 2. Conversion of solid tissues to a fluid or semifluid state.

liquescent (lĭk-wĕs′sĕnt) [L. *liquescere*, to become liquid]. Becoming liquid. SYN: *deliquescent.*

liqueur (lĭ-kĕr′) [Fr.]. Alcoholic beverage, aromatically flavored, often colored, and sweetened. A cordial.

liquid (lĭk′wĭd) [L. *liquere*, to flow]. 1. Flowing easily. 2. State of matter where a substance flows without being melted. SEE: *emulsion; liquefacient; liquefaction.*

liquid air therapy. Therapeutic application of air that is so cold as to be liquefied. SEE: CO_2 *therapy; cryotherapy; hypothermia.*

liquid crystals. Substances that alter their color or change from opaque to transparent when subjected to changes in temperature, electric current, pressure, electromagnetic waves, or when impurities are present. They have been used to detect temperature fluctuation in infants. Liquid crystals are of two general classes: cholestric, which change color, and nematic, which can change back and forth from transparent to opaque.

liquid diet. Coffee with hot milk; tea; water; milk in all forms; milk and cream mixtures; cocoa; strained cream soups; fruit juices; meat juices; beef tea; clear broths; gruels; strained meat soups; eggnogs. SEE: *fluid diet.*

liquid measure. Measure of liquid capacity.

liquor (lĭk′ĕr) [L.]. 1. Any liquid or fluid. 2. An alcoholic beverage. 3. Solution of medicinal substance in water.

   l. amnii. The amniotic fluid, a clear watery fluid that surrounds the fetus in the amniotic sac. SEE: *hydramnion.*

   l. folliculi. The fluid contained in the graafian follicle.

   l. sanguinis. Blood serum or plasma.

liquor solutions. Aqueous solutions of nonvolatile substances presenting the greatest variety in strength, character, and method of preparation. They are usually very active medicinal preparations.

Lisch nodules [K. Lisch, contemporary Ger. scientist]. Melanocytic hamartomas projecting from the surface of the iris of the eye. They are well-defined, dome-shaped elevations that are clear to yellow or brown. These growths, which do not cause ophthalmologic complications, may be seen without magnification, but examination with use of a slit lamp will be needed to differentiate them from nevi of the iris. Lisch nodules are found only in patients with neurofibromatosis, Type 1, q.v.

Lisfranc's ligament (lĭs-frănks') [Jacques Lisfranc, Fr. surgeon, 1790–1847]. The ligament joining the first cuneiform bone of the ankle to the second metatarsal.

lisping (lĭsp'ĭng) [AS. *wlisp,* lisping]. Substitution of sounds due to defect in speech, as of "th" sound for "s" and "z."

lissencephalous (lĭs″sĕn-sĕf′ă-lŭs) [Gr. *lissos,* smooth, + *enkephalos,* brain]. Pert. to condition in which the brain is smooth owing to failure of development of cerebral gyri.

lissotrichy (lĭs-sŏt′rĭ-kē) [″ + *thrix,* hair]. Condition of having straight hair.

Lister, Baron Joseph (lĭs′tĕr). British surgeon, 1827–1912, who developed the technique of antiseptic surgery. Without this, modern surgery would not be possible.

listeriosis, listerosis (lĭs-tĕr″ē-ō′sĭs, lĭs″tĕr-ō′sĭs). A disease affecting many domestic animals, wild animals, and humans. Caused by *Listeria monocytogenes,* a soil saprophyte that becomes pathogenic for animals or humans under favorable circumstances, e.g., pregnancy, immunosuppression, or extremes of age. The most common manifestation in the adult is meningitis. It may be transmitted transplacentally to the fetus, in which case it may cause abortion. In newborns, the disease is much more serious than in the adult. The mortality may be 100% when it occurs in the first four days. Although man has a high degree of resistance to the bacteria, hygienic precautions should be taken when handling infected animals.

TREAT: Initially, treat with ampicillin and an aminoglycoside antibiotic. If patient is allergic to penicillin, use trimethoprim sulfamethoxazole.

lisuride. A drug used in treating parkinsonism. Its action is similar to that of bromocriptine.

liter (lē′tĕr) [Fr. *litre,* liter]. Metric fluid measure; equivalent to 1000 milliliters (ml), 270 fl. drams, 61 cu. in., 33.8 fl. oz, or 1.0567 qt. The volume occupied by 1 kg of water at 4°C and 760 mmHg pressure. SEE: *metric system.*

NOTE: It is common to define a liter as 1000 cubic centimeters (cc). This is almost but not quite correct because 1 ml is equal to 1.000028 cc. Thus liquid volume should be expressed in ml rather than cc.

literate. Being able to read and write, and to use written language as in understanding graphs, charts, tables, maps, symbols, and formulae.

lithagogue (lĭth′ă-gŏg) [Gr. *lithos,* stone, + *agogos,* leading]. 1. Agent that expels calculi. 2. Expelling calculi.

Lithane. Trade name for lithium carbonate, USP.

lithectasy (lĭth-ĕk′tă-sē) [″ + *ektasis,* dilatation]. Removal of a calculus from the bladder through the dilated urethra.

lithectomy (lĭ-thĕk′tō-mē) [″ + *ektome,* excision]. Surgical removal of a calculus.

lithemia (lĭth-ē′mē-ă) [″ + *haima,* blood]. Excess of lithic or uric acid in the blood due to imperfect metabolism of the nitrogenous substances.

lithiasis (lĭth-ī′ă-sĭs). 1. Formation of calculi and concretions. 2. Uric acid diathesis.

l. biliaris. Gallstones.

l. nephritica. Stone formation in the kidneys. SYN: *nephrolithiasis.* SEE: *calculus, renal.*

l. renalis. Kidney stones. SEE: *calculus, renal.*

lithic acid (lĭth′ĭk). Uric acid.

lithicosis (lĭth″ĭ-kō′sĭs) [Gr. *lithikos,* made of stone]. Stone cutters' silicosis; pneumoconiosis.

lithium (lĭth′ē-ŭm) [Gr. *lithos,* stone]. SYMB: Li. At. wt. 6.941; at. no. 3. A metallic element.

l. carbonate. USP. A drug that is particularly useful in treating the manic phase of manic-depressive illness. Trade names are Eskalith, Lithane, Lithonate, and Lithotabs. Given orally it is readily absorbed and eliminated at a fast rate for 5 to 6 hours and eliminated at a much slower rate over the next 24 hours. It is essential to monitor the blood level of the drug in patients on this therapy; samples should be taken 8 to 10 hours after the last dose and at intervals after medication.

A dose of 1200 mg each day is initially given and adjusted as needed to produce a plasma level of 0.8 mEq per liter. When the dose has been found to produce the optimal plasma concentration, blood analysis is done every three months. Plasma levels of 2 or more mEq per liter cause serious toxic effects including stupor or coma, muscular rigidity, marked tremor, and in some cases epileptic seizure.

Side effects including fatigue, weakness,

fine tremor of the hands, nausea and vomiting, thirst, and polyuria may be noticed in the first week of therapy. If these are mild, most will disappear, but the thirst, polyuria, and tremor tend to persist.

Caution: Decreased dietary sodium intake lowers the excretion rate of lithium. It should not be administered to patients on a salt-free diet.

litho-, lith- [Gr. *lithos,* stone]. Prefixes pert. to stone or calculus.

lithocenosis (lĭth″ō-sĕn-ō′sĭs) [″ + *kenosis,* evacuation]. Removal of crushed fragments of calculi from the bladder.

lithoclast (lĭth′ō-klăst) [″ + *klastos,* broken]. Forceps for breaking up large calculi.

lithoclasty (lĭth′ō-klăs″tē). The crushing of a stone into fragments that may pass through natural channels.

lithoclysmia (lĭth-ō-klĭz′mē-ă) [″ + *klysma,* a clyster]. Injection into urinary bladder of substances that have the ability to dissolve calculi.

NOTE: There are no such substances that are both effective and safe to use.

lithocystotomy (lĭth″ō-sĭs-tŏt′ō-mē) [″ + *kystis,* bladder, + *tome,* incision]. Incision of the bladder to remove a calculus.

lithodialysis (lĭth″ō-dī-ăl′ĭ-sĭs) [″ + *dialyein,* to dissolve]. Fragmentation or dissolution of calculi by injection of a solvent. SYN: *litholysis.*

lithogenesis (lĭth″ō-jĕn′ĕ-sĭs) [″ + *gennan,* to produce]. Formation of calculi.

lithokelyphopedion (lĭth″ō-kĕl″ĭ-fō-pē′dē-ŏn) [″ + *kelyphos,* sheath, + *paidion,* child]. Calcification of both the fetus and the membranes of a lithopedion.

lithokelyphos (lĭth″ō-kĕl′ĭ-fŏs) [″ + *kelyphos,* sheath]. A type of lithopedion in which only the membranes are calcified.

lithokonion (lĭth″ō-kō′nē-ŏn) [″ + *konios,* dusty]. Instrument for pulverizing vesical calculi. SYN: *lithomyl.*

litholabe (lĭth′ō-lāb) [″ + *lambanein,* to hold]. Device for holding a calculus during its removal.

litholapaxy (lĭth-ŏl′ă-păks″ē) [Gr. *lithos,* stone, + *lapaxis,* evacuation]. The operation of crushing a stone in the bladder followed by immediate washing out of the crushed fragments through a catheter. SEE: *percutaneous ultrasonic lithotriptor.*

lithology (lĭth-ŏl′ō-jē) [″ + *logos,* word, reason]. The science dealing with calculi.

litholysis (lĭth-ŏl′ĭ-sĭs) [″ + *lysis,* dissolution]. Dissolving of calculi. SYN: *lithodialysis.*

lithometer (lĭth-ŏm′ĕ-tĕr) [″ + *metron,* measure]. Instrument for estimating the size of calculi.

lithometra (lĭth-ō-mē′tră) [″ + *metra,* uterus]. Uterine tissue ossification.

lithomyl (lĭth′ō-mĭl) [″ + *myle,* mill]. Instrument for crushing a vesical stone. SYN: *lithokonion.*

Lithonate. Trade name for lithium carbonate, USP.

lithonephritis (lĭth″ō-nĕ-frī′tĭs) [″ + *nephros,* kidney, + *itis,* inflammation]. Inflammation of the kidney due to a calculus.

lithonephrotomy (lĭth″ō-nē-frŏt′ō-mē) [″ + *nephros,* kidney, + *tome,* incision]. Incision of kidney for removal of renal calculus.

lithontriptic (lĭth-ŏn-trĭp′tĭk) [″ + *tribein,* to rub]. An agent or instrument that dissolves or crushes calculi. SYN: *lithotriptic.*

lithopedion (lĭth″ō-pē′dē-ŏn) [″ + *paidion,* child]. A uterine or extrauterine fetus that has died and become calcified. SYN: *ostembryon; osteopedion.*

lithophone (lĭth′ō-fōn) [″ + *phone,* sound]. Instrument for determining the presence of calculi in the bladder by sound.

lithoscope (lĭth′ō-skōp) [″ + *skopein,* to examine]. Instrument for examining calculi in the bladder.

Lithotabs. Trade name for lithium carbonate, USP.

lithotome (lĭth′ō-tōm) [″ + *tome,* incision]. Instrument for performing lithotomy.

lithotomy (lĭth-ŏt′ō-mē) [″ + *tome,* incision]. Incision of a duct or organ, esp. of the bladder, for removal of a calculus.

NURSING IMPLICATIONS: Assess dietary history for factors contributing to stone formation. Relieve pain by using prescribed noninvasive measures and analgesics; encourage fluid intake to 4000 ml per day unless contraindicated by cardiac status; and strain all urine for evidence of stones. Monitor intake and output. Monitor vital signs and laboratory studies for infection, and administer antibiotics as prescribed. Assess any incisions for drainage and healing. Based on analysis of calculus, teach patient about dietary regimens to change urine pH as indicated.

l., bilateral. Lithotomy performed with the incision across the perineum.

l., high. Lithotomy performed through a suprapubic incision.

l., lateral. Lithotomy performed with incision from front of the rectum to one side of the raphe.

l., median. Lithotomy performed with incision in median line in front of the anus.

l., rectal. Lithotomy performed through the rectum.

l., vaginal. Lithotomy performed with

incision through the vaginal wall.

lithotomy position. Position in which the patient lies supine with thighs flexed upon abdomen and legs upon thighs, which are abducted. SYN: *dorsosacral position.* SEE: *position* for illus.

lithotony (lĭth-ŏt′ō-nē) [Gr. *lithos*, stone, + *teinein*, to stretch]. Removal of a calculus through a small incision that is instrumentally dilated.

lithotresis (lĭth″ō-trē′sĭs) [″ + *tresis*, boring]. Drilling or boring of holes in a calculus to facilitate crushing.

lithotripsy (lĭth′ō-trĭp″sē) [″ + *tribein*, to rub]. Crushing of a calculus in the bladder or urethra.

lithotriptic (lĭth-ō-trĭp′tĭk). 1. Pert. to lithotripsy. SEE: *lithontriptic.* 2. An agent that dissolves calculi.

NOTE: There are no substances that have this capability and are harmless to the patient.

lithotriptor (lĭth′ō-trĭp″tor) [″ + *tripsis*, friction]. A device for breaking up renal calculi. SEE: *percutaneous ultrasonic lithotriptor.*

lithotriptoscopy (lĭth″ō-trĭp-tŏs′kō-pē) [″ + ″ + *skopein*, to examine]. Crushing of a renal calculus under direct vision by using a lithotriptoscope.

lithotrite (lĭth′ō-trīt) [″ + *tribein*, to rub]. Instrument for crushing bladder stones. SEE: *lithotrity.*

lithotrity (lĭth-ŏt′rĭ-tē). Crushing of a stone to small fragments in the bladder.

lithous (lĭth′ŭs) [Gr. *lithos*, stone]. Rel. to a calculus or stone. SYN: *calculous.*

lithoxiduria (lĭth″ŏks-ĭ-dū′rē-ă) [″ + L. *oxidum*, oxide, + Gr. *ouron*, urine]. Presence of xanthic oxide in the urine.

lithuresis (lĭth″ū-rē′sĭs) [″ + *ouresis*, urination]. Passage of calculus through the urethra during urination.

lithureteria (lĭth″ū-rē-tē′rē-ă) [″ + *oureter*, ureter]. Disease of the ureter due to presence of calculi.

lithuria (lĭth-ū′rē-ă) [″ + *ouron*, urine]. Excess of uric acid or of urates in the urine.

litigation. A lawsuit or legal action that determines legal rights and remedies of the person or party.

litmus (lĭt′mŭs). A blue dyestuff made by treating coarsely powdered lichens, such as those of the genus *Roccella,* with ammonia.

litmus paper. Chemically prepared blue paper that is turned red by acids and remains blue in alkali solutions; pH range is 4.5 to 8.5. SEE: *indicator.*

litter (lĭt′tĕr) [O. Fr. *litiere*, offspring at birth, bed]. 1. A stretcher for carrying the wounded or the sick. 2. The young produced at one birth by a multiparous mammal.

Little's disease [William John Little, Brit. physician, 1810–1894]. Congenital spastic paralysis on both sides (diplegia), although it may be paraplegic or hemiplegic in form. SYN: *cerebral spastic diplegia.*

SYM: Child may be delayed in developing sphincter control and is usually mentally normal. Stiff, awkward movements, legs crossed and pressed together, arm adducted, forearm flexed, hand pronated, scissors gait.

ETIOL: Unknown. Efforts to implicate hypoxemia in utero have not been successful.

little league elbow [Little League Baseball, an international baseball league for children 8 to 12 years of age, founded in 1939]. A form of overuse syndrome in which there is inflammation of the medial condyle of the elbow. Seen in adolescent baseball players, esp. in pitchers. Little League Baseball regulations limit the time pitchers may play in any one game.

Littre's glands (lē′trz) [Alexis Littre, Fr. surgeon, 1658–1725]. Urethral glands.

littritis (lĭt-trī′tĭs). Inflammation of the urethral glands.

Litzmann's obliquity [Karl K. T. Litzmann, Ger. gynecologist, 1815–1890]. Posterior parietal presentation of the fetal head during labor. SYN: *asynclitism, posterior.*

live birth. A term used for statistical purposes indicating an infant born with signs of life such as heartbeat, respiration, or movement of voluntary muscle. In some countries a live birth is considered not to have occurred if the infant dies in the 24 hours following delivery. Obviously, which of these two definitions is used has considerable effect on various vital statistics concerned with the viability of the fetus at time of delivery.

lived experience. Refers to the subjective perception of one's health or illness experience. The term is associated with Rosemary Parse's nursing theory of Man-Living-Health and emphasizes the nurse's need to understand the personal health experience of patients, rather than to collect data from patients as objects.

livedo (lĭv-ē′dō) [L. *livedo*, lividness]. Patchy or general bluish discoloration of the skin, as a bruise. SYN: *lividity.*

l. reticularis. Semipermanent bluish mottling of the skin of the legs and hands. Aggravated by exposure to cold.

livedoid vasculitis. Vascular inflammation combined with intravascular thrombosis. These purpuric lesions are slow to heal. The cause in most cases in unknown, but they may be associated with diseases such as systemic lupus or scleroderma. SYN: *atrophie blanche.*

liver (lĭv′ĕr) [AS. *lifer*]. Largest organ in the

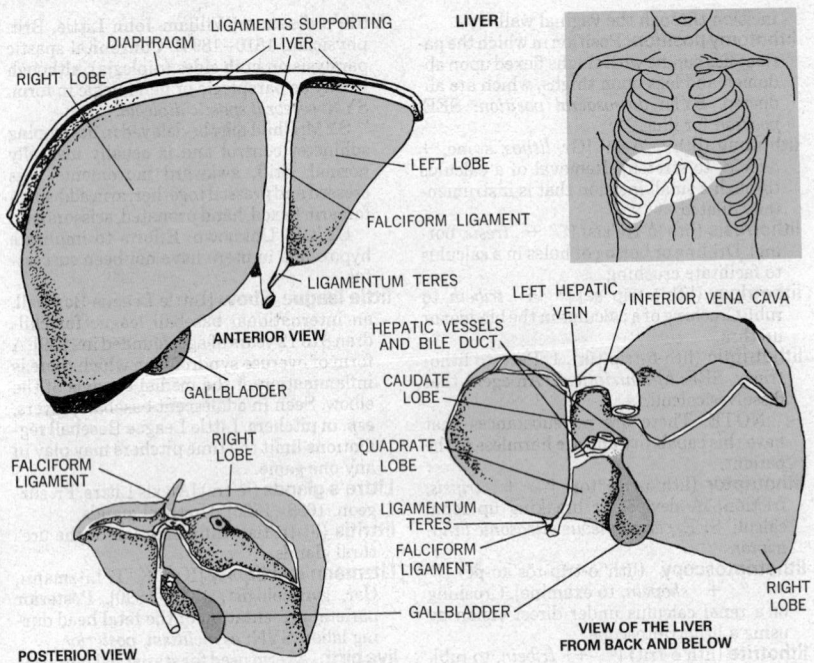

ANTERIOR VIEW

POSTERIOR VIEW

VIEW OF THE LIVER FROM BACK AND BELOW

body, approx. 21 to 22.5 cm in its greatest transverse diameter, 15 to 17.5 cm in its greatest vertical height, and 10 to 12.5 cm in its anteroposterior depth, weighing 1200 to 1600 gm, situated on right side beneath the diaphragm; occupies the right hypochondrium, epigastrium, and part of left hypochrondrium; level with bottom of sternum; undersurface concave; covers stomach, duodenum, hepatic flexure of colon, right kidney, and suprarenal capsule; secretes bile and is the site of a great many metabolic functions. SEE: illus.

ANAT: Completely covered by a tough fibrous sheath, Glisson's capsule, which is thickest at the transverse fissure. At this point the capsule carries the blood vessels and hepatic duct, which enter the organ at the hilus. Strands of connective tissue originating from the capsule enter the liver parenchyma and form the supporting network of the organ and separate the functional units of the liver, the hepatic lobules.

The many intrahepatic bile passages converge and anastomose, finally leading into the hepatic duct, the excretory channel of the liver. This structure receives the cystic duct, on the end of which is situated the gallbladder. The union of the cystic and the he-

patic ducts forms the common bile duct or the ductus choledochus, which enters the duodenum at the papilla of Vater. A ring of smooth muscle at the terminal portion of the choledochus, the sphincter of Oddi, permits the passage of bile into the duodenum by relaxing. The bile leaving the liver enters the gallbladder, where it undergoes concentration principally through loss of fluids absorbed by the gallbladder mucosa. When bile is needed in the small intestine for digestive purposes, the gallbladder contracts and the sphincter relaxes, thus permitting escape of the viscid gallbladder bile. Ordinarily, the sphincter of Oddi is contracted, shutting off the duodenal entrance and forcing the bile to enter the gallbladder after leaving the liver.

Within the sinusoids of the liver and attached to their walls are found the cells of Kupffer, which are highly phagocytic. They remove cellular detritus, bacteria, and other foreign particulate substances from the bloodstream.

The liver has four lobes, five ligaments, five fissures; derives its blood supply from the hepatic artery and portal vein; and secretes 800 to 1000 ml of bile in 24 hours. The rate of bile secretion is greatly increased during digestion.

BLOOD SUPPLY: From the hepatic artery, a branch of the celiac artery and the hepatic portal vein, which drains the intestine.

NERVE SUPPLY: Parasympathetic fibers from the vagi and sympathetic fibers from celiac plexus via hepatic artery.

FUNCT: The liver receives blood from the portal vein and thus is the first organ to receive blood from the intestines, where the blood has absorbed the final products of digestion and decomposition products. From this blood the liver removes glucose, from which it synthesizes glycogen, which it stores. Glucose not stored as glycogen or used to form amino acids is converted to fatty acids, carbon dioxide, and water. It deaminizes amino acids with the resultant formation of ammonia, which is converted into urea. Hippuric acid and uric acid are synthesized in the liver. The liver incorporates amino acids into proteins. It probably makes such proteins as albumin, prothrombin component, fibrinogen, transferrin, and glycoprotein. The liver is important in the biotransformation (i.e., so-called detoxification) of such substances as indole and skatole, which may be absorbed into the blood from the intestine.

The liver excretes bile pigments bilirubin and biliverdin, formed in the cells of the reticuloendothelial system in various parts of the body from hemoglobin derived from effete (exhausted and no longer functioning) red corpuscles. It synthesizes fibrinogen and prothrombin, blood constituents essential for clotting. It is the source of heparin, an anticoagulant, and of red blood cells in the fetus, and is the main site for the production of plasma proteins. Reticuloendothelial cells (Kupffer cells), present in the linings of the sinusoids, act to filter out and destroy bacteria present in the bloodstream.

The liver also performs the following functions. It is a storage place for vitamin B_{12} (the antipernicious anemia factor) and the fat-soluble vitamins A, D, E, and K. It plays a role in the regulation of blood volume and is one of the main sources of body heat. It is important in lipid metabolism. Cholesterol, which is found in most body cells and is a major constituent of bile, is manufactured mainly in the liver. SEE: *hepatitis*.

l., abscess of. SYM: Temperature elevated in evening, low in morning; sweats and chills; liver enlarged, painful, tender, may be bulging and fluctuating. Pus may be detected by aspiration.

ETIOL: Pathogenic bacteria, esp. pyogenic organisms such as those of *Streptococ-*

cus and *Staphylococcus;* trauma; infection by *Entamoeba histolytica*.

PROG: Embolic (multiple) abscesses are generally fatal. Traumatic abscesses, or those due to an amebic dysentery, may terminate favorably after spontaneous or induced evacuation.

l., acute yellow atrophy of. A rare and grave disease, characterized anatomically by a rapid destruction of the liver tissues, and manifested by jaundice and hemorrhages, a reduction in size of liver, and marked cerebral phenomena. Usually due to viral hepatitis B infection or toxic reaction to a drug. SYN: *hepatitis, fulminant.* SEE: *asterixis; hepatic coma.*

SYM: Malaise, slight fever, nausea, vomiting, jaundice, severe headache, tremor, delirium, convulsions, and coma. Urine is scanty, contains albumin, blood, and casts; renal failure may occur. Hemorrhages are common, the skin may be covered with ecchymoses, and bleeding from the mucous membranes may occur. Hepatic dullness diminished; splenic dullness increased.

TREAT: Symptomatic.

PROG: Generally fatal.

l., amyloid. An enlargement of liver due to the deposition of an albuminoid substance.

SYM: Failure of general health with anemia. Liver is enlarged, smooth, firm, and painless. Spleen and kidneys share in the degeneration, so the spleen is enlarged and the urine albuminous.

TREAT: Therapy must be directed to the causal disease, usually prolonged suppuration, syphilis, tuberculosis, or chronic malaria.

PROG: Unfavorable.

l., biliary cirrhotic. Cirrhosis of liver due to fibrous tissue formed as a result of infection or obstruction of the bile ducts.

l., cancer of. Male sex and heredity are predisposing factors. Malignancy in the liver as a result of spread from a primary source is many times more frequent than primary tumor of the liver. The liver is the most usual site of metastatic spread of tumors that disseminate through the bloodstream.

SYM: Severe pain and tenderness; cachexia, i.e., loss of weight; pressure symptoms; jaundice common; liver enlarged, surface is nodular and a central depression or umbilications can often be detected; symptoms of the primary growth. Fever generally absent, but secondary perihepatitis or suppuration of cancerous nodules may produce it.

TREAT: Symptomatic.

PROG: Fatal; duration from few months

to 1 year.

l., cirrhosis of. Generalized pathology of the liver with disturbed normal architecture of the lobes due to infiltration of fibrous tissue and nodule formation. These changes are accompanied by impaired liver function. Spider nevi may be present on the skin. The disease can progress to the stage of complete liver failure. SEE: *asterixis; hepatic coma; spider nevus.*

SYM: Abdominal swelling due to ascites, jaundice, weakness, weight loss, anorexia, nausea, fetor hepaticus, and mild continuous fever. As cirrhosis progresses, portal blood finds new channels, and the superficial abdominal veins enlarge, notably about the umbilicus, forming the so-called caput medusae; hemorrhoids and esophageal varices result from the same cause. In the final stages, hepatic encephalopathy develops. This is due in part to substances including ammonia absorbed from the intestines that have not been metabolized by the liver. These reach the brain and produce encephalopathy. Clinically, the patient is mentally dulled, may have hallucinations and a peculiar type of flapping tremor. SEE: *asterixis.*

ETIOL: In the U.S., the most frequent cause is chronic alcoholism. About 20% of those who drink alcohol heavily for a 5- to 10-year period develop cirrhosis. It may occur in individuals with no history of alcoholism. It can develop due to contact with toxic substances such as methotrexate, methanol, halothane, or oxyphenisatin. Other causes include infectious hepatitis; metabolic disorders, including glycogen storage diseases, tyrosinosis, thalassemia, and hemochromatosis; heart disease with chronic passive congestion of the liver; biliary obstruction; and as a complication of intestinal bypass surgery.

TREAT: Depends on the etiology. Major complications that occur regardless of etiology include portal hypertension, upper gastrointestinal tract bleeding, ascites, and hepatic coma.

PROG: Unfavorable except in first stages.

l., cysts of. May be simple cysts, usually small and single; hydatid cysts; or cysts associated with hydatid disease of the liver, a rare condition usually associated with congenital cystic kidneys. SEE: *Echinococcus granulosus; hydatid.*

l., fatty. Degenerative changes in liver cells due to fat deposits in the cells.

l., floating. An easily displaced liver.

l., foamy. Presence of gas bubbles in the liver as a result of infection with anaerobic bacteria. This produces a honeycomb appearance in the liver tissue.

l., hobnail. Degeneration of the liver characterized by fatty changes, fibrous scarring, nodular degeneration, and atrophy of the liver with the surface covered with brown or yellow nodules. Seen in chronic alcoholism and malnutrition.

l., inflammation of. The usual cause of inflammation is the same as that of viral hepatitis. The clinical picture may be so mild as to be almost unnoticed or may be so severe that the jaundice is followed rapidly by hepatic encephalopathy and death. SYN: *hepatitis.*

TREAT: Treated as if the condition were going to progress to the severe form; bedrest; diet as requested by patient but should be high caloric; cortisone should not be given routinely. There is no specific treatment and in general the disease is self-limiting.

l., lardaceous. L., amyloid, q.v.

l., nutmeg. Chronic passive congestion of the liver, which produces a reddened central portal area and a yellowish periportal zone.

l., wandering. L., floating, q.v.

liver, words pert. to: bile; -acids; -calculi; -colic; -pigments; "bili-" words; capsule, Glisson's; cardiohepatic; choleresis; cirrhosis; facies hepatica; flexure; "glyco-" words; "hepa-" words; jaundice; perihepatitis; transplant.

liver extract. A dry brown powder obtained from mammalian livers that contains the hematinic factor (antianemic factor), which stimulates erythropoiesis. Was important in treatment of pernicious anemia until vitamin B_{12} was discovered.

liver failure. Inability of the liver to function because of a disease process within the liver or because of demands beyond its capability.

liver flap. A characteristic flapping type of tremor of the hands seen in patients with severe impairment of liver function. SYN: *asterixis.*

liver fluke, human. *Clonorchis sinensis*, common in Far East. Adults infest biliary and pancreatic ducts. Eggs pass from the body with feces and continue development in snails of the subfamily Buliminae (family Hydrobiidae). Cercariae emerge and infest numerous species of freshwater fishes in which they encyst. Infestation results from eating raw fish containing encysted metacercariae.

liver spots. Yellow-brown spots on skin. SYN: *chloasma hepaticum.*

liver transplantation. Transplantation of the liver. This can be done so that the transplanted organ is an auxiliary at an ectopic site to the host's liver or in the usual location after the removal of the host's liver. The procedure has been used to treat a number of benign diseases and to replace cirrhotic livers.

livid (lĭv'ĭd) [L. *lividus*, lead-colored]. 1. Ashen, cyanotic. 2. Discolored, black and blue.

lividity (lĭ-vĭd'ĭ-tē). 1. Skin discoloration, as from a bruise or venous congestion. 2. State of being livid.

   l., postmortem. Livedo, q.v., that may be present beginning after death.

living will. A statement prepared at a time when the individual was well. It attests to the wish that heroic measures such as use of life-support devices not be used to prolong life when it is obvious that such actions will not permit recovery from the condition. SEE: *advance directive; hopelessly ill patients.*

livor (lī'vor) [L., a black-and-blue spot]. Lividity.

   l. mortis. Cutaneous dark spot on dependent portion of a cadaver due to gravitational pooling of blood.

lixiviation (lĭks″ĭv-ē-ā'shŭn) [L. *lixivia*, lye]. Separation of soluble from insoluble substances by washing and filtration. SYN: *leaching.*

L.L.E. *left lower extremity.*

LLQ. *left lower quadrant* (of abdomen).

L.M.A. *left mentoanterior* fetal position.

L.M.P. *left mentoposterior* fetal position.

L.M.T. *left mentotransverse* fetal position.

L.O.A. *left occipitoanterior* fetal position.

load. 1. The weight supported or force imposed. 2. A substance given to test body function, esp. metabolic function. SEE: *loading test.*

loading, carbohydrate. SEE: *carbohydrate loading.*

loading test. Administration of a substance in order to determine individual's ability to metabolize or excrete it. Thus a glucose tolerance test is one form of this test.

loaiasis. Loiasis, q.v.

Loa loa (lō'ă) [W. African]. The African eyeworm, a species of filarial worm that infests the subcutaneous tissues and conjunctiva of humans. Its migration causes itching and a creeping sensation. Sometimes it causes itchy edematous areas known as Calabar swellings. It is transmitted by flies of the genus *Chrysops.*

lobar (lō'băr) [Gr. *lobos*, lobe]. Pert. to a lobe.

lobar pneumonia. Inflammation of one or more lobes of the lungs. SEE: *pneumonia, lobar.*

lobate (lō'bāt) [L. *lobatus*, lobed]. 1. Pert. to a lobe. 2. Having a deeply undulated border. 3. Producing lobes.

lobe (lōb) [Gr. *lobos*, lobe]. 1. A fairly well-defined part of an organ separated by boundaries, especially glandular organs and the brain. 2. A major part of a tooth formed by a separate calcification center.

   l., anterior, of hypophysis. Anterior portion of the hypophysis or pituitary gland, consisting of the pars distalis and pars tuberalis.

   l., azygos. An anomalous lobe at the apex of the right lobe of the lung.

   l., caudate, of liver. Lobe on the posterior surface of the liver. SYN: *l., spigelian.*

   l., central. Island of Reil, which forms the floor of the lateral cerebral fossa.

   l., flocculonodular. Lobe of the cerebellum consisting of the flocculi, nodulus, and their connecting peduncles.

   l., frontal. That part of a cerebral hemisphere in front of the central and sylvian fissures.

   l.'s, hepatic. Lobes of the liver.

   l., insular. L., central.

   l.'s, lateral, of prostate. The portions on each side of the urethra.

   l.'s, lateral, of thyroid gland. The two main portions, one on each side of the trachea, united below by the thyroid isthmus.

   l., limbic. Marginal section of the cerebral hemisphere on the medial aspect. SYN: *gyrus fornicatus.*

   l., occipital. Caudal region of either hemicerebrum.

   l.'s of cerebrum. Frontal, parietal, occipital, and temporal lobes and the insula or island of Reil (central lobe).

   l. of ear. Lower portion of the auricle having no cartilage.

   l.'s of lungs. Large divisions of the lungs: superior and inferior lobes of the left lung; superior, middle, and inferior lobes of the right lung.

   l. of mamma. One of the 15 to 20 divisions of the glandular tissue of the breast separated by connective tissue and each possessing a duct (lobar duct) opening via the nipple.

   l.'s of pancreas. Round aggregations of glandular tissue separated by connective tissue.

   l. of parotid, accessory. A small lobe, variable in size, on the anterior surface of the parotid gland superior to the exit of the parotid duct.

   l.'s of prostate. The lateral lobes and the middle lobe of the prostate gland.

   l., olfactory. A series of convolutions below the horizontal portion of the intraparietal fissure of the cerebrum, containing the olfactory bulb. SYN: *rhinencephalon.*

   l.'s, orbital. The convolutions above the orbit.

   l., parietal. Upper and lateral portion of the hemisphere of the cerebrum.

   l., posterior, of hypophysis. The posterior portion of the pituitary gland, consisting of the pars intermedia and the processus infundibuli (pars nervosa).

l., prefrontal. The frontal portion of the frontal lobe of the brain.

l., pyramidal, of thyroid. A portion of the thyroid gland extending upward from the isthmus. It is extremely variable in size.

l., quadrate, of liver. An oblong elevation on the lower surface of the liver.

l., Riedel's. An anomalous tonguelike extension from the right lobe of the liver to the gallbladder.

l., spigelian. Irregular quadrangular portion of liver behind fissure for portal vein and between fissures for vena cava and ductus venosus. SYN: *l, caudate.*

l., temporal. The portion of the cerebral hemisphere lying below the lateral fissure of Sylvius. It is continuous posteriorly with the occipital lobe.

lobectomy (lō-běk'tō-mē) [Gr. *lobos,* lobe, + *ektome,* excision]. Surgical removal of a lobe of any organ or gland.

lobelia (lō-bē'lē-ă). Substance obtained from the dried leaves and tops of the herb *Lobelia inflata.* The chief constituent, lobeline, has the same action as nicotine but is less potent. SYN: *Indian tobacco.*

lobeline (lŏb'ĕ-lēn). The chief constituent of lobelia, q.v.

lobi. Pl. of lobus.

lobitis (lō-bī'tĭs) [" + *itis,* inflammation]. Inflammation of a lobe.

Loboa loboi. Fungus that causes keloidal blastomycosis (Lobo's disease). It has been identified in tissues but has not been cultured.

Lobo's disease. Keloidal blastomycosis. SEE: *blastomycosis.*

lobotomy (lō-bŏt'ō-mē) [Gr. *lobos,* lobe, + *tome,* incision]. Incision of a lobe. An operation that is performed for relief of some forms of mental disturbances that do not respond to other treatments. It is accomplished by a small bilateral trephination in the plane of the coronal suture through which the white matter of the brain is sectioned; the diencephalon, esp. the hypothalamic area, is disconnected from the prefrontal cortex by section of the white fiber connecting pathways subcortically in a plane passing adjacent to the anterior tip of the lateral ventricle and the posterior margin of the sphenoid wing.

Lobstein's disease (lōb'stīnz) [John Georg Friedrich Lobstein, Ger. surgeon, 1777–1835]. Osteogenesis imperfecta, q.v.

lobular (lŏb'ū-lăr) [L. *lobulus,* small lobe]. Composed of small lobes; pert. to a lobule. SYN: *lobulate.*

lobulate, lobulated (lŏb'ū-lāt, -lāt-ĕd). 1.

Consisting of lobes or lobules. 2. Pert. to lobes or lobules. 3. Resembling lobes. SYN: *lobular.*

lobule (lŏb'ūl) [L. *lobulus,* small lobe]. A small lobe or primary subdivision of a lobe. Typical of pancreas and major salivary glands and may be represented on the surface by bumps or bulges as seen on the thyroid gland.

l., central, of cerebellum. A small lobe at anterior part of the superior vermiform process.

l.'s of epididymis. Conelike divisions of the head of the epididymis formed by the much coiled distal ends of the efferent ducts of the testis.

l. of kidney. Subdivision of the renal cortex consisting of a medullary ray and surrounding glandular tissue.

l. of liver. Structural unit consisting of hepatic cells arranged in irregular, branching, and interconnected groups and anastomosing blood channels (sinusoids) surrounding a central vein. Polyhedral in shape with branches of portal vein, hepatic artery, and interlobular bile ducts at its periphery.

l.'s of lung. Physiological units of the lung consisting of a respiratory bronchiole and its branches (alveolar ducts, alveolar sacs, and alveoli).

l.'s of testis. Pyramidal divisions separated from each other by incomplete partitions called septula. Each consists of one to three coiled seminiferous tubules.

l.'s of thymus. Subdivisions of a lobe, each consisting of a cortex and medulla.

l., paracentral. Superior convolution of ascending frontal and parietal convolutions of the brain, forming a union of both.

l., parietal. One of two subdivisions of the parietal lobe of the brain. The superior parietal lobule comprises the posterior part of the upper portion, and the inferior parietal lobule comprises a lateral area continuous with temporal and occipital lobes.

l., primary pulmonary. The functional unit of the lung. Included are the respiratory bronchiole, alveolar ducts, sacs, and alveoli. SYN: *respiratory lobe.*

lobuli. Pl. of lobulus.

lobulus (lŏb'ū-lŭs) [L.] (pl. *lobuli*). [NA] A lobule or small division of a lobe.

lobus (lō'bŭs) [L.] (pl. *lobi*). [NA] Lobe.

L.O.C. *level of consciousness.*

local (lō'kăl) [L. *locus,* place]. Limited to one place or part.

localization (lō-kăl-ĭ-zā'shŭn). 1. Limitation to a definite area. 2. Determination of the site of an infection. 3. Relation of a sensation to its point of origin.

l., cerebral. Determination of centers of various faculties and functions in particular parts of the brain.

localized (lō'kăl-īzd). Restricted to a limited region.

localizer. Apparatus used for locating solid opaque bodies in the eye or other areas by roentgenographic examination.

locator (lō'kā-tĕr). Device for locating or discovering an object such as a foreign body.

lochia (lō'kē-ă) [Gr. *lochia*]. The discharge from the uterus of blood, mucus, and tissue during the puerperal period. The first six days it is distinctly blood-tinged and is known as lochia rubra or lochia cruenta; the following three or four days the discharge becomes brown and is known as lochia serosa; after this it becomes yellow, turning to white, and is known as lochia alba. It is diminished or suppressed in high fever. If the odor is offensive, it is the result of contamination with saprophytic organisms. Position the patient to favor drainage.

   l. alba. The white postpartum vaginal discharge that is no longer blood-tinged.

   l. cruenta. The bloody postpartum vaginal discharge.

   l. purulenta. L. alba, q.v.

   l. rubra. L. cruenta, q.v.

   l. serosa. A thin, watery postpartum vaginal discharge.

lochial (lō'kē-ăl). Pert. to the lochia.

lochiocolpos (lō″kē-ō-kŏl'pŏs) [Gr. *lochia*, discharge following childbirth, + *kolpos*, vagina]. Distention of the vagina due to retention of lochia.

lochiometra (lō″kē-ō-mē'tră) [″ + *metra*, uterus]. Retention of lochia in the uterus.

lochiometritis (lō″kē-ō-mē-trī'tĭs) [″ + ″ + *itis*, inflammation]. Puerperal inflammation of the uterus.

lochiorrhagia (lō′kē-ō-rā'jē-ă) [″ + *rhegnynai*, to break forth]. Excessive flow of lochia.

lochiorrhea (lō″kē-ō-rē'ă) [″ + *rhoia*, flow]. Abnormal flow of lochia.

lochioschesis (lō″kē-ŏs'kĕ-sĭs) [″ + *schesis*, retention]. Retention or suppression of the lochia.

lochometritis (lō″kō-mē-trī'tĭs) [″ + *metra*, uterus, + *itis*, inflammation]. Puerperal inflammation of uterus.

loci [L.]. Pl. of locus.

locked-in syndrome. Pseudocoma in patients who are awake but have no means of communication. They cannot talk or move limbs or face muscles. This is due to infarction or hemorrhage into the brain in the central pons area. The ability to move the eyes vertically and to blink are generally normal, and those movements may be used to give signals and respond to questions.

Locke's solution, Locke-Ringer's solution [Frank S. Locke, Brit. physician, 1871–

1949; Sydney Ringer, Brit. physiologist, 1835–1910]. A solution used in experiments in physiology. It contains sodium, potassium, calcium, and magnesium chlorides; sodium bicarbonate, dextrose, and water.

lockjaw. Tonic spasm of muscles of jaw. SEE: *tetanus.*

Lockwood's ligament [Charles B. Lockwood, Brit. surgeon, 1856–1914]. The suspensory ligament of the eyeball.

loco (lō'kō) [Sp., cracked brain]. 1. Locoweed disease, a nervous disorder that affects cattle that eat the locoweed. 2. Slang for insane.

locomotion (lō″kō-mō'shŭn) [L. *locus*, place, + *movere*, to move]. Movement or power of movement from one place to another.

locomotor (lō″kō-mō'tor). Pert. to locomotion.

locomotor ataxia. A sclerosis affecting the posterior columns of the spinal cord. SEE: *ataxia, locomotor; Charcot's joint.*

locomotorium (lō″kō-mō-tō'rē-ŭm). The locomotor apparatus of the body.

locular (lŏk'ū-lăr) [L. *loculus*, a small space]. Divided into small cavities.

loculated (lŏk'ū-lāt-ĕd). Containing or divided into loculi. SYN: *locular.*

loculi (lŏk'ū-lī). Pl. of loculus.

loculus (lŏk'ū-lŭs) [L.] (pl. *loculi*). A small space or cavity.

locum tenens (lō'kŭm tĕn'ĕns) [L. *locus*, place, + *tenere*, to hold]. A substitute. Physician who temporarily substitutes for another.

locus (lō'kŭs) [L. *locus*, a place] (pl. *loci*). 1. A spot or place. 2. In genetics, the site of a gene on a chromosome.

   l. ceruleus. [NA] A dark-colored depression in floor of 4th ventricle of the brain at its upper part.

   l. niger. Gray matter separating the crusta and tegmentum of the crura cerebri of the brain. SYN: *substantia nigra* [NA].

locus of control. Refers to an individual's sense of mastery or control over events. Persons with an internal locus of control are more apt to believe that they can influence events while those with an external locus of control tend to believe that events are dictated by fate. These respective orientations can influence a person's practice of health-related behaviors.

Loeffler's bacillus (lĕf'lĕrz) [Friedrich August Johannes Loeffler (Loffler), Ger. bacteriologist, 1852–1915]. The bacillus of diphtheria, *Corynebacterium diphtheriae.* SYN: *Klebs-Loeffler bacillus.* SEE: *diphtheria.*

Löffler's endocarditis (lĕf'lĕrz) [Wilhelm Löffler, Swiss physician, b. 1887]. Endocarditis associated with eosinophilia and fibroplastic thickening of the endocardium. The

cause is unknown.

logadectomy (lŏg″ă-dĕk′tō-mē) [Gr. *logades,* the whites of the eyes, + *ektome,* excision]. Excision of a portion of the conjunctiva.

logaditis (lŏg″ă-dī′tĭs) [″ + *itis,* inflammation]. Inflammation of the sclerotic coat of the eye. SYN: *scleritis.*

logagnosia (lŏg″ăg-nō′sē-ă) [Gr. *logos,* word, reason, + *a-,* not, + *gnosis,* knowledge]. A type of aphasia in which words are seen but not identified with respect to their meaning. SEE: *aphasia.*

logagraphia (lŏg-ă-grăf′ē-ă) [″ + ″ + *graphein,* to write]. Loss of ability to express ideas in writing. SYN: *agraphia.*

logamnesia (lŏg-ăm-nē′zē-ă) [″ + *amnesia,* forgetfulness]. Aphasia of a sensory character. Inability to recognize spoken or written words.

logaphasia (lŏg″ă-fā′zē-ă) [″ + *a-,* not, + *phasis,* speaking]. Motor aphasia, usually due to a cerebral lesion.

logasthenia (lŏg″ăs-thē′nē-ă) [″ + ″ + *sthenos,* strength]. Mental impairment characterized by defective ability to understand the spoken word.

logoklony (lŏg′ō-klŏn-ē) [″ + *klonein,* to agitate]. Intermittent repetition of the last syllable of a word.

logokophosis (lŏg″ō-kō-fō′sĭs) [″ + *kophosis,* deafness]. Inability to understand spoken language; word deafness. SYN: *Wernicke's aphasia.*

logomania (lŏg-ō-mā′nē-ă) [″ + *mania,* madness]. Repetitious, continuous, and excessive flow of speech in monomania.

logoneurosis (lŏg″ō-nū-rō′sĭs) [″ + *neuron,* nerve, + *osis,* condition]. Any neurosis marked by speech disorders.

logopathia (lŏg-ō-păth′ē-ă) [″ + *pathos,* disease, suffering]. Any disorder of speech arising from derangement of the central nervous system.

logopedia (lŏg″ō-pē′dē-ă) [″ + *pais,* child]. Science dealing with speech defects and their correction.

logoplegia (lŏg-ō-plē′jē-ă) [″ + *plege,* stroke]. Paralysis of the speech organs.

logorrhea (lŏg″ō-rē′ă) [″ + *rhoia,* flow]. Unusual loquacity seen in insanity. SYN: *logomania.*

logospasm (lŏg′ō-spăzm) [″ + *spasmos,* a convulsion]. Spasmodic word enunciation.

-logy [Gr. *logos,* word, reason]. Suffix meaning discourse, science or study of.

loiasis (lō-ī′ă-sĭs). Infestation with *Loa loa,* q.v.

loin (loyn) [O. Fr. *loigne,* long part]. Lower part of back and sides between the ribs and pelvis. SYN: *lumbus* [NA].

lolism. Poisoning by the seeds of *Lolium*

temulentum, darnel ryegrass.

lomustine (lō-mŭs′tēn). A chemotherapeutic agent used in treating certain neoplastic conditions. Also called CCNU.

loneliness. Literally, the condition of being alone. Medically, it is the important state of being frightened, anxious, depressed, or sad because of the lack of companionship, esp. of a particular person or group; i.e., one may experience loneliness even though in the presence of people.

Long, Crawford Williamson. U.S. physician, 1815–1878, who in 1842 first administered an anesthetic during surgery.

long-acting thyroid stimulator. ABBR: LATS. A serum globulin that causes hyperfunction of the thyroid. There are probably other similar substances involved in affecting the thyroid gland in thyrotoxicosis.

longevity (lŏn-jĕv′ĭ-tē) [L. *longaevus,* aged]. Long duration of life. Age was reckoned by the Romans in six stages: *pueritia,* childhood, to 5 years; *adolescentia,* youth, to 18 years; *juventus,* young man, to 25 years; *majores,* man, to 50 years; *senectus,* old man, to 60 years; *crepita aetas,* decrepit, 60 years to death.

longevity record. In 1987 the average life expectancy of a newborn was 75 years. For males it was 71.4 years and 78.4 years for females.

longing. A persistent desire or craving for something, usually that which is remote or unattainable.

longissimus (lŏn-jĭs′ĭ-mŭs) [L.]. Anatomical term indicating a long structure.

longitudinal (lŏn″jĭ-tū′dĭ-năl) [L. *longitudo,* length]. Parallel to the long axis of the body or part.

longsightedness. Farsightedness. SYN: *hyperopia.*

longus (lŏng′gŭs) [L.]. Anatomical term indicating a long structure.

loop [ME. *loupe*]. A curve or bend in a cord or cordlike structure, forming roughly an oval.

  l., cervical. The part of an enamel organ in which the inner enamel epithelium is continuous with the outer enamel epithelium. This establishes the limit of enamel formation and therefore represents the site of the cementoenamel junction. The cells of the cervical loop become Hertwig's epithelial root sheath, induce dentinogenesis, and determine the number, size, and shape of the tooth roots.

  l., closed. A biological system in which a substance produced affects the output of the substance by a feedback mechanism.

  l., Henle's. The descending and ascending loops of the renal tubule.

  l., Lippes. Lippes loop, q.v.

  l.'s of capillary. Minute blood vessels in

the papillae of the skin.

loosening of association. A sign of disordered thought processes in which the person speaks with frequent changes of subject, and the content is only obliquely related, if at all, to the subject matter. This may be seen in mania or schizophrenia.

loose-packed position. Position of a joint where it is unlocked and free to move.

loose-packed position, maximum. Position where maximum joint play occurs. The position where ligaments and capsule have the least amount of tension. Also known as resting position.

L.O.P. *left occipitoposterior* fetal position.

loperamide hydrochloride. Generic name for Imodium.

lophotrichea (lŏf-ō-trĭk′ē-ă) [Gr. *lophos,* tuft, + *thrix,* hair]. Microorganisms possessing flagella in tufts.

lophotrichous (lŏf-ŏt′rĭ-kŭs). Having bunches of flagella at one end.

lordoscoliosis (lor″dō-skō″lē-ō′sĭs) [Gr. *lordosis,* bending, + *skoliosis,* curvation]. Forward curvature of the spine complicated by lateral curvature.

lordosis (lor-dō′sĭs) [Gr.]. Abnormal anterior convexity of the spine.

Lorfan. Trade name for levallorphan tartrate, USP.

L.O.T. *left occipitotransverse* fetal position.

lotio (lō′shē-ō) [L.]. Lotion.

   l. alba. Lotion, white, q.v.

lotion (lō′shŭn) [L. *lotio*]. Liquid medicinal preparation for local application to, or bathing of, a part.

   l., calamine. SEE: *calamine.*

   l., white. A combination of 4% zinc sulfate with 4% sulfurated potash.

Lotrimin. Trade name for clotrimazole.

Lotusate. Trade name for talbutal.

loudness. Sound intensity. SEE: *decibel.*

Louis-Bar syndrome (loo-wē′băr) [Denise Louis-Bar, 20th century European physician]. Ataxia-telangiectasia, q.v.

loupe (loop) [Fr.]. A magnifying lens used in the form of a monocular or binocular lens. Surgeons, dentists, jewelers, and watchmakers frequently use this device.

louse (laus) [AS. *lus*] (pl. *lice*). A small wingless insect that lives as an ectoparasite on birds and mammals. Sucking lice belong to the order Anoplura; biting or chewing lice belong to the order Mallophaga. Lice that are parasitic on humans are the primary transmitters of epidemic typhus, trench fever, and relapsing fever. They may also be the mechanical transmitters of other diseases such as plague. SYN: *pediculus.* SEE: illus.; *Pediculus.*

   l., body. Pediculus humanus corporis; lives principally in or on clothing.

LOUSE

PUBIC LOUSE
(PHTHIRUS
PUBIS)

BODY LOUSE
(PEDICULUS
HUMANUS)

   l., crab. Phthirus pubis; lives principally in hair in pubic region but also found in beard, eyebrows, and eyelashes.

   l., head. Pediculus humanus capitis; lives in hair of the head. For treatment, SEE: *pediculosis capitis.*

lousiness. State of being infested with lice. SYN: *pediculosis.*

lovastatin. A drug used to control the level of cholesterol in the blood. It inhibits synthesis of cholesterol. Trade name is Mevacor.

love [ME.]. 1. Concern and affection for another person. This may be to such a degree as to cause individuals to risk losing their lives in their concern for the safety, care, and well-being of another. 2. In psychiatry, love may be equated to pleasure, particularly as it applies to the gratifying sexual experiences between individuals.

Loven's reflex (lō-vānz′) [Otto Christian Loven, Swed. physician, 1835–1904]. Vasodilation with corresponding increase in size of organ resulting from stimulation of afferent nerve or organ.

low birth weight. Abnormally low weight of a newborn. It is usually less than 2500 gm. A 280-gm infant has survived, but with physical and mental impairment.

lower motor neuron lesion. Injury occurring in the anterior horn cells, nerve roots, or peripheral nervous system that results in diminished reflexes, flaccid paralysis, and atrophy.

Lowe's syndrome (lōz) [Charles U. Lowe, U.S. pediatrician, b. 1921]. Oculocerebrorenal dystrophy characterized by hypotonia, loss of reflexes, mental deterioration, glaucoma, cataracts, and renal tubular dysfunction. Transmitted as a sex-linked recessive.

low-level radiation. SEE: *radiation, lowlevel.*

low-protein diet. Diet that contains limited amount of protein. The principal sources of food energy are fats and carbohydrates. Used in treating hepatic coma.

low-salt diet. Diet in which no salt is allowed on patient's tray and no salty foods are served. Used in treating hypertension as well as congestive heart failure.

lox. *liquid oxygen.*

loxarthron (lŏks-ăr′thrŏn) [Gr. *loxos,* slanting, + *arthron,* joint]. Oblique deformity of a joint without dislocation.

loxia (lŏks′ē-ă) [Gr., slanting]. Stiff neck caused by spasmodic contraction of the neck muscles drawing the head to one side with the chin pointing to the other side. SYN: *torticollis; wryneck.*

Loxosceles (lŏks-ŏs′-sĕ-lēz). A genus of spiders.

loxoscelism (lŏk-sŏs′sĕ-lizm). The disease produced by the bite of the brown spider, *Loxosceles laeta* or *L. reclusa.* Symptoms include a painful red vesicle that eventually becomes gangrenous and sloughs.

loxotic (lŏks-ŏt′ĭk) [Gr. *loxos,* slanting]. Distorted in an awry manner.

loxotomy (lŏks-ŏt′ō-mē) [″ + *tome,* incision]. Amputation by oblique section.

lozenge (lŏz′ĕnj) [Fr.]. Small, dry, medicinal solid to be held in mouth until it dissolves. SYN: *troche.*

Lp(a). *lipoprotein (a).*

L-phase variants. L-forms, q.v.

L.P.N. *licensed practical nurse.*

LPO. *left posterior oblique* position.

Lr. Chem. symb. for the element lawrencium.

L.R.C.P. *licentiate of the Royal College of Physicians.*

L.R.C.S. *licentiate of the Royal College of Surgeons.*

LRF. *luteinizing hormone releasing factor.*

L.S.A. *left sacroanterior* fetal position.

L.Sc.A. *left scapuloanterior* fetal position.

L.Sc.P. *left scapuloposterior* fetal position.

LSD. *lysergic acid diethylamide,* a derivative of an alkaloid in ergot. LSD is used legally only for experimental purposes. It is used ille-

gally for its hallucinogenic effects.

LSI. *life satisfaction index.*

L.S.P. *left sacroposterior* fetal position.

L/S ratio. *lecithin/sphingomyelin ratio,* q.v.

L.S.T. *left sacrotransverse* fetal position.

LTC. *long-term care.*

LTH. *luteotropic hormone.*

Lu. Chem. symb. for the element lutetium.

lubb-dupp (lŭb-dŭp′). The two sounds heard in auscultation marking a complete cycle of the heart. Pause following the cycle is slightly longer than that between the two sounds. SEE: *heart, auscultation of.*

lubricant (loo′brĭ-kănt) [L. *lubricans*]. Agent, usually a liquid oil, that reduces friction between parts that brush against each other as they move. Joints are lubricated by synovial fluid.

lubricating enema. Enema given to soften feces and lubricate anal canal after hemorrhoidectomy, or to soften fecal impaction. SEE: *enema, lubricating.*

Lucas-Championnière's disease (lū-kă′ shaw″pē-ŏn-ē-ayrz′) [J. M. M. Lucas-Championnière, Fr. surgeon, 1843–1913]. Pseudomembranous bronchitis.

lucent [L. *lucere,* to shine]. Shining, translucent, clear.

lucid (lū′sĭd) [L. *lucidus,* clear]. Clear, esp. applied to clarity of the mind.

lucid interval. Period of normal mental functioning between attacks of mental illness or cerebral trauma. In head trauma, the period of being awake following injury until coma develops. A lucid interval is common in epidural and subdural hematomas.

lucidity (lū-sĭd′ĭ-tē). Quality of clearness or brightness, esp. with regard to mental conditions.

luciferase (loo-sĭf′ĕr-ās). An enzyme that acts on luciferins to oxidize them and cause bioluminescence. It is present in certain organisms, such as the firefly, or insects, that emit light either continuously or intermittently.

luciferin (loo-sĭf′ĕr-ĭn). General term for substances present in some organisms. It becomes luminescent when acted upon by luciferase.

lucifugal (loo-sĭf′ū-găl) [L. *lux,* light, + *fugere,* to flee from]. Being repelled by bright light.

lucipetal (loo-sĭp′ĭ-tăl) [″ + *peter,* to seek]. Being attracted by bright light.

lucotherapy (lū″kō-thĕr′ă-pē) [″ + Gr. *therapeia,* treatment]. Therapeutic use of light rays. SYN: *phototherapy.*

Ludwig's angina (lūd′vĭgz) [Wilhelm F. von Ludwig, Ger. surgeon, 1790–1865]. A suppurative inflammation of subcutaneous connective tissue adjacent to a submaxillary gland.

L.U.E. *left upper extremity.*

Luer-Lok syringe (lū'ĕr-lŏk'). A syringe made to permit rapid and firm attachment of the needle.

lues (lū'ēz) [L.]. Syphilis.

luetic (lū-ĕt'ĭk). 1. Pert. to syphilis. 2. Affected with syphilis. SYN: *syphilitic.*

Lugol's solution (lū'gŏlz) [Jean G. A. Lugol, Fr. physician, 1786–1851]. Strong iodine solution used in iodine therapy. Iodine 5 gm, potassium iodide 10 gm, and water to make 100 ml.

LUL. *left upper lobe* (of the lung).

lumbago (lŭm-bā'gō) [L. *lumbus*, loin]. A general nonspecific term for dull, aching pain in the lumbar region of the back.

lumbar (lŭm'băr) [L. *lumbus*, loin]. Pert. to the loins; the part of the back between the thorax and pelvis.

lumbarization (lŭm″băr-ĭ-zā'shŭn). The first sacral vertebra is not fused with the sacrum and, therefore, functions as a 6th lumbar vertebra.

lumbar nerves. Five pairs of nerves, corresponding with the lumbar vertebrae.

lumbar plexus. A nerve plexus formed by the ventral branches of the second to fifth lumbar nerves.

lumbar puncture. Puncture made by placing an aspiration needle into the subarachnoid space of the spinal cord. Usually done in the lumbar area at the level of the 4th intervertebral space. SYN: *spinal puncture.* SEE: *cerebrospinal fluid; cisternal puncture; headache; Queckenstedt's sign; spinal puncture.*

PURPOSE: For the removal of spinal fluid for diagnostic purposes, and for the injection of an anesthetic solution.

NOTE: May be lethal if done in the presence of increased intracranial pressure. The brain stem may, upon decrease of pressure in the spinal canal, herniate into the foramen magnum of the base of the skull.

PROCEDURE: Medication, dissolved in previously removed cerebrospinal fluid, or anesthetics for cord blocking may be cautiously introduced. The area is cleansed and painted with antiseptic. A sterile puncture needle of small gauge (22) is then readily passed directly into the midline, to and through the dura. When the stylet is removed, spinal fluid will escape and can be collected in two or three tubes for examination. When procedure is completed, instruct the patient to lie flat in a prone position for 6 to 12 hours. This will greatly reduce the possibility of developing a headache. Post-lumbar puncture headache is related to continued leakage of fluid from the spinal canal. The use of a small-gauge needle will lessen the chance that spinal fluid will continue to seep from the spinal canal after the needle is removed, and thus the possibility of development of post-spinal tap headache will be diminished.

NURSING IMPLICATIONS: Explain the procedure and reassure patient. Patient should be turned on side near edge of the bed with back to operator. Thighs are flexed on trunk and head is lowered to chest with back bowed as far as possible. Nurse holds patient in this position. Alternatively, the patient may be in a sitting position with head, neck, and thoracic spine flexed. The legs are allowed to dangle over the side of the bed or table. The nurse stands in front of the patient to provide support in this position.

After the procedure, assess the vital signs and neurological status, looking particularly for signs of paralysis, weakness, and loss of sensation in the legs or trunk. In order to decrease the chance of the development of a headache, instruct the patient to remain in bed in a prone position. The head may be moved from side to side but not elevated.

ARTICLES NECESSARY: Sterilized lumbar puncture needles, gloves for physician, antiseptic for skin, sterilized gauze and sponge, sterile towel, 5 ml of 0.5% solution of procaine hydrochloride, two sterile test tubes. If spinal fluid pressure is to be determined, sterile manometer tubes and a 3-way stopcock adapter for connecting the manometer to the spinal puncture needle will be required.

lumbar reflex. Irritation of the skin over the erector spinae muscles, causing contraction of muscles of the back.

lumbar region. Each side of umbilical region above the iliac region and below the hypochondriac region.

lumbar stenosis. Overgrowth of the laminae of the vertebrae so that the spinal canal is narrowed. This causes back and leg pain especially when walking. SYN: *lumbar canal stenosis.* SEE: *back pain.*

lumbar vertebrae. Five bones of the spinal column between the sacrum and thoracic vertebrae. SEE: *spinal column* for illus.

lumbo- [L. *lumbus*, loin]. Combining form pert. to the loins.

lumboabdominal (lŭm″bō-ăb-dŏm'ĭ-năl) [″ + *abdomen*, belly]. Concerning the lateral and frontal areas of the abdomen.

lumbocolostomy (lŭm″bō-kō-lŏs'tō-mē) [″ + Gr. *kolon*, colon, + *stoma*, mouth]. Colostomy by lumbar incision.

lumbocolotomy (lŭm″bō-kō-lŏt'ō-mē) [″ + ″ + *tome*, incision]. Incision into the colon through the lumbar region.

lumbocostal (lŭm″bō-kŏs′tăl) [″ + *costa*, rib]. Rel. to the loins and ribs.

lumbodynia (lŭm″bō-dĭn′ē-ă) [″ + Gr. *odyne*, pain]. Pain and rigidity in the loins. SYN: *lumbago*.

lumboiliac (lŭm″bō-ĭl′ē-ăk) [″ + *iliacus*, pert. to ilium]. Concerning the lumbar and inguinal areas.

lumboinguinal (lŭm″bō-ĭng′gwĭ-năl) [″ + *inguinalis*, pert. to the groin]. Lumboiliac, q.v.

lumbosacral. Pert. to the lumbar vertebrae and the sacrum.

lumbosacral plexus. Nerve plexus formed by union of lumbar, sacral, and coccygeal nerves.

lumbrical (lŭm′brĭ-kăl) [L. *lumbricus*, earthworm]. Like a worm. SYN: *vermiform*.

lumbrical bar. A component of a hand splint which rests on the dorsal surface of the proximal phalanges for the purpose of preventing hyperextension of the metacarpophalangeal joints.

lumbricalis. One of the muscles of the hand or foot that are wormlike in shape.

lumbricide (lŭm′brĭ-sīd) [″ + *caedere*, to kill]. An agent that kills lumbricoid worms, i.e., ascarides or intestinal worms.

lumbricoid (lŭm′brĭ-koyd) [″ + Gr. *eidos*, form, shape]. Resembling a roundworm.

lumbricosis (lŭm″brĭ-kō′sĭs) [″ + Gr. *osis*, condition]. State of being infested with lumbricoid worms.

Lumbricus (lŭm-brĭ′kŭs). A genus of worms that includes earthworms.

lumbricus (lŭm-brĭ′kŭs). *Ascaris lumbricoides.*

lumbus [L.]. [NA] The loin; part of back between thorax and pelvis.

lumen (lū′mĕn) [L., light] (pl. *lumina*). 1. The space within an artery, vein, intestine, or tube. 2. Unit of light, the amount of light emitted in a unit solid angle by a uniform point source of one international candle. SEE: *light unit; candela.*

Luminal. Trade name for phenobarbital, USP.

luminal (lū′mĭ-năl). Rel. to lumen of tubular structure, such as a blood vessel.

Luminal Sodium. Trade name for phenobarbital sodium, USP.

luminescence (loo″mĭ-nĕs′ĕns). 1. Production of a light without production of heat. SEE: *bioluminescence.* 2. In radiology, the light produced by a fluorescent phosphor when exposed to radiation.

luminiferous (loo″mĭ-nĭf′ĕr-ŭs) [L. *lumen*, light, + *ferre*, to bear]. Producing or conveying light.

luminophore (loo′mĭ-nō-for″) [″ + Gr. *phoros*, bearing]. A chemical present in organic compounds that permits luminescence of those compounds.

luminous (loo′mĭ-nŭs). Emitting light.

lumirhodopsin (loo″mĭ-rō-dŏp′sĭn). In the retina of the eye, an intermediate between rhodopsin and all-*trans*-retinal, and opsin during bleaching of rhodopsin by light.

lumpectomy (lŭm-pĕk′tō-mē) [*lump* + Gr. *ektome*, excision]. Surgical removal of a tumor from the breast, esp. to remove only the tumor and no other tissue or lymph nodes.

lunacy (lū′nă-sē) [L. *luna*, moon]. Obsolete term for insanity. Insanity was formerly thought to be affected by the moon.

lunar. Pert. to the moon, a month, or silver.

lunate. 1. Moon-shaped or crescent. 2. A bone in the proximal row of the carpus. SYN: *semilunar bone.*

lunatic (lū′nă-tĭk) [L. *luna*, moon]. Obsolete term for an insane person. SEE: *lunacy.*

lunatomalacia (loo-nă″tō-mă-lā′shē-ă). Kienböck's disease, q.v.

lung (lŭng) [AS. *lungen*]. One of two cone-shaped spongy organs of respiration contained within the pleural cavity of the thorax. SEE: illus.; *alveolus* for illus.

ANAT: Connected with the pharynx through the trachea and larynx. The base rests on the diaphragm and the apex rises from 2.5 to 5 cm above the sternal end of the first rib, the collarbone, supported by its attachment to the hilum or root structures. The lungs include the lobes, lobules, bronchi, bronchioles, infundibula, and alveoli or air cells.

The right lung has three lobes and the left two. Approx. weight in the adult male: right lung 625 gm, left 570 gm. The lungs contain 300,000,000 alveoli and their respiratory surface is about 70 square meters. Averages 18 respirations per minute in adult. The total capacity of the lung varies from 3.6 to 9.4 liters in adult men and 2.5 to 6.9 in adult women.

The left lung has an indentation, called the cardiac depression, for the normal placement of the heart. Behind this is the hilum, through which the blood vessels, lymphatics, and bronchi enter and leave the lung.

Air travels from the mouth and nasal passage to the pharynx and the trachea. Two main bronchi, one on each side, extend from the trachea. The main bronchi divide into smaller bronchi, one for each of five lobes. These further divide into a great number of smaller bronchioles. The pattern of distribution of these into the segments of each lobe is important in pulmonary and thoracic surgery. There are 10 bronchopulmonary segments in the right lung and 8 in the left, but the number varies. There are 50 to 80

LUNGS

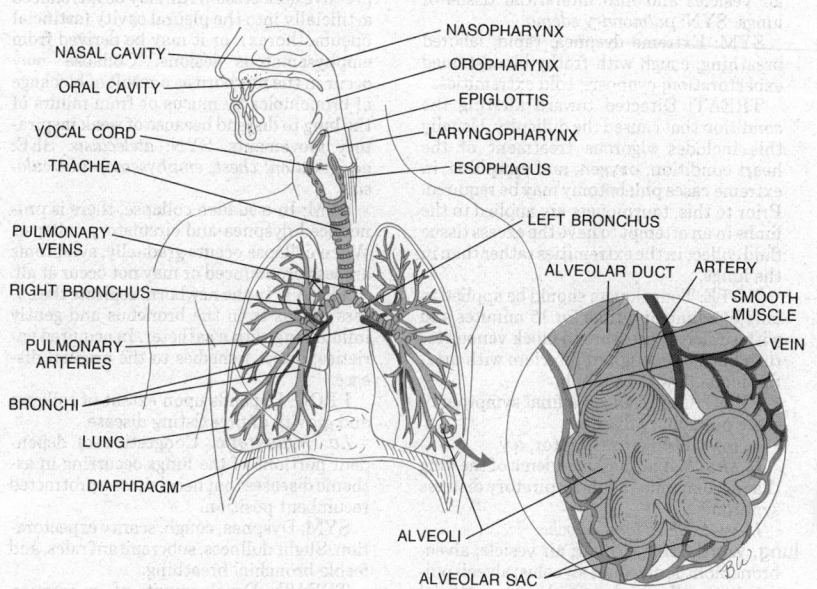

NASOPHARYNX

OROPHARYNX

EPIGLOTTIS

LARYNGOPHARYNX

ESOPHAGUS

LEFT BRONCHUS

ALVEOLAR DUCT   ARTERY

SMOOTH MUSCLE

VEIN

ALVEOLI

ALVEOLAR SAC

NASAL CAVITY

ORAL CAVITY

VOCAL CORD

TRACHEA

PULMONARY VEINS

RIGHT BRONCHUS

PULMONARY ARTERIES

BRONCHI

LUNG

DIAPHRAGM

terminal bronchioles in each lobe. Each of these divides into two respiratory bronchioles, which in turn divide to form 2 to 11 alveolar ducts. The alveolar sacs and alveoli arise from these ducts. The spaces between the alveolar sacs and alveoli are called atria.

The alveolus is the point at which the blood and inspired air are separated only by a very thin wall or membrane that allows O_2 and nitrogen to diffuse into the blood and CO_2 and other gases to pass from the blood into the alveoli. This wall is so thin (0.07 to 2.0 micrometers) that it is best seen by using an electron microscope. The alveoli contain small pores that serve to connect adjacent alveoli to each other.

NERVE SUPPLY: Parasympathetic fibers via vagus nerve and sympathetic fibers from anterior and posterior pulmonary plexuses.

BLOOD VESSELS: Bronchial and pulmonary arteries and pulmonary veins. Blood passing through lungs gives off carbon dioxide and receives oxygen.

FUNCT: The primary purpose of the lung is to bring air and blood into intimate contact so that oxygen can be added to the blood and carbon dioxide can be removed. This is

achieved by two pumping systems, one moving a gas and the other a liquid. The blood and air are brought together so closely that approximately one micrometer (10^{-6} meter) of tissue separates them. The volume of the pulmonary capillary circulation is 150 ml, but this is spread out over a surface area of approx. 750 sq feet (69.68 sq meters). This capillary surface area surrounds 300 million air sacs called alveoli. The blood that is low in oxygen but high in CO_2 is in contact with the air that is high in oxygen and low in CO_2 for less than one second. SEE: *respiratory defense function.*

l., blast. The shredding-type effect that takes place in the alveolar surfaces of the lung caused by the shock of an explosion or blast, which can cause alveolar contusion.

l.'s, compliance of. A measure of the distensibility of the lungs. It is expressed as the change in volume of the lungs in liters when the transpulmonary pressure is changed by 1 cm of water pressure. Normally it is between 0.08 and 0.33 liters/cm H_2O. It is reduced by anything that obstructs the normal flow of air in and out of the lung, whether due to changes in the airway or the mechanical forces that move the ribs and diaphragm.

l., edema of. Effusion of serous fluid into air vesicles and into interstitial tissue of lungs. SYN: *pulmonary edema.*

SYM: Extreme dyspnea; rapid, labored breathing; cough with frothy bloodstained expectoration; cyanosis; cold extremities.

TREAT: Directed toward altering the condition that caused the difficulty. Usually this includes vigorous treatment of the heart condition, oxygen, and morphine; in extreme cases phlebotomy may be required. Prior to this, tourniquets are applied to the limbs in an attempt to have the excess tissue fluid collect in the extremities rather than in the lungs.

NOTE: Tourniquets should be applied to only one limb at a time for 15 minutes and with sufficient pressure to block venous return but not enough to interfere with arterial blood flow to the limb.

PROG: Grave. Often a final symptom of some pulmonary disease.

l., iron. Drinker respirator, q.v.

l., shock. The massive edema of the lung that accompanies adult respiratory distress syndrome.

l., wet. SEE: *lung, shock.*

lung, words pert. to: air; air vesicle; alveobronchiolitis; alveolar; alveolus; alveoli pulmonis; anthracosis; anthrax; artificial pneumothorax; asbestosis; atelectasis; auscultation; "bronch-" words; byssinosis; cardiopulmonary; chest; embolism; emphysema; hilum; pectoriloquy; "pleur-" words; "pneum-" words; pulmonary; rales; siderosis; silicosis; tuberculosis.

lung abscess. Circumscribed suppuration of lung.

SYM: High and irregular fever, rigors, sweats, and pallor. Dyspnea, cough, and purulent expectoration. May be bubbling rales and later cavernous breathing and pectoriloquy.

TREAT: Nutritious food. Remedies called for by general condition. Abscess should be opened and drained.

PROG: Fair, except in embolic abscesses.

lung cancer. Cancer that may appear in trachea, air sacs, and other lung tubes. It may appear as an ulcer in the windpipe, as a nodule or small flattened lump, or on the surface blocking air tubes. It may extend into lymphatics and into blood vessels.

lung collapse. Condition resulting from a lowering of intrapulmonic pressure or an increase in intrathoracic pressure. It may be focal, involving only a few lobules, or massive, in which an entire lobe or the complete lung is involved. It may result from obstruction of the bronchial tubes (obstructive atelectasis) or pressure upon the lung by air or

fluid in the pleural cavity, an intrathoracic tumor, or a greatly enlarged heart (compressive atelectasis). Air may be introduced artificially into the pleural cavity (artificial pneumothorax), or it may be derived from emphysematous lesions. Collapse may occur in the newborn as a result of blockage of bronchioles by mucus or from failure of the lung to distend because of weak inspiratory movements. SYN: *atelectasis.* SEE: *auscultation; chest; emphysema; tuberculosis.*

SYM: In a sudden collapse, there is pronounced dyspnea and circulatory collapse. When collapse occurs gradually, symptoms are less pronounced or may not occur at all.

TREAT: In the newborn, aspirate the excess mucus from the bronchus and gently inflate lung with a catheter. In acquired varieties, direct remedies to the original disease.

PROG: Depends upon extent of collapse and gravity of preexisting disease.

l.c., hypostatic. Congestion of dependent portions of the lungs occurring in asthenic diseases that necessitate a protracted recumbent position.

SYM: Dyspnea, cough, scanty expectoration. Slight dullness, subcrepitant rales, and feeble bronchial breathing.

TREAT: Development of congestion should be prevented by frequent change in position, by deep breathing exercises, and by assisted ventilation if required.

l.c., passive. Results from obstruction to the flow of blood from the lungs to the heart.

SYM: Dyspnea, hard cough, mucous expectoration containing pigmented cells, and rales. Slight dullness, feeble breathing.

lung fluke. *Paragonimus westermani.*

lung hemorrhage. Hemoptysis.

lung inflammation. Pneumonia.

lungmotor. An apparatus designed for forcing air or a mixture of air and oxygen into the lungs.

lung surfactant. A substance in the lung that acts to regulate the amount of surface tension of the fluid lining the alveoli. Synthetic lung surfactant has been produced and is being investigated as therapy for infants with respiratory distress syndrome.

lung transplantation. Transplantation of a lung into patients with end-stage lung disease. The majority of patients who have a single-lung or double-lung transplant will survive.

lungworm (lŭng′wĕrm). Nematodes that infest the lungs of humans and animals.

lunula (lū′nū-lă) [L., little moon] (pl. *lunulae*). [NA] A crescent-shaped area.

l. of valves of heart. One of two narrow

portions on the free edges of the semilunar valves on each side of the nodulus.

lupiform (lū′pĭ-form) [L. *lupus,* wolf, + *forma,* shape]. Resembling lupus.

lupoid (loo′poyd) [″ + Gr. *eidos,* form, shape]. 1. Resembling lupus. 2. Boeck's sarcoid.

lupous (lū′pŭs) 1. Pert. to lupus. 2. Affected with lupus.

lupus (lū′pŭs) [L., wolf]. Originally any chronic, progressive, usually ulcerating, skin disease. In current usage when the word is used alone, it has no precise meaning.

   l. erythematosus, discoid. ABBR: DLE. A chronic disease of the skin characterized by remissions and exacerbations of a scaling, red, macular rash. These lesions contain plugged follicles and are atrophic. In one form, the lesions are above the chin, and in the second form, they are on the rest of the body. The disease is limited to the skin in 90% of patients, but may eventually develop into systemic lupus erythematosus, q.v. Thought to be an autoimmune disorder, it is approximately five times more common in females than in males.

   TREAT: Avoid exposure to sun. Treat skin lesions with topical corticosteroids, but avoid overuse of these preparations.

   l. erythematosus, systemic. A chronic inflammatory disease of connective tissue that causes injury to the skin, joints, kidneys, nervous system, and mucous membranes. A characteristic butterfly rash or erythema may be present on the malar areas and across the nose. The disease may begin acutely with fever, joint pain, and malaise or smolder over a period of years with intermittent fever and malaise. Symptoms from any organ system may be present. The disease occurs most frequently in young women. It's etiology is unknown. Antinuclear antibodies and the L.E. cell factor, q.v., are usually present but are not required for a positive diagnosis. SEE: *Nursing Diagnoses* in *Appendix.*

   DIAG: Diagnosis can be made if four or more of the following are present either at one time or sequentially: butterfly rash; characteristic discoid skin lesion; Raynaud's phenomenon; alopecia; photosensitivity; oral or nasopharyngeal ulceration; arthritis without deformity; L.E. cells; chronic pleuritis or pericarditis; chronic false-positive serological test for syphilis; over 35 grams of protein in the urine in 24 hr; cellular casts in the urine; psychosis or convulsions; hemolytic anemia, less than 4000 white blood cells/cu. mm, thrombocytopenia of less than 100,000/cu. mm.

   TREAT: In mild cases, salicylates or indomethacin if fever and joint pain are present. For severe cases, antimalarial therapy such as hydroxychloroquine, chloroquine, or quinacrine is indicated, as are corticosteroids. It is preferable to give corticosteroids on alternate days if this will control symptoms. Dosage is determined by the patient's response. Immunosuppressive agents are useful when life-threatening or severe crippling disease is present, or when there is failure to respond to conventional therapy, or when intolerable side effects have developed. When antimalarials are used, the patient must be closely observed for retinal damage. In general, patients should not be exposed to the sun, and intercurrent infections should be treated early and vigorously.

   l. pernio. Skin lesions sometimes present in sarcoidosis. They are hard, blue-purple, swollen, shiny lesions of the nose, cheeks, lips, ears, fingers, and knees.

   l. vulgaris. Tuberculosis of the skin. Characterized by patches that break down and ulcerate, leaving scars on healing.

LUQ. *left upper quadrant* of abdomen.

Luque wires. Wires used in surgical procedure for the stabilization of scoliosis. Transverse traction on each vertebra is accomplished by wrapping flexible wires around the affected vertebrae and attaching the wires to flexible rods.

Lust's reflex (lŭsts) [Franz Alexander Lust, Ger. pediatrician, b. 1880]. Dorsal flexion and abduction of foot resulting from percussion of external branch of sciatic nerve.

lusus naturae (loo′sŭs nä-chū′rē). A congenital anomaly.

luteal [L. *luteus,* yellow]. Pert. to the corpus luteum, its cells, or its hormone.

luteal hormone. Progesterone, q.v. Secreted by the corpus luteum. SEE: *corpus luteum; endocrine; estrogen; hormone; ovary.*

lutein (lū′tē-ĭn). Yellow pigment derived from corpus luteum, egg yolk, and fat cells or lipochromes.

lutein cells. Ovarian cells that contain a yellow pigment and are involved in the formation of the corpus luteum. They are of two types: granulosa-lutein cells of follicular origin and theca-lutein cells from the theca interna.

luteinic (loo″tē-ĭn′ĭk). Concerning the corpus luteum of the ovary.

luteinization (lū″tē-ĭn-ī-zā′shŭn). Process of development of the corpus within a ruptured graafian follicle.

luteinizing hormone. ABBR: LH. Hormone secreted by anterior lobe of the hypophysis that stimulates development of the corpus luteum.

luteinizing hormone releasing hormone.

ABBR: LHRH. A hormone produced in the hypothalamus. It controls the release and synthesis of luteinizing hormone.

Lutembacher's syndrome (loo"tĕm-băk"ĕrz) [René Lutembacher, Fr. physician, 1884–1916]. Atrial septal defect of the heart with mitral stenosis.

luteolysin (loo"tē-ō-lī'sĭn) [L. *luteus*, yellow, + Gr. *lysis*, dissolution]. Something that promotes death of the corpus luteum.

luteoma (lū"tē-ō'mă) [L. *luteus*, yellow, + Gr. *oma*, tumor]. An ovarian tumor containing lutein cells.

luteotropin (loo"tē-ō-trō'pĭn). The luteotropic hormone of the anterior pituitary. SYN: *prolactin*.

lutetium (lū-tē'shē-ŭm). SYMB: Lu. At. wt. 174.97; at. no. 71. A rare element.

luteum (lū'tē-ŭm) [L.]. Yellow.

   l., corpus. Yellow cellular mass in the ovary that forms after the graafian follicle has erupted. It persists and enlarges if pregnancy occurs. SEE: *ovary* for illus.

Lutz-Splendore-Almeida disease [A. Lutz, Brazilian physician, 1855–1940; A. Splendore, contemp. Italian physician; Floriano P. de Almeida, Brazilian physician, b. 1898]. Brazilian or South American blastomycosis, paracoccidioidomycosis, q.v.

lux (lŭks) [L., light]. A unit of light intensity equivalent to one lumen per square meter.

luxation (lŭks-ā'shŭn) [L. *luxatio*, dislocation]. 1. Displacement of organs or articular surfaces; dislocation of a joint. SEE: *subluxation.* 2. In dentistry, injury to supporting tissues that results in loosening of the teeth with rotation or partial displacement.

luxus (lŭks'ŭs) [L.]. Excess of anything.

Luys' body (lū-ēz') [Jules-Bernard Luys, Fr. physician, 1828–1898]. Small mass of gray matter lying on the dorsal surface of the peduncle dorsolateral to the substantia nigra of the brain. Luys' nucleus is located in the posterior portion of the thalamus.

LV. *left ventricle.*

L.V.N. *licensed vocational nurse.*

lyase (lī'ās). The class name for enzymes that remove chemical groups other than by hydrolysis. Ex.: decarboxylase, aldolase, and synthases.

lycanthropy (lī-kăn'thrō-pē) [Gr. *lykos*, wolf, + *anthropos*, man]. Mania in which one believes oneself to be a wild beast, esp. a wolf.

lycopene (lī'kō-pēn). The red carotenoid pigment found in tomatoes. It is also present in other red fruits and berries.

lycopenemia (lī"kō-pĕ-nē'mē-ă) [*lycopene* + Gr. *haima*, blood]. A type of carotenemia, q.v., caused by eating excessive amount of foods that contain lycopene, q.v.

lycoperdonosis (lī"kō-pĕr"dŏn-ō'sĭs) [Gr.

lykos, wolf, + *perdesthai*, to break wind, + *osis*, condition]. Respiratory disease caused by inhaling large quantities of spores from the mature mushroom commonly called puffball. *Lycoperdon* is the genus of fungi to which most puffballs belong.

lycopodium (lī-kō-pō'dē-ŭm). A yellow powder formed from spores of *Lycopodium clavatum*, a club moss. Used as a dusting powder and as a desiccant and absorbent.

lye (lī) [AS. *leag*]. 1. Liquid from leaching of wood ashes. 2. Any strong alkaline solution, esp. sodium or potassium hydroxide. SEE: *alkali; potassium hydroxide; sodium hydroxide.*

lye poisoning. SEE: *Poisons and Poisoning* in *Appendix.*

lying-in. 1. The puerperal state. 2. Being hospitalized for the purpose of childbearing.

Lyme disease, Lyme arthritis [Lyme, Connecticut, U.S.A., where the disease was originally described]. ABBR: LD. A recurrent inflammatory disorder accompanied by distinctive skin lesions, erythema chronicum migrans (ECM), polyarthritis, and involvement of the heart and nervous system. The onset, usually in the summer, consists of a red macule or papule that expands to a large annular lesion (ECM). There may be several of these lesions. They are associated with fever, fatigue, malaise, headache, and a stiff neck that lasts several weeks. Within the next few days or as late as two years later, polyarthritis without joint swelling develops. This develops into chronic arthritis within weeks or months after the skin lesion. Neurological symptoms of neuritis of cranial and somatic nerves appear. These may last months. The cardiac abnormalities including myopericarditis and cardiomegaly develop within weeks of the initial skin lesion. SYN: *Lyme borreliosis.*

   ETIOL: A spirochete, *Borrelia burgdorferi,* transmitted by a very small tick, *Ixodes dammini,* and similar ticks.

   TREAT: For adults, tetracycline or doxycycline for early infection; ceftriaxone or penicillin G for neurologic abnormalities. If patient is allergic to either of the latter, use doxycycline or erythromycin. For children less than 8 years of age, use amoxicillin or penicillin V. If child is allergic to penicillin, use erythromycin.

lymph (lĭmf) [L. *lympha*]. An alkaline fluid found in the lymphatic vessels and the cisterna chyli. It is usually a clear, transparent, colorless fluid; however, in vessels draining the intestines it may appear milky owing to presence of absorbed fats. It differs from blood in that red blood corpuscles are absent and the protein content is lower. Osmotic pressure is slightly higher than in blood plasma; viscosity, slightly less. Sp. gr. 1.016 to 1.023.

Lymph may vary considerably in composition in different parts of the body. In peripheral vessels, it is similar to blood plasma except that the protein content is usually much lower. Lymph contains proteins (serum albumin, serum globulin, serum fibrinogen), salts, organic substances (urea, creatinine, neutral fats, glucose), and water. Cells present are principally lymphocytes, formed in lymph nodes and other lymphatic organs. Lymph from the intestine (called chyle) contains fats and other substances absorbed from the intestine.

Lymph is formed in tissue spaces all over the body and is gathered into small vessels that carry it centrally. All lymph eventually enters into either the thoracic duct or right lymph duct, each terminating at the junction of the internal jugular and subclavian veins, where the lymph re-enters the bloodstream. The thoracic duct commences in the abdomen as a dilated sac, the cisterna (receptaculum) chyli, which receives lymph vessels from the lower limbs and pelvis and from the intestines and digestive organs. It continues upward through the thorax, receiving intercostal lymph vessels, and near its termination, it receives the left subclavian trunk, draining the left upper extremity, and the left jugular trunk, draining the left side of head and neck. The right lymph duct drains the right sides of the thorax, head, and neck. SEE: *lymphatic system* for illus.

Lymph, in passing from any region of the body to the main lymph ducts, must pass through lymph vessels that lead to regional lymph nodes. These filter the lymph, freeing it of foreign particulate matter, esp. bacteria.

The absorption of fatty matter chiefly takes place through the epithelial cells of the intestines and those of the villi. These cells carry it to the lacteals, the lymph vessels of the small intestine.

Absorption is most active in the alimentary canal, the digested material passing into the bloodstream through the vessels of the portal circulation and into the lacteals.

l., animal. Lymph or vaccine from an animal.

l., inflammatory. Exudate due to inflammation.

l., intercellular. Tissue fluid.

lymphadenectasis (lĭm-făd″ĕ-nĕk′tă-sĭs) [L. *lympha*, lymph, + Gr. *aden*, gland, + *ektasis*, dilatation]. Dilatation or distention of a lymph node.

lymphadenectomy (lĭm-făd″ĕ-nĕk′tō-mē) [″ + ″ + *ektome*, excision]. Surgical

removal of a lymph node.

lymphadenia (lĭm″fă-dē′nē-ă). Hyperplasia affecting lymph nodes.

l. ossea. Bone marrow hyperplasia accompanied by Bence Jones protein in urine.
SYM: Neuralgic pains followed by painful swellings on ribs and skull and possible occurrence of spontaneous fractures. SYN: *myeloma, multiple.*

lymphadenitis (lĭm-făd″ĕn-ī′tĭs) [″ + ″ + *itis*, inflammation]. Inflammation of the lymph nodes. SYN: *adenolymphitis.*
SYM: Marked increase of tissue; possible suppuration. Swelling, pain, tenderness. Usually accompanies lymphangitis.
ETIOL: Drainage of bacteria or toxic substances into lymph nodes. May be specific, as when caused by the organisms of typhoid, syphilis, or tuberculosis, or nonspecific, in which causative organism is not identified.
TREAT: Hot, moist dressings; incision and drainage if abscesses occur. Antibiotics as indicated.

l., tuberculous. Tuberculosis of lymph nodes.
SYM: Possible loss of weight and strength; gradual onset and enlargement of lymph nodes; may become adherent, necrotic, and discharge pus through skin.
ETIOL: *Mycobacterium tuberculosis.*
TREAT: Antituberculosis drugs.

lymphadenocele (lĭm-făd′ĕ-nō-sēl″) [″ + ″ + *kele*, tumor, swelling]. Cyst of a lymph node.

lymphadenogram (lĭm-făd′ĕ-nō-grăm″) [″ + ″ + *gramma*, something written]. Roentgenogram of a lymph gland.

lymphadenography (lĭm-făd″ĕ-nŏg′ră-fē) [″ + ″ + *graphein*, to write]. Radiography of lymph glands after injection of radiopaque material.

lymphadenoid (lĭm-făd′ĕ-noyd) [″ + ″ + *eidos*, form, shape]. Resembling a lymph node or lymph tissue.

lymphadenopathy (lĭm-făd″ĕ-nŏp′ă-thē) [″ + ″ + *pathos*, disease]. Disease of the lymph nodes.

l., dermatopathic. Widespread lymphadenopathy secondary to various skin disorders.

lymphadenosis benigna cutis (lĭm-făd″ĕ-nō′sĭs) [″ + ″ + *osis*, condition]. A benign collection of lymphocytes in the skin.

lymphadenotomy (lĭm-făd″ĕ-nŏt′ō-mē) [″ + ″ + *tome*, incision]. Surgical incision of a lymph node.

lymphadenovarix (lĭm-făd″ĕ-nō-vā′rĭks) [″ + ″ + L. *varix*, a twisted vein]. Enlargement of lymph nodes due to increased pressure in the lymph vessels.

lymphagogue (lĭmf′ă-gŏg) [″ + Gr.

agogos, leading]. An agent that stimulates the production or flow of lymph.

lymphangial (lĭm-făn'jē-ăl) [" + Gr. *angeion*, vessel]. Concerning lymph vessels.

lymphangiectasis (lĭm-făn"jē-ĕk'tă-sĭs) [" + " + *ektasis*, dilatation]. Dilatation of lymphatic vessels. SYN: *lymphectasia*.

lymphangiectomy (lĭm-făn"jē-ĕk'tō-mē) [" + " + *ektome*, excision]. Surgical removal of lymph vessels.

lymphangiitis (lĭm-făn"jē-ī'tĭs) [" + " + *itis*, inflammation]. Inflammation of lymph vessels.

lymphangioendothelioma (lĭm-făn"jē-ō-ĕn"dō-thē-lē-ō'mă) [" + " + *endon*, within, + *thele*, nipple, + *oma*, tumor]. Endothelioma originating from lymph vessels. SYN: *lymphendothelioma*.

lymphangiofibroma (lĭm-făn"jē-ō-fī-brō'mă) [" + Gr. *angeion*, vessel, + L. *fiber*, fiber, + Gr. *oma*, tumor]. Fibroma and lymphangioma combined.

lymphangiogram (lĭm-făn'jē-ō-grăm) [" + " + *gramma*, something written]. Roentgenogram of the lymph vessels.

lymphangiography (lĭm-făn"jē-ŏg'ră-fē) [" + " + *graphein*, to write]. Roentgenography of the lymph vessels after a radiopaque substance has been injected into the vessels.

lymphangiology (lĭm-făn"jē-ŏl'ō-jē) [" + " + *logos*, word, reason]. The branch of medical science concerned with the lymphatic system.

lymphangioma (lĭm-făn"jē-ō'mă) [" + " + *oma*, tumor]. Tumor composed of lymphatic vessels.

l., cavernous. Dilated lymph vessels filled with lymph.

l., cystic. Multilocular cysts filled with lymph. The condition is usually congenital.

lymphangiophlebitis (lĭm-făn"jē-ō-flĕ-bī'tĭs) [" + " + *phleps*, vein, + *itis*, inflammation]. Inflammation of lymphatic vessels and veins.

lymphangioplasty (lĭm-făn'jē-ō-plăs"tē) [" + Gr. *angeion*, vessel, + *plassein*, to form]. Formation of artificial lymphatics.

lymphangiosarcoma (lĭm-făn"jē-ō-săr-kō'mă) [" + " + *sarx*, flesh, + *oma*, tumor]. A malignant neoplasm that develops from the endothelial lining of lymphatics.

lymphangiotomy (lĭm-făn"jē-ŏt'ō-mē) [" + " + *tome*, incision]. 1. Dissection of the lymphatics. 2. Anatomy of the lymphatics. SYN: *lymphotomy*.

lymphangitis (lĭm"făn-jī'tĭs) [" + Gr. *angeion*, vessel, + *itis*, inflammation]. Inflammation of lymphatic channels or vessels.

SYM: Onset of chill and high fever, mod-

erate swelling and pain. Deep general flush with raised border on affected area if infection is in deep layers of skin. The red inflamed area is commonly called blood poisoning by lay persons.

ETIOL: May be due to a variety of organisms but is frequently due to streptococci.

NURSING IMPLICATIONS: Elevate affected area. If affected area is an extremity, elevate above the level of the heart. Apply warm moist dressings as ordered. Administer antibiotics as prescribed. Force fluids. Dispose of dressings in an appropriate waste container. Monitor vital signs and assess inflammatory site, noting changes.

lymphatic (lĭm-făt'ĭk) [L. *lymphaticus*]. 1. Of or pert. to lymph. 2. A lymph vessel.

ANAT: A lymph vessel conveys toward the heart; contains valves like the veins. The intestinal parts of the lymphatics that take up some of the products of digestion are called lacteals. After the chyle enters the lacteals, it is known as lymph. The lymphatics, or lacteals, carry the food material in the form of lymph, which has not hitherto been taken directly into the blood vessels of the alimentary canal, into the bloodstream.

Fluids exuded from the blood vessels into the tissues are collected and returned to the blood via the lymphatics. They appear like small veins with thin walls, and they are provided with valves. They commence as lymph capillaries, microscopic in size, and empty into two trunks that open into the large veins near the heart.

Unlike blood, the fluid contained in the lymphatics flows only in one direction from the small capillaries to the main trunk (the thoracic duct and a smaller duct on the right side) and then to the large veins. When the lymph enters the blood, it becomes part of its constituents.

RS: angiolymphitis; angiolymphoma; bubo; chylangioma; varix; "vas-" words.

l., afferent. Any of the small vessels carrying lymph to a lymph node.

l., efferent. Any of the small vessels carrying lymph from a lymph node.

lymphatic blockade. Local defense mechanism in which minute bits of material, such as fibrinous exudate from injured tissue, enter local lymphatic vessels, tending to obstruct them and thus prevent foreign substances, esp. bacteria, from passing to other parts of the body.

lymphatic capillary. The smallest lymph vessel. A minute tube consisting of a single layer of endothelium ending blindly in a swollen or rounded end. Tissue fluid enters the lymphatic system through the lymph capillaries. In intestinal villi they are called lacteals.

lymphatic organ. A structure composed principally of lymphatic tissue. Includes lymph nodes, spleen, tonsil, and thymus.

lymphaticostomy (lĭm-făt″ĭ-kŏs′tō-mē) [L. *lymphaticus,* lymphatic, + Gr. *stoma,* mouth]. Making of a permanent aperture into a lymphatic duct.

lymphatic system. That system including all structures involved in the conveyance of lymph from the tissues to the bloodstream. It includes the lymph capillaries, lacteals, lymph nodes, lymph vessels, and main lymph ducts (thoracic and right lymphatic ducts). SEE: illus.; *lymph.*

lymphatic vessels. Thin-walled vessels conveying lymph from the tissues. They resemble veins in structure, possessing three layers: the intima, media, and adventitia. They possess paired valves.

lymphatism (lĭm′fă-tĭzm) [″ + Gr. *-ismos,* condition]. Condition of an excess of lymphatic or tonsillar tissue.

lymphatitis (lĭm″fă-tī′tĭs) [″ + Gr. *itis,* inflammation]. Inflammation of the lymphatic system.

lymphatology (lĭm″fă-tŏl′ō-jē) [″ + Gr. *logos,* word, reason]. Study of the lymphatic system.

lymphatolysis (lĭm″fă-tŏl′ĭ-sĭs) [″ + Gr. *lysis,* dissolution]. Destruction of lymphatic vessels or tissue.

lymphatolytic (lĭm″fă-tō-lĭt′ĭk). Destructive to lymphatics.

lymph cell. Lymphocyte.

lymph channel. Lymph sinus.

lymphectasia (lĭmf″ĕk-tā′zē-ă) [L. *lympha,* lymph, + Gr. *ektasis,* dilatation]. Dilatation of the lymphatics. SYN: *lymphangiectasis.*

lymphedema (lĭmf-ĕ-dē′mă) [″ + Gr. *oidema,* swelling]. Edema due to obstruction of lymphatics. SEE: *phlegmasia alba dolens.*

    l., congenital. Chronic pitting edema of the lower extremities. SYN: *Meige-Milroy's disease.*

lymphemia (lĭm-fē′mē-ă) [″ + Gr. *haima,* blood]. An increased number of lymphocytes in the blood.

lymphendothelioma (lĭmf″ĕn-dō-thē-lē-ō′mă) [″ + Gr. *endon,* within, + *thele,* nipple, + *oma,* tumor]. Tumor from proliferation and dilatation of lymphatics with overgrowth of myxomatous tissue.

lymphenteritis (lĭmf″ĕn-tĕr-ī′tĭs) [″ + Gr. *enteron,* intestine, + *itis,* inflammation]. Serous infiltration accompanying inflammation of bowels.

lymph follicle. An irregular and inconstant aggregation of lymphocytes, usually seen in the lamina propria of a mucosal layer; an old term for lymph node.

lymphization (lĭm″fĭ-zā′shŭn). Production of lymph.

lymph node. A rounded body consisting of accumulations of lymphatic tissue found at intervals in the course of lymphatic vessels. Lymph nodes vary in size from a pinhead to an olive and may occur singly or in groups. One side bears an indentation, the hilum, from which blood vessels enter and leave and efferent lymph vessels leave. Afferent vessels enter on the side opposite from the hilum.

    The node is enclosed in a capsule, from which trabeculae project inwardly, dividing the node into compartments called ampullae or alveoli. An outer compact region comprises the cortex; the inner diffuse portion is the medulla. The cortex is tightly packed with lymph nodules, which are separated from the capsule by the cortical sinus. The lymphatic tissue of the medulla is arranged in the form of medullary cords. Irregular tortuous spaces, called lymph sinuses, are present throughout the node. The nodes are aggregated in regions, the principal ones of which are in the neck (cervical), the armpit (axillary), and the groin (inguinal). Lymph nodes as well as vessels are divided into superficial and deep groups. Among the deep groups are those draining lymph from the visceral organs of the thorax and abdomen. SEE: illus.

    FUNCT: Lymph nodes produce lymphocytes and monocytes. They act as filters keeping particulate matter, esp. bacteria, from gaining entrance to the bloodstream. They may stop cancer cells, but in turn may become a metastatic site.

lymphnoditis (lĭmf″nō-dī′tĭs) [″ + *nodus,* knot, + Gr. *itis,* inflammation]. Inflamed condition of a lymph node.

lymph nodule. A small, compact, densely staining mass of cells, each containing a lighter-staining central area in which lymphocytes are formed. They constitute the structural unit of lymphatic tissue. May occur singly, in groups as in Peyer's patches, or in encapsulated organs as lymph nodes.

lymphoblast (lĭm′fō-blăst) [″ + Gr. *blastos,* germ]. An immature cell that gives rise to a lymphocyte.

lymphoblastic (lĭm″fō-blăs′tĭk) [″ + Gr. *blastos,* germ]. Concerning a lymphoblast.

lymphoblastoma (lĭm″fō-blăst-ō′mă) [″ + ″ + *oma,* tumor]. Tumor composed of lymphocytes. SYN: *lymphosarcoma.*

lymphoblastomatosis (lĭm″fō-blăs″tō-mă-tō′sĭs) [″ + ″ + *oma,* tumor, + *osis,* condition]. Condition produced by lymphoblastomas.

lymphoblastosis (lĭm″fō-blăs-tō′sĭs) [″ + ″ + *osis,* condition]. Excessive number of lymphoblasts in the blood.

LYMPHATIC DRAINAGE OF ABDOMINAL AND THORACIC AREA

SUBMANDIBULAR NODES

RIGHT LYMPH DUCT

DEEP CERVICAL NODES

THORACIC DUCT

LEFT SUBCLAVIAN VEIN

CENTRAL AXILLARY DUCT

THYMUS

THORACIC DUCT

SPLEEN

AXILLARY NODES

CISTERNA CHYLI

LARGE INTESTINE

APPENDIX

INGUINAL NODES

BONE MARROW

SMALL INTESTINE

PEYER'S PATCH

LUMBAR NODES

ILIAC NODES

SACRAL NODES

LYMPH NODE

CAPSULE

B-LYMPHOCTYES

AFFERENT LYMPHATIC VESSEL

FOLLICLE

MEDULLARY

ZONES OF
LYMPHOCYTE
PACKING

EFFERENT
LYMPHATIC
VESSEL

ZONE
3
2
1

DISTRIBUTION
OF B & T
LYMPHOCYTES

B CELLS

T CELLS

B CELLS
(PLASMOCYTES)

VALVE

HILUM

ARTERY

VEIN

CIRCULATION
OF
LYMPHOCYTE

MEDULLA

PARACORTEX

RETICULUM
MATRIX

DENDRITIC CELL

VASCULAR
PATTERN

CORTEX

CAPSULE

SINUS

CORTICLE
SINUS

MARGINAL ZONE

SUBSCAPSULAR
SINUS

MACROPHAGE

ENDOTHELIAL
CELL

GERMINAL CENTRE

lymphocele (lǐm'fō-sēl) [L. *lympha*, lymph, + Gr. *kele*, tumor, swelling]. A cyst that contains lymph.

lymphocytapharesis [" + Gr. *aphairesis*, removal]. Removal of lymphocytes from the blood after it has been withdrawn. The blood is then returned to the donor. SYN: *lymphapheresis*.

lymphocyte (lǐm'fō-sīt) [L. *lympha*, lymph, + Gr. *kytos*, cell]. Cell present in the blood and lymphatic tissue. Less than 1% are present in the circulating blood. These cells travel from the blood to the lymph and lymph nodes and back into the circulation. Small lymphocytes are 6 to 9 micrometers and the largest ones are 9 to 15 micrometers in diameter. There are a number of different types of lymphocytes with respect to function, but these cannot be differentiated by microscopic examination.

Lymphocytes are derived from the stem cells from which all blood cells arise. They are the main means of providing the body with immune capability. This is done by means of humoral immunity produced by B cells and cell-mediated immunity produced by T cells.

The total cell mass of lymphocytes is about equivalent to that of the liver. In the circulating blood, lymphocytes constitute 20% to 44% of the total white cells. SEE: *blood cell* for illus.; *cells, plasma; immunity, cell-mediated; immunity, humoral.*

l., activated. Lymphocyte that has been stimulated by exposure to a specific antigen or by macrophage processing so that it is capable of responding to a foreign antigen by neutralizing or eliminating it.

l., B. Lymphocyte formed from pluripotent stem cells in the bone marrow that migrates to the spleen, lymph nodes, and other peripheral lymphoid tissue where it comes in contact with foreign antigens and becomes a mature functioning cell. Mature B cells are able to independently identify foreign antigens and differentiate into antibody-producing plasma cells or memory cells; their activity also may be stimulated by IL-2 (previously called B cell growth factor). Plasma cells are the only source of immunoglobulins (antibodies), q.v. Memory cells enable the body to quickly produce antibodies when it is invaded by the same organism at a later date. SYN: *B cell.* SEE: *B cell mediated immunity; immune response.*

l., T. Lymphocyte that develops in the bone marrow and then migrates to the thymus, where it begins to mature. T cells circulate throughout the body and are essential for the specific immune response, q.v. Subpopulations of T cells include helper/T4 cells, suppressor/T8 cells, and two types of cytotoxic cells, natural killer cells and cytotoxic T cells. SYN: *T cell.* SEE: *immune response; T cell mediated immunity.*

lymphocyte activation. Use of an antigen (or mitogen, q.v., in vitro) to stimulate lymphocyte metabolic activity.

lymphocyte mitogenic factor. ABBR: LMF. A lymphokine, q.v., that stimulates protection of lymphocytes and other lymphokines.

lymphocythemia (lǐm"fō-sī-thē'mē-ă) [" + Gr. *kytos*, cell, + *haima*, blood]. Excess of lymph cells in the blood. SYN: *lymphocytosis.*

lymphocytoblast (lǐm"fō-sī'tō-blăst") [" + " + *blastos*, germ]. Lymphoblast.

lymphocytopenia (lǐm"fō-sīt"ō-pē'nē-ă) [" + " + *penia*, lack]. Less than normal number of lymphocytes in the blood.

lymphocytopoiesis (lǐm"fō-sīt"ō-poy-ē'sǐs) [" + " + *poiesis*, production]. Lymphocyte production.

lymphocytosis (lǐm"fō-sī-tō'sǐs) [" + " + *osis*, condition]. Excess of lymph cells. SYN: *lymphocythemia.*

lymphocytotoxin (lǐm"fō-sīt"ō-tŏks'ǐn) [" + " + *toxikon*, poison]. A toxin destructive to lymphocytes.

lymphoduct (lǐm'fō-dŭkt) [" + *ducere*, to lead]. A lymph vessel.

lymphoepithelioma (lǐm"fō-ĕp"ǐ-thē-lē-ō'mă) [" + Gr. *epi*, at, + *thele*, nipple, + *oma*, tumor]. A poorly differentiated squamous cell carcinoma that involves the lymphoid tissue of the tonsils and nasopharynx.

lymphogenesis (lǐm"fō-jĕn'ĕ-sǐs) [" + Gr. *genesis*, generation, birth]. Production of lymph.

lymphogenous (lǐm-fŏj'ĕn-ŭs) [" + Gr. *gennan*, to produce]. 1. Forming lymph. 2. Derived from lymph.

lymphoglandula (lǐm"fō-glăn'dū-lă) [" + *glandula*, little gland]. Lymph gland.

lymphogram (lǐm'fō-grăm) [" + Gr. *gramma*, something written]. Roentgenogram of a lymph vessel and nodes. SYN: *lymphangiogram.*

lymphogranuloma inguinale. Previous term for lymphogranuloma venereum.

lymphogranulomatosis (lǐm"fō-grăn-ū-lō"mă-tō'sǐs) [" + *granulum*, granule, + Gr. *oma*, tumor, + *osis*, condition]. 1. Infectious granuloma of the lymphatics. 2. Hodgkin's disease.

lymphogranuloma venereum (lǐm"fō-grăn"ū-lō'mă) [" + " + Gr. *oma*, tumor]. ABBR: LGV. An infectious venereal disease. SYN: *lymphogranuloma inguinale; lymphopathia venereum.*

SYM: From 7 to 12 days after exposure, a

vesicle similar to that caused by herpes will appear, usually on the genitals. This ruptures and heals painlessly. Then from 1 to 8 weeks later, the regional lymph nodes enlarge, become tender, and may suppurate. These enlarged glands are called buboes. They heal and leave scars that may obstruct lymph channels. The perirectal lymph nodes in women may scar and cause rectal obstruction.

ETIOL: Group A *Chlamydiae* (C. *trachomatis*) and rarely group B (C. *psittaci*).

DIAG: Usually by clinical findings, but a skin reaction to injected killed organisms may help to confirm the clinical evidence.

TREAT: Tetracyclines cure the acute clinical signs but do not affect the previous scarring.

lymphogranuloma venereum antigen. USP. An antigen used in a skin test for lymphogranuloma venereum.

lymphography (lĭm-fŏg′ră-fē) [L. *lympha*, lymph, + Gr. *graphein*, to write]. Roentgenography of a lymph vessel and nodes after a radiopaque substance has been injected in the lymphatic system.

lymphoid (lĭm′foyd) [″ + Gr. *eidos*, form, shape]. Resembling lymph or lymph tissue.

lymphoid cells. Lymphocytes.

lymphoidectomy (lĭm″foyd-ĕk′tō-mē) [″ + ″ + *ektome*, excision]. Surgical removal of lymphoid tissue.

lymphoidocyte (lĭm-foyd′ō-sīt) [″ + ″ + *kytos*, cell]. A hemocytoblast.

lymphokines (lĭm′fō-kīnz). Substances released by sensitized lymphocytes when they contact specific antigens. They help to produce cellular immunity by stimulating macrophages and monocytes. Included in this group of materials are interleukins 1, 2, and 3; interferon-gamma; tumor necrosis factor; colony stimulating factor; B-cell growth factor; lymphotoxin; migration inhibition factor; leukocyte migration inhibition factor; macrophage chemotactic factor; macrophage activating factor; lymphocyte mitogenic factor; soluble immune response suppressor; and T-cell replacement factor. SEE: *cytokines*.

lymphokinesis (lĭm″fō-kĭ-nē′sĭs) [″ + Gr. *kinesis*, motion]. 1. Circulation of lymph in the lymphatic system. 2. Movement of lymph in the semicircular canals of the inner ear.

lymphology (lĭm-fŏl′ō-jē) [″ + Gr. *logos*, word, reason]. Science of the lymphatics.

lymphoma, Burkitt's. A form of malignant, non-Hodgkin's lymphoma that causes bone-destroying lesions of the jaw. The Epstein-Barr virus is the causative agent. Initially reported from central Africa.

lymphoma, non-Hodgkin's. ABBR: NHL.

A group of malignant solid tumors of lymphoid tissues.

SYM: Painless lymphadenopathy in two-thirds of patients is the most frequent presenting symptom. Others have fever, night sweats, loss of 10% or more of body weight in the 6 months prior to presenting with symptoms of infiltration into nonlymphoid tissue. Additional involvement is in peripheral areas such as epitrochlear nodes, the tonsillar area, and bone marrow. NHL is 50% more frequent in males than in females of similar age. In most cases the cause of NHL is unknown, but patients who have received immunosuppressive agents have a more than 100 times greater chance of developing NHL. This is most probably due to the immunosuppressive agents activating tumor viruses. Some patients taking a hydantoin anticonvulsant develop pseudolymphomas. These resolve when the drug is stopped.

Classification of NHL is unsettled, but includes various types of malignant lymphomas, including low grade, intermediate grade, high grade, and miscellaneous. The last category includes, among others, mycosis fungoides.

TREAT: Specific therapy depends upon the type, grade, and stage of the NHL. Radiation and combinations of chemotherapy are of benefit. Monoclonal antibodies to remove NHL tumor cells are used. SEE: *Hodgkin's disease*.

lymphoma, non-Hodgkin's, T cell. Lymphomas that arise directly from the thymus.

lymphomatoid (lĭm-fō′mă-toyd) [L. *lympha*, lymph, + Gr. *oma*, tumor, + *eidos*, form, shape]. Resembling lymphoma.

lymphomatosis (lĭm″fō-mă-tō′sĭs) [″ + ″ + *osis*, condition]. General lymphatic engorgement; deposition of lymphomata throughout the body.

lymphomatous (lĭm-fō′mă-tŭs). 1. Pert. to a lymphoma. 2. Affected with lymphomata.

lymphomyxoma (lĭm″fō-mĭk-sō′mă) [″ + Gr. *mys*, muscle, + *oma*, tumor]. A soft, nonmalignant tumor that contains lymphoid tissue.

lymphonodus (lĭm″fō-nō′dŭs) [″ + *nodus*, knot]. Lymphatic node.

lymphopathia venereum. Venereal disease marked by ulceration and enlargement of lymph nodes in inguinal area. SYN: *lymphogranuloma venereum*.

lymphopathy (lĭm-fŏp′ă-thē) [″ + Gr. *pathos*, disease]. Any disease of the lymphatic system.

lymphopenia (lĭm-fō-pē′nē-ă) [″ + Gr. *penia*, a lack]. Deficiency of lymphocytes in the blood.

lymphoplasmapheresis [″ + Gr. *aphair-*

esis, removal]. Removal of lymphocytes and plasma from the blood after it has been withdrawn. The blood is then returned to the donor.

lymphoplasty (lĭm'fō-plăs"tē) [" + Gr. *plassein,* to form]. Lymphoangioplasty, q.v.

lymphopoiesis (lĭm"fō-poy-ē'sĭs) [" + Gr. *poiesis,* production]. Formation of lymphocytes or of lymphoid tissue.

lymphopoietic (lĭm"fō-poy-ĕt'ĭk) [" + Gr. *poiein,* to produce]. Forming lymphocytes.

lymphoproliferative (lĭm"fō-prō-lĭf'ĕr-ă-tĭv). Concerning proliferation of lymphoid tissue.

lymphoproliferative syndrome, HTLV-1 induced. Disease seen in persons infected with human T cell leukemia-lymphoma virus (HTLV-1). Clinical signs are lymphadenopathy, hepatomegaly, splenomegaly, cutaneous infiltration with neoplastic T cells, hypercalcemia, lymphocytosis, and skeletal changes. Most patients develop T cell leukemia.

TREAT: Combination chemotherapy. Median duration of remission is 12 months.

lymphoprotease. Protein-splitting enzyme secured from a suspension of lymphatic tissue.

lymphoreticular (lĭm"fō-rĕ-tĭk'ū-lăr) [" + *reticula,* net]. Pert. to reticuloendothelial cells of the lymph node.

lymphoreticular disorders. A great variety of poorly understood and inadequately classified diseases of the lymphoreticular system. Included are self-limited proliferation of lymph glands, lymphocytes, and monocytes; infectious mononucleosis; benign abnormalities of immunoglobulin synthesis; leukemias; lymphomas such as Hodgkin's disease, lymphosarcoma, reticulum cell sarcoma, and mycosis fungoides; malignant proliferative response or abnormal immunoglobulin synthesis such as plasma cell myeloma, macroglobulinemia, and amyloidosis; histiocytosis and lipid storage disease.

lymphoreticular system. In general, the lymphatic tissue and the reticuloendothelial system. Specifically the system includes fixed and mobile cellular tissue involved in body defense by macrophage activity and immunologic mechanisms but does not include the granulocytic cells of the blood, i.e., neutrophils, eosinophils, and basophils.

lymphoreticulosis, benign, of inoculation (lĭm"fō-rĕ-tĭk"ū-lō'sĭs) [" + " + Gr. *osis,* condition]. A benign self-limited granulomatous lymphadenitis transmitted by cat scratches. A pustular lesion appears about 10 days after the cat scratch. Then regional lymph nodes enlarge and may progress to suppuration. The causative orga-

nism is unknown, and there is no specific treatment. SYN: *cat scratch disease.*

lymphorrhagia (lĭm"fō-rā'jē-ă) [" + Gr. *rhegnynai,* to burst forth]. Flow of lymph from ruptured lymph vessels. SYN: *lymphorrhea.*

lymphorrhea (lĭm"fō-rē'ă) [" + Gr. *rhoia,* flow]. Internal or external discharge of lymph through a wound. SYN: *lymphorrhagia.*

lymphorrhoid (lĭm'fō-royd). Dilated lymph channels that resemble hemorrhoids.

lymphosarcoma (lĭm"fō-săr-kō'mă) [" + Gr. *sarx,* flesh, + *oma,* tumor]. A malignant disease of lymphatic tissue. Clinically it may be quite similar to Hodgkin's disease. Diagnosis is made by biopsy rather than by clinical examination.

lymphosarcomatosis (lĭm"fō-săr"kō-mă-tō'sĭs) [" + " + " + *osis,* condition]. Condition characterized by the development of lymphosarcoma.

lymphostasis (lĭm"fōs'tă-sĭs) [" + Gr. *stasis,* a stoppage]. Stoppage of flow of lymph.

lymphotaxis (lĭm"fō-tăk'sĭs) [" + Gr. *taxis,* arrangement]. The effect of attracting or repelling lymphocytes.

lymphotome (lĭm'fō-tōm) [" + Gr. *tome,* incision]. Instrument for removing glandular growths from tonsils and adenoids.

lymphotomy (lĭm-fŏt'ō-mē) [" + Gr. *tome,* incision]. Lymphangiotomy, q.v.

lymphotoxin (lĭm"fō-tŏk'sĭn) [" + Gr. *toxikon,* poison]. A lymphokine, q.v., that is produced by activated lymphocytes. The toxin affects a variety of cells.

lymphotrophy (lĭm-fŏt'rō-fē) [" + Gr. *trophe,* nourishment]. Lymph nourishment of cells in regions devoid of blood vessels.

lymphotropic. Being attracted to lymph cells, e.g., human immunodeficiency virus and human T cell leukemia virus are lymphotropic for CD4+ lymphocytes and Epstein-Barr virus is lymphotropic for B lymphocytes.

lymph sinus. One of several irregular tortuous vessels found in lymphatic organs. Lined with cells belonging to the reticuloendothelial system. SYN: *lymph channel.*

lymph spaces. Spaces in connective tissue filled with lymph.

lymphuria (lĭm-fū'rē-ă) [" + Gr. *ouron,* urine]. Lymph in the urine.

lymph vascular (lĭmf-văs'kū-lăr) [" + *vasculus,* a little vessel]. Rel. to the lymphatic vessels.

lynestrenol (lĭn-ĕs'trĕ-nŏl). A progestational agent.

lyo- [Gr. *lyein,* to dissolve]. Combining form meaning dissolved or loose.

lyochrome (lī'ō-krōm) [" + *chroma,* color].

Flavin.

lyoenzyme (lī″ō-ĕn′zīm) [″ + *en*, in, + *zyme*, leaven]. An extracellular enzyme.

lyogel (lī′ō-jĕl). A gel containing much water.

Lyon hypothesis (lī′ŏn) [Mary Lyon, Brit. geneticist, b. 1925]. The idea that one of the X chromosomes of the female is inactivated during embryogenesis and becomes hyperpyknotic. This chromosome forms, in the cell nucleus, the sex chromatin mass, or Barr body, q.v. This X chromosome remains in this state throughout the cell's progeny so that in the adult only one X chromosome is active in each cell.

lyophil(e) (lī′ō-fĭl, -fīl) [″ + *philos*, love]. Lyophilic, q.v.

lyophilic (lī″ō-fĭl′ĭk). Concerning a colloid that forms a stable colloidal solution. It is not easily precipitated, but once precipitated, the action is readily reversed.

lyophilization (lī-ŏf″ĭ-lĭ-zā′shŭn). Process of rapidly freezing a substance at an extremely low temperature and then dehydrating in a high vacuum. SYN: *freeze-drying*.

lyophobe, lyophobic (lī′ō-fōb, lī″ō-fō′bĭk) [Gr. *lyein*, to dissolve, + *phobos*, fear]. Tending not to go into solution; applied to colloidal systems in which there is no strong affinity between dispersed phase and dispersion medium.

lyosorption (lī″ō-sorp′shŭn) [″ + *sorbere*, to suck in]. The absorption, in a colloid, of a substance on the surface of the particles in the dispersed phase.

lyotrope (lī′ō-trōp) [″ + *tropos*, a turning]. A substance that goes into solution readily. Opposite of lyophobe.

lyotropic (lī″ō-trŏp′ĭk) [″ + *tropikos*, turning]. Lyophilic, q.v.

lypressin (lī-prĕs′ĭn). USP. A posterior pituitary hormone obtained from the pituitary gland of healthy pigs. Used as an antidiuretic. It is also used in treating some variants of von Willebrand's disease. Trade name is Diapid. SEE: *vasopressin*.

lyra (lī′ră) [L., Gr., *lyre*]. One of several anatomical structures so called because of their resemblance to the shape of a lyre.

lysate (lī′sāt). 1. The products of hydrolysis. 2. Material produced when cells are lysed by the actions of agents such as chemicals, enzymes, or physical agents.

lyse (līz) [Gr. *lysis*, dissolution]. To cause lysis.

lysemia (lī-sē′mē-ă) [″ + *haima*, blood]. Lysis of red blood cells with release of hemoglobin into the plasma.

lysergic acid diethylamide. *LSD.*

lysimeter (lī-sĭm′ĕ-tĕr) [Gr. *lysis*, dissolution, + *metron*, measure]. Apparatus for determining solubilities of various substances.

lysin (lī′sĭn). A specific antibody acting de-

structively upon cells and tissues. SEE: *antibody*.

lysine (lī′sēn). An amino acid that is a hydrolytic cleavage product of digested protein. It is essential for growth and repair of tissues.
    l. acetate. USP. An amino acid.
    l. hydrochloride. USP. An amino acid.

lysinogen (lī-sĭn′ō-jĕn) [Gr. *lysis*, dissolution, + *gennan*, to produce]. An antibody that forms lysins.

lysis (lī′sĭs) [Gr., dissolution]. 1. The gradual decline of a fever or disease. Opposite of crisis. 2. Destruction of blood cells by a lysin, as when rabbit's red corpuscles are dissolved by dog's serum.

-lysis. 1. Combining form meaning dissolution or decomposition of. 2. Combining form indicating, in medicine, reduction or relief of.

lysocephalin (lī″sō-sĕf′ă-lĭn). Partial hydrolysis of a cephalin. It can be caused by the action of cobra venom.

Lysodren. Trade name for mitotane, USP.

lysogen (lī′sō-jĕn) [″ + *gennan*, to produce]. Something capable of producing a lysin.

lysogenesis (lī″sō-jĕn′ĕ-sĭs) [″ + *genesis*, generation, birth]. The production of cell-dissolving substances known as lysin.

lysogenic (lī-sō-jĕn′ĭk) [″ + Gr. *gennan*, to produce]. Producing lysins.

lysogeny (lī-sŏj′ĕ-nē). A special type of virus-bacterial cell interaction maintained by a complex cellular regulatory mechanism. Bacterial strains freshly isolated from their natural environment may contain a low concentration of bacteriophage. This phage will lyse other related bacteria. Cultures that contain these substances are said to be lysogenic.

Lysol (lī′sŏl). A proprietary preparation of a mixture of cresols. Because of its potential for causing toxicity, its use should be confined to disinfecting inanimate objects, feces, and urine. SEE: *Lysol poisoning*.

lysolecithin (lī″sō-lĕs′ĭ-thĭn). A substance obtained from lecithin through the action of an enzyme present in cobra venom. Exerts a powerful hemolytic action.

Lysol poisoning. When swallowed, Lysol causes corrosion, edema of the lungs, immobility of pupils, and collapse. Vomiting may occur; death sometimes occurs after symptoms have abated.
    TREAT: Prompt emptying of the stomach by emesis and lavage if the esophagus is not injured. Treat shock and convulsions symptomatically. Correct acidosis and maintain airway. Do tracheotomy if indicated.

lysosomal storage diseases. Diseases that occur as a result of deficiency of specific lysosomal enzymes that normally degrade glycoproteins, glycolipids, or mucopolysaccharides. Thus, the substances that cannot be catabolized accumulate in lysosomes. Specific enzymes account for specific storage diseases. Included in this group of diseases are Gaucher's; Hurler's; Tay-Sachs; Niemann-Pick; Fabry; Morquio; Scheie; and Maroteaux-Lamy.

lysosome (lī′sō-sōm). Part of an intracellular digestive system that exists as separate particles in the cell. Inside their limiting membrane, they contain a number of hydrolytic enzymes capable of breaking down proteins and certain carbohydrates. Even though their importance in health and disease is certain, all of the precise ways in which lysosomes effect changes are not understood.

lysozyme (lī′sō-zīm) [Gr. *lysis*, dissolution,

+ *zyme*, leaven]. An enzyme that is now called muramidase.

lyssa (lis′sä) [Gr., frenzy]. An acute infectious disease, transferable by inoculation, attacking the nervous system in particular. SYN: *hydrophobia; rabies.*

Lyssavirus. The genus of the family Rhabdoviridae. The previous term was rabies virus.

lyssoid (lis′oyd) [Gr. *lyssa*, frenzy, + *eidos*, form, shape]. Resembling lyssa or rabies.

lyssophobia (lis-ō-fō′bē-ä) [″ + *phobos*, fear]. 1. Hysteria resembling rabies. 2. Fear of rabies.

lyterian (lī-tēr′ē-ăn) [Gr. *lyein*, to dissolve]. Indicative of the lessening of a disease process.

lytic (lit′ik). Rel. to lysis or a lysin.

lyze (līz) [Gr. *lysis*, dissolution]. To bring about lysis.

M

μ [*mu*, the twelfth letter of the Greek alphabet]. Symbol for micro-, a prefix indicating one-millionth (10^{-6}) of the quantity, e.g., microgram or 0.000001 gram.

$\mu\mu$. Symbol for micromicro.

μm. Symbol for micrometer.

mμ. Symbol for millimicron.

M. *master* or *medicine* in professional titles; *mille*, a thousand; *misce*, mix; *molar*.

m. *meter* and *minim;* in chemistry, for *meta-*, and for *mol* or *mole*.

MA. *mental age*.

M.A. *Master of Arts*.

ma. *milliampere*.

Maalox. Trade name for magnesia and alumina tablets.

MAC. *maximum allowable concentration*.

Mace. A proprietary substance for which the name is an acronym for *m*ethylchloroform chloro-*ace*tophenone, a chemical compound used at one time in riot control because of its ability to irritate the eyes. Now it is considered too toxic for that purpose. SEE: *IDU.*

TREAT: Instillation of 0.1% aqueous solution of idoxuridine (IDU) into the eye. Contact lenses must be removed immediately.

mace (mās) [L. *macis*]. A spice from the outer covering of the nutmeg; employed as a condiment.

macerate (măs′ĕr-āt). To soften by steeping or soaking in water. Usually pertains to the skin.

maceration (măs-ĕr-ā′shŭn) [L. *macerare*, to make soft]. Process of softening a solid by steeping in a fluid.

Mache unit (mă′kĕ) [Heinrich Mache, Austrian physicist, 1876–1954]. ABBR: M.u., or German, M.E. Unit of measurement of concentration of radium emanation.

machine. Any mechanical device or apparatus.

macho [L. *masculus*, male]. Exhibition of masculine pride, strength, and power. Often a "posture" assumed by one who does not, in effect, have those characteristics.

Machover test [Karen Alper Machover, U.S. psychologist, b. 1902]. SYN: *Draw-a-Person test*, q.v.

macies (mā′shē-ēz) [L., wasting]. Atrophy, wasting, emaciation.

macrencephalia, macrencephaly (măk-rĕn″sĕ-fā′lē-ă, -sĕf′ă-lē) [Gr. *makros*, large, + *enkephalos*, brain]. Abnormally large size of the brain.

macro-, macr- [Gr. *makros*, large]. Combining forms meaning large or long.

macroamylase (măk″rō-ăm″ĭ-lās). A form of amylase with a molecular weight much greater than ordinary amylase. The macroamylase molecule is too large to be excreted by the glomerulus of the kidney. Clinically important because routine blood amylase study of an individual with macroamylase in the blood would indicate amylase to be elevated. This could lead the physician to believe that the patient required therapy for disease of the pancreas or the gastrointestinal tract. In such a patient the urinary amylase would be within normal limits, which would not be true if the elevation of blood amylase were due to an actual increase in amylase present.

macroamylasemia (măk″rō-ăm″ĭl-ă-sē′mē-ă). Macroamylase in the serum. The presence of increased amounts of macroamylase in the blood has not been correlated with a specific single disease state.

macrobiosis (măk″rō-bī-ō′sĭs) [Gr. *makros*, large, + *biosis*, life]. Longevity.

macrobiota (măk″rō-bī-ō′tă). The macroscopic living organisms, flora and fauna, of an area.

macrobiotic diet. Diet consisting of unprocessed foods, vegetables, beans, whole grains, and some fish and fruits.

macroblepharia (măk″rō-blĕ-fā′rē-ă) [Gr. *makros*, large, + *blepharon*, eyelid]. Abnormal largeness of eyelid.

macrobrachia (măk″rō-brā′kē-ă) [″ + *brachion*, arm]. Abnormal size or length of the arm.

macrocardius (măk″rō-kăr′dē-ŭs) [″ + *kardia*, heart]. Individual with an abnormally large heart caused by congenital heart disease.

macrocephalia (măk″rō-sĕ-fā′lē-ă) [″ + *kephale*, head]. Abnormal largeness of head. SYN: *macrocephaly.*

ETIOL: Found in acromegaly, hydrocephalus, rickets, osteitis deformans, leontiasis ossea, myxedema, leprosy, and pituitary disturbances.

macrocephalic. Megalocephalic, q.v.

macrocephalous (măk″rō-sĕf′ă-lŭs). Pert. to or having an excessively large head.

macrocephaly (măk-rō-sĕf′ă-lē). Abnormal largeness of the head. SYN: *macrocephalia.*

macrocheilia (măk″rō-kī′lē-ă) [″ + *cheilos*, lip]. Abnormal size of lip characterized by swelling of glands of lip. It is a congenital condition. SYN: *macrolabia.*

macrocheiria (măk-rō-kī′rē-ă) [″ + *cheir*, hand]. Excessive size of the hands.

macrochemistry. Use of chemical tests that produce changes detectable by the unaided eye.

macrocnemia (măk″rŏk-nē′mē-ă) [″ + kneme, shin]. Condition in which the legs below the knees are excessively large.

macrocolon (măk″rō-kō′lŏn) [″ + kolon, colon]. Megacolon.

macroconidium (măk″rō-kō-kō-nĭd′ē-ŭm). A large conidium or exospore.

macrocornea (măk-rō-kor′nē-ă) [″ + L. cornu, horn]. Abnormal size of the cornea. SYN: *megalocornea.*

macrocyst (măk′rō-sĭst) [″ + kystis, bladder]. A large cyst.

macrocyte [″ + kytos, cell]. Abnormally large erythrocyte exceeding 10 microns in diameter.

macrocythemia, macrocytosis (măk″rō-sī-thē′mē-ă, măk″rō-sī-tō′sĭs) [″ + ″ + haima, blood]. Condition in which erythrocytes are larger than normal.

macrodactylia (măk″rō-dăk-tĭl′ē-ă) [″ + daktylos, finger]. Excessive size of one or more of the digits.

Macrodantin. Trade name for nitrofurantoin.

Macrodex. Trade name for dextran 70.

macrodontia (măk″rō-dŏn′shē-ă) [″ + odous, tooth]. Abnormal increase in size of the teeth.

macroesthesia (măk″rō-ĕs-thē′zē-ă) [Gr. makros, large, + aisthesis, sensation]. State in which objects seen or felt appear to be greatly magnified.

macrofauna (măk″rō-faw′nă). In a particular location or area, the animal life visible to the naked eye.

macroflora (măk″rō-flō′ră). In a particular area or location, the plant life visible to the naked eye.

macrogamete (măk″rō-găm′ĕt) [″ + gamete, wife]. A large immobile reproductive cell formed in certain protozoa and simple plants. Corresponds to the ovum in higher forms.

macrogametocyte (măk″rō-gă-mē′tō-sīt). A large nonmotile reproductive cell developing from the merozoite of certain protozoans. Red blood cell infected with female form of the malarial parasite. SEE: *Plasmodium.*

macrogenitosomia praecox (măk″rō-jĕn″ĭ-tō-sō′mē-ă prē′kŏks) [″ + L. genitalis, genital, + Gr. soma, body, + L. praecox, early]. Abnormal size of genitalia due to excess androgens (male hormones) from the fetal adrenal. In the female this causes pseudohermaphroditism and in the male enlarged external genitalia.

macrogingivae (măk″rō-jĭn-jī′vē) [″ + L. gingiva, gum]. Hypertrophy of the gums.

macroglia (măk-rŏg′lē-ă) [″ + glia, glue]. Astrocyte.

macroglobulin (măk″rō-glŏb′ū-lĭn). A globulin of high molecular weight of about 400 kilodaltons normally present in the blood but increased in disease states such as multiple myeloma, collagen disorders, cirrhosis of the liver, and amyloidosis.

macroglobulinemia (măk-rō-glŏb″ū-lĭn-ē′mē-ă). ABBR: WM. Presence of globulins of high molecular weight in serum.

m., Waldenström′s. Excessive number of plasma cells, which are responsible for synthesis of IgM globulins. This causes excess production of IgM globulins. Patients are usually middle-aged or elderly, and the frequency is slightly higher in men than in women. Anemia due to infiltration of the bone marrow with lymphocytes and plasma cells, weight loss, neurologic disturbances, blurred vision, bleeding tendency (epistaxis), cold sensitivity, generalized lymphadenopathy, chronic lymphocytic leukemia, and hyperviscosity of the blood are present.

TREAT: Plasmaphoresis to remove the excess IgM from the blood. This may require removing 4 to 6 units of plasma a day until blood viscosity returns to normal, and it needs to be continued until chemotherapy is effective. Reduce tumor mass by use of cytotoxic agents; symptomatic therapy for complications.

macroglossia [Gr. makros, large, + glossa, tongue]. Hypertrophied condition of the tongue; a congenital disorder.

macrognathia (măk-rō-nă′thē-ă) [″ + gnathos, jaw]. Abnormal size of the jaw.

macrography (măk-rō-rŏg′ră-fē) [″ + graphein, to write]. Writing with large letters.

macrogyria [″ + gyros, circle]. Excessively large size of convolutions (gyri) of cerebral hemispheres.

macrolabia (măk-rō-lā′bē-ă) [″ + L. labium, lip]. Abnormal size of lip. SYN: *macrocheilia.*

macroleukoblast (măk″rō-lū′kō-blăst) [″ + leukos, white, + blastos, germ]. A large leukoblast.

macrolymphocyte (măk″rō-lĭmf′ō-sīt) [″ + L. lympha, lymph, + Gr. kytos, cell]. A large lymphocyte.

macromania (măk″rō-mā′nē-ă) [″ + mania, madness]. 1. Megalomania, q.v. 2. The delusion that the affected individual or his or her parts or surroundings are extremely large.

macromastia (măk-rō-măs′tē-ă) [″ + mastos, breast]. Abnormally large breasts.

macromelia [″ + melos, limb]. Excessive size of an organ or a part, esp. an extremity.

macromelus (măk-rŏm′ē-lŭs) [″ + melos, limb]. An individual with abnormally large extremities.

macromere (măk′rō-mēr) [″ + *meros*, a part]. Blastomere of large size.

macromethod (măk′rō-měth″ŏd). Chemical examinations or analyses wherein ordinary quantities of the material being studied are used.

macromolecule (măk″rō-mŏl′ĕ-kūl). A large molecule such as a protein, polymer, or polysaccharide.

macromonocyte (măk″rō-mŏn′ō-sīt). A large monocyte.

macromyeloblast (măk″rō-mī′ĕ-lō-blăst) [″ + *myelos*, marrow, + *blastos*, germ]. A large myeloblast.

macronormoblast (măk″rō-nor′mō-blăst) [″ + L. *norma*, rule, + Gr. *blastos*, germ]. Large nucleated red blood corpuscle.

macronucleus (măk″rō-nū′klē-ŭs). A nucleus that occupies most of the cell.

macronychia (măk″rō-nĭk′ē-ă) [″ + *onyx*, nail]. Abnormal length or thickness of the fingernails or toenails.

macropathology (măk″rō-pă-thŏl′ō-jē). Pathological changes in gross anatomical structures.

macrophage, macrophagus (măk′rō-fāj, măk-rŏf′ă-gŭs) [″ + *phagein*, to eat]. A monocyte, q.v., that has left the circulation and settled and matured in a tissue. Macrophages are found in large quantities in the spleen, lymph nodes, alveoli, and tonsils. Approximately 50% of all macrophages are found in the liver as Kupffer cells. They are also present in the brain, serous cavities, breast, and placenta. Along with neutrophils, macrophages are the major phagocytic cells of the immune system. They have the ability to recognize and ingest all foreign antigens through receptors on the surface of their cell membranes; these antigens are then destroyed by lysosomes, q.v. Their placement in the peripheral lymphoid tissues enables macrophages to serve as the major scavengers of the blood, clearing it of abnormal or old cells and cellular debris as well as pathogenic organisms. Macrophages have a life span of several months.

Macrophages also serve a vital role by processing antigens and presenting them to T cells, activating the specific immune response, q.v. They also release many chemical mediators that are involved in the body's defenses, including IL-1, q.v., coagulation proteins, complement, q.v., and erythropoietin, q.v. SEE: illus.; *macrophage processing; monocyte; phagocytosis; tumor-necrosis factor*.

macrophage activating factor. ABBR: MAF. A lymphokine, q.v., that stimulates macrophages to change in appearance and metabolic activities and to become more ef-

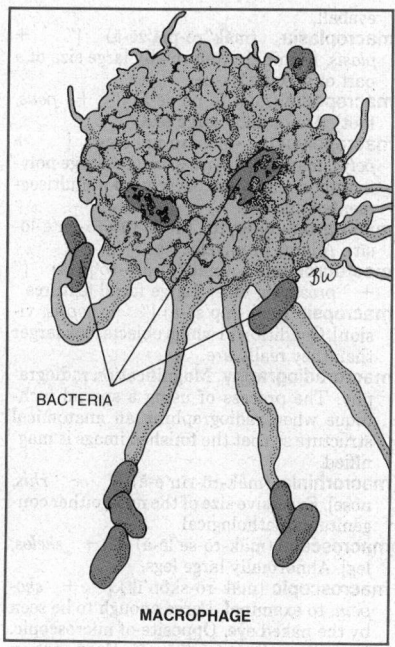

BACTERIA

MACROPHAGE

fective killers of certain microbial cells. Macrophages stimulated by MAF can kill tumor cells.

macrophage chemotactic factor. ABBR: MCF. A lymphokine, q.v., released by T and B cell lymphocytes in response to an antigen. MCF attracts macrophages to the site of the invading antigen.

macrophage migration inhibiting factor. ABBR: MIF. A lymphokine that blocks the migration of macrophages in culture.

macrophage processing. The mechanism by which foreign antigens are taken into the macrophage by phagocytosis and broken up. Part of the antigen is then displayed on the surface of the macrophage next to a histocompatibility or "self" antigen, q.v., activating T lymphocytes and the specific immune response. T lymphocytes are unable to recognize or respond to most antigens without macrophage assistance.

macrophagocyte (măk″rō-făg′ō-sīt). A large phagocyte.

macrophallus (măk″rō-făl′ŭs) [Gr. *makros*, large, + *phallos*, penis]. Abnormally large penis.

macrophthalmia (măk″rŏf-thăl′mē-ă) [″ + *ophthalmos*, eye]. Abnormally large eyeball.

macroplasia (măk″rō-plā′zē-ă) [″ + *plasis*, forming]. Abnormally large size of a part or specific tissue.

macropodia (măk-rō-pō′dē-ă) [″ + *pous*, foot]. Abnormally large feet.

macropolycyte (măk″rō-pŏl′ē-sīt) [″ + *polys*, many, + *kytos*, cell]. A large polymorphonuclear leukocyte with a multisegmented nucleus.

macropromyelocyte (măk″rō-prō-mī′ē-lō-sīt). A large promyelocyte.

macroprosopia (măk″rō-prō-sō′pē-ă) [″ + *prosopon*, face]. Large facial features.

macropsia (măk-rŏp′sē-ă) [″ + *opsis*, vision]. Condition in which objects look larger than they really are.

macroradiography. Magnification radiography. The process of using a special technique when radiographing an anatomical structure so that the finished image is magnified.

macrorhinia (măk-rō-rīn′ē-ă) [″ + *rhis*, nose]. Excessive size of the nose, either congenital or pathological.

macroscelia (măk-rō-sē′lē-ă) [″ + *skelos*, leg]. Abnormally large legs.

macroscopic (măk-rō-skŏp′ĭk) [″ + *skopein*, to examine]. Large enough to be seen by the naked eye. Opposite of microscopic.

macroscopy (măk-rŏs′kŏ-pē). Examination of an object with the naked eye.

macrosigmoid (măk″rō-sĭg′moyd). Abnormally large sigmoid colon.

macrosis (mă-krō′sĭs) [″ + *osis*, condition]. Increase in size.

macrosmatic (măk″rŏs-măt′ĭk) [″ + *osmasthai*, to smell]. Indicating an abnormally keen sense of smell.

macrosomatia, macrosomia (măk″rō-sō-mā′shē-ă, măk-rō-sō′mē-ă) [Gr. *makros*, large, + *soma*, body]. Abnormally large body.

macrospore (măk′rō-spor). In certain fungi and protozoa with two spores, the larger of the two.

macrostereognosis (măk″rō-stē″rē-ō-nō′sĭs) [″ + *stereos*, solid, + *gnosis*, knowledge]. A misperception that objects appear to be larger than they are.

macrostomia (măk-rō-stō′mē-ă) [″ + *stoma*, mouth]. Excessively large mouth.

macrostructure (măk′rō-strŭk″tūr). The gross structure of an entity.

macrothrombocytes [″ + *thrombos*, clot, + *kytos*, cell]. Large platelets. These are seen in some rare disorders of platelets.

macrothrombocytopenia [″ + ″ + ″ + *penia*, lack]. Deficiency of macrothrombocytes. SEE: *Alport's syndrome.*

macrotia (măk-rō′shē-ă) [″ + *ous*, ear]. Abnormally large ears.

macrotome (măk′rō-tōm) [″ + *tome*, incision]. Device for cutting large anatomical sections. SEE: *microtome.*

macrotooth. Abnormally enlarged tooth.

macula (măk′ū-lă) [L., spot] (pl. *maculae*). 1. [NA] A small spot or colored area. SEE: *roseola.* 2. A macule.

maculae acusticae. Thickened oval areas in the saccule and utricle in which fibers of the vestibular branch of the acoustic nerve terminate. They are sensory receptors containing hair cells that respond to movement of the endolymph. They include macula sacculi and macula utriculi.

m. albida. White mark found on the visceral layer of the peritoneum or epicardium in some contagious diseases.

m. atrophica. Glistening white spot on skin due to atrophy.

m. caerulea. Steel-gray or blue stain of epidermis without elevation. It does not disappear on pressure and occurs esp. with pediculosis pubis or flea bites.

m., cerebral. Reddened line that becomes deeper and persists for some time when the fingernail is drawn across the skin, esp. in tuberculous meningitis. SYN: *tache cérébrale.*

m. corneae. Opaque spot in cornea.

m. cribrosa. [NA] One of several tiny foramina in the wall of the vestibule of the bony labyrinth of the ear through which pass filaments of the acoustic nerve.

m. densa. Closely packed cells in the distal tubular epithelium of each nephron. These cells are close to the juxtaglomerular apparatus and may function as chemoreceptors.

m. flava laryngis. A small yellow spot at the ventral end of each vocal cord formed by a small mass of elastic tissue or, sometimes, cartilage.

m. folliculi. The point on the ovarian follicle where it ruptures.

m. germinativa. The germinal area in eggs with large yolks.

m. gonorrhoeica. Red spot at orifice of Bartholin's gland. Seen in gonorrheal vulvitis.

m. lutea retinae. A yellow spot in the center of the retina approx. 2 mm lateral to the exit of optic nerve. Contains a pit, fovea centralis, where the retina is reduced to a layer of closely packed cones, which functions as the area of most acute vision (central vision).

m. sacculi. [NA] Thickened area in the saccule where vestibular impulses are received and transmitted.

m. utriculi. [NA] Thickened area in the utricle where vestibular impulses are received and transmitted.

macular (măk′ū-lăr) [L. *macula,* spot]. 1. Rel. to macules. 2. Having macules.

macular atrophies. A disease of the skin in which there are localized areas of flaccid, saclike lesions. The skin is not atrophied; thus, the name is a misnomer. These permanent lesions are due to circumscribed loss of skin elasticity.

TREAT: Excise cosmetically unattractive areas. SYN: *anetoderma,* q.v.

macular degeneration. Degeneration of the macular area of the retina of the eye. Even though this may be related to the toxic effects of drugs such as chloroquine or phenothiazine, the cause of the most common type — age-related macular degeneration (ARMD) — is unknown. This condition, the most common cause of visual impairment in persons over age 50, can lead to loss of central vision.

If this condition is due to growth of blood vessels under the retina and it is diagnosed early, the loss of vision can be arrested by using laser therapy to destroy the vessels. Test for loss of central vision may be done by using the Amsler grid, q.v. The patient looks at the grid with each eye separately. If central vision is impaired, the lines will appear wavy instead of straight. SEE: *Amsler grid.*

maculate(d) (măk′ū-lāt, -lāt-ĕd). Spotted, as with macules.

maculation (măk-ū-lā′shŭn) [L. *macula,* spot]. Process of becoming maculate; development of macules.

macule (măk′ūl) [L. *macula,* spot]. Discolored spot or patch on the skin, neither elevated nor depressed, of various colors, sizes, and shapes. Macules include hyperemia, roseola, erythema, telangiectasis, nevi vasculosi, areola, achromia, chloasma, purpura, petechiae, ecchymoses, vibices, albinism, vitiligo, lentigines, nevi pigmentosi, nevi spili, and discolorations.

Macules occur in pellagra, pityriasis rosea, pediculosis corporis, rubella, scurvy, serum sickness, peliosis, anemia, leukemia, cancer, infectious diseases, erysipelas, acne rosacea, nevus pigmentosus, vitiligo, leprosy, morphea, and facial hemiatrophy. SYN: *macula.*

maculocerebral (măk″ū-lō-sĕr′ē-brăl) [″ + *cerebrum,* brain]. Concerning the macula of the retina and the brain.

maculopapular (măk″ū-lō-păp′ū-lăr). Consisting of or pert. to macules and papules. An eruption consisting of both macules and papules.

maculopathy (măk″ū-lŏp′ă-thē) [″ + Gr. *pathos,* disease]. Retinal pathology involving the macula of the eye.

mad. 1. Not rational. SYN: *insane.* 2. Angry. 3. Rash, foolish, frantic. 4. Suffering from infection with rabies. SYN: *rabid.*

madarosis (măd-ă-rō′sĭs) [Gr. *madaros,* bald]. Loss of eyelashes or eyebrows.

madder (măd′ĕr). Root of the plant *Rubia tinctoria,* a source of the red dye alizarin.

Madelung's deformity [Otto W. Madelung, Strasbourg surgeon, 1846–1926]. Displacement of the hand to the radial side due to relative overgrowth of the ulna.

Madelung's disease. Generalized symmetrical deposits of fatty tissue, lipomata, on the upper back, shoulders, and neck. SYN: *Madelung's neck.*

madescent (măd-ĕs′ĕnt) [L. *madescere,* to become moist]. Slightly moist or becoming so.

madidans (măd′ĭ-dăns) [L. *madidus,* wet]. Exuding moisture as in some skin lesions.

Madura foot [from Madur district in India where disease was first described in 1842]. A local painless lesion — called a mycetoma — of an exposed area, such as bare feet. It consists of swollen tissue, sinuses filled with pus, and microbial colonies (called grains) embedded in the pustular tissues. Mycetomas may occur in any body part. It is usually found in adult males who work outside and have poor or no medical care for wounds.

ETIOL: Various fungi including eumycetoma and actinomycetes. In the U.S. the most frequent cause is *Pseudallescheria boydii.*

TREAT: The antibiotic given depends upon the specific organism involved. Streptomycin, dapsone, sulfamethoxazole, and trimethoprim are used for actinomycetoma. Ketoconazole has been used in eumycetomas. Surgery should not be necessary, but treatment will be needed for at least 10 months. SYN: *maduromycosis.*

maduromycosis (măd-ū″rō-mī-kō′sĭs). Chronic infection of the foot or hand characterized by marked swelling and development of nodules, vesicles, abscesses, and sinuses. A type of mycetoma, q.v.

ETIOL: Various fungi.

mafenide acetate (măf′ĕn-īd). USP. An antibacterial drug of the sulfonamide class, used topically in cream form for treating burns.

magaldrate (măg′ăl-drāt). USP. A complex of magnesium oxide and aluminum oxide, used as a gastric antacid. Trade name is Riopan.

Magendie's foramen (mă-jĕn′dēz) [François Magendie, Fr. physiologist, 1783–1855]. The median of three openings in the roof of the 4th ventricle. It is in front of the cerebellum and behind the pons varolii, connecting the ventricle with the subarachnoid space.

magenblase syndrome [Ger. *Magen,* stomach, + *Blase*, bubble]. Accumulation of swallowed air in the stomach that leads to postprandial fullness and pressure. Radiograph of the stomach will reveal a large gastric bubble.

magenstrasse (măg"ĕn-străs'ē) [" + *strasse*, street]. A groove along the lesser curvature of the stomach from cardia to pylorus.

magenta (mă-jĕn'tă). The dye basic fuchsin.

Magill forceps. Angulated forceps used during direct laryngoscopy to remove foreign body from an obstructed airway.

maggot. Larva of an insect, esp. the softbodied footless larva of flies (order Diptera). Many are parasitic, giving rise to myiasis, q.v.

maggot treatment. A method of treating septic wounds. In the 1930s, scientific studies indicated that neglected and infected compound fractures were aided in healing when blowfly maggots accidentally infested the wounds. The maggots removed necrotic tissue and left healthy granulating tissue. Modern therapy, including antibiotics, has made this method of treating wounds and osteomyelitis obsolete. Nevertheless, it is possible to culture sterile blowfly maggots for this use. In severe skin infections when all other forms of therapy have failed, this method has been used.

magic thinking. The feeling that thoughts or actions have the ability to cause actions or effects which would defy the normal laws of cause and effect.

magistery (măj'ĭs-tĕr"ē) [L. *magister*, master]. 1. Specially compounded remedy. 2. A precipitate.

magistral (măj'ĭs-trăl). Concerning medicines prescribed by a physician for a particular case. SEE: *officinal.*

magma (măg'mă) [Gr.]. 1. Mass left after extraction of principal. 2. Salve or paste. 3. A suspension of finely divided material in a small amount of water.

magnesia (măg-nē'zē-ă) [magnetic stone found in Magnesia, region of ancient Thessaly]. Magnesium oxide. MgO.

m., milk of. Aperient composed of magnesium hydroxide and water.

magnesia and alumina (tablets). An antacid preparation composed of aluminum hydroxide and magnesium hydroxide. Trade name is Maalox.

magnesium [L.]. SYMB: Mg. At. wt. 24.312; at. no. 12; sp. gr. 1.738. A white mineral element found in soft tissue, muscles, bones, and to some extent in the body fluids. It is a naturally occurring element on earth, being extracted from well and sea water. The human body contains approx. 25 gm of magnesium, most of which is in the bones.

Muscles contain less of it than they do of calcium. Concentration of magnesium in the blood serum is between 1.5 and 2.5 mEq/liter.

Magnesium is widely distributed in foods; therefore, deficiency rarely occurs. It is obtained in sufficient quantities in whole grains, fruits, and vegetables. A typical diet contains 200 to 400 mg, but very little of this is absorbed. Deficiency may be present in patients with chronic diarrhea or diseases that interfere with absorption.

FUNCT: Magnesium activates enzymes that catalyze reactions between phosphate ions and adenosine triphosphate (ATP). It is also associated with regulation of body temperature, neuromuscular contraction, and synthesis of protein.

DEFICIENCY SYM: Tetany quite similar to that produced by hypocalcemia, weakness, and mental depression.

m. carbonate. USP. $MgCO_3 \cdot 3H_2O$. A bulky, white, odorless powder. Taken by mouth to neutralize acid in stomach.

m. chloride. USP. $MgCl_2 \cdot 6H_2$. It is used in treating electrolyte disturbances and in dialysis solutions.

m. citrate oral solution. USP. A solution containing an amount of magnesium citrate corresponding to approx. 1.6% magnesium oxide. Used as a purgative. Trade name is Evac-Q-Mag.

m. gluconate. USP. A medicine used to replace magnesium in the body.

m. hydroxide. $Mg(OH)_2$. USP. A bulky white powder that, in aqueous suspension, is milk of magnesia. Used as a laxative and an antacid.

m. oxide. USP. MgO. Calcined magnesia. Light magnesia. A white, very bulky powder. In Great Britain called light magnesium oxide. Used as an antacid and laxative.

m. phosphate. USP. A white, odorless powder. Used as an antacid and a laxative.

m. salicylate. USP. An antipyretic and analgesic drug. Trade name is Magan.

m. stearate. USP. Compound of magnesium and palmitic and stearic acids. Used in manufacture of pharmaceutical tablets.

m. sulfate. USP. $MgSO_4 \cdot 7H_2O$. Small colorless crystals with a bitter saline taste. SYN: *epsom salt.* Used as a cathartic, anticonvulsant and topically as an anti-inflammatory agent.

INCOMPAT: Ammonium chloride, soapsuds enema, quinine, ferric chloride, sulfanilamide.

m. trisilicate. USP. Magnesium oxide, silicon dioxide, and water. Used as an antacid. Trade names are Azolid-A and Trimax.

magnet [Gr. *magnes*, magnet]. Any body that has the property of attracting iron. This may be a natural iron oxide or a mass of iron or steel that has this property given to it artificially. A piece of iron may be magnetized by passage of an electric current through an insulated wire wound around it.

    m., horseshoe. Magnet in shape of a horseshoe.

magnetic. Pert. to a magnet or having magnetism.

magnetic field. The space permeated by the magnetic lines of force surrounding a permanent magnet or coil of wire carrying electric current.

magnetic lines of force. The lines indicating the direction of the magnetic force in the space surrounding a magnet or constituting a magnetic field.

magnetic microspheres. In autologous bone marrow transplant, use of microscopic magnetic particles coated with or coupled to antibodies which, when exposed to certain types of malignant cells, can bind to them. The microspheres so bound can be removed by passing the cells through a magnetic field. This technique is experimental.

magnetic resonance imaging. ABBR: MRI. When certain atomic nuclei with an odd number of protons or neutrons or both are subjected to a strong magnetic field, they absorb and re-emit electromagnetic energy. Analysis of the net magnetization vector's deflection by application of a radiofrequency pulse provides image information. This technique is valuable in providing images of the heart, large blood vessels, brain, and soft tissues. It does not involve exposure to ionizing radiation, nor is there need to inject a contrast medium. Nevertheless, it is expensive and necessitates keeping the patient immobile for a lengthy period. It is contraindicated in patients with cardiac pacemakers or ferromagnetic aneurysmal clips in place.

magnetism (măg′nĕ-tĭzm) [Gr. *magnes*, magnet, + *-ismos*, condition]. The property of repulsion and attraction of certain substances that have magnetic properties. SEE: *magnet.*

magnetoelectricity (măg-nē″tō-ē″lĕk-trĭs′ĭ-tē) [″ + *elektron*, amber]. Electricity generated by use of magnets.

magnetometer (măg″nĕ-tŏm′ĕ-tĕr) [″ + *metron*, measure]. Device for measuring magnetic fields.

magneton (măg′nĕ-tŏn). The unit of nuclear magnetic force.

magnetotherapy (măg-nē″tō-thĕr′ă-pē) [″ + *therapeia*, treatment]. Application of magnets or magnetism in treating diseases. There is no evidence that such therapy is effective.

magnetropism (măg-nĕt′rō-pĭzm) [″ + *trope*, a turn]. The change in direction of growth of a plant or organism in response to the action of a magnetic field.

magnification (măg-nĭ-fĭ-kā′shŭn) [L. *magnus*, great, + *facere*, to make]. Process of increasing apparent size of an object, esp. under a microscope.

magnitude. Size, extent, or dimensions.

magnum [L.]. 1. Large or great. 2. Old term for capitate bone (os magnum), the largest of the carpals.

Mahaim fibers [I. Mahaim, contemporary Fr. physician]. Fibers for conducting cardiac impulses. They connect the proximal main atrioventricular bundle to the septal myocardium and permit ventricular pre-excitation with resultant tachycardia.

maidenhead. Lay term for the thin crescentic fold surrounding or covering vaginal opening. At one time considered to be a sign of virginity. However, it may be present in those who have had sexual intercourse and may be absent in those who have never experienced sexual intercourse. SYN: *hymen.*

maim (mām) [ME. *maymen*, to cripple]. 1. To injure seriously; to disable. 2. To deprive of the use of a part, such as an arm or leg.

main (măn) [Fr.]. Hand.

    m. en griffe. Flexion and atrophy of the hand in a claw shape. SYN: *clawhand.*

mainstreaming. Term referring to the philosophy of educating children with disabling conditions in natural settings so as not to deprive them of normal social experiences and conditions.

maintainer. Something that supports or keeps another thing in existence or continuity.

    m., space. Device fashioned to keep teeth separated when placed across an edentulous segment of the dental arch. It may consist of bands, bars, springs, etc., and is cemented or soldered to orthodontic bands or crowns on the adjacent teeth.

Majocchi's disease (mă-yŏk′ēz) [Domenico Majocchi, It. physician, 1849–1929]. Ring-shaped purple eruption of lower limbs. SYN: *purpura annularis telangiectodes.*

Majocchi's granuloma. Allergic granulomata of the skin due to fungal infections.

major histocompatibility complex. ABBR: MHC. The chromosomal region that controls strong transplantation antigens. These are called histocompatibility locus antigens (HLA) in man. In humans, antibodies to HLA-controlled antigens have been found in sera from women with multiple pregnancies and from persons who have received multiple blood transfusions. Investigation of these antigens led to the work indicating that these antigens are controlled by genes at loci on chromosome 6. These loci have been designated HLA-A, HLA-B, and HLA-C, which are universally distributed, and HLA-D and HLA-DR, which are restricted to immunoregulatory genes. HLA indicates human leukocyte associated antigen. In choosing donors of organs to be transplanted, it is essential that the recipient match the HLA type of the donor. SEE: *human leukocyte associated antigens.*

makro- [Gr.]. SEE: words beginning with *macro-*.

mal-. Combining form meaning ill, bad, poor.

mal (măl) [Fr., from L. *malum,* an evil]. A sickness or disorder.

    m. de Cayenne. Elephantiasis.

    m. de mer. Seasickness.

    m. perforant. A perforating ulcer of the foot.

    m. perforant palatin. A perforating ulcer of the palate.

mala (mā'lă) [L.]. 1. [NA] The cheek. 2. The cheekbone.

malabsorption syndrome. Disordered or inadequate absorption of nutrients from the intestinal tract, esp. the small intestine. May be associated with or due to a number of diseases, including those affecting the intestinal mucosa, such as infections, tropical sprue, gluten enteropathy, pancreatic insufficiency, or lactase deficiency. May also be due to surgery such as gastric resection and ileal bypass or to antibiotic therapy such as neomycin. SEE: *gluten-induced enteropathy; irritable bowel syndrome; lactose intolerance.*

malacia (mă-lā'shē-ă) [Gr. *malakia,* softening]. Abnormal softening of tissues of an organ or of tissues themselves.

malacoma (măl-ă-kō'mă). Softening of an organ or part of the body. SYN: *malacia; malacosis.*

malacoplakia (măl"ă-kō-plā'kē-ă) [Gr. *malakos,* soft, + *plax,* plaque]. Existence of soft patches in mucous membrane of a hollow organ.

    m. vesicae. Soft, funguslike patches on mucosa of the bladder and ureters.

malacosarcosis (măl"ă-kō-săr-kō'sĭs) [" + *sarx,* flesh, + *osis,* condition]. Softness of tissue, esp. muscular.

malacosis (măl-ă-kō'sĭs) [" + *osis,* condition]. Abnormal softening of an organ or tissue. SYN: *malacia; malacoma.*

malacosteon (măl-ă-kŏs'tē-ŏn) [" + *osteon,* bone]. Softening of the bones. SYN: *mollities ossium; osteomalacia.*

malacotic (măl-ă-kŏt'ĭk). 1. Soft. 2. Affected with malacia. 3. Rel. to malacia.

malacotomy (măl-ă-kŏt'ō-mē) [Gr. *malakos,* soft, + *tome,* incision]. Incision of soft

areas of the body, esp. of the abdominal wall.

malactic (mă-lăk'tĭk) [Gr. *malakos,* soft]. Emollient.

maladie de Roger (măl'ă-dē') [Henry L. Roger, Fr. physician, 1809–1891]. Congenital interventricular septal defect.

maladjusted. Poorly adjusted; unhappy or unsuccessful because of inability or failure to adjust to life stresses. Marked by depression, anxiety, and irritability.

malady (măl'ă-dē) [Fr. *maladie,* illness, from L. *malum,* an evil]. A disease or disorder. SYN: *disease.*

malaise (mă-lāz') [Fr.]. Discomfort, uneasiness, or indisposition, often indicative of infection.

malalignment (măl"ă-līn'měnt). Improper alignment of structures such as teeth or the portions of a fractured bone. SEE: *malocclusion.*

malar (mā'lăr) [L. *mala,* cheek]. Pert. to the cheek or cheekbones.

malar bone. A four-pointed bone on each side of the face, uniting the frontal and superior maxillary bones with the zygomatic process of the maxilla. SYN: *cheekbone; mala; zygoma; zygomatic bone.*

malaria (mă-lā'rē-ă) [It. *malaria,* bad air]. An acute and sometimes chronic infectious disease due to the presence of protozoan parasites within red blood cells. Malaria is transmitted to the human by the bite of an infected female anopheles mosquito. The mosquito becomes infected by ingesting the blood of a human infected with malaria. SEE: *Anopheles.*

Of the 1.8 billion persons at risk of malaria worldwide, 200 million become infected each year. It is therefore one of the most important infectious diseases in the world.

The parasites undergo an asexual cycle in man and a sexual cycle in the mosquito. Sporozoites injected by the bite of a mosquito or by blood transfusion go through an exoerythrocytic cycle in tissue cells, such as liver cells, where they undergo schizogony. After an interval of 7 to 10 days, they invade erythrocytes in which they undergo several divisions (schizogony), forming many merozoites. These break free and invade other corpuscles. The destruction of corpuscles with liberation of pigment and waste products brings on the characteristic paroxysms of chills and fever. This occurs at 48-hour intervals in tertian malaria and 72-hour intervals in quartan malaria.

After several generations of schizonts, some merozoites develop into micro- and macrogametocytes, which, when sucked up by a mosquito feeding on the patient, undergo further development. The microgametocytes produce several flagellated bodies that unite with a macrogamete to form a zygote. This elongates, forming a vermicule or ookinete, which penetrates the stomach wall of the mosquito, forming an oocyst in which sporozoites develop. The oocyst bursts when mature, liberating sporozoites into the body cavity through which the sporozoites then make their way to salivary glands. They are discharged through salivary ducts when the mosquito bites a person.

SYM: Characterized by periodicity of chills, fever, and sweats in that order. There are signs and symptoms of progressive anemia, splenic enlargement, and deposition in various organs of a melanin, resulting from biological activity of *Plasmodium* species. *P. vivax* and *P. ovale* have dormant forms that may initiate a relapse. *P. falciparum* and *P. malariae* have no such dormant forms.

ETIOL: Four species of a sporozoan, *Plasmodium* (*P. vivax*, *P. falciparum*, *P. malariae*, *P. ovale*). The causative organism is transmitted through bites of infected female mosquitoes of the genus *Anopheles*. It is a rare occurrence, but malaria may be transmitted by blood transfusion.

DIAG: Identification of the parasites in the blood.

PROPHYLAXIS: When traveling to areas where falciparum malaria is endemic, adults should take 500 mg of chloroquine phosphate (which contains 300 mg of base) orally once a week beginning one week prior to arrival in the area, and continue that dose once a week while in the malarious area; and for 4 weeks after leaving the area. Children are given a dose appropriate for their weight.

In areas where chloroquine-resistant falciparum malaria occurs, adults should take 250 mg of mefloquine orally once a week beginning one week prior to arrival in the area. One should continue that weekly dose during the stay and for 4 weeks after leaving the area. Mefloquine should not be used during pregnancy.

Prevention of other forms of malaria requires the addition of primaquine phosphate to the chloroquine regimen.

INCUBATION: Average 12 days for *P. falciparum*, 14 days for *P. vivax* and *P. ovale*, and 30 days for *P. malariae*.

TREAT: Chloroquine phosphate is indicated in all types of malaria except that due to drug-resistant *P. falciparum*. In drug-resistant *P. falciparum*, treatment with combinations of quinine, pyrimethamine, and a sulfonamide is indicated. Malaria due to other species should be treated with both chloroquine and primaquine in a dose of 15 mg of the base each day for 14 days. This may be given at the same time as the chloroquine. Persons with glucose-6-phosphate-dehydrogenase deficiency may develop hemolysis of red blood cells, but this is a rare complication.

Severe malaria due to *P. falciparum* with evidence of cerebral involvement may be treated with continuous infusion of quinidine gluconate and exchange transfusion.

m., cerebral. Falciparum malaria in which the brain is affected due to tendency of parasites to agglutinate, resulting in clogging of capillaries, which leads to coma or sometimes sudden death.

m., falciparum. Malaria caused by *Plasmodium falciparum*. More prevalent in the tropics. Symptoms more severe than in other types but runs a shorter course without relapses.

m., quartan. Malaria with short and less severe paroxysms. Sporulation occurs each 72 hours, causing seizures every 4 days. Caused by *Plasmodium malariae*.

m., quotidian. Malaria in which paroxysms occur with daily periodicity due to 24-hour sporulation of two groups of *P. vivax*. Abrupt rise and fall of temperature.

m., tertian. Malaria in which sporulation occurs each 48 hours. Symptoms more common during the day. Paroxysms divided into chill, fever, and sweating stages. Cold stage usually is 10 to 15 minutes but may last an hour or more. Febrile stage varies from 4 to 6 hours. Benign tertian malaria is caused by *Plasmodium vivax*, malignant tertian malaria by *Plasmodium falciparum*.

m., vivax. Malaria caused by *Plasmodium vivax*. It is the most common form of malaria. Marked by frequent recurrence.

malariacidal (mă-lā″rē-ă-sī′dăl) [It. *malaria*, bad air, + L. *caedere*, to kill]. Having the property of killing malaria parasites.

malarial (mă-lăr′ē-ăl) [It. *malaria*, bad air]. 1. Affected with malaria. 2. Causing malaria. 3. Resembling malaria. 4. Pert. to malaria. SYN: *malarious*.

malariology (mă-lăr-ē-ŏl′ō-jē). The scientific study of malaria.

malariotherapy (mă-lăr-ē-ō-thĕr′ă-pē). A now obsolete method of treating syphilis of the central nervous system by injecting malarial organisms into the body. The organisms produce hyperthermia, which is then terminated by administration of an antimalarial.

malarious (mă-lăr′ē-ŭs). Of the nature of, or afflicted with malaria. SYN: *malarial*.

Malassezia (măl″ă-sē′zē-ă) [Louis Charles Malassez, Fr. physiologist, 1842–1909]. A genus of fungi.

malassimilation (măl″ă-sĭm-ĭ-lā′shŭn) [L. *malus,* ill, + *assimilatio,* making like]. Defective, incomplete, or faulty assimilation, esp. of nutritive material. SEE: *malabsorption syndrome.*

malate (mā′lāt). A salt or ester of malic acid.

malathion (măl″ă-thī′ŏn). An effective pesticide.

malaxate (măl′ăk-sāt) [L. *malaxare,* to soften]. To knead, as in massaging a part.

malaxation (măl-ăks-ā′shŭn). Kneading movement used in massage.

maldigestion (măl″dī-jĕs′chŭn). Disordered digestion.

male [O. Fr.]. 1. Masculine. 2. The sex that has organs for producing sperm for fertilization of ova.

    RS: female; organ; penis; sperm; testicle; virile; virilescence; virilism; virility.

malemission (măl″ē-mĭsh′ŭn) [L. *malus,* evil, + *e,* out, + *mittere,* to send]. Failure of semen to be ejaculated from the urinary meatus during coitus.

maleruption (măl-ē-rŭp′shŭn). Incorrect eruption of teeth.

malformation (măl-for-mā′shŭn) [″ + *formatio,* a shaping]. Deformity; abnormal shape or structure, esp. congenital.

    m., tooth. Abnormalities of size and shape that usually occur during the morphodifferentiation stage of tooth formation. Incomplete matrix formation or mineralization will also result in defective teeth that may or may not be abnormal in shape initially.

malfunction (măl-fŭnk′shŭn). Defective function.

malic (mā′lĭk, măl′ĭk) [L. *malum,* apple]. Pert. to apples.

malic acid. An acid found in some fruits, such as apples. SEE: *acid, malic.*

malice (măl′ĭs) [L. *malus,* bad]. Desire or intent to harm someone or to see others suffer.

malign (mă-līn′) [ME. *maligne*]. Tending to injure or harm; malignant.

malignancy (mă-lĭg′năn-sē) [L. *malignus,* of bad kind]. 1. State of being malignant. 2. A neoplasm or tumor that is cancerous as opposed to benign. SYN: *virulence.*

malignant (mă-lĭg′nănt). Growing worse; resisting treatment, said of cancerous growths. Tending or threatening to produce death; harmful. SYN: *virulent.*

malinger (mă-lĭng′ĕr) [Fr. *malingre,* weak, sickly]. To feign illness, usually to arouse sympathy, to escape work, or to continue to receive compensation. SEE: *factitious disorder; Munchausen syndrome.*

malingerer (mă-lĭng′gĕr-ĕr). 1. One who pretends to be ill or suffering from a nonexistent disorder to arouse sympathy. 2. One who pretends slow recuperation from a disease once suffered in order to continue to receive benefits of medical insurance and work absence.

malinterdigitation (măl″ĭn-tĕr-dĭj″ĭ-tā′shŭn). Abnormal intercuspal relation of the upper and lower teeth.

malleable (măl′ē-ă-b′l) [L. *mallere,* to hammer]. Having the property of being shaped by pressure.

malleation (măl-lē-ā′shŭn). Spasmodic action of the hands in which they seem drawn to strike any near object, as spasmodic rapping against thighs or furniture. SEE: *tic.*

malleoincudal (măl″ē-ō-ĭng′kū-dăl) [L. *malleus,* hammer, + *incus,* anvil]. Concerning or pert. to the malleus and incus.

malleolar (măl-ē-ō′lăr) [L. *malleolus,* little hammer]. Concerning the malleolus.

malleolus (măl-ē′ō-lŭs) [L.] (pl. *malleoli*). The protuberance on both sides of the ankle joint, the lower extremity of the fibula being known as the lateral malleolus and lower end of the tibia as the medial malleolus.

    m., external. Process on outer edge of fibula at lower end.

    m., internal. Round process on inner edge of tibia at lower end.

malleotomy (măl″ē-ŏt′ō-mē) [″ + Gr. *tome,* incision]. 1. Division of the malleus of the inner ear. 2. Severing the ligaments attached to the malleoli of the ankle.

mallet. A hammerlike tool to condense amalgam or direct filling gold. The hammer head is of wood or plastic so that when driving another tool it will leave no mark or imprint.

mallet finger. Flexion deformity of the distal joint of a finger. It is caused by avulsion of the extensor tendon. SYN: *hammer finger.*

mallet toe. Abnormal flexion or loss of power of extension of a toe. SYN: *hammertoe.*

malleus (măl′ē-ŭs) [L., hammer] (pl. *mallei*). [NA] The largest of the three auditory ossicles in the middle ear, attached to the eardrum, and articulating with the incus. SEE: *ear.*

Mallophaga (măl-ŏf′ă-gă) [Gr. *mallos,* wool, + *phagein,* to eat]. An order of insects that includes biting lice.

Mallory-Weiss syndrome [G. Kenneth Mallory, U.S. pathologist, b. 1900; Soma Weiss, U.S. internist, 1898–1942]. Hemorrhage from the upper gastrointestinal tract due to a tear in the mucosa of the esophagus or gastroesophageal junction. The syndrome is associated with chronic alcoholism and is usually preceded by severe vomiting. SEE: *cirrhosis; esophageal varices; Müller maneuver.* SEE: *Nursing Diagnoses in Appendix.*

malnutrition (măl″nū-trĭ′shŭn). Lack of necessary or proper food substances in the body or improper absorption and distribution of

Physical Signs of Malnutrition and Deficiency State

Infants and Children	Adolescents and Adults
Lack of subcutaneous fat	Red swollen lingual papillae
Wrinkling of skin on light stroking	Glossitis
Poor muscle tone	Papillary atrophy of tongue
Pallor	Stomatitis
Rough skin (toad skin)	Spongy, bleeding gums
Hemorrhage of newborn, vitamin K deficiency	Muscle tenderness in extremities
Bad posture	Poor muscle tone
Nasal area is red and greasy	Loss of vibratory sensation
Sores — at angles of mouth, cheilosis	Increase or decrease of tendon reflexes
Rapid heartbeat	Hyperesthesia of skin
Red tongue	Bilateral symmetrical dermatitis
Square head, wrists enlarged, rib beading	Purpura
Vincent's angina, thrush	Dermatitis: facial butterfly, perineal, scrotal, vulval
Serious dental abnormalities	Thickening and pigmentation of skin over bony prominences
Corneal and conjunctival changes	Nonspecific vaginitis
	Follicular hyperkeratosis of extensor surfaces of extremities
Adolescents and Adults	Rachitic chest deformity
	Anemia not responding to iron
Nasolabial sebaceous plugs	Fatigue of visual accommodation
Sores at corners of mouth, cheilosis	Vascularization of cornea
Vincent's angina	Conjunctival changes
Minimal changes in tongue color or texture	

Source: Committee on Medical Nutrition, National Research Council.

them. Any disorder of nutrition; may be due to a deficient diet or deficient breakdown, assimilation, or utilization of food. SEE: table.

m., protein-energy. Malnutrition due to inadequate intake of calories or protein or both. Usually seen in children less than age five. SYN: *protein-calorie malnutrition.* SEE: *kwashiorkor.*

malocclusion. Malposition and imperfect contact of the mandibular and maxillary teeth.

m., classification of. The designation by Angle of the types of malocclusion based on the relative positions of the first molar in the two arches when in occlusion: *Class I* — normal anteroposterior relationship but with crowding and rotated teeth. *Class II* — the lower arch is distal to the upper arch on one or both sides; the lower first molar is

distal to the upper first molar. *Class III* — the lower arch is anterior to the upper arch on one or both sides; the lower first molar is anterior to the upper first molar.

malonylurea (măl″ō-nĭl-ū′rē-ă). Barbituric acid. SEE: *acid, barbituric.*

malpighian body (măl-pĭg′ē-ăn) [Marcello Malpighi, It. anatomist, founder of histology, 1628–1694]. 1. A malpighian capsule, q.v. 2. A splenic nodule; a spherical, ovoid body found in the white pulp of the spleen. Similar in structure to a lymphatic nodule.

malpighian capsule. A spherical body found in cortex of kidney consisting of a glomerulus and Bowman's capsule.

malpighian layer. Includes both stratum germinativum and stratum spinosum.

malpighian pyramid. A renal pyramid.

malposition (măl-pō-zĭ′shŭn) [L. *malus,* evil, + *positio,* placement]. Faulty or abnormal position or placement, esp. of the body or one of its parts.

malpractice [" + Gr. *praxis*, an action]. Incorrect or negligent treatment of a patient by persons responsible for health care, such as physicians, dentists, and nurses.

malpresentation [" + *praesentatio*, a presenting]. Abnormal position of fetus rendering natural delivery difficult or impossible.

malrotation (măl″rō-tā′shŭn). During embryogenesis, failure of normal rotation of the viscera or a portion of them.

malt [AS. *mealt*]. Germinated grain, usually barley, used in manufacture of ale and beer. Contains carbohydrates (dextrin, maltose), a diastase, and proteins. Used as a food, esp. in wasting diseases.

Malta fever. Brucellosis, q.v.

maltase (mawl′tās) [AS. *mealt*, grain]. A salivary and pancreatic enzyme that acts on maltose, converting it by hydrolysis to glucose. SEE: *digestion; enzyme.*

malt extract. A viscous, light brown fluid obtained from malt steeped in water.

maltose (mawl′tōs). $C_{12}H_{22}O_{11}$. A disaccharide present in malt, malt products, and sprouting seeds. It is formed by the hydrolysis of starch and is converted into glucose by the enzyme maltase. SYN: *malt sugar.* SEE: *carbohydrate.*

maltosuria (mawl″tō-sūr′ē-ă) [" + Gr. *ouron*, urine]. Presence of maltose in urine.

malt sugar. Maltose.

malturned. Abnormally turned, said of a tooth turned on its long axis.

malum (mă′lŭm) [L., an evil]. A disease.

   m. articulorum senilis. Arthritis in the aged.

   m. coxae senilis. Hip disease in the aged, esp. osteoarthritis.

   m. perforans pedis. Perforating ulcer of the foot. Begins with thickening epidermis.

   m. venereum. Syphilis.

malunion [L. *malus*, evil, + *unio*, oneness]. Growth of the fragments of a fractured bone in a faulty position, forming an imperfect union.

mamanpian (mă-măn″pē-ăn′) [Fr. *maman*, mother, + *pian*, yaw]. A mother yaw.

mamelon (măm′ē-lŏn) [Fr., nipple]. One of three rounded protuberances present on the cutting edge of an incisor tooth when it erupts. These are worn away by use.

mamill-. SEE: words beginning with *mamill-.*

mamma (măm′ă) [L., breast] (pl. *mammae*). [NA] Cutaneous glandular structure in the female that secretes milk. In the human female, there are two, situated over the anterolateral area between the 3rd and 6th ribs. SYN: *breast; mammary gland.*

mammal (măm′ăl). An animal of the class Mammalia. Characterized by having breasts from which milk is available for the nourishment of the newborn.

mammalgia (măm-ăl′jē-ă) [L. *mamma*, breast, + Gr. *algos*, pain]. Pain in the breast. SYN: *mastalgia; mastodynia.*

mammaplasty (măm′ă-plăs″tē) [" + Gr. *plassein*, to form]. Plastic surgery of the breast.

   m., augmentation. Plastic surgical procedure to increase the size of the breast(s) or to make an artificial breast to replace one surgically removed. This is usually done by implanting a soft plastic material in an impervious cover or by implanting a gel.

Caution: The long-term health risks of some of the implant materials is unknown.

---

mammary (măm′ă-rē) [L. *mamma*, breast]. Pert. to the breast.

mammary glands. Compound glands of the female breast that can secrete milk. They are made up of lobes and lobules bound together by areolar tissue. The main ducts number 15 to 20 and are known as lactiferous ducts, each one discharging through a separate orifice upon the surface of the nipple. The dilatations of the ducts form reservoirs for the milk during lactation, q.v. The pink, or dark-colored, skin around the nipple is called the areola, q.v. SYN: *mammae.*

   RS: breast; caked breast; galactagogue; gynecomastia; mammectomy; mastectomy; mastopathy; nipple.

mammectomy (măm-mĕk′tō-mē) [" + Gr. *ektome*, excision]. Removal of the breast. SYN: *mastectomy.*

mammilla (mă-mĭl′lă) [L., nipple]. 1. Nipple. 2. Any structure resembling a nipple.

mammillary (măm′ĭl-lăr-ē) [L. *mammilla*, nipple]. Shaped like or concerning a nipple.

mammillated (măm′mĭl-lā-tĕd). Having protuberances like a nipple.

mammillation (măm-ĭl-lā′shŭn). 1. Condition of having a granulated appearance or nipplelike projections. 2. A nipplelike protuberance.

mammilliform (măm-mĭl′ĭ-form) [" + *forma*, shape]. Shaped like a nipple.

mammilliplasty (măm-mĭl′ĭ-plăs″tē) [" + Gr. *plassein*, to form]. Plastic operation on a nipple. SYN: *theleplasty.*

mammillitis (măm″mĭl-ī′tĭs) [" + Gr. *itis*, inflammation]. Inflammation of a nipple. SYN: *acromastitis; thelitis.*

mammitis (măm-ī′tĭs) [L. *mamma*, breast, + Gr. *itis*, inflammation]. Inflamed condition of the breast. SYN: *mastitis.*

mammogen (măm′ō-jĕn) [" + Gr. *gennan*, to produce]. Prolactin, q.v.

mammogram (măm′ō-grăm) [" + Gr. *gramma*, something written]. X-ray of the breast.

mammography (măm-ŏg′ră-fē) [" + Gr. *graphein*, to write]. Use of radiography of the breast to diagnose breast cancer. This technique has increased the rate of early detection. Mammography is capable of detecting 85% to 90% of existing breast cancers. Despite the increased exposure to radiation, mammography is recommended as a screening technique for breast cancer. Women in the high-risk group for breast cancer (ages 40 to 49) should have the examination every one to two years. Women over age 50 should have the examination every year. Use of mammography as a diagnostic tool does not mean that a careful periodic physical examination should be omitted. This is esp. true for women with dense, fibrous breast tissue, in which lesions are difficult to detect.

mammoplasty (măm′ō-plăs″tē) [" + Gr. *plassein*, to form]. Surgical reconstruction of the breasts; sometimes augmented by substances such as fat tissue or silicone to alter the size and shape.

    m., augmentation. Plastic surgery of the breast involving increase of size.

    m., reduction. Plastic surgery of the breast in order to decrease and reshape the breast(s).

mammose (măm′ōs) [L. *mammosus*]. 1. Having unusually large breasts. 2. Shaped like a breast.

mammotomy (măm-ŏt′ō-mē) [L. *mamma*, breast, + Gr. *tome*, incision]. Surgery of a breast. SYN: *mastotomy*.

mammotrophic (măm″ō-trŏf′ĭk) [" + Gr. *trophe*, nourishment]. To have the effect of stimulating size or function of the breast.

man [AS. *mann*]. 1. Member of the human species; *Homo sapiens*. 2. Male member of the species as distinguished from female. 3. The human race, collectively; mankind. SEE: words beginning with *anthro-*.

manchette (măn-chĕt′) [Fr., a cuff]. A circular band consisting of microtubules around the caudal pole of the developing sperm.

manchineel (măn″kĭ-nēl′) [Sp. *manzanilla*, small apple]. A tropical tree native to America, *Hippomane mancinella*, that contains a milky, poisonous sap. Contact with the sap causes blistering of the skin. The fruit is also poisonous.

mancinism (măn′sĭn-ĭzm) [L. *mancus*, crippled]. State of being left-handed.

Mandelamine Trade name for methenamine mandelate, USP.

mandelic acid. $C_8H_8O_3$. A colorless hydroxy acid, q.v. Its salt is used in urinary tract infections.

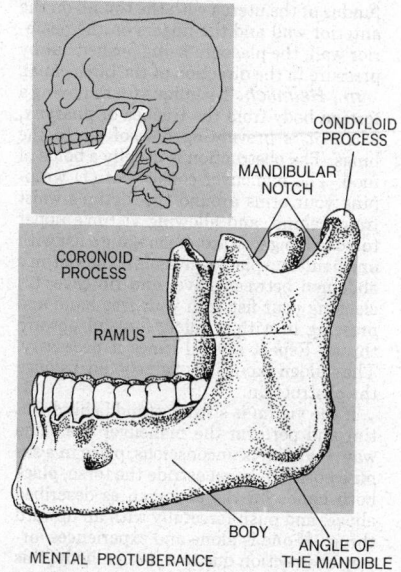

CONDYLOID PROCESS

MANDIBULAR NOTCH

CORONOID PROCESS

RAMUS

BODY

ANGLE OF THE MANDIBLE

MENTAL PROTUBERANCE

MANDIBLE—LEFT LATERAL VIEW

mandible (măn′dĭ-bl) [L. *mandibula*, lower jawbone]. The horseshoe-shaped bone forming the lower jaw. SEE: illus. SYN: *mandibula* [NA].

mandibula (măn-dĭb′ū-lă) [L.] (pl. *mandibulae*). [NA] The bone of the lower jaw, having a horseshoe shape.

mandibular (măn-dĭb′ū-lăr). Rel. to the lower jaw.

mandibular reflex. Clonic movement resulting from percussing or stroking lower jaw.

mandibulopharyngeal (măn-dĭb″ū-lō-fă-rin′jē-ăl) [" + Gr. *pharynx*, throat]. Concerning the mandible and pharynx.

mandrel, mandril (măn′drĕl). Handle that holds a dental tool so that it may be rotated. A spindle or shaft designed to fit a dental handpiece for the purpose of using a variety of tools for grinding, polishing or buffing.

mandrin (măn′drĭn) [Fr.]. A guide or stylet for a flexible catheter.

maneuver [Fr. *manoeuvre*, from L. *manu operari*, to work by hand]. 1. Any dextrous or skillful procedure. 2. In obstetrics, manipulation of the fetus to aid in delivery. SEE: *labor*.

    m., Crede's. Method of expressing the placenta in which the hand is placed on the fundus of the uterus with the thumb on the anterior wall and the fingers on the posterior wall, the placenta being pushed out by pressure in the direction of the birth canal.

m., Heimlich. Technique for removing a foreign body from the trachea or pharynx, where it is preventing flow of air to the lungs. The obstruction is usually a bolus of food. The maneuver consists of (1) wrapping your arms around the victim's waist from behind, and allowing victim's upper torso to hang forward; (2) making a fist with one hand and placing it against the victim's abdomen between navel and rib cage; (3) clasping your fist with your free hand and pressing in with a quick, forceful upward thrust. Repeat several times if necessary. The sudden expulsion of air should dislodge the obstruction.

If the victim is sitting, stand behind victim and perform the maneuver the same way. If victim is unconscious, place in a supine position, kneel astride the torso, place both hands on the abdomen as described above, and push forcefully with an upward thrust. If one is alone and experiences airway obstruction due to a foreign body, this technique could be self-applied.

This treatment is quite effective in dislodging the obstruction by forcing air against the mass much as pressure from a carbonated beverage will forcibly remove a cork or cap from a bottle. SEE: *Heimlich maneuver* for illus.

m., Leopold's. SEE: *Leopold's maneuver.*

m., Mauriceau-Smellie-Veit. Method employed to deliver the aftercoming head in breech presentation. The baby is held over the right arm, and the index finger of the right hand is introduced into the mouth of the child and applied over the maxilla; two fingers of the other hand are then hooked over the neck, grasping the shoulders. Downward traction is made until the occiput appears under the symphysis pubis. The body of the child is then raised up toward the mother's abdomen and the mouth, nose, brow, and occiput are successively brought over the perineum.

m., Müller's. Inspiratory effort with a closed glottis at the end of expiration. This produces negative intrathoracic pressure and may cause engorgement of blood vessels and thus allow those structures to be better visualized during radiographic studies. Esp. useful in demonstrating esophageal varices.

m., Munro Kerr. Method for determining the presence of disproportion between the fetal head and the maternal pelvis. The fetal head is pushed into the pelvis with the right hand on the abdomen while, with two fingers of the left hand in the vagina, the possibilities of engagement of the head are noted. At the same time the thumb of the left hand feels over the brim of the pelvis to determine the degrees of overlapping.

m., Pinard's. Method used in breech presentation. Fingers are placed behind the fetal knee, pushing it toward and past the fetal body, causing flexion of the knee. The foot is then grasped and brought down.

m., Prague. Method for the delivery of the aftercoming head in a breech delivery when the occiput is posterior.

m., Scanzoni. Double application of forceps in posterior position of the occiput.

m., Valsalva's. Forcible expiration against the closed glottis with both mouth and nose closed. This produces increased intrathoracic pressure and also increases the pressure in the eustachian tube. If the tubes are patent, air will be forced into the middle ear. A useful maneuver in "clearing" ears that have become blocked during a descent from altitude.

manganese (măn′gă-nēz) [L. *manganesium*]. SYMB: Mn. At. wt. 54.938; at. no. 25; sp. gr. 7.21. A metal element found in many foods, some plants, and in the tissues of the higher animals. An essential element needed for normal bone metabolism and many enzyme reactions. Deficiency in humans has not been demonstrated.

SOURCES: Bananas, bran, beans, beets, blueberries, chard, chocolate, peas, leafy vegetables, and whole grains.

manganese poisoning. A rather uncommon cause of toxicity in workers exposed to manganese on a regular basis.

SYM: Muscular weakness, peculiar gait, tremors, central nervous system disturbances, salivation.

mange (mānj). A cutaneous communicable disease of domestic animals, including dogs and cats. A number of mites, such as *Chorioptes, Demodex, Psoroptes,* and *Sarcoptes* are causative agents. In man, this condition is known as scabies, q.v.

mania (mā′nē-ă) [Gr., madness]. 1. Mental disorder characterized by excessive excitement. 2. A form of psychosis characterized by exalted feelings, delusions of grandeur, elevation of mood, psychomotor overactivity, and overproduction of ideas. SEE: *psychosis, manic-depressive.* 3. Used as combining form to signify obsessive preoccupation.

m., puerperal. A form of mental disorder that occurs occasionally following childbirth.

m., religious. Mania resulting from excessive religious fervor.

m., transitory. Attacks of severe frenzy, of short duration.

m., unproductive. Behavior characteristic of mania with lack of spontaneity in speech or muteness, sometimes seen in manic-depressive psychosis. SEE: *alcoholism.*

maniac (mā'nē-ăk). Person afflicted by mania.

maniacal (mă-nī'ă-kl). 1. Rel. to or characterized by mania. 2. Afflicted with mania.

manic (măn'ĭk). Mood state characterized by excessive energy, poor impulse control, psychosis, agitation, flight of ideas, frenzied movement, and decreased sleep.

manic-depressive psychosis. Bipolar affective disorder characterized by severe alterations in mood that are usually episodic and recurrent; mood fluctuates between depression and mania.

manifest. To reveal in an obvious manner.

manifestation. The demonstration of the presence of a sign, symptom, or alteration, esp. one that is associated with a disease process.

manifest squint. Tropia, q.v.

manikin [D. *manneken,* little man]. A model of the human body or its parts, used esp. in teaching anatomy and nursing procedures.

maniphalanx (măn"ĭ-fā'lănks) [L. *manus,* hand, + Gr. *phalanx,* closely knit row]. A phalanx, or finger, of the hand. SEE: *pediphalanx.*

manipulation [L. *manipulare,* to handle]. 1. Conscious or unconscious process by which one person attempts to influence another person in order to get his or her own needs or desires met. 2. A joint mobilization technique, usually involving a rapid thrust or stretching a joint with the patient under anesthesia. SEE: *joint manipulation.* 3. A method of realigning a fractured long bone with manual pressure, traction or angulation.

manipulative surgery. Use of manipulation in surgery or bone-setting.

manna (măn'ă) [L.]. 1. The sweet juice obtained from the flowering ash, *Fraxinus ornus.* 2. General term applied to sweetish juices obtained from a variety of plants.

mannans (măn'ănz). Polysaccharides of mannose.

mannerism. A peculiar modification or exaggeration of style or habit of dress, speech, or action.

mannitol (măn'ĭ-tŏl). USP. A carbohydrate that may be obtained from plant sources. It is used as an osmotic diuretic and to reduce cerebrospinal fluid pressure, and in prophylaxis of acute renal failure. Trade names are Osmitrol and Resectisol.

Mannkopf's sign [Emil W. Mannkopf, Ger. physician, 1836–1918]. Pulse acceleration exhibited on pressing a painful point. Not present in feigned pain.

mannose (măn'ōs). A polysaccharide present in certain plants. It is an aldohexose.

mannoside (măn'ō-sīd). A glycoside of mannose.

mannosidosis (măn"ōs-ĭ-dō'sĭs). An inborn error of metabolism in which the deficiency of α-mannosidase is associated with mental deficiency, kyphosis, enlarged tongue, abnormal lymphocytes, and accumulation of mannose in tissues.

manometer (măn-ŏm'ĕt-ĕr) [Gr. *manos,* thin, + *metron,* measure]. Device for determining liquid or gaseous pressure such as blood, spinal fluid, or atmospheric. The measurement is expressed in millimeters of either mercury or water, or in torr.

m., saline. Manometer that utilizes a special hollow tube shaped like a U with both ends open. This is called a U tube and is partially filled with saline. Pressure is determined by connecting one end of the U tube to the system in which pressure is to be measured. The pressure, in millimeters of saline, is the measured distance between the fluid level in one side of the U tube and that in the other side.

Mansonella (măn"sō-nĕl'ă). A genus of filarial nematodes.

M. ozzardi. A filaria that occurs in Central and South America and the Caribbean. They are unsheathed and usually harmless, but they may cause hydrocele or lymphadenopathy.

mansonelliasis (măn"sō-nĕl-ĭ'ă-sĭs) [*Mansonella* + Gr. *-iasis,* condition]. Infection in man with *Mansonella ozzardi.*

Mansonia (măn-sō'nē-ă). A genus of mosquitoes in tropical countries; transmits microfilaria to man.

mantle [AS. *mentel,* a garment]. A covering structure or layer.

m., dentin. The narrow zone of dentin that is first formed in the crown and root of a tooth.

Mantoux test (măn-tū') [Charles Mantoux, Fr. physician, 1877–1947]. Intracutaneous injection of one-tenth ml of intermediate strength Purified Protein Derivative (PPD). Remove the needle after a brief delay in order to minimize leakage of the PPD at the puncture site. Within 24 to 72 hours the injected area becomes hard (indurated) and 10 mm is diameter if either an active or inactive tuberculous infection is present. Induration of 5 to 10 mm is doubtful and a reaction of less than 5 mm is considered to be negative. SEE: *tuberculosis.*

manual (măn'ū-ăl) [L. *manus,* hand]. 1. Pert. to the hands. 2. Performed by or with the hands.

manual muscle test. A manual technique for

estimating the relative strength of specific muscles. Rating categories and values include normal (5), good (4), fair (3), poor (2), trace (1), and zero (0). A grade of fair (3) is based on the ability of the muscle to move the bone through its full range of motion against gravity; poor (2) is through the range with gravity eliminated. Higher grades are then based on the muscles' ability to maintain an isometric contraction against resistance.

manubrium (mă-nū′brē-ŭm) [L., handle] (pl. *manubria*). Any handle-shaped structure.

   m. sterni. [NA] The upper segment of the sternum articulating with the clavicle and first pair of costal cartilages.

manudynamometer (măn″ū-dī″nă-mŏm′ĕ-tĕr) [L. *manus*, hand,   +   Gr. *dynamis*, force,   +   *metron*, measure]. A device for measuring the force of a thrust.

manus (mā′nŭs) [L.] (pl. *manus*). [NA] The hand.

MAO. *monoamine oxidase.*

map. A graphic presentation in two dimensions of the location of items.

   m., genetic. SEE: *gene map.*

   m., linkage. Map of chromosomes indicating the relationship of genes to each other on the chromosome.

maple bark disease. A pneumonitis caused by inhalation of spores from the mold *Cryptostroma corticale,* which is present in the bark of maple trees.

maple syrup urine disease. An inherited metabolic disease involving defective amino acid metabolism; so named because of the characteristic odor of the urine and sweat. The amino acids involved are leucine, isoleucine, valine, and alloisoleucine. Clinically, in the first few months of life, there is rapid deterioration of the nervous system and then death at an early age.

   TREAT: Controlling the intake of these amino acids; exchange transfusion; and peritoneal dialysis.

mapping. Location of the genes on a chromosome.

marantic (mă-răn′tĭk) [Gr. *marantikos,* wasting away]. 1. Pert. to marasmus. 2. Wasting away. SYN: *marasmic.*

marantology (mă″răn-tŏl′ō-jē) [Gr. *marasmos,* a dying away,   +   *logos,* word, reason]. Study, care, and treatment of debilitated, elderly, and chronically ill patients whose outlook for recovery is poor.

marasmic (mă-răz′mĭk) [Gr. *marasmos,* a dying away]. Affected with marasmus; wasting away. SYN: *marantic.*

marasmoid (mă-răz′moyd) [″   +   *eidos,* form, shape]. Similar to marasmus.

marasmus (măr-ăz′mŭs). Emaciation and wasting in an infant due to malnutrition.

Caused by caloric deficiency secondary to acute diseases, esp. diarrheal diseases of infancy. May also be due to deficiency in nutritional composition, inadequate food intake, malabsorption, child abuse, failure to thrive syndrome, deficiency of vitamin D, or scurvy. Most common in children over two years.

SYM: Extreme wasting. Failure to gain weight is followed by a loss of weight. Brain and skeletal growth continues, resulting in a long body and a large head in proportion to weight. Subcutaneous fat is minimal, the eyes are sunken, and tissue turgor is lost. The skin appears loose and sags. The infant is not active, muscles are flabby and relaxed, and the cry is weak and shrill.

TREAT: Initial feedings should be small and low in calories because digestive capacity is poor. Diluted formula or breast milk is best. The amount of calories and protein, carbohydrates, and fat should be increased gradually. The goal for protein intake is 5 gm/kg of body weight per day. If diarrhea due to disaccharidase deficiency is present, a low-lactose diet will be of benefit. Parenteral fluid therapy is indicated if shock or fluid and electrolyte imbalance exists.

PROG: Death will occur in 40% of the children. SYN: *wasting.*

marble bones. Abnormally calcified bones with spotted appearance on roentgenogram. SEE: *Albers-Schönberg disease; osteopetrosis.*

Marburg virus disease [Marburg, Germany]. Clinically this disease, caused by a virus classed as a member of the family *Filoviridae,* is identical to that caused by the Ebola virus. SEE: *Ebola virus disease.*

marc (märk) [Fr.]. The remaining substance after a drug has been percolated.

Marchiafava-Micheli syndrome (măr″kēă-fă′vă-mē-kā′lē) [Ettore Marchiafava, It. pathologist, 1847–1935; F. Micheli, It. clinician, 1872–1937]. A rare hemolytic anemia associated with paroxysmal nocturnal hemoglobinuria.

marcid (măr′sĭd) [L. *marcere,* to waste away]. 1. Wasted or emaciated. 2. Exhausted.

Marcus Gunn pupil [Robert Marcus Gunn, Brit. ophthalmologist, 1850–1909]. A pupil of the eye that responds by constricting more to an indirect than a direct light.

Marcus Gunn syndrome [Robert Marcus Gunn]. A congenital condition in which a ptotic eyelid retracts briefly when the mouth is opened or the jaw moved to one side. The person appears to wink each time the jaw is opened. SEE: *jaw winking.*

Marezine Hydrochloride. Trade name for cyclizine hydrochloride, USP.

Marfan's syndrome [Bernard-Jean Antonin

Marfan, Fr. physician, 1858–1942]. A hereditary condition of connective tissue, bones, muscles, ligaments, and skeletal structures.

SYM: Irregular and unsteady gait, a tall lean body type with long extremities including fingers and toes. There are abnormal joint flexibility, flat feet, stooped shoulders, and dislocation of the optic lens. The aorta will usually be dilated and may become sufficiently weakened to allow an aneurysm to develop. SEE: *arachnodactyly.*

margarine. Artificial butter substitute made from refined vegetable oils or a combination of vegetable oils and fats. Coloring material and vitamins A and D are added. Contains 7.2 Cal per gram. SYN: *oleomargarine.*

margin [L. *marginalis,* border]. 1. A boundary, such as the edge of a structure of the anatomy. SYN: *margo.* 2. In dentistry, the apical extent or boundary of enamel adjacent to cementum of the tooth root; the junction of a restoration with the cavosurface angle of a prepared cavity in enamel.

marginal (măr′jĭn-ăl). Concerning a margin or border. SYN: *limbic.*

margination (măr″jĭ-nā′shŭn). Adhesion of leukocytes to walls of blood vessel in first stages of inflammation.

marginoplasty (mar-jĭn′ō-plăs″tē) [L. *marginalis,* border, + Gr. *plassein,* to mold]. Plastic surgery of a border, as of an eyelid.

margo (măr′gō) [L.] (pl. *margines*). [NA] A border or edge.

m. acutus. A sharp margin of the heart extending from the apex to the right.

m. obtusus. Portion of a line extending from apex to root of the pulmonary artery that lies along the rounded left side of the left ventricle.

Marie′s ataxia (mă-rēz′) [Pierre Marie, Fr. neurologist, 1853–1940]. Hereditary cerebellar ataxia caused by bilateral cortical atrophy of the cerebellum.

Marie′s disease. Chronic condition with enlargement of bones and soft tissues of hands, feet, and face. SYN: *acromegaly,* q.v.

Marie′s sign. Hand tremor seen in exophthalmic goiter.

marijuana, marihuana (măr″ĭ-wă′nă). The dried flowering tops of the *Cannabis sativa* (hemp) plant.

There is controversy over the effects of marijuana. This substance has dose-related effects on mood, perception, and psychomotor coordination. Driving and other machine-operating skills may therefore be seriously affected. Users have impairment of short-term memory and its use slows learning. Depending on the dose of the drug and the underlying psychological conditions of the user, marijuana may cause transient episodes of confusion, anxiety, or even frank toxic delirium. Use may exacerbate pre-existing mental illness, esp. schizophrenia. Long-term, relatively heavy use may be associated with behavioral disorders and a kind of ennui called the amotivational syndrome, but it is not known whether use of the drug is a cause or a result of this condition. Transient symptoms occur on withdrawal, indicating that the drug can lead to physical dependence. Research has demonstrated a significant correlation between heavy marijuana use by pregnant women and impaired fetal growth and development.

Because marijuana smoke contains many of the components of tobacco smoke, prolonged heavy smoking of marijuana leads to impaired pulmonary function. The possibility that chronic marijuana use is associated with an increased risk of developing lung cancer exists, but it has not been proved because most people who smoke marijuana also smoke cigarettes.

Marijuana, its constituents or its derivatives may be useful in the acute treatment of glaucoma and in the control of the severe nausea and vomiting caused by cancer chemotherapy.

One of the most important constituents of marijuana is delta-9-tetrahydrocannabinol (THC). Synthetic THC, dronabinol, is approved for use as an antiemetic in treating cancer. Trade names of synthetic THC are Deltanyne and Marinol. SYN: *cannabis.* SEE: *hashish.*

Marinol. Trade name of synthetic delta-9-tetrahydrocannabinol. SEE: *marijuana.*

mark [AS. *mearc*]. Any nevus, bruise, cut, or spot on the surface of a body.

m., birth-. Blemish on the skin at birth. SYN: *nevus.*

m., port-wine. A congenital hemangioma or nevus vascularis.

m., strawberry. Nevus vascularis.

marker. 1. A device or substance used to indicate or mark something. 2. An identifying characteristic or trait that allows apparently similar materials or disease conditions to be differentiated.

m., fecal. A substance, such as carmine, ingested to mark the beginning and end of fecal collection periods.

Marlex mesh. A monofilament, biologically inert mesh used in surgical procedures to help cover or strengthen areas as in hernia repair.

Marplan. Trade name for isocarboxazid.

marrow [AS. *mearh*]. The soft tissue occupying the medullary cavities of long bones, some haversian canals, and spaces between trabeculae of cancellous or spongy bone.

Marrow is of two types: red and yellow. The yellow marrow is found esp. in medullary cavity of long bones, and the red in spongy bones.

m., gelatinous. Yellow marrow of old or emaciated persons, almost devoid of fat and having a gelatinous consistency.

m., red. Marrow found in cancellous tissue of bone. Concerned with the production of blood cells and hemoglobin, i.e., hematopoiesis.

m., spinal. The spinal cord.

m., yellow. Marrow found in the medullary canal of long bones. Consists principally of fat cells and connective tissue. It does not participate in hematopoiesis.

marrow aspiration. Procedure using a special aspirating needle to obtain a specimen of bone marrow for examination. The material is usually obtained from the upper portion of the sternum or the iliac crest. Examination of the stained marrow is helpful in diagnosing a great number of blood disorders, infections, and malignant diseases.

marrow transplantation. SEE: *bone marrow transplant.*

marsh fever. Malaria.

marsh gas. Methane.

Marsh's test [James Marsh, Brit. chemist, 1789–1846]. A test to detect the presence of arsenic.

marsupialization (măr-sū″pē-ăl-ĭ-zā′shŭn) [L. *marsupium*, pouch]. Process of raising the borders of an evacuated tumor sac to the edges of the abdominal wound and stitching them there to form a pouch. The interior of the sac suppurates and gradually closes by granulation.

marsupium (măr-sū′pē-ŭm) [L., pouch]. 1. Scrotum. 2. A sac or pouch that serves to hold the young of a marsupial.

MAS. *milliamperage seconds.*

masculation (măs-kū-lā′shŭn) [L. *masculus*, a male]. Development of male secondary sexual characteristics.

masculine (măs′kū-lĭn). 1. Pert. to the male sex. 2. Having male characteristics. SYN: *virile.*

masculinization. 1. The normal development of secondary male sex characteristics that occur at puberty. 2. The abnormal development of masculine characteristics in the female. This may be caused by certain testosterone-producing tumors, medication that contains testosterone, or anabolic steroids. SYN: *virilization.*

masculinovoblastoma (măs″kū-lĭn-ō″vō-blăs-tō′mă). A benign ovarian tumor that microscopically resembles adrenocortical tissue. Usually results in masculinization.

maser. Acronym for *m*icrowave *a*mplification by *s*timulation *e*mission of *r*adiation. A device that produces a small, nondiverging radiation beam. SEE: *laser.*

mask [Fr. *masque*]. 1. A covering for the face, as the mask of a surgeon, dentist, or nurse. SEE: *Universal Precautions in Appendix.* 2. The countenance or appearance of the face such as occurs in certain pathological conditions. 3. To conceal or prevent detection.

m., BLB. Mask for administering oxygen to aviators or to patients during anesthesia. Invented by Boothby, Lovelace, and Bulbulian, working at the Mayo Clinic.

m., death. A plaster cast of the face molded soon after death.

m., ecchymotic. Cyanotic facies accompanying traumatic asphyxia.

m., Hutchinson's. A feeling of compression over face as though one is wearing a mask.

m., luetic. Blotchy brown pigmentation of cheeks, forehead, and temples, seen in tertiary syphilis.

m. of pregnancy. Pigmented areas seen on the face of some pregnant women. SYN: *chloasma gravidarum.*

m., Parkinson's. Immobile facial appearance as a result of paralysis agitans (Parkinson's disease). The face is devoid of expression.

masked. Concealed, esp. as in masked infection.

Ex.: women exposed to rubella during the first trimester of pregnancy may be given immune globulin. This may prevent clinical symptoms of rubella in the mother, yet the fetus may be adversely affected and born with congenital defects.

masochism (măs′ō-kĭzm) [Leopold von Sacher-Masoch, Austrian novelist, 1835–1895]. A general orientation to life that suffering relieves guilt and leads to a reward. Opposite of sadism. SEE: *algolagnia; flagellation.*

m., sexual. Sexual excitement produced in an individual by his or her own suffering. The individual with this condition usually prefers to be bound, beaten, or made to suffer or be humiliated.

masochist (măs′ō-kĭst). A person addicted to masochism.

mass [L. *massa*]. 1. A quantity of material, such as cells that unite or adhere to each other. 2. Soft solid preparation for internal use and of such consistency that it may be molded into pills. It is frequently prescribed alone or with other agents and may be given in pill form or put into capsules. 3. A fundamental scalar property of an object that describes the amount of acceleration an object will have when a given force is applied to it. The metric unit of mass is the kilogram. One kilogram equals 2.205 pounds. SEE: *weight.*

m., cell. An aggregation of cells that serves as the primordium (anlage) of a future organ or part.

m., epithelial. Inner portion of a developing gonad enclosed within the germinal epithelium.

m., inner cell. Mass of cells within the blastocyst, q.v., from which the embryo, yolk sac, and amnion develop.

m., intermediate cell. A plate of nonsegmented mesoderm lying lateral to the segments (somites) and connecting them to the nonsegmented lateral mesoderm. SYN: nephrotome.

massa [L.] (pl. *massae*). [NA] Mass.

m. intermedia. The middle commissure of the brain, an inconstant mass of gray matter extending across the third ventricle and connecting adjacent surfaces of the thalami.

massage [Gr. *massein*, to knead]. Manipulation, methodical pressure, friction, and kneading of the body.

RS: anatripsis; effleurage; flagellation; friction; frolement; fustigation; kneading; malaxation; masseur; petrissage; Swedish gymnastics; tapotement; vibration.

m., auditory. Massage of the eardrum.

m., cardiac. Manual compression of the heart to restore heartbeat after heart has stopped. Accomplished either through an incision in the chest wall or over the sternum. This forces blood out of the heart and, when pressure is removed, allows the heart to fill as if it were beating.

m., electrovibratory. Massage by means of an electric vibrator.

m., general. Centripetal stroking in connection with some muscular kneading from the toes upward. Principally used for nervousness, being an important part of the well-known rest cure. Useful in connection with certain baths, duration 30 to 40 minutes. As soon as a part is massaged, it should be given a few passive rotary movements and afterwards covered up.

m., introductory. Massage consisting of centripetal strokings around the affected part.

Ex.: an affection of the knee joint, where introductory massage should be used on lower part of thigh and somewhat below the knee. Very useful in cases in which it is impossible for operator to apply treatment directly to diseased parts.

m., local. Massage confined to particular parts.

m., tremolo. A type of mechanical massage.

m., vapor. Treatment of a cavity by a medicated and nebulized vapor under interrupted pressure.

m., vibratory. Massage by rapidly repeated tapping of the affected surface by means of a vibrating hammer or sound.

masseter (măs-sē′tĕr) [Gr. *maseter*, chewer]. The muscle that closes the mouth and is the principal muscle in mastication.

masseur (mă-soor′) [Fr.]. 1. A man who gives massages. 2. An instrument for massaging.

masseuse (mă-sooz′) [Fr.]. A woman who gives massages.

massive (măs′siv) [Fr. *massif*]. Bulky; consisting of a large mass; huge.

massive collapse of the lung. Dyspnea, cyanosis, shock, and pain in chest, esp. in patients who have suffered severe shock and collapse after abdominal operation or thyroidectomy. Collapse is due to obstruction of a main bronchus by a mucous plug, foreign body, or a tension pneumothorax. SEE: lung.

TREAT: If caused by mucus: CO_2 inhalation and breathing exercises, antibiotics, and oxygen. If due to foreign body: remove the foreign body.

mass number. Total number of neutrons and protons in the nucleus of an atom.

massotherapy (măs-ō-thĕr′ă-pē) [Gr. *massein*, to knead, + *therapeia*, treatment]. Use of massage in treatment of disease.

mass psychogenic illness. The occurrence of psychogenic illnesses in a related group of people over a short period of time. Historical sources described tarantism, the dancing mania reported in Italy in the 15th to 17th centuries; dancing mania in Germany and the Netherlands. The condition is poorly understood but somatic complaints, e.g., headache, dizziness, nausea, dry mucous membranes, sleepiness, weakness, numbness, and chest tightness, are frequently reported. SYN: *mass hysteria; mass panic; mental epidemic; group pathology.* SEE: *hysteria, epidemic; mass sociogenic illness.*

mass sociogenic illness. ABBR: MSI. A self-limiting illness characterized by onset of a group of symptoms in persons in a social setting such as a school, work place, church, or military group. The onset is usually rapid and may include dizziness, weakness, headache, abdominal pain, rash, itching, blurred vision, nausea and vomiting, and fainting. There are no laboratory studies to confirm an etiologic agent. Resolution of the mass illness occurs when those affected are reassured that it is not due to a toxic substance. SEE: *mass psychogenic illness.*

MAST. *military antishock trousers.* SEE: *anti-G suit.*

mastadenitis (măst-ăd-ĕ-nī′tĭs) [Gr. *mastos*, breast, + *aden*, gland, + *itis*, inflammation]. A mammary gland inflammation.

mastadenoma (măst″ă-dĕ-nō′mă) [″ + ″

+ *oma*, tumor]. A tumor of the breast.

mastalgia (măst-ăl′jē-ă) [″ + *algos*, pain]. Pain in the breast. SYN: *mammalgia; mastodynia.*

mastatrophia, mastatrophy (măst-ă-trō′fē-ă, măst-ăt′rō-fē) [″ + *atrophia*, want of nourishment]. Atrophy of breasts.

mastauxe (măs-tawk′sē) [″ + *auxe*, increase]. Enlargement of the breast.

mast cells [Gr. *masten*, to feed]. Cells resident in connective tissue just below epithelial surfaces, serous cavities, and around blood vessels, including those in bone marrow. They synthesize and store histamine. When stimulated they release mediators of inflammation, including leukotrienes. They are also important in producing the signs and symptoms of immediate hypersensitivity reactions, e.g., drug anaphylaxis, urticaria, insect stings, allergic reactions, and certain forms of asthma.

mastectomy (măs-těk′tō-mē) [Gr. *mastos*, breast, + *ektome*, excision]. Excision of the breast.

NURSING IMPLICATIONS: Provide emotional support for the woman undergoing diagnostic studies, and encourage discussion of treatment options. Postoperatively, monitor vital signs and wound drainage quantity and character. Position patient with affected arm elevated on pillow until drain is removed, then teach and encourage active exercise of the arm to prevent shoulder joint contracture and muscle shortening. Provide pain medication as ordered; support patient and family in coping with diagnosis and grief response; assist patient with problems related to changed body image and self-concept; teach the patient protective measures for lymphedema; and offer information about breast prostheses and reconstructive surgery. SEE: *Nursing Diagnoses* in *Appendix.*

m., radical. Treatment of breast cancer in which the breast, involved skin, pectoral muscles, axillary lymph nodes, and subcutaneous fat are removed. SEE: *lumpectomy.*

m., simple. Treatment of breast cancer in which the breast, nipple, areola, and the involved overlying skin is removed. SEE: *lumpectomy.*

Master two-step test [Arthur Matthew Master, U.S. physician, 1895–1973]. A standardized exercise test used to assess cardiac function. The patient participates in a standardized exercise of repeatedly walking up and down on a step. The electrocardiogram is monitored during the study, and the exercise is stopped if abnormal changes appear. Though useful, the test has been replaced with use of a treadmill. SEE: *exercise tolerance test.*

masthelcosis (măs″thěl-kō′sĭs) [Gr. *mastos*, breast, + *helkosis*, ulceration]. Ulcerated condition of the breast.

mastic (măs′tĭk). A resin obtained from the tree *Pistacia lentiscus*. It has been used in industry and in coating tablets.

mastication (măs-tĭ-kā′shŭn) [L. *masticare*, to chew]. Chewing. The comminution and insalivation of the food in the mouth is the first stage of digestion. Certain muscles close the mouth, raise and lower the mandible, tense the cheeks, and accomplish the highly coordinated movements of the tongue. The smell and taste of food stimulate sensory nerves, which reflexively elicit both motor and secretory activity in various digestive organs. Thus the salivary glands begin to secrete at once, and both the glands and the musculature of the stomach gradually become active. The saliva dissolves some substances, dilutes materials too concentrated for the stomach, hydrolyzes (due to the salivary enzyme ptyalin) some of the starch to maltose, and lubricates material to be swallowed.

RS: absorption; amaseis; digestion; enzyme.

masticatory (măs′tĭk-ă-tō″rē) [L. *masticare*, to chew]. 1. Pert. to mastication. 2. Any substance chewed to stimulate secretion of saliva.

Mastigophora (măs″tĭ-gŏf′ō-ră). A subphylum of protozoa characterized by the possession of one or more flagella. Includes both free-living and parasitic forms.

mastigote (măs′tĭ-gōt). A member of the protozoan class Mastigophora.

mastitis (măs-tī′tĭs) [Gr. *mastos*, breast, + *itis*, inflammation]. Inflammation of the breast. Most common in women during lactation but it may occur at any age. SEE: *Nursing Diagnoses* in *Appendix.*

SYM: The earliest sign is a triangular flush generally underneath the breast. There may be a high temperature and pulse rate.

ETIOL: May be due to entry of disease-producing germs through the nipple. In most cases there is a crack or abrasion of the nipple. Infection begins in one lobule but may extend to other areas.

m., cystic. Mastitis resulting in formation of cysts that give the breast a nodular feeling upon palpation.

m., interstitial. Inflammation of connective tissue of the breast.

m., parenchymatous. Inflammation of the secreting tissue of the breast.

m., puerperal. Mastitis in later portion of puerperium and often accompanied by suppuration. Breast may become indurated due to retention of milk.

m., stagnation. Painful distention of breast occurring during early lactation. SYN: *caked breast.*

mastocarcinoma (măst″ō-kär-sĭn-ō′mă) [″ + *karkinos*, crab, + *oma*, tumor]. Carcinoma of the breast.

mastochondroma (măst″ō-kŏn-drō′mă) [″ + *chondros*, cartilage, + *oma*, tumor]. Cartilaginous breast tumor.

mastocyte (măs′tō-sīt) [Gr. *masten*, to feed, + *kytos*, cell]. Mast cell.

mastocytoma (măs″tō-sī-tō′mă) [″ + ″ + *oma*, tumor]. An accumulation of mast cells that resembles a neoplasm.

mastocytosis (măs″tō-sī-tō′sĭs) [″ + ″ + *osis*, condition]. A general term for a variety of rare disorders in which there is proliferation of mast cells in the skin and systemically. Lesions present on the skin are termed urticaria pigmentosa. Firm stroking of the skin lesion will cause the area to become raised and pruritic with surrounding erythema; this is Darier's sign.

Systemic mastocytosis in addition to the skin manifestations is marked by infiltration of mast cells into the bone marrow, abdominal organs, and lymph nodes. Many of the signs and symptoms of this illness are due to the mast cells releasing their granules that contain histamine, prostaglandins, and leukotrienes. Their release may be triggered by ingestion of alcohol, aspirin, morphine, codeine, nonsteroidal anti-inflammatory agents, certain foods, and exposure to cold.

mastodynia (măst-ō-dĭn′ē-ă) [Gr. *mastos*, breast, + *odyne*, pain]. Pain in the breast. SYN: *mammalgia; mastalgia.*

mastography [″ + *graphein*, to write]. Roentgenography of the breasts.

mastoid (măs′toyd) [″ + *eidos*, form, shape]. 1. Formed like a breast. 2. Pert. to mastoid process of the temporal bone. 3. The mastoid process of temporal bone.

mastoidal (măs-toy′dăl). Rel. to mastoid process.

mastoidale (măs-toy-dā′lē). The lowest point of the mastoid process.

mastoidalgia (măs-toyd-ăl′jē-ă) [Gr. *mastos*, breast, + *eidos*, form, shape, + *algos*, pain]. Pain in the mastoid.

mastoid antrum. Small chamber through which the mastoid cells communicate with the tympanic cavity.

mastoid cells. Air spaces in the mastoid process of the temporal bone.

mastoidectomy [″ + ″ + *ektome*, excision]. Excision of mastoid cells. Rarely indicated since advent of antibiotics. May be simple, involving exenteration of the air cells of the mastoid process alone, or radical involving the middle ear.

NURSING IMPLICATIONS: Inspect dressing at frequent intervals, reinforcing as necessary. Utilize aseptic technique during dressing changes. Observe for bright red drainage, neck stiffness, vomiting, dizziness, disorientation, headache, and facial paralysis. If any of above symptoms occur, notify physician immediately. Deafness will be present in the affected ear if the ossicles were removed during surgery. SEE: *Nursing Diagnoses* in *Appendix.*

mastoideocentesis (măs-toyd″ē-ō-sĕn-tē′sĭs) [″ + ″ + *kentesis*, puncture]. Surgical puncture of the mastoid process and subsequent paracentesis of mastoid cells.

mastoiditis (măs-toyd-ī′tĭs) [″ + ″ + *itis*, inflammation]. Inflammation of the air cells of the mastoid process.

SYM: Fever, chills, tenderness over emissary vein, leukocytosis, sepsis.

TREAT: Surgical. Myringotomy and antibiotics, mastoidectomy.

COMPLICATIONS: Perisinuous abscess, periphlebitis, lateral sinus thrombosis. Involvement is metastatic through blood vessels without erosion of sinus plate or extension of suppuration directly through sinus plate into the sinus.

m., Bezold's. Abscess underneath insertion of sternocleidomastoid muscle due to pus breaking through the mastoid tip.

m. externa. Inflammation of the periosteum of the mastoid process.

m., sclerosing. Mastoiditis in which there is thickening and hardening of trabeculae between mastoid cells.

mastoidotomy (măs-toyd-ŏt′ō-mē) [″ + *tome*, incision]. Incision into the mastoid process.

mastoid portion of temporal bone. Portion of the temporal bone lying behind the external opening of the ear and below the temporal line. Contains mastoid cells and antrum, and its inner surface bears a deep, curved, sigmoid groove that contains a part of the transverse sinus. The opening of the mastoid foramen is visible in it.

mastoid process. Nipple-shaped process of mastoid portion of temporal bone extending downward and forward behind the external auditory meatus. Serves for attachment of sternocleidomastoid, splenius capitis, and longissimus capitis muscles.

mastology (măs-tŏl′ō-jē) [″ + *logos*, word, reason]. The branch of medicine concerned with study of the breast.

mastomenia (măs-tō-mē′nē-ă) [″ + *menes*, menses]. Vicarious menstruation from the breast.

mastoncus (măst-ŏng′kŭs) [″ + *onkos*, bulk]. Any tumor of the breast.

masto-occipital (măs″tō-ŏk-sĭp′ĭ-tăl). Rel.

to the mastoid process and occipital bone.

mastoparietal (măs″tō-pă-rī′ĕ-tăl). Concerning the mastoid process and the parietal bone.

mastopathy (măs-tŏp′ă-thē) [Gr. *mastos*, breast, + *pathos*, disease]. Any disease of the mammary glands.

mastopexy (măs′tō-pěks-ē) [″ + *pexis*, fixation]. Correction of a pendulous breast by surgical fixation and plastic surgery. SYN: *mazopexy*.

mastoplasia (măst-ō-plā′zē-ă) [″ + *plassein*, to form]. Hyperplasia of mammary gland tissue. SYN: *mazoplasia*.

mastoplasty (măs′tō-plăs″tē) [″ + *plassein*, to form]. Plastic surgery of the breast.

mastoptosis (măs″tō-tō′sĭs) [″ + *ptosis*, a dropping]. Pendulous breasts.

mastorrhagia (măs-tor-ā′jē-ă) [″ + *rhegnynai*, to burst forth]. Hemorrhage from the breast.

mastoscirrhus (măs-tō-skĭr′ŭs) [″ + *skirros*, hardness]. A hardening of the breast.

mastosquamous (măs-tō-skwā′mŭs). Relating to the mastoid process and the squamous portion of the temporal bone.

mastostomy (măs-tŏs′tō-mē) [″ + *stoma*, mouth]. Incision into the breast in order to drain a cyst or obtain tissue for microscopic study.

mastotomy (măs-tŏt′ō-mē). Surgical incision of a breast. SYN: *mammotomy*.

masturbate (măs′těr-bāt) [L. *masturbari*, fr. *manus*, hand, + *stuprare*, to defile]. 1. To induce sexual self-excitement through manipulation of the genital organs or other erogenous areas. 2. To perform masturbation on another.

masturbation (măs″těr-bā′shŭn). Stimulation of genitals or other erogenous areas, usually to orgasm, by some means other than sexual intercourse.

At one time practicing masturbation was believed to cause a great variety of mental and physical disorders. There is no scientific basis for such beliefs. It has also been reported that masturbation is practiced by an increasing number of persons of all ages and of both sexes. This interest probably reflects a fear of contracting AIDS from casual sexual contact. SEE: *AIDS; safe sex.*

match [ME. *macche*, lamp wick]. A narrow strip of wood tipped with a compound that ignites by friction. Lucifer matches usually are made of phosphorus, q.v., and potassium chlorate. Safety matches contain antimony, sulfide, and potassium chlorate and must be lit by striking a rough surface.

matching. 1. Comparison in order to select objects with similar characteristics. 2. Being identical, equal, or exactly alike.

m., cross. Technique of determining the compatibility of the patient's blood with that of blood being considered for use in transfusion. SEE: *blood groups.*

m. of blood. Technique and procedure for determining the immunologic and genetic characteristics of the patient's blood so that appropriate blood may be used for transfusion. SEE: *blood groups.*

match poisoning. SYM: Gastrointestinal irritation with blood changes.

F.A.: Wash out stomach with water or very dilute potassium permanganate. Repeated catharsis. SEE: *phosphorus poisoning.*

maté (mă-tā′) [Sp., vessel for preparing leaves]. Tea made from the leaves of *Ilex paraguayensis*. Contains caffeine and tannin.

USES: Diaphoretic and diuretic when taken in large quantities.

mater (mā′tŭr) [L. mother]. The tissue coverings of the brain and spinal cord. SYN: *meninges*.

m., dura. SEE: *dura mater.*

m., pia. SEE: *pia mater.*

materia alba (mă-tē′rē-ă ăl′bă) [L., white matter]. White cheeselike deposit along gum line about the necks of teeth, consisting of mucus, epithelial cells, food particles, leukocytes, and microorganisms.

material. The substance from which something may be made, constructed, or created.

m., base. The basic ingredient in a denture. It may be a polymer, shellac, or metal.

m., impression. Any material used to make an impression of teeth.

material safety data sheet. ABBR: MSDS. A descriptive sheet that accompanies a chemical or a chemical mixture. The sheet provides: identity of the material; physical hazard, such as flammability; acute and chronic health hazards associated with contact with or exposure to the compound. It is estimated that there are almost 600,000 hazardous chemical products in American workplaces. SEE: *right to know law.*

materia medica (mă-tē′rē-ă mĕd′ĭ-kă) [L., medical matter]. 1. That branch of science dealing with all drugs used in treatment of diseases, their source, preparation, dosage, and use. SYN: *pharmacology*. 2. A substance used to prepare a medicine.

maternal [L. *maternus*]. 1. Rel. to the mother. 2. From a mother.

maternal deprivation syndrome. As a result of the premature loss or absence of the mother, emotional, physical, and nutritional neglect of an infant or young child. Children suffering from this are emotionally disturbed, withdrawn, apathetic, and retarded in growth and development. The lack of expected growth and development is due to a combination of nutritional and emotional neglect.

maternal mortality rate. SEE: *rate, maternal mortality.*

maternity (mă-tĕr′nĭ-tē). 1. The condition of motherhood. 2. The obstetrical department of a hospital.

mating [ME. *mate,* companion]. Pairing of male and female, esp. for reproduction.

   m., assortative. Pairing of male and female that is not random.

   m., random. Pairing of male to female when each individual has the same chance of mating with those of other genetic makeup.

matricide [L. *mater,* mother, + *caedere,* to kill]. Killing one's mother.

matrilineal (mă″trĭ-lĭn′ē-ăl) [L. *mater,* mother, + *linea,* line]. Concerning descent through the female line.

matrix (mā′trĭks) [L.] (pl. *matrices*). 1. The womb. 2. The basic substance from which a thing is made or develops. 3. The intercellular material of a tissue. 4. Mold for casting amalgams in dental restoration. 5. The arrangement of pixels (picture elements) that make up the computerized image.

   m. unguis. [NA] Nailbed.

matrixitis (mā-trĭks-ī′tĭs). Inflammation of the nailbed. SYN: *onychia.* SEE: *paronychia.*

matter. 1. Anything that occupies space. May be gaseous, liquid, or solid. 2. Pus.

   m., gray. The gray substance of the spinal cord and brain, consisting principally of nerve-cell bodies, dendrites, and portions of axons. Also found in peripheral ganglia and retina of eye. SYN: *substantia grisea.*

   m., white. The white substance of spinal cord and brain, consisting principally of nerve fibers (myelinated and unmyelinated). SYN: *substantia alba.*

Matulane. Trade name for procarbazine hydrochloride, USP.

maturate (măt′ū-rāt) [L. *maturus,* ripe]. 1. To ripen; to mature. 2. To suppurate.

maturation (măt″ū-rā′shŭn). 1. Maturing; ripening, as a graafian follicle. 2. Suppuration. 3. The process in the development of germ cells (spermatozoa and ova) occurring in spermatogenesis or oogenesis in which the number of chromosomes is reduced from the diploid number to the haploid number (one half of diploid). Includes two cell divisions. SEE: *oogenesis; spermatogenesis.* 4. The completion of the mineralization pattern or crystalline structure of calcified tissues.

   m., enamel. The process of changing from approximately 30% inorganic mineral in enamel matrix to the 96% inorganic content in mature enamel; maturation is accomplished by the ameloblast cells over a long period of time, with a decrease in water and organic content, and an increase in mineral content and size or density of hydroxyapatite crystals.

mature (mă-tūr′). 1. Fully developed or ripened. 2. To become fully developed.

mature minor rule. Regulations in some states that allow the practitioner treatment of minors without parental consent if the minor is deemed to be capable of understanding the nature and consequences of the treatment and if the treatment is of benefit to the minor.

maturity. State of completed growth; fully developed; time when an individual becomes capable of reproducing.

matutinal (mă-tū′tĭ-năl) [L. *matutinalis,* morning]. Pert. to or occurring early in the day, as morning sickness.

matzoon (măt-zūn′) [Armenian]. Milk with a ferment containing lactic acid, bacilli, and other organisms. Similar to yogurt.

Maurer's dots (mow′ĕrz) [Georg Maurer, Ger. physician in Sumatra, b. 1909]. In malaria due to *Plasmodium falciparum,* coarse stippling of the red cells.

Maxidex. Trade name for dexamethasone, USP.

maxilla [L., jawbone] (pl. *maxillae*). [NA] A paired bone with several processes that form the skeletal base of most of the upper face, roof of the mouth, sides of the nasal cavity, and floor of the orbit. The alveolar process of the maxilla supports the teeth, which is the basis for calling the maxilla the upper jaw. SEE: *skeleton.*

maxillary (măk′sĭ-lĕr″ē). Pert. to the upper jaw.

maxillary sinus. The antrum of Highmore, air cavity in maxilla opening into middle meatus of nose.

maxillitis (măks″ĭl-ī′tĭs) [L. *maxilla,* jawbone, + Gr. *itis,* inflammation]. Inflammation of the maxilla.

maxillodental (măk-sĭl″ō-dĕn′tăl) [″ + *dens,* tooth]. Concerning the maxilla and teeth it contains.

maxillofacial (măks-ĭl″ō-fā′shăl). Pert. to the maxilla and face.

maxillofacial syndrome. A syndrome of facial defects resulting from improper ossification of the fetal cartilages of the facial area.

maxillojugal (măk-sĭl″ō-jū′găl). Concerning the maxilla and zygomatic bone.

maxillomandibular (măk-sĭl″ō-măn-dĭb′ū-lăr) [″ + *mandibula,* lower jawbone]. Concerning the maxilla and mandible.

maxillopalatine (măk-sĭl″ō-păl′ă-tĭn). Concerning the maxilla and palatine bone.

maxillotomy (măk″sĭ-lŏt′ō-mē) [″ + Gr. *tome*, incision]. Surgical incision of the maxilla.

maxima (măk′sĭ-mă) [L.]. Pl. of maximum.

maximal (măks′ĭ-măl) [L. *maximus*, greatest]. Greatest possible; highest. Opposite of minimal.

maximum (măks′ĭ-mŭm) [L.] (pl. *maxima*). 1. The greatest quantity or effect. 2. Height of a disease.

maximum allowable concentration. ABBR: MAC. The upper limit of concentration of certain atmospheric contaminants allowed in the workplace.

maximum breathing capacity. The greatest amount of air that can be breathed in a specified period of time, usually 30 seconds. It is expressed in liters of air/minute.

maximum permissible dose. ABBR: MPD. Maximum dose of radiation allowed a person occupationally exposed over a stated length of time.

Mayo-Robson's point [Arthur Mayo-Robson, Brit. surgeon, 1853–1933]. A point just above and to right of the umbilicus where pressure causes tenderness in pancreatic disease.

maze. A labyrinth of communicating paths.

mazindol. USP. An anorexic drug. Trade name is Sanorex.

mazopexy (mā″zō-pĕk″sē) [Gr. *mazos*, breast, + *pexis*, fixation]. Correction of a pendulous breast by surgical fixation and plastic surgery. SYN: *mastopexy*.

mazoplasia (mā″zō-plā′zē-ă) [″ + *plassein*, to form]. Degenerative hyperplasia of mammary gland tissue. SYN: *mastoplasia*.

M.B. *Bachelor of Medicine.*

m.b. Prescription sign meaning L. *misce bene*, mix well.

MBC. *maximum breathing capacity.*

M.B.D. *minimal brain dysfunction.*

µc. *microcurie.*

M.C. 1. *Master of Surgery.* 2. *Medical Corps.*

Mc. *megacurie.*

mc. Former abbreviation for *millicurie.*

McArdle's disease [Brian McArdle, Brit. pediatrician, b. 1911]. One of the glycogen storage diseases (type V) in which there is an abnormal accumulation of glycogen in muscle tissue due to deficiency of myophosphorylase B.
    SYM: Pain, fatiguability, and muscle stiffness after prolonged exertion.

McBurney's incision [Charles McBurney, U.S. surgeon, 1845–1913]. Abdominal incision employed in appendectomy. An incision is made parallel to path of external oblique muscle, 1 to 2 in. (2.5 to 5.1 cm) away from the anterosuperior spine of the right ilium, incision through the external oblique

to the internal oblique and transversalis, separating their fibers.

McBurney's point. Point of tenderness in acute appendicitis, situated on a line between the umbilicus and the right anterosuperior iliac spine, about 1 or 2 in. (2.5–5.1 cm) above the latter.

McBurney's sign. Tenderness and rigidity at McBurney's point, which may be indicative of appendicitis.

McCarthy's reflex [Daniel J. McCarthy, U.S. neurologist, 1874–1958]. Contraction of orbicularis palpebrarum with closure of lids resulting from percussion above the supraorbital nerve.

McCormac's reflex. Adduction of one leg resulting from percussion of the patellar tendon of the opposite leg.

mcg. *microgram.*

MCH. *mean corpuscular hemoglobin.*

mc.h. *millicurie hour.*

MCHC. *mean corpuscular hemoglobin concentration*, average hemoglobin concentration in each red blood cell, expressed as a percentage value.

µCi. *microcurie.*

mCi. *millicurie.*

McMurray's sign [Thomas P. McMurray, Brit. orthopedic surgeon, 1887–1949]. Manipulation of the tibia, with the leg flexed, produces a pronounced click if the meniscus has been injured.

M.C.P. *metacarpophalangeal joint.*

MCV. *mean corpuscular volume.* Expressed as the average volume of individual cells in cubic microns.

M.D. [L. *Medicinae*, Doctor]. *Doctor of Medicine.* Often shortened to Doctor, but this usage leads to confusion. Doctor may mean dentist, veterinarian, or other persons possessing a doctoral degree (e.g., Ph.D., Doctor of Philosophy). Thus, the word *physician* is preferred over *doctor* when doctor of medicine is intended.

Md. Chem. symb. for the element mendelevium.

MDR. *multiple drug resistance.*

meal (mēl) [AS. *mael*, measure, meal]. 1. Portion of food eaten at a particular time to satisfy the appetite. 2. The edible portion of any cereal grain that has been coarsely ground, as in corn meal.

mean. In statistics, the arithmetic mean, q.v., or average of the values. SEE: *median.*

    m., arithmetic. The result obtained by adding all of the values given and dividing by the number of items which were added. SYN: *average; mean.* SEE: *median.*

mean corpuscular hemoglobin. ABBR: MCH. A measure of hemoglobin content of red corpuscles. The formula for determining this is

$$MCH = \frac{\text{hemoglobin in grams/1000 ml of blood}}{\text{red cell count in millions/cubic micrometers}}$$

Ex.: if the hemoglobin is 13.6 gm per 100 ml and the red cell count is 3,600,000, then

$$MCH = \frac{13.6 \times 10}{3.6} = 37.8$$

This is the amount of hemoglobin in each red cell.

mean corpuscular hemoglobin concentration. ABBR: MCHC. A measure of concentration of hemoglobin in the average red cell. The formula used is

$$\frac{\text{hemoglobin, gm/100 ml} \times 100}{\text{vol. of packed red cells, ml/100 ml}}$$

Ex.: if the hemoglobin is 13.6 gm and the volume of packed red cells (hematocrit) is 39.2 ml per 100 ml, then

$$MCHC = \frac{13.6 \times 100}{39.2} = 35\%$$

mean corpuscular volume. ABBR: MCV. A measure of the volume of red corpuscles expressed in cubic micrometers. The formula for determining this is

$$\frac{\text{vol. of packed red cells/1000 ml of blood}}{\text{red cell count in millions/cubic millimeter}}$$

Ex.: if the volume of packed red cells (hematocrit) is 39.2 per 100 ml and the red cell count is 3,600,000, then

$$MCV = \frac{39.2 \times 10}{3.6} = 108.9 \text{ cubic millimeters}$$

measles (mē′zls) [Dutch *maselen*]. A highly communicable disease characterized by fever, general malaise, sneezing, nasal congestion, brassy cough, conjunctivitis, spots on the buccal mucosa (Koplik's spots), and a maculopapular eruption over the entire body caused by the rubeola virus. It is most common in school-age children with outbreaks occurring in the winter and spring. The occurrence of measles before the age of six months is relatively uncommon, because of passively acquired maternal antibodies from the immune mother.

An attack of measles almost invariably confers permanent immunity. Active immunization can be produced by administration of measles vaccine, preferably that containing the live attenuated virus, although measles vaccine containing the inactivated virus is available for individuals in whom the live attenuated type is contraindicated. Passive immunization is afforded by ad-

ministration of gamma globulin. SYN: *rubeola.*

SYM: Onset gradual; coryza, rhinitis, drowsiness, loss of appetite, gradual elevation of temperature for first two days, when fever may rise to 101° to 103°F (38.3° to 39.4°C). Koplik's spots appear on the buccal mucosa opposite the molars on the second or third day. Photophobia and cough soon develop, although some recession in the temperature may occur. About the fourth day, fever usually reaches a higher elevation than previously, at times as high as 104° to 106°F (40° to 41.1°C). With this recurrence the rash appears.

Eruption first appears on face, being seen early as small maculopapular lesions that increase rapidly in size and coalesce in places, often causing a swollen, mottled appearance. The rash extends to the body and extremities and in some areas may resemble the rash of scarlet fever.

A cough, present at this time, is due to bronchitis produced by the inflammatory condition of the mucous membranes which undoubtedly corresponds to the rash seen on the skin. Ordinarily, the rash lasts from 4 to 5 days; as it subsides, the temperature declines. Consequently, 5 days after the appearance of the rash, the temperature should be normal or approx. normal in uncomplicated cases. Early in the disease leukopenia, esp. of polymorphonuclear cells, may be present.

COMPLICATIONS: Encephalitis is a grave complication. Of those who develop encephalitis about one in eight will die, approx. half will have permanent central nervous system injury, and the remainder will recover completely. Bronchopneumonia is a serious complication of measles. Otitis media, followed by mastoiditis, brain abscess, or even meningitis, is not rare. Cervical adenitis with marked cellulitis sometimes leads to fatal consequences. Tracheitis and laryngeal stenosis, due to edema of glottis, are sometimes seen in the course of measles. Eye complications are not common in measles, although a marked conjunctivitis usually occurs.

DIFF. DIAG: Scarlet fever and German measles. If the measles patient is observed prior to the appearance of a rash, or sometimes even after a rash has developed, a definite decision may be based on the presence of Koplik's spots, q.v.

Hemorrhagic spots are also seen on the hard palate and mucous membrane many times before a rash is evident on the skin. These spots probably correspond to the typical maculopapular eruption of the disease.

INCUBATION: From 10 to 21 days.

PROG: While usually favorable in the well-nourished child, the seriousness of the possible complications of measles should not be minimized.

PREVENTION: All children who have not had measles or who have not been vaccinated previously should be immunized with live attenuated measles vaccine at 9 months of age and again at or about 15 months.

Live attenuated vaccine is contraindicated in pregnancy, leukemia, lymphomas, and other generalized neoplasms; when agents that depress resistance such as steroids and antimetabolites are being given; during severe illness; in active tuberculosis that is not being treated; in individuals with neomycin, duck, or egg sensitivity; and after blood transfusion or injection of immune serum globulin. In these latter two cases wait 12 weeks before administering vaccine.

Persons who were born after 1956 who are traveling to foreign countries should be vaccinated with live attenuated measles vaccine one to two weeks prior to departure.

Measles immune serum globulin is effective in preventing measles if it is given not later than 5 days after exposure. SYN: *rubeola.*

NURSING IMPLICATIONS: Maintain bedrest and provide quiet activities for child. If photophobia occurs, keep room dimly lit. Remove eye secretions with warm saline or water. Encourage child not to rub eyes. Promote adequate hydration. Administer antipyretics and tepid sponge baths as ordered. Use cool mist vaporizer to relieve cough and coryza. Apply antipruritic medication as ordered to prevent itching. Isolate child until fifth day of rash, teaching parents about importance of handwashing and care of contaminated articles. Assess for complications of otitis media, pneumonia, bronchiolitis, laryngotracheitis with obstructive edema, and encephalitis. SEE: *Nursing Diagnoses* in *Appendix.*

    m., black. A severe form of measles in which the eruption is dark in color due to an effusion of blood into the skin. SYN: *m., hemorrhagic.*

    m., German. Rubella.

    m., hemorrhagic. M., black.

measles and mumps virus vaccine, live. A standardized vaccine containing live measles and mumps viruses.

measles and rubella virus vaccine, live. A standardized vaccine containing live measles and rubella viruses.

measles, mumps, and rubella virus vaccine, live. A standardized vaccine containing live measles, mumps, and rubella viruses.

measles virus vaccine, live. USP. A standardized live virus vaccine for use in immunizing against measles. Trade name is Attenuvax.

measly (mē′zlē). Description of pork that is infected with the cysticerci of *Taenia solium* or *saginata.*

measure (mĕ′zhŭr) [L. *mensura*, a measuring]. 1. The dimensions, capacity, or quantity of anything that can be so evaluated. Length, area, volume, and mass are basic properties of matter and materials that can be measured. 2. To determine the extent of length, area, mass, or volume of a substance or object. SEE: *mensuration.* 3. A device used in measuring, for ex., a marked tape or a graduated beaker. SEE: *Metric System; Weights and Measures* in *Appendix.*

Measurin. Trade name for aspirin.

meat [AS. *mete*, food]. 1. The edible portion of anything. 2. The flesh of animals, including poultry, that is used for food.

Meat from animals is a source of vitamins, esp. those of the B complex (thiamine, riboflavin, niacin). Pork is especially rich in thiamine. Liver has an unusually high vitamin content, esp. of vitamin A. The glandular organs such as liver and kidney contain a considerably higher percentage of certain mineral elements and vitamins than are found in other forms of meat.

Most meats have the same nutritive value but differ greatly in flavor and tenderness. Muscle contains about 20% protein, 20% fat, and 60% water. Lean meat is rich in phosphorus, potassium, and iron; it has a good percentage of other minerals but is deficient in calcium. In all meats the acid-forming elements are decidedly in excess of those that are base-forming.

Many myths about meat have been repudiated. For instance, one kind of meat is as easily digested as another and tough meat is just as nutritious as tender meat.

meatal (mē-ā′tăl) [L. *meatus*, passage]. Pert. to a meatus or passage.

meatometer (mē-ă-tŏm′ĕt-ĕr) [″ + Gr. *metron*, measure]. Device for measuring the size of a passage or opening.

meatorrhaphy (mē″ă-tor′ăf-ē) [″ + Gr. *rhaphe*, seam, ridge]. Suture of the severed end of the urethra to the glans penis following surgical procedure to enlarge the meatus.

meatoscope (mē-ăt′ō-skōp) [″ + Gr. *skopein*, to examine]. A speculum for examining a meatus.

meatoscopy (mē-ă-tŏs′kō-pē) [″ + Gr. *skopein*, to examine]. Instrumental examination of a meatus, esp. the meatus of the urethra.

meatotome (mē-ăt'ŏ-tōm) [" + Gr. *tome*, incision]. Knife with probe or guarded point for enlarging a meatus by direct incision.

meatotomy (mē"ă-tŏt'ō-mē). Incision of urinary meatus to enlarge the opening.

meatus (mē-ā'tŭs) [L.] (pl. *meatus*). [NA] A passage or opening.

    m. acusticus externus. [NA] External auditory canal from the eardrum to the external ear.

    m. acusticus internus. [NA] Canal in the petrous portion of temporal bone, through which pass the cochlear and vestibular nerves.

    m., external auditory. The lateral, outer opening of the external auditory canal.

    m., internal auditory. The most medial opening of the internal auditory canal, located on the posterior surface of the petrous portion of the temporal bone.

    m. nasi communis. Common nasal cavity on either side of septum, into which three meatus open.

    m. nasi inferior. [NA] Space beneath inferior turbinate of the nose.

    m. nasi medius. [NA] Space beneath middle turbinate or concha of the nose.

    m. nasi superior. [NA] Space beneath superior turbinate or concha of the nose.

    m. nasopharyngeus. [NA] Posterior portion of nasal cavity, which communicates with the nasopharynx.

    m. urinarius. External opening of the urethra.

Mebaral. Trade name for mephobarbital, USP.

mebendazole (mē-bĕn'dă-zōl). A broadspectrum antihelmintic drug. It is used in treating tapeworm infections and is the drug of choice in treating *Ascaris lumbricoides*, *Trichuris trichuria*, hookworm, and *Strongyloides stercoralis*. Trade name is Vermox.

Caution: This drug should not be used during pregnancy.

---

mebutamate (mē-bū'tă-māt). A sedative-hypnotic drug that also has antihypertensive action.

mecamylamine hydrochloride (mĕk"ă-mil'ă-mĭn). USP. An antihypertensive drug of the ganglionic blocking agent type. Trade name is Inversine.

mechanical rectifier. A device that, by changing contacts at the proper moment in a cycle, changes alternating current into pulsating direct current.

mechanics [Gr. *mechane*, machine]. Science of force and matter.

mechanism. 1. Involuntary and consistent response to a stimulus. 2. A habit or response pattern to achieve a result. 3. A machine or machinelike structure.

    m., countercurrent. Mechanism used by the kidneys in making it possible to excrete excess solutes in the urine with little loss of water from the body.

    m., defense. The means utilized in coping with stress. Included are denial, rationalization, repression, sublimation, and conversion.

    m., Duncan's. Delivery of the placenta from the uterus with the rough side presenting first.

    m. of injury. The manner by which an injury occurred. The most common type of injuries are due to movement or motion: rapid forward deceleration, rapid vertical deceleration, and projectile penetration.

mechanoreceptor (mĕk"ă-nō-rē-sĕp'tor). A receptor that receives mechanical stimuli such as pressure from sound or touch.

mechanotherapy (mĕk"ăn-ō-thĕr'ă-pē) [Gr. *mechane*, machine, + *therapeia*, treatment]. Use of various types of mechanical apparatus to perform passive movements and to exercise various parts of the body.

mechlorethamine (mĕk"lor-ĕth'ă-mēn). USP. A cytotoxic drug of the nitrogen mustard type. Trade name is Mustargen.

Mecholyl test. A test of parasympathetic nervous system function. A 2% solution of methacholine (Mecholyl) is instilled in the conjunctival sac. The pupil constricts if the patient has a parasympathetic disorder, such as familial dysautonomia.

mecism (mē'sizm) [Gr. *mekos*, length]. Abnormal lengthening of the body.

Meckel, Johann Friedrich [the elder] (mĕk'ĕl). German anatomist, 1724–1774.

    M.'s ganglion. Ganglion located in the sphenomaxillary fossa giving off nerves to eyes, nose, and palate. SYN: *sphenopalatine ganglion*.

    M.'s space. Area in dura holding the gasserian ganglion.

Meckel, Johann Friedrich [the younger] (mĕk'ĕl). German anatomist, 1781–1833, grandson of J. F. Meckel, the elder.

    M.'s cartilage. A cartilaginous bar about which the mandible develops.

    M.'s diverticulum. A congenital sac or blind pouch sometimes found in lower portion of the ileum. It represents the persistent proximal end of the yolk stalk. Sometimes it is continued to the umbilicus as a cord or as a tube forming a fistulous opening at the umbilicus. Strangulation may cause intestinal obstruction. SEE: *diverticulitis; diverticulum*.

meckelectomy (mĕk-ĕl-ĕk'tō-mē). Excision of Meckel's ganglion.

meclizine hydrochloride (měk′lĭ-zēn). USP. Antiemetic esp. effective for control of nausea and vomiting of motion sickness. Trade names are Antivert and Bonine.

meclocycline sulfosalicylate. USP. An antibacterial drug used topically. Trade name is Meclan cream.

meconium (mē-kō′nē-ŭm) [Gr. *mekonion,* poppy juice]. 1. Opium; poppy juice. 2. First feces of a newborn infant, made up of salts, liquor amnii, mucus, bile and epithelial cells. Greenish black to light brown, almost odorless and of a tarry consistency. The first meconium stool should appear during the first 24 hours and persist for about 3 days.

meconium aspiration syndrome. ABBR: MAS. The aspiration of meconium, q.v., by the newborn prior to delivery. The presence of meconium in the trachea or a chest x-ray consistent with the appearance of aspirated meconium with overdistention of the chest establishes the diagnosis.

　　TREAT: At time of birth, remove pharyngeal and tracheal meconium by use of gentle suction; assisted pulmonary ventilation as needed.

meconium ileus. Ileus due to impacted meconium in the intestines. It is usually associated with newborn children with cystic fibrosis.

meconium staining or show. Fetal defecation while in utero at time of labor that occurs with fetal distress. It is composed of thick, mucus-pasty material which must be suctioned before newborn takes first breath or the material may be aspirated.

mecystasis (mē-sĭs′tă-sĭs). Process in which a muscle maintains its original degree of tension although its length is increased.

M.E.D. *minimal effective dose; minimal erythemal dosage.*

medi- [L.]. Prefix indicating middle.

media (mē′dē-ă) [L.]. 1. Pl. of medium. 2. Middle or muscular coat of an artery. SYN: *tunica media.*

mediad (mē′dē-ăd) [L. *medium,* middle, + *ad,* toward]. Toward the median line or plane of the body.

medial [L. *medialis*]. 1. Pert. to middle. 2. Nearer the medial plane.

medialis (mē″dē-ā′lĭs) [L.]. Term indicating something is close to the midline of the body.

medial tibial syndrome. Shin splints, q.v.

median (mē′dē-ăn) [L. *medianus*]. 1. Middle; central. 2. In statistics, a number obtained by arranging the given series in order of magnitude and taking the middle number; one then has an equal number of values above and below that number. Thus, in the series 5, 7, 8, 9, 10, the median is 8. SYN: *mesial.* SEE: *mean.*

median line. An imaginary line extending longitudinally on the anterior or posterior surface of the body marking the edges of the median plane.

median nerve. A combined motor and sensory nerve having its origin in the brachial plexus.

median plane. A vertical plane through the trunk and head dividing the body into right and left halves. SYN: *midsagittal plane.* SEE: *plane* for illus.

mediastinal (mē″dē-ăs-tī′năl) [L. *mediastinalis*]. Rel. to the mediastinum.

mediastinitis (mē″dē-ăs″tī-nī′tĭs) [″ + Gr. *itis,* inflammation]. Inflammation of tissue of the mediastinum.

mediastinography (mē″dē-ăs″tī-nŏg′ră-fē) [″ + Gr. *graphein,* to write]. X-raying of the mediastinum.

mediastinopericarditis (mē-dē-ăs″tī-nō-pĕr″ĭ-kăr-dī′tĭs) [″ + Gr. *peri,* around, + *kardia,* heart, + *itis,* inflammation]. Inflammatory condition of the mediastinum and pericardium.

mediastinoscopy (mē″dē-ăs″tī-nŏs′kō-pē) [″ + *skopein,* to examine]. Endoscopic examination of the mediastinum.

mediastinotomy (mē″dē-ăs″tī-nŏt′ō-mē) [″ + *tome,* incision]. Surgical incision of the mediastinum.

mediastinum (mē″dē-ăs-tī′nŭm) [L., in the middle] (pl. *mediastina*). 1. A septum or cavity between two principal portions of an organ. 2. The mass of organs and tissues separating the lungs. It contains the heart and its large vessels, trachea, esophagus, thymus, lymph nodes, and connective tissue.

　　m. testis. [NA] The thickened portion of the tunica albuginea on posterior surface of the testis. SYN: *corpus highmorianum.*

mediate (mē′dē-āt). 1. Accomplished by indirect means. 2. Between two parts or sides.

mediation (mē″dē-ā′shŭn). The action of an intermediary, i.e., mediating, substance.

mediator (mē′dē-ā′tŏr). That which acts to mediate. The mediator may be a person, a nerve, a chemical substance, or a cellular substance.

medic. A member of the medical team in the U.S. Armed Forces. SYN: *medical corpsman.*

medicable (mĕd′ĭ-kă-bl) [L. *medicari,* to heal]. Possibly responsive to therapy; curable.

Medicaid. In the U.S., a government program for providing medical care for the poor. The program is jointly funded by the federal and state governments.

medical (mĕd′ĭ-kăl). 1. Pert. to medicine or the study of the art and science of caring for those who are ill. 2. Requiring therapy with

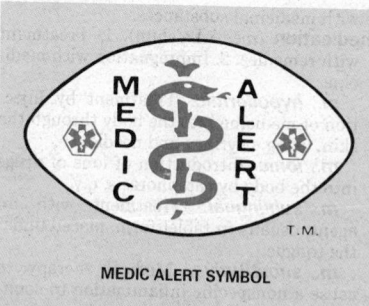

MEDIC ALERT SYMBOL

Source: Medic Alert Foundation International, P.O. Box 1009, Turlock, CA 95381, with permission.

medicines as distinct from surgical treatment.

medical access. The right or ability of an individual to obtain medical and health care services.

medical assistant. An individual who assists a qualified physician in an office or other clinical setting, performing administrative tasks (such as those of a secretary, receptionist, or bookkeeper) and technical duties (vital signs, height, weight, laboratory tests) as delegated and in accordance with state laws governing medical practice.

medical audit. A systematic approach to reviewing, analyzing, and evaluating medical care in order to identify discrepancies in the quality of care and to provide a mechanism for improving that quality. SEE: *medical outcomes study.*

medical corpsman. An enlisted man in the U.S. Armed Forces who works as a member of the medical team. SYN: *corpsman; medic.*

Medic Alert. A nonprofit organization that provides a bracelet or pendant with an emblem on which is contained information and a warning in case of emergency. The company also keeps a file of the medical information and provides an emergency phone number that medical personnel can call collect. The purpose is the prevention of a serious or fatal mistake in rendering aid or medical care to an injured or unconscious person who may have an additional condition or allergy, e.g., diabetes, penicillin allergy. Applications may be obtained from Medic Alert, P.O. Box 1009, Turlock, CA 95381. Persons wishing to donate organs may also acquire an emblem from the Medic Alert company stating that fact. SEE: illus.

medical examiner. A physician who is trained and qualified for the task of investigating the cause of death and the circumstances surrounding it. Training usually includes study of pathology and forensic medicine. The examiner is empowered by governmental agencies to represent them, and is expected to make a comprehensive report of findings to judicial or police authorities. The skill of a medical examiner is especially important in investigating deaths wherein malpractice, homicide, suicide or other criminal actions are suspected of being a contributing factor. SEE: *coroner; death investigation; forensic medicine.*

medical grand rounds. A medical education procedure, used esp. in teaching hospitals, in which all aspects of a patient's condition, management, and problems encountered are presented to faculty members and medical students. This provides an opportunity for all concerned to ask questions and provide comments on the patient's diagnosis, care, and clinical program. The patient is usually, but not always, present during the conference. This method of teaching was begun in America by Sir William Osler at Johns Hopkins Hospital, Baltimore, Maryland. SEE: *clinical pathological conference.*

medical history. That portion of a patient's life history, including ancestry and social, occupational, and medical information, that is important in diagnosing and caring for the medical or surgical condition or conditions present. This information, which is recorded in the patient's permanent record, may be obtained from all available sources if for some reason the patient isn't able or willing to provide full details. The importance of an accurate and complete medical history for proper care of the patient cannot be overestimated. SEE: *history, dental;* Nursing Assessment Tool illus.

medical informatics. The application of information technology and processing to all aspects of medical knowledge, practice, and management including medical education and research. This process is facilitated by using computer technology.

medical jurisprudence. Principles of medicine in their application to questions of law.

medical outcomes study. ABBR: MOS. Studies designed to provide valid comparisons between medical care processes and outcomes as they are affected by system of care, clinician's specialty, as well as by patients' diagnoses and the levels of severity of the illness. Thus, MOS provides a model for monitoring the results of medical care. SEE: *medical audit.*

medical preparations. SOLID SUBSTANCES: Capsule or capsula, confection, extract, lozenge, lamella, ointment, plaster, powder or pulvis, pill or pilula, paper, suppository or suppositorium, tablet or tabella.
    FLUIDS: Fluidextract, tincture infusion,

decoction, wine, oleoresin.

SUSPENSIONS: Mixture, emulsion.

SOLUTIONS: Water, mucilage, solution or liquor, elixir, syrup, spirit, glycerite, vinegar.

MISC: Liniment or linimentum, oleate or oleatum.

RS: active principle; alkaloid; antidote; dosage; drug action; drug administration; names of individual drugs; names of individual poisons; poison; poisoning; prescription writing.

medical problems of musicians. SEE: *musicians, medical problems of.*

medical record. Transcript of information obtained from a patient, guardian, or professionals and presented in tabular, outline, or written form. It may contain history, diagnoses, treatment, prognosis, etc. Utilized by the school, place of employment, personal physician, hospital, etc.

medical record, problem-oriented. A technique of clinical record keeping described by Lawrence Weed, a contemporary U.S. physician. The patient's record is organized in a logical and efficient manner, including a list of problems and flow charts determining diagnostic and therapeutic plans and indicating what has been done.

medical records librarian. An individual trained and experienced in maintaining, storing, and retrieving the medical records collected for the patients treated at a medical care facility.

medical transcriptionist. A person who makes a typed record from the data and information available from the physician's dictated material concerning the patient's medical records. An individual who has met the requirements of the American Association of Medical Transcription is certified by that body as a Certified Medical Transcriptionist.

medical waste. Infectious or physically dangerous medical or biological waste. Included are discarded blood and blood products; waste from pathology department, including body parts, tissues or fluids discarded during surgery or at autopsy; contaminated animal carcasses; animal body parts and bedding; sharps; discarded preparations made from genetically altered living organisms and their products. SEE: *sharps; Universal Precautions* in *Appendix.*

medicament [L. *medicamentum*]. A medicine or remedy.

medicamentosus (měd″ĭ-kă-měn-tō′sŭs). Concerning drugs.

Medicare. Federal medical and hospital care program, in the U.S., for the elderly.

medicate (měd′ĭ-kāt) [L. *medicatus*]. 1. To treat a disease with drugs. 2. To permeate

with medicinal substances.

medication (měd-ĭ-kā′shŭn). 1. Treatment with remedies. 2. Impregnation with medicine.

    m., hypodermic. Treatment by injection of medicine into the body through the skin, using a syringe and needle.

    m., ionic. Introduction of ions of drugs into the body by cataphoresis, q.v.

    m., sublingual. Treatment with an agent, usually in tablet form, placed under the tongue.

    m., substitutive. Medical therapy to cause a nonspecific inflammation to counteract a specific one.

medication errors. Administering the wrong medicine, administering an incorrect dose of a medicine, failing to administer a prescribed medicine, or administering the medicine either at the incorrect time or via the incorrect route. Every effort should be made to prevent errors in medication. It is essential that the nurse, physician, and pharmacist cooperate and communicate concerning medication. In addition, the following will help to avoid errors: Administer no drug without an order; identify drug and amount in each dose unit; be certain the name of the medicine ordered is spelled precisely as that on the label — if in doubt, do not administer until the question is resolved; do not use outdated medicines; if drug appears unusual due to discoloration or precipitation, do not use; administer medicine at the time specified or as close to that time as possible — if there is a delay, document it; identify patient; do not leave medication at bedside; permit patient to self-administer medicines only if permitted by physician's written order; unless authorized by physician, do not use drugs patient brought to hospital; if an alert patient questions the drug's identity or appropriateness for use, recheck the identity of the patient and the drug; if patient refuses medication, document this on chart and notify the physician responsible for the care of the patient at that time.

medication route. The way that a drug is introduced into the body. The route of administration is chosen according to the speed of absorption desired and the site of action of the medication. Some medications are formulated for a specific route only and must be given in that manner. It is important that medicines be administered as directed by the manufacturer. Various routes of administration used are as follows:

    Oral and *enteral* administration require that the medication not be destroyed by the environment of the stomach and digestive enzymes. It is too slow if rapid absorption is required, and cannot be used if the patient is vomiting. Rectal administration in the form of liquids or suppositories circumvents this problem in enteral administration.

Mucosal routes of administration other than the above include absorption through the nasal mucosa, the buccal mucosa, sublingually, or the bronchioles, the latter usually achieved through inhalation of an aerosol. Vaginal administration is also a mucosal route of medication.

Percutaneous administration is used for iontophoresis or by direct absorption through the skin.

Parenteral administration is used when a drug cannot be given by mouth. The speed of absorption varies greatly with the specific route used, which may be subcutaneous, intravenous, intramuscular, intra-arterial, intraperitoneal, intrathecal, intracardiac, or intrasternal.

medicinal (mĕ-dĭ′sĭn-ăl) [L. *medicina*, medicine]. Pert. to medicine.

medicinal enema. An enema to which some drug or medication has been added, for retention or absorption, particularly in cases in which medication cannot be administered by mouth. SEE: *enema, medicinal; medication route.*

medicine. 1. A drug or remedy. 2. The act of maintenance of health, and prevention and treatment of disease and illness. 3. Treatment of disease by medical, as distinguished from surgical, treatment.

   m., aerospace. Branch of medicine concerned with the selection of individuals for duty as pilots or crew members for flight and space missions. Includes study of the pathology and physiology of persons and animals who travel in airplanes and spacecraft in the earth's atmosphere and in outer space.

   m., alternative. SEE: *alternative medicine.*

   m., clinical. Observation and treatment at the bedside; the practice of medicine in the clinical setting as distinguished from laboratory science.

   m., community. Medical care directed toward service of the entire population of the community, with emphasis on preventive medicine.

   m., "cookbook." SEE: *"cookbook" medicine.*

   m., dental. Branch of medicine concerned with the preservation and treatment of the teeth and other orofacial tissues. It includes preventive measures such as oral hygiene, as well as restorative procedures or prostheses and surgery. The results are widespread, including better nutrition and digestion from restored and balanced occlusion, and improved mental health from the

control of oral and dental infections which often are overlooked but jeopardize the success of other medical treatments.

   m., disaster. Large-scale application of emergency medical services in a community following a natural or man-made catastrophe. The aim is to save lives and restore every survivor to maximum health as promptly as possible. Its success depends upon prompt sorting of patients according to their immediate needs and prognosis. SEE: *triage.*

   m., emergency. The medical specialty concerned with those who are acutely ill or suddenly injured and thus require immediate care.

   m., environmental. Branch of medicine concerned with the effects of the environment (temperature, population size, pollution, radiation) on man.

   m., experimental. The scientific study of disease or pathological conditions through experimentation upon laboratory animals or through clinical research.

   m., family. Area of medical specialization concerned with providing or supervising the medical care of all members of the family.

   m., folk. Use of home remedies for treatment of diseases.

   m., forensic. Application of medical knowledge to legal affairs. SYN: *m., legal.* SEE: *forensic medicine.*

   m., group. 1. Practice of medicine by a group of physicians, usually consisting of specialists in various fields who pool their services and share laboratory and roentgenography facilities. Such a group is commonly called a clinic. 2. Securing of medical services by a group of individuals who, upon paying definite sums of money, are entitled to certain medical services or hospitalization in accordance with prearranged rules and regulations.

   m., industrial. M., occupational, q.v.

   m., internal. 1. Branch of medicine that treats diseases of the internal organs by other than surgical means. 2. Treatment of diseases nonsurgical in nature. SEE: *internal medicine.*

   m., legal. M., forensic.

   m., nuclear. Branch of medicine involved with the use of radioactive substances for diagnosis, therapy, and research.

   m., occupational. ABBR: OC. The branch of medical specialization in which the object is to investigate, prevent and treat diseases peculiar to persons whose environment includes the work space(s). OC is a form of environmental medicine.

   m., patent. Medicine for which a patent has been granted. May be purchased without a physician's prescription. SEE: *patent medicine*.

  m., physical. Treatment of disease by physical agents such as heat, cold, light, electricity, manipulation, or the use of mechanical devices.

  m., preclinical. 1. Preventive medicine, q.v. 2. Term used to indicate the first two years of medical school training, during which there is little or no exposure to patients for teaching purposes.

  m., preventive. Study and practice of preventing disease.

  m., proprietary. Medicine in which exclusive interests have been secured by patent, copyright of labels, or secrecy of composition. SEE: *proprietary medicine*.

  m., psychosomatic. Branch of medicine that recognizes the importance of mind-body interrelationship in all illnesses and in which therapy and management are based on this fact.

  m., socialized. Practice of medicine under control and direction of a government agency. The cost of medical care under this plan usually is financed by levying taxes or through a national medical insurance program.

  m., sports. Field of medicine concerned with all aspects of physiology, pathology, and psychology as they apply to persons who participate in sports whether at the recreational, amateur, or professional level. An important facet of sports medicine is the application of medical knowledge to the prevention of injuries in those who participate in sports.

  m., tropical. Branch of medical science that deals principally with diseases common in tropical or subtropical regions, esp. diseases of parasitic origin.

  m., veterinary. Branch of medical science that deals with diagnosis and treatment of diseases of animals.

medicine man. Shaman, q.v.

medicinerea (mĕd″ĭ-sĭn-ē′rē-a) [L. *medius*, middle, + *cinerea*, ashen]. Internal gray matter of the claustrum and lenticula of the brain.

medicochirurgical (mĕd″ĭ-kō-kī-rŭr′jĭ-kăl) [L. *medicus*, medical, + Gr. *cheir*, hand, + *ergon*, work]. Concerning both medicine and surgery.

medicolegal (mĕd″ĭ-kō-lē′găl) [″ + *legalis*, legal]. Rel. to medical jurisprudence or forensic medicine.

medicomechanical (mĕd″ĭ-kō-mĕ-kăn′ĭ-kăl). Concerning both medical and mechanical aspects of treating patients.

medicopsychology (mĕd″ĭ-kō-sī-kŏl′ō-jē). The relationship of medicine with the mind or with mental illness.

medicopter. Helicopter equipped for emergency care of sick or injured while they are being evacuated to a hospital.

medicornu (mĕd″ĭ-kor′nū) [L. *medius*, middle, + *cornu*, horn]. The inferior horn of the lateral ventricle of the brain.

Medihaler-Epi. Trade name for epinephrine bitartrate, USP.

Medina worm. *Dracunculus medinensis*.

medio- [L. *medius*, middle]. Prefix meaning middle.

mediocarpal (mē″dē-ō-kăr′păl). Concerning the middle part of the carpal bone.

mediolateral (mē″dē-ō-lăt′ĕr-ăl). Concerning the middle and side of a structure.

medionecrosis (mē″dē-ō-nē-krō′sĭs) [″ + *nekrosis*, state of death]. Necrosis of the tunica media of a blood vessel.

mediopontine (mē″dē-ō-pŏn′tĭn) [″ + *pons*, bridge]. Rel. to center of the pons varolii.

mediotarsal (mē″dē-ō-tăr′săl). Rel. to the middle of the tarsus.

medisect (mē′dĭ-sĕkt) [″ + *secare*, to cut]. To cut on the median line of the body or structure.

meditation. The act of contemplative thinking. SEE: *meditation, transcendental*.

  m., transcendental. ABBR: TM. A type of meditation based on ancient Hindu practices in which an individual tries to relax by sitting quietly for regular periods while repeating a mantra. The value of TM in treating various conditions is under investigation. SEE: *relaxation response*.

Mediterranean anemia. A hereditary anemia due to an abnormality in the synthesis of hemoglobin. Usually occurs in Mediterranean populations. There is no specific therapy. SYN: *Cooley's anemia; thalassemia*.

Mediterranean fever, familial. A disease originally common in people of the Middle East, but now seen in various parts of the world. This familial disease is characterized by short attacks of fever, signs of peritonitis, pleuritis, and arthritis. The most frequent cause of death is amyloidosis, which occurs as the disease progresses. There is no specific diagnostic test. SYN: *polyserositis, recurrent*.

  TREAT: Symptomatic.

medium (mēd′ē-ŭm) (pl. *media*). 1. An agent through which an effect is obtained. 2. Substance used for the cultivation of microorganisms or cellular tissue. SYN: *culture medium*. 3. Substance through which impulses are transmitted.

  m., clearing. A substance that renders histological specimens transparent.

  m., contrast. A substance used in radiology which, when introduced into the body, changes the density of the anatomic structure.

m., culture. A substance or mixture used to support growth.

m., defined. SEE: *defined medium.*

m., nutrient. A fortified culture medium with added nutrient materials.

m., radiolucent. A substance injected into an anatomical structure to decrease the density which will increase the radiographic detail for diagnostic purposes.

m., radiopaque. A substance injected into a cavity or region or passed through the gastrointestinal tract to increase the density and radiographic detail for diagnostic purposes. SYN: *contrast medium.*

m., refracting. The fluids and transparent tissues of the eye refract the light rays passing through them toward the retina. Also called dioptric medium.

m., separating. In dentistry, a substance applied to the surface of an impression or mold to prevent interaction of the materials and to facilitate their separation after casting. Also called separating agent.

medium-chain triglycerides. Triglycerides with 8 to 10 carbon atoms. They are digested and absorbed differently than the usual dietary fats and, for that reason, have been useful in treating malabsorption.

medius (mē′dē-ŭs) [L.]. Middle. Indicating the middle one of three similar structures.

MEDLARS [*Medical Literature Analysis and Retrieval System*]. Acronym indicating the U.S. National Library of Medicine's system of computerized bibliography. Index Medicus is produced by this system. A MEDLARS search is use of this system to retrieve medical references of specific interest.

MEDLINE [*MED*LARS on *line*]. The system in which telephone lines may be linked to the MEDLARS system so that bibliographic data may be transmitted from the National Library of Medicine to a great number of locations.

medrogestone (měd-rō-jěs′tōn). A progestin.

Medrol. Trade name for methylprednisolone.

medroxyprogesterone acetate (měd-rŏk″sē-prō-jěs′těr-ōn). USP. A progestational agent. It is used intramuscularly in appropriate dose. It is effective for as long as 90 days. Trade names are Depo-Provera and Provera.

medrysone (měd′rĭ-sōn). USP. An adrenal corticosteroid drug. Trade name is HMS Liquifilm.

medulla (mě-dŭl′lă) [L.] (pl. *medullae*). [NA] 1. The marrow. 2. Inner or central portion of an organ in contrast to the outer portion or cortex. 3. Medulla oblongata.

m., adrenal. Inner portion of the adrenal gland composed of chromaffin tissue. Secretes epinephrine. SEE: *adrenal gland.*

m. nephrica. Pyramids of kidneys.

m. oblongata. [NA] Enlarged portion of spinal cord in cranium after it enters the foramen magnum of the occipital bone; the lower portion of the brain stem.

m. of hair. Central axis of a hair.

m. of kidneys. Renal pyramids. SEE: *pyramid, renal.*

m. of ovary. Central portion of the ovary composed of loose connective tissue, blood vessels, lymphatics, and nerves.

m. ossium. [NA] Marrow in bone.

m. spinalis. [NA] Spinal cord.

medullary (měd′ū-lār-ē) [L. *medullaris*]. Concerning marrow or medulla.

medullated (měd′ū-lāt″ěd). Covered by or containing marrow or medulla; myelinated.

medullated nerve fiber. A nerve fiber possessing a myelin or medullary sheath; a myelinated nerve fiber.

medullation. Acquiring a myelin sheath.

medullectomy (měd″ū-lěk′tō-mē) [L. *medulla*, marrow, + Gr. *ektome*, excision]. Surgical excision of a part of the medulla of the brain.

medullitis (měd-ū-lī′tĭs) [″ + Gr. *itis*, inflammation]. Inflammation of marrow. SYN: *myelitis.*

medullization (měd″ū-lī-zā′shŭn). Abnormal conversion to marrow.

medulloadrenal (mě-dŭl″ō-ă-drē′năl) [″ + *ad*, to, + *ren*, kidney]. Concerning the medulla of the adrenal gland.

medulloarthritis (mě-dŭl″ō-ăr-thrī′tĭs) [L. *medulla*, marrow, + Gr. *arthron*, joint, + *itis*, inflammation]. Inflammation of marrow elements of bone ends.

medulloblast (mě-dŭl′ō-blăst) [″ + Gr. *blastos*, germ]. An immature cell of the neural tube that may develop into either a nerve or neuroglial cell.

medulloblastoma (mě-dŭl″ō-blăs-tō′mă) [″ + Gr. *blastos*, germ, + *oma*, tumor]. A soft infiltrating malignant tumor of the roof of the 4th ventricle and cerebellum. Often invades the meninges.

medulloepithelioma (mě-dŭl″ō-ěp″ĭ-thěl-ē-ō′mă) [″ + Gr. *epi*, upon, + *thele*, nipple, + *oma*, tumor]. Tumor composed of retina epithelium and of neuroepithelium. SYN: *glioma; neuroepithelioma.*

Mees lines. Transverse white lines that appear above the lunula of the fingernails about 5 weeks after exposure to arsenic.

mefenamic acid. An analgesic and antipyretic drug that also has anti-inflammatory action. Trade name is Ponstel.

mega- [Gr. *megas*, large]. 1. Combining form that means great or large. 2. Indicates one million (10^6) when used in combination with terms indicating units of measure; thus megaton is one million tons. SEE: words beginning with *megalo-*.

megabladder (mĕg″ă-blăd′ĕr) [″ + AS. *blaedre*, bladder]. Permanent abnormal distention of the urinary bladder. SYN: *megalocystis*.

megacardia (mĕg″ă-kăr′dē-ă). Enlargement of the heart. SYN: *cardiomegaly*.

Megace. Trade name for megestrol acetate.

megacephalic (mĕg-ă-sĕf-ăl′ĭk). Having an abnormally large head. SYN: *macrocephalous*.

megacolon (mĕg-ă-kō′lŏn) [″ + *kolon*, colon]. Extremely dilated colon. Usually congenital but occurs also in infancy or childhood. SEE: *Hirschsprung's disease*.

m., toxic. Acute dilatation of the colon that may progress to rupture. Seen in acute attacks of ulcerative colitis.

megacurie (mĕg″ă-kū′rē) [″ + *curie*]. ABBR: Mc. A unit of radioactivity equal to 10^6 curies.

megadontia (mĕg″ă-dŏn′shē-ă) [″ + *odous, odont-*, tooth]. Possessing very large teeth.

megadyne (mĕg′ă-dīn). A unit equal to one million dynes. SEE: *dyne*.

megaesophagus (mĕg″ă-ē-sŏf′ă-gŭs) [″ + *oisophagos*, esophagus]. A grossly dilated esophagus, usually associated with achalasia.

megahertz (mĕg′ă-hĕrtz). ABBR: MHz. One million, 10^6, cycles per second (i.e., hertz).

megakaryoblast (mĕg″ă-kăr′ē-ō-blăst). An immature megakaryocyte.

megakaryocyte (mĕg″ă-kăr′ē-ō-sīt″) [″ + *karyon*, nucleus, + *kytos*, cell]. Large bone marrow cell with large or multiple nuclei which gives rise to blood platelets essential for the clotting mechanism of blood. SYN: *giant cell; myeloplax*.

megakaryocytosis (mĕg″ă-kăr″ē-ō-sī-tō′sĭs) [″ + ″ + ″ + *osis*, condition]. An increased number of megakaryocytes in the bone marrow; presence of megakaryocytes in the blood.

megalencephaly (mĕg″ăl-ĕn-sĕf′ă-lē) [″ + *enkephalos*, brain]. Abnormally large size of the brain, usually accompanied by mental deficiency.

megalgia (mĕg-ăl′jē-ă) [″ + *algos*, pain]. Very severe pain.

megalo- [Gr. *megas*, large]. Combining form meaning of great size.

megaloblast (mĕg′ă-lō-blăst) [″ + *blastos*, germ]. A large, nucleated abnormal red blood corpuscle, from 11 to 20 microns in diameter, oval and slightly irregular. Found in the blood in cases of pernicious anemia.

megalocardia (mĕg″ă-lō-kăr′dē-ă) [″ + *kardia*, heart]. Cardiac hypertrophy. SYN: *cardiomegaly*.

megalocephalic (mĕg-ă-lō-sĕf-ăl′ĭk) [″ + *kephale*, head]. Having an abnormally large skull. SYN: *megacephalic; macrocephalic*.

megalocephaly (mĕg″ă-lō-sĕf′ă-lē) [″ + *kephale*, head]. 1. Abnormal size of the head. SYN: *macrocephaly*. 2. A rare disease characterized by hyperostosis of bones of the skull. SYN: *leontiasis ossea*.

megalocheiria (mĕg″ă-lō-kī′rē-ă) [″ + *cheir*, hand]. Abnormally large hands.

megalocornea (mĕg″ă-lō-kor′nē-ă) [″ + L. *cornu*, horn]. An enlarged cornea due to a developmental anomaly. SYN: *macrocornea*.

megalocystis (mĕg″ă-lō-sĭs′tĭs) [″ + *kystis*, bladder]. Abnormal permanent enlargement of the bladder. SYN: *megabladder*.

megalocyte (mĕg′ă-lō-sīt) [″ + *kytos*, cell]. A larger than average red blood corpuscle.

megalodactylous (mĕg″ă-lō-dăk′tĭl-ŭs) [″ + *daktylos*, finger]. Having very large fingers or toes.

megalodontia (mĕg″ă-lō-dŏn′shē-ă) [″ + *odous*, tooth]. Abnormally large teeth.

megaloesophagus (mĕg″ă-lō-ē-sŏf′ă-gŭs) [″ + *oisophagos*, esophagus]. Megaesophagus, q.v.

megalogastria (mĕg″ă-lō-găs′trē-ă) [″ + *gaster*, belly]. Excessive size of stomach. SYN: *gastromegaly*.

megaloglossia (mĕg″ă-lō-glŏs′sē-ă) [″ + *glossa*, tongue]. Enlargement of the tongue. SYN: *macroglossia*.

megalographia (mĕg″ă-lō-grā′fē-ă) [″ + *graphein*, to write]. Macrography, q.v.

megalohepatia (mĕg″ă-lō-hĕ-păt′ē-ă) [″ + *hepar*, liver]. Abnormal enlargement of the liver. SYN: *hepatomegaly*.

megalokaryocyte (mĕg″ă-lō-kăr′ē-ō-sīt) [″ + *karyon*, nucleus, + *kytos*, cell]. A large bone marrow cell with multiple nuclei. SYN: *megakaryocyte*.

megalomania (mĕg″ă-lō-mā′nē-ă) [″ + *mania*, madness]. A psychosis characterized by ideas of personal exaltation and delusions of grandeur.

megalomelia (mĕg′ă-lō-mēl′ē-ă) [″ + *melos*, limb]. Abnormally large size of the limbs. SYN: *macromelia*.

megalonychosis (mĕg″ă-lō″nĭ-kō′sĭs) [″ + *onyx*, nail]. Hypertrophy of the nails.

megalopenis (mĕg″ă-lō-pē′nĭs) [″ + L. *penis*, penis]. Abnormally large penis. SYN: *macrophallus*.

megalophthalmus (mĕg″ă-lŏf-thăl′mŭs) [″ + *ophthalmos*, eye]. Abnormally large eyes.

megalopodia (mĕg″ă-lō-pō′dē-ă) [″ + *pous*, foot]. Abnormally large feet.

megalopsia (mĕg″ă-lŏp′sē-ă) [″ + *opsis,* vision]. An affection of the eyes in which objects appear enlarged. SYN: *macropsia.*

megaloscope (mĕg′ă-lō-skōp″) [″ + *skopein,* to examine]. A large magnifying lens; a speculum fitted with a magnifying lens.

megalosplenia (mĕg″ă-lō-splēn′ē-ă) [″ + *splen,* spleen]. Hypertrophy of the spleen. SYN: *splenomegaly.*

megalospore (mĕg′ă-lō-spor″). Macrospore, q.v.

megalosyndactyly (mĕg′ă-lō-sĭn-dăk′tĭl-ē) [″ + *syn,* with, + *daktylos,* finger]. A condition of large and webbed digits.

megaloureter (mĕg″ă-lō-ū-rē′tĕr, -ūr′ē-tĕr) [″ + *oureter,* ureter]. Increase in diameter of the ureter.

-megaly [Gr. *megas,* abnormally large]. Suffix indicating large.

megaprosopous (mĕg″ă-prŏs′ō-pŭs) [″ + *prosopon,* face]. Possessing a large face.

megarectum (mĕg-ă-rĕk′tŭm) [″ + L. *rectum,* straight]. Excessive dilatation of the rectum.

megaseme (mĕg′ă-sēm) [″ + *sema,* sign]. Having an orbital aperture with an index exceeding 89, said of a skull.

megavitamin (mĕg″ă-vī′tă-mĭn). A dose of one or more vitamins that is in huge excess of the normal daily requirements.

megavolt (mĕg′ă-vōlt). One million, 10^6, volts.

megestrol acetate (mĕ-jĕs′trōl). A synthetic progestin that is also used in treating certain neoplasms. Trade name is Megace.

meglumine (mĕg′lū-mēn). USP. A radiopaque compound used in x-ray studies.

    m. antimonate. A drug used in treating leishmaniasis.

megohm (mĕg′ōm). One million, 10^6, ohms.

megophthalmos (mĕg-ŏf-thăl-mōs) [″ + *ophthalmos,* eye]. Abnormally large eyes. SYN: *megalophthalmus.*

meibomian cyst (mī-bō′mē-ăn) [Heinrich Meibom, Ger. anatomist, 1638–1700]. Small tumor on eyelid, the result of inflammation of a meibomian gland. SYN: *chalazion.*

meibomian gland. One of the sebaceous glands between the tarsi and conjunctiva of eyelids. SYN: *tarsal gland.*

meibomitis (mī-bō″mī′tĭs). Inflammation of the meibomian glands.

Meigs′ syndrome [Joe V. Meigs, U.S. gynecologist, 1892–1963]. Benign tumor of the ovary associated with ascites and pleural effusion.

meio- [Gr. *meioun,* diminution]. Combining form indicating decrease in size or number. SEE: words beginning with *mio-.*

meiogenic (mī″ō-jĕn′ĭk) [Gr. *meiosis,* diminution, + *gennan,* to produce]. Causing meiosis.

meiosis (mī-ō′sĭs) [Gr., diminution]. A type of cell division of germ cells (sperm or ova) in which two successive divisions of the nucleus produce cells that contain half the number of chromosomes present in somatic cells. When fertilization occurs, the nuclei of the sperm and ovum fuse and produce a zygote with the full chromosome complement. SEE: *chromosome; mitosis.*

Meissner′s corpuscles (mīs′nĕrz) [Georg Meissner, Ger. histologist, 1829–1905]. An encapsulated end-organ of touch found in dermal papillae close to epidermis. Each is an ovoid body containing endings of myelinated and unmyelinated nerve fibers. Most numerous in hairless portion of skin, esp. volar surface of hands, fingers, feet, and toes; also present in lips, eyelids, tip of tongue, and nipple.

Meissner′s plexus. Small aggregations of ganglion cells located in submucosa of intestine.

mel [L.]. Honey.

melagra (mĕl-ā′gră) [Gr. *melos,* limb, + *agra,* seizure]. Muscular pain in the limbs.

melalgia (mĕl-ăl′jē-ă) [″ + *algos,* pain]. Pain of neural origin in the limbs.

melancholia (mĕl-ăn-kō′lē-ă) [Gr. *melankholia,* sadness]. A severe depression with a dull, uninterested affect and lack of interest in activities that would normally be pleasurable. There may be agitation or retardation. Weight loss, anorexia, insomnia, and worsening of the symptoms may occur in the early morning.

    m., affective. Melancholia observed in depressed phase of manic-depressive psychoses. SEE: *psychosis, manic-depressive.*

    m. agitata. Agitated depression.

    m., climacteric. Melancholia occurring at the time of menopause.

    m., involutional. Despondency, suicidal tendencies, feelings of unworthiness and mental agitation occurring in late middle age.

    m., panphobic. Melancholia characterized by dread of everything.

    m., sexual. Melancholia associated with fear of impotence, venereal disease, unsatisfied sexual desires.

    m., simplex. A mild form of melancholia, without delusions or great excitement.

    m. stuporosa. Melancholia in which patient lies silent and motionless, indifferent to surroundings.

    m., suicidal. Impulse to commit suicide combined with melancholia.

melanedema (mĕl-ăn-ĕ-dē′mă) [Gr. *melas,* black, + *oidema,* swelling]. Black deposit in the lungs; melanosis of the lungs. SYN: *anthracosis.*

melanemia (mĕl-ăn-ē'mē-ă) [" + *haima*, blood]. Unnaturally dark color of blood, due to presence of free dark pigment. Seen mainly in pernicious anemia.

melanephidrosis, melanidrosis (mĕl"ăn-ĕf"ĭ-drō'sĭs, mĕl"ăn-ĭd-rō'sĭs) [" + *ephidrosis*, sweating]. A form of chromhidrosis in which the sweat is black.

melaniferous (mĕl"ăn-ĭf'ĕr-ŭs) [" + L. *ferre*, to carry]. Containing melanin or some other black pigment.

melanin [Gr. *melas*, black]. The pigment that gives color to hair, skin, the substantia nigra of the brain, and the choroid of the eye. Exposure to sunlight stimulates melanin production. It can be prepared chemically. It is present in some cancers such as melanoma.

melanism (mĕl'ăn-ĭzm) [" + *-ismos*, condition]. Abnormal black pigmentation of the organs and tissues. SYN: *melanosis*.

melano- [Gr. *melas*, black]. Prefix meaning black or darkness.

melanoameloblastoma (mĕl"ă-nō-ă-mĕl"ō-blăs-tō'mă) [" + O. Fr. *amel*, enamel, + Gr. *blastos*, germ, + *oma*, tumor]. Melanotic neuroectodermal tumor.

melanoblast (mĕl'ăn-ō-blăst", mĕl-ăn'ō-blăst) [" + *blastos*, germ]. A cell originating from the neural crest that differentiates into a melanocyte.

melanoblastoma (mĕl"ă-nō-blăs-tō'mă) [" + " + *oma*, tumor]. A tumor containing melanin.

melanocarcinoma (mĕl"ă-nō-kăr-sĭn-ō'mă) [" + *karkinos*, cancer, + *oma*, tumor]. Malignant melanoma.

melanocyte (mĕl'ăn-ō-sīt, mĕl-ăn'ō-sīt) [" + *kytos*, cell]. Melanin-forming cell.

melanocyte-stimulating hormone. ABBR: MSH. Hormone that regulates skin pigmentation in man.

melanocytoma (mĕl"ă-nō-sī-tō'mă) [" + *kytos*, cell, + *oma*, tumor]. A rare pigmented benign tumor of the optic disk.

melanoderma (mĕl"ăn-ō-dĕr'mă). A patchy or generalized skin discoloration caused by either an increase in the production of melanin by the normal number of melanocytes or an increase in the number of melanocytes. SYN: *melanopathy*.

melanodermatitis (mĕl"ă-nō-dĕr"mă-tī'tĭs) [" + " + *itis*, inflammation]. Dermatitis in which an excess of melanin is deposited in the involved area.

melanoepithelioma (mĕl"ăn-ō-ĕp"ĭ-thē-lē-ō'mă) [" + *epi*, upon, + *thele*, nipple, + *oma*, tumor]. A malignant epithelioma containing melanin.

melanogen (mĕ-lăn'ō-jĕn) [" + *gennan*, to produce]. A colorless substance that may be converted into melanin.

melanogenesis (mĕl"ăn-ō-jĕn'ĕ-sĭs) [" + *genesis*, generation, birth]. Formation of melanin.

melanoglossia (mĕl"ăn-ō-glŏs'ē-ă) [" + *glossa*, tongue]. Black tongue. SYN: *glossophytia*.

melanoid (mĕl'ă-noyd) [" + *eidos*, form, shape]. 1. Concerning or resembling melanin. 2. Artificial melanin that is chemically prepared.

melanoleukoderma (mĕl"ăn-ō-lū"kō-dĕr'mă) [" + *leukos*, white, + *derma*, skin]. Mottled skin.
  m. colli. Mottled skin of the neck sometimes seen in syphilis. SYN: *collar of Venus; venereal collar.*

melanoma (mĕl"ă-nō'mă) [" + *oma*, tumor]. A malignant, darkly pigmented mole or tumor of the skin. Malignant melanoma was the cause of death of 5800 persons in the U.S. in 1988.
  ETIOL: Excessive exposure to the sun, esp. in light-skinned people; but having dark or black skin in no guarantee of protection against melanoma. Heredity may also be important. The lesion of melanoma is characterized by its asymmetry, irregular border, and lack of uniform color. The diameter is usually greater than 6 mm (about ¼ inch). Also, the following should be considered as a warning of melanoma: change in surface appearance or size of a mole; scaliness; oozing; bleeding; itchiness, tenderness, or pain of the area.
  PREVENTION: Avoid sun or, if exposure is necessary, limit it by using sunscreen on exposed areas of skin.
  TREAT: Early detection is essential; surgical removal.

melanomatosis (mĕl"ă-nō"mă-tō'sĭs) [" + " + *osis*, condition]. Formation of numerous melanomas on or beneath the skin.

melanonychia (mĕl"ă-nō-nĭk'ē-ă) [" + *onyx*, nail]. Black pigmentation of the nails.

melanopathy (mĕl"ă-nŏp'ă-thē) [" + *pathos*, disease]. 1. Dark pigmentation of skin. 2. Any disease with dark pigmentation of the skin. SYN: *melanoderma*.

melanophage (mĕl'ă-nō-fāj") [" + *phagein*, to eat]. A phagocytic cell that contains ingested melanin.

melanophore (mĕl'ăn-ō-for) [" + *phoros*, bearing]. Cell containing dark pigment.

melanoplakia (mĕl"ăn-ō-plă'kē-ă) [" + *plax*, a flat plain]. Condition marked by pigmented patches on the tongue and buccal mucosa.

melanorrhagia, melanorrhea (mĕl"ăn-ō-rā'jē-ă, mĕl"ăn-ō-rē'ă) [" + *rhegnynai*, to burst forth]. Black feces. SYN: *melena.*

melanosarcoma (mĕl"ă-nō-săr-kō'mă) [" + *sarx*, flesh, + *oma*, tumor]. Sarcoma containing melanin.

melanoscirrhus (měl″ă-nō-skĭr′ŭs) [Gr. *melas*, black, + *skirros*, hardness]. Black-pigmented cancer; an unusual form of melanoma. SYN: *melanocarcinoma*.

melanosis (měl-ăn-ō′sĭs) [″ + *osis*, condition]. 1. Unusual deposit of black pigment in different parts of body. 2. Disorder of pigment metabolism.

 m. lenticularis. Rare skin disease beginning in early youth and characterized by scattered pigment discolorations, ulcers, and atrophy. SYN: *Kaposi's disease; xeroderma pigmentosum.*

 m., pustular. A benign lesion that is present at birth as a vesiculopustular eruption around the chin, neck, back, extremities, and palms or soles, and lasts 2 to 3 days. Seen predominantly in black neonates.

melanosome (měl′ă-nō-sōm″) [″ + *soma*, body]. The pigment granule produced by melanocytes.

melanotic. 1. Black in color. 2. Pert. to melanosis.

 NOTE: Not to be confused with melenic, q.v. or melenotic.

melanotic macule. A small, usually less than 1 cm in diameter, brown to black lesion of the oral mucosa which is usually solitary and asymptomatic. In most instances, this type of macule is benign and requires no therapy. It can, however, be due to melanoma, which will require vigorous therapy without delay. When it is benign it may be due to Peutz-Jeghers syndrome, q.v., physiologic pigmentation, Addison's disease, healing of traumatic lesions, or secondary to a variety of medications.

melanotrichia linguae (měl″ăn-ō-trĭk′ē-ă lĭng′gwē) [″ + *thrix*, hair, + L. *linguae*, tongue]. Black, hairy tongue.

melanotroph (měl′ă-nō-trōf″) [″ + *trophe*, nutrition]. A cell of the pituitary that produces melanocyte-stimulating hormone.

melanuria (měl-ăn-ū′rē-ă) [″ + *ouron*, urine]. Dark pigment in urine.

melasma (měl-ăz′mă) [Gr., a black spot]. Any discoloration of the skin.

 m. gravidarum. Discoloration of the skin during pregnancy.

melatonin (mel″ă-tō′nĭn). Hormone produced by the pineal gland in mammals.

melena (měl′ĕ-nă, měl-ē′nă) [Gr. *melaina*, black]. Black, tarry feces due to action of intestinal secretions on free blood. Common in the newborn.

 m. neonatorum. Melena in the newborn.

melenic (měl-ĕ′nĭk) [Gr. *melaina*, black]. Concerning melena, i.e., black, tarry stools. SYN: *melenotic.*

melicera, meliceris (měl-ĭ-sēr′ă, -ĭs) [Gr. *meli*, honey, + *keros*, wax]. 1. Cyst containing matter of honeylike consistency. 2. Viscid, syrupy.

melioidosis (mē″lē-oy-dō′sĭs) [Gr. *melis*, a distemper of asses, + *eidos*, form, shape, + *osis*, condition]. An acute or chronic disease due to *Pseudomonas pseudomallei* (formerly called *Malleomyces pseudomallei*). Acute form causes pneumonia, multiple abscesses, septicemia, and possibly death.

melissophobia (mē-lĭs″ō-fō′bē-ă) [Gr. *melissa*, bee, + *phobia*, fear]. Abnormal fear of bee or wasp stings.

melitagra. Eczema with honeycomb crusting.

melitemia (měl-ĭ-tē′mē-ă) [Gr. *meli*, honey, + *haima*, blood]. Abnormal amount of sugar in the blood.

melitensis (měl-ĭ-těn′sĭs). Undulant fever; brucellosis.

melitis (měl-ĭ′tĭs) [Gr. *melon*, cheek, + *itis*, inflammation]. Inflammation of the cheek.

melitoptyalism (měl″ĭ-tō-tī′ăl-ĭzm) [″ + *ptyalon*, saliva]. Saliva containing glucose. SYN: *glycoptyalism.*

melituria (měl-ĭ-tū′rē-ă) [″ + *ouron*, urine]. Presence of sugar in the urine.

Mellaril. Trade name for thioridazine hydrochloride, USP.

mellitum (mě-lĭ′tŭm) [L.]. A pharmaceutical preparation with honey as the vehicle or excipient.

melo-, mel-. 1. [Gr. *melon*, cheek]. Combining form meaning cheek. 2. [Gr. *melos*, limb]. Combining form meaning extremity.

melomelus (mē-lŏm′ē-lŭs) [Gr. *melos*, limb, + *melos*, limb]. A malformed fetus with rudimentary limb attached to normal limb.

meloncus (měl-ŏn′kŭs) [Gr. *melon*, cheek, + *onkos*, bulk]. Tumor of the cheek.

melonoplasty (měl′ŏn-ō-plăs″tē) [″ + *plassein*, to form]. Plastic surgery of the cheek.

meloplasty (měl′ō-plăs-tē) 1. [″ + *plassein*, to form]. Plastic surgery of the face. 2. [Gr. *melos*, limb, + *plassein*, to form]. Reparative surgery of the extremities.

melorheostosis (měl″ō-rē″ŏs-tō′sĭs) [Gr. *melos*, limb, + *rhein*, to flow, + *osteon*, bone, + *osis*, condition]. A rare disease of long bones in which new bone is formed so that the bone looks like candle wax had dripped down the sides.

melosalgia (měl″ō-săl′jē-ă) [″ + *algos*, pain]. Pain in the lower limbs.

meloschisis (mě-lŏs′kĭ-sĭs) [Gr. *melon*, cheek, + *schistos*, divided]. A congenitally cleft cheek.

melotia (mě-lō′shē-ă) [″ + *ous*, ear]. Congenital displacement of the ear on the cheek.

melphalan (měl′fă-lăn). USP. A cytotoxic drug of the nitrogen mustard class. Trade name is Alkeran.

melting point. Temperature at which conversion of a solid to a liquid begins.

member [L. *membrum*]. An organ or part of the body, esp. a limb.

membrane (mĕm′brān) [L. *membrana*]. A thin, soft, pliable layer of tissue that lines a tube or cavity, covers an organ or structure, or separates one part from another.

    m., alveolocapillary. Very thin tissue that separates the air inside the pulmonary alveolus from blood in the surrounding capillaries.

    m., alveodental. Periodontium, q.v.

    m., arachnoid. Middle layer of membranes covering brain and spinal cord.

    m., atlanto-occipital. A single midline ligamentous structure that extends from the arch of the atlas to borders of the foramen magnum.

    m., basement. A delicate, noncellular membrane underlying a layer of epithelial cells and serving for their support and attachment. SYN: *basement lamina.*

    m., basilar. Membrane extending from the tympanic lip of the osseous spiral lamina to the crest of the spiral ligament in the cochlea of the ear. It separates the scala tympani from the cochlear duct and forms supporting structure for the organ of Corti.

    m., Bowman's. Thin homogeneous membrane separating corneal epithelium from proper substance of the cornea.

    m., Bruch's. Inner layer of the choroid of the eye. SYN: *lamina basalis of choroid.*

    m., buccopharyngeal. In the embryo, the membrane that separates the oral cavity from the foregut until the fourth week of development. SYN: *m., oral; m., pharyngeal.*

    m., cell. Surface layer of the cytoplasm of a cell. SYN: *m., plasma.*

    m., choroid. The choroid, the portion of the vascular tunic or uvea of the eye that extends posteriorly from the ora serrata.

    m., costocoracoid. Dense fascia between the pectoralis minor and subclavius muscles.

    m., cricothyroid. Membrane connecting thyroid and cricoid cartilages of the larynx.

    m., croupous. False yellow-white membrane in the larynx during croup.

    m., decidual. One of the membranes formed in the endometrium of a pregnant uterus. Includes the decidua basalis, decidua capsularis, and decidua parietalis.

    m., Descemet's. Elastic membrane forming the lining surface of the cornea. SYN: *m., vitreous.*

    m., diphtheritic. Fibrinous false membrane on mucous surfaces in diphtheria.

    m., drum. Tympanic membrane.

    m., egg. One of the protective membranes or envelopes enclosing an ovum. May be primary (formed by egg itself, e.g., vitelline membrane); secondary (formed by follicle cells, e.g., zona pellucida); or tertiary (formed by oviduct or uterus, e.g., albumin and shell of hen's egg).

    m., elastic. One of several membranes formed of elastic connective tissue fibers.

    m., enamel. 1. Cuticula dentis. 2. Thin internal layer of cells of the enamel organ.

    m., false. Fibrinous exudate on a mucous surface of a membrane, as in diphtheria.

    m., fenestrated. A layer of elastic connective tissue possessing minute round or oval openings. Found in tunica intima and tunica media of medium-sized and large arteries. SYN: *m., Henle's elastic.*

    m., fetal. One of the membranous structures that serve to protect and support the embryo. The structures are yolk sac, allantois, amnion, chorion, decidua, and placenta.

    m., fibrous. Membrane composed entirely of connective tissue. Examples include the fasciae, aponeuroses, perichondrium, periosteum, dura mater, and capsules of some organs.

    m., glassy. 1. Transparent capsule that separates membrana granulosa from the theca of the graafian follicle. 2. Internal layer of a hair follicle separating the epithelial and connective tissues.

    m., glial cell. Extremely delicate membrane, formed of foot plates of astrocytes, that surrounds all blood vessels in the brain, spinal cord, and in lining of pia mater separating these vessels from nervous tissue proper. Thought to be one of the components of the blood-brain barrier, q.v.

    m., Henle's elastic. M., fenestrated.

    m., homogeneous. A fine membrane covering villi of the placenta.

    m., Huxley's. SEE: *layer, Huxley's.*

    m., hyaline. 1. Basement lamina. 2. Membrane between outer root sheath of a hair follicle and inner fibrous layer.

    m., hyaloid. Membrane investing the vitreous humor of the eye, seen on longitudinal section.

    m., hyoglossal. A transverse fibrous lamella uniting tongue to hyoid bone.

    m., interosseous. 1. A fibrous membrane in the arm connecting ulna to radius. 2. A fibrous membrane in the leg connecting tibia to fibula.

    m., Krause's. Dark membranous band limiting the sarcomere in striated muscle. SYN: *myofibril; Z disk.*

    m., laryngeal mucous. The mucous membrane, glands, and cilia that characterize the surface covering within the larynx.

    m., limiting, external. 1. Outer layer of

cells of the embryonic neural tube. 2. Membrane in retina of eye separating rods and cones from their cell bodies.

m., limiting, internal. 1. Inner layer of ependymal cells lining embryonic neural tube. 2. Glial membrane forming innermost layer of the retina and of the iris.

m., lingual mucous. Mucosa covering the tongue.

m., masticatory mucous. The mucosa of the mouth involved in the masticatory process; it is characterized by a keratinized surface epithelium and includes hard palate, gingiva, and the dorsum of the tongue.

m., medullary. Endosteum.

m., mucous. Membrane lining cavities and canals communicating with the air and kept moist by secretion of mucus.

m., nasal mucous. Mucosa lining the nasal cavity and characterized by pseudostratified ciliated columnar epithelium with goblet mucous gland cells.

m., Nasmyth's. A thin cuticle that consists of the cellular remnants of the enamel organ and the mucopolysaccharide basement membrane that attaches them to the enamel surface. This covering is very friable and usually lost after eruption of the tooth into the oral cavity but may persist in protected areas, such as the labial surface of maxillary incisors. SYN: *m., enamel.*

m., nictitating. A third eyelid present in lower vertebrates and represented in man by a fold of the conjunctiva, the plica semilunaris.

m., nuclear. A two-layered membrane surrounding the nucleus, q.v. Prior to electron microscopy, the nucleus was thought to be surrounded by a single thin membrane.

m., obturator. Fibrous membrane closing the obturator foramen.

m., olfactory. The olfactory portion of the membrane lining the nasal fossa.

m., oral. The buccopharyngeal membrane. SYN: *m., pharyngeal.*

m., oronasal. A double epithelial layer separating the nasal pits from the embryonic oral cavity.

m., otolithic. A layer of gelatinous substance containing otoconia or otoliths, found on the surface of maculae in the inner ear.

m., palatal mucous. Mucosa covering the hard and soft palatal surfaces within the mouth. The hard palate has heavily keratinized epithelium and copious mucous glands or fat in the submucosa, whereas, being mobile, the soft palate contains muscle as well as mucous glands and is much less keratinized on the surface.

m., peridental. Connective tissue between the root of a tooth and the alveolar bone.

m., periodontal. An obscure term used inaccurately to indicate periodontal ligament or the several tissues surrounding the tooth, none of which is a membrane. SYN: *periodontium.*

m., permeable. Membrane that permits the passage of water and certain substances in solution. SEE: *m., selectively permeable; m., semipermeable.*

m., pharyngeal. The buccopharyngeal membrane. SYN: *m., oral.*

m., pharyngeal mucous. The mucosa that lines the funnel-shaped pharynx. The mucosa varies according to the adjacent area with pseudostratified epithelium in the region of the nasal cavity, stratified squamous epithelium near the oral cavity, and ciliated stratified columnar or pseudostratified in the region of the laryngeal opening. The lower pharynx is lined by stratified squamous epithelium as it is continuous with the esophagus.

m., placental. Membrane of the placenta that separates the maternal blood from fetal blood.

m., plasma. M., cell.

m., pseudoserous. Membrane resembling a serous membrane but differing in structure as the endothelium.

m., pupillary. Transparent membrane closing the fetal pupil. If it persists after birth, it is known as persistent pupillary membrane.

m., pyogenic. Granular lining of an abscess or fistula.

m., quadrangular. Upper portion of the elastic membrane of the larynx.

m., Reissner's. Delicate membrane separating cochlear canal from scala vestibuli.

m., Ruysch's. Middle layer of the choroid membrane of the eye, composed of a close capillary network. SYN: *lamina choriocapillaris* [NA].

m., Scarpa's. Membrane that covers the opening to the fenestra cochleae of the inner ear.

m., schneiderian. Mucosa of the nasal fossae.

m., Schwann's. The neurilemma or cell membrane of a neuron.

m., selectively permeable. Membrane that allows a substance such as water to pass through more readily than another, such as salt or sugar.

m., semipermeable. Membrane that allows passage of water but not substances in solution.

m., serous. Membrane consisting of mesothelium lying on thin layer of connective tissue that lines the closed cavities (peritoneal, pleural, and pericardial) of the body.

Surface is moistened by a thin fluid similar to lymph.

m., Shrapnell's. That portion of the tympanic membrane filling the notch of Rivinus.

m., submucous. A layer of connective tissue, often quite elastic, which attaches the mucosal layer to subjacent tissues. It contains sizable blood vessels and nerves and, in some areas, many glands. Also called submucosa.

m., synovial. Membrane lining a joint and secreting synovia.

m., tectorial. Thin, jellylike membrane projecting from vestibular lip of osseous spiral lamina and overlying the spiral organ of Corti of the ear.

m., thyrohyoid. Membrane joining the hyoid bone and the thyroid cartilage.

m., tympanic. Membrane separating the tympanic cavity from the external auditory canal. SYN: m., drum.

m., unit. A thin intracellular plasma membrane that has three layers. It can be visualized only by use of electron microscopy.

m., vestibular mucous. The mucosa of the oral vestibule with its nonkeratinized stratified squamous epithelium, elastic lamina propria, and seromucous labial glands.

m., virginal. The hymen.

m., vitelline. Membrane that forms the surface layer of an ovum.

m., vitreous. Descemet's membrane.

m., yolk. Membrane surrounding the ovum. SYN: *vitelline membrane; zona pellucida.*

membranectomy (měm″brăn-něk′tō-mē) [L. *membrana,* membrane, + Gr. *ektome,* excision]. Surgical removal of a membrane.

membranelle (měm″bră-něl′ă). A thin membrane composed of fused cilia.

membrane potential. The electrical potential difference across the membrane of a cell.

membraniform (měm-brā′nĭ-form). Resembling or of the nature of a membrane. SYN: *membranoid; membranous.*

membranocartilaginous (měm″brăn-ō-kăr-tĭ-lăj′ĭ-nŭs). 1. Pert. to both membrane and cartilage. 2. Derived from both membrane and cartilage.

membranoid (měm′bră-noyd) [L. *membrana,* membrane, + Gr. *eidos,* form, shape]. Resembling a membrane. SYN: *membraniform; membranous.*

membranous. Rel. to or resembling a membrane. SYN: *membraniform, membranoid.*

membrum muliebre (měm′brŭm mū-lē-ě′brē) [L., female member]. The clitoris.

membrum virile (měm′brŭm vĭr-ĭl′ē) [L., male member]. The penis.

memory [L. *memoria*]. The mental registration, retention, and recall of past experience, knowledge, ideas, sensations, and thoughts. Registration of experience is favored by clear comprehension during intense consciousness. Memory for specific details differs greatly with individuals and with the content of the event. Thus, exciting, unusual, or novel events are easily remembered, but those that are dull or ordinary are quickly forgotten. Memory recall, esp. its intentional recall, means the reproduction of a memory in consciousness. Clear comprehension greatly favors retention. Recall may fail because the memory has been obliterated or because one does not wish to remember the stream of ideas. Various memory defects occur in many diseases.

In general, disease states in the aged are more important in having an adverse affect on memory than is merely having attained advanced age.

Memory is confused or obliterated in maniacal states, lively in paranoia, abolished in senile psychosis and organic brain disease, but undisturbed in depressions. In dementia from senile causes, there is accurate memory for remote events but little or none for recent occurrences.

The precise neurophysiological, biochemical, molecular, and emotional factors important in memory are being investigated; but so far, how the individual stores and recalls material in and from the brain is poorly understood.

Helpful in maintaining the quality of memory is the use of various methods and systems of exercising memory, e.g., establish habits with respect to writing things down; keep all essential items such as keys and eyeglasses in the same place; and, most important of all, keep your memory exercised by being mentally active and willing to abandon old habit patterns. Remember that forgetting is a natural event at any age and, in time, the item you are attempting to recall will probably come to you. If it doesn't, just admit you have forgotten and don't make a fuss about it.

RS: amnesia; anamnesis; association; consciousness; lethologica; mnemic; mnemonics; recall; retention; retention defect; subconscious.

m., anterograde. Ability to remember events occurring in the remote past but lacking ability to remember recent events. SYN: *amnesia, anterograde.*

m., long-term. Recall of experiences, or of information gained, in the distant past.

m., retrograde. Ability to recall events of recent occurrence but lacking ability to recall knowledge with which patient had previously been familiar. SYN: *amnesia, retrograde.*

m., selective. Choice an older individual makes to remember only the pleasant memories of the past or those which are ego-protective.

menacme (măn-ăk′mē) [Gr. *men*, month, + *akme*, top]. The height of the menstrual activity of a woman.

menadiol sodium diphosphate. USP. A synthetic water-soluble vitamin, having same activity as natural vitamin K. Used as an antihemorrhagic agent in hypoprothrombinemia or hemorrhagic disorders due to hypoprothrombinemia. Trade name is Synkayvite.

menadione (měn′ă-dī′ōn). USP. A synthetic drug that acts like vitamin K. It is used parenterally in oil, or orally in tablet form.

Caution: Menadione powder is irritating to the respiratory tract and skin. In alcoholic solution, it is a vesicant.

---

m. sodium bisulfite. USP. Synthetic vitamin K. Trade name is Hykinone.

menarchal, menarcheal, menarchial. Pert. to menarche.

menarche (měn-är′kē) [Gr. *men*, month, + *arche*, beginning]. The initial menstrual period. Occurs normally between the 9th and 17th year. The average age of menarche in the U.S. is 12.8 years. SEE: *puberty; adrenarche.*

mendelevium (měn-dě-lē′vē-ūm). SYMB: Md. At. wt. 257.0956; at no. 101. A transuranium element.

mendelism (měn′děl-īzm). The principles of heredity expressed in Mendel's laws.

Mendel's laws [Gregor Johann Mendel, Austrian monk, 1822–1884]. Mendel carefully studied the heredity characteristics of garden peas, and was able to explain the transmission of certain traits from one generation to the next.

Some inherited characteristics are controlled by the combination of two units, genes, from the reproductive cells of each parent. Each of these cells, gametes, has a pair of chromosomes that contain the genes for a specific trait at paired locations. Alternate forms of the gene for a specific trait are called alleles. During meiosis, q.v., the cells of each parent divide and contribute half their chromosome complement to the offspring. SEE: *allele; chromosome; gamete; gene.*

Mendel's law of segregation states that as the gametes are formed, the gene pairs separate and do not influence each other.

Mendel's law of dominance resulted from his observation that crossing a tall strain of peas with a short strain resulted in the expression of the dominant trait, in this case tallness. Thus, some alleles will dominate others in physical expression.

Mendel's law of independent assortment states that traits controlled by different gene pairs (such as height and color) pass to the offspring independently of each other.

Mendel's reflex [Kurt Mendel, Ger. neurologist, 1874–1946]. Dorsal flexion of second to fifth toes upon percussion of the dorsum of the foot.

Ménétrier's disease (mān″ā-trē-ārz′) [Pierre Ménétrier, Fr. physician, 1859–1935]. Diffuse giant hypertrophic gastritis of unknown etiology.

menhidrosis, menidrosis (měn-hī-drō′sĭs, měn″ĭ-drō′sĭs) [Gr. *men*, month, + *hidros*, sweat]. Vicarious menstruation through the sweat glands.

Ménière's disease (mān″ē-ārz′) [Prosper Ménière, Fr. physician, 1799–1862]. A recurrent and usually progressive group of symptoms including progressive deafness, ringing in the ears, dizziness, and a sensation of fullness or pressure in the ears. SYN: *vertigo, labyrinthine.*

ETIOL: Unknown, but edema of the membranous labyrinth has been found in autopsy studies.

TREAT: In acute attacks, bedrest is the most effective treatment. Also antihistamines; discontinuation of smoking; rarely, surgical treatment.

meningeal (měn-ĭn′jē-ăl). Rel. to the meninges.

meningeocortical (mě-nĭn″jē-ō-kor′tĭ-kăl) [Gr. *meninx*, membrane, + L. *corticalis*, pert. to cortex]. Concerning the meninges and cortex of the brain.

meningeorrhaphy (mě-nĭn″jē-or′ă-fē) [″ + *rhaphe*, seam, ridge]. Suture of membranes, esp. those of the brain and spinal cord.

meninges (měn-ĭn′jēz) [Gr.] (sing. *meninx*). 1. Membranes. 2. [NA] The three membranes investing the spinal cord and brain: the dura mater (external), the arachnoid middle), and pia mater (internal).

meningioma (měn-ĭn″jē-ō′mă) [Gr. *meninx*, membrane, + *oma*, tumor]. A slow-growing tumor that originates in the arachnoidal tissue.

meningiomatosis (mě-nĭn″jē-ō-mă-tō′sĭs) [″ + ″ + *osis*, condition]. Multiple meningomas.

meningism (měn-ĭn′jĭzm) [″ + *-ismos*, condition]. Irritation of the brain and spinal cord with symptoms simulating meningitis, but without actual inflammation.

meningismus. Meningism.

meningitic (měn-ĭn-jĭt′ĭk) [Gr. *meninx*, membrane]. Pert. to meningitis.

meningitis (měn-ĭn-jī′tĭs) [″ + *itis*, inflammation] (pl. *meningitides*). Inflammation of the membranes of the spinal cord or brain. SEE: *choriomeningitis; Kernig's sign; leptomeningitis; pachymeningitis; Universal Precautions* in *Appendix*.

　　m., acute aseptic. A nonpurulent form of meningitis usually running a short, benign course with recovery. Usually due to viral infection.

　　m., acute meningococcal. SYM: Moderate, irregular fever; loss of appetite; constipation; intense headache; intolerance to light and sound; contracted pupils; delirium; retraction of head; convulsions; and coma.

　　ETIOL: Various serogroups of *Neisseria meningitidis*, gram-negative cocci.

　　TREAT: Intravenous penicillin G; if patient is allergic to penicillin, chloramphenicol with appropriate monitoring for abnormal blood changes, or cephalosporins such as cefotaxime or ceftriaxone.

　　Supportive measures for shock and other complications such as disseminated intravascular coagulation (DIC), congestive heart failure, and metabolic acidosis. Patient will need cardiac vascular monitoring in an intensive care unit.

　　A potentially lethal complication is acute adrenal insufficiency, Waterhouse-Friderichsen syndrome, q.v.

　　DIET: A fluid diet is necessary during the acute stage, but later a general diet should be given. Tube feeding is necessary with stuporous patients; and children and some adults may have to be fed with a spoon or a medicine dropper.

　　PROG: Favorable with prompt diagnosis and appropriate therapy. SEE: *Waterhouse-Friderichsen syndrome.*

　　PREVENTION: For epidemic control, measures may be initiated by using chemoprophylaxis, i.e., use of sulfadiazine, rifampin, or minocycline for close contacts of the patients; polyvalent polysaccharide vaccines containing A, C, Y, and W135 are highly effective in preventing the disease.

Caution: The meningococci may be resistant to sulfonamides. Minocycline may cause ototoxicity. The vaccines are of little benefit in children under age 2. SEE: *Universal Precautions* in *Appendix*.

NURSING IMPLICATIONS: Isolate patient for at least 24 hours following initiation of antibiotic therapy. If causative organism is meningococcus, follow strict isolation techniques. Force fluids; provide high-protein diet. Administer antipyretics and tepid sponge baths as ordered. Dispose of contaminated articles using double-bagging technique. Monitor neurologic status for changes in level of consciousness and increases in intracranial pressure. Provide personal hygiene and intervene to prevent complications related to immobility. Change position gently to reduce excessive stimulation. Have artificial airway, suction, and oxygen readily available. Provide dark, quiet atmosphere. Pad siderails. Administer analgesics and apply cool compresses to forehead to relieve headache. Administer intravenous fluids or tube feedings as ordered and monitor intake and output. Assess for complications that may include shock, respiratory distress, and disseminated intravascular coagulation. SEE: *Nursing Diagnoses* in *Appendix*.

　　m., aseptic. Inflammation of the meninges not due to microorganisms. May be due to injection of air or drugs into subarachnoid space.

　　m., basal. Inflammation of the meninges at base of brain, usually due to tuberculosis.

　　m., cerebral. Acute or chronic meningitis of the brain.

　　m., cerebrospinal. Meningitis of brain and spinal cord.

　　m., pneumococcal. Meningitis caused by the pneumococcus. Common in young children.

　　m., serosa circumscripta. Meningitis accompanied by the formation of cystic accumulations of fluid that simulate tumors.

　　m., serous. Meningitis with serous exudation into the cerebral ventricles.

　　m., spinal. Meningitis of spinal cord membranes.

　　m., sterile. m., aseptic, q.v.

　　m., traumatic. Meningitis resulting from trauma to the meninges.

　　m., tuberculous. An acute inflammation of the cerebral meninges caused by the tubercle bacillus.

　　SYM: Loss of weight, gradual wasting of strength, evening rise of temperature, restlessness, irritability, and sleeplessness may exist for some time before acute symptoms come on. These are severe headache, occasional convulsions, delirium, vomiting, fever, optic neuritis.

meningitophobia (měn″ĭn-jĭt″ō-fō′bē-ă) [Gr. *meninx*, membrane, + *phobos*, fear]. A condition that simulates meningitis and is caused by fear of meningitis.

meningo- (měn-ĭn′gō) [Gr. *meninx*, membrane]. A combining form that denotes relationship to the membranes covering the spinal cord or brain.

meningoarteritis (měn-ĭn″gō-ăr″tĕr-īt′ĭs) [″ + *arteria*, artery, + *itis*, inflammation]. Inflammatory condition of the meningeal arteries.

meningocele (měn-ĭn′gō-sēl) [″ + *kele*, tumor, swelling]. Congenital hernia in which the meninges protrude through an opening of the skull or spinal column.

meningococcal vaccines. Meningococcal polysaccharide vaccines A, C, Y, and W135 are available for treating those serogroups. A vaccine for meningococcal serogroup B is not available. SEE: *meningitis, acute meningococcal.*

meningococcemia (měn-ĭn″gō-kŏk-sē′mē-ă) [″ + *kokkyx*, coccyx, + *haima*, blood]. Meningococci in the circulating blood.

meningococci (měn-ĭn″gō-kŏk′sī) Pl. of meningococcus.

meningococcidal (mě-nĭng″gō-kŏk-sī′dăl) [″ + ″ + L. *caedere*, to kill]. Lethal to meningococci.

meningococcus (měn-ĭn″gō-kŏk′ŭs) (pl. *meningococci*). A microorganism of *Neisseria meningitidis*, the causative agent of epidemic cerebral meningitis (cerebrospinal fever, spotted fever).

meningocortical (měn-ĭn″gō-kor′tĭ-kăl). Pert. to the meninges and the cortex of the brain.

meningocyte (mě-nĭng′gō-sīt) [″ + *kytos*, cell]. A macrophage of the meninges of the brain.

meningoencephalitis (měn-ĭn″gō-ĕn-sĕf″ă-lī′tĭs) [″ + *enkephalos*, brain, + *itis*, inflammation]. Inflammation of the brain and its meninges. The usual cause is a bacterial infection, but free-living amebae such as the species of *Naegleria* and *Acanthamoeba*, have also caused this condition.

   m. due to Naegleria and Acanthamoeba. Disease of brain and meninges caused by free-living amebae ordinarily found in water, soil, and decaying vegetation. Organisms that can cause this include *Naegleria fowleri, Acanthamoeba culbertsoni,* and other species of *Acanthamoeba.* SYN: *m., primary amoebic.*

   SYM: Similar to those of acute meningoencephalitis.

   TREAT: For *Naegleria* infections, amphotericin B, miconazole, tetracycline, and rifampin. All are effective, but only a few patients survive. *Acanthamoeba* species are sensitive to sulfonamides, clotrimazole, and polymyxin B sulfate.

meningoencephalocele (měn-ĭn″gō-ĕn-sĕf″ăl-ō-sēl) [″ + ″ + *kele*, tumor, swelling]. Hernial protrusion of brain and meninges through a defect in the skull.

meningoencephalomyelitis (měn-ĭn″gō-ĕn-sĕf″ăl-ō-mī-ĕl-ī′tĭs) [″ + ″ + *myelos*, marrow, + *itis*, inflammation]. Inflammation of the brain, spinal cord, and their meninges.

meningoencephalopathy (mě-nĭng″gō-ĕn-sĕf″ă-lŏp′ă-thē) [″ + ″ + *pathos*, disease]. Disease of the meninges and brain.

meningomalacia (měn-ĭn″gō-mă-lā′shē-ă) [″ + *malakia*, softening]. Softening of any membrane.

meningomyelitis (měn-ĭn″gō-mī″ĕl-ī′tĭs) [″ + *myelos*, marrow, + *itis*, inflammation]. Inflammation of spinal cord and its enveloping arachnoid and pia mater, and, less commonly, of the dura mater.

meningomyelocele (měn-ĭn″gō-mī-ĕl′ō-sēl) [″ + ″ + *kele*, tumor, swelling]. Hernia of the spinal cord and membranes through a defect in the vertebral column.

meningomyeloradiculitis (mě-nĭng″gō-mī″ĕ-lō-ră-dĭk″ū-lī′tĭs) [″ + ″ + L. *radicula*, radicle, + Gr. *itis*, inflammation]. Inflammation of the meninges, spinal cord, and brain.

meningo-osteophlebitis (mě-nĭng″gō-ŏs″tē-ō-flĕ-bī′tĭs) [″ + *osteon*, bone, + *phleps*, vein, + *itis*, inflammation]. Parosteitis and inflammation of the veins of the bone.

meningopathy (měn-ĭn-gŏp′ă-thē) [″ + *pathos*, disease, suffering]. Any pathological condition of the meninges.

meningoradicular (mě-nĭng″gō-ră-dĭk′ū-lăr) [″ + L. *radicula*, radicle]. Concerning the meninges and spinal and cerebral nerve roots.

meningoradiculitis (mě-nĭng″gō-ră-dĭk″ū-lī′tĭs) [″ + ″ + Gr. *itis*, inflammation]. Inflammation of the meninges and roots of the spinal nerves.

meningorrhachidian (měn-ĭn″gō-ră-kĭd′ē-ăn) [″ + *rhachis*, spine]. Concerning the spinal cord and meninges.

meningorrhagia (měn-ĭn″gō-rā′jē-ă) [″ + *rhegnynai*, to burst forth]. Hemorrhage of the cerebral or spinal membrane.

meningorrhea (měn-ĭn″gō-rē′ă) [″ + *rhoia*, flow]. Effusion of blood on or between the meninges.

meningosis (měn″ĭn-gō′sĭs) [″ + *osis*, condition]. The fibrous tissue union of some bones.

meningotyphoid (měn-ĭn″gō-tī′foyd). Typhoid fever with symptoms of meningitis.

meningovascular (měn-ĭn″gō-văs′kū-lăr). Pert. to blood vessels of the meninges.

meninguria (měn″ĭn-gū′rē-ă) [Gr. *meninx*, membrane, + *ouron*, urine]. Presence of membraniform shreds in urine.

meninx (mē′nĭnks) [Gr., membrane] (pl. *meninges*). [NA] Any membrane, but esp. one of the coverings of the brain or spinal cord.

meniscectomy (měn″ĭ-sěk′tō-mē) [″ + *ektome*, excision]. Removal of meniscus cartilage of the knee. SEE: *Nursing Diagnoses* in *Appendix.*

menisci (měn-ĭs′ē). Pl. of meniscus.

meniscitis (měn″ĭ-sī′tĭs) [Gr. *meniskos*, crescent, + *itis*, inflammation]. Inflamed condition of an interarticular cartilage, esp. the semilunar cartilage of the knee joint.

meniscocyte (měn-ĭs′kō-sīt) [″ + *kytos*, cell]. A crescent-shaped red blood cell. SYN: *sickle cell.*

meniscocytosis (měn-ĭs″kō-sī-tō′sĭs) [″ + ″ + *osis*, intensive]. Sickle cell anemia.

meniscus (měn-ĭs′kŭs) [Gr. *meniskos*, crescent] (pl. *menisci*). 1. Concavoconvex lens. 2. Interarticular fibrocartilage of crescent shape, found in certain joints, esp. the lateral and medial menisci (semilunar cartilages) of the knee joint. 3. The curved upper surface of a liquid in a container. The surface is convex if the liquid does not wet the container and concave if it does.

    m. articularis. [NA] Crescent-shaped interarticular fibrocartilage found in certain synovial joints.

Menkes disease. Metabolic defect blocking the absorption of copper in the gastrointestinal tract. Referred to as "kinky hair" or "steely hair" disease.

meno-. Pert. to menses or menstruation.

menometrorrhagia (měn″ō-mět-rō-rā′jē-ă) [Gr. *men*, month, + *metra*, womb, + *rhegnynai*, to burst forth]. Irregular or excessive menstrual bleeding. SEE: *menorrhagia; metrorrhagia.*

menopause (měn′ō-pawz) [″ + *pausis*, cessation]. That period which marks the permanent cessation of menstrual activity. Usually occurs between the ages of 35 and 58. The menses may stop suddenly, there may be a decreased flow each month until a final cessation, or the interval between periods may be lengthened until complete cessation is accomplished.

    Natural menopause will occur in 25% of women by age 47, in 50% by age 50, 75% by age 52, and in 95% by age 55. Menopause due to surgical removal of the ovaries has occurred in almost 30% of U.S. women who are 50 years of age or older. Women with short menstrual cycles may reach menopause as much as two years earlier than women with long cycles. SYN: *change of life; climacteric.* SEE: *osteoporosis.*

    SYM: The symptoms that may be associated with menopause begin soon following the cessation of ovarian function. This is true whether menopause occurs naturally or is due to surgical removal of the ovaries or failure of the pituitary gland to function.

Symptoms that may last from a few months to years vary from being hardly noticeable to severe. Included are symptoms of vasomotor instability, nervousness, hot flashes, chills, excitability, fatigue, apathy, mental depression, crying following circumstances that would not normally cause that reaction, insomnia, palpitation, vertigo, headache, numbness, tingling, myalgia, urinary disturbances such as frequency and incontinence, and various disorders of the gastrointestinal system.

    Hot flashes, or hot flushes, may start with an aura followed by a feeling of discomfort in the abdominal area, perhaps a chill quickly followed by a feeling of heat moving toward the head. Next the face becomes red, and sweating is followed by exhaustion. The cause, or causes, of hot flashes is not completely understood and is controversial.

    Even though the popular myth is that sexual desire and activity inevitably decrease following menopause, there is little to support this. Sexual desire may remain at the pre-menopause level or be increased due to the lack of fear of pregnancy. If sexual activity decreases, it is most probably due to the lack of a socially acceptable, sexually capable partner.

    TREAT: Hormone replacement as required. However, the use of estrogen or estrogen combined with a progestogen as a cure-all in treating the symptoms of menopause has been seriously questioned due to the possibility of undesired side effects. Hormonal replacement therapy is contraindicated in those with a history of an estrogen-dependent breast tumor, thromboembolic disease, or acute liver disease. The long-term use of estrogens in order to prevent osteoporosis, q.v., is questionable. If menopause is the result of surgical removal of the ovaries, it is possible that estrogen therapy will reduce the risk of coronary disease. Yearly pelvic examination should include Papanicolaou test for cancer of the uterus and cervix.

    NURSING IMPLICATIONS: As women may experience a variety of symptoms during this period, determine their nature and severity and the impact on the individual. Explain the process of menopause as a normal phase in the reproductive cycle. If symptoms are severe, assessment by a physician may be indicated. Encourage a well-balanced diet high in calcium, vitamins and minerals. Discuss advantages and disadvantages of estrogen replacement therapy. Offer support and emotional reassurance, as symptoms can be distressing and frightening to women. Refer to written information and self-help resources.

m., artificial. Menopause occurring subsequent to surgical castration, x-ray irradiation, or radium implantation into the uterus.

m., male. SEE: *climacteric.*

m., premature. Natural or artificial menopause occurring before age 35.

m., surgical. A form of artificial menopause that follows surgical removal of the ovaries.

menophania (měn-ō-fā'nē-ä) [" + *phainesthai,* to appear]. First appearance of the menses at puberty.

menoplania (měn-ō''plā'nē-ä) [" + *plane,* deviation]. Menstruation through other than the normal outlet, as through the nose. SYN: *vicarious menstruation.*

menorrhagia (měn''ō-rā'jē-ä) [" + *rhegnynai,* to burst forth]. Excessive bleeding at the time of a menstrual period, either in number of days or amount of blood or both. SEE: *hemorrhage, uterine.*

ETIOL: Endocrine disturbances: pituitary gland, thyroid, and ovary. General systemic diseases: hypertension, diabetes mellitus, blood dyscrasias, chronic nephritis. Malpositions of the uterus: retroversion and retroflexion. New growths of the uterus: particularly fibroids of the intramural and submucous types, adenomyosis of the uterus, fibrosis of the uterus with hyperplastic changes of the endometrium. Conditions of the cervix uteri: erosions or polyps. Inflammations in the pelvis: acute salpingitis, acute metritis, acute endometritis, chronic metritis, and endometritis.

menorrhalgia (měn-ō-răl'jē-ä) [" + *rhoia,* flow, + *algia,* pain]. Painful menstruation or pelvic pain accompanying menstruation, sometimes a symptom of endometriosis. SYN: *dysmenorrhea.*

menorrhea (měn''ō-rē'ä). 1. Normal menstruation. 2. Free or profuse menstruation. SYN: *menorrhagia.*

menostasis (měn-ŏs'tă-sĭs) [" + *stasis,* standing still]. Suppression of the menses.

menostaxis (měn''ō-stăk'sĭs) [" + *staxis,* dripping]. Prolonged menstruation.

menotropins (měn''ō-trō'pĭns). USP. Combination of follicle-stimulating and luteinizing hormones (FSH and LH) used to promote growth and maturation of the follicle of the ovary. Menotropins is obtained from the urine of postmenopausal women, and a standard extract is used with human chorionic gonadotropin (HCG) to induce ovulation. Trade name is Pergonal.

menoxenia (měn-ŏk-sē'nē-ä) [" + *xenos,* strange]. Abnormal menstruation.

menses (měn'sēz) [L., month]. Monthly flow of bloody fluid from the uterine mucous membrane.

menstrual (měn'stroo-äl) [L. *menstrualis*]. Pert. to menstruation. SYN: *catamenial.*

menstrual cramps. Abdominal cramps associated with menstruation. SEE: *dysmenorrhea.*

menstrual cycle. The periodically recurrent series of changes occurring in the uterus and associated sex organs (ovaries, cervix, and vagina) associated with menstruation and the intermenstrual period. The human cycle averages 28 days in length, measured from the beginning of menstruation. The menstrual cycle is, however, quite variable in length even in the same person from month to month. Variations in the length of the cycle are due principally to variation in the length of the proliferative phase.

The menstrual cycle is divided into four phases characterized by histological changes that take place in the uterine endometrium. They are:

Proliferative Phase: Uterine epithelium is restored to normal; endometrium becomes thicker and more vascular; glands elongate. During this period the ovarian follicle is maturing and secreting estrogens. Period is terminated by rupture of follicle and liberation of ovum at about 14 days before next menstrual period begins.

Luteal or Secretory Phase: Endometrium increases in thickness; glands become more tortuous and produce an abundant secretion containing glycogen. Coiled arteries make their appearance; endometrium becomes edematous; stroma becomes compact. During this period the corpus luteum in an ovary is developing and secreting progesterone. Lasts 10 to 14 days.

Premenstrual or Ischemic Phase: A day or two before menstruation, coiled arteries constrict and endometrium becomes anemic and shrinks. Corpus luteum of ovary begins involution. Phase lasts about two days and is terminated by opening up of constricted arteries, the breaking off of small patches of necrotic endometrium, and the beginning of menstruation with the flow of menstrual fluid.

Menstruation: Period of uterine bleeding accompanied by shedding of the endometrium. Averages 4 to 5 days in length.

The menstrual cycle in normal individuals may be altered by taking birth control pills or by using an intrauterine device. In general, the former decreases the amount of flow and the latter increases it.

menstrual epilepsy. Epileptic convulsions that tend to occur at certain times during the menstrual period. SEE: *epilepsy.*

menstrual extraction. Vacuum or suction curettage of the uterus done just prior to the date of the next menstrual period. The procedure, performed using carefully controlled suction and a soft flexible catheter, is used to be certain the menstrual period is induced, even though in a sexually active individual the uterus may contain a fertilized ovum.

menstrual regulation. Vacuum or suction curettage of the uterus done within the first two weeks following the expected date of the onset of menstruation. If the amenorrhea was due to pregnancy, the procedure is classed as a form of fertility control.

menstrual synchrony. The valid observation that women living in close association, as in dormitories, may develop menstrual cycles in which the various phases are synchronized for that group.

menstruant (měn'stroo-ănt) [L. *menstruare,* to discharge the menses]. 1. In the condition of menstruating. 2. One who menstruates.

menstruate (měn'stroo-āt). To discharge menses.

menstruation (měn-stroo-ā'shŭn) [L. *menstruare,* to discharge the menses]. The periodic discharge of a bloody fluid from the uterus, occurring at more or less regular intervals during the life of a woman from age of puberty to menopause. The discharge contains altered blood with normal, hemolyzed, and sometimes agglutinated, red blood cells; disintegrated endometrial and stroma cells; and secretions of glands. In general, menstrual blood does not coagulate, but the passage of occasional clots is not unusual. Menstruation is brought on by the reduction in production of ovarian hormones, esp. progesterone, that results from involution of the corpus luteum following failure of the ovum to become fertilized. SEE: *lactation amenorrhea method; menstrual cycle; ovary* for illus.

Menstruation has its onset at puberty (9 to 17 years of age). Length of flow varies from 3 to 7 days (av. 4 to 5 days). It occurs on an average every 27 to 28 days, although time may vary from 18 to 40 days. Menstruation ceases during pregnancy; may or may not cease during lactation; and ceases permanently with the completion of menopause. Its failure to occur may result from congenital abnormalities, physical disorders (disease, obesity, malnutrition), emotional or hormonal disturbances, esp. diseases involving the ovaries, hypophysis, thyroid, or adrenal glands.

Menstrual irregularities: Absence of flow when normally expected is called *amenorrhea;* scanty flow is known as *oligomenorrhea;* painful menstruation is *dysmenorrhea.* Excessive loss of blood is termed *menorrhagia;* loss of blood during intermenstrual periods is known as spotting or *me-*

trorrhagia.

   m., anovulatory. Menstruation occurring without discharge of ovum from ovary, i.e., without ovulation.

   m., retrograde. Backflow of menstrual fluid through fallopian tubes into peritoneal cavity.

   m., suppressed. Failure of menstruation to occur when normally expected.

   m., vicarious. Menstruation from site other than the uterus when menstrual flow is expected.

menstruous (měn'stroo-ŭs). Rel. to menstruation.

menstruum (měn'stroo-ŭm) [L. *menstruus,* menstrual fluid; once it was believed that this fluid had solvent qualities]. A solvent; a medium. SEE: *vehicle.*

mensual (měn'sū-ăl) [L. *mensis,* month]. Monthly.

mensuration (měn-sū-rā'shŭn) [L. *mensuratio*]. The process of measuring.

mental. 1. [L. *mens,* mind] Rel. to the mind. 2. [L. *mentum,* chin]. Rel. to the chin.

mental age. ABBR: MA. Age of a person with respect to the intellectual development as contrasted with the chronological age.

mental deficiency. Mental retardation.

mental disorder. An imprecise and quite general term that may be described briefly as a clinically significant behavioral or psychological syndrome or pattern typically associated with either a distressing symptom or impairment of function. It is important to bear in mind that different individuals described as having the same mental disorder are not alike in the way they react to their illness and how they will need to be treated.

mental fog. Clouding of consciousness, usually with some loss of memory.

mental health. In general, mental health is the absence of mental illness. This definition, of course, is vague because of the difficulty of providing a comprehensive definition of mental illness. Nevertheless, individuals who have adjusted to life in such a way that they feel comfortable about their life situation and, at the same time, are able to live so that their behavior is not in conflict with either their associates or society are considered mentally healthy. Inherent to this, for most individuals, are a feeling of self-worth and accomplishment and the ability to be gainfully employed with sufficient reward for that employment to satisfy the economic needs required for their life situations. One can be mentally healthy without being physically healthy.

mental hygiene. Science of maintaining healthy mental and emotional responses and preventing development of psychoses.

mental illness. Any disorder that affects the

mind or behavior.

mentality. Mental power or activity.

Mental Measurements Yearbook. A widely used index of commercially published, standardized tests.

mental retardation. Below normal intellectual function that has its cause or onset during the developmental period and usually in the first years after birth. There is impaired learning, social adjustment, and maturation. The causes may be but do not have to be genetic. Rubella in the first trimester of pregnancy may be associated with mental retardation. Intrauterine trauma or infection may also cause this condition. The degree of intellectual impairment is classed on the basis of the Wechsler IQ scale as follows: 1. Mild, IQ 69–55. These children are educable. 2. Moderate, IQ 54–40. These children are trainable. 3. Severe, IQ 39–25. 4. Profound, IQ below 25. SEE: *Nursing Diagnoses* in *Appendix.*

Caution: Because the measurement of IQ may be inaccurate, its value should not be the sole basis for classifying an individual's intellectual state or potential.

mental status. The functional state of the mind as judged by the individual's behavior, appearance, responsiveness to stimuli of all kinds, speech, memory, and judgment.

mentation (měn-tā′shŭn). Mental activity. During sleep it is possible to determine the level of mental activity by studying eye movements observed through the closed eyelids and by monitoring the electrical activity of the brain by use of electroencephalography. SEE: *REM.*

Mentha [L.]. Mint; a genus of labiate plants.

　M. piperita. Peppermint.

　M. pulegium. Pennyroyal.

　M. spicata. Spearmint.

menthol. USP. $C_{10}H_{20}O$. An alcohol obtained from oil of peppermint or other mint oils. May be prepared synthetically. Occurs in crystalline form. It is an antipruritic.

menton (měn′tŏn) [L. *mentum,* chin]. A craniometric landmark, being the lowest point of the mandibular symphysis seen in a lateral radiograph. Similar to but not necessarily the same as gnathion, which is the lowest point of the mandible in the midline as palpated in the living.

mentor. A long-term relationship between a novice and an expert. The relationship is mutual and usually directed toward professional advancement and growth. The relationship may be harmonious and lead to the development of both the mentor and the protege, or it may decompensate into a state of dependency and exploitation.

mentulagra (měn″tū-lăg′ră) [L. *mentula,* penis, + Gr. *agra,* seizure]. Painful involuntary erection of the penis, sometimes curved. SYN: *priapism.* SEE: *chordee; Peyronie's disease.*

mentulate (měn′tū-lāt) [L. *mentula,* penis]. Possessing a large penis.

mentulomania (měn″tū-lō-mā′nē-ă) [″ + Gr. *mania,* madness]. Mental state characterized by addiction to masturbation.

mentum [L.]. [NA] The chin. SYN: *genion.*

mepacrine hydrochloride (měp′ă-krĭn). Quinacrine hydrochloride, USP. An antimalarial drug. Trade name is Atabrine.

mepazine (měp′ă-zēn). An antipsychotic drug.

mepenzolate bromide (mě-pěn′zō-lāt). USP. An anticholinergic drug used as an antispasmodic in treating peptic ulcer. Its action mimics belladonna. Trade name is Cantil.

meperidine hydrochloride (mě-pěr′ĭ-dēn). USP. A narcotic analgesic sold under the trade name of Demerol.

mephenesin (mě-fěn′ě-sĭn). Chemical formerly used as a skeletal muscle relaxant.

mephentermine sulfate (mě-fěn′těr-měn). USP. A drug used for its pressor effect in treating hypotension. Trade name is Wyamine Sulfate.

mephenytoin (mě-fěn′ĭ-tō-ĭn). USP. An anticonvulsive drug that is used in the lowest concentration possible in combination with other drugs. This is done because of its toxicity. Trade name is Mesantoin.

mephitic [L. *mephiticus, mephitis,* foul exhalation]. Noxious, foul, as a poisonous odor.

mephobarbital (měf″ō-bär′bĭ-tăl). USP. A hypnotic and sedative drug of the barbiturate class. Trade names are Mebaral and Menta-Bal.

Mephyton. Trade name for phytonadione, USP.

mepivacaine hydrochloride (mě-pĭv′ă-kān). USP. A local anesthetic drug. Trade name is Carbocaine.

meprednisone (mě-prěd′nĭ-sōn). USP. An adrenocorticosteroid drug. Trade name is Betapar.

meprobamate (mě-prō′bă-māt). USP. A tranquilizing agent, used for relief of anxiety and mental tension. Trade names are Equanil, Miltown, and Meprospan. SEE: *Poisons and Poisoning* in *Appendix.*

Meprospan. Trade name for meprobamate, USP.

meprylcaine hydrochloride (měp′rĭl-kān). USP. A local anesthetic drug.

mEq. *milliequivalent.*

meralgia (měr-ăl′jē-ă) [Gr. *meros,* thigh, + *algos,* pain]. Pain in the thigh.

　m. paresthetica. Pain and hyperesthesia on the outer femoral surface from lesion or disease of the external cutaneous nerve of the thigh.

merbromin (měr-brō'mǐn). An organic mercury compound used as a topical antiseptic. Its effectiveness is doubtful. Trade name is Mercurochrome.

mercaptan (měr-kăp'tăn). Any organic chemical that contains the —SH radical. It is formed when the oxygen of an alcohol is replaced by sulfur.

mercaptomerin sodium injection (měrkăp″tō-měr'ĭn). A diuretic of the organomercurial type.

mercaptopurine (měr-kăp″tō-pū'rēn). USP. An antineoplastic and immunosuppressive agent used in treating acute leukemia. Trade name is Purinethol.

Mercier's bar (měr-sē-āz') [Louis A. Mercier, Fr. urologist, 1811–1882]. A curved fold at neck of bladder forming posterior margin of trigonum vesicae.

mercurial (měr-kū'rē-ăl) [L. *mercurialis*]. 1. Pert. to mercury. 2. A substance containing mercury.

mercurial diuretics. A class of organic mercurial compounds that produce diuresis.

mercurialism (měr-kū'rē-ăl-ĭzm) [L. *mercurius*, mercury, + Gr. *-ismos*, condition]. Chronic poisoning by mercury. Seen as a result of continuous administration of mercury or occurs in persons who work with the metal or inhale its vapors.

    SYM: Soreness of gums and loosening of teeth; increased salivation; fetor of breath; griping, and diarrhea.

mercurialized (měr-kū'rē-ăl-īzd). 1. Impregnated with mercury. 2. Influenced by or treated with mercury.

mercurial palsy. Paralysis induced by mercury poisoning.

mercurial rash. Rash caused by local application of mercurial preparations.

mercuric (měr-kū'rĭk). Rel. to bivalent mercury.

    m. chloride. $HgCl_2$. A common compound of mercury used in the past as a topical antiseptic.

    m. oxide, yellow. HgO. A powder, usually yellow in color. Previously used in ointments as an antibacterial agent.

mercuric chloride poisoning. SYM: *Acute:* Those of any severe gastrointestinal irritation with pain, cramping, constriction of the throat, vomiting, and a metallic taste in the mouth. Stronger solution causes a white coating due to coagulation. Abdominal pain may be so severe as to cause fainting, bloody diarrhea, bloody vomitus, scanty urine, prostration, convulsions, and unconsciousness. Death is the usual outcome unless treatment is begun immediately.

    Chronic: Halitosis, loosening of teeth, fever, urinary difficulties, nausea, diarrhea, sore tongue, paralysis, weakness, and death.

    F.A.: Evacuate stomach, wash out with milk or with a baking soda solution made by dissolving a teaspoonful of sodium bicarbonate in 6 oz (177 ml) of water. Treatment with BAL (British antilewisite) should begin as soon as possible after poisoning has occurred. Maintain fluid and electrolyte balance. SEE: *Poisons and Poisoning* in *Appendix.*

Mercurochrome. SEE: *merbromin.*

mercurous (měr-kū'rŭs, měr'kū-rŭs). Rel. to monovalent mercury.

    m. chloride. HgCl. A heavy white powder used in small doses in medicine as a laxative. It is used in powder form as an application in ulcers and skin rashes.

mercurous chloride poisoning. SYM: Salivation, abdominal discomfort, and diarrhea. SEE: *mercuric chloride* in *Poisons and Poisoning* in *Appendix.*

mercury (měr'kū-rē) [L. *mercurius*]. SYMB: Hg. At. wt. 200.59; at. no. 80. A metallic element. Insoluble in ordinary solvents but soluble in hydrochloric acid upon boiling. It is a silvery liquid at room temperature. Forms two series of salts: mercurous, in which it has a valence of one (univalent), and mercuric, in which it has a valence of two (bivalent). SYN: *hydrargyrum; quicksilver.*

    NOTE: Metallic mercury swallowed in small quantities, as from a broken thermometer, is not harmful.

    m., ammoniated. USP. A topical antiseptic used in treating certain skin diseases.

Caution: Chronic use can cause mercury poisoning.

---

    m. bichloride. $HgCl_2$. Corrosive sublimate that is no longer used in medicine.

    m. chloride, mild. Mercurous chloride. SYN: *calomel.*

mercury in amalgam (dental) fillings. SEE: *amalgam, mercury in.*

mercury poisoning. SYM: In large doses, increased salivation, abdominal cramps, and interference with kidney function. SEE: *mercuric chloride; mercuric chloride* in *Poisons and Poisoning* in *Appendix.*

mercy (měr'sē) [L. *merces*, reward]. In medicine, the compassionate provision for relief or mitigation of physical pain, mental suffering, or psychological distress. Mercy is not being utilized if patients in pain are given narcotics or analgesics "by the clock"; i.e., even though the patient is in obvious pain, the prescribed narcotic is not given until the dictated amount of time has elapsed since the last dose. SEE: *TLC.*

meridian (mĕ-rĭd′ē-ăn). An imaginary line encircling a globular body at right angles to its equator and passing through the poles, or a half of such a line.

   m. of eye. A circle passing through anterior and posterior poles of the eyeball.

merinthophobia (mĕr-ĭn″thō-fō′bē-ă) [Gr. *merinthos,* a cord, + *phobia,* fear]. Morbid fear of being tied.

merispore (mĕr′ĭ-spor) [Gr. *meros,* a part, + *sporos,* seed]. A secondary spore resulting from the division of another spore.

meristic (mĕr-ĭs′tĭk) [Gr. *meristikos,* fit for dividing]. Bilaterally symmetrical.

mero- [Gr. *meros*]. Combining form meaning a part.

meroacrania (mĕr″ō-ă-krā′nē-ă) [″ + *a-,* not, + *kranion,* skull]. Congenital absence of a part of the cranium.

meroblastic (mĕr-ō-blăst′ĭk) [″ + *blastos,* germ]. Pert. to a type of ovum containing considerable yolk or a type of cleavage in which cleavage divisions are restricted to the protoplasmic region of the animal pole. SEE: *holoblastic ova.*

merocele (mĕr′ō-sēl) [″ + *kele,* tumor, swelling]. Femoral hernia.

merocoxalgia (mĕr″ō-kŏk-săl′jē-ă) [″ + L. *coxa,* hip, + Gr. *algos,* pain]. Painful condition of the thigh and hip.

merocrine (mĕr′ō-krĭn) [″ + *krinein,* to separate]. Pert. to a type of secretion in which the glandular cell remains intact during the process of elaborating and discharging its product. SEE: *apocrine; eccrine; holocrine.*

merodiastolic (mĕr″ō-dī-ă-stŏl′ĭk). Concerning a part of diastole of the cardiac cycle.

meroergasia (mĕr″ō-ĕr-gā′zē-ă) [Gr. *meros,* a part, + *ergasia,* work]. Partial mental disorder with symptoms of emotional instability. SEE: *holergastic.*

merogenesis (mĕr″ō-jĕn′ē-sĭs) [″ + *genesis,* generation, birth]. Multiplication or reproduction by segmentation.

merogony (mĕ-rŏg′ō-nē) [″ + *gonos,* procreation]. Incomplete development of fragments of an ovum.

meromelia (mĕr″ō-mē′lē-ă) [″ + *melos,* limb]. Partial absence of a limb.

meromicrosomia (mĕr″ō-mī″krō-sō′mē-ă) [″ + *mikros,* small, + *soma,* body]. Abnormal smallness of some part or structure of the body.

meromyosin (mĕr″ō-mī′ō-sĭn). That produced by tryptic digestion of myosin.

meronecrosis (mĕr″ō-nĕk-rō′sĭs) [″ +

nekrosis, state of death]. Death of cells.

meropia (mĕr-ō′pē-ă) [″ + *ops,* vision]. Partial blindness.

merorrhachischisis (mĕ″rō-ră-kĭs′kĭ-sĭs) [″ + *rhachis,* spine, + *schisis,* a splitting]. Fissure of a portion of the spinal cord.

merosmia (mĕr-ŏs′mē-ă) [″ + *osme,* odor]. Inability to detect certain odors.

merosystolic (mĕr″ō-sĭs-tŏl′ĭk) [″ + *systole,* a contraction]. Rel. to a portion of the systole.

merotomy (mĕr-ŏt′ō-mē) [″ + *tome,* incision]. Division into sections or segments.

merozoite (mĕr″ō-zō′ĭt) [″ + *zoon,* animal]. A body formed by segmentation or breaking up of schizont in asexual reproduction of certain sporozoans such as *Plasmodium.* Merozoites when formed are liberated and invade other corpuscles, where they repeat the process of schizogony, or develop into gametocytes.

merozygote (mĕr″ō-zī′gōt) [″ + *zygotos,* yoked together]. A bacterial mechanism of gene transfer in which part of the genome, or chromosome complement, is transferred into an intact recipient cell.

Merthiolate. Trade name for thimerosal.

Meruvax. Trade name for rubella virus vaccine, live.

mesad (mē′săd) [Gr. *mesos,* middle, + L. *ad,* toward]. Toward a median point, line, or plane.

mesal (mē′săl). Toward the middle point or midline plane. SYN: *mesial.*

mesangium (mĕs-ăn′jē-ŭm). The suspensory structure of the renal glomerulus.

Mesantoin. Trade name for mephenytoin, USP.

mesaortitis (mĕs″ā-or-tī′tĭs) [″ + *aorte,* aorta + *itis,* inflammation]. Inflammation of the middle aortic coat.

mesaraic, mesareic (mĕs-ă-rā′ĭk, -rī′ĭk) [Gr. *mesaraion,* the mesentery]. Rel. to the mesentery. SYN: *mesenteric.*

mesarteritis (mĕs-ăr-tĕr-ī′tĭs). Inflammation of the tunica media or middle coat of an artery.

mesaticephalic (mĕs-ăt″ĭ-sĕf-ăl′ĭk) [Gr. *mesatos,* medium, + *kephale,* brain]. Having a skull with a cephalic index of 75 to 79.9.

mesatipellic, mesatipelvic (mĕs-ăt″ĭ-pĕl′lĭk, -pĕl′vĭk) [″ + *pella,* bowl]. Having a pelvis with an index between 90 and 95.

mescaline (mĕs′kă-lēn). A poisonous alkaloid, the active ingredient of the mescal buttons of the cactus plant *Lophophora williamsii,* which causes hallucinations, esp. those involving color and music.

mescalism (mĕs′kă-lĭzm). Intoxication produced by ingesting mescal.

mesectoderm (mĕs-ĕk′tō-derm). Migratory

cells derived from ectoderm, esp. from the neural crest of the cephalic area in young embryos; they become pigment cells.

mesencephalitis (mĕs″ĕn-sĕf″ă-lī′tĭs) [″ + *enkephalos,* brain, + *itis,* inflammation]. Inflammation of the mesencephalon.

mesencephalon (mĕs-ĕn-sĕf′ă-lŏn) [″ + *enkephalos,* brain]. [NA] The midbrain, one of three primitive cerebral vesicles from which develop the corpora quadrigemina, the crura cerebri, and the aqueduct of Sylvius.

mesencephalotomy (mĕs″ĕn-sĕf″ă-lŏt′ō-mē) [″ + ″ + *tome,* incision]. Surgical incision of the midbrain. Usually done to relieve intractable pain.

mesenchyme (mĕs′ĕn-kīm) [″ + *enchyma,* infusion]. A diffuse network of cells forming the embryonic mesoderm and giving rise to connective tissues, blood and blood vessels, the lymphatic system, and cells of the reticuloendothelial system.

mesenchymoma (mĕs″ĕn-kī-mō′mă). A neoplasm containing a mixture of mesenchymal and fibrous tissue.

mesenterectomy (mĕs″ĕn-tĕ-rĕk′tō-mē) [″ + *enteron,* intestine, + *ektome,* excision]. Surgical removal of the mesentery.

mesenteric (mĕs″ĕn-tĕr′ĭk) [Gr. *mesenterikos*]. Pert. to the mesentery. SYN: *mesaraic.*

mesenteriolum (mĕs-ĕn″tĕr-ī′ō-lŭm) [L.]. A small mesentery, as that of a diverticulum of the intestine.

mesenteriopexy (mĕs″ĕn-tĕr′ē-ō-pĕk″sē) [″ + *enteron,* intestine, + *pexis,* fixation]. Operation for attaching a torn mesentery.

mesenteriorrhaphy (mĕs″ĕn-tĕr-ē-or′ă-fē) [″ + ″ + *rhaphe,* seam, ridge]. Suturing of the mesentery. SYN: *mesorrhaphy.*

mesenteriplication (mĕs″ĕn-tĕr″ĭ-plĭ-kā′shŭn) [″ + ″ + L. *plicare,* to fold]. Shortening the mesentery by taking tucks in it surgically.

mesenteritis (mĕs″ĕn-tĕr-ī′tĭs) [″ + ″ + *itis,* inflammation]. Inflamed condition of the mesentery.

mesenterium (mĕs″ĕn-tē′rē-ŭm). Mesentery.

mesenteron (mĕs-ĕn′tĕr-ŏn). Middle portion of the embryonic digestic tract.

mesentery (mĕs′ĕn-tĕr″ē) [″ + *enteron,* intestine]. A peritoneal fold encircling the greater part of the small intestines and connecting the intestine to the posterior abdominal wall.

MESH. *M*edical *S*ubject *H*eadings. A list of the medical words used in storing and retrieving medical references by the U.S. National Library of Medicine. SEE: *MEDLARS.*

mesiad (mē′zē-ăd) [″ + L. *ad,* toward].

Toward the median plane of a body or part. SYN: *mesad.*

mesial (mē′zē-ăl). Toward the middle point or midline plane. In dentistry, ventral or nearer to the center of the dental arch.

mesial drift. The natural tendency for teeth to move in a mesial direction within the dental arch to maintain tight interproximal contacts between adjacent teeth. Also called physiological tooth movement. SEE: *tooth migration, pathologic; tooth migration, physiologic; tooth movement.*

mesio- [Gr. *mesos,* middle]. A combining form meaning toward the middle. In dentistry, pertaining to the ventral surface of teeth or ventrally toward the center of the dental arch.

mesiobuccal (mē″zē-ō-bŭk′kăl). Concerning the mesial and buccal surfaces of a tooth or the surfaces involved in a cavity in the tooth.

mesiobucco-occlusal (mē″zē-ō-bŭk″kō-ō-kloo′zăl). Concerning the mesial, buccal, and occlusal surfaces of a tooth.

mesiobuccopulpal (mē″zē-ō-bŭk″kō-pŭl′păl). Concerning the mesial, buccal, and pulpal sides of a tooth cavity.

mesiocervical (mē″zē-ō-sĕr′vĭ-kăl). Concerning the mesial surface of the neck of a tooth.

mesioclusion (mē″zē-ō-kloo′zhŭn). Malocclusion of the lower teeth. They are positioned in front of their normal position with respect to the upper teeth.

mesiodens (mē′zē-ō-dĕnz). A supernumerary tooth, often paired, that has a small, cone-shaped crown and a short root and appears between the maxillary central incisors.

mesiodistal (mē″zē-ō-dĭs′tăl). Concerning the mesial and distal surfaces of a tooth.

mesiogingival (mē″zē-ō-jĭn′jĭ-văl). Concerning the mesial and gingival walls of a tooth cavity.

mesiolabial (mē″zē-ō-lā′bē-ăl). Concerning the mesial and labial surfaces of a tooth or cavity.

mesiolingual (mē″zē-ō-lĭng′gwăl). Concerning the mesial and lingual surfaces of a tooth or cavity.

mesiolinguo-occlusal (mē″zē-ō-lĭng′gwō-ō-kloo′zăl). Concerning the mesial, lingual, and occlusal surfaces of a tooth.

mesiolinguopulpal (mē″zē-ō-lĭng′gwō-pŭl′păl). Concerning the mesial, lingual, and pulpal sides of a tooth cavity.

mesion (mē′sē-ŏn) [Gr. *mesos,* middle]. The imaginary plane dividing the body into right and left symmetric halves. SYN: *meson* (def. 2).

mesiopulpal (mē″zē-ō-pŭl′păl). Concerning the mesial and pulpal sides of a tooth cavity.

mesioversion (mē″zē-ō-vĕr′zhŭn). Displacement of a tooth posteriorly in the dental arch.

mesiris (měs-ī′rĭs). Middle portion of the iris.

mesmeric (měs-měr′ĭk) [Franz Anton Mesmer, Austrian physician, 1734–1815]. Rel. to or induced by hypnotism.

mesmerism (měs′měr-ĭzm). Originally Mesmer's theory of animal magnetism, it now means therapeutics employing hypnotism or hypnotic suggestion.

mesna. A synthetic sulfhydryl compound used with ifosamide in treating metastatic germ-cell testicular cancer. Trade name is Mesnex. SEE: *ifosfamide; testicular cancer, germ-cell.*

meso- [Gr. *mesos,* middle]. Combining form meaning (1) middle; (2) in anatomy, pert. to a mesentery; (3) in medicine, secondary or partial.

mesoappendicitis. Inflamed condition of the mesoappendix.

mesoappendix (měs″ō-ă-pěn′dĭks) [Gr. *mesos,* middle, + L. *appendix,* an appendage]. [NA] Mesentery of the vermiform appendix.

mesoarium (měs″ō-ā′rē-ŭm). Mesovarium, q.v.

mesoblast (měs′ō-blăst) [″ + *blastos,* germ]. Mesoderm.

mesobronchitis (měs″ō-brŏng-kī′tĭs). Inflammation of the middle layer of the bronchi.

mesocardia (měs″ō-kăr′dē-ă) [″ + *kardia,* heart]. Location of the heart in the middle line of the thorax, being a normal position in fetal stage but a malposition after birth.

mesocardium (měs-ō-kăr′dē-ŭm). An embryonic mesentery supporting the heart. The dorsal mesocardium connects the heart to the foregut, and the ventral mesocardium connects the heart to the central body wall.

mesocarpal (měs″ō-kăr′păl). Mediocarpal.

mesocecum (měs″ō-sē′kŭm) [″ + L. *caecum,* blindness]. Part of the mesentery that connects the cecum to the right iliac fossa.

mesocele (měs′ō-sēl) [″ + *koilia,* hollow]. Sylvian aqueduct in the brain.

mesocephalic (měs″ō-sě-făl′ĭk) [″ + *kephale,* head]. 1. Pert. to the midbrain. 2. Having a medium-sized head, with a cranial index of 76.0 to 80.9.

mesocephalon (měs″ō-sěf′ă-lŏn). The mesencephalon, q.v.

mesocolic (měs″ō-kŏl′ĭk). Concerning the mesocolon.

mesocolon (měs″ō-kō′lŏn) [″ + *kolon,* colon]. [NA] Mesentery connecting the colon with the posterior abdominal wall.

mesocolopexy (měs″ō-kō′lō-pěk″sē) [″ + ″ + *pexis,* fixation]. The taking of tucks in the mesocolon and then suturing it to shorten it in order to correct unneeded mobility and ptosis.

mesocoloplication (měs″ō-kō″lō-plĭ-kā′shŭn) [″ + ″ + L. *plicare,* to fold]. Plication of the mesocolon in order to stabilize it.

mesocord. A portion of umbilical cord attached to the placenta by means of an amniotic fold.

mesocuneiform (měs″ō-kū′nē-ĭ-form). The intermediate cuneiform bone of the ankle.

mesoderm (měs′ō-děrm) [″ + *derma,* skin]. A primary germ layer of the embryo lying between ectoderm and entoderm. From it arise all connective tissues; muscular, skeletal, circulatory, lymphatic, and urogenital systems; and the linings of the body cavities. SEE: *ectoderm; entoderm.*

m., axial. Portion of the mesoderm that gives rise to the notochord and prechordal plate.

m., extraembryonic. Mesoderm lying outside the embryo proper. It is involved in formation of amnion, chorion, yolk sac, and body stalk.

m., intermediate. Mesoderm lying between somite and lateral mesoderm. Gives rise to embryonic and definitive kidneys and their ducts. SYN: *mesomere; nephrotome.*

m., lateral. Unsegmented mesoderm lying lateral to the intermediate mesoderm. In it develops a cavity, the coelom, separating it into layers, the somatic and splanchnic mesoderm. SYN: *hypomere.*

m., paraxial. Mesoderm lying immediately lateral to the neural tube and notochord.

m., somatic. Outer layer of lateral mesoderm. Becomes intimately associated with ectoderm, forming the somatopleure, from which ventral and lateral walls of the embryo develop.

m., splanchnic. Inner layer of lateral mesoderm. Becomes intimately associated with entoderm, forming the splanchnopleure, from which the gut and lungs and their coverings arise.

mesodiastolic (měs″ō-dī″ă-stŏl′ĭk). In middiastole of the heartbeat sequence.

mesodont (měs′ō-dŏnt). Having teeth of medium size; a dental index of 42 to 43.9.

mesoduodenum (měs″ō-dū″ō-dē′nŭm). Mesentery connecting the duodenum to the abdominal wall.

mesoepididymis (měs″ō-ěp″ĭ-dĭd′ĭ-mĭs). A fold of the tunica vaginalis that is not always present. It binds the epididymis to the testicle.

mesogastric (měs″ō-găs′trĭk). 1. Pert. to umbilical region. 2. Pert. to the mesogastrium.

mesogastrium (mĕs″ō-găs′trē-ŭm) [″ + *gaster,* belly]. 1. [NA] The umbilical region. 2. The part of the mesentery of the embryo attached to the primitive stomach.

mesoglia (mĕ-sŏg′lē-ă). Phagocytes present in the neuroglia. They probably arise in the mesoderm.

mesogluteal (mĕs″ō-gloo′tē-ăl). Concerning the gluteus medius muscle.

mesogluteus (mĕs″ō-gloo′tē-ŭs). The gluteus medius muscle.

mesognathion (mĕs-ŏg-nā′thē-ŏn). A point in the lateral portion of the intermaxillary bone or premaxilla.

mesognathous. Having a facial profile that protrudes slightly from the vertical line between nasion and gnathion. Also called mesognathic. SEE: *prognathous.*

mesohyloma (mĕs″ō-hī-lō′mă) [″ + *hyle,* matter, + *oma,* tumor]. Tumor derived from the mesothelium.

mesoileum (mĕs″ō-ĭl′ē-ŭm). Mesentery of the ileum.

mesojejunum (mĕs″ō-jē-jū′nŭm). Mesentery of the jejunum.

mesolymphocyte (mĕs″ō-lĭm′fō-sīt). A moderate-sized lymphocyte.

mesomere (mĕs′ō-mēr) [″ + *meros,* part]. 1. Portion of the mesoderm between epimere and hypomere. SYN: *nephrotome; mesoderm, intermediate.* 2. A blastomere that is intermediate in size between a micromere and a macromere.

mesometritis (mĕs-ō-mē-trī′tĭs) [″ + *metra,* uterus, + *itis,* inflammation]. Inflammation of the uterine musculature. SYN: *myometritis.*

mesometrium (mĕs″ō-mē′trē-ŭm). 1. The uterine musculature. 2. [NA] The broad ligament below the mesovarium.

mesomorph (mĕs′ō-morf). Body build characterized by predominance of tissues derived from the mesoderm; a well-proportioned individual. SEE: *ectomorph; endomorph; somatotype.*

meson (mĕs′ŏn, mē′sŏn) [Gr. *mesos,* middle]. 1. Particle of mass intermediate between that of the electron and proton. Mesons of more than one variety and of both positive and negative charge occur. SYN: *mesotron.* 2. Mesion.

mesonasal (mĕs″ō-nā′zăl). In the middle of the nose.

mesonephric (mĕs″ō-nĕf′rĭk) [″ + *nephros,* kidney]. Pert. to the mesonephros.

mesonephric duct. Embryonic duct that gives rise in the male to reproductive ducts (ductus epididymidis, ductus deferens, seminal vesicle, and ejaculatory duct). In the female, it gives rise to Gartner's duct of the epoophoron, a rudimentary structure. SYN: *wolffian duct.*

mesonephric tubules. Embryonic tubules consisting of two groups, cranial and caudal. The cranial group gives rise in the male to the efferent ductules of the testes and appendix epididymis; in the female, it gives rise to the epoophoron and vesicular appendices. The caudal group gives rise in the male to the paradidymis and aberrant ductules; in the female, it gives rise to the paroophoron. All structures except the efferent ductules of the testes are vestigial. SYN: *wolffian tubules.*

mesonephroma (mĕs″ō-nē-frō′mă) [″ + *nephros,* kidney, + *oma,* tumor]. A relatively rare tumor derived from mesonephric cells developing in reproductive organs, esp. ovary or genital tract.

mesonephros (mĕs″ō-nĕf′rŏs) (pl. *mesonephroi*). [NA] A type of kidney that develops in all vertebrate embryos of classes above the Cyclostomes. It is the permanent kidney of fishes and amphibians but is replaced by the metanephros in reptiles and mammals. SYN: *wolffian body.*

mesoneuritis (mĕs-ō-nū-rī′tĭs) [″ + *neuron,* nerve, + *itis,* inflammation]. Inflammation of the substance of a nerve or of its lymphatics.

meso-ontomorph (mĕs″ō-ŏn′tō-morf). A broad, husky body type.

mesopexy (mĕs′ō-pĕks″ē) [″ + *pexis,* fixation]. Surgery to attach a torn mesentery.

mesophilic (mĕs-ō-fĭl′ĭk) [″ + *philein,* to love]. Preferring moderate temperature, as some bacteria, which develop best at temperatures between 15° and 43°C.

mesophlebitis (mĕs″ō-flĕ-bī′tĭs). Inflammation of the medial layer of the wall of a vein.

mesophragma (mĕs″ō-frăg′mă) [″ + *phragmos,* a fencing in]. A band in the center of the A-band in the myofibrils of a striated muscle.

mesophryon (mĕs-ŏf′rē-ŏn) [″ + *ophrys,* eyebrow]. Midpoint in smooth space between the eyebrows. SEE: *glabella.*

mesopic (mĕs-ŏp′ĭk). Pert. to vision at low levels of light, e.g., at twilight.

mesopneumon (mĕs″ō-nū′mŏn) [″ + *pneumon,* lung]. Meeting point of two pleural layers at the hilus of the lung.

mesoporphyrin. $C_{34}H_{38}O_4N_4$. An iron-free derivative of hemin.

mesoprosopic (mĕs″ō-prō-sŏp′ĭk) [″ + *prosopon,* face]. Pert. to a face of moderate width; a facial index of 90.

mesopulmonum (mĕs″ō-pŭl-mō′nŭm). The mesentery of the lung.

mesorchium (mĕs-or′kē-ŭm) [″ + *orchis,* testicle]. [NA] Peritoneal fold that holds fetal testes in place.

mesorectum (mĕs″ō-rĕk′tŭm). Mesentery of

the rectum.

mesoridazine besylate (měs″ō-rĭd′ă-zēn). USP. A drug used in treating psychoses.

mesoropter (měs-ō-rŏp′tĕr) [″ + *horos*, boundary, + *opter*, observer]. Normal eye position with muscles at rest.

mesorrhachischisis (měs″ō-ră-kĭs′kĭ-sĭs) [″ + *rhachis*, spine, + *schisis*, a splitting]. Fissure of a portion of the spinal cord. SYN: *merorrhachischisis*.

mesorrhaphy (měs-or′ă-fē) [″ + *rhaphe*, seam, ridge]. Suture of the mesentery. SYN: *mesenteriorrhaphy*.

mesorrhine (měs′ō-rīn) [″ + *rhis*, nose]. With a nasal index variously quoted to range between 48 and 53.

mesosalpinx (měs″ō-săl′pĭnks) [″ + *salpinx*, tube]. [NA] The free margin of the upper division of the broad ligament within which lies the oviduct.

mesoseme (měs′ō-sēm) [″ + *sema*, sign]. Possessing an orbital index between 83 and 89.

mesosigmoid (měs-ō-sĭg′moyd). Mesentery of the sigmoid flexure.

mesosigmoiditis (měs″ō-sĭg″moy-dī′tĭs). Inflammation of the sigmoid colon.

mesosigmoidopexy (měs″ō-sĭg-moy′dō-pĕk″sē). Surgical fixation of the sigmoid colon.

mesoskelic (měs-ō-skěl′ĭk) [″ + *skelos*, leg]. Legs of normal length.

mesosome (měs′ō-sōm) [″ + *soma*, body]. In some bacteria, one or more large irregular convoluted invaginations of the cytoplasmic membrane. Mesosomes are larger in gram-positive than in gram-negative bacteria. Their function in the cell is not well understood.

mesosternum (měs″ō-stěr′nŭm) [″ + *sternon*, chest]. The middle or second section of the sternum. SYN: *gladiolus*.

mesosystolic (měs″ō-sĭs-tŏl′ĭk). Midsystolic portion of the cardiac cycle.

mesotarsal (měs″ō-tăr′săl). Mediotarsal, q.v.

mesotendineum (měs″ō-tĕn-dĭn′ē-ŭm). The part of the synovial sheath of a tendon that connects the lining of the tendon sheath to the fibrous sheath covering the tendon.

mesotendon. Tissue lining a fibrous sheath attaching the sheath to the tendon.

mesothelial (měs″ō-thē′lē-ăl). Concerning the mesothelium.

mesothelioma (měs″ō-thē-lē-ō′mă). A rare malignant tumor of the mesothelium of the pleura, pericardium, or peritoneum.

mesothelium (měs″ō-thē′lē-ŭm) [″ + *epi*, at, + *thele*, nipple]. [NA] The layer of cells derived from the mesoderm lining the primitive body cavity. In the adult it be-

comes the epithelium covering the serous membranes.

mesothenar (měs″ō-thē′năr) [″ + *thenar*, palm]. The adductor pollicis muscle.

mesothorium (měs″ō-thō′rē-ŭm). The first two disintegration products of thorium.

mesotron. A subatomic particle of weight intermediate between light particles (electrons) and heavy particles (protons). SYN: *meson* (def. 1).

mesouranic (měs″ō-ū-răn′ĭk). Having a palatal index between 110 and 114.9.

mesovarium (měs″ō-vā′rē-ŭm). [NA] The portion of the peritoneal fold that connects the anterior border of the ovary to the posterior layer of the broad ligament.

Mestinon. Trade name for pyridostigmine bromide, USP.

mestranol (měs′trä-nōl). USP. An estrogen used in combination with progestational drugs in some birth control pill formulations.

MET. *metabolic equivalent.*

meta- (mět′ă) [Gr. *meta*, after, beyond, over]. 1. Prefix denoting change, transformation, or following something in a series. 2. In chemistry, prefix indicating the 1,3 position of benzene derivatives.

meta-analysis. A statistical procedure for combining data from a number of studies and investigations in order to analyze the therapeutic effectiveness of specific treatments and plan future studies. Data obtained from combined studies must be compatible in order to be evaluated by this method.

metabiosis (mět′ă-bī-ō′sĭs) [″ + *biosis*, way of life]. Dependence of an organism for its existence upon another. SYN: *commensalism*. SEE: *symbiosis*.

metabolic (mět″ă-bŏl′ĭk) [Gr. *metaballein*, to change]. Pert. to metabolism.

metabolic balance. Comparison of the intake and excretion of a specific nutrient. The balance may be negative when an excess of the nutrient is excreted or positive when more is taken in than excreted.

metabolic body size. Body weight in kilograms to the three-fourths power ($kg^{0.75}$), representative of the active tissue mass or metabolic mass of an individual.

metabolic equivalent. ABBR: MET. Unit used to estimate the metabolic cost of physical activity. One MET equals the uptake of 3.5 ml of oxygen per kilogram of body weight per minute.

metabolic failure. Rapid failure of physical and mental functions ending in death.

metabolic gradient. A gradient in metabolic activity that exists in certain structures such as the small intestine from duodenum to ileum or in embryos from animal to vegetal poles in which metabolic activity is highest in one region and becomes progressively lower away from this region.

metabolic rate. The rate of utilization of energy. This is usually measured at a time when the subject is completely at rest and in a fasting state. Energy used is calculated from the amount of oxygen used during the test. The clinical usefulness of this test is doubtful. SEE: *basal metabolic rate; metabolism, basal.*

metabolimeter (mĕt″ă-bō-lĭm′ĕ-tĕr) [Gr. *meta,* after, beyond, over, + *biosis,* way of life, + *metron,* measure]. Device for measuring the metabolic rate.

metabolism [″ + *-ismos,* state of]. The sum of all physical and chemical changes that take place within an organism; all energy and material transformations that occur within living cells. It includes material changes, i.e., changes undergone by substances during all periods of life (growth, maturity, senescence) and energy changes, i.e., all transformations of chemical energy of foodstuffs to mechanical energy or heat. It involves two fundamental processes: anabolism (assimilation or building-up processes) and catabolism (disintegration or tearing-down processes). Anabolism is the conversion of ingested substances into the constituents of protoplasm; catabolism is the breakdown of substances into simpler substances, the end products usually being excreted.

Inborn errors of metabolism are a group of inherited metabolic diseases caused by the absence of deficiency of specific enzymes essential to the metabolism of basic substances such as amino acids, carbohydrates, vitamins, or essential trace elements. Examples include phenylketonuria and hereditary fructose intolerance.

     m., basal. Lowest level of energy expenditure. It is determined when the body is at complete rest. For an average person, this is, in terms of Cal, approx. 1500 to 1800 per day; in terms of body weight, 1 Cal per kilogram per hour; in terms of body surface, 40 Cal per sq. meter per hour.

     m., carbohydrate. All carbohydrates are digested to monosaccharides and absorbed as such principally in the form of hexoses, of which glucose is the principal one. In the liver and muscles, glucose is converted to glycogen or it may be oxidized to carbon dioxide and water, the ultimate fate of all carbohydrates. These reactions require the presence of insulin and other hormones. In the process, many intermediate compounds are formed, among them lactic acid. The basic reaction is

$$C_6H_{12}O_6 + 6O_2 \rightarrow 6CO_2 + 6H_2O$$

which is the basis for the determination of the respiratory quotient (R.Q.). SEE: *quotient, respiratory.*

     m., constructive. The building-up processes by which complex substances are synthesized. SYN: *anabolism; assimilation.*

     m., destructive. The breakdown or decomposition of substances into their simple constituents. SYN: *catabolism.*

     m., fat. Fats are digested to fatty acids and glycerol. Following absorption they may be reconverted to neutral fats and stored as adipose tissue or oxidized to CO_2 and H_2O. Fats may be formed from carbohydrates or proteins. In the utilization of fats, the liver plays an important role in the desaturation of fatty acids. Fat metabolism also involves the formation and utilization of substances related to fats, such as sterols and phospholipids.

     m., general. Includes all processes involved in utilization of substances entering the body.

     m., muscle. SEE: *muscle metabolism.*

     m., protein. Proteins are digested to amino acids and absorbed as such. In the body these are synthesized into body proteins, which form an integral part of protoplasm; thus, they are essential for normal growth, development, and repair of tissues. Those not utilized thus are deaminized; i.e., the amino, NH, group is removed. This results in the production of urea, which is excreted; the remainder, a fatty acid residue (COOH), may be oxidized or converted to glucose, which may be stored as glycogen or converted to fat.

     m., purine. Metabolism involving nucleic acids, present in nuclei of cells, in which they are combined with proteins to form nucleoproteins. In the breakdown of nucleic acid, uric acid, one of the end products, is formed.

     m., special. Applies to all changes involved in utilization of particular substances such as carbohydrates, proteins, fats, minerals, or water. Referred to as carbohydrate metabolism, protein metabolism, etc.

metabolite (mĕ-tăb′ō-līt). Any product of metabolism.

metabolize (mĕ-tăb′ō-līz) [Gr. *metaballein,* to change]. To alter the character of a food substance by metabolic reactions.

metacarpal [Gr. *meta,* after, beyond, over, + *karpos,* wrist]. Pert. to the bones of the metacarpus or bones of the hand. SEE: *skeleton.*

metacarpectomy (mĕt″ă-kăr-pĕk′tō-mē) [″

+ " + *ektome*, excision]. Surgical excision or resection of one or more wrist bones.

metacarpophalangeal (mĕt″ă-kăr″pō-fă-lăn′jē-ăl). Concerning the metacarpus and the phalanges.

metacarpus (mĕt″ă-kăr′pŭs) [" + *karpos*, wrist]. [NA] The five metacarpal bones of the palm of the hand. SEE: *carpometacarpal.*

metacentric (mĕt″ă-sĕn′trĭk). Term indicating a chromosome with the centromere in the median position. Thus the arms of the chromosome are of equal length.

metacercaria (mĕt″ă-sĕr-kā′rē-ă). The encysted stage in the life history of a trematode. This stage occurs in an intermediate host prior to transfer to the definitive host.

metachromasia, metachromatism (mĕt″ă-krō-mā′zē-ă, -krōm′ă-tĭzm) [Gr. *meta*, change, + *chroma*, color]. Condition in which different components of the same tissue assume different colors or shades of color. The colors are different from those of the dye used.

metachromatic (mĕt″ă-krō-măt′ĭk). Pert. to metachromatism.

metachromatic granules. Granules that stain a different color from that of the dye used.

metachromatic leukodystrophy. A fatal disease of infancy, caused by a deficiency of the enzyme aryl sulfatase A. Metachromatic material is deposited in the brain, peripheral nerves, liver, kidney, and frequently the urine. This material, sulfated lipids, would normally be degraded to cerebrosides. There is no specific therapy.

metachromophil (mĕt-ă-krōm′ō-fĭl) [" + *chroma*, color, + *philein*, to love]. Not reacting normally to staining.

metachrosis (mĕt-ă-krō′sĭs). Change of color in animal life, as in the chameleon.

metacone [Gr. *meta*, after, beyond, over, + *konos*, cone]. The distobuccal cusp of an upper molar tooth.

metaconid (mĕt-ă-kŏn′ĭd). The mesiolingual cusp of a lower molar tooth.

metaconule (mĕt-ă-kŏn′ūl). The distal intermediate cusp of an upper molar tooth.

metacyesis (mĕt-ă-sī-ē′sĭs) [" + *kyesis*, pregnancy]. Extrauterine gestation.

metagenesis [" + *genesis*, generation, birth]. Alternation of generations, esp. involving regular alternation of sexual with asexual reproduction. Seen in some fungi.

metagglutinin (mĕt″ă-gloo′tĭn-ĭn) [" + L. *agglutinare*, glue]. A partial agglutinin; an agglutinin present in immune serum that acts on organisms closely related to the one acting as the specific antigen.

Metagonimus (mĕt″ă-gŏn′ĭ-mŭs) [" +

gonimos, productive]. A genus of flukes belonging to the family Heterophyidae.

M. yokogawai. A species of intestinal flukes common in the Middle and Far East. Normally infests the intestines of dogs, cats, and other animals, but commonly found in man also. Intermediate hosts: snails and fish, esp. a species of trout, *Plecoglossus altivelis.*

Metahydrin. Trade name for trichlormethiazide.

metainfective (mĕt″ă-ĭn-fĕk′tĭv). Occurring subsequent to an infection.

metakinesis (mĕt″ă-kĭ-nē′sĭs). Moving apart, esp. the moving of the two chromatids of each chromosome away from each other as they move to opposite poles in the anaphase of mitosis.

metalbumin (mĕt-ăl-bū′mĭn). The mucin present in ovarian cysts. SYN: *pseudomucin.*

metal fume fever. A syndrome resembling influenza produced by inhalation of excessive concentrations of metallic oxide fumes such as zinc oxide or antimony, arsenic, cadmium, cobalt, copper, iron, lead, magnesium, manganese, mercury, nickel, or tin. Occurs in persons whose occupations lead to exposure to these metals. SEE: *polymer fume fever.*

SYM: Onset of symptoms is usually delayed. Chills, weakness, lassitude, profound thirst, followed after some hours by sweating and anorexia; occasionally there is mild inflammation of the eyes and respiratory tract. The symptoms are more acute at the beginning of the work week than at the end. This is felt to be due to the individual's adapting to the fumes as exposure continues.

F.A.: Fresh air and symptomatic treatment.

metallesthesia (mĕt″ăl-ĕs-thē′sē-ă) [Gr. *metallon*, metal, + *aisthesis*, sensation]. Recognition of metals by touching them.

metallic. 1. Pert. to metal. 2. Composed of or resembling a metal.

metallic tinkling. A peculiar ringing or bell-like auscultatory sound in pneumothorax over large pulmonary cavities.

metalloenzyme (mĕ-tăl″ō-ĕn′zīm). An enzyme that contains a metal ion in its structure.

metalloid (mĕt′ăl-loyd) [" + *eidos*, form, shape]. Resembling a metal.

metallophilia (mĕ-tăl″ō-fĭl′ē-ă) [" + *philein*, to love]. The property of some tissues of binding certain metal salts.

metallophobia (mĕ″tăl-ō-fō′bē-ă) [" + *phobos*, fear]. Abnormal fear of metals and metallic objects and of touching them.

metalloporphyrin (mĕ-tăl″ō-por′fĭ-rĭn). Porphyrin combined with a metal. Ex.: iron with heme to form hemoglobin; magnesium in chlorophyll.

metalloprotein (mĕ-tăl″ō-prō′tē-ĭn). A protein bound with metal ions.

metalloscopy (mĕt-ăl-ŏs′kō-pē) [″ + *skopein*, to examine]. Determination of the effects of applying metals to the body and the body's sensitivity to them.

metallotherapy (mĕt″ăl-ō-thĕr′ă-pē) [″ + *therapeuein*, to heal]. Treatment of disease by applying metals to the affected part.

metallurgy (mĕt″ăl-ŭr′jē) [″ + *ergon*, work]. Science of obtaining metals from their ores, refining them, and making them into various shapes and forms.

metamer (mĕt′ă-mĕr). Something similar to but different from something else. Ex.: isomers of chemical compounds.

metamere (mĕt′ă-mēr) [Gr. *meta*, after, beyond, over, + *meros*, part]. One of a series of similar segments arranged in a linear series and making up the body of an animal such as an earthworm.

metameric (mĕt-ă-mĕr′ĭk). Rel. to metamerism. SYN: *isomeric.*

metamerism (mĕ-tăm′ĕr-ĭzm). 1. Isomerism, q.v. 2. Isomerism consisting of segments or metameres.

metamorphopsia (mĕt″ă-mor-fŏp′sē-ă) [Gr. *meta*, after, beyond, over, + *morphe*, form, + *opsis*, vision]. In ophthalmology, visual distortion of objects; found in refractive errors, esp. astigmatism, retinal disease, choroiditis, detachment of retina, and tumors of retina and choroid.

metamorphosis (mĕt″ă-mor′fō-sĭs) [″ + *morphosis*, bringing into shape]. 1. A change in form or structure, esp. the transition from one form to another as in complete metamorphosis of an insect (egg, larva, pupa, adult). 2. In pathology, a degenerative change.

    m., fatty. Transformation of fat by infiltration or degeneration.

    m., platelet. Fusion of platelets during blood coagulation.

    m., retrograde. Degeneration.

    m., structural. M., platelet, q.v.

    m., viscous. M., platelet, q.v.

Metamucil. Trade name for psyllium husk.

metamyelocyte (mĕt″ă-mī-ĕl′ō-sīt). A transitional cell intermediate in development between a myelocyte and a mature granular leukocyte. SYN: *juvenile cell.*

Metandren. Trade name for methyltestosterone.

metanephrine (mĕt″ă-nĕf′rĭn). An inactive metabolite of epinephrine.

metanephrogenic (mĕt″ă-nĕf″rō-jĕn′ĭk) [″ + *nephros*, kidney, + *gennan*, to pro-

duce]. The part of the caudal mesoderm of the embryo that forms metanephric tubules of the kidney.

metanephros (mĕt″ă-nĕf′rŏs) [″ + *nephros*, kidney] (pl. *metanephroi*). The permanent kidney of amniotes (reptiles, birds, and mammals). Part of it develops from the caudal portion of the intermediate cell mass or nephrotome; the remaining portion is derived from a bud of the mesonephric duct.

metaneutrophil (mĕt-ă-nū′trō-fĭl) [″ + L. *neuter*, neither, + Gr. *philein*, to love]. Not reacting normally with neutral dyes.

metaphase (mĕt′ă-fāz) [″ + *phasis*, an appearance]. Stage in mitosis in which the chromosomes are arranged in an equatorial plane prior to separation. Follows the prophase and precedes the anaphase in which longitudinal halves of chromosomes diverge. SEE: *mitosis.*

metaphrenia (mĕt″ă-frē′nē-ă) [″ + *phren*, mind]. The mental status of turning away from family interests toward personal goals such as business.

metaphysis (mĕ-tăf′ĭ-sĭs) [Gr. *meta*, after, beyond, over, + *phyein*, to grow] (pl. *metaphyses*). Portion of a developing long bone between the diaphysis or shaft and epiphysis; the growing portion of a bone.

metaphysitis (mĕt″ă-fĭs-ī′tĭs) [″ + ″ + *itis*, inflammation]. Inflammation of the metaphysis of a bone.

metaplasia (mĕt″ă-plā′zē-ă) [″ + *plassein*, to form]. Conversion of one kind of tissue into a form that is not normal for that tissue.

    m., myeloid. Development of marrow tissue at sites at which it would not normally occur.

metaplastic (mĕt-ă-plăs′tĭk) [″ + *plastikos*, formed]. Pert. to or formed by metaplasia.

metapophysis (mĕt″ă-pŏf′ĭ-sĭs) [″ + *apophysis*, a process]. Mammillary process on the superior articular processes of a vertebra.

Metaprel. Trade name for metaproterenol sulfate.

metaprotein. Derived protein resulting from the action of acids or alkalies, in which the molecule is changed to form protein insoluble in neutral solvents but soluble in alkalies and weak acids. SEE: *protein.*

metaproterenol sulfate (mĕt″ă-prō-tĕr′ĕ-nŏl). An adrenergic stimulant used to treat bronchospasm and bronchial asthma. It is effective when given by inhalation. Trade name is Metaprel.

metaraminol bitartrate (mĕt″ă-răm′ĭ-nŏl). USP. A drug used for its pressor effect in treating hypotension. Trade names are Aramine and Pressonex Bitartrate.

metarteriole (mĕt″ăr-tē′rē-ōl). A small vessel connecting an arteriole to a venule from which true capillaries are given off. SYN: *precapillary.*

metastasis (mĕ-tăs′tă-sis) [″ + *stasis,* stand] (pl. *metastases*). 1. Movement of bacteria or body cells (esp. cancer cells) from one part of the body to another. 2. Change in location of a disease or of its manifestations or transfer from one organ or part to another not directly connected.

    The usual application is to the manifestation of a malignancy as a secondary growth arising from the primary growth in a new location. Disease may spread through the lymphatic circulation, the bloodstream, or avenues such as the cerebrospinal fluid.

metastasize (mĕ-tăs′tă-sīz). To invade by metastasis.

metastatic (mĕt″ă-stăt′ĭk). Pert. to metastasis.

metastatic survey. Procedure in which various structures of the body are investigated, esp. by x-ray or imaging, to demonstrate any spread of cancer.

metasternum (mĕt″ă-stĕr′nŭm). Xiphoid process of the sternum.

metatarsal (mĕt″ă-tăr′săl). Concerning the metatarsal arch of the foot.

metatarsalgia (mĕt″ă-tăr-săl′jē-ă) [″ + *tarsos,* a broad flat surface, + *algos,* pain]. Severe pain or cramp in anterior portion of metatarsus. SEE: *Morton's disease, syndrome.*

metatarsectomy (mĕt″ă-tăr-sĕk′tō-mē) [″ + ″ + *ektome,* excision]. Removal of the metatarsus or a metatarsal bone.

metatarsophalangeal (mĕt″ă-tăr″sō-fă-lăn′jē-ăl) [″ + ″ + *phalanx,* closely knit row]. Concerning the metatarsus and phalanges of the toes.

metatarsus (mĕt″ă-tăr′sŭs) [″ + *tarsos,* a broad flat surface]. [NA] The region of the foot between the tarsus and phalanges that includes the five metatarsal bones.

metatarsus primus varus. Inturning of the first metatarsal bone of the foot.

metatarsus varus. A congenital deformity of the foot involving adduction of the forefoot. When the child walks, the foot toes in. SEE: illus.

metathalamus (mĕt″ă-thăl′ă-mŭs) [″ + *thalamos,* a chamber]. [NA] The posterior part of the thalamus including the two geniculate bodies.

metathesis (mĕ-tăth′ĕ-sĭs) [″ + *thesis,* placement]. 1. A changing of places. 2. Forcible transference of a disease process from one part to another where it will be more accessible for treatment or where it causes less inconvenience. 3. Double decomposition of two chemical compounds.

metatrophia (mĕt-ă-trō′fē-ă) [″ + *trophe,* nourishment]. 1. A wasting due to malnutrition. 2. A change in diet.

metatypical (mĕt″ă-tĭp′ĭ-kăl). Tissue elements similar to those of other tissues at that site, but the components are not in a normal pattern.

metaxalone (mĕ-tăks′ă-lōn). A centrally acting muscle relaxant. Trade name is Skelaxin.

Metazoa [″ + *zoon,* animal]. Division of the animal kingdom that includes all multicellular forms, in contrast to unicellular forms or Protozoa.

Metchnikoff's theory (mĕch′nĭ-kŏfs) [Elie Metchnikoff, Russian biologist and zoologist in France, 1845–1916]. The theory that the body is protected against infection by cells such as leukocytes and phagocytes that attack and destroy invading microorganisms. SEE: *phagocytosis.*

metencephalon (mĕt″ĕn-sĕf′ă-lŏn) [Gr. *meta,* after, beyond, over, + *enkephalos,* brain]. [NA] The anterior portion of the embryonic rhombencephalon, from which the cerebellum and pons arise. SYN: *hindbrain.*

meteorism (mē′tē-or-ĭzm) [Gr. *meteorizein,* to raise up]. Distention by gas in the abdomen or intestines. SYN: *tympanites.*

meteoropathy (mē″tē-ĕ-rŏp′ă-thē) [″ + *pathos,* disease, suffering]. Illness due to climatic conditions.

meteorotropic (mē″tē-ĕ-rō-trŏp′ĭk) [″ + *trope,* a turn]. Pert. to diseases that are affected in their occurrence rate by weather.

meteorotropism (mē″tē-ĕ-rŏt′rō-pĭzm). The influence of meteorological events on biological conditions and events such as death rate, disease incidence, and birth rate.

meter [Gr. *metron,* measure]. A linear standard of measurement in the SI measurement system that is equal to about 39.37 inches. Also spelled *metre* in certain European countries.

metergasis (mĕt″ĕr-gā′sĭs) [Gr. *meta,* change, + *ergon,* work]. Change or alteration in function.

metestrus (mĕ-tĕs′trŭs) [″ + L. *oistros,* mad desire]. Period following estrus and preceding diestrus. SEE: *estrus.*

methacholine chloride (mĕth″ă-kō′lēn). USP. A cholinergic drug that is rarely used because of the unpredictability of the intensity of response.

methacycline hydrochloride. USP. An antibacterial drug. Trade name is Rondomycin.

methadone hydrochloride. USP. A synthetic analgesic drug with potency equal to that of morphine, but the narcotic action is weaker than that of morphine. Methadone

METATARSUS VARUS
LEFT FOOT

TARSAL AREA FLEXED

FOOT AND ANKLE
TURNED TOWARD MIDLINE

is a habit-forming agent, and its use should be carefully supervised. Used experimentally in treatment of drug dependence due to use of opium derivatives. Trade names are Dolophine Hydrochloride and Methadose.

methallenestril (mĕth″ăl-ĕ-nĕs′trĭl). A nonsteroidal estrogenic substance.

methamphetamine hydrochloride (mĕth″ăm-fĕt′ă-mēn). A sympathomimetic agent that is now used principally as a drug of abuse. SEE: *"ice."*

methane. CH₄. A colorless, odorless, inflammable gas. It is produced as a result of putrefaction and fermentation of organic matter. SYN: *marsh gas.*

methandriol (mĕth-ăn′drē-ŏl). An anabolic steroid drug.

methandrostenolone (mĕth-ăn′drō-stĕn′ō-lōn). An anabolic steroid used as replacement therapy in treating deficient endocrine function of the testes.

methanol. CH₃OH. A poisonous, volatile, inflammable alcohol that may be mistaken for ethyl alcohol. If ingested, it can cause blindness and death. SYN: *methyl alcohol; wood alcohol.*

methantheline bromide (mĕ-thăn′thĕ-lēn). USP. An anticholinergic drug that acts similarly to belladonna. Trade name is Banthine.

methapyrilene fumarate (mĕth″ă-pĭr′ĭ-lēn). An antihistamine drug.

methaqualone hydrochloride (mĕ-thă′-

kwă-lōn). A hypnotic and sedative drug that has become a drug of abuse. Because of the illegal and abused use of this drug, it is no longer distributed in the United States.

metharbital (mĕ-thär′bĭ-tăl). USP. An anticonvulsant drug of the barbiturate class. Trade name is Gemonil.

methazolamide (mĕth″ă-zō′lă-mīd). USP. A carbonic acid inhibitor used in treating glaucoma. Trade name is Neptazane.

methdilazine (mĕth-dī′lă-zēn). USP. An antihistamine drug. Trade name is Tacaryl.

methemalbumin (mĕt″hĕm-ăl-bū′mĭn). The abnormal combination of heme with albumin instead of globulin. It is present in blackwater fever and paroxysmal nocturnal hemoglobinuria.

methemoglobin (mĕt-hē″mō-glō′bĭn) [Gr. *meta*, across, + *haima*, blood, + L. *globus*, globe]. A form of hemoglobin in which the ferrous iron has been oxidized to ferric iron. Methemoglobin cannot transport oxygen. This may be due to toxic substances such as aniline dyes, potassium chlorate, or nitrate-contaminated water. Methemoglobin is also present when there is a hereditary deficiency of NADH-diaphorase, q.v.

    m. reductase. Nicotinamide adenine dinucleotide-diaphorase. SYN: *NADH-diaphorase,* q.v.

methemoglobinemia (mĕt″hē-mō-glōb″ĭ-nē′mē-ă) [″ + ″ + ″ + *haima,* blood]. The clinical condition in which more than 1% of hemoglobin in blood has been oxidized to the ferric (Fe^{+++}) form. The principal sign is cyanosis because the oxidized hemoglobin is incapable of transporting oxygen.

m., congenital. Condition due to a hereditary deficiency of NADH-diaphorase.

methemoglobinuria (mĕt″hē-mō-glŏb″ĭ-nū′rē-ă) [" + " + " + ouron, urine]. Presence of methemoglobin in the urine.

methenamine (mĕth-ĕn′ă-mēn). USP. A urinary antiseptic drug. Previously used name was hexamethylenamine.

m. mandelate. USP. A urinary antiseptic that derives its activity from the release of formaldehyde. Trade name is Mandelamine.

USES: In the treatment of urinary tract infection, esp. pyelitis and cystitis. It is necessary that the acidity of the urine be controlled: thus an acidifying agent, such as ammonium chloride, usually is required to maintain a urine pH of 5.5. This drug should not be used as the sole therapeutic agent in acute urinary tract infections.

methene. Methylene, q.v.

Methergine. Trade name for methylergonovine maleate, USP.

methicillin-resistant Staphylococcus aureus. ABBR: MRSA. *Staphylococcus aureus* organisms that are resistant to the antibacterial action of methicillin, a form of penicillin.

methicillin sodium (mĕth″ĭ-sĭl′ĭn). USP. A semisynthetic penicillinase-resistant penicillin. Trade names are Azapen, Celbenin, and Staphcillin.

methimazole (mĕth-īm′ă-zōl). USP. An antithyroid drug. Trade name is Tapazole.

methiodal sodium (mĕth-ī′ŏ-dăl). USP. A radiopaque compound used in x-ray examination of the urinary tract. Trade name is Skiodan Sodium.

methionine (mĕth-ī′ŏ-nīn). USP. $C_5H_{11}NO_2S$. A sulfur-bearing compound; an essential amino acid.

methisazone (mĕ-thĭs′ă-zōn). An antiviral agent.

methixene hydrochloride (mĕ-thĭks′ēn). A smooth muscle relaxant drug.

methocarbamol (mĕth″ō-kăr′bă-mōl). USP. A centrally acting muscle relaxant drug. Trade name is Robaxin.

method [Gr. *methodos*]. The systematic manner, procedure, or technique in performing details of an operation, tests, treatment, or any act. SEE: *algorithm; maneuver; stain; test; treatment.*

methodology (mĕth″ō-dŏl′ō-jē) [" + logos, word, reason]. The system of principles and procedures used in scientific endeavors.

methohexital sodium (mĕth″ō-hĕk′sĭ-tăl). USP. An ultrashort-acting barbiturate. Used in anesthesia. Trade name is Brevital Sodium.

methotrexate (mĕth″ō-trĕk′sāt). USP. An antimetabolite that acts as a folic acid antagonist. It is used in treating acute lymphoblastic leukemia in children, and in treating choriocarcinoma and psoriasis. Previously used name was amethopterin. Trade names are Mexate and Folex.

methotrimeprazine (mĕth″ō-trī-mĕp′ră-zēn). USP. A tranquilizer and analgesic drug. Trade name is Levoprome.

methoxamine hydrochloride (mĕ-thŏk′să-mēn). USP. An adrenergic drug used to maintain blood pressure in hypotensive states by causing vasoconstriction. It is also used to end attacks of paroxysmal atrial tachycardia. Trade name is Vasoxyl.

methoxsalen (mĕ-thŏk′să-lĕn). USP. A psoralen used in treating vitiligo, eczema, mycosis fungoides, and psoriasis. Trade name is Oxsoralen. SEE: *psoralen; PUVA therapy; trioxsalen.*

methoxyflurane (mĕ-thŏk″sē-floo′rān). USP. A general anesthetic administered by inhalation. Its renal toxicity prevents its being used for prolonged anesthesia. Trade name is Penthrane.

methoxyphenamine hydrochloride (mĕthŏk″sē-fĕn′ă-mēn). USP. A sympathomimetic drug used in treating bronchospasm.

methscopolamine bromide (mĕth″skō-pŏl′ă-mēn). USP. An anticholinergic drug used in treating gastric hyperacidity and hypermotility. Trade name is Pamine.

methsuximide (mĕth-sŭk′sĭ-mīd). USP. An anticonvulsant drug used in treating epilepsy. Trade name is Celontin.

methyclothiazide (mĕth″ĭ-klō-thī′ă-zīd). USP. An antihypertensive and diuretic drug. Trade names are Aquatensen and Enduron.

methyl (mĕth′ĭl) [Gr. *methy*, wine, + *hyle*, wood]. In organic chemistry, the radical CH_3, seen, for instance, in the formula for methyl alcohol, CH_3OH.

m. alcohol. A colorless liquid with an alcoholic odor. It is largely used as a solvent for paints or varnishes.

m. ether. An anesthetic gas without color.

m. orange. A dye used as a pH indicator.

m. purine. An oxidation product of purine. Includes caffeine, theophylline and theobromine. SEE: *aminopurine; oxypurine.*

m. salicylate. Oil of wintergreen, oil of gaultheria. Produced from distillation of leaves of sweet birch; it has a characteristic odor.

ACTION/USES: Commonly used in preparations in the form of liniment or ointment for topical use as an analgesic balm and counterirritant.

m. violet. Stain employed in histology and bacteriology.

methyl alcohol poisoning. Symptoms are different from those of ordinary alcoholism. Depression, weakness, nausea, headache, abdominal cramping, difficult breathing, cold sweats, coma, and convulsions. May be confused with cerebrovascular accident. Blindness, which often follows, may appear in several hours or not for several days; it may be permanent.

TREAT: Gastric lavage, q.v., or induce vomiting. This is effective only if given within two hours after ingestion. Intravenous alkali solution (5% sodium bicarbonate) in large amounts; supportive therapy. To prevent formation of formic acid, give ethanol in a 5% dextrose and water solution. This is continued in adults until a blood level of about 100 mg/dl of ethanol is obtained; and it is maintained at that level. This ethyl alcohol will help to prevent metabolism of methyl alcohol to its toxic and acid metabolites. Hemodialysis may be necessary. SEE: *Poisons and Poisoning* in *Appendix.*

methylate (měth′ĭ-lāt). 1. To introduce the methyl group, CH_3, into a chemical compound. 2. To mix with methyl alcohol. 3. A compound of methyl alcohol and a base.

methylation (měth″ĭ-lā′shŭn). The addition of methyl groups to a compound.

methylatropine nitrate (měth″ĭl-ăt′rō-pēn). A quaternary ammonium derivative of atropine, with action similar to that drug. Trade name is Eumydrin.

methylbenzethonium chloride (měth″ĭl-běn″zĕ-thō′nē-ŭm). USP. A deodorant used topically. It acts by reducing the number of resident bacteria on the skin. Trade name is Diaparene.

methylcellulose. USP. A tasteless powder that becomes swollen and gummy when wet. Used as a bulk substance in foods and laxatives, also as an adhesive or emulsifier. Trade names are Cologel and Methocel A.

methylcytosine (měth″ĭl-sī′tō-sĭn). A derivative of pyrimidine present in some nucleic acids.

methyldopa (měth″ĭl-dō′pă). USP. An antihypertensive drug used in treating essential hypertension. Previously used name was alpha-methyldopa. Trade name is Aldomet.

methyldopate hydrochloride (měth″ĭl-dō′pāt). USP. An antihypertensive drug used in treating essential hypertension.

Trade name is Aldomet Ester Hydrochloride.

methylene (měth′ĭ-lēn). The chemical radical $=CH_2$.

methylene blue (měth′ĭ-lēn). A dark green crystalline powder, producing a distinct blue stain.

methylenophil (měth″ĭ-lēn′ō-fĭl). Something that stains easily with methylene blue.

methylergonovine maleate (měth″ĭl-ĕr″gō-nō′vĕn). USP. A drug of the ergot alkaloid type. It is used to stimulate uterine contractions and in the treatment of migraine. Trade name is Methergine.

methylmalonic acidemia. An inherited metabolic disease caused by inability to convert methylmalonic acid to succinic acid. Clinically there are failure to grow, mental retardation, and severe metabolic acidosis. One form of the disease will respond to vitamin B_{12} given either in utero or to the mother prior to delivery.

methylparaben (měth″ĭl-păr′ă-běn). An antifungal agent used as a preservative in pharmaceuticals.

methylphenidate hydrochloride (měth″ĭl-fĕn′ĭ-dāt). USP. A drug that is chemically related to amphetamine. It is used in treating narcolepsy. Trade name is Ritalin Hydrochloride.

methylprednisolone (měth″ĭl-prĕd′nĭ-sō-lōn). USP. An adrenal corticosteroid drug. Trade name is Medrol.

methylrosaniline chloride (měth″ĭl-rō-zăn′ĭ-lĭn). Previously used name for gentian violet, q.v.

methyltestosterone (měth″ĭl-tĕs-tŏs′tĕr-ōn). USP. An androgenic steroid hormone. Trade names are Metandren, Oreton Methyl, and Testred.

methylthiouracil (měth″ĭl-thī″ō-ū′ră-sĭl). USP. An antithyroid drug used in treating hyperthyroidism.

methyltransferase (měth″ĭl-trăns′fĕr-ās). An enzyme that catalyzes the transfer of a methyl group from one compound to another.

methyprylon (měth″ĭ-prī′lŏn). USP. A sedative and hypnotic drug. Trade name is Noludar.

methysergide maleate (měth″ĭ-sĕr′jĭd). USP. A vasoconstrictor drug used in treating migraine. Trade name is Sansert. SEE: *carcinoid syndrome; serotonin.*

Meticorten. Trade name for prednisone, USP.

Meti-Derm. Trade name for prednisolone, USP.

metmyoglobin (mĕt-mī″ō-glō′bĭn). Myoglobin with the ferrous ion in the heme oxidized to the ferric ion.

metocurine iodide (mĕt″ō-kū′rĕn). USP. A

drug that relaxes skeletal muscle. It is used as an adjuvant in surgical anesthesia. Previously used name was dimethyl tubocurarine iodide. Trade name is Metubine Iodide.

Caution: An overdose may be lethal due to prolonged apnea and cardiac collapse. This drug should be used only by those familiar with its pharmacology and where facilities and staff for respiratory and cardiovascular resuscitation are immediately available.

metonymy (mĕ-tŏn'ĭ-mē) [Gr. *meta,* after, beyond, over, + *onyma,* name]. Mental confusion exhibited by the patient's use of a word that is not the precise term intended but of similar meaning.
Ex.: rifle in place of war; apple in place of ball.

metopagus (mĕ-tŏp'ă-gŭs) [Gr. *metopon,* forehead, + *pagos,* thing fixed]. Conjoined twins united at the forehead.

metopic (mĕ-tŏp'ĭk) [Gr. *metopon,* forehead]. Rel. to the forehead.

metopion (mĕ-tō'pē-ŏn). Craniometric point in forehead midway between frontal eminences. SYN: *glabella.*

metopism (mĕt'ō-pĭzm). Persistence of the metopic suture in an adult.

metopodynia (mĕt″ō-pō-dĭn'ē-ă) [″ + *odyne,* pain]. Frontal headache.

metoprolol tartrate. USP. An antiadrenergic drug. Trade name is Lopressor.

metoxenous (mĕt″ŏk-sē'nŭs) [Gr. *meta,* change, + *xenos,* host]. Denoting a parasite that spends each of its two cycles on a different host. SYN: *heteroecious.*

metoxeny (mĕt-ŏk'sĕ-nē). Condition of being metoxenous.

metra (mē'tră) [Gr.]. Combining form meaning the uterus. SEE: *metro-.*

metralgia (mē-trăl'jē-ă) [Gr. *metra,* uterus, + *algos,* pain]. Pain in the uterus. SYN: *metrodynia.*

metratome (mē'tră-tōm) [″ + *tome,* incision]. Instrument for incising the uterus.

metratomy (mē-trăt'ō-mē). Surgical incision of the uterus. SYN: *hysterotomy; metrotomy.*

metratonia (mē″tră-tō'nē-ă). Uterine atony occurring after childbirth.

metratrophia (mē″tră-trō'fē-ă). Atrophy of the uterus.

metre (mē'tĕr) [Gr. *metron,* measure]. Meter.

metrectasia (mē″trĕk-tā'zē-ă) [Gr. *metra,* uterus, + *ektasis,* extension]. Dilatation of nonpregnant uterus.

metrectopia (mē″trĕk-tō'pē-ă) [″ + *ektopos,* displaced]. Displacement of the uterus.

metreurynter (mē-troo-rĭn'tĕr) [″ + *eu-*

rynein, to stretch]. An inflatable bag that is inserted in the os uteri and distended to dilate the cervix.

metreurysis (mē-troo'rĭ-sĭs). Dilatation of the cervix uteri with the metreurynter.

metria (mē'trē-ă). Inflammation of the uterus during pregnancy.

metric system. A system of weights and measures based upon the meter (about 39.37 in.) as the unit of measurement; the gram (about 15.432 gr) as the unit of weight; the liter (about 1.057 qt. liquid or 0.908 qt. dry measure) as the unit of volume.
CONVERSION RULES: (Approximate) To change grams (gm) to grains (gr), multiply grams by 15. To change gr to gm, divide by 15. To change gm to avoirdupois ounces (oz), divide by 28.35. To change fluid oz to ml, multiply by 30. SEE: *avoirdupois; SI units; troy weight; Weights and Measures* in *Appendix.*

metriocephalic (mĕt″rē-ō-sĕ-făl'ĭk) [Gr. *metrios,* moderate, + *kephale,* head]. A skull with a vertical index of 72 to 76.9.

metritis (mē-trī'tĭs) [Gr. *metra,* uterus, + *itis,* inflammation]. Inflammation of the uterus. Designated endometritis if the endometrium is involved and myometritis if the musculature (myometrium) is involved.
m., chronic. Condition in which there is an increase in fibrous tissue and infiltration of lymphocytes.

metrizamide. A water-soluble contrast medium used for the radiographic examinations of the spinal cord and canal.

metro- [Gr. *metra,* uterus]. Combining form meaning rel. to the uterus.

metrocarcinoma (mē″trō-kăr-sĭ-nō'mă) [″ + *karkinos,* cancer, + *oma,* tumor]. Uterine carcinoma.

metrocele (mē'trō-sēl) [″ + *kele,* tumor, swelling]. Uterine hernia.

metrocolpocele (mē″trō-kŏl'pō-sēl) [″ + *kolpos,* vagina, + *kele,* tumor, swelling]. Protrusion of the uterus into the vagina, which pushes the vaginal wall downward. SEE: *procidentia.*

metrocystosis (mē″trō-sĭs-tō'sĭs) [″ + *kystis,* cyst, + *osis,* intensive]. Formation of uterine cysts.

metrodynia (mē″trō-dĭn'ē-ă) [″ + *odyne,* pain]. Uterine pain. SYN: *metralgia.*

metrofibroma (mē-trō-fī-brō'mă) [″ + L. *fibra,* fiber, + *oma,* tumor]. Uterine fibroma.

metromalacia (mē″trō-măl-ā'shē-ă) [″ + *malakia,* softness]. Softening of the uterus.

metromalacosis (mē″trō-măl-ă-kō'sĭs) [″ + ″ + *osis,* condition]. Malacia or softening of uterine tissues.

metronidazole. USP. Medicine used in treating infections due to *Trichomonas vag-*

inalis or *Giardia lamblia,* and in treating amebiasis. Trade name is Flagyl.

Caution: This drug may depress the level of white blood cells. Drinking alcohol while taking it may cause abdominal pain, nausea, or vomiting; and central nervous system symptoms such as vertigo, dizziness, and ataxia.

---

metronome (mĕt′rō-nōm) [Gr. *metron,* measure, + *nomos,* law]. Apparatus for recording intervals or periods of time.

metronoscope (mĕ-trŏn′ō-skōp). A device for exposing written material to the eye at timed intervals in order to facilitate development of reading skills and speed.

metroparalysis (mĕ″trō-pă-răl′ĭ-sĭs) [Gr. *metra,* uterus, + *paralyein,* to disable]. Uterine paralysis during or immediately following childbirth.

metropathia hemorrhagica (mĕ″trō-păth′ē-ă hĕm″ō-răj′ĭk-ă) [″ + *pathos,* disease, + *haima,* blood, + *rhegnynai,* to burst forth]. Condition of the uterus characterized by hemorrhage, usually accompanied by hypertrophy of the uterine mucous membranes and ovarian cystic disease.

metropathic (mĕ″trō-păth′ĭk). Pert. to or caused by uterine disease.

metropathy (mē-trŏp′ă-thē). Any uterine disease.

metroperitoneal (mĕ″trō-pĕr″ĭ-tō-nē′ăl) [″ + *peritonaion,* peritoneum]. Concerning the uterus and the peritoneum.

metroperitonitis (mĕ″trō-pĕr″ĭ-tō-nī′tĭs) [″ + ″ + *itis,* inflammation]. Inflamed condition of uterus and peritoneum.

metrophlebitis (mĕ″trō-flē-bī′tĭs) [″ + *phleps,* vein, + *itis,* inflammation]. Inflamed condition of the uterine veins.

metroplasty (mĕ″trō-plăs′tē) [″ + *plastikos,* formed]. Any plastic operation on the uterus.

metroptosis (mē-trō-tō′sĭs) [″ + *ptosis,* a dropping]. Downward displacement or prolapse of the uterus.

metrorrhagia (mĕt″rō-rā′jē-ă) [″ + *rhegnynai,* to burst forth]. Bleeding from the uterus, esp. at any time other than during the menstrual period. May be caused by lesions of the cervix uteri. Its occurrence should lead one to suspect and search for a malignancy in the genital tract, specifically cancer of the cervix. SEE: *menorrhagia.*

metrorrhea (mĕ″trō-rē′ă) [″ + *rhoia,* flow]. Abnormal uterine discharge.

metrorrhexis (mĕ″trō-rĕk′sĭs) [″ + *rhexis,* rupture]. Rupture of the uterus.

metrosalpingitis (mĕ″trō-săl″pĭn-jī′tĭs) [″ + *salpinx,* tube, + *itis,* inflammation]. Inflamed condition of uterus and oviducts.

metrosalpingography (mĕ″trō-săl″pĭng-gŏg′ră-fē) [″ + ″ + *graphein,* to write]. Radiography of the uterus and the fallopian tubes after the injection of air or an opaque medium into them.

metrostaxis (mĕ″trō-stăk′sĭs) [″ + *staxis,* a dripping]. Persistent but slight hemorrhage from the uterus.

metrostenosis (mĕ″trō-stĕn-ō′sĭs) [″ + *stenosis,* contraction]. Contraction or narrowing of the uterine cavity.

metrotherapy [Gr. *metron,* measure, + *therapeia,* treatment]. Judging the result of treatment of a condition by measurement.
    Ex.: in restoration of joint function following injury, measurement of the angle of joint motion and recording the progress has a psychological effect on the patient.

metrotome (mĕ″trō-tōm) [Gr. *metra,* uterus, + *tome,* incision]. Instrument used in incising the uterus.

metrotomy (mē-trŏt′ō-mē). Incision of the uterus. SYN: *hysterotomy; metratomy.*

metrourethrotome (mĕt″rō-ū-rē′thrō-tōm) [Gr. *metron,* measure, + *ourethra,* urethra, + *tome,* incision]. Device for incising the urethra and measuring depth to be incised.

-metry [Gr. *metrein,* to measure]. Suffix meaning to measure.

metyrapone (mĕ-tēr′ă-pōn). USP. A drug that reduces adrenocortical secretion from the adrenal gland. It is used to treat excessive adrenocortical hormone secretion and to test the function of the adrenal gland.

metyrapone test. Diagnostic test to assess ACTH and cortisol production.

mev. *million electron volts.*

Mexate. Trade name for methotrexate sodium.

Meynert's commissure (mī′nĕrts) [Theodor H. Meynert, Austrian neurologist, 1833–1892]. Fibrous tract extending from subthalamic body to base of 3rd ventricle.

Meynet's nodosities (mā-nāz′) [Paul C. H. Meynet, Fr. physician, 1831–1892]. In rheumatic disease, nodules attached to the tendon sheaths and joints.

M.F.D. *minimum fatal dose.*

μg. *microgram.*

Mg. Chem. symb. for the element magnesium.

mg. *milligram.*

mgh. *milligram hour.* Dosage of radiation obtained by application of 1.0 mg radium for 1 hour.

MHC. *major histocompatibility complex.*

mho (mō). Ohm spelled backwards. Siemens, q.v.

MHz. *megahertz.*

MI. *myocardial infarction.*

miasm, miasma (mī′ăzm, mī-ăz′mă) [Gr. *miasma*, stain]. A foul emanation or odor from the earth. Formerly thought to cause disease endemic to certain regions, esp. fevers such as malaria.

miasmatic (mī′′ăz-măt′ĭk). Pert. to miasm.

mica (mī′kă) [L.]. 1. A crumb. 2. A mineral composed of various silicates of metals. It occurs in thin, laminated scales.

mication (mī-kā′shŭn). A sudden movement such as eye blinking.

micella, micelle (mī-sĕl′ă, mī-sĕl′). One of the ultramicroscopic units of protoplasm.

miconazole nitrate (mī-kŏn′ă-zōl). An antifungal agent used as a vaginal cream. Trade names are Monistat-Derm and Monistat Cream.

micra. Pl. of micron.

micracusia (mī′′kră-kū′zē-ă) [Gr. *mikros*, small, + *akousis*, hearing]. An auditory illusion in which sounds appear to be remote. May occur at the onset of an epileptic seizure.

micrencephalon (mī′′krĕn-sĕf′ă-lon) [Gr. *mikros*, small, + *enkephalos*, brain]. 1. Cerebellum. 2. Smallness of the brain; cretinism, q.v.

micrencephalous (mī′′krĕn-sĕf′ă-lŭs). Possessing a small brain.

micrencephaly (mī′′krĕn-sĕf′ă-lē). Abnormal smallness of the brain.

micro-, micr- [Gr. *mikros*, small]. Combining forms denoting small size or extent. Indicates one-millionth of a unit; thus microgram is one-millionth of a gram. SYMB: μ.

microabscess (mī′′krō-ăb′sĕs) [″ + L. *abscessus*, a going away]. A very small abscess.

microaerophilic (mī′′krō-ā′ĕr-ō-fĭl′ĭk) [″ + *aer*, air, + *philein*, to love]. Growing at low amounts of oxygen; said of certain bacteria.

microanalysis. Analytical examination of tiny granules.

microanatomy. Microscopic anatomy; histology.

microaneurysm (mī′′krō-ăn′ū-rĭzm) [″ + *aneurysma*, a widening]. A microscopic aneurysm.

microangiitis (mī′′krō-ăn′′jē-ī′tĭs). Inflammation of very small blood vessels.

microangiopathy (mī′′krō-ăn′′jē-ŏp′ă-thē) [″ + *angeion*, vessel, + *pathos*, disease, suffering]. Pathology of small blood vessels.

   m., thrombotic. Formation of thrombi in small blood vessels.

microangioscopy (mī′′krō-ăn′′jē-ŏs′kō-pē) [″ + ″ + *skopein*, to examine]. Use of microscopy to diagnose pathological changes in capillaries.

microbalance (mī′krō-băl′′ăns). A scale or balance for measuring very small weight changes.

microbe (mī′krōb) [″ + *bios*, life]. 1. A minute one-celled form of life not distinguishable as to its vegetable or animal nature. 2. Bacteria, germs producing fermentation, putrefaction, and disease. SYN: *microorganism.*

microbial (mī-krō′bē-ăl). Rel. to microbes. SYN: *microbian; microbic.*

microbic (mī-krōb′ĭk). Concerning microbes. SYN: *microbial; microbian.*

microbicidal (mī-krō′′bĭ-sī′dăl) [″ + *bios*, life, + L. *cidus*, kill]. Lethal to microbes.

microbicide (mī-krō′bĭ-sīd). An agent that kills microbes.

microbiological antagonism. The action of certain bacteria in interfering with or preventing the growth and development of other microorganisms. SEE: *opportunistic infections.*

microbiology (mī′′krō-bī-ŏl′ō-jē) [″ + *bios*, life, + *logos*, word, reason]. Scientific study of microorganisms.

microbiophobia (mī′′krō-bī′′ō-fō′bē-ă) [″ + ″ + *phobos*, fear]. An abnormal fear of germs. SYN: *microphobia* (def. 1).

microbiota (mī′′krō-bī-ō′tă). Microscopic organisms of an area. SEE: *macrobiota.*

microbiotic (mī′′krō-bī-ŏt′ĭk). Pertinent to microbial forms of life.

microbism (mī′krōb-īzm) [″ + *bios*, life, + *ismos*, state of]. Infection with microbes.

microblast (mī′krō-blăst) [″ + *blastos*, germ]. Minute red blood corpuscle.

microblepharism, microblephary (mī′′krō-blĕf′ăr-ĭzm, -ăr-ē) [″ + *blepharon*, eyelid]. Condition of having abnormally small eyelids.

microbodies. Small, spherical, cytoplasmic bodies approx. 0.5 μm in diameter. They have been found in the cells of the liver and kidney tubule.

microbrachia (mī′′krō-brā′kē-ă) [″ + *brachion*, arm]. Abnormally small arms.

microbrachius (mī′′krō-brā′kē-ŭs) [″ + *brachion*, arm]. A fetus with very small arms.

microcardia (mī′′krō-kăr′dē-ă) [Gr. *mikros*, small, + *kardia*, heart]. Unusually small heart.

microcaulia (mī′′krō-kaw′lē-ă) [″ + *kaulos*, penis]. Unusually small size of penis. SYN: *microphallus.*

microcentrum (mī′′krō-sĕn′trŭm) [″ + *kentron*, center]. 1. Centrosome. 2. Motor or dynamic center of a cell.

microcephalia (mī′′krō-sĕf-ā′lē-ă) [″ + *kephale*, head]. Abnormal smallness of the head. SYN: *microcephalism; microcephaly.*

microcephalic (mī″krō-sĕf-ăl′ĭk). Having or pert. to small head; one below 1350 cc capacity.

microcephalous (mī″krō-sĕf′ă-lŭs). Having an abnormally small head. SYN: *microcephalic.*

microcephalus (mī″krō-sĕf′ă-lŭs). Individual with an exceptionally small head.

microcephaly (mī″krō-sĕf′ă-lē). Abnormal smallness of head often seen in mental retardation; it is congenital.

microcheilia (mī″krō-kī′lē-ă) [Gr. *mikros,* small, + *cheilos,* lip]. Abnormal smallness of lips.

microchemistry (mī″krō-kĕm′ĭs-trē) [″ + *chemeia,* chemistry]. Chemical analysis of specimens of very small quantity.

microchiria, microcheiria (mī″krō-kī′rē-ă) [″ + *cheir,* hand]. Abnormal smallness of the hand.

microcinematography (mī″krō-sĭn″ē-mă-tŏg′ră-fē) [″ + *kinema,* motion, + *graphein,* to write]. Motion pictures of microscopic objects.

microcirculation (mī″krō-sĭr″kū-lā′shŭn). Blood or lymph flow in the very small vessels.

Micrococcaceae (mī″krō-kŏk-ā′sē-ē). A family of bacteria belonging to the order Eubacteriales. Contains the genera *Micrococcus, Sarcina,* and *Staphylococcus.*

Micrococcus (mī″krō-kŏk′ŭs) [Gr. *mikros,* small, + *kokkos,* berry]. A genus of spherical gram-positive bacteria belonging to the family Micrococcaceae. Cells occur singly or in irregular groups.

micrococcus (mī″krō-kŏk′ŭs). An organism of the genus *Micrococcus.*

microcolon. Abnormally small colon.

microcoria (mī″krō-kō′rē-ă) [″ + *kore,* pupil]. Smallness of the pupil of the eye.

microcornea. Abnormally small cornea.

microcoulomb (mī″krō-koo′lŏm). A microunit of quantity of current electricity; one-millionth part (10^{-6}) of a coulomb, q.v.

microcrystalline (mī″krō-krĭs′tăl-ĭn, -ēn). Composed of microscopic crystals.

microcurie. Measure of radiation. One-millionth of a curie.

microcurie-hour. The radiation produced by radioactive decay at the rate of 3.7×10^4 atoms per second.

microcyst (mī′krō-sĭst). A very small cyst.

microcyte. A small erythrocyte or red blood corpuscle; one less than 5 microns in diameter.

microcythemia (mī″krō-sī-thē′mē-ă) [″ + ″ + *haima,* blood]. Smallness of the red blood cells.

microcytosis. Condition characterized by presence of abnormal numbers of micro-

cytes in the blood.

microdactylia (mī″krō-dăk-tĭl′ē-ă) [″ + *daktylos,* digit]. Abnormal smallness of the digits.

microdetermination. The chemical examination of extremely minute quantities of a substance.

microdissection (mī″krō-dī-sĕk′shŭn) [″ + L. *dissectio,* a cutting apart]. Dissection with the aid of a microscope, esp. by utilization of a micromanipulator.

microdont (mī′krō-dŏnt) [″ + *odous,* tooth]. Possessing very small teeth.

microdontia (mī″krō-dŏn′shē-ă) [″ + *odous,* tooth]. Abnormal smallness of the teeth or a single tooth.

microdontism (mī″krō-dŏn′tĭzm) [″ + ″ + *-ismos,* condition]. Unusual smallness of the teeth.

microdose. Minute dose.

microelectrophoresis. Electrophoresis of minute quantities of a solution.

microembolus (mī″krō-ĕm′bō-lŭs) [″ + *embolos,* plug]. A very small embolus.

microencephaly (mī″krō-ĕn-sĕf′ă-lē) [″ + *enkephalos,* brain]. Having a very small head.

microenvironment. The environment at the microscopic or cellular level.

microerythrocyte (mī″krō-ē-rĭth′rō-sīt) [″ + *erythros,* red, + *kytos,* cell]. Microcyte, q.v.

microfarad (mī-krō-făr′ăd). A microunit of electrical capacity; one-millionth of a farad, q.v.

microfauna (mī″krō-faw′nă). In a specific location, the animal life that is microscopic in size.

microfibril (mī″krō-fī′brĭl). A very small fibril.

microfiche (mī″krō-fēsh″) [Gr. *mikros,* small, + Fr. *fiche,* index card]. A sheet of microfilm that enables a large number of library data and medical records to be stored in a small space.

microfilament (mī″krō-fīl′ă-mĕnt). Submicroscopic elements of the cell.

microfilaremia (mī″krō-fīl″ă-rē′mē-ă). Microfilaria in the blood.

microfilaria (mī″krō-fī-lā′rē-ă). The embryos of filarial worms. They are present in the blood and tissues and are of importance in the diagnosis of filarial infections.

microfilm. A film containing a greatly reduced photoimage of printed or graphic matter.

microflora (mī″krō-flō′ră). In a specific area, the plant life that is visible by use of a microscope.

microgamete (mī-krō-găm′ēt) [″ + *gametes,* spouse]. Male element in conjugation of protozoa.

microgametocyte (mī″krō-gă-mē′tō-sīt) [″ + ″ + *kytos*, cell]. Mother cell of the microgamete.

microgamy (mī-krŏg′ă-mē). Union of male and female cells in certain lower forms.

microgastria (mī″krō-găs′trē-ă) [″ + *gaster*, stomach]. Unusual smallness of the stomach.

microgenia (mī″krō-jĕn′ē-ă) [″ + *geneion*, chin]. Abnormal smallness of the chin.

microgenitalism (mī″krō-jĕn′ĭ-tăl-īzm) [″ + L. *genitalia*, genitals, + Gr. *-ismos*, condition]. Abnormal smallness of the external genitals.

microglia (mī-krŏg′lē-ă) [″ + *glia*, glue]. Neuroglia tissue probably derived from the mesoderm, forming a portion of the adventitial structure of the central nervous system.

microgliacyte (mī″krŏg′lē-ă-sīt) [″ + ″ + *kytos*, cell]. An embryonic cell of the microglia.

microglioma (mī″krō-glī-ō′mă) [″ + ″ + *oma*, tumor]. A tumor composed of microglial cells.

microglossia (mī-krō-glŏs′ē-ă) [″ + *glossa*, tongue]. Abnormally small tongue.

micrognathia (mī-krō-nă′thē-ă) [″ + *gnathos*, jaw]. Abnormal smallness of jaws, esp. the lower jaw.

microgonioscope (mī″krō-gō′nē-ō-skōp) [″ + *gonia*, angle, + *skopein*, to examine]. Device for measuring the angles of the anterior chamber of the eye. Used in studying glaucoma.

microgram. ABBR: μg or mcg. One-millionth part of a gram. One-thousandth of a milligram.

micrograph (mī′krō-grăf) [Gr. *mikros*, small, + *graphein*, to write]. 1. Apparatus for magnifying and recording minute movements. 2. Photograph of an object through a microscope. SYN: *photomicrograph*.

micrography (mī-krŏg′ră-fē). 1. Study of physical appearance and characteristics of microscopic objects. 2. Very minute writing, engraving, etc. 3. Study of an object by use of a microscope.

microgyria (mī-krō-jīr′ē-ă) [″ + *gyros*, circle]. Smallness of cerebral convolutions.

microgyrus (mī″krō-jī′rŭs) [″ + *gyros*, circle]. A small, malformed gyrus of the brain.

microhematocrit (mī″krō-hē-măt′ō-krĭt). Packed red cell volume of blood determined by using very small amount of blood collected in a capillary tube and placed in high-speed centrifuge.

microhepatia (mī″krō-hē-păt′ē-ă) [″ + *hepar*, liver]. Abnormally small size of the liver.

microhm (mī′krōm). A microunit of electrical resistance; one-millionth of an ohm.

microincineration. Determination of presence and distribution of inorganic matter in tissues by subjecting a microscopic section of tissue to a high temperature, which destroys organic matter and leaves mineral matter as ash.

microinjection. Injection of substances into cells or minute vessels by means of a micropipette.

microinvasion (mī″krō-īn-vā′zhŭn). Invasion of the cellular tissue adjacent to a carcinoma in situ.

microleakage. The seepage of oral fluids containing bacteria and debris between the walls of a tooth cavity and the restoration or cement layer.

microlentia (mī″krō-lĕn′shē-ă). Possessing a very small crystalline lens.

microlesion (mī″krō-lē′zhŭn). A very small lesion.

microleukoblast [″ + *leukos*, white, + *blastos*, germ]. A small leukoblast. SYN: *myeloblast*.

microliter (mī′krō-lē″tĕr). One-millionth part of a liter.

microlith (mī′krō-līth) [″ + *lithos*, stone]. A very tiny calculus.

microlithiasis (mī″krō-lĭ-thī′ă-sĭs) [″ + ″ + *-iasis*, process]. The development of very minute calculi.
   m., pulmonary alveolar. Deposition of microscopic granules of bone throughout the lungs.

micromanipulator. Apparatus by which extremely minute pipettes or needles can be manipulated under a microscope for microinjection or microsurgery.

micromastia (mī-krō-măs′tē-ă). Micromazia.

micromazia (mī-krō-mā′zē-ă) [Gr. *mikros*, small, + *mazos*, breast]. Abnormally small size of the breasts.

micromelia (mī″krō-mē′lē-ă) [″ + *melos*, limb]. Abnormally small or short limbs.

micromelus (mī-krŏm′ē-lŭs) [″ + *melos*, limb]. One who has micromelia.

micromere (mī′krō-mēr) [″ + *meros*, part]. A small blastomere.

micrometer. 1. (mī′krō-mē-ter) ABBR: μm. One-millionth part of a meter (10^{-6}); one-thousandth part of a millimeter (0.001 mm). SEE: *micron*. 2. (mī-krŏm′ē-tĕr) Device for measuring small distances.

micromethod (mī′krō-mĕth′ŏd). Any chemical or physical method involving small amounts of material or very small tissues, respectively.

micrometry (mī-krŏm′ē-trē) [″ + *metron*, measure]. Use of device, esp. a micrometer, to measure small objects or thickness.

micromicro- (μμ). Prefix formerly used to indicate one trillionth (10^{-12}). The term currently used is *pico*.

micromicrogram (mī″krō-mī′krō-grăm). ABBR: *μμg*. One-millionth of a microgram. Now called a picogram, or 10^{-12} gram.

micromicron (mī″krō-mī′krŏn). ABBR: *μμ*. Former name for picometer or 10^{-12} meter.

micromillimeter (mī-krō-mĭl′ĭ-mē-tĕr). ABBR: *μmm*. One-millionth part of a millimeter. SYN: *millimicron*.

micromole (mī′krō-mōl). One-millionth, 10^{-6}, of a mole. SEE: *mole* (def. 2).

micromolecular (mī″krō-mō-lĕk′ū-lăr). Composed of small molecules.

Micromonospora (mī″krō-mō-nŏs′por-ä). A genus of fungi belonging to the family Streptomycetaceae.

micromyces (mī-krŏm′ĭ-sēs) [Gr. *mikros*, small, + *mykes*, fungus] (pl. *micromycetes*). Minute fungus.

micromyelia (mī″krō-mī-ē′lē-ä) [″ + *myelos*, marrow]. Abnormally small size of spinal cord.

micromyeloblast (mī-krō-mī′ĕl-ō-blăst) [″ + *myelos*, marrow, + *blastos*, germ]. A small, immature myelocyte; often the predominating cell in myeloblastic leukemia.

micromyelolymphocyte (mī″krō-mī″ē-lō-lĭm′fō-sīt) [″ + ″ + L. *lympha*, lymph, + Gr. *kytos*, cell]. Micromyeloblast, q.v.

micron (pl. *micra, microns*). Unit of linear measure; equal to .001 millimeter (10^{-3} mm). In the International System (SI) of units, micron has been designated micrometer. The abbr. for micrometer is *μm*.

microne (mī′krŏn). A colloid particle that is distinguishable with the microscope.

microneedle. Extremely minute needle used in a micromanipulator for microdissection.

micronize. To pulverize a substance into particles only a few micra in size.

micronodular (mī″krō-nŏd′ū-lăr). Having small nodules.

micronucleus (mī-krō-nū′klē-ŭs) [″ + L. *nucleus*, kernel] (pl. *micronuclei*). 1. A small nucleus. 2. The smaller of the two nuclei of Ciliata considered as containing the inheritable germ substance.

micronutrient (mī″krō-nū′trē-ĕnt). An essential nutrient required only in small amounts.

micronychia (mī″krō-nĭk′ē-ä) [″ + *onyx*, nail]. Possessing abnormally small nails.

microorganism (mī-krō-or′găn-ĭzm) [″ + *organon*, organ, + *-ismos*, condition]. Minute living body not perceptible to the naked eye, esp. a bacterium or protozoon.

Microorganisms may be carried from one host to another as follows:

Animal sources: Some organisms are pathogenic for animals as well as man and may be communicated to man through direct, indirect, or intermediary hosts.

By air: Pathogenic microorganisms in the respiratory tract may be discharged from the mouth or nose and settle on food, dishes, or clothing. They may carry infection if they resist drying.

Contact infections: These are the result of direct transmission of bacteria from one to another, as in venereal diseases.

Food-borne: Food and water may contain pathogenic organisms acquired from infected persons handling the food or through fecal or insect contamination.

Fomites: Inanimate objects such as linens, books, cooking utensils, or clothing that will harbor microorganisms and could serve to transport them from one location to another.

Human carriers: Persons who have recovered from an infectious disease remain carriers of the organism causing the infection and may transfer the organism to another host.

Insects: They may be physical carriers, such as the housefly, or act as intermediate hosts, such as the Anopheles mosquito.

Soil-borne: Spore-forming organisms in the soil may enter the body through a cut or wound. Vegetables and fruits, esp. root crops, need thorough cleansing before being eaten raw.

m., pathologic. Any disease-causing microorganism. Includes rickettsias, bacteria, spirochetes, yeasts, molds, protozoons, and some helminths.

micropannus. A pathological condition in which a vascular sheet of tissue covers the corner of the eye.

microparasite (mī″krō-păr′ă-sīt). A parasitic microorganism.

micropathology (mī″krō-păth-ŏl′ō-jē) [Gr. *mikros*, small, + *pathos*, disease, + *logos*, word, reason]. The use of a microscope to study diseases caused by microorganisms.

micropenis (mī″krō-pē′nĭs). A very small penis.

microphage, microphagus (mī′krō-fāj, mī-krŏf′ă-gŭs) [″ + *phagein*, to eat]. A small phagocyte.

RS: bacteria; bacteriolysin; leukocyte; opsonic index; opsonin.

microphagocyte (mī″krō-făg′ō-sīt) [″ + ″ + *kytos*, cell]. Microphage.

microphakia (mī″krō-fā′kē-ä) [″ + *phakos*, lens]. Abnormally small crystalline lens.

microphallus (mī-krō-făl′ŭs) [″ + *phallos*, penis]. Abnormally small size of penis. SYN: *microcaulia*.

microphobia (mī-krō-fō′bē-ä) [″ + *phobos*, fear]. 1. Psychopathic fear of microbes. 2. Morbid dread of small objects. SYN: *microbiophobia*.

microphone (mī′krō-fōn) [″ + *phone*, voice]. Device for detecting and transmitting sound.

microphonia (mī-krō-fō′nē-ă). Weakness of the voice.

microphonoscope (mī″krō-fō′nō-skōp) [Gr. *mikros*, small, + *phone*, voice, + *skopein*, to examine]. Form of binaural stethoscope for magnifying sound.

microphotograph (mī″krō-fō′tō-grăf) [″ + *phos*, light, + *graphein*, to write]. 1. A photograph of extremely small size. 2. A photograph on microfilm. 3. A photomicrograph.

microphthalmia (mī-krŏf-thăl′mē-ă) [″ + *ophthalmos*, eye]. Abnormally small size of one or both eyes.

microphthalmus (mī-krŏf-thăl′mŭs). 1. Person with unusually small eyes. 2. Condition characterized by abnormally small eyes.

microphyte (mī′krō-fīt) [″ + *phyton*, plant]. Any microscopic plant, esp. if parasitic.

micropia (mī-krō′pē-ă) [″ + *opsis*, vision]. A condition in which objects seem diminished in size. SYN: *micropsia*.

micropipette. An extremely small pipette used for measuring small amounts of fluid substances.

microplasia (mī″krō-plā′zē-ă) [″ + *plassein*, to form]. Failure to attain full size, as in dwarfism.

microplethysmography (mī″krō-plĕth″ĭs-mŏg′ră-fē) [″ + *plethysmos*, increase, + *graphein*, to write]. Detection of small changes in the volume of a part due to alteration in blood flow.

micropodia (mī-krō-pō′dē-ă) [″ + *pous*, feet]. Unusually small size of the feet.

micropolariscope (mī″krō-pōl-ăr′ĭ-skōp). A microscope with a polarizer.

microprobe (mī′krō-prōb). A very small probe, suitable for use in microsurgery.

microprojection. Projection of images of microscopic objects upon a screen.

microprosopia (mī″krō-prō-sō′pē-ă) [″ + *prosopon*, face]. Abnormal smallness of the face.

micropsia (mī-krŏp′sē-ă) [″ + *opsis*, vision]. Condition in which objects seem smaller than they usually are. Seen in paralysis of accommodation, retinitis, and choroiditis. SYN: *micropia*.

micropuncture (mī″krō-pŭnk′chŭr). A very small incision or puncture of a structure such as a single cell.

micropus (mī-krō′pŭs) [″ + *pous*, feet]. One with unusually small feet.

micropyle (mī′krō-pīl) [″ + *pyle*, gate]. The opening in the ovum for entrance of the spermatozoon. Seen in ovum of some animals.

microradiography (mī″krō-rā″dē-ŏg′ră-fē). Technique of x-raying microscopic objects. The pictures are usually enlarged.

microrefractometer (mī″krō-rē″frăk-tŏm′ĕ-tĕr). Refractometer used to study cells, esp. red blood cells.

microrespirometer (mī″krō-rĕs″pĭ-rŏm′ĕ-tĕr). Device for measuring oxygen consumption of very small bits of tissue.

microrhinia (mī″krō-rĭn′ē-ă) [″ + *rhis*, nose]. Abnormal smallness of the nose.

microscelous (mī-krŏs′kĕ-lŭs) [″ + *skelos*, leg]. Possessing short legs.

microscope (mī′krō-skōp) [″ + *skopein*, to examine]. Optical instrument that greatly magnifies very minute objects.

m., binocular. Microscope possessing two eyepieces or oculars.

m., compound. Microscope with two or more lenses or lens systems for use in observing very small bodies.

m., dark-field. Microscope using darkfield illumination. SYN: *ultramicroscope*. SEE: *illumination, dark-field.*

m., electron. A microscope that utilizes streams of electrons deflected from their course by an electrostatic or electromagnetic field for the magnification of objects. The final image is viewed on a fluorescent screen or recorded on a photographic plate. Because of greater resolving power, images may be magnified up to 400,000 diameters. SEE: *m., scanning electron.*

m., light. Microscope that uses visible light to allow viewing of the object.

m., operating. Microscope designed for use during surgery involving small tissue such as vessels, the inner ear, or fallopian tubes. SEE: *microsurgery.*

m., phase. A compound microscope to which two elements have been added, namely, a diffraction or phase plate and a specialized condenser diaphragm. This makes it possible to view details of objects characterized by differences in refractive index and thus delineates a change of phase such as brightness or color. Particularly useful for viewing living cells, observing cytoplasmic organelles. Buccal smears of desquamated epithelial cells, food debris, and spirochetes easily convinces dental patients that better oral hygiene is essential.

m., polarization. Microscope for examining specimens that polarize light or have double refraction.

m., scanning electron. ABBR: SEM. An electron microscope that scans the image point-by-point and displays the image on a photographic film or television screen. The SEM, unlike other types of microscopes, allows a three-dimensional view of the tissue and tissues do not need to be extensively handled and prepared in order to be visualized. The magnification ranges from 20 to 100,000 times.

m., simple. Microscope with a simple or single lens; magnifying glass.

m., slit-lamp. Microscope with slit illumination for examining the eye, esp. the cornea.

m., stereoscopic. A binocular microscope with an objective lens for each eyepiece. This permits the object to be viewed stereoscopically.

m., ultraviolet. Microscope utilizing ultraviolet radiations as a light source and having an optical system for transmitting them. Used in observing a specimen that fluoresces such as tissues stained with a fluorescent dye.

m., x-ray. Microscope for utilizing x-rays to reveal structure of objects through which light cannot pass. The image is usually reproduced on film.

microscopic, microscopical (mī-krō-skŏp′ĭk, -ĭ-kăl). 1. Pert. to the microscope. 2. Visible only by using the microscope.

microscopy (mī-krŏs′kŏp-ē). Inspection with the microscope.

microsecond (mī′krō-sĕk″ŭnd). One-millionth of a second; 10^{-6} second.

microseme (mī′krō-sēm) [Gr. *mikros*, small, + *sema*, sign]. Possessing an orbital index of less than 83.

microsmatic (mī″krŏs-măt′ĭk) [″ + *osmasthai*, to smell]. Having a poorly developed sense of smell.

microsoma (mī″krō-sō′mă) [″ + *soma*, body]. Unusually small stature.

microsome (mī′krō-sōm). One of the particles derived from the endoplasmic reticulum of cell nuclei which consist mainly of RNA. Obtained when cells are broken up by centrifuging with a force 100,000 times that of gravity. Microsomes can be seen only by use of electron microscopy.

microsomia (mī-krō-sō′mē-ă). Abnormally small size of body.

microspectrophotometry (mī″krō-spĕk″trō-fō-tŏm′ĕ-trē). Method for the histochemical study of substances present in cells, such as nucleic acid, based on absorption in the ultraviolet spectrum. Permits quantitative and qualitative studies of certain cellular components.

microspectroscope [″ + L. *spectrum*, image, + Gr. *skopein*, to examine]. A combined spectroscope and microscope.

microspheres. Minute containers suitable for implantation or injection into the body or circulatory system. They may be used for delivering medicines to certain sites or, if radioactive, to study the blood flow to an area. If microspheres are used as a drug-de-

livery system, the container is designed to be dissolved in body fluids.

microspherocyte (mī″krō-sfē′rō-sīt) [″ + *sphaira*, globe, + *kytos*, cell]. Red blood cells, small and shaped like spheres. Seen in certain kinds of anemia.

microspherocytosis (mī″krō-sfē″rō-sī-tō′sĭs) [″ + ″ + *osis*, condition]. Spherocytosis.

microsplanchnic (mī″krō-splănk′nĭk). Having an abdominal cavity relatively small compared to the rest of the body.

microsplenia (mī-krō-splē′nē-ă) [″ + *splen*, spleen]. Abnormal smallness of the spleen.

microsporid (mī-krŏs′pō-rĭd). A skin eruption distant from the site of infection with *Microsporum*, and due to hypersensitivity to the organism.

microsporosis (mī″krō-spō-rō′sĭs). Ringworm infection due to fungi of the genus *Microsporum*.

Microsporum (mī″krŏs′por-ŭm). A genus of ringworm fungi that causes disease of the skin, hair, and nails.

M. audouini. Causative agent of tinea capitis (ringworm of scalp), q.v.

M. canis. Cause of ringworm of cats and dogs. May be transmitted to children.

microstomia (mī-krō-stō′mē-ă) [″ + *stoma*, mouth]. Unusual smallness of the mouth.

microstrabismus (mī″krō-stră-bĭs′mŭs) [″ + *strabismos*, a squinting]. Movement of the eyes in divergent directions or at different speeds. These movements are too small and too quick to be seen, but they have been detected through analysis of high-speed motion pictures.

microsurgery. Surgery in which various types of magnification, specialized instrumentation, fine sutures, and meticulous techniques are used to repair, anastomose, or restore tissues.

microsyringe. A special syringe for injecting very small quantities of solutions.

microthelia (mī″krō-thē′lē-ă) [″ + *thele*, nipple]. Very small nipples.

microtia (mī-krō′shē-ă) [″ + *ous*, ear]. Unusually small size of the auricle or external ear.

microtome (mī′krō-tōm) [″ + *tome*, incision]. Instrument for preparing thin sections of tissue for microscopic study.

m., freezing. Microtome equipped to cut frozen tissues.

m., sliding. Microtome in which the tissue being sectioned slides along a track.

microtomy (mī-krŏt′ō-mē). The process of incising thin sections of tissues.

microtonometer (mī″krō-tō-nŏm′ĕ-tĕr). Device for determining oxygen and carbon dioxide concentration in blood.

microtrauma (mī″krō-traw′mä). A very small lesion.

microtropia (mī″krō-trō′pē-ă) [″ + *trope*, a turning]. Strabismus with very small deviation, usually less than 4°.

microtubule (mī″krō-tū′būl). An elongated (200 to 300 angstrom), hollow or tubular structure present in the cell. Microtubules are important in helping certain cells maintain their rigidity in converting chemical energy into work, and in providing a means of transporting substances in different directions in a cell. They increase in number during mitosis.

microtus (mī-krō′tŭs) [″ + *ous*, ear]. Individual with very small ears.

microvascular (mī″krō-văs′kū-lăr). Pert. to the very fine blood vessels of the body.

microvilli (mī″krō-vil′ī) [L., tufts of hair] (sing. *microvillus*). Microscopic projections from the free surface of cell membranes. They greatly increase the exposed surface area of the cell. SEE: *border, brush.*

microvolt. One-millionth part of a volt.

microwave (mī′krō-wāv). That portion of the radio wave spectrum between a wavelength of 1 mm and 30 cm.

microxycyte (mī-krŏk′sī-sīt) [Gr. *mikros*, small, + *oxys*, sharp, + *kytos*, cell]. Any cell containing fine granules.

microzoon (mī″krō-zō′ŏn) [″ + *zoon*, animal]. Microscopic animal.

miction (mĭk′shŭn). Urination.

micturate (mĭk′tū-rāt) [L. *micturire*]. To pass the urine. SYN: *urinate.*

micturition (mĭk-tū-rĭ′shŭn). The voiding of urine. SYN: *urination.*

micturition syncope. The abrupt loss of consciousness during micturition. It usually occurs in men who get up at night to urinate. The pathophysiology of this is not understood. Recovery is uneventful.

MICU. *medical intensive care unit.*

MID. *minimum infective dose.*

midazolam hydrochloride. A benzodiazepine used to produce sedation for brief diagnostic or endoscopic procedures and as sedation prior to general anesthesia. Trade name is Versed.

midbody (mĭd′bŏd-ē). Microtubules that appear as a granule between daughter cells during telophase of mitosis.

midbrain [AS. *mid*, middle, + *braegen*, brain]. The corpora quadrigemina, the crura cerebri, and aqueduct of Sylvius, which connect the pons and cerebellum with the hemispheres of the cerebrum. SYN: *mesencephalon.*

midcarpal (mĭd-kăr′păl). 1. Between the two rows of carpal bones. 2. Mediocarpal.

middle age. A vague term indicating someone

is between 40 and 60 years of age, approximately. SEE: *chronologically enhanced.*

middle lobe syndrome. Atelectasis, bronchiectasis, or chronic pneumonitis of the right middle lobe of the lung. May be due to calcified lymph nodes compressing the right middle lobe bronchus.

midge (mĭj) [ME. *migge*]. Small, gnatlike flies including those from the families Chironomidae and Ceratopogonidae. Some cause painful bites.

midget. A non-technical term for a very small person; an adult who is perfectly formed but has not attained and will not attain normal size.

midgut [AS. *mid*, middle, + *gut*, intestine]. The midportion of the embryonic gut that opens ventrally into the yolk stalk.

midline (mĭd′līn). Any line that bisects a structure that is bilaterally symmetrical.

midoccipital (mĭd″ŏk-sĭp′ĭ-tăl). In the middle of the occiput.

midpain (mĭd′pān). Intermenstrual pain. SEE: *mittelschmerz.*

midplane (mĭd′plān). 1. The plane bisecting a symmetrical structure. 2. In obstetrics, the plane of least dimensions in the pelvic outlet.

midriff (mĭd′rĭf) [″ + *hrif*, belly]. The diaphragm; the middle region of the torso.

midsection (mĭd-sĕk′shŭn) [″ + L. *secare*, to cut]. A section through the middle of a structure.

midsternum (mĭd-stĕr′nŭm). The largest and middle portion of the sternum.

midstream specimen. A urine specimen collected during the passage of the urine after the flow has begun and prior to the end. It is done to obtain a specimen with little urethral contamination.

midtarsal (mĭd-tăr′săl). Between the two rows of bones that make up the tarsus of the foot.

midwife [″ + *wif*, wife]. A female who delivers babies. She may or may not have received formal training in this field.

m., nurse-. A nurse who has received special training in obstetrics and is qualified to deliver infants.

midwifery (mĭd-wĭf′ĕr-ē). The art of assisting at childbirth. SYN: *obstetrics.*

mifepristone. An antiprogesterone steroid used as an abortifacient. SYN: RU-486.

migraine (mī′grān) [Fr. from Gr. *hemikrania*, half skull]. Paroxysmal attacks of headache, frequently unilateral, usually accompanied by disordered vision and gastrointestinal disturbances. Thought to be the result of vasodilation of extracerebral cranial arteries. An estimated 8 million people in the U.S. suffer from migraine headaches. SEE: *Nursing Diagnoses* in Appendix.

SYM: Headaches associated with the sensation of seeing zigzags of light, called scintillating scotomata, vomiting, and at times diplopia, unilateral sweating, and focal symptoms. Sharp stabbing pains frequently in temporofrontal region.

ETIOL: Unknown but a family history of migraine will be found in over half of the patients. It may be precipitated by allergic hypersensitivity or emotional disturbances. At one time it was believed that red wine was less likely than white wine to be tolerated by persons with migraine because of a higher concentration of tyramine in red wine. It is now known that tyramine is present in about the same concentration in both red and white wine. However, phenolic flavonoids are much higher in red wine than in white wine. This may account for persons with migraine tolerating white wine better than red wine.

DIAG: It must be distinguished from other types of headache, but the history, the course of the disorder, and the peculiar combination of symptoms rarely permit much uncertainty. The frequency may vary from several times a week to several times a year and tends to decrease with age.

TREAT: The best therapy is prevention. The patient can help prevent migraines by avoiding conditions that he or she has learned will cause an attack. In addition, persons with frequent attacks may use propanolol (Inderal) daily. A dose of 20 mg three times a day may be increased to a total dose of as much as 240 mg in 1 day. Methysergide (Sansert), an ergot derivative, also may be used to prevent migraines. For infrequent mild attacks, 0.6 gm of aspirin or a small dose of codeine may suffice. For severe attacks, the patient should hold a 2-mg tablet of ergotamine tartrate under the tongue until it dissolves; this should be repeated every half hour until the headache is relieved or until 8 mg has been taken. A single dose of promethazine (Phenergan) will help prevent side effects and relax the patient. If this regimen fails, codeine or Demerol will control the pain. Pregnant patients and those with vascular disease should not be given ergotamine because of the danger of arterial spasm.

Sumatriptan, an expensive drug, is effective in treating migraines. It may be approved for use in the U.S.

migration (mī-grā′shŭn) [L. *migrare*, to move from place to place]. Passage of cells from one position to another.

Ex.: migration of an ovum from the ovary into the fallopian tube; movement of leukocytes through the wall of a blood vessel into surrounding tissues.

m., internal, of ovum. Passage of the ovum through the uterine (fallopian) tube to the uterus.

m. of leukocytes. Passage of white blood corpuscles through walls of capillaries. SYN: *diapedesis.*

m. of testicle. Descent of testicle into the scrotum. SYN: *descensus testis.*

migratory. 1. Pert. to migration. 2. Changing or capable of changing positions.

mikro-. SEE: words beginning with *micro-*.

Mikulicz′s drain (mĭk′ū-lĭch″ĕs) [Johann von Mikulicz-Radecki, Polish surgeon, 1850–1905]. Drain formed by pushing a single layer of gauze into a cavity or wound, then packing with several layers of gauze as the original layer is pushed farther and farther into the defect.

Mikulicz′s mask. Gauze-covered frame worn over nose and mouth during performance of operation.

Mikulicz′s pad. Folded gauze pad for packing off the viscera in abdominal operations and used as a sponge in general.

Mikulicz′s syndrome. Chronic infiltration with lymphocytes and painless enlargement of lacrimal and salivary glands.

mildew [AS. *mildeaw*]. Lay term for a discoloration or superficial coating on various materials caused by the growth of fungi. Occurs in damp conditions.

milia (mĭl′ē-ă). Pl. of milium.

miliaria (mĭl-ē-ā′rē-ă) [L. *milium,* millet]. Vesicles caused by obstruction of ducts of sweat glands. Acute inflammation of the sweat glands will result if the obstruction persists. The three forms of miliaria (sudamina, rubra, and profunda) represent different levels of obstruction of the sweat ducts. Occurs most commonly in infants, the obese, and in those exposed to excessive heat for prolonged periods. Excessive clothing and hyperhidrosis are contributing factors. SYN: *miliaria rubra; prickly heat.*

SYM: Sudden appearance of red patches of small papules. Vesicles are discrete and accompanied by red areolae. They usually appear on the trunk and are accompanied by itching, burning, and fever of short duration. They occur in hot weather, in tropical countries, and in individuals sweating profusely. Papules may become eczematous if irritated.

ETIOL: Exposure to excessive heat, skin irritants, and tendency to hyperhidrosis.

TREAT: The only effective treatment and prevention is avoidance of further sweating. Calamine lotion helps to relieve symptoms.

m., apocrine. SEE: *Fordyce-Fox disease.*

m. crystallina. Sweat escaped into or just below the stratum corneum. SYN: *su-*

Composition of Whole Milk

	Human Milk	Cow's Milk
Water	87%–88%	85%–88%
Minerals	0.2%	0.8%
Protein	1.1%	3.3%
Fat	3.8%	3.7%
Sugar (lactose, carbohydrate)	6.5%–7.0%	4.8%
Sodium	7 mEq/liter	25 mEq/liter
Potassium	14 mEq/liter	35 mEq/liter
Calories	22 kcal/oz	20 kcal/oz

damen.

m. profunda. Nearly always follows attacks of miliaria rubra. Seen almost exclusively in the tropics. Area is covered with pale, firm papules 1 to 3 mm across. These are painless and do not cause itching.

miliary (mĭl′ē-ă-rē) [L. *miliaris,* like a millet seed]. Characterized by presence of small nodules or lesions resembling millet seed.

miliary tubercles. Small gray nodules in first stage of tuberculosis.

miliary tuberculosis. Acute, generalized tuberculosis with minute tubercles in the affected part or organ.

milieu (mē-lyū′) [Fr.]. Environment.

m. interieur. Internal environment of extracellular fluids of the body.

milieu therapy. A method of psychotherapy that controls the environment of the patient to provide interpersonal contacts that will develop trust, assurance, and personal autonomy.

military antishock trousers. ABBR: MAST. SEE: *anti-G suit.*

milium (mĭl′ē-ŭm) [L., millet seed] (pl. *milia*). White pinhead-size papules occurring on face, and sometimes the trunk of a newborn, and usually disappearing in several weeks; keratin-filled cysts.

TREAT: Mechanical keratolytics (pumice stone, soap), salicylic acid and sulfur ointment, or incision and expression of contents.

m., colloid. Tiny papule formed beneath the epidermis due to colloid degeneration.

milk [AS. *meolc*]. A secretion of the mammary glands for feeding the young. The constituent food substances vary from animal to animal.

COMP: Milk from cows consists of water, organic substances, and mineral salts. SEE: table. *Organic substances:* Proteins: The principal proteins are caseinogen, lactoalbumin, and lactoglobulin; in the presence of calcium ions, soluble caseinogen is converted into insoluble casein by the action of

acids, rennet, or pepsin. This brings about the curdling of milk. Lactoglobulin is identical with serum globulin of blood and hence contains maternal antibodies. Carbohydrates: Lactose or milk sugar is the principal sugar, although small quantities of other sugars are present. Fats: The principal fats are glycerides of oleic, palmitic, and myristic acids. Smaller quantities of stearic acid and short-chain fatty acids with carbon chains of C_4 to C_{24} are present. Sterols and phosphatides (lecithin and cephalin) are also present. Churning causes the fat globules to unite into a solid mass and separate from the whey to form butter. *Mineral salts:* The principal cations are calcium, potassium, and sodium; the principal anions are phosphate and chloride. Citrates and lactates are present in small quantities. Milk is low in iron and magnesium.

Vitamins: Vitamin A and those of the B complex (thiamine, riboflavin, and pantothenic acid) are present in adequate quantities to meet the needs of a growing child. Milk is low in vitamins C and D.

On standing at room temperature, milk sours as a result of the action of lactic acid bacilli on lactose converting it into lactic acid. When the pH reaches 5.34, coagulation occurs, resulting in production of a curd. The remaining watery portion is called whey.

Milk contains antibodies that are present in the mother's blood and a number of enzymes (catalase, oxidase, reductase, phosphatase).

m., acidophilus. Milk inoculated with *Lactobacillus acidophilus,* a bacterium that grows best in an acid medium. Used to modify the bacterial flora of the digestive tract.

m., breast. Milk obtained from the breast, esp. the human breast.

m., breast, storage of. Human breast milk that is collected and refrigerated immediately may be used for up to 5 days. If it is collected, frozen, and stored at −17.7°C

(0°F), it is safe for 6 months.

m., butter-. That portion of milk left after removal of butter following churning.

m., casein. Milk prepared with a large quantity of casein and fat but little sugar and salts.

m., certified. Milk certified by a milk commission as pure.

m., condensed. Partly evaporated and sweetened milk.

m., cow's. For composition, SEE: table.

m., evaporated. Cow's milk that has been concentrated by evaporating some of the water. It can be canned after pasteurization, q.v., and stored for long periods of time. SEE: *milk, lactic acid evaporated.*

m., filled. A product made by combining fats or oils other than milk fat with milk solids. The product resembles milk.

m., fortified. Milk enriched by the addition of cream, albumin, or vitamins.

m., homogenized. Milk that has been processed so that fats are combined with the body of the milk; thus the cream does not separate.

m., instant dry nonfat. Dried skimmed milk. It may be stored at room temperature until needed. Reconstituted by adding water to the granules.

m., lactic acid evaporated. Evaporated milk to which sugar and lactic acid have been added. To prepare this milk, add 17 oz (503 ml) of water to 13 oz (384 ml) of evaporated milk, 2 level tbsp (1 oz or 28 gm) of granulated sugar, and 3 tbsp (45 ml) of vinegar. This mixture contains 77 Cal per 100 ml.

May be used for normal infants from birth to 12 months. For older children omit the sugar. This reduces the Cal to about 67 per 100 ml (20 per oz).

m., low fat, 1%. Cow's milk with 1% fat, which represents 22% of the calories.

m., low fat, 2%. Cow's milk with 2% fat, which represents 35% of the calories.

m., modified. Milk altered so that its composition more closely approximates that of human milk.

m., mother's. Milk from the mammary glands of a woman.

m., nonfat. M., skim.

m. of bismuth. USP. A suspension of bismuth hydroxide and bismuth subcarbonate in water. It is an antacid. Previously used name was bismuth magma.

m., pasteurized. Milk heated to a specified temperature for a precise length of time and then cooled rapidly. This process kills pathogenic bacteria without appreciably altering the taste of the milk. SEE: *pasteurization.*

m., protein. Milk with high protein and low carbohydrate and fat content.

m., red. Milk contaminated by blood, chromogenic bacteria, or plant pigments.

m., ropy. Milk that has become viscid due to formation of vegetable gums from carbohydrates or mucinlike substances from proteins as a result of bacterial action.

m., skim. Cow's milk that contains a small amount of fat. The percentage of calories from fat is 4%.

m., sour. Milk with lactic acid caused by lactic acid bacteria.

m., sterilized. Milk that has been boiled to kill bacteria.

m., uterine. A white fluid found between villi in placenta of pregnant uterus.

m., vegetable. 1. The latex of plants. 2. A synthetic milk prepared from juices of various plants, such as soybean.

m., vitamin D. Milk in which vitamin D content has been increased by addition of concentrates, ultraviolet irradiation, or by feeding irradiated yeast to milk-producing animals.

m., whole. Milk that has not been altered except for pasteurization. The fat content is 3.3%, which represents 51% of the calories present.

m., witch's. Milk secreted in the breast of the newborn.

milk-alkali syndrome. Elevated blood calcium without an increase in calcium or phosphate in the urine, renal insufficiency, and alkalosis due to prolonged intake of excessive amounts of milk and soluble alkali. This condition is usually found as an undesired side effect in conjunction with treating a peptic ulcer. SYN: *Burnett's syndrome.*

milker's nodules. Painless smooth or warty lesions on the hands and arms, produced by the virus that causes paravaccinia, a viral disease that affects the udders of cows and may be transmitted to man. SEE: *paravaccinia.*

milk fever. Fever during the puerperium due to infection.

milking. Removal of the contents of a tubular structure by compressing the tube with the fingers and moving them along the course of the tube. This maneuver forces material out of the tube which might not otherwise be seen or available for study.

Ex.: milking to express purulent material from the urethra. SEE: *strip.*

milk leg. Thrombosis of the iliac or femoral vein followed by swelling of the leg. So named because it is often a complication of puerperium. SYN: *phlegmasia alba dolens.*

Milkman's syndrome (milk'mănz) [Louis A. Milkman, U.S. roentgenologist, 1895–1951]. Failure of reabsorption of phosphate by the renal tubules. This causes a special type of demineralization of bones that produces a transverse striped area of multiple pseudofractures in roentgenograms of the bones.

milk of magnesia. USP. Magnesium hydroxide in suspension, used as an antacid and a cathartic. Previously used name was magnesia magma. Trade name is Mint-O-Mag.

milk teeth. The first or deciduous teeth.

milk tumor. Retention of milk in the mammary gland.

Miller-Abbott tube [Thomas Grier Miller, U.S. physician, b. 1886; William Osler Abbott, U.S. physician, 1902–1943]. A double-channel intestinal tube used to relieve intestinal distention. Inserted through a nostril, the tube is passed through the stomach into the small intestine.

Miller Assessment for Preschoolers [Lucy Jane Miller, Ph.D., contemporary occupational therapist]. ABBR: M.A.P. A widely used standardized developmental screening test for youngsters from 2 to 5 years of age. It contains sensory, motor and cognitive performance items.

milli- [L. *milli,* thousand]. Prefix used in metric system to denote one-thousandth (10^{-3}).

milliammeter. Ammeter registering in milliamperes. SEE: *ammeter.*

milliamperage seconds. ABBR: MAS. In radiography, the milliamperage of the exposure multiplied by the time of the exposure in seconds. This factor determines the exposure of the radiograph.

milliampere (mĭl″ē-ăm′pēr). ABBR: ma. One-thousandth of an ampere.

milliampere minute. An electrical unit of quantity, equivalent to that delivered by 1 milliampere in 1 minute.

milliampere-seconds. Product of the time of radiation exposure and the milliamperage used.

millibar (mĭl′ĭ-băr). One-thousandth of a bar, which is 100 newtons per square meter. The normal atmospheric pressure of 14.7 pounds per square inch is equal to 1013 millibars.

millicoulomb (mĭl″ĭ-koo′lŏm). A unit of electric current, one-thousandth (10^{-3}) of a coulomb.

millicurie (mĭl″ĭ-kū′rē). ABBR: mc. One-thousandth of a curie. A practical unit of dosage for a radioactive source: 1 mc of a radioactive substance applied for one hour.

millicurie hour. A practical unit of dosage for radon: 1 mc of radon applied for one hour. The biological effect depends on time, filtration, and distance.

milliequivalent. ABBR: mEq. The concentration of electrolytes in a certain volume of solution. Usually expressed as milliequivalent per liter (mEq/L). It is calculated by multiplying the milligrams per liter by the

valence of the chemical and dividing by the molecular weight of the substance:

$$mEq/L = \frac{(mg/L) \times valence}{molecular\ weight}$$

For gases, it is known that a quantity of gas equal in weight to its molecular weight in grams occupies 22.4 liters under standard conditions. The concentration is expressed as millimoles (mM) per liter. For example: if the carbon dioxide (CO_2) present in a sample is 60.5 volume percent, the calculation would be

$$\frac{60.5 \times 10}{22.4} = 27\ mM/L$$

The concentration 60.5 volume percent was multiplied by 10 in order to obtain the amount of CO_2 in one liter. SEE: Appendix, *Normal Ranges of Laboratory Values.*

milligram (mĭl′ĭ-grăm). ABBR: mg. One-thousandth of a gram.

millilambert (mĭl″ĭ-lăm′bĕrt). A unit of light intensity, one-thousandth of a lambert. About one foot-candle, but more accurately, it is 0.929 lumens per square foot.

milliliter. ABBR: ml. One-thousandth of a liter. For practical purposes it is equivalent to one cubic centimeter. The term milliliter (ml) is used when referring to *liquid* volume; cubic centimeter (cc) is used when referring to the volume of a gas.

millimeter. ABBR: mm. One-thousandth of a meter.

millimicro- (mμ). Prefix formerly used to indicate one billionth (10^{-9}). The term currently used is *nano.*

millimicrocurie (mĭl″ĭ-mī″krō-kū′rē). A nanocurie or 10^{-9} curie.

millimicrogram (mĭl″ĭ-mī′krō-grăm). A nanogram or 10^{-9} gram.

millimicron (mĭl-ĭ-mī′krŏn). ABBR: mμ or mmm. One-thousandth of a micron; one-millionth of a millimeter.

millimole (mĭl′ĭ-mōl). ABBR: mM. One-thousandth of a mole.

milling-in. A method of adjusting the occlusion of teeth by moving them against each other while an abrasive substance is between them.

millinormal (mĭl″ĭ-nor′măl). Strength of a solution equal to one-thousandth normal.

milliosmole (mĭl″ē-ŏs′mōl). The osmotic pressure equal to one-thousandth of the molecular weight of a substance divided by the number of ions that the substance forms in a liter of solution.

millipede (mĭl′ĭ-pēd). A wingless, wormlike insect with a pair of legs on each body segment. Some produce an irritating venom.

millisecond (mĭl″ĭ-sĕk′ŏnd). One-thousandth of a second.

millivolt (mĭl'ĭ-vōlt). One-thousandth of a volt.

Milontin. Trade name for phensuximide.

milphae (mĭl'fē) [Gr. *milphai*]. Loss of eyebrow hair.

milphosis (mĭl-fō'sĭs) [Gr.]. Loss of eyebrows or eyelashes.

Milroy's disease (mĭl'roys) [William Forsyth Milroy, U.S. physician, 1855–1942]. Chronic hereditary edema of the legs.

Miltown. Trade name for meprobamate, USP.

Milwaukee brace. A brace made of strong, lightweight materials. It extends from a chin cup with neck pad to the pelvis, used to correct minimal curve scoliosis.

mimesis [Gr.]. Imitation, mimicry. Term applied to a disease that exhibits symptoms of another disease or to conditions in hysteria that simulate organic disease.

mimetic, mimic (mī-mĕt'ĭk, mĭm'ĭk) [Gr. *mimetikos*]. Imitative.

mimmation (mĭ-mā'shŭn). A form of stuttering in which the "m" sound is inappropriately used.

mimosis (mī-mō'sĭs). Mimesis, q.v.

min. *minim; minute.*

Minamata disease (mĭn"ă-maw'tă). Neurological disease due to ingestion of alkyl mercury, an organic mercury compound used in industrial processes. Present in fish taken from Minamata Bay, Japan. SYN: *yushi.*

SYM: Paresthesias, loss of peripheral vision, dysarthria, ataxia, tremors, excessive salivation, sweating, and mental disturbances.

PROG: Poor. Death may occur.

mind [AS. *gemynd*]. Integration and organization of functions of the brain resulting in the ability to perceive surroundings, to have emotions, imagination, memory, and will, and to process information in an intelligent manner. The quality and quantity of the functions of the mind vary with experience and development.

mineral [L. *minerale*]. 1. An inorganic element or compound occurring in nature, esp. one that is solid. 2. Inorganic; not of animal or plant origin. 3. Impregnated with minerals, as mineral water. 4. Pert. to minerals.

mineral acid. An acid containing no carbon atoms. SYN: *inorganic acid.*

mineral compounds. Compounds of mineral elements. Many such chemicals are present in the body. SEE: *acid-base balance; buffer; Elements* in *Appendix.*

FUNCT: Minerals are essential constituents of all cells; they form the greater portion of the hard parts of the body (bone, teeth, nails); they are essential components of respiratory pigments, enzymes, and en-

zyme systems; they regulate the permeability of cell membranes and capillaries; they regulate the excitability of muscular and nervous tissue; they are essential for regulation of osmotic pressure equilibria; they are necessary for maintenance of proper acid-base balance; they are essential constituents of secretions of glands; they play an important role in water metabolism and regulation of blood volume.

Mineral salts and water are excreted daily from the body. These must be replaced through food intake. Daily requirements for principal minerals for a normal adult are as follows: calcium and phosphorus, 800 to 1200 mg; copper, 1.5 to 3 mg; iodine, 150 μg (micrograms); magnesium, 280 to 400 mg; potassium, 2000 mg; sodium, about 500 mg. Daily intake of sodium chloride should be limited to 6 gm (2.4 gm of sodium) or less each day. Requirements are greater for growing children and pregnant women and in certain pathological conditions. SEE: *Recommended Daily Dietary Allowances* in *Appendix.*

mineralization (mĭn"ĕr-ăl-ī-zā'shŭn). Normal or abnormal deposition of minerals in tissues.

mineralocorticoid (mĭn"ĕr-ăl-ō-kor'tĭkoyd). A biologically active principle of the adrenal cortex predominantly involved in the regulation of fluid and electrolytes by its effects on ion transport and on the renal tubules.

mineral oil. USP. Liquid petrolatum.

mineral spring. A spring in which water contains mineral salts thought to have a therapeutic value in certain diseases, but usually the principal action is as a cathartic. SYN: *spa.*

mineral water. Water that contains sufficient inorganic salts to cause it to have characteristic properties.

minification. In radiography, the reduction in the size of a fluoroscopic image to intensify the brightness of that image.

minim (mĭn'ĭm) [L. *minimum*, least]. ABBR: m., min. One-sixtieth part of a fluidram or 0.06 milliliter.

minimal (mĭn'ĭ-măl). Least; the smallest possible.

minimal brain damage. SEE: *attention deficit disorder.*

minimal brain dysfunction. ABBR: MBD. A poorly defined concept rather than a specific diagnosis. SEE: *attention deficit disorder.*

minimal cerebral dysfunction. SEE: *attention deficit disorder.*

minimal change disease. SEE: *nephrosis, lipoid.*

minimal dose. Smallest dose producing an

effect.

minimum (mĭn′ĭ-mŭm) (pl. *minima*). Least quantity or lowest limit. SEE: *threshold*.

minimum daily requirements. ABBR: MDR. The daily requirements of vitamins and minerals needed to prevent symptoms of deficiency. SEE: *Recommended Daily Dietary Allowances* in *Appendix*.

minimum lethal dose. Smallest quantity of a substance capable of producing death.

Minin light (mĭn′ĭn) [A.V. Minin, Russian surgeon]. A special light that produces violet or ultraviolet light.

Minipress. Trade name for prazosin hydrochloride.

mini-stroke. Transient ischemic attack, q.v.

Minnesota Multiphasic Personality Inventory. ABBR: MMPI. SEE: *personality testing*.

Minocin. Trade name for minocycline hydrochloride, USP.

minocycline hydrochloride (mĭ-nō-sī′klēn). USP. An antibiotic of the tetracycline class. Trade name is Minocin.

minor. Person not of legal age and thus requiring consent for medical, surgical, or dental care. Legal age in the U.S. varies from state to state.

    m., emancipated. A person not of legal age who is either in the armed services, married or mother of a child whether married or not, or has left home and is self-sufficient. Some state legislatures do not require such an individual to have parental consent in order to receive medical or surgical care.

Minot-Murphy diet (mī′nŏt) [George R. Minot, U.S. physician, 1885–1950; William P. Murphy, U.S. physician, b. 1892]. Diet for pernicious anemia containing large quantities of liver.

minoxidil. USP. A drug approved for use in promoting hair growth. Trade name is Rogaine.

Mintezol. Trade name for thiabendazole, USP.

minute volume. Volume of air breathed in a minute.

mio- (mī′ō) [Gr. *meion*, less]. Combining form meaning less, smaller.

miocardia (mī-ō-kär′dē-ă) [″ + *kardia*, heart]. Lessening of heart's volume during systolic contraction. SYN: *systole*.

Miochol. Trade name for acetylcholine chloride.

miodidymus (mī″ō-dĭd′ĭ-mŭs) [″ + *didymos*, twin]. A fetus with two heads joined at the occiput.

miolecithal (mī″ō-lĕs′ĭ-thăl) [″ + *lekithos*, egg yolk]. Pert. to an egg with a small amount of yolk.

miopragia (mī-ō-prā′jē-ă) [Gr. *meion*, less,

    + *prassein*, to perform]. Decrease of functional activity.

miopus (mī′ō-pŭs) [″ + *ops*, face]. Conjoined twins with one having a rudimentary face.

miosis (mī-ō′sĭs) [Gr. *meiosis*, a lessening]. 1. Abnormal contraction of the pupils.

    ETIOL: May be due to irritation of the oculomotor system, or paralysis of dilators. Occurs in certain fevers, congestion of iris, in typhus, in early stages of meningitis, and in some forms of drug poisoning. Also seen in brain lesions and sunstroke.

    2. The stage of disease during which intensity of signs and symptoms diminishes.

Miostat. Trade name for carbachol.

miotic. 1. An agent that causes the pupil to contract, such as eserine or pilocarpine. 2. Pert. to or causing contraction of the pupil. 3. Diminishing. SYN: *myotic*.

miracidium (mī″ră-sĭd′ē-ŭm) [Gr. *meirakidion*, lad] (pl. *miracidia*). A ciliated free-swimming larva of a digenetic fluke. On emerging from an ovum, it penetrates a snail of a particular species and metamorphoses into a sporocyst. SEE: *fluke*.

miracle, medical. The unexplained spontaneous regression of a medical condition thought to be invariably fatal or incurable or both. Such miracles have been claimed after sick persons have visited the shrine in Lourdes, France. The Roman Catholic Church has carefully investigated alleged miracles at Lourdes and has found that, since 1858 when the story of Lourdes began, some of the spontaneous regressions meet their criteria for classification as miracles.

    Miracles may be negative in that healthy persons may become ill and die without any reasonable explanation. SEE: *voodoo*.

mire (mēr) [L. *mirari*, to look at]. A test object on the ophthalmometer, the images of which denote the amount of astigmatism.

mirror [Fr. *miroir*]. A polished surface that reflects rays of light and thus reproduces visible images of objects in front of it.

    m., dental. A dental instrument commonly used for viewing occlusal and distal surfaces of teeth and for retracting soft tissues from the field of operation. SYN: *mouth mirror*.

mirror writing. Writing so that letters and words are reversed and appear as in a mirror.

miryachit (mĭr-ē′ă-chĭt) [Russian]. A type of "jumping disorder" seen in Siberia. It is similar to the Jumping Frenchmen of Maine, q.v. SYN: *saltatory spasm*.

mis- [AS. *mis*, wrong]. Prefix implying bad, wrong, improper, or negative.

misandry [Gr. *miso*, hatred, + *andros*, man]. Hatred of males. SEE: *misogyny*.

misanthropia (mĭs"ăn-thrō'pē-ă) [" + Gr. *anthropos,* man]. Hatred of mankind.

miscarriage [" + L. *carrus,* cart]. Lay term for termination of pregnancy at any time before the fetus has attained extrauterine viability. Usually refers specifically to expulsion of fetus in period between fourth month and viability. SYN: *abortion.*

misce (mĭs'ē) [L., mix]. ABBR: M. A direction given on prescriptions, instructing the pharmacist to mix the ingredients.

miscegenation (mĭs"ē-jē-nā'shŭn) [L. *miscere,* to mix, + *genus,* race]. Sexual relations or marriage between those of different races.

miscible (mĭs'ĭ-bl). Capable of being mixed.

misery. Extreme mental or emotional unhappiness.

misinformation. Data or information concerning a patient that may be assumed erroneously to be accurate, e.g., laboratory data that are inaccurate, historical data from the patient or the family that are unreliable, and transcription errors in recording data. In some instances, the misinformation is knowingly presented to or withheld from the physician by the patient in order to conceal something that would be personally embarrassing or incriminating.

misocainia (mĭs-ō-kī'nē-ă) [Gr. *miseio,* to hate, + *kainos,* new]. Aversion to new ideas. SYN: *misoneism.*

misogamy (mĭ-sŏg'ă-mē) [" + *gamos,* marriage]. Aversion to marriage.

misogynist (mĭs-ŏj'ĭ-nĭst) [" + *gyne,* woman]. One who hates women.

misogyny (mĭs-ŏj'ĭn-ē). Aversion to or hatred of women.

misologia (mĭs-ō-lō'jē-ă) [Gr. *miseio,* to hate, + *logos,* word, reason]. Aversion to mental activity.

misoneism (mĭ-sō-nē'ĭzm) [" + *neos,* new]. Aversion to new things or new ideas; conservatism. SYN: *misocainia.*

misopedia (mĭ-sō-pē'dē-ă) [" + Gr. *pais,* child]. Abnormal dislike of children or the young.

Mist., mist. *mistura.*

mister. In England and other parts of the British Commonwealth, the title of address of a surgeon.

mistura (mĭs-tū'ră) [L.]. Mixture. Preparation intended for internal use and containing suspended insoluble substances that do not unite chemically. Should always be shaken before being used.

Mitchell's disease (mĭch'ĕlz) [Silas Weir Mitchell, U.S. neurologist, 1829–1914]. Erythromelalgia, q.v.

mite (mīt) [AS.]. A minute arachnid, a member of the order Acarina. Some are parasitic and are the cause of conditions such as asthma, mange, and scabies. Some serve as vectors of disease organisms and as intermediate hosts for certain Cestodes.

Asthma has a higher prevalence rate in households with a large number of dust mites. SEE: *Demodex folliculorum.*

m., follicle. Mite that lives in hair follicles and sebaceous glands. SYN: *Demodex folliculorum.*

m., harvest. SEE: *harvest mite.*

m., itch. *Sarcoptes scabiei.* SEE: *scabies.*

m., mange. Mites belonging to the families Sarcoptidae and Psoroptidae. The cause of mange and scabies in many species of animals. SEE: *mange; scabies.*

m., red. Redbugs or chiggers, members of the family Thrombiculidae. SEE: *chiggers.*

mitella (mī-tĕl'ă) [L.]. A sling for the arm.

Mithracin. Trade name for plicamycin, USP.

mithramycin (mĭth"ră-mī'sĭn). Previously used name for plicamycin.

mithridatism (mĭth'rĭ-dāt"ĭzm) [Mithridates, king of Pontus, 132–63 B.C., supposed to have acquired immunity in this fashion]. Immunity to a poison acquired by taking it in doses of gradually increasing size.

miticide (mī'tĭ-sīd) [AS. *mite,* mite, + L. *caedere,* to kill]. A substance that kills mites.

mitigated (mĭt'ĭ-gāt-ĕd) [L. *mitigare,* to soften.]. Diminished in severity. SYN: *allayed; moderated.*

mitis (mī'tĭs) [L.]. Mild.

mitochondria (mīt"ō-kŏn'drē-ă) [Gr. *mitos,* thread, + *chondros,* cartilage] (sing. *mitochondrion*). Slender microscopic filaments or rods 0.5 micrometer in diameter that can be seen in cells by using phase-contrast microscopy or electron microscopy. They are the source of energy in the cell and are involved in protein synthesis and lipid metabolism. SEE: *cell; organelle* for illus.

mitogen (mī'tō-jĕn). A protein substance derived from plants that is used in the laboratory to stimulate cells to divide (mitosis). Frequently used in vitro, q.v., to study the proliferation of lymphocytes from blood drawn during a research study. The most commonly used mitogens are phytohemagglutinin and concanavalin A. SEE: *concanavalin A; lectin; phytohemagglutinin; pokeweed.*

m., pokeweed. ABBR: PWM. A mitogen isolated from the pokeweed plant, *Phytolacca americana.* It has, in the presence of T lymphocytes, the capacity to induce primed B lymphocytes to proliferate and differentiate to plasma cells. The B lymphocytes are also influenced by PWM.

mitogenesis (mī"tō-jĕn'ē-sĭs) [" + *osis,* condition, + *genesis,* generation, birth]. To cause cell mitosis.

mitoma, mitome [Gr. *mitos,* thread]. A fine

network support or framework of protoplasm in a cell.

mitomycin (mī″tō-mī′sĭn). USP. An antibiotic with antineoplastic action. Trade names are Mitocin-C and Mutamycin.

mitoplasm (mī′tō-plăzm) [″ + *plassein*, to form]. The chromatic substance in a cell nucleus.

mitosis (mī-tō′sĭs) [″ + *osis*, condition] (pl. *mitoses*). Type of cell division of somatic cells in which each daughter cell contains the same number of chromosomes as the parent cell. It is the process by which the body grows, and by which somatic cells are replaced. SEE: *cell division* for illus.; *meiosis*.

Mitosis is a continuous process divided into four phases:

Prophase: the chromatin granules of the nucleus stain more densely and become organized into chromosomes that first appear as long, delicate, spiral structures, each consisting of two spiral filaments called chromatids. Each chromosome possesses a clear region (centromere) usually in the midregion. As the prophase progresses, the chromosomes become shorter, more compact, and stain densely; the nuclear membrane and the nucleoli disappear. At the same time, the centriole divides and the two daughter centrioles, each surrounded by a centrosphere, move to opposite poles of the cell. They are connected by fine protoplasmic fibrils that form the achromatic spindle.

Metaphase: the chromosomes (paired chromatids) arrange themselves in an equatorial plane midway between the two centrioles forming the equatorial plate.

Anaphase: the chromatids (now called daughter chromosomes) diverge and move toward their respective centrosomes. The end of their migration marks the beginning of the next phase.

Telophase: the chromosomes at each pole of the spindle undergo changes the reverse of those in the prophase, each becoming a long, loosely spiraled thread. The nuclear membrane reforms and nucleoli reappear. Outlines of chromosomes disappear and chromatin appears as granules scattered throughout nucleus and connected by a lightly staining net. The cytoplasm becomes separated into two parts, resulting in two complete cells. This is accomplished in animal cells by constriction in the equatorial region; in plant cells, a cell plate that gives rise to the cell membrane forms in a similar position. The period between two successive divisions is called interphase.

Mitosis is of particular significance in that genes are distributed equally to each daughter cell and a fixed number of chromosomes is maintained in all somatic cells of an organism.

   m., heterotypic. The first or reduction division in the maturation of germ cells.

   m., homeotypic. The second or equational division in the maturation of germ cells.

mitosome (mī′tō-sōm) [Gr. *mitos*, thread, + *soma*, body]. 1. A body giving rise to the middle piece of the spermatozoon. 2. Chromatin mass in a cellular nucleus.

mitotane (mī′tō-tān). USP. A drug that selectively acts against the cells of the adrenal cortex. It is used in treating inoperable adrenal cortical carcinoma. Previously named was *o,p′*-DDD. Trade name is Lysodren.

mitotic (mī-tŏt′ĭk). Pert. to mitosis.

mitral (mī′trăl). Pert. to the bicuspid or mitral valve. SEE: *facies mitralis.*

mitral commissurotomy. Surgical procedure for treating stenosis of the mitral valve of the heart.

mitral disease. Disease of the mitral valve. SEE: *heart.*

mitralization (mī″trăl-ī-zā′shŭn). In the roentgenogram of the heart, straightening of the left border, as seen in the anterior-posterior view, due to mitral valve disease.

mitral murmur. Murmur produced at the mitral valve.

mitral orifice. Left atrioventricular aperture.

mitral regurgitation. Backflow of blood from the left ventricle into the left atrium due to failure of the valve to close completely.

mitral stenosis. Narrowing orifice of the mitral valve obstructing free flow from atrium to ventricle. SEE: *Nursing Diagnoses* in *Appendix.*

mitral valve. Bicuspid valve, q.v.; valvula bicuspidalis.

mitral valve prolapse. A common and occasionally serious condition in which the cusp or cusps of the mitral valve prolapse into the left atrium during systole. In patients without evidence of mitral regurgitation, q.v., there are usually no symptoms; but in some patients, nonanginal chest pain, palpitations, dyspnea, and fatigue may be present. Upon auscultation, there is a murmur at the apex that is present during all of systole (holosystolic). Sometimes, only a midsystolic click and late systolic murmur are heard. SYN: *floppy valve syndrome.*

   TREAT: Simple prolapse requires no therapy, but if mitral regurgitation is present, antibiotic prophylaxis is indicated during surgical and dental procedures. If heart failure develops, surgery should be considered.

mittelschmerz (mĭt′ĕl-shmărts) [Ger.]. Abdominal pain midway between menstrual periods, occurring at time of ovulation and from the ovulation site.

Mittendorf's dot [20th century U.S. physician]. A gray dot on the posterior lens capsule. It is the remnant of the fetal hyaloid artery of the eye.

mix (mĭks) [L. *mixtus*, to mix]. 1. To put things, substances, or people together in solution, a collection, or an assembly. 2. The act of mixing. 3. A mixture of materials, as a cement mix, available in various proportions of ingredients.

mixed [L. *mixtus*]. Consisting of two or more intermingling substances.

mixed infection. An infectious disease process caused by the patient being infected at the same time by two or more microorganisms. SYN: *multiple infection.*

mixed lymphocyte culture or reaction. A laboratory test in which lymphocytes from different individuals are mixed to identify the presence of particular Class II HLA antigens. The T cells from the "responder" will synthesize DNA and proliferate only if they do not have the same histocompatibility antigens as the "donor cells," homozygous cells with known HLA types. The donor cells are irradiated to prevent their proliferation during the test.

mixoscopia [Gr. *mixis*, intercourse, + *skopein*, to examine]. Sexual perversion in which sexual gratification is obtained through observation of others in coition.

mixture (mĭks'tūr) [L. *mistura*]. A combination of two or more substances without chemical union. SEE: *mistura.*

MKS, mks. *meter-kilogram-second.* Indicates measurements used with meter for length, kilogram for weight, and second for time.

ml. *milliliter.*

M.L.D., m.l.d. *minimum lethal dose.*

mM. *millimole.*

mm. *millimeter.*

mmm. *millimicron.*

MMPI. *Minnesota Multiphasic Personality Inventory.*

MMPR. *medical malpractice payment report.*

MMWR. *Morbidity and Mortality Weekly Report.*

Mn. Chem. symb. for the element manganese.

mnemasthenia (nē″măs-thē′nē-ă) [Gr. *mneme*, memory, + *a-*, not, + *sthenos*, strength]. Poor memory not resulting from organic disease.

mnemic (nē′mĭk). Rel. to memory.

mnemonics (nē-mŏn′ĭks) [Gr. *mnemonikos*, pert. to memory]. The art of improving or assisting memory. A device to help recall a series of related data, names, or anatomical terms.

MNL. *Mononuclear leukocytes,* e.g., monocytes and macrophages.

M.O. *Medical Officer.*

Mo. Chem. symb. for the element molybdenum.

mo. *month.*

mobile [L. *mobilis*]. Movable.

mobile arm support. A device for support of the forearm, usually mounted on a wheelchair, that assists weak shoulder and elbow muscles in positioning the hand, as in feeding. Also: *ball bearing feeder; ball bearing forearm orthosis.*

mobile spasm. Tonic spasm with irregular, slow movements of limbs following hemiplegia. SYN: *athetosis.*

mobility [L. *mobilitas*]. State or quality of being mobile; facility of movement.

   m., abnormal tooth. Excessive tooth movement within the bony socket due to degenerative changes in the supporting alveolar bone and periodontal ligament as a result of poor oral hygiene, hormone balance changes, or trauma. SEE: *tooth movement.*

   m., tooth. Normal movement of teeth horizontally and, to a lesser extent, occlusally in response to various forces. Also called physiological tooth mobility or normal tooth mobility.

mobility training. That category of activities necessary for teaching blind and partially sighted persons techniques for successfully moving about in indoor and outdoor environments.

mobilization (mō″bĭl-ĭ-zā′shŭn). 1. The making of a fixed or ankylosed part movable. 2. Restoration of motion to a joint. 3. Freeing an organ or making it movable. 4. The freeing, or making available, of substances held in reserve as glycogen or fat.

   m., stapes. Surgical treatment to restore mobility to the stapes. Used in treatment of deafness.

mobilize (mō′bĭl-īz). 1. To incite to physiological action. 2. To render movable; to put in movement.

Möbius' disease (mē′bē-ŭs) [Paul J. Möbius, Ger. neurologist, 1853–1907]. Migraine accompanied by paralysis of the oculomotor nerves.

Möbius' sign. A symptom of Graves' disease in which one eye converges and the other diverges when one looks at the tip of one's nose.

modal (mōd′l) [L. *modus*, mode]. Pert. to, or characteristic of, a mode. In statistics, pert. to the most frequent, common or typical.

modality. 1. Quality of being modal. 2. A method of application or the employment of any therapeutic agent; limited usually to physical agents and devices. 3. Any specific sensory stimulus such as taste, touch, vision, pressure, or hearing.

Modane. Trade name for danthron.

Modane Soft. Trade name for docusate sodium.

mode (mōd). In statistics, the value or item of the class occurring most frequently in a series of variables.

model. 1. The pattern or form to be used in duplicating or constructing something. In dentistry, the cast or impression of teeth or a single tooth or cavity. 2. The ideal that would be used as a guide for action or imitation, e.g., model conduct or behavior.

m., animal. The study of anatomy, physiology, or pathology in an animal with respect to the possibility of applying the information obtained to human function and disease.

m., study. A diagnostic cast of an impression of a part or the complete dental arches, trimmed with the arches articulated and the edges perpendicular to the occlusal plane. It serves as the basis for construction of dental appliances, dentures or orthodontic treatment.

modeling. Acquisition of social behavior, and mental response by following the example of associates, esp. parents and siblings. To the extent this behavior is socially acceptable, it is rewarded and reinforced by the group.

model trimmer. A water-bathed grinding wheel to trim plaster or dental stone models for diagnostic purposes.

modem. *modulator-demodulator.* In computers, a device that allows data to be transmitted in serial form over conventional phone lines.

moderated. Mitigated, q.v.

modification (mŏd″ĭ-fĭ-kā′shŭn). The result of having changed something such as the shape or character of an object or structure.

modified jaw thrust. Airway maneuver used to open the airway of an unconscious patient which omits hyperextension in cases where possible cervical spine injury has occurred. The jaw is jutted forward, moving the tongue away from the hypopharynx.

modiolus (mō-dī′ō-lŭs) [L., hub]. [NA] Central pillar or axial part of cochlea extending from the base to the apex.

modulation (mŏd″ū-lā′shŭn). 1. The alteration in function or status of something in response to a stimulus or altered chemical or physical environment. 2. In electronics, a term used to describe the manner in which a signal is used to vary either the amplitude, frequency, or phase of a normally constant carrier signal. A method of coding information onto a carrier.

modulus (mŏj′ū-lŭs) [L., a small measure]. In physics, a constant or coefficient that indicates to what extent a substance possesses some property.

modus [L.]. A method or a mode.

modus operandi. Method of performing an act.

Moebius syndrome. Maldevelopment of the cranial nerves resulting in unbalanced movements of the facial muscles.

mogilalia (mōj-ĭ-lā′lē-ă) [Gr. *mogis*, with difficulty, + *lalia*, chatter]. Any speech defect, as stuttering.

mogiphonia (mōj-ĭ-fō′nē-ă) [″ + *phone*, voice]. Difficulty in emitting vocal sounds.

Mohrenheim's space (mor′ĕn-hīmz) [Baron J. J. Freiherr von Mohrenheim, Austrian surgeon, 1759–1799]. Space between the pectoralis major and deltoid muscles just beneath the clavicle.

Mohs' chemosurgery technique [Frederic Edward Mohs, U.S. surgeon, 1910–1979]. A method of excising tumors of the skin. The tumor tissue is fixed in place and a layer is removed. That portion is then examined microscopically. This procedure is repeated until the entire tumor is removed. Use of this technique ensures complete removal. It is esp. useful in treating basal cell epitheliomas.

moiety (moy′ĕ-tē) [Fr. *moitié*, fr. L. *medietas*, middle]. 1. One of two equal parts. 2. A portion of something that has been divided.

moist (moyst). Damp, wet.

mol. Mole, def. 2, q.v.

molal (mō′lăl). One mole of solute per kilogram of solvent. SEE: *molar.*

molality (mō-lăl′ĭ-tē). The number of moles of a solute per kilogram of solvent.

molar. 1. [L. *molaris*, grinding] A grinding or back tooth, one of three on each side of each jaw. The first permanent molar erupts between 6 and 7 years; the second between the 13th and 16th years. The third molars (wisdom teeth) are extremely variable, usually erupting between 18th and 25th years; however, they may erupt later or not at all. SEE: *dentition* for table; *teeth.* 2. [L. *moles*, a mass] Pert. to a mass; not molecular. 3. Pert. to a mole (def. 3). 4. Gram-molecule. SYN: *mole* (def. 3).

m., impacted. A tooth which is unable to erupt into its place in normal occlusion, usually due to crowding by other teeth. Commonly related to the third molar or wisdom tooth.

m., mulberry. A malformed first molar with dwarfed cusps and aggregations of enamel globules around the surface so that the crown has the appearance of a berry. Seen in congenital syphilis and other diseases.

molariform (mōl-ăr′ĭ-form). Resembling a molar tooth.

molarity. The number of gram molecular weights (moles) of a substance per liter of solution. Thus 1/M (also expressed as 1 M) means one mole of a substance per liter, and

0.1/M indicates 0.1 mole per liter.

molar solution. One in which there is one mole of the solute dissolved in each liter of the solution.

mold. 1. A fuzzy coating due to growth of a fungus on the surface of decaying vegetable matter or on nonorganic objects. 2. Any one of a group of parasitic or saprophytic fungi that causes mold, such as black molds (Mucorales) and blue and green molds (Aspergillales). The latter include *Penicillium,* the source of the antibiotic penicillin. 3. To shape a mass, as a pill. 4. To shape the fetal head, adapting it to the pelvic inlet.

molding. 1. Shaping of the fetal head, adapting itself to the pelvic inlet. 2. A protective border, used in plastic surgery. 3. Casting of a reproduction.

    m., border. In dentistry, the shaping of impression material at the edges by the oral tissues.

mole (mōl). 1. [AS. *mael*] A congenital discolored spot elevated above the surface of the skin. SYN: *nevus.* SEE: *racemose; melanoma.*

    ETIOL: Not clear. Harmless unless irritated.

    TREAT: Protect against irritation.

Caution: Do not attempt to remove a mole by tying a thread around it. Removal should be done by a physician.

---

    2. [L. *moles,* a shapeless mass] A uterine mass arising from a poorly developed or degenerating ovum. 3. [Ger. *Mol,* abbr. for *Molekulargewicht,* molecular weight] In the SI system, one mole of a substance contains as many atoms as exist in 0.012 kg of carbon-12.

    m., blood. A mass made up of blood clots, membranes, and placenta, retained following abortion.

    m., Breus'. Malformation of the ovum, a decidual tuberous subchorional hematoma.

    m., carneous. Blood mole that assumes a fleshlike appearance when retained in uterus for some time. SYN: *m., fleshy.*

    m., false. Mole formed from a uterine tumor or polypus.

    m., fleshy. M., carneous.

    m., hydatid. A polycystic mass in which the chorionic villi have undergone cystic degeneration.

    m., pigmented. Nevus pigmentosus.

    m., stone. A fleshy mole that has undergone calcareous degeneration in the uterus.

    m., true. Mole representing the degenerated embryo or fetus.

    m., vascular. A hemangioma.

    m., vesicular. M., hydatid.

molecular (mō-lĕk′ū-lăr) [L. *molecula,* little mass]. Pert. to a molecule.

molecular biology. Branch of biology dealing with analysis of the structure and development of biological systems with respect to the chemistry and physics of their molecular constituents.

molecular disease. Disease due to a defect in a single molecule. The abnormal hemoglobin molecule found in persons with sickle cell anemia causes the abnormally shaped red cells characteristic of this disease.

molecular layer. 1. Cortical layer of cerebellar or cerebral substance. 2. (Inner). Inner retinal plexiform layer. 3. (Outer). Outer retinal plexiform layer.

molecular lesion. Defect or absence of a basic organic molecule that is of sufficient importance to cause disease. Sickle cell anemia is an example of this type of lesion.

molecular weight. ABBR: mol. wt. Weight of a molecule attained by totaling the atomic weight of its constituent atoms. SEE: *atomic weight.*

molecule (mŏl′ĕ-kūl) [L. *molecula,* little mass]. 1. The smallest quantity into which a substance may be divided without loss of its characteristics. 2. Any small portion of a substance. 3. A chemical combination of two or more atoms that form a specific chemical compound; the chemical elements are formed by the combination of atoms.

    Combinations of dissimilar atoms form chemical compounds. In normal molecules the positive and negative electrical charges balance exactly. Excess or deficiency of either positive or negative charge by the loss or acquisition of electrons results in the formation of an ion.

    The molecule is designated by the number of atoms it contains, as monatomic (one atom); diatomic (two); triatomic (three); tetratomic (four); pentatomic (five); or hexatomic (six). SEE: *cleavage.*

molimen (mō-lī′mĕn) [L., effort] (pl. *molimina*). Effort to establish any normal function, esp. that necessary to establish the menstrual flow.

Mol-Iron. Trade name for ferrous sulfate, USP.

Moll's glands [Jacob Anthoni Moll, Dutch ophthalmologist, 1832–1914]. Modified sweat glands at border of eyelids. SYN: *ciliary glands.*

mollities (mōl-ĭsh′ē-ēz) [L.]. Abnormal softening of a part.

    m. ossium. Softening of the bones. SYN: *malacosteon; osteomalacia.*

mollusc, mollusk. Any member of the phylum Mollusca.

Mollusca. A phylum of animals that includes

the bivalves (mussels, oysters, clams), slugs, and snails. Snails serve as intermediate hosts of many parasitic flukes. Oysters and clams may transmit the virus of infectious hepatitis, esp. if improperly cooked.

molluscous (mŏ-lŭs'kŭs). Concerning molluscum.

molluscum (mŏ-lŭs'kŭm) [L., soft]. A mildly infective skin disease characterized by tumor formations on the skin.

m. contagiosum. The usual mildly contagious form of molluscum that affects mainly children and young adults.

SYM: Characterized by small waxy globular epithelial tumors that are umbilicated and contain semifluid caseous matter or solid masses. They heal without scarring, though they may suppurate and break down, commonly on face, eyelids, breasts, genitalia, and inner surface of thigh. These may only be a few millimeters in diameter, but are sometimes 2 or 3 cm wide. On pressure a substance resembling sebum is expressed.

ETIOL: A large virus of the pox group.

TREAT: Incision, expression of contents, followed by application of tincture of iodine.

m. fibrosum. A form of molluscum showing masses of fibrocellular tissue.

molt. To shed a covering such as feathers or skin that is replaced by new growth.

mol. wt. *molecular weight.*

molybdenum (mŏ-lĭb'dĕ-nŭm). SYMB: Mo. At. wt. 95.94; at. no. 42. A hard, heavy, metallic element.

molysmophobia (mō-lĭz″mŏ-fō'bē-ă) [Gr. *molysma*, stain, + *phobia*, fear]. Morbid fear of contamination or infection. SYN: *mysophobia.*

momentum (mō-mĕn'tŭm) [L.]. 1. In physics, the description of a quantity obtained by multiplying the mass of a body by its linear velocity. 2. Force of motion acquired by a moving object as a result of continuance of its motion; impetus.

momism [Coined in 1922 by Phillip Wylie in his book *A Generation of Vipers*]. In American culture, undue dependence on one's mother, esp. in very early life. This was alleged to cause the individual to be immature.

monad [Gr. *monas*, a unit]. 1. A univalent element. 2. A unicellular organism. 3. One of the four components of a tetrad.

monamide (mŏn-ăm'ĭd). An amide with one amide group.

monamine (mŏn-ăm'ĭn). An amine with one amine group.

monarthric (mŏn-ăr'thrĭk) [Gr. *monos*, single, + *arthron*, joint]. Concerning a single joint.

monarthritis (mŏn″ăr-thrī'tĭs) [″ + ″ + *itis*, inflammation]. Arthritis affecting a single joint.

monarticular (mŏn-ăr-tĭk'ŭ-lăr). Concerning or affecting one joint.

monaster (mŏn-ăs'tĕr) [″ + *aster*, star]. Single starlike figure formed in mitosis.

monathetosis (mŏn″ăth-ē-tō'sĭs) [″ + *athetos*, not fixed, + *osis*, condition]. Athetosis affecting a single part of the body.

monatomic (mŏn″ă-tŏm'ĭk) [″ + *atomos*, indivisible]. 1. Concerning a single atom. 2. Univalent.

monaural (mŏn-aw'răl). Concerning an ear.

monaxonic (mŏn″ăk-sŏn'ĭk) [″ + Gr. *axon*, axis]. A neuron with one axon.

Mondonesi's reflex (mŏn-dō-nā'zēz) [Filippo Mondonesi, It. physician]. In coma, contraction of facial muscles following pressure on eyeball. SYN: *bulbomimic reflex; facial reflex.*

Mondor's disease (mŏn'dorz) [Henri Mondor, Fr. physician, 1885–1962]. Thrombosis and sclerosis of a subcutaneous vein or veins in the breast area of either sex. May occur after trauma or appear without apparent cause. The long, firm, tender cord or string like structure extends from the breast up into the axilla or down toward the epigastrium. It is a benign, self-limiting disease that is important because its appearance may be confused with cancer of the breast.

monecious (mŏn-ē'shŭs). Monoecious, q.v.

monesthetic (mŏn″ĕs-thĕt'ĭk) [Gr. *monos*, single, + *aisthesis*, sensation]. Affecting only one of the senses.

monestrous (mŏn-ĕs'trŭs). Having a single estrous cycle in a single sexual season.

Monge's disease [Carlos Monge, Peruvian pathologist, 1884–1970]. Chronic mountain sickness. SEE: *mountain sickness, chronic.*

mongolian spots (mŏn-gō'lē-ăn). Blue-gray areas of discoloration of the skin of the lower back, thighs, and sometimes the shoulders of the newborn. They gradually fade. Eighty percent of nonwhite and 10% of white infants have these benign spots.

mongolism. An inappropriate term for Down syndrome, q.v.

mongoloid (mŏn'gŏ-loyd). 1. Concerning Mongols. 2. Characterized by mongolism, i.e., Down syndrome.

monilethrix (mŏn-ĭl'ē-thrĭks) [L. *monile*, necklace, + Gr. *thrix*, hair]. A genetic defect of the hair shaft in which the hair becomes beaded and brittle. The defect usually appears by the second month of life. No effective treatment.

Monilia [L. *monile*, necklace]. Former name for the genus of fungi now called *Candida,* q.v.

monilial (mō-nĭl′ē-ăl). Concerning *Monilia*.

moniliasis (mō″nĭ-lī′ă-sĭs). Infection of the skin or mucous membranes by yeastlike fungi. Usually localized in skin, nails, mouth, vagina, bronchi, or lungs, but may invade bloodstream. SYN: *candidiasis*.

ETIOL: Various species of *Candida* but chiefly *C. albicans*.

moniliform (mō-nĭl′ĭ-form) [″ + *forma*, shape]. Resembling a necklace or string of beads.

moniliid (mō-nĭl′ē-ĭd). A skin eruption due to hypersensitivity to a *Monilia* infection in another part of the body.

moniliosis (mō-nĭl-ē-ō′sĭs). Moniliasis.

monitor (mŏn′ĭ-tor) [L., one who warns]. 1. One who observes an operation, procedure, or apparatus, esp. one responsible for detecting and preventing malfunction. 2. A device that provides a warning if that which is being observed fails or malfunctions. 3. To check by using an electronic device.

m., apnea. SEE: *apnea monitoring.*

m., blood pressure. Monitor that provides a record of systolic and diastolic blood pressure.

m., cardiac. Monitor of heart function, providing visual and audible record of heartbeat.

m., fetal. 1. Monitor that detects and displays fetal heartbeat. 2. Assessment of fetus in utero with respect to its heart rate by use of electrocardiogram or by chemical analysis of the amniotic fluid or fetal blood. SEE: *apnea monitoring.*

m., Holter. SEE: *Holter monitor.*

m., personal radiation. Small device carried by an individual to measure the accumulated radiation dosage over a period of time. SEE: *dosimeter.*

m., respiratory. SEE: *respiratory function monitoring.*

m., temperature. Monitor for measuring and recording temperature of the body or some particular portion of the body.

mono-, mon- [Gr. *monos*, single]. Prefix designating one, single.

monoacidic (mŏn″ō-ă-sĭd′ĭk). Having one replaceable hydroxyl (OH) group.

monoamide. Monamide.

monoamine. Containing one amine radical.

monoamine oxidase inhibitors. ABBR: MAO inhibitors. A group of drugs that are effective in treating depression. Their mode of action in addition to inhibiting monoamine oxidase is not clearly understood. Because of their toxic potential, they should be used with caution. Hypertensive crises have been observed in persons who eat certain kinds of cheese or chicken liver or drink chianti wine while taking MAO inhibitors.

SEE: *tyramine.*

monoanesthesia (mŏn″ō-ăn-ĕs-thē′sē-ă). Anesthesia of a single member or organ.

monobacillary (mŏn″ō-băs′ĭ-lā″rē). Concerning a single species of bacilli.

monobacterial (mŏn″ō-băk-tē′rē-ăl). Concerning a single species of bacteria.

monobasic (mŏn-ō-bā′sĭk) [″ + *basis*, a base]. Having one hydrogen atom replaceable by a metal or positive radical.

monobenzone (mŏn″ō-bĕn′zōn). USP. A drug used in treating hyperpigmentation conditions. Trade name is Benoquin.

monoblast (mŏn′ō-blăst) [″ + *blastos*, germ]. A cell that gives rise to a monocyte.

monoblastoma (mŏn″ō-blăs-tō′mă) [″ + ″ + *oma*, tumor]. A neoplasm that contains both monoblasts and monocytes.

monoblepsia (mŏn-ō-blĕp′sē-ă) [″ + *blepsis*, sight]. 1. Condition in which vision is more distinct when only one eye is used, hence tendency to close one eye to see clearly. 2. A type of color blindness in which only one color can be seen.

monobrachius (mŏn″ō-brā′kē-ŭs) [″ + *brachion*, arm]. 1. State of having only one arm. 2. Fetus with only one arm.

monobromated (mŏn″ō-brō′măt-ĕd). Pert. to chemical compound with only one atom of bromine in each molecule.

monocalcic (mŏn-ō-kăl′sĭk). Pert. to a chemical compound containing only one atom of calcium in the molecule.

monocardian (mŏn-ō-kăr′dē-ăn) [″ + *kardia*, heart]. Individual possessing a heart with only one atrium and one ventricle.

monocelled (mŏn′ō-sĕld). Composed of a single cell.

monocephalus (mŏn″ō-sĕf′ă-lŭs) [″ + *kephale*, head]. A congenitally deformed fetus with duplicated parts except for the head. SYN: *syncephalus.*

monochord (mŏn′ō-kord) [″ + *chorde*, cord]. A single-string instrument for testing upper tone audition.

monochorea (mŏn″ō-kō-rē′ă) [″ + *choreia*, dance]. Chorea that affects a single part or extremity.

monochorionic (mŏn-ō-kor″ē-ŏn′ĭk). Possessing a single chorion, as in the case of identical twins.

monochromasy (mŏn″ō-krō-mā′sē) [″ + *chroma*, color]. Color blindness in which all colors are perceived as shades of gray.

monochromatic (mŏn″ō-krō-măt′ĭk). 1. Having one color. 2. A color-blind person to whom all colors appear to be of one hue.

monochromatism (mŏn″ō-krō′mă-tĭzm) [Gr. *monos*, single, + *chroma*, color, + *-ismos*, condition]. Complete color blindness.

monochromatophil (mŏn″ō-krō-măt′ō-fĭl)

[" + " + *philein*, to love]. A cell or tissue that accepts only one stain.

monochromator (mŏn-ō-krō'mă-tor). Instrument for selective transmission of homogeneous radiant energy.

Monoclate. A drug used to treat hemophilia type A.

monoclinic (mŏn"ō-klin'ĭk) [" + *klinein*, to incline]. Pert. to crystals in which the vertical axis is inclined to one lateral axis but at right angles to the other.

monoclonal (mŏn"ō-klōn'ăl). Arising from a single cell.

monoclonal antibodies. Antibodies derived from hybridoma cells, q.v. Such antibodies are of exceptional purity and specificity; they are being used to identify antigens on a number of viruses, and bacteria; in addition, they are used in tissue and blood typing, in identifying hormones such as human chorionic gonadotropin, in diagnosis of infectious diseases, and in identifying tumor antigens. These antibodies are being studied extensively for their potential for treating cancer.

monococcus (mŏn-ō-kŏk'ŭs) [" + *kokkos*, berry]. A form of coccus existing singly instead of as part of the usual group or chain.

monocontaminated (mŏn"ō-kŏn-tăm"ĭnāt"ĕd). Infected with a single species of organism.

monocrotic (mŏn"ō-krŏt'ĭk) [" + *krotos*, beat]. Indicating a single pulse wave with no notches in it.

monocular (mŏn-ŏk'ū-lar) [" + L. *oculus*, eye]. 1. Concerning or affecting but one eye. 2. Possessing a single eyepiece as in a monocular microscope.

monoculus (mŏn-ŏk'ū-lŭs). 1. A bandage for shielding one eye. 2. A fetus with only one eye. SYN: *cyclops*.

monocyclic (mŏn"ō-sī'klĭk). Concerning one cycle.

monocyesis (mŏn"ō-sī-ē'sĭs) [" + *kyesis*, pregnancy]. Pregnancy with a single fetus.

monocyte (mŏn'ō-sīt) [" + *kytos*, cell]. A mononuclear phagocytic white blood cell derived from the myeloid stem cells. Monocytes are short-lived, with a half-life of approximately 1 day. They circulate in the blood stream from which they move into tissues, at which point they mature into macrophages, q.v., which are long-lived. Monocytes and macrophages are one of the first lines of defense in the inflammatory process. This network of fixed and mobile phagocytes that engulf foreign antigens and cell debris is commonly called the reticuloendothelial system, q.v. SEE: *blood cell* for illus.; *macrophage*.

monocytic (mŏn-ō-sĭt'ĭk). Concerning or resembling monocytes.

monocytopenia (mŏn"ō-sī"tō-pē'nē-ă) [" + *kytos*, cell, + *penia*, lack]. Diminished number of monocytes in the blood.

monocytosis (mŏn"ō-sī-tō'sĭs) [" + " + *osis*, condition]. Excessive number of monocytes in the blood.

monodactylism (mŏn-ō-dăk'tĭl-ĭzm) [" + *daktylos*, digit]. Condition, usually congenital, of having only one digit on a hand or foot.

monodal (mŏn-ō'dăl) [" + *hodos*, road]. Connected with one terminal of a resonator so that the patient acts as a capacitor for entrance and exit of high-frequency currents.

monodermoma (mŏn"ō-dĕr-mō'mă) [" + *derma*, skin, + *oma*, tumor]. A neoplasm originating in one germinal layer.

monodiplopia (mŏn"ō-dĭ-plō'pē-ă) [" + *diploos*, double, + *ops*, eye]. Double vision in one eye only.

monodromia. Condition of muscles or nerves in which conduction occurs in one direction only.

monoecious (mŏn-ē'shŭs) [" + *oikos*, house]. Pert. to the presence of functioning male and female sex organs in the same individual.

monogamy (mō-nŏg'ă-mē) [" + *gamos*, marriage]. The practice of being married to only one person at a time.

monogenesis (mŏn"ō-jĕn'ĕ-sĭs) [Gr. *monos*, single, + *genesis*, generation, birth]. 1. Production of offspring of only one sex. 2. The theory that all organisms arise from a single cell. 3. Asexual reproduction.

monogerminal (mŏn"ō-jĕr'mĭ-năl). Produced from a single ovum.

monogony (mŏn-ŏg'ō-nē) [" + *gone*, seed]. Asexual reproduction.

monograph (mŏn'ō-grăf) [" + *graphein*, to write]. A treatise dealing with a single subject.

monogyny (mō-nŏj'ă-nē) [" + *gyne*, woman]. Condition in which a male has only one female mate.

monohybrid [" + L. *hybrida*, mongrel]. Offspring of a cross between parents differing in a single character.

monohydrated (mŏn-ō-hī'drăt-ĕd) [" + *hydor*, water]. United with only one molecule of water.

monohydric (mŏn"ō-hī'drĭk). Having a single replaceable hydrogen atom.

monoideaism, monoideism (mŏn"ō-ī-dē'ăĭzm, -dē'ĭzm) [" + *idea*, idea]. Preoccupation with only one idea; a slight degree of monomania.

monoinfection (mŏn"ō-ĭn-fĕk'shŭn). Infection with a single species of organism.

monoiodotyrosine (mŏn"ō-ī-ō"dō-tī'rō-sēn). An amino acid intermediate in the synthesis of thyroxine and triiodothyronine.

monokine. A chemical mediator released by monocytes and macrophages during the immune response. Monokines affect the growth and activity of other white blood cells. Interleukin-1, q.v., is the most important monokine. SEE: *autocrine; cytokines; inflammation; interleukin-1; lymphokines; paracrine.*

monolayer (mŏn'ō-lā'ĕr). Having a single layer, esp. of cells growing in culture.

monolocular (mŏn''ō-lŏk'ū-lar) ['' + L. *loculus,* a small chamber]. Having only one cell or cavity. SYN: *unilocular.*

monomania (mŏn-ō-mā'nē-ă) ['' + *mania,* madness]. Mental illness characterized by distortion of thought processes concerning a single subject or idea.

monomaniac. One afflicted with monomania.

monomastigote (mŏn-ō-măs'tĭ-gōt) ['' + *mastix,* whip]. Possessing only one flagellum.

monomelic (mŏn-ō-mĕl'ĭk) ['' + *melos,* limb]. Affecting a single limb.

monomer (mŏn'ō-mĕr). Any molecule that can be bound to similar molecules to form a polymer.

monomeric (mŏn-ō-mĕr'ĭk) ['' + *meros,* part]. Consisting of, or affecting, a single piece or segment of a body.

monometallic (mŏn''ō-mĕ-tăl'ĭk). Containing a single atom of a metal in the formula.

monomicrobic (mŏn''ō-mī-krō'bĭk). Concerning organisms of a single species.

monomolecular (mŏn''ō-mō-lĕk'ū-lăr). Concerning one molecule.

monomorphic (mŏn-ō-mor'fĭk) ['' + *morphe,* form]. Unchangeable in form; keeping the same form throughout every stage of development.

monomyoplegia (mŏn''ō-mī''ō-plē'jē-ă) ['' + *mys,* muscle, + *plege,* stroke]. Paralysis of only one muscle.

monomyositis (mŏn''ō-mī-ō-sī'tĭs) ['' + '' + *itis,* inflammation]. Inflamed condition of only one muscle.

mononeural (mŏn-ō-nū'răl) ['' + *neuron,* nerve]. Supplied by or concerning a single nerve.

mononeuritis (mŏn''ō-nū-rī'tĭs) ['' + '' + *itis,* inflammation]. Inflamed condition of a single nerve.

   m. **multiplex.** Inflammation of nerves in separate body areas.

mononeuropathy (mŏn''ō-nū-rŏp'ă-thē) ['' + '' + *pathos,* disease, suffering]. Disease of a single nerve.

mononoea (mŏn''ō-nē'ă) ['' + *nous,* mind]. Mental fixation on a single subject.

mononuclear (mŏn-ō-nū'klē-ăr) ['' + L. *nucleus,* kernel]. Having one nucleus, par-

ticularly a blood cell such as a monocyte or lymphocyte. SYN: *uninuclear.*

mononuclear phagocyte system. ABBR: MPS. The modern name for reticuloendothelial system, q.v.

mononucleosis (mŏn-ō-nū''klē-ō'sĭs) ['' + *nucleus,* kernel, + *osis,* condition]. Presence of an abnormally high number of mononuclear leukocytes in the blood.

   m., infectious. An acute infectious disease that affects lymphoid tissue primarily. Characterized by fever, usually a skin rash, enlarged and often tender lymph nodes, and enlarged spleen with great increase of atypical or abnormal mononuclear leukocytes in the blood. Abnormal liver function test will be found in about 90% of cases. Clinical manifestations are highly variable. The disease is caused by the Epstein-Barr virus, a herpesvirus. Incubation period may be as long as 4 to 7 weeks. SEE: *Nursing Diagnoses* in Appendix.

   SYM: Constitutional symptoms, fever, sore throat, and generalized lymphadenopathy; hyperplasia of lymphatic tissue. Blood contains heterophil antibodies.

   DIAG: Serologic testing for heterophil antibody. This test is often negative in children less than 4 years of age but will identify about 90% of cases of adults with the Epstein-Barr virus.

   TREAT: There is no specific therapy but, for serious complications (for example, hemolytic anemia, pharyngeal swelling interfering with swallowing), cortisone is indicated.

mononucleotide (mŏn''ō-nū'klē-ō-tīd''). A product resulting from hydrolysis of nucleic acid. Contains phosphoric acid combined with a glucoside or pentoside. SYN: *nucleotide.*

monoparesis (mŏn-ō-păr-ē'sĭs) [Gr. *monos,* single, + *paresis,* weakness]. Paralysis of a single part of the body.

monoparesthesia (mŏn''ō-păr-ĕs-thē'sē-ă) ['' + *para,* beside, + *aisthesis,* sensation]. Paresthesia of only one region or limb.

monopathy (mō-nŏp'ă-thē) ['' + *pathos,* disease, suffering]. A disease attacking only one part of the body.

monophagia (mŏn-ō-fā'jē-ă) ['' + *phagein,* to eat]. 1. Appetite for only one kind of food. Said especially of insects. 2. The habit of eating only one meal a day.

monophasia (mŏn-ō-fā'zē-ă) ['' + *phasis,* speech]. Inability to utter anything but one word or phrase repeatedly.

monophobia (mŏn-ō-fō'bē-ă) ['' + *phobos,* fear]. Abnormal fear of being alone.

monophthalmus (mŏn''ŏf-thăl'mŭs) ['' + *ophthalmos,* eye]. A cyclops, q.v.

monophyletic (mŏn''ō-fĭl-ĕt'ĭk) ['' +

phyle, tribe]. Originating from a single source. Opposite of polyphyletic.

monophyletism (mŏn"ō-fī'lĕ-tizm). Concerning the concept that all blood cells are derived from a single stem cell.

monophyodont (mŏn"ō-fī'ō-dŏnt) [" + *phyein*, to grow, + *odous*, tooth]. Having a single set of teeth, which are permanent.

monoplasmatic (mŏn"ō-plăz-măt'ĭk) [" + LL. *plasma*, form, mold]. Made up of a single substance or tissue.

monoplast (mŏn"ō-plăst) [" + *plastos*, formed]. A single-cell type of organism that does not change during its life cycle.

monoplegia (mŏn-ō-plē'jē-ă) [" + *plege*, stroke]. Paralysis of a single limb or a single group of muscles.

monopodia (mŏn"ō-pō'dē-ă) [" + *pous*, foot]. Condition of having only one foot; usually the two feet are fused.

monopolar (mŏn-ō-pōl'ăr) [" + L. *polus*, pole]. Using one terminal only, the ground acting as the second terminal. SYN: *monoterminal*.

monops (mŏn'ŏps) [" + *ops*, eye]. Cyclops, q.v.

monopsychosis (mŏn"ō-sī-kō'sĭs) [Gr. *monos*, single, + *psyche*, mind, + *osis*, condition]. Monomania, q.v.

monopus (mŏn'ō-pŭs) [" + *pous*, foot]. Individual exhibiting monopodia, q.v.

monorchia (mŏn-or'kē-ă). Monorchism.

monorchid (mŏn-or'kĭd) [" + *orchis*, testicle]. Person having only one testicle or ovary.

monorchidism, monorchism (mŏn-or'kĭd-ĭzm, mŏn'or-kĭzm). Condition in which there is only one descended testicle.

monorhinic (mŏn"ō-rĭn'ĭk) [" + *rhis*, nose]. 1. Having a single nose as conjoined twins. 2. Having a single fused nasal cavity.

monosaccharide (mŏn-ō-săk'ă-rĭd) [" + Sanskrit *sarkara*, sugar]. A simple sugar that cannot be decomposed by hydrolysis, such as fructose, galactose, or glucose.

monosodium glutamate ABBR: MSG. $C_5H_8NNaO_4$. H_2O. Sodium salt of glutamic acid. A white crystalline substance that has a meatlike taste. Used to flavor foods, esp. in the Orient. When ingested in large amounts, it causes chest pain, a sensation of facial pressure, headaches, burning sensation, and excessive sweating. This has been termed the Chinese restaurant syndrome, q.v. Its use to enhance the flavor of foods prepared for infants is questionable. Manufactured and sold under various names as Ajinomoto, Accent, Vetsin.

monosome (mŏn'ō-sōm) [" + *soma*, body]. An accessory chromosome that, without dividing, goes into only one of the daughter cells. The unpaired sex chromosome.

monosomy (mŏn'ō-sō"mē). Condition of having one member of a chromosome pair missing.

monospasm (mŏn'ō-spăzm) [" + *spasmos*, convulsion]. Spasm of a single limb or part.

monospermy (mŏn'ō-spĕr"mē) [" + *sperma*, seed]. Fertilization by a single spermatozoon entering an ovum.

monostotic (mŏn"ŏs-tŏt'ĭk) [" + *osteon*, bone]. Concerning a single bone.

monostratal (mŏn"ō-strā'tăl). Consisting of a single layer.

monosubstituted (mŏn"ō-sŭb'stĭ-tūt"ĕd). Having only a single molecule replaced.

monosymptomatic (mŏn"ō-sĭmp-tō-măt'ĭk) [" + *symptomatikos*, pert. to symptom]. Having only one dominant symptom.

monosynaptic (mŏn"ō-sĭ-năp'tĭk). Transmitted through only a single synapse.

monosyphilide (mŏn-ō-sĭf'ĭl-id) [" + Fr. *syphilide*, syphilitic lesion]. Characterized by a single syphilitic lesion.

monoterminal [" + *terma*, a limit]. Using one terminal only in the giving of treatments, the ground acting as the second terminal for the completion of the electrical circuit. SYN: *monopolar*.

monothermia (mŏn-ō-thĕrm'ē-ă) [" + *therme*, heat]. Condition in which body temperature is stable; absence of rise in evening temperature.

monotocous (mō-nŏt'ō-kŭs) [Gr. *monos*, single, + *tokos*, birth]. Production of a single offspring at birth.

Monotricha (mō-nŏt'rĭ-kä) [" + *thrix*, hair]. Bacteria having a single flagellum at one pole.

monotrichous (mŏn-ŏt'rĭ-kŭs). Pert. to or having a single flagellum.

monovalent (mŏn-ō-vā'lĕnt) [" + L. *valere*, to have power]. Having the combining power of a single hydrogen atom. SYN: *univalent*.

monoxenous (mō-nŏks'ĕn-ŭs) [" + *xenos*, stranger]. Said of a parasite that requires only one species as a host.

monoxide (mŏn-ŏk'sīd). An oxide having only one atom of oxygen.

monozygotic (mŏn"ō-zī-gŏt'ĭk) [" + *zygotos*, yoked]. Originating from a single fertilized ovum, said of identical twins.

monozygotic twins. Two offspring developed from a single fertilized ovum. At an early stage the ovum separates into independent cells that develop into offspring of the same sex with identical genetic characteristics. SEE: *twins*.

Monro's foramen (mŏn-rōz') [Alexander Monro (Secundus), Scot. anatomist, 1733-1817]. Point of communication between 3rd and lateral ventricles of the brain.

Monro's sulcus. Sulcus on lateral wall of 3rd ventricle from the foramen interventriculare to the aditus ad aquaeductum cerebri.

mons (mŏns) [L., mountain] (pl. *montes*). An anatomical eminence above the surface of the body.

     m. pubis. [NA] Pubic eminence. SYN: *mons veneris.*

     m. veneris. A pad of fatty tissue and coarse skin overlying the symphysis pubis. After puberty it is covered with hair. SYN: *mons pubis.*

monster [L. *monstrum*]. A grossly deformed fetus or infant, usually due to faulty development; is usually nonviable. The term should never be used when discussing such a patient with those who are emotionally attached to him or her. Terms such as handicapped, congenitally deformed, or abnormal are more appropriate.

monstriparity (mŏn″strĭ-păr′ĭ-tē) [″ + *parere*, to give birth to]. Giving birth to an abnormally formed infant.

monstrosity [L. *monstrositas*]. A congenitally deformed child or infant.

.onteggia's fracture (mŏn-tĕj′ăz) [Giovanni B. Monteggia, It. surgeon, 1762–1815]. Fracture of the upper portion of the ulna with dislocation of the radial head.

Montgomery's glands [William F. Montgomery, Ir. obstetrician, 1797–1859]. Small prominences around the nipple of the breast that enlarge during pregnancy and lactation. SEE: *areola; mamma.*

Montgomery straps. Adhesive straps affixed to the skin arranged opposite to each other, and with the middle ends turned back on each other, so that gauze straps can be placed between holes of each end of the middle of the paired tapes. This provides a method of securing a bandage and subsequently changing it without having to replace the tape each time. SEE: illus.

monticulus (mŏn-tĭk′ū-lŭs) [L., little mountain] (pl. *monticuli*). A protuberance.

     m. cerebelli. In the cerebellum, protuberance of the superior vermis, the anterior portion of which is called the culmen and the posterior portion, the declive.

mood [AS. *mod*, mind, feeling]. A pervasive and sustained emotion that may have a major influence on a person's perception of the world. Examples of mood include depression, joy, elation, anger, and anxiety. SEE: *affect.*

mood disorders. A group of disorders in which the disturbance of mood is accompanied by full or partial manic or depressive syndrome.

mood swings. Periods of variation in how one feels, changing from a sense of well-be-

ing to one of depression. This occurs normally, but may become abnormally intense in persons with manic depressive states.

moon face. The development of a round full face in response to excess secretion of adrenal cortical hormone or prolonged therapy with this hormone.

Moore's lightning streaks [Robert F. Moore, Brit. ophthalmologist, 1878–1963]. The perception of zigzag flashes of light in the peripheral field of vision that occurs in the dark, esp. in older persons. These are due to vitreous tags on the retina. The condition is benign. SEE: *coruscation.*

Moraxella lacunata (mor-ăx-ĕl′ă). A gram-negative coccobacillus that is a rare cause of conjunctivitis.

morbid (mor′bĭd) [L. *morbidus*, sick]. 1. Diseased. 2. Pert. to disease. 3. Preoccupied with unwholesome ideas and circumstances.

morbidity [L. *morbidus*, sick]. 1. State of being diseased. 2. The number of sick persons or cases of disease in relationship to a specific population. SEE: *incidence.*

Morbidity and Mortality Weekly Report. The weekly report published by the Centers for Disease Control, Atlanta, Georgia, of illness and death rates for a variety of diseases. Prominent in the material are statistics on communicable diseases in each state, territory, and 121 major cities in the United States. Articles concerning outbreaks of disease or accidents appear in it. These may include reports of public health importance from international events.

morbidity rate. Number of cases of a specific disease in a specified period of time (usually a year) per unit of population (usually 1000, 10,000 or 100,000) alive.

morbific (mor-bif′ĭk) [″ + *facere*, to make]. Causing or producing disease.

morbilli (mor-bĭl′ī) [L. *morbillus*, little disease]. Measles.

morbilliform [″ + *forma*, shape]. Like measles or its rash.

morbillous (mor-bĭl′ŭs). Concerning measles.

morbus [L.]. Disease.

     m. caeruleus. Cyanosis that is congenital.

     m. miseriae. Any condition due to neglect and want.

morcellation, morcellement (mor-sĕl-ā′shŭn, -ā-mŏn′) [Fr. *morceller*, to subdivide]. Method of removing a fetus, tumor, or organ by pieces.

mordant (mor′dănt) [L. *mordere*, to bite]. A substance that fixes a stain or dye, as alum and phenol.

mores (mō′rāz) [L.]. Habits and customs of society. Usually those that come to be re-

MONTGOMERY STRAPS
(TWO METHODS)

TAPE STUCK TO THE SKIN

STRIPS OF ADHESIVE TAPE.
THEY ARE FOLDED BACK SO THAT
A SMALL HOLE MAY BE PLACED
THROUGH THE DOUBLE THICKNESS.

GAUZE OR COTTON STRING IS
THREADED THROUGH THE HOLES
SO THAT THE STRAPS MAY BE
PULLED SNUG AND THUS HOLD
THE DRESSING IN PLACE.

ADHESIVE
SIDE

SMALL
ROD

THE STRAP IS MADE AS SHOWN,
THEN TURNED OVER AND
APPLIED TO THE SKIN.

THE OPPOSING STRAPS CAN BE
CONNECTED BY COTTON TAPE
OR RUBBER BANDS AROUND
THE RODS.

garded as being essential to the survival and well-being of the society.

Morgagni, Giovanni B. (mor-găn′yē). Italian pathological anatomist, 1682–1771.

M.'s caruncle. The middle prostatic lobe.

M.'s cataract. Cataract that is hypermature with a softened cortex and a hard nucleus. SEE: *cataract.*

M.'s hydatid. Cystlike remains of müllerian duct attached to testicle or oviduct.

M.'s hyperostosis. Hyperostosis of the frontal bones of the head. Associated with obesity, headache, amenorrhea, diabetes, multiple endocrine abnormalities, and various neuropsychiatric disturbances.

M.'s ventricle. Ventriculus laryngis. SEE: *ventricle of larynx.*

morgagnian (mor-găn′yē-ăn). Pert. to or described by Morgagni, q.v.

morgagnian cyst. Cystlike remnant of the müllerian duct that is attached to the fallopian tube.

Morganella morganii. Bacterial species that may cause urinary tract infections, wound infections, bacteremia, meningitis, keratitis, and acute enteritis.

morgue (morg) [Fr.]. A place for holding dead bodies until they are identified or buried.

moria (mō′rē-ă) [Gr. *moria,* folly]. 1. Simple dementia. 2. Foolishness. SEE: *witzelsucht.*

moribund (mor′ĭ-bŭnd) [L. *moribundus*]. In a dying condition; dying.

morning care. Care provided for a patient which includes taking temperature, pulse, and respiration, oral hygiene, bath, change of linen on bed, and breakfast.

morning sickness. The nausea and vomiting that affect some women during first few months of pregnancy, particularly in the morning. Headache, dizziness, and exhaustion also may be experienced. It may clear up after the 3rd month. SEE: *hyperemesis gravidarum.*

Occurs usually about the 5th or 6th week, and symptoms vary from simple morning sickness to pernicious vomiting of pregnancy. Usually clears up without treatment in 1 to 3 weeks. Occurs in about 50% of pregnancies.

TREAT: Dietary management will help in most cases. Frequent small feedings of bland foods such as crackers, broths, and clear soups will be beneficial. If the sickness persists, an antinausea medicine suitable for use during pregnancy is usually effective.

Caution: The use of any drug during pregnancy should be carefully evaluated prior to its administration to avoid possible damage to the fetus.

morning stiffness. Generalized joint and muscle stiffness that is present upon awakening. It tends to subside as activity is increased during the day. The stiffness is associated with various types of inflammatory arthritis.

moron [Gr. *moros,* stupid]. A feebleminded person, not beyond the intellectual development level of age 12, having the mentality ordinarily attained between 7 and 12, or an IQ of 50 to 70. The term implies no moral defect. SEE: *mental retardation.*

Moro reflex [Ernst Moro, Ger. pediatrist, 1874–1951]. A reflex seen in infants in response to a variety of stimuli, such as movement of the surface on which the infant rests, blowing in the face, or tapping the abdomen. The infant responds by rapid abduction and extension of the arms followed by an embracing motion (adduction) of the arms. SYN: *embrace reflex; startle reflex.*

morphea (mor-fē′ă) [Gr. *morphe,* form]. A rare skin disease of unknown etiology, characterized by sclerosis of the skin which may be localized or widespread. There is no specific treatment, but physical therapy or infiltration with cortisone solution may help to prevent contractures.

   m., generalized. A severe form of localized morphea. There are multiple indurated plaques, hyperpigmentation, and possible muscle atrophy. It is not associated with systemic disease. The disease may become inactive in 3 to 5 years.

   m., localized (mor-fē′ă) [Gr. *morphe,* form]. Localized form of scleroderma that does not progress to the systemic form of the disease. A rare skin disease of unknown etiology, characterized by sclerosis of the skin. There is no specific treatment.

morpheme (mor′fēm). The smallest meaningful unit in phonetics. SEE: *phoneme.*

morphia. Morphine.

morphine (mor′fēn) [L. *morphina,* from *Morpheus,* god of sleep]. Main alkaloid found in opium, occurring in bitter colorless crystals. Widely used as an analgesic and sedative.

   m. sulfate. USP. The sulfate of an alkaloid obtained from opium and occurring as feathery white crystals, incompatible with alkalies, tannic acid, and iodides. Loses water of crystallization when exposed to air. Trade name is Epimorph.

   ACTION/USES: Hypnotic and analgesic.

Caution: Morphine sulfate is used by drug addicts due to its action on the central nervous system. For this reason, its security in the hospital and pharmacy must be strictly maintained.

morphine poisoning. Brief mental exhilaration; languor; followed by weariness, sleepiness, pinpoint pupils; rapid forcible pulse that becomes slow and feeble. Respiration slow and shallow. Unconsciousness from which patient may be aroused with difficulty. Muscles become relaxed, reflexes diminished, and temperature low. The skin is pale, cold, and moist, and the pupils dilated. If dose is large enough, coma and death follow.

   TREAT: Establish airway and provide ventilation. Give a narcotic antagonist such as naloxone, which is the treatment of choice, in small doses and repeat if necessary at 30-minute intervals. Pulmonary edema may occur; treat with positive-pressure respiration. SEE: *Poisons and Poisoning* in *Appendix.*

morphinism (mor′fĭn-ĭzm) [L. *morphina,* morphine, + *-ismos,* condition]. Morbid condition due to habitual or excessive use of morphine. Morphine habit. SEE: *morphine poisoning.*

morphinomania, morphiomania (mor″fĭn-ō-mā′nē-ă, -fē-ō-mā′nē-ă) [″ + *mania,* madness]. 1. Morbid craving for morphine. 2. Insanity resulting from use of morphine.

morphodifferentiation. The stage of tooth formation that determines the shape and size of the tooth crown. SEE: *enamel organ.*

morphogenesis (mor″fō-jĕn′ĕ-sĭs) [Gr. *morphe,* form, + *genesis,* generation, birth]. Various processes occurring during development by which the form of the body and its organs is established.

morphogenetic (mor″fō-jĕn-ĕt′ĭk). Stimulating growth and development of form.

morphogenetic processes. Processes by which morphogenesis is accomplished. Include cell migration, cell aggregation, localized growth, splitting including delamination and cavitation, folding including invagination and evagination.

morphogenetic substance. Chemical substance present in eggs or early embryos that induces morphologic differentiation. SEE: *induction.*

morphography (mor-fŏg′ră-fē) [″ + *graphein,* to write]. The classification of organisms by describing their form and structure.

morphology (mor-fŏl′ō-jē) [Gr. *morphe,* form, + *logos,* word, reason]. Science of structure and form without regard to function.

morphometry (mor-fŏm′ĕ-trē) [″ + *metron*, measure]. The measurement of forms of organisms.

morphosis (mor-fō′sĭs) [Gr., a shaping]. The formation of a structure.

morphovar [morphological variation]. Variants within a species defined by variation in morphological characteristics. SEE: *biovar; serovar.*

morpio, morpion (mor′pē-ō, -pē-ŏn) [L.] (pl. *morpiones*). The crab louse, *Phthirus pubis*, which infests the pubic area. SEE: *lice.*

Morquio′s syndrome (mor-kē′ōz) [Louis Morquio, Uruguayan physician, 1867–1935]. Mucopolysaccharidosis IV.

morrhuate sodium injection (mor′ū-āt). USP. A sclerosing agent used to obliterate varicose veins.

mors [L.]. Death.
    m. putativa. Apparent death.
    m. subita. Sudden death.

morsal (mor′săl) [L. *morsus*, bite]. Involved in biting and chewing, as the occlusal surfaces of teeth.

morsulus (mor′sū-lŭs) [L. dim. of *morsus*, bite]. Troche, q.v.

mortal [L. *mortalis*]. 1. Causing death. 2. Subject to death. 3. Human.

mortality. 1. State of being mortal. 2. The death rate; ratio of number of deaths to a given population.

mortar [L. *mortarium*]. Vessel with a smooth interior in which crude drugs are crushed or ground with a pestle.

mortician [L. *mors*, death]. Undertaker; person trained to attend to the dead.

mortification (mor″tĭ-fĭ-kā′shŭn) [″ + *facere*, to make]. Death or failure of a tissue, organ, or part. SYN: *gangrene; necrosis.*

mortinatality (mor″tĭ-nā-tăl′ĭ-tē) [″ + *natus*, birth]. Ratio of stillbirths to general birth rate. SYN: *natimortality.*

mortise joint. Ankle joint.

Morton′s disease, syndrome (mor′tŭnz) [Dudley J. Morton, U.S. orthopedist, 1884–1960]. The condition of having a short hypertrophied second metatarsal bone with tenderness over the head of that bone, callosities under the second and third metatarsals, and pain and tenderness of the metatarsal area.

Morton′s foot syndrome. SEE: *Morton′s disease, syndrome.*

Morton′s neuralgia [Thomas G. Morton, U.S. surgeon, 1835–1903]. Pain in the metatarsal area due to a fallen transverse arch with pressure on the lateral plantar nerve. SYN: *Morton′s metatarsalgia.*

Morton′s neuroma. A neuromalike mass of

the neurovascular bundle of the intermetatarsal spaces.

mortuary (mor′chū-ā-rē) [L. *mortuarium*, a tomb]. 1. Temporary place for keeping dead bodies before burial. SYN: *morgue.* 2. Rel. to the dead or to death.

morula (mor′ū-lă) [L. *morus*, mulberry]. Solid mass of cells, resembling a mulberry, resulting from cleavage of an ovum. SEE: *fertilization* for illus.

morulation (mor″ū-lā′shŭn). The formation of morula.

moruloid (mor′ū-loyd) [″ + Gr. *eidos*, form, shape]. 1. A bacterial colony made up of a mass resembling a mulberry. 2. Resembling a mulberry.

Morvan′s disease (mor′vănz) [Augustin M. Morvan, Fr. physician, 1819–1897]. A form of syringomyelia, q.v., in which there are trophic changes in the extremities with formation of slowly healing lesions.

MOS. *medical outcomes study.*

mosaic. 1. A picture or design made of many small colored pieces interspersed in some other material. 2. An individual whose tissues are of different genetic kinds even though they were derived from the same cell. Caused by a genetic mutation. 3. Spotted condition in plants as in tobacco mosaic, a disease caused by a virus.

mosaic bone. Bone appearing as small pieces fitted together, characteristic of Paget′s disease.

mosaicism (mō-zā′ĭ-sĭzm). Presence of cells of two different genetic materials in the same individual.

mosquito [Sp., little fly] (pl. *mosquitoes*). A blood-sucking insect belonging to the order Diptera, family Culicidae, q.v. Important genera are *Anopheles, Culex, Aedes, Haemagogus, Mansonia,* and *Psorophora.* They serve as transmitting agents of many diseases, including malaria, filariasis, yellow fever, dengue, viral encephalitis, and dermatobiasis.

mosquitocide [″ + L. *caedere*, to kill]. An agent that is lethal to mosquitoes or their larvae.

mosquito forceps. A very small, delicately pointed hemostat. SYN: *Halsted′s forceps.*

moss. 1. Any low-growing green plant of the class Musci. 2. In general, any one of a number of lichens and seaweeds.
    m., sphagnum. Peat moss. It has been used as a surgical bandage and by some primitive people for menstrual protection.

mossy cell. A protoplasmic astrocyte, a neuroglia cell with many branching processes. SEE: *neuroglia.*

mossy fibers. Afferent fibers to the cerebellar cortex. They give off many collaterals, each ending in a glomerulus.

mother [AS. *modor*]. 1. Female parent. 2. A structure that gives rise to others.

> **m., biological.** SEE: *biological mother; surrogate parenting.*

> **m., surrogate.** SEE: *surrogate mother.*

mother cell. A cell that, by fission or budding, gives rise to similar cells.

mother cyst. An echinococcus cyst enveloping smaller ones.

mother liquor. Portion left after removal of crystals from a solution.

mother's mark. A birthmark. SEE: *mark.*

motile (mō'tĭl) [L. *motilis*, moving]. Able to move spontaneously.

motility (mō-tĭl'ĭ-tē). Power to move spontaneously.

motion (mō'shŭn) [L. *motio*, movement]. 1. A change of place or position; movement. 2. Evacuation of the bowels. 3. Matter evacuated from bowels. SEE: words beginning with *cine-* and *kine-*.

> **m., active.** Movement caused by the patient's own intention.

> **m., passive.** Movement as the result of the attendant's causing the part to be moved.

motion sickness. Drowsiness, dizziness, nausea, and vertigo induced by irregular or rhythmic movements of a vehicle being used for transportation, such as a car, airplane, or boat.

> Ex.: seasickness, airsickness, car sickness, swing sickness.

> TREAT: Transdermal scopolamine, q.v., is helpful in preventing motion sickness. The treatment should be started several hours prior to exposure to the motion. The use of wristbands to apply pressure to an acupressure point to treat motion sickness is being investigated.

motivation (mō"tĭ-vā'shŭn). The internal drive or externally arising stimulus to action or thought.

motive (mō'tĭv). The mental condition or state that affects, alters, or stimulates behavior.

motofacient (mō"tō-fā'shĕnt). Producing motion.

motolin. A gastrointestinal hormone that stimulates intestinal motor activity.

motoneuron (mō"tō-nū'rŏn). A motor neuron.

> **m.'s, lower.** Peripheral motor neurons that originate in the ventral gray columns of the spinal cord and terminate in skeletal muscles.

> **m.'s, peripheral.** Motor neurons that transmit stimuli to skeletal muscles.

> **m.'s, upper.** Neurons of the cerebral cortex that conduct stimuli from the motor cortex of the brain to motor nuclei of cere-

bral nerves or the ventral gray columns of the spinal cord.

motor [L. *motus*, moving]. 1. Causing motion. 2. A part or center that induces movements, as nerves or muscles.

motor aphasia. Condition in which patients understand but cannot express themselves in words or cannot read aloud.

motor area. Posterior part of frontal lobe anterior to the central sulcus, from which impulses for volitional movement arise.

motor endplate. Flat expansion ending a motor nerve fiber where it connects with a muscle fiber.

motor fibers. Axons of motor neurons that innervate skeletal muscles.

motorial (mō-tor'ē-ăl) [L. *motus*, moving]. Concerning motion or a motor center.

motoricity (mō-tor-ĭs'ĭ-tē). Capability of movement.

motor nerve. A nerve composed entirely of motor fibers.

motor neuron. 1. A neuron that innervates muscle tissue. 2. A neuron that carries impulses initiating muscle contraction.

motor neuron disease. One of several types of disease of the motor neurons: progressive muscle atrophy, progressive bulbar palsy, and amyotrophic lateral sclerosis. These diseases are characterized by degeneration of anterior horn cells of the spinal cord, the motor cranial nerve nuclei, and the pyramidal tracts. They occur principally in males. In the U.S., amyotrophic lateral sclerosis is better known as Lou Gehrig's disease. Gehrig was a well-known athlete whose baseball career and life were prematurely ended as a result of this disease. SEE: *amyotrophic lateral sclerosis.*

motorpathy (mō-tor'păth-ē) [L. *motus*, moving, + Gr. *pathos*, disease, suffering]. Treatment of a condition by prescribed movements. SYN: *kinesitherapy; kinetotherapy.*

motor points. Points where the motor nerve enters the muscle and where visible contraction can be elicited with a minimal amount of stimulation.

motor sense. The kinesthetic sense.

motor speech area. Area in the hemisphere of the brain that controls movements of the tongue, lips, and vocal cords. In right-handed people, this area is in the left hemisphere; and in left-handed persons, in the right hemisphere. Loss of speech may follow hemorrhage into this area. SYN: *Broca's area.*

motor unit. A single motor neuron and the muscle fibers its branches innervate.

Motrin. Trade name for ibuprofen.

mottled enamel. Condition in which the enamel of the teeth becomes discolored.

Often associated with excessive fluorine or fluoride in drinking water. Also it may be caused in the child by prolonged administration of tetracyclines during the first half of pregnancy or while the teeth are developing in children. SEE: *fluorosis.*

mottling (mŏt′lĭng) [ME. *motteley,* many colored]. Condition that is marked by discolored areas.

moulage (moo-lăzh′) [Fr.]. 1. A wax model or reproduction of the configuration of some part of the anatomy such as the face or nose, or of a pathological skin lesion. 2. Molding of a wax model.

mounding [origin uncertain]. The rising of a lump, as the mounding of a wasting muscle when struck a quick, firm blow. SYN: *myoedema.*

mount (mownt) [ME. *mounten,* to mount]. 1. To climb onto. 2. To place on a support or backing. 3. To place specimens or sections in special containers or on slides for study.

m., x-ray. A stiff cardboard folder with windows in which radiographs of teeth in the dental arches are placed in sequence for examination and diagnosis.

mountain fever. Condition occurring in individuals ascending to high altitudes (over 10,000 ft or 3,048 meters) or to those subjected to rarefied atmospheres. Due to anoxia resulting from reduced oxygen tension. SEE: *bends.*

SYM: euphoria, tachycardia, headache, nausea, increased respiratory rate, fatigue, and cerebral disorders (loss of memory, errors of judgment).

mountain sickness, chronic. The slow onset of symptoms in persons who reside at high altitude for several years. Included are florid color that turns to cyanosis during mild exertion; apathy, fatigue, and headache. Persons between ages 40 and 60 are most likely to be affected. The symptoms subside when the person returns to sea level. SYN: *Monge's disease; seroche.*

mountant. A medium used to embed specimens or thin sections on microscope slides for study. It is usually a synthetic or natural resin but may be glycerin or some water-soluble material for fresh or frozen sections. Also called mounting medium.

mounting (mownt′ĭng). 1. The arrangement of specimens on slides, frames, chart boards, display boards, or any background for study. 2. In dentistry, attaching a cast of the mandible or maxilla to an articulator.

mourning [AS. *murnan*]. Normal grief usually produced by the death of a loved one. Not synonymous with depression or melancholia.

mouse (mows). 1. A small rodent of the genus *Mus.* Used extensively in research. 2. A small piece of tissue that has become free or unattached, esp. in a body cavity or joint.

m., joint. Pieces of synovial membrane or cartilage that because of trauma or osteoarthritis are free in the joint space.

m., NZB. SEE: *NZB mouse.*

mouse unit. The smallest amount of estrogen that will produce cornified cells in the vaginal epithelium of a spayed mouse. SYN: *Allen-Doisy unit.*

mouth [AS. *muth*]. 1. The opening of any cavity. SYN: *buccal cavity; cavity, oral.* 2. The cavity within the cheeks, containing the tongue and teeth and communicating with the pharynx. SEE: illus.

ABNORM: *Tongue:* dry, coated, smooth, strawberry, large, pigmented, geographic, deviated, tremulous, sore. *Gums and teeth:* gingivitis, sordes, lead line, pyorrhea, atrophy, hypertrophy, dental caries, alveolar abscesses. *Mucous membranes and other parts of mouth:* eruptions accompanying exanthematous diseases, stomatitis, canker sores, herpes simplex, thrush, trench mouth, cysts, tumors, carcinoma, lesions of syphilis such as chancre, mucous patches gumma, lesions of tuberculosis, abscesses.

Disorders of the mouth cavity may be indications of purely local diseases or they may be symptoms of systemic disturbances such as dehydration, pernicious anemia, nutritional deficiencies, esp. avitaminoses.

Rashes of the mouth may indicate stomatitis, measles, or scarlet fever. Rashes on lips may indicate typhoid fever, meningitis, or pneumonia. In secondary syphilis, chancre, cancer, and epithelioma, mucous patches appear.

EXAM: In addition to visual examination, careful digital examination should be made because it reveals areas of tenderness and alterations of texture characteristic of leukoplakia, cancer, cystic swellings, and lymphadenopathy.

Excessive moisture of the mouth is seen in stomatitis, irritation of the vagus nerve, ingestion of irritating drugs or foods, nervous disorders, teething, seeing appetizing foods, and smelling pleasant odors. SEE: *burning mouth syndrome.*

RS: antitrismus; bucca; cancrum oris; canker; catarrh; chalinoplasty; Escherich's reflex; glossodynia; glossopyresis; mandible; maxilla; oral; orifice; palate; palatine; stoma; stomatitis; tongue; xerostomia.

m., trench. SEE: *trench mouth.*

mouth guard. A removable dental appliance used to protect the teeth and investing tissues during contact sports. SEE: *occlusal guard.*

mouthrinse. A medicated solution used to cleanse or treat diseases of the oral tissues,

MOUTH, TONGUE, AND PHARYNX

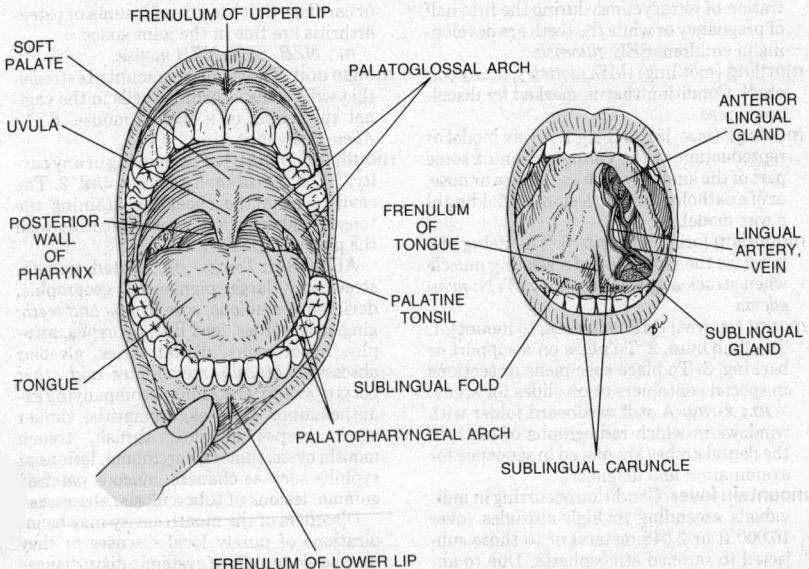

reduce halitosis, or add fluoride to the teeth for dental caries control or prevention. SYN: *mouthwash; oral rinse.*

mouthstick. Adapted device consisting of a stick attached to a molded dental mouthpiece that permits page-turning and other tasks through head movement.

mouthwash. A medicated solution to cleanse or treat diseases of the oral mucosa. It may contain various chemical compounds, such as fluoride or zinc chlorides, alcohol, glycerin, detergents, essential oils for flavoring, and coloring agents. According to the composition and proposed function, mouthwashes may be described as antibacterial, astringent, buffered, concentrated, cosmetic, deodorizing, or therapeutic. Also called oral rinse or dental rinse.

movement [L. *movere,* to move]. 1. Act of passing from place to place or changing position of body or its parts. 2. Evacuation of feces.

   m., active. Voluntary movement accomplished without external assistance.

   m., ameboid. Movement resembling that of an ameba in which the protoplasm of a cell flows into a projection of the cell membrane forming a pseudopodium. Characteristic of leukocytes and certain protozoa.

   m., angular. Voluntary muscular movement resulting in change in the angle between the involved bones.

   m., associated. Involuntary movement of a part occurring coincident with and subsequent to the movement of another part, as in the eyes.

   m., autonomic. Spontaneous, involuntary movement independent of external stimulation.

   m., bodily. Movement of tooth by natural or orthodontic forces so that the crown and root maintain their same vertical axis. SEE: *m., rotational; m., tipping.*

   m., brownian. The peculiar jiggling or dancing movement of minute particles suspended in liquids or gases when observed under the microscope due to bombardment of the particles by molecules of their surrounding medium.

   m., ciliary. Rhythmic movement of the cilia of a ciliated cell or epithelium. SYN: *m., vibratile.*

   m., circus. A phenomenon after injury to a corpus striatum, optic thalamus, or crus cerebri, causing an odd circular gait.

   m., disorders of. May be due to injury or disease of muscle, nerve ending, motor nerve, spinal cord, or the brain. Types are hemiplegia, ataxia, monoplegia, tremors, rigors, chorea, athetosis, convulsions, spasm (clonic or tonic), reflex (hysterical, habit spasm, tics), and spastic paralysis.

m.'s, fetal. Muscular movements performed by the fetus in utero.

m., gliding. Movement of one surface over another without angular or rotatory movement, as well. This type of movement occurs in the temporomandibular joint after opening when the condyles and discs move forward, as in protrusion of the jaw.

m., hinge. Movement in a joint around a transverse axis, as occurs in the lower compartment of the temporomandibular joints at the beginning of jaw opening when the occluding teeth are separated or in the final stage of wide opening of the mouth.

m., jaw. Movement of the mandible. SEE: *m., gliding; m., hinge.*

m., masticatory. One of the movements of the jaw which result in the cutting and grinding of food. It may involve unilateral chewing, alternating bilateral chewing according to the learned automatic pattern of activity, or consciously initiated movements.

m., molecular. Movement of molecules of a substance, the basis of the kinetic theory of matter. SEE: *m., brownian.*

m. of restitution. A partial rotation of the fetal head in cases of head presentation.

m., orthodontic. Movement of teeth by orthodontic appliances for aesthetics or to correct malocclusions. Such movement depends on remodeling of the bony socket which usually occurs without resorption of the tooth root unless excessive forces have been used.

m., passive. Movement of the body or a part due to outside forces.

m.'s, pendular. Swaying movements of the intestines caused by rhythmic contractions of the longitudinal muscles of the walls of the intestines.

m., peristaltic. Peristalsis.

m., respiratory. Any movement resulting from the contraction of respiratory muscles or occurring passively as a result of elasticity of the thoracic wall or lungs. SEE: *compliance,* def. 1; *expiration; inspiration; respiration.*

m., rotational. Movement around an axis, as in hinge movement of the temporomandibular joint or rotation of a tooth around its longitudinal axis in tooth movement or extraction. SEE: *m., bodily; m., tipping.*

m.'s, saccadic. Jerky movements of the eyes as they move from one point of fixation to another.

m., segmenting. Movement of the in-

testine in which annular constrictions occur, dividing intestine into ovoid segments.

m., tipping. Movement of a tooth crown while the root apex remains essentially stationary, resulting in an inclination of the axis of the tooth in one direction. SEE: *m., bodily; m., rotational.*

m., vermicular. Intestinal peristalsis.

m., vibratile. M., ciliary.

moxa (mŏk'sa) [Japanese]. A soft, combustible substance to be burned on skin, popular in the Orient as a cautery and counterirritant. SEE: *moxibustion.*

moxalactam disodium. An antibacterial drug. Trade name is Moxam.

Moxam. Trade name for moxalactam disodium.

moxibustion (mŏks-ĭ-bŭs'chŭn) [" + L. *combustus,* burned]. Cauterization by means of a cylinder or cone of cotton wool, called a moxa, placed on the skin and fired at the top. Used to produce counterirritation.

Mozart ear [Wolfgang Amadeus Mozart, Austrian composer, 1756–1791. Alleged to have had this deformity]. Deformity of the ear in which the antehelix is fused with the crura of the helix.

M.P.D. *maximum permissible dose.*

M.P.H. *Master of Public Health.*

M.P.N. *most probable number* (of bacteria present in a quantity of solution, esp. water).

MPS *mucopolysaccharidosis,* q.v.

MR. *magnetic resonance.*

mR. *milliroentgen.*

MRI. *magnetic resonance imaging.*

M.R.L. *medical records librarian.*

mRNA. *messenger RNA.*

MS. *multiple sclerosis.*

M.S. *Master of Surgery; Master of Science.*

ms. *millisecond.*

msec. *millisecond.*

MSH. *melanocyte-stimulating hormone.*

M.S.N. *Master of Science in Nursing.*

M.T. *medical technologist.*

M.u. *Mache unit.*

m.u. *mouse unit.*

mu (mū) [Gr. μ, letter m]. SYMB: μ; u. Symb. used for the prefix *micro-* which stands for multiplication by 10^{-6}. Thus, μm would stand for 10^{-6} meter.

mucedin (mū'sĕ-dĭn) [L. *mucedo,* mucus]. A substance obtained from gluten.

muciferous (mū-sĭf'ĕr-ŭs) [L. *mucus,* mucus, + *ferre,* to carry]. Secreting or producing mucus. SYN: *mucigenous; muciparous.*

muciform (mū'sĭ-form) [" + *forma,* shape]. Appearing similar to mucus.

mucigen (mū'sĭ-jĕn) [" + Gr. *gennan,* to produce]. A substance present in mucous cells that, upon being extruded from the cell, is converted into mucin.

mucigenous (mū-sĭj'ĕn-ŭs). Producing mucus. SYN: *muciferous; muciparous.*

mucilage (mū'sĭ-lĭj) [L. *mucilago,* moldy juice]. Vegetable preparation used in pharmaceuticals. SEE: *mucilago.*

mucilaginous (mū-sĭl-ăj'ĭn-ŭs). Resembling mucilage; slimy; sticky.

mucilago. Thick, viscid, adhesive liquid, containing gum or mucilaginous principles dissolved in water, usually employed to hold insoluble substances in suspension in aqueous liquids or as a demulcent.

mucilloid (mū'sĭl-loyd). A mucilaginous preparation.

    m., psyllium hydrophilic. Mucilloid prepared from psyllium seeds. It is used as a bulk-type laxative.

mucin (mū'sĭn) [L. *mucus,* mucus]. A glycoprotein found in mucus. It is present in saliva and bile, in salivary glands, and in the skin, connective tissues, tendon, and cartilage. It is formed from mucigen and in water forms a slimy solution.

    m., gastric. A commercial preparation made from the gastric mucosa of the hog and used in the treatment of ulcers of the digestive tract. It forms a protective coating over the ulcer or erosion, which prevents irritation from the passing of bile and acid secretions in the duodenum and from acid conditions irritating peptic ulcer of the stomach.

mucinase (mū'sĭ-nās). Any enzyme that acts on mucin.

mucinemia (mū"sĭn-ē'mē-ă) [" + Gr. *haima,* blood]. Mucin in the blood. SYN: *myxemia.*

mucinogen (mū-sĭn'ō-jĕn) [" + Gr. *gennan,* to produce]. A glycoprotein that forms mucin.

mucinoid (mū'sĭn-oyd) [" + Gr. *eidos,* form, shape]. Appearing similar to mucin.

mucinolytic (mū"sĭ-nō-lĭt'ĭk) [" + Gr. *lysis,* dissolution]. Hydrolyzing or dissolving mucin.

mucinuria (mū-sĭn-ū'rē-ă) [" + Gr. *ouron,* urine]. Presence of mucin in the urine.

muciparous (mū-sĭp'ăr-ŭs) [" + *parere,* to bring forth, to bear]. Producing or secreting mucus. SYN: *muciferous; mucigenous.*

muco- [L. *mucus,* mucus]. Combining form indicating rel. to mucus.

mucocele (mū'kō-sēl) [" + Gr. *kele,* tumor, swelling]. 1. Enlargement of the lacrimal sac. 2. A mucous cyst. 3. A mucous polypus. 4. Cystic disease of the air cavities of the cranial bones causing erosion of the bone.

mucocolpos (mū"kō-kŏl'pŏs) [" + Gr. *kolpos,* vagina]. Accumulation of mucus in the vagina.

mucocutaneous (mū"kō-kū-tā'nē-ŭs) ["

+ *cutis,* skin]. Concerning mucous membrane and the skin. SYN: *mucodermal.*

mucocutaneous lymph node syndrome. SEE: *Kawasaki disease.*

mucodermal (mū-kō-dĕr'măl) [" + Gr. *derma,* skin]. Pert. to the mucous membranes and skin. SYN: *mucocutaneous.*

mucoenteritis (mū"kō-ĕn-tĕr-ī'tĭs) [" + Gr. *enteron,* intestine, + *itis,* inflammation]. Inflammation of intestinal mucosa.

mucoglobulin (mū"kō-glŏb'ū-lĭn) [" + *globulus,* globule]. A type of glycoprotein, q.v.

mucoid (mū'koyd) [" + Gr. *eidos,* form, shape]. 1. Glycoprotein similar to mucin. 2. Muciform similar to mucus.

mucomembranous (mū"kō-mĕm'bră-nŭs) [" + *membrana,* membrane]. Concerning mucous membrane.

mucoperiosteum (mū"kō-pĕr"ē-ŏs'tē-ŭm). Periosteum that has a mucous surface; or mucous and periosteal surfaces combined to form a membrane.

mucopolysaccharidase (mū"kō-pŏl"ē-săk'ă-rī-dās). An enzyme that catalyzes the hydrolysis of polysaccharides.

mucopolysaccharide (mū"kō-pŏl"ī-săk'ă-rĭd). Polysaccharides that form chemical bonds with water. They contain hexosamine and sometimes proteins. Thick gelatinous material that is found many places in the body; it forms intercellular ground substance and basement membranes of cells; it is in mucous secretions and synovial fluid. SYN: *glycosaminoglycans.*

mucopolysaccharidosis. ABBR: MPS. A group of inherited disorders characterized by a deficiency of enzymes that are essential for the degradation of the mucopolysaccharides heparan sulfate, dermatan sulfate, and keratan sulfate. These chemicals are excreted in excess quantities in the urine; and they usually accumulate in reticuloendothelial cells, endothelial cells, intimal smooth muscle cells, and fibroblasts throughout the body. Clinically, these disorders include some or all of the following: coarse facies, corneal clouding, hepatosplenomegaly, joint stiffness, hernias, skeletal dysplasia, and mental deficiency. The changes are not usually apparent at birth; but the inherited defect can be diagnosed prior to birth by culturing amniotic fluid cells and testing them for specific enzyme activity. The test may yield either false-positive or false-negative results. After birth the conditions may be diagnosed by testing cultured skin fibroblasts for specific enzymes. The MPS disorders have been classified as follows:

    MPS IH. Hurler's syndrome. A type of MPS due to a deficiency of the enzyme alpha-L-iduronidase with accumulation of dermatan sulfate and heparan sulfate. Clinically characterized by lens opacities, coarse facies, skeletal dysplasia, hepatosplenomegaly, and mental deficiency.

MPS IS. Scheie's syndrome. An MPS due to the same enzyme defect as MPS IH and with similar clinical characteristics except mental deficiency is absent.

MPS IHS. Hurler-Scheie. An intermediate syndrome between MPS IH and MPS IS. It is due to the same enzyme deficiency. Mental development may be normal.

MPS II. Hunter syndrome. An MPS due to a deficiency of the enzyme L-iduronosulfate sulfatase. Clinically, there is retinal degeneration but no corneal clouding; mental retardation, joint stiffness, skeletal dysplasia, cardiac lesions, and deafness.

MPS III. Sanfilippo syndrome. This MPS has been further differentiated into Sanfilippo A, B, C, or D, on the basis of the specific enzyme deficiency present in each form. Clinically, it may not be possible to distinguish the types. Present are moderate coarse facies, severe mental deficiency, and mild hepatosplenomegaly. Corneal clouding is absent and growth is normal.

MPS IV. Morquio's syndrome. MPS due to a deficiency of the enzyme N-acetylgalactosamine-6-sulfatase. Clinically, there are dwarfism, thoracolumbar gibbus (hunchback), kyphoscoliosis, coarse facies, cardiac lesions, moderate hepatosplenomegaly, and joint hypermobility.

MPS V. Now classed as MPS IS, q.v.

MPS VI. Maroteaux-Lamy syndrome. MPS due to a deficiency of the enzyme N-acetylgalactosamine-4-sulfatase. Clinically, there is normal intelligence, and is otherwise similar to MPS IH, q.v.

MPS VII. Glucuronidase deficiency disease. MPS due to a deficiency of beta-glucuronidase. Clinically quite similar to MPS IH, q.v., except intelligence may be normal.

mucopolysacchariduria (mū″kō-pŏl″ē-săk′ă-rĭ-dū′rē-ă). Mucopolysaccharides in the urine.

mucoprotein (mū″kō-prō′tē-ĭn). A complex of protein and mucopolysaccharide. Usually the polysaccharide contains hexosamine.

m., Tamm-Horsfall [Igor Tamm, Russian-born U.S. virologist, 1922–1971; Frank L. Horsfall, Jr., U.S. physician, 1906–1971]. A normal mucoprotein in the urine. It is not derived from plasma, but is produced by the ascending limb of the loop of Henle. When this protein is concentrated at low pH, it forms gel. These conditions may be met when the urine is exposed to myoglobin, hemoglobin, albumin, Bence-Jones protein, and pyelographic contrast media. This protein is contained in most urinary casts and is identical to *uromedulin, human,* q.v.

mucopurulent (mū-kō-pūr′ū-lĕnt) [L. *mucus,* mucus, + *purulentus,* made up of pus]. Consisting of mucus and pus.

mucopus (mū′kō-pŭs). Mucus combined with or resembling pus.

Mucor (mū′kor) [L.]. A genus of mold fungi seen on dead and decaying matter. Sometimes responsible for infections of external ear, skin, and respiratory passageways. SEE: *mucormycosis.*

mucoriferous (mū″kor-ĭf′ĕr-ŭs) [L. *mucor,* mold, + *ferre,* to carry]. Covered with mold or a moldlike substance.

mucormycosis (mū″kor-mī-kō′sĭs) [″ + Gr. *mykes,* fungus, + *osis,* condition]. A group of mycoses usually caused by fungi of the family Mucoraceae of the class Zygomycetes. These fungi have an affinity for blood vessels in which they cause thrombosis and infarction. The disease in the form that affects the head and face usually causes paranasal sinus infections, esp. during periods of ketoacidosis in persons with diabetes mellitus. Also, it may disseminate to the brain. The pulmonary form of the disease causes infarcts of the lung; and in the gastrointestinal form, mucosal ulcers and gangrene of the stomach may occur. The disease is contracted by inhalation or ingestion of the fungus by susceptible individuals. Most persons have a natural resistance to the fungus, accounting for the rarity of the disease. SYN: *zygomycosis.*

TREAT: Control of or prevention of diabetic acidosis; amphotericin B; and resection of necrotic tissue.

mucorrhea [″ + *rhoia,* to flow]. Increased cervical discharge at ovulation. Usually covers a 3- to 4-day span and has character and appearance of raw egg white. SEE: *spinnbarkeit.*

mucosa (mū-kō′să) [L., mucous] (pl. *mucosae*). A mucous membrane or the moist tissue layer that lines a hollow organ or body cavity. Specifically, it consists of an epithelial covering with its basement membrane, a connective tissue layer often called lamina propria, and may have smooth muscle present, which is called the muscularis mucosae. The type of epithelium, thickness, and presence or absence of glands varies with the function or location of the mucosa.

m., alveolar. A thin, nonkeratinized, mucosal layer that covers the alveolar processes and is continuous with the mucosa of the cheek, lips, tongue, and palate.

m., buccal. The lining of the cheeks of the oral cavity. It is characterized by stratified squamous non-keratinized epithelium which may become keratinized in local areas due to cheek-biting. It may also contain ectopic sebaceous glands. SEE: *Fordyce disease.*

m., lingual. The keratinized, papillated covering of the dorsum of the tongue which contains nerve endings for the sense of taste.

m., masticatory. Those areas of the mucosa of the mouth that have become keratinized due to the friction and abrasion of the masticatory process, especially the gingivae and hard palate.

m., nasal. The mucosa lining the nasal cavity and paranasal sinuses, characterized by pseudostratified ciliated columnar epithelium with goblet cells and functions to warm and hydrate the air inspired and by ciliary action to exteriorize mucous-entrapped dust and debris.

m., oral. The mucous membrane lining the oral cavity and described by its location on the gingiva, hard palate, soft palate, cheek, vestibule, lip, tongue, and pharyngeal area.

mucosal (mū-kō′săl). Concerning any mucous membrane.

mucosanguineous (mū″kō-săn-gwĭn′ē-ŭs) [″ + *sanguineus,* bloody]. Containing mucus and blood.

mucosedative (mū″kō-sĕd′ă-tĭv) [″ + *sedativus,* allaying]. Soothing to mucosae of the body. SYN: *demulcent.*

mucoserous (mū″kō-sēr′ŭs). Composed of mucus and serum.

mucosin (mū′kō-sĭn). Mucin found in thick sticky mucus.

mucositis (mū″kō-sī′tĭs) [″ + Gr. *itis,* inflammation]. Inflammation of a mucous membrane.

mucosocutaneous (mū-kō″sō-kū-tā′nē-ŭs). Concerning mucous membrane and skin.

mucostatic (mū″kō-stăt′ĭk) [″ + *statikos,* standing]. Stopping the secretion of mucus.

mucous (mū′kŭs). 1. Having the nature of or resembling mucus. 2. Secreting mucus. 3. Depending on presence of mucus.

mucous colitis. Inflammation of the mucosa of the colon. SEE: *colitis; irritable bowel syndrome.*

mucous membrane. Membrane lining passages and cavities communicating with the air. Consists of a surface layer of epithelium, a basement membrane, and an underlying layer of connective tissue, the lamina propria. Mucus-secreting cells or glands usually are present in the epithelium but may be absent. Examination should reveal degree of moisture, cyanosis, pallor, hyperemia, pigmentation, lesions or their absence, and hemorrhage. Pallor is seen in all anemias. If temporary, it may indicate shock or vaso-

motor spasm, or it may occur in severe hemorrhages. Blanching and flushing alternately accompanies aortic regurgitation.

Hyperemia or excessive redness of the mucous membranes is indicative of certain pathological changes in particular tissues. For example:

Buccal mucous membrane: Due to decayed teeth, traumatism, stomatitis. SEE: *mouth.*

Nasal mucosa: Ulceration of nose, rhinitis, inflammation. SEE: *nose.*

Eyes (local irritation): Foreign body, ulcer, inflammation. SEE: *jaundice.*

Dryness is seen in fevers, chronic gastritis, some liver disturbances, excitement, shock, prostration, fatigue, thirst, and certain drugs.

mucous polypus. Small growth from mucous lining of the cervix or uterus.

mucoviscidosis (mū″kō-vĭs″ĭ-dō′sĭs). Cystic fibrosis, q.v.

mucus (mū′kŭs) [L.]. A viscid fluid secreted by mucous membranes and glands, consisting of mucin, leukocytes, inorganic salts, water, and epithelial cells. A good example is the almost ropy secretion from the sublingual and submandibular glands.

RS: amyxorrhea, expectorant; expectoration; glairy; goblet cell; "blenn-" and "muc-" words.

mulatto (mū-lăt′tō) [Sp. *mulato,* of mixed breed]. A person with one black parent and one white parent; popularly, anyone of mixed white and black ancestry.

muliebria (mū″lē-ĕb′rē-ă) [L.]. The female genitalia.

muliebrity (mū″lē-ĕb′rĭ-tē) [L. *muliebritas*]. 1. Femininity; womanliness. The assumption of womanly qualities at puberty. 2. The assumption of female characteristics by a male.

mull (mŭl). 1. To grind or pulverize. 2. A type of soft muslin.

Müller, Heinrich (mĭl′ĕr). German anatomist, 1820–1864.

M.'s fibers. Fine fibers of neuroglia cells that form supporting elements of the retina.

M.'s muscle. 1. Circular fibers of ciliary muscle. 2. The superior tarsal muscle of the eyelid. 3. Smooth muscle covering the sphenomaxillary fissure.

M.'s trigone. Portion of tuber cinereum folding over the optic chiasm.

Müller, Johannes P. (mĭl′ĕr). German physician, 1801–1858.

M.'s ducts. Embryonic tubes from which the oviducts, uterus, and vagina develop in the female; in the male, they atrophy.

M. maneuver. A maneuver to produce negative intrathoracic pressure. To do this, the patient exhales and makes an inspiratory effort while the glottis is closed. This technique is used during fluoroscopy to attempt to visualize esophageal varices. SEE: *esophageal varices; Valsalva's maneuver.*

M.'s ring. Muscular ring at the junction of the cervical canal and the gravid uterus.

M.'s tubercle. Projection on the dorsal wall of the cloaca at which Müller's ducts terminate.

mult-, multi- [L. *multus*]. Prefixes indicating many or much.

multangular. Having many angles.

multangular bone, greater. The first or outermost of the distal row of carpal bones. SYN: *trapezium.*

multangular bone, lesser. The second in distal row of carpal bones. SYN: *trapezoid bone.*

multiallelic (mŭl″tē-ă-lĕl′ĭk). Concerning a large number of genes affecting hereditary characteristics.

multiarticular (mŭl″tē-ăr-tĭk′ū-lăr) [L. *multus*, many, + *articulus*, joint]. Concerning, having, or affecting many joints. SYN: *polyarticular.*

multicapsular (mŭl″tĭ-kăp′sū-lăr) [″ + *capsula*, a little box]. Composed of many capsules.

multicellular (mŭl″tĭ-sĕl′ū-lăr) [″ + *cellula*, small chamber]. Consisting of many cells.

Multiceps. A genus of tapeworms.

multicuspid, multicuspidate (mŭl″tĭ-kŭs′pĭd, -pĭ-dāt) [″ + *cuspis*, point]. Having several cusps.

multidisciplinary. Refers to multiple disciplines involved in the care of patients. The term *multidisciplinary* suggests that the various disciplines are working in collaboration, but in a parallel mode of interaction. In that situation, each distinctive discipline is accountable and responsible for its tasks and functions regarding patient care.

multifactorial. The result of many factors, as in a disease resulting from the combined effects of several factors.

multifamilial (mŭl″tĭ-fă-mĭl′ē-ăl). Concerning a familial disease that affects children in several generations.

multifid (mŭl′tĭ-fĭd) [″ + *fidus*, from *findere*, to split]. Divided into many sections.

multifocal (mŭl″tĭ-fō′kăl). Concerning many foci.

multiform (mŭl′tĭ-form) [″ + *forma*, shape]. Having many forms or shapes. SYN: *polymorphic; polymorphous.*

multiglandular (mŭl″tĭ-glănd′ū-lăr) [″ + *glandula*, a little acorn]. Concerning several glands.

multigravida (mŭl″tĭ-grăv′ĭ-dă) [″ + *gravida*, pregnant]. A woman who has been preg-nant two or more times. May be written as gravida II or III, etc., according to the number of pregnancies. SEE: *multipara.*

multi-infarct dementia. A dementia resulting from damage to the cerebral blood vessels characterized by facial presentation of aphasia, apraxia, alexia. The onset occurs in middle age after an episode of hypertension or stroke.

multi-infection (mŭl″tĭ-ĭn-fĕk′shŭn) [L. *multus*, many, + *infectio*, an infection]. A mixed infection with several organisms developing at the same time.

multilobular (mŭl″tĭ-lŏb′ū-lar) [″ + *lobulus*, a small lobe]. Formed of or possessing many lobules.

multilocular (mŭl″tĭ-lŏk′ū-lăr) [″ + *loculus*, a cell]. Having many cells or compartments. SYN: *multicellular.*

multimammae (mŭl″tĭ-măm′mē) [″ + *mamma*, breast]. Condition of possessing more than the normal number of breasts. SYN: *polymastia.*

multinodal (mŭl-tĭ-nō′dăl). Having many nodes or knots.

multinodular (mŭl-tĭ-nŏd′ū-lar) [″ + *nodulus*, little knot]. Possessing many nodules or small knots.

multinuclear, multinucleate (mŭl-tĭ-nū″klē-ăr, -āt). Possessing several nuclei. SYN: *polynuclear.*

multipara (mŭl-tĭp′ă-rä) [″ + *parere*, to bring forth, to bear]. A woman who has borne more than one viable fetus, whether or not the offspring were alive at birth. May be written para II or III, and so on, according to the number of deliveries. SEE: *multigravida.*

m., grand. A woman who has given birth seven or more times.

multiparity (mŭl-tĭ-păr′ĭ-tē). 1. Condition of having borne more than one child. 2. Production of more than one child at one birth.

multiparous (mŭl-tĭp′ăr-ŭs). 1. Having borne more than one child. 2. Producing more than one child at birth.

multiphasic screening. Attempting to determine an individual's health through a variety of methods and techniques. Usually consists of one or more of the following: self-completed medical history, variety of laboratory examinations of urine and blood, chest x-ray, serological test for syphilis, Papanicolaou smear, tonometry, pulmonary vital capacity, electrocardiogram, breast examination, height, weight, vision test, blood pressure. The cost-effectiveness of this approach in screening the apparently well has not been demonstrated.

multiple (mŭl′tĭ-pl) [L. *multiplex*, many folded]. 1. Consisting of or containing more than one; manifold. 2. Occurring simultaneously in various parts of the body.

multiple drug resistance. In cancer therapy, resistance to a wide range of unrelated drugs after resistance to a single agent has developed. SEE: *gene amplification.*

multiple endocrine neoplasia. ABBR: MEN. An inherited genetic defect that produces hyperplasia or malignant tumors in several endocrine glands. This group of diseases has been classed according to the glands affected:

   MEN type I (MEN I). Tumors of the parathyroids, pancreatic islet cells, adrenal cortex, and thyroid. SYN: *Wermer's syndrome. MEN type II (MEN II).* Medullary thyroid carcinoma, pheochromocytoma, and parathyroid hyperplasia. SYN: *Sipple syndrome. MEN type III (MEN III).* Quite similar to MEN II but there are marked facial aberrations with neuromas of the conjunctiva, labial mucosa, tongue, larynx, and gastric intestinal tract.

multiple malformation syndrome. Developmental anomalies of two or more systems in the fetus. These may be caused by chromosome and genetic abnormalities, and by teratogens including certain drugs and chemicals. In attempting to determine the etiology, it is important to obtain a complete family history and history of exposure to known teratogens and infectious diseases. SEE: *amniotic band disruption sequence syndrome.*

multiple myeloma. SEE: *myeloma, multiple.*

multiple personality. Condition in which the subject may develop two or more personalities. SEE: *dissociation of personality; dual personality.*

multiple sclerosis. ABBR: MS. An inflammatory disease of the central nervous system in which infiltrating lymphocytes, predominantly T cells and macrophages, degrade the myelin sheath of nerves. It is suspected that the cause is an autoimmune disease somehow linked to a viral infection. The symptoms were once thought to develop gradually, but this is not necessarily true. In about 40% of cases the onset may occur in less than a few hours. The disease is rare in children; and, in about two-thirds of cases, it begins between ages 20 and 40. The prevalence is less than one in 100,000 in the tropics; 6 to 14 in 100,000 in southern Europe and the southern U.S.; 30 to 80 in 100,000 in Canada, northern Europe and the northern U.S. Blacks are at less risk than whites. SEE: *Nursing Diagnoses in Appendix.*

   SYM: At onset and in about one-half the patients, the symptoms and signs are weakness or numbness or both in one or more limbs; later, the tendon reflexes become hy-peractive. In about one-quarter of patients, the initial manifestation is retrobulbar or optic neuritis. Other clinical findings at onset include unsteady gait, diplopia, vertigo, vomiting, and difficulty urinating. Nystagmus may be present. In the established stage of the disease, various clinical syndromes are present. They may be mostly due to optic nerve, brain stem, cerebellar, and spinal cord involvement or combinations of these. At one time, euphoria was thought to be a frequent finding, but emotional disturbances, including depression, irritability, and being short tempered, are not unusual.

   Clinically, MS is of the exacerbating-remitting type in which episodes of neurologic dysfunction are followed by recovery; or the chronic progressive type in which there is a steady progression of neurologic dysfunction. The duration of the disease is variable; some patients die a few months after onset; the average duration is more than 30 years. As many as one-third of surviving patients may still be working at the end of 25 years, and two-thirds will be ambulating. The availability of home and office computers with electronic keyboards and ocular-, voice-, and breath-activated devices has made it possible for patients with MS to be employable and to lead productive and more enjoyable lives.

   TREAT: There is no specific therapy, but short-term administration of ACTH and prednisone will benefit patients, although their use does not alter the eventual course of the disease process. Otherwise, the disease is treated symptomatically, particular care being taken to prevent bed sores in bed-ridden patients. Patients often benefit from referral to occupational or physical therapy, or both.

Multiple Sleep Latency Test. SEE: *narcolepsy.*

multiple systems organ failure. ABBR: MSOF. Acute, usually generalized clinical conditions that lead to progressive failure of two or more organ systems mediated by the body's inability to control its defense mechanisms. Organs fail because of this generalized defense system malfunction, rather than as isolated incidents. The clinical signs will be consistent with failure of organ systems such as the lungs, kidneys, circulatory system, liver, central nervous system, gastrointestinal system, or hematologic system. SYN: *hypermetabolic organ failure; multiple systems organ failure; sequential organ failure.* SEE: *disseminated intravascular coagulation.*

   NURSING IMPLICATIONS: Closely monitor patients at risk (those experiencing sepsis, perfusion deficits, or persistent inflammatory states), and help to prevent MSOF by prompt recognition and correction of perfusion problems, infection, and organ dysfunction. Assess for indicators of hypermetabolic hyperdynamic state as body tries to compensate for initial insult. This will be followed by a hypodynamic, decompensated state with imbalances in oxygen supply and demand, maldistribution of circulating volume and metabolic abnormalities, resulting in organs beginning to fail. Common problems are pulmonary, cardiovascular, renal, and hepatic, often followed or accompanied by gram-negative sepsis and disseminated intravascular coagulation (DIC). Appropriate medical interventions will be initiated for each failing system's problems. Nursing responsibilities include monitoring vital signs and assessing diagnostic study results, coordinating and carrying out prescribed therapies and evaluating patient responses while simultaneously assessing for adverse effects, protecting the patient from nosocomial infections and environmental stressors, and providing emotional support for patient and family through this type of devastating illness, which has a 90% mortality rate.

multiplexor. In computers and instrumentation, a circuit that allows a single processor to sample multiple input channels by sequencing them.

multipolar (mŭl-tĭ-pōl′ăr) [L. *multus,* many, + *polus,* a pole]. 1. Possessing more than two poles. 2. Possessing more than two processes, said of neurons.

multirooted. In dentistry, a tooth having several roots.

multisynaptic (mŭl″tē-sĭ-năp′tĭk). Polysynaptic.

multiterminal [″ + Gr. *terma,* a limit]. Providing several sets of terminals, making possible the use of several electrodes.

multivalent (mŭl-tĭ-vā′lĕnt) [″ + *valere,* to have power]. 1. Having ability to combine with more than two atoms of a univalent element or radical 2. Active against several strains of an organism.

mummification (mŭm″mĭ-fĭ-kā′shŭn) [Arabian *mumiyaa,* mummy, + L. *facere,* to make]. 1. Mortification producing a hard, dry mass. SYN: *gangrene, dry.* 2. Drying and shriveling of a body, as a dead fetus.

mumps (mŭmps). An acute, contagious, febrile disease characterized by inflammation of the parotid glands and other salivary glands. SYN: *parotitis.* SEE: *Nursing Diagnoses* in Appendix.

SYM: Onset gradual. There may be chilliness, malaise, headache, pain below ears, moderate fever of 101° to 102°F (38.3° to

38.9°C) or higher followed by swelling of one or both parotid glands. Usually swelling in one gland is subsiding as other swells. Swelling is below and in front of the ear. The lobe of the ear is sometimes pushed forward, surrounding tissues are edematous, and the features may be greatly distorted. Movements of the jaw are painful and restricted. Saliva may be increased or diminished. In a third of cases only one parotid is involved. Occasionally the parotid glands seem to escape, and swelling is confined to the submaxillary gland. Swelling usually lasts from 5 to 7 days.

ETIOL: Mumps virus.

COMPLICATIONS: Complications usually develop about the time the swelling in the parotids subsides. The most common complication in the postpubertal male is orchitis, which occurs in about 20% to 30% of cases; in the female, oöphoritis and mastitis. In rare cases permanent impairment of hearing follows an attack of mumps. Meningoencephalitis has been estimated to occur in 10% of patients.

DIFF. DIAGNOSIS: Cases of symptomatic parotitis may be excluded. Instances of trauma, infections about teeth and mouth, or a blocking of Stensen's duct may be suggestive of mumps.

TREAT: Rest in bed, a soft diet, and analgesics for headache and general malaise. Cold local applications may control swelling of testicles in orchitis.

PROG: Favorable, although the possibility of sexual sterility may occur in rare instances of bilateral orchitis.

mumps skin test antigen. USP. A standardized suspension of sterile formaldehyde-inactivated mumps virus. It is used in diagnosing mumps.

Mumpsvax. Trade name for mumps virus vaccine live, USP.

mumps virus vaccine live. USP. A sterile preparation of live mumps virus used to immunize against mumps. Trade name is Mumpsvax.

Munchausen syndrome (mĕn-chow′zĕn) [Baron Karl F. H. von Munchausen, fictional 18th century baron created by Rudolph Raspe]. A type of malingering or factitious disorder in which the patient may practice self-multilation and deception in order to feign illness. When detected, such patients leave one hospital and appear in the emergency room of another. Patients of this type are seldom recognized in time to receive psychiatric diagnoses and therapy, which they need.

mural (mū′răl) [L. *murus,* a wall]. Pert. to a wall of an organ or part.

muramidase. An enzyme found in blood cells

of the granulocytic and monocytic series. Its serum and urine level is increased in patients with acute or chronic leukemia. It is also normally present in saliva, sweat, and tears. Formerly called lysozyme.

Murchison-Pel-Ebstein fever (mŭr'chĭ-sŏn-pĕl-ĕb'stĭn) [Charles Murchison, Brit. physician, 1830–1879; Pieter K. Pel, Dutch physician, 1852–1919; Wilhelm Ebstein, Ger. physician, 1836–1912]. SEE: *Pel-Ebstein fever.*

murdering while asleep. The act of killing while asleep and not being conscious of the action. Persons who commit such an act cannot be held legally responsible for their action.

muriate (mūr'ē-āt) [L. *muria*, brine]. Former term for chloride.

muriatic acid (mū"rē-ăt'ĭk). Commercial hydrochloric acid.

murine (mū'rĭn) [L. *mus*, mouse]. Concerning rodents, esp. rats and mice.

murmur [L.]. A soft blowing or rasping sound heard on auscultation. An adventitious sound heard on auscultation of the heart. It results from vibrations produced by movement of the blood within the heart and adjacent large blood vessels. May be heard during systole, diastole, or both. Two of the valves give forth a "lubb" sound and the other two a "dupp" sound, known as the first and second heart sounds. A blowing sound is heard if the valve does not close tightly, indicating an incompetent valve. A great vessel irregularity, such as an aortic aneurysm, or the flow of blood through a narrowed orifice, as in aortic or mitral stenosis, may produce a murmur.

A murmur does not necessarily indicate organic pathology, and heart disease may not result in any murmur; this may also be true in angina pectoris and coronary artery disease. Air in the lungs may simulate sounds similar to heart murmurs.

RS: auscultation; bruit; circulation of blood; heart; hum, venous.

m., anemic. Murmur, hemic, q.v.

m., aneurysmal. Whizzing systolic sound heard over an aneurysm.

m., aortic obstructive. Harsh systolic murmur heard with and after the first heart sound. Loudest at the base.

m., aortic regurgitant. Blowing and hissing following second heart sound.

m., apex. Inorganic murmur over apex of heart.

m., arterial. Soft flowing murmur, synchronous with pulse.

m., Austin Flint. A presystolic or late diastolic heart murmur best heard at the apex of the heart. It is present in some cases of aortic insufficiency and is thought to be due

to the vibration of the mitral valve caused by the backward-flowing blood from the aorta meeting the blood flowing in from the left atrium.

m., bronchial. Murmur heard over large bronchi, resembling respiratory laryngeal murmur.

m., cardiac. A sound arising due to blood flow through the heart.

m., cardiopulmonary. Murmur caused by movement of heart against lungs.

m., continuous. A continuous murmur that extends through systole and diastole.

m., crescendo. Murmur that builds up in intensity and subsides.

m., Cruveilhier-Baumgarten. Murmur, heard on the abdominal wall, from the collateral veins connecting the caval and portal veins.

m., diastolic. Murmur during dilation of heart.

m., Duroziez'. A diastolic and systolic murmur heard over peripheral arteries of patients with aortic insufficiency.

m., ejection. A systolic murmur that is most intense at the time of maximum flow of blood from the heart; associated with pulmonary and aortic stenosis.

m., endocardial. Abnormal sound produced by any cause and arising within the heart.

m., exocardial. A cardiac murmur produced outside the cavities of the heart.

m., extracardiac. Murmur, exocardial, q.v.

m., Flint's. M., Austin Flint, q.v.

m., friction. Murmur caused by rubbing of two inflamed mucous surfaces.

m., functional. Murmur occurring in the absence of any pathological change in structure of heart valves or orifices. It does not indicate organic disease of the heart. It may disappear upon a return to health. It must not be mistaken for true pathological murmurs.

m., Gibson. A continuous, machinery-like murmur heard in patent ductus arteriosus.

m., Graham Steell's. An early systolic murmur associated with pulmonic insufficiency caused by pulmonary hypertension.

m., heart. Cardiac murmur.

m., hemic. Sound heard on auscultation of anemic persons without a valvular lesion. Result of an abnormal, usually anemic, blood condition.

m., holosystolic. Murmur, pansystolic, q.v.

m., machinery. A continuous rough murmur heard in patients with a patent ductus arteriosus.

m., mitral. Murmur produced at orifice

of mitral or bicuspid valve.

m., musical. A cardiac murmur that occurs when the sounds have an intermittent harmonic pattern.

m., organic. Murmur due to structural changes.

m., pansystolic. A heart murmur heard throughout systole.

m., pericardial. A friction sound produced within the pericardium.

m., physiologic. M., functional.

m., prediastolic. Systolic murmur.

m., presystolic. Murmur occurring just before systole, due to mitral or tricuspid obstruction.

m., pulmonary. Murmur produced at the orifice of the pulmonary artery.

m., regurgitant. Murmur due to leakage or backward flow of blood current through a dilated valvular orifice.

m., seagull. Murmur that mimics the cry of a seagull.

m., Still's. A benign, functional midsystolic murmur heard in children. The maximum sound is heard over the left lower sternal border.

m., systolic. Murmur heard during contraction of heart due to obstruction of flow of blood at one or several of the heart valves or in the aorta.

m., to-and-fro. Pericardial murmur heard during both systole and diastole.

m., tricuspid. Murmur produced at orifice of tricuspid valve, caused by disease.

m., vascular. Murmur occurring within a blood vessel.

m., vesicular. Normal breathing sounds.

Murphy's button [John B. Murphy, U.S. surgeon, 1857–1916]. Mechanical device used for intestinal anastomosis. Consists of two buttonlike hollow cylinders, each one sutured to an open end of the intestine and fitted together. After firm union of intestines, the sutures separate and the cylinders are passed in stools.

Murphy's sign. When the inflamed gallbladder is palpated by pressing the fingers under the rib cage, deep inspiration causes pain because the gallbladder is forced down to touch the fingers.

Mus (mŭs) [L., mouse]. A genus of rodents including mice and rats.

M. musculus. The common house mouse.

Musca (mŭs′kă) [L., fly]. A genus of flies belonging to the order Diptera, family Muscidae.

M. domestica. The common house fly, the transmitting agent for causative organisms of typhoid fever, bacillary and amebic dysentery, cholera, trachoma, and many other diseases.

muscae volitantes (mŭs′sē vōl-ĭ-tăn′tēz) [L., flitting flies]. Black specks seen floating in the vitreous humor of the eye. They are sometimes apparent to the individual. This benign phenomenon is present in most individuals.

muscarine (mŭs′kă-rĭn) [L. muscarius, pert. to flies]. A highly toxic organic compound present in Amanita muscaria, a form of mushroom. SEE: Amanita in Poisons and Poisoning in Appendix; mushroom and toadstool poisoning; Poison Control Centers in Appendix.

muscegenetic (mŭs″ē-jě-nět′ĭk) [L. musca, fly, + Gr. genesis, generation, birth]. Causing muscae volitantes, q.v.

muscicide (mŭs′ĭ-sīd) [″ + cidus, killing]. Lethal to flies.

muscle (mŭs′ĕl) [L. musculus]. A type of tissue composed of contractile cells or fibers that effects movement of an organ or part of the body. The outstanding characteristic of muscular tissue is its ability to shorten or contract. It also possesses the properties of irritability, conductivity, and elasticity. Muscle tissue possesses little intercellular material, hence its cells or fibers lie close together. SYN: musculus [NA]. SEE: illus.; arm; cell; face; leg for illus.

TYPES: Three types of muscle differentiated on basis of histologic structure occur in the body, namely, smooth, striated, and cardiac. SEE: table; Muscles in Appendix.

Smooth, Nonstriated: Cells are fusiform or spindle-shaped, each containing a central nucleus. Cells usually arranged in sheets or layers but may occur as isolated units in connective tissue. Called involuntary because they are not under conscious control. Found principally in the internal organs, esp. digestive tract, respiratory passages, urinary and genital ducts, urinary bladder and gallbladder, and walls of blood vessels. Smooth muscle lacks the cross striations characteristic of other types of muscle.

Striated, Skeletal: The cytoplasm (sarcoplasm) contains numerous myofibrillae. The cytoplasmic cell membrane is called the sarcolemma. Muscle fibers are grouped into bundles called fasciculi, each of which is surrounded by a sheath or connective tissue called perimysium. The fibers within a fasciculus are surrounded by and held together by delicate reticular fibrils forming the endomysium. Striated muscle is found in all skeletal muscles, and movement is under conscious control. It also occurs in the tongue, pharynx, and upper portion of esophagus.

Cardiac: Fibers branch and anastomose, forming a continuous network or syncy-

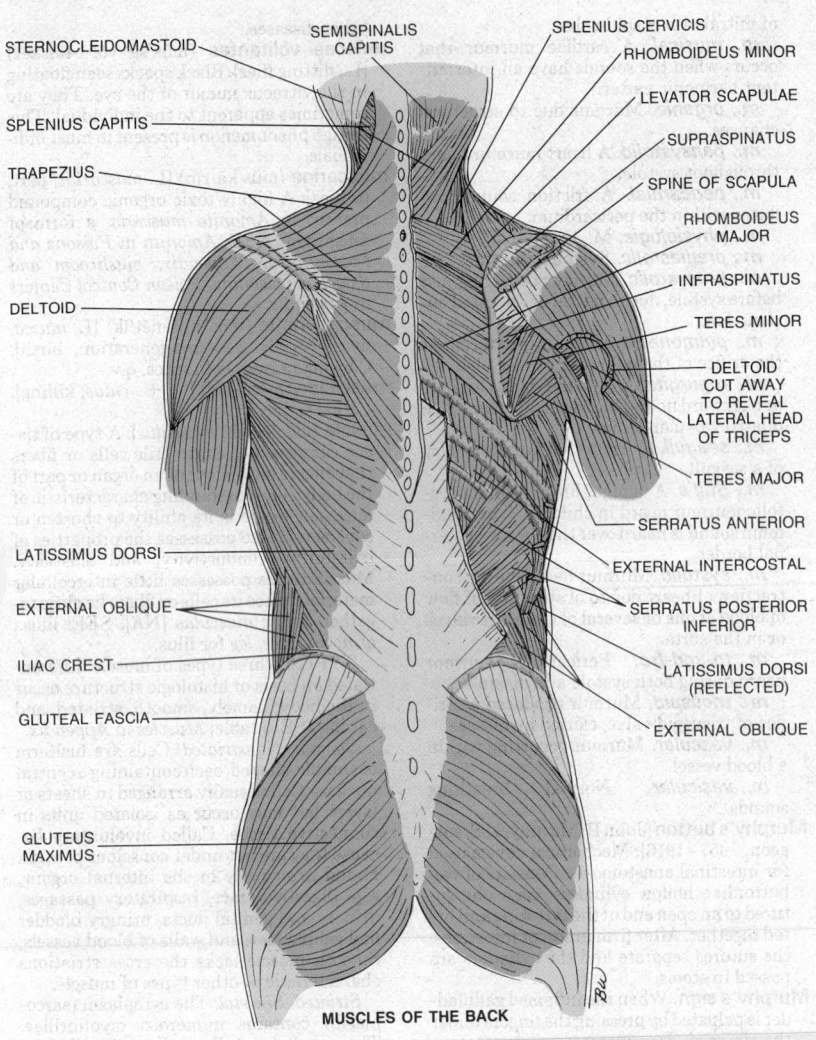

STERNOCLEIDOMASTOID

SEMISPINALIS CAPITIS

SPLENIUS CERVICIS

RHOMBOIDEUS MINOR

LEVATOR SCAPULAE

SPLENIUS CAPITIS

SUPRASPINATUS

TRAPEZIUS

SPINE OF SCAPULA

RHOMBOIDEUS MAJOR

INFRASPINATUS

DELTOID

TERES MINOR

DELTOID CUT AWAY TO REVEAL LATERAL HEAD OF TRICEPS

TERES MAJOR

SERRATUS ANTERIOR

LATISSIMUS DORSI

EXTERNAL INTERCOSTAL

EXTERNAL OBLIQUE

SERRATUS POSTERIOR INFERIOR

ILIAC CREST

LATISSIMUS DORSI (REFLECTED)

GLUTEAL FASCIA

EXTERNAL OBLIQUE

GLUTEUS MAXIMUS

MUSCLES OF THE BACK

tium. At intervals, prominent bands or intercalated disks cross the fibers. Certain fibers, called Purkinje fibers, form the impulse-conducting system of the heart.

ANAT: A contractile organ consisting of muscle tissue, which effects movements of parts of the body, esp. a structure composed of striated muscle and attached to a part of the skeleton. A typical muscle consists of a central fleshy portion or belly and its attachments. One end called the head is at-

tached to a fixed structure termed the origin; the other end is attached to a movable part called the insertion. Some muscles are spindle-shaped; others form flat sheets or bands. Muscles may be attached directly to the periosteum of bones, or they may be attached by means of tough cords of connective tissue (tendons) or broad flat sheets (aponeuroses). The connective tissue enclosing a muscle is called epimysium; it is continuous with the deep fascia.

Comparison of Properties of Three Types of Muscle

	Smooth	Cardiac	Striped
Synonyms	Involuntary Nonstriated Visceral Plain	Myocardium	Voluntary Skeletal Striated
Fibers:			
Length (in micrometers)	50–200		25,000
Thickness (in micrometers)	4–8		75
Shape	Spindles		Cylinders
Marking	No striation	Striation	Marked striation
Nuclei	Single	Single	Multiple
Speed of contraction	Very slow	Moderate	Very quick
Effects of cutting related nerve	Slight	Slight	Complete paralysis

BLOOD SUPPLY: Obtained from small blood vessels that enter the muscular tissue and subdivide into capillaries that permeate throughout.

NERVE SUPPLY: *Voluntary:* From branches of the peripheral cerebrospinal nervous system. It is because of this that the skeletal muscles are under conscious control. *Involuntary:* Smooth and cardiac muscles receive their nerve supply from autonomic nervous system and function involuntarily without conscious control.

m., abductor. Muscle that draws away from the midline.

m., adductor. Muscle that draws toward the midline.

m., agonist. Muscle which is the prime mover.

m., antagonistic. Muscle that counteracts the action of another muscle.

m.'s, antigravity. Muscles that pull against the constant force of gravity to maintain posture.

m., appendicular. One of the skeletal muscles of the limbs.

m., arrector pili. SEE: *arrectores pilorum.*

m., articular. Muscle attached to capsule of a joint.

m., axial. A skeletal muscle of the head or trunk.

m., bipennate. Muscle in which the fibers converge toward a central tendon on both sides.

m., constrictor, of pharynx. Muscle that constricts the pharynx.

m., digastric. Muscle that lowers the jaw.

m., extensor. Muscle that extends a part.

m.'s, extraocular eye. SEE: *extraocular eye muscles.*

m., extrinsic. Muscle whose origin lies outside the part moved.

m., fixation. Muscle that acts to steady a part in order that more precise movements in a related structure may be accomplished.

m., flexor. Muscle that bends a part.

m., fusiform. Muscle resembling a spindle.

m., intrinsic. Muscle that has both its origin and insertion within a structure, as intrinsic muscles of the tongue, eye, hand, or foot.

m., involuntary. Muscle not under conscious control; mainly smooth muscle.

m.'s, mastication. The four pairs of muscles that move the mandible and provide the primary forces of mastication; the masseter, temporalis, medial pterygoid, and lateral pterygoid muscles.

m.'s, mimetic. Superficial muscles of the facial region that by skin movements produce the facial expressions. Also: *muscles of facial expression.*

m., multipennate. Muscle with several tendons of origin and several tendons of insertion in which fibers pass obliquely from a tendon of origin to a tendon of insertion on each side.

m., nonstriated. M., smooth.

m., papillary. Muscle on inner surface of ventricle of heart to which chordae tendineae are attached.

m., pectinate. Muscle on inner surface of right atrium, giving it a ridged appearance.

m., postaxial. Muscle on the posterior or dorsal aspect of a limb.

m., preaxial. Muscle on the anterior or

1254

ventral aspect of a limb.

m., skeletal. Muscle that is connected with a bone; mainly striated.

m., smooth. Muscle tissue that lacks cross striations on its fibers; involuntary in action and found principally in visceral organs. SYN: *m., nonstriated.*

m., somatic. Muscle derived from mesodermal somites. Includes most skeletal muscle.

m., sphincter. Muscle that encircles a duct, tube, or orifice, thus controlling its opening.

m., sphincter, of urinary bladder. Muscle fibers around the origin of the urethra. They are effective in helping to control urination.

m., stabilizer. Muscle which acts to support a body segment so muscles attached to it can function.

m., striated. Muscle fibers that possess alternate light and dark bands or striations; mainly voluntary and comprise skeletal muscles.

m.'s, synergistic. Muscles aiding one another in function.

m., unipennate. Muscle whose fibers converge on only one side of a tendon.

m., unstriated. Muscle without markings; mainly involuntary. SYN: *m., smooth.*

m., voluntary. Muscle whose action is controlled by will. Except for the cardiac muscle, all striated muscles are voluntary.

muscle compartment syndrome. The production of nerve damage, ischemia, edema, and muscle contractures by compression of nerves, vessels, and tissue within a fascial compartment. SEE: *carpal tunnel syndrome.*

muscle contraction, concentric. Muscle contraction in which the extended muscle contracts and is shortened. An example would be pulling the body up by grasping a bar over the head.

muscle contraction, eccentric. Contraction of a muscle in which the tensed muscle lengthens. An example would be the lowering of the body from a position in which the body was supported by the flexed arms, i.e., holding on to a bar above the head.

muscle cramps. Painful involuntary contractions of muscles. They may be due to ischemia of the muscle(s), dehydration, or electrolyte imbalance.

Cramps associated with exercise may be alleviated, if not abolished, by flexing (stretching) the involved muscle group. At the same time, gentle massage to the area will help.

Nocturnal cramps may be prevented by use of quinine. There is not enough quinine in tonic water to make it effective.

muscle fiber types, fast twitch and slow twitch. Types of fibers found in skeletal muscle. Fast twitch fibers are more abundant in muscles requiring intensive activity for short periods of time. Slow twitch oxidative fibers resist fatigue and are able to carry on sustained activities as needed to maintain posture or aerobic exercise.

muscle metabolism. All cells, including those of muscle tissue, consume energy in order to perform work. The source of chemical energy, adenosine triphosphate (ATP), is metabolized to adenosine diphosphate (ADP). If the energy requirement is short term, the ADP is converted back to ATP. This process goes at a rate too slow to keep up with energy demands during long-term exercise, thus consumption of other fuels is required. The main sources of fuel for muscles are carbohydrates and lipids. Prior to being available for intracellular metabolism, glycogen is obtained when glucose is converted to glycogen. The main lipid fuel is free fatty acids present in plasma. Carbohydrates can be metabolized in either the presence (aerobically) or absence (anerobically) of oxygen, but lipids can be metabolized only aerobically. During light exercise or when the body is at rest, muscle metabolism is usually entirely aerobic and the source of fuel is the free fatty acids in plasma. During intense exercise, metabolism of the fatty acids cannot keep up with the demand, thus glycogen is utilized. However, as intense exercise continues, glycogen stores are exhausted and free fatty acids become the principal source of energy. Trained athletes have an increased ability to metabolize fatty acids as compared to sedentary individuals. This permits athletes to exercise longer and at higher work rates than would be the case if they were not trained. Athletic trainers found that muscle glycogen stores could be increased by a regimen known as carbohydrate loading, q.v. That regimen will permit the athlete to exercise for a much longer period than would be possible if carbohydrate loading had not been done prior to exercising.

muscle soreness. The onset of muscular discomfort within 24 to 48 hours following unaccustomed exercise or of exercise of greater intensity than usual.

muscular [L. *muscularis*]. 1. Pert. to muscles. 2. Possessing well-developed muscles.

muscular contractions, graduated. 1. The mechanism by which all smooth, coordinated muscle activity occurs. Normally controlled involuntarily by the central nervous system, motor units are recruited and stimulated at an intensity needed to accomplish a desired activity. 2. Accomplished by use of electric current of varying strength and duration. Used in muscles with an intact nerve supply when muscles are atonic, wasted away, or when voluntary exercise is not feasible; and in denervated muscles as in cases following nerve injury or poliomyelitis.

muscular dystrophy. Wasting away and atrophy of muscles. SEE: *dystrophy, progressive muscular.*

muscularis (mŭs-kū-lā'rĭs) [L.]. Muscular layer of an organ or tubule.

   m. mucosae. Unstriated muscular tissue layer of mucous membrane.

muscularity. State or quality of being muscular.

muscularize (mŭs'kū-lăr-īz). To change into muscle tissue.

musculature [L. *musculus,* muscle]. The arrangement of muscles in the body or its parts.

musculo- [L. *musculus,* muscle]. Combining form pert. to a muscle.

musculoaponeurotic (mŭs-kū-lō-ăp″ō-nū-rŏt'ĭk). Composed of muscle and an aponeurosis of fibrous connective tissue.

musculocutaneous (mŭs″kū-lō-kū-tān'ē-ūs) [″ + *cutis,* skin]. 1. Pert. to the muscles and skin. 2. Supplying or affecting the muscles and skin. 3. The specific nerve from the brachial plexus that innervates the coracobrachialis, biceps branchii, and brachialis muscles and provides cutaneous sensory distribution to the forearm.

musculofascial (mŭs″kū-lō-făsh'ē-ăl). Composed of muscle and fascia.

musculomembranous (mŭs″kū-lō-měm'brăn-ūs). Pert. to or consisting of muscle and membrane.

musculophrenic (mŭs″kū-lō-frěn'ĭk). Pert. to muscles of the diaphragm.

musculoskeletal (mŭs″kū-lō-skěl'ě-tăl). Pert. to the muscles and skeleton.

musculospiral (mŭs″kū-lō-spī'răl) [″ + *spira,* coil]. Concerning the musculospiral (radial) nerve.

musculotendinous. Composed of both muscle and tendon.

musculotropic (mŭs″kū-lō-trŏp'ĭk) [″ + Gr. *tropikos,* turning]. Affecting, acting on, or having an affinity for muscular tissue.

musculus [L.] (pl. *musculi*). [NA] Muscle.

mushroom [Fr. *mousseron*]. Umbrella-shaped fungus, belonging to the Basidiomycetes, that grows on decaying vegetable matter; common in woods and damp places. Some of the poisonous varieties are commonly called toadstools. SEE: *Amanita* in *Poisons and Poisoning* in *Appendix; toadstool.*

COMP: Low in carbohydrates and fats; high in protein. Their relationship and similarity to poisonous fungi are so close that only those who are thoroughly capable of distinguishing the poisonous varieties from the edible ones should attempt to gather and eat them.

mushroom and toadstool poisoning. Poisoning resulting from ingestion of mushrooms such as *Amanita muscaria,* which contains muscarine, or other species that contain phalloidine, a component of the amanita toxin. SEE: *Amanita* in *Poisons and Poisoning* in *Appendix.*

musicians, medical problems of. The most common medical problems of musicians are overuse injuries involving muscle-tendon units. The pain associated with this may be mild or severe enough to prevent use of the affected part. Those who play string instruments have more difficulty than those who use percussion instruments; women are more commonly affected than men. Focal dystonias may involve the hands or the muscles of the face and lips, and may be severe. Stress and anxiety may interfere with or prevent performing.

   TREAT: Rest for physical difficulties; beta adrenergic blocking agents for stress and anxiety.

musicogenic (mū″zĭ-kō-jěn'ĭk) [L. *musica,* music, + *gennan,* to produce]. Caused by music, esp. epileptic convulsions.

musicogenic epilepsy. Epilepsy in which the convulsive attacks are induced by music. SEE: *epilepsy.*

musicomania [″ + Gr. *mania,* madness]. Insane love of music.

musicotherapy [″ + *therapeia,* treatment]. Treatment of disease with music.

musk (mŭsk) [Sanskrit *muska,* testicle]. An oily secretion obtained from the musk bag, a gland beneath the abdominal skin of the male musk deer. Has a very strong odor. Used in manufacturing perfume.

mussel. A freshwater bivalve mollusc belonging to the class Pelecypoda.

mussel poisoning. Poisoning common on the Pacific coast of the United States resulting from eating mussels or clams that have ingested a poisonous dinoflagellate. Occurs from June to October. The poison is not destroyed by cooking.

Musset's sign (mū-sāz') [Louis C. A. de Musset, Fr. poet, 1810–1857]. Repetitive jerking movements of the head and neck in synchrony with ventricular contractions of the heart. Seen in advanced aortic incompetence or aortic aneurysm.

mussitation (mŭs-sĭ-tā'shŭn) [L. *mussitare,* to matter]. The muttering of delirium or the moving of the lips without sound.

mustard [Fr. *moustarde*]. Yellow powder of mustard seed used as a counterirritant, rubefacient, emetic, stimulant, and condiment. SEE: *plaster.*

m., nitrogen. SEE: *nitrogen mustards.*

mustard gas. Dichlorodiethyl sulfide, a war gas that causes burns and destruction of tissue either topically or if inhaled.

Mustargen. Trade name for mechlorethamine hydrochloride, USP.

mutacism (mū″tă-sĭzm). A form of speech impediment in which the "m" sound is often substituted for other sounds.

mutagen (mū″tă-jĕn) [L. *mutare*, to change, + Gr. *gennan*, to produce]. Any agent that causes genetic mutations. Many medicines, chemicals, and physical agents such as ionizing radiations and ultraviolet light have this ability. SEE: *teratogen.*

mutagenesis (mū″tă-jĕn′ĕ-sĭs). The induction of genetic mutation. SEE: *mutation* (defs. 2 and 3); *teratogenesis.*

mutagenicity (mū″tă-jĕ-nĭs′ĭ-tē). Property of causing genetic mutation.

mutant (mū′tănt) [L. *mutare*, to change]. A variation of genetic structure that breeds true.

mutase (mū′tās) [″ + *ase*, enzyme]. 1. Enzyme that accelerates oxidation-reduction reactions through activation of oxygen and hydrogen. 2. A food preparation made from leguminous plants high in protein content.

mutation (mū-tā′shŭn). 1. Change; transformation; instance of such change. 2. Permanent variation in genetic structure with offspring differing from parents in a characteristic. Differentiated from gradual variation through many generations. 3. A change in a gene potentially capable of being transmitted to offspring.

m., induced. Mutation resulting from exposure to x-rays, radioactive substances, and certain drugs and chemicals.

m., natural. Mutation occurring without artificial external intervention; thought to be a primary factor in evolutionary change.

m., somatic. Mutation occurring in somatic cells.

mute (mūt) [L. *mutus*, dumb]. 1. One who is unable to speak. 2. Dumb, without ability to speak.

m., deaf. Individual who is unable to hear or to speak.

mutilate [L. *mutilatus*, to maim]. To deprive of a limb or a part; to maim or disfigure.

mutilation (mū″tĭ-lā′shŭn). Maiming; the act of removing or destroying a conspicuous or essential part or organ.

mutism (mū′tĭzm) [L. *mutus*, dumb]. 1. Condition of being unable to speak. 2. Persistent inhibition to speech; seen in some severe forms of mental disorder.

m., akinetic. Syndrome consisting of mutism, loss of physical movement, and apparent loss of feeling.

m., hysterical. Inability to speak due to hysteria.

mutualism (mū″tū-ăl-ĭzm) [L. *mutuus*, exchanged]. A form of symbiosis in which organisms of two different species live in close association to the mutual benefit of each.

mutualist (mū″tū-ăl-ĭst). Organism associated with another organism to the mutual benefit of each.

M.V. *Medicus Veterinarius.* Latin for veterinary physician.

mv. *millivolt.*

M.W.I.A. *Medical Women's International Association.*

my-, myo- [Gr. *mys*, muscle]. Prefix denoting rel. to muscle.

myalgia (mī-ăl′jē-ă) [″ + *algos*, pain]. Tenderness or pain in the muscles; muscular rheumatism. SYN: *myodynia.*

m., tension. SEE: *fibromyalgia.*

Myambutol. Trade name for ethambutol hydrochloride.

myasis (mī-ā′sĭs) [Gr. *myia*, a fly]. Condition that arises from infestation with larvae of flies or maggots in the body or upon mucous membranes. SYN: *myiasis.*

myasthenia (mī-ăs-thē′nē-ă) [Gr. *mys*, muscle, + *astheneia*, weakness]. Muscular weakness and abnormal fatigue.

m., angiosclerotic. Vascular changes producing excessive muscular fatigue.

m. gastrica. Loss of muscular tone in coats of the stomach.

m. gravis. A disease characterized by great muscular weakness (usually without atrophy) and progressive fatigability. Power is restored with rest. Marked improvement in strength following administration of anticholinesterase drugs. It is due to a functional abnormality, lack of acetylcholine or excess of cholinesterase at the myoneural junction, in which nerve impulses fail to induce normal muscle contractions. SEE: *edrophonium test.* SEE: *Nursing Diagnoses* in *Appendix.*

SYM: Abnormal fatigability and weakness of muscles. Muscles of the face and neck primarily involved, those of the trunk and extremities secondarily. Onset gradual; symptoms worse in the evening. Patient complains of difficulty in chewing, swallowing, and talking. Expressionless facies, drooping of the eyelids, and intermittent dyplopia are usually present.

ETIOL: An autoimmune mechanism causes the disease. More common in females if onset is at an age less than 40. Occurs most frequently between ages of 20 and 50.

TREAT: Restricted activity; complete rest in severe cases. Soft or liquid diet; tube feedings sometimes essential. Physostigmine and neostigmine given intramuscularly or orally are effective. Potassium chloride, ephedrine, and guanidine are also used as adjuvants of pyridostigmine bromide (Mestinon), the drug of choice. If a thymoma is present, the thymus is removed. Corticosteroids are effective in patients who have not been aided by thymectomy. In severe cases, use of plasmapheresis may be life-saving. Immunosuppression is a useful adjunct to alternate-day therapy with corticosteroids.

PROG: Some cases mild; others rapidly fatal, death resulting from respiratory failure. Course is variable. Prolonged remissions may occur.

NURSING IMPLICATIONS: Following diagnosis, explain the nature of the disease process and treatment required. Provide emotional support and reassurance. Encourage patient to conserve energy and plan type and amount of activity which will be realistic in terms of patient's capabilities. Reinforce individual's coping abilities. Urge regular medical follow-up and early reporting of any untoward symptoms. Encourage family assistance and support.

myasthenic. Marked by muscular weakness.

myatonia (mī-ă-tō'nē-ă). Deficiency or loss of muscular tone.

m. congenita. A noninherited but sometimes familial disease characterized by absence of muscular development, with the lower extremities being the first involved. It is seen shortly after birth. SYN: *amyotonia congenita; Oppenheim's disease.*

myatrophy (mī-ăt'rō-fē). Muscular wasting.

myc-, myco- [Gr. *mykes,* fungus]. Combining form meaning fungus.

mycelioid (mī-sē'lē-oyd) [" + *helos,* nail, + *eidos,* form, shape]. Moldlike; resembling mold colonies in which filaments radiate from a center, said of bacterial colonies.

mycelium (mī-sē'lē-ŭm) [Gr. *mykes,* fungus, + *helos,* nail]. The mass of filaments (hyphae) that constitutes the vegetative body of fungi such as molds.

mycetes (mī-sē'tēz). The fungi.

mycethemia (mī-sĕ-thē'mē-ă) [" + *haima,* blood]. Fungi in the blood. SYN: *mycohemia.*

mycetism, mycetismus (mī'sĕ-tĭzm, mī-sĕ-tĭz'mŭs) [" + *-ismos,* condition]. Poisoning from eating fungi, esp. poisonous mushrooms.

mycetogenetic (mī-sē''tō-jĕn-ĕt'ĭk) [" + *gennan,* to produce]. Induced by fungi.

mycetoma (mī-sĕ-tō'mă) [" + *oma,* tumor]. A syndrome caused by a variety of aerobic actinomycetes and fungi. It is characterized by swelling and suppuration of subcutaneous tissues; and formation of

sinus tracts, with granules present in the pus draining from the sinus tracts. These tracts usually appear on the lower body.

TREAT: Sulfones, trimethoprimsulfamethoxazole, or sulfonamides may benefit lesions caused by actinomycetes. If lesions are due to fungi, there is no specific therapy.

Mycifradin. Trade name for neomycin sulfate, USP.

mycobacteriosis (mī''kō-băk-tē''rē-ō'sĭs). An infection caused by any mycobacterium.

Mycobacterium [" + *bakterion,* little rod]. A genus of acid-fast organisms belonging to the Mycobacteriaceae family that includes the causative organisms of tuberculosis and leprosy. They are slender, nonmotile, grampositive rods and do not produce spores or capsules.

Species include: *M. avium intracellulare, M. chelonei, M. fortuitum, M. gastri, M. gordonae, M. kansasii, M. marinum, M. scrofulaceum, M. terrae, M. triviale, M. smegmatis,* and *M. xenopi.*

M. bovis. Organism that causes tuberculosis in cows.

M. kansasii. A cause of tuberculosis-like pulmonary disease in humans.

M. leprae. Causative agent of leprosy.

M. marinum. An atypical mycobacterium that produces skin infection resembling sporotrichosis. The organism has been cultured from tropical fish aquariums. SEE: *swimming pool granuloma.*

M. tuberculosis. Causative agent of tuberculosis in mammals.

mycocidin (mī''kō-sī'dĭn). An antibiotic derived from molds of the family Aspergillaceae.

mycoderma [Gr. *mykos,* mucus, + *derma,* skin]. Mucous membrane.

mycohemia (mī''kō-hē'mē-ă) [Gr. *mykes,* fungus, + *haima,* blood]. Mycethemia, q.v.

mycoid (mī'koyd) [" + *eidos,* form, shape]. Funguslike.

mycology (mī-kŏl'ō-jē) [" + *logos,* word, reason]. Science of fungi.

mycomyringitis (mī''kō-mĭr-ĭn-jī'tĭs) [" + L. *myringa,* drum membrane, + *itis,* inflammation]. Fungus inflammation of the tympanic membrane SYN: *myringomycosis; otomycosis.*

mycophthalmia (mī-kŏf-thăl'mē-ă). Ophthalmia resulting from fungus infection.

mycoplasmas. A group of very small organisms in which the ability to form a cell wall has been lost. There are more than 70 organisms in this group, including 12 species that infect man, including *M. hominis* and *M. pneumoniae.* The former can cause genital tract infections; the latter, infections of the upper respiratory tract and the lungs, i.e., mycoplasma pneumonia.

TREAT: Tetracycline or erythromycin for *M. pneumoniae* and *M. hominis* infections.

mycoprecipitin (mī″kō-prē-sĭp′ĭ-tĭn). A precipitin for extracts of yeast and fungi.

mycosis (mī-kō′sĭs) [″ + *osis,* condition]. Any disease induced by a fungus.

    m. fungoides. A rare, poorly understood, malignant, cutaneous T-cell lymphoma.

    SYM: Urticarial, erythematous, or eczematous patches of irregular shape and size, with well-defined margins usually upon scalp and skin of trunk. Itching intense; frequently the patches become hypertrophic and firm. Hard nodules varying from size of pea to apple, either sessile or pedunculated, develop on them. These eventually break down and form ulcers that contain sensitive, fungating granulation tissue, and discharge thin pus and serum. This progression of the disease may take many years.

    In addition to the cutaneous changes, lesions may be present throughout the body. Death may be due to infection of the lesions.

    TREAT: Electron beam radiation and cytotoxic agents have produced a good response but they have produced no significant improvement in either disease-free or overall survival.

    m., superficial. A dermatomycosis; a fungus infection of the skin. Includes erythrasma; tinea barbae, tinea capitis, tinea corporis, tinea cruris, tinea favosa, tinea pedis, tinea unguium; trichomycosis axillaris.

    m., systemic. A deep mycosis; a fungus infection involving various bodily systems or regions. Includes aspergillosis, blastomycosis, chromoblastomycosis, coccidioidomycosis, cryptococcosis, geotrichosis, histoplasmosis, maduromycosis, moniliasis, mucormycosis, nocardiosis, penicilliosis, rhinosporidiosis, sporotrichosis.

mycostasis (mī-kŏs′tă-sĭs) [Gr. *mykes,* fungus, + *stasis,* standing]. Stopping the growth of fungi.

mycostat (mī′kō-stăt) [″ + *statikos,* standing]. Anything that stops the growth of fungi.

Mycostatin. Trade name for nystatin, USP.

mycotic (mī-kŏt′ĭk). Caused by or affected with microorganisms; concerning mycosis.

mycotoxicosis (mī″kō-tŏk″sĭ-kō′sĭs) [″ + *toxikon,* poisoning, + *osis,* condition]. Disease either caused by toxins on molds or produced by molds.

mycotoxinization (mī″kō-tŏk″sĭn-ī-zā′shŭn). Inoculation with a fungal toxin.

mycotoxins. Substances, produced by mold growing in food or animal feed, that cause illness or death when ingested by man or an-

imals. SEE: *ergotism.*

mycterophonia (mĭk″tĕr-ō-fō′nē-ă) [Gr. *mykter,* nostril, + *phone,* voice]. Phonation in which the voice possesses a nasal quality.

mydaleine (mĭd-ā′lē-ēn) [Gr. *mydaleos,* moldy]. A poisonous ptomaine from putrefied visceral organs, acting mainly on the heart.

Mydfrin. Trade name for phenylephrine hydrochloride, USP.

Mydriacyl. Trade name for tropicamide, USP.

mydriasis (mĭd-rī′ă-sĭs) [Gr.]. Pronounced or abnormal dilation of the pupil.

    ETIOL: Fright, sudden emotion, first and third stages of anesthesia, drugs, coma, hysteria, botulism, or irritation of cervical sympathetic nerve.

    m., alternating. Mydriasis that affects one eye, then the other.

    m., paralytic. Mydriasis resulting from paralysis of oculomotor nerve.

    m., spastic. Mydriasis resulting from overactivity of dilator muscle of iris or of sympathetic nerves supplying that muscle.

    m., spinal. Mydriasis resulting from a lesion of, or irritation of, ciliospinal center of spinal cord.

mydriatic (mĭd-rē-ăt′ĭk). 1. Causing pupillary dilatation. 2. Any drug that dilates the pupil. In certain eye diseases it is essential that the pupil be dilated during the course of treatment to prevent adhesions of the pupils.

    Ex.: atropine, cocaine, ephedrine, euphthalmine, homatropine.

myectomy (mī-ĕk′tō-mē) [Gr. *mys,* muscle, + *ektome,* excision]. Excision of a portion of a muscle.

myectopia (mī-ĕk-tō′pē-ă) [″ + *ek,* out, + *topos,* place]. Muscle dislocation.

myelalgia (mī-ĕl-ăl′jē-ă) [Gr. *myelos,* marrow, + *algos,* pain]. Pain of the spinal cord or its membranes.

myelapoplexy (mī″ĕl-ăp′ō-plĕks-ē) [″ + *apoplexia,* stroke]. Hemorrhagic effusion into the spinal cord.

myelatelia (mī″ĕl-ă-tē′lē-ă) [″ + *ateleia,* imperfection]. Myelodysplasia, q.v.

myelauxe (mī-ĕl-awks′ē) [″ + *auxe,* increase]. Abnormal enlargement of spinal cord.

myelencephalon (mī″ĕl-ĕn-sĕf′ă-lŏn) [Gr. *myelos,* marrow, + *enkephalos,* brain]. [NA] The most posterior portion of the embryonic hindbrain (rhombencephalon), which gives rise to the medulla oblongata.

myelic. Pert. to the spinal cord.

myelin. 1. A fatlike substance forming a sheath around the axons of certain nerves. Composed of lipids and protein. 2. A complex lipoid substance present in the brain in small quantities.

myelination (mī″ĕl-ĭn-ā′shŭn) [Gr. *myelos*, marrow]. Process of acquiring a myelin sheath. SYN: *myelinization*.

myelinic (mī-ĕl-ĭn′ĭk). Concerning or composed of myelin.

myelinization (mī″ĕl-ĭn-ĭ-zā′shŭn). Acquisition of myelin sheath for nerve fibers. SYN: *myelination*.

myelinoclasis (mī″ĕ-lĭn-ŏk′lă-sĭs) [″ + *klasis*, breaking]. Destruction of myelin.

myelinogenesis (mī″ĕ-lĭn″ō-jĕn′ĕ-sĭs) [″ + *genesis*, generation, birth]. Myelinization.

myelinogenetic (mī″ĕl-ĭn-ō-jĕn-ĕt′ĭk) [″ + *gennan*, to produce]. Producing myelin or a myelin sheath.

myelinolysis (mī″ĕ-lĭn-ŏl′ĭ-sĭs) [″ + *lysis*, dissolution]. Destructive of the myelin sheaths of nerves.

myelinosis (mī″ĕl-ĭn-ō′sĭs) [″ + *osis*, condition]. Fatty degeneration during which myelin is produced.

myelitic (mī-ĕl-ĭt′ĭk). Concerning myelitis.

myelitis (mī-ĕ-lī′tĭs) [″ + *itis*, inflammation]. 1. Inflammation of bone marrow. 2. Inflammation of the spinal cord.

SYM: Moderate fever (101° to 103°F or 38.3° to 39.4°C), loss of appetite and constipation, followed by pain in back radiating into the limbs. Various forms of paresthesia, such as numbness, tingling, or burning, may be present. Frequently a sense of painful constriction, girdle pain, also develops. Paralysis soon develops and may become more or less complete. At first there may be retention of feces, later incontinence. Decubiti (bedsores) are likely to develop if care is not taken to prevent them. Death may result in a few days from upward extension and involvement of respiratory muscles. In rare cases, a spontaneous arrest of inflammation and slow recovery follow, attended with partial paralysis. SEE: *osteomyelitis; poliomyelitis.*

    m., acute. Simple acute form of myelitis that develops following injury.

    m., ascending, acute. Myelitis that moves progressively upward in the spinal cord.

    m., bulbar. Myelitis involving the medulla oblongata.

    m., central. 1. Inflammation of the spinal cord. 2. Inflammation of the bone marrow.

    m., compression. Myelitis caused by pressure on the spinal cord, as by a hemorrhage or tumor.

    m., descending. Myelitis affecting successively lower areas of the spinal cord.

    m., disseminated. Inflammation of several separate areas of the spinal cord.

    m., focal. Myelopathy, q.v., of small areas of the spinal cord.

    m., hemorrhagic. Myelitis with hemorrhage.

    m., sclerosing. Myelopathy wherein there is hardening of the spinal column.

    m., transverse. Myelitis involving the whole thickness of the spinal cord, but limited longitudinally.

    m., transverse, acute. Acute form of myelitis involving entire thickness of spinal cord, developing subsequent to injury to spinal cord.

    m., traumatic. Myelitis due to spinal cord injury.

myelo- [Gr. *myelos*, marrow]. Prefix denoting the spinal cord or bone marrow.

myeloblast (mī′ĕl-ō-blăst) [″ + *blastos*, germ]. Immature bone marrow cell that develops into a myelocyte. It matures to develop into a promyelocyte, and eventually the granular leukocyte. SYN: *microleukoblast.*

myeloblastemia (mī″ĕl-ō-blăst-ē′mē-ă) [″ + ″ + *haima*, blood]. Occurrence of myeloblasts in the blood.

myeloblastoma (mī″ĕl-ō-blăst-ō′mă) [″ + ″ + *oma*, tumor]. Tumor containing myeloblasts, seen in the myelogenic form of leukemia.

myeloblastosis (mī″ĕ-lō-blăs-tō′sĭs) [″ + ″ + *osis*, condition]. Excess production of myeloblasts and their presence in circulating blood.

myelocele (mī′ĕ-lō-sēl). [″ + *kele*, tumor, swelling]. A form of spina bifida with spinal cord protrusion.

myelocyst (mī′ĕl-ō-sĭst) [″ + *kystis*, bladder]. Cyst arising from the rudimentary medullary canal of the spinal cord.

myelocystocele (mī″ĕl-ō-sĭst′ō-sēl) [″ + ″ + *kele*, tumor, swelling]. Cystic tumor of spinal cord substance through a defect in the canal.

myelocystomeningocele (mī″ĕl-ō-sĭst″ō-mĕn-ĭn′gō-sēl) [″ + *kystis*, bladder, + *meninx*, membrane, + *kele*, tumor, swelling]. Combined myelocystocele and meningocele.

myelocyte (mī′ĕl-ō-sīt) [″ + *kytos*, cell]. A large cell in red bone marrow from which leukocytes are derived.

myelocythemia (mī″ĕl-ō-sī-thē′mē-ă) [″ + ″ + *haima*, blood]. Presence of an excess number of myelocytes in the blood. SYN: *myelemia; myelocytosis.*

myelocytic (mī″ĕl-ō-sĭt′ĭk). Characterized by presence of, or pert. to, myelocytes.

myelocytosis (mī″ĕl-ō-sī-tō′sĭs) [″ + *osis*, condition]. Myelocytes in large quantities in the blood. SYN: *myelemia; myelocythemia.*

myelodiastasis (mī″ĕl-ō-dī-ăs′tă-sĭs) [Gr. *myelos,* marrow, + *diastasis,* separation]. Destruction and disintegration of spinal cord.

myelodysplasia (mī″ĕl-ō-dĭs-plă′zē-ă) [″ + *dys,* bad, + *plassein,* to form]. Defective formation of the spinal cord.

myeloencephalic (mī″ĕl-ō-ĕn-sĕf-ăl′ĭk) [″ + *enkephalos,* brain]. Concerning the spinal cord and brain.

myeloencephalitis (mī″ĕl-ō-ĕn-sĕf″ă-lī′tĭs) [″ + ″ + *itis,* inflammation]. Inflamed condition of spinal cord and brain.

myelofibrosis (mī″ĕ-lō-fī-brō′sĭs). Replacement of bone marrow by fibrous tissue.

myelogenesis (mī″ĕl-ō-jĕn′ĕ-sĭs) [″ + *genesis,* generation, birth]. 1. Development of brain and spinal cord. 2. Development of the myelin sheath of nerve fiber.

myelogenic, myelogenous (mī-ĕ-lō-jĕn′ĭk, -lŏj′ĕn-ŭs) [″ + *gennan,* to produce]. Producing or originating in marrow.

myelogeny (mī″ĕ-lŏj′ĕ-nē). Maturation of the myelin sheaths during the development of the central nervous system.

myelogram (mī′ĕ-lō-grăm) [″ + *gramma,* something written]. 1. Roentgenogram of the spinal canal after injection of a radiopaque dye. 2. Differential count of bone marrow cells.

myelography (mī-ĕ-lŏg′ră-fē) [″ + *graphein,* to write]. Roentgenographic inspection of the spinal cord by use of a radiopaque medium injected into the intrathecal space.

   m., air. Myelography in which oxygen or air is used instead of radiopaque dye.

myeloid (mī′ĕ-loyd) [″ + *eidos,* form, shape]. 1. Medullary; like marrow. 2. Resembling a myelocyte, but not necessarily originating from bone marrow.

myeloidosis (mī″ĕ-loy-dō′sĭs) [″ + ″ + *osis,* condition]. Development of myeloid tissue.

myelolymphangioma (mī″ĕ-lō-lĭm-făn″jē-ō′mă). Elephantiasis.

myelolymphocyte (mī″ĕ-lō-lĭmf′ō-sīt) [″ + L. *lympha,* lymph, + Gr. *kytos,* cell]. Tiny lymphocyte formed abnormally in bone marrow.

myelolysis (mī″ĕ-lŏl′ĭs-sĭs) [″ + *lysis,* dissolution]. Dissolution of myelin.

myeloma (mī-ĕ-lō′mă) [″ + *oma,* tumor]. A tumor originating in cells of the hematopoietic portion of bone marrow.

   m., multiple. A neoplastic disease characterized by the infiltration of bone and bone marrow by myeloma cells forming multiple tumor masses. Usually progressive and generally fatal. Accompanied by anemia, renal lesions, and high globulin levels in blood. Common in sixth decade of life. More frequent in males by ratio of 3 : 1. Bone marrow transplantation therapy promises to improve the prognosis for these patients. SYN: *myelomatosis.*

myelomalacia (mī″ĕ-lō-mă-lā′sē-ă) [Gr. *myelos,* marrow, + *malakia,* softening]. Abnormal softening of spinal cord.

myelomatosis (mī″ĕl-ō-mă-tō′sĭs) [″ + *oma,* tumor, + *osis,* intensive]. Myeloma, multiple.

myelomeningocele (mī″ĕ-lō-mĕn-ĭn′gō-sēl) [″ + ″ + *kele,* tumor, swelling]. Spina bifida with portion of cord and membranes protruding.

myelomere (mī′ĕ-lō-mēr) [″ + *meros,* part]. A segment of the developing spinal cord.

myelomyces (mī″ĕ-lō-mī′sēs) [″ + *mykes,* fungus]. Malignant growth resembling brain substance. SYN: *encephaloma.*

myeloneuritis (mī″ĕ-lō-nū-rī′tĭs) [″ + *neuron,* nerve, + *itis,* inflammation]. Multiple neuritis and myelitis combined.

myelopathy (mī-ĕ-lŏp′ă-thē) [″ + *pathos,* disease, suffering]. Any pathological condition of the spinal cord.

   m., ascending. Myelopathy that ascends along the spinal cord toward the head.

   m., descending. Myelopathy that descends along the spinal cord toward the feet.

   m., focal. Myelopathy of small areas.

   m., sclerosing. Myelopathy in which there is hardening of the spinal cord.

   m., transverse. Myelopathy extending across the spinal cord.

   m., traumatic. Myelopathy due to trauma to the spinal cord.

myelopetal (mī-ĕ-lŏp′ĕt-ăl) [″ + L. *petere,* to seek for]. Proceeding toward the spinal cord, said of certain nerve impulses.

myelophage (mī′ĕ-lō-fāj) [″ + *phagein,* to eat]. A macrophage that ingests myelin.

myelophthisis (mī-ĕ-lŏf′thĭ-sĭs) [″ + *phthisis,* a wasting]. 1. Atrophy of the spinal cord. SYN: *myelanalosis.* 2. Replacement of the bone marrow by a disease process such as a neoplasm.

myeloplast (mī′ĕl-ō-plăst) [″ + *plastos,* formed]. A leukocyte cell of the bone marrow.

myeloplegia (mī″ĕl-ō-plē′jē-ă) [Gr. *myelos,* marrow, + *plege,* stroke]. Paralysis of spinal origin.

myelopoiesis (mī″ĕl-ō-poy-ē′sĭs) [″ + *poiein,* to form]. Development of bone marrow or formation of cells derived from bone marrow.

   m., ectopic. M., extramedullary.

   m., extramedullary. Development of myeloid elements (erythrocytes and granular leukocytes) in regions other than bone marrow. SYN: *m., ectopic.*

myelopore. An opening in the spinal cord.

myeloproliferative (mī″ĕ-lō-prō-lif″ĕr-ā′tĭv). Concerning proliferation of bone marrow either in the bone marrow or extramedullary.

myeloradiculitis (mī″ĕ-lō-ră-dĭk″ū-lī′tĭs) [″ + L. *radiculus,* rootlet, + Gr. *itis,* inflammation]. Inflammation of the spinal cord and dorsal roots of spinal nerves.

myeloradiculodysplasia (mī″ĕ-lō-ră-dĭk″ū-lō-dĭs-plā″sē-ă) [″ + ″ + Gr. *dys,* bad, + *plassein,* to form]. Congenital abnormality of the spinal cord and spinal nerve roots.

myeloradiculopathy (mī″ĕ-lō-ră-dĭk″ū-lŏp′ă-thē) [″ + ″ + Gr. *pathos,* disease, suffering]. Disease of the spinal cord and spinal nerves.

myelorrhagia (mī-ĕ-lō-rā′jē-ă) [″ + *rhegnynai,* to burst forth]. Hemorrhage into the spinal cord.

myelorrhaphy (mī-ĕl-or′ă-fē) [″ + *rhaphe,* seam, ridge]. Suture of a cut or wound of the spinal cord.

myelosarcoma (mī″ĕl-ō-săr-kō″mă) [″ + *sarx,* flesh, + *oma,* tumor]. Sarcoma composed of bone marrow cells and tissue. SYN: *osteosarcoma.*

myelosarcomatosis (mī″ĕ-lō-săr-kō″mă-tō′sĭs) [″ + ″ + ″ + *osis,* condition]. Disseminated myelosarcomas.

myeloschisis (mī″ĕ-lŏs′kĭ-sĭs) [″ + *schisis,* a splitting]. Cleft spinal cord resulting from failure of neural tube to close. SEE: *rachischisis; spina bifida cystica.*

myelosclerosis (mī″ĕ-lō-sklĕr-ō′sĭs) [″ + *sklerosis,* hardening]. Sclerosis of the spinal cord.

myelosis (mī-ĕ-lō′sĭs) [″ + *osis,* condition]. Formation of a myeloma or medullary tumor.

    m., erythremic. A malignancy involving the erythropoietic tissue. Symptoms and signs include anemia, fever, hepatosplenomegaly, bleeding tendency, and abnormal cells in the circulating blood.

myelospongium (mī″ĕ-lō-spŏn′jē-ŭm) [Gr. *myelos,* marrow, + *spongos,* sponge]. Embryonic network from which the neuroglia arises.

myelosuppressive (mī″ĕ-lō-sŭ-prĕs′ĭv). Concerning inhibition of bone marrow function.

myelosyphilis (mī″ĕ-lō-sĭf′ĭ-lĭs). Syphilis of the spinal cord.

myelosyringosis (mī″ĕ-lō-sĭr″ĭng-gō′sĭs) [″ + *syrinx,* pipe, + *osis,* condition]. Syringomyelia.

myelotome (mī-ĕl′ō-tōm) [″ + *tome,* incision]. Instrument used to dissect the spinal cord.

myelotomy (mī-ĕl-ŏt′ō-mē). Surgical sever-

ance of nerve fibers of the spinal cord.

myelotoxic (mī-ĕl-ō-tŏk′sĭk) [″ + *toxikon,* poison]. 1. Destroying bone marrow. 2. Pert. to or arising from diseased bone marrow.

myelotoxin (mī″ĕl-ō-tŏk′sĭn). Toxin that destroys marrow cells.

myenteric (mī″ĕn-tĕr′ĭk) [Gr. *mys,* muscle, + *enteron,* intestine]. Concerning the myenteron.

myenteric reflex. Intestinal contraction above and relaxation below the point of stimulation.

myenteron (mī-ĕn′tĕr-ŏn). Muscular coat of the intestine.

Myerson's sign. In Parkinson's disease, inability to stop blinking in response to tapping the forehead, nasal bridge, or maxilla.

myesthesia (mī″ĕs-thē′zē-ă) [″ + *aisthesis,* sensation]. Muscle sense; consciousness of muscle contraction.

myiasis (mī′ă-sĭs) [Gr. *myia,* fly, + *-sis,* condition]. Condition resulting from infestation by the larvae (maggots) of flies. Infestation may be cutaneous, intestinal, atrial (within a cavity such as mouth, nose, eye, sinus, vagina, urethra), via a wound, or external.

myiocephalon (mī″yō-sĕf′ă-lŏn) [″ + *kephale,* head]. Extrusion of a part of the iris through a tear in the cornea.

myiodesopsia (mī″ē-ō-dĕs-ŏp′sē-ă) [Gr. *myiodes,* flylike, + *opsis,* vision]. Condition in which spots are seen before the eyes. SEE: *muscae volitantes.*

myiosis (mī-yō′sĭs) [″ + *osis,* condition]. Myiasis.

myitis (mī-ī′tĭs) [Gr. *mys,* muscle, + *itis,* inflammation]. Inflamed condition of a muscle. SYN: *myositis.*

Mylaxen. Trade name for hexafluorenium bromide.

Myleran. Trade name for busulfan, USP.

Mylicon. Trade name for simethicone.

mylodus. A molar tooth.

mylohyoid (mī″lō-hī′oyd) [Gr. *myle,* mill, + *hyoid,* U-shaped]. 1. Pert. to the hyoid bone and the molar teeth. 2. The paired muscles attached to the mandible that fuse in the midline and form the floor of the mouth.

myo- [Gr. *mys,* muscle]. Combining form pert. to muscle.

myoalbumin (mī″ō-ăl-bū′mĭn) [″ + L. *albus,* white]. Albumin found in muscular tissue.

myoalbumose (mī″ō-ăl′bū-mōs). A protein derived from muscle.

myoarchitectonic (mī″ō-ăr″kĭ-tĕk-tŏn′ĭk) [Gr. *mys,* muscle, + *architekton,* master workman]. Pert. to or resembling structural arrangement of muscle or of fibers.

myoatrophy (mī-ō-ăt′rō-fē). Muscular wasting.

myoblast (mī′ō-blăst) [″ + *blastos*, germ]. An embryonic cell that develops into muscle fiber cell.

myoblastoma (mī″ō-blăs-tō′mă) [″ + ″ + *oma*, tumor]. A tumor consisting of cells resembling myoblasts.

myobradia (mī″ō-brā′dē-ă) [″ + *bradys*, slow]. Slow muscular reaction to stimulation.

myocardial, myocardiac (mī-ō-kăr′dē-ăl, -ăk) [″ + *kardia*, heart]. Concerning the myocardium.

myocardial infarction. ABBR: MI. Condition caused by partial or complete occlusion of one or more of the coronary arteries. The symptoms include prolonged heavy pressure or squeezing pain in the center of the chest behind the sternum. Typically the patient will describe this by clenching a fist and holding it over the heart to demonstrate the character of the pain. The pain may spread or be localized to the shoulder, neck, arm, and fourth and fifth fingers of the left hand; to the back, to the teeth, or to the jaw. These symptoms may be accompanied by nausea and vomiting, sweating, and shortness of breath. About 15% to 20% of MIs are painless.

It is imperative that medical care be instituted without delay. Many myocardial infarction patients not treated prior to reaching the hospital die. Delaying specific therapy may cause loss of life.

TREAT: Therapy should be in a coronary care unit. Complete bed rest initially; monitor ECG; oxygen therapy if indicated. Treat pain with morphine I.V., supplemented with continuous drip I.V. nitroglycerine if pain continues. Treat arrhythmias with appropriate drugs. Be prepared to institute life support measures immediately. Treat hypotension by elevating foot of bed or use of vasopressors or both.

Attempt without delay to remove blockage of coronary artery(s). This can be done by immediate use of thrombolytic agents such as streptokinase or tissue plasminogen activator (tPA). After the patient's condition is stabilized, percutaneous transluminal angioplasty may be done. SYN: *heart attack.* SEE: *angina; artificial respiration; cardiopulmonary resuscitation; reperfusion.*

NURSING IMPLICATIONS: Briefly explain all diagnostic and treatment procedures to help reduce stress and anxiety. Monitor cardiac rhythm, rate, and conduction on a lead that provides easily identified P and R waves (include a 12-lead ECG). Assess for and document chest pain regarding locations and radiation, quality and severity, and temporal elements. Administer pre-

scribed oxygen and analgesic medications (mainly I.V.) and evaluate response. Monitor vital signs and hemodynamic parameters according to agency protocol or patient need, and oversee follow-up diagnostic studies, including serial ECGs and serum enzymes. Establish and maintain a venous access for emergency therapy, and be prepared to administer antidysrhythmics, other cardiac and diuretic drugs, and emergency measures, following protocol or as prescribed for individual patient problems. Promote physical and emotional rest for the patient, and provide support to patient throughout the acute illness period. Teach patient and family about required modifications in lifestyle and diet and about long-term drug regimens. Assist patient with and teach about cardiac rehabilitation program, evaluating response to gradual increases in cardiac work. Explain stress-testing, and encourage rehabilitation participation after discharge. Assist patient with grief related to changes in health and self-concept. SEE: *Nursing Diagnoses* in *Appendix.*

myocardial insufficiency. Inability of the heart to perform its usual function. Eventually this results in cardiac failure.

myocardial ischemia. This condition, inadequate flow of blood to the heart, leads to angina pectoris, q.v., and, if untreated, to myocardial infarction, q.v. About half of the deaths that occur in the U.S. each year are caused by ischemic heart disease, and about half of these deaths occur suddenly. Myocardial ischemia may be treated by use of drugs, i.e., nitroglycerin, beta adrenergic blockers, calcium entry blockers, by the use of surgical procedures such as coronary artery bypass, or by dilating the coronary arteries by use of the procedure of percutaneous transluminal coronary angioplasty. SEE: *angina pectoris, stable; angina pectoris, unstable; Prinzmetal's angina.*

myocardiograph (mī″ō-kăr′dē-ō-grăf) [″ + ″ + *graphein*, to write]. Instrument for recording heart movements.

myocardiopathy (mī″ō-kăr″dē-ŏp′ă-thē) [″ + ″ + *pathos*, disease, suffering]. Any disease of the myocardium.

myocarditis (mī″ō-kăr-dī′tĭs) [″ + *kardia*, heart, + *itis*, inflammation]. Inflammation of the myocardium.

SYM: Apex beat is extremely weak and rapid; pulse is irregular and weak; tenderness over precordium, percussion is negative, auscultation reveals first sound of heart resembling second heart sound, being high pitched and wanting in muscular quality. The ECG may be normal or show only non-specific ST-T wave abnormalities.

ETIOL: Associated with a number of conditions including many types of bacterial, fungal, protozoal, and viral infections, heat stroke, and ionizing radiation. Occurs commonly after rheumatic fever and diphtheria. The cause may be unknown. SEE: *cardiomyopathy.*

NURSING IMPLICATIONS: Initially establish complete bedrest as ordered until symptoms have resolved. Provide light diet, stress-free environment, and a diet to help prevent constipation. Monitor ECG and assess cardiac status at frequent intervals for signs of increased cardiac workload and fatigue. If these occur, provide more rest periods. Administer ordered antibiotics, and treat progressive or life-threatening dysrhythmias immediately. Increase activity gradually after acute phase. In period of recuperation, avoid travel to high altitudes, frequent stair climbing, and mental stress. SEE: *Nursing Diagnoses* in *Appendix.*

myocardium (mī-ō-kăr′dē-ŭm) [″ + *kardia,* heart]. [NA] The middle layer of the walls of the heart, composed of cardiac muscle.

myocele (mī′ō-sēl) [″ + *kele,* tumor, swelling]. 1. Muscular protrusion through a muscle sheath. 2. Cavity within a somite of an embryo.

myocelialgia (mī″ō-sē-lē-ăl′jē-ă) [″ + *koilia,* belly, + *algos,* pain]. Abdominal muscle pain.

myocelitis (mī″ō-sē-lī′tĭs) [″ + ″ + *itis,* inflammation]. Inflamed condition of abdominal muscles.

myocellulitis (mī″ō-sĕl-ū-lī′tĭs) [″ + L. *cellula,* little chamber, + Gr. *itis,* inflammation]. Myositis combined with cellulitis.

myoceptor (mī′ō-sĕp″tor) [″ + L. *capere,* to take]. The endplates of a nerve supplying a muscle.

myocerosis (mī″ō-sē-rō′sĭs) [″ + *keros,* wax]. Waxy degeneration of a muscle.

myochorditis (mī″ō-kor-dī′tĭs) [″ + *chorde,* cord, + *itis,* inflammation]. Inflammation of the muscles of the vocal cord.

myochrome (mī′ō-krōm) [″ + *chroma,* color]. 1. Any muscle pigment. 2. Cytochrome C.

myochronoscope (mī″ō-krō′nō-skōp) [″ + *chronos,* time, + *skopein,* to examine]. Device for determining time for producing a muscular contraction.

myocinesimeter (mī″ō-sĭn″ē-sĭm′ē-tĕr). Device for measuring muscle activity.

myoclonia (mī-ō-klō′nē-ă) [″ + *klonos,* tumult]. Condition of intermittent clonic spasm or twitching of a muscle or muscles.

myoclonus (mī-ōk′lō-nŭs). Twitching or clonic spasm of a muscle or group of muscles.

m. multiplex. Condition marked by persistent and continuous muscular spasms in unrelated muscles. SYN: *paramyoclonus multiplex.*

m., palatal. Rapid clonus of one or both sides of the palate.

myocoele (mī′ō-sēl) [″ + *koila,* hollow]. Cavity within a somite of an embryo.

myocolpitis (mī″ō-kōl-pī′tĭs) [″ + *kolpos,* vagina, + *itis,* inflammation]. Inflammation of vaginal muscular tissue.

myocomma (mī-ō-kŏm′mă) [″ + *komma,* cut] (pl. *myocommata*). Septum dividing the myotomes.

myocrismus (mī-ō-krĭs′mŭs) [″ + *krizein,* to creak]. A peculiar crackling sound sometimes heard in auscultation resulting from contraction of a muscle.

myocyte (mī′ō-sīt) [″ + *kytos,* cell]. A muscular tissue cell.

myocytoma (mī″ō-sī-tō′mă) [″ + ″ + *oma,* tumor]. Tumor containing muscle cells.

myodemia (mī-ō-dē′mē-ă) [″ + *demos,* fat]. Fatty degeneration of muscular tissue. Muscular fiber cells become filled with fat granules and are ultimately destroyed.

myodesopsia (mī″ō-dēs-ŏp′sē-ă) [Gr. *myiodes,* flylike, + *opsis,* vision]. The presence of muscae volitantes.

myodiastasis (mī″ō-dī-ăs′tă-sĭs) [Gr. *mys,* muscle, + *diastasis,* separation]. Division or rupture of a muscle.

myodiopter (mī″ō-dī-ŏp′tĕr). The force of the ciliary muscle to increase the refraction of the eye one diopter more than when the eye is at rest.

myodynamia (mī″ō-dī-năm′ē-ă) [″ + *dynamis,* force]. Muscular force or strength.

myodynamometer (mī″ō-dī″nă-mŏm′ĕt-ĕr) [″ + ″ + *metron,* measure]. Device for measurement of muscular strength.

myodynia (mī″ō-dĭn′ē-ă) [″ + *odyne,* pain]. Muscle pain. SYN: *myalgia.*

myodystonia (mī″ō-dĭs-tō′nē-ă) [″ + *dys,* bad, + *tonos,* tension]. Disorder of muscle tone.

myodystrophy (mī″ō-dĭs′trō-fē) [″ + ″ + *trophe,* nutrition]. Muscular dystrophy.

myoedema (mī″ō-ĕ-dē′mă) [″ + *oidema,* swelling]. 1. Lumping in a wasting muscle when struck. May also be seen in normal muscle. SYN: *mounding.* 2. Edema of a muscle.

myoelastic. Pert. to muscle and elastic tissue.

myoelectric. Pert. to electrical properties of muscles.

myoelectric prosthesis. An advanced prosthetic device operated by battery-powered electric motors that are activated through electrodes by the myoelectric potentials provided by muscles.

myoendocarditis (mī″ō-ĕn″dō-kăr-dī′tĭs) [″

+ *endon,* within, + *kardia,* heart, + *itis,* inflammation]. Inflammation of the cardiac muscular wall and membranous lining.

myoepithelial (mī″ō-ĕp″ĭ-thē′lē-ăl). Pert. to contractile epithelial cells.

myoepithelial cells. Spindle-shaped or branched contractile epithelial cells found between glandular cells and basement membrane of sweat, mammary, and salivary glands.

myoepithelioma (mī″ō-ĕp″ĭ-thē″lē-ō′mă) [″ + *epi,* upon, + *thele,* nipple, + *oma,* tumor]. A slow-growing tumor of the sweat gland.

myoepithelium (mī″ō-ĕp″ĭ-thē′lē-ŭm) [″ + ″ + *thele,* nipple]. Tissue containing contractile epithelial cells.

myofasciitis (mī″ō-făs″ē-i′tĭs) [″ + L. *fascia,* band, + Gr. *itis,* inflammation]. Inflammation of a muscle and its fascia.

myofibril, myofibrilla (mī-ō-fī′brĭl, -fī-brĭl′lă) [″ + L. *fibrilla,* a small fiber] (pl. *myofibrillae*). A tiny fibril found in muscular tissue, running parallel to the cellular long axis, from one cell to another. May be the contractile element.

myofibroma (mī″ō-fī-brō′mă) [″ + L. *fibra,* fiber, + Gr. *oma,* tumor]. Tumor containing muscular and fibrous tissue.

myofibrosis (mī″ō-fī-brō′sĭs) [″ + ″ + Gr. *osis,* condition]. Increase of connective or fibrous tissue with degeneration of muscular tissue.

myofibrositis (mī″ō-fī″brō-sī′tĭs) [Gr. *mys,* muscle, + L. *fibra,* fiber, + Gr. *itis,* inflammation]. Inflammation of the perimysium, the fibrous tissue that encloses muscle tissue.

myofilament (mī″ō-fīl′ă-mĕnt). Filament in the fine structure of muscles. Thick ones contain myosin and thin ones actin. These are seen by use of electron microscopy.

myofunctional (mī″ō-fŭnk′shŭn-ăl). Concerning muscle function.

myogelosis (mī″ō-jĕ-lō′sĭs) [″ + L. *gelare,* to congeal]. Hardening of a portion of muscle.

myogenesis (mī-ō-jĕn′ĕ-sĭs) [″ + *genesis,* generation, birth]. Formation of muscular tissue, esp. in embryos.

myogenetic, myogenic (mī-ō-jĕn′ĕt′ĭk, mī-ō-jĕn′ĭk) [″ + *gennan,* to produce]. Having origin in muscle.

myoglia (mī-ŏg′lē-ă) [″ + *glia,* glue]. A fibrous network in muscular tissue resembling neuroglia in appearance.

myoglobin. Myohemoglobin.

myoglobinuria (mī″ō-glō″bĭn-ū′rē-ă). Myoglobin in the urine. It may occur following muscular activity, trauma, or as a result of a deficiency of muscle phosphorylase.

myoglobulin (mī″ō-glŏb′ū-lĭn) [″ + L. *globulus,* globule]. A coagulable globulin present in muscular tissue.

myognathus (mī-ŏg′nă-thŭs) [″ + *gnathos,* jaw]. Deformed individual with a rudimentary conjoined twin.

myogram [″ + *gramma,* something written]. Tracing made by the myograph of muscular contractions.

myograph (mī′ō-grăf) [″ + *graphein,* to write]. Instrument for tracing movements caused by muscular contractions.

myographic (mī-ō-grăf′ĭk). Pert. to a myograph or the tracings made by it.

myographic tracing. A myogram or muscular tracing.

myography (mī-ŏg′ră-fē). 1. Recording of muscular contractions by a myograph. 2. Description of the muscles and their action.

myohematin (mī″ō-hĕm′ă-tĭn). Cytochrome C.

myohemoglobin (mī″ō-hē″mō-glō′bĭn). ABBR: MHb. A respiratory pigment in muscle tissue that serves as an oxygen carrier. SYN: *myoglobin.*

myohysterectomy (mī″ō-hĭs-tĕr-ĕk′tō-mē) [Gr. *mys,* muscle, + *hystera,* womb, + *ektome,* excision]. Excision of the body of the uterus, leaving the cervix in place. SYN: *hysterectomy, subtotal.*

myoid (mī′oyd) [″ + *eidos,* form, shape]. Resembling muscle.

myoidema (mī-oy-dē′mă) [″ + *oidema,* swelling]. Myoedema.

myoischemia (mī″ō-ĭs-kē′mē-ă) [″ + *ischein,* to hold back, + *haima,* blood]. Localized deficiency of blood supply in muscle tissue.

myokerosis (mī″ō-kē-rō′sĭs) [″ + *keros,* wax, + *osis,* intensive]. Waxy degeneration of muscle or muscular tissue.

myokinase (mī″ō-kĭn′ās). An enzyme present in muscle that catalyzes the synthesis of adenosine triphosphate.

myokinesimeter (mī″ō-kĭn″ĕ-sĭm′ĕ-tĕr) [″ + *kinesis,* movement, + *metron,* measure]. Myocinesimeter, q.v.

myokinesis (mī″ō-kĭn-ē′sĭs) [″ + *kinesis,* movement]. 1. Muscular activity. 2. Surgical displacement of muscular fibers.

myokymia (mī-ō-kĭm′ē-ă) [″ + *kyma,* wave]. Twitching of fibers of a muscle. It may be functional and is also seen in organic affections and general paresis. SYN: *kymatism.*

myolemma (mī″ō-lĕm′ă) [″ + *lemma,* sheath]. Sarcolemma, q.v.

myolipoma (mī″ō-lī-pō′mă) [″ + *lipos,* fat, + *oma,* tumor]. Muscle tissue tumor containing fatty elements.

myology (mī-ŏl′ō-jē) [″ + *logos,* word, reason]. The science or study of the muscles and their parts.

myolysis (mī-ŏl'ĭ-sĭs) [" + *lysis*, dissolution]. Fatty degeneration and infiltration with destruction of muscular tissue accompanied by separation and disappearance of muscle cells.

myoma (mī-ō'mă) [" + *oma*, tumor] (pl. *myomas* or *myomata*). A tumor containing muscle tissue. SEE: *chondromyoma*.

    m., nonstriated. A tumor of unmarked muscle tissue. SYN: *leiomyoma*.

    m. striocellulare. Fibroma with striated muscular fibers. SYN: *rhabdomyoma*.

    m. telangiectodes. Coiled blood vessel tumor in muscular fibers. SYN: *angiomyoma*.

    m. uteri. Fibroid tumor of the uterus.

myomalacia (mī"ō-mă-lā'sē-ă) [Gr. *mys*, muscle, + *malakia*, softening]. Softening of muscular tissue.

    m. cordis. Softening of the heart muscle.

myomatosis (mī"ō-mă-tō'sĭs) [" + *oma*, tumor, + *osis*, condition]. The development of multiple myomata.

myomatous (mī-ō'mă-tŭs). Pert. to or resembling a myoma.

myomectomy (mī"ō-měk'tō-mē) [" + *oma*, tumor, + *ektome*, excision]. 1. Removal of a portion of muscle or muscular tissue. 2. Removal of a myomatous tumor, generally uterine, usually by abdominal section, leaving the uterus in place. SYN: *myomotomy*.

myomelanosis (mī"ō-měl-ă-nō'sĭs) [" + *melanosis*, blackening]. Abnormal darkening of muscle tissue.

myomere (mī'ō-mēr) [" + *meros*, part]. Myotome.

myometer (mī-ŏm'ět-ěr) [" + *metron*, measure]. Device for measurement of muscular contractions.

myometrial. Concerning the myometrium.

myometritis (mī"ō-mē-trī'tĭs) [" + *metra*, uterus, + *itis*, inflammation]. Inflamed condition of the muscular wall of the uterus. SYN: *mesometritis*.

myometrium (mī"ō-mē'trē-ŭm). [NA] Muscular wall of the uterus forming the main mass of the uterus.

myomohysterectomy (mī-ō"mō-hĭs-těr-ěk'tō-mē) [" + *oma*, tumor, + *hystera*, womb, + *ektome*, excision]. Hysterectomy performed to remove a myomatous uterus.

myomotomy (mī"ō-mŏt'ō-mē) [" + " + *tome*, excision]. Excision of a myoma, usually uterine. SYN: *myomectomy* (def. 2).

myon [Gr. *mys*, muscle]. A single muscle unit.

myonecrosis (mī"ō-ně-krō'sĭs) [" + *nekrosis*, state of death]. Necrosis of muscle tissue.

myonephropexy (mī"ō-něf'rō-pěk"sē) [" + *nephros*, kidney, + *pexis*, fixation]. Fixation of a movable kidney by attaching it to a portion of muscular tissue with sutures.

myoneural. Pert. to muscle and nerve, esp. nerve terminations in muscles.

myoneuralgia (mī"ō-nū-răl'jē-ă) [" + *neuron*, nerve, + *algos*, pain]. Muscle pain.

myoneural junction. Ending of a nerve in a muscle. SEE: *motor endplate*.

myoneurasthenia (mī"ō-nūr"ăs-thē'nē-ă) [" + " + *astheneia*, weakness]. Relaxed condition of muscular system associated with neurasthenia.

myoneuroma (mī"ō-nū-rō'mă) [" + " + *oma*, tumor]. Neuroma partially composed of muscular elements.

myonosus (mī-ŏn'ō-sŭs) [" + *nosos*, disease]. Disease of muscular tissue. SYN: *myopathy*.

myonymy (mī-ŏn'ĭ-mē) [" + *onoma*, name]. Nomenclature of muscles.

myopachynsis (mī"ō-păk-ĭn'sĭs) [" + *pachynsis*, thickening]. Abnormal thickening of muscle tissue.

myopalmus (mī-ō-păl'mŭs) [" + *palmos*, a twitching]. Twitching of muscles.

myoparalysis (mī"ō-pă-răl'ĭ-sĭs). Paralysis of a muscle.

myoparesis (mī"ō-păr'ē-sĭs). Weakness or incomplete paralysis of a muscle.

myopathic (mī-ō-păth'ĭk) [" + *pathos*, disease, suffering]. 1. Pert. to muscular disease. 2. One suffering from a muscular disease.

myopathic facies. Facial expression caused by relaxation of facial muscles.

myopathy (mī-ŏp'ă-thē). Any disease or abnormal condition of striated muscle.

    m., centronuclear. Myopathy in which the muscle fibers resemble those seen in fetal development. The nuclei of the cells are surrounded by a clear zone. SYN: *m., myotubular*.

    m., distal. Myopathy of the hands.

    m., myotubular. M., centronuclear, q.v.

    m., nemaline. Congenital nonprogressive weakness, esp. of the proximal muscles. The muscles are thin and resemble rods.

    m., ocular. Hereditary dystrophy of the extraocular muscles. This may progress to complete paralysis of these muscles.

    m., thyrotoxic. A chronic disease characterized by progressive muscular weakness and atrophy and hyperthyroidism.

myope (mī'ōp) [Gr. *myein*, to shut, + *ops*, eye]. One afflicted with myopia or nearsightedness.

myopericarditis (mī"ō-pěr-ĭ-kar-dī'tĭs) [Gr. *mys*, muscle, + *peri*, around, + *kardia*, heart, + *itis*, inflammation]. Inflammation of the pericardium and cardiac muscular wall.

myophage (mī'ō-fāj) [" + *phagein,* to eat]. A macrophage that destroys muscular tissue.

myophone (mī'ō-fōn) [" + *phone,* voice]. Device for amplifying the sound of muscular contractions.

myopia [Gr. *myein,* to shut, + *ops,* eye]. Defect in vision in which parallel rays come to a focus in front of the retina; objects can be seen distinctly only when very close to the eyes. SYN: *nearsightedness.* SEE: *emmetropia* for illus.

    m., axial. Myopia due to elongation of the axis of the eye.

    m., chromic. Color blindness only when viewing distant objects.

    m., curvature. Myopia due to curvature of the eye's refracting surfaces.

    m., index. Myopia resulting from abnormal refractivity of the media.

    m., malignant. Progressive myopia leading to retinal detachment and blindness. SYN: *m., pernicious.*

    m., pernicious. M., malignant.

    m., prodromal. Myopia in which reading without glasses becomes possible; seen in incipient cataract.

    m., progressive. Myopia that increases steadily during adult life.

    m., space. Myopia occurring when the eye is attempting to focus on an object but all that is visible is a complete noncontrasting material such as may occur when looking into dense fog, e.g., while piloting an airplane. No image is produced on the retina.

    m., stationary. Myopia that ends after adult growth is attained.

    m., transient. Myopia seen in spasm of accommodation, as in acute iritis or iridocyclitis.

myopic (mī-ŏp'ĭk). Pert. to or affected with myopia.

myopic crescent. Posterior crescentic protrusion seen in myopia.

myoplasm (mī'ō-plăzm) [Gr. *mys,* muscle, + LL. *plasma,* form, mold]. The contractile part of the muscle cell, as differentiated from the sarcoplasm.

myoplastic (mī'ō-plăs'tĭk) [" + *plassein,* to form]. Pert. to plastic use of muscle tissue or plastic surgery on muscles.

myoplasty (mī-ō-plăs"tē). Plastic surgery of muscle tissue.

myopolar (mī"ō-pō'lăr). The muscle tissue between electrodes.

myoporthosis (mī"ŏp-or-thō'sĭs). Correction of myopia or nearsightedness.

myoprotein (mī"ō-prō'tēn). Any of several proteins present in muscle tissue.

myopsis (mī-ŏp'sĭs). Myodesopsia, q.v.

myopsychopathy (mī"ō-sī-kŏp'ă-thē) ["

+ *psyche,* mind, + *pathos,* disease, suffering]. Any muscle dysfunction associated with mental disorder.

myoreceptor (mī"ō-rē-sĕp'tor). A proprioceptor in the muscle.

myorrhaphy (mī-or'ă-fē) [Gr. *mys,* muscle, + *rhaphe,* a sewing]. Suture of a muscle wound.

myorrhexis (mī-or-ĕk'sĭs) [" + *rhexis,* a rupture]. Rupture of a muscle.

myosalgia (mī-ō-săl'jē-ă) [" + *algos,* pain]. Pain in a muscle. SYN: *myalgia.*

myosalpingitis (mī"ō-săl-pĭn-jī'tĭs) [" + *salpinx,* tube, + *itis,* inflammation]. Inflamed condition of muscular tissue of a fallopian tube.

myosarcoma (mī"ō-sar-kō'mă) [" + *sarx,* flesh, + *oma,* tumor]. A malignant tumor derived from myogenic cells.

myosclerosis (mī"ō-sklĕr-ō'sĭs) [" + *skleros,* hardening]. Hardening of muscle.

myosin [Gr. *mys,* muscle]. A protein present in muscle fibrils and constituting about 65% of total muscle protein. It consists of long chains of polypeptides joined to each other by side chains. The molecular structure of myosin is thought to be responsible for the properties of muscle tissue, namely, birefringence, double refraction, contractility, and elasticity. Myosin combines with another muscle protein, actin, to form actomyosin.

myosinose (mī-ŏs'ĭn-ōs). A proteose resulting from the hydrolysis of myosin.

myosinuria (mī"ō-sĭn-ū'rē-ă). The occurrence of myosin in the urine. SYN: *myosuria.*

myositis (mī-ō-sī'tĭs) [" + *itis,* inflammation]. Inflammation of muscle tissue, esp. voluntary muscles. SYN: *myitis.* SEE: *fibrositis.*

    ETIOL: Infection, trauma, diathetic states, or infestation by parasites.

    m., epidemic. Epidemic pleurodynia.

    m. fibrosa. Myositis accompanied by infiltration of fibrous tissue.

    m., interstitial. Myositis with hyperplasia of connective tissue.

    m., multiple. Polymyositis.

    m. ossificans. Myositis marked by ossification of muscles.

    m., parenchymatous. Myositis of substance of a muscle.

    m. purulenta. Suppurative myositis with abscesses; caused by bacterial infection.

    m., traumatic. May be simple with pain and swelling or may be suppurative.

    m. trichinosa. Myositis due to infestation with trichinae. SYN: *trichinous myositis.*

myospasm (mī'ō-spăzm) [" + *spasmos,* a

convulsion]. Spasmodic contraction of a muscle.

myosteoma (mī-ŏs"tē-ō'mă) [" + *osteon*, bone, + *oma*, tumor]. A bony growth found in muscle tissue.

myosthenometer (mī"ō-sthĕn-ŏm'ĕ-tĕr) [" + *sthenos*, strength, + *metron*, measure]. Device for measuring muscle power.

myostroma (mī"ō-strō'mă) [" + *stroma*, mattress]. The framework of muscle tissue.

myosuria (mī-ō-sū'rē-ă) [" + *ouron*, urine]. Presence of myosin in the urine. SYN: *myosinuria*.

myosuture (mī"ō-sū'chūr) [" + L. *sutura*, sewing]. Stitching of a muscle.

myotactic (mī"ō-tăk'tĭk) [" + L. *tactus*, touch]. Pert. to muscle or kinesthetic sense.

myotasis (mī-ŏt'ă-sĭs) [" + *tasis*, stretching]. Stretching of a muscle.

myotatic. Pert. to the stretching of muscles.

myotatic reflex. Stretch reflex.

myotenontoplasty (mī"ō-tĕn-ŏn'tō-plăst"ē) [" + *tenon*, tendon, + *plassein*, to form]. Plastic operation involving muscles and tendons. SYN: *tenomyoplasty; tenonto-myoplasty.*

myotenositis (mī"ō-tĕn-ō-sī'tĭs) [" + " + *itis*, inflammation]. Inflamed condition of a muscle and its tendon.

myotenotomy (mī"ō-tĕn-ŏt'ō-mē) [" + " + *tome*, incision]. Division of the tendon of a muscle.

myotherapy. A method for relaxing muscle spasm, improving circulation, and alleviating pain. Pressure is held for several seconds to fingers and joints, including elbows, to defuse "trigger points." The success of this method depends upon the use of specific corrective exercises of the freed muscles. The method was developed by Bonnie Pruden in 1976.

myothermic (mī"ō-thĕrm'ĭk) [Gr. *mys*, muscle, + *therme*, heat]. Pert. to rise in muscle temperature due to its activity.

myotic (mī-ŏt'ĭk). Miotic, q.v.

myotome (mī'ō-tōm) [" + *tome*, incision]. 1. Knife for cutting muscles. 2. That portion of an embryonic somite that gives rise to somatic (striated) muscles. SYN: *myomere.*

myotomy (mī-ŏt'ō-mē). Surgical division or anatomical dissection of muscles.

myotonia (mī"ō-tō'nē-ă) [" + *tonos*, tension]. Tonic spasm of a muscle or temporary rigidity after muscular contraction.

  m. atrophica. M. dystrophica.

  m. congenita. A benign disease characterized by tonic spasms of the muscles induced by voluntary movements; usually congenital and transmitted from one generation to another. SYN: *Thomsen's disease.*

  SYM: Disease appears in early childhood, is manifested by a tonic spasm of the mus-

cles every time they are used. In a few minutes, rigidity wears away and the movements become free from repeated contractions, the muscles becoming firm and extremely well developed.

  TREAT: Quinine or procainamide for relief of myotonia. Avoid obesity. Neostigmine is contraindicated.

  PROG: Incurable but may improve with age.

  m. dystrophica. A hereditary disease characterized by muscular wasting, myotonia, and cataract. SYN: *myotonia atrophica; Steinert's disease.*

myotonic. Pert. to tonic muscular spasm, as differentiated from myokinetic spasm.

myotonoid (mī-ŏt'ō-noyd). Similar to myotonia.

myotonus (mī-ŏt'ō-nŭs). A tonic muscle spasm with temporary rigidity.

myotony (mī-ŏt'ō-nē). Myotonia.

myotrophy (mī-ŏt'rō-fē) [" + *trophe*, nourishment]. Nutrition of muscle tissues.

myotropic (mī"ō-trŏp'ĭk) [" + *trope*, a turn]. Attracted to muscle tissue.

myotube (mī'ō-tūb). The developing stage of skeletal muscle. The central nucleus occupies most of the cell.

myovascular (mī"ō-văs'kū-lăr). Concerning muscles and blood supply to them.

myriachit (mĭr-ē'ă-chĭt) [Russian]. SEE: *miryachit.*

Myriapoda (mĭr-ē-ăp'ō-dă) [Gr. *myrios*, numberless, + *pous*, foot]. Group of arthropods including millipedes and centipedes.

myriapodiasis (mĭr"ē-ăp-ō-dī'ă-sĭs). Infestation with one of the Myriapoda class of arthropods.

myricin (mĭr'ĭ-sĭn). A chemical obtained from beeswax.

myringa (mĭr-ĭn'gă) [L.]. The tympanic membrane.

myringectomy (mĭr-ĭn-jĕk'tō-mē) [" + Gr. *ektome*, excision]. Myringodectomy.

myringitis (mĭr-ĭn-jī'tĭs) [L. *myringa*, drum membrane, + Gr. *itis*, inflammation]. Inflammation of the tympanum or eardrum.

  m. bullosa. Myringitis with serous or hemorrhagic blebs or vesicular inflammation of the eardrum and adjacent wall.

myringodectomy (mĭr-ĭn"gō-dĕk'tō-mē) [" + Gr. *ektome*, excision]. Excision of a part of or the entire tympanic membrane. SYN: *myringectomy.*

myringomycosis (mĭr-ĭn"gō-mī-kō'sĭs) [" + Gr. *mykes*, fungus, + *osis*, condition]. Inflammation of the tympanic membrane resulting from infection by parasitic fungi. SYN: *mycomyringitis; otomycosis.*

myringoplasty (mĭr-ĭn'gō-plăst"ē) [" + Gr. *plassein*, to form]. Plastic operation of the tympanic membrane.

myringoscope (mĭr-ĭn'gō-skōp) [″ + Gr. *skopein*, to examine]. Instrument used for examination of the eardrum.

myringotome (mĭ-rĭn'gō-tōm) [″ + Gr. *tome*, incision]. Knife for incising the tympanic membrane.

myringotomy (mĭr-ĭn-gŏt'ō-mē). Incision of the tympanic membrane. SEE: *Nursing Diagnoses* in *Appendix.*

myrmecia (mŭr-mē'shē-ă) [Gr. *myrmex*, ant]. A dome-shaped wart.

myrmecology. Study of ants.

myrrh (mŭr) [Gr. *myrra*]. A gum resinous substance used by man for many centuries. In antiquity, cherished as a constituent of incense and perfume; most important use today is as an aromatic astringent mouthwash. Tincture of myrrh provides symptomatic relief when applied to canker sores.

mysophilia (mī″sō-fīl'ē-ă). Erotic interest in body excretions.

mysophobia (mī″sō-fō'bē-ă) [Gr. *mysos*, filth, + *phobos*, fear]. Abnormal aversion to dirt or contamination. SYN: *molysmophobia.*

mytacism (mī'tă-sĭzm) [Gr. *mytakismos* from Gr. letter μ]. Excessive or incorrect use of the letter *m* or the *m* sound, in writing or speaking.

mythomania (mĭth″ō-mā'nē-ă) [Gr. *mythos*, myth, + *mania*, madness]. Abnormal tendency to lie and exaggerate.

mythophobia (mĭth″ō-fō'bē-ă) [″ + *phobos*, fear]. Abnormal dread of making a false or incorrect statement.

mytilotoxin (mĭt″ĭ-lō-tŏk'sĭn). A neurotoxin present in certain mussels.

myxadenitis (mĭks″ăd-ĕn-ī'tĭs) [Gr. *myxa*, mucus, + *aden*, gland, + *itis*, inflammation]. Inflammation of mucous gland or glands.

    m. labialis. Painless inflammation of the mucous glands of the lips. SYN: *cheilitis glandularis.*

myxadenoma (mĭks″ăd-ē-nō'mă) [″ + ″ + *oma*, tumor]. 1. A tumor with the structure of a mucous gland. SYN: *myxoadenoma.* 2. A tumor of glandular structure containing mucous elements.

myxangitis (mĭks″ăn-jī'tĭs) [″ + *angeion*, vessel, + *itis*, inflammation]. Inflammation of mucous gland ducts.

myxasthenia (mĭks″ăs-thē'nē-ă) [″ + *astheneia*, weakness]. Imperfect or insufficient secretion of mucus.

myxedema (mĭks-ē-dē'mă) [Gr. *myxa*, mucus, + *oidema*, swelling]. Condition resulting from hypofunction of the thyroid gland. Occurs in older children and adults. SEE: *Nursing Diagnoses* in *Appendix.*

    SYM: Decreased metabolic rate, low ra-

dioactive iodine uptake by thyroid, decreased protein-bound iodine, anemia, myxedematous facies, large tongue, slow speech, puffiness of hands and face, coarse and thickened edematous skin, loss and dryness of hair, mental apathy, drowsiness, and sensitivity to cold.

    ETIOL: Iodine deficiency in diet; surgical excision or atrophy of thyroid gland; excessive use of antithyroid drugs. May occur secondary to hypofunction of anterior pituitary and is complicated by adrenal and gonadal deficiencies.

    TREAT: Thyroid hormone replacement.

    m., childhood. Myxedema occurring before puberty.

    m., operative. Myxedema following removal of thyroid gland. SYN: *cachexia strumipriva.*

    m., pituitary. Myxedema occurring secondary to anterior pituitary hypofunction.

    m., pretibial. Edema of the anterior surface of the legs following hyperthyroidism and exophthalmos.

myxedematoid (mĭks-ĕ-dēm'ă-toyd) [Gr. *myxa*, mucus, + *oidema*, swelling, + *eidos*, form, shape.]. Resembling myxedema.

myxedematous (mĭks-ĕ-dēm'ă-tŭs). Concerning or marked by myxedema.

myxemia (mĭks-ē'mē-ă) [″ + *haima*, blood]. Accumulation of mucin in the blood. SYN: *mucinemia.*

myxiosis (mĭks-ē-ō'sĭs) [″ + *osis*, condition]. A mucous discharge or secretion.

myxo-, myx- [Gr. *myxa*]. Combining form designating rel. to mucus.

myxoadenoma (mĭks″ō-ăd-ē-nō'mă) [″ + *aden*, gland, + *oma*, tumor]. Myxadenoma.

Myxobacterales (mĭks″ō-băk-tē-rā'lēz). An order of bacteria found in soil and dung. Characterized by a slimy spreading colony.

myxochondrofibrosarcoma (mĭks″ō-kŏn″drō-fī″brō-săr-kō'mă). A malignant tumor composed of myxomatous, chondromatous, fibrous, and sarcomatous elements.

myxochondroma (mĭks″ō-kŏn-drō'mă). A benign tumor composed of myxomatous and chondromatous elements.

myxocystoma (mĭks″ō-sĭs-tō'mă) [Gr. *myxa*, mucus, + *kystis*, cyst, + *oma*, tumor]. A benign cystic tumor containing mucus.

myxocyte (mĭk'sō-sīt) [″ + *kytos*, cell]. A characteristic cell of mucous tissue.

myxoedema (mĭks″ē-dē'mă) [″ + *oidema*, swelling]. Myxedema.

myxoenchondroma (mĭks″ō-ĕn-kŏn-drō'mă) [″ + *en*, in, + *chondros*, cartilage, + *oma*, tumor]. A cartilaginous tissue tumor that has undergone partial mucous degeneration.

myxofibroma (mĭks″ō-fī-brō′mă) [″ + L. *fibra*, fiber, + Gr. *oma*, tumor]. Tumor composed of mucous and fibrous elements. SYN: *myxoinoma*.

myxofibrosarcoma (mĭk″sō-fī″brō-săr-kō′mă) [″ + ″ + Gr. *sarx*, flesh, + *oma*, tumor]. Fibrosarcoma that contains primitive mesenchymal tissue.

myxoglioma (mĭk″sō-glī-ō′mă) [Gr. *myxa*, mucus, + *glia*, glue, + *oma*, tumor]. Tumor composed of myxomatous and gliomatous elements.

myxoid (mĭk′soyd) [″ + *eidos*, form, shape]. Similar to or resembling mucus.

myxoinoma (mĭk″sō-ĭn-ō′mă). A myxofibroma.

myxolipoma (mĭk″sō-lĭ-pō′mă) [″ + *lipos*, fat, + *oma*, tumor]. Mucous tumor with fatty tissue elements in it. SYN: *lipomyxoma*.

myxoma (mĭk-sō′mă) [″ + *oma*, tumor] (pl. *myxomas* or *myxomata*). Tumor composed of mucous connective tissue similar to that present in the embryo or umbilical cord. Cells are stellate or spindle-shaped and separated by mucoid tissue. The tumors are usually soft, gray, lobulated, and translucent and are not completely encapsulated. May be pure or of mixed types involving other types of tissue.

　　m., cartilaginous. Chondromyxoma.

　　m., cystic. Tumor with parts fluid enough to resemble cysts.

　　m., enchondromatous. Tumor with nodules of hyaline cartilage.

　　m., erectile. Myxoma containing an excess of vessels, resembling an angioma.

　　m., fibrous. Fibromyxoma.

　　m., intracanalicular, of mamma. Myxoma that develops in the interstitial connective tissue of the breasts.

　　m., odontogenic. Tumor of the jaw that appears to arise from mesenchymal tissue.

　　m., telangiectatic, vascular. Myxoma of highly vascular structure.

myxomatosis (mĭk″sō-mă-tō′sĭs) [″ + + *osis*, condition]. 1. Formation of multiple myxomas. 2. Myxomatous degeneration.

Myxomycetes (mĭk″sō-mī-sē′tēz) [Gr.

myxa, mucus, + *mykes*, fungus]. A group of organisms of uncertain classification, but thought to be funguslike. Includes slime molds. SEE: *Myxobacterales*.

myxomyoma (mĭks-ō-mī-ō′mă) [″ + *mys*, muscle, + *oma*, tumor]. Muscle tissue tumor that has undergone mucous degeneration.

myxoneuroma (mĭks″ō-nū-rō′mă) [″ + *neuron*, nerve, + *oma*, tumor]. Tumor composed of mucous and nerve tissue elements.

myxopapilloma (mĭk″sō-păp″ĭl-ō′mă) [″ + L. *papilla*, nipple, + Gr. *oma*, tumor]. Combination of myxomatous and papillomatous tumor or tumors.

myxopoiesis (mĭk″sō-poy-ē′sĭs) [″ + *poiesis*, creation]. Formation of mucus.

myxorrhea (mĭk-sō-rē′ă) [″ + *rhoia*, flow]. Free discharge from mucous surfaces. SYN: *blennorrhea*.

　　m. gastrica. Excessive mucous secretion in the stomach.

　　m. intestinalis. Secretion of mucus from the bowel in neurotic persons in times of mental stress.

myxosarcoma (mĭk″sō-săr-kō′mă) [″ + *sarx*, flesh, + *oma*, tumor]. Mixed tumor, partly myxomatous and partly sarcomatous, having undergone partial degeneration.

myxosarcomatous (mĭk″sō-săr-kō′mă-tŭs). Pert. to or of the nature of myxosarcoma.

myxospore (mĭks′ō-spor) [″ + *sporos*, seed]. Spore embedded in a gelatinous mass, seen in some fungi and protozoa.

Myxosporidia (mĭks-ō-spor-ĭd′ē-ă). Parasitic sporozoans, most commonly found in epithelial cells of lower vertebrates.

myxoviruses. Family of viruses including those that cause influenza. SEE: *paramyxoviruses.*

Myzomyia (mī″zō-mī′ă) [Gr. *myzan*, to suck, + *myia*, fly]. Subgenus of anopheline mosquitoes. Some species transmit malarial parasites.

Myzorhynchus (mī″zō-rĭng′kŭs) [″ + *rhynchos*, snout]. Subgenus of anopheline mosquitoes. Some species transmit malarial parasites.

N

N. 1. Chem. symb. for the element nitrogen. 2. *normal,* esp. with reference to solutions.

n. 1. Symb. for *index of refraction.* 2. *nasal; number.*

n₁, n₂, n₃ . . . nₙ. In statistical terminology, the notations used for subjects, i.e., n_1 is subject number one, n_2 subject number two, and the last subject n_n, where the subscript n would be the last subject in the series.

¹⁵N. Symb. for radioactive isotope of nitrogen.

NA. *nicotinic acid; Nomina Anatomica; numerical aperture; nurse's aide.*

Na [L. *natrium*]. Chem. symb. for the element sodium.

N.A.A.C.O.G. *Nurses Association of the American College of Obstetricians and Gynecologists.*

nabothian cysts (nă-bō'thē-ăn). Retention cysts formed by the nabothian glands at the neck of the uterus.

ETIOL: Due to closing of mouths of glands by new epithelium of a healed ectropion. The cysts always denote that an ectropion has been present.

NaBr. Sodium bromide.

NaCl. Sodium chloride.

NaClO. Sodium hypochlorite.

Na₂CO₃. Sodium carbonate.

nacreous (nā'krē-ŭs) [L. *nacer,* mother of pearl]. Having an iridescent pearl-like luster, as bacterial colonies.

NAD. *nicotinamide adenine dinucleotide.*

NAD⁺. Oxidized form of NAD. This enzyme is important in accepting electrons in the course of metabolic reactions. When NAD⁺ gives up its electron, it is converted to the reduced form, NADH.

N.A.D. *no appreciable disease.*

NADH. The reduced form of NAD⁺. SYN: *TPN; coenzyme.*

NADH-diaphorase. The reduced form of the enzyme nicotinamide adenine dinucleotide-diaphorase. It is important in reducing the ferric iron (Fe^{+++}) to its ferrous (Fe^{++}) form; thus it is one of the enzymes that converts methemoglobin (which is unable to transport oxygen) to hemoglobin (which can transport oxygen). Deficiency of NADH-diaphorase causes congenital methemoglobinemia. SYN: *methemoglobin reductase.*

NADP. *nicotinamide adenine dinucleotide phosphate,* reduced form of NADP⁺, an enzyme important in accepting electrons in the course of metabolic reactions.

NADP⁺. Oxidized form of NADP.

Naegele's obliquity (nā'gĕ-lēz) [Franz Carl Naegele, Ger. obstetrician, 1777–1851].

Anterior parietal presentation of the fetal head in labor. SYN: *asynclitism, anterior.*

Naegele's pelvis. An obliquely contracted pelvis, caused by disease in infancy.

Naegele's rule. A system to estimate the date of onset of labor: count back exactly 90 days from the day the last menstrual period began and add seven days to that date.

Naegleria. A genus of protozoa present in soil, ground water, and sewage. One species, *N. fowleri,* is the causative agent of a lethal form of meningoencephalitis. SEE: *acanthamebiasis.*

N.A.E.M.T. *National Association of Emergency Medical Technicians.*

NaF. Sodium fluoride.

Nafcil. Trade name for nafcillin sodium, USP.

nafcillin sodium (năf-sĭl'ĭn). USP. A semisynthetic penicillin that is penicillinase-resistant. Trade names are Nafcil and Unipen.

NaHCO₃. Sodium bicarbonate.

NaHSO₃. Sodium bisulfite.

nail [AS. *naegel*]. 1. A rod made of metal, bone, or solid material used to attach the ends or pieces of broken bones. 2. A horny cell structure of the epidermis forming flat plates upon the dorsal surface of the terminal phalanges. Called toenail and fingernail on the toes and fingers, respectively. SYN: *unguis* (def. 1) (L.); *onyx* (def. 1) (Gr.).

A nail consists of a body, composed of keratin, the exposed portion, and a root, the proximal portion hidden by the nail fold, both of which rest on the nailbed or matrix. The latter consists of epithelium and corium continuous with the epidermis and dermis of the skin of the nail fold. The crescent-shaped white area near the root is the lunula. The epidermis extending from the margin of the nail fold over the root is called eponychium; that underlying the free border of the distal portion is called hyponychium.

A nail grows in length and thickness through activity of cells in the stratum germinativum of the root. Average rate of growth in fingernails is about 1 mm per week. It is slower in toenails and slower in summer than in winter. Nail growth varies with age and is affected by disease and certain hormone deficiencies.

The onset of a disease that briefly interferes with nail growth and development may be estimated by measuring the distance of the line (Beau's line) across the nail from the root of the nail.

DIFF. DIAG: Changes in the nails, such as ridges, may occur in defective nutrition or after a serious illness. In achlorhydria and hypochromic anemia, excessively spoon-shaped nails, which are depressed in the center, may occur. In chronic pulmonary conditions and congenital heart disease, spongy excess of soft tissue at base of nails may be associated with clubbed fingers.

Atrophy may occur as a result of hereditary or congenital tendencies. Permanent atrophy may follow injuries, scars from disease, frostbite, nerve injuries, and hyperthyroidism. Nail shedding is due to the same causes.

Nails that are fragile or split often may occur as a congenital condition or may be due to prolonged contact with chemicals or too frequent manicuring.

Dry, malformed nails may be due to trophic changes resulting from injury to nerve or finger, neuritis, Raynaud's disease, pulmonary osteoarthropathy, syphilis, onychia, scleroderma, acrodermatitis, and granuloma fungoides of the fingers.

Transverse lines (Beau's lines) may result from previous interference of nail matrix growth. May be caused by local or systemic conditions. Approximate date of lesion may be determined, because it takes 4 to 6 months for the fingernail to be replaced.

Chancre may be suspected if a small indolent ulcer appears near the nail, esp. if indurated and associated with enlarged lymph glands above the inner condyle.

Quincke's capillary pulsation, indicated by a rhythmic flushing and blanching under the nails, is seen most frequently in aortic regurgitation and often in anemia.

Discolorations: Black: In diabetes and other forms of gangrene. Blue-black: Common condition, usually due to hemorrhage, bleeding diseases such as hemophilia, or trauma. May be painful and can be relieved by drilling a small hole in the nail at the site of hemorrhage. A dental drill, the heated tip of a paper clip, or a similar rigid wire of small diameter may be used. Brown: May be due to arsenical poisoning. Brownish-black: This discoloration often indicates chronic mercurial poisoning due to formation of sulfide of mercury in the tissues. Cyanosis: Usually indicates anemia, poor circulation, or venous stasis. Green: Staining of the nail fold or under the nail associated with growth of *Pseudomonas* in a wet area. Slate: This is an early manifestation of argyria, and administration of silver should be stopped at once. White spots: Striate lesions may be due to trauma and are more frequent in women. Transverse white bands in all nails may be a sign of acute or chronic arsenical

poisoning or, rarely, of thallium acetate poisoning. SEE: *Mees lines.*

n., clubbing of. SEE: *clubbing.*

n., eggshell. A condition in which the nail plate is soft and semitransparent, bends easily, and splits at the end. Associated with arthritis, peripheral neuritis, leprosy, and hemiplegia. May be the only visible sign of late syphilis.

n., fungal infections of. Infections of the nails by one of a number of fungi. Systemic therapy with griseofulvin is helpful but may need to be used 6 to 12 months for fingernails and 12 to 18 months for toenails.

n., habit deformity. Disruption of the nail surface by the habit of abrading or stroking that area. This produces a wavy or washboard-like nail surface.

n., hang. Broken epidermis at edge of the nail.

n., ingrown. Growth of the nail edge into the soft tissue, thus causing inflammation and sometimes an abscess. May be due to improper paring of the nail or pressure on the nail edge from improperly fitted shoes. In many cases, this condition may be prevented by cutting the nail(s) straight across rather than curved.

n., intermedullary. Surgical rod inserted into the intermedullary canal to act as an immobilization device to hold the two ends of a fractured long bone in position.

n., reedy. Nail marked by longitudinal fissures.

n., Smith-Petersen. A three-flanged nail employed to fix fractures of the neck of the femur.

n., splitting. A troublesome condition in which the brittle nails split easily. Polishing, buffing, or abrading the nail surface will weaken the nail; thus, these practices should be discouraged. Brittle nails should be soaked prior to cutting them. A bath oil soak is best for this.

n., spoon. Nail with central portion depressed and lateral edges elevated. May follow trauma to the nail fold or iron deficiency anemia, or may be present in normal persons. SYN: *koilonychia.*

nailbed. The portion of a finger or toe covered by the nail. SYN: *nail matrix.*

nail biting. A nervous affliction or neurosis in which the free edges of the nails are bitten down. SYN: *onychophagy.*

nail fold. Groove in the cutaneous tissue surrounding the margins and proximal edges of the nail.

nail groove. Space between the nail wall and the nailbed.

nailing. Fixing fragments of bone by use of a nail.

nail matrix. Nailbed.

...ycho-osteodys-

... of nail covered by

...overing edges of the
...nguis.

...dian cobra, a poisonous

na... ... AS *naced*, nude]. Uncovered, exp... ...w, nude, bare, devoid of clothing.

Nalfon. Trade name for fenoprofen calcium.

nalidixic acid. USP. An antibiotic used in treating certain urinary tract infections. Trade names are NegGram, Wintomylon, and Cybis.

nalorphine hydrochloride (năl-or′fēn). USP. A narcotic antagonist used in treatment of certain kinds of narcotic overdose, esp. with morphine.

naloxone hydrochloride (năl-ŏks′ōn). USP. A drug that prevents or reverses the action of morphine and other opioid drugs. Its most important use is treatment of narcotic overdose. Trade name is Narcan.

NANDA. *North American Nursing Diagnosis Association.*

nandrolone decanoate (năn′drō-lōn). USP. An anabolic androgenic steroid. Trade name is Deca-Durabolin.

nandrolone phenpropionate. USP. An anabolic androgenic steroid. Trade name is Durabolin.

nanism (nā′nĭzm) [L. *nanus*, dwarf, + Gr. *-ismos*, condition]. Condition of being dwarflike in build. SYN: *nanosomia.*

n., symptomatic. Nanism with deficient dentition, sexual development, and ossification.

nano- (nā′nō) [L. *nanus*, dwarf]. Prefix indicating one billionth (10^{-9}) of the unit following; thus, a nanogram is one billionth (10^{-9}) of a gram.

nanocephalism (nā-nō-sĕf′ăl-ĭzm) [″ + Gr. *kephale*, head, + *-ismos*, condition]. Condition of having an abnormally small head.

nanocephalous (nā-nō-sĕf′ă-lŭs). Having an abnormally small head.

nanocormia (nā″nō-kor′mē-ă) [L. *nanus*, dwarf, + Gr. *kormos*, trunk]. Abnormally dwarfed thorax or body.

nanocurie (nā″nō-kū′rē). A unit of radioactivity equal to 10^{-9} curie.

nanogram. One billionth (10^{-9}) of a gram. SEE: *picogram.*

nanoid (nā′noyd) [″ + Gr. *eidos*, form, shape]. Dwarflike.

nanomelus (nă-nŏm′ĕ-lŭs) [″ + Gr. *melos*, limb]. Fetus with congenital deformity characterized by undersized extremities.

nanometer (nā″nō-mē′tĕr). A unit of length

equal to 10^{-9} meter.

nanophthalmos (năn″ŏf-thăl′mŭs) [″ + Gr. *ophthalmos*, eye]. Abnormal smallness of one or both eyes. SYN: *microphthalmia.*

nanosecond (nā″nō-sĕk′ŏnd). A unit of time measurement equal to 10^{-9} second.

nanosoma, nanosomia (nā″nō-sō′mă, nā-nō-sō′mē-ă) [L. *nanus*, dwarf, + Gr. *soma*, body]. State of being a dwarf. SYN: *nanism.*

nanosomus (nā-nō-sō′mŭs). A person of stunted size; a dwarf.

nanous (nā′nŭs) [L. *nanus*, dwarf]. Dwarfed or stunted.

nanukayami (nā″nū-kă-yă′mē). A form of leptospirosis present in Japan.

nanus (nā′nŭs) [L.]. 1. A dwarf. 2. Stunted; dwarflike.

NaOH. Sodium hydroxide.

nap (năp) [AS. *hnappian*, nap]. 1. To slumber. 2. A short sleep; a doze. SEE: *sleep.*

napalm (nā′pălm) [from *naphthene* + *palmitate*]. Gasoline made thick or jelly-like for use in incendiary bombs and flame throwers.

napalm burn. Burn due to use of napalm, usually during war.

nape (năp, năp) [origin uncertain]. Back of neck. SYN: *nucha; scruff.*

napex (nā′pĕks) [origin uncertain]. Scalp beneath the occipital protuberance.

naphazoline hydrochloride (năf-ăz′ō-lēn). USP. A vasoconstrictor drug used topically esp. on nasal mucosa. Trade names are Privine Hydrochloride, Albalon Liquifilm, and Vasocon.

naphtha (năf′thă). 1. A volatile inflammable liquid distilled from carbonaceous substances. 2. Petroleum, esp. more volatile varieties.

naphthalene (năf′thă-lēn). $C_{10}H_8$. A hydrocarbon, one of principal constituents of coal tar. SEE: *Poisons and Poisoning* in Appendix.

USES: As a disinfectant, in moth balls, and in manufacture of dyes and explosives.

naphthol (năf′thōl). $C_{10}H_8O$. Petroleum substance used as an antiseptic and in certain dyes. It is prepared from naphthalene.

napiform (nā′pĭ-form) [L. *napus*, turnip, + *forma*, shape]. In bacteriology, formed like a turnip, as gelatin liquefaction in a culture.

N.A.P.N.A.P. *National Association of Pediatric Nurse Associates and Practitioners.*

N.A.P.N.E.S. *National Association for Practical Nurse Education and Services.*

Naprosyn. Trade name for naproxen, USP.

N.A.P.T. *National Association of Physical Therapists.*

Naqua. Trade name for trichlormethiazide.

Narcan. Trade name for naloxone hydrochloride, USP.

narcissism (năr'sĭs-ĭzm) [Narcissus, a Gr. mythical character who fell in love with his own reflection]. 1. Self-love or self-admiration. 2. Sexual pleasure derived from observing one's own naked body.

narcissistic (năr-sĭs-sĭst'ĭk). Pert. to narcissism.

narcissistic object choice. Selection of another like one's own self as the object of love, friendship, or liking.

narco- [Gr. *narke*, numbness]. Combining form meaning numbness, stupor.

narcoanalysis (năr"kō-ă-năl'ĭ-sĭs) [" + *analysis*, a dissolving]. A form of psychotherapy in which light anesthesia is produced by use of I.V. barbiturates. Patients are encouraged to talk about their experiences and may discuss events that would ordinarily be suppressed.

narcoanesthesia (nar"kō-ăn-ĕs-thē'zē-ă). Anesthesia produced by a narcotic, as scopolamine and morphine.

narcohypnia (năr"kō-hĭp'nē-ă) [Gr. *narke*, numbness, + *hypnos*, sleep]. Numbness following sleep.

narcohypnosis (năr"kō-hĭp-nō'sĭs). Stupor or deep sleep produced by hypnosis.

narcolepsy (năr'kō-lĕp"sē) [Gr. *narke*, numbness, + *lepsis*, seizure]. A chronic ailment consisting of recurrent attacks of drowsiness and sleep during daytime. More than 125,000 people in the U.S. have narcolepsy. The patient is unable to control these spells of sleep but is easily awakened. These attacks may be distinguished from ordinary drowsiness following a meal by the frequency of occurrence of attacks in narcolepsy, their irresistibility, and their happening in unusual circumstances, such as while eating, standing, or conversing.

About 40% of these patients will have some form of cataplexy, i.e., sudden loss of muscle tone brought on by some strong emotion such as laughter, surprise, or anger. The knees may buckle, the head will fall forward, and the person may fall to the ground but remain conscious.

DIAG: Results of the Multiple Sleep Latency Test are positive in that the patient falls asleep within less than 5 minutes if asked to try to sleep at 2-hour intervals throughout the day. In addition, there will be abnormalities of rapid eye movement (REM) sleep during at least two of these sleep periods.

Narcolepsy occurs in families and is probably controlled by a specific gene. It is also present as a familial disorder in cats, certain breeds of dogs, ponies, quarterhorses, and Brahma bulls. Except for frequent sleep patterns, the electroencephalogram is normal. SEE: *sleep, disorders of.*

TREAT: Symptomatic with dr... as ephedrine or dextroamphetamine su... or methylphenidate hydrochloride. In addition, 15-minute naps planned to coincide with known time of occurrence of drowsiness will help.

Caution: Patients with this illness must be warned to avoid participation in activities that require constant alertness, i.e., driving, or employment in security guard jobs. Drivers with narcolepsy should, at the first sign of drowsiness, park the vehicle and take a nap.

narcoleptic (năr-kō-lĕp'tĭk) [" + *lepsis*, seizure]. Pert. to or marked by an overwhelming desire to sleep.

narcomatous (năr-kō'mă-tŭs) [Gr. *narke*, numbness, + *koma*, coma]. Pert. to a state of stupor from use of narcotics.

narcosis [Gr. *narkosis*, a benumbing]. Unconscious state due to narcotics. SYN: *narcotism.*

    n., basal. Initial narcosis produced by sedatives used prior to administration of a general anesthetic.

    n., medullary. General anesthesia induced by a local anesthetic injected in the sheath of the spinal cord in lumbar region. SYN: *spinal anesthesia.*

narcosynthesis (năr"kō-sĭn'thĕ-sĭs) [" + *synthesis*, synthesis]. Narcoanalysis.

narcotic [Gr. *narkotikos*, benumbing]. 1. Producing stupor or sleep. 2. A drug that in moderate doses depresses the central nervous system, thus relieving pain and producing sleep, but that in excessive doses produces unconsciousness, stupor, coma, and possibly death. SEE: *pain.* Ex.: opium, morphine, codeine, papaverine, heroin, and many synthetics. Most are habit-forming. 3. Anything that soothes, relieves, or lulls. 4. One addicted to the use of narcotics.

    RS: drug action; drug addiction; drug dependence; drug reaction; drugs and their administration; narcotism; overdose (O.D.).

narcotic addict. One who has become physiologically or psychologically dependent upon narcotics. SEE: *drug addiction.*

narcotic poisoning. Caused by narcotic or sleep-producing poisons such as opium and its derivatives, chloral combinations, or barbital and its myriad subvarieties.

    SYM: Depression, slowing of heart rate and respiration, and sleep, followed by coma.

    F.A.: Remove poison by gastric lavage. Administer nalorphine if poisoning is due to a derivative of opium such as morphine.

narcotism (năr'kō-tĭzm) [Gr. *narke*, stupor, + *-ismos*, condition]. 1. State of stupor induced by a narcotic. SYN: *narcosis.* 2. An addiction to the use of narcotics. Addiction may be said to exist when discontinuance causes abstinence symptoms that are speedily relieved by a dose of the drug.

TREAT: Ordinarily successful only during hospitalization. Relapses are frequent, and the adoption of an alternate philosophy of life is of prime importance.

narcotize [Gr. *narkotikos,* benumbing]. To place under the influence of a narcotic.

Nardil. Trade name for phenelzine sulfate.

naris (nā′rĭs) [L.] (pl. *nares).* [NA] The nostril. SEE: *nose.*

     n., anterior. External nostril.

     n., posterior. The opening between the nasal cavity and the nasopharynx.

     RS: anosmia; epistaxis; hyperosmia; nasal; parosmia; septum; smell.

narrowing. Decreasing the width or diameter of some space or channel, e.g., narrowing of the size of the coronary arteries, usually due to some pathological process.

NASA. *National Aeronautics and Space Administration.*

nasal (nā′zl) [L. *nasus,* nose]. 1. Pert. to the nose. 2. Uttered through the nose. 3. A nasal bone.

nasal bleeding. SEE: *epistaxis.*

nasal bones. The two small bones forming the arch of the nose.

nasal cartilages. Cartilages forming the principal portion of the framework of the external nose.

nasal cavity. Cavity between floor of cranium and roof of mouth. SEE: illus.

nasal concha (pl. *nasal conchae).* SEE: *concha, nasal.*

nasal douche. Injection of fluid into nostril with fluid escaping by way of the nasopharynx out of the mouth. Patient should keep mouth open and glottis closed to prevent fluid from entering the throat and bronchus. Force must not be great. Atomized spray is faster. Container should not be suspended more than 6 in. (9.2 cm) above patient, who should not blow the nose during treatment.

nasal feeding. Administration of liquid foods through a tube passing through the nose to the stomach. It is employed when this route is the only one available or when the patient refuses to eat. SYN: *nasal gavage.* SEE: *feeding, tube.*

nasal fossa. One of the two halves of the nasal cavity.

nasal gavage. Nasal feeding, q.v.

nasal height. Distance between lower border of nasal aperture and the nasion.

nasal index. The greatest width of the nasal aperture in relation to a line from the lower edge of the nasal aperture to the nasion.

nasal line. Line from lower edge of the ala nasi curving to outer side of the orbicularis oris muscle. SEE: *Jadelot's line.*

nasal meatus. SEE: *meatus.*

nasal obstruction. Commonest causes: irregular septum; enlarged turbinates; nasal polypi; in children, foreign bodies such as food, buttons, or pins. Complications such as infections, sinusitis, and otitis may develop.

TREAT: Nasal douches, inhalations, and operative care: resection of septum; turbinectomy; removal of polypi; opening and draining sinuses; removal of foreign body.

nasal reflex. Sneezing resulting from irritation of nasal mucosa.

nasal septum. A wall or septum between the two nasal cavities. SEE: *nasal cavity* for illus.

nasal sinuses, accessory. The paranasal sinuses, q.v. SEE: *sinuses, accessory nasal.*

nasal width. Maximum width of nasal aperture.

nascent (năs′ĕnt; nā′sĕnt) [L. *nascens,* born]. 1. Just born; incipient or beginning. 2. Pert. to a substance being set free from a compound.

nasioiniac (nā″zē-ō-ĭn′ē-ăk) [L. *nasus,* nose, + Gr. *inion,* back of the head]. Concerning the nasion and inion.

nasion (nā′zē-ŏn) [L. *nasus,* nose]. The point at which the nasofrontal suture is cut across by the median anteroposterior plane.

nasitis (nā-zī′tĭs) [″ + Gr. *itis,* inflammation]. Inflammation of the nose. SEE: *rhinitis.*

Nasmyth's membrane (năz′mĭths) [Alexander Nasmyth, Scottish dental surgeon, died 1847]. Epithelial membrane that envelops the enamel of a tooth for a short period after birth.

naso- [L. *nasus,* nose]. Combining form pert. to the nose.

nasoantral (nā″zō-ăn′trăl) [″ + Gr. *antrum,* cavity]. Concerning the nose and maxillary antrum, or sinus.

nasoantritis (nā″zō-ăn-trī′tĭs) [″ + ″ + *itis,* inflammation]. Inflammation of the nose and antrum of Highmore.

nasociliary (nā″zō-sĭl′ē-ār-ē). Pert. to the nose, eyebrow, and eyes. Applied esp. to nerve supplying these structures.

nasofrontal [″ + *frontalis,* forehead]. Pert. to nasal and frontal bones.

nasogastric tube (nā″zō-găs′trĭk) [″ + Gr. *gaster,* belly]. A tube inserted through the nose and extending into the stomach. It may be used for emptying the stomach of gas and liquids or for administering liquids to the patient.

nasolabial [″ + *labium,* lip]. Connected with or rel. to the nose and lip.

nasolacrimal (nā″zō-lăk′rĭm-ăl) [″ + *lac-*

TWO VIEWS OF NASAL CAVITY

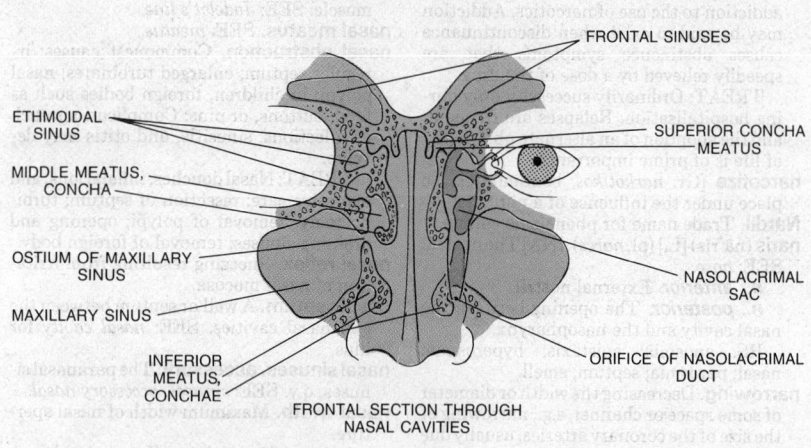

FRONTAL SINUSES

ETHMOIDAL SINUS

SUPERIOR CONCHA
MEATUS

MIDDLE MEATUS, CONCHA

OSTIUM OF MAXILLARY SINUS

NASOLACRIMAL SAC

MAXILLARY SINUS

INFERIOR MEATUS, CONCHAE

ORIFICE OF NASOLACRIMAL DUCT

FRONTAL SECTION THROUGH NASAL CAVITIES

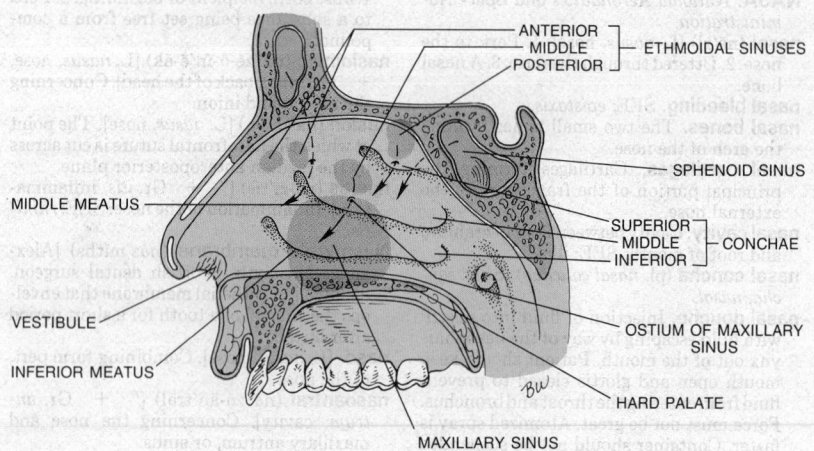

ANTERIOR
MIDDLE — ETHMOIDAL SINUSES
POSTERIOR

SPHENOID SINUS

MIDDLE MEATUS

SUPERIOR
MIDDLE — CONCHAE
INFERIOR

VESTIBULE

OSTIUM OF MAXILLARY SINUS

INFERIOR MEATUS

HARD PALATE

MAXILLARY SINUS

VIEW TOWARD NASAL SEPTUM FROM LATERAL AREA OF THE NOSE

rima, tear]. Pert. to the nose and lacrimal apparatus.

nasology (nā-zŏl′ō-jē) [″ + Gr. *logos*, word, reason]. Study of the nose and its diseases.

nasomental (nā″zō-mĕn′tăl) [″ + *mentum*, chin]. Pert. to the nose and chin.

nasomental reflex. Contraction of mentalis muscle with elevation of lower lip and wrinkling of skin of chin. Elicited by percussion of side of nose.

naso-oral (nā″zō-ō′răl) [″ + *oralis*, pert. to

the mouth]. Concerning the nose and oral cavity.

nasopalatine (nā″zō-păl′ă-tĭn) [L. *nasus*, nose, + *palatum*, palate]. Pert. to both nose and palate.

nasopharyngeal (nā″zō-făr-ĭn′jē-ăl) [″ + Gr. *pharynx*, throat]. Pert. to the pharynx and nose.

nasopharyngeal airway, maintenance of. By means of a flexible tube that is inserted into the nose of an unresponsive patient and rests above the hypopharynx, the airway is maintained. Used in patients with intact gag reflexes to prevent retching during attempt to maintain an air passage.

nasopharyngitis (nā″zō-făr-ĭn-jī′tĭs) [″ + ″ + *itis,* inflammation]. Inflamed condition of the nasopharynx.

nasopharyngography. Radiographic examination of the nasopharynx.

nasopharyngoscope. Device used to visualize the nasal passage and pharynx.

nasopharynx (nā″zō-făr′ĭnks) [L. *nasus,* nose, + Gr. *pharynx,* throat]. Part of pharynx situated above the soft palate (postnasal space).

nasorostral (nā″zō-rŏs′trăl) [″ + *rostralis,* resembling a beak]. Concerning the rostrum of the nose.

nasoscope (nā′zō-skōp) [″ + Gr. *skopein,* to examine]. Instrument for examination of the nasal cavity.

nasoseptitis (nā″zō-sĕp-tī′tĭs) [″ + *saeptum,* partition, + Gr. *itis,* inflammation]. Inflamed condition of the nasal septum.

nasosinusitis (nā″zō-sī″nū-sī′tĭs) [″ + *sinus,* cavity]. Inflammation of the nasal accessory sinuses and cavities.

nasospinale (nā″zō-spīn′ăl-ē). Point at which median sagittal plane intersects line joining lowest points on nasal margins.

nasotracheal intubation. Insertion of an endotracheal tube via the nose. Unlike orotracheal intubation, the tube is passed "blindly" without using a laryngoscope to visualize the glottic opening. It is useful in cases of cervical spinal trauma because it can be done without hyperextension, and also in patients who have clenched teeth.

nasus (nā′sŭs) [L.]. [NA] The nose, organ for respiration and sense of smell. SEE: *nose.*

Natacyn. Trade name for natamycin, USP.

natal (nā′tăl). 1. [L. *natus,* birth]. Pert. to birth or the day of birth. 2. [L. *nates,* buttocks]. Pert. to the buttocks.

natality [L. *natalis,* birth]. The birth rate; ratio of births to population of a given community.

natamycin (năt″ă-mī′sĭn). USP. An antibiotic agent used topically. Trade name is Natacyn.

natant (nā′tănt) [L. *natare,* to swim]. Floating; swimming.

nates (nā′tēz) [L.] (sing. *natis*). 1. [NA] Gluteal region; fleshy prominences on the lower back formed by the gluteal muscles with a covering of fat and skin. SYN: *buttocks.* 2. The anterior, superior, or upper two corpora quadrigemina.

natimortality (nā″tĭ-mor-tăl′ĭ-tē) [L. *natus,* birth, + *mortalitas,* death]. Rate of stillbirths in proportion to birth rate.

National Formulary. ABBR: NF. Formulary originally issued by the American Pharmaceutical Association. Now published by the U.S. Pharmacopeial Convention, Inc. Included in it are drugs of established usefulness that are not in the U.S. Pharmacopeia.

National League for Nursing. An organization originally formed from three other nursing organizations that merged. The principal interest of the League is in the areas of nursing education and service.

National Institute on Aging. ABBR: NIA. An institute created in 1974 by Congress. Under the National Institutes of Health, the NIA conducts and supports biomedical, social, and behavioral research and training related to aging.

National Practitioner Data Bank. ABBR: NPDB. The mandatory reporting in the U.S. of all payments by or on behalf of physicians as a result of medical malpractice settlements or judgments. The NPDB collects information regarding the professional conduct and competence of physicians (MD and DO), dentists, and in some cases other licensed health care professionals. The data are collected from a medical malpractice payment report (MMPR) which the physician or insurance company must submit within 30 days from the date payment is made. If a physician pays a patient in response to the patient's oral demand for money, the MMPR is not prepared.

Nationally Registered Emergency Medical Technician. ABBR: N.R.E.M.T. This designation is awarded after successful completion of written, practical and oral examination.

National Marrow Donor Program. ABBR: NMDP. Coordinating center for bone marrow donors. Phone 1-800-654-1247.

National Organization for Rare Disorders. ABBR: NORD. An organization created by a group of voluntary agencies, medical researchers, and individuals concerned about orphan diseases and orphan drugs. Orphan diseases are rare, debilitating illnesses that strike small numbers of people. Orphan drugs are therapies that alleviate symptoms of some rare diseases, but have not been developed by the pharmaceutical industry because they are unprofitable.

Rare Disease Database articles are available from NORD. Persons with personal computers may access the database directly through the NORD services section of CompuServe by typing "GO RDB" at any prompt on the CompuService Information System.

NORD's address is P.O. Box 8423, New Fairfield, CT 06812, phone (203) 746-6518.

native (nā′tĭv) [L. *nativus*]. 1. Born with; inherent. 2. Natural, normal. SYN: *indige-*

nous. 3. Belonging to, as place of one's birth.

Native American. An American Indian.

natremia (nă-trē′mē-ă) [L. *natrium*, sodium, + Gr. *haima*, blood]. Sodium in the blood.

natrium (nā′trē-ŭm) [L.]. SYMB: Na. Sodium.

natriuresis (nā″trē-ū-rē′sĭs) [″ + Gr. *ouresis*, make water]. The excretion of abnormal amounts of sodium in the urine. SEE: *aldosterone*.

natriuretic (nā″trē-ūr-ĕt′ĭk). A drug that increases rate of excretion of sodium in the urine. SEE: *diuretic*.

natron. Sodium carbonate.

natural [L. *natura*, nature]. Not abnormal or artificial.

natural childbirth. SEE: *childbirth, natural*.

natural killer cells. ABBR: NK cells. Large granular lymphocytes that bond to cells and lyse them by releasing cytotoxins. NK cells are known to be effective against cells infected with viruses and some types of tumor cells. Proliferation of NK cells is produced by gamma interferon, interleukin-2, antibodies, retinoic acid, and prostaglandin-E.

natural selection. A mechanism of evolution, q.v., proposed by Charles Darwin. It states that the tendency for survival and reproduction of organisms is most likely to occur in those who are best adapted to their environment.

nature and nurture. The combination of an individual's genetic constitution and the environmental conditions to which he or she is exposed. The interplay of these effects produces physical and mental characteristics that make each human being different from another. In many cases, it is not readily apparent which of these effects is the more important in producing a particular characteristic.

Naturetin. Trade name for bendroflumethiazide, USP.

naturopath (nā′tūr-ō-păth) [″ + Gr. *pathos*, disease, suffering]. One who practices naturopathy.

naturopathy (nā″tūr-ŏp′ă-thē). A therapeutic system that does not use drugs but employs natural forces such as light, heat, air, water, and massage.

nausea (naw′sē-ă) [Gr. *nausia*, seasickness]. Unpleasant sensation usually preceding vomiting. It is present in seasickness, early pregnancy, diseases of the central nervous system, neurasthenia, or hysteria. It may be due to the sight or odor of obnoxious matter or conditions or to mental images of same. It may be present, without vomiting, in certain gallbladder disturbances, in carsickness, and in other types of motion sickness.

NURSING IMPLICATIONS: Remove any materials or environmental factors that precipitate the nausea. Note frequency, time, amount, and characteristics of emesis. Test vomitus for blood when indicated. Record and report any pertinent factors to physician. Provide oral hygiene and comfort measures to patient. SEE: *vomitus*.

n. gravidarum. Morning sickness of pregnancy.

n. navalis. Seasickness. SYN: *mal de mer*.

nauseant (naw′shē-ănt, naw′sē-ănt). 1. Provoking nausea. 2. That which causes nausea.

nauseate (naw′shē-āt, naw′sē-āt). To cause nausea.

nauseous (naw′shŭs, naw′shē-ŭs). 1. Producing nausea, disgust, or loathing. 2. Affected with nausea.

Navane Hydrochloride. Trade name for thiothixene hydrochloride.

navel (nā′vĕl) [AS. *nafela*]. The depression or scar in the center of the abdomen where the umbilical cord was attached to the fetus. SYN: *umbilicus*.

navicula (nă-vĭk′ū-lă) [L. *navicula*, boat]. Fossa navicularis, q.v.

navicular (nă-vĭk′ū-lăr). 1. Shaped like a boat. 2. Scaphoid bones in the carpus (wrist) and in the tarsus (ankle). SEE: *skeleton*.

navicular fossa. Fossa navicularis.

Nb. Chem. symb. for the element niobium (formerly columbium).

nc. *nanocurie*.

N.C.A.P. *National Coalition for Action in Politics*.

N.C.I. *National Cancer Institute*.

NCLEX. *National Council Licensure Examination*.

Nd. Chem. symb. for the element neodymium.

N.D.A. *National Dental Association*.

Ne. Chem. symb. for the element neon.

near-death experience. ABBR: NDE. The account of their perceptions by persons who have experienced actually coming close to death. Some of these persons believe that they have had a glimpse of the situation of life after death. These accounts may reveal more about psychological events than death. SEE: *out-of-body experience*.

near-drowning. Persons who live following an immersion incident that could have produced fatal drowning. SEE: *drowning*.

near point. ABBR: n.p. Closest point of distinct vision with maximum accommodation. It recedes with age, varying from about 3 in. (7.62 cm) at 2 yr to 40 in. (101.60 cm) at 60 yr. SYN: *punctum proximum*.

nearsight. Ability to see clearly only those objects held close to the eye. SYN: *myopia*. SEE: *nearsighted*.

nearsighted. Able to see clearly only those objects held close to the eye. Caused by error in refraction in which rays are focused in front of the retina. A negative (concave) lens of proper strength will correct this condition. SYN: *myopic*.

RS: eye; eyeball; farsightedness; hypermetropia; hyperopia; lens; presbyopia.

nearsightedness. Error in refraction in which rays are focused in front of the retina; thus the person is able to see distinctly for only a short distance. A negative (concave) lens of proper strength will correct this condition. SYN: *myopia*.

nearthrosis (nē″ăr-thrō′sĭs) [Gr. *neos*, new, + *arthron*, joint, + *osis*, condition]. A false joint or abnormal articulation. SYN: *neoarthrosis*.

Nebcin. Trade name for tobramycin sulfate (sterile).

nebula (nĕb′ū-lă) [L., mist, cloud] (pl. *nebulae*). 1. Slight haziness on the cornea. 2. Cloudiness in urine. 3. Aqueous or oily substance for use in an atomizer.

nebulization. Production of particles such as a spray or mist from liquid. The size of particles produced depends upon the method used. SEE: *nebulizer*.

nebulizer (nĕb′ū-lī″zĕr) [L. *nebula*, mist]. An apparatus for producing a fine spray or mist. This may be done by rapidly passing air through a liquid or by vibrating a liquid at a high frequency so that the particles produced are extremely small. SEE: *aerosol; atomizer; vaporizer*.

NEC. *necrotizing enterocolitis*.

Necator (nē-kā′tor) [L., murderer]. A genus of nematode hookworms belonging to the family Ancylostomidae.

    N. americanus. A species of hookworm widely distributed in tropical regions and common in the southern United States. Adults live in the small intestine of man attached to mucosa by their mouths. Adults lay eggs, which pass out with feces and under proper conditions of warmth and moisture hatch within 24 hours into rhabditiform larvae. After two molts, the larvae become strongyliform. After two more molts occurring within five days, they become infective larvae. They enter the body through the skin, enter the venous system, and are carried to the lungs. Here they burrow into air spaces, from which they pass via bronchial tubes and trachea to the pharynx, from which they are expectorated or swallowed. If swallowed, they reach the intestine, bury themselves among the villi, molt again, acquire a mouth part, and attach themselves to the mucosa. Worms may live 5 years. Disease is contracted by walking barefoot or otherwise exposing the skin to soil that has been contaminated by feces of persons infected with the worm.

    SYM: Anemia, weakness, failure to grow.

LATERAL ASPECT OF THE NECK

    DIAG: Microscopic examination of preparation of feces reveals eggs of the worm.

    TREAT: Mebendazole (trade name Vermox) is the drug of choice. Pyrantel pamoate is also effective. If anemia is severe blood transfusion may be required.

    RS: Ancylostoma; ancylostomiasis; hookworm.

necatoriasis (nē-kā″tō-rī′ă-sĭs). Infestation by *Necator americanus*. SEE: *ancylostomiasis*.

neck [AS. *hnecca*, nape]. 1. Part of body between the head and shoulders. SEE: illus.; *muscle* for illus. 2. The constricted portion of an organ, or that resembling a neck. 3. Region between crown and root of a tooth.

    n., anatomical, of humerus. Constriction just below the head of the humerus.

    n., Madelung's. Diffuse lipoma of the neck.

    n. of femur. The heavy column of bone that connects the head of the femur to the shaft.

    n. of mandible. The constricted area below the articular condyle, the area of attachment for the articular capsule and the lateral pterygoid muscle.

    n. of tooth. The constricted area that

connects the crown of a tooth to the root of a tooth.

n. of uterus. The cervix uteri.

n., surgical, of humerus. Narrow part of humerus below the tuberosity. Fracture here is common.

n., webbed. A broad neck as seen anteriorly or posteriorly. The breadth is due to a fold of skin that extends from the clavicle to the head. This is present in Turner's syndrome.

n., wry-. Torsion of the neck caused by contracted muscles. SYN: *torticollis.*

neck conformer. Splint, usually fabricated of thermoplastic material, that positions the neck to prevent flexion contractures due to burns of the anterior neck.

necklace, Casal's. In pellagra, a ring of pigmented, reddened skin around the neck.

neck-righting reflex. SEE: *reflex, neck-righting.*

necrectomy (nĕ-krĕk'tō-mē) [Gr. *nekros,* corpse, + *ektome,* excision]. Surgical removal of necrotic tissue.

necro- [Gr. *nekros,* corpse]. Combining form meaning pert. to death, dead cells or tissue.

necrobiosis (nĕk-rō-bī-ō'sĭs) [" + *biosis,* life]. Gradual degeneration and swelling of collagen bundles in the dermis. SEE: *necrosis.*

n. lipoidica diabeticorum. A skin disease characterized by necrobiosis of connective and elastic tissue and discoloration of skin. Common in diabetics.

necrobiotic (nĕ"krō-bī-ŏt'ĭk). Pert. to or affected by necrobiosis.

necrocytotoxin (nĕk"rō-sī'tō-tŏks'ĭn). A toxin that causes death of cells.

necrogenic, necrogenous (nĕ-krō-jĕn'ĭk, -krŏj'ĕn-ŭs) [" + *gennan,* to produce]. Caused by, pert. to, or originating in dead matter.

necrologist (nĕk-rŏl'ō-jĭst) [" + *logos,* word, reason]. A student of mortality statistics.

necrology (nĕk-rŏl'ō-jē). The study of mortality statistics.

necrolysis (nĕ-krŏl'ĭ-sĭs) [" + *lysis,* dissolution]. Necrosis and dissolution of tissue.

necromania (nĕk-rō-mā'nē-ă) [" + *mania,* madness]. Abnormal interest in dead bodies or in death.

necromimesis (nĕk"rō-mī-mē'sĭs) [" + *mimesis,* imitation]. A delusion in which one believes oneself to be dead or acts as though one were dead.

necronectomy (nĕk-rō-nĕk'tō-mē) [" + *ektome,* excision]. Excision of a necrotic part, esp. of necrotic ossicles.

necroparasite (nĕk"rō-păr'ă-sīt) [" + *para,* beside, + *sitos,* food]. Saprophyte.

necrophagous (nĕ-krŏf'ă-gŭs) [" + *pha-*

gein, to eat]. Feeding or existing on dead bodies or matter.

necrophile (nĕk'rō-fīl) [" + *philein,* to love]. One who has a morbid interest in dead bodies or who has intercourse with corpses.

necrophilia (nĕk"rō-fīl'ē-ă) [" + *philein,* to love]. 1. Abnormal concern with corpses. 2. Sexual intercourse with a dead body.

necrophilic (nĕk"rō-fīl'ĭk) [" + *philein,* to love]. 1. Concerning necrophilism. 2. Descriptive of bacteria that prefer dead tissue.

necrophilism (nĕk-rŏf'ĭl-ĭzm). Sexual perversion in which there is insane love for, or intercourse with, the dead.

necrophilous (nĕk-rŏf'ĭl-ŭs). 1. Having a morbid fondness for, or feeding on, dead tissue. 2. Pert. to or affected with necrophilism.

necrophobia (nĕk-rō-fō'bē-ă) [" + *phobos,* fear]. 1. Abnormal aversion to dead bodies. 2. Insane dread of death. SYN: *thanatophobia.*

necropneumonia (nĕk"rō-nū-mō'nē-ă) [" + *pneumon,* lung]. Pulmonary gangrene.

necropsy (nĕk'rŏp-sē) [" + *opsis,* view]. Examination of a dead body to determine cause of death or pathological conditions. SYN: *autopsy; necroscopy; postmortem examination.*

necrosadism (nĕk"rō-sā'dĭzm) [" + *sadism*]. Sexual gratification derived from the mutilation of dead bodies.

necroscopy (nĕ-krŏs'kō-pē) [" + *skopein,* to examine]. Examination of a dead body to find cause of death or pathological condition. SYN: *autopsy; necropsy; postmortem examination.*

necrose (nĕk-rōs') [Gr. *nekroun,* to make dead]. To cause or to undergo necrosis.

necrosis (nĕ-krō'sĭs) [Gr. *nekrosis,* state of death] (pl. *necroses*). Death of areas of tissue or bone surrounded by healthy parts; death in mass as distinguished from necrobiosis, which is a gradual degeneration. The dead part in bone is called a sequestrum; in soft tissue it is called a slough or sphacelus. Term is usually applied to bone destruction or small areas of tissue, while gangrene is generally applied to destruction of specific parts or larger areas. SYN: *gangrene; mortification.*

ETIOL: Insufficient blood supply; physical agents such as trauma, radiant energy (electricity, infrared, ultraviolet, roentgen, and radium rays); chemical agents acting locally, acting internally following absorption, or placed into the wrong tissue. For example, some medicines cause necrosis if injected into the tissues rather than the vein, and iron dextran causes necrosis if injected into areas other than deep muscle or vein.

n., anemic. Necrosis caused by disturbed circulation in a part.

n., aseptic. Necrosis occurring without infection.

n., Balser's fatty. Pancreatitis with gangrenous areas in the fatty tissues.

n., caseous. N., cheesy.

n., central. Necrosis that affects only the center of a part.

n., cheesy. Necrosis with soft, dry, cheeselike formation. Usually seen in tuberculosis or syphilis. SYN: *n., caseous.*

n., coagulation. Necrosis occurring esp. in infarcts in which coagulation occurs in necrotic area, converting it into a homogenous mass and depriving the organ or tissue of blood. SYN: *n., fibrinous.*

n., colliquative. Necrosis caused by liquefaction of tissue due to autolysis or bacterial putrefaction. SYN: *n., liquefactive.*

n., dry. Necrosis with dryness of the sequestrum.

n., embolic. Necrosis resulting from an embolus, which causes anemic necrosis.

n., fat. Necrosis in small scattered areas in the fatty tissue.

n., fibrinous. N., coagulation.

n., focal. Necrosis in small scattered areas, often seen in infection.

n., gummatous. Necrosis resulting from syphilis forming a dry rubbery mass.

n., ischemic. N., coagulation.

n., liquefactive. N., colliquative.

n., medial. Necrosis of cells in tunica media of an artery.

n., moist. Necrosis with softening and moist condition of the dead tissue.

n., postpartum pituitary. Necrosis of the pituitary gland following childbirth. The cause of Sheehan's syndrome, q.v.

n., putrefactive. Necrosis caused by bacterial decomposition.

n., subcutaneous fat, of newborn. An inflammatory disorder of fat tissue that may occur in the newborn at the site of application of forceps during delivery, and occasionally in premature infants. The cause is unknown.

n., superficial. Necrosis affecting only the outer layers of bone or any tissue.

n., thrombotic. Necrosis due to thrombus formation.

n., total. Necrosis affecting an entire organ or part.

n., Zenker's. SEE: *Zenker's degeneration.*

necrospermia (nĕk-rō-spĕr′mē-ă) [″ + *sperma,* seed]. Condition in which spermatozoa in the ejaculate are immobile or lifeless.

necrotic [Gr. *nekrosis,* state of death]. Rel. to death of a portion of tissue.

necrotizing (nĕk′rō-tīz″ĭng). Causing necrosis.

necrotomy (nĕ-krŏt′ō-mē) [″ + *tome,* incision]. 1. Dissection of a cadaver. 2. Excision of a sequestrum or other necrotic tissue.

necrotoxin (nĕk″rō-tŏk′sĭn) [″ + *toxikon,* poison]. A general term for any toxin that causes necrosis.

need. Something required or wanted, a requisite. Certain elements are essential for the physical and mental health of humans. Included in physical needs are oxygen, water, food, shelter, freedom from fear and physical harm, usually some form of acceptable human (loving) relationship, and stress in its positive sense. Not an absolute need, but highly desirable, is that each individual has some goal no matter how trivial or grandiose, and the feeling that the goal is being attained. Most human beings seem to need some form of physical exercise over and above that required for ordinary daily living.

needle [AS. *naedl*]. A pointed instrument for stitching, ligaturing, or puncturing. It may be straight, half-curved, full-curved, semicircular, double-curved (sometimes called "S-" or sigmoid-shaped), or double-ended. There are two classifications: cutting edge and round point. Cutting edge needles are used in skin and dense tissue, while round point needles are used for more delicate operations.

n., aneurysm. A blunt, curved needle with an eye in tip; used for passing a suture around a vessel.

n., aspirating. A hollow needle, usually fitted to a syringe, for withdrawing fluids from a cavity.

n., atraumatic. Needle of smaller diameter than the suture material. Use of this type of needle causes minimal damage to the tissue being sutured.

n., cataract. Needle used in removing a cataract.

n., discission. A special cataract needle for making multiple cuts into the lens capsule.

n., Hagedorn. A curved, flattened needle with a cutting edge near the end.

n., hypodermic. A hollow needle for administration of hypodermic solutions.

n., knife. A narrow needle-pointed knife.

n., ligature. N., aneurysm, q.v.

n., obturator. Device that fits into the lumen of a needle to prevent blockage during the puncture procedure.

n., Reverdin's. Needle used to carry a suture. It has an eye at the tip that can be opened and closed by use of a lever.

n., stop. Needle with an eye at its tip and a flange or shelf extending out from its shank end. This prevents the needle being inserted any farther than the shelf.

needle-stick injuries. Health care workers are especially at risk for injuring themselves while handling needles. Prevention of this is very important because such injury may expose those involved to infection from diseases transmitted by blood, e.g., AIDS, hepatitis B. SEE: *sharps; Universal Precautions* in *Appendix.*

NEF. *Nurses' Educational Funds.*

NEFA. *nonesterified fatty acids.*

negation (nē-gā′shŭn) [L. *negare,* to deny]. Denial.

negative (nĕg′ă-tĭv) [L. *negare,* to deny]. 1. Possessing a numerical value that is less than zero. 2. Lacking results or indicating an absence, as in a test result. 3. Marked by resistance or retreat.

negative culture. A culture that does not reveal the suspected organism.

negative electrode. The pole by which electric current leaves the generating source.

negative glow. The luminous glow that is adjacent to the cathode in a vacuum tube through which an electrical discharge is passing.

negative sign. Minus sign (−) used in subtraction and to indicate a lack.

negative studies. Investigations in which only negative results are obtained. Such studies may be important in disproving myths or contrary evidence about a drug or therapy.

negativism. Behavior peculiarity marked by not performing suggested actions (passive negativism) or in doing the opposite (active negativism), as seen in some forms of mental illness. A patient may refuse to respond to suggestions because of sluggish mental reflexes or from fear. Retardation may be slow, or sudden and intense, as in manic-depressive insanity. Opposition caused by fear must be considered apart from dementia praecox, in which the patient performs acts directly contrary to those suggested.

negatron (nĕg′ă-trŏn). Negative electron.

NegGram. Trade name for nalidixic acid, USP.

negligence. In forensic medicine, the failure to act as a reasonably prudent person with the same knowledge, experience and background would do under similar circumstances, which causes injury or damage to a person. There are four elements of negligence: duty owed; breach of duty or standard of care; proximate cause or causal connection (between the breach and damages); and damages or injuries. Nurses are legally liable for their own negligence, as well as the negligence of others of which they have knowledge but do not report.

Negri bodies (nā′grē) [Adelchi Negri, It. phy-

sician, 1876–1912]. Very minute bodies formed in nerve cells of the brain of one affected by rabies.

Negro. In anthropology, an individual classified as being a member of the Negro race. Physical characteristics include brown or black skin, dark eyes, and curly hair.

Neisseria (nī-sē′rē-ă) [Albert Neisser, Ger. physician, 1855–1916]. A genus of bacteria belonging to the family Neisseriaceae. They are gram-negative and usually occur in pairs with flattened sides but may occur singly or in irregular groups. The two species most often associated with disease in man are *Neisseria meningitidis* and *Neisseria gonorrhoeae,* which cause meningitis and gonorrhea, respectively.

   N. catarrhalis. SEE: *Branhamella (Neisseria) catarrhalis.*

   N. gonorrhoeae. Species causing gonorrhea. SYN: *gonococcus.* SEE: *gonorrhea.*

   N. meningitidis. Species causing epidemic cerebrospinal meningitis, usually called meningococcal meningitis.

   N. sicca. Species found in mucous membrane of respiratory tract. Occasionally may cause bacterial endocarditis.

Neisseriaceae (nīs-sē′′rē-ā′sē-ē). A family of bacteria that are spherical, gram-negative, and nonmotile. The two genera are *Neisseria* and *Veillonella.*

Nélaton's line (nā-lă-tŏnz′) [Auguste Nélaton, Fr. surgeon, 1807–1873]. Line from the anterior superior spine of the ilium to tuberosity of the ischium.

nemathelminth (nĕm′′ă-thĕl′mĭnth) [Gr. *nema,* thread, + *helmins,* worm]. A roundworm belonging to the phylum Nemathelminthes.

Nemathelminthes (nĕm′′ă-thĕl-mĭn′thēz). The phylum of the roundworm.

nematocide (nĕm′ă-tō-sīd′′) [Gr. *nema,* thread, + L. *caedere,* to kill]. An agent that kills nematode worms.

nematocyst (nĕm′ă-tō-sĭst) [′′ + *kystis,* bladder]. A small stinger present in the cnidoblasts of some coelenterates, including jellyfish and Portuguese man-of-war. It can penetrate the skin upon contact.

Nematoda (nĕm′′ă-tō′dă) [′′ + *eidos,* form, shape]. A class of the phylum Nemathelminthes that includes the true roundworms or threadworms, many species of which are parasitic. They are cylindrical or spindle-shaped worms that possess a resistant cuticle, have a complete alimentary canal, and lack a true coelom. The sexes usually separate, and development usually is direct and simple.

nematode (nĕm′ă-tōd) [Gr. *nema,* thread, + *eidos,* form, shape]. A member of the class Nematoda.

nematodiasis (nĕm″ă-tō-dī′ă-sĭs) [″ + ″ + -iasis, condition]. Infestation by a parasite belonging to the class Nematoda.

nematoid (nĕm′ă-toyd). Threadlike, like a nematode.

nematology (nĕm″ă-tŏl′ō-jē). The division of parasitology that deals with worms belonging to the class Nematoda.

nematospermia (nĕm″ă-tō-spĕr′mē-ă) [″ + sperma, seed]. Spermatozoa with long tails.

Nembutal (nĕm′bū-tăl). Trade name for pentobarbital sodium. It is a short-acting drug used as a preanesthetic, sedative, and hypnotic.

neo- [Gr. neos]. Combining form meaning new or recent.

neoadjuvant therapy. In treating cancer, the use of chemotherapy prior to or immediately after curative resection of malignancy.

neoantigen (nē″ŏ-ăn′tĭ-jĕn) [″ + anti, against, + gennan, to produce]. A nonspecific term for various tumor antigens.

neoarthrosis (nē″ŏ-ăr-thrō′sĭs) [″ + arthron, joint, + osis, condition]. A false joint. SYN: nearthrosis.

Neo-Betalin 12. Trade name for hydroxocobalamin (vitamin B$_{12}$), USP.

neobiogenesis (nē″ŏ-bī″ō-jĕn′ē-sĭs) [″ + bios, life, + genesis, generation, birth]. The theory that life can arise from inorganic compounds.

Neobiotic. Trade name for neomycin sulfate, USP.

neoblastic [″ + blastos, germ]. Pert. to, or constituting, a new growth of tissue.

neocerebellum (nē″ŏ-sĕr-ĕ-bĕl′ŭm) [Gr. neos, new, + L. cerebellum, little brain]. The portion of the corpus cerebelli of the cerebellum that lies between the primary and prepyramidal fissures. Consists principally of the ansiform lobules. Phylogenetically, it develops last, in conjunction with cerebral cortex, and is concerned with the integration of voluntary movements. It is the posterior lobe of the cerebellum.

neocinetic (nē″ŏ-sī-nĕt′ĭk) [″ + kinetikos, pert. to movement]. Concerning the portion of the nervous system that regulates voluntary muscular control. SYN: neokinetic.

neocortex (nē″ŏ-kor′tĕks). Neopallium.

neodymium (nē″ŏ-dĭm′ē-ŭm). SYMB: Nd. At. wt. 144.24; at. no. 60. A shiny, silvery, rare-earth chemical element.

neofetus (nē-ŏ-fē′tŭs) [″ + L. foetus, offspring]. Embryo during eighth or ninth week of intrauterine life.

neoformation (nē″ŏ-for-mā′shŭn) [″ + L. formatio, a shaping]. 1. Regeneration. 2. A neoplasm or new growth.

neogala (nē-ŏg′ă-lă) [″ + gala, milk]. The first milk following childbirth. SEE: colostrum.

neogenesis (nē-ō-jĕn′ē-sĭs) [″ + genesis, generation, birth]. Regeneration or reformation, as of tissue.

neogenetic (nē″ŏ-jĕn-ĕt′ĭk). Newly formed; rel. to new formations.

neohymen (nē-ō-hī′mĕn) [Gr. neos, new, + hymen, membrane]. A false or new membrane. SYN: pseudomembrane.

neolalism (nē″ō-lăl′ĭzm) [″ + laleo, to chatter]. Use of neologisms in speech. This may be associated with schizophrenia.

neologism (nē-ŏl′ō-jĭzm) [″ + logos, word, reason, + -ismos, state]. 1. A new word or phrase, or a new meaning attached to an old word or phrase. 2. A mental condition in which the patient coins new words that are meaningless or words to which he or she gives special significance without being aware of their normal significance.

neomembrane (nē-ō-mĕm′brăn) [″ + L. membrana, membrane]. A false or a new membrane. SYN: pseudomembrane.

neomorph (nē′ō-morf) [″ + morphe, form]. A new formation or development that is not inherited from a similar structure in an ancestor.

neomycin sulfate (nē″ŏ-mī′sĭn) [″ + mykes, fungus]. USP. An antibiotic from a species of Streptomyces, isolated from soil. Active against gram-positive and gram-negative bacteria, as well as streptomycin-resistant strains of Mycobacterium tuberculosis. It is toxic to kidneys and to the eighth nerve and may cause hearing difficulties. Trade names are Neobiotic and Mycifradin.

neon (nē′ŏn) [Gr. neos, new]. SYMB: Ne. At. wt. 20.183; at no. 10. A rare, inert, gaseous element in the air. Only 18 parts per million parts of air are neon.

neonatal (nē″ŏ-nā′tăl) [″ + L. natus, born]. Concerning the first six weeks after birth.

neonatal mortality rate. SEE: rate, neonatal mortality.

neonate (nē′ŏ-nāt). A newborn infant up to six weeks of age.

neonate, killing of a. SEE: infanticide.

neonatologist (nē″ŏ-nā-tŏl′ō-jĭst) [″ + ″ + Gr. logos, word, reason]. A physician who specializes in the study, care, and treatment of neonates.

neonatology (nē″ŏ-nā-tŏl′ō-jē). The study, care, and treatment of neonates.

neon gas. Colorless gas that makes a reddish-orange glow when an electric charge strikes it.

neopallium (nē″ŏ-păl′ē-ŭm) [Gr. neos, new, + L. pallium, cloak]. That portion of cerebral hemisphere not belonging to the rhinencephalon or corpus striatum, comprising most of the convoluted cortex and its associated white fibers. Phylogenetically, it is the new part of the pallium. SYN: *isocortex; neocortex.*

neopathy (nē-ŏp'ă-thē) [" + *pathos,* disease, suffering]. 1. A newly found disease. 2. A new complication or new condition of a disease.

neophilism (nē-ŏf'ĭl-ĭzm) [" + *philein,* to love, + *-ismos,* condition]. Morbid love of novelty and new persons and scenes.

neophobia (nē"ō-fō'bē-ă) [" + *phobos,* fear]. Fear of new scenes or novelties; aversion to all that is unknown or not understood.

neophrenia (nē"ō-frē'nē-ă) [" + *phren,* mind]. Mental deterioration in early youth.

neoplasia (nē"ō-plā'zē-ă) [" + *plassein,* to form]. The development of neoplasms.

neoplasia, cervical intraepithelial. SEE: *cervical intraepithelial neoplasia.*

neoplasm (nē'ō-plăzm) [" + LL. *plasma,* form, mold]. A new and abnormal formation of tissue, as a tumor or growth. It serves no useful function, but grows at the expense of the healthy organism.

   n., benign. Growth not spreading by metastases or infiltration of tissue.

   n., histoid. Neoplasm in which structure resembles the tissues and elements that surround it.

   n., malignant. Growth that infiltrates tissue, metastasizes, and often recurs after attempts at surgical removal. SYN: *cancer.*

   n., mixed. Neoplasm composed of tissues from two of the germinal layers.

   n., multicentric. Growth arising from a number of distinct groups of cells.

   n., organoid. Neoplasm in which the structure is similar to some organ of the body.

   n., unicentric. Growth having origin in one group of cells.

neoplastic (nē"ō-plăs'tĭk) [Gr. *neos,* new, + *plastikos,* formed]. Pert. to, or of the nature of, new, abnormal tissue formation.

neoplasty (nē'ō-plăs-tē) [" + *plassein,* to form]. Surgical formation or restoration of parts.

neostigmine (nē-ō-stĭg'mĭn). A cholinergic drug used clinically in the form of a bromide or methylsulfate.

   n. bromide. USP. A preparation of neostigmine used for oral administration in the treatment of myasthenia gravis. Ophthalmic solution used for glaucoma. Trade name is Prostigmin.

   n. methylsulfate. USP. A preparation of neostigmine used for parenteral administration in treatment of myasthenia gravis. Trade name is Prostigmin.

neostomy (nē-ŏs'tō-mē) [" + *stoma,* mouth]. Surgical formation of artificial

opening into an organ or between two organs.

neostriatum (nē"ō-strī-ā'tŭm) [" + L. *striatum,* grooved]. The caudate nucleus and the putamen considered together.

Neo-Synephrine Hydrochloride (nē"ō-sĭn-ĕf'rĭn). Trade name for phenylephrine hydrochloride, USP.

neoteny (nē-ŏt'ĕ-nē) [" + *teinein,* to extend]. In zoology, maturation during the larval stage.

neothalamus (nē"ō-thăl'ă-mŭs) [" + L. *thalamus,* thalamus]. The lateral and dorsomedial nuclei of the thalamus.

nephelometer (nĕf"ĕl-ŏm'ĕ-ter) [Gr. *nephele,* mist, + *metron,* measure]. Apparatus for measuring the turbidity of a fluid. It also may be used in estimating the degree of contamination of air by particulate matter.

nephelometry (nĕf"ĕl-ŏm'ĕ-trē). The employment of the nephelometer.

nephelopia (nĕf"ĕ-lō'pē-ă) [Gr. *nephele,* mist, + *ops,* eye]. Dim or cloudy vision from lessened transparency of the ocular media.

nephr- [Gr. *nephros,* kidney]. Combining form pert. to the kidney.

nephradenoma (nĕf"răd-ĕ-nō'mă) [Gr. *nephros,* kidney, + *aden,* gland, + *oma,* tumor]. Renal adenoma.

nephralgia (nĕ-frăl'jē-ă) [" + *algos,* pain]. Renal pain. In absence of other symptoms, may alone be symptomatic of an obstructive renal process, but commonly presents a problem in differential diagnosis.

nephralgic (nĕ-frăl'jĭk). Pert. to renal pain.

nephrapostasis (nĕf"ră-pŏs'tă-sĭs) [" + *apostasis,* suppuration]. Renal abscess or purulent inflammation of the kidney.

nephratony (nĕ-frăt'ō-nē) [" + *a,* not, + *tonos,* tension]. Lack of normal renal tone. SYN: *nephratonia.*

nephrauxe (nĕf-rawks'ē) [" + *auxe,* increase]. Renal enlargement.

nephrectasia, nephrectasis, nephrectasy (nĕf-rĕk-tā'zē-ă, -rĕk'tă-sĭs, -tă-sē) [Gr. *nephros,* kidney, + *ektasis,* distention]. Distention of the kidney.

nephrectomize (nĕ-frĕk'tō-mīz) [" + *ektome,* excision]. To remove, surgically, one or both kidneys.

nephrectomy (nĕ-frĕk'tō-mē) [" + *ektome,* excision]. Removal of a kidney.

   NURSING IMPLICATIONS: Provide adequate pre- and post-operative instruction. Physically prepare the patient according to prescribed protocol such as skin preparation, laboratory studies, and preoperative medications. Provide activities that are interesting but not tiring. Prevent or control complications of fluid or electrolyte imbalance and weigh daily. Encourage verbalization of feelings and concerns, and provide reassurance and support.

Postop: Check vital signs every 2 to 4 hours. Administer analgesics and other prescribed medications. Report and record any excessive bleeding. Turn patient so entire dressing area can be viewed. Assist with cough and deep breathing exercises at frequent intervals. Turn and position frequently, observing operative site, and change dressing as necessary. Institute range of motion exercises. Check drainage tubes at frequent intervals to be certain they are functioning. Monitor and record intake and output. Change position frequently to prevent complications (operative side may be most comfortable). Provide frequent mouth care while the patient is not taking anything by mouth. Encourage progressive diet upon return of bowel sounds. Establish discharge teaching plan including diet, activities, incision care, and medications. Instruct patient concerning engaging in activities that could injure the remaining kidney.

SEE: *Nursing Diagnoses* in *Appendix.*

COMPLICATIONS: Spontaneous pneumothorax and secondary hemorrhage.

n., abdominal. Nephrectomy through an incision in the abdominal wall.

n., paraperitoneal. Removal of a kidney through an extraperitoneal incision.

nephrelcosis (nĕf-rĕl-kō′sĭs) [Gr. *nephros*, kidney, + *helkosis*, ulceration]. Ulceration of the mucosa of the kidney.

nephrelcus (nĕf-rĕl′kŭs). Renal ulcer.

nephremia (nĕf-rē′mē-ă) [″ + *haima*, blood]. Congested state of kidney.

nephremphraxis (nĕf″rĕm-frăks′ĭs) [″ + *emphraxis*, obstruction]. Obstruction in the renal vessels.

nephric (nĕf′rĭk) [Gr. *nephros*, kidney]. Pert. to the kidney or kidneys. SYN: *renal.*

nephridium (nĕ-frĭd′ē-ŭm) [Gr. *nephridios*, pert. to the kidney]. A segmented excretory tubule present in many invertebrates.

nephritic (nĕ-frĭt′ĭk). 1. Rel. to the kidney. 2. Pert. to nephritis. 3. An agent used in nephritis.

nephritis (nĕf-rī′tĭs) [Gr. *nephros*, kidney, + *itis*, inflammation]. (pl. *nephritides*) Inflammation of the kidney. The glomeruli, tubules, and interstitial tissue may be affected. It may be either acute or chronic.

ETIOL: Bacteria or their toxins; streptococcal infections; diphtheria; septicemia; or toxic drugs such as mercury, arsenic, or alcohol.

NURSING IMPLICATIONS: Assess renal function and report signs of renal failure (oliguria, azotemia, acidosis), monitor hemoglobin, hematocrit, and electrolytes.

Use aseptic technique in handling catheters. Observe, record, and report hematuria. Monitor blood pressure using same arm, same cuff, same position each time. Observe or question concerning headache, restlessness, lethargy, convulsions, tachycardia, arrhythmias. Administer antihypertension drugs as prescribed. Maintain adequate hydration and prescribed dietary restrictions. Carefully monitor and record intake of prescribed I.V. fluids. Anticipate and attempt to avoid complications of hypertension.

RS: arteriosclerosis; glomerulonephritis; kidney; nephritic syndrome; nephrosclerosis; nephrotic syndrome.

n., acute. Inflammatory form of nephritis involving the glomeruli, the tubules, or the entire kidney. It is of various types depending on the portion of the kidney involved: degenerative, diffuse, suppurative, hemorrhagic, interstitial, and parenchymatous.

n., analgesic. Chronic nephritis caused by excess intake of almost any of the antiinflammatory analgesics, e.g., salicylates, acetaminophen, nonsteroidal anti-inflammatory agents. The pathological lesion is chronic tubulointerstitial nephritis with renal papillar necrosis. The reason these drugs adversely affect some and not others is unknown.

n., chronic. Progressive form of nephritis in which entire structure of kidney or only the glomerular or tubular processes may be affected. One variety of nephritis may merge with another, causing a diffuse nephritis. Symptoms depend upon the tissues involved.

n., glomerular. Glomerulonephritis, q.v.

n., interstitial. Nephritis associated with pathological changes in the renal interstitial tissue that in turn may be primary or due to a toxic agent such as a drug or chemical. The end result is that the nephrons are destroyed and renal function is seriously impaired.

n., scarlatinal. Acute glomerulonephritis complicating scarlet fever.

n., suppurative. Nephritis associated with abscesses in the kidney.

n., transfusion. Renal failure and tubular disease caused by transfusion of incompatible blood.

nephritogenic (nĕ-frĭt″ō-jĕn′ĭk) [″ + *gennan*, to produce]. Causing nephritis.

nephro- [Gr. *nephros*, kidney]. Combining form pert. to the kidney.

nephroabdominal (nĕf″rō-ăb-dŏm′ĭ-năl) [″ + L. *abdominalis*, abdomen]. Concerning the kidney and abdomen.

nephroblastoma (nĕf″rō-blăs-tō′mă) [″

+ *blastos,* germ, + *oma,* tumor]. Wilms' tumor, q.v.

nephrocalcinosis (nĕf-rō″kăl″sĭn-ō′sĭs) [″ + L. *calx,* lime, + Gr. *osis,* condition]. Calcinosis of the kidney characterized by deposits of calcium phosphate in renal tubules.

nephrocapsectomy (nĕf″rō-kăp-sĕk′tō-mē) [″ + L. *capsula,* capsule, + Gr. *ektome,* excision]. Renal decapsulation.

nephrocardiac (nĕf″rō-kăr′dē-ăk) [″ + *kardia,* heart]. Concerning the heart and kidney.

nephrocele (nĕf′rō-sēl) [″ + *kele,* tumor, swelling]. Renal hernia.

nephrocolic (nĕf″rō-kŏl′ĭk) [Gr. *nephros,* kidney, + *kolikos,* colic]. 1. Severe colicky pain in ureter due to passage of stone. 2. Concerning the colon and kidney.

nephrocolopexy (nĕf″rō-kŏl′ō-pĕks″ē) [″ + *kolon,* colon, + *pexis,* fixation]. Surgical suspension of the kidney and colon using the nephrocolic ligament.

nephrocoloptosis (nĕf″rō-kō″lŏp-tō′sĭs) [″ + ″ + *ptosis,* a dropping]. Condition in which the kidney and colon are displaced downward.

nephrocystanastomosis (nĕf″rō-sĭst-ă-năs″tō-mō′sĭs) [″ + *kystis,* bladder, + *anastomosis,* outlet]. Surgical formation of an artificial connection between the kidney and bladder in permanent ureteral obstruction.

nephrocystitis (nĕf″rō-sĭs-tī′tĭs) [″ + ″ + *itis,* inflammation]. Inflamed condition of the kidneys and bladder.

nephrocystosis (nĕf″rō-sĭs-tō′sĭs) [″ + ″ + *osis,* condition]. Formation of renal cysts.

nephroerysipelas (nĕf″rō-ĕr″ĭ-sĭp′ĕ-lăs) [″ + *erythros,* red, + *pella,* skin]. Acute nephritis occurring as a complication of erysipelas.

nephrogenetic (nĕf″rō-jĕn-ĕt′ĭk) [″ + *gennan,* to produce]. Arising in or from the renal organs; capable of giving rise to kidney tissue. SYN: *nephrogenic; nephrogenous.*

nephrogenic. Nephrogenetic, q.v.

nephrogenous (nĕ-frŏj′ĕ-nŭs). Arising from the kidney.

nephrogram. A roentgenogram of the kidney.

nephrography (nĕ-frŏg′ră-fē) [″ + *graphein,* to write]. Roentgenography of the kidney.

nephrohydrosis (nĕf″rō-hī-drō′sĭs) [″ + *hydor,* water, + *osis,* condition]. Accumulation of urine in renal pelvis and calyces due to obstruction. SYN: *hydronephrosis; nephrydrosis.*

nephrohypertrophy (nĕf″rō-hī-pĕr′trō-fē) [″ + *hyper,* over, + *trophe,* nourishment]. Increased size of kidneys.

nephroid (nĕf′royd) [″ + *eidos,* form, shape]. Resembling a kidney; kidney-shaped. SYN: *reniform.*

nephrolith (nĕf′rō-lĭth) [″ + *lithos,* stone]. Stone in the kidney.

nephrolithiasis (nĕf″rō-lĭth-ī′ă-sĭs). The presence of calculi in the kidney. SEE: *calculus, renal.*

nephrolithotomy (nĕf″rō-lĭth-ŏt′ō-mē) [″ + *lithos,* stone, + *tome,* incision]. Renal incision for removal of calculus.

nephrology (nĕ-frŏl′ō-jē) [″ + *logos,* word, reason]. Science of the structure and function of the kidney.

nephrolysine (nĕ-frŏl′ĭ-sĭn) [″ + *lysis,* dissolution]. A toxic substance, esp. an antigen, that can destroy renal tissue.

nephrolysis (nĕ-frŏl′ĭ-sĭs) [″ + *lysis,* dissolution]. 1. Surgical detachment of an inflamed kidney from paranephric adhesions. 2. Destruction of kidney tissue by action of a nephrotoxin.

nephroma (nĕ-frō′mă) [″ + *oma,* tumor]. Renal tumor.

nephromalacia (nĕf″rō-mă-lā′sē-ă) [″ + *malakia,* softening]. Abnormal renal softness or softening.

nephromegaly (nĕf″rō-mĕg′ă-lē) [″ + *megas,* great]. Extreme enlargement of one or both kidneys.

nephromere (nĕf′rō-mēr) [″ + *meros,* part]. Segment in embryo from which kidney develops; the intermediate mesoderm in an embryo from which the kidney develops. SYN: *nephrotome.*

nephron (nĕf′rŏn) [Gr. *nephros,* kidney]. The structural and functional unit of the kidney, consisting of a renal (malpighian) corpuscle (a glomerulus enclosed within Bowman's capsule), and its attached tubule, consisting of the proximal convoluted portion, loop of Henle, and distal convoluted portion. These connect by arched collecting tubules with straight collecting tubules. Urine is formed by filtration in renal corpuscles, and selective reabsorption and secretion by cells of the renal tubule. There are approximately one million nephrons in each kidney. SYN: *renal tubule.* SEE: *kidney* for illus.; *malpighian corpuscle; urine.*

nephroncus (nĕf-rŏn′kŭs) [″ + *onkos,* tumor]. A renal tumor.

nephroparalysis (nĕf″rō-păr-ăl′ĭ-sĭs) [″ + *paralyein,* to disable]. Paralyzed renal function.

nephropathy (nĕ-frŏp′ă-thē) [″ + *pathos,* disease, suffering]. Disease of the kidney. This term includes inflammatory (nephritis), degenerative (nephrosis), and sclerotic (arteriosclerotic) lesions of the kidney.

    n., analgesic. SEE: *nephritis, analgesic.*

n., hypercalcemic. Renal damage due to hypercalcemia. It is usually caused by hyperparathyroidism, sarcoidosis, excess vitamin D intake, excess ingestion of milk and alkali, multiple myeloma, malignant disease, and occasionally immobilization or Paget's disease. If the underlying cause is allowed to persist, the damage to the renal tubules may be permanent.
TREAT: Correction of the primary disease.

n., hypokalemic. Renal damage due to abnormal depletion of potassium regardless of the basic cause of the electrolyte abnormality. Characteristically, there are multiple vacuoles in microscopic sections of the renal tubular epithelium. Clinically, the patient is unable to concentrate urine.
TREAT: Therapy for the primary cause of the hypokalemia may allow the kidney lesions to become completely reversed.

n., membranous. A glomerular disease of unknown etiology that produces the nephrotic syndrome, q.v. It may be distinguished from lipoid nephrosis by the use of immunofluorescence and electron microscopy. SEE: *glomerular disease; nephrotic syndrome.*
TREAT: High-protein diet and diuretics. Adrenocortical hormones may be of benefit in young patients.

n., radiocontrast-induced. In some individuals, especially those with conditions that cause diminished renal blood flow, diabetic renal failure, jaundice, or multiple myeloma, use of radio contrast media may cause acute renal failure. In normal patients, use of such agents rarely causes nephropathy.

nephropexy (nĕf′rō-pĕks-ē) [″ + *pexis*, fixation]. Surgical attachment of a floating kidney.

nephrophthisis (nĕ-frŏf′thĭ-sĭs) [″ + *phthisis*, a wasting]. 1. Tuberculosis of the kidney with caseous degeneration. 2. Suppurative nephritis with wasting of the kidney substance.

nephroptosis (nĕf′rŏp-tō′sĭs) [″ + *ptosis*, a dropping]. Prolapse or downward displacement of the kidney.

nephropyelitis (nĕf″rō-pī-ĕl-ī′tĭs) [″ + *pyelos*, pelvis, + *itis*, inflammation]. Inflammation of the renal pelvis and parenchyma of kidney. SYN: *pyelonephritis.*

nephropyelography (nĕf″rō-pī″ē-lŏg′ră-fē) [″ + *pyelos*, pelvis, + *graphein*, to write]. Roentgenogram of the kidney and renal pelvis.

nephropyeloplasty (nĕf″rō-pī″ē-lō-plăs″tē) [″ + ″ + *plassein*, to form]. Plastic surgery on the kidney and renal pelvis.

nephropyosis (nĕf″rō-pī-ō′sĭs) [″ + *pyosis*, suppuration]. Purulence of a kidney.

nephrorrhagia (nĕf-ror-ā′jē-ă) [″ + *rhegnynai*, to burst forth]. Renal hemorrhage into the pelvis and tubules.

nephrorrhaphy (nĕf-ror′ă-fē) [″ + *rhaphe*, seam, ridge]. Surgical procedure of suturing the kidney.

nephros (nĕf′rŏs) [Gr.]. The kidney.

nephrosclerosis (nĕf″rō-sklĕ-rō′sĭs) [″ + *sklerosis*, a hardening]. Renal sclerosis or hardening.

n., arterial. Arteriosclerosis of kidney arteries. Results in ischemia, atrophy of parenchyma, and fibrosis of kidney.

n., arteriolar. Sclerosis of the smaller renal arterioles, esp. the afferent glomerular arterioles with resulting fibrosis, ischemic necrosis, and glomerular degeneration and failure. Occurs in most cases of essential hypertension.

n., malignant. Nephrosclerosis that develops rapidly in patients with severe hypertension. SEE: *hypertension, malignant.*

nephrosis (nĕf-rō′sĭs) [Gr. *nephros*, kidney, + *osis*, condition] (pl. *nephroses*). 1. Condition in which there are degenerative changes in the kidneys, esp. the renal tubules, without the occurrence of inflammation. 2. Clinical classification of kidney disease in which protein loss is so extensive that edema and hypoproteinemia are produced. SEE: *nephrotic syndrome, idiopathic.*

n., lipoid. SEE: *nephrotic syndrome, idiopathic.*

nephrosonephritis (nĕ-frō″sō-nĕ-frī′tĭs) [″ + *osis*, condition, + *nephros*, kidney, + *itis*, inflammation]. Renal disease with characteristics of nephritis and nephrosis.

nephrospasis (nĕf″rō-spăs′ĭs) [″ + *span*, to draw]. A kidney with poor supporting tissue. It may be suspended by its pedicle.

nephrostoma (nĕ-frŏs′tō-mă) [″ + *stoma*, mouth]. The internal orifice of a wolffian tubule, connected with the coelom in the human embryo.

nephrostomy (nĕ-frŏs′tō-mē). Formation of an artificial fistula into the renal pelvis.

nephrotic (nĕ-frŏt′ĭk) [Gr. *nephros*, kidney]. Rel. to, or caused by, nephrosis.

nephrotic syndrome. ABBR: NS. The end result of a variety of diseases that damage the capillary wall of the arteries of the glomerulus. Clinically, this leads to loss of a large amount of protein in the urine, which in turn results in hypoalbuminemia and edema. Hyperlipidemia also develops in many cases. Factors causing NS include any disorder that may affect the glomerulus, immunologic disorders, toxic injury to the kidneys, neoplasms, metabolic abnormalities, biochemical defects, multisystem diseases, infections, and diseases of the vascular system.

TREAT: Management of this condition and the complication of venous and arterial thromboembolism requires use of diuretics and medicines to reduce the lipid levels in the blood. Long-term use of anticoagulants may be needed for the complication of chronic renal vein thrombosis. If NS is secondary to a specific disease, infection, certain forms of cancer, specific drugs, or any of the other diseases known to be associated with NS, then those are treated appropriately. Adrenal cortical steroid hormones have a dramatic, immediate effect on the condition, but their use does not alter the survival rate.

NURSING IMPLICATIONS: Monitor side effects of proteinuria and fluid and electrolyte balance (intake and output, weight). Provide and encourage adequate nutritional intake as ordered. Assist the patient with hygienic care, and prevent skin trauma. Plan patient activities to provide periods of rest and prevent fatigue and weakness, and protect the patient from infection. Support the patient experiencing grief and difficulties in coping with changes in body image and self-concept. SEE: *Nursing Diagnoses* in *Appendix.*

n.s., idiopathic. This condition is diagnosed when the known causes of nephrotic syndrome (NS) have been excluded. It is usually diagnosed in adults by use of renal biopsy. Causes are classified according to the changes found in the capillaries of the glomerulus when examined by use of electron microscopy. Clinical features are similar to those of NS, but hematuria is also present.

TREAT: Use of corticosteroids and therapy for associated conditions or complications. Depending on severity of NS and the cellular changes in the glomerulus, 5% to 50% of cases of idiopathic NS may be treated without the need for renal dialysis or transplantation.

nephrotome (nĕf″rō-tōm) [″ + *tome*, incision]. Embryonic bridge of cells connecting primitive segments along neural tube to the somatic and splanchnic mesoderm from which arises the urogenital system. SYN: *mesomere; nephromere.*

nephrotomogram (nĕf″rō-tō′mō-grăm). A tomogram of the kidney.

nephrotomography (nĕf″rō-tō-mŏg′ră-fē) [″ + ″ + *graphein*, to write]. Tomograph, q.v., of the kidney after the intravenous injection of a radiopaque contrast medium that is excreted by the kidney.

nephrotomy (nĕ-frŏt′ō-mē) [″ + *tome*, incision]. Surgical incision of the kidney.

nephrotoxin (nĕf″rō-tŏk′sĭn) [″ + *toxikon*,

poison]. A toxic substance that damages kidney tissues.

nephrotresis (nĕf-rō-trē′sĭs) [″ + *tresis*, piercing]. Formation of a permanent excretory opening in the kidney through the loin.

nephrotropic (nĕf″rō-trŏp′ĭk) [″ + *tropos*, turning]. 1. Affecting the kidneys. 2. An agent or drug that exerts its effect principally on the kidney or renal function.

nephrotuberculosis (nĕf″rō-tū-bĕr″kū-lō′sĭs) [″ + *tuberculum*, a little swelling, + *osis*, condition]. Infection of the kidney due to *Mycobacterium tuberculosis.*

nephrotyphoid (nĕf″rō-tī′foyd) [″ + *typhos*, stupor, + *eidos*, form, shape]. Renal disease complicating typhoid fever.

nephroureterectomy (nĕf″rō-ū-rē″tĕr-ĕk′tō-mē) [″ + *oureter*, ureter, + *ektome*, excision]. Surgical excision of the kidney with the ureter or part of it.

nephrourography. Radiographic examination of the nephron phase during urography.

nephrydrosis (nĕf″rĭ-drō′sĭs) [″ + *hydor*, water, + *osis*, condition]. Distention and dilatation of renal pelvis resulting from obstruction. SYN: *hydronephrosis; nephrohydrosis.*

Neptazane. Trade name for methazolamide, USP.

neptunium [planet Neptune]. SYMB: Np. At. wt. 237; at. no. 93. An element obtained by bombarding uranium with neutrons.

nerve [L. *nervus*, sinew; Gr. *neuron*, sinew]. A bundle or a group of bundles of nerve fibers outside the central nervous system that connect the brain and spinal cord with various parts of the body. Nerves conduct afferent impulses centrally from receptor organs and efferent impulses peripherally to effector tissues and organs. The fibers of peripheral nerves are the processes of neurons whose cell bodies are located within the brain or spinal cord, or in ganglia. A bundle of nerve fibers is called a fasciculus, q.v. The fibers within a fasciculus are surrounded and held together by delicate connective tissue fibers forming the endoneurium. Each fasciculus is surrounded by a sheath of connective tissue, the perineurium. The entire nerve is enclosed in a thick sheath of connective tissue, the epineurium, which may contain numerous fat cells. Small nerves may lack an epineurium. SYN: *nervus* [NA]. SEE: *cell* and *nerve cell* for illus.; *Nerves* in *Appendix.*

Test for loss of function: It is important to know the extent of peripheral nerve damage and to follow the course of healing. This may be done for injury of nerves of the hand by observing the wrinkling of the hand when it is soaked in warm water for 30 minutes. If the nerve supply is intact, skin of the fingers shows characteristic wrinkling; however, the fingers remain unwrinkled over the area in which the nerve supply is absent.

n.'s, accelerator. Nerves to the heart that carry sympathetic fibers that convey impulses. These impulses, when stimulated, accelerate the heartbeat.

n., acoustic. Eighth cranial nerve. SEE: *vestibulocochlear nerve* for illus.

n., adrenergic. A sympathetic nerve that liberates norepinephrine at a synapse when it transmits a stimulus.

n., afferent. Any nerve that transmits impulses from the periphery to the central nervous system.

n., autonomic. Nerve of the autonomic nervous system, q.v.

n., cerebrospinal. Nerve originating from the brain or spinal cord.

n., cholinergic. A parasympathetic nerve that liberates acetylcholine when it transmits a stimulus.

n., cranial. One of the 12 pairs of nerves arising from the brain. They exit through foramina of the cranium. SEE: *cranial nerves; Cranial Nerves* in *Appendix.*

n., depressor. Any afferent nerve that, when stimulated, depresses the activity of an organ or nerve center.

n., efferent. Nerve that transmits impulses from a nerve center to the periphery. SYN: *n., motor.*

n., excitatory. Nerve that transmits impulses that stimulate function.

n., excitoreflex. A visceral nerve that, when stimulated, causes reflex action.

n., facial. Seventh cranial nerve. SEE: *facial nerve* for illus.

n., gangliated. Any sympathetic nervous system nerve.

n., glossopharyngeal. Ninth cranial nerve. SEE: *glossopharyngeal nerve* for illus.

n., inhibitory. A nerve that, upon stimulation, lessens activity in a part.

n., mixed. Nerve containing both afferent (sensory) and efferent (motor) fibers.

n., motor. Nerve containing motor fibers and conveying motor impulses. SYN: *efferent nerve.*

n.'s, olfactory. First pair of cranial nerves. SEE: *olfactory nerves* for illus.

n., optic. Second cranial nerve.

n., parasympathetic. Nerve of the parasympathetic division of the autonomic nervous system. SEE: *parasympathetic nervous system.*

n., peripheral. Any nerve that connects the brain or spinal cord with peripheral receptors or effectors. SEE: illus.

n., pilomotor. Nerve that innervates the arrectores pilorum muscles of hair follicles.

n., pressor. An afferent nerve that, when stimulated, excites the vasoconstrictor center and thus increases blood pressure.

n., secretory. Nerve whose stimulation excites secretion in a gland or a tissue.

n., sensory. Nerve that conducts afferent impulses from sensory receptors to the brain or spinal cord. SYN: *afferent nerve.*

n., somatic. Nerve that innervates somatic structures, i.e., those of the body wall and extremities.

n., spinal. One of 31 pairs of peripheral nerves that connect with the spinal cord. Includes 8 cervical, 12 thoracic, 5 lumbar, 5 sacral, 1 coccygeal. SEE: *cranial nerves.*

n., splanchnic. One of the nerves that supply the visceral organs.

n., sudomotor. One of the nerves that supply sweat glands.

n., sympathetic. Nerve of the sympathetic division of the autonomic nervous system. SEE: *autonomic nervous system.*

n., trigeminal. The fifth cranial and the most important sensory and motor nerve of the oral area. SEE: *cranial nerves; trigeminal nerve.*

n., trophic. Any nerve involved in regulating nutrition of tissues.

n., vagus. Tenth cranial nerve. SEE: *vagus* for illus.

n., vasoconstrictor. Nerve that conducts impulses that bring about constriction of a blood vessel.

n., vasodilator. Nerve that conducts impulses that bring about dilation of a blood vessel.

n., vasomotor. Nerve that controls the caliber of a blood vessel. A vasoconstrictor or vasodilator nerve.

n., vasosensory. Any nerve providing sensory fibers for a vessel.

nerve block. The induction of regional anesthesia by preventing sensory nerve impulses from reaching centers of consciousness. This is usually done on a temporary basis, by using chemical or electrical means. In the former case, it is accomplished by injecting an anesthetic solution, such as procaine, around the nerve but some distance from the region, or by anesthetizing nerve endings in the region itself (infiltration).

nerve cell. A neuron, q.v.; consists of a cell body and its processes, an axon and one or more dendrites. SEE: illus.

nerve ending. The termination of a nerve fiber (axon or dendrite) in a peripheral structure. May be sensory (receptor) or motor (effector). Sensory endings can be nonencapsulated, such as free nerve endings, peritrichal endings, or tactile corpuscles of Merkel, or they can be encapsulated as in the end-bulbs of Krause, Meissner's corpuscles, Vater-Pacini corpuscles, or neu-

PERIPHERAL CUTANEOUS NERVES

TRIGEMINAL NERVE:

GREATER OCCIPITAL N. (C-2)

LESSER OCCIPITAL N. (C2,3)

OPTHALMIC DIVISION I

MAXILLARY DIVISION II

AURICULOTEMPORAL N.
(MANDIBULAR DIV.III OF TRIGEMINAL N.)

DORSAL DIVISIONS OF 3RD-8TH
CERVICAL NN. (C3-8)

DORSAL DIVISIONS OF 1ST-12TH
THORACIC NN.TH1-12

GREAT AURICULAR N. (C3)

ANTERIOR CUTANEOUS N.
OF NECK (C3)

LATERAL CUTANEOUS N.
OF ARM

INTERCOSTOBRACHIAL N.

MEDIAL CUTANEOUS
NERVE OF ARM

POSTERIOR SUPRACLAVICULAR
NN. (C3,4)

LATERAL CUTANEOUS N. OF
ARM (C8,TH1)

POSTERIOR CUTANEOUS
N. OF ARM (C5, TH1)

ILIOHYPOGASTRIC N.
(TH12,L1)

CUTAN. BRANCH
OF NERVES OF
FOREARM:

POSTERIOR

MEDIAL

LATERAL

MEDIAN N.

POSTERIOR CUTANEOUS N. OF
FOREARM
(RADIAL N. C5-TH1)

MEDIAL CUTANEOUS
N. OF FOREARM
(C8-TH1)

DORSAL BRANCH
OF ULNAR N.

LATERAL CUTANEOUS
N. OF FOREARM
(MUSCULOCUTANEOUS)
N. C5-7

POSTERIOR BRANCHES OF:
LUMBAR NN.L1-3
SACRAL NN.S1-3

LATERAL CUTAN. N.
OF THIGH (L2,3)

OBTURATOR N.

POSTERIOR CUTAN.
N. OF THIGHS (S1-3)

LATERAL CUTAN. N. OF CALF
(COMMON PERONEAL N.)

MEDIAL CUTAN. N.
OF CALF (TIBIAL N.)

INTERNAL SAPHENOUS N.
(FEMORAL N. L3,4)

SURAL N.

LATERAL BRANCH
OF SURAL N.

CUTANEOUS BRANCHES OF
FEMORAL N. (L2-4)

LATERAL CUTANEOUS
N. OF THIGH (L2,3)

DEEP PERONEAL N.

SUPERFICIAL PERONEAL N.

SURAL N.

POST. CUTAN. N. OF THIGH (S1-3)

GLUTEAL BR. OF POST. CUTAN. N.
OF THIGH (S2,3)

PUDENDAL N. (S3)

GENITOFEMORAL N. (L1,2)

LATERAL BRANCH OF
SUPERFICIAL
PERONEAL N.

MEDIAL PLANTAR N.

MEDIAL PLANTAR N.
(TIBIAL N.)

LATERAL PLANTAR N.
(TIBIAL N.)

INTERNAL
SAPHENOUS N.

SURAL N.

POSTERIOR VIEW

PERIPHERAL CUTANEOUS NERVES

TRIGEMINAL N.:
OPTHALMIC DIVISION I
MAXILLARY DIVISION II
MANDIBULAR DIVISION III

MEDIAL AND LATERAL
SUPRACLAVICULAR NN.(C3,4)
LATERAL CUTANEOUS N. OF ARM,
(AXILLARY N. C5-7)
INTERCOSTOBRACHIAL N.
POSTERIOR CUTANEOUS N.
OF ARM (RADIAL N. C5-TH1)
MEDIAL CUTANEOUS
N. OF ARM (C8,TH1)
POSTERIOR CUTANEOUS
N. OF FOREARM
MEDIAL CUTANEOUS
N. OF FOREARM
(C8, TH1)
LATERAL CUTANEOUS
N. OF FOREARM
(MUSCULOCUTANEOUS)
N. C5-7)
DORSAL BRANCH
OF ULNAR N.
ULNAR N.
MEDIAN N.
SUPERFICIAL BRANCH OF
RADIAL N.(C5-TH1)
POSTERIOR CUTANEOUS N.
OF THIGH (S1-3)
INTERNAL SAPHENOUS N.
(FEMORAL N. L3-4)
MEDIAL CUTANEOUS N.
OF CALF (TIBIAL N.)
SUPERFICIAL PERONEAL N.
SURAL N.
PLANTAR N.

GREATER OCCIPITAL N.(C2)
LESSER OCCIPITAL N. (C2,3)
AURICULOTEMPORAL N.
(MANDIBULAR N.)
GREAT AURICULAR N. (C3)
ANTERIORCUTANEOUS N.
OF NECK (C3)
MEDIAN N.
PALMAR BRANCH OF
ULNAR N.
(C8-TH1)
PALMAR BRANCH
MEDIAN N.
(C5, TH1)
POSTERIOR
CUTANEOUS
N. OF ARM
LATERAL CUTANEOUS
N. OF FOREARM
MEDIAL CUTANEOUS
N. OF FOREARM
INTERCOSTOBRACHIAL N.
MEDIAL CUTANEOUS N. OF ARM
INTERCOSTAL NN. OR VENTRAL
BRANCHES OF THORACIC
NN. (TH 1-12)
LATERAL CUTANEOUS BRANCHES
OF INTERCOSTAL NN.
VENTRAL CUTAN. BRANCHES OF
INTERCOSTAL NN.
ILIOHYPOGASTRIC N. (TH 12,L1)
ILIO-INGUINAL N. (L1)
LATERAL CUTANEOUS N.
OF THIGH (L2,3)
GENITOFEMORAL N. (L1,2)
CUTANEOUS BRANCHES OF
FEMORAL N. (L2-4)
PUDENDAL N.
OBTURATOR N. (L2-4)
LATERAL CUTANEOUS N.
OF CALF (COMMONPERONEAL N.)
INTERNAL SAPHENOUS N. (L3,4)
SURAL N.
LATERAL BRANCH OF SURAL N.
MEDIAL TERMINAL BRANCH OF
ANTERIOR TIBIAL N.
(DEEP PERONEAL N.)
LATERAL BRANCH OF SUPERFICIAL
PERONEAL N.

ANTERIOR VIEW

TERMINAL BRANCHES
OF DENDRITE NEAR
SURFACE OF BRAIN

ASCENDING
DENDRITE

BRANCHES OF
AXON THAT
COMMUNICATE
WITH OTHER
NERVES

AXON

WHITE
SUBSTANCE
OF BRAIN

**NERVE CELL FROM
CEREBRAL CORTEX**

romuscular and neurotendinous spindles.

nerve entrapment syndrome. Compression of a nerve or nerves to the extent that the nerve is damaged. This may cause anesthesia if a sensory nerve is affected and paralysis if a motor nerve is involved. The compression may be due to physical pressure on the nerve, i.e., sleeping in a position in which a nerve is pressed upon by surrounding tissue; or to swelling of tissue in a compartment through which the nerve passes. SEE: *carpal tunnel syndrome; muscle compartment syndrome.*

nerve fiber. An elongated process of a nerve cell or neuron, usually the axon, concerned primarily with the transmission of impulses. Nerve fibers form the major portion of the white matter of the brain and spinal cord and all nerves. Most fibers in peripheral nerves are myelinated (also called medullated, which means they are covered by a noncellular sheath of myelin, a fatty substance). The myelin sheath is interrupted at intervals by the nodes of Ranvier. Outside the myelin sheath and closely investing it is another sheath, the neurilemma or sheath of Schwann. Between the two sheaths are Schwann cells, thin cells having flat, oval-shaped nuclei. One Schwann cell occurs at each internode length. Fibers lacking a myelin sheath are called nonmedullated (unmyelinated). The neurilemma is lacking in all fibers of the central nervous system.

   n.f., adrenergic. Nerve fiber that liberates norepinephrine at its synapse when an impulse is transmitted. Includes most postganglionic fibers of the sympathetic division.

   n.f., arcuate. Arch-shaped nerve fiber in the medulla. They comprise three groups, the external dorsal, external ventral, and internal.

   n.f., association. Nerve fiber that connects one region of the cerebral cortex with another region in the same hemisphere.

   n.f., cholinergic. Nerve fiber that liberates acetylcholine at its synapse when an impulse is transmitted. Includes preganglionic fibers ending in sympathetic ganglia, postganglionic parasympathetic fibers, and efferent somatic fibers ending in skeletal muscle.

   n.f.'s, climbing, of cerebellum. 1. Afferent nerve fibers entering the cortex and synapsing with dendrites of Purkinje cells. SYN: *mossy fibers.* 2. Collateral branches of Purkinje cell axons that return to molecular layer terminating about Purkinje or basket cell dendrites.

   n.f., collateral. A small branch of nerve fibers extending at a right angle from an axon.

n.f., commissural. Nerve fiber that passes from one cerebral hemisphere to the other.

n.f., myelinated. Nerve fiber possessing a myelin sheath.

n.f., nonmedullated. Nerve fiber containing only an axis cylinder and a neurilemma.

n.f., postganglionic. Nerve fiber of the autonomic nervous system that terminates in smooth or cardiac muscle or a gland. Its cell body lies in an autonomic ganglion.

n.f., preganglionic. Nerve fiber of the autonomic nervous system that terminates and synapses in one of the autonomic ganglia. Its cell body lies in the brain or spinal cord.

n.f., projection. 1. Nerve fiber arising in the diencephalon and passing to the cerebral cortex. 2. Nerve fiber arising in the cerebral cortex and terminating in lower portions of the brain or in the spinal cord.

nerve fibril. A fine fiber in the cytoplasm and cell processes of a neuron. SYN: *neurofibrilla.*

nerve gas. Gaseous materials used in chemical warfare. The agents may actually be in liquid form but are aerosolized at the time of use. These chemicals are readily absorbed through the skin. Some forms, organophosphates that inhibit acetylcholinesterase, cause copious secretions from the nose, eyes, mouth, lungs, and intestines. Muscle fasiculations, twitching, and miosis are present. A large dose may cause sudden unconsciousness, convulsions, flaccid paralysis, apnea, and death. With some agents, only a few breaths of the vapor may cause death. SYN: *nerve agents.*

PROTECTION: Charcoal-lined suits. The agents will penetrate ordinary clothing worn with a gas mask.

TREAT: Pretreatment with pyridostigmine and concurrent treatment at the time of exposure with atropine, pralidoxime, and diazepam may be life-saving. Decontaminate skin with household bleach diluted 1:10 or soap and water. Irrigate eyes with plain water. Military personnel carry small towels impregnated with chloramine, hydroxide, and phenol.

Caution: Gas masks should cover face and eyes and be proven to be adequately effective. Persons treating patients must protect themselves from the nerve agents.

---

nerve growth factor. ABBR: NGF. A protein necessary for the growth and maintenance of sympathetic and certain sensory neurons.

nerve impulse. The excitatory process that travels along a nerve fiber when stimulated. SEE: *impulse, nervous.*

nerve plexus. A network of nerves.

nerve trunk. The main stem of a peripheral nerve.

nervi. Pl. of nervus.

n. terminales. [NA] Terminal nerves, accompanying the olfactory nerve to the brain. Consist principally of sensory fibers from mucosa of nasal septum.

nervimotility (nĕr″vĭ-mō-tĭl′ĭ-tē) [L. *nervus,* nerve, + *motilis,* moving]. Capability for motion or movement in response to nervous stimulation.

nervimotor (nĕr″vĭ-mō′tor) [″ + *motus,* moving]. Concerning a motor nerve.

nervo- [L. *nervus,* nerve]. Combining form pert. to a nerve.

nervone. A cerebroside present in brain tissue; contains nervonic acid.

nervous [L. *nervosus*]. 1. Anxious. 2. Characterized by excitability. 3. Pert. to the nerves.

nervous breakdown. A lay term for any mental illness, esp. one with acute onset, that interferes with normal function, thought, or action.

nervous debility. Nervous fatigue with resultant physical exhaustion. SYN: *neurasthenia.*

nervous impulse. The excitatory process set up in nerve fibers by stimuli. It is probably in the nature of a wave of electrochemical charges traveling at the comparatively slow rate (even in fastest conducting mammalian nerves) of 50 to 80 meters per second. The velocity varies in different fibers according to the diameter. SEE: *impulse, nervous.*

nervousness. State of being nervous.

nervous prostration. Neurasthenia, q.v.

nervous system. A system of extremely delicate nerve cells, elaborately interlaced with each other. Made up collectively of the brain, cranial nerves, spinal cord, spinal nerves, autonomic ganglia, ganglionated trunks and nerves, maintaining the vital function of reception and response to stimuli. The nervous system regulates and coordinates body activities and brings about responses by which the body adjusts to changes of environment, either external or internal. These changes constitute stimuli that initiate impulses in receptors or sense organs. The principal organs of this group are the eye, ear, the organs of taste and smell, and sensory receptors located in the skin, joints, muscles, and various parts of the body.

The nervous system consists of two divisions: the central nervous system, which includes the brain and spinal cord; and the peripheral nervous system, which includes all the other neural elements. SEE: *autonomic nervous system; central nervous system; parasympathetic nervous system; sympathetic nervous system.*

nervous tissue. Tissue that makes up the nervous system. Includes the nervous elements proper (neurons) and the interstitial tissue (neuroglia, neurilemma cells, and satellite cells).

nervus [L.] (pl. *nervi*). [NA] Nerve. SEE: *Nerves* in *Appendix.*

    n. erigens. [NA] A scattered bundle of craniosacral autonomic fibers originating from the 2nd to 4th sacral nerves and passing to terminal ganglia from which postganglionic fibers pass to the pelvic organs (bladder, colon, rectum, prostate gland, seminal vesicles, external genitalia).

    n. intermedius. [NA] A branch of the facial nerve consisting principally of sensory fibers.

    n. nervorum. Nerve fibers that innervate sheaths of nerves.

    n. vasorum. Nerve fibers that innervate the walls of blood vessels.

Nesacaine. Trade name for chloroprocaine hydrochloride, USP.

nesidiectomy (nē-sĭd″ē-ĕk′tō-mē) [Gr. *nesidion*, islet, + *ektome*, excision]. Surgical excision of islet-cell tissue of the pancreas.

nesidioblastoma (nē-sĭd″ē-ō-blăs-tō′mă) [″ + *blastos*, germ, + *oma*, tumor]. Islet-cell tumor of the pancreas.

nesslerize (nĕs′lĕr-īz). To test with Nessler's reagent.

Nessler's reagent (nĕs′lĕrz) [A. Nessler, Ger. chemist, 1827–1905]. A solution used to test for ammonia. It contains potassium iodide, mercuric chloride, and potassium hydroxide.

nest. A small mass of cells that resembles a bird's nest and is alien to the surrounding tissue.

    n., cancer. Nest of cells extending from a common center; seen in cancerous growths.

    n., cell. Nest of epithelial cells set apart from surrounding cells by connective tissue.

nesteostomy (nĕs″tē-ŏs′tō-mē) [Gr. *nestis*, jejunum, + *stoma*, mouth]. Jejunostomy, q.v.

nestiatria (nĕs″tē-ā′trē-ă) [Gr. *nestis*, fasting, + *iatreia*, medical treatment]. Fasting therapy.

n. et m. *nocte et mane*, night and morning.

net reproductive rate. ABBR: NRR. A measure of whether a population is reproducing at a greater or lesser rate than needed for its replacement. It is determined by calculating the average number of surviving daughters born to the women in that population during their reproductive years. An NRR of 1 indicates that each woman in the population has one surviving daughter during her lifetime.

ne tr. s. num. *ne tradas sine nummo*, do not deliver unless paid.

nettle. Plants of the genus *Urtica*. Their sawtoothed leaves contain hairs that secrete a fluid that irritates the skin.

nettle rash [AS. *netel*]. Skin rash with intense itching, resembling condition produced by stinging with nettles. SYN: *hives; urticaria.*

network [AS. *net*, net, + *wyrcan*, to work]. Fiber arrangement in a structure resembling a net. SYN: *rete; reticulum.*

Neumann's disease (noy′mănz) [Isidor Neumann, Austrian dermatologist, 1832–1906]. Pemphigus vegetans.

neur-, neuri-, neuro-. Combining form concerning a nerve or the nervous system.

neurad (nū′răd) [Gr. *neuron*, nerve, sinew, + L. *-ad*, toward]. Toward a nerve or its axis.

neuragmia (nū-răg′mē-ă) [Gr. *neuron*, nerve, sinew, + *agmos*, break]. The tearing or rupturing of a nerve trunk.

neural (nū′răl) [L. *neuralis*]. Pert. to nerves or connected with the nervous system.

neural crest. A band of cells extending longitudinally along the neural tube of an embryo from which cells forming cranial, spinal, and autonomic ganglia arise. They also give rise to cells (ectomesenchyme) that migrate into the forming facial region and become odontoblasts, which form the dentin of the tooth.

neural fold. One of two longitudinal elevations of the neural plate of an embryo that unite to form the neural tube.

neuralgia (nū-răl′jē-ă) [Gr. *neuron*, nerve, sinew, + *algos*, pain]. Severe sharp pain along the course of a nerve. SYN: *neurodynia*. SEE: *sciatica and low back pain.*

    ETIOL: Pressure on nerve trunks, faulty nerve nutrition, toxins, neuritis. Usually no morphologic changes can be detected.

    n., cardiac. Angina pectoris.

    n., degenerative. Neuralgia caused by degenerative changes in the nerves or nerve cells; occurs in the elderly.

    n., facial. N., trigeminal.

    n. facialis vera. N., geniculate.

    n., Fothergill's. N., trigeminal.

    n., geniculate. Neuralgia characterized by pain over all or any part supplied by sensory fibers of facial nerve. Pain may be deep in facial muscles, within the ear, or in pharynx. SYN: *n., Hunt's.*

    n., glossopharyngeal. Neuralgia along the course of the glossopharyngeal nerve, characterized by severe pain in back of the throat, tonsils, and middle ear.

    n., hallucinatory. Impression of local pain without an actual stimulus to cause the pain.

    n., Hunt's. N., geniculate.

n., idiopathic. Neuralgia without structural lesion or pressure from a lesion.

n., intercostal. Neuralgia in which pain follows course of intercostal nerves; frequently associated with eruption of herpes zoster. Spots of tenderness near vertebral column, in middle of nerve, and near sternum. May be dependent upon spinal caries or thoracic aneurysm. SYN: *pleuralgia.*

n., mammary. Neuralgia of the breast. SYN: *mastodynia.*

n., Morton's. Neuralgia of joint of third and fourth toes. SYN: *metatarsalgia.*

n., nasociliary. Neuralgia of eyes, brows, and root of nose.

n., occipital. Neuralgia involving upper cervical nerves. A spot of tenderness found between mastoid process and upper cervical vertebrae. May be due to spinal caries.

n., otic. N., geniculate.

n., reminiscent. Continued mental perception of pain after neuralgia has ceased.

n., sphenopalatine. Neuralgia of the sphenopalatine ganglion, causing pain in the area of the upper jawbone and radiating into the neck and shoulders.

SYM: Pain on one side of face radiating to eyeballs, ear, and occipital and mastoid areas of skull; sometimes to nose, upper teeth, and shoulder of same side.

PROG: Good.

n., stump. Neuralgia due to pressure on nerves at site of amputation.

n., symptomatic. Neuralgia not primarily involving the nerve structure but occurring as a symptom of local or systemic disease.

n., trifacial. Old term for trigeminal neuralgia.

n., trigeminal. Neuralgia involving the gasserian ganglion or one or more branches of the trigeminal nerve. SYN: *n., facial; n., Fothergill's; tic douloureux.* SEE: *Nursing Diagnoses* in *Appendix.*

SYM: Tender points corresponding to supraorbital, infraorbital, and mental foramina. Often violent spasm of muscles. In long-standing cases, hair on affected side sometimes becomes coarse and bleached.

ETIOL: Unknown. Attacks often precipitated by initiation of pain by obvious stimuli on certain hypersensitive areas called trigger zones of face, lips, or tongue.

TREAT: Drugs such as phenytoin or dibenzazepine have been useful in suppressing or shortening attacks. Their use for temporary relief may permit spontaneous remission. If, however, the syndrome persists, then the nerve is injected with alcohol or phenol, or it is surgically sectioned.

neuralgic (nū-răl′jĭk) [Gr. *neuron,* nerve, sinew, + *algos,* pain]. Of, or concerning, neuralgia.

neuralgiform (nū-răl′jĭ-form) [″ + ″ + L. *forma,* form]. Similar to neuralgia.

neural grafting. An experimental procedure for transplanting tissue into the brain and spinal cord. Possible sources of material to be used include human fetal tissue, cultured and genetically engineered cells, and tissues from the patient's own body.

neural network, artificial. A group of interconnected mathematic equations that accept input data and that calculate an output based on this input. This system has been used to predict both the presence and the absence of acute myocardial infarction. In one study, use of this method was better than the physicians caring for the patients in the Emergency Department.

neural plate. A thickened band of ectoderm along the dorsal surface of an embryo. The nervous system develops from this tissue.

neural spine. Spinous vertebral process.

neural tube. Tube formed from fusion of the neural folds from which the brain and spinal cord arise.

neural tube defects. ABBR: NTD. Defective closures of the neural tube during early embryogenesis. Included are fetal anencephaly, spina bifida, lumbar meningomyelocele, and meningocele. The tendency for this condition to be present may be inherited. The overall incidence is 1 to 2 in every 1000 live births. If the defect is of the type with an open tube, the levels of maternal and fetal serum alpha-fetoprotein (AFP) are elevated.

The alleged association of NTD with vitamin use around the time of conception has not been validated.

neuramebimeter (nū″răm-ē-bĭm′ĕt-ēr) [″ + *amoibe,* response, + *metron,* measure]. Device for determining time of response of a nerve to a stimulus.

neuraminidase (nūr-ăm′ĭn-ĭ-dās″). An enzyme present on the surface of influenza virus particles. Activity of this enzyme enables the virus particle to separate itself from cells. Persons with increased levels of antibodies against neuraminidase in their serum may have increased resistance to influenza infection.

neuranagenesis (nū″răn-ă-jĕn′ē-sĭs) [″ + *anagennan,* to regenerate]. Regeneration of a nerve.

neurapophysis (nū″ră-pŏf′ĭ-sĭs) [″ + *apo,* from, + *physis,* growth]. Either of the two sides of a vertebra that unite to form the neural arch.

neurapraxia (nū″ră-prăks′ē-ă) [″ + *apraxia,* nonactive]. Cessation in function of a peripheral nerve without degenerative changes occurring. Recovery is the usual outcome.

neurarchy (nū′rär-kē) [″ + *arche*, rule]. The domination of the nervous system over the body.

neurarthropathy (nū″rär-thrŏp′ă-thē) [″ + *arthron*, joint, + *pathos*, disease, suffering]. Neuroarthropathy, q.v.

neurasthenia (nū″răs-thē′nē-ă) [″ + *astheneia*, weakness]. A term previously used for persons with unexplained chronic fatigue and lassitude. Accompanying these symptoms were usually nervousness, irritability, anxiety, depression, headache, insomnia, and sexual disorders. Those individuals are now diagnosed according to their total condition, such as some form of psychiatric illness, esp. anxiety neurosis or tension state.

neurasthenic (nū-răs-thē′nĭk). 1. Individual suffering from neurasthenia. 2. Suffering from or concerning neurasthenia.

neuratrophia, neuratrophy (nū-ră-trō′fē-ă, -răt′rō-fē) [″ + *atrophia*, a wasting]. Atrophy of the nervous tissue or deficient nutrition of the nervous system.

neuraxis (nū-răk′sĭs) [″ + L. *axon*, axis]. The cerebrospinal axis.

neuraxitis (nū-răks-ī′tĭs) [″ + ″ + Gr. *itis*, inflammation]. Encephalitis.

n., epidemic. Epidemic encephalitis.

neuraxon(e) (nū-răks′ōn). The axis cylinder process of a nerve cell. SYN: *axon*. SEE: *nerve fiber*.

neurectasia, neurectasis, neurectasy (nū″rĕk-tā′sē-ă, -rĕk′tă-sĭs, -rĕk′tă-sē) [″ + *ektasis*, a stretching]. Surgical nerve stretching. SYN: *neurotension*.

neurectomy (nū-rĕk′tō-mē) [″ + *ektome*, excision]. Partial or total excision or resection of a nerve.

n., presacral. Severing or removing the presacral nerve. A surgical procedure that has been used in treating severe dysmenorrhea.

neurectopia, neurectopy (nū-rĕk-tō′pē-ă, nūr-ĕk′tō-pē) [″ + *ek*, out, + *topos*, place]. Displacement or abnormal position of a nerve.

neurenteric (nū-rĕn-tĕr′ĭk) [″ + *enteron*, intestine]. Rel. to the neural canal and intestinal tube of the embryo.

neurenteric canal. Temporary canal of the embryo, between the neural and intestinal tubes. In human development, the temporary communication between cavities of the yolk sac and the amnion.

neurepithelium (nūr″ĕp-ĭ-thē′lē-ŭm) [″ + *epi*, upon, + *thele*, nipple]. 1. Epithelial structures forming the terminations of nerves of special sense. 2. Embryonic layer from which arises the cerebrospinal axis. SYN: *neuroepithelium*.

neurergic (nū-rĕr′jĭk) [″ + *ergon*, work]. Concerning the activity of a nerve.

neurexeresis (nūr″ĕks-ĕr′ĕ-sĭs) [″ + *exairein*, to draw out]. Ripping or tearing out of a nerve to relieve neuralgia.

neuriatry (nū-rī′ă-trē) [″ + *iatreia*, medication]. Neurology, q.v.

neurilemma (nū″rĭ-lĕm″mă) [″ + *lemma*, husk]. A thin membranous sheath enveloping a nerve fiber. SYN: *neurolemma; sheath of Schwann*. SEE: *nerve fiber*.

neurilemmitis (nū″rĭ-lĕm-mī′tĭs) [″ + ″ + *itis*, inflammation]. Inflamed condition of a neurilemma.

neurilemmosarcoma (nū″rĭ-lĕm″ō-săr-kō′mă). A malignant neurilemoma.

neurilemoma, neurilemmoma (nū″rĭ-lĕm-ō′mă) [″ + *eilema*, tight sheath, + *oma*, tumor]. A firm, encapsulated fibrillar tumor of peripheral nerves. SYN: *neurinoma; neurofibroma; peripheral glioma; schwannoma*.

neurimotility (nū″rĭ-mō-tĭl′ĭ-tē) [″ + *motilus*, moving]. Nervimotility, q.v.

neurimotor [″ + L. *motor*, a mover]. Concerning a motor nerve.

neurinoma (nū-rĭ-nō′mă) [″ + *oma*, tumor]. A peripheral glioma. A tumor of a peripheral nerve arising from endoneurium or sheath of Schwann. SYN: *neurilemmoma; neurofibroma; schwannoma*.

neurinomatosis (nū″rĭ-nō-mă-tō′sĭs) [″ + ″ + *osis*, condition]. Condition of having multiple neurinomas on nerve fibers. SYN: *neurofibromatosis*.

neurite (nū′rīt) [Gr. *neuron*, nerve, sinew]. The axis cylinder process of a neuron. Both axons and dendrites are neurites. SYN: *neuraxon*.

neuritis (nū-rī′tĭs) [″ + *itis*, inflammation]. Inflammation of a nerve or nerves, usually associated with a degenerative process. SEE: *Guillain-Barré syndrome; polyneuritis*.

SYM: Neuralgia in part affected; hyperesthesia, paresthesia, dysesthesia, hypesthesia, or anesthesia; muscular atrophy of part supplied by affected nerve; paralysis; lack of reflexes.

ETIOL: Mechanical factors: compression, contusion, trauma. Infections: localized involving direct infection of nerves or may accompany diseases such as leprosy, tetanus, tuberculosis, malaria, or measles. Toxins: esp. poisoning by heavy metals (arsenic, lead, mercury), alcohol, or carbon tetrachloride. Metabolic factors: as in thiamine deficiency, gastrointestinal dysfunction, diabetes, or toxemias of pregnancy. Vascular: as in neuritis accompanying peripheral vascular disease.

NURSING IMPLICATIONS: Monitor

changes in motor and sensory function. Relieve pain with correct positioning and prescribed analgesic drugs. Promote physical and emotional rest for the patient, and rest affected extremities by limiting use and by using supportive appliances. Prevent contracture formation with passive range-of-motion exercises. Provide skin care. Promote proper nutrition and dietary therapy for metabolic disorders. Remove causative factors or counsel patient about their avoidance. After pain subsides, support use of prescribed activity: massage, electrostimulation, exercise. SEE: *Nursing Diagnoses* in *Appendix.*

n., adventitial. Inflammation of nerve sheath.

n., ascending. Neuritis moving upward along a nerve trunk away from periphery.

n., axial. Inflammation of inner portion of a nerve.

n., degenerative. Neuritis with rapid degeneration of nerve.

n., descending. Neuritis that leads away from the central nervous system.

n., dietetic. Beriberi.

n., diphtheritic. Neuritis following diphtheria.

n., disseminated. Neuritis involving a large group of nerves.

n., endemic. Beriberi.

n., interstitial. Neuritis involving connective tissue of a nerve.

n., intraocular. Neuritis of retinal fibers of optic nerve.

SYM: Disturbed vision, contracted field, enlarged blind spot, fundus findings such as exudates, hemorrhages, and abnormal condition of blood vessels.

TREAT: Depends on etiology such as brain tumors, meningitis, syphilis, nephritis, diabetes.

n. migrans. Neuritis that passes along a nerve trunk, affecting one area and then another. May be ascending or descending.

n., multiple. Simultaneous impairment of a number of peripheral nerves. SYN: *polyneuritis.*

SYM: Related to suddenness of onset and severity; usually lower limbs are affected first with weakness that may progress until the entire body is affected. Muscle strength, deep tendon reflexes, sensory nerves, and autonomic nerves become involved.

ETIOL: Infectious diseases such as diphtheria; metabolic disorders including alcoholism, diabetes, pellagra, beriberi, and sprue; various poisons, including lead. In some instances the disease arises without apparent cause.

TREAT: Remove causative factors if possible. Skilled nursing with particular

care taken to prevent bedsores. Dietary therapy depending upon the etiology.

n. nodosa. Neuritis with formation of nodes on nerves.

n., optic. Neuritis of optic nerve.

n., parenchymatous. Neuritis of nerve fiber substance.

n., peripheral. Neuritis of terminal nerves or end organs.

n., retrobulbar. Neuritis of optic nerve behind the eyeball.

SYM: Acute loss of vision in one or both eyes. Pain may be absent or unbearable and may last for days or only a brief period.

ETIOL: May be caused by a variety of illnesses but is most frequently caused by multiple sclerosis.

n., rheumatic. Neuritis with symptoms of rheumatism.

n., sciatic. Inflammation of the sciatic nerve. SEE: *sciatica and low back pain.*

n., segmental. Neuritis affecting segments of a nerve interspersed with healthy segments.

n., senile. Neuritis in the elderly, usually affecting the extremities.

n., sympathetic. Neuritis of the opposite nerve without attack of nerve center.

n., tabetic. Neuritis in locomotor ataxia. Caused by syphilis.

n., toxic. Neuritis resulting from poisons. Metallic poisons such as arsenic, mercury, and thallium or nonmetallic poisons such as various hydrocarbons and organic solvents can cause this.

n., traumatic. Neuritis following an injury.

neuro- [Gr. *neuron*, nerve, sinew]. Combining form pert. to a nerve, nervous tissue, or nervous system.

neuroallergy (nū″rō-ăl′ĕr-jē) [″ + *allos*, other, + *ergon*, work]. Allergy in nervous tissue.

neuroanastomosis (nū″rō-ă-năs″tō-mō′sĭs) [″ + *anastomosis*, opening]. Surgical attachment of one end of a severed nerve to the other end.

neuroanatomy (nū″rō-ăn-ăt′ō-mē). Study of anatomy of the nervous system.

neuroarthropathy (nū″rō-ăr-thrŏp′ă-thē) [″ + ″ + *pathos*, disease, suffering]. Disease of a joint combined with disease of the central nervous system.

neuroastrocytoma (nū″rō-ăs″trō-sī-tō′mă) [″ + *kytos*, cell, + *oma*, tumor]. A tumor of the central nervous system composed of neurons and glial cells.

neurobiology (nū″rō-bī-ŏl′ō-jē) [″ + *bios*, life, + *logos*, word, reason]. Biology of the nervous system.

neurobiotaxis (nū″rō-bī-ō-tăk′sĭs) [″ + *bios*, life, + *taxis*, order]. The phenomenon involving growth of dendrites and migration of nerve-cell bodies during development toward the region from which their dominant impulses are initiated.

neuroblast (nū′rō-blăst) [″ + *blastos*, germ]. An embryonic cell derived from neural tube or neural crest, giving rise to a neuron.

neuroblastoma (nū″rō-blăs-tō′mă) [″ + ″ + *oma*, tumor]. A malignant hemorrhagic tumor composed principally of cells resembling neuroblasts that give rise to cells of the sympathetic system, esp. adrenal medulla. Occurs chiefly in infants and children. Primary sites are in the mediastinal and retroperitoneal regions.

neurocanal (nū″rō-kă-năl′) [″ + L. *canalis*, passage]. The central canal of the spinal cord.

neurocardiac (nū″rō-kăr′dē-ăk) [″ + *kardia*, heart]. 1. Pert. to the nerves supplying the heart or nervous system and the heart. 2. Concerning a cardiac neurosis.

neurocele (nū′rō-sēl) [″ + *koilia*, cavity]. Ventricles and cavities in the cerebrospinal axis.

neurocentral (nū′rō-sĕn′trăl) [″ + *kentron*, center]. Pert. to the centrum of a vertebra and the neural arch.

neurocentrum (nū′rō-sĕn′trŭm). The body of a vertebra.

neurochemistry (nū″rō-kĕm′ĭs-trē). Physiological chemistry dealing with nervous tissue.

neurochorioretinitis (nū″rō-kō″rē-ō-rĕ″tĭn-ī′tĭs) [Gr. *neuron*, nerve, sinew, + *chorion*, skin, + L. *retina*, retina, + Gr. *itis*, inflammation]. Inflammation of choroid and retina combined with optic neuritis.

neurochoroiditis (nū″rō-kō-roy-dī′tĭs) [″ + ″ + *eidos*, form, shape, + *itis*, inflammation]. Inflamed condition of the choroid coat and optic nerve.

neurocirculatory (nū″rō-sŭr′kū-lă-tō″rē) [″ + L. *circulatio*, circulation]. Pert. to circulation and the nervous system.

neurocirculatory asthenia. A combination of functional nervous and circulatory disturbances with fatigue and precordial pain.

neurocladism (nū-rŏk′lă-dĭzm) [″ + *klados*, a young branch, + *-ismos*, condition]. Phenomenon occurring after a nerve is severed, where an outgrowth of fibrils closes the gap and begins the process of nerve repair. SYN: *odogenesis.*

neuroclonic (nū″rō-klŏn′ĭk) [″ + *klonos*, spasm]. Marked by spasms of nervous origin.

neurocoele (nū′rō-sēl) [″ + *koilia*, cavity]. System of cavities in cerebrospinal axis. SYN: *neurocele.*

neurocranium (nū″rō-krā′nē-ŭm) [″ + *kranion*, skull]. The part of the skull enclosing the brain.

neurocrine (nū′rō-krĭn) [″ + *krinein*, to secrete]. 1. Indicating an endocrine influence on nerves or the influence of nerves on endocrine tissue. 2. A chemical transmitter.

neurocutaneous (nū″rō-kū-tā′nē-ŭs) [″ + L. *cutis*, skin]. Pert. to the nervous system and skin.

neurocyte (nū′rō-sīt) [″ + *kytos*, cell]. A nerve cell. SYN: *neuron.*

neurocytolysis (nū″rō-sī-tŏl′ĭ-sĭs) [″ + *kytos*, cell, + *lysis*, dissolution]. Dissolution or destruction of nerve cells.

neurocytoma (nū″rō-sī-tō′mă) [″ + ″ + *oma*, tumor]. A tumor formed of cells, usually ganglionic, of nervous origin. SEE: *neuroma.*

neurodealgia (nū-rō″dē-ăl′jē-ă) [Gr. *neurodes*, retina, + *algos*, pain]. Pain in the retina.

neurodegenerative. Concerning degeneration of tissue of the nervous system.

neurodendrite, neurodendron (nū″rō-dĕn′drīt, -drŏn) [Gr. *neuron*, nerve, sinew, + *dendron*, tree]. Protoplasmic branched process of a nerve cell. SYN: *dendrite; dendron.* SEE: *dendrite* and *nerve cell* for illus.

neurodermatitis (nū″rō-dĕr-mă-tī′tĭs) [″ + *derma*, skin, + *itis*, inflammation]. Cutaneous inflammation with itching that is associated with, but not entirely due to, emotional disturbance. Circumscribed neurodermatitis is used as a synonym for lichen simplex.

> *n., disseminated.* Chronic superficial inflammation of skin characterized by thickening, excoriation, and lichenification, usually beginning in infancy. Common in families with high familial incidence of allergic diseases. SYN: *dermatitis, atopic.*

neurodermatosis (nū″rō-dĕr-mă-tō′sĭs) [″ + ″ + *osis*, condition]. Any skin disease of neural origin. Includes neurofibromatosis (von Recklinghausen's disease), von Hippel-Lindau disease, Sturge-Weber syndrome, and tuberous sclerosis. SYN: *phacomatosis.*

neurodermatrophia (nū″rō-dĕrm″ă-trŏf′ē-ă). Atrophy of the skin from nervous disease.

neurodevelopmental treatment [Karel and Bertha Bobath, Brit. neuropsychiatrist and physiotherapist, respectively]. ABBR: NDT. A rehabilitation treatment approach for cerebral palsy, hemiplegia, and other CNS deficits that emphasizes the use of carefully considered treatment handling to inhibit abnormal reflexes and movement patterns and facilitate higher level reactions and patterns in order to attain normal movement.

neurodiagnosis (nū″rō-dī-ăg-nō'sĭs). Diagnosis of nervous disorders.

neurodynamic (nū″rō-dī-năm'ĭk). Concerning nervous force or energy.

neurodynia (nū″rō-dĭn'ē-ă) [Gr. *neuron*, nerve, + *odyne*, pain]. Pain in a nerve or nerves. SYN: *neuralgia*.

neuroectoderm (nū″rō-ĕk'tō-dĕrm) [″ + *ektos*, outside, + *derma*, skin]. The embryonic tissue that gives rise to nerve tissue.

neuroencephalomyelopathy (nū″rō-ĕn-sĕf″ă-lō-mī″ĕ-lŏp'ă-thē) [″ + *enkephalos*, brain, + *myelos*, marrow, + *pathos*, disease, suffering]. Disease of the brain, spinal cord, and nerves.

neuroendocrine (nū″rō-ĕn'dō-krĭn). Pert. to the nervous and endocrine systems as an integrated functioning mechanism.

neuroendocrine carcinoma. A diverse group of tumors such as carcinoid, islet cell tumors, neuroblastoma, and small-cell carcinomas of the lung. All have dense core granules and produce polypeptides that can be identified by immunochemical methods.

neuroendocrinology (nū″rō-ĕn″dō-krī-nŏl'ō-jē) [″ + *endon*, within, + *krinein*, to secrete, + *logos*, word, reason]. Study of the relationship between the nervous and endocrine systems.

neuroenteric (nū″rō-ĕn-tĕr'ĭk). Concerning the nervous system and intestines.

neuroepidermal (nū″rō-ĕp-ĭ-dĕr'măl) [″ + *epi*, upon, + *derma*, skin]. Pert. to or giving rise to the nervous system and epidermis.

neuroepithelioma (nū″rō-ĕp″ĭ-thē-lē-ō'mă) [″ + ″ + *thele*, nipple, + *oma*, tumor]. A relatively rare tumor of neuroepithelium in a nerve of special sense.

neuroepithelium (nū″rō-ĕp″ĭ-thē'lē-ŭm). 1. A specialized epithelial structure forming the termination of a nerve of special sense. Includes gustatory cells, olfactory cells, hair cells of inner ear, and rods and cones of retina. 2. Embryonic layer of the epiblast from which the cerebrospinal axis is developed. SYN: *neurepithelium*.

neurofibril, neurofibrilla (nū-rō-fī'brĭl, -fī-brĭl'ă) [″ + L. *fibrilla*, a small fiber] (pl. *neurofibrils, neurofibrillae*). Many tiny fibrils that extend in every direction in the cytoplasm of the nerve cell body. They extend into the axon and dendrites of the cell. SEE: *neuron*.

neurofibroma (nū″rō-fī-brō'mă) [Gr. *neuron*, nerve, + L. *fibra*, fiber, + Gr. *oma*, tumor] (pl. *neurofibromata* or *-mas*). A tumor of connective tissue of a nerve including medullated layer of a nerve fiber. May occur in mouth, pleura, or stomach. SYN: *pseudoneuroma*.

neurofibromatosis (nū″rō-fī-brō″mă-tō'sĭs) [″ + ″ + ″ + *osis*, condition]. A genetic disorder that affects cell growth of neural tissues.

n., Type 1. ABBR: NF-1. Previously known as von Recklinghausen's neurofibromatosis, NF-1 affects about 1 in 4000 persons. Clinically, there are multiple hyperpigmented areas. These appear shortly after birth and may be present any place on the body. Multiple cutaneous and subcutaneous tumors appear in late childhood. There may be a few or thousands. When the tumors are pressed, they pass through a small opening in the skin, leaving the space vacant where the tumor was in the skin. This characteristic, called buttonholing, helps to distinguish these tumors from lipomas. In about 2% to 5% of cases, the tumors become malignant. There is no cure, and tumors that give rise to symptoms or those that become malignant need to be excised. If the tumor is on a vital nerve, excision may be impossible. Radiation therapy is of benefit.

n., Type 2. ABBR: NF-2. A genetic disorder that affects 1 in 50,000 persons. Most tumors form in the 8th cranial nerve, but may also be present in other intracranial and intraspinal locations. These are treated by use of microsurgical technique in an attempt to remove the tumor(s) and preserve hearing. SYN: *acoustic neuroma*.

neurofibrosarcoma (nū″rō-fī″brō-săr-kō'mă) [″ + ″ + Gr. *sarx*, flesh, + *oma*, tumor]. A malignant neurofibroma. SYN: *neurogenic sarcoma*.

neurofibrositis (nū″rō-fī″brō-sī'tĭs) [″ + ″ + Gr. *itis*, inflammation]. Inflammation of nerve fibers and sensory nerve fibers in muscular tissue.

neurogangliitis (nū″rō-găn-glē-ī'tĭs) [″ + *ganglion*, knot, + *itis*, inflammation]. Inflamed condition of a neuroganglion.

neuroganglion (nū″rō-găn'glē-ŏn). A mass of nervous tissue.

neurogastric (nū″rō-găs'trĭk) [″ + *gaster*, belly]. Concerning the nerves of the stomach.

neurogenesis (nū″rō-jĕn'ĕ-sĭs) [″ + *genesis*, generation, birth]. 1. Growth or development of nerves. 2. Development from nervous tissue.

neurogenetic (nū″rō-jĕn-ĕt'ĭk). 1. Pert. to nerve formation. 2. Pert. to origin in nerves.

neurogenic, neurogenous (nū-rō-jĕn'ĭk, -rŏj'ĕn-ŭs). 1. Originating from nervous tissue. 2. Due to or resulting from nervous impulses.

neuroglia (nū-rŏg'lē-ă) [″ + *glia*, glue]. The tissue that forms the interstitial or supporting elements — cells and fibers — of the nervous system. Neuroglia, also called glia, includes astrocytes, oligodendroglias, microglia (mesoglia), ependyma, neurilemma sheath cells or nerve fibers (cells of Schwann), and satellite (capsule) cells surrounding cranial and spinai ganglia. All except the microglia are of ectodermal origin. Neuroglia acts as connective or supporting tissue and also plays an important role in the reaction of the nervous system to injury or infection.

neurogliacyte (nū-rŏg′lē-ă-sīt) [″ + ″ + kytos, cell]. Any one of the cells found in neuroglial tissue. SYN: *glia cell.*

neuroglial (nū-rŏg′lē-ăl). Pert. to the neuroglia.

neuroglioma (nū″rō-glī-ō′mă) [Gr. *neuron,* nerve, + *glia,* glue, + *oma,* tumor]. Tumor of neuroglial tissue. SYN: *glioma.*

    n. ganglionare. Glioma with ganglion cells.

neurogliomatosis (nū″rō-glī″ō-mă-tō′sĭs) [″ + ″ + ″ + *osis,* condition]. Multiple glioma formation in the nervous system.

neurogliosis (nū-rŏg″lē-ō′sĭs) [″ + ″ + *osis,* condition]. Development of numerous neurogliomas.

neurogram (nū′rō-grăm). Engram, q.v.

neurohistology (nū″rō-hĭs-tŏl′ō-jē) [″ + *histos,* tissue, + *logos,* study]. Study of the microscopic anatomy of nervous tissue.

neurohormone (nū-rō-hor′mōn) [″ + *hormon,* urging on]. Substances released as minute secretory granules from neurons. In contrast to the method of action of neurotransmitters, q.v., these materials affect distant cells via the bloodstream. SEE: *neuromodulator.*

neurohypophysis (nū″rō-hī-pŏf′ĭs-ĭs) [″ + *hypo,* under, + *physis,* growth]. Posterior portion or pars nervosa of the pituitary gland.

neuroid (nū′royd) [″ + *eidos,* form, shape]. Similar to a nerve.

neuroinduction (nū″rō-ĭn-dŭk′shŭn) [″ + L. *inductus,* leading]. Mental suggestion.

neurokeratin (nū″rō-kĕr′ă-tĭn) [″ + *keras,* horn]. The type of keratin found in myelinated nerve fibers.

neurokyme (nū′rō-kīm) [″ + *kyma,* wave]. A nerve process or action.

neurolemma. Neurilemma, q.v.

neurolemmitis (nū″rō-lĕ-mī′tĭs) [″ + *lemma,* husk, + *itis,* inflammation]. Neurilemmitis, q.v.

neurolemmoma (nū″rō-lĕ-mō′mă) [″ + ″ + *oma,* tumor]. Neurilemoma, q.v.

neuroleptanesthesia (nū″rō-lĕp″tăn-ĕs-thē′zēă) [″ + *leptos,* slender, + *-an,* not, + *aisthesis,* sensation]. General anesthesia involving intravenous administration of a neuroleptic drug and an analgesic.

neuroleptic (nū″rō-lĕp′tĭk) [″ + *lepsis,* a taking hold]. 1. An agent or drug that modifies psychotic behavior. In general, the term is synonymous with antipsychotic. 2. Indicating a condition produced by a neuroleptic agent.

neuroleptic anesthesia. SEE: *anesthesia, neuroleptic.*

neuroleptic drugs. Medicines that produce symptoms resembling those of diseases of the nervous system.

neuroleptic malignant syndrome. ABBR: NMS. The combination of catatonic rigidity, stupor, unstable blood pressure, hyperthermia, profuse sweating, dyspnea, and incontinence that occurs as a toxic reaction to use of potent neuroleptic (antipsychotic) agents in therapeutic doses. The condition lasts 5 to 10 days after discontinuation of the drug(s). The mortality rate may be as high as 20%. Bromocriptine and dantrolene have been used to treat NMS if the usual treatment for hyperthermia is ineffective. SEE: *hyperpyrexia, malignant.*

neurologic, neurological (nū-rō-lŏj′ĭk, -ĭ-kăl) [″ + *logos,* word, reason]. Pert. to the study of nervous diseases.

neurologist (nū-rŏl′ō-jĭst). A specialist in diseases of the nervous system.

neurology (nū-rŏl′ō-jē) [″ + *logos,* word, reason]. The branch of medicine that deals with the nervous system and its diseases. SEE: *psychiatry and neurology, words pert. to.*

    n., clinical. The branch of medicine that is concerned with study and treatment of diseases of the nervous system.

neurolymphomatosis (nū″rō-lĭm″fō-mă-tō′sĭs) [″ + L. *lympha,* lymph, + Gr. *oma,* tumor, + *osis,* condition]. Malignant lymphoma involving the nervous system.

neurolysin (nū-rŏl′ĭ-sĭn) [″ + *lysis,* dissolution]. A substance that destroys nerve cells.

neurolysis (nū-rŏl′ĭs-ĭs). 1. Stretching of a nerve to relieve tension. 2. Loosening of adhesions surrounding a nerve. 3. Disintegration or destruction of nerve tissue.

neurolytic (nū-rō-lĭt′ĭk). Concerning neurolysis.

neuroma (nū-rō′mă) [″ + *oma,* tumor]. Former term for any type of tumor composed of nerve cells. New growth of nerves is now categorized with respect to the specific portion of the nerve involved. SEE: *ganglioneuroma; neurilemoma.*

    n., acoustic. A benign tumor of the eighth cranial nerve. The symptoms may include hearing loss, balance disturbances, pain, headache, and tinnitus.

    n., amputation. Neuroma occurring on a stump after amputation.

n., amyelinic. Neuroma composed principally of unmyelinated nerve fibers.

n., appendiceal. Neuroma found in mucosa and submucosa of the appendix.

n. cutis. Neuroma in the skin.

n., cystic. Neuroma with cystic formations.

n., false. Tumor arising from connective tissue of nerves, including the myelin sheath. SYN: *neurofibroma; pseudoneuroma.*

n., ganglionated. Neuroma composed of true nerve cells.

n., multiple. Neurofibromatosis.

n., myelinic. Neuroma composed of medullated nerve fibers.

n., plexiform. Neuroma of nerve trunks that appear to be twisted.

n. telangiectodes. Neuroma with an abundance of blood vessels contained within it.

n., traumatic. Unorganized mass of nerve fibers occurring in wounds or on an amputation stump; result of accidental or intentional incision of the nerve.

neuromalacia (nū″rō-măl-ā′sē-ă) [″ + *malakia*, softening]. Pathological softening of neural tissue.

neuromatosis (nū-rō″mă-tō′sĭs) [″ + *oma*, tumor, + *osis*, condition]. Multiple neuromas occurring in the body.

neuromatous (nū-rō′mă-tŭs). Rel. to a neuroma.

neuromechanism (nū″rō-mĕk′ăn-ĭzm). The neural structure controlling organic and systemic function.

neuromere (nū′rō-mēr) [″ + *meros*, part]. One of a series of segmental elevations on the ventrolateral surface of the rhombencephalon.

neuromimesis (nū″rō-mĭ-mē′sĭs) [″ + *mimesis*, imitation]. Hysterical or neurotic simulation of organic disease.

neuromodulator. Biologically active substances produced by neurons that enhance or diminish the effects of neurotransmitters. Some neuromodulators are substance P, cholecystokinin, and somatostatin. SEE: *neurohormone; neuron; neurotransmitter.*

neuromuscular (nū″rō-mŭs′kū-lăr) [″ + L. *musculus*, a muscle]. Concerning both nerves and muscles.

neuromyasthenia (nū″rō-mī″ăs-thē′nē-ă) [″ + *mys*, muscle, + *astheneia*, weakness]. Muscular weakness usually due to an emotional disorder.

neuromyelitis (nū″rō-mī-ĕl-ī′tĭs) [″ + *myelos*, marrow, + *itis*, inflammation]. Inflammation of nerves and the spinal cord.

n. optica. A syndrome resulting from demyelinization occurring in the spinal cord, optic nerves, and chiasma. Etiology is unknown. May be a variant form of multiple sclerosis.

neuromyopathic (nū″rō-mī″ō-păth′ĭk) [″ + *mys*, muscle, + *pathos*, disease, suffering]. Pert. to pathological conditions involving both muscles and nerves.

neuromyositis (nū″rō-mī″ō-sī′tĭs) [″ + ″ + *itis*, inflammation]. Neuritis complicated by inflammation of muscles that come in contact with affected nerves.

neuron (nū′rŏn) [Gr. *neuron*, nerve, sinew]. A nerve cell, the structural and functional unit of the nervous system. A neuron consists of a cell body or perikaryon and its processes, an axon, and one or more dendrites. Neurons function in initiation and conduction of impulses. In addition, the brain cells influence cells by secreting neurotransmitters that function to alter the affected cell by actually physically contacting it. Alternatively, a neuron may release neurohormones, q.v., into the bloodstream. SEE: *nerve; nervous impulse; nervous system; neurohormone; neuromodulator; neurotransmitter.*

n., afferent. Neuron that conducts impulses toward the brain or spinal cord.

n., associative. Neuron that mediates impulses between a sensory and a motor neuron.

n., bipolar. Neuron that bears two processes.

n., central. Neuron confined entirely to central nervous system.

n., commissural. Neuron whose axon crosses to opposite side of the brain or spinal cord.

n., efferent. Neuron that conducts impulses away from the brain or spinal cord.

n., motor. Neuron that conveys impulses initiating muscle contraction. SEE: illus.

n., motor, lower. Neuron whose cell body lies in anterior gray column of spinal cord. Its axon innervates striated muscle fibers.

n., motor, upper. Neuron whose cell body lies in motor area of cerebral cortex. Its axon passes down spinal cord and synapses with lower motor neurons.

n., multipolar. Neuron with one axon and many dendrites.

n., peripheral. Neuron whose process constitutes a part of the peripheral nervous system (cranial, spinal, or sympathetic nerves).

n., postganglionic. Neuron whose body lies in an autonomic ganglion and whose axon terminates in an effector organ (smooth or cardiac muscle or glands).

n., preganglionic. Neuron of autonomic nervous system whose cell body lies in cen-

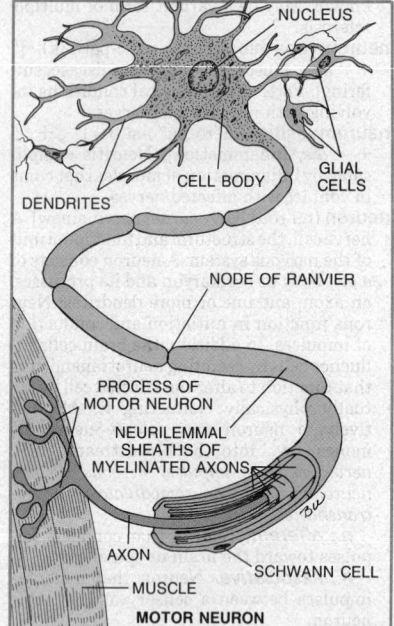

NUCLEUS

GLIAL CELLS

CELL BODY

DENDRITES

NODE OF RANVIER

PROCESS OF MOTOR NEURON

NEURILEMMAL SHEATHS OF MYELINATED AXONS

AXON

SCHWANN CELL

MUSCLE

MOTOR NEURON

tral nervous system and axon terminates in peripheral ganglia.

n., sensory. An afferent neuron that conveys impulses that give rise to sensations.

n., unipolar. Neuron whose cell body bears one process.

neuronal (nū′rō-năl). Pert. to one or more neurons.

neurone (nū′rōn). Neuron.

neuronephric (nū″rō-něf′rĭk) [″ + *nephros*, kidney]. Concerning the nervous and renal systems.

neuronevus (nū″rō-nē′vŭs). Intradermal nevus.

neuronitis (nū-rō-nī′tĭs) [Gr. *neuron*, nerve, + *itis*, inflammation]. Inflammation or degenerative inflammation of nerve cells.

neuronophage (nū-rŏn′ō-fāj) [″ + *phagein*, to eat]. A phagocyte that destroys tissue in the nervous system.

neuronophagia, neuronophagy (nū-rŏn″ō-fā′jē-ă, -ŏf′ă-jē). Destruction of nerve cells by phagocytes.

neuro-ophthalmology (nū″rō-ŏf″thăl-mŏl′ō-jē) [″ + *ophthalmos*, eye, + *logos*, word, reason]. The branch of ophthalmology concerned with the neurology of the vi-

sual system.

neuro-optic (nū″rō-ŏp′tĭk) [″ + *optikos*, pert. to vision]. Concerning the central nervous system and the eye.

neuropacemaker. An implantable device for electrical stimulation of the dorsal column of the spinal tract. The electrical energy is provided in pulses at an appropriate rate in order to inhibit perception of pain.

neuropapillitis (nū″rō-păp″ĭ-lī′tĭs) [″ + L. *papilla*, nipple, + Gr. *itis*, inflammation]. Optic neuritis.

neuroparalysis (nū″rō-pă-răl′ĭ-sĭs) [″ + *paralyein*, to disable]. Paralysis due to disease of the nervous system.

neuropathic (nū-rō-păth′ĭk) [″ + *pathos*, disease, suffering]. Rel. to neuropathy.

neuropathogenesis (nū″rō-păth″ō-jĕn′ĕ-sĭs) [″ + ″ + *genesis*, generation, birth]. The origin and development of a neural disease.

neuropathogenicity (nū″rō-păth″ō-jĕ-nĭs′ĭ-tē) [″ + *pathos*, disease, suffering, + *gennan*, to produce]. The ability to cause pathological changes in nerves.

neuropathology (nū″rō-pă-thŏl′ō-jē) [″ + ″ + *logos*, word, reason]. The study of diseases of the nervous system and structural and functional changes occurring in them. The diseases are divided into (1) congenital defects in development, those in which a degeneration reveals itself only after a period of time, and (2) those in which destructive influences act upon a brain that was normal initially. The latter are mainly inflammatory, toxic, traumatic, mechanical, or neoplastic in type. Circulatory impairment as well as failure to use elements of the nervous system will cause impaired function.

neuropathy (nū-rŏp′ă-thē). Any disease of the nerves.

n., ascending. Pathological condition of the nervous system that ascends from the lower body to the upper.

n., descending. Pathological condition of the nervous system that descends from the upper part of the body to the lower.

n., entrapment. Pathological changes in a nerve due to its inflammation in a confined space, such as the median nerve in the carpal tunnel.

n., hypertrophic mono-. Neuropathy associated with enlargement and tenderness of two or three nerves of the head and neck area. The nerves may appear to be a neurofibroma, but biopsy will provide the correct diagnosis.

n., optic. SEE: *optic neuropathy.*

neuropharmacology (nū″rō-făr″mă-kŏl′ō-jē) [″ + *pharmakon*, drug, + *logos*, word, reason]. The branch of pharmacology concerned with the effects of drugs on the nervous system.

neurophilic (nū″rō-fĭl′ĭk) [″ + philos, fond]. Having an affinity for nervous tissue.

neurophonia (nū″rō-fō′nē-ă) [Gr. neuron, nerve, + phone, voice]. A tic or spasm of muscles of speech resulting in an involuntary cry or sound.

neurophthalmology (nū″rŏf-thăl-mŏl′ō-jē) [″ + ophthalmos, eye, + logos, word, reason]. Neuro-ophthalmology, q.v.

neurophysin (nū″rō-fī′zĭn). Neurosecretory material in the hypothalamus. Neurophysins are proteins and are involved in the transport of oxytocin and vasopressin.

neurophysiological treatment approach. In occupational and physical therapy, various techniques used in sensorimotor rehabilitation that rely on voluntary and involuntary activation, facilitation, and inhibition of muscle action through the reflex arc.

neurophysiology (nū″rō-fĭz-ē-ōl′ō-jē) [″ + physis, growth, + logos, word, reason]. Physiology of the nervous structure of the body.

neuropil (nū′rō-pĭl) [″ + pilos, felt]. Network of unmyelinated fibrils into which nerve processes of central nervous system divide.

neuroplasm (nū′rō-plăzm) [″ + LL. plasma, form, mold]. The undifferentiated cytoplasmic substance of a neuron that surrounds and separates the neurofibrils.

neuroplasmic (nū″rō-plăz′mĭk). Concerning the protoplasm of a neuron.

neuroplasty (nū′rō-plăs″tē) [″ + plassein, to form]. Reparative surgery of the nerves.

neuropodia (nū″rō-pō′dē-ă) [″ + podion, little feet] (pl. of neuropodium). Small bulb-like expansions of axon terminals at a synaptic junction.

neuropore (nū′rō-por″) [″ + poros, an opening]. Embryonic opening from neural canal to exterior.

neuropotential (nū″rō-pō-tĕn′shăl) [″ + L. potentia, power]. Nerve energy.

neuropsychiatrist (nū″rō-sī-kī′ă-trĭst) [″ + psyche, mind, + iatreia, healing]. A specialist in neuropsychiatry.

neuropsychiatry (nū″rō-sī-kī′ă-trē). The branch of medicine pert. to study and treatment of nervous and mental diseases.

neuropsychopathy (nū″rō-sī-kŏp′ăth-ē) [″ + ″ + pathos, disease, suffering]. Disease of the nerves combined with mental disorder.

neuropsychopharmacology (nū″rō-sī″kō-făr″mă-kŏl′ō-jē) [″ + ″ + pharmakon, drug, + logos, word, reason]. The study of the effects of drugs on mental illness.

neuroradiography (nū″rō-rā″dē-ŏg′ră-fē) [″ + L. radius, ray, + Gr. graphein, to write]. Radiography of the structures of the nervous system.

neuroradiology (nū″rō-rā″dē-ŏl′ō-jē) [″ + ″ + Gr. logos, word, reason]. The branch of medicine that utilizes radiography for diagnosis of pathology of the nervous system.

neurorelapse (nū″rō-rē-lăps′) [Gr. neuron, nerve, sinew, + L. relapsus, fallen back]. Reappearance of neurological symptoms in syphilis subsequent to institution of therapy.

neuroretinitis (nū″rō-rĕt″ĭn-ī′tĭs) [″ + L. retina, retina, + Gr. itis, inflammation]. Inflamed condition of optic nerve and retina.

neuroretinopathy (nū″rō-rĕt″ĭ-nŏp′ă-thē) [″ + ″ + Gr. pathos, disease, suffering]. Pathology of the retina and optic nerve.

neuroroentgenography (nū″rō-rĕnt″gĕn-ŏg′ră-fē) [″ + roentgen + Gr. graphein, to write]. Neuroradiology, q.v.

neurorrhaphy (nū-ror′ă-fē) [″ + rhaphe, seam, ridge]. Suturing of ends of a severed nerve. SYN: neurosuture.

neurosarcokleisis (nū″rō-săr″kō-klī′sĭs) [″ + sarx, flesh, + kleisis, closure]. Operation for relief of neuralgia by resection of a wall of the osseous canal carrying a nerve and by transplanting the nerve to soft tissues.

neurosarcoma (nū″rō-săr-kō′mă) [″ + ″ + oma, tumor]. A sarcoma containing neuromatous components.

neuroscience (nū″rō-sī′ĕns). Any one of the various branches of science such as embryology, anatomy, physiology, histopathology, biochemistry, and pharmacology concerned with growth, development, and function of the nervous system.

neurosclerosis (nū″rō-sklĕ-rō′sĭs) [″ + sklerosis, a hardening]. Hardening of nervous tissue.

neurosecretion (nū″rō-sē-krē′shŭn) [″ + L. secretio, separation]. The elaboration and discharge of a chemical substance by a neuron.
Ex.: secretion of hormones by cells of the hypothalamus.

neurosensory (nū″rō-sĕn′sō-rē) [″ + L. sensorius, pert. to a sensation]. Concerning a sensory nerve.

neurosis (nū-rō′sĭs) [″ + osis, condition] (pl. neuroses). The definition of this term is controversial. Some feel its use should be limited to describing an unpleasant mental symptom in an individual with intact reality testing; others would have it apply to the etiological process, i.e., unconscious conflict that arouses anxiety and leads to maladaptive use of defensive mechanisms that result in symptom formation. Alternatively, some consider the neuroses to have a physical basis. To further confuse the picture, some would entirely abandon the terms neurosis and psychoneurosis and replace them with anxiety disorders (panic states, phobias, and obsessive-compulsive neuroses) and somatoform disorders (hysteria, conversion symptoms, and hypochondriasis). The various neuroses listed below are of both the descriptive and etiological types. SYN: *psychoneurosis*. SEE: *neurotic disorder*.

TREAT: Psychotherapy, tranquilizers, and sedatives. It must be remembered that in general, a symptom due to a neurotic reaction to a situation is just as real to the patient as if it were due to organic disease. Usually such a symptom is much more difficult to treat than it would be if due to organic disease.

n., accident. A nervous disorder caused by injury or an accident. SYN: *n., traumatic*.

n., anxiety. Neurosis in which vague anxiety or apprehension is the essential symptom to the point where it interferes with daily living.

n., association. Neurosis in which association of ideas causes mental repetition of an experience.

n., cardiac. Neurocirculatory asthenia.

n., compensation. Neurosis that develops after an accident in people who think they can obtain compensation by appearing to be ill. SYN: *n., pension*.

n., compulsion. Neurosis marked by overpowering impulse to perform acts against the will.

n., craft. N., occupational.

n., expectation. Condition in which anticipation of an occurrence produces nervous symptoms.

n., fatigue. Neurasthenia.

n., obsessional. Neurosis in which uncontrollable obsessions dominate the victim's behavior.

n., occupational. Neurosis due to the occupation or profession of a patient. SYN: *n., craft*.

n., pension. N., compensation.

n., sexual. Neurosis involving sexual function.

n., traumatic. N., accident.

n., war. Neurosis brought on by conditions of war, seen in soldiers.

neuroskeletal (nū″rō-skĕl′ĕ-tăl) [Gr. *neuron*, nerve, + *skeleton*, a dried-up body]. Concerning the skeletal and nervous systems.

neuroskeleton (nū″rō-skĕl′ĕ-tŏn) [″ + *skeleton*, a dried-up body]. That portion of the skeleton that surrounds and protects the nervous system, i.e., the cranium, and spinal column.

neurosome (nū′rō-sōm) [″ + *soma*, body]. 1. The body of a neuron. 2. One of the minute granules in the protoplasm of nerve cells.

neurospasm (nū′rō-spăzm) [″ + *spasmos*, a convulsion]. Spasmodic muscular twitching due to a nervous disorder.

neurosplanchnic (nū″rō-splăngk′nĭk) [″ + *splanchnikos*, pert. to the viscera]. Concerning the sympathetic and cerebrospinal nervous system.

neurospongioma (nū″rō-spŏn″jē-ō′mă) [″ + *spongos*, sponge, + *oma*, tumor]. Spongioblastoma.

Neurospora (nū-rŏs′pō-ră). Genus of fungi belonging to the Ascomycetes class. Includes certain bread molds.

neurosurgeon (nū″rō-sŭr′jŭn). A physician specializing in surgery of the nervous system.

neurosurgery [Gr. *neuron*, nerve, sinew, + L. *chirurgia*, hand, + *ergon*, work]. Surgery of the nervous system.

neurosuture (nū″rō-soo′chŭr) [″ + L. *sutura*, a stitch]. Stitching of ends of a cut nerve. SYN: *neurorrhaphy*.

neurosyphilis (nū″rō-sĭf′ĭ-lĭs). Syphilis affecting the nervous structures. SEE: *dementia paralytica*.

n., asymptomatic. Neurosyphilis showing no symptoms and preceding symptomatic neurosyphilis. Diagnosed by changes in spinal fluid.

n., meningovascular. A form of neurosyphilis involving the meninges and vascular structures in the brain or spinal cord, or in both.

n., paretic. Dementia paralytica.

n., tabetic. Tabes dorsalis.

neurotendinous (nū″rō-tĕn′dĭ-nŭs) [″ + L. *tendinosus*, tendinous]. Concerning a nerve and tendon.

neurotension (nū″rō-tĕn′shŭn) [″ + L. *tensio*, a stretching]. Operative stretching of a nerve. SYN: *neurectasia*.

neurothecitis (nū″rō-thē-sī′tĭs) [″ + *theke*, sheath, + *itis*, inflammation]. Inflamed condition of a nerve sheath.

neurothele (nū″rō-thē′lē) [″ + *thele*, nipple]. A nerve papilla.

neurotherapeutics (nū″rō-thĕr-ă-pū′tĭks) [″ + *therapeutike*, treatment]. Treatment of disorders of the nervous system. SYN: *neurotherapy*.

neurotherapy (nū″rō-thĕr′ă-pē) [″ + *therapeia*, treatment]. Treatment of nervous disorders. SYN: *neurotherapeutics*.

neurotic (nū-rŏt′ĭk) [Gr. *neuron*, nerve, sinew]. 1. One suffering from a neurosis. 2. Pert. to neurosis. 3. Nervous.

neurotic disorder. A mental disorder in which the predominant disturbance is a symptom or group of symptoms that is distressing the individual and is recognized by that person as being unacceptable, undesirable, and alien (ego-dystonic). Reality testing is grossly intact and behavior is socially acceptable. This disorder is chronic unless treated. This term does not imply that there is a special etiological process. SEE: *neurosis*.

neuroticism (nū-rŏt′ĭ-sĭzm) [″ + *-ismos*, condition]. A condition or trait of neurosis.

neurotization (nū″rŏt-ĭ-zā′shŭn) [Gr. *neuron*, nerve, sinew]. 1. Regeneration of a nerve after division. 2. Surgical introduction of a nerve into a paralyzed muscle.

neurotmesis (nū″rŏt-mē′sĭs) [″ + *tmesis*, cutting]. Nerve injury with complete loss of function of the nerve even though there is little apparent damage anatomically.

neurotology (nū″rŏ-tŏl′ō-jē) [″ + *ous*, ear, + *logos*, word, reason]. The division of otology that deals with the inner ear, esp. its nerve supply, nerve connections with the brain, and auditory and labyrinthine pathways and centers within the brain. SYN: *otoneurology*.

neurotome (nū′rŏ-tōm). Fine knife used in the division of a nerve.

neurotomy (nū-rŏt′ō-mē) [″ + *tome*, an incision]. Division or dissection of a nerve.

neurotonic (nū″rŏ-tŏn′ĭk) [″ + *tonos*, tension]. 1. Concerning neural stretching. 2. Having a stimulating effect upon nerves or the nervous system.

neurotony (nū-rŏt′ō-nē). Nerve stretching, usually to ease pain.

neurotoxic (nū″rŏ-tŏks′ĭk) [″ + *toxikon*, poison]. Poisonous to the nerve cells.

neurotoxicity (nū″rŏ-tŏk-sĭs′ĭ-tē) [″ + *toxikon*, poison]. Having the capability of harming nerve tissue.

neurotoxin (nū″rŏ-tŏks′ĭn). A toxin that attacks nerve cells. SYN: *neurolysin*.

neurotransmitter (nū″rŏ-trăns′mĭt-ĕr). Substance such as norepinephrine, acetylcholine, and dopamine that is released when the axon terminal of a presynaptic neuron is excited. The substance then travels across the synapse to act on the target cell to either inhibit or excite it. Disorders in the brain physiology of neurotransmitters have been implicated in the pathogenesis of a variety of psychiatric illnesses. SEE: *substance P*.

neurotrauma (nū-rŏ-traw′mă) [″ + *trauma*, wound]. Injury of a nerve.

neurotripsy (nū″rŏ-trĭp′sē) [″ + *tripsis*, a rubbing]. Surgical crushing of a nerve.

neurotrophic. Pert. to the influence of nervous impulses upon the nutrition and function of an organ or structure.

neurotrophy (nū-rŏt′rō-fē). Nutrition and maintenance of nervous tissue.

neurotropism (nū-rŏt′rō-pĭzm) [Gr. *neuron*,

nerve, + *trope*, a turning, + *-ismos*, condition]. Attraction that materials including nutritive elements, basic dyes, and microorganisms have for nervous tissue.

neurotropy (nū-rŏt′rō-pē). Neurotropism.

neurotrosis (nū″rŏ-trō′sĭs) [″ + *trosis*, a wound]. Injury of a nerve.

neurotubule (nū″rŏ-too′būl) [″ + L. *tubulus*, a tubule]. A microtubule seen by use of electron microscopy in nerve cells, dendrites, and axons.

neurovaccine (nū″rŏ-văk′sĭn). A standardized vaccine virus of specific strength. Usually prepared by cultivation in a rabbit's brain.

neurovaricosis (nū″rŏ-văr″ĭ-kō′sĭs) [″ + L. *varicosus*, pert. to a swollen vein, + Gr. *osis*, condition]. Multiple swellings along the pathway of a nerve.

neurovascular (nū″rŏ-văs′kū-lăr) [″ + L. *vasculus*, a small vessel]. Concerning both the nervous and vascular systems.

neurovegetative (nū″rŏ-vĕj′ĕ-tā″tĭv). Concerning the autonomic nervous system.

neurovirus (nū″rŏ-vī′rŭs). Virus that has been modified by its growing in nervous tissue. Used in preparing a vaccine.

neurovisceral (nū″rŏ-vĭs′ĕr-ăl) [″ + L. *viscera*, body organs]. Neurosplanchnic, q.v.

neurula (nū′roo-lă). Stage in development of an embryo, esp. amphibian embryos, during which the neural plate develops and axial embryonic nervous structures are elaborated.

neurulation (nū″roo-lā′shŭn). Formation of the neural plate in the embryo and development and closure of the neural tube.

neutral (nū′trăl) [L. *neutralis*, neither]. 1. Neither alkaline nor acid. 2. Indifferent; having no positive qualities or opinions.

neutral fat. One of the lipids commonly found in the tissues; an ester of fatty acids with glycerol. Ex.: tristearin; triolein; tripalmitin.

neutralization (nū″trăl-ĭ-zā′shŭn). 1. The opposing of one force or condition with an opposite force or condition to such degree as to cause counteraction that permits neither to dominate. 2. In chemistry, the process of destroying the peculiar properties or effect of a substance, e.g., the neutralization of an acid with a base or vice versa. 3. In medicine, the process of checking or counteracting the effects of any agent that produces a morbid effect.

neutralize (nū′trăl-īz). 1. To counteract and make ineffective. 2. In chemistry, to destroy peculiar properties or effect; to make inert.

neutral point. A point on the pH scale (pH 7.0) that represents neutrality, i.e., the solution is neither acid or alkaline in reaction.

neutral red. A dye used as an indicator and as

a vital stain.

neutral warmth. A technique used in neuromuscular rehabilitation that relies on the body's own heat for the purposes of normalizing muscle tone.

neutrino (nū-trē′nō). In physics, subatomic particle with no mass, at rest, and no electric charge. These particles are constantly flowing through the universe, including the Earth. They are not known to affect the matter through which they pass.

neutroclusion (nū″trō-kloo′zhŭn) [L. *neuter*, neither, + *occludo*, to close]. State in which the anteroposterior occlusal positions of the teeth or the mesiodistal positions are normal but malocclusion of the other positions exists.

neutrocytopenia (nū″trō-sī″tō-pē′nē-ă) [″ + Gr. *cytos*, cell, + *penia*, poverty]. Neutropenia.

neutrocytosis (nū″trō-sī-tō′sĭs) [″ + ″ + *osis*, condition]. Neutrophilia.

neutron (nū′trŏn) [L. *neuter*, neither]. Subatomic particle equal in mass to a proton but without an electric charge. It is believed to be a particle of all nuclei of mass number greater than one. As a free particle, it has an average life of about 12 minutes.

neutron capture analysis. Use of the ability of a neutron to be absorbed (i.e., captured) by an atomic nucleus to detect the presence of various substances.

neutropenia (nū-trō-pē′nē-ă) [″ + Gr. *penia*, lack]. Abnormally small number of neutrophil cells in the blood.

n., malignant. Agranulocytosis.

neutrophil(e) (nū′trō-fĭl, -fīl) [″ + Gr. *philein*, to love]. The most common type of granulocytic white blood cell, neutrophils are responsible for much of the body's protection against infection. They play the primary role in inflammation, q.v., easily recognizing foreign antigens and destroying them through phagocytosis. An inadequate number of neutrophils (neutropenia) leaves the body at high risk for infection from many sources and requires protective precautions on the part of health care workers. Patients with leukemia receiving chemotherapy, which destroys all leukocytes, become neutropenic and can die from infection before the bone marrow produces additional leukocytes.

Neutrophils may overreact to stimuli and become involved in tissue destruction. Notable examples include neutrophil activity in rheumatoid arthritis, myocardial reperfusion injury, respiratory distress syndrome, and ulcerative colitis. Considerable research is now directed toward determining methods of controlling the tissue-destructive properties of neutrophils. SYN:

polymorphonuclear leukocytes. SEE: *blood cell* for illus.

neutrophilia (nū″trō-fĭl′ē-ă). Increase in the number of neutrophilic leukocytes in the blood.

neutrophilic, neutrophilous (nū-trō-fĭl′ĭk, -trŏf′ĭ-lŭs) [″ + Gr. *philein*, to love]. Staining readily with neutral dyes.

neutrotaxis (nū″trō-tăk′sĭs) [*neutrophil* + Gr. *taxis*, arrangement]. The phenomenon in which neutrophils are repelled from or attracted to something.

nevocarcinoma (nē″vō-kăr″sĭ-nō′mă) [L. *naevus*, birthmark, + Gr. *karkinos*, crab, + *oma*, tumor]. Malignant melanoma.

nevoid (nē′voyd) [″ + Gr. *eidos*, form, shape]. Resembling a nevus.

nevolipoma (nē″vō-lĭ-pō′mă) [″ + Gr. *lipos*, fat, + *oma*, tumor]. Rare lipoma containing numerous blood vessels and fatty tissue, probably a degenerated nevus. SYN: *nevus lipomatodes.*

nevose (nē′vōs) [L. *naevus*, birthmark]. Spotted or marked with nevi. SEE: *nevus.*

nevoxanthoendothelioma (nē″vō-zăn″thō-ĕn″dō-thē″lē-ō′mă) [″ + Gr. *xanthos*, yellow, + *endon*, within, + *thele*, nipple, + *oma*, tumor]. Juvenile xanthogranuloma. SEE: *xanthogranuloma, juvenile.*

nevus (nē′vŭs) [L. *naevus*, birthmark] (pl. *nevi*). 1. A congenital discoloration of a circumscribed area of the skin due to pigmentation. SYN: *birthmark; mole.* 2. Circumscribed vascular tumor of the skin, usually congenital, due to hyperplasia of the blood vessels. SEE: *angioma.*

n. angiectodes. N. vascularis.

n. angiomatodes. Extensive diffuse angiomatous condition of the subcutaneous tissues.

n. araneus. Acquired or congenital dilatation of the capillaries, marked by red lines radiating from a central red dot. SYN: *n., spider.*

n., blue. A dark blue nevus covered by smooth skin. It is composed of melanin-pigmented spindle cells in the mid-dermis.

n., blue rubber bleb. A rubbery blue cavernous hemangiomatous nodule that is erectile and easily compressed. Present in the skin and gastrointestinal tract.

n., capillary. Nevus of dilated capillary vessels, elevated above the skin. Usually treated by ligature and excision.

n. comedonicus. A horny nevus that contains a hard plug of keratin. Caused by failure of the pilosebaceous follicles to develop normally.

n., connective tissue. Nevus composed of collagenous tissue.

n., cutaneous. Nevus formation on the

skin.

   n., epidermal. Raised lesions present at birth; they may be hyperkeratotic and widely distributed.

   n. flammeus. Red discoloration of the face or neck, usually not elevated above the skin. A serious deformity due to its large size and color. SYN: *port-wine stain.*

   n., hairy. Nevus, usually pigmented, from which hair grows.

   n., halo. Papular brown nevus with oval halo occurring in first three decades of life. Usually benign, but needs to be evaluated for malignancy.

   n., intradermal. Nevus in which the melanocytes are found in nests in the dermis and have no connection with the deeper layers from which they were formed.

   n., Ito's. A mongolian spot, q.v., innervated by lateral branches of the supraclavicular nerve and the lateral cutaneous nerve of the arm.

   n., junction. Nevus in the basal cell zone at the junction of the epidermis and dermis. They are slightly raised, do not contain hair, and are pigmented. These may become malignant.

   n. lipomatodes. Fatty connective tissue tumor, probably a degenerated nevus containing numerous blood vessels. SYN: *nevolipoma.*

   n. maternus. A birthmark; congenital angioma.

   n., melanocytic. Any nevus that contains melanocytes.

   n., nevocytic. A common mole. They may appear at any age. They are classified according to their stage of growth and as to whether or not they are still growing.

   n., Ota's. A mongolian spot, q.v., occurring in the skin surrounding the eye.

   n. pigmentosus. Congenital pigment spot varying in color from light yellow to black. Intradermal, or common moles, are benign. Other types are or may become malignant.

   TREAT: Malignant or suspicious lesions should be treated by wide surgical excision. Benign lesions do not require treatment except when located at sites of friction causing bleeding or ulceration. Some are removed for cosmetic reasons.

   n. pilosus. Nevus covered with hair.

   n., sebaceous. Nevus composed of sebaceous-gland tissue.

   n., spider. N. araneus.

   n. spilus. Pigmented nevus with smooth surface.

   n. spongiosus albus mucosae. A white, spongy nevus that may occur in the mouth, labia, vagina, or rectum.

   n., strawberry. N. vascularis.

   n., telangiectatic. Nevus containing dilated capillaries.

   n. unius lateris. Congenital nevus that occurs in streaks or linear bands on one side of the body. They usually occur between the neurotomes of the lumbar or sacral area.

   n. vascularis. Nevus in which superficial blood vessels are enlarged. Nevi are usually congenital and of variable size and shape; slightly elevated; red or purple; on face, head, neck, and arms, though no region is exempt. Usually disappear spontaneously, but wrinkling, pigmentation, and scarring are sometimes seen. SYN: *nevus angiectodes; strawberry mark.*

   n. venosus. Nevus formed of dilated venules.

   n. verrucosus. Nevus with a raised wartlike surface.

   n., white sponge. N. spongiosus albus mucosae.

newborn. Born recently. Term applied to human infants less than one month old. SYN: *neonate.*

Newcastle disease (nū′kăs-ĕl) [Newcastle, England]. An acute viral disease of birds, particularly chickens. It occasionally produces accidental infections in man, usually a mild conjunctivitis.

new growth. Any new growth of tissue. Usually considered to be abnormal but not always so; the normal fetus is in fact a new growth. SYN: *neoplasm.*

newton. SYMB: N. The name of a measure of force derived from the base units used in SI units of measurement. It is equal to the force that will accelerate one kilogram a meter per second squared, 10^5 dynes. SEE: *SI Units in Appendix.*

newton meter. SYMB: Nm. In SI units, one newton per square meter. This is called one pascal (Pa). Thus $1\ Pa = 1N/M^2$.

nexus (nĕk′sŭs) [L., bond] (pl. *nexus*). A connection or link; a binding together. Used to designate a bond between components of a group.

NF. *National Formulary.*

N.F.L.P.N. *National Federation of Licensed Practical Nurses.*

ng. *nanogram.*

NG tube. *nasogastric* tube.

NH₃. Ammonia.

NH₄⁺. The univalent ammonium radical.

NH₄Br. Ammonium bromide.

NH₄Cl. Ammonium chloride.

N.H.I. *National Heart Institute.*

NHL. *non-Hodgkin's lymphoma.*

N.H.L.I. *National Heart and Lung Institute.*

NH₄NO₃. Ammonium nitrate.

NH₄OH. Ammonium hydroxide. SYN: *ammonia water; aqua ammonia.*

Ni. Chem. symb. for the element nickel.

NIA. *National Institute on Aging.*
niacin (nī′ă-sĭn). USP. Nicotinic acid. A vitamin used in preventing and treating pellagra. Trade names are Nicobid, Nicocap, and Nicolar.

Caution: Niacin has been used as a self-medication by persons seeking to control hypercholesterolemia. Taken in excess, niacin can cause hyperglycemia, dry skin, itching, flushing, and abnormal liver function tests.

---

niacinamide (nī″ă-sĭn-ăm′īd). USP. A niacin derivative used in the prophylaxis and treatment of pellagra. SYN: *nicotinamide.*
N.I.A.I.D. *National Institute of Allergy and Infectious Diseases.*
N.I.A.M.D. *National Institute of Arthritis and Metabolic Diseases.*
nib (nĭb). In dentistry, the smooth or serrated blade of a condensing instrument that contacts the restorative material placed in a cavity preparation. Also called condenser point.
nicardipine. A calcium entry blocker, q.v. Trade name is Cardene.
niche (nĭch) [Fr.]. A depression or recess on a smooth surface, esp. an erosion in the wall of a hollow organ, detected by roentgenography.
   n., enamel. One of two depressions that develop between the dental lamina and the enamel organ.
N.I.C.H.H.D. *National Institute of Child Health and Human Development.*
nickel. SYMB: Ni. At. wt. 58.70, at. no. 28. Metallic element.
   n. carbonyl. Ni(CO)₄. An industrial chemical used in plating metals. It is toxic when inhaled, causing pulmonary edema.
nicking. 1. Compression of the retinal vessels of the eye at the point where a vein and an artery cross. Seen in hypertensive cardiovascular disease. 2. To notch a tissue.
niclosamide (nĭ-klō′să-mĭd). A teniacide esp. effective against the cestodes that infect humans. Trade names are Niclocide and Yomesan.
Nicobid. Trade name for niacin, USP.
Nicolar. Trade name for niacin, USP.
Nicolas-Favre disease (nē″kō-lă-făv′r) [Josef Nicolas, b. 1868, and M. Favre, 1876–1954, Fr. physicians]. Venereal disease marked by involvement of inguinal lymph glands with an exuding lesion. SYN: *lymphogranuloma venereum.*
nicotinamide (nĭk″ō-tĭn′ă-mĭd). Member of vitamin B complex, used in management or prevention of pellagra. The peripheral flush that often accompanies therapy with nico-

tinic acid, q.v., is avoided with nicotinamide. SYN: *niacinamide.*
   n. adenine dinucleotide. SEE: *NAD⁺.*
   n. adenine dinucleotide-dehydrogenase. SYN: *nicotinamide adenine dinucleotide diaphorase; methemoglobin reductase.* SEE: *NADH-diaphorase.*
   n. adenine dinucleotide-diaphorase. SEE: *NADH-diaphorase.*
   n. adenine dinucleotide phosphate. A coenzyme that contains adenine, nicotinamide, D-ribose, and phosphoric acid. It serves as an electron carrier in catabolic and anabolic reactions.
   n. adenine diphosphate. SEE: *NADP.*
nicotine (nĭk′ō-tēn, -tĭn) [L. *nicotiana*, tobacco]. A poisonous alkaloid found in all parts of the tobacco plant, but esp. in the leaves. When pure, it is a colorless oily fluid with little odor but a sharp burning taste. On exposure to air or in crude materials, it becomes deep brown with the characteristic tobacco-like smell. Nicotine is one of the most toxic and addicting of all poisons. Cigarette tobacco contains varying amounts of nicotine per cigarette. SEE: *nicotine chewing gum; nicotine poisoning, acute.*
nicotine chewing gum. Incorporation of nicotine in a chewing gum. This is an aid in smoking cessation programs, or it may be used alone to help those who wish to discontinue use of tobacco products. The effectiveness of this approach, even though questionable, is worth trying. Trade name is Nicorette. SEE: *tobacco.*
nicotine poisoning, acute. Nicotine is an extremely toxic substance that acts as swiftly as cyanide. The fatal dose for an adult is estimated to be less than 5 mg/kg body weight.
   SYM: Nausea, salivation, abdominal pain, vomiting, diarrhea, sweating, dizziness, and mental confusion. If dose is sufficient, the patient will collapse, develop shock, convulse, and die of respiratory failure due to paralysis of respiratory muscles. For treatment, SEE: *Poisons and Poisoning* in *Appendix.*
   TREAT: If patient is conscious, oral administration of universal antidote, q.v., tannic acid, activated charcoal, or strong tea, followed by gastric lavage or an emetic. If patient is unconscious, use gastric lavage. Keep patient warm with external heat and maintain the airway. Artificial or mechanical respiration and oxygen therapy if necessary. If convulsions are severe or persist, intravenous barbiturates in small doses are indicated.
nicotinic acid (nĭk″ō-tĭn′ĭk). The antipellagra principle of vitamin B complex. Occurs

naturally in liver, yeast, milk, cheese, and cereals. Used orally or parenterally for treatment of pellagra. SYN: *niacin.*

nicotinism (nĭk'ō-tĭn-ĭzm). Poisoning from excessive use of tobacco or nicotine.

nictation [L. *nictitare*, to wink]. Involuntary winking. SYN: *nictitation.*

nictitate (nĭk'tĭ-tāt). To wink.

nictitating (nĭk'tĭ-tāt-ĭng). Winking.

nictitating membrane. SEE: *membrane, nictitating.*

nictitating spasm. Clonic spasm of eyelid with continuous winking.

nictitation [L. *nictitare*, to wink]. Involuntary winking. SYN: *nictation.*

nidal (nī'dăl) [L. *nidus*, nest]. Pert. to a nidus.

nidation (nī-dā'shŭn). Implantation of the fertilized ovum in the lining of the uterus (endometrium).

NIDA. *National Institute on Drug Abuse.*

NIDDM. *non-insulin dependent diabetes mellitus.*

N.I.D.R. *National Institute of Dental Research.*

N.I.D.R.R. *National Institute of Disability and Rehabilitation Research.*

nidus (nī'dŭs) [L., nest] (pl. *nidi*). 1. A cluster; nestlike structure. 2. Focus of infection. 3. A nucleus or origin of a nerve.

    n. avis cerebelli. A deep sulcus on each side of the inferior vermis, separating it from adjacent lobes of hemispheres.

    n. hirundinis. Swallow's nest, q.v.

Niemann-Pick disease (nē'măn-pĭk) [Albert Niemann, Ger. pediatrician, 1880–1921; Ludwig Pick, Ger. physician, 1868–1944]. A disturbance of sphingolipid metabolism characterized by enlargement of liver and spleen (hepatosplenomegaly), anemia, lymphadenopathy, and progressive mental and physical deterioration. A hereditary disease, its onset is in early infancy. Death usually occurs before the third year. Typical cell, having a foamy appearance and filled with a lipoid believed to be sphingomyelin, can be found in bone marrow, spleen, or lymph nodes and aids in establishing the diagnosis.

night blindness. Decreased ability to see at night. Caused by lack of visual purple in the rods or by its slowness in regenerating after exposure to light. May result from vitamin A deficiency or hereditary factors. SYN: *nyctalopia.* SEE: *night vision.*

nightguard. A dental prosthesis worn at night to prevent trauma to the teeth by grinding them during sleep. SEE: *bruxism; occlusal guard.*

Nightingale, Florence (nīt'ĭn-gāl). British philanthropist, 1820–1910, who was founder of modern nursing and reformer of

hospital conditions. Served as a nurse in Crimean War. Founded a training school for nurses.

Nightingale Pledge. An oath used universally by nurses upon capping or graduation as a pledge of ethical standards of their profession. The pledge was formulated by a committee of the Farrand School of Nursing, Harper Hospital, Detroit, Michigan.

"I solemnly pledge myself before God and in the presence of this assembly to pass my life in purity and to practice my profession faithfully. I will abstain from whatever is deleterious and mischievous, and will not take or knowingly administer any harmful drug. I will do all in my power to maintain and elevate the standard of my profession, and will hold in confidence all personal matters committed to my keeping and all family affairs coming to my knowledge in the practice of my calling. With loyalty will I endeavor to aid the physician in his work, and devote myself to the welfare of those committed to my care." SEE: *Declaration of Hawaii; Declaration of Geneva; Hippocratic Oath; Prayer of Maimonides.*

nightmare (nīt'mār) [AS. *nyht*, night, + *mara*, a demon]. A bad dream accompanied by great fear. SYN: *incubus; oneirodynia.* SEE: *paralysis, sleep; sleep, disorders of.*

nightshade (nīt'shād) [AS. *nihtscada*]. Any of several of the plants of the genus *Solanum.* SEE: *belladonna.*

    n., deadly. Belladonna, q.v.

night sweat [AS. *nyht*, night, + *swat*, sweat]. Profuse sweating during sleep at night. Often it is an early sign of disease, esp. with intermittent fever. In children, it occurs in rickets and in debilitated states. Patient should be rubbed down, sponged, and changed into dry clothing.

night terrors [″ + L. *terrere*, to frighten]. Form of nightmare in children causing them to awaken in terror, screaming. Fear continues for a period after the return to consciousness. SYN: *pavor nocturnus.* SEE: *sleep, disorders of.*

night vision. The ability to see at night or in light of low intensity. Results from dark adaptation in which pupil dilates, visual purple increases, and intensity threshold of the retina is lowered. Any decrease in oxygen content of the blood is accompanied by some loss of night vision. Thus, smoking cigarettes or being in an atmosphere with decreased oxygen content decreases night vision. SYN: *scotopic vision.*

nightwalking. State in which individual habitually walks about while sleeping. SYN: *somnambulism.*

night work, maladaption to. In the U.S.

about 7.3 million people work at night. Thus, they are forced to attempt to readjust their day-night schedule for working and sleeping. Adaptation may be facilitated by making the work space as light as possible and scheduling the sleep period, 8 hours, in a totally dark environment. SEE: *circadian; clock, biological; shift work.*

N.I.G.M.S. *National Institute of General Medical Sciences.* A division of the National Institutes of Health of the U.S. Department of Health and Human Services.

nigra (nī′grä) [L., black]. Mass of gray matter between the dorsal and pedal parts of the crus cerebri. SYN: *substantia nigra.*

nigri-, nigro- [L. *nigra,* black]. Combining forms pert. to blackness.

nigricans (nī′grĭ-kănz). Blackened.

nigrities (nī-grĭsh′ĭ-ēz). Blackness; black pigmentation.

   n. linguae. A black pigmentation of the tongue.

nigrosin (nī′grō-sĭn). An aniline dye used to stain nervous tissue and certain bacteria, and to discriminate between live and dead cells.

nigrostriatal (nī″grō-strī-ā′tăl). Concerning a bundle of nerve fibers that connect the substantia nigra of the brain to the corpus striatum.

NIH. *National Institutes of Health* (of the U.S. Department of Health and Human Services).

nihilism (nī′ĭ-lĭzm) [L. *nihil,* nothing, + Gr. *-ismos,* condition]. 1. Disbelief in efficacy of medical therapy. 2. A delusion in which everything is unreal or does not exist.

nikethamide (nĭ-kĕth′ă-mīd). A drug that is supposed to selectively stimulate central respiratory centers. Use for this purpose in treating respiratory depression due to poisoning from sedative-hypnotic drugs is ineffective. Trade name is Coramine.

Nikolsky's sign (nĭ-kŏl′skēz) [Pyotr Nikolsky, Russ. dermatologist, 1855–1940]. Condition of the external layer of the skin in which it can be rubbed off by slight friction or injury. Seen in pemphigus.

Nilstat. Trade name for nystatin, USP.

N.I.M.H. *National Institute of Mental Health.* A division of the National Institutes of Health of the U.S. Department of Health and Human Services.

N.I.N.D.B. *National Institute of Neurological Diseases and Blindness.* A division of the National Institutes of Health of the U.S. Department of Health and Human Services.

ninth cranial nerve. Glossopharyngeal nerve. SEE: *glossopharyngeal nerve* for illus.; *Cranial Nerves* in Appendix.

niobium (nī-ō′bē-um) [Legendary Gr.

woman, Niobe, who was turned into stone]. SYMB: Nb. At. wt. 92.906; at. no. 41. A chemical element formerly called columbium.

niphablepsia (nĭf″ă-blĕp′sē-ă) [Gr. *nipha,* snow, + *ablepsia,* blindness]. Blindness caused by light glare on snow. SYN: *niphotyphlosis; snowblindness.*

niphotyphlosis (nĭf″ō-tĭf-lō′sĭs) [″ + *typhlosis,* blindness]. Snow blindness. SYN: *niphablepsia.*

nipple (nĭp′l) [AS. *neble,* a little protuberance]. 1. The conical protuberance in each breast from which the lactiferous ducts discharge in the female. SYN: *mammilla; papilla mamma* [NA]; *teat.* 2. Artificial substitute for female nipple to be used on a nursing bottle.

The nipple contains erectile tissue and is surrounded by a pigmented area called the areola. The areola may be darker in those who have borne children. It is supplied with a row of small sebaceous glands around its base, called areolar glands, which secrete an oily substance to keep it supple. SEE: *breast* for illus.

NURSING IMPLICATIONS: *Postpartum:* Wash with warm water and pat dry. Gently massage a nonalcoholic lubricant such as lanolin or liquid petrolatum into the nipples, and allow to air dry for 20 to 30 minutes if possible. Instruct mother to position areola in infant's mouth properly and limit length of early feeding periods to prevent trauma. Cracked or eroded nipples require further intervention and maternal support if breast feeding is to be successful.

RS: acromastitis; areola; breast; halo; mamma; mammary glands; mammillation; Paget's disease of nipple; "thel-" words.

   n., crater. N., retracted.

   n., retracted. Nipple whose tip lies below the level of the surrounding skin. Caused by deficiency of muscle tissue or flattening of erectile tissue.

nipple shield. A device consisting of an artificial nipple used by some nursing mothers to protect the natural nipple.

Nipride. Trade name for sodium nitroprusside, USP.

Nisentil. Trade name for alphaprodine hydrochloride.

Nissl bodies (nĭs′l) [Franz Nissl, Ger. neurologist, 1860–1919]. Chromophil substance in the form of granules found in the cell bodies and dendrites of neurons but lacking in the most peripheral region of the nerve cell cytoplasm and the area where the axis cylinder (axon hillock) originates and from the axon cylinder. They are stained selectively by toluidine and other basic aniline dyes. They consist principally of the ribose type of nucleic acid and nucleoprotein.

They are concerned with protein synthesis and metabolism; their condition varies with physiological and pathological conditions. In fatigue and certain pathological states, they may dissolve and disappear, a phenomenon called chromatolysis. SYN: *tigroid bodies*.

nisus (nī'sŭs) [L.]. Effort, exertion, or a strong force.

nit (nĭt) [AS. *hnitu*]. The egg of a louse or any other parasitic insect. SEE: *pediculosis; Pediculus*.

niter (nī'tĕr) [Gr. *nitron*, salt]. Sodium nitrate or potassium nitrate (saltpeter).

niton (nī'tŏn). Radon.

nitr- [Gr. *nitron*, salt]. Combining form denoting combination with nitrogen or presence of the group NO_2.

nitrate (nī'trāt) [L. *nitratum*]. A salt of nitric acid.

nitrated. Combined with nitric acid or a nitrate.

nitration. Combination with nitric acid or a nitrate.

nitre (nī'tĕr) [Fr.]. British spelling of niter, q.v.

nitremia (nī-trē'mē-ă). Azotemia.

nitric acid. HNO_3. A colorless, corrosive, poisonous liquid in concentrated form, employed as a caustic. It is widely used in industry and in chemical laboratories.

    n.a., fuming. Concentrated nitric acid, which emits toxic fumes that cause choking if inhaled. SEE: *fumes*.

nitric acid poisoning. Symptoms are essentially the same as those produced by sulfuric acid poisoning, q.v. Pain, burning, vomiting, thirst, and shock.

    TREAT: Dilute with large volumes of water. Neutralize with weak alkalies; give magnesium oxide, milk of magnesia, milk, or egg white in large amounts. Avoid emetics and stomach tubes because they may cause rupture of the esophagus or stomach.

nitridation (nī-trĭ-dā'shŭn). Combination with nitrogen to form a nitride.

nitride (nī'trīd). A binary compound formed by direct combination of nitrogen with another element, e.g., lithium nitride (Li_3N), formed from nitrogen and lithium.

nitrification (nī″trĭ-fĭ-kā'shŭn). The process by which the nitrogen of ammonia or other compounds is oxidized to nitric or nitrous acid or their salts (nitrates, nitrites). Takes place continually in the soil through the action of nitrifying bacteria.

nitrifying (nī'trĭ-fī″ĭng). The process of nitrification.

nitrifying bacteria. Bacteria that induce nitrification. Include the nitrite bacteria of the genus *Nitrosomonas*, which convert ammonia to nitrites, and nitrate bacteria of the genus *Nitrobacter*, which convert nitrites to nitrates.

nitrile (nī'tril). An organic compound in which trivalent nitrogen is attached to a carbon atom.

nitrite (nī'trīt) [Gr. *nitron*, salt]. A salt of nitrous acid. Nitrites dilate blood vessels, reduce blood pressure, depress motor centers of the spinal cord, and act as antispasmodics. Principal nitrites used in medicine are amyl nitrite, ethyl nitrite, potassium nitrite, and sodium nitrite, q.v.

nitritoid (nī'trĭ-toyd) [″ + *eidos*, form, shape]. Resembling a nitrite.

    n. crisis. A syndrome resembling symptoms produced by the use of a nitrite, usually occurring after arsphenamine injection.

nitrituria (nī-trĭ-tū'rē-ă) [″ + *ouron*, urine]. Nitrites present in the urine.

nitro- [Gr. *nitron*, salt]. Combining form denoting combination with nitrogen or presence of the group NO_2.

nitrobenzene (nī″trō-bĕn'zēn). A toxic derivative of benzene. It is used in making aniline.

nitroblue tetrazolium test. A test of the ability of leukocytes to transform nitroblue tetrazolium from a colorless state to deep blue. Failure to produce this reaction indicates that the leukocytes do not have the capability of reacting in a normal manner to the ingestion of the particular bacteria used in the test.

nitrocellulose (nī″trō-sĕl'ū-lōs). Pyroxylin, q.v.

nitrofurantoin (nī″trō-fū-răn'tō-ĭn). USP. An antibacterial drug used in treating certain urinary tract infections. Trade names are Dantafur, Furadantin, and Macrodantin.

nitrofurazone (nī″trō-fū'ră-zōn). USP. An antibacterial agent used topically. Trade names are Amifur and Furacin.

nitrogen (nī'trō-jĕn) [Fr. *nitrogene*]. SYMB: N. At. wt. 14.0067; at. no. 7. A colorless, odorless, tasteless, gaseous element occurring free in the atmosphere, forming approx. 80% of its volume.

    A component of all proteins, nitrogen is essential to plant and animal life for tissue building. Generally it is found in organic nature only in the form of compounds such as ammonia, nitrites, and nitrates. These are transformed by plants into proteins and, being consumed by animals, are converted into animal proteins of the blood and tissues. SYN: *azote*.

    n. monoxide. N_2O. Laughing gas; nitrous oxide.

    n. mustards. 1. A term embracing certain therapeutic mustard compounds that act as alkylating agents and therefore have the ability to disturb cell growth during a cell's growth phase. Used to destroy lymphoid tissue in Hodgkin's disease. They are also used in treating lymphosarcoma, giant follicular lymphoblastoma, chronic lymphoid myeloid leukemia, rheumatoid arthritis, and nephritis. Nitrogen mustards include mechlorethamine, cyclophosphamide, uracil mustard, melphalan, and chlorambucil. 2. Gases used in chemical warfare. SEE: *gas, mustard; gas, vesicant.*

n., nonprotein. Nitrogen that appears in food, blood, or other substance but is not present as a protein.

nitrogenase (nī′trō-jĕn-ās) [*nitrogen* + *-ase*, enzyme]. An enzyme that catalyzes the reduction of nitrogen to ammonia.

nitrogen balance. The difference between the amount of nitrogen ingested and that excreted each day. If intake is greater, a positive balance exists; if less, there is a negative balance. SEE: *nitrogen equilibrium.*

nitrogen cycle. A natural cycle in which nitrogen is discharged from animal life into the soil; it is then taken up from soil into plants for their nourishment; and in turn nitrogen returns to animal life through plants eaten.

nitrogen equilibrium. Condition during which nitrogen excreted in the urine, feces, and sweat equals amount taken in by the body in food.

nitrogen fixation. Conversion of atmospheric nitrogen into nitrates through the action of bacteria in the soil.

nitrogen lag. Extent of time required after a given protein is ingested before an amount of nitrogen equal to that in protein has been excreted.

nitrogen narcosis. Condition of euphoria, impaired judgment, and decreased coordination and motor ability seen in persons exposed to high air pressure such as divers and submariners. The effects, caused by the increased concentration of nitrogen gas in body tissues, including the brain, are similar to those produced by alcoholic intoxication.

nitrogenous (nī-trŏj′ĕn-ŭs). Pert. to or containing nitrogen. Foods that contain nitrogen are the proteins; those that do not contain nitrogen are the fats and carbohydrates. The retention of nitrogenous products in the blood is marked in kidney diseases.

nitroglycerin (nī″trō-glĭs′ĕr-ĭn) [Gr. *nitron,* salt, + *glycerin*]. Any nitrate of glycerol. Specifically the trinitrate—a heavy, oily, explosive, colorless liquid obtained by treating glycerol with nitric and sulfuric acids. Even though it is the explosive constituent of dynamite, it is not used medically in an explosive form. In medicine it has the action of nitrites and is a vasodilator. Used esp. in angina pectoris.

Persons who use nitroglycerin regularly should be told that the tablets must be stored in a tightly sealed dark-tinted glass (not plastic) container without a cotton plug. Nitroglycerin ointment is available for treatment of angina. It is especially helpful when used in the prophylactic treatment of angina. It is used in a 2% ointment rubbed into the chest wall. A long-term transdermal delivery system is also available for nitroglycerin.

nitroglycerin tablets. USP. A standardized preparation of nitroglycerin, q.v. Trade names are Klavikordal, Nitrospan, Nitrostat, and Nitrong. Previously used name was glyceryl trinitrate.

nitromersol (nī″trō-mĕr′sŏl). USP. An organic mercurial antiseptic used topically. It penetrates poorly and the mercury is fixed by tissues so that its bacteriostatic action is prevented.

nitrometer (nī-trŏm′ĕ-tĕr) [*nitrogen* + Gr. *metron,* measure]. Device for measuring the amount of nitrogen produced in a chemical reaction.

nitromuriatic acid (nī″trō-mū-rē-ăt′ĭk) [″ + L. *muriaticus,* briny]. A mixture of one part nitric acid and three parts hydrochloric acid used in commercial industries because it dissolves all the metals including platinum and gold. SYN: *aqua regia.*

Nitrong. Trade name for nitroglycerin, USP.

Nitropress. Trade name for sodium nitroprusside, USP.

Nitrosomonas. A genus of gram-negative, aerobic bacteria that oxidize ammonia to nitrate.

nitrous (nī′trŭs) [Gr. *nitron,* salt]. Containing nitrogen in its lowest valency.

nitrous acid. HNO_2. A chemical reagent used in biological laboratories.

nitrous oxide. USP. N_2O. Colorless sweet-tasting gas with pleasing smell causing temporary general anesthesia when inhaled in proper concentration. It is given in various amounts with oxygen and is used as an adjuvant with other anesthetic agents. It should not be used as the sole anesthetic agent because the concentration required to produce anesthesia is close to the concentration that would also lead to hypoxia. Its action as an anesthetic can be potentiated by other classes of drugs—barbiturates, narcotics, and tranquilizers. Nitrous oxide is not flammable, but it will support combustion when it is present in proper concentration with a flammable anesthetic. SYN: *laughing gas.*

Nitrous oxide has little or no effect on body temperature, blood pressure, volume or composition of blood, metabolism, or the genitourinary system. Diaphoresis, increased muscle tone, or both may occur with induction of anesthesia with nitrous oxide.

Asphyxiation may occur if it is not administered properly. Prolonged administration of nitrous oxide will cause depression of bone marrow.

SYM: Signs of deep nitrous oxide anesthesia include a slight increase in respirations and some dyspnea. Cyanosis becomes deeper; eyeballs are fixed either upward or downward. There is muscular rigidity; cyanosis increases to a grayish pallor; pupils become fixed in a dilated form; and respirations cease.

TREAT: The patient who suffers from an overdose should be resuscitated and given oxygen under pressure.

Nix Creme Rinse. Trade name for Permethrin.

NK cells. SEE: *natural killer cells.*

N.L.N. *National League for Nursing.*

nm. *nanometer.*

N.M.D.P. National Marrow Donor Program.

NMRI. *Naval Medical Research Institute* (U.S. Navy); *nuclear magnetic resonance imaging.*

NMR spectroscopy. *nuclear magnetic resonance spectroscopy.* Uses the characteristic absorption of nuclei inside a strong magnetic field to identify and characterize molecules.

N.M.S.S. *National Multiple Sclerosis Society.*

N.N.D. *New and Nonofficial Drugs,* a former publication of the American Medical Association, which described new drugs that had not been admitted to the U.S. Pharmacopeia.

N₂O. Nitrous oxide.

N₂O₃. Nitrogen trioxide.

N₂O₅. Nitrogen pentoxide.

No. Chem. symb. for the element nobelium.

no. [L. *numero*]. Abbreviation meaning *to the number of.*

nobelium (nō-bē′lē-ŭm) [Named for Nobel Institute, where it was first isolated]. SYMB: No. At. wt. of the most stable isotope is 254 (other isotopes vary in weight from 252 through 256); at. no. 102. Element obtained from bombardment of curium.

Nobel prize [Alfred B. Nobel, Swedish chemist and philanthropist, 1833–1896, whose will provided funds for awarding the annual prizes]. Awards consisting of a medal and monetary prize of over $250,000 usually awarded annually to those selected for excellence in the fields of chemistry, literature, medicine, physics, and physiology. The first prizes were awarded in 1901. A prize in economics has also been established.

Nocardia [Edmund I. E. Nocard, Fr. veterinary pathologist, 1850–1903]. A genus of gram-positive aerobic bacteria. Some species are acid-fast and thus when stained may be confused with the causative organism for tuberculosis. Species pathogenic for humans cause the disease nocardiosis.

    N. asteroides. Species pathogenic for humans. The invasion site may be the lungs or skin. Abscesses called mycetomas arise in the skin.

    N. brasiliensis. Species pathogenic for humans. Chronic subcutaneous abscesses are formed.

nocardial (nō-kăr′dē-ăl). Concerning *Nocardia.*

nocardiosis. Pathological condition resulting from infection by any species of *Nocardia.* May occur as a pulmonary infection that spreads, resulting in abscesses in the skin, brain, or other areas. May also give rise to tumors that occur most frequently in lower extremities, esp. the foot, in which case it is called maduromycosis or Madura foot. Nocardiosis is distinguishable from actinomycosis by identification of organism.

    TREAT: Sulfadiazine daily for several months.

noci- (nō′sē) [L. *nocere*, to injure]. A combining form indicating pain or injury.

nociassociation (nō″sē-ă-sō″sē-ā′shŭn) [" + *ad,* to, + *socius,* companion]. The involuntary release of nervous energy during surgical shock or following trauma.

nociceptive (nō″sĭ-sĕp′tĭv) [" + *ceptus,* receiving]. Pert. to stimuli to the brain.

nociceptive impulses. Impulses giving rise to sensations of pain.

nociceptive reflex. A reflex initiated by painful stimuli.

nociceptor (nō″sē-sĕp′tor) [" + *receptor,* receiver]. A nerve for receiving and transmitting painful stimuli.

noci-influence (nō″sē-ĭn′floo-ĕns) [" + *influence*]. Injurious or harmful influence.

nociperception (nō″sĭ-pĕr-sĕp′shŭn) [" + *perceptio,* apprehension]. The perception by the nerve centers of injurious influences or painful stimuli.

"no code" orders. An indication on the chart of a terminally ill patient that he or she does not want heroic and life-saving measures to be instituted at the time when death is imminent. SEE: *hopelessly ill patients.*

noct. L. *nocte,* night.

noctalbuminuria (nŏk″tăl-bū-mĭn-ū′rē-ă) [L. *nocte,* at night, + *albumen,* white of egg, + Gr. *ouron,* urine]. Excess of albumin voided in urine at night. SYN: *nyctalbuminuria.*

noctambulation (nŏk″tăm-bū-lā′shŭn) [″ + *ambulare,* to move about]. Sleepwalking.

noctambulism (nŏk-tăm′bū-lĭzm) [″ + ″ + Gr. *-ismos,* state of]. Sleepwalking. SYN: *somnambulism.*

Noctec. Trade name for chloral hydrate, USP.

noctiphobia (nŏk″tĭ-fō′bē-ă) [″ + Gr. *phobos,* fear]. Fear of the night and darkness. SYN: *nyctophobia; scotophobia.*

nocturia (nŏk-tū′rē-ă) [″ + Gr. *ouron,* urine]. Urination, esp. excessive, during the night. May be due to excessive fluid intake before going to bed, prostatic disease, urinary tract infection, or impaired renal function which results in excretion of urine with low specific gravity. SYN: *nycturia.* SEE: *enuresis.*

nocturnal [L. *nocturnus,* at night]. Pert. to or occurring in the night. Opposed to diurnal. SEE: words beginning with *nyct-.*

nocturnal emission. Harmless involuntary discharge of semen during sleep. Usually occurs in conjunction with an erotic dream. SYN: *wet dream.*

nocturnal enuresis. Urinary incontinence during sleep at night. SYN: *bedwetting.* SEE: *enuresis.*

nocturnal penile tumescence. ABBR: NPT. In the normal male, erections occur during sleep beginning in early childhood and continuing to at least the eighth decade. The total time of NPT averages 100 minutes per night. In evaluating impotence, if the patient confirms that NPT occurs, then the cause of the impotence is probably due to a psychiatric disorder.

nocuous (nŏk′ū-ŭs) [L. *nocuus*]. Noxious, injurious, harmful, poisonous.

nodal (nō′dăl) [L. *nodus,* knot]. Pert. to a protuberance.

nodal points. A pair of points situated on the axis of an optical system so that any incident ray sent through one will produce a parallel emergent ray sent through the other.

nodal rhythm. Cardiac rhythm with origin at atrioventricular node.

nodding (nŏd′ĭng). Involuntary allowing of head to fall downward as when momentarily dozing. SYN: *nutation.*

nodding spasm. Nodding of the head due to spasm of the sternomastoid muscles. SYN: *salaam convulsion.*

node (nōd) [L. *nodus,* knot]. 1. A knot, knob, protuberance, or swelling. 2. A constricted region. 3. A small rounded organ or structure.

    n., Aschoff′s. Atrioventricular node of the heart.

    n., atrioventricular. A tangled mass of Purkinje fibers located in the lower part of the interatrial septum from which the atrioventricular bundle (bundle of His) arises. SEE: *bundle, atrioventricular.*

    n., A-V. N., atrioventricular.

    n., Bouchard′s. In osteoarthritis, bony enlargement of the proximal interphalangeal joints. SEE: *n.′s, Heberden′s.*

    n., Flack′s. The sinoatrial node of the heart.

    n.′s, Haygarth′s. Joint swelling in arthritis deformans.

    n.′s, Heberden′s. Nodes on fingers seen in osteoarthritis, usually on the terminal phalangeal joints.

    n., hemal. A lymphoid structure in which blood sinuses are present instead of lymph sinuses. These structures occur in animals but most probably not in humans.

    n., Hensen′s. Mass of rapidly proliferating cells at the anterior end of the primitive streak of the embryo.

    n., lymph. Mass of lymphoid tissue along the course of lymphatic vessels.

    n.′s, Meynet′s. Nodes in capsules of joints and in tendons in rheumatism, esp. in children.

    n.′s of Ranvier. Constrictions of the myelin sheath of a myelinated nerve fiber.

    n.′s, Osler′s. Tender cutaneous nodes, usually in fingers and toes, that may be seen with subacute bacterial endocarditis.

    n.′s, Parrot′s. Osteophytes around anterior fontanel seen in hereditary syphilis.

    n., piedric. Node on the hair shaft seen in piedra, q.v.

    n., Schmorl′s. Node seen in roentgenograms of the spine. They are caused by prolapse of the nucleus pulposus into the endplate of the vertebra.

    n., sentinel. N., signal. SEE: *sentinel node.*

    n., signal. Enlargement of one of the supraclavicular lymph nodes. Usually indicative of primary carcinoma of thoracic or abdominal organs.

    n., singer′s. Small white node that develops on vocal cords caused by overuse or improper use of the voice. SEE: *chorditis nodosa.*

    n., sinoatrial. Node in wall of right atrium near entrance of superior vena cava, consisting of dense network of Purkinje fibers. Source of impulses initiating heartbeat. SYN: *pacemaker* (def. 2); *n., sinoauricular; n., sinus.*

    n., sinoauricular. N., sinoatrial.

    n., sinus. N., sinoatrial.

    n., syphilitic. Circumscribed swelling at end of long bones due to congenital syphilis. Sensitive and painful during inflammation, esp. at night. SEE: *n.′s, Parrot′s.*

n., teacher's. N., singer's.

n., Troisier's. An enlarged node above the clavicle. It is caused by metastasis usually from an intrathoracic neoplasm.

n., Virchow. N., signal.

nodi (nō'dī) Plural of nodus.

no diagnosis. The condition when a patient is studied extensively but no evidence of mental or physical disease can be established.

nodose (nō'dōs) [L. *nodosus*, knotted]. Swollen or knotlike at intervals; marked by nodes or projections.

nodosity (nō-dŏs'ĭ-tē) [L. *nodositas*, a knot]. 1. A protuberance or knot. 2. Condition of having nodes.

nodular (nŏd'ū-lăr). Containing or resembling nodules.

nodular elastosis. A severe form of elastosis caused by a history of prolonged exposure to the sun. Elastotic material accumulates in the skin and forms cysts and comedones around the face. Occurs almost exclusively in white men of middle age or older.

TREAT: Remove cysts and evacuate comedones, followed by application of retinoic acid cream to the area nightly for 6 to 8 weeks. Avoidance of sun exposure to prevent recurrence.

nodulation (nŏd"ū-lā'shŭn). Formation of nodules.

nodule (nŏd'ūl) [L. *nodulus*, little knot]. 1. A small node. 2. A small aggregation of cells.

  n.'s, aggregate. A group of solitary lymph nodules, such as Peyer's patches of the small intestine.

  n.'s, Albini's. Nodules sometimes seen on free edges of atrioventricular valves of the heart in infants.

  n., apple jelly. The jelly-like lesion of lupus vulgaris.

  n.'s, Arantius'. Central fibrous tubercles in segments of semilunar valves. SYN: *corpora arantii; n.'s, Morgagni.*

  n., Aschoff's. Nodule found in myocardium, a characteristic lesion of rheumatic carditis.

  n.'s, cortical. Lymph nodules located in cortex of a lymph node.

  n., lymph. A mass of densely packed lymphocytes forming the structural unit of lymphatic tissue. Each contains a germinal center where new lymphocytes are formed.

  n., lymphatic. N., lymph.

  n., milker's. Nodule due to poxvirus that is transmitted from the udder of infected cows to the hands of milkers.

  n.'s, Morgagni. N.'s, Arantius'.

  n.'s of semilunar valve. N.'s, Arantius'.

  n., rheumatic. Subcutaneous nodes of fibrous tissue that may be present in patients with rheumatic fever.

  n., Schmorl's. Nodule seen in roentgen-

ograms of the spine. They are caused by prolapse of the nucleus pulposus into the endplate of the vertebra.

  n.'s, siderotic. Small brown nodules, seen in spleen and other organs, consisting of necrotic tissue encrusted by iron salts.

  n., Sister Mary Joseph. A hard, periumbilical lymph node sometimes present when pelvic or gastrointestinal tumors have metastasized.

  n., solitary. An isolated nodule of lymphatic tissue such as occurs in mucous membranes.

  n.'s, subcutaneous. Small, non-tender swellings resembling Aschoff bodies and found over bony prominences on hands and feet, occurring in persons with rheumatic fever.

  n.'s, surfer's. Surfer's knots, q.v.

  n.'s, typhoid. Nodules characteristic of typhoid fever and found in the liver.

  n.'s, typhus. Small nodules of the skin seen in typhus. They are composed of mononuclear cell infiltration around vessels.

nodulus (nŏd'ū-lŭs) [L.] (pl. *noduli*). [NA] 1. Nodule. 2. Anterior portion of vermis of the cerebellum.

nodus (nō'dŭs) [L.] (pl. *nodi*). [NA] Node; anatomically, a small circumscribed mass of undifferentiated tissue.

noematachograph (nō-ē"mă-tăk'ō-grăf) [Gr. *noema*, thought, + *tachys*, swift, + *graphein*, to write]. Device for recording time taken in mental activity.

noematic (nō"ē-măt'ĭk) [Gr. *noema*, thought]. Concerning the mental process of thinking.

noesis (nō-ē'sĭs) [Gr. *noesis*, thought]. The act of thinking; cognition.

Noguchia (nō-goo'chē-ă) [Hideyo Noguchi, Japanese bacteriologist in U.S., 1876–1928]. A genus of microorganisms of the family Brucellaceae. They are slim, gram-negative, flagellated rods present in the conjunctiva of humans and animals with follicular conjunctivitis.

noise [O. Fr. *noise*, strife, brawl]. 1. Sound of any sort, including that which is loud, harsh, confused, or senseless. SEE: *acoustic trauma; pollution, noise.* 2. In electronics or physics, any electronic disturbance that interferes with the signal being recorded or monitored. In electrocardiography, the 60-cycle alternating current used to power the machine may be inadvertently recorded. This obscures the signal from the electrical activity of the heart. 3. Unwanted information on a radiograph caused by fogging, scattered radiation, and quantum mottle.

noli me tangere (nō"lē-mē-tăn'jĕ-rē) [L., touch me not]. Cancerous ulcer, generally of

Typical Noise Levels in Decibels and Their Effect

Situation	Level Decibels	Effect
Jet engine (close by)*	140	Harmful to hearing
Jet takeoff*	130	
Propeller aircraft*	120	
Live rock band	110	Risk hearing loss
Jackhammer	100	
Heavy duty truck	90	
Private car; business office	70	Probably no risk of permanent damage to hearing
Wooded residential area	50	No harm
Whisper	30	No harm
Rustle of leaf	10	No harm

* Outside aircraft

the face, which eats away bone and soft tissue; rodent ulcer.

Noludar. Trade name for methyprylon, USP.

Nolvadex. Trade name for tamoxifen citrate.

noma (nō′mă) [Gr. *nome*, a spreading]. A gangrenous progressive condition, generally found in undernourished children, spreading rapidly from the mucous membrane of the cheek or gum to the cutaneous surface. SYN: *cancrum oris; gangrenous stomatitis.*

    n. pudendi. An ulcerative condition affecting the labia majora, esp. in young children.

nomadism [Gr. *nomas*, roaming about]. Impulse to wander about aimlessly; restlessness.

nomenclature (nō′měn-klā″chūr) [L. *nomen*, name, + *calare*, to call]. Classified system of technical or scientific names. SYN: *terminology.*

    n., binomial. The system of classifying plants and animals by the use of two Latin-derived words to indicate the genus and species.

Nomina Anatomica (nō′mĭ-nă ăn-ă-tŏm′-ĭ-kä) [″ + Gr. *anatome*, dissection]. ABBR: NA. Anatomical terminology adopted as official by the International Congress of Anatomists at various meetings since 1955. The 11th International Congress was held in Mexico City in 1980. The 1983 publication *Nomina Anatomica*, containing the nomenclature, is published by Williams & Wilkins, Baltimore and London.

nomogram (nŏm′ō-grăm) [Gr. *nomos*, law, + *gramma*, something written]. Representation by graphs, diagrams, or charts of the relationship between numerical variables.

nomography (nō-mŏg′ră-fē) [″ + *gra-*

phein, to write]. A graphic representation of the relationship between numerical variables.

nomotopic (nō-mō-tŏp′ĭk) [″ + *topos*, place]. Occurring at the normal site.

non- [L.]. Prefix denoting negation or absence.

nona-, non [L. *nonus*, ninth]. Prefix meaning ninth.

nonan (nō′năn). Having increased symptoms or reappearing every ninth day, as the paroxysms of malaria.

noncompliance. The failure of the patient to cooperate by carrying out that portion of the medical care plan under his or her control, e.g., not taking prescribed medicines or not adhering to the diet ordered.

non compos mentis (nŏn kŏm′pŏs měn′tĭs) [L.]. Not of sound mind; mentally incompetent to handle one's affairs.

nonconductor [L. *non*, not, + *con*, with, + *ductor*, a leader]. Any substance that does not transmit heat, sound, or electricity or that conducts it with difficulty. Strictly speaking, there is no perfect nonconductor. On the application of a sufficiently high voltage, current may be caused to flow through materials usually spoken of as nonconductors. SYN: *insulator.*

nondisjunction. Failure of a pair of chromosomes to separate at meiosis. This allows one daughter cell to have two chromosomes and the other to have none.

nonelectrolyte [″ + Gr. *elektron*, amber, + *lytos*, dissolved]. A solution that will not conduct electricity because its chemical constituents are not sufficiently dissociated into ions.

nongonococcal urethritis. SEE: *urethritis, nongonococcal.*

non-Hodgkin's lymphoma. SEE: *lymphoma, non-Hodgkin's.*

nonigravida (nō″nĭ-grā′vĭ-dă) [L. *nonus,* ninth, + *gravida,* pregnant]. A woman pregnant for the ninth time. Written gravida IX. SEE: *nonipara.*

noninvasive. 1. Not tending to spread as certain tumors. 2. Devices or procedures that do not require entering the body or puncturing the skin.

noninvasive neoplasm. A tumor that has not spread or does not spread.

nonipara (nō-nĭp′ăr-ă) [″ + *parere,* to bring forth, to bear]. A woman who has given birth nine times. Written para IX.

nonlaxative diet. Low-residue diet with boiled milk and toasted crackers. No strained oatmeal, vegetable juice, or fruit juice given. Fats and concentrated sweets are restricted.

nonmedullated (nŏn-mĕd′ū-lāt″ĕd) [L. *non,* not, + *medulla,* marrow]. Containing no myelin.

nonmyelinated (nŏn-mī′ĕ-lĭ-nāt″ĕd) [″ + Gr. *myelos,* marrow]. Containing no myelin.

non-nucleated (nŏn-nū′klē-āt″ĕd) [″ + *nucleatus,* having a kernel]. Containing no nucleus.

nonocclusion (nŏn″ŏ-kloo′zhŭn) [″ + *occlusio,* occlusion]. A type of malocclusion in which the teeth fail to make contact.

nonopaque (nŏn″ō-pāk′). Not opaque, esp. to x-rays.

nonose (nō′ōs) [L. *nonus,* ninth]. A nine-carbon carbohydrate.

nonoxynol (nō-nŏks′ĭ-nŏl). A general class of surface-active agents with the basic formula of $C_{15}H_{24}O(C_2H_4O)_n$; they are named with respect to the value of *n.* Thus nonoxynol 10 is $C_{15}H_{24}O(C_2H_4O)_{10}$.
   n. 9. A spermicide.

nonparous (nŏn-păr′ŭs) [L. *non,* not, + *parere,* to bear]. Nulliparous.

nonpolar [″ + *polus,* a pole]. Not having separate poles; sharing electrons.

nonpolar compound. Compound formed by the sharing of electrons.

nonproprietary name. The name of a drug other than its proprietary or trademarked name. The nonproprietary name for a new drug is usually the same as that selected by United States Adopted Name (USAN) Council. The official names for older drugs may differ from the nonproprietary names. In some cases, the generic name is the same as the nonproprietary name. Drugs also have chemical names, and in most cases those names are too long and complex to permit their use. Thus the use of a USAN-selected name simplifies and standardizes drug nomenclature. SEE: *proprietary medicine.*

nonprotein [L. *non,* not, + Gr. *protos,* first]. Any substance not a protein.

nonprotein nitrogen. 1. A nitrogenous constituent of blood that is not a protein. 2. Sum of all nonprotein nitrogen in the blood. SEE: *nitrogen.*

non rep. [L. *non repetatur*]. Abbreviation meaning *do not repeat.*

nonrestraint (nŏn″rē-strānt′) [L. *non,* not, + *re,* back, + *stringere,* to bind back]. Treatment of the insane without using mechanical repression.

nonrotation (nŏn″rō-tā′shŭn) [″ + *rotare,* to turn]. Failure of a part or organ to rotate, esp. during embryological development.
   n. of intestine. In embryonic development, the intestines fail to rotate, so that the descending colon is on the left side of the abdominal cavity instead of the right.

nonsecretor (nŏn″sē-krē′tor) [″ + *secretio,* separation]. An individual whose saliva does not contain the ABO blood antigens.

nonseptate (nŏn-sĕp′tāt) [″ + *septum,* a partition]. Having no dividing walls.

nonsexual (nŏn-sĕk′shū-ăl). Without sex. SYN: *asexual.*

nonspecific. Term used in reference to the cause of a disease when the exact organism or agent has not been identified.

nonspecific urethritis. Urethritis not due to a provable specific virus or bacteria.

nonsteroidal anti-inflammatory drugs. ABBR: NSAID. A group of drugs that have analgesic, anti-inflammatory, and antipyretic action. They are similar to aspirin and aspirin-like drugs. These drugs have been used extensively in treating arthritis, dysmenorrhea, and inflammation in general. Even though effective as analgesics and in moderating inflammation, there is no evidence that the pathological progression of a disease such as rheumatoid arthritis is altered. As many as 10-15% of patients will experience side effects, esp. gastrointestinal irritation and hemorrhage of such severity as to require discontinuing the use of NSAIDs. Anti-ulcer therapy is ineffective in preventing gastrointestinal ulcers in those who develop this condition while taking NSAIDs. Hepatotoxicity is a rare but important undesired side effect of NSAID use. SEE: *nephritis, analgesic.*

nontoxic (nŏn-tŏk′sĭk) [L. *non,* not, + Gr. *toxikon,* poison]. Not poisonous or productive of poison.

nontoxic substances. Characteristic of being nontoxic as ordinarily encountered. For those involved in patient care, it is important to know that some of the common materials that children and adults can accidentally ingest are not toxic. A list of substances considered to be generally nontoxic is provided in the Appendix. SEE: *Nontoxic Substances* in *Appendix*.

nonunion (nŏn-ūn′yŭn) [″ + *unio*, oneness]. Failure of fragments of a fractured bone to knit together.

Diagnosis of nonunion is established when a minimum of nine months has elapsed since injury and the fracture site shows no progressive signs of healing for a minimum of three months and is not complicated by a synovial pseudoarthrosis. SEE: *bone fracture, nonunion, electrical stimulation for.*

nonus [L.]. 1. Ninth. 2. Hypoglossal nerve, formerly regarded as ninth cranial nerve.

nonvalent (nŏn-vā′lĕnt) [L. *non*, not, + *valens*, powerful]. Having no chemical valency.

nonviable (nŏn-vī′ă-b′l) [″ + *via*, life]. Incapable of life or of living; frequently used to indicate a fetus that has died in utero, born prior to 20th week of gestation.

nonyl. A univalent radical, $CH_3(CH_2)_8$, that contains nine carbon atoms.

nookleptia (nō-ō-klĕp′tē-ă) [Gr. *nous*, mind, + *kleptein*, to steal]. An obsession that one's thoughts are being stolen by others.

Noonan's syndrome [Jacqueline A. Noonan, U.S. cardiologist, b. 1921]. A syndrome quite similar to Turner's, q.v. There are low-set ears, webbing of the neck, congenital heart disease, cubitum valgum, and in some cases severe mental retardation.

noopsyche (nō′ō-sī″kē) [Gr. *nous*, mind, + *psyche*, soul]. Mental processes.

noradrenalin bitartrate (nor″ă-drĕn′ă-lĭn). Norepinephrine bitartate, USP.

NORD. *National Organization for Rare Disorders,* q.v.

nordefrin hydrochloride (nor-dĕf′rĭn). A vasoconstrictor drug. Trade name is Cobefrin.

norepinephrine (nor-ĕp″ĭ-nĕf′rĭn). 1. A hormone produced by the adrenal medulla, similar in chemical and pharmacological properties to epinephrine, but chiefly a vasoconstrictor with little effect on cardiac output. 2. A catecholamine. A disturbance in its metabolism at important brain sites has been implicated in affective disorders.

    n. bitartrate. USP. A standardized preparation of norepinephrine, q.v. Trade name is Levophed. Previously used name was levarterenol bitartrate.

norethandrolone (nor″ĕth-ăn′drō-lōn). An anabolic steroid.

norethindrone (nor-ĕth′ĭn-drōn). USP. A steroid hormone similar in action to progesterone. Used in progestational agents for birth control. Trade names are Micronor, Nor-Q.D., and Norlutin.

norethynodrel (nor″ĕ-thī′nō-drĕl). USP. A progestational agent used in certain birth control pills.

Norflex. Trade name for orphenadrine citrate, USP.

norflurane (nor-floor′ān). An inhalation anesthetic.

norgestrel (nor-jĕs′trĕl). USP. A progestational agent used in certain birth control pills. Trade names are Microlut and Ovrette.

Norisodrine Aerotrol. Trade name for isoproterenol hydrochloride, USP.

Norlutate. Trade name for norethindrone acetate, USP.

Norlutin. Trade name for norethindrone, USP.

norm [L. *norma*, rule]. 1. A standard or ideal for a specific group. 2. Normal.

norma [L., rule]. A view or aspect, esp. with reference to the skull.

    n., anterior. N. frontalis.

    n., basilaris. N. ventralis.

    n. facialis. N. frontalis.

    n. frontalis. Outline of the skull viewed from the front. SYN: *n., anterior; n. facialis.*

    n., inferior. N. ventralis.

    n. lateralis. View of skull as seen from the side; a profile view.

    n. occipitalis. View of skull as seen from behind.

    n. sagittalis. View as seen in sagittal section.

    n., superior. N. verticalis.

    n. ventralis. View of inferior surface of skull. SYN: *n., inferior; n. basilaris.*

    n. verticalis. View of skull as seen from above. SYN: *n., superior.*

normal (nor′măl) [L. *normalis*, according to pattern]. 1. Standard; performing proper functions; natural; regular. 2. In biology, not affected by experimental treatment; occurring naturally and not because of disease or experimentation. 3. In psychology, free from mental disorder; or of average development or intelligence. 4. In chemistry, a term used to describe a solution so made that 1 liter contains 1 gram equivalent of the solute.

normal distribution. In statistics, the smooth, bell-shaped, hypothetical curve made by a frequency distribution diagram in which the occurrences are plotted on the vertical axis (ordinate), and the values of the variable are plotted on the horizontal axis (abscissa). SYN: *bell-shaped curve; gaussian curve.* SEE: *frequency distribution.*

normalization (nor″măl-ĭ-zā′shŭn) [L. *normalis*, according to pattern]. Modification or reduction to the normal standard.

normal salt. An ionic compound containing no replaceable hydrogen or hydroxyl ions.

normal solution. SEE: *normal* (def. 4).

normergic (nor-mĕr′jĭk). Reacting, or pert. to

that which reacts, in a normal manner.

normetanephrine (nor-mĕt″ă-nĕf′rĭn). A metabolite of epinephrine.

normo- [L. *norma*, rule]. A combining form indicating normal or usual.

normoblast (nor′mō-blăst) [″ + Gr. *blastos*, germ]. A nucleated red blood corpuscle similar in size to an ordinary erythrocyte.

normoblastosis (nor″mō-blăs-tō′sĭs) [″ + ″ + *osis*, condition]. Increased production of normoblasts.

normocalcemia (nor″mō-kăl-sē′mē-ă). Normal level of blood calcium.

normocapnia (nor″mō-kăp′nē-ă). Presence of carbon dioxide in the blood and serum in normal concentration.

normocapnic (nor″mō-kăp′nĭk). Having a normal amount of carbon dioxide in the blood.

normocholesterolemia (nor″mō-kō-lĕs′tĕr-ō-lē′mē-ă). Presence of cholesterol in the blood in normal concentration.

normochromasia (nor″mō-krō-mā′zē-ă) [″ + Gr. *chroma*, color]. Average staining capacity in a cell or tissue.

normochromia (nor″mō-krō′mē-ă). Blood possessing normal color and hemoglobin content.

normocyte (nor′mō-sīt) [″ + Gr. *kytos*, cell]. An average-sized red blood corpuscle. SYN: *erythrocyte; normoerythrocyte.*

normocytosis (nor″mō-sī-tō′sĭs) [″ + ″ + *osis*, condition]. A normal state of the corpuscular elements of the blood.

normoerythrocyte (nor″mō-ĕ-rĭth′rō-sīt) [″ + Gr. *erythros*, red, + *kytos*, cell]. Normocyte.

normoglycemia (nor″mō-glī-sē′mē-ă) [″ + Gr. *glykys*, sweet, + *haima*, blood]. Normal state of sugar content of the blood.

normoglycemic (nor″mō-glī-sē′mĭk). Having a normal amount of sugar in the blood.

normokalemia (nor″mō-kă-lē′mē-ă). Normal level of blood potassium.

normo-orthocytosis (nor″mō-or″thō-sī-tō′sĭs) [L. *norma*, rule, + Gr. *orthos*, correct, + *kytos*, cell, + *osis*, condition]. Increase of the number of leukocytes in the blood but with normal proportion of the different varieties.

normoskeocytosis (nor″mō-skē″ō-sī-tō′sĭs) [″ + Gr. *skaios*, left, + *kytos*, cell, + *osis*, condition]. Normal number of the leukocytes of the blood with shift to the left, i.e., with immature forms present.

normospermic (nor″mō-spĕr′mĭk) [″ + Gr. *sperma*, seed]. The production of normal spermatozoa.

normosthenuria (nor″mō-sthĕn-ū′rē-ă) [″ + Gr. *sthenos*, strength, + *ouron*, urine]. Urination of normal amount and specific gravity.

normotensive (nor″mō-tĕn′sĭv). 1. Normal blood pressure. 2. A person with normal blood pressure.

normothermia (nor″mō-thĕr′mē-ă) [″ + Gr. *therme*, heat]. Normal body temperature.

normotonic (nor″mō-tŏn′ĭk) [″ + Gr. *tonos*, tension]. 1. Having normal muscular tonus. 2. One who has normal muscle tonus.

normotopia (nor″mō-tō′pē-ă) [″ + Gr. *topos*, place]. Situation in the regular place.

normotopic (nor″mō-tŏp′ĭk). In the right location; pert. to the normal situation.

normovolemia (nor″mō-vō-lē′mē-ă) [″ + *volumen*, volume, + Gr. *haima*, blood]. Normal state of blood volume.

Norpace. Trade name for disopyramide phosphate, USP.

Norplant. A contraceptive for women that prevents pregnancy for up to five years. It consists of a fan-like arrangement of six silicone rubber capsules containing levonorgestrel that are of the diameter of matchsticks and that are implanted beneath the skin of a woman's inner arm, just above the elbow. The procedure takes approximately 15 minutes and is performed in a physician's office under a local anesthetic. When the rods are removed, fertility is restored.

Use of Norplant, like all drugs, is not free of side effects. Some users report amenorrhea, menstrual irregularities, weight change, mood swings, and headache. Some of these side effects are the same as would serve to identify early pregnancy. Thus, tests should be performed whenever pregnancy is suspected.

Norpramin. Trade name for desipramine hydrochloride, USP.

Norrie's disease [Gordon Norrie, Danish ophthalmologist, 1855–1941]. A rare form of sex-linked hereditary blindness. Also present are peripheral vascular pathology, retinal malformation, vitreous opacities, microphthalmia, and sometimes mental retardation and loss of hearing.

nortriptyline hydrochloride (nor-trĭp′tĭ-lēn). USP. An antidepressant drug of the tricyclic class. Trade names are Aventyl Hydrochloride and Pamelor.

Norwalk agent [virus first identified in Norwalk, Ohio, U.S.A.]. The viral agent that is the causative organism in over half of the reported cases of epidemic viral gastroenteropathy.

Norwegian itch. Severe form of scabies marked by pustules and crusts.

noscapine (nŏs′kă-pēn). A naturally occurring opium alkaloid that is used as an antitussive in cough preparations.

nose [AS. *nosw*]. Projection in center of face; the organ of olfaction and the entrance that warms, moistens, and filters the air as it passes through to the respiratory tract. SYN: *nasus* [NA]; *organum olfactus.*

ANAT: The external portion of the nose is a triangle of cartilage and bone covered with skin and lined with mucous membrane. Internally, a septum divides the nose into two chambers. Each chamber contains three meatus, which are found underneath the corresponding turbinates. Orifices of frontal, anterior, ethmoid, and maxillary sinuses are in middle meatus. Orifices of posterior ethmoids and sphenoids are in superior meatus.

Communicating sinuses: Ethmoidal, frontal, maxillary, and sphenoidal. *Nerves:* Facial, olfactory, ophthalmic, and maxillary. *Blood supply:* External and internal maxillary arteries from the external carotid artery and ethmoidal artery from the internal carotid artery.

EXAM: Note shape, size, color, state of the alae nasi, discharge, interference with respiration, evidence of injury, deflected or perforated septum, enlarged turbinates, and tenderness over frontal and maxillary sinuses.

DIAG: *Chronic red nose:* Dilated capillaries as a result of alcoholism, lupus erythematosus, acne rosacea, pustules, and boils. *Superficial ulceration:* Tuberculous ulcer, epithelioma, syphilis. *Broad and coarse:* Cretinism, myxedema, acromegaly. *Sunken:* Syphilis or injury. *Pinched with small nares:* Hypertrophied adenoid tissue or chronic obstructions; tumors. *Inoffensive watery discharge:* Nasal catarrh, early stages of measles, hay fever, acute irritation of lining membranes. *Offensive discharge:* Nasopharyngeal diphtheria, lupus, local infection, impacted foreign bodies, caries, rhinitis, glanders, syphilitic infection.

n., bridge of. Superior portion of external nose formed by union of the two nasal bones.

n., foreign body in. Irritation of nose resulting in coughing or watery or purulent discharge. Occasionally pain and obstruction of nose. If not recognized immediately, it often causes a foul discharge on the affected side of the nose. There may be obstruction to breathing in one nostril. If the foreign body is very small, symptoms may be absent.

TREAT: Take the patient to a physician. Vigorous blowing of the nose is dangerous because it may spread infection to the various cavities and sinuses about the nose or to the middle ear. Attempts to dislodge it may cause it to slip further into the nose or down the throat and into the windpipe.

n., hammer. Rhinophyma.

n., saddle. Nose with depressed bridge that is seen in tertiary syphilis and is due to gummatous destruction of septal supporting structure, and seen following operations that are complicated by suppuration and destruction of supporting framework.

nose, words pert. to: ala nasi; alinasal; anosmia; bulb, olfactory; choana; columella nasi; epistaxis; hyperosmia; Kiesselbach's area; naris; nasal; nostril; parosmia; rhinalgia; septum, nasal; sinuses, accessory nasal; sinusitis; smell; vestibule of nose; vibrissae; vomer; and "nas-" and "rhino-" words.

nosebleed. Hemorrhage from nose. SEE: illus.; *epistaxis; Kiesselbach's area.*

Nosema (nō-sē'mă). A genus of parasites of the order Microsporidia.

nosepiece (nōz'pēs). The portion of a microscope to which the objective lenses attach.

nosh. 1. Between-meal snacks. 2. To eat or nibble between meals.

noso- [Gr. *nosos,* disease]. Combining form pert. to disease.

nosochthonography (nŏs″ŏk-thō-nŏg'ră-fē) [″ + *chthon,* earth, + *graphein,* to write]. Study of geographical distribution of diseases; medical geography. SYN: *nosogeography.*

nosocomial (nŏs″ō-kō'mē-ăl) [Gr. *nosokomos,* one who tends the sick]. Pert. to a hospital or infirmary.

nosocomial infection. Infection acquired in a hospital.

nosography (nō-sŏg'ră-fē) [Gr. *nosos,* disease, + *graphein,* to write]. The written description of a disease.

nosology (nō-sŏl'ō-jē) [″ + *logos,* word, reason]. The science of description or classification of diseases.

nosomycosis (nŏs″ō-mī-kō'sĭs) [″ + *mykes,* fungus, + *osis,* condition]. Any disease caused by a parasitic fungus or schizomycete.

nosophilia (nŏs″ō-fĭl'ē-ă) [″ + *philein,* to love]. An abnormal desire to be ill.

nosophobia (nō″sō-fō'bē-ă) [″ + *phobos,* fear]. Abnormal aversion to illness or to a particular affection.

nosophyte (nŏs'ō-fīt) [″ + *phyton,* plant]. A disease-causing plant microorganism.

Nosopsyllus (nŏs″ō-sĭl'ŭs) [″ + *psylla,* flea]. A genus of fleas belonging to the order Siphonaptera.

N. fasciatus. A species of rat fleas responsible for transmission of murine typhus and perhaps of plague.

nosotherapy (nŏs″ō-thĕr'ă-pē) [″ + *therapeia,* treatment]. Treatment of one disease by voluntarily introducing another microorganism into the body.

Ex.: In the past, the use of malaria parasites to cause fever in treatment of central

TECHNIQUE FOR CONTROL OF HEMORRHAGE FROM POSTERIOR NASAL CAVITY

A.
INSERT SOFT FLEXIBLE CATHETER
INTO NOSE AND BRING DISTAL TIP
OUT THROUGH THE MOUTH. ATTACH
MOISTENED PACK TO CATHETER

B.
BY PULLING ON CATHETER
DRAW PACK IN PLACE SO IT IS
PLACED SECURELY IN POSTERIOR
NASAL CAVITY

C.
REMOVE CATHETER AND USE STRING
TO ATTACH TO A SOFT CUSHION OF
SUFFICIENT SIZE TO PREVENT ITS
PASSING INTO THE NOSTRIL

D.
ALTERNATIVELY, A FOLEY CATHETER
MAY BE USED. THE INFLATED TIP IS
HELD SECURELY IN PLACE AS IN
PREVIOUS ILLUSTRATIONS

nervous system syphilis.

nosotoxic (nŏs″ō-tŏk′sĭk) [″ + *toxikon*, poison]. Anything that produces a disease-causing toxin.

nosotoxicosis (nŏs″ō-tŏk″sĭ-kō′sĭs) [″ + ″ + *osis*, condition]. Any disease caused by poisoning.

nosotrophy (nō-sŏt′rō-fē) [″ + *trophe*, nourishment]. Nursing care and feeding of the sick.

nosotropic (nō″sō-trŏp′ĭk) [″ + *tropos*, turning]. Directed against the symptoms or effects of a disease. Opposite of etiotropic.

nostalgia (nŏs-tăl′jē-ă) [Gr. *nostos*, a return home, + *algos*, pain]. Homesickness; longing to return home.

nostril [AS. *nosu*, nose, + *thyrel*, a hole]. One of the external apertures of the nose. SYN: *naris*. SEE: *nose*.

nostril reflex. Reduction of opening of naris on affected side in lung disease in proportion to lessened alveolar air capacity on affected side.

nostrum (nŏs′trŭm) [L., our]. A patent, secret, or quack remedy.

notal (nō′tăl) [Gr. *noton*, back]. Concerning the back. SYN: *dorsal*.

notalgia (nō-tăl′jē-ă) [″ + *algos*, pain]. Painful condition of the back. SYN: *dorsalgia*.

notancephalia (nō″tăn-sě-fā′lē-ă) [″ + *-an*, not, + *kephale*, head]. Congenital absence of the back of the skull.

notanencephalia (nō″tăn-ěn-sě-fā′lē-ă) [″ + ″ + *enkephalos*, brain]. Absence of the cerebellum.

notch (nŏch). A rather deep indentation or narrow gap in the edge of a structure. SYN: *incisura* [NA].

    n., acetabular. Notch in inferior border of acetabulum. SYN: *n., cotyloid.*

    n., aortic. Notch in sphygmogram from rebound at aortic valve closure.

    n., cardiac. Concavity on anterior border of left lung into which the heart projects.

    n., cerebellar, anterior and posterior. Deep notches separating the hemispheres of the cerebellum.

    n., clavicular. Notch at the upper angle of the sternum with which the clavicle articulates.

    n., costal. One of seven pairs of indentations on lateral surfaces of the sternum, for articulation with costal cartilages.

    n., cotyloid. N., acetabular.

    n., ethmoidal. Notch separating the two orbital portions of frontal bone.

    n., frontal. Notch on supraorbital arch that transmits frontal artery and nerve.

    n., interclavicular. A rounded notch at the top of the manubrium of the sternum, between surfaces articulating with the clavicles.

    n., jugular (of occipital bone). Notch that forms the posterior and middle portions of jugular foramen.

    n., jugular (of sternum). Notch on upper surface of manubrium between the two clavicular notches.

    n., labial. Notch in the labial flange of a denture at the point where it crosses the frenum.

    n., mandibular. Notch on superior border of ramus of mandible separating coronoid and condyloid processes.

    n., manubrial. Depression on the superior edge of the sternum.

    n., nasal. 1. A deep notch on anterior surface of maxilla, forming lateral border of piriform aperture. 2. Notch between internal angular processes of frontal bone.

    n. of Rivinus. N., tympanic.

    n., pancreatic. Notch on lateral surface of head of pancreas for superior mesenteric artery and vein. It separates uncinate process of head from remaining portion.

    n., parotid. The space between the ramus of the mandible and the mastoid process of the temporal bone.

    n., radial. Notch on lateral surface of coronoid process of ulna for receiving circumference of head of radius.

    n., scapular. A deep notch on superior border of scapula. Transmits suprascapular nerve.

    n., sciatic, greater. A large notch on the posterior border of the hip bone between the posterior inferior iliac spine and the spine of ischium.

    n., sciatic, lesser. Notch immediately below the spine of the ischium on the posterior border of the hip bone. Converted into a foramen by the sacrotuberous ligament.

    n., semilunar. Notch on anterior aspect of proximal end of ulna for articulation with trochlea of humerus.

    n., sphenopalatine. Notch between orbital and sphenoidal processes of palatine bone.

    n., tentorial. Notch in free border of tentorium cerebelli through which brain stem passes.

    n., thyroid. A deep notch on superior border of thyroid cartilage of larynx separating the two laminae.

    n., tympanic. Notch in superior portion of the tympanic ring. SYN: *n. of Rivinus.*

    n., ulnar. Notch on distal end of radius that receives head of ulna.

    n., umbilical. Notch on anterior border of liver where it is crossed by falciform ligament.

    n., vertebral. Concavity on inferior surface of root of vertebral arch. When two vertebrae are in position, the notches form the intervertebral foramina.

note [L. *nota*, a mark]. 1. A sound of definite pitch. 2. A brief comment or condensed report.

note blindness. Inability to recognize musical notes; due to a central lesion.

notencephalocele (nŏ″tĕn-sĕf′ăl-ō-sēl) [Gr. *noton*, back, + *enkephalos*, brain, + *kele*, tumor, swelling]. Protrusion of brain substance at the back of the head.

notencephalus (nŏ″tĕn-sĕf′ă-lŭs) [″ + *enkephalos*, brain]. A deformed fetus with notencephalocele.

nothing by mouth. An instruction used in patient care to indicate that the patient is to take or receive no food, liquid, or medicine, i.e., *nothing*, by mouth. Usually abbreviated n.p.o.

notifiable diseases. The laws of the various states require that occurrence of certain diseases shall be reported to the local health authorities, such as a board of health. A fine may be levied for not doing so. Among the diseases that may be required to be reported are all communicable or contagious diseases such as scarlet fever, diphtheria; enteric fevers such as typhoid fever; cholera; typhus; meningococcal meningitis; AIDS; acute anterior poliomyelitis; polioencephalitis; encephalitis lethargica; tuberculosis; epidemic of acute diarrheal disease; rubella; chickenpox; gonorrhea; syphilis. SEE: *quarantine; reportable diseases.*

noto- [Gr. *noton*, back]. Combining form indicating a relationship to the back.

notochord (nō′tō-kord) [″ + *chorde*, cord]. A rod of cells lying dorsal to the intestine and extending from anterior to posterior end. It forms axial skeleton in embryos of all chordates. In vertebrates it is replaced partially or completely by the bodies of vertebrae. A remnant persists in man as a portion of nucleus pulposus of intervertebral disk.

notogenesis (nō″tō-jĕn′ē-sĭs) [″ + *genesis*, generation, birth]. Development of the notochord.

notomelus (nō-tŏm′ē-lŭs) [″ + *melos*, limb]. A deformed fetus with one or more accessory limbs attached to the back.

noumenal (nū′mē-năl) [Gr. *nooumenon*, a thing perceived]. Pert. to noumenon, q.v. Pert. to that which arises because of intellectual intuition rather than sensory perception.

noumenon (nū′mē-nŏn) [Gr. *nooumenon*]. That which one knows or perceives by intellectual intuition alone, as distinguished from something perceived through sensory perception.

nourishment [L. *nutrire*, to nurse]. 1. Act of

nourishing or of being nourished. 2. Sustenance; nutriment. SEE: *center, trophic; trophic.*

Novafed. Trade name for pseudoephedrine hydrochloride, USP.

Novocain. Trade name for procaine hydrochloride, USP.

noxa (nŏk′să) [L., injury] (pl. *noxae*). Anything harmful to health.

noxious (nŏk′shŭs) [L. *noxius*, injurious]. Harmful; not wholesome.

NP. *nucleoprotein; nurse practitioner; nursing practice; nursing procedure; neuropsychiatrist; neuropsychiatry.*

Np. Chem. symb. for the element neptunium.

NPC. *nodal premature complex.* Ectopic cardiac beat originating in the atrioventricular node.

NPDB. *National Practitioner Data Bank.*

NPH insulin. *neutral protamine Hagedorn* insulin.

NPN. *nonprotein nitrogen.*

n.p.o. [L.] *non per os,* nothing by mouth.

NPT. *nocturnal penile tumescence.*

n.p.t. *normal pressure and temperature.*

NR. *nodal rhythm.*

NREM sleep. *Nonrapid eye movement* sleep. SEE: *sleep, NREM.*

N.R.E.M.T. *Nationally Registered Emergency Medical Technician.*

N.R.M.S. *National Registry of Medical Secretaries.*

ns. 1. *nanosecond.* 2. *nonsignificant.*

NSA. *Neurosurgical Society of America.*

NSAID. *nonsteroidal anti-inflammatory drug.*

NSCC. *National Society for Crippled Children.*

NSD. *nominal standard dose* in ret. Ret indicates radiation equivalent *t*herapy, which is analogous to the rem (roentgen equivalent [in] *m*an) used in radiation protection.

nsec. *nanosecond.*

N.S.N.A. *National Student Nurses' Association.*

NSPB. *National Society for the Prevention of Blindness.*

NSR. *normal sinus rhythm.*

NT. *nodal tachycardia.*

Nt. Chem. symb. for niton.

nth (ĕnth). Used in medical statistics to indicate the continuation of data or subjects to large numbers in a progression or series. Thus, one would indicate patients numbered P1, P2, P3, and so forth through P nth. P nth would be the last patient indicated.

Nubain. Trade name for nalbuphine hydrochloride.

nubecula (nū-bĕk′ū-lă) [L., little cloud]. Cloudiness of the cornea or the urine.

nubile (nū′bĭl) [L. *nubere,* to marry]. Pert. to a girl who has attained puberty.

nubility (nū-bĭl′ĭ-tē). Marriageableness, said of the female.

nucha (nū′kă) [L.]. [NA] Nape of neck.

nuchal (nū′kăl) [L. *nucha*, back of neck]. Pert. to the neck or nucha.

Nuck's canal (nŭks) [Anton Nuck, Dutch anatomist, 1650–1692]. An anomalous peritoneal pouch extending for a variable distance into the labium of the external female genitalia. Homologous to processus vaginalis of the male.

nuclear (nū′klē-ăr) [L. *nucleus*, a kernel]. Resembling or concerning a nucleus.

nuclear antigen. Antigen present in the cells of patients with certain types of connective tissue disorders. Corticosteroids are very helpful in treating patients with high concentrations of extractable nuclear antigen.

nuclear arc. Spiral patterns on the surface of the lens due to concentric pattern of fiber growth.

nuclear envelope. Two parallel membranes enclosing a narrow perinuclear space, enveloping the nucleus. Prior to electron microscopy, the nucleus of a cell was thought to be surrounded by a single, thin membrane.

nuclear family. The basic family unit consisting of parents and their children.

nuclear magnetic resonance imaging. ABBR: NMRI. SEE: *magnetic resonance imaging.*

nuclear medicine. That branch of medicine concerned with the diagnostic, therapeutic, and investigative use of radionuclides, q.v.

nuclear medicine scanning tests. The use of radioactive substances injected in the body or inhaled to diagnose certain conditions. The dose of radiation is minimal and the substances used either lose their radioactivity in a short time or are excreted. This technique called a "scan" may be used to diagnose tumors, biliary disease, gastrointestinal emptying or bleeding, coronary artery disease, valvular heart disease, red blood cell survival time, renal dysfunction, deep vein thrombosis, and thyroid function.

nuclear winter. The proposition that nuclear war would cause an accumulation of pollution in the atmosphere sufficient to act as a barrier to sunlight and heat. This would cause the land temperature to decrease to a point at which agriculture would be destroyed, and the area under the polluted air would be enveloped in nearly total darkness. How long this condition would last is unknown.

nuclease (nū′klē-ās) [L. *nucleus*, kernel, + *-ase*, enzyme]. Any enzyme in animals and plants that facilitates hydrolysis of nuclein and nucleic acids.

nucleate (nū′klē-āt) [L. *nucleatus*, having a kernel]. 1. Having a nucleus. 2. To form a

nucleus. 3. A salt or ester of nucleic acid.

nucleic acid. A group of high-molecular-weight substances found in cells of all living things. They have a complex chemical structure, being formed of sugars (pentoses), phosphoric acid, and nitrogen bases (purines and pyrimidines). Most important are deoxyribonucleic acid, q.v., and ribonucleic acid, q.v.

nucleiform (nū′klē-ĭ-form) [L. *nucleus*, kernel, + *forma*, shape]. Shaped like a nucleus.

nuclein (nū′klē-ĭn) [L. *nucleus*, a kernel]. A normal chemical constituent of a cell nucleus; a colorless, shapeless substance obtained by hydrolysis of nucleoproteins to form nucleic acid and proteins.

nuclein bases. Bases formed from decomposition of nuclein.
    Ex.: adenine, guanine, xanthine, hypoxanthine.

nucleo- [L. *nucleus*, kernal]. Pert. to a nucleus.

nucleocapsid (nū″klē-ō-kăp′sĭd). In a virus, the protein coat and the viral nucleic acid.

nucleochylema (nū″klē-ō-kī-lē′mă). [″ + Gr. *chylos*, juice]. Karyolymph or nuclear sap.

nucleochyme (nū′klē-ō-kīm) [″ + Gr. *chymos*, juice]. Karyolymph.

nucleofugal (nū-klē-ŏf′ū-găl) [″ + *fugere*, to flee]. Directed or moving away from a nucleus in the cell.

nucleohistone (nū″klē-ō-hĭs′tŏn, -tōn) [″ + Gr. *histos*, tissue]. A substance composed of nuclein and histone, found in sperm of various animals.

nucleoid (nū′klē-oyd) [″ + Gr. *eidos*, form, shape]. Resembling a nucleus.

nucleolar (nū-klē′ō-lăr) [L. *nucleolus*, a little kernel]. Pert. to a nucleolus.

nucleoli (nū-klē′ō-lī). Pl. of nucleolus.

nucleoliform (nū-klē-ō′lĭ-form) [″ + *forma*, shape]. Like a nucleolus.

nucleoloid (nū′klē-ō-loyd). Similar to a nucleus.

nucleolonema (nū″klē-ō″lō-nē′mă) [″ + Gr. *nema*, thread]. A fine network in the nucleolus of a cell.

nucleolus (nū-klē′ō-lŭs) [L., little kernel] (pl. *nucleoli*). A spherical body made up of dense fibers and granules within the cell nucleus.

nucleomicrosome (nū″klē-ō-mī′krō-sōm) [L. *nucleus*, kernel, + Gr. *mikros*, tiny, + *soma*, body]. Any one of the minute granules that make up nuclear fibers.

nucleons (nū′klē-ŏnz). Collective name of the particles that make up the nucleus of an atom.

nucleopetal (nū-klē-ŏp′ĕ-tăl) [L. *nucleus*, kernel, + *petere*, to seek]. Seeking or moving toward the nucleus.

nucleophilic (nū″klē-ō-fīl′ĭk) [″ + Gr. *philein*, to love]. Having an attraction to nuclei.

nucleoplasm (nū′klē-ō-plăzm″) [″ + LL. *plasma*, form, mold]. The protoplasm of a cell nucleus.

nucleoplasmic. Pert. to nucleoplasm.

nucleoplasmic index. The ratio of nuclear volume to cytoplasmic volume, expressed thus:

$$NP = \frac{\text{vol. of nucleus}}{\text{vol. of cell} - \text{vol. of nucleus}}$$

nucleoprotein (nū″klē-ō-prō′tē-ĭn) [″ + Gr. *protos*, first]. The combination of one of the proteins with nucleic acid to form a conjugated protein found in cell nuclei.

nucleoreticulum (nū″klē-ō-rē-tĭk′ū-lŭm) [″ + *reticulum*, network]. Any mesh framework in a nucleus.

nucleosidase (nū″klē-ō-sī′dās). Enzyme that catalyzes the hydrolysis of nucleosides.

nucleoside. A glycoside formed by the union of a purine or pyrimidine base with a sugar (pentose).

nucleospindle (nū″klē-ō-spĭn′d′l). Spindle-shaped body occurring in karyokinesis, q.v.

nucleotidase (nū″klē-ŏt′ĭ-dās). Enzyme (nucleophosphatase) that splits phosphoric acid from nucleotides leaving a nucleoside.

5′-nucleotidase. Enzyme present in serum. Its serum level is increased in carcinoma of the pancreas when there is common bile duct obstruction or metastasis to the liver.

nucleotide (nū′klē-ō-tīd) [L. *nucleus*, kernel]. A compound formed of phosphoric acid, a sugar, and a base (purine or pyrimidine), all of which constitute the structural unit of nucleic acid. SYN: *mononucleotide*.

nucleotidyl (nū″klē-ō-tīd′ĭl). The residue of a nucleotide.

nucleotidyltransferase (nū″klē-ō-tīd″ĭl-trăns′fĕr-ās). Enzyme that transfers nucleotidyls from nucleosides into dimer or polymer forms.

nucleotoxin [″ + Gr. *toxikon*, poison]. A toxin acting upon or produced by cell nuclei.

nucleus (nū′klē-ŭs) [L., kernel] (pl. *nuclei*). 1. A central point about which matter is gathered, as in a calculus. 2. The vital body in the protoplasm of a cell; the essential agent in growth, metabolism, reproduction, and transmission of characteristics of a cell. SEE: *cell*. 3. [NA] Group of nerve cells or mass of gray matter in the central nervous system, esp. the brain. 4. In chemistry, a heavy central atomic particle in which most of the mass and total positive electric charge are concentrated.

n. abducens. A gray nucleus, the origin of the abducens nerve, on the floor of the 4th ventricle, behind the trigeminal nucleus.

n., ambiguous. Nucleus of the glossopharyngeal and vagus nerves in medulla oblongata. Lies in lateral half of reticular formation.

n., amygdaloid. Nucleus projecting into inferior cornua of lateral ventricle. Constitutes part of basal ganglia.

n., angular. The superior vestibular nucleus. SYN: *n., Bechterew's.* SEE: *n., vestibular.*

n., anterior, of thalamus. Nucleus located in rostral part of thalamus. Receives fibers of mamillothalamic tract.

n., arcuate. 1. Nucleus located on basal aspect of pyramid of medulla. 2. The posteromedial ventral nucleus of the thalamus.

n., atomic. The central part of an atom, which contains protons and electrons.

n., auditory. Nest of nerve cells where auditory nerves arise.

n., Bechterew's, Bekhterev's. N., angular.

n., caudate. A comma-shaped mass of gray matter forming part of the corpus striatum. Constitutes part of the basal ganglia. SYN: *n., intraventricular.*

n., central, of thalamus. A group of nuclei in middle part of thalamus. SYN: *n., centromedian.*

n., centromedian. N., central, of thalamus.

n., cerebellar. One of the nuclei of the cerebellum.

n., cochlear, dorsal. Nucleus in medulla oblongata lying dorsal to restiform body. Receives fibers of cochlear nerve.

n., cochlear, ventral. Nucleus in medulla oblongata lying anterior and lateral to restiform body. Receives fibers from cochlear nerve.

n., cornucommissural, posterior. A column of cells that extends the entire length of the spinal cord and lies along the medial border of the posterior column near the posterior gray commissure.

n., cuneate. Nucleus in inferior portion of medulla oblongata in which fibers of the fasciculus cuneatus terminate. SYN: *n. of Burdach.*

n., Deiters′. Lateral vestibular nucleus. SEE: *n., vestibular.*

n., dentate. Large convoluted mass of gray matter in lateral portion of cerebellum. It is folded so as to enclose some of the central white matter. Gives rise to fibers of the superior cerebellar peduncle.

n., diploid. Nucleus containing the normal double complement of chromosomes.

n., dorsal, of spinal cord. A column of gray matter lying at base of dorsal horn of the gray matter and extending from 7th cervical to 3rd lumbar segments. Cells give rise to fibers of the dorsal spinocerebellar tract. SYN: *Clarke's column.*

n., dorsal motor, of vagus. A column of cells in medulla oblongata lying lateral to hypoglossal nucleus. Its cells give rise to most of the efferent fibers of vagus nerve.

n., dorsal sensory, of vagus. Nucleus lying lateral to dorsal motor nucleus of vagus. Receives fibers of solitary tract.

n., ectoblastic. Nucleus in cells of the epiblast.

n., Edinger-Westphal. Nucleus of midbrain located dorsomedially to oculomotor nucleus. Gives rise to visceral efferent fibers terminating in ciliary ganglion, axons from which the ciliary muscle and the sphincter iridis are innervated.

n., emboliform. Nucleus of cerebellum lying between dentate and globose nuclei. Receives axons of Purkinje cells and sends efferent fibers into brachium conjunctivum.

n., facial motor. Nucleus in medulla oblongata in floor of 4th ventricle giving rise to efferent fibers of facial nerve.

n., fastigial. Nucleus in medullary portion of cerebellum. Receives afferent fibers from vestibular nerve and superior vestibular nucleus. Afferent fibers form fasciculus uncinatus and fastigiobulbar tract.

n., fertilization. Nucleus produced by the joining of the male and female nuclei in fertilization of the ovum.

n., free. Nucleus that is no longer surrounded by the other cellular elements.

n. funiculi gracilis. Elongated mass of gray matter in dorsal pyramid of medulla oblongata.

n., germinal. Nucleus resulting from union of male and female pronuclei.

n., globose. Nucleus of the cerebellum located medial to the emboliform nucleus.

n., gonad. Micronucleus (def. 1).

n. gracilis. [NA] Nucleus in medulla oblongata in which fibers of the fasciculus gracilis terminate.

n., habenular. Nucleus of the diencephalon located in the habenular trigone. Functions as an olfactory correlation center.

n., haploid. Cell nucleus with half the normal number of chromosomes. This is true for germ cells, i.e., ova or sperm, following the normal reduction divisions in gametogenesis.

n., hypoglossal. An elongated mass of gray matter in the medulla oblongata in floor of 4th ventricle. Gives rise to motor fibers of hypoglossal nerve.

n., hypothalamic. One of the nuclei occurring in four groups found in the hypothalamus. Includes the following nuclei: dorsomedial, intercalatus, lateral, mamillary (lateral and medial), paraventricular, posterior, supraoptic, tuberal, ventromedial. Cells of these nuclei, esp. the supraoptic and paraventricular, in addition to serving a neural function, are secretory and produce the vasopressor oxytocin as well as antidiuretic principles of the hypophysis. These hormones pass through efferent fibers of the infundibular stalk to the pars nervosa (posterior lobe) of the hypophysis, where they are stored and liberated.

n., interpeduncular. Nucleus of the midbrain near superior border of pons. Receives fibers of the habenulopeduncular tract.

n., interstitial, of Cajal. Nucleus in superior portion of midbrain. Receives fibers from vestibular nuclei, basal ganglia, and occipital regions of cerebral cortex. Efferent fibers pass to ipsilateral and contralateral fasciculi and interstitiospinal tracts.

n., intraventricular. N., caudate.

n., lenticular. One of the nuclei forming part of the basal ganglia of the cerebrum. Consists of globus pallidus and putamen. With the caudate nucleus, it forms the corpus striatum.

n. lentis. [NA] The core or inner dense section of the crystalline lens.

n., masticatory. The motor nucleus of the trigeminal nerve.

n., mesencephalic tract. The only site of primary sensory neurons within the central nervous system for proprioceptive impulses from the trigeminal nerve.

n., mother. Nucleus that divides into two or more parts to form daughter nuclei.

n., motor. Nucleus giving rise to motor fibers of a nerve.

n., motor, of trigeminal nerve. Nucleus in medulla oblongata near first margin of superior part of 4th ventricle. Gives rise to motor fibers of trigeminal nerve, which innervates the muscles of mastication, tensor tympani, tensor palatini, and the anterior digastric muscle. Also called masticatory nucleus.

n., oculomotor. Nucleus in central gray matter of midbrain lying below rostral end of cerebral aqueduct.

n. of Burdach. N., cuneate.

n. of origin. Any collection of nerve cells giving rise to fibers of a nerve or nerve tract.

n. of termination. Clusters of cells in the brain and medulla in which fibers of a nerve or nerve tract terminate.

n., olivary, inferior. A large convoluted mass of cells lying in ventral part of medulla oblongata and forming part of the reticular system. Gives rise to fibers of the olivocerebellar tract.

n., olivary, superior. A small nucleus located in mid-lateral tegmental region of pons. Receives fibers from ventral cochlear nucleus.

n., paraventricular. Nucleus of hypothalamus lying in supraoptic portion. Its axons with those of supraoptic nucleus form supraopticohypophyseal tract. SEE: *n., hypothalamic.*

n., pontine. One of several groups of nerve cells located in the pons. Receives afferent fibers from cerebral cortex; efferent fibers pass through brachium pontis to cerebellum.

n., principal trigeminal sensory. The site of sensory neurons of the trigeminal nerve associated with discriminatory touch. It is located in the pons. Also called superior sensory nucleus of trigeminal nerve.

n. pulposus. [NA] The center cushioning gelatinous mass lying within an intervertebral disk; remains of the notochord.

n., pyramidal. Band of gray matter near olivary nucleus in the medulla.

n., red. Large oval pigmented mass in upper portion of midbrain and extending upward into subthalamus. Receives fibers from cerebral cortex and cerebellum; efferent fibers give rise to rubrospinal tracts.

n., reproductive. Micronucleus (def. 2).

n., reticular. A column of neurons in spinal cord, brain stem, and thalamus affecting local reflex activity, muscle tone, and wakefulness.

n. ruber. [NA] Mass of red-colored gray matter in crus cerebri located in the anterior portion of the tegmentum and extending into the posterior portion of the subthalamic region.

n., salivatory, inferior. Nucleus located in pons near level of dorsal motor nucleus of the vagus. Gives rise to preganglionic parasympathetic fibers that pass to otic ganglion via hypoglossal nerve. Impulses regulate secretion of parotid gland.

n., salivatory, superior. An ill-defined nucleus in pons lying dorsomedial to facial nucleus. Gives rise to preganglionic parasympathetic fibers passing through chorda tympani and lingual nerve to submaxillary ganglion. Impulses regulate secretion of submaxillary and sublingual glands.

n., segmentation. Nucleus of zygote formed by fusion of male and female pronuclei.

n., sensory. Nucleus of termination, q.v., of afferent fibers of a peripheral nerve.

n., sensory, of trigeminal nerve. A group of nuclei in pons and medulla oblongata consisting of the spinal nucleus, which extends inferiorly into the spinal cord; the main nucleus, which lies dorsal and lateral to the motor nucleus; and the mesencephalic nucleus, which lies in the lateral wall

of the 4th ventricle.

n., sperm. The head of the sperm.

n., subthalamic. N., hypothalamic.

n., supraoptic. Nucleus of the hypothalamus lying above rostral ends of the optic tracts and lateral to the optic chiasma. SEE: *n., hypothalamic.*

n., thalamic. Any of the nuclei of the thalamus. Include a large number belonging to the following groups: anterior, intralaminar, lateral, and medial thalamic nuclei.

n., thoracic. A column of large neurons in the posterior gray column of the spinal cord. These cells give rise to the dorsal spinocerebellar tract on the same side.

n., trigeminal spinal. The site of sensory neurons of the trigeminal nerve associated with pain, temperature, and light touch. It is located in the pons and upper spinal tract. Also called inferior sensory nucleus of trigeminal nerve.

n., vesicular. Nucleus having deeply staining membrane and a pale center.

n., vestibular. One of four nuclei in medulla oblongata in which fibers of the vestibular nerve terminate. Includes medial (Schwalbe's), superior (Bechterew's), lateral (Deiters'), and inferior nuclei.

n., vitelline. Nucleus formed by union of male and female pronuclei within the vitellus. SYN: *n., yolk.*

n., white. Central white substance of corpus dentatum or olive.

n., yolk. A part of the cytoplasm of an ovum in which the initial process of accumulation of food supplies is probably located. SYN: *n., vitelline.*

nuclide (nū'klīd). Any atomic nucleus identified by its atomic number, mass, and energy state.

nude [L. *nudus,* naked]. 1. Bare; naked; unclothed. 2. An unclothed body.

nude mice. Mice that are devoid of hair. These T lymphocyte deficient animals are used in immunological investigations.

nudism. 1. In psychiatry, morbid desire to remove clothing. 2. The cult or practice of living in a nude condition.

nudo- [L. *nudus*]. Combining form denoting uncovered, naked.

nudomania (nū"dō-mā'nē-ă) [" + Gr. *mania,* madness]. Abnormal desire to be nude.

nudophobia (nū"dō-fō'bē-ă) [" + Gr. *phobos,* fear]. Abnormal fear of being unclothed. SEE: *gymnophobia.*

Nuel's space (nū'ĕlz) [Jean-Pierre Nuel, Belg. physician, 1847–1920]. Space in organ of Corti between outer pillar and outer phalangeal cells (Deiters' cells).

NUG. *necrotizing ulcerative gingivitis.*

Nuhn's glands (noonz) [Anton Nuhn, Ger.

anatomist, 1814–1889]. Anterior lingual glands on each side of frenum of the tongue. SYN: *Blandin's glands.*

null cell. A white blood cell that is a lymphocyte but does not have the characteristics of either a T cell or a B cell.

null hypothesis. The assumption or hypothesis that the observed difference between two groups of patients studied is accidental or due to chance and is not due to one of the groups having received a specific treatment.

nulligravida. A woman who never conceived a child.

nullipara (nŭl-ĭp'ă-ră) [L. *nullus,* none, + *parere,* to bear]. A woman who has never produced a viable offspring.

nulliparity (nŭl"ĭ-păr'ĭ-tē). Condition of not having given birth to a child.

nulliparous (nŭl-lĭp'ăr-ŭs). Never having borne a child.

nullisomatic (nŭl"ĭ-sō-măt'ĭk) [" + Gr. *soma,* body]. Lacking one pair of chromosomes.

numb (nŭm). 1. Insensible; lacking in feeling as from cold. 2. Deadened or lacking in power to move, as numb with cold.

number [L. *numerus,* number]. 1. A total of units. 2. A symbol graphically representing an arithmetical sum.
RS: mean; median; modality; mode; numeral.

    n., atomic. The numeral indicating the number of negatively charged electrons in an uncharged atom, or the number of protons in the nucleus. This number determines the position of elements in the periodic table of elements.

    n., Avogadro's. Number of molecules, 6.0221367×10^{23}, in one gram-molecular weight of a compound.

    n., hardness. SEE: *hardness number.*

    n., mass. The mass of the atom of a specific isotope relative to the mass of hydrogen. In general, this number is equal to the total of the protons and electrons in the atomic nucleus of that specific isotope.

numbness. Lack of sensation in a part, esp. from cold. SEE: *narcohypnia; obdormition.*

numeral (nū'mĕr-ăl) [L. *numerus,* number]. 1. Denoting or pert. to a number. 2. A conventional symbol expressing a number.

nummiform (nŭm'mĭ-form) [L. *nummus,* a coin, + *forma,* shape]. 1. Coin-shaped, said of some mucous sputum. 2. Arranged like a stack of coins.

nummular (nŭm'ū-lăr) [L. *nummus,* coin]. 1. Coin-shaped. 2. Stacked like coins, as in a rouleau, q.v., of red blood cells.

nummulation (nŭm-ū-lā'shŭn). The formation of a coin-shaped mass.

Numorphan. Trade name for oxymorphone hydrochloride, USP.

nunnation (nŭn-ā'shŭn) [Heb. *nun,* letter N]. Frequent and abnormal use of the "n" sound.

Nuremberg Code. Set of principles established after World War II to protect the rights of research participants, i.e., subjects.

nurse [L. *nutrix,* nurse]. 1. An individual who provides health care. The extent of participation varies from simple patient-care tasks to the most expert professional techniques necessary in acute life-threatening situations. The ability of a nurse to function in making self-directed judgments and to act independently will depend on his or her professional background, motivation, and opportunity for professional development. The health care team includes the technical nurse, who is technique-oriented, deals with commonly recurring nursing problems, and knows standardized procedures and medically delegated techniques. Also included in the team is the professional nurse, who is prepared to assume responsibility for the care of individuals and groups through a colleague relationship with a physician. The roles of nurses constantly change in response to the growth of biomedical knowledge, changes in patterns of demand for health services, and the evolution of professional relationships among nurses, physicians, and other health care professionals. 2. To feed an infant at the breast. 3. To perform the duties of caring for an invalid. 4. To care for a young child.

    n., charge. N., head.

    n., clinical (nurse) specialist. Nurse with particular competence in certain areas such as intensive care, cardiology, oncology, obstetrics, or psychiatry. A clinical nurse specialist holds a master's degree in nursing, preferably with emphasis in clinical nursing.

    n., community health. Nurse who combines principles and practices of nursing and public health to provide care to people in a community rather than an institution.

    n., dental. A dental auxiliary trained to provide oral hygiene instruction and dental health care to school children. Formerly, the term applied to dental hygienists, but now it refers to persons trained according to a program developed in New Zealand.

    n., epidemiologist. Registered nurse with special training and certification in the prevention of hospital-acquired infections in patients. SEE: *n., infection control.*

    n., flight. Nurse who cares for patients being transported in an aircraft.

    n., general duty. Nurse not specializing in a particular field but available for any duty.

    n., graduate. Nurse who is a graduate of

an accredited school of nursing.

n., head. Nurse in charge of a group of patients, usually a unit within an institution, and the nursing staff required to care for the patients.

n., health. A community or visiting nurse whose duty is to give information on hygiene and prevention of disease. SEE: *n., community health.*

n., infection control. Registered nurse employed by an agency to monitor the rate and causes of nosocomial infections and to promote measures to prevent such infections.

n., licensed practical. Nurse who has graduated from a school of practical nursing and has passed the practical nursing state board examination.

n., practical. Nurse who is licensed to administer care, usually working under direction of a licensed physician or a registered nurse. May be a graduate of an accredited school for practical nursing.

n., prescribing. SEE: *prescribing nurse.*

n., private duty. Nurse who on a fee-for-service basis cares for one or two patients, usually in an institution. The nurse is not a staff member of the institution.

n.'s, probationer. Student nurses who are on probation until the instructors have had sufficient time to determine their suitability for the nursing profession.

n., public health. N., community health.

n., registered. Nurse who has graduated from a state-approved school of nursing, has passed the professional nursing state board examination, and has been granted a license to practice within a given state.

n., school. Nurse who is responsible for the health of children, adolescents, and young adults in school.

n., scrub. Nurse who assists at surgery primarily by passing instruments and supplies to the surgeon(s).

n., special. N., private duty.

n., specialist. Clinical nurse specialist.

n., student. An individual enrolled in a school of nursing.

n., trained. N., graduate.

n., visiting. N., community health.

n., wet. A woman who breast-feeds a child that is not her own.

nurse anesthetist. A registered nurse who administers anesthesia to patients in the operating room and delivery room. The knowledge and skill required to provide this service are attained through an organized program of study recognized by the American Association of Nurse Anesthetists.

nurse clinician. A registered nurse with preparation in a specialized educational program. The nurse clinician is capable of

working independently in solving patient-care problems and is able to teach and work successfully with others on the medical care team. Term was first used by Frances Reiter, R.N., M.A., Dean, Graduate School of Nursing, New York Medical College.

nurse-midwife. A registered nurse who manages the care of mothers and babies throughout the maternity cycle including the postpartum period. The knowledge and skill required to provide this service are attained through an organized program of study recognized by the American College of Nurse-Midwives.

nurse practitioner. A registered nurse with advanced preparation in the care of particular types of patients with whom the emphasis is on primary care. This nurse includes medical skills in his or her practice of nursing.

nursery. A hospital department in which the newborn are cared for.

n., day. A nursery in which children, usually of preschool age, are cared for during the day. SYN: *day care center.*

nurse's aide. An individual who assists nurses by performing the patient-care procedures that do not require special technical training, such as feeding and bathing patients, and by taking temperature, pulse, and respiration.

nursing. 1. The profession of practicing the art and science of being a nurse. The American Nurses' Association defines nursing as "the diagnosis and treatment of human responses to actual or potential health problems." 2. Breast feeding. 3. Lactation.

nursing assessment. The initial step in the nursing process, q.v. It consists of obtaining a careful and complete history from the patient. If this cannot be done because the mental or physical condition of the patient makes communication impossible, the nursing history is obtained from those who have information about the patient and the reason(s) for his or her need of medical and nursing care. Obtaining an accurate and comprehensive history requires skill in communicating with individuals who are ill and who may feel that obtaining a history of their illness is not what they need at that time. The skilled nurse will be able to obtain the essential information despite resistance. Next in the assessment is the physical examination of the patient in order to determine how the disease has altered physical and mental status. To do this requires that the nurse be capable of performing visual and tactile inspection, palpation, percussion, and auscultation and have knowledge of what represents deviation from the norm and how disease and trauma alter the physical and mental condition of a patient. After these two steps have been completed, the nurse will be able to establish a nursing diagnosis.

It is important to realize the difference between the nursing diagnosis and the medical diagnosis. Nursing diagnosis is the statement of the patient's mental and physical condition that can be ameliorated or resolved by appropriate action(s) of the nurse or nursing team. SEE: *evaluation; nursing intervention; nursing process; planning; problem-oriented medical record.*

nursing audit. A procedure to evaluate the quality of nursing care provided for a patient. Established criteria for care are the yardstick for the evaluation of the care.

nursing diagnosis. Nurses, esp. those involved in patient care, are in virtually constant need to make decisions and diagnoses based on their clinical experience and judgment. In many instances, that process dictates a course of action for the nurse that is of vital importance to the patient. As the nursing profession evolves and develops, nursing diagnosis will be defined, and indeed specified, in accordance with the specialized training and experience of nurses, particularly for nurse practitioners and clinical nurse specialists.

nursing histories. The assessment stage of the nursing process that leads to development of a nursing care plan. Valuable information can be obtained from this history, and reactions to previous hospitalization can be recorded and utilized in managing the patient's care during the current stay. SEE: illus.

nursing home. An extended care facility for persons who need medical attention of the type and complexity not requiring hospitalization. Well-run and properly designed and staffed nursing homes will provide a fall- and restraint-free environment; careful attention to the nutritional needs of patients; facility for tube feeding; ability to manage urinary incontinence; prevention of decubitus ulcers; a competent plan for controlling infectious disease; recreational activity; and a pleasant, clean, mentally stimulating environment.

In 1990, it was estimated that 43% of all Americans who turn 65 will use a nursing home at leat once before they die. It is also estimated that by the year 2020 there will be 1.7 million Americans aged 65 who eventually will enter a nursing home.

nursing intervention. In the nursing process, q.v., the next step after planning, q.v. This step involves all aspects of actual caring for the patient and requires full knowledge of the assessment and planning stages of the nursing process. The goals of nursing intervention will have been stated in the planning step of the nursing process. Included in this step are patient care in the areas of hygiene, mental and physical comfort, assistance in feeding and elimination; controlling the physical aspects of the patient's environment; and instructing the patient about the factors important to his or her care and what actions to take to facilitate recovery. After the patient's acute and immediate needs are met, he or she should be instructed concerning actions that could be taken to help prevent a recurrence of the condition. SEE: *evaluation; nursing assessment; nursing process; planning; problem-oriented medical record.*

nursing process. An orderly, logical approach to administering nursing care so that the patient's needs for such care are met comprehensively and effectively. The goal of health care is to provide total, comprehensive care of patients. Nursing has always been dedicated to this concept and, from the holistic viewpoint, has formalized the scientific processes that contribute to the prevention of illness as well as restoration and maintenance of health. In so doing, the traditional approaches used in problem-solving have been utilized. Thus, the nurse will need skills in the following five areas in order to provide comprehensive care of patients: (1) *Assessment:* Systemic collection of all data and information relevant to the patients, their problems, and needs. (2) *Problem identification:* Interpretation of the information obtained during assessment. (3) *Planning:* Utilization of skills to choose the optimum course of action in order to solve the problem. (4) *Implementation:* The process of putting the plan into action. (5) *Evaluation:* The ongoing process of assessing the effectiveness of the plan and altering it as the need arises. SEE: *evaluation; nursing assessment; nursing intervention; planning; problem-oriented medical record.*

nursing theorist. An individual who develops theories regarding the purpose, meaning, structure, and functions of the profession and discipline of nursing. Nursing theories explore, describe, and analyze the epistemological origins of nursing knowledge.

nutation (nū-tā'shŭn) [L. *nutare,* to nod]. Nodding, as of the head. SEE: *nodding.* 2. A complex movement of the sacrum.

nutgall (nŭt'gawl). A growth on certain oak trees. It is produced by insect eggs and larvae in the twigs of the tree. Gallic and tannic acids are obtained from these growths.

Nutracort. Trade name for hydrocortisone,

NURSING ASSESSMENT TOOL (Medical/Surgical)

This is a suggested guide/tool for development by an individual/institution to create a data base reflecting Diagnostic Divisions of Nursing Diagnoses. Although the divisions are alphabetized for ease of presentation, they can be prioritized or rearranged to meet individual needs.

Name: _____
Age: _____ DOB: _____ Sex: _____ Race: _____
Admission date: _____ Time: _____ From: _____
Source of information: _____ Reliability (1–4): _____
Family member/Significant other: _____

ACTIVITY/REST
Reports (Subjective)

Occupation: _____ Usual activities/Hobbies: _____
Leisure time activities: _____
Complaints of boredom: _____
Limitations imposed by condition: _____

Sleep: Hours: _____ Naps: _____ Aids: _____
    Insomnia: _____ Related to: _____
    Rested upon awakening: _____

Exhibits (Objective)

Observed response to activity: Cardiovascular: _____
                  Respiratory: _____
Mental status (i.e., withdrawn/lethargic): _____
Neuromuscular assessment:
    Muscle mass/tone: _____
    Posture: _____ Tremors: _____
    ROM: _____ Strength: _____
    Deformity: _____ Other: _____

CIRCULATION
Reports (Subjective)

History of: Hypertension: _____ Heart trouble: _____
          Rheumatic fever: _____ Ankle/leg edema: _____
          Phlebitis: _____ Slow healing: _____
          Claudication: _____ Other: _____
Extremities: Numbness: _____ Tingling: _____
Cough/hemoptysis: _____
Change in frequency/amount of urine: _____

Exhibits (Objective)

BP: R: Lying: _____ Sitting: _____ Standing: _____
    L: Lying: _____ Sitting: _____ Standing: _____
    Pulse pressure: _____ Auscultatory gap: _____
Pulse (palpation): Carotid: _____ Temporal: _____
                Jugular: _____ Radial: _____
                Femoral: _____ Popliteal: _____
                Post Tibial: _____ Dorsalis pedis: _____
Cardiac (palpation): PMI: _____
    Thrill: _____ Heaves: _____
Heart sounds: Rate: _____ Rhythm: _____ Quality: _____
    Friction rub: _____ Murmur: _____

Adapted from: Nursing Care Plans, Guidelines for Planning Patient Care, Ed.2, Marilynn E. Doenges, Mary Frances Moorehouse, Alice C. Geissler, FA Davis Pub Co Phila.

NURSING ASSESSMENT TOOL (Medical/Surgical) — continued

Breath sounds: _____
Vascular bruit: (specify): _____
Jugular vein distention: _____
Extremities: Temperature: _____ Color: _____
    Capillary refill: _____
    Homan's sign: _____ Varicosities: _____
    Nails (describe abnormalities): _____
    Distribution/quality of hair: _____
Color/cyanosis: Overall: _____ Mucous membranes: _____ Lips: _____
    Nail beds: _____ Conjunctiva: _____ Sclera: _____

EGO INTEGRITY

Reports (Subjective)

Report of stress factors: _____
Ways of handling stress: _____
Financial concerns: _____
Relationship status: _____
Cultural factors: _____
Religion: _____ Practicing: _____
Lifestyle: _____ Recent changes: _____
Feelings of: Helplessness: _____ Hopelessness: _____
    Powerlessness: _____

Exhibits (Objective)

Emotional status (check those that apply):
    Calm: _____ Anxious: _____ Angry: _____
    Withdrawn: _____ Fearful: _____ Irritable: _____
    Restive: _____ Euphoric: _____ Other (specify): ___
Observed physiologic response(s): _____

ELIMINATION

Reports (Subjective)

Usual bowel pattern: _____ Laxative use: _____
Character of stool: _____ Last BM: _____
History of bleeding: _____ Hemorrhoids: _____
Constipation: _____ Diarrhea: _____
Usual voiding pattern: _____ Incontinence: _____ When: _____
    Urgency: _____ Frequency: _____ Retention: _____
Character of urine: _____
Pain/burning/difficulty voiding: _____
History of kidney/bladder disease: _____

Exhibits (Objective)

Abdomen: Tender: _____ Soft/Firm: _____
    Palpable mass: _____ Size/girth: _____
    Bowel sounds: _____
Hemorrhoids (per rectal exam): Internal: _____ External: _____
Bladder palpable: _____ Overflow voiding: _____

FOOD/FLUID

Reports (Subjective)

Usual diet (type): _____ No. meals daily: _____
Last meal/intake: _____ Dietary pattern: _____
Loss of appetite: _____ Nausea/vomiting: _____
Heartburn/indigestion: _____ Related to: _____ Relieved by: _____
Allergy/Food intolerance: _____
Mastication/swallowing problems: _____
    Dentures: Upper: _____ Lower: _____

NURSING ASSESSMENT TOOL (Medical/Surgical) — continued

Usual weight: _____ Changes in weight: _____
Use of diuretics: _____

Exhibits (Objective)

Current weight: _____ Height: _____ Body build: _____
Skin turgor: _____ Mucous membranes moist/dry: _____
Hernia/masses: _____
Edema: General: _____ Dependent: _____
      Periorbital: _____ Ascites: _____
Jugular vein distention: _____
Thyroid enlarged: _____ Halitosis: _____
Condition of teeth/gums: _____
Appearance of tongue: _____
    Mucous membranes: _____
Bowel sounds (previously assessed): _____
Breath sounds (previously assessed): _____
Urine S/A or Chemstix: _____

HYGIENE

Reports (Subjective)

Activities of daily living: Independent: _____
    Dependent (specify): Mobility: _____ Feeding: _____
                    Hygiene: _____ Dressing: _____
                    Toileting: _____ Other: _____
    Equipment/prosthetic devices required: _____
    Assistance provided by: _____
    Preferred time of bath: _____ AM _____ PM

Exhibits (Objective)

General appearance: _____
Manner of dress: _____ Personal habits: _____
Body odor: _____ Condition of scalp: _____
Presence of vermin: _____

NEUROSENSORY

Reports (Subjective)

Fainting spells/dizziness: _____
Headaches: Location: _____ Frequency: _____
Tingling/Numbness/Weakness (location): _____
Stroke (residual effects): _____
Seizures: _____ Aura: _____ How controlled: _____
Eyes: Vision loss: R: _____ L: _____
    Glaucoma: _____ Cataract: _____
Ears: Hearing loss: R: _____ L: _____
Nose: Epistaxis: _____ Sense of smell: _____

Exhibits (Objective)

Mental status:
    Oriented/disoriented: Time: _____
                      Place: _____
                      Person: _____
    Alert: _____ Drowsy: _____ Lethargic: _____
    Stuporous: _____ Comatose: _____ Other: _____
    Cooperative: _____ Combative: _____ Delusions: _____
    Hallucinations: _____ Affect (describe): _____
Memory: Recent: _____ Remote: _____
Speech pattern: _____ Content: _____
    Word choice: _____ Congruence: _____
Glasses: _____ Contacts: _____ Hearing Aids: _____
Pupil size/reaction: R: _____ L: _____

NURSING ASSESSMENT TOOL (Medical/Surgical) — continued

Facial droop: _____ Swallowing: _____
Handgrip/release: R: _____ L: _____ Posturing: _____
Deep tendon reflexes: _____ Paralysis: _____

PAIN/COMFORT
Reports (Subjective)

Location: _____ Intensity (1–10): _____ Frequency: _____
Quality: _____ Duration: _____ Radiation: _____
Precipitating factors: _____
How relieved: _____

Exhibits (Objective)

Facial grimacing: _____ Guarding affected area: _____
Emotional response: _____ Narrowed focus: _____

RESPIRATION
Reports (Subjective)

Dyspnea (related to): _____
Cough/sputum: _____
History of Bronchitis: _____ Asthma: _____
    Tuberculosis: _____ Emphysema: _____
    Recurrent pneumonia: _____ Other: _____
    Exposure to noxious fumes: _____
Smoker: _____ Packs/day: _____ Number of years: _____
Use of respiratory aids: _____ Oxygen: _____

Exhibits (Objective)

Respiratory: Rate: _____ Depth: _____ Symmetry: _____
Use of accessory muscles: _____ Nasal flaring: _____
Fremitis: _____
Breath sounds: _____
Egophony: _____
Cyanosis: _____ Clubbing of fingers: _____
Sputum characteristics: _____
Mentation/restlessness: _____
Other: _____

SAFETY
Reports (Subjective)

Allergies/Sensitivity: _____ Reaction: _____
Previous alteration of immune system: _____ Cause: _____
History of sexually transmitted disease (date/type): _____
Blood transfusion: _____ When: _____
    Reaction (describe): _____
History of accidental injuries: _____
Fractures/dislocations: _____
Arthritis/Unstable joints: _____
Back problems: _____
Changes in moles: _____ Enlarged nodes: _____
Impaired: Vision: _____ Hearing: _____
Prosthesis: _____ Ambulatory devices: _____
Expressions of ideation of violence (self/others): _____

Exhibits (Objective)

Temperature: _____ Diaphoresis: _____
Skin integrity: _____
    Scars: _____ Rashes: _____
    Lacerations: _____ Ulcerations: _____
    Ecchymosis: _____ Blisters: _____

NURSING ASSESSMENT TOOL (Medical/Surgical) — continued

Burns (degree/percent): _____
Mark location of above on diagram:

General strength: _____ Muscle tone: _____
Gait: _____ ROM: _____
Paresthesia/Paralysis: _____

SEXUALITY

Sexual concerns: _____

Female

Reports (Subjective)

Age at menarche: _____ Length of cycle: _____ Duration: _____
Last menstrual period: _____ Menopause: _____
Vaginal discharge: _____ Bleeding between periods: _____
Practices breast self-exam: _____ Last PAP smear: _____
Method of birth control: _____

Exhibits (Objective)

Breast exam: _____
Vaginal warts/lesions: _____

Male

Reports (Subjective)

Penile discharge: _____ Prostate disorder: _____
Vasectomy: _____ Use of condoms: _____
Practices self-exam: Breast: _____ Testicles: _____
Last proctoscopic exam: _____ Last prostate exam: _____

Exhibits (Objective)

Exam: Breast: _____ Testicles: _____

SOCIAL INTERACTION

Reports (Subjective)

Marital status: _____ Years in relationship: _____
 Living with: _____
 Concerns/Stresses: _____
Extended family: _____
Other support person(s): _____
Role within family structure: _____
Report of problems related to illness/condition: _____

NURSING ASSESSMENT TOOL (Medical/Surgical) — continued

Coping behaviors: _____
Do others depend on you for assistance? _____
   How are they managing? _____
Frequency of social contacts (other than work): _____

Exhibits (Objective)

Speech: Clear: _____ Slurred: _____
   Unintelligible: _____ Aphasic: _____
   Unusual speech pattern/impairment: _____
   Laryngectomy: _____ Speech aids: _____
Verbal/nonverbal communication with family/SO(s): _____
_____
Family interaction (behavioral) pattern: _____

TEACHING/LEARNING

Reports (Subjective)

Dominant language (specify): _____
Education level: _____
Learning disabilities (specify): _____
Cognitive limitations (specify): _____
Health beliefs/practices: _____
Special health care practices: _____
Familial risk factors (indicate relationship):
   Diabetes: _____ Tuberculosis: _____
   Heart disease: _____ Strokes: _____
   High BP: _____ Epilepsy: _____
   Kidney disease: _____ Cancer: _____
   Mental illness: _____ Other (specify): _____
Prescribed medications (circle last dose):

Drug	Dose	Times	Takes regularly	Purpose

Nonprescription drugs: OTC: _____
   Street drugs: _____ Smokeless tobacco: _____
Use of alcohol (amount/frequency): _____
Admitting diagnosis (physician): _____
Reason for hospitalization (patient): _____
History of current complaint: _____
Patient expectations of this hospitalization: _____
Previous illnesses and/or hospitalizations/surgeries: _____
_____
Evidence of failure to improve: _____
Last complete physical exam: _____ By: _____

Discharge Plan Considerations

Date data obtained: _____
1. Anticipated date of discharge: _____
2. Resources available: Persons: _____
   Financial: _____
3. Do you anticipate changes in your living situation after discharge? ____
4. If Yes: Areas that may require alteration/assistance:
   Food preparation: _____ Shopping: _____
   Transportation: _____ Ambulation: _____
   Medication/IV therapy: _____ Treatments: _____
   Wound care: _____ Supplies: _____
   Self-care assistance (specify): _____
   Physical layout of home (specify): _____
   Homemaker assistance (specify): _____
   Living facility other than home (specify): _____

USP.

nutrient (nū'trē-ĕnt) [L. *nutriens*]. 1. Food or any substance that supplies the body with elements necessary for metabolism. 2. Nourishing; supplying nutriment.

Certain nutrients (carbohydrates, fats, proteins, and alcohol) provide energy; other nutrients (water, electrolytes, minerals, and vitamins) are essential to the metabolic process. Those containing carbon are organic food nutrients. Organic food nutrients may or may not contain nitrogen.

RS: calorie; carbohydrate; fat; food; mineral; nitrogen; protein; vitamin.

nutrilite (nū'trĭ-līt). Any essential nutrient, esp. ones that are required by bacteria in only trace quantities.

nutriment (nū'trĭ-mĕnt) [L. *nutrimentum*, nourishment]. That which nourishes; nutritious substance.

nutrition (nū-trĭ'shŭn) [L. *nutritio*, nourish]. All the processes involved in the taking in and utilization of food substances by which growth, repair, and maintenance of activities in the body as a whole or in any of its parts are accomplished. Includes ingestion, digestion, absorption, and metabolism (assimilation). Some nutrients are capable of being stored by the body in various forms and drawn upon when the food intake is not sufficient. An example of a nutrient that is not stored is vitamin C.

nutritional (nū-trĭsh'ŭn-ăl). Rel. to nutrition.

nutritional adequacy. The relationship between intake of nutrients and individual requirements.

nutritious (nū-trĭsh'ŭs) [L. *nutritius*]. Affording nutriment. SYN: *nutritive.*

nutritive (nū'trĭ-tĭv). Pert. to the process of assimilating food; having the property of nourishing.

nutritive enema. Enema containing easily assimilated foods to give sustenance to a patient unable to take nourishment in the usual way.

nutriture (nū'trĭ-tūr). The state of body nutrition.

nux vomica (nŭks vŏm'ĭ-kă). A poisonous seed from an East Indian tree, containing several alkaloids, the principal ones being brucine and strychnine, q.v.

nyctalbuminuria (nĭk"tăl-bū"mĭn-ū'rē-ă) [Gr. *nyx*, night, + L. *albus*, white, + Gr. *ouron*, urine]. A cyclic albuminuria occurring at night. SYN: *noctalbuminuria.*

nyctalgia (nĭk-tăl'jē-ă) [" + *algos*, pain]. Pain during the night.

nyctalopia (nĭk-tă-lō'pē-ă) [" + *alaos*, blind, + *ops*, eye]. 1. A condition in which the individual cannot see well in a faint light or at night. Occurs in retinitis pigmentosa and choroidoretinitis. Also may be due to vi-

tamin A deficiency. Smoking tobacco impairs ability to see at night. Hypoxia associated with being above sea level in an aircraft will also decrease night vision. SYN: *night blindness.* 2. Incorrectly used to indicate the condition of having better sight at night or in semidarkness than by day; night vision. SEE: *hemeralopia.*

nyctamblyopia (nĭk"tăm-blē-ō'pē-ă) [Gr. *nyx*, night, + *amblyopia*, poor sight]. Poor vision at night without visible eye changes.

nyctaphonia (nĭk-tă-fō'nē-ă) [" + *a*, not, + *phone*, voice]. Hysterical loss of voice during the night.

nycterine (nĭk'tĕr-īn) [Gr. *nykterinos*, by night]. 1. Taking place at night. SYN: *nocturnal.* 2. Obscure.

nycthemerus (nĭk-thĕm'ĕ-rŭs) [Gr. *nychthemeros*]. 1. Space of a day and a night. 2. Pert. to a night and day.

nycto-, nyct- (nĭk'tō) [Gr. *nyx*, night]. Combining form indicating night or darkness.

nyctohemeral (nĭk"tō-hĕm'ĕr-ăl). Rel. to both day and night.

nyctophilia (nĭk"tō-fĭl'ē-ă) [Gr. *nyx*, night, + *philein*, to love]. Abnormal preference for darkness or night. SYN: *scotophilia.*

nyctophobia (nĭk"tō-fō'bē-ă) [" + *phobos*, fear]. Abnormal dread of the night or of darkness. SYN: *scotophobia.*

nyctophonia (nĭk"tō-fō'nē-ă) [" + *phone*, voice]. Loss of voice only at night.

nyctotyphlosis (nĭk"tō-tĭf-lō'sĭs) [" + *typhlosis*, blindness]. Poor vision at night. SYN: *night blindness; nyctalopia.*

nycturia (nĭk-tū'rē-ă) [" + *ouron*, urine]. Nocturia, q.v.

Nydrazid. Trade name for isoniazid, USP.

nylidrin hydrochloride (nĭl'ĭ-drĭn). USP. A drug used to produce peripheral vasodilation. Trade name is Arlidin.

nymph (nĭmf) [Gr. *nymphe*, a maiden]. The immature stage of insect development in which wings and genitalia have not fully developed.

nympha [Gr. *nymphe*, a maiden] (pl. *nymphae*). One of the labia minora, q.v., the small folds of mucous membrane forming the inner lips of the vulva. So called from the nymphs or goddesses of the fountain. SYN: *labium minus pudendi.*

nymphectomy (nĭm-fĕk'tō-mē) [" + *ektome*, excision]. Excision of hypertrophied nymphae.

nymphitis (nĭm-fī'tĭs) [" + *itis*, inflammation]. Inflamed condition of the nymphae.

nympho- (nĭm'fō) [Gr. *nymphe*, a maiden]. A combining form indicating relationship to the labia minora.

nymphocaruncular sulcus (nĭm"fō-kăr-ŭn' kū-lăr sŭl'kŭs) [" + L. *caruncula*, little mass of flesh, + *sulcus*, a groove]. The depression between the caruncula of the hymen and the labium minus.

nymphohymenal sulcus (nĭm″fō-hī′mĕn-ăl sŭl′kŭs) [″ + *hymen*, membrane, + *sulcus*, a groove]. Trench between the labium minus and the hymen on either side.

nympholepsy (nĭm′fō-lĕp″sē) [″ + *lepsis*, a seizure]. 1. Frenzied ecstasy, usually erotic in nature. 2. Obsession for something that is unattainable.

nymphomania (nĭm″fō-mā′nē-ă) [″ + *mania*, madness]. Abnormally excessive sexual desire in a female. SYN: *furor femininus*. SEE: *satyriasis*.

nymphomaniac (nĭm″fō-mā′nē-ăk) [″ + *mania*, madness]. 1. Woman who is afflicted with excessive sexual desire. 2. Affected by excessive sexual desire.

nymphoncus (nĭm-fŏn′kŭs) [″ + *onkos*, a swelling]. Swelling or tumor of the nymphae.

nymphotomy (nĭm-fŏt′ō-mē) [″ + *tome*, incision]. 1. Removal of the nymphae. SYN: *nymphectomy*. 2. Incision into a nympha or clitoris.

nystagmic (nĭs-tăg′mĭk) [Gr. *nystagmos*, to nod]. Rel. to or suffering from condition of involuntary eyeball movements.

nystagmiform (nĭs-tăg′mĭ-form) [″ + L. *forma*, shape]. Like or resembling nystagmus. SYN: *nystagmoid*.

nystagmograph (nĭs-tăg′ĭ-grăf) [″ + *graphein*, to write]. Apparatus for recording the oscillations of the eyeball in nystagmus.

nystagmoid (nĭs-tăg′moyd) [″ + *eidos*, form, shape]. Similar to or resembling nystagmus.

nystagmus (nĭs-tăg′mŭs) [Gr. *nystagmos*, to nod]. Constant, involuntary, cyclical movement of the eyeball. Movement may be in any direction. SEE: *saccadic*.

    ETIOL: May be congenital and inapparent to the patient; seen in bilateral amblyopia; occupational, as in miners and train dispatchers; labyrinthine irritability; neurologic diseases.

    n., aural. Nystagmus due to disorder in the labyrinth of the ear. Eye movement is spasmodic.

    n., Cheyne's. Rhythmic nystagmus that resembles the rhythm of Cheyne-Stokes breathing, q.v.

    n., convergence. Slow abduction of eyes followed by rapid adduction. Usually accompanies other types of nystagmus.

    n., dissociated. Nystagmus in one eye that is not synchronized with that in the other eye.

    n., end-position. Nystagmus that occurs when eyes are turned to extreme positions.

May occur normally in debilitation or fatigue. May be due to pathology of the subcortical centers for conjugate gaze.

    n., fixation. Nystagmus that occurs only when the eyes gaze at an object.

    n., jerk. N., rhythmic.

    n., labyrinthine. Nystagmus due to disease of the labyrinthine vestibular apparatus.

    n., latent. Nystagmus that occurs only when one eye is covered.

    n., lateral. Horizontal movement of eyes from side to side.

    n., miner's. Nystagmus occurring in those who work in comparative darkness for long periods.

    n., opticokinetic. A rhythmic jerk nystagmus occurring while looking at constantly moving objects, such as telephone poles from a moving car or train.

    n., pendular. Nystagmus characterized by movement that is approximately equal in both directions. Usually seen in those who have congenital absence of central vision or who lost it prior to the age of two.

    n., postrotatory. A form of vestibular nystagmus which occurs when the body is rotated and then the rotation is stopped. If, while sitting upright in a chair that can be swiveled, the body is rapidly rotated to the right, the nystagmus during rotation has its slow component to the left. When the rotation stops, the slow component is to the right. Stimulation of the semicircular canals causes this type of nystagmus, and it is a normal reaction.

    n., retraction. Nystagmus associated with drawing of the eye backward into the orbit. SYN: *nystagmus retractorius*.

    n., rhythmic. Nystagmus in which the eyes move slowly in one direction and then are jerked back rapidly. SYN: *n., jerk*.

    n., rotatory. Nystagmus in which eyes rotate about the visual axis. Voluntary nystagmus, q.v.

    n., vertical. Up-and-down ocular movements.

    n., vestibular. Nystagmus either caused by disease of the vestibular apparatus of the ear or due to normal stimuli produced when the semicircular canals are tested by rotating the body. SEE: *n., postrotatory*.

    n., voluntary. A rare type of pendular nystagmus in persons who have learned to oscillate their eyes rapidly, usually by extreme convergence. It is an acquired art that has no clinical significance.

nystatin (nĭs′tă-tĭn). USP. An antifungal agent. Trade names are Mycostatin and O-V Statin.

nystaxis (nĭs-tăk′sĭs) [Gr.]. Nystagmus.

Nysten's law (nē-stănz′) [Pierre Hubert Nysten, Fr. pediatrician, 1774–1817]. Law stating that rigor mortis begins with muscles of mastication and progresses from the head down the body, affecting legs and feet last. SEE: *rigor mortis*.

nyxis (nĭk′sĭs) [Gr.]. Puncture or piercing. SYN: *paracentesis*.

NZB mouse [*New Zealand black mouse*]. A mouse bred for the genetic trait of spontaneously developing autoimmune hemolytic anemia.

O

O. 1. Chem. symb. for the element oxygen. 2. *octarius*, pint; *oculus*, eye. 3. Symb. for a particular blood type.

o-. *ortho-*, prefix commonly used in chemical terminology.

O₂. Symb. for the molecular formula for oxygen.

O₃. Chem. symb. for ozone.

O.A. *occiput anterior.*

OAF. *osteoclast activating factor.*

oakum (ō′kŭm) [AS. *acumba*, tow]. Loose fiber obtained from old hemp ropes, formerly used as a surgical dressing.

oarialgia (ō″ār-ē-ăl′jē-ă) [Gr. *oarion*, little egg, + *algos*, pain]. Ovarian pain. SYN: *oophoralgia; ovaralgia.*

oario-, oari- [Gr. *oarion*, little egg]. Prefix pert. to the ovary. SEE: words beginning with *ovario-* or *oophor-*.

oasis (ō-ā′sĭs) [Gr., a fertile area in an arid region] (pl. *oases*). Area of healthy tissue surrounded by a diseased portion.

oasthouse urine disease. Methionine malabsorption syndrome, which is associated with mental retardation, diarrhea, convulsions, phenylketonuria, and a peculiar odor. The odor is due to the absorption from the intestinal tract of fermentation products of methionine. SYN: *Smith-Strang disease.*

oat [AS. *ate*, oat]. Grain or seed of a cereal grass used as food.

oath [AS. *ooth*]. A solemn attestation or affirmation. SEE: *Hippocratic oath; Nightingale Pledge.*

oatmeal [AS. *ate*, oat, + *mele*, meal]. A meal made from oats. Usually cooked to make porridge. Oatmeal is sometimes used in a tepid bath to sooth inflamed or irritated skin.

OB. *obstetrics.*

ob- [L.]. Combining form meaning toward, against, in the way of.

obdormition (ŏb-dor-mĭsh′ŭn) [L. *ob*, toward, + *dormire*, to sleep]. Numbness followed by tingling in an extremity produced by pressure on the nerve trunk supplying it. Limb is commonly referred to as being asleep.

obelion (ō-bē′lē-ŏn) [Gr. *obelos*, a spit]. A craniometric point on the sagittal suture between the two parietal foramina.

obese (ō-bēs′) [L. *obesus*]. Extremely fat. SYN: *corpulent.*

obesity (ō-bē′sĭ-tē) [L. *obesitas*, corpulence]. Abnormal amount of fat on the body. The term is usually not employed unless the individual is from 20% to 30% over average weight for his or her age, sex, and height.

It is estimated that 34 million adults in the U.S. are overweight. Obese individuals have an increased risk of developing chronic disease such as diabetes mellitus, hypertension, and some types of cancer. In addition, obesity is associated with increased risk of developing osteoarthritis of the knees.

An accepted technical definition of obesity in adults is, in males, a body mass index greater than 27.8 kg/m²; and for females, greater than 27.3 kg/m². SYN: *adiposity; corpulence; overweight.* SEE: *body mass index; Recommended Daily Dietary Allowances* in *Appendix; weight, set point.* SEE: *Nursing Diagnoses in Appendix.*

ETIOL: Obesity is the result of an imbalance between food eaten and energy expended, but the underlying cause usually is quite complex and difficult to diagnose and treat.

Nevertheless, there is evidence that genetic factors have a role in determining whether or not an individual is or will become obese.

TREAT: Prophylaxis in children of families with a tendency to obesity in the form of establishing moderate eating and exercise habits; dieting. SEE: *gastroplasty.*

DIET: Caloric intake should be less than maintenance requirements, but all other essential nutrients must be included. Maintenance requirements are based on what the average or desired weight should be. A slow reduction regimen, depending on ideal body weight considerations, is 1200 to 1600 Cal per day; 1000 to 1200 Cal will provide a more rapid loss of weight.

The average basic reducing diet is about 9 Cal per pound of ideal body weight per day. Thus, a 160-pound (72.6-kg) person whose ideal weight is 135 pounds (61.2 kg) should maintain a diet of about 1200 Cal a day. These calories should be obtained from foods that would provide adequate protein, carbohydrates, fats, minerals, and vitamins, and not from a fad diet. Adherence to this diet should cause the person to lose the excess weight. After that the diet is adjusted so that caloric intake is just equal to total energy required. Obviously this is different for each individual.

Losing weight by fasting is effective but is not recommended unless done under strict medical and nursing supervision. Death has occurred in persons fasting without medical care.

RS: anorexia nervosa; bulimia; caloric excess; carbohydrate; diet; dietetics; emaciation; fat; mineral compounds; protein; starch; starvation; sugar; vegan; vitamin; weight.

o., endogenous. Obesity associated with some metabolic or endocrine abnormality within the body.

o., exogenous. Obesity due to excessive intake of food.

o., hypothalamic. Obesity resulting from dysfunction of hypothalamus, esp. the appetite-regulating center.

o., morbid. Obesity of such degree as to interfere with normal activities, including respiration. SEE: *pickwickian syndrome.*

obex (ō'bĕks) [L., a band]. [NA] A thin, crescent-shaped band of tissue covering the calamus scriptorius, q.v., at the point of convergence of nervous tissue at the caudal end of the fourth ventricle.

obfuscation (ŏb-fŭs-kā'shŭn) [L. *obfuscare,* to darken]. 1. The act of making obscure or confusing. 2. Mental confusion.

OB/GYN. *obstetrics* and *gynecology.*

object [L. *objectus*]. That which is visible or tangible to the senses.

object, sex. 1. An individual regarded as being of little interest except for providing sexual pleasure. 2. A person to whom one is sexually attracted.

object blindness. Affection in which brain fails to recognize things even though the eyes are functioning normally. SEE: *apraxia.*

objective (ŏb-jĕk'tĭv). 1. Perceptible to other persons, said of symptoms. Opposite of subjective. 2. Directed toward external things. 3. The lens of a microscope that is closest to the object.

o., achromatic. A microscope objective in which chromatic aberration is corrected for red and blue light.

o., apochromatic. A microscope objective in which chromatic aberration is corrected for red, blue, and green light.

o., immersion. A microscope objective designed so that the space between the objective lens and the specimen is filled with oil or water.

objective sign. In physical diagnosis, a sign that can be seen, heard, smelled, tasted, stimulated (or fail to be stimulated), measured, or felt by the diagnostician. Finding of such a sign(s) can be used to confirm or deny the diagnostician's impressions of the disease suspected of being present.

objective symptoms. Symptoms apparent to physical means of diagnosis.

object permanence. Thought process whereby infants perceive that objects have constancy. Normally develops by 6 to 12 months. First described by Piaget.

object relations. Emotional attachment for other persons or objects.

object span test. A test of temporal-sequential organization, wherein the child is asked to point to or tap a series of objects in the order demonstrated by the examiner. SEE: *digit span test; temporal-sequential organization.*

obligate (ŏb'lĭ-gāt) [L. *obligatus*]. To make necessary or require; without alternative. SEE: *anaerobe, obligatory.*

oblique (ō-blēk', ō-blīk') [L. *obliquus*]. Slanting, diagonal.

obliquimeter (ŏb''lĭ-kwĭm'ĕt-ĕr) ['' + Gr. *metron,* measure]. Apparatus for indicating the angle of the pelvic brim with the upright body.

obliquity (ŏb-lĭk'wĭ-tē) [L. *obliquus,* slanting]. The state of being oblique or slanting.

o., Litzmann's. Inclining of the fetal head until the posterior parietal bone presents to the uterine canal.

o., Naegele's. Presentation of the fetal head with anterior parietal bone toward the uterine canal with oblique biparietal diameter in relation to the pelvic brim.

o. of pelvis. Inclination of pelvis.

o., Roederer's. Presentation of fetal head with occiput at pelvic brim.

obliquus (ŏb-lĭk'wŭs) [L.]. Oblique.

obliquus reflex. Contraction of the entire external obliquus muscle on application of stimulus to skin of thigh below Poupart's ligament.

obliteration (ŏb-lĭt''ĕr-ā'shŭn) [L. *obliterare,* to remove]. Extinction or complete occlusion of a part by degeneration, disease, or surgery.

Oblomov syndrome [After Ilya Ilych Oblomov, a character in Ivan Goncharov's 19th century novel who would not get out of bed]. Refusal to resume normal activity after an illness or during depression.

oblongata (ŏb''lŏng-gā'tă) [L. *oblongus,* long]. Oblong. Sometimes used to designate the cylindrical extension of the spinal cord as it enters the brain. It is about an inch long, reaches to the pons, and forms part of the base of the fourth ventricle. SYN: *medulla oblongata.*

obmutescence (ŏb''mū-tĕs'ĕns) [L. *obmutescere,* to become dumb]. Loss of vocal power. SYN: *aphonia.*

obscure (ŏb-skūr') [L. *obscurus,* hide]. 1. Hidden, indistinct, as the cause of a condition. 2. To make less distinct or to hide.

observerscope (ŏb-zĕr'vĕr-skōp). Type of endoscope designed so that two persons can view the site simultaneously.

obsession [L. *obsessus,* besiege]. The neurotic mental state of having an uncontrollable desire to dwell on an idea or an emotion. The patient is usually aware of the abnormality and attempts to resist these thoughts. SEE: *obsessive-compulsive disorder.*

obsessive-compulsive disorder. ABBR: OCD. Recurrent obsessions or compulsions severe enough to cause distress because of time consumed or interference with an individual's normal routine. Obsessions manifest as persistent ideas, thoughts, or impulses that the patient may attempt to ignore. Examples would be thoughts of violence, fear of being contaminated and, therefore, being afraid of shaking hands. Compulsions are repetitive, purposeful, and intentional stereotyped behavior in response to an obsession. Examples are hand washing, counting, checking, or touching. Individuals with OCD experience a sense of tension when they attempt to resist a compulsion. Associated with OCD are depression and anxiety. OCD is estimated to affect 2% of the population.

TREAT: The antidepressant clomipramine has been of great benefit in treating OCD. SEE: *Gilles de la Tourette's syndrome; trichotillomania.*

obsolescence [L. *obsolescere,* to grow old]. The condition of becoming useless, or out of date.

obstetric (ŏb-stĕt'rĭk) [L. *obstetrix,* midwife]. Pert. to obstetrics or midwifery.

obstetrician (ŏb-stĕ-trĭsh'ăn). A physician who treats women during pregnancy and parturition and delivers infants.

obstetrics (ŏb-stĕt'rĭks) [L. *obstetrix,* midwife]. Branch of medicine that concerns management of women during pregnancy, childbirth, and the puerperium.

RS: ballottement; breech presentation; brow presentation; cesarean section; childbirth; childbirth, prepared; delivery; fetus; gestation; labor; maneuver; midwife; nurse-midwife; parturition; position; postpartum hemorrhage; pregnancy; puerpera; puerperal.

obstipation (ŏb″stĭ-pā'shŭn) [L. *obstipatio*]. Obstinate or extreme constipation

obstruction (ŏb-strŭk'shŭn). 1. Blockage of a structure that prevents it from functioning normally. 2. A thing that impedes; an obstacle.

o., aortic. Blockage of the aorta, thereby preventing the flow of blood.

o., intestinal. Blockage of the lumen of the intestine.

obstructive lung disease, chronic. ABBR: COLD. Increased resistance to the passage of air in and out of the lung due to narrowing of the bronchial tree. It is diagnosed by determining that the amount of air forcibly expired from the lung in one second is less than normal. The disease process may be caused by a number of irritants or diseases that damage the bronchial tree, including pulmonary tuberculosis, cigarette smoking, and silicosis.

NURSING IMPLICATIONS: Teach breathing with coughing exercises to decrease the work of breathing and improve breathing pattern. Encourage participation in pulmonary rehabilitation program, including smoking cessation and avoiding other respiratory irritants. Warn patient to avoid contact with others with respiratory infections, and educate patient about use of antibiotic and bronchodilator therapy.

Teach breathing, postural drainage, and coughing exercises to strengthen respiratory muscles and mobilize secretions. Educate patient about rationale for low concentration oxygen therapy. Encourage frequent small meals and adequate fluid intake. Help patient plan a schedule that alternates periods of activity with periods of rest. Assist patient and family with lifestyle changes imposed by disease limitations, and encourage expression of feelings and concerns.

obstruent (ŏb'stroo-ĕnt) [L. *obstruens*]. 1. Blocking up. 2. That which closes a normal passage in the body. 3. Any agent or agency causing obstruction.

obtund (ŏb-tŭnd') [L. *obtundere,* to beat against]. To dull or blunt, as sensitivity or pain. SEE: *consciousness, levels of.*

obtundent (ŏb-tŭn'dĕnt) [L. *obtundens*]. 1. Having the capacity to deaden sensibility of a part or reduce irritability. 2. A soothing remedy.

obturation (ŏb-tūr-ā'shŭn) [L. *obturare,* to stop up]. Closure of a passage or opening, as in intestinal obstruction.

obturator (ŏb'tū-rā″tor). 1. Anything that obstructs or closes a cavity or opening. 2. Rel. to the obturator membrane. 3. Bridge for spanning the gap in the cleft palate.

obturator foramen. Obturator in the anterior part of the os innominatum between the pubis and ischium.

obturator membrane. Strong obturator occluding the obturator foramen.

obturator muscles. Two muscles on each side of the pelvic region that rotate the thighs outward. SEE: *Muscles* in *Appendix.*

obturator sign. Obturator test of inward rotation of the hip so that the obturator internus muscle is stretched. This test result may be positive in acute appendicitis.

obtuse (ŏb-tūs') [L. *obtusus*]. 1. Not pointed or acute; dull or blunt. 2. Of dull mentality.

obtusion (ŏb-tū'zhŭn). Blunting or weakening of normal sensation, as in certain diseases.

O.C. *oral contraceptive.*

Occam's razor (ŏck'hăms) [William of Occam, or Ockham, Brit. Franciscan and philosopher, c. 1285–1349]. The concept that entities do not have to be proved beyond the point of proof; or "what can be done with fewer (assumptions) is done in vain with more."

occipital (ŏk-sĭp'ĭ-tăl) [L. *occipitalis*]. Concerning the back part of the head.

occipital bone. Bone in lower back part of skull between the parietal and temporal bones.

occipitalis (ŏk-sĭp"ĭ-tā'lĭs) [L.]. Posterior portion of the occipitofrontalis muscle at the back of the head.

occipitalization (ŏk-sĭp"ĭ-tăl-ĭ-zā'shŭn). Fusion of the atlas and occipital bones.

occipital lobe. Posterior lobe of the cerebral hemisphere that is shaped like a three-sided pyramid.

occipito- [L. *occiput*]. Combining form showing relationship between the occiput and another part.

occipitoatloid (ŏk-sĭp"ĭ-tō-ăt'loyd). Concerning the occipital and atlas bones.

occipitoaxoid (ŏk-sĭp"ĭ-tō-ăk'soyd). Concerning the occipital and axis bones.

occipitobregmatic (ŏk-sĭp"ĭ-tō-brĕg-măt'ĭk). Concerning the occiput and bregma.

occipitocervical (ŏk-sĭp"ĭ-tō-sĕr'vĭ-kăl). Concerning the occiput and neck.

occipitofacial (ŏk-sĭp"ĭ-tō-fā'shăl). Concerning the occiput and face.

occipitofrontal (ŏk-sĭp"ĭ-tō-frŏn'tăl). Concerning the occiput and forehead.

occipitomastoid (ŏk-sĭp"ĭ-tō-măs'toyd). Concerning the occiput and mastoid process.

occipitomental (ŏk-sĭp"ĭ-tō-mĕn'tăl). Concerning the occiput and chin.

occipitoparietal (ŏk-sĭp"ĭ-tō-pă-rī'ē-tăl). Concerning the occiput and parietal bones or lobes of the brain.

occipitotemporal (ŏk-sĭp"ĭ-tō-tĕm'pō-răl). Concerning the occiput and temporal bones.

occipitothalamic (ŏk-sĭp"ĭ-tō-thă-lăm'ĭk). Concerning the occiput and thalamus.

occiput (ŏk'sĭ-pŭt) [L.]. [NA] The back part of the skull.

occlude (ŏ-klūd') [L. *occludere*, to shut up]. To close up, obstruct, or join together, as bringing the biting surfaces of opposing teeth together.

occlusal (ŏ-kloo'zăl). Pert. to the closure of an opening.

occlusal adjustment. Reshaping the occlusal surface of teeth by grinding to create a harmonious contact relationship between upper and lower teeth. This is done to equalize the stress of occlusal forces on the supporting tissues of the teeth, thereby eliminating pain, root resorption, and periodontal problems.

occlusal equilibration. The modification of occlusal forms of teeth by grinding with the intent of equalizing occlusal forces or producing simultaneous occlusal contacts and harmonious cuspal relations.

occlusal guard. A removable dental appliance that covers one or both arches and is designed to minimize the damaging effects of bruxism, contact sports, or any occlusal habits that are detrimental.

occlusal plane. The imaginary surface extending from the tip of the mandibular incisors back along the cusp tips of the mandibular molar teeth to contact the cranium; more precise points are used for some dental records but generally the occlusal plane is considered a curve of the occlusal surface rather than a true plane.

occlusal surface. The masticating surface of the premolar and molar teeth.

occlusal wear. The attritional loss of substance on opposing occlusal surfaces in natural or artificial teeth; the modification of tooth cusps, ridges, and grooves by functional use.

occlusion (ŏ-kloo'zhŭn) [L. *occlusio*]. 1. The closure, or state of being closed, of a passage. May be acquired or congenital. SYN: *imperforation*. 2. Absorption of gas by a substance that does not thereby lose its characteristic property. 3. Alignment of the mandibular and maxillary teeth when the jaw is closed or in functional contact, i.e., dental occlusion. SEE: *malocclusion*.

o., abnormal. Malocclusion of the teeth.

o., adjusted. The alteration of occlusal contacts by dental restorations in order to achieve a balanced or functional occlusion.

o., balanced. The ideal and equal contact of the teeth of the working side of the jaw by the complementary contact of the teeth on the opposite side of the jaw. SYN: *balanced bite.*

o., centric. The position of the mandible, both vertical and horizontal, that produces maximal interdigitation of the cusps of the maxillary and mandibular teeth. The ideal position or type of occlusion. Also described as intercuspal position, tooth-to-tooth position, habitual centric, or acquired centric.

o., coronary. Obstruction of a coronary vessel by thrombosis or as a result of spasm. SYN: *coronary thrombosis.* SEE: *myocardial infarction.*

o., eccentric. Any occlusion other than centric.

o., habitual. The usual relationship between the teeth of the maxilla and mandible that represents the maximum contact; this varies from individual to individual and is seldom ideal or true centric occlusion.

o., traumatic. Injury to the tissues that support the teeth due to malocclusion, missing teeth, improper chewing habits, or some pathological condition that causes an individual to chew in an abnormal way.

o., working. The usual method of contact of teeth as the mandible is moved to one side during chewing. SYN: *working bite.*

occlusive (ŏ-kloo'sĭv). Concerning occlusion.

occlusive dressing. SEE: *dressing, occlusive.*

occlusometer (ŏk"loo-sŏm'ĕ-tĕr). Device for measuring the force exerted during forcible occlusion of the teeth. SYN: *gnathodynamometer.*

occult (ŭ-kŭlt') [L. *occultus*]. Obscure; concealed, as a hemorrhage.

occult blood. Blood in such minute quantity that it can be recognized only by microscopic examination or by chemical means.

occult blood test. A chemical test or microscopic examination for blood, esp. in feces, that is not apparent on visual inspection.

occupational medicine. SEE: *medicine, occupational.*

occupational neurosis. A functional disorder that may develop in persons in certain occupations. SEE: *neurosis.*

occupational performance. A term used by occupational therapists to refer to a person's ability to perform the required activities, tasks, and roles of living.

occupational therapist. One who provides assessment and intervention to ameliorate physical and psychological deficits which interfere with the performance of activities and tasks of living.

occupational therapist assistant. One who works under the supervision of an occupational therapist in evaluating clients and in planning and implementing programs designed to restore or develop a client's skills for self-care, work, play, or leisure time tasks. Although requiring supervision in conducting a remedial program, the assistant can function independently when conducting a maintenance program.

occupational therapy. Therapeutic use of work, self-care, and play activities to increase independent function, enhance development, and prevent disability; may include adaptation of task or environment to achieve maximum independence and to enhance quality of life.

occupational therapy aide. An individual with on-the-job training or experience in occupational therapy who performs routine tasks under the direction of an occupational therapist.

ochlesis (ŏk-lē'sĭs) [Gr., crowding]. Any disease caused by conditions of overcrowding.

ochlophobia (ŏk"lō-fō'bē-ă) [Gr. *ochlos*, crowd, + *phobos*, fear]. Abnormal dread of crowds or populated places.

ochrometer (ō-krŏm'ĕt-ĕr) [Gr. *ochros*, pale yellow + *metron*, measure]. Device for estimating the capillary blood pressure by recording the pressure required to compress a finger until the skin becomes blanched.

ochronosis (ō-krō-nō'sĭs) [" + *nosos*, disease]. A rare condition marked by dark pigmentation of the ligaments, cartilage, fibrous tissues, skin, and urine. May be caused by an inborn error of metabolism, alkaptonuria. This allows formation of homogentisic acid, part of which is excreted in the urine and part of which is stored in the tissues. The condition also may be caused by chronic phenol poisoning.

OCT. *oxytocin challenge test.*

octa-, octo- [Gr. *okto*, L. *octo*]. Combining forms meaning eight.

octahedron (ŏk-tă-hē'drŏn). An eight-sided solid figure.

octan (ŏk'tăn) [L. *octo*, eight]. Reappearing on every eighth day, as a fever.

octane (ŏk'tān). C_8H_{18}. A hydrocarbon of the paraffin series.

octapeptide (ŏk"tă-pĕp'tĭd). A peptide that contains eight amino acids.

octaploid (ŏk'tă-ployd). 1. Concerning octaploidy. 2. Having eight pairs of chromosomes.

octaploidy (ŏk'tă-ploy'dē). The condition of having eight sets or pairs of chromosomes.

octarius (ŏk-tā'rē-ŭs) [L.]. ABBR: O. Pint.

octavalent (ŏk"tă-vā'lĕnt) [L. *octo*, eight, + *valeo*, to have power]. Having a valency of eight.

octigravida (ŏk"tĭ-grăv'ĭ-dă) [" + *gravida*, pregnant]. One who has been pregnant eight times.

octipara (ŏk-tĭp'ă-ră) [" + L. *parere*, to bring forth, to bear]. A woman who has given birth to eight children.

octogenarian (ŏk"tō-jĕn-ĕr'ē-ĕn) [L. *octogenarius*, containing eighty]. A person who is in his or her eighties.

octreotide acetate. A synthetic drug that mimics the action of somatostatin. Used in treating malignant carcinoid. Trade name is Sandostatin.

ocular (ŏk'ū-lăr) [L. *oculus*, eye]. 1. Concerning the eye or vision. 2. Eyepiece of a microscope.

ocularist. An allied health specialist who is prepared by training and experience to make an artificial eye to match, as nearly as possible, the remaining eye or the eye or eyes removed.

oculi (ŏk'ū-lī). Pl. of oculus.

oculinium. A botulin-derived drug used experimentally to alter nerve impulses to muscles. It has been used for that purpose in treating blepharospasm and strabismus.

oculist (ŏk'ū-lĭst). Former term for ophthalmologist, a physician who is a specialist in diseases of the eye.

oculo- (ŏk'ū-lō) [L. *oculus*, eye]. Combining form indicating relationship to the eye.

oculocardiac reflex. Slowing of the pulse following pressure applied to the eyeball or carotid sinus. SYN: *Aschner's phenomenon.*

oculocephalic reflex (ŏk"ū-lō-sĕf'ă-lĭk). The deviation of the neonate's eyes to the opposite side when the head is rotated. SYN: *doll's eye reflex.*

oculocerebrorenal syndrome. A sex-linked condition characterized by hydrophthalmia, cataracts, mental retardation, aminoaciduria, impaired renal ammonia production, and vitamin D-resistant rickets.

oculocutaneous (ŏk"ū-lō-kū-tā'nē-ŭs). Concerning the eye and skin.

oculofacial (ŏk"ū-lō-fā'shē-ăl). Concerning the eye and face.

oculogyration (ŏk"ū-lō-jī-rā'shŭn) [" + Gr. *gyros*, circle]. Circular motion of the eyeball around its anterior-posterior axis. SEE: *nystagmus.*

oculogyria (ŏk"ū-lō-jĭ'rē-ă). The limits of rotation of the eyeballs.

oculogyric (ŏk"ū-lō-jĭ'rĭk). Producing or concerning movements of the eye. SYN: *oculomotor; ophthalmogyric.*

oculogyric crisis. Attack of involuntary deviation and fixation of the eyeballs, usually upward. It may last for several minutes or hours. May be seen with postencephalitic parkinsonism or encephalitis lethargica.

oculomotor (ŏk"ū-lō-mō'tor) [" + *motor*, mover]. Rel. to eye movements. SYN: *oculogyric.*

oculomotorius (ŏk"ū-lō-mō-tō'rē-ŭs) [L.]. Oculomotor nerve.

oculomotor nerve. Nerve that originates in the medial surface of the cerebral peduncle of the midbrain and consists of general somatic efferent, general visceral efferent, and general somatic afferent fibers. It is distributed through all extrinsic muscles of the eye except the exterior rectus and superior oblique, through the levator palpebrae superioris of the eyelid, through the ciliary muscle, and through the sphincter muscle of the iris. Its function is primarily motor, but it also contains proprioceptive fibers. SYN: *third cranial nerve.* SEE: *Cranial Nerves* in *Appendix.*

oculomycosis (ŏk"ū-lō-mī-kō'sĭs) [" + Gr. *mykes*, fungus, + *osis*, condition]. Any disease of the eye or its parts caused by fungus.

oculonasal (ŏk"ū-lō-nā'săl) [" + *nasus*, nose]. Concerning both the eye and nose.

oculopupillary (ŏk"ū-lō-pū'pĭ-lăr-ē). Concerning the pupil of the eye.

oculoreaction (ŏk"ū-lō-rē-ăk'shŭn) [L. *oculus*, eye, + *re*, back, + *actus*, acting]. A reaction observed in the conjunctiva of the eye when toxins of tuberculosis and typhoid are instilled into the conjunctival space. Of diagnostic value. SYN: *ophthalmic reaction; ophthalmoreaction.*

oculozygomatic (ŏk"ū-lō-zī"gō-măt'ĭk) [" + Gr. *zygon*, yoke]. Pert. to the eye and zygoma.

oculozygomatic line. Line appearing between the inner canthus of eye and cheek, supposedly indicative of neural disorders.

oculus (ŏk'ū-lŭs) [L.] (pl. *oculi*). [NA] Eye; the organ of vision made up of the eyeball and optic nerve.

  o. dexter. ABBR: O.D. or o.d. The right eye.

  o. sinister. ABBR: O.S. The left eye.

  o. uterque. Each eye.

O.D., o.d. *Doctor of Optometry; overdose;* [L.] *oculus dexter,* right eye. SEE: *O.S., o.s.*

OD'd. Street term for a death due to a drug overdose, esp. a drug of abuse.

odaxesmus (ō"dăk-sĕz'mŭs) [Gr. *odaxesmos,* an irritation]. The biting of the tongue, lip, or cheek during an epileptic attack.

odaxetic (ō"dăk-sĕt'ĭk). Producing a stinging or itching sensation.

Oddi's sphincter (ŏd'ēz) [Ruggero Oddi, It. physician, 1864–1913]. A sphincter at the opening of the common bile duct into the duodenum at the papilla of Vater.

odditis (ŏd-dī'tĭs) [*Oddi* + Gr. *itis,* inflammation]. Inflammation of the sphincter of Oddi.

odogenesis (ō"dō-jĕn'ē-sĭs) [Gr. *hodos,* pathway, + *genesis,* generation, birth]. The branching and growth of axons from the proximal end of a severed nerve. It allows the space between the nerves to be bridged and thus repaired. SYN: *neurocladism.*

odont-, odonto- [Gr. *odous,* tooth]. Combining form rel. to the tooth or teeth.

odontagra (ō-dŏn-tă'grā) [Gr. *odous,* tooth, + *agra,* seizure]. Toothache, esp. when originating from gout.

odontalgia (ō-dŏn-tăl'jē-ă) [" + *algos,* pain]. Toothache. SYN: *odontia; odontodynia.*

  o., phantom. Pain felt in the area from which a tooth has been pulled.

odontatrophy (ō"dŏn-tăt'rō-fē) [" + *atrophia,* atrophy]. Imperfect development of the teeth.

odontectomy (ō-dŏn-tĕk'tō-mē) [" + *ektome,* excision]. Surgical removal of a tooth.

odonterism (ō-dŏn'tĕr-ĭzm) [" + *erismos,* quarrel]. Chattering of the teeth.

odontia (ō-dŏn'shē-ă) [Gr. *odous,* tooth]. 1. Pain in a tooth. SYN: *odontalgia; odontodynia.* 2. Condition or abnormality of the teeth.

odontic (ō-dŏn′tĭk) [Gr. *odous*, tooth]. Concerning the teeth.

odontitis (ō″dŏn-tī′tĭs) [″ + *itis*, inflammation]. Inflammation of a tooth.

odontoblast (ō-dŏn′tō-blăst) [″ + *blastos*, germ]. One of the cells forming the surface layer of the dental papilla that is responsible for the formation of the dentin of a tooth. After a tooth is formed, the odontoblasts line the pulp cavity and continue to produce dentin for years after the tooth has erupted.

odontoblastoma [″ + ″ + *oma*, tumor]. A tumor composed principally of odontoblasts.

odontobothrion (ō-dŏn″tō-bŏth′rē-ōn) [″ + *bothrion*, pit]. Socket of a tooth.

odontobothritis [″ + ″ + *itis*, inflammation]. Inflammation of alveolar process of the tooth.

odontocele (ō-dŏn′tō-sēl) [″ + *kele*, tumor, swelling]. An alveolodental cyst.

odontochirurgical (ō-dŏn″tō-kĭ-rŭr′jĭ-kăl) [″ + *chirurgia*, surgery]. Pert. to dental surgery.

odontoclasis (ō″dŏn-tŏk′lă-sĭs) [″ + *klasis*, fracture]. The breaking or fracture of a tooth.

odontoclast. A cell that brings about the absorption of the roots of deciduous teeth.

odontodynia (ō-dŏn″tō-dĭn′ē-ă) [″ + *odyne*, pain]. Toothache. SYN: *odontalgia; odontia*.

odontogenesis, odontogeny (ō-dŏn″tō-jĕn′ĕ-sĭs, -tŏj′ĕn-ē) [″ + *genesis*, generation, birth]. The origin and formation of the teeth.

   o. imperfecta. A congenital anomaly of the developing teeth in which there is deficient production of enamel and dentin in affected teeth. There is decreased density of the teeth and enlarged pulp chambers.

odontograph (ō-dŏn′tō-grăf) [″ + *graphein*, to write]. Device for determining the degree of uneven surface of tooth enamel.

odontography (ō-dŏn-tŏg′ră-fē). Descriptive anatomy of the teeth.

odontoid (ō-dŏn′toyd) [″ + *eidos*, form, shape]. Toothlike.

odontoid process. The toothlike projection from upper surface of the body of the second cervical vertebra.

odontolith (ō-dŏn′tō-lĭth) [″ + *lithos*, stone]. The accretion of a calcareous substance on the teeth; tartar.

odontologist (ō″dŏn-tŏl′ō-jĭst). A dentist or dental surgeon.

odontology (ō″dŏn-tŏl′ō-jē) [″ + *logos*, word, reason]. The art and science of dentistry, q.v.

odontolysis (ō-dŏn-tŏl′ĭ-sĭs) [″ + *lysis*, dissolution]. Loss of calcium from a tooth.

odontoma (ō″dŏn-tō′mă) [″ + *oma*, tumor]. Tumor of a tooth or tumor originating in the dental tissue.

   o., ameloblastic. Neoplasm that contains enamel, dentin, and odontogenic tissue that does not develop to form enamel.

   o., composite. Odontoma in which the epithelial and mesenchymal cells are completely differentiated. This causes enamel and dentin to be formed in an abnormal manner.

   o., coronary. Bony tumor at the crown of a tooth.

   o., follicular. Bony shell in gums below the tooth margin, usually after the second dentition. SYN: *cyst, dentigerous.*

   SYM: Crepitating to pressure. Tumor often involves one or more teeth.

   ETIOL: Excessive number of dental follicles.

   o., radicular. Odontoma close to or on the root of a tooth.

odontonecrosis (ō-dŏn″tō-nĕ-krō′sĭs) [″ + *nekros*, corpse, + *osis*, condition]. Extensive decay of a tooth.

odontonomy (ō″dŏn-tŏn′ō-mē) [″ + *onoma*, name]. Dental nomenclature.

odontopathy (ō-dŏn-tŏp′ă-thē) [″ + *pathos*, disease, suffering]. Any disease of the teeth.

odontophobia (ō-dŏn″tō-fō′bē-ă) [″ + *phobos*, fear]. 1. Abnormal aversion to the sight of teeth. 2. Abnormal fear of dental surgery.

odontoprisis (ō-dŏn″tō-prī′sĭs) [″ + *prisis*, sawing]. Grinding of the teeth. SYN: *bruxism.*

odontorrhagia (ō-dŏn″tō-rā′jē-ă) [″ + *rhegnynai*, to burst forth]. Hemorrhage from a tooth socket following extraction.

odontoschism (ō-dŏn″tō-skĭzm) [″ + *schisma*, cleft]. Fissure of a tooth.

odontoscopy (ō″dŏn-tŏs′kō-pē) [″ + *skopein*, to examine]. 1. Examination of the teeth and oral cavity by use of an odontoscope. 2. An impression made of the biting marks made by teeth. These are used as a means of identification.

odontosis (ō-dŏn-tō′sĭs) [″ + *osis*, condition]. 1. Development of teeth. 2. Eruption of teeth.

odontotherapy (ō-dŏn″tō-thĕr′ă-pē) [″ + *therapeia*, treatment]. Care of diseased teeth.

odor (ō′dĕr) [L.]. 1. That quality of a substance that renders it perceptible to sense of smell. 2. Any smell. 3. Any sensation of sense of smell.

   Each odoriferous substance causes its own sensations, the description of which is complex and subjective. Odors have been classed as (1) pure, (2) those mixed with sensations from the mucous membrane, and (3) those mixed with the sensation of taste. A suggested classification of odors includes aromatic, burning, fragrant, fetid, nauseating, and repulsive. Another classification is spicy, flowery, fruity, resinous, foul, and scorched. Although classification attempts are useful, it is important to realize that most complex substances do not produce a single odor.

RS: "brom-" words; deodorant; effluvium; nose; olfactology; olfactory; osmolagnia; "osmo-" words; osphresiolagnia; osphresiometer; pungent; smell; taste.

odorant (ō'dor-ănt). Something that stimulates the sense of smell.

odoriferous (ō″dor-ĭf′ĕ-rŭs) [L. *odor*, smell, + *ferre*, to bear]. Bearing scent, having an odor; fragrant; perfumed.

odorimetry. The measurement of the ability of a substance to induce olfactory sensations.

odoriphore (ō-dor′ĭ-for) [″ + Gr. *phoros*, bearing]. The portion of a molecule that imparts odor to the substance.

odorography (ō″dor-ŏg′ră-fē) [″ + Gr. *graphein*, to write]. Description of odors.

odorous [L. *odor*, smell]. Having an odor, scent, or fragrance.

odynacusis (ō″dĭn-ă-kū′sĭs) [Gr. *odyne*, pain, + *akousis*, hearing]. A condition in which noises cause pain in the ear.

-odynia, odyno- (ō-dĭn′ē-ă, ō-dĭn′ō) [Gr. *odyne*, pain]. Combining form concerning pain.

odynometer (ō″dĭn-om′ĕt-ĕr) [″ + *metron*, measure]. Device for measuring pain.

odynophagia (ŏd″ĭn-ō-fā′jē-ă) [″ + *phagein*, to eat]. Pain upon swallowing.

odynophobia (ŏd″ĭn-ō-fō′bē-ă) [″ + *phobos*, fear]. Abnormal dread of pain.

Oedipus complex (ĕd′ĭ-pŭs) [Oedipus, a character in Gr. tragedy who unwittingly fell in love with his mother, Jocasta, killed his father in jealousy, and married his mother]. Abnormally intense love of the child for parent of the opposite sex. This love continues in adulthood. Usually involves jealous dislike of the other parent. Most commonly love of a son for his mother. SEE: *Electra complex; Jocasta complex.*

oenology (ē-nŏl′ō-jē) [Gr. *oinos*, wine, + *logos*, word, reason]. The science of production and evaluation of wine.

oersted (ĕr′stĕd) [Hans Christian Oersted, Danish physicist, 1777–1851]. A unit of magnetic field intensity. An oersted is the magnetism that exerts a force of one dyne on a unit magnetic pole.

oesophagostomiasis (ē-sŏf″ă-gō-stō-mī′ă-sĭs) [Gr. *oisophagos*, esophagus, + *stoma*, mouth, + *-iasis*, state]. Infection with the nematode of the genus *Oesophagostomum*.

Oesophagostomum (ē-sŏf″ă-gŏs′tō-mŭm) [Gr. *oisophagos*, esophagus, + *stoma*, mouth]. A genus of nematodes belonging to the suborder Strongylata; parasitic in the intestinal walls of animals and humans.

O. apiostomum. The nodular nematode worm parasitic to monkeys. Occasionally infests humans.

oestrus. Estrus.

Oestrus ovis. A botfly that may cause ocular myiasis in humans.

O.F.D. *object film distance.* Distance from the radiographic film to the object being radiographed.

official. Said of medicines authorized as standard in the U.S. Pharmacopeia and in the National Formulary.

officinal (ŏf-ĭs′ĭn-ăl) [L. *officina*, shop]. Regularly kept in a druggist's stock. SEE: *magistral.*

off-label drug use. In cancer treatment, the prescribing of drugs that lack evidence of effectiveness for Food and Drug Administration approval. The oncologists who prescribe such drugs feel that the drugs are effective and that the long approval process makes it necessary to use the drugs without delay.

Ogen. Trade name for estropipate, USP.

Ogilvie's syndrome [Sir William Heneage Ogilvie, Brit. physician, 1887–1971]. Acute intestinal pseudo-obstruction. There is acute intestinal dilatation, mostly of the colon. These patients have usually recently undergone severe surgical or medical stress, such as myocardial infarction, sepsis, or respiratory failure; they may be on a respirator, have metabolic and electrolyte disturbances, and have received narcotics.

TREAT: Therapy for the underlying disease; correct electrolyte disturbances; avoid drugs that inhibit intestinal motility; intubate small intestine for decompression. Cecostomy may be required in order to avoid ischemic necrosis and perforation of the bowel.

Oguchi's disease (ō-goot′chēz) [Chuta Oguchi, Japanese ophthalmologist, 1875–1945]. Hereditary night blindness with onset in infancy. Commonly found in Japan; rare in the United States.

OH⁻. Chemical symbol for the hydroxyl ion.

ohm (ōm). Unit of electrical resistance equal to that of a conductor in which a current of one ampere is produced by a potential of one volt across the terminals. SEE: *electromotive force.*

ohmammeter (ōm′ăm-mē″tĕr). Combined ohmmeter and ammeter.

Ohm's law [Georg S. Ohm, Ger. physicist, 1789–1854]. The strength of an electric current, expressed in amperes, is equal to the electromotive force, expressed in volts, divided by the resistance, expressed in ohms. SEE: *electricity*.

ohmmeter (ōm'mē-tĕr). Device for determining the electrical resistance of a conductor.

-oid [Gr. *eidos*, form, shape]. Suffix indicating resemblance to the item designated in the first part of the word.

oikofugic (oy"kō-fū'jĭk) [Gr. *oikos*, house, + L. *fugere*, to flee]. Having a compulsion to leave home.

oikomania (oy"kō-mā'nē-ă) [" + *mania*, madness]. Nervous disorder induced by unhappy home surroundings.

oikophobia (oy"kō-fō'bē-ă). Morbid dislike of the home.

oil (oyl) [L. *oleum*]. A greasy liquid not miscible with water, usually obtained from and classified as mineral, vegetable, or animal. According to character, oils are subdivided principally as fixed (or fatty) and volatile (or essential).
Ex.: *Fixed:* castor oil, olive oil, cod liver oil. *Volatile:* oils of mustard, peppermint, rose.
RS: oleaginous; oleate; oleic, olein; "oleo-" words; oleum; unctuous.

o.'s, essential. Volatile oils, esp. those that have an odor and produce taste sensations, obtained from certain plants by various means of extraction. Some of these oils have been used since antiquity as preservatives and antiseptics, e.g., thymol and eugenol. Also, they are used in flavorings, perfumes, and medicines. They are usually complex chemicals that are difficult to purify. SYN: *volatile oil*.

o.'s, fixed. Oils in plants and animals that are glyceryl esters of fatty acids. These oils serve as food reserves in animals. They are nonvolatile and contain no acid.

o., volatile. Essential oil, q.v.

ointment (oynt'mĕnt) [Fr. *oignement*]. A medicated, fatty, soft substance for external application to the body, having antiseptic, cosmetic, or healing properties. Usually its base is petroleum jelly or lanolin to which the medicament is added. These forms are not water soluble. However, some ointments are composed of ingredients that are water soluble. SYN: *salve; unguent*.

o., hydrophilic. USP. A standardized ointment preparation used topically as an emollient.

o., white. USP. Ointment containing white wax and white petrolatum.

o., yellow. USP. Ointment containing yellow wax and petrolatum.

O.L. L. *oculus laevus*, left eye.

ol. L. *oleum*, oil.

-ol. Suffix indicating a substance is an alcohol or phenol.

O.L.A. L. *occipito laevo anterior*, fetal presentation with the occiput toward the maternal left acetabulum. SYN: *L.O.A.* SEE: *position*.

old age. An imprecise term. SEE: *age is not a diagnosis; chronologically enhanced*.

olea (ō'lē-ă) [L.]. 1. Olive. 2. Pl. of oleum.

oleaginous (ō-lē-ăj'ĭ-nŭs) [L. *oleaginus*]. Greasy; oily; unctuous.

oleander (ō"lē-ăn'dĕr). An ornamental evergreen shrub, *Nerium oleander*. It is toxic.

oleate (ō'lē-āt) [L. *oleatum*]. 1. Any salt of oleic acid. 2. Salt of oleic acid dissolved in an excess of the acid. Used as an ointment.

oleatum (ō-lē-ā'tŭm) [L.]. Preparation made by dissolving metallic salts or alkaloids in oleic acid. SYN: *oleate*.

olecranal (ō-lĕk'răn-ăl) [Gr. *olekranon*, elbow]. Concerning the elbow.

olecranarthritis (ō-lĕk"răn-ăr-thrī'tĭs) [" + *arthron*, joint, + *itis*, inflammation]. Inflamed condition of the elbow joint.

olecranarthrocace (ō-lĕk"răn-ăr-thrŏk'ă-sē) [" + " + *kake*, badness]. Tuberculous ulceration of the elbow joint.

olecranarthropathy (ō-lĕk"răn-ăr-thrŏp'ă-thē) [" + " + *pathos*, disease, suffering]. Any disease of the elbow joint.

olecranoid (ō-lĕk'ră-noyd) [" + *eidos*, form, shape]. Similar to the olecranon.

olecranon (ō-lĕk'răn-ŏn) [Gr., elbow]. [NA] A large process of the ulna projecting behind the elbow joint and forming the bony prominence of the elbow. SEE: *elbow; skeleton; ulna*.

o., fracture of. In treating this type of injury, prevent spasm of triceps muscle to avoid separation of fragments. The latter may have to be wired.
TREAT: Prevent spasm of the triceps by either placing the arm in a sling or bandaging the arm to the side.

oleic (ō-lē'ĭk) [L. *oleum*, oil]. Derived from or pert. to oil.

oleic acid. $C_8H_{34}O_2$. A colorless oily liquid prepared from tallow and other fats, the salts of which are oleates.

olein (ō'lē-ĭn) [L. *oleum*, oil]. An oleate of glyceryl found in nearly all fixed oils and fats; an important part of oils. SYN: *triolein*.

oleo- [L. *oleum*, oil]. Combining form meaning oil.

oleoarthrosis (ō"lē-ō-ăr-thrō'sĭs) [" + Gr. *arthron*, joint, + *osis*, condition]. Therapeutic introduction of oil into a joint.

oleogranuloma (ō"lē-ō-grăn"ū-lō'mă) [" + L. *granulum*, little grain, + Gr. *oma*, tumor]. A granuloma caused by continuous contact with oil, or at sites of subcutaneous injection of oily substances.

oleoinfusion (ō"lē-ō-ĭn-fū'zhun) [" + *in*,

into, + *fusus*, poured]. A formulation of a drug in oil.

oleoma (ō″lē-ō′mă) [" + Gr. *oma*, tumor]. Oleogranuloma.

oleomargarine (ō″lē-ō-măr′jă-rin) [" + *margarine*]. Butter substitute that may be salted or plain. It is made from refined vegetable and animal fats. These may be saturated or polyunsaturated. Vitamins, preservatives, and coloring agents usually are included. Caloric content is 7.2 Calories per gram. SYN: *margarine*.

oleometer (ō″lē-ŏm′ĕ-tĕr). Device for testing the purity of oil.

oleoresin (ō″lē-ō-rĕz′ĭn) [" + *resina*, resin]. Extract of plant containing resinous substance and oil, prepared by dissolving the crude drug in ether, acetone, or alcohol.

oleosaccharum (ō-lē-ō-săk′ă-rŭm) [" + *saccharum*, sugar]. A substance compounded by sugar and volatile oil.

oleostearate (ō″lē-ō-stē′ăr-āt). A combination of a base with oleic and stearic acids.

oleosus (ō″lē-ō′sŭs) [L.]. Greasy.

oleotherapy (ō″lē-ō-thĕr′ă-pē) [L. *oleum*, oil, + Gr. *therapeia*, treatment]. Therapeutic injection of oil. SYN: *eleotherapy*.

oleothorax (ō-lē-ō-thō′răks) [" + Gr. *thorax*, chest]. Therapeutic injection of oil into the pleural cavity, as in pulmonary tuberculosis.

oleovitamin (ō″lē-ō-vī′tă-mĭn). A vitamin preparation in an edible oil.

   o. A and D. USP. A standardized preparation of vitamins A and D.

oleum (ō′lē-ŭm) [L.] (pl. *olea*). Oil.

   o. morrhuae. Cod liver oil.

   o. olivea. Olive oil.

   o. percomorphum. Mixture of oils from livers of various members of order Percomorphi. More potent in vitamins A and D than cod liver oil.

   o. ricini. Castor oil.

olfactie (ōl-făk′tē). Unit of smell; the threshold of olfactory stimulation determined by the distance at which an odor may be detected.

olfaction (ōl-făk′shŭn) [L. *olfacere*, to smell]. 1. The sense of smell. 2. The act of smelling.

olfactive (ōl-făk′tĭv) [L. *olfacere*, to smell]. Pert. to the sense of smell. SYN: *olfactory*.

olfactology (ōl-făk-tŏl′ō-jē) [" + Gr. *logos*, word, reason]. Scientific investigation of sense of smell.

olfactometer (ōl″făk-tŏm′ĕt-ĕr) [" + Gr. *metron*, measure]. Apparatus for testing the power of the sense of smell.

olfactory (ōl-făk′tō-rē). Pert. to smell.

olfactory area. Area in the hippocampal convolution, the anterior portion of the callosal gyrus and the uncus of the brain. Includes the olfactory bulb, tract, and trigone and is perforated by many blood vessels.

olfactory bulb. Enlarged anterior extremity of the olfactory tract.

olfactory cortex. Portion of the cerebral cortex concerned with the olfactory sense. Includes the pyriform lobe and the hippocampal formation.

olfactory esthesioneuroma. Slowly growing malignant tumor of the nasal fossa, developing from epithelial and neural tissues of the olfactory mucosa.

olfactory lobe. A cranial lobe projecting from the anterior lower part of each cerebral hemisphere.

olfactory membrane. Membrane in the upper part of the nasal cavity that contains olfactory receptors.

olfactory nasal sulcus. An anterior-posterior groove in the wall of the nasal cavity. It passes from the anterior area to the lamina cribrosa.

olfactory nerves. The nerves supplying the nasal olfactory mucosa. Consist of delicate bundles of unmyelinated fibers, the fila olfactoria, that pass through cribriform plate and terminate in olfactory glomeruli of olfactory bulb. The fila are central processes of bipolar receptor neurons of olfactory mucous membrane. SEE: illus.; *cranial nerves*.

olfactory organ. The nose.

olfactory striae. Three bands of fibers (lateral, intermediate, and medial) that form the roots of the olfactory tract.

olfactory tract. Band of fibers that extends posteriorly from the olfactory bulb to the anterior perforated substance. Here it enlarges and divides into the olfactory striae.

olfactory trigone. Small triangular area between lateral and medial olfactory striae.

olfactory tubercle. An elevation at rostral end of anterior perforated substance. Well developed in lower mammals but rudimentary in humans.

oligemia (ōl-ĭg-ē′mē-ă) [Gr. *oligos*, little, + *haima*, blood]. Deficient volume of blood in the body. SYN: *oligohemia*.

oligo-, olig- [Gr. *oligos*, little]. Combining form meaning small or few.

oligoamnios (ōl″ĭ-gō-ăm′nē-ŏs) [" + *amnion*, lamb]. Oligohydramnios, q.v.

oligochylia (ōl″ĭ-gō-kī′lē-ă) [" + *chylos*, juice]. Deficiency of gastric juice.

oligocystic (ōl-ĭ-gō-sĭs′tĭk) [" + *kystis*, a bladder]. Having just a few cysts.

oligodactylia (ōl-ĭ-gō-dăk-tĭl′ē-ă) [" + *daktylos*, digit]. Subnormal number of fingers or toes.

oligodendroblast (ōl″ĭ-gō-dĕn′drō-blăst) [" + Gr. *dendron*, tree, + *blastos*, germ]. A primitive precursor cell of the oligodendrocyte.

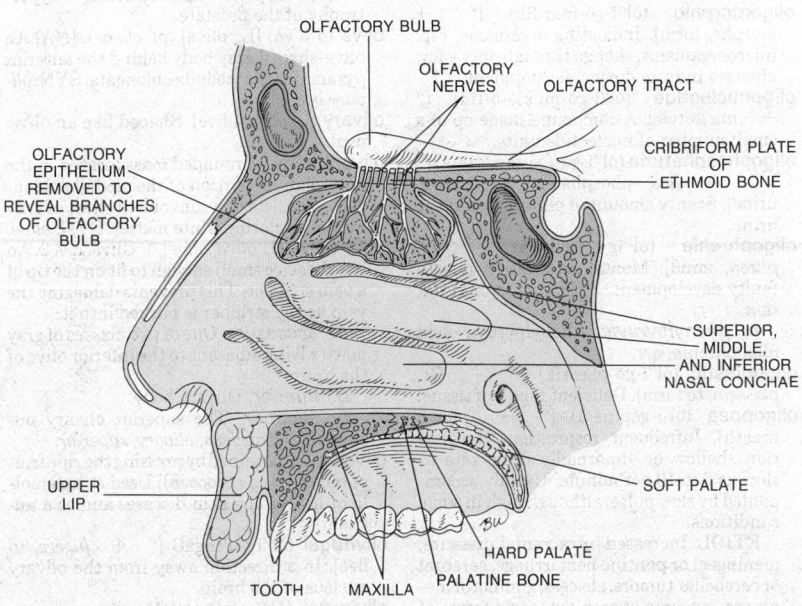

RIGHT OLFACTORY NERVE
(1st CRANIAL)

OLFACTORY BULB

OLFACTORY NERVES

OLFACTORY TRACT

OLFACTORY EPITHELIUM REMOVED TO REVEAL BRANCHES OF OLFACTORY BULB

CRIBRIFORM PLATE OF ETHMOID BONE

SUPERIOR, MIDDLE, AND INFERIOR NASAL CONCHAE

SOFT PALATE

UPPER LIP

HARD PALATE

TOOTH   MAXILLA   PALATINE BONE

oligodendroblastoma (ŏl″ĭ-gō-dĕn″drō-blăs-tō′mă) [″ + ″ + ″ + *oma*, tumor]. A neoplasm derived from oligodendroblasts.

oligodendrocyte [″ + ″ + *kytos*, cell]. Neuroglial cells having few and delicate processes.

oligodendroglia (ŏl″ĭ-gō-dĕn-drŏg′lē-ă) [″ + ″ + *glia*, glue]. The neuroglial cell of ectodermal origin that functions in the central nervous system to form or maintain the myelin sheath of neural processes. The cells have long, slender processes and are often found associated with nerve cells or satellites.

oligodendroglioma (ŏl″ĭ-gō-dĕn″drō-glī-ō′mă) [″ + ″ + ″ + *oma*, tumor]. A malignant tumor occurring principally in the cerebrum, consisting mostly of oligodendrocytes. Frequently calcification occurs. Etiology is unknown.

oligodipsia (ŏl″ĭ-gō-dĭp′sē-ă) [″ + *dipsa*, thirst]. Abnormal absence of desire for fluids.

oligodontia (ŏl″ĭ-gō-dŏn′shē-ă) [″ + *odont*, tooth]. A hereditary developmental anomaly characterized by fewer teeth than normal.

oligodynamic (ŏl″ĭ-gō-dī-năm′ĭk) [″ +

dynamis, power]. Effective in a small quantity.

oligogalactia (ŏl″ĭ-gō-găl-ăk′tē-ă) [″ + *galaktos*, milk]. Deficient milk secretion.

oligohemia (ŏl″ĭ-gō-hē′mē-ă) [″ + *haima*, blood]. Insufficiency in the amount of blood in the body. SYN: *oligemia*.

oligohydramnios (ŏl″ĭg-ō-hī-drăm′nē-ŏs) [″ + *hydor*, water, + *amnion*, amnion]. Abnormally small amount of amniotic fluid. Amount of amniotic fluid may be only 100 to 200 ml. It is associated with fetal renal agenesis or postmaturity. If it occurs early in the pregnancy, the amnion may stick to the fetus, or amniotic bands may form around the extremities with resultant deformities. Fetal hypoxia may occur because of cord compression.

oligolecithal (ŏl″ĭg-gō-lĕs′ĭ-thăl) [″ + *lethikos*, yolk]. Pert. to an egg with a small yolk.

oligoleukocythemia (ŏl″ĭ-gō-lū″kō-sī-thē′mē-ă) [Gr. *oligos*, little, + *leukos*, white, + *kytos*, cell, + *haima*, blood]. Reduction in leukocytic content of blood. SYN: *leukopenia*.

oligomastigate (ŏl″ĭ-gō-măs′tĭ-gāt) [″ + *mastix*, whip]. Characterized by two flagella.

oligomenorrhea (ŏl″ĭ-gō-mĕn″ō-rē′ă) [″

+ *men,* month, + *rhoia,* flow]. Scanty or infrequent menstrual flow.

oligomorphic (ŏl″ĭ-gō-mor′fĭk) [″ + *morphe,* form]. Indicating organisms, esp. microorganisms, that go through only a few changes in form during development.

oligonucleotide (ŏl″ĭ-gō-nū′klē-ō-tīd) [″ + *nucleotide*]. A compound made up of a small number of nucleotide units.

oligophosphaturia (ŏl″ĭ-gō-fŏs-fă-tū′rē-ă) [″ + *phosphas,* phosphate, + *ouron,* urine]. Scanty amount of phosphates in the urine.

oligophrenia (ŏl″ĭg-ō-frē′nē-ă) [″ + *phren,* mind]. Mental retardation due to faulty development. SYN: *mental retardation.*

   o., phenylpyruvic. Phenylpyruvic acid oligophrenia, q.v.

oligoplastic (ŏl″ĭ-gō-plăs′tĭk) [″ + Gr. *plassein,* to form]. Deficient repair of tissue.

oligopnea (ŏl-ĭ-gŏp′nē-ă) [″ + *pnoia,* breath]. Infrequent respiration. Respiration shallow or abnormally deep; rate as slow as 6 to 10 per minute. Usually accompanied by slow pulse, although high in some conditions.

   ETIOL: Increased intracranial pressure, meningeal or pontine hemorrhage, cerebral or cerebellar tumors, abscess, gumma of meninges, osteoma of cranium, some forms of meningitis, trauma of brain, drug poisoning, shock, or constitutional diseases.

oligoptyalism (ŏl-ĭ-gō-tī′ă-lĭzm) [″ + *ptyalon,* saliva]. Insufficient secretion of saliva. SYN: *oligosialia.*

oligosaccharide (ŏl″ĭ-gō-săk′ă-rīd). A compound made up of a small number of monosaccharide units.

oligosialia (ŏl″ĭ-gō-sī-ā′lē-ă) [Gr. *oligos,* little, + *sialon,* saliva]. Scanty salivary secretion. SYN: *oligoptyalism.*

oligospermia (ŏl″ĭ-gō-spĕr′mē-ă) [″ + *sperma,* seed]. Deficient amount of spermatozoa in seminal fluid. It may be temporary or permanent.

oligosynaptic (ŏl″ĭ-gō-sĭn-ăp′tĭk) [″ + Gr. *synapsis,* point of contact]. Nerve conducting pathways involving only a few synapses.

oligotrichia (ŏl″ĭ-gō-trĭk′ē-ă) [″ + *thrix,* hair]. Congenital scantiness of hair.

oligozoospermatism, oligozoospermia (ŏl″ĭ-gō-zō″ō-spĕr′mă-tĭzm, -spĕr′mē-ă). Oligospermia, q.v.

oliguresis (ŏl-ĭg-ū-rē′sĭs) [″ + *ouresis,* urination]. Scantiness of urine or infrequent urination. SYN: *oliguria.*

oliguria (ŏl-ĭg-ū′rē-ă) [″ + *ouron,* urine]. Diminished amount of urine formation.

   ETIOL: Seen after profuse perspiration, bleeding, diarrhea, and renal failure due to any disease. Also in retention of urine due to

disease of the central nervous system, shock, drug poisoning, deep coma, or hypertrophy of the prostate.

oliva (ō-lī′vă) [L., olive] (pl. *olivae*). [NA] An olive-shaped gray body behind the anterior pyramid of the medulla oblongata. SYN: *olivary body.*

olivary [L. *oliva,* olive]. Shaped like an olive; oval.

olivary body. A rounded mass located in the anterolateral portion of the medulla oblongata. Consists of a convoluted sheet of gray matter enclosing white matter. SYN: *oliva.*

olive (ŏl′ĭv) [L. *oliva,* olive]. 1. Oliva, q.v. 2. An ovoid device small enough to fit on the tip of a vein stripper. This prevents damaging the vein as the stripper is pushed into it.

   o., accessory. One of two masses of gray matter lying adjacent to the inferior olive of the brain.

   o., inferior. Olivary body.

   o., superior. The superior olivary nucleus. SEE: *nucleus, olivary, superior.*

olive oil. Oil obtained by pressing the ripe fruit of olives (*Olea europaea*). Used as an emollient in treating skin diseases and as a nutrient.

olivifugal (ŏl″ĭ-vĭf′ū-găl) [″ + *fugere,* to flee]. In a direction away from the olivary nucleus of the brain.

olivipetal (ŏl″ĭ-vĭp′ē-tăl) [″ + *peter,* to seek]. In a direction toward the olivary nucleus of the brain.

olivopontocerebellar (ŏl″ĭ-vō-pŏn″tō-sĕr″ē-bĕl′ăr). Concerning the olivary nucleus, the pons, and the cerebellum of the brain.

Ollier, Louis Xavier Edouard (ŏl″ē-ā′). French surgeon, 1830–1900.

   O.'s disease. Chondrodysplasia, q.v.

   O. layer. The deepest layer of the periosteum closest to the bone. The osteoblasts are in this layer.

   O.- Thiersch graft [Karl Thiersch, Ger. surgeon, 1822–1895]. A split-thickness skin graft that is quite thin.

-ology [Gr. *logos,* word, reason]. Suffix pert. to study of, knowledge of, or science of.

O.L.P. L. *occipitolaeva posterior,* fetal presentation with its occiput toward the left posterior quadrant of the pelvis. SYN: *L.O.P.* SEE: *position.*

olsalazine. A drug used to treat ulcerative colitis. It is esp. useful in treating adult patients who cannot tolerate sulfasalazine. Trade name is Dipentum.

o.m. L. *omni mane,* every morning.

-oma [Gr.]. Suffix denoting a tumor.

omagra (ō-mă′gră) [Gr. *omos,* shoulder, + *agra,* seizure]. Attack of gout in the shoulder.

omalgia (ō-măl′jē-ă) [″ + *algos,* pain]. Neuralgia of the shoulder.

omasitis (ō-mă-sī'tĭs). Inflammation of the omasum, q.v.

omasum (ō-mā'sŭm) [L.]. The third division of a ruminant's stomach.

ombrophobia (ŏm-brō-fō'bē-ă) [Gr. *ombros*, rain, + *phobos*, fear]. Fear and anxiety induced by storms, threatening clouds, or rain.

ombudsman. In medicine, an advocate, esp. for the elderly in a nursing home. A volunteer trained by the state to receive complaints from nursing home residents. The ombudsman verifies complaints and advocates for their resolution.

omega-3 fatty acids (ω3). SEE: *acids, omega-3 fatty.*

omenta (ō-měn'tă) [L.]. Pl. of omentum.

omental (ō-měn'tăl) [L. *omentum*, covering]. Pert. to the omentum, the peritoneal fold supporting the viscera.

omental bursa. A cavity within the layers of peritoneum forming the great omentum. Its opening into the main peritoneal cavity is the epiploic foramen (foramen of Winslow).

omentectomy (ō-měn-těk'tō-mē) [" + Gr. *ektome*, excision]. Surgical removal of a portion of the omentum.

omentitis (ō-měn-tī'tĭs) [" + Gr. *itis*, inflammation]. Inflamed condition of omentum.

omentofixation (ō-měn"tō-fĭk-sā'shŭn). Omentopexy, q.v.

omentopexy (ō-měn'tō-pěks"ē) [" + Gr. *pexis*, fixation]. Fixation of the omentum to the abdominal wall or adjacent organ.

omentoplasty (ō-měn'tō-plăs"tē) [L. *omentum*, covering, + Gr. *plassein*, to form]. Use of tissue from the greater omentum as a graft in rejoining tissues.

omentorrhaphy (ō-měn-tor'ră-fē) [" + Gr. *rhaphe*, seam, ridge]. Suturing of the omentum.

omentosplenopexy (ō-měn"tō-splē'nō-pěks-ē) [" + Gr. *splen*, spleen, + *pexis*, fixation]. Fixation of the spleen and omentum. Combined omentopexy and splenopexy.

omentotomy (ō-měn-tŏt'ō-mē) [" + Gr. *tome*, incision]. Incision of the omentum.

omentovolvulus (ō-měn"tō-vŏl'vū-lŭs) [" + *volvere*, to roll]. Volvulus, i.e., twisting, of the omentum.

omentum (ō-měn'tŭm) [L., a covering] (pl. *omenta*). A double fold of peritoneum attached to the stomach and connecting it with certain of the abdominal viscera. It contains a cavity, the omental bursa (lesser peritoneal cavity). The omenta are the greater or gastrocolic omentum and the lesser or gastrohepatic omentum. SEE: illus.

PALPATION: Infiltration of the omen-

tum by any kind of new growth, either inflammatory or malignant, can be distinguished by the fact that upon palpation the changes found are limited to the omentum and thus do not extend to the posterior portion of the abdominal cavity, but extend across the abdomen, cannot be traced backward, do not ascend behind the ribs, and are rough, hard, and uneven.

RS: abdomen; caul; epiploon; kidney; ovary; spleen.

   o., gastrocolic. O., greater, q.v.

   o., gastrohepatic. O., lesser, q.v.

   o., greater. Portion of the omentum that is suspended from the greater curvature of the stomach and covers the intestines like an apron. It dips in among the folds of the intestines and is attached to the transverse colon and mesocolon. It contains fat, aids in keeping the intestines warm, prevents friction, and aids in localizing infections.

   o., lesser. Portion of the omentum that passes from the lesser curvature of the stomach to the transverse fissure of the liver.

omentumectomy (ō-měn"tŭm-ěk'tō-mē) [" + Gr. *ektome*, excision]. Omentectomy, q.v.

omeprazole. A potent inhibitor of formation of gastric acid. Trade name is Losec.

omitis (ō-mī'tĭs) [Gr. *omos*, shoulder, + *itis*, inflammation]. Inflamed condition of the shoulder.

OML. *orbitomeatal line.*

Ommaya reservoir [A.K. Ommaya, contemporary U.S. neurosurgeon]. A mushroom-shaped reservoir with a self-sealing plastic dome to which a catheter is attached. The device is implanted over the frontal lobe under a skin flap. The catheter is guided through a bur hole in the skull into the lateral ventricle. The reservoir may be implanted for months. It is available for obtaining samples of cerebrospinal fluid (CSF), measuring CSF pressure, and administering drugs intrathecally via the plastic dome.

omn. bih. L. *omni bihora,* every two hours.

omn. hor. L. *omni hora,* every hour.

omni- (ŏm'nĭ) [L. *omnis*]. Prefix designating all.

Omnipen. Trade name for ampicillin, USP.

Omnipen-N. Trade name for ampicillin sodium, USP.

omnipotence of thought. In psychiatry, infantile concept of reality in which one expects all of one's wishes to be instantly accomplished.

Ex: Children who gain their objectives through crying come to believe in their own omnipotence because of a parent's surrender to their demands.

RELATIONSHIP OF GREATER OMENTUM TO ABDOMINAL ORGANS

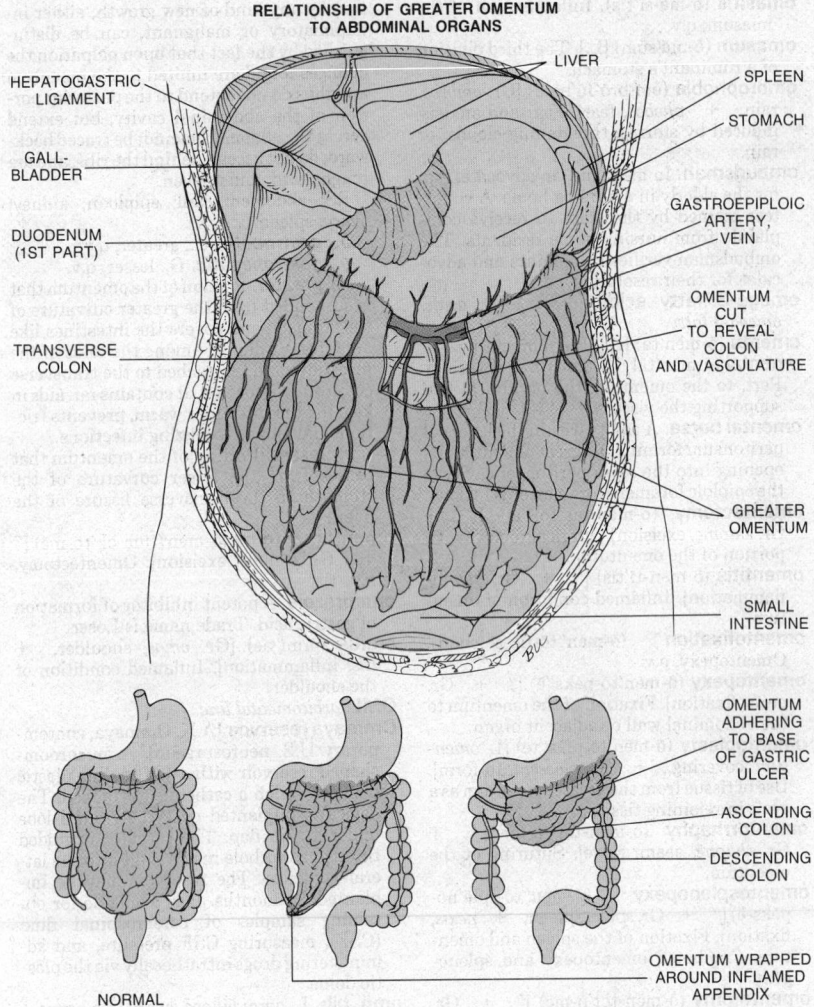

HEPATOGASTRIC LIGAMENT

GALL-BLADDER

DUODENUM (1ST PART)

TRANSVERSE COLON

LIVER

SPLEEN

STOMACH

GASTROEPIPLOIC ARTERY, VEIN

OMENTUM CUT TO REVEAL COLON AND VASCULATURE

GREATER OMENTUM

SMALL INTESTINE

OMENTUM ADHERING TO BASE OF GASTRIC ULCER

ASCENDING COLON

DESCENDING COLON

NORMAL

OMENTUM WRAPPED AROUND INFLAMED APPENDIX

omnivorous (ŏm-nĭv′ō-rŭs) [L. *omnis*, all, + *vorare*, to eat]. Eating both vegetable and animal foods.

omn. noct. L. *omni nocte*, every night.

omn. quad. hor. L. *omni quadrante hora*, every quarter of an hour.

omo- [Gr. *omos*, shoulder]. Combining form pert. to the shoulder.

omoclavicular (ō″mō-klă-vĭk′ū-lăr). Concerning the shoulder and clavicle.

omodynia (ō-mō-dĭn′ē-ă) [Gr. *omos*, shoulder, + *odyne*, pain]. Pain of the shoulder.

omohyoid (ō-mō-hī′oyd). 1. Concerning the scapula and the hyoid bone. 2. Muscle attached to the hyoid bone and the scapula. SEE: *Muscles* in *Appendix*.

omophagia (ō-mō-fā′jē-ă) [Gr. *omos*, raw, + *phagein*, to eat]. The custom of eating raw foods, esp. flesh.

omphal-, omphalo- [Gr. *omphalos*, navel]. Combining form designating relationship to the navel.

omphalectomy (ŏm-făl-ĕk′tō-mē) [″ + *ektome*, excision]. Surgical removal of the umbilicus.

omphalelcosis (ŏm″făl-ĕl-kō′sĭs) [″ + *helkosis*, ulceration]. Ulceration of the umbilicus.

omphalic (ŏm-făl′ĭk) [Gr. *omphalos*, navel]. Concerning the umbilicus.

omphalitis (ŏm-făl-ī′tĭs) [″ + *itis*, inflammation]. Inflamed condition of the navel.

omphaloangiopagus (ŏm″fă-lō-ăn″jē-ŏp′ă-gŭs) [″ + *angeion*, vessel, + *pagos*, thing fixed]. Conjoined twins united by vessels of the umbilical cord.

omphalocele (ŏm-făl′ō-sēl) [″ + *kele*, tumor, swelling]. Congenital hernia of the navel. SEE: *hernia.*

omphalochorion (ŏm″fă-lō-kō′rē-ŏn). A chorion supplied with blood by the omphalomesenteric blood vessels of the yolk sac.

omphalomesenteric (ŏm″făl-ō-mĕs-ĕn-tĕr′ĭk) [″ + *mesenterion*, mesentery]. Concerning the umbilicus and mesentery.

omphaloncus (ŏm″făl-ŏn′kŭs) [″ + *onkos*, tumor]. Umbilical tumor or swelling.

omphalopagus (ŏm″fă-lŏp′ă-gŭs) [″ + *pagos*, thing fixed]. Conjoined twins joined at the abdomen.

omphalophlebitis (ŏm″făl-ō-flē-bī′tĭs) [″ + *phleps*, vein, + *itis*, inflammation]. Inflamed condition of umbilical veins.

omphalorrhagia (ŏm″făl-ō-rā′jē-ă) [″ + *rhegnynai*, to burst forth]. Umbilical hemorrhage.

omphalorrhea (ŏm″făl-ō-rē′ă) [″ + *rhoia*, flow]. Discharge of lymph at the navel.

omphalorrhexis (ŏm″făl-ō-rĕk′sĭs) [″ + *rhexis*, rupture]. Rupture of the navel.

omphalos (ŏm′făl-ŏs) [Gr.]. Umbilicus. SYN: *navel.*

omphalosite (ŏm″fă-lō-sīt″) [″ + *sitos*, food]. The underdeveloped twin of the omphaloangiopagus twins.

omphalospinous (ŏm″făl-ō-spī′nŭs) [″ + L. *spina*, thorn]. Concerning the navel and the anterior superior spine of the ilium.

omphalotomy (ŏm-făl-ŏt′ō-mē) [″ + *tome*, incision]. Division of umbilical cord at birth.

omphalotripsy (ŏm″făl-ō-trĭp′sē) [″ + *tripsis*, a rubbing]. Severing of the umbilical cord by a crushing method.

omphalus (ŏm′fă-lŭs) [Gr. *omphalos*]. The navel.

ON. *orthopedic nurse.*

o.n. L. *omni nocte*, every night.

onanism (ō′năn-ĭzm) [So named because it was practiced by the Biblical character Onan, son of Judah]. Coitus interruptus; withdrawal before ejaculation. Term was previously used erroneously to designate masturbation, q.v.

onanist (ō′nă-nĭst). One who practices coitus interruptus. Erroneously used to indicate one who masturbates.

Onanoff's reflex (ŏn-ă-nŏfs′) [Jacques Onanoff, Fr. physician, b. 1859]. Contraction of bulbocavernous muscle resulting from compression of glans penis.

Onchocerca (ŏng″kō-sĕr′kă) [Gr. *onkos*, hook, + *kerkos*, tail]. A genus of filarial worms. They live in subcutaneous and connective tissues and usually are enclosed in fibrous cysts or nodules.

   O. volvulus. A species of *Onchocerca* that infests humans, frequently invading the tissues of the eye. Transmitted by species of the black fly *Simulium* and *Eusimulium.*

onchocerciasis (ŏng″kō-sĕr-kī′ă-sĭs) [″ + *iasis*, infestation]. Condition produced by infestation with one of the filarial worms of the genus *Onchocerca.* It is characterized by a nodular swelling over the coiled parasite. The microfilariae present in the nodules eventually affect the eye and cause blindness.

   The disease is spread by the bites of black flies of the genus *Simulium.* In some areas of Africa, half or more of the middle-aged men are blind from this disease. The men, working in fields, are exposed more than women, who are working at home. SYN: *river blindness.*

   TREAT: Ivermectin.

onco- [Gr. *onkos*, bulk, mass]. Combining form pert. to a tumor, swelling, or mass.

Oncocerca. *Onchocerca.*

oncocercosis. Onchocerciasis.

oncocyte (ŏn′kō-sīt) [″ + *kytos*, cell]. A large columnar cell with granular, acidophilic cytoplasm and a large number of mitochondria. They may become neoplastic.

oncocytoma (ŏng″kō-sī-tō′mă) [″ + ″ + *oma*, tumor]. A benign adenoma composed of eosinophilic epithelial cells, esp. one of the salivary or parathyroid glands.

oncofetal (ŏng″kō-fē′tăl). Concerning tumors in the fetus.

oncogene (ŏng′kō-jēn) [″ + *gennan*, to produce]. A gene in a virus that has the ability to induce a cell to become malignant. Oncogenes have been identified in human tumors. In addition to genes that can induce tumor formation, there are anti-oncogenes that suppress tumors.

oncogenesis (ŏng″kō-jĕn′ĕ-sĭs) [″ + *genesis*, generation, birth]. Tumor formation and development.

oncogenic (ŏng″kō-jĕn′ĭk). Giving rise to tumors, esp. malignant tumors.

oncogenic virus. Virus that produces tumors. Although there is a relationship between viruses and human cancer, their exact role is not fully understood.

oncograph (ŏng′kō-grăf) [Gr. *onkos*, bulk,

mass, + *graphein*, to write]. Device attached to oncometer for recording the size and configuration of internal organs.

oncoides (ŏng-koy′dēz) [″ + *eidos*, form, shape]. Turgescence.

oncologist [Gr. *onkos*, bulk, + *logos*, word]. A scientist who specializes in oncology.

oncology (ŏng-kŏl′ō-jē) [″ + *logos*, word, reason]. The branch of medicine dealing with tumors.

oncolysis (ŏng-kŏl′ĭ-sĭs) [″ + *lysis*, dissolution]. The absorption or dissolution of tumor cells.

oncolytic (ŏng″kō-lĭt′ĭk). Destructive to tumor cells.

oncometer (ŏng-kŏm′ĕt-ĕr) [″ + *metron*, measure]. Apparatus for measurement of variations in size of internal organs. SEE: *plethysmograph*.

oncometric (ŏng″kō-mĕt′rĭk). Pert. to oncometry.

oncometry. The measurement of variations in size of internal organs.

oncornaviruses. A group of RNA viruses that can cause cancer in humans or animals.

oncosis (ŏng-kō′sĭs) [″ + *osis*, condition]. 1. A condition characterized by the development of tumors. 2. A swelling or tumor.

oncosphere (ŏng′kō-sfēr) [″ + *sphaira*, sphere]. Embryonic stage of a tapeworm in which it has hooks.

oncotherapy (ŏng″kō-thĕr′ă-pē) [″ + *therapeia*, treatment]. Treatment of tumors.

oncothlipsis (ŏng″kō-thlĭp′sĭs) [″ + *thlipsis*, pressure]. Pressure caused by presence of a tumor.

oncotic (ŏng-kŏt′ĭk) [Gr. *onkos*, bulk, mass]. Concerning, caused, or marked by swelling.

oncotic pressure, colloidal. The total influence of the protein on the osmotic activity of plasma water.

oncotomy (ŏng-kŏt′ō-mē) [″ + *tome*, incision]. The incision of a tumor, abscess, or boil.

oncotropic (ŏng″kō-trŏp′ĭk) [″ + *tropos*, a turning]. Possessing special attraction for tumor cells.

Oncovin. Trade name for vincristine sulfate, USP.

oncovirus (ŏn′kō-vī″rŭs) [″ + *virus*]. Any virus that causes malignant neoplasms.

Ondine's curse [Fr. Undine, mythical water nymph whose human lover was cursed to continuous sleep]. 1. Primary alveolar hypoventilation due to reduced responsiveness of the respiratory center to carbon dioxide. 2. Loss of automatic respiratory function due to a lesion in the cervical portion of the spinal cord.

oneir(o)- (ō-nī′rō) [Gr. *oneiros*, dream]. Combining form indicating or concerning dreams.

oneiric (ō-nī′rĭk) [Gr. *oneiros*, dream]. Resembling, rel. to, or accompanied by dreams.

oneirism (ō-nī′rĭzm) [″ + *-ismos*, state of]. Dreamlike hallucination in a waking state.

oneirodynia (ō-nī″rō-dĭn′ē-ă) [″ + *odyne*, pain]. Painful dreaming; nightmare.

oneirogmus (ō″nī-rŏg′mŭs) [Gr. *oneirogmos*, an effusion during sleep]. Emission of semen during an erotic dream. SYN: *wet dream*.

oneirology (ō″nī-rŏl′ō-jē) [Gr. *oneiros*, dream, + *logos*, word, reason]. The scientific study of dreams.

oniomania (ō″nē-ō-mā′nē-ă) [Gr. *onios*, for sale, + *mania*, madness]. A psychoneurotic urge to spend money.

onion (ŭn′yŭn) [AS. *oignon*]. The edible bulb of the onion plant, cultivated as a vegetable. Latin name for the common onion is *Allium cepa*. The characteristic odor of onions is due to several volatile chemicals, some of which contain sulfur. The ability of onions to cause persons who peel them to shed tears is probably caused by the chemical propanethial S-oxide. When this material comes in contact with tears, sulfuric acid is formed.

onkinocele (ŏng-kin′ō-sēl) [Gr. *onkos*, bulk, mass, + *inos*, fiber, + *kele*, tumor, swelling]. Inflammation with swelling of a tendon sheath.

onlay. 1. A graft applied to the surface of a tissue, esp. a bone graft applied to bone. 2. In dentistry, a cast metal restoration that overlays the cusps of the tooth, thereby providing additional strength to the restored tooth.

onomatology (ŏn″ō-mă-tŏl′ō-jē) [Gr. *onoma*, name, + *logos*, word, reason]. Science of names. SYN: *nomenclature; terminology*.

onomatomania (ŏn″ō-mă″tō-mā′nē-ă) [″ + *mania*, madness]. A mental illness characterized by an abnormal impulse to dwell upon or repeat certain words by attaching significance to their imagined hidden meanings or by trying frantically to recall a particular word.

onomatophobia (ŏn″ō-mă″tō-fō′bē-ă) [″ + *phobos*, fear]. Abnormal fear of hearing a certain name or word because of an imaginary dreadful meaning attached to it.

onomatopoiesis (ŏn″ō-mă″tō-poy-ē′sĭs) [Gr. *onoma*, name, + *poiein*, to make]. In psychiatry, created, usually meaningless, imitative words and sounds formed by the psychotic.

ontogenesis (ŏn″tō-jĕn′ē-sĭs). Ontogeny.

ontogenetic (ŏn″tō-jĕ-nĕt′ĭk). Concerning ontogeny.

ontogeny (ŏn-tŏj′ĕn-ē) [Gr. *on*, being, + *gennan*, to produce]. The history of the development of an individual. SYN: *ontogene-*

sis.

onych(o)- [Gr. *onyx,* nail]. Combining form indicating a relationship to fingernails or toenails.

onychalgia (ŏn″ĭ-kăl′jē-ă) [″ + *algos,* pain]. Pain in the nails.

o. nervosa. Extreme sensitivity of nails.

onychatrophia (ŏ″nĭk-ă-trō′fē-ă) [″ + *trophe,* nourishment]. Atrophy of the nails.

onychauxis (ŏn″ĭ-kawk′sĭs) [″ + *auxein,* to increase]. Overgrowth of the nails.

onychectomy (ŏn″ĭ-kĕk′tō-mē) [″ + *ektome,* to cut]. Surgical removal of the nail of a finger or toe.

onychia (ō-nĭk′ē-ă) [Gr. *onyx,* nail]. Inflammation of the nailbed with suppuration and frequently loss of the nail. SYN: *matrixitis; onychitis; onyxitis.* SEE: *paronychia.*

o. craquele. Fragility of nails.

o. lateralis. Suppuration of tissues in the area lateral to the fingernail. SYN: *paronychia.*

o. maligna. Type of onychia in debilitated persons in which there is fetid ulceration and loss of the nail.

o. parasitica. Any parasitic disease of the nails. SYN: *onychomycosis.*

o., piannic. Hyperkeratotic plaques that occur in the periungual region and cause deformities of the nail fold. ETIOL: Yaws.

o. punctata. Condition in which a nail possesses small punctiform depressions.

onychitis (ŏn″ĭ-kī′tĭs) [″ + *itis,* inflammation]. Inflammation of the nailbed. SYN: *onychia.*

onychocryptosis (ŏn″ĭ-kō-krĭp-tō′sĭs) [″ + *kryptein,* to conceal]. Ingrowing of the toenail.

onychodystrophy (ŏn″ĭ-kō-dĭs′trō-fē) [″ + *dys,* bad, + *trophe,* nutrition]. Any maldevelopment of a nail.

onychogenic (ŏn″ĭ-kō-jĕn′ĭk) [″ + *gennan,* to produce]. Concerning nail formation.

onychograph (ŏn-ĭk′ō-grăf) [″ + *graphein,* to write]. Device for making record of capillary blood pressure under the fingernails.

onychogryposis (ŏn″ĭ-kō-grĭ-pō′sĭs) [″ + *gryposis,* a curving]. Abnormal overgrowth of the nails with inward curvature.

onychoheterotopia (ŏn″ĭ-kō-hĕt″ĕr-ō-tō′pē-ă) [″ + *heteros,* other, + *topos,* place]. Abnormally located nails.

onychoid (ŏn′ĭ-koyd) [″ + *eidos,* form, shape]. Similar to a nail, esp. a fingernail.

onycholysis (ŏn″ĭ-kŏl′ĭ-sĭs) [″ + *lysis,* dissolution]. Loosening or detachment of the nail from the nailbed. SEE: *photo-onycholysis.*

onychoma (ŏn-ĭ-kō′mă) [″ + *oma,* tumor].

Tumor of the nail or nailbed.

onychomadesis (ŏn″ĭ-kō-mă-dē′sĭs) [Gr. *onyx,* nail, + *madesis,* loss of hair]. Complete loss of nails.

onychomalacia (ŏn″ĭ-kō-mă-lă′sē-ă) [″ + *malakia,* softening]. Abnormal softening of the nails. SYN: *hapalonychia.*

onychomycosis (ŏn″ĭ-kō-mī-kō′sĭs) [″ + *mykes,* fungus, + *osis,* condition]. Disease of the nails due to a parasitic fungus.

onycho-osteodysplasia (ŏn″ĭ-kō-ŏs″tē-ō-dĭs-plā′zē-ă). A genetic disease involving ectodermal and mesodermal tissues. The nails and patellae may be absent, and other bones and joints are affected. SYN: *nail-patella syndrome.*

onychopathology (ŏn″ĭ-kō-pă-thŏl′ō-jē) [″ + *pathos,* disease, suffering, + *logos,* word, reason]. Study of diseases of the nails.

onychopathy (ŏn-ĭ-kŏp′ăth-ē) [″ + *pathos,* disease, suffering]. Any disease of the nails. SYN: *onychosis.*

onychophagy (ŏn-ĭ-kŏf′ă-jē) [″ + *phagein,* to eat]. The practice of nail biting.

onychophosis (ŏn″ĭk-ō-fō′sĭs). Accumulation of horny layers of epidermis under the toenail.

onychophyma (ŏn″ĭ-kō-fī′mă) [″ + *phyma,* a growth]. Painful degeneration of the nail with hypertrophy.

onychoptosis (ŏn″ĭk-ŏp-tō′sĭs) [″ + *ptosis,* a dropping]. Dropping off of the nails.

onychorrhexis (ŏn″ĭ-kō-rĕk′sĭs) [″ + *rhexis,* a rupture]. Abnormal brittleness and nail splitting. SYN: *fragilitas unguium.*

onychoschizia (ŏn″ĭ-kō-skĭz′ē-ă) [″ + *schizein,* to split]. Loosening and eventual separation of the nail from its bed.

onychosis (ŏn-ĭ-kō′sĭs) [″ + *osis,* disease]. Any diseased condition of the nails. SYN: *onychopathy.*

onychotillomania (ŏn″ĭ-kō-tĭl″ō-mā′nē-ă) [″ + *tillein,* to pluck, + *mania,* insanity]. A neurotic tendency to pick the nails.

onychotomy (ŏn″ĭ-kŏt′ō-mē) [″ + *tome,* incision]. Surgical incision of a fingernail or toenail.

onychotrophy (ŏn-ĭ-kŏt′rō-fē) [″ + *trophe,* nourishment]. Nourishment of the nails.

onyx (ŏn′ĭks) [Gr., nail]. 1. A fingernail or toenail. 2. Pus collection between the corneal layers of the eye. SYN: *hypopyon.*

onyxis (ō-nĭk′sĭs). Ingrowing of the nails.

onyxitis (ŏn-ĭk-sī′tĭs) [Gr. *onyx,* nail, + *itis,* inflammation]. Onychia.

oo- (ō-ō) [Gr. *oon,* egg]. Combining form denoting an egg or the primordial cell that develops into an ovule. SEE: words beginning with *ovo-.*

ooblast (ō′ō-blăst) [″ + *blastos,* germ]. The primitive cell from which the ovum is developed.

oocyesis (ō″ō-sī-ē′sĭs) [″ + *kyesis*, pregnancy]. Ectopic pregnancy in the ovary.

oocyst (ō′ō-sĭst) [Gr. *oon*, egg, + *kystis*, bladder]. The encysted form of a fertilized gamete (zygote) occurring in certain sporozoa. SEE: *ookinete*.

oocyte (ō′ō-sīt) [″ + *kytos*, cell]. The early or primitive ovum before it has developed completely.

   o., primary. Oocyte at end of growth period of oogonium and before first maturation division has occurred.

   o., secondary. The larger of two oocytes resulting from first maturation division. SEE: *body, polar.*

oogenesis (ō″ō-jĕn′ĕ-sĭs) [″ + *genesis*, generation, birth]. Formation and development of the ovum. SYN: *ovigenesis.*

oogenetic (ō″ō-jĕ-nĕt′ĭk). Concerning oogenesis.

oogonium (ō″ō-gō′nē-ŭm) [″ + *gone*, seed] (pl. *oogonia*). 1. The primordial cell from which an oocyte originates. 2. Descendant of the primordial cell from which the oocyte arises.

ookinesis (ō″ō-kĭn-ē′sĭs) [″ + *kinesis*, movement]. Mitotic phenomena taking place within an ovum during maturation and fertilization.

ookinete (ō″ō-kī-nēt′) [″ + *kinetos*, motile]. An elongated motile zygote occurring in the life cycle of certain sporozoan parasites, esp. those of the genus *Plasmodium*. It penetrates the stomach wall of a mosquito and gives rise to an oocyst.

oolemma (ō″ō-lĕm′ă) [″ + *lemma*, sheath]. The plasma membrane of the oocyte.

oophagy (ō-ŏf′ă-jē) [″ + *phagein*, to eat]. Eating of eggs.

oophor- [Gr. *oophoros*, bearing eggs]. Combining form pert. to the ovary.

oophoralgia (ō″ŏf-ō-răl′jē-ă) [″ + *algos*, pain]. Pain in an ovary. SYN: *oarialgia; ovarialgia.*

oophorauxe (ō″ŏf-ō-rawks′ē) [″ + *auxein*, to increase]. Ovarian enlargement.

oophorectomy (ō″ŏf-ō-rĕk′tō-mē) [″ + *ektome*, excision]. Excision of an ovary. SYN: *ovariectomy.*

oophoritis (ō″ŏf-ō-rī′tĭs) [″ + *itis*, inflammation]. Inflamed condition of the ovary. SYN: *ovaritis.*

   o., follicular. Inflammation of the graafian follicles.

oophorocystectomy (ō-ŏf″ō-rō-sĭs-tĕk′tō-mē) [″ + *kystis*, cyst, + *ektome*, excision]. Surgical removal of an ovarian cyst.

oophorocystosis (ō-ŏf″ō-rō-sĭs-tō′sĭs) [Gr. *oophoros*, bearing eggs, + *kystis*, cyst, + *osis*, condition]. Development of an ovarian cyst.

oophorohysterectomy (ō-ŏf″ō-rō-hĭs″tĕr-ĕk′tō-mē) [″ + *hystera*, womb, + *ektome*, excision]. Surgical removal of the uterus and ovaries. SYN: *oothecohysterectomy; ovariohysterectomy.*

oophoroma (ō-ŏf″ō-rō′mă) [″ + *oma*, tumor]. Malignant ovarian tumor.

oophoron (ō-ŏf′ō-rŏn) [Gr. *oophoros*, bearing eggs]. An ovary. SYN: *ootheca.*

oophoropathy (ō-ŏf″or-ŏp′ă-thē) [″ + *pathos*, disease, suffering]. Any pathological condition of the ovary.

oophoropeliopexy (ō-ŏf″ō-rō-pē′lē-ō-pĕk″sē) [″ + *pellis*, pelvis, + *pexis*, fixation]. Suture of a displaced ovary to the pelvic wall.

oophoropexy (ō-ŏf″ō-rō-pĕk′sē) [″ + *pexis*, fixation]. Fixation of a displaced ovary. SYN: *oophoropeliopexy.*

oophoroplasty (ō-ŏf″ō-rō-plăs″tē) [″ + *plassein*, to form]. Plastic surgery on the ovary.

oophorosalpingectomy (ō-ŏf″ō-rō-săl-pĭn-jĕk′tō-mē) [″ + *salpinx*, tube, + *ektome*, excision]. Excision of an oviduct and ovary. SYN: *ovariosalpingectomy.*

oophorosalpingitis (ō-ŏf″or-ō-săl″pĭn-jī′tĭs) [″ + ″ + *itis*, inflammation]. Inflammation of the ovary and oviduct.

oophorostomy (ō-ŏf″ō-rŏs′tō-mē) [″ + *stoma*, mouth]. Creation of an artificial opening into the ovarian cyst for drainage.

oophorotomy (ō-ŏf″ō-rŏt′ō-mē) [″ + *tome*, incision]. Surgical incision of the ovary.

oophorrhagia (ō″ŏf-ō-rā′jē-ă) [″ + *rhegnynai*, to burst forth]. Hemorrhage from an ovulatory site severe enough to cause clinical symptoms or signs.

oophorrhaphy (ō-ŏf-or′ă-fē) [″ + *rhaphe*, seam, ridge]. Suture of a displaced ovary to the pelvic wall.

ooplasm (ō′ō-plăzm) [Gr. *oon*, egg, + LL. *plasma*, form, mold]. The cytoplasm of an ovum.

oosperm (ō′ō-spĕrm) [″ + *sperma*, seed]. Cell formed by union of the spermatozoon with the ovum; the fertilized ovum. SYN: *zygote.*

oosporangium (ō″ō-spō-răn′jē-ŭm). The female portion in the sexual formation of oospores.

oospore (ō′ō-spor) [″ + *sporos*, seed]. Spore formed by the union of opposite sexual elements.

ootheca (ō-ō-thē′kă) [Gr. *ootheke*, ovary]. An ovary. SYN: *oophoron.*

oothecohysterectomy (ō-ō-thē″kō-hĭs″tĕr-ĕk′tō-mē) [Gr. *ootheke*, ovary, + *hystera*, womb, + *ektome*, excision]. Excision of the uterus and ovaries. SYN: *oophorohys-*

terectomy; ovariohysterectomy.

ootid (ō'ō-tĭd). The ripe ovum after first maturation has been completed and the second has begun.

OP. *operative procedure; outpatient.*

O.P. *occiput position.*

opacification (ō-păs"ĭ-fĭ-kā'shŭn) [L. *opacitas,* shadiness, + *facere,* to make]. 1. Process of making something opaque. 2. Formation of opacities.

opacity (ō-păs'ĭ-tē) [L. *opacitas,* shadiness]. 1. State of being opaque. 2. An opaque area or spot. 3. The ratio of incident light to transmitted light in a specific area or a radiograph.

opalescent (ō"păl-ĕs'ĕnt). Similar to an opal with respect to colors produced.

opaque (ō-pāk') [L. *opacus,* dark]. 1. Impenetrable by visible light rays or by other forms of radiant energy such as x-rays. 2. Not transparent. 3. Dense or slow to learn.

OPC. *outpatient clinic.*

OPD. *outpatient department.*

open [AS.]. 1. Not shut. 2. Uncovered, exposed, as a wound to air. 3. To puncture, as to open a boil. 4. Interrupted, as in an electric circuit when current cannot pass because a switch is open.

open heart surgery. Surgery involving the heart, either the myocardium itself, the coronary arteries, or the heart valves. The term open refers to the chest, not to the heart itself.

opening. 1. A hole or aperture or the entrance to a hole. 2. An open space that serves as an entrance to a tissue or organ. 3. The act of becoming open.

    o., aortic. Opening in the diaphragm through which the aorta passes.

    o., cardiac. Opening of the esophagus into the cardiac end of the stomach.

    o., pyloric. Opening between the stomach and duodenum.

open-label study. An experimental study involving the use of a medicine, the identity of which is known to the patient.

open reduction. In orthopedics, realigning the fractured segments after incising the skin and tissues in order to expose the fractured bone. SEE: *reduction of fractures, closed.*

operable (ŏp'ĕr-ă-bl) [L. *operor,* to work]. 1. Practicable. 2. Admitting of treatment by surgery with reasonable expectation of cure.

operant. Producing effects.

operant conditioning. Conditioning or influencing behavior by rewarding an individual for certain forms of behavior. This reward, also called reinforcement, induces the person to act in such a way as to receive the award.

operate (ŏp'ĕr-āt) [L. *operatus,* worked]. 1. To

perform an excision or incision, or to make a suture on the body or any of its organs or parts to restore health. 2. To produce an effect, as a drug.

operation (ŏp-ĕr-ā'shŭn) [L. *operatio,* a working]. 1. The act of operating. 2. A surgical procedure. 3. The effect or method of action of any type of therapy. SEE: *surgery.*

    Preoperative shaving of the skin over the surgical site may be unnecessary insofar as bacterial considerations are concerned; nevertheless, it is still utilized in order to facilitate access to the operative site.

    o., ablative. Operation in which a part is removed.

    o., cosmetic. Operation for the purpose of improving the appearance of some part of the body.

    o., exploratory. Operation performed for diagnostic purposes.

    o., flap. Surgical procedure in which a flap of tissue or periosteum is raised. An amputation flap is a tissue flap produced to cover the amputation stump.

    o., major. Operation involving a considerable hazard to the patient.

    o., minor. Operation not serious or risking life.

    o., plastic. Operation for reconstruction and repair of surface and other structures.

    o., radical. Operation performed to remove a large amount of damaged or neoplastic tissue.

    o., reconstructive. Operation to repair a loss or defect.

    o., second-look. Surgery some months or as much as a year after the original operation for cancer. The second look is to detect recurrences, if any.

    o., subtotal. Operation in which only a portion of the organ is removed, as subtotal removal of the thyroid gland.

operative (ŏp'ĕr-ă-tĭv) [L. *operativus,* working]. 1. Effective, active. 2. Pert. to or brought about by an operation.

operative dentistry. The area of dentistry concerned with operations to restore or replace the hard dental tissues by silver amalgam, gold, porcelain, or a variety of plastic dental materials. Such operations are necessitated by caries, trauma, or malocclusions. SYN: *restorative dentistry.*

opercular (ō-pĕr'kū-lär) [L. *operculum,* a cover]. Concerning a covering structure.

operculitis (ō-pĕr"kū-lī'tĭs) [" + Gr. *itis,* inflammation]. Inflammation of the gingiva over a partially erupted tooth.

operculum (ō-pĕr'kū-lŭm) [L., a cover] (pl. *opercula*). 1. Any covering. 2. Plug of mucus that fills up the opening of the cervix upon impregnation. 3. [NA] Convolutions of the cerebrum, the margins of which are separated by the lateral cerebral (sylvian) fissure. The opercula cover the insula.

   o., dental. The soft tissue overlying the crown of a partially erupted tooth.

   o., trophoblastic. The plug of fibrin that covers the opening in the endometrium made by the implanting ovum.

operon (ŏp′ĕr-ŏn). In genetics, a group of linked genes and regulatory elements that functions as a unit of transcription.

ophiasis (ō-fī′ă-sĭs) [Gr. *ophis*, snake]. Baldness occurring in winding streaks across the head.

ophidiasis (ō-fī-dī′ă-sĭs). Ophidism, q.v.

ophidiophobia (ō-fĭd″ē-ō-fō′bē-ă) [Gr. *ophidion*, snake, + *phobos*, fear]. Abnormal fear of snakes.

ophidism (ō′fĭd-ĭzm) [″ + *-ismos*, condition]. Poisoning from snake bite.

ophiotoxemia (ō″fē-ō-tŏk-sē′mē-ă) [″ + *toxikon*, poison, + *haima*, blood]. Poisoning due to venom injected by a snake.

ophritis, ophryitis (ŏf-rī′tĭs, -rē-ī′tĭs) [Gr. *ophrys*, eyebrow, + *itis*, inflammation]. Inflammation of the eyebrow.

ophryon (ŏf′rē-ŏn). Meeting point of the facial median line with a transverse line across the forehead's narrowest portion.

ophryosis (ŏf″rē-ō′sĭs) [″ + *osis*, condition]. Eyebrow spasm.

Ophthaine. Trade name for proparacaine hydrochloride, USP.

Ophthalgan. Trade name for glycerin, USP.

ophthalmagra (ŏf″thăl-măg′ră) [Gr. *ophthalmos*, eye, + *agra*, seizure]. Sudden development of eye pain.

ophthalmalgia (ŏf″thăl-măl′jē-ă) [″ + *algos*, pain]. Pain in the eye. SYN: *ophthalmodynia.*

ophthalmatrophy (ŏf-thăl-măt′rō-fē) [″ + *atrophia*, a wasting]. Atrophy of eyeball.

ophthalmectomy (ŏf-thăl-mĕk′tō-mē) [″ + *ektome*, excision]. Surgical excision of an eye.

ophthalmencephalon (ŏf″thăl-mĕn-sĕf′ă-lŏn) [″ + *enkephalos*, brain]. The vision apparatus from the retina, to the optic nerves, optic chiasm, optic tract, and the visual centers of the brain.

ophthalmia (ŏf-thăl′mē-ă) [Gr. *ophthalmos*, eye]. Severe inflammation of the eye, usually including the conjunctiva.

   o., catarrhal. Conjunctivitis of a severe, frequently purulent, form.

   o., Egyptian. Granular conjunctivitis. SYN: *trachoma.*

   o., electric. Ophthalmia marked by pain in the eye, intolerance to light, and tearing (lacrimation). Occurs following exposure, usually prolonged, to intense light such as that in arc welding.

   o., gonorrheal. Severe purulent conjunctivitis due to infection with gonococcus.

   o., granular. Severe purulent conjunctivitis with formation of granules on the eyelids. SYN: *trachoma.*

   o., metastatic. Sympathetic inflammation of the choroid due to pyemia or metastasis.

   o. neonatorum. Severe purulent conjunctivitis in the newborn.

   ETIOL: Infection of the birth canal at the time of delivery. *Neisseria gonorrhoeae* and *Chlamydia trachomatis* are responsible for the great majority of cases. Symptoms present 12 to 48 hours after birth when due to gonorrhea; and one week or more after birth for chlamydia infections.

   PROPHYLAXIS: Introduction of two drops of a 1% silver nitrate solution into each eye of a newborn at birth for infections with gonococcal organisms. For chlamydial infections, systemic erythromycin for 3 weeks. SEE: *Credé's method* (def. 2).

   o., neuroparalytic. Ophthalmia resulting from injury or disease involving semilunar ganglion or branches of the trigeminal nerve supplying eyeball.

   o., phlyctenular. Vesicular formations on epithelium of conjunctiva or cornea. SYN: *o., scrofulous.*

   o., purulent. Purulent inflammation of eye, usually due to gonococcus.

   o., scrofulous. O., phlyctenular.

   o., spring. Conjunctivitis in the spring of the year, usually an allergic reaction to pollen. SYN: *conjunctivitis, vernal.*

   o., sympathetic. Rare bilateral granulomatous inflammation of the entire uveal tract of both eyes. Occurs in the untraumatized eye following perforation of the globe of the other eye.

   SYM: Photophobia, lacrimation, pain, blurring of vision, eyeball tenderness, deposits on posterior surface of cornea. Exudate appears in pupillary area with posterior synechia, seclusio pupillae, secondary atrophy with blindness.

   TREAT: Mydriatics, analgesics, steroids, other anti-inflammatory therapy. Sympathetic ophthalmia does not occur immediately following injury; thus it is not necessary to remove the injured eye as an emergency procedure.

   o., varicose. Ophthalmia seen in varicose veins of the conjunctiva.

ophthalmiatrics (ŏf″thăl-mē-ăt′rĭks) [″ + *iatreia*, treatment]. The treatment of eye diseases.

ophthalmic (ŏf-thăl′mĭk). Pert. to the eye.

ophthalmic nerve. A branch of the trigeminal (5th cranial) nerve. It is sensory and its branches are the lacrimal, frontal, and nasociliary.

ophthalmic reaction. Reaction of the eye following instillation into the eye of toxins of typhoid or tuberculosis. SYN: *Calmette's reaction; oculoreaction; ophthalmoreaction.*

ophthalmitis (ŏf″thăl-mī′tĭs) [″ + *itis,* inflammation]. Inflamed condition of the eye.

ophthalmo- [Gr. *ophthalmos,* eye]. Combining form pert. to the eye.

ophthalmoblennorrhea (ŏf-thăl″mō-blĕn″ō-rē′ă) [″ + *blenna,* mucus, + *rhoia,* flow]. Purulent inflammation of the eye or conjunctiva, usually due to gonococcus.

ophthalmocele (ŏf-thăl′mō-sēl) [″ + *kele,* tumor, swelling]. Abnormal protrusion of the eyeballs. SYN: *exophthalmos.*

ophthalmocopia (ŏf-thăl″mō-kō′pē-ă) [″ + *kopos,* fatigue]. Ocular fatigue; eyestrain. SYN: *asthenopia.*

ophthalmodesmitis (ŏf-thăl″mō-dĕs-mī′tĭs) [″ + *desmos,* ligament, + *itis,* inflammation]. Inflammation of tendons of the eye.

ophthalmodiagnosis (ŏf-thăl″mō-dī″ăg-nō′sĭs) [″ + *dia,* through, + *gnosis,* knowledge]. Diagnosis of eye conditions by means of the ophthalmoreaction, q.v.

ophthalmodiaphanoscope (ŏf-thăl″mō-dī-ă-făn′ō-skōp) [″ + ″ + *phainein,* to appear, + *skopein,* to examine]. Device for examining the retina by transillumination, the source of which may be a light in the oral cavity.

ophthalmodonesis (ŏf-thăl″mō-dō-nē′sĭs) [″ + *donesis,* trembling]. Tremor or oscillatory movement of the eye.

ophthalmodynamometer (ŏf-thăl″mō-dī″nă-mŏm′ĕ-tĕr) [″ + *dynamis,* power, + *metron,* measure]. Instrument for determining pressure in ophthalmic arteries. Device is placed against conjunctiva of eye. If pressure is higher on one side than the other, appropriate studies to attempt to define the cause are indicated.

ophthalmodynamometry (ŏf-thăl″mō-dī″nă-mŏm′ĕ-trē). Determination of pressure in the ophthalmic artery by use of an instrument that produces pressure on the eyeball until pulsations in the ophthalmic artery are seen through the ophthalmoscope. That pressure is diastolic. As the pressure is increased, the vessel collapses; this is systolic pressure.

ophthalmodynia (ŏf-thăl″mō-dĭn′ē-ă) [″ + *odyne,* pain]. Pain in the eye. SYN: *ophthalmalgia.*

ophthalmoeikonometer (ŏf-thăl″mō-ī″kō-nŏm′ĕ-tĕr) [″ + *eikon,* image, + *metron,* measure]. Device for measuring the relative size of the two ocular images.

ophthalmofundoscope (ŏf-thăl″mō-fŭn′dō-skōp) [″ + L. *fundus,* base, + Gr. *skopein,* to examine]. Apparatus used in examining the fundus of the eye.

ophthalmography (ŏf″thăl-mŏg′ră-fē) [″ + *graphein,* to write]. Description of the eye.

ophthalmogyric (ŏf-thăl″mō-jī′rĭk) [″ + *gyros,* circle]. Causing or concerning concentric ocular movements. SYN: *oculogyric; oculomotor.*

ophthalmolith (ŏf-thăl′mō-lĭth) [″ + *lithos,* stone]. A calculus of the lacrimal duct.

ophthalmologist (ŏf-thăl-mŏl′ō-jĭst) [″ + *logos,* word, reason]. A physician who specializes in the treatment of disorders of the eye; an oculist.

NOTE: The preferred term for a physician who treats and studies diseases of the eye is ophthalmologist. An optometrist is not a physician, but one who is skilled in testing visual acuity and prescribing corrective lenses. An optician sells or makes optical materials.

ophthalmology (ŏf-thăl-mŏl′ō-jē) [″ + *logos,* word, reason]. The science dealing with the eye and its diseases.

ophthalmomalacia (ŏf-thăl″mō-măl-ā′sē-ă) [″ + *malakia,* softening]. Abnormal shrinkage or softening of the eye. SYN: *ophthalmophthisis.*

ophthalmometer (ŏf-thăl-mŏm′ĕt-ĕr) [″ + *metron,* measure]. 1. Instrument for measuring error of refraction. 2. Instrument for measuring the volume of various chambers of the eye. 3. Instrument for measuring the anterior curvatures of the eye. 4. Device for measuring the size of the eye.

ophthalmometry (ŏf-thăl-mŏm′ĕ-trē). Measurement of the ocular defects and refractive powers.

ophthalmomycosis (ŏf-thăl″mō-mī-kō′sĭs) [″ + *mykes,* fungus, + *osis,* condition]. Any fungus disease of the eye.

ophthalmomyiasis (ŏf-thăl″mō-mī-ī′yă-sĭs) [Gr. *ophthalmos,* eye, + *myia,* a fly, + *-iasis,* condition]. Eye infestation by larvae of the fly *Oestrus ovis.*

ophthalmomyitis (ŏf-thăl″mō-mī-ī′tĭs) [″ + *mys,* muscle, + *itis,* inflammation]. Inflammation of the ocular muscles.

ophthalmomyositis (ŏf-thăl″mō-mī″ō-sī′tĭs). Ophthalmomyitis.

ophthalmomyotomy (ŏf-thăl″mō-mī-ŏt′ō-mē) [″ + *mys,* muscle, + *tome,* incision]. Surgical section of the muscles of the eyes.

ophthalmoneuritis (ŏf-thăl″mō-nū-rī′tĭs) [″ + *neuron,* sinew, + *itis,* inflammation]. Inflamed condition of the optic nerve.

ophthalmopathy, Graves'. SEE: *Graves' ophthalmopathy.*

ophthalmophlebotomy (ŏf-thăl″mō-flĕ-bŏt′ō-mē) [″ + *phleps,* vein, + *tome,* incision]. Incision of the eye to overcome congestion of conjunctival veins.

ophthalmophthisis (ŏf″thăl-mŏf′thĭ-sĭs) [″ + *phthisis*, wasting]. Ophthalmomalacia.

ophthalmoplasty (ŏf-thăl′mō-plăs″tē) [″ + *plassein*, to form]. Ocular plastic surgery.

ophthalmoplegia (ŏf-thăl″mō-plē′jē-ă) [″ + *plege*, stroke]. Paralysis of ocular muscles.

   o. externa. Paralysis of extraocular muscles.

   o. interna. Paralysis of the iris and ciliary muscle.

   o., nuclear. Ophthalmoplegia due to lesion of nuclei of origin of the ocular motor nerves.

   o., Parinaud's. Paralysis of conjugate movement of the eyes upward. Convergence is not affected. The pathological lesion is in the midbrain.

   o. partialis. Incomplete paralysis, involving only one or two of the ocular muscles.

   o. progressiva. Form of ophthalmoplegia in which all muscles become involved slowly, caused by deterioration of the motor nerve nuclei.

   o. totalis. Paralysis that affects both internal and external ocular muscles.

ophthalmoptosis (ŏf-thăl″mŏp-tō′sĭs) [″ + *ptosis*, a dropping]. Protrusion of the eyeball. SYN: *exophthalmos.*

ophthalmoreaction (ŏf-thăl″mō-rĕ-ăk′shŭn) [″ + L. *re*, back, + *actus*, acted]. Reaction of the conjunctiva following instillation of a drop of tuberculin or typhoid fever toxin into the eye of persons suffering from tuberculosis or typhoid diseases. Of diagnostic value. SYN: *oculoreaction; ophthalmic reaction.*

ophthalmorrhagia (ŏf-thăl″mō-rā′jē-ă) [″ + *rhegnynai*, to burst forth]. Ocular hemorrhage.

ophthalmorrhea (ŏf-thăl″mō-rē′ă) [″ + *rhoia*, flow]. Discharge from the eye.

ophthalmorrhexis (ŏf-thăl″mō-rĕk′sĭs) [″ + *rhexis*, rupture]. Rupture of an eyeball.

ophthalmoscope (ŏf-thăl′mō-skōp) [″ + *skopein*, to examine]. Instrument for examining interior of the eye, esp. the retina.

ophthalmoscopy (ŏf-thăl-mŏs′kō-pē). Examination of the interior of the eye.

   o., medical. Use of ophthalmoscopy to diagnose systemic disease.

   o., metric. 1. Use of the ophthalmoscope to determine the refractive error of the lens of the eye. 2. Use of ophthalmoscopy to measure the height of the head of the optic nerve in cases of papilledema.

ophthalmospasm (ŏf-thăl′mō-spăsm). Spasm of ocular muscles.

ophthalmostasis (ŏf″thăl-mŏs′tă-sĭs) [Gr. *ophthalmos*, eye, + *stasis*, standing]. Fixation of the eyeball during surgery on it.

ophthalmostat (ŏf-thăl′mō-stăt) [″ + *statikos*, standing]. Instrument used to hold the eye still during an operation.

ophthalmostatometer (ŏf-thăl″mō-stăt-ŏm′ĕ-tĕr) [″ + ″ + *metron*, measure]. Instrument for ascertaining position of eyes.

ophthalmosynchysis (ŏf-thăl″mō-sĭn′kĭ-sĭs) [″ + *synchisis*, a mixing]. Effusion into one of the cavities of the eye.

ophthalmothermometer (ŏf-thăl″mō-thĕr-mŏm′ĕ-tĕr) [″ + *therme*, heat, + *metron*, measure]. Instrument for determining local temperature in eye diseases.

ophthalmotomy (ŏf″thăl-mŏt′ō-mē) [″ + *tome*, incision]. Surgical incision of the eyeball.

ophthalmotonometer (ŏf-thăl″mō-tō-nŏm′ĕ-tĕr) [″ + *tonos*, tension, + *metron*, measure]. Instrument for determining tension within the eye.

ophthalmotoxin (ŏf-thăl″mō-tŏk′sĭn) [″ + *toxikon*, poison]. Any substance that has a toxic effect on the eyes.

ophthalmotrope (ŏf-thăl′mō-trōp) [″ + *trope*, a turning]. Instrument or model of the eye used to demonstrate movements of the extraocular muscles.

ophthalmotropometer (ŏf-thăl″mō-trō-pŏm′ĕ-tĕr) [″ + ″ + *metron*, measure]. Instrument for measuring the eye movements.

ophthalmovascular (ŏf-thăl″mō-văs′kū-lăr) [″ + L. *vasculum*, a small vessel]. Pert. to blood vessels of the eye.

ophthalmoxerosis (ŏf-thăl″mō-zē-rō′sĭs) [″ + *xeros*, dry, + *osis*, condition]. Xerophthalmia, q.v.

ophthalmoxyster (ŏf-thăl″mŏks-īs′tĕr) [″ + *xyster*, scraper]. Instrument used to scrape the conjunctiva.

Ophthetic. Trade name for proparacaine hydrochloride, USP.

-opia. Suffix concerning vision.

opiate (ō′pē-āt). Any drug containing or derived from opium.

opiate abstinence syndrome. The drug-dependent individual whose choice of drug has been one derived from opium will, upon stopping its use, undergo withdrawal symptoms ranging from restlessness, depression, and mild disturbances in function of the autonomic nervous system, to chills, nausea, vomiting, and diarrhea. Emotional reactions may be pronounced.

opiate poisoning. Toxic reaction to an overdose of an opium-derived drug.

   SYM: Acute poisoning causes euphoria, flushing, itching of the skin, miosis, drowsiness, decreased respiratory rate and depth, bradycardia, hypotension, and a decrease in body temperature. If condition is untreated, death may be the outcome. SEE: *morphine* in *Poisons and Poisoning* in *Appendix.*

opiate receptor. Specific sites on cell surfaces that interact in a highly selective fashion with opiate drugs. These receptors mediate the major known pharmacological actions of opiates and the physiologic functions of the endogenous opiatelike substance, endorphins and enkephalins, q.v.

opioid (ō'pē-oyd) [L. *opium,* opium, + Gr. *eidos,* form, shape]. 1. Non-opium-derived synthetic narcotics. 2. Indicating substances such as enkephalins or endorphins occurring naturally in the body that act on the brain to decrease the sensation of pain.

opioid peptides, endogenous. A group of more than 15 substances present in the brain, certain endocrine glands, and the gastrointestinal tract. They have morphinelike analgesic properties, behavioral effects, and neurotransmitter and neuromodulator functions. Included in this group of chemicals are endorphins, enkephalins, dynorphin, and *d*-neoendorphin.

opiomania (ō"pē-ō-mā'nē-ă) [" + Gr. *mania,* madness]. Insane craving for opium or its derivatives.

opiophagism (ō"pē-ŏf'ă-jĭzm) [" + Gr. *phagein,* to eat]. Addiction to the use of opium, esp. the eating of it.

opisthenar (ō-pĭs'thē-năr) [Gr. *opisthen,* behind, in the rear, + *thenar,* palm]. Back of the hand.

opisthiobasial (ō-pĭs"thē-ō-bā'sē-ăl). Concerning the opisthion and basion of the skull.

opisthion (ō-pĭs'thē-ŏn) [NL. fr. Gr. *opisthen,* back, in the rear]. Craniometric point at middle of lower border of the foramen magnum.

opisthionasial (ō-pĭs"thē-ō-nā'zē-ăl). Concerning the opisthion and nasion of the skull.

opistho-, opisth- [Gr. *opisthen,* behind, in the rear]. Combining form meaning backward or indicating behind.

opisthognathism (ō"pĭs-thŏg'nă-thĭzm) [" + *gnathos,* jaw, + *-ismos,* state of]. Skull abnormality marked by a receding lower jaw.

opisthoporeia (ō-pĭs"thō-pō-rē'ă) [" + *poreia,* walk]. Involuntary walking backward due to loss of motor control.

opisthorchiasis (ō"pĭs-thor-kī'ă-sĭs). Infestation of the liver by flukes of the genus *Opisthorchis.*

Opisthorchis (ō"pĭs-thor'kĭs) [" + *orchis,* testicle]. A genus of parasitic flukes characterized by having testicles near the posterior end of the tapered body.

O. felineus. A species of liver flukes in dogs, cats, foxes. Occasionally infests humans through raw or partially cooked fish.

O. sinensis. A common liver fluke in humans, esp. in the Far East. It develops in those who eat inadequately cooked fish that are infected with the larval form.

opisthotic (ō"pĭs-thŏt'ĭk) [Gr. *opisthen,* behind, in the rear, + *ous,* ear]. Located behind the ear or in the interior ear.

opisthotonoid (ō"pĭs-thŏt'ō-noyd) [" + *tonos,* tension, + *eidos,* form, shape]. Resembling opisthotonos.

opisthotonos (ō"pĭs-thŏt'ō-nŏs) [" + *tonos,* tension]. Form of spasm in which head and heels are bent backward and body is bowed forward. Caused by a tetanic spasm. Seen in strychnine poisoning, tetanus, hysteria, epilepsy, the convulsions of rabies, and in severe cases of meningitis. In the latter case, the patient's neck is rigid and the head retracted, seeming to press into the pillow. SEE: illus.; *emprosthotonos; pleurothotonos.*

opium (ō'pē-ŭm) [L.]. 1. The substance obtained by air-drying of the juice from the unripe capsule of the poppy, *Papaver somniferum L.* It contains a number of important alkaloids such as morphine, codeine, heroin, and papaverine. The growing and transportation of the poppy as well as the manufacture of drugs from the juice are controlled by national and international laws. 2. USP. A standardized preparation of the air-dried milky exudate from unripe capsules of the poppy, *Papaver somniferum* or *P. album.* It contains not less than 9.5% anhydrous morphine.

opiumism (ō'pē-ŭm-ĭzm). 1. Opium habit; addiction to use of opium. 2. Physical condition resulting from overuse of opium.

opium poisoning. SEE: *morphine* in *Poisons and Poisoning* in *Appendix.*

opo- [Gr. *opos,* juice]. Prefix meaning derived from juice; used in trade names of some organic extracts.

opocephalus (ō"pō-sĕf'ă-lŭs) [Gr. *ops,* face, + *kephale,* head]. A congenitally deformed fetus without nose or mouth, fused at the ears. There is either a single orbit or two orbits very close together.

opodidymus (ō"pō-dĭd'ĭ-mŭs) [" + *didymos,* twin]. Congenitally deformed twins in which there is a single body, two fused heads, and partial fusion of the sense organs.

Oppenheim's disease (ŏp'ĕn-hīmz) [Hermann Oppenheim, Ger. neurologist, 1858–1919]. A noninherited but sometimes familial disease, characterized by absence of

OPISTHOTONOS

muscular development, with the lower extremities being the first involved. It is first seen at, or shortly after, birth. SYN: *myotonia congenita.*

Oppenheim's gait. Gait in which there is a wide swinging motion of the head, body, and extremities. It is a variation of the gait seen in multiple sclerosis.

opponens (ō-pō'něns) [L.]. Opposing, a term applied to muscles of hand or foot by which one of the lateral digits may be opposed to one of the other digits. SEE: *Muscles* in *Appendix.*

opponens splint. A splint designed to maintain the thumb in a position to oppose the other fingers.

opportunistic infections. Infections that result from a defective immune system that cannot defend against pathogens normally found in the environment. Common types include bacterial (*Clostridium difficile*), fungal (*Histoplasma capsulatum*), and protozoan (*Pneumocystis carinii*). Seen in patients receiving large doses of steroids or other immunosuppressive drugs, or in patients with acquired immunodeficiency syndrome (AIDS). SEE: *AIDS; immunocompromised.*

opposition. The ability to move the thumb into contact with the other fingers.

opsialgia (ŏp"sē-ăl'jē-ă) [Gr. *ops*, face, + *algos*, pain]. Neuralgic pain of the face.

opsin (ŏp'sĭn). The protein portion of the rhodopsin molecule.

opsinogen (ŏp-sĭn'ō-jěn). An antigen that causes the production of opsonins.

opsinogenous (ŏp"sĭn-ŏj'ěn-ŭs). Capable of forming opsonins.

opsiometer (ŏp"sē-ŏm'ě-těr). Optometer, q.v.

opsiuria (ŏp-sē-ū'rē-ă) [Gr. *opse*, late, + *ouron*, urine]. Condition in which excretion of urine is more rapid during fasting than after a meal.

opsoclonus. Conjugate irregular and non-rhythmical jerking movements of the eyes. The eyes move in any linear or rotating direction at a speed of up to 10 times per second. Any one of several areas of the brain, including the cerebellum and brain stem, may be diseased and cause this sign.

opsogen (ŏp'sō-jěn). An opsinogen, q.v.

opsomania (ŏp"sō-mā'nē-ă) [Gr. *opson*, food, + *mania*, madness]. Craving for some special article of food.

opsonic (ŏp-sŏn'ĭk) [Gr. *opsonein*, to purchase food]. Pert. to opsonins or their use in therapy.

opsonification (ŏp-sŏn"ĭ-fĭ-kā'shŭn). Effect of opsonins in rendering cells or bacteria phagocytized more readily.

opsonin (ŏp-sō'nĭn) [Gr. *opsonein*, to purchase food]. A substance that coats foreign antigens, making them more susceptible to macrophages and other leukocytes, thus increasing phagocytosis of the organism. Complement and antibodies are the two main opsonins in human blood.

    o., immune. Opsonin formed after stimulation by a specific antigen.

opsonization (ŏp"sō-nī-zā'shŭn). Action of opsonins to facilitate phagocytosis. SYN: *opsonification.*

opsonize (ŏp'sō-nīz) [Gr. *opsonein*, to purchase food]. To facilitate phagocytosis.

opsonocytophagic (ŏp"sŏn-ō-sī"tō-fā'jĭk) [" + *kytos*, cell, + *phagein*, to eat]. Pert. to phagocytic action of blood when serum opsonins are present.

opsonometry (ŏp-sō-nŏm'ě-trē) [" + *metron*, measure]. Estimation of amount of opsonins in the blood serum. SEE: *index, opsonic.*

opsonophilia (ŏp"sō-nō-fĭl'ē-ă) [" + *philein*, to love]. Attraction for opsonins.

opsonophilic. Having attraction to opsonins.

opsonotherapy (ŏp"sō-nō-thěr'ă-pē). Treatment by stimulation of a specific opsonin with bacterial vaccines. SEE: *vaccine.*

Optacon II. Acronym for *Optical to Tactile Converter*, a proprietary name of a portable electronic reading device for use by the blind. It translates printed material to patterns of raised pins under the user's fingers. It is manufactured by TeleSensory, 455 N. Bernardo Ave., Mountain View, CA 94043; (800) 227-8418 or (415) 960-0920.

optic (ŏp'tĭk) [Gr. *optikos*]. Pert. to the eye or the sight.

optical (ŏp'tĭ-kăl) [Gr. *optikos*; L. *opticus*]. Pert. to vision, the eye, or optics.

optical activity. In chemistry, the property of rotating the plane of polarized light. Measurement of this property, called polarimetry, is useful in the determination of optically active substances such as dextrose. Sugars are classified according to this criterion. Optical activity of a substance in solution can be detected by placing it between polarizing and analyzing prisms.

optical tweezers. A laser device used to alter or manipulate microorganisms, molecules, or living cells.

optic chiasm. An X-shaped crossing of the optic nerve fibers in the brain. Past this point, the fibers travel in optic tracts. Fibers that originated in the outer half of the retina end up on the same side of the brain; those from the inner half cross over.

optic disk. Area in retina for entrance of optic nerve; the blind spot, q.v. SYN: *optic papilla.*

optic foramen. Groove for optic nerve and ophthalmic artery at the orbit's apex.

optician (ŏp-tĭsh'ăn). One who is a specialist in the making of optical apparatus.

opticianry (ŏp-tĭsh'ăn-rē). The science and art of optics applied to filling optical prescriptions for ordinary glasses as well as contact lenses.

opticist (ŏp'tĭ-sĭst). One trained in and capable in the science of optics.

optic nerve. The nerve carrying impulses for the sense of sight. It originates in the lateral geniculate body of the thalamus and travels by the optic tract and optic chiasma, where it enters the retina through the optic disk. SYN: *second cranial nerve.* SEE: *Cranial Nerves in Appendix.*

optic neuropathy. Pathological change in the optic nerves or the blood supply to them. Usually only one eye is affected. Several forms have been described: ischemic, which if prolonged leads to blindness in the affected eye; optic neuritis due to acute demyelination of optic nerve fibers; infiltrative, in which the optic nerve(s) is compressed by a tumor or aneurysm; and that due to toxic nutritional factors, e.g. methanol or a combined nutritional and vitamin deficiency.

optico- [Gr. *optikos*]. Combining form pert. to the eye or vision.

opticociliary (ŏp″tĭ-kō-sĭl'ē-ăr-ē). Concerning the optic and ciliary nerves.

opticokinetic (ŏp″tĭ-kō-kĭ-nĕt'ĭk) [″ + *kinesis,* movement]. Concerning the movement of the eye.

opticonasion (ŏp″tĭ-kō-nā'sē-ŏn). Length of an imaginary line drawn from the posterior edge of the optic foramen to the nasion.

opticopupillary (ŏp″tĭ-kō-pū'pĭl-ĕr″ē). Concerning the optic nerve and pupil.

optic papilla. Optic disk.

optics (ŏp'tĭks) [Gr. *optikos,* pert. to vision]. The science dealing with light and its relationship to vision.

optic tract. Fibers of the optic nerve that continue beyond the optic chiasma, most of which terminate in the lateral geniculate body of the thalamus. Some continue to the superior colliculus of the midbrain; others enter the hypothalamus and terminate in the supraoptic and medial nuclei.

Optimine. Trade name for azatadine maleate, USP.

optimism. The characteristic of regarding only the bright side of a condition or event. SEE: *pessimism.*

optimum (ŏp'tĭ-mŭm) [L. *optimus,* best] (pl. *optima*). Condition that is most conducive to a function or functions such as growth and development.

optimum temperature. Temperature that is most suitable for a procedure or operation, esp. the development of bacterial cultures.

opto- [Gr. *optos,* seen]. Combining form meaning vision or eye.

optogram (ŏp'tō-grăm) [Gr. *optos,* seen, + *gramma,* something written]. Image of external object fixed on the retina by photochemical bleaching action of light on the visual purple.

optokinetic (ŏp″tō-kĭ-nĕt'ĭk) [″ + *kinesis,* movement]. Concerning the appearance of twitching of the eye, as in nystagmus when the eyes gaze at moving objects.

optometer (ŏp-tŏm'ĕ-tĕr) [″ + *metron,* measure]. Instrument for measurement of the eye's refractive power. SYN: *opsiometer.*

optometrist (ŏp-tŏm'ĕ-trĭst). Doctors of optometry are primary health care providers who diagnose, manage, and treat conditions and diseases of the human eye and visual system as regulated and permitted by state laws. Persons who have completed the required course of training in optometry are awarded the D.O. degree. SEE: *optometry.*

optometry (ŏp-tŏm'ĕ-trē). The science of diagnosing, managing, and treating conditions and diseases of the human eye and visual system. Persons who practice optometry, doctors of optometry (D.O.), are professionally trained health care providers licensed and regulated by state laws. Most but not all states permit optometrists to prescribe drugs for the treatment of certain eye diseases.

optomyometer (ŏp″tō-mī-ŏm′ĕ-tĕr) [″ + *mys*, muscle, + *metron*, a measure]. Instrument for determining strength of the muscles of the eye.

optophone (ŏp′tō-fōn) [″ + *phone*, voice]. Instrument converting light energy into sound waves. Used by the blind.

optostriate (ŏp-tō-strī′āt) [″ + L. *striatus*, grooved]. Concerning the optic thalamus and the corpus striatum.

optotype (ŏp′tō-tīp). The test type used in determining visual acuity.

OPV. *oral poliovirus vaccine.*

OR. *operating room.*

ora (ō′ră) [L.]. 1. Pl. of os. 2. (pl. *orae*) A border or margin.

    o. serrata retinae. [NA] Notched anterior edge of sensory portion of retina.

orad (ō′răd) [L. *oris*, mouth, + *ad*, toward]. Toward the mouth or oral region.

Oragrafin Sodium. Trade name for ipodate sodium, which is used for radiographic examinations of the biliary system.

oral (or′ăl) [L. *oralis*]. 1. Concerning the mouth. 2. In dental anatomy, describes the surface of the tooth towards the oral cavity or tongue and the opposite of the buccal or facial tooth surface.

oral contraceptive. SEE: *contraceptive.*

oral diagnosis. The procedure or special area of dentistry devoted to the compilation and study of the patient's dental history, and a detailed clinical examination of the oral tissues and radiographs to assess the level of oral health, with the object of developing a treatment plan to restore tooth structure and proper occlusion, and to promote healing and better oral health.

orale (ō-ra′lē). Point on hard palate in the midsagittal plane where lines drawn tangent to the lingual margins of the alveoli of the medial incisor teeth intersect.

orality (ō-răl′ĭ-tē). The oral stage of psychosexual development, which involves sucking, or chewing on objects other than food.

oralogy (ō-răl′ō-jē) [L. *oralis*, oral, + Gr. *logos*, word, reason]. 1. The science of dentistry or stomatology. 2. Study of diseases of the mouth. SYN: *dentistry; stomatology.*

oral rehydration solutions. ABBR: ORS. Solutions used in oral rehydration therapy, q.v. The World Health Organization recommends that the solution contain the following amounts of electrolytes and glucose: 3.5 gm sodium chloride; 2.9 gm potassium chloride; 2.9 gm trisodium citrate; and 1.5 gm glucose dissolved in each liter (approximately one quart) of drinking water.

oral rehydration therapy. ABBR: ORT. The administration by mouth of a solution of electrolytes in sufficient quantity to correct the deficits produced by dehydration due to diarrhea. The earlier this therapy is begun, the more effective it is; i.e., fluid should be started before the infant is dehydrated. Because this therapy is simple, is economical, and can be supervised by nonprofessionals, it has been extremely effective in treating infantile diarrhea in countries lacking economic resources and health care professionals.

    In many parts of the world, commercially prepared ORT solutions are not available or are too expensive. In these areas, very inexpensive and effective solutions can be prepared from sources such as cooled water from a pot in which rice is boiled; two pinches of salt added to a quart (in Bangladesh, a "seer") of water and a fistful of molasses (estimated one ounce). SEE: *epidemic viral gastroenteritis; oral rehydration solutions.*

orange, methyl. A chemical used as an indicator in acid-base titrations.

Orasone. Trade name for prednisone, USP.

Ora-Testryl. Trade name for fluoxymesterone, USP.

orb [L. *orbis*, circle, disk]. A spherical body, esp. the eyeball.

orbicular (or-bĭk′ū-lăr) [L. *orbiculus*, a small circle]. Circular.

orbicular bone. The rounded end of the long process of the incus, a middle ear ossicle. It probably represents a secondary ossification center in the long or lenticular process. SYN: *orbiculare.*

orbicularis sign. SEE: *wink.*

orbicular muscle. Muscle encircling an opening.

orbicular process. End of long process of the incus. SYN: *process, lenticular.*

orbiculus (or-bĭk′ū-lŭs) [L., little circle] (pl. *orbiculi*). Muscle surrounding an orifice; a sphincter muscle.

    o. ciliaris. Ciliary muscles of the eye. SYN: *ring, ciliary.*

    o. oculi. Measure encircling the opening or orbit of the eye.

    o. oris. Circular muscle surrounding the mouth.

orbit (or′bĭt) [L. *orbita*, track]. The bony pyramid-shaped cavity of the skull that contains and protects the eyeball. It is pierced posteriorly by the optic foramen, which transmits the optic nerve and ophthalmic artery, the superior and inferior orbital fissures, and several foramina. It is formed by the frontal, malar, ethmoid, maxillary, lacrimal, sphenoid, and palatine bones.

orbita (or′bĭ-tă) [L.] (pl. *orbitae*). [NA] Orbit.

tion elsewhere in the body.

SYM: Swelling, severe pain, possibly gangrene, chills, fever, vomiting, hiccough, delirium. May end in atrophy of organ.

TREAT: Confine patient to bed first eight days, immobilize organ, and use ice bag.

o., gonorrheal. Orchitis due to gonococcus.

o., metastatic. Orchitis due to infection from organisms in bloodstream.

o., syphilitic. Orchitis due to syphilis.

SYM: Usually begins painlessly in body of gland but apt to be bilateral. Causes dense, irregular, knotty induration but little enlargement in size.

o., tuberculous. Form of orchitis generally arising in the epididymis. It may be accompanied by formation of chronic sinuses, and destruction of tissues.

SYM: Little or no pain. Begins as hard, irregular enlargement at lower and posterior aspect of gland, gradually increases, and sometimes extends along vas deferens. Later whole gland undergoes caseous degeneration.

orchitolytic (or″kĭt-ō-lĭt′ĭk) [″ + *lysis,* dissolution]. Destructive to testicular tissue.

orchotomy (or-kŏt′ō-mē) [″ + *tome,* incision]. Incision, but not excision, of a testicle.

orcin, orcinol (or′sĭn, -ōl). A white, crystalline substance derived from lichens and used as a reagent.

order [L. *ordo,* a row, series]. 1. An arrangement or sequence of events; rules; regulations; procedures. 2. In biological classification, the main division under class, superior to family.

orderly (or′dĕr-lē). An attendant in a hospital who does general work to assist nurses. Responsible for lifting and transporting patients and preparing them for surgery (shaving, catheterizing, or administering enemas).

ordinate (or′dĭ-năt). In a graph in which horizontal and perpendicular lines are crossed in order to provide a frame of reference, the ordinate is a vertical line parallel to the y-axis. The abscissa, q.v., is a horizontal line parallel to the x-axis. SEE: *abscissa* for illus.

ordure (or′dūr). Feces or other excrement.

Oretic. Trade name for hydrochlorothiazide, USP.

Oreton-Methyl. Trade name for methyltestosterone, USP.

orexia (ō-rĕk′sē-ă) [Gr. *orexis*]. Appetite.

orexigenic (ō-rĕk″sĭ-jĕn′ĭk) [Gr. *orexis,* appetite, + *gennan,* to produce]. Stimulating the appetite.

oreximania (ō-rĕk″sĭ-mā′nē-ă) [″ + *mania,* madness]. Abnormal desire for food because of fear of becoming thin.

orf. A contagious pustular dermatitis mainly affecting lambs and occurring in the spring. The disease rarely occurs in humans. When it does, it usually is confined to a single pustular lesion on a finger, which encrusts and finally heals. Antibiotics are not indicated except for secondary bacterial infections.

ETIOL: Orf virus, a DNA virus of the *Parapoxvirus* genus, which is related to the vaccinia-variola subgroup of poxviruses.

organ (or′găn) [Gr. *organon;* L. *organum*]. A part of the body having a special function. Many organs are in pairs. In such pairs, one organ may be extirpated and the remaining one can perform all necessary functions peculiar to it. One third to two fifths of some organs may be removed without loss of function necessary to support life. SEE: table.

o., accessory. Organ that has a subordinate function.

o., acoustic. Organ of Corti.

o., enamel. A knoblike thickening that develops on dental lamina, giving rise to a double-walled cup-shaped organ that encloses the dental papilla. It functions in the shaping of the tooth and the formation of enamel.

o., end. The specialized termination of a sensory nerve fiber that serves as a receptor. May be nonencapsulated or encapsulated.

o., excretory. Organ that is concerned with the excretion of waste products from the body. SEE: *excretion.*

o., Golgi tendon. A spindle-shaped structure at junction of a muscle and tendon. Functions as a receptor for proprioceptive sense.

o., gustatory. Organ that controls the sense of taste; a taste bud. SYN: *organum gustus* [NA].

o. of Corti. Terminal acoustic apparatus in the cochlea. SYN: *organum spirale.* SEE: *Claudius' cells; ear.*

o. of Giraldés. A small body on the spermatic cord above the epididymis. SYN: *paradidymis.*

o. of Jacobson. A blind tubular sac that develops in the medial wall of the nasal cavity. Becomes a functional olfactory organ in lower animals but degenerates or remains rudimentary in humans. SYN: *o., vomeronasal.*

o. of Ruffini. Sensory receptor of warmth located principally at tips of fingers. SYN: *Ruffini's corpuscles.*

o.'s of Zuckerkandl. A pair of organs containing chromaffin tissue present in the embryo and persisting until shortly after birth. Located adjacent to the anterior surface of the abdominal aorta. The cells secrete epinephrine. SYN: *corpora paraaor-*

Size, Weight, and Capacity of Various Organs and Parts of the Adult Body
♂ male ♀ female

Description	Size	Weight	Capacity
Adrenal gland	5 cm high 3 cm across 1 cm thick	5.0 gm	
Bladder	12 cm in diameter		50 ml (when moderately full)
Blood volume			♂ 4680 ml ♀ 3400 ml
Brain		♂ 1240–1680 gm ♀ 1130–1570 gm	
Ear, external canal	2.5 cm long (from concha)		
Esophagus	23–25 cm		
Eye	23.5 mm vertical diameter 24 mm anteroposterior diameter		
Fallopian tube	10 cm		
Gallbladder	7–10 cm long 3 cm wide		30–50 ml
Heart	12 × 8–9 × 6 cm	♂ 280–340 gm ♀ 230–280 gm	
Intestines — small	Quite variable 6–7 meters long		
Intestines — large	1.5 meters long		
Intestines — vermiform appendix	2–20 cm long Average 9 cm		
Intestines — rectum	12 cm long		
Kidney	11 cm long 6 cm broad 3 cm thick	♂ 150 gm ♀ 135 gm	
Larynx	♂ 44 × 43 × 36 mm ♀ 36 × 41 × 26 mm		
Liver		♂ 1.4–1.8 kg ♀ 1.0–2.5 kg	6500 cc
Lung		Rt. 625 gm Lt. 565 gm	
Ovaries	3 × 1.5 × 1 cm	2–3.5 gm	
Pancreas	15 cm long	♂ 74–106 gm ♀ 70–100 gm	
Parathyroid	6 × 3–4 × 1–2 mm	50 mg	
Pharynx	12.5 cm long		
Prostate	2 × 4 × 3 cm	8 gm	

Size, Weight, and Capacity of Various Organs and Parts of the Adult Body
♂ male ♀ female *(Continued)*

Description	Size	Weight	Capacity
Skeleton		Average adult male, 4957 gm	
Skull		Average (without teeth), 642 gm	♂ 406 ml ♀ 207 ml
Spinal cord	42–45 cm long	30 gm	
Spleen	12 × 7 × 3–4 cm	150 gm Range 80–300 gm Decreases with age	
Stomach	Quite variable 25 cm long 10 cm wide		Quite variable 1500 ml
Testes	4–5 × 2.5 × 3.0 cm	10.5–14 gm	
Thoracic duct	38–45 cm long		
Thymus		Newborn, 10.9 gm 10–15 yr, 29.5 gm 20–25 yr, 18.6 gm	
Thyroid	Each lobe 5 × 3 × 2 cm	30 gm total	
Trachea	11 cm long 2–2.5 cm in diameter		
Ureter	28–34 cm long		
Urethra	♂ 17.5–20 cm long ♀ 4 cm long		
Uterus	7.5 × 5.0 × 2.5 cm	30–40 gm (nonpregnant)	
Vagina	Anterior wall length 7.5 cm Posterior wall length 9.0 cm		

Source: Adapted from Gray's Anatomy, ed 27. Lea & Febiger, Philadelphia, 1959; Gray's Anatomy, ed 37. Churchill Livingstone, London, 1987; Growth, Federation of American Societies for Experimental Biology, Washington, DC, 1962; Jandl, JH, Blood. Little, Brown and Co., Boston, 1987.

tica.

o., reproductive. Any organ concerned with the production of offspring. Includes the primary organs (testes and ovaries) and accessory structures (penis and spermatic cord in the male and fallopian tubes, uterus, and vagina in the female). SYN: *o., sex.*

o., sense. A sensory receptor; a structure consisting of specialized sensory nerve endings that are capable of reacting to a stimulus (an environmental change) by giving rise to nerve impulses that pass through afferent nerves to the central nervous system. These impulses may give rise to sensations or reflexly bring about responses in the body.

o., sex. O., reproductive.

o.'s, special sense. Organs of smell, taste, sight, and hearing.

o., spiral. The spiral organ of the inner ear, which contains the special sensory apparatus for hearing.

o., target. Organ upon which a chemical

ORGANELLE

GOLGI COMPLEX

MITOCHONDRION

CENTRIOLES

ENDOPLASMIC
RETICULUM

or hormone acts.

    o., vestigial. Organ that is immature or underdeveloped in humans but is fully functional in some animals.

    o., vomeronasal. O. of Jacobson.

    o., Weber's. Residual prostatic pouch in the male, the remains of the müllerian ducts.

organelle (or″găn-ĕl′). A specialized part of a cell that performs a definite function. Ex.: mitochondria; Golgi apparatus; endoplasmic reticulum; lysosomes; and cell centriole. SEE: illus.

organic (or-găn′ĭk) [Gr. *organikos*]. 1. Pert. to an organ or organs. 2. Structural. 3. Pert. to or derived from animal or vegetable forms of life. 4. Denoting chemical substances containing carbon.

organic acid. Acid containing one or more —COOH, i.e., carboxyl groups. Acetic, formic, lactic, and all fatty acids are organic.

organic brain syndromes. A large group of acute and chronic mental disorders associated with brain damage or impaired cerebral function.

    SYM: The clinical characteristics vary not only with the nature and severity of the underlying organic disorder but also from time to time in each individual. The following functions may be impaired: consciousness, orientation, memory, intellect, judgment and insight, and thought content such as hallucinations, illusions, and mood.

    ETIOL: Any acute or chronic disease or injury that interferes with cerebral function such as infection, intoxication, trauma, circulatory disturbance, epilepsy, metabolic and endocrine diseases, or intracranial neoplasms.

    DIAG: May be difficult because of the possibility of attributing all of the signs and symptoms to a psychiatric disorder and ignoring the organic disease or vice versa.

    TREAT: Treat basic organic disease and provide psychiatric care.

organic chemistry. Branch of chemistry dealing with substances containing carbon compounds.

organic disease. A disease associated with observable or detectable changes in the organs or tissues of the body.

organic dust toxic syndrome. ABBR: ODTS. A nonallergic, noninfectious, respiratory illness caused by inhalation of organic dust from moldy silage, hay, or other agricultural products.

    SYM: Fever, muscle pain, and cough.

organicism (or-găn′ĭ-sĭzm). The theory that all diseases are due to organic disease.

organicist (or-găn′ĭ-sĭst). One who believes in organicism.

organic psychoses. A general term applied to those psychoses induced by structural brain changes. In general, a character change is manifested in behavior and disposition. Emotional instability, irritability, and angry outbursts become frequent. Attention fluctuates widely; gradually the patient deteriorates. At any time in the course of the disease, memory, comprehension, ideation, and orientation may become defective.

    ETIOL: Alcohol, narcotics, trauma, syphilis, drugs, poisons, chronic infections, encephalitis, and brain tumors among many others.

organism (or′găn-ĭzm) [Gr. *organon,* organ, + *-ismos,* condition]. Any living thing, plant, or animal. May be unicellular (bacteria, yeasts, protozoa) or multicellular (all complex organisms including humans).

    o., fastidious. A microorganism for which the requirements for growth are complex.

organization (or″găn-ĭ-zā′shŭn). 1. Process of becoming organized. 2. Systematic arrangement. 3. That which is organized; an organism.

organization center. 1. An embryonic group of cells, which induces the development of another structure. 2. A region in an ovum that is responsible for the mode of development of the fertilized ovum.

organize (or′găn-īz). To develop from an amorphous state to that having structure and form.

organo- (or′gă-nō). A combining form indicating a relationship to an organ.

organoferric (or″gă-nō-fēr′ĭk). Concerning iron and an organic molecule.

organogel (or-găn′ō-jĕl). A gel in which the continuous phase is an organic liquid instead of water.

organogenesis (or″găn-ō-jĕn′ĕ-sĭs) [″ + genesis, generation, birth]. The formation and development of body organs from embryonic tissues.

It is important that the fetus not be exposed to harmful chemicals. This is particularly important during organogenesis. The first critical period for the effects of teratogenic drugs on the human fetus is between the 13th and 56th day of gestation. The second period of high risk is during the last trimester when metabolic enzyme systems are beginning to be defined. The third period is during labor when the physiologic changes required for transition of the fetus to life outside the womb are taking place. SYN: *organogeny.*

organogeny (or″gă-nŏj′ĕ-nē). Organogenesis, q.v.

organography (or-găn-ŏg′ră-fē) [″ + graphein, to write]. 1. The description of the body organs. 2. Roentgenographic visualization of the organs of the body.

organoid [″ + eidos, form, shape]. 1. Resembling an organ. 2. An organelle.

organoleptic (or″găn-ō-lĕp′tĭk) [″ + lepsis, a seizure]. 1. Affecting an organ, esp. the organs of special sense. 2. Susceptible to sensory impressions.

organology (or-gă-nŏl′ō-jē) [″ + logos, word, reason]. The science dealing with the body organs.

organoma (or-gă-nō′mă) [″ + oma, tumor]. A neoplasm containing cellular elements that can be definitely identified as being specific to certain tissues and organs.

organomegaly (or″gă-nō-mĕg′ă-lē) [″ + megas, large]. Enlargement of visceral organs.

organomercurial (or″gă-nō-mĕr-kū′rē-ăl). Any organic mercurial compound.

organometallic (or-gă-nō-mĕ-tăl′ĭk). A compound containing a metal combined with an organic molecule.

organon (or′gă-nŏn) [Gr.] (pl. organa). Organum, q.v.

organonomy (or″gă-nŏn′ō-mē) [″ + nomos, law]. The laws regulating the biological processes of living organisms.

organopathy (or″gă-nŏp′ă-thē) [″ + pathos, disease, suffering]. Any disease affecting an organ of the body.

organopexy (or′găn-ō-pĕk″sē) [″ + pexis, fixation]. Surgical fixation of an organ that is detached from its proper position.

organophilic (or″gă-nō-fĭl′ĭk) [″ + philos, to love]. Organotropism, q.v.

organoscopy (or-gă-nŏs′kō-pē) [″ + skopein, to examine]. Examination of abdominal organs of the body by means of an endoscope.

organotherapy (or″găn-ō-thĕr′ă-pē) [″ + therapeia, treatment]. The treatment of disease by preparations of the endocrine glands of animals or by extracts made from the same.

organotrope, organotropic (or-găn′ō-trōp, -găn-ō-trŏp′ĭk) [″ + tropos, turning]. Having affinity for tissues or certain organs.

organotrophic (or″gă-nō-trŏf′ĭk) [″ + trophe, nutrition]. Concerning the nutrition of organs.

organotropism (or″gă-nŏt′rō-pĭzm) [″ + trope, a turn, + -ismos, condition]. The attraction or affinity of chemicals or biological agents for body organs or tissues.

organ perfusion system. A mechanical device equipped to supply metabolic, oxygen, and electrolyte needs in order to keep viable for transplantation an organ obtained from a cadaver or donor. The organ and the perfusion solution pumped through it can be kept at the ideal temperature for organ survival. Together they can be transported by any means required to deliver the organ to the recipient.

organ-specific (or′găn-spē-sif′ĭk). Originating in a single organ or affecting only one specific organ.

organum [L.] (pl. organa). [NA] An organ.

    o. auditus. O. vestibulocochleare.

    o. gustus. [NA] Organ of taste.

    o. olfactus. [NA] Organ of smell; olfactory region in the nasal cavity.

    o. spirale. [NA] Spiral organ in the cochlea. SYN: *organ of Corti.*

    o. vestibulocochleare. [NA] Organ of hearing. SYN: *organum auditus.* SEE: *ear.*

    o. visus. [NA] Organ of sight; the eye and its adnexa.

    o. vomeronasale. [NA] Canal opening into the nasal septum. SYN: *organ of Jacobson.*

orgasm (or′găzm) [Gr. orgasmos, swelling]. A state of physical and emotional excitement, esp. that which occurs at the climax of sexual intercourse. In the male it is accompanied by the ejaculation of semen. SYN: *climax.*

Oriental sore. An ulcerating, chronic, nodular skin lesion prevalent in the Orient and tropics and due to infection with *Leishmania tropica.* SYN: *Aleppo boil; leishmaniasis, cutaneous.*

orientation (or″ē-ĕn-tā′shŭn) [L. *oriens,* to arise]. Ability to comprehend and to adjust oneself in an environment with regard to time, location, and identity of persons. Partially or completely absent in some psychoses.

orifice (or′ĭ-fĭs) [L. *orificium*]. Mouth, entrance, or outlet of any aperture.

  o., anal. The anus.

  o., atrioventricular. Opening between the atrium and the ventricle on each side of the heart.

  o., cardiac. Opening of esophagus into the stomach.

  o., mitral. Opening between the atrium and ventricle.

  o., oral. The opening into the mouth. Also called rima oris; oral fissure.

  o., pyloric. Opening from the stomach into the duodenum. SEE: *pylorus.*

  o., ureteric. Opening of ureter into the bladder.

  o., urethral, external. Exterior opening of the urethra. In male, located at tip of glans penis; in female, located anterior and cephalad to vaginal opening.

  o., urethral, internal. Opening from which urethra makes its exit from bladder.

orificial (or″ĭ-fĭ′shăl) [L. *orificium,* outlet]. Pert. to or forming an orifice.

orificium (or″ĭ-fĭsh′ē-ŭm) [L.]. An opening or orifice.

origin (or′ĭ-jĭn) [L. *origo,* beginning]. 1. The source of anything; a starting point. 2. The beginning of a nerve. 3. The more fixed attachment of a muscle.

  o., deep. The region within the brain where the fibers that make up a cranial nerve terminate.

  o., superficial. Point where a cranial nerve exits from the brain.

Orimune. Trade name for poliovirus vaccine, live oral, USP.

Orinase. Trade name for tolbutamide, USP.

Ormond's disease. Retroperitoneal fibrosis causing ureteral obstruction.

ornithine (or′nĭ-thĭn). An amino acid formed when arginase hydrolyzes arginine. It is not present in proteins.

Ornithodoros (or″nĭ-thŏd′ō-rŏs). A genus of ticks belonging to the family Argasidae, which infest mammals, including humans. Several species serve as transmitters of the causative agents of disease, including spotted fever, tick fever, Q fever, tularemia, Russian encephalitis, and relapsing fever.

ornithosis (or″nĭ-thō′sĭs) [Gr. *ornithos,* bird, + *osis,* condition]. An acute generalized infectious disease of birds and domesticated

fowls, communicated to humans. SYN: *psittacosis.*

  SYM: Headache, chills and fever, anorexia, myalgia, sore throat, nausea, and vomiting.

  ETIOL: *Chlamydia psittaci.*

  TREAT: Tetracyclines continued for 10 to 14 days after temperature returns to normal.

oro-. Combining form denoting the mouth.

orodiagnosis (or″ō-dī-ăg-nō′sĭs) [Gr. *oros,* serum, + *dia,* through, + *gnosis,* knowledge]. Diagnosis by using serums or serum reactions.

orofacial (or″ō-fā′shē-ăl) [L. *oris,* mouth, + *facies,* face]. Concerning the mouth and face.

orofaciodigital syndrome. The condition of mental retardation and deformities of the mouth, tongue, fingers, and sometimes the face.

orogastric hose. Large-bore (36 to 40 French size in an adult) tube used to perform gastric lavage. A smaller size (as in nasogastric tube) will be inadequate for removing pills or pill fragments. SEE: *gastric lavage.*

orolingual (or″ō-lĭng′gwăl) [L. *oris,* mouth, + *lingua,* tongue]. Concerning the mouth and tongue.

oromeningitis (or″ō-mĕn″ĭn-jī′tĭs) [″ + Gr. *meninx,* membrane, + *itis,* inflammation]. Orrhomeningitis, q.v.

oronasal (or″ō-nā′zăl) [″ + *nasus,* nose]. Concerning the mouth and nose.

oropharyngeal airway. Firm airway tube that is inserted into the mouth of an unconscious patient and prevents the flaccid tongue from blocking the airway.

oropharynx (or″ō-făr′ĭnks) [″ + Gr. *pharynx,* throat]. Central portion of the pharynx lying between the soft palate and upper portion of the epiglottis.

orosomucoid (or″ō-sō-mū′koyd). An alpha 1-globulin in plasma.

orotic acid. Uracil-6-carboxylic acid. It is a precursor in the formation of pyrimidine nucleotides.

orotic aciduria. An inherited disorder of pyrimidine metabolism in which orotic acid accumulates in the body. Clinically, children fail to grow and have megaloblastic anemia and leukopenia. The disease responds to administration of uridine or cytidine.

Oroya fever [Oroya, a region of Peru]. An acute infectious disease endemic in Peru and other South American countries. The first clinical stage of bartonellosis. SYN: *bartonellosis; Carrion's disease.*

  SYM: Intermittent fever; lymphadenopathy; severe anemia and pains in joints and long bones.

TREAT: SEE: *bartonellosis*.

orphan [L. *orphanus*, destitute, without parents]. A child whose parents have died or are unknown.

orphan disease. A type of illness that, because of its rarity, has received minimal attention from medical researchers. SEE: *National Organization for Rare Disorders*.

orphan drugs. Drugs that are effective for certain illnesses but, for a variety of reasons, are not profitable for manufacturers to produce. SEE: *National Organization For Rare Disorders*.

orphenadrine citrate (or-fĕn′ă-drēn). USP. An antiparkinsonism drug. Trade names are Banflex and Norflex.

orrhology (or-ŏl′ō-jē) [Gr. *orrhos*, blood serum, + *logos*, word, reason]. The study of serums and their reactions. SYN: *serology*.

orrhomeningitis (or″ō-mĕn″ĭn-jī′tĭs) [″ + *meninx*, membrane, + *itis*, inflammation]. Inflammation of a serous membrane.

orrhorrhea (or″ō-rē′ă) [″ + *rhein*, to flow]. Any watery, thin, colorless discharge from a body structure. Usually it is the result of inflammation.

orris root (or′ĭs). The powder made from the root of certain varieties of iris. It is used in making some types of cosmetics. It is a sensitizer by either contact or inhalation.

ORT. *oral rehydration therapy*.

orthergasia (or″thĕr-gā′zē-ă) [Gr. *orthos*, straight, + *ergon*, work]. The state of normal mental condition.

orthesis (or-thē′sĭs). Orthosis, q.v.

orthetics (or-thĕt′ĭks). Orthotics, q.v.

orthetist (or′thĕ-tĭst). Orthotist, q.v.

ortho- [Gr. *orthos*, straight]. Combining form meaning straight, correct, normal, in proper order.

orthoacid (or″thō-ăs′ĭd). An acid with as many hydroxyl groups as the number of valences of the acid-forming portion of the molecule.

orthobiosis (or″thō-bī-ō′sĭs) [″ + *bios*, life]. Right living. A term used by Metchnikoff to encompass all the factors that may affect longevity and well-being.

orthocephalic (or″thō-sĕ-făl′ĭk) [″ + *kephale*, head]. Having a well-proportioned head; having a head with a height-length index between 70 and 75.

orthochorea (or″thō-kō-rē′ă) [″ + *choreia*, dance]. A type of chorea in which attacks appear mainly when the person is in an erect position.

orthochromatic (or″thō-krō-măt′ĭk) [″ + *chroma*, color]. Having normal color or staining normally.

orthochromophil (or″thō-krō′mō-fĭl) [″ + ″ + *philein*, to love]. Staining normally with neutral dyes.

orthodentin (or″thō-dĕn′tĭn). Tubular dentin as in human teeth.

orthodiagraph (or″thō-dī′ă-grăf) [″ + *dia*, through, + *graphein*, to write]. An instrument for accurate recording of the outlines and positions of organs or foreign bodies as seen by radiographic apparatus.

orthodigita (or″thō-dĭj′ĭ-tă) [″ + L. *digitus*, finger]. Division of podiatry that deals with the correction of deviated toes; the prevention and correction of deformities of the fingers or toes.

orthodontia (or″thō-dŏn′shē-ă) [″ + *odous*, tooth]. Division of dentistry dealing with prevention and correction of abnormally positioned or aligned teeth. SYN: *orthodontics*.

orthodontics (or″thō-dŏn′tĭks). Orthodontia, q.v.

orthodontist. A dentist who is an expert in orthodontia.

orthodromic (or″thō-drŏm′ĭk) [Gr. *orthodromein*, to run straight forward]. Concerning an impulse moving in the normal direction via a nerve. SEE: *antidromic*.

orthogenesis (or″thō-jĕn′ĕ-sĭs) [Gr. *orthos*, straight, + *genesis*, generation, birth]. A biological principle that evolution of an animal species is in a given direction, governed by intrinsic factors, and independent of external factors.

orthogenic. Pert. to, or related to, the correction, treatment, or rehabilitation of children with mental or emotional difficulties.

orthogenics (or″thō-jĕn′ĭks). Eugenics, q.v.

orthograde (or′thō-grād) [″ + L. *gradi*, to walk]. Walking with the body vertical or upright; pert. to bipeds, esp. humans. Opposite of pronograde.

orthokeratology. Use of special contact lenses to treat myopia by altering the curvature of the cornea. The lens presses on the center of the cornea, thus decreasing the protrusion.

orthokinetic cuff. An elastic device fitted around a muscle and employing the principle that tactile stimulation over a muscle belly will facilitate contraction in the muscle or inhibit contraction in its antagonist.

orthokinetics. Various tactile stimulation techniques to stimulate the proprioceptors of muscles and tendons and thereby enhance motor performance in rehabilitation.

orthomelic (or″thō-mē′lĭk) [″ + *melos*, limb]. Correcting deformed arms and legs.

orthometer (or-thŏm′ĕ-tĕr) [″ + *metron*, measure]. Device for determining the degree of protrusion or retraction of the eyeballs.

orthomolecular (or″thō-mō-lĕk′ū-lăr). Indicating the normal chemical constituents of the body or the restoration of those constituents to normal.

orthomolecular psychiatry. Theoretical school of thought proposing that mental illness is due to biochemical abnormalities resulting in increased requirements for specific substances, such as vitamins and minerals.

orthomyxoviruses (or″thō-mĭk″sō-vī′rŭs-ĕs). Influenza viruses.

Ortho-Novum. Trade name for an estrogen combined with a progestogen.

orthopedia (or″thō-pē′dē-ă) [Gr. *orthos*, straight, + *pais*, child]. Orthopedics.

orthopedic (or″thō-pē′dĭk). Concerning orthopedics; prevention or correction of deformities.

orthopedics (or″thō-pē′dĭks) [″ + *pais*, child]. Branch of medical science that deals with prevention or correction of disorders involving locomotor structures of the body, esp. the skeleton, joints, muscles, fascia, and other supporting structures such as ligaments and cartilage.

orthopedic surgery. Surgical prevention and correction of musculoskeletal deformities.

orthopedist (or″thō-pē′dĭst). A specialist in orthopedics.

orthopercussion (or″thō-pĕr-kŭsh′ŭn) [″ + L. *percussio*, a striking]. Percussion with the distal phalanx of the percussing finger held perpendicularly to the surface percussed.

orthophoria (or″thō-fō′rē-ă) [″ + *pherein*, to bear]. Parallelism of visual axes, the normal muscle balance.

orthophrenia (or″thō-frē′nē-ă) [″ + *phren*, mind]. The normal mental state in social relations.

orthopnea (or″thŏp′nē-ă) [″ + *pnoia*, breath]. Respiratory condition in which there is discomfort in breathing in any but erect sitting or standing position.

SYM: Respiratory rate, slow or rapid; sitting or standing posture necessary; muscles of respiration forcibly used; patients feel necessity of bracing themselves in order to breathe. Anxious expression, face cyanosed. Struggle to inhale and exhale.

ETIOL: Seen in heart failure, bronchial and cardiac asthma, pulmonary edema, severe emphysema, pneumonia, angina pectoris, spasmodic cough.

RS: dyspnea; hyperpnea; oligopnea; posture; respiration.

orthopneic position (or″thŏp-nē′ĭk). The upright or nearly upright position of the upper trunk of a patient in a bed or chair. It facilitates breathing in those with congestive heart failure and some forms of pulmonary disease.

Orthopoxvirus. A genus of virus that includes the virus of smallpox, variola, and monkeypox.

orthopraxis (or″thō-prăk′sĭs) [″ + *prassein*, to make]. Mechanical or surgical correction of deformities.

orthopsychiatry (or″thō-sī-kī′ă-trē) [″ + *psyche*, soul, + *iatreia*, treatment]. Branch of psychiatry dealing with mental and emotional development; it encompasses child psychiatry and mental hygiene.

orthoptic (or-thŏp′tĭk) [″ + *optikos*, pert. to vision]. Pert. to or producing normal binocular vision.

orthoptics. 1. The science of correcting defects in binocular vision resulting from defects in optic musculature. 2. The technique of eye exercises for correcting faulty eye coordination affecting binocular vision.

orthoptic training. Eye muscle exercises for the purpose of correcting squint. SYN: *orthoptics*.

orthoroentgenography (or″thō-rĕnt-gĕn-ŏg′ră-fē). Accurate measurement of size and position of internal organs, using radiographic apparatus. A radiographic procedure used for the accurate measurement of long bones. SEE: *orthodiagraph*.

orthoscopic (or″thō-skŏp′ĭk). 1. Having correct and undistorted vision. 2. Made to correct optical distortion.

orthoscopy (or-thŏs′kō-pē). Ocular examination with an orthoscope.

orthosis [Gr., straightening]. Any device added to the body to stabilize or immobilize a body part, prevent deformity, protect against injury, or assist with function. Orthotic devices range from arm slings to corsets and finger splints. They may be made from a variety of materials, including rubber, leather, canvas, rubber synthetics, and plastic. SYN: *orthotic*.

orthostatic (or″thō-stăt′ĭk) [Gr. *orthos*, straight, + *statikos*, causing to stand]. Concerning an erect position. SYN: *orthotic*.

orthostatic hypotension. Postural hypotension, q.v.

orthostatic vital signs determination. Measurement of blood pressure and pulse rate in supine and erect positions. A significant change in vital signs signifies hypovolemia or dehydration. A positive test occurs if the patient becomes dizzy, has a pulse increase of 20 or more beats per minute, or a systolic blood pressure decrease of 20 or more mmHg (millimeters of mercury). Also known as tilt test or postural vital signs.

orthostatism (or′thō-stăt″ĭzm) [″ + ″ + -ismos, condition]. An upright standing position of the body.

orthotast (or′thō-tăst) [″ + *tassein*, to arrange]. Instrument for straightening bone curvatures.

ORTHOTONOS

orthotic [Gr. *orthosis*, straightening]. 1. Rel. to orthosis. 2. Orthostatic.

orthotics (or-thŏt'ĭks). 1. The science pert. to mechanical appliances for orthopedic use. 2. The use of orthopedic appliances.

orthotist (or'thō-tĭst) [Gr. *orthosis*, straightening]. One skilled in orthotics.

orthotonos, orthotonus (or-thŏt'ō-nŏs, -nŭs) [" + *tonos*, tension]. Tetanic spasm marked by rigidity of the body in a straight line. SEE: illus.

orthotopic (or"thō-tŏp'ĭk). In the correct place. Graft of an organ to a site where that organ would normally be present.

orthovoltage (or"thō-vōl'tĭj). Median voltage used in x-ray therapy. Approx. 250 kilovolts.

orthropsia (or-thrŏp'sē-ă) [Gr. *orthros*, time near dawn, + *opsis*, sight]. Characteristic of human vision by which sight is better at dawn or dusk than in bright sunlight.

orthuria (orth-ū'rē-ă) [Gr. *orthos*, normal, + *ouron*, urine]. Normal frequency of urination.

Ortolani's sign. Assessment maneuver designed to detect subluxation or dislocation of the hip. The examiner places the infant on the back with hips and knees flexed while abducting and lifting the femurs. A palpable click will be felt as the femur enters the dysplastic joint.

O.S., o.s. L. *oculus sinister*, left eye. SEE: *O.D., o.d.*

Os. Chem. symb. for the element osmium.

os (ōs) [L.] (pl. *ora*). [NA] Mouth, opening.
  o. uteri. Mouth of the uterus.
  o. uteri externum. The opening of the cervical canal of the uterus into the vagina.
  o. uteri internum. The internal opening of the cervical canal into the uterus.
  o. ventriculi. The cardia of the stomach.

os (ōs) [L] (pl. *ossa*). [NA] Bone.
  o. calcis. [NA] Heel bone. SYN: *calcaneus* [NA].

  o. coxae. [NA] Hip bone.
  o. hamatum. [NA] Hooked bone in second row of carpus (wrist). SYN: *unciform bone.*
  o. hyoideum. [NA] U-shaped bone at the base of the tongue. SYN: *hyoid bone.*
  o. ilii. [NA] The ilium.
  o. innominatum. Hip bone.
  o. magnum. A carpal bone, the third in the second distal row. SYN: *capitatum.*
  o. orbiculare. Tiny bone in the ear that becomes attached to the incus, forming the lenticular process.
  o. peroneum. Bone occasionally found in the tendon of peroneus longus muscle.
  o. planum. 1. Flat bone; any bone that has a slight thickness only. 2. Orbital plate of ethmoid bone.
  o. pubis. [NA] The pubic bone; anteroinferior part of the hip bone. In the adult, it unites the innominate bone with the ilium and ischium to form the pelvis. It is irregular in shape, divided into a horizontal, ascending, and descending ramus. The outer extremity constitutes approx. one fifth of the acetabulum. The inner ramus forms the symphysis pubis.
  o. scaphoideum. [NA] Scaphoid, q.v.
  o. temporale. Temporal bone, q.v.
  o. trigonum. [NA] Bone of foot that develops from an extra center of ossification along posterior surface of the talus.
  o. unguis. Lacrimal bone.
  o. vesalianum. Bone that develops from ossification of the posterior tubercle of the fifth metatarsal.

osazone (ō'să-zōn). Any of a series of compounds resulting from heating sugars with acetic acid and phenylhydrazine.

oscedo (ŏs-sē'dō) [L.]. 1. Yawning. 2. White spots on the mucosa of the mouth. SYN: *aphtha.*

oscheal (ŏs'kē-ăl) [Gr. *oscheon*, scrotum]. Concerning the scrotum.

oscheitis (ŏs-kē-ī′tĭs) [″ + *itis*, inflammation]. Inflamed condition of the scrotum. SYN: *oschitis*.

oschelephantiasis (ŏsk″ĕl-ĕ-făn-tī′ă-sĭs). Elephantiasis of the scrotum.

oscheo- [Gr. *oscheon*]. Combining form meaning the scrotum.

oscheocele (ŏs′kē-ō-sēl) [″ + *kele*, tumor, swelling]. A scrotal swelling or tumor. SYN: *oscheoma*.

oscheohydrocele (ŏs″kē-ō-hī′drō-sēl) [″ + *hydor*, water, + *kele*, tumor, swelling]. Scrotal hydrocele; collection of fluids in the sac of a scrotal hernia.

oscheolith (ŏs′kē-ō-lĭth) [″ + *lithos*, stone]. A concretion in the scrotal sebaceous glands.

oscheoma (ŏs-kē-ō′mă) [″ + *oma*, tumor]. Scrotal tumor. SYN: *oscheoncus*.

oscheoncus (ŏs″kē-ŏng′kŭs) [″ + *onkos*, mass, bulk]. A tumor of the scrotum. SYN: *oscheoma*.

oscheoplasty (ŏs′kē-ō-plăs″tē) [″ + *plassein*, to form]. Plastic surgical repair of the scrotum.

oschitis (ŏs-kī′tĭs). Oscheitis.

oscillation (ŏs″sĭl-ā′shŭn) [L. *oscillare*, to swing]. A swinging, pendulumlike movement; a vibration; fluctuation.

oscillator (ŏs′ĭ-lā″tor). 1. Device for producing oscillations. 2. An electronic circuit that will produce an oscillating current of a certain frequency.

oscillogram (ŏs′ĭl-ō-grăm) [″ + Gr. *gramma*, something written]. Graphic record made by the oscillograph.

oscillograph (ŏs′ĭl-ō-grăf) [″ + Gr. *graphein*, to write]. An electronic device for detecting and recording variations in electrical phenomena. In medicine, it is used for recording electrical activity of the heart and other muscular tissues. Electrocardiographs and electroencephalographs are examples of the application of this technique. SEE: *oscilloscope*.

oscillometer (ŏs-ĭl-ŏm′ĕt-ĕr) [″ + Gr. *metron*, measure]. Machine to measure oscillations, esp. those of the bloodstream.

oscillometry (ŏs-ĭl-ŏm′ĕ-trē). The measurement of oscillations with a machine.

oscillopsia. Sensation of oscillation or swinging of the visual field. It is illusory and may be associated with a severe form of labyrinthine nystagmus.

oscilloscope (ŏ-sĭl′ō-skōp) [L. *oscillare*, to swing, + Gr. *skopein*, to examine]. An instrument for making visible the presence, nature, and form of oscillations or irregularities of an electric current. SEE: *oscillograph*.

Oscinidae. The eye flies. A family of small hairless flies that includes the genera *Hippelates, Siphunculina,* and *Oscinis*. They are serious pests and transmit a number of infectious diseases.

oscitation (ŏs-ĭ-tā′shŭn) [L. *oscitatio*]. Yawning, gaping.

osculation [L. *osculum*, little mouth, kiss]. 1. The union of two vessels or structures by their mouths. 2. Kissing.

osculum (ŏs′kū-lŭm) [L.] (pl. *oscula*). Any tiny aperture or pore.

-ose. 1. Chemical suffix indicating that the substance is a carbohydrate, as glucose. 2. Suffix indicating a primary alteration product of a protein, as proteose.

Osgood-Schlatter disease (ŏz-good-shlăt′ĕr) [Robert B. Osgood, U.S. orthopedist, 1873–1956; Carl Schlatter, Swiss surgeon, 1864–1934]. Osteochondritis of the epiphysis of the tibial tuberosity.

OSHA. *Occupational Safety and Health Administration*. A U.S. governmental regulatory agency that is concerned with the health and safety of workers.

-osis [Gr.]. Suffix added to words of Greek origin. Indicates the condition, status, or process. Usually denotes an increase in the condition. SEE: *-sis*.

Osler, Sir William (ŏs′lĕr). Canadian-born physician, 1849–1919. In his career he was associated with McGill, Johns Hopkins, and Oxford Universities. During that time, he prepared a number of editions of his monumental *The Principles and Practice of Medicine.*

   O.'s disease. Disease of the blood in which the red cells are increased in number, the spleen becomes enlarged, and the face is a deep red rather than truly cyanotic. SYN: *erythremia; polycythemia vera; Vaquez's disease.*

   O.'s maneuver. An attempt to compress the radial artery sufficiently to prevent palpation of the radial pulse past the point of compression. If this pulse is still palpable, then the artery is sclerosed. This could lead to the diagnosis of hypertension when, in fact, the blood pressure could be normal.

   O.'s nodes. A small, raised, red, tender area present in the pads of the fingers and toes in bacterial endocarditis. The areas are due to infected emboli from the heart.

   O.- Vaquez disease. Polycythemia vera.

   O.- Weber-Rendu disease [Frederick Parkes Weber, Brit. physician, 1863–1962; Henri Jules Louis Marie Rendu, Fr. physician, 1844–1902]. A hereditary disease of capillaries. SEE: *telangiectasia, hereditary hemorrhagic.*

osmate. A salt of osmic acid.

osmatic (ŏz-măt′ĭk) [Gr. *osmasthai*, to smell]. Pert. to, or having, a keen sense of smell.

osmesis (ŏz-mē′sĭs) [Gr. *osmesis*, smelling].

1. The sense of smell. 2. The act of smelling. SYN: *olfaction.*

osmesthesia (ŏz″mĕs-thē′zē-ă) [Gr. *osme,* odor, + *aisthesis,* sensation]. Olfactory sensibility; power of perceiving and distinguishing odors.

osmic acid (ŏz′mĭk). OsO₄. Volatile colorless compound formed by heating osmium in air. Used as a caustic, stain for fats, tissue fixative for electron microscopy. SYN: *osmium tetroxide.*

Caution: Vapors are extremely toxic to eyes, skin, and respiratory tract. Container must not be opened without safeguarding eyes from vapors released from uncapping and possible spilling.

---

osmicate (ŏz′mĭ-kāt). To impregnate or stain with osmic acid.

osmics (ŏz′mĭks) [Gr. *osme,* odor]. The science of odors.

osmidrosis (ŏz-mĭ-drō′sĭs) [″ + *hidros,* sweat]. Condition in which perspiration has a very strong odor. SYN: *bromidrosis.*

osmiophilic (ŏz″mē-ō-fĭl′ĭk). Having an affinity for the staining material osmium tetroxide.

osmiophobic (ŏz″mē-ō-fō′bĭk). Having resistance to the staining material osmium tetroxide.

Osmitrol. Trade name for mannitol, USP.

osmium (ŏz′mē-ŭm) [Gr. *osme,* smell]. SYMB: Os. At. wt. 190.2; at. no. 76. A metallic element.

   o. tetroxide. OsO₄. Osmic acid.

osmo-. 1. [Gr. *osme,* odor]. Combining form indicating relationship to odor or smell. 2. [Gr. *osmos,* impulse]. Combining form indicating a thrusting forth. 3. [Gr. *osmos,* impulse]. Pert. to osmosis.

osmodysphoria (ŏz-mō-dĭs-fō′rē-ă) [Gr. *osme,* odor, + *dys,* bad, + *pherein,* to bear]. Deep-seated and abnormal dislike of certain odors.

osmolagnia (ŏz″mō-lăg′nē-ă) [″ + *lagneia,* lust]. Erotic satisfaction derived from odors, usually of the body. SYN: *osphresiolagnia.*

osmolality (ŏs″mō-lăl′ĭ-tē). Osmotic concentration, the characteristic of a solution determined by the ionic concentration of the dissolved substances per unit of solvent.

   o., serum. The osmotic concentration of the serum.

   o., urine. The osmotic concentration of the urine.

osmolar (ŏz-mō′lăr). Concerning the osmotic concentration of a solution.

osmolarity (ŏs″mō-lăr′ĭ-tē). Concentration of osmotically active particles in solution.

osmology (ŏz-mŏl′ō-jē). 1. [Gr. *osme,* odor,

+ *logos,* word, reason]. The study of odors. SYN: *osphresiology.* 2. [Gr. *osmos,* impulse, + *logos,* word, reason]. Study of osmosis.

osmometer (ŏz-mŏm′ĕt-ĕr). 1. [Gr. *osme,* odor, + *metron,* measure]. Device for measuring acuity of sense of smell. 2. [Gr. *osmos,* impulse, + *metron,* measure]. A device for measuring osmotic pressure.

osmonosology (ŏz″mō-nō-sŏl′ō-jē) [Gr. *osme,* odor, + *nosos,* disease, + *logos,* word, reason]. Branch of medicine dealing with diseases and disorders of the organs of smell.

osmophilic (ŏz″mō-fĭl′ĭk) [Gr. *osmos,* impulse, + *philos,* to love]. The character that promotes osmosis.

osmophore (ŏz″mō-for) [Gr. *osme,* odor, + *phoros,* bearing]. The portion of a chemical that is responsible for the odor of the compound.

osmoreceptor (ŏz″mō-rē-sĕp′tor). 1. A receptor in the hypothalamus that is sensitive to the osmotic pressure of the serum. 2. A receptor in the brain that is sensitive to olfactory stimuli.

osmoregulation (ŏz″mō-rĕg″ū-lā′shŭn). The regulation of osmotic pressure.

osmose (ŏz′mōs) [Gr. *osmos,* impulse]. 1. To subject to osmosis. 2. To undergo osmosis.

osmosis (ŏz-mō′sĭs) [Gr. *osmos,* impulse, + *osis,* condition]. The passage of solvent through a semipermeable membrane that separates solutions of different concentrations. The solvent, usually water, passes through the membrane from the region of lower concentration of solute to that of a higher concentration of solute, thus tending to equalize the concentrations of the two solutions. The rate of osmosis is dependent primarily upon the difference in osmotic pressures of the solutions on the two sides of a membrane, the permeability of the membrane, and the electric potential across the membrane and charge upon walls of the pores in it. SEE: illus.

   RS: absorption; dialysis; diffusion; hypotonic; isotonic solution.

osmotherapy (ŏz″mō-thĕr′ă-pē) [″ + *therapeia,* treatment]. Intravenous administration of hypertonic solutions in order to increase the osmolar concentration of the serum. This is used in treating cerebral edema.

osmotic (ŏz-mŏt′ĭk) [Gr. *osmos,* impulse]. Pert. to osmosis.

osmotic pressure. 1. Pressure that develops when two solutions of different concentrations are separated by a semipermeable membrane. 2. Pressure that would develop if a solution were enclosed in a membrane impermeable to all solutes present and surrounded by pure solvent. Osmotic pres-

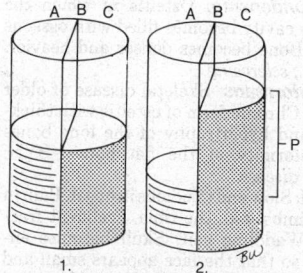

A. CHAMBER CONTAINING WATER.

B. MEMBRANOUS PARTITION
SEPARATING TWO CHAMBERS.

C. CHAMBER CONTAINING
A SOLUTION OF SALT IN WATER.

1. MEMBRANE B IS PERMEABLE
TO WATER AND SALT.

2. MEMBRANE B IS SEMIPERMEABLE
IN THAT IT IS IMPERMEABLE TO
SALT BUT PERMEABLE TO WATER.

P. OSMOTIC PRESSURE CAUSES
THE DIFFERENCE IN LEVELS
BETWEEN CHAMBERS A AND C
WHEN SEPARATED BY A
SEMIPERMEABLE MEMBRANE.

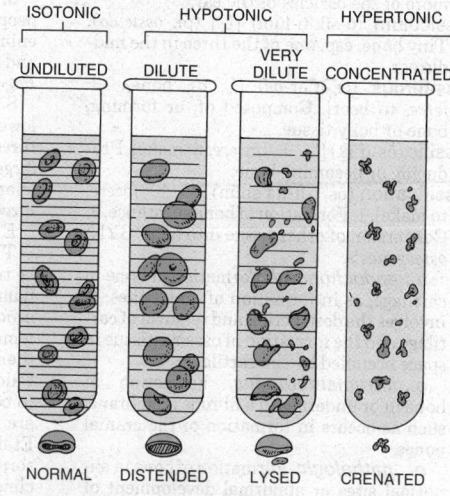

OSMOSIS

OSMOSIS IN WHOLE BLOOD AND IN SALT SOLUTIONS THAT
HAVE INCREASED OR DECREASED SALT CONCENTRATION

ISOTONIC   HYPOTONIC   HYPERTONIC

UNDILUTED   DILUTE   VERY DILUTE   CONCENTRATED

NORMAL   DISTENDED   LYSED   CRENATED

THE ERYTHROCYTES SWELL IN HYPOTONIC AND CONTRACT
(BECOME CRENATED) IN HYPERTONIC SALT SOLUTIONS.

sure varies with concentration of the solution and with temperature increase. Animal cells have an osmotic pressure approximately equal to that of the circulating fluid, the blood. Solutions exerting this osmotic pressure are said to be isotonic or isosmotic; stronger solutions that cause cells to shrink are hypertonic; weaker solutions that cause cells to swell are hypotonic.

osphresiolagnia (ŏs-frē″zē-ō-lăg′nē-ă) [Gr. *osphresis*, smell, + *lagneia*, lust]. Excitement of an erotic nature produced by odors. SYN: *osmolagnia*.

osphresiology (ŏs″frē-zē-ŏl′ō-jē) [″ + *logos*, word, reason]. Science of odors and the sense of smell. SYN: *osmology*.

osphresiometer (ŏs″frē-zē-ŏm′ĕ-tĕr) [″ + *metron*, measure]. Apparatus for measuring the acuteness of the sense of smell. SYN: *osmometer*.

osphresis (ŏs-frē′sīs) [Gr.]. The sense of smell. SYN: *olfaction*.

osphretic (ŏs-frĕt′ĭk). Concerning the sense of smell. SYN: *olfactory*.

osphus (ŏs′fŭs) [Gr. *osphys*]. Loin.

osphyalgia (ŏs-fē-ăl′jē-ă) [″ + *algos*, pain]. Pain in the loins or hips. SEE: *lumbago; sciatica and low back pain*.

osphyitis (ŏs-fē-ī′tĭs) [″ + *itis*, inflamma-

tion]. Inflammation of the lumbar region.

osphyomyelitis (ŏs″fē-ō-mī″ĕl-ī′tĭs) [″ + *myelos*, marrow, + *itis*, inflammation]. Inflamed condition of the lumbar region of the spinal cord.

ossa (ŏs′ă) [L., bones]. Pl. of os.

ossein (ŏs′ē-ĭn) [L. *ossa*, bones]. The collagen of bone. It forms the framework of bone.

osseocartilaginous (ŏs″ē-ō-kăr″tĭ-lăj′ĭ-nŭs). Concerning bone and cartilage.

osseofibrous (ŏs″ē-ō-fī′brŭs) [″ + *fibra*, fiber]. Composed of bone and fibrous tissue.

osseointegration. In dental implants, difficulty in removing a chamber that apparently has bonded to bone.

osseomucin (ŏs″ē-ō-mū′sĭn). Ground substance of bone.

osseous (ŏs′ē-ŭs) [L. *osseus*, bony]. Bonelike; concerning bones. SYN: *bony*.

ossicle (ŏs′ĭ-kl) [L. *ossiculum*, little bone]. Any small bone, esp. one of the three bones of the ear.

o.′s, auditory. The three bones of the inner ear: incus, malleus, and stapes. SEE: *ear* for illus.

ossicula (ŏ-sĭk′ū-lă) [L.] (sing. *ossiculum*). Little bones.

ossiculectomy (ŏs″ĭk-ū-lĕk′tō-mē) [L. *ossiculum*, little bone, + Gr. *ektome*, excision]. Excision of an ossicle, esp. one of the ear.

ossiculotomy (ŏ″sĭk-ū-lŏt′ō-mē) [″ + Gr. *tome*, incision]. Surgical incision of one or more of the ossicles of the ear.

ossiculum (ō-sĭk′ū-lŭm) [L.] (pl. *ossicula*). Tiny bone, esp. one of the three in the middle ear.

ossiferous (ŏs-ĭf′ĕr-ŭs) [L. *os*, bone, + *ferre*, to bear]. Composed of, or forming, bone or bony tissue.

ossific (ŏs-ĭf′ĭk) [″ + *facere*, to make]. Producing or becoming bone.

ossification (ŏs″ĭ-fĭ-kā′shŭn) [″ + *facere*, to make]. 1. Formation of bone substance. 2. Conversion of other tissue into bone. SYN: *osteogenesis*.

   o., endochondral. Formation of bone in cartilage, as in formation of long bones. It involves the destruction and removal of cartilage and the formation of osseous tissue in space occupied by the cartilage.

   o., intramembranous. Formation of bone in or underneath a fibrous membrane, such as occurs in formation of the cranial bones.

   o., pathologic. Formation of bone in abnormal sites or abnormal development of bone.

   o., periosteal. Formation of successive thin layers of bone by osteoblasts between the underlying bone or cartilage and the cellular and fibrous layer that covers the forming bone. Also called subperiosteal ossification.

ossifluence (ŏ-sĭf′lū-ĕns). Osteolysis or softening of bone.

ossiform (ŏs′ĭ-form). Resembling bone. SYN: *osteoid*.

ossify (ŏs′ĭ-fī) [″ + *facere*, to make]. To turn into bone.

ostalgia (ŏs-tăl′jē-ă) [Gr. *osteon*, bone, + *algos*, pain]. Pain in a bone. SYN: *osteodynia*.

osteal (ŏs′tē-ăl). Pert. to bone.

ostealgia (ŏs′tē-ăl′jē-ă) [″ + *algos*, pain]. Bone pain.

osteanagenesis (ŏs″tē-ăn-ă-jĕn′ĕ-sĭs) [″ + *ana*, on, + L. *genesis*, generation, birth]. Regeneration or re-formation of bone.

ostearthrotomy (ŏs″tē-ăr-thrŏt′ō-mē) [″ + *arthron*, joint, + *tome*, incision]. Surgical excision of the articular end of a bone. SYN: *osteoarthrotomy*.

ostectomy, osteectomy (ŏs-tĕk′tō-mē, -tē-ĕk′tō-mē) [″ + *ektome*, excision]. Surgical excision of a bone or a portion of one.

osteectopia (ŏs″tē-ĕk-tō′pē-ă) [″ + *ektopos*, out of place]. Displacement of a bone.

osteitis (ŏs-tē-ī′tĭs) [″ + *itis*, inflammation]. Inflammation of a bone.

   o., condensing. Osteitis in which the marrow cavity becomes filled with osseous tissue. Bone becomes denser and heavier. SYN: *o., sclerosing*.

   o. deformans. Skeletal disease of older people. Chronic form of osteitis with thickening and hypertrophy of the long bones and deformity of the flat bones. SYN: *Paget's disease*.

   SYM: Slow and insidious in onset. Pain in lower limbs, esp. the tibia. Frequent fractures. Waddling gait. Skull becomes enlarged, so that the face appears small and triangular in shape with the head pushed forward. Stature shortens.

   ETIOL: Unknown.

   TREAT: Asymptomatic cases should not be treated. Aspirin or nonsteroidal anti-inflammatory drugs are given for pain. There is no specific curative therapy, but male and female sex hormones, fluoride, and x-ray therapy have been used to control the pain. Calcitonin and mithramycin have been used to control the resorption of bone and thus are of assistance in alleviating bone pain. Etidronate sodium has reduced bone resorption in most patients and produced clinical improvement in some.

   o. fibrosa cystica generalisata. A condition resulting from overactivity of the parathyroid glands with resulting disturbances in calcium and phosphorus metabolism. Characterized by decalcification and softening of bone, nephrolithiasis, and elevation of blood calcium and lowering of blood phosphorus. Cysts form and tumors may develop. SYN: *hyperparathyroidism*.

   o. fragilitans. Osteogenesis imperfecta, q.v.

   o., gummatous. Chronic osteitis associated with syphilis and characterized by the formation of gummas.

   o., rarefying. Form of osteitis in which inorganic matter is lessened and bone tissue becomes latticelike in structure. SYN: *osteoporosis*.

   o., sclerosing. O., condensing.

ostembryon (ŏs-tĕm′brē-ŏn) [Gr. *osteon*, bone, + *embryon*, something that swells in the body]. A fetus that has become ossified. SYN: *lithopedion; osteopedion*.

ostemia (ŏs-tē′mē-ă) [″ + *haima*, blood]. Congestion of blood in a bone.

ostempyesis (ŏs″tĕm-pī-ē′sĭs) [″ + *empyesis*, suppuration]. Purulent inflammation within a bone.

osteo- [Gr. *osteon*, bone]. Combining form indicating relationship to a bone.

osteoanagenesis (ŏs″tē-ō-ăn″ă-jĕn′ĕ-sĭs) [″ + Gr. *ana*, again, + L. *genesis*, generation, birth]. Regeneration of bone.

osteoanesthesia (ŏs″tē-ō-ăn″ĕs-thē′zē-ă) [″

+ *an-*, not, + *aisthesis*, sensation]. The condition of the bone being insensitive, esp. to stimuli that would normally produce pain.

osteoaneurysm (ŏs″tē-ō-ăn′ū-rĭzm) [″ + *aneurysma*, a widening]. Aneurysm, or dilatation of a blood vessel filled with clotted blood, occurring within a bone.

osteoarthritis (ŏs″tē-ō-ăr-thrī′tĭs) [″ + *arthron*, joint, + *itis*, inflammation]. A chronic disease involving the joints, esp. those bearing weight. Characterized by destruction of articular cartilage, overgrowth of bone with lipping and spur formation, and impaired function.

This disease is an almost inevitable consequence of aging and is a major cause of severe chronic disability, affecting nearly 10% of the population over age 60. SYN: *arthritis, degenerative*.

NURSING IMPLICATIONS: Plan with patient to provide rest following activity and to pace activities to prevent excessive fatigue or irritation to joints. Support patient in coping with limitations of mobility. Teach exercise and treatment regimens specific to affected joints, including application of moist heat, range-of-motion exercises to limit of pain, maintenance of correct body weight and posture, use of supportive appliances and devices, and home safety measures as ordered. SEE: *Nursing Diagnoses* in *Appendix*.

osteoarthropathy (ŏs″tē-ō-ăr-thrŏp′ă-thē) [″ + ″ + *pathos*, disease, suffering]. Any disease involving the joints and bones, accompanied by severe pain.

 o., hypertrophic pulmonary. An affection characterized by enlargement of distal phalanges of fingers and toes and a thickening of their distal ends, accompanied by a peculiar longitudinal curving of nails. Wrist and interphalangeal joints may become enlarged, as may distal ends of tibia and fibula and the jaw.

ETIOL: Found in pulmonary tuberculosis, chronic bronchitis, bronchiectasis, and congenital heart disease.

osteoarthrosis (ŏs″tē-ō-ăr-thrō′sĭs) [″ + ″ + *osis*, condition]. Osteoarthritis.

osteoarthrotomy (ŏs″tē-ō-ăr-thrŏt′ō-mē) [″ + ″ + *tome*, incision]. Excision of joint end of a bone. SYN: *ostearthrotomy*.

osteoblast (ŏs′tē-ō-blăst) [Gr. *osteon*, bone, + *blastos*, germ]. A cell of mesodermal origin that is concerned with the formation of bone.

osteoblastoma (ŏs″tē-ō-blăs-tō′mă) [″ + ″ + *oma*, tumor]. A large benign tumor of osteoblasts in a patchy osteoid matrix. It occurs mostly in the vertebral columns of young people.

osteocampsia (ŏs″tē-ō-kămp′sē-ă) [″ + *kamptein*, to bend]. Curvature of a bone, as in osteomalacia.

osteocarcinoma (ŏs″tē-ō-kăr-sĭn-ō′mă) [″ + *karkinos*, cancer, + *oma*, tumor]. 1. Combined osteoma and carcinoma. 2. Carcinoma of a bone.

osteocartilaginous (ŏs″tē-ō-kăr″tĭ-lăj′ĭ-nŭs). Concerning bone and cartilage.

osteocele (ŏs′tē-ō-sēl) [″ + *kele*, tumor, swelling]. 1. A testicular or scrotal tumor that contains bony tissue. 2. A bone-containing hernia.

osteocephaloma (ŏs″tē-ō-sĕf″ă-lō′mă) [″ + *kephale*, head, + *oma*, tumor]. Encephaloma, a malignant neoplasm of brain-like texture in a bone.

osteochondral (ŏs″tē-ō-kŏn′drăl). Concerning bone and cartilage.

osteochondritis (ŏs″tē-ō-kŏn-drī′tĭs) [″ + *chondros*, cartilage, + *itis*, inflammation]. Inflammation of bone and cartilage.

 o. deformans juvenilis. Chronic inflammation of the head of the femur in children. Results in atrophy and shortening of the neck of femur with a wide flat head. SYN: *Waldenström's disease.*

 o. dissecans. Condition affecting a joint in which a fragment of cartilage and its underlying bone become detached from articular surface. Occurs commonly in the knee joint.

osteochondrodystrophy (ŏs″tē-ō-kŏn″drō-dĭs′trō-fē) [″ + ″ + *dys*, bad, + *trephein*, to nourish]. A disorder of skeletal growth resulting from bone and cartilage malformation. Produces a form of dwarfism. SYN: *Morquio's syndrome.*

 o., familial. Morquio's syndrome. SEE: *mucopolysaccharidosis IV.*

osteochondrolysis (ŏs″tē-ō-kŏn-drŏl′ĭ-sĭs) [″ + ″ + *lysis*, dissolution]. Osteochondritis dissecans.

osteochondroma (ŏs″tē-ō-kŏn-drō′mă) [″ + ″ + *oma*, tumor]. Tumor composed of both cartilaginous and bony substance.

osteochondromatosis (ŏs″tē-ō-kŏn″drō-mă-tō′sĭs) [″ + ″ + ″ + *osis*, condition]. A disease in which there are multiple osteochondromata.

osteochondrosarcoma (ŏs″tē-ō-kŏn″drō-săr-kō′mă) [″ + ″ + *sarx*, flesh, + *oma*, tumor]. Chondrosarcoma occurring in bone.

osteochondrosis (ŏs″tē-ō-kŏn-drō′sĭs) [″ + ″ + *osis*, condition]. Degenerative changes in the ossification centers of the epiphyses of bones, particularly during periods of rapid growth in children. The process continues to the stage of avascular and aseptic necrosis and then there is slow healing and repair.

NURSING IMPLICATIONS: Encourage bedrest and support patient through disruption of normal activity. Teach correct use of crutches. Evaluate neurocirculatory function distal to supportive device (splint, elastic support, or cast). Evaluate joint mobility and limitation of motion daily.

o. deformans tibiae. Degeneration or aseptic necrosis of the medial condyle of the tibia.

osteochondrous (ŏs″tē-ō-kŏn′drŭs). Containing bone and cartilage.

osteoclasia, osteoclasis (ŏs″tē-ō-klā′zē-ă, -ŏk′lă-sĭs) [″ + klasis, a breaking]. 1. Surgical fracture of a bone in order to remedy a deformity. SYN: *diaclasis.* 2. Bony tissue absorption and destruction.

osteoclast (ŏs′tē-ō-klăst) [″ + klan, to break]. 1. Device for fracturing bones for therapeutic purposes. 2. Giant multinuclear cell formed in bone marrow of growing bones. Found in depressions (called Howship's lacunae) on the surface of the bone. Concerned with absorption and removal of unwanted tissue.

osteoclast activating factor. ABBR: OAF. A lymphokine produced in certain conditions associated with resorption of bone. Periodontal disease and lymphoid proliferative diseases such as multiple myeloma and malignant lymphoma are included. Interleukin-1 is an OAF, as are other substances produced by T lymphocytes and prostaglandins.

osteoclastic (ŏs″tē-ō-klăs′tĭk). Concerning osteoclasts.

osteoclastoma (ŏs″tē-ō-klăs-tō′mă) [″ + ″ + oma, tumor]. Giant cell tumor of bone.

osteoclasty (ŏs′tē-ō-klăs″tē). Osteoclasis.

osteocope (ŏs′tē-ō-kōp) [″ + kopos, pain]. Extreme pain in the bones, esp. in syphilitic bone disease.

osteocopic (ŏs″tē-ō-kŏp′ĭk). Concerning severe pain in the bone.

osteocranium (ŏs″tē-ō-krā′nē-ŭm) [″ + kranion, skull]. The portion of the cranium formed of membrane bones in contrast to that formed of cartilage (chondrocranium).

osteocystoma (ŏs″tē-ō-sĭs-tō′mă) [″ + kystis, sac, bladder, + oma, tumor]. Cystic tumor of a bone.

osteocyte (ŏs′tē-ō-sīt″) [″ + kytos, cell]. A mesodermal bone-forming cell that has become entrapped within the bone matrix; it lies within a lacuna with processes extending outward through canaliculi and, by its metabolic activity, helps to maintain bone as a living tissue.

osteodensitometer. Device for determining the density of bones. Usually x-ray technique is used.

osteodentin. Dentin that forms very rapidly or in response to severe trauma so that cells and blood vessels are incorporated, resembling bone.

osteodermia (ŏs″tē-ō-dĕr′mē-ă) [″ + derma, skin]. The formation of bony deposits in the skin.

osteodesmosis (ŏs″tē-ō-dĕs-mō′sĭs) [″ + desmos, tendon, + osis, condition]. Transformation of tendon into bone.

osteodiastasis (ŏs″tē-ō-dī-ăs′tă-sĭs) [″ + diastasis, separation]. Separation of two adjacent bones.

osteodynia (ŏs″tē-ō-dĭn′ē-ă) [″ + odyne, pain]. Persistent pain in a bone. SYN: *ostealgia.*

osteodystrophia (ŏs″tē-ō-dĭs-trō′fē-ă) [″ + dys, ill, + trophe, nourishment]. Defective bone development. SYN: *osteodystrophy.*

osteodystrophy (ŏs″tē-ō-dĭs′trō-fē). Defective bone development.

o., renal. Generalized pathological changes in bone with resemblance to osteitis fibrosa cystica, osteomalacia, and osteoporosis. These changes are associated with renal failure. The serum phosphorus is elevated, calcium is low or normal, and there is increased parathyroid gland activity.

osteoectomy (ŏs″tē-ō-ĕk′tō-mē) [″ + ektome, excision]. Ostectomy, q.v.

osteoepiphysis (ŏs″tē-ō-ē-pĭf′ĭs-ĭs) [″ + epi, upon, + physis, growth]. A small piece of bone that is separated in childhood from the larger bone by cartilage; during later growth, the two bones join.

osteofibroma (ŏs″tē-ō-fī-brō′mă) [″ + L. fibra, fiber, + Gr. oma, tumor]. Tumor of bony and fibrous tissues. SYN: *fibro-osteoma.*

osteogen (ŏs′tē-ō-jĕn) [″ + gennan, to produce]. Substance of the inner periosteal layer from which bone is formed.

osteogenesis, osteogeny (ŏs″tē-ō-jĕn′ē-sĭs, -ŏj′ē-nē). Formation and development of bone taking place in connective tissue or in cartilage. SYN: *ossification.*

o. imperfecta. An inherited disorder of connective tissue characterized by defective bone matrix with calcification occurring normally on whatever matrix is present. Clinical findings are multiple fractures with minimal trauma, blue sclerae, early deafness, opalescent teeth, tendency to capillary bleeding, translucent skin, and joint instability. Although the disease is heterogeneous, two different classifications of osteogenesis imperfecta are still used for clinical distinction: osteogenesis imperfecta congenita, with early fractures occurring even in utero; and osteogenesis imperfecta tarda, with delayed onset of fracturing and much milder manifestations. Healing of bone fractures progresses normally. Later in life, the tendency to fracture decreases and often disappears. The vast majority of cases are inherited as an autosomal dominant trait, although a small percentage of congenital cases are transmitted as an autosomal recessive. There is no known cure for osteogenesis imperfecta; therefore, treatment is supportive and palliative. Definition provided by the American Brittle Bone Society, Inc.

osteogenic. Pert. to osteogenesis.

osteography (ŏs″tē-ŏg′răf-ē) [Gr. *osteon*, bone, + *graphein*, to write]. Descriptive treatise on the bones.

osteohalisteresis (ŏs″tē-ō-hăl-ĭs″tĕr-ē′sĭs) [″ + *hals*, salt, + *sterein*, to deprive]. Softening of the bones, caused by deficiency of mineral constituents of the bone.

osteoid (ŏs′tē-oyd) [″ + *eidos*, form, shape]. 1. Resembling bone; ossiform. 2. The noncalcified matrix of bone. Also called prebone.

osteokinematics. Description of bone movement when a bone swings through a range of motion around the axis in a joint, such as with flexion, extension, abduction, adduction, or rotation.

osteolipochondroma (ŏs″tē-ō-lĭ-pō″kŏn-drō′mă) [″ + *lipos*, fat, + *chondros*, cartilage, + *oma*, tumor]. A chondroma containing fatty and bony tissue.

osteologist (ŏs″tē-ŏl′ō-jĭst) [″ + *logos*, word, reason]. A specialist in the study of bone.

osteology (ŏs-tē-ŏl′ō-jē) [″ + *logos*, word, reason]. The science of structure and function of bones.

osteolysis (ŏs″tē-ŏl′ĭ-sĭs) [″ + *lysis*, dissolution]. A softening and destruction of bone without osteoclastic activity; it occurs within compact bone and results from a breakdown of the organic matrix and subsequent leaching out of the inorganic fraction, probably caused by localized metabolic disturbances, vascular changes, or release of hydrolytic enzymes by osteocytes.

osteolytic (ŏs″tē-ō-lĭt′ĭk). Causing osteolysis.

osteoma (ŏs-tē-ō′mă) [″ + *oma*, tumor] (pl. *osteomata*). A benign bony tumor; a bonelike structure that develops on a bone or, occasionally, at other sites. SYN: *exostosis; osteoncus.*

   o., cancellous. A soft and spongy tumor. Its thin and delicate trabeculae enclose large medullary spaces similar to that in cancellous bone.

   o., cavalryman's. Bony outgrowth of femur at the insertion of the adductor

femoris longus.

   o. cutis. Benign formation of bone nodules in the skin.

   o., dental. A bony outgrowth or exostosis of the root of a tooth.

   o. durum, o. eburneum. A very hard osteoma in which the bone is ivorylike.

   o. medullare. Osteoma containing medullary spaces.

   o., osteoid. A rare benign tumor of bone composed of sheets of osteoid tissue partially calcified and ossified. Occurs esp. in extremities of young.

   o. spongiosum. Spongy tumor in the bone. SYN: *osteospongioma.*

osteomalacia (ŏs″tē-ō-măl-ā′shē-ă) [Gr. *osteon*, bone, + *malakia*, softening]. A disease marked by increasing softness of the bones, so that they become flexible and brittle, thus causing deformities. Osteomalacia is the adult form of rickets, q.v.

SYM: Rheumatic pains in the limbs, spine, thorax, and esp. the pelvis; anemia and signs of deficiency disease; progressive weakness.

ETIOL: Deficiency or loss of calcium salts due to vitamin D deficiency.

TREAT: If the diet contains an adequate amount of calcium and phosphorus, a daily dose of 1600 I.U. of vitamin D for about a month will cause great improvement. The dose can then be gradually decreased to the normal daily requirement for vitamin D.

osteomalacic (ŏs″tē-ō-măl-ā′sĭk) [″ + *malakia*, softening]. Concerning or characterized by softening of the bone.

osteomatoid (ŏs-tē-ō′mă-toyd) [″ + *oma*, tumor, + *eidos*, form, shape]. Resembling a bonelike tumor.

osteomatosis (ŏs″tē-ō″mă-tō′sĭs) [″ + ″ + *osis*, condition]. Formation of multiple osteomas.

osteomere (ŏs′tē-ō-mēr) [″ + *meros*, part]. One in a series of similar bony segments, as the vertebrae.

osteometry (ŏs-tē-ŏm′ĕt-rē) [″ + *metron*, measure]. The study of the measurement of parts of the skeletal system.

osteomyelitis (ŏs″tē-ō-mī″ĕl-ī′tĭs) [″ + *myelos*, marrow, + *itis*, inflammation]. Inflammation of bone, esp. the marrow, caused by a pathogenic organism. SEE: *Nursing Diagnoses in Appendix.*

SYM: Pain in the affected part, fever, sweats, leukocytosis, overlying muscles usually rigid, skin inflamed, pain on pressure over affected part. Suppuration may occur.

TREAT: Prompt and adequate doses of antibiotics; sedation for pain and anxiety; aspiration of abscess; immobilization of affected extremity; surgery if abscess persists.

SEE: *bone scan.*

osteomyelodysplasia (ŏs″tē-ō-mī″ĕ-lō-dĭs-plā′sē-ă) [″ + ″ + *dys*, bad, + *plassein*, to form]. Condition in which the marrow space of the bones is increased, the bony tissue becomes thin, and there are leukopenia and fever.

osteon (ŏs′tē-ŏn) [Gr., bone]. The microscopic bone unit of compact bone, consisting of the haversian canals and the surrounding lamellae.

osteoncus (ŏs-tē-ŏng′kŭs) [″ + *onkos*, bulk, mass]. A bone tumor. SYN: *exostosis; osteoma.*

osteonecrosis (ŏs″tē-ō-nē-krō′sĭs) [″ + *nekrosis*, state of death]. Generalized death of bone tissue rather than isolated areas of necrosis.

osteonectin. A glycoprotein present in the noncollagenous portion of the matrix of bone.

osteoneuralgia (ŏs″tē-ō-nū-răl′jē-ă) [″ + *neuron*, nerve, + *algos*, pain]. Pain of a bone.

osteopath (ŏs′tē-ō-păth) [″ + *pathos*, disease]. A practitioner of osteopathy.

osteopathic (ŏs″tē-ō-păth′ĭk). Concerning osteopathy.

osteopathology (ŏs″tē-ō-păth-ŏl′ō-jē) [″ + *pathos*, disease, + *logos*, word, reason]. 1. Any bone disease. SYN: *osteopathy* (def. 1). 2. Study of bone diseases.

osteopathy (ŏs-tē-ŏp′ă-thē) [″ + *pathos*, disease, suffering]. 1. Any bone disease. 2. A system of medicine based upon the theory that the normal body is a vital mechanical organism in which structural and functional states are of equal importance and that the body is able to rectify itself against toxic conditions when it has favorable environmental circumstances and satisfactory nourishment. Therefore, it is the osteopathic physician's responsibility to remove any internal or external abnormalities of the system. Although using manipulation for the most part to restore structural and functional balance, osteopaths also rely upon physical, medicinal, and surgical methods. Osteopathy, which was founded by Dr. Andrew Taylor Still (1828–1917), is recognized as a standard method or system of medical and surgical care.

Physicians with a degree in osteopathy use the designation D.O.

osteopecilia (ŏs″tē-ō-pĕ-sĭl′ē-ă) [″ + *poikilia*, spottedness]. Osteopoikilosis, q.v.

osteopedion (ŏs″tē-ō-pē′dē-ŏn) [″ + *paidion*, child]. A calcified or hardened fetus. SYN: *lithopedion; ostembryon.*

osteopenia (ŏs″tē-ō-pē′nē-ă) [″ + *penia*, lack]. 1. Condition of diminished amount of bone tissue, without respect to cause. 2. De-creased bone density caused by failure of rate of osteoid tissue synthesis to keep up with the normal rate of bone lysis. SEE: *osteoporosis.*

osteoperiosteal (ŏs″tē-ō-pĕr″ē-ŏs′tē-ăl) [″ + *peri*, around, + *osteon*, bone]. Concerning bone and its periosteum, the protective connective tissue covering bone.

osteoperiostitis (ŏs″tē-ō-pĕr″ē-ŏs-tī′tĭs) [″ + ″ + ″ + *itis*, inflammation]. Inflammation of a bone and its protective membrane, the periosteum.

osteopetrosis (ŏs″tē-ō-pĕ-trō′sĭs) [″ + *petra*, stone, + *osis*, condition]. Hereditary condition marked by excessive calcification of bones causing spontaneous fractures and marblelike appearance. SYN: *Albers-Schönberg disease; osteosclerosis fragilis.* SEE: *marble bones.*

osteophage (ŏs′tē-ō-fāj) [″ + *phagein*, to eat]. Large multinuclear cell that causes absorption of bone. SEE: *osteoclast.*

osteophagia (ŏs″tē-ō-fā′jē-ă). In animals, a craving to eat bones, caused by a calcium or phosphorus deficiency.

osteophlebitis (ŏs″tē-ō-flē-bī′tĭs) [″ + *phleps, phleb-*, vein, + *itis*, inflammation]. Inflammation of veins of a bone.

osteophone (ŏs′tē-ō-fōn″) [Gr. *osteon*, bone, + *phone*, voice]. Device used by the deaf for conducting sound through facial bones.

osteophony (ŏs″tē-ŏf′ō-nē). Bone conduction of sound.

osteophore (ŏs′tē-ō-for) [″ + *pherein*, to carry]. A forceps for crushing bone.

osteophyma (ŏs″tē-ō-fī′mă) [″ + *phyma*, growth]. A swelling or growth of bone.

osteophyte (ŏs′tē-ō-fīt) [″ + *phyton*, plant]. A bony excrescence or outgrowth, usually branched in shape.

osteoplaque (ŏs′tē-ō-plăk). A layer of bone.

osteoplast (ŏs′tē-ō-plăst) [″ + *plastos*, formed]. Osteoblast.

osteoplastic (ŏs″tē-ō-plăs′tĭk) [″ + *plastikos*, formed]. 1. Pert. to bone repair by plastic surgery or grafting. 2. Concerning bone formation.

osteoplasty (ŏs′tē-ō-plăs″tē) [″ + *plassein*, to form]. Plastic repair of the bones.

osteopoikilosis (ŏs″tē-ō-poy″kĭ-lō′sĭs) [″ + *poikilos*, spotted]. Hereditary disease of bones marked by excessive calcification in spots less than 1 cm in diameter. It is a benign disease.

osteoporosis (ŏs″tē-ō-por-ō′sĭs) [″ + *poros*, a passage, + *osis*, condition]. A general term for describing any disease process that results in reduction in the mass of bone per unit of volume. The reduction is sufficient to interfere with the mechanical support function of bone. This term does not indicate a specific etiological agent; indeed, many conditions and diseases may be involved in the process. The condition becomes apparent when the osteoporosis has progressed to the stage at which the bone fractures in a situation that would not normally cause damage to the skeleton, i.e., a pathological fracture. The bones that are most frequently involved are the vertebrae of the lower dorsal and lumbar areas. Osteoporosis may affect any bone, including those of the jaw. Bone loss is a universal concomitant of advanced age, but it proceeds at a faster rate in women, esp. following menopause. This condition is more likely to occur in sedentary individuals.

TREAT: Supplemental calcium and vitamin D are indicated and may help to stop the rate of bone loss. In menopausal women, therapy with estrogen decreases the rate of bone resorption, but bone formation does not increase; thus, skeletal mass is not increased.

Prevention of osteoporosis should begin prior to bone loss, because there has been little success in therapy aimed at restoring bone. Exercise is important in arresting the rate of bone loss. Regular exercise has been shown to reduce the risk of hip fracture by about one half. Quitting smoking is another important preventive measure. SEE: illus.; *bone scan; hip, fracture of.*

NURSING IMPLICATIONS: Teach the patient the importance of an exercise program, including mechanics and range of motion. Use a firm mattress and assistive safety devices at home. Explain and encourage a diet high in vitamin D, calcium, and protein to prevent further bone loss. Encourage gynecologic follow-up examinations if the patient is being maintained on estrogen therapy. SEE: *Nursing Diagnoses* in *Appendix.*

o. circumscripta cranii. Localized osteoporosis of the skull associated with Paget's disease of bone.

o. of disuse. Osteoporosis due to lack of stress to the bones. It may occur while in bed for a prolonged period or while flying in outer space in a weightless condition.

o., posttraumatic. Loss of bone tissue following trauma, esp. when there is damage to a nerve supplying the injured area. The condition may also be caused by disuse.

osteoporotic (ŏs″tē-ō-por-ŏt′ĭk). Concerning a porous condition of the bones.

osteoradionecrosis (ŏs″tē-ō-rā″dē-ō-nĕ-krō′sĭs) [Gr. *osteon*, bone, + L. *radiatio*, radiation, + Gr. *nekrosis*, state of death]. Death of bone following irradiation.

osteorrhagia (ŏs″tē-ō-rā′jē-ă) [″ + *rhegnynai*, to burst forth]. Hemorrhagic flow of blood from a bone.

osteorrhaphy (ŏs-tē-or′ă-fē) [″ + *rhaphe*, seam, ridge]. Suture of bone or the wiring of bone fragments. SYN: *osteosuture.*

osteosarcoma (ŏs″tē-ō-săr-kō′mă) [″ + *sarx*, flesh, + *oma*, tumor]. A malignant sarcoma of the bone. SYN: *myelosarcoma.*

osteosarcomatous (ŏs″tē-ō-săr-kō′măt-ŭs). Concerning or like an osteosarcoma.

osteosclerosis (ŏs″tē-ō-sklĕ-rō′sĭs) [″ + *skleros*, hard, + *osis*, condition]. Abnormal increase in thickening and density of bone.

o. fragilis. Osteopetrosis, q.v.

osteoscope (ŏs′tē-ō-skōp) [″ + *skopein*, to examine]. Appliance used to test x-ray machines by observing certain bones of the forearm that are considered as a standard.

osteoseptum (ŏs″tē-ō-sĕp′tŭm) [″ + L. *septum*, a partition]. The bony area of the nasal septum.

osteosis (ŏs″tē-ō′sĭs) [″ + *osis*, condition]. Presence of bone-containing nodules in the skin.

o. cutis. Diffuse thickening of skin and subcutaneous tissue.

osteospongioma (ŏs″tē-ō-spŏn″jē-ō′mă) [″ + *spongos*, sponge, + *oma*, tumor]. A spongy neoplasm of bone. SYN: *osteoma spongiosum.*

osteosteatoma (ŏs″tē-ō-stē″ă-tō′mă) [″ + *stear*, fat, + *oma*, tumor]. A benign fatty tumor with bony elements.

osteostixis (ŏs″tē-ō-stĭk′sĭs) [″ + *stixis*, a puncture]. Therapeutic diagnostic puncture of a bone.

osteosuture (ŏs″tē-ō-sū′chŭr) [″ + L. *sutura*, a stitch]. Suture or wiring of bone fragments. SYN: *osteorrhaphy.*

osteosynovitis (ŏs″tē-ō-sĭn″ō-vī′tĭs) [″ + *syn*, with, + *oon*, egg, + *itis*, inflammation]. Inflammation of a synovial membrane and the surrounding bones.

osteosynthesis (ŏs″tē-ō-sĭn′thĕ-sĭs) [″ + *synthesis*, a joining]. Surgical fastening of the ends of a fractured bone by mechanical means.

osteotelangiectasia (ŏs″tē-ō-tĕl-ăn″jē-ĕk-tă′zē-ă) [″ + *telos*, end, + *angeion*, vessel, + *ektasis*, a stretching]. Sarcomatous tumor of the bone containing dilated blood vessels.

osteothrombosis (ŏs″tē-ō-thrŏm-bō′sĭs) [″ + *thrombosis*, a clotting]. Clot formation in the veins of a bone.

osteotome (ŏs′tē-ō-tōm) [″ + *tome*, incision]. A chisel beveled on both sides for cutting through bones.

osteotomoclasis (ŏs″tē-ō-tō-mŏk′lă-sĭs) [Gr. *osteon*, bone, + *tomos*, section, + *klasis*, breaking]. Correction of a pathologically curved bone by bending it after a wedge has been chiseled out of it by use of an osteo-

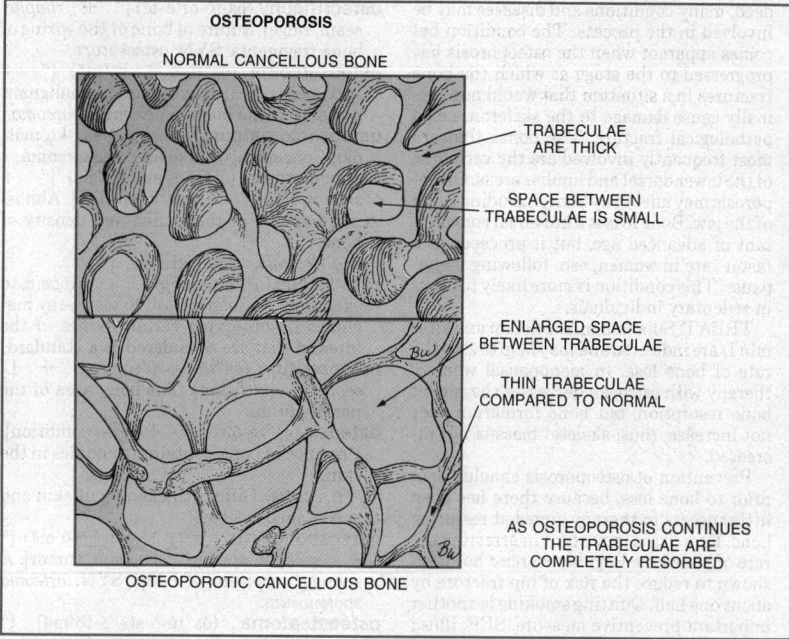

OSTEOPOROSIS

NORMAL CANCELLOUS BONE

TRABECULAE ARE THICK

SPACE BETWEEN TRABECULAE IS SMALL

ENLARGED SPACE BETWEEN TRABECULAE

THIN TRABECULAE COMPARED TO NORMAL

AS OSTEOPOROSIS CONTINUES THE TRABECULAE ARE COMPLETELY RESORBED

OSTEOPOROTIC CANCELLOUS BONE

tome.

osteotomy (ŏs-tē-ŏt′ō-mē) [″ + *tome*, incision]. The operation for cutting through a bone.

o., C-form. A C-shaped cut through the ramus of the mandible to allow forward placement of the mandible in correcting a retrognathic condition.

o., condylar neck. Surgery on the condylar neck of the mandible to correct prognathism.

o., cuneiform. The excision of a wedge of bone.

o., linear. Lengthwise division of a bone.

o., Macewen′s. Supracondylar section of the femur for correction of knock-knee.

o., subtrochanteric. Division of shaft of femur below lesser trochanter to correct ankylosis of hip joint.

o., transtrochanteric. Section of the femur through the lesser trochanter for deformity about the hip joint.

osteotribe (ŏs′tē-ō-trīb″) [″ + *tribein*, to rub]. A bone rasp.

osteotrite (ŏs′tē-ō-trīt) [″ + *tribein*, to grind or rub]. Instrument used to scrape away diseased bone.

osteotrophy (ŏs-tē-ŏt′rō-fē) [″ + *trophe*, nutrition]. Bone nutrition.

osteotylus (ŏs″tē-ŏt′ĭ-lŭs) [″ + *tylos*, callus]. The callus around the ends of bones that have been fractured.

osteotympanic (ŏs″tē-ō-tĭm-păn′ĭk). Craniotympanic, q.v.

ostial (ŏs′tē-ăl) [L. *ostium*, a little opening]. Concerning an orifice.

ostitis (ŏs-tī′tĭs) [Gr. *osteon*, bone, + *itis*, inflammation]. Inflammation of a bone. SYN: *osteitis.*

ostium (ŏs′tē-ŭm) [L.] (pl. *ostia*). [NA] Small opening, esp. one into a tubular organ.

o. abdominale tubae uterinae. [NA] Fimbriated end of fallopian tube.

o. arteriosum. [NA] Arterial orifice of ventricle of the heart into the aorta or pulmonary artery.

o. internum. Uterine end of a fallopian tube.

o. pharyngeum. Pharyngeal opening of the auditory (eustachian) tube.

o. primum. Primary opening in the lower part of the septum of the atria of the embryonic heart. This closes shortly after birth.

o. primum defect. Atrial septal defect located low in septum.

o. secundum. Opening in the higher part of the septum of the atria of the embryonic heart. This closes shortly after birth.

o. secundum defect. Atrial septal defect located high in septal wall.

o. tympanicum. Tympanic opening of the auditory (eustachian) tube.

o. urethrae externum. [NA] External opening of the urethra.

o. uteri. [NA] Opening from the uterus to the vagina. SYN: *cervical os.*

o. uterinum tubae. [NA] Opening of the uterine tube into the uterus.

o. vaginae. [NA] External opening of the vagina.

ostomate (ŏs'tō-māt) [L. *ostium,* little opening]. One who has a surgically formed fistula connecting the bowel or intestine to the outside, usually through the abdominal wall. Thus an artificial anus exists at the ostomy site. SEE: *colostomy; ileostomy.*

ostomy (ŏs'tō-mē). The surgically formed artificial opening that serves as the exit site for connections that the surgeon has made from the bowel or intestine to the outside. SEE: *colostomy; ileostomy.*

OSTOMY CARE: Whether the ostomy is temporary or permanent, assure the patient that it will be possible to carry on normal activities with a minimum of inconvenience. Prior to being discharged from the hospital, the patient should be provided full explanation and demonstration of ostomy care. It is esp. important to have the patient and family become involved in ostomy care as soon as possible. This will promote confidence that a normal life will be possible. Consultation with another patient who has become competent in ostomy care will be esp. helpful. Those individuals may be contacted through ostomy clubs that have been organized in various cities. The patient should be provided with precise directions concerning places that sell ostomy care equipment. Detailed instructions for care and use of ostomy devices are included in the package.

Specific care involves the stoma (enterostomal care) and irrigation of the bowel leading from the stoma. In caring for a double-barrel colostomy, it is important to irrigate only the proximal stoma.

STOMA CARE: Character of material excreted through the stoma will depend on the portion of the bowel to which it is attached; excretions from the ileum will be fluid and quite irritating to skin; those from the upper right colon will be semifluid; those from the upper left colon are mushy; and those from the sigmoid colon will tend to be solid. Care of the stoma, whether for ileostomy or colostomy, is directed toward maintaining the peristomal skin and mucosa of the stoma in a healthy condition. This is more difficult to achieve with an ileostomy

than with a lower colon colostomy. The skin surrounding the stoma can be protected by use of commercially available discs, or washers, made of karaya gum or hypoallergenic skin shields. The collecting bag or pouch can be attached to the karaya gum washer or skin shield so that a watertight seal is made. The karaya gum washers can be used on weeping skin, but the skin shields cannot. New skin will grow beneath the karaya gum. The stoma may require only a gauze pad covering in the case of a sigmoid colostomy that is being irrigated daily or every other day. If a plastic bag is used for collecting drainage, it will need to be emptied periodically and changed as directed. At each change of the bag, meticulous but gentle skin care will be given. The stoma should not be manually dilated except by those experienced in enterostomal care.

IRRIGATION OF COLOSTOMY: Many individuals will be able to regulate the character of their diet so that the feces may be removed from the colon at planned intervals. The stoma is attached to a plastic bag held in place with a self-adhering collar or a belt. The irrigating fluid, tap water, or saline solution (1 tsp or 4 gm of salt to 1 pint or 500 ml of water) at 40°C (104°F) is introduced slowly through a soft rubber catheter. Catheter is inserted about 10 to 15 cm, and container for irrigating fluid is hung at height that will allow fluid to flow slowly. The return from the irrigation may be collected in a closed or open-ended bag. The latter will allow the return to empty into a basin or toilet. The return of fluid and feces should be completed in less than one-half hour after irrigating fluid has entered bowel.

At the completion, clean the skin and stoma carefully and replace the dressing or the pouch. Then clean equipment thoroughly and store in a dry, well-ventilated space. When irrigation of ostomy is provided for a hospitalized patient, chart amount and kind of fluid instilled, amount and character of return, care provided for stoma and condition of stoma. If pouch or bag is attached, note whether or not it was replaced.

MISCELLANEOUS CONSIDERATIONS: Odor may be controlled by avoiding foods that the individual finds to cause undesirable odors. Gas may be controlled by avoiding foods known to produce gas, which will vary from patient to patient. Diet should be planned to provide stool consistency that will be neither hard and constipating nor loose and watery. The patient may learn this by trial and error and by consulting with nutritionists and ostomy club members. Daily physical activity, sexual relations, and swimming are all possible.

ostosis (ŏs-tō′sĭs). Osteogenesis.

ostraceous (ŏs-trā′shŭs). Shaped like an oyster shell.

ostraco-, ostrac- [Gr. *ostrakon*, shell]. Combining form meaning hard shell.

ostreotoxismus (ŏs″trē-ō-tŏks-ĭz′mŭs) [Gr. *ostreon*, oyster, + *toxikon*, poison]. Poisoning from eating contaminated oysters.

O.T. *occupational therapy.*

otacoustic (ō″tă-koo′stĭk) [Gr. *otakousteo*, to listen]. 1. Aiding or concerning the hearing. 2. Device to aid hearing; an ear trumpet.

otalgia (ō-tăl′jē-ă) [Gr.]. Pain in the ear. SYN: *earache; otodynia; otoneuralgia.*

TREAT: Local: Heat in the form of compresses, hot water bottle, or warm glycerin dropped in ear. General: Nasal astringents to help maintain patency of the eustachian tube; relieve pain; use appropriate systemic antibiotic if there is an infection.

otantritis (ō″tăn-trī′tĭs) [Gr. *otos*, ear, + L. *antrum*, sinus, + Gr. *itis*, inflammation]. Inflammation of the mastoid antrum.

O.T.(C). An occupational therapist who is a member of the Canadian Association of Occupational Therapists.

O.T.C. *over the counter.* Refers to drugs and devices available without a prescription.

OTD. *organ tolerance dose.* Limitation of radiation tolerated by particular tissues.

otectomy (ō-tĕk′tō-mē) [Gr. *otos*, ear, + *ektome*, excision]. Surgical excision of the contents of the middle ear.

othelcosis (ō-thĕl-kō′sĭs) [″ + *helkosis*, ulceration]. Ulceration or suppuration of the ear.

othematoma (ŏt″hē-mă-tō′mă) [″ + *haima*, blood, + *oma*, tumor]. Effusion of blood, causing a hard swelling between perichondrium and cartilage of pinna. Common in fighters and wrestlers. SYN: *hematoma auris.* SEE: *cauliflower ear.*

otic (ō′tĭk) [Gr. *otikos*]. Concerning the ear.

otitic (ō-tĭt′ĭk). Concerning inflammation of the ear.

otitis (ō-tī′tĭs) [Gr. *otos*, ear, + *itis*, inflammation]. Inflamed condition of the ear. It is differentiated as externa, media, and interna, depending upon which portion of the ear is inflamed.

   o., aero-. Otitis resulting from pressure changes when auditory tubes are obstructed. Occurs commonly in aviators and divers.

   o., aviation. Barotitis, q.v.

   o. externa. Inflammation of the external auditory canal.

   o., furuncular. Furuncle formation in the external meatus of the ear.

   o. interna, labyrinthica. Labyrinthitis, q.v.

   o. labyrinthica. Inflammation of the labyrinth of the ear.

   o. mastoidea. Inflammation of the middle ear that involves the mastoid spaces.

   o. media. Inflammation of the middle ear.

   o. media with effusion. Chronic otitis characterized by the secretion of a serous fluid into the middle ear due to obstruction of the eustachian tube. This causes retraction of the eardrum; and, upon examination, a level of air fluid may be seen through the tympanic membrane. The serous fluid may be sterile or it may be infected with pathogenic organisms. The cause of the obstruction may be enlarged adenoid tissue in the pharynx, inflammation in the pharynx, tumors in the pharyngeal area, or allergy.

TREAT: Nasal decongestants may afford symptomatic relief. The use of antibiotics is controversial. Adenoidectomy and bilateral myringotomy may be necessary if conservative measures, including insertion of a ventilation or tympanostomy tube, are not effective. SYN: *allergic otitis media; non-suppurative otitis media; secretory otitis media.* SEE: *tympanostomy tubes.*

   o. mycotica. Inflammation of the ear caused by a fungal infection.

   o. parasitica. Inflammation of the ear caused by a parasite.

   o. sclerotica. Inflammation of the inner ear accompanied by hardening of the aural structures.

oto-, ot- [Gr. *otos*, ear]. Combining form rel. to the ear.

otoantritis (ō″tō-ăn-trī′tĭs) [″ + *antron*, cavity, + *itis*, inflammation]. Inflamed condition of the mastoid antrum and tympanic attic.

otoblennorrhea (ō″tō-blĕn″ō-rē′ă) [″ + *blenna*, mucus, + *rhoia*, flow]. Mucous discharge from the ear.

otocatarrh (ō″tō-kă-tăr′) [″ + *katarrhein*, to flow down]. Catarrhal discharge of the ear.

otocephalus (ō″tō-sĕf′ă-lŭs). One with otocephaly.

otocephaly (ō″tō-sĕf′ă-lē) [″ + *kephale*, head]. Congenital absence of the lower jaw and fusion or near fusion of the ears on the front of the neck.

otocleisis (ō-tō-klī′sĭs) [″ + *kleisis*, closure]. Occlusion of any auditory passages.

otoconium (ō″tō-kō′nē-ŭm) [″ + *konis*, dust] (pl. *otoconia*). Minute particle, composed chiefly of calcium carbonate, found in otolithic membrane on surface of maculae of inner ear. SYN: *ear dust; otolith.*

otocyst (ō′tō-sĭst) [″ + *kystis*, sac, bladder]. Primordial chamber from which arises the membranous labyrinth.

otodynia (ō″tō-dĭn′ē-ă) [″ + *odyne*, pain]. Pain in the ear; earache. SYN: *otalgia; otoneuralgia.*

otoganglion (ō″tō-găng′glē-ŏn) [″ + *ganglion*, ganglion]. The otic ganglion.

otogenic, otogenous (ō″tō-jĕn′ĭk, ō-tŏj′ĕn-ŭs) [″ + *gennan*, to produce]. Having its origin in the ear.

otolaryngologist (ō″tō-lar″ĭn-gŏl′ō-jĭst) [″ + *larynx*, larynx, + *logos*, word, reason]. A specialist in otolaryngology.

otolaryngology (ō″tō-lar″ĭn-gŏl′ō-jē). The division of medical science that includes otology, rhinology, and laryngology.

otolith (ō′tō-lĭth) [″ + *lithos*, stone]. Otoconium.

otological (ō″tō-lŏj′ĭ-kăl) [″ + *logos*, word, reason]. Rel. to study of diseases of the ear.

otologist (ō-tŏl′ō-jĭst). One knowledgeable in the anatomy, physiology, and pathology of the ear. A specialist in diseases of the ear.

otology (ō-tŏl′ō-jē) [Gr. *otos*, ear, + *logos*, word, reason]. The science dealing with the ear, its function, and its diseases.

otomassage [″ + *massein*, to knead]. Massage of the tympanic membrane and bones of the middle ear by means such as sound waves, puffs of air in the ear canal, or vibratory percussion of the tympanic membrane.

otomucormycosis (ō″tō-mū″kor-mī-kō′sĭs) [″ + L. *mucor*, mold, + Gr. *mykes*, fungus, + *osis*, condition]. Mucormycosis, q.v., of the ear.

otomyces (ō″tō-mī′sēz) [″ + *mykes*, fungus]. Any fungus infection of the ear.

otomycosis (ō″tō-mī-kō′sĭs) [″ + ″ + *osis*, condition]. An infection of the external auditory meatus of the ear caused by a fungus infestation. SYN: *mycomyringitis; myringomycosis; otitis mycotica.*

otoncus (ō-tŏng′kŭs) [″ + *onkos*, tumor]. Tumor of the ear.

otonecrectomy, otonecronectomy (ō″tō-nē-krĕk′tō-mē, ō″tō-nē″krō-nĕk′tō-mē) [″ + *nekros*, corpse, + *ektome*, excision]. Excision of necrosed areas from the ear.

otoneuralgia (ō″tō-nū-răl′jē-ă) [″ + *neuron*, sinew, + *algos*, pain]. Pain in the ear. SYN: *otalgia; otodynia.*

otoneurasthenia (ō″tō-nū″răs-thē′nē-ă) [″ + ″ + *astheneia*, weakness]. Neurasthenia caused by ear disease.

otoneurology (ō″tō-nū-rŏl′ō-jē) [″ + ″ + *logos*, word, reason]. The division of otology that deals with the inner ear, esp. its nerve supply, nerve connections with the brain, and auditory and labyrinthine pathways and centers within the brain. SYN: *neurotology.*

otopathy (ō-tŏp′ă-thē) [″ + *pathos*, dis-ease, suffering]. Any diseased condition of the ear.

otopharyngeal (ō″tō-făr-ĭn′jē-ăl) [″ + *pharynx*, throat]. Concerning the ear and pharynx.

otopharyngeal tube. Passage between the tympanic cavity and the pharynx. SEE: *eustachian tube.*

otoplasty (ō′tō-plăs″tē) [″ + *plassein*, to form]. Plastic surgery of the ear to correct defects and deformities.

otopyorrhea (ō″tō-pī″ō-rē′ă) [″ + *pyon*, pus, + *rhein*, to flow]. Purulent discharge from the ear.

otopyosis (ō″tō-pī-ō′sĭs) [″ + ″ + *osis*, infection]. Ear disease marked by discharge of pus.

otorhinolaryngology (ō″tō-rī″nō-lăr″ĭn-gŏl′ō-jē) [″ + *rhis*, nose, + *larynx*, larynx, + *logos*, word, reason]. The science of ear, nose, and larynx and of their functions and diseases.

otorhinology (ō″tō-rī-nŏl′ō-jē) [″ + ″ + *logos*, word, reason]. Branch of medicine dealing with the ear and nose and their diseases.

otorrhea (ō″tō-rē′ă) [″ + *rhein*, flow]. Inflammation of ear with purulent discharge. SEE: *otitis.*

otosalpinx (ō″tō-săl′pĭnks) [″ + *salpinx*, tube]. Passage connecting pharynx and tympanic cavity. SYN: *eustachian tube; otopharyngeal tube.*

otoscleronectomy (ō″tō-sklē″rō-nĕk′tō-mē) [″ + *skleros*, hard, + *ektome*, excision]. Surgical excision of sclerosed and ankylosed ear ossicles.

otosclerosis (ō″tō-sklē-rō′sĭs) [″ + *sclerosis*, hardening]. Condition characterized by chronic progressive deafness, esp. for low tones. Caused by formation of spongy bone, esp. around the oval window with resulting ankylosis of stapes. In late stages, atrophy of the organ of Corti may occur. More common in females. May be made worse by pregnancy.

ETIOL: Unknown. In some cases, condition is familial.

TREAT: Various surgical procedures including stapedectomy, q.v., have been used with considerable improvement in hearing. It is also possible to remove the diseased stapes and replace it with a prosthesis that transmits sound waves to the inner ear.

otoscope (ō′tō-skōp) [″ + *skopein*, to examine]. Device for examination of the ear.

otoscopy (ō-tŏs′kō-pē). Use of the otoscope in examining the ear.

otosis (ō-tō′sĭs) [″ + *osis*, condition]. Mishearing or misunderstanding of spoken sounds.

otosteal (ō-tŏs′tē-ăl) [″ + *osteon*, bone].

Concerning the bones or ossicles of the ear.

ototomy (ō-tŏt'ō-mē) [" + *tome,* incision]. Incision into or dissection of the ear.

ototoxic (ō"tō-tŏk'sĭk) [" + *toxikon,* poison]. Having a detrimental effect on the eighth nerve or the organs of hearing.

ototoxicity (ō"tō-tŏks-ĭs'ĭ-tē). The quality of being ototoxic.

O.T.R. *occupational therapist, registered.*

Otrivin Hydrochloride. Trade name for xylometazoline hydrochloride, USP.

Otto pelvis (ŏt'ō) [Adolph W. Otto, Ger. surgeon, 1786–1845]. Protrusion of the acetabulum into the pelvic cavity. This may occur in association with severe osteoarthritis of the hip.

O.U., o.u. L. *oculus uterque,* each eye.

ouabain (wă-bā'ĭn). A glycoside prepared from *Strophanthus gratus.* Its action is similar to that of digitalis.

oulitis (oo-lī'tĭs) [Gr. *oulon,* gum, + *itis,* inflammation]. Inflammation of the gums.

oulorrhagia (oo-lō-rā'jē-ă) [" + *rhegnynai,* to burst forth]. Hemorrhage from the gums. SYN: *ulorrhagia.*

ounce (owns) [L. *uncia,* a twelfth]. ABBR: oz. A measure of weight and liquid volume used in the apothecaries' system. When used in the avoirdupois system, ounce indicates only a unit of weight.

Apothecaries' or *troy* weight: SYMB: ℥. Equivalent to ½ pound, 480 grains, 31.103 grams. When used in U.S. Pharmacopeia, 1 oz contains 8 drams.

Avoirdupois measure: Equivalent to 1⁄16 pound, 437.5 grains, 28.349 grams.

o., fluid-. Apothecaries' measure for liquid medicines, 8 fluidrams (1⁄16 pint, 29.6 milliliters).

-ous. Suffix indicating possessing, full of.

outbreak. Sudden increase in the incidence of a disease or condition in a specific area.

outcome. The result of an action.

outcome criteria. Criteria in quality assurance programs in which the adequacy of the programs is judged by the achievement of predetermined outcomes.

outflow. In neurology, the passage of impulses outwardly from the central nervous system.

o., craniosacral. Impulses passing through parasympathetic nerves.

o., thoracolumbar. Impulses passing through sympathetic nerves.

"outing." The practice of forcing persons with alternate sexual preferences, i.e., homosexual and bisexual individuals, to publicly declare their preference(s).

outlet. A vent or opening for something to escape.

o., pelvic. SEE: *pelvic outlet.*

out-of-body experience. Concerning the

perception of being away from and overlooking oneself. The feeling is that the mind and soul have departed and the body is acting on its own.

outpatient. One who receives treatment at a hospital, clinic, or dispensary but is not hospitalized.

outpocketing. Evagination, q.v.

output (owt'poot). That which is produced, ejected, or expelled.

o., cardiac. Volume of blood pumped into the arterial system per unit of time. The stroke volume multiplied by the heart rate per minute gives the cardiac output. Normal value in healthy adults is 2.5 to 6.0 liters per minute.

o., energy. Work expended per unit of time by the body.

o., stroke. Amount of blood pumped in a single heartbeat.

o., urinary. Amount of urine produced by the kidneys.

outrigger. An attachment for hand splints that permits the fingers to be placed in elastic traction.

ova (ō'vă) [L. *ovum,* egg]. Pl. of ovum.

oval (ō'văl) [L. *ovalis,* egg shaped]. 1. Concerning an ovum, the reproductive cell of the female. 2. Having an elliptical shape like an egg.

ovalbumin (ō"văl-bū'mĭn) [" + *albumen,* white of egg]. Albumin occurring in egg white.

ovalocyte (ō'văl-ō-sīt") [" + Gr. *kytos,* cell]. Elliptical red blood corpuscle.

ovalocytosis (ō-văl"ō-sī-tō'sĭs) [" + " + *osis,* condition]. Abnormally large amount of elliptical red blood corpuscles in the blood.

oval window. Oval-shaped aperture in the middle ear into which fits the base of the stapes.

ovaralgia, ovarialgia (ō"văr-ăl'jē-ă, -ē-ăl'jē-ă) [LL. *ovarium,* ovary, + Gr. *algos,* pain]. Ovarian pain. SYN: *oarialgia, oophoralgia.*

ovarian (ō-vā'rē-ăn) [LL. *ovarium,* ovary]. Concerning or resembling the ovary.

ovarian cyst. A sac that develops in the ovary proper. It consists of one or more chambers containing fluid. These loculi, or chambers, may contain an enormous amount of fluid. Although nonmalignant, the cyst may have to be removed surgically because of twisting of the pedicle, which causes gangrene, or because of pressure. SEE: *polycystic ovary syndrome.*

ovariectomy (ō"vă-rē-ĕk'tō-mē) [" + Gr. *ektome,* excision]. Excision of an ovary or a portion of it. SYN: *oophorectomy.*

ovario- [LL. *ovarium,* ovary]. Combining form indicating relationship to the ovary.

ovariocele (ō-vā'rē-ō-sēl) [" + Gr. *kele,*

tumor, swelling]. Ovarian tumor or hernia.

ovariocentesis (ō-vā″rē-ō-sĕn-tē′sĭs) [″ + Gr. *kentesis*, puncture]. Surgical puncture and drainage of an ovarian cyst.

ovariocyesis (ō-vā″rē-ō-sī-ē′sĭs) [″ + Gr. *kyesis*, pregnancy]. Pregnancy in the ovary. SEE: *gestation, ectopic.*

ovariodysneuria (ō-vā″rē-ō-dĭs-nū′rē-ă) [″ + Gr. *dys*, ill, + *neuron*, sinew]. Neuralgia in an ovary.

ovariogenic (ō-vā″rē-ō-jĕn′ĭk) [″ + *gennan*, to produce]. Originating in the ovary.

ovariohysterectomy (ō-vā″rē-ō-hĭs″tĕr-ĕk′tō-mē) [″ + Gr. *hystera*, womb, + *ektome*, excision]. Excision of the ovaries and uterus. SYN: *oophorohysterectomy; oothecohysterectomy.*

ovariopathy (ō-vā″rē-ŏp′ă-thē) [″ + *pathos*, disease, suffering]. Disease of the ovary.

ovariopexy (ō-vā″rē-ō-pĕk′sē) [″ + *pexis*, fixation]. Surgical fixation of the ovary to the abdominal wall.

ovariorrhexis (ō-vā″rē-ō-rĕk′sĭs) [″ + Gr. *rhexis*, a rupture]. Rupture of an ovary.

ovariosalpingectomy (ō-vā″rē-ō-săl″pĭn-jĕk′tō-mē) [″ + Gr. *salpinx*, tube, + *ektome*, excision]. Removal of an ovary and oviduct. SYN: *oophorosalpingectomy.*

ovariosteresis (ō-vā″rē-ō-stĕr-ē′sĭs) [″ + Gr. *steresis*, loss]. Removal of an ovary.

ovariostomy (ō-vā″rē-ŏs′tō-mē) [″ + Gr. *stoma*, mouth]. Creation of an opening in an ovarian cyst for the purpose of drainage.

ovariotexy. Surgical procedure for encompassing the ovaries in a Silastic bag in order to prevent contact of the ovum with sperm.

ovariotomy (ō-vā″rē-ŏt′ō-mē) [LL. *ovarium*, ovary, + Gr. *tome*, incision]. 1. Incision into, or removal of, an ovary. 2. Removal of a tumor of the ovary.

ovariotubal (ō-vā″rē-ō-tū′băl) [″ + *tuba*, a narrow duct]. Concerning the ovary and oviducts.

ovariprival (ō-vā″rĭ-prī′văl) [″ + *privare*, to remove]. Resulting from loss of the ovaries.

ovaritis (ō″vă-rī′tĭs) [″ + Gr. *itis*, inflammation]. Inflamed condition of an ovary. Usually involved secondarily in inflammation of the oviducts or pelvic peritoneum. May involve the substance of the organ (oophoritis) or its surface (perioophoritis), and may be acute or chronic.

ovarium (ō-vā′rē-ŭm) [LL.] (pl. *ovaria*). [NA] The ovary.

ovary (ō′vă-rē) [LL. *ovarium*, ovary]. One of two glands in the female that produce the reproductive cell, the ovum, and two known hormones. The ovaries are almond-shaped bodies lying in the fossa ovarica on either side of the pelvic cavity, attached to the uterus by the utero-ovarian ligament and lying close to the fimbria ovarica of the fallopian tube. About 4 cm long, 2 cm wide, and 8 mm thick. Each ovary is attached to the broad ligament by the mesovarium and to the side of the pelvis by the suspensory ligament. The surface of the ovary in early life is smooth and in later life is markedly pitted as an end result of the atrophy of corpora lutea.

Each ovary consists of two parts, an outer portion or cortex, which encloses a central medulla. The medulla consists of a stroma of connective tissue containing nerves, blood, and lymphatic vessels, and some smooth muscle tissue at region of hilus. The cortex consists principally of follicles in various stages of development (primary, growing, and mature or graafian). Its surface is covered by a single layer of cells, the germinal epithelium, beneath which is a layer of dense connective tissue, the tunica albuginea. Other structures (corpus luteum, corpus albicans, q.v.) may be present. SEE: illus.

BLOOD SUPPLY: Mainly derived from the ovarian artery, which reaches the ovary through the infundibulopelvic ligament.

PHYS: 1. The production of ova. 2. The production of hormones, among which are estrogen, secreted by the follicles, and progesterone, secreted by the corpus luteum. These hormones are responsible for development and maintenance of secondary sexual characteristics, preparation of uterus for pregnancy, and development of the mammary gland.

Functional activity of the ovary is controlled primarily by gonadotropins of the hypophysis, esp. the follicle-stimulating hormone (FSH) and luteinizing hormone (LH) or interstitial cell hormone (ICH).

ovary, words pert. to: adnexitis; albuginea; castrate; cell, interstitial; conception; corpus albicans; facies ovarina; fertilization; fimbria ovarica; folliculoma; graafian follicle; hyperovaria; Krukenberg's tumor; menstrual cycle; menstruation; mesosalpinx; mesovarium; oarialgia; polycystic ovaries; pyoovarium; spay; spermatozoon; teratoma; tunica albuginea; and words beginning with "oophor-" and "ov-".

Ovcon. Trade name for an estrogen combined with a progestogen.

overbite. The vertical extension of the incisal ridges of the upper teeth over the incisal ridges of the lower anterior teeth when the jaws are in occlusion.

overclosure. A form of defective bite in which the mandible closes too far before the teeth make contact.

overcompensation. The process by which a person substitutes an opposite trait or

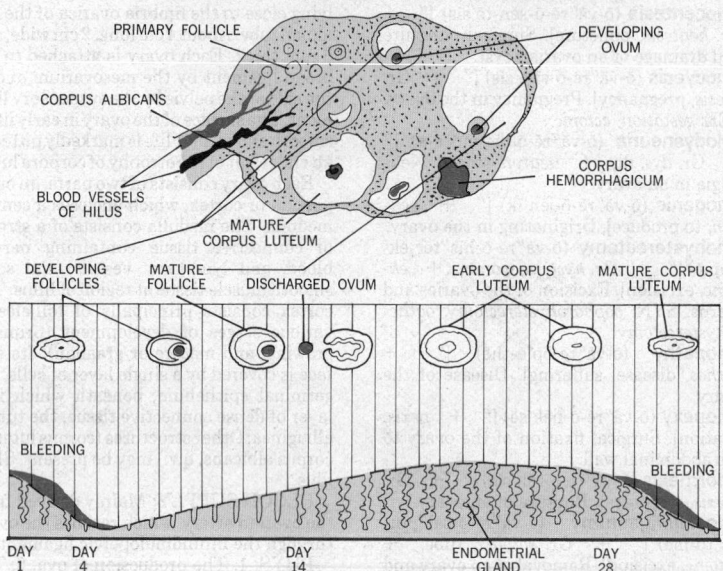

OVARY WITH DEVELOPING FOLLICLES AND CORPUS LUTEUM

PRIMARY FOLLICLE

DEVELOPING OVUM

CORPUS ALBICANS

CORPUS HEMORRHAGICUM

BLOOD VESSELS OF HILUS

MATURE CORPUS LUTEUM

DEVELOPING FOLLICLES   MATURE FOLLICLE   DISCHARGED OVUM   EARLY CORPUS LUTEUM   MATURE CORPUS LUTEUM

BLEEDING

BLEEDING

DAY 1   DAY 4   DAY 14   ENDOMETRIAL GLAND   DAY 28

ENDOMETRIAL CYCLE CORRELATED WITH FOLLICLE, AND CORPUS LUTEUM DEVELOPMENT

exerts effort in excess of that needed to compensate for, or conceal, a psychological feeling of guilt, inadequacy, or inferiority. May lead to maladjustment.

overcorrection. The use of too powerful a lens to correct the defect in refractive power of the eye.

overdenture. A denture supported by the soft tissue and whatever natural teeth remain. These have been altered so the denture will fit over them.

overdetermination. The idea in psychoanalysis that every symptom and dream may have several meanings, being determined by more than a single association.

overdose. ABBR: O.D. A dose of a drug, esp. a drug of abuse, sufficient to cause an acute reaction such as coma, mania, hysteria, or even death.

overeruption. Condition in which the occluding surface of a tooth projects beyond the line of occlusion.

overexertion. Physical exertion to a state of abnormal exhaustion.

overextension. 1. Extension beyond that which usually occurs. SYN: *hyperextension.* 2. In dentistry, the assessment of the vertical extent of a root canal filling, denoting an extrusion beyond the apical foramen.

overflow. The continuous escape of fluid from a vessel or viscus, as of urine or tears.

overgrowth. 1. Excessive growth. SYN: *hyperplasia; hypertrophy.* 2. In bacteriology, the growth of one type of microorganism on a culture plate so that it covers and obscures the growth of other types.

overhang. The extension beyond the margins of a cavity of the excess filling material used. This is not the desired outcome.

overhydration. An excess of fluids in the body.

overjet. Horizontal overlap of the teeth.

overlap. Something that covers the tissue or object but also extends past the border.

overlay. 1. An addition superimposed upon an already existing state. 2. In dentistry, a cast restoration for the occlusal surface of one or more cusps of a tooth but not a three-quarter- or full-cast crown.

　　o., psychogenic. The emotional component of a symptom or illness that has an organic basis.

overmedication. The practice of taking more medicines than are needed. This is esp. important in elderly patients who have several conditions that require medication. The patient may forget which pill to take and at what frequency. Often this is complicated by the patient's being under the care of two or more physicians who do not coordinate their management of the patient and the drugs prescribed. Drug interaction, both with prescribed and over-the-counter drugs, is an important possibility in any patient taking a variety of drugs. Therefore, it is important that one individual have full knowledge of all the medicines a patient is taking.

overpressure. A force applied passively to a joint and surrounding soft tissue at the end of the range of motion in order to determine the end feel of the tissues.

overproduction. Excessive output of an organic element during the reparative process, as excessive callous development after a bone fracture. SEE: *keloid.*

overresponse. An abnormally intense reaction to a stimulus; inappropriate degree of response.

overriding. The slipping of one end of a fractured bone past the other part.

overshoot. A response to a stimulus that is greater than would normally be expected.

overtoe. Hallux varus of the great toe to the extent that it rests over the other toes.

overtone. In music and acoustics, a harmonic.

overuse syndrome. Excessive use of a body part whereby microtrauma occurs with a cumulative effect, so that in time there is tissue breakdown with pain and inflammation. The result may be a stress fracture, tendonitis, myofascitis, shin splints, bursitis, chronic recurring pain, or traumatic arthritis.

overvalued idea. An unreasonable and strongly held belief or idea that is maintained with less than delusional intensity. Such a belief is beyond the norm of beliefs held or accepted by other members of the person's culture or subculture.

overventilation. Hyperventilation, q.v.

ovi- [L. *ovum,* egg]. Combining form meaning egg.

ovi albumin (ō′vē-ăl-bū′mĭn) [L.]. White of egg. SYN: *ovalbumin.*

ovicide (ō′vĭ-sīd) [L. *ovum,* egg, + *caedere,* to kill]. An agent destructive to ova.

oviduct (ō′vĭ-dŭkt) [″ + *ductus,* a path]. One of two tubes extending laterally from superior angles of the uterus; serves to convey the ovum from the ovary to the uterus. Each oviduct consists of the infundibulum, expanded portion surrounding the ostium or opening through which the ovum enters, bearing many fingerlike processes called fimbriae; the ampulla, the tube itself; and the isthmus, a straight narrow portion that connects with the uterus.

Each oviduct is a muscular tube consisting of three layers: mucosa, muscular layer, and serosa. The mucosa consists of columnar epithelial cells, some ciliated, others glandular. In addition to conveying the ovum, the oviduct provides a passageway through which sperm travel from the uterus toward the ovary. It is the usual site of fertilization of the ovum. SYN: *fallopian tube; uterine tube.*

oviferous (ō-vĭf′ĕr-ŭs) [″ + *ferre,* to bear]. Containing or producing ova.

oviform (ō′vĭ-form) [″ + *forma,* shape]. 1. Having the shape of an egg. SYN: *ovoid.* 2. Resembling an ovum.

ovigenesis [″ + Gr. *gennan,* to produce]. Oogenesis.

ovigerm (ō′vĭ-jĕrm) [″ + *germen,* a bud]. The cell that produces or develops into an ovum.

ovination (ō″vĭ-nā′shŭn) [L. *ovinus,* of a sheep]. Inoculation with the virus of sheeppox.

ovine (ō′vīn) [L. *ovinus,* of a sheep]. Concerning sheep.

ovinia (ō-vĭn′ē-ă) [L. *ovinus,* of a sheep]. Sheep-pox.

oviparity (ō″vĭ-păr′ĭ-tē). Quality of being oviparous.

oviparous (ō-vĭp′ăr-ŭs) [L. *ovum,* egg, + *parere,* to produce]. Producing eggs that are hatched outside the body; egg laying. Opposite of ovoviviparous.

oviposition [″ + *ponere,* to place]. The laying of eggs as in oviparous reproduction.

ovipositor (ō″vĭ-pŏs′ĭ-tor). A specialized tubular structure found in many female insects, through which they lay their eggs in plants or soil.

ovisac (ō′vĭ-săk). The graafian follicle.

ovo- [L. *ovum,* egg]. Combining form indicating rel. to an egg.

ovocenter. The centrosome of a fertilized ovum.

ovocyte (ō′vō-sīt) [″ + *kytos,* cell]. Oocyte.

ovoflavin (ō′vō-flā′vĭn) [″ + *flavus,* yellow]. A flavin derived from eggs; identical to riboflavin.

ovogenesis (ō″vō-jĕn′ĕ-sĭs) [″ + Gr. *genesis,* generation, birth]. Production of ova. SYN: *oogenesis.*

ovoglobulin (ō″vō-glŏb′ū-lĭn) [″ + *globulus,* globule]. The globulin found in egg white. SEE: *albumin; protein, simple.*

ovogonium (ō″vō-gō′nē-ŭm). Oogonium.

ovoid (ō′voyd) [L. *ovum,* egg, + Gr. *eidos,* form, shape]. Egg shaped. SYN: *oviform.*

ovomucin (ō″vō-mū′sĭn). A glycoprotein in the white of an egg.

ovomucoid (ō″vō-mū′koyd) [″ + *mucus,* mucus, + Gr. *eidos,* form, shape]. A glycoprotein principle derived from egg white.

ovoplasm (ō′vō-plăzm) [″ + LL. *plasma,* form, mold]. Protoplasm of an unfertilized

o., alecithal. Ovum with a small yolk portion that is distributed throughout the protoplasm.

o., centrolecithal. Ovum having a large central food yolk, as in a bird's egg.

o., holoblastic. Ovum that undergoes complete cleavage.

o., human. The female reproductive cell that develops within the graafian follicle of the ovary. It develops from an oogonium that undergoes a process of maturation (oogenesis), during which primary and secondary oocytes are produced, finally giving rise to the mature ovum. During this process, the number of chromosomes is reduced from 46 to 23 and the egg is prepared for fertilization.

A mature ovum is approximately 0.130 to 0.140 mm (0.0051 to 0.0055 in.) in diameter. Each contains a spherical nucleus, bounded by a nuclear membrane, enclosing chromatin material and one or more nucleoli. The cytoplasm is granular and contains yolk granules or deuteroplasm and other characteristic organoids of cells. Its surface layer is the vitelline membrane. When liberated from the ovary as a primary oocyte, it is surrounded by a clear layer, zona pellucida, and several layers of adhering follicular cells, the latter constituting the corona radiata.

The length of time a human ovum retains its ability to be fertilized and develop is not known precisely, but it is probably at least 48 hours. If fertilized, it undergoes development. If not fertilized, it degenerates. SEE: *cleavage; conception; embryo, development of; fertilization; follicle; menstruation; ovulation; spermatozoon.*

o., isolecithal. O., alecithal.

o., meroblastic. Ovum in which only the protoplasmic region undergoes cleavage; characteristic in ova containing a large amount of yolk.

o., permanent. Ovum that is ready for fertilization.

o., primordial. Germ cell that arises very early in development of the embryo, usually in the yolk sac endoderm, migrates into the urogenital ridge, and possibly serves as progenitor of functional sex cell.

o., telolecithal. Ovum in which yolk is fairly abundant and tends to concentrate in one hemisphere.

Owren's disease [Paul A. Owren, Norwegian hematologist, b. 1905]. Factor V deficiency (parahemophilia). SEE: *parahemophilia.*

ox-. Combining form indicating presence of oxygen.

oxa-. Combining form indicating presence of oxygen in place of carbon.

oxacillin (ŏks″ă-sĭl′ĭn). A semisynthetic penicillin.

o. sodium. USP. An antibiotic drug. Trade names are Prostaphlin and Bactocill.

oxal-, oxalo-. Combining forms indicating derivation from oxalic acid.

oxalacetic acid (ŏks″ăl-ă-sē′tĭk). A product of carbohydrate metabolism $HOOC \cdot CH_2 \cdot CO \cdot COOH$ resulting from oxidation of malic acid. May be derived from other sources.

oxalate (ŏk′să-lāt) [Gr. *oxalis*, sorrel]. A salt of oxalic acid.

o., potassium. The potassium salt of oxalic acid.

oxalemia (ŏk″să-lē′mē-ă) [″ + *haima*, blood]. Excess oxalates in the blood.

oxalic acid (ŏks-ăl′ĭk). A white crystalline powder often used about the home as a stain remover or bleach, resembling epsom salts in appearance. SYN: *ethanedioic acid.*

SOURCES: Cranberries, chard, rhubarb, gooseberries, spinach, beet leaves. When eaten, they should be accompanied by liberal portions of calcium foods, such as eggs, beans, and milk.

oxalic acid poisoning. Acute poisoning occurs when oxalic acid is accidentally ingested or when large quantities of foods rich in oxalic acid are eaten. Ingestion of 5 grams of oxalic acid may be fatal. Chronic poisoning may result from inhalation of vapors. SEE: *Poisons and Poisoning* in *Appendix.*

SYM: Corrosive action on mucosa of mouth, esophagus, and stomach; sour taste; burning in mouth, throat, and stomach; great thirst; bloody vomitus; collapse; sometimes convulsions and coma.

TREAT: Prompt treatment with any soluble calcium salt such as powdered chalk in water or milk, lime water, or calcium lactate. This procedure inactivates the acid by precipitating it as an insoluble calcium salt. Careful gastric lavage with dilute lime water. Do not induce vomiting. Intravenous calcium gluconate or calcium chloride to treat tetany. Morphine may be required for pain.

oxalism (ŏks-ăl-ĭzm) [Gr. *oxalis*, sorrel, + *-ismos*, condition]. Poisoning from oxalic acid or an oxalate.

oxalosis. An autosomal recessive hereditary disease due to faulty metabolism of glyoxylic acid. Oxalic acid is elevated in the urine due to increased production of oxalic acid. Calcium oxalate is deposited in body tissues, esp. in the kidneys.

oxaluria (ŏk-să-lū′rē-ă) [″ + *ouron*, urine]. Excess excretion of oxalates in the urine, esp. calcium oxalate.

oxalylurea (ŏk″săl-ĭl-ū-rē′ă). An oxidation product of uric acid.

oxandrolone (ŏk-săn′drō-lōn). USP. An anabolic steroid. Trade name is Anavar.

oxazepam (ŏks-ăz′ē-păm). USP. A short-acting, benzodiazepine, antianxiety drug. Trade name is Serax.

oxidant (ŏk′sĭ-dănt). In oxidation-reduction reactions, the acceptor of an electron.

oxidase (ŏk′sĭ-dās) [Gr. *oxys*, sharp]. A class of enzymes present in animal and vegetable life. It catalyzes an oxidation reaction; a respiratory enzyme.

    o., cytochrome. An enzyme present in most cells that oxidizes reduced cytochrome back to cytochrome.

oxidation (ŏk′sĭ-dā′shŭn) [Gr. *oxys*, sharp]. 1. The process of a substance combining with oxygen. 2. The loss of electrons in an atom with an accompanying increase in positive valence. SEE: *reduce* (def. 2).

oxidation-reduction reaction. Chemical interaction in which one substance is oxidized and loses electrons, and thus is increased in positive valence, while another substance gains an equal number of electrons by being reduced. This is called a redox system or reaction.

oxide (ŏk′sīd). Any chemical compound in which oxygen is the negative radical.

oxidize (ŏk′sĭ-dīz). 1. To combine with oxygen. 2. To increase the positive valence, or to decrease the negative valence, by bringing about a loss of electrons. SYN: *oxygenize.* SEE: *oxidation-reduction reaction.*

oxidoreductase (ŏk′sĭ-dō-rē-dŭk′tās). An enzyme that catalyzes oxidation-reduction reactions.

oxim, oxime (ŏk′sĭm). Any compound produced by the action of hydroxylamine on an aldehyde or ketone. When an aldehyde is involved, the general formula RCH = NOH is produced. When a ketone is acted upon, $R_2CH = NOH$ is produced.

oximeter (ŏk-sĭm′ē-ter) [Gr. *oxys*, sharp, + *metron*, measure]. Photoelectric apparatus for determining the amount of oxygen in the blood. Usually done by measuring the amount of light transmitted through a translucent part of the skin.

    o., ear. Oximeter that attaches to the pinna of the ear to determine the degree of oxygen saturation of blood flowing through the ear.

    o., finger. An oximeter that attaches to the finger.

oxisensor. A noninvasive device used to determine the oxygen saturation. It is usually applied to a readily accessible site such as the nose, earlobe, toe, or finger. SEE: *oximeter.*

oxonemia (ŏk″sō-nē′mē-ă) [L. *oxone*, acetone, + Gr. *haima*, blood]. Excess of acetone bodies found in the blood. SYN: *acetonemia.*

oxophenarsine hydrochloride. An antitrypanosomal compound containing 30% arsenic.

oxprenolol hydrochloride (ŏks-prĕn′ō-lōl). A beta-adrenergic blocking agent. It is used as a coronary vasodilator.

oxtriphylline (ŏks-trĭf′ĭ-lēn). USP. A drug that resembles theophylline in its actions. Trade name is Choledyl.

oxy- [Gr. *oxys*]. Combining form indicating (1) sharp, keen, acute, acid, pungent; (2) presence of oxygen in a compound; (3) presence of a hydroxyl group.

oxyacoia (ŏk″sē-ă-koy′ă). Oxyecoia, q.v.

oxyacusis (ŏk″sē-ă-kū′sis) [Gr. *oxys*, sharp, + *akousis*, hearing]. Abnormally acute hearing. SYN: *hyperacusis.*

oxybenzene (ŏk″sē-bĕn′zēn). Phenol.

oxybenzone (ŏk″sē-bĕn′zōn). USP. A sunscreen agent used topically. Trade name is Spectra-Sorb UV9.

oxyblepsia (ŏk″sē-blĕp′sē-ă) [Gr. *oxys*, sharp, + *blepsis*, vision]. Extraordinary acuteness of vision.

oxybutyria (ŏk″sē-bū-tĭr′ē-ă). Oxybutyric acid in the urine.

oxycalcium (ŏk″sē-kăl′sē-ŭm). Of or pert. to oxygen and calcium.

Oxycel. Trade name for cellulose, oxidized, USP.

oxycellulose. Cellulose that has undergone oxidation.

oxycephalous (ŏk-sē-sĕf′ă-lŭs) [Gr. *oxys*, sharp, + *kephale*, head]. Denoting a head that is pointed and conelike.

oxycephaly (ŏk″sē-sĕf′ă-lē). State of having a high and pointed skull.

oxychloride (ŏk″sē-klō′rĭd) [Gr. *oxys*, sharp, + *chloros*, green]. A compound consisting of an element or radical combined with oxygen and chlorine or the hydroxyl radical (OH) and chlorine.

oxychromatic (ŏk″sē-krō-măt′ĭk) [″ + *chroma*, color]. Staining readily with acid dyes.

oxychromatin (ŏk″sē-krō′mă-tĭn). That part of chromatin that stains readily with acid dyes.

oxycinesia (ŏk″sē-sī-nē′zē-ă) [″ + *kinesis*, movement]. The experiencing of pain when movement occurs.

oxyecoia (ŏk″sē-ē-koy′ă) [″ + *akoe*, hearing]. Abnormal sensitivity to noises.

oxyesthesia (ŏk″sē-ĕs-thē′zē-ă) [″ + *aisthesis*, sensation]. Abnormal acuteness of sensation. SYN: *algesia; hyperesthesia.*

oxygen (ŏk′sĭ-jĕn) [Gr. *oxys*, sharp, + *gennan*, to produce]. USP. 1. A standardized preparation of oxygen used as a medicinal gas. 2. SYMB: O. At. wt. 15.9994; at. no. 8. A nonmetallic element occurring free in the atmosphere as a colorless, odorless, tasteless gas. It is a constituent of animal, vegetable, and mineral substances. Oxygen is essential to respiration of most forms of animal and plant life and is the most important and abundant element. At sea level, it represents 10% to 16% of venous and 17% to 21% of arterial blood.

It is the only element that enters the animal organism in a free state. It is absorbed by plants in the form of water and carbon dioxide, converted by them into organic substances that are used as food by humans, and returned to the atmosphere by humans in the form of waste products of water and carbon dioxide. Thus the balance of oxygen and carbon dioxide in the atmosphere is maintained.

When oxygen combines with another substance, the process is called oxidation. When combination takes place rapidly enough to produce light and heat, the process is called burning or combustion. Oxygen combines readily with other elements to form oxides.

USES: In conditions in which there is insufficient oxygen carried by the blood to the tissues. Therefore oxygen is used in cases of severe anemia, shock or circulatory collapse, pulmonary edema, pneumonia; or by mountain climbers, astronauts, or aviators when at heights where the amount of oxygen present in the atmosphere is insufficient to support life.

Frequently oxygen is employed with agents used for the induction of general anesthesia. Following extensive surgery, it reduces reactions to the anesthetic. Also employed in septicemia, gas gangrene, peritonitis, and intestinal obstruction.

Oxygen is used in pressure chambers for cardiac surgery; in treating aerobic infections such as gas gangrene; vascular disorders; bends, q.v.; carbon monoxide poisoning; and in connection with radiation therapy for tumors. When oxygen is administered in this manner, it is called hyperbaric oxygenation.

ADM: Oxygen is administered by mask, nasal tube, tent, or by placing the patient in an airtight chamber in which pressure may be increased. No matter how much oxygen is given, it is important to have it adequately humidified. It is desirable to administer oxygen at whatever rate is necessary to increase the oxygen content of inspired air to 50%. SEE: *hypoxia*.

Caution: Inhalation of high concentrations of oxygen, esp. at pressures of more than one atmosphere, may produce deleterious effects such as irritation of respiratory tract, reduced

vital capacity, and sometimes neurological symptoms. Serious eye defects may result if premature infants are exposed as part of their therapy to a high concentration of oxygen. SEE: *retrolental fibroplasia*.

Because oxygen provides perfect support of combustion, it should not be used in the presence of oil, lighted cigarettes or open flames, or where there is the possibility of electrical or spark hazards.

oxygen, transtracheal. Delivery of oxygen to the lungs via a transtracheal tube.
oxygenase (ŏk′sĭ-jĕn-ās″) [Gr. *oxys*, sharp, + *gennan*, to produce, + *-ase*, enzyme]. An enzyme that enables an organism to use atmospheric oxygen in respiration.
oxygenate (ŏk′sĭ-jĕn-āt). To combine or supply with oxygen.
oxygenation (ŏk″sĭ-jĕn-ā′shŭn). Saturation or combination with oxygen, as the aeration of the blood in the lungs.
   o., hyperbaric. Administration of oxygen under increased pressure while the patient is in an airtight chamber. Used for certain surgical procedures, treatment of aerobic infections such as gas gangrene, and in conjunction with radiation therapy of tumors.
oxygenator (ŏk″sĭ-jĕ-nā′tor). A device for mechanically oxygenating anything, but esp. blood. When used to oxygenate blood, it is usually used during thoracic surgery or open-heart surgery.
   o., bubble. Device for bubbling oxygen through the blood during extracorporeal circulation.
   o., rotating disk. Device for oxygenating blood during extracorporeal circulation. A thin film of blood attaches to a disk as it dips into the blood flow. The portion of the disk not in the blood is rotating in an atmosphere of oxygen.
   o., screen. During extracorporeal circulation, the blood passes over a series of screens that are in an oxygen atmosphere. Oxygen is exchanged in the thin film of blood on the screens.
oxygen capacity. The maximum amount of oxygen expressed in volume percent (cc per 100 ml) that a given amount of blood will absorb. For normal blood it is about 20 cc.
oxygen content. The amount of oxygen in volume percent that is present in the blood at any one moment.
oxygen debt or deficit. After strenuous (i.e., anaerobic) physical activity, the oxygen required in the recovery period, in addition to that required while resting, to oxidize the excess lactic acid produced and to replenish the depleted stores of adenosine triphosphate and phosphocreatinase.

oxygen-derived free radicals. Reactive oxygen metabolites produced in neurophils and macrophages. These may be released from the cell as part of the response to cellular damage or inflammation. SEE: *superoxide.*

oxygenic (ŏk″sĭ-jĕn′ĭk) [″ + *gennan,* to produce]. Concerning, resembling, containing, or consisting of oxygen.

oxygenize. Oxidize.

oxygen radicals. Incomplete reduction of oxygen produces hydrogen peroxide (H_2O_2) or the superoxide radical ($:O_2^-$). Oxygen free radicals are released during the "respiratory burst" phase of phagocytosis by neutrophils and macrophages during the inflammatory process. They cause direct cell damage, increase vascular permeability through damage to the capillary endothelium, and promote chemotaxis, q.v. Oxygen free radicals are normally contained by antioxidant protective measures; however, with severe inflammation they cause significant damage. They are believed to be responsible for much of the cellular damage involved in adult respiratory distress syndrome (ARDS), in which massive neutrophil aggregation and phagocytosis occur.

oxygen saturation. Oxygen content of blood divided by oxygen capacity and expressed in volume percent.

oxygen tent. An airtight enclosure for a patient's head and shoulders in which the oxygen content of the air can be raised above normal.

oxygen therapy. The administration of oxygen for the treatment of conditions resulting from oxygen deficiency. It is used to combat acute arterial anoxia that may result from pneumonia, pulmonary edema, or obstruction to breathing. It is also employed in congestive heart failure, coronary thrombosis, and following surgery. It may be administered by nasal catheter, mask (nasal or oronasal), funnel or cone, oxygen tent, or special oxygen chamber, and usually in a concentration of 70% to 100%. It is important that the oxygen be humidified by bubbling it through water. This will prevent drying of the mucosal epithelium of the upper respiratory tract. Supplemental oxygen is available through a method called molecular sieve, in which a device removes nitrogen from room air. The oxygen remaining is available for use just as if it were stored in a cylinder. SEE: *hyperbaric oxygen; oximeter.*

   o.t., transtracheal. Delivery of oxygen via a small plastic cannula inserted directly into the trachea. SEE: illus.

oxygen toxicity. Progressive failure of ventilation of the lungs that develops when pure

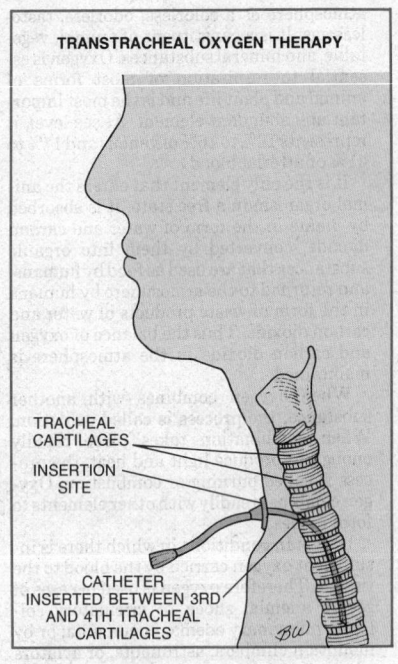

TRANSTRACHEAL OXYGEN THERAPY

TRACHEAL CARTILAGES

INSERTION SITE

CATHETER INSERTED BETWEEN 3RD AND 4TH TRACHEAL CARTILAGES

oxygen is breathed for a prolonged period. Failure of ventilation leads to decreased oxygen tension in the blood.

oxygeusia (ŏk″sē-gū′sē-ă) [Gr. *oxys,* sharp, + *geusis,* taste]. Abnormally keen sense of taste.

oxyhematin (ŏk″sē-hĕm′ă-tĭn). An iron compound that constitutes the coloring matter in oxyhemoglobin. When oxidized, it yields hematinic acid; when reduced, hematoporphyrin.

oxyhematoporphyrin (ŏk″sē-hĕm″ă-tō-por′fĭ-rĭn). A derivative of hematoporphyrin sometimes present in urine.

oxyhemoglobin (ŏk″sē-hē″mō-glō′bĭn) [″ + *haima,* blood, + L. *globus,* a sphere]. The combined form of hemoglobin with oxygen. Hemoglobin with oxygen is found in arterial blood and is the oxygen carrier to the body tissues.

oxyhemoglobin dissociation curve. A curve that shows relationship between partial pressure of oxygen and the percentage saturation of hemoglobin with oxygen, i.e., the proportion of oxyhemoglobin to reduced hemoglobin. Factors that favor shift of curve to the right, accelerating the decomposition of hemoglobin, are a rise in temper-

OXYHEMOGLOBIN DISSOCIATION CURVE

ALKALOSIS

ACIDOSIS

PERCENTAGE SATURATION OF HEMOGLOBIN

100
80
60
40
20

0   20   40   60   80 100 120
OXYGEN TENSION (mmHG)

ature and an increase of H ions that results from liberation of CO_2 and formation of lactic acid. SEE: illus.

oxyhemoglobinometer (ŏk″sē-hē″mō-glō″bĭn-ŏm′ĕ-tĕr) [″ + ″ + ″ + Gr. *metron*, measure]. Apparatus for measurement of amount of oxygen in the blood.

oxyhydrocephalus (ŏk″sē-hī-drŏ-sĕf′ăl-ŭs) [″ + *hydor*, water, + *kephale*, brain]. Type of hydrocephalus in which the head has a pointed shape.

oxyiodide (ŏk″sē-ī′ō-dīd) [″ + *ioeides*, violet colored]. Compound of iodine and oxygen with an element or radical.

oxylalia (ŏk″sē-lā′lē-ă) [″ + *lalein*, to speak]. Abnormal rapidity of speech.

Oxylone. Trade name for fluorometholone, USP.

oxymetazoline hydrochloride (ŏk″sē-mĕt-ăz′ō-lēn). USP. A vasoconstrictor drug used topically for nasal decongestion. Trade names are Afrin and Duration.

oxymetholone (ŏk″sē-mĕth′ō-lōn). USP. An anabolic steroid. Trade name is Anadrol.

oxymorphone hydrochloride (ŏk″sē-mor′fōn). USP. A semisynthetic analgesic narcotic similar in action to morphine. Trade name is Numorphan.

oxymyoglobin (ŏk″sē-mī″ō-glō′bĭn). The compound formed when myoglobin is exposed to air.

oxyntic (ŏk-sĭn′tĭk) [Gr. *oxynein*, to make acid]. Producing or secreting acid.

oxyopia (ŏk″sē-ō′pē-ă) [Gr. *oxys*, sharp, + *ops*, sight]. Unusual acuteness of vision.

oxyopter (ŏk″sē-ŏp′tĕr). A unit of measuring visual acuity; the reciprocal of the visual angle expressed in degrees.

oxyosmia (ŏk″sē-ŏz′mē-ă) [″ + *osme*, odor]. Unusual acuity of sense of smell.

oxyosphresia (ŏk″sē-ŏs-frē′zē-ă) [″ + *osphresis*, smell]. Abnormal acuity of the sense of smell.

oxypathia, oxypathy (ŏk″sē-păth′ē-ă, -sĭp′ă-thē) [″ + *pathos*, disease, suffering]. 1. Unusual acuity of sensation. 2. An acute condition. 3. Condition in which the body is unable to eliminate unoxidizable acids, which combine with fixed alkalies of the tissues and harm the organism.

oxyperitoneum (ŏk″sĭ-pĕr-ĭ-tō-nē′ŭm) [″ + *peritonaion*, peritoneum]. Introduction of oxygen into the peritoneal cavity.

oxyphenbutazone (ŏk″sē-fĕn-bū′tă-zōn). USP. Anti-inflammatory and antipyretic drug similar in action to phenylbutazone.

oxyphencyclimine hydrochloride (ŏk″sē-fĕn-sī′klĭ-mēn). USP. A belladonna-like drug. Trade name is Daricon.

oxyphil(e) (ŏk′sē-fĭl, -fīl) [″ + *philein*, to love]. 1. Staining readily with acid dyes. 2. A cell that stains readily with acid dyes.

oxyphilous (ŏk-sĭf′ĭl-ŭs). Having an affinity for acid dyes. SYN: *oxyphil*.

oxyphonia (ŏk″sē-fō′nē-ă). An abnormally sharp or shrill pitch to the voice.

oxypurine (ŏk″sē-pū′rēn) [″ + L. *purus*, pure, + *urina*, urine]. An oxidation product of purine. Includes hypoxanthine, xanthine, and uric acid. SEE: *aminopurine; methyl purine.*

oxyrhine (ŏk′sē-rīn) [″ + *rhis*, nose]. 1. Having a sharp-pointed nose. 2. Possessing an acute sense of smell.

oxytalan (ŏks-ĭt′ă-lăn). A type of connective tissue fiber present in periodontal tissues.

oxytetracycline (ŏks″ē-tĕt″ră-sī′klēn). USP. One of a group of broad-spectrum antibiotic substances called tetracyclines. Combines with sites of calcification so that teeth forming in children or the unborn fetus may be stained as a result of extensive medication with this group of antibiotics. Originally obtained from a strain of *Streptomyces*, it is now prepared synthetically. Trade name is Terramycin.

oxytocia (ŏk″sē-tō′sē-ă) [″ + *tokos*, childbirth]. Unusual rapidity of childbirth.

oxytocic (ŏk″sē-tō′sĭk). 1. Agent that stimulates uterine contractions. 2. Accelerating childbirth.

oxytocic principle. A hormone stored in the posterior lobe of the hypophysis that acts specifically on the smooth musculature of the uterus, therefore increasing tone of, and inducing, uterine contractions. SYN: *oxytocin.*

oxytocin [injection] (ŏk″sē-tō′sĭn). USP. A pituitary hormone that stimulates the uterus to contract, thus inducing parturition. It also acts on the mammary gland to stimulate the release of milk. Trade names are Syntocinon and Pitocin.

oxytocin challenge test. I.V. infusion of 10 very small doses of oxytocin in order to determine whether contraction of the uterus in response to the oxytocin will cause signs of fetal distress. The results of the test provide a basis of making a decision concerning continuation of high-risk pregnancies. Also known as contraction stress test or CST.

NURSING IMPLICATIONS: Explain the test and support patient throughout. Piggyback solution into tubing of main I.V., and deliver via infusion pump or controller to ensure accurate dose. Monitor uterine contractions and fetal heart rate until three uterine contractions of good quality are observed within a ten-minute period. The fetal heart rate pattern is then interpreted for the absence or presence of late decelerations. Discontinue the infusion of oxytocin, remove the I.V., and assist the patient with discharge preparations.

oxyuriasis (ŏk″sē-ū-rī′ăs-ĭs) [Gr. *oxys*, sharp, + *oura*, tall, + *iasis*, infection]. Infestation with *Enterobius vermicularis* (pinworm), q.v. SYN: *enterobiasis*.

oxyuricide (ŏk″sē-ū′rĭ-sīd) [″ + ″ + L. *caedere*, to kill]. An agent that is destructive to pinworms.

oxyurid (ŏk″sē-ūr′ĭd). Pinworm or seatworm. SEE: *Enterobius vermicularis*.

Oxyuris [″ + *oura*, tail]. Former name for genus of nematode intestinal worms that includes the pinworms or seatworms. SEE: *Enterobius*.

    O. vermicularis. Enterobius vermicularis.

Oxyuroidea (ŏk″sē-ū″roy-dē′ă). A superfamily of nematodes that includes the pinworm *Enterobius vermicularis*.

oyster [AS. *oistre*]. Shellfish eaten raw or cooked. When eaten raw or partially cooked, it may be source of infectious hepatitis virus

and other pathogens.

oz. *ounce.*

oz. ap. *ounce apothecaries'* (pharmaceutical term).

oz. av. *ounce avoirdupois.*

ozena (ō-zē′nă) [Gr. *oze*, stench]. Disease of the nose characterized by atrophy of the turbinates and mucous membrane accompanied by considerable crusting, discharge, and a very offensive odor. It is present in various forms of rhinitis.

ozochrotia (ō″zō-krō′shē-ă) [″ + *chros*, skin]. Strong odor given off by the skin. SYN: *bromidrosis*.

ozonator (ō′zō-nā″tor). Device for generating ozone.

ozone (ō′zōn) [Gr. *ozein*, to smell]. A form of oxygen in which three atoms of the element combine to form the molecule O_3. In even very low concentration in inhaled air, ozone is toxic. Ozone is present in the stratosphere. It is constantly being formed by the action of ultraviolet light on oxygen. Ozone is essential to life on earth because it absorbs harmful wavelengths of ultraviolet radiation from the sun.

ozonization (ō″zō-nī-zā′shŭn). The act of converting to, or impregnating with, ozone.

ozonize (ō′zō-nīz) [Gr. *ozein*, to smell]. 1. To convert oxygen to ozone, q.v. 2. To impregnate the air of a substance with ozone.

ozonometer (ō″zō-nŏm′ĕ-tĕr) [Gr. *oze*, stench, + *metron*, measure]. An apparatus for estimating the quantity of ozone in the atmosphere.

ozonoscope (ō-zō′nō-skōp) [″ + *skopein*, to examine]. A device for showing the presence or amount of ozone.

ozostomia (ō″zō-stō′mē-ă) [″ + *stoma*, mouth]. Fetid breath, halitosis.

P

P. 1. *position; posterior; postpartum; pressure; pulse; pupil.* 2. Chem. symb. for the element phosphorus.

p. *page; probability* (in statistics); *pupil.*

p-. *para-* in chemical formulas.

p. *after-* or *post-.*

P₁. *first parental generation* (in genetics); *first pulmonic heart sound.*

P₂. *pulmonic second sound.*

³²P. Chem. symb. for radioactive isotope of phosphorus.

PA. *pulmonary artery.*

P.A. *physician's assistant.*

Pa. Chem. symb. for the element protactinium.

P-A, p-a. *posteroanterior.*

P & A. *percussion and auscultation.*

PABA. Trade name for para-aminobenzoic acid, previously used name for aminobenzoic acid.

Pabanol. Trade name for para-aminobenzoic acid, previously used name for aminobenzoic acid.

Pablum (păb′lŭm). Trade name for a cereal food for infants.

pabular (păb′ū-lăr) [L. *pabulum,* food]. Pert. to nourishment.

pabulum (păb′ū-lŭm) [L.]. Food; nourishment.

PAC. *premature atrial contraction.*

PA catheter. I.V. catheter with the tip in the pulmonary artery.

pacchionian bodies (păk″ē-ō′nē-ăn) [Antonio Pacchioni, It. anatomist, 1665–1726]. Enlarged villi, small pedunculated or rounded growths of fibrous tissue along longitudinal fissure of the cerebrum growing on arachnoid membrane of the brain.

pacchionian depressions. Small pits produced on inner surface of skull by protuberance of the pacchionian bodies.

pacemaker (pās′māk-ĕr) [L. *passus,* a step, + AS. *macian,* to make]. 1. Anything that influences the rate and rhythm of occurrence of some activity or process. 2. In cardiology, a specialized cell or group of cells that automatically generates impulses that may spread to other regions of the heart. The normal cardiac pacemaker is the sinoatrial node, a group of cells in the atrium near the entrance of the superior vena cava into the right atrium.

   p., cardiac, artificial. An electrical device that can substitute for a defective natural pacemaker and control the beating of the heart by a series of rhythmic electrical discharges. If the electrodes that deliver the discharges to the heart are placed on the outside of the chest, the device is called an external pacemaker. If the electrodes are placed within the chest wall, the device is called an internal pacemaker.

   These devices are powered by batteries that last 16 years or longer. SEE: *pacemaker syndrome; pacing code; sick sinus syndrome.*

Caution: Older models of pacemakers were sensitive to outside electrical and electromagnetic devices, such as microwave ovens. Exposure to those devices could cause malfunction of the pacemaker. The modern pacemaker is shielded from such interference.

   NURSING IMPLICATIONS: *Preop:* Monitor cardiac rate and rhythm for evidence of failure of the heart's pacemaker, and treat using hospital protocol. Teach the patient and family about cardiac function and pacemaker insertion and function. Encourage verbalization of fears and concerns, answer questions, and dispel myths and correct misconceptions. Provide routine preoperative preparation.

   Postop: Ascertain type of pacemaker employed and expectations for its function. Monitor cardiac rate and rhythm for evidence of pacemaker function. Assess patient for evidence of pacemaker failure or noncapture (vertigo, loss of consciousness, hypotension, chest discomfort, dyspnea) and evaluate patient for effects on cardiac output. Teach patient technique and rationale for monitoring own pulse rate, and care and protection of insertion site. Counsel concerning telephone monitoring check-up, battery replacement, medication regimen, physical activity, and follow-up care. Encourage patient to wear or carry medical identification and information indicating presence and type of pacemaker implanted, along with electrocardiogram (ECG) rhythm strip showing pacemaker activity and capture. Pacemaker patients who travel extensively should be cautioned to have spare batteries available.

   p., demand. An implanted pacemaker that is designed to permit its electrical output to be inhibited by the heart's electrical impulses. This decreases the chances for the pacemaker to induce ventricular fibrillation.

   p., double-chamber, artificial. Also known as an atrioventricular (A-V) sequential pacemaker because both atria and ventricles are stimulated sequentially.

p., ectopic. Any endogenous cardiac pacemaker other than the sinoatrial node.

p., external. An artificial cardiac pacemaker that is located outside the body. The electrodes for delivering the stimulus are located on the chest wall or may be introduced through an intravenous catheter.

p., failure of artificial. Defect in pacemaker device caused by either a failure to sense the patient's intrinsic beat or failure to pace. Failure to pace can be caused by a worn-out battery, fracture or displacement of the electrode, or pulse generator defect.

p., fixed rate. An artificial pacemaker that stimulates the heart at a fixed rate.

p., implanted. A pacemaker device implanted beneath the skin.

p., mediastinal. Cardiac pacemaker using pacing electrodes surgically implanted through the mediastinum.

p., permanent. Cardiac pacemaker implanted inside the body of the patient for permanent use.

p., programmable. Electronic permanent pacemaker in which one or more settings can be changed from outside the patient by use of an electronic device.

p., temporary. Electronic cardiac pacemaker external to the patient's body, usually connected to a transvenous pacing electrode. It is intended for temporary use.

p., transthoracic. Cardiac pacemaker using pacing electrodes passed through the chest wall. Usually used only in emergency situations, on a temporary basis.

p., transvenous. Cardiac pacemaker using a pacing electrode or wire passed through a vein into the chambers of the heart. May be permanent or temporary.

p., uterine. One or more areas in the uterus that stimulate contraction of the myometrium.

p., ventricular, artificial. Most commonly inserted type in which electrode rests in right ventricle.

p., wandering. A cardiac arrhythmia in which the site of origin of the pacemaker stimulus shifts from one site to another, usually from the atrioventricular (A-V) node to some other part of the atrium.

pacemaker syndrome. Lightheadedness or syncope due to long intervals of asynchronous stimulation of the heart. Also included are symptoms of angina associated with inadequate cardiac output.

pacer. Pacemaker.

pachismus (păk-ĭz′mŭs) [Gr. *pachys*, thick, + *-ismos*, condition]. Condensation or thickening of an organ or part.

pachy-, pach- [Gr.*pachys*, thick]. Combining form meaning thick, large, heavy, massive.

pachyacria, pachyakria (păk″ē-ā′krē-ă) [Gr.*pachys*, thick, + *akron*, end]. Hypertrophy of soft portions of the extremities.

pachyblepharon (păk″ē-blĕf′ă-rŏn) [″ + *blepharon*, eyelid]. A thickening of the border of the eyelid.

pachyblepharosis (păk″ē-blĕf″ă-rō′sĭs). Chronic thickening of the eyelid.

pachycephalic (păk″ē-sĕ-făl′ĭk) [″ + *kephale*, brain]. Possessing an abnormally thick skull. SYN: *pachycephalous.*

pachycephalous (păk″ē-sĕf′ă-lŭs). Thick-skulled. SYN: *pachycephalic.*

pachycephaly (păk″ē-sĕf′ă-lē). Unusual thickness of the walls of the skull.

pachycheilia (păk″ē-kī′lē-ă) [″ + *cheilos*, lip]. Unusual thickness of the lips.

pachycholia (păk″ē-kō′lē-ă) [″ + *chole*, bile]. Thickening or inspissation of the bile.

pachychromatic (păk″ē-krō-măt′ĭk) [″ + *chroma*, color]. Possessing a coarse chromatin network.

pachycolpismus (păk″ē-kŏl-pĭz′mŭs) [″ + *kolpos*, vagina, + *-ismos*, condition]. Chronic inflammation of the vagina with thickened vaginal walls. SYN: *pachyvaginitis.*

pachydactylia, pachydactyly (păk″ē-dăk-tĭl′ē-ă, -dăk′tĭ-lē) [″ + *daktylos*, digit]. Condition marked by unusually large fingers and toes.

pachyderma (păk-ē-dĕr′mă) [″ + *derma*, skin]. Unusual thickness of the skin. SYN: *pachydermatosis.* SEE: *elephantiasis.*

p. circumscripta. P. laryngis, q.v.

p. laryngis. Irregular thickening and hypertrophy of mucous membrane in the larynx, seen in chronic laryngitis.

p. lymphangiectatica. Diffuse form of skin thickening due to blocked or defective lymph drainage.

p., occipital. Disease in which the skin of the scalp, esp. in the occipital region, falls into thickened folds.

p. vesicae. Condition in which there is a thickened mucous membrane in the urinary bladder.

pachydermatocele (păk″ē-dĕr-măt′ō-sēl) [″ + ″ + *kele*, tumor, swelling]. 1. A pendulous state of the skin with thickening. SYN: *cutis laxa; dermatolysis.* 2. Huge neurofibroma.

pachydermatosis (păk″ē-dĕr″mă-tō′sĭs) [″ + ″ + *osis*, condition]. Unusual thickness of the skin. SYN: *pachyderma; pachydermia.*

pachydermatous (păk-ē-dĕr′mă-tŭs) [″ + *derma*, skin]. Possessing a thick skin.

pachydermoperiostosis (păk″ē-dĕr″mō-pĕr″ē-ŏs-tō′sĭs). Hereditary form of osteoarthropathy with marked thickening of the skin over the face and extremities. It is self-limiting with an active progressive phase during adolescence.

pachyemia (păk-ē-ē'mē-ă) [Gr. *pachys*, thick, + *haima*, blood]. Thickness of the blood.

pachyglossia (păk″ē-glŏs'sē-ă) [″ + *glossa*, tongue]. Unusual thickness of the tongue.

pachygnathous (pă-kĭg'năth-ŭs) [″ + *gnathos*, jaw]. Having a thick or large jaw.

pachygyria (păk-ē-jī'rē-ă) [″ + *gyros*, a circle]. Flat, broad formation of the cerebral convolutions.

pachyhematous (păk-ē-hĕm'ă-tŭs) [″ + *haima*, blood]. Having, or pert. to, thickened blood.

pachyleptomeningitis (păk-ē-lĕp″tō-mĕn″ĭn-jī'tĭs) [″ + *leptos*, thin, + *meninx*, membrane, + *itis*, inflammation]. Inflammation of pia and dura of the brain and spinal cord.

pachymenia (păk-ē-mē'nē-ă) [″ + *hymen*, membrane]. Thickening of the skin or membranes.

pachymeningitis (păk-ē-mĕn″ĭn-jī'tĭs) [″ + *meninx*, membrane, + *itis*, inflammation]. Inflamed condition of the dura mater. Inflammation of any of three membranes — the pia, dura, or arachnoid — is sure to extend to one or both of the other two membranes, and the consequence in any form is suppuration, abscess, effusion into the ventricles, and softening of cerebral tissue if brain is involved. SYN: *perimeningitis*.

   p., external. Inflammation of outer layer of dura mater.

   p., hemorrhagic. Circumscribed effusion of blood on inner surface of dura with inflammation.

   SYM: Intermittent headache, choked optic disks, hemiparesis, dilated pupil, unconsciousness.

   ETIOL: Usually the result of trauma, such as a blow, resulting in a venous tear. Blood oozes into subdural space, and a blood clot is formed, becomes encysted, and gives rise to a hematoma. SEE: *hematoma, subdural.*

   p., internal. Inflammation of inner layer of dura mater.

   p., spinal. Inflammation of the dura of the spinal cord.

pachymeningopathy (păk″ē-mĕn″ĭn-gŏp'ă-thē) [″ + ″ + *pathos*, disease]. Any noninflammatory disease of the dura mater.

pachymeninx (păk-ē-mē'nĭnks) [″ + *meninx*, membrane]. The dura mater.

pachymeter [″ + *metron*, to measure]. Device to determine the thickness of a material or object.

pachynema (păk-ē-nē'mă) [″ + *nema*, thread]. Pachytene, q.v.

pachyonychia (păk″ē-ō-nĭk'ē-ă) [Gr. *pachys*, thick, + *onyx*, nail]. Abnormal thickening of fingernails or toenails.

   p. congenita. A congenital condition characterized by thickening of the nails, thickening of the skin on palms of hands and soles of feet, follicular keratosis at knees and elbows, and corneal dyskeratosis.

pachyostosis (păk″ē-ŏs-tō'sĭs) [″ + *osteon*, bone, + *osis*, condition]. A benign condition of thickening of the bones.

pachyotia (păk-ē-ō'shē-ă) [″ + *ous*, ear]. Abnormal thickness of the ears.

pachypelviperitonitis (păk″ē-pĕl″vĭ-pĕr″ĭ-tō-nī'tĭs) [″ + L. *pelvis*, basin, + Gr. *peritonaion*, peritoneum, + *itis*, inflammation]. Inflammation of the pelvic and peritoneal membranes with hypertrophy and thickening of their surfaces.

pachyperiostitis (păk″ē-pĕr″ē-ŏs-tī'tĭs) [″ + *periosteon*, periosteum, + *itis*, inflammation]. Thickening of the periosteum due to inflammation.

pachyperitonitis (păk″ē-pĕr″ī-tō-nī'tĭs) [″ + ″ + *itis*, inflammation]. Inflammation of the peritoneum with thickening of the membrane.

pachypleuritis (păk-ē-plū-rī'tĭs) [″ + *pleura*, side, + *itis*, inflammation]. Inflamed condition of the pleura with thickening.

pachypodous (pă-kĭp'ō-dŭs) [″ + *pous*, foot]. Having abnormally thick feet.

pachyrhinic (păk″ē-rī'nĭk) [″ + *rhis*, nose]. Having a thick, flat nose.

pachysalpingitis (păk″ē-săl″pĭn-jī'tĭs) [″ + *salpinx*, tube, + *itis*, inflammation]. Chronic inflammation of an oviduct with thickening of the walls.

pachysalpingoovaritis (păk″ē-săl-pĭng″gō-ō″văr-ī'tĭs) [″ + ″ + LL. *ovarium*, ovary, + Gr. *itis*, inflammation]. Chronic inflamed condition of an ovary and oviduct with thickening of the membranes.

pachysomia (păk-ē-sō'mē-ă) [Gr. *pachys*, thick, + *soma*, body]. Pathological thickening of the soft parts of the body.

pachytene (păk'ē-tēn) [″ + *tainia*, band]. The stage in meiosis, or cell division, in which the paired homologous chromosomes contract due to their becoming intertwined in a spiral fashion and then become much thicker than in the preceding leptotene and zygotene stages.

pachytrichous. Presence of enlarged hair fibers.

pachyvaginalitis (păk″ē-văj″ĭn-ă-lī'tĭs) [″ + L. *vagina*, sheath, + Gr. *itis*, inflammation]. Inflamed condition of the tunica vaginalis of the testes.

pachyvaginitis (păk″ē-văj″ĭn-ī′tĭs). Chronic inflammation of the vagina with thickening of the vaginal walls. SYN: *pachycolpismus.*

pacifier. An artificial nipple, usually made of plastic, provided for infants in order to satisfy their need for something to suck on.

pacing (pās′ĭng) [L. *passus,* a step]. Setting the rate or pace of an event, esp. the heartbeat. SEE: *pacemaker.*

pacing code. A three-letter code for describing pacemaker type and function. The first letter indicates the chamber or chambers paced: V for ventricle, A for atrium, or D (dual) for pacing of both chambers. The second letter, which may also be V, A, or D, indicates the chamber from which electrical activity is sensed. The third letter indicates the response to the sensed electrical activity. O indicates no response to the electrical activity sensed; I indicates inhibition of the pacing action; and T represents triggering of the pacemaker function; D indicates that a dual response of spontaneous atrial and ventricular activity will inhibit atrial and ventricular pacing. SEE: *pacemaker; pacemaker, cardiac, artificial.*

pacing wire. Pacemaker electrode.

pacinian corpuscles (pă-sĭn′ē-ăn) [Filippo Pacini, It. anatomist, 1812–1883]. Encapsulated sensory nerve endings found in subcutaneous tissue and many other parts of the body (pancreas, penis, clitoris, nipple). These corpuscles are sensitive to deep or heavy pressure. SYN: *Vater's corpuscles.*

pack (păk) [AS. *pak*]. 1. A dry or moist, hot or cold blanket or sheet wrapped around a patient and used for treatment. 2. The procedure in which one enwraps a person. 3. To fill up a cavity with cotton, gauze, or a similar substance.

p., cold. A physiological sedative and hypnotic employed for relief of restlessness and insomnia; used extensively in psychiatric conditions. Patient is wrapped in two or more sheets that have been placed in cold water and wrung out before application. The patient's body is then wrapped in heavy blankets to prevent loss of cooling and evaporation of moisture.

p., dry. Procedure used in combination with hot bath to induce perspiration. When leaving the hot bath, the patient is placed in a dry warm sheet and wrapped in several warm blankets.

p., full. Any pack that enwraps the entire body.

p., half. Wet-sheet pack extending from the axillae to below the knees.

p., hot. A type of superficial moist heat applied to reduce pain and promote muscle relaxation. The pack usually has a canvas cover and is filled with a silicon dioxide gel.

The pack is heated to 65° to 90°C in hot water.

p., ice. A substitute for an ice bag; a local cold application made by folding a soft towel so that it will fit the area and filling it with crushed ice.

p., one-sheet. Wet-sheet pack in which only one large sheet, 84 × 96 in. (213.4 × 243.8 cm), is used.

p., partial. Wet pack that covers a portion of the body.

p., periodontal. A surgical dressing applied over an area involved in periodontal surgery to enhance healing and tissue recovery. Components may include eugenol, resin zinc oxide, tannic acid, cocoa butter, paraffin, olive oil, and an antibiotic.

p., posterior nasal. SEE: *epistaxis.*

p., three-quarter. Pack that uses same temperatures as the wet-sheet pack but envelops the body upward as far as the armpits.

p., umbrella. Pack inserted through the abdominal incision following hysterectomy to stop arterial bleeding. The pack itself consists of a piece of absorbent cloth about 24 in. (61 cm) square into the middle of which is placed about 60 ft (18.28 meters) of 2-in. (5-cm) gauze. The tails of the pack are pulled through the vagina from below, and the corners of the cloth are brought together to form the tail of the pack. After placement, the tail is pulled firmly, and the bolus of gauze in the cloth exerts enough pressure against the blood vessels to stop arterial bleeding. In Greece it is known as the Logothetopulos tampon, named after the physician who developed it in 1926.

p., wet-dry. Pack placed in a healing area, esp. an ulcer to facilitate debridement. The pack, which may contain a topical antiseptic, is moistened, placed in the ulcer, and changed when it becomes dry. SYN: *wet-dry dressing.*

p., wet-sheet. The envelopment of a patient in one, two, or three linen or soft cotton sheets that have been wrung out of water. They are held against the body by large woolen blankets. Temperature of the water used for the sheets varies, depending upon the purpose.

package insert. An informational leaflet placed inside the container or package of prescription drugs. The Food and Drug Administration requires that the drug's generic name, indications, contraindications, adverse effects, dosage, and route of administration be described in the leaflet.

packed cells. Red blood cells that have been separated from the plasma. Used in treating conditions that require red blood cells but not the liquid components of whole blood.

This prevents excess hydration of the vascular system.

packer (păk'ĕr). Device for packing a cavity or a wound.

packing (păk'ĭng). 1. Process of filling a cavity or wound with gauze sponges or gauze strips. 2. Material used to fill a cavity or wound.

PaCO₂. Partial pressure of carbon dioxide in the arterial blood. Arterial carbon dioxide concentration or tension. Usually expressed in millimeters of mercury (mm Hg).

pad (păd). 1. Cushion of soft material used to apply pressure, relieve pressure, or support an organ or part. Usually cotton or rayon. 2. A fleshlike or fatty mass.

p., abdominal. Dressing for absorbing discharges from surgical wounds of the abdomen.

p., dinner. Pad placed on stomach prior to application of a plaster cast. Pad is then removed, leaving space from abdominal distention after meals.

p., fat. 1. The sucking pad in the infant's cheek. 2. Pad of fat behind and below the patella.

p., kidney. Air or water pad fixed on abdominal belt for compression over a movable kidney.

p.'s, knuckle. Congenital condition in which small nodules appear on dorsal side of fingers.

p., Malgaigne's. Mass of fat in knee joint on either side of the patella's upper end.

p., Mikulicz's. Pad of folded gauze used in surgery.

p., perineal. Pad covering the perineum. Used to cover a wound or to absorb the menstrual flow.

p., sucking. Pad of fat seen inside the cheeks of infants.

p., surgical. Soft rubber pad with apron and inflatable rim for drainage of escaping fluids. Used in surgery and obstetrics.

paed-, paedo-. SEE: words beginning with *ped-, pedia-, pedo-*.

Paget, Sir James (păj'ĕt). British surgeon, 1814–1899.

P.'s disease. Skeletal disease of the elderly with chronic inflammation of bones, resulting in thickening and softening of bones, and bowing of long bones. SYN: *osteitis deformans.*

TREAT: Asymptomatic cases should not be treated. There is no specific curative therapy, but vitamin D three times a week and anabolic hormones may be of help in treating osteoporosis. Calcitonin, etidronate disodium, and mithramycin have been used to control resorption of bone and thus are of assistance in alleviating bone pain.

P.'s disease, extramammary. A plaque with a definite margin found in the anogenital area and in the axilla. It is a rare malignant disease.

TREAT: Surgical excision.

P.'s disease, mammary. Carcinoma of the mammary ducts.

pagetoid (păj'ĕ-toyd) [*Paget* + Gr. *eidos*, form, shape]. Similar to Paget's disease.

page turner. An adaptive device for persons with limited or absent upper extremity movement. It is used to turn the pages of a book.

Pagitane Hydrochloride. Trade name for cycrimine hydrochloride.

pagophagia [Gr. *pagos*, frost, + *phagein*, to eat]. A form of pica, q.v., characterized by the deliberate eating of large quantities of ice. This condition may be associated with iron deficiency anemia.

-pagus [Gr. *pagos*, thing fixed]. A terminal combining form indicating twins joined together at the site indicated in the initial part of the word. SEE: *craniopagus*.

PAH, PAHA. *para-aminohippuric acid.*

pain (pān) [L. *poena*, a fine, a penalty, punishment]. The International Association for the Study of Pain defines pain as the sensory and emotional experience associated with actual or potential tissue damage. Thus, pain includes not only the perception of an uncomfortable stimulus but also the response to that perception. Approximately one half of the persons who seek medical help do so because of the primary complaint of pain. In the U.S. each year 155 million persons experience at least one episode of acute pain, and one third of that number reported pain that was severe. An estimated 700 million workdays, at a cost of $60 billion, are lost annually in the U.S. due to chronic pain.

Experiencing pain is influenced by a great number of interacting physical, mental, biochemical, physiologic, psychologic, social, cultural, and emotional factors. All of these interactions are dynamic and constantly changing. Thus, the pain that is perceived to be of a certain intensity at one time may, at another time, be perceived as being either less or more intense, even though all other factors appear to be the same.

Acute pain is to be distinguished from chronic pain. Acute pain warns the patient that something is wrong, but persistent acute pain may interfere with the healing and recovery process. Thus, the pain of myocardial infarction or postoperative pain may cause a series of reflexes that prevent optimum function of the heart and lungs as well as other essential body systems.

The signs of pain include increased heart

rate and output, increased blood pressure, pupillary dilatation, palmar sweating, hyperventilation, hypermotility, escape behavior, and anxiety state.

Acute pain is managed by diagnosing the underlying cause and attempting to remove it or decrease its intensity; use of drugs appropriate for the severity and type of pain; use of noninvasive measures such as application of heat, cold, manipulation, or splint; transcutaneous electrical nerve stimulation (T.E.N.S.), q.v.; relaxation therapy; and biofeedback to attempt to prevent the development of chronic pain at this stage.

In treating pain, it is not unusual for analgesics to be administered in accordance with the time specified to have elapsed between doses. This practice is neither humane nor merciful. It stems from an obsession with the possibility of causing addiction to the drug. Investigators have reported that creation of physical dependence requires the regular routine administration of therapeutic doses of narcotics four to six times a day for six weeks. Also, the incidence of addiction has been found to be 1 per 4000 hospitalized patients who have received narcotics.

When pain persists beyond the expected time required for healing of an injury or after the expected course of an acute disease, it is considered to be chronic. There is no evidence that most chronic pain stems from an apparent or treatable cause. For this reason chronic pain is considered to be a separate disease entity.

With respect to chronic intractable pain, however, there are known causes, including carcinomatosis; invasion or compression syndromes due to cancer; mental illness; neurologic disorders such as neuralgias, phantom limb pain, nerve entrapment syndromes, spinal cord damage, myofascial syndromes, or thalamic syndrome pain.

The signs of chronic pain include sleep disturbance, irritability, appetite disturbance, constipation, psychomotor retardation, decreased pain tolerance, social withdrawal, and mental depression. The management of chronic pain is similar to that given for acute pain, but the goal is to decrease the use of analgesics. Encourage the patient concerning eventual success of therapy, but at the same time set realistic therapeutic goals, and inform the patient that he or she and the treating physician should be prepared to accept the possibility that some pain is likely to continue.

It is important for those responsible for treating neonates to be aware that the mechanism for pain perception is fully developed and functioning by the time the fetus is born. Thus, the decision to use analgesics and local anesthesia or general anesthesia should be based on the same principles as those used in decisions involving adult patients. SEE: table; *endorphins; mercy; patient-controlled analgesia; substance P; T.E.N.S.*

NURSING IMPLICATIONS: Evaluate pain characteristics to determine the location and radiation, quality, severity (on a scale of 1 to 10), temporal qualities (onset and duration), any associated symptoms experienced, any known exacerbators, and treatments the person has used to obtain relief. Believe that the patient's pain exists, because pain is a subjective phenomenon and only the individual experiencing it can know its characteristics. When using prescribed medications for relief, remember the time lag before they become effective.

p., abdominal. Pain in the abdomen that usually increases with respiration. Experienced in a great variety of conditions including appendicitis; broken ribs; intercostal neuralgia; wounds; herpes zoster; pleurisy; pleurodynia; myalgia; periostitis; acute peritonitis; sickle cell anemia crisis; colic; hepatic, gastric, or renal ulcer; gallbladder disorders; carcinoma in late stages; and gummata of this region.

p., aching. Generalized aching that may accompany infectious disease such as influenza, smallpox, or rheumatic fever. It is also found in myalgia and various headaches.

p., acute. A short, sharp, cutting pain. Usually associated with acute inflammation or inflammation of serous membranes as in pleurisy and pericarditis; also posterior spinal-root pains. SYN: *p., lancinating.*

p., adnexal. Pain arising from the fallopian tubes and ovaries. Most commonly due to infection of those structures.

p.'s, after-. Pains following labor, caused by contraction of uterine muscles during their involution.

p., agonizing. Intense, torturing pain of mind or body. May be due to coronary thrombosis, angina pectoris, aortic aneurysm, mediastinitis. May occur in milder form in asthma or tracheobronchitis, or it may be due to referred pain from gallbladder, intestinal obstruction, diaphragmatic hernia, pancreatitis, or a perforated ulcer.

p., angina pectoris. Severe paroxysmal pain due to decreased blood supply to the myocardium, radiating through the shoulder down arm, or rarely from the heart to the abdomen, ear, or back. At the same time, the patient may experience a feeling that the chest is being crushed or compressed. Lasts from a few seconds to several minutes. SEE: *angina pectoris.*

Usual Doses and Intervals of Drugs for Relief of Pain

Nonnarcotic Analgesics

Generic Name	PO Dose, mg	Interval	Comments
Acetylsalicylic acid	650	4 hr	Enteric-coated preparations available
Acetaminophen	650	4 hr	Side effects uncommon
Ibuprofen	400	4–6 hr	Available without prescription
Indomethacin	25–50	8 hr	Gastrointestinal side effects common
Naproxen	250–500	12 hr	Delayed effects may be due to long half-life
Suprofen	200	6 hr	Little anti-inflammatory effect
Trisalicylate	1000–1500	12 hr	Fewer gastrointestinal or platelet effects

Narcotic Analgesics

Generic Name	Parenteral Dose, mg	PO Dose, mg	Comments
Codeine	30–60 every 4 hr	30–60 every 4 hr	Nausea common
Hydromorphone	1–2 every 4 hr	2–4 every 4 hr	Shorter acting than morphine sulfate
Levorphanol	2 every 6–8 hr	4 every 6 hr	Longer acting than morphine sulfate; absorbed well PO
Methadone	10 every 6–8 hr	20 every 6–8 hr	Delayed sedation due to long half-life
Meperidine	75–100 every 3–4 hr	300 every 4 hr	Poorly absorbed PO; normeperidine a toxic metabolite
Morphine	10 every 4 hr	60 every 4 hr	
Morphine, sustained release	90 every 12 hr	Oral slow-release preparation	
Oxycodone	—	5–10 every 4–6 hr	Usually available with acetaminophen or aspirin

Source: Adapted from Braunwald, E, et al: Harrison's Principles of Internal Medicine, ed 12. McGraw-Hill, New York, 1991.

p., appendicitis. If the attack is acute, there is pain, usually severe, generally through the abdomen, followed by localization of pain in lower right quadrant of abdomen with tenderness over right rectus muscle with rigidity. Rebound pain at McBurney's point is a classic symptom. SEE: *appendicitis.*

p.'s, bearing-down. Pain and pressure of the second stage of labor that causes the female to strain or bear down as one does to defecate.

p., boring. Pain deep in tissues that gives the sensation of being produced by a boring instrument.

p., Brodie's. Pain caused near a joint affected with neuralgia when the skin is folded near it.

p., burning. Pain experienced in heat burns, superficial skin lesions, herpes zoster, and in circumscribed neuralgias.

p., causalgic. Spontaneous pain, esp. burning in character, when associated with anesthesia or hyperesthesia in a given nerve. SYN: *causalgia.*

p., central. Pain due to a lesion in the central nervous system.

p., chest. Severe pain in chest from exercise; may be due to heart disease. If due to pleurisy, it comes with a deep breath. If pain accompanies stiff shoulder or neck, it may be due to arthritis or fibrositis. If it comes when patient is bending over after a meal, it may be due to diaphragmatic or hiatal hernia.

p., chronic. The persistence of pain beyond the usual or expected course of an acute disease or after a reasonable time for an injury to heal has elapsed. SEE: *pain.*

p., chronic intractable. Chronic pain due to a known cause, such as malignancy, mental illness, or a neurological disorder.

p., cramplike. Muscular spasm such as epigastric pain. Significance depends upon location of pain. Menstrual pain is often cramplike. SEE: *cramp; muscle cramps.*

p., dental. Pain in the oral area in general may be of two origins. Soft tissue pain may be acute or chronic, and a burning pain is due to surface lesions and usually can be discretely localized; pulpal pain or tooth pain varies according to whether it is acute or chronic, but often is difficult to localize.

p.'s, dilating. Rhythmic pains occurring during the first stage of labor accompanying dilatation of the cervix.

p., dull. Continuous mild throbbing.

p., ear. May indicate inflammation of the external auditory canal or mastoid area. Also may indicate a furuncle in the meatus or middle ear disease. SYN: *earache; otalgia; otodynia.*

p., eccentric. Pain occurring in peripheral structures due to a lesion involving posterior roots of spinal nerves.

p., epigastric. Severe pain occurring in paroxysms in gastric disorders. In general, may accompany any gastric or intestinal disorder, or some pleural and cardiac affections. SYN: *p., gastralgic.* SEE: *cardialgia.*

p.'s, expulsive. Pains of the second and third stages of labor.

p., false. Pain mistaken for a true labor pain; an ineffective pain of labor. Braxton-Hicks contractions are often confused with labor, particularly by the female experiencing her first pregnancy. SEE: Braxton-Hicks sign.

p., fulgurant. P., lightning.

p., gallbladder. Pain in upper right abdominal quadrant, dull pain just below the last rib in infection, or sharp pain in same area radiating to the back and up under the right shoulder, esp. if calculi are present.

p., gas. Pain in the intestines due to accumulation of gas therein.

p., gastralgic. Severe pain occurring in paroxysms in gastric disorders. SYN: *p., epigastric.*

p., girdle. Pain resembling sensation of a constricting cord around the waist, occurring in spinal cord disease.

p.'s, growing. Pains felt in the joints or limbs of growing children; may be rheumatic. An imprecise term indicating ill-defined pains in the muscular system of young persons. There is no evidence that the pains are related to rapid growth.

p., head. Ache or pain located in the head, esp. one experienced in region of cranial vault. Headache may be a symptom of acute systemic infections; intracranial tumors; infections; vascular lesions; hypertension; acute and chronic infections of the nose, sinuses, pharynx, eye, and ear; and toxic states such as alcoholism or uremia. Headache may occur after the injection of histamine, following a lumbar puncture, in infections of the meninges, and in subarachnoid hemorrhages. Headache occurs in many febrile diseases, in anemia, hypoxia, and following head injuries

(post-traumatic). Migraine, q.v., is a common cause of headache. SYN: *cephalalgia; headache.*

p., heterotopic. P., referred.

p., homotopic. Pain felt at the point of injury.

p., hunger. Pain due to need for food; coincides with powerful contractions of the stomach. May be indicative of gastric disorder. SEE: *hunger.*

p., hypogastric. Pain in the hypogastrium.

p., inflammatory. Pain in presence of inflammation that is increased by pressure.

p., intermenstrual. Pelvic pain arising during the cycle between the menses; may accompany ovulation. SEE: *mittelschmerz.*

p., intractable. Pain that cannot be easily relieved, as that occurring from certain neoplastic invasions.

p.'s, labor. Rhythmical uterine contractions at childbirth; increasing in frequency and severity, climaxing in vaginal delivery.

p., lancinating. A short, sharp, cutting pain. SYN: *p., acute.*

p., lightning. A sudden brief pain that may be repetitive. It is usually in the legs but may be at any location. These pains are associated with tabes dorsalis.

p., lingual. Pain in tongue that may be due to local lesions, glossitis, fissures, or pernicious anemia.

p., lung. Sharp pain in the region of the lungs. SYN: *p., pulmonary.*

p., menstrual. Pain, usually cramping, occurring just prior to onset of or during the menstrual period. SYN: *dysmenorrhea.*

p., mental. Pain of psychic origin such as mental distress or grief. If persistent, it may cause true physical pain.

p., middle. Pain between menstrual periods. SYN: *p., intermenstrual.* SEE: *mittelschmerz.*

p., migraine. Headache accompanied by nausea and vomiting. It may arise from a number of causes, esp. when it is of neurological origin. SEE: *migraine.*

p., mind. Pain of mental origin or occurring subsequent to mental effort, noted esp. in melancholia.

p., mobile. Pain that moves from one area to another.

p., movement. Kinesalgia, q.v.

p., neuralgic. Pain, frequently paroxysmal, occurring along the branches of a nerve. Temporarily relieved by heat or pressure. May be rheumatic in origin.

p., night. Musculoskeletal pain which awakens the patient at night or interferes with sleep. May be due to infection, inflammation, neurovascular compromise, or severe structural damage. Night pain is a frequent occurrence in patients with arthritis or bursitis of the shoulder.

p., noise. Pain of ear caused by noise. SYN: *odynacusis.*

p., objective. Pain induced by some external or internal irritant, by inflammation, or by injury to nerves, organs, or other tissues that interferes with the function, nutrition, or circulation of the affected part. Usually traceable to a definite pathological process.

p., paresthesic. Stinging or tingling sensation manifested in central and peripheral nerve lesions. SEE: *paresthesia.*

p., periodontal. A discrete, well-localized pain due to inflammation of tissues surrounding a tooth. This may be contrasted with the throbbing, nonlocalized pain typical of a toothache or pulpal pain.

p., phantom limb. Pain that seems to be in a certain limb following amputation of that limb. SEE: *phantom limb.*

p., postprandial. Abdominal pain after eating.

p., precordial. The sensation of pain over the heart.

p., premonitory. Ineffective contractions of the uterus prior to the beginning of true labor.

p., pseudomyelic. False sensation of movement in a paralyzed limb or of no movement in a moving limb. Not a true pain.

p., psychogenic. Pain having mental origin as opposed to organic origin.

p., rectal, constant. Pain in rectal area. Usually aggravated by defecation. May be due to ischiorectal abscess, anal abscess, inflamed or strangulated hemorrhoids, carcinoma, periproctitis, prostatic abscess, seminal vesiculitis, fecal impaction, acute salpingitis, tabes dorsalis, irritation from diarrhea, foreign bodies, fissures, rectal polyps, or adenoma. Pain during defecation may result from anal fissure, ulcer, hemorrhoids, anal abscess, stenosis, stricture, dysentery, impaction, foreign body, or any inflammation. SEE: *proctalgia fugax.*

p., referred. Pain seeming to arise in an area other than its origin, as pain from appendicitis, which often seems to occur in areas other than that of the appendix. SYN: *p., heterotopic; p., sympathetic; synalgia.*

p., remittent. Pain with temporary abatements in severity. Characteristic of neuralgia and colic.

p., rest. Pain due to ischemia that comes on when sitting or lying.

p., root. Cutaneous pain caused by disease of sensory nerve roots.

p., shooting. Pain that seems to travel like lightning from one place to another.

p.'s, spot. Pains that seem to be located in patches of the skin.

p.'s, starting. Pains accompanied by muscular spasm during early stages of sleep.

p., subdiaphragmatic. A sharp stitch-like pain occurring during breathing. When the breath is held, the pain ceases. Pressure against the lower rib cage eases the pain.

p., subjective. Pain with no apparent physical basis for its existence. It may be found among the highly imaginative neurotics in whom mild sensations are perceived as pain.

p., sympathetic. P., referred.

p., tenesmic. Pain accompanying urination or defecation. SEE: *tenesmus.*

p., terebrant. Boring or piercing type of pain.

p., thalamic. SEE: *thalamic syndrome.*

p., thermalgesic. Pain caused by heat.

p., thoracic. Sharp pain over the sternum, primarily in the chest or thoracic region, often running down the arm to the elbow. May be indicative of angina pectoris, although it must not be confused with pain from gastric pressure in the region of the heart, caused by an accumulation of gas. It is increased with respiration. It is experienced in connection with broken ribs; intercostal neuralgia; wounds; herpes zoster; pleurisy; pleurodynia; myalgia; periostitis; acute peritonitis; colic; hepatic, gastric, or renal ulcer; gallbladder disorders; carcinoma in late stages.

p., throbbing. Pain found in dental caries, headache, and localized inflammation.

p., tongue. P., lingual.

p., tracheal. Trachealgia.

p., wandering. Pain that changes its location repeatedly.

painful arc. During active movement of an extremity, a portion of the range of motion where the patient experiences pain. Pain is usually due to pinching of soft tissues at only a specific portion of the range of motion. A painful arc may be caused by tendonitis or bursitis.

pain relief, standards for. In 1991, the American Pain Society developed Standards for the Relief of Acute Pain and Cancer Pain. These are summarized as follows:

1. Acute pain and cancer pain are recognized and effectively treated. Essential to this process is the development of a clinically useful and easy to use scale for rating pain and its relief. Patients will be evaluated according to the scales and the results recorded as frequently as needed.
2. Information about analgesics is readily available. This includes data concerning

the effectiveness of various agents in controlling pain and the availability of equianalgesic charts wherever drugs are used for pain.

3. Patients are informed on admission of the availability of methods of relieving pain, and that they must communicate the presence and persistence of pain to the health care staff.

4. Explicit policies for use of advanced analgesic technologies are defined. These advances include patient-controlled analgesia, epidural analgesia, and regional analgesia. Specific instructions concerning use of these techniques need to be available for the medical care staff.

5. Adherence to standards is monitored by an interdisciplinary committee. The committee is responsible for overseeing the activities related to implementing and evaluating the effectiveness of these pain standards.

paint (pānt). 1. A solution of medication for application to skin. 2. To apply a medicated liquid to the skin.

p., Castellani's. A germicide consisting of phenol, resorcinol, boric acid, acetone, and basic fuchsin.

painters' colic. Colic accompanying lead poisoning. SEE: *lead* in Poisons and Poisoning in Appendix.

pair. Two of anything similar in shape, size, and conformation.

p., base. Pair of nucleotides, one a purine and the other a pyrimidine, joined by hydrogen bonds. These pairs make up deoxyribonucleic acid (DNA), q.v.

PAL. *posterior axillary line.*

palatable (păl'ăt-ă-b'l) [L. *palatum,* palate]. Pleasing to the palate or taste, as food.

palatal (păl'ă-tăl). Pert. to the roof of the mouth, the palate.

palatal reflex. Swallowing induced by stimulation of the soft palate.

palate (păl'ăt) [L. *palatum,* palate]. The horizontal structure separating the mouth and the nasal cavity; the roof of the mouth. SEE: *mouth* for illus.

DIFF. DIAG: *Koplik's spots:* A rash frequently seen upon the palate in measles. *Secondary syphilis:* Indicated by mucous patches on the palate. *Herpes of the throat:* Shown by vesicles in the circles upon the pharyngeal walls and soft palate. *Swelling of uvula:* Noted in inflammations of pharynx and tonsil, in nephritis, severe anemia, angioneurotic edema, and general debility. In diphtheria and Vincent's angina, a membranous exudate appears. In purpura hemorrhagica and some hemorrhagic diatheses, bloody extravasation appears. *Paralysis:* May result from diphtheria, bulbar paraly-

sis, neuritis, basal meningitis, tumor at base of brain. *Anesthesia:* Seen in pathological conditions of second division of the 5th nerve.

RS: Avellis' paralysis syndrome; Bednar's aphthae; cheilognathopalatoschisis; cleft; "palat-," "staphyl-," "uran-," "uvul-" words.

p., artificial. Prosthetic device molded to fill a cleft in the palate.

p., bony. P., hard, q.v.

p., cleft. Palate with a congenital opening.

p., falling. Abnormally long uvula.

p., gothic. An excessively high palatal arch.

p., hard. Anterior part of the palate supported by the maxillary and palatine bones.

p., pendulous. Uvula.

p., primary. In the embryo, the partition between the nasal cavities and mouth.

p., secondary. In the embryo, the palate formed from the maxillary arches and frontonasal process.

p., soft. Posterior musculomembranous fold partly separating the mouth and pharynx. SYN: *velum palatinum* [NA].

palate bones. Bones forming the posterior part of the hard palate and lateral nasal wall between the interior pterygoid plate of the sphenoid bone and maxilla.

palatiform (pă-lăt'ĭ-form) [L. *palatum,* palate, + *forma,* form]. Resembling the palate.

palatine (păl'ă-tīn) [L. *palatinus*]. 1. Concerning the palate. 2. The palate bones.

palatine arches. Two archlike folds of mucous membrane (glossopalatine and pharyngopalatine arches) that form the lateral margins of faucial and pharyngeal isthmuses. They are continuous above with the soft palate.

palatine artery, greater. Branch of the maxillary artery that supplies the palate, upper pharynx, and pharyngotympanic tube.

palatine bone. Palate bones.

palatitis (păl-ăt-ī'tĭs) [L. *palatum,* palate, + Gr. *itis,* inflammation]. Inflamed condition of the palate.

palatoglossal (păl''ă-tō-glŏs'ăl). Concerning the palate and tongue.

palatoglossus (păl''ă-tō-glŏs'ŭs) [" + Gr. *glossa,* tongue]. Muscle arising from sides and undersurface of the tongue. Fibers pass upward through glossopalatine arch and are inserted in palatine aponeurosis. It constricts faucial isthmus by raising the root of tongue and drawing sides of soft palate downward. SYN: *glossopalatinus.*

palatognathous (păl''ă-tŏg'nă-thŭs) [" + Gr. *gnathos,* jaw]. Having a congenital cleft in the palate.

palatograph (păl′ă-tō-grăf). Device that records the movements of the palate during speech.

palatography (păl″ă-tŏg′ră-fē) [″ + Gr. *graphein*, to write]. 1. Recording of the movements of the palate in speech. 2. Radiographic examination of the soft palate after injection of a contrast medium.

palatomaxillary (păl″ă-tō-măk′sĭ-lĕr″ē). Concerning the palate and maxilla.

palatomyograph (păl″ă-tō-mī′ō-grăf) [″ + Gr. *mys*, muscle, + *graphein*, to write]. Palatograph, q.v.

palatonasal (păl″ă-tō-nā′zăl). Concerning the palate and nasal cavity.

palatopharyngeal (păl″ă-tō-fă-rĭn′jē-ăl). Concerning the palate and pharynx.

palatopharyngeus (păl″ăt-ō-fă″rĭn′jē-ŭs) [″ + Gr. *pharynx*, throat]. Muscle arising from thyroid cartilage and pharyngeal wall, extending upward in posterior pillar, and inserting into aponeurosis of soft palate. Constricts pharyngeal isthmus, raises larynx, and depresses soft palate.

palatopharyngoplasty. Plastic surgical procedure for decreasing the nasopharyngeal passageway. It has been used in treating chronic snoring.

palatoplasty (păl″ăt-ō-plăs″tē) [″ + Gr. *plassein*, to form]. Plastic surgery of the palate, usually to correct a cleft. SYN: *staphylorrhaphy; uranoplasty.*

palatoplegia (păl″ă-tō-plē′jē-ă) [″ + Gr. *plege*, stroke]. Paralysis of muscles of the soft palate. SEE: *palate.*

palatorrhaphy (păl-ă-tor′ă-fē) [″ + Gr. *rhaphe*, seam, ridge]. Operation for uniting of a cleft palate. SYN: *staphylorrhaphy.*

palatosalpingeus (păl″ă-tō-săl-pĭn′jē-ŭs) [″ + Gr. *salpinx*, tube]. The tensor veli palatini muscle.

palatoschisis (păl-ă-tŏs′kĭ-sĭs) [″ + *schisis*, a splitting]. Palate with cleft in it.

palatum (păl-ă′tŭm) [L.] (pl. *palata*). [NA] The palate.

paleencephalon, paleoencephalon (pā″lē-ĕn-sĕf′ă-lŏn, -ō-ĕn-sĕf′ă-lŏn) [Gr. *palaios*, old, + *enkephalos*, brain]. Phylogenetically older portion of the brain; includes all of it except the cerebral cortex and its allied structures.

paleo- [Gr. *palaios*, old, ancient]. Combining form meaning old or ancient.

paleocerebellum (păl″ē-ō-sĕr″ē-bĕl′ŭm) [Gr. *palaios*, old, + L. *cerebellum*, little brain]. Phylogenetically, the older portion of the cerebellum including the flocculi, certain parts of the vermis (lingula, nodulus, uvula), and the lobulus centralis (culmen, pyramis, uvula, and simple lobule). These parts are concerned primarily with equilibrium and movements of locomotion.

paleogenesis (pā″lē-ō-jĕn′ē-sĭs) [″ + *genesis*, generation, birth]. Reproduction of ancestral characteristics, esp. abnormalities, without change in a later generation. SYN: *atavism; palingenesis.*

paleogenetic (pā″lē-ō-jĕn-ĕt′ĭk) [″ + *gennan*, to produce]. Having origin in a previous generation.

paleokinetic (pā″lē-ō-kĭ-nĕt′ĭk) [″ + *kinetikos*, concerning movement]. Noting a peripheral motor nervous system controlling automatic associated movements. It is older phylogenetically than the system controlling voluntary movement.

paleontology (pā″lē-ŏn-tŏl′ō-jē) [″ + *onta*, existing things, + *logos*, word, reason]. Branch of biology dealing with ancient plant and animal life of the earth.

paleopathology (pā″lē-ō-pă-thŏl′ō-jē) [″ + *pathos*, disease, + *logos*, word, reason]. Study of diseases in remains of bodies and fossils of ancient times.

paleostriatal (pā″lē-ō-strī-ā′tăl) [″ + L. *striatus*, ridged]. Concerning the primitive portion of the corpus striatum.

paleostriatum (pā″lē-ō-strī-ā′tŭm). Primitive portion of corpus striatum, the globus pallidus. SEE: *neostriatum.*

paleothalamus (pā″lē-ō-thăl′ă-mŭs) [″ + *thalamos*, chamber]. Medial portion of thalamus (the medullary or noncortical part), which is older phylogenetically. SEE: *thalamus.*

pali-, palin- [Gr. *palin*, backward, again]. Prefix meaning recurrence or repetition.

palikinesia (păl″ĭ-kĭn-ē′zē-ă) [″ + *kinesis*, movement]. Continued, involuntary, repetitious movements.

palilalia (păl-ĭ-lā′lē-ă) [″ + *lalein*, to speak]. Pathological repetitious use of words and phrases with increasing rapidity. SYN: *paliphrasia.*

palinal (păl′ĭn-ăl) [Gr. *palin*, backward]. Moved or moving backward.

palindromia (păl-ĭn-drō′mē-ă) [″ + *dromos*, a running]. The recurrence of a disease or a relapse.

palindromic (păl-ĭn-drŏm′ĭk). Recurring, as the symptoms of a disease. SYN: *relapsing.*

palindromic arthritis or rheumatism. A disease of unknown etiology characterized by intermittent joint pain with tenderness, heat, and swelling that lasts from a few hours to as long as a week. The knees or fingers are most often involved, but the disease does not necessarily return to the same joint(s). Between attacks there is no evidence of the disease. Symptomatic treatment is usually sufficient.

palinesthesia (păl″ĭn-ĕs-thē′zē-ă) [Gr. *palin*, again, + *aisthesis*, sensation]. Return of power of sensation, as after recovery from anesthesia or coma.

palingenesis (păl″ĭn-jĕn′ĕ-sĭs) [″ + *genesis*, generation, birth]. 1. Regeneration or restoration of an organism or part of one. 2. Reappearance of ancestral characteristics, esp. abnormal ones, in successive generations. SYN: *atavism; paleogenesis.*

palingraphia (păl″ĭn-grăf′ē-ă) [″ + *graphein*, to write]. Pathological repetition of words or phrases in writing.

palinopsia [″ + *opsis*, vision]. Persistence of a visual image after the object has been removed. It may be associated with a lesion in the occipital lobe of the brain. SEE: *afterimage.*

paliphrasia (păl-ĭ-frā′zē-ă) [″ + *phrasis*, speech]. Pathological condition in which there is coherent speech but certain words or phrases frequently are repeated. SYN: *palilalia.*

palladium (pă-lā′dē-ŭm) [L.]. SYMB: Pd. At. wt. 106.4; at. no. 46. Metallic element used in dentistry and surgical instruments.

pallanesthesia (păl″ăn-ĕs-thē′zē-ă) [Gr. *pallein*, to shake, + *anaisthesia*, anesthesia]. Loss of ability to sense vibrations. SYN: *apallesthesia.* SEE: *pallesthesia.*

pallesthesia (păl-ĕs-thē′zē-ă) [Gr. *pallein*, to shake, + *aisthesis*, sensation]. The sensation of vibration felt in skin or bones, as that produced by a tuning fork held against the body.

palliate (păl′ē-āt) [L. *palliatus*, cloaked]. To ease or reduce effect or intensity, esp. of a disease; to allay temporarily, as pain, without curing.

palliative (păl′ē-ā″tĭv). 1. Serving to relieve or alleviate, without curing. 2. An agent that alleviates or eases.

pallid (păl′ĭd) [L. *pallidus*, pale]. Lacking color, pale, wan.

pallidal (păl′ĭ-dăl). Concerning the pallidum of the brain.

pallidectomy (păl″ĭ-dĕk′tō-mē) [L. *pallidum*, pallidum, + Gr. *ektome*, excision]. Surgical, chemical, or cryogenic removal or inactivation of the globus pallidus of the brain.

pallidoansotomy (păl″ĭ-dō-ăn-sŏt′ō-mē) [″ + *ansa*, a handle, + Gr. *tome*, incision]. Production of lesions in the globus pallidus and ansa lenticularis of the brain.

pallidotomy (păl″ĭ-dŏt′ō-mē) [″ + Gr. *tome*, incision]. Surgical destruction of the globus pallidus done to treat involuntary movements or muscular rigidity.

pallidum (păl′ĭ-dŭm) [L.]. The globus pallidus of the lenticular nucleus in the corpus striatum.

pallium (păl′ē-ŭm) [L., cloak]. [NA] The cerebral cortex with its adjacent white substance, considered as a cover for the rest of the brain.

pallor (păl′or) [L.]. Lack of color; paleness. SEE: *skin.*

palm [L. *palma*, hand]. Anterior or flexor surface of the hand from wrist to fingers. SYN: *vola manus.* SEE: *antithenar; thenar.*

palma (păl′mă) [L.]. The palm of the hand.

palmar (păl′măr). Concerning the palm of the hand.

palmar cuff. A band of fabric, usually elasticized, fitted around the palm of the hand for the purpose of attaching utensils and tools for persons with limited or absent function of the hand and wrist. SYN: *universal cuff.*

palmar grasp reflex. SEE: *reflex, palmar grasp.*

palmaris (păl-mā′rĭs). [NA] One of two muscles, palmaris brevis and palmaris longus. SEE: *Muscles* in *Appendix.*

palmar reflex. SEE: *reflex, palmar grasp.*

palmature (păl′mă-tūr) [L. *palma*, hand]. The pathological condition in which the fingers are joined or united.

palm-chin reflex. When the thenar eminence is scratched with a sharp object, contraction of the superficial muscles of the eye and chin is produced on the same side as the palmar area that was stimulated.

palmic (păl′mĭk) [Gr. *palmikos*]. 1. Concerning palpitation or pulse. 2. Concerning palmus.

palmitic acid (păl-mĭt′ĭk). $C_{16}H_{32}O_2$. A fatty acid found in palm oil, solid fats, some waxes, and many fatty oils. It is one of the basic building blocks from which long-chain fatty acids are constructed.

palmitin (păl′mĭ-tĭn). An ester of glycerol and palmitic acid, derived from fat of both animal and vegetable origin.

palmomental reflex. Palm-chin reflex, q.v.

palmoplantar (păl″mō-plăn′tăr). Pert. to the palms of the hands and soles of the feet.

palmus (păl′mŭs) [Gr. *palmos*, pulsation, quivering]. 1. Palpitation; a throb. 2. Jerking; a disease with convulsive nervous twitching of the leg muscles, similar to jumping. 3. Heartbeat.

palpable (păl′pă-b′l) [L. *palpabilis*, stroke, touch]. Perceptible, esp. by touch.

palpate (păl′pāt) [L. *palpare*, to touch]. To examine by touch; to feel.

palpation (păl-pā′shŭn) [L. *palpatio*]. Process of examining by application of the hands or fingers to the external surface of the body to detect evidence of disease or abnormalities in the various organs.

    p., light-touch. Determining the outline of abdominal organs by lightly palpating the abdominal wall with the fingers.

palpatopercussion (păl″pă-tō-pĕr-kŭsh′ŭn). Palpation combined with percussion.

palpebra (păl′pĕ-bră) [L.] (pl. *palpebrae*). An eyelid.

p. inferior. [NA] The lower eyelid.

p. superior. [NA] The upper eyelid.

palpebral (păl′pē-brăl). Concerning an eyelid.

palebral cartilages. Thin plates of condensed tissue resembling cartilage that form the framework of the eyelid. SYN: *tarsal cartilages.*

palpebral commissure. The union of the eyelids at each end of the palpebral fissure.

palpebral fissure. The opening between the eyelids.

palpebral ligament. One of two ligamentous structures (medial and lateral) that fix the two ends of the tarsi to the orbital wall.

palpebral muscles. 1. Palpebral portion of musculus orbicularis oculi. 2. Musculus levator palpebrae superioris.

palpebrate (păl′pē-brāt). 1. [L. *palpebrare*]. To wink. 2. [L. *palpebra*, eyelid]. Possessing eyelids.

palpebritis (păl″pē-brī′tĭs) [L. *palpebra*, eyelid, + Gr. *itis*, inflammation]. Blepharitis, q.v.

palpitant (păl′pĭ-tănt) [L. *palpitare*, to quiver]. Throbbing; trembling.

palpitate (păl′pĭ-tāt) [L. *palpitatus*, throbbing]. 1. To cause to throb. 2. To throb or beat intensely or rapidly, usually said of the heart.

palpitation (păl-pĭ-tā′shŭn). Rapid, violent, or throbbing pulsation, as an abnormally rapid throbbing or fluttering of the heart. The palpitation is perceptible to the patient. SEE: *heart.*

    p., arterial. Palpitation felt in course of an artery.

PALS. *pediatric advanced life support.*

palsy (pawl′zē) [ME. *palesie*, from L. *paralysis*]. Temporary or permanent loss of sensation or loss of ability to move or to control movement. SYN: *paralysis.*

    p., Bell's. Paralysis of the facial nerve in its peripheral distribution. Muscles of unaffected side of face pull the face into a distorted position.

    p., birth. Palsy arising from an injury received at birth.

    p., bulbar. Palsy caused by degeneration of the nuclear cells of the lower cranial nerves. This causes progressive muscular paralysis.

    p., cerebral. A nonprogressive paralysis resulting from developmental defects in brain or trauma at birth. SEE: *Nursing Diagnoses* in *Appendix.*

    p., crutch. Paralysis resulting from pressure on nerves in the axilla from use of a crutch.

    p., diver's. Paralysis caused by decompression illness, q.v. SEE: *bends; caisson disease.*

    p., Erb's. Paralysis of the deltoid, biceps, long supinator, and brachialis anticus muscles due to a lesion of the brachial plexus or of the fifth and sixth cervical nerves.

    p., facial. P., Bell's, q.v.

    p., lead. Paralysis of extremities in lead poisoning.

    p., night. Form of paresthesia in which numbness is a symptom, esp. at night.

    p., progressive supranuclear. Chronic progressive degenerative disease of the central nervous system that has its onset in middle age. There are conjugate ocular palsies, dystonia of the neck, and widespread rigidity.

    p., Saturday night. SEE: *paralysis, musculospiral.*

    p., scrivener's. Writer's cramp.

    p., shaking. Progressive muscular weakness and tremor with impaired voluntary motion. SYN: *paralysis agitans; Parkinson's disease.*

    p., wasting. Chronic condition in which there are atrophy and paralysis of muscles; grows progressively worse. SYN: *progressive muscular atrophy.*

paludal (păl′ū-dăl) [L. *palus*, a marsh]. Concerning, or originating in, marshes. SYN: *malarial.*

paludism (păl′ū-dĭzm) [″ + Gr. *-ismos*, condition]. Swamp fever. SYN: *malaria.*

palynology [Gr. *palumein*, to sprinkle, + *logos*, word, reason]. Study of pollens, spores, or microscopic segments of organisms present in sediments.

Pamelor. Trade name for nortriptyline hydrochloride.

pamidronate disodium. A drug used to treat hypercalcemia associated with malignancy, with or without bone metastases. In the U.S. it is approved for I.V. use. Oral forms are available in Europe.

Pamine. Trade name for methscopolamine bromide.

pampiniform (păm-pĭn′ĭ-form) [L. *pampinus*, tendril, + *forma*, shape]. Convoluted like a tendril.

pampiniform plexus. 1. A mesh of spermatic or ovarian veins. 2. Network of nerves supplying the testicles.

pampinocele (păm-pĭn′ō-sēl) [″ + Gr. *kele*, tumor, swelling]. A swollen, painful condition of the veins of the spermatic cord. SYN: *varicocele.*

pan- [Gr.]. Combining form indicating all.

panacea (păn-ă-sē′ă) [Gr. *panakeia*, universal remedy]. A remedy for all ills; cure-all.

panagglutinable (păn″ă-gloo′tĭ-nă-b′l) [Gr. *pan*, all, + L. *agglutinare*, to glue to]. Blood cells that are agglutinable by every blood group serum of the species.

panagglutinin (păn″ă-glū′tĭn-ĭn) [Gr. *pan*,

all, + L. *agglutinare,* to glue to]. Substance capable of agglutinizing corpuscles of every blood group.

panangiitis (păn″ăn-jē-ī′tĭs) [″ + *angeion,* vessel, + *itis,* inflammation]. Inflammation of all the coats of a blood vessel.

panaris (păn′ă-rĭs) [L. *panaricium,* disease of the fingernail]. Inflammation of the skin fold surrounding the nail. SYN: *paronychia.*

panarteritis (păn″ăr-tĕ-rī′tĭs) [Gr. *pan,* all, + *arteria,* artery, + *itis,* inflammation]. 1. Inflammation of all the coats of an artery.

panarthritis (păn″ăr-thrī′tĭs) [″ + *arthron,* joint, + *itis,* inflammation]. 1. Inflammation of all parts of a joint. 2. Inflamed condition of all the joints of the body.

panasthenia (păn″ăs-thē′nē-ă) [″ + *astheneia,* weakness]. Generalized weakness or exhaustion without evidence of organic disease. SYN: *neurasthenia.*

panatrophy (păn-ăt′rō-fē) [″ + *a-,* not, + *trophe,* nourishment]. Wasting away of an entire structure; generalized wasting away of the body.

panblastic (păn-blăs′tĭk) [″ + *blastos,* germ]. Concerning all the layers of the blastoderm.

pancarditis (păn-kăr-dī′tĭs) [″ + *kardia,* heart, + *itis,* inflammation]. Inflamed condition involving all the structures of the heart.

panchreston (păn-krē′stŏn) [″ + *chrestos,* useful]. A remedy for every disease. SYN: *panacea.*

panchromia (păn-krō′mē-ă) [″ + *chroma,* color]. Power of staining with numerous dyes.

Pancoast syndrome [Henry Khunrath Pancoast, U.S. physician, 1875–1939]. Production of Horner's syndrome, q.v., by a malignant neoplasm of the cervical area with involvement of the brachial plexus and cervical sympathetic nerves. The neoplasm is called Pancoast's tumor.

pancolectomy (păn″kō-lĕk′tō-mē) [Gr. *pan,* all, + *kolon,* colon, + *ektome,* excision]. Surgical excision of the entire colon.

pancreas (păn′krē-ăs) [″ + *kreas,* flesh] (pl. *pancreata*). [NA] A compound acinotubular gland situated behind the stomach in front of the 1st and 2nd lumbar vertebrae in a horizontal position, its head attached to the duodenum and its tail reaching to the spleen. The portion between the head and the tail constitutes the body.

The gland is composed of lobules that form lobes connected by strands of tissue with ducts that lead from the lobules into a main one, the pancreatic duct or duct of Wirsung. This duct is connected with the duodenum. Scattered throughout the sub-

stance are differentiated masses of cells that are the islets of Langerhans. An accessory pancreatic duct or duct of Santorini frequently is present. It is smaller than the main duct and opens into the duodenum cephalad to the main duct with which it communicates. SEE: illus.

FUNCT: The pancreas produces both an external and an internal secretion. It has, therefore, an exocrine and endocrine function. The external secretion, called pancreatic juice, q.v., passes through the pancreatic ducts into the duodenum, where it plays an important role in the digestion of all classes of foods.

The internal secretion, elaborated by the beta cells of the islets of Langerhans, includes the hormones insulin and glucagon (hyperglycemic-glycogenolytic factor) secreted by the alpha cells. These hormones, in conjunction with hormones from other endocrine glands (adrenal cortex, medulla, anterior hypophysis), play a primary role in the regulation of carbohydrate metabolism.

Pancreatic peptide (PP) cells have an exocrine function by stimulating the secretion of gastric and intestinal enzymes and inhibiting intestinal motility.

Delta cells contain somatostatin, which suppresses the release of both insulin and glucagon.

Diminished secretion of insulin by the islets of Langerhans results in diabetes mellitus, q.v. In this disease there are disturbances in the metabolism of carbohydrates and fats resulting in the elevation of blood glucose, cholesterol, and ketone bodies.

Excessive secretion of insulin, called hyperinsulinism, q.v., may sometimes occur. This results in marked lowering of blood sugar (hypoglycemia, q.v.). SEE: *diabetes mellitus; insulin; pancreatic function tests.*

   p., accessory. Small mass of pancreatic tissue close to the pancreas but detached from it.

   p., annular. An anomalous condition in which a portion of the pancreas encircles the duodenum.

   p. divisum. A congenital anomaly in which the two portions of the embryonic pancreas fail to unite. SYN: *divided pancreas.*

   p., dorsal. A dorsal outpocketing of the embryonic gut that gives rise to the body and tail of the adult pancreas.

   p., lesser. Semi-detached lobular part of the posterior surface of a head of the pancreas, sometimes having a separate duct opening into the principal one. SYN: *p., Willis'.*

   p., transplantation of. The implantation of a part of the pancreas or the entire

PANCREAS AND ITS RELATIONSHIP TO THE DUODENUM

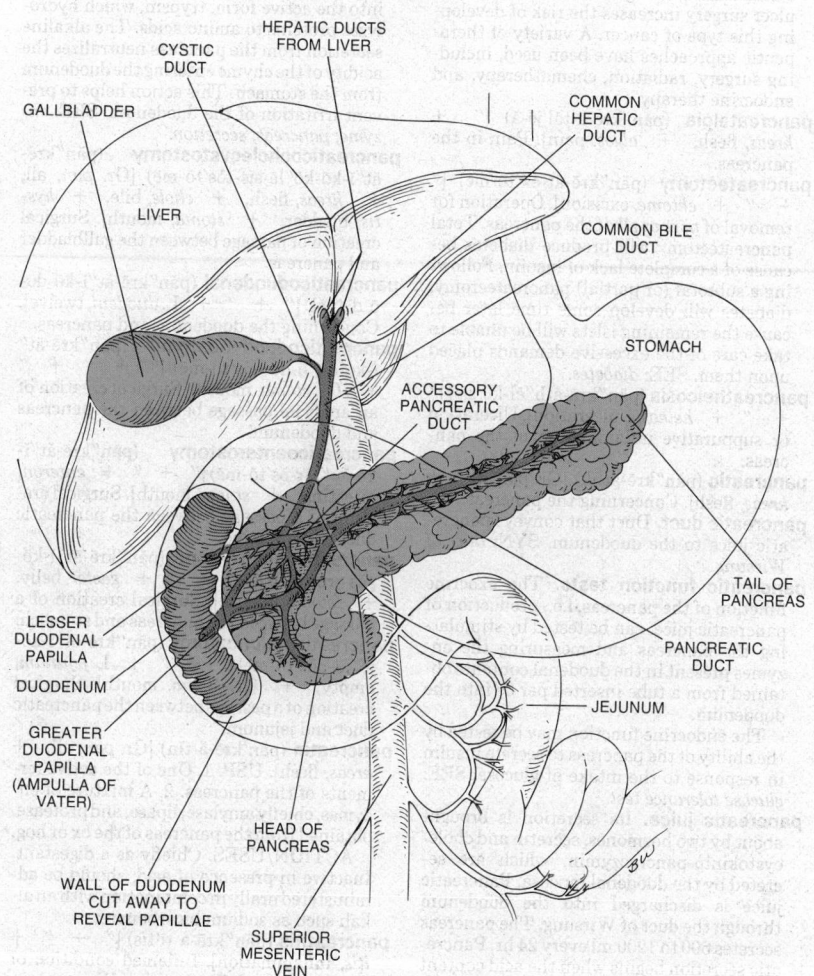

HEPATIC DUCTS FROM LIVER

CYSTIC DUCT

GALLBLADDER

COMMON HEPATIC DUCT

LIVER

COMMON BILE DUCT

STOMACH

ACCESSORY PANCREATIC DUCT

TAIL OF PANCREAS

LESSER DUODENAL PAPILLA

PANCREATIC DUCT

DUODENUM

JEJUNUM

GREATER DUODENAL PAPILLA (AMPULLA OF VATER)

HEAD OF PANCREAS

WALL OF DUODENUM CUT AWAY TO REVEAL PAPILLAE

SUPERIOR MESENTERIC VEIN

gland from a donor into a patient whose own pancreas is no longer functioning. Survival of the transplanted tissue for one year is about 50%.

Transplantation of islet cells is being actively investigated.

p., ventral. An outgrowth at the angle of the hepatic diverticulum and the embryonic gut that migrates and fuses with the dorsal pancreas. It forms the head of the definitive organ.

p., Willis'. P., lesser.

pancreas, carcinoma of. Twenty-two percent of deaths from gastrointestinal cancer are due to cancer of the pancreas. The prognosis is extremely poor in that only 3% of patients are alive 5 years after the diagnosis is made. This cancer occurs more frequently in men than women. The cause of this type of cancer is unknown, but two risk factors are important: cigarette smoking and a high intake of fat or meat, or both. There is no statistically significant association between coffee consumption and cancer of the pancreas. Having had gastric cancer or peptic ulcer surgery increases the risk of developing this type of cancer. A variety of therapeutic approaches have been used, including surgery, radiation, chemotherapy, and endocrine therapy.

pancreatalgia (păn″krē-ă-tăl′jē-ă) [″ + *kreas*, flesh, + *algos*, pain]. Pain in the pancreas.

pancreatectomy (păn″krē-ăt-ĕk′tō-mē) [″ + ″ + *ektome*, excision]. Operation for removal of part or all of the pancreas. Total pancreatectomy will produce diabetes because of a complete lack of insulin. Following a subtotal (or partial) pancreatectomy, diabetes will develop some time later because the remaining islets will be unable to take care of the excessive demands placed upon them. SEE: *diabetes*.

pancreathelcosis (păn″krē-ăth″ĕl-kō′sĭs) [″ + ″ + *helkosis*, ulceration]. Ulceration or suppurative inflammation of the pancreas.

pancreatic (păn″krē-ăt′ĭk) [Gr. *pan*, all, + *kreas*, flesh]. Concerning the pancreas.

pancreatic duct. Duct that conveys pancreatic juice to the duodenum. SYN: *duct of Wirsung.*

pancreatic function tests. The exocrine function of the pancreas, i.e., production of pancreatic juice, can be tested by stimulating the pancreas and measuring the enzymes present in the duodenal contents obtained from a tube inserted per os into the duodenum.

The endocrine function may be tested by the ability of the pancreas to secrete insulin in response to the intake of glucose. SEE: *glucose tolerance test.*

pancreatic juice. Its secretion is brought about by two hormones, secretin and cholecystokinin-pancreozymin, which are secreted by the duodenal mucosa. Pancreatic juice is discharged into the duodenum through the duct of Wirsung. The pancreas secretes 500 to 1200 ml every 24 hr. Pancreatic secretion begins when the acid content of the stomach passes through the pylorus. It is a clear, viscid, alkaline fluid (pH 8.4 to 8.9) resembling saliva in consistency. It contains water, protein, inorganic salts, and enzymes. Among the enzymes are the following: trypsinogen, which by the action of intestinal enterokinase is converted into trypsin, a proteolytic enzyme; chymotrypsinogen, which is converted by trypsin into chymotrypsin, a milk-curdling enzyme; amylopsin, a maltase that acts on carbohydrates; and steapsin, a lipase that acts on fats. Amylopsin hydrolyzes starch to maltose; steapsin hydrolyzes fats to fatty acids and glycerol; trypsinogen, by the action of

enterokinase in the duodenum, is converted into the active form, trypsin, which hydrolyzes proteins to amino acids. The alkaline secretion from the pancreas neutralizes the acidity of the chyme entering the duodenum from the stomach. This action helps to prevent irritation of the duodenum. SEE: *enzyme; pancreas; secretion.*

pancreaticocholecystostomy (păn″krē-ăt″ĭ-kō-kō″lē-sĭs-tŏs′tō-mē) [Gr. *pan*, all, + *kreas*, flesh, + *chole*, bile, + *kystis*, bladder, + *stoma*, mouth]. Surgical creation of passage between the gallbladder and pancreas.

pancreaticoduodenal (păn″krē-ăt″ĭ-kō-dū-ō-dē′năl) [″ + ″ + L. *duodeni*, twelve]. Concerning the duodenum and pancreas.

pancreaticoduodenostomy (păn″krē-ăt″ĭ-kō-dū″ō-dē-nŏs′tō-mē) [″ + ″ + ″ + Gr. *stoma*, mouth]. Surgical creation of an artificial passage between the pancreas and duodenum.

pancreaticoenterostomy (păn″krē-ăt″ĭ-kō-ĕn″tĕr-ŏs′tō-mē) [″ + ″ + *enteron*, intestine, + *stoma*, mouth]. Surgical creation of a passage between the pancreatic duct and intestine.

pancreaticogastrostomy (păn″krē-ăt″ĭ-kō-găs-trŏs′tō-mē) [″ + ″ + *gaster*, belly, + *stoma*, mouth]. Surgical creation of a passage between the pancreas and stomach.

pancreaticojejunostomy (păn″krē-ăt″ĭ-kō-jē″jū-nŏs′tō-mē) [″ + ″ + L. *jejunum*, empty, + Gr. *stoma*, mouth]. Surgical creation of a passage between the pancreatic duct and jejunum.

pancreatin (păn′krē-ă-tĭn) [Gr. *pan*, all, + *kreas*, flesh]. USP. 1. One of the active ferments of the pancreas. 2. A mixture of enzymes, chiefly amylase, lipase, and protease, obtained from the pancreas of the ox or hog.

ACTION/USES: Chiefly as a digestant. Inactive in presence of acid; should be administered orally in combination with an alkali such as sodium bicarbonate.

pancreatitis (păn′krē-ă-tī′tĭs) [″ + ″ + *itis*, inflammation]. Inflamed condition of the pancreas. SEE: *Nursing Diagnoses in Appendix.*

p., acute. Form of pancreatitis characterized by necrosis, suppuration, gangrene, and hemorrhage. Characterized by sudden onset of abdominal pain, nausea, and vomiting.

SYM: Sudden and intense pain in epigastric region, vomiting, belching of gas, sometimes hiccough, collapse. Rigidity and tenderness over umbilicus. Constipation, slow pulse, possible jaundice.

p., acute hemorrhagic. Form of pancreatitis with hemorrhage into pancreatic tissue.

SYM: Paroxysms of deep-seated pain in epigastrium, nausea, retching, constipation. Slight rise in temperature, blood and mucus in vomitus, delirium, tympanites, jaundice, hiccough, cyanosis, collapse.

   p., calcareous. Pancreatitis accompanied by calculi formation.

   p., centrilobar. Pancreatitis located around divisions of the pancreatic duct.

   p., chronic. Form of pancreatitis marked by formation of scar tissue associated with malfunction.

   SYM: Pain, mild, or severe. Pain has tendency to radiate to the back. Jaundice, weakness, emaciation, diarrhea.

   p., interstitial. Pancreatitis with overgrowth of interacinar and intra-acinar connective tissue.

   p., perilobar. Fibrosis of the pancreas between acinous groups.

   p., purulent. Pancreatitis with suppuration.

   p., suppurative. Form of pancreatitis marked by development of many small abscesses. Symptoms may be those of acute or chronic form.

pancreatoduodenectomy (păn″krē-ă-tō-dū″ō-dē-něk′tō-mē) [Gr. *pan*, all, + *kreas*, flesh, + L. *duodeni*, twelve, + Gr. *ektome*, excision]. Excision of the head of the pancreas and the adjacent portion of the duodenum.

pancreatoduodenostomy (păn″krē-ă-tō-dū″ō-dē-nŏs′tō-mē) [″ + ″ + ″ + *stoma*, mouth]. Surgical anastomosis of the pancreatic duct, or a pancreatic fistula, to the duodenum.

pancreatogenic, pancreatogenous (păn″krē-ă-tō-jĕn′ĭk, -tŏj′ĕ-nŭs) [″ + ″ + *gennan*, to produce]. Produced in or by the pancreas; originating in the pancreas.

pancreatography (păn″krē-ă-tŏg′ră-fē) [″ + ″ + *graphein*, to write]. Combined surgical and radiographic procedure in which a roentgenogram of the pancreas is taken after iodinated contrast medium is injected into the duct of Wirsung.

pancreatolith (păn″krē-ăt′ō-lĭth) [″ + ″ + *lithos*, stone]. A calculus within the pancreas.

pancreatolithectomy (păn″krē-ăt-ō-lĭth-ĕk′tō-mē) [″ + ″ + ″ + *ektome*, excision]. Removal of a calculus from the pancreas. SYN: *pancreatolithotomy; pancreolithotomy.*

pancreatolithiasis (păn″krē-ă-tō-lĭ-thī′ă-sĭs) [″ + ″ + ″ + *-iasis*, condition]. Calculi in the duct system of the pancreas.

pancreatolithotomy (păn″krē-ăt-ō-lĭ-thŏt′ō-mē) [″ + ″ + ″ + *tome*, incision]. Removal of a calculus from the pancreas. SYN: *pancreatolithectomy; pancreoli-*

thotomy.

pancreatolysis (păn″krē-ă-tŏl′ĭ-sĭs) [″ + ″ + *lysis*, dissolution]. Destruction of the pancreatic substance by pancreatic enzymes.

pancreatolytic (păn″krē-ăt-ō-lĭt′ĭk). Destructive to the pancreatic tissues. SYN: *pancreolytic.*

pancreatomy (păn-krē-ăt′ō-mē) [″ + ″ + *tome*, incision]. Pancreatotomy, q.v.

pancreatoncus (păn-krē-ăt-ŏng′kŭs) [″ + ″ + *onkos*, tumor]. A pancreatic tumor.

pancreatopathy (păn″krē-ă-tŏp′ă-thē) [″ + ″ + *pathos*, disease, suffering]. Any pathological state of the pancreas. SYN: *pancreopathy.*

pancreatotomy (păn″krē-ă-tŏt′ō-mē) [″ + ″ + *tome*, incision]. Surgical incision into the pancreas. SYN: *pancreatomy.*

pancreatotropic (păn-krē″ă-tō-trŏp′ĭk) [″ + ″ + *tropikos*, turning]. Having an affinity for or action on the pancreas.

pancreectomy (păn″krē-ĕk′tō-mē) [″ + *ektome*, excision]. Partial or total excision of the pancreas.

pancrelipase (păn″krē-lī′pās). USP. A standardized preparation of enzymes, principally lipase, with amylase and protease, obtained from the pancreas of the hog. Used in treating conditions associated with deficient secretion from the pancreas. Trade names are Accelerase, Cotazym, and Ilozyme.

pancreolithotomy (păn″krē-ō-lĭ-thŏt′ō-mē) [″ + *kreas*, flesh, + *lithos*, stone, + *tome*, incision]. Surgical removal of a pancreatic concretion. SYN: *pancreatolithectomy; pancreatolithotomy.*

pancreolysis (păn″krē-ŏl′ĭ-sĭs) [″ + ″ + *lysis*, dissolution]. Enzymatic destruction of the pancreas.

pancreolytic (păn″krē-ō-lĭt′ĭk) [″ + *lysis*, dissolution]. Destructive to the pancreas. SYN: *pancreatolytic.*

pancreopathy (păn″krē-ŏp′ă-thē) [″ + ″ + *pathos*, disease, suffering]. Any diseased condition of the pancreas. SYN: *pancreatopathy.*

pancreoprivic (păn″krē-ō-prĭv′ĭk). Having no pancreas.

pancuronium bromide (păn″kū-rō′nē-ŭm). A neuromuscular blocking agent. Trade name is Pavulon.

pancytopenia (păn″sī-tō-pē′nē-ă) [″ + *kytos*, cell, + *penia*, poverty]. A reduction in all cellular elements of the blood. SEE: *anemia, aplastic.*

pandemia (păn-dē′mē-ă) [″ + *demos*, the people]. Epidemic affecting the major portion of the population of a district.

pandemic (păn-dĕm′ĭk). A disease affecting

the majority of the population of a large region, such as dental caries or periodontal disease, or one that is epidemic at the same time in many different parts of the world.

pandiculation (păn″dĭk-ū-lā′shŭn) [L. *pandiculari,* to stretch one's self]. Stretching of the limbs and yawning, as on awakening from normal sleep.

panel. 1. A number of patients or normal subjects who participate in medical investigations, esp. studies in which new drugs, devices, or procedures are tested. SEE: *informed consent; institutional review board.* 2. The list of patients who obtain their primary medical care from the physician to whom they are assigned. This system is used in some health care plans.

panencephalitis (păn″ĕn-sĕf″ă-lī′tĭs) [Gr. *pan,* all, + *enkephalos,* brain, + *itis,* inflammation]. A cerebral degenerative disease thought to be secondary to entrance of the measles virus into the brain. The first signs are due to a progressive decrease in higher cerebral functions, usually manifested as failure to progress in school. There are personality changes, emotional instability, and generalized myoclonic jerks. In late stages, dementia and generalized rigidity occur. There is no treatment, and most patients die of the disease. SYN: *subacute sclerosing panencephalitis.*

panendoscope (păn-ĕn′dō-skōp) [″ + *endon,* within, + *skopein,* to view]. A cystoscope that gives a wide view of the bladder.

panesthesia (păn″ĕs-thē′zē-ă) [″ + *aisthesis,* sensation]. The sum of all of the stimuli and sensations coming from the body at one time.

Paneth, cells of (pă′nät) [Josef Paneth, Ger. physician, 1857–1890]. Large secretory cells, containing coarse granules, found at the blind end of the crypts of Lieberkühn (the intestinal glands).

pang. 1. A paroxysm of extreme agony. 2. A sudden attack of any emotion.

pangamic acid. A substance of disputed composition with no known therapeutic or nutritional properties. SYN: *"vitamin B₁₅."*

pangenesis (păn″jĕn′ĕ-sĭs) [Gr. *pan,* all, + *genesis,* generation, birth]. The discredited hypothesis that each cell of the parent is represented by a particle in the reproductive cell, and thus each part of the organism reproduces itself in the progeny.

panglossia (păn-glŏs′sē-ă) [Gr.]. Excessive talkativeness, esp. in psychotic persons.

panhidrosis (păn″hĭd-rō′sĭs) [Gr. *pan,* all, + *hidros,* sweat]. Perspiration over the entire surface of the body.

panhyperemia (păn″hī-pĕr-ē′mē-ă) [″ + *hyper,* over, + *haima,* blood]. Widespread or complete hyperemia.

panhypopituitarism (păn-hī″pō-pī-tū′ĭ-tăr-ĭzm) [″ + *hypo,* under, + L. *pituita,* mucus, + Gr. *-ismos,* condition]. Defective or absent function of the entire pituitary gland. SEE: *Simmonds' disease.*

panhysterectomy (păn″hĭs-tĕr-ĕk′tō-mē) [″ + *hystera,* womb, + *ektome,* excision]. Excision of entire uterus including the cervix uteri. SEE: *hysterectomy.*

panhysterocolpectomy (păn-hĭs″tĕr-ō-kŏl-pĕk′tō-mē) [″ + ″ + *kolpos,* vagina, + *ektome,* excision]. Total excision of the uterus and vagina.

panhystero-oophorectomy (păn-hĭs″tĕr-ō-ō″ŏf-ō-rĕk′tō-mē) [″ + ″ + *oophoros,* bearing eggs, + *ektome,* excision]. Excision of uterus, cervix uteri, and one or both ovaries.

panhysterosalpingectomy (păn-hĭs″tĕr-ō-săl″pĭn-jĕk′tō-mē) [″ + ″ + *salpinx,* tube, + *ektome,* excision]. Surgical removal of the uterus, cervix, and fallopian tubes.

panhysterosalpingo-oophorectomy (păn-hĭs″tĕr-ō-săl″pĭng-gō-ō″ŏf-ō-rĕk′tō-mē) [″ + ″ + ″ + *oophoros,* bearing eggs, + *ektome,* excision]. Excision of entire uterus, including the cervix, ovaries, and uterine tubes.

panic (păn′ĭk). Acute anxiety, terror, or fright that is usually of sudden onset, may be uncontrollable, and may require sedation. Because it is difficult to know the cause of this reaction, it is quite difficult to evaluate the response. If hyperventilation and tetany are present, the patient should breathe with the mouth closed and one nostril held closed. This will alleviate the symptoms in a short time.

    p., homosexual. An acute anxiety syndrome due to unconscious homosexual conflicts. Symptoms include fear, paranoid ideas, and excitement, and sometimes hallucinations and combative behavior are present.

panic attack. Acute intense anxiety; symptoms include dyspnea, sweating, vertigo, palpitations, chest pain, nausea, blurred vision, dread, feeling that there will be loss of mental control, and feeling of approaching death.

panic disorder. An anxiety disorder characterized by panic attacks; an example is agoraphobia with panic attacks.

panimmunity (păn″ĭ-mū′nĭ-tē) [″ + L. *immunitas,* immunity]. General immunity to a large number of bacterial diseases.

panis (păn′ĭs) [L.]. Bread.

Panmycin. Trade name for tetracycline hydrochloride, USP.

panmyeloid (păn-mī′ĕ-loyd) [Gr. *pan,* all, + *myelos,* marrow, + *eidos,* form, shape]. Concerning all of the elements of the bone marrow.

panmyelophthisis (păn″mī-ĕl-ŏf′thĭ-sĭs) [″ + *myelos,* marrow, + *phthisis,* a wasting]. 1. General wasting away of the bone marrow. 2. Aplastic anemia.

panmyelosis (păn″mī-ĕl-ō′sĭs) [″ + ″ + *osis,* condition]. Increase in all the elements of the bone marrow.

panneuritis (păn″ū-rī′tĭs) [″ + *neuron,* sinew, + *itis,* inflammation]. Generalized neuritis.

p. epidemica. Deficiency disease in which there is lack of vitamin B₁. SYN: *beriberi.*

panniculitis (păn-ĭk″ū-lī′tĭs) [L. *panniculus,* a small piece of cloth, + *itis,* inflammation]. Inflamed condition of a layer of fatty connective tissue in the anterior wall of the abdomen.

SYM: Pain, tenderness, and hypertrophy of tissue in parts where fat is the thickest.

p., nodular nonsuppurative. A rare disease of unknown etiology characterized by intermittent fever and groups of tender nodules in the subcutaneous fat tissue. SYN: *Weber-Christian disease.*

p., relapsing febrile nodular nonsuppurative. P., nodular nonsuppurative, q.v.

panniculus (păn-ĭk′ū-lŭs) [L., a small piece of cloth]. Any clothlike sheet or layer of tissue.

p. adiposus. [NA] The subcutaneous layer of fat, esp. where fat is abundant; the superficial fascia that is heavily laden with fat cells.

p. carnosus. Thin layer of muscular tissue in the superficial fascia. SEE: *platysma myoides.*

pannus (păn′nŭs) [L., cloth]. 1. Newly formed superficial vascular tissue over the cornea. The area is cloudy, and its surface is uneven because it is covered with a film of new capillary blood vessels. May cover the entire cornea. May be seen in trachoma, acne rosacea, eczema, and as a result of irritation in granular conjunctivitis. 2. Inflamed synovial granulation tissue seen in chronic rheumatoid arthritis. SEE: *micropannus.*

p. carateus. Pinta.

p. carnosus. P. crassus.

p., corneal. An overgrowth of vascular tissue in the periphery of the cornea. This is in response to inflammation of the cornea, esp. in trachoma, q.v.

p. crassus. Pannus that is highly vascularized, thick, and opaque. SYN: *p. carnosus.*

p. degenerativus. P. siccus.

p., phlyctenular. Pannus that occurs in conjunction with phlyctenular conjunctivitis.

p. siccus. Pannus accompanying xerophthalmia. It is composed principally of connective tissue, poorly vascularized, and dry. SYN: *p. degenerativus.*

p. tenuis. Pannus that is thin, poorly vascularized, and slightly opaque.

panodic (pă-nŏd′ĭk). Radiating in all directions, esp. said of a nerve impulse.

panography (păn-ŏg′ră-fē). Radiographic procedure that provides a panoramic view of an entire dental arch on one film.

panophobia (păn-ō-fō′bē-ă) [Gr. *pan,* all, + *phobos,* fear]. Morbid fear of some unknown evil or of everything in general; general apprehension. SYN: *pantophobia.*

panophthalmia, panophthalmitis (păn-ŏf-thăl′mē-ă, -thăl-mī′tĭs) [″ + *ophthalmos,* eye, + *itis,* inflammation]. Inflammation of entire eye.

panoptic (păn-ŏp′tĭk) [″ + *optikos,* vision]. Making every part visible.

panoptic stain. Stain that causes every part of the tissue to be differentiated.

panoptosis (păn-ŏp-tō′sĭs) [″ + *ptosis,* a dropping]. General prolapse of the abdominal organs.

pan-oral radiography. Radiographic procedure that provides a panoramic view of an entire dental arch on one film.

panosteitis (păn″ŏs-tē-ī′tĭs) [Gr. *pan,* all, + *osteon,* bone, + *itis,* inflammation]. Inflammation of every structure of a bone.

panotitis (păn-ō-tī′tĭs) [″ + *ous,* ear, + *itis,* inflammation]. Inflammation involving all the parts of the ear.

Panoxyl. Trade name for benzoyl peroxide, USP.

panphobia (păn-fō′bē-ă) [″ + *phobos,* fear]. Groundless fear of everything. SYN: *pantophobia.*

panplegia (păn-plē′jē-ă) [″ + *plege,* stroke]. Total paralysis.

pansclerosis (păn″sklē-rō′sĭs) [″ + *sklerosis,* hardening]. Hardening of all of an organ.

pansinusitis (păn″sī-nŭs-ī′tĭs) [″ + L. *sinus,* curve, hollow, + *itis,* inflammation]. Inflammation of all of the paranasal sinuses.

pansphygmograph (păn-sfĭg′mō-grăf) [″ + *sphygmos,* pulse, + *graphein,* to write]. Apparatus for registering cardiac movements, the pulse wave, and chest movements at the same time.

Panstrongylus (păn-strŏn′jĭ-lŭs). A genus of insects belonging to the order Hemiptera, family Reduviidae.

P. megistus. Species that serves as vector for *Trypanosoma cruzi,* the causative agent of Chagas' disease.

pansystolic. Occurring throughout systole of the heart. Used to describe that type of cardiac murmur.

pant [ME. *panten*]. 1. To gasp for breath. 2. A short and shallow breath.
  ETIOL: Produced by physical overexertion, as in running, or from fear.

pant-, panto- [Gr. *pantos*, all]. Combining form indicating all or the whole of something.

pantachromatic (păn″tă-krō-măt′ĭk) [″ + *achromatos*, colorless]. Entirely colorless.

pantalgia (păn-tăl′jē-ă) [″ + *algos*, pain]. Pain felt over the entire body.

pantamorphia (păn″tă-mor′fē-ă) [″ + *a-*, not, + *morphe*, form]. Generalized malformation.

pantanencephaly (păn″tăn-ĕn-sĕf′ă-lē) [″ + *an-*, not, + *enkephalos*, brain]. Complete absence of the brain in the fetus.

pantankyloblepharon (păn-tăng″kĭ-lō-blĕf′ă-rŏn) [″ + *ankyle*, noose, + *blepharon*, lid]. Generalized adhesion of the eyelids to the eyeball.

pantatrophia, pantatrophy (păn-tă-trō′fē-ă, -tăt′rō-fē) [″ + *atrophia*, atrophy]. General wasting and atrophy.

Panteric. Trade name for pancreatin.

pantetheine (păn-tē-thē′ĭn). The naturally occurring amide of pantothenic acid. It is a growth factor for *Lactobacillus bulgaricus.*

panthodic (păn-thŏd′ĭk) [″ + *hodos*, way]. Radiating to all parts of the body, esp. applied to nervous impulses.

panting (pănt′ĭng) [ME. *panten*]. Short, shallow, rapid respirations.

pantograph (păn′tō-grăf) [Gr. *pantos*, all, + *graphein*, to write]. A device that will reproduce, through a system of levers connected to a stylus, a duplicate of whatever figure or drawing is being copied by the device.

pantomography (păn″tō-mŏg′ră-fē). Tomography of curved surfaces.

pantomorphia (păn″tō-mor′fē-ă) [″ + *morphe*, form]. 1. State of being symmetrical. 2. Being able to assume any shape.

Pantopaque. Trade name for iophendylate; used for radiographic examinations of the spinal cord and canal.

pantophobia (păn-tō-fō′bē-ă) [″ + *phobos*, fear]. Morbid, groundless fear of everything in general. SYN: *panphobia.*

pantoscopic (păn″tō-skŏp′ĭk) [″ + *skopein*, to examine]. Adjusted to view both close and distant objects.

pantoscopic glasses. Glasses with two segments of different focal lengths for near and far objects. SYN: *lenses, bifocal.*

pantothenate (păn-tō′thĕn-āt). A salt of pantothenic acid.

pantothenic acid (păn-tō-thĕn′ĭk). $C_9H_{17}NO_5$. A vitamin of the B-complex group widely distributed in nature, occur-

ring naturally in yeast, liver, heart, salmon, eggs, and various grains. It was synthesized in 1940.

pantothermia (păn″tō-thĕr′mē-ă) [″ + *therme*, heat]. Condition in which there is a variation in body temperature without any apparent reason.

pantropic (păn-trō′pĭk, -trŏp′ĭk) [″ + *tropos*, turning]. Showing affinity to many organs, as pantropic viruses. SYN: *polycytotropic.*

panturbinate (păn-tŭr′bĭ-nāt) [″ + L. *turbinatus*, shaped like a top]. All of the turbinate structures of the nose; the nasal conchae.

Panwarfin. Trade name for warfarin sodium, USP.

panzootic (păn″zō-ŏt′ĭk) [″ + *zoon*, animal]. Any animal disease that is widespread.

PaO₂. The partial pressure of oxygen in arterial blood. Arterial oxygen concentration, or tension. Usually expressed in millimeters of mercury (mm Hg).

pap (păp) [L. *pappa*, infant's sound for food]. Any soft, semiliquid food.

papain (pă-pā′ĭn). USP. Proteolytic enzyme obtained from the fruit of the papaya, *Carica papaya.* Used to tenderize meat. Trade name is Caroid.

Papanicolaou test [George Nicholas Papanicolaou, Gr.-born U.S. scientist, 1883–1962]. ABBR: Pap smear; Pap test. A study for early detection of cancer cells. It involves collecting material from areas of the body that shed cells or in which shed cells collect, esp. the cervix and vagina. This material is then prepared for microscopic study by special staining. Analysis of the cells is extremely helpful in diagnosing cancer.

papaverine hydrochloride (pă-păv′ĕr-ēn) [L., poppy]. USP. The salt of an alkaloid obtained from opium. Used as a smooth muscle relaxant, esp. in gastric and intestinal distress. It is used in bronchial spasm. Trade names are Cerespan and Pavabid.

papaya (pă-pā′yă) [Sp. Amerind.]. 1. A tropical tree, *Carica papaya.* 2. Large, oblong, edible fruit from that tree. Source of papain, q.v.

paper [L. *papyrus*, paper]. 1. Cellulose pulp prepared in thin sheets from fibers of wood, rags, and other substances. 2. A piece of paper prepared with a medicinal solution. SYN: *charta.* 3. Thin sheet of cellulosic material impregnated with specific chemicals that react in a definite manner when exposed to certain solutions. This permits use of these papers for testing purposes.
  p., articulating. Paper coated on both sides with a pigment that marks the teeth when their occlusal surfaces contact the paper. This allows the contact points of the

teeth to be demonstrated.

p., bibulous. Paper that absorbs water readily.

p., blistering. Paper saturated with a substance that causes vesiculation when applied to the skin, such as cantharides.

p., filter. A porous, unglazed paper used for filtration.

p., indicator. Paper saturated with an indicator solution of known strength and then dried. Used for testing the pH (acidity or alkalinity) of a solution.

p., litmus. An indicator paper impregnated with litmus, which turns blue in alkaline solutions and turns red in acidic solutions.

p., occluding. P., articulating, q.v.

p., test. Paper impregnated with a substance that will change color when exposed to solutions of a certain pH, or to specific chemicals.

papilla (pă-pĭl'ă) [L.] (pl. *papillae*). [NA] A small, nipple-like protuberance or elevation.

p., acoustic. The spiral organ of the ear.

p., Bergmeister's. A veil in front of the retina of the eye. It is made of a conical mass of glial elements that are the developmental tissue of the eye that has not been reabsorbed.

p., circumvallate. One of the large papillae near the base on the dorsal aspect of the tongue, arranged in a V-shape. The taste buds are located in the epithelium of the trench surrounding the papilla.

p., clavate. P., fungiform.

p., conical. 1. Papillae on the dorsum of the tongue. 2. Papillae in the ridgelike projections in the corium of the surface of the skin.

p., dental. A mass of connective tissue that becomes enclosed by the developing enamel organ. It gives rise to dentin and dental pulp.

p., dermal. Small elevations of the corium that indent the inner surface of the epidermis.

p., douodenal. P. of Vater.

p., filiform. One of the very slender papillae at the tip of the tongue.

p., foliate. Folds, which are rudimentary papillae, in the sides of the tongue.

p., fungiform. One of the broad flat papillae resembling a fungus, chiefly found on the dorsal central area of the tongue.

p., gingival. The gingiva that fills the space between adjacent teeth.

p., gustatory. Taste papilla of tongue; one of those possessing a taste bud.

p., incisive. Projection on the anterior portion of the raphe of the palate.

p., interdental. The triangular part of

the gingivae that fits between adjacent teeth, including both free gingiva and attached gingiva.

p., interproximal. The gingival papillae between adjacent teeth. These include the projections seen from the lingual, buccal, or labial sides.

p., lacrimal. An elevation in medial edge of each eyelid, in the center of which is the opening of the lacrimal duct.

p., lenticular. A small rounded elevation underlying lymphatic nodules in mucosa of the root of the tongue.

p., lingual. Any one of the tiny eminences covering the anterior two thirds of the tongue, including circumvallate, filiform, fungiform, and conical papillae.

p., mammae. [NA] The nipple of the mammary gland.

p. of corium. P., conical (def. 2).

p. of hair. A conical process of the corium that projects into undersurface of a hair bulb. It contains capillaries through which a hair receives its nourishment.

p. of Vater. The duodenal end of the drainage systems of the pancreatic and common bile ducts. Commonly, but inaccurately, called ampulla of Vater. SYN: *p., duodenal.*

p., optic. Point at which optic nerve fibers leave the eyeball. SYN: *blind spot; optic disk.*

p., palatine. P., incisive.

p., parotid. The projections around the opening of the parotid duct into the mouth.

p. pili. P. of hair.

p., renal. Apex of a malpighian pyramid in the kidney.

p., tactile. A dermal papilla that contains a sensory end organ for touch.

p., taste. P., gustatory.

p., urethral. The small projection in the vestibule of the vagina at the entrance of the urethra.

p., vallate. P., circumvallate.

papillary (păp'ĭ-lăr-ē) [L. *papilla*, nipple]. 1. Concerning a nipple or papilla. 2. Resembling or composed of papillae.

papillary ducts of Bellini. Short ducts that open on tip of renal papillae. They are formed by union of the straight collecting tubules.

papillary layer. The layer of the corium that adjoins the epidermis. SYN: *stratum papillare.*

papillary muscles. Muscular eminences in ventricles of the heart.

papillary tumor. Neoplasm composed of or resembling enlarged papillae. SEE: *papilloma.*

papillate (păp'ĭ-lāt) [L. *papilla*, nipple]. Having nipple-like growths on the surface, as a culture in bacteriology.

papillectomy (păp″ĭ-lĕk′tŏ-mē) [″ + Gr. *ektome*, excision]. Excision of any papilla or papillae.

papilledema (păp″ĭl-ĕ-dē′mă) [″ + Gr. *oidema*, swelling]. Edema and inflammation of the optic nerve at its point of entrance into the eyeball. SYN: *choked disk.*

ETIOL: Intracranial pressure, often caused by tumor of the brain pressing on optic nerve.

PROG: Blindness may result very rapidly unless relieved.

papilliferous (păp″ĭ-lĭf′ĕr-ŭs) [″ + *ferre*, to carry]. Having or containing papillae.

papilliform (pă-pĭl′ĭ-form) [″ + *forma*, shape]. Having the characteristics or appearance of papillae.

papillitis (păp-ĭ-lī′tis) [″ + Gr. *itis*, inflammation]. Inflammation of the optic disk, usually accompanied by swelling. SYN: *choked disk.*

papilloadenocystoma (păp″ĭl-ō-ăd″ē-nō-sĭs-tō′mă) [″ + Gr. *aden*, gland, + *kystis*, a cyst, + *oma*, tumor]. A tumor composed of elements of papilloma, adenoma, and cystoma.

papillocarcinoma (păp″ĭl-ō-kăr-sĭ-nō′mă) [″ + Gr. *karkinos*, crab, + *oma*, tumor]. 1. A malignant tumor of hypertrophied papillae. 2. Carcinoma with papillary growths.

papilloma (păp-ĭ-lō′mă) [″ + Gr. *oma*, tumor]. 1. Any benign epithelial tumor. 2. Epithelial tumor of skin or mucous membrane consisting of hypertrophied papillae covered by a layer of epithelium. Included in this group are warts, condylomas, and polyps. SEE: *acanthoma; papillomaviruses.*

p. durum. A hardened papilloma, as a wart or corn.

p., fibroepithelial. A skin tag containing fibrous tissue.

p., hard. Papilloma that develops from squamous epithelium.

p., Hopmann's. Papillomatous overgrowth of the nasal mucosa. SYN: *Hopmann's polyp.*

p., intracystic. Papilloma within a cystic adenoma.

p., intraductal. A solitary neoplasm of the breast that occurs in the large, lactiferous ducts. A distinct neoplasm that displays a papillary histologic pattern.

p. molle. Papilloma with only a thin, horny layer covering it. SYN: *condyloma.*

p., soft. Papilloma formed from columnar epithelium; applies to any small, soft growth.

p., villous. Papilloma with thin, long excrescences present in the urinary bladder, breast, intestinal tract, or choroid plexus of the cerebral ventricles.

papillomatosis (păp″ĭ-lō-mă-tō′sĭs) [″ + Gr. *oma*, tumor, + *osis*, condition]. 1. Widespread formation of papillomas. 2. Condition of being afflicted with many papillomas.

papillomaviruses. Viruses that cause papillomas or warts in humans and animals. They belong to the papovavirus family or group. SEE: *wart, genital.*

papilloretinitis (păp″ĭ-lō-rĕt-ĭn-ī′tĭs) [″ + *rete*, net, + Gr. *itis*, inflammation]. Inflamed condition of the papilla and retina extending to the optic disk.

papovaviruses (păp″ō-vă-vī′rŭs-ĕs) [*papilloma*, + *polyoma*, + *vacuolating* agent + *virus*]. A group of viruses important in investigating viral carcinogenesis. Included are polyoma virus, simian virus 40 (SV 40), and papillomaviruses.

pappataci fever. Sandfly fever.

pappose (păp′pōs) [L. *pappus*, down]. Covered with fine, downy hair.

pappus [L.]. The first growth of beard hair appearing on the cheeks and chin as fine, downy hair.

paprika (păp′rĭ-kă, păp-rē′kă) [Gr. *peperi*, pepper]. A mild, powdered seasoning made from sweet red peppers. Also used to color food.

Pap smear; Pap test. Papanicolaou test, q.v.

papula (păp′ū-lă) [L.]. A small, inflammatory, congested spot on the skin; a pimple. SYN: *papule.*

papular (păp′ū-lĕr). Concerning an eruption of the nature of papules.

papular fever. Mild fever with maculopapular eruptions and rheumatoid pains.

papulation (păp-ū-lā′shŭn). 1. The development of papules. 2. The stage of pimple formation in a disease.

papule (păp′ūl) [L. *papula*, pimple]. Red elevated area on the skin, solid and circumscribed. Papules often precede vesicular or pustular formation and may appear in erythema multiforme, eczema papulosum, prurigo, syphilis, measles, and smallpox, and they may develop after use of bromides, iodides, or coal tar preparations.

DIFF. DIAG: In measles they are small and run together. In smallpox they are hard and feel like pellets, terminating in umbilicated vesicles that itch. In prurigo they are small, pale, deep-seated, and accompanied by intense itching. In syphilis they are dark and widely distributed, esp. on the trunk and surfaces of the extremities; they do not cause itching. In eczema they are small, are often associated with pustules and vesicles, and are closely aggregated; there is intense itching and the skin is thickened. In erythema multiforme they are found with macules and tubercles and are bright red or purple and flat, appearing esp. on the extremities; they do not suppurate or cause itching.

p., dry. Hard papule that is primary lesion of syphilis, occurring at site of infection. SYN: *chancre.*

p., moist. A syphilitic eruption of papules with flat tops. SYN: *condyloma latum; p., mucous.*

p., mucous. P., moist.

p.'s, split. Fissures at the corners of the mouth. Seen in some cases of secondary syphilis.

papuliferous (păp″ū-lĭf′ĕr-ŭs) [L. *papula,* pimple, + *ferre,* to bear]. Having papules or pimples.

papulo- [L. *papula,* pimple]. Combining form indicating a pimple or a papule.

papuloerythematous (păp″ū-lō-ĕr″ĕ-thĕm′ă-tŭs) [″ + Gr. *erythema,* redness]. Denoting occurrence of papules on an erythematous surface.

papulopustular (păp″ū-lō-pŭs′tū-lăr) [″ + *pustula,* blister]. Denoting presence of both pustules and papules.

papulosis (păp-ū-lō′sĭs) [″ + Gr. *osis,* condition]. Presence of numerous and generalized papules.

papulosquamous (păp″ū-lō-skwā′mŭs) [″ + *squamosus,* scalelike]. Denoting presence of both papules and scales.

papulovesicular (păp″ū-lō-vē-sĭk′ū-lăr) [″ + *vesicula,* tiny bladder]. Denoting presence of both papules and vesicles.

papyraceous (păp-ĭ-rā′shŭs) [L.]. Parchment-like. In obstetrics, it denotes a fetus that is retained in the uterus beyond natural term and has a mummified appearance.

par [L., equal]. A pair, esp. a pair of cranial nerves.

para [L. *parere,* to bring forth, to bear]. A woman who has produced a viable infant (weighing 500 grams or more, or of over 20 weeks gestation) regardless of whether the infant is alive at birth. Multiple births are considered to be single parous experience. The term is used with numerals to designate the number of pregnancies. Ex.: para 0 (nullipara), para 1 (primipara), para 2 (secundipara), para 3 (tertipara). SEE: *gravida.*

para-, par- [Gr. *para,* beyond; L. *par,* equal, pair]. ABBR: *p-* when used in chemistry to indicate *para-.* Combining forms meaning near, beside, past, beyond, the opposite, abnormal; irregular, or two like parts.

para-actinomycosis. Pseudoactinomycosis.

para-aminobenzoic acid (păr″ă-ăm″ĭ-nō-bĕn-zō′ĭk). ABBR: PABA. Previously used name for aminobenzoic acid.

para-aminohippuric acid. ABBR: PAHA. A derivative of aminobenzoic acid. The salt, para-aminohippurate, is used to test the excretory capacity of the renal tubules.

para-aminosalicylic acid (păr″ă-ăm″ĭ-nō-săl″ĭ-sĭl′ĭk). USP. ABBR: PAS. $C_7H_7NO_3$. A white or nearly white and practically odorless powder that darkens when exposed to air or light. It is an antituberculosis drug, and its effectiveness is greatly enhanced when used in combination with streptomycin and isoniazid; it is believed to delay development of bacterial resistance. SYN: *aminosalicylic acid.*

para-anesthesia (păr″ă-ăn-ĕs-thē′zē-ă) [Gr. *para,* beside, + *an-,* negative, + *aisthesis,* sensation]. Anesthesia of two corresponding sides, esp. of lower half of body.

para-aortic bodies. Small masses of chromaffin tissue along the abdominal aorta. They secrete epinephrine.

parabionts (păr-ăb′ē-ŏnts) [″ + *bioun,* to live]. Two individuals living in the condition of parabiosis, q.v.

parabiosis (păr″ă-bī-ō′sĭs) [″ + *biosis,* living]. 1. Joining together of two individuals. It may occur congenitally as with Siamese twins or may be produced surgically for experimentation in animals. 2. Temporary suppression of excitability of a nerve.

parabiotic (păr″ă-bī-ŏt′ĭk). Concerning parabiosis.

parablepsia, parablepsis (păr″ă-blĕp′sē-ă, -sĭs) [Gr. *para,* beside, + *blepsis,* vision]. Abnormality of vision, e.g., visual hallucinations.

paracanthoma (păr″ă-kăn-thō′mă) [Gr. *para,* beside, + *akantha,* thorn, + *oma,* tumor]. A tumor involving the prickle-cell layer of the epidermis.

paracasein (păr-ă-kā′sē-ĭn). A substance formed when rennin or pepsin acts on the casein of milk. In the presence of calcium ions, an insoluble protein is formed, resulting in the curdling of milk.

Paracelsus (păr-ă-sĕl′sŭs) [Philippus Aureolus Theophrastus Bombastus von Hohenheim, 1493–1541]. Swiss alchemist and physician who introduced several chemicals (lead, sulfur, iron, and arsenic) into pharmaceutical chemistry. Remembered because of his independent spirit, observant mind, and fearlessness in breaking with traditional practice.

paracenesthesia (păr″ă-sē″nĕs-thē′zē-ă) [Gr. *para,* beside, + *koinos,* common, + *aisthesis,* sensation]. Decrease in the sense of well-being.

paracentesis (păr″ă-sĕn-tē′sĭs) [Gr. *para,* beside, + *kentesis,* a puncture]. Puncture of a cavity with removal of fluid, as in pleural effusion or ascites.

NURSING IMPLICATIONS: Explain procedure to patient, and have patient void prior to treatment. Provide emotional support for patient during the procedure, and provide an opportunity for patient to express feelings. Position patient as directed by physician. Assist physician during procedure. Monitor vital signs and observe for signs of shock (such as cold and clammy skin). Measure and record amount of fluid removed, and describe its appearance, odor, specific gravity, and whether or not it clots upon standing. Observe and redress puncture site as necessary. Send specimens to laboratories as directed. Document procedure and patient's response.

p., abdominal. Paracentesis of the abdominal cavity.

p. capitis. Paracentesis of the cranium.

p. cordis. Surgical puncture of the heart.

p. pericardii. Puncture of the pericardial sac.

p. pulmonis. Removal of fluid from a lung.

p. thoracis. Drainage of fluid from the cavity of the chest. SEE: *aspiration*.

p. tunicae vaginalis. Puncture of the tunica vaginalis.

p. tympani. Drainage or irrigation through incision of the tympanic membrane.

p. vesicae. Puncture of the wall of the urinary bladder.

paracentetic (păr″ă-sĕn-tĕt′ĭk). Concerning paracentesis.

paracentral (păr″ă-sĕn′trăl) [″ + L. *centralis*, center]. Located near the center.

paracentral lobule. Cerebral convolution on mesial surface joining the upper terminations of the ascending parietal and frontal convolutions.

paracephalus (păr″ă-sĕf′ă-lŭs) [″ + *kephale*, head]. A parasitic placental twin with a small rudimentary head.

parachlorophenol (păr″ă-klō″rō-fē′nŏl). USP. A drug that has the same actions and uses as phenol, q.v.

p., camphorated. USP. A mixture of parachlorophenol, q.v., and camphor. Its activity as a topical antiseptic in root canal therapy is markedly decreased by blood and necrotic tissue.

paracholera (păr″ă-kŏl′ĕr-ă) [″ + L. *cholera*, cholera]. A disease resembling cholera, but caused by vibriones other than true *Vibrio cholerae*.

paracholia (păr″ă-kō′lē-ă) [″ + *chole*, bile]. Condition of disturbed bile secretion.

parachordal (păr-ă-kor′dăl) [Gr. *para*, beside, + *chorde*, cord]. Lying alongside the anterior portion of the notochord in the embryo.

parachordal cartilage. One of a pair of cartilages in the cephalic portion of the notochord of the embryo that unite in humans to form a single basal plate that is the forerunner of the occipital bone.

parachromatism (păr″ă-krō′mă-tĭzm) [″ + *chroma*, color, + *-ismos*, condition]. Incorrect perception of colors but not true color blindness.

parachromatopsia (păr″ă-krō-mă-tŏp′sē-ă) [″ + ″ + *opsis*, vision]. Color blindness.

parachute reflex (reaction). SEE: *reflex, parachute*.

paracinesia, paracinesis (păr″ă-sĭ-nē′zē-ă, -sĭs) [″ + *kinesis*, movement]. Condition in which there is perversion of motor powers; motor abnormality. SYN: *parakinesia*.

paracme (păr-ăk′mē) [″ + *akme*, point]. Denoting the stage at which symptoms or a fever begins to decline.

Paracoccidioides (păr″ă-kŏk-sĭd″ē-oy′dēz). A genus of yeastlike fungi.

P. brasiliensis. The causative agent of paracoccidioidomycosis. SYN: *Blastomyces brasiliensis*.

paracoccidioidomycosis (păr″ă-kŏk-sĭd″ē-ŏy″dō-mī-kō′sĭs). A chronic granulomatous disease of the skin caused by *Paracoccidioides brasiliensis*. SYN: *South American blastomycosis*.

paracolitis (păr″ă-kō-lī′tĭs). Inflammation of the tissue surrounding the colon.

paracolpitis (păr″ă-kŏl-pī′tĭs) [″ + *kolpos*, vagina, + *itis*, inflammation]. Inflammation of tissues surrounding the vagina.

paracolpium (păr″ă-kŏl′pē-ŭm). The connective tissue adjacent to the vagina.

paracone (păr′ă-kōn) [″ + *konos*, cone]. The mesiobuccal cusp of an upper molar tooth.

paraconid (păr″ă-kō′nĭd). The mesiobuccal cusp of a lower molar tooth.

paracousis (păr″ă-koo′sĭs). Paracusis, q.v.

paracrine. Secretion of a hormone from a source other than an endocrine gland.

paracrine control. A general form of bioregulation in which one cell type in a tissue selectively influences the activity of an adjacent cell type by secreting chemicals that diffuse into the tissue and act specifically on cells in that area. SEE: *autocrine factor*.

paracrisis (păr-ăk′rĭ-sĭs, păr″ă-krī′sĭs) [″ + *krinein*, to secrete]. Any abnormality of body secretions.

paracusia, paracusis (păr″ă-kū′sē-ă, -kū′sĭs) [″ + *akousis*, hearing]. Any abnormality or disorder of the sense of hearing.

p. acris. Excessively acute hearing.

p. duplicata. The hearing of one sound as two. SYN: *diplacusis*.

p. loci. Difficulty in locating the direction of sound.

p. willisiana. An apparent ability to hear

better in a noisy place, found in deafness due to stapes fixation and adhesive processes.

paracystic (păr″ă-sĭs′tĭk) [Gr. *para*, beside, + *kystis*, bladder]. Located close to a bladder, esp. the urinary bladder.

paracystitis (păr″ă-sĭs-tī′tĭs) [″ + ″ + *itis*, inflammation]. Inflamed condition of connective tissues and other structures around the urinary bladder.

paracystium (păr-ă-sĭs′tē-ŭm). The connective tissue surrounding the urinary bladder.

paracytic (păr″ă-sĭt′ĭk) [″ + *kytos*, cell]. Concerning cells other than those normally present in a specific location.

paradenitis (păr″ăd-ĕn-ī′tĭs) [″ + *aden*, gland, + *itis*, inflammation]. Inflammation of tissues around a gland.

paradental (păr″ă-dĕn′tăl) [″ + L. *dens*, tooth]. 1. Concerning the practice of dentistry. 2. Periodontal, q.v.

paradentium (păr″ă-dĕn′shē-ŭm). Periodontium, q.v.

paradidymal (păr″ă-dĭd′ĭ-măl) [″ + *didymos*, testicle]. 1. Concerning the paradidymis. 2. Adjacent to the testis.

paradidymis (păr-ă-dĭd′ĭ-mĭs) [″ + *didymos*, testicle]. [NA] The atrophic remnants of the tubules of the wolffian body, situated on the spermatic cord above the epididymis. SYN: *organ of Giraldès.*

paradigm. An example that serves as a model.

Paradione. Trade name for paramethadione.

paradipsia (păr″ă-dĭp′sē-ă) [″ + *dipsa*, thirst]. Perverted desire for fluids irrespective of the need for liquids.

paradox [Gr. *paradoxos*, unbelievable]. Something that seems untrue, and even absurd and inconsistent with a logical explanation of the true condition, but in fact is actually true.

p., Weber's. A muscle loaded beyond its ability to contract may elongate.

paradoxic, paradoxical (păr″ă-dŏk′sĭk, -sĭkăl) [Gr. *paradoxos*, conflicting with expectation]. Seemingly contradictory but demonstrably true.

paradoxical respiration. 1. Respiration occurring in open pneumothorax in which lung fills on expiration and deflates on inspiration. 2. Condition seen in paralysis of diaphragm in which diaphragm ascends during inspiration.

paraequilibrium (păr″ă-ē″kwĭ-lĭb′rē-ŭm). Vertigo caused by disease or malfunction of the vestibular apparatus of the ear. Sometimes accompanied by nystagmus and nausea.

paraffin (păr′ă-fĭn) [L. *parum*, too little, + *affinis*, neighboring]. 1. A waxy, white, tasteless, odorless mixture of solid hydrocarbons obtained from petroleum. Used as ointment base or wound dressing. SEE: *pet-*

rolatum. 2. One of a series of saturated aliphatic hydrocarbons having the formula C_nH_{2n+2}. Paraffins constitute the methane or paraffin series. 3. A series of solid waxes prepared according to their melting point, to be used to infiltrate and embed tissues for sectioning in the preparation of microscope slides.

p., hard. Solid paraffin with a melting point between 45°C and 60°C.

p., liquid. Liquid hydrocarbon. Mineral oil.

p., soft. A semisolid paraffin. Petrolatum.

p., white soft. White petrolatum. SEE: *petrolatum.*

p., yellow soft. Petrolatum, q.v.

paraffinoma (păr″ă-fĭn-ō′mă) [″ + ″ + Gr. *oma*, tumor]. A tumor that arises at site of injection of paraffin.

Paraflex. Trade name for chlorzoxazone.

paraformaldehyde (păr″ă-for-măl′dĕ-hīd). A white, powdered antiseptic and disinfectant, a polymer of formaldehyde.

paragammacism (păr″ă-găm′mă-sĭzm) [Gr. *para*, beside, + *gamma*, Gr. letter G, + *-ismos*, condition]. Inability to pronounce "g," "k," and "ch" sounds, with substitution of other consonants such as "d" or "t."

paraganglia (păr″ă-găng′lē-ă) [″ + *ganglion*, knot] (sing. *paraganglion*). [NA] Groups of chromaffin cells, similar in staining reaction to cells of the adrenal medulla, associated anatomically and embryologically with the sympathetic system. They are located in various organs and parts of the body.

paraganglioma (păr″ă-găng-lē-ō′mă) [″ + ″ + *oma*, tumor]. A tumor derived from chromaffin cells. Includes tumors of the adrenal medulla and the paraganglia. SYN: *chemodectoma.* SEE: *pheochromocytoma.*

paraganglion (păr″ă-găng′lē-ŏn) [″ + *ganglion*, knot]. Sing. of paraganglia.

parageusia, parageusis (păr-ă-gū′sē-ă, -sĭs) [″ + *geusis*, taste]. Disorder or abnormality of the sense of taste.

paraglossa (păr-ă-glŏs′să) [″ + *glossa*, tongue]. 1. Enlargement of the tongue. 2. Congenital hypertrophy of the tongue.

paraglossia (păr-ă-glŏs′sē-ă). Inflammation of the tissues underlying the tongue.

paragnathus (păr-ăg′nă-thŭs) [″ + *gnathos*, jaw]. 1. A congenital deformity in which there is an accessory jaw. 2. A parasitic fetus attached to the outer part of the jaw of the autosite.

paragonimiasis (păr″ă-gŏn″ĭ-mī′ă-sĭs) [*Paragonimus* + *-iasis*, condition]. Infection with worms of genus *Paragonimus.* The clinical signs depend on the path the worm takes in migrating through the body, after the larvae contained in partially cooked freshwater crabs or crayfish are eaten. The larvae migrate from the duodenum to various organs, including the lungs, intestinal wall, lymph nodes, brain, subcutaneous tissues, and genitourinary tract. When the lungs are involved, the symptoms are cough and hemoptysis. In peritoneal infections, there may be an abdominal mass, pain, and dysentery. When the larvae invade the brain, paralysis, epilepsy, homonymous hemianopsia, optic atrophy, and papilledema are common. In some cases, the infected person may appear to be well.

TREAT: Praziquantel.

Paragonimus (păr″ă-gŏn′ĭ-mŭs). Genus of trematode worms.

P. westermani. The lung fluke, a common parasite of certain mammals including humans, dogs, cats, pigs, and minks. Human infestation occurs through eating partially cooked crabs or crayfish, the second intermediate host. Infestation endemic in certain parts of Asia.

paragrammatism. A speech defect characterized by improper use of words and inability to arrange them grammatically.

paragranuloma (păr″ă-grăn″ū-lō′mă) [Gr. *para*, beside, + L. *granulum*, little grain, + Gr. *oma*, tumor]. A benign form of Hodgkin's disease usually limited to lymph nodes.

paragraphia (păr-ă-grăf′ē-ă) [″ + *graphein*, to write]. The writing of letters or words other than those intended.

parahemophilia (păr-ă-hē″mō-fīl′ē-ă) [″ + *haima*, blood, + *philein*, to love]. A rare, congenital, idiopathic disorder due to deficiency of coagulation factor V, characterized by prolonged prothrombin and coagulation times. SYN: *Factor V deficiency.*

parahepatic (păr″ă-hē-păt′ĭk) [″ + *hepar*, liver]. Adjacent to the liver.

parahepatitis (păr″ă-hĕp″ă-tī′tĭs) [″ + ″ + *itis*, inflammation]. Inflamed condition of parts immediately adjacent to the liver.

parahormone [″ + *hormaein*, to set in motion]. A substance that, like hormones, is conveyed through the circulatory system and exerts a stimulating effect, yet does not originate in endocrine tissue. Carbon dioxide is an example.

parahypnosis [″ + *hypnos*, sleep]. Abnormal or disordered sleep.

parahypophysis (păr″ă-hī-pŏf′ĭ-sĭs) [″ + *hypophysis*, an undergrowth]. Accessory to the pituitary tissue.

parainfection [″ + L. *in*, into, + *facere*, to make]. The symptomatology of an infectious disease without evidence of the presence of the microorganisms causing the disease.

parainfluenza viruses. A group of viruses that cause acute respiratory infections in humans, esp. in children. Virtually all children in the U.S. have been infected by age six.

parakeratosis (păr″ă-kĕr″ă-tō′sĭs) [″ + *keras*, horn, + *osis*, condition]. The persistence of nuclei within the keratinocytes of the stratum corneum of epidermis or mucosal layers, which indicates a partial keratinization process; a general term applied to disorders of the keratinized layer of the skin.

p. ostracea. Parakeratosis scutularis, q.v.

p. psoriasiformis. Scab formation resembling that of psoriasis.

p. scutularis. Scalp disease with hairs encircled by epidermic crust formation.

parakinesia. Paracinesia.

Paral. Trade name for paraldehyde.

paralalia (păr″ă-lā′lē-ă) [″ + *lalein*, to babble]. Any speech defect characterized by sound distortion.

p. literalis. Stammering.

paralambdacism (păr″ă-lăm′dă-sĭzm) [″ + *lambda*, Gr. letter L, + *-ismos*, condition]. Inability to sound the letter "l" correctly, substituting some other letter for it.

paraldehyde (păr-ăl′dĕ-hīd). USP. $C_6H_{12}O_3$. A liquid polymer of acetaldehyde that is colorless. It has an unpleasant taste and a characteristic odor. Made by action of hydrochloric acid on acetic aldehyde. Trade name is Paral.

ACTION/USES: Hypnotic, having low toxicity and prompt action as a sedative. Useful in treating acute alcoholism and delirium tremens. Sometimes used as an analgesic in obstetrics, esp. in combination with rectal ether.

Caution: Do not dispense paraldehyde from a bottle that has been open for longer than 24 hours. In partially filled containers, oxidation occurs, forming acetic acid.

---

paraldehyde poisoning. Symptoms resemble those of chloral hydrate: cardiac and respiratory depression, dizziness, collapse with partial or complete anesthesia. Odor on the breath is a constant distinct sign.

F.A.: Maintain airway and physiological responses by use of tracheostomy, artificial ventilation, and oxygen. If poisoning is mild, induce vomiting. Because of the danger of asphyxiation, gastric lavage is dangerous unless the airway is protected.

paraldehydism (păr-ăl′dĕ-hīd″ĭzm). Poisoning from an overdose of paraldehyde, q.v.

paralepsy (păr″ă-lĕp″sē) [″ + *lepsis*, seizure]. Temporary attack of mental inertia and hopelessness, or sudden alteration in mood or mental tension. SYN: *psycholepsy*.

paralexia (păr″ă-lĕk′sē-ă) [″ + *lexis*, speech]. Inability to comprehend printed words or sentences, together with substitution of meaningless combinations of words.

paralgesia (păr″ăl-jē′zē-ă) [″ + *algesis*, sense of pain]. Any unusual sensation that is painful. SYN: *paralgia*.

paralgia (păr-ăl′jē-ă) [″ + *algos*, pain]. An abnormal sensation that is painful.

paralipophobia. Fear of omitting or neglecting a duty.

parallactic. Concerning parallax.

parallagma (păr″ăl-ăg′mă) [Gr., alternation]. Overlapping or displacement of the fragments of a fractured bone.

parallax (păr′ă-lăks) [Gr. *parallaxis*, change of position]. The apparent movement or displacement of objects caused by change in the observer's position or by movement of the head or eyes.

    p., binocular. The basis of stereoscopic vision. The difference in the angles formed by the lines of sight to two objects at different distances from the eyes. This is important in depth perception.

    p., heteronymous. When one eye is closed, the object viewed appears to move closer to the closed eye.

    p., homonymous. When one eye is covered, the object viewed appears to move closer to the uncovered eye.

parallelism (păr′ă-lĕl″ĭzm). Condition of being parallel.

parallelometer (păr″ă-lĕl-ŏm′ĕ-tĕr). Device used in dentistry to determine whether or not lines and tooth surfaces are parallel to each other.

parallel play. Stage in social development in which a child plays alongside, but not with, other children. Characteristic of toddlers.

parallergic (păr″ă-lĕr′jĭk). Concerning parallergy.

parallergy (păr-ăl′ĕr-jē). Condition of being allergic to nonspecific stimuli after having been sensitized with a specific allergen.

paralogia (păr″ă-lō′jē-ă) [Gr. *para*, beside, + *logos*, word, reason]. A disorder of the reasoning.

    p., benign. Disordered thinking and communication of thought. Delusions, bizarre thoughts, hallucinations, and regressive behavior are absent. The patient is not severely incapacitated and should not be considered to have schizophrenia.

paralogy (pă-răl′ō-jē). Paralogia, q.v.

paralysis (pă-răl′ĭ-sĭs) [Gr. *paralyein*, to disable]. (pl. *paralyses*) Temporary suspension or permanent loss of function, esp. loss of sensation or voluntary motion.

Any voluntary movement depends on the integrity of two types of motor neurons: one, the upper motor neurons, arising in the motor cortex, coursing through the brain stem, and ending in the anterior gray horn of the spinal cord; and the lower neurons, arising in the anterior horn cell and passing to the muscle. If the latter are destroyed, the muscle loses tone, atrophies (withers away), and shows reaction of degeneration (RD).

The flaccidity and absent muscular reflexes reveal the loss of tonus. If the upper neuron is paralyzed, the patient is equally unable to move the affected part, but the intact lower neuron may permit other motor centers to act on the muscle. In addition, tone is increased, there is no RD, and there is no atrophy except that of disuse. So-called pathological reflexes may appear in addition to the increase of normal deep reflexes.

Paralyses are divided into two groups: *spastic* when due to lesion of upper motor neuron and *flaccid* when due to lesion of lower motor neuron. Psychic inhibition of motor function occurs most characteristically in hysteria, but the evidence of organic disease is always lacking in these hysterical paralyses.

NURSING IMPLICATIONS: Refer to physical therapy for evaluation of motor and sensory capabilities (muscle size, tone and strength, involuntary movement, response to touch or to painful stimulus). Position the patient to prevent deformities, and see that extremities are moved through their range of motion to prevent contractures. Massage or electrical stimulation is given as prescribed. Evaluate local and systemic responses, including fatigue. Evaluate and attend to self-care deficits that may be present. Support patient and family in dealing with psychological concerns and grief and loss responses. Assist the patient in achieving optimal level of function and in adapting to the disability.

    p., acoustic. Deafness.

    p. agitans. A disease of middle and late life producing a picture of rigid tremulousness, progressive in its course and marked by weakness, delay of voluntary motion, a peculiar festinating gait, and muscular contraction, causing peculiar and characteristic positions of the limbs and head. While movement is slow, there is no true paralysis. The face appears expressionless, there is general flexion attitude, the balance tends to be lost (in a forward direction). Sometimes occurs following encephalitis lethargica; at other times is due to an unknown cause. SYN: *palsy, shaking; Parkinson's disease.*

    p., alcoholic. Paralysis due to the toxic

effect of alcohol on nerve tissue.

p., anesthesia. Paralysis that develops following administration of anesthesia.

p., arsenical. Paralysis due to the toxic effect of arsenic.

p., Bell's. Facial paralysis.

SYM: One side of entire face may be affected, corner of mouth may drop, or eyelid may droop or be unable to close. Patient may be unable to close lips or to speak, or may lose ability to close the eye.

ETIOL: Lesion of the facial nerve or of its nucleus; a neuritis of this nerve. Pressure on the nerve as it reaches the face through its bony canal near the ear.

p., birth. Paralysis caused by injury received at birth.

p., brachial. Paralysis of one or both arms.

p., brachiofacial. Paralysis of the face and an arm.

p., bulbar. Paralysis caused by changes in the motor centers of the brain stem.

p., complete. Paralysis in which there is total loss of function and sensation.

p., compression. Paralysis due to prolonged pressure on a nerve, as by improper use of a crutch or during sleep.

p., conjugate. Paralysis of the conjugate movement of the eyes in all directions even though the fixation axis remains parallel.

p., crossed. Paralysis affecting one side of the face and limbs of the opposite side of the body.

p., crutch. Paralysis due to pressure on nerves in the axilla caused by improper use of a crutch.

p., decubitus. Paralysis due to pressure on a nerve from lying in one position for a long time, as in sleep or while in a coma.

p., diphtheritic. Paralysis of the muscles of the palate, eyes, limbs, diaphragm, and intercostal muscles that occurs as a complication of diphtheria. It is caused by a toxin produced by the diphtheria bacillus.

p., diver's. Paralysis due to decrease in pressure after a deep-sea diver has been exposed to pressure greater than atmospheric pressure. SYN: *bends; caisson disease.*

p., Duchenne-Erb. Paralysis of the muscles of the upper arm due to injury of the upper nerves, the fifth and sixth cervical roots, of the brachial plexus. The hand muscles are unaffected.

p., facial. P., Bell's.

p., flaccid. Paralysis in which there is loss of muscle tone, loss or reduction of tendon reflexes, atrophy and degeneration of muscles, and reaction of degeneration. Due to lesions of lower motor neurons of spinal cord.

p., general. Progressive loss of power

and mental faculties resulting eventually in dementia and death. SYN: *paresis.*

p., ginger. P., Jamaica ginger.

p., glossolabial. Paralysis of the tongue and lips. Occurs in bulbar paralysis.

p., Gubler's. A form of alternate hemiplegia in which a brain stem lesion causes paralysis of the cranial nerves on one side and of the body on the opposite side.

p., histrionic. Paralysis of certain facial muscles, producing a fixed facial expression of a certain emotion.

p., hyperkalemic. A rare form of periodic paralysis characterized by brief, 1- to 2-hour attacks of limb weakness. In some cases, respiratory muscles are involved. The term hyperkalemic is misleading, in that the potassium levels may be normal. However, an attack is precipitated by administration of potassium. Thus, this form of paralysis should be termed potassium-sensitive periodic paralysis.

TREAT: Emergency treatment is seldom necessary. Oral glucose will hasten recovery. In addition, attacks may be prevented by use of acetazolamide or thiazide diuretics.

p., hypokalemic periodic. A form of periodic paralysis with onset usually prior to adulthood. An attack typically comes on during sleep, after strenuous exercise during the day. The weakness may be so pronounced as to prevent the patient's being able to call for help. The attack may last from several hours to a day or more. The diagnosis is established by determining that the serum potassium level is decreased during an attack.

TREAT: Oral potassium salts will improve the paralysis. If the patient is too weak to swallow, intravenous potassium salts will be required. Attacks may be prevented by oral administration of 5 to 10 grams of potassium chloride daily.

p., hysterical. Apparent loss of movement that may simulate any form of paralysis. There is no organic cause. SEE: *Hoover sign.*

p., immunological. Inability to form antibodies after exposure to large doses of the antigen.

p., incomplete. Partial paralysis of the body or a part.

p., infantile. Motor paralysis in children with atrophy of a group of muscles, following an acute infectious disease that is transmitted by a filtrable virus. SYN: *poliomyelitis, acute anterior.*

p., infantile cerebral ataxic. SEE: *palsy, cerebral.*

p., ischemic. Paralysis resulting from impaired blood supply. SYN: *Volkmann's* contracture.

p., jake. P., Jamaica ginger.

p., Jamaica ginger. Paralysis due to polyneuropathy that affects the muscles of the distal portions of the limbs. It is caused by drinking an alcoholic beverage called Jamaica ginger that contains the toxic substance triorthocresylphosphate.

p., Klumpke's. Wasting paralysis of the arms and hands, often resulting from birth injury.

p., Landry's. Flaccid paralysis that begins in the lower extremities and rapidly ascends to the trunk.

p., lead. Paralysis due to lead poisoning.

p., local. Paralysis of a single muscle or one group of muscles.

p., mimetic. Paralysis of the facial muscles.

p., mixed. Paralysis of motor and sensory nerves.

p., muscular. Loss of the capacity of muscles to contract. May be due to a structural or functional disorder in the muscle at the myoneural junction, in efferent nerve fibers, in cell bodies of nuclei of origin of brain or gray matter of spinal cord, in conducting pathways of brain or spinal cord, or in motor centers of the brain.

p., musculospiral. Paralysis due to prolonged ischemia of the musculospiral nerve incident to compressing an arm against a hard edge. It occurs if the patient has been comatose or in a stupor or has fallen asleep with the arm hanging over the edge of a bed or chair. Sometimes called Saturday night paralysis because in some cultures individuals traditionally become intoxicated on Saturday night; while stuporous, they may remain in a position that allows the nerve to be compressed.

p., nuclear. Paralysis caused by lesion of nuclei in the central nervous system.

p., obstetrical. P., birth.

p., ocular. Paralysis of the extraocular and intraocular muscles.

p. of accommodation. Inability of the eye to adjust itself to various distances due to paralysis of ciliary muscles.

p., postdiphtheritic. P., diphtheritic.

p., posticus. Paralysis of the posterior cricothyroid muscles.

p., Pott's. Paralysis of the lower part of the body due to tuberculosis of the spine (Pott's disease).

p., primary periodic. The occurrence of intermittent weakness, usually following rest or sleep, and almost never during vigorous activity. The condition usually begins in early life and rarely has its onset after age 25. The attacks may last from a few hours to a day or more. The patient is alert during an attack.

The causes include hypokalemia, hyperkalemia, thyrotoxicosis, and a form of paramyotonia. Both forms of the disease in which potassium regulation is a factor respond to acetazolamide; the thyrotoxicosis-related disorder is treated by correcting the underlying thyrotoxicosis. In cases of paramyotonia congenita with periodic paralysis, the treatment is spironolactone.

p., progressive bulbar. P., bulbar.

p., pseudobulbar. Paralysis caused by cerebral center lesions, simulating the bulbar types of paralysis.

p., pseudohypertrophic muscular. SEE: *dystrophy, pseudohypertrophic muscular.*

p., radial. P., musculospiral.

p., Saturday night. P., musculospiral.

p., sensory. Loss of sensation. May be due to a structural or functional disorder of the sensory end organs, sensory nerves, conducting pathways of spinal cord or brain, or sensory centers in the brain.

p., sleep. SEE: *sleep, disorders of.*

p., spastic. Paralysis usually involving groups of muscles. Characterized by excessive tone and spasticity of muscles, exaggeration of tendon reflexes but loss of superficial reflexes, positive Babinski reflex, no atrophy or wasting except from prolonged disuse, and absence of reaction of degeneration. Due to lesions of upper motor neurons or cerebrum.

p., spinal. Paralysis due to injury or disease of the spinal cord.

p., supranuclear. Paralysis resulting from disorders in pathways or centers above nuclei of origin.

p., tick-bite. Paralysis resulting from bites of certain species of ticks, esp. of the genera *Ixodes* and *Dermacentor*, presumably due to a toxin present in saliva of tick. Affects domestic animals and humans, esp. children. Causes a progressive ascending, flaccid, motor paralysis. Recovery usually occurs after removal of ticks.

p., tourniquet. Paralysis, esp. of the arm, resulting from a tourniquet being applied for too long a time.

p., vasomotor. Paralysis of vasomotor centers resulting in lack of tone and dilation of blood vessels.

p., vocal. Paralysis of vocal cords.

p., Volkmann's. Volkmann's contracture, q.v.

p., wasting. Progressive wasting away of the muscles. SYN: *atrophy, progressive muscular.*

paralytic (păr″ă-lĭt′ĭk) [Gr. *paralyein*, to disable]. 1. Concerning paralysis. 2. One afflicted with paralysis.

paralytic dementia. Progressive paralysis with mental deterioration. SYN: *paresis.*

paralytic ileus. Paralysis of intestines, usually temporary, with distention and symptoms of acute obstruction. May occur after any abdominal surgery. It can be a rare anticholinergic side effect of certain psychotropic drugs.

paralyzant (păr′ă-līz″ănt) [Fr. *paralyser,* paralyze]. 1. Causing paralysis. 2. A drug or other agent that induces paralysis.

paralyze (păr′ă-līz) [Fr. *paralyse*]. 1. To cause temporary or permanent loss of muscular power or sensation. 2. To render ineffective.

paralyzer (păr′ă-līz″ēr). 1. That which causes paralysis. 2. A substance that inhibits a chemical reaction.

paramagnetic (păr″ă-măg-nĕt′ĭk). Anything that is attracted by the poles of a magnet and becomes parallel to the lines of magnetic force.

paramania (păr″ă-mā′nē-ă) [Gr. *para,* beside, + *mania,* madness]. A type of emotional disturbance in which the individual derives pleasure from complaining.

paramastigote (păr″ă-măs′tĭ-gōt) [″ + *mastix,* lash]. Having a small supernumerary flagellum next to a larger one.

paramastitis (păr″ă-măs-tī′tĭs) [″ + *mastos,* breast, + *itis,* inflammation]. Inflammation around the breast.

paramastoid (păr″ă-măs′toyd) [″ + ″ + *eidos,* form, shape]. Next to the mastoid.

paramedian (păr″ă-mē′dē-ăn) [″ + L. *medianus,* median]. Close to the midline.

paramedian incision. A surgical incision, esp. of the abdominal wall, close to the midline.

paramedic (păr″ă-mĕd′ĭk) [Gr. *para,* beside, + L. *medicus,* doctor]. A trained medical assistant who participates in rescue operations or assists a physician. SEE: *emergency medical technician.*

paramedical. Supplementing the work of medical personnel in related fields: social work; physical, occupational, and speech therapy.

paramedical personnel. Health care workers who are not physicians. These include medical technicians, emergency medical technicians, and physician's assistants. SEE: *allied health professional.*

paramenia (păr″ă-mē′nē-ă) [″ + *meniaia,* menses]. Irregular, abnormal, or difficult menstruation.

paramesial (păr″ă-mē′sē-ăl) [″ + *mesos,* middle]. Paramedian, q.v.

parameter (păr-ăm′ĕ-tĕr) [″ + *metron,* measure]. 1. In mathematics, an arbitrary constant, each value of which determines the specific form of the equation in which it appears. Often misused to indicate a variable. 2. In biostatistics, the term pertains to a measurement taken on a population, which consists of all the subjects in a defined group.

paramethadione (păr″ă-mĕth″ă-dī′ōn). USP. Anticonvulsive drug used in treating absence seizures. Trade name is Paradione.

paramethasone acetate (păr″ă-mĕth′ă-sōn). USP. A glucocorticosteroid drug. Trade names are Haldrone and Stemex.

parametric (păr′ă-mĕt′rĭk) [Gr. *para,* beside, + *metra,* uterus]. 1. Concerning the area near the uterus. 2. Rel. to the parametrium, the tissue surrounding the uterus. 3. [Gr. *para,* beside, + *metron,* measure] Adjectival form of parameter, q.v.

parametric statistics. That class of statistics based on the assumption that the samples measured are from normally distributed populations.

parametritic (păr″ă-mĕ-trĭt′ĭk). Concerning parametritis, q.v.

parametritis (păr″ă-mĕ-trī′tĭs) [″ + *metra,* uterus, + *itis,* inflammation]. Inflamed condition of parametrium, the cellular tissue adjacent to the uterus. SYN: *cellulitis, pelvic.*

parametrium (păr-ă-mē′trē-ŭm) [″ + *metra,* uterus]. [NA] Loose connective tissue around the uterus.

paramimia (păr″ă-mĭm′ē-ă) [″ + *mimeisthai,* to imitate]. Use of gestures that are inappropriate to the spoken words that they accompany.

paramnesia (păr″ăm-nē′zē-ă) [″ + *amnesia,* loss of memory]. 1. Use of words without meaning. 2. Distortion of memory in which there is inability to distinguish imaginary or suggested experiences from those that have actually occurred. 3. Seeming recall of events that never have occurred.

paramolar (păr″ă-mō′lăr). A supernumerary tooth close to a molar.

paramorphia (păr″ă-mor′fē-ă) [″ + *morphe,* form]. Abnormality of shape or structure.

paramucin (păr″ă-mū′sĭn). A glycoprotein found in ovarian and some other cysts.

paramusia (păr″ă-mū′zē-ă) [″ + *mousa,* music]. A form of aphasia in which the ability to render music correctly is lost.

paramyloidosis (păr-ăm″ĭ-loy-dō′sĭs) [″ + L. *amylum,* starch, + Gr. *eidos,* form, shape, + *osis,* condition]. The presence and build-up of atypical amyloid in tissues.

paramyoclonus multiplex (păr-ă-mī-ŏk′lō-nŭs mŭl′tĭ-plĕks) [″ + *mys,* muscle, + *klonos,* tumult]. Sudden and frequent shocklike contractions usually affecting muscles of both legs, and trunk muscles particularly. The contractions, which disappear during sleep and motion, may occur 10 to 50 times each minute. Usually the condition develops spontaneously, but it has been known to follow fright, trauma, infectious diseases, and poliomyelitis.

paramyosinogen (păr″ă-mī″ō-sĭn′ō-jĕn) [Gr. *para*, beside, + *myosin*, protein globin of muscle, + *gennan*, to produce]. Protein derived from muscle plasma.

paramyotonia (păr″ă-mī″ō-tō′nē-ă) [″ + *mys*, muscle, + *tonos*, tone]. Disorder marked by muscular spasms and abnormal muscular tonicity.

   p., ataxic. Tonic muscular spasm with slight ataxia or paresis during any attempt at movement.

   p. congenita. Congenital condition of tonic muscular spasms when body is exposed to cold. SYN: *Eulenburg's disease.*

   p., symptomatic. Temporary muscular rigidity when one first tries to walk, as in paralysis agitans.

paramyotonus (păr″ă-mī-ŏt′ō-nŭs) [″ + ″ + *tonos*, tone]. Condition in which there is tonic muscular spasm.

paramyxoviruses. A subgroup of the myxoviruses that are similar in physical, chemical, and biological characteristics. However, they are quite different pathogenetically. Includes parainfluenza, measles, mumps, Newcastle disease, and respiratory syncytial viruses.

paranalgesia (păr″ăn-ăl-jē′sē-ă) [″ + *an-*, not, + *algos*, pain]. Analgesia of the lower half of the body.

paranasal (păr″ă-nā′săl) [″ + L. *nasalis*, pert. to nose]. Situated near or along the nasal cavities.

paranasal sinuses. Accessory nasal sinuses that open into the nasal cavities. They are the frontal, ethmoidal, sphenoidal, and maxillary. All are lined with a ciliated mucous membrane continuous with that of the nasal cavities.

paraneoplastic syndromes. Term used to describe indirect effects of neoplasms that may be so severe as to be the actual cause of death, rather than the tumor itself being the cause. These include endocrine effects of neoplasms of the lungs or kidneys, and various neoplasms of the endocrine glands.

paranephric (păr″ă-nĕf′rĭk) [″ + *nephros*, kidney]. 1. Close to the kidney. 2. Concerning the adrenal glands.

paranephritis (păr″ă-nĕ-frī′tĭs) [″ + ″ + *itis*, inflammation]. 1. Inflamed condition of the suprarenal capsules. 2. Inflammation of connective tissue about kidney. SYN: *perinephritis.*

paranephros (păr-ă-nĕf′rŏs). A suprarenal or adrenal capsule.

paranesthesia (păr″ăn-ĕs-thē′zē-ă) [″ + *an-*, not, + *aisthesis*, sensation]. Paraanesthesia, q.v.

paraneural (păr″ă-nū′răl) [″ + *neuron*, nerve]. Adjacent to a nerve.

paranoia (păr″ă-noy′ă) [Gr. *para*, beside, + *nous*, mind]. This term indicates patients who show persistent persecutory delusions or delusional jealousy; emotion and behavior appropriate to the content of the delusional system; the disorder has been present at least one week; symptoms of schizophrenia such as bizarre delusions or incoherence are present; no prominent hallucinations; a full depressive or manic syndrome is either not present or is of brief duration; the illness is not due to organic disease of the brain.

This disorder, which usually occurs in middle or late adult life and may be chronic, often includes resentment and anger that may lead to violence. These patients rarely seek medical attention. They are brought for care by associates or relatives.

   p., erotomanic type. A form of paranoid delusion that one is loved by another. The delusion is more nearly one of romantic or spiritual love, rather than physical; the object is usually someone who is of a higher status or famous, but may be a complete stranger.

   p., jealous type. The unfounded conviction that the patient's spouse or lover is unfaithful.

   p., litigious. Paranoia in which the patient institutes or threatens to institute legal action because of the imagined persecution.

   p., somatic. The delusion that one's body is malodorous, or is infested with an internal or external parasite, or that the body is physically misshapen or unduly ugly.

paranoiac (păr-ă-noy′ăk). 1. Concerning or afflicted with paranoia. 2. One suffering from paranoia.

paranoid (păr′ă-noyd) [″ + *nous*, mind, + *eidos*, form, shape]. 1. Resembling paranoia. 2. A person afflicted with paranoia.

paranoid ideation. Suspicious thinking that is persecutory, accompanied by feelings that one is being harassed, treated wrongly, or being judged critically.

paranoid reaction type. Individual who has fixed systematized delusions, is suspicious, has a persecution complex, is resentful and bitter, and is a megalomaniac. Many states approach true paranoia and resemble it but lack one or more of its distinguishing features. Some of these are transitory paranoid states due to toxic conditions, a paranoid type of schizophrenia, and paranoid states due to alcoholism.

paranomia (păr″ă-nŏ′mē-ă) [″ + *onoma*, name]. Form of aphasia in which there is inability to remember correct names of objects shortly after seeing or using them.

paranormal. 1. Pert. to claimed experiences that are not within the range of normal experiences or are not scientifically explainable. SEE: *extrasensory perception; psychokinesis.* 2. Moderately abnormal.

paranuclear (păr″ă-nū′klē-ăr). Adjacent to the nucleus of a cell.

paranucleate (păr″ă-nū′klē-āt). Concerning or having a paranucleus.

paranucleolus (păr″ă-nū-klē′ō-lŭs). A small basophil body in the sac enclosing the nucleus.

paranucleus (păr″ă-nū′klē-ŭs) [Gr. *para*, beside, + L. *nucleus*, a kernel]. A small body lying close to a cell nucleus.

paraomphalic (păr″ă-ŏm-făl′ĭk) [″ + *omphalos*, navel]. Adjacent to the navel. SYN: *paraumbilical.*

paraoperative (păr″ă-ŏp′ĕr-ă-tĭv) [″ + L. *operari*, to work]. Concerning all the details and accessories of surgery and preparation of the patient.

paraosteoarthropathy (păr″ă-ŏs″tē-ō-ăr-thrŏp′ă-thē) [″ + *osteon*, bone, + *arthron*, joint, + *pathos*, disease, suffering]. Paralysis of lower portion of the body in addition to bone and joint disease.

parapancreatic (păr″ă-păn″krē-ăt′ĭk) [″ + *pan*, all, + *kreas*, flesh]. Located close to the pancreas.

paraparesis (păr″ă-păr-ē′sĭs, -păr′ē-sĭs) [″ + *parienai*, to let fall]. Partial paralysis affecting the lower limbs.

parapedesis (păr″ă-pĕd-ē′sĭs) [″ + *pedesis*, leaping]. Secretion or excretion through other than normal channels.

parapeptone (păr″ă-pĕp′tōn) [″ + *peptein*, to digest]. Intermediate digestion product of albumin. SEE: *peptone.*

paraperitoneal (păr″ă-pĕr″ĭ-tō-nē′ăl) [″ + *peritonaion*, peritoneum]. Near the peritoneum.

paraphasia (păr-ă-fā′zē-ă) [″ + *aphasis*, speech loss]. The misuse of spoken words or word combinations; a form of aphasia. SEE: *paraphrasia.*

paraphemia (păr″ă-fē′mē-ă) [″ + *pheme*, speech]. A disorder marked by consistent use of the wrong words, or mispronunciation of words.

paraphilia [″ + *philein*, to love]. A psychosexual disorder in which unusual or bizarre imagery or acts are necessary for realization of sexual excitement. Included in this disorder are bestiality, fetishism, transvestism, zoophilia, pedophilia, exhibitionism, voyeurism, sexual masochism, and sexual sadism.

paraphimosis (păr″ă-fĭ-mō′sĭs) [″ + *phimoun*, to muzzle, + *osis*, condition]. Strangulation of glans penis due to retraction of narrowed or inflamed foreskin.

paraphimosis oculi. Retraction of the eyelid behind a protruding eyeball.

paraphobia (păr″ă-fō′bē-ă) [″ + *phobos*, fear]. A mild form of phobia.

paraphrasia (păr-ă-frā′zē-ă) [Gr. *para*, beside, + *phrasis*, speech]. Condition characterized by loss of the ability to use words correctly and coherently. The words spoken are so jumbled and misused as to make speech unintelligible. SYN: *paraphasia.*

paraphrenitis (păr″ă-frē-nī′tĭs) [″ + *phren*, diaphragm, + *itis*, inflammation]. Inflammation of the tissues around the diaphragm.

paraphyseal (păr″ă-fĭz′ē-ăl). Concerning the paraphysis.

paraphysis (pă-răf′ĭ-sĭs) [Gr., offshoot]. The vestigial structure that originates from the roof plate of the telencephalon. Presumably the colloid cyst of the third ventricle arises from it. A midline organ that develops from the roof plate of the diencephalon of some lower vertebrates.

paraplasm (păr′ă-plăzm) [Gr. *para*, beside, + LL. *plasma*, form, mold]. 1. Any abnormal new formation or malformation. 2. The fluid portion of protoplasm. SYN: *hyaloplasm.*

paraplastic (păr″ă-plăs′tĭk) [″ + *plastikos*, formed]. 1. Misshapen; deformed. 2. Pert. to fluid portion of protoplasm.

paraplectic (păr″ă-plĕk′tĭk) [Gr. *paraplektikos*, striking at the side]. Afflicted with paralysis of lower extremities. SYN: *paraplegic.*

paraplegia (păr-ă-plē′jē-ă) [Gr. *paraplegia*, stroke on one side]. Paralysis of lower portion of the body and of both legs. SEE: *Nursing Diagnoses* in *Appendix.*

ETIOL: A lesion involving the spinal cord that may be due to the following: maldevelopment, epidural abscess, hematomyelia, acute transverse myelitis, spinal neoplasms, multiple sclerosis, syringomyelia, or trauma.

    p., alcoholic. Paraplegia of spinal origin due to excessive use of alcohol.

    p., ataxic. Lateral and posterior sclerosis of the spinal cord characterized by slowly progressing ataxia and paresis.

    p., cerebral. Paraplegia from a bilateral cerebral lesion.

    p., congenital spastic. P., infantile spastic.

    p. dolorosa. Paraplegia due to pressure of a neoplasm on the posterior spinal cord and nerve roots. Extremely painful despite paralysis.

p., infantile spastic. Spastic paraplegia that occurs in infants. It is usually due to birth injury. SEE: *p., spastic.*

p., peripheral. Paraplegia due to pressure on, injury to, or disease of peripheral nerves.

p., Pott's. Paraplegia associated with tuberculosis of the spine.

p., senile. Paraplegia resulting from sclerosis of arteries supplying spinal cord.

p., spastic. Paraplegia characterized by increased muscular tone and accentuated tendon reflexes. Seen in multiple sclerosis and other conditions involving the pyramidal tracts. SYN: *p., tetanoid.*

p., spastic, primary. Paraplegia from degeneration in pyramidal tracts.

p., superior. Paralysis of both arms.

p., tetanoid. P., spastic.

paraplegic (păr-ă-plē'jĭk) [Gr. *paraplegia,* stroke on one side]. Pert. to, or affected with, paraplegia. SYN: *paraplectic.*

paraplegiform (păr"ă-plĕj'ĭ-form) [" + L. *forma,* form]. Similar to paraplegia.

parapleuritis (păr"ă-plū-rī'tĭs) [Gr. *para,* beside, + *pleura,* side, + *itis,* inflammation]. 1. Inflammation in the thoracic wall. 2. Mild inflammation of the pleura. 3. Pain in the pleura. SYN: *pleurodynia.*

parapoplexy (păr-ăp'ō-plĕk"sē) [" + *apoplessein,* to cripple by a stroke]. A mild or slight apoplexy with partial stupor; a stupor resembling apoplexy. SYN: *pseudoapoplexy.*

parapraxia (păr-ă-prăk'sē-ă) [" + *praxis,* doing]. Disturbed mental processes producing inaccuracy, forgetfulness, and tendency to misplace things and make slips of speech or pen. SYN: *parapraxis.*

paraproctitis (păr"ă-prŏk-tī'tĭs) [Gr. *para,* beside, + *proktos,* anus, + *itis,* inflammation]. Inflamed condition of tissues near the rectum.

paraproctium (păr"ă-prŏk'shē-ŭm) [" + *proktos,* anus]. The connective tissue around the anus and rectum.

paraprostatitis (păr"ă-prŏs"tă-tī'tĭs) [" + *prostates,* prostate, + *itis,* inflammation]. Inflammation of the tissues around the prostate.

paraprotein (păr"ă-prō'tē-ĭn). An abnormal plasma protein, such as a macroglobulin, cryoglobulin, or the protein present in myeloma.

paraproteinemia. The presence of abnormal immunoglobulins or antibodies in the serum or urine of patients with various disease states which, as a group, are called plasma cell dyscrasias. Paraproteins are a monoclonal antibody (cloned from a single lymphoid cell). Paraproteinemias include various forms of lymphoid malignancies, amyloidosis, and benign disorders associated with drug administration. SEE: *Bence Jones protein.*

parapsoriasis (păr"ă-sō-rī'ă-sĭs) [" + *psoriasis,* an itching]. A chronic disorder of the skin marked by scaly red lesions.

p. en plaque. A form of parapsoriasis that is often the precursor of mycosis fungoides.

p. lichenoides chronica. A form of parapsoriasis that forms a widespread network over the extremities and trunk. It is red to blue in color and sometimes resembles psoriasis and at other times lichen planus.

parapsychology (păr"ă-sī-kŏl'ō-jē). The division of psychology that deals with extrasensory perception, telepathy, psychokinesis, clairvoyance, and associated phenomena.

paraquat (păr'ă-kwăt). A toxic chemical used in agriculture to kill certain weeds. It damages the skin on contact and if ingested may cause liver, renal, and pulmonary disease. This chemical is sometimes present as a contaminant in marijuana.

TREAT: Remove from stomach and gastrointestinal tract by emesis, gastric lavage, and catharsis. A slurry of clay and charcoal should be administered to absorb the poison. Cortisone I.V. and hemodialysis are helpful.

pararectal (păr"ă-rĕk'tăl) [" + L. *rectum,* straight]. Close to the rectum.

parareflexia (păr"ă-rē-flĕk'sē-ă). An abnormal condition of the reflexes.

pararenal (păr"ă-rē'năl) [" + L. *ren,* kidney]. Near the kidneys.

pararhotacism (păr"ă-rō'tă-sĭzm) [" + *rho,* Gr. letter R, + *-ismos,* condition]. Constant erroneous use of letter "r" or the placing of undue emphasis on letter "r."

pararrhythmia (păr"ă-rĭth'mē-ă) [" + *a-,* not, + *rhythmos,* rhythm]. A cardiac rhythm caused by action of two pacemakers at different sites. It is not caused by a disturbance of the normal conducting pathways.

pararthria (păr-ăr'thrē-ă) [" + *arthron,* articulation]. A speech disorder characterized by difficulty in uttering sounds.

parasacral (păr"ă-sā'krăl) [" + L. *sacrum,* sacred]. Close to the sacrum.

parasalpingitis (păr"ă-săl-pĭn-jī'tĭs) [" + *salpinx,* tube, + *itis,* inflammation]. Inflamed condition of tissues around an oviduct or a eustachian tube.

parasecretion (păr"ă-sē-krē'shŭn) [" + L. *secretio,* secretion]. 1. An abnormality in secretion. 2. A substance abnormally secreted.

parasexuality (păr"ă-sĕks"ū-ăl'ĭ-tē) [" + L. *sexus,* sex]. Any sexually deviant act.

parasigmatism (păr"ă-sĭg'mă-tĭzm) [" +

sigma, Gr. letter S, + *-ismos,* condition]. Imperfect pronunciation of the letters "s" and "z." SYN: *lisping.*

parasinoidal (păr″ă-sī-noy′dăl) [″ + L. *sinus,* a curve]. Close to a sinus.

parasite (păr′ă-sīt) [″ + *sitos,* food]. 1. An organism that lives within, upon, or at expense of another organism, known as the host, without contributing to survival of the host. 2. The smaller or incomplete element of conjoined twins that is attached to and dependent upon the more nearly normal twin, called the autosite.

　　p., accidental. Parasite infesting a host that is not its normal host. SYN: *p., incidental.*

　　p., external. Parasite that lives on the outer surface of its hosts, such as fleas, lice, mites, or ticks. SYN: *ectoparasite.*

　　p., facultative. Parasite capable of living independently of its host at times. Opposite of obligate parasite.

　　p., incidental. P., accidental.

　　p., intermittent. Parasite that visits its host at intervals for nourishment. SYN: *p., occasional.*

　　p., internal. Parasite such as a protozoon or worm that lives within the body of the host, occupying the digestive tract or body cavities, or living within body organs, blood, tissues, or even cells.

　　p., malarial. Any one of the four species of *Plasmodium* that can cause malaria. SEE: *malaria.*

　　p., obligate. Parasite completely dependent on its host. Opposite of facultative parasite.

　　p., occasional. Parasite that seeks its host at intervals to obtain nourishment. SYN: *p., intermittent.*

　　p., periodic. Parasite that lives upon the host for short periods of time.

　　p., permanent. Parasite, such as a fluke or an itch mite, that lives upon its host until maturity or spends its entire life upon its host.

　　p., specific. Parasite that requires a specific host in order to complete its life cycle.

　　p., temporary. Parasite that is free-living during a part of its life cycle.

parasitemia (păr″ă-sī-tē′mē-ă) [″ + *haima,* blood]. Presence of parasites in the blood.

parasitic (păr″ă-sīt′ĭk) [Gr. *para,* beside, + *sitos,* food]. Like, caused by, or concerning a parasite.

parasitic disease drug service. The Centers for Disease Control (CDC), Public Health Service, U.S. Department of Health and Human Services, maintains a supply of antiparasitic agents which otherwise are difficult to obtain. These drugs are available to licensed physicians by writing or calling the Centers for Disease Control, Drug Service, Atlanta, GA, 30333, U.S.A. Phone (404) 639-3670 during working hours; otherwise, and on holidays, phone (404) 639-2888.

Drugs not available commercially or from CDC may be available from the National Institute of Allergy and Infectious Diseases, phone 1-800-537-9979. SEE: table.

parasiticide (păr″ă-sīt′ĭ-sīd) [″ + ″ + L. *caedere,* to kill]. 1. Destructive to parasites. 2. An agent that will kill parasites.

parasitism (păr′ă-sīt″ĭzm) [″ + ″ + *-ismos,* condition]. 1. The state or condition of being infected or infested with parasites. 2. The behavior of a parasite.

parasitize (păr′ă-sīt-īz″, -sīt-īz″). To infest or infect with a parasite.

parasitogenic (păr″ă-sī″tō-jĕn′ĭk) [″ + *gennan,* to produce]. 1. Caused by parasites. 2. Favoring parasitic development.

parasitologist (păr″ă-sī-tŏl′ō-jĭst) [″ + *logos,* word, reason]. One who specializes in the science of parasitology.

parasitology (păr″ă-sī-tŏl′ō-jē) [″ + *logos,* word, reason]. The study of parasites and parasitism.

parasitophobia (păr″ă-sī″tō-fō′bē-ă) [″ + ″ + *phobos,* fear]. Unusual fear of parasites.

parasitosis (păr″ă-sī-tō′sĭs) [″ + ″ + *osis,* condition]. A disease or condition resulting from parasitism.

parasitotropic (păr″ă-sī″tō-trŏp′ĭk) [″ + ″ + *tropos,* turning]. Having attraction for parasites, esp. certain drugs that act chiefly upon parasites in the body.

parasitotropism (păr″ă-sī-tŏt′rō-pĭzm) [″ + ″ + ″ + *-ismos,* condition]. The special affinity of drugs or other agents for parasites.

parasitotropy (păr″ă-sī-tŏt′rō-pē). Parasitotropism, q.v.

parasomnias (păr″ă-sŏm′nē-ăz) [″ + L. *somnus,* sleep]. An abnormal event that occurs during sleep. SEE: *sleep, disorders of.*

paraspadia (păr-ă-spā′dē-ă) [Gr. *paraspadein,* to draw aside]. Condition in which the urethra has an opening through one side of the penis.

paraspasm (păr′ă-spăzm) [L. *paraspasmus*]. 1. Muscular spasm of the lower extremities. 2. Spastic paralysis of the lower extremities.

parasteatosis (păr″ă-stē″ă-tō′sĭs) [Gr. *para,* beside, + *steatos,* fat, + *osis,* condition]. Any disordered condition of the sebaceous secretions.

parasternal (păr-ă-stĕrn′ăl) [″ + *sternon,* chest]. Beside the sternum.

parasternal line. Imaginary vertical line running midway between sternal margin and line passing through the nipple.

Partial List of Antiparasitic Drugs

* albendazole — Zentel (SKF)
  amphotericin B — Fungizone (Squibb)
** benznidazole — Rochagan (Roche)
† bithionol — Bitin (Tanabe, Japan)
  chloroquine — Aralen (Winthrop-Breon);
    others
  crotamiton — Eurax (Westwood)
† dehydroemetine — Meban (Hoffmann-
    LaRoche, Switzerland)
* diethylcarbamazine — Hetrazan (Lederle)
† diloxanide furoate — Furamide (Boots,
    England)
* eflornithine (difluoromethylornithine;
    DFMO) — Ornidyl (Merrell Dow)
  emetine — (Lilly)
** flubendazole — (Janssen)
  furazolidone — Furoxone (Norwich Eaton)
  hydroxychloroquine — Plaquenil
    (Winthrop-Breon)
  iodoquinol (diiodohydroxyquin) —
    Yodoxin (Glenwood); others
* itraconazole — Sporanox (Janssen)
† ivermectin — Mectizan (Merck)
  ketoconazole — Nizoral (Janssen)
  lindane (gamma benzene hexachloride) —
    Kwell (Reed and Carnrick); others
  malathion — Ovide (GenDerm)
  mebendazole — Vermox (Janssen)
  mefloquine — Lariam (Roche)
† melarsoprol — Arsobal (Rhône Poulenc,
    France)
** metrifonate — Bilarcil (Bayer, Germany)
  metronidazole — Flagyl (Searle); others
  niclosamide — Niclocide (Miles)
† nifurtimox — Lampit (Bayer, Germany)
** ornidazole — Tiberal (Hoffmann-
    LaRoche, Switzerland)
  oxamniquine — Vansil (Pfizer)

  paromomycin — Humatin (Parke-Davis)
  pentamidine isethionate — Pentam 300
    (LyphoMed)
  permethrin — Nix (Burroughs Wellcome);
    Elimite (Herbert)
  piperazine — many manufacturers
  praziquantel — Biltricide (Miles)
  primaquine phosphate — (Winthrop-
    Breon)
** proguanil — Paludrine (Ayerst, Canada;
    ICI, England)
  pyrantel pamoate — Antiminth (Pfizer)
  pyrethrins and piperonyl butoxide — RID
    (Pfizer); others
  pyrimethamine — Daraprim (Burroughs
    Wellcome)
  pyrimethamine-sulfadoxine — Fansidar
    (Roche)
  quinacrine — Atabrine (Winthrop-Breon)
  quinidine gluconate — many manufacturers
† quinine dihydrochloride
  quinine sulfate — many manufacturers
** spiramycin — Rovamycine (Poulenc, Can-
    ada)
† stibogluconate sodium (antimony sodium
    gluconate) — Pentostam (Burroughs
    Wellcome, England)
† suramin — Germanin (Bayer, Germany)
  thiabendazole — Mintezol (Merck)
** tinidazole — Fasigyn (Pfizer)
  trimethoprim-sulfamethoxazole — Bactrim
    (Roche); Septra (Burroughs Wellcome);
    others
‡ trimetrexate (Parke-Davis)
** tryparsamide

* Available in the USA only from manufacturer
** Not available in the USA
† Available from the CDC Drug Service, Centers for Disease Control, Atlanta, Georgia 30333; 404-639-3670
  (evenings, weekends, or holidays: 404-639-2888)
‡ Available from the National Institute of Allergy and Infectious Diseases, 1-800-537-9978
NOTE: Name of drug manufacturer is in parentheses.

parasternal region. Area between the sternal margin and parasternal line.

parasthenia (păr″ăs-thē′nē-ă) [″ + sthenos, strength]. Condition characterized by abnormal functioning of organic tissue at odd intervals.

parastruma (păr″ă-stroo′mă) [″ + L. struma, goiter]. Goiter-like tumor due to hypertrophy of a parathyroid gland.

parasympathetic (păr″ă-sĭm″pă-thĕt′ĭk) [″ + sympathetikos, sympathetic nerve]. Of or pert. to the craniosacral division of the autonomic nervous system.

parasympathetic nervous system. The craniosacral division of the autonomic nervous system. Preganglionic fibers originate from nuclei in the midbrain, medulla, and sacral portion of the spinal cord. They pass through the 3rd, 7th, 9th, and 10th cranial nerves and the 2nd, 3rd, and 4th sacral nerves, and synapse with postganglionic neurons located in autonomic (terminal) ganglia that lie in the walls of or near the organ innervated.

Some effects of parasympathetic stimulation are constriction of pupil, contraction of smooth muscle of alimentary canal, constriction of bronchioles, slowing of heart rate, and increased secretion by glands, except sweat glands. Parasympathetic effects are specific rather than general. SEE: *autonomic nervous system; sympathetic nervous system.*

parasympathicotonia (păr″ă-sĭm-păth″ĭk-ō-tō′nē-ă) [″ + *sympathetikos,* sympathetic nerve, + *tonos,* tension]. Condition in which there is an imbalance in functioning of the autonomic nervous system, the parasympathetic division dominating over the sympathetic. SYN: *vagotonia.*

parasympatholytic (păr″ă-sĭm″pă-thō-lĭt′ĭk) [″ + ″ + *lytikos,* dissolving]. Having a destructive effect on or blocking parasympathetic nerve fibers.

parasympathomimetic (păr″ă-sĭm″pă-thō-mĭm-ĕt′ĭk) [″ + ″ + *mimetikos,* imitative]. Producing effects similar to those resulting from stimulation of parasympathetic nervous system.

parasynapsis (păr″ă-sĭ-năp′sĭs) [″ + *synapsis,* conjunction]. The side-to-side union of chromosomes in the process of reduction division of meiosis.

parasynovitis (păr″ă-sĭn″ō-vī′tĭs) [″ + *syn,* with, + *oon,* egg, + *itis,* inflammation]. Inflamed condition of tissues around a synovial sac.

parasystole (păr-ă-sĭs′tō-lē) [″ + *systole,* contraction]. An ectopically originating cardiac rhythm independent of the normal sinus rhythm.

paratarsium (păr-ă-tăr′sē-ŭm) [″ + *tarsos,* tarsus]. The covering and connective tissues of the tarsus of the feet.

paratenon (păr″ă-tĕn′ŏn) [″ + *tenon,* tendon]. Fatty and areolar tissue that surrounds the tendon and fills the spaces around the tendon.

paratereseomania (păr″ă-tĕr-ē″sē-ō-mā′nē-ă) [Gr. *paratereesis,* observation, + *mania,* madness]. Insane desire to investigate new scenes and subjects.

parathion (păr″ă-thī′ŏn). An agricultural insecticide, highly toxic to humans and animals.

parathion poisoning. Contracted by accidental inhalation or ingestion while working with the pesticide or by inadvertent contamination of food products. SEE: *Poisons and Poisoning in Appendix.*

SYM: Shortly after exposure, headache, sweating, salivation, lacrimation, vomiting, diarrhea, muscular twitching, convulsions, dyspnea, and blurred vision occur.

parathormone (păr″ă-thor′mōn) [Gr. *para,* beside, + *thyreos,* shield, + *eidos,* form, shape, + *hormaein,* to excite]. Hor-

mone secreted by the parathyroid glands that regulates calcium and phosphorus metabolism. Deficiency results in tetany, carpopedal spasm, wheezing, muscle cramps, urinary frequency, mood changes, and lassitude. An extract from fresh or frozen parathyroid glands of domestic animals that contains the active principle or principles of these glands is used therapeutically. SYN: *hormone, parathyroid.* SEE: *parathyroid.*

parathymia (păr″ă-thī′mē-ă) [″ + *thymos,* mind, spirit]. Disordered or inappropriate mood.

parathyroid (păr-ă-thī′royd) [″ + *thyreos,* shield, + *eidos,* form, shape]. 1. Located close to the thyroid gland. 2. One of four small endocrine glands about 6 mm long by 3 to 4 mm broad on the back of, and at lower edge of, the thyroid gland, or embedded within its substance. These glands secrete a hormone, parathyroid hormone (parathormone), that regulates calcium and phosphorus metabolism.

ABNORM: Hypoparathyroidism or hyposecretion results in neuromuscular hyperexcitability manifested by convulsions and tetany, carpopedal spasm, wheezing, muscle cramps, urinary frequency, mood changes, and lassitude. Blood calcium falls and blood phosphorus rises. Other symptoms include blurring of vision due to cataracts, poorly formed teeth if onset was in childhood, maldevelopment of hair and nails, and dry and scaly skin. Hyperparathyroidism or hypersecretion results in a rise in blood calcium and fall in blood phosphorus. Calcium is removed from bones, resulting in increased fragility. Muscular weakness, reduced muscular tone, and general neuromuscular hypoexcitability occur. Generalized osteitis fibrosa, or osteitis fibrosa cystica, is a clinical entity associated with hyperplasia and resulting hypersecretion of the parathyroids. Parathormone, q.v., secreted by these glands, contains the active principle or principles.

parathyroidectomy (păr″ă-thī-royd-ĕk′tō-mē) [″ + ″ + ″ + *ektome,* excision]. Excision of one or more of the parathyroid glands. SEE: *Nursing Diagnoses in Appendix.*

parathyroid injection. USP. A standard preparation of the water-soluble hormone obtained from the parathyroid glands of mammals used for food by humans. It acts to increase the calcium content of the blood.

parathyroprivia (păr″ă-thī′rō-prĭ′vē-ă) [″ + ″ + L. *privus,* deprived of]. Condition that results when the parathyroids are removed or cease functioning.

parathyroprivic (păr″ă-thī′rō-prĭv′ĭk). Resulting from loss of function of, or removal of, parathyroid glands.

parathyrotropic (păr″ă-thī-rō-trŏp′ĭk) [″ + ″ + *tropikos*, turning]. Having an affinity for the parathyroid gland.

paratonsillar (păr″ă-tŏn′sĭl-ăr) [″ + L. *tonsillaris*, pert. to tonsil]. Near or about the tonsil.

paratope (păr′ă-tōp) [″ + *topos*, a place]. The site on an antibody to which an antigen attaches. SEE: *epitope*.

paratrichosis (păr″ă-trĭ-kō′sĭs) [″ + *trichosis*, being hairy]. Abnormality of hair or its location.

paratripsis (păr″ă-trĭp′sĭs) [″ + *tribein*, to rub]. Rubbing, chafing.

paratrophic (păr″ă-trō′fĭk) [″ + *trophe*, nourishment]. 1. Requiring living substances for food; parasitic. 2. Pert. to abnormal nutrition.

paratyphlitis (păr″ă-tĭf-lī′tĭs) [″ + *typhlos*, blind, + *itis*, inflammation]. Inflammation of the connective tissue close to the cecum.

paratyphoid (păr-ă-tī′foyd) [″ + *typhos*, fever, + *eidos*, form, shape]. Similar to typhoid.

paratyphoid fever. An infectious fever resembling typhoid.

SYM: Fever with gastroenteritis. Incubation period may be less than in typhoid. Usually patient's condition is less severe than that found in typhoid fever, but symptoms vary from a mild transient diarrhea to those quite similar to typhoid fever, q.v.

ETIOL: Bacteria of the genus *Salmonella*, esp. the species *S. paratyphi* (A and B strains) and *S. schottmülleri*. However, any species of *Salmonella* pathogenic to humans may cause a similar disease.

paratypic (păr″ă-tĭp′ĭk) [″ + *typos*, type]. Diverging from a type.

paraumbilical (păr″ă-ŭm-bĭl′ĭk-ăl) [″ + L. *umbilicus*, navel]. Close to the navel.

paraurethral (păr″ă-ū-rē′thrăl) [″ + *ourethra*, urethra]. Located close to the urethra.

parauterine (păr″ă-ū′tĕr-ĭn) [″ + L. *uterus*, womb]. Located close to or around the uterus.

paravaccinia (păr″ă-văk-sĭn′ē-ă). A viral disease that affects the udders of cows and may be transmitted to humans. In humans, the virus produces painless, smooth or warty lesions, called "milker's nodules," on the hands and arms. SEE: *milker's nodules*.

paravaginal (păr″ă-văj′ĭn-ăl) [″ + *vagina*, sheath]. Located close to or around the vagina.

paravaginitis (păr″ă-văj-ĭn-ī′tĭs) [″ + ″ + *itis*, inflammation]. Inflammation of the tissue surrounding the vagina.

paravenous (păr″ă-vē′nŭs) [″ + L. *vena*, vein]. Close to a vein.

paravertebral (păr″ă-vĕr′tĕ-brăl) [″ + L. *vertebralis*, pert. to vertebrae]. Alongside or near the vertebral column.

paravertebral anesthesia. Injection of a local anesthetic at roots of spinal nerves.

paravesical (păr″ă-vĕs′ĭk-ăl) [″ + L. *vesica*, bladder]. Near the urinary bladder.

paravitaminosis (păr″ă-vī″tă-mĭ-nō′sĭs). 1. Any disease indirectly associated with a vitamin deficiency. 2. A disease that mimics avitaminosis but is not due to a vitamin deficiency.

paraxial (păr-ăk′sē-ăl) [″ + L. *axis*, axis]. On either side of the axis of the body or one of its parts.

paraxon (păr-ăk′sŏn) [″ + *axon*, axis]. A collateral branch of an axon.

parazoon (păr″ă-zō′ŏn) [″ + *zoon*, animal]. An animal that lives as a parasite upon another animal.

parched [ME. *parchen*]. Extremely dry.

Paré, Ambroise (păr-ā′). French surgeon, 1510–1590, who instituted certain refined techniques into surgery and obstetrics.

parectasia, parectasis (păr″ĕk-tā′sē-ă, -tă-sĭs) [Gr. *para*, beside, + *ektasis*, stretching]. Excessive dilatation or stretching of a structure.

parectropia (păr″ĕk-trō′pē-ă) [″ + *ek*, out, + *trope*, a turn]. Apraxia, q.v.

paregoric (păr-ĕ-gor′ĭk) [L. *paregoricus*, soothing]. 1. USP. Camphorated tincture of opium, a narcotic-containing drug that in large doses is poisonous. Used in the symptomatic treatment of diarrhea. 2. Soothing.

paregoric poisoning. SEE: *morphine poisoning*.

parelectronomic (păr″ē-lĕk″trō-nŏm′ĭk) [Gr. *para*, beside, + *elektron*, amber, + *nomos*, law]. Not stimulated by an electric stimulus.

parencephalia (păr″ĕn-sĕ-fā′lē-ă) [″ + *enkephalos*, brain]. Congenital defect of the brain.

parencephalocele (păr″ĕn-sĕf′ă-lō-sēl) [″ + ″ + *kele*, tumor, swelling]. Herniation of the cerebellum through a defect in the cranium.

parencephalous (păr″ĕn-sĕf′ă-lŭs) [″ + *enkephalos*, brain]. A fetus with imperfect development of the cranium.

parenchyma (păr-ĕn′kĭ-mă) [Gr. *parenkheim*, to pour in beside] [NA] The essential parts of an organ that are concerned with its function in contradistinction to its framework.

p. testis. [NA] The functional portion of the testis, including the seminiferous tubules within the lobules.

parenchymatitis (păr″ĕn-kĭm″ă-tī′tĭs) [″ + *itis*, inflammation]. Inflamed condition of parenchyma or substance of a gland.

parenchymatous (păr″ĕn-kĭm′ă-tŭs). Concerning the essential substances of an organ.

parent [L. *parens*]. A father or a mother; one who begets offspring.

parentage, determination of. SEE: *paternity test.*

parental leave. Policy of allowing both parents to have leave from work following the birth of their child.

parenteral (păr-ĕn′tĕr-ăl) [Gr. *para*, beside, + *enteron*, intestine]. Denoting any medication route other than the alimentary canal, such as intravenous, subcutaneous, intramuscular, or mucosal. SEE: *medication routes.*

parenteral digestion. Digestion of foreign substances by body cells as opposed to enteral digestion, which occurs in the alimentary canal.

parenteral nutrition. SEE: *total parenteral nutrition.*

parenting. 1. Caring for and raising a child or children. 2. Producing offspring.

p., surrogate. An alternative method of childbearing for an infertile couple in which the wife is unable to bear a child. The surrogate mother agrees to be artificially inseminated by the husband's sperm and to relinquish the baby to the couple. Another approach is to retrieve eggs from the infertile wife and have them impregnated in vitro by her husband. The fertilized ovum is then implanted in the surrogate mother. SEE: *fertilization, in vitro; GIFT; surrogate parenting.*

parepididymis (păr″ĕp-ĭ-dĭd′ĭ-mĭs). Paradidymis, q.v.

parepithymia (păr″ĕp-ĭ-thī′mē-ă) [″ + *epithymia*, desire]. Abnormal desire or craving.

paresis (păr′ĕ-sĭs, pă-rē′sĭs) [Gr. *parienai*, to let fall]. 1. Partial or incomplete paralysis. SEE: *paralysis.* 2. An organic mental disease with somatic, irritative, and paralytic focal symptoms and signs running a slow, chronic, progressive course. SYN: *dementia paralytica.*

SYM: May simulate any psychoneurosis or psychosis. Pupillary changes, facial tremors, tremors of the lips and tongue, speech disturbances. Usually Argyll Robertson pupil, impaired vision, headache, speech slurred with letters and syllables often omitted. As the disease progresses, the patient demonstrates a disregard for social convention and moral standards. Memory is defective; depression and dementia are present; epileptic convulsions; unequal exaggeration of the reflexes. Always present is a positive serologic test for syphilis in the spinal fluid with increase of protein and lymphocytes.

ETIOL: Diffuse and focal involvement of brain and spinal cord due to syphilis, usually occurring 5 to 15 years after primary infection.

PATH: A diffuse meningoencephalitis with degenerative changes dependent upon vascular and toxic factors.

TREAT: Penicillin.

p., juvenile. General paresis due to congenital syphilis; seen in children.

paresthesia (păr″ĕs-thē′zē-ă) [Gr. *para*, beside, + *aisthesis*, sensation]. Sensation of numbness, prickling, or tingling; heightened sensitivity. Experienced in central and peripheral nerve lesions and in locomotor ataxia.

p., Berger's. Paresthesia of the legs that occurs in young people.

paretic (pă-rĕt′ĭk, pă-rē′tĭk) [Gr. *parienai*, to let fall]. Affected with or concerning paresis.

pareunia [Gr. *pareunos*, lying beside]. Sexual intercourse. SEE: *dyspareunia.*

Parfuran. Trade name for nitrofurantoin.

pargyline hydrochloride (păr′gĭ-lēn). USP. An antihypertensive drug. Trade name is Eutonyl.

parhidrosis (păr″hī-drō′sĭs) [Gr. *para*, beside, + *hidrosis*, sweat]. Any disordered secretion of perspiration.

paries (pā′rē-ēs) [L., a wall] (pl. *parietes*). [NA] The enveloping wall of any structure; applied esp. to hollow organs.

parietal (pă-rī′ĕ-tăl) [L. *parietalis*]. 1. Pert. to, or forming, the wall of a cavity. 2. Pert. to the parietal bone.

parietal bone. One of two bones that together form the roof and sides of the skull.

parietal cells. Large cells on margin of the peptic glands of the stomach. SYN: *cell, oxyntic.*

parietal lobe. The division of each side of the brain lying beneath each parietal bone.

parietes (pă-rī′ĕ-tēs) [L.]. Pl. of paries; walls of an organ or hollow part.

parietofrontal (pă-rī″ĕ-tō-frŏn′tăl). Concerning the parietal or frontal bones or lobes.

parietography (pă-rī″ĕ-tŏg′ră-fē) [″ + Gr. *graphein*, to write]. X-ray study of the walls of an organ.

parieto-occipital (pă-rī″ĕ-tō-ŏk-sĭp′ĭ-tăl). Concerning the parietal and occipital bones or lobes.

parietosplanchnic (pă-rī″ĕ-tō-splănk′nĭk). Parietovisceral, q.v.

parietosquamosal (pă-rī″ĕ-tō-skwă-mō′săl). Concerning the parietal bone and squamous part of the temporal bone.

parietotemporal (pă-rī″ĕ-tō-tĕm′pō-răl). Concerning the parietal and temporal bones or lobes.

parietovisceral (pă-rī″ĕ-tō-vĭs′ĕr-ăl). Concerning the wall of a body cavity and the viscera within.

Parinaud, Henri (pă-rĭ-nō′). French ophthalmologist, 1844–1905.

P.'s oculoglandular syndrome. Conjunctivitis with palpable preauricular lymph nodes.

P.'s ophthalmoplegia syndrome. Palsy of vertical gaze that may or may not be associated with pupillary or oculomotor nerve paresis. It is caused by a lesion at the level of the anterior corpora quadrigemina of the brain.

pari passu (pă′rē-păs′ū) [L., with equal speed]. Occurring at the same time or at the same rate; side by side.

parity (păr′ĭ-tē). 1. [L. *par*, equal] Equality, similarity. 2. [L. *parere*, to bring forth, to bear] The condition of having carried pregnancy to a point of viability (500 gm birth weight or 20 weeks gestation), regardless of the outcome. SEE: *multiparity; nulliparity; primiparity; secundiparity.*

Parkinson, James. British physician, 1755–1824.

P.'s disease. A chronic nervous disease characterized by a fine, slowly spreading tremor, muscular weakness and rigidity, and a peculiar gait. SYN: *paralysis agitans; shaking palsy.*

SYM: Onset may be abrupt; generally insidious. First symptom is a fine tremor beginning in hand or foot that may spread until it involves all the members. At first paroxysmal but becomes almost continuous. Face becomes expressionless. Slow and measured speech; later muscular rigidity. Head bowed, body bent forward, arms flexed, thumbs turned into palms, knees slightly bent. Gait characteristic by this time: steps grow faster and faster, body inclines more and more forward until patient falls and seeks some support; this is termed festination. Occasionally a tendency to fall backwards, retropulsion, replaces festination. Numbness, tingling, and sensation of heat may be present.

TREAT: General supportive measures plus medicines to combat muscle rigidity and lethargy. Drugs used include anticholinergics, antidepressants, antihistamines, dopa inhibitor combined with levodopa (sinemet), dopamine agonists such as bromocriptine or pergolide, monoamine oxidase-B inhibitor (deprenyl). Patients often benefit from referral to occupational or physical therapy, or both.

PROG: Recovery rarely, if ever, occurs. Duration indefinite.

NURSING IMPLICATIONS: Adminis-

ter prescribed drugs, evaluate patient response, and teach patient to do both so that side effects can be minimized by adjustment of dosages. Teach patient and family safety measures to prevent injury, about drug-related dietary restriction, and about administering needed fluids, calories, and dietary bulk by offering frequent but smaller feedings. Help patient to plan daily activities to prevent fatigue. Encourage participation in local support groups. Physical therapy and occupational therapy consultations are advisable. Refer him or her to national organizations for further information. SEE: *Nursing Diagnoses* in *Appendix.*

P.'s facies. The immobile, masklike facies characteristic of parkinsonism.

P.'s mask. Expressionless appearance of the face. Eyebrows are raised, wrinkles are smoothed out, and there is immobility of the facial muscles. A typical symptom seen in Parkinson's disease and in post-encephalitic states.

parkinsonian (păr″kĭn-sōn′ē-ăn). Concerning parkinsonism.

parkinsonism (păr′kĭn-sŏn-ĭzm″). Parkinson's disease.

Parlodel. Trade name for bromocriptine mesylate.

Parnate. Trade name for tranylcypromine sulfate.

PAR nurse. *Postanesthesia recovery room nurse.*

paroccipital (păr-ŏk-sĭp′ĭt-ăl) [Gr. *para*, beside, + L. *occiput*, occiput]. 1. Close to the occipital bone. 2. The paramastoid process.

parodontitis (păr″ō-dŏn-tī′tĭs) [″ + *odous*, tooth, + *itis*, inflammation]. Inflamed condition of tissues around a tooth.

parodontium (păr″ō-dŏn′shē-ŭm). Periodontium.

parodynia (păr-ō-dĭn′ē-ă) [L. *parere*, to bring forth, to bear, + Gr. *odyne*, pain]. 1. Labor pains. 2. Difficult or abnormal labor or birth. SYN: *dystocia.*

p. perversa. Presentation with fetus lying transversely across the uterus.

parole [Fr. *parole*, short for *parole d'honneur*, word of honor]. In psychiatry, the release of a patient from the hospital on a trial basis.

parolivary (păr-ŏl′ĭ-vă″rē) [Gr. *para*, beside, + L. *oliva*, olive]. Situated close to the olivary body.

parolivary bodies. Nuclei in medulla oblongata, lying close to the olivary bodies.

paromomycin sulfate (păr′ō-mō-mī″sĭn). USP. An aminoglycoside antibiotic used in treating intestinal amebiasis and various tapeworms. It is not effective against extraintestinal infections with amebae. Trade name is Humatin.

paromphalocele (păr″ŏm-făl′ō-sēl″) [″ +

omphalos, navel, + *kele,* tumor, swelling]. Hernia or tumor close to the umbilicus.

paroniria (păr-ō-nī'rē-ă) [" + *oneiros,* dream]. Abnormal or terrifying dreams.

    p. ambulans. Sleepwalking.

    p. salax. Restlessness in sleep with lascivious dreams and nocturnal emissions.

paronychia (păr-ō-nĭk'ē-ă) [" + *onyx,* nail]. Acute or chronic infection of marginal structures about the nail. SYN: *felon; panaris; runaround; whitlow.*

    ETIOL: Trauma, infection.

    SYM: Redness, swelling, and suppuration around nail edge.

    TREAT: Application of heat to area unless there is inadequate blood supply; surgery in severe cases.

    p. tendinosa. Inflammation of sheath of a digital tendon due to sepsis.

paronychomycosis (păr"ō-nĭk"ō-mī-kō'sĭs) [" + " + *mykes,* fungus, + *osis,* condition]. Fungus infection about the nails.

paronychosis (păr-ō-nĭ-kō'sĭs). Growth of a nail in an abnormal position.

paroophoritis (păr"ō-ŏf-ō-rī'tĭs) [" + *oophoros,* bearing eggs, + *itis,* inflammation]. Inflammation of the tissues around the ovary.

paroophoron (păr-ō-ŏf'ō-rŏn) [" + *oophoros,* bearing eggs]. A group of minute tubules located in the mesosalpinx between the uterus and ovary. It is a vestigial structure consisting of the remains of the caudal group of mesonephric tubules and is a homologue of the paradidymis of the male.

parophthalmia (păr-ŏf-thăl'mē-ă) [" + *ophthalmos,* eye]. Inflamed condition of tissue around the eye.

parophthalmoncus (păr"ŏf-thăl-mŏn'kŭs) [" + " + *onkos,* mass]. A tumor located near the eye.

parorchidium (păr-or-kĭd'ē-ŭm) [" + *orchis,* testicle]. Abnormal position, or nondescent, of a testicle. SYN: *ectopia testis.*

parorexia (păr-ō-rĕk'sē-ă) [" + *orexis,* appetite]. An abnormal or perverted craving for special or strange foods. SEE: *appetite, perverted; taste.*

parosmia (păr-ŏz'mē-ă) [" + *osme,* odor]. Any disorder or perversion of the sense of smell; a false sense of odors or perception of those that do not exist. Agreeable odors are considered offensive, and disagreeable ones are accepted as pleasant. SYN: *parosphresia.* SEE: *cacosmia; kakosmia.*

parosphresia, parosphresis (păr"ŏs-frē'zē-ă, -sĭs) [" + *osphresis,* smell]. Disordered sense of smell. SYN: *parosmia.*

parosteal (păr-ŏs'tē-ăl). Concerning the outermost layer of the periosteum.

parosteitis, parostitis (păr-ŏs-tē-ī'tĭs, -tī'tĭs) [Gr. *para,* beside, + *osteon,* bone, + *itis,* inflammation]. Inflammation of tissues next to the bone.

parosteosis, parostosis (păr"ŏs-tē-ō'sĭs, -tō'sĭs) [" + *osteon,* bone, + *osis,* condition]. 1. Bone formation outside of the periosteum. 2. Bone development in an unusual location.

parotic (pă-rŏt'ĭk) [" + *ous,* ear]. Near the ear.

parotid (pă-rŏt'ĭd). Located near the ear; esp. the parotid gland.

parotid duct. Approx. 2 in. (5.1 cm) long. Extends from anterior border of the parotid gland, crossing the masseter muscle and piercing the buccinator muscle, and then runs between the buccinator muscle and the mucous membrane. It opens into the mouth opposite the 2nd upper molar. The transverse facial artery is above the duct, and the buccal branch of the 7th cranial nerve is below. The duct transports secretions from the parotid gland to the oral cavity. Stenosis of the duct causes pain and swelling in the parotid gland. SYN: *Stensen's duct.* SEE: *saliva.*

parotidectomy (pă-rŏt"ĭ-dĕk'tō-mē) [" + *ous,* ear, + *ektome,* excision]. Excision of the parotid gland.

parotid gland. A nearly pure serous gland, its secreting tubules and acini being long and branched. It is enclosed in a sheath, the parotid fascia. It is one of the salivary glands of the mouth. The secretion helps to lubricate food and makes it easier to chew and swallow. SEE: *mumps.*

parotidoscirrhus (pă-rŏt"ĭd-ō-skĭr'ŭs) [" + " + *skirrhos,* hardness]. 1. Hardening of the parotid gland. 2. A scirrhous cancer of the parotid area.

parotitis (pă"rō-tī'tĭs) [" + *ous,* ear, + *itis,* inflammation]. Inflammation of the parotid gland.

parous (păr'ŭs) [L. *pario,* to bear]. Parturient; fruitful; having borne at least one child.

parovarian (păr-ō-vā'rē-ăn) [Gr. *para,* beside, + LL. *ovarium,* ovary]. 1. Situated near or beside the ovary. 2. Pert. to the parovarium, a residual structure in the broad ligament.

parovariotomy (păr"ō-vā"rē-ŏt'ō-mē) [" + " + Gr. *tome,* incision]. Removal of a parovarian cyst.

parovaritis (păr"ō-vă-rī'tĭs) [" + LL. *ovarium,* ovary, + Gr. *itis,* inflammation]. Inflammation of the epoophoron.

parovarium (păr"ō-vā'rē-ŭm). Lateral portion of the vestigial remains of the mesonephric tubules. Located in the mesosalpinx between the ovary and the fallopian tube. SYN: *epoophoron* [NA].

paroxysm (păr'ŏk-sizm) [Gr. *paroxysmos,* irritation]. 1. A sudden, periodic attack or recurrence of symptoms of a disease; an exacerbation of the symptoms of a disease. 2. A sudden spasm or convulsion of any kind. 3. Sudden emotional state, as of fear, grief, or joy.

paroxysmal (păr″ŏk-sĭz′măl). 1. Occurring in or concerning paroxysms. 2. Of the nature of a paroxysm.

paroxysmal cold hemoglobinuria. ABBR: PCH. A rare form of an acquired hemolytic syndrome that occurs idiopathically, in association with syphilis, or following viral or presumed viral diseases such as measles, mumps, chickenpox, infectious mononucleosis, and influenza.

SYM: Acute onset of back and extremity pain and abdominal cramps following chilling. Hemoglobinuria if sufficient numbers of red blood cells have been destroyed. Fever may be as high as 40°C (104°F).

TREAT: Therapy of primary disease; otherwise, protection from the cold is the only practical therapy in the idiopathic form. In general, once the cold exposure terminates, therapy is not needed.

paroxysmal nocturnal dyspnea. SEE: *dyspnea, paroxysmal nocturnal.*

parricide (păr′ĭ-sīd) [L. *parricida*]. The murdering of one's own parent or a close relative. SYN: *patricide.*

Parrot, Joseph Marie Jules (păr-ō′). French physician, 1829–1883.
  P.'s disease. 1. Osteochondritis that occurs in infants with congenital syphilis. 2. A form of dwarfism that is transmitted as an autosomal dominant.
  P.'s nodes. Bony nodules on the skull of infants with congenital syphilis. SYN: *P.'s sign.*
  P.'s pseudoparalysis. Pseudoparalysis caused by syphilitic osteochondritis.
  P.'s sign. P.'s nodes.
  P.'s ulcer. Lesions seen in thrush or stomatitis.

Parry's disease (păr′ēz) [Caleb H. Parry, Brit. physician, 1755–1822]. Hyperthyroidism.

pars (părz) [L.] (pl. *partes*). [NA] A part; portion of a larger structure.
  p. basilaris ossis occipitalis. [NA] Basilar process of the occipital bone.
  p. buccalis hypophyseos. Developmental protrusion in primitive buccal cavity of anterior lobe of hypophysis.
  p. caeca oculi. The optic disk.
  p. caeca retinae. The parts of the retina not sensitive to light (pars ciliaris retinae and pars iridica retinae).
  p. cephalica et cervicalis systematis autonomici. Cranial and cervical portion of autonomic nervous system.
  p. ciliaris retinae. [NA] Portion of the

retina situated in front of the ora serrata and covering the ciliary body.
  p. distalis adenohypophyseos. That part of the hypophysis forming the major portion of the anterior lobe. SEE: *pituitary gland.*
  p. flaccida membranae tympani. Portion of the membrane of the eardrum that fills the notch of Rivinus. This portion of the drum is not taut. SYN: *Shrapnell's membrane.*
  p. interarticularis. The region between the superior and inferior articulating facets of the vertebra. Region where fracture frequently occurs with spondylolysis.
  p. intermedia adenohypophyseos. The intermediate lobe of the hypophysis cerebri. SEE: *pituitary gland.*
  p. iridica retinae. [NA] Portion of the retina on the posterior surface of the iris.
  p. mastoidea ossis temporalis. The mastoid portion of the temporal bone.
  p. membranacea urethrae masculinae. The membranous portion of the urethra. It extends from the prostate to the bulb of the penis. SEE: *p. spongiosa urethrae masculinae.*
  p. nervosa hypophyseos. Posterior lobe of the pituitary gland.
  p. optica hypothalami. The optic chiasm.
  p. optica retinae. [NA] The sensory portion of the retina, extending from the optic disk to the ora serrata.
  p. petrosa ossis temporalis. The petrous portion of the temporal bone.
  p. plana corporis ciliaris. Ciliary ring of the eye.
  p. radiata lobuli corticalis renis. SEE: *ray, medullary.*
  p. spongiosa urethrae masculinae. [NA] Portion of the male urethra included from the point of entrance to the bulb of the penis to its termination at the end of the penis. The bulbourethral glands empty into it via their ducts just after the urethra passes the perineal membrane.
  p. squamosa ossis temporalis. The flat portion of the temporal bone that forms part of the lateral wall of the skull.
  p. tensa membranae tympani. The larger portion of the tympanic membrane, a tightly stretched membrane lying inferior to the malleolar folds. SEE: *p. flaccida membranae tympani.*
  p. tuberalis adenohypophyseos. Portion of the anterior lobe of the hypophysis cerebri that invests the infundibular stalk.
  p. tympanica ossis temporalis. The tympanic portion of the temporal bone.

pars planitis (părs plă-nī′tĭs). Inflammation of the peripheral retina characterized by aggregations of inflammatory cells on the anterior inferior retina. These are called "snowbanks." This chronic condition, which occurs mostly in the young, is of unknown etiology. It may cause loss of vision.

TREAT: Corticosteroids administered systemically or by injection behind the eye.

part. aeq. *partes aequales,* in equal parts.

partes (păr′tēs). Pl. of pars.

parthenogenesis (păr″thĕn-ō-jĕn′ĕ-sĭs) [Gr. *parthenos,* virgin, + *genesis,* generation, birth]. Reproduction arising from a female egg that has not been fertilized by the male; unisexual reproduction.

parthenophobia (păr″thĕ-nō-fō′bē-ă) [″ + *phobos,* fear]. Fear of virgins or girls.

participant observation. A method of field research whereby the investigator observes and records information about the characteristics of a setting through his or her experiences as a participant in that setting.

particle [L. *particula*]. 1. A very small piece or part of matter; a tiny fragment or trace. 2. One of several subatomic components of the nuclei of radioactive matter, such as alpha and beta particles. 3. Attraction particle or centriole, q.v., of the nucleus of a cell. 4. Viral particle or virion, q.v.

p., alpha. A charged particle emitted from a radioactive substance made up of a helium nucleus consisting of two protons and two electrons. The particle has very low penetrability.

p., beta. A high-speed electron emitted during the decay of an atom.

p., Dane. A very small, round particle present in the serum of some patients with viral hepatitis.

p., elementary. The subatomic parts of the atomic nucleus.

p., elementary, of the mitochondria. A surface particle on the mitochondrial cristae.

particulate (păr-tĭk′ū-lāt). Made up of particles.

parts per million. ABBR: PPM; ppm. Phrase used with a number to indicate the concentration of one substance with respect to another. For example, a chemical substance may be said to be present in air at a level of 50 parts per million (parts of air). The units also may be expressed as weight of one substance to the weight of another. This is called weight-to-weight comparison, or the concentration may be expressed as volume-to-volume.

parturient (păr-tū′rē-ĕnt) [L. *parturiens,* in labor]. Concerning childbirth or parturition; giving birth.

parturifacient (păr-tū-rĭ-fā′shĕnt) [″ + *facere,* to make]. 1. Inducing or accelerating labor. 2. Drug used to cause or hasten delivery of the fetus.

parturiometer (păr″tū-rē-ŏm′ĕ-tĕr) [″ + Gr. *metron,* measure]. A device for determining the force of uterine contractions during childbirth.

parturiphobia [″ + Gr. *phobos,* fear]. Fear of childbirth.

parturition (păr-tū-rĭsh′ŭn) [L. *parturitio*]. Act of giving birth to young. SYN: *childbirth; delivery.*

parturition, words pert. to: accouchement; accoucheur; accoucheuse; afterbirth; afterpains; amniocentesis; ante partum; axis traction; bag of waters; ballottement; bipara; bradytocia; breech presentation; cephalic version; cephalotomy; cesarean section; childbirth; dystocia; hourglass contraction; labor; maneuver; multipara; nullipara; obstetrics; oxytocia; parturient; parturifacient; partus; placenta; placenta previa; postpartum; puerperium; Rh; uterus.

part. vic. *partitis vicibus,* in divided doses.

parueresis. Difficulty initiating urination, esp. in the presence of strangers.

parulis (păr-ū′lĭs) [Gr. *para,* beside, + *oulon,* gum]. Abscess of a gum. SYN: *gumboil.*

parumbilical (păr″ŭm-bĭl′ĭ-kăl) [″ + L. *umbilicus,* navel]. Close to the navel.

paruria (păr-ū′rē-ă) [Gr. *para,* beside, + *ouron,* urine]. Any abnormality in discharge of urine.

parvicellular (păr-vĭ-sĕl′ū-lăr) [L. *parvus,* small, + *cellula,* little box]. Concerning, or composed of, tiny cells.

parvoline (păr′vō-lĭn). A ptomaine formed in decaying fish.

parvovirus (păr″vō-vī′rŭs) [″ + *virus,* poison]. A group of viruses similar to adeno-associated viruses. They are pathogenic in animals and humans. Parvovirus B-19 causes erythema infectiosum, q.v.

parvovirus B-19. The cause of a usually benign disease, erythema infectiosum or fifth disease, q.v. In immunocompromised patients, infection with this virus may cause aplastic anemia, and complications may lead to death.

parvule (păr′vūl) [L. *parvulus,* very small]. A small pill, pellet, or granule.

PAS, PASA. *para-aminosalicylic acid.*

pascal. A unit of pressure equal to the force of one newton acting uniformly over one square meter. SEE: *newton; SI Units* in *Appendix.*

Paschen bodies (pä′shĕn) [Enrique Paschen, Ger. pathologist, 1860–1936]. Particles thought to be the pathogenic virus of vaccinia and variola found in great numbers in skin exanthemas.

PASG. *pneumatic anti-shock garment.* SEE:

MAST.

passage (păs'ăj) [ME., to pass]. 1. A channel between cavities and body structures or with the external surface of an organ. 2. Act of passing. 3. An evacuation of the bowels. 4. Introduction of a probe or catheter. 5. Incubation of a pathogenic organism, esp. a virus, in one or a series of tissue cultures or living organisms.

passion (păsh'ŭn) [L. *passio*, suffering]. 1. Suffering. 2. Great emotion or zeal; frequently associated with sexual excitement.

passional (păsh'ŭn-ăl). Concerning any passion. SEE: *emotional.*

passive (păs'ĭv) [L. *passivus*, capable of suffering]. Submissive; acted upon; not active.

passive-aggressive type personality disorder. A personality disorder seen in persons who are dependent and lack self-confidence and who have no insight into the fact that their own actions cause this difficulty. The signs and symptoms include procrastination, irritability, sulkiness, slowness at work, unreasonable protests that others make demands on them, avoidance of obligations by claiming to have forgotten, having an unrealistic opinion of the high quality of their work, obstruction of the work of others by failing to do their share of the work, and constant criticism and demeaning of those in authority.

passive congestion. Congestion due to obstruction in venous return or, if general, due to myocardial insufficiency.

passive exercise. A therapeutic exercise technique used to move a patient's joints through a range of motion without any effort on the part of the patient. Accomplished by use of a machine, a therapist, or an assistant. SYN: *passive motion; passive movement.*

passive hyperemia. Increased blood in an area or part due to decreased outflow.

passive motion. Passive exercise.

passive movement. Passive exercise.

passive restraint device. A safety device used in automobiles to automatically restrain a person at the moment a crash occurs. This may be a seat belt or an air bag, q.v.

passive smoking. Breathing the smoke produced by persons smoking in one's immediate environment. This type of exposure to smoked tobacco is hazardous to the health of those exposed.

It is estimated that from 9 to 12 million children in the U.S. under the age of 5 are exposed to passive smoke.

passivism (păs'ĭ-vĭzm) [" + Gr. *-ismos*, condition]. 1. Passive behavior or character. 2. Sexual perversion with subjugation of the will to another.

passivity (păs-sĭv'ĭ-tē) [L. *passivus*, capable of suffering]. In psychiatry, the condition of being dependent on others and a reluctance to be assertive or to be responsible.

pasta. 1. Paste. 2. Any dough prepared from a mixture of flour and eggs and made into a great variety of forms. Originally of Italian origin.

paste. A semisolid gelatinous substance usually intended for external application. It may contain specific active ingredients or simple materials such as oils, waxes, and starch.

Pasteur, Louis (păs-stěr'). French chemist and bacteriologist, 1822–1895, who founded the science of microbiology. His greatest accomplishments were in the fields of bacteriology and immunology. He developed the technique of immunization and produced vaccines.

   P. effect. Inhibition of fermentation by bacteria when oxygen is abundant.

   P. treatment. Used for the prevention of rabies. Daily injection of increasingly virulent suspensions prepared from the brains or spinal cords of rabbits that have died of rabies. The treatment is continued for 21 days. Suspension is treated so as to kill or inactivate the virus. This treatment is no longer used but is presented for historical purposes. SEE: *rabies.*

Pasteurella (păs-těr-ěl'ă) [Louis Pasteur]. A genus of bacteria that at one time included the species *P. pestis, P. tularensis, P. multocida,* and *P. pseudotuberculosis. P. pestis,* the organism that causes plague, is now classed as *Yersinia pestis. P. tularensis,* the causative organism of tularemia, is now classed as *Francisella tularensis. P. pseudotuberculosis,* which can cause acute mesenteric lymphadenitis or enterocolitis, is now classed as *Yersinia pseudotuberculosis.*

   P. canis. Previous name for *P. multocida.*

   P. multocida. A small nonmotile gram-negative coccobacillus that can cause disease in animals and humans. The infection may be transmitted to humans by animal bites. In other cases the organism can cause cellulitis, abscesses, osteomyelitis, pneumonia, peritonitis, or meningitis.

   TREAT: Penicillin.

pasteurellosis (păs"těr-ě-lō'sĭs). Disease caused by infection with bacteria of the genus *Pasteurella.*

pasteurization (păs"tūr-ĭ-zā'shŭn) [Louis Pasteur]. The process of heating a fluid at a moderate temperature for a definite period of time in order to destroy undesirable bacteria without changing to any extent its chemical composition.

In pasteurization of milk, pathogenic bacteria are destroyed by heating at 62°C for 30 minutes, or by "flash" heating to higher temperatures for less than 1 minute. The pasteurization process, reducing total bacterial count of the milk by 97% to 99%, is effective because the common milk-borne pathogens (tubercle bacillus, and *Salmonella*, *Streptococcus*, and *Brucella* organisms) do not form spores and are quite sensitive to heat. However, pasteurization should not be considered a substitute for hygienic practices in milk production. SEE: *milk*.

pastille (păs-tĕl′, -tĭl′) [L. *pastillus*, a little roll]. 1. A medicated disk used for local action on the mucosa of the throat and mouth. SYN: *lozenge; troche.* 2. A small cone used to fumigate or scent the air of a room.

past-pointing. Term used to describe the inability to place finger or some other part of the body accurately on a selected point. Seen in certain neurologic disorders.

PAT. *paroxysmal atrial tachycardia.*

patagia (pă-tā′jē-ă) [L.]. Pl. of patagium.

patagium (pă-tā′jē-ŭm) [L.] (pl. *patagia*). A weblike membrane. SEE: *pterygium*.

patch (păch) [ME. *pacche*]. A small circumscribed area distinct from surrounding surface in character and appearance.

   p., cotton-wool. The appearance of exudative areas in the retina. Usually seen in connection with hypertensive retinopathy.

   p., herald. Solitary oval patch of efflorescence showing before the general eruption of pityriasis rosea, often several days before.

   p., Hutchinson's. Salmon-yellow area seen on cornea in syphilitic keratitis.

   p., mucous. A syphilitic eruption having an eroded, moist surface; generally on mucous membrane of mouth or external genitals, or on surface subject to moisture and heat.

   p., opaline. White patch in mouth sometimes present in syphilis.

   p., Peyer's. Aggregation of lymph nodules found in the mucosal and submucosal layers of the small intestine. SEE: *Peyer's patch; typhoid fever.*

   p., salmon. Salmon-colored area of cornea seen in interstitial keratitis due to syphilis.

   p., smoker's. Leukoplakia of the oral mucosa.

   p., soldier's. SEE: *spot, milk.*

   p., white. A white, thickened area of oral mucosa that will not rub off and represents a benign hyperkeratosis. SYN: *leukoplakia.*

patch test. SEE: *test, patch.*

patefaction (păt″ĕ-făk′shŭn) [L. *patefacere*, to lay open]. A laying open.

patella (pă-tĕl′ă) [L., a small pan] (pl. *patellae*). [NA] A lens-shaped sesamoid bone sit-

uated in front of the knee in the tendon of the quadriceps femoris muscle. SYN: *kneecap.* SEE: *osteochondritis dissecans.*

   p. alta. A high-riding patella (high positioning of patella). When a person is standing, the patella rests in a more superior position than normal.

   p. baja. A low-riding patella (low positioning of patella). When a person is standing, the patella rests in a more inferior position than normal.

   p., bipartite. Bipartite patella, q.v.

   p., floating. Patella that rides up from the condyles due to a large effusion in the knee.

   p., fracture of. TREAT: Suture of bone fragments. A plaster cast is applied from the toes to the groin, remaining on for 6 to 8 weeks. Following removal of cast, gradual exercise and weight upon the leg for a few weeks, after which the patient may walk.

   p., rider's painful. Tenderness and pain in patella from horseback riding.

   p., squinting. A disorder in which the patella appears to be pointing inward when the patient is standing. This is caused by excessive femoral anteversion.

patellapexy (pă-tĕl′ă-pĕk″sē) [L. *patella*, small pan, + Gr. *pexis*, fixation]. Fixation of the patella to the lower end of the femur to stabilize the joint.

patellar (pă-tĕl′ăr). Concerning the patella.

patellar ligament. The ligamentous continuation of the tendon of the quadriceps muscle of the thigh to extend beyond the distal portion of the patella to attach to the tuberosity of the tibia.

patellar reflex. Involuntary jerk of leg due to sudden spasm of quadriceps muscle following percussion of patellar ligament. SYN: *knee-jerk reflex.* SEE: *Jendrassik's maneuver.*

patellectomy (păt″ĕ-lĕk′tō-mē) [″ + Gr. *ektome*, excision]. Surgical removal of the patella.

patelliform (pă-tĕl′ĭ-form) [″ + *forma*, shape]. Shaped like the patella.

patellofemoral (pă-tĕl″ō-fĕm′ō-răl). Concerning the patella and femur.

patellometer (păt″ĕ-lŏm′ĕ-tĕr) [″ + Gr. *metron*, measure]. Device for measuring the patellar reflex.

patency (pā′tĕn-sē) [L. *patens*, open]. The state of being freely open.

patent (păt′ĕnt, pā′tĕnt). Wide open; evident; accessible.

patent ductus arteriosus. Persistence of a communication between the main pulmonary artery and the aorta, after birth.

   The condition of patent and persistent ductus arteriosus in preterm infants has been treated successfully by using drugs, such as indomethacin, that inhibit prostaglandin synthesis. SEE: *prostaglandins.*

patent medicine. A drug or medical preparation that is protected by patent and sold without a physician's prescription. The law requires that it be labeled with names of active ingredients, the quantity or proportion of the contents, and directions for its use, and that it not have misleading statements as to curative effects on the label. This term is rarely used. SEE: *nonproprietary name; prescription; proprietary medicine.*

paternal (pă-tĕr′năl) [L. *paternis,* fatherly]. Of, pert. to, or inherited from the father.

paternity analysis. SEE: *paternity test.*

paternity test. Because paternity is a clinical estimate, there is the need to have tests to determine whether it would be possible for an individual to have fathered a specific child. At one time, the tests used to prove or exclude the possibility of paternity utilized blood type data from the child and the suspected father. Tests involving the technique of molecular genetic fingerprinting and of determining genetic markers are available and have the ability to exclude almost all non-fathers. Use of these techniques makes it possible to distinguish differences between the genotype of all individuals except identical twins. SYN: *paternity analysis.*

path. A particular course that is followed or traversed. SEE: *pathway.*

p., condyle. Path traversed by the condyle during various mandibular movements.

p., incisor. Arc described by the incisal edge of the lower incisors when the mandible closes to normal occlusion.

p. of closure. Path traversed by the mandible as it closes when its neuromuscular mechanisms are in a balanced functional state.

path-, patho- [Gr. *pathos,* disease, suffering]. Combining form indicating disease or suffering.

pathetic (pă-thĕt′ĭk) [L. *patheticus*]. 1. Pert. to, or arousing, the emotions of pity, sympathy, or tenderness. 2. Pert. to trochlear nerve.

pathfinder [AS. *paeth,* road, + *findan,* to locate]. 1. Instrument for locating stricture of the urethra. 2. Dental instrument for tracing the course of root canals.

-pathic (pă′thĭk). Combining form concerning disease or suffering.

Pathilon. Trade name for tridihexethyl chloride.

pathoamine (păth″ō-ăm′ĭn). A toxic ptomaine.

pathoanatomy (păth″ō-ă-năt′ō-mē). Anatomical pathology.

pathobiology (păth″ō-bī-ŏl′ō-jē). Pathology.

Pathocil. Trade name for dicloxacillin sodium.

pathoclisis (păth″ō-klĭs′ĭs). A specific tendency to be sensitive to certain toxins.

pathocrine (păth′ō-krĭn, -krēn, -krĭn) [Gr. *pathos,* disease, suffering, + *krinein,* to secrete]. Concerning an endocrine disorder.

pathodontia (păth″ō-dŏn′shē-ă) [″ + *odous* tooth]. The science of dental pathology.

pathogen (păth′ō-jĕn) [″ + *gennan,* to produce]. A microorganism or substance capable of producing a disease.

p., opportunistic. SEE: *opportunistic infections.*

pathogenesis (păth″ō-jĕn′ĕ-sĭs). Origin and development of a disease.

pathogenetic, pathogenic (păth″ō-jĕn-ĕt′ĭk, -jĕn′ĭk). Productive of disease. SYN: *morbific.*

pathogenicity (păth″ō-jĕ-nĭs′ĭ-tē) [″ + *gennan,* to produce]. The state of producing or being able to produce pathological changes and disease.

pathogeny (păth-ŏj′ĕn-ē). Origin and development of a disease. SYN: *pathogenesis.*

pathognomonic (păth″ŏg-nō-mŏn′ĭk) [Gr. *pathognomonikos,* skilled in diagnosing]. Indicative of a disease, esp. its characteristic symptoms.

pathognomy (păth-ŏg′nō-mē) [Gr. *pathos,* disease, suffering, + *gnome,* a means of knowing]. Diagnosing the cause of an illness after careful study of the signs and symptoms of a disease.

pathognostic (păth″ŏg-nŏs′tĭk) [″ + *gnosis,* knowledge]. Pathognomonic, q.v.

pathography (păth-ŏg′ră-fē) [″ + *graphein,* to write]. A narrative description of disease, esp. one written by a person who experiences the disease.

pathologic, pathological (păth-ō-lŏj′ĭk, -ĭ-kăl) [Gr. *pathos,* disease, suffering, + *logos,* word, reason]. 1. Concerning pathology. 2. Diseased; due to a disease. SYN: *morbid.*

pathological reaction to alcohol. An exceedingly severe reaction to ingestion of alcohol, esp. to small amounts. Manifested by irrational violent behavior followed by exhaustion, sleep, and loss of recall of the event. Patient may not be intoxicated. SEE: *alcoholism.*

ETIOL: Unknown but is associated with hypoglycemia, exhaustion, and stress.

pathologist (pă-thŏl′ō-jĭst) [″ + *logos,* word, reason]. A specialist in diagnosing the abnormal changes in tissues removed at operations and postmortem examinations.

pathology (pă-thŏl′ō-jē) [Gr. *pathos,* disease, suffering, + *logos,* word, reason]. 1. Study of the nature and cause of disease, which involves changes in structure and function. 2. Condition produced by disease.

p., anatomic. Field of pathology that deals with structural changes in disease.

p., cellular. Pathology based upon microscopic changes in body cells produced by disease.

p., chemical. Study of chemical changes that occur in disease.

p., clinical. Pathology as it is used to aid in the diagnosis of disease and care for patients.

p., comparative. The observation of pathological condition, spontaneous or artificial, in the lower animals or in vegetable organisms as compared with those of the human body.

p., dental. The science of diseases of the mouth.

p., experimental. Study of diseases induced artificially and intentionally, esp. in animals.

p., functional. Study of alterations of functions that occur in disease processes without associated structural changes.

p., geographical. Pathology in its relationship to climate and geography.

p., humoral. Pathology of the fluids of the body.

p., medical. Pathology of disorders that are not accessible for surgical procedures.

p., molecular. Study of the pathological effects of specific molecules.

p., oral. P., dental, q.v.

p., special. Pathology of particular diseases or organs.

p., surgical. Application of pathological procedures and techniques for investigating tissues removed surgically.

pathomimesis (păth″ō-mĭm-ē′sĭs) [Gr. *pathos*, disease, suffering, + *mimesis*, imitation]. Intentional (conscious or unconscious) imitation of a disease. SYN: *malingering; pathomimicry.*

pathomimicry (păth″ō-mĭm′ĭ-krē). Pathomimesis.

pathomorphism (păth″ō-mor′fĭzm) [″ + *morphe*, form, + *-ismos*, condition]. Study of abnormal form and structure of organisms.

pathonomia (păth-ō-nō′mē-ă) [″ + *nomos*, law]. Study of the laws of disease processes.

pathophobia (păth-ō-fō′bē-ă) [″ + *phobos*, fear]. Morbid fear of disease.

pathophysiology (păth″ō-fĭz″ē-ŏl′ō-jē) [″ + *physis*, nature, + *logos*, word, reason]. Study of how normal physiological processes are altered by disease.

pathopsychology (păth″ō-sī-kŏl′ō-jē) [″ + *psyche*, soul, + *logos*, word, reason]. The branch of psychology dealing with mental processes during disease.

pathway. 1. A path or a course; more specifically, a pathway formed by neurons (cell bodies and their processes) over which impulses pass from their point of origin to their destination. 2. A chemical or metabolic pathway; the various chemical reactions that occur in metabolism as specific substances are absorbed, metabolized, and altered as they undergo biotransformation in the body.

p., afferent. Pathway leading from a receptor to the spinal cord and/or brain.

p., biosynthetic. The chemical and metabolic events that lead to the formation of substances in the body.

p., central. Pathway within the brain or spinal cord.

p., conduction. A group of fibers in a nerve, spinal cord, or brain over which impulses are conducted.

p., efferent. Pathway from the central nervous system to an effector.

p., Embden-Myerhof. The anaerobic series of enzymatic reactions involved in the metabolism of glucose to form lactic acid, and to produce adenosine triphosphate, which releases energy for muscular and other cellular activity.

p., metabolic. The sequence of chemical reactions that occur as a substance is metabolized.

p., motor. Pathway over which motor impulses are conveyed from a motor center to muscles.

p. of incidence. Path of a penetrating foreign object from the point of entry into the body to the point where it stops; e.g., path of a bullet from where it enters the body to where it lodges.

p., pentose phosphate. Pathway of glucose metabolism in tissues during which five-carbon sugars are formed. SYN: *hexose monophosphate shunt.*

p., sensory. Pathway over which sensory impulses are conveyed from sense organs or receptors to sensory or reflex centers of the spinal cord or brain.

-pathy. Combining form used as a suffix indicating illness, disease, or suffering.

patient (pā′shĕnt) [L. *patiens*]. 1. One who is sick with, or being treated for, an illness or injury. 2. An individual receiving medical care. Included are persons with no demonstrable illness who are being investigated for signs of insidious pathology such as altered blood chemical values or physical changes such as asymptomatic cardiovascular abnormalities.

patient advocate. A person who acts to ensure that a patient is served adequately by the health care system.

patient-controlled analgesia. ABBR: PCA. A drug administration method that permits the patient to control the rate of drug delivery for the control of pain. It is usually accomplished by the use of an infusion pump. The patient must have complete understanding of the system and be willing to use it. It is essential that the system be designed so that the patient will be unable to administer an overdose of the analgesic; also, as with all narcotics, the system has to be designed to prevent its theft.

patient day. The basic unit for calculating the cost of keeping a patient in a hospital for one day.

patient delay. Delay on the part of the patient in seeking medical attention; or delay in taking prescribed medicines or advice.

patient dumping. SEE: *dumping.*

patient mix. The numbers and types of patients served by a hospital or other health program.

patricide (păt′rĭ-sīd) [L. *patricida*]. Parricide.

Patrick's test (păt′riks) [Hugh Talbot Patrick, U.S. neurologist, 1860–1939]. A test for arthritis of the hip. The thigh and knee of the supine patient are flexed, and the external malleolus of the ankle is placed over the patella of the opposite leg. The test is positive if depression of the knee produces pain.

patrilineal (păt-rĕ-lĭn′ē-ăl) [L. *pater,* father, + *linea,* line]. Tracing descent through the father.

patten (păt′ĕn) [Fr. *patin,* wooden shoe]. Support applied under one shoe as part of the treatment for hip disease or unequal length of the legs. The device may be attached to a leg caliper.

pattern. 1. A design, figure, model, or example. 2. In psychology, a set or arrangement of ideas or behavior reactions.

   p., occlusal. The appearance and anatomic location of the occluding surfaces of teeth.

   p., trabecular. The arrangement of the trabeculae of bone in relation to marrow spaces.

   p., wax. A molded or carved pattern in wax used extensively in dentistry and jewelry-making whereby casts are made using the lost wax technique.

   p., wear. The location of tooth wear as determined by the wear characteristics of the facets of the teeth.

patterning. A therapeutic method used in treating children and adults with brain damage. The patient is guided through movements such as creeping or crawling, based on the theory that undamaged sections of the brain will develop the ability to perform these functions.

patulous (păt′ū-lŭs) [L. *patulus*]. Open, dis-

tended, spread apart. SYN: *patent.*

pauciarticular. A classification of juvenile rheumatoid arthritis that indicates that four or fewer joints are affected at the time of onset of the disease.

Paul-Bunnell test [John R. Paul, U.S. physician, 1893–1971; Walls W. Bunnell, U.S. physician, b. 1902]. Test for heterophil antibodies in the serum of patients thought to have infectious mononucleosis.

pause [ME.]. An interruption; a temporary cessation of activity.

   p., compensatory. The long interval following an extrasystole, so called because its duration is such that the next beat occurs at the exact time of the succeeding normal beat.

Pavabid. Trade name for papaverine hydrochloride.

pavementing. Condition occurring during inflammation in which leukocytes adhere to the linings of capillaries.

Pavlik harness. A device used to stabilize the hip in neonates with congenital hip dislocation.

Pavlov, Ivan Petrovich (păv′lŏv). Russian physiologist, 1849–1936; winner of Nobel prize in medicine in 1904. He is remembered particularly for his work on conditioned response. SEE: *reflex, conditioned.*

pavor (pā′vor) [L.]. Anxiety, dread.

   p. diurnus. Attacks of terror or fright during the day, esp. in children.

   p. nocturnus. Night terror during sleep in children and the aged.

Pavulon. Trade name for pancuronium bromide.

P.B. *Pharmacopoeia Britannica,* British pharmacopeia.

Pb [L. *plumbum*]. Chem. symb. for the element lead.

PBI. *protein-bound iodine.*

P.B.W. *posterior bitewing* in dentistry.

PBZ. *pyribenzamine.*

p.c. L. *post cibum,* after a meal.

PCG. *phonocardiogram.*

pCO$_2$. Symb. for *partial pressure of carbon dioxide.*

PCV. *packed cell volume.*

Pd. Chem. symb. for the element palladium.

p.d. *prism diopter; pupilla diameter; pupillary distance.*

PDA. *patent ductus arteriosus.*

PDR. *Physicians' Desk Reference.*

peanut oil. A refined oil obtained from the seed kernels of one or more of the cultivated varieties of *Arachis hypogaea.* May be used as a solvent for some medicines that are injected intramuscularly.

pearl [ME. *perle*]. 1. Small, tough mass in sputum in asthma. 2. Small capsule containing a medicinal fluid for inhalation. Capsule is crushed in handkerchief and inhaled. 3. Small mass of cells.

p.'s, enamel. Small rounded globules of highly mineralized material seen near or attached to the enamel margin or furcation of the tooth roots. These are formed by aberrant ameloblasts and hypermineralization.

p., epithelial. Concentric squamous epithelial cells in carcinoma.

p., gouty. Sodium urate concretion on cartilage of the ear seen in people with gout.

p., Laënnec's. A mucous cast of the bronchus or bronchiole sometimes present in the sputum of asthmatic patients.

pearly penile papules. Asymptomatic white papules with a pink, white, or pearly surface on the dorsum of the penis of blacks and uncircumcised men. No treatment is indicated, just reassurance.

peau d'orange (pō″dō-ränj′) [Fr., orange skin]. Dimpled skin condition that resembles an orange. Seen in lymphatic edema, and may be present over the area of carcinoma of the breast.

peccant (pĕk′änt) [L. *peccans*, sinning]. 1. Corrupt; producing disease. 2. Sinning, or violating a law. SYN: *morbid; pathogenic; unhealthy*.

peccatiphobia (pĕk″ät-ĭ-fō′bē-ă) [″ + Gr. *phobos*, fear]. Abnormal fear of sinning.

pecilo-. SEE: words beginning with *poikilo-*.

pecten (pĕk′tĕn) [L., comb] (pl. *pectines*). 1. A comblike organ. 2. The pubic bone. 3. Middle portion of the anal canal.

p. ossis pubis. [NA] A sharp ridge on the superior ramus of the pubis that forms the pubic portion of the terminal (iliopectineal) line.

pectenosis (pĕk″tĕ-nō′sĭs) [″ + Gr. *osis*, condition]. Narrowing of the anal canal.

pectic acid (pĕk′tĭk) [Gr. *pektos*, congealed]. An acid derived from pectin by hydrolyzing the methyl ester group and found in many fruits.

pectin (pĕk′tĭn) [Gr. *pektos*, congealed]. USP. Purified carbohydrate obtained from peel of citrus fruits, or from apple pulp. When pectin is cooked with sugar at the proper pH, a gel forms. SEE: *pectose*.

pectinase (pĕk′tĭ-nās). An enzyme that catalyzes the formation of sugars and galacturonic acid from pectin.

pectinate (pĕk′tĭ-nāt) [L. *pecten*, comb]. Having teeth like a comb. SYN: *pectiniform*.

pectineal (pĕk-tĭn′ē-ăl). Rel. to the os pubis or the pectineal muscle.

pectineal line. The line or ridge on the os pubis separating the true from the false pelvis.

pectineus (pĕk-tĭn-ē′ŭs) [L. *pecten*, comb]. A flat quadrangular muscle at the upper and inner part of the thigh, arising from the superior ramus of pubis and inserted between the lesser trochanter and linea aspera of the femur, which flexes and adducts the thigh. SEE: *Muscles* in *Appendix*.

pectiniform (pĕk-tĭn′ĭ-form) [″ + *forma*, shape]. Toothed like a comb. SYN: *pectinate*.

pectization (pĕk-tĭ-zā′shŭn) [Gr. *pektos*, congealed]. In colloidal chemistry, the conversion of a substance from sol to gel state.

pectora (pĕk′tor-ă) [L.]. Pl. of pectus.

pectoral (pĕk′tō-răl) [L. *pectoralis*]. 1. Concerning the chest. 2. Efficacious in relieving chest conditions, as a cough.

pectoralgia (pĕk″tō-răl′jē-ă) [L. *pectoralis*, chest, + Gr. *algos*, pain]. Neuralgic pain in the chest.

pectoralis (pĕk″tō-rā′lĭs) [L.]. 1. Pert. to the breast or chest. 2. One of four muscles of the anterior upper portion of the chest.

p. major. A large triangular muscle that extends from the anterior chest wall to the humerus and functions to flex, horizontally adduct, and internally rotate the arm, and aids in chest expansion when the upper extremities are stabilized.

p. minor. A muscle beneath the pectoralis major, attached to the coracoid process of the scapula that depresses as well as causes anterior tipping of the scapula.

pectoriloquy (pĕk″tō-rĭl′ō-kwē) [L. *pectoralis*, chest, + *loqui*, to speak]. The distinct transmission of vocal sounds to the ear through the chest wall in auscultation, q.v. The words seem to emanate from the spot that is auscultated. Heard over cavities that communicate with a bronchus and areas of consolidation near a large bronchus, over pneumothorax when the opening in the lung is patulous, and over some pleural effusions. SYN: *pectorophony*. SEE: *chest*.

p., aphonic. In auscultation, whispered sound heard over a lung with a cavity or pleural effusion.

p., whispering. Sound heard over a lung with a cavity of limited extent when patient whispers, in auscultation of the chest.

pectorophony (pĕk″tō-rŏf′ō-nē) [″ + Gr. *phone*, voice]. Exaggeration of vocal sounds heard on auscultation of the chest. SYN: *pectoriloquy*.

pectose (pĕk′tōs) [Gr. *pektos*, congealed]. A substance found in some fruits and vegetables. It yields pectin when boiled.

pectunculus (pĕk-tŭn′kū-lŭs) [L., little comb]. One of the tiny longitudinal ridges on the sylvian aqueduct of the brain.

pectus (pĕk′tŭs) [L.] (pl. *pectora*). [NA] The chest, breast, or thorax.

p. carinatum. Abnormal prominence of the sternum. SYN: *chicken breast; pigeon* breast.

p. excavatum. Congenital condition in which sternum is abnormally depressed. SYN: *funnel breast.*

p. recurvatum. P. excavatum, q.v.

ped- [L.]. Combining form denoting foot.

pedal (pĕd'l) [L. *pedalis*]. Concerning the foot.

pedal spasm. Involuntary contractions of the muscles of the feet.

pedarthrocace (pē″där-thrŏk'ă-sē) [Gr. *paidos,* child, + *arthron,* joint, + *kakos,* bad]. Carious condition of joints of children.

pedatrophy (pē-dăt'rō-fē) [Gr. *pais,* child, + *atrophia,* want of nourishment]. 1. Marasmus. 2. Any wasting disease in children. 3. Tabes mesenterica.

pederast (pĕd'ĕr-ăst) [Gr. *paiderastes,* a lover of boys]. A male who indulges in anal intercourse with young boys.

pederasty (pĕd'ĕr-ăs″tē). Anal intercourse between a man and a young boy.

pedes (pē'dēz). Pl. of pes.

pedesis (pē-dē'sĭs) [Gr., leaping]. The incessant dancing or to-and-fro movements of particles in a colloidal system or of minute particles of any substance in a liquid or gaseous medium. SYN: *brownian movement.* SEE: *diapedesis.*

pedi- (pĕd'ĭ) [L. *pedalis*]. Combining form denoting foot.

pedia- [Gr. *pais,* child]. Combining form denoting relationship to a child.

Pediaflor. Trade name for sodium fluoride.

pedialgia (pĕd-ē-ăl'jē-ă, pē-dē-) [Gr. *pedion,* foot, + *algos,* pain]. Pain of the foot.

Pediamycin. Trade name for erythromycin ethylsuccinate.

pediatric (pē-dē-ăt'rĭk) [Gr. *pais,* child, + *iatreia,* treatment]. Concerning the treatment of children.

pediatric advanced life support. ABBR: PALS. The treatment measures, including basic and advanced life support, needed to stabilize a critically ill or injured child.

pediatrician (pē-dē-ă-trĭsh'ăn) [″ + *iatrikos,* healing]. A specialist in treatment of children's diseases. SYN: *pediatrist.*

Pediatric Nurse Practitioner. A registered nurse who provides primary health care to children. Special preparation is required. Abbreviation is P.N.P. and is used after one's name, e.g., Jane Grey, R.N., P.N.P.

pediatrics (pē-dē-ăt'rĭks) [Gr. *pais,* child, + *iatreia,* treatment]. Medical science relating to care of children and treatment of their diseases. SYN: *pediatry.*

pediatric trauma score. ABBR: PTS. A method for scoring and quantifying the severity of trauma in pediatric patients. SYN: *revised trauma score.*

pediatrist (pē″dē-ăt'rĭst) [″ + *iatrikos,*

healing]. Physician who specializes in treatment of children's diseases. SYN: *pediatrician.*

pediatry (pĕd″ē-ăt'rē, pē'dē-ăt″rē). The treatment of children's diseases. SYN: *pediatrics.*

pedicel (pĕd'ĭ-sĕl). 1. Foot process or footplate. 2. A secondary process of a podocyte that in conjunction with other podocytes helps form the visceral capsule of a renal corpuscle.

pedicellation (pĕd″ĭ-sĕl-ā'shŭn) [L. *pediculus,* a little foot; stalk]. Formation and development of a pedicle.

pedicle (pĕd'ĭ-k'l). 1. The stem that attaches a new growth. 2. The bony process that projects backward from the body of a vertebra, connecting with the lamina on each side. Forms the root of the vertebral arch. SYN: *peduncle.*

pedicle flap. In plastic surgery, a type of flap that is attached by a pedicle to its source of blood supply. The other end may be attached to a site from which a new blood supply will develop. This permits the eventual severance of the original pedicle, so the flap may be moved step by step to where it is needed in the plastic surgical procedure.

pedicterus (pē-dĭk'tĕr-ŭs) [Gr. *pais,* child, + *ikteros,* jaundice]. Jaundice of the newborn. SYN: *icterus neonatorum.*

pedicular (pē-dĭk'ū-lar). 1. [L. *pediculus,* a louse] Infested with or concerning lice. 2. [L. *pediculus,* a little foot] Concerning a stalk or stem.

pediculate (pē-dĭk'ū-lāt) [L. *pediculus,* a little foot]. Having a pedicle or stem. SYN: *pedunculate.*

pediculation (pē-dĭk″ū-lā'shŭn) [L. *pediculatio*]. 1. Infestation with lice. 2. Development of a pedicle.

pediculicide (pē-dĭk'ū-lĭ-sīd) [L. *pediculus,* a louse, + *caedere,* to kill]. Destroying, or that which destroys, lice.

Pediculidae. A family of lice belonging to the order Anoplura. Includes the species parasitic on primates including humans. SEE: *Pediculus.*

pediculophobia (pē-dĭk″ū-lō-fō'bē-ă) [″ + Gr. *phobein,* to fear]. Abnormal dread of lice. SYN: *phthiriophobia.*

pediculosis (pē-dĭk″ū-lō'sĭs) [″ + Gr. *osis,* condition]. Lousiness; infestation with lice. SEE: *Pediculus.*

p. capitis. Pediculosis due to infestation with the head louse, *Pediculus humanus capitis.* Transmission is by personal contact or common use of brushes, combs, or headgear.

SYM: Itching and eczematous dermatitis. In long-standing, neglected cases, scratching may result in marked inflammation and secondary infection by bacteria may occur with formation of pustules, crusts, and suppuration. Hair may become matted and malodorous.

TREAT: Shampoo the hair, dry it, and apply 25 to 50 ml of 1% permethrin creme or enough to wet the hair and scalp. Leave on the head for 10 minutes, and rinse off with clear water; or apply 1% gamma benzene hexachloride to the scalp or affected areas once each day for 2 days. Repeat this in 10 days to destroy nits that may have survived. All possible sources of infection should be examined and treated if necessary. Headgear, combs, and brushes should be disinfected by heat or use of disinfection solutions. If lice have infested the eyelashes and eyelids, the lice will have to be removed with forceps.

p. corporis. Pediculosis due to infestation with body louse, *Pediculus humanus corporis,* q.v. Transmitted by direct contact or use of infested wearing apparel. Occurs as a result of crowding or unhygienic conditions.

SYM: Intense itching. In heavy infestations there is generalized red skin eruption, mild fever, tiredness, irritability, and in severe cases, weakness and debility.

TREAT: As for pediculosis capitis, q.v. In addition, clothing and bedding should be sterilized by dry heat (140°F or 60°C for 5 min), by hot water (075°F or 65.6°C for 5 min), or by dry cleaning.

p. palpebrarum. Infestation by lice of the eyebrows and eyelashes.

p. pubis. Pediculosis due to infestation with the crab louse, *Phthirus pubis,* q.v. Generally confined to hairs of genital region but hair of the axilla, eyebrows, eyelashes, beard, and in hairy individuals body surface may be involved. Lice may be acquired through personal contact, by wearing contaminated clothing, from toilet seats, or from bed clothes. For treatment, SEE: *p. capitis.*

SYM: Itching and irritation of the external genital area (not introital), esp. the mons. The pubic louse bite produces in light-skinned individuals blue- or slate-colored macules that do not blanch when pressure is applied.

p. vestimenti. Infestation by lice of the clothing.

pediculous (pĕ-dĭk'ū-lŭs). Infested with lice.

Pediculus (pĕ-dĭk'ū-lŭs). A genus of parasitic insects commonly called lice that infest humans and other primates. Lice are sucking insects belonging to the family Pediculidae, order Anoplura. They are of medical importance in that they are the transmitters of the causative organisms of epidemic typhus, trench fever, and relapsing fever.

They may serve as mechanical transmitters of bubonic plague and possibly other diseases.

P. humanus capitis. The head louse that lives in fine hair of the head, although beard and eyebrows may be infested. Its eggs, commonly called nits, are glued to hairs and frequently form nests in the vicinity of the ears. Cause of pediculosis capitis, q.v.

P. humanus corporis. The body louse that inhabits the seams of clothing worn next to the body and feeds on regions of the body covered by that clothing. Eggs are attached to fibers of the clothing. The cause of pediculosis corporis, q.v.

pediculus (pē-dĭk'ū-lŭs) [L.] (pl. *pediculi*). 1. A little foot. 2. Louse. SEE: *Pediculus.*

pedicure (pĕd'ĭ-kūr) [L. *pes,* foot, + *cura,* care]. 1. Care of the feet. 2. Cosmetic care of the feet and toenails. 3. A podiatrist.

pediform (pĕd'ĭ-form) [" + *forma,* shape]. Having the shape of a foot.

pedigree. A chart, diagram, or table of an individual's ancestors used in human genetics in the analysis of mendelian inheritance.

pedionalgia (pē"dē-ō-năl'jē-ă) [Gr. *pedion,* metatarsus, + *algos,* pain]. Neuralgic pain in the sole of the foot.

pediophobia (pē"dē-ō-fō'bē-ă) [Gr. *pais,* child, + *phobos,* fear]. Unnatural dread of young children or of dolls.

pediphalanx (pĕd"ĭ-fā'lănks) [L. *pes,* foot, + Gr. *phalanx,* closely knit row]. Phalanx of the foot. SEE: *maniphalanx.*

pedobaromacrometer (pē"dō-băr"ō-mă-krŏm'ĕ-tĕr) [Gr. *pais,* child, + *baros,* weight, + *makros,* long, + *metron,* measure]. Apparatus for determining measurement and weight of infants.

pedodontia, pedodontics (pē"dō-dŏn'shē-ă, -tĭks) [Gr. *pais,* child, + *odous,* tooth]. Phase of dentistry dealing with care of children's teeth.

pedodontist (pē"dō-dŏn'tĭst). Dentist who specializes in care of children's teeth.

pedodynamometer (pĕd"ō-dī-nă-mŏm'ĕ-tĕr) [L. *pes,* foot, + Gr. *dynamis,* power, + *metron,* measure]. Device for measuring the strength of the leg muscles.

pedograph (pĕd'ō-grăf) [" + Gr. *graphein,* to write]. Imprint of the foot on paper.

pedologist (pē-dŏl'ō-jĭst) [Gr. *pais,* child, + *logos,* word, reason]. One who has made a study of children and their development.

pedology (pē-dŏl'ō-jē). The study of children and their development.

pedometer. 1. (pĕd'ĕ-tĕr) [Gr. *pais,* child, + *metron,* measure] Device for measurement of infants. 2. (pĕd-ŏm'ĕ-tĕr) [L. *pes,* foot, + Gr. *metron,* measurement] Instrument that indicates number of steps taken while walking.

pedomorphism (pē″dō-mor′fĭzm) [Gr. *pais*, child, + *morphe*, form, + *-ismos*, condition]. Retention of juvenile characteristics in the adult.

pedophilia (pē″dō-fĭl′ē-ă) [″ + *philein*, to love]. 1. Fondness for children. 2. In psychology, an unnatural desire for sexual relations with children.

peduncle (pĕ-dŭn′kl) [L. *pedunculus*, a little foot]. 1. A stem or stalk. SYN: *pedicle*. 2. A brachium of the brain; a band connecting parts of the brain. SYN: *pedunculus*. SEE: *cimbia; crus; sessile*.

p., cerebellar, inferior. A band of fibers running along the lateral border of the 4th ventricle, connecting spinal cord and medulla with the cerebellum. SYN: *restiform body*.

p., cerebellar, middle. A band of fibers connecting cerebellum with basilar portion of the pons. SYN: *brachium pontis*.

p., cerebellar, superior. A band of fibers connecting cerebellum with midbrain. SYN: *brachium conjunctivum*.

p., cerebral. A pair of white bundles from upper part of the pons to the cerebrum. It constitutes the ventral portion of the midbrain. SYN: *crus cerebri*.

p., mamillary. A band of fibers extending from tegmentum of midbrain to mamillary body.

p. of flocculus. A band of fibers connecting flocculus of cerebellum with vermis.

p. of superior olive. A slender band of fibers extending from the superior olivary nucleus in the medulla to the nucleus of the abducens nerve.

p., olfactory. The long stalk of the olfactory bulb.

p., pineal. A band from either side of the pineal gland to the anterior pillars of the fornix.

p., thalamic. One of four groups of fibers known as thalamic radiations which connect thalamus with the cerebral cortex. SEE: *radiation, thalamic*.

peduncular (pĕ-dŭn′kū-lăr) [L. *pedunculus*, a little foot]. Concerning a peduncle.

pedunculate, pedunculated (pĕ-dŭn′kū-lāt, -ĕd). Possessing a stalk or peduncle. SYN: *pediculate*.

pedunculotomy (pĕ-dŭng″kū-lŏt′ō-mē) [″ + Gr. *tome*, incision]. Surgical section of a cerebral peduncle. This is done in treating involuntary movement disorders.

pedunculus (pĕ-dŭng′kū-lŭs) [L.]. Peduncle.

peeling [ME. *pelen*, to peel]. Shedding of surface layer of skin. SYN: *desquamation*.

peeling, chemical. Chemicals applied to skin to produce a mild, superficial burn. Done to remove wrinkles.

peenash (pē′năsh) [Indian]. Rhinitis due to insect larvae in the nose.

PEEP. *positive end-expiratory pressure*.

peer (pēr). 1. [ME.] One who has an equal standing with another in age, class, or rank. 2. To observe closely.

peer review. The evaluation of the quality of the work effort of an individual by his or her peers. It could involve evaluation of articles submitted for publication or the quality of medical care administered by an individual, group, or hospital.

peg, rete. SEE: *rete ridge*.

Pegademase. Trade name for adenosine deaminase conjugated with polyethylene glycol.

Peganone. Trade name for ethotoin.

peg tooth. An abnormally shaped tooth of genetic origin. Usually noted as a maxillary lateral incisor with a smaller cone-shaped crown.

pejorative (pĭ-jor′ă-tĭv, pē″jă-rā′tĭv) [L. *pejor*, worse]. 1. Tending to become or make worse. 2. Being disparaging or belittling, e.g.,in making a less than flattering remark about something or someone. SEE: *honorific*.

PEL. *permissible exposure limits*.

pelade (pĕl-ăd′) [Fr., to remove hair]. Loss of body hair in patchy areas. SYN: *alopecia areata*.

pelage (pĕl′ĭj) [Fr.]. The collective hair of the body.

Pel-Ebstein fever [Pieter K. Pel, Dutch physician, 1852–1919; Wilhelm Ebstein, Ger. physician, 1836–1912]. Cyclic fever occurring in Hodgkin's disease in which periods of fever lasting from 3 to 10 days are separated by an afebrile period of about the same length.

Pelger-Huët anomaly (pĕl″jĕr hū′ĕt) [Karel Pelger, Dutch physician, 1885–1931; Gauthier Jean Huët, Dutch physician, 1879–1970]. Granulocytes of the blood with rodlike, dumbbell, peanut-shaped, and spectacle-like nuclei. The chromatin of the nuclei is unusually coarse. The condition is inherited as a non-sex-linked dominant. The cells function in a normal manner and carriers have no demonstrably lowered resistance to infection.

pelioma (pē-lē-ō′mă) [Gr.]. A livid cutaneous patch. SYN: *ecchymosis*.

peliosis (pē-lē-ō′sĭs) [Gr.]. A disease marked by purple patches on the mucous membranes and skin. SYN: *purpura*.

SYM: Sore throat, urticaria, moderate fever, and purpuric spots over extremities or trunk. Tenderness, swelling, and pain in joints.

p. hepatis. The presence of blood-filled lakes in the body of the liver. The condition may be associated with use of oral contraceptive drugs or anabolic steroids. It has also been reported in patients with human immunodeficiency virus infection.

pellagra (pĕl-ă′gră, pĕ-lăg′ră) [L. *pellis*, skin, + Gr. *agra*, rough]. A deficiency disease or syndrome endemic in certain parts of the world, characterized by cutaneous, gastrointestinal, mucosal, neurologic, and mental symptoms.

SYM: In advanced cases, scarlet stomatitis and glossitis, diarrhea, dermatitis, and central nervous system involvement. Cutaneous lesions include erythema followed by vesiculation, crusting, and desquamation. Skin may become dry, scaly, and atrophic. The mucous membranes of mouth, esophagus, and vagina may undergo atrophy; ulcers and cysts may develop. Anemia is common. Nausea, vomiting, and diarrhea occur, the last being characteristic. Involvement of the central nervous system is first manifested by neurasthenia, followed by organic psychosis characterized by disorientation, impairment of memory, and confusion. Later, delirium and clouding of consciousness may occur.

ETIOL: Due to deficiency in diet or failure of body to absorb niacin (nicotinic acid) or its amide (niacinamide, nicotinamide). Usually associated with a deficiency of tryptophan-containing proteins, such as occurs in a high-corn diet. Pellagra may occur secondary to gastrointestinal diseases or alcoholism.

TREAT: A diet adequate in all vitamins, minerals, and amino acids supplemented by 500 to 1000 mg of niacinamide given orally three times daily. If there is any doubt about the ability of the intestinal tract to absorb vitamins, the vitamins should be given parenterally.

pellagrazein (pĕl-ă-grā′zē-ĭn). Poisonous substance in decomposed cornmeal. At one time was regarded erroneously as the cause of pellagra.

pellagrin (pĕ-lā′grĭn, -lăg′rĭn). A person afflicted with pellagra.

pellagroid (pĕ-lăg′royd, -lăg′royd) [L. *pellis*, skin, + Gr. *agra*, rough, + *eidos*, form, shape]. Resembling pellagra.

pellagrous (pĕ-lā′grŭs, -lăg′rŭs). Concerning or affected with pellagra.

Pellegrini's disease, Pellegrini-Stieda disease (pĕl″ă-grē′nē-stē′dă) [Augusto Pellegrini, It. surgeon, b. 1877; Alfred Stieda, Ger. surgeon, 1869–1945]. Following trauma, ossification of the superior portion of the medial collateral ligament of the knee.

pellet (pĕl′ĕt) [Fr. *pelote*, a ball]. A tiny pill or small ball of medicine or food.

p., cotton. A small rolled cotton ball, less than ⅜ inch (about 1 cm) in diameter, used

for desiccation or topical application of medicaments, particularly in dentistry. Also called pledgets.

p., foil. Loosely rolled gold foil used for direct filling in dental restoration. SEE: *foil.*

pellicle (pĕl′ĭ-k'l) [L. *pellicula*, a little skin]. 1. A thin piece of cuticle or skin. 2. Film or surface on a liquid. 3. A thin nonliving sheath forming the surface layer of certain one-celled animals. SYN: *scum.*

p., salivary. The thin layer of salivary proteins and glycoproteins that quickly adhere to the tooth surface after the tooth has been cleaned; this amorphous, bacteria-free layer may serve as an attachment medium for bacteria, which in turn form plaque. SYN: *acquired pellicle.*

pellucid (pĕl-lū′sĭd) [L. *pellucidus*]. Translucent; transparent.

pellucid zone. Clear layer covering the oocyte. SYN: *zona pellucida.*

pelotherapy (pĕ″lō-thĕr′ă-pē) [Gr. *pelos*, mud, + *therapeia*, treatment]. Therapeutic use of mud, peat, moss, or clay applied to all or part of the body.

pelvic (pĕl′vĭk) [L. *pelvis*, basin]. Pert. to a pelvis, usually the bony pelvis.

pelvic bone. Os coxae, which is the hip bone. This includes the ilium, ischium, and pubis.

pelvic diameter. Any one of several diameters of the pelvis. SEE: *diameter of pelvis.*

pelvicephalography (pĕl″vē-sĕf″ă-lŏg′ră-fē) [″ + Gr. *kephale*, head, + *graphein*, to write]. X-ray study and measurement of the fetal head and the pelvic outlet.

pelvicephalometry (pĕl″vē-sĕf″ă-lŏm′ĕ-trē) [″ + ″ + *metron*, measure]. Measurement of the diameters of the fetal head and comparison of these with the diameters of the maternal pelvis.

pelvic examination. Physical examination of the vagina and adjacent organs by palpation by means of fingers of one hand placed intravaginally. The other hand is placed on the abdominal wall, and tissues between the fingers of the two hands may be palpated. This is called a bimanual examination. Visual examination of the vagina and cervix is made by use of a speculum inserted intravaginally.

pelvic girdle. Arch made by the innominate bones.

pelvic inflammatory disease. ABBR: PID. Ascending infection from the vagina or cervix to the uterus, fallopian tubes, and broad ligaments. SEE: *Nursing Diagnoses* in *Appendix.*

SYM: A mucopurulent vaginal discharge caused by cervicitis; there may be associated dysuria, due to urethritis; anorectal pain and bleeding due to proctitis are sometimes present; the abdominal pain may be in the midline, or bilateral in the lower abdominal area; when salpingitis is present, the pain and tenderness are severe and usually accompanied by nausea and vomiting.

ETIOL: Almost any bacterium may cause PID, but the most frequent agents are *Neisseria gonorrhoeae* and *Chlamydia trachomatis*.

DIAG: History of previous PID or of sexual intercourse with a man with urethritis; insertion of an IUD; abortion; childbirth; fever and increased white blood count; severe pain during pelvic examination when the cervix is moved or the adnexa are moved; and lower genital tract infection as evidenced by the preponderance of white blood cells in the vaginal fluid. Laparoscopy and ultrasonography may also be useful in making the diagnosis. PID must be distinguished from ectopic pregnancy and other pelvic disease, esp. surgical emergencies such as acute appendicitis.

PREVENT: SEE: *safe sex*.

TREAT: Early therapy with appropriate antibiotics is important if subsequent infertility due to occlusion of the fallopian tubes by adhesions is to be prevented. Pelvic and tubal abscesses may need to be drained but may subside with conservative therapy. All sexual partners should be examined for evidence of sexually transmitted diseases and, if positive, treated with the appropriate antibiotic. PID patients should be followed for several days after discontinuation of therapy to be certain that they are cured as judged by culture of the cervix and vagina.

pelvic inlet. Upper pelvic entrance between the sacral promontory and the superior aspect of the symphysis pubis.

pelvic outlet. Lower pelvic opening between the tip of the coccyx, the ischial tuberosities, and the lower margin of the symphysis pubis.

pelvic pain, chronic idiopathic. Unexplained pelvic pain in the female that persists for more than 2 to 6 months. It is essential that a complete medical, social, and sexual history be obtained. In an experimental study, women with this illness reported a higher number of sexual partners, having had significantly more spontaneous abortions, having undergone previous nongynecologic surgery, and were more likely to have experienced previous significant psychosexual trauma.

TREAT: If medical management fails to alleviate the condition, presacral neurectomy may be of benefit.

pelvic relaxation. Diminished support of the pelvic tissues and organs, esp. in the female. This is usually due to childbirth or aging. The organs affected and the pathological conditions associated with the relaxation are bladder and cystocele; rectum and rectocele; uterus and uterine prolapse; small intestine with production of enterocele; urethra with protrusion of urethra into the vagina. Symptoms are related to the organ(s) affected. Treatment is determined by the severity of the relaxation. Surgery may be required.

pelvifixation (pĕl″vē-fĭk-sā′shŭn) [″ + *fixatio*, fixation]. Surgical stabilization of loose pelvic organs.

pelvilithotomy (pĕl″vĭ-lĭ-thŏt′ō-mē) [″ + Gr. *lithos*, stone, + *tome*, incision]. Surgical removal of a stone from the renal pelvis. SYN: *nephrolithotomy; pelviolithotomy; pyelolithotomy.*

pelvimeter (pĕl-vĭm′ĕ-tĕr) [″ + Gr. *metron*, measure]. Device for measuring the pelvis.

pelvimetry (pĕl-vĭm′ĕ-trē). Measurement of the pelvic dimensions or proportions. Helps determine whether or not it will be possible to deliver a fetus through the normal route. Done by various methods including manual or x-ray. SEE: *pelvis*.

pelviolithotomy (pĕl″vē-ō-lĭ-thŏt′ō-mē) [L. *pelvis*, basin, + Gr. *lithos*, stone, + *tome*, incision]. Incision of the renal pelvis to remove a calculus.

pelvioplasty (pĕl″vē-ō-plăs′tē) [″ + Gr. *plassein*, to form]. 1. Enlargement of the pelvic outlet to facilitate childbirth. SYN: *pelviotomy* (def. 1); *pubiotomy; symphysiotomy.* 2. Plastic surgical procedure on the pelvis of the kidney.

pelvioscopy (pĕl″vē-ŏs′kō-pē) [L. *pelvis*, basin, + Gr. *skopein*, to examine]. Inspection of the pelvis.

pelviotomy (pĕl-vē-ŏt′ō-mē) [″ + Gr. *tome*, incision]. 1. Enlargement of the pelvic outlet to facilitate childbirth. 2. Incision of the renal pelvis. Usually done in order to remove a calculus.

pelviperitonitis (pĕl″vĭ-pĕr-ĭ-tō-nī′tĭs) [″ + Gr. *peritonaion*, peritoneum, + *itis*, inflammation]. Inflammation of the peritoneum lining the pelvic cavity.

pelvirectal (pĕl″vē-rĕk′tăl) [″ + *rectum*, straight]. Concerning the pelvis and rectum.

pelvis (pĕl′vĭs) [L., basin] (pl. *pelves*). 1. [NA] Any basin-shaped structure or cavity. 2. The bony structure formed by the innominate bones, the sacrum, the coccyx, and the ligaments uniting them. The structure serves as a support for the vertebral column and for articulation with the lower limbs. SEE: illus. 3. The cavity included within the innominate bones, the sacrum, and the coccyx.

ANAT: The pelvis is separated into a false or superior pelvis and a true or inferior

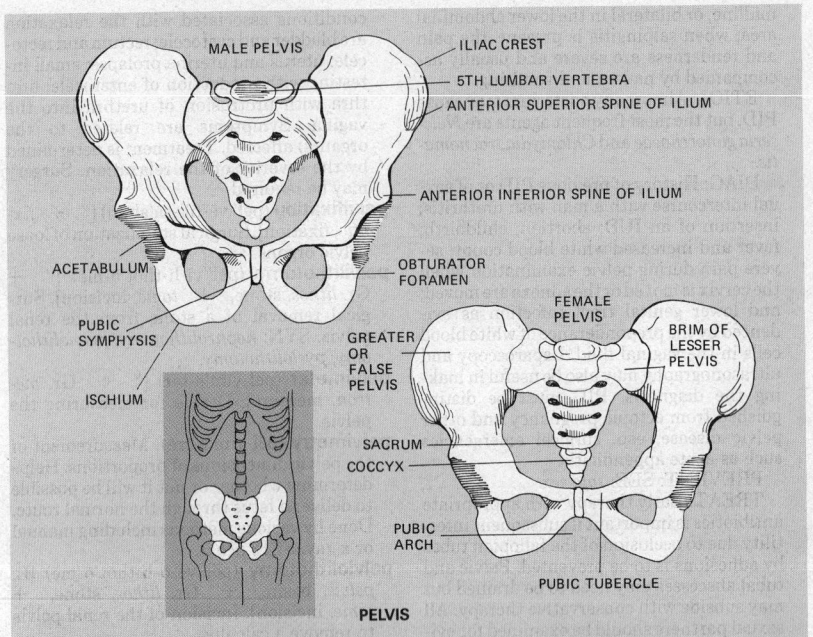

PELVIS

pelvis by the iliopectineal line and the upper margin of the symphysis pubis. The circumference of this area constitutes the inlet of the true pelvis. The lower border of the true pelvis, termed the outlet, is formed by the coccyx, the protuberances of the ischia, the ascending rami of the ischia, and the descending rami of the ossa pubis and the sacrosciatic ligaments. The floor of the pelvis is formed by the perineal fascia, the levator ani, and the coccygeus muscles. All diameters normally are larger in the female than in the male.

EXTERNAL DIAMETERS: *Interspinous:* Distance between outer edges of the anterosuperior iliac spines, diameter normally measuring 26 cm (10¼ in.). *Intercristal:* Distance between outer edges of the most prominent portion of the iliac crests, diameter normally being 28 cm (11 in.). *Intertrochanteric:* Distance between most prominent points of the femoral trochanters, 32 cm (12½ in.). *Oblique* (right and left): Distance from one posterosuperior iliac spine to the opposite anterosuperior iliac spine, 22 cm (8½ in.), right being slightly greater than the left. *External conjugate:* Distance from the undersurface of the spinous process of last lumbar vertebra

to the upper margin of anterior surface of the symphysis pubis, 20 cm (7⅞ in.). SYN: *Baudelocque's diameter.*

INTERNAL DIAMETERS: *True conjugate:* Anteroposterior diameter of the pelvic inlet, 11 cm (4¼ in.), the most important single diameter of the pelvis. *Diagonal conjugate:* Distance between the promontory of the sacrum to undersurface of symphysis pubis, 13 cm (5⅛ in.). Two cm (¾ in.) is deducted for the height and inclination of symphysis pubis to obtain diameter of conjugate. *Transverse:* Distance between ischial tuberosities, 11 cm (4¼ in.). *Anteroposterior* (of outlet): Distance between the lower border of symphysis pubis and tip of sacrum, 11 cm (4¼ in.). *Anterior sagittal:* Distance from undersurface of symphysis pubis to center of line between the ischial tuberosities, 7 cm (2¾ in.). *Posterior sagittal:* Distance from the center of line between ischial tuberosities to the tip of the sacrum, 10 cm (4 in.).

RS: acanthopelvis; brim; cavity, pelvic; Claudius' fossa; conjugate diameter of pelvis; endopelvic fasciae; pelvic; "pelvi-" words; sacrum; symphysis pubis.

p. aequabiliter justo major. Pelvis that is symmetrically larger than the standard in all its dimensions. SYN: *pelvis, giant.*

p. aequabiliter justo minor. Pelvis with all its dimensions uniformly smaller than the standard. SYN: *p., reduced.*

p., android. A female pelvis that resembles that of a male. SYN: *p., masculine.*

p., anthropoid. A female pelvis that is long and narrow.

p., assimilation. Abnormal pelvis in which the transverse processes of the last lumbar vertebra are fused with the sacrum, or the last sacral vertebra is fused with the coccyx.

p., beaked. Pelvis with the pelvic bones laterally compressed and pushed forward so that the outlet is narrow and long. SYN: *p., rostrate; p., triradiate.*

p., brachypellic. An oval pelvis in which the transverse diameter is at least 1 cm longer, but no more than 3 cm longer, than the anteroposterior diameter of the pelvis.

p., brim of. Inlet of pelvis. SEE: *brim* (def. 2).

p., contracted. Pelvis in which one or more of the principal diameters is reduced to a degree that parturition is impeded.

p., cordate. Pelvis possessing a heart-shaped inlet.

p., coxalgic. Pelvis deformed subsequent to hip joint disease.

p., dolichopellic. An abnormal pelvis in which the anteroposterior diameter is greater than the transverse diameter.

p., dwarf. An aequabiliter justo minor pelvis, reduced in all its diameters and resembling an infantile pelvis. Bones usually united by cartilage. SYN: *p. nana.*

p., elastic. P., osteomalacic.

p., extrarenal. When there is obstruction of the uteropelvic junction of the ureter, the renal pelvis may be outside the kidney.

p., false. Portion above the iliopectineal line. SYN: *p. major.*

p. fissa. P., split.

p., fissured. A rachitic pelvis with ilia pushed forward so as to be almost parallel.

p., flat. Pelvis in which the anteroposterior diameters are shortened.

p., frozen. Fixation of the pelvic organs in the pelvis due to infection or neoplastic infiltration.

p., funnel-shaped. Pelvis in which the outlet is considerably contracted but the inlet dimensions are normal.

p., giant. P. aequabiliter justo major.

p., gynecoid. The normal female pelvis.

p., halisteretic. Deformed pelvis resulting from softening of bones.

p., infantile. An adult pelvis that retains its infantile characteristics.

p. justo major. An unusually large pelvis.

p. justo minor. An unusually small pelvis.

p., juvenile. P., infantile.

p., Kilian's. P., osteomalacic.

p., kyphoscoliotic. Deformed pelvis due to rickets.

p., kyphotic. Deformed pelvis characterized by increase of the conjugate diameter at the brim with reduction of the transverse diameter at the outlet.

p., large. P. justo major.

p., lordotic. Deformed pelvis in which the spinal column has an anterior curvature in the lumbar region.

p. major. [NA] P., false.

p., malacosteon. P., rachitic.

p., masculine. A female pelvis that resembles a male pelvis, esp. in that it is narrower, more conical, and heavier-boned and has a heart-shaped inlet. SYN: *p., android.*

p., mesatipellic. P., round.

p. minor. [NA] P. justo minor.

p., Naegele's. An obliquely contracted pelvis in which the conjugate diameter assumes an oblique direction.

p. nana. P., dwarf.

p. obtecta. Deformed pelvis in which the vertebral column extends across the pelvic inlet.

p., osteomalacic. Pelvis distorted as a consequence of osteomalacia, q.v. SYN: *p., elastic; p., rubber.*

p., Otto. Pelvis in which the acetabulum is depressed. This allows the head of the femur to extend into the pelvis.

p. plana. P., flat.

p., platypellic. Pelvis in which there are short anteroposterior and wide transverse diameters.

p., Prague. P., spondylolisthetic.

p., pseudo-osteomalacic. A rachitic pelvis similar to that of a person with osteomalacia.

p., rachitic. Pelvis deformed from rickets. SYN: *p., malacosteon.*

p., reduced. P., aequabiliter justo minor.

p., renal. [NA] The expanded proximal end of the ureter. It lies within the renal sinus of the kidney and receives the urine through the major calyces.

p., reniform. Pelvis shaped like a kidney.

p., Robert's. Pelvis with an embryonic sacrum and narrowing of the transverse and oblique diameters.

p., Rokitansky. P., spondylolisthetic.

p., rostrate. P., beaked.

p. rotunda. A tympanic depression in the inner wall, at the bottom of which is the fenestra rotunda.

p., round. Pelvis with a circular inlet.

p., rubber. P., osteomalacic.

p., scoliotic. Deformed pelvis resulting from spinal curvature.

p., simple flat. Pelvis with a shortened anteroposterior diameter.

p., small. P. justo minor.

p. spinosa. A rachitic pelvis with a pointed pubic crest.

p., split. Pelvis with a congenital division at the symphysis pubis.

p., spondylolisthetic. Pelvis in which the last lumbar vertebra is dislocated in front of the sacrum, causing occlusion of the brim.

p. spuria. P. justo major.

p., triangular. Pelvis whose inlet is triangular.

p., triradiate. P., beaked.

p., true. The part of the pelvis below the iliopectineal line.

pelvitherm (pĕl′vĭ-thĕrm) [L. *pelvis,* basin, + Gr. *therme,* heat]. Device for applying heat to the pelvis through the vagina.

pelvoscopy (pĕl-vŏs′kō-pē) [″ + Gr. *skopein,* to examine]. Inspection of pelvis.

pelvospondylitis (pĕl″vō-spŏn″dĭ-lī′tĭs) [″ + Gr. *spondylos,* vertebra, + *itis,* inflammation]. Inflammation of the pelvic portion of the spine.

p. ossificans. Rheumatoid spondylitis.

pemoline (pĕm′ō-lĕn). USP. A central nervous system stimulating drug that is used in treating children with hyperkinesis and minimal brain damage. Trade name is Cylert.

pemphigoid (pĕm′fĭ-goyd) [Gr. *pemphigodes,* breaking out in blisters]. A skin condition similar to pemphigus.

p., bullous. A chronic bullous eruption over many sites. In contrast to pemphigus, the lesions, though large and leaving denuded areas when they burst, do heal. It is rarely fatal.

    TREAT: Corticosteroids and immunosuppressive agents.

pemphigus (pĕm′fĭ-gŭs) [Gr. *pemphix,* a blister]. An acute or chronic autoimmune disease principally of adults, but occurring sometimes in children, characterized by occurrence of successive crops of bullae that appear suddenly on apparently normal skin and disappear, leaving pigmented spots. A characteristic sign is a positive Nikolsky sign: when pressure is applied to an area as if trying to push the skin parallel to the surface, the skin will detach from the lower layers.

p., erythematous. Scaling, erythematous macules and blebs of the scalp, face, and trunk. The lesions have a "butterfly" distribution over the face. The disease resembles pemphigus foliaceus.

p. foliaceus. Pemphigus with a chronic course and in which bullous lesions may be absent. Once lesions develop, they may spread to the entire body and mimic generalized exfoliative dermatitis. The positive Nikolsky sign helps to make the correct diagnosis.

p. vegetans. A form of pemphigus vulgaris characterized by pustules instead of bullae. Pustules are followed by warty vegetations. Prognosis, even prior to therapy with corticosteroids, has been good.

p. vulgaris. The most common form of pemphigus. Lesions develop suddenly and are round or oval, thin-walled, tense, and translucent with contents bilateral in distribution. The lesions have little tendency to heal and bleed easily when they burst. Since the introduction of corticosteroids, the prognosis is favorable, but the mortality rate is still high. Immunosuppressive agents are used with corticosteroid therapy. SEE: *photochemotherapy.*

Pen A/N. Trade name for ampicillin sodium.

Penapar VK. Trade name for penicillin V potassium.

pencil. A material rolled into cylindrical form. May contain a caustic substance or a therapeutic paste or ointment.

pendular (pĕn′dū-lĕr) [L. *pendulus*]. Hanging so as to swing by an attached part; oscillating like a pendulum.

pendulous (pĕn′dū-lŭs). Swinging freely like a pendulum; hanging.

penetrance. 1. The frequency of manifestation of a hereditary condition in individuals. In theory, if the genotype is present, penetrance should be 100%. That is not usually the case, and the cause is attributed to the modifying effects of other genes. 2. The extent to which something enters an object.

penetrate (pĕn′ĕ-trāt) [L. *penetrare*]. To enter or force into the interior; pierce.

penetrating (pĕn′ĕ-trāt-ĭng). Entering beyond the exterior.

penetrating power. Penetrating capacity of a lens.

penetrating wound. Wound entering the interior of an organ or cavity.

penetration (pĕn″ĕ-trā′shŭn) [L. *penetrare,* to go within]. 1. Process of entering within a part. 2. Capacity to enter within a part. 3. Power of a lens to give a clear focus at varying depths. 4. Ability of radiation to pass through a substance.

penetrometer (pĕn″ĕ-trŏm′ĕ-tĕr) [″ + Gr. *metron,* measure]. An instrument that compares roughly the comparative absorption of roentgen rays in various metals, esp. silver, lead, and aluminum; hence, it gives a rough estimation of the ability of x-rays to penetrate tissues. SYN: *qualimeter.*

-penia (pē′nē-ă) [Gr. *penia,* lack]. Combining

form indicating a decrease from normal, or a deficiency.

penicillamine (pĕn″ĭ-sĭl′ă-mēn). USP. A hydrolytic degradation product of penicillin. It is used to treat copper, mercury, zinc, or lead poisoning. It promotes the urinary excretion of these metals. Trade names are Cuprimine and Depen.

penicillic acid. $C_8H_{10}O_4$. An antibiotic produced by some species of *Penicillium*.

penicillin (pĕn-ĭ-sĭl′ĭn). One of a group of antibiotics biosynthesized by several species of molds, esp. *Penicillium notatum* and *P. chrysogenum*. Penicillin is bactericidal, inhibiting the growth of most gram-positive bacteria and certain gram-negative forms. It is effective also against certain molds, spirochetes, and rickettsiae. There are many different penicillins, including synthetic ones, and their effectiveness varies for different organisms. SEE: *penicillin allergy or sensitivity.*

p., beta-lactamase resistant. Synthetic penicillins that resist the action of the enzyme beta-lactamase, produced by some organisms. Bacteria that produce the enzyme are not susceptible to the action of non-beta-lactamase resistant penicillins.

p. G benzathine. USP. An antibiotic of the penicillin class. It is available in a variety of dosage forms. It is used orally and parenterally. Trade names are Bicillin L-A and Permapen.

p. V potassium. USP. An antibiotic of the penicillin class. It is relatively stable in an acid medium and is therefore not inactivated by gastric acid when taken orally. Trade names are Ledercillin VK, Pfizerpen VK, Robincillin-VK, SK-Penicillin VK, Uticillin VK, and V-Cillin K.

penicillin allergy or sensitivity. Penicillin frequently causes allergy. If anaphylaxis occurs, immediate therapy with subcutaneous epinephrine is indicated. If the allergic response is not acute and penicillin therapy is needed to treat infection with a life-threatening organism for which no alternative antibiotic is available, it is possible to desensitize the patient by giving very small doses by mouth in gradually increasing doses. This should be done by a clinician experienced in this technique and with the materials needed to treat anaphylaxis.

penicillinase (pĕn-ĭ-sĭl′ĭ-nās). A bacterial enzyme that inactivates most but not all penicillins.

penicillinase-producing Neisseria gonorrhoeae. ABBR: PPNG. Penicillin-resistant strains of *Neisseria gonorrhoeae*.

penicilliosis (pĕn″ĭ-sĭl″ē-ō′sĭs) [L. *penicillum*, brush, + *osis*, condition]. Infection with the fungi of the genus *Penicillium*.

Penicillium (pĕn″ĭ-sĭl′ē-ŭm) [L. *penicillum*, brush]. A genus of molds belonging to the Ascomycetes (sac fungi). They form the blue molds that grow on fruits, bread, and cheese. A number of species *(P. chrysogenum, P. notatum)* are the source of penicillin. Occasionally in humans they produce infections of the external ear, skin, or respiratory passageways. They are common allergens.

penicilloyl-polylysine (pĕn″ĭ-sĭl′oyl-pŏl″ĕ-lī′sēn). A substance used to determine sensitivity to some forms of penicillin. When it is injected intradermally into a sensitive individual, a wheal appears within 20 minutes.

penicillus (pĕn″ĭ-sĭl′ŭs) [L., paint brush] (pl. *penicilli*). [NA] A group of the branches of arteries in the spleen that are arranged like the bristles of a brush. Each consists of successive portions: the pulp arteries, sheathed arteries, and terminal arteries.

penile (pē′nĭl, -nīl) [L. *penis*, penis]. Pert. to the penis. SEE: *penile prosthesis.*

penile prosthesis. Device implanted in the penis that assists it to become erect. The device is used in patients with impotence due to such organic causes as trauma, postprostatectomy, or diabetes. It is usually in the form of inflatable plastic cylinders implanted in each corpus cavernosum of the penis. These cylinders are attached to a pump embedded in the scrotal pouch. A reservoir for the fluid used to fill the cylinders is implanted behind the rectus muscle. This system allows the cylinders to be filled when an erection is desired and the fluid to be drained back into the reservoir when the need for the erection has passed. In most patients, this device permits the attaining of a nearly physiologic erection. SEE: *Peyronie's disease.*

penile reflex. 1. Sudden downward movement of penis when the prepuce or gland of a completely relaxed penis is pulled upward. 2. Contraction of bulbocavernous muscle on percussing dorsum of penis. 3. Contraction of bulbocavernous muscle resulting from compression of glans penis.

penile ring. A ring made of metal, plastic, or leather. When placed around the flaccid penis, it is small enough to prevent venous return. Use of the device assists in causing and maintaining erection of the penis and delaying orgasm. In practice the ring is removed prior to the penis becoming so large that it is impossible to remove. If this is not done, the ring has to be cut off to prevent gangrene of the penis.

penis (pē′nĭs) [L.] (pl. *penises* or *penes*). [NA] The male organ of copulation and, in mammals, urination. It is a cylindrical pendulous organ suspended from the front and sides of

PENIS, INCLUDING TESTICLES AND SCROTUM

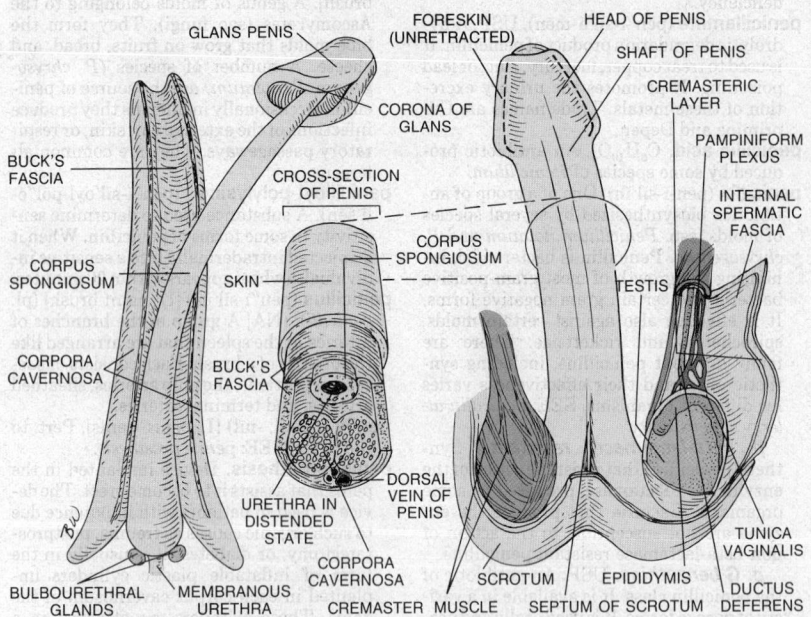

the pubic arch. It is homologous to the clitoris in the female. Contrary to popular myths, the size of the normal penis has no physical bearing on the male's or female's enjoyment of sexual intercourse.

ANAT: The penis is composed mainly of erectile tissue arranged in three columns, the whole being covered with skin. The two lateral columns are the corpora cavernosa penis. The third or median column, known as the corpus spongiosum, contains the urethra. The body is attached to the descending portion of the pubic bone or the crura of the penis. The cone-shaped head of the penis, the glans penis, contains the urethral orifice. It is covered with a movable hood known as the foreskin or prepuce, under which is secreted the substance called smegma.

Hyperemia of the genitals fills the corpora cavernosa with blood as the result of sexual excitement or stimulation, thus causing an erection. The hyperemia subsides following orgasm and ejaculation of the seminal fluid. The organ then returns to its flaccid condition. The size of the flaccid penis does not necessarily correlate with that of the erect penis. SEE: illus., *circumcision; pearly penile papules; penile prosthesis;*

Peyronie's disease; priapism.

   p. captivus. During sexual intercourse, the locking of a couple together due to the penis being entrapped in the vagina. Even though this is quite common in dogs, the evidence that it occurs in human beings for more than a few moments, if ever, is lacking.

   p., clubbed. Condition in which the penis is curved during erection.

   p., double. A congenital deformity in which the penis in the embryo is completely divided by the urethral groove.

   p. lunatus. Painful curved erection in gonorrhea. SYN: *chordee.*

   p. palmatus. Penis enclosed by the scrotum.

   p., webbed. P. palmatus.

penis, words pert. to: balanitis; cavernitis; cavernosum; chordee, circumcision; condyloma; cord, spermatic; corpus cavernosum; Cowper's glands; ductus deferens; epispadias; erection; foreskin; frenulum preputii; genitalia, male; gonorrhea; hypospadia; nervus erigens; pearly penile papules; penile prosthesis; peotillomania; Peyronie's disease; prepuce; priapism; prostate; scrotum; seminal vesicle; smegma; testes; Tyson's glands; urethra; vas deferens; "balano-" and "phall-" words.

penischisis (pě-nǐs′kǐ-sǐs) [L. *penis*, penis, + Gr. *schisis*, a splitting]. Epispadias, hypospadias, paraspadias, or any fissured condition of the penis.

penis envy. In psychoanalysis, the female's desire to have a penis. The validity of this concept is controversial.

penitis (pě-nī′tǐs) [″ + Gr. *itis*, inflammation]. Inflammation of the penis.

pennate (pěn′āt) [L. *penna*, feather]. An object in which parts extend at an angle from a central portion, as the barbs do from a feather.

penniform (pěn′ǐ-form) [″ + *forma*, shape]. Feather-shaped.

pennyroyal (pěn′ǐ-roy′ǎl). Name for various plants, esp. those of the genera *Hedeoma* and *Mentha*, that yield commercial oil used as a carminative and stimulant.

pennyweight. Troy weight containing 24 grains or 1/20 of a troy ounce. Equal to 1.555 grams. Commonly used for describing the quantities of precious metals, as the amount of gold needed for dental restorations.

penoscrotal (pē″nō-skrō′tǎl). Concerning the penis and scrotum.

pension neurosis. A form of malingering that develops subsequent to an injury in the belief that financial or other forms of compensation can be obtained or will be continued by being ill. SEE: *neurosis, compensation.*

pent-, penta- [Gr. *pente*, five]. Combining form meaning five.

pentabasic (pěn″tǎ-bā′sǐk). 1. A compound that contains five replaceable hydrogen atoms. 2. An alcohol that contains five hydroxyl groups.

pentachlorophenol. C_6HCl_5O. A chemical used as a wood preservative for termite control and as a defoliant. It is extremely toxic on its own, but some grades are contaminated with dioxin, q.v.

pentad (pěn′tǎd) [Gr. *pente*, five]. 1. A radical or element with a valence of five. 2. Group of five.

pentadactyl (pěn″tǎ-dǎk′tǐl) [″ + *daktylos*, finger]. Having five digits on each hand and foot.

pentaerythritol tetranitrate (pěn″tǎ-ě-rǐth′rǐ-tōl). USP. An organic nitrate drug used in treating angina pectoris. Trade names are Pentritol and Peritrate.

pentagastrin (pěn″tǎ-gǎs′trǐn). A synthetic gastrin that may be administered to test the ability of the stomach to secrete hydrochloric acid.

pentalogy (pěn-tǎl′ō-jē). The occurrence of five factors in combination, e.g., symptoms or signs of a disease.

pentamethylenediamine (pěn″tǎ-měth″ǐl-ěn-dī′ǎ-měn). A ptomaine occurring in tissue decomposed by certain bacteria.

pentamidine (pěn-tǎm′ǐ-děn). A drug used in treating leishmaniasis, early cases of Gambian and Rhodesian trypanosomiasis, and pneumonia due to *Pneumocystis carinii.* This drug is available in the U.S. only from the Centers for Disease Control, Drug Service, Atlanta, Georgia, 30333, (404) 633-3311.

pentane (pěn′tān). C_5H_{12}. One of the hydrocarbons of the methane series. A product of petroleum distillation.

pentapeptide (pěn″tǎ-pěp′tǐd). A polypeptide with five amino acid groups.

pentaploid (pěn′tǎ-ployd) [″ + *ploos*, a fold, + *eidos*, form, shape]. Having five sets of chromosomes.

pentastomiasis (pěn″tǎ-stō-mī′ǎ-sǐs). Infection with certain genera of Pentastomida, the tongue worms. The larval forms usually live in the bodies of lower animals but have been reported in humans.

pentatomic (pěn″tǎ-tǒm′ǐk) [″ + *atomos*, indivisible]. 1. Containing five atoms in the molecule. 2. An alcohol with five hydroxyl groups.

pentavalent (pěn″tǎ-vā′lěnt, -tǎv′ǎ-lěnt) [Gr. *pente*, five, + L. *valens*, having power]. Having a chemical valence of five.

pentazocine (pěn-tǎz′ō-sēn). USP. An analgesic drug that is effective orally and parenterally. Originally thought to be nonaddicting, but it is potentially addicting. Prolonged use of the drug may cause a woody sclerosis of the skin and subcutaneous tissues around injection sites. The lesions may appear on other areas of the skin also. Ulcers surrounded by areas of hyperpigmentation may develop. Skin changes do not develop in short-term users of the drug. Trade names are Talwin and Fortral.

Pentids. Trade name for penicillin G potassium.

pentobarbital (pěn″tō-bǎr′bǐ-tǎl). USP. A hypnotic sedative drug of the barbiturate class.

p. sodium. A barbituric acid derivative used as an oral or intravenous hypnotic agent in preanesthetic medication. Used in labor with or without scopolamine. Trade name is Nembutal Sodium.

pentosazon (pěn″tō-sā′zǒn). Crystalline compound formed when a pentose is treated with phenylhydrazine. It is not normally present in urine.

pentose (pěn′tōs) [Gr. *pente*, five]. $C_5H_{10}O_5$. A simple sugar with five atoms of carbon in the molecule.

pentosemia (pěn″tō-sē′mē-ǎ). Pentose in the blood.

pentoside (pěn″tō-sīd). Pentose combined with some other substance. Pentoses combined with purine or pyrimidine bases are present in nucleic acid.

pentostam. A drug used in leishmaniasis and available in the U.S. only from the Centers for Disease Control, Drug Service, Atlanta, Georgia 30333, (404) 633-3311.

pentosuria (pĕn″tō-sū′rē-ă). A condition in which pentose is found in the urine.

Pentothal Sodium. Trade name for thiopental sodium.

pentoxide (pĕn-tŏk′sīd). A chemical molecule containing five atoms of oxygen.

pentoxifylline. A drug used to increase peripheral tissue blood flow. Trade name is Trental.

Pen-Vee-K. Trade name for penicillin V potassium.

peonin (pē′ō-nĭn). A dye used as a hydrogen ion concentration test.

peotillomania (pē″ō-tĭl″ō-mā′nē-ă) [Gr. *peos*, penis, + *tillein*, to pull, + *mania*, madness]. A nervous habit or tic consisting of constant pulling at the penis.

peotomy (pē-ŏt′ō-mē) [″ + *tome*, incision]. Surgical removal of the penis.

pepo (pē′pō) [L., pumpkin]. Pumpkin seed.

pepper (pĕp′ĕr) [ME. *peper*]. A spice that is used as a condiment, stimulant, carminative, and counterirritant. The dried berries of the fruit of plants of the genus *Piper*. These are ground or used whole to season foods. Even though pepper irritates the oral mucosa and produces a burning sensation, evidence that its use causes peptic ulcers is lacking.

peppermint spirit. USP. The leaves and tops of the plant *Mentha piperita,* from which oil of peppermint is derived.

USES: Aromatic stimulant, carminative, and flavoring agent.

pepsic (pĕp′sĭk) [Gr. *peptein*, to digest]. Peptic.

pepsin (pĕp′sĭn) [Gr. *pepsis*, digestion]. The chief enzyme of gastric juice, which converts proteins into proteoses and peptones. It is formed by the chief cells of gastric glands and produces its maximum activity at a pH of 1.5 to 2. It is obtainable in granular form. In the presence of hydrochloric acid it will digest proteins in vitro.

pepsinogen (pĕp-sĭn′ō-jĕn) [″ + *gennan*, to produce]. The antecedent of pepsin existing in the form of granules in the chief cells of gastric glands.

pepsinuria (pĕp″sĭ-nū′rē-ă) [″ + *ouron*, urine]. Excretion of pepsin in the urine.

peptic (pĕp′tĭk) [Gr. *peptikos*]. 1. Concerning digestion. 2. Concerning pepsin.

peptic ulcer. An ulcer occurring in the lower end of the esophagus; in the stomach usually along the lesser curvature; in the duodenum; or on the jejunal side of a gastrojejunostomy.

SYM: Pain is the most characteristic symptom, tending to be of uniform quality and usually described as "gnawing." It is localized in the epigastrium and exhibits a rhythmicity and periodicity usually appearing one to three hours after a meal. It is usually absent before breakfast but may occur during the night. Usually, but not always, the pain is relieved by food and alkalies. The pain lasts for minutes rather than hours, and the clusters of pain may be present for days or weeks followed by long symptom-free periods.

Other symptoms include dyspepsia, heartburn, acid eructations, nausea, vomiting, and anorexia. In some cases, physical signs may be absent, the first indication of the condition being hemorrhage or perforation.

ETIOL: The usual but not the only cause is the action of gastric acid and peptic activity on the mucosa of the esophagus, stomach, or duodenum. Ulcers may form in other situations where the mucosal defenses are overcome by forces that can damage the mucosa. SEE: *ulcer, Curling's; ulcer, stress.*

The importance of the bacterium *Helicobacter pylori* (formerly named *Campylobacter pylori*) in causing peptic ulcers is being investigated.

TREAT: Symptoms may disappear and the ulcer may heal without benefit of any medical therapy, and symptoms may subside without evidence of healing by x-ray evaluation.

Medical therapy: Consists of giving agents to reduce the levels of acid and pepsin in the stomach, and use of drugs to enhance mucosal defense. Thus, histamine-blocking agents, q.v., that interfere with the formation of histamine and lower gastric acid are of great benefit. Also, antacids are used to neutralize gastric acidity.

Diet has not proven to be as effective in treating peptic ulcer as previously thought. Cessation of tobacco and alcohol use is beneficial in treating peptic ulcer. Some analgesics can cause peptic ulcers; they should be discontinued.

Coating agents: Several agents that are used in treating peptic ulcer act by coating the ulcer and preventing further harm from the acid-peptic digestion process normally present in the stomach and duodenum. These substances include sucralfate, q.v., and bismuth colloids, q.v.

Surgery: Surgical therapy including vagotomy and subtotal gastric resection may be needed if hemorrhage, perforation, or intractable bleeding occurs.

Psychotherapy: Some patients will need extensive psychotherapy in order to change lifestyles or situations from those that are stressful to those less likely to cause stress. SEE: *nonsteroidal anti-inflammatory agents; Zollinger-Ellison syndrome.*

NURSING IMPLICATIONS: Reduce emotional stress. Provide physical rest. Control gastric acidity with prescribed medications.

In the acute state, test vomitus and stools for blood. Observe for complications such as perforation or hemorrhage. Prevent injuries that may occur due to drowsiness associated with use of sedatives and tranquilizers.

Develop coping mechanism to relieve anxiety. Advise that all activities should be done in moderation. Establish teaching plan including prescribed medications; drugs to avoid because of gastric irritation; discontinuation of or decreased smoking; and significance of follow-up care.

peptidase. An enzyme that converts peptides to amino acids.

peptide (pĕp'tīd) [Gr. *peptein*, to digest]. Compound formed by hydrolytic cleavage of peptones and containing two or more amino acids. A class of substances prepared by synthesis from amino acids and intermediate in molecular weight and chemical properties between the amino acids, which can be made artificially, and the proteins, which cannot.

RS: dipeptide; polypeptide; tripeptide.

peptidoglycan. The dense material consisting of cross-linked polysaccharide chains that make up the cell wall of most bacteria. This membrane is much thicker in gram-positive bacteria than it is in gram-negative organisms.

peptidolytic (pĕp'tĭ-dō-lĭt'ĭk) [" + *lytikos*, dissolving]. Causing the splitting up or digestion of peptides.

peptinotoxin (pĕp'tĭn-ō-tŏk'sĭn) [" + *toxikon*, poison]. Poisonous ptomaine found in the body as a result of disordered or defective digestion.

peptization (pĕp'tĭ-zā'shŭn) [Gr. *peptein*, to digest]. In the chemistry of colloids, the process of making a colloidal solution more stable; conversion of a gel to a sol.

Pepto-Bismol. Trade name for bismuth subsalicylate.

Peptococcaceae. A family of bacteria that includes the genus *Peptococcus.* These gram-positive anaerobic cocci may be normal or pathologic inhabitants of the respiratory and intestinal tracts.

Peptococcus (pĕp'tō-kŏk'ŭs). Strictly anaerobic gram-positive cocci that are normally present in the oral cavity, on the skin, and in the intestinal and urinary tracts. They are usually associated with infections, in which they act synergistically with other organisms.

peptogenic, peptogenous (pĕp-tō-jĕn'ĭk, -tŏj'ĕn-ŭs) [" + *gennan*, to produce]. 1. Producing peptones and pepsin. 2. Promoting digestion.

peptoid (pĕp'toyd) [" + *eidos*, form, shape]. A product of protein digestion that does not give the biuret reaction.

peptolysis (pĕp-tŏl'ĭ-sĭs) [Gr. *peptein*, to digest, + *lysis*, dissolution]. The splitting up or hydrolysis of peptones. SYN: *peptonolysis.*

peptolytic (pĕp-tō-lĭt'ĭk). Pert. to the splitting up of peptone.

peptone (pĕp'tōn) [Gr. *pepton*, digesting]. A secondary protein formed by the action of proteolytic enzymes, acids, or alkalies on certain proteins. Peptones are nitrogenous compounds soluble in water; they are not coagulated by boiling.

peptonemia (pĕp'tō-nē'mē-ă) [" + *haima*, blood]. Peptones in the blood.

peptonization (pĕp'tō-nĭ-zā'shŭn) [Gr. *pepton*, digesting]. Process of changing protein substance into peptones by action of proteolytic enzymes.

peptonize. To convert into peptones; to predigest with pepsin.

peptonolysis (pĕp'tō-nŏl'ĭ-sĭs) [Gr. *pepton*, digesting, + *lysis*, dissolution]. The breakdown of peptones into simpler products (peptides or amino acids). SYN: *peptolysis.*

peptonuria (pĕp'tō-nū'rē-ă) [" + *ouron*, urine]. Excretion of peptones in the urine.

Peptostreptococcus (pĕp'tō-strĕp'tō-kŏk'ŭs). A genus of bacteria of the *Peptococcaceae* family. These organisms may be normal or pathologic inhabitants of the intestinal and respiratory tracts. They are also important as opportunistic pathogens.

peptotoxin (pĕp'tō-tŏk'sĭn) [" + *toxikon*, poison]. Any toxin produced from a peptone.

per [L. *per*, through]. 1. A word used as a prefix or by itself meaning through, by, or by means of. 2. In chemistry, the highest valence of an element. 3. For each unit or entity, e.g., milligrams per kilogram, usually written as *mg/kg.*

per-. A prefix indicating throughout, through, utterly, or intense.

peracephalus (pĕr'ă-sĕf'ă-lŭs) [" + Gr. *a-*, not, + *kephale*, head]. A parasitic twin of the placenta. It does not contain a head or arms, and the thorax is malformed.

peracid (pĕr-ăs'ĭd). 1. An acid that contains the highest valence possible. 2. An acid containing the peroxide group, $O-OH$.

peracidity (pĕr'ă-sĭd'ĭ-tē) [L. *per*, through, + *acidus*, sour]. Abnormal acidity.

peracute (pĕr'ă-kūt') [" + *acutus*, keen].

Very acute or violent.

per anum (pĕr ā'nŭm) [L.]. Through or by way of the anus.

perarticulation (pĕr″är-tĭk″ū-lā'shŭn) [L. *per,* through, + *articulatio,* joint]. Diarthrosis, q.v.

percent. Per hundred. For or out of each hundred. Its symbol, %, is used to indicate that the preceding number is a percentage.

percentile (pĕr-sĕn'tīl). One of 100 equal divisions of a series of items or data. Thus if a value such as a test score is higher than 92% of all the other test scores, that result is above the 92nd percentile of the range of scores.

percept (pĕr'sĕpt). The mental image of an object seen.

perception (pĕr-sĕp'shŭn) [L. *percepitio,* perceive]. 1. Process of being aware of objects; consciousness. 2. Process of receiving sensory impressions. 3. The elaboration of a sensory impression; the ideational association modifying, defining, and usually completing the primary impression or stimulus. Vague or inadequate association occurs in confused and depressed states.

   p., depth. Term used in evaluating visual function. The ability to recognize that an object has depth as well as height and width. It is generally believed that both eyes must function normally for a person to have normal ability to perceive depth. Sometimes this is true, but most persons with the use of only one eye learn to judge depth quite accurately.

   p., extrasensory. ABBR: ESP. Perception not through the recognized senses.

   p., stereognostic. Recognition of objects by touch.

perceptivity (pĕr-sĕp-tĭv'ĭ-tē). Power to receive sense impressions.

percolate (pĕr'kō-lāt) [L. *percolare,* to strain through]. 1. To allow a liquid to seep through a powdered substance. 2. Any fluid that has been filtered or percolated. 3. To strain a fluid through powdered substances in order to impregnate it with soluble principles of such substances.

percolation (pĕr″kō-lā'shŭn) [L. *percolatio*]. 1. Filtration. 2. Process of extracting soluble portions of a drug of powdered composition by filtering a liquid solvent through it.

percolator (pĕr'kō-lā″tor). Apparatus used for extraction of a drug with a liquid solvent.

per contiguum (pĕr kŏn-tĭg'ū-ŭm) [L.]. Touching, as in the spread of an inflammation from one part to an adjacent structure.

per continuum (pĕr kŏn-tĭn'ū-ŭm) [L.]. Continuous, as the spread of an inflammation from part to part.

percuss (pĕr-kŭs') [L. *percutere*]. To tap parts of the body to aid diagnosis by sound emit-ted.

percussible (pĕr-kŭs'ĭ-b'l). Able to be detected by percussion.

percussion (pĕr-kŭsh'ŭn) [L. *percussio,* a striking]. 1. Use of the fingertips to tap the body lightly but sharply to determine position, size, and consistency of an underlying structure and the presence of fluid or pus in a cavity. These conditions are established by alterations felt and heard in resonance and pitch of the sound emitted, vibration elicited, or resistance encountered. 2. A technique used with postural drainage to mobilize secretions by mechanically dislodging viscous or adherent secretions in the lungs by manually cupping over the chest wall. SEE: *cystic fibrosis.*

   RS: abdomen; bladder; box-note; chest; heart; intestines; kidney; liver; ovary; palpation; spleen; uterus.

   p., auscultatory. Percussion combined with auscultation.

   p., bimanual. P., mediate.

   p., deep. Forceful percussion used to elicit a note from a deeply seated tissue or organ.

   p., direct. P., immediate.

   p., finger. Striking of the finger resting upon the body with a finger of the other hand.

   p., immediate. Percussion performed by striking the surface directly with the fingers. SYN: *p., direct.*

   p., indirect. P., mediate.

   p., mediate. Percussion performed by using fingers of one hand as a plexor and those of the opposite hand as a pleximeter. SYN: *p., indirect.*

   p., palpation. Percussion in which the fingers perceive the tactile impression rather than the examiner relying on the sounds produced.

   p., threshold. Percussing lightly with the fingers on a glass-rod pleximeter, the far end of which is covered with a rubber cap. The cap is usually placed on an intercostal space. This technique is used to confine the percussion to a very small area. SYN: *Goldscheider's percussion.*

percussor (pĕr-kŭs'or) [L., striker]. Device used for diagnosis by percussion, consisting of a hammer with a rubber or metal head.

percutaneous (pĕr″kū-tā'nē-ŭs) [L. *per,* through, + *cutis,* skin]. Effected through the skin. Describes the application of a medicated ointment by friction, or the removal or injection of a fluid by needle.

percutaneous balloon valvuloplasty. The percutaneous insertion of one or more balloons across a stenotic heart valve. Inflating the balloons decreases the constriction. This technique has been especially helpful in treating pulmonic stenosis.

percutaneous endoscopic gastrostomy. ABBR: PEG. A feeding ostomy. PEG tubes are inserted through the esophagus into the stomach with the aid of an endoscope and then pulled through a stab wound made in the abdominal wall.

percutaneous transhepatic cholangiography. ABBR: PTC. Direct percutaneous puncture of an intrahepatic duct by a needle inserted through the 8th or 9th intercostal space into the center of the liver. Radiopaque material is injected into the dilated intrahepatic biliary tree. The procedure is useful in determining the cause of jaundice. SEE: *endoscopic retrograde cholangiopancreatography; jaundice.*

percutaneous transluminal coronary angioplasty. ABBR: PTCA. A method of treating localized coronary artery narrowing. A special double-lumen catheter is designed so that a cylindrical balloon surrounds a portion of it. Inflation of the balloon with pressure of up to 90 p.s.i. dilates the narrowed vessel. This technique may be used on narrowed arteries other than the coronaries. SEE: *angioplasty, laser coronary.*

NURSING IMPLICATIONS: *Preop:* Reinforce cardiologist's explanation of procedure. Encourage verbalization of feelings and concerns, clarifying misconceptions. Prepare patient physically according to surgeon's orders. Gather baseline data that will be needed for comparison with postoperative status.

Postop: Monitor vital signs, cardiac rate and rhythm, neurovascular status distal to catheter insertion site. Use a Doppler stethoscope if peripheral pulses are difficult to palpate. Inspect catheter insertion site periodically for hematoma formation, ecchymosis, or hemorrhage, marking dressing and notifying surgeon of any rapid expansion. Apply direct pressure to catheter site if bleeding occurs. Instruct patient to keep leg straight and to limit head elevation to no more than 15 degrees in order to prevent hip flexion and potential catheter migration. Assess for chest pain which may indicate vasospasm or reocclusion of ballooned vessel. Administer I.V. fluids as prescribed, at least 100 ml/hr to promote excretion of contrast medium. Monitor for signs or symptoms of fluid overload (dyspnea, pulmonary crackles, distended neck veins, tachycardia, bounding pulse, hypertension, gallop rhythms. Continue pharmacologic therapy as prescribed (I.V. nitroglycerin, heparin). Explain catheter removal to patient, and assist physician by applying direct pressure to insertion site for 30 minutes, then applying

pressure dressing. Continue monitoring vital signs until certain no occult hemorrhage is occurring. Provide discharge instructions to patient and family regarding check-up appointment with cardiologist, follow-up exercise, thallium-stress testing, or angiography, and any exercise prescriptions or activity restrictions (usually, patient can walk 24 hours following procedure, return to work in 2 weeks). Reinforce importance of continuing drug regimen, stressing action of each drug and the importance of reporting any side effects.

percutaneous ultrasonic lithotriptor. Device that employs ultrasound to break up kidney stones and gallstones. The sound waves are applied to the outside of the body.

per diem cost. Hospital or other inpatient institutional cost per day.

perencephaly (pĕr″ĕn-sĕf′ă-lē) [Gr. *pera,* pouch, + *enkephalos,* brain]. Porencephaly, q.v.

Perez reflex. A mass reflex present at birth which consists of extension of the head and spine, flexion of the knees on the chest, a cry, and emptying of the bladder. Absence of the reflex during the first 3 months of life indicates severe cerebral insult, injury to the upper cervical cord, advanced anterior horn disease, or severe myopathy.

perfectionism (pĕr-fĕk′shŭn-ĭzm). A type of neurosis in which the individual attempts to achieve goals of behavior or performance that are unrealistic or unnecessary.

perflation (pĕr-flā′shŭn) [L. *perflatio*]. The process of blowing air into a cavity to expand its walls or to force out secretions or other matter.

perforans (pĕr′fō-răns) [L.]. Perforating or penetrating, as a nerve or muscle.

perforate (pĕr′fō-rāt) [L. *perforatus,* pierced with holes]. 1. To puncture or to make holes. 2. Pierced with holes.

perforation (pĕr″fō-rā′shŭn). 1. The act or process of making a hole, such as that caused by ulceration. 2. The hole made through a substance or part.

    p., Bezold's. Perforation on the inner surface of the mastoid bone.

    p., tooth. An opening through the wall of a tooth, produced by pathological processes or accidentally, thereby exposing the dental pulp. Also called pulp exposure.

perforation of stomach or intestine. Abdominal crisis due to escape of contents of the perforated viscus into the peritoneal cavity. Peritonitis is certain to develop unless there is immediate surgical intervention. SEE: *intestinal perforation; peritonitis.*

    SYM: Onset is accompanied by acute pain, which begins over perforated area and spreads all over the abdomen, which has become rigid. Face is anxious with beads of perspiration on it. Nausea and vomiting will occur. Pulse rapid and feeble and respiration rapid and shallow. Temperature drops, but rises as peritonitis sets in, and pulse becomes stronger.

TREAT: Surgical. Pending operation, give no fluids. Complete rest.

perforator (pĕr'fō-rā-tor) [L., a piercing device]. Instrument for piercing the skull and other bones.

p., tympanum. Instrument for perforating the tympanum.

perforatorium (pĕr"fō-ră-tō'rē-ŭm). The pointed tip of the acrosome of the spermatozoa.

performance. The act of performing, i.e., the undertaking and completing of, either mental or physical work. Thus, a person's performance is observed and measured in order to determine functional capability.

perfrication (pĕr-frĭ-kā'shŭn) [L. perfricare, to rub]. Thorough rubbing with an ointment. SYN: inunction.

perfrigeration (pĕr-frĭj"ĕr-ā'shŭn) [L. per, through, + frigere, to be cold]. Frostbite.

perfusate (pĕr-fū'zāt). The fluid used to perfuse a tissue or organ.

perfusion (pĕr-fū'zhŭn) [L. perfundere, to pour through]. 1. Passing of a fluid through spaces. 2. Pouring of a fluid. 3. Supplying an organ or tissue with nutrients and oxygen by injecting blood or a suitable fluid into an artery.

perfusionist. Perfusionists assist the physician in all aspects of managing the equipment and techniques used during extracorporeal circulation. They may also be involved in inducing prescribed hypothermia.

Pergonal. Trade name for menotropins.

perhydrocyclopentanophenanthrene (pĕr-hī"drō-sī"klō-pĕn-tăn"ō-phĕn-ăn'thrĕn). Name of the ring structure of the chemical nucleus of the steroids. SEE: steroid hormones for illus.

peri- [Gr.]. Prefix meaning around or about.

periacinal, periacinous (pĕr"ē-ăs'ĭ-năl, -nŭs) [Gr. peri, around, + L. acinus, grape]. Placed around a saclike dilation.

Periactin. Trade name for cyproheptadine hydrochloride.

periadenitis (pĕr"ē-ă"dĕ-nī'tĭs) [" + aden, gland, + itis, inflammation]. Inflamed condition of tissues surrounding a gland.

p. mucosa necrotica recurrens. Recurring necrotic or ulcerative lesions on the buccal and pharyngeal mucosa. These start as small hard nodules that ulcerate and leave a deep crater. These may be associated with Behçet's syndrome.

perialienitis (pĕr"ē-ā"lē-ĕn-ī'tĭs) [" + L.

alienus, foreign, + Gr. itis, inflammation]. Noninfectious inflammation around a foreign body. SYN: perixenitis.

periamygdalitis (pĕr"ē-ăm-ĭg"dăl-ī'tĭs) [" + amygdale, tonsil, + itis, inflammation]. Inflammation of connective tissue around the tonsil. SYN: peritonsillitis.

perianal (pĕr"ē-ā'năl) [" + L. anus, anus]. Around or close to the anus.

periangiitis (pĕr"ē-ăn"jē-ī'tĭs) [" + angeion, vessel, + itis, inflammation]. Inflamed condition of tissue around a blood or lymphatic vessel.

periangiocholitis (pĕr"ē-ăn"jē-ō-kō-lī'tĭs) [" + " + chole, bile, + itis, inflammation]. Inflamed condition of tissues around the bile ducts. SYN: pericholangitis.

periaortic (pĕr"ē-ā-or'tĭk) [" + aorte, aorta]. Around the aorta.

periaortitis (pĕr"ē-ā-or-tī'tĭs) [" + aorte, aorta, + itis, inflammation]. Inflamed condition of adventitia and tissues around the aorta.

periapex (pĕr"ē-ā'pĕks) [" + L. apex, tip]. Area around the apex of a tooth.

periapical (pĕr"ē-ăp'ĭ-kăl) [" + L. apex, tip]. Around the apex of the root of a tooth.

periappendicitis (pĕr"ē-ă-pĕn"dĭ-sī'tĭs) [" + L. appendix, appendage, + Gr. itis, inflammation]. Inflamed condition of the appendix and its surrounding tissues.

p. decidualis. Condition in which there are decidual cells in the peritoneum of the appendix vermiformis in cases of tubal pregnancy due to adhesions between fallopian tubes and the appendix.

periappendicular (pĕr"ē-ăp"ĕn-dĭk'ū-lăr) [" + L. appendix, appendage]. Surrounding an appendix.

periarterial (pĕr"ē-ăr-tē'rē-ăl) [" + arteria, artery]. Placed around an artery.

periarteritis (pĕr"ē-ăr-tĕr-ī'tĭs) [" + " + itis, inflammation]. Inflammation of the external coat of an artery.

p. gummosa. Gummas in the blood vessels in syphilis.

p. nodosa. Polyarteritis nodosa, q.v. SEE: Nursing Diagnoses in Appendix.

periarthric (pĕr"ē-ăr'thrĭk) [" + arthron, joint]. Surrounding a joint. SYN: circumarticular; periarticular.

periarthritis (pĕr"ē-ăr-thrī'tĭs) [" + " + itis, inflammation]. Inflammation of area around a joint.

periarticular (pĕr"ē-ăr-tĭk'ū-lăr) [Gr. peri, around, + L. articulus, a joint]. Surrounding a joint. SYN: circumarticular; periarthric.

periatrial (pĕr"ē-ā'trē-ăl) [" + L. atrium, corridor]. Around the atria, or auricles, of the heart.

periauricular. Around the ear.

periaxial (pĕr-ē-ăk'sē-ăl) [" + *axon*, axis]. Located around an axis.

periaxillary (pĕr"ē-ăk'sĭl-ĕ"rē) [" + L. *axilla*, armpit]. Occurring around the axilla.

periaxonal (pĕr"ē-ăk'sō-năl) [" + *axon*, axis]. Around an axon.

periblast (pĕr'ĭ-blăst) [" + *blastos*, germ]. That portion of the yolk surface adjacent to the blastoderm in telolecithal eggs.

peribronchial (pĕr"ĭ-brŏng'kē-ăl) [" + *bronchos*, windpipe]. Surrounding a bronchus.

peribronchiolar (pĕr"ĭ-brŏng-kī'ō-lăr) [" + L. *bronchiolus*, bronchiole]. Surrounding a bronchiole.

peribronchiolitis (pĕr"ĭ-brŏng"kē-ō-lī'tĭs) [" + Gr. *itis*, inflammation]. Inflammation of area around the bronchioles.

peribronchitis (pĕr"ĭ-brŏng-kī'tĭs) [" + *bronchos*, windpipe, + *itis*, inflammation]. Inflammation of all tissues surrounding the bronchi or bronchial tubes.

peribulbar (pĕr"ĭ-bŭl'băr) [" + L. *bulbus*, bulbous root]. Surrounding a bulb, esp. the bulb of the eye.

peribursal (pĕr"ĭ-bĕr'săl) [" + *bursa*, leather sack]. Around a bursa.

pericanalicular (pĕr"ĭ-kăn"ă-lĭk'ū-lăr) [" + L. *canaliculus*, small canal]. Around a canaliculus.

pericardiac, pericardial (pĕr-ĭ-kăr'dē-ăk, -ăl) [" + *kardia*, heart]. Concerning the pericardium.

pericardial rub. A friction sound heard when the inflamed or roughened pericardial surfaces rub against each other.

pericardicentesis, pericardiocentesis (pĕr"ĭ-kăr"dĭ-sĕn-tē'sĭs, -kăr"dē-ō-sĕn-tē'sĭs) [" + " + *kentesis*, puncture]. Surgical perforation of the pericardium.

pericardiectomy (pĕr"ĭ-kăr-dē-ĕk'tō-mē) [" + " + *ektome*, excision]. Excision of part or all of the pericardium.

pericardiolysis (pĕr"ĭ-kăr"dē-ŏl'ĭ-sĭs) [" + " + *lysis*, dissolution]. Separation of adhesions between the visceral and parietal pericardium.

pericardiomediastinitis (pĕr"ĭ-kăr"dē-ō-mē-dē-ăs"tĭ-nī'tĭs) [" + " + L. *mediastinum*, + Gr. *itis*, inflammation]. Inflamed condition of the pericardium and mediastinum.

pericardiopexy [" + " + *pexis*, fixation]. Surgical procedure designed to increase the blood supply to the heart by joining the pericardium to an adjacent tissue.

pericardiophrenic (pĕr-ĭ-kăr"dē-ō-frĕn'ĭk) [" + *kardia*, heart, + *phren*, diaphragm]. Concerning the pericardium and diaphragm.

pericardiopleural (pĕr"ĭ-kăr"dē-ō-ploo'răl) [" + " + *pleura*, rib]. Concerning the pericardium and pleura.

pericardiorrhaphy (pĕr"ĭ-kăr"dē-or'ă-fē) [" + " + *rhaphe*, seam, ridge]. Suture of a wound in the pericardium.

pericardiostomy (pĕr"ĭ-kăr"dē-ŏs'tō-mē) [" + *kardia*, heart, + *stoma*, mouth]. Formation of an opening into the pericardium for drainage.

pericardiosymphysis (pĕr"ĭ-kăr"dē-ō-sĭm'fĭ-sĭs) [" + " + *symphysis*, a joining]. Adhesion between the layers of the pericardium.

pericardiotomy (pĕr"ĭ-kăr-dē-ŏt'ō-mē) [" + " + *tome*, incision]. Incision of the pericardial sac around the heart.

pericarditic (pĕr"ĭ-kăr-dĭt'ĭk). Concerning the pericardium.

pericarditis (pĕr-ĭ-kăr-dī'tĭs) [" + *kardia*, heart, + *itis*, inflammation]. Inflammation of the pericardium. SEE: *Nursing Diagnoses* in *Appendix*.

SYM: Moderate fever, precordial pain and tenderness, dry cough, dyspnea, and palpitation. Pulse is first rapid and forcible, then weak and irregular.

First stage: Auscultation reveals to-and-fro friction sound heard over 4th left intercostal space near sternum. Inspection and palpation sometimes reveal a diffuse apex beat. Friction rub may sometimes be palpated.

Second stage: Serofibrinous effusion. Bulging of precordium. Increased area of dullness, triangular in shape, base down. Heart sounds muffled, distant, feeble. Purulent effusion yields similar signs, but in addition high, irregular fever; sweats; chills, and progressive pallor; sometimes edema over the precordium.

ETIOL: Tuberculosis, mycoses, infection by pyogenic organisms, collagen disease, uremia, myocardial infarction, neoplasms, trauma.

TREAT: *General:* Absolute bedrest, light diet. For relief of pain apply ice bag over precordium or administer pain-relieving drugs, depending on its intensity. *Specific:* Appropriate antibiotic for specific organisms involved. If purulent effusion occurs, aspiration or surgical drainage. If gallop rhythm or signs of heart failure occur, restrict fluids and salt. For chronic constrictive pericarditis, resection of pericardium.

PROG: Fair in early stages but extremely grave in purulent and fibrinous stages.

p., acute fibrinous. Pericarditis characterized by fibrinous exudation.

p., acute nonspecific. A disease of unknown etiology usually following respiratory infections. SYN: *p., idiopathic.*

p., adhesive. Form of pericarditis in

which the layers of pericardium adhere.

  p., constrictive. Pericarditis in which adhesions form between visceral and parietal layers of the pericardium.

  p., external. Inflammation of exterior surface of the pericardium.

  p., fibrinous. Pericarditis in which the membrane is covered with butter-like exudate that organizes and unites the pericardial surfaces.

  SYM: Precordial bulging, a weak apex beat with loud sounds, a systolic retraction at apex and over a large part of the precordium, peculiar diastolic collapse of jugular veins, feeble apex beat with a forcible impulse over body of the heart. Signs of heart failure, as dyspnea, generalized edema, cyanosis.

  p., hemorrhagic. Pericarditis in which the exudate contains blood.

  p., idiopathic. P., acute nonspecific.

  p., ischemic. Pericarditis resulting from myocardial infarction.

  p., neoplastic. Pericarditis due to invasion of the pericardium by malignant tumors of adjoining structures.

  p. obliterans. Pericardial inflammation causing adhesions and obliteration of the pericardial cavity.

  p., serofibrinous. Pericarditis in which there is a considerable quantity of serous exudate but little fibrin.

  p., uremic. Pericarditis resulting from uremia.

pericardium (pĕr″ĭ-kăr′dē-ŭm) [Gr. *peri*, around, + *kardia*, heart]. [NA] The double membranous fibroserous sac enclosing the heart and the origins of the great blood vessels. It is composed of an inner serous layer (visceral pericardium or epicardium) and an outer fibrous layer (parietal pericardium). The space between the two constitutes the pericardial cavity, which is normally filled with a small amount of serous fluid. Its base is attached to the diaphragm, its apex extending upward as far as the first subdivision of the great blood vessels. It is attached in front to the sternum, laterally to the mediastinal pleura, and posteriorly to the esophagus, trachea, and principal bronchi. Normally, the pericardium contains a thin serous fluid.

  p., adherent. Condition in which fibrous bands form between the two layers of the pericardium, obliterating the pericardial cavity. SEE: *pericarditis, constrictive.*

  p., bread-and-butter. Condition seen in fibrinous pericarditis in which the pericardium has a peculiar appearance due to fibrinous deposits on the two opposing surfaces.

  p. externum. Outer fibrous layer of the pericardium. SYN: *p., parietal.*

  p., fibrous. Strong fibrous tissue on the outer surface of the pericardial sac.

  p. internum. Serous inner layer of the pericardium.

  p., parietal. Outer fibrous layer of the pericardium. SYN: *p. externum.*

  p., serous. Smooth lining of the pericardial sac.

  p., shaggy. Condition occurring in fibrinous pericarditis in which loose shaggy deposits of fibrin are seen on the surfaces of the pericardium.

  p., visceral. Serous inner layer of the pericardium.

pericardotomy (pĕr″ĭ-kăr-dŏt′ō-mē) [Gr. *peri*, around, + *kardia*, heart, + *tome*, incision]. Incision of the pericardium.

pericecal (pĕr″ĭ-sē′kăl) [″ + L. *caecum*, blind]. Situated around the cecum.

pericecitis (pĕr″ĭ-sē-sī′tĭs) [″ + ″ + Gr. *itis*, inflammation]. Inflamed condition of area around the cecum.

pericellular (pĕr″ĭ-sĕl′ū-lăr) [″ + L. *cellula, cell*]. Around a cell.

pericemental (pĕr″ĭ-sē-mĕn′tăl) [″ + L. *caementum*, cement]. Concerning the pericementum, i.e., the periodontal ligament.

pericementitis (pĕr″ĭ-sē-mĕn-tī′tĭs) [″ + ″ + Gr. *itis*, inflammation]. Progressive necrosis of the alveoli of the teeth. SYN: *periodontitis.*

  p., apical. Apical abscess of the tooth.

pericementoclasia (pĕr″ĭ-sē-mĕn″tō-klā′zē-ă) [″ + ″ + Gr. *klasis*, a breaking]. Dissolution of the pericementum with alveolar absorption. SYN: *pyorrhea alveolaris.*

pericementum (pĕr″ĭ-sē-mĕn′tŭm). Fibrous tissue covering the root of a tooth. SYN: *periodontal ligament.*

pericentral (pĕr″ĭ-sĕn′trăl) [″ + *kentron*, center]. Around the center.

pericholangitis (pĕr″ĭ-kō-lăn-jī′tĭs) [Gr. *peri*, around, + *chole*, bile, + *angeion*, vessel, + *itis*, inflammation]. Inflammation of tissues surrounding a bile duct. SYN: *periangiocholitis.*

pericholecystitis (pĕr″ĭ-kō-lē-sĭs-tī′tĭs) [″ + ″ + *kystis*, a sac, + *itis*, inflammation]. Inflammation of tissues situated around the gallbladder.

perichondral, perichondrial (pĕr-ĭ-kŏn′drăl, -drē-ăl) [″ + *chondros*, cartilage]. Concerning the membrane that covers cartilage.

perichondritis (pĕr-ĭ-kŏn-drī′tĭs) [″ + ″ + *itis*, inflammation]. Inflamed condition of the perichondrium.

perichondrium (pĕr-ĭ-kŏn′drē-ŭm) [″ + *chondros*, cartilage]. [NA] Membrane of fibrous connective tissue around the surface of cartilage.

perichondroma (pĕr″ĭ-kŏn-drō′mă) [″ + ″ + *oma*, tumor]. A tumor arising from fibrous tissue that covers cartilage.

perichord (pĕr′ĭ-kord) [″ + *chorde*, cord]. The sheath of the notochord.

perichordal (pĕr-ĭ-kor′dăl) [″ + *chorde*, cord]. Placed around the notochord.

perichorioidal, perichoroidal (pĕr″ĭ-kō-rē-oy′dăl, -roy′dăl) [″ + *chorioeides*, skinlike]. Situated around the choroid coat.

pericolic (pĕr-ĭ-kō′lĭk) [″ + *kolon*, colon]. Around or encircling the colon.

pericolitis (pĕr″ĭ-kō-lī′tĭs) [″ + ″ + *itis*, inflammation]. Inflammation of area around the colon.

pericolonitis (pĕr″ĭ-kō-lŏn-ī′tĭs). Inflamed condition of region around the colon.

pericolpitis (pĕr″ĭ-kŏl-pī′tĭs) [Gr. *peri*, around, + *kolpos*, vagina, + *itis*, inflammation]. Inflammation of connective tissues surrounding the vagina.

periconchal (pĕr-ĭ-kŏng′kăl) [″ + *konche*, concha]. Around the concha of the ear.

pericorneal (pĕr″ĭ-kor′nē-ăl) [″ + L. *cornu*, horn]. Placed around the cornea.

pericoronal (pĕr″ĭ-kor′ō-năl) [″ + *korone*, crown]. Around the crown of a tooth.

pericoronitis (pĕr″ĭ-kor″ō-nī′tĭs) [″ + ″ + *itis*, inflammation]. Inflammation around the crown of a tooth.

pericranial (pĕr″ĭ-krā′nē-ăl) [″ + *kranion*, skull]. Pert. to the periosteum of the skull.

pericranitis (pĕr″ĭ-krā-nī′tĭs) [″ + ″ + *itis*, inflammation]. Inflamed condition of pericranium.

pericranium (pĕr″ĭ-krā′nē-ŭm). [NA] Fibrous membrane surrounding the cranium; periosteum of the skull.

    p. internum. Lining surface of the cranium. SYN: *endocranium.*

pericystic (pĕr″ĭ-sĭs′tĭk) [″ + *kystis*, bladder]. Surrounding a cyst.

pericystitis (pĕr″ĭ-sĭs-tī′tĭs) [″ + ″ + *itis*, inflammation]. Inflamed condition of tissues about the bladder.

pericystium (pĕr″ĭ-sĭs′tē-ŭm) [″ + *kystis*, bladder]. 1. The vascular wall surrounding a cyst. 2. Tissues around the urinary bladder or gallbladder.

pericyte (pĕr′ĭ-sīt) [″ + *kytos*, cell]. A flat, undifferentiated, contractile connective tissue cell around the capillary walls.

pericytial (pĕr-ĭ-sĭsh′ăl) [″ + *kytos*, cell]. Placed around a cell.

peridectomy (pĕr″ĭ-dĕk′tō-mē) [″ + *ektome*, excision]. Peritectomy, q.v.

peridendritic (pĕr″ĭ-dĕn-drĭt′ĭk) [″ + *dendron*, a tree]. Surrounding a dendrite of a nerve cell.

peridens (pĕr″ĭ-dĕns) [″ + L. *dens*, tooth]. A supernumerary tooth not situated in the dental arch.

peridental (pĕr″ĭ-dĕn′tăl) [″ + L. *dens*, tooth]. Surrounding a tooth or part of one. SYN: *periodontal.*

peridentitis (pĕr″ + ″ + *itis*, inflammation]. Inflammation of tissues surrounding a tooth. SYN: *periodontoclasia.*

peridentium (pĕr″ĭ-dĕn′shē-ŭm) [″ + L. *dens*, tooth]. Periodontium, q.v.

periderm [″ + *derma*, skin]. Thin layer of flattened cells forming a transient layer of embryonic epidermis. SYN: *epitrichial layer; epitrichium.*

peridesmitis (pĕr″ĭ-dĕz-mī′tĭs) [″ + *desmion*, band, + *itis*, inflammation]. Inflammation of the areolar tissue around a ligament.

peridesmium (pĕr″ĭ-dĕz′mē-ŭm). The connective tissue membrane sheathing a ligament.

perididymis (pĕr″ĭ-dĭd′ĭ-mĭs) [″ + *didymos*, testicle]. The tunica vaginalis of the testicle.

perididymitis (pĕr″ĭ-dĭd″ĭ-mī′tĭs) [″ + ″ + *itis*, inflammation]. Inflammation of the perididymis.

peridiverticulitis (pĕr″ĭ-dī″vĕr-tĭk″ū-lī′tĭs) [″ + L. *diverticulare*, to turn aside, + Gr. *itis*, inflammation]. Inflammation of tissues situated around an intestinal diverticulum.

periductal (pĕr-ĭ-dŭk′tăl) [″ + L. *ductus*, a passage]. Situated around a duct.

periduodenitis (pĕr″ĭ-dū″ō-dĕ-nī′tĭs) [″ + L. *duodeni*, twelve, + Gr. *itis*, inflammation]. Inflammation around the duodenum, often causing adhesions attaching it to the peritoneum.

peridural (pĕr″ĭ-dū′răl) [″ + L. *durus*, hard]. Outside the dura mater of the spinal cord.

periencephalitis (pĕr″ē-ĕn-sĕf″ă-lī′tĭs) [″ + *enkephalos*, brain, + *itis*, inflammation]. Inflamed condition of the surface of the brain.

periencephalomeningitis (pĕr″ē-ĕn-sĕf″ă-lō-mĕn″ĭn-jī′tĭs) [″ + ″ + *meninx*, membrane, + *itis*, inflammation]. Inflamed condition of cerebral cortex and the meninges.

periendothelioma (pĕr″ē-ĕn″dō-thē″lē-ō′mă) [″ + *endon*, within, + *thele*, nipple, + *oma*, tumor]. A tumor arising from the endothelium of the lymphatics and the perithelium of blood vessels.

perienteric (pĕr″ē-ĕn-tĕr′ĭk) [Gr. *peri*, around, + *enteron*, intestine]. Around the intestines.

perienteritis (pĕr″ē-ĕn″tĕr-ī′tĭs) [″ + ″ + *itis*, inflammation]. Inflammation of the intestinal peritoneum.

perienteron (pĕr″ē-ĕn′tĕr-ŏn) [″ + *enteron*, intestine]. The peritoneal cavity of the embryo.

periependymal (pĕr″ē-ĕp-ĕn′dĭ-măl) [″ + *ependyma*, an upper garment]. Around the ependyma.

periesophagitis (pĕr″ē-ē-sŏf″ă-jī′tĭs) [″ + *oisophagos*, esophagus, + *itis*, inflammation]. Inflamed condition of tissues around the esophagus.

perifistular (pĕr-ĭ-fĭs′tū-lĕr) [″ + L. *fistula*, pipe]. Located around a fistula.

perifocal (pĕr″ĭ-fō′kăl) [″ + L. *focus*, hearth]. Around a focus, esp. around an infected focus.

perifollicular (pĕr″ĭ-fŏl-lĭk′ū-lăr) [″ + L. *folliculus*, a little sac]. Around a follicle.

perifolliculitis (pĕr″ĭ-fō-lĭk″ū-lī′tĭs) [″ + ″ + Gr. *itis*, inflammation]. Inflamed condition of area around the hair follicles.

perigangliitis (pĕr″ĭ-găng′lē-ī′tĭs) [″ + *ganglion*, knot, + *itis*, inflammation]. Inflamed condition of region around a ganglion.

periganglionic (pĕr″ĭ-găng′glē-ŏn′ĭk) [″ + *ganglion*, knot]. Around a ganglion.

perigastric (pĕr″ĭ-găs′trĭk) [″ + *gaster*, belly]. Around the stomach.

perigastritis (pĕr″ĭ-găs-trī′tĭs) [″ + ″ + *itis*, inflammation]. Inflammation of peritoneal covering of the stomach.

perigemmal (pĕr″ĭ-jĕm′ăl) [″ + L. *gemma*, bud]. Around any bud, esp. a taste bud.

periglandulitis (pĕr″ĭ-glăn″dū-lī′tĭs) [″ + L. *glandula*, small gland, + Gr. *itis*, inflammation]. Inflammation of tissues around a gland.

periglottic (pĕr″ĭ-glŏt′ĭk) [″ + *glotta*, tongue]. Around the base of the tongue and epiglottis.

perihepatic (pĕr″ĭ-hē-păt′ĭk) [Gr. *peri*, around, + *hepar*, liver]. Around the liver.

perihepatitis (pĕr″ĭ-hĕp-ă-tī′tĭs) [″ + ″ + *itis*, inflammation]. Inflammation of peritoneal covering of the liver, usually occurring in circumscribed areas.

perihernial (pĕr″ĭ-hĕr′nē-ăl) [″ + L. *hernia*, rupture]. Around a hernia.

perijejunitis (pĕr″ĭ-jē-jū-nī′tĭs) [″ + L. *jejunum*, empty, + Gr. *itis*, inflammation]. Inflamed condition of tissues around the jejunum.

perikaryon (pĕr″ĭ-kăr′ē-ŏn) [″ + *karyon*, nucleus]. The cell body of a neuron.

perikeratic (pĕr″ĭ-kĕr-ă′tĭk) [″ + *keras*, horn]. About the cornea. SYN: *pericorneal.*

perikymata (pĕr″ĭ-kī′mă-tă) [″ + *kyma*, wave]. The transverse wavelike grooves most apparent in surface enamel of newly erupted anterior teeth; they are more pronounced at eruption and are reduced in depth with wear in advancing age.

perilabyrinthitis (pĕr″ĭ-lăb″ĭr-ĭn-thī′tĭs) [″ + *labyrinthos*, a maze of canals, + *itis*,

inflammation]. Inflammation of tissues around the labyrinth.

perilaryngeal (pĕr″ĭ-lă-rĭn′jē-ăl) [″ + *larynx*, larynx]. Around the larynx.

perilaryngitis (pĕr″ĭ-lăr″ĭn-jī′tĭs) [″ + ″ + *itis*, inflammation]. Inflamed condition of tissues around the larynx.

perilenticular (pĕr″ĭ-lĕn-tĭk′ū-lăr) [″ + L. *lenticularis*, pert. to a lens]. Around the lens of the eye.

periligamentous (pĕr″ĭ-lĭg″ă-mĕn′tŭs) [″ + L. *ligamentum*, a band]. Around a ligament.

perilymph, perilympha (pĕr′ĭ-lĭmf, pĕr″ĭ-lĭm′fă) [″ + L. *lympha*, serum]. The pale limpid fluid contained in the space between the membranous and bony labyrinth of the internal ear.

perilymphangeal (pĕr″ĭ-lĭm-făn′jē-ăl) [″ + ″ + Gr. *angeion*, vessel]. Around a lymphatic vessel.

perilymphangitis (pĕr″ĭ-lĭmf-ăn-jī′tĭs) [″ + ″ + ″ + *itis*, inflammation]. Inflammation of tissues around a lymphatic vessel.

perimastitis (pĕr″ĭ-măs-tī′tĭs) [″ + *mastos*, breast, + *itis*, inflammation]. Inflammation of the fibrous tissue around a breast.

perimeningitis (pĕr″ĭ-mĕn″ĭn-jī′tĭs) [Gr. *peri*, around, + *meninx*, membrane, + *itis*, inflammation]. Inflamed condition of the dura mater. SYN: *pachymeningitis.*

perimeter (pĕr-ĭm′ĕ-tĕr) [″ + *metron*, measure]. 1. The outer edge or periphery of a body or measure of the same. 2. Device for determining the extent of the field of vision. SEE: *perimetry.*

perimetric (pĕr″ĭ-mĕt′rĭk). 1. [″ + *metron*, measure] Concerning perimetry, q.v. 2. [″ + *metra*, uterus] Around the uterus.

perimetritic (pĕr″ĭ-mē-trĭt′ĭk) [″ + *metra*, uterus, + *itis*, inflammation]. Concerning perimetritis.

perimetritis (pĕr″ĭ-mē-trī′tĭs) [″ + ″ + *itis*, inflammation]. Inflammation of the peritoneal covering of the uterus. May be associated with parametritis.

perimetrium (pĕr-ĭ-mē′trē-ŭm). [NA] Serous coat of the uterus.

perimetry (pĕr-ĭm′ĕ-trē) [″ + *metron*, measure]. 1. Circumference, edge, border of a body. 2. Measurement of the scope of the field of vision with a perimeter.

perimyelis (pĕr″ĭ-mī′ĕ-lĭs) [″ + *myelos*, marrow]. Endosteum.

perimyelitis (pĕr″ĭ-mī″ĕ-lī′tĭs) [″ + ″ + *itis*, inflammation]. 1. Inflammation of the pia mater and arachnoid of the brain or spinal cord. SYN: *leptomeningitis.* 2. Inflammation of the endosteum or membrane around medullary cavity of a bone.

perimyelography (pĕr″ĭ-mī″ĕ-lŏg′ră-fē) ["
+ ″ + *graphein*, to write]. X-ray examination of the area around the spinal cord.

perimyoendocarditis (pĕr″ĭ-mī″ō-ĕn″dō-
kăr-dī′tĭs) [″ + *mys*, muscle, + *endon*,
within, + *kardia*, heart, + *itis*, inflam-
mation]. Inflammation of the muscular wall
of the heart, its endothelial lining, and the
pericardium.

perimyositis (pĕr″ĭ-mī″ō-sī′tĭs) [″ + ″
+ *itis*, inflammation]. Inflammation of
the connective tissue around a muscle.

perimysia (pĕr″ĭ-mĭs′ē-ă). Pl. of perimysium.

perimysial (pĕr-ĭ-mĭs′ē-ăl). Concerning, or of
the nature of, the fibrous sheath of a muscle.

perimysiitis (pĕr″ĭ-mĭs″ē-ī′tĭs) [″ + *mys*,
muscle, + *itis*, inflammation]. Inflamed
condition of the perimysium, the sheath
surrounding a muscle.

perimysium (pĕr″ĭ-mĭs′ē-ŭm) (pl. *perimysia*). [NA] Connective tissue sheath that envelops each primary bundle of muscle fibers.
Sometimes called perimysium internum.
   p. externum. The epimysium.

perinatal (pĕr″ĭ-nā′tăl) [Gr. *peri*, around, +
L. *natalis*, birth]. Concerning the period beginning after the 28th week of pregnancy
through 28 days following birth.

perinatal mortality rate. SEE: *rate, perinatal
mortality.*

perinatology. Study of the fetus and infant
during the perinatal period. SEE: *perinatal.*

perineal (pĕr″ĭ-nē′ăl) [Gr. *perinaion*, peri-
neum]. Concerning, or situated on, the perineum.

perineal body. Mass of tissue composed of
skin, muscle, and fascia between the vagina
and rectum in the female and the penis and
rectum in the male.

perineal fascia. Three layers of tissue between the muscles of the perineum.

perineal hernia. Hernia perforating the perineum. SYN: *perineocele.*

perineal section. Surgical incision through
the perineum. SYN: *perineotomy.*

perineo- [Gr. *perinaion*]. Combining form
pert. to the perineum.

perineocele (pĕr″ĭ-nē′ō-sēl) [Gr. *perinaion*,
perineum, + *kele*, tumor, swelling]. Hernia in the region of the perineum, between
the rectum and vagina or between the rectum and prostate.

perineocolporectomyomectomy (pĕr″ĭ-
nē-ō-kŏl″pō-rĕk″tō-mī″ō-mĕk′tō-mē) [″
+ *kolpos*, vagina, + L. *rectus*, straight,
+ Gr. *mys*, muscle, + *oma*, tumor, +
ektome, excision]. Excision of a myoma by
incising the perineum, vagina, and rectum.

perineometer (pĕr″ĭ-nē-ŏm′ĕ-ter) [Gr. *perinaion*, perineum, + *metron*, measure].
Apparatus for measuring pressure or force
that is produced in the vagina when pubo-

coccygeus and levator ani muscles are contracted voluntarily. SEE: *Kegel exercises.*

perineoplasty (pĕr″ĭ-nē′ō-plăs″tē) [″ +
plassein, to form]. Reparative surgery on the
perineum.

perineorrhaphy (pĕr″ĭ-nē-or′ă-fē) [″ +
rhaphe, a sewing]. Suture of the perineum to
repair a laceration that occurs or is made
during the delivery of the fetus.

   NURSING IMPLICATIONS: Prevent
infection by thorough irrigation of the perineum with warm, sterile saline following
urination and defecation. Be certain washing solution drains down toward the anal
area. Gently blot the area dry with sterile
cotton. Keep sutures dry and clean. Assess
perineum daily for signs of infection. Use a
heat lamp several times a day to dry area and
to promote healing. Application of an ice
bag so that the weight is on the bed and not
the vulva may help to relieve pain. Encourage ambulation. Check for daily bowel
movement, and adjust diet and fluid intake
to prevent constipation.
   p., anterior. Surgical repair of anterior
perineum and vaginal wall to correct a cystocele.
   p., colpo-. Removal of part of posterior
vaginal wall and suturing of torn perineal
body.
   p., posterior. Removal and repair of rectocele.

perineoscrotal (pĕr″ĭ-nē-ō-skrō′tăl) [″ +
L. *scrotum*, a bag]. Concerning the perineum
and scrotum.

perineotomy (pĕr″ĭ-nē-ŏt′ō-mē) [″ +
tome, incision]. Surgical incision into the
perineum. SYN: *perineal section.*

perineovaginal (pĕr″ĭ-nē″ō-văj′ĭn-ăl) [″
+ L. *vagina*, sheath]. Concerning the perineum and vagina.

perinephrial (pĕr″ĭ-nĕf′rē-ăl). Concerning
the perinephrium.

perinephric (pĕr″ĭ-nĕf′rĭk) [Gr. *peri*, around,
+ *nephros*, kidney]. Located or occurring
around the kidney.

perinephric abscess. Abscess formation in
the peritoneal membrane surrounding the
kidney.

perinephritis (pĕr″ĭ-nē-frī′tĭs) [″ + ″ +
itis, inflammation]. Inflammation of peritoneal tissues around the kidney. SYN: *paranephritis.*

perinephrium (pĕr″ĭ-nĕf′rē-ŭm). The connective and fatty tissue surrounding the
kidney.

perineum (pĕr″ĭ-nē′ŭm) [Gr. *perinaion*]. 1.
[NA] The structures occupying the pelvic
outlet and constituting the pelvic floor. 2.
The external region between the vulva and
anus in a female or between the scrotum and
anus in a male. It is made up of skin, muscle,

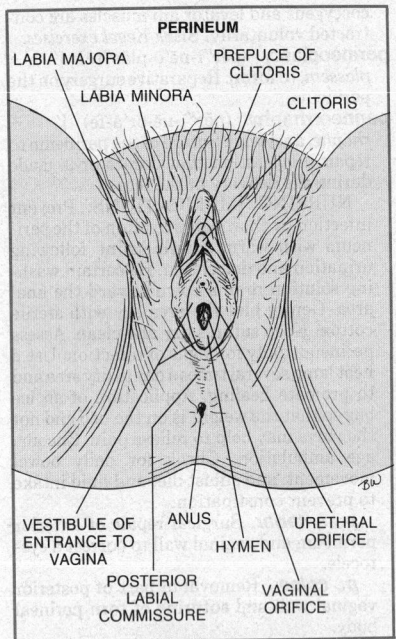

PERINEUM

LABIA MAJORA
PREPUCE OF CLITORIS
LABIA MINORA
CLITORIS
VESTIBULE OF ENTRANCE TO VAGINA
ANUS
HYMEN
URETHRAL ORIFICE
POSTERIOR LABIAL COMMISSURE
VAGINAL ORIFICE

and fasciae. The muscles of the perineum are the anterior portion of the intact levator ani muscle, the transverse perineal muscle, and the pubococcygeus muscle. SEE: illus.; body, perineal; "perine-" words.

perineum, tears of the. There are four degrees of severity caused by overstretching of the vagina and perineum in delivery. Fetal malposition increases the chance of tears occurring.

A first-degree tear involves superficial tissues of the perineum and vaginal mucosa but does not injure muscular tissue. A second-degree tear involves those tissues included in a first-degree tear and the muscles of the perineum but not the muscles of the anal sphincter. A third-degree tear involves all of the tissues of the second-degree tear and the muscles of the anal sphincter. A fourth-degree tear extends completely through the perineal skin, vaginal mucosa, perineal body, anal sphincter muscles, and the rectal mucosa.

COMPLICATIONS: Hemorrhage, infection, cystocele, rectocele, descent of uterus, perhaps loss of bowel control.

TREAT: Surgery.

perineural (pĕr″ĭ-nū′răl) [Gr. peri, around, + neuron, nerve]. Around a nerve.

perineurial (pĕr″ĭ-nū′rē-ăl) [″ + neuron, sinew]. Concerning the perineurium, the sheath around a bundle of nerve fibers.

perineuritis (pĕr″ĭ-nū-rī′tĭs) [″ + ″ + itis, inflammation]. Inflammation of the sheath enveloping nerve fibers.

perineurium (pĕr″ĭ-nū′rē-ŭm) [″ + neuron, sinew]. A connective tissue sheath investing a fasciculus or bundle of nerve fibers.

perinuclear (pĕr″ĭ-nū′klē-ăr) [″ + L. nucleus, a kernel]. Around a nucleus.

periocular (pĕr″ē-ŏk′ū-lăr) [″ + L. oculus, eye]. Located around the eye. SYN: circumocular.

period [L. periodus]. 1. The interval of time between two successive occurrences of any regularly recurring phenomenon or event; a cycle. 2. The menses. 3. Time occupied by a disease in running its course, or by a stage of a disease, such as an incubation period.

p., absolute refractory. Following contraction of a muscle, the period in which a stimulus, no matter how strong, will not elicit a response.

p., childbearing. Period in the female during which she is capable of procreation; puberty to the menopause.

p., critical. SEE: critical period.

p., effective refractory. Used in electrocardiography. The interval during which a second action potential cannot occur in an excitable fiber, unless there is a much stronger than normal action potential, because the membrane is still depolarized from the preceding action potential.

p., ejection. P., sphygmic, q.v.

p., fertile. The time during the menstrual cycle when the ovum can be fertilized.

p., gestation. Period of pregnancy; time from conception to parturition. Average length is 10 lunar months or 280 days measured from onset of last menstrual period. Length varies from 250 to 310 days. SEE: gestation; pregnancy for table.

p., incubation. Time from moment of infection to appearance of first symptom.

p., isoelectric. Period in an ECG or other electrical record when either no electrical current is being produced or those positive charges are exactly equal to the negative ones being produced. Thus the tracing is flat.

p., isometric. P., postsphygmic, q.v.

p., latency. Time from the stimulus to the response of the tissue stimulated.

p., latent. Time between stimulation and the resulting response.

p., menstrual. Menstruation.

p., missed. Menstruation not occurring at the time it was expected.

p., monthly. Time of menstrual flow.

p., neonatal. The first 30 days of infant life.

p., patent. Time in a parasitic disease during which organisms are demonstrable in the body.

p., postsphygmic. The short period in diastole when the ventricles are relaxed and no blood is entering. This lasts until the atrioventricular valves open.

p., presphygmic. The short period in systole beginning with closing of the atrioventricular valves and ending with opening of the valves connecting the right and left ventricles to the pulmonary artery and aorta, respectively.

p., puerperal. Interval of time from birth of a child to approximately six weeks later, at which time complete involution of the uterus has occurred.

p., relative refractory. Period after activation of a nerve or muscle, during recovery, when it can be excited only by a stronger than normal stimulus.

p., safe. Time during the menstrual cycle when conception is allegedly not possible. Because of the great variability of the menstrual cycle, it is extremely difficult to predict the portion of the cycle in which intercourse may take place and be "safe" from conception.

p., silent. 1. Time in the course of a disease in which the signs and symptoms are so mild as to be difficult to detect. 2. A pause in normally continuous electrical events such as an ECG or EEG.

p., sphygmic. Period in the cardiac cycle when the blood is being ejected into the arterial system.

p., Wenckebach. Time when a systolic beat of the heart is skipped. This follows a series of ever-lengthening P-R intervals.

periodic (pĕr-ē-ŏd'ĭk) [Gr. *periodikos*]. Recurring after definite intervals.

periodic health examination. The effectiveness of providing a periodic health examination for healthy individuals is controversial. This is not the case for individuals who have a family history of a potentially lethal disease such as colorectal cancer.

As medical progress occurs and techniques employed in this type of examination are refined and have greater degrees of sensitivity and specificity, the periodic health examination will have greater importance.

periodicity (pĕr″ē-ō-dĭs′ĭ-tē). 1. State of being regularly recurrent. 2. The rate of rise and fall or interruption of a unidirectional current in physical therapy.

periodic law. Law stating that the chemical and physical properties of the chemical elements are periodic functions of their atomic numbers.

periodic table. A chart with the chemical elements arranged by their atomic numbers according to the periodic law, q.v.

periodontal (pĕr″ē-ō-dŏn′tăl) [Gr. *peri*, around, + *odous*, tooth]. Located around a tooth. SYN: *peridental*.

periodontal abscess. A localized area of acute or chronic inflammation with pus formation found in the gingiva, periodontal pockets, or periodontal ligament.

periodontal disease. Disease of supporting structures of the teeth, the periodontium, q.v., including alveolar bone to which the teeth are anchored. The most common symptom is bleeding gums, but loosening of the teeth, receding gums, abscesses in pockets between the gums and the teeth, and necrotizing ulcerative gingivitis may be present as the disease process continues. Proper dental hygiene, including proper brushing of the teeth, use of dental floss, and periodic removal of plaque, q.v., by a dentist or dental hygienist, will help to prevent periodontal disease.

TREAT: In the early stages of the disease, curettage of the irritating material, i.e., plaque and calculus (tartar), from the crown and root surfaces of the teeth may be the only treatment required. In more advanced stages, procedures such as gingivectomy, gingivoplasty, and correction of the bony architecture of the teeth may be required. Adjustment of the occlusion of the teeth and orthodontic treatment may be used in order to help prevent recurrences. SEE: *plaque; teeth; tooth; toothbrush and toothbrushing.*

periodontal ligament. The structural unit of oriented collagen fiber bundles that attaches the tooth to the surrounding alveolar bone proper and gingiva; may be subdivided into gingival ligament, alveolodental ligament, and interdental ligament according to the attachment of its fibers.

periodontal pocket. A gingival sulcus, q.v., enlarged beyond normal limits as a result of poor oral hygiene; the space bordered on one side by the tooth and the other side by ulcerated sulcular epithelium; it will be several millimeters deep when probed and limited at its apex by attachment epithelium.

periodontia (pĕr″ē-ō-dŏn′shē-ă) [Gr. *peri*, around, + *odous*, tooth]. 1. Plural of periodontium. 2. The study and treatment of diseases of the periodontal tissues.

periodontics (pĕr″ē-ō-dŏn′tĭks) [″ + *odous*, tooth]. The branch of dentistry concerned with study and treatment of the periodontal tissues.

periodontitis (pĕr″ē-ō-dŏn-tī′tĭs) [″ + ″ + *itis*, inflammation]. Inflammation or degeneration, or both, of the dental periosteum, alveolar bone, cementum, and adjacent gingiva. Suppuration usually occurs, supporting bone is resorbed, teeth become loose, and recession of gingivae occurs. Usually follows chronic gingivitis, Vincent's infection, or poor dental hygiene. Systemic factors may predispose. SYN: *pyorrhea alveolaris; Riggs' disease.*

p., apical. Periodontitis of periapical region usually leading to formation of periapical abscess.

periodontium (pĕr-ē-ō-dŏn'shē-ŭm). [NA] The structures that support the teeth, cushion the shock of chewing, and keep the teeth firmly anchored in the bone. These structures are the gingivae, periodontal membrane or ligament, cementum, and alveolar bone.

periodontoclasia (pĕr″ē-ō-dŏn″tō-klā′zē-ă) [″ + *odous,* tooth, + *klasis,* breaking]. Condition characterized by inflammation accompanied by degenerative and retrogressive changes in the periodontium. SYN: *peridentitis.*

periodontology (pĕr″ē-ō-dŏn-tŏl′ō-jē) [″ + ″ + *logos,* word, reason]. Branch of dentistry dealing with treatment of diseases of the tissues around the teeth.

periodontosis (pĕr″ē-ō-dŏn-tō′sĭs) [″ + ″ + *osis,* condition]. Any degenerative disease of the periodontal tissues.

periodoscope (pĕr″ē-ŏd′ō-skōp) [LL. *periodus,* interval of time, + *skopein,* to examine]. Table or dial for calculation of expected date of delivery. SEE: *pregnancy* for table.

periomphalic (pĕr″ē-ŏm-făl′ĭk) [Gr. *peri,* around, + *omphalos,* navel]. Located around or near the umbilicus.

periontogenic [″ + *on,* existing, + *gennan,* to produce]. Diseases caused by the environment.

perionychia (pĕr″ē-ō-nĭk′ē-ă) [″ + *onyx,* nail]. Inflammation around a nail.

perionychium (pĕr″ē-ō-nĭk′ē-ŭm). The epidermis surrounding a nail.

perionyx (pĕr″ē-ō′nĭks) [″ + *onyx,* nail]. The remnant of the eponychium that persists as a band across the root of the nail.

perionyxis (pĕr″ē-ō-nĭk′sĭs). Inflammation of epidermis surrounding a nail.

perioophoritis (pĕr″ē-ō-ŏf″ō-rī′tĭs) [″ + *oophoron,* ovary, + *itis,* inflammation]. Inflammation of the surface membrane of the ovary. SYN: *perioothecitis.*

perioophorosalpingitis (pĕr″ē-ō-ŏf″ō-rō-săl″pĭn-jī′tĭs) [″ + ″ + *salpinx,* tube, + *itis,* inflammation]. Inflamed condition of tissues around an ovary and oviduct. SYN: *perioothecosalpingitis; perisalpingoovaritis.*

perioothecitis (pĕr″ē-ō″ō-thē-sī′tĭs) [″ + *oon,* egg, + *theke,* box, + *itis,* inflammation]. Inflammation of the tissues

around the ovary. SYN: *perioophoritis.*

perioothecosalpingitis (pĕr″ē-ō″ō-thē″kō-săl-pĭn-jī′tĭs) [″ + ″ + ″ + *salpinx,* tube, + *itis,* inflammation]. Inflammation of peritoneal membrane around the ovary and oviduct. SYN: *perioophorosalpingitis; perisalpingoovaritis.*

perioperative. Occurring in the period immediately before, during, and immediately after surgery.

periophthalmic (pĕr″ē-ŏf-thăl′mĭk) [″ + *ophthalmos,* eye]. Around the eye.

perioptometry (pĕr″ē-ŏp-tŏm′ē-trē) [″ + *optos,* visible, + *metron,* measure]. Measurement of the visual field. SYN: *perimetry.*

perioral (pĕr″ē-or′ăl) [″ + L. *oralis,* mouth]. Surrounding the mouth. SYN: *circumoral.*

periorbita (pĕr″ē-or′bĭ-tă) [″ + L. *orbita,* orbit]. [NA] Connective tissue covering the socket of the eye.

periorbital (pĕr″ē-or′bĭ-tăl). Surrounding the socket of the eye. SYN: *circumorbital.*

periorbititis (pĕr″ē-or″bĭ-tī′tĭs) [″ + L. *orbita,* orbit, + Gr. *itis,* inflammation]. Inflamed condition of the periorbita.

periorchitis (pĕr″ē-or-kī′tĭs) [″ + *orchis,* testicle, + *itis,* inflammation]. Inflamed condition of the tissues investing a testicle.

p. hemorrhagica. Chronic hematocele of the tunica vaginalis coat of the testis.

periosteal (pĕr-ē-ŏs′tē-ăl) [″ + *osteon,* bone]. Concerning the periosteum. SYN: *periosteous.*

periosteitis (pĕr″ē-ŏs″tē-ī′tĭs) [″ + ″ + *itis,* inflammation]. Inflammation of membrane investing a bone, the periosteum. SYN: *periostitis.*

periosteoedema (pĕr″ē-ŏs″tē-ō-ē-dē′mă) [Gr. *peri,* around, + *osteon,* bone, + *oidema,* swelling]. Edema of the periosteum, the membrane surrounding a bone.

periosteoma (pĕr″ē-ŏs-tē-ō′mă) [″ + ″ + *oma,* tumor]. 1. An abnormal growth surrounding a bone. 2. Tumor of the periosteum, the tissue surrounding a bone.

periosteomyelitis (pĕr″ē-ŏs″tē-ō-mī″ē-lī′tĭs) [″ + ″ + *myelos,* marrow, + *itis,* inflammation]. Inflammation of bone, including the periosteum and marrow.

periosteophyte (pĕr″ē-ŏs′tē-ō-fīt) [″ + *osteon,* bone, + *phyton,* growth]. Abnormal bony growth on periosteum, or arising from it.

periosteorrhaphy (pĕr″ē-ŏs″tē-or′ă-fē) [″ + ″ + *rhaphe,* seam, ridge]. Joining by suture the margins of a severed periosteum.

periosteosis (pĕr″ē-ŏs″tē-ō′sĭs) [″ + ″ + *osis,* condition]. Periostosis, q.v.

periosteotome (pĕr″ē-ŏs′tē-ō-tōm) [″ + *osteon,* bone, + *tome,* incision]. Instrument for cutting the periosteum or removing it from the bone.

periosteotomy (pĕr″ē-ŏs-tē-ŏt′ō-mē). Incision into the periosteum.

periosteous (pĕr″ē-ŏs′tē-ŭs) [″ + *osteon*, bone]. Concerning, or of the nature of, periosteum. SYN: *periosteal.*

periosteum (pĕr-ē-ŏs′tē-ŭm) [Gr. *periosteon*]. [NA] The fibrous membrane that forms the investing covering of bones except at their articular surfaces. Consists of a dense external layer containing numerous blood vessels and an inner layer of connective tissue cells that function as osteoblasts when the bone is injured and then participate in new bone formation. Periosteum serves as a supporting structure for blood vessels nourishing bone and for attachment of muscles, tendons, and ligaments. It extends over the whole surface except at the cartilaginous articulations.

　　p., alveolar. The periodontal ligament.

　　p. externum. Periosteum covering external surfaces of bones.

　　p. internum. Interior periosteum lining the medullary canal of a bone.

periostitis (pĕr″ē-ŏs-tī′tĭs) [″ + *itis*, inflammation]. Inflamed condition of periosteum, the membrane investing a bone.

　　SYM: Pain over part, esp. under pressure, fever, sweats, leukocytosis, skin inflamed, rigidity of overlying muscles.

　　ETIOL: Infectious diseases, esp. syphilis; also trauma.

　　p., albuminous. Periostitis with albuminous serous fluid exudate beneath the membrane affected.

　　p., alveolar. Inflammation of the peridental membrane. SYN: *periodontitis.*

　　p., diffuse. Periostitis of the long bones.

　　p., hemorrhagic. Periostitis with extravasation of blood under the periosteum.

periostoma (pĕr″ē-ŏs-tō′mă) [Gr. *peri*, around, + *osteon*, bone, + *oma*, tumor]. A bony neoplasm around a bone or arising from its membranous sheath.

periostomedullitis (pĕr″ē-ŏs″tō-mĕd-ū-lī′tĭs) [″ + ″ + L. *medulla*, marrow, + Gr. *itis*, inflammation]. Inflammation of the marrow or sheath of a bone. SYN: *periosteomyelitis.*

periostosis (pĕr″ē-ŏs-tō′sĭs) [″ + ″ + *osis*, condition]. A bony neoplasm around a bone or arising from it.

periostosteitis (pĕr″ē-ŏs-tŏs″tē-ī′tĭs) [″ + ″ + *osteon*, bone, + *itis*, inflammation]. Osteoperiosteitis, q.v.

periostotome (pĕr″ē-ŏs′tō-tōm) [″ + ″ + *tome*, incision]. A device for cutting the periosteum. SYN: *periosteotome.*

periostotomy (pĕr″ē-ŏs-tŏt′ō-mē) [″ + ″ + *tome*, incision]. Incision of the perios-

teum, the sheath covering a bone. SYN: *periosteotomy.*

periotic (pĕr-ē-ō′tĭk) [″ + *ous*, ear]. Situated around the ear, esp. the internal ear.

periotic bone. The mastoid and petrous portions of the temporal bone.

periovaritis (pĕr″ē-ō″vă-rī′tĭs) [″ + L. *ovarium*, ovary, + Gr. *itis*, inflammation]. Perioophoritis, q.v.

periovular (pĕr″ē-ō′vū-lăr) [″ + L. *ovulum*, little egg]. Around an ovum.

peripachymeningitis (pĕr″ĭ-pak″ē-mĕn″in-jī′tĭs) [″ + *pachys*, thick, + *meninx*, membrane, + *itis*, inflammation]. Inflamed condition of connective tissue between the dura mater and the bone that encloses the central nervous system.

peripancreatitis (pĕr″ĭ-păn″krē-ă-tī′tĭs) [″ + *pankreas*, pancreas, + *itis*, inflammation]. Inflammation of tissues about or around the pancreas.

peripapillary (pĕr″ĭ-păp′ĭ-lĕr″ē) [″ + L. *papilla*, nipple]. Around a papilla.

peripatetic (pĕr″ĭ-pă-tĕt′ĭk) [L. *peripateticus*, to walk about while teaching]. Moving from place to place.

peripenial (pĕr″ĭ-pē′nē-ăl) [Gr. *peri*, around, + L. *penis*, penis]. Around the penis.

periphacitis (pĕr-ĭ-fă-sī′tĭs) [″ + *phakos*, lens, + *itis*, inflammation]. Inflamed condition of the capsule of the crystalline lens of the eye.

periphakus (pĕr″ĭ-fā′kŭs). The elastic capsule surrounding the crystalline lens.

peripharyngeal (pĕr″ĭ-fă-rĭn′jē-ăl) [″ + *pharynx*, throat]. Around the pharynx.

peripherad (pĕr-ĭf′ĕr-ăd) [″ + *pherein*, to bear, + L. *ad*, to]. In the direction of the periphery.

peripheral (pĕr-ĭf′ĕr-ăl). Located at, or pert. to, the periphery; occurring away from the center.

peripheral nervous system. That portion of the nervous system outside the central nervous system. Included are the 12 pairs of cranial nerves, 31 pairs of spinal nerves, and their branches to the entire body. Also included are all sensory nerves, the sympathetic and parasympathetic nerves.

peripheral vascular disease. An imprecise term indicating diseases of the arteries and veins of the extremities, esp. those conditions that interfere with adequate flow of blood to or from the extremities, such as atherosclerosis with narrowing of the arterial lumen. SEE: *Nursing Diagnoses* in *Appendix.*

peripheraphose (pĕr-ĭf′ĕr-ă-fōs). Subjective sensation of darkness or shadow that originates in peripheral optic structures (optic nerve or eyeball).

peripherocentral (pĕ-rĭf″ĕr-ō-sĕn′trăl) [″

+ *pherein*, to bear, + *kentron*, center].
Concerning both the periphery and central
part of an organ.

peripherophose (per-ĭf'ĕr-ō-fōs). A subjective sensation of light or color that originates in peripheral optic structures (optic nerve or eyeball).

periphery (pĕr-ĭf'ĕ-rē) [Gr. *periphereia*].
Outer part or surface of a body; the part away from the center.

periphlebitis (pĕr″ĭ-flĕ-bī'tĭs) [Gr. *peri*, around, + *phleps*, vein, + *itis*, inflammation]. Inflamed condition of external coat of a vein or tissues around it.

periphoria (pĕr-ĭ-fō'rē-ă) [″ + *phoros*, bearing]. Tendency of the axis of the eye to deviate from the normal due to weakness of oblique muscles. SYN: *cyclophoria*.

periphrastic (pĕr″ĭ-frăs'tĭk) [Gr. *periphrastikos*]. Rel. to the use of superfluous words in expressing a thought. Appears in the writings and speech of some schizophrenics.

periphrenitis (pĕr″ĭ-frĕ-nī'tĭs) [Gr. *peri*, around, + *phren*, diaphragm, + *itis*, inflammation]. Inflamed condition of the structures around the diaphragm.

Periplaneta (pĕr″ĭ-plă-nē'tă). A genus of cockroaches belonging to the order Orthoptera. Roaches contaminate food by mechanically transporting disease-producing bacteria, ova, and protozoa to the food.

    P. americana. The American cockroach.

    P. australasiae. The Australian cockroach.

periplasmic vesicles. A specialized apparatus in bacteria for excreting certain substances such as penicillinase.

periplast (pĕr'ĭ-plăst) [″ + *plassein*, to form]. Peripheral protoplasm of a cell exclusive of the nucleus.

peripleural (pĕr'ĭ-plū'răl) [″ + *pleura*, rib]. Encircling the pleura.

peripleuritis (pĕr-ĭ-plū-rī'tĭs) [″ + ″ + *itis*, inflammation]. Inflamed condition of the connective tissues between the pleura and wall of the chest.

peripolar (pĕr″ĭ-pō'lăr) [″ + L. *polus*, pole]. Around a pole.

peripolesis (pĕr″ĭ-pō-lē'sĭs) [Gr., a going about]. In tissue culture, the collecting of lymphocytes around macrophages.

periporitis (pĕr″ĭ-por-ī'tĭs) [Gr. *peri*, around, + L. *porus*, pore, + Gr. *itis*]. Multiple abscesses around sweat glands, esp. as a complication of malaria in children.

periportal (pĕr″ĭ-por'tăl) [″ + L. *porta*, gate]. Around the portal vein and its branches.

periproctic (pĕr″ĭ-prŏk'tĭk) [″ + *proktos*, anus]. Around the anus.

periproctitis (pĕr″ĭ-prŏk-tī'tĭs) [″ + ″ + *itis*, inflammation]. Inflammation of

areolar tissues in region of the rectum and anus. SYN: *perirectitis*.

periprostatic (pĕr″ĭ-prŏs-tăt'ĭk) [″ + *prostates*, prostate]. Surrounding or occurring about the prostate.

periprostatitis (pĕr″ĭ-prŏs-tă-tī'tĭs) [″ + ″ + *itis*, inflammation]. Inflamed condition of tissues surrounding the prostate.

peripylephlebitis (pĕr″ĭ-pī″lĕ-flĕ-bī'tĭs) [″ + *pyle*, gate, + *phlebos*, vein, + *itis*, inflammation]. Inflamed condition of tissues about the portal vein.

peripyloric (pĕr″ĭ-pī-lor'ĭk) [″ + *pyloros*, pylorus]. Extending around the pylorus.

periradicular. Around a root or rootlike process, especially relating to a tooth.

perirectal (pĕr″ĭ-rĕk'tăl) [″ + L. *rectus*, straight]. Extending around the rectum.

perirectitis (pĕr″ĭ-rĕk-tī'tĭs) [″ + ″ + Gr. *itis*, inflammation]. Inflamed condition of tissues about rectum and anus. SYN: *periproctitis*.

perirenal (pĕr″ĭ-rē'năl) [″ + L. *ren*, kidney]. Extending around the kidney. SYN: *circumrenal; perinephric*.

perirhinal (pĕr″ĭ-rī'năl) [″ + *rhis*, nose]. Located about the nose or nasal fossae.

perirhizoclasia (pĕr″ĭ-rī″zō-klā'zē-ă) [″ + *rhiza*, root, + *klasis*, destruction]. Inflammation and destruction of tissues extending around the roots of a tooth.

perisalpingitis (pĕr″ĭ-săl″pĭn-jī'tĭs) [″ + *salpinx*, tube, + *itis*, inflammation]. Inflamed condition of peritoneal coat about the oviduct. SYN: *perioophorosalpingitis; perioothecosalpingitis*.

perisalpingooscaritis (pĕr″ĭ-săl-pĭn″gō-ō″vār-ī'tĭs) [″ + ″ + L. *ovarium*, ovary, + Gr. *itis*, inflammation]. Inflammation of peritoneal tissues surrounding the fallopian tubes and ovaries. SYN: *perioophorosalpingitis; perioothecosalpingitis*.

perisalpinx (pĕr″ĭ-săl'pĭnks) [″ + *salpinx*, tube]. The peritoneum covering the upper borders of the uterine tubes.

perisclerium (pĕr″ĭ-sklē'rē-ŭm) [″ + *skleros*, hard]. Fibrous tissue encircling ossifying cartilage.

periscopic (pĕr″ĭ-skŏp'ĭk) [″ + *skopein*, to examine]. Viewing on all sides; providing a wide range of vision.

perish (pĕr'ĭsh) [ME. *perisshen*]. To die, esp. by other than natural causes.

perisigmoiditis (pĕr″ĭ-sĭg″moy-dī'tĭs) [Gr. *peri*, around, + *sigma*, Gr. letter S, + *eidos*, form, shape, + *itis*, inflammation]. Inflamed condition of peritoneal tissues around the sigmoid flexure of the colon.

perisinuous. Adjacent to or around a sinus.

perisinusitis (pĕr″ĭ-sī″nŭ-sī'tĭs) [″ + L. *sinus*, cavity, + Gr. *itis*, inflammation]. Inflammation of membranes about a sinus, esp. a venous sinus of the dura mater.

perispermatitis (pĕr″ĭ-spĕr″mă-tī′tĭs) [″ + *sperma*, seed, + *itis*, inflammation]. Inflamed condition of tissues about the spermatic cord.

   p. serosa. Hydrocele of spermatic cord.

perisplanchnic (pĕr″ĭ-splănk′nĭk) [″ + *splanchnon*, viscus]. Extending around a viscus or the viscera.

perisplanchnitis (pĕr″ĭ-splănk-nī′tĭs) [″ + ″ + *itis*, inflammation]. Inflamed condition of the tissues around the viscera. SYN: *perivisceritis.*

perisplenic (pĕr″ĭ-splĕn′ĭk) [″ + *splen*, spleen]. Near or around the spleen.

perisplenitis (pĕr″ĭ-splē-nī′tĭs) [″ + ″ + *itis*, inflammation]. Inflammation of peritoneal coat of the spleen, the splenic capsule.

   p. cartilaginea. Inflammation of capsule of the spleen resulting in thickening and hardening.

perispondylic (pĕr″ĭ-spŏn-dĭl′ĭk) [Gr. *peri*, around, + *spondylos*, vertebra]. Around a vertebra.

perispondylitis (pĕr″ĭ-spŏn-dĭl-ī′tĭs) [″ + ″ + *itis*, inflammation]. Inflamed condition of the parts around a vertebra.

perissodactylous (pĕr-ĭs″sō-dăk′tĭ-lŭs) [Gr. *perissos*, odd, + *daktylos*, digit]. Having an odd number of digits on a hand or foot. SYN: *imparidigitate.*

peristalsis (pĕr-ĭ-stăl′sĭs) [Gr. *peri*, around, + *stalsis*, contraction]. A progressive wavelike movement that occurs involuntarily in hollow tubes of the body, esp. the alimentary canal. It is characteristic of tubes possessing longitudinal and circular layers of smooth muscle fibers.

   Peristalsis is induced reflexly by distention of the walls of the tube. The wave consists of contraction of the circular muscle above the distention with relaxation of the region immediately distal to the distended portion. The simultaneous contraction and relaxation progresses slowly for a short distance as a wave that causes the contents of the tube to be forced onward.

   p., mass. Forced peristaltic movements of short duration in which contents are moved from one section of the colon to another, occurring three or four times daily.

   p., reverse. Peristalsis in a direction opposite to the normal direction. SYN: *antiperistalsis.*

peristaltic (pĕr″ĭ-stăl′tĭk). Concerning, or of the nature of, peristalsis.

peristaphyline (pĕr″ĭ-stăf′ĭ-lĭn) [″ + *staphyle*, uvula]. About the uvula.

peristasis (pĕr-rĭs′tă-sĭs) [″ + *stasis*, standing]. 1. In the early stage of inflammation, the decrease in blood flow in the af-

fected area. 2. Environment.

peristomatous (pĕr″ĭ-stŏm′ă-tŭs) [″ + *stoma*, mouth]. Around the mouth.

peristome (pĕr″ĭ-stōm) [″ + *stoma*, mouth]. Channel leading to the cytosome or mouth in certain types of protozoa.

peristrumitis (pĕr″ĭ-stroo-mī′tĭs) [″ + L. *struma*, goiter, + *itis*, inflammation]. Inflamed condition of tissues around a goiter. SYN: *perithyroiditis.*

peristrumous (pĕr″ĭ-stroo′mŭs) [″ + L. *struma*, goiter]. Around a goiter.

perisynovial (pĕr″ĭ-sĭ-nō′vē-ăl) [Gr. *peri*, around, + L. *synovia*, joint fluid]. Extending around a synovial structure.

perisystole (pĕr″ĭ-sĭs′tō-lē) [″ + *systole*, contraction]. The period preceding the systole in the cardiac rhythm. SYN: *presystole.*

peritectomy (pĕr″ĭ-tĕk′tō-mē) [″ + *ektome*, excision]. Surgical removal of a ring of conjunctiva around the cornea.

peritendineum (pĕr″ĭ-tĕn-dĭn′ē-ŭm) [″ + L. *tendo*, tendon]. [NA] A sheath of fibrous connective tissue investing a fiber bundle of a tendon.

peritendinitis, peritenonitis (pĕr″ĭ-tĕn″dĭ-nī′tĭs, -tĕn″ō-nī′tĭs) [″ + ″ + Gr. *itis*, inflammation]. Inflamed condition of the sheath of a tendon. SYN: *tenosynovitis.*

   p. calcarea. The deposition of calcareous material in tendons and associated regions, characterized by pain, tenderness, and limitation of motion.

   p. serosa. Peritendinitis with effusion into the sheath.

peritenon (pĕr″ĭ-tē′nŏn) [″ + *tenon*, tendon]. 1. The sheath of a tendon. 2. Peritendineum.

perithelioma (pĕr″ĭ-thē-lē-ō′mă) [″ + *thele*, nipple, + *oma*, tumor]. A tumor derived from the perithelial layer of the blood vessels.

perithelium (pĕr″ĭ-thē′lē-ŭm). Fibrous outer layer of the smaller blood vessels and capillaries.

   p., Eberth's. An incomplete layer of cells covering capillaries.

perithoracic (pĕr″ĭ-thō-răs′ĭk) [″ + *thorax*, chest]. Around the thorax.

perithyroiditis (pĕr″ĭ-thī-roy-dī′tĭs) [″ + *thyreos*, shield, + *eidos*, form, shape, + *itis*, inflammation]. Inflammation of capsule or tissues sheathing the thyroid gland. SYN: *peristrumitis.*

peritomy (pĕr-ĭt′ō-mē) [″ + *tome*, incision]. 1. Excision of narrow strip of conjunctiva around the cornea in treatment of pannus. SYN: *syndectomy.* 2. Circumcision.

peritoneal (pĕr″ĭ-tō-nē′ăl) [Gr. *peritonaion*, peritoneum]. Concerning the peritoneum.

peritoneal cavity. A potential space between layers of the parietal and visceral perito-

PERITONEAL AND PLEURAL FLUID
INDICATING LOCATION OF INCREASED AMOUNTS (ASCITES)

POSTERIOR PLEURAL SPACE

PELVIC CAVITY

neum. A small amount of fluid is contained in the space. Thus friction is minimized as the viscera glide on each other, or against the wall of the abdominal cavity.

peritoneal chemotherapy. Intraperitoneal injection of antineoplastic drugs.

peritoneal dialysis. Removal of toxic substances from the body by perfusing specific warm sterile chemical solutions through the peritoneal cavity. Used in treating renal failure and in certain poisonings. Some of the drugs and chemicals that may be so removed are salicylates, barbiturates, meprobamate, amphetamines, bromide, methanol, boric acid, sulfonamide, and various antibiotics.

This technique, using chilled, sterile isotonic saline, has been used in treating heatstroke.

Caution: Peritoneal dialysis may be dangerous and may cause death if not done with adequate supervision of body fluid and electrolyte balance.

---

p.d., continuous ambulatory. SEE: *dialysis, continuous ambulatory peritoneal.*

peritoneal fluid. The clear straw-colored serous fluid secreted by the cells of the peritoneum. The few milliliters present in the peritoneal cavity moisten the surfaces of the viscera and allow them to glide over each other as the intestinal tract changes shape during the process of digestion and absorption. In certain disease states the amount of peritoneal fluid is increased. If this is not due to inflammation, the fluid is called ascitic fluid. SEE: illus.; *ascites.*

peritonealgia (pĕr″ĭ-tō″nē-ăl′jē-ă) [″ + *algos,* pain]. Pain of the peritoneum.

peritonealize. During abdominal surgery, to cover a tissue with peritoneum.

peritoneo-. Combining form concerning the peritoneum.

peritoneocentesis (pĕr″ĭ-tō″nē-ō-sĕn-tē′sĭs) [Gr. *peritonaion,* peritoneum, + *kentesis,* puncture]. Piercing of the peritoneal cavity to obtain fluid. SEE: *paracentesis.*

peritoneoclysis (pĕr″ĭ-tō″nē-ō-klī′sĭs) [″ + *klysis,* a washing out]. Introduction of fluid into the peritoneal cavity.

peritoneopathy (pĕr″ĭ-tō-nē-ŏp′ă-thē) [″ + *pathos,* disease, suffering]. Any disordered condition of the peritoneum.

peritoneopericardial (pĕr″ĭ-tō-nē″ō-pĕr″ĭ-kăr′dē-ăl) [″ + *peri,* around, + *kardia,* heart]. Concerning the peritoneum and pericardium.

peritoneopexy (pĕr″ĭ-tō′nē-ō-pĕks″ē) [Gr. *peritonaion,* peritoneum, + *pexis,* fixation]. Fixation of the uterus by way of the vagina.

peritoneoplasty (per″ĭ-tō′nē-ō-plăs″tē) [″ + *plassein,* to form]. Reparative surgery to prevent re-formation of loosened adhesions.

peritoneoscope (pĕr″ĭ-tō′nē-ō-skōp″) [Gr. *peritonaion,* peritoneum, + *skopein,* to examine]. Long, slender periscope or telescope device with a light at one end and an eyepiece at the other. Used to inspect the peritoneal and abdominal cavities through a small incision in the abdominal wall.

peritoneoscopy (pĕr″ĭ-tō″nē-ŏs′kŏ-pē). Examination of peritoneal cavity with the peritoneoscope.

peritoneotomy (pĕr″ĭ-tō″nē-ŏt′ō-mē). Process of incising the peritoneum.

peritoneum (pĕr″ĭ-tō-nē′ŭm) [LL., Gr. *peritonaion*]. [NA] The serous membrane reflected over the viscera and lining the abdominal cavity.

PALPATION: If palmar surface of hand is applied to side of abdomen at level of the liquid in ascites and light percussion is performed on the opposite side, a sense of fluctuation will be communicated to the hand.

p., parietal. Peritoneum lining abdominal and pelvic walls and undersurface of diaphragm.

p., visceral. Peritoneum that invests the abdominal organs. The peritoneum holds the viscera in position by its folds.

peritonism (pĕr′ĭ-tō-nĭzm) [Gr. *peritonaion*, peritoneum, + *-ismos*, condition]. 1. The clinical signs of shock and peritonitis but without inflammation of the peritoneum. 2. A neurosis in which the patient's complaints are consistent with peritonitis.

peritonitic (pĕr″ĭ-tō-nĭt′ĭk) [″ + *itis*, inflammation]. Affected with or concerning peritonitis.

peritonitis (pĕr″ĭ-tō-nī′tĭs) [″ + *itis*, inflammation]. Inflammation of the peritoneum, the membranous coat lining the abdominal cavity and investing the viscera. SEE: *Nursing Diagnoses* in *Appendix*.

ETIOL: Infectious organisms that gain access by way of rupture or perforation of viscus or associated structures, via the female genital tract, by piercing of abdominal wall, via the bloodstream or lymphatic vessels, via surgical incisions, and by failure to practice aseptic techniques during surgery. Prophylactic measures to prevent development of peritonitis are of utmost importance in the care of all patients.

TREAT: Antibiotic therapy.

p., acute diffuse. Generalized peritonitis of a large area.

SYM: Chill; fever, 102° to 103°F (38.9° to 39.4°C); rapid pulse rate; abdominal pain and tenderness so intense that abdominal respiration and bodily movement are inhibited; patient on back with thighs flexed; facial features pinched and anxious; vomiting persistent; bowels usually constipated; hiccough; abdominal distention.

ETIOL: Rupture of an intra-abdominal viscus, as the appendix or stomach. Infection may take place directly from an adjacent organ that is inflamed or from the bloodstream in patients with septicemia.

TREAT: Surgical intervention. Absolute bedrest; sips of water by mouth; saline or glucose solution, blood, or plasma parenterally; analgesics for pain; suction of gastrointestinal tract; antibiotic therapy.

PROG: Guarded.

p., adhesive. Peritonitis in which the visceral and parietal layers stick together by means of adhesions.

p., aseptic. Peritonitis due to causes other than bacterial infection, such as trauma, presence of chemicals produced naturally or introduced from without, or irradiation.

p., benign paroxysmal. Familial paroxysmal polyserositis. SEE: *familial Mediterranean fever.*

p., bile. Peritonitis caused by the escape of bile into the peritoneal cavity.

p., chemical. Peritonitis due to presence of chemicals such as intestinal juices, pancreatic secretions, or bile in the peritoneal cavity.

p., chronic. Peritonitis that is usually due to tuberculosis or cancer.

SYM: Fever slight or absent. Pain not severe; paroxysms; usually diffuse tenderness; anemia and emaciation may be marked.

TREAT: Rest; paracentesis. Laparotomy.

PROG: Guarded.

p., circumscribed. P., localized.

p. deformans. Chronic peritonitis with thickened membrane and adhesions contracting and causing retraction of the intestines.

p., diaphragmatic. Peritonitis in which the peritoneal surface of the diaphragm is mainly affected.

p., diffuse. Peritonitis that is widespread, involving most of the peritoneum. SYN: *p., generalized.*

p. encapsulans. A localized abscess in the peritoneal cavity. This may occur after generalized peritonitis has subsided.

p., fibrocaseous. Peritonitis with fibrosis and caseation. Usually due to tuberculosis.

p., gas. Peritonitis in which gas is present in the peritoneal cavity.

p., generalized. P., diffuse.

p., localized. Peritonitis in which only a small area is involved. SYN: *peritonitis, circumscribed.*

p., meconium. Peritonitis in the newborn due to perforation of the gastrointestinal tract in utero. Neonatal intestinal obstruction may be present. In males a soft hydrocele or scrotal mass may be found.

p., pelvic. Peritonitis involving peritoneum of the pelvic region, usually the sequela of uterine tube infection in female.

p., periodic. Familial Mediterranean fever, q.v.

p., primary. Peritonitis resulting from infectious organisms transmitted through blood or lymph.

p., puerperal. Peritonitis that develops following childbirth.

p., secondary. Peritonitis resulting from extension of infection from adjoining structures, rupture of a viscus, abscess, or trauma.

p., septic. Peritonitis caused by a pyogenic bacterium.

p., serous. Peritonitis in which there is copious liquid exudation.

p., silent. Peritonitis in which there are no signs or symptoms.

p., talc. Peritonitis due to particles of talcum powder in the peritoneal cavity. Talc was present due to its having been used as a powder on surgeon's gloves. Talc is no longer used for that purpose.

p., traumatic. Acute peritonitis due to injury or wound infection.

p., tuberculous. Peritonitis caused by numerous tubercle bacilli on the peritoneum.

peritonize (pĕr'ĭ-tō-nīz) [Gr. *peritonaion*, peritoneum]. Peritonealize, q.v.

peritonsillar (pĕr''ĭ-tŏn'sĭ-lăr) [Gr. *peri*, around, + L. *tonsilla*, tonsil]. Extending around a tonsil.

peritonsillitis (pĕr''ĭ-tŏn''sĭ-lī'tĭs) [" + " + Gr. *itis*, inflammation]. Inflamed condition of tissues around the tonsils. SYN: *periamygdalitis.*

peritracheal (pĕr''ĭ-trā'kē-ăl) [" + *tracheia*, trachea]. Around the trachea.

Peritrate. Trade name for pentaerythritol tetranitrate.

Peritricha (pĕr-ĭt'rĭ-kă) [Gr. *peri*, around, + *thrix*, hair]. A group of protozoa having flagella over the entire surface.

peritrichal, peritrichic (pĕ-rĭt'rĭ-kăl, pĕr''ē-trĭk'ĭk) [" + *thrix*, hair]. Uniform distribution of flagellae over a cell, usually a bacterial cell. SYN: *peritrichous.*

peritrichous (pĕ-rĭt'rĭk-ŭs) [" + *thrix*, hair]. Indicating microorganisms that have cilia or flagella covering the entire surface.

peritrochanteric (pĕr''ĭ-trō''kăn-tĕr'ĭk) [" + *trokhanter*, runner]. Around a trochanter.

perityphlic (pĕr''ĭ-tĭf'lĭk) [" + *typhlon*, cecum]. Around the cecum.

perityphlitis (pĕr''ĭ-tĭf-lī'tĭs) [" + " + *itis*, inflammation]. Inflamed condition of tissues around the cecum and appendix. SYN: *appendicitis.*

periumbilical (pĕr''ē-ŭm-bĭl'ĭ-kăl) [" + L. *umbilicus*, a pit]. Around the navel, i.e., umbilicus.

periungual (pĕr''ē-ŭng'gwăl) [" + L. *unguis*, nail]. Around a nail.

periureteral (pĕr''ē-ū-rē'tĕr-ăl) [" + *oureter*, ureter]. Around the ureter.

periureteritis (pĕr''ē-ū-rē''tĕr-ī'tĭs) [" + " + *itis*, inflammation]. Inflamed condition of parts about the ureter.

periurethral (pĕr''ē-ū-rē'thrăl) [" + *ourethra*, urethra]. Located about the urethra.

periurethritis (pĕr''ē-ū''rē-thrī'tĭs) [" + " + *itis*, inflammation]. Inflammation of the tissues around the urethra.

periuterine (pĕr''ē-ū'tĕr-ĭn) [" + L. *uterus*, womb]. Located about the uterus. SYN: *perimetric.*

periuvular (pĕr''ē-ū'vū-lăr) [" + L. *uvula*, little grape]. Around the uvula.

perivaginal (pĕr''ĭ-văj'ĭ-năl) [" + L. *vagina*, sheath]. Around the vagina.

perivaginitis (pĕr''ĭ-văj''ĭ-nī'tĭs) [" + " + Gr. *itis*, inflammation]. Inflammation of region around the vagina. SYN: *pericolpitis.*

perivascular (pĕr''ĭ-văs'kū-lăr) [" + L. *vasculus*, a little vessel]. Located around a vessel, esp. a blood vessel.

perivasculitis (pĕr''ĭ-văs''kū-lī'tĭs) [" + " + Gr. *itis*, inflammation]. Inflamed condition of tissues surrounding a blood vessel. SYN: *periangiitis.*

perivenous (pĕr''ĭ-vē'nŭs) [" + L. *vena*, vein]. Surrounding or occurring around a vein.

perivertebral (pĕr''ĭ-vĕr'tĕ-brăl) [" + L. *vertebra*, vertebra]. Around a vertebra.

perivesical (pĕr''ĭ-vĕs'ĭ-kăl) [" + L. *vesicula*, little bladder]. Around the urinary bladder.

perivesiculitis (pĕr''ĭ-vĕ-sĭk''ū-lī'tĭs) [" + " + Gr. *itis*, inflammation]. Inflammation of tissues around a seminal vesicle.

perivisceral (pĕr''ĭ-vĭs'ĕr-ăl) [" + L. *viscera*, internal organs]. Around the viscera or a seminal vesicle.

perivisceritis (pĕr''ĭ-vĭs''ĕr-ī'tĭs) [" + " + Gr. *itis*, inflammation]. Inflamed condition of the tissues surrounding the viscera.

perivitelline (pĕr''ĭ-vĭ-tĕl'ēn) [" + L. *vitellus*, yolk]. Around a vitellus or yolk.

perixenitis (pĕr''ĭ-zē-nī'tĭs) [" + *xenos*, strange, + *itis*, inflammation]. Inflammation occurring around a foreign body in a tissue or organ. SYN: *perialienitis.*

perle (pĕrl) [Fr., pearl]. A soft capsule containing medicine.

perlèche (pĕr-lĕsh') [Fr.]. Disorder marked by fissures and epithelial desquamation at corners of the mouth, esp. seen in children. May be due to oral candidiasis or may be a symptom of dietary deficiency, esp. riboflavin deficiency.

perlingual (pĕr-lĭng'gwăl) [L. *per*, through, + *lingua*, tongue]. By way of the tongue; method of administering medicines.

permanent (pĕr'mă-nĕnt) [" + *manere*, to remain]. Enduring; without change.

permanent teeth. Teeth developing at the second dentition. SEE: *dens permanens; teeth, permanent* for illus.

permanganate (pĕr-măn'gă-nāt). Any one of the salts of permanganic acid.

Permapen. Trade name for penicillin G benzathine.

permeability (pĕr''mē-ă-bĭl'ĭ-tē) [LL. *permeabilis*]. The quality of being permeable; that which may be traversed.

p., capillary. The condition of the capillary wall that enables substances in the blood to diffuse into tissue spaces or into cells, or vice versa.

permeable (pĕr″mē-ă-b'l). Capable of allowing the passage of fluids or substances in solution.

permeation (pĕr″mē-ā′shŭn) [L. *permeare*, permeate]. Penetration of and spreading throughout an organ, tissue, or space.

permethrin. A pediculocide used in treating head lice. Trade name Nix Creme Rinse.

permissible exposure limits. The limits, usually expressed as a combination of time and concentration, to which humans may be safely exposed to physical agents, ionizing radiations, or chemical substances in the environment in general and in work areas specifically. SEE: *hazardous material; health hazard; maximum allowable concentration; right to know law; toxic substance.*

Permitil. Trade name for fluphenazine hydrochloride.

permutation (pĕr″mū-tā′shŭn) [L. *per*, completely, + *mutare*, to change]. Transformation; complete change; act of altering objects in a group.

perniciosiform (pĕr-nĭsh″ē-ō′sĭ-form) [L. *perniciosus*, destructive, + *forma*, form]. Pert. to a condition that is apparently but not actually pernicious.

pernicious (pĕr-nĭsh′ŭs) [L. *perniciosus*, destructive]. Destructive; fatal; harmful.

pernicious anemia. Severe form of blood disease marked by progressive decrease in red blood corpuscles, muscular weakness, and gastrointestinal and neural disturbances. May be fatal if not treated with vitamin B_{12}, iron, and diet. SEE: *anemia, pernicious.*

pernicious trend. A psychological term indicating an abnormal departure from conventional ideas and social interests.

pernio (pĕr′nē-ō) [L.]. Chilblain. Congestion and swelling of the skin due to cold.

　　SYM: Attended with severe burning or itching; ulceration may result from vesicles and bullae that sometimes form.

pero- [Gr. *peros*, maimed]. Combining form meaning deformed.

perobrachius (pē″rō-brā′kē-ŭs) [″ + *brachion*, arm]. An individual with congenitally deformed forearms and hands.

perocephalus (pē″rō-sĕf′ă-lŭs) [″ + *kephale*, head]. An individual with a congenitally defective head.

perochirus (pē″rō-kī′rŭs) [″ + *cheir*, hand]. An individual with congenitally deformed hands.

perocormus (pē″rō-kor′mŭs) [″ + *kormos*, trunk]. An individual with a congenitally deformed trunk.

perodactylia (pē″rō-dăk-tĭl′ē-ă) [″ + *daktylos*, finger]. Condition in which one or more fingers or toes are deformed.

perodactylus (pē″rō-dăk′tĭ-lŭs) [″ + *dak-*

tylos, finger]. An individual with congenitally deformed fingers or toes.

peromelia (pē″rō-mē′lē-ă) [″ + *melos*, limb]. Birth defect with absence or deformity of the terminal part of a limb or limbs.

peromelus (pē-rŏm′ē-lŭs) [″ + *melos*, limb]. At birth, an individual with malformation of extremities, including absence of hand or foot.

perone (pĕr-ō′nē) [Gr. *perone*, pin]. The fibula.

peroneal (pĕr″ō-nē′ăl) [Gr. *perone*, pin]. Concerning the fibula.

peroneal sign. In patients with tetany, tapping on the fibular side over the peroneal nerve causes eversion and dorsiflexion of the foot.

peroneo- [Gr. *perone*, pin]. Combining form pert. to the fibula.

peroneotibial (pĕr″ō-nē″ō-tĭb′ē-ăl) [″ + L. *tibia*, shinbone]. Concerning the fibula and tibia.

peroneus (pĕr″ō-nē′ŭs) [Gr. *perone*, pin]. One of several muscles of the leg that act to move the foot.

peronia (pē-rō′nē-ă) [Gr. *peros*, maimed]. Malformation.

peropus (pē′rō-pŭs) [″ + *pous*, foot]. An individual with congenitally deformed feet.

peroral (pĕr-or′ăl) [L. *per*, through, + *oris*, mouth]. Administered through the mouth.

per os [L.]. By mouth. Through mouth.

perosomus (pē″rō-sō′mŭs) [Gr. *peros*, maimed, + *soma*, body]. An individual with a congenitally defective body.

perosplanchnia (pē″rō-splănk′nē-ă) [″ + *splanchnon*, viscus]. Congenital malformation of the viscera.

perosseous (pĕr-ŏs′ē-ŭs) [L. *per*, through, + *os*, bone]. Through bone.

peroxidase (pĕr-ŏk′sĭ-dās) [″ + Gr. *oxys*, acid, + *-ase*, enzyme]. An enzyme that hastens the transfer of oxygen from peroxide to a tissue that requires oxygen. This process is essential to intracellular respiration.

peroxide (pĕr-ŏk′sīd). In chemistry, a compound containing more oxygen than the other oxides of the element in question.

　　Ex.: peroxides of hydrogen, H_2O_2; sodium, Na_2O_2; magnesium, MgO_2; and nitrogen, NO_2.

peroxisome (pĕr-ŏks′ĭ-sōm). A microbody present in vertebrate animal cells. Peroxisomes contain a great number and variety of enzymes important in cell metabolism.

perphenazine (pĕr-fĕn′ă-zēn). USP. An antipsychotic drug that is also used as an antiemetic. Trade name is Trilafon.

perplication (pĕr-plĭ-kā′shŭn) [″ + *plicare*, to fold]. Inserting the cut end of an artery through an incision in its own wall to arrest bleeding.

per primam intentionem (pĕr prī′măm ĭn-tĕn-shē-ō′nĕm) [L.]. By first intention. SEE: *healing.*

per rectum (pĕr rĕk′tŭm) [L.]. By the rectum; through the rectum.

PERRLA. *pupils equal, regular, react to light and accommodation.*

Persadox. Trade name for benzoyl peroxide.

persalt (pĕr′sawlt). In chemistry, a salt containing the largest possible amount of an acid radical.

Persantine. Trade name for dipyridamole.

per secundam intentionem (pĕr sē-kŭn′ dăm) [L.]. By second intention. SEE: *healing.*

perseveration (pĕr-sĕv″ĕr-ā′shŭn) [L. *perseverare,* to persist]. Continued repetition of a meaningless word or phrase, or repetition of answers that are not related to successive questions asked.

person. A human being.

persona (pĕr-sō′nă) [L., mask]. The outer attitude or appearance a person presents to others.

personal [L. *personalis*]. Characteristic of an individual.

personal equation. A personal bias or peculiarity that may explain a difference in approach or interpretation.

personality [LL. *personalitas*]. The unique organization of traits, characteristics, and modes of behavior of an individual, setting the individual apart from others and at the same time determining how others react to the individual. Personality refers to the mental aspects of an individual, in contrast to physique. SEE: *personality testing.*

RS: consciousness; dissociation; somnambulism; vigilambulism.

p., alternating. SEE: *p., multiple.*

p., antisocial. A type of personality disorder characterized by disregard of the rights of others. It usually begins prior to age 15. In early childhood there are lying, stealing, fighting, truancy, and disregard of authority. In adolescence there are usually aggressive sexual behavior, excessive use of alcohol, and use of drugs of abuse. In adulthood these behavior patterns continue with the addition of poor work performance, inability to function responsibly as a parent, and inability to accept normal restrictions imposed by laws. This type of personality disorder is not due to mental retardation, schizophrenia, or manic episodes. It is much more common in males than females.

p., borderline. Individuals who have difficulty maintaining a consistent stable mood and self-image. This manifests as unpredictable and impulsive behavior, outbursts of anger, irritability, sadness, and

fear. Self-mutilation or suicidal behavior may be present. Some of these individuals have a chronic feeling of emptiness or boredom.

p., compulsive. A type of personality disorder in which there is inability to express warm and tender emotions. The individual's perfectionism, q.v., interferes with ability to consider the entire situation. Instead, the individual is preoccupied with trivial details, rules, orderliness, organization, schedules, and lists. These individuals resist the authority of others but insist that others conform to their wishes. The desire for work and productivity precludes enjoying a vacation or warm interpersonal relations. Because of fear of making a mistake, decision-making is difficult. This disorder may be incapacitating with respect to success in an occupation.

p., double. P., dual.

p., dual. Mental dissociation in which one individual shows in alternation two very different personalities. SEE: *dual personality.*

p., extroverted. Personality in which activities or libido is directed to other individuals or the environment.

p., histrionic. A disorder in which the individuals are active and dramatic, draw attention to themselves, are prone to exaggerate, and are subject to emotional excitability such as irrational, angry outbursts or tantrums. They are bored with normal routines and crave novelty and excitement. Even though these individuals are usually attractive and productive, their behavior in interpersonal relationships is perceived to be shallow, vain, demanding, dependent, and constantly seeking reassurance.

p., inadequate. Personality in which the individual is ineffective and is physically and emotionally unstable to the extent of being unable to cope with the normal stress of living.

p., introverted. Personality in which activities or libido is directed to the individual himself or herself.

p., multiple. State in which three or more personalities alternate in the same individual, usually with each personality unaware of the others.

p., neurotic. Personality characterized by behavior intermediate between normal and that of a neurotic individual.

p., obsessive-compulsive. SEE: *p., compulsive.*

p., paranoid. A disorder characterized by a continuing and unwarranted suspiciousness, mistrust of people, and hypersensitivity. It is not a psychosis but those affected have great difficulty with interpersonal relations. They are quite critical of others but virtually unable to accept criticism.

p., passive-aggressive. Personality in which individuals resist demands for adequate performance in work and social situations. The resistance is indirectly expressed. This is done by misplacing work assignments, or being late to appointments or forgetting them. Persons with this type of personality are ineffective at work and socially.

p., psychopathic. An obsolete term. SEE: *p., antisocial.*

p., schizoid. Personality characterized by shyness, oversensitivity, seclusiveness, dissociation from close interpersonal or competitive relationships, eccentricity, daydreaming, and inability to express hostility and aggression in situations that would call for such reactions.

personality disorders. These conditions exist when an individual repeatedly uses certain coping mechanisms in an inappropriate, stereotyped, or maladaptive fashion. A large number of personality disorders are recognized. Some of these are paranoid, schizoid, histrionic, narcissistic, antisocial, borderline, avoidant behavior, dependent behavior, compulsive, and passive-aggressive personality disorders.

TREAT: Psychotherapy or psychopharmacologic drugs, or combinations of these approaches. SEE: *coping.*

personality pattern, type A. SEE: *behavior patterns, types A and B.*

personality pattern, type B. SEE: *behavior patterns, types A and B.*

personality testing. A number of tests are available that attempt to evaluate an individual's personality dysfunction and stress. A test that has been found to be useful in the fields of mental health, medicine, education, job placement, and counseling is the copyrighted Minnesota Multiphasic Personality Inventory (MMPI). It contains 550 statements that describe a wide variety of thoughts, feelings, attributes, and life experiences. The test requires the individual to answer "true" or "false" to each statement. Their responses are measured against the response of "normal" adults or adolescents.

persons in need of supervision. ABBR: PINS. A legal term for children who because of behavioral problems require supervision, usually in an institution.

person-years of life lost. A calculation of the impact of a disease on society due to premature death from the specific disease, i.e., the number of years the person would have been alive if the disease had not occurred. SEE: *cancer, person-years of life lost due to.*

perspiration (pĕr″spĭr-ā′shŭn) [L. *perspirare,* breathe through]. Salty fluid secreted through the sweat glands of the skin; sweat. Essentially, it is a weak solution of sodium chloride, but it also contains potassium, lactate, and urea. Perspiration is a means of removing heat from the body. This is best accomplished by sweat evaporating from the skin rather than dripping off. Evaporation of one liter of sweat removes 580 Cal of heat from the body. Sweat loss will vary from 100 to 1000 ml/hr but may be more than that in a hot climate.

Perspiration is increased by temperature and humidity of the atmosphere, exercises, pain, nausea, nervousness, mental excitement, dyspnea, diaphoretics, and shock. It is decreased by cold, diarrhea, voiding large quantities of urine, and using certain drugs.

p., insensible. Evaporation of water vapor from the body without appearing as moisture on the skin.

p., sensible. Perspiration that forms moisture on the skin.

perspiration, words pert. to: adiaphoresis; anhidrosis; apocrine gland; bromidrosis; bromohyperhidrosis; chromidrosis; diaphoresis; eccrine gland; polyhidrosis; secretion; sudor; sweat; sweating; transpiration.

perspire (pĕr-spīr′) [L. *perspirare,* breathe through]. To excrete fluid through the pores of the skin. SYN: *sweat.*

persuasion (pĕr-swā′zhŭn). In psychiatry, the attempt to influence behavior by authority, reason, or argument.

persulfate (pĕr-sŭl′fāt). One of a series of sulfates containing more sulfuric acid than the others in the same series.

per tertiam intentionem (pĕr tĕr′shē-ăm ĭn-tĕn-shē-ō′nĕm) [L.]. By third intention. SEE: *healing.*

Perthes' disease (pĕr′tēz) [Georg C. Perthes, Ger. surgeon, 1869–1927]. Disease in which changes take place in bone at the head of the femur with deformity resulting. SYN: *osteochondritis deformans juvenilis.*

SYM: Similar to tuberculous hip joint disease.

Pertofrane. Trade name for desipramine hydrochloride.

per tubam (pĕr tū′băm) [L.]. Through a tube.

perturbation (pĕr″tĕr-bā′shŭn) [L. *perturbare,* thoroughly disordered]. State of being greatly disturbed or agitated; uneasiness of mind.

pertussis (pĕr-tŭs′ĭs) [L. *per,* through, + *tussis,* cough]. An acute, infectious disease characterized by a catarrhal stage, followed by a peculiar paroxysmal cough, ending in a whooping inspiration. Pertussis may be prevented by immunization of infants beginning at 3 months of age. SYN: *whooping* *cough.*

SYM: Elevated white blood count with marked lymphocytosis. May be in excess of 30,000 per cubic millimeter.

Often divided into the following three stages: *Catarrhal:* At this time the symptoms are chiefly suggestive of the common cold — slight elevation of fever, sneezing, rhinitis, and dry cough; irritability and loss of appetite.

Paroxysmal: Sets in after approx. 2 weeks. The cough is more violent and consists of a series of several short coughs, followed by long drawn inspiration during which the typical whoop is heard, this being occasioned by the spasmodic contraction of the glottis. Often with the beginning of each paroxysm, the patient assumes a worried expression, sometimes even one of terror. The face becomes cyanosed, eyes injected, veins distended. With conclusion of the paroxysm, vomiting is common. Also at this time there may be epistaxis, subconjunctival hemorrhages, or hemorrhages in other portions of body. Number of paroxysms in 24 hours may vary from 3 to 4 up to 40 to 50. Cough is precipitated by eating, drinking, or pressing on the trachea. It is associated often with vomiting.

Decline: Begins after an indefinite period of several weeks. Paroxysms grow less frequent and less violent. Nutrition of child improves, and after a period that may be prolonged for several months, the cough finally ceases.

ETIOL: Due to a small, nonmotile, gram-negative bacillus, *Bordetella pertussis.*

INCUB: Seven to 10 days.

TREAT: Symptomatic and supportive.

pertussis immune globulin. USP. A sterile solution of globulins derived from the blood of adults who have been immunized with pertussis vaccine. Used to produce passive immunity to pertussis.

pertussis vaccine. USP. Sterile bacterial fraction of killed pertussis bacilli. Used for active immunization against pertussis.

pertussoid (pĕr-tŭs'oyd) [L. *per,* through, + *tussis,* cough, + Gr. *eidos,* form, shape]. 1. Of the nature of whooping cough. 2. A cough generally similar to that of whooping cough.

per vaginam (pĕr vă-jī'năm) [L.]. Through the vagina.

perversion (pĕr-vĕr'zhŭn) [L. *perversus,* perverted]. Deviation from the normal path, whether it be in the area of one's intellect, emotions, actions, or reactions. SEE: *paraphilia.*

p., sexual. Maladjustment of sexual life in which satisfaction is sought in ways deviating from the accepted norm. In judging

the sexual actions of individuals, it is important to remember that what is normal behavior in one society may be regarded as grossly abnormal or perverted in another.

pervert [L. *pervetere,* to turn the wrong way]. 1. (pĕr-vĕrt') To turn from the normal; to misuse. 2. (pĕr'vĕrt) One who has turned from the normal or socially acceptable path, esp. sexually.

per vias naturales (pĕr vē'ăs năt"ū-rā'lēz) [L.]. Through natural ways.

pervious (pĕr'vē-ŭs) [L. *pervius*]. 1. Capable of being penetrated. SYN: *permeable.* 2. Penetrating.

pes (pĕs) [L.] (pl. *pedes*). [NA] The foot or a footlike structure.

p. abductus. Talipes valgus, q.v.

p. adductus. Talipes varus, q.v.

p. anserinus. 1. Three primary branches of the facial nerve after leaving the stylomastoid foramen. 2. The tendinous expansions of the sartorius, gracilis, and semitendinosus muscles at the medial border of the tibia's tuberosity.

p. cavus. Abnormal hollowness or concavity of the sole of the foot. An excessively high longitudinal arch in the foot.

p. contortus. Clubfoot. SYN: *talipes.*

p. equinovalgus. Talipes equinovalgus. The heel is elevated and turned laterally.

p. equinovarus. Talipes equinovarus. The heel is turned inward and the foot is plantar flexed.

p. equinus. Deformity marked by walking without touching the heel to the ground. SYN: *talipes equinus.*

p. gigas. An abnormally large foot. SYN: *macropodia.*

p. hippocampi. [NA] Lower portion of the hippocampus major.

p., infraorbital. Terminal radiating branches of the infraorbital nerve after exit from the infraorbital canal.

p. planus. Flatfoot.

p. valgus. Clubfoot in which sole turns outward. SYN: *talipes valgus.*

p. varus. Clubfoot in which sole turns inward. SYN: *talipes varus.*

Peseshet. An Egyptian physician who practiced about 2500 B.C. She is assumed to be the earliest known female physician.

pessary (pĕs'ă-rē) [L. *pessarium*]. Device inserted into the vagina to function as a supportive structure for the uterus.

p., cup. Pessary that has a cup-shaped hollow that fits over the os uteri.

p., diaphragm. Cup-shaped rubber pessary used as a contraceptive device.

p., Gariel's. Inflatable hollow rubber pessary.

p., Hodge's. Pessary used to correct retrodeviations of the uterus.

p., lever. Pessary designed according to the principles of a lever.

p., Menge's. A ring pessary with a fixed crossbar to which a detachable stem may be affixed.

p., ring. Round pessary.

p., stem. Pessary with stem that fits into the uterine canal.

pessimism. The characteristic of regarding events and situations from the darkest possible aspect. SEE: *optimism.*

p., therapeutic. Tendency not to believe in the effectiveness of therapeutic measures, esp. of drugs.

pest (pĕst) [L. *pestis*, plague]. 1. Fatal epidemic disease, esp. plague. 2. A noxious, destructive insect.

pesticemia (pĕs″tĭ-sē′mē-ă) [″ + Gr. *haima*, blood]. Presence of plague organisms in the blood.

pesticide (pĕs′tĭ-sīd) [″ + *cida*, killer]. Any chemical used to kill pests, esp. rodents and insects.

pesticide residue. The amount of any pesticide remaining on or in food or beverages intended for human consumption.

pestiferous (pĕs-tĭf′ĕr-ŭs) [L. *pestiferus*]. Producing a pestilence; carrying infection. SYN: *pestilential.*

pestilence (pĕs′tĭl-ĕns) [L. *pestilentia*]. 1. An epidemic contagious disease. 2. An epidemic caused by such a disease.

pestilential (pĕs-tĭ-lĕn′shăl). Concerning or causing a pestilence. SYN: *pestiferous.*

pestis (pĕs′tĭs) [L.]. Plague.

p. ambulans. Ambulatory plague.

p. fulminans. The most severe form of plague.

p. major. P. fulminans, q.v.

p. minor. P. ambulans, q.v.

p. siderans. Septicemic plague.

p. variolosa. Smallpox.

pestle (pĕs′l) [L. *pistillum*]. Device for macerating drugs in a mortar.

PET. *positron emission tomography.*

-petal [L. *petere*, to seek]. Combining form indicating seeking or moving toward.

petechiae (pē-tē′kē-ē) [It. *petecchia*, skin spot] (sing. *petechia*). 1. Small, purplish, hemorrhagic spots on the skin that appear in certain severe fevers and are indicative of great prostration, as in typhus. May be due to abnormality of blood-clotting mechanism. Also applied to similar spots occurring on mucous membranes or serous surfaces. 2. Red spots from bite of a flea.

petechial (pē-tē′kē-ăl). Marked by presence of petechiae.

pethidine hydrochloride (pĕth′ĭ-dīn). The international nonproprietary name for meperidine hydrochloride, q.v.

petiole (pĕt′ē-ōl) [LL. *petiolus*]. A slender stalk or stem, as petiole of the epiglottic cartilage.

petiolus (pĕ-tī′ō-lŭs) [LL.]. The stalk or stem of a fruit. A pedicle.

p. epiglottidis. The pedicle of the cartilage of the epiglottis. It is attached to the superior notch of the thyroid cartilage.

Petit, François Pourfour du (pĕt-ē′). French anatomist and surgeon, 1664–1741.

P.'s canal. A space or cleft encircling lens between points of attachment of fibers of suspensory ligament. SYN: *zonular spaces.*

P.'s sinuses. Hollows in aortic and pulmonary arteries behind semilunar valves.

Petit, Jean Louis (pĕt-ē′). French surgeon, 1674–1750.

P.'s ligament. The uterosacral ligament.

P.'s triangle. Area on lateral abdominal wall bounded by crest of ilium, posterior margin of external oblique muscle, and lateral margin of latissimus dorsi muscle. SYN: *trigonum lumbale.*

petit mal (pĕt-ē′ mäl′) [Fr., little illness]. SEE: *epilepsy; pyknolepsy.*

Petri dish (pā′trē) [Julius Petri, Ger. bacteriologist, 1852–1921]. A shallow dish made of plastic or glass with a cover. Used to hold solid media for culturing bacteria.

petrifaction (pĕt-rĭ-făk′shŭn) [L. *petra*, stone, + *facere*, to make]. Process of changing into stone or hard substance.

petrified (pĕt′rĭ-fīd). Changed into stone; rigid.

petrify (pĕt′rĭ-fī). To convert into stone; make rigid.

pétrissage (pā″trē-săzh′) [Fr.]. A kneading movement in massage. Performed generally by the tips of the thumbs, with index finger and thumb, or with palm of hand. It is used principally on the extremities. The operator picks up a special muscle or tendon and, placing one finger on each side of the part, proceeds in centripetal motion with a firm pressure. SYN: *kneading.*

petro- [L. *petra*, stone]. Combining form meaning stone. Pert. to the petrous portion of the temporal bone.

petrolatoma (pĕt″rō-lă-tō′mă) [L. *petrolatum*, petroleum]. Tumor or swelling caused by introduction of liquid petrolatum under the skin.

petrolatum (pĕt″rō-lā′tŭm) [L.]. USP. A purified semisolid mixture of hydrocarbons obtained from petroleum. SYN: *paraffin, soft.*

ACTION/USES: As a base for ointments. It is not suitable for use as a vaginal lubricant because it is not miscible in body secretion.

p., liquid. A mixture of liquid hydrocarbons obtained from petroleum.

ACTION/USES: A vehicle for medicinal substances for local applications. Light petrolatum is employed as a topical spray while heavy petrolatum is given internally in treatment of constipation.

p., white. USP. Purified mixture of semisolid hydrocarbons obtained from petroleum. It is decolorized and may contain a suitable stabilizer. Trade name is Moroline.

petroleum (pĕ-trō'lē-ŭm) [L. *petra*, stone, + *oleum*, oil]. An oily inflammable liquid found in the upper strata of the earth; a hydrocarbon mixture.

petromastoid (pĕt"rō-măs'toyd). Pert. to the petrous and mastoid portions of the temporal and occipital bones.

petro-occipital (pĕt"rō-ŏk-sĭp'ĭ-tăl) [" + *occipitalis*, occipital]. Concerning the petrous portion of the temporal bone and the occipital bone.

petropharyngeus (pĕt"rō-făr-rĭn'jē-ŭs) [" + Gr. *pharynx*, throat]. A small muscle joining the lower surface of the petrous portion of the temporal bone and the pharynx. It helps to constrict the pharynx.

petrosa (pĕ-trō'să) [L. *petrosus*, stony]. The petrous part of the temporal bone.

petrosal (pĕt-rō'săl) [L. *petrosus*, stony]. Of, pert. to, or situated near the petrous portion of the temporal bone.

petrosalpingostaphylinus (pĕt"rō-săl-pĭng"gō-stăf"ĭ-lī'nŭs) [L. *petra*, stone, + Gr. *salpinx*, tube, + *staphyle*, uvula]. Musculus levator veli palatini.

petrositis (pĕt"rō-sī'tĭs) [" + Gr. *itis*, inflammation]. Inflamed condition of the petrous region of the temporal bone.

petrosomastoid (pĕ-trō"sō-măs'toyd) [" + Gr. *mastos*, breast, + *eidos*, form, shape]. Concerning the petrous portion of the temporal bone and its mastoid process.

petrosphenoid (pĕt"rō-sfē'noyd) [" + Gr. *sphen*, wedge, + *eidos*, form, shape]. Pert. to the petrous portion on the temporal and sphenoid bones.

petrosquamous (pĕt"rō-skwă'mŭs) [" + *squamosus*, scaly]. Pert. to the petrous and squamous portions of the temporal bones.

petrostaphylinus (pĕt"rō-stăf"ĭ-lī'nŭs) [" + Gr. *staphyle*, uvula]. Musculus levator veli palatini.

petrous (pĕt'rŭs) [L. *petrosus*]. 1. Resembling stone. 2. Rel. to the petrous portion of the temporal bone. SYN: *petrosal*.

petrous ganglion. Inferior ganglion of the glossopharyngeal nerve.

Peutz-Jeghers syndrome (pūtz-jā'kĕrs) [Johannes Laurentius Augustinus Peutz, Dutch physician, 1886–1957; Harold J. Jeghers, U.S. physician, b. 1904]. Polyps of the small intestine and melanin pigmenta-

tion of the lips, mucosa, fingers, and toes. Anemia due to bleeding from the intestinal polyps is a common finding. It is an inherited disorder.

pexin (pĕk'sĭn). Rennet.

pexis [Gr., fixation]. Fixation of material in the tissue.

-pexy [Gr. *pexis*, fixation]. A combining form meaning fixation.

Peyer's patch (pī'ĕrz) [Johann Conrad Peyer, Swiss anatomist, 1653–1712]. An aggregation of lymph nodules found chiefly in the ileum near its junction with the colon. They are circular or oval, about 1 cm wide, and 2 to 3 cm long. They lie in the mucosal and submucosal layers and always occur on side of intestine opposite to attachment of mesentery. In typhoid fever, they undergo hyperplasia and often become ulcerated. SYN: *aggregated follicles*.

peyote (pā-ō'tē). 1. The cactus plant, *Lophophora williamsii*, from which the hallucinogen mescaline is obtained. 2. The drug from the flowering heads, buttons, of *L. williamsii*, used by some Indians of the North American continent to produce altered states of consciousness. In certain tribes the buttons are used in religious ceremonies. For that reason, members of that tribe are permitted to use this substance even though the drug is classed as a narcotic and its use is otherwise restricted to research.

Peyronie's disease (pā-rō-nēz') [François de la Peyronie, Fr. surgeon, 1678–1747]. Hardening of the corpora cavernosa of the penis. This condition, which may be painful, causes distortion and curvature of the penis, esp. when erect.

TREAT: The disease is self-limiting in many instances. Persistence or progression of the penile deformity requires therapy, but of the several medical, surgical, and radiological approaches, none seem to be completely effective. There are devices that will assist the individual with the disease in participating in sexual intercourse. SEE: *penile prosthesis*.

Pfeiffer, Emil (fī'fĕr). German physician, 1846–1921.

P.'s disease. Infectious mononucleosis, q.v.

Pfeiffer, Richard F. (fī'fĕr). German bacteriologist, 1858–1945.

P.'s bacillus. *Haemophilus influenzae.*

P.'s phenomenon. A discovery announced in 1894 stating that serum of guinea pigs immunized with cholera vibrios destroyed cholera organisms in peritoneal cavity of immune and nonimmune guinea pigs and that the same reaction occurred in vitro. Also, that same lytic reaction occurred with typhoid and colon bacteria.

pH of Some Fluids

Material	pH
Decinormal HCl	1.0
Gastric juice	1.0–5.0
Thousandth-normal HCl	3.0
Pure water (neutral) at 25°C	7.0
Blood plasma	7.35–7.45
Pancreatic juice	8.4–8.9
Thousandth-normal NaOH	11.0
Decinormal NaOH	13.0

PG. *prostaglandin.*

pg. *picogram.*

PGA. *pteroylglutamic acid.*

Ph. 1. *Pharmacopoeia.* SEE: *pharmacopeia.* 2. Chem. symb. for phenyl.

pH. *potential of hydrogen.* In chemistry, the degrees of acidity or alkalinity of a substance are expressed in pH values. The neutral point, where a solution would be neither acid nor alkaline, is pH 7. Increasing acidity is expressed as a number less than 7, and increasing alkalinity as a number greater than 7. Maximum acidity is pH 0 and maximum alkalinity is pH 14. Because each unit on the scale represents a logarithm, there is a tenfold difference between each unit.

Ex.: pH 5 is 10 times as acid as pH 6 and pH 4 is 100 times as acid as pH 6. Expressed mathematically, pH is logarithm of the hydrogen ion concentration divided into one, i.e.,

$$\text{Log } \frac{1}{H^+}$$

The pH of a solution may be determined electrically by a pH meter or colorimetrically by the use of indicators. A list of indicators and the pH range registered by each is given under indicator, q.v. SEE: table.

PHA. *phytohemagglutinin.*

phacitis (fă-sī'tĭs) [Gr. *phakos*, lens, + *itis*, inflammation]. Inflamed condition of the crystalline lens. SYN: *phakitis; lentitis.*

phaco- [Gr. *phakos*]. Prefix pert. to lens of the eye.

phacoanaphylaxis (făk″ō-ăn″ă-fĭ-lăk'sĭs) [Gr. *phakos*, lens, + *ana*, excessive, + *phylaxis*, protection]. Hypersensitivity to protein of the crystalline lens.

phacocele (făk'ō-sēl) [" + *kele*, tumor, swelling]. Displacement of the crystalline lens into the interior chamber of the eye. SYN: *phacometachoresis.*

phacocyst (făk'ō-sĭst) [Gr. *phakos*, lens, + *kystis*, a sac]. Capsule of the crystalline lens.

phacocystectomy (făk″ō-sĭs-tĕk'tō-mē) [" + " + *ektome*, excision]. Surgical excision of part of crystalline lens capsule for treatment of cataract.

phacocystitis (făk″ō-sĭs-tī'tĭs) [" + " + *itis*, inflammation]. Inflamed condition of the capsule of the crystalline lens.

phacoemulsification (făk″ō-ē-mŭl'sĭ-fĭ-kā″shŭn). A method of treating cataracts of the crystalline lens of the eye. An ultrasonic device is used to disintegrate the cataract, which is then aspirated and removed.

phacoerysis (făk″ō-ĕr-ē'sĭs) [" + *eresis*, removal]. Removal of the lens of the eye by attaching a suction device, an erysiphake, to it. SEE: *erysiphake.*

phacoglaucoma (făk″ō-glaw-kō'mă) [" + *glaukos*, green, + *oma*, tumor]. Glaucoma and the changes it induces in the crystalline lens. SEE: *glaucoma.*

phacohymenitis (făk″ō-hī″mĕn-ī'tĭs) [" + *hymen*, membrane, + *itis*, inflammation]. Inflamed condition of the capsule of the crystalline lens.

phacoid (făk'oyd) [" + *eidos*, form, shape]. Lentil- or lens-shaped.

phacoiditis (făk″oy-dī'tĭs) [" + " + *itis*, inflammation]. Phakitis, q.v.

phacoidoscope (fă-koyd'ō-skōp) [" + " + *skopein*, to examine]. Instrument for observing accommodative changes of the lens. SYN: *phacoscope.*

phacolysis (făk-ŏl'ĭ-sĭs) [" + *lysis*, dissolution]. 1. Dissection and removal of the lens of the eye in treatment of cataract. 2. Any dissolution or disintegration of the crystalline lens.

phacoma (fă-kō'mă) [" + *oma*, tumor]. Phakoma, q.v.

phacomalacia (făk″ō-mă-lā'shē-ă) [" + *malakia*, softening]. A softening of the lens usually due to a soft cataract.

phacomatosis (fă″kō-mă-tō'sĭs) [" + *oma*, tumor, + *osis*, condition]. One of a group of diseases that are congenital and probably hereditary in origin, manifested by cutaneous and neurological syndromes. They include the following: neurofibromatosis (von Recklinghausen's disease); von Hippel-Lindau disease; Sturge-Weber syndrome; and tuberous sclerosis. SYN: *neurodermatosis.*

phacometachoresis (făk″ō-mĕt″ă-kō-rē'sĭs) [" + *metachoresis*, displacement]. Dislocation of the crystalline lens. SYN: *phacocele.*

phacometer (făk-ŏm'ĕ-tĕr) [Gr. *phakos*, lens, + *metron*, measure]. Device for ascertaining refractive power of a lens.

phacoplanesis (făk″ō-plăn-ē'sĭs) [" + *planesis*, wandering]. Abnormal mobility of the crystalline lens.

phacosclerosis (făk″ō-sklĕr-ō'sĭs) [" +

sklerosis, a hardening]. Hardening of crystalline lens of the eye.

phacoscope (făk′ō-skōp) [″ + *skopein,* to examine]. Instrument for observing change of curvature of crystalline lens during accommodation.

phacoscotasmus (făk″ō-skō-tăs′mŭs) [″ + *skotasmos,* clouding]. Clouding of crystalline lens of the eye.

phacotoxic (făk′ō-tŏk′sĭk) [″ + *toxikon,* poison]. Concerning the toxicity of material in the lens of the eye.

Phaedra complex [Wife of King Theseus of Athens]. The love and attraction between a stepparent and a stepchild. So named because of Phaedra's tragic love for the son (Hippolytus) of her husband by a previous marriage.

phag-, phago- [Gr. *phagein,* to eat]. Combining form meaning eating, or pert. to ingestion, or engulfing.

phage (fāj) [Gr. *phagein,* to eat]. A virus with a specific affinity for inducing lysis of certain bacterial cells. Phages are widely distributed in nature and have been isolated in feces, sewage, and polluted surface waters. They are regarded as bacterial viruses, the phage particle consisting of a head composed of RNA or DNA and a tail by which it attaches to host cells. SYN: *bacteriophage.*

phagedena (făj-ě-dē′nǎ) [Gr. *phagedaina*]. A sloughing ulcer that spreads rapidly.

    p., sloughing. Hospital gangrene; bedsores.

phagedenic (făj-ě-děn′ĭk). Concerning, or of the nature of, phagedena.

phage typing. A method of identifying particular strains of bacteria that are lysed only by strain-specific bacteriophages.

phagocyte (făg′ō-sīt) [Gr. *phagein,* to eat, + *kytos,* cell]. A cell that has the ability to ingest and destroy particulate substances such as bacteria, protozoa, cells and cell debris, dust particles, and colloids by ingesting them.

    Ex.: Cells of the reticuloendothelial system (macrophages or histiocytes, reticular cells of lymph nodes, Kupffer's cells of liver, dust cells of lung) and leukocytes. SEE: *cytokine; endocytosis; histiocyte; macrophage; phagolysome; phagosome; pinocytosis; reticuloendothelial system.*

phagocytic (făg′ō-sīt′ĭk). Concerning phagocytes or phagocytosis.

phagocytic index. The average number of bacteria ingested by each leukocyte after incubation of the bacteria in a mixture of serum and bacterial culture. SEE: *index, opsonic.*

phagocytize (făg′ō-sīt″īz). To ingest bacteria and foreign particles by phagocytosis.

phagocytoblast (făg″ō-sī′tō-blăst) [″ + ″

+ *blastos,* germ]. A cell that develops into a phagocyte.

phagocytolysis (făg″ō-sī-tŏl′ĭ-sĭs) [″ + *kytos,* cell, + *lysis,* dissolution]. Destruction or disintegration of phagocytes. SYN: *phagolysis.*

phagocytolytic (făg″ō-sī″tō-lĭt′ĭk). Destroying phagocytes.

phagocytose (făg″ō-sī′tōs) [″ + *kytos,* cell]. Phagocytize, q.v.

phagocytosis (făg″ō-sī-tō′sĭs) [″ + ″ *osis,* condition]. Ingestion and digestion of bacteria and particles by phagocytes. SEE: illus.; *autophagocytosis; endocytosis; heterophagocytosis; phagolysome; phagosome; pinocytosis.*

    p., induced. Phagocytosis that is aided or stimulated by the effect of serum opsonins or bacteria.

    p., spontaneous. Phagocytosis occurring in an indifferent medium such as physiologic salt solution.

phagodynamometer (făg″ō-dī″nă-mŏm′ě-těr) [″ + *dynamis,* power, + *metron,* measure]. Device that measures energy expended in chewing food.

phagokaryosis (făg″ō-kăr″ē-ō′sĭs) [″ + *karyon,* nucleus, + *osis,* condition]. Phagocytic action that is performed by a cell nucleus.

phagolysis (făg-ŏl′ĭ-sĭs) [″ + *lysis,* dissolution]. Disintegration of phagocytes. SYN: *phagocytolysis.*

phagolysosome (făg″ō-lī′sō-sōm) [″ + *lysis,* dissolution, + *soma,* body]. The body formed when the membrane-bound phagosome inside a macrophage fuses with a lysosome. SYN: *secondary lysosome.* SEE: *phagosome.*

phagomania (făg″ō-mā′nē-ă) [″ + *mania,* madness]. Abnormal craving for food.

phagophobia (făg″ō-fō′bē-ă) [″ + *phobos,* fear]. Dread of being eaten.

phagopyrism (făg″ō-pī′rĭzm) [″ + *pyr,* fever, + *-ismos,* condition]. Hypersensitivity to certain foods, causing symptoms of poisoning upon ingestion.

phagosome (făg′ō-sōm) [″ + *soma,* body]. A membrane-bound vacuole inside a phagocyte that contains material waiting to be digested. Digestion is facilitated by the fusion of the vacuole with the lysosome. The phagosome is then called a phagolysosome or secondary lysosome. After the material is digested, it is extruded from the phagosome to the exterior of the cell. SEE: *phagocytosis.*

phagotherapy (făg″ō-thĕr′ă-pē) [″ + *therapeia,* treatment]. Treatment by feeding or overfeeding.

phagotype (făg′ō-tīp) [″ + *typos,* mark]. Classification of bacteria by their sensitivity to phage types. SEE: *phage typing.*

PARTICLE TO BE INGESTED BY CELL | BEGINNING OF INGESTION | INGESTION CONTINUES | INGESTION COMPLETE

PHAGOCYTOSIS

phakitis (făk-ī'tĭs) [Gr. *phakos,* lens, + *itis,* inflammation]. Inflamed condition of the crystalline lens of the eye. SYN: *phacitis; lentitis.*

phakolysis (făk-ŏl'ĭ-sĭs) [" + *lysis,* dissolution]. Disintegration or removal of the crystalline lens of the eye. SYN: *phacolysis.*

phakoma (fă-kō'mă) [" + *oma,* tumor]. 1. Microscopic gray white tumor present in the retina in tuberous sclerosis. 2. Area of myelinated nerve fibers rarely seen in the retina in association with neurofibromatosis.

phalangeal (fă-lăn'jē-ăl) [Gr. *phalanx,* closely knit row]. Concerning a phalanx.

phalangeal cells, inner. A row of cells along surface of inner pillar cells in the organ of Corti.

phalangeal cells, outer. Cells arranged in rows that support the outer hair cells in the organ of Corti. SYN: *Deiters' cells.*

phalangectomy (făl-ăn-jěk'tō-mē) [" + *ektome,* excision]. Excision of one or more phalanges.

phalanges (fă-lăn'jēz) (sing. *phalanx*). [NA] Bones of a finger or toe. SEE: *skeleton.*

phalangette (făl"ăn-jět'). The distal phalanx of a digit.

   p., drop. Falling of the distal phalanx of a digit with loss of power to extend it when the hand is prone. This is due to trauma or overstretching of the extensor tendon.

phalangitis (făl"ăn-jī'tĭs) [Gr. *phalanx,* closely knit row, + *itis,* inflammation]. Inflamed condition of one or more phalanges.

phalanx (făl'ănks) [Gr., closely knit row] (pl. *phalanges*). 1. [NA] Any one of the bones of the fingers or toes. 2. One of a set of plates formed of phalangeal cells (inner and outer) forming the reticular membrane of the organ of Corti.

   p., distal. Phalanx most remote from the metacarpus or metatarsus. SYN: *p., terminal; p., ungual; p., unguicular.*

   p., metacarpal. Any phalanx that articulates with a metacarpal bone. SYN: *p., proximal.*

   p., metatarsal. Any phalanx that articulates with a metatarsal bone. SYN: *p., proximal.*

   p., middle. When there are three phalanges, the phalanx intermediate between distal and proximal phalanges.

   p., proximal. Any phalanx that articulates with a metacarpal or metatarsal bone.

   p., terminal. P., distal.

   p., ungual. P., distal. SYN: *p., terminal.*

phall- [Gr. *phallos,* penis]. Combining form indicating penis.

phallalgia (făl-ăl'jē-ă) [Gr. *phallos,* penis, + *algos,* pain]. Pain in the penis.

phallectomy (făl-ĕk'tō-mē) [" + *ektome,* excision]. Surgical removal of the penis.

phallic (făl'ĭk). Concerning the penis.

phalliform (făl'ĭ-form) [" + L. *forma,* form]. Shaped like a penis.

phallitis (făl-ī'tĭs) [" + *itis,* inflammation]. Inflamed condition of the penis.

phallocampsis (făl-ō-kămp'sĭs) [" + *kampsis,* a bending]. Painful downward curvature of the penis when erect.

phallocrypsis (făl"ō-krĭp'sĭs) [" + *krypsis,* hiding]. Contraction of the penis so that it is almost invisible.

phallodynia (făl-ō-dĭn'ē-ă) [" + *odyne,* pain]. Pain in the penis. SYN: *phallalgia.*

phalloid (făl'oyd) [" + *eidos,* form, shape]. Similar to a penis.

phalloidin (fă-loyd'ĭn). A poisonous peptide from the mushroom *Amanita phalloides.* Death can be caused by ingestion of this material.

phalloncus (făl-ŏn'kŭs) [" + *onkos,* mass]. Tumor or swelling on the penis.

phalloplasty (făl'ō-plăs"tē) [" + *plassein,* to form]. Reparative or plastic surgery on the penis.

phallorrhagia (făl-ō-rā'jē-ă) [" + *rheg-*

nynai, to burst forth]. Hemorrhage from the penis.

phallus (făl′ŭs) [Gr. *phallos*, penis]. 1. The penis. 2. An artificial penis, used as a symbol. 3. Embryonic structure developing at tip of the genital tubercle that in the male develops into the penis and in the female, the clitoris.

phanero-, phaner- [Gr. *phaneros*, visible]. Combining forms meaning evident, visible.

phanerogenic (făn″ĕr-ō-jĕn′ĭk) [″ + *gennan*, to produce]. Indicating a disease with a known cause.

phaneromania (făn″ĕr-ō-mā′nē-ă) [″ + *mania*, madness]. Abnormal tendency to bite the nails or pick, scratch, or pull a pimple, wart, hair, beard, or mustache.

phanerosis (făn″ĕr-ō′sĭs) [Gr.]. The process of becoming visible.

phanic (făn′ĭk) [Gr. *phainein*, to show]. Manifest; apparent.

phantasia (făn-tā′zē-ă) [Gr.]. An appearance that is imaginary.

phantasm (făn′tăzm) [Gr. *phantasma*]. An optical illusion; an apparition, or illusion of something that does not exist.

phantasmagoria [Gr. *phantasma*, an appearance, + *agora*, assembly, gathering]. A series of phantasms, deceptive illusions, either imagined or remembered from a dream.

phantasmology (făn″tăz-mŏl′ō-jē) [″ + *logos*, word, reason]. Study of dreams, phantoms, and spiritually derived apparitions.

phantasy (făn′tă-sē) [Gr. *phantasia*, imagination]. A daydream. Phantasy-thinking is a form of wish fulfillment, a disregard for reality, from which one would escape through reveling in imaginative possibilities.

RS: delirium; delusion; hallucination; hysteria; illusion; phobia.

phantogeusia (făn-tō-gū′sē-ă) [″ + *geusis*, taste]. An intermittent or persistent taste sensation in the mouth not produced by an external stimulus.

phantom (făn′tŭm) [Gr. *phantasma*, an appearance]. 1. An apparition. 2. A model of the body or of one of its parts.

phantom corpuscle. A colorless erythrocyte.

phantom limb. A sensation, following amputation of a limb, that the limb still exists. The sensation that pain exists in the removed part is known as phantom-limb pain.

phantom tumor. An apparent tumor due to muscular contractions or flatus seen in hysteria.

phantom vision. An experience, usually transient, of visual sensations in the area from which an eye has been surgically removed.

phantosmia (făn-tŏs′mē-ă) [″ + *osme*, smell]. Intermittent or persistent perception of odor when no odor is inhaled.

pharmacal (făr′mă-kăl) [Gr. *pharmakon*, drug]. Concerning pharmacy.

pharmaceutical (făr-mă-sū′tĭ-kăl) [Gr. *pharmakeutikos*]. Concerning drugs or pharmacy.

pharmaceutical chemistry. The chemistry of medicines, their composition, synthesis, analysis, storage, and actions.

pharmaceutics (făr-mă-sū′tĭks). Science of dispensing medicines. SYN: *pharmacy*.

pharmacist (făr′mă-sĭst) [Gr. *pharmakon*, drug]. A druggist; one licensed to prepare and dispense drugs. SYN: *apothecary*.

pharmaco- [Gr. *pharmakon*, drug]. Combining form meaning drug, medicine, poison.

pharmacochemistry (făr″mă-kō-kĕm′ĭs-trē) [″ + *chemeia*, chemistry]. Pharmaceutical chemistry, q.v.

pharmacodiagnosis (făr″mă-kō-dī″ăg-nō′sĭs) [″ + *dia*, through, + *gnosis*, knowledge]. Use of drugs in making a diagnosis.

pharmacodynamics (făr″mă-kō-dī-năm′ĭks) [″ + *dynamis*, power]. Study of drugs and their actions on living organisms.

pharmacoendocrinology (făr″mă-kō-ĕn″dō-krī-nŏl′ō-jē) [″ + *endon*, within, + *krinein*, to secrete, + *logos*, word, reason]. The pharmacology of the function of endocrine glands.

pharmacoepidemiology. Application of the science of epidemiology to the study of the effects of drugs, desired and undesired, and uses of drugs in human populations.

pharmacogenetics (făr″mă-kō-jĕn-ĕt′ĭks) [″ + *genesis*, generation, birth]. Study of the influence of hereditary factors on response of individual organisms to drugs.

pharmacognosy (făr″mă-kŏg′nō-sē) [″ + *gnosis*, knowledge]. The science of natural drugs and their physical, botanical, and chemical properties.

pharmacography (făr″mă-kŏg′ră-fē) [″ + *graphein*, to write]. Treatise on the properties of drugs.

pharmacokinetics (făr″mă-kō-kĭ-nĕt′ĭks). Study of the metabolism and action of drugs with particular emphasis on the time required for absorption, duration of action, distribution in the body, and method of excretion.

pharmacologist (făr″mă-kŏl′ō-jĭst). An individual who by training and experience is a specialist in pharmacology.

pharmacology (făr″mă-kŏl′ō-jē) [″ + *logos*, word, reason]. Study of drugs and their origin, nature, properties, and effects upon living organisms.

pharmacomania (făr″mă-kō-mā′nē-ă) [″ + *mania*, madness]. Abnormal desire for giving or taking medicines.

pharmacopedia (făr″mă-kō-pē′dē-ă) [″ +

paideia, education]. Information concerning drugs and their preparation.

pharmacopeia (fär″mă-kō-pē′ă) [Gr. *pharmakopoeia*, preparation of drugs]. Authorized treatise on drugs and their preparation, esp. a book containing formulas and information that provide a standard for preparation and dispensation of drugs.

Pharmacopeia, United States. ABBR: USP. A pharmacopeia issued every five years, but with periodic supplements, prepared under supervision of a national committee of pharmacists, pharmacologists, physicians, chemists, biologists, and other scientific and allied personnel. The United States Pharmacopeia was adopted as standard in 1906. Beginning with the U.S. Pharmacopeia XIX, 1975, the National Formulary has been included in that publication.

pharmacophilia (fär″mă-kō-fil′ē-ă) [Gr. *pharmakon*, drug, + *philos*, love]. Pathological fondness for drugs and medicines.

pharmacophobia (fär″mă-kō-fō′bē-ă) [″ + *phobos*, fear]. Abnormal fear of taking medicines.

pharmacophore (fär′mă-kō-for) [″ + *phoros*, bearing]. The particular group or arrangement of atoms in a molecule that gives the material its medicinal activity.

pharmacopsychosis (fär″mă-kō-sī-kō′sĭs) [″ + *psyche*, soul, + *osis*, condition]. Mental disorder associated with addiction to drugs or alcohol.

pharmacotherapy (fär″mă-kō-thĕr′ă-pē) [″ + *therapeia*, treatment]. Use of medicine in treatment of disease.

pharmacy (fär′mă-sē) [Gr. *pharmakon*, drug]. 1. The practice of compounding and dispensing medicinal preparations. 2. A drugstore.

Pharm.D. *Doctor of Pharmacy.*

pharyngalgia (fär″ĭn-găl′jē-ă) [Gr. *pharynx*, throat, + *algos*, pain]. Pain in the pharynx. SYN: *pharyngodynia.*

pharyngeal (fär-ĭn′jē-ăl) [L. *pharyngeus*]. Concerning the pharynx.

pharyngeal bursa. A small blind sac often present in lower portion of pharyngeal tonsil.

pharyngeal hypophysis. A small structure anterior to pharyngeal bursa. It is derived from the lower portion of Rathke's pouch and occasionally gives rise to a cyst or tumor.

pharyngeal reflex. Attempt to swallow following any application of stimulus to pharynx.

pharyngeal suction (Yankaner) catheter. Rigid tube used to suction the pharynx during direct visualization.

pharyngeal tonsil. Lymphoid tissue on posterior superior wall of the pharynx. When hypertrophied, it is called an adenoid, q.v.

pharyngectomy (fär-ĭn-jĕk′tō-mē) [Gr. *pharynx*, throat, + *ektome*, excision]. Partial excision of the pharynx to remove growths or abscesses.

pharyngemphraxis (fär″ĭn-jĕm-fräk′sĭs) [″ + *emphraxis*, stoppage]. Pharyngeal obstruction.

pharyngismus (fär″ĭn-jĭz′mŭs) [″ + *-ismos*, condition]. Spasm of the muscles in the pharynx. SYN: *pharyngospasm.*

pharyngitis (fär″ĭn-jī′tĭs) [″ + *itis*, inflammation]. Inflammation of pharynx.

    p., acute. Inflammation of the pharynx with pain in the throat.

    SYM: Malaise, fever, dysphagia, pain in throat, postnasal secretion.

    TREAT: *Local:* Gargles, lozenges, topical application to oral pharynx. *General:* Bedrest, adequate fluids, analgesics. Appropriate antibiotic after material has been taken for bacterial study, esp. for beta-hemolytic streptococci.

    p., atrophic. Chronic form of pharyngitis with some atrophy of mucous glands and abnormal secretion. SYN: *p. sicca.*

    p., chronic. Pharyngitis associated with pathology in nose and sinuses, mouth breathing, excessive smoking, and chronic tonsillitis.

    SYM: Dryness and irritation of throat; cough.

    TREAT: Intranasal medication and removal of pathological factors in sinuses; tonsillectomy.

    p., croupous. Pharyngitis with the false membrane of croup.

    p., diphtheritic. Sore throat with general symptoms of diphtheria and formation of a true membrane.

    p., follicular. P., granular.

    p., gangrenous. Gangrenous inflammation of mucous membrane of the pharynx. SYN: *angina maligna.*

    p., granular. Chronic pharyngitis with granulations seen on the pharynx. SYN: *p., follicular.*

    p. herpetica. Pharyngitis characterized by formation of vesicles and ulcers.

    p., hypertrophic. Chronic pharyngitis with thickened red mucous membrane on each side with a glazed central portion.

    p., membranous. Pharyngitis in which a membranous exudate forms a false membrane.

    p. sicca. P., atrophic.

    p. ulcerosa. Pharyngitis with fever, pain, and the formation of ulcerations.

pharyngo- [Gr. *pharynx*, throat]. Combining form pert. to the pharynx.

pharyngoamygdalitis (fă-rĭn″gō-ă-mĭg″dăl-ī′tĭs) [″ + *amygdale*, tonsil, + *itis*, inflammation]. Inflamed condition of the pharynx and tonsil.

pharyngocele (far-ĭn'gō-sēl) [" + *kele*, tumor, swelling]. Hernia through pharyngeal wall.

pharyngoceratosis (fă-rĭng″gō-sĕr″ă-tō'sĭs) [" + *keras*, horn, + *osis*, condition]. Pharyngokeratosis, q.v.

pharyngoconjunctival fever, acute. ABBR: APC. An acute disease consisting of fever, pharyngitis, and conjunctivitis.
    ETIOL: Adenovirus type 3. It is particularly predisposed to occur in children in summer camp and may temporarily disable more than half of the campers in a few weeks.
    TREAT: Symptomatic.

pharyngodynia (far-ĭn″gō-dĭn'ē-ă) [" + *odyne*, pain]. Pain in the pharynx. SYN: *pharyngalgia*.

pharyngoepiglottic, pharyngoepiglottidean (fă-rĭng″gō-ĕp″ĭ-glŏt'ĭk, -glŏ-tĭd'ē-ăn) [" + *epi*, upon, + *glottis*, glottis]. Concerning the pharynx and glottis.

pharyngoesophageal (fă-rĭng″gō-ē-sŏf'ă-jē″ăl) [" + *oisophagos*, esophagus]. Concerning the pharynx and esophagus.

pharyngoglossal (fă-rĭng″gō-glŏs'ăl) [" + *glossa*, tongue]. Concerning the pharynx and tongue.

pharyngography. Radiographic examination of the pharynx after ingestion of a contrast medium.

pharyngokeratosis (far-ĭn″gō-kĕr″ă-tō'sĭs) [" + *keras*, horn, + *osis*, condition]. Thickening and hardening of mucous lining of the pharynx.

pharyngolaryngeal (fă-rĭng″gō-lă-rĭn'jē-ăl) [" + *larynx*, larynx]. Concerning the pharynx and larynx.

pharyngolaryngitis (far-ĭn″gō-lăr-ĭn-jī'tĭs) [" + " + *itis*, inflammation]. Inflamed condition of the pharynx and larynx. SYN: *laryngopharyngitis*.

pharyngolith (far-ĭn'gō-lĭth) [" + *lithos*, stone]. Concretion in pharyngeal walls.

pharyngology (far″ĭn-gŏl'ō-jē) [" + *logos*, word, reason]. Branch of medicine dealing with the pharynx.

pharyngolysis (far″ĭn-gŏl'ĭ-sĭs) [" + *lysis*, dissolution]. Paralysis of the pharynx.

pharyngomaxillary (fă-rĭng″gō-măk'sĭ-lĕr″ē) [" + L. *maxilla*, jawbone]. Concerning the pharynx and maxillae.

pharyngomycosis (far-ĭn″gō-mī-kō'sĭs) [" + *mykes*, fungus, + *osis*, condition]. Disease of the pharynx due to fungi.

pharyngonasal (fă-rĭng″gō-nā'săl) [" + L. *nasus*, nose]. Concerning the pharynx and nose.

pharyngo-oral (fă-rĭng″gō-or'ăl) [" + L. *os*, mouth]. Concerning the pharynx and mouth.

pharyngopalatine (fă-rĭng″gō-păl'ă-tīn) [" + L. *palatum*, palate]. Concerning the pharynx and palate.

pharyngoparalysis (far-ĭn″gō-păr-ăl'ĭ-sĭs) [" + *paralysis*, a loosening at the side]. Paralysis of the muscles of the pharynx. SYN: *pharyngoplegia*.

pharyngopathy (far″ĭn-gŏp'ă-thē) [" + *pathos*, disease, suffering]. Any disorder of the pharynx.

pharyngoperistole (far-ĭn″gō-pĕr-ĭs'tō-lē) [" + *peristole*, contracture]. Narrowing or stricture of the lumen of the pharynx.

pharyngoplasty (far-ĭn'gō-plăs″tē) [" + *plassein*, to form]. Reparative surgery of the pharynx.

pharyngoplegia (far-ĭn″gō-plē'jē-ă) [" + *plege*, a stroke]. Paralysis of muscles of the pharynx. SYN: *pharyngoparalysis*.

pharyngorhinitis (far-ĭn″gō-rī-nī'tĭs) [" + *rhis*, nose, + *itis*, inflammation]. Inflamed condition of the nasopharynx.

pharyngorhinoscopy (far-ĭn″gō-rī-nŏs'kō-pē) [" + " + *skopein*, to examine]. Inspection of the nasopharynx and posterior nares.

pharyngorrhea (far″ĭn-gō-rē'ă) [" + *rhoia*, flow]. Discharge of mucus from the pharynx.

pharyngoscleroma (far-rĭng″gō-sklē-rō'mă) [" + *skleroma*, induration]. An indurated patch, or scleroma, in the pharynx.

pharyngoscope (far-ĭn'gō-skōp) [" + *skopein*, to examine]. Instrument for visual examination of the pharynx.

pharyngoscopy (far″ĭn-gŏs'kō-pē). Visual examination of the pharynx.

pharyngospasm (far-ĭn'gō-spăzm) [" + *spasmos*, a convulsion]. Spasmodic contraction of muscles of the pharynx. SYN: *pharyngismus*.

pharyngostenosis (fă-rĭng″gō-stē-nō'sĭs) [" + *stenosis*, narrowing]. Narrowing or stricture of the pharynx.

pharyngotherapy (far-ĭn″gō-thĕr'ă-pē) [" + *therapeia*, treatment]. Treatment of pharyngeal disturbances or diseases.

pharyngotome (far-ĭn'gō-tōm) [" + *tome*, incision]. Instrument for incision of the pharynx.

pharyngotomy (far-ĭn-gŏt'ō-mē). Incision of the pharynx.

pharyngotonsillitis (fă-rĭng″gō-tŏn″sĭ-lī'tĭs) [" + L. *tonsilla*, almond, + Gr. *itis*, inflammation]. Inflammation of the pharynx and tonsils.

pharyngoxerosis (fă-rĭng″gō-zē-rō'sĭs) [" + *xerosis*, dryness]. Dryness of the pharynx.

pharynx (far'ĭnks) [Gr.] (pl. *pharynges*). [NA] Passageway for air from nasal cavity to larynx and food from mouth to esophagus. Also acts as a resonating cavity. A musculomembranous tube extending from base of skull to level of the 6th cervical vertebra, where it becomes continuous with the esophagus. Upper portion is lined with pseudostratified ciliated epithelium, middle portion with stratified columnar epithelium, and lower portion with stratified squamous epithelium.

Communicates with the posterior nares, eustachian tube, mouth, esophagus, and larynx. The nasopharynx is the section above the palate, the oropharynx lies between the palate and the hyoid bone, and the laryngopharynx is below the hyoid bone.

Nerve supply is from the autonomic system, the vagus, and glossopharyngeal. Blood vessels branch from the exterior carotid artery. Veins form an extensive pharyngeal plexus and drain into the interior jugular vein. SEE: *mouth* for illus.

phase (fāz) [Gr. *phasis,* an appearance]. 1. A stage of development. 2. A transitory appearance. 3. The state of a component of a heterogeneous system, as when oil is mixed with water, which is homogeneous throughout itself and bounded by an interface with other phases of the system.

p., aqueous. The water portion of a mixture of liquids and solids.

p., continuous. State of substance in a heterogeneous system in which particles are continuous.

Ex.: The water particles in which oil has been dispersed.

p., disperse. State of a substance in a heterogeneous system in which particles are separated from each other.

Ex.: Oil particles in water.

phasic (fā'sĭk). Of, or pert. to, a phase.

phatnorrhagia (făt″nō-rā'jē-ă) [Gr., socket of a tooth, + *rhegnynai,* to burst forth]. Hemorrhage from the socket of a tooth.

Ph.D. *Doctor of Philosophy.*

phenacaine hydrochloride (fĕn'ă-kān). USP. A local anesthetic drug used in ophthalmology.

phenacemide (fĕ-năs'ĕ-mīd). USP. An anticonvulsive drug. Serious adverse side effects limit its usefulness. Trade name is Phenurone.

phenacetin (fĕ-năs'ĕ-tĭn). An odorless, white, crystalline substance derived from coal tar. An antipyretic and analgesic. Combined with aspirin and caffeine in some common headache tablets. Excessive use can be toxic and may cause hemolysis of red blood cells. Prolonged use causes serious damage to the kidneys. SYN: *acetophenetidin.* SEE: *Poisons and Poisoning* in *Appendix.*

phenakistoscope (fĕ″nă-kĭs′tō-skōp) [Gr. *phenakistos,* deceiver, + *skopein,* to view]. A device that produces a stroboscopic-like view of the figures seen through slits that revolve in the same direction. The figures are seen in a mirror, and they appear to move.

phenanthrene (fĕ-năn′thrēn). $C_{14}H_{10}$. A coal tar derivative that is carcinogenic.

Phenaphen. Trade name for acetaminophen.

phenate (fē'nāt). A salt of phenic acid (phenol).

phenazopyridine hydrochloride (fĕn″ă-zō-pĕr′ĭ-dēn). USP. A drug with analgesic action on the urinary tract. It causes a red or orange color of the urine. Trade name is Pyridium.

phencyclidine hydrochloride. An anesthetic used in veterinary medicine. It is also used illegally as a hallucinogen, referred to as PCP or angel dust. Moderate doses cause elevated blood pressure, rapid pulse, increased skeletal muscle tone and sometimes, myoclonic jerks. Large doses can cause seizures, ataxia, nystagmus, respiratory depression, and death. Pupils are usually of normal size or small.

TREAT: For agitation caused by acute intoxication, diazepam is indicated. After initial therapy the patient should be observed in a quiet room. Efforts to "talk down" the patient are contraindicated.

phenelzine sulfate (fĕn′ĕl-zēn). USP. An antidepressant drug. Trade name is Nardil.

Phenergan. Trade name for promethazine hydrochloride, USP.

phenethicillin potassium (fĕ-nĕth″ĭ-sĭl′ĭn). A penicillin that may be used orally because its activity is not appreciably affected by gastric acid. Trade names are Syncillin and Maxipen.

phenformin hydrochloride (fĕn-for′mĭn). An oral hypoglycemic agent no longer marketed in the U.S. because of its tendency to cause lactic acidosis.

phenic acid (fē'nĭk). Phenol.

phenindione (fĕn″ĭn-dī′ōn). USP. An anticoagulant drug.

pheniramine maleate (fĕn-ĭr′ă-mēn). An antihistamine drug.

phenmetrazine hydrochloride (fĕn-mĕt′ră-zēn). USP. A sympathomimetic drug. Its effectiveness in treating obesity is unpredictable. Trade name is Preludin.

phenobarbital (fē″nō-bǎr′bǐ-tǎl). USP. Phenylethylbarbituric acid, a white crystalline substance soluble in alcohol. Trade names are Luminal Sodium, and Sulfoton.

ACTION/USES: A hypnotic, long-acting sedative, and anticonvulsant. Used, often in combination with diphenylhydantoin sodium, in treatment of epilepsy because it has a depressive effect on motor areas of the cerebral cortex.

p., sodium. USP. Soluble phenobarbital. More rapidly absorbed than phenobarbital but has the same uses. Trade name is Luminal Sodium.

phenocopy (fē′nō-kŏp″ē) [Gr. *phainein*, to show, + *copy*]. An individual with a biochemical or physical characteristic that resembles that produced by a genetic mutation but is instead due to an environmental condition.

phenol (fē′nōl). USP. C_6H_5OH. 1. A crystalline, colorless or light pink solid, melting at 43°C, obtained from the distillation of coal tar. It has a characteristic odor and is dangerous because of its rapid corrosive action on tissues. When used carefully and properly diluted, it is effective as a bacteriostatic agent. SYN: *carbolic acid; phenic acid.* 2. Any of the aromatic derivatives of benzene with one or more hydroxyl groups attached.

p. red. An indicator used in determining hydrogen ion concentration.

Phenolax. Trade name for phenolphthalein.

phenolemia (fē″nō-lē′mē-ă) [*phenol* + Gr. *haima*, blood]. Presence of phenol in the blood.

phenology (fē-nŏl′ō-jē) [Gr. *phainesthai*, to appear, + *logos*, word, reason]. Study of the effects of climate on living things.

phenolphthalein (fē″nŏl-thăl′ē-ĭn, fē″nŏl-thăl′ēn). USP. A white or yellow crystalline powder, produced by the interaction of phenol and phthalic anhydride. Trade names are Phenolax and Evac-Q-Tabs.

Sometimes self-administration of phenolphthalein is done to induce diarrhea. This occurs more frequently in females. If this is suspected, it may be validated by the pink color of a stool specimen that has been made alkaline.

ACTION/USES: Laxative.

phenol poisoning. Phenol is rapidly corrosive on tissues.

SYM: Strong solutions cause burning pain and, later, anesthesia. The skin and mucous membrane first become pale, then gray-white, opalescent, and finally brown to black. Even a 1% solution may cause local gangrene. It is absorbed from intact skin wounds and mucous membrane to cause general effects, including collapse and coma. When taken by mouth, it causes whitish discoloration of mucous membranes, intense burning, nausea and rarely vomiting, followed shortly by faintness, weakness, and collapse. Pulse slow and weak and hypothermia with respiratory arrest may be present. Perspiration is increased and there is renal damage. Profound coma may occur within 30 minutes of exposure of skin to phenol.

PROG: A guarded prognosis should always be given because, although the patient may improve at first, damage to the mucous membrane and absorption of phenol may lead to serious complications later.

NURSING IMPLICATIONS: Remove poison from stomach as soon as possible. While waiting to do this, administer 5 to 6 tsp (25 to 30 ml) of activated charcoal in water. Turn the patient from side to side to ensure that all portions of the stomach come in contact with the charcoal.

A well-lubricated gastric tube should be used with caution. Give extensive lavage with charcoal. If this isn't available, use olive oil, leaving some in the stomach. If olive oil is not available, use cottonseed oil or water. Do not use ethyl alcohol as lavage fluid because it speeds absorption of phenol. Demulcents such as egg whites or milk may be left in the stomach when lavage is finished.

Remove contaminated clothing instantly, and wash external burns with large amounts of water or with olive oil. Use external heat, oxygen therapy, and morphine as required. SEE: *Poisons and Poisoning* in *Appendix.*

phenolsulfonphthalein (fē″nŏl-sŭl″fŏn-thăl′ē-ĭn). USP. A dye that is given parenterally. It is used to test renal function.

phenoluria (fē″nŏl-ū′rē-ă). Elimination of phenols in the urine.

phenomenology (fē-nŏm″ĕ-nŏl′ō-jē) [Gr. *phainomenon*, appearing, + *logos*, word, reason]. The study and classification of phenomena.

phenomenon (fē-nŏm′ĕ-nŏn) [Gr. *phaino-menon*, appearing] (pl. *phenomena*). A change, perceivable by the senses, that occurs in an organ or vital function; an objective symptom.

p., Bell's. Rolling of the eyeball upward and outward when an attempt is made to close the eye on the side of the face affected in peripheral facial paralysis.

p., breakaway. Persons flying in outer space may experience the sensation of losing contact with all other human beings. SYN: *breakoff phenomenon.*

p., déjà vu. SEE: *déjà vu.*

phenothiazine (fē″nō-thī′ă-zēn). An organic compound used in manufacturing a certain class of tranquilizers and in the production of insecticides, anthelmintics for livestock, and dyes.

Caution: Overdose may cause severe postural hypotension, drowsiness, tachycardia, nausea, drying of the mouth, ataxia, fever, tremor, blurring of vision, and occasionally paralytic ileus.

TREAT: Symptomatic therapy; remove drug from stomach by gastric lavage. SEE: *chlorpromazine* in *Poisons and Poisoning* in *Appendix.*

phenotype (fē'nō-tīp) [Gr. *phainein*, to show, + *typos*, type]. 1. The physical appearance or makeup of an individual. Some phenotypes, such as the blood groups, are completely determined by heredity, while others are readily altered by environmental agents. 2. A group of individuals who resemble each other in appearance. SEE: *genotype.*

phenoxybenzamine hydrochloride (fē-nŏk"sē-bĕn'ză-mēn). USP. An alpha-adrenergic blocking agent used to produce peripheral vasodilation. Trade name is Dibenzyline.

phenozygous (fē-nŏz'ĭ-gŭs) [" + *zygon*, yoke]. Possessing a cranium much narrower than the face.

phenprocoumon (fĕn-prō'koo-mŏn). USP. An anticoagulant drug.

phensuximide (fĕn-sŭk'sĭ-mīd). USP. An anticonvulsant drug used in treating absence seizures. Trade name is Milontin.

phentermine (fĕn'tĕr-mēn). A sympathomimetic drug used as an anorexic.

phentolamine hydrochloride (fĕn-tŏl'ă-mēn). USP. An α-adrenergic blocking agent used in diagnosing pheochromocytoma. Trade name is Regitine Hydrochloride.

Phenurone. Trade name for phenacemide.

phenyl (fĕn'ĭl, fē'nĭl). The univalent radical of phenol, C_6H_5.

phenylalanine (fĕn"ĭl-ăl'ă-nīn). An essential amino acid formed from protein.

phenylamine. C_6H_7N. The simplest aromatic amine, an oily liquid derived from benzene. Used in manufacture of dyes for medical and industrial purposes. SYN: *aminobenzene.*

phenylbutazone (fĕn"ĭl-bū'tă-zōn). USP. An antiarthritic and anti-inflammatory drug originally developed for use in various forms of arthritis. Because of the possibility of serious side effects, the drug is used only when it is possible to supervise the patient carefully. Its long-term unsupervised use is contraindicated. Trade names are Azolid and Butazolidin.

phenylephrine hydrochloride. USP. Adrenergic compound used in a suitably weak concentration to produce nasal decongestion. May also be used in ophthalmic solutions.

phenylethyl alcohol. USP. An antibacterial agent that has been used as a preservative in ophthalmic solutions.

phenylhydrazine (fĕn"ĭl-hī'dră-zēn). Oily nitrogenous base used as a test for presence

of sugar in the urine.

phenylketonuria (fĕn"ĭl-kē"tō-nū're-ă). ABBR: PKU. 1. Phenylpyruvic acid in the urine. 2. A recessive hereditary disease caused by the body's failure to oxidize an amino acid (phenylalanine) to tyrosine, because of a defective enzyme. If the disease is not treated early, brain damage may occur, causing severe mental retardation. Test for phenylketonuria should be made at birth; some states require it. The disease is seen equally in the sexes, and in the U.S. the incidence is approximately 1 : 14,000 births.

Adult women who have PKU, plan to become pregnant, and have an elevated level of phenylalanine should start a low-phenylalanine diet prior to pregnancy. The level of phenylalanine should be kept below 10 mg/dl throughout pregnancy.

SYM: Tremor, spasticity, convulsions, hyperactivity, mental deficiency, eczema, unusual hand posturing, and offensive odor of urine and sweat.

TREAT: Low-phenylalanine diet.

PROG: Excellent if treatment is started early postnatally. If started after three years, no improvement will occur, because of brain damage.

phenylmercuric acetate (fĕn"ĭl-mĕr-kū'rĭk). A bacteriostatic agent that also acts as a fungicide and herbicide.

phenylmercuric nitrate. A bacteriostatic agent that has been used in treating wounds and as a preservative for intravenous solutions.

phenylpropanolamine hydrochloride (fĕn"ĭl-prō"pă-nŏl'ă-mēn). USP. A sympathomimetic drug used to produce bronchodilation.

phenylpyruvic acid (fĕn"ĭl-pī-roo'vĭk). A metabolic derivative of phenylalanine.

phenylpyruvic acid oligophrenia. A form of inherited mental deficiency resulting from phenylketonuria.

phenylthiocarbamide (fĕn"ĭl-thī"ō-kăr'bă-mīd). ABBR: PTC. A chemical used in studying medical genetics to detect the presence of a marker gene. About 70% of the population inherit the ability to note the taste of phenylthiocarbamide to be extremely bitter. To the remainder of the population, it is tasteless. The inheritance of this trait is due to a single dominant gene pair.

phenylthiourea (fĕn"ĭl-thī"ō-ū-rē'ă). Phenylthiocarbamide, q.v.

phenytoin (fĕn'ĭ-tō-ĭn). USP. An anticonvulsant drug. Trade name is Dilantin.

A very small number of patients using this anticonvulsant will develop benign pseudolymphoma that may resemble Hodgkin's disease. SYN: *diphenylhydantoin.*

SEE: *Dupuytren's contracture.*

pheochrome (fē″ō-krōm) [Gr. *phaios,* dusky, + *chroma,* color]. Staining darkly with chrome salts.

pheochromoblast (fē″ō-krō′mō-blăst) [″ + ″ + *blastos,* germ]. Embryonic cells that develop into pheochromocytes.

pheochromoblastoma (fē″ō-krō″mō-blăs-tō′mă) [″ + ″ + + *oma,* tumor]. Pheochromocytoma, q.v.

pheochromocyte (fē″ō-krō′mō-sīt) [″ + ″ + *kytos,* cell]. A chromaffin cell, such as one of those in the adrenal medulla, that gives a positive chromaffin reaction, i.e., it gives a yellowish reaction with chrome salts.

pheochromocytoma (fē-ō-krō″mō-sī-tō′mă) [″ + ″ + ″ + *oma,* tumor]. A chromaffin cell tumor of the sympathoadrenal system that produces catecholamines, i.e., norepinephrine and epinephrine. Although the tumor usually is benign, it produces hypertension that may be paroxysmal in about half the patients. The patient will complain of attacks of pounding headaches, sweating, palpitation, apprehension, flushing of the face, nausea and vomiting, and tingling of the extremities. SYN: *paraganglioma.* SEE: *Nursing Diagnoses* in *Appendix.*

TREAT: Surgical removal of the tumor.

pheomelanins (fē-ō-mĕl′ă-nĭnz) [″ + Gr. *melas,* black]. Yellow-brown, sulfur-containing pigments present as the pigment in human red hair.

pheresis. Removal of blood from the individual, separating certain elements, e.g., cells such as platelets or red blood cells, and reintroducing the remaining components into the patient. SYN: *apheresis.* SEE: *leukapheresis; plateletpheresis; plasmapheresis.*

pheromone (fĕr′ō-mōn). A substance that provides chemical means of communication between animals, and between certain insects, of the same species. It is probably detected by smell. May affect development, reproduction, or behavior of other individuals.

Ph.G. *German Pharmacopeia; Graduate in Pharmacy.*

phial (fī′ăl) [Gr. *phiale,* a bowl]. A small vessel for medicine; a vial.

Philadelphia chromosome. Abnormal chromosome 22 in which there is translocation of the distal portion of its long arm to chromosome 9. Found in leukocyte cultures of many patients with chronic myelocytic leukemia.

-philia, -phil, -philic (fĭl′ē-ă) [Gr. *philein,* to love]. Combining form meaning love for, tendency towards, craving for.

philiater (fi-lī′ă-tĕr) [″ + *iatreia,* healing]. A student of medicine.

philoneism (fĭ-lō′nē-ĭzm) [Gr. *philein,* to love, + *neos,* new, + *-ismos,* condition]. Excessive love or fondness for newness or change. Opposed to misoneism.

philoprogenitive (fĭ″lō-prō-jĕn′ĭ-tĭv) [″ + *pro,* for, + *gennan,* to produce]. Producing a large number of offspring. SYN: *prolific.*

philter, philtre [Gr. *philtron*]. A potion or drug that is supposed to induce love or promote sexual activity.

philtrum. [NA] The median groove on the external surface of the upper lip.

phimosis (fī-mō′sĭs) [Gr., a muzzling]. Stenosis or narrowness of preputial orifice so that the foreskin cannot be pushed back over the glans penis.

TREAT: Circumcision.

p. vaginalis. Narrowness or closure of the vaginal orifice.

pHisoHex (fī′sō-hĕks). Trade name for an antibacterial skin cleanser containing hexachlorophene as the main ingredient.

phlebalgia (flĕ-băl′jē-ă) [Gr. *phlebos,* vein, + *algos,* pain]. Pain arising from a vein.

phlebangioma (flĕb″ăn-jē-ō′mă) [″ + *angeion,* vessel, + *oma,* tumor]. An aneurysm occurring in a vein.

phlebarteriectasia (flĕb″ăr-tē″rē-ĕk-tā′zē-ă) [″ + *arteria,* artery, + *ektasis,* dilatation]. Dilatation of blood vessels.

phlebarteriodialysis (flĕb″ăr-tē″rē-ō-dī-ăl′ĭ-sĭs) [″ + ″ + *dialysis,* separation]. Arteriovenous aneurysm.

phlebectasia, phlebectasis (flĕb-ĕk-tā′zē-ă, -ĕk′tă-sĭs) [″ + *ektasis,* dilatation]. Venous dilatation. SYN: *varicosity.*

phlebectomy (flĕb-ĕk′tō-mē) [″ + *ektome,* excision]. Surgical removal of a vein or part of a vein.

phlebectopia (flĕb″ĕk-tō′pē-ă) [″ + *ek,* out, + *topos,* place]. Abnormal position of a vein.

phlebemphraxis (flĕb″ĕm-frăk′sĭs) [″ + *emphraxis,* stoppage]. Artificial obstruction of a vein.

phlebismus (flĕb-ĭz′mŭs) [″ + *-ismos,* condition]. Venous congestion and dilatation.

phlebitis (flĕ-bī′tĭs) [″ + *itis,* inflammation]. Inflammation of a vein. SYN: *milk leg; phlegmasia alba dolens; thrombophlebitis.* SEE: *Nursing Diagnoses* in *Appendix.*

SYM: Pain and tenderness along course of vein; discoloration of skin; inflammatory swelling and acute edema below obstruction; rapid pulse; mild elevation of temperature; pain in joints.

ETIOL: Unknown. May occur in acute or chronic infections or following operations or childbirth.

NURSING IMPLICATIONS: In acute

phase, direct efforts toward reducing inflammation and preventing emboli by ensuring rest, elevation of affected limb, and use of antiembolic stockings. Administer analgesics and anticoagulants as ordered. Observe patient carefully for bleeding in nose, gums, urine, and feces.

Prevention: Teach individual to avoid long periods of standing or sitting with little body movement; also avoid pressure behind the knees such as that produced by crossing the legs. If oral anticoagulants are being taken, advise discussion with physician relative to contraindicated medications such as aspirin. Advise against smoking because of negative effects on cardiovascular system. Encourage use of elastic stockings if indicated. Reinforce long-term medical follow-up if patient has had episodes of phlebitis.

p., adhesive. Phlebitis in which vein tends to become obliterated. SYN: *p., plastic; p., proliferative.*

p., migrating. A transitory phlebitis that appears in a portion of a vein, then clears up only to reappear later in another location.

p. nodularis necrotisans. Circumscribed inflammation of cutaneous veins resulting in nodules that ulcerate.

p., obliterative. Phlebitis in which the lumen of a vein becomes permanently closed.

p., plastic. P., adhesive.

p., proliferative. P., adhesive.

p., puerperal. Venous inflammation following childbirth.

p., sclerosing. Phlebitis in which the veins become obstructed and hardened.

p., sinus. Inflammation of a sinus of the cerebrum.

p., suppurative. Phlebitis characterized by the formation of pus.

phlebo- [Gr. *phleps, phlebos*]. Combining form meaning vein.

phlebogram (flĕb′ō-grăm) [Gr. *phlebos*, vein, + *gramma*, something written]. A tracing of the venous pulse.

phlebograph (flĕb′ō-grăf). Device for recording the venous pulse.

phlebography (flĕ-bŏg′ră-fē) [″ + *graphein*, to write]. A study of the structure and function of the veins.

phleboid (flĕb′oyd) [″ + *eidos*, form, shape]. Pert. to, resembling, or of the nature of a vein; venous.

phlebolith, phlebolite (flĕb′ō-lĭth, -līt) [″ + *lithos*, a stone]. A calcareous concretion in a vein.

phlebolithiasis (flĕb″ō-lĭ-thī′ă-sĭs) [″ + *lithiasis*, forming stones]. The formation of phleboliths in veins.

phlebology (flĕb-ŏl′ō-jē) [″ + *logos*, word,

reason]. The science of veins and their diseases.

phlebomanometer (flĕb″ō-mă-nŏm′ĕ-tĕr) [″ + *manos*, thin, + *metron*, measure]. Device for direct measurement of venous pressure.

phlebometritis (flĕb″ō-mĕ-trī′tĭs) [″ + *metra*, uterus, + *itis*, inflammation]. Inflammation of uterine veins.

phlebomyomatosis (flĕb″ō-mī″ō-mă-tō′sĭs) [″ + *mys*, muscle, + *oma*, tumor, + *osis*, condition]. Thickening of the tissue of a vein from overgrowth of muscular fibers.

phlebopexy (flĕb′ō-pĕk″sē) [″ + *peksis*, fixation]. Extraserous transplantation of the testes for varicocele, with preservation of venous network.

phlebophlebostomy (flĕb″ō-flē-bŏs′tō-mē) [″ + *phlebos*, vein, + *stoma*, mouth]. Surgical anastomosis of veins.

phleboplasty (flĕb′ō-plăs″tē) [″ + *plassein*, to form]. Plastic repair of an injured vein.

phleborrhagia (flĕb″ō-rā′jē-ă) [″ + *rhegnynai*, to burst forth]. Bleeding from a vein.

phleborrhaphy (flĕb-or′ă-fē) [″ + *rhaphe*, seam, ridge]. Suturing of a vein.

phleborrhexis (flĕb″ō-rĕk′sĭs) [″ + *rhexis*, rupture]. Rupture of a vein.

phlebosclerosis (flĕb″ō-sklē-rō′sĭs) [″ + *sklerosis*, hardening]. Fibrous hardening of a vein's walls.

phlebostasia, phlebostasis (flĕb-ō-stā′zē-ă, -ŏs′tă-sĭs) [″ + *stasis*, stoppage]. Compression of veins temporarily to restrict an amount of blood from the general circulation. SYN: *phlebotomy, bloodless.*

phlebostenosis (flĕb″ō-stĕ-nō′sĭs) [″ + *stenosis*, narrowing]. Constriction of a vein.

phlebothrombosis (flĕb″ō-thrŏm-bō′sĭs) [″ + *thrombos*, a clot]. Clotting in a vein; phlebitis with secondary thrombosis.

phlebotome (flĕb′ō-tōm) [″ + *tome*, incision]. Lancet used in incising a vein.

phlebotomist (flĕ-bŏt′ō-mĭst) [″ + *tome*, incision]. One who practices venesection, i.e., draws blood by use of a syringe and needle.

phlebotomize (flĕ-bŏt′ō-mīz). To take blood from a person.

Phlebotomus (flĕ-bŏt′ō-mŭs) [″ + *tome*, incision]. A genus of insects, the sandflies, belonging to the family Psychodidae, order Diptera. The bloodsucking insects are annoying and transmit various forms of leishmaniasis, sandfly (pappataci) fever, and Oroya fever.

P. argentipes. In India, the transmitter of *Leishmania donovani*, causative agent of kala-azar.

P. chinensis. Transmitter of kala-azar in China.

P. papatasii. Transmitter of the causative agent of sandfly fever. The virus is capable of being transmitted through the offspring of flies.

P. sergenti. Transmitter of kala-azar in Middle East and India.

P. verrucarum. The transmitter of *Bartonella bacilliformis,* causative agent of Oroya fever (Carrion's disease), in South America.

phlebotomus fever (flĕ-bŏt′ō-mŭs). Sandfly fever, q.v.

phlebotomy (flĕ-bŏt′ō-mē) [" + *tome,* incision]. Surgical opening of a vein to withdraw blood. SYN: *venesection.*

p., bloodless. Compression of veins of the extremities, restricting some of the blood from the general circulation. SYN: *phlebostasia.*

phlegm (flĕm) [Gr. *phlegma*]. 1. Thick mucus, esp. that from the respiratory passages. 2. One of the four "humors" of early physiology.

phlegmasia (flĕg-mā′zē-ă) [Gr. *phlegmasia*]. Inflammation.

p. alba dolens. Acute edema, esp. of the leg, from venous obstruction, usually a thrombosis. SYN: *milk leg; white leg.*

SYM: Usually begins with slight fever, esp. in women who have recently given birth. Pain in lower part of abdomen follows, extends to hips and back, passes under Poupart's ligament, then down the thigh and into the calf of the leg. Sometimes proceeds from calf upwards. Whole extremity becomes excessively swollen, hot, and painful, but not red, hence the name.

Tenderness on pressure most marked along course of the femoral vein, and veins of the affected region together with associated lymphatics may be felt to be hard and cordlike. Sometimes marked by faint red line. Progress is rapid, frequently doubling size of limb in 24 hours or less. Often, there is difficulty in evacuating the bladder and rectum, glands in the groin sometimes swell and suppurate, and abscesses may form in different parts of the limb.

TREAT: Elevate limb, protect with a cradle, and apply heat. Anticoagulants to prevent clot formation. Vasodilator drugs and paracervical block may be used to combat vasospasm. Ligation of main venous channel proximal to thrombus may be done to prevent embolus.

NURSING IMPLICATIONS: Maintain strict bedrest, and elevate and immobilize the affected limb. Utilize leg and foot cradle to protect limb from pressure by bed linens. Apply pneumatic or elastic anti-embolic dressings as prescribed to unaffected limb. Apply intermittent or continuous warm,

moist compresses to affected limb as prescribed to resolve inflammation. Administer anticoagulant and analgesic drug therapies as prescribed, and evaluate patient and laboratory study responses. Teach patient about importance of bedrest in preventing embolization of thrombi, and assess for embolic complications; and about concerns related to smoking and use of oral birth control drugs, and explain importance of walking rather than standing, and long-term use of oral anticoagulant drug regimen and antiembolic stockings in preventing recurrence.

p., cellulitic. Septic inflammation of connective tissue of the leg following childbirth.

phlegmatic (flĕg-măt′ĭk) [Gr. *phlegmatikos*]. Of sluggish or dull temperament; apathetic.

phlegmon (flĕg′mŏn) [Gr. *phlegmone,* inflammation]. Acute suppurative inflammation of subcutaneous connective tissue, esp. a pyogenic inflammation that spreads along fascial planes or other natural barriers.

p., diffuse. Diffuse inflammation of subcutaneous tissues with sepsis.

p., gas. Gas gangrene.

phlegmonous (flĕg′mŏn-ŭs). Pert. to inflammation of subcutaneous tissues.

phlogistic (flō-jĭs′tĭk) [Gr. *phlogistos*]. Pert. to, or inducing, inflammation.

phlogogenic, phlogogenous (flō-gō-jĕn′ĭk, -gŏj′ĕn-ŭs) [Gr. *phlogosis,* inflammation, + *gennan,* to produce]. Producing or exciting inflammation.

phlorhizin (flō-rī′zĭn). A glycoside present in the bark of some fruit trees. It is a powerful inhibitor of sugar transport in some animals.

phlyctena (flĭk-tē′nă) [Gr. *phlyktaina*] (pl. *phlyctenae*). A vesicle, esp. one of many after a first-degree burn.

phlyctenar (flĭk′tē-năr). Concerning a vesicle.

phlyctenoid (flĭk′tē-noyd) [Gr. *phlyktaina,* a blister, + *eidos,* form, shape]. Resembling a blister or pustule.

phlyctenosis (flĭk″tē-nō′sĭs) [" + *osis,* condition]. Appearance of blisters or pustules.

phlyctenula (flĭk-tĕn′ū-lă) [L.] (pl. *phlyctenulae*). A tiny vesicle or pustule, esp. that seen on the cornea.

phlyctenular (flĭk-tĕn′ū-lăr). Resembling or pert. to vesicles or pustules.

phlyctenule (flĭk′tĕn-ūl) [Gr. *phlyktaina,* a blister; L. *phlyctenula*]. A small vesicle or blister, as on cornea or conjunctiva.

phlyctenulosis (flĭk-tĕn-ū-lō′sĭs) [" + *osis,* condition]. The formation of many phlyctenules.

phobia (fō′bē-ă) [Gr. *phobos,* fear]. Any persistent and irrational fear of a specific object, activity, or situation that results in a compelling desire to avoid the feared or phobic stimulus. Phobias are classified into three types: agoraphobias, social phobias, and simple phobias. SEE: *Phobias in Appendix.* SEE: *Nursing Diagnoses in Appendix.*

p., social. Avoidance of social situations in which the individual would be noticed or would attract attention to himself or herself, e.g., speaking or lecturing in public.

-phobia [Gr.]. Suffix indicating abnormal fear of, or aversion to, a subject.

phobic (fō′bĭk) [Gr. *phobos,* fear]. Concerning a phobia.

phobic desensitization. Method of treating phobias in which the patient is taught to relax while slowly re-entering the phobic situation, first in imagination and then in real life. Anxiety and fear are kept to a minimum at all times. SEE: *implosion flooding.*

phobophobia (fō″bō-fō′bē-ă) [″ + *phobos,* fear]. Morbid fear of acquiring a phobia.

phocomelia (fō″kō-mē′lē-ă) [Gr. *phoke,* seal, + *melos,* limb]. A congenital malformation in which the proximal portions of the extremities are poorly developed or absent. Thus the hands and feet are attached to the trunk directly or by means of a poorly formed bone. In some cases this condition was due to the administration of thalidomide, a sleeping pill, during early pregnancy. That drug is no longer approved for such use.

phocomelus (fō-kŏm′ē-lŭs). A person with phocomelia, q.v.

phon-. SEE: *phono-.*

phonacoscope (fō-năk′ō-skōp) [Gr. *phone,* voice, + *skopein,* to examine]. Device for increasing the percussion note or voice sounds.

phonacoscopy (fō-nă-kŏs′kō-pē). Inspection of the chest with the phonacoscope.

phonal (fō′năl) [Gr. *phone,* voice]. Concerning the voice.

phonasthenia (fōn-ăs-thē′nē-ă) [″ + *asthenia,* weakness]. Vocal weakness or hoarseness due to straining the voice.

phonation (fō-nā′shŭn). Process of uttering vocal sounds.

phonatory (fō′nă-tō″rē) [Gr. *phone,* voice]. Concerning utterance of vocal sounds.

phonautograph (fōn-aw′tō-grăf) [″ + *autos,* self, + *graphein,* to write]. Device for registering the voice's vibrations.

phone (fōn) [Gr. *phone,* voice]. An element of speech; a single speech sound.

-phone [Gr. *phone,* voice]. Combining form indicating sound or voice.

phoneme (fō′nēm) [Gr. *phonema,* an utterance]. In linguistics, the smallest unit of

speech that distinguishes one sound from another.

phonendoscope (fō-něn′dō-skōp) [Gr. *phone,* voice, + *endon,* within, + *skopein,* to examine]. A stethoscope that intensifies sounds.

phonendoskiascope (fō-něn″dō-skī′ă-skōp) [″ + ″ + *skia,* shadow, + *skopein,* to examine]. Device for observing the cardiac movements and for hearing heart sounds.

phonetics (fō-nět′ĭks) [Gr. *phonetikos,* spoken]. Science of speech and pronunciation. SYN: *phonology.*

phoniatrics (fō″nē-ăt′rĭks) [Gr. *phone,* voice, + *iatrikos,* treatment]. The study of the voice and treatment of its disorders.

phonic (fō′nĭk). Concerning the voice or sound.

phonism (fō′nĭzm) [″ + *-ismos,* condition]. An auditory sensation occurring when another sense is stimulated. SEE: *synesthesia.*

phono- [Gr. *phone,* voice]. Combining form indicating sound, voice.

phonocardiogram (fō″nō-kăr′dē-ō-grăm) [″ + *kardia,* heart, + *gramma,* something written]. Graphic recording of the heart sounds.

phonocardiography (fō″nō-kăr″dē-ŏg′ră-fē) [″ + *graphein,* to write]. Mechanical or electronic registration of heart sounds.

phonocatheter (fō″nō-kăth′ě-těr) [″ + *katheter,* something inserted]. A catheter with a microphone at its end.

phonogram (fō′nō-grăm) [″ + *gramma,* something written]. A graphic curve indicating intensity and duration of a sound.

phonograph (fō′nō-grăf) [″ + *graphein,* to write]. Instrument used for reproduction of sounds.

phonology (fō-nŏl′ō-jē) [″ + *logos,* word, reason]. Science of vocal sounds. SYN: *phonetics.*

phonomania (fŏn″ō-mā′nē-ă) [Gr. *phonos,* murder, + *mania,* madness]. Mental illness characterized by tendency to commit murder.

phonomassage (fō″nō-mă-sahzh′) [Gr. *phone,* voice, + *massein,* to knead]. Exciting movements of the ossicles of the ear by means of noise or alternating suction and pressure directed through the external auditory meatus.

phonometer (fō-nŏm′ě-těr) [″ + *metron,* measure]. Device for determining intensity of vocal sounds.

phonomyoclonus (fō″nō-mī-ŏk′lō-nŭs) [″ + *mys,* muscle, + *klonos,* a contraction]. Invisible fibrillary muscular contractions revealed by auscultation.

phonomyogram (fō″nō-mī′ō-grăm) [″ + ″

+ *gramma*, something written]. A recording of sound produced by action of a muscle.

phonomyography (fō″nō-mī-ŏg′ră-fē) [″ + ″ + *graphein*, to write]. The recording of sounds made by contracting muscular tissue.

phonopathy (fō-nŏp′ă-thē) [″ + *pathos*, disease, suffering]. Any disease of organs affecting speech.

phonophobia (fō″nō-fō′bē-ă) [″ + *phobos*, fear]. 1. Morbid fear of sound or noise. 2. Fear of speaking or hearing one's own voice.

phonophoresis. The use of ultrasound to introduce medication into a tissue. This has been used in treating injuries to soft tissues. Not all medicines are suitable for application using this technique.

Caution: Use of phonophoresis should be supervised by persons skilled in using the technique.

---

phonophotography. Photography of the vibrations produced by speech.

phonopsia (fō-nŏp′sē-ă) [″ + *opsis*, vision]. The subjective perception of sensations upon hearing certain sounds.

phonoreceptor. A receptor for sound waves.

phonorenogram (fō″nō-rē′nō-grăm) [″ + L. *ren*, kidney, + Gr. *gramma*, something written]. A recording of the pulse in the renal artery.

phonoscope (fō′nō-skōp) [″ + *skopein*, to examine]. Device for recording heart sounds.

phonoscopy (fō-nŏs′kō-pē). A recording made by use of a phonoscope.

-phoresis (fō-rē′sĭs) [Gr. *phoresis*, being borne]. A word termination denoting the migration of ions through a membrane by the action of an electric current. The direction of movement is distinguished by the use of prefixes, as in cataphoresis and anaphoresis for migrations toward cathode and anode, respectively.

-phoria [Gr. *phoresis*, being borne]. In ophthalmology, a combining form meaning a turning with reference to the visual axis, such as cyclophoria, q.v.

Phormia (for′mē-ă). A genus of blowflies belonging to the family Calliphoridae. Their larvae normally live in decaying flesh of dead animals, but they may infest neglected wounds or sores, giving rise to myiasis.

phorotone (fō′rō-tōn) [Gr. *phora*, motion, + *tonos*, tension]. Device for exercising eye muscles.

phorozoon (fō″rō-zō′ŏn) [Gr. *phoros*, fruitful, + *zoon*, animal]. The nonsexual stage of an animal that in its life cycle passes through several stages.

phose (fōz) [Gr. *phos*, light]. A subjective sensation of light or color. SEE: *centraphose; centrophose; chromophose; erythrophose.*

phosgene (fŏs′jēn) [″ + *genes*, born]. COCl₂. Carbonyl chloride, a poisonous gas causing nausea and suffocation when inhaled. Used in chemical warfare, esp. during World War I.

phosphagen (fŏs′fă-jĕn). Several chemicals, including phosphocreatine, that release energy when split. They are high-energy phosphate compounds.

Phosphaljel. Trade name for aluminum phosphate.

phosphatase (fŏs′fă-tās). One of a group of enzymes that catalyze the hydrolysis of phosphoric acid esters. They are of importance in absorption and metabolism of carbohydrates, nucleotides, and phospholipids and are essential in the calcification of bone.

  p., acid. Phosphatase whose optimum pH is between 4.0 and 5.4. Present in kidney, semen, serum, and prostate gland, and particularly in osteoclasts or odontoclasts in which it is associated with demineralization or resorption of bone and teeth.

  p., alkaline. Phosphatase whose optimum pH is about 9.0 and which functions in the mineralization process of bone. Present in teeth, developing bone, plasma, kidney, and intestine. It is excreted by the liver and hence increases in blood in obstructive jaundice. It is also elevated in diseases of the pancreas, lung, and bone, in some malignancies without metastases, and in pregnancy; in the first month of life, it may be as high as six times the normal level in adults. The level gradually decreases during childhood and puberty. Alkaline phosphatase can by use of special techniques be separated into bone, intestinal, and placental fractions.

phosphate (fŏs′fāt) [Gr. *phosphas*]. Any salt of phosphoric acid containing the radical PO₄. Phosphates are important in maintenance of acid-base balance of the blood, the principal ones being monosodium and disodium phosphate. The former is acid, the latter alkaline. In the blood, because of their low concentration, they exert a minor buffering action. In the formation of urine, through alteration of the proportions of acid and alkaline phosphates, an acid urine is formed, and the body's fixed base, chiefly sodium but also potassium, magnesium, and calcium, is conserved.

  Decreased phosphate excretion in urine occurs when alkaline reserve is high; in nephritis, tetany (hypoparathyroidism), adrenal cortical deficiency, and certain bone diseases.

  Increased phosphate excretion in urine occurs when alkali reserve is low, and in starvation, hyperparathyroidism, high-protein diet, and extreme muscular exercise.

p., acid. Phosphate in which only one or two hydrogen atoms of phosphoric acid have been replaced by a metal.

p., calcium. Any one of three salts of calcium and phosphate. Used as an antacid and as a dietary supplement.

p., creatine. Phosphocreatine, q.v.

p., normal. Phosphate in which all three hydrogen atoms of phosphoric acid have been replaced by metals.

p., triple. Calcium, ammonium, and magnesium phosphate.

phosphate-bond energy. Energy derived from phosphorylated compounds such as adenosine triphosphate (ATP) and creatine phosphate.

phosphatemia (fŏs″fă-tē′mē-ă) [Gr. *phosphas*, phosphate, + *haima*, blood]. Phosphates in the blood.

phosphatide (fŏs′fă-tīd). A phospholipid.

phosphaturia (fŏs″fă-tū′rē-ă) [″ + *ouron*, urine]. Excessive amount of phosphates in the urine. Often causes renal calculi. SYN: *phosphoruria; phosphuria.*

SYM: Cloudy, opaque, and pale urine. Alkaline reaction. Pearly or pink-white deposits of phosphates in standing urine.

phosphene (fŏs′fēn) [Gr. *phos*, light, + *phainein*, to show]. A subjective sensation of light caused by pressure upon the eyeball.

p., accommodation. Phosphene resulting from contraction of ciliary muscles in accommodation. Seen esp. in the dark.

phosphide (fŏs′fīd) [″ + *phorein*, to carry]. Binary compound of phosphorus with an element or radical.

phosphite (fŏs′fīt). A salt of phosphoric acid.

phosphoamidase (fŏs″fō-ăm′ĭ-dās). An enzyme that catalyzes the conversion of phosphocreatine to creatine and orthophosphate.

phosphocreatine (fŏs″fō-krē′ă-tĭn). A compound found in muscle. It is important in muscle metabolism, yielding inorganic phosphate and creatine in this process.

phosphofructokinase (fŏs″fō-frŭk″tō-kī′nās). A glycolytic enzyme that catalyzes phosphorylation of fructose-6-phosphate by adenosine triphosphate.

Pholine Iodide. Trade name for echothiophate iodide.

phospholipase (fŏs″fō-lĭp′ās). An enzyme that catalyzes hydrolysis of a phospholipid.

phospholipid (fŏs″fō-lĭp′ĭd) [Gr. *phos*, light, + *phorein*, to carry, + *lipos*, fat]. A lipoid substance containing phosphorus, fatty acids, and nitrogenous base, as lecithin. SYN: *phosphatide; phospholipin.*

phospholipin (fŏs″fō-lĭp′ĭn). A lipoid compound containing phosphorus. SYN: *phosphatide; phospholipid.*

phosphonecrosis (fŏs″fō-ně-krō′sĭs) [″ + *phorein*, to carry, + *nekros*, dead, + *osis*, condition]. Necrosis of the alveolar process in persons working with phosphorus.

phosphonuclease (fŏs″fō-nū′klē-ās). An enzyme that catalyzes the hydrolysis of nucleotides to nucleosides and phosphoric acid.

phosphopenia (fŏs″fō-pē′nē-ă) [″ + *phorein*, to carry, + *penia*, lack]. Deficiency of phosphorus in the body.

phosphoprotein (fŏs″fō-prō′tē-ĭn) [″ + ″ + *protos*, first]. One of a group of proteins in which the protein is combined with a phosphorus-containing compound. Caseinogen and vitellin are examples. Formerly called nucleoalbumin.

phosphor. Substance in the fluoroscopic image intensifier that converts photons of energy into light.

p., rare earth. Elements such as yttrium, gadolinium, and lanthanum, which are used for ultra-high-speed radiographic intensification screens.

phosphorated (fŏs″fō-rā′tĕd) [″ + *phorein*, to carry]. Impregnated with phosphorus.

phosphorescence (fŏs″fō-rĕs′ĕns). The induced luminescence that persists after cessation of the irradiation that caused it. The emission of light without appreciable heat.

phosphorhidrosis (fŏs″for-hĭd-rō′sĭs) [″ + *phorein*, to carry, + *hidrosis*, sweating]. Secretion of luminous perspiration. SYN: *phosphoridrosis.*

phosphoribosyltransferase (fŏs″fō-rī″bō-sĭl-trăns′fĕr-ās). An enzyme that catalyzes reconversion to the ribonucleotide stage of the purine bases, hypoxanthine and guanine. The deficiency is inherited as an X chromosome-linked trait.

phosphoric acid (fŏs-for′ĭk). H_3PO_4. Orthophosphoric acid, a tribasic acid. Used as a 30% to 50% solution to etch enamel of teeth in preparation for bonding of resin dental restorations. SEE: *etching.*

phosphoridrosis (fŏs″for-ĭd-rō′sĭs) [″ + *phorein*, to carry, + *hidrosis*, sweat]. Secretion of perspiration that is luminous. SYN: *phosphorhidrosis.*

phosphorism (fŏs″for-ĭzm) [″ + ″ + *-ismos*, condition]. Chronic poisoning from phosphorus.

phosphorolysis (fŏs″fō-rŏl′ĭ-sĭs). The chemical reaction of incorporating phosphoric acid into a molecule.

phosphorous acid (fŏs-fō′rŭs, fŏs′for-ŭs) [″ + *phoros*, carrying]. H_3PO_3. Crystalline acid formed when phosphorus is oxidized in moist air.

phosphoruria (fŏs″for-ū′rē-ă) [″ + *phorein*, to carry, + *ouron*, urine]. Phosphorus in the urine in excess of normal. SYN: *phosphaturia; phosphuria.*

phosphorus (fŏs′fō-rŭs) [Gr. *phos*, light, + *phoros*, carrying]. SYMB: P. At. wt. 30.9738; at. no. 15. A nonmetallic element not found in a free state but in combination with alkalies.

The adult body contains from 600 to 900 gm of phosphorus in various forms: 70% to 80% in bones and teeth, principally combined with calcium; 10% in muscle; and 1% in nerve tissue. Minimum daily requirement is approx. 800 mg. Amount should be increased during pregnancy and lactation. Vitamin D is important in the absorption and metabolism of phosphorus. Excesses of phosphorus are excreted by kidney and intestine, about 60% being excreted in urine principally as phosphates.

Phosphorus compounds (adenosine triphosphate and phosphocreatine) are the principal sources of energy in muscle contraction, and phosphorus is essential in the conversion of glycogen to glucose.

SOURCE: Phosphorus is found in many foods. Excellent sources are almonds, beans, barley, bran, cheese, cocoa, chocolate, eggs, lentils, liver, milk, oatmeal, peanuts, peas, walnuts, whole wheat, and rye. Good sources are asparagus, beef, cabbage, carrots, celery, cauliflower, chard, chicken, clams, corn, cream, cucumbers, eggplant, fish, figs, meat, prunes, pineapples, pumpkin, raisins, and string beans.

DEFICIENCY SYM: Perverted appetite, retarded growth, loss of weight, weakness, rickets, imperfect bone and teeth development.

phosphorus poisoning. Prior to the introduction of safety matches (which contain no yellow phosphorus), phosphorus poisoning was quite common. However, acute phosphorus poisoning still is seen following ingestion of rat and roach poisons, which contain yellow phosphorus. Yellow phosphorus is also used in manufacturing fireworks and fertilizers.

SYM: Acute irritation of gastrointestinal tract followed by symptoms resembling acute yellow atrophy of liver and marked blood changes. Bloody vomitus, garlic odor of breath, cramps, headache, liver and kidney damage. Profound weakness, hemorrhage, heart failure. Occasionally, nervous symptoms predominate.

NURSING IMPLICATIONS: *Ingestion:* Gastric lavage is preferred to induce emesis if phosphorus was swallowed. Protect airway by cuffed endotracheal intubation or left lateral decubitus position. Administer charcoal slurry and a cathartic. The patient requires close monitoring for delayed effects for at least 24 hours. SEE: *Poisons and Poisoning* in *Appendix.*

phosphoryl (fŏs′for-ĭl). The radical [PO]≡.

phosphorylase (fŏs-for′ĭ-lās). An enzyme that catalyzes the formation of glucose-1-phosphate from glycogen.

phosphorylation (fŏs″for-ĭ-lā′shŭn). The combining of a phosphate with an organic compound.

phosphuria (fŏs-fū′rē-ă) [Gr. *phos*, light, + *phoros*, a bearer, + *ouron*, urine]. Excess of phosphorus in the urine. SYN: *phosphaturia; phosphoruria.*

phot (fŏt) [Gr. *photos*, light]. ABBR: ph. The unit of photochemical energy equal to 1 lumen per square centimeter or about 929 foot-candles.

phot-. SEE: words beginning with *photo-*.

photalgia (fō-tăl′jē-ă) [Gr. *photos*, light, + *algos*, pain]. Pain produced by light. SYN: *photodynia.*

photaugiaphobia (fō-taw″jē-ă-fō′bē-ă) [Gr. *photaugeia*, glare, + *phobos*, fear]. Intolerance of bright light.

photechy (fō′tĕk-ē) [Gr. *photos*, light, + *echo*, echo]. The acquisition of radioactivity by having been exposed to a radioactive source.

photesthesis (fō″tĕs-thē′sĭs) [″ + *aisthesis*, sensation]. Sensitivity to light.

photic (fō′tĭk). 1. Concerning light. 2. In biology, pert. to the production of light by certain organisms.

photic driving. In neurology, altering the electroencephalogram by intermittently flashing light into the eyes.

photic epilepsy. Convulsive attacks that occur as a result of intermittent light stimulus. SEE: *epilepsy.*

photic sneezing. Sneezing initiated or hastened in its onset by light stimulus. Sometimes due to light causing tears, which upon draining into the nasal area cause sneezing.

photism (fō′tĭzm) [″ + *-ismos*, condition]. A subjective sensation of color or light produced by a stimulus of another sense, such as smell, hearing, taste, or touch. SEE: *synesthesia.*

photo- [Gr. *photos*]. Combining form indicating light.

photoactinic (fō″tō-ăk-tĭn′ĭk). Emitting both luminous and actinic rays.

photoaged skin. Skin changes caused by chronic sun exposure. This condition has been treated with topical tretinoin.

photoallergic contact dermatitis. Inflammation of the skin due to substances made allergenic by the effect of ultraviolet or light in the visible spectrum. SEE: *photoallergy.*

photoallergy (fō″tō-ăl′ĕr-jē) [Gr. *photos*,

light, + *allos,* other, + *ergon,* work]. An immunological reaction produced by interaction of light rays and certain chemicals. It is a form of contact allergic reaction in which light is necessary to cause the sensitivity reaction. Some of the photocontact allergens are phenothiazine, sulfonamides, hexachlorophene, sunscreen agents, optical bleaches, and topical antihistamines. SEE: *photosensitivity; phototoxic.*

photobacterium (fō″tō-băk-tē′rē-ŭm). A bacterium that produces light.

photobiology (fō″tō-bī-ŏl′ō-jē) [″ + *bios,* life, + *logos,* word, reason]. Study of the effect of light on living things.

photobiotic (fō″tō-bī-ŏt′ĭk) [″ + *bios,* life]. Capable of living only in the light.

photocatalysis (fō″tō-kă-tăl′ĭ-sĭs) [″ + *katalysis,* dissolution]. Catalysis of a chemical reaction by light.

photoceptor (fō″tō-sĕp′tor) [″ + L. *ceptor,* a receiver]. A nerve ceptor receiving light ray sensations.

photochemistry (fō″tō-kĕm′ĭs-trē) [″ + *chemeia,* chemistry]. Branch of chemistry concerned with the effects of light rays. SYN: *actinochemistry.*

photochemotherapy. Use of light and chemicals together to treat certain conditions.

    p., extracorporeal. Administering drugs in the usual manner and then exposing the blood to ultraviolet A radiation. The blood is returned to the body. The combination of 8-methoxypsoralen and light has been used in treating drug-resistant pemphigus vulgaris.

photochromic glass. SEE: *glass, photochromic.*

photochromogen [″ + *chroma,* color, + *gennan,* to produce]. Certain microorganisms in which a pigment develops when it is grown in the presence of light, such as *Mycobacterium kansasii.*

photocoagulation. Alteration of proteins in tissue by the use of light energy in the form of ordinary light rays or a laser beam. Used esp. in treating retinal detachments or bleeding from the retina.

photodermatitis (fō″tō-dĕr-mă-tī′tĭs) [″ + *dermatos,* skin, + *itis,* inflammation]. Sensitivity of the epithelium to light. May be due to photoallergy, q.v., or to phototoxic, q.v., reaction.

photodynamic (fō″tō-dī-năm′ĭk) [″ + *dynamis,* force]. Pert. to the energy or force effected by light on organisms.

photodynamic action. Action exerted by certain dyes, such as methylene blue and eosin, on certain biological systems when subjected to light.

photodynia (fō″tō-dĭn′ē-ă) [″ + *odyne,* pain]. Pain produced by rays of light. SYN: *photalgia.*

photodysphoria (fō″tō-dĭs-for′ē-ă) [″ + *dysphoria,* distress]. Extreme intolerance of light. SEE: *photophobia.*

photoelectricity (fō″tō-ē-lĕk-trĭ′sĭ-tē) [″ + *elektron,* amber]. Electricity formed by action of light.

photoelectron (fō″tō-ē-lĕk′trŏn) [″ + *elektron,* amber]. An electron that is ejected from its orbit around the nucleus of an atom by interaction with a photon of energy (light, x radiation, etc.).

photoerythema (fō″tō-ĕr′ĭ-thē′mă) [″ + *erythema,* redness]. Erythema of the skin caused by light.

photofluorography (fō″tō-flū″ĕr-ŏg′ră-fē). Photographing the images seen during fluoroscopic examination.

photogastroscope (fō″tō-găs′trō-skōp) [″ + *gaster,* belly, + *skopein,* to view]. Device for viewing and taking photographs of the interior of the stomach.

photogene (fō′tō-jēn) [″ + *gennan,* to produce]. Prolonged retinal image. SYN: *afterimage.*

photogenic, photogenous (fō″tō-jĕn′ĭk, -tŏj′ĕn-ŭs). Induced by, or inducing, light.

photogenic epilepsy. Epileptic seizures induced by the intermittent flashing of light into the eyes.

photographic radiometer. An instrument containing a half-tone color index for strips of photographic paper after exposure to roentgen rays; after development, it is used to estimate the quantity of roentgen rays.

photohemotachometer (fō″tō-hĕm″ō-tăk-ŏm′ĕ-tĕr) [″ + *haima,* blood, + *tachys,* swift, + *metron,* measure]. Device for photographing rate of blood flow.

photokinetic (fō″tō-kĭn-ĕt′ĭk) [″ + *kinetikos,* motion]. Reacting with motion to stimulus of light.

photokymograph (fō″tō-kī′mō-grăf) [″ + *kyma,* wave, + *graphein,* to write]. Device for making continuous photographs of a physiologic event.

photolabile. The characteristic of being destroyed or inactivated by light.

photoluminescence (fō″tō-lū-mĭ-nĕs′ĕns) [″ + L. *lumen,* light]. The power of an object to become luminescent when acted on by light.

photolysis (fō-tŏl′ĭ-sĭs) [″ + *lysis,* dissolution]. Dissolution or disintegration under stimulus of light rays.

photolyte (fō′tō-līt). A substance decomposed by light.

photolytic (fō″tō-lĭt′ĭk). Dissolved by stimulus of light rays.

photomania (fō″tō-mā′nē-ă) [″ + *mania,* madness]. 1. A psychosis produced by prolonged exposure to intense light. 2. A psychotic desire for light.

photomedicine. Use of light to treat certain conditions. SEE: *hemolytic disease of the newborn; phototherapy; psoriasis.*

photometer (fō-tŏm′ĕ-tĕr) [″ + *metron,* measure]. Device for measuring the intensity of light.

photometry (fō-tŏm′ĕ-trē). Measurement of light rays.

photomicrograph (fō″tō-mī′krō-grăf) [″ + *mikros,* small, + *graphein,* to write]. Photograph of an object under the microscope.

photomotor. Pert. to muscular contraction induced by light.

photon (fō′tŏn) [Gr. *photos,* light]. A light quantum or unit of energy of a light ray or other form of radiant energy. Generally considered to be a discrete particle with zero mass, with no electric charge, and of indefinitely long life.

photo-onycholysis. Separation of the nail from the distal nailbed in conjunction with sun exposure and simultaneous use of drugs such as antibiotics.

photo-ophthalmia, photophthalmia (fō″tō-ŏf-thăl′mē-ă, fō″tŏf-thăl′mē-ă) [″ + *ophthalmos,* eye]. Keratoconjunctivitis produced by excess exposure to intense light rays.

photopathy (fō-tŏp′ă-thē) [″ + *pathos,* disease, suffering]. Pathologic effect produced by light.

photoperceptive (fō″tō-pĕr-sĕp′tĭv) [″ + L. *percipere,* to receive]. Capable of perceiving light.

photoperiod (fō″tō-pēr′ē-ŏd) [″ + L. *periodus,* period]. The daily duration of exposure to light of a living thing.

photoperiodism (fō″tō-pēr′ē-ō-dĭzm) [″ + ″ + Gr. *-ismos,* condition]. The periodic occurrence of biological phenomena in relationship to the presence or absence of light. In most animals, the sleep-wake cycle is a form of photoperiodism.

photophilic (fō-tō-fĭl′ĭk) [″ + *philein,* to love]. Seeking, or fond of, light.

photophobia (fō″tō-fō′bē-ă) [″ + *phobos,* fear]. Unusual intolerance of light. Occurs in measles and rubella, meningitis, and inflammation of the eyes.

photophone (fō′tō-fōn) [″ + *phone,* voice]. Device for production of sound by action of light.

photophoresis. SEE: *photochemotherapy.*

photopia. Adjustment of the eye for vision in bright light. Opposite of scotopia.

photopic (fō-tō′ĭk). Pert. to bright light.

photopsia, photopsy (fō-tŏp′sē-ă, fō-tŏp′sē) [Gr. *photos,* light, + *opsis,* vision]. Subjective sensation of sparks or flashes of light in retinal, optic, or brain diseases.

photopsin (fō-tŏp′sĭn). The protein portion or opsin of the pigment in the cover of the retina of the eye.

photoptarmosis (fō″tō-tär-mō′sĭs) [″ + *ptarmosis,* sneezing]. Sneezing caused by the effect of light. SYN: *photic sneezing.*

photoptometer (fō-tŏp-tŏm′ĕ-tĕr) [″ + *opsis,* vision, + *metron,* measure]. Device for determining the smallest amount of light that will make an object visible.

photoptometry (fō″tŏp-tŏm′ĕ-trē). Measurement of light perception.

photoradiometer (fō″tō-rā″dē-ŏm′ĕ-tĕr) [″ + L. *radius,* ray, + Gr. *metron,* measure]. Device for determining the ability of ionizing radiation to penetrate substances.

photoreaction (fō″tō-rē-ăk′shŭn) [″ + LL. *reactus,* reacted]. A chemical reaction produced or influenced by light.

photoreactivation (fō″tō-rē-ăk″tĭ-vā′shŭn). Enzymatic repair of lesions such as can be produced in DNA by ultraviolet light.

photoreception (fō″tō-rē-sĕp′shŭn) [″ + L. *recipere,* to receive]. The perception of light rays in the visible light spectrum.

photoreceptive (fō″tō-rē-sĕp′tĭv) [″ + L. *receptor,* a receiver]. Capable of perceiving light rays.

photoreceptor (fō″tō-rē-sĕp′tor). Sensory nerve endings or cells that are capable of being stimulated by light. In humans, rods and cones of the retina.

photoretinitis (fō″tō-rĕt″ĭ-nī′tĭs) [Gr. *photos,* light, + L. *retina,* retina, + Gr. *itis,* inflammation]. Damage to the macula of the eye due to exposure to intense light. SEE: *blindness, eclipse.*

photoscan. A representation of the concentration of a radioisotope outlining an organ in the body. The map is printed on photographic paper. SEE: *scintiscan.*

photosensitivity [″ + L. *sensitivus,* feeling]. Sensitivity to light. SEE: *photoallergy.*

photosensitization (fō″tō-sĕn″sĭ-tĭ-zā′shŭn). Condition in which the skin reacts abnormally to light, esp. ultraviolet radiations or sunlight; due to the presence of drugs, hormones, or heavy metals in the system. SEE: *photoallergy.*

photosensitizer (fō″tō-sĕn′sĭ-tī″zĕr). Substance that, in combination with light, will cause a sensitivity reaction in the substance or organism.

photosensor. A device that detects light. SYN: *photodetector.*

photostable (fō′tō-stā″b′l) [″ + L. *stabilis,* stable]. Uninfluenced by exposure to light.

photosynthesis (fō″tō-sĭn′thĕ-sĭs) [″ + *synthesis,* placing together]. The process by which plants are able to manufacture carbohydrates by combining carbon dioxide from the air with water from the soil, utilizing light energy in the presence of chlorophyll.

The basic chemical reaction is as follows:

$$6CO_2 + 6H_2O + \text{light energy} \rightarrow$$
$$C_6H_{12}O_6 + 6O_2$$

Only plants containing chlorophyll are capable of thus producing sugars. The red and blue waves of the spectrum are absorbed by the chlorophyll, but all other rays are reflected.

When simple sugar is formed, the plant utilizes the light energy plus water and carbon dioxide to form carbohydrate. The sources of energy for this synthesis are the blue and red rays that are absorbed by the plant. To make 1 gm of natural sugar, the plant uses 750 cu. ft (21.24 cu. meters) of carbon dioxide.

phototaxis (fō″tō-tăk′sĭs) [Gr. *photos*, light, + *taxis*, arrangement]. The reaction and movement of cells and microorganisms under the stimulus of light.

phototherapy (fō″tō-thĕr′ă-pē) [″ + *therapeia*, treatment]. 1. Exposure to sunlight or artificial light for therapeutic purposes. 2. Use of light to treat certain conditions. Hemolytic jaundice of the newborn, q.v., is treated with either exchange transfusion or phototherapy, or with both. Phototherapy is used by exposing the jaundiced newborn to either natural sunlight or fluorescent light (blue light). The exposure is continuous; the infant is turned frequently for maximal exposure to the light. Use of phototherapy has decreased the need for exchange transfusion in infants with hemolytic disease of the newborn. SEE: *exchange transfusion; hemolytic disease of the newborn; icterus neonatorum; kernicterus; photomedicine; psoriasis.*

Caution: The infant's eyes must be protected from the light, but the pressure from the eye bandage should not be so tight as to prevent opening of the eyes under the bandage. Also, shield the infant from bulb breakage and monitor temperature. The dose of light must be known and kept within the limits prescribed.

---

photothermal (fō″tō-thĕr′măl) [″ + *therme*, heat]. Concerning heat produced by light.

photothermal radiation. Radiation of heat by a source of light, as that from an electric bulb.

phototimer. Device that automatically terminates a radiographic exposure after a preset amount of radiation has reached it.

phototonus (fō-tŏt′ō-nŭs) [″ + *tonos*, tension]. Sensitivity in an organism produced by exposure to light.

phototopia (fō″tō-tō′pē-ă). A subjective sensation of light.

phototoxic (fō″tō-tŏk′sĭk) [″ + *toxikon*, poison]. Pert. to the harmful reaction produced by light energy, esp. that produced in the skin. Simple sunburn of the skin is an example of phototoxicity.

phototoxis (fō″tō-tŏk′sĭs). Disorder produced by effects of overexposure to light or radiation.

phototrophic (fō″tō-trŏf′ĭk) [″ + *trophe*, nutrition]. Concerning the ability to use light in metabolism.

phototropism (fō-tŏt′rō-pĭzm) [″ + *tropos*, turning, + *-ismos*, condition]. A tendency exhibited by green plants and some microorganisms to turn toward or grow toward light.

photuria (fō-tū′rē-ă) [″ + *ouron*, urine]. Excretion of phosphorescent urine.

phren (frĕn, frēn) [Gr.]. 1. The mind. 2. The diaphragm.

phrenalgia (frĕ-năl′jē-ă). 1. [Gr. *phren*, mind, + *algos*, pain] Pain of hysterical origin. 2. [Gr. *phren*, diaphragm, + *algos*, pain] Pain in the diaphragm.

phrenectomy (frĕ-nĕk′tō-mē) [Gr. *phren*, diaphragm, + *ektome*, excision]. 1. Surgical excision of all or part of the diaphragm. 2. Surgical resection of part of the phrenic nerve.

phrenemphraxis (frĕn″ĕm-frăk′sĭs) [″ + *emphraxis*, stoppage]. Crushing of the phrenic nerve in order to induce temporary paralysis of the diaphragm; a therapeutic measure that was previously employed in treatment of pulmonary tuberculosis.

phrenetic (frĕn-ĕt′ĭk) [Gr. *phren*, mind]. 1. Maniacal; frenzied. 2. A maniac.

-phrenia. Combining form indicating mental disorder.

phrenic (frĕn′ĭk). 1. [Gr. *phren*, diaphragm] Concerning the diaphragm, as the phrenic nerve. 2. [Gr. *phren*, mind] Concerning the mind.

phrenic avulsion. Elevation of a side of the diaphragm and semi-collapse of the corresponding lung by means of excision of part of the phrenic nerve.

phrenicectomy (frĕn-ĭ-sĕk′tō-mē) [Gr. *phren*, diaphragm, + *ektome*, excision]. Resection of a part of the phrenic nerve. Used to collapse the lung on one side by paralyzing the diaphragm.

phreniclasia (frĕn″ĭ-klā′zē-ă) [″ + *klasis*, destruction]. Phrenemphraxis, q.v.

phrenic nerve. Nerve arising in the cervical plexus, entering the thorax, and passing to the diaphragm. A motor nerve to the diaphragm with sensory fibers to the pericardium.

phrenicoexeresis (frĕn″ĭ-kō-ĕk-sĕr′ĕ-sĭs) [″

+ *exairesis*, taking out]. Excision of part of the phrenic nerve.

phreniconeurectomy (frĕn″ĭ-kō-nū-rĕk′tō-mē) [" + *neuron*, nerve, + *ektome*, excision]. Excision of part of the phrenic nerve.

phrenicotomy (frĕn″ĭ-kŏt′ō-mē) [" + *tome*, incision]. Cutting of the phrenic nerve to produce immobilization of a lung by inducing paralysis of one side. This causes the diaphragm to rise; it compresses the lung and diminishes respiratory movement, thus resting the lung on that side.

phrenicotripsy (frĕn″ĭ-kō-trĭp′sē) [" + *tripsis*, a crushing]. Crushing of the phrenic nerve.

phrenitis (frē-nī′tĭs) [Gr. *phren*, mind, + *itis*, inflammation]. 1. Acute delirium or frenzy. 2. Inflammation of the brain. SYN: *encephalitis*. 3. [Gr. *phren*, diaphragm, + *itis*, inflammation] Inflammation of the diaphragm.

phreno- [Gr. *phren*, mind; L. *phrenicus*, diaphragm]. Combining form meaning mind or diaphragm.

phrenocolic (frĕn″ō-kŏl′ĭk) [Gr. *phren*, diaphragm, + *kolon*, colon]. Concerning the diaphragm and colon.

phrenocolopexy (frĕn″ō-kō′lō-pĕk″sē) [" + *kolon*, colon, + *pexis*, fixation]. Suture of the transverse colon to the diaphragm.

phrenodynia (frĕn″ō-dĭn′ē-ă) [" + *odyne*, pain]. Pain in the diaphragm.

phrenogastric (frĕn″ō-găs′trĭk) [" + *gaster*, belly]. Concerning the diaphragm and stomach.

phrenoglottic (frĕn″ō-glŏt′ĭk) [" + *glottis*, back of tongue]. Concerning the diaphragm and glottis.

phrenograph (frĕn′ō-grăf) [" + *graphein*, to write]. Device for registering movements of the diaphragm.

phrenohepatic (frĕn″ō-hĕ-păt′ĭk) [" + *hepar*, liver]. Concerning the diaphragm and liver.

phrenologist (frĕ-nŏl′ō-jĭst) [Gr. *phren*, mind, + *logos*, word, reason]. A person who claims to use the shape of the head to diagnose and predict mental capabilities. There is no evidence that such efforts have been scientifically validated.

phrenology (frĕ-nŏl′ō-jē) [" + *logos*, study]. The imagined ability to predict mental capabilities and personality traits by studying the shape of the head.

phrenopericarditis (frē″nō-pĕr″ĭ-kăr-dī′tĭs) [Gr. *phren*, diaphragm, + *peri*, around, + *kardia*, heart, + *itis*, inflammation]. Attachment of the heart by adhesions to the diaphragm.

phrenoplegia (frĕn-ō-plē′jē-ă) 1. [Gr. *phren*,

mind, + *plege*, stroke]. A sudden attack of mental illness. 2. [Gr. *phren*, diaphragm, + Gr. *plege*, stroke] Paralysis of the diaphragm.

phrenoptosis (frĕn″ŏp-tō′sĭs) [Gr. *phren*, diaphragm, + *ptosis*, a dropping]. Downward displacement of the diaphragm.

phrenosin (frĕn′ō-sĭn). A cerebroside isolated from brain tissue.

phrenospasm (frĕn′ō-spăzm) [" + *spasmos*, a convulsion]. Spasm of the diaphragm.

phrenosplenic (frĕn″ō-splĕn′ĭk) [" + *splen*, spleen]. Concerning the diaphragm and spleen.

phrenotropic (frĕn″ō-trŏp′ĭk) [Gr. *phren*, mind, + *tropikos*, turning]. Affecting the brain.

phrictopathic (frĭk-tō-păth′ĭk) [Gr. *phriktos*, shuddering, + *pathos*, disease, suffering]. Pert. to or having a shuddering sensation.

phrynoderma (frĭn-ō-dĕr′mă) [Gr. *phryne*, toad, + *derma*, skin]. A form of follicular keratosis of unknown etiology but thought to be related to one of several vitamin deficiencies.

phthiriasis (thĭr-ī′ă-sĭs) [Gr. *phtheiriasis*]. Condition of being infested with lice. SYN: *pediculosis*.

phthiriophobia (thĭr″ē-ō-fō′bē-ă) [Gr. *phtheir*, louse, + *phobos*, fear]. Abnormal dread of lice. SYN: *pediculophobia*.

Phthirus (thĭr′ŭs) [Gr. *phtheir*, louse]. A genus of sucking lice belonging to the order Anoplura.

    P. pubis. The crab louse. Infests primarily the pubic region but is also found in armpits, beard, eyebrows, and eyelashes. SEE: *pediculosis pubis*.

phyco- [Gr. *phykos*, seaweed]. Combining form concerning seaweed.

phycobilin (fī″kō-bĭl′ĭn). A chemical that acts as a light absorber in algae.

phycochrome (fī′kō-krōm) [Gr. *phykos*, seaweed, + *chroma*, color]. A blue-green pigment present in algae.

phycocyanin (fī″kō-sī′ăn-ĭn). A blue pigment present in blue-green algae.

phycoerythrin (fī″kō-ĕr′ĭ-thrĭn). A red pigment present in the chloroplasts of some red algae.

phycology (fī-kŏl′ō-jē) [Gr. *phykos*, seaweed, + *logos*, word, reason]. Study of algae.

Phycomycetes (fī″kō-mī-sē′tēz) [" + *mykes*, fungus]. A class of fungi, several genera which consist of organisms that occasionally cause disease in humans.

phycomycosis (fī″kō-mī-kō′sĭs) [" + " + *osis*, condition]. A disease caused by the Phycomycetes fungi. Those of the genus *Rhizopus* are the most common cause of disease in humans, but fungi of the genera *Ab-*

sidia, Mortierella, and *Basidiobolus* may also cause infection.

Infection is contracted through inhalation of the spores, but may also enter the body through breaks in the skin or mucous membranes. Patients with poorly controlled diabetes can contract severe infection of the central nervous system from fungi of the group Phycomycetes. Visceral infections can occur secondary to severe malnutrition, uremia, or liver failure, or in patients on corticosteroid or broad-spectrum antibiotic therapy. Infection spreads to adjacent areas by direct contact.

TREAT: Therapy for the primary condition and administration of amphotericin B.

phylactic (fĭ-lăk′tĭk) [Gr. *phylaktikos,* preservative]. Concerning or producing phylaxis.

phylaxis (fĭ-lăk′sĭs) [Gr., protection]. The active defense of the body against infection.

phyletic (fĭ-lĕt′ĭk) [Gr. *phyletikos*]. Pert. to a phylum or race. SYN: *phylogenetic.*

phyllo- [Gr. *phyllon,* leaf]. Combining form meaning leaf.

phylloquinone (fĭl′ō-kwĭn′ōn). Phytonadione, q.v.

phylogenesis (fī″lō-jĕn′ĕ-sĭs) [Gr. *phyle,* tribe, + *genesis,* generation, birth]. The evolutionary development of a group, race, or species. SEE: *phylogeny.*

phylogenetic (fī″lō-jĕ-nĕt′ĭk). Concerning the development of a race or group.

phylogeny (fī-lŏj′ĕ-nē). Development and growth of a race or group of animals. SEE: *ontogeny.*

phylum (fī′lŭm) [Gr. *phylon,* tribe] (pl. *phyla*). One of the primary divisions of the animal or plant kingdom, one division higher than a class.

physaliform, physalliform (fĭ-săl′ĭ-form) [Gr. *physallis,* bubble, + L. *forma,* shape]. Resembling a bleb or bubble.

physaliphore (fĭ-săl′ĭ-for) [″ + *phorein,* to carry]. Physaliphorous cell.

physaliphorous (fĭs″ă-lĭf′ō-rŭs). Pert. to a highly vacuolated cell present in a chordoma.

physalis (fĭs′ă-lĭs) [Gr. *physallis,* bubble]. A large vacuole present in the cell of certain malignancies such as a chondroma.

Physaloptera (fĭs″ă-lŏp′tĕr-ă) [″ + *pteron,* wing]. A genus of nematode worms belonging to the suborder Spiruata.

P. caucasica. Species that occurs in and damages the upper gastrointestinal tract.

physiatrics (fĭz″ē-ăt′rĭks) [Gr. *physis,* nature, + *iatrikos,* treatment]. The curing of disease by natural methods, esp. physical therapy.

physiatrist (fĭz″ē-ăt′rĭst). A physician who specializes in physical medicine.

physic (fĭz′ĭk) [Gr. *physikos,* natural]. 1. The

art of medicine and healing. 2. A medicine, esp. a cathartic.

physical (fĭz′ĭ-kăl). 1. Of or pert. to nature or material things. 2. Concerning or pert. to the body; bodily.

physical activity and exercise. A general term for any sort of muscular effort but esp. the kinds intended to train, condition, or increase flexibility of the muscular and skeletal systems of the body.

physical examination. Examination of the body by auscultation, palpation, percussion, inspection, and smelling.

physical fitness. The ability to carry out daily tasks with vigor and alertness, without undue fatigue, and with ample energy to enjoy leisure-time pursuits and meet unforeseen emergencies. It is the ability to withstand stress and persevere under difficult circumstances where an unfit person would quit. Implied in this is more than lack of illness; it is a positive quality that everyone has to some degree. Physical fitness is minimal in the severely ill and maximal in the highly trained athlete.

physical sign. An abnormal finding observed during physical examination of a patient.

physical therapist. An individual who has successfully completed an accredited physical therapy education program and has passed a licensing examination, and who is then legally responsible for evaluating, planning, conducting, and supervising a physical therapy program.

physical therapy. Rehabilitation concerned with restoration of function and prevention of disability following disease, injury, or loss of body part. The therapeutic properties of exercise, heat, cold, electricity, ultraviolet radiation, and massage are used to improve circulation, strengthen muscles, encourage return of motion, and train or retrain an individual to perform the activities of daily living.

physical therapy assistant. A technical health care worker trained to use and apply physical therapy procedures such as exercise and physical agents under the supervision of a physical therapist.

physical therapy diagnosis. Physical therapists are in need of making decisions of appropriate treatment for patients requiring rehabilitation and education. As the physical therapy profession evolves and develops, physical therapy diagnoses are becoming accepted in accordance with specialized training and experience. Frequently, functional definitions of problems can be used as diagnostic statements for specific physical therapy intervention. This is not meant to replace or supersede medical or pathologic diagnosis.

physician (fĭ-zĭsh′ŭn) [O. Fr. *physicien*]. A person who has successfully completed the prescribed course of studies in medicine in a medical school officially recognized by the country in which it is located, and who has acquired the requisite qualifications for licensure in the practice of medicine.

   p., attending. Physician who is on the staff of a hospital and regularly cares for patients therein.

   p., family. SEE: *p., primary care.*

   p., primary care. Physician to whom a family or individual goes initially when ill or for a periodic health check. This physician assumes medical coordination of care with other physicians for the patient with multiple health concerns.

   p., resident. Physician who works full or part time in a hospital to continue training after internship. Commonly called resident.

physician accountability. SEE: *accountability.*

physician's assistant. ABBR: P.A. A specially trained and (when necessary) licensed individual who performs tasks usually done by physicians and works under the direction of a supervising physician. Physician's assistants are usually salaried rather than reimbursed on a fee-for-service basis, although the supervising physician may receive fees based on his or her services.

Physicians' Desk Reference. ABBR: PDR. An annual compendium of information concerning drugs, primarily prescription and diagnostic products. The information is largely that included by the manufacturer in the labeling or package insert as required by the Food and Drug Administration: indications for use, effects, dosages, administration, warnings, hazards, contraindications, drug interactions, side effects, and precautions.

physician shortage area. An area with an inadequate supply of physicians, usually with a physician-to-population ratio of less than 1:4000.

physicist (fĭz′ĭ-sĭst) [L. *physics*, natural sciences]. A specialist in the science of physics.

physico- [Gr. *physikos*]. Combining form indicating physical or natural.

physicochemical (fĭz″ĭ-kō-kĕm′ĭ-kăl) [″ + *chemeia*, chemistry]. Concerning the application of the laws of physics to chemical reactions.

physics (fĭz′ĭks) [Gr. *physis*, nature]. The study of the laws of matter and their interactions with energy. Included are the fields of acoustics, optics, mechanics, electricity, and thermodynamics, and the study of ionizing radiation.

physio- [Gr. *physis*]. Combining form indicat-

ing relationship to nature.

physiochemical (fĭz″ē-ō-kĕm′ĭ-kăl) [Gr. *physis*, nature, + *chemeia*, chemistry]. Concerning clinical chemistry.

physiocogenic (fĭz″ē-ō-kō-jĕn′ĭk) [″ + *gennan*, to produce]. Originating from physical causes.

physiocopyrexia (fĭz″ē-ō-kō″pī-rĕk′sē-ă) [″ + *pyressein*, feverish]. Fever produced artificially by physical means.

physiognomy (fĭz″ē-ŏg′nō-mē) [Gr. *physis*, nature, + *gnomon*, a judge]. 1. The countenance. 2. Assumed ability to judge the mental or moral character and qualities by the face.

physiognosis (fĭz″ē-ŏg-nō′sĭs) [″ + *gnosis*, knowledge]. Diagnosis determined from one's facial expression and appearance of the eyes.

physiological (fĭz″ē-ō-lŏj′ĭ-kăl) [Gr. *physis*, nature, + *logos*, word, reason]. Concerning body function.

physiological salt solution. ABBR: P.S.S. A sterile solution consisting of 0.85% sodium chloride in distilled water. It is isotonic to body fluids. A teaspoonful of table salt in a pint of water approximates a physiological salt solution. Used in irrigating mucous membranes and raw surfaces, in replenishing body water in dehydration, and in restoring circulating blood volume during shock or hemorrhage. SEE: *saline solution.*

physiological tooth movement. SEE: *tooth movement.*

physiologic movement. Movements that are normally executed by muscles that are under voluntary control such as flexion, extension, abduction, adduction, and rotation. Also known as physiologic motion. SEE: *accessory motion.*

physiologicoanatomical (fĭz″ē-ō-lŏj″ĭ-kō-ăn″ă-tŏm′ĭ-kăl) [″ + ″ + *anatome*, dissection]. Concerning physiology and anatomy.

physiologist (fĭz″ē-ŏl′ō-jĭst). A person trained in and capable in the field of physiology.

physiology (fĭz″ē-ŏl′ō-jē) [Gr. *physis*, nature, + *logos*, study]. The science of the functions of the living organism and its components and of the chemical and physical processes involved.

   p., cell. The physiology of cells.

   p., comparative. Study and comparison of the physiology of different species.

   p., general. The broad scientific basis of physiology.

   p., pathologic. The physiological explanation of pathological events.

   p., special. Physiology of special organs or systems.

physiomedical (fĭz″ē-ō-mĕd′ĭ-kăl) [″ + L.

medicina, medicine]. Practice of medicine utilizing only bland plant-derived medicines.

physiopathologic (fĭz″ē-ō-păth″ō-lŏj′ĭk) [″ + *pathos,* disease, suffering, + *logos,* word, reason]. 1. Concerning physiology and pathology. 2. Pertaining to a pathological alteration in a normal function.

physiotherapy (fĭz″ē-ō-thĕr′ă-pē) [″ + *therapeia,* treatment]. Treatment by physical and mechanical means, as massage or electricity. SYN: *physical therapy.*

physique (fĭ-zēk′) [Fr.]. Body build; the structure and organization of the body.

physo- [Gr. *physa,* air]. Combining form indicating air or gas.

physocele (fī′sō-sēl) [Gr. *physa,* air, + *kele,* tumor, swelling]. 1. A tumor filled with gas or circumscribed swelling due to gas. 2. A gas-distended hernial sac.

physometra (fī″sō-mē′tră) [″ + *metra,* uterus]. Air or gas in the uterine cavity.

physopyosalpinx (fī″sō-pī″ō-săl′pĭnks) [″ + *pyon,* pus, + *salpinx,* tube]. Pus and gas in the fallopian tube.

physostigmine salicylate (fī″sō-stĭg′mĕn săl-ĭs′ĭl-āt). USP. The salicylate of an alkaloid usually obtained from the dried ripe seed of *Physostigma venenosum.* Trade names are Antilirium and Isopto Eserine.

ACTION/USES: Cholinergic. It inactivates cholinesterase, thus prolonging and intensifying the action of acetylcholine. It improves the tone and action of skeletal muscle; it increases intestinal peristalsis through its effects on the parasympathetic nervous system; and it acts as a miotic in the eye. It is used in tetanus and strychnine poisoning and in the treatment of myasthenia gravis.

phytalbumose (fī-tăl′bū-mōs) [Gr. *phyton,* plant, + L. *albumen,* white of egg]. An albumose found in plants and vegetables.

phytase (fī′tās) [″ + *ase,* enzyme]. An enzyme found in grains and present in the kidneys; important in splitting phytin or phytic acid into inositol and phosphoric acid.

phytin (fī′tĭn). A calcium or magnesium salt of inositol and hexaphosphoric acid, present in cereals. SEE: *inositol.*

phyto-, phyt- [Gr. *phyton*]. Combining forms indicating a plant or that which grows.

phytoagglutinin (fī″tō-ă-gloo′tĭ-nĭn) [Gr. *phyton,* plant, + L. *agglutinans,* gluing]. A lectin that agglutinates red blood cells and leukocytes.

phytoalexins. Substances produced by plants. These counteract plant infections.

phytobezoar (fī″tō-bē′zor) [″ + Arabic *bazahr,* protecting against poison]. A mass composed of vegetable matter found in the stomach. SYN: *food ball.* SEE: *bezoar.*

phytochemistry (fī″tō-kĕm′ĭs-trē) [″ + *chemeia,* chemistry]. Study of plant chemistry.

phytocholesterol (fī″tō-kō-lĕs′tĕr-ŏl) [″ + *chole,* bile, + *stereos,* solid]. Phytosterol, q.v.

phytogenesis (fī″tō-jĕn′ĕ-sĭs) [″ + *genesis,* generation, birth]. The origin and development of plants. SYN: *phytogeny.*

phytogenous (fī-tŏj′ĕ-nŭs) [″ + *gennan,* to produce]. Arising in or caused by plants.

phytohemagglutinin (fī″tō-hĕm-ă-glū′tĭ-nĭn) [″ + *haima,* blood, + L. *agglutinare,* to glue to]. ABBR: PHA. A substance derived from red kidney beans that agglutinates red blood cells and is a mitogen, q.v., that stimulates T lymphocytes.

phytoid (fī′toyd) [″ + *eidos,* form, shape]. 1. Plantlike. 2. Any disease of vegetable parasitic origin. 3. The production of a disease by plant parasites. 4. The presence of plant parasites in an organism.

phytomenadione (fī″tō-mĕn″ă-dī′ōn). Phytonadione, q.v.

phytonadione (fī″tō-nă-dī′ōn). 1. USP. Synthetic vitamin K₁. Used as a prothrombogenic agent. 2. USP. An anticoagulant drug that is little used because of its toxicity. Trade names are Aquamephyton, Konakion, and Mephyton.

phytoparasite (fī″tō-păr′ă-sīt) [Gr. *phyton,* plant, + *parasitos,* fellow guest]. A vegetable parasite.

phytopathogenic (fī″tō-păth″ō-jĕn′ĭk) [″ + *pathos,* disease, suffering + *gennan,* to produce]. Causing disease in plants.

phytopathology (fī″tō-pă-thŏl′ō-jē) [″ + ″ *logos,* word, reason]. Study of plant diseases.

phytophagous (fī-tŏf′ă-gŭs) [″ + *phagein,* to eat]. 1. Plant-eating. 2. Vegetarian.

phytopharmacology (fī″tō-făr″mă-kŏl′ō-jē) [″ + *pharmakon,* drug, + *logos,* word, reason]. The study of the effects of drugs and chemicals on plants.

phytophotodermatitis (fī″tō-fō″tō-dĕr″mă-tī′tĭs) [″ + *photos,* light, + *derma,* skin, + *itis,* inflammation]. A dermatitis produced by exposure to certain plants and then sunlight.

phytoplankton (fī″tō-plănk′tŏn) [″ + *planktos,* wandering]. Plankton that are classed as vegetable life rather than animal.

phytoplasm (fī′tō-plăzm) [″ + LL. *plasma,* form, mold]. Vegetable protoplasm.

phytoprecipitin (fī″tō-prē-sĭp′ĭ-tĭn). A precipitin produced by immunization with a plant protein.

phytosis (fī-tō′sĭs) [″ + *osis,* condition]. 1. A disease caused by a vegetable parasite. 2. Presence of vegetable parasites.

phytosterol (fī″tō-stē′rŏl). Any sterol present in vegetable oil or fat.

phytotoxic (fī″tō-tŏk′sĭk). 1. Concerning a substance poisonous to plants. 2. Concerning a phytotoxin.

phytotoxin (fī″tō-tŏk′sĭn) [Gr. *phyton*, plant, + *toxikon*, a poison]. A toxin produced by or derived from a plant. SEE: *ricin.*

pl. The pH of the isoelectric point of a substance in solution.

pia (pē′ă) [L.]. Tender, soft.

pia-arachnitis (pē″ă-ăr″ăk-nī′tĭs). Piarachnitis.

pia-arachnoid. Piarachnoid.

Piaget, Jean. Swiss philosopher and psychologist, 1896–1980, whose work provided understanding of how children's thinking differs from adults' and of how children learn. Concerning education, he explained, "The goal of education is not to increase the amount of knowledge but to create the possibilities for a child to invent and discover, to create men who are capable of doing new things."

pial (pī′ăl). Concerning the pia mater.

pia mater (pē′ă mă′tĕr) [L. *pia*, soft, + *mater*, mother]. A thin vascular membrane closely investing the brain and spinal cord and proximal portions of the nerves. Innermost of the three meninges. The other portions of the covering are dura mater and the arachnoid. SEE: *meninges.*

pian (pē-ăn′) [Fr.]. Contagious skin disease of the tropics. SYN: *yaws.*

pianists' cramp. Spasm, or occupational neurosis, of muscles of fingers and forearms from piano playing.

piarachnitis (pī″ăr-ăk-nī′tĭs) [L. *pia*, tender, + Gr. *arachne*, spider, + *itis*, inflammation]. Inflammation of the arachnoid and pia mater. SYN: *leptomeningitis.*

piarachnoid (pī″ăr-ăk′noyd) [″ + ″ + *eidos*, form, shape]. The pia mater and arachnoid membranes when regarded as one structure. SYN: *leptomeninges.*

piblokto, pibloktog [Inuit]. A syndrome, apparently culturally specific for Eskimo women, in which the individual screams, removes or tears off her clothes, and runs naked in the snow. She has no memory of these events.

pica (pī′kă) [L., magpie]. An eating disorder manifested by a craving to ingest any material not fit for food, including starch, clay, ashes, toy balloons, crayons, cotton, grass, cigarette butts, soap, twigs, wood, paper, metal, or plaster. Condition seen in pregnancy, chlorosis, hysteria, helminthiasis, and certain psychoses. This condition may also be associated with iron deficiency anemia.

    The importance of this condition, the etiology of which is unknown, stems from the toxicity of ingested material (e.g., paint that contains lead) or from ingesting materials in place of essential nutrients.

    The inclusion of compulsive ingestion of non-food and food items such as licorice, croutons, chewing gum, coffee grounds, or oyster shells as examples of pica is controversial. SEE: *appetite; geophagia; taste.*

piceous (pī′sē-ŭs) [L. *piceus*, pitch]. Like pitch.

pick. 1. A sharp, pointed, curved dental instrument used to explore tooth surfaces and restorations for defects. 2. To remove bits of food from teeth.

Pick, Arnold. Czechoslovakian physician, 1851–1924.

    P.'s disease. A form of presenile dementia due to atrophy of the frontal and temporal lobes. Usually occurs between the ages of 40 and 60, more often in women than men. Involves progressive, irreversible loss of memory, deterioration of intellectual functions, disordered emotions, apathy, speech disturbances, and disorientation. Course may take from a few months to 4 or 5 years to progress to complete loss of intellectual function. SEE: *Alzheimer's disease.*

Pick, Friedel. Czechoslovakian physician, 1867–1926.

    P.'s disease. Nonrheumatic chronic pericarditis of unknown etiology.

Pick, Ludwig. German physician, 1868–1944.

    P.'s cells. A foamy, lipid-filled cell present in the spleen and bone marrow in Niemann-Pick disease. SYN: *cell, Niemann-Pick.*

    P.'s disease. Niemann-Pick disease, q.v.

pickling. 1. A method of preserving and flavoring food in which the food is soaked in a solution of salt and vinegar. 2. Use of a chemical solution to remove scales and oxides from metals after casting or prior to plating them.

pickwickian syndrome [Inspired by Joe, an obese character in Pickwick Papers by Charles Dickens]. Obesity, decreased pulmonary function, and polycythemia.

pico- [It. *pico*, small]. Combining form used to indicate a unit of measurement that is one trillionth of the basic unit. This is 10^{-12} of the basic unit. Thus a picogram is:

$$\frac{1}{10^{12}} \text{ or } 0.000000000001 \text{ gram}$$

picogram. ABBR: pg. 1×10^{-12} gram or one trillionth of a gram.

picornaviruses (pī-kor″nă-vī′rŭ-sĕs) [″ + *RNA*, ribonucleic acid, + L. *virus*, virus]. Very small viruses that are insoluble in a lipid solvent such as ether. Those that affect humans have been classified into two species: enteroviruses, which include the polio, coxsackie, and ECHO viruses; and rhinoviruses.

picrate (pĭk′rāt). A salt of picric acid.

picric acid. SEE: *acid, picric.*

picro-, picr- [Gr. *pikros*, bitter]. Combining forms meaning bitter.

picrocarmine (pĭk″rō-kăr′mĭn). A stain used in microscopy.

picroformal (pĭk″rō-for′măl). Solution of picric acid, formaldehyde, and water, used as a fixing agent.

picrotoxin (pĭk″rō-tŏk′sĭn) [″ + *toxikon*, poison]. A stimulant to the central nervous system, obtained from the seed of *Anamirta cocculus*, a shrub. It is no longer used as a stimulant.

pictograph (pĭk′tō-grăf). A set of test pictures used for testing vision in children and illiterate adults.

PID. *pelvic inflammatory disease*, q.v.

piebald skin (pī′băld) [ME. *pie*, magpie, + *ballede*, bald]. Skin with spots of pigmentation, or patches with loss of pigment. SEE: *leukoderma; vitiligo.*

piedra (pē-ā′drä) [Sp., stone]. A fungus disease that affects only the hair and in which hard nodules form on the hair shafts. Black piedra is caused by the fungus *Piedraia hortae* and white piedra by *Trichosporon beigelii.* Either form of the disease is cured by shaving the hair. SYN: *tinea nodosa.*

Pierre Robin syndrome [Pierre Robin, French physician, 1867–1950]. Unusual smallness of the jaw combined with cleft palate, downward displacement of the tongue, and an absent gag reflex.

piesesthesia (pī-ē″zĕs-thē′zē-ă) [Gr. *piesis*, pressure, + *aisthesis*, sensation]. Sensitivity to pressure.

piesimeter, piesometer (pī″ē-sĭm′ĕ-tĕr, -sŏm′ĕ-tĕr) [″ + *metron*, measure]. Device for measurement of skin's sensitiveness to pressure.

-piesis. Combining form used at the end of a word to indicate pressure.

piezochemistry (pī-ē′zō-kĕm″ĭs-trē) [Gr. *piezein*, to squeeze, + *chemeia*, chemistry]. The study of the effect of high pressure on chemical reactions.

piezoelectricity [″ + *elektron*, amber]. Production of an electric current by application of pressure to certain crystals such as mica, quartz, or Rochelle salt. SEE: *triboluminescence.*

piezogenic pedal papules (pī-ē′zō-jĕn″ĭk) [″ + *gennan*, to produce]. Soft painful skin-colored papules present on the non-weight-bearing portion of the heel. They disappear when weight is taken off the foot and heel. Caused by herniation of fat through connective tissue defects.

piezometer (pī″ē-zŏm′ĕ-tĕr) [″ + *metron*, measure]. Piesimeter, q.v.

PIF. *proliferation inhibiting factor.* SEE: *factor, proliferation inhibiting.*

pigeon breast. Deformity in which the sternum projects anteriorly. Caused by rickets or obstructed respiration in childhood. SYN: *chicken breast.*

pigeon-breeder's disease. Attacks of chills, fever, and cough with shortness of breath in persons who are closely associated with birds such as pigeons and parakeets. In some patients the onset is slow rather than acute. The symptoms are due to antigenic substances in the bird's excreta. Symptoms usually subside when exposure to the birds ceases.

pigeon-toed. Walking with feet turned inward.

pigment (pĭg′mĕnt) [L. *pigmentum*, paint]. Any organic coloring matter in the body. SEE: *albino;* words beginning with *chrom-.*

    p.'s, bile. Complex, highly colored substances found in bile derived from the red pigment (hemoglobin) of the blood and imparting brown color to intestinal contents and feces. Included are bilirubin, biliverdin and their derivatives (urobilinogen, urobilin, bilicyanin, and bilifuscin).

    p., blood. Pigment in blood (hemoglobin) or a derivative of it (hematin, hemin, methemoglobin, hemosiderin).

    p., endogenous. Pigment produced within the body, as melanin.

    p., exogenous. Pigment produced outside the human body.

    p., hematogenous. Pigment from hemoglobin of the erythrocytes.

    p., hepatogenous. Pigment from hemoglobin destruction in the liver. SYN: *bile pigment.*

    p., respiratory. Any pigment such as hemoglobin, myoglobin, or cytochrome that has a part in oxidative processes of the body.

    p., skin. Melanin, melanoid, and carotene.

    p., urinary. Urochrome and sometimes urobilin.

    p., uveal. Pigment found in cells on the inner or posterior surface of the iris, choroid, and ciliary processes.

pigmentary (pĭg′mĕn-tĕr″ē) [L. *pigmentum*, paint]. Concerning, or like, a pigment.

pigmentation (pĭg″mĕn-tā′shŭn). Coloration due to deposition of pigments. SEE: *albinism; carotenemia;* words beginning with *chrom.*

    p., hematogenous. Pigmentation produced by the collection of hemoglobin, or pigment carried to a site through the blood.

pigmented (pĭg'mĕnt-ĕd). Colored by a pigment.

pigmentolysin (pĭg″mĕn-tŏl'ĭ-sĭn) [″ + Gr. *lysis*, dissolution]. A substance that destroys a pigment.

pigmentophage (pĭg-mĕn'tō-fāj) [″ + Gr. *phagein*, to eat]. Any cell that ingests a pigment.

pigmentophore (pĭg-mĕn'tō-for) [″ + Gr. *phorein*, to carry]. A cell that carries pigment.

pigmentum nigrum (pĭg-mĕn'tŭm nī'grŭm) [L., black paint]. The black pigment of the lamina vitrea or the choroid of the eye.

piitis (pī-ī'tĭs) [L. *pia*, tender, + Gr. *itis*, inflammation]. Inflamed condition of the pia mater.

pil. L. *pilula*, pill, or *pilulae*, pills.

pila (pī'lă) [L., pillar] (pl. *pilae*). A pillarlike structure in spongy bone.

pilar, pilary (pī'lăr, pĭl'ă-rē) [L. *pilaris*]. Concerning, or covered with, hair.

pilaster (pĭ-lăs'tĕr) [L. *pilastrum*, small pillar]. A prominent ridge sometimes seen on the femur.

pile [L. *pila*, a ball, a pillar]. 1. A single hemorrhoid. SEE: *piles*. 2. The hair. 3. A battery for production of electricity. 4. An apparatus for producing and regulating a nuclear chain-reaction fission process.

   p., sentinel. A localized thickening of the mucous membrane at the distal end of an anal fissure.

pileous (pī'lē-ŭs) [L. *pilus*, hair]. Hairy; hirsute.

piles (pīls) [L. *pila*, a mass]. Dilated blood vessels in the rectal mucosa forming a vascular tumor. SYN: *hemorrhoid*.

pileum (pī'lē-ŭm) [L., a cap]. 1. A membrane or portion of the amnion sometimes covering a baby's head at birth. SYN: *caul; pileus* (def. 2). 2. Great omentum.

pileus (pī'lē-ŭs) [L., a cap]. 1. A hemisphere of the cerebellum. 2. Membrane that sometimes covers the head of an infant at birth. SYN: *caul; pileum* (def. 1).

pili (pī'lē) (sing. *pilus*). Hairs.

   In bacteria, filamentous appendages of which there may be hundreds on a single cell. One function of pili is to attach the bacterium to cells of the host; another is to propel the bacterial cell.

   p. incarnati. Condition of ingrowing hair, esp. in the beard area.

   p. tactiles. Sensitive or tactile hairs.

   p. torti. Condition in which hairs are broken and twisted.

piliation (pī-lē-ā'shŭn) [L. *pilus*, hair]. Formation and development of hair.

piliform (pī'lĭ-form) [″ + *forma*, shape]. Hairlike.

pilimiction (pī″lĭ-mĭk'shŭn) [″ + *mictio*,

micturition]. Passing of urine containing hairlike or filamentous substances.

pill (pĭl) [L. *pilula*, small mass]. 1. Medicine in the form of a tiny solid mass or pellet to be swallowed or chewed. May be coated. 2. Term used to designate a hormonal contraceptive drug that is taken orally. SYN: *"the pill."*

   p., morning-after. A pill containing an estrogen or synthetic estrogen that can be taken after intercourse to prevent pregnancy.

pillar (pĭl'ĕr) [L. *pila*, a column]. An upright support, column, or structure resembling a column.

   p.'s, anterior, of fornix. Two diverging columns extending downward from anterior extremity of body of the fornix of cerebrum.

   p.'s of Corti. Two layers resting on membrana basilaris in the ear. SYN: *rods of Corti.*

   p.'s of diaphragm. Crura of diaphragm, two bundles of muscle fibers extending from lumbar vertebrae to the central tendon and forming sides of hiatus aorticus.

   p.'s of fauces. Folds of mucous membrane, one on each side of the fauces, q.v., and between which is situated the tonsil. SYN: *arches, glossopalatine; arches, pharyngopalatine.*

pillar cells. Two groups of cells (inner and outer) resting on basement membrane of organ of Corti in which elongated bodies (pillars) develop. These enclose the inner tunnel (Corti's tunnel).

pillet (pĭl'ĕt). A small pill.

pillion (pĭl'yŭn) [L. *pellis*, skin]. Temporary form of artificial leg, esp. a peg-leg type of stump.

pilo- [L. *pilus*]. Combining form indicating hair.

pilobezoar (pī″lō-bē'zor) [″ + Arabic *bazahr*, protecting against poison]. Trichobezoar, q.v.

pilocarpine hydrochloride (pī″lō-kăr'pĭn). USP. $C_{11}H_{16}N_2O_2 \cdot HCl$. Hydrochloride of an alkaloid obtained from leaflets of *Pilocarpus jaborandi* and *P. microphyllus*. Trade names are Almocarpine and Isopto Carpine.

   ACTION/USES: Cholinergic. Causes contraction of the pupil. Used topically as a miotic, esp. in glaucoma.

pilocarpine nitrate. USP. Nitrate of the alkaloid obtained from leaves of the jaborandi tree.

   ACTION/USES: Same as pilocarpine hydrochloride.

pilocystic (pī″lō-sĭs'tĭk) [L. *pilus*, hair, + Gr. *kystis*, bladder]. Encysted and containing hair, said of a dermoid cyst.

piloerection. Hair erection or apparent stiffening due to stimulation and contraction of the arrector pili muscles. SYN: *goose flesh.*

pilojection [" + *jacere,* to throw]. Introduction of hairs, by use of a pneumatic gun, into an aneurysm to induce clotting in the aneurysmal sac. Has been used in treating intracranial aneurysms.

pilomatrixoma. Benign calcifying tumor of the skin. It is small and firm with normal skin over it.

pilomotor (pī″lō-mō′tor) [" + *motor,* mover]. Causing movements of hairs, as the arrectores pilorum, q.v.

pilomotor nerve. A nerve that stimulates an arrector pili muscle. SEE: *arrectores pilorum.*

pilomotor reflex. Goose flesh formation when skin is cooled or as a result of emotional reaction.

pilonidal (pī″lō-nī′dăl) [" + *nidus,* nest]. Containing hairs in a dermoid cyst in nest formation.

pilonidal cyst. A cyst in the sacrococcygeal region, usually at the upper end of the intergluteal cleft. The cyst is due to a developmental defect that permits epithelial tissue to be trapped below the skin. May become symptomatic in early adulthood when an infected draining sinus forms.

pilonidal fistula. Fistula beneath the skin at the lower end of the spinal column resulting from a pilonidal cyst.

pilonidal sinus. SEE: *pilonidal cyst.*

pilose (pī′lōs) [L. *pilosus*]. Hairy, downy.

pilosebaceous (pī″lō-sē-bā′shŭs) [" + *sebaceus,* fatty]. Concerning the hair and sebaceous glands.

pilosis (pī-lō′sĭs) [L. *pilosus,* hairy, + Gr. *osis,* condition]. Excessive formation of hair.

pilosity (pī-lŏs′ĭ-tē). Hairiness.

pilous (pī′lŭs) [L. *pilus,* hair]. Covered with hair; hirsute.

Piltz's reflex (pilts′ēz) [Jan Piltz, Polish neurologist, 1870–1931]. Change in size of pupil on sudden fixation of attention. SYN: *pupillary reflex.*

pilula (pĭl′ū-lă) [L., pill] (pl. *pilulae*). A small amount of medicine intended to be swallowed whole and to produce medicinal action.

pilular (pĭl′ū-lar). Pert. to, or of the nature of, pills.

pilule (pĭl′ūl) [L. *pilula*]. A small pill.

pilus (pī′lŭs) [L.] (pl. *pili*). [NA] A hair.

    p. **cuniculatus.** A hair that burrows into the skin.

    p. **incarnatus.** An ingrown hair.

    p. **tortus.** A twisted hair.

pimel-, pimelo [Gr. *pimele,* fat]. Combining form or prefix indicating an association with fat.

pimeloma (pĭm″ē-lō′mă) [Gr. *pimele,* fat,

+ *oma,* tumor]. A fatty tumor. SYN: *lipoma.*

pimelopterygium (pĭm″ē-lō-tĕ-rĭj′ē-ŭm) [" + *pterygion,* wing]. A fatty outgrowth of the conjunctiva.

pimelorthopnea (pĭm″ĕl-or-thŏp′nē-ă) [" + *orthos,* straight, + *pnoia,* breath]. Difficulty in breathing when lying down, resulting from obesity.

pimelosis (pĭm″ē-lō′sĭs) [" + *osis,* condition]. 1. Conversion into fat. 2. Fatty degeneration of any tissue. 3. Corpulence; obesity.

pimple (pĭm′pl) [ME. *pinple*]. A papule or pustule of the skin, sometimes going on to suppuration. Often seen in clusters on skin of the adolescent with acne. Patients should be warned not to pick at pimples because infection may result.

pin. A short, slim piece of wire, plastic, or metal. It may or may not have one end blunt and the other sharp.

    p., **endodontic.** A straight or threaded pin that is passed through the root canal to the alveolar bone beyond the apex of the tooth root.

    p., **self-threading.** A pin screwed through a small hole into dentin.

    p., **Steinmann.** A metal rod used for internal fixation of the adjacent sections of a fractured bone.

pincement (păns-mŏn′) [Fr.]. Pinching or nipping of the flesh in massage.

pinch. A type of hand prehension. The pinch of the human hand is achieved principally through holding objects between the thumb and index finger or the index and long fingers.

Hand pinch is classified according to the anatomical parts involved, as follows:

Pinch, finger tip—pinch using the tips of strongly arched digits, primarily the thumb and index finger. Used to pick up very small objects such as pins and needles.

Pinch, palmar tripod or three jaw chuck—pinch using the palmar pads of the thumb and index and long fingers.

Pinch, lateral—pinch accomplished by clamping the palmar surface of the distal portion of the thumb against the side of the index finger.

pinch meter. Device for objectively measuring the strength of hand pinch in grams or pounds.

pindolol (pĭn′dō-lōl). A β-adrenergic blocking agent.

pineal (pĭn′ē-ăl) [Fr., pine cone]. 1. Shaped like a pine cone. 2. Pert. to the pineal body.

pineal body (gland). A glandlike structure in the brain, shaped like a pine cone, and located in a pocket near the splenium of the corpus collosum. It appears to be the major site of melatonin biosynthesis in most mammals and in humans. The effect of melatonin on the human and the exact function of the pineal body remain unknown.

There is evidence that inhibition of secretion from the pineal gland is associated with the onset of puberty.

pinealectomy (pĭn″ē-ăl-ĕk′tō-mē) [L. *pineus*, of the pine, + Gr. *ektome*, excision]. Removal of the pineal body.

pineal gland. SEE: *pineal body*.

pinealism (pĭn′ē-ăl-ĭzm) [″ + Gr. -*ismos*, condition]. Disorder caused by abnormal secretion of the pineal body.

pinealoblastoma (pĭn″ē-ă-lō-blăs-tō′mă) [″ + Gr. *blastos*, germ, + *oma*, tumor]. Pineoblastoma, q.v.

pinealocyte (pĭn′ē-ă-lō-sĭt″) [″ + Gr. *kytos*, cell]. The principal cell of the pineal body. It contains pale-staining cytoplasm and has long processes that terminate in bulbous expansions.

pinealoma (pĭn″ē-ă-lō′mă) [″ + Gr. *oma*, tumor]. A tumor of the pineal body, usually encapsulated. Often associated with precocious puberty.

pinealopathy (pĭn″ē-ă-lŏp′ă-thē) [″ + Gr. *pathos*, disease, suffering]. Any disorder of the pineal gland.

Pinel, Philippe (pē-nĕl′). French psychologist, 1745–1826, who developed a method or system of treating the mentally ill without the use of restraint, at a time when use of restraint was the accepted form of therapy.

pineoblastoma (pĭn″ē-ō-blăs-tō′mă) [L. *pineus*, of the pine, + Gr. *blastos*, germ, + *oma*, tumor]. A blastoma of the pineal body.

pine tar. USP. A product obtained from the distillation of pine wood. Used as an expectorant and in certain skin preparations.

ping-ponging. The transmission of an infectious disease, esp. a sexually transmitted one, between two people. After the first person has been cured, the second person reinfects the first.

pinguecula (pĭn-gwĕk′ū-lă) [L. *pinguiculus*, fatty]. Yellow thickening of bulbar conjunctiva, triangular in shape, on inner and outer margins of the cornea. The base of the triangle is toward the limbus. Yellow color is due to increase in elastic fibers.

pinhole (pĭn′hōl) [AS. *pinn*, pin, + *hol*, hole]. Small perforation made by, or size of that made by, a pin.

pinhole os. A very small opening to the uterus from the vagina. It may be present in very young women.

pinhole pupil. Extreme contraction of the iris. The condition is seen in locomotor ataxia, after use of miotics, in some brain diseases, and in opium and morphine poisoning.

piniform (pĭn′ĭ-form) [L. *pinea*, pine cone, + *forma*, shape]. Conical; shaped like a pine cone.

pink disease. Acrodynia, q.v.

pinkeye [D. *pinck oog*]. Epidemic form of acute conjunctivitis caused by various organisms. Sporadic noninfectious cases may result from irritation by various agents such as intense light, or they may accompany exanthematous disease such as measles.

pinna (pĭn′ă) [L., feather] (pl. *pinnae*). 1. The auricle or projected part of the exterior ear. It collects and directs sound waves into the external acoustic meatus and then to the tympanic membrane. 2. A feather, fin, wing, or similar appendage.

p. nasi. Protruding cartilaginous extension on each nostril. SYN: *ala nasi* [NA].

pinnal (pĭn′ăl). Concerning pinna.

pinocyte (pī′nō-sĭt) [Gr. *pinein*, to drink, + *kytos*, cell]. A cell that exhibits pinocytosis.

pinocytosis (pī″nō-sī-tō′sĭs) [″ + ″ + *osis*, condition]. Process by which cells absorb or ingest nutrients and fluid. A hollowed-out portion of the cell membrane is filled with liquid, and the area closes to form a small sac or vacuole. The nutrient, now inside, is available for use in the cell's metabolism. SEE: illus.

pinosome (pī′nō-, pĭn′ō-sōm) [″ + *soma*, body]. The fluid-filled vacuole formed during pinocytosis, q.v.

pinprick test. A test for cutaneous pain receptors. A small, clean, sharp object such as a pin or needle is gently applied to the skin and the patient is asked to describe the sensation. Be certain the patient is reporting the sensation of pain rather than that of pressure. Usually, application of the sharp object is interspersed with application of a dull object, and the patient is asked to state whether a sharp or dull sensation was sensed. The patient is not, of course, allowed to observe the test procedure.

Caution: The sharp object should not penetrate the dermis, and in order to prevent passage of infectious material from one patient to another, the test objects should be either discarded after use or sterilized prior to their use on another patient.

PINS. *persons in need of supervision*, q.v.

Pins' sign [Emil Pins, Aust. physician, 1845–1913]. In pericarditis, the disappearance of symptoms of pleurisy when patient assumes knee-chest position.

pint (pīnt) [ME. *pinte*]. ABBR: pt. In the U.S. a measure of capacity equal to ½ qt.; 16 fl. oz; 473.2 ml. SEE: *Weights and Measures* in *Appendix*.

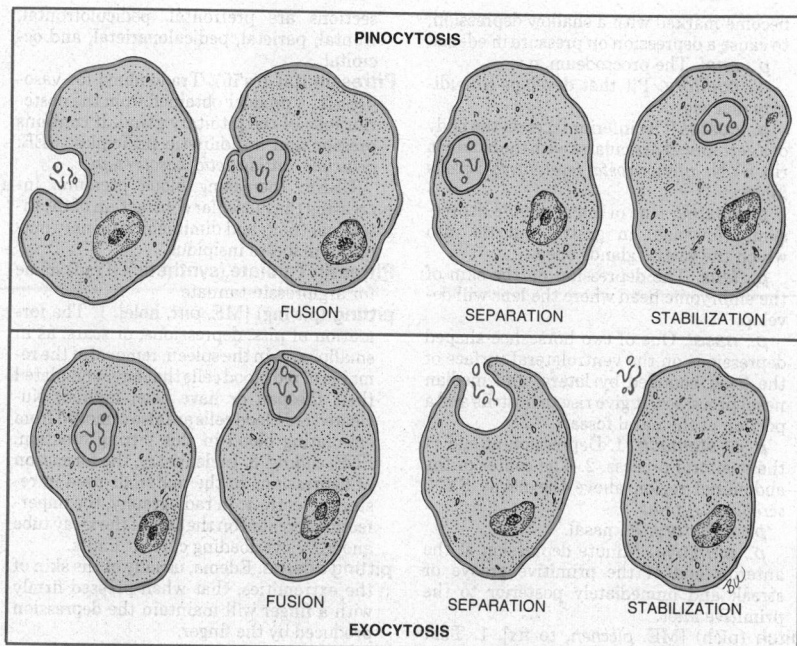

PINOCYTOSIS

FUSION | SEPARATION | STABILIZATION

FUSION | SEPARATION | STABILIZATION

EXOCYTOSIS

pinta (pēn'tă) [Sp., paint]. A nonvenereal disease caused by the spirochete *Treponema carateum.* This infection is spread by body contact. Manifested by depigmented spots or patches.
  TREAT: penicillin.
pintid (pĭn'tĭd). A flat red skin lesion present in the second stage of pinta, q.v.
pinus (pī'nŭs) [L., pine]. Pertaining to the pineal gland.
pinworm. A parasitic nematode, *Enterobius vermicularis,* q.v., causing enterobiasis, infection of intestines and rectum.
pioepithelium (pī″ō-ĕp″ĭ-thē'lē-ŭm) [Gr. *pion,* fat, + *epi,* upon, + *thele,* nipple]. Epithelium that contains fat globules.
pion therapy. Experimental use of the subatomic particle, the pion, in treating cancer.
Piper (pī'pĕr) [L.]. Genus of plants that produce pepper.
piperacetazine (pĭp″ĕr-ă-sĕt'ă-zēn). USP. An antipsychotic drug.
piperazine (pī-pĕr'ă-zēn). USP. A white crystalline powder used in the treatment of ascariasis and enterobiasis.
piperoxan (pī″pĕr-ŏks'ăn). An α-adrenergic blocking agent effective in inhibiting response to catecholamines.
pipet, pipette (pī-pĕt') [Fr. *pipette,* tiny pipe].

Narrow glass tube with both ends open for transferring and measuring liquids by sucking them into the tube.
pipobroman (pī″pō-brō'măn). USP. A cytotoxic drug that has been used in treating certain blood diseases. Trade name is Vercyte.
piptonychia (pĭp″tō-nĭk'ē-ă) [Gr. *piptein,* to fall, + *onyx,* nails]. The shedding of nails.
piriform (pĭr'ĭ-form) [L. *pirum,* pear, + *forma,* shape]. Pear-shaped. Also spelled *pyriform.*
Pirogoff's amputation (pĭr″ō-gŏfs') [Nikolai Ivanovich Pirogoff, Russ. surgeon, 1810–1881]. Foot amputation at the ankle, removing a portion of the os calcis.
Pirquet's test (pĕr-kāz') [Clemens Peter Johann von Pirquet, Austrian pediatrician, 1874–1929]. Test for tuberculosis by means of a skin reaction, used esp. in children.
piscicide (pĭs'ĭ-sīd) [L. *piscis,* fish, + *caedere,* to kill]. An agent that kills fish.
pisiform (pī'sĭ-form) [L. *pisum,* pea, + *forma,* shape]. 1. Pea-shaped. 2. The smallest carpal bone, located in the flexor carpi ulnaris tendon as a sesamoid bone, on the ulnar side in the proximal row of carpals.
pit (pĭt) [ME. *pitt,* hole]. 1. A tiny hollow or pocket. SYN: *depression; fossa.* 2. To be or

become marked with a shallow depression; to cause a depression on pressure in edema.

p., anal. The proctodeum, q.v.

p., auditory. Pit that develops in auditory placode.

p., costal. The inferior facet on the body of a vertebra. It articulates with the head of a rib. SYN: *inferior costal facet; fovea costalis inferior.*

p., gastric. One of many minute depressions (foveolae) in gastric mucosa into which the gastric glands open.

p., lens. The depression on the skin of the embryonic head where the lens will develop.

p., nasal. One of two horseshoe-shaped depressions on the ventrolateral surface of the head bounded by lateral and median nasal processes. It give rise to nostrils and a portion of the nasal fossa.

p. of stomach. 1. Depression at end of the ensiform process. 2. The center of the abdominal region above the navel. SYN: *scrobiculus cordis.*

p., olfactory. P., nasal.

p., primitive. Minute depression at the anterior end of the primitive groove or streak and immediately posterior to the primitive knot.

pitch (pĭch) [ME. *picchen*, to fix]. 1. That quality of the sensation of sound that enables one to classify it in a scale from high to low. It is dependent principally on frequency of vibrations. 2. Residue obtained from distillation of coal or wood tar.

pitchblende (pĭch′blĕnd). Uraninite, the principal source of uranium. It is a mineral that resembles pitch.

pith (pĭth). 1. The center of a hair or the soft material in the stalk of a plant. 2. Destruction of a part of the central nervous system of an animal being prepared for certain experiments. A blunt probe is inserted in the brain through a foramen.

pithecoid (pĭth′ē-koyd) [Gr. *pithekos*, ape, + *eidos*, form, shape]. Apelike; resembling an ape.

pithing (pĭth′ĭng) [ME. *pithe*]. Destruction of the central nervous system by the piercing of brain or spinal cord, as in vivisection. Done on experimental animals to render them insensible to pain and to inhibit controlling effects of the central nervous system during research and experimentation. SEE: *decerebration.*

pithode (pī′thōd) [Gr. *pithose*, wine cask, + *eidos*, form, shape]. The barrel-shaped spindle formed during karyokinesis.

Pitocin. Trade name for oxytocin.

Pitres′ sections (pē-trĕs′) [Jean A. Pitres, Fr. physician, 1848–1927]. Series of six coronal vertical sections of the brain for study. The sections are prefrontal, pediculofrontal, frontal, parietal, pediculoparietal, and occipital.

Pitressin (pĭt-rĕs′ĭn). Trade name for vasopressin, a product obtained from the posterior lobe of the pituitary gland. It contains pressor and antidiuretic principles. SEE: *principle, antidiuretic; vasopressin.*

USES: Increasing blood pressure, increasing the muscular contraction of the intestinal tract, and diminishing urinary output in diabetes insipidus.

Pitressin Tannate (synthetic). Trade name for argipressin tannate.

pitting (pĭt′ĭng) [ME. *pitt*, hole]. 1. The formation of pits, depressions, or scars, as in smallpox. 2. In the spleen, removal of the remains of red blood cells that have completed their lifespan or have been injured. Nucleated red blood cells are also removed from circulating blood in this pitting function. SEE: *culling.* 3. In dentistry, the formation of depressions in the materials used in restoring teeth. 4. In radiography, the imperfections created on the face of the x-ray tube anode by overloading current limits.

pitting edema. Edema, usually of the skin of the extremities, that when pressed firmly with a finger will maintain the depression produced by the finger.

pituicyte (pĭ-tū′ĭ-sīt) [L. *pituita*, phlegm, + Gr. *kytos*, cell]. A modified branched neuroglia cell characteristic of pars nervosa of the posterior lobe of the pituitary gland. Also present in the infundibular stalk.

pituita (pĭ-tū′ĭ-tă) [L., phlegm]. Gluelike mucus.

pituitarism (pĭ-tū′ĭ-tă-rĭzm) [″ + Gr. *-ismos*, condition]. Any disorder of the pituitary gland and its function.

pituitarium (pĭ-tū″ĭ-tăr′ē-ŭm) [L.]. Pituitary.

pituitary (pĭ-tū′ĭ-tār″ē) [L. *pituitarius*, phlegm]. 1. Concerning phlegm. 2. The pituitary body or gland. SYN: *hypophysis.* SEE: *hormone, releasing; hormone, inhibiting; pituitary gland.*

p., anterior. Preparation consisting of dried, defatted, powdered anterior lobe of the pituitary gland of domestic animals.

p., posterior. Dried, powdered posterior lobe of the pituitary gland of animals used as food by humans.

p., whole. Dried, defatted, powdered entire pituitary gland of domestic animals.

pituitary gland. A small, gray, rounded body attached to the base of the brain by the infundibular stalk, a downward extension of the floor of the third ventricle. It averages $1.3 \times 1.0 \times 0.5$ cm in size and 0.55 to 0.6 gm in weight. SYN: *hypophysis cerebri.* SEE: illus.

FUNCT: The pituitary is an endocrine

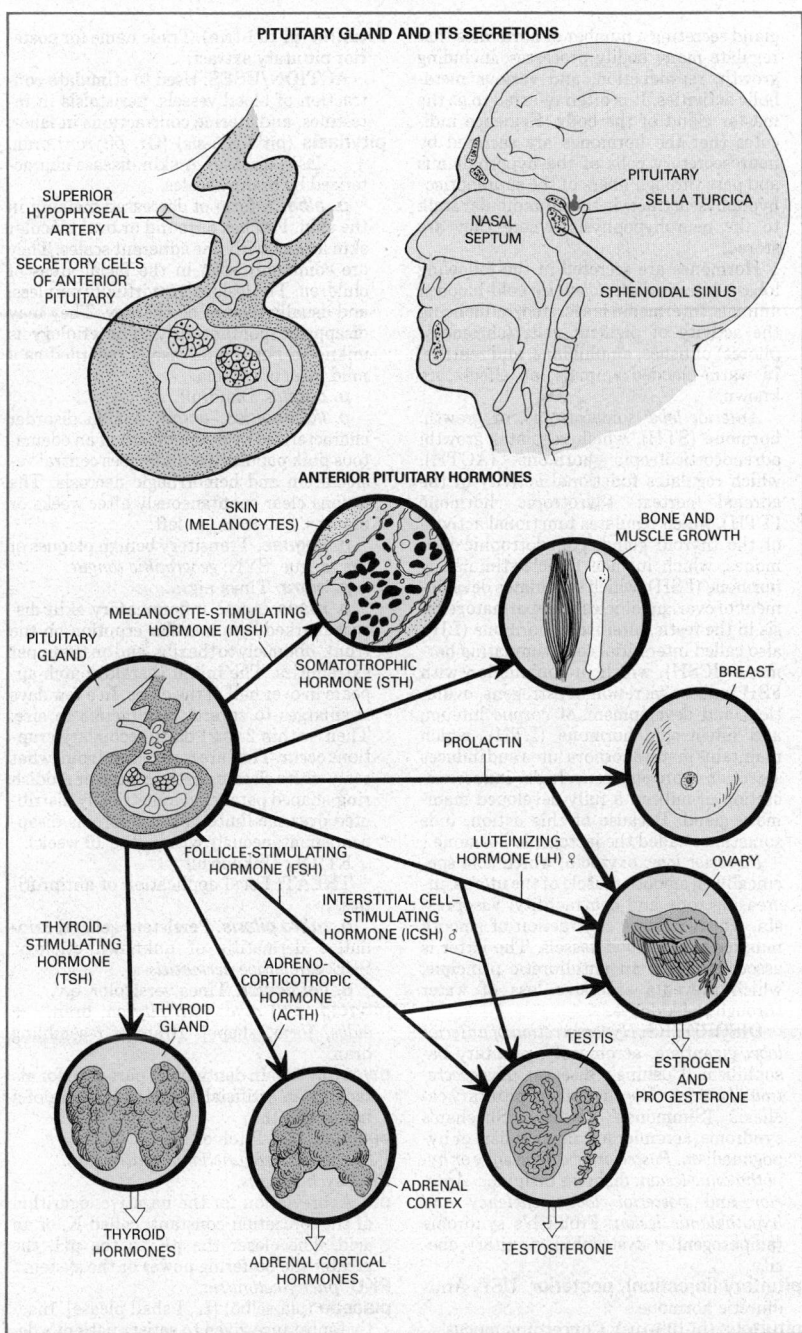

PITUITARY GLAND AND ITS SECRETIONS

SUPERIOR HYPOPHYSEAL ARTERY

SECRETORY CELLS OF ANTERIOR PITUITARY

PITUITARY

SELLA TURCICA

NASAL SEPTUM

SPHENOIDAL SINUS

ANTERIOR PITUITARY HORMONES

SKIN (MELANOCYTES)

BONE AND MUSCLE GROWTH

PITUITARY GLAND

MELANOCYTE-STIMULATING HORMONE (MSH)

SOMATOTROPHIC HORMONE (STH)

BREAST

PROLACTIN

LUTEINIZING HORMONE (LH) ♀

OVARY

FOLLICLE-STIMULATING HORMONE (FSH)

INTERSTITIAL CELL–STIMULATING HORMONE (ICSH) ♂

THYROID-STIMULATING HORMONE (TSH)

ADRENO-CORTICOTROPIC HORMONE (ACTH)

THYROID GLAND

TESTIS

ESTROGEN AND PROGESTERONE

ADRENAL CORTEX

THYROID HORMONES

ADRENAL CORTICAL HORMONES

TESTOSTERONE

gland secreting a number of hormones that regulate many bodily processes, including growth, reproduction, and various metabolic activities. It is often referred to as the master gland of the body. Evidence indicates that the hormones are secreted by neurosecretory cells of the hypothalamus and pass through fibers of the supraoptico-hypophyseal tracts in the infundibular stalk to the neurohypophysis, where they are stored.

Hormones are secreted in the following lobes: *Intermediate lobe:* In cold-blooded animals, intermedin is secreted, influencing the activity of pigment cells (chromatophores) of fishes, amphibians, and reptiles. In warm-blooded animals, no effects are known.

Anterior lobe: somatotropic, or growth, hormone (STH), which regulates growth; adrenocorticotropic hormone (ACTH), which regulates functional activity of the adrenal cortex; thyrotropic hormone (TTH), which regulates functional activity of the thyroid gland; gonadotrophic hormones, which include follicle-stimulating hormone (FSH), which stimulates development of ovarian follicles and spermatogenesis in the testis, luteinizing hormone (LH), also called interstitial cell-stimulating hormone (ICSH), which in conjunction with FSH induces secretion of estrogens, ovulation, and development of corpus luteum, and luteotropic hormone (LTH), which maintains mature corpora lutea and induces secretion of progesterone. It also induces secretion of milk in a fully developed mammary gland. Because of this action, it is sometimes called the lactogenic hormone.

Posterior lobe: oxytocin, which acts specifically on smooth muscle of the uterus, increasing tone and contractility; vasopressin, which induces contraction of smooth muscles of the blood vessels. The latter is associated with an antidiuretic principle, which prevents excessive loss of water through the kidneys.

DISORDERS: *Hypersecretion of anterior lobe:* gigantism, acromegaly, pituitary basophilism (Cushing's disease). *Hyposecretion of anterior lobe:* dwarfism, pituitary cachexia (Simmonds' disease). Sheehan's syndrome, acromicria, eunuchoidism or hypogonadism. *Posterior lobe deficiency or hypothalamic lesion:* diabetes insipidus. *Anterior* and *posterior lobe deficiency and hypothalamic lesion:* Frohlich's syndrome (adiposogenital dystrophy), pituitary obesity.

pituitary (injection), posterior. USP. Antidiuretic hormone.

pituitous (pĭ-tū′ĭ-tŭs). Concerning mucus.

Pituitrin (pĭ-tū′ĭ-trĭn). Trade name for posterior pituitary extract.

ACTION/USES: Used to stimulate contraction of blood vessels, peristalsis in intestines, and uterine contractions in labor.

pityriasis (pĭt″ĭ-rī′ă-sĭs) [Gr. *pityron,* bran, + *-iasis,* disease]. A skin disease characterized by branny scales.

   p. alba. A form of decreased melanin in the skin. Patches of round or oval macular skin lesions with fine adherent scales. They are commonly seen in the facial areas of children. The lesions are virtually painless, and usually require no therapy. They may disappear spontaneously. The etiology is unknown but the disease is regarded as a mild form of eczema.

   p. capitis. Dandruff.

   p. lichenoides, acute. A skin disorder characterized by development of an edematous pink papule that undergoes central vesiculation and hemorrhagic necrosis. The lesions clear spontaneously after weeks or months, but scars are left.

   p. linguae. Transitory benign plaques of the tongue. SYN: *geographic tongue.*

   p. nigra. Tinea nigra.

   p. rosea. Acute inflammatory skin disease marked by a macular eruption on the trunk, obliquely to the ribs, and on the upper extremities. The initial (herald) patch appears in over half of the cases. In a few days it enlarges to several centimeters in size. Then, within 2 to 21 days, secondary eruptions occur. They are rose red and somewhat scaly with a clearing in the center, or reddish ring-shaped patches symmetrically distributed over the limbs. The symptoms disappear spontaneously within 2 to 10 weeks.

   ETIOL: Unknown.

   TREAT: Local application of antipruritics.

   p. rubra pilaris. Persistent general exfoliative dermatitis of unknown etiology. SEE: *exfoliative dermatitis.*

   p. versicolor. Tinea versicolor, q.v.

pityroid (pĭt′ĭ-royd) [Gr. *pityron,* bran, + *eidos,* form, shape]. Branny; resembling bran.

pivot (pĭv′ŭt). In dentistry, a part used for attaching an artificial crown to the base of a natural tooth.

pix (pĭks) [L.]. Pitch or tar.

PJC. *premature junctional contraction.*

PK. *psychokinesis.*

pK. Abbreviation for the negative logarithm of the ionization constant, called K, of an acid. The closer the pK to the pH, the greater the buffering power of the system.

PKU. *phenylketonuria.*

placebo (plă-sē′bō) [L., I shall please]. Inactive substance given to satisfy patient's de-

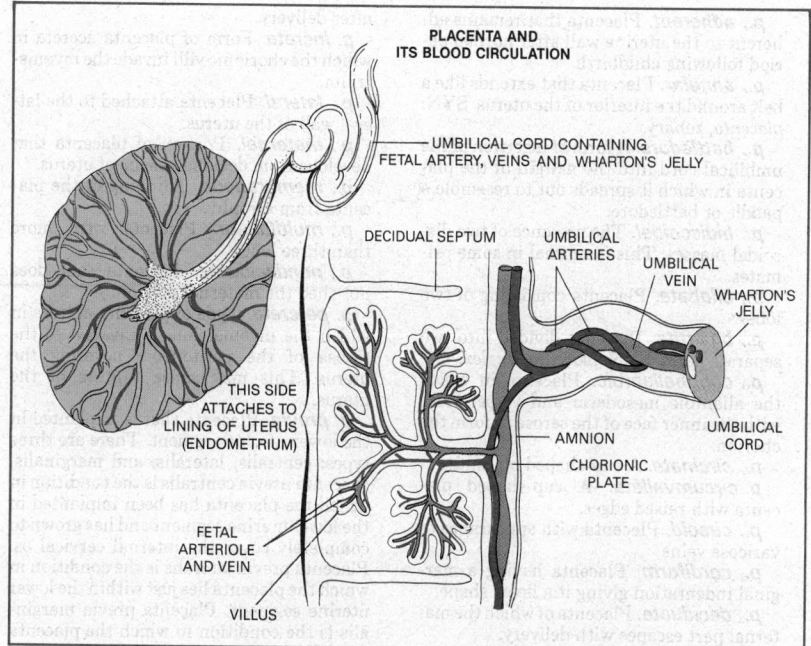

PLACENTA AND ITS BLOOD CIRCULATION

UMBILICAL CORD CONTAINING FETAL ARTERY, VEINS AND WHARTON'S JELLY

DECIDUAL SEPTUM

UMBILICAL ARTERIES

UMBILICAL VEIN

WHARTON'S JELLY

THIS SIDE ATTACHES TO LINING OF UTERUS (ENDOMETRIUM)

UMBILICAL CORD

AMNION

CHORIONIC PLATE

FETAL ARTERIOLE AND VEIN

VILLUS

mand for medicine. Also used in controlled studies of drugs. The placebo is given to a group of patients and the drug being tested is given to a similar group; then the results obtained in the two groups are compared. SEE: *double-blind technique.*

placenta (plă-sĕn′tă) [L., a flat cake] (pl. *placentae, placentas*). [NA] The oval or discoid spongy structure in the uterus of eutherian mammals through which the fetus derives its nourishment. SEE: illus.

ANAT: The placenta consists of a fetal portion, the chorion frondosum, bearing many chorionic villi that interlock with the decidua basalis of the uterus, which constitutes the maternal portion. The chorionic villi lie in spaces in the uterine endometrium, where they are bathed in maternal blood and lymph. Groups of villi are separated by placental septa forming about 20 distinct lobules called cotyledons.

Attached to the margin of the placenta is a membrane that encloses the embryo. It is a composite of several structures (decidua parietalis, decidua capsularis, chorion laeve, and amnion). At the center of the concave side is attached the umbilical cord through which the umbilical vessels (two arteries and one vein) pass to the fetus. The cord is approx. 50 cm long at full term.

The mature placenta is 15 to 18 cm (6 to 7 in.) in diameter and weighs about 450 gm (approx. 1 lb). When expelled following parturition, it is known as the afterbirth.

Maternal blood enters the intervillous spaces of the placenta through spiral arteries, branches of the uterine arteries. It bathes the chorionic villi and flows peripherally to the marginal sinus, which leads to uterine veins. Food substances, oxygen, and antibodies pass into fetal blood of the villi; metabolic waste products pass from fetal blood into the mother's blood. In general, there is no admixture of fetal and maternal blood. The placenta also serves as an endocrine organ. It produces chorionic gonadotropins, the presence of which in urine is the basis of one type of pregnancy test. Estrogen and progesterone are also secreted by the placenta.

   p., abruption of. Premature separation of placenta. SYN: *abruptio placentae.*

   p., accessory. Placenta separate from the main placenta.

   p. accreta. Placenta in which the cotyledons have invaded the uterine musculature and, as a result of this, separation of the placenta is very difficult or impossible.

p., adherent. Placenta that remains adherent to the uterine wall after normal period following childbirth.

p., annular. Placenta that extends like a belt around the interior of the uterus. SYN: *placenta, zonary.*

p., battledore. A form of insertion of the umbilical cord into the margin of the placenta in which it spreads out to resemble a paddle or battledore.

p., bidiscoidal. The presence of two discoidal masses. This is normal in some primates.

p., bilobate. Placenta consisting of two lobes.

p., bipartite. Placenta divided into two separate parts. SYN: *placenta, duplex.*

p., chorioallantoic. Placenta in which the allantoic mesoderm and vessels fuse with the inner face of the serosa to form the chorion.

p., circinate. A cup-shaped placenta.

p. circumvallata. A cup-shaped placenta with raised edges.

p., cirsoid. Placenta with appearance of varicose veins.

p., cordiform. Placenta having a marginal indentation giving it a heart shape.

p., deciduate. Placenta of which the maternal part escapes with delivery.

p., dimidiate. P., bilobate, q.v.

p., discoid. Placenta that constitutes practically one mass, circumscribed and circular in form.

p., double. A placental mass of the two placentae of a twin gestation.

p., duplex. P., bipartite.

p., endotheliochorial. Placenta in which the syncytial trophoblasts of the chorion penetrate to the blood vessels of the uterus.

p., epitheliochorial. Placenta in which the chorion is next to the lining of the uterus but does not invade or erode the lining.

p. fenestrata. Placenta in which there is thinning or absence of placental tissue.

p., fetal. That part of the placenta formed by aggregation of chorionic villi in which the umbilical vein and arteries ramify.

p., fundal. Placenta attached to the uterine wall within the fundal zone.

p., hemochorial. Placenta in which the maternal blood is in direct contact with the chorion. The human placenta is of this type.

p., hemoendothelial. Placenta in which the maternal blood is in contact with the endothelium of the chorionic vessels.

p., horseshoe. A formation in which the two placentae of a twin gestation are united.

p., incarcerated. Placenta retained in the uterus by irregular uterine contractions after delivery.

p. increta. Form of placenta accreta in which the chorionic villi invade the myometrium.

p., lateral. Placenta attached to the lateral wall of the uterus.

p., maternal. Portion of placenta that develops from decidua basalis of uterus.

p., membranous. Thinning of the placenta from atrophy.

p., multilobate. Placenta with more than three lobes.

p., nondeciduate. Placenta that does not shed the maternal portion.

p. percreta. Type of placenta accreta in which the myometrium is invaded to the serosa of the peritoneum covering the uterus. This may cause rupture of the uterus.

p. previa. Placenta that is implanted in the lower uterine segment. There are three types: centralis, lateralis, and marginalis. Placenta previa centralis is the condition in which the placenta has been implanted in the lower uterine segment and has grown to completely cover the internal cervical os. Placenta previa lateralis is the condition in which the placenta lies just within the lower uterine segment. Placenta previa marginalis is the condition in which the placenta partially covers the internal cervical os. SEE: *Nursing Diagnoses* in *Appendix.*

SYM: Slight hemorrhage, recurrent with greater severity, appears 7th or 8th month; gradual anemia, pallor, rapid weak pulse, air hunger, low blood pressure.

DIAG: Painless bleeding during last 3 months; placenta in lower portion of uterus.

TREAT: Conserve blood supply during delivery and before; prevent and control postpartum hemorrhage; combat anemia before and after labor; prevent sepsis.

PROG: Depends upon control of hemorrhage and asepsis.

p. previa partialis. Placenta that only partially covers the internal os of the uterus.

p. reflexa. An abnormal placenta in which the margin is thickened and appears to turn back on itself.

p., reniform. A kidney-shaped placenta.

p., retained. Placenta not expelled for two hours after second stage of labor.

p. spuria. An outlying portion of the placenta that has not maintained its vascular connection with the decidua vera.

p., succenturiate. An accessory placenta that has a vascular connection to the main part of the placenta.

p., trilobate. A placenta with three lobes.

p., tripartite. A three-lobed placenta attached to a single fetus.

p., triple. A placental mass of three lobes

in a triple gestation.

p. uterina. The uterine part of the placenta.

p., velamentous. Placenta with the umbilical cord attached to the membrane a short distance from the placenta, the vessels entering the placenta at its margin.

p., villous. Placenta in which the chorion forms villi.

p., zonary. P., annular.

placental (plă-sĕn′tăl) [L. *placenta*, a flat cake]. Rel. to the placenta.

placental souffle. Sound heard in auscultation over the placenta in pregnancy; due to circulation of the blood.

placentation (plă″sĕn-tā′shŭn). The process of formation and attachment of the placenta.

placentitis (plă″sĕn-tī′tĭs) [″ + Gr. *itis*, inflammation]. Inflamed condition of the placenta.

placentography (plă″sĕn-tŏg′ră-fē) [″ + Gr. *graphein*, to write]. Examination of the placenta by roentgenography.

p., indirect. Measurement of the space between the placenta and the head of the fetus by means of x-ray. It is done to diagnose placenta previa.

placentoid (plă-sĕn′toyd) [″ + Gr. *eidos*, form, shape]. Like the placenta.

placentolysin (plă″sĕn-tŏl′ĭ-sĭn) [″ + Gr. *lysis*, dissolution]. A lysin obtained by injecting placental tissue into an animal, the serum thus obtained being destructive to placental cells of the species of animal from which the placenta was originally taken.

placentoma (plă″sĕn-tō′mă) [″ + Gr. *oma*, tumor]. A neoplasm derived from retained placental tissue.

placentotherapy (plă-sĕn″tō-thĕr′ă-pē) [″ + Gr. *therapeia*, treatment]. Therapeutic use of placental extract.

Placido's disk (plă-sē′dōz) [Antonio Placido, Portuguese ophthalmologist, 1848–1916]. A disk marked with black and white circles used in determining the amount and character of corneal astigmatism.

Placidyl. Trade name for ethchlorvynol.

placing reflex. SEE: *reflex, placing.*

placode (plăk′ōd) [Gr. *plax*, plate, + *eidos*, form, shape]. In embryology, a platelike thickening of epithelium, usually ectoderm, that serves as the anlage of an organ or structure.

p., auditory. A dorsolateral placode located alongside hindbrain that gives rise to the otocyst, which in turn develops into the internal ear.

p., lens. Placode developing in the ectoderm directly overlying the optic vesicle. Forms the lens vesicle, which becomes enclosed in the optic cup and eventually becomes the lens of the eye.

p., olfactory. Placode that gives rise to the olfactory pit and finally the major portion of the nasal cavity.

placoid (plăk′oyd) [″ + *eidos*, form, shape]. Platelike.

pladaroma (plăd-ă-rō′mă) [Gr. *pladaros*, damp, + *oma*, tumor]. A soft growth like a wart on the eyelid.

pladarosis (plăd-ă-rō′sĭs) [″ + *osis*, condition]. Condition of pladaroma.

plagio- [Gr. *plagios*, slanting or sideways]. Combining form concerning slanting or oblique.

plagiocephalic (plā-jē″ō-sĕ-făl′ĭk) [Gr. *plagios*, oblique, + *kephale*, head]. Marked by or rel. to plagiocephaly.

plagiocephalism (plā″jē-ō-sĕf′ă-lĭzm). Plagiocephaly.

plagiocephaly (plā″jē-ō-sĕf′ă-lē). Malformation of the skull producing the appearance of a twisted and lopsided head. Due to irregular closure of the cranial sutures.

plague (plăg) [ME., calamity]. A word once used to describe any widespread contagious disease associated with a high death rate. Now applied specifically to the highly fatal disease caused by *Yersinia pestis* (previously classed as *Pasteurella pestis*) infection.

SYM: High fever, restlessness, staggering gait, mental confusion, prostration, delirium, shock, and coma. Exists in several forms: bubonic with acutely inflamed lymph nodes (buboes); septicemic with absence of buboes; primary pneumonic characterized by pulmonary symptoms. The pneumonic form may be spread from person to person.

TREAT: Streptomycin, tetracyclines, and chloramphenicol are effective in treating plague.

p., ambulatory. Mild but often fatal form of bubonic plague.

p., black. SEE: *black death.*

p., bubonic. The most common form of plague marked by formation of buboes.

p., hemorrhagic. A severe form of bubonic plague in which there is hemorrhage into the skin.

p., murine. Plague infecting rats.

p., pneumonic. A highly virulent form of plague with extensive involvement of the lungs. Occurs as sequela of bubonic plague or as a primary infection.

p., septicemic. Plague characterized by septicemia before the formation of buboes.

p., sylvatic. Plague infecting various species of rodents.

p., white. Tuberculosis.

plague vaccine. USP. A standard preparation of specific plague bacilli that have been killed by the addition of formaldehyde.

plaintiff. The person or party who sues or brings a legal action against another and seeks damages or other legal relief. SEE: *defendant.*

plan. The conscious design of desired future states and of the goals, objectives, and activities required.

  p., dental care. 1. The statement of the goals, objectives, and procedures related to the dentist's care for the patient, based on the medical history, oral examination, and oral radiographs. 2. Third party insurance that covers part or all of the cost for regular dental care. SYN: *dental health insurance.*

  p., medical care. The goals and objectives of the physician's care and the treatment instituted to accomplish them.

  p., nursing care. The statement of the goals and objectives of the nursing care provided for the patient and the activities or tasks required to accomplish the plan, including the criteria to be utilized to evaluate the effectiveness and appropriateness of the plan.

planaria (plă-năr′ē-ă). Free-living flatworms of the Turbellaria class. They are used extensively in studying regeneration.

planchet (plăn′chĕt). A small flat container or dish upon which a radioactive sample is placed.

plane (plān) [L. *planus*]. 1. A flat or relatively smooth surface. SYN: *planum.* 2. A flat surface formed by making a cut, imaginary or real, through the body or a part of it. Planes are used as points of reference by which positions of parts of the body are indicated. In the human subject, all planes are based on the body being in an upright anatomic position. SEE: illus.; *position, anatomic.* 3. A certain stage, as in levels of anesthesia. 4. To smooth a surface or rub away.

  p.'s, Addison's. Planes used as landmarks in thoracoabdominal topography.

  p., Aeby's. Plane perpendicular to the median plane of the cranium through the basion and nasion.

  p., alveolocondylar. Plane tangent to the alveolar point with most prominent points on lower aspects of condyles of the occipital bone.

  p., axiolabiolingual. Plane that passes through an incisor or canine tooth parallel to the long axis of the tooth and in a labiolingual direction.

  p., axiomesiodistal. Plane that passes through a tooth parallel to the axis and in a mesiodistal direction.

  p., Baer's. Plane through upper border of the zygomatic arches.

  p., bite. Plane formed by the biting surfaces of the teeth.

  p., coccygeal. The fourth parallel plane of the pelvis.

  p., coronal. Vertical plane at right angles to a sagittal plane. It divides the body into anterior and posterior portions. SYN: *p., frontal.*

  p., datum. Assumed horizontal plane from which craniometric measurements are taken.

  p., Daubenton's. Plane passing through the opisthion and inferior bones of the orbits.

  p.'s, focal. Two planes through the anterior and posterior principal foci of a dioptric system and perpendicular to the line connecting the two.

  p., Frankfort horizontal. Cephalometric plane joining porion and orbitale, the upper part of the ear openings and the lowest margin of the orbit, to establish a reproducible position of the head for radiographic and cephalometric studies.

  p., frontal. P., coronal.

  p., Hodge's. Plane running parallel to the pelvic inlet and passing through the 2nd sacral vertebra and upper border of the os pubis.

  p., horizontal. Transverse plane at right angles to the vertical axis of the body. SYN: *p., transverse.*

  p.'s, inclined, of pelvis. Anterior and posterior inclined planes of the pelvic cavity, two unequal sections divided by the sciatic spines. In the larger, anterior section, the lateral walls slope toward the symphysis and arch of the pubes; and the posterior walls slope in the direction of the sacrum and coccyx. The anterior inclined planes are the declivities over which rotation of the occiput takes place in the mechanism of normal labor.

  p., intertubercular. Horizontal plane passing through the tubercles of the crests of the ilia. Lies approx. at level of the 5th lumbar vertebra.

  p., Listing's. Transverse vertical plane lying perpendicular to the anteroposterior axis of the eye and containing the center of motion of the eyes. In it also lie the transverse and vertical axes of voluntary ocular rotation.

  p., Meckel's. Plane through the auricular and alveolar points.

  p., median. Anteroposterior plane dividing a body or organ into two equal and symmetrical parts. The median plane of the body is known as the mesion.

  p., midsagittal. Vertical plane dividing the body into symmetrical right and left halves.

  p., Morton's. Plane passing through the most projecting points of the parietal and occipital protuberances.

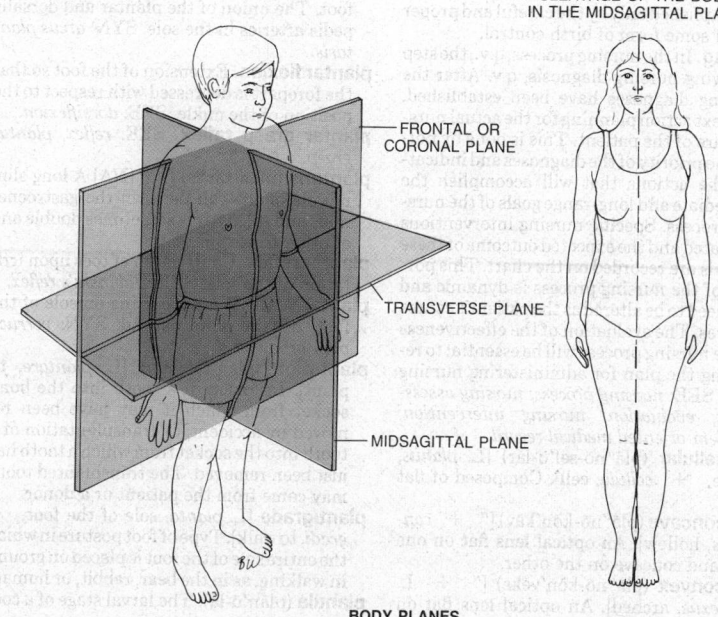

CLEAVAGE OF THE BODY
IN THE MIDSAGITTAL PLANE

FRONTAL OR CORONAL PLANE

TRANSVERSE PLANE

MIDSAGITTAL PLANE

BODY PLANES

p., occlusal. Imaginary plane extending from the incisal edge of the incisors along the tips of the cusps of the posterior teeth to contact the cranium; it is not a true plane but represents the mean of the curvature of the occlusal surface.

p.'s of pelvis. Imaginary planes touching the same parts of the pelvic canal on both sides.

p. of refraction. Plane passing through a refracted ray of light and drawn perpendicular to the surface at which refraction takes place.

p. of regard. Plane through the fovea of the eye; fixation point.

p.'s, parallel, of pelvis. Planes intersecting the axis of the pelvic canal at right angles. The first plane is that of the superior strait. The second plane is that extending from the middle of the sacral vertebra to the level of the subpubic ligament. The third plane is at the level of the spines of the ischia and the fourth plane is at the outlet.

p., sagittal. Vertical plane parallel to the midsagittal plane. One that divides the body into right and left portions.

p., subcostal. Horizontal plane passing through the lowest points of the 10th costal cartilages. Lies approx. at level of 3rd lumbar vertebra.

p., transverse. P., horizontal.

p., vertical. Any body plane perpendicular to a horizontal plane.

p., visual. Plane passing the visual axis of the eye.

planigram (plă'nĭ-grăm) [L. *planus*, plane, + Gr. *gramma*, something written]. A radiographic photograph of a layer or section of the body.

planigraphy (plă-nĭg'ră-fē) [" + Gr. *graphein*, to write]. Body section radiography.

planimeter (plă-nĭm'ĕ-tĕr) [" + Gr. *metron*, measure]. Apparatus used to measure the area of a plane figure by passing a tracer around the boundaries.

planing (plā'nĭng). 1. Dermabrasion, q.v. 2. In dentistry, a meticulous treatment procedure designed to remove calculus, diseased cementum or dentin, microbial flora, and bacterial toxins on the root surface of a tooth or in a gingival pocket. SYN: *root planing.*

plankton (plănk'tŏn) [Gr. *planktos*, wandering]. Free-floating marine life including diatoms, algae, copepods, and some crustacea, protozoa, and worms.

planned parenthood. The concept that a couple or a woman may choose when to conceive and give birth. This can, of course, be accomplished only by the careful and proper use of some form of birth control.

planning. In the nursing process, q.v., the step following nursing diagnosis, q.v. After the nursing diagnoses have been established, the next action planning for the actual nursing care of the patient. This is done by noting the priority of the diagnoses and indicating the actions that will accomplish the immediate and long-range goals of the nursing process. Specific nursing interventions indicated and the expected outcome of these actions are recorded on the chart. This portion of the nursing process is dynamic and will need to be altered as the patient's course evolves. The evaluation of the effectiveness of the nursing process will be essential to restating the plan for administering nursing care. SEE: *nursing process; nursing assessment; evaluation; nursing intervention; problem-oriented medical record.*

planocellular (plă"nō-sĕl'ū-lăr) [L. *planus,* plane, + *cellula,* cell]. Composed of flat cells.

planoconcave (plă"nō-kŏn'kāv) [" + *concavus,* hollow]. An optical lens flat on one side and concave on the other.

planoconvex (plă"nō-kŏn'vĕks) [" + L. *convexus,* arched]. An optical lens flat on one side and convex on the other.

planography (plă-nŏg'ră-fē) [" + Gr. *graphein,* to write]. Planigraphy, q.v.

planomania (plă"nō-mā'nē-ă) [Gr. *plane,* wandering, + Gr. *mania,* madness]. Morbid desire to wander and to be free of social restraints.

Planorbis (plăn-or'bĭs). A genus of freshwater snails serving as intermediate hosts for certain species of blood flukes (*Schistosoma*).

planotopokinesia (plă"nō-tŏp"ō-kī-nē'zē-ă) [" + *topos,* place, + *kinesis,* movement]. Loss of orientation in space.

plant (plănt) [L. *planta,* a sprout]. An organism that contains chlorophyll and manufactures carbohydrates from carbon dioxide and water or, if lacking these characteristics, is similar in structure and life history to those organisms that do possess chlorophyll and manufacture food. SEE: *chlorophyll.*

planta pedis (plăn'tă pē'dŭs) [L.] (pl. *plantae*). [NA] The sole of the foot.

plantago seed (plăn-tă'gō). USP. The cleaned, dried, ripe seed of *Plantago psyllium* or *P. indica.* It is used as a cathartic, but usually in a powdered form rather than in the form of whole seeds.

plantalgia (plăn-tăl'jē-ă) [L. *planta,* sole of the foot, + Gr. *algos,* pain]. Pain in the sole of the foot.

plantar (plăn'tăr). Concerning the sole of the foot.

plantar arch. Vascular arch in the sole of the foot. The union of the plantar and dorsalis pedis arteries in the sole. SYN: *arcus plantaris.*

plantar flexion. Extension of the foot so that the forepart is depressed with respect to the position of the ankle. SEE: *dorsiflexion.*

plantar grasp reflex. SEE: *reflex, plantar grasp.*

plantaris (plăn-tăr'ĭs) [L.]. [NA] A long slim muscle of the calf between the gastrocnemius and soleus. It is sometimes double and at other times missing.

plantar reflex. Contraction of toes upon irritation of the sole. SEE: *Babinski's reflex.*

plantar wart. Wart occurring on sole of the foot; usually quite painful. SYN: *verruca plantaris.*

plantation (plăn-tā'shŭn) [L. *plantare,* to plant]. Insertion of a tooth into the bony socket from which it may have been removed by accident; or transplantation of a tooth into the socket from which a tooth has just been removed. The transplanted tooth may come from the patient or a donor.

plantigrade [L. *planta,* sole of the foot, + *gradi,* to walk]. Type of foot posture in which the entire sole of the foot is placed on ground in walking, as in the bear, rabbit, or human.

planula (plăn'ū-lă). The larval stage of a coelenterate.

planum (plā'nŭm) [L.] (pl. *plana*). A flat or relatively smooth surface. A plane.

  p., nuchal. Outer surface of occipital bone between the foramen magnum and superior nuchal line.

  p., occipital. Outer surface of occipital bone lying above the superior nuchal line.

  p., orbital. Portion of maxilla that forms greater part of floor of orbit.

  p., popliteal. Smooth triangular area on posterior surface of distal end of femur. Bordered by medial and lateral supracondylar lines and forms floor of popliteal fossa.

  p., sternal. Anterior or ventral surface of sternum.

  p., temporal. Depressed area on side of skull below inferior temporal line. Underlies the temporal fossa.

planuria (plă-nū'rē-ă) [Gr. *plane,* wandering, + *ouron,* urine]. The voiding of urine from an abnormal passage of the body.

plaque (plăk) [Fr., a plate]. 1. A patch on the skin or on a mucous surface. 2. A blood platelet.

  p., atheromatous. A yellow swollen area of the lining of an artery. It is formed by deposition of lipid in the area.

  p., bacterial. P., dental, q.v.

  p., dental. A gummy mass of microorganisms that grows on the crowns and spreads along the roots of teeth. It usually is too small to be seen and is both colorless and transparent. Dental plaques are the forerunners of dental caries and periodontal disease. They may be prevented by proper daily self-care of the teeth. SEE: *caries; periodontal disease; periodontitis; pyorrhea alveolaris; tooth; toothbrush and toothbrushing; teeth.*

p., Hollenhorst. Orange-yellow emboli in the retinal vessels.

p., mucous. Condyloma latum, q.v.

Plaquenil Sulfate. Trade name for hydroxychloroquine sulfate, USP.

-plasia [Gr. *plasis,* molding]. Combining form indicating growth or cellular proliferation.

plasm (plăzm) [LL. *plasma,* form, mold]. Plasma.

plasm- [Gr. *plasma,* anything formed]. Combining form concerning living substance or tissue.

plasma (plăz′mă) [LL. *plasma,* form, mold]. 1. The liquid part of the lymph and of the blood. 2. Protoplasm, cell substance outside the nucleus. 3. An ointment base of glycerol and starch.

In the blood, corpuscles and platelets are suspended in plasma. The plasma consists of serum, protein, and chemical substances in aqueous solution. The aqueous solution also contains solids and dissolved gases. Among the chemical materials are electrolytes, glucose, proteins including enzymes and hormones, fats, bile pigments, and bilirubin.

Plasma serves as the medium for transporting the substances previously mentioned to various structures and, at the same time, transports waste products to various sites of clearance, that is, lungs, liver, kidneys, and spleen.

Different constituents of plasma have specific functions within the blood. Proteins, bicarbonates, carbon dioxide, chlorides, phosphates, and ammonia serve to keep the acid-base equilibrium of the blood constant when acid or base substances are added to it. Proteins, esp. albumin, by virtue of their osmotic pressure, tend to prevent undue leakage of fluids out of the capillaries and to maintain a proper exchange of fluid between capillaries and tissues.

Normal plasma is thin and colorless when free from corpuscles, or it has a faint yellow tinge when seen in thick layers.

After clotting of the blood, the liquid squeezed out by the clot is called blood serum. If whole blood is prevented from clotting either by chilling it or by adding anticoagulants, such as sodium citrate, it can be centrifuged. The clear fluid that then occupies the upper half of the centrifuge tube is called plasma. SEE: *blood; coagulation,*

blood; serum.

p., antihemophilic factor. Human plasma in which the antihemophilic globulin has been preserved. It is used to correct temporarily the bleeding tendency in some forms of hemophilia. SEE: *antihemophilic factor.*

p., blood. Fluid in which cellular elements of the blood are suspended.

p., fresh frozen. SEE: *fresh frozen plasma.*

p., hyperimmune. Plasma with a high titer of a specific antibody. It is administered in order to create passive immunity to the antigen.

p., lymph. Lymph without its corpuscles.

p., normal human. Pooled plasma from a number of human donors. The plasma is sterile and the donors are free from diseases that could be transmitted by transfusion.

plasmablast (plăz′mă-blăst) [LL. *plasma,* form, mold, + Gr. *blastos,* germ]. The primitive cell that is the precursor of the plasma cell.

plasmacyte (plăz′mă-sīt) [″ + Gr. *kytos,* cell]. A plasma cell, one of those found in connective tissue, with an eccentrically placed round nucleus and filled with a chromatin mass that stains deeply.

plasmacytoma (plăz″mă-sī′tō′mă) [″ + ″ + *oma,* tumor]. A plasma cell myeloma occurring in bone marrow. SEE: *myeloma, multiple.*

plasmacytosis (plăz″mă-sī-tō′sĭs) [″ + ″ + *osis,* condition]. An excess of plasma cells in the blood.

plasma exchange therapy. Removal of several liters of plasma from a patient and replacing it with normal plasma. This is used experimentally to treat certain diseases, esp. neurological ones. SEE: *plasmapheresis.*

plasmagel (plăz′mă-jĕl″) [″ + L. *gelare,* to congeal]. The peripheral portion of the endoplasm of a cell, such as in an ameba. It is immobile and has the consistency of a gel.

plasmagene (plăz′mă-jēn″) [″ + Gr. *gennan,* to produce]. A cytoplasmic hereditary determiner.

plasmalemma (plăz″mă-lĕm′ă) [″ + Gr. *lemma,* husk]. Plasma, or cell, membrane.

Plasmanate. Trade name for plasma protein fraction.

plasmapheresis (plăz″mă-fĕr-ē′sĭs) [″ + Gr. *aphairesis,* separation]. Removing blood from the body and centrifuging it in order to separate the cellular elements from the plasma. The packed red cells then are suspended in a physiological solution. They may be reinjected into the donor or injected into a patient who requires red cells rather than whole blood.

plasma protein fraction. USP. A standard sterile preparation of serum albumin and globulin obtained by fractionating blood, serum, or plasma from healthy human donors and testing for absence of hepatitis B surface antigen. Used as a blood volume expander. Trade names are Plasmanate, Plasma-Plex, Plasmatein, and Protenate.

plasmasome (plăz′mă-sōm) [″ + Gr. *soma*, body]. A leukocyte granule; nucleolar substance (nonchromatin-staining) in the cytoplasm.

Plasmatein. Trade name for plasma protein fraction.

plasmatherapy (plăz″mă-thĕr′ă-pē) [″ + Gr. *therapeia*, service]. The use of blood plasma for therapeutic purposes, as injection in treatment of shock.

plasmatic (plăz-măt′ĭk). 1. Rel. to plasma. 2. Formative or plastic.

plasmatogamy (plăz″mă-tŏg′ă-mē) [″ + Gr. *gamos*, marriage]. The union of the cytoplasm of two or more cells without joining of the nuclei.

plasmatorrhexis (plăz″mă-tō-rĕk′sĭs) [″ + Gr. *rhexis*, rupture]. Rupture of a cell with loss of its plasma, caused by internal pressure due to swelling.

plasma volume extender. A nontoxic substance composed of high-molecular-weight compounds in a solution suitable for intravenous use. The materials such as dextran or certain proteins are used in treating shock due to loss of blood volume.

plasmic (plăz′mĭk) [LL. *plasma*, form, mold]. Concerning protoplasm.

plasmid. A diverse group of extrachromosomal genetic elements. They are circular double-stringed DNA molecules present intracellularly and symbiotically in most bacteria. They reproduce inside the bacterial cell but are not essential to its viability. Plasmids have the capability of influencing a great number of bacterial functions including resistance to antibiotics, production of enzymes that produce some antibiotics; the ability of the cell to detoxify harmful materials; production of bacteriocins, q.v. Plasmids are gained or lost depending on their value to the bacterial cell in a specific circumstance. SEE: *bacteriocin; transposon.*

plasmin (plăz′mĭn). Fibrinolytic enzyme derived from its precursor plasminogen.

plasminogen (plăz-mĭn′ō-jĕn). A protein found in many tissues and body fluids. It is important in preventing fibrin clot formation.

plasmocyte (plăz′mō-sīt) [″ + Gr. *kytos*, cell]. Cells found in bone marrow, connective tissue, and sometimes in blood plasma. Considered by some to be abnormal leuko-

cytes. They are numerous in plasma cell myeloma.

plasmocytoma (plăz″mō-sī-tō′mă) [″ + ″ + *oma*, tumor]. Plasmacytoma, q.v.

plasmodesma (plăz″mō-dĕz′mă). Singular of plasmodesmata.

plasmodesmata (plăz″mō-dĕz′mă-tă) [″ + Gr. *desmos*, bond]. Tunnels in plant cells. These facilitate communication between cells.

plasmodial (plăz-mō′dē-ăl). Concerning *Plasmodia.*

plasmodicidal (plăz″mō-dĭ-sī′dăl) [″ + Gr. *eidos*, form, shape, + L. *caedere*, to kill]. Lethal to plasmodia.

Plasmodium (plăz-mō′dē-ŭm). A genus of protozoa belonging to subphylum Sporozoa, class Telosporidia. Includes causative agents of malaria in humans and lower animals. SEE: *malaria; mosquito.*

   P. falciparum. Causative agent for malignant tertian (estivoautumnal) malaria.

   P. malariae. Causative agent for quartan malaria.

   P. ovale. Causative agent for benign tertian or ovale malaria.

   P. vivax. Causative agent for benign tertian or vivax malaria.

plasmodium (plăz-mō′dē-ŭm) [LL. *plasma*, form, mold, + Gr. *eidos*, form, shape] (pl. *plasmodia*). 1. A multinucleate mass of naked protoplasm, occurring commonly among slime molds. 2. An organism in the genus *Plasmodium.*

plasmogamy (plăs-mŏg′ă-mē) [″ + Gr. *gamos*, marriage]. The fusion of cells.

plasmolysis (plăz-mŏl′ĭ-sĭs) [″ + Gr. *lysis*, dissolution]. Shrinking of cytoplasm in a living cell due to loss of water by osmosis.

plasmolyzable (plăz″mō-līz′ă-b′l). Capable of being plasmolyzed.

plasmolyze (plăz′mō-līz). To bring about loss of water by osmosis.

plasmoma (plăz-mō′mă) [″ + Gr. *oma*, tumor]. 1. A collection of plasma cells. 2. Plasmacytoma.

plasmon (plăz′mŏn). The genetic portion of the cell cytoplasm.

plasmoptysis (plăz-mŏp′tĭ-sĭs) [″ + Gr. *ptyein*, to spit]. Escape of cytoplasm from a cell.

plasmorrhexis (plăz″mō-rĕk′sĭs) [″ + Gr. *rhexis*, rupture]. Rupture of a cell with loss of plasma. SYN: *erythrocytorrhexis; erythrorrhexis; plasmatorrhexis.*

plasmoschisis (plăz-mŏs′kĭ-sĭs) [″ + Gr. *schisis*, a splitting]. The splitting of a cell.

plasmotomy (plăz-mŏt′ō-mē) [″ + Gr. *tome*, incision]. Mitosis in which the cytoplasm divides into two or more masses.

plasson (plăs′sŏn) [Gr. *plasson*, forming]. Primitive protoplasm in cytode or nonnucleated cell stage.

plastein (plăs'tē-ĭn). Proteins or polypeptides synthesized by proteolytic enzymes following the peptic digestion of proteins.

plaster [Gr. *emplastron*]. 1. Material, usually plaster of paris, that is applied to a part and allowed to harden in order to immobilize the part or to make an impression. 2. External medicinal preparation in which the constituents are formed into a tenacious mass of substance harder than an ointment and spread upon muslin, linen, skin, or paper.

  p., adhesive. Plaster made of a strong cloth coated on one side with an adhesive substance. Used to immobilize a part, to relieve pressure upon sutures, to protect wounds, to secure traction in fractures, to exert pressure, or to hold dressings in place. Hair on the area should be removed before applying any plaster. Plaster should never be applied to abraded or raw surfaces. In reapplying, dead skin should be removed. Surface should be dry and clean.

  p., dental. A semi-solid paste which hardens to form a stone-like investment or model material. It is composed of a hemihydrate of gypsum ($CaSO_4 \cdot 2H_2O$), which differs in compression strength and expansion coefficient according to how it is treated and rehydrated. There are four classes of dental plaster, with differing uses as materials for casts, impressions, or stone models, based on the differences of characteristics.

  p., mustard. Plaster made of powdered mustard paste spread on cloth; used as a rubefacient. SYN: *sinapism.*

  p. of paris. Gypsum cement, hemihydrated calcium sulfate ($CaSO_4 \cdot 2H_2O$), mixed with water to form a paste that sets rapidly; used to make casts and stiff bandages.

  p., salicylic acid. A uniform mixture of salicylic acid spread on an appropriate base such as paper, cotton, or fabric. It is applied topically for use as a keratolytic agent.

plaster cast. Rigid dressing made of gauze impregnated with plaster of paris, used to immobilize an injured part, esp. in bone fractures.

  NURSING IMPLICATIONS: Monitor neurovascular status of the casted part. Do this hourly for 24 hours, then every four hours, and teach patient about assessment concerns. Assess for pressure areas (burning sensation) and skin irritation at least daily. Once the cast is dry, unfinished edges may be covered with adhesive tape or moleskin strips to prevent irritation. Assess for indications of infection. If patient's complaints of discomfort are not relieved by repositioning or comfort measures, report these immediately; cast removal, bivalving, or windowing may be necessary. Encourage physical mobility as permitted or prescribed, teaching the patient preventive measures related to immobility hazards and safety measures to prevent further injury. Instruct patient never to insert anything under the cast to attempt to relieve itching, as further irritation or infection may result. Assist the patient with self-care as required, and teach measures to avoid wetting or soiling the cast. Monitor respiratory, nutritional, and elimination status, and provide respiratory toilet. Prepare the patient for the cast removal procedure and the appearance of the casted area.

plastic (plăs'tĭk) [Gr. *plastikos*, fit for molding]. 1. Capable of being molded. 2. Contributing to building tissues.

plastic and reconstructive surgery. Surgery for the restoration, repair, or reconstruction of body structures. SEE: *surgery, cosmetic; surgery, plastic; tissue expansion, soft.*

plastic bronchitis. Bronchitis with fibrin exudate adhering in the form of a cast to the bronchial tubes.

plasticity (plăs-tĭs'ĭ-tē). The ability to be molded.

plastid (plăs'tĭd) [Gr. *plastos*, formed]. A cytoplasmic organoid found in plant cells. Includes chloroplasts (which contain chlorophyll), leukoplasts (colorless), chromoplasts (which contain pigment), and amyloplasts (which store starch). Plastids are centers of chemical activity involved in cell metabolism.

plastogamy (plăs-tŏg'ă-mē) [″ + *gamos*, marriage]. Plasmatogamy, q.v.

plastron [Fr., breastplate]. The sternum and attached cartilages.

-plasty [Gr. *plastos*, formed]. A word ending meaning molding or surgically forming.

plate (plāt) [Gr. *plate*, flat]. 1. A thin flattened part or portion, such as a flattened process of a bone. SYN: *lamella; lamina.* 2. An incorrect reference to a full denture. 3. A shallow covered dish for culturing microorganisms. 4. To inoculate and culture microorganisms in a culture plate.

  p., approximation. A disk of decalcified bone used in intestinal surgery.

  p., auditory. Bony roof of the external auditory meatus.

  p., axial. The primitive streak of the embryo.

  p., base-. SEE: *baseplate.*

  p., bite. In dentistry a plate made of some suitable plastic material into which the patient bites in order to have a record of the relationship between the upper and lower jaw. The device may be reinforced with wire and used as a splint in the mouth or to treat temporomandibular joint difficulties.

p., blood. Platelet.

p., bone. Flat, round or oval, decalcified bone or metal disk, employed in pairs, used in approximation.

p., cortical. The compact layers of bone forming the surfaces of the alveolar processes of the mandible and maxilla.

p., cribriform. SEE: *cribriform plate.*

p., deck. The roof plate of the embryonic neural tube.

p., dental. An old term for the denture base of metal or acrylic material that rests on the oral mucosa and to which artificial teeth are attached; by extension, *incorrectly* used to mean the complete denture.

p., dorsal. One of two prominences of the notochord in the embryo.

p., end-. The terminal mass of a nerve fiber ending on a muscle cell.

p., epiphyseal. The thin layer of cartilage between the epiphysis and the shaft of a bone. Growth in length of the bone occurs at this layer.

p., equatorial. The platelike mass of chromosomes at the equator of the spindle in cell division.

p., floor. The floor of the embryonic neural tube.

p., foot-. [NA] Flat portion of stapes.

p., medullary. Central portion of the ectoderm in the embryo developing into the neural canal. SYN: *p., neural.*

p., muscle. In the somite, the myotome from which the striated muscles are formed.

p., neural. P., medullary.

p., palate. Part of the palate bone forming the dorsal half of roof of the mouth. SYN: *horizontal palatine plate.*

p., polar. In some cells, the flattened platelike bodies seen at the end of the spindle during mitosis.

p., pterygoid. Either of a pair of thin, bony processes that arise from the sphenoid bone. They are termed medial and lateral pterygoid plates on each side and serve to bound the infratemporal fossa and give origin to muscles of mastication.

p., roof. P., deck, q.v.

p., tarsal. Plate of dense fibrous tissue inside of and supporting each eyelid.

p., tympanic. Bony plate between the anterior wall of the external auditory meatus and the tympanum.

p., ventral. P., floor, q.v.

plateau. 1. An elevated and usually flat area. A steady and consistent fever appears as a plateau on the patient's chart of vital signs. 2. The stage in training or skill acquisition when progress occurs at a very slow or flat rate in comparison with earlier phases.

p., ventricular. The flat portion of the record of intraventricular pressure during the end of the ejection phase of ventricular systole.

platelet (plāt′lĕt) [Gr. *plate*, flat]. A round or oval disk, 2 to 4 micra (micrometers) in diameter, found in the blood of vertebrates. Platelets number 200,000 to 300,000/cu. mm. They contain no hemoglobin. SYN: *thrombocyte.* SEE: *blood.*

FUNCT: Platelets play an important role in blood coagulation, hemostasis, and blood thrombus formation. When a small vessel is injured, platelets adhere to each other and the edges of the injury and form a plug that covers the area. This leads to enhancement of the coagulation mechanism and deposition of fibrin. The plug or blood clot formed soon retracts and stops the loss of blood. The actions of platelets, though quite beneficial in initiating the reaction to injury, may actually be harmful in conditions such as coronary occlusion. In that case, platelet function may delay reperfusion and help to cause reocclusion of the vessel.

DISORDERS OF: Thrombocytopenia (reduced platelet count) occurs in acute infections, anaphylactic shock, and certain hemorrhagic diseases and anemias. Thrombocytosis (increased platelet count) occurs after operations, esp. splenectomy, and following violent exercise and tissue injury.

platelet concentrate. USP. Platelets prepared from a single unit of whole blood or plasma and suspended in a specific volume of the original plasma. This blood fraction must be used prior to the indicated expiration date on its label. Platelets are stored at room temperature (22°C) either in plasma or in a concentrated form as platelet-rich plasma.

plateletpheresis. The process of treating donor blood to remove platelets and then returning the remaining blood to the donor.

plating. In bacteriology, inoculation of liquefiable, solid media (gelatin or agar) with microorganisms and pouring of medium into a shallow flat dish.

platinic (plă-tĭn′ĭk). Pert. to a compound containing quadrivalent platinum.

Platinol. Trade name for cisplatin.

platinosis. Cutaneous and respiratory allergic reactions to exposure to complex salts of platinum.

platinous (plăt′ĭ-nŭs). A compound containing divalent platinum.

platinum (plăt′ĭ-nŭm) [Sp. *platina*]. SYMB: Pt. At. wt. 195.09; at. no. 78; sp. gr. 21.45. Heavy silver-white metal.

platy- [Gr. *platys*, broad]. Combining form meaning broad.

platybasia (plăt″ē-bā′sē-ă). A developmental

defect of the skull in which the floor of the posterior fossa of the skull around the foramen magnum protrudes upward.

platycelous (plăt-ē-sē′lŭs) [Gr. *platys*, broad, + *koilos*, hollow]. Concave ventrally and convex dorsally, said of vertebrae.

platycephalic, platycephalous (plăt″ē-sē-făl′ĭk, -sĕf′ă-lŭs) [″ + *kephale*, head]. Having a wide skull with vertical index less than 70.

platycephaly (plăt″ē-sĕf′ă-lē). Flattening of the skull.

platycnemia (plăt-ĭk-nē′mē-ă) [″ + *kneme*, leg]. 1. Condition of having an unusually broad tibia. 2. Broad-legged condition.

platycnemic (plăt″ĭk-nē′mĭk). Having an unusually broad tibia.

platycnemism (plăt″ĭk′nē-mĭzm). Platycnemia.

platycoria, platycoriasis (plăt″ē-kor-ē′ă, -kor-ī′ă-sĭs) [″ + *kore*, pupil]. Dilatation of the pupil. SYN: *mydriasis*.

platycrania (plăt″ē-krā′nē-ă) [″ + *kranion*, skull]. Platycephaly, q.v.

platyglossal (plăt″ē-glŏs′ăl) [Gr. *platys*, broad, + *glossa*, tongue]. Having a broad, flat tongue.

platyhelminth (plăt″ē-hĕl′mĭnth). Common name for any flatworm.

Platyhelminthes (plăt″ē-hĕl-mĭn′thēz) [″ + *helmins*, worm]. A phylum of flatworms including the classes Turbellaria, Trematoda (flukes), and Cestoidea (tapeworms). The last two are parasitic and include many species of medical importance. SEE: *Cestoda; Cestoidea; fluke; tapeworm; trematode*.

platyhieric (plăt″ē-hī-ĕr′ĭk) [″ + *hieron*, sacrum]. Having a broad sacrum with a sacral index over 100.

platymeric (plăt″ē-mĕr′ĭk) [″ + *meros*, thigh]. Having an unusually broad femur.

platymorphia (plăt″ē-mor′fē-ă) [″ + *morphe*, form]. Having an eye with a shortened anteroposterior diameter. Results in hyperopia, q.v.

platyopia (plăt″ē-ō′pē-ă) [″ + *ops*, face]. Having a very broad face, the nasomalar index being less than 107.5.

platyopic (plăt″ē-ŏp′ĭk). Having a broad, flattened face.

platypellic, platypelvic (plăt″ē-pĕl′ĭk, -vĭk) [″ + *pella*, a basin]. Having a broad pelvis.

platypnea (plă″tĭp′nē-ă) [″ + *pnoia*, breath]. Shortness of breath, dyspnea, only when the patient is upright or seated. SEE: *orthopnea*.

platypodia (plăt″ē-pō′dē-ă) [″ + *pous*, foot]. Condition of being flatfooted.

platyrrhine (plăt″ĭr-īn) [″ + *rhis*, nose]. 1. Having a very wide nose in proportion to length. 2. Pert. to a skull with a nasal index

between 51.1 and 58.

platysmal reflex (plăt-tĭz′măl rē′flĕks). Dilation of pupil resulting from sharp pinching of platysma myoides.

platysma myoides (plă-tĭz′mă mī-oy′dēz) [Gr. *platysma*, plate, + *mys*, muscle, + *eidos*, form, shape]. Broad, thin, platelike layer of muscle that extends from the fascia of both sides of the neck to jaw and muscles around the mouth. Acts to wrinkle the skin of the neck and to depress the jaw.

platyspondylia (plăt″ē-spŏn-dĭl′ē-ă). Platyspondylisis, q.v.

platyspondylisis (plăt″ĭ-spŏn-dĭl′ĭ-sĭs) [Gr. *platys*, flat, + *spondylos*, vertebra]. Flatness of the vertebral bodies.

platystencephaly (plăt″ĭ-stĕn-sĕf′ă-lē) [″ + *kephale*, head]. Having a skull wide at the occiput.

play. Involvement in a sport, amusement, or any form of recreation, esp. an activity other than that in which one is usually engaged as an occupation. What is play to one individual might be considered work to another. From the medical standpoint, it is important that the recreational activity be enjoyable and that participation in it be safe and satisfactory. From the medical aspect, the value of engaging in a sport or recreation that causes frustration, anger, or uncontrolled stress to the extent that the activity is no longer fun is questionable.

pleasure [L. *placere*, to please]. Being delighted or pleased.

pleasure principle. In psychology, the avoidance of pain and the seeking of pleasure, indicative of the early stages of human development. SYN: *hedonism*.

pledget (plĕj′ĕt) [origin uncertain]. 1. Small, flat compress, usually of gauze or absorbent cotton, used to apply or absorb fluid, to protect, or to exclude air. 2. A small spherical mass of cotton about ⅛ in. (3 mm) in diameter that is used with forceps for topical application of medicinal substances, particularly in dentistry.

plegaphonia (plĕg″ă-fō′nē-ă) [Gr. *plege*, stroke, + *a-*, not, + *phone*, voice]. A sound produced in percussion of the larynx when the glottis is open during auscultation of the chest.

-plegia (plē′jē-ă) [Gr. *plege*, stroke]. Suffix meaning paralysis or stroke.

Plegine. Trade name for phendimetrazine tartrate.

pleio-, pleo-, plio- [Gr. *pleion, pleon*, more]. Combining forms meaning more.

pleiotropia (plī″ō-trō′pē-ă) [Gr. *pleion*, more, + *trope*, turn]. The ability of a gene to have many effects.

pleiotropism (plī-ŏt′rō-pĭzm) [″ + ″ + *-ismos*, condition]. Pleiotropia, q.v.

pleochroic (plē″ō-krō′ĭk) [Gr. *pleon*, more, + *chroia*, color]. Pleochromatic.

pleochroism (plē-ŏk′rō-ĭzm) [″ + ″ + *-ismos*, condition]. The property of a crystal that produces different colors when light passes through it at different angles.

pleochromatic (plē″ō-krō-măt′ĭk) [″ + *chroma*, color]. Pert. to the property of crystals and some other bodies that show different colors when seen from different axes. SYN: *pleochroic*.

pleocytosis (plē″ō-sī-tō′sĭs) [″ + *kytos*, cell, + *osis*, condition]. Increased number of lymphocytes in the cerebrospinal fluid.

pleomastia, pleomazia (plē″ō-măs′tē-ă, -mā′zē-ă) [Gr. *pleon*, more, + *mastos*, *mazos*, breast]. The state of having more than two mammae. SYN: *polymastia*.

pleomorphic (plē-ō-mor′fĭk) [″ + *morphe*, form]. Having many shapes.

pleomorphism (plē-ō-mor′fĭzm) [″ + ″ + *-ismos*, condition]. 1. Property of crystallizing into two or more different forms. 2. Occurrence of more than one form in a life cycle. SYN: *polymorphism*.

pleomorphous (plē-ō-mor′fŭs). Having many shapes or crystallizing into several forms.

pleonasm (plē′ō-năzm) [Gr. *pleonasmos*, exaggeration]. 1. State of having more than normal number of organs or parts. 2. Using more words than necessary to express an idea.

pleonexia (plē″ō-nĕk′sē-ă) [Gr.]. Having morbid desire for possession of material things; greediness.

pleonosteosis (plē″ŏn-ŏs″tē-ō′sĭs) [Gr. *pleon*, more, + *osteon*, bone, + *osis*, condition]. Premature and excessive ossification of bones.

    p., Leri's. A hereditary syndrome manifesting as pleonosteosis of the long bones, esp. of the digits, with short stature, and mongolian facies. It is apparent during the first year of age and is inherited as an autosomal dominant trait.

pleoptics (plē-ŏp′tĭks) [″ + *optikos*, sight]. A method of eye exercises created to stimulate and train an amblyopic eye.

plerocercoid. The solid wormlike larva of certain tapeworms. Plerocercoids develop in secondary hosts.

plesiomorphism (plē″sē-ō-mor′fĭzm) [Gr. *plesios*, close, + *morphe*, form, + *-ismos*, condition]. Similarity of form.

plesiomorphous (plē″sē-ō-mor′fŭs) [″ + *morphe*, form]. Of, like, or nearly the same in form.

plesiopia (plē″sē-ō′pē-ă) [″ + *ops*, eye]. Increase in convexity of lens of eye.

plessesthesia (plĕs″ĕs-thē′zē-ă) [Gr. *ples-*

sein, to strike, + *aisthesis*, sensation]. Palpatory percussion with the left middle finger pressed against body and the right index finger percussing in contact with the left finger.

plessimeter (plĕs-sĭm′ĕ-tĕr) [″ + *metron*, measure]. A disk that is struck in mediate percussion while being held over the surface of the body. SYN: *pleximeter*.

plessor (plĕs′or) [Gr. *plessein*, to strike]. A hammer for performing percussion. SYN: *plexor*.

plethora (plĕth′ō-ră) [Gr. *plethore*, fullness]. 1. Overfullness of blood vessels or of the total quantity of any fluid in the body. SEE: *sanguine*. 2. Congestion causing distention of blood vessels.

plethoric (plĕ-thor′ĭk, plĕth′ō-rĭk). Pert. to, or characterized by, plethora; overfull.

plethysmograph (plĕ-thĭz′mō-grăf) [Gr. *plethysmos*, to increase, + *graphein*, to write]. Device for finding variations in size of a part due to variations in amount of blood passing through or contained in the part.

plethysmography (plĕth″ĭz-mŏg′ră-fē). Use of a plethysmograph to record the changes in volume of an organ or extremity.

pleur-, pleuro- [Gr. *pleura*, rib, side]. Prefix indicating rel. to the pleura, the side, or a rib.

pleura (ploo′ră) [Gr., side] (pl. *pleurae*). [NA] Serous membrane that enfolds both lungs and is reflected upon the walls of the thorax and diaphragm. The pleurae are moistened with a serous secretion that reduces friction during respiratory movements of the lungs. SEE: *effusion, pleural; mediastinum; thorax.*

    p., costal. P., parietal.

    p. diaphragmatica. [NA] Part of the pleura covering the upper surface of the diaphragm. SYN: *p. phrenica.*

    p., mediastinal. Portion of the parietal pleura that extends to cover the mediastinum.

    p., parietal. Portion of the pleura that extends from the roots of the lungs and covers the sides of the pericardium to chest wall and backward to the spine. The visceral and costal pleural layers are separated only by a lubricating secretion. These layers may become adherent or separated by fluid or air in diseased conditions. SYN: *pleura, costal.*

    p. pericardiaca. Portion of the pleura covering the pericardium.

    p. phrenica. P. diaphragmatica [NA].

    p. pulmonalis. [NA] Pleura investing the lungs and fissures between the lobes.

    p., visceral. Pleura that invests the lungs and enters into and lines the interlobar fissures. It is loose at the base and at sternal and vertebral borders to allow for lung expansion.

pleuracentesis (ploor"ă-sĕn-tē'sĭs) [Gr. *pleura*, side, + *kentesis*, puncture]. Thoracentesis.

pleuracotomy (ploor"ă-kŏt'ō-mē) [" + *tome*, incision]. Incision into the pleura through the chest wall.

pleural (ploo'răl) [Gr. *pleura*, side]. Concerning the pleura.

pleural cavity. Space between the parietal and visceral layers of the pleura.

pleural effusion. SEE: *effusion, pleural.*

pleural fibrosis. Condition occurring in pulmonary tuberculosis in which the pleura becomes thickened and the pleural cavity often is obliterated.

pleuralgia (ploo-răl'jē-ă) [" + *algos*, pain]. Pain in the pleura, or in the side. SYN: *neuralgia, intercostal.*

pleurapophysis (ploo-ră-pŏf'ĭ-sĭs) [" + *apo*, from, + *physis*, a growth]. A rib or a vertebral lateral process.

pleurectomy (ploo-rĕk'tō-mē) [" + *ektome*, excision]. Excision of part of the pleura.

pleurisy (ploo'rĭs-ē) [Gr. *pleuritis*]. Inflammation of the pleura. It may be primary or secondary; unilateral, bilateral, or local; acute or chronic; fibrinous, serofibrinous, or purulent.

NURSING IMPLICATIONS: Assess and monitor respiratory function using percussion, auscultation, and arterial blood gas values. Position the patient in high Fowler's position to facilitate chest expansion. Encourage deep breathing and coughing every one to two hours to prevent atelectasis. Splint the chest as necessary during coughing and employ analgesic drugs and noninvasive measures, such as local application of warm or cool compresses, to reduce pain. Provide respiratory toilet and avoid antitussives if secretions are present. Encourage and promote physical and emotional rest. Carry out prescribed medical regimens and evaluate patient response. SEE: *Nursing Diagnoses in Appendix.*

p., acute. Chilliness, stabbing pain or stitch in affected side, intensified by coughing or deep breathing. Fever of 101° to 103°F (38.3° to 39.4°C); a short, dry, partially suppressed cough; pale, anxious face; patient usually lies on affected side. An effusion of fluid that remains unabsorbed in the pleural space characterizes chronic pleurisy.

p., adhesive. Pleurisy in which the exudate causes the parietal pleura to adhere to the visceral. If this is extensive, the pleural space is obliterated.

p., diaphragmatic. Inflammation of the diaphragmatic pleura.

SYM: Intense pain under margin of the ribs, sometimes referred into abdomen, with tenderness on pressure; thoracic breathing; tenderness over the phrenic nerve referred to the supraclavicular region in the neck or same side; hiccough; extreme dyspnea.

p., dry. Condition in which the pleural membrane is covered with a fibrinous exudate. It clings together, causing pain during respiration. There is slight pain when apical pleura is inflamed, but there is acute stabbing pain in costal or diaphragmatic pleural inflammation.

p., encysted. Pleurisy with effusion limited by adhesions.

p., fibrinous. Pleurisy with severe and continuous pain. Aspiration gives negative results, later much retraction of affected side.

p., hemorrhagic. Pleurisy with hemorrhage.

p., interlobar. Pleurisy in interlobar spaces.

p., plastic. P., dry.

p., pulmonary. Inflammation of the pleura covering the lung.

p., purulent. Pleurisy with high, irregular fever; sweats; chills; anemia; purulent effusion found on aspiration. SYN: *empyema; p., suppurative.*

p., sacculated. Pleurisy in which there are inflammatory areas, sealed off and filled with fluid.

p., serofibrinous. Pleurisy with fibrinous exudate and serous effusion.

p., serous. Pleurisy with a serous effusion.

p., suppurative. P., purulent.

p., tuberculous. Inflammation of the pleura as a result of tuberculosis. The effusion may be bloody.

p., typhoid. Pleurisy with symptoms of typhoid.

p., visceral. P., pulmonary.

p., wet. P., serous, q.v.

p. with effusion. P., serous, q.v.

pleuritic (ploo-rĭt'ĭk) [Gr. *pleuritis*, pleurisy]. Rel. to, or like, pleurisy.

pleuritis (ploo-rī'tĭs) [Gr.]. Inflammation of the pleura. SYN: *pleurisy.*

pleuritogenous (ploor"ĭ-tŏj'ĕ-nŭs) [" + *gennan*, to produce]. Causing pleurisy.

pleurocele (ploo'rō-sēl) [Gr. *pleura*, side, + *kele*, tumor, swelling]. 1. Hernia of the lungs or pleura. 2. A serous pleural effusion.

pleurocentesis (ploo"rō-sĕn-tē'sĭs) [" + *kentesis*, a piercing]. Surgical puncture of the pleural cavity. SYN: *thoracentesis; thoracocentesis.*

pleurocentrum (ploo"rō-sĕn'trŭm) [" + *kentron*, center] (pl. *pleurocentra*). The lateral half of the centrum of a vertebra.

pleurocholecystitis (ploo"rō-kō"lē-sĭst-ī'

tĭs) [" + *chole*, bile, + *kystis*, bladder, + *itis*, inflammation]. Inflamed condition of the pleura and gallbladder.

pleuroclysis (ploo-rŏk′lĭ-sĭs) [" + *klysis*, a washing]. Injection of fluid into the pleural cavity to wash it out.

pleurodesis (ploo″rŏ-dē′sĭs) [" + *desis*, binding]. Production of adhesions between the parietal and visceral pleura. Usually done surgically. Method is useful in treating recurrent pneumothorax.

pleurodynia (ploo″rŏ-dĭn′ē-ă) [" + *odyne*, pain]. Pain of sharp intensity in the intercostal muscles due to chronic inflammatory changes in the chest fasciae; pain of the pleural nerves.

    p., epidemic. An epidemic disease caused by coxsackie B virus. Characterized by sudden onset of pain in the chest and fever. SYN: *Bornholm disease.*

pleurogenic (ploo″rŏ-jĕn′ĭk) [" + *gennan*, to produce]. Arising in the pleura. SYN: *pleurogenous.*

pleurogenous (ploo-rŏj′ĕn-ŭs). Having origin in the pleura. SYN: *pleurogenic.*

pleurography (ploo-rŏg′ră-fē) [" + *graphein*, to write]. X-ray examination of the lungs and pleura.

pleurohepatitis (ploo″rŏ-hĕp″ă-tī′tĭs) [" + *hepatos*, liver, + *itis*, inflammation]. Inflammation of the pleura and liver.

pleurolith (ploo′rŏ-lĭth) [" + *lithos*, stone]. A calculus in the pleura.

pleurolysis (ploo-rŏl′ĭ-sĭs) [" + *lysis*, dissolution]. Loosening of parietal pleura from intrathoracic fascia to facilitate contraction of the lung or artificial pneumothorax.

pleuromelus (ploor″ŏ-mē′lŭs) [" + *melos*, limb]. A congenital anomaly in which an accessory limb arises from the thorax or flank.

pleuroparietopexy (ploo″rŏ-păr-ī′ĕt-ō-pĕk″sē) [" + L. *parietalis*, wall, + Gr. *pexis*, fixation]. Fastening of the lung to the wall of the chest by binding the visceral pleura to the wall of its cavity.

pleuropericardial (ploor″ŏ-pĕr-ĭ-kăr′dē-ăl) [" + *peri*, around, + *kardia*, heart]. Concerning the pleura and pericardium.

pleuropericarditis (ploo″rŏ-pĕr″ĭ-kăr-dī′tĭs) [" + " + " + *itis*, inflammation]. Pleuritis accompanied by pericarditis.

pleuroperitoneal (ploo″rŏ-pĕr″ĭ-tō-nē′ăl) [" + *peritonaion*, peritoneum]. Rel. to the pleura and peritoneum.

pleuroperitoneal cavity. The body cavity. SYN: *celom.*

pleuropneumonia (ploo″rŏ-nū-mō′nē-ă) [" + *pneumon*, lung]. Pleurisy accompanied by pneumonia.

pleuropneumonia-like organisms. ABBR: PPLO. The name once given organisms that are now called mycoplasmas, q.v.

pleuropneumonolysis (ploo″rŏ-nū″mŏn-ŏl′ĭ-sĭs) [Gr. *pleura*, side, + *pneumon*, lung, + *lysis*, a loosening]. Resection of one or more ribs from one side to collapse the lung in unilateral pulmonary tuberculosis. This procedure is rarely necessary.

pleuropulmonary (ploor″ŏ-pŭl′mō-nĕr″ē) [" + L. *pulmo*, lung]. Concerning the pleura and lung.

pleurorrhea (ploor″ŏ-rē′ă) [" + *rhoia*, flow]. Effusion of fluid into the pleura.

pleuroscopy (ploo-rŏs′kŏ-pē) [" + *skopein*, to examine]. Inspection of the pleural cavity through an incision into the thorax.

pleurosoma (ploor″ŏ-sō′mă) [" + *soma*, body]. A fetus with a cleft in the abdominal wall and thorax with protrusion of the contents of the thoracic and abdominal cavities.

pleurothotonos (ploo″rŏ-thŏt′ŏ-nŏs) [Gr. *pleurothen*, from the side, + *tonos*, tension]. Tetanic spasm in which the body is arched to one side.

    RS: emprosthotonos; opisthotonos; orthotonos; position; posture.

pleurotomy (ploo-rŏt′ŏ-mē) [Gr. *pleura*, side, + *tome*, incision]. Incision of the pleura.

pleurotyphoid (ploo″rŏ-tī′foyd) [" + *typhos*, fever, + *eidos*, form, shape]. Typhoid fever with pleural involvement.

pleurovisceral (ploo″rŏ-vĭs′ĕr-ăl) [" + L. *viscera*, viscera]. Concerning the pleura and viscera.

plexal (plĕk′săl) [L. *plexus*, a braid]. Pert. to, or of the nature of, a plexus.

plexectomy (plĕk-sĕk′tŏ-mē) [" + Gr. *ektome*, excision]. Surgical removal of a plexus.

plexiform (plĕk′sĭ-form) [" + *forma*, shape]. Resembling a network or plexus.

pleximeter (plĕks-ĭm′ĕ-tĕr) [Gr. *plexis*, stroke, + *metron*, measure]. Device for receiving the blow of the percussion hammer. SYN: *plessimeter.*

plexitis (plĕk-sī′tĭs) [L. *plexus*, a braid, + Gr. *itis*, inflammation]. Inflammation of a nerve plexus.

plexometer (plĕk-sŏm′ĕ-tĕr). Pleximeter, q.v.

plexor (plĕks′or). Hammer or other device for striking upon the pleximeter in percussion. SYN: *plessor.*

plexus (plĕks′ŭs) [L., a braid] (pl. *plexus* or *plexuses*). [NA] A network of nerves or of blood or lymphatic vessels. SEE: *rete*; *Nerve Plexuses* in *Appendix*.

    p., autonomic. An extensive network of nerve fibers and nerve cell bodies belonging to the sympathetic or parasympathetic nervous system. SEE: *Nerve Plexuses* in *Appendix*.

    p., cavernous. Plexus of a cavernous part of the body. The following are included.

Of the nose: a venous plexus in the mucosa covering the superior and middle conchae. Of the penis: nerve plexus at the base of the penis giving rise to large and small cavernous nerves. Of the clitoris: nerve plexus at the base of the clitoris, formed of fibers from the uterovaginal plexus. Of the cavernous sinus: a sympathetic plexus that supplies fibers to the internal carotid artery and its branches within the cranium.

p., choroid. SEE: *choroid plexus.*

p., dental. A network of sensory nerve fibers that are distributed to the teeth. The inferior alveolar nerve is distributed to the mandibular teeth; the anterior, middle, and posterior superior alveolar nerves contribute fibers to innervate the maxillary teeth.

p., enteric. One of two plexuses of nerve fibers and ganglion cells that lie in the wall of the alimentary canal. These are the myenteric (Auerbach's) and submucosal (Meissner's) plexuses.

p., myenteric. One of the two plexuses in the wall of the alimentary canal. SYN: *Auerbach's plexus.*

p., nerve. Plexus made of nerve fibers. SEE: *Nerve Plexuses* in *Appendix.*

p., pampiniform. In the male, a complicated network of veins lying in the spermatic cord and draining the testis. In the female, a network of veins lying in the mesovarium and draining the ovary.

p., prevertebral. One of three plexuses of autonomic nerve division that lie in body cavities. These are the cardiac, celiac, and hypogastric (pelvic) plexuses. SEE: *Nerve Plexuses* in *Appendix.*

pliability (plī″ă-bĭl′ĭ-tē) [O. Fr. *pliant*, bend, + L. *abilis*, able]. Capacity of being bent or twisted easily.

plica (plī′kă) [L.] (pl. *plicae*). [NA] A fold. SEE: *fold.*

p., circular. One of the transverse folds in the small intestine. SYN: *Kerckring's folds.*

p., epiglottic. One of three folds of mucosa between the tongue and the epiglottis.

p., lacrimal. Mucosal fold at the lower orifice of the nasolacrimal duct.

p., palmate. Radiating fold in the uterine mucosa on the anterior and posterior walls of the cervical canal.

p. polonica. Tangled matted hair in which crusts and vermin are embedded.

p., semilunar, of colon. Transverse fold of mucosa of the large intestine lying between sacculations.

p., semilunar, of conjunctiva. Mucosal fold at the inner canthus of the eye.

p., synovial. A fold of synovial membrane that projects into a joint cavity.

p., transverse, of rectum. One of the mucosal folds in the rectum.

plicamycin. An antineoplastic agent that has been used in treating Paget's disease of the bone. Trade name is Mithracin.

plicate (plī′kāt) [L. *plicatus*]. Braided or folded.

plication (plī-kā′shŭn) [L. *plicare*, to fold]. The stitching of folds or tucks in an organ's walls to reduce its size.

p. of stomach. Surgical creation of tucks in the wall of the stomach. This technique has been used experimentally in treating obesity.

plicotomy (plī-kŏt′ō-mē) [″ + Gr. *tome*, incision]. Section of the posterior fold of the tympanic membrane.

pliers. Commonly, a scissor-action, pointed-jawed tool for bending or cutting metal wires or grasping small objects. In dentistry, a variety of instruments which have been shaped or adapted for special uses such as cutting arch wires or metal clasps, shaping metal crown details, applying cotton pledgets or rolls, carrying metal foils, tying ligatures, and placing or removing matrix bands.

plinth [Gr. *plinthos*, tile]. A table, seat, or apparatus that a patient lies or sits on while doing remedial exercise.

-ploid [Gr. *ploos*, fold]. Suffix indicating the number of chromosome pairs of the root word to which it is added.

ploidy (ploy′dē) [Gr. *ploos*, a fold, + *eidos*, form, shape]. The number of chromosome sets in a cell, e.g., haploidy, diploidy, and triploidy for one, two, and three sets, respectively, of chromosomes.

plombage (plŏm-băzh′) [Fr. *plomber*, to plug]. A method of collapsing the apex of the lung by stripping the parietal pleura from the chest wall at the site of desired collapse and packing the space between the lung and the chest wall with an inert substance such as small balls made of certain plastic materials.

plototoxin (plō″tō-tŏk′sĭn). A toxic substance present in catfish, *Plotosus lineatus.*

plug (plŭg) [MD. *plugge*]. A mass obstructing a hole or intended for closing a hole.

p., Dittrich's. A mass of foul-smelling bacteria, and fatty acid crystals, in the sputum in bronchiectasis or gangrenous bronchitis.

p., epithelial. A mass of epithelial cells temporarily plugging an orifice in the embryo, esp. the nasal openings.

p., mucous. A mass of cells and mucus that closes the cervical canal of the uterus during pregnancy and between menstrual periods.

p., Traube's. P., Dittrich's, q.v.

p., vaginal. Closed tube for maintaining

patency of the vagina following operation for fistula.

plugger. A hand- or machine-operated device for condensing amalgam, or gold foil, in the cavity of a tooth.

    p., automatic. Plugger that is run by a machine rather than by hand.

    p., back-action. Plugger with a bent shank so that the pressure applied is back toward the operator.

    p., foot. Plugger having a broad, foot-shaped tip.

plumbic (plŭm′bĭk) [L. *plumbicus*, leaden]. Pert. to, or containing, lead.

plumbism (plŭm′bĭzm) [L. *plumbum*, lead, + Gr. *-ismos*, condition]. Poisoning from lead.

plumbum (plŭm′bŭm) [L.]. Lead; a bluish-white metal. SEE: *lead.*

Plummer-Vinson syndrome (plŭm′ĕr-vĭn′sŏn) [Henry S. Plummer, U.S. physician, 1874–1937; Porter P. Vinson, U.S. surgeon, 1890–1959]. Iron-deficiency anemia, associated with dysphagia, gastric achlorhydria, splenomegaly, spooning of the nails due to an esophageal web. It occurs most commonly in premenopausal women. Treatment consists of disrupting the web. SEE: *esophageal web.*

plumose (plŭ′mōs) [L. *plumosus*]. Having a delicate, feathery growth.

plumper (plŭm′pĕr) [Middle Low Ger. *plump*, to fill]. Pad for filling out sunken cheeks, sometimes in form of a flange or extension from artificial dentures.

pluri- [L. *plus*, more]. Prefix meaning several or more.

pluriceptor (ploo′rĭ-sĕp′tor) [L. *plus*, more, + *ceptor*, a receiver]. A receptor that has more than two groups uniting with the complement.

pluriglandular (ploo″rĭ-glănd′ū-lăr) [″ + *glandula*, gland]. Pert. to several glands. SYN: *polyglandular.*

plurigravida (ploo″rĭ-grăv′ĭ-dă) [″ + *gravida*, pregnant]. A pregnant woman who has had three or more pregnancies.

plurilocular (ploo″rĭ-lŏk′ū-lăr) [″ + *loculus*, a cell]. Composed of several compartments or cavities. SYN: *multilocular.*

plurinuclear (ploo″rĭ-nū′klē-ăr) [″ + *nucleus*, kernel]. Having a number of nuclei.

pluripara (ploo-rĭp′ă-ră) [″ + *parere*, to bring forth, to bear]. A woman who has given birth three or more times.

pluriparity (ploo″rĭ-păr′ĭ-tē). Condition of having three or more pregnancies that have reached a point of viability regardless of the outcome.

pluripotent, pluripotential (ploo-rĭp′ō-tĕnt, ploor″ĭ-pō-tĕn′shăl) [″ + *potentia*, power]. 1. Concerning an embryonic cell that can form different kinds of cells. 2. Having a number of different actions.

pluripotentiality (ploor″ĭ-pō-tĕn″shē-ăl′ĭ-tē). The potential for developing in several ways or acting in different ways.

pluriresistant (ploor″ĭ-rē-zĭs′tănt) [″ + *resistens*, standing back]. Resistant to several drugs, esp. antibiotics.

plutomania (ploo″tō-mā′nē-ă) [Gr. *ploutos*, wealth, + *mania*, madness]. Delusion that one is very rich.

plutonium (ploo-tō′nē-ŭm) [Named after the planet Pluto]. SYMB: Pu. At. wt. of the most stable isotope is 244; at. no. 94. A chemical element obtained from neptunium, which in turn is obtained from uranium.

Pm. Chem. symb. for the element promethium.

PML. *progressive multifocal leukoencephalopathy.* SEE: *leukoencephalopathy, progressive multifocal.*

PMS. *premenstrual syndrome,* q.v.

PMSG. *pregnant mare serum gonadotropin.* SEE: *gonadotropin, chorionic.*

PMT. *premenstrual tension.*

PNC. *premature nodal contraction* or *complex.*

pneo- (nē′ō) [Gr. *pnein*, to breathe]. Combining form meaning pert. to breath or breathing. SEE: words beginning with *pneum-*.

pneocardiac reflex (nē″ō-kăr′dē-ăk) [Gr. *pnein*, to breathe, + *kardia*, heart]. Change in rate and rhythm of heart and blood pressure when an irritant vapor is inhaled.

pneopneic reflex (nē-ŏp-nē′ĭk) [″ + *pnein*, to breathe]. Change in respiratory depth and rate, coughing, suffocation, and pulmonary edema when an irritant vapor is inhaled.

pneum-, pneuma-, pneumato- [Gr. *pneuma, pneumatos*, air, breath]. Combining form meaning pert. to air or gas, or respiration.

pneumarthrogram (nū-măr′thrō-grăm) [Gr. *pneuma*, air, + *arthron*, joint, + *gramma*, something written]. Roentgenogram of a joint into which air has been injected.

pneumarthrography (nū″măr-thrŏg′ră-fē) [″ + ″ + *graphein*, to write]. X-ray study of a joint into which air has been injected.

pneumarthrosis (nū-măr-thrō′sĭs) [″ + ″ + *osis*, condition]. Accumulation of gas or air in a joint.

pneumatic (nū-măt′ĭk) [Gr. *pneumatikos*, pert. to air]. 1. Concerning gas or air. 2. Rel. to respiration. 3. Rel. to rarefied or compressed air.

pneumatics (nū-măt′ĭks). The branch of physics that is concerned with the physical and mechanical properties of gases and air.

pneumatinuria (nū″măt-ĭn-ū′rē-ă) [″ + *ouron*, urine]. Excretion of urine containing free gas. SYN: *pneumaturia.*

pneumatization (nū″mă-tĭ-zā′shŭn). The formation of air-filled cells or cavities, usually in bone, e.g., the paranasal sinuses and mastoid processes.

pneumatized (nū′mă-tīzd). Filled with air.

pneumatocardia (nū″măt-ō-kăr′dē-ă) [″ + *kardia*, heart]. Air or gas in the heart chambers.

pneumatocele (nū-măt′ō-sēl) [″ + *kele*, tumor, swelling]. 1. Hernia protuberance of lung tissue. 2. A swelling containing gas or air, esp. a swelling of the scrotum. SYN: *pneumocele; pneumonocele.*

    p., extracranial. A collection of gas under the scalp, caused by a fracture of the skull that communicates with a paranasal sinus.

    p., intracranial. A collection of gas within the skull.

pneumatodyspnea (nū″măt-ō-dĭsp′nē-ă) [″ + *dys*, bad, + *pneia*, breath]. Dyspnea caused by pulmonary emphysema.

pneumatology (nū″mă-tŏl′ō-jē) [″ + *logos*, word, reason]. Science of gases and air and their chemical properties and use in treatment.

pneumatorrhachis (nū″măt-or′ă-kĭs) [″ + *rhachis*, spine]. Air in the spinal canal.

pneumatosis (nū″mă-tō′sĭs) [Gr. *pneumatosis*]. Presence of air or gas in an abnormal location in the body.

    p. abdominis. Air in the peritoneal cavity. SYN: *pneumoperitoneum.*

    p. cystoides intestinalis. Presence of thin-walled gas-filled cysts in the intestines. The cause is unknown. The cysts usually disappear but occasionally rupture and cause pneumoperitoneum.

pneumatotherapy (nū″măt-ō-thĕr′ă-pē) [Gr. *pneumatos*, air, + *therapeia*, treatment]. 1. Treatment of diseases by use of rarefied or condensed air. 2. Treatment of diseases of the lungs. SYN: *pneumotherapy.*

pneumatothorax (nū″măt-ō-thō′răks) [″ + *thorax*, chest]. Air or gas accumulation in the pleural cavity. SYN: *pneumothorax.*

pneumaturia (nū″măt-ū′rē-ă) [Gr. *pneuma*, air, + *ouron*, urine]. Excretion of urine containing gas. SYN: *pnematinuria.*

pneumatype (nū′mă-tīp) [″ + *typos*, type]. Deposit of moisture on glass from the breath exhaled through the nostrils with the mouth closed for purpose of comparing the airflow through the nostrils.

pneumectomy (nū-měk′tō-mē) [Gr. *pneumon*, lung, + *ektome*, excision]. Excision of all or part of a lung.

pneumo-, pneumono- [Gr. *pneumon*, lung].

Combining forms meaning air; lung.

pneumoangiography (nū″mō-ăn″jē-ŏg′ră-fē) [Gr. *pneumon*, lung, + *angeion*, vessel, + *graphein*, to write]. X-ray study of the vessels of the lungs, usually performed using a contrast medium.

pneumoarthrography (nū″mō-ăr-thrŏg′ră-fē) [″ + *arthron*, joint, + *graphein*, to write]. Pneumarthrography, q.v.

pneumobulbar (nū″mō-bŭl′băr) [″ + L. *bulbus*, bulbous root]. Concerning the lungs and respiratory center in the medulla oblongata of the brain.

pneumocardial (nū″mō-kăr′dē-ăl) [″ + *kardia*, heart]. Concerning the lungs and heart.

pneumocele (nū′mō-sēl). Pneumatocele.

pneumocentesis (nū″mō-sěn-tē′sĭs) [″ + *kentesis*, a piercing]. Paracentesis, q.v., or surgical puncture of a lung to evacuate a cavity.

pneumocephalus (nū″mō-sěf′ă-lŭs) [Gr. *pneuma*, air, + *kephale*, head]. Gas or air in the cavity of the cranium.

pneumocholecystitis (nū″mō-kō″lē-sĭs-tī′tĭs) [″ + *chole*, bile, + *kystis*, bladder, + *itis*, inflammation]. Cholecystitis with gas in the gallbladder.

pneumococcal (nū″mō-kŏk′ăl) [″ + *kokkos*, berry]. Concerning or caused by pneumococci.

pneumococcal vaccine, polyvalent. A vaccine that contains 23 of the known 83 pneumococcal capsular polysaccharides. The vaccine induces immunity for 3 to 5 years. This vaccine is estimated to protect against 90% of the pneumococcal types that produce serious disease in patients over 2 years of age. Children at high risk can be vaccinated at 6 months of age and reinoculated at 2 years. The vaccine is particularly indicated in high-risk groups such as persons with sickle cell diseases, the elderly, and persons with chronic debilitating disease or with immunologic defects.

pneumococcemia (nū″mō-kŏk-sē′mē-ă). Presence of pneumococci in the blood.

pneumococci (nū″mō-kŏk′sī). Pl. of pneumococcus.

pneumococcidal (nū″mō-kŏk-sī′dăl) [″ + ″ + L. *cidus*, killing]. Killing pneumococci.

pneumococcolysis (nū″mō-kŏk-ŏl′ĭ-sĭs) [″ + *kokkos*, berry, + *lysis*, dissolution]. Destruction or lysis of pneumococci.

pneumococcus (nū″mō-kŏk′ŭs) [″ + *kokkos*, berry] (pl. *pneumococci*). An oval-shaped, encapsulated, non-spore-forming, gram-positive organism occurring usually in pairs (diplococcus) having lancet-shaped ends. There are more than 80 serological types of pneumococci. In addition to causing pneumonia, pneumococci are found to cause infections such as otitis media, mastoiditis, meningitis, bronchitis, bloodstream infections, keratitis, and conjunctivitis. A pneumococcal vaccine is available. Pneumococcal infections are effectively treated with penicillin. Erythromycin may be used if the patient is allergic to penicillin. SYN: *Streptococcus pnemoniae*. SEE: *pneumococcal vaccine, polyvalent; pneumonia.*

pneumocolon (nū″mō-kō′lŏn) [″ + *kolon*, colon]. Air in the colon. This may be introduced as an aid in radiological diagnosis.

pneumoconiosis (nū″mō-kō″nē-ō′sĭs) [″ + *konis*, dust, + *osis*, condition]. A condition of the respiratory tract due to inhalation of dust particles. An occupational disorder such as that caused by mining or stonecutting. SEE: *bituminosis*.

RS: anthracosis; chalicosis; coal worker's pneumoconiosis; pneumomelanosis; siderosis; silicosis.

pneumocranium (nū″mō-krā′nē-ŭm) [″ + *kranion*, skull]. Pneumocephalus, q.v.

Pneumocystis carinii (nū″mō-sĭs′tĭs). The causative organism of pneumocystis carinii pneumonia, q.v. SEE: *AIDS*.

pneumocystis carinii pneumonia. An acute interstitial plasma cell pneumonia characterized by slight if any fever, nonproductive cough, tachypnea, and dyspnea. It is caused by *Pneumocystis carinii*, an organism thought to be a protozoon. This disease is seen in marasmic and other debilitated children, and in immunodeficient adults. SYN: *pneumonia, interstitial plasma cell*. SEE: *AIDS*.

DIAG: Established by demonstration of the organism in tissue obtained by lung biopsy, in aspirations from the lung, or in smears of tracheobronchial mucus.

TREAT: Intravenous sulfamethoxazole-trimethoprim. Pentamidine by inhalation. If the pneumonia is untreated, mortality is quite high.

pneumocystography (nū″mō-sĭs-tŏg′ră-fē) [Gr. *pneuma*, air, + *kystis*, bladder, + *graphein*, to write]. Cystogram done after air has been introduced into the urinary bladder.

pneumocystosis (nū″mō-sĭs-tō′sĭs). SEE: *pneumocystis carinii pneumonia*.

pneumocyte. Pneumonocyte, q.v.

pneumoderma (nū″mō-dĕr′mă) [″ + *derma*, skin]. Emphysema under the skin.

pneumodynamics (nū″mō-dī-năm′ĭks) [″ + *dynamis*, force]. Branch of science dealing with force employed in respiration.

pneumoempyema (nū″mō-ĕm-pī-ē′mă) [″ + *en*, in + *pyon*, pus]. Empyema accompanied by an accumulation of gas.

pneumoencephalitis (nū″mō-ĕn-sĕf″ă-lī′

tĭs) [″ + *enkephalos*, brain, + *itis*, inflammation]. Newcastle disease, q.v.

pneumoencephalogram (nū″mō-ĕn-sĕf″ă-lō-grăm) [″ + ″ + *gramma*, something written]. Roentgenogram of the brain during pneumoencephalography, q.v.

pneumoencephalography (nū″mō-ĕn-sĕf″ă-lŏg′ră-fē) [″ + ″ + *graphein*, to write]. Roentgenographic examination of ventricles and subarachnoid spaces of the brain following withdrawal of cerebrospinal fluid and injection of air or gas via lumbar puncture.

pneumoenteritis (nū″mō-ĕn″tĕr-ī′tĭs) [″ + *enteron*, intestine, + *itis*, inflammation]. Pneumonia and enteritis combined.

pneumofasciogram (nū″mō-făs′ē-ō-grăm) [″ + L. *fascia*, a band, + Gr. *gramma*, something written]. Roentgenogram of fascial tissues and spaces after air has been injected in the fascia.

pneumogalactocele (nū″mō-găl-ăk′tō-sēl) [″ + *gala*, milk, + *kele*, tumor, swelling]. A breast tumor containing milk and gas.

pneumogastric (nū″mō-găs′trĭk) [Gr. *pneumon*, lung, + *gaster*, stomach]. Pert. to the lungs and stomach.

pneumogastric nerve. Term formerly used for the vagus nerve.

pneumogastrography (nū″mō-găs-trŏg′ră-fē) [Gr. *pneuma*, air, + *gaster*, stomach, + *graphein*, to write]. X-ray study of the stomach after air has been introduced into it.

pneumogram (nū′mō-grăm) [″ + *gramma*, something written]. 1. A record of respiratory movements. 2. A roentgenogram following injection of air. SYN: *pneumatogram*.

pneumograph (nū′mō-grăf) [″ + *graphein*, to write]. A device for recording frequency and intensity of respiration.

pneumography (nū-mŏg′ră-fē). 1. Anatomical description or illustration of the lung. 2. Recording of respiratory movements on a graph. 3. Roentgenography of a part or organ after air is injected.

p., pelvic. Roentgenography of the pelvis after CO_2 has been injected into the peritoneal cavity.

pneumohemia (nū″mō-hē′mē-ă) [″ + *haima*, blood]. Presence of air or gas in blood vessels.

pneumohemopericardium (nū″mō-hēm″ō-pĕr-ĭ-kăr′dē-ŭm) [Gr. *pneumon*, lung, + *haima*, blood, + *peri*, around, + *kardia*, heart]. The accumulation of air and blood in the pericardium.

pneumohemorrhagica (nū″mō-hēm-ō-rā′jĭ-kă) [″ + ″ + *rhegnynai*, to burst forth]. Hemorrhage into pulmonary air cells; apoplexy of the lungs.

pneumohemothorax (nŭ″mō-hēm″ō-thō′ răks) [″ + ″ + *thorax*, chest]. Gas or air and blood collected in the pleural cavity.

pneumohydrometra (nŭ″mō-hī″drō-mē′ trä) [″ + *hydor*, water, + *metra*, uterus]. The accumulation of gas and fluid in the uterus.

pneumohydropericardium (nŭ″mō-hī″drō-pĕr-ĭ-kăr′dē-ŭm) [″ + *hydor*, water, + *peri*, around, + *kardia*, heart]. Air and fluid accumulated in the pericardium.

pneumohydrothorax (nŭ″mō-hī″drō-thō′ räks) [″ + ″ + *thorax*, chest]. Gas or air and fluid in the pleural cavity.

pneumohypoderma (nŭ″mō-hī″pō-dĕr′mă) [″ + *hypo*, under, + *derma*, skin]. Air in the tissues under the skin.

pneumokidney (nŭ″mō-kĭd′nē) [″ + ME. *kidenei*, kidney]. Air in the pelvis of the kidney.

pneumolith (nŭ″mō-lĭth) [″ + *lithos*, stone]. A pulmonary calculus.

pneumolithiasis (nŭ″mō-lĭth-ī′ăs-ĭs) [″ + ″ + *-iasis*, condition]. Formation of concretions in the lungs.

pneumology (nū-mŏl′ŏ-jē) [″ + *logos*, word, reason]. The scientific study of diseases of the lungs and air passages.

pneumolysin (nū-mŏl′ĭ-sĭn). A hemolytic toxin produced by pneumococci.

pneumolysis (nū-mŏl′ĭs-ĭs) [″ + *lysis*, dissolution]. Separation of an adherent lung from costal pleura. SYN: *pneumonolysis.*

pneumomalacia (nŭ″mō-mă-lā′shē-ă) [″ + *malakia*, a softening]. Abnormal softening of the lung.

pneumomassage (nŭ″mō-mă-săzh′) [Gr. *pneuma*, air, + *massein*, to knead]. Massage of the tympanum with air to cause movement of the ossicles of the inner ear.

pneumomediastinum (nŭ″mō-mē″dē-ăs-tī′nŭm) [″ + L. *mediastinum*, in the middle]. Presence of air or gas in the mediastinal tissues. It may be present due to disease or following injection of air into the area for diagnostic purposes.

pneumomelanosis (nŭ″mō-mĕl-ăn-ō′sĭs) [Gr. *pneumon*, lung, + *melano*, black, + *osis*, condition]. Pigmentation of the lung seen in pneumoconiosis, q.v.

pneumometer (nū-mŏm′ĕt-ĕr) [Gr. *pneuma*, air, + *metron*, measure]. Instrument for measuring the amount of air inspired and expired in respiration. SYN: *spirometer.*

pneumomycosis (nŭ″mō-mī-kō′sĭs) [Gr. *pneumon*, lung, + *mykes*, fungus, + *osis*, condition]. A fungal pulmonary disease. SYN: *pneumonomycosis.*

pneumomyelography (nŭ″mō-mī-ĕl-ŏg′rä-fē) [Gr. *pneuma*, air + *myelos*, marrow, + *graphein*, to write]. X-ray inspection of

the spinal canal following injection of air or gas.

pneumonectasia, pneumonectasis (nŭ″ mŏn-ĕk-tā′zē-ă, -ĕk′tă-sĭs) [″ + *ektasis*, dilatation]. Distention of lungs with air.

pneumonectomy (nŭ″mŏn-ĕk′tō-mē) [Gr. *pneumon*, lung, + *ektome*, excision]. Removal of a lung. SYN: *pneumectomy; pulmonectomy.*

pneumonia (nū-mō′nē-ă) [Gr.]. Inflammation of the lungs caused primarily by bacteria, viruses, and chemical irritants. There are more than 50 causes; the most common ones are listed in the accompanying table.

SYM: Pneumonia caused by pneumococci, staphylococci, streptococci, or bacilli often begins suddenly. Chills, high fever, pain in the chest, cough, purulent and often bloody sputum. Mortality is high unless treated with an appropriate antibiotic. SEE: *pneumococcal vaccine, polyvalent.*

NURSING IMPLICATIONS: Identify patients at risk for pneumonia. Encourage immunization for aged individuals or those with chronic illness. Provide supportive care for the patient with pneumonia to reduce oxygen demand, remove secretions, and improve gas exchange (position changes; deep breathing, effective coughing, respiratory toilet; active and passive limb exercise; assistance with self-care). Monitor patient's respiratory status via chest assessment and arterial blood gas studies for indications of respiratory failure; e.g., hypoxemia, hypercapnia, deteriorating level of consciousness; and assess for sepsis and shock. Administer prescribed analgesics. Carry out the prescribed medical regimen and evaluate patient response. Encourage patient to verbalize concerns, and explain diagnostic studies and therapeutic measures. Teach patient the importance of follow-up care. SEE: *Nursing Diagnoses* in *Appendix.*

p., abortive. Mild pneumonia with a brief course.

p., acute lobar. Pneumonia caused by pneumococci. SYN: *p., croupous.*

p. alba. A fatal pneumonia of the newborn caused by congenital syphilis.

p., anthrax. Anthrax that affects the lungs.

p., apex, apical. Pneumonia limited to the apices of the lungs; a form of lobar pneumonia.

p., aspiration. Pneumonia after inhaling foreign matter into the lungs.

p., bronchial. A general classification that defines pneumonia due to mixed bacterial infections usually associated with a complication of surgery, aspiration, anesthesia, chronic illnesses, or chronic pulmo-

Pneumonias

Specific Microbial Causes	Disease That May Be Accompanied by Pneumonia	Pneumonia Not Caused by Infections
Viruses	Tularemia	Oil aspiration
Adenoviruses	Brucellosis	Radiation
Influenza	Rheumatic fever	Chemicals
Rhinoviruses	Syphilis	Vegetable dusts
Respiratory syncytial	Typhus	Silo-filler's disease
Coxsackieviruses	Typhoid	
Coronaviruses	Rocky Mountain fever	
	Q fever	
Mycoplasmas	Acute viral respiratory disease	
Mycoplasma pneumoniae	Infectious mononucleosis	
	Trichiniasis	
Cocci	Acquired immune deficiency	
Pneumococcus	syndrome (AIDS)	
Staphylococcus	Psittacosis	
Hemolytic *Streptococcus*	Plague	
	Legionnaires' disease	
Protozoan (probable)	Rickettsial diseases	
Pneumocystis carinii		
Bacilli		
Hemophilus influenzae		
Mycobacterium tuberculosis		
Klebsiella pneumoniae		
(Friedländer's bacillus)		
Gram-negative bacilli		
Chlamydiae		
Chlamydia trachomatis		
C. psittaci		
Fungi		
Histoplasma capsulatum		
Coccidioides immitis		
Rickettsiae		
Rickettsia rickettsii		
R. burnetii		

nary diseases such as bronchiectasis or emphysema. SYN: *bronchopneumonia*.

p., caseous. Pneumonia associated with tuberculosis, in which the lung has undergone necrosis and appears to be cheeselike.

p., central. P., lobar, q.v.

p., congenital aspiration. Pneumonia that existed prior to birth or is due to aspiration during the birth process.

p., contusion. P., traumatic, q.v.

p., croupous. P., acute lobar.

p., deglutition. P., aspiration, q.v.

p., desquamative interstitial. Pneumonia accompanied by cellular infiltration or fibrosis in the pulmonary interstitium. The cause is unknown.

SYM: Progressive dyspnea and nonproductive cough. Clubbing of the fingers is a common finding. Diffusion of oxygen and carbon dioxide is abnormal. Diagnosis is made by lung biopsy.

TREAT: Corticosteroids.

p., double. Pneumonia that involves both lungs.

p., Eaton agent. Pneumonia caused by *Mycoplasma pneumoniae*.

p., embolic. Pneumonia following embolization of a pulmonary blood vessel.

p., eosinophilic. Inflammation of the lung characterized by transient or prolonged pulmonary changes. Principal known causes are parasites such as roundworms or filariae; fungus infection; drugs or chemicals such as nickel, penicillin, aminosalicylic acid, nitrofurantoin, and sulfonamides. In most cases, however, the cause is unknown.

p., fibrinous. Acute lobar pneumonia.

p., fibrous. Pneumonia followed by formation of scar tissue.

p., Friedländer's. A form of lobar pneumonia caused by the specific organism *Klebsiella pneumoniae.*

p., gangrenous. Pulmonary gangrene.

p., giant cell. An interstitial pneumonitis of infancy and childhood. The lung tissue contains multinucleated giant cells. The disease often occurs in connection with measles. SYN: *Hecht pneumonia.*

p., hypostatic. Pneumonia occurring in the elderly or debilitated patient who constantly remains in the same position. Posterior and lower areas of the lung are poorly aerated and collapse due to lack of deep breathing and pressure from nearby tissues and organs, and gravity contributes to local alveolar fluid congestion and capillary pooling. Congestion contributes to infection, by tending to promote the development of bacterial or viral pneumonia.

NURSING IMPLICATIONS: Prevention is the most important factor, especially in the elderly and those who are immobile. SEE: *pneumonia.*

p., influenza. 1. Pneumonia that occurs in association with influenza. The disease may be fatal. 2. Pneumonia caused by *Haemophilus influenzae.*

p., interstitial. Pneumonia with inflammation of the tissues surrounding the air passages rather than the bronchi, bronchioles, and alveoli themselves.

p., interstitial plasma cell. Pneumocystis carinii pneumonia, q.v.

p., intrauterine. Pneumonia contracted in utero.

p., Legionella. An acute lobar pneumonia caused by *Legionella pneumophila.* SEE: *Legionnaires' disease.*

p., lipid. Pneumonia after aspiration of oily substances such as oily nose drops or mineral or other bland oil.

p., lobar. Pneumonia infecting one or more lobes of the lung. It is usually caused by *Streptococcus pneumoniae.* The pathological changes are, in order, first congestion; then redness and firmness due to exudate and red blood cells in the alveoli; and, finally, gray hepatization as the exudate degenerates and is absorbed.

p., migratory. Pneumonia in which infected area shifts from one part of the lung to another part.

p., pneumocystis carinii. SEE: *pneumocystis carinii pneumonia.*

p., primary atypical. A relatively mild pneumonia characterized by cough, fever, pharyngitis, and radiological evidence of lung infiltration out of proportion to the minimal findings upon examining the lungs.

Caused by *Mycoplasma pneumoniae.*

TREAT: Tetracyclines and erythromycin are effective.

p., secondary. Pneumonia that occurs in connection with a specific systemic disease such as typhoid, diphtheria, or plague.

p., staphylococcal. Pneumonia due to infection with staphylococci.

p., streptococcal. Pneumonia due to infection with *Streptococcus pneumoniae.*

p., terminal. Lethal pneumonia that occurs secondary to another disease.

p., traumatic. Pneumonia that occurs after trauma to the lung or the thoracic cage. SYN: *p., contusion.*

p., tuberculous. Pneumonia caused by the tubercle bacilli. May result in rapid and widespread inflammatory exudation. If untreated, it may run a malignant course, ending fatally, or may subside and become chronic.

p., tularemic. Pneumonia caused by *Francisella tularensis.* May be primary or associated with tularemia, q.v.

p., typhoid. Pneumonia complicating typhoid fever.

p. varicella. Pneumonia complicating chickenpox.

p., viral. An acute systemic disease caused by a variety of viruses, including those that cause childhood exanthems. Symptoms vary, ranging from those of the common cold to those of progressive respiratory insufficiency. Prognosis is influenced by the type of viral agent, age of the patient, extent of pulmonary involvement, and underlying systemic disease. SEE: *influenza.*

p., woolsorter's. Pulmonary anthrax.

pneumonic (nū-mŏn'ĭk) [Gr. *pneumon,* lung]. Concerning the lungs or pneumonia.

pneumonitis (nū″mō-nī'tĭs) [″ + *itis,* inflammation]. Inflammation of the lung. SYN: *pneumonia.*

p., hypersensitivity. A diffuse granulomatous lung disease caused by hypersensitivity to inhalation of organic dusts. Usually occurs in those with a hobby or occupation that involves heavy exposure to dust. SYN: *allergic alveolitis.* SEE: *bagassosis; farmer's lung.*

p., mycoplasma. Pneumonia caused by mycoplasma organisms. SYN: *pneumonia, primary atypical.*

p., pneumococcal. Pneumonia in which the causative agent is pneumococci, q.v. A vaccine is available for this form of pneumonia. Its effectiveness is much greater in young persons than in those who are elderly. SEE: *pneumococcal vaccine, polyvalent.*

pneumono- [Gr. *pneumon,* lung]. Combining form pert. to the lung.

pneumonocele (nū-mŏn′ō-sēl) [″ + *kele*, tumor, swelling]. A pulmonary hernia. SYN: *pneumatocele; pneumocele.*

pneumonocentesis (nū-mō″nō-sĕn-tē′sĭs) [″ + *kentesis*, a piercing]. Pneumocentesis, q.v.

pneumonoconiosis (nū-mō″nō-kō″nē-ō′sĭs) [″ + *konis*, dust, + *osis*, condition]. Fibrous inflammation or chronic induration of the lungs resulting from inhalation of dust. SYN: *pneumoconiosis.*

pneumonocyte. Alveolar cell of the lung. It may function as an epithelial cell or as a macrophage.

pneumonograph (nū-mŏn′ō-grăf) [″ + *graphein*, to write]. A roentgenogram of the lungs.

pneumonography (nū″mŏn-ŏg′ră-fē). Roentgenography of the lungs.

pneumonolysis (nū″mŏn-ŏl′ĭs-ĭs) [″ + *lysis*, dissolution]. Loosening of an adherent lung from the chest wall to induce collapse of lung. SYN: *pneumolysis.*

    p., extrapleural. Separation of parietal pleura from the chest wall. SEE: *apicolysis.*

    p., intrapleural. Separation of adhering visceral and parietal layers of pleura.

pneumonomelanosis (nū″mō-nō-mĕl″ăn-ō′sĭs) [″ + *melano*, black, + *osis*, condition]. Darkening of the lung tissue as a result of inhalation of black dust particles such as coal dust. SYN: *pneumomelanosis.*

pneumonomycosis (nū-mŏn″ō-mī-kō′sĭs) [″ + *mykes*, fungus, + *osis*, condition]. Disease of the lungs caused by fungi. SYN: *pneumomycosis.*

pneumonopathy (nū″mō-nŏp′ăth-ē) [″ + *pathos*, disease, suffering]. Any diseased condition of the lung.

pneumonoperitonitis (nū″mō-nō-pĕr″ĭ-tō-nī′tĭs) [″ + *peritonaion*, peritoneum, + *itis*, inflammation]. Peritonitis with gas in the peritoneal cavity.

pneumonopexy (nū-mō″nō-pĕk′sē) [″ + *pexis*, fixation]. Surgical attachment of the lung to the chest wall. SYN: *pneumopexy.*

pneumonopleuritis (nū-mō″nō-ploo-rī′tĭs) [Gr. *pneumon*, lung, + *pleura*, side, + *itis*, inflammation]. Pneumopleuritis, q.v.

pneumonorrhapy (nū″mō-nor′ă-fē) [″ + *rhaphe*, seam, ridge]. Suture of a lung.

pneumonosis (nū-mō-nō′sĭs) [″ + *osis*, condition]. Any noninfective disease or disorder of the lungs, esp. those resulting from degenerative processes.

pneumonotherapy. Pneumotherapy, q.v.

pneumonotomy (nū-mō-nŏt′ō-mē) [″ + *tome*, incision]. Incision into the lung. SYN: *pneumotomy.*

pneumoparotiditis. Aeroparotiditis, q.v.

pneumopathy (nū-mŏp′ă-thē) [″ + *pathos*, disease]. Any disease of the lungs.

pneumopericardium (nū″mō-pĕr-ĭ-kăr′dē-ŭm) [Gr. *pneuma*, air, + *peri*, around, + *kardia*, heart]. Air or gas in the pericardial sac.

    ETIOL: Trauma or pathological communication between the esophagus, stomach, or lungs and the pericardium.

    SYM: Unusual metallic heart sounds, tympany over precordial area.

pneumoperitoneography. Radiographic examination of the peritoneum and internal organs after introduction of sterile air into the peritoneal cavity.

pneumoperitoneum (nū″mō-pĕr-ĭ-tō-nē′ŭm) [″ + *peritonaion*, peritoneum]. Condition in which air or gas is collected in the peritoneal cavity. May be artificially induced to treat tuberculous peritonitis. SYN: *pneumatosis abdominis.*

pneumoperitonitis (nū″mō-pĕr-ĭ-tō-nī′tĭs) [″ + *peritonaion*, peritoneum, + *itis*, inflammation]. Peritonitis with gas accumulation.

pneumopexy (nū′mō-pĕks″ē) [Gr. *pneumon*, lung, + *pexis*, fixation]. Surgical attachment of a lung to the thoracic wall. SYN: *pneumonopexy.*

pneumopleuritis (nū″mō-ploo-rī′tĭs) [″ + *pleura*, a side, + *itis*, inflammation]. Inflamed condition of lungs and pleura.

pneumopleuroparietopexy (nū″mō-ploo″rō-pă-rī″ĕt-ō-pĕk″sē) [″ + ″ + L. *paries*, wall, + Gr. *pexis*, fixation]. The operation of attaching the lung with its parietal pleura to the border of the thoracic wound.

pneumopyelography (nū″mō-pī-ĕ-lŏg′ră-fē) [Gr. *pneuma*, air, + *pyelos*, pelvis, + *graphein*, to write]. X-ray examination of the renal pelvis and ureters after they are injected with oxygen.

pneumopyopericardium (nū″mō-pī″ō-pĕr-ĭ-kar′dē-ŭm) [″ + *pyon*, pus, + *peri*, around, + *kardia*, heart]. Air, gas, and pus collected in the pericardial sac.

pneumopyothorax (nū″mō-pī″ō-thō′răks) [″ + ″ + *thorax*, chest]. Air and pus collected in the pleural cavity.

pneumoradiography (nū″mō-rā-dē-ŏg′ră-fē) [″ + L. *radius*, ray, + Gr. *graphein*, to write]. Injection of air into a part for the purpose of taking an x-ray picture.

pneumoretroperitoneum (nū″mō-rĕt″rō-pĕr″ĭ-tō-nē′ŭm) [″ + L. *retro*, backwards, + Gr. *peritonaion*, peritoneum]. Air or gas in the retroperitoneal space.

pneumorrhachis (nū″mō-rā′kĭs) [Gr. *pneumon*, lung, + *rhachis*, spine]. Gas accumulation in the spinal canal.

pneumorrhagia (nū″mō-rā′jē-ă) [Gr. *pneumon*, lung, + *rhegnynai*, to burst forth]. Pulmonary hemorrhage. SYN: *hemptysis.*

pneumoserothorax (nū″mō-sē-rō-thō′răks) [Gr. *pneuma,* air, + L. *serum,* whey, + Gr. *thorax,* chest]. Air or gas and serum collected in the pleural cavity.

pneumosilicosis (nū″mō-sĭl″ĭ-kō′sĭs) [Gr. *pneumon,* lung, + L. *silex,* flint, + Gr. *osis,* condition]. Silicosis, q.v.

pneumotachograph (nū″mō-tăk′ō-grăf) [Gr. *pneuma,* air, + *tachys,* swift, + *graphein,* to write]. Device for registering velocity of inspired air.

pneumotachometer (nū″mō-tăk-ŏm′ĕ-tĕr) [″ + *tachos,* speed, + *metron,* measure]. Device for measuring expired air flow.

pneumotaxic (nū″mō-tăk′sĭk) [″ + *taxis,* arrangement]. Concerning the regulation of breathing.

pneumotherapy (nū-mō-thĕr′ă-pē). 1. [Gr. *pneumon,* lung, + *therapeia,* treatment] Treatment of diseases of the lungs. 2. [Gr. *pneuma,* air, + *therapeia,* treatment] Treatment of diseases by the use of rarefied or condensed gases. SYN: *pneumonotherapy.*

pneumothermomassage (nū″mō-thĕr″mō-măs-ăzh′) [Gr. *pneuma,* air, + *therme,* heat, + *massein,* to knead]. Application to the body of air of varying temperature and pressure.

pneumothorax (nū-mō-thō′răks) [″ + *thorax,* chest]. A collection of air or gas in the pleural cavity. The gas enters as the result of a perforation through the chest wall or the pleura covering the lung (visceral pleura). This perforation may be the result of an injury or of the rupture of an emphysematous bleb or superficial lung abscess. The most common cause of the last condition is a tuberculous abscess in the presence of pulmonary tuberculosis. SYN: *aeropleura; aerothorax; pneumatothorax.* SEE: illus. SEE: *Nursing Diagnoses* in Appendix.

SYM: The onset is sudden, usually with a severe sharp pain in the side and marked dyspnea. Fluid very frequently is found, developing within 48 hours (hydropneumothorax). The physical signs are those of a distended unilateral chest, tympanitic resonance, absence of breath sounds, and if fluid is present, a splashing sound on succussion (or shaking) of the patient.

NURSING IMPLICATIONS: Explain the procedure for chest tube insertion to the patient and assist as necessary. Assess vital signs, breath sounds, chest expansion, chest tube site, drainage, and blood gas analysis. Administer oxygen as prescribed. Implement coughing and deep breathing and chest physical therapy. Place patient in semi-Fowler's position to promote drainage, comfort, and ease of breathing. Provide adequate rest periods. Establish range of motion exercises and activity as tolerated. Administer medications as prescribed (analgesics, antibiotics, expectorants). Monitor intake and output. Maintain adequate nutrition and fluid intake to promote tissue healing and repair and to promote secretion liquefaction. Observe catheter site daily and redress daily or as necessary. Have patient avoid excessive exercise and avoid smoking. Stress the importance of follow-up examination. Teach patient care of the insertion site after discharge.

p., artificial. Pneumothorax induced intentionally by artificial means, employed in the treatment of pulmonary tuberculosis or pneumonia. Pneumothorax gives the diseased lung temporary rest. The lung collapses when the air enters the pleural space.

Scattered adhesions may afford only a partial collapse. Effusion may occur in about one-third of the cases. Hazards are minimal.

p., extrapleural. Formation of a pneumothorax by introducing air into the space between the pleura and the inside of the rib cage.

p., open. Pneumothorax in which the pleural cavity is exposed to the atmosphere through an open wound in the chest wall.

p., spontaneous. Spontaneous entrance of air into the pleural cavity. The pressure may collapse the lung and displace the mediastinum away from the side of the lesion. SYM: Sudden sharp pain, dyspnea, and cough. Pain may be referred to the shoulder. Majority of cases are mild and require only rest. Rarely shock and collapse occur.

p., tension. A type of pneumothorax in which air can enter the pleural space but cannot escape via the route of entry. This leads to an increase of pressure in the pleural space with collapse of the lung.

NURSING IMPLICATIONS: Assess for pallor, gasping respirations, and sudden, sharp chest pain. Auscultate for decreased breath sounds over area of collapsed lung, and inspect for mediastinal shift (deviation of trachea away from affected side). Assess vital signs for hypotension, tachypnea and tachycardia, ominous signs indicating need for immediate water-seal chest tube drainage.

p., therapeutic. P., artificial, q.v.

p., valvular. Pneumothorax characterized by an opening through the pleura, which has a slit with a valvelike action, allowing the air to pass in but not out. SYN: *tension pneumothorax.*

pneumotomy (nū-mŏt′ō-mē) [Gr. *pneumon,* lung, + *tome,* incision]. Incision of the lung.

pneumotoxin (nū″mō-tŏks′ĭn) [″ + *toxi-*

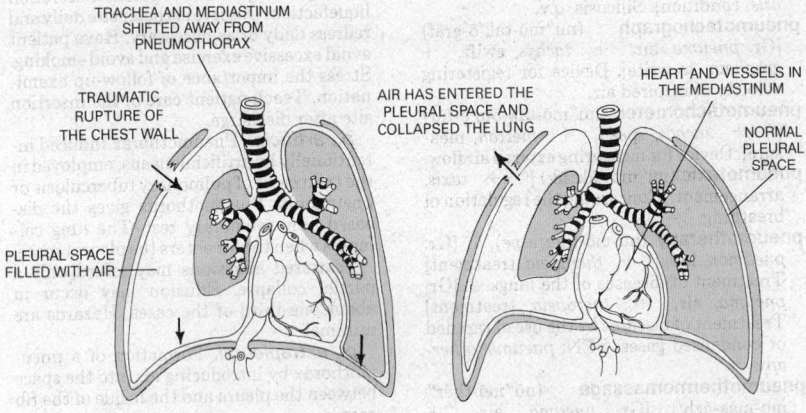

PNEUMOTHORAX
(OPEN—THE CHEST WALL INJURY PERMITS
AIR TO FLOW IN AND OUT OF THE PLEURAL
SPACE ON THE AFFECTED SIDE)

TRACHEA AND MEDIASTINUM
SHIFTED AWAY FROM
PNEUMOTHORAX

TRAUMATIC
RUPTURE OF
THE CHEST WALL

AIR HAS ENTERED THE
PLEURAL SPACE AND
COLLAPSED THE LUNG

HEART AND VESSELS IN
THE MEDIASTINUM

NORMAL
PLEURAL
SPACE

PLEURAL SPACE
FILLED WITH AIR

INHALATION: AIR ENTERS THE INJURED
SIDE, CAUSING COLLAPSE OF THE LUNG
AND SHIFT OF THE MEDIASTINUM AND
HEART TOWARD THE UNAFFECTED SIDE

EXHALATION: THE AIR IS PARTIALLY
FORCED FROM THE AFFECTED SIDE
PLEURAL SPACE AND THE MEDIASTINUM
SHIFTS TOWARD THE AFFECTED SIDE

kon, poison]. A toxin produced by pneumo-coccus.

pneumotyphus (nū″mō-tī′fŭs) [″ + *typhos*, fever]. 1. Typhoid fever with pneumonia at onset. 2. Development of pneumonia during typhoid fever.

pneumouria (nū″mō-ū′rē-ă) [Gr. *pneuma*, air, + *ouron*, urine]. Excretion of urine with free gas. SYN: *pneumaturia*.

pneumoventricle (nū″mō-vĕn′trĭ-kl) [″ + L. *ventriculus*, little belly]. Air accumulation in the cerebral ventricles.

pneumoventriculography (nū″mō-vĕn-trĭk″ū-lŏg′ră-fē) [″ + ″ + Gr. *graphein*, to write]. Radiography of the ventricles of the brain after the injection of air.

pneusis (nū′sĭs) [Gr. *pnein*, to breathe]. 1. Respiration. 2. Panting.

pnigophobia (nī″gŏ-fō′bē-ă) [Gr. *pnigos*, choking, + *phobos*, fear]. Morbid fear of choking; sometimes experienced in angina pectoris.

Po. Chem. symb. for the element polonium.

Po₂. Abbr. for *partial pressure of oxygen*.

p.o. L. *per os*, i.e., by mouth.

pock (pŏk) [AS. *poc*, pustule]. A pustule of an eruptive fever, esp. of smallpox.

pocket (pŏk′ĕt) [ME. *poket*, pouch]. A saclike cavity.

p., gingival. A gingival sulcus of abnormal depth. SYN: *periodontal pocket*.

p., pseudo-. Pocket that results from gingival inflammation with edema that produces an apparent abnormal depth of the gingival sulcus without apical movement of the bottom of the sulcus; a false pocket.

pocket face mask. Folding mask with oxygen inlet valve that can be carried in a pocket and used for artificial ventilation.

pocketing. Method of treating the pedicle in ovariotomy by enclosing it within the edges of the wound.

pockmarked. Pitted or marked with cicatrices from healed pustules, esp. those due to smallpox.

poculum diogenis (pŏk′ū-lŭm dī-ōj′ĕ-nĭs) [L. *poculum*, cup, + Diogenes, Gr. philosopher, 4th century B.C.]. The concavity formed by contracting the muscles of the hand so the palm becomes cupped instead of flat.

podagra (pō-dăg′ră) [Gr. *podos*, foot, + *agra*, seizure]. Gout, esp. of the joints of the foot or of the great toe.

podalgia (pō-dăl′jē-ă) [″ + *algos*, pain]. Pain in the feet.

podalic (pō-dăl′ĭk) [Gr. *podos*, foot]. Pert. to the feet.

podalic version. Shifting position of a fetus to bring the feet to the outlet in labor.

podarthritis (pŏd″ăr-thrī′tĭs) [″ + *arthron*, joint, + *itis*, inflammation]. Inflammation of any tarsal or metatarsal joints of the feet. SYN: *podagra.*

podedema (pŏd″e-dē′mă) [″ + *oidema*, swelling]. Edema of the feet.

podencephalus (pŏd″ĕn-sĕf′ă-lŭs) [″ + *enkephalos*, brain]. A deformed individual in whom most of the brain is outside the skull and is attached by a thin pedicle.

podiatrist (pō-dī′ă-trĭst″) [″ + *iatreia*, treatment]. A health professional responsible for the examination, diagnosis, prevention, treatment, and care of conditions and functions of the human foot. A podiatrist performs surgical procedures and prescribes corrective devices, drugs, and physical therapy as legally authorized in the state in which he or she is practicing. SYN: *chiropodist.*

podiatry (pō-dī′ă-trē). The diagnosis, treatment, and prevention of conditions of human feet. SYN: *chiropody.*

podium (pō′dē-ŭm) [Gr. *podos*, foot]. A footlike projection.

podo-, pod- [Gr. *pous, podos*, foot]. Combining forms rel. to the foot or resemblance to a foot.

podobromidrosis (pŏd″ō-brō″mĭ-drō′sĭs) [″ + *bromos*, stench, + *hidros*, sweat]. Offensive perspiration of the feet.

podocyte (pŏd′ō-sīt) [″ + *kytos*, cell]. A special epithelial cell that forms an incomplete covering for the glomerulus of the kidney.

pododynamometer (pŏd″ō-dī″nă-mŏm′ĕ-tĕr) [″ + *dynamis*, force, + *metron*, measure]. Device for testing strength of the leg and foot muscles.

pododynia (pŏd″ō-dĭn′ē-ă) [″ + *odyne*, pain]. Pain in the feet, esp. a neuralgic pain in the heel with swelling and redness.

podogram (pŏd′ō-grăm) [″ + *gramma*, something written]. An imprint or outline of the sole of the foot.

podograph (pŏd′ō-grăf) [″ + *graphein*, to write]. Device for taking an imprint of the sole of the foot.

podology (pŏd-ŏl′ō-jē) [″ + *logos*, word, reason]. The study of the anatomy and physiology of the foot.

podophyllum (pŏd-ō-fĭl′ŭm) [″ + *phyllon*, leaf]. USP. The dried rhizome and roots of *Podophyllum peltatum.* Used for treating, by direct application, certain papillomas such as verruca acuminata. SEE: *verruca acuminata.*

podophyllum resin (pŏd″ō-fĭl′ŭm). USP. The resinous extract from podophyllum, q.v.

pogoniasis (pŏ″gō-nī′ă-sĭs) [Gr. *pogon*, beard, + *-iasis*, disorder]. 1. Excessive growth of the beard. 2. Growth of a beard in a woman.

pogonion (pō-gō′nē-ŏn). The most anterior projecting midpoint of the chin.

-poiesis [Gr.]. Suffix meaning pertaining to formation or production, as in hematopoiesis.

-poietic [Gr.]. Suffix meaning pertaining to making or producing something.

poikilo- [Gr. *poikilos*, spotted, varied or mottled]. Combining form concerning state of being irregular or mottled.

poikiloblast (poy′kĭ-lō-blăst″) [Gr. *poikilos*, varied, + *blastos*, germ]. A nucleated red cell of irregular shape.

poikilocyte (poy′kĭl-ō-sīt) [″ + *kytos*, cell]. SEE: *dacryocyte.*

poikilocytosis (poy″kĭl-ō-sī-tō′sĭs) [″ + ″ + *osis*, condition]. Term used to describe variations in shape of red blood corpuscles. Examples are elliptocytes, spherocytes, dacryocytes, sickle cells, schizocytes, echinocytes, and acanthocytes.

poikilodentosis (poy″kĭ-lō-dĕn-tō′sĭs) [″ + L. *dens*, tooth, + Gr. *osis*, condition]. Mottling of the teeth usually due to an excess of fluoride in the drinking water.

poikiloderma (poy-kĭl-ō-dĕr′mă) [″ + *derma*, skin]. A skin disorder characterized by pigmentation, telangiectasia, purpura, pruritus, and atrophy.

    p. atrophicans vasculare. A generalized dermatitis of unknown cause. It is symmetrical and occurs almost exclusively in adults. There is widespread telangiectasia, pigmentation, and atrophy of the skin.

    p. of Civatte. Reticulated pigmentation and telangiectasia of the sides of the face and neck. Seen quite commonly in middle-aged women.

poikilonymy (poy″kĭ-lŏn′ĭ-mē) [″ + *onoma*, name]. The use of terms from several nomenclature systems.

poikilotherm (poy-kĭl′ō-thĕrm) [″ + *therme*, heat]. An animal whose body temperature varies according to the temperature of the environment. SYN: *allotherm.* SEE: *homotherm.*

poikilothermal, poikilothermic (poy″kĭ-lō-thĕr′măl, -mĭk). Concerning poikilothermy.

poikilothermy (poy″kĭ-lō-thĕr′mē). The condition of having the temperature of the organism or animal match the temperature of the environment. Reptiles have this property. SEE: *homoiotherm.*

poikilothrombocyte (poy-kĭl″ō-thrŏm′bō-sīt) [″ + *thrombos*, clot, + *kytos*, cell]. A blood platelet of abnormal shape.

point (poynt) [O.Fr., a prick, a dot]. 1. The sharp end of any object. 2. Stage at which the surface of an abscess is about to rupture. 3. A minute spot. 4. Position in space, time, or degree.

p., absorbent. A cone of paper used in drying or in keeping liquid medicines in a root canal of a tooth.

p., acupuncture. Specific anatomical locations where needles are inserted and stimulated to achieve anesthesia or pain relief by the acupuncture method.

p., auricular. Center of the external orifice of the auditory canal. SYN: *p., Broca's.*

p., Boas'. A tender spot left of the 12th thoracic vertebra in patients with gastric ulcer.

p., boiling. The temperature at which a liquid will boil.

p., Broca's. P., auricular.

p.'s, Capuron's. Four fixed points in the pelvic inlet, the two iliopectineal eminences and the two sacroiliac joints. SYN: *p.'s, cardinal* (def. 2).

p.'s, cardinal. 1. Six points determining the direction of light rays emerging from and entering the eye. SEE: *p.'s, nodal; p.'s, principal.* 2. P.'s, Capuron's.

p., cold rigor. The temperature at which cell activity ceases.

p., contact. Point on a tooth that touches an opposed tooth.

p., convergence. 1. Point to which rays of light converge. 2. The closest point to the patient on which the eyes can converge as the object is moved closer and closer.

p., corresponding. Point in the retina of each eye that, when stimulated simultaneously, results in a single visual sensation.

p., craniometric. One of the fixed points of the skull used in craniometry.

p., critical, of gases. Temperature at or above which a gas is no longer liquefied by pressure.

p., critical, of liquids. Temperature above which no pressure may retain a substance in a liquid form.

p.'s, deaf, of ear. Several points or areas close to the external auditory meatus where a vibrating tuning fork will not be heard.

p., dew. The temperature at which moisture begins to be condensed and deposited as dew.

p.'s, disparate. Points on the retinae unequally paired.

p., end-. The point or time at which a reaction or activity is completed.

p., Erb's. Point on the side of the neck, 2 to 3 cm above the clavicle and in front of the transverse process of the sixth cervical vertebra. Electrical stimulation over this area causes various arm muscles to contract.

p., external orbital. The prominent point at outer edge of orbit above the frontomalar suture.

p., far. Point (20 ft [6.1 meters] or more) at which distinct vision is possible without aid of the muscles of accommodation. It may be nearer than 20 ft (6.1 meters) according to degree of myopia. There is no far point in the hypermetropic eye.

p., fixation. Point at which the two visual axes converge.

p., flash. The lowest temperature at which a volatile liquid will ignite.

p., focal. Point at which a group of light rays converge.

p., freezing. Temperature at which liquids become solid.

p., fusion. Melting point.

p., Guéneau de Mussy's. Pressure on this point causes pain in cases of diaphragmatic pleurisy. The point is located at the junction of a line extending down from the left border of the sternum with a horizontal line at the level of the bony part of the anterior portion of the tenth rib.

p., gutta-percha. Cone made of guttapercha combined with other material that is used in filling root canals of teeth.

p., Halle's. Point at the intersection of a horizontal line drawn from the anterior superior iliac spines and an angled line extending up from the pubic spine. At that point, the ureter is palpable as it crosses the pelvic brim.

p., hot. A spot on the skin that perceives hot but not cold stimuli.

p.'s, hysterogenic. Circumscribed areas of the body that produce symptoms of a hysterical aura, and eventually a hysterical attack, when rubbed or pressed.

p., ice. The temperature at which there is equilibrium between ice and air-saturated water at one atmosphere of pressure.

p.'s, identical retinal. Points in the two retinae upon which the images are seen as one.

p., isoelectric. The particular pH of a solution of an amphoteric electrolyte such as an amino acid or protein in which the charged molecules do not migrate to either electrode. Proteins are least soluble at this point. Thus at the appropriate pH, proteins may be precipitated.

p., isoionic. The pH at which a solution of ionized material has as many negative as positive ions.

p., jugal. Posterior border of frontal process of the malar bone where cut by a line tangent to upper border of zygoma.

p., lacrimal. Outlet of lacrimal canaliculus. SYN: *punctum lacrimale* [NA].

p., Lanz's. Point on the line between the

two anterior superior iliac spines, one-third of the distance from the right spine, indicating origin of the vermiform appendix.

p., Lian's. Point at junction of outer and middle thirds of a line from the umbilicus to the anterior superior spine of ilium where a trocar may be introduced safely for paracentesis.

p., malar. The most prominent point on the external tubercle of the malar bone.

p., maximum occipital. The point on the occipital bone farthest from the glabella.

p., McBurney's. Point 1½ to 2 in. (4.1 to 5.1 cm) above the anterosuperior spine of the ilium, on a line between the ilium and umbilicus, where pressure produces tenderness in acute appendicitis.

p., median mandibular. Point on the anterior-posterior center of the mandibular ridge in the median sagittal plane.

p., melting. The temperature at which a solid becomes a liquid. This is a constant for each material.

p., mental. The most anterior point of the midline of the chin. SYN: *pogonion.*

p., metopic. Glabella, q.v.

p., motor. Point usually about the middle of a muscle where a motor nerve enters the muscle at which a minimal electrical stimulus to the overlying skin will elicit a visible contraction.

p., Munro's. Point halfway between the left anterior iliac spine and the umbilicus.

p., nasal. Nasion, q.v.

p., near. Nearest point at which the eye can accommodate for distinct vision.

p.'s, nodal. An anterior and a posterior cardinal point on the surface of lens of the eye so related that every ray directed toward the anterior point is represented after refraction by a ray emanating from the posterior point.

p., occipital. The most posterior point on the occipital bone.

p. of maximal impulse. ABBR: P.M.I. Point on the chest wall over the heart at which the contraction of the heart is best seen or felt. Normally at the 4th to 5th intercostal space in the midclavicular line.

p. of regard. Point at which the eye is looking.

p.'s, painful. Points over which a neuralgic nerve is tender on pressure. SYN: *p.'s, Valleix's.*

p., preauricular. Point immediately in front of the auricular point.

p.'s, pressure. 1. Points on the skin that, when stimulated, give rise to sensation of pressure. 2. Points where arteries come near the surface and at which pressure may be applied to stop arterial bleeding.

p.'s, principal. Two points so situated that the optical axis is cut by the two principal planes.

p., silver. An elongated, tapered silver plug used to fill the root canal in the endodontic treatment of teeth.

p., spinal. P., subnasal, q.v.

p., subnasal. Center of the root of the anterior nasal spine.

p., supra-auricular. Point on the skull on the posterior root of the zygomatic process of the temporal bone, directly above the auricular point.

p., supranasal. P., supraorbital, q.v.

p., supraorbital. 1. Point on the skull in the midline of the forehead, just above the glabella. SYN: *ophryon.* 2. A neuralgic point just above the supraorbital notch.

p., thermal death. The temperature required to kill all of the organisms in a culture in a specified time.

p., trigger. A spot at which the application of pressure will cause pain. The pain is not necessarily in the area of the pressure.

p., triple. The temperature and pressure at which a substance that can exist in three phases, liquid, solid, and gas, is at equilibrium.

p.'s, Trousseau's apophysiary. Sensitive points over the dorsal and lumbar vertebrae in neuralgia.

p.'s, Valleix's. Tender spots upon pressure over the course of a nerve in neuralgia. SYN: *p.'s, painful.*

p., vital. Point in the medulla oblongata close to the floor of the fourth ventricle, puncture of which causes instant death due to destruction of the respiratory center.

p., Voillemier's. Point on the linea alba of the abdominal wall about 6 to 7 cm below a line connecting the anterior superior iliac spines. Suprapubic puncture of the bladder may be made at this point in obese or edematous individuals.

pointillage (pwän″tĭ-yäzh′) [Fr.]. Massage with finger tips.

pointing. Reaching a point.

poise (poyz) [J. M. Poiseuille]. The unit of viscosity. The tangential shearing force required to be applied to an area of 1 square cm between two parallel planes of 1 square cm in area and 1 cm apart in order to produce a velocity of flow of the liquid of 1 cm per second.

Poiseuille's law (pwă-zŭ′yĕz) [Jean Marie Poiseuille, Fr. physiologist, 1799–1869]. A law that states that the rapidity of the capillary current is in direct proportion to the fourth power of the radius of the capillary tube, the pressure on the fluid, and indirectly to the viscosity of the liquid and length of the tube. The formula is:

$$\text{rate of flow} = \frac{\pi p r^4}{8ln}$$

where $\pi = 3.1416$; p = pressure; r = radius of tube; l = length of tube; and n = coefficient of viscosity of the liquid.

Poiseuille's space. The inert capillary current in which leukocytes close to the wall of the vessel move slowly; the erythrocytes travel more rapidly in the middle current.

POISINDEX®. A computerized database of information, revised quarterly, on over 300,000 commercial compounds. For information, contact Micromedex Inc., 600 Grant St., Denver, CO 80203; (800) 525-9083.

poison (poy'zn) [L. *potio,* a poisonous draft]. Any substance taken into the body by ingestion, inhalation, injection, or absorption that interferes with normal physiological functions. Virtually any substance can be poisonous if consumed in sufficient quantity; therefore the term poison more often implies an excessive degree of dosage rather than a specific group of substances. Aspirin is not usually thought of as a poison, but overdoses of this drug kill more children accidentally each year than any of the traditional poisons. Because the list of poisonous substances is infinite, it defies classification in any simple way. For a list of commonly encountered hazardous substances in the home, SEE: *Poisons and Poisoning* in *Appendix.*

    p., cellular. Anything that damages or kills cells.

    p., pesticidal. Chemicals whose toxic properties are commercially exploited in agriculture, industry, or commerce to increase quantity, improve quality, or generally promote consumer acceptability of a variety of products. Common types include insecticides, rodenticides, herbicides, defoliants, fungicides, insect repellants, molluscicides, and some kinds of food additives. The wide variety of poisons commonly found in and around the home constitutes an important source of accidental poisonings. SEE: *Poisons and Poisoning* in *Appendix.*

poison control center. A facility meeting the staffing and equipment standards of the American Association of Poison Control Centers and recognized to be able to give information on, or treatment to patients suffering from, poisoning. A poison information center consists only of a reference library and does not have treatment facilities. Over 400 poison centers of these two types are scattered throughout the U.S. Staffed largely by volunteer personnel, they offer 24-hour service. By virtue of their function, they are commonly associated with or are part of large hospitals or medical schools. A government agency—the Bureau of Drugs Division of the Poison Control Branch of the Food and Drug Administration, U.S. Department of Health and Human Services—is also active in poison control programs and in coordinating the efforts of individual centers. For address and telephone number of state or province control center, SEE: *Poison Control Centers* in *Appendix.*

poisoning [L. *potio,* a poisonous draft]. 1. The state produced by introduction of a poison into the body. 2. Administration of a poison. Symptoms of poisoning vary widely with the agent. SEE: *Poisons and Poisoning* in *Appendix.*

    NURSING IMPLICATIONS: Identify the poison and contact the local poison control center for directions. In certain types of poisons, a physical, mechanical, or physiological antidote will help to decrease absorption, protect body tissues, or reverse the effects of the poison.

    Establish and maintain the airway; administer oxygen as ordered. If indicated and safe to do so, induce vomiting by tickling the back of the throat or administering large quantities of water, saline, milk, soap solution, or ipecac syrup.

    Support the patient physically and psychologically. Hospitalize for treatment and close observation. Treat for shock. Keep the patient warm. Provide appropriate nursing measures to the convulsing patient to prevent injury. Monitor intake and output. Monitor fluid and electrolyte balance. Reduce elevated temperature by use of cool or alcohol sponge bath and use of antipyretics. Assist with medical procedures such as dialysis.

    Teach patient and family methods to avoid food contamination, to place toxic substances in a safe place out of children's reach, and to place the poison control center's telephone number with the list of emergency numbers. Instruct the family to have ipecac syrup in the household.

    NOTE: Do not be hasty in concluding that a patient has been poisoned. Many disease states mimic the symptoms of poisoning. Cerebral hemorrhage, epilepsy, overdose of insulin, diabetic coma, meningitis, thrombosis, and uremia may simulate poisoning. Acute indigestion, appendicitis, gastritis, renal colic, or peptic ulcer may mimic poisoning by corrosive substances.

    p., arsenic. In acute poisoning, symptoms may appear in a few minutes. When arsenic is ingested with solid food, symptoms may not appear for many hours. Symptoms are metallic taste and odor of garlic on breath, burning pain throughout gastrointestinal tract, vomiting and purging, dehydration, shock syndrome, coma, convulsions, paralysis, and death.

F.A.: Lavage stomach with copious amounts of water. If this cannot be done, induce vomiting. Administer dimercaprol (British antilewisite).

TREAT: After first aid, maintain fluid and electrolyte balance. Morphine for pain. Treat for shock and pulmonary edema. Blood transfusion may be required. SEE: *arsenic* at *Poisons and Poisoning* in *Appendix*.

p., blood. Presence of pathogenic bacteria in the blood. If allowed to progress, the organisms may multiply and cause an overwhelming infection and death. Symptoms and signs usually include chills and fever, petechiae, purpuric pustules, and abscesses. SYN: *septicemia*.

p., convulsive. Common convulsive poisons are strychnine and infrequently used drugs such as picrotoxin. For symptoms and treatment, SEE: *convulsant poisons*.

p., corrosive. Poisoning by strong acids, alkalies, strong antiseptics including bichloride of mercury, carbolic acid (phenol), Lysol, cresol compounds, tincture of iodine, and arsenic compounds. These are destructive and cause tissue damage similar to that caused by burns. If the substances have been swallowed, any part of the alimentary canal may be affected. Tissues involved are easily perforated. Death comes very shortly from shock or swelling of throat and pharynx, which causes choking, or by closure of esophagus, causing slow starvation. For symptoms and treatment, SEE: *corrosive poisoning*.

p., fish. A form of food poisoning caused by eating fish that are inherently poisonous or that are poisonous because they had decomposed, become infected, or been feeding on other poisonous life forms. For symptoms and treatment, SEE: *fish poisoning*.

p., food. Illness resulting from ingestion of foods containing poisonous substances. These include mushrooms; shellfish; foods contaminated with pesticides, lead, or mercury; milk from cows that have fed on poisonous plants; or foods that have putrefied or decomposed due to bacterial action.

p., lead. Symptoms of acute poisoning include a metallic taste in mouth, burns in throat and pharynx, and later abdominal cramps and prostration. Chronic lead poisoning is characterized by anorexia, nausea, vomiting, excess salivation, anemia, a lead line on the gums, abdominal pains, muscle cramps, and pains in the joints.

F.A.: In acute poisoning, wash out stomach. Administration of magnesium sulfate (epsom salts) or sodium sulfate, which precipitates the lead, and helps to remove it by purging. Give 10% dextrose in water intravenously to increase urine flow.

TREAT: If children have signs of lead encephalopathy, administer dimercaprol 4 mg/kg I.M. every four hours for 30 doses. Four hours after the last of that series of doses give calcium disodium edetate, 12.5 mg/kg I.M. every four hours in a 20% solution with 0.5% procaine added for a total of 30 doses. Adults with signs of acute encephalopathy should be given the same therapy. Treatment for chronic poisoning depends on the severity of the symptoms.

p., mercury. Mercury per se, i.e., mass of mercury, is not poisonous, but its bivalent salt, mercuric chloride ($HgCl_2$), is highly poisonous. Symptoms of acute poisoning include severe gastrointestinal irritation with pain, cramping, constriction of the throat, vomiting, and a metallic taste in the mouth. A stronger solution causes a white coating due to coagulation. Abdominal pain is very severe, bloody diarrhea and vomitus appear, urine flow is scanty. Prostration, convulsions, unconsciousness, and death occur. Chronic poisoning is characterized by bad breath, loosening of teeth, fever, urinary difficulties, nausea, diarrhea, sore tongue, paralysis, weakness, and death.

F.A.: Evacuate stomach, wash out with milk or with a solution of a teaspoon of sodium bicarbonate dissolved in 6 oz (177 ml) of water. Treatment with dimercaprol (British antilewisite) should be instituted immediately. Maintain fluid and electrolyte balance. SEE: *mercuric chloride* at *Poisons and Poisoning* in *Appendix*.

p., mushroom. Ingestion of mushrooms such as *Amanita muscaria*, which contains muscarine, or species that contain phalloidin, a component of the amanita toxin, cause poisoning. The nearest poison control center should be called for emergency treatment. SEE: *amanita* at *Poisons and Poisoning* in *Appendix*.

p., potato. Poisoning due to ingestion of potatoes that contain excess amounts of solanine, q.v. This toxic substance is present in the potato peel and in the green sprouts. Potatoes usually contain about 7 mg of solanine per 100 grams; the toxic dose of solanine is about 20 to 25 grams. Boiling but not baking removes most of the solanine from the potato. Symptoms of poisoning include headache, vomiting, abdominal pain, diarrhea, and fever. Neurological disturbances include apathy, restlessness, drowsiness, confusion, stupor, hallucinations, and visual disturbances.

TREAT: There is no specific therapy.

PROG: With appropriate supportive and symptomatic therapy, prognosis is good.

p., unknown substances. Cases in which there is no information concerning the nature of the poison taken, and the signs and symptoms are not recognized as being due to any particular substance. Specific antidotes cannot be given in this situation. There are, however, certain agents that act in a general manner and may be efficacious.

One of these is activated charcoal, which is available from many sources. Although a slurry of this in water is messy and offensive to the patient, it is a highly effective adsorbent for certain kinds of poisons. Another substance is referred to as the universal antidote. It consists of a mixture of 2 parts activated charcoal, 1 part magnesium oxide, and 1 part tannic acid. The universal antidote has been used empirically for a number of years and prepackaged units now are available commercially. It is doubtful if this mixture offers any real advantage over activated charcoal, which has a proven effectiveness against many substances. Each of these materials may be given as a slurry made from several heaping teaspoonsful in a glass of water. Because the ingredients are essentially harmless and the efficiency is increased by increasing the amount of adsorbent relative to the amount of poison, the dose may be repeated several times.

poison ivy. A climbing vine, *Rhus toxicodendron*, which on contact produces a severe form of dermatitis. *Rhus* species contain urushiol, an extremely irritating oily resin. Urushiol may also be a potent sensitizer since in many cases subsequent contacts produce increasingly severe reactions. SEE: illus.

poison ivy dermatitis. Dermatitis resulting from irritation or sensitization of the skin by urushiol, the toxic resin of the poison ivy plant. There is no absolute immunity, although susceptibility varies greatly, even in the same individual.

Persons sensitive to poison ivy may also react to contact with other plants such as the mango rind and cashew oil. These plants contain chemicals that cross-react with the *Rhus* sap present in poison ivy. SYN: *ivy poisoning; Rhus.*

SYM: An interval of time between skin contact of poison and first appearance of symptoms, varying from a few hours to several days and depending on sensitivity of the patient and possibly condition of the skin. Moderate itching or burning sensation soon followed by small blisters; later manifesta-

POISON IVY - POISON OAK
POISON SUMAC
(FROM TOP TO BOTTOM)

tions vary. Blisters usually rupture and are followed by oozing of serum and subsequent crusting.

PREVENTION: Certain substances, including organoclay compounds, have been useful in preventing poison ivy dermatitis. They are sprayed on the skin, where they serve as a barrier to prevent the irritating agent, urushiol, from bonding with the skin. Organoclay compounds are present in some spray deodorants.

TREAT: In mild dermatitis, a lotion to relieve itching is usually sufficient. In severe dermatitis, cool, wet dressings or compresses, potassium permanganate baths, and perhaps a course of intramuscular or oral corticosteroid therapy will be required. Sedation is also necessary in some cases.

Tepid water is used to provide symptomatic relief from itching and burning. The affected area is massaged with water as hot as can be tolerated for 1 or 2 minutes. The relief from itching is dramatic and may last several hours.

NURSING IMPLICATIONS: Teach the patient how to recognize the plant, how to avoid contact with it, and what to wear (long-sleeved shirts and long pants) in wooded areas. If contact occurs, wash with soap and water immediately to remove the toxic oil. Apply antipruritic lotion (e.g., calamine) or a cool wet dressing of aluminum acetate (Burow's) solution or epsom salts. Cover this with plastic wrap to retain moisture.

poison oak. A climbing vine, *Rhus radicans* or *R. diversiloba,* closely related to poison ivy and containing the same active principle. The symptoms and treatment of poison oak dermatitis are identical with those of poison ivy dermatitis, q.v. SEE: illus.

poisonous (poy′zŏn-ŭs) [L. *potio,* a poisonous draft]. Having the properties or qualities of a poison. SYN: *toxic; venomous.*

poisonous plants. *Do not eat:* castor bean, chinaberry, European bittersweet, wild or black cherry, horse chestnuts, poison hemlock, laurel, death cup, black nightshade or deadly nightshade, jimsonweed. *Do not touch:* poison ivy, poison oak, poison sumac.

poison sumac. A shrublike plant, *Toxicodendron vernix,* widely distributed in the U.S. Because it contains the same active principle as poison ivy, the symptoms and treatment of poison sumac dermatitis are the same as for poison ivy dermatitis, q.v. SEE: illus.

poker back. Stiffness of the spine. May result from spondylitis, q.v., or rheumatoid arthritis. SEE: *arthritis, rheumatoid.*

pokeroot (pōk′root). The dried root of *Veratrum viride,* used internally as an antihypertensive agent.

pokeroot poisoning. Poisoning resulting from ingestion of pokeroot.

    SYM: Nausea, vomiting, drowsiness, vertigo, and possibly convulsions and respiratory paralysis.

    TREAT: Emetic or lavage.

pokeweed mitogen. ABBR: PWM. A derivative of the pokeweed plant that stimulates both T and B cell proliferation in vitro. SEE: *phytohemagglutinin.*

polar [L. *polaris*]. Concerning a pole.

polarimeter (pō″lär-ĭm′ĕ-tĕr) [″ + Gr. *metron,* measure]. Instrument for measuring amount of polarization of light or rotation of polarized light.

polarimetry (pō″lär-ĭm′ĕ-trē). Measurement of the amount and rotation of polarized light.

polariscope (pō-lăr′ĭ-skōp) [L. *polaris,* pole, + Gr. *skopein,* to examine]. Apparatus used in measurement of polarized light.

polariscopy (pō″lär-ĭs′kō-pē). Study of polarized light by use of a polariscope.

polarity (pō-lăr′ĭ-tē). 1. The quality of having poles. 2. The exhibition of opposite effects at the two extremities in physical therapy. 3. The positive or negative state of an electrical battery. 4. In cell division, the relation of

cell constituents to the poles of the cell.

polarization (pō″lär-ĭ-zā′shŭn) [L. *polaris,* pole]. 1. Condition in a ray of light in which vibrations occur in only one plane. 2. In a galvanic battery, collection of hydrogen bubbles on negative plate and oxygen on the positive plate, whereby generation of current is impeded. 3. Condition in which ions of opposite charges are separated by a semipermeable membrane such as a cell membrane.

polarizer (pō′lă-rīz″ĕr). The part of a polariscope that polarizes light.

poldine methylsulfate (pōl′dēn). USP. An anticholinergic drug with action similar to belladonna.

pole (pōl) [L. *polus*]. 1. The extremity of any axis about which forces acting on it are symmetrically disposed. SYN: *polus.* 2. One of two points in a magnet, cell, or battery having opposite physical qualities.

    p., animal. Pole opposite the yolk in an ovum. At this point, polar bodies are formed and pinched off and protoplasm is concentrated and has its greatest activity.

    p., frontal. Farthest projecting part of the anterior extremity of both cerebral hemispheres.

    p., germinal. Pole of an ovum at which the development begins.

    p., occipital. The posterior extremity of the occipital lobe.

    p.'s of eye. The anterior and posterior extremities of the optic axis.

    p.'s of kidney. The upper and lower extremities of the kidney.

    p.'s of testicle. The upper and lower extremities of a testicle.

    p., pelvic. Breech of a fetus.

    p., placental, of chorion. Spot at which the domelike placenta is situated.

    p., temporal. The anterior extremity of the temporal lobe.

    p., vegetal. Part of the egg containing the food yolk.

policlinic (pŏl″ĭ-klĭn′ĭk) [Gr. *polis,* city, + *kline,* bed]. Polyclinic, q.v.

polio. poliomyelitis, *acute anterior.*

polio- [Gr. *polios,* gray]. Combining form indicating rel. to the gray matter of the nervous system.

polioclastic (pŏl″ē-ō-klăs′tĭk) [″ + *klastos,* breaking]. Destructive to gray matter of the nervous system.

polioencephalitis (pŏl″ē-ō-ĕn-sĕf″ă-lī′tĭs) [″ + *enkephalos,* brain, + *itis,* inflammation]. Condition characterized by inflammatory lesions of the gray matter of the brain.

    p., anterior superior. A disease involving necrotic changes in gray matter about the 3rd ventricle, anterior portion of the 4th ventricle, and aqueduct of Sylvius. Characterized by ocular abnormalities, mental disturbances, and ataxia. Of nutritional origin, probably thiamine (vitamin B₁) deficiency. SYN: *Wernicke's syndrome.*

    p. hemorrhagica. Polioencephalitis accompanied by hemorrhagic lesions.

    p., posterior. Polioencephalitis involving gray matter about the 4th ventricle.

polioencephalomeningomyelitis (pōl″ē-ō-ĕn-sĕf″ăl-ō-mĕn-in″gō-mī-ĕl-ī′tĭs) [″ + ″ + *meninx,* membrane, + *myelos,* marrow, + *itis,* inflammation]. Inflammation of the gray matter of the brain and spinal cord and their meninges.

polioencephalomyelitis (pōl″ē-ō-ĕn-sĕf″ăl-ō-mī″ĕl-ī′tĭs). Inflamed condition of the gray matter of the brain and spinal cord.

polioencephalopathy (pōl″ē-ō-ĕn-sĕf″ăl-ŏp′ă-thē) [Gr. *polios,* gray, + *enkephalos,* brain, + *pathos,* disease, suffering]. Diseased condition of the gray matter of the brain.

poliomyelencephalitis (pōl″ē-ō-mī″ĕl-ĕn-sĕf″ăl-ī′tĭs) [″ + *myelos,* marrow, + *enkephalos,* brain, + *itis,* inflammation]. Poliomyelitis with polioencephalitis.

poliomyelitis (pōl″ē-ō-mī″ĕl-ī′tĭs) [″ + ″ + *itis,* inflammation]. Inflammation of the gray matter of the spinal cord. An acute viral disease characterized by fever, sore throat, headache, vomiting, and often stiffness of the neck and back. There may also be subsequent atrophy of groups of muscles ending in contraction and permanent deformity.

    p., abortive. Poliomyelitis in which illness is mild with no involvement of central nervous system.

    p., acute anterior. An acute infectious inflammation of the anterior horns of the gray matter of the spinal cord. This is an acute, systemic, infectious disease in which paralysis may or may not occur. In the majority of patients, the disease is mild, being limited to respiratory and gastrointestinal symptoms, such constituting the minor illness or the abortive type, which lasts only a few days. In the major illness, paralysis or weakness of muscles occurs with loss of superficial and deep reflexes. In such cases characteristic lesions are found in the gray matter of the spinal cord, medulla, motor area of cerebral cortex, and cerebellum. SEE: *postpoliomyelitis muscular atrophy.*

    SYM: Onset often is abrupt, although the ordinary manifestations of a severe cold or some gastrointestinal disturbances may come on gradually, accompanied by slight elevation of temperature, frequently enduring for not more than three days. At the end of this period, paralysis may or may not develop. The extent of any paralysis necessarily depends upon degree of nerve involvement. Consequently, paralysis may be confined to one small group of muscles or affect one or all extremities. In some instances, the respiratory muscles also are involved and it is in these cases that death is so likely to ensue. In the average paralytic case it is the extensor muscles in particular that are affected.

    ETIOL: Causative agent is a virus consisting of particles from 270 to 300 angstrom units in diameter. The virus that is excreted in the feces is resistant and stable, remaining viable for months outside the body. Three immunologic types exist.

    DIFF. DIAG: Among the diseases confused with this infection are the various types of meningitis, postinfection encephalomyelitis, and hysteria.

    PROPHYLAXIS: Active immunization with either poliovirus vaccine live oral (USP) or poliovirus vaccine inactivated (USP) has greatly reduced the incidence of paralytic poliomyelitis. The oral vaccine containing all three types of the virus should be given to young infants beginning at 6 to 12 weeks, with a second dose about 2 months later and then a third dose 8 to 12 months later. Older children who have not been previously immunized with trivalent oral poliovirus vaccine should be given two doses at 8-week intervals and a third dose 6 months to 1 year later. SEE: *poliovirus vaccine, inactivated.*

    INCUBATION: Ranges from 5 to 35 days, but usually 7 to 12 days.

    COMPLICATIONS: Paralysis, atrophy of muscles, and ultimate deformities. Aside from bronchopneumonia, which may develop in very severe cases, other complications are surprisingly few.

    PROG: Ordinarily the outcome as to life is good. It is only the bulbar and respiratory types in which death is likely to occur. These two types constitute nearly all of the fatal cases. Even when paralysis develops, 50% of the patients make a full recovery and about 25% have mild permanent paralysis. In the more severe types, however, some paralysis may remain.

    Progressive paralysis may occur years after the acute attack. This recently described syndrome may be due to a combination of aging and atrophy of anterior horn cells.

    INCIDENCE: Poliomyelitis is endemic throughout the world but occurs in epidemics in certain countries, including the U.S. However, the disease in the U.S. has been brought under almost complete control by vaccination. In countries where polio vaccine has not been used extensively, epidemics are seasonal, occurring in summer and fall. Children are more susceptible than adults. Infection is spread by direct contact, the virus probably entering the body via the mouth. It reaches the central nervous system through the blood.

PREDISPOSING: Tonsillectomy and other nose and throat operations, routine immunizations, excessive physical strain, and fatigue. Pregnant women are especially susceptible during epidemics.

NURSING IMPLICATIONS: Encourage immunization at an early age to prevent disease. Enforce isolation with concurrent disinfection of throat discharge and feces to prevent transmission of polio virus. Maintain a calm, reassuring manner. Maintain a patent airway and observe closely for respiratory distress; administer oxygen as necessary; and keep a tracheostomy tray at the bedside.

Maintain strict bedrest during the acute phase. Alleviate muscle pain by gentle, passive range-of-motion exercises and application of hot moist packs at 20-minute intervals or tub baths for children. Maintain proper body alignment and turn frequently to prevent deformity and decubiti. Administer mild sedative or analgesic to decrease pain and anxiety and to promote rest. Observe for distended bladder due to transitory paralysis. Promote personal hygiene, and provide oral hygiene. Provide appetizing food because anorexia is common. Administer antipyretic to reduce fever. Closely monitor fluid and electrolyte balance and elimination. Use footboard to prevent foot drop. Provide emotional support to the patient who is coping with loss of body function and paralysis. SEE: *post-polio syndrome.*

p., anterior. Inflamed state of the anterior horns of the spinal cord.

p., ascending. Poliomyelitis in which paralysis begins in the lower extremities and progresses up the legs, thighs, trunk, and finally involves respiratory muscles.

p., bulbar. Poliomyelitis in which gray matter of the medulla oblongata is involved, resulting in paralysis and usually respiratory failure. SEE: *poliomyelitis, acute anterior.*

p., chronic anterior. Progressive wasting of the muscles. Myelopathic progressive muscular atrophy.

p., nonparalytic. Pain and stiffness in the muscles of the axial skeleton, esp. of the neck and back; mild fever; increased proteins and leukocytes in the cerebrospinal fluid. Diagnosis depends on the isolation of the virus and serological reactions.

p., paralytic. Poliomyelitis with a variable combination of signs of damage of the central nervous system. These include weakness, incoordination, muscle tenderness and spasms, flaccid paralysis, and disturbance of consciousness.

poliosis (pŏl″ē-ō′sĭs) [Gr. *polios,* gray, + *osis,* condition]. Whiteness of the hair, esp. when due to a hereditary condition or as a result of infection. SYN: *canities.*

poliovirus (pō″lē-ō-vī′rŭs). Etiological agent of poliomyelitis, q.v., separable into three serotypes based on the specificity of the neutralizing antibody. The three serotypes are type I, II, and III. A virus found worldwide, it spreads directly or indirectly from infected persons or convalescent carriers. Epidemics of poliomyelitis that were characteristic of infections with this virus have been virtually eliminated by poliovirus vaccine. SEE: *poliovirus vaccine, inactivated.*

poliovirus vaccine, inactivated. ABBR: IPV. USP. A poliovirus vaccine recommended for prevention of paralytic poliomyelitis. The vaccine contains inactivated types I, II, and III polioviruses. It is suitable for parenteral administration to all infants and children.

Infants should be given three doses, the first at 2 months of age, followed by two more doses at 8-week intervals. A fourth dose should be given at 18 months unless poliomyelitis is endemic in the area, in which case the fourth dose is given at 6 to 12 months after the third. Additional doses are recommended prior to school entry and then every 5 years until age 18.

poliovirus vaccine, live oral. USP. ABBR: OPV. A standard preparation of one type or a combination of the three types of live, attenuated polioviruses. It is suitable for immunizing children and adults against all three types of poliovirus, but the inactivated poliovirus vaccine is preferred for adults because of the slightly high risk of vaccine-associated paralysis. The schedule for infants is first dose at 6 to 12 weeks, the second about 2 months later, a third 8 to 12 months after the second. No additional "boosters" are recommended. For children and adolescents not previously immunized prior to age 18, two doses are given 8 weeks apart and a third dose is given 6 to 12 months later. Trade name is Orimune.

polishing (pŏl′ĭsh-ĭng). Producing a smooth, glossy finish on a denture or a dental restoration.

Politzer bag (pŏl′ĭt-zěr) [Adam Politzer, Hungarian otologist, 1835–1920]. Soft rubber bag with rubber tip for inflating the middle ear by increasing the pressure in the nasopharynx.

politzerization (pŏl″ĭt-sěr-ĭ-zā′shŭn). The

inflation of the middle ear by means of a Politzer bag, q.v.

pollakiuria (pŏl″ă-kē-ū′rē-ă) [Gr. *pollakis*, often, + *ouron*, urine]. Abnormally frequent passage of urine.

pollen (pŏl′ĕn) [L., dust]. The microspores of a seed plant that develop in the anther at the tip of the stamen. Each pollen grain develops a pollen tube and constitutes the male gametophyte. Within it develops a tube nucleus and two sperm nuclei, the latter constituting the male reproductive elements. Many airborne pollens are allergens, q.v. SEE: *hay fever.*

pollenogenic (pŏl″ĕn-ō-jĕn′ĭk) [″ + Gr. *gennan*, to produce]. Caused by the pollen of plants, or producing plant pollen.

pollenosis (pŏl″ĕn-ō′sĭs) [″ + Gr. *osis*, condition]. Pollinosis.

pollex (pŏl′ĕks) [L.] (pl. *pollices*). [NA] The thumb.

    p. extensus. Backward deviation of the thumb.

    p. flexus. Permanent flexion of the thumb.

    p. valgus. Abnormal deviation of the thumb toward the ulnar side.

    p. varus. Abnormal deviation of the thumb toward the radial side.

pollicization (pŏl″ĭs-ĭ-zā′shŭn) [L. *pollex*, thumb]. The plastic surgical procedure of constructing a thumb from adjacent tissues.

pollinosis (pŏl-ĭn-ō′sĭs) [L. *pollen*, dust, + Gr. *osis*, disease]. Nasal congestion of mucous membranes due to contact with pollen. SYN: *hay fever.*

pollodic (pŏl-lŏ′dĭk) [Gr. *polloi*, many, + *hodos*, way]. Concerning nerve stimuli that originate from one center.

pollution (pŭ-loo′shŭn) [ME. *polluten*]. State of making impure or defiling.

    p., noise. A level of noise in the environment, no matter what its source, of such nature or intensity as to cause mental or physical discomfort or damage to the hearing system.

polocyte (pō′lō-sīt) [Gr. *polos*, pole, + *kytos*, cell]. Body, polar, q.v.

polonium (pō-lō′nē-ŭm). [L. *Polonia*, Poland, native country of its discoverers, the Curies]. SYMB: Po. At. wt. 210; at. no. 84. Radioactive element isolated from pitchblende.

poltophagy (pŏl-tŏf′ă-jē) [Gr. *poltos*, porridge, + *phagein*, to eat]. Thorough chewing of food so that it is reduced to a finely divided mass. SEE: *fletcherism.*

polus (pō′lŭs) [L.] (pl. *poli*). [NA] The extremity of an organ. SYN: *pole.*

poly (pŏl′ē). *polymorphonuclear leukocyte.*

poly- [Gr. *polys*, many]. Prefix indicating many or much.

polyacid (pŏl″ē-ăs′ĭd). An alcohol or a base with two or more hydroxyl groups that will combine with an acid.

polyadenitis (pŏl″ē-ăd″ē-nī′tĭs) [″ + Gr. *aden*, gland, + *itis*, inflammation]. Condition of inflamed lymph nodes, esp. the cervical lymph nodes.

polyadenomatosis (pŏl″ē-ăd″ē-nō-mă-tō′sĭs) [″ + ″ + *oma*, tumor, + *osis*, condition]. Adenomas in many glands.

polyadenopathy (pŏl″ē-ăd″ē-nŏp′ă-thē) [″ + ″ + *pathos*, disease, suffering]. Any disease in which many glands are involved.

polyadenous (pŏl″ē-ăd′ē-nŭs). Involving or rel. to many glands.

polyagglutination. Red cells that are agglutinated by a large proportion of adult human sera regardless of blood group.

polyalgesia (pŏl″ē-ăl-jē′zē-ă) [″ + *algesis*, sense of pain]. A single stimulus of a part, producing sensation in many parts.

polyandry (pŏl″ē-ăn′drē) [Gr. *polyandria*]. The practice of having more than one husband at the same time. SEE: *polygamy.*

polyangiitis (pŏl″ē-ăn″jē-ī′tĭs) [Gr. *polys*, many, + *angeion*, vessel, + *itis*, inflammation]. Inflammation of a number of blood vessels.

polyarteritis (nodosa) (pŏl″ē-ăr″tĕr-ī′tĭs) [″ + *arteria*, artery, + *itis*, inflammation]. A disease of medium and small arteries, particularly at the point of bifurcation and branching. Segmental inflammation, infiltration with fibrinoid, and necrosis of the vessel lining and walls lead to a diminished flow of blood to the areas normally supplied by these arteries. Signs and symptoms depend on the location of the affected vessels and may affect any organ or body system. SYN: *periarteritis nodosa.* SEE: *collagen disease.* SEE: *Nursing Diagnoses* in *Appendix.*

    ETIOL: Unknown, but associated with hypersensitivity. Drug therapy, vaccines, bacterial and viral infections have been associated with the onset of polyarteritis.

    TREAT: Corticosteroids in large doses initially, then tapered off, may be of benefit. General supportive therapy. The value of immunosuppressive therapy is questionable.

    PROG: Without therapy, only one person in eight will live 5 years. Death is due to failure of a function of a vital organ such as the heart or kidney; hemorrhage from the gastrointestinal tract; or a ruptured aneurysm.

polyarthric (pŏl″ē-ăr′thrĭk) [″ + *arthron*, joint]. Affecting or pert. to several joints.

polyarthritis (pŏl-ē-ăr-thrī′tĭs) [″ + ″ + *itis*, inflammation]. Inflammation of more than one joint. The role of infection in this disease is being investigated.

p., chronic villous. Chronic inflammation of the synovial membrane of several joints.

p. rheumatica, acute. Acute rheumatic fever.

polyarticular (pŏl″ē-är-tĭk′ū-lăr) [″ + L. *articulus*, a joint]. Affecting many joints. SYN: *multiarticular*.

polyatomic (pŏl″ē-ă-tŏm′ĭk) [″ + *atomon*, atom]. 1. Having several atoms. 2. Having more than two replaceable hydrogen atoms.

polyavitaminosis (pŏl″ē-ā-vī″tă-mĭn-ō′sĭs) [″ + *a-*, not, + L. *vita*, life, + *amine* + Gr. *osis*, condition]. A deficiency of more than one vitamin.

polybasic (pŏl″ē-bā′sĭk) [Gr. *polys*, many, + *basis*, base]. Pert. to an acid with two or more hydrogen ions that will combine with a base.

polyblast (pŏl′ē-blăst) [″ + *blastos*, a germ]. Large mononuclear phagocyte that is derived from an embryonic wandering cell and is present in inflammation.

polyblennia (pŏl″ē-blĕ′nē-ă) [″ + *blennos*, mucus]. Secretion of an abnormal amount of mucus.

polycarbophil (pŏl″ē-kär′bō-fĭl). A hydrophilic substance that is used as a bulk-forming laxative. Trade name is Mitrolan.

polycentric (pŏl″ē-sĕn′trĭk) [″ + *kentron*, center]. Condition of having many centers.

polycheiria (pŏl″ē-kī′rē-ă) [″ + *cheir*, hand]. Having more than two hands.

polychemotherapy (pŏl″ē-kē″mō-thĕr′ă-pē) [″ + *chemeia*, chemistry, + *therapeia*, treatment]. Treatment with several chemotherapeutic agents at once.

polychlorinated biphenyls. ABBR: PCBs. A group of complex chemicals classed as chlorinated aromatic hydrocarbons. They were widely used in industry as a component of transformers and capacitors; in paints and hydraulic systems; and in carbonless NCR paper. Because of their extremely low rate of biodegradation, accumulation in animal tissues (particularly in adipose tissue), and their potential for chronic or delayed toxic effects, the manufacture of PCBs was discontinued in the U.S. in 1977. PCBs were sold in the U.S. under the trade name Aroclor.

polycholia (pŏl″ē-kō′lē-ă) [″ + *chole*, bile]. Abnormal secretion of bile.

polychondritis (pŏl″ē-kŏn-drī′tĭs) [″ + *chondros*, cartilage, + *itis*, inflammation]. Inflammation of several cartilages of the body.

p., chronic atrophic relapsing. A degenerative disease of cartilage associated with polyarthritis, involvement of the cartilage of the nose, ears, joints, bronchi, and trachea. The cause is unknown and there is no specific therapy. Because of the collapse of the bronchial walls, repeated infections of the lungs will occur and death may result from these infections.

polychrest (pŏl′ē-krĕst) [″ + *chrestos*, useful]. A medicine useful in many diseases.

polychromasia (pŏl″ē-krō-mā′zē-ă) [″ + *chroma*, color]. Quality of having many colors.

polychromatic (pŏl″ē-krō-măt′ĭk). Multicolored.

polychromatocyte (pŏl″ē-krō-măt′ō-sīt) [″ + ″ + *kytos*, cell]. A cell that has an affinity for various stains. SEE: *polychromatophilia* (def. 1).

polychromatophil(e) (pŏl″ē-krō-măt′ō-fĭl) [Gr. *polys*, many, + *chroma*, color, + *philein*, to love]. A cell, esp. an erythrocyte, that is stainable with more than one kind of stain.

polychromatophilia (pŏl″ē-krō-măt″ō-fĭl′ē-ă). 1. The quality of being stainable with more than one stain. 2. Excess of polychromatophils in the blood.

polychromophilia (pŏl″ē-krō-mō-fĭl′ē-ă) [″ + ″ + *philos*, to love]. Polychromatophilia, q.v.

polychylia (pŏl″ē-kī′lē-ă) [″ + *chylos*, juice]. Excessive secretion of chyle.

Polycillin-N. Trade name for ampicillin sodium.

polyclinic (pŏl″ē-klĭn′ĭk) [″ + *kline*, bed]. Hospital or clinic treating patients with various medical and surgical conditions; a general hospital.

polyclonal (pŏl″ē-klōn′ăl). Arising from different cell lines.

polyclonia (pŏl″ē-klō′nē-ă) [″ + *klonos*, tumult]. A disease characterized by many clonic spasms, but distinct from chorea or tic.

polycoria (pŏl″ē-kō′rē-ă) [″ + *kore*, pupil]. The state of having more than one pupil in one eye.

polycrotic (pŏl″ē-krŏt′ĭk) [″ + *krotos*, beat]. Having several pulse waves for each heartbeat.

polycrotism (pŏl-ĭk′rō-tĭzm) [″ + ″ + *-ismos*, condition]. Condition of having several pulse waves for each heartbeat.

polycyesis (pŏl″ē-sī-ē′sĭs) [″ + *kyesis*, pregnancy]. Multiple pregnancy.

polycystic (pŏl″ē-sĭs′tĭk) [″ + *kystis*, cyst]. Composed of many cysts.

polycystic ovary syndrome. An endocrine disturbance associated with primary anovulation and polycystic ovaries. One possible explanation for this condition is the continued stimulation of the ovary by pituitary luteinizing hormone. SYN: *Stein-Leventhal syndrome*.

TREAT: Clomiphene, gonadotropins, or

polyethylene glycol electrolyte for
gastrointestinal lavage solution
polycythemia   **1552**

wedge resection of the ovary.

polycythemia (pŏl″ē-sī-thē′mē-ă) [″ + *kytos,* cell, + *haima,* blood]. An excess of red blood cells. SYN: *erythrocytosis; polyemia; polyhemia.*

  p., compensatory. P., secondary, q.v.

  p., myelopathic. P. vera.

  p., primary. P. vera.

  p., relative. Relative increase in number of erythrocytes that occurs in hemoconcentration.

  p. rubra; p. rubra vera. P. vera, q.v.

  p., secondary. Polycythemia resulting from some physiological condition that stimulates erythropoiesis, such as lowered oxygen tension in blood. SYN: *erythrocytosis.*

  p., splenomegalic. P. vera.

  p. vera. A chronic, life-shortening myeloproliferative disorder involving all bone marrow elements. Characterized by an increase in red blood cell mass and hemoglobin concentration. SYN: *erythremia.* SEE: *Nursing Diagnoses* in *Appendix.*

  SYM: Weakness, fatigue, vertigo, tinnitus, irritability, enlarged spleen, flushing of face, redness and pain of extremities, black-and-blue spots. Bone marrow shows increased cellularity.

  ETIOL: Unknown.

  TREAT: Permanent cure cannot be achieved today, but remissions of many years can be produced. Phlebotomy and radioactive phosphorus (^{32}P) are effective. Phlebotomy followed by chemotherapy with either chlorambucil or cyclophosphamide has been used, but requires much closer follow-up than phlebotomy and use of ^{32}P.

polycytotropic. Pantropic, q.v.

polydactylism (pŏl″ē-dăk′tĭ-lĭzm) [Gr. *polys,* many, + *daktylos,* digit, + *-ismos,* condition]. State of having supernumerary fingers or toes.

polydactyly (pŏl″ē-dăk′tĭ-lē) [″ + *daktylos,* finger]. Condition of having more than the normal number of fingers and toes.

polydentia (pŏl″ē-dĕn′shē-ă) [″ + L. *dens,* tooth]. Polyodontia, q.v.

polydipsia (pŏl″ē-dĭp′sē-ă) [″ + *dipsa,* thirst]. Excessive thirst.

polydrug use. In drug abusers, the practice of concurrent use of several dissimilar drugs. Thus, alcohol, cocaine, opiates, and other drugs may be used at the same time. The toxic potential of multiple drug use is increased as compared with use of a single drug.

polydysplasia (pŏl″ē-dĭs-plā′zē-ă) [″ + *dys,* bad, + *plassein,* to form]. Condition of having multiple developmental abnormalities.

polydystrophic (pŏl″ē-dĭs-trō′fĭk). Concerning or having polydystrophy.

polydystrophy (pŏl″ē-dĭs′trō-fē) [″ + ″ + *trophe,* nourishment]. Condition of having multiple congenital anomalies of the connective tissues.

polyendocrine (pŏl″ē-ĕn′dō-krĭn) [″ + *endon,* within, + *krinein,* to secrete]. Concerning several endocrine glands.

polyendocrine deficiency syndromes. *Type I:* A disease that begins at about age 12, characterized by hypoparathyroidism, primary adrenal insufficiency, and mucocutaneous candidiasis. Alopecia, pernicious anemia, malabsorption, and chronic hepatitis may also be present. *Type II:* A disease whose average age of onset is about 30 years and which is characterized by primary adrenal insufficiency, autoimmune thyroid disease, and insulin-dependent diabetes mellitus. SYN: *Schmidt's syndrome.*

polyene (pŏl-ē′ēn). An organic compound containing alternating, or conjugate, double bonds. An example is butadiene, $CH_2{=}CHCH{=}CH_2$.

polyergic (pŏl″ē-ĕr′jĭk) [″ + *ergon,* work]. Having the ability to act in several different ways.

polyesthesia (pŏl″ē-ĕs-thē′zē-ă) [″ + *aisthesis,* sensation]. Abnormal sensation of touch in which a single stimulus is felt at two or more places.

polyesthetic (pŏl″ē-ĕs-thĕt′ĭk). 1. Pert. to polyesthesia. 2. Pert. to several senses or sensations.

polyestrous (pŏl″ē-ĕs′trŭs) [″ + *oistros,* mad desire]. Having two or more estrous cycles in each mating season.

polyethylene (pŏl″ē-ĕth′ĭ-lēn). A polymerized resin of ethylene. Used to make a wide variety of products, including tubing used in intravenous sets.

  p. glycol 400. A polymer consisting of ethylene oxide and water. The formula is $H(OCH_2CH_2)_nOH$, in which the value of n is from 8.2 to 9.1. Used as a water-soluble ointment base.

  p. glycol 4000. A polymer consisting of ethylene oxide and water. The formula is $H(OCH_2CH_2)_nOH$, in which the value of n is from 68 to 84. Used as a water-soluble ointment base.

  p. glycol electrolyte for gastrointestinal lavage solution. A white powder added to water to make a volume of 4 liters. It is an isosmotic solution for oral administration. Contains 236 gm of polyethylene glycol 3350; 23.74 gm of sodium sulfate; 6.74 gm of sodium bicarbonate; 5.86 gm of sodium chloride; and 2.97 gm of potassium chloride. For adults the 4 liters are given at the rate of 8 oz (240 ml) every 10 minutes until completed. This solution is given prior to colonoscopy and barium enema examinations. The bowel will be cleansed within 3 to 4 hours. Trade name is Golytely.

polygalactia (pŏl″ē-gă-lăk′shē-ă) [Gr. *polys,* many, + *gala,* milk]. Excessive secretion or flow of milk.

polygalacturonase (pŏl″ē-gă-lăk-tū′rō-nās). An enzyme present in plant tissues that hydrolyzes pectins to cause them to form gels.

polygamy (pō-lĭg′ă-mē) [″ + *gamos,* marriage]. Practice of having several wives, husbands, or mates at the same time. SEE: *polyandry; polygyny.*

polyganglionic (pŏl″ē-găng″glē-ŏn′ĭk) [″ + *ganglion,* ganglion]. 1. Concerning many ganglia. 2. Affecting many glands.

polygastria (pŏl″ē-găs′trē-ă) [″ + *gaster,* stomach]. Excessive secretion or flow of gastric juice.

polygen (pŏl′ē-jĕn). 1. An element that has more than one valency and that can form more than one series of compounds. 2. An antigen that will cause the formation of two or more specific antibodies.

polygenic (pŏl″ē-jĕn′ĭk) [″ + *gennan,* to produce]. Pert. to or caused by several genes.

polyglandular (pŏl″ē-glăn′dū-lăr) [″ + L. *glandula,* a little kernel]. Pert. to or affecting many glands. SYN: *pluriglandular.*

polyglycolic acid. A polymer of glycolic acid anhydride units. It is used in manufacturing surgical sutures.

polygnathus (pō-lĭg′nă-thŭs) [″ + *gnathos,* jaw]. Conjoined twins of unequal size in which the smaller is attached to the jaw of the larger.

polygram (pŏl′ē-grăm) [″ + *gramma,* something written]. A tracing or record made by a polygraph.

polygraph (pŏl′ē-grăf) [″ + *graphein,* to write]. Device that records simultaneously tracings of several different pulsations, as arterial and venous pulse waves, and the apex beat of the heart. Has been used as a so-called lie detector. The scientific basis for the validity of this test is disputed. SYN: *sphygmograph.* SEE: *lie detector.*

polygyny. The practice of having more than one female mate at a time. SEE: *polygamy.*

polygyria (pŏl″ē-jī′rē-ă) [″ + *gyros,* circle]. Excess of the normal number of convolutions in the brain.

polyhedral (pŏl″ē-hē′drăl) [Gr. *polys,* many, + *hedra,* base]. Having many surfaces.

polyhemia (pŏl″ē-hē′mē-ă) [″ + *haima,* blood]. Abnormal increase in amount of the blood. SYN: *polycythemia; polyemia.*

polyhidrosis (pŏl″ē-hī-drō′sĭs) [″ + *hidrosis,* sweat]. Excessive perspiration.

polyhistor (pŏl″ē-hĭs′tŭr) [″ + *histor,* learned]. A scholar or physician who has great and varied abilities and knowledge. SYN: *polymath.*

Ex.: Hippocrates, Galen, Paracelsus, Leonardo da Vinci, Boerhaave, Richard Mead, and Thomas Jefferson.

polyhybrid (pŏl″ē-hī′brĭd) [″ + L. *hybrida,* mongrel]. The offspring of parents that are different with respect to three or more characteristics.

polyhydramnios (pŏl″ē-hī-drăm′nē-ŏs) [″ + *hydor,* water, + *amnion,* amnion]. An excess of amniotic fluid in the bag of waters in pregnancy. SEE: *amnion.*

polyhydric (pŏl″ē-hī′drĭk). Containing more than two hydroxyl groups.

polyhydruria (pŏl″ē-hī-droo′rē-ă) [″ + ″ + *ouron,* urine]. Excessive amount of water in the urine.

polyhypermenorrhea (pŏl″ē-hī″pĕr-mĕn″ō-rē′ă) [″ + *hyper,* over, + *men,* month, + *rhoia,* flow]. Frequent menstruation with excessive discharge.

polyhypomenorrhea (pŏl″ē-hī″pō-mĕn″ō-rē′ă) [″ + *hypo,* under, + *men,* month, + *rhoia,* flow]. Frequent menstruation with scanty discharge.

Poly I:C. A complex of synthetic polyriboinosinic and polyribocytidylic acids. They are a form of double-stranded ribonucleic acids that may help to induce resistance to virus infection. Poly I:C stimulates production of interferon, q.v.

polyidrosis (pŏl″ē-ĭd-rō′sĭs) [″ + *hidrosis,* sweat]. Hyperhidrosis, q.v.

polyinfection (pŏl″ē-ĭn-fĕk′shŭn) [″ + ME. *infecten,* infect]. Infection with two or more microorganisms. SYN: *multi-infection.*

polykaryocyte (pŏl″ē-kăr′ē-ō-sīt) [″ + *karyon,* nucleus, + *kytos,* cell]. A cell possessing several nuclei.

polyleptic (pŏl″ē-lĕp′tĭk) [″ + *lepsis,* a seizure]. Characterized by numerous remissions and exacerbations, as malaria.

polylysine (pŏl″ē-lī′sĭn). A polypeptide in which two lysine molecules are joined by a peptide linkage.

polymastia (pŏl″ē-măs′tē-ă) [Gr. *polys,* many, + *mastos,* breast]. Condition of having more than two breasts. SYN: *multimammae; polymazia.*

polymastigote (pŏl″ē-măs′tĭ-gōt) [″ + *mastix,* whip]. Possessing several flagella.

polymath. Polyhistor, q.v.

polymazia [″ + *mazos,* breast]. Condition of having more than two breasts. SYN: *multimammae; polymastia.*

polymelia (pŏl″ē-mē′lē-ă) [″ + *melos,* limb]. A congenital abnormality in which there are supernumerary limbs.

polymelus (pō-lĭm′ē-lŭs) [″ + *melos,*

limb]. One having polymelia.

polymenia (pŏl″ē-mē′nē-ă) [″ + *men*, month]. Polymenorrhea.

polymenorrhea (pŏl″ē-mĕn-ō-rē′ă) [″ + ″ + *rhoia*, to flow]. Menstrual periods occurring with abnormal frequency. SYN: *polymenia*.

polymer (pŏl′ĭ-mĕr) [″ + *meros*, a part]. A natural or synthetic substance formed by a combination of two or more molecules (and up to millions) of the same substance.

Ex.: paraformaldehyde (HCHO)₃ formed from three molecules of formaldehyde, HCHO; starch and cellulose formed from a large number of D-glucose molecules. SEE: *polysaccharide*.

polymerase (pŏl-ĭm′ĕr-ās). An enzyme that catalyzes polymerization of nucleosides to form DNA.

polymerase chain reaction. ABBR: PCR. A process that permits making, in vitro, unlimited numbers of copies of genes. This is done beginning with a single molecule of the genetic material, DNA. One hundred billion similar molecules can be generated within a few hours. The practical importance of this method of investigating genetic material is enormous. Thus, the technique can be used in investigating and diagnosing bacterial diseases, viruses associated with cancer, genetic diseases such as diabetes mellitus, pemphigus vulgaris, and various diseases of the blood, e.g., sickle cell anemia, and of muscles.

polymer fume fever. Condition resulting from breathing fumes produced by certain polymers when they are heated to 300° to 700°C or higher. SEE: *metal fume fever*.

SYM: Tight gripping sensation of the chest associated with shivering, sore throat, fever, and weakness.

TREAT: Discontinue exposure to fumes.

polymeria (pŏl-ĭ-mē′rē-ă). Condition of having supernumerary parts of the body. SYN: *polymerism*.

polymeric (pŏl″ĭ-mĕr′ĭk). 1. Having the characteristics of a polymer. 2. Muscles derived from more than one myotome.

polymerid (pō-lĭm′ĕr-ĭd). A polymer.

polymerism (pŏl′ĭ-mĕr″ĭzm, pō-lĭm′ĕr-ĭzm) [″ + *meros*, part, + *-ismos*, condition]. Condition of having more than normal number of parts. SYN: *polymeria*.

polymerization (pŏl″ĭ-mĕr″ĭ-zā′shŭn). Process of changing a simple chemical substance or substances into another compound having the same elements usually in the same proportions but with a higher molecular weight.

polymerize (pŏl′ĭ-mĕr-īz). To cause polymerization.

polymicrobial (pŏl″ē-mī-krō′bē-ăl) [Gr. *polys*, many, + *mikros*, small, + *bios*, life]. Concerning a number of species of microorganisms.

polymicrobic infections. Bacterial infections caused by two or more different microorganisms.

polymicrogyria (pŏl″ē-mī″krō-jī′rē-ă) [″ + ″ + *gyros*, convolution]. A malformed brain in which multiple small convolutions have developed.

polymitus (pō-lĭm′ĭ-tŭs) [″ + *mitos*, thread]. Stage in reproduction of microorganisms in which threads of protoplasm, now being detached, constitute the microgamete.

polymorph (pŏl′ē-morf) [″ + *morphe*, form]. A polymorphonuclear leukocyte.

polymorphic. Occurring in more than one form. SYN: *multiform; polymorphous*.

polymorphism [″ + *morphe*, form, + *-ismos*, condition]. 1. Capacity for appearing in many forms. 2. Existence of several types in the same group or species. SYN: *pleomorphism*.

polymorphocellular (pŏl″ē-mor″fō-sĕl′ū-lăr) [″ + ″ + L. *cellula*, a small chamber]. Composed of cells of many forms.

polymorphonuclear (pŏl″ē-mor″fō-nū′klē-ăr) [″ + ″ + L. *nucleus*, a kernel]. Possessing a nucleus consisting of several parts or lobes connected by fine strands.

polymorphonuclear leukocyte. A white blood cell that possesses a nucleus composed of two or more lobes or parts. Also called a *granulocyte* (neutrophil, eosinophil, basophil). Neutrophils, the most populous polymorphonuclear leukocytes, are the most important phagocytic cells in the body. Clinically, polymorphonuclear leukocytes are often referred to as "polys."

polymorphous (pŏl″ē-mor′fŭs). Appearing in many forms. SYN: *multiform; polymorphic*.

Polymox. Trade name for amoxicillin.

polymyalgia arteritica (pŏl″ē-mī-ăl′jē-ă) [″ + *mys*, muscle, + *algos*, pain]. Polymyalgia rheumatica, q.v.

polymyalgia rheumatica. A poorly understood condition almost always found in patients over 50 years of age and found four times more frequently in women. It is characterized by the following: pain in the muscles of the shoulder and pelvic girdle; marked elevation of erythrocyte sedimentation rate; morning stiffness, and jelling after prolonged sitting; absence of evidence of inflammatory arthritis of any kind; absence of signs of muscle disease such as atrophy, weakness, or fibrillation; and prompt and dramatic response to low doses of corticosteroid therapy.

Corticosteroids relieve symptoms and the

sedimentation rate approaches normal. Temporal and cranial arteritis may be associated with this disease.

polymyoclonus (pŏl"ē-mī-ŏk'lō-nŭs) [" + " + *klonos*, tumult]. A shocklike muscular contraction occurring in various parts at the same time. SYN: *myoclonus multiplex; paramyoclonus multiplex.*

polymyopathy (pŏl"ē-mī-ŏp'ă-thē) [" + " + *pathos*, disease, suffering]. Disease that affects several muscles.

polymyositis (pŏl"ē-mī"ō-sī'tĭs) [" + " + *itis*, inflammation]. A rare, inflammatory disease of skeletal muscle tissue characterized by symmetric weakness of proximal muscles of the limbs, neck and pharynx. Some patients will have arthralgias, erythematous rash, Raynaud's syndrome, and dysphagia.

The disease has been classified as Type I, adult polymyositis; Type II, dermatomyositis; Type III, myositis with malignancy; Type IV, childhood myositis; and Type IV, myositis associated with other connective tissue diseases.

ETIOL: Etiology is unknown, but an autoimmune mechanism is the most likely cause.

TREAT: Corticosteroids combined with azathioprine. Maintenance therapy may be needed for years.

PROG: The 5-year survival rate is about 80%.

polymyxin (pŏl"ē-mĭks'ĭn). One of several closely related antibiotics isolated from various strains of *Bacillus polymyxa* and designated polymyxins A, B, C, D, and E. Most polymyxins cause renal toxicity.

p. B. Least toxic of the antibiotic fractions of polymyxin, and the only one used therapeutically for treating infection.

p. B sulfate. USP. An antibiotic substance produced by *Bacillus polymyxa.* Trade name is Aerosporin.

polynesic (pŏl"ē-nē'sĭk) [" + *nesos*, island]. Appearing in many separate locations or foci.

polyneural (pŏl"ē-nū'răl) [" + *neuron*, nerve, sinew]. Pert. to, innervated, or supplied by many nerves.

polyneuralgia (pŏl"ē-nū-răl'jē-ă) [" + " + *algos*, pain]. Neuralgia in several nerves.

polyneuritic (pŏl"ē-nū-rĭt'ĭk) [" + " + *itis*, inflammation]. Inflammation of several nerves at once.

polyneuritis (pŏl"ē-nū-rī'tĭs) [" + " + *itis*, inflammation]. A neuritis involving two or more nerves, usually a large number. SYN: *neuritis, multiple.*

p., acute idiopathic. Landry-Guillain-Barré syndrome.

p., diabetic. Polyneuropathy, diabetic, q.v.

p., Jamaica ginger. Polyneuritis, esp. of the nerves of the extremities following ingestion of Jamaica ginger beverage. SYN: *ginger paralysis.*

p., metabolic. Polyneuritis resulting from metabolic disorders such as nutritional deficiency, esp. the lack of thiamine; gastrointestinal disorders; or pathological conditions such as diabetes, pernicious anemia, and toxemias of pregnancy.

p., toxic. Polyneuritis resulting from poisons such as heavy metals, alcohol, carbon monoxide, or various organic compounds.

polyneuromyositis (pŏl"ē-nū"rō-mī"ō-sī'tĭs) [" + " + *mys*, muscle, + *itis*, inflammation]. Disease in which polyneuritis and polymyositis occur together.

polyneuropathy (pŏl"ē-nū-rŏp'ă-thē) [Gr. *polys*, many, + *neuron*, nerve, sinew, + *pathos*, disease, suffering]. Term applied to any disorder or affection of peripheral nerves, but preferably restricted to those of a noninflammatory nature. SYN: *neuritis, multiple; polyneuritis.*

p., amyloid. Polyneuropathy characterized by deposition of amyloid in nerves.

p., buckthorn. A symmetrical progressive polyneuropathy that starts in the lower limbs and ascends until there is respiratory paralysis when the brain stem becomes affected. If the patient survives, improvement is slow but may progress to almost complete functional recovery. There is no specific therapy.

Disease is due to ingestion of the fruit of the poisonous shrub of the buckthorn (*Rhamnus* genus). This plant grows in central and northern Mexico, Texas, and New Mexico.

p., diabetic. The most common disabling chronic complication of diabetes mellitus, affecting up to 50% of patients with either type of diabetes. The neuropathy may be symmetrical or asymmetrical, and affects peripheral nerves as well as the autonomic nervous system and cranial nerves. Clinically, neuropathic ulcers may develop, esp. on the feet. Thus, patients should be instructed to examine their feet daily for evidence of trauma, callous formation, and blisters. SYN: *diabetic polyneuritis.*

TREAT: Supportive with emphasis on preventing tissue damage.

p., porphyric. Polyneuropathy resulting from acute porphyria, characterized by pains and paresthesias in the extremities and by flaccid paralysis.

p., progressive hypertrophic. A rare familial disease beginning in childhood and characterized by increased size of peripheral nerves due to multiplication and hypertrophy of cells of the sheath of Schwann.

polyneuroradiculitis (pŏl″ē-nū″rō-ră-dĭk″ū-lī′tĭs) [″ + ″ + *radix*, root, + *itis*, inflammation]. Inflammation of the nerve roots, the peripheral nerves, and spinal ganglia.

polynuclear (pŏl″ē-nū′klē-ăr) [″ + L. *nucleus*, a kernel]. Possessing more than one nucleus. SYN: *multinuclear.*

polynucleate (pŏl″ē-nū′klē-āt). Having many nuclei.

polynucleotidase (pŏl″ē-nū″klē-ō′tĭ-dās). An enzyme present in intestinal mucosa and intestinal juice that catalyzes the breakdown of nucleic acid to nucleotides.

polynucleotide (pŏl″ē-nū′klē-ō-tīd). Nucleic acid composed of two or more nucleotides.

polyodontia (pŏl″ē-ō-dŏn′shē-ă) [″ + *odous*, tooth]. State of having supernumerary teeth.

polyomavirus (pŏl″ē-ō-mă-vī′rŭs). A virus of the papovirus family that produces malignancies in lower animals.

polyonychia (pŏl″ē-ō-nĭk′ē-ă) [″ + *onyx*, nail]. Having supernumerary nails.

polyopia, polyopsia (pŏl″ē-ō′pē-ă, -ŏp′sē-ă) [″ + *opsis*, vision]. Multiple vision; perception of more than one image of the same object.

polyorchidism (pŏl″ē-or′kĭ-dĭzm) [″ + *orchis*, testicle, + *-ismos*, condition]. Condition of having more than two testicles.

polyorchis (pŏl″ē-or′kĭs). An individual with more than two testicles.

polyorchism (pŏl″ē-or′kĭzm) [″ + *orchis*, testicle, + *-ismos*, condition]. Having more than two testicles.

polyostotic (pŏl″ē-ŏs-tŏt′ĭk) [″ + *osteon*, bone]. Concerning many bones.

polyotia (pŏl″ē-ō′shē-ă) [″ + *ous*, ear]. State of having more than two ears.

polyovulatory (pŏl″ē-ŏv′ū-lă-tō″rē) [″ + L. *ovulum*, little egg]. Releasing several ova in a single ovulatory cycle.

polyoxyl stearate (pŏl″ē-ŏks′ĭl). Any of several polyoxyethylene stearates. They have varying lengths of the polymer chain; e.g., polyoxyl 8 stearate and polyoxyl 40 stearate (trade name Myrj 52) have polymer lengths of 8 and 40 respectively. They are nonionic surface-active agents that are useful emulsifiers. SYN: *polyoxyethylene stearate.*

polyp (pŏl′ĭp) [Gr. *polypous*, many-footed]. A tumor with a pedicle. Commonly found in vascular organs such as the nose, uterus, and rectum. Polyps bleed easily; if there is a possibility that they will become malignant, they should be removed surgically. SYN: *polypus.*

p., adenomatous. Benign neoplastic tissue originating in glandular epithelium.

p., aural. Polypoid granulation tissue in the external canal of the ear attached to the tympanic membrane or middle ear structures.

p., bleeding. Angioma of the nasal mucous membrane.

p., cardiac. A pedunculated tumor attached to the inside of the heart. If situated close to a valve, it may cause blockage of the valve intermittently.

p., cervical. A fibrous or mucous polyp of the cervical mucosa.

p., choanal. Nasal polyp that extends into the pharynx.

p.'s, colonic. Polyps of the colon. They are usually benign but may undergo malignant transformation.

p., fibrinous. Polyp containing fibrin and blood, and located in the uterine cavity.

p., fibroepithelial. A smooth-surfaced polyp of the oral mucosa. These usually come on after trauma to the area. SEE: *acrochordon.*

p., fleshy. A submucous myoma in the uterus.

p., gelatinous. 1. Polyp made up of loose swollen edematous tissue. 2. Myxoma.

p., Hopmann's. A papillary growth of the nasal mucosa.

p., hydatid. A cystic polyp.

p., juvenile. A benign rounded mucosal hamartoma of the large bowel. These polyps may be present in large numbers in an infant and are commonly associated with rectal bleeding.

p., laryngeal. Polyp attached to the vocal cords and extending to the air passageway.

p., lymphoid. Benign lymphoma of the rectum.

p., mucous. Polyp of soft or jellylike consistency and exhibiting mucoid degeneration.

p., nasal. A pedunculated polyp of the nasal mucosa.

p., placental. Polyp composed of retained placental tissue.

p., retention. P., juvenile, q.v.

p., vascular. A pedunculated angioma.

polypapilloma (pŏl″ē-păp″ĭ-lō′mă) [Gr. *polys*, many + L. *papilla*, nipple, + Gr. *oma*, tumor]. Yaws, q.v.

polyparesis (pŏl″ē-pă-rē′sĭs) [″ + *parienai*, to let fall]. General progressive paralysis of paralytic dementia.

polypathia (pŏl″ē-păth′ē-ă) [″ + *pathos*, disease, suffering]. In the same person, the presence of several diseases at one time.

polypectomy (pŏl″ĭ-pĕk′tō-mē) [″ + *pous*, foot, + *ektome*, excision]. Surgical removal of a polyp.

polypeptidase (pŏl″ē-pĕp′tī-dās). An enzyme that catalyzes the hydrolysis of peptides.

polypeptide (pŏl″ē-pĕp′tīd) [″ + *peptein*, to digest]. A union of two or more amino acids. SEE: *peptide*.

polypeptidorrhachia (pŏl″ē-pĕp″tī-dō-rā′kē-ă) [″ + ″ + *rhachis*, spine]. Presence of polypeptides in the cerebrospinal fluid.

polyphagia (pŏl″ē-fā′jē-ă) [Gr. *polys*, many, + *phagein*, to eat]. Eating abnormally large amounts of food at a meal.

RS: acoria; anorexia; bulimia; parorexia; taste.

polyphalangism (pŏl″ē-fă-lăn′jĭzm) [″ + *phalanx*, closely knit row, + *-ismos*, condition]. An extra number of phalanges on a hand or foot.

polypharmacy (pŏl″ē-făr′mă-sē) [″ + *pharmakon*, drug]. 1. Excessive use of drugs or overdose of a drug. 2. Prescribing many drugs to be given at one time.

polyphenoloxidase (pŏl″ē-fē″nŏl-ŏk′sĭ-dās). An enzyme present in bacteria, fungi, and some plants that catalyzes the oxidation of polyphenols, but not monophenols such as tyrosine, to quinones.

polyphobia (pŏl″ē-fō′bē-ă) [Gr. *polys*, many, + *phobos*, fear]. Excessive or abnormal fear of a number of things.

polyphrasia (pŏl″ē-frā′zē-ă) [″ + *phrasis*, speech]. Excessive talkativeness, a manifestation of mental illness.

polyphyletic (pŏl″ē-fī-lĕt′ĭk) [″ + *phyle*, tribe]. Having more than one origin. Opposed to monophyletic.

polyphyodont (pŏl″ē-fī′ō-dŏnt) [″ + *phyein*, to produce, + *odous*, tooth]. Developing more than two sets of teeth at intervals during a lifetime.

polypiform (pō-lĭp′ĭ-form) [″ + *pous*, foot, + L. *forma*, form]. Resembling a polyp.

polyplastic (pŏl″ē-plăs′tĭk) [″ + *plastos*, formed]. 1. Having had many evolutionary modifications. 2. Having many substances in cellular composition.

polyplegia (pŏl″ē-plē′jē-ă) [″ + *plege*, stroke]. Paralysis affecting several muscles.

polyploid (pŏl′ē-ployd). 1. Characterized by polyploidy. 2. An individual in which the chromosome number is two or more times the normal haploid number.

polyploidy (pŏl′ē-ploy″dē). Condition in which the chromosome number is two or more times the normal haploid number found in gametes.

polypnea (pŏl″ĭp-nē′ă) [″ + *pnoia*, breath]. Very rapid breathing. SYN: *panting*.

polypodia (pŏl″ē-pō′dē-ă) [″ + *pous*, foot].

Possession of more than the normal number of feet.

polypoid (pŏl′ē-poyd) [″ + ″ + *eidos*, form, shape]. Like a polyp.

polyporous (pŏl-ĭp′ō-rŭs) [″ + *poros*, pore]. Possessing many small openings or pores.

polyposia (pŏl″ē-pō′zē-ă) [″ + *posis*, drinking]. Sustained ingestion of large amounts of fluid.

polyposis (pŏl″ē-pō′sĭs) [″ + *pous*, foot, + *osis*, condition]. The presence of numerous polyps.

    p. coli. Polyposis of the large intestine.

    p., familial. A rare familial condition in which the mucosa of the colon is covered with polyps. This causes rectal bleeding and the passage of polyps that come loose. These may become infected and cause chronic intussusception of the colon. The polyps may become malignant.

    p., multiple intestinal. Polyps or tumors that are derived from mucous membrane and are scattered throughout the intestine and rectum. They may undergo degeneration.

    p. ventriculi. Presence of numerous polyps in the stomach, sometimes involving entire mucosa, accompanied by chronic atrophic gastritis.

polypotome (pŏl-ĭp′ō-tōm) [″ + ″ + *tome*, incision]. Instrument for excision of polyps.

polypotrite (pō-lĭp′ō-trīt) [″ + ″ + L. *terere*, to crush]. A device for crushing polyps.

polyptychial (pŏl″ē-tī′kē-ăl) [″ + *ptyche*, fold]. Arranged in several layers, as is the case in some glands.

polypus (pŏl′ĭ-pŭs) [L.] (pl. *polypi*). A polyp.

polyradiculitis (pŏl″ē-ră-dĭk′ū-lī′tĭs) [″ + L. *radix*, root, + Gr. *itis*, inflammation]. Inflammation of nerve roots, esp. those of spinal nerves. SEE: *Nursing Diagnoses* in *Appendix.*

polyradiculoneuritis (pŏl″ē-ră-dĭk″ū-lō-nū-rī′tĭs) [″ + ″ + Gr. *neuron*, nerve, + *itis*, inflammation]. Inflammation of the peripheral nerves and spinal ganglia.

polyradiculoneuropathy (pŏl″ē-ră-dĭk″ū-lō-nū-rŏp′ă-thē) [″ + ″ + ″ + *pathos*, disease, suffering]. Guillain-Barré syndrome, q.v.

polyribosome (pŏl″ē-rī′bō-sōm). A cluster or group of ribosomes, q.v. They are important in transmitting genetic information and in protein synthesis. SYN: *polysome.*

polyrrhea, polyrrhoea (pŏl″ē-rē′ă) [″ + *rhoia*, flow]. Excessive secretion of fluid.

polysaccharide (pŏl″ē-săk′ă-rīd) [″ + Sanskrit *sarkara*, sugar]. One of a group of carbohydrates that upon hydrolysis yield more than two molecules of simple sugars. They are complex carbohydrates of high molecular weight, usually insoluble in water, but when soluble, they form colloidal solutions. Their basic formula is $(C_6H_{12}O_6)_n$. They include two groups: starch (e.g., starch, inulin, glycogen, dextrin) and cellulose (e.g., cellulose and hemicelluloses). The hemicelluloses include the pentosans (e.g., gum arabic), hexosans (e.g., agar-agar), and hexopentosans (e.g., pectin). SEE: *carbohydrates; disaccharide; monosaccharide.*

p.'s, immune. Polysaccharides in bacteria, esp. in the cell wall, that are antigenic.

polysaccharose (pŏl″ē-săk′ă-rōs). A polysaccharide.

polyscelia (pŏl″ē-sē′lē-ă) [″ + *skelos*, leg]. Condition of having more than the normal number of legs.

polyscelus (pŏ-lĭs′ē-lŭs). One having polyscelia, q.v.

polyserositis (pŏl″ē-sē-rō-sī′tĭs) [″ + L. *serum*, whey, + *itis*, inflammation]. Familial Mediterranean fever.

p., familial paroxysmal. SEE: *familial Mediterranean fever.*

polysialia (pŏl″ē-sī-ă′lē-ă) [″ + *sialon*, saliva]. Ptyalism, q.v.

polysinusitis, polysinuitis (pŏl″ē-sī″nŭs-ī′tĭs, -nū-ī′tĭs) [″ + L. *sinus*, a hollow, + Gr. *itis*, inflammation]. Inflammation of several sinuses simultaneously.

polysomaty (pŏl″ē-sō′mă-tē) [″ + *soma*, body]. Having reduplicated chromatin in the nucleus.

polysome. Polyribosome.

polysomia (pŏl″ē-sō′mē-ă) [″ + *soma*, body]. Having more than one body, as in the doubling of the body of a fetus.

polysorbates (pŏl″ē-sor′bāts). Nonionic surface-active agents composed of polyoxyethylene esters of sorbitol. They usually contain associated fatty acids. The series includes polysorbates 20, 40, 60, and 80, which are used in preparing pharmaceuticals. These polysorbates have the trade names of Tween 20, Tween 40, etc.

polyspermia (pŏl″ē-spĕr′mē-ă) [Gr. *polys*, many, + *sperma*, seed]. 1. Excessive secretion of seminal fluid. 2. Entrance of several spermatozoa into one ovum. SYN: *polyspermism.*

polyspermism (pŏl″ē-spĕrm′ĭzm). Polyspermia.

polyspermy (pŏl″ē-spĕr′mē). Fertilization of an ovum by multiple spermatozoa.

polystichia (pŏl″ē-stĭk′ē-ă) [″ + *stichos*, a row]. Condition in which there are two or more rows of eyelashes.

polystomatous (pŏl″ē-stō′mă-tŭs) [″ + *stoma*, mouth]. Possessing many mouths or openings.

polystyrene (pŏl″ē-stī′rēn). A synthetic resin produced by the polymerization of styrene from ethylene and benzene. The formula is $(CH_2CHC_6H_5)_n$. It is used in the plastics industry.

polysynaptic (pŏl″ē-sĭ-năp′tĭk) [″ + *synapsis*, point of contact]. Pert. to nerve pathways involving multiple synapses.

polysyndactyly (pŏl″ē-sĭn-dăk′tĭl-ē) [″ + *syn*, together, + *daktylos*, finger]. Multiple syndactyly.

polytendinitis (pŏl″ē-tĕn″dĭ-nī′tĭs) [″ + L. *tendo*, tendon, + Gr. *itis*, inflammation]. Inflammation of several tendons.

polytene (pŏl′ē-tēn) [″ + *tainia*, band]. Composed of many filaments of chromatin.

polyteny (pŏl″ē-tē′nē) [″ + *tainia*, band]. Multiple lateral duplication of the chromosome. This produces a giant chromosome.

polytetrafluoroethylene. ABBR: PTFE. A synthetic material that has slippery, nonsticking properties. It is used in a variety of products, including frying pan coatings and, in manufacturing, the fabric known by its trade name, Gore-Tex, q.v. The expanded form has the property of becoming "fatter" when it is stretched, rather than thinner. Trade name is Teflon.

polythelia (pŏl″ē-thē′lē-ă) [″ + *thele*, nipple, + *-ismos*, condition]. Presence of more than one nipple on a mamma. SYN: *polythelism.*

polythelism (pŏl″ē-thē′lĭzm). Polythelia.

polythiazide (pŏl″ē-thī′ă-zīd). USP. A diuretic drug. Trade name is Renese.

polytocous (pō-lĭt′ō-kŭs) [″ + *tokos*, birth]. Producing several offspring at one time.

polytrichia (pŏl″ē-trĭk′ē-ă) [″ + *thrix*, hair]. Hypertrichosis.

polytrichosis (pŏl″ē-trĭ-kō′sĭs) [″ + ″ + *osis*, condition]. Excessive growth of hair. SYN: *hypertrichosis.*

polytrophia (pŏl″ē-trō-fē-ă) [″ + *trophe*, nourishment]. Excessive or abundant nutrition. SYN: *polytrophy.*

polytrophy (pō-lĭt′rō-fē). Polytrophia.

polytropic (pŏl″ē-trŏp′ĭk) [″ + *trope*, a turning]. Affecting more than one type of cell, said of viruses, or affecting more than one type of tissue, said of certain poisons.

polyunguia (pŏl″ē-ŭng′gwē-ă) [″ + L. *unguis*, nail]. Polyonychia, q.v.

polyunsaturated. In chemistry, rel. to long-chain carbon compounds, esp. fats that have many carbon atoms joined by double or triple bonds.

polyuria (pŏl″ē-ū′rē-ă) [″ + *ouron*, urine]. Excessive secretion and discharge of urine. The urine does not, as a rule, contain abnormal constituents. Several liters in excess of normal may be voided each day. The urine is virtually colorless. Sp. gr. 1.000 to 1.002 and higher in diabetes.

ETIOL: Occurs in diabetes insipidus; diabetes mellitus; chronic nephritis; nephrosclerosis; following edematous states, esp. those induced by heart failure treated with diuretics; in hyperthyroidism; and following excessive intake of liquids.

polyvalent (pŏl"ē-vā'lĕnt, pō-lĭv'ă-lĕnt) [" + L. *valere*, to be strong]. Multivalent; having a combining power of more than two atoms of hydrogen.

polyvalent serum. Serum with antibodies produced by injecting several strains of microorganisms of the same species, or by injecting different species.

polyvalent vaccine. Vaccine produced from cultures of a number of strains of the same species.

polyvinyl alcohol (pŏl"ē-vī'nĭl). USP. A water-soluble synthetic resin used in preparing medicines, esp. ophthalmic solutions.

polyvinyl chloride. ABBR: PVC. A thermoplastic polymer formed from vinyl chloride. It is used in the manufacture of many products such as rainwear, garden hoses, phonograph records, and floor tiles.

NOTE: Exposure to toxic fumes of PVC can cause respiratory arrest due to oxygen deprivation. The reaction to PVC is delayed for 6 to 24 hr after exposure. Patients with suspected exposure should be closely monitored.

polyvinylpyrrolidone (pŏl"ē-vī"nĭl-pĕr-rŏl'ĭ-dōn). ABBR: PVP. Previously used name for povidone, q.v.

pomade (pō-mād') [Fr. *pommade*]. A perfumed ointment, esp. one for the hair. SYN: *pomatum.*

pomatum (pō-mā'tŭm). A medicinal ointment, esp. one used on the hair. SYN: *pomade.*

Pompe's disease. Glycogen storage disease, type II, q.v.

pompholyx. Deep-seated vesicles of the hands and feet, esp. the palms and soles. The condition may be chronic and produce itching. Cause is unknown, but it may be associated with contact allergy or a fungal infection. Condition is treated with cortisone combined with diiodohydroxyquin ointment applied under an occlusive dressing. This is worn at night. Even though pompholyx is often considered to be due to dyshidrosis, q.v., sweating may be normal, decreased, or increased. SEE: *hyperhidrosis.*

pomphus (pŏm'fŭs) [L.] (pl. *pomphi*). A blister or a circumscribed elevation on the skin; a wheal.

POMR. *problem-oriented medical record.*

pomum (pō'mŭm) [L.]. An apple.

p. adami. Prominence in the middle line of the throat, caused by junction of two lateral wings of the thyroid cartilage. SYN: *Adam's apple.*

ponderal (pŏn'dĕr-ăl) [L. *pondus*, weight]. Rel. to weight.

ponderal index. The ratio of an individual's height to the cube root of his or her weight; used to determine body mass. Expressed as:

$$\frac{\text{height (in inches)}}{\sqrt[3]{\text{weight (in pounds)}}}$$

SEE: *Quatelet index.*

Pondimin. Trade name for fenfluramine hydrochloride.

ponograph (pō'nō-grăf) [Gr. *ponos*, pain, fatigue, + *graphein*, to write]. Device for measuring and registering sensitiveness to pain or fatigue.

ponophobia (pō"nō-fō'bē-ă) [" + *phobos*, fear]. 1. Abnormal distaste for exerting oneself. 2. Dread of pain.

pons (pŏnz) [L., bridge] (pl. *pontes*). 1. A process of tissue connecting two or more parts. 2. [NA] Pons varolii.

p. cerebelli. Pons varolii.

p. hepatis. Part of liver sometimes present that extends from the quadrate lobe to the left lobe across the umbilical fissure.

p. varolii [Costanzo Varolio (Varolius), It. anatomist, 1543–1575]. A rounded eminence on the ventral surface of the brain stem. It lies between the medulla and cerebral peduncles, and appears externally as a broad band of transverse fibers. It is connected to the cerebellum by the midcerebellar peduncle, or brachium pontis. It contains fiber tracts connecting the medulla oblongata and cerebellum with upper portions of the brain. The origins of the abducens, facial, trigeminal, and cochlear divisions of the 8th (vestibulocochlear) nerve are at the borders of the pons. SYN: *pons* (def. 2) [NA]; *p. cerebelli.*

Ponstel. Trade name for mefenamic acid.

pontic (pŏn'tĭk) [L. *pons, pontis,* bridge]. An artificial tooth set in a bridge.

ponticulus (pŏn-tĭk'ū-lŭs) [L., little bridge]. An obsolete term for a little ridge.

pontile (pŏn'tēl). Pert. to the pons varolii.

pontile hemiplegia. Hemiplegia due to lesion of the pons. The arm and leg on one side and the face on the opposite side are affected.

pontile nuclei. The gray matter in the pons.

pontine (pŏn'tēn). Pert. to the pons varolii.

pontobulbar (pŏn"tō-bŭl'bar). Pert. to the pons and medulla oblongata.

Pontocaine. Trade name for tetracaine.

Pontocaine Hydrochloride (pŏn'tō-kān). Trade name for tetracaine hydrochloride. Is available in several forms for use as a topical or spinal anesthetic.

pool. 1. To mix blood from several donors. 2. Accumulation of blood in a body site.

p., abdominal. The accumulation of blood in the visceral organs of the abdominal cavity. This may occur during shock.

p., gene. The sum of the genetic material in the members of a specified population.

p., metabolic. All of the chemical compounds included in metabolic processes in the body.

p., vaginal. The mucus and cells that are present in the posterior fornix of the vagina when the patient is in a supine position. Material obtained from this site is used in cancer detection and in evaluating the character of the vaginal fluid in investigating infertility problems.

poples (pŏp′lēz) [L., ham of the knee]. The popliteal or posterior region of the knee.

popliteal (pŏp″lĭt-ē′ăl, pŏp-lĭt′ē-ăl) [L. *poples*, ham of the knee]. Concerning the posterior surface of the knee.

popliteus (pŏp-lĭt″ē-ŭs, -lĭt-ē′ŭs). Muscle located in hind part of the knee joint that flexes the leg and aids it in rotating. SEE: *Muscles* in *Appendix*.

poppy. Any of the several plants of the genus *Papaver*. Opium is obtained from the juice of the unripe pods of *Papaver somniferum*.

population dynamics. The concept that certain factors influence changes in the numbers of persons in a population.

population of world. A variable depending upon the rate at which the number of people on earth increases. The number of people on earth has never been known with any degree of accuracy due to the difficulty of obtaining accurate worldwide census data. It is estimated that there were 250 million people on earth in the year A.D. 1; 500 million by the early 17th century; 3.2 billion by 1964; and 5.8 billion in 1975. It is estimated that there will be 8.5 billion people on earth by the year 2025. Population of the world increases by an estimated 150 persons a minute, and the estimated U.S. population will be 262.5 million by the year 2000.

POR. *problem-oriented record.*

poradenitis (por″ăd-ĕ-nī′tĭs) [Gr. *poros*, passage, + *aden*, gland, + *itis*, inflammation]. Formation of small abscesses in the iliac glands.

porcelain (por′sĕ-lĭn). A hard, translucent ceramic made by fusing clay. It is colored by glazing with fusible pigments. It is used in dentistry.

porcelaneous, porcelanous (por″sĕ-lā′nē-ŭs, -sĕl′ăn-ŭs) [Fr. *porcelaine*]. Translucent or white like porcelain, as the skin.

porcine (por′sīn) [L. *porcus*, pig]. Piglike.

pore (por) [Gr. *poros*, passage.]. 1. A minute opening, esp. one on an epithelial surface. SYN: *porus* [NA]. 2. Opening of the excretory duct of a sweat gland. SEE: *skin; stoma; sweat glands.*

p., alveolar. A minute opening that is thought to exist between adjacent alveoli of the lung.

p., gustatory. P., taste.

p., taste. The external opening of a taste bud. SYN: *p., gustatory.* SEE: *taste.*

porencephalia, porencephaly (por″ĕn-sĕf-ă′lē-ă, por″ĕn-sĕf′ă-lē) [″ + *enkephalos*, brain]. An anomalous condition in which the ventricles of the brain are connected with the subarachnoid space.

porencephalitis (por″ĕn-sĕf″ă-lī′tĭs) [″ + ″ + *itis*, inflammation]. Inflammation of the brain with development of cavities communicating with the subarachnoid space.

porencephalous. Pert. to porencephalia.

pores of Kohn [Hans Kohn, Ger. pathologist, b. 1866]. Passageway for gas from one alveolus of the lung to an adjacent one. These may be of assistance in preventing atelectasis. SEE: *canals of Lambert.*

pori. Pl. of porus.

poriomania [Gr. *poreia*, walking, + *mania*, madness]. Morbid desire to wander from home.

porion (pō′rē-ŏn) [Gr. *poros*, passage]. The midpoint of the upper margin of the auditory meatus.

pornography (por-nŏg′ră-fē) [Gr. *porne*, prostitute, + *graphein*, to write]. Written or graphic forms of communication that are intended to, or may, incite sexual interest.

pornolagnia [Gr. *porno*, prostitute]. Sexual attraction to prostitutes.

porocele (pō′rō-sēl) [Gr. *poros*, passage, + *kele*, tumor, swelling]. A herniation into the scrotal sac. This causes hardening and thickening of the scrotum.

porocephaliasis, porocephalosis (pō″rō-sĕf″ă-lī′ă-sĭs, -lō′sĭs) [″ + *kephale*, head, + *-iasis*, state or condition of]. Infection with a species of *Porocephalus.*

Porocephalus (pō″rō-sĕf′ă-lŭs). A genus of wormlike arthropods found commonly in snakes. The young sometimes infest mammals, including humans.

porokeratosis (pō″rō-kĕr″ă-tō′sĭs) [″ + *keras*, horn, + *osis*, condition]. A rare skin disease marked by thickening of the stratum corneum in linear arrangement, followed by its atrophy. Porokeratosis appears on smooth areas. It is irregular in form and size with a circumscribed outline and affects hands and feet, forearms and legs, the face, neck, and scalp.

poroma (pō-rō′mă) [Gr.]. 1. A callosity. 2. A tumor of cells lining the opening of the sweat glands.

p., cerebral. At postmortem examination, the presence of cavities in the brain substance due to gas-forming bacteria.

p., eccrine. A tumor arising from the duct of an eccrine gland. It usually occurs on the palm or sole.

porosis (pō-rō'sĭs) [Gr. *poros,* passage, + *osis,* condition]. Formation of callus in repair of fractured bone. SEE: *callus.*

porosity (pō-rŏs'ĭ-tē) [Gr. *poros,* passage]. The state of being porous.

porotomy (pō-rŏt'ō-mē) [" + *tome,* incision]. Incision of the urethral meatus.

porous (pō'rŭs). Full of pores; able to admit passage of a liquid.

porphin (por'fĭn). The basic ring structure forming the framework of all porphyrins. Consisting of four pyrrole rings united by methene, —CH₂—, couplings.

porphobilinogen (por″fō-bĭ-lĭn'ō-jĕn). An intermediate product in heme synthesis sometimes found in the urine of patients with acute porphyria. The urine may appear to be normal when fresh, but will change to a Burgundy wine color or even to black when heated with dilute hydrochloric acid to 100°C.

porphyria (por-fĭ'rē-ă, por-fĭr'ē-ă) [Gr. *porphyra,* purple]. A group of disorders that result from a disturbance in porphyrin metabolism, causing increased formation and excretion of porphyrin or its precursors.

p., acute intermittent. A rare metabolic disorder characterized by excessive excretion of porphyrins, acute abdominal pain, and neurological disturbances, inherited as an autosomal dominant trait. Sometimes precipitated by excessive use of sulfonamides, barbiturates, or other drugs. Sensitivity to light is characteristic.

p., congenital erythropoietic. A rare condition characterized by severe skin lesions, hemolytic anemia, and splenomegaly. Inherited as an autosomal recessive trait.

p. cutanea tarda hereditaria. Porphyria inherited as an autosomal dominant characteristic. Onset of symptoms usually occurs between the ages of 10 and 30.

p. erythropoietica. Mild form of porphyria characterized by cutaneous lesions and excess protoporphyrin in erythrocytes and feces.

p. hepatica. Porphyria due to disturbance in liver metabolism such as occurs following hepatitis, poisoning by heavy metals, certain anemias, and other conditions.

p., South African genetic. P., variegate, q.v.

p., variegate. A form of hepatic porphyria in which there are recurrent episodes of abdominal pain and neuropathy. The skin is especially fragile.

porphyrin (por'fĭ-rĭn) [Gr. *porphyra,* purple]. Any of a group of nitrogen-containing organic compounds that occur in protoplasm and form the basis of animal and plant respiratory pigments, obtained from hemoglobin and chlorophyll.

porphyrinuria (por″fĭ-rĭ-nū'rē-ă) [" + *ouron,* urine]. Excretion of an increased amount of porphyrin in the urine. SYN: *porphyruria.*

porphyrization (por″fĭr-ĭ-zā'shŭn). Process of pulverizing.

porphyruria (por″fĭr-ū'rē-ă) [" + *ouron,* urine]. Excretion of an increased amount of porphyrin in urine. SYN: *porphyrinuria.*

Porro's operation (por'ōz) [Eduardo Porro, It. obstetrician, 1842–1902]. Cesarean section followed by removal of the uterus, the ovaries, and fallopian tubes. SYN: *cesarean hysterectomy.*

porta [L., gate] (pl. *portae*). The point of entry of nerves and vessels into an organ or part.

p. hepatis. [NA] The fissure of the liver where the portal vein and hepatic artery enter and the hepatic duct leaves.

p. lienis. Hilus of the spleen where vessels enter and leave. SYN: *hilum splenicum.*

p. pulmonis. Pulmonary hilus for entry and exit of the bronchi, nerves, and vessels. SYN: *hilum pulmonis.*

p. renis. Hilus of the kidney, the site of entry and leaving of vessels. SYN: *hilum renalis.*

portacaval (por″tă-kā'văl). Concerning the portal vein and the vena cava.

portacaval shunt. Surgical joining of the portal vein and the inferior vena cava.

portal [L. *porta,* gate]. 1. An entryway. 2. Concerning a porta or entrance to an organ, esp. that through which the blood is carried to the liver.

p., intestinal. The opening of the midgut or yolk sac into the foregut or hindgut of an embryo.

p. of entry. The avenue by which infectious organisms gain access to the body.

portal circulation. The circulation of blood into the liver by the portal vein and out by the hepatic vein.

portal hypertension. Increased pressure in the portal vein as a result of obstruction of the flow of blood through the liver.

portal system. The portal vein and its branches by which blood is collected from abdominal viscera and conveyed to the sinusoids of the liver, from which it passes through the hepatic veins to the inferior vena cava.

portal-systemic encephalopathy. ABBR: PSE. Related to the presence of shunting of blood around the liver and hepatic insufficiency. Substances that are toxic to the brain are not metabolized by the liver. PSE includes dementia as well as neuromuscular abnormalities, metabolic slowing of electroencephalogram, and elevated ammonia levels. SEE: *asterixis; hepatic coma.*

portal vein. Vein formed by the veins of the splanchnic area that conveys its blood into the liver. It is made of the combined superior and inferior mesenteric, splenic, gastric, and cystic veins.

portio (por′shē-ō) [L.] (pl. *portiones*). [NA] A part. In anatomy, it designates a certain portion of a structure or organ.

    p. dura. The seventh cranial nerve; the facial nerve.

    p. intermedia. Nervus, intermedius, q.v.

    p. vaginalis. The part of the cervix within the vagina.

portogram (por′tō-grăm) [L. *porta*, gate, + Gr. *gramma*, something written]. Roentgenogram of the portal vein.

portography (por-tŏg′ră-fē) [″ + Gr. *graphein*, to write]. Roentgenography of the portal vein while an opaque medium is in it.

    p., portal. Portography after injection of opaque material into the superior mesenteric vein. This is usually done during laparotomy.

    p., splenic. Roentgenography of the splenic and portal veins after injection of opaque material into the spleen.

portosystemic (por″tō-sĭs-tĕm′ĭk). Joining the portal and systemic venous circulation.

Portuguese man-of-war. A type of jellyfish, *Physalia physalis*, whose tentacles contain a neurotoxin that produces a burning sensation on contact. For treatment, SEE: *bites or stings.*

port-wine mark, stain. A superficial purplered birthmark. In children, these have been treated with the flashlamp-pulsed tunable dye laser. SYN: *nevus flammeus.*

porus (pō′rŭs) [L.] (pl. *pori*). A meatus or foramen; a tiny aperture in a structure; a pore.

    p. acusticus externus. [NA] The outer opening of the external acoustic meatus.

    p. acusticus internus. [NA] Opening of the internal acoustic meatus into the cranial cavity.

    p. gustatorius. The small taste pore openings in the taste buds of the tongue.

    p. lactiferous. Opening of a lactiferous duct on the tip of the nipple of the mammary gland.

    p. opticus. Opening in center of the optic disk through which retinal vessels (central artery and vein) reach retina through the lamina cribrosa of the sclera.

    p. sudoriferus. [NA] Opening of a sweat gland.

Positions of Fetus in Utero

Vertex Presentation (point of designation — occiput):

Left occiput anterior	LOA
Right occiput posterior	ROP
Right occiput anterior	ROA
Left occiput posterior	LOP
Right occiput transverse	ROT
Occiput anterior	OA
Occiput posterior	OP

Breech presentation (point of designation — sacrum):

Left sacroanterior	LSA
Right sacroposterior	RSP
Right sacroanterior	RSA
Left sacroposterior	LSP
Sacroanterior	SA
Sacroposterior	SP
Left sacrotransverse	LST
Right sacrotransverse	RST

Face Presentation (point of designation — chin [mentum]):

Left mentoanterior	LMA
Right mentoposterior	RMP
Right mentoanterior	RMA
Left mentoposterior	LMP
Mentoposterior	MP
Mentoanterior	MA
Left mentotransverse	LMT
Right mentotransverse	RMT

Transverse presentation (point of designation — scapula of presenting shoulder):

Left scapuloanterior	LScA
Right scapuloposterior	RScP
Right scapuloanterior	RScA
Left scapuloposterior	LScP

position (pō-zĭsh′ŭn) [L. *positio*]. 1. Place in which a thing is put. 2. Manner in which a body is arranged, as by the nurse or physician for examination. 3. In obstetrics, the relation of some arbitrarily chosen portion of the child in the pelvis to the right or left side of the mother, the occiput, chin, sacrum, and scapula being the points of reference that are most commonly used. SEE: table; *presentation* for illus.

    p., anatomic. Position assumed when a person is standing erect with arms at the sides, palms forward. SYN: *p., orthograde.*

    p., Bonnet's. In inflammation of the hip joint, the flexion, abduction, and outward rotation of the thigh, which produces relief.

    p., Bozeman's. The knee-elbow position in which the patient is strapped to supports.

p., Brickner. A method of obtaining traction, abduction, and external rotation of the shoulder by tying the patient's wrists to the head of the bed.

p., centric. The most posterior position of the mandible in relation to the maxilla.

p., decubitus. Position of the patient on a flat surface. The exact position is indicated by which surface of the body is closest to the flat surface, i.e., in left or right lateral decubitus, the patient is flat on the left or right side, respectively; in dorsal or ventral decubitus, the patient is on the back or abdomen, respectively.

p., dorsal. Position in which the patient is on back. SYN: *supine.*

p., dorsal elevated. Position with patient lying on back with head and shoulders elevated at an angle of 30° or more. Employed in digital examination of genitalia and in bimanual examination of the vagina.

p., dorsal recumbent. Position of patient on back with lower extremities moderately flexed and rotated outward. Employed in application of obstetrical forceps, repair of lesions following parturition, vaginal examination, and bimanual palpation. SEE: illus.

p., dorsosacral. P., lithotomy. SEE: illus.

p., Edebohls'. P., Simon's.

p., Elliot's. Position in which supports are placed under the small of the patient's back so that patient resembles a double inclined plane.

p., English. P., left lateral recumbent.

p., Fowler's. Position in which the head of the patient's bed is raised about 1½ ft (46 cm), and knees are elevated. SEE: illus.; *Fowler's position.*

p., genucubital. Position with patient on knees, thighs upright, body resting on elbows, head down on hands. Employed when it is not possible to use the classic knee-chest position. SYN: *p., knee-elbow.*

p., genupectoral. Position with patient on knees, thighs upright, head and upper part of chest resting on table, arms crossed above head. Employed in displacement of prolapsed fundus, dislodgment of impacted head of fetus, management of transverse presentation, replacement of retroverted uterus or displaced ovary, or flushing of intestinal canal. SYN: *p., knee-chest.* SEE: illus.

p., horizontal. Position with patient lying supine with feet extended. Employed in palpation, in auscultation of fetal heart, and in operative procedures.

p., horizontal abdominal. Position with patient flat on abdomen, feet extended. Employed in examination of back and spinal column.

p., jackknife. Position with patient on back, shoulders elevated, legs flexed on thighs, thighs at right angles to abdomen. Employed when passing urethral sound. SYN: *p., reclining.*

p., knee-chest. P., genupectoral. SEE: illus.

p., knee-elbow. P., genucubital.

p., laterosemiprone. P., Sims'.

p., left lateral recumbent. Position with patient on left side, right knee and thigh drawn up. Employed in vaginal examination.

p., lithotomy. Position with patient on back, thighs flexed on abdomen, legs on thighs, thighs abducted. Employed in operation on genital tract, in vaginal hysterectomy, and diagnosis and treatment of diseases of urethra and bladder. SYN: *p., dorsosacral.* SEE: illus.

p., Noble's. Position in which the patient is standing, leaning forward, and supporting the upper body by bracing the arms against the wall or a chair. This position is useful in examining the kidney.

p., obstetrical. P., left lateral recumbent.

p., orthograde. P., anatomic.

p., orthopneic. Sitting erect or propped up in bed by use of pillows or bed angulation. Position is for those who have difficulty breathing.

p., PA. In radiology, a position in which the central ray enters the posterior surface of the body and exits the anterior surface.

p., physiologic rest. In dentistry, position of the mandible at rest when the patient is sitting upright and the condyles are in an unstrained position. The jaw muscles are relaxed.

p., prone. Position in which patient is lying face downward. SEE: illus.

p., reclining. P., jackknife.

p., rest. In dentistry, the position of the mandible when the jaws are at rest. The masticatory musculature is relaxed, and the teeth are slightly separated.

p., Rose's. In repairing a laceration of the upper lip or mouth; the patient's head is extended and hangs over the end of the table. This permits blood to flow down and not into the patient's mouth.

p., side, semiprone. P., Sims'.

p., Simon's. Exaggerated lithotomy position. Patient flat on back, legs flexed on thighs, thighs on abdomen, hips somewhat elevated, thighs strongly abducted. Employed in vaginal operations.

p., Sims'. Position with patient on left side, right knee and thigh drawn well up above left, left arm back of patient and

POSITIONS

DORSAL RECUMBENT POSITION

KNEES MAY BE BENT

FOWLER'S POSITION

KNEE-CHEST OR GENUPECTORAL POSITION

LITHOTOMY OR DORSOSACRAL POSITION

POSITIONS

PRONE POSITION

SIMS' POSITION

SHOULDER BRACE

TRENDELENBURG POSITION

RIGHT LATERAL RECUMBENT POSITION

hanging over edge of table, chest inclined forward so that patient rests upon it. Employed in curettement of uterus, intrauterine irrigation after labor, tamponade of vagina, rectal exploration, and operations on cervix. SYN: *p., laterosemiprone.* SEE: illus.

p., Trendelenburg. Dorsal position in which patient's body is supine on a bed tilted at about 45° angle with the head low. Employed in abdominal surgery to favor gravitation upward of abdominal viscera and in treating cardiovascular shock. SEE: illus.

p., unilateral recumbent. Position in which patient is on right side, used in acute pleurisy, lobar pneumonia of the right side, and in a greatly enlarged liver; position in which patient is on left side, used in lobar pneumonia, pleurisy on that side, and in large pericardial effusions. SEE: illus.

positioner (pō-zīsh'ŭn-ĕr). Apparatus for holding or placing the body or part, esp. the head, in a certain position.

positioning. In rehabilitation, a term used to refer to placing the body and extremities so as to aid treatment by inhibiting undesirable reflexes and preventing deformities. In treatment of children with developmental disabilities involving neuromotor function, the position of the body affects the presence of some primitive reflexes which can affect muscle tone. Alignment of the head, neck, and trunk is therefore thought to be important to reduce unnecessary influences on muscle tone, and the careful placement of the limbs is important to reduce or prevent contractions and deformities.

positive (pŏz'ĭ-tĭv) [L. *positivus*, ruling]. 1. Definite; affirmative; opposed to negative. 2. Indicating an abnormal condition in examination and diagnosis. 3. Having a value greater than zero.

Often in laboratory findings and mathematical expressions, positive is indicated by a plus (+) sign.

positive end-expiratory pressure. ABBR: PEEP. In respiratory medicine, a method of holding alveoli open during expiration. This is done by gradually increasing the expiratory pressure. When PEEP is used, it is important that pulmonary capillary wedge pressure be monitored by use of a Swan-Ganz catheter in the pulmonary artery. The goal is to achieve adequate arterial oxygenation without using toxic levels of inspired oxygen, and without compromising cardiac output.

Caution: The patient must be carefully monitored during the therapy to ensure compliance and to allow observation for undesired side effects such as pneumomediastinum, subcuta-

neous emphysema, and pneumothorax.

positron (pŏz'ĭ-trŏn). A particle having the same mass as a negative electron, but possessing a positive charge.

positron emission tomography. ABBR: PET. Reconstruction of brain sections by using positron-emitting radionuclides. By using several different radionuclides, researchers can measure regional cerebral blood flow, blood volume, oxygen uptake, and glucose transport and metabolism, and they can locate neurotransmitter receptors.

posological (pŏ"sō-lŏj'ĭ-kăl) [Gr. *posos*, how much, + *logos*, word, reason]. Concerning dosage of medicines.

posology (pō-sŏl'ō-jē). Branch of scientific study dealing with dosage of medicines.

possessed. Obsessed, or as if controlled by an outside spirit or force.

possession (pō-zĕsh'ŭn) [ME. *possessen*]. Psychological state of being dominated by an idea, a passion, or a mental obsession.

p., demoniacal. Belief of being controlled by an evil spirit or demon.

Possum (pŏs'ŭm) [*p*atient *o*perated *s*elector *m*echanism]. Device that permits a disabled individual to control and operate various machines such as switches, telephones, and typewriters by breathing into the master control of the apparatus.

post. In dentistry, a dowel or pin which is anchored in an upright position in a tooth or bone for the attachment of a dental crown or prosthesis.

post- [L.]. A prefix meaning behind, after, or posterior.

postabortal (pōst"ă-bor'tăl) [L. *post*, behind, after, + *abortus*, abortion]. Happening subsequent to abortion.

postacetabular (pōst"ăs-ĕ-tăb'ū-lăr) [" + *acetabulum*, a little saucer for vinegar]. Behind the acetabulum.

postadolescent (pōst"ăd-ō-lĕs'ĕnt) [" + *adolescens*, to grow up]. An individual who has passed adolescence.

postanal (pōst-ā'năl) [" + *anus*, anus]. Located behind the anus.

postanesthesia recovery room nurse. ABBR: PAR nurse. Nurses who have received special training in caring for patients who have come from surgery and are recovering from the effects of anesthesia.

postanesthetic (pōst"ăn-ĕs-thĕt'ĭk) [" + Gr. *an-*, not, + *aisthesis*, sensation]. Pert. to the period following anesthesia.

postapoplectic (pōst"ăp-ō-plĕk'tĭk) [" + Gr. *apoplessein*, to cripple by a stroke]. Pert. to the period immediately following a stroke or apoplexy.

postaxial (pōst-ăk'sē-ăl) [" + Gr. *axon*,

axis]. Situated or happening behind an axis.

postbrachial (pŏst-brā'kē-ăl) [" + *brachiolis*, arm]. Pert. to the posterior portion of the upper arm.

postcapillary (pŏst-kăp'ĭl-lā-rē). A terminal vessel of a capillary network that leads to a venule. SYN: *capillary, venous.*

postcardial (pŏst-kăr'dē-ăl) [" + Gr. *kardia*, heart]. Behind the heart.

postcardiotomy (pŏst-kăr"dē-ŏt'ō-mē) [" + " + *tome*, incision]. The period after open-heart surgery.

postcaval. Concerning the postcava, the ascending or inferior vena cava.

postcentral (pŏst-sĕn'trăl) [" + Gr. *kentron*, center]. 1. Situated or happening behind a center. 2. Located behind the fissure of Rolando.

postcibal (pŏst-sī'băl) [" + *cibum*, food]. Occurring after meals.

postclavicular (pŏst"klā-vĭk'ū-lăr) [" + *clavicula*, a little key]. Located or occurring behind the clavicle.

postclimacteric (pŏst"klī-măk-tĕr'ĭk, -măk'tĕr-ĭk) [" + Gr. *klimakter*, rung of a ladder]. Occurring after the menopause.

postcoital (pŏst-kō'ĭt-ăl) [" + *coitio*, a coming together]. Subsequent to sexual intercourse.

postconnubial (pŏst"kŏn-ū'bē-ăl) [" + *connubium*, marriage]. Occurring after marriage.

postconvulsive (pŏst"kŏn-vŭl'sĭv) [" + *convulsus*, pull violently]. Occurring after a convulsion.

postdiastolic (pŏst"dī-ăs-tŏl'ĭk) [" + Gr. *diastole*, expansion]. Occurring after the cardiac diastole.

postdicrotic (pŏst"dī-krŏt'ĭk) [" + Gr. *dikrotos*, beating double]. Occurring after the dicrotic pulse wave.

postdicrotic wave. A recoil or second wave (not always present) in a sphygmographic tracing.

postdiphtheritic (pŏst"dĭf-thĕr-ĭt'ĭk). Following diphtheria.

postencephalitis (pŏst"ĕn-sĕf-ă-lī'tĭs) [" + Gr. *enkephalos*, brain, + *itis*, inflammation]. Occurring after encephalitis; an abnormal state remaining after the acute stage of encephalitis has passed.

postepileptic (pŏst"ĕp-ĭ-lĕp'tĭk) [" + Gr. *epi*, upon, + *lepsis*, a seizure]. Following an epileptic seizure. SEE: *postictal.*

posterior (pŏs-tē'rē-or) [L. *posterus*, behind]. [NA] 1. Toward the rear or caudal end; opposed to anterior. 2. In humans, toward the back; dorsal. 3. Situated behind; coming after.

posterior central gyrus. Gyrus, postcentral, q.v.

posterior chamber (of the eye). In the eye, the space behind the iris and in front of the vitreous body. It is occupied by the lens, its zonules, and the aqueous humor. SEE: *chamber, anterior; eye* for illus.

posterior drawer sign or test. With the knee flexed to a right angle, there is increased posterior glide of the tibia in posterior cruciate ligament rupture. SEE: *anterior drawer sign or test.*

posterior pituitary injection. USP. A standard preparation of the polypeptide hormones obtained from the posterior lobe of the pituitary body of healthy domestic animals used for food by humans. Trade name is Pituitrin.

postero- (pŏs'tĕr-ō) [L.]. Prefix indicating posterior, situated behind, or towards the back.

posteroanterior (pŏs"tĕr-ō-ăn-tēr'ē-or) [L. *posterus*, behind, + *anterior*, anterior]. Term indicating the flow or movement from back to front.

posteroexternal (pŏs"tĕr-ō-ĕks-tĕr'năl) [" + *externus*, outer]. Toward the back and outer side.

posteroinferior (pŏs"tĕr-ō-ĭn-fēr'ē-or) [" + *inferus*, below]. Posterior and inferior.

posterointernal [" + *internus*, inner]. Toward the back and inner side.

posterolateral [" + *lateralis*, side]. Located behind and at the side of a part.

posteromedial (pŏs"tĕr-ō-mē'dē-ăl) [" + *medius*, middle]. Toward the back and toward the median plane.

posteromedian. Situated posteriorly and in the median plane.

posteroparietal (pŏs"tĕr-ō-pă-rī'ĕ-tăl) [" + *paries*, a wall]. Located at the back of the parietal bone.

posterosuperior (pŏs"tĕr-ō-sū-pē'rē-or) [" + *superior*, upper]. Located behind and above a part.

posterotemporal (pŏs"tĕr-ō-tĕm'pō-răl) [" + *temporalis*, temporal]. Located at the back of the temporal bone.

post eruption. The stage of tooth eruption in which the tooth has reached the occlusal plane and is functional, but continues to erupt to compensate for loss of tooth substance due to wear. SEE: *eruption; pre-eruption.*

postesophageal (pŏst"ē-sŏf"ă-jē'ăl) [L. *post*, behind, after, + Gr. *oisophagos*, gullet]. Located behind the esophagus.

postethmoid (pŏst-ĕth'moyd) [" + Gr. *ethmos*, sieve, + *eidos*, form, shape]. Located behind the ethmoid bone.

postfebrile (pŏst-fē'brĭl) [" + *febris*, fever]. Occurring after a fever.

postganglionic (pŏst"găn-glē-ŏn'ĭk) [" +

Gr. *ganglion*, knot]. Situated posterior or distal to a ganglion.

postganglionic fiber. The axon of a postganglionic neuron that passes from an autonomic ganglion to a visceral effector.

postganglionic neuron. The second of a series of efferent neurons that transmit impulses from the central nervous system to a visceral effector. Its cell body lies in one of the autonomic ganglia.

posthemiplegic (pŏst″hĕm-ĭ-plē′jĭk) [″ + Gr. *hemi*, half, + *plege*, a stroke]. Occurring after hemiplegia.

posthemorrhagic (pŏst-hĕm″ō-răj′ĭk) [″ + Gr. *haima*, blood, + *rhegnynai*, to burst forth]. Occurring after hemorrhage.

posthepatitic (pŏst″hĕp-ă-tĭt′ĭk) [″ + Gr. *hepar*, liver, + *itis*, inflammation]. Occurring after hepatitis.

posthetomy (pŏs-thĕt′ō-mē) [Gr. *posthe*, foreskin, + *tome*, incision]. Surgical removal of all or part of the foreskin. SYN: *circumcision*.

posthioplasty (pŏs′thē-ō-plăs″tē) [″ + *plastos*, formed]. Plastic surgery of the prepuce or foreskin.

posthitis (pŏs-thī′tĭs) [″ + *itis*, inflammation]. Inflammation of the foreskin. SYN: *acrobystitis; acroposthitis*.

posthumous (pŏs′tū-mŭs) [L. *postumus*, last]. 1. Occurring after death. 2. Born after death of father. 3. Said of a child taken by cesarean section after death of mother.

posthypnotic (pŏst″hĭp-nŏt′ĭk) [L. *post*, behind, after, + Gr. *hypnos*, sleep]. Occurring or performed subsequent to the hypnotic state.

posthypnotic suggestion. Suggestion given during the hypnotic state influencing a later action when individual returns to normal state.

posthypoxia syndromes. Having experienced severe hypoxia may lead to a variety of syndromes including: persistent coma or stupor; dementia; visual agnosia; parkinsonism; choreoathetosis; cerebral ataxia; inattention or action myoclonus; amnesic state. SEE: *hypoxia*.

postictal (pŏst-ĭk′tăl) [″ + *ictus*, a blow or stroke]. Following a sudden attack or stroke, as an epileptic seizure or apoplexy.

postictal confusion. Confusion following a minor seizure lasts only a few seconds, and after a major seizure usually resolves in an hour unless complicated by head injury, hypoxia, or status epilepticus. SEE: *epilepsy*.

posticteric (pŏst″ĭk-tĕr′ĭk) [″ + Gr. *ikteros*, jaundice]. Following jaundice.

postmalarial (pŏst″mă-lā′rē-ăl) [″ + It. *malaria*, bad air]. Occurring after malaria.

postmature (pŏst″mă-tūr′) [″ + *maturus*, ripe]. 1. Pert. to an infant born after the cal-

culated due date. 2. Pert. to an infant born after 42 weeks of gestation.

postmaturity (pŏst″mă-tū′rĭ-tē) [″ + *maturus*, ripe]. Overdevelopment, as in a postmature infant.

postmediastinal (pŏst″mē-dē-ăs′tĭ-năl) [″ + *mediastinum*, in the middle]. Behind the mediastinum.

postmenopausal (pŏst″mĕn-ō-paw′zăl) [″ + Gr. *men*, month, + *pausis*, cessation]. Occurring after the menopause.

post mortem [L.]. After death.

postmortem [L.]. Occurring or performed after death. SEE: *autopsy*.

postmortem examination. Examination of the organs and tissue of a body to determine the cause of death or pathological conditions. SYN: *autopsy*.

postmyocardial infarction syndrome. A syndrome described in France originally in 1953 and again in 1958. Chest pain similar to that of pericarditis appears in the second week following onset of myocardial infarction. The pain is aggravated by deep breathing, swallowing, and change in body position. Usually present are fever and a pericardial friction rub. The white blood cell count and sedimentation rate may be elevated. The pathological mechanism of this syndrome is unknown.

TREAT: Aspirin for pain; drain pleural effusion; if pain and effusion persist, administer adrenal cortical hormones.

postnasal (pŏst-nā′zăl) [L. *post*, behind, after, + *nasus*, nose]. Located behind the nose.

postnatal [″ + *natus*, birth]. Happening after birth.

postnecrotic (pŏst″nĕ-krŏt′ĭk) [″ + Gr. *nekros*, corpse]. After death of a tissue or a part.

postneuritic (pŏst″nū-rĭt′ĭk) [″ + Gr. *neuron*, nerve, + *itis*, inflammation]. Occurring after neuritis.

postocular (pŏst-ŏk′ū-lar) [″ + *oculus*, eye]. Behind the eye.

postocular neuritis. Inflammation of the optic nerve behind the eyeball.

postolivary (pŏst-ŏl′ĭ-vā-rē) [″ + *oliva*, olive]. Behind the olivary body; back of the anterior pyramid of the medulla.

postoperative care [″ + *operatus*, work]. Care after or following a surgical operation.

NURSING IMPLICATIONS: Prior to discharge from the recovery room, the following criteria should be met: recovery from the effects of anesthesia; stable vital signs; no excessive drainage from any site or body cavity; satisfactory level of consciousness; essential orders must be completed; adequate urine output (30 ml per hour); and notification of the nursing unit receiving the patient regarding his or her status and essential equipment needed to care for the patient.

The common problems that may be associated with postoperative discomfort that require monitoring and care include nausea, vomiting, headache, sore throat, paresthesias, atelectasis, abdominal gas, muscle aches, and urinary retention.

Throughout the postoperative period, the nurse must monitor vital signs at indicated intervals, obtain necessary equipment and supplies, observe patient for adequate circulatory function, provide for adequate nutrition and elimination, maintain fluid and electrolyte balance, check wounds and tubes for drainage, administer analgesics as prescribed, provide comfort by properly positioning the patient. If guard rails are indicated, be certain they are in place; also, all electrical devices used must be properly grounded. Provide sufficient rest periods, provide wound care, establish range of motion exercises progressing to ambulation as indicated, prevent and recognize postoperative complications, and prepare patient and family for discharge with pertinent discharge instruction.

postoperculum (pŏst-ō-pŭr'kū-lŭm) [" + operculum, a covering]. The fold covering the insula that is formed of part of the superior temporal gyrus of the brain.

postoral (pōst-or'ăl) [" + os, mouth]. Behind, or in the posterior part of, the mouth.

postorbital (pōst-or'bĭ-tăl) [" + orbita, track]. Behind the orbit of the eye.

postpalatine (pōst-păl'ă-tĭn) [" + palatum, palate]. Behind the palate.

postpallium (pōst-păl'ē-ŭm) [" + pallium, cloak]. That part of the cerebral cortex behind the fissure of Rolando.

postpaludal (pōst-păl'ū-dăl) [" + palus, swamp]. After a malarial attack.

postparalytic (pōst"păr-ă-lĭt'ĭk) [" + para, beside, + lyein, to loosen]. Subsequent to an attack of paralysis.

post partum (pōst-păr'tŭm) [L. post, after, + partus, birth]. After childbirth.

postpartum. Occurring after childbirth.

postpartum blues. The "let-down" feeling experienced during the postpartum period for no apparent reason. The mother becomes tearful and irritable, loses her appetite, and finds sleeping difficult. This temporary state may occur during the hospital stay or after. It is thought to be due to hormonal changes as well as emotional needs during this period. This occurs in 70% to 80% of mothers.

postpartum depression. The most common neurotic reaction during the puerperal period is depression. The symptoms are tear-

fulness, despondency, a feeling of hopelessness, inadequacy, inability to cope with infant care, mood swings, extreme anxiety over the baby, guilt of not loving the baby enough, irritability, fatigue, loss of normal interests, and insomnia. This depression occurs in about 3% of women; and it may occur in other family members, including the father.

postpartum hemorrhage. Hemorrhage that occurs after childbirth. It is usually defined as loss of more than 500 ml of blood following delivery.

Caution: Universal precautions are essential. SEE: *Universal Precautions* in *Appendix.*

ETIOL: Uterine atony; retained placental fragments; lower genital tract lacerations; uterine inversion; uterine rupture; or blood coagulation disorder.

NURSING IMPLICATIONS: During the first postpartum hour, the chance of hemorrhage is the greatest. To prevent hemorrhage, check the mother's fundus at least every 5 minutes and massage it. Check the mother's vital signs and vaginal discharge at least every 15 minutes.

If hemorrhage begins, elevate and hold the uterus up out of the pelvis by pushing the lower hand onto the abdomen above the symphysis pubis and massaging the fundus with the upper hand to initiate and maintain a firmly contracted organ. If softness begins to occur, massage is immediately reinstituted. A hand is kept on the uterus during the treatment of hemorrhage in order to assess its condition and to massage it as indicated. Overmassage is contraindicated. The mother's bladder should be kept empty. I.V. oxytocic drugs, plasma, or blood may be prescribed by the physician.

When ordered, administer well-diluted oxytocic drug therapy by I.V. push followed by continuous I.V. oxytocic therapy in solution over 3 to 4 hours as prescribed. Methylergonovine or prostaglandin $F_{2\alpha}$ may be ordered. Blood transfusions may be required to treat shock. Prepare the patient for and assist the obstetrician with examination of the interior of the uterus for removal of retained products of conception or repair of lacerations. Be aware that if the blood being lost fails to clot, a coagulopathy may have developed, requiring prompt, life-saving, appropriate treatment.

It is important to provide support and comfort for such a patient, who is understandably quite apprehensive. Assure her that during this period the newborn is well taken care of.

postpartum pituitary necrosis. Sheehan's

syndrome, q.v.

postpartum psychosis. A psychosis that develops during the six months following childbirth, the highest incidence being in the third to sixth day after delivery through the first month postpartum. The symptoms and signs include: hallucinations, delusions, preoccupation with death, self-multilation, infanticide, distorted reality, extreme dependency, and a demanding attitude. This psychosis may become a chronic condition, but for most women it becomes an isolated event in their lives.

postpharyngeal (pōst-fă-rĭn'jē-ăl) [L. *post*, after, + Gr. *pharynx*, throat]. Behind the pharynx.

postpneumonic (pōst″nū-mŏn'ĭk) [″ + Gr. *pneumon*, lung]. Occurring after pneumonia.

postpoliomyelitis muscular atrophy. ABBR: PPMA. The development of new neuromuscular symptoms, including muscle weakness, many years after recovery from acute paralytic poliomyelitis. This may occur in muscles that were previously affected by polio and recovered or in muscles that were clinically unaffected by the acute disease. There is no treatment for this slowly progressing atrophy, but the unaffected muscles remain strong. The disease is not thought to be related to amyotrophic lateral sclerosis. SEE: *poliomyelitis, acute anterior.*

post-polio syndrome. A variety of musculoskeletal symptoms and muscular atrophy that create new difficulties with activities of daily living 25 to 30 years after the original attack of acute paralytic poliomyelitis.

postpontile (pōst-pŏn'tĭl) [″ + *pons*, bridge]. Situated behind the pons varolii.

postprandial (pōst-prăn'dē-ăl). Following a meal.

postprandial dumping syndrome. Dumping syndrome, q.v.

postprandial (reactive) hypoglycemia syndrome. A controversial disorder in which the symptoms of weakness, nausea, hunger, sweating, and difficulty concentrating are not correlated with detectable hypoglycemia. Use of a glucose tolerance test is of little diagnostic benefit.

postpubertal (pōst-pū'bĕr-tăl) [″ + *pubertas*, puberty]. Concerning the period following puberty.

postpuberty (pōst-pū'bĕr-tē). The period after puberty.

postpubescent (pōst″pū-bĕs'ĕnt) [″ + *pubescens*, becoming hairy]. Following puberty.

postpyramidal (pōst-pĭ-răm'ĭd-ăl). Behind a pyramidal tract.

postpyramidal nucleus. Mass of gray matter in posterior column of the medulla. SYN: *nucleus funiculi gracilis.*

postradiation (pōst″rā-dē-ā'shŭn). Occurring after exposure to ionizing radiation.

postsacral (pōst-sā'krăl) [″ + *sacrum*, sacred]. Below the sacrum.

postscapular (pōst-skăp'ū-lăr) [″ + *scapula*, shoulder blade]. Below or behind the scapula.

postscarlatinal (pōst″skăr-lă-tī'năl) [″ + *scarlatina*, scarlet fever]. Following scarlet fever.

postsphygmic (pōst-sfĭg'mĭk) [″ + Gr. *sphygmus*, pulse]. Following the pulse wave.

postsplenic (pōst-splĕn'ĭk) [″ + Gr. *splen*, spleen]. Behind the spleen.

poststenotic (pōst″stĕ-nŏt'ĭk) [″ + Gr. *stenosis*, act of narrowing]. Distal to a stenosed or constricted area, esp. of an artery.

postsynaptic (pōst″sĭ-năp'tĭk) [″ + Gr. *synapsis*, point of contact]. Located distal to a synapse.

post-tarsal (pōst-tăr'săl) [″ + Gr. *tarsos*, a broad, flat surface]. Behind the tarsus.

post-term pregnancy. An infant born after the beginning of the 42nd week (294 days) of gestation as counted from the first day of the last normal menstrual period. This occurs in an estimated 3% to 12% of pregnancies. Complications include oligohydramnios, meconium passage, macrosomia, and dysmaturity. All of these may lead to poor pregnancy outcome.

TREAT: Delivery of fetus to be effected if any sign of fetal compromise is detected.

post-tibial (pōst-tĭb'ē-ăl) [″ + *tibia*, shinbone]. Behind the tibia.

post-transfusion syndrome. Condition of fever, splenomegaly, atypical lymphocytes, abnormal liver function tests, and occasionally a skin rash that develops following blood transfusion or perfusion of an organ during surgery. The syndrome appears three to five weeks after transfusion or perfusion with fresh (less than 24-hour-old) blood, usually in large quantities. The causative agent is thought to be cytomegalovirus.

post-traumatic (pōst″traw-măt'ĭk) [″ + Gr. *traumatikos*, traumatic]. Following an injury or traumatic event.

post-traumatic stress disorder. ABBR: PTSD. The development of characteristic symptoms after a psychologically traumatic event that is generally outside the range of usual human experience. It is important to remember that the reaction to stress is highly individualized; and, because of that, the stress that would cause this syndrome in one individual might have little if any effect on another.

The symptoms include re-experiencing

the traumatic event; avoidance of stimuli associated with the trauma; numbing of general responsiveness; and symptoms related to increased arousal, including insomnia, recurrent nightmares, hypervigilance; exaggerated startle response; and changes in aggression.

The disorder may last for decades. It is estimated that 15% of male and 9% of female Vietnam combat veterans have PTSD.

postulate (pŏs′tū-lāt) [L. *postulare*, to request]. A supposition or view, usually self-evident, that is assumed without proof. SEE: *Koch's law.*

postural (pŏs′tū-răl) [L. *postura*, position]. Pert. to or affected by posture.

postural drainage. Drainage of secretions from the bronchi or a cavity in the lung by having the patient positioned so that gravity will allow drainage of the particular lobe or lobes of the lung involved. Used in bronchiectasis and before operation for lobectomy. The position aggravates coughing, resulting in expectoration of much sputum, 5 to 10 oz. (148 to 296 ml) in severe cases. Five to 10 minutes morning and evening is recommended. High-protein diet to replace protein lost. SEE: illus.

NURSING IMPLICATIONS: If procedure is used, evaluate patient's physical tolerance. Teach and assist the patient in the procedure, as ordered, by positioning for effective drainage, encouraging the patient to mechanically remove secretions with forceful cough, and caution the patient not to perform procedure after meals, in order to prevent aspiration.

postural hypotension. Decrease in blood pressure upon assuming erect posture. This is normal, but may be of such degree as to cause fainting, esp. in persons who first stand up after having been flat in bed for several days. SYN: *orthostatic hypotension.* SEE: *blackout.*

posture (pŏs′tūr) [L. *postura*]. Attitude or position of the body.

 p., coiled. Body on one side with legs drawn up to meet the trunk. Noted in cerebral diseases and in hepatic, intestinal, and renal colic.

 p., dorsal rigid. Patient on back with both legs drawn up. Seen in peritonitis, meningitis, ascites, tympanites. In appendicitis the right leg is drawn up; this also occurs in pelvic inflammation or peritonitis of right side, renal calculus in right ureter, and in psoas abscess.

 p., orthopnea. Patient sitting upright, hands or elbows resting upon some support. Seen in spasmodic asthma, emphysema, dyspnea, ascites, effusions into the pleural and pericardial cavities, and in late stages of diseases of the heart.

 p., orthotonos. Neck and trunk extended rigidly in straight line; seen in tetanus, strychnine poisoning, rabies, and meningitis.

 p., prone. Posture assumed after abdominal colic or because of tuberculosis of the spine, eroded vertebrae, abdominal pain, or gastric ulcer.

 p., semireclining. Posture used for patients with diseases of heart and interference with respiration in asthma and pleural effusions.

postuterine (pōst-ū′tĕr-ĭn) [L. *post*, behind, after, + *uterus*, womb]. Situated behind the uterus.

postvaccinal (pōst-văk′sĭ-năl) [″ + *vaccinus*, pert. to cows]. Following vaccination for smallpox.

postviral fatigue syndrome. Chronic disability following a presumed viral infection. The most characteristic and persistent feature of the disease is muscle fatiguability unrelieved by rest. Other symptoms and signs include low-grade fever, headache, blurred vision or diplopia, stiff neck, vertigo, nausea and vomiting, lymphadenopathy, emotional lability, insomnia, urinary frequency, and either deafness or hyperacusis. In addition, psychological disturbances are usually present. These include mild depression, anxiety, or severe behavioral abnormalities. There is no effective treatment, but the usual course is slow recovery. SYN: *epidemic neuromyasthenia; Iceland disease; myalgic encephalomyelitis; Royal Free disease.*

potable (pō′tă-bl) [LL. *potabilis*]. Suitable for drinking, esp. pert. to water free of harmful organic or inorganic ingredients.

Potain's apparatus (pō-tănz′) [Pierre C. E. Potain, Fr. physician, 1825–1901]. A form of aspirator.

Potain's sign. In dilatation of the aorta, there will be dullness on percussion over the area extending from the manubrium sterni toward the third costal cartilage on the right, and to the base of the sternum.

potamophobia (pŏt″ă-mō-fō′bē-ă) [Gr. *potamos*, river, + *phobos*, fear]. A morbid fear of large bodies of water.

potash (pŏt′ăsh) [Obsolete Dutch, *potasschan*]. Potassium carbonate.

 p., caustic. Potassium hydroxide.

 p., sulfurated. Liver-colored or green-yellow substance made up of potassium thiosulfate and potassium polysulfides and containing 12.8% sulfur as a sulfide. A principal ingredient of white lotion.

potassemia (pŏt-ă-sē′mē-ă) [NL. *potassa*, potash, + Gr. *haima*, blood]. Presence of excessive quantity of potassium in the

POSTURAL DRAINAGE OF LUNGS

DRAINAGE OF UPPER LOBES

APICAL SEGMENTS

RIGHT AND LEFT   RIGHT AND LEFT

RIGHT AND LEFT   ANTERIOR SEGMENTS

LEFT   POSTERIOR SEGMENTS

POSTERIOR SEGMENTS   RIGHT

DRAINAGE OF MIDDLE LOBES

LINGULAR

RIGHT

DRAINAGE OF LOWER LOBES

SUPERIOR SEGMENTS   RIGHT AND LEFT

DRAINAGE OF LOWER LOBES

RIGHT AND LEFT ANTERIOR

BASAL SEGMENTS

RIGHT AND LEFT POSTERIOR

BASAL SEGMENTS

LEFT

LATERAL SEGMENTS

LATERAL SEGMENTS

RIGHT

blood.

potassic (pō-tăs′ĭk). Composed of or containing potash.

potassium (pō-tăs′ē-ŭm) [NL. *potassa*, potash]. SYMB: K. At. wt. 39.098; at. no. 19; sp. gr. 0.86. Mineral element found in combination with other elements in the body and constituting 0.35% of body weight. SYN: *kalium.*

SOURCES: Found in most foods. Excellent sources are cereals, dried peas and beans, fresh vegetables, fresh or dried fruits, fruit juices such as orange or prune, sunflower seeds, watermelon, nuts, molasses, cocoa, fresh fish, beef, ham, and poultry.

FUNCT: Potassium is the principal cation in intracellular fluid and is of primary importance in its maintenance. In conjunction with sodium and chloride, it aids in regulation of osmotic pressure and acid-base balance. A proper balance of potassium, calcium, and magnesium ions is essential for normal excitability of muscle tissue, esp. cardiac muscle, and it plays a role in the conduction of nerve impulses.

The usual intake of potassium is 50 to 150 mEq/day. Intake must be monitored carefully to be certain it is adequate in prolonged intravenous feeding, during severe diarrhea or diabetic acidosis, and in patients receiving diuretics. In these conditions an intake of 1 to 3 mEq/kg/day usually is adequate.

DEFICIENCY SYM: Muscle weakness, dizziness, thirst, mental confusion, and changes in the electrocardiogram.

EXCESS: Extracellular potassium is increased in renal failure; in destruction of cells with release of intracellular potassium in burns, crushing injuries, or severe infection; in adrenal insufficiency; in overtreatment with potassium salts; and in metabolic acidosis. This causes weakness and paralysis, impaired electrical conduction in the heart and eventually ventricular fibrillation and death. Hyperkalemia can be treated by withholding potassium, by using drugs such as sodium polystyrene sulfonate, a cation exchange resin, to lower the potassium concentration in cells, and by using calcium gluconate to counteract the effects on the heart.

Caution: Rapid infusion of potassium intravenously may cause severe hyperkalemia and cardiac arrest.

p. acetate. USP. $C_2H_3KO_2$. A white powder or crystalline flakes. Used to replenish potassium.

p. alum. Aluminum potassium sulfate; strongly astringent, used topically as a styptic. SEE: *alum.*

p. aminosalicylate. Para-aminosalicylic acid, q.v.

p. arsenite solution. An arsenical solution containing 0.95 to 1.4 gm of arsenic trioxide in each 100 ml of solution. SYN: *Fowler's solution.*

p. bicarbonate. USP. $KHCO_3$. White crystals or powder. Used to neutralize acid of the stomach and to treat acid-base imbalance. Trade name is K-Lyte.

p. bitartrate. $C_4H_5KO_6$. White powder or crystalline salt, used as a dusting powder in place of starch for surgical gloves. SYN: *cream of tartar.*

p. bromide. White cubical crystals of powder, used as a sedative.

p. carbonate. K_2CO_3. A white crystalline powder used in pharmaceutical and chemical preparations. SYN: *potash.*

p. chlorate. $KClO_3$. An explosive white crystalline salt, soluble in water. Formerly used internally in treatment of pharyngitis and stomatitis but its use has been discontinued because of destructive effect on red blood cells.

p. chloride. USP. KCl. A white crystalline salt, soluble in water. One of the three chlorides used in preparation of Ringer's solution. Used in treatment of potassium deficiencies and digitalis intoxication. Trade names are K-Lor, K-Lyte/Cl, Kaochlor, Kaon-Cl, Kay Ciel, and Slow-K.

p. chromate. K_2CrO_4. Lemon-yellow crystals used as a dye and furniture stain, in manufacture of batteries, in photography, and in laboratories to preserve tissue.

p. citrate. USP. $C_6H_5K_3O_7 \cdot H_2O$. Transparent prismatic crystals. Used as an alkalizer.

INCOMPAT: Caffeine sodium benzoate.

p. cyanide. KCN. A highly poisonous compound used as a fumigant.

p. gluconate. USP. $C_6H_{11}KO_7$. A drug used orally to replenish loss of potassium ion. Trade name is Kaon.

p. guaiacolsulfonate. USP. $C_7H_7KO_5S \cdot$ ½H_2O. An expectorant.

p. hydroxide. KOH. Gray-white compound used in preparation of soap and as a chemical reagent. SYN: *potash, caustic.*

p. iodide. USP. KI. Colorless or white crystals having a faint odor of iodine. Used as an expectorant.

This form of potassium is recommended for use following exposure to radioactive iodides downwind from a nuclear reactor accident. The rationale is that it would block the uptake of radioactive iodides by the thyroid gland, thus preventing or decreasing the chance of developing cancer of the thyroid many years later.

p. nitrite. KNO_2. Medicine formerly used as a diuretic.

p. permanganate. USP. $KMnO_4$. Crystals of dark purple prisms, odorless, with sweet taste. Used as a topical astringent and antiseptic, as an oxidizing agent, and as an antidote in phosphorus poisoning. Concentrated solutions irritate and even corrode the skin and, when swallowed, induce gastroenteritis. The solutions have considerable power as disinfectants, because their oxidizing ability destroys bacteria. They fail to penetrate deeply in an active form and this renders them of less value than many other disinfectants, except for use in very superficial infections.

p. phosphate, dibasic. USP. K_2HPO_4. A drug used to treat calcium imbalance.

p. sodium tartrate. $C_4H_4KNaO_6 \cdot 4H_2O$. USP. A saline cathartic.

p. sulfate. K_2SO_4. Has been used as a laxative, but because of its irritant qualities it is not recommended.

p. tartrate. $C_4H_4K_2O_6$. A medicine used as a cathartic.

potassium chlorate poisoning. Large doses cause abdominal discomfort, vomiting, diarrhea, hematuria with nephritis, and disturbances of the blood. Stomach should be washed out; other treatment is symptomatic.

Caution: Do not induce vomiting.

---

potassium chromate poisoning. May be contracted by inhalation or from touching the nose with contaminated fingers, causing deep indolent ulcers.

SYM: When taken by mouth has a disagreeable taste, causes cramping, pain, vomiting, diarrhea, slow respiration; may affect liver and kidneys.

Caution: Do not induce vomiting.

NURSING IMPLICATIONS: For ingestion, treat as if poisoned with a strong acid. Dilute with water and milk. BAL or penicillamine may be used.

potassium hydroxide poisoning. Characterized by nausea, soapy taste, and burning pain in mouth; bloody, slimy vomitus; abdominal cramping; bloody purging and prostration.

Caution: Do not induce vomiting.

NURSING IMPLICATIONS: The patient will require hospitalization, morphine for pain, and most probably treatment for shock. If airway has been burned, tracheostomy may be required. Corticosteroids and antibiotics may be given.

potbelly. Slang term for the selective deposition of adipose tissue in the abdominal subcutaneous tissue. This condition usually occurs in middle-aged persons who have sedentary occupations. It is accentuated by weakening of the anterior abdominal musculature and lumbar lordosis.

TREAT: Weight reduction; exercises to strengthen abdominal muscles; and therapy for lordosis.

potency (pō'tĕn-sē) [L. *potentia,* power]. 1. Strength; force; power. 2. Strength of a medicine. 3. Ability of male to perform coitus.

potent (pō'tĕnt) [L.*potens,* powerful]. 1. Powerful. 2. Highly effective medicinally. 3. Having power of procreation.

potentia coeundi (pō-tĕn'shē-ă kō-ē-ŭn'dī) [L.]. Ability to perform sexual intercourse in a normal manner.

potential. 1. Latent; existing in possibility. 2. In electricity, voltage or electrical pressure; a condition in which a state of tension or pressure, capable of doing work, exists. When two electrically charged bodies of different potentials are brought together, an electric current passes from the body of high potential to that of low.

p., action. ABBR: A.P. The change in electrical potential of nerve or muscle fiber when it is stimulated.

p., after. The period occurring subsequent to the spike potential, q.v.

p., demarcation. The difference in potential between an intact longitudinal surface and the injured end of a muscle or nerve. SYN: *p., injury.*

p., injury. P., demarcation.

p., membrane. The electrical charge or potential difference between the inside and outside of a cell membrane.

p., resting. The potential difference in electrical charge between the inside and outside of a cell at rest.

p., spike. A change in potential that occurs when a cell membrane is stimulated.

potentiate (pō-tĕn'shē-āt). To augment or increase the potency or action.

potentiation (pō-tĕn''shē-ā'shŭn). The synergistic action of two substances, such as hormones or drugs, in which the total effects are greater than the sum of the independent effects of the two substances.

potentiometer (pō-tĕn''shē-ŏm'ĕ-tĕr). A voltmeter.

p., calibration. A mechanically adjusted resistance used as calibration controls on many instruments. It adjusts a voltage or current within the device.

potion (pō'shŭn) [L. *potio,* draft]. A drink or draft; a dose of poison or liquid medicine.

Pott's disease [Percivall Pott, Brit. surgeon, 1713–1788]. Caries or osteitis of the vertebrae, usually of tuberculous origin; tubercular inflammation of bodies of the vertebrae. The disease occurs primarily in children and in adults up to age 40. Destruction and compression of affected vertebrae often results in kyphosis with resulting compression of spinal cord and nerves. Often infection spreads to paravertebral tissues giving rise to paravertebral abscesses. SYN: *spondylitis, tuberculous.* SEE: *kyphosis.*

SYM: Patient will complain of pain in region supplied by the nerves arising from affected segment of the cord—if disease is lumbar, pains are abdominal and apt to be associated with vesical irritability; if dorsal, pains are epigastric or intercostal, and respiration sometimes irregular and hurried from failure of respiratory muscles to function adequately; if cervical, neuralgic pain or numbness in hands, a tickling cough, and difficult swallowing. Pains apt to be symmetrical.

Increase of pain on jumping, flexing, or rotating spine is extremely significant. If patient can jump painlessly from chair to floor, it is almost certain that inflammation of the body of a vertebra is not present. If vertebrae are compressed by pressure on head or shoulders while the patient sits or stands or while he or she lies face downward across the knees of the surgeon, pain is much increased. If patient is placed in traction to elongate spine, relief is obtained.

Involuntary immobilization of spine, as a result of pain on movement, gives an exaggerated characteristic military posture, i.e., stiff and straight. If asked to look at something behind him or her, the patient turns the whole trunk. If requested to pick up something from the floor, he or she stoops by bending the thighs upon the trunk and knees upon the thighs, never by flexing the spinal column in the usual way.

In walking, the patient moves as if on ice, sliding or shuffling along so as to avoid the jar of successive steps. In standing, he or she fixes the upper portion of the column by aid of the trapezii and other scapular muscles, the action of which at the same time raises shoulders and throws arms out from sides. In standing or sitting, there is an involuntary transfer of the weight of head and shoulders and parts above diseased area to the pelvis, by means of the upper extremities. Hands placed upon the hips and arm muscles are tense. In walking about the room, he or she holds on to furniture for aid. Spinal abscess occurs later, location varying with seat of caries. Paralysis may occur, always motor at first, not affecting sensation at all.

TREAT: Endeavor to secure resolution of the tuberculous osteitis. Limit destruction of tissue and resulting deformity. Promote ankylosis if indicated. Evacuate abscess. Remove a sequestrum or the focus of carious bone. Rest in bed in recumbent position. Adequate diet and exercise care to prevent development of decubitus ulcers. Chemotherapy as for pulmonary tuberculosis.

Pott's fracture. Fracture of the lower end of the fibula and medial malleolus of the tibia with dislocation of foot outward and backward. After reduction, foot and leg are put in a cast in which a walking iron is incorporated. The patient is able to walk, and cast is removed in about six weeks.

pouch (powch) [ME. *pouche*]. Any pocket or sac.

   p., branchial. P., pharyngeal.

   p., Broca's. A sac in tissues of the labia majora.

   p., Heidenhain. A small, surgically constructed pouch of the stomach that is denervated and separated from the stomach and drained to the outside of the body. Used to study the physiology of the stomach.

   p., laryngeal. Blind pouch of mucosa entering the ventral portion of the ventricle of the larynx.

   p. of Douglas. P., rectouterine.

   p., Pavlov. A stomach pouch formed surgically for the experimental study of gastric secretion. A section of the stomach is separated from the main stomach except for the vagal nerves. Named after I. P. Pavlov, who devised the pouch in order to investigate gastric function and conditioned reflexes.

   p., pharyngeal. One of a series of five pairs of entodermal outpocketings that develop in lateral walls of the pharynx of the embryo. SYN: *p., branchial.*

   p., Prussak's. The anterior recess of the tympanic membrane.

   p., Rathke's. An outpocketing of the roof of embryonic stomodeum. Gives rise to the anterior lobe of the hypophysis cerebri.

   p., rectouterine. Pouch between the anterior rectal wall and posterior uterine wall. SYN: *cul-de-sac; p. of Douglas.*

   p., rectovesical. A fold of peritoneum that in the male extends downward between bladder and rectum.

pouchitis. Acute inflammation of the surgically produced pouch used in restorative proctocolectomy.

poudrage (pū-dräzh') [Fr.]. Application of an irritating, but otherwise nontoxic, powder to the pleural space of the lung in order to produce pleural adhesions.

poultice (pōl'tĭs) [L. *pultes,* thick paste]. A hot, moist mass of linseed, mustard, or soap and oil between two pieces of muslin applied to the skin to relieve congestion or pain, to stimulate absorption of inflammatory products, and to act as a counterirritant. SEE: *plaster.*

pound (pownd) [L. *pondus,* weight]. SYMB: lb. A measure of weight of the avoirdupois and the apothecaries' systems that is equal to 16 ounces. SEE: *Weights and Measures* in *Appendix.*

   p., avoirdupois. Sixteen ounces, equal to 453.59 gm.

   p., foot. Work expended when one pound is moved a distance of one foot in the direction of the force.

   p., troy. Twelve ounces, 5760 grains, and equal to 373.242 gm.

Poupart's ligament (pū-pärz') [François Poupart, Fr. anatomist, 1661–1708]. The ligament forming the lower border of aponeurosis of external oblique muscle between the anterosuperior spine of the ilium and spine of the pubis. SYN: *inguinal ligament.*

poverty. The condition of having an inadequate supply of money, resources, or means of subsistence. Poverty is sometimes defined on the basis of income and sometimes on budget for an urban family's modest but adequate standard of living. Poverty levels are used to establish eligibility for federal and state aid, such as aid to dependent children, supplemental security income, or food stamps.

It is estimated that 20% of children in the U.S. live in families with incomes below the poverty line.

poverty of thought. The mental state of being devoid of thought and having a feeling of emptiness.

povidone (pō'vĭ-dōn). USP. A synthetic polymer used as a dispersing and suspending agent in manufacturing drugs. The name previously used was polyvinylpyrrolidone. Trade name is Plasdone.

povidone-iodine. USP. A complex of iodine with povidone. It contains not less than 9% and not more than 12% available iodine. This iodophor is used in dilute concentration as a surgical scrub, in aerosol spray, in vaginal douche solutions, and in ointments and gels. Trade names are Betadine and PVP-Iodine.

powder [ME. *poudre*]. 1. Aggregation of fine particles of one or more substances that may be passed through fine meshes. 2. A dose of such a powder, contained in a paper.

power [ME. *power*]. 1. Rate at which work is done. Power may be calculated by multiplying force times velocity. The metric unit for power is the watt. One watt equals one newton meter per second, or 0.7376 foot pounds per second. Sometimes power is measured in horsepower. A horsepower unit equals 745.7 watts or 550 footpounds per second. 2. Capacity for action. 3. In optics, the degree to which a lens or optical instrument magnifies. 4. In microscopy, the number of times the diameter of an object is magnified, indicated by placing an × after the number. Ex.: 10× indicates magnification of ten times. 5. In mathematics and in scientific nomenclature, the number of times a value is to be multiplied by itself, i.e., $10^2 = 10 \times 10 = 100$; $10^3 = 10 \times 10 \times 10 = 1000$. A negative power, e.g., 10^{-2}, indicates the reciprocal of that value. For example, $10^{-2} = \frac{1}{10}^2 = \frac{1}{100}$.

pox (pŏks) [ME. *pokkes*, pits]. 1. An eruptive, contagious disease. 2. A papular eruption that becomes pustular. SEE: *chickenpox; smallpox.*

poxvirus (pŏks'vī-rŭs). One of a group of DNA viruses that produce characteristic spreading vesicular lesions, often called pocks. It is the largest of the true viruses and includes viruses responsible for smallpox, vaccinia, molluscum contagiosum, and orf. Lower animals are also susceptible to the poxvirus.

p.p. *punctum proximum,* near point of accommodation (in vision).

ppb. *parts per billion.*

P.P.D. *purified protein derivative,* substance used in intradermal test for tuberculosis.

PPLO. *pleuropneumonia-like organisms,* now called mycoplasmas. SEE: *mycoplasmas.*

ppm. *parts per million.*

ppt. *parts per trillion; precipitate; prepared.*

Pr. 1. *presbyopia.* 2. Chem. symb. for the element praseodymium.

p.r. L. *punctum remotum,* far point of visual accommodation.

practical nurse. SEE: *nurse, licensed practical.*

practice (prăk'tĭs) [Gr. *praktike,* business]. The use, by a health care professional, of knowledge and skill to provide a service in the prevention, diagnosis, and treatment of illness, and the maintenance of health.

practitioner (prăk-tĭsh'ŭn-ĕr). One who has met the professional and legal requirements necessary to provide a health care service, such as a physician, nurse, dentist, or physical therapist.

Practitioners' Reporting Network, USP. ABBR: USP-PRN. Three separate programs designed to collect practitioners' experience with unreliable drug products, defective medical devices, and medication errors. Practitioners and pharmacists report their experience to the United States Pharmacopeia, 12601 Twinbrook Parkway, Rockville, MD 20852. The USP receives the reports and publishes the results. Drug problem reports and medical device and laboratory product problem reports may be made by calling (800) 638-6725; medication errors may be reported by calling (800) 23ERROR.

prae-. SEE: words beginning with *pre-.*

praecox (prē'kŏks) [L.]. Early.

praevia, praevius (prē'vē-ă, prē'vē-ŭs) [L.]. Going before in time or place.

pragmatagnosia (prăg″măt-ăg-nō'zē-ă) [Gr. *pragma,* object, + *agnosia,* lack of recognition]. Inability to recognize objects once familiar.

pragmatamnesia (prăg″măt-ăm-nē'zē-ă) [″ + *amnesia,* forgetfulness]. Inability to recall the appearance of an object.

   p., visual. Name for the mental condition making possible pragmatamnesia.

pragmatic (prăg-măt'ĭk) [Gr. *pragma,* a thing done]. Pert. to, or concerned with, the practical side of anything.

pragmatism (prăg'mă-tĭzm) [″ + *-ismos,* condition]. A belief that the practical application of a principle should be the determining factor.

pragmatist (prăg'mă-tĭst). A person whose goals are achieved or attempted from a practical concept, action or approach; a practical person.

pralidoxime chloride (prăl″ĭ-dŏks'ēm). USP. A cholinesterase reactivator used in treating poisoning due to certain pesticides or drugs with anticholinesterase activity. Trade name is Protopam Chloride.

pramoxine hydrochloride (prăm-ŏk'sēn). USP. A topical anesthetic. It is too irritating to be used on the eye or in the nose. Trade names are Tronolane and Tronothane HCl.

prandial (prăn'dē-ăl) [L. *prandium,* breakfast]. Rel. to a meal.

Prantal. Trade name for diphemanil methylsulfate.

praseodymium (prā″sē-ō-dĭm'ē-ŭm) [Gr. *prasios,* leek-green, + *didymium*]. SYMB: Pr. At. wt. 140.907; at. no. 59. A metallic element obtained from rare earth.

Prausnitz-Küstner reaction (prows'nĭts-kĭst'nĕr) [Carl Willi Prausnitz, Ger. bacteriologist, b. 1876; Heinz Küstner, Ger. gynecologist, b. 1897]. Intracutaneous injection of a hypersensitive patient's serum into a nonallergic person; then 24 to 48 hours later, the suspected antigen is applied to the injected site. If a wheal and flare occur, there is evidence that the suspected antigen is causing the hypersensitivity. Because of the danger of transmitting viral hepatitis and AIDS, this test is no longer used. SYN: *passive transfer test.*

praxinoscope (prăk-sĭn'ō-skōp) [Gr. *praxis,* action, + *skopein,* to examine]. Contrivance for studying the larynx.

praxiology (prăk″sē-ŏl′ō-jē) [″ + *logos*, word, reason]. Study of behavior.

praxis (prăk′sĭs) [Gr., action]. The ability to plan and execute coordinated movement.

-praxis [Gr., action]. Combining form indicating: 1. Act or activity. 2. Practice, use.

Prayer of Maimonides [Rabbi Moses ben Maimon, Jewish philosopher and physician in Egypt, 1135–1204]. A prayer used at graduation ceremonies by some medical schools.

"Thy eternal providence has appointed me to watch over the life and health of Thy creatures. May the love for my art actuate me at all times; may neither avarice nor miserliness, nor thirst for glory, or for a great reputation engage my mind; for the enemies of truth and philanthropy could easily deceive me and make me forgetful of my lofty aim of doing good to Thy children.

"May I never see in the patient anything but a fellow creature in pain.

"Grant me strength, time, opportunity always to correct what I have acquired, always to extend its domain; for knowledge is immense and the spirit of man can extend indefinitely to enrich itself daily with new requirements.

"Today he can discover his errors of yesterday and tomorrow he can obtain a new light on what he thinks himself sure of today. Oh, God, Thou has appointed me to watch over the life and death of Thy creatures; here am I ready for my vocation and now I turn unto my calling." SEE: *Declaration of Geneva; Declaration of Hawaii; Hippocratic oath; Nightingale Pledge.*

prazepam (prǎ′zĕ-păm). USP. An anti-anxiety medicine. Trade name is Centrax.

praziquantel. USP. A broad-spectrum antischistosomal drug that is very useful in treating infections with helminths such as *Hymenolepis nana*, and *Taenia saginata*. It is also quite effective in treating infections with *Diphyllobothrium latum*. Trade names are Biltricide and Droncit.

prazosin hydrochloride. USP. Drug used in treating hypertension. It acts as an alpha-adrenergic receptor blocker. Trade name is Minipress.

pre- [L. *prae*, before]. Prefix indicating before or in front of.

preadmission certification. Review of the need for proposed inpatient services prior to the time of admission to an institution.

preagonal (prē-ăg′ō-năl) [L. *prae*, before, in front of, + Gr. *agonia*, agony]. Pert. to condition immediately before death agony.

prealbuminuric (prē″ăl-bū″mĭn-ū′rĭk) [″ + *albumen*, white of egg]. Before the appearance of albuminuria.

preanal (prē-ā′năl) [″ + *anus*, anus]. In front of the anus.

preanesthesia (prē″ăn-ĕs-thē′zē-ă). A light anesthesia produced by medication given prior to the anesthesia.

preanesthetic (prē″ăn-ĕs-thĕt′ĭk) [″ + Gr. *anaisthesia*, lack of sensation]. Preliminary drug given to facilitate induction of general anesthesia.

preantiseptic (prē″ăn-tĭ-sĕp′tĭk) [″ + Gr. *anti*, against, + *sepsis*, putrefaction]. Before the adoption of antisepsis in surgery.

preaortic (prē″ā-or′tĭk) [″ + Gr. *aorte*, aorta]. Located in front of the aorta.

preataxic (prē-ă-tăk′sĭk) [″ + Gr. *ataxia*, lack of order]. Before the onset of ataxia.

preauricular (prē″aw-rĭk′ū-lăr) [″ + *auricula*, little ear]. Located in front of the ear.

preaxial (prē-ăk′sē-ăl) [″ + Gr. *axon*, axis]. In front of the axis of a limb or of the body.

precancer (prē′kăn-sĕr) [″ + *cancer*, crab]. A condition that tends to become malignant.

precancerous (prē-kăn′sĕr-ŭs) [″ + *cancer*, crab]. Said of a growth that is not yet, but probably will become, cancerous.

precapillary [″ + *capillaris*, hairlike]. An arterial capillary; one that branches from an arteriole or venule. SYN: *metarteriole.*

precautions, universal. SEE: *Universal Precautions* in *Appendix.*

precava (prē-kā′vă) [″ + *cavus*, hollow]. The descending or superior vena cava. SEE: *vena cava superior* [NA].

precentral (prē-sĕn′trăl) [″ + Gr. *kentron*, center]. In front of a center, as the central fissure of the brain.

precentral convolution. The ascending frontal convolution of the brain.

prechordal (prē-kor′dăl) [″ + Gr. *chorde*, cord]. In front of the notochord.

precipitable (prē-sĭp′ĭ-tă-b′l). Capable of being precipitated.

precipitant (prē-sĭp′ĭ-tănt) [L. *praecipitare*, to cast down]. A substance bringing about precipitation.

precipitate (prē-sĭp′ĭ-tāt). 1. A deposit separated from a suspension or solution by precipitation, the reaction of a reagent that causes the deposit to fall to the bottom or float near the top. 2. To separate as a precipitate. 3. Occurring suddenly or unexpectedly.

precipitation (prē-sĭp″ĭ-tā′shŭn) [L. *praecipitatio*]. 1. Process of a substance being separated from a solution by action of a reagent so that a precipitate forms. 2. The sudden and unprepared-for delivery of an infant. SEE: *delivery, precipitate.*

precipitation test. Test in which positive reaction is indicated by formation of a precipitate in the solution being tested.

precipitin (prē-sĭp'ĭ-tĭn). An antibody formed in the blood serum of an animal due to presence of a soluble antigen, usually a protein. When added to a solution of the antigen, it brings about precipitation. The injected protein is called the antigen, and the antibody produced is the precipitin. It was originally thought that these antibodies were members of a unique class, but most antibodies are capable of precipitating when combined with their antigens. SEE: *autoprecipitin; precipitinogen.*

precipitinogen (prē-sĭp''ĭ-tĭn'ō-jĕn). Any protein that, acting as an antigen, stimulates the production of a specific precipitin.

precipitinoid (prē-sĭp'ĭt-ĭn-oyd). Precipitin that can no longer cause precipitation when mixed with its antigen, but that retains its affinity to the antigen.

precipitin test. The formation of a precipitate in a solution containing a soluble antigen upon addition of serum containing the specific precipitin. The reaction is specific. The test is used for identification of unknown proteins; determination of types of pneumococci and meningococci; and determination of types of blood stains, whether human or animal.

precipitophore (prē-sĭp'ĭt-ō-for''). The part of a precipitin that produces the actual precipitation.

precipitum (prē-sĭp'ĭ-tŭm). The precipitate produced by action of a precipitin.

preclinical (prē-klĭn'ĭ-kăl) [L. *prae*, before, in front of, + Gr. *klinike*, medical treatment in bed]. Occurring before diagnosis of a definite disease is possible.

preclinical dental training. Study and mastery of the theory and techniques related to the various dental procedures required prior to treating human patients.

preclinical technique. In dentistry, the use of manikins, mechanical articulator, artificial or extracted teeth, and the variety of dental instruments and materials to study and master the techniques necessary to do clinical dentistry.

preclival (prē-klī'văl) [" + *clivus*, slope]. In front of the cerebellar clivus.

precocious (prē-kō'shŭs) [L. *praecox*, ripening early]. Either mental or physical development earlier than would be expected.

precocity (prē-kŏs'ĭ-tē). Premature development of physical or mental traits.

p., sexual. Premature genital maturation; precocious sexual maturity.

precognition (prē''kŏg-nĭsh'ŭn) [L. *prae*, before, in front of, + *cognoscere*, to know]. Prior knowledge that an event will occur even though there is no rational explanation of why one would have that knowledge.

precoital (prē-kō'ĭ-tăl) [" + *coitio*, a going together]. Prior to sexual intercourse.

precoma (prē-kō'mă) [" + Gr. *koma*, a deep sleep]. The mental state immediately prior to a coma.

preconscious (prē-kŏn'shŭs) [" + *conscius*, aware]. Not present in consciousness but able to be recalled as desired.

preconvulsive (prē''kŏn-vŭl'sĭv) [" + *convulsio*, pulling together]. Before a convulsion.

precordia (prē-kor'dē-ă) [L. *praecordia*]. The precordium.

precordial (prē-kor'dē-ăl). Pert. to the precordium or epigastrium.

precordialgia (prē''kor-dē-ăl'jē-ă) [L. *praecordia*, precordia, + Gr. *algos*, pain]. Pain in the chest or precordial area.

precordium (prē-kor'dē-ŭm). The area on the anterior surface of the body overlying the heart and lower part of the thorax. SYN: *antecardium; precordia.*

precornu (prē-kor'nū) [L. *prae*, before, in front of, + *cornu*, horn]. Anterior horn of lateral ventricle of the brain.

precostal (prē-kŏs'tăl) [" + Gr. *costa*, rib]. In front of the ribs.

precritical (prē-krĭt'ĭ-kăl) [" + Gr. *kritikos*, critical]. Prior to the occurrence of a crisis.

precuneus (prē-kū'nē-ŭs) [" + *cuneus*, wedge]. [NA] The division of the mesial surface of a cerebral hemisphere between the cuneus and the paracentral lobule.

precursor. A substance that precedes another substance.

predentin. Uncalcified dentinal matrix.

prediabetes (prē-dī''ă-bē'tēz) [" + Gr. *diabetes*, passing through]. The condition prior to the development of clinical diabetes.

prediastole (prē''dī-ăs'tō-lē) [" + Gr. *diastellein*, to expand]. The period in the cardiac cycle immediately prior to diastole.

prediastolic (prē''dī-ă-stōl'ĭk) [" + Gr. *diastole*, expansion]. Before the diastole, or interval in the cardiac cycle that precedes it.

predicrotic (prē''dī-krŏt'ĭk) [" + Gr. *dikrotos*, beating double]. Preceding the dicrotic wave of the sphygmographic tracing.

prediction rules. Identifying predictive factors important in establishing a diagnosis and giving each of them a certain "weight." That information is used to establish the probability of various diagnoses being present.

predigestion (prē''dī-jĕs'chŭn) [" + *digestio*, carrying apart]. Artificial proteolysis or digestion of proteins and amylolysis of starches before ingestion.

predisposing (prē''dĭs-pōz'ĭng) [" + *disponere*, to dispose]. Indicating a tendency to, or susceptibility to, disease.

predisposition (prē″dĭs-pō-zĭsh′ŭn). The potential to develop a certain disease or condition in the presence of specific environmental stimuli.

prednisolone (prĕd-nĭs′ō-lōn). USP. A glucocorticosteroid drug. It is available in a variety of dosage forms. Trade names are Delta-Cortef, Meti-Derm, and Sterane.

prednisone (prĕd′nĭ-sōn). USP. A steroid hormone with the same effects as cortisone. Trade names are Deltasone, Meticorten, Orasone, and SK-Prednisone.

predormition (prē-dor-mĭ′shŭn) [″ + *dormire*, to sleep]. State of unconsciousness immediately preceding actual sleep.

pre-eclampsia (prē″ē-klămp′sē-ă) [″ + Gr. *ek*, out, + *lampein*, to flash]. A toxemia of pregnancy characterized by increasing hypertension, headaches, albuminuria, and edema of the lower extremities. If this condition is neglected or not treated properly, the patient may develop true eclampsia. SEE: *eclampsia.* SEE: *Nursing Diagnoses* in *Appendix.*

pre-embryos. Frozen, fertilized ova. These are stored for future use by the woman. This practice has led to legal difficulties in couples who provided the ova and sperm and later were divorced.

pre-eruption (prē″ē-rŭp′shŭn) [″ + *eruptio*, a breaking out]. 1. Before an eruption. 2. Stage of tooth eruption when the tooth bud is in the bony socket prior to root formation. SEE: *eruptive stage.*

pre-excitation, ventricular (prē-ĕk″sī-tā′shŭn) [″ + *excitare*, to arouse]. Premature excitation of the ventricle by an impulse that traveled a path other than through the atrioventricular node. This produces a short P-R interval. SEE: *Wolff-Parkinson-White syndrome.*

pre-existing condition. Any injury, disease, or physical condition occurring prior to an arbitrary date; usually used in reference to the issuance of a health insurance policy. This often results in an exclusion from coverage for costs resulting from the injury, disease, or condition.

preferred provider organization. ABBR: PPO. A form of health-care delivery in which a group of health providers agrees to supply services to a defined group of patients at an agreed-upon fee-for-service rate.

Prefrin Liquifilm. Trade name for phenylephrine hydrochloride.

prefrontal (prē-frŏn′tăl) [″ + *frons*, front]. 1. The middle portion of the ethmoid bone. 2. In anterior part of the frontal lobe of the brain.

preganglionic (prē″găng-lē-ŏn′ĭk) [″ + Gr. *ganglion,* knot]. Situated in front of or

anterior to a ganglion.

preganglionic fiber. The axon of a preganglionic neuron.

preganglionic neuron. The first of a series of two efferent neurons that transmit impulses to visceral effectors. Its cell body lies in the central nervous system. Its axon terminates in an autonomic ganglion.

pregenital (prē-jĕn′ĭ-tăl) [″ + *genitalia,* genitals]. In psychology, rel. to that period when erotic interest in the reproductive organs and functions is not yet organized.

pregnancy (prĕg′năn-sē) [L. *praegnans*]. The condition of carrying a developing embryo in the uterus. SEE: table. SEE: *Nursing Diagnoses* in *Appendix.*

SYM: Presumptive signs are amenorrhea, nausea and vomiting, inordinate appetite, pigmentation of the areola of the breasts, the development of Montgomery's tubercles around the nipple, changes in the cervix and uterus (softening and progressive enlargement), vaginal and cervical discoloration, and frequent urination.

Positive signs are hearing and counting the fetal heartbeat, detection of movements of the fetus, and use of ultrasound to detect the fetal outline. The various immunodiagnostic tests for pregnancy are 90% to 95% accurate. These tests are based on various methods of detecting human chorionic gonadotropin (HCG) in the urine or serum.

The duration of pregnancy is approximately 280 days. To estimate the day of delivery, count back 3 months from the day of onset of the last menstrual period and then add 7 days. For example, if the last menstrual period began June 10, subtracting 3 months leaves March 10, and adding 7 days indicates the expected day of delivery would be March 17 of the next year. This method assumes all months have the same number of days; thus the date determined will not agree exactly with that found by using the Pregnancy Table.

PHYSICAL CHANGES: *Uterus:* Changes shape, size, and consistency; lining undergoes changes; peritoneal covering enlarges; muscle mass increases enormously.

Vaginal Canal: Elongation caused by rising of uterus in pelvis; mucosa thickens; secretion increased; increased vascularity and elasticity; cervix, vagina, and vulva become softer.

Abdominal: Growing distention and flattened navel; striae gravidarum.

Breasts: Enlarged and tender; skin thin and sensitive; nipple erectile and areola enlarged and darker; escape of colostrum; tingling sensation.

Endocrine Glands: Thyroid increases in size and activity; parathyroids enlarge and

Pregnancy Table for Expected Date of Delivery

Find the date of the last menstrual period in the top line (light-face type) of the pair of lines.
The dark number (bold-face type) in the line below will be the expected day of delivery.

| Jan. | 1 | 2 | 3 | 4 | 5 | 6 | 7 | 8 | 9 | 10 | 11 | 12 | 13 | 14 | 15 | 16 | 17 | 18 | 19 | 20 | 21 | 22 | 23 | 24 | 25 | 26 | 27 | 28 | 29 | 30 | 31 | | | | | | | |
| Oct. | 8 | 9 | 10 | 11 | 12 | 13 | 14 | 15 | 16 | 17 | 18 | 19 | 20 | 21 | 22 | 23 | 24 | 25 | 26 | 27 | 28 | 29 | 30 | 31 | (1 | 2 | 3 | 4 | 5 | 6 | 7 | | | | | Nov. | | |

| Feb. | 1 | 2 | 3 | 4 | 5 | 6 | 7 | 8 | 9 | 10 | 11 | 12 | 13 | 14 | 15 | 16 | 17 | 18 | 19 | 20 | 21 | 22 | 23 | 24 | 25 | 26 | 27 | 28 | | | | | | |
| Nov. | 8 | 9 | 10 | 11 | 12 | 13 | 14 | 15 | 16 | 17 | 18 | 19 | 20 | 21 | 22 | 23 | 24 | 25 | 26 | 27 | 28 | 29 | 30 | (1 | 2 | 3 | 4 | 5 | | | | | Dec. | |

| Mar. | 1 | 2 | 3 | 4 | 5 | 6 | 7 | 8 | 9 | 10 | 11 | 12 | 13 | 14 | 15 | 16 | 17 | 18 | 19 | 20 | 21 | 22 | 23 | 24 | 25 | 26 | 27 | 28 | 29 | 30 | 31 | | | | |
| Dec. | 6 | 7 | 8 | 9 | 10 | 11 | 12 | 13 | 14 | 15 | 16 | 17 | 18 | 19 | 20 | 21 | 22 | 23 | 24 | 25 | 26 | 27 | 28 | 29 | 30 | 31 | (1 | 2 | 3 | 4 | 5 | | Jan. | |

| April | 1 | 2 | 3 | 4 | 5 | 6 | 7 | 8 | 9 | 10 | 11 | 12 | 13 | 14 | 15 | 16 | 17 | 18 | 19 | 20 | 21 | 22 | 23 | 24 | 25 | 26 | 27 | 28 | 29 | 30 | | | | |
| Jan. | 6 | 7 | 8 | 9 | 10 | 11 | 12 | 13 | 14 | 15 | 16 | 17 | 18 | 19 | 20 | 21 | 22 | 23 | 24 | 25 | 26 | 27 | 28 | 29 | 30 | 31 | (1 | 2 | 3 | 4 | | Feb. | |

| May | 1 | 2 | 3 | 4 | 5 | 6 | 7 | 8 | 9 | 10 | 11 | 12 | 13 | 14 | 15 | 16 | 17 | 18 | 19 | 20 | 21 | 22 | 23 | 24 | 25 | 26 | 27 | 28 | 29 | 30 | 31 | | | |
| Feb. | 5 | 6 | 7 | 8 | 9 | 10 | 11 | 12 | 13 | 14 | 15 | 16 | 17 | 18 | 19 | 20 | 21 | 22 | 23 | 24 | 25 | 26 | 27 | 28 | (1 | 2 | 3 | 4 | 5 | 6 | 7 | Mar. | |

| June | 1 | 2 | 3 | 4 | 5 | 6 | 7 | 8 | 9 | 10 | 11 | 12 | 13 | 14 | 15 | 16 | 17 | 18 | 19 | 20 | 21 | 22 | 23 | 24 | 25 | 26 | 27 | 28 | 29 | 30 | | | |
| Mar. | 8 | 9 | 10 | 11 | 12 | 13 | 14 | 15 | 16 | 17 | 18 | 19 | 20 | 21 | 22 | 23 | 24 | 25 | 26 | 27 | 28 | 29 | 30 | 31 | (1 | 2 | 3 | 4 | 5 | 6 | April | |

| July | 1 | 2 | 3 | 4 | 5 | 6 | 7 | 8 | 9 | 10 | 11 | 12 | 13 | 14 | 15 | 16 | 17 | 18 | 19 | 20 | 21 | 22 | 23 | 24 | 25 | 26 | 27 | 28 | 29 | 30 | 31 | | |
| April | 7 | 8 | 9 | 10 | 11 | 12 | 13 | 14 | 15 | 16 | 17 | 18 | 19 | 20 | 21 | 22 | 23 | 24 | 25 | 26 | 27 | 28 | 29 | 30 | (1 | 2 | 3 | 4 | 5 | 6 | 7 | May |

| Aug. | 1 | 2 | 3 | 4 | 5 | 6 | 7 | 8 | 9 | 10 | 11 | 12 | 13 | 14 | 15 | 16 | 17 | 18 | 19 | 20 | 21 | 22 | 23 | 24 | 25 | 26 | 27 | 28 | 29 | 30 | 31 | | |
| May | 8 | 9 | 10 | 11 | 12 | 13 | 14 | 15 | 16 | 17 | 18 | 19 | 20 | 21 | 22 | 23 | 24 | 25 | 26 | 27 | 28 | 29 | 30 | 31 | (1 | 2 | 3 | 4 | 5 | 6 | 7 | June |

| Sept. | 1 | 2 | 3 | 4 | 5 | 6 | 7 | 8 | 9 | 10 | 11 | 12 | 13 | 14 | 15 | 16 | 17 | 18 | 19 | 20 | 21 | 22 | 23 | 24 | 25 | 26 | 27 | 28 | 29 | 30 | | | |
| June | 8 | 9 | 10 | 11 | 12 | 13 | 14 | 15 | 16 | 17 | 18 | 19 | 20 | 21 | 22 | 23 | 24 | 25 | 26 | 27 | 28 | 29 | 30 | (1 | 2 | 3 | 4 | 5 | 6 | 7 | July | |

| Oct. | 1 | 2 | 3 | 4 | 5 | 6 | 7 | 8 | 9 | 10 | 11 | 12 | 13 | 14 | 15 | 16 | 17 | 18 | 19 | 20 | 21 | 22 | 23 | 24 | 25 | 26 | 27 | 28 | 29 | 30 | 31 | | |
| July | 8 | 9 | 10 | 11 | 12 | 13 | 14 | 15 | 16 | 17 | 18 | 19 | 20 | 21 | 22 | 23 | 24 | 25 | 26 | 27 | 28 | 29 | 30 | 31 | (1 | 2 | 3 | 4 | 5 | 6 | 7 | Aug. |

| Nov. | 1 | 2 | 3 | 4 | 5 | 6 | 7 | 8 | 9 | 10 | 11 | 12 | 13 | 14 | 15 | 16 | 17 | 18 | 19 | 20 | 21 | 22 | 23 | 24 | 25 | 26 | 27 | 28 | 29 | 30 | | | |
| Aug. | 8 | 9 | 10 | 11 | 12 | 13 | 14 | 15 | 16 | 17 | 18 | 19 | 20 | 21 | 22 | 23 | 24 | 25 | 26 | 27 | 28 | 29 | 30 | 31 | (1 | 2 | 3 | 4 | 5 | 6 | | Sept. | |

| Dec. | 1 | 2 | 3 | 4 | 5 | 6 | 7 | 8 | 9 | 10 | 11 | 12 | 13 | 14 | 15 | 16 | 17 | 18 | 19 | 20 | 21 | 22 | 23 | 24 | 25 | 26 | 27 | 28 | 29 | 30 | 31 | | |
| Sept. | 7 | 8 | 9 | 10 | 11 | 12 | 13 | 14 | 15 | 16 | 17 | 18 | 19 | 20 | 21 | 22 | 23 | 24 | 25 | 26 | 27 | 28 | 29 | 30 | (1 | 2 | 3 | 4 | 5 | 6 | 7 | Oct. |

secretion increases; pituitary increases its activity; placenta produces hormones, affecting ovaries and corpus luteum.

Circulatory System: Increased activity; increased blood volume; blood pressure should be normal; varicose veins may be present.

Skeletal: Pelvic joints soften; pelvic joints more movable; bones and teeth affected.

Respiratory: Full ventilation of the lungs may be diminished in late pregnancy; breathing is more frequent.

Digestive Tract: Nausea and vomiting in early pregnancy; appetite affected; loss of weight in early pregnancy; metabolism increased in later pregnancy; constipation frequent.

Liver: Displaced in late pregnancy.

Skin: Sudoriparous and sebaceous glands very active; deposit of brown pigment on face (mask of pregnancy); linea nigra.

Weight: In normal-size individuals, the weight gain is 2 to 3 pounds (907 to 1361 grams) per month of pregnancy. Weight gain above 30 pounds (13.6 kg) is not desired.

Posture: Changes as enlargement of abdomen advances; sacroiliac joints and symphysis pubis more movable; painful locomotion and back pain; gait may be altered.

Urinary Tract: Increased kidney activity; failure of kidneys produces nephritic toxemia; ureters, esp. right one, dilated; pressure on bladder; frequent urination in late pregnancy; bladder lifted into abdomen and pressure diminished. Bladder later pressed upon by presenting part; urinary output varies; presence of albumin abnormal.

DISORDERS OF: *Nausea and vomiting:* May be noted when stomach is empty, but may occur at any time. Four or five small meals per day may control this.

Constipation and flatulence: Pressure of uterus on intestines may be a cause; stool softeners and an increase in fiber content of diet may help; intestinal stasis may cause flatulence; gas-forming foods should be avoided.

Muscular cramps: Rest between periods of standing. Tetany may ensue because of deficient calcium supply; calcium and vitamin D supplement indicated.

Pressure edema: May occur at end of pregnancy with condition better in morning and worse at end of day. Frequent rest and elevation of limbs indicated. May be due to calcium deficiency. Toxemia must be considered. The blood pressure and weight should be recorded, and a urinalysis done at each prenatal visit. All of these will help to alert the physician to the possible development of toxemia of pregnancy.

Headache: Cause may be sinusitis or toxemia.

Toothache: May be due to caries induced by deficient calcium. Frequent dental examinations desirable.

Back pain: Abnormal balance caused by protruding abdomen; proper shoes indicated. Intra-abdominal pressure may be a cause; flatulence aggravates; enemas may help.

Dyspnea: Pressure of uterus upward on transverse colon and stomach; aggravated by flatulence, esp. when lying down. Alkalies may help; pillows under head and shoulder indicated; re-examination of heart indicated.

Vaginal discharge: Routine perineal hygiene but douches are not indicated. Foul, blood-tinged, or profuse discharge should be reported.

Pruritus: Breasts, abdomen, and vulva may be affected; stretching of skin of abdomen a cause in that area. If general, a toxic or nervous origin may be cause. Diabetes mellitus may cause pruritus of vulva.

Heartburn: Hyperacidity or nervous tension may be responsible. Sedation, frequent small meals, no highly seasoned foods.

Varicose veins: Aggravated by pregnancy. May occur in pelvis, vulva, and legs. Avoid tight garters, tight clothing, and standing. Rest and support stockings indicated; elevation of lower limbs while sleeping; Sims' position, pillow under hips to shift uterus.

Hemorrhoids: Avoid constipation. Ointments, wet compresses, suppositories on physician's orders; surgical therapy may be required.

p., abdominal. Pregnancy with implantation of the ovum in the abdominal cavity. SYN: *p., extrauterine; p., ectopic.*

p., ampullar. Pregnancy in the ampulla of the uterine tube.

p., bigeminal. Pregnancy with twins in utero.

p., cervical. Pregnancy with implantation of the ovum in the cervical canal.

p., cornual. Pregnancy in one of the horns of the bicornuate uterus.

p., ectopic. Pregnancy in which ovum develops outside the uterus. SEE: illus.

p., extrauterine. Pregnancy in which ovum develops outside the uterine cavity. SYN: *p., ectopic.*

p., false. P., phantom.

p., heterotopic. Combined intrauterine and extrauterine pregnancies.

p., hydatid. Pregnancy giving rise to a hydatidiform mole. SEE: *hydatid mole.*

p., interstitial. Pregnancy that occurs in the uterine wall where the oviduct is formed. SYN: *p., intramural.*

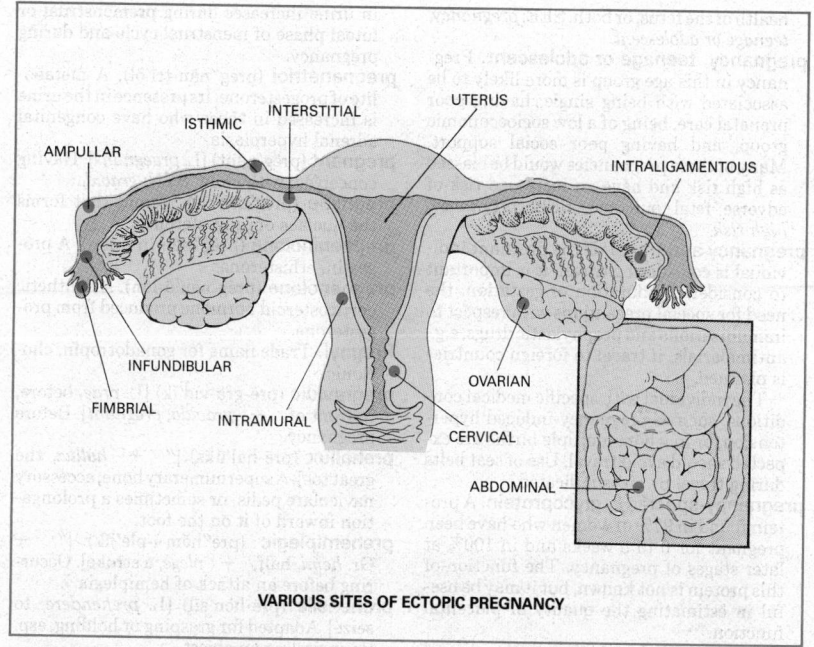

ISTHMIC · INTERSTITIAL · UTERUS · AMPULLAR · INTRALIGAMENTOUS · INFUNDIBULAR · FIMBRIAL · INTRAMURAL · CERVICAL · OVARIAN · ABDOMINAL

VARIOUS SITES OF ECTOPIC PREGNANCY

p., intraligamentary. Pregnancy that occurs within the broad ligament.

p., intramural. P., interstitial.

p., mask of. Area of brown pigmentation sometimes appearing on the face during pregnancy. SYN: *chloasma gravidarum.*

p., membranous. Pregnancy in which the amniotic sac ruptures and fetus comes to lie in direct contact with the uterine wall.

p., mesenteric. P., tuboligamentary.

p., molar. Pregnancy in which instead of the ovum developing into an embryo, it develops into a mole.

p., multiple. State of having more than one fetus in the uterus during the same pregnancy.

p., mural. P., interstitial, q.v.

p., ovarian. Implantation of the fertilized ovum in the substance of the ovary.

p., phantom. Enlargement of the abdomen, simulating pregnancy. SYN: *p., false; pseudopregnancy.* SEE: *pseudocyesis.*

p., postdate. Pregnancy that extends beyond 42 weeks of gestation. An average of 10% of normal pregnancies are so classified. SYN: *post-term pregnancy.*

p., tubal. Form of ectopic pregnancy in which the embryo develops in the fallopian tube.

p., tuboabdominal. Pregnancy in which part of the fetus is in the uterine tube and part in the abdominal cavity.

p., tuboligamentary. Pregnancy occurring in the uterine tube and extending into the broad ligament. SYN: *p., mesenteric.*

p., tubo-ovarian. Pregnancy in which development of the fetus occurs in both the uterine tube and the ovary.

p., uteroabdominal. Twin pregnancy with one embryo in the uterus and the other in the abdominal cavity.

pregnancy, coitus during. Sexual intercourse during pregnancy. There is no evidence that this has adverse effects on the pregnancy or the infant, i.e., perinatal mortality. Also, sexual intercourse does not initiate labor.

pregnancy, exercise during. SEE: *exercise during pregnancy.*

pregnancy, high risk. Pregnancy wherein factors such as diabetes, hypertension, kidney disease, viral infections, vaginal bleeding, multiple pregnancies, and certain lifestyle and environmental factors such as drug, alcohol, or cigarette abuse, or exposure to toxic chemicals are present. Pregnancy in association with these conditions produces a greater risk to the mother's health, the health of the fetus, or both. SEE: *pregnancy, teenage or adolescent.*

pregnancy, teenage or adolescent. Pregnancy in this age group is more likely to be associated with being single, having poor prenatal care, being of a low socioeconomic group, and having poor social support. Many of these pregnancies would be classed as high risk and have an increased risk of adverse fetal outcome. SEE: *pregnancy, high risk.*

pregnancy and travel. If the pregnant individual is considering travel, it is important to consider the duration of gestation, the need for special precautions with respect to immunizations and prophylactic drugs, e.g., antimalarials, if travel to foreign countries is planned.

The individual with specific medical conditions, such as pregnancy-induced hypertension, or in whom multiple births are expected should avoid travel. Use of seat belts during travel by air is indicated.

pregnancy-specific β_1 glycoprotein. A protein found in 97% of women who have been pregnant for 6 to 8 weeks and in 100% at later stages of pregnancy. The function of this protein is not known, but it may be useful in estimating the quality of placental function.

pregnancy test. In addition to the clinical signs and symptoms of pregnancy, almost none of which are reliable within the first several weeks of pregnancy, there are chemical tests done in the physician's office that are quite accurate by as early as the time the first menstrual period is missed. There are also test kits available for purchase without a prescription. If that type of test is used, it is very important to follow the directions carefully.

A major class of pregnancy tests is those using immunodiagnostic procedures. They are: hemagglutination inhibition test, which requires a sample of urine; radioreceptor assay, which requires blood from the patient; radioimmunoassay, which requires a blood sample; and monoclonal antibody determination, which requires a sample of urine. In general, these tests are accurate beginning the 40th day following the first day of the last menstrual period; the monoclonal antibody test is somewhat more sensitive. Reliability of the test methods increases as pregnancy continues.

pregnane (prĕg'nān). The organic compound that is a precursor of two series of steroid hormones: the progesterones and several adrenal cortical hormones.

pregnanediol (prĕg''nān-dī'ŏl). $C_{21}H_{36}O_2$. The inactive end product of metabolism of progesterone present in the urine. Amount in urine increases during premenstrual or luteal phase of menstrual cycle and during pregnancy.

pregnanetriol (prĕg''nān-trī'ŏl). A metabolite of progesterone. Its presence in the urine is increased in those who have congenital adrenal hyperplasia.

pregnant (prĕg'nănt) [L. *praegnans*]. Having conceived; with child. SYN: *gravid.*

pregnene (prĕg'nēn). A steroid that forms the nucleus of progesterone.

pregneninolone (prĕg''nēn-in'ō-lōn). A progestin, ethisterone.

pregnenolone (prĕg-nĕn'ō-lōn). A synthetic corticosteroid hormone produced from progesterone.

Pregnyl. Trade name for gonadotropin, chorionic.

pregravidic (prē-gră-vĭd'ĭk) [L. *prae*, before, in front of, + *gravida, pregnant*]. Before pregnancy.

prehallux (prē-hăl'ŭks) [" + *hallux*, the great toe]. A supernumerary bone, accessory naviculare pedis, or sometimes a prolongation inward of it on the foot.

prehemiplegic (prē''hĕm-ĭ-plē'jĭk) [" + Gr. *hemi*, half, + *plege*, a stroke]. Occurring before an attack of hemiplegia.

prehensile (prē-hĕn'sĭl) [L. *prehendere*, to seize]. Adapted for grasping or holding, esp. by encircling an object.

prehension (prē-hĕn'shŭn) [L. *prehensio*]. The primary function of the hand; includes pinching, grasping, and seizing.

prehormone. A precursor of a hormone.

pre-hospital care. The care a patient receives from emergency medical service before arriving at the hospital. This is usually done by emergency medical technicians and paramedics.

prehyoid (prē-hī'oyd) [L. *prae*, before, in front of, + Gr. *hyoeides*, U-shaped]. In front of the hyoid bone.

prehypophysis (prē''hī-pŏf'ĭ-sĭs) [" + Gr. *hypophysis*, an undergrowth]. Anterior lobe of the pituitary gland.

preictal (prē-ĭk'tăl) [" + *ictus*, stroke]. The period just prior to a stroke or convulsion.

preicteric (prē-ĭk-tĕr'ĭk) [" + *ikteros*, jaundice]. In liver disease, the period prior to the appearance of jaundice.

preimmunization (prē-ĭm''ū-nĭ-zā'shŭn) [" + *immunis*, safe]. Immunization produced artificially in very young infants.

preinvasive (prē''ĭn-vā'sĭv) [" + *in*, into, + *vadere*, to go]. A stage of development of a malignancy in which the neoplastic cells have not invaded adjacent tissues.

Preiser's disease (prī'zĕrz) [Georg K.F. Preiser, Ger. orthopedic surgeon, 1879–1913]. Osteoporosis caused by trauma and affecting the scaphoid bone of the wrist.

prekallikrein. A cofactor in blood coagulation. SEE: *coagulation, blood.*

preleukemia. A group of nondiagnostic physical and blood abnormalities that may indicate leukemia will develop later. They include unexplained anemia, purpura, susceptibility to infections, or slow healing of skin and mucous membrane lesions. Possible laboratory findings are anemia, neutropenia, sometimes a relative lymphopenia, and marked monocytosis. In general, the diagnosis of preleukemia is made in retrospect because all of the findings and signs may be reversible abnormalities that occur in patients with various other illnesses.

preload. In cardiac physiology, the end-diastolic stretch of the muscle fiber. In the intact ventricle, this is approximately equal to the end-diastolic volume or pressure. SEE: *afterload.*

Preludin. Trade name for phenmetrazine hydrochloride.

premaniacal (prē″mā-nī′ă-kăl) [L. *prae*, before, in front of, + Gr. *mania*, madness]. Prior to an attack of mania.

Premarin. Trade name for conjugated estrogens.

premature (prē-mă-chūr′) [L. *praematurus*, ripening early]. Not mature; before term or full development.

premature beat. A cardiac contraction occurring before the normal one. SYN: *extrasystole.*

premature ejaculation. An imprecise term. Usually indicates ejaculation very shortly after the onset of sexual excitement. Also indicates ejaculation prior to orgasm by the partner.

premature infant. An infant who at birth is not fully developed because of curtailed gestation, low birth weight, or both. Birth weight of 2500 gm (5.5 lb) or less is considered to be evidence of premature birth. SEE: *prematurity.*

premature labor. Onset of labor before full term.

premature rupture of membranes. ABBR: PROM. Rupture of the fetal membranes prior to the onset of labor. This occurs in about 10% of patients. PROM is the single most common diagnosis leading to admission of the newborn to intensive care nursing.

PROM is more common among those of poor socioeconomic groups, teenagers, single women, smokers, and in women who have virtually any sexually transmitted organism cultured from the cervix or vagina in the first half of pregnancy. SEE: *prematurity.*

premature ventricular contraction. ABBR: PVC. The contraction of the cardiac ventricle prior to the normal time. This is caused by an electrical impulse to the ventricle arising from a site other than the sinoatrial node. The PVC may be a single event or occur several times in a minute or in pairs or strings. PVCs of such duration as to cause ventricular tachycardia may lead to death.

prematurity. The state of an infant born any time prior to completion of the 37th week of gestation. The normal gestation period for the human being is 40 weeks. Because of the difficulty of obtaining accurate and objective data on the exact length of gestation, a birth weight of 2500 gm (5.5 lb) or less has been accepted internationally as the clinical criterion of prematurity regardless of the period of gestation. Other measures suggestive of prematurity are crown-heel length (47 cm or less), crown-rump length (32 cm or less), occipitofrontal circumference (33 cm or less), occipitofrontal diameter (11.5 cm or less), and ratio of the thorax circumference to the head circumference (less than 93%).

The use of a single-criterion measure (birth weight) imposes limitations in accurately identifying those infants born before adequate development of body organs and systems has been achieved; it can easily include mature infants who are of low birth weight for reasons other than a shortened gestation period. The Expert Committee on Prematurity of the World Health Organization (1961) recommended that the concept of prematurity in the international definition be replaced by that of low birth weight. This term, low birth weight, more accurately describes infants weighing less than 2500 gm at birth than does the term prematurity; the latter should be reserved for those neonates within the low birth weight group with evidence of incomplete development.

In the United States approx. 7.1% white liveborn and 13.4% nonwhite infants weighed 2500 gm or less. Chances of survival depend upon degree of maturity achieved, general condition, and quality of care received.

Prematurity is the leading cause of death in the neonatal period; mortality among infants weighing less than 2500 gm at birth is 17 times greater than among infants with birth weight above 2500 gm. Chief causes of mortality are abnormal pulmonary ventilation, infection, intracranial hemorrhage, abnormal blood conditions, and congenital anomalies.

ETIOL: The incidence of neonates of low birth weight is more frequent among the female sex, nonwhite races, plural births, and the first- and fifth- (and over) born infants. Delivery of infants of low birth weight is reported to be more frequent among women with one or more of the following character-istics: having their children at either a very young age or between ages 45 and 49; being unmarried; having children closely spaced, i.e., less than 2 to 4 years between births; living in a large urban area.

Another factor associated with low birth weight is the socioeconomic status of the family as measured by the mother's educational attainment. The proportion of infants of low birth weight born to mothers with 16 years or more of education was half of that of infants born to mothers with less than 9 years of education. Low birth weight is also associated with generally elevated risk of infant mortality, congenital malformations, mental retardation, and various other physical and neurological impairments.

COMPLICATIONS: Frequently, premature infants are handicapped by a number of anatomical and physiological limitations. These limitations vary in direct proportion to the degree of immaturity present. Limitations include weakness of the sucking and swallowing reflexes, small capacity of stomach, impairment of renal function, incomplete development of capillaries of the lungs, immature alveoli of the lungs, weakness of the cough and gag reflexes, weakness of the thoracic cage muscles and muscles used in respiration, inadequate regulation of body temperature, incomplete or poorly developed enzyme systems, hepatic immaturity, and deficient placental transfer and antenatal storage of minerals, vitamins, and immune substances. SEE: *intrauterine growth retardation; premature rupture of membranes.*

NURSING IMPLICATIONS: Perform a physical assessment that is correlated with expected maturation at the fetal age; this will include neurological evaluation; perform Apgar rating; provide: a proper environmental temperature, proper fluid and caloric intake, appropriate parental bonding and support; assess laboratory reports; monitor intake and output; notify the nursery of the birth of the possible premature infant; weigh infant daily without clothing and on the same scale and at the same time; monitor oxygen concentration at frequent intervals; hold and cuddle infant during feedings; cover sufficiently when removing infant from isolette; and provide adequate time for feeding.

Care of low-birth-weight infants: Care of low-birth-weight infants should be individualized and reflect the needs of the developing organism in relation to the presence of anatomical and physiological handicaps. Evaluation for degree of immaturity present

and the identification of special problems appearing after birth will dictate care required by these infants. In general, care revolves around the prevention of infection, stabilization of body temperature, maintenance of respiration, provision for adequate nutrition and hydration.

Aseptic technique is required. An incubator or heated bed provides a suitable environment for maintenance of body temperature. A high-humidity environment may be of value in respiratory difficulties. Gentle nasal and pharyngeal suctioning will aid to keep airways clear. Use of oxygen should be restricted to those minimal amounts required for survival of infant. Because of the danger of retrolental fibroplasia, the oxygen concentration should not exceed 30%.

Depending upon the ability of the infant to suck and swallow, gavage feedings may be necessary. Some of these infants may not be given anything by mouth for as long as 72 hours following birth. Caloric and fluid intakes are gradually increased until 100 to 120 Cal/kg and 140 to 150 ml/kg, respectively, in 24 hr are reached. The time required to achieve these intakes depends upon the size and condition of the newborn baby. Small, frequent feedings may be needed to cope with the small capacity of the stomach, to prevent vomiting and distention, and to meet caloric and fluid requirements of the body. Overfeeding should be avoided. During early days of life, clyses sometimes are administered to maintain adequate hydration.

The infant should not be allowed to become fatigued either from excessive handling, prolonged feeding procedures, or too much crying. Body position should be changed every 2 to 4 hours. Minimal handling regimen should not be used indiscriminately; gentle handling, rather than minimal handling, should be practiced. It is essential that the newborn and infant be cuddled at least several times a day.

Because of the possibility of retinal damage, premature infants should not be exposed to excessively bright light.

premaxilla (prē″măk-sĭl′ă) [L. *prae*, before, in front of, + *maxilla*, jawbone]. A separate element, derived from the median nasal process embryologically, that fuses with the maxilla in humans; formerly called the incisive bone.

premaxillary (prē-măk′sĭ-lĕr″ē). Located before the maxilla.

premedication (prē″mĕd-ĭ-kā′shŭn) [″ + *medicari*, to heal]. 1. Administration of drugs before treatment to enhance the therapeutic effect and safety of a given procedure. 2. Induction of unconsciousness by drugs prior to administration of inhalation anesthesia. SYN: *prenarcosis.*

premenarchal (prē″mĕ-năr′kăl) [″ + Gr. *men,* mouth, + *arche,* beginning]. The time prior to the first menstrual period, i.e., prior to menarche.

premenstrual (prē-mĕn′stroo-ăl) [″ + *menstruare,* to discharge the menses]. Before menstruation.

premenstrual tension syndrome. ABBR: PMS. A syndrome that occurs several days prior to the onset of menstruation and ends a short time after the onset of menstruation. A great number of symptoms involving almost every organ system have been attributed to PMS. The most common are irritability, emotional tension, anxiety, mood changes, esp. depression, headache, breast tenderness with or without swelling, and water retention, which may be sufficient enough to cause edema. The reason most individuals with PMS seek medical assistance is related to changes in mood.

It is estimated that 2% to 8% of women with PMS have severe symptoms. SEE: *Nursing Diagnoses* in *Appendix.*

ETIOL: Unknown, but may be related to the alterations of estrogen and progesterone during the menstrual cycle. Consumption of caffeine-containing beverages may be causally related to PMS.

TREAT: Depends on the severity of symptoms. Mild analgesics may be helpful, but in severe cases restriction of salt intake and use of a diuretic to control fluid retention are indicated. In severe cases, therapy to prevent ovulation may be necessary.

premenstruum (prē-mĕn′stroo-ŭm) [″ + *menstruus,* menstrual fluid]. The period of time prior to menstruation.

premolar (prē-mō′lĕr) [″ + *moles,* a mass]. The permanent teeth which erupt to replace the deciduous molars. They are often called bicuspid teeth, for the maxillary premolars have two cusps, whereas the mandibular premolars may have from one to three cusps. They are located between the canine and first molar of each quadrant of the dental arches. SEE: *dentition.*

premonition (prĕm″ĕ-, prē-mĕ-nĭsh′ŭn) [L. *praemonere,* to warn beforehand]. A feeling of an impending event.

premonitory (prē-mŏn′ĭ-tō-rē) [LL. *praemonitorius*]. Giving a warning, as an early symptom.

premonocyte (prē-mŏn′ō-sīt) [L. *prae,* before, in front of, + Gr. *monos,* alone, + *kytos,* cell]. An embryonic cell transitional in development prior to a monocyte.

premorbid (prē-mor′bĭd) [″ + *morbidus,* sick]. Prior to the development of disease.

premunition (prē″mū-nĭsh′ŭn) [″ + *mu-*

nitio, a fortification]. Immunity depending upon existence of a long-continued latent infection.

premyeloblast (prē-mī′ĕ-lō-blăst) [″ + Gr. *myelos,* marrow, + *blastos,* germ]. A precursor of the mature myeloblast.

premyelocyte (prē-mī′ĕl-ō-sīt) [″ + ″ + *kytos,* cell]. The cell that is the immediate precursor of a myelocyte.

prenarcosis (prē-năr-kō′sĭs) [″ + Gr. *narkosis,* a benumbing]. Induction of unconsciousness by drugs before administration of a general inhalation anesthetic. SYN: *premedication.*

prenares (prē-nā′rēz) [″ + *naris,* nostril]. The nostrils.

prenatal (prē-nā′tl) [″ + *natalis,* birth]. Before birth.

prenatal care. Care of the woman during the period of gestation. It consists of periodic examinations for determination of blood pressure, weight, changes in the size of the uterus, condition of the fetus; urinalysis; instruction in nutritional requirements, preparation for labor and delivery, care of the newborn; and provision of suggestions and support to deal with the discomforts of pregnancy.

Scheduled visits at regular intervals offer the opportunity to detect any untoward changes in the condition of the mother so that necessary treatment can be instituted.

prenatal diagnosis. Diagnosis of disease or developmental defects while the infant is in utero. A great number of pathological conditions can be diagnosed prenatally by use of tests such as ultrasound, amniocentesis, q.v., chorionic villus sampling, q.v., embryoscopy, q.v., and fetoscopy. Thus the sex of the child and information provided by study of the physical and chemical characteristics of the placenta, fetus, and inherited characteristics can be determined in the early months of pregnancy. If the results of these tests indicate the presence of a treatable disease, the indicated therapy can sometimes be instituted prenatally and, if needed, on the first day of life. If the tests indicate an incurable condition, genetic counseling is advisable. SEE: *prenatal surgery.*

prenatal surgery. Intrauterine surgical procedures. These techniques have been used to repair heart defects and anatomical defects of other organs. SEE: *prenatal diagnosis.*

preneoplastic (prē″nē-ō-plăs′tĭk) [″ + *neos,* new, + *plassein,* to form]. Prior to the development of a tumor.

preoperative care (prē-ŏp′ĕr-ă-tĭv) [″ + *operatus,* work]. Care preceding an operation.

NURSING IMPLICATIONS: Allow for time to discuss meaning of procedure with patient and to allow patient to express concerns and fears. Instruct the patient to cough, breathe deeply (splinting incision as necessary), turn, and exercise extremities at frequent intervals. Prepare the operative site as prescribed; prepare the gastrointestinal tract as indicated (restrict food and fluids as ordered); promote rest and sleep; review laboratory results; administer preoperative medications as prescribed after the patient has voided. Have patient perform oral hygiene, and remove dentures. Remove jewelry and make-up, apply a patient gown, and verify proper identification on the patient identification bracelet. If patient is menstruating, be certain that appropriate chart notation is made concerning type of menstrual protection used and be certain tampons or pads are changed, at least every 4 to 6 hours in the case of tampons.

Counsel patient concerning the timing of prescribed activities including return to work and athletic endeavors, when sexual activity may be resumed, whether or not there will be postoperative restriction on driving automobiles.

preoptic area. The anterior portion of the hypothalamus. It is above the optic chiasma and on the sides of the third ventricle.

preoral (prē-ō'răl) [L. *prae*, before, in front of, + *os*, mouth]. In front of the mouth.

preoxygenation. Breathing of 100% oxygen via a face mask by the fully conscious patient prior to induction of anesthesia. Duration is 2 to 7 minutes. In that time the nitrogen is washed out of the lungs and oxygen replaces it.

This same procedure is used for a longer period of time in persons prior to exposure to very low atmospheric pressure, e.g., aviators prior to flying to high altitudes, or to very high atmospheric pressure, e.g., divers descending to a great depth in water. In both cases, the goal is to rid the body of nitrogen to prevent bends, q.v.

prep (prěp) [*prepare; preparation*]. Used esp. when referring to preparation for surgery. SEE: *preoperative care.*

prepalatal (prē-păl'ă-tăl) [L. *prae*, before, in front of, + *palatum*, plate]. Located in front of the teeth.

preparalytic (prē″păr-ă-lĭt'ĭk) [″ + Gr. *para*, at the side, + *lyein*, to loosen]. Before the appearance of paralysis.

preparation (prĕp-ă-rā'shŭn) [L. *praeparatio*]. 1. The making ready, esp. of a medicine for use. 2. A specimen set up for demonstration in anatomy, pathology, or histology. 3. A medicine made ready for use.

p., corrosion. In anatomical and pathology investigations, hollow organs and structures such as vessels are filled with a liquid substance that hardens. Then the surrounding tissues are dissolved by use of suitable chemicals. This leaves a cast of the structures.

p., heart-lung. In animal studies and in open-heart surgery, the use of devices that take over the function of the heart and lungs while those organs are being treated or possibly replaced.

p.'s, rectal. Chloral hydrate: 0.5 to 1.0 gm dissolved in 90 ml of warmed olive oil, or 90 ml of very warm milk, or 90 ml of thin, boiled cornstarch water. This makes a good preparation or a base in which to hold the medicine in suspension. The patient's pulse should be taken 5 minutes before and 5 minutes after the administration. If adverse effects are noticed, action may be taken to prevent further absorption.

Paraldehyde: 1 to 4 ml may be mixed with water in the proportion of 1:8, and in this ratio it may be mixed with thin starch water for rectal medication. There should be about 90 ml of starch water.

prepatellar (prē″pă-tĕl'ăr) [L. *prae*, before, in front of, + *patella*, pan]. In front of the patella.

prepatellar bursitis. Inflammation of the bursa in front of the patella. SYN: *housemaid's knee.* SEE: *bursitis.*

prepatent. Before becoming evident or manifest.

prepatent period. Period between the time of introduction of parasitic organisms into the body and their appearance in the blood or tissues.

preperception (prē″pĕr-sĕp'shŭn) [″ + *percepitio*, to perceive]. The anticipation of a perception. This intensifies the response to the perception.

preperitoneal (prē″pĕr-ĭ-tō-nē'ăl) [″ + Gr. *peritonaion*, peritoneum]. Located in front of the peritoneum.

preplacental (prē″plă-sĕn'tăl) [″ + *placenta*, a flat cake]. Occurring prior to formation of the placenta.

prepotent (prē-pō'tĕnt) [″ + *potentia*, power]. Pert. to the greater power of one parent to transmit inherited characteristics to the offspring.

preprandial (prē-prăn'dē-ăl) [″ + *prandium*, breakfast]. Prior to a meal.

prepuberal, prepubertal (prē-pū'bĕr-ăl, -tăl) [″ + *pubertas*, puberty]. Prior to puberty.

prepubescent (prē″pū-bĕs'ĕnt) [″ + *pubescens*, becoming hairy]. Pert. to the period just prior to puberty.

prepuce (prē'pūs) [L. *praeputium*, prepuce]. The foreskin or fold of skin over the glans penis in the male. Excision constitutes circumcision, a common religious practice, but also performed in cases of phimosis and for hygienic purposes. A sebaceous secretion under the prepuce is called smegma.

RS: acroposthitis; aposthia; circumcision; frenulum; penis; phimosis; smegma; urethra.

p. of clitoris. Fold of the labia minora that covers the clitoris. SEE: *clitoris*.

preputial (prē-pū'shăl). Concerning the prepuce.

preputial glands. Small sebaceous glands of the corona of the penis that secrete an odoriferous discharge. SYN: *Tyson's glands*.

preputiotomy (prē-pū"shē-ŏt'ō-mē) [" + Gr. *tome*, incision]. Incision of the prepuce of the penis to relieve phimosis.

preputium (prē-pū'shē-ŭm) (pl. *preputia*). [NA] The fold of skin that covers the glans penis. SYN: *prepuce*.

p. clitoridis. [NA] Prepuce of the clitoris, a fold overhanging the glans clitoridis formed by the union of the two labia minora.

p. penis. [NA] Fold of skin covering the glans penis. SYN: *foreskin*.

prepyloric (prē"pī-lor'ĭk). Anterior to, or preceding, the pylorus of the stomach.

prerectal (prē-rĕk'tăl) [L. *prae*, before, + *rectus*, straight]. Located in front of the rectum.

prerenal (prē-rē'năl) [" + *ren*, kidney]. 1. Located in front of the kidney. 2. Occurring prior to reaching the kidney, such as changes in consistency of the blood prior to its flow to the kidney.

preretinal (prē-rĕt'ĭ-năl) [" + *retina*, retina]. In front of the retina of the eye.

presacral (prē-sā'krăl) [" + *sacrum*, sacred]. In front of the sacrum.

presacral neurectomy. Surgical procedure for removing the hypogastric (presacral) nerve plexus. This is done to treat conditions such as dysmenorrhea and chronic idiopathic pelvic pain.

presby- [Gr. *presbys*, old]. Combining form concerning old age.

presbyacusia, presbyacousia (prĕz"bē-ă-kū'sē-ă) [Gr. *presbys*, old, + *akousis*, hearing]. Progressive loss of hearing ability due to the normal aging process. SYN: *presbycusis*.

presbyatrics, presbyatry (prĕz-bē-ăt'rĭks, prĕz'bē-ăt-rē) [" + *iatrikos*, healing]. That branch of medicine dealing with the diseases of old age. SYN: *geriatrics; presbytiatrics*.

presbycardia (prĕz-bī-kăr'dē-ă) [" + *kardia*, heart]. Disease or decreased functional capacity of the heart associated with aging.

presbycusis, presbykousis (prĕz-bī-kū'sĭs) [" + *akousis*, hearing]. Impairment of hearing in old age. SYN: *presbyacusia*.

presbyope (prĕs'bē-ōp) [" + *ops*, eye]. A person who is presbyopic.

presbyopia (prĕz-bē-ō'pē-ă) [" + *ops*, eye]. Defect of vision in advancing age involving loss of accommodation or recession of near point. Due to loss of elasticity of crystalline lens. The onset usually occurs between 40 and 45 years of age. SEE: *farsightedness*.

presbyopic (prĕs"bē-ŏp'ĭk). Concerning presbyopia.

presbytiatrics (prĕz"bī-tē-ăt'rĭks) [" + *iatrikos*, healing]. Science of old age and its management. SYN: *geriatrics; presbyatrics; presbyatry*.

prescribe (prē-skrīb') [L. *praescriptio*, prescription]. To indicate the medicine to be administered. This can be done orally but is usually done by writing a prescription or an order in the patient's hospital chart.

prescribing errors. An error in prescribing medications. Included are incorrect dose or medicine, duplicate therapy, incorrect route of administration, or wrong patient. In one extensive study of prescriptions written by physicians in a tertiary-care teaching hospital, 0.3% were erroneous and over half of these were rated as having potential for adverse consequences. Monitoring of medications and patients is thought to be helpful in limiting these errors.

prescribing nurse. A nurse who is allowed to prescribe drugs. Certain states in the U.S. permit nurses to prescribe only certain types and classes of drugs; most states require that prescribing nurses work with a supervising or collaborating physician; and approval for prescribing is granted only to nurse practitioners.

prescription (prē-skrĭp'shŭn) [L. *praescriptio*]. A written direction or order for dispensing and administering drugs. It is signed by a physician, dentist, or other practitioner licensed by law to prescribe such a drug. Historically, a prescription consists of four main parts.

Superscription: Represented by the symbol Rx, which signifies Recipe, from the Latin *recipere*, meaning to take.

Inscription: Containing the ingredients. This is generally constructed of four parts: the basis or principal drug; the adjuvant, which assists the action of the basis; the corrective, which diminishes unpleasant taste or pain or griping, etc.; the vehicle to hold the drugs either in solution or suspension.

Subscription: Directions to the dispenser as to the manner of preparation of the drugs.

Signature: Directions to the patient with regard to the manner of taking dosage; finally the physician's signature, address, telephone number, date, and whether or not the prescription may be refilled. When applicable, the physician's narcotics registry number must be included. Also, some states require that the prescriber indicate on the prescription whether or not a generic drug may be substituted for the trade name equivalent.

Caution: Unused prescription pads should be kept in a secure place in order to prevent their being misused or stolen; also number each prescription consecutively; never sign a prescription blank in advance; use ink to prevent changes being made; and do not use prescription pads for writing notes or memos.

---

p., shotgun. Indiscriminate prescription for a large number of drugs in the hope that at least one of them will accomplish the desired effect.

prescription drug. A drug available to the public only upon prescription written by a physician, dentist, or other practitioner licensed to do so.

prescription writing. Modern practice is to write prescriptions entirely in the language of the country in which written (as English in the United States) and to use few, if any, abbreviations. All drug quantities should be shown by using the metric system of weights and measures (grams, milligrams, liters, milliliters, etc.). SEE: *Prescription Writing, Abbreviations,* in *Appendix.*

The following classical presentation of the art of prescription writing is included primarily for its historical interest: An official Latin name in the nominative case. Drugs are written in the genitive case because the prescription is an order, meaning "take thou." The word "of" is not written in Latin but is indicated by the ending of a word: *quinina* means *quinine,* but changing the termination to "ae," we have *quininae,* meaning *of quinine.*

ALKALOIDS: Written the same as in English, except that the final "e" is changed to "a" to form the nominative case, as *quinina,* for the English quinine. To form the genitive case, the final "e" is changed to "ae," as *quininae.*

ACTIVE PRINCIPLES: These, such as glucosides, resinoids, and others, add "um" to the nominative and "i" to the genitive, so that strophanthin becomes *strophanthinum* to form the Latin nominative, and *strophanthini,* to form the Latin genitive.

ACIDS: The names of these are formed in the same way as those of alkaloids, except that the adjective is formed in the same way and follows the nominative, as *acidum hydrochloricum,* or the genitive, *acidi hydrochlorici.*

METALS: Latin names of metals, except those of a few known to the ancients, are the same as English forms ending in "um," as in *sodium,* forming the Latin nominative, but ending in "i" to form the genitive, *sodii.*

SALTS: Written first with the name of the base in its genitive form, next the acid radical in the nominative, followed by the qualitative adjective in the nominative, as *ferri sulfas exsiccatus,* exsiccated sulfate of iron.

NAMES OF PREPARATIONS: Show the class to which it belongs first, the name of the ingredient next, and the qualifying adjective last, as *syrupus scillae compositus* (compound syrup of squills). First and last words are in nominative case and middle one in genitive.

DRUGS WITH TWO NAMES: Both should be in the genitive, as *liquor potassi arsenitis.* (-ate endings): The Latin nominative ends in "as," as *sulfas,* for sulfate; and the genitive in "atis," as *sulfatis.* (-ite endings): If the English word ends in "ite," as *sulfite,* the Latin nominative ends in "is," as *sulfis,* and the genitive in "itis," as *sulfitis.* (-ide endings): If an English word has this ending, as "bromide," the Latin nominative ends in "um," dropping the final "e" in the English form, as *bromidum;* the genitive dropping the "um" to add "i," as *bromidi.* (-a, -us, -um endings): English words with these endings are the same in the Latin nominative, but the genitive is formed by changing "a" to "ae," or the "us" or "um" to "i." (-in endings): An English word having this ending adds "um" (usually) to form the Latin nominative as benzoin and *benzoinum,* the genitive being formed by merely adding "i," as *benzoini.* (-ol endings): The Latin nominative is the same as the English, as in phenol, but "is" is added to form the genitive, as *phenolis.* (-al endings): To form the Latin nominative, "um" is added, as chloral and *chloralum.* To form the genitive, "i" is added to the English form, as *chlorali.*

There are, of course, exceptions to the foregoing. Many Latin words have the same form as in English.

RS: active principle; antidotes; dosage; drug action; drugs and their administration; names of individual drugs in alphabetical order; names of poisons; poison; poisoning; preparations often given rectally.

presenile (prē-sē′nīl) [L. *prae,* before, in front of, + *senilis,* old]. Premature old age as judged by mental or physical condition but usually the former. Dementia may appear as early as age 40 to 45 and is characterized by personality disintegration as well as loss of intellectual functioning. Alzheimer's disease, Pick's disease, and Creutzfeldt-Jakob disease are characterized as presenile dementias.

presenium (prē-sē'nē-ŭm) [" + *senium,* old age]. Just prior to the onset of senility.

present [L. *praesent,* to be present before others]. The presence of the patient for examination.

presentation (prē"zĕn-tā'shŭn) [L. *praesentatio*]. 1. In obstetrics, term applied to the manner of the fetus presenting itself to the examining finger in the vagina or rectum. Thus longitudinal (normal) and transverse (pathological) presentation. 2. Relationship of the long axis of fetus to that of mother; also called *lie.* SEE: illus.; *position* for table.

p., breech. When buttocks of fetus present. Breech presentation is of three types: complete breech, when the thighs of the fetus are flexed on the abdomen and the legs flexed upon the thighs; frank breech, when the legs of the fetus are extended over the anterior surface of the body; and footling, when a foot or feet present. Footling can be single, double, or if the leg remains flexed, knee presentation. SEE: illus.

p., brow. When the brow of the fetus presents. SEE: illus.

p., cephalic. Presentation of the head of the fetus in any position.

p., compound. A prolapsed limb that is alongside the main presenting part.

p., face. When the head of the fetus is sharply extended so that the face presents. SEE: illus.

p., footling. A fetus presenting feet first. SEE: *p., breech.*

p., funic; p., funis. Appearance of the umbilical cord during labor.

p., longitudinal. Presentation in which the long axis of the fetus is parallel to the long axis of the mother.

p., oblique. Presentation in which the long axis of the fetus is oblique to that of the mother.

p., pelvic. P., breech.

p., placental. Presentation of the placenta first. SYN: *placenta previa.*

p., shoulder. Presentation in which the shoulder of the fetus is the presenting part.

p., transverse. Presentation with fetus lying crosswise. SEE: illus.

p., vertex. Presentation of the upper and back part of the fetal head. SEE: illus.

preservative (prē-zĕr'vă-tiv) [L. *prae,* before, in front of, + *servare,* to keep]. A substance added to medicines or foods to prevent them from spoiling. It may act by interfering with certain chemical reactions or with the growth of molds, fungi, bacteria, or parasites. Some common preservatives are sugar, salt, vinegar, ethyl alcohol, sulfur dioxide, and benzoic acid.

presomite (prē-sō'mīt) [" + Gr. *soma,* body]. The embryonic stage prior to the formation of somites.

presphenoid (prē-sfē'noyd) [" + Gr. *sphen,* wedge, + *eidos,* form, shape]. Anterior region of the body on the sphenoid bone.

presphygmic (prē-sfĭg'mĭk) [" + Gr. *sphygmos,* pulse]. Pert. to the period preceding the pulse wave.

prespinal (prē-spī'năl) [" + *spina,* thorn]. In front of the spine, or ventral to it.

prespondylolisthesis (prē-spŏn"dĭl-ō-lĭs-thē'sĭs) [" + Gr. *spondylos,* vertebra, + *olisthanein,* to slip]. A congenital defect of both pedicles of the fifth lumbar vertebra without displacement. This predisposes to spondylolisthesis.

pressor (prĕs'or) [O. Fr. *presser,* to press]. 1. Stimulating, increasing the activity of a function, esp. of vasomotor activity, as a nerve. 2. Inducing an elevation in blood pressure.

pressor base. One of several amines or nitrogenous bases of plant or animal origin that, when injected, have the ability to increase blood pressure.

pressoreceptive (prĕs"ō-rē-sĕp'tĭv). Sensitive to pressure stimuli.

pressoreceptor (prĕs"ō-rē-sĕp'tor). Sensory nerve ending, such as those in the aorta and carotid sinus, that is stimulated by changes in blood pressure.

pressor nerves. Nerves that when stimulated bring about an increase in blood pressure.

pressor reflex. Any reflex in which the response to stimulation is increased by blood pressure.

pressosensitive (prĕs"ō-sĕn'sĭ-tĭv). Pressoreceptive, q.v.

pressure (prĕsh'ŭr) [L. *pressura*]. 1. A compression. 2. Stress or force exerted on a body, as by tension, weight, or pulling. 3. In psychology, quality of sensation aroused by moderate compression of the skin. 4. In physics, the quotient obtained by dividing a force by the area of the surface on which it acts.

RS: atmosphere; blood; hypertonic; isotonic.

p., after-. A feeling of pressure that remains for a few seconds after removal of a weight or other pressure.

p., arterial. Pressure of blood in the arteries. For a normal young person at physical and mental rest and in sitting position, systolic blood pressure averages about 120 mmHg; diastolic pressure about 80 mmHg. A wide range of normal variation is due to constitutional, physical, and psychic factors. For women the figures are slightly lower. For older people they are higher. Nor-

PRESENTATIONS OF FETUS

ATTITUDES OF THE FETUS

A—VERTEX PRESENTATION; B—SINCIPUT PRESENTATION;
C—BROW PRESENTATION; D—FACE PRESENTATION*

BROW PRESENTATION

A—ANTERIOR VIEW; B—SAGITTAL VIEW*

FACE PRESENTATIONS

L.M.A. R.M.A. R.M.P. L.M.P.

LEFT MENTOANTERIOR (L.M.A.); RIGHT MENTOANTERIOR (R.M.A.);
RIGHT MENTOPOSTERIOR (R.M.P.); LEFT MENTOPOSTERIOR (L.M.P.)*

*Reproduced with permission from Bonica, J.: Principles and Practice of Obstetric Analgesia and Anesthesia. F.A. Davis, Philadelphia, 1972.

PRESENTATIONS OF FETUS

TYPES OF BREECH PRESENTATIONS

A—FRANK; B—COMPLETE; C—INCOMPLETE; D—FOOTLING*

TRANSVERSE PRESENTATION

A—RIGHT SCAPULOANTERIOR;
B—PROLAPSE OF AN ARM IN TRANSVERSE LIE*

SYNCLITISM (A) AND ASYNCLITISM (B AND C)

A. Sagittal suture of the fetus lies exactly midway between the symphysis and the sacral promontory. B. Sagittal suture is close to the sacrum, and the anterior parietal bone is felt by the examining finger (anterior asynclitism of Nägele's obliquity). C. Posterior parietal presentation of posterior asynclitism (Litzmann's obliquity).*

*Reproduced with permission from Bonica, J.: *Principles and Practice of Obstetric Analgesia and Anesthesia.* F.A. Davis, Philadelphia, 1972.

mally there is little difference in the blood pressure recorded in the two arms. SEE: *blood pressure.*

p., atmospheric. Pressure of weight of atmosphere; at sea level it averages about 760 mmHg.

p., back. Pressure resulting from interference in flow of blood from the ventricles, such as occurs in valvular disorders. Results in reduced venous return to the heart and consequent venous engorgement.

p., biting. Pressure exerted on the teeth during biting.

p., blood. Pressure exerted by blood against the walls of blood vessels. SEE: *blood pressure.*

p., capillary. Blood pressure in capillaries.

p., central venous. Pressure in the right atrium of the heart. It is determined by inserting a catheter into the heart via a vein, usually in the arm. The catheter is attached to a manometer.

p., cerebrospinal. Pressure of the cerebrospinal fluid. This varies with body position.

p., diastolic. Arterial pressure during diastole or dilatation of heart chambers.

p., effective osmotic. That portion of the total osmotic pressure of a solution that determines the tendency of the solvent to pass through a membrane, usually one that is semipermeable. The tendency is for the solvent to pass from a solution containing a high concentration of the solute to the side of the membrane with the low concentration.

p., end-diastolic. Blood pressure in a ventricle of the heart at the end of diastole.

p., endocardiac. Blood pressure within the heart.

p., hydrostatic. Pressure exerted by a fluid within a closed system.

p., intra-abdominal. Pressure within the abdominal cavity, such as that caused by descent of the diaphragm.

p., intracranial. Pressure of the cerebrospinal fluid in the subarachnoid space between the skull and the brain. The pressure is normally the same as that found during lumbar puncture.

p., intraocular. Normal tension within the eyeball, equal to approximately 12 to 20 mm Hg.

p., intrathoracic. Pressure within the thorax.

p., intraventricular. Pressure within the ventricles of the heart during different phases of diastole and systole.

p., negative. Any pressure less than that of the atmosphere, or less than that pressure to which the initial pressure is being compared.

p., occlusal. P., biting, q.v.

p., oncotic. Osmotic pressure exerted by colloids in a solution.

p., osmotic. The force with which a solvent, usually water, passes through a semipermeable membrane separating solutions of different concentrations. It is measured by determining the hydrostatic (mechanical) pressure that must be opposed to the osmotic force to bring the passage to a standstill.

p., partial. In a gas containing several different components, the pressure exerted by each component.

p., positive. Pressure greater than atmospheric or greater than the pressure to which the initial pressure is being compared.

p., positive end-expiratory. ABBR: PEEP. The application of slight positive pressure at the end of expiration while intermittent positive pressure is being used. This increases the amount of air remaining in the lungs at the end of expiration.

p., preload filling. Amount of pressure or volume in the ventricle at end diastole, measured by central venous pressure (right ventricular end-diastolic pressure) or pulmonary capillary wedge pressure (left ventricular end-diastolic pressure).

p., pulse. The difference between systolic and diastolic pressures.

p., solution. Pressure that tends to dissolve a solid present in a solution.

p., static. SEE: *static pressure.*

p., systolic. Arterial pressure at time of the contraction of the ventricles, or the ventricular systole.

p., venous. Pressure of the blood within the veins. It is highest near the periphery, diminishing progressively from capillaries to the heart. Near the heart the pressure may be below zero (negative pressure) due to negative intrathoracic pressure.

p., wedge. Pressure determined by use of a fluid-filled catheter wedged in the distal end of a branch of the pulmonary artery. This provides an indirect measurement of the pressure in the left atrium of the heart.

pressure of speech. Loud and emphatic speech that is increased in amount, accelerated, and usually difficult or impossible to interrupt. The speech is not in response to a stimulus and may continue even though no one is listening. May be present in manic episodes, organic brain disease, depression with agitation, psychotic disorders, and sometimes as an acute reaction to stress.

pressure palsy. Temporary paralysis due to pressure on a nerve trunk.

pressure paralysis. Paralysis due to pressure

on the spinal cord or a nerve.

ETIOL: Injury, tumor, gummata.

pressure points. Areas for exerting pressure to control bleeding. For control of hemorrhage, pressure above bleeding point when an artery passes over a bone may be sufficient. Principal pressure points follow.

Common carotid artery, 2 in. (5 cm) above clavicle, press backwards against spine. Temporal artery, at side of face in front of ear. Occipital artery, behind mastoid process. Subclavian artery, behind clavicle, pressing down onto first rib. Axillary artery, by compression in axilla. Brachial artery, compressed by pressure at inner edge of biceps muscle halfway down arm and also above bend of elbow before artery divides into radial and ulnar arteries. Radial artery, press on thumb side of wrist against radius. Ulnar artery, press on little finger side of wrist against ulna. Deep palmar arch, in thumb opposite root of abducted thumb. Abdominal artery, may be compressed against lumbar vertebrae to left of middle line when patient lies on back. Femoral artery, by abduction and external rotation of thigh, bringing head of femur forward into groin and compressing artery against it. Popliteal artery, in popliteal space over artery. Anterior tibial artery, at front of bend of ankle. Posterior tibial artery, behind internal malleolus as it passes into foot. SEE: *bleeding* for table.

pressure ulcer or sore. A sore caused by pressure from a splint or other appliance, or from the body itself when it has remained immobile in bed for extended periods of time. The likelihood of a patient developing a pressure ulcer or sore is increased if urinary incontinence is present. In actual practice, the tendency is to speak of decubitus ulcers as being synonymous with pressure sores. However, the latter is due to pressure on the skin, even when the patient is not lying down. Nevertheless, the operative force is pressure, leading to inadequate blood supply of the area, and if continued, a sore or ulcer develops. SEE: *decubitus ulcer.*

SEE: *Nursing Diagnoses in Appendix.*

presternum (prē-stěr′nŭm) [L. *prae,* before, in front of, + Gr. *sternon,* chest]. The upper part of the sternum. SYN: *manubrium sterni* [NA].

presuppurative (prē-sŭp′ū-rā″tĭv) [″ + *sub,* under, + *puris,* pus]. Rel. to period of inflammation before suppuration.

presylvian fissure (prē-sĭl′vē-ăn). The anterior division of the sylvian fissure.

presymptomatic (prē″sĭmp-tō-măt′ĭk). The state of health prior to the clinical appearance of the signs and symptoms of a disease.

presynaptic (prē″sĭ-năp′tĭk) [″ + Gr. *syn-*

apsis, point of contact]. Located before the nerve synapse.

presystole (prē-sĭs′tō-lē) [L. *prae,* before, in front of, + Gr. *systole,* contraction]. The period in the heart's cycle just before the systole. SYN: *perisystole.*

presystolic (prē-sĭs-tŏl′ĭk). Before the systole of the heart.

pretarsal (prē-tär′săl) [″ + Gr. *tarsos,* a broad flat surface]. In front of the tarsus.

preterm. In obstetrics, events occurring prior to the 37th week of gestation.

preterm birth. Delivery occurring before 37 weeks of gestation. Despite intensive study of causes and methods of preventing preterm birth, progress has been slow. SEE: *prematurity.*

pretibial (prē-tĭb′ē-ăl) [″ + *tibia,* shinbone]. In front of the tibia.

pretibial fever. A form of leptospirosis caused by one of the several serotypes of the autumnalis serogroup. It is characterized by fever, rash on legs, prostration, splenomegaly, and respiratory disturbances. SYN: *Fort Bragg fever.*

pretympanic (prē″tĭm-păn′ĭk) [″ + *tympanon,* drum]. Located in front of the tympanic membrane.

preurethritis (prē″ū-rē-thrī′tĭs) [″ + Gr. *ourethra,* urethra, + *itis,* inflammation]. Inflammation around the urethral orifice of the vaginal vestibule.

prevalence (prěv′ă-lěns) [L. *praevalens,* prevail]. The number of cases of a disease present in a specified population at a given time. SEE: *incidence.*

preventive (prē-věn′tĭv) [ME. *preventen,* to anticipate]. Hindering the occurrence of something, esp. disease. SYN: *prophylactic.*

preventive dentistry. That phase of dentistry concerned with the maintenance of the normal masticatory apparatus by teaching good oral hygiene and dietary practice, and preserving dental health by early restorative procedures.

preventive medicine. The branch of medicine concerned with preventing the occurrence of both mental and physical illness and disease.

There are three levels of preventive effort. Primary preventive medicine is concerned with preventing the development of disease in a susceptible or potentially susceptible population. These efforts include general promotion of health and specific protection such as immunization. Secondary preventive medicine involves early diagnosis and prompt therapy to shorten duration of illness, reduce the severity of disease, reduce possibility of contagion, and limit sequelae. Tertiary preventive medicine is important in limiting the degree of disability and promoting rehabilitation in chronic and irreversible diseases.

preventive nursing. The nurse is an essential part of the health care team and has the opportunity to emphasize and indeed implement health care services to promote health and prevent disease. Nursing expertise and general professional competence can also be utilized in supporting community action at all levels for promoting public health measures. There are three levels of preventive nursing:

A. Primary. The goal of primary prevention is general health promotion. This includes whatever intervention is required to provide a health-promoting environment at home, in the schools, and in the workplace by ensuring good nutrition, adequate clothing and shelter, rest and recreation, and health education (including sex education and, for the aging, realistic plans for retirement). Areas of emphasis are specific protective measures such as immunizations, environmental sanitation, accident prevention, and protection from occupational hazards. Changes in lifestyle through behavior therapy, though difficult, must be attempted with respect to those areas known to represent major health risk factors, i.e., smoking, obesity, sedentary lifestyle, improper diet, alcohol and drug abuse, sexual promiscuity, and falls. Major efforts must be made to prevent automobile accidents.

B. Secondary. Nursing care aimed at early recognition and treatment of disease. It includes general nursing interventions and teaching of early signs of disease conditions. Disease such as infectious diseases, glaucoma, and cancer fall in this category.

C. Tertiary. Nursing care for patients with incurable diseases, and patient instruction concerning how to manage those conditions and diseases. Parkinson's disease, multiple sclerosis, and diabetes are conditions that lend themselves to tertiary prevention. The goal is to prevent further deterioration of physical and mental function, and to have the patient utilize whatever residual function is available for maximum enjoyment of and participation in life's activities. Rehabilitation is of course an essential part of tertiary prevention.

prevertebral (prē-vĕr'tē-brăl) [L. *prae,* before, in front of, + *vertebra,* vertebra]. In front of a vertebra.

prevertebral ganglia. Ganglia of the sympathetic division of the autonomic nervous system, located near origins of the celiac and mesenteric arteries. These include the celiac and mesenteric ganglia. SYN: *collateral ganglia.*

prevertiginous (prē-vĕr-tĭj'ĭ-nŭs) [" +

vertigo, a turning round]. Having a tendency to fall forward.

prevesical (prē-vĕs'ĭ-kl) [" + *vesica,* bladder]. Located in front of the bladder.

previa, praevia (prē'vē-ă) [L.]. Appearing before or in front of.

previable. Pert. to a fetus not sufficiently mature to survive outside the uterus.

prevocational evaluation. In rehabilitation, the assessment of those interests, aptitudes, abilities, and behavioral traits which are necessary for developing or performing specific job skills.

prezonular. Pert. to the posterior chamber of the eye, the space between the iris and ciliary zonule (suspensory ligament).

prezygotic (prē-zī-gŏt'ĭk) [" + *zygotos,* yoked]. Happening prior to fertilization of the ovum.

priapism (prī'ă-pĭzm) [LL. *priapismus*]. Abnormal, painful, and continued erection of the penis due to disease, and usually without sexual desire. SEE: *erection; gonorrhea.*

ETIOL: May be due to lesions of the cord above the lumbar region, or turgescence of the corpora cavernosa without erection may exist. It may be reflex from peripheral sensory irritants, from organic irritation of nerve tracts or nerve centers when libido may be lacking. Sometimes seen in patients with acute leukemia.

p., stuttering. Painful, recurrent attacks of priapism that last two to six hours. The condition is seen in some patients with homozygous sickle cell disease.

priapitis (prī-ă-pī'tĭs) [Gr. *priapos,* phallus, + *itis,* inflammation]. Inflammation of the penis.

priapus (prī'ă-pŭs) [Gr. *priapos*]. The penis.

prickle cell (prĭk'l). A cell with rod-shaped processes, intercellular bridges connecting with similar adjoining cells.

prickly heat. The blockage of sweat pores due to bacterial damage of cells in the lumen. This causes sweat to escape into the epidermis. The tiny blisters that form may go unnoticed; but, as the sweat penetrates deeper in the epidermis, the area becomes painful and itching is intense. SYN: *miliaria.*

TREAT: Cool and dry the area, and avoid conditions that cause sweating.

prilocaine hydrochloride (prĭl'ō-kān). USP. A local anesthetic. It may cause methemoglobinemia. Trade name is Citanest.

primal scene. In psychiatry, the term for a child's first observation of sexual intercourse, real or imagined.

primaquine phosphate (prĭm'ă-kwĭn). USP. An antimalarial drug.

primary (prī'mă-rē) [L. *primarius,* principal]. First in time or order. SYN: *principal.*

primary amputation. Amputation performed before inflammation has set in.

primary bubo. Inflamed lymph node that represents the initial lesion following exposure to a venereal disease, esp. to syphilis. Also called *bubon d'emblée.*

primary care. Basic or general health care provided at the person's first contact with the health care system. Usually this contact is for common illnesses. The primary health care provider assumes ongoing responsibility for health maintenance and therapy for illness, including consultation with specialists.

primary cell. In physical therapy, a device consisting of a container, two solid conducting elements, and an electrolyte for the production of electric current by chemical energy.

primary hemorrhage. Bleeding at time of an injury.

primary lesion. 1. An original lesion from which a second one originates. 2. Lesion of syphilis, a chancre, q.v.

primary nursing. The nursing practice system in which the entire nursing care of a patient is managed and coordinated by one nurse for a 24-hour period. The nurse is involved in, manages, and coordinates all aspects of the patient's case in that period. This includes scheduling of activities, tests, and procedures.

primary physician. The physician to whom a family or individual goes initially for medical care and the management of their care even if eventually referred to other physicians.

primary radiation. That radiation being emitted directly to the patient from the x-ray source.

primary sore. The initial sore or hard chancre of syphilis.

primate (prī'māt) [L. *primus,* first]. A member of the order Primates.

Primatene Mist. Trade name for epinephrine.

Primates (prī-mā'tēz). An order of vertebrates belonging to the class Mammalia, subclass Theria. Includes the lemurs, tarsiers, monkeys, apes, and humans. This order is most highly developed with respect to the brain and nervous system.

prime (prīm) [L. *primus,* first]. 1. Period of greatest health and strength. 2. To give an initial treatment in preparation for either a larger dose of the same medicine, or a different medicine.

primidone (prim'ĭ-dōn). USP. An anticonvulsive drug used in treating epilepsy. Trade name is Mysoline.

primigravida (prī-mĭ-grăv'ĭ-dă) [" + *gravida,* pregnant]. A woman during her first pregnancy.

p., elderly. SEE: *elderly primigravida.*

primipara (prī-mĭp'ă-ră) [" + *parere,* to bring forth, to bear]. A woman who has been delivered of one infant of 500 grams (or of 20 weeks' gestation), regardless of whether it is alive or dead.

primiparity (prī"mĭ-păr'ĭ-tē). Condition of having given birth to only one infant of 500 grams (or 20 weeks' gestation), regardless of its viability.

primiparous (prī-mĭp'ă-rŭs). Pert. to a primipara.

primitiae (prī-mĭsh'ē-ē) [L. *primus,* first]. Liquor amnii appearing just before birth of the fetus. SEE: *amnion; bag of waters; labor; liquor amnii.*

primitive (prim'ĭ-tĭv) [L. *primitivus*]. Original; early in point of time; embryonic.

primitive groove. The longitudinal depression in the dorsum of the embryonic area.

primitive streak. A dark, thickened longitudinal band that forms at caudal end of the embryonic disk, consisting of a surface layer of ectoderm overlying a thickened mass of mesoderm cells. It marks the future longitudinal axis of the embryo.

primordial (prī-mor'dē-ăl) [L. *primordialis*]. 1. Existing first. 2. Existing in an undeveloped, primitive, or early form.

primordium (prī-mor'dē-ŭm) [L., origin] (pl. *primordia*). The first accumulation of cells in an embryo that constitutes the beginning of a future tissue, organ, or part. SYN: *anlage.*

primum non nocere (prī"mŭm nōn nō'sĕ-rā) [L.]. "First do no harm." No one's condition should be made worse because of having visited a physician. This is an idealistic but virtually unattainable goal, because there is no medical procedure, operation, or drug that does not have the potential for harm. SEE: *risk-benefit analysis.*

princeps (prin'sĕps) [L., chief]. 1. Original; first. 2. The name of certain arteries. Ex.: princeps cervicis. 3. Chief, principal.

principal (prin'sĭ-păl). 1. Chief. 2. Outstanding.

principal fibers of the periodontal ligament. ABBR: PDL. The oriented bundles of collagen fibers that by their attachments and position within the periodontal ligament space are recognized as specific parts of the alveolodental ligament; bundles of PDL fibers named according to orientation and attachment.

principle (prin'sĭ-pl) [L. *principium,* foundation]. 1. A constituent of a compound representing its essential properties. 2. A fundamental truth. 3. An established rule of action.

p., active. The portion of a pharmaceutical preparation that produces the therapeutic action.

p., antianemic. A substance stored in the liver that is essential for the normal development of red blood cells in the bone marrow. It is formed in the stomach and intestine by the interaction of an extrinsic factor, vitamin B_{12}, and an intrinsic factor present in gastric juice. It is used in the treatment of pernicious anemia. SYN: *factor, antianemic.*

p., antidiuretic. The antidiuretic hormone (ADH) present in extracts of the posterior lobe of the pituitary gland.

p.'s, gastrointestinal. Substances, secreted by mucosa of stomach and intestine, that are absorbed by the blood and act as hormones. SEE: *cholecystokinin-pancreozymin; gastrin; secretin.*

p., oxytocic. A hormone in extracts of the posterior lobe of the hypophysis that stimulates contraction of uterine muscle.

p., pleasure. In psychoanalysis, the idea that unconsciously the individual is striving to attain pleasure and avoid painful situations.

p., proximate. A substance that may be extracted from its complex form without destroying or altering its chemical properties.

p., purpura-producing. A toxic substance produced when pneumococci are autolyzed. This causes dermal and internal hemorrhages when injected into rabbits.

p., reality. In psychoanalysis, the idea that the striving for pleasure is balanced by the situations produced by the real world.

Prinzmetal's angina [Myron Prinzmetal, U.S. cardiologist, b. 1908]. An atypical form of angina pectoris, q.v., thought to be due to vasospasm of otherwise normal coronary arteries. Pain is experienced at rest and sometimes while in bed rather than during activity. The electrocardiogram taken during an attack will indicate S – T segment elevation rather than depression. Nitroglycerin and drugs that influence calcium metabolism by the myocardium are of benefit. SYN: *angina, variant.*

prion [*proteinaceous infection* particle]. A small proteinaceous infection particle that is resistant to most procedures that modify nucleic acid. It is felt to be important in the transmission of certain slow viral infections, including these neurologic diseases: Creutzfeldt-Jakob disease and kuru, q.v., in humans; and scrapie in sheep.

Priscoline Hydrochloride. Trade name for tolazoline hydrochloride.

prism (prizm) [Gr. *prisma*]. A transparent solid, three sides of which are parallelograms. The bases, perpendicular to the three sides, are triangles. A transverse section of the solid is a triangle. Light rays

going through a prism are deflected toward the base of the triangle and at the same time are split into the primary colors.

p., enamel. A minute rod of calcareous material deposited at the end of an ameloblast in the formation of the enamel of a tooth.

p., Maddox. Two base-together prisms used in testing for cyclophoria or torsion of the eyeball.

p., Nicol. Prism made by splitting a prism of Icelandic spar and rejoining the cut surfaces. This causes the light passing through to be split. Ordinary light rays are reflected by the joined surfaces, and polarized light is transmitted.

p., Risley's rotary. Prism mounted in a device that allows it to be rotated. This is used in testing eye muscle imbalance.

prismatic (priz-măt′ĭk). 1. Shaped like a prism. 2. Produced by a prism.

prismoid (priz′moyd) [″ + *eidos*, form, shape]. Resembling a prism.

prismoptometer (priz-mŏp-tŏm′ĕ-tĕr) [″ + *opsis*, vision, + *metron*, measure]. Device for estimating abnormal refraction of the eye by using prisms.

prisoners, medical care of. In the U.S., standards for medical care of prisoners are mandated by legislation. That these are ignored is evidenced by the placement of mentally disabled prisoners in jails, where they are kept without medical care.

privacy. In the medical context, the rights of a patient to control the distribution and release of data concerning his or her illness. This includes information the patient has provided to the health care professionals and all additional information contained in the chart, medical records, and laboratory data. Failure to observe this aspect of a patient's rights is classed as an invasion of privacy. SEE: *Hippocratic oath.*

private patient. Patient whose care is the responsibility of one identifiable health care professional, usually a physician or dentist. The health care professional is paid directly, either by the patient or by the patient's insurer.

private practice. Practice by a health care professional, usually a physician or dentist, in a setting in which the practice and the practitioner are independent of external policy control other than ethics of the professional and state licensing laws.

privileged communication. Confidential information furnished (in order to facilitate diagnosis and treatment) by the patient to a professional authorized by law to care for him or her. In some states the person who has received this communication cannot be made to divulge it. When this is the case, communication between the patient and the recipient is classed as privileged.

Information given by the patient with the family present may not be considered privileged.

Privine Hydrochloride. Trade name for naphazoline hydrochloride.

p.r.n. L. *pro re nata,* as circumstance may require; as necessary. Frequently used in prescription and order writing.

pro- [L., Gr. *pro,* before]. Prefix indicating for, in front of, before, from, in behalf of, on account of.

proaccelerin. The fifth factor (factor V) in blood coagulation. SEE: *coagulation factors.*

proactinomycin (prō-ăk″tĭ-nō-mī′sĭn). An antibiotic obtained from *Nocardia gardneri.* Effective against gram-positive bacteria.

proagglutinoid (prō″ă-gloo′tĭ-noyd). An agglutinoid having a greater affinity for the agglutinogen than that possessed by the agglutinin.

proal (prō′ăl) [Gr. *pro,* before]. Concerning forward movement.

proamnion (prō-ăm′nē-ŏn) [Gr. *pro,* before, + *amnion,* amnion]. A region anterior to the head in a vertebrate embryo in which mesoderm is lacking.

proantithrombin (prō″ăn-tĭ-thrŏm′bĭn). A substance present in blood plasma or serum which, through the action of heparin, is converted into antithrombin.

proatlas (prō-ăt′lăs) [″ + *atlas,* a support]. A rudimentary vertebra in front of the atlas of small animals. It may be present as an anomaly in the understructure of the occipital bone in humans.

probability. The ratio that expresses the likelihood of the occurrence of a specific event. The probability of a tossed coin landing head side up is one-half or 50%, as is the probability of the tail side landing up. This 50% probability remains the same each time a coin is tossed. Probability ratios based on sophisticated techniques are used for estimating the chance of occurrence of diseases in a population and in projecting vital statistics such as birth and death rates.

proband [L. *probare,* to test]. The initial subject presenting a mental or physical disorder, who causes a study of his or her heredity in order to determine if other members of the family have had the same disease or carry it. SYN: *propositus.*

probang (prō′băng). A slim, flexible rod with a sponge or similar material attached to the end. Used for determining the location of strictures in the larynx or esophagus and for removing objects from the trachea. Medicines may also be applied to these areas by use of this device.

Pro-Banthine. Trade name for propantheline bromide.

probationary (prō-bā′shŭn-ăr-ē) [L. *probatio,* probation]. One who is in a trial period waiting, as for admission or for a test.

probationer (prō-bā′shŭn-ĕr). A person working during a trial period, as a student nurse just after entering training.

probe (prōb) [L. *probare,* to test]. An instrument, usually flexible, for exploring the depth and direction of a wound or sinus.

p., dental. A sharp, pointed hand instrument used to examine the surface features of teeth and dental restorations for irregularities, cracks, and soft or carious enamel. SYN: *dental explorer.*

p., periodontal. A fine-caliber probe, calibrated in millimeters, designed and used to measure the depth and extent of the gingival sulcus and periodontal pockets present.

probenecid. USP. A benzoic acid derivative useful in treating gout. In large doses it prevents reabsorption of uric acid by the kidney and retards the excretion of penicillin in the urine. Trade names are Benemid and SK-Probenecid.

problem-oriented medical record. ABBR: POMR. Method of establishing and maintaining the patient's medical record so that problems are clearly stated, usually in order of importance, and a rational plan for dealing with them is stated. These data are kept at the front of the chart and are evaluated as frequently as indicated with respect to recording changes in the patient's problems as well as progress made in solving the problems. Use of this system may bring a degree of comprehensiveness to total patient care that might not be possible with conventional medical records.

problem-oriented record. ABBR: POR. SEE: *problem-oriented medical record.*

probucol (prō′bū-kōl). An antihypercholesteremic drug. Trade name is Lorelco.

procainamide hydrochloride. USP. A drug used in treating cardiac arrhythmias, particularly those that originate in the ventricle. Trade names are Procan and Pronestyl.

procaine hydrochloride (prō′kān). USP. White, colorless, crystalline compound. Trade name is Novocain.

ACTION/USES: A safe, local anesthetic, less toxic than cocaine. Used in infiltration anesthesia, nerve block, and spinal anesthesia. Its effect is prolonged by simultaneous injection of epinephrine.

Procan. Trade name for procainamide hydrochloride.

procarbazine hydrochloride (prō-kär′bă-zēn). USP. A cytotoxic drug used in treating Hodgkin's disease and certain other neoplastic diseases. Trade name is Matulane.

procarboxypeptidase (prō″kăr-bŏk″sē-pĕp′tǐ-dās). Inactive precursor of carboxypeptidase. Trypsin activates it.

procaryote (prō-kăr′ē-ōt) [Gr. *pro*, before, + *karyon*, nucleus]. Prokaryote, q.v.

procedure (prō-sē′dūr) [L. *procedere*, to proceed]. A particular way of accomplishing a desired result.

procelous (prō-sē′lŭs) [Gr. *pro*, before, + *koilos*, hollow]. Concave anteriorly.

procentriole (prō-sĕn′trē-ōl). The early form of the centrioles and ciliary basal bodies in the cell. SEE: *centriole.*

procephalic (prō″sē-fāl′ĭk) [″ + *kephale*, head]. Of, or relating to, the anterior part of the head.

procercoid (prō-sĕr′koyd). The first larval stage in the development of certain cestodes belonging to the order Pseudophyllidea. It is an elongated structure that develops in crustaceans.

procerus muscle. [NA] A muscle that arises in the skin over the nose and is connected to the forehead. It acts to draw the eyebrows down.

process (prŏs′ĕs) [L. *processus*, going before]. 1. A method of action. 2. State of progress of a disease. 3. A projection or outgrowth of bone or tissue. SYN: *processus* [NA]. 4. Series of steps or events that lead to achievement of specific results.

 p., acromion. The acromion.

 p., alar. Process of cribriform plate of the ethmoid bone that articulates with the frontal bone.

 p., alveolar. 1. The inferior border of the maxilla containing sockets for upper teeth. 2. The superior border of body of mandible containing sockets for lower teeth.

 p., articular, of vertebra. One of four processes (two superior and two inferior) by which vertebrae articulate with each other.

 p., basilar. Narrow part of the base of the occipital bone, in front of the foramen magnum, articulating with the sphenoid bone. SYN: *pars basilaris ossis occipitalis.*

 p., caudate. Process of the caudate lobe of the liver extending under the right lobe.

 p., ciliary. One of about 70 prominent meridional ridges projecting from the corona ciliaris of the choroid coat of the eye to which the suspensory ligament of the lens is attached.

 p., clinoid. The three processes of the sphenoid bone: anterior, middle, and posterior clinoid.

 p., condyloid. Posterior process on superior border of the ramus of the mandible that articulates with the temporal bone.

 p., coracoid. A beak-shaped process extending upward and laterally from the neck of the scapula.

 p., coronoid. 1. Process extending upward from the anterior portion of the ramus of the mandible. 2. Sharp projection forming the anterior and lower border of the semilunar notch of the ulna.

 p., ensiform. The xiphoid process of the sternum.

 p., ethmoidal. Small process on superior border of the inferior concha that articulates with the uncinate process of the ethmoid.

 p., falciform. An extension of the posterior edge of the sacrotuberous ligament to the ramus of the ischium.

 p., frontal. Upward projection of maxilla that articulates with the frontal bone. Forms part of the orbit and nasal fossa.

 p., frontonasal. In the area of the primitive mouth of the embryo, a median swelling that is the anlage of the nose, upper lip, and front part of the palate.

 p., frontosphenoidal. Upward projecting process of the zygomatic bone.

 p., head. An axial strand of cells in vertebrate embryos extending forward from the primitive knot. Forms primitive axis about which the embryo differentiates. SYN: *notochordal plate.*

 p., infraorbital. Medially projecting process of the zygomatic bone that articulates with the maxilla. Forms inferior lateral margin of orbit.

 p., jugular. Process of occipital bone lying lateral to the occipital condyle.

 p., lacrimal. A short process of inferior concha that articulates with the lacrimal bone.

 p., lenticular. A knob on the malleus in the ear that articulates with the stapes.

 p., malar. Projection from the maxilla that articulates with the zygomatic bone.

 p., mandibular. Posterior portion of the first branchial arch from which the lower jaw develops.

 p., mastoid. Projection of the mastoid portion of the temporal bone.

 p., maxillary. 1. Anterior portion of the first branchial arch, which, with medial nasal processes, forms the upper jaw. 2. Process of inferior nasal concha extending laterally and covering the orifice of the antrum. 3. Process on the anterior border of the perpendicular portion of the palatine bone.

 p., nursing. SEE: *nursing process.*

 p., odontoid. Toothlike process extending upward from the axis and about which the axis rotates. SYN: *dens.*

 p., olecranon. The olecranon, q.v., an extension at the proximal end of the ulna.

 p., orbital. 1. Process at tip of the perpendicular portion of the palatine bone directed upward and backward. 2. Process of the zygomatic bone that forms the anterior boundary of the temporal fossa.

p., palatine. Process extending transversely from the medial surface of the maxilla. With the corresponding process from the other side, it forms the major portion of the hard palate.

p., postglenoid. Process of the temporal bone separating the mandibular fossa from the external acoustic meatus.

p., pterygoid. Process of sphenoid bone extending downward from junction of the body and great wing. Consists of the lateral and medial pterygoid plates.

p., spinous, of vertebrae. The posterior-most part of a vertebra. This spine projects back and serves as a point of attachment for muscles of the back.

p., styloid. Styloid process.

p., transverse. Process extending laterally and dorsally from the arch of a vertebra.

p., uncinate, of ethmoid bone. A sickle-shaped bony process on the medial wall of the ethmoidal labyrinth below the concha.

p., vermiform. Vermiform appendix.

p., vocal. Process of arytenoid cartilage that serves for attachment of the vocal ligament.

p., xiphoid. Thin, elongated process extending caudally from the body of the sternum. SYN: p., ensiform.

p., zygomatic. SEE: zygomatic process.

processus (prō-sĕs'ŭs) [L.] (pl. processus). [NA] Process, q.v., or processes.

p. cochleariformis. [NA] Curved portion of a thin plate of bone separating the eustachian tube from the canal for the tensor tympani muscle over which the tendon of the muscle passes before insertion into the manubrium of the malleus.

p. retromandibularis. Wedge-shaped portion of the parotid gland that projects medially toward the pharynx.

p. uncinatus. [NA] 1. Curved process of ethmoid labyrinth projecting from the lateral wall of the middle meatus that forms the inferior border of hiatus semilunaris. 2. A hooklike portion of the head of the pancreas that curves around the superior mesenteric vessels.

procheilon (prō-kī'lŏn) [Gr. pro, before, + cheilon, lip]. Prominence in central portion of the upper lip.

prochlorperazine (prō″klor-pĕr'ă-zēn). USP. A phenothiazine-type drug used in treating nausea and vomiting. Trade name is Compazine.

prochondral (prō-kŏn'drăl) [″ + chondros, cartilage]. Preceding the formation of cartilage.

prochordal (prō-kor'dăl) [″ + chorde, cord]. In front of the notochord.

procidentia (prō″sī-dĕn'shē-ă) [L.]. A complete prolapse, esp. of the uterus, to such an extent that the uterus lies outside of the vulva with everted vaginal walls.

ETIOL: Generally due to relaxation of the tissues that provide support for the pelvic organs.

procoagulant factor. A lymphokine, q.v., that can assume the role of Factor VIII, antihemolytic factor, in coagulation cascade.

procollagen (prō-kŏl'ă-jĕn) [″ + kolla, glue, + gennan, to produce]. Precursor of collagen.

proconvertin (prō″kŏn-vĕr'tĭn). Coagulation factor VII, q.v.

procreate [L. procreare]. To beget; to be the parents of an infant.

procreation (prō″krē-ā'shŭn). The act or state of conceiving and giving birth to an infant. SYN: reproduction.

procreative (prō'krē-ā″tiv). Concerning procreation.

proctagra (prŏk-tăg'ră) [Gr. proktos, anus, + agra, seizure]. Sudden rectal pain.

proctalgia (prŏk-tăl'jē-ă) [″ + algos, pain]. Pain in or about the anus and rectum.

p. fugax. Rectal pain that occurs usually nocturnally. The pain is usually of short duration, and even though its cause is unknown, it is not considered to be due to organic disease. In some individuals, having an orgasm or a bowel movement will alleviate the pain.

proctatresia (prŏk″tă-trē'zē-ă) [″ + atresis, imperforation]. Imperforation of the anus.

proctectasia (prŏk″tĕk-tā'sē-ă) [″ + ektasis, dilatation]. Dilatation of the anus or rectum.

proctectomy (prŏk-tĕk'tō-mē) [″ + ektome, excision]. Excision of the rectum or anus. SYN: rectectomy.

proctenclisis (prŏk″tĕn-klī'sĭs) [″ + enkleiein, to shut in]. Stricture of the anus or rectum.

procteurynter (prŏk″tū-rĭn″tĕr) [″ + eurynein, to widen]. Instrument for dilation of the anus or rectum.

proctitis [″ + itis, inflammation]. Inflammation of rectum and anus. It may be acute or chronic with rectal discomfort and repeated urge to evacuate the rectum accompanied by inability to pass feces. Mucus, blood, or pus may be present in the stools and there may be tenesmus. SYN: rectitis.

ETIOL: Infectious organisms; trauma; radiation injury; drugs, esp. broad-spectrum antibiotics; allergy.

p., diphtheritic. Proctitis in which a diphtheritic and albuminous membrane forms over the surface of mucous membrane. There is headache with roaring in ears; constipation, gas, and bloating; neurasthenia.

p., dysenteric. Proctitis resulting from ordinary diarrhea. May produce ulcers and scarring of the rectum and anus.

p., gonorrheal. Gonorrheal infection around the rectum and anus.

p., traumatic. Proctitis with pain, pressure as if bowels were going to move; irritation; mucous membrane red, eroded. Surface tissues sensitive to touch. Chronic constipation.

procto-, proct- [Gr. *proktos*, anus]. Combining forms indicating relationship to the anus and rectum.

proctocele (prŏk'tō-sēl) [" + *kele*, tumor, swelling]. A protrusion of the rectal mucosa into the vagina. SYN: *rectocele*.

proctoclysis (prŏk-tŏk'lĭ-sĭs) [" + *klysis*, a washing]. A continuous infusion into the rectum and colon. SEE: *enteroclysis*.

THERAP. EFFECT: To supply fluid in postoperative cases when fluids cannot be taken otherwise; to supply the body with fluid as in hemorrhage, vomiting, or diarrhea; to relieve thirst as in persistent vomiting; to lower body temperature by giving ice water enemas.

SOLUTIONS: The fluid usually consists of a normal saline solution, a sodium bicarbonate solution, or plain tap water at body temperature. Normal salt solution at half strength frequently is used. This need not be a sterile solution unless so ordered. Sodium bicarbonate of 2% to 5% strength or a glucose solution of 2% to 5%, but no stronger, may be used. A combination of these may also be ordered as a normal saline with glucose and sodium bicarbonate, 5% and 2%, respectively, or other combinations may be used.

NURSING IMPLICATIONS: A cleansing enema is given prior to beginning proctoclysis; when the bowel is completely evacuated, fluid at body temperature is introduced through a lubricated rectal catheter inserted to approx. 4 in. (10 cm). The liquid is given at a rate of 40 to 60 drops/min. If given faster, the bowel will be stimulated. Do not give more than 6 oz (180 ml) in a single continuous proctoclysis. Turn the patient frequently during the treatment. If rectal gas needs to be passed, clamp the tube temporarily. Discontinue if pain or distention develops.

proctococcypexia, proctococcypexy (prŏk"tō-kŏk-sĭ-pĕk'sē-ă, -kŏk'sĭ-pĕk"sē) [" + *kokkyx*, coccyx, + *pexis*, fixation]. Suture of rectum to the coccyx.

proctocolitis (prŏk"tō-kō-lī'tĭs) [" +

kolon, colon, + *itis*, inflammation]. Inflamed condition of colon and rectum.

proctocolonoscopy (prŏk"tō-kō"lŏn-ŏs'kō-pē) [" + " + *skopein*, to examine]. Examination of interior of rectum and lower colon.

Proctocort. Trade name for hydrocortisone.

proctocystoplasty (prŏk"tō-sĭs'tō-plăs"tē) [Gr. *proktos*, anus, + *kystis*, bladder, + *plastos*, formed]. Plastic surgery involving the rectum and bladder.

proctocystotomy (prŏk"tō-sĭs-tŏt'ō-mē) [" + *kystis*, bladder, + *tome*, incision]. Incision into the bladder through the rectum.

proctodeum (prŏk-tō-dē'ŭm) [" + *hodaios*, a way]. An ectodermal depression located caudally that upon rupture of the cloacal membrane forms the anal canal.

proctodynia (prŏk"tō-dĭn'ē-ă) [" + *odyne*, pain]. Pain in the rectum or about the anus.

proctologic (prŏk"tō-lŏj'ĭk) [" + *logos*, word, reason]. Concerning proctology.

proctologist (prŏk-tŏl'ō-jĭst) [" + *logos*, word, reason]. One who specializes in diseases of the colon, rectum, and anus.

proctology (prŏk-tŏl'ō-jē). Phase of medicine dealing with treatment of diseases of the colon, rectum, and anus.

proctoparalysis (prŏk"tō-păr-ăl'ĭ-sĭs) [" + *para*, at the side, + *lyein*, to loosen]. Paralysis of the anal sphincter muscle. SYN: *proctoplegia*.

proctoperineoplasty (prŏk"tō-pĕr"ĭ-nē'ō-plăs"tē) [" + *perinaion*, perineum, + *plassein*, to form]. Plastic surgery of the anus and rectum.

proctoperineorrhaphy (prŏk"tō-pĕr"ĭ-nē-or'ă-fē) [" + " + *rhaphe*, seam, ridge]. Proctoperineoplasty, q.v.

proctopexia, proctopexy (prŏk-tō-pĕk'sē-ă, prŏk'tō-pĕk"sē) [" + *pexis*, fixation]. Suture of the rectum to some other part.

proctophobia (prŏk"tō-fō'bē-ă) [" + *phobos*, fear]. Abnormal apprehension in those suffering from rectal disease.

proctoplasty (prŏk'tō-plăs"tē) [" + *plastos*, formed]. Plastic surgery of the anus or rectum.

proctoplegia (prŏk"tō-plē'jē-ă) [" + *plege*, a stroke]. Paralysis of the anal sphincter. SYN: *proctoparalysis*.

proctopolypus (prŏk"tō-pŏl'ĭ-pŭs) [" + *polys*, many, + *pous*, foot]. Polyp of the rectum.

proctoptosis (prŏk"tŏp-tō'sĭs) [" + *ptosis*, a dropping]. Prolapse of the anus and rectum. SEE: *procidentia*.

proctorrhagia (prŏk"tō-rā'jē-ă) [" + *rhegnynai*, to burst forth]. Bleeding from the rectum.

proctorrhaphy (prŏk-tor'ă-fē) [" + *rhaphe*, seam, ridge]. Suturing of the rectum or anus.

proctorrhea (prŏk-tōr-ē′ă) [″ + *rhoia*, flow]. Mucous discharge from the anus.

proctoscope [″ + *skopein*, to examine]. Instrument for inspection of the rectum.

proctoscopy (prŏk-tŏs′kō-pē). Instrumental inspection of the rectum.

proctosigmoidectomy (prŏk″tō-sĭg″moy-dĕk′tō-mē) [″ + *sigma*, Gr. letter S, + *eidos*, form, shape, + *ektome*, excision]. Surgical removal of the anus, rectum, and sigmoid flexure of the colon.

proctosigmoiditis (prŏk″tō-sĭg″moyd-ī′tĭs) [″ + ″ + *eidos*, form, shape, + *itis*, inflammation]. Inflamed condition of the rectum and sigmoid.

proctosigmoidoscopy (prŏk″tō-sĭg-moyd-ŏs′kō-pē). Visual examination of the rectum and sigmoid colon by use of a sigmoidoscope.

proctospasm [″ + *spasmos*, a convulsion]. Rectal spasm.

proctostasis (prŏk″tō-stā′sĭs) [″ + *stasis*, stoppage]. Constipation resulting from failure of rectum to respond to defecation stimulus.

proctostenosis (prŏk″tō-stĕn-ō′sĭs) [″ + *stenosis*, act of narrowing]. Stricture of the anus or rectum.

proctostomy (prŏk-tŏs′tō-mē) [″ + *stoma*, mouth]. Surgical creation of a permanent opening into the rectum.

proctotome (prŏk′tō-tōm) [″ + *tome*, incision]. Knife for incision into rectum.

proctotomy (prŏk-tŏt′ō-mē). Incision of the rectum or anus.

NURSING IMPLICATIONS: Assess the dressing at frequent intervals for the presence and amount of bleeding and drainage, and record. Dressings should be changed or reinforced as prescribed by the physician. A T binder (female) or split-T binder (male) is advantageous to insure proper dressing placement.

proctotresia (prŏk-tō-trē′sē-ă) [″ + *tresis*, a perforation]. Surgical correction of an imperforate anus.

proctovalvotomy (prŏk″tō-văl-vŏt′ō-mē) [″ + L. *valva*, leaf of a folding door, + Gr. *tome*, incision]. Incision of the rectal valves.

procumbent [L. *procumbens*, lying down]. Lying face down. SYN: *prone*.

procursive (prō-kŭr′sĭv) [L. *procursivus*]. Having an involuntary tendency to run forward.

procurvation (prō″kŭr-vā′shŭn) [L. *procurvare*, to bend forward]. A bending forward.

procyclidine hydrochloride (prō-sī′klī-dēn). USP. An antiparkinsonism drug. Trade name is Kemadrin.

prodromal (prō-drō′măl) [Gr. *prodromos*, running before]. Pert. to the initial stage of a disease; the interval between the earliest symptoms and the appearance of the rash or fever.

prodromal rash. A rash that precedes the true rash of an infectious disease.

prodrome (pl. *prodromes, prodromata*). A symptom indicative of an approaching disease.

prodromic (prō-drō′mĭk). Prodromal, q.v.

prodrug. An inert drug that becomes active after biotransformation.

product (prŏd′ŭkt) [L. *productum*]. Anything that is made. Also, the resulting compound after the reaction of two chemical substances.

production (prō-dŭk′shŭn). Development or formation of a substance.

productive (prō-dŭk′tĭv). Forming, esp. new tissue.

productive inflammation. Inflammation producing new tissue with or without an exudate.

proencephalus (prō″ĕn-sĕf′ă-lŭs) [Gr. *pro*, before, + *enkephalos*, brain]. A deformed fetus in which the brain protrudes through a fissure in the frontal area of the skull.

proenzyme (prō-ĕn′zīm) [″ + *en*, in, + *zyme*, a leaven]. The inactive form of an enzyme found within a cell, which, upon leaving the cell, is converted into the active form, such as pepsinogen.

proerythroblast (prō″ē-rĭth′rō-blăst) [″ + *erythros*, red, + *blastos*, germ]. The earliest cells that show differentiation in the direction of erythrocyte formation.

proestrus (prō-ĕs′trŭs). The period preceding estrus in females, characterized by development of ovarian follicles and uterine endometrium.

proferment [Gr. *pro*, before, + L. *fermentum*, leaven]. An inactive precursor of a ferment. SYN: *proenzyme*.

professional (prō-fĕsh′ŭn-ăl) [ME. *profession*, sacred vow]. Pert. to a profession.

professional liability. The obligation of health care providers or their insurers to pay for damages resulting from the providers' acts of omission or commission in treating patients.

professional liability insurance. A type of insurance contract that provides compensation for a person or party injured by a professional's acts or omissions. Two common types of policies are: 1. *claims made*. The claim for damages by the injured party must be made during the policy coverage period in order for the professional to be covered and represented by the insurance company. 2. *occurrence*. The claim for damages by the injured party is covered by the insurance company as long as the act of professional liability occurs during the policy coverage period, even though the claim is filed after the coverage period ends.

Professional Standards Review Organization. ABBR: PSRO. Peer review at the local level required by Public Law 92-603 of the U.S. for the services provided under the Medicare, Medicaid, and maternal and child health programs funded by the federal government.

profibrinolysin (prō″fī-brī-nō-lī′sĭn) [Gr. *pro*, before, + L. *fibra*, fiber, + Gr. *lysis*, dissolution]. The inactive precursor of the proteolytic enzyme fibrinolysin.

profile (prō′fīl) [L. *pro*, forward, + *filare*, to draw a line]. 1. An outline of the side view of an object, esp. the human head. 2. A summary, graph, or table presenting a subject's most notable characteristics and achievements.

profluvium (prō-floo′vē-ŭm) [L.]. An excessive flow or discharge; a flux.

    p. lactis. Excessive flow of milk.

    p. seminis. Flow of semen from the vagina deposited during coition.

profunda [L.]. Deep seated; term applied to certain deeply located blood vessels.

profundus (prō-fŭn′dŭs) [L.]. Located deeper than the indicated reference point.

progastrin (prō-găs′trĭn). The inactive precursor of gastrin.

progenitor (prō-jĕn′ĭ-tor) [L.]. An ancestor.

progeny (prŏj′ĕ-nē) [ME. *progenie*]. Offspring.

progeria (prō-jē′rē-ă) [Gr. *pro*, before, + *geras*, old age]. Premature senility occurring in childhood.

    SYM: Small stature, face looks old and wizened, skin is dry and thin, hair is scanty, and sex organs are infantile.

    ETIOL: Unknown.

progestational (prō″jĕs-tā′shŭn-ăl). Concerned with the luteal phase of the menstrual cycle, at which time, by the action of the hormone progesterone, q.v., the endometrium is further prepared for implantation of the fertilized ovum.

progestational agent. Any one of several chemical substances that have the effect of progesterone. They are usually synthetic and may be used in birth control pills. SYN: *progestin.*

progesterone (prō-jĕs′tĕr-ōn). USP. $C_{21}H_{30}O_2$. A steroid hormone obtained from the corpus luteum and placenta. It is responsible for changes in the endometrium in the second half of the menstrual cycle preparatory for implantation of the blastocyst, development of maternal placenta after implantation, and development of mammary glands.

    USES: In treatment of menstrual disorders (amenorrhea, dysmenorrhea) and threatened abortion.

progestin (prō-jĕs′tĭn). 1. A corpus luteum hormone that prepares the endometrium for implantation of the fertilized ovum. SYN: *progesterone.* 2. Term used to cover a large group of synthetic drugs that have a progesteronelike effect on the uterus.

progestogen (prō-jĕs′tō-jĕn). Any natural or synthetic hormonal substance that produces effects similar to those due to progesterone, q.v.

proglossis (prō-glŏs′ĭs) [Gr.]. Tip of the tongue.

proglottid. Proglottis.

proglottis (prō-glŏt′tĭs) [Gr. *pro*, before, + *glossa*, tongue] (pl. *proglottides*). A segment of a tapeworm, containing both male and female reproductive organs. SEE: *Cestoda; tapeworm.*

Proglycem. Trade name for diazoxide.

prognathic (prŏg-nă′thĭk) [″ + *gnathos*, jaw]. Prognathous, q.v.

prognathism (prŏg′nă-thĭzm) [″ + *gnathos*, jaw + *-ismos*, condition]. Projection of jaws beyond projection of forehead.

prognathous (prŏg′nă-thŭs). Having jaws projecting forward beyond rest of the face.

prognose (prŏg-nōs′). To predict the course of disease.

prognosis (prŏg-nō′sĭs) [Gr., foreknowledge]. Prediction of course and end of disease, and the estimate of chance for recovery.

prognostic. Rel. to prediction of outcome of a disease.

prognosticate (prŏg-nŏs′tĭ-kāt) [Gr. *prognostikon*, knowing before]. To make a statement on the probable outcome of an illness.

prognostician (prŏg″nŏs-tĭsh′ăn). One skilled in making prognoses.

progonoma (prō″gō-nō′mă) [Gr. *pro*, before, + *gonos*, sperm, + *oma*, tumor]. A tumor that develops from displacement of embryonic cells that resemble ancestral forms of the species. An example is a hairy mole.

progranulocyte (prō-grăn′ū-lō-sīt) [″ + L. *granula*, granule, + Gr. *kytos*, cell]. A promyelocyte.

progravid (prō-grăv′ĭd) [″ + L. *gravidus*, pregnant]. Preceding pregnancy.

progress [L. *progressus*, a going forward]. The ongoing sequence of events of an illness.

progression (prō-grĕsh′ŭn) [L. *progressus*]. Advancing or moving forward.

progressive (prō-grĕs′ĭv). Advancing, as a disease from bad to worse.

progressive muscular atrophy. Gradual advancing atrophy of groups of muscles due to spinal cord degeneration. SYN: *paralysis, wasting.* SEE: *atrophy, muscular.*

progressive ossifying myositis. Tendency

to bony deposits in the muscles with chronic inflammation.

progressive resistive exercise. ABBR: PRE. A form of active resistive exercise based on a principle of gradual increases in the amount of resistance in order to achieve maximum strength.

progress notes. Notes made on the chart by those involved in caring for the patient. Physicians, nurses, consultants, and therapists may record their notes concerning the progress or lack of progress made by the patient in the interim between the previous note and the time of the most recent note. In patients who are not critically ill, a note concerning progress might be made daily or less frequently; in critical care situations, notes could be made hourly.

progress report. The written or verbal account of a patient's present condition, esp. as compared to the previous state.

prohormone (prō-hor′mōn). Precursor of a hormone.

proinsulin. Precursor of insulin produced in the beta cells of the pancreas.

projectile vomiting. Vomiting in which the stomach contents are ejected with great force.

projection (prō″jĕk′shŭn) [Gr. *pro*, before, + *jacere*, to throw]. 1. The act of throwing forward. 2. A part extending beyond the level of its surroundings. 3. The mental process by which sensations are referred to the sense organs or receptors stimulated, or outside the body to the object that is the stimulus. 4. Distortion of a perception as a result of its repression, resulting in such a phenomenon as hating without cause one who has been dearly loved, or attributing to others one's own undesirable traits. Characteristics of the paranoid reaction.

projective technique. Any one of several forms of psychological assessment or evaluation. Using ambiguous activities and tasks which encourage self-expression, the products or results and the individual's verbalizations about them are evaluated and interpreted to determine indications of unconscious needs, thoughts or concerns.

prokaryon (prō-kăr′ē-ŏn) [″ + *karyon*, nucleus]. 1. Nuclear material that is spread throughout the cell cytoplasm and is not bounded by a membrane. 2. Prokaryote, q.v.

prokaryote (prō-kăr′ē-ōt) [″ + *karyon*, nucleus]. Organism with a single, circular chromosome, without a nuclear membrane, or membrane-bound organelles, i.e., mitochondria and lysosomes. Included in this classification are bacteria and blue-green algae. SEE: *eukaryote*.

Proklar. Trade name for sulfamethizole.

prolabium (prō-lā′bē-ŭm) [″ + *labium*, lip]. The entire central portion of the upper lip.

prolactin (prō-lăk′tĭn) [″ + *lac*, milk]. A hormone produced by the pituitary gland. In humans, prolactin in association with estrogen and progesterone stimulates breast development and the formation of milk during pregnancy. The act of sucking is an important stimulus for the production of prolactin in the postpartum period. Some of the metabolic effects of prolactin resemble those of growth hormone. In the female this includes amenorrhea, galactorrhea, and infertility. In the male it may cause impotence. Hyperprolactinemia may be associated with amenorrhea in women and reduced sexual potency in men. Thyrotropin-releasing hormone and stress of all kinds can stimulate prolactin release.

prolactinoma. An adenoma of the pituitary that produces prolactin. The excess prolactin, q.v., secreted may be treated by the use of a dopamine agonist, bromocriptine. In some cases, surgical removal of the tumor may be necessary.

prolamin(e) (prō-lăm′ĭn, prō′lă-mĭn). Any one of a class of proteins found in seeds.

prolapse (prō-lăps′) [L. *prolapsus*]. A falling or dropping down of an organ or internal part, such as the uterus or rectum. SEE: *procidentia; ptosis.*

   p. of anus. Protrusion of lower portion of the digestive tract through external sphincter of anus.

   p. of cord. Expulsion of umbilical cord prematurely. SEE: *labor.*

   p. of iris. Protrusion of iris through an injury in the cornea.

   p. of rectum. Protrusion of rectal mucosa through the anus.

   p. of uterus. Downward displacement of uterus, the cervix sometimes protruding from the vaginal orifice. The causes include age with weakening of pelvic musculature, traumatic vaginal delivery, chronic straining in association with coughing or difficult bowel movements, and pelvic tumors that push the uterus down. SEE: *Kegel exercises.*

prolapsus [L.]. A falling or downward displacement of some part of the body, as the uterus. SYN: *prolapse.*

prolepsis [Gr. *pro*, before, + *lepsis*, a seizure]. Return of paroxysmal attacks at successively shorter intervals.

proleptic. Recurring before the time expected, said of paroxysms. SEE: *subintrant.*

proleukocyte (prō-lū′kō-sīt) [″ + *leukos*, white, + *kytos*, cell]. An undeveloped leukocyte.

proliferate (prō-lĭf′ĕr-āt) [L. *proles*, offspring, + *ferre*, to bear]. To increase by reproduction of similar forms.

proliferation (prō-lĭf″ĕr-ā′shŭn). 1. Reproduction rapidly and repeatedly of new parts, as by cell division. 2. Process or result of rapid reproduction.

proliferous. 1. Multiplying, as by formation of new tissue cells. 2. Bearing offspring.

proliferous cyst. Cyst with epithelial lining, proliferating and projecting from its inner surface.

prolific [L. *prolificus*]. Fruitful; reproductive. SYN: *fertile*.

prolinase. An enzyme that is found in animal tissues and yeast and that hydrolyzes proline peptides to simpler peptids and proline.

proline (prō′lēn). C₄H₈NCOOH. An important amino acid formed by decomposition of protein.

Prolixin Enanthate. Trade name for fluphenazine enanthate.

Proloid. Trade name for thyroglobulin.

Proloprim. Trade name for trimethoprim.

prolymphocyte (prō″lĭmf′ō-sīt) [″ + L. *lympha*, lymph, + Gr. *kytos*, cell]. A cell intermediate between a lymphoblast and lymphocyte.

Promapar. Trade name for chlorpromazine hydrochloride.

promazine hydrochloride (prō′mă-zēn). USP. An antipsychotic drug. Trade name is Sparine.

promegakaryocyte (prō-mĕg″ă-kăr′ē-ō-sīt) [″ + *megas*, big, + *karyon*, nucleus, + *kytos*, cell]. Cell from which a megakaryocyte develops.

promegaloblast (prō-mĕg′ă-lō-blast″) [″ + ″ + *blastos*, germ]. Cell of the erythrocyte series preceding the megaloblast.

prometaphase (prō-mĕt′ă-fāz) [″ + *meta*, change, + *phasis*, to appear]. Stage of mitosis in which the nuclear membrane disintegrates, and the chromosomes move toward the equatorial plate.

promethazine hydrochloride (prō-mĕth′ă-zēn). USP. An antihistamine drug. Trade names are Anergan 25 and Remsed.

promethium (prō-mē′thē-ŭm). SYMB: Pm. At. wt. 144.9128; at. no. 61. A radioactive element of the rare earth series.

promine. A tissue extract that promotes growth of certain tumors in mice.

prominence (prŏm′ĭ-nĕns) [L. *prominens*, project]. A projection or protrusion. SEE: *prominentia*.

prominentia (prŏm″ĭ-nĕn′shē-ă) [L.] (pl. *prominentiae*). [NA] A projection.

   p. laryngea. [NA] The laryngeal prominence; Adam's apple. SYN: *promum adami*.

   p. spiralis. [NA] A small ridge extending entire length of the cochlea located on inner surface of spiral ligament. It projects slightly into cochlear canal and contains blood vessels, including the vas prominens.

promonocyte (prō-mŏn′ō-sīt) [Gr. *pro*, before, + *monos*, single, + *kytos*, cell]. In the development of white blood cells, the precursor of the monocyte. It is between the monoblast and monocyte.

promontory (prŏm′ŏn-tor″ē) [L. *promontorium*]. A projecting process or part.

   p. of sacrum. The anterior projecting portion of the pelvic surface of the base of the sacrum. With the 5th lumbar vertebra, it forms the sacrovertebral angle.

   p. of tympanic cavity. Projection on medial wall of the tympanic cavity produced by first turn of the cochlea.

promoter (prō-mō′tĕr). A substance that assists a catalyst to act.

promyelocyte (prō-mī′ĕl-ō-sīt) [Gr. *pro*, before, + *myelos*, marrow, + *kytos*, cell]. 1. A large mononuclear myeloid cell seen in the blood in leukemia. 2. Cell development between myeloblast and a myelocyte, resembling a myeloblast.

pronate (prō′nāt). To place in a prone position.

pronation (prō-nā′shŭn) [L. *pronus*, prone]. 1. The act of lying prone or face downward. 2. The act of turning the hand so that the palm faces downward or backward. SEE: *supination*.

pronator. A muscle that pronates. SEE: *Muscles* in *Appendix*.

pronator syndrome. A neurological disorder caused by entrapment of the median nerve at the elbow. Symptoms and signs include aching pain in the wrist with a subjective feeling of poor coordination; paresthesias extending into the hand; paresis of the thumb muscles; pain on pronation of the forearm and flexion of the wrist against resistance; and tenderness in the proximal thenar muscles. A positive Tinel's sign over the pronator teres muscles may be present. The disease usually affects the dominant arm of males. Corticosteroid injection into the site is usually effective.

pronaus, pronaeus (prō-nā′ŭs) [Gr. *pro*, before, + *naos*, temple]. The vagina or vestibule of the vagina.

prone (prōn) [ME.]. 1. Lying horizontal with face downward. 2. Denoting the hand with the palm turned downward. Opposite of supine.

pronephric (prō-nĕf′rĭk) [Gr. *pro*, before, + *nephros*, kidney]. Pert. to the pronephros.

pronephric duct. Duct that connects posteriorly to the cloaca and to which pronephric tubules are connected.

pronephric tubules. Several pairs of segmentally arranged tubules that open into the cranial portion of the pronephric duct. They communicate with coelom through a ciliated funnel-shaped nephrostome. They are vestigial in higher vertebrates.

pronephros, pronephron (prō-nĕf'rŏs, -rŏn). The earliest and simplest type of excretory organ of vertebrates, functional in simpler forms (cyclostomes), and serving as a provisional kidney in some fishes and amphibians. In reptiles, birds, and mammals, it appears in the embryo as a temporary, functionless structure.

Pronestyl. Trade name for procainamide hydrochloride.

prong (prŏng). A conically shaped body such as the root of a tooth.

pronograde (prō'nō-grād) [L. *pronus*, prone, + *gradus*, a step]. In animals, walking on hands and feet or resting with the body in a horizontal position. Opposite of orthograde.

pronometer (prō-nŏm'ĕ-tĕr) [" + Gr. *metron*, measure]. Device for showing amount of pronation or supination of forearm.

pronormoblast (prō-nor'mō-blăst) [Gr. *pro*, before, + L. *norma*, rule, + Gr. *blastos*, germ]. An early precursor of the red blood cell.

pronucleus (prō-nū'klē-ŭs) [Gr. *pro*, before, + *nucleus*, little kernel]. Nucleus of the ovum (the female pronucleus) or of the spermatozoon (the male pronucleus) after fertilization of the ovum.

prootic (prō-ŏt'ĭk, -ō'tĭk) [" + *ous*, ear]. In front of the ear.

prop. A device of sturdy material used to support or hold something in place.

 p., mouth. A metal or rubber device inserted between the jaws to maintain the mouth in an open position. SYN: *bite block; jaw brace.*

propagation (prŏp-ă-gā'shŭn) [L.]. Act of reproducing or giving birth. SYN: *generation; reproduction.*

propagative (prŏp'ă-gā"tĭv). Pert. to or taking part in reproduction.

propalinal (prō-păl'ĭ-năl) [Gr. *pro*, before, + *palin*, back]. Applied to a backward and forward movement, as of the jaws.

propane (prō'pān). C_3H_8. A hydrocarbon that is present in natural gas. It is odorless and colorless. When it is to be used in dwellings, as a fuel, to produce heat, or in hot air balloons, an odoriferous substance is added so that a leak that could go undetected would be obvious because of the odor.

propantheline bromide (prō-păn'thĕ-lēn). USP. An anticholinergic drug that acts like belladonna. Trade name is Pro-Banthine.

proparacaine hydrochloride (prō-păr'ă-kān). USP. A topical anesthetic drug used in ophthalmology. Trade names are Alcaine, Ophthaine, and Ophthetic.

propepsin (prō-pĕp'sĭn). Pepsinogen.

propeptone (prō-pĕp'tōn) [" + *peptein*, to digest]. An intermediate product in the digestive conversion of protein into peptone. SYN: *hemialbumose.*

propeptonuria (prō"pĕp-tō-nū'rē-ă) [" + " + *ouron*, urine]. Excretion of propeptone in the urine. SYN: *hemialbumosuria.*

properdin (prō-pĕrd'ĭn). A serum protein that, in the presence of magnesium ions and complement, has the ability to help destroy various bacteria and viruses. SEE: *complement.*

prophase (prō'fāz) [" + *phasis*, an appearance]. First stage of indirect cell division. SEE: *centriole; metaphase; mitosis.*

prophylactic (prō-fĭ-lăk'tĭk) [Gr. *prophylaktikos*, guarding]. 1. Any agent or regimen that contributes to the prevention of infection and disease. 2. Popular term for a condom.

prophylaxis (prō-fĭ-lăk'sĭs, prō-fĭl-ăks'ĭs) [Gr. *prophylassein*, to guard against]. Observance of rules necessary to prevent disease.

 p., oral. The removal of calculus and stains from the exposed and unexposed surfaces of the teeth by scaling and polishing as a preventive measure for the control of local irritational factors.

propiolactone (prō"pē-ō-lăk'tōn). A disinfectant used in preparing certain viral and bacterial vaccines. Trade name is Betaprone. SYN: *β-propiolactone,* or *beta-propiolactone.*

propiomazine hydrochloride (prō"pē-ō-mă'zĕn). USP. A sedative drug. Trade name is Largon.

propionic acid. C_2H_5COOH, methylacetic acid, which is present in sweat.

Propionibacterium acnes. (Formerly *Corynebacterium acnes.*) A gram-positive rod bacterium that may be part of the normal skin flora, but can also be pathogenic in wounds and infected prosthetic devices.

proplasmacyte (prō-plăz'mă-sīt) [Gr. *pro*, before, + LL. *plasma*, form, mold, + Gr. *kytos*, cell]. The precursor of the plasma cell.

proplastid (prō-plăs'tĭd). The cytoplasmic body from which a plastid is formed.

Proplex. Trade name for factor IX complex.

propolis [Gr. *pro*, before, + *polis*, city]. A sticky resin present in the buds and bark of certain trees and plants. It is collected by bees for the purpose of repairing combs, filling cracks, and making the entrance to the hive waterproof. There is anecdotal evidence that propolis may be of benefit in treating certain diseases. Scientific, in vitro investigations indicate that the material inhibits the reproduction of certain viruses. These studies employed propolis as well as the resin obtained from poplar trees and then refined. SYN: *bee glue.*

propositus (prō-pŏz′ĭ-tŭs) [L. *proponere*, to put on view]. The initial individual whose condition led to investigation of a hereditary disorder. SYN: *index case; proband.*

propoxycaine hydrochloride (prō-pŏk′sē-kān). USP. A local anesthetic drug. Trade names are Blockaine Hydrochloride and Ravocaine Hydrochloride.

propoxyphene hydrochloride (prō-pŏk′sē-fēn). USP. An analgesic drug available in a variety of dosage forms and combinations. Trade names are Darvon, Dolene, and SK 65.

propranolol hydrochloride. USP. A β-adrenergic blocking agent used in treating hypertension; for prevention of angina pectoris; and for treating certain cardiac arrhythmias, esp. those caused by overdose of digitalis. Trade name is Inderal.

Caution: Persons with asthma should not be treated with this drug.

proprietary medicine (prō-prī′ĕ-tăr″ē) [L. *proprietarius*, pert. to property]. Any chemical, drug, or similar preparation used in the treatment of diseases, if such article is protected against free competition as to name, product, composition, or process of manufacture by secrecy, patent or copyright, or by another means. SEE: *nonproprietary name; patent medicine.*

proprioception (prō″prē-ō-sĕp′shŭn) [L. *proprius*, one's own, + *capio*, to take]. The awareness of posture, movement, and changes in equilibrium and the knowledge of position, weight, and resistance of objects in relation to the body.

proprioceptive (prō″prē-ō-sĕp′tĭv). Pert. to proprioception.

proprioceptive impulses. Afferent impulses arising in a proprioceptor, q.v.

proprioceptive sense. The correlation of unconscious sensations from the skin and joints that allows conscious appreciation of the position of the body.

proprioceptor (prō″prē-ō-sĕp′tor) [″ + *ceptor*, a receiver]. A receptor that responds to stimuli originating within the body itself, esp. one that responds to pressure, position, or stretch.

Ex.: muscle spindles, pacinian corpuscles, and labyrinthine receptors.

propriospinal (prō″prē-ō-spī′năl) [″ + *spina*, thorn]. Concerned exclusively with the spinal cord.

proptometer (prŏp-tŏm′ē-tĕr) [Gr. *proptosis*, protrusion, + *metron*, a measure]. An instrument for measuring extent of exophthalmos.

proptosis (prŏp-tō′sĭs). A downward displacement such as the uterus or the eyeball in exophthalmic goiter or in inflammatory conditions of the orbit.

propulsion (prō-pŭl′shŭn) [L. *propulsus*, driven forward]. 1. A tendency to push or fall forward in walking. 2. A condition seen in paralysis agitans. SEE: *festination.*

propyl (prō′pĭl). The radical of propyl alcohol or propane, $CH_3—CH_2—CH_2—$.

propylene glycol (prŏp′ĭ-lēn). USP. A demulcent agent used as a solvent for medicines, and in cosmetics.

propylhexedrine (prō″pĭl-hĕk′sē-drēn). USP. A sympathomimetic drug usually dispensed in an inhaler to produce nasal decongestion. Trade name is Benzedrex.

propyliodone (prō″pĭl-ī′ō-dōn). USP. A radiopaque dye used in x-ray studies of the bronchi.

propylparaben (prō″pĭl-păr′ă-bĕn). Propyl *p*-hydroxybenzoate, $C_{10}H_{12}O_3$, a chemical used as an antifungal agent and as a preservative in pharmaceuticals.

propylthiouracil (prō″pĭl-thī″ō-ū′ră-sĭl). USP. Antithyroid drug used in treatment of hyperthyroidism, thyroiditis, and thyrotoxicosis. Also employed for preoperative therapy and in cases in which surgery is contraindicated.

pro re nata (prō rē nā′tă) [L.]. ABBR: p.r.n. According to the circumstances; as necessary.

prorrhaphy (prō′ră-fē) [Gr. *pro*, before, + *rhaphe*, seam, ridge]. Surgical movement of a muscle or tendon insertion to a point farther away. Done to change the action of a muscle. SYN: *advancement.*

prorsad (pror′săd). In a forward direction.

prorubricyte (prō-roo′brĭ-sīt). A basophilic normoblast.

prosecretin (prō″sē-krē′tĭn) [″ + *secretio*, separation]. Substance present in the duodenal mucosa that, when acted on by hydrochloric acid in chyme, is converted into secretin. SEE: *secretin.*

prosection (prō-sĕk′shŭn) [″ + L. *sectio*, a cutting]. Dissection for the purpose of demonstrating anatomic structure.

prosector (prō-sĕk′tor) [L.]. One who prepares cadavers for dissection or dissects for demonstration.

prosencephalon (prŏs″ĕn-sĕf′ă-lŏn) [Gr. *proso*, before, + *enkephalos*, brain]. The embryonic forebrain, which gives rise to the telencephalon and diencephalon, q.v.

proso- [Gr. *proso*, forward]. Combining form indicating forward or anterior.

prosodemic (prŏs″ō-dĕm′ĭk) [″ + *demos*, people]. Spread by individual contact; said of a disease. SEE: *epidemic.*

prosody (prŏs′ă-dē) [L. *prosodia*, accent of a syllable]. The normal rhythm, melody, and articulation of speech.

prosopagnosia (prŏs″ō-păg-nō′sē-ă) [Gr. *prosopon*, face, + *a-*, not, + *gnosis*, recognition]. Inability to recognize faces, even one's own face.

prosopalgia (prŏs″ō-păl′jē-ă) [″ + *algos*, pain]. Neuralgic pain in the trigeminal nerve and its branches. SYN: *prosopodynia; prosoponeuralgia; tic douloureux.*

prosopectasia (prŏs″ō-pĕk-tā′zē-ă) [″ + *ektasis*, dilatation]. Abnormal enlargement of the face.

prosopic (prō″sŏp′ĭk). Pert. to face or facial skeleton that is convex anteriorly.

prosoplasia (prŏs″ō-plā′sē-ă) [Gr. *proso*, forward, + *plassein*, to form]. Progressive transformation of cells until they develop into cells with a higher degree of function.

prosopoanoschisis (prŏs″ō-pŏ″ă-nŏs′kĭ-sĭs) [Gr. *prosopon*, face, + *ana*, up, + *schisis*, a splitting]. Oblique facial cleft, a slanting furrow extending from mouth to eye.

prosopodiplegia (prŏs″ō-pō-dī-plē′jē-ă) [″ + *dis*, twice, + *plege*, a stroke]. Paralysis on both sides of the face.

prosopodynia (prŏs″ō-pō-dĭn′ē-ă) [″ + *odyne*, pain]. Pain in the face. SYN: *prosoponeuralgia; tic douloureux.*

prosoponeuralgia (prŏs″ō-pō-nū-răl′jē-ă) [″ + *neuron*, sinew, + *algos*, pain]. Facial neuralgia. SYN: *prosopalgia; tic douloureux.*

prosopopagus (prŏs″ō-pŏp′ă-gŭs) [″ + *pagos*, a thing fixed]. Unequal conjoined twins in which the parasite is attached to some part of the face other than the jaw.

prosopoplegia (prŏs″ō-pō-plē′jē-ă) [″ + *plege*, stroke]. Facial paralysis. SYN: *facioplegia.*

prosoposchisis (prŏs-ō-pŏs′kĭ-sĭs) [Gr. *prosopon*, face, + *schisis*, a splitting]. Congenital cleft of the face.

prosopospasm (prŏs′ō-pō-spăzm) [″ + *spasmos*, a convulsion]. Facial spasm.

prosopothoracopagus (prŏs″ō-pō-thō″ră-kŏp′ă-gŭs) [″ + *thorax*, chest, + *pagos*, a thing fixed]. Conjoined twins joined in the frontal area between the face and the chest.

prosopotocia (prŏs″ō-pō-tō′shē-ă) [″ + *tokos*, birth]. Presentation of the face in parturition.

prosopus varus (prŏs″ō-pŭs vā′rŭs) [Gr. *prosopon*, face, + L. *varus*, crooked]. Congenital obliquity of the face due to atrophy of one side of the head.

prospective payment system. A reimbursement method used in which a fixed, predetermined amount is allocated for treating patients with a specific diagnosis when an individual is hospitalized. Originally developed for use with Medicare recipients. Also referred to as payment-by-diag-

nosis.

prospective study. A clinical or epidemiological investigation of patients or health subjects with respect to the medical, social, and environmental factors encountered from the time of the beginning of the study until the investigation is terminated. SEE: *retrospective study.*

prostacyclin. Prostaglandin GI_2, q.v.

prostaglandin GI_2. ABBR: PGI_2. A compound formed from the metabolism of arachidonic acid. It is a potent vasodilator and inhibitor of platelet aggregation.

prostaglandin inhibitor. A substance which inhibits the production of prostaglandins. Nonsteroidal and steroid anti-inflammatory agents are two major categories which inhibit prostaglandins.

prostaglandins (prŏs″tă-glănd′ĭns). ABBR: PG. A large group of biologically active, carbon-20, unsaturated fatty acids that represent some of the metabolites of arachidonic acid. They are local short-range autocoids which are formed rapidly, exert their effects locally, and then decay or are destroyed enzymatically. Some of the physiologically important are PGD_2, PGE_2, $PGF_{2\alpha}$, and PGI_1. The PGs have a wide assortment of biological effects that are not mediated via the plasma, but they act as local intercellular or intracellular modulators of the biochemical activity of the tissues in which they are formed. Thus, they are classed as autocoids rather than as hormones.

Some physiologic actions influenced by PGs include lipolysis, fluid balance, platelet aggregation, blood flow, gastrointestinal function and activity, neurotransmission, pancreatic endocrine function, and corpus luteum regression. Increased production of PGs is important in causing bone resorption and dysmenorrhea, and in influencing glucose metabolism. The normal closure of the patent ductus arteriosus is inhibited if endogenous PG production is enhanced. In some types of congenital heart disease, it is important to maintain the patency of the ductus until the appropriate surgical procedure can be performed. Conversely, if the heart is normal except for delayed closure of the patent ductus, then PG inhibitors may be given to hasten the closing. SEE: *arachidonic acid; nonsteroidal anti-inflammatory drugs; patent ductus arteriosus.*

prostanoids. The name of the end products of the cyclo-oxygenase pathway of the metabolism of arachidonic acid. These are prostaglandins and thromboxanes. SEE: *eicosanoids; prostaglandins; thromboxane A_2.*

Prostaphlin. Trade name for oxacillin sodium.

prostatalgia (prŏs-tă-tăl′jē-ă) [Gr. *prostates*,

prostate, + *algos,* pain]. Pain of the prostate gland.

prostate (prŏs′tāt) [Gr. *prostates*]. A gland that surrounds the neck of the bladder and the urethra in the male. It is partly muscular and partly glandular, with ducts opening into the prostatic portion of the urethra. Consists of a median lobe and two lateral lobes. About $2 \times 4 \times 3$ cm, and weighing about 20 gm, it is enclosed in a fibrous capsule containing smooth muscle fibers in its inner layer. Muscle fibers also separate the glandular tissue and encircle the urethra. The gland secretes a thin, opalescent, slightly alkaline fluid that forms part of the seminal fluid.

PATH: Inflammation of the prostate may occur, often the result of gonorrheal urethritis. Enlargement of the prostate is common, esp. after middle age. This results in urethral obstruction, impeding urination and sometimes leading to retention. Benign and malignant tumors, calculi, and nodular hyperplasia are common, particularly in men past 60. SEE: *benign prostatic hypertrophy.*

prostate, balloon dilatation of. SEE: *benign prostatic hypertrophy.*

prostate, transrectal ultrasonography of the. The use of an ultrasonic detection device placed in the rectum in order to guide biopsy of the prostate.

prostate cancer. Malignant neoplasm, usually adenocarcinoma, of the prostate gland. This form of cancer is a major cause of cancer in males. An estimated 28,500 men died of this disease in 1989. Its occurrence in men under 50 is unusual, but 8.7% of white males and 9.4% of non-white males will develop cancer of the prostate. There is no evidence that benign prostatic hypertrophy (BPH) develops into prostate cancer.

SYM: Early in the disease there may be no symptoms, but as the disease progresses signs of urinary outflow obstruction or bone pain occur.

DIAG: Early detection of this disease may be possible by digital rectal examination (DRE). Every male over 40 years of age should have an annual rectal examination. If there is clinical suspicion of cancer, several means of diagnosing the disease are available: ultrasound-guided needle biopsy of the gland, determination of level of prostate specific antigen and acid phosphatase, and transrectal ultrasound.

TREAT: Prostatectomy, q.v., orchiectomy, estrogen therapy or use of other agents that interfere with metabolism of testosterone may be useful especially if the cancer has spread. The drug flutamide, an oral antiandrogen, has been approved for treatment of metastatic prostate cancer. SEE: *benign prostatic hypertrophy; prostatectomy; prostate-specific antigen.*

prostatectomy (prŏs″tă-tĕk′tō-mē) [Gr. *prostates,* prostate, + *ektome,* excision]. Excision of part or all of the prostate gland. The operation may be performed through an incision in the perineum (perineal prostatectomy), into the bladder (suprapubic prostatectomy), or through the urethra (transurethral prostatectomy, TUP). After prostatectomy the libido is unaffected, but during ejaculation sperm enters the bladder rather than the urethra. In the past about 90% of patients who had prostatectomy became impotent. New surgical techniques, however, have made it possible to preserve the autonomic nerves to the corpora cavernosa of the penis. When this procedure is used, about 70% of patients are potent postoperatively. SEE: *Nursing Diagnoses* in *Appendix.*

COMPLICATIONS: Retention of urine, hematuria, cystitis, infection of kidney, pyelitis, infective nephritis, renal failure.

NURSING IMPLICATIONS: *Preop:* Prepare the patient for surgery and the postoperative period by explaining the procedure. Encourage verbalization of feelings and concerns, recognizing that patient may fear loss of sexual erectile function (sometimes more than he fears cancer). Explain the type of prostatectomy planned and the positive results expected; also help the patient to understand what occurs in retrograde ejaculation. Prepare the patient physically according to the urologist's protocol.

Postop: Monitor vital signs closely for indications of hemorrhage or shock. Manage any dressings and drainage tubes, protecting skin from excoriation and assessing incisions or tube insertion wounds for signs of infection. If suprapubic tube is present, monitor patency and drainage, which should be amber to pink-tinged. Monitor patency of urinary catheter, and maintain intermittent or continuous bladder irrigation as prescribed, usually via three-channel indwelling catheter. Keep irrigation rate fast enough to limit drainage color change to amber to pink-tinged, rather than red, increasing rate if color deepens or clots appear. Keep careful track of volume of irrigant instilled and amount of drainage obtained, subtracting the former from the latter to determine urinary output. Compare this resulting figure with intake to assess fluid balance. Document findings and report any abnormalities in drainage color, output volume, or patient's response to surgery. Traction may be applied to catheter as directed to provide tamponade if bleeding increases. Provide belladonna and opium suppositories to reduce bladder spasm and pain as prescribed and required. Sitz baths also may be used to relieve pain and discomfort.

When catheter is removed, encourage patient to void every 2 hours, and monitor serial urines for color, time and amount of each voiding. Encourage fluid intake of 2 to 3 quarts per day (unless restricted by cardiac or renal deficits), mainly as water, avoiding caffeine. Explain that patient may experience urinary frequency temporarily, and that dribbling may occur, but that he can regain control of urinary function with the help of Kegel exercises, q.v. Explain that urine may be blood-tinged for a few weeks, but that he should report any bright bleeding and fever, chills or other signs of infection. Teach patient to avoid straining at stool (stool softeners often are prescribed), lifting more than 10 pounds, long automobile trips, and other strenuous exercise for several weeks. Walking is usually considered acceptable exercise. Sexual intercourse should be delayed until patient has been seen at follow-up visit and has physician's permission for such activity. Patient also should continue prescribed medications, at least until this return visit, and should be instructed to have annual prostatic examinations if removal was partial.

prostate-specific antigen. An antigen in blood that may be indicative of cancer of the prostate. Measurement of this antigen plus information obtained by rectal examination of the prostate and use of ultrasound study of the prostate greatly increases the chance of diagnosing cancer of the prostate. SEE: *prostate cancer.*

prostathelcosis (prŏs″tă-thĕl-kō′sĭs) [″ + *helkosis*, ulceration]. Ulceration of the prostate gland.

prostatic (prŏs-tăt′ĭk) [Gr. *prostates*, prostate]. Concerning the prostate gland.

prostatic calculus. A stone in the prostate.

prostatic plexus. 1. Veins around the base and neck of the bladder and prostate gland. 2. Nerves from the pelvic plexus to the prostate gland, erectile tissue of the penis, and the seminal vesicles.

prostatic syncope. Fainting during examination of the prostate. It is a rare occurrence that usually can be avoided by examining the patient in the lateral recumbent position.

prostatic urethra. That part of the urethra surrounded by the prostate gland.

prostatism (prŏs′tă-tĭzm) [″ + *-ismos*, condition]. Any condition of the prostate gland that interferes with the flow of urine from the bladder.

SYM: Frequent uncomfortable urination, nocturia. Retention of urine may occur with development of uremia.

ETIOL: Benign hypertrophy, carcinoma, prostatitis, nodular hyperplasia.

prostatitis (prŏs″tă-tī′tĭs) [″ + *itis*, inflammation]. Inflamed condition of the prostate gland. May be a complication of gonorrheal infection.

   p., acute. Discomfort and pain in the perineal area. Frequent urination; later, retention of urine. If severe, marked malaise, rise of temperature, constipation, chills, and vomiting.

   p., chronic. Dull, aching pain in perineal region. Discharge from the penis.

   p., chronic bacterial. ABBR: CBP. Inflammation of the prostate due to long-standing bacterial infection. Clinical symptoms of fever, pain, and dysuria may be relatively mild as compared with the acute infection. Therapy depends upon the causative organism and in addition to antibiotics may involve treatment of prostatic hypertrophy.

prostatocystitis (prŏs″tă-tō-sĭs-tī′tĭs) [Gr. *prostates*, prostate, + *kystis*, bladder, + *itis*, inflammation]. Inflammation of the prostatic urethra involving the bladder.

prostatocystotomy (prŏs″tă-tō-sĭs-tŏt′ō-mē) [″ + ″ + *tome*, incision]. Surgical incision of the prostate and bladder.

prostatodynia (prŏs″tă-tō-dĭn′ē-ă) [″ + *odyne*, pain]. Condition of having the symptoms and signs of prostatitis but no evidence of inflammation of the prostate, with negative urine culture. Use of antibiotics in these patients is contraindicated. SYN: *prostatalgia.*

prostatography (prŏs″tă-tŏg′ră-fē) [″ + *graphein*, to write]. Radiographic examination of the prostate gland after introduction of a contrast medium.

prostatolith (prŏs-tăt′ō-lĭth) [″ + *lithos*, stone]. A calculus of the prostate gland.

prostatolithotomy (prŏs-tăt″ō-lĭ-thŏt′ō-mē) [″ + ″ + *tome*, incision]. Incision of the prostate in order to remove a calculus.

prostatomegaly (prŏs″tă-tō-mĕg′ă-lē) [″ + *megas*, large]. Enlargement of the prostate gland.

prostatomy, prostatotomy (prŏs-tăt′ō-mē, prŏs″tă-tŏt′ō-mē) [″ + *tome*, incision]. Incision into the prostate.

prostatomyomectomy (prŏs″tă-tō-mī″ō-mĕk′tō-mē) [″ + *mys*, muscle, + *ektome*, excision]. Surgical excision of a prostatic myoma.

prostatorrhea (prŏs″tă-tō-rē′ă) [″ + *rhoia*, flow]. Abnormal discharge from the prostate gland.

prostatosis (prŏs″tă-tō′sĭs) [″ + *osis*, condition]. General term indicating nonmalignant and noninflammatory disorder of the prostate gland.

prostatovesiculectomy (prŏs"tă-tō-vē-sīk"ū-lĕk'tō-mē) [Gr. *prostates*, prostate, + L. *vesiculus*, a little sac, + Gr. *ektome*, excision]. Removal of the prostate gland and seminal vesicles.

prostatovesiculitis (prŏs"tă-tō-vē-sīk"ū-lĭ'tĭs) [" + " + Gr. *itis*, inflammation]. Inflammation of the seminal vesicles and prostate gland.

prosternation (prō"stĕr-nā'shŭn) [Gr. *pro*, before, + *sternon*, chest]. Deformity characterized by habitual flexion of the trunk forward when the individual is erect. SYN: *camptocormia*.

prostheon (prŏs'thē-ŏn) [Gr. *prosthios*, foremost]. The alveolar point; midpoint of lower border of upper alveolar arch of the jaw.

prosthesis (prŏs'thē-sĭs) [Gr. *prosthesis*, an addition] (pl. *prostheses*). 1. Replacement of a missing part by an artificial substitute, such as an artificial extremity. 2. An artificial organ or part. Advances in bioengineering have enabled scientists to develop artificial extremities, including arms, hands, and portions of legs. SEE: *Boston arm*. 3. Device to augment performance of a natural function, such as a hearing aid.

p., dental. Replacement of a tooth or of a section of teeth by partial or full dentures.

p., maxillofacial. Repair and artificial replacement of face and jaw missing because of disease or injury.

p., penile. SEE: *penile prosthesis.*

prosthetic group (prŏs-thĕt'ĭk). The nonamino acid component of a conjugated protein. Usually that portion of an enzyme which is not an amino acid. SEE: *apoenzyme; holoenzyme.*

prosthetics (prŏs-thĕt'ĭks). Branch of surgery dealing with replacement of missing parts.

p., externally powered. Any prosthesis in which a small electric motor has been incorporated for the purpose of providing force to control various functions.

prosthetist (prŏs'thē-tĭst). 1. Specialist in artificial dentures. 2. Maker of artificial limbs.

prosthetosclerokeratoplasty (prŏs"thē-tō-sklē"rō-kĕr'ă-tō-plăs"tē). Surgical procedure for replacement of diseased scleral and corneal tissue with a transparent prosthesis.

prosthion (prŏs'thē-ŏn) [Gr. *prosthios*, foremost]. The lowest joint on the alveolar process of the maxilla.

prosthodontics (prŏs"thō-dŏn'tĭks) [" + *odous*, tooth]. Branch of dentistry dealing with construction of artificial appliances for the mouth.

prosthodontist (prŏs"thō-dŏn'tĭst). A dentist who specializes in the mechanics of making and fitting artificial teeth.

prosthokeratoplasty (prŏs"thō-kĕr'ă-tō-plăs"tē) [" + *keras*, horn, + *plassein*, to form]. Surgical replacement of diseased or scarred corneal tissue with a transparent prosthesis.

Prostigmin. Trade name for neostigmine bromide.

Prostin E₂. Trade name for dinoprostone.

Prostin F₂ Alpha. Trade name for dinoprost tromethamine.

Prostin/15M. Trade name for carboprost tromethamine.

prostitute (prŏs'tĭ-tūt) [L. *prostituere*, to prostitute]. 1. A person who solicits or accepts payment for sexual relations. 2. To sell oneself basely, such as to prostitute one's talents.

prostitution (prŏs"tĭ-tū'shŭn). Act or practice of prostituting. Prostitution is a major cause of the spread of venereal disease and may be a mode of transmission of AIDS.

prostrate (prŏs'trāt) [Gr. *pro*, before, + L. *sternere*, stretch out]. 1. Lying with body extended. 2. To deprive of strength or to exhaust.

prostrated. Depleted of strength; exhausted.

prostration (prŏs-trā'shŭn). Absolute exhaustion.

p., heat. Exhaustion resulting from exposure to excessive heat.

p., nervous. General physical and nervous exhaustion. SYN: *neurasthenia.*

protactinium (prō"tăk-tĭn'ē-ŭm). SYMB: Pa. At. wt. 231; at. no. 91. A radioactive element.

protal (prō'tăl) [Gr. *protos*, first]. Existing from time of birth or before. SYN: *congenital.*

protamine (prō'tă-mĭn). 1. One of a class of simple proteins that are strongly basic, noncoagulable in heat, and yield diamino acids when hydrolyzed. 2. An amine, $C_{16}H_{32}O_2N_9$, isolated from spermatozoa and spawn of fish. Found in fish sperm and named from the fish from which it is derived. SEE: *salmin(e); sturine.*

p. insulin. Preparations of insulin that are more slowly dissolved and absorbed by body tissues than ordinary insulin. Acts longer than ordinary insulin and lowers the blood sugar for 20 to 24 hours.

p. sulfate. USP. A purified form of protamine used to neutralize the anticoagulant action of heparin.

protanope (prō'tă-nōp) [Gr. *protos*, first, + *an-*, not, + *opsis*, vision]. A person with protanopia, q.v.

protanopia (prō-tăn-ō'pē-ă) [" + " + *opsis*, vision]. Red blindness; color blindness in which there is a defect in the perception of red. SEE: *color blindness.*

protean (prō'tē-ăn) [Gr. *Proteus,* a god who could change his form]. Having ability to change form, as the ameba. Variable.

protease inhibitors. Substances that act to inhibit the action of enzymes.

proteases (prō'tē-ās) [Gr. *protos,* first, + -*ase,* enzyme]. A class of enzymes that break down, or hydrolyze, the peptide bonds that join the amino acids in a protein. The protein is broken down into its basic building blocks, i.e., amino acids. SEE: *digestion.*

protective (prō-tĕk'tĭv) [L. *protectus,* shielding]. 1. Covering, preventing infection, providing immunity. 2. An agent that will mechanically protect the part to which applied such as collodion or plaster. SYN: *dressing.*

protective isolation. Isolation in which the patient is being protected from potentially harmful bacteria in the environment. This is particularly important in caring for immunodeficient patients such as those undergoing transplantation surgery. SYN: *reverse isolation.*

proteidogenous (prō"tē-ĭd-ŏj'ĕn-ŭs). Producing proteins.

protein (prō'tē-ĭn, prō'tēn) [Gr. *protos,* first]. One of a class of complex nitrogenous compounds that occur naturally in plants and animals and yield amino acids when hydrolyzed. Proteins provide the amino acids essential for the growth and repair of animal tissue.

COMP: Proteins, composed of carbon, hydrogen, oxygen, nitrogen, phosphorus, sulfur, and iron, make up the greater part of plant and animal tissue. Amino acids represent the basic structure of proteins. Foods containing protein consist of different numbers and kinds of amino acids. A complete protein is one that contains all the essential amino acids (tryptophan, lysine, methionine, valine, leucine, isoleucine, phenylalanine, threonine, arginine, and histidine). They are necessary for growth and maintenance of body weight.

SOURCES: Milk, eggs, cheese, meat, fish, and some vegetables such as soybeans are the best sources. Proteins are found in both vegetable and animal sources of food. Many "incomplete" proteins are found in vegetables; they contain some of the essential amino acids. A vegetarian diet can make up for this by combining vegetable groups that complement each other in their basic amino acid groups. This provides the body with complete protein.

Principal animal proteins are ovalbumin in eggs; lactalbumin in milk; serum albumin in serum; myogen or myosinogen in striated muscle tissue; fibrinogen in blood; ovo-

globulin in eggs; lactoglobulin in milk; serum globulin in serum; myosin in striated muscle tissue; thyroglobulin in thyroid; globin in blood; thymus histones in thymus; collagen and gelatin in connective tissue; elastin; and keratin. Nucleoprotein is found in the thymus, pancreas, liver, animal cells, and glands; chondroprotein is found in tendons and cartilage; mucin and mucoids are found in various secreting glands and animal mucilaginous substances; caseinogen in milk; vitellin in egg yolk; hemoglobin in blood; and lecithoprotein in blood, brain, and bile.

FUNCT: Proteins are a source of heat and energy to the body. They are essential for growth, the building of new tissue, and the repair of injured or broken-down tissue. They form an integral part of the protoplasm of every cell. When they are oxidized in the body, heat is liberated. One gm supplies 4 Cal.

Infants and children require from 2 to 2.2 gm of protein per kilogram of body weight per day. This should be calculated on the basis of ideal, rather than actual, weight of the child. Age also is a factor in determining protein requirements, the amount decreasing with age. Physical work, menstruation, pregnancy, lactation, and convalescence require increased protein intake. Excess protein in the diet results in increased nitrogen excretion in the urine.

p., Bence Jones. An abnormal protein that occurs in urine. Its presence is symptomatic of certain pathologic conditions: multiple myeloma, lymphosarcoma, leukemia, or Hodgkin's disease.

p.'s, blood. Proteins present in blood include hemoglobin in red blood cells and serum proteins. Normal values are: hemoglobin, 13–18 gm/dl in men and 12–16 gm/dl in women; albumin, 3.5–5.0 gm/dl of serum; globulin, 2.3–3.5 gm/dl of serum. The amount of albumin in relation to the amount of globulin is referred to as the albumin-globulin (A/G) ratio, which is normally 1.5:1 to 2.5:1.

p., carrier. Protein that elicits an immune response when coupled with a hapten.

p.'s, complete. Protein containing all the essential amino acids.

p.'s, conjugated. Proteins containing the protein molecule with some other molecule or molecules. *Chromoproteins:* Ex.: hemoglobin. *Glycoproteins:* Ex.: mucin. *Lecithoproteins:* Compounds of lecithins or similar substances with the protein molecule. *Nucleoproteins. Phosphoproteins:* Ex.: casein.

p., C-reactive. SEE: *C-reactive protein.*

p., denatured. Protein in which the

amino acid composition and stereochemical structure have been altered by physical or chemical means.

p., derived. Derivatives of protein molecules obtained by the action of chemical alteration or a physical agent such as heat.

p.'s, immune. Proteins that serve to protect the body against antigens. Immunoglobulins are immune proteins.

p., incomplete. Protein lacking one or more of the essential amino acids. SEE: *amino acid, essential.*

p., native. Protein in its natural state; one that has not been denatured.

p.'s, plasma. Proteins present in blood plasma, such as albumin or globulin.

p.'s, serum. Proteins present in the serum part of the blood.

p.'s, simple. Those proteins that produce alpha amino acids on hydrolysis. *Albumins:* Soluble in water and coagulated by heat. Ex.: egg albumin. *Globulins:* Insoluble in water, soluble in salt solutions, coagulated by heat. Ex.: edestin from hemp seed. *Glutelins, Prolamines:* alcohol-soluble proteins. Ex.: gliadin from wheat. *Albuminoids:* Ex.: keratin from corn. *Histones, Protamines:* Ex.: salmine from the ripe sperm of salmon.

proteinaceous (prō″tē-in-ā′shŭs). Concerning or resembling proteins.

proteinase (prō′tē-in-ās) [Gr. *protos*, first, + *lase*, enzyme]. A proteolytic enzyme; an enzyme that catalyzes the breakdown of native proteins.

protein balance. Equilibrium between protein intake and anabolism, and protein catabolism and elimination of nitrogenous products. SEE: *nitrogen equilibrium.*

protein C. A protein in the blood that, after conversion, inhibits coagulation of blood. Deficiency of this protein causes thrombosis.

protein-calorie malnutrition. Malnutrition usually seen in infants and young children whose diets are deficient in both proteins and calories. Clinically the condition may be precipitated by other factors such as infection or intestinal parasites. SEE: *kwashiorkor.*

proteinemia (prō″tē-in-ē′mē-ă) [″ + *haima*, blood]. An excess of protein in the blood.

protein hydrolysate injection. USP. A sterile solution of amino acids and short-chain peptides. They represent the approximate nutritive equivalent of casein, lactalbumin, plasma, fibrin, or other suitable proteins from which the hydrolysate is derived by acid, enzymatic, or other method of hydrolysis. It may contain alcohol, dextrose, or other carbohydrate suitable for intravenous

infusion. It is used intravenously in the treatment of hypoproteinemia in patients who are unable to eat or absorb food. Trade name is Travamin.

proteinic (prō″tē-in′ĭk). Rel. to protein.

protein kinase. An enzyme important in regulating many cellular processes.

protein-losing enteropathy. Abnormal loss of protein into the gastrointestinal tract. May be due to any disease that causes extensive ulceration of the intestinal mucosa.

proteinogenous (prō″tē-in-ŏj′ĕn-ŭs) [″ + *gennan*, to produce]. Developing from a protein.

proteinophobia (prō″tē-ĭn-ō-fō′bē-ă) [″ + *phobos*, fear]. Aversion to foods containing protein.

proteinosis (prō″tē-ĭn-ō′sĭs) [″ + *osis*, condition]. Accumulation of excess proteins in the tissues.

p., lipoid; p., lipid. A rare hereditary condition resulting from an undefined metabolic defect. Yellow deposits of a mixture of protein and lipoid occur, esp. on the mucous surface of the mouth and tongue. Nodules may appear on the face, extremities, and on the epiglottis and vocal cords. This latter abnormality produces hoarseness.

p., pulmonary alveolar. SEE: *pulmonary alveolar proteinosis.*

protein sensitization. Condition in which a patient is hypersensitive to foreign proteins, so that a severe reaction occurs when they are administered.

protein sparer. A substance in the diet such as carbohydrate or fat that prevents the utilization of protein for energy needs.

proteinuria (prō″tē-in-ū′rē-ă) [″ + *ouron*, urine]. Protein, usually albumin, in the urine. This finding may be transient and entirely benign. In other cases, proteinuria may be a sign of severe renal disease. SYN: *albuminuria.*

p., orthostatic. Appearance of protein in the urine when the patient has been standing but not while reclining.

p., postural. Protein in the urine in relation to bodily position.

Protenate. Trade name for plasma protein fraction.

proteoclastic (prō″tē-ō-klăs′tĭk) [Gr. *protos*, first, + *klasis*, a breaking]. Splitting up proteins.

proteolipid (prō″tē-ō-lĭp′ĭd). A lipid-protein complex that is insoluble in water. It is found principally in the brain.

proteolysin (prō″tē-ŏl′ĭ-sĭn) [″ + *lysis*, dissolution]. A specific substance causing decomposition of proteins.

proteolysis (prō″tē-ŏl′ĭ-sĭs). The hydrolysis of proteins, usually by enzyme action, into simpler substances.

proteolytic (prō″tē-ō-lĭt′ĭk). Hastening the hydrolysis of proteins.

proteometabolism (prō″tē-ō-mĕ-tăb′ō-lĭzm) [″ + *metabole*, change, + *-ismos*, condition]. Digestion, absorption, and assimilation of proteins.

proteopepsis (prō″tē-ō-pĕp′sĭs) [″ + *peptein*, to digest]. The digestion of proteins.

proteopeptic (prō″tē-ō-pĕp′tĭk) [″ + *peptein*, to digest]. Pert. to the digestion of protein.

proteopexic (prō-tē-ō-pĕks′ĭk) [″ + *pexis*, fixation]. Pert. to fixation of proteins within the organism.

proteopexy (prō″tē-ō-pĕks′ē). The fixation of proteins within the body.

proteose (prō′tē-ōs) [Gr. *protos*, first]. One of the class of intermediate products of proteolysis between protein and peptone.

> **p., primary.** First products formed during proteolysis of proteins.

> **p., secondary.** Protein resulting from further hydrolysis of primary proteoses.

proteosuria (prō″tē-ōs-ū′rē-ă) [″ + *ouron*, urine]. Proteose in urine. SYN: *albumosuria.*

proteuria (prō″tē-ū′rē-ă). Proteins in the urine. SYN: *proteinuria.*

Proteus (prō′tē-ŭs) [Gr. *Proteus*, a god who could change his form]. A genus of enteric bacilli, found in intestines and decaying material, causing protein decomposition.

> **P. mirabilis.** Species abundant in nature but only rarely is it a human pathogen.

> **P. morganii.** Previous name of *Morganella morganii,* q.v.

> **P. vulgaris.** An essentially saprophytic species that may produce urinary tract infections.

prothrombin. A chemical substance existing in circulating blood that, through the medium of thrombokinase, interacts with calcium salts to produce thrombin. SEE: *coagulation factors.*

prothrombinase. An enzyme important in blood coagulation. In a reaction with activated factors X (Xa) and V (Va) in the presence of calcium and platelets, prothrombinase catalyzes the conversion of prothrombin to thrombin.

prothrombinemia (prō-thrŏm″bĭn-ē′mē-ă) [Gr. *pro*, before, + *thrombos*, clot, + *haima*, blood]. Presence of prothrombin in the blood.

prothrombinogenic (prō-thrŏm″bĭ-nō-jĕn′ĭk) [″ + ″ + *gennan*, to produce]. Promoting the formation of prothrombin.

prothrombinopenia (prō-thrŏm″bĭ-nō-pē′nē-ă) [″ + ″ + *penia*, lack]. Deficiency of prothrombin in the blood. SYN: *hypoprothrombinemia.*

prothrombin time. A test of clotting time made by determining the time for clotting to occur after thromboplastin and calcium are added to decalcified plasma. Test is used to evaluate the effect of administration of anticoagulant drugs.

prothymocytes. Precursor cells that mature and differentiate into functioning T cells in the thymus gland. SEE: *T cells.*

protide (prō′tĭd). Protein.

protist (prō′tĭst). Any member of the Protista kingdom.

Protista (prō-tĭs′tă) [LL., simplest organisms]. Term applied to kingdom of organisms including the simpler unicellular animals and plants. Includes bacteria, some algae, spirochetes, protozoa, and other forms not easily classified as being either plants or animals. SEE: *eukaryote; prokaryote.*

protistologist (prō-tĭs-tŏl′ō-jĭst) [″ + *logos*, word, reason]. One who studies the Protista, the unicellular organisms.

protistology (prō-tĭs-tŏl′ō-jē). The science of Protista or unicellular plants and microorganisms. SYN: *microbiology.*

protium (prō-tē-ŭm). Hydrogen with atomic weight of one.

proto- [Gr. *protos*, first]. 1. Prefix signifying first. 2. The lowest of a series of compounds having the same elements.

protobiology (prō″tō-bī-ŏl′ō-jē) [″ + *bios*, life, + *logos*, word, reason]. The phase of science dealing with life forms more minute than bacteria, i.e., the ultraviruses and bacteriophages.

protoblast (prō′tō-blăst) [″ + *blastos*, germ]. 1. A naked cell with an unformed cell wall. 2. Blastomere of segmenting ovum that is parent cell of a part or organ.

protoblastic (prō″tō-blăs′tĭk). Pert. to a protoblast.

protocol (prō′tō-kŏl) [Gr. *protokollon*, first notes glued to manuscript]. 1. A clinical report from first notes taken. 2. Minutes of a meeting. 3. Description of steps to be taken in an experiment.

protodiastole (prō″tō-dī-ăs′tō-lē) [Gr. *protos*, first, + *diastole*, expansion]. The first of four phases of ventricular diastole characterized by drop in intraventricular pressure and closure of semilunar valves. Occurs immediately after second heart sound.

protoduodenum (prō″tō-dū-ō-dē′nŭm) [″ + L. *duodeni*, twelve]. The upper half of the duodenum. It is derived from the embryonic foregut.

protogaster (prō″tō-găs′tĕr) [″ + *gaster*, belly]. The archenteron or gastrocele; the cavity in a gastrula or developing embryo from which the digestive tract develops.

protoleukocyte (prō″tō-lū′kō-sīt) [″ + *leukos*, white, + *kytos*, cell]. A minute lymphoid cell in red bone marrow and in the spleen.

Protomastigida (prō″tō-măst-ĭj′ĭ-dä) [″ + *mastix*, whip, + *eidos*, form, shape]. An order of flagellate protozoa. It contains several pathogenic genera including *Leishmania* and *Trypanosoma*.

proton (prō′tŏn) [Gr. *protos*, first]. A positively charged particle forming the nucleus of hydrogen and present in the nuclei of all elements, the atomic number of the element indicating the number of protons present. Its mass is 1836 times that of an electron. SEE: *atom; atomic theory; electron; element*.

protoneuron (prō″tō-nū′rŏn) [″ + *neuron*, nerve]. The initial neuron in a reflex arc.

Protopam Chloride. Trade name for pralidoxime chloride.

protopathic [″ + *pathos*, disease, suffering]. Primitive, undiscriminating, esp. with respect to sensing and localizing pain stimuli. SEE: *sensibility*.

protoplasia (prō-tō-plā′zē-ä) [″ + *plassein*, to form]. The primary formation of tissue.

protoplasm (prō′tō-plăzm) [″ + LL. *plasma*, form, mold]. A thick, viscous colloidal substance that constitutes the physical basis of all living activities, exhibiting the properties of assimilation, growth, motility, secretion, irritability, and reproduction. It is a complex mixture of heterogeneous substances surrounded by a chemically active membrane that regulates the interchange of substances with the surrounding medium. It possesses the physical properties of a colloidal mass, the medium of dispersion being water. SEE: *cell; cytoplasm; nucleus*.

Protoplasm consists of inorganic substances (water, mineral compounds) and organic substances (proteins, carbohydrates, and lipids). The principal elements present are oxygen, carbon, hydrogen, nitrogen, calcium, and phosphorus, which constitute about 99% of protoplasm. Others present in small amounts are potassium, sulfur, chlorine, sodium, magnesium, and iron, together with trace elements (copper, cobalt, manganese, zinc, and others).

protoplasmic (prō-tō-plăz′mĭk). Pert. to protoplasm, or composed of it.

protoplast (prō′tō-plăst) [″ + *plassein*, to form]. In bacteriology, the sphere remaining after gram-positive bacteria have had their cell contents lysed. The bacterial cell wall constituents are absent. In gram-negative organisms these spheres retain an outer wall layer and are called spheroplasts.

protoporphyria (prō″tō-por-fĭr′ē-ä). Porphyria erythropoietica, q.v.

protoporphyrin (prō″tō-por-fī′rĭn). A derivative of hemoglobin containing four pyrrole nuclei; $C_{34}H_{34}N_4O_4$. Formed from heme (ferriprotoporphyrin) by deletion of an atom of iron. Occurs naturally.

protoporphyrinuria (prō″tō-por″fī-rĭn-ū′rē-ä). Protoporphyrin in the urine.

protoproteose (prō″tō-prō′tē-ōz). A primary proteose that, upon further digestion, is converted to deuteroproteose.

protospasm (prō′tō-spăzm) [Gr. *protos*, first, + *spasmos*, a convulsion]. A spasm beginning in one area and extending to other parts.

prototroph (prō′tō-trōf). An organism with the same nutritional requirements as its ancestors.

prototrophic (prō″tō-trō′fĭk) [″ + *trophe*, nourishment]. Requiring simple inorganic elements as food.

prototype (prō′tō-tīp). An original or initial model or type from which subsequent types arise.

protovertebra (prō″tō-věr′tě-brä) [″ + L. *vertebra*, vertebra]. Primitive vertebra in the notochord.

protoxide (prō-tŏk′sīd). Of the series of oxides of a metal, the one with the least amount of oxygen.

Protozoa [″ + *zoon*, animal]. The phylum of the animal kingdom that includes the simplest animals. Most are unicellular, although some are colonial. Reproduction usually asexual by fission, although conjugation and sexual reproduction occur.

protozoa. Pl. of protozoon.

protozoacide (prō-tō-zō′ă-sīd) [″ + *zoon*, animal, + L. *cidus*, kill]. Destructive to, or that which kills, protozoa.

protozoal (prō″tō-zō′ăl). Pert. to protozoa, unicellular organisms.

protozoal diseases. Diseases produced by single-celled organisms, such as amebic dysentery, sleeping sickness, and malaria. SEE: table.

protozoan (prō″tō-zō′ăn) [″ + *zoon*, animal]. Concerning protozoa.

protozoiasis (prō″tō-zō-ī′ă-sĭs) [″ + ″ + *-iasis*, condition]. A disease caused by protozoa.

protozoology (prō″tō-zō-ŏl′ō-jē) [Gr. *protos*, first, + *zoon*, animal, + *logos*, word, reason]. Phase of science dealing with study of protozoa.

protozoon (pl. *protozoa*). Unicellular organism. SEE: *Protozoa*.

protozoophage (prō″tō-zō′ō-fāj) [″ + *zoon*, animal, + *phagein*, to eat]. A phagocyte that ingests protozoa.

protraction (prō-trăk′shŭn) [″ + L. *protractus*, dragged out]. The extension forward or drawing forward of a part of the

Table of Pathogenic Protozoa

Subphylum	Genus and Species	Disease Caused
Mastigophora	*Borrelia recurrentis*	Relapsing fever
Locomotion by flagella	*Borrelia duttonii*	Relapsing fever
	Borrelia bronchialis	Bronchial infection
	Borrelia vincentii	Vincent's disease
	Giardia lamblia	Gastroenteritis
	Leptospira icterohaemorrhagiae	Weil's disease
	Leishmania donovani	Kala-azar
	Leishmania braziliensis	American leishmaniasis
	Leishmania tropica	Oriental sore
	Trypanosoma gambiense	Sleeping sickness
	Trypanosoma rhodesiense	Sleeping sickness
	Trypanosoma cruzi	Chagas' disease
Sarcodina	*Dientamoeba fragilis*	Diarrhea, fever
Locomotion by pseudopodia	*Entamoeba histolytica*	Amebic dysentery
Sporozoa	*Plasmodium malariae*	Quartan malaria
No locomotion in adult stage	*Plasmodium falciparum*	Malignant tertian malaria
	Plasmodium vivax	Benign tertian malaria
	Plasmodium ovale	Ovale malaria
Ciliophora	*Balantidium coli*	Balantidiasis
Possess cilia in some stage of life cycle		

body such as the mandible.

protractor (prō-trăk'tor) [L. *protractus*, dragged out]. 1. Instrument for removing foreign bodies from wounds. 2. A muscle that draws a part forward. Opposed to retractor.

protriptyline hydrochloride (prō-trǐp'tǐ-lēn). USP. An antidepressant drug. Trade name is Vivactil.

protrude [L. *protrudere*]. To project; to extend beyond a border or limit.

protrusion (prō-troo'zhŭn). State or condition of being thrust forward or projecting. In dentistry, particularly related to the position of the mandible, as opposed to retrusion.

protuberance (prō-tū'bĕr-ăns) [Gr. *pro*, before, + L. *tuber*, bulge]. A part that is prominent beyond a surface, like a knob.

protuberantia (prō-tū''bĕr-ăn'shē-ă). A protuberance, eminence, or projection.

proud flesh. A mass of excessive granulation formed when a wound shows no other sign of healing or tendency to cicatrization.

Provera. Trade name for medroxyprogesterone acetate.

provertebra (prō-vĕr'tĕ-bră). Protovertebra, q.v.

provirus (prō-vī'rŭs). The precursor of a virus.

provisional (prō-vĭzh'ŭn-ăl) [L. *provisio*, provision]. Serving a temporary use pending permanent arrangements.

provitamin (prō-vī'tă-mĭn) [L. *pro*, before, + *vita*, life, + *amine*]. An inactive substance that can be transformed in the body to a corresponding active vitamin and thus function as a vitamin.

   p. A. Carotene, the precursor of vitamin A.

proximad (prŏk'sĭm-ăd) [L. *proximus*, next, + *ad*, toward]. Toward the proximal or central point.

proximal (prŏk'sĭm-ăl). Nearest the point of attachment, center of the body, or point of reference. Opposite of distal.

proximalis (prŏk''sĭ-mā'lĭs). Proximal.

proximate (prŏk'sĭm-āt). Closely related with respect to space, time, or sequence. Next to, or nearest.

proximate cause. A legal concept that means there is a causal connection between the breach of the standard of care or negligence on the part of defendant and the injury sustained by plaintiff.

proximoataxia (prŏk''sĭ-mō-ă-tăk'sē-ă) [" + Gr. *ataxia*, lack of order]. Lack of coordination in muscles of the proximal area of an extremity, as the arm, forearm, thigh, or leg.

proximobuccal (prŏk''sĭ-mō-bŭk'ăl) [" + *bucca*, cheek]. Concerning the proximal and buccal surfaces of a tooth.

proximolabial (prŏk''sĭ-mō-lā'bē-ăl) [" +

labialis, pert. to the lips]. Concerning the proximal and labial surfaces of a tooth.

proximolingual (prŏk″sĭ-mō-lĭng′gwăl) [″ + *lingua*, tongue]. Concerning the proximal and lingual surfaces of a tooth.

Prozac. Trade name for fluoxetine hydrochloride.

prozone. That portion of the low dilution range of a homologous serum that fails to agglutinate bacteria that are agglutinated by the same serum in a higher dilution.

prozymogen (prō-zī′mō-jĕn) [Gr. *pro*, before, + *zyme*, leaven, + *gennan*, to produce]. An intranuclear substance that is a precursor of zymogen.

prune (proon) [L. *pruna*]. A dried plum, rich in carbohydrate. Contains a substance that is useful in stimulating the bowel, esp. for those who suffer from chronic constipation. The ability of prunes and prune juice to exert a laxative effect is due to the presence of dihydroxyphenyl isatin.

prune-belly defect. A nonstandard, but descriptive, term for children with congenital absence of one or more layers of abdominal muscles.

pruriginous (proo-rĭj′ĭ-nŭs) [L. *prurigo*, itch]. Pert. to, or of the nature of, prurigo.

prurigo (proo-rī′gō) [L., the itch]. A chronic skin disease marked by constantly recurring, discrete, pale, deep-seated, intensely itchy papules on extensor surfaces of limbs. Superimposed exanthematous manifestations may mask the true nature. This term is used by dermatologists throughout the world, but it has not received a universally acceptable definition. SYN: *pruritus*.

ETIOL: Exciting cause unknown.

TREAT: Constitutional and local. Antipruritics locally.

PROG: Guarded. Prurigo begins in childhood and may last a lifetime.

   p. agria. A severe type of prurigo that starts in childhood and persists. The skin becomes thickened and pigmented. Because of the severe itching and scratching, secondary pustules, boils, and abscesses may develop.

   p. estivalis. A form of polymorphic light eruption characterized by prurigo and photodermatitis. Recurring every summer and continuing during hot weather.

   p., Hebra's. P. mitis, q.v.

   p. mitis. Mild prurigo.

   p., pregnancy. A form of prurigo that usually has its onset in the middle trimester of pregnancy or later. The lesions occur on the proximal portion of the limbs and upper part of the trunk. The skin lesions usually improve spontaneously before term or rapidly after delivery.

   p., simple acute. Simple form of prurigo

with recurring tendency. Thought to be caused by reaction to bites in sensitive subjects.

   p. simplex. Urticaria papulosa, q.v.

pruritic. Concerning pruritus.

pruritogenic (proo″rĭ-tō-jĕn′ĭk) [L. *pruritus*, itching, + *gennan*, to produce]. Causing pruritus.

pruritus (proo-rī′tŭs) [L., itching]. Severe itching. May be a symptom of a disease process such as allergic response, or may be due to emotional factors. SEE: *Nursing Diagnoses* in *Appendix*.

ETIOL: Predisposing factor is cutaneous hyperesthesia. Localized causes are present in pruritus ani, pruritus vulvae, intestinal parasites (pinworms), and mycotic infection.

TREAT: Exciting or contributory cause located and removed. Hygienic regimen. In anal and vulvar pruritus, examination by competent gynecologist or proctologist before cutaneous therapy is instituted. In bath avoid too sudden changes of temperature. For dry skins, avoid frequent soap and water bathing. Soft, nonirritating underclothing and soothing lotions are of benefit.

   p. ani. Itching about the anus. May be due to poor perineal hygiene; perianal skin damage caused by scratching, or abrasion due to use of harsh, dry paper; excess moisture due to wearing tight, nonporous clothing; decreased resistance to fungi and yeasts during steroid therapy; ingestion of dietary irritants; pinworms; fistula in anus, hemorrhoids; or contact with soap or detergents that remain in underclothing following improper washing.

TREAT: Remove or avoid primary cause. Keep anus scrupulously clean by use of mild soap, and avoid applications of drugs that produce sensitivity and irritation. It is not possible to adequately cleanse the anal area by use of toilet tissue. SEE: *bidet*.

   p., aquagenic. Pruritus produced by contact with water.

   p., emperor of. SEE: *emperor of pruritus*.

   p., essential. Pruritus without apparent skin lesion.

   p. estivalis. Pruritus with prickly heat occurring in hot weather.

   p. hiemalis. Pruritus that occurs in cold weather and is provoked by cooling of the skin.

   p. senilis. Pruritus in aged with degenerative skin changes.

   p. vulvae. Disorder marked by severe itching of external female genitalia. Often an early sign of diabetes mellitus. May be associated with vaginitis.

Prussak's space (proo′săks) [Alexander

Prussak, Russ. otologist, 1839–1897]. Tiny space in middle ear between Shrapnell's membrane laterally and neck of malleus medially.

prussic acid (prŭs'ĭk). A rapidly acting poison. SYN: *acid, hydrocyanic*.

psalterium (săl-tē'rē-ŭm) [Gr. *psalterion*, harp]. 1. Omasum, or third division of the stomach of a ruminant. 2. Commissure of the fornix of the brain.

psammoma (săm-ō'mă) [Gr. *psammos*, sand, + *oma*, tumor]. A small tumor of the brain, the choroid plexus, and other areas, containing calcareous particles.

psammoma bodies. Laminated concretions often found in the pineal body. SYN: *brain sand; corpora arenacea.*

psammosarcoma (săm"ō-săr-kō'mă) [" + *sarx*, flesh, + *oma*, tumor]. A sarcoma in which psammoma bodies are present.

psammotherapy (săm"ō-thĕr'ă-pē) [" + *therapeia*, treatment]. The application of sand baths in treatment.

psammous (săm'ŭs). Sandy, gritty.

psellism, psellismus (sĕl'ĭzm, sĕl-ĭz'mŭs) [Gr. *psellisma*, stammer]. Defective pronunciation, stuttering, or stammering.

    p. mercurialis. Jerking, hurried, unintelligible speech present as part of the tremor that accompanies mercury poisoning.

pseudacousma (soo"dă-kooz'mă) [Gr. *pseudes*, false, + *akousma*, a thing heard]. Condition in which all sounds are heard falsely, seeming to be altered in quality of pitch, or imaginary sounds are heard. SYN: *pseudacusis.*

pseudacusis (soo"dă-kū'sĭs). State in which sounds are heard falsely or imagined. SYN: *pseudacousma.*

pseudagraphia (soo"dă-grăf'ē-ă) [" + *a-*, not, + *graphein*, to write]. A form of agraphia in which a person is unable to write independently, but is able to copy words or letters. SYN: *pseudoagraphia.*

pseudarthritis (soo"dăr-thrī'tĭs) [" + *arthron*, joint, + *itis*, inflammation]. Condition that imitates arthritis.

pseudarthrosis (soo"dăr-thrō'sĭs) [" + *arthron*, joint, + *osis*, condition]. A false joint developing after a fracture that has not united.

pseudencephalus (soo"dĕn-sĕf'ă-lŭs) [" + *enkephalos*, brain]. A congenital deformity in which the cranium is open and contains poorly organized vascular tissue.

pseudesthesia (soo"dĕs-thē'zē-ă) [" + *aisthesis*, sensation]. 1. An imaginary or false sensation, as that felt in the lost part after amputation. 2. Sense of feeling not caused by external stimulation.

pseudo- (soo'dō) [Gr. *pseudes*, false]. A prefix meaning false.

pseudoacanthosis nigricans (soo"dō-ăk"ăn-thō'sĭs) [" + *akantha*, thorn, + *osis*, condition]. Velvety, pigmented thickening of the flexural surfaces. This occurs in dark-skinned obese persons.

pseudoacephalus (soo"dō-ă-sĕf'ă-lŭs) [" + *a-*, not, + *kephale*, head]. A parasitic twin that has a rudimentary cranium.

pseudoagglutination (soo"dō-ă-glū"tĭ-nā'shŭn). The clumping together of red blood cells as in the formation of rouleaux, but differing from true agglutination in that they can be dispersed by shaking.

pseudoagraphia. Pseudagraphia.

pseudoalbinism (soo"dō-ăl'bĭ-nĭzm) [" + L. *albus*, white, + Gr. *-ismos*, condition]. Loss of pigment of the skin, as occurs in leukopathia or vitiligo.

pseudoalleles (soo"dō-ă-lēlz') [" + *allelon*, of one another]. A set of genes that seem to be present in the same locus in certain conditions and in closely situated loci in other conditions.

pseudoanemia (soo"dō-ă-nē'mē-ă) [" + *an-*, not, + *haima*, blood]. Pallor of mucous membranes and skin without other signs of true anemia.

pseudoaneurysm (soo"dō-ăn'ū-rĭzm) [" + *aneurysma*, a widening]. A dilation or tortuosity in a vessel that gives the impression of an aneurysm.

pseudoangina (soo"dō-ăn'jĭ-nă, -ăn-jī'nă) [" + L. *angina*, a choking]. False symptoms of nervous origin, resembling angina pectoris.

    SYM: Functional attacks of pain in cardiac region but not associated with any disease of the heart or its vessels.

pseudoankylosis (soo"dō-ăng"kĭ-lō'sĭs) [" + *ankyle*, stiff joint, + *osis*, condition]. A false joint.

pseudoapoplexy (soo"dō-ăp'ŏ-plĕk"sē). A mild condition simulating apoplexy, but not accompanied by cerebral hemorrhage. SYN: *parapoplexy*. SEE: *transient ischemic attack.*

pseudoataxia (soo"dō-ă-tăk'sē-ă) [" + *ataxia*, lack of order]. Condition resembling ataxia, but not due to tabes dorsalis.

pseudoblepsia, pseudoblepsis (soo"dō-blĕp'sē-ă, -sĭs) [" + *blepsis*, sight]. False or imaginary vision. SYN: *parablepsia; pseudopsia.*

pseudobulbar paralysis (soo"dō-bŭl'bĕr) [" + *bolbos*, a swollen end]. Paralysis resembling bulbar paralysis, but due to lesion of cortical centers.

pseudocartilaginous (soo"dō-kăr"tĭ-lăj'ĭ-nŭs) [" + L. *cartilago*, gristle]. Pert. to, or formed of, a substance resembling cartilage.

pseudocast (soo″dō-kăst) [″ + ME. *casten,* to carry]. A sediment in urine resembling a true cast; a false cast.

pseudocele (soo′dō-sēl) [″ + *koilos,* hollow]. The cavity of the septum pellucidum, the so-called 5th ventricle. SYN: *pseudocoele.*

pseudochancre (soo″dō-shăng′kĕr) [″ + Fr. *chancre,* ulcer]. A lesion resembling the chancre produced by syphilis.

pseudocholesteatoma (soo″dō-kō″lĕs-tē-ă-tō′mă) [″ + *chole,* bile, + *steatos,* fat, + *oma,* tumor]. Hard epithelium present as a mass in the tympanic cavity in association with chronic inflammation of the middle ear.

pseudocholinesterase (soo″dō-kō″lĭn-ĕs′tĕr-ās). A nonspecific cholinesterase that hydrolyzes noncholine esters as well as acetylcholine. Found in blood serum and pancreatic tissue.

pseudochorea (soo″dō-kō-rē′ă) [″ + *choreia,* dance]. Hysterical state resembling chorea.

pseudochromesthesia (soo″dō-krō″mĕs-thē′zē-ă) [″ + *chroma,* color, + *aisthesis,* sensation]. Condition in which sounds, esp. of the vowels, seem to induce a sensation of a distinct visual color. SEE: *phonism; photism; synesthesia.*

pseudochromidrosis (soo″dō-krō″mĭd-rō′sĭs) [″ + ″ + *hidros,* sweat, + *osis,* condition]. Appearance of colored sweat, in which the sweat acquires its color after it is excreted.

pseudocirrhosis (soo″dō-sĭr-ō′sĭs) [″ + *kirrhos,* orange yellow, + *osis,* disease]. Condition with symptoms of cirrhosis of liver, due to any process that causes obstruction of venous flow from the liver. Constrictive pericarditis can cause this condition.

SYM: Cyanosis, ascites, dyspnea.

pseudocoele (soo′dō-sēl) [″ + *koilos,* hollow]. The 5th ventricle of the brain. SYN: *cavum septi pellucidi; pseudocele.* SEE: *cavum septi pellucidi.*

pseudocolloid (soo″dō-kŏl′oyd) [″ + *kollodes,* glutinous]. A mucoid substance present in various locations and in ovarian cysts.

p. of lips. Fordyce's spots, q.v.

pseudocoloboma (soo″dō-kŏl-ō-bō′mă) [″ + *koloboma,* a mutilation]. A scarcely noticeable scar on the iris from an embryonic fissure.

pseudocoma. Locked-in syndrome, q.v.

pseudocoxalgia (soo″dō-kŏk-săl′jē-ă) [″ + L. *coxa,* hip, + Gr. *algos,* pain]. Osteochondrosis of the head of the femur, in children. SYN: *Legg-Calvé-Perthes disease.*

pseudocrisis (soo-dō-krī′sĭs) [″ + *krisis,* turning point]. A false crisis; a temporary fall of body temperature, which may be followed by a rise.

pseudocroup (soo-dō-kroop′). False croup. SYN: *laryngismus stridulus.*

pseudocyesis (soo″dō-sī-ē′sĭs) [″ + *kyesis,* pregnancy]. Condition in which a patient has nearly all of the usual signs and symptoms of pregnancy such as enlargement of abdomen, weight gain, cessation of menses, and morning sickness, but is not pregnant. Usually seen in women who either are very desirous of having children or wish to avoid pregnancy.

Treatment usually is done by psychiatric means. Pseudocyesis also occurs in men. SYN: *phantom pregnancy; pseudopregnancy.*

pseudocylindroid (soo″dō-sī-lĭn′droyd) [″ + *kylindros,* cylinder, + *eidos,* form, shape]. A shred of mucus in the urine that resembles a cast.

pseudocyst (soo′dō-sĭst) [″ + *kystis,* bladder]. A dilatation resembling a cyst.

pseudodementia (soo″dō-dē-mĕn′shē-ă) [″ + L. *dementare,* to make insane]. Exaggerated indifference to environment without impairment of mental capacity. Symptoms mimic dementia and are sometimes evident in the older, depressed individual.

pseudodiphtheria (soo″dō-dĭf-thē′rē-ă) [″ + *diphthera,* membrane]. Condition resembling diphtheria, but not due to *Corynebacterium diphtheriae.*

pseudoedema (soo″dō-ē-dē′mă) [″ + *oidema,* a swelling]. A puffy condition of the skin simulating edema.

pseudoemphysema (soo″dō-ĕm-fĭ-zē′mă) [″ + *emphysema,* an inflation]. A bronchial condition simulating emphysema, due to temporary blockage of the bronchi.

pseudoencephalitis (soo″dō-ĕn-sĕf″ă-lī′tĭs) [″ + *enkephalos,* brain, + *itis,* inflammation]. A false encephalitis due to profuse diarrhea.

pseudoephedrine hydrochloride (soo″dō-ĕ-fĕd′rĭn). USP. A sympathomimetic drug, an isomer of ephedrine, that has actions similar to ephedrine. Trade names are Sudafed and Novafed.

pseudoerysipelas (soo″dō-ĕr-ĭ-sĭp′ĕ-lăs) [″ + *erythros,* red, + *pella,* skin]. An inflammation of subcutaneous cellular tissue simulating erysipelas.

pseudoesthesia (soo″dō-ĕs-thē′zē-ă) [″ + *aisthesis,* sensation]. An imaginary or false sensation. SYN: *pseudesthesia.*

pseudofracture (soo″dō-frăk′chūr). A ribbonlike zone of decalcification seen in certain types of osteomalacia.

pseudoganglion (soo″dō-găn′glē-ŏn) [″ + *ganglion,* knot]. A slight thickening of a nerve, resembling a ganglion.

pseudogeusesthesia (soo″dō-gūs″ĕs-thē′zē-ă) [″ + *geusis,* taste, + *aisthesis,* sensation]. A sense of taste stimulated by one of the other senses.

pseudogeusia (soo″dō-gū′sē-ă). A subjective sensation of taste not produced by external stimulus.

pseudoglioma (soo″dō-glī-ō′mă) [″ + *glia,* glue, + *oma,* tumor]. Inflammatory changes occurring in the vitreous body that simulate glioma of retina, but are due to iridochoroiditis.

pseudoglobulin (soo″dō-glŏb′ū-lĭn) [″ + L. *globulus,* little globe]. One of a class of globulins characterized by being soluble in salt-free water. SEE: *euglobulin.*

pseudoglottis (soo″dō-glŏt′ĭs) [″ + *glottis,* back of tongue]. Area between false vocal cords.

pseudogout (soo′dō-gowt″). Chronic recurrent arthritis clinically similar to gout. The crystals found in synovial fluid are calcium pyrophosphate dihydrate and not urate crystals. Also, the most commonly involved joint is the knee and not small joints as in gout. SYN: *chondrocalcinosis.*
  TREAT: Joint aspiration, phenylbutazone or salicylates.

pseudogynecomastia (soo″dō-jĭn″ĕ-kō-măs′tē-ă) [Gr. *pseudes,* false, + *gyne,* woman, + *mastos,* breast]. Excess adipose tissue in the male breast, but with no increase in glandular tissue.

pseudohematuria (soo″dō-hē″mă-tū′rē-ă) [″ + *haima,* blood, + *ouron,* urine]. A red pigment in the urine than makes the urine appear to have blood in it.

pseudohemophilia (soo″dō-hē″mō-fĭl′ē-ă) [″ + ″ + *philos,* to love]. Von Willebrand's disease, q.v.

pseudohemoptysis (soo″dō-hē-mŏp′tĭ-sĭs) [″ + *haima,* blood, + *ptyein,* to spit]. Spitting of blood that does not arise from the bronchi or the lungs.

pseudohermaphrodite (soo″dō-hĕr-măf′rō-dīt). An individual having the sex glands of only one sex but having some of the physical appearances of an individual of the opposite sex.

pseudohermaphroditism (soo″dō-hĕr-măf′rō-dīt″izm) [″ + *Hermaphroditos,* mythical two-sexed god, + *-ismos,* condition]. A congenital abnormality of the external genitalia and of the body in which one possesses sex glands of one sex but genitalia of the opposite sex. SYN: *hermaphroditism, false.* SEE: *intersex.*
  p., female. Condition in a female marked by a large clitoris, resembling the penis, and hypertrophied labia majora, resembling the scrotum, thus producing re-

semblance to male genitalia. Can be caused by disease of the adrenal gland.
  p., male. Condition in a male marked by a small penis, perineal hypospadias, and scrotum without testes, thereby resembling the vulva. Can be due to disease of the adrenal gland or a feminizing tumor of the undescended testis.

pseudohernia (soo″dō-hĕr′nē-ă) [″ + L. *hernia,* rupture]. Inflammation in the scrotal area resembling a hernia.

pseudohypertension. The observation of elevated blood pressure when taken by conventional means, i.e., sphygmomanometer, that is in reality not elevated when compared with the actual pressure in the artery when it is determined by more nearly accurate methods. True blood pressure may be obtained directly by use of an intra-arterial catheter or by use of an infrasonic recorder. The latter method is almost as accurate as the direct intra-arterial method. Pseudohypertension is more likely to be found in elderly patients. SEE: *blood pressure, indirect determination of; hypertension; infrasonic recorder.*

pseudohypertrophic (soo″dō-hī-pĕr-trō′fĭk) [″ + *hyper,* above, + *trophe,* nourishment]. Pert. to a false hypertrophy.

pseudohypertrophy (soo″dō-hī-pĕr′trō-fē). Increase in size of an organ or structure due to hypertrophy or hyperplasia of tissue other than parenchyma. Often accompanied by diminution of function.

pseudohypoparathyroidism (soo″dō-hī″pō-păr″ă-thī′royd-ĭzm). Hereditary disease resembling hypoparathyroidism but caused by an inadequate response to parathyroid hormone rather than a deficiency of the hormone. Some of the patients will be obese with short, stocky build and moonfaced. Mental deficiency may be present along with cataracts, strabismus, tetany, stridor, convulsions, and muscular cramps.

pseudoicterus (soo″dō-ĭk′tĕr-ŭs) [″ + *ikteros,* jaundice]. Pseudojaundice.

pseudoisochromatic (soo″dō-ī″sō-krō-măt′ĭk) [″ + *isos,* equal, + *chroma,* color]. Seemingly of the same color; colors used in charts testing for color blindness.

pseudojaundice (soo″dō-jawn′dĭs) [″ + Fr. *jaune,* yellow]. Pigment in the skin, such as in carotenemia, that resembles jaundice, but is not due to jaundice. SEE: *carotenemia.*

pseudologia (soo-dō-lō′jē-ă) [″ + *logos,* word, reason]. Falsification in writing or in speech, a form of pathological lying.
  p. fantastica. Pathological lying; one of the forms of the psychopathic state.

pseudomania (soo-dō-mā′nē-ă) [″ + *mania,* madness]. 1. A psychosis in which patients falsely accuse themselves of crimes that they think they have committed. 2. Pathological lying.

pseudomasturbation (soo″dō-măs-tŭr-bā′shŭn) [″ + L. *manus*, hand, + *stuprare*, to rape]. A nervous habit of pulling at the penis. SYN: *peotillomania.*

pseudomelanosis (soo″dō-měl-ă-nō′sĭs) [″ + *melas*, black, + *osis*, condition]. Discoloration of tissues after death.

pseudomembrane (soo″dō-měm′brān) [″ + L. *membrana*, membrane]. A false membrane, as in diphtheria.

pseudomembranous (soo″dō-měm′brănŭs). Pert. to, or marked by, false membranes.

pseudomeningitis (soo″dō-měn-ĭn-jī′tĭs) [″ + *meninx*, membrane, + *itis*, inflammation]. A condition resembling symptoms of meningitis without lesions of meningeal inflammation.

pseudomenstruation (soo″dō-měn″strū-ā′shŭn) [″ + L. *menstruare*, menstruate]. Bleeding from the uterus not accompanied by the usual changes in the endometrium.

pseudomnesia (soo″dŏm-nē′zē-ă) [″ + *mnesis*, memory]. A memory perversion in which patient remembers that which never occurred.

Pseudomonas (soo-dō-mō′năs) [″ + *monas*, single]. A genus of small, motile, gram-negative bacilli with polar flagella. Most are saprophytic, living in soil and decomposing organic matter. Some produce blue and yellow pigments.

P. aeruginosa. Species that is sometimes pathogenic for humans. May cause urinary tract infections, otitis externa, or folliculitis, including the inflammation that may follow use of a "hot tub."

P. mallei. Species that causes glanders in horses.

P. maltophilia. A species potentially pathogenic for humans. It is found in plants, soil, water, sewage, and raw milk.

P. pseudomallei. Species that causes melioidosis, q.v., in humans and animals.

pseudomucin (soo-dō-mū′sĭn) [″ + L. *mucus*, mucus]. A variety of mucin found in ovarian cysts.

pseudomyopia (soo″dō-mī-ō′pē-ă) [″ + *myein*, to shut, + *ops*, eye]. Condition in which defective vision causes persons to hold objects close in order to see them. However, these individuals do not have myopia.

pseudomyxoma (soo″dō-mĭk-sō′mă) [″ + *myxa*, mucus, + *oma*, tumor]. A peritoneal tumor resembling a myxoma and containing a thick viscid fluid.

p. peritonei. A type of tumor that develops in the peritoneum from implantation metastases resulting from rupture of ovar-

ian cystadenoma or cells escaping during surgical removal. Numerous papillomas develop attached to the abdominal wall and intestine, and the peritoneal cavity becomes filled with mucuslike fluid.

pseudoneoplasm (soo-dō-nē′ō-plăsm) [″ + *neos*, new, + LL. *plasma*, form, mold]. A false or phantom tumor. A temporary swelling that simulates a tumor, usually of an inflammatory nature.

pseudoneuritis (soo″dō-nū-rī′tĭs) [″ + *neuron*, nerve, + *itis*, inflammation]. Reddening and blurring of the optic disk that resembles optic neuritis.

pseudoneuroma (soo″dō-nū-rō′mă) [″ + ″ + *oma*, tumor]. A mass of interlacing, coiled fibers, cells of Schwann, and fibrous tissue forming a mass at end of amputation stump. Also called amputation or traumatic neuroma. It is not a true neuroma.

pseudonucleolus (soo″dō-nū″klē-ōl′ŭs) [″ + L. *nucleus*, a nut]. The false nucleolus or karyosome.

pseudopapilledema (soo″dō-păp″ĭ-lě-dē′mă) [″ + *papilla*, nipple, + *oidema*, swelling]. Swelling of the optic nerve head that is not caused by optic neuritis.

pseudoparalysis (soo″dō-pă-răl′ĭ-sĭs) [″ + *para*, at the side, + *lyein*, to loosen]. Loss of muscular power not due to lesion of the nervous system. SYN: *pseudoplegia.*

pseudoparaplegia (soo″dō-păr-ă-plē′jē-ă) [″ + ″ + *plege*, a stroke]. Seeming paralysis of the lower extremities without impairment of the reflexes.

pseudoparasite (soo″dō-păr′ă-sīt) [″ + ″ + *sitos*, food]. 1. Anything resembling a parasite. 2. Organism that can live as a parasite, although it is normally not one. SEE: *parasite, facultative.*

pseudoparesis (soo″dō-păr-ē′sĭs, -păr′ē-sĭs) [″ + *parienai*, to let fall]. Condition simulating paresis but unlike the ordinary forms and due to hysteria.

pseudopelade (soo″dō-pē′lăd) [″ + Fr. *pelade*, to remove hair]. A type of alopecia, of unknown etiology, associated with scarring.

Pseudophyllidea (soo″dō-fĭ-lĭd′ē-ă). An order belonging to the class Cestoidea, subclass Cestoda. Includes tapeworms with scolex bearing two lateral (or one terminal) sucking grooves (bothria). Includes *Diphyllobothrium latum*, the fish tapeworm of humans.

pseudoplegia (soo″dō-plē′jē-ă) [″ + *plege*, a stroke]. Paralysis of hysterical origin. SYN: *pseudoparalysis.*

pseudopod (soo″dō-pŏd) [″ + *pous*, foot]. Temporary protruding protoplasmic process in protozoa for the purpose of taking up food and aiding in locomotion. SYN: *pseudopodium.*

pseudopodium (soo″dō-pō′dē-ŭm) (pl. *pseudopodia*). 1. A temporary protruding process of a protozoan or ameboid cell, such as a leukocyte, that aids in locomotion and the engulfing of food particles or foreign substances, as in phagocytosis. SYN: *pseudopod*. 2. An irregular projection at the edge of a wheal.

pseudopolyp (soo″dō-pŏl′ĭp) [″ + *polys*, many, + *pous*, foot]. A hypertrophied area of mucous membrane resembling a polyp.

pseudopolyposis (soo″dō-pŏl″ĭ-pō′sĭs) [″ + ″ + ″ + *osis*, condition]. A large number of pseudopolyps in the colon due to chronic inflammation.

pseudopregnancy (soo″dō-prĕg′năn-sē) [Gr. *pseudes*, false, + L. *praegnans*, with child]. 1. Condition in lower animals following sterile matings in which anatomical and physiological changes, similar to those of pregnancy, occur. 2. Pseudocyesis.

pseudo-pseudohypoparathyroidism (soo″dō-soo″dō-hī″pō-păr″ă-thī′royd-ĭzm) [″ + *pseudes*, false, + *hypo*, under, + *para*, beside, + *thyreos*, shield, + *eidos*, form, shape + *-ismos*, condition]. Pseudohypoparathyroidism in which most of the clinical but none of the biochemical changes are present.

pseudopsia (soo-dŏp′sē-ă) [″ + *opsis*, vision]. Visual hallucinations or false perceptions. SYN: *pseudoblepsis*.

pseudopterygium (soo″dō-tĕr-ĭj′ē-ŭm) [″ + *pterygion*, wing]. A scar on the conjunctiva of the eye that is firmly attached to the underlying tissue.

pseudoptosis (soo-dō-tō′sĭs) [″ + *ptosis*, a dropping]. Apparent ptosis of the eyelid, resulting from a fold of skin or fat projecting below the edge of the eyelid.

pseudorabies (soo″dō-rā′bēz) [″ + L. *rabere*, to rage]. A rabieslike disease in animals that is due to a type of herpesvirus. It causes death within several days.

pseudoreaction (soo″dō-rē-ăk′shŭn). A false reaction. A response to injection of a test substance into the tissues due to presence of an allergen other than one for which test is made.

pseudorickets (soo″dō-rĭk′ĕts). Rickets, renal, q.v.

pseudoscarlatina (soo″dō-skăr-lă-tē′nă). A septic febrile condition with rash resembling scarlatina.

pseudosclerosis (soo″dō-sklē-rō′sĭs) [″ + *sklerosis*, a hardening]. A condition with the symptoms, but without the lesions, of multiple sclerosis of the nervous system.

p., Westphal-Strümpell. Hepatolenticular degeneration, q.v.

pseudosmia (soo-dŏz′mē-ă) [″ + *osme*, smell]. An olfactory hallucination or perversion of the sense of smell.

pseudostoma (soo-dŏs′tō-mă) [″ + *stoma*, mouth]. An apparent aperture between endothelial cells that have been stained.

pseudostratified (soo-dō-străt′ĭ-fĭd) [″ + L. *stratificare*, to arrange in layers]. Apparently composed of layers.

pseudostratified epithelium. Epithelium in which basal ends of all cells rest on basement membrane but distal ends may or may not reach the surface. Their nuclei lie at different levels, giving the appearance of being stratified.

pseudosyphilis (soo″dō-sĭf′ĭ-lĭs). A nonspecific condition resembling syphilis.

pseudotabes (soo″dō-tā′bēz) [Gr. *pseudes*, false, + L. *tabes*, wasting away]. A neural disease simulating tabes dorsalis.

pseudotetanus (soo″dō-tĕt′ă-nŭs) [″ + *tetanos*, stretched]. Persistent muscular contractions resembling tetanus.

pseudotruncus arteriosus (soo″dō-trŭnk′ŭs ăr-tē″rē-ō′sŭs). The severest form of tetralogy of Fallot.

pseudotuberculosis (soo″dō-tū-ber″kū-lō′sĭs) [″ + L. *tuberculus*, tubercle, + Gr. *osis*, condition]. A group of diseases that resemble tuberculosis but are due to an organism other than the tubercle bacillus. In humans the most common cause is *Yersinia pseudotuberculosis*, a gram-negative organism.

pseudotumor cerebri (soo″dō-tū′mor sĕr′ĕ-brī). Benign intracranial hypertension. This diagnosis is made after exclusion of tumors, obstruction of the ventricles, intracranial infection, and vascular hypertensive encephalopathy. The cause may be due to a variety of disorders, but in most cases the etiology is unknown. The prognosis is for spontaneous recovery.

pseudotympany (soo″dō-tĭm′pă-nē) [″ + *tympanon*, drum]. Flattening of arch of diaphragm and swelling of abdomen with increased respiration. It disappears under anesthesia and is of purely nervous origin.

pseudoxanthoma (soo″dō-zăn-thō′mă) [″ + *xanthos*, yellow, + *oma*, tumor]. Condition resembling xanthoma.

p. elasticum. Chronic degenerative cutaneous disease marked by yellow patches and stretching of skin. Associated with hypertension and degeneration of elastic coat of arteries. Angioid streaks in retina are common.

p.s.i. *pounds per square inch.*

psilocin (sī′lō-sĭn). A hallucinogen similar to psilocybin.

psilocybin (sī″lō-sī′bĭn). A hallucinogen obtained from a particular mushroom.

psi phenomena. Occurrences, events, or actions that have no logical explanation.

Ex.: extrasensory perception, clairvoyance, precognition, psychokinesis, and telepathy.

psittacosis (sĭt-ă-kō′sĭs) [Gr. *psittakos*, parrot, + *osis*, condition]. An infectious disease, caused by *Chlamydia psittaci*, of parrots and other birds that may be transmitted to humans. Tetracyclines, erythromycin, and penicillin are effective in treatment. SYN: *ornithosis; parrot fever*. SEE: *Chlamydia*.

SYM (in humans): Headache, epistaxis, nausea, chill followed by fever, constipation, sometimes pulmonary disorders.

psoas (sō′ăs) [Gr. *psoa*]. One of two muscles of the loins. SEE: *Muscles* in *Appendix*.

psoas abscess. A cold abscess in sheath of the psoas major muscle. It follows the sheath of this muscle until it reaches the surface and points. Generally it occurs above Poupart's ligament in the iliac fossa or near the attachment of the psoas muscle to the femur.

ETIOL: Usually tuberculous disease of the vertebrae.

psoitis (sō-ī′tĭs) [Gr. *psoa*, muscle of the loin, + *itis*, inflammation]. Inflammation of the psoas muscles or of the area of the loins.

psomophagia (sō″mō-fā′jē-ă) [Gr. *psomos*, morsel, + *phagein*, to eat]. The habit of swallowing food without thoroughly chewing it. SEE: *fletcherism*.

psoralen. One of a group of substances derived from plants, some of which are capable of causing a phototoxic dermatitis when applied to the skin and exposed to sunlight or artificial ultraviolet wavelengths. Methoxsalen, USP, is a psoralen, and trioxsalen, USP, is a synthetic psoralen. SEE: *psoriasis; PUVA therapy; vitiligo*.

psorelcosis (sō″rĕl-kō′sĭs) [″ + *helkosis*, ulceration]. Ulceration occurring as a result of scabies.

psorenteritis (sō″rĕn-tĕr-ī′tĭs) [″ + *enteron*, intestine, + *itis*, inflammation]. Inflammation of the intestines seen in Asiatic cholera.

psoriasis (sō-rī′ă-sĭs) [Gr., an itching]. A common, chronic disease of the skin consisting of erythematous papules which coalesce to form plaques with distinct borders. As the disease progresses and if it is untreated, a silvery, yellow-white scale develops. New lesions tend to appear at sites of trauma; they may be in any location, but frequently are located on the scalp, knees, elbows, umbilicus, and genitalia.

The clinical course is variable but less than one-half of the patients followed for a prolonged period will have prolonged remis-

sions. Severity may range from a minimal cosmetic problem to a life-threatening emergency. In about 5% of psoriasis patients, arthritis will develop, and in most of these, joint involvement will occur after the onset of the skin lesions. The course of the arthritis is mild, affects only a few joints, and spontaneous remissions occur. Most of the skin changes, with the exception of inflammation, may be explained by the rapid turnover of the epidermis. Normal skin produces about 1250 cells a day for each square cm, and these come from 27,000 cells; psoriatic skin produces 35,000 new cells each day for each square cm, and these come from 52,000 cells. The normal duration of the cell cycle of skin is 311 hours, but is reduced to 36 hours for psoriatic skin. SEE: *Nursing Diagnoses* in *Appendix*.

ETIOL: The cause of psoriasis is unknown, but a genetic factor is present; certain conditions, e.g., infection, some drugs, climate, and perhaps hormonal factors and smoking, may trigger attacks.

TREAT: General care, including explanation of what is known about the course and treatment of the disease, and reassurance. Remove keratolytics, emollients, and corticosteroids. The last should be used under occlusive polyethylene covering, and their long-term use is inadvisable because of undesired side effects. Long-wave ultraviolet light (330-360 nm) combined with topical psoralens has been effective. For severe, life-threatening cases that have failed to respond to other treatment, the systemic drugs methotrexate or etretinate are effective.

Caution: The use of ultraviolet light is contraindicated in patients with a history of cancer of the skin. All male psoriasis patients treated with ultraviolet light should be protected in the genital area from the ultraviolet light. The use of methotrexate requires that the patient be carefully monitored for renal, hematological, or hepatic changes.

NURSING IMPLICATIONS: Teach patient about prescribed therapy to soften and remove scales, relieve pruritus, reduce pain and discomfort, retard rapid cell proliferation, and help induce remission, monitoring for adverse effects. Assist them to gain confidence in managing these largely palliative treatments, many of which require special instructions for application and removal. Help patient to protect against and minimize skin trauma. Evaluate ability to manage therapies and whether desired results occur. Assist patient to recognize stressors that seem to exacerbate condition (cold weather, emotional stress, infection), and to avoid or reduce these as possible. Suggest participation in a smoking cessation program if this is a factor. Help patient who is young at onset (20 to 30) to deal with body image changes and resultant effects on self-esteem, encouraging verbalization of feelings and supporting patient through loss and grief. Refer patient for psychological counseling or cosmetic concealment therapy as appropriate.

p. annularis. Circular or ringlike lesions of psoriasis.

p. arthropica. Psoriasis associated with arthritis. SYN: *psoriatic arthropathy.*

p. buccalis. Leukoplakia of the oral mucosa.

p., elephantine. A rare, but persistent, psoriasis that occurs on the back, thighs, and hips in thick scaling plaques.

p., guttate. Psoriasis characterized by small distinct lesions that generally occur over the body. They appear particularly in the young after acute streptococcal infections.

p., nummular. The most common form of psoriasis with discs and plaques of varying sizes on the extremities and trunk. There may be a great number of lesions or a solitary lesion.

p., pustular. Psoriasis in which small sterile pustules form, dry up, and then form a scab.

p., rupioid. Psoriasis with hyperkeratotic lesions on the feet.

p. universalis. Severe generalized psoriasis.

psorophthalmia (sō″rŏf-thăl′mē-ă) [Gr.]. Marginal inflammation of the eyelids with ulceration.

psorous (sō′rŭs) [Gr. *psoros*]. Rel. to, or affected with, itch.

P.S.P. *phenolsulfonphthalein;* a substance used to test kidney function.

PSRO. *Professional Standards Review Organization.*

PSVT. *paroxysmal supraventricular tachycardia.*

psych-, psycho- [Gr. *psyche*, mind]. Combining form indicating relationship to the mind or mental processes.

psychagogy (sī″kă-gō′jē) [Gr. *psyche*, soul, mind, + *agein*, to lead]. A psychotherapeutic re-educational procedure that stresses proper social adjustment of the individual.

psychalgia (sī-kăl′jē-ă) [″ + *algos*, pain]. 1. Pain of hysterical origin. 2. Mental distress characterized by auditory and visual hallucinations, often associated with melancholia.

psychanopsia (sī-kăn-ŏp′sē-ă) [″ + *an-,*

not, + *opsis*, vision]. Condition in which the patient sees objects but perceives an erroneous concept of their size and three-dimensional relationships. SYN: *psychic blindness.*

psychataxia (sī″kă-tăk′sē-ă) [″ + *ataxia*, lack of order]. Disordered power of concentration.

psychauditory (sīk-aw′dĭ-tor-ē) [″ + L. *auditorius*, hearing]. Pert. to the perception and interpretation of sounds.

psyche (sī′kē) [Gr. *psyche*, soul, mind]. All that constitutes the mind and its processes.

psychedelic (sī″kĕ-dĕl′ĭk) [″ + *delos*, manifest]. Originally used in 1963 to mean mind-manifesting. Now used by lay persons to describe some of the subjective aspects of intoxication, particularly with a drug such as lysergic acid diethylamide (LSD) or other drugs that produce visual hallucinations.

psychiatric (sī-kē-ă′trĭk) [″ + *iatrikos*, healing]. Pert. to psychiatry, the science concerned with the study, diagnosis, and prevention of mental illness.

psychiatric disorders. Unlike diseases in which a specific function, or lack of it, overreaction, or inhibition of a function can be observed objectively and tested by use of more or less precise techniques, aberrations of the function of the human mind are difficult to quantify, esp. when the definitions of the items that need to be measured are controversial, arbitrary, and most probably subjective. Nevertheless, it is of little benefit to attempt to categorize diseases with respect to whether or not the process is physical, i.e., organic, or functional. It is not possible to have any disorder of the psyche that does not influence the body. The patient must be regarded as a complex psychobiological unit functioning in relationship to the immediate physical and social environment. It is in this context that diseases that affect the human psyche, whether "organic" or "functional," must be considered by the thoughtful physician and, indeed, all involved in patient care.

psychiatrist (sī-kī′ă-trĭst). A physician who specializes in study, treatment, and prevention of mental disorders.

psychiatry (sī-kī′ă-trē). The branch of medicine that deals with diagnosis, treatment, and prevention of mental illness.

p., descriptive. A system of psychiatry concerned with the readily observable external factors that influence the mental state of an individual. SEE: *p., dynamic.*

p., dynamic. The study of the origin, influence, and control of emotions. This involves investigating the factors both from within and without that alter emotions and motivation. Such analysis provides a basis for judging regression or progression.

p., emergency. The emergency therapy and intervention in patients who are suicidal, homicidal, or are perpetrators or victims of child abuse, spouse abuse, or incest. Most of these individuals see a physician within hours or days of their violent or abusive act. Many physician training programs fail to prepare a student for managing patients who need this emergency service.

p., forensic. Use of psychiatry in legal matters, esp. in determining social adaptability of an individual suspected of insanity; or the presence or absence of insanity, esp. at the time the individual committed a crime.

p., orthomolecular. The concept that mental illness may be treated by determining and treating abnormalities of body chemistry.

psychiatry and neurology, words pert. to:
aberration; abreaction; abulia; acathisia; affect; agnosia; agraphia; agoraphobia; akinesia; alcoholism; alexia; alliteration; Alzheimer's disease; ambivalence; amentia; amnesia; amok; amusia; anal erotism; anhedonia; anomia; anorexia; apathy; aphasia; aphonia; aphrasia; aphrenia; apraxia; apsychosis; association; astereognosis; asyllabia; asymbolia; asynesia; atactilia; atavism; ataxia; ataxiaphasia; ateliosis; attitude; autism; autistic child; automatism; autoecholalia; autophagia; autophobia; autopsychosis; autosuggestion; blocking; bradylalia; bradylexia; catatonia; catharsis; cenesthesia; chorea; claustrophilia; claustrophobia; compulsion; conation; condensation; conditioning; confabulation; conflict; coprolagnia; coprolalia; coprophilia; cretinism; deafness; delire de toucher; delirium; delusion; dementia; depersonalization; depression; dereistic; determinism; disorientation; displacement; dissociation; distractibility; dysbulia; dyscinesia; dyslexia; dysmnesia; echolalia; echomimia; ego; egocentric; electroconvulsive therapy; electroencephalogram; emotion; emotivity; empathy; erethism; ergasiomania; ergasiophobia; eroticism; erotomania; erythrophobia; exhibitionism; extrasensory perception; extrovert; fabrication; fastidium; fear; fixation; folie; free association; fugue; furor; Ganser's syndrome; geophagia; hallucination; hallucinosis; heterolalia; homosexual; hyperhedonia; hyperselephesia; hypersthenia; hyperthymia; hypnagogic; hypnogenic zones; hypnosis; hypnotic; hypnotism; hypochondria; hypochondriac; hypochondriasis; hysteria; id; idea; illusion; image; imago; incoherence; incompetent; infantilism; inhibition; insanity; instinct; integration; intelligence; intrapsychic; introjection; intro-

version; introvert; kinesthesia; Korsakoff's syndrome; latent content; lesbian; lethargy; libido; locked-in syndrome; malingerer; masochism; melancholia; mental deficiency; mesmerism; mind; narcissism; negativism; neologism; neurology; neurosis; noctambulism; non compos mentis; nymphomania; object choice; obsession; oligopnea; organic psychoses; orthopsychiatry; overtone; paragraphia; paralexia; paralogia; paramimia; paramnesia; paranoia; paranomia; paranormal; parapathia; paraphasia; parent fixation; paresis; pedophilia; periphrastic; perseveration; personality; phantasia; phantasm; phantasy; phantom; phoneme; pica; pleasure principle; post-traumatic stress disorder; poverty of thought; pragmatism; preconscious; projection; psychosexual disorders; rationalization; reaction; reactive depression; reading disorders; reality principle; recapitulation theory; repression; resistance; restraint; retardation; Rorschach; sadism; satyriasis; schizoid; schizophrenia; stereotypy; stupor; subconscious; subjective; sublimation; subliminal; suggestion; superego; surrogate; sycophancy; symbiosis; symbol; symbolism; syntonic; transfer; transvestism; trend; unconscious; verbigeration; vigil; vision; voice; word blindness; **words beginning with "psyche-" or "neuro-".**

psychic (sī′kĭk) [Gr. *psychikos*]. 1. Concerning the mind or psyche. 2. One said to be endowed with semisupernatural powers, such as the ability to read the minds of others or to foresee coming events; one apparently sensitive to nonphysical forces.

psychic blindness. Sight without recognition of that which is seen. SYN: *psychanopsia*.

psychic contagion. Communication of another's nervous disorder by imitation.

psychic deafness. Inability to recognize sounds heard.

psychic determinism. The theory that mental processes are determined by conscious or unconscious motives, and are never irrelevant.

psychic force. Force generated apart from physical energy.

psychoactive (sī″kō-ăk′tĭv) [″ + L. *actio*, action]. Affecting the mental state, such as a drug that has that action.

psychoanaleptic (sī″kō-ăn″ă-lĕp′tĭk) [″ + *analepsis*, a taking up]. Having a stimulating effect upon the mind.

psychoanalysis (sī″kō-ă-năl′ĭ-sĭs) [″ + *analysis*, a dissolving]. Method of obtaining a detailed account of past and present mental and emotional experiences and repressions in order to determine the source and to eliminate or diminish the undesirable effects of unconscious conflicts by making the patient aware of their existence, origin, and inappropriate expression in emotions and behavior. It is largely a system that was the creation of Sigmund Freud, q.v., and was originally the outgrowth of his observations of neurotics. Frequently the term is used synonymously with freudianism, but more commonly it is used for a more extensive system of psychological fact and theory applying both to normal and abnormal groups.

Psychoanalysis is based upon the theory that abnormal phenomena are caused by repression of painful or undesirable past experiences that, although totally forgotten, later manifest themselves in various abnormal ways. Psychoanalysis includes a study of the ego in relationship to reality, and more particularly the herd and the conflicting goals so created. This conflict is solved by repressing one component. This repressed or censored emotion-laden complex of ideas exists in the subconscious, manifesting itself in the hidden content of dreams, in neuroses, and tension states. Anger outbursts, rationalization of unfair attitudes, or slips of the tongue occur because the patient is unaware of the influence of the subconscious.

Repressed material is largely sexual, and the peculiar conditioning of the patient is determined chiefly by emotional experiences of earlier years. Reactions of inferiority may result in a compensatory reaction of goodness or ambition. Sublimation is the escape of creative interest on levels not socially taboo. Therefore, psychoanalysis makes an effort to bring forgotten memories into the conscious mind. The patient thus is enabled to view the occurrence in its true perspective, and to minimize its harm.

In addition to the freudian method, other schools of thought or disciplines utilized in analysis of the psyche include analytical psychology (Jung), psychobiology (Meyer), and individual psychology (Adler).

psychoanalyst (sī″kō-ăn′ă-list) [Gr. *psyche*, mind, + *analysis*, a dissolving]. One who practices psychoanalysis.

psychobiology (sī″kō-bī-ŏl′ō-jē) [″ + *bios*, life, + *logos*, word, reason]. 1. The study of the biology of the psyche, including the anatomy, physiology, and pathology of the mind. SYN: *biopsychology*. 2. A method of psychoanalysis employing distributive analysis, which includes a study of all mental and physical factors involved in the growth and development of an individual.

p., objective. Psychobiology in which special emphasis is placed on the relationship of the individual to his or her environment.

psychocatharsis (sī″kō-kă-thăr′sĭs) [″ + *katharsis*, purification]. The bringing of so-called traumatic experiences and their affective associations into consciousness by interview, hypnosis, or by use of drugs such as sodium amytal. SEE: *catharsis.*

psychochrome (sī′kō-krōm) [″ + *chroma*, color]. Color impression resulting from sensory stimulation of a part other than the visual organ.

psychochromesthesia (sī″kō-krōm″ĕs-thē′zē-ä) [″ + ″ + *aisthesis*, sensation]. Color sensation produced by the stimulus of a sense organ other than that of vision. SEE: *pseudochromesthesia.*

psychocoma (sī″kō-kō′mä) [″ + *koma*, a deep sleep]. Condition of mental stupor.

psychocortical (sī″kō-kor′tĭ-kăl) [″ + L. *cortex*, rind]. Pert. to the cerebral cortex as the seat of sensory, motor, and psychic functions.

psychodiagnosis (sī″kō-dī″ăg-nō′sĭs) [″ + *diagignoskein*, to discern]. Use of psychological tests to assist in diagnosing diseases, esp. mental illness.

psychodiagnostics (sī″kō-dī″ăg-nŏs′tĭks). Use of psychological testing as an aid in diagnosing mental disorders.

Psychodidae (sī″kŏd′ĭ-dē). A family of the order Diptera, characterized by minute size, long legs, and hairy bodies and wings. Includes moth flies, owl midges, and sandflies. SEE: *Phlebotomus.*

psychodometry (sī″kō-dŏm′ĕ-trē) [″ + *hodos*, way, + *metron*, measure]. Measurement of rate of mental activity.

psychodrama (sī″kō-dräm′ä) [″ + L. *drama*, drama]. A form of group psychotherapy. Patients act out assigned roles and, in so doing, are able to gain insight into their own mental disturbances.

psychodynamics (sī″kō-dī-năm′ĭks) [″ + *dynamis*, power]. The scientific study of mental action or force.

psychogalvanic reflex. Variation in the electrical resistance of the skin in response to emotional stimuli.

psychogalvanometer (sī″kō-găl″vă-nŏm′ĕ-tĕr) [″ + *galvanism* + Gr. *metron*, measure]. Device for determining the changes in the electrical resistance of the skin in response to emotional stimuli.

psychogenesis (sī″kō-jĕn′ĕ-sĭs) [″ + *genesis*, generation, birth]. 1. The origin and development of mind; the formation of mental traits. 2. Origin within the mind or psyche.

psychogenetic (sī″kō-jĕn-ĕt′ĭk). 1. Originating in the mind, as a disease. 2. Concerning formation of mental traits.

psychogenic (sī-kō-jĕn′ĭk) [″ + *gennan*, to produce]. 1. Of mental origin. 2. Concerning the development of the mind. SYN: *psy-*

chogenetic.

psychogenic fever. SEE: *fever, factitious; fever, psychogenic.*

psychogenic vomiting. Occasional or persistent vomiting associated with severe emotional stress. Each person has the potential for this reaction to emotional stress, but the threshold varies from one person to another.

psychogeriatric. Concerning elderly patients who have a psychiatric disorder.

psychogeusic (sī″kō-gū′sĭk) [″ + *geusis,* taste]. Pert. to perception of taste.

psychogram (sī′kō-grăm) [Gr. *psyche,* mind, + *gramma,* something written]. A subjective visualization of a mental concept.

psychograph (sī′kō-grăf) [″ + *graphein,* to write]. 1. A chart that lists personality traits. 2. A history of the personality of an individual.

psychokinesis (sī″kō-kĭ-nē′sĭs) [″ + *kinesis,* movement]. 1. Explosive or impulsive maniacal action caused by defective inhibition. 2. In parapsychology, claimed or alleged influence exerted on a physical object by a subject without any intermediate physical energy or instrumentation. SEE: *paranormal; psi phenomena.*

psycholagny (sī″kō-lăg′nē) [″ + *lagneia,* lust]. Sexual excitation brought about by mental imagery; psychic or mental masturbation.

psycholinguistics (sī″kō-lĭng-gwĭs′tĭks). The study of linguistics as it relates to human behavior.

psychological (sī″kō-lŏj′ĭ-kăl) [″ + *logos,* word, reason]. Pert. to study of the mind in all of its relationships, normal and abnormal.

psychologist (sī-kŏl′ō-jĭst). One who is trained in methods of psychological analysis, therapy, and research.

psychology (sī-kŏl′ō-jē) [″ + *logos,* word, reason]. The science dealing with mental processes, both normal and abnormal, and their effects upon behavior. There are two main approaches to the study: introspective, looking inward or self-examination of one's own mental processes, and objective, i.e., studying the minds of others. SEE: words beginning with *psych-.*

    p., abnormal. The study of deviational behavior and the mental phenomena associated with such.

    p., analytic. Psychoanalysis based on the concepts of Carl Jung, de-emphasizing sexual factors in motivation and emphasizing the "collective unconscious" and "psychological types" (introvert and extrovert).

    p., animal. The study of animal behavior.

    p., applied. The application of the principles of psychology to special fields, such as clinical, industrial, educational, nursing, or pastoral applications.

    p., clinical. The branch of psychology concerned with diagnosing and treating mental disorders.

    p., criminal. The branch of psychology concerned with the behavior and therapy of criminals.

    p., dynamic. Psychology of motivation; that which seeks the causes of mental phenomena.

    p., experimental. The study of mental acts by tests and experiments.

    p., genetic. The branch of psychology concerned with the evolution of and inheritance of psychological characteristics.

    p., gestalt. Psychology that emphasizes the wholeness of psychological processes and behavior, maintaining that such cannot be adequately explained by breaking down into constituent parts.

    p., individual. A system of psychological thinking developed by Alfred Adler in which an individual is regarded as having three life goals: physical security, sexual satisfaction, and social integration. Self-evaluations lead to feelings of inferiority and inadequacy, which often lead to overcompensation or a striving for superiority.

    p., physiologic. Psychology that deals with the structure and function of the nervous system and other bodily organs and their relationship to behavior.

    p., social. The branch of psychology concerned with study of groups and their influence on the individual's actions and mental processes.

psychometrician (sī″kō-mĕ-trĭsh′ăn) [Gr. *psyche,* mind, + *metron,* measure]. 1. A person skilled in psychometry, q.v. 2. A person skilled in the application of statistical analysis to psychological data.

psychometry (sī-kŏm′ĕ-trē) [″ + *metron,* measure]. The measurement of psychological variables, such as intelligence, aptitude, behavior, and emotional reactions.

psychomotor (sī″kō-mō′tor) [″ + L. *motor,* a mover]. Concerning or causing physical activity associated with mental processes.

psychomotor and physical development of infant. It is important that all concerned with the care of the newborn through infancy have guidelines for comparing the growth and development of an individual with normal standards. The charts provided will be of assistance in this.

    Certain activities of infants serve as general indicators of normal psychomotor development. The average ages for certain of these activities are shown in the accompa-

psychomotor and physical
development of infant   1629   psychomotor and physical
development of infant

Psychomotor and Physical Development
Birth to One Year

		Physical Development			
		Length Range		Weight Range	
		in.	cm	lb	kg
Birth	boys	$18\frac{1}{4}-21\frac{1}{2}$	46.4–54.4	$5\frac{1}{2}-9\frac{1}{4}$	2.54–4.15
	girls	$17\frac{3}{4}-20\frac{3}{4}$	45.4–52.9	$5\frac{1}{4}-8\frac{1}{2}$	2.36–3.81
1 Month	boys	$19\frac{3}{4}-23$	50.4–58.6	$7-11\frac{3}{4}$	3.16–5.38
	girls	$19\frac{1}{4}-22\frac{1}{2}$	49.2–56.9	$6\frac{1}{2}-10\frac{3}{4}$	2.97–4.92
3 Months	boys	$22\frac{1}{4}-25\frac{3}{4}$	56.7–65.4	$9\frac{3}{4}-16\frac{1}{4}$	4.43–7.37
	girls	$21\frac{3}{4}-25$	55.4–63.4	$9\frac{1}{4}-14\frac{3}{4}$	4.18–6.74
6 Months	boys	$25-28\frac{1}{2}$	63.4–72.3	$13\frac{3}{4}-20\frac{3}{4}$	6.20–9.46
	girls	$24\frac{1}{4}-27\frac{3}{4}$	61.8–70.2	$12\frac{3}{4}-19\frac{1}{4}$	5.79–8.73
9 Months	boys	$26\frac{3}{4}-30\frac{1}{4}$	68.0–77.1	$16\frac{1}{2}-24$	7.52–10.93
	girls	$26-29\frac{1}{2}$	66.1–75.0	$15\frac{1}{2}-22\frac{1}{2}$	7.0–10.17
12 Months	boys	$28\frac{1}{4}-32$	71.7–81.2	$18\frac{1}{2}-26\frac{1}{2}$	8.43–11.99
	girls	$27\frac{1}{2}-31\frac{1}{4}$	69.8–79.1	$17\frac{1}{4}-24\frac{3}{4}$	7.84–11.24

Psychomotor Development

Birth Through 1st Month — Ability to suck, swallow, gag, cry, and maintain eye contact with a person. The head needs to be supported. Loud noises may cause a startle reflex.

2nd Month — May turn to either side when on their backs; will follow moving objects; able to lift head but not for a sustained period; begin to smile, frown, and turn away.

3rd Month — Greater movement and vocal response to stimuli; notice own hands and suck on them; head will be steady while in a supported position.

4th and 5th Months — Able to lift head higher when lying on stomach; will reach for objects and may be able to encircle a bottle with both hands; may drool a lot; attempt to put all kinds of objects in mouth.

6th–9th Month — Develop ability to grasp and pick up food; are able to pull themselves up to a sitting position and eventually will crawl; they begin to make noises that sound like words and to recognize certain words; will play peek-a-boo.

9th–11th Month — Develop ability to handle food and to drink from a cup; may imitate sounds and say certain words; crawl by pulling body along with arms, and pull themselves to a standing position; they will point at objects and throw things; they want to feed themselves and to help with dressing and undressing; they will walk while holding a person's hand.

12th Month — Can eat food alone and drink from a cup with assistance; able to move around easily, and crawl up stairs, and out of crib.

nying table.

Appearance and loss of certain reflexes and reactions: The Moro reflex is present at birth and disappears by 3 months; the stepping and placing reflexes are present at birth and are no longer obtainable by 6 weeks; the tonic neck reflex is usually present at 2 months and is gone by 6 months; neck righting appears at 4 to 6 months and is gone by 24 months; the parachute reaction is present at 9 months and persists; sucking and rooting are present at birth and are usually gone by 4 months if tested while awake and by 7 months if tested while the infant is asleep; palmar grasp is present from birth to 6 months; plantar grasp is present from birth to 10 months. SEE: *arousal level.*

psychomotor epilepsy. Epilepsy, temporal lobe, q.v.

psychomotor retardation. A generalized slowing of physical and mental reactions; seen frequently in depression.

psychoneuroimmunology. The study of the relationships that exist between the central nervous system, autonomic nervous sytem, endocrine system and immune system. Social scientists use the data gathered from studies in psychoneuroimmunology as they examine the impact of psychosocial stressors and the psychophysiologic stress response on the development of disease.

psychoneurosis (sī″kō-nū-rō′sĭs) [″ + *neuron,* sinew, + *osis,* condition]. Emotional maladaptation due to unresolved unconscious conflicts. This leads to disturbances in thought, feelings, attitudes, and behavior. There is little, if any, loss of contact with reality, but the patient's effectiveness in performing his or her usual responsibilities is handicapped. Psychoneurosis is a major category in classifying mental illness and is classified according to the symptoms that predominate. The patient usually recognizes that the altered thoughts and feelings are abnormal and indeed unwelcome. This is in contrast to the patient with a psychosis or character disorder. SYN: *neurosis.*

    p., anxiety reaction. Anxiety with apprehension out of proportion to any obvious external cause. SEE: *anxiety neurosis.*

    p., conversion reaction. Psychoneurosis in which unacceptable unconscious impulses are converted into hysterical somatic symptoms. Although the symptoms have a specific symbolic meaning to the patient, their interpretation is different in each individual.

    p., depressive reaction. Psychoneurosis marked by depression out of proportion to any obvious cause.

    p., dissociated reaction. Psychoneurosis characterized by dissociated behavior such as amnesia, fugue, sleepwalking, and dream states. Important to differentiate from schizophrenia, q.v.

    p., obsessive-compulsive reaction. Persistent, repetitive impulses to perform certain acts or rituals, such as handwashing, touching something, or counting.

    p., phobic reaction. Irrational fear of any of a variety of situations, persons, or objects.

psychoneurotic (sī″kō-nū-rŏt′ĭk) [Gr. *psyche,* mind, + *neuron,* sinew]. 1. Pert. to a functional disorder of mental origin. 2.

A person suffering from a psychoneurosis.

psychopath (sī′kō-păth) [″ + *pathos,* disease, suffering]. Individual with a psychopathic personality. SEE: *personality, psychopathic.*

psychopathia. Psychopathy.

psychopathic (sī″kō-păth′ĭk). 1. Concerning or characterized by a mental disorder. 2. Concerning treatment of mental disorders. 3. Abnormal.

psychopathology (sī″kō-păth-ŏl′ō-jē) [″ + *pathos,* disease, suffering + *logos,* word, reason]. The study of the causes and nature of mental disease or abnormal behavior.

psychopathy (sī-kŏp′ă-thē). Any mental disease, esp. one associated with defective character or personality. SEE: *personality, psychopathic.*

psychopharmacology (sī″kō-făr″mă-kŏl′ō-jē). The science of drugs having an effect on psychomotor behavior and emotional states.

psychophysical (sī″kō-fĭz′ĭ-kăl) [″ + *physikos,* natural]. Concerning the relationship of the physical and the mental. SEE: *childbirth, natural; psychoprophylactic childbirth.*

psychophysics (sī″kō-fĭz′ĭks). 1. The study of mental processes in relationship to physical processes. 2. The study of stimuli in relationship to the effects they produce.

psychophysiologic (sī″kō-fĭz-ē-ō-lŏj′ĭk). Pert. to psychophysiology, q.v.

psychophysiologic disorders. Term applied to a large number of disorders of organs and viscera innervated by the autonomic nervous system in which emotional factors are a primary contributing factor. Formerly called psychosomatic disease or disorder.

psychophysiology (sī″kō-fĭz″ē-ŏl′ō-jē). Physiology of the mind; science of the correlation of body and mind.

psychoplegic (sī″kō-plē′jĭk) [″ + *plege,* a stroke]. An agent reducing excitability of the mental processes.

psychoprophylactic preparation for childbirth. Mental and physical training of the mother in preparation for delivery. The goals of the preparation are the dispelling of the fear of pain and the delivery of a healthy child. SEE: *childbirth, natural; childbirth, prepared; Lamaze technique or method.*

psychoprophylaxis (sī″kō-prō″fĭ-lăk′sĭs). In obstetrics, a method of mental and physical preparation for natural childbirth. SEE: *childbirth, natural; Lamaze technique or method.*

psychorhythmia (sī″kō-rĭth′mē-ă) [″ + *rhythmos,* rhythm]. Mental condition in which involuntary repetition of previous voluntary actions occurs.

psychorrhea (sī″kō-rē′ă) [″ + *rhoia*, flow]. Mental condition characterized by an incoherent stream of thought resulting in vague and often bizarre theories and ideas.

psychosensory (sī″kō-sĕn′sō-rē) [″ + L. *sensorius*, organ of sensation]. 1. Understanding and interpreting sensory stimuli. 2. Concerning perceptions not arising in sensory organs, as hallucinations.

psychosexual (sī″kō-sĕks′ū-ăl) [Gr. *psyche*, soul, mind, + L. *sexus*, sex]. Concerning the emotional components of sexual instinct.

psychosexual development. Evolution of personality through infantile and pregenital periods to sexual maturity.

psychosexual disorders. Disorders of sexual function not due to organic causes. Included are gender identity disorders, transsexualism, paraphilias, transvestism, zoophilia, pedophilia, exhibitionism, voyeurism, and sexual sadism.

psychosine (sī′kō-sēn). A cerebroside present in brain tissue.

psychosis (sī-kō′sĭs) [″ + *osis*, condition] (pl. *psychoses*). A term formerly applied to any mental disorder, but now generally restricted to those disturbances of such magnitude that there is personality disintegration and loss of contact with reality. The disturbances are of psychogenic origin, or without clearly defined physical cause or structural change in the brain. They usually are characterized by delusions and hallucination, and hospitalization generally is required.

This condition is manifest in the behavior, emotional reaction, and ideation of the patient, who fails to mirror reality as it is, reacts erroneously to it, and builds up false concepts regarding it. Behavior responses are peculiar, abnormal, inefficient, or definitely antisocial.

All this does not include amentia because defective intelligence merely lessens comprehension of reality but does not distort it. The psychopathic personality reacts badly because of intrinsic emotional differences playing upon an undistorted world of reality.

p., alcoholic. Psychosis resulting from chronic alcoholism. SEE: *delirium tremens; Korsakoff's syndrome.*

p., depressive. Psychosis characterized by extreme depression, melancholia, and feelings of unworthiness.

p., drug. Psychosis caused by ingestion of a drug.

p., exhaustion. Acute state of confusion and delirium that occurs in relation to extreme fatigue, chronic illness, prolonged sleeplessness, or tension.

p., functional. Psychosis that is not due to an organic disease.

p., gestational. Psychosis that occurs during pregnancy.

p., involutional. Psychosis occurring during involutional period of bodily and intellectual decline.

p., Korsakoff's. Korsakoff's syndrome, q.v.

p., manic-depressive. Ordinarily a series of periods of psychotic depression or excessive well-being, appearing in any sequence and alternating with longer periods of relative normalcy. Though intensity may vary greatly, the manic shows an elated though unstable mood, a flight of ideas, and great physical activity. In primary depression, the victim finds all exertion exhausting; there is difficulty in thinking or acting, and the victim is very unhappy. SYN: *bipolar affective disorder.*

p., organic. Psychosis resulting from a pathological condition of the central nervous system, such as paresis, q.v.

p., polyneuritic. Korsakoff's syndrome, q.v.

p., postinfectious. Psychosis following an infectious disease such as meningitis, pneumonia, typhoid fever.

p., postpartum. Psychosis occurring in the period following childbirth. SEE: *postpartum psychosis.*

p., puerperal. Postpartum psychosis, q.v.

p., senile. Psychosis in which onset occurs in an aged individual.

p., situational. Psychosis due to excessive stress in an unbearable environmental situation.

p., toxic. Psychosis resulting from toxic agents.

p., traumatic. Psychosis resulting from head injuries and belonging to the organic group.

psychosocial (sī″kō-sō′shăl). Related to both psychological and social factors.

psychosomatic (sī″kō-sō-măt′ĭk) [Gr. *psyche*, mind, + *soma*, body]. Pert. to the relationship of the mind and body.

Disorders that have a physiological component but are thought to originate in the emotional state of the patient are termed psychosomatic. When so used, the impression is created that the mind and body are separate entities and that a disease may be purely somatic in its effect or entirely emotional. This partitioning of the human being is not possible; thus no disease is limited to only the mind or the body. A complex interaction is always present even though in specific instances a disease might on superficial examination appear to involve only the

Psychotherapeutic Drugs and Agents

Indication	Drugs	Clinical Use	Note
Antianxiety	Benzodiazepines Sedatives/hypnotics	Anxiety Nervousness Psychoneuroses Insomnia	Patients may become tolerant to the drug or abuse the drug and become addicted. Use may delay definitive therapy.
Antidepressants	Tricyclic compounds Monoamine oxidase inhibitors Lithium carbonate (not to be used in patients on a salt-free diet) Electroconvulsive therapy	Depression	Patients must be closely monitored with respect to the possibility of self-destruction (suicide) while waiting for medicines to have their effect.
Antipsychotics	Phenothiazines (chlorpromazine, thioridazine, trifluoperazine) Thioxanthenes Butyrophenones Dihydroindolone Dibenzoxazepine	Schizophrenic reactions Excitement	May have long-term undesired side effects on the autonomic nervous system and extrapyramidal tract.

body or the mind. SEE: *psychophysiologic disorders.*

psychosomatic medicine. Branch of medicine that recognizes the importance of mind-body interrelationships in all illnesses and in which therapy and management are based on this fact.

psychosurgery (sī″kō-sur′jĕr-ē) [″ + L. *chirurgia,* surgery]. Surgical intervention for mental disorders, esp. for certain types of violent or antisocial behavior.

psychotechnics (sī″kō-tĕk′nĭks) [″ + *techne,* art]. Use of psychological methods in the study of economic and social problems.

psychotherapeutic drugs. Drugs that are used because of their effects in ameliorating the principal symptoms that occur in mentally disturbed persons, such as anxiety, depression, and psychosis. SEE: table.

psychotherapy (sī-kō-thĕr′ă-pē) [Gr. *psyche,* mind, + *therapeia,* treatment]. A method of treating disease, esp. nervous disorders, by mental means rather than physical.

Ex.: suggestion, re-education, hypnotism, psychoanalytic therapy.

psychotic (sī-kŏt′ĭk). Pert. to or affected by psychosis.

psychotogenic (sī-kŏt″ō-jĕn′ĭk) [″ + *gen-*

nan, to produce]. Producing a psychosis, usually temporary and due to certain powerful drugs.

psychotomimetic (sī-kŏt″ō-mĭ-mĕ′tĭk) [″ + *mimetikos,* imitative]. A hallucinogen producing weird illusions.

psychotropic drugs [″ + *trope,* a turning]. Drugs that affect psychic function, behavior, or experience. Many drugs can be classed as being intentionally psychotropic, but many other drugs also occasionally may produce undesired psychotropic side effects.

psychro- [Gr. *psychros,* cold]. Combining form concerning cold.

psychroalgia (sī″krō-ăl′jē-ă) [Gr. *psychros,* cold, + *algos,* pain]. Painful sensation of cold.

psychroesthesia (sī″krō-ĕs-thē′zē-ă) [″ + *aisthesis,* sensation]. A sensation of cold in a part of the body, although it is warm.

psychrometer (sī-krŏm′ĕ-tĕr) [″ + *metron,* measure]. Device for measuring relative humidity of the atmosphere. Calculations are made utilizing the readings of two thermometers, one with a dry bulb and one with a wet bulb.

psychrophilic (sī-krō-fĭl′ĭk) [″ + *philein,*

to love]. Preferring cold, as bacteria that thrive at low temperatures, between 0° and 30°C (32° and 86°F).

psychrophobia (sī-krō-fō′bē-ă) [″ + *phobos*, fear]. Abnormal aversion or sensitiveness to cold.

psychrophore (sī′krō-for) [″ + *phorein*, to carry]. A double-lumen catheter for applying cold to the urethra or any canal.

psychrotherapy (sī″krō-thěr′ă-pē) [″ + *therapeia*, treatment]. Treatment of disease by use of cold.

psyllium seed (sĭl′ē-ŭm). The dried ripe seed of the psyllium plant, grown in France, Spain, and India. Used as a mild laxative.

PT. *prothrombin time; physical therapist.*

Pt. Chem. symb. for the element platinum.

pt. *pint.*

PTA. *plasma thromboplastin antecedent; physical therapy assistant.*

ptarmic (tăr′mĭk) [Gr. *ptarmikos*, causing to sneeze]. 1. Causing sneezing. 2. Agent that causes sneezing. SYN: *sternutatory.*

ptarmus (tar′mŭs). Spasmodic sneezing.

PTC. *plasma thromboplastin component; phenylthiocarbamide; percutaneous transhepatic cholangiography.*

PTCA. *percutaneous transluminal coronary angioplasty.*

pterion (tē′rē-ŏn) [Gr. *pteron*, wing]. Point of suture of frontal, parietal, temporal, and sphenoid bones.

pternalgia (tĕr-năl′jē-ă) [Gr. *pterna*, heel, + *algos*, pain]. Pain in the heel.

pteroylglutamic acid. Folic acid.

pterygium (tĕr-ĭj′ē-ŭm) [Gr. *pterygion*, wing]. Triangular thickening of bulbar conjunctiva extending from inner canthus to border of the cornea with apex toward pupil.

    p. colli. A congenital band of fascia extending from the mastoid process of the temporal bone to the clavicle.

    p., progressive. Stage in which the growth extends toward center of cornea.

pterygoid (tĕr′ĭ-goyd) [Gr. *pterygoeides*]. Wing shaped. SYN: *alate.*

pterygoid hamulus. A small bony projection, just medial to the pterygoid process, which serves as attachment for the tensor veli palatini muscle.

pterygoid process. One of two large processes of the sphenoid bone extending downward from the junction of the body and great wings, each consisting of lateral and medial pterygoid plates.

pterygomandibular (tĕr″ĭ-gō-măn-dĭb′ū-lăr) [″ + L. *mandibula*, lower jawbone]. Concerning the pterygoid process of the sphenoid bone and mandible.

pterygomaxillary (tĕr″ĭ-gō-măk′sĭ-lĕr″ē) [″ + L. *maxillaris*, upper jaw]. Concerning the pterygoid process and upper jaw.

pterygopalatine (tĕr″ĭ-gō-păl′ă-tĭn) [″ + L. *palatinus*, palate]. Rel. to the pterygoid process and the palate bone.

PTFE. *polytetrafluoroethylene* (Teflon).

PTH. *parathyroid hormone.*

ptilosis (tĭ-lō′sĭs) [Gr.]. Loss of eyelashes.

ptomaine (tō′mān, tō-mān′) [Gr. *ptoma*, dead body]. One of a class of nitrogenous organic bases formed in the action of putrefactive bacteria on proteins and amino acids.

    Ex.: cadaverine, $NH_2(CH_2)_5NH_2$.

ptosed (tōst). Having ptosis.

ptosis (tō′sĭs) [Gr. *ptosis*, a dropping]. Dropping or drooping of an organ or part, as the upper eyelid from paralysis, or the visceral organs from weakness of the abdominal muscles.

    p., abdominal. Sagging of the transverse colon, sometimes almost to the pelvic floor.

    ETIOL: Obesity or lack of abdominal muscle tone.

    TREAT: A properly adjusted abdominal belt may help. This is contraindicated if the patient shows dependence upon belt instead of exercising and developing abdominal muscles.

    p., morning. Difficulty in raising the eyelids upon awakening.

    p., waking. P., morning, q.v.

ptotic (tŏt′ĭk). Concerning ptosis.

ptyalagogue (tī-ăl′ă-gŏg) [Gr. *ptyalon*, saliva, + *agogos*, leading]. Causing, or that which causes, a flow of saliva. SYN: *sialogogue.*

ptyalectasis (tī″ă-lĕk′tă-sĭs) [″ + *ektasis*, dilation]. Surgical dilation of a salivary duct.

ptyalin (tī′ă-lĭn). A salivary enzyme that hydrolyzes starch and glycogen to maltose and a small amount of glucose. The optimum pH for ptyalin activity is 6.9. SYN: *amylase, salivary.* SEE: *enzyme; ptyalism; saliva.*

ptyalism (tī′ă-lĭzm) [″ + -*ismos*, condition]. Excessive secretion of saliva. SYN: *salivation.* SEE: *xerostomia.*

    ETIOL: May be due to pregnancy, stomatitis, rabies, exophthalmic goiter, menstruation, epilepsy, hysteria, nervous conditions, and gastrointestinal disorders. May be induced by mercury, iodides, pilocarpine, and other drugs.

ptyalith (tī′ă-lĭth) [″ + *lithos*, stone]. A calculus in a salivary gland.

ptyalocele (tī-ăl′ō-sēl) [″ + *kele*, tumor, swelling]. A salivary cystic tumor or cystic dilatation of a salivary duct.

ptyalogenic (tī″ăl-ō-jĕn′ĭk) [Gr. *ptyalon*, saliva, + *gennan*, to produce]. Of salivary origin.

ptyalogogue (tī″ăl′ō-gŏg) [″ + *agogos*, leading]. An agent that causes the flow of saliva. SYN: *sialogogue.*

ptyalography (tī-ăl-ŏg′ră-fē) [″ + *gra-*

phein, to write]. Roentgenography of the salivary glands and ducts. SYN: *sialography.*

ptyalolith (tī′ă-lō-lĭth) [″ + *lithos,* stone]. A salivary concretion.

ptyalolithiasis (tī″ă-lō-lĭ-thī′ă-sĭs). Presence of a concretion in a salivary gland or duct.

ptyalolithotomy (tī″ăl-ō-lĭ-thŏt′ō-mē) [Gr. *ptyalon,* saliva, + *lithos,* stone, + *tome,* incision]. Surgical removal of a concretion from a salivary duct or gland.

ptyaloreaction (tī″ă-lō-rē-ăk′shŭn). A reaction occurring in saliva.

ptyalorrhea (tī″ă-lō-rē′ă) [″ + *rhoia,* flow]. An excessive flow of saliva.

ptyocrinous (tī-ŏk′rĭ-nŭs). A type of glandular secretion in which the contents of the cell are discharged.

ptysis (tī′sĭs) [Gr.]. Spitting; the ejection of saliva from the mouth.

Pu. Chem. symb. for the element plutonium.

pubarche (pū-băr′kē) [L. *puber,* grown up, + Gr. *arche,* beginning]. 1. The beginning of puberty. 2. Beginning development of pubic hair. SEE: *semenarche; thelarche.*

puber (pū′bĕr) [L., grown up]. One at onset of puberty.

puberal (pū′bĕr-ăl) [L. *pubertas,* puberty]. Concerning puberty.

pubertal. Pert. to puberty.

pubertas (pū′bĕr-tăs) [L.]. Puberty.

    p. praecox. Precocious puberty or puberty at an early age.

puberty (pū′bĕr-tē). Period in life at which members of both sexes become functionally capable of reproduction. A period of rapid change occurs between the ages of 13 and 15 in boys and 9 to 16 in girls, ending in the attainment of sexual maturity.

    There is evidence that the onset of puberty is related to a decrease in secretion of the pineal gland.

    p., onset of. *Boys:* Between the ages of 13 and 15, a relatively rapid increase in height and weight occurs with broadening of the shoulders and increase in size of the penis and testicles. Pubic hair and the beard begin to grow. Endocrine and sebaceous gland activity is increased. Nocturnal emissions usually occur. Young boys should be assured that the size of the penis is not related to the degree of masculinity and is not an important factor in experiencing or providing sexual gratification.

    Girls: Between the ages of 9 and 16, a marked increase in growth rate is accompanied by breast enlargement and appearance of pubic hair. Within one to two years after these changes, underarm hair grows and the normal whitish vaginal secretion (physiological leukorrhea) characteristic of the adult female is noticed. Several months later the first menstrual period (menarche) occurs. Each individual will vary somewhat from this schedule. The young girl should be told prior to puberty about menstruation and the technique of menstrual protection through use of perineal pads or tampons. In addition, she should be told that a certain amount of intermenstrual vaginal discharge (leukorrhea) is normal but if the secretion is malodorous or causes irritation of the vulva, a physician should be consulted. SEE: *menstruation.*

    p., precocious. Onset of puberty at an age much earlier than normal. Gonadotropin-releasing hormone (GnRH) has been used to treat this condition.

pubes (pū′bēz) [L., grown up] (sing. *pubis*). 1. Anterior part of innominate bone. SYN: *os pubis* [NA]. 2. The pubic region. 3. [NA] Hair of the pubic region.

pubescence (pū-bĕs′ĕns) [L. *pubescens,* becoming hairy]. 1. Puberty or its approach. 2. Covering of fine, soft hairs on the body. SYN: *lanugo.*

pubescent (pū-bĕs′ĕnt). 1. Reaching puberty. 2. Covered with downy hair.

pubetrotomy (pū″bĕ-trŏt′ō-mē) [NL. *(os) pubis,* bone of the groin, + Gr. *etron,* belly, + *tome,* incision]. Section through the os pubis and lower abdominal wall.

pubic (pū′bĭk) [L. *pubes,* pubic hair]. Concerning the pubes.

pubic bone. The lower anterior part of the innominate bone. SYN: *os pubis* [NA].

pubic hair. Hair over the pubes, which appears at onset of sexual maturity. The distribution is somewhat different in men as compared with women.

pubio-, pubo- [L. *pubes,* pubic hair]. Combining form meaning the pubic hair or the pubic bone or region.

pubiotomy (pū-bē-ŏt′ō-mē) [L. *pubes,* pubic region, + *tome,* incision]. Incision across the pubis in order to enlarge the pelvic passage, facilitating the delivery of the fetus when pelvis is malformed. SYN: *hebosteotomy; hebotomy.*

pubis (pū′bĭs) [NL. *(os) pubis,* bone of the groin] (pl. *pubes*). Pubic bone; os pubis.

public health. The science of providing protection and promotion of community health through organized community effort.

Public Health Service Act. One of the principal laws of Congress giving the authority for federal health activities. First enacted July 1, 1944, it provided a complete codification of all the federal public health laws. Many of the health laws since 1944 have actually been amendments to the PHS act that have revised, extended, or given new authority to the act.

pubococcygeal (pū″bō-kŏk-sĭj′ē-ăl) [″ +

Gr. *kokkyx*, coccyx]. Concerning the pubis and coccyx.

pubofemoral (pū″bō-fĕm′or-ăl) [″ + *femur*, thigh bone]. Pert. to the os pubis and femur.

pubomadesis [L. *pubes*, pubic hair, + Gr. *madesis*, baldness]. Loss of or absent pubic hair.

puboprostatic (pū″bō-prŏs-tăt′ĭk) [″ + Gr. *prostates*, prostate]. Rel. to the os pubis and prostate gland.

puborectal (pū″bō-rĕk′tăl) [″ + *rectus*, straight]. Concerning the pubis and rectum.

pubovaginal device. Apparatus that is fitted for use in the vagina to help prevent urinary incontinence.

pubovesical (pū″bō-vĕs′ĭ-kl) [″ + *vesiculus*, a little sac]. Pert. to the os pubis and bladder.

pudenda (pū-dĕn′dă) [L.] (sing. *pudendum*). The external genitalia, esp. of the female. SYN: *vulva*.

pudendagra (pū″dĕn-dăg′ră) [″ + Gr. *agra*, seizure]. Pain in the external genitals.

pudendal (pū-dĕn′dăl) [L. *pudenda*, external genitals]. Rel. to the external genitals of the female. SYN: *pudic*.

pudendum (pū-dĕn′dŭm) [L.] (pl. *pudenda*). The external genitals, esp. those of the female. SYN: *vulva*.

   p. femininum. Vulva, q.v.

   p. muliebre. External genitals of the female.

pudic (pū′dĭk) [L. *pudicus*, modest]. Concerning external female genitalia. SYN: *pudendal*.

puerile (pū′ĕ-rĭl) [L. *puerilis*]. Concerning a child; childlike.

puerilism (pū′ĕr-ĭl-ĭzm) [″ + Gr. *-ismos*, condition]. Childishness; second childhood.

puerpera (pū-ĕr′pĕr-ă) [L. *puer*, child, + *parere*, to bring forth, to bear]. A woman during puerperium.

puerperal (pū-ĕr′pĕr-ăl) [L. *puerperalis*]. Concerning puerperium.

puerperal eclampsia. Convulsions and eclampsia during puerperium.

puerperal fever. Septicemia following childbirth. SYN: *childbed fever; puerperal sepsis.*

puerperalism (pū-ĕr′pĕr-ăl-ĭzm) [L. *puer*, child, + *parere*, to bring forth, to bear, + Gr. *-ismos*, condition]. Pathological condition accompanying childbirth.

puerperal period. Period immediately following childbirth.

puerperal sepsis. Any infection of the genital tract occurring during the puerperium or as a complication of abortion. This disease is presumed to be present when the temperature is 38°C (100.4°F) on any two consecutive days, exclusive of the first 24 hours postpartum, if no other causes of fever are apparent. The causative organisms, which are usually streptococci or clostridia, are introduced from the outside in the majority of cases. The establishment of careful techniques of asepsis and hygiene in maternity wards has effectively reduced the importance of this disease as a cause of death in the puerperium.

   DIAG: Made on the basis of clinical findings consistent with infection of the genital tract, including fever and pain and tenderness of the lower abdominal area and genital tract.

   TREAT: Appropriate antibiotic, incision and drainage if abscess forms, and supportive therapy.

puerperant (pū-ĕr′pĕr-ănt). A woman in labor, or one who has recently given birth.

puerperium (pū″ĕr-pē′rē-ŭm) [L.]. The period of 42 days following childbirth and expulsion of the placenta and membranes. The generative organs usually return to normal during this time.

puerperous (pū-ĕr′pĕr-ŭs) [″ + *parere*, to bring forth, to bear]. In the period following childbirth. SYN: *puerperal.*

PUFA. *polyunsaturated fatty acids.* SEE: *acid, fatty.*

puff. A soft, short, blowing sound heard on auscultation.

Pulex (pū′lĕks) [L., flea]. A genus of fleas belonging to the order Siphonaptera.

   P. irritans. The human flea, which also infests dogs, hogs, and other mammals. May serve as intermediate host of the tapeworms *Dipylidium caninum* and *Hymenolepis diminuta.* SEE: *flea.*

pulicatio (pū″lĭ-kā′tē-ō). Infested with fleas.

Pulicidae (pū-lĭs′ĭ-dē). A family of fleas belonging to the order Siphonaptera. Pulicidae includes the genera *Pulex, Echidnophaga, Ctenocephalides,* and *Xenopsylla.* SEE: *flea.*

pulicide (pū′lĭ-sīd) [L. *pulex*, flea, + *caedere*, to kill]. An agent that kills fleas.

pullulate (pŭl″ū-lāt) [L. *pullulare*, to sprout]. To bud or germinate.

pullulation (pŭl″ū-lā′shŭn). The act of budding or germinating, as seen in yeast plant.

pulmo- (pŭl′mō-, pool′mō-) [L. *pulmo*, lung]. Combining form meaning lung.

pulmoaortic (pŭl″mō-ā-or′tĭk) [″ + Gr. *aorte*, aorta]. 1. Concerning the lungs and the aorta. 2. Rel. to the pulmonary artery and aorta.

pulmometer (pŭl-mŏm′ĕ-tĕr) [″ + Gr. *metron*, measure]. Device for measuring lung capacity. SYN: *spirometer.*

pulmometry (pŭl-mŏm′ĕ-trē). Determination of capacity of the lungs.

pulmonary (pŭl′mō-nĕ-rē) [L. *pulmonarius*]. Concerning or involving the lungs.

pulmonary alveolar proteinosis. Disease of unknown cause in which eosinophilic material is deposited in the alveoli. Principal symptom is dyspnea. Death from pulmonary insufficiency may occur, but complete recovery has been observed. There is no specific treatment, but general supportive measures including antibiotics and bronchopulmonary lavage have helped. SEE: *bronchoalveolar lavage.*

In about 25% of cases the disease will clear spontaneously, but in the majority of untreated cases the disease is progressive and leads to respiratory failure.

pulmonary arterial webs. Weblike deformities seen in pulmonary angiograms at the site of previous pulmonary thromboembolism.

pulmonary artery. The artery leading from the right ventricle of the heart to the lungs.

pulmonary artery wedge pressure. ABBR: PAWP. Pressure measured in the pulmonary artery at its capillary end. The catheter is positioned in the pulmonary artery, and the distal portion of the catheter is isolated from pressure behind it in the artery by inflating a balloon with air. This allows the catheter to float into a wedged position, and permits transmission of pressures ahead of the catheter (in the pulmonary capillary bed) by the transducer. Since no valve is present between this location and the left atrium, the measurement reflects left atrial pressure, and, in the presence of a competent mitral valve, the measurement provides an indication of left ventricular end-diastolic pressure. The balloon is then passively deflated, allowing the catheter to drift back into the main pulmonary artery where it measures pulmonary artery forward pressure. SYN: *wedge pressure.* SEE: *Swan-Ganz catheter.*

NURSING IMPLICATIONS: Prepare and set up transducer equipment to monitor pulmonary artery pressure and PAWP alternately, following agency protocol and manufacturer's instructions. Balance and calibrate transducer as required (every 4 to 8 hours). Monitor hemodynamic status and document findings, including pulmonary artery pressure (normally 20 to 30 mm Hg systolic and 8 to 12 mm Hg diastolic), every hour or as directed. To measure pulmonary capillary wedge pressure (PCWP), every 1 to 4 hours as directed, inflate balloon with 0.75 to 1.5 cc of air depending on balloon size (never inflate balloon with fluid), watching for change in wave form that indicates wedging. Assess for balloon rupture (lack of resistance on inflation, with absence of wedging). If this occurs, discontinue wedging procedure (concern for air embolism) and manage therapy based on pulmonary artery diastolic pressures. Read and document PCWP (normally 4 to 12 mm Hg). Correlate to clinical findings and other hemodynamic values, and report abnormal findings as directed. Remove syringe and permit passive deflation of balloon, observing for reappearance of pulmonary artery pressure wave-form. If balloon remains inflated, patient is at risk for pulmonary artery necrosis. Position on right side, and encourage to take deep breaths and cough as you mobilize the right arm. Notify physician if balloon remains wedged. Adjust fluid volume and diuretic therapy based on PCWP and other values as prescribed.

pulmonary circulation. Passage of blood from the heart to the lungs for purification and the return to the heart. The blood flows from the right cardiac ventricle through to the lungs, there to be oxygenated, then back to the left cardiac atrium. SEE: *circulation, pulmonary; circulation, coronary,* for illus.

pulmonary edema. Lung, edema of, q.v.

pulmonary embolism. Embolism, pulmonary, q.v.

pulmonary emphysema. SEE: *emphysema* (def. 2).

pulmonary function tests. A number of different tests used to determine the ability of the lungs to exchange oxygen and carbon dioxide. These are done by measuring the amount of air that can be maximally exhaled after a maximum inspiration and the time required for that expiration; and by determining the ability of the alveolar capillary membrane to transport oxygen into the blood and carbon dioxide from the blood into the expired air. SEE: FEV_1.

pulmonary insufficiency. Failure of the pulmonary valve to close properly.

pulmonary mucociliary clearance. The removal of inhaled particles, endogenous cellular debris, and excessive secretions from the tracheobronchial tree by the action of the ciliated cells that live in the respiratory tract. The cilia of these cells beat and are therefore able to propel mucus and debris upward and out of the tracheobronchial tree. This action is one of the most important defenses of the respiratory tract.

pulmonary stenosis. Narrowing of the opening into the pulmonary artery from the right cardiac ventricle.

pulmonary surfactant. A phospholipid substance important in controlling the surface tension of the air-liquid emulsion that is present in the lungs. Abnormalities in this surfactant have been noted in prematurity, respiratory distress syndrome, and pulmonary edema.

pulmonary valve. The valve between the

right ventricle and the opening into the pulmonary artery.

pulmonary vein. The vein draining the lungs and returning the blood to the left atrium of the heart.

pulmonectomy (pŭl″mō-nĕk′tō-mē) [L. *pulmonis*, lung, + Gr. *ektome*, excision]. Removal of part or all of a lung's tissue. SYN: *pneumonectomy.*

pulmonic (pŭl-mŏn′ĭk). 1. Concerning the lungs. 2. Concerning the pulmonary artery.

pulmonitis (pŭl-mō-nī′tĭs) [″ + Gr. *itis*, inflammation]. Inflamed condition of the lung. SYN: *pneumonia.*

pulmotor (pŭl′mō-tor) [″ + *motor*, mover]. Apparatus for inducing artificial respiration by forcing air or oxygen into the lungs.

pulp [L. *pulpa*, flesh]. 1. The soft part of fruit. 2. The soft part of an organ. 3. Mass of partly digested food passed from stomach to duodenum. SYN: *chyme.* 4. In dentistry, the soft vascular portion of the center of a tooth.

   p., coronal. That portion of the dental pulp in the crown of the pulp cavity.

   p., dead. Devitalized or necrotic dental pulp.

   p., dental. The connective tissues that fill the pulp cavity enclosed by dentin of the tooth; it includes a vascular and nerve network, a peripheral layer of odontoblasts involved with dentin formation, and other cellular and fibrous components.

   p., devitalized. A dead or necrotic dental pulp as indicated by a vitalometer used for pulp testing.

   p., digital. Elastic, soft prominence on the palmar or plantar surface of the last phalanx of a finger or toe.

   p., enamel. Cells forming a stellate reticulum lying between outer and inner layers of the enamel organ of a tooth.

   p., exposed. Pulp that due to disease is exposed to the air and saliva in the mouth.

   p., nonvital. P., dead.

   p., putrescent. Dead pulp that has a foul odor due to the action of putrefactive bacteria.

   p., radicular. Pulp that is in the root canal of a tooth.

   p., red. The portion of splenic pulp consisting of venous sinuses plus pulp cords.

   p., splenic. Soft spongelike tissue-forming substance of the spleen.

   p., vertebral. Nucleus pulposus, q.v., of the intervertebral disk.

   p., vital. Dental pulp that is alive and thus normal.

   p., white. Portion of splenic pulp consisting of a compact type of lymphatic tissue that forms a sheath about certain arteries.

pulpa (pŭl′pă) [L., flesh]. Pulp.

pulpal (pŭl′păl). Rel. to pulp.

pulpalgia (pŭl-păl′jē-ă) [″ + Gr. *algos*, pain]. Pain in the pulp of a tooth.

pulp amputation. The technique of removing the coronal portion of an exposed or involved vital pulp in an effort to retain the radicular pulp in a healthy, vital condition.

pulp capping. The technique and material for covering and protecting from external conditions a vital, exposed pulp while the pulp heals and secondary or tertiary dentin forms to cover it.

pulpectomy (pŭl-pĕk′tō-mē) [″ + Gr. *ektome*, excision]. Pulp extirpation, q.v.

pulpefaction (pŭl-pĭ-făk′shŭn) [L. *pulpa*, pulp, + *facere*, to make]. Conversion into pulpy substance.

pulp extirpation. The complete removal of the pulp tissue from the pulp chamber and root canal, irrespective of the state of health of the pulp.

pulpitis (pŭl-pī′tĭs) [″ + *itis*, inflammation] (pl. *pulpitides*). Inflammation of the pulp of a tooth.

pulpotomy (pŭl-pŏt′ō-mē) [″ + Gr. *tome*, incision]. Pulp amputation, q.v.

pulpy (pŭl′pē). Resembling pulp; flabby. SYN: *pultaceous.*

pulsate (pŭl′sāt) [L. *pulsare*]. To throb or beat in rhythm.

pulsatile (pŭl′să-tĭl). Pulsating; characterized by a rhythmic beat. SYN: *throbbing.*

pulsation (pŭl-sā′shŭn) [L. *pulsatio*, a beating]. The rhythmic beat, as of the heart and blood vessels; a throbbing. SEE: *pulse.*

   ABNORMAL CENTERS OF PULSATION: *Epigastric:* May result from forceful action of heart from any cause; enlargement of right ventricle; pulsating aorta noted in certain anxious persons and in anemic patients; aortic aneurysm; tumors of left lobe of liver resting on the aorta. *Left axillary region:* May result from enlargement of heart; a tense purulent effusion in left pleural sac (pulsating empyema); aneurysm; chronic disease of left lung and pleura associated with retraction of the lung. *Carotids:* May result from strong heartbeat from any cause; exophthalmic goiter; anemia; valvular disease, esp. aortic regurgitation; aneurysm or dilatation of the vessels; unnatural elasticity of the vessels noted in certain nervous and anemic patients. *Jugular:* Often becomes distended in forced expiration and coughing; sometimes noted in adherent pericardium. A true rhythmical venous pulsation usually results from tricuspid regurgitation. A pulsation may be transmitted to the jugular vein from the underlying carotid, but this false pulsation will continue when light pressure is made on the vein of the neck, while the true venous pulse will cease.

pulse (pŭls) [L. *pulsus*, beating]. 1. Rate,

rhythm, condition of arterial walls, compressibility and tension, and size and shape of the fluid wave of blood traveling through the arteries as a result of each heartbeat. 2. Rhythmical throbbing. 3. Throbbing caused by the regular contraction and alternate expansion of an artery as the wave of blood passes through the vessel; the periodic thrust felt over arteries in time with the heartbeat.

A tracing of this is called a sphygmogram and consists of a series of waves in which the upstroke is called the anacrotic limb, and the downstroke (on which is normally seen the dicrotic notch), the catacrotic limb.

Normal pulse rate of the adult is about 72 in men and 80 in women. It is usually felt in the radial artery of the wrist.

POINTS TO BE OBSERVED: Hour, frequency, pressure, regularity, force. Temperature and respiration are of clinical importance to the physician. Right and left radial arteries are usually tested and differences, if any, or absence of either pulse should be noted. If pressure of finger on artery is too great, the vessel will be collapsed and the pulse will not be discernible. The thumb should not be used because the examiner may be counting the pulse in his or her own thumb rather than patient's. Count for at least half a minute.

The rate of the pulse depends upon sex, age, exertion, position of body, and state of general health. It is higher in children and increases with very old age. It is slower in tall persons than it is in short persons. It is about 10 to 12 beats more frequent during standing than sitting. Physical exertion will increase it normally to as much as 200 beats per minute in young healthy persons. Eating and drinking also increase heart action. Pulse rate decreases during sleep, relaxation, and rest.

p., abdominal. A palpable pulse in the abdominal area. This is produced by the pulse of the abdominal aorta.

p., accelerated. A common symptom in most fevers. The pulse of the adult rarely exceeds 150 beats per minute even in acute inflammatory infections; when it exceeds 170, it may portend a fatal outcome. If such an acceleration does not diminish within a short time, it is esp. unfavorable. When quick and bounding, it indicates acute fever or inflammation, or it may result from a toxic goiter; organic heart disease; pressure at the base of the brain sufficient to paralyze the phrenic nerve as in clot, tumor, and advanced meningitis; shock; rheumatoid arthritis; or the use of certain drugs such as belladonna, nitrites, or alcohol. SYN: *p., rapid; tachycardia.*

p., alternating. Pulse with alternating weak and strong pulsations.

p., anacrotic. Pulse showing a secondary wave on ascending limb of the main wave.

p., anadicrotic. A pulse wave with two small notches on the ascending portion.

p., apical. Pulse felt or heard over the apex of the heart.

p., asymmetrical radial. Pulse in which beats vary in force. SYN: *p., unequal.*

p., bigeminal. Pulse in which two regular beats are followed by a longer pause. It has the same significance as an irregular pulse.

p., bounding. Pulse that reaches a higher intensity than normal, then disappears quickly. Best detected when arm is held aloft. Due to shortened ventricular systole and reduced peripheral pressure. SYN: *p., collapsing.*

p., brachial. Pulse felt in the brachial artery.

p., capillary. Alternating redness and pallor of capillary region, as in the matrices beneath the nails, occurring chiefly where an excessive cardiac impulse coincides with general arterial narrowing. SYN: *p., Quincke's.*

p., carotid. Pulse felt in the carotid artery.

p., catacrotic. Pulse showing one or more secondary waves on descending limb of the main wave.

p., catadicrotic. A pulse wave with two small notches on the descending portion.

p., central. Pulse recorded near the origin of the carotid or subclavian arteries.

p., collapsing. Pulse feebly striking the finger, then subsiding abruptly and completely. SYN: *p., bounding.*

p., Corrigan's. Short, forceful, bounding pulse characteristic of aortic insufficiency. SEE: *p., waterhammer.*

p., coupled. P., bigeminal, q.v.

p., deficit. Condition in which the number of pulse beats counted at the wrist is less than those counted in the same period of time at the heart. Seen in atrial fibrillation.

p., dicrotic. Pulse with a double beat, one heartbeat for two arterial pulsations, or a seemingly weak wave between the usual heartbeats. This weak wave should not be counted as a regular beat. It is indicative of low arterial tension and is noted in fevers.

p., dorsalis pedis. Pulse felt over the dorsalis pedis artery of the foot.

p., entoptic. Intermittent subjective sensations of light that accompany the heartbeat.

p., febrile. A full, bounding pulse at onset of fever, becoming feeble and weak when fever subsides.

p., femoral. Pulse felt over the femoral artery.

p., filiform. P., thready.

p., full. A distended pulse in an artery, giving a tense feeling. Observed in inflammation.

p., hard. Pulse with sensation of hardness due to changes in the arterial wall or to vascular distention.

p., hepatic. Pulse due to expansion of veins of the liver at each ventricular contraction.

p., high-tension. Pulse in which force of beat is relatively increased. The force may be roughly estimated by noting the amount of pressure of the fingers that is required to arrest the beat. It is observed in many conditions: cardiac diseases, such as hypertrophy; chronic nephritis; cerebral affections; high fever; irritation of the vasomotor center as in apoplexy, tumors, and beginning meningitis; after the use of certain drugs such as digitalis, ergot, and alcoholic stimulants; chills; angina pectoris; epileptic and hysterical seizures; gout; and uremia.

p., intermediate. Pulse recorded in proximal portions of carotid, femoral, and brachial arteries.

p., intermittent. Pulse in which occasional beats are skipped. Caused by an apparent drop of a heartbeat. It is not inconsistent with health, yet it is commonly an indication of disease, frequently from gastric, hepatic, uterine, and renal causes. It is common in fatty degeneration of the heart and is habitual in certain people after exercise, eating, or excitement.

p., irregular. Pulse with a variation in force and frequency. Has same significance as intermittent pulse. Common in myocarditis and valvular diseases, esp. in mitral regurgitation. Heart trouble may be noted by long-continued irregular pulse.

p., jerky. Pulse characteristic of aortic regurgitation, because from a state of emptiness, the artery is suddenly filled with blood.

p., jugular. Venous pulse felt in the jugular vein.

p., Kussmaul's. P., paradoxical, q.v.

p., long. Pulse in which duration of the systolic wave is comparatively long.

p., low-tension. Pulse with sudden onset, short duration, and rapid decline, esp. noted in heart failure, collapse, debility, and fevers.

p., monocrotic. Pulse in which the sphygmogram shows a simple ascending and descending uninterrupted line and no dicrotism.

p., nail. Visible pulsation in the capillaries under the nails.

p., paradoxical. Pulse that is more or less suppressed at close of each full inspiration. Thought to be due to compression of the great vessels by inflammatory adhesions, the latter being stretched during act of inspiration. Frequently noted in adherent pericarditis.

p. parvus [pulse + L. *parvus*, small]. A weak, small pulse. Present in patients with diminished left ventricular stroke volume, narrow pulse pressure, and increased peripheral vascular resistance.

p., peripheral. Pulse recorded in arteries (radial or pedal) in distal portion of limbs.

p., pistol-shot. Pulse resulting from rapid distention and collapse of an artery as occurs in aortic regurgitation.

p., plateau. Pulse associated with an increase in pressure that slowly rises but is maintained.

p., popliteal. Pulse felt over the popliteal artery.

p., Quincke's. P., capillary.

p., radial. Pulse felt over the radial artery.

p., rapid. P., accelerated.

p., regular. Pulse felt when the force and frequency are the same, i.e., when the length of beat and number of beats per minute and the strength are the same.

p., respiratory. Alternate dilatation and contraction of the large veins of the neck occurring simultaneously with inspiration and expiration.

p., Riegel's. Diminution of the pulse during expiration.

p., running. A weak, rapid pulse with one wave continuing into the next.

p., senile. Pulse characteristic of the aged. The sphygmogram shows a high position of the secondary waves in descent with increased amplitude of the first secondary wave as compared with the second.

p., short. Pulse with a short, quick systolic wave.

p., slow. A very slow pulse, fully accentuated, often found among the aged. It is a habitual rate among those inclined to be slow and easy in their actions and is found in the highly conditioned athlete. Such a pulse rate ranges between 40 and 60 beats per minute.

p., small. SEE: *pulse parvus.*

p., soft. Pulse that may be stopped by moderate digital compression.

p., tense. A full but not bounding pulse.

p., thready. A fine, scarcely perceptible pulse. SYN: *p., filiform.*

p., tremulous. Pulse in which a series of oscillations is felt with each beat.

p., tricrotic. Pulse with three separate expansions during each heartbeat.

p., trigeminal. Pulse in which a pause follows three regular beats.

p., triphammer. P., Corrigan's, q.v.

p., undulating. Pulse that seems to have several successive waves.

p., unequal. Pulse in which beats vary in force. SYN: *p., asymmetrical radial.*

p., vagus. A slow pulse resulting from vagus inhibition of the heart.

p., venous. Pulse in a vein, esp. one of the large veins near the heart, such as the internal or external jugular. Normally it is undulating and scarcely palpable. In conditions such as tricuspid regurgitation, it is pronounced.

p., vermicular. A small, frequent pulse with a wormlike feeling.

p., waterhammer. Pulse characterized by a short, powerful, jerky beat that suddenly collapses. The peculiar pulsation may be distinctly visible, not only in the carotids but throughout the brachial artery. It is diagnostic of aortic regurgitation during the period of compensation, and its force is due to excessive ventricular hypertrophy and to the large amount of blood expelled with each systole; its sudden recession is due to the incompetent valves failing to support the column of blood. SYN: *p., Corrigan's.*

p., wiry. A tense pulse that feels like a wire or firm cord.

pulse, words pert. to: acrotic; acrotism; Adams-Stokes syndrome; anacrotic; arrhythmia; artery; asphyctic; bisferious; bradycrotic; diastole; diastolic pressure; dicrotic; heart; hemisystole; murmur; phlebogram; pulsate; pulsation; pulsus; respiration; sphygmomanometer; systole; systolic pressure; thermometry; vein.

pulse generator. Device for producing an intermittent electrical discharge in order to serve as a cardiac pacemaker.

pulseless disease. Progressive arterial disease that obliterates the arteries leading to the brain and the arms. This causes absent pulses in the carotid and brachial arteries and ischemia of the areas supplied. SYN: *Takayasu's arteritis.*

pulse pressure. The difference between the systolic and the diastolic pressure. This is really expressive of the tone of the arterial walls. Ex.:

systolic pressure is	120
diastolic pressure is	100
pulse pressure is	20

systolic pressure is	130
diastolic pressure is	90
pulse pressure is	40

Normal pulse pressure: The systolic pressure is normally about 40 points greater than the diastolic. *Abnormal pulse pressure:* A pulse pressure over 50 points or under 30 points is considered abnormal.

pulse wave. A wave in the blood column and the arterial walls that is initiated by the ejection of blood from the left ventricle into the aorta. The velocity in the aorta may be as high as 500 cm/sec; and as low as 0.07 cm/sec in capillaries.

pulsimeter (pŭl-sĭm'ĕt-ĕr) [L. *pulsus*, a beat, + Gr. *metron*, measure]. Device for measuring frequency and force of the pulse. SYN: *sphygmometer.*

pulsing electromagnetic field. ABBR: PEMF. The production of a pulsing electromagnetic field applied to a fractured bone in order to induce healing. The electric field is applied externally to the affected leg and does not involve invasion of the tissue. This treatment is esp. useful in treating fractures that have previously failed to heal. Direct-current stimulation has also been used in treating these conditions.

pulsion (pŭl'shŭn). Driving or propelling in any direction.

p., lateral. Movement, particularly walking as if pulled to one side.

pulsus (pŭl'sŭs) [L.]. Pulse.

p. alternans. A weak pulse alternating with a strong one.

p., bigeminus. Pulse, bigeminal, q.v.

p. celer. Quick pulse that rises and falls suddenly.

p. differens. Condition in which the pulses on either side of the body are of unequal intensity.

p. paradoxus. Pulse, paradoxical, q.v.

p. parvus et tardus. Pulse that is small and rises and falls slowly.

p. tardus. An abnormally slow pulse.

pulv. L. *pulvis*, powder.

pulverization (pŭl"vĕr-ĭ-zā'shŭn) [L. *pulvis*, powder]. The crushing of any substance to powder or tiny particles.

pulverulent (pŭl-vĕr'ū-lĕnt). Of the nature of, or resembling, powder.

pulvinar (pŭl-vī'năr) [L., cushioned seat]. [NA] Part of the thalamus comprising a portion of the posterior nuclei. Projects posteriorly and medially, partially overlying midbrain.

pulvinate (pŭl'vĭ-nāt) [L. *pulvinus*, cushion]. Convex; shaped like a cushion.

pulvis [L.]. Powder.

pumice (pŭm'ĭs). USP. A substance derived from volcanic material. It contains chiefly complex silicates of aluminum, potassium, and sodium. Used as an abrasive, esp. in dental prophylaxis.

pump [ME. *pumpe*]. 1. Apparatus that transfers fluids or gases by pressure or suction. 2. To force air or fluid along a certain pathway, as the heart pumps blood.

p., air. Device for forcing air in or out of a chamber.

p., blood. Device for pumping blood. It is attached to an extracorporeal circulation system.

p., breast. Apparatus for removing milk from the breasts.

p., dental. Apparatus for removing saliva from the mouth during operation on teeth or jaws.

p., sodium. The biological system that permits the flow or transport of sodium across a membrane even though the sodium concentration is higher on the side of the membrane to which the sodium is flowing.

p., stomach. Apparatus for removing contents from the stomach.

pump-oxygenator. Device that pumps blood and oxygenates it.

puna (poo'nä). Mountain sickness.

punch. An instrument for making a small circular hole in material or tissue, esp. the skin.

punchdrunk. 1. A concussion syndrome present in persons who have boxed and experienced multiple episodes of trauma to the head. If severe, both the cognitive and memory functions of the brain are affected. At autopsy, there is evidence of multiple scars of the cerebral tissue. 2. One who is punchdrunk.

punched out. Appears as if holes have been made; used to describe appearance of bones (as seen on x-ray film) in certain pathological states.

puncta (pŭnk'tä) [L.] (sing. *punctum*). Points.

punctate (pŭnk'tāt) [L. *punctum,* point]. Having pinpoint punctures or depressions on the surface; marked with dots.

punctate keratoses. Discrete yellow-to-brown firm keratotic papules of the palms and soles. Most probably due to the performing of manual labor.

punctate pits. Depressed areas of the skin, esp. of the palmar creases of the hands and soles.

punctate rash. Rash with minute red points.

punctiform (pŭnk'tĭ-form) [" + *forma,* shape]. 1. Formed like a point. 2. In bacteriology, referring to pinpoint colonies of less than 1 mm in diameter.

punctio (pŭnk'shē-ō) [L. *punctura,* a point]. The act of puncturing or pricking.

punctum (pŭnk'tŭm) [L.] (pl. *puncta*). Point.

p. caecum. Spot in fundus of the eyeball where the optic nerve enters. SYN: *blind spot.*

puncta dolorosa. Painful points in the course of, or at the exit of, nerves affected by neuralgia.

p. lacrimale. [NA] Outlet of lacrimal canaliculus.

p. nasale inferius. Lower portion of suture joining the nasal bones. SYN: *rhinion.*

p. proximum. ABBR: P.P. Visual accommodation near-point.

p. remotum. ABBR: P.R. Visual accommodation far-point.

p. saliens. First trace of the embryonic heart.

puncta vasculosa. Minute red areas that mark the cut surface of white central substance of the brain, caused by blood escaping from divided blood vessels.

puncture (pŭnk'chŭr) [L. *punctura,* prick]. 1. A hole or wound made by a sharp pointed instrument. 2. To make a hole with such an instrument.

p., cisternal. Puncture of the cerebromedullary cisterna by introducing a needle in the midline through the suboccipital tissue. This is done in order to obtain a sample of cerebrospinal fluid.

Caution: This procedure may be lethal if not done by one skilled in this technique.

p., diabetic. Puncture in floor of the 4th ventricle, which results in glycosuria. This lesion was produced experimentally by the French physiologist Claude Bernard, 1813–1878. SYN: *Bernard's puncture.*

p., exploratory. Piercing of a cavity or cyst for purpose of examining fluid or pus removed.

p., lumbar. Puncture of the subarachnoid space at the lumbar level of the spinal cord. This is done to obtain a sample of spinal fluid and to measure the pressure in the cerebrospinal fluid. SEE: *cerebrospinal fluid; cisternal puncture; lumbar puncture.*

p., Quincke's. P., lumbar, q.v.

p., spinal. P., lumbar, q.v.

p., sternal. Puncture of the manubrium sternum by use of a needle, the purpose of which is to obtain a bone marrow specimen.

p., ventricular. Puncture of a ventricle of the brain for purpose of withdrawing fluid or introducing air for ventriculography.

puncture wound. A wound made by piercing with a sharp instrument. SEE: *wound, puncture.*

pungency (pŭn'jĕn-sē) [L. *pungens,* prick]. Quality of being sharp, strong, or bitter, as an odor or taste.

pungent (pŭn'jĕnt). Acrid or sharp, as applied to an odor or taste.

P.U.O. *pyrexia of unknown origin.*

pupa (pū'pă) [L., girl]. Stage in complete metamorphosis of an insect that follows the larva and precedes the adult or imago. The insect does not feed in this stage and usually is inactive.

pupil (pū'pĭl) [L. *pupilla*]. The contractile opening at the center of the iris of the eye. It contracts when exposed to strong light and when the focus is on a near object. It dilates in the dark and when the focus is on a distant object. Average diameter is 4 to 5 mm. The pupils should be equal.

DIFF. DIAG: Constriction of the pupil occurs in old age and in photophobia. It is induced by morphine, pilocarpine, physostigmine, eserine, and other miotic drugs.

Dilation of the pupil may occur in blindness or deficient sight from any cause; from distress or strong emotion; in fevers, comatose states, oculomotor nerve paralysis, and glaucoma. May be induced by belladonna (atropine), cocaine, homatropine, hyoscine (scopolamine), and other mydriatic drugs.

RS: accommodation; adaptation; anisocoria; ciliospinal center; corectasia; eye; hippus; iris; iridoplegia; isocoria; miosis; miotic; mydriasis; mydriatic; myosis; reflex; seclusio pupillae.

p., Adie's. SEE: *Adie's syndrome.*

p., Argyll Robertson. Pupil that reacts to accommodation but not to light. Seen occasionally in diseases affecting the midbrain.

p., artificial. Pupil made by iridectomy when normal pupil is occluded.

p., bounding. Rapid dilatation of pupil alternating with contraction.

p., Bumke's. Dilatation of the pupil due to psychic stimulus.

p., cat's-eye. Pupil that is narrow and slitlike.

p., cornpicker's. Dilated pupils found in agricultural workers who are exposed to dust from jimsonweed. The dust contains stramonium, a mydriatic.

p., fixed. Pupil that does not react to stimuli.

p., Hutchinson's. Condition in which one pupil is dilated and the other is not. The pupil on the side of the lesion is dilated and the other is contracted. This condition is usually due to compression of the third cranial nerve in meningitis.

p., keyhole. Pupil with an artificial coloboma at the pupillary margin.

p., Marcus Gunn. SEE: *Marcus Gunn pupil.*

p., occlusion of. Pupil with opaque membrane shutting off the pupillary area.

p., pinhole. Pupil of minute size; one excessively constricted. Seen after use of miotics, in opium poisoning, and in certain brain disorders.

p., stiff. P., Argyll Robertson, q.v.

p., tonic. Pupil that reacts slowly in accommodation-convergence reflexes.

pupilla (pū-pĭl'ă) [L., pupil]. Pupil of the eye.

pupillary (pū'pĭ-lĕr-ē) [L. *pupilla*, pupil]. Concerning the pupil.

pupillary reflex. 1. Constriction of pupil upon stimulation of retina by light. 2. Constriction of pupil upon accommodation for near vision, and dilatation upon accommodation for far vision. SYN: *accommodation reflex.* 3. Constriction of pupil of one eye in response to stimulation of the other by light. SYN: *consensual light reflex.* 4. Constriction of pupil upon attempted closure of eyelids that are held apart. SEE: *ciliospinal reflex; hippus.*

pupillography. Recording movements of the pupil of the eye.

pupillometer (pū-pĭl-ŏm'ĕ-tĕr) [" + Gr. *metron*, measure]. Device for measurement of diameter of a pupil.

pupillometry (pū-pĭl-lŏm'ĕ-trē) [" + *metron*, measure]. Measurement of the diameter of the pupil.

pupillomotor reflex. Purkinje phenomenon, q.v.

pupilloplegia (pū"pĭ-lō-plē'jē-ă) [" + *plege*, stroke]. Slow reaction of the pupil of the eye.

pupilloscopy (pū-pĭl-ŏs'kō-pē) [" + Gr. *skopein*, to examine]. 1. Measurement of eye refraction by effect of light and shadow on the retina. SYN: *retinoscopy; skiascopy.* 2. Examination of the pupil.

pupillostatometer (pū"pĭl-ō-stă-tŏm'ĕ-tĕr) [" + Gr. *statos*, placed, + *metron*, measure]. Device for measuring distance between centers of the pupils.

pure (pūr) [ME.]. Free from pollution; uncontaminated.

pure line. 1. The progeny of a single homozygous individual obtained by self-fertilization. 2. The progeny of an individual reproducing asexually by simple fission, or by buds, runners, stolons, etc. 3. The progeny of two homozygous individuals reproducing sexually.

purgation (pŭr-gā'shŭn) [L. *purgatio*]. 1. Cleansing. 2. Evacuation of bowels by action of a purgative medicine. SYN: *catharsis.*

purgative (pŭr'gă-tĭv) [L. *purgativus*]. 1. Cleansing. 2. An agent that will stimulate the production of bowel movements. SEE: *catharsis; cathartic.*

p., cholagogue. Purgative that stimulates flow of bile, producing green stools.

p., drastic. Purgative that produces violent bowel movements.

p., saline. Purgative that produces

copious watery discharges.

purgative enema. A strong, high colonic purgative that is used when other enemas fail. SEE: *enema.*

purge (pŭrj) [L. *purgare,* to cleanse]. 1. To evacuate the bowels by means of a cathartic. 2. A drug that causes evacuation of the bowels. 3. Removal of malignant or other pathological cells from bone marrow that has been removed from a patient so that it could be purged and then reinfused in the same patient. This technique is experimental. SEE: *bone marrow transplant, autologous; magnetic microscopheres.*

puriform (pū'rĭ-form) [L. *pus,* pus, + *forma,* shape]. Resembling pus. SYN: *puruloid.*

purinase (pū'rĭ-nās). An enzyme that catalyzes purine metabolism.

purine (pū'rēn") [L. *purum,* pure, + *uricus,* uric acid]. Parent compound of purine bases, as adenine, guanine, xanthine, caffeine, and uric acid. Purines are the end products of nucleoprotein digestion. They may be synthesized in the body. They break down to form uric acid. SEE: *aminopurine; oxypurine; methyl purine.*

   p., endogenous. Purine originating from nucleoproteins within the tissues.

   p., exogenous. Purine present in, or derived from, foods. SEE: table.

purine base. Xanthine base, q.v.

purine-free diet. Diet that excludes the following: meat, esp. sweetbreads, liver, kidney; poultry; fish; condiments; alcohol; concentrated sweets, rich pastries, and fried foods.

purine-low diet. Diet that excludes foods such as meat, fish, fowl, spinach, lentils, mushrooms, peas, asparagus.

purinemia (pū"rĭ-nē'mē-ă) [*purine,* + Gr. *haima,* blood]. Purine in the blood.

Purinethol. Trade name for mercaptopurine.

purity [L. *puris,* clean, pure, unmixed]. The state of being clean and free of contamination.

Purkinje, Johannes E. von (pŭr-kĭn'jē). Bohemian anatomist and physiologist, 1787–1869.

   P. cells. Large neurons that have dendrites extending to the molecular layer of the cerebellar cortex and into the white matter of the cerebellum.

   P. fibers. Atypical muscle fibers lying beneath the endocardium. They form the electrical impulse-conducting system of the heart.

   P. figures. Shadows of blood vessels perceived when light is projected out of focus or obliquely onto the retina.

   P. network. Fibrous network of large muscle cells found in cardiac muscle beneath the endocardium.

   P. phenomenon. A phenomenon of adjustment of the pupil of the eye to light intensity. When the eye adapts from light to dark conditions, the maximum pupillary movement is caused by green instead of yellow light. SYN: *pupillomotor reflex.*

   P.-Sanson images [Louis J. Sanson, Fr. physician, 1790–1841]. Three images of the same object, produced by reflections from the surface of the cornea and the anterior and posterior surfaces of the lens. For the most part, the viewer adapts to this phenomenon and ignores these normal images.

   P. vesicle. The nuclear portion of an ovum. SYN: *germinal vesicle.*

purohepatitis (pū"rō-hĕp"ă-tī'tĭs) [L. *pus,* pus + Gr. *hepar,* liver, + *itis,* inflam-

Purines in Food

Group A: High concentration (150 to 1000 mg per 100 gm)	
Liver	Sardines (in oil)
Kidney	Meat extracts
Sweetbreads	Consommé
Brains	Gravies
Heart	Fish roes
Anchovies	Herring

Group B: Moderate amounts (50 to 150 mg per 100 gm)	
Meat, game, and fish other than those mentioned in Group A	
Fowl	Asparagus
Lentils	Cauliflower
Whole grain cereals	Mushrooms
Beans	Spinach
Peas	

Group C: Very small amounts. Need not be restricted in diet of persons with gout.	
Vegetables other than those mentioned above	
Fruits of all kinds	Coffee
Milk	Tea
Cheese	Chocolate
Eggs	Carbonated beverages
Refined cereals, spaghetti, macaroni	Tapioca
Butter, fats, nuts, peanut butter*	Yeast
Sugars and sweets	
Vegetable soups	

* Fats interfere with the urinary excretion of urates and thus should be limited if you are attempting to promote excretion of uric acid.

mation]. Purulent inflammation of the liver.

puromucous (pū″rō-mū′kŭs) [″ + *mucus*, mucus]. Mucopurulent, containing both mucus and pus.

purple. Color formed by mixing red with blue.

p., visual. Rhodopsin.

purposeful movement. Motor activity requiring the planned and consciously directed involvement of the patient. It is hypothesized that evoking cortical involvement in movement patterns during sensorimotor rehabilitation will enhance the development of coordination and voluntary control.

purpura (pŭr′pū-ră) [L., purple]. Condition with various manifestations and diverse causes, characterized by hemorrhages into the skin, mucous membranes, internal organs, and other tissues. Hemorrhage into the skin shows red, darkening into purple, then brownish-yellow and finally disappearing in 2 to 3 weeks. Areas of discoloration do not disappear under pressure.

p., allergic. A group of purpuras due to a variety of agents, including bacteria, drugs, and food.

p., anaphylactoid. P., Schönlein-Henoch, q.v.

p. annularis telangiectodes. Eruption of ring-shaped spots on lower limbs with pronounced telangiectasia. SYN: *Majocchi's disease.*

p., fibrinolytic. Purpura resulting from excess fibrinolytic activity of blood.

p. fulminans. A rapidly progressing form of purpura occurring principally in children; of short duration and frequently fatal.

p., hemorrhagic. P., idiopathic thrombocytopenic, q.v.

p., Henoch. P., Schönlein-Henoch, q.v., with acute vomiting, diarrhea, and renal colic, but without joint involvement.

p., idiopathic thrombocytopenic. ABBR: ITP. A hemorrhagic disorder in which there is a pronounced reduction in circulating blood platelets, due to presence in blood plasma of a substance that agglutinates platelets. Primary cause unknown. SEE: *Nursing Diagnoses* in *Appendix.*

SYM: Bleeding from mouth and skin upon slight injury. Bleeding may also occur from mucous membranes, in serous membranes, and sometimes into brain. Increased bleeding time and reduced platelet count. Clot is nonretractile, but the coagulation time is normal.

p. nervosa. P., Henoch, q.v.

p., nonthrombocytopenic. P., allergic.

p. rheumatica. Purpura with joint pain, colic, bloody stools, and vomiting of blood.

p., Schönlein-Henoch. Purpura due to

vasculitis. It was first described by William Heberden prior to 1800, by Schönlein in 1830, and by Henoch in the 1870s. The skin lesions are obvious, but the visceral lesions are difficult to diagnose and are very serious. The cause is unknown, but allergy or drug sensitivity is important in some cases. There is no specific treatment unless a specific allergen can be proved and then removed.

p., senile. Purpura occurring in debilitated and aged persons with ecchymoses and petechiae on legs.

p. simplex. Purpura that is not associated with systemic illness.

p., thrombocytopenic. P., idiopathic thrombocytopenic.

p., thrombopenic. P., idiopathic thrombocytopenic, q.v.

p., thrombotic thrombocytopenic. A rare disease characterized by embolism and thrombosis of the small blood vessels of the brain. Shifting neurological signs such as aphasia, blindness, and convulsions are present. Therapy has been of little value, but adrenal corticosteroids in large doses have been tried. Exchange transfusions have been of some help in treating this disease.

purpureaglycosides A and B (pŭr-pū″rē-ă-glī′kō-sīds). True cardiac glycosides present in the leaves of *Digitalis purpurea*, foxglove.

purpuric (pŭr-pū′rĭk) [L. *purpura*, purple]. Pert. to, resembling, or suffering from purpura.

purpurin (pŭr′pū-rĭn). 1. An acid dye used to stain nuclei. 2. A red pigment sometimes present in urine. SYN: *uroerythrin.*

purpurinuria (pŭr″pū-rĭn-ū′rē-ă) [″ + Gr. *ouron*, urine]. Purpurin in urine.

purpuru. Pinta, q.v.

purring thrill. Thrill or vibration, like a cat's purring, due to mitral stenosis, aneurysm, or valvular disease of the heart; felt by palpation over the precordium.

purulence (pūr′ū-lĕns) [L. *purulentus*, full of pus]. The state of containing pus. SYN: *suppuration.*

purulency (pūr′ū-lĕn″sē). Purulence.

purulent (pūr′ū-lĕnt) [L. *purulentus*, full of pus]. Suppurative; forming or containing pus. SEE: *sputum.*

puruloid (pūr′ū-loyd) [L. *pus*, pus, + Gr. *eidos*, form, shape]. Like pus. SYN: *puriform.*

pus (pŭs) [L.]. Liquid product of inflammation composed of albuminous substances, a thin fluid, and leukocytes; generally yellow in color. If red, it suggests rupture of small vessels. If blue or green, it indicates presence of *Pseudomonas aeruginosa.*

ETIOL: Streptococci, staphylococci,

gonococci, pneumococci, and other species of bacteria.

p., blue. Purulence with a blue tint; usually associated with infection due to *Pseudomonas aeruginosa.*

p., cheesy. Very thick pus.

p., ichorous. Pus that is thin with shreds of sloughing tissue. It may have a fetid odor.

pus, words pert. to: cell; empyema; pyemia; resorption; suppurate; suppuration; "pyo-" words.

pus cells. Leukocytes that are dead or show degenerative changes. Found in suppurative inflammation.

pus in urine. Condition in which there are more than the normal number of white blood cells in the urine. It may be due to cystitis, pyelitis, urethritis, tuberculosis of the kidney, infection of the genitourinary tract, or trauma. Freshly passed urine may be cloudy due to presence of phosphates or pus. If the former, the addition of acid will cause the urine to clear; if pus is present, it will not clear but may become gelatinous. SYN: *pyuria.*

pustula (pŭs'tū-lȧ) [L., blister]. Pustule.

pustulant (pŭs'tū-lȧnt) [L. *pustula*, blister]. 1. Causing pustules. 2. Agent that produces the formation of pustules.

pustular (pŭs'tū-lĕr) [L. Pert. to, or characterized by, pustules.

pustulation (pŭs″tū-lā'shŭn). The development of pustules.

pustule (pŭs'tūl) [L. *pustula*, blister]. Small elevation of skin filled with lymph or pus. Pustules may be circumscribed, flat, rounded, or umbilicated. They occur in eczema pustulosum, acne vulgaris, dermatitis herpetiformis, impetigo simplex, ecthyma, varicella, syphilis, and smallpox. SEE: *pus; pustulant.*

pustulocrustaceous (pŭs″tū-lō-krŭs-tā'shŭs) [″ + *crusta*, shell]. Characterized by formation of pustules and crusts.

pustulosis (pŭs″tū-lō'sĭs) [″ + Gr. *osis*, condition]. A generalized eruption of pustules.

p., infantile acro-. SEE: *acropustulosis, infantile.*

putamen (pū-tā'mĕn) [L., shell]. [NA] The darker outer layer of the lenticular nucleus.

Putnam-Dana syndrome (pŭt'năm-dā'nă) [James J. Putnam, U.S. neurologist, 1846–1918; Charles L. Dana, U.S. neurologist, 1852–1935]. Subacute combined degeneration of the spinal cord that may be present in patients with untreated pernicious anemia.

putrefaction (pū″trĕ-făk'shŭn) [L. *putrefactio*]. Decomposition of animal matter, esp. protein associated with malodorous and poisonous products such as the ptomaines, mercaptans, and hydrogen sulfide, caused

by certain kinds of bacteria and fungi. Decomposition occurring spontaneously in sterile tissue after death is called autolysis. SEE: *sepsis.*

putrefactive (pū″trĕ-făk'tĭv) [L. *putrefacere*, to putrefy]. 1. Causing, or pert. to, putrefaction. 2. Agent promoting putrefaction.

putrefy (pū'trĕ-fī) [L. *putrefacere*, to putrefy]. To undergo putrefaction.

putrescence (pū-trĕs'ĕns) [L. *putrescens*, grow rotten]. Decay; rottenness.

putrescine (pū-trĕs'īn). A poisonous polyamine formed by bacterial action on the amino acid arginine.

putrid (pū'trĭd) [L. *putridus*]. Decayed; rotten; foul.

PUVA therapy [psoralen + *ultraviolet A*]. Therapy of psoriasis by use of a psoralen and high-intensity long-wave ultraviolet light. SEE: *psoralen; psoriasis.*

PVC. *polyvinyl chloride; premature ventricular contraction.*

PVP. *polyvinylpyrrolidone.*

PVP-iodine. *povidone-iodine.*

PWA. *person with AIDS.*

pyarthrosis (pī″ăr-thrō'sĭs) [Gr. *pyon*, pus, + *arthron*, joint, + *osis*, condition]. Pus in the cavity of a joint.

pycno- (pĭk'nō) [Gr. *pyknos*, thick]. Combining form meaning dense or thick. SEE: words beginning with *pykno-.*

pyecchysis (pī-ĕk'ĭ-sĭs) [Gr. *pyon*, pus, + *ek*, out, + *chein*, to pour]. An effusion of pus.

pyelectasia, pyelectasis (pī″ĕ-lĕk-tā'zē-ȧ, -lĕk'tăs-ĭs) [Gr. *pyelos*, pelvis, + *ektasis*, dilatation]. Dilatation of the renal pelvis.

pyelitic (pī″ĕ-lĭt'ĭk). Rel. to, or affected with, pyelitis.

pyelitis (pī″ĕ-lī'tĭs) [Gr. *pyelos*, pelvis, + *itis*, inflammation]. Inflammation of the pelvis of the kidney and its calices.

p., calculous. Pyelitis resulting from a calculus.

p. cystica. Pyelitis associated with multiple small cysts in the mucosa of the renal pelvis.

pyelo- [Gr. *pyelos*, pelvis]. Combining form meaning the pelvis.

pyelocaliectasis (pī″ĕ-lō-kăl″ē-ĕk'tȧ-sĭs) [″ + *kalyx*, cup, + *ektasis*, dilation]. Dilation of the pelvis and calyces of the kidney.

pyelocystitis (pī″ĕ-lō-sĭs-tī'tĭs) [″ + *kystis*, bladder, + *itis*, inflammation]. Inflamed condition of the renal pelvis and bladder.

pyelocystostomosis (pī″ĕ-lō-sĭs″tō-stō-mō'sĭs) [″ + + *stoma*, mouth, + *osis*, condition]. Establishment of surgical communication between the kidney and bladder.

pyelogram (pī′ĕ-lō-grăm) [Gr. *pyelos*, pelvis,

+ *gramma*, something written]. A roentgenogram of the ureter and renal pelvis.

p., intravenous. Pyelogram in which a radiopaque material is given intravenously. A roentgenogram of the urinary tract taken while the material is excreted provides important information about the structure and function of the kidney, ureter, and bladder. Any blockage along this tract will be readily detected by this examination.

pyelography (pī″ĕ-lŏg′ră-fē) [″ + *graphein*, to write]. Roentgenography of the renal pelvis and ureter.

pyelolithotomy (pī″ĕ-lō-lĭth-ŏt′ō-mē) [″ + *lithos*, stone, + *tome*, incision]. Removal of calculus from the pelvis of a kidney through an incision.

pyelonephritis (pī″ĕ-lō-nĕ-frī′tĭs) [″ + *nephros*, kidney, + *itis*, inflammation]. Inflammation of kidney substance and pelvis. SEE: *Nursing Diagnoses* in *Appendix*.

SYM: Sudden onset of chilliness and fever with dull pain in the flank over either or both kidneys. There is tenderness when the kidney is palpated. Usually there are signs of cystitis, i.e., pyuria, urgency with burning and frequency of urination.

ETIOL: Usually due to bacteria that have ascended from the bladder after entering through the urethra. *Escherichia coli* is the cause in 85% of cases.

TREAT: Recognition and removal of cause; measures to increase resistance of patient; bedrest. Avoidance of alcohol and drugs irritating to kidney. Apply heat to flanks; administer antipyretic drugs and an appropriate antibiotic. If there is urinary tract obstruction, surgery may be indicated.

PROG: Depends upon character and virulence of infection, accessory etiological factors, drainage of kidney, presence or absence of complications, and general physical condition. SEE: *glomerulonephritis.*

pyelonephrosis (pī″ĕ-lō-nĕ-frō′sĭs) [″ + ″ + *osis*, condition]. Disease of the pelvis of the kidney.

pyelopathy (pī″ĕ-lŏp′ăth-ē) [″ + *pathos*, disease, suffering]. Any disease of the pelvis of the kidney. SYN: *pyelonephrosis.*

pyeloplasty (pī″ĕ-lō-plăs″tē) [″ + *plastos*, formed]. Reparative surgery on the pelvis of the kidney.

pyeloplication (pī″ĕ-lō-plĭ-kā′shŭn) [″ + L. *plicare*, to fold]. Shortening of the wall of a dilated renal pelvis by taking tucks in it.

pyeloscopy (pī″ĕl-ŏs′kō-pē) [″ + *skopein*, to examine]. Examination of the pelvis of the kidney using fluoroscopy. The pelvis is filled with a radiopaque material.

pyelostomy (pī″ĕ-lŏs′tō-mē) [″ + *stoma*, mouth]. Creation of an opening into the renal pelvis.

pyelotomy (pī″ĕ-lŏt′ō-mē) [″ + *tome*, incision]. Incision of renal pelvis.

NURSING IMPLICATIONS: Secure all catheters to the patient to prevent dislodgement. Assess and record the appearance of the urine, including color, consistency, and amount. Catheter drainage tubing must be kept free of kinks. Catheters should never be clamped. Monitor and record intake and output. After removal of the catheter, use stoma-bag collection device to collect any drainage and maintain skin integrity while the wound heals.

pyeloureterectasis. Dilatation of the pelvis of the kidney and ureter.

pyemesis (pī-ĕm′ĭ-sĭs) [Gr. *pyon*, pus, + *emein*, to vomit]. Vomiting of pus.

pyemia (pī-ē′mē-ă) [″ + *haima*, blood]. A form of septicemia due to presence of pus-forming organisms in the blood, manifested by formation of multiple abscesses of a metastatic nature.

SYM: High intermittent temperature with recurrent chills; metastatic processes in various parts of the body, esp. in lungs; septic pneumonia, empyema. May be fatal.

TREAT: Antibiotics. Prophylactic treatment consists in prevention of suppuration.

p., arterial. Pyemia resulting from dissemination of emboli from a thrombus in cardiac vessels.

p., cryptogenic. Pyemia, the origin of which is hidden in the deeper tissues.

p., metastatic. Multiple abscesses resulting from infected pyemic thrombi.

p., portal. Suppurative inflammation of the portal vein.

pyemic (pī-ē′mĭk) [Gr. *pyon*, pus, + *haima*, blood]. Rel. to, or affected with, blood poisoning.

Pyemotes (pī-ĕ-mō′tēz). A genus of mites parasitic on the larvae of insects.

P. ventricosus. A mite present in the straw of some cereals. Contact with it causes a vesiculopapular dermatitis in humans. This is called grain itch.

pyencephalus (pī″ĕn-sĕf′ă-lŭs) [″ + *enkephalos*, brain]. A brain abscess with suppuration within the cranium. SYN: *pyocephalus.*

pyesis (pī-ē′sĭs). Formation of pus. SYN: *suppuration.*

pygal (pī′găl) [Gr. *pyge*, rump]. Concerning the buttocks. SEE: *steatopygia.*

pygalgia (pī-găl′jē-ă) [″ + *algos*, pain]. Pain in the buttocks.

pygmalionism (pĭg-mā′lē-ŏn-ĭzm) [named for Pygmalion, a sculptor and king in Gr. mythology, who fell in love with a figure he carved]. Psychopathic condition in which a person is in love with a creation of his own.

pygmy (pĭg'mē). A very small person, a dwarf.

pygo- [Gr. *pyge*, rump]. Combining form meaning the rump.

pygoamorphus (pī″gō-ă-mor'fŭs) [″ + *a-*, not, + *morphe*, form]. Conjoined twins in which the parasite, joined to the buttocks, is an amorphous mass of tissue, or a teratoma.

pygodidymus (pī″gō-dĭd'ĭ-mŭs) [″ + *didymos*, twin]. Conjoined twins with fusion of the cephalothoracic area, but with doubling of the pelvis and extremities.

pygomelus (pī-gŏm'ĕ-lŭs) [″ + *melos*, limb]. Unequal conjoined twins with the parasite represented by an accessory limb attached to the pelvic area.

pyknic (pĭk'nĭk) [Gr. *pyknos*, thick]. Pert. to a body type characterized by roundness of the extremities, stockiness, large chest and abdomen, and tendency to obesity.

pykno- [Gr. *pyknos*, thick]. Combining form meaning thick, compact, dense, frequent. SEE: words beginning with *pycn-*.

pyknocardia (pĭk-nō-kăr'dē-ă) [″ + *kardia*, heart]. Rapid pulse. SYN: *tachycardia*.

pyknocyte (pĭk'nō-sīt) [″ + *kytos*, cell]. A form of spiculed red cell. SEE: *spiculed red cell*.

pyknodysostosis (pĭk″nō-dĭs″ŏs-tō'sĭs) [″ + *dys*, bad, + *osteon*, bone, + *osis*, condition]. An autosomal recessive disease that affects bones and resembles osteopetrosis, but the disease is mild and not associated with hematologic or neurologic abnormalities. The children have short stature, open fontanels, frontal bossing, hypoplastic facial bones, and dental abnormalities. There may be double rows of malformed teeth. The only treatment is surgical correction of deformities and fractures.

pyknometer (pĭk-nŏm'ĕ-tĕr) [″ + *metron*, measure]. Device for determining specific gravity of liquids.

pyknomorphous (pĭk″nō-morf'ŭs) [″ + *morphe*, form]. Characterized by compact arrangement of the stainable portions, said esp. of certain nerve cells.

pyknophrasia (pĭk″nō-frā'zē-ă) [″ + *phrasis*, speech]. Thickness of words uttered in speech.

pyknosis (pĭk-nō'sĭs) [″ + *osis*, condition]. Thickness, esp. shrinking of cells through degeneration. SYN: *inspissation*.

pyle- [Gr. *pyle*, gate]. Combining form meaning orifice, esp. that of the portal vein.

pylemphraxis (pī″lĕm-frăk'sĭs) [″ + *emphraxis*, stoppage]. Occlusion of the portal vein.

pylephlebectasia, pylephlebectasis (pī″lē-flē-bĕk-tā′zē-ă, -bĕk′tă-sĭs) [″ + *phleps*, vein, + *ektasis*, dilatation]. Distention of the portal vein.

pylephlebitis (pī″lē-flē-bī'tĭs) [″ + ″ + *itis*, inflammation]. Inflamed condition of the portal vein, generally suppurative.

   p., adhesive. Thrombosis of the portal vein.

   p. obturans. Pylephlebitis with obstructed flow in the portal vein.

pylethrombophlebitis (pī″lē-thrŏm″bō-flē-bī'tĭs) [″ + *thrombos*, clot, + *phleps*, vein, + *itis*, inflammation]. Thrombosis and inflammation of the portal vein.

pylethrombosis (pī″lē-thrŏm-bō'sĭs) [Gr. *pyle*, gate, + *thrombos*, clot, + *osis*, condition]. Occlusion of portal vein by a thrombus.

pylon (pī'lŏn). A temporary artificial leg.

pyloralgia (pī″lō-răl'jē-ă) [Gr. *pyloros*, gatekeeper, + *algos*, pain]. Pain around the pylorus, distal aperture of the stomach.

pylorectomy (pī″lō-rĕk'tō-mē) [″ + *ektome*, excision]. Surgical removal of the pylorus.

pyloric (pī-lor'ĭk) [Gr. *pyloros*, gatekeeper]. Pert. to the opening between the stomach and duodenum.

pyloric antrum. The first part of the pyloric portion of the stomach; portion leading to pyloric canal.

pyloric canal. The narrow constricted region of the pyloric portion of the stomach that opens through the pylorus into the duodenum.

pyloric cap. First part of the duodenum.

pyloric gland. A gland of the stomach near the pylorus.

pyloric obstruction and dilatation. Pyloric obstruction increases the resistance offered to the expulsion of food from the stomach. In its efforts to overcome this, the stomach first becomes hypertrophied, then dilated. Causes of dilatation are pyloric obstruction, laxness of walls from simple atony, or excessive ingestion of food or drink.

   SYM: The general symptoms of dyspepsia and the following symptoms relating to vomiting. Vomiting occurs long after eating, sometimes several hours or days. Amount is often excessive, sometimes several quarts; it is sour and fermented, and on standing it separates into a sediment of undigested food and a turbid, frothy liquid. Ejected fluid is rich in torulae and sarcinae, forms of bacteria. Obstinate constipation.

   Bulging over epigastrium; in thin subjects, the outline of stomach may be visible. Palpation gives a splashing fremitus. In percussion there is an increased area of gastric tympany. In auscultation, splashing sounds often are audible at some distance.

   TREAT: Diet light, nutritious, not bulky, and should be given in small amounts at frequent intervals.

   PROG: Guarded but depends upon the

cause. More favorable in dilatation without obstruction.

pyloric orifice. Opening or passage between the stomach and duodenum.

pyloric stenosis. Narrowing of the pyloric orifice. May be due to excessive thickening of the circular muscle of the pylorus (hypertrophic pyloric stenosis) or hypertrophy and hyperplasia of mucosa and submucosa.

TREAT: Surgical section of the thickened muscle around the pylorus.

NURSING IMPLICATIONS: *Preop:* Position the infant to prevent aspiration; feed and observe; obtain accurate daily weights; record vomitus; provide pacifier as needed; monitor and record administration of parenteral fluids; chart intake and output; and instruct parents concerning surgery.

Postop: Administer parenteral fluids as prescribed; continue nothing by mouth for 12 to 24 hours; instruct parents concerning deep-breathing exercises; turn and position at scheduled intervals. Increase oral feedings gradually; position infant in upright position for one hour after feeding to prevent aspiration; include instruction for the parents in the care of the infant; provide visual stimulation for infant. Prior to discharge, teach parents to meet infant's needs at home, and establish schedule for follow-up at home.

pyloristenosis (pī-lor″ĭ-stĕn-ō′sĭs) [Gr. *pyloros,* gatekeeper, + *stenos,* narrow]. Constriction of the pylorus.

pyloritis (pī″lō-rī′tĭs) [″ + *itis,* inflammation]. Inflamed condition of the pylorus.

pyloro- [Gr. *pyloros,* gatekeeper]. Combining form meaning gatekeeper; applied to the pylorus.

pylorodiosis (pī-lō″rō-dī-ō′sĭs) [″ + *diosis,* pushing under]. Dilation of the pylorus of the stomach.

pyloroduodenitis (pī-lor″ō-dū″ō-dē-nī′tĭs) [″ + L. *duodeni,* twelve, + Gr. *itis,* inflammation]. Inflammation of the mucosa of the pyloric outlet of the stomach and duodenum.

pylorogastrectomy (pī-lor″ō-găs-trĕk′tō-mē) [″ + *gaster,* belly, + *ektome,* excision]. Excision of pyloric portion of the stomach.

pyloromyotomy (pī-lor″ō-mī-ŏt′ō-mē) [″ + *mys,* muscle, + *tome,* incision]. Incision and suture of the pyloric sphincter.

pyloroplasty (pī-lor′ō-plăs″tē) [″ + *plassein,* to form]. Operation to repair the pylorus, esp. one to increase the caliber of the pyloric opening by stretching.

   p., Finney. Surgical procedure for enlarging the opening from the stomach to the duodenum.

   p., Heineke-Mikulicz. Surgical procedure for correcting a pyloric stricture. The stricture is incised longitudinally and closed transversely.

pyloroscopy (pī-lō-rŏs′kō-pē) [Gr. *pyloros,* gatekeeper, + *skopein,* to examine]. Fluoroscopic examination of the pylorus.

pylorospasm (pī-lor′ō-spăzm) [″ + *spasmos,* a convulsion]. Spasmodic contraction of the pyloric orifice. Usually due to a disturbance in the motor mechanism of the pylorus. May occur secondary to lesions of the stomach and duodenum near the pylorus.

pylorostenosis (pī-lor″ō-stĕn-ō′sĭs) [″ + *stenos,* narrow]. Abnormal narrowing or stricture of the pyloric orifice. SEE: *pyloric stenosis.*

pylorostomy (pī-lor-ŏs′tō-mē) [″ + *stoma,* mouth]. Formation of an opening through the abdominal wall into the pylorus.

pylorotomy (pī-lor-ŏt′ō-mē) [″ + *tome,* incision]. Incision of the pyloric submucosa to relieve hypertrophic stenosis.

pylorus (pī-lor′ŭs) [Gr. *pyloros,* gatekeeper]. The lower orifice of the stomach opening into the duodenum. The pylorus is closed most of the time but opens at intervals, permitting acid chyme to enter the duodenum. The primary factor in the opening of the pylorus is elevation of gastric pressure over duodenal pressure.

pyo-, py- [Gr. *pyon,* pus]. Combining forms meaning pus.

pyocele (pī′ō-sēl) [Gr. *pyon,* pus, + *kele,* tumor, swelling]. A hernia or distended cavity containing pus.

pyocelia (pī″ō-sē′lē-ă) [″ + *koilia,* cavity]. Pus formation in the abdominal cavity.

pyocephalus (pī″ō-sĕf′ă-lŭs) [″ + *kephale,* head]. Effusion of purulent nature within the cranium.

   p., circumscribed. Brain abscess.

   p., external. Suppuration of the meninges.

   p., internal. Pus in the cerebrospinal fluid.

pyochezia (pī″ō-kē′zē-ă) [Gr. *pyon,* pus, + *chezein,* to go to stool]. Pus in the feces.

pyococcus (pī″ō-kŏk′ŭs) [″ + *kokkos,* berry]. A micrococcus that causes pus formation, such as *Streptococcus pyogenes.*

pyocolpocele (pī″ō-kŏl′pō-sēl) [″ + *kolpos,* vagina, + *kele,* tumor, swelling]. A vaginal tumor containing pus. SEE: *pyocolpos.*

pyocolpos (pī″ō-kŭl′pōs). Accumulation of pus in the vagina.

pyocyanic (pī″ō-sī-ăn′ĭk) [″ + *kyanos,* dark blue]. Pert. to pyocyanin or blue pus.

pyocyst (pī′ō-sĭst) [″ + *kystis,* sac]. A cyst containing pus.

pyoderma (pī-ō-dĕr′mă) [″ + *derma,*

skin]. Any acute, inflammatory, purulent bacterial dermatitis.

p. gangrenosum. Pyoderma usually associated with ulcerative colitis or any severe chronic disease that leads to wasting. Occurs principally on the trunk.

pyodermatitis (pī″ō-dĕr″mă-tī′tĭs) [″ + ″ + *itis*, inflammation]. Pyogenic infection of the skin causing a dermatitis.

pyodermatosis (pī″ō-dĕr″mă-tō′sĭs) [″ + ″ + *osis*, condition]. Any skin condition of pyogenic origin. SYN: *pyodermia.*

pyodermia (pī″ō-dĕr′mē-ă). Any suppurative skin disease.

pyofecia (pī″ō-fē′sē-ă) [Gr. *pyon*, pus, + L. *faeces*, refuse]. Pus in the stools.

pyogenesis (pī″ō-jĕn′ĕ-sĭs) [″ + *genesis*, generation, birth]. The formation of pus. SYN: *pyopoiesis; suppuration.*

pyogenic (pī-ō-jĕn′ĭk) [″ + *gennan*, to produce]. Producing pus.

pyogenic microorganisms. Microorganisms that form pus. The principal ones are *Staphylococcus aureus, Staphylococcus epidermidis, Streptococcus hemolyticus, Bacillus anthracis, B. subtilis, Clostridium perfringens, Pseudomonas aeruginosa,* and *Neisseria gonorrhoeae.* These pathogens also stimulate a huge influx of neutrophils, q.v., to the site. The pus is formed from dead organisms, white blood cells, and other cells destroyed during the immune response.

pyohemia (pī″ō-hē′mē-ă) [″ + *haima*, blood]. Pyemia.

pyohemothorax (pī″ō-hē″mō-thō′răks) [″ + *haima*, blood, + *thorax*, chest]. Pus and blood in the pleural cavity.

pyoid (pī′oyd) [″ + *eidos*, form, shape]. Resembling pus.

pyolabyrinthitis (pī″ō-lăb″ĭ-rĭn-thī′tĭs) [″ + *labyrinthos*, maze, + *itis*, inflammation]. Inflammation with suppuration of the labyrinth of the ear.

pyometra (pī″ō-mē′tră) [″ + *metra*, uterus]. Retained pus accumulation in the uterine cavity.

pyometritis (pī″ō-mē-trī′tĭs) [″ + ″ + *itis*, inflammation]. Purulent inflammation of the uterus.

pyonephritis (pī″ō-nĕf-rī′tĭs) [″ + *nephros*, kidney, + *itis*, inflammation]. Inflammation of the kidney, suppurative in character.

pyonephrolithiasis (pī″ō-nĕf″rō-lĭth-ī′ă-sĭs) [″ + ″ + *lithos*, stone, + *-iasis*, condition]. Pus and calculi in the kidney.

pyonephrosis (pī″ō-nĕf-rō′sĭs) [″ + ″ + *osis*, condition]. Pus accumulation in the pelvis of the kidney.

pyoovarium (pī″ō-ō-vă′rē-ŭm) [″ + LL. *ovarium*, ovary]. Abscess formation in an ovary.

Pyopen. Trade name for carbenicillin disodium.

pyopericarditis (pī″ō-pĕr″ĭ-kăr-dī′tĭs) [″ + *peri*, around, + *kardia*, heart, + *itis*, inflammation]. Pericarditis with suppuration.

pyopericardium (pī″ō-pĕr″ĭ-kăr′dē-ŭm). Pus formation in the pericardium.

pyoperitoneum (pī″ō-pĕr″ĭ-tō-nē′ŭm) [Gr. *pyon*, pus, + *peritonaion*, peritoneum]. Pus formation in the peritoneal cavity.

pyoperitonitis (pī″ō-pĕr″ĭ-tō-nī′tĭs) [″ + ″ + *itis*, inflammation]. Purulent inflammation of the lining of peritoneum.

pyophthalmia (pī″ōf-thăl′mē-ă) [″ + *ophthalmos*, eye]. Suppurative inflamed condition of the eye. SYN: *pyophthalmitis.*

pyophthalmitis (pī″ōf-thăl-mī′tĭs) [″ + ″ + *itis*, inflammation]. Suppurative inflamed condition of the eye. SYN: *pyophthalmia.*

pyophylactic (pī″ō-fī-lăk′tĭk) [″ + *phylaxis*, protection]. Protective against formation of pus.

pyophylactic membrane. Lining membrane of an abscess cavity separating it from healthy tissue.

pyophysometra (pī″ō-fī″sō-mē′tră) [″ + *physa*, air, + *metra*, uterus]. Pus and gas accumulation in the uterus.

pyoplania (pī″ō-plā′nē-ă) [″ + *planos*, wandering]. Spreading of pus by infiltration into other tissue.

pyopneumocholecystitis (pī″ō-nū″mō-kō-lē-sĭs-tī′tĭs) [″ + *pneuma*, air, + *chole*, bile, + *kystis*, sac, + *itis*, inflammation]. Distention of the gallbladder with air and pus.

pyopneumocyst (pī″ō-nū′mō-sĭst) [″ + ″ + *kystis*, bladder]. A cyst enclosing pus and gas.

pyopneumohepatitis (pī″ō-nū″mō-hĕp″ă-tī′tĭs) [″ + *pneuma*, air, + *hepar*, liver, + *itis*, inflammation]. Liver abscess with gas in the abscess cavity.

pyopneumopericardium (pī″ō-nū″mō-pĕr″ĭ-kăr′dē-ŭm) [″ + ″ + *peri*, around, + *kardia*, heart]. Pus and air or gas in the pericardium.

pyopneumoperitoneum (pī″ō-nū″mō-pĕr″ĭ-tō-nē′ŭm) [″ + ″ + *peritonaion*, peritoneum]. Peritonitis with gas and pus in the peritoneal cavity.

pyopneumoperitonitis (pī″ō-nū″mō-pĕr″ĭ-tō-nī′tĭs) [″ + ″ + ″ + *itis*, inflammation]. Pus and air in the peritoneal cavity complicating peritonitis.

pyopneumothorax (pī″ō-nū″mō-thō′răks) [″ + ″ + *thorax*, chest]. Presence of pus and gas in the pleural cavity.

pyopoiesis (pī″ō-poy-ē′sĭs) [″ + *poiein*, to make]. Formation of pus. SYN: *pyogenesis;*

suppuration.

pyopoietic (pī″ō-poy-ĕt′ĭk). Pert. to formation of pus. SYN: *suppurative.*

pyoptysis (pī-ŏp′tĭ-sĭs) [″ + *ptysis*, spitting]. Spitting of pus.

pyopyelectasis (pī″ō-pī″ĕ-lĕk′tă-sĭs) [″ + *pyelos*, pelvis, + *ektasis*, dilation]. Purulent fluid in the dilated renal pelvis.

pyorrhea (pī″ō-rē′ă) [″ + *rhoia*, flow]. A discharge of purulent matter.

   p. alveolaris. An archaic term no longer considered proper to describe the several types of periodontal disease known.

pyosalpingitis (pī″ō-săl″pĭn-jī′tĭs) [Gr. *pyon*, pus, + *salpinx*, tube, + *itis*, inflammation]. Retained pus in the oviduct with inflammation.

pyosalpingo-oophoritis (pī″ō-săl-pĭn″gō-ō″ŏf-ō-rī′tĭs) [″ + ″ + *oon*, ovum, + *phoros*, a bearer, + *itis*, inflammation]. Inflammation of ovary and oviduct, with suppuration.

pyosalpinx (pī″ō-săl′pĭnks). Pus in the fallopian tube.

pyosemia (pī″ō-sē′mē-ă) [Gr. *pyon*, pus, + L. *semen*, seed]. Pus in the semen.

pyostatic (pī″ō-stăt′ĭk) [″ + *statikos*, standing]. 1. Preventing pus formation. 2. Agent preventing the development of pus.

pyothorax (pī″ō-thō′răks) [″ + *thorax*, chest]. Pus in the pleural cavity. SYN: *empyema.*

pyotorrhea (pī″ō-tō-rē′ă) [″ + *ous*, ear, + *rhoia*, flow]. Purulent discharge from the ear.

pyoturia (pī″ō-tū′rē-ă) [″ + *ouron*, urine]. Pus cells in the urine. SYN: *pyuria.*

pyourachus (pī″ō-ū′ră-kŭs) [″ + *ourachos*, fetal urinary canal]. Accumulation of pus in the urachus, q.v.

pyoureter (pī″ō-ū-rē′tĕr) [″ + *oureter*, ureter]. Pus collection in the ureter.

pyovesiculosis (pī″ō-vĕ-sĭk″ū-lō′sĭs) [″ + L. *vesiculus*, a small vessel, + Gr. *osis*, condition]. Pus collection in the seminal vesicles.

pyoxanthin(e) (pī″ō-zăn′thĭn) [″ + *xanthos*, yellow]. A yellow pigment resulting from oxidation of pyocyanin. Sometimes present in pus.

pyramid (pĭr′ă-mĭd) [Gr. *pyramis*, a pyramid]. 1. A solid on the base with three or more triangular sides that meet at an apex. 2. Any part of the body resembling a pyramid. 3. A compact bundle of nerve fibers in the medulla oblongata. 4. Petrous portion of temporal bone. SYN: *pyramis.*

   p., malpighian. P., renal.

   p. of cerebellum. A median ventral projection of vermis of cerebellum lying between tuber and uvula.

   p. of light. The triangular light reflex

from the typanic membrane of the ear.

   p. of medulla. One of a pair of elongated tapering prominences on the anterior surface of the medulla oblongata, composed of descending corticospinal fibers.

   p. of temporal bone. The pyramis or petrous portion of the temporal bone.

   p. of thyroid. A conical process sometimes present, extending cephalad from the isthmus of the thyroid gland.

   p. of tympanum. A hollow projection on the inner wall of the tympanum through which passes the stapedius muscle.

   p., renal. One of a number of cone-shaped structures making up the medulla of the kidney along with renal columns. Each pyramid has an external base in the kidney's boundary with an apex that projects as a renal papilla into the renal sinus. The pyramids converge. SYN: *pyramid, malpighian.*

pyramidal (pĭ-răm′ĭ-dăl) [L. *pyramidalis*]. In the shape of a pyramid.

pyramidal cell. Pyramid-shaped cell of cerebral cortex.

pyramidalis (pĭ-răm″ĭ-dăl′ĭs) [L.]. The muscle that arises from the crest of the pubis and is inserted into the linea alba upward about halfway to the navel.

   p. auriculae. Small muscle inserted into the auricle of the ear. It is often absent.

pyramidal tract. One of three descending tracts (lateral, ventral, ventrolateral) of the spinal cord. Consists of fibers arising from giant pyramidal cells of Betz present in the motor area of the cerebral cortex. SYN: *corticospinal tract.*

pyramidotomy (pēr″ăm-ĭ-dŏt′ō-mē) [Gr. *pyramis*, a pyramid, + *tome*, incision]. Excision of the pyramidal tracts of the spinal cord in order to alleviate involuntary muscular movements.

pyramis (pĭr′ă-mĭs) [Gr., a pyramid] (pl. *pyramides*). A general term for a structure resembling a pyramid.

pyran (pī′răn). The compound C_5H_6O, the ring structure of which consists of five carbon atoms and one oxygen atom.

pyranose (pī′ră-nōs). A cyclic sugar or glycoside with a structure similar to a pyran, q.v.

pyrantel pamoate (pĭ-răn′tĕl). USP. A drug used in treating the parasitic diseases ascariasis and enterobiasis, as well as those caused by *Ancylostoma, Necator americanus,* and *Trichostrongylus.* Trade name is Antiminth.

pyrazinamide (pī″ră-zĭn′ă-mīd). USP. A drug used in treating tuberculosis. It is used in treating persons who are resistant to usually effective agents.

pyrectic (pī-rĕk′tĭk). Concerning fever.

pyrenemia (pī″rĕ-nē′mē-ă) [Gr. *pyren*, fruit stone, + *haima*, blood]. Condition in which there are nucleated red cells in the blood.

pyretherapy (pī''rĕ-thĕr'ă-pē) [Gr. *pyr*, fever, + *therapeia*, treatment]. Artificial fever treatment. SEE: *pyretotherapy*.

pyrethrins (pī-rē'thrĭnz). General name of substances derived from pyrethrum flowers (chrysanthemums). Used as insecticides.

pyretic (pī-rĕt'ĭk) [Gr. *pyretos*, fever]. Concerning fever.

pyretic therapy. Treatment of disease by artificial induction of fever, either by heat or by the inoculation of malarial organisms.

pyreticosis (pī-rĕt''ĭ-kō'sĭs) [" + *osis*, condition]. Any condition characterized by fever.

pyreto- (pī-rĕt'ō) [Gr. *pyretos*, fever]. Prefix indicating relationship to fever.

pyretogen (pī-rĕt'ō-jĕn) [" + *gennan*, to produce]. A substance producing fever.

pyretogenesia, pyretogenesis (pī''rē-tō-jĕn-ē'zē-ă, -jĕn'ē-sĭs) [" + *genesis*, generation, birth]. Origin and production of fever.

pyretogenic (pī''rĕt-ō-jĕn'ĭk). Producing or causing fever.

pyretogenic bacteria. Pathogenic bacteria causing fever.

pyretogenic stage. Period during which a fever is rising slowly.

pyretogenous (pī''rĕ-tŏj'ĕn-ŭs). 1. Producing or causing fever. 2. Caused by fever.

pyretolysis (pī''rĕ-tŏl'ĭ-sĭs) [" + *lysis*, dissolution]. 1. Reduction of fever. 2. Lysis of symptoms of disease process that is accelerated by fever.

pyretotherapy (pī''rē-tō-thĕr'ă-pē) [" + *therapeia*, treatment]. 1. Treatment by artificially raising the patient's temperature. 2. Treatment of fever.

pyretotyphosis (pī''rĕ-tō-tī-fō'sĭs) [" + *typhosis*, delirium]. The delirious or stuporous condition characteristic of high fever.

pyrexia (pī-rĕk'sē-ă) [Gr. *pyressein*, to be feverish]. Condition in which the temperature is above normal. SYN: *fever*.

pyrexial (pī-rĕk'sē-ăl). Concerning fever.

pyrexin (pī'rĕks'ĭn). A substance extracted from inflammatory exudates that induces fever.

Pyribenzamine Hydrochloride. Trade name for tripelennamine hydrochloride.

pyridine (pĕr'ĭ-dēn). A colorless, volatile liquid with a charred odor. It is obtained by dry distillation of nitrogen-containing organic matter. It is used as an industrial solvent.

Pyridium. Trade name for phenazopyridine hydrochloride.

pyridostigmine bromide (pĕr''ĭ-dō-stĭg'mēn). USP. An anticholinesterase drug used in treating myasthenia gravis. Trade names are Mestinon and Regonol.

pyridoxal 5-phosphate. A derivative of pyri-

doxine. It serves as a coenzyme of certain amino-acid decarboxylases in bacteria, and in animal tissues of 3,4-dihydroxyphenylalanine (dopa) decarboxylase.

pyridoxamine (pĭr''ĭ-dŏks'ă-mĭn). One of the vitamin B_6 group; a 4-aminoethyl analog of pyridoxine.

4-pyridoxic acid (pĭr''ĭ-dŏks'ĭk). The principal end product of pyridoxine metabolism excreted in human urine.

pyridoxine hydrochloride (pĭ-rĭ-dŏks'ēn). USP. One of a group of substances, including pyridoxal and pyridoxamine, that make up vitamin B_6. Trade names are Hexa-Betalin and Beesix. SEE: *vitamin B_6* in *Vitamins* in *Appendix*.

pyriform (pĭr'ĭ-form) [L. *pirum*, pear, + *forma*, shape]. Shaped like a pear. Also spelled piriform.

pyrilamine maleate (pĕr-ĭl'ă-mēn). USP. A histamine antagonist drug used in treating certain allergic diseases.

pyrimethamine (pĕr''ĭ-mĕth'ă-mēn). USP. An antimalarial drug used in prophylaxis against malaria rather than in treatment of an acute attack. Trade name is Daraprim.

pyrimidine (pĭ-rĭm'ĭd-ĭn). The parent of a group of heterocyclic nitrogen compounds, $C_4H_4N_2$, including uracil, cytosine, and thymine, some of which are components of nucleic acid.

pyrithiamine (pĭr''ĭ-thī'ă-mĭn). A synthetic analog of thiamine that acts as an antithiamine substance. When administered, it produces many of the symptoms of thiamine deficiency.

pyro- (pī'rō) [Gr. *pyr*, fire]. Prefix meaning heat or fire.

pyrogallol (pī''rō-găl'ŏl). $C_6H_6O_3$. A toxic chemical derived from gallic acid.

pyrogen (pī'rō-jĕn) [Gr. *pyr*, fire, + *gennan*, to produce]. Any substance that produces fever.

Caution: Do not give a fluid intravenously that has been opened previously and allowed to stand, even though the top may have been closed tightly, because pyrogens will have formed.

p., leukocytic. A substance found in blood during fever that acts upon the thermoregulatory centers of the hypothalamus.

pyrogenic (pī''rō-jĕn'ĭk) [Gr. *pyr*, fire, + *gennan*, to produce]. Producing fever.

pyroglobulinemia (pī''rō-glŏb''ū-lĭ-nē'mē-ă) [" + *globulus*, globule, + *haima*, blood]. Presence of an abnormal globulin in the blood of patients with multiple myeloma and certain other diseases. The globulin is irreversibly precipitated when heated to

56°C.

pyrolagnia (pī″rō-lăg′nē-ă) [″ + *lagneia*, lust]. Insane desire to see or produce fires; accompanied by sexual gratification. SEE: *pyromania*.

pyrolysis (pī-rŏl′ĭ-sĭs) [″ + *lysis*, dissolution]. Decomposition of organic matter when there is a rise in temperature.

pyromania (pī″rō-mā′nē-ă) [″ + *mania*, madness]. Fire madness; mania for setting fires or seeing them.

pyrometer (pī-rŏm′ĕ-tĕr) [″ + *metron*, measure]. Device for measuring temperature.

pyronine (pī′rō-nĭn). A histologic stain used to demonstrate the presence of RNA and DNA.

pyronyxis (pī″rō-nĭk′sĭs) [″ + *nyxis*, a piercing]. Treatment or cauterization by puncturing a part with hot needles. SYN: *ignipuncture*.

pyrophobia (pī″rō-fō′bē-ă) [″ + *phobos*, fear]. Abnormal fear of fire.

pyrophosphatase (pī″rō-fŏs′fă-tās). An enzyme that catalyzes splitting of phosphoric groups.

pyrophosphate (pī″rō-fŏs′fāt). Any salt of phosphoric acid.

pyroptothymia (pī″rŏp-tō-thī′mē-ă) [″ + *ptoein*, to scare, + *thymos*, mind]. A psychosis in which one imagines himself or herself surrounded by flames.

pyropuncture (pī″rō-pŭnk′chūr) [″ + L. *punctura*, piercing]. Treatment by puncture of a part with hot needles. SEE: *counterirritation*.

pyrosis (pī-rō′sĭs) [Gr. *pyrosis*, burning]. A burning sensation in the epigastric and sternal region with raising of acid liquid from stomach. SYN: *heartburn*.

NURSING IMPLICATIONS: Assess what the term means to the patient, exact location, time of occurrence in relation to food intake, duration, if position changes exaggerate discomfort, precipitating factors (such as type and amount of food), method of relief, and factors that aggravate the discomfort.

pyrotic (pī-rŏt′ĭk) [Gr. *pyrotikos*]. 1. Caustic; burning. 2. Pert. to pyrosis.

pyrotoxin (pī″rō-tŏk′sĭn) [Gr. *pyr*, fire, + *toxikon*, poison]. A toxin produced during a febrile disease.

pyroxylin (pī-rŏk′sĭ-lĭn). USP. A substance obtained by the action of a mixture of nitric and sulfuric acids on cotton. It consists chiefly of cellulose tetranitrate. It is combined with ether and alcohol to form collodion, q.v. SYN: *gun cotton*.

Caution: Pyroxylin and collodion are exceedingly flammable.

pyrrobutamine phosphate (pĕr″rō-bū′tă-mēn). USP. An antihistamine drug.

pyrrol cells. Cells of the reticuloendothelial system, so called because of their ability to ingest colloidal dyes (pyrrol blue). SYN: *histiocytes*.

pyrrole (pĕr′ōl). A heterocyclic substance that provides the building blocks for a large number of vital compounds such as hemoglobin, chlorophyll, and bile acids. It is a colorless liquid with the odor of chloroform.

pyrrolidine (pĭ-rŏl′ĭ-dĭn). Tetramethylamine, $(CH_2)_4NH$. It may be obtained from pyrrole or tobacco, which contains pyrrole.

pyruvate (pī′roo-vāt). A salt or ester of pyruvic acid.

pyruvic acid (pī-roo′vĭk). $CH_3CO \cdot COOH$. An organic acid that plays an important role in Krebs cycle, q.v. It is an intermediate product in the metabolism of carbohydrates, fats, and amino acids. It increases in quantity in the blood and tissues in thiamine deficiency because thiamine is essential for its oxidation.

pyrvinium pamoate (pĭr-vĭn′ē-ŭm). USP. A cyanine dye drug used in treating pinworms.

pythogenesis (pī″thō-jĕn′ē-sĭs) [Gr. *pythein*, to rot, + *genesis*, generation, birth]. Originating in decaying matter.

pythogenic [Gr. *pythein*, to rot]. Decay caused by filth or decomposition.

pyuria (pī-ū′rē-ă) [Gr. *pyon*, pus, + *ouron*, urine]. Pus in the urine; evidence of renal disease. Condition in which there are more than the normal number of pus or white blood cells in the urine. Freshly passed urine may be cloudy due to presence of phosphates or pus. If the former, the addition of acid will cause it to clear; if pus is present, it will not clear but may become gelatinous.

ETIOL: Lesion of urethra, ureters, bladder, kidneys; infection.

RS: cystitis; kidney; pyelitis, ureteritis; urethritis.

PZI. *protamine zinc insulin.* SEE: *insulin.*

Q

Q. 1. quantity. 2. Symb. for coulomb.

Q angle. The acute angle formed by a line from the anterior superior iliac spine of the pelvis through the center of the patella and a line from tibial tubercle through the patella. The angle describes the tracking of the patella in the trochlear groove of the femur. Normal angle is around 15 degrees. It is usually greater in females.

QCO₂. Number of microliters of CO_2 given off per milligram of dry weight of tissue per hour.

q.d. L. *quaque die*, every day.

Q disk. A dark, doubly refractile, anisotropic band of a striated muscle myofibril. SYN: *disk, anisotropic.*

Q fever [Q is for *query* because its etiology was unknown]. All acute infectious disease characterized by headache, fever, severe sweating, malaise, myalgia, and anorexia. Caused by the rickettsial organism, *Coxiella burnetii*. Contracted by inhaling infected dusts, drinking unpasteurized milk from infected animals, or by handling infected animals such as goats, cows, or sheep. Transmission by human contact is rare but has occurred. An effective vaccine is available for prevention of infection in persons who have a good chance of being exposed to the disease. Tetracyclines are effective in treating Q fever.

q.h. L. *quaque hora*, every hour.

q.i.d. L. *quater in die*, four times 〈

q.l. L. *quantum libet*, as much as on⌒ ⌒⌒es.

Q law. As temperature decreases, chemical activity decreases.

Qo₂. Number of microliters of O_2 taken up per milligram of dry weight of tissue per hour.

q.q.h. L. *quaque quarta hora*, every four hours.

QRS complex. The Q, R, and S waves or deflections of an electrocardiogram produced during the transmission of the excitation wave through the conductile tissue of the heart. Consists of an initial downward deflection (Q wave), a large upward deflection (R wave), and a second downward deflection (S wave) that represents the spread of the electrical impulse from the Purkinje fibers to the ventricular muscle. This initiates ventricular depolarization. Normal duration is 0.06 to 0.08 seconds.

QRST complex. The Q, R, S, and T waves of an electrocardiogram. Duration is approx. same as that of mechanical systole. The T wave, which follows the QRS complex, reflects ventricular depolarization. During the T wave, the ventricles are in their recovery period. Between the QRS complex and the T wave is the ST segment, which represents the completion of depolarization and the beginning of repolarization of the ventricles; this being the time of ventricular contraction. SEE: *electrocardiogram* for illus.

q.s. L. *quantum sufficit*, as much as suffices.

qt. *quart.*

Q-T segment. Portion of cardiac complex on the ECG that extends from the beginning of the Q wave and ends with the end of the T wave.

Quaalude. Trade name for methaqualone hydrochloride. Because of the illegal use and abuse of this drug, it is no longer distributed in the United States.

quack (kwăk) [D. *kwaksalven*, to peddle salve]. One who pretends to have knowledge or skill in medicine. SYN: *charlatan.*

quad. Medical "shorthand" for quadriceps, quadrilateral, quadrant, quadriplegia.

quadrangular (kwŏd-răng'ū-lĕr) [L. *quadri*, four, + *angulus*, angle]. Having four angles.

quadrangular lobe. A region forming the superior portion of each cerebellar hemisphere.

quadrangular membrane. The upper portion of the elastic membrane of the larynx. Extends from the aryepiglottic folds above to the level of the ventricular folds below.

quadrant (kwŏd'rănt) [L. *quadrans*, a fourth]. 1. The quarter or fourth of a circle. 2. One of four corresponding regions, as of the abdomen, divided for descriptive and diagnostic purposes.

 q., dental. One-quarter of the mouth. Each arch is divided in half so that one can easily describe the location of teeth or soft tissue observations. Quadrants are labeled as maxillary right and left or mandibular right and left and are shown in diagram form for dental records.

quadrantanopia (kwŏd″rănt-ă-nō′pē-ă) [″ + Gr. *an-*, not, + *opsis*, vision]. Blindness or diminished visual acuity in one-fourth of the visual field.

quadrantanopsia (kwŏd″rănt-ăn-ŏp′sē-ă) [″ + ″ + *opsis*, vision]. Loss of sight in approximately one-fourth of the visual field.

quadrate (kwŏd′rāt) [L. *quadratus*, squared]. Square, or having four equal sides.

quadrate lobe. A small lobe of liver located on the visceral surface and lying in contact with the pylorus and duodenum.

quadrate lobule. The square lobule of the

upper surface of the cerebellum.

quadri-, quadr- [L. *quattuor,* four]. Combining forms meaning having four or consisting of four.

quadribasic (kwŏd″rĭ-bā′sĭk). Having four replaceable atoms of hydrogen.

quadriceps (kwŏd′rĭ-sĕps) [″ + *caput,* head]. Four-headed, as a quadriceps muscle.

quadriceps femoris. A large muscle on the anterior surface of the thigh composed of four muscles: rectus femoris, vastus lateralis, vastus medialis, and vastus intermedius. These muscles are inserted by a common tendon on the tuberosity of the tibia. Quadriceps femoris is an extensor of the leg. SEE: *Muscles* in *Appendix.*

quadricepsplasty (kwŏd″rĭ-sĕps′plăs-tē) [″ + ″ + Gr. *plassein,* to form]. Plastic surgery for adhesions and scars around the quadriceps femoris muscle in order to restore function.

quadriceps reflex. Extension of the leg following contraction of the quadriceps muscle resulting from a quick tap of the patellar tendon. SYN: *knee-jerk reflex; patellar reflex.* SEE: *Jendrassik's maneuver.*

quadricuspid (kwŏd″rĭ-kŭs′pĭd) [″ + *cuspis,* point]. Having four cusps, as a heart valve or a tooth.

quadridigitate (kwŏd″rĭ-dĭj′ĭ-tāt). Having only four fingers on a hand or four toes on a foot.

quadrigemina (kwŏd″rĭ-jĕm′ĭn-ă) [″ + *geminus,* twin]. The corpora quadrigemina. SEE: *colliculus inferior; colliculus superior.*

quadrigeminal (kwŏd″rĭ-jĕm′ĭn-ăl). Fourfold; having four symmetrical parts. Pert. to the corpora quadrigemina, q.v.

quadrigeminum (kwŏd″rĭ-jĕm′ĭ-nŭm). One of the four quadrigeminal bodies of the brain.

quadrigeminus (kwŏd″rĭ-jĕm′ĭ-nŭs). Composed of four parts.

quadrilateral (kwŏd″rĭ-lăt′ĕr-ăl) [″ + *latus,* side]. Having four sides.

quadrilocular (kwŏd″rĭ-lŏk′ū-lăr) [″ + *loculus,* a small space]. Having four chambers, cavities, or spaces.

quadripara (kwŏd-rĭp′ă-ră) [″ + *parere,* to bring forth, to bear]. A woman who has had four pregnancies that have continued beyond the 20th week of gestation. SYN: *quartipara.* SEE: *para.*

quadripartite (kwŏd″rĭ-păr′tĭt) [″ + *partire,* to divide]. Divided into four parts.

quadriplegia (kwŏd″rĭ-plē′jē-ă) [″ + Gr. *plege,* stroke]. Paralysis of all four extremities and usually the trunk.

ETIOL: Injury to the spinal cord in the cervical spine. The higher the injury, the less function is available in the arms. Injury above the 3rd cervical vertebra requires a mechanical respiratory device to maintain life.

EMERGENCY CARE: When a fracture of a cervical vertebra is suspected, the injured patient's head and neck should be held steady with applied traction during transportation.

TREAT: Initial treatment includes immobilization with the use of Crutchfield tongs and antibiotic therapy. When the fracture has healed, physical and occupational therapy are instituted.

NURSING IMPLICATIONS: In accordance with prescribed procedure, immobilize the patient's neck. Establish and maintain a patent airway, and monitor respiratory status for signs of insufficiency (hypoxemia, hypercapnia, and acidemia). Assess bowel sounds for development of paralytic ileus. Apply full-length antithromboembolic stockings to legs; when positioning patient upright, monitor blood pressure for evidence of orthostatic hypotension. If that condition is present, an abdominal binder may be helpful. If injury is above T-4, assess for hypertension, a sign of autonomic dysreflexia. Assist patient with self-care deficits, including skin and oral care, feeding and nutrition, elimination, respiratory toilet, positioning, and exercise. When assisting with activities of daily living, be sure urinary catheter is patent and provide fluids and bulk in diet to prevent fecal impaction. Encourage patient and family to verbalize their concerns and support them through their grief and loss. Assist family to plan realistically for the future regarding changed functional abilities, body image, and self concept. Involve the patient in a rehabilitation program as soon as he is stabilized. SEE: *Nursing Diagnoses* in *Appendix.*

quadripolar (kwŏd″rĭ-pō′lăr). Pert. to a cell having four poles.

quadrisect (kwŏd′rĭ-sĕkt) [″ + *sectio,* a cutting]. To divide into four parts.

quadrisection (kwŏd″rĭ-sĕk′shŭn). Dividing into four sections or parts.

quadritubercular (kwŏd″rĭ-tū-bĕr′kū-lĕr) [″ + *tuberculum,* a little swelling]. Having four tubercles or cusps.

quadrivalent (kwŏd″rĭ-vā′lĕnt) [″ + *valens,* powerful]. Having ability to replace four atoms of hydrogen in a compound, i.e., a chemical valence of four.

quadruped (kwŏd′roo-pĕd″) [″ + *pes,* foot]. 1. Four-footed animal. 2. Assuming a position with hands and feet on floor.

quadrupedal reflex (kwŏd-roop′ĕd-ăl). Extension of flexed arm on assuming quadrupedal posture.

quadruplet (kwŏd′roo-plĕt, kwŏ-droo′plĕt) [L. *quadruplus,* fourfold]. One of four children born of the same mother in the same confinement. SEE: *Hellin's law.*

quail poisoning. Acute myoglobinuria following ingestion of quail. It is postulated that the actual cause of the poisoning is a toxic substance the quail has ingested, perhaps hemlock. Fatigued persons who presumably have an enzymatic abnormality in their muscular tissue are susceptible to this type of poisoning. It has been suggested that this type of poisoning accounts for a plague associated with eating quails mentioned in the Holy Bible (Numbers 11:31-35).

quale (kwā'lē) [L. *qualis,* of what kind]. The quality of anything, esp. of a sensation.

qualimeter (kwŏl-ĭm'ĕt-ĕr) [″ + Gr. *metron,* measure]. Device for measuring the quality of roentgen rays. SEE: *penetrometer.*

qualitative (kwŏl'ĭ-tā″tĭv) [L. *qualitativus*]. Referring to the quality of anything. SEE: *quantitative.*

qualitative analysis. In chemistry, an analysis that determines the nature of the elements of a compound, or the identity of the components of a mixture. SEE: *quantitative.*

quality (kwŏl'ĭ-tē) [L. *qualitas,* quality]. That which constitutes or characterizes a thing; the natural character.

quality-adjusted life-years. ABBR: QALY. A term used in economic analyses to provide a numerical description of the value of a medical procedure or service to groups of patients with similar medical conditions. This attempt to quantify the outcome of medical procedures is predicated on a number of difficult-to-measure assumptions. The validity and, therefore, the usefulness of this concept is controversial.

quality assurance. Activities and programs designed to achieve a desired degree or grade of care in a defined medical, nursing, or health-care setting or program. The quality assurance program must include evaluation and educational components to identify and correct problems. Such programs are required for funding by the Public Health Act.

The Quality Assurance Program for Medical Care in the Hospital (QAP) is a guide developed by the American Hospital Association for development of such programs by hospital administrators and medical staffs.

quality of life. A concept that differs for each person and may vary for the same individual as that person's life situation changes. The holistic treatment of a patient requires that the health-care team assess what is most important to that individual. In some cases, it is not possible to establish a situation in which there is complete freedom from the

signs and symptoms of disease. In those cases, the goal is to have the quality of life be as good as possible despite the disease. Also, in persons who have suffered disabilities or loss of mental or physical skills, it is important to emphasize the positive features of their remaining capabilities rather than to dwell on the negative aspects of what has been lost.

quanta (kwŏn'tă) [L.]. Pl. of quantum.

quantimeter (kwŏn-tĭm'ĕt-ĕr) [L. *quantus,* how great, + Gr. *metron,* measure]. Device for measuring quantity of roentgen rays to which a subject is exposed.

quanti-Pirquet (kwŏn″tĭ-pēr-kā') [Clemens Peter Johann von Pirquet, Austrian pediatrician, 1874 – 1929]. Quantitative cutaneous test of amount of sensitiveness to tuberculin by use of graduated dilutions.

quantitative (kwŏn″tĭ-tā'tĭv) [LL. *quantitativus*]. Concerning quantity. SEE: *qualitative.*

quantitative analysis. Analysis that determines the proportionate parts of elements in a compound, or the percentage of components of a mixture. SEE: *qualitative.*

quantity (kwŏn'tĭ-tē) [L. *quantitas,* quantity]. Amount; portion.

quantivalence. The number of hydrogen atoms with which an element or radical will combine.

quantum (kwŏn'tŭm) [L., how much]. (pl. *quanta*) 1. A definite amount. 2. A unit of radiant energy.

quantum libet (kwŏn'tŭm lĭ'bĕt) [L.]. ABBR: q.l. As much as desired.

quantum mottle. A variation in the number of x-ray photons that strike the radiographic film during an exposure. This phenomenon causes a non-uniform intensity over the areas of similar densities on the film.

quantum sufficit (kwŏn'tŭm sŭf'fi-sĭt) [L.]. ABBR: q.s. As much as suffices.

quantum theory. Theory stating that radiation is an intermittent, not continuous, emission of energy in varying multiples of quanta action.

quarantine (kwor'ăn-tēn″) [It. *quarantina,* 40 days]. 1. The period during which entry to a country is prohibited or the period of isolation of persons exposed to infectious diseases — formerly 40 days. 2. Period of isolation from public communication following onset of a contagious disease.

Complete quarantine is limitation of freedom of movement of healthy persons or domestic animals that have been exposed to a communicable disease for a period of time equal to the longest incubation period of the disease, in such a manner as to prevent effective contact with those not so exposed.

SEE: *contagious; isolation.*

quart (kwort) [L. *quartus,* a fourth]. ABBR: qt. A unit of fluid equal to one fourth of a gallon, or 2 pints, or 946 ml; in dry measure, one eighth of a peck.

quartan (kwor'tăn) [L. *quartana,* of the fourth]. 1. Occurring every fourth day. 2. Malarial fever with a paroxysm every fourth day, figuring from and including the first day of paroxysm. SEE: *fever; malaria.*

   q., double. Malaria in which two concurrent cycles result in fever occurring on two successive days.

   q., triple. Malaria in which three concurrent cycles result in fever occurring every day.

quartile (kwor'tĭl) [L. *quartus,* a fourth]. One of the two middle values of each half of a series of variables.

quartipara (kwor-tĭp'ă-ră) [" + *parere,* to bring forth, to bear]. A woman who has had four pregnancies that have continued beyond the 20th week of gestation. SYN: *quadripara.* SEE: *para.*

quartisect (kwor'tĭ-sĕkt) [" + *sectio,* a cutting]. To cut into four parts.

quartz (kwärts) [Ger. *quarz*]. Silicon dioxide, the principal ingredient of sandstone (crystallized silica; rock crystal). When crystal is clear and colorless, it permits the passage of large amounts of ultraviolet radiations.

quartz applicator. Quartz rod of various shapes and angles to conduct, by total internal reflection, ultraviolet radiation from a water-cooled mercury arc quartz lamp.

quartz glass. Crystalline quartz is used for prisms and lenses; fused quartz for windows, through which ultraviolet radiations are freely transmitted.

Quarzan. Trade name for clidinium bromide.

quassation (kwă-sā'shŭn) [L. *quassatio*]. A beating, a shaking; breaking up of crude materials into small pieces.

quassia (kwŏsh'ă, kwŏsh'ē-ă) [*Quassi,* Surinam inhabitant who discovered its medicinal value]. The wood of a tree, *Quassia amara,* grown in tropical America. Once considered valuable as a bitter tonic, and in an enema for certain intestinal parasites.

Quatelet index. An index for estimating obesity. The weight in kilograms is divided by the height in meters squared:

$$\frac{W}{H^2}$$

SYN: *body mass index.* SEE: *ponderal index.*

quater in die (kwŏ'tĕr ĭn dē'ă) [L.]. ABBR: q.i.d. Four times a day.

quaternary (kwŏ-tĕr'nă-rē) [L. *quaternarius,* of four]. 1. The fourth in order. 2. Composed of four elements.

Queckenstedt's sign (kwĕk'ĕn-stĕts) [Hans Queckenstedt, Ger. physician, 1876–1918]. Upon compression of the veins of the neck, unilaterally or bilaterally, cerebrospinal fluid pressure rises rapidly in healthy persons; this disappears when pressure is released. In vertebral canal block, the pressure is scarcely affected by this procedure.

quenching (kwĕnch'ĭng). 1. Cooling something that is hot; or decreasing the radioactive energy released. 2. In toxicology, the effect of a material to decrease the toxicity of some of the chemical or chemicals in the compound.

   q., fluorescence. A technique for investigating antigen-antibody reactions by measuring the light absorbed by antigen mixed with fluorescent-labeled antibody.

querulent (kwĕr'ū-lĕnt) [L. *querulus,* complaining]. 1. Complaining; fretful. 2. One who is dissatisfied, complaining, and suspicious.

Quervain's disease (kār'vănz). [Fritz de Quervain, Swiss surgeon, 1868–1940]. Chronic tenosynovitis of the abductor pollicis longus and extensor pollicis brevis muscles.

questionnaire. A list of questions submitted to a patient or research subject in order to obtain data for analysis.

Questran. Trade name for cholestyramine resin.

quick (kwĭk) [ME. *quicke,* alive]. 1. A part susceptible to keen feeling, esp. part of a finger or toe to which nail is attached. 2. Pregnant and experiencing fetal movements.

quickening (kwĭk'ĕn-ĭng). First movements of the fetus felt in utero. Occurs from 18th to 20th week of pregnancy. Movements have been felt as early as the tenth week and in rare cases are not felt during the entire pregnancy.

quicklime. CaO. Calcium oxide, unslaked lime. Forms calcium hydroxide when water is added to it.

quicksilver [ME. *quicke,* alive, + *silver,* silver]. The metal mercury.

Quick's test (kwĭks) [Armand James Quick, U.S. physician, 1894–1978]. 1. A liver function test that measures the amount of hippuric acid excreted after a dose of sodium benzoate is given. 2. A test for the amount of prothrombin present in blood plasma.

quiescent. The condition of being inactive or at rest. SYN: *dormant; latent.*

quinacrine hydrochloride. USP. An agent used in the treatment of malaria. Also used in infestations of *Giardia lamblia,* a parasite. Trade name is Atabrine Hydrochloride.

Quinaglute. Trade name for quinidine gluconate, USP.

Quincke's disease (kwĭnk'ēz). [Heinrich I.

Quincke, Ger. physician, 1842–1922]. Angioneurotic edema of skin; urticaria; giant hives.

Quincke's pulse. A sign of aortic insufficiency, seen under fingernails and indicated by alternate reddening and blanching. SYN: *pulse, capillary.*

Quincke's puncture. Lumbar puncture to determine tension of spinal fluid, or to remove some of the spinal fluid.

Quine. Trade name for quinine sulfate.

quinestrol (kwĭn-ĕs'trōl). USP. An estrogen. Trade name is Estrovis.

quinethazone (kwĭn-ĕth'ă-zōn). USP. A diuretic. Trade name is Hydromox.

quingestanol acetate (kwĭn-jĕs'tă-nōl). A progestational drug. SEE: *progestational agent.*

quinic acid. A substance present in some plants, including cinchona bark, and berries.

Quinidex. Trade name for quinidine sulfate.

quinidine sulfate (kwĭn'ĭ-dēn). USP. The sulfate of an alkaloid obtained from cinchona bark; a white, crystalline substance with a bitter taste. Trade names are Quinidex, Cin-Quin, and SK-Quinidine Sulfate.

ACTION/USES: To regulate heart rhythm, esp. to prevent fibrillation.

quinine (kwī'nīn″, kwĭ-nēn′) [Sp. *quina*]. Bitter white crystalline alkaloid derived from cinchona bark.

USES: Antimalarial. Usually administered in the form of its salts.

q. bisulfate. The acid sulfate of quinine. Used the same as quinine sulfate, but has greater solubility.

q. dihydrochloride. The dihydrochloride of quinine, freely soluble in water, 1 gm dissolving in 0.6 ml of water. Suitable for intravenous injection.

q. hydrochloride. The hydrochloride of quinine. Used in treatment of malaria.

q. sulfate. USP. The sulfate of an alkaloid obtained from cinchona. Used to treat malaria. Trade names are Coco-Quinine, Quinamm, and Quine.

quinine and urea hydrochloride. Combination used, in dilute solutions, as a sclerosing agent for injection treatment of hemorrhoids and varicose veins.

quininism (kwī'nīn-izm, kwĭ-nēn′izm) [Sp. *quina*, quinine, + Gr. *-ismos*, condition]. Poisoning by cinchona or its alkaloids. SYN: *cinchonism.*

quinolones. A general class of broad-spectrum antibiotics that are readily absorbed from the gastrointestinal tract and have a low incidence of adverse reactions.

quinone (kwĭn'ōn). 1. Yellow crystalline oxidation product of quinic acid. 2. Class of organic compounds in which two atoms of hydrogen are replaced by two oxygen atoms.

quinqu- [L. *quinque*]. Combining form meaning five.

Quinquaud's disease (kăn-kōz′). [Charles E. Quinquaud, Fr. physician, 1841–1894] Purulent inflammation of the hair follicles of the scalp, resulting in bald patches. SEE: *folliculitis.*

quinquetubercular (kwĭn″kwē-tū-bĕr′kū-lăr). Having five cusps or tubercles.

quinquevalent (kwĭng″kwĕ-vā′lĕnt). Pert. to a radical or element with a valence of five.

quinquina (kwĭn-kwī′nă, kĭn-kē′nă). Cinchona, q.v.

quinsy (kwĭn′zē) [ME. *quinesye*, sore throat]. Abscess of tonsil capsule due to bacterial inflammation. Abscess may rupture spontaneously; if not, surgical incision may be required. SYN: *abscess, peritonsillar.*

quintan (kwĭn′tăn) [L. *quintanus*, of a fifth]. 1. Occurring every fifth day. 2. Intermittent fever, the paroxysms occurring every fifth day with intermission of three days.

quinti- [L. *quintus*, fifth]. Combining form meaning fifth.

quintipara (kwĭn-tĭp′ă-ră) [″ + *parere*, to bear]. A woman who has had five pregnancies that have continued beyond the 20th week of gestation. SEE: *para.*

quintuplet (kwĭn′tū-plĕt, kwĭn-tŭp′lĕt) [LL. *quintuplex*, fivefold]. One of five children born of one mother during the same confinement. SEE: *Hellin's law.*

quotidian (kwō-tĭd′ē-ăn) [L. *quotidianus*, daily]. Occurring daily.

quotidian fever. A malarial fever characterized by daily paroxysms.

quotient (kwō′shĕnt) [L. *quotiens*, how many times]. Number of times one number is contained in another.

q., achievement. A percentile rating of a child's score on a test with respect to age, level of education, and peer performance.

q., intelligence. Division of an individual's mental age by the actual age.

q., respiratory. The result of dividing the amount of carbon dioxide in expired air by the oxygen inhaled, normally 0.9.

q.v. L. *quantum vis*, as much as you please; *quod vide*, which see.

Q wave. A downward or negative wave of an electrocardiogram following the P wave. It is usually not prominent and may be absent without significance.

R

R. 1. *respiration; right; roentgen.* 2. In chem., a radical.

R−. Abbr. used in organic chemistry to indicate part of a molecule.

−R. Rinne negative. SEE: *Rinne's test.*

+R. Rinne positive. SEE: *Rinne's test.*

℞. Symb. for L. *recipe*, take. SEE: *prescription.*

RA. *rheumatoid arthritis; right atrium.*

Ra. Chem. symb. for the element radium.

rabbetting (răb'ĕt-ĭng) [Fr. *raboter*, to plane]. Interlocking of the jagged edges of a fractured bone.

rabbit fever. Tularemia.

rabbitpox. An acute viral disease of laboratory rabbits.

rabiate (rā'bē-āt) [L. *rabies,* rage]. Suffering from rabies. SYN: *rabid.*

rabic (răb'ĭk). Concerning rabies.

rabicidal (răb-ĭ-sī'dăl) [L. *rabies,* rage, + *cidus,* kill]. Destructive to causative virus of rabies.

rabid (răb'ĭd). Pert. to, or affected with, rabies. SYN: *rabiate.*

rabies (rā'bēz) [L. *rabere,* to rage]. An acute infectious disease of warm-blooded mammals, esp. carnivores. Wildlife, esp. bats, skunks, foxes, and raccoons, have been found to have rabies; dogs, cats, and cattle are the domestic animals particularly susceptible. Rabbits, squirrels, chipmunks, rats, and mice are rarely infected. Characterized by involvement of central nervous system, resulting in paralysis and finally death. May be communicated to man through the bite of a rabid animal. The virus can also be transmitted to man or other animals from bats without a direct bite. It is assumed that this transmission occurs through inhalation of infectious aerosols. However, this mode of transmission is rare. The virus can be transmitted as if the conjunctiva, mucous membranes, or scratches were contaminated with saliva from a rabid animal. SYN: *hydrophobia; lyssa.*

SYM: The site of the bite is painful, tingles, and is sensitive to changes in temperature. Attempts to drink water produce laryngeal spasm. Behavior is restless and abnormal, and convulsions may be produced by sensory stimuli. Fever, muscle twitches, hyperventilation, and excess saliva may be present during an acute attack.

ETIOL: A neurotropic filterable virus present in saliva of rabid animals.

DIAG: No tests are available to diagnose rabies in humans before the onset of clinical disease.

The most reliable test for rabies in patients who have clinical signs of the disease is direct immunofluorescent study of a full thickness biopsy of the skin taken from the back of the neck above the hair line.

The rapid fluorescent focus inhibition test (RFFIT) is used to measure rabies-neutralizing antibodies in serum. This test has the advantage of providing results within 24 hours. Other tests of antibodies may take as long as 14 days.

True rabies must be distinguished from rabies hysteria, a psychological condition in persons who think they have been bitten by a rabid animal.

INCUB: Usually 2 to 8 weeks but may be as short as 10 days or as long as a year, or even longer, depending on depth of laceration and site of wound. The virus moves along nerve axons passively at about 3 millimeters per hour. It is not known how the virus remains viable or where it is located during prolonged incubation periods.

PREVENTION: The most important preventive measure is to provide rabies vaccination for domestic animals, esp. house pets. Thoroughly clean all bites or scratches made by any animal with strong (20%) medicinal soap solution. Deep puncture wounds should be opened to permit access of solution.

Report rabid domestic or wild animals to proper authorities.

TREAT: If the attack by the animal was unprovoked, the animal was not caught, and rabies is present in that species in the geographic area, give rabies immune globulin and vaccine immediately. If the animal is available and the owner and the health authorities agree, the animal may be killed and the brain examined by fluorescent-antibody technique to determine the need for anti-rabies treatment. Valuable or loved animals may be confined and observed for 10 days. If this is done, the decision to treat the patient is based on the behavior of the animal while observed, the presence of rabies in the area, and the circumstances of the bite.

The wound should be treated as soon as possible with virus-destroying solutions such as soap and water, alcohol, iodine, and quaternary-ammonium disinfectants. The wound should be sutured only if absolutely required. Tetanus prophylaxis is included in the treatment, as is the use of antibiotics when indicated.

Human diploid cell rabies vaccine

(HDCV) and rabies immune globulin (RIG) are available. These should be given as soon as possible after exposure to the bite of an animal known to be rabid. Some of the RIG is infiltrated around the bite and the rest is given intramuscularly. If the animal is not caught and rabies is known to be present in the area, start HDCV and RIG immediately, following the schedule enclosed in the vaccine package.

PROG: As of 1990 there were only three reported cases in which patients recovered from rabies. Each of those patients had received either pre-exposure or postexposure prophylactic treatment prior to the onset of clinical illness.

NURSING IMPLICATIONS: Administer prescribed rabies vaccine, treating local erythema, pruritus, or pain symptomatically. Administer antibiotics and other drug therapy as prescribed. Assess, cleanse, and redress the wounds as needed. If rabies develops, isolate the patient in a dark, quiet room. Use universal precautions in handling saliva and saliva-contaminated articles. Monitor and support cardiac and pulmonary function. Provide psychologic support to the patient and the family regarding impending death. Help prevent rabies by educating the public to the need for vaccination of family pets. Warn people to avoid all contact with wild animals because they may have rabies. SEE: *Nursing Diagnoses* in *Appendix.*

rabies immune globulin. USP. ABBR: RIG. A standardized preparation of globulins derived from the blood plasma or serum from selected human donors who have been immunized with rabies vaccine and have developed high titers of rabies antibody. It is used to produce passive immunity in persons bitten by animals. Trade name is Hyperab. SEE: *rabies.*

rabies virus group. A genus of virus, the official designation of which is *Lyssavirus.* The virus that causes human rabies is included in this group.

rabiform (rā′bĭ-form) [″ + *forma,* shape]. Resembling rabies.

raccoon sign [raccoons have distinctive periorbital coloration]. Periorbital ecchymosis. May be present in patients who have a basilar skull fracture.

race (rās) [Fr.]. 1. A distinct ethnic group characterized by traits that are transmitted through the offspring. 2. A group of individuals with the same characteristics who originated from a common ancestor. 3. A taxonomic classification of individuals within the same species who show distinct genetic characteristics.

racemase (rā′sē-mās). An enzyme that cata-

lyzes racemization, i.e., the production of an optically active compound.

racemate (rā′sē-māt). A racemic compound.

racemic (rā-sē′mĭk). A mixture that is optically inactive.

racemization (rā″sē-mĭ-zā′shŭn). The production of a racemic form of an optically active compound.

racemose (răs′ē-mōs) [L. *racemosus,* full of clusters]. Resembling a clustered bunch of grapes, as a gland, divided and subdivided, ending in a bunch of follicles.

rachi-, rachio- [Gr. *rhachis,* spine]. Combining forms indicating spine.

rachial (rā′kē-ăl) [Gr. *rhachis,* spine]. Concerning the spine. SYN: *rachidial.*

rachicele (rā′kĭ-sēl) [″ + *kele,* tumor, swelling]. Protrusion of contents of spinal canal in spina bifida cystica.

rachidial (ră-kĭd′ē-ăl). Concerning the spine.

rachidian (ră-kĭd′ē-ăn). Rel. to the spinal column.

rachigraph (rā′kĭ-grăf) [″ + *graphein,* to write]. Device for outlining the curves of the spine.

rachilysis (ră-kĭl′ĭ-sĭs) [″ + *lysis,* dissolution]. Mechanical treatment of lateral curvature of the spine through traction and pressure.

rachiocampsis (rā-kē-ō-kămp′sĭs) [″ + *kampsis,* a bending]. Curvature of spine.

rachiometer (rā-kē-ŏm′ē-tĕr) [″ + *metron,* measure]. Instrument for measuring a curvature of the spine.

rachiomyelitis (rā″kē-ō-mī″ĕ-lī′tĭs) [″ + *myelos,* marrow, + *itis,* inflammation]. Inflammation of the spinal cord.

rachiopagus (rā″kē-ŏp′ă-gŭs) [″ + *pagos,* thing fixed]. A conjoined twin deformity in which the two are joined at the vertebral column.

rachiopathy (rā″kē-ŏp′ă-thē) [″ + *pathos,* disease]. Disease of the spine.

rachioplegia (rā-kē-ō-plē′jē-ă) [″ + *plege,* a stroke]. Paralysis due to a lesion in the spinal cord.

rachioscoliosis (rā″kē-ō-skō′lē-ō′sĭs) [″ + *skoliosis,* curvature]. Lateral curvature of the spine.

rachiotome (rā′kē-ō-tōm″) [″ + *tome,* incision]. Instrument for dividing the vertebrae.

rachiotomy (rā″kē-ŏt′ō-mē). Surgical cutting of the vertebral column.

rachis (rā′kĭs) [Gr. *rhachis*] (pl. *rachises*). The spinal column.

rachischisis (ră-kĭs′kĭ-sĭs) [″ + *schisis,* a splitting]. Congenital spinal column fissure. SYN: *spina bifida.*

r., posterior. Spina bifida.

rachitic (ră-kĭt′ĭk). Pert. to, or affected with, rickets.

rachitic rosary. Widening of the ends of the ribs, creating a beaded tract running down either side of the anterior chest wall in the person with rickets.

rachitis (rä-kī′tĭs) [″ + *itis*, inflammatory]. 1. Inflammation of the spine. 2. Rickets.

     r. fetalis annularis. Congenital enlargement of epiphyses of long bones.

     r. fetalis micromelica. A congenital shortness of the bones.

rachitism (răk′ĭ-tĭsm). Tendency to rickets.

rachitogenic (ră-kĭt″ō-jĕn′ĭk) [″ + *genesis*, generation, birth]. Causing or inducing development of rickets.

rachitome (răk′ĭ-tōm″) [″ + *tome*, incision]. Instrument employed for opening spinal canal.

rachitomy (ră-kĭt′ō-mē) [″ + *tome*, incision]. Rachiotomy, q.v.

raclage (ră-klŏzh′) [Fr.]. Destruction and removal of a soft growth by scraping or rubbing. SEE: *curettage.*

rad. *radiation absorbed dose.*

radectomy (rā-dĕk′tō-mē) [L. *radix*, root, + Gr. *ektome*, excision]. Surgical removal of all or a portion of the root of a tooth.

radiability (rā″dē-ă-bĭl′ĭ-tē) [L. *radius*, ray, + *habilitas*, able]. Capability of being penetrated readily by roentgen ray.

radiable. The property of being penetrable by x-rays.

radiad (rā′dē-ăd) [L. *radialis*, radial, + *ad*, toward]. In the direction of the radial side.

radial (rā′dē-ăl). 1. Radiating out from a given center. 2. Pert. to the radius.

radialis (rā″dē-ā′lĭs) [L.]. Concerning the radius bone.

radial reflex. Flexion of forearm resulting when lower end of radius is percussed.

radian (rā′dē-ăn). 1. A unit of angular measurement equivalent to 57.295 degrees. It is subtended at the center of a circle by an arc the length of the radius of a circle. 2. In ophthalmometry, a lens of one radian would have one plane surface equal in length to the radius of curvature of the curved surface.

radiant (rā′dē-ănt) [L. *radians*, radiate]. 1. Emitting beams of light. 2. Transmitted by radiation. 3. Emanating from a common center. SEE: *energy; heat; radiation.*

radiate (rā′dē-āt) [L. *radiatre*, to emit rays]. To spread from a common center.

radiatio (rā-dē-ā′shē-ō) [L.]. An anatomical structure, esp. a neurological one, that by means of radiating fibers forms interconnections between parts.

radiation (rā-dē-ā′shŭn) [L. *radiatio*, to radiate]. 1. Process by which energy is propagated through space or matter. 2. Emission of rays in all directions from a common center. 3. Ionizing radiation used for diagnostic or therapeutic purposes. 4. A general term for any form of radiant energy emission or divergence, as of energy in all directions from luminous bodies, roentgen ray tubes, radioactive elements, and fluorescent substances. 5. In neurology, a group of fibers that diverge from a common origin.

     r., acoustic. R., auditory.

     r., auditory. A band of fibers that connect auditory areas of cerebral cortex with the medial geniculate body of the thalamus. SYN: *r., acoustic.*

     r., corpuscular. Radiation composed of discrete elements or particles such as elements of atomic nuclei, i.e., alpha, beta, neutron, positron, or proton particles.

     r., electromagnetic. Rays that travel at the speed of light. They exhibit both magnetic and electrical properties. SEE: *electromagnetic spectrum* for table.

     r., heterogeneous. Radiation containing waves of various wavelengths.

     r., homogeneous. Radiation containing waves of only one wavelength.

     r., infrared. Invisible heat rays beyond the red end of the spectrum. Near or short infrared extends from 7200 to 14,000 angstrom units (A.U.); far or long infrared extends from 15,000 to 120,000 A.U. SEE: *infrared rays.*

     r., interstitial. Radiation accomplished by insertion of radium or radon directly into tissues.

     r., ionizing. Radiation that either directly or indirectly induces ionization of radiation-absorbing material. SEE: *radiation injury, ionizing.*

     r., irritative. Overdose of ultraviolet irradiation resulting in erythema and, in exceptional cases, blister formation.

     r., low-level. Radiation, usually nonionizing, emitted by the magnetic fields produced by electrical currents. Included would be power lines and electrical appliances such as electric blankets, television sets, and computer terminals. Even though evidence that these levels of radiation are harmful is controversial, it would be prudent to avoid exposure to these sources of radiation as much as possible.

     r., nonionizing. ABBR: NIR. SEE: *radiation, low-level.*

     r., occipitothalamic. R., optic.

     r. of corpus callosum. Total of fibers radiating from corpus callosum into each cerebral hemisphere.

     r., optic. A system of fibers extending from the lateral geniculate body of the thalamus through the sublenticular portion of the internal capsule to the calcarine occipital cortex (striate area). SYN: *geniculocalcarine tract; r., occipitothalamic.*

     r., photochemical. From a therapeutic

standpoint, the electromagnetic spectrum is divided into photothermal and photochemical radiations. Photochemical radiations penetrate tissues only fractions of a millimeter, are absorbed by protoplasm, and cause physical and biological changes. Photothermal radiation does not penetrate the skin but causes surface heating. A heating pad provides photothermal, i.e., infrared, heat.

r., pyramidal. Radiation of fibers from the cerebral cortex to the pyramidal tract.

r.'s, solar. Radiations of the sun, 60% in infrared region and 40% visible and ultraviolet.

r., striatomesencephalic. Fibers originating in corpus striatum and terminating principally in substantia nigra of midbrain.

r., striatosubthalamic. A system of fibers consisting of three groups emerging from medial aspect of lentiform nucleus and entering subthalamic region, most terminating there but some continuing into the midbrain. SYN: *ansa lenticularis.*

r., striatothalamic. Groups of fibers connecting the corpus striatum with the thalamus and subthalamus.

r., thalamic. Groups of fibers that connect the thalamus with cerebral hemispheres. Include frontal, centroparietal, occipital, and optic radiations.

r., ultraviolet. Radiant energy extending from 3900 to 200 angstrom units (A.U.) Divided into near ultraviolet, which extends from 3900 to 2900 A.U., and far ultraviolet, which extends from 2900 to 200 A.U.

r., visible. Visible spectrum may be broken up into different wavelengths representing different colors:

    Violet, 3900 – 4550 angstrom units (A.U.)
    Blue, 4550 – 4920 A.U.
    Green, 4920 – 5770 A.U.
    Yellow, 5770 – 5970 A.U.
    Orange, 5970 – 6220 A.U.
    Red, 6220 – 7700 A.U.

    SEE: *heliotherapy; helium; spectrum.*

radiation absorbed dose. The quantity of ionizing radiation that is absorbed by any material per unit mass of matter.

radiation accidents, emergency handling of. As the field of nuclear energy expands into industry, medicine, and university studies, it is to be expected that there will be a rise in contamination accidents.

The U.S. Energy Research and Development Administration has regional offices for information and assistance on radiological emergencies. Contacts may be made in person or by phone.

Emergency handling of radiation exposure or radioactive contamination cases should not be feared. The handling of these cases is a matter involving common sense, cleanliness, and good housekeeping. Radiation accident problems have parallels in other conditions handled frequently by emergency rooms and rescue squads.

Radiation can be detected and measured by a simple instrument, a survey meter. The hospital or medical team can be involved by following these simple rules.

There are four types of radiation accident patients. The first type is the individual who has received whole or partial external body radiation and may have received a lethal dose of radiation, but is no hazard to attendants, other patients, or the environment. This patient is no different from the radiation therapy or diagnostic x-ray patient.

The second type is the individual who has received internal contamination by inhalation or ingestion. This patient also is no hazard to attendants, other patients, or the environment. Following cleansing of minor amounts of contaminated material deposited on the body surface during airborne exposure, this individual is similar to the patient with chemical poisoning, such as lead. Body wastes should be collected and saved for measurements of the amount of nuclides to assist in determination of appropriate therapy.

External contamination of body surface and clothing by liquids or by dirt particles presents a third type, with problems similar to vermin infestation. Surgical isolation technique to protect attendants, and cleansing to protect other patients and the hospital environment, must take place to confine and remove a potential hazard.

In the fourth type, when external contamination is complicated by a wound, care must be taken not to cross-contaminate surrounding surfaces from the wound and vice versa. The wound and surrounding surfaces are cleansed separately and sealed off when clean. When crushed dirty tissue is involved, early preliminary wet debridement following wound irrigation may be indicated. Further debridement and more definitive therapy can await sophisticated measurement and consultant guidance.

STANDING ORDERS FOR EMERGENCY HANDLING: If the ambulance or rescue squad that picks up the radiation accident case has a radio or telephone, the crew should alert the Emergency Room to expect a patient who may have had radiation exposure or radioactive contamination.

On receipt of notification of the momentary arrival of a case involving radiation exposure or contamination, it is the responsibility of the senior person (nurse or physician) on duty in the hospital Emergency Room to take the following steps:

1. Notify responsible staff physician or nurse and aides (trained health physicists or technologists from the nuclear medicine or x-ray department).

2. Get appropriate survey meter if one is on hand in the hospital. If the hospital has no meter, notify the hospital administrator or responsible hospital official so that a survey meter and other pertinent equipment may be obtained by calling the police department.

3. Notify the hospital administrator so he or she can seek expert professional consultation for technical management of the case.

4. Prepare separate space if contamination is suspected, using either isolation room or cubicle if available. Some hospitals use the morgue, since the autopsy table lends itself to washing. The morgue entrance, rather than the Emergency Room, would then be used. When the morgue is used, the patient and family must be reassured as to why that space is used. If no separate space is available, cover a floor area immediately adjacent to the entrance to the Emergency Room with absorbent paper—the area should be adequate for stretcher-cart, disposal hampers, and working space for professional attendants. Mark and close off this area. If dust is involved, be prepared to shut off the air-circulation system to prevent spread of contamination.

Upon arrival of the ambulance, the responsible physician or nurse in the Emergency Room should:

1. Check patient on stretcher for contamination (preferably as stretcher is removed from the ambulance) by use of a survey meter.

2. If patient is seriously injured, give emergency lifesaving assistance immediately.

3. Handle contaminated patient and wound as one would a surgical procedure, with gown, gloves, cap, and mask.

4. If possible external contamination is involved, save all clothing and bedding from ambulance, as well as blood, urine, stool, vomitus, and all metal objects (such as jewelry, belt buckles, dental plates). Label with name, body location, time, and date. Save each in appropriate containers; mark containers clearly, "Radioactive—Do Not Discard."

5. If physical status permits, start decontamination by cleansing and scrubbing the area of highest contamination. If an extremity alone is involved, clothing may serve as an effective barrier and the affected limb alone may be scrubbed and cleansed.

Initial cleansing should be done with soap and warm water. If the body as a whole is involved or clothing is generally permeated by contaminated material, showering and scrubbing will be necessary. Pay special attention to hair-covered areas, body orifices, and body folds. Remeasure radiation contamination and record measurement after each washing or showering.

If a wound is involved, prepare and cover the wound with self-adhering disposable surgical drape. Cleanse neighboring surfaces of skin. Seal off cleansed areas with self-adhering disposable surgical drapes. Remove wound covering and irrigate wound with sterile water, catching the irrigating fluid in a basin or can to be marked and handled as described in rule 4 above. Each step in the decontamination should be preceded and followed by monitoring and recording of the location and extent of contamination.

6. Save physicians', nurses', and attendants' scrub or protective clothing, as described in rule 4 for patients' clothing. Doctors, nurses, and attendants must follow the same monitoring and decontamination routine as the patients.

7. If the Emergency Room staff is confronted with a grossly contaminated wound with dirt particles and crushed tissue, they should be prepared to do a preliminary simple wet debridement. Further measurements may necessitate sophisticated wound counting detection instruments supplied by the consultant who will advise if further definitive debridement is necessary.

When the accident has occurred at a plant, university, or medical group regularly working with nuclear material, the health physicist, supervisor, coworker, and patient should be able to inform the rescue squad of the nature of the accident, type of radiation exposure or radioactive contamination involved, and possible body areas that may be affected.

radiation biology. The scientific study of the effects of radiation on living organisms.

radiation injury, ionizing. Injury to cell life because of therapeutic radiation. Ionizing radiation has the ability to penetrate cells and deposit energy within them in a random fashion, unaffected by the usual cellular barriers. This form of energy, when sufficiently intense, kills cells by inhibiting their division. The sensitivity of cells to ionizing radiation varies considerably in different stages of cell life. Because of this effect of ionizing radiation, the amount of exposure to all forms of it, including x-rays, radioisotopes, and other radioactive sources, is limited to a certain amount each year and to a specific total lifetime dose.

UNIVERSAL RADIATION SYMBOL
(PURPLE PROPELLER ON A YELLOW BACKGROUND)

In sufficient dosage, radiation damages DNA and can inhibit the cells' capacity to divide. When the dose is experienced during fetal development, selective cell killing leads to the teratogenic and somatic effects of radiation. SEE: *radiation accidents, emergency handling of; radiation, low-level.*

radiation protection. There is no substitute for prevention. The only effective preventive measures are shielding the source and the operator, handlers, and patients; maintaining appropriate distance from the source; and limiting the time and amount of exposure. In general the use of drugs to protect against radiation is not practical because of their toxicity. An exception is the use of orally administered potassium iodide to protect the thyroid from radioactive iodine.

radiation sickness. Radiation syndrome.

radiation symbol. A universal symbol used to indicate radioactive sources, containers for radioactive materials, and areas where radioactive materials are stored and used. Presence of the symbol notes the need for caution in order to prevent contamination with or undue exposure to atomic radiation. The symbol consists of a purple propeller on a yellow field. SEE: illus.

radiation syndrome. 1. Illness resulting from exposure of body tissue to ionizing radiations from radioactive substances (radium, radon) or roentgen rays. Mild acute illness is manifested by anorexia, headache, nausea, vomiting, and diarrhea. Delayed effects resulting from repeated or prolonged exposure may result in amenorrhea, sterility, disturbances in blood cell formation, cataract formation, carcinogenesis, and leukemia. 2. Illness resulting from effects of explosion of an atomic bomb. Effects include destruction of lymphatic tissue, extensive hemorrhages, aplastic bone marrow, prolonged clotting and bleeding times, loss of hair and teeth,

and possible genetic changes. In massive exposure to radiation, such as would occur in persons close to the center of an atomic bomb explosion, death may occur within several weeks among individuals who do not die immediately from the physical effects of the explosion. SYN: *radiation sickness.*

radiation therapy. The branch of medicine that utilizes ionizing radiation in the treatment of malignant neoplasms.

radiator (rā'dē-ā"tor) [LL. *radiatus,* radiate]. Device for radiating heat or light.

   r., infrared. Device for transmitting infrared rays.

radical (răd'ĭ-kăl) [LL. *radicalis,* having roots]. 1. In chemistry, a group of atoms acting as a single unit, passing without change from one compound to another, but not able to exist in a free state. 2. Oriented toward the origin or root. 3. A foundation or principle.

   r., acid. The electronegative portion of a molecule when the acid hydrogen is removed.

   r., alcohol. The portion of an alcohol molecule left when the hydrogen of the OH group is removed.

   r., color. Any group that when introduced into an organic compound causes it to become colored.

   r., free. A molecule containing an odd number of electrons. These molecules contain an open bond or a half bond and are highly reactive. The odd electron is represented in chemical formulae by a dot. If two radicals react, both are eliminated; and if a radical reacts with a nonradical, another free radical must be produced. This type of reaction may become a chain reaction. In ischemic injury to tissues, e.g., myocardial infarction, free radical production may play an important role at certain stages in progression of the injury. SEE: *superoxide.*

radical treatment. Treatment that seeks an absolute cure, as radical surgery; not palliative. Opposite of conservative treatment.

radices (răd'ĭ-sēz) [L.]. Pl. of radix.

radiciform. Resembling a root.

radicle (răd'ĭ-kl) [L. *radicula,* little root]. A structure resembling a rootlet, as a radicle of a nerve or vein.

radicotomy (răd"ĭ-kŏt'ō-mē) [L. *radix,* root, + Gr. *tome,* incision]. Section of spinal nerve roots. SYN: *rhizotomy.* SEE: *radiculectomy.*

radicula (ră-dĭk'ū-lă) [L.]. Radicle, q.v.

radiculalgia (ră-dĭk"ū-lăl'jē-ă) [L. *radix,* root, + Gr. *algos,* pain]. Neuralgia of roots of nerves.

radicular (ră-dĭk'ū-lăr) [L. *radix,* root]. 1. Concerning a root or radicle. 2. The tissues on or around a tooth root, e.g., radicular dentin, radicular bone.

radiculectomy (ră-dĭk″ū-lĕk′tō-mē) [″ + Gr. *ektome*, excision]. 1. Excision of a spinal nerve root. 2. Resection of posterior spinal nerve root. SEE: *radicotomy.*

radiculitis (ră-dĭk″ū-lī′tĭs) [L. *radicula*, little root, + Gr. *itis*, inflammation]. Inflammation of spinal nerve roots, accompanied by pain and hyperesthesia.

radiculoganglionitis (ră-dĭk″ū-lō-găng″glē-ō-nī′tĭs) [″ + Gr. *ganglion*, knot, + *itis*, inflammation]. Inflammation of posterior spinal roots and their ganglia.

radiculomedullary (ră-dĭk″ū-lō-mĕd′ū-lĕr″ē) [″ + *medullaris*, marrow]. Concerning the nerve roots and the spinal cord.

radiculomeningomyelitis (ră-dĭk″ū-lō-mĕ-nĭn″gō-mī-ĕl-ī′tĭs) [″ + Gr. *meninx*, membrane, + *myelos*, marrow, + *itis*, inflammation]. Inflamed condition of nerve roots, meninges, and spinal cord.

radiculomyelopathy (ră-dĭk″ū-lō-mī″ĕ-lŏp′ă-thē) [″ + Gr. *myelos*, marrow, + *pathos*, disease, suffering]. Any diseased condition involving the spinal cord and roots of spinal nerves.

radiculoneuritis (ră-dĭk″ū-lō″nū-rī′tĭs) [L. *radicula*, little root, + Gr. *neuron*, sinew, + *itis*, inflammation]. Inflammation of roots of spinal nerves.

radiculoneuropathy (ră-dĭk″ū-lō-nū-rŏp′ă-thē) [″ + ″ + *pathos*, disease, suffering]. Pathological condition of the nerve roots and nerve.

radiculopathy (ră-dĭk″ū-lŏp′ă-thē) [″ + Gr. *pathos*, disease, suffering]. Any diseased condition of roots of spinal nerves.

radiectomy (rā″dē-ĕk′tō-mē) [L. *radix*, root, + Gr. *ektome*, excision]. Surgical removal of the root of a tooth.

radiferous (ră-dĭf′ĕr-ŭs). Containing radium.

radii (rā′dē-ī) [L.]. Plural of radius.

radio- [L. *radius*, ray]. 1. Combining form indicating relationship to radiant energy or radioactive substances. 2. As a prefix to a chemical element indicating a radioactive isotope.

radioactinium (rā″dē-ō-ăk-tĭn′ē-ŭm). A radioactive product formed from disintegration of the element actinium.

radioactive (rā″dē-ō-ăk′tĭv) [L. *radius*, ray, + *activus*, acting]. Capable of emitting radiant energy.

radioactive decay. The decrease with passage of time in the number of radioactive atoms in a radioactive substance. This occurs when the nuclei disintegrate spontaneously by emitting radiant energy.

radioactive patient. An individual who originally was treated or accidentally contaminated with radioactive materials and who continues to be radioactive. If still emitting radiation when discharged from the hospi-

tal, the patient should be told how long to avoid close contact with children and pregnant women. SEE: *radiation accidents, emergency handling of.*

radioactive tracer. An atom that has been made radioactive so that its course may be followed in the body.

radioactivity (rā″dē-ō-ăk″tĭv′ĭ-tē). The ability of a substance to emit rays or particles (alpha, beta, gamma) from its nucleus.

    r., artificial. Radioactivity resulting from bombardment of a substance with high-energy particles in a cyclotron, betatron, or other apparatus.

    r., induced. Temporary radioactivity of a substance that has been within the sphere of influence of a radioactive element.

    r., natural. Radioactivity possessed by a number of elements that are continuously disintegrating and emitting alpha particles (helium nuclei) or beta particles (electrons) atom by atom. Radium is an example.

radioallergosorbent test (rā″dē-ō-ăl″ĕr-gō-sor′bĕnt). ABBR: RAST. Blood test for allergy. It is capable of measuring minute quantities of immunoglobulin E (IgE) in blood. Persons who are allergic to foreign substances will develop antibodies that can be detected by use of this test.

radioautogram (rā″dē-ō-aw′tō-grăm) [″ + Gr. *autos*, self, + *gramma*, something written]. Autoradiogram, q.v.

radioautograph (rā″dē-ō-aw′tō-grăf) [″ + ″ + *graphein*, to write]. A photograph of a histologic section of a tissue showing the distribution of radioactive substances in the tissue.

radioautography (rā″dē-ō-aw-tŏg′ră-fē). Autoradiography, q.v.

radiobicipital (rā″dē-ō-bī-sĭp′ĭ-tăl). Concerning the radius and biceps muscle of the arm.

radiobiology (rā″dē-ō-bī-ŏl′ō-jē). Branch of biology that deals with the effects of ionizing radiations on living organisms.

radiocalcium (rā″dē-ō-kăl′sē-ŭm). A radioisotope of calcium; ^{45}Ca and ^{47}Ca are used in medical studies.

radiocarbon (rā″dē-ō-kăr′bŏn). Radioactive isotope of carbon; ^{11}C and ^{14}C are used in medical studies.

radiocardiogram (rā″dē-ō-kăr′dē-ō-grăm) [L. *radius*, ray, + Gr. *kardia*, heart, + *gramma*, something written]. The record or film obtained during radiocardiography.

radiocardiography (rā″dē-ō-kăr″dē-ŏg′ră-fē) [″ + ″ + *graphein*, to write]. The investigation of the anatomy and function of the heart by obtaining a record or film of a radioactive substance as it travels through the heart.

radiocarpal (rā″dē-ō-kăr′păl) [″ + Gr.

karpos, wrist]. Concerning the radius and carpus.

radiochemistry [" + Gr. *chemeia,* chemistry]. The phase of chemistry dealing with radioactive phenomena.

radiochroism (rā″dē-ō-krō′ĭzm) [" + Gr. *chroa,* color]. The ability of a substance to absorb radioactive rays.

radiochrometer (rā″dē-ō-krŏm′ĕ-tĕr) [" + Gr. *chroma,* color, + *metron,* measure]. Device for measuring penetrating powers of x-rays and the character of roentgen tubes. SEE: *penetrometer.*

radiocinematograph (rā″dē-ō-sĭn″ē-măt′ō-grăf) [" + Gr. *kinema,* motion, + *graphein,* to write]. Simultaneous recording of the picture provided during fluoroscopy of organs of the body.

radiocurable (rā″dē-ō-kūr′ă-bl). Curable by use of radiation therapy.

radiocystitis (rā″dē-ō-sĭs-tī′tĭs) [" + Gr. *kystis,* bladder, + *itis,* inflammation]. Inflammation of the bladder following treatment by radium or roentgen rays.

radiode (rā′dē-ōd) [" + Gr. *hodos,* way]. Metal container for radium used in therapeutic application.

radiodensity. Property of substances that does not allow the passage of x-rays.

radiodermatitis (rā″dē-ō-dĕr″mă-tī′tĭs) [" + Gr. *derma,* skin, + *osis,* condition]. Inflammation of the skin caused by exposure to roentgen rays or radioactive elements.

radiodiagnosis (rā″dē-ō-dī″ăg-nō′sĭs) [" + Gr. *dia,* through, + *gnosis,* knowledge]. Diagnosis by means of roentgen rays.

radiodigital (rā″dē-ō-dĭg′ĭ-tăl). Concerning the radius of the arm and the fingers.

radiodontia (rā″dē-ō-dŏn′shē-ă) [" + Gr. *odous,* tooth]. Roentgenography of the teeth.

radioecology (rā″dē-ō-ē-kŏl′ō-jē) [" + Gr. *oikos,* house, + *logos,* word, reason]. Investigation of the effect of radiation on the living organisms in the environment.

radioelectrocardiogram (rā″dē-ō-ē-lĕk″trō-kär′dē-ō-grăm). The record obtained by radioelectrocardiography.

radioelectrocardiography (rā″dē-ō-ē-lĕk″trō-kär″dē-ŏg′ră-fē) [L. *radius,* ray, + Gr. *elektron,* amber, + *kardia,* heart, + *graphein,* to write]. Recording of changes in heartbeats by radio wave from subject to receiver without direct attachment of apparatus, thus allowing recordings to be made during normal life activities of the patient. SEE: *telemetry.*

radioelement (rā″dē-ō-ĕl′ĕ-mĕnt) [" + *elementum,* a rudiment]. Any of the elements possessing power of radioactivity.

radioencephalogram (rā″dē-ō-ĕn-sĕf′ă-lō-grăm″) [" + Gr. *enkephalos,* brain, + *gramma,* something written]. The record obtained when a radioactive tracer passes through the cerebral blood vessels.

radioencephalography (rā″dē-ō-ĕn-sĕf″ă-lŏg′ră-fē) [" + " + *graphein,* to write]. The recording of radio waves transmitted from the brain to a receiver but without use of electrodes placed on the scalp.

radioepidermitis (rā″dē-ō-ĕp″ĭ-dĕr-mī′tĭs) [" + Gr. *epi,* upon, + *derma,* skin, + *itis,* inflammation]. Destructive changes in the skin caused by radioactive rays.

radioepitheliitis (rā″dē-ō-ĕp″ĭ-thē-lē-ī′tĭs) [" + " + *thele,* nipple, + *itis,* inflammation]. Disintegration of epithelium due to exposure to irradiation.

radiofrequency electrophrenic respiration. Method of stimulating respiration in cases of respiratory paralysis from injury of the spinal cord at the cervical level. Electrical stimuli to the phrenic nerves are supplied by a radiofrequency transmitter implanted subcutaneously. The diaphragmatic muscles contract in response to intermittent electrical stimuli.

radiogenesis (rā″dē-ō-jĕn′ĕ-sĭs) [" + Gr. *genesis,* generation, birth]. Production of radiant energy.

radiogenic (rā″dē-ō-jĕn′ĭk) [" + *gennan,* to produce]. 1. Producing radiation. 2. Caused by radiation. SYN: *actinogenic.*

radiogold (rā′dē-ō-gōld). A radioisotope of gold.

radiograph (rā′dē-ō-grăf) [" + Gr. *graphein,* to write]. 1. The film on which an image is produced through exposure to x-radiation. 2. To make a radiograph.

   r., bitewing. SEE: *bitewing radiograph.*

   r., dental. R., periapical, q.v.

   r., interproximal. An intraoral radiograph taken using bitewing film to show the interproximal surfaces of teeth and the interdental bone.

   r., lateral cephalometric. A film of the entire head, taken from the side with the head in a known, fixed position for the purpose of making definitive observations or measurements.

   r., panoramic. A type of extraoral body-section radiograph that shows the entire upper and lower jaws in a continuous single film.

   r., periapical. An intraoral film that depicts the tooth and surrounding tissues extending to the apical region. SYN: *r., dental.*

radiography (rā-dē-ŏg′ră-fē). The making of x-ray pictures. SYN: *roentgenography.*

radiohumeral (rā″dē-ō-hū′mĕr-ăl) [" + *humerus,* upper arm]. Concerning the radius and humerus.

radioimmunity (rā″dē-ō-ĭ-mū′nĭ-tē) [″ + *immunitas,* immunity]. Apparent decreased sensitivity to radiation that may follow repeated radiation therapy.

radioimmunoassay (rā″dē-ō-ĭm″ū-nō-ăs′ā). ABBR: RIA. A very sensitive method of determining the concentration of substances, particularly the protein-bound hormones, in blood plasma. The procedure is based on the competitive inhibition of binding of radioactively labeled hormones to a specific antibody. Concentrations of protein in the picogram (10^{-12} gm) range can be measured by using this technique.

radioimmunodiffusion (rā″dē-ō-ĭm″ū-nō-dĭf-fū′zhŭn) [″ + ″ + *dis,* apart, + *fundere,* to pour]. Study of antigen-antibody interaction by use of radioisotope-labeled antigens or antibodies diffused through a gel.

radioimmunoelectrophoresis (rā″dē-ō-ĭm″ū-nō-ē-lĕk″trō-fō-rē′sĭs) [″ + ″ + Gr. *elektron,* amber, + *phoresis,* bearing]. Electrophoresis involving the use of radioisotope-labeled antigen or antibody. An autoradiograph is taken of the electrophoretic pattern produced.

radioiodine (rā″dē-ō-ī′ō-dīn). A radioactive isotope of iodine. Used in the diagnosis and treatment of thyroid disorders. The most commonly used isotope is ^{131}I.

radioiron (rā″dē-ō-ī′ĕrn). A radioactive isotope of iron; ^{55}Fe and ^{59}Fe are used in medical studies.

radioisotope (rā″dē-ō-ī′sō-tōp). A radioactive form of an element.

radiolead (rā″dē-ō-lĕd′). A radioactive isotope of lead.

radiolesion (rā″dē-ō-lē′zhŭn). A lesion or injury caused by radiation.

radioligand (rā″dē-ō-lī′gănd, răd″dē-ō-lĭg′ănd). A molecule, esp. an antigen or antibody, with a radioactive tracer attached to it.

radiological emergency assistance. SEE: *radiation accidents, emergency handling of.*

radiologic technologist. An individual who maintains and safely uses equipment and supplies necessary to produce images of the human body on x-ray film or fluoroscopic screen for diagnostic purposes. This individual may also supervise or teach others. Radiologic technology programs approved by the American Medical Association Council on Medical Education are conducted in hospitals, medical schools, and colleges with hospital affiliations.

radiologist (rā-dē-ōl′ō-jĭst) [L. *radius,* ray, + Gr. *logos,* word, reason]. A physician who practices diagnosis and treatment by use of radiant energy.

radiology (rā-dē-ōl′ō-jē). The branch of med-

icine concerned with radioactive substances, including x-rays, radioactive isotopes, and ionizing radiations, and the application of this information to prevention, diagnosis, and treatment of disease.

radiolucency (rā″dē-ō-lū′sĕn-sē) [″ + *lucere,* to shine]. Property of being partly or wholly permeable to radiant energy.

radiolucent (rā″dē-ō-lū′sĕnt) [″ + *lucere,* to shine]. Allowing x-rays to pass through. Appears as a dark area on the radiograph.

radiolus (rā-dē′ō-lŭs) [L., a little ray]. A sound or probe.

radiometer (rā-dē-ŏm′ĕ-tĕr) [″ + Gr. *metron,* measure]. Instrument for measuring intensity of radiation.

radiomicrometer (rā″dē-ō-mī-krŏm′ĕ-tĕr) [″ + Gr. *mikros,* small, + *metron,* measure]. An instrument for measuring small changes in radiation.

radiomimetic (rā″dē-ō-mĭm-ĕt′ĭk) [″ + Gr. *mimetikos,* imitation]. Imitating the biological effects of radiation. Alkylating agents are examples of substances with this property. SEE: *alkylating agent.*

radiomuscular (rā″dē-ō-mŭs′kū-lăr). Concerning the radius or radial artery and muscles of the arm.

radiomutation. Permanent alteration of the genetic material of a cell due to the effects of ionizing radiation.

radion (rā′dē-ŏn) [″ + Gr. *on,* being]. One of the radioactive particles given off by radioactive matter.

radionecrosis (rā″dē-ō-nĕ-krō′sĭs) [″ + Gr. *nekrosis,* state of death]. Disintegration of tissue due to exposure to radiant energy.

radioneuritis (rā″dē-ō-nū-rī′tĭs) [″ + Gr. *neuron,* sinew, + *itis,* inflammation]. Neuritis caused by exposure to radioactive substance.

radionitrogen (rā″dē-ō-nī′trō-jĕn). A radioisotope of nitrogen.

radionuclide (rā″dē-ō-nū′klīd). Atom that disintegrates by emission of electromagnetic radiation.

radiopacity (rā″dē-ō-pās′ĭ-tē). Condition of being radiopaque.

radiopaque (rā-dē-ō-pāk′) [″ + *opacus,* dark]. Impenetrable to the x-ray or other forms of radiation. Appears as a light area on the radiograph.

radioparency (rā″dē-ō-păr′ĕn-sē). Condition of being radiolucent or radioparent.

radioparent (rā″dē-ō-păr′ĕnt) [″ + *parere,* to appear]. Penetrable by radioactive rays.

radiopathology (rā″dē-ō-pă-thŏl′ō-jē) [″ + Gr. *pathos,* disease, suffering, + *logos,* word, reason]. Study of pathological changes induced by radiation.

radiopelvimetry (rā″dē-ō-pĕl-vĭm′ĕt-rē) [″ + *pelvis,* basin, + Gr. *metron,* measure]. Measurement of the pelvis by use of x-rays.

radiopharmaceuticals (rā″dē-ō-färm″ă-sū′tĭ-kăls). Radioactive chemicals either in the form of individual elements or elements attached to other substances called carriers. They are used in testing the location, size, outline, or function of tissues, organs, vessels, or body fluids. The presence and location of radiopharmaceutical substances in the body are detected by special methods or apparatus that record the radioactivity being emitted. These compounds may also be used to treat certain diseases.

Caution: Radiopharmaceuticals must be handled in accordance with prescribed methods in order to prevent the patient or those treating the patient from being exposed to unnecessary ionizing radiation.

---

radiophobia (rā″dē-ō-fō′bē-ă) [″ + Gr. *phobos,* fear]. Abnormal fear of x-rays and radiation.

radiophosphorus (rā″dē-ō-fŏs′fō-rŭs). A radioactive isotope of phosphorus; ^{32}P is used in medical studies.

radiopotassium (rā″dē-ō-pō-tăs′ē-ŭm). A radioactive isotope of potassium; ^{42}K is used in medical studies.

radiopotentiation (rā″dē-ō-pō-tĕn″shē-ā′shŭn) [″ + *potentia,* power]. The action of potentiating the effect of radiation. This may be produced by certain drugs and by oxygen.

radioprotective drugs. Drugs that protect man against the damaging or lethal effects of ionizing radiation. Example: Lugol's solution or a saturated solution of potassium iodide will block the uptake of inhaled or ingested radioactive iodine by the thyroid.

radiopulmonography (rā″dē-ō-pŭl″mō-nŏg′ră-fē) [″ + *pulmo,* lung, + Gr. *graphein,* to write]. Use of radioactive materials to measure the flow of (or lack of) gases through the lung during respiration.

radioreaction (rā″dē-ō-rē-ăk′shŭn). The reaction of the body to radiation.

radioreceptor (rā″dē-ō-rē-sĕp′tor). Something that receives radiant energy such as light, heat, or x-ray.

radioresistant. Resistant to the action of radiation, esp. said of a tumor that cannot be destroyed by treatment with radiation.

radioresponsive (rā″dē-ō-rē-spŏn′sĭv). Radiosensitive, q.v.

radioscopy (rā-dē-ŏs′kō-pē) [L. *radius,* ray, + Gr. *skopein,* to examine]. Inspection and examination of the inner structures of the body by means of roentgen rays. SYN: *fluoroscopy.*

radiosensibility. Radiosensitivity, q.v.

radiosensitivity (rā″dē-ō-sĕn″sĭ-tĭv′ĭ-tē). Reactiveness or responsiveness of a cell to radiation.

radiosodium (rā″dē-ō-sō′dē-ŭm). A radioisotope of sodium; ^{24}Na and ^{22}Na are used in medical studies.

radiostrontium (rā″dē-ō-strŏn′shē-ŭm). A radioisotope of strontium.

radiosulfur (rā″dē-ō-sŭl′fŭr). A radioisotope of sulfur.

radiosurgery (rā″dē-ō-sŭr′jĕr-ē) [″ + Gr. *cheirurgia,* handwork]. The use of high-energy protons and alpha particles in the form of beams, as an atomic knife in treating diseases such as cancer or in selectively destroying an overactive endocrine gland.

radiotelemetry (rā″dē-ō-tĕl-ĕm′ē-trē) [″ + Gr. *tele,* distant, + *metron,* measure]. Transmission of data, including biological data, via radio from a patient to a remote monitor or recording device for storage, analysis, and interpretation.

radiotherapeutics (rā″dē-ō-thĕr″ă-pū′tĭks). 1. Radiotherapy. 2. Study of radiotherapeutic agents.

radiotherapist (rā″dē-ō-thĕr′ă-pĭst) [″ + Gr. *therapeia,* treatment]. One trained in use of radiant energy for therapeutic purposes.

radiotherapy (rā″dē-ō-thĕr′ă-pē). The treatment of disease by application of roentgen rays, radium, ultraviolet, and other radiations.

radiothermy (rā″dē-ō-thĕr′mē) [″ + Gr. *therme,* heat]. 1. Use of radiant heat or heat from radioactive substances for therapeutic purposes. 2. Short-wave diathermy.

radiothorium (rā″dē-ō-thō′rē-ŭm). A radioisotope of thorium.

radiotoxemia (rā″dē-ō-tŏk-sē′mē-ă) [″ + Gr. *toxikon,* poison, + *haima,* blood]. Toxemia produced by exposure to radioactive substance. SEE: *radiation syndrome.*

radiotransparent (rā″dē-ō-trăns-păr′ĕnt) [″ + *trans,* across, + *parere,* to appear]. Penetrable by radiation.

radiotropic (rā″dē-ō-trŏp′ĭk) [″ + Gr. *tropos,* turning]. Affected by radiation.

radioulnar (rā″dē-ō-ŭl′năr) [″ + *ulna,* arm]. Concerning the radius and ulna.

radium (rā′dē-ŭm) [L. *radius,* ray]. SYMB: Ra. At. no. 88. There are more than a dozen isotopes, but radium with a half-life of 1622 years and an atomic weight of 226 is the most common. A metallic element found in very small quantities in pitchblende. It is radioactive and fluorescent.

There are three kinds of radiation: alpha (α-rays); beta (β-rays); and gamma (γ-rays), which are analogous to x-rays. SEE: words beginning with *actin-.*

radium needles. Slender containers for radium. These are inserted into tissue in order to kill malignant cells.

radium therapy [″ + Gr. *therapeia*, treatment]. The treatment of disease by means of radium or radon, its emanation, or its active deposit. SYN: *radiotherapy*.

radius [L., ray] (pl. *radii*). 1. A line extending from a circle's center point to its circumference. 2. [NA] The outer and shorter bone of the arm, which revolves partially about the ulna. Its head articulates with the capitulum of the humerus. Its lower portion articulates by the ulnar notch with the ulna, and by another articulation with the navicular (scaphoid) and lunate bones of the wrist.

r., fracture of. A fracture and dislocation of the lower end of the radius, generally caused by falling on the outstretched hand. SEE: *Colles' fracture.*

radix (rā′dĭks) [L., root] (pl. *radices*). [NA] 1. The root portion of a cranial or spinal nerve. 2. The root of a plant.

radon (rā′dŏn) [L. *radius*, ray]. SYMB: Rn. At. wt. 222; at. no. 86. A radioactive gaseous element resulting from disintegration of radium. Because radium is present in the earth's crust, radon accumulates in caves, mines, houses, and any space not freely exchanging the air contained in it with the outside air. Thus, radon and its disintegration products may accumulate in houses, particularly those that are energy efficient. The level of radon in a house may be measured, and if it exceeds acceptable limits, steps should be taken to reduce it. Radon exposure is estimated to cause 5% to 10% of the lung cancers occurring in the general population.

raffinose (răf′ĭ-nōs). A trisaccharide, melitose, present in certain plants, cereals, and fungi. Hydrolysis yields fructose and melibiose.

rage (rāj′) [ME.]. Violent anger.

r., sham. A rage reaction produced by stimuli to decorticated animals.

ragsorters' disease. A febrile pulmonary disease that may occur in persons who sort paper and rags. It is caused by the anthrax bacillus.

ragweed. One of several species of the genus *Ambrosia*, whose pollen is an important allergen. Pollen-producing period of grasses is, in temperate zones, from middle of August to the first hard frost, usually the middle of October. SEE: *allergy.*

Raillietina (rī″lē-ē-tī′nă). A genus of tapeworms belonging to family Davaineidae.

R. demerariensis. A species that infests humans, reported from several S. American countries, esp. Ecuador.

railway sickness. Motion sickness resulting from riding on a train.

Raimiste's phenomenon or sign. An associated reaction in hemiplegia whereby resistance to hip abduction or adduction in the non-involved extremity evokes the same motion in the involved extremity.

raised (rāzd) [ME. *reisen*, to rise]. In bacteriology, having a thick elevated growth with terraced edges.

rale (răl) [Fr., rattle]. An abnormal sound heard on auscultation of the chest, produced by passage of air through bronchi that contain secretion or exudate or that are constricted by spasm or a thickening of their walls. May be heard on inspiration or expiration.

CLASSIF: There is no general agreement as to classification of the sounds. They are designated moist and dry. Moist rales are also called crackling, and these in turn may be coarse, medium, or dry. If loud and sharp, they are consonating. Dry rales are sometimes designated musical and may be tinkling, sonorous, snoring, or low pitched, or they may be whistling, piping, and high pitched.

r., amphoric. The musical sound heard by auscultation of the chest when a fluid-containing cavity communicates with a bronchus.

r., atelectatic. Transitory rale that disappears upon deep breathing or coughing.

r., bronchiectatic. Rale heard over bronchiectatic cavities filled with accumulated secretion. Disappears with expectoration.

r., bubbling. Rale heard in inspiration and expiration, produced by passage of air through mucus in the larger tubes. May be classified as small or medium.

r., cavernous. Rale heard in inspiration and expiration, produced by passage of air through a small cavity with flaccid walls that collapse with expiration. Hollow and metallic.

r., clicking. Rale heard in inspiration only, produced by passage of air through softening material in smaller bronchi. Small, sticky. Heard in pulmonary tuberculosis, early stage.

r., coarse. Rale that originates in the larger bronchi.

r., consonating. A loud, sharp rale sounding close to the ear. Usually associated with consolidation of tissues about bronchial tubes.

r., crackling. Rale heard chiefly in inspiration, produced by fluid in the finer bronchi. May be classified as small or medium. Heard in softening of the tubercular deposit or pneumonic exudation.

r., crepitant. Rale heard at end of inspiration, produced by passage of air into collapsed vesicles containing fibrinous exudation, usually at base of lungs. Heard in early-stage edema of lungs and in hypostatic pneumonia. It is localized in pulmonary tuberculosis. SYN: *r., vesicular.*

r., dry. Rale heard in inspiration and expiration, produced by narrowing of the bronchial tubes from thickening of their mucous lining, from spasmodic contraction of the muscular coat, viscid mucus within, or pressure from without. Large and sonorous, small, hissing or whistling. Heard in bronchitis, asthma, and localized in beginning pulmonary tuberculosis.

r., gurgling. Rale heard in inspiration and expiration, produced by passage of air through fluid in cavities of large bubbles. Heard in pulmonary tuberculosis after formation of cavities.

r., moist. Rale produced by passage of air through bronchi containing fluid.

r. redux. Rale heard in inspiration and expiration, produced by passage of air through fluid in bronchial tubes. Crackling, unequal. Heard in pneumonia in the stage of resolution.

r., sibilant. High-pitched, whistling, and frequent rale heard at the end of inspiration.

r., sonorous. Low snoring rale that continues during inspiration.

r., subcrepitant. Rale heard in inspiration and expiration, produced by passage of air through mucus in the capillary bronchial tubes. Small, moist. Heard in capillary bronchitis.

r., vesicular. R., crepitant.

ramal (rā'măl) [L. *ramus,* branch]. Concerning a ramus.

rami (rā'mī) [L.]. Pl. of ramus.

ramicotomy (răm″ĭ-kŏt'ō-mē) [L. *ramus,* branch, + Gr. *tome,* incision]. Ramisection, q.v.

ramification (răm″ĭ-fĭ-kā'shŭn) [L. *ramificare,* to make branches]. 1. Process of branching. 2. A branch. 3. Arrangement in branches.

ramify (răm'ĭ-fī). To branch; to spread out in different directions.

ramisection (răm'ĭ-sĕk″shŭn) [L. *ramus,* branch, + *sectio,* a cutting]. Surgical division of a ramus communicans between a spinal nerve and a ganglion of the sympathetic trunk.

ramisectomy (răm-ĭs-ĕk'tō-mē) [″ + Gr. *ektome,* excision]. Excision of a ramus, specifically ramus communicans. SEE: *ramisection.*

ramitis (răm-ī'tĭs) [″ + Gr. *itis,* inflammation]. Inflammation of a ramus.

ramollissement (ră″mŏl-ēs-mŏn') [Fr.]. Pathological softening of some organ or tissue, esp. of brain.

ramose (rā'mōs) [L. *ramus,* branch]. Branching; having many branches.

ramulus [L.] (pl. *ramuli*). A small branch or ramus.

ramus (rā'mŭs) [L., branch] (pl. *rami*). [NA] A branch; one of the divisions of a forked structure.

r., anterior. A primary division of a spinal nerve that supplies the lateral and ventral portions of body wall, the limbs, and perineum.

r., bronchial. Collateral branches of each primary bronchus.

r. communicans. [NA] One of the primary branches of a spinal nerve that connects with a sympathetic ganglion. Each consists of a white portion (white ramus communicans) of myelinated preganglionic sympathetic fibers and a gray portion (gray ramus communicans) composed of unmyelinated postganglionic fibers.

r., mandibular. The vertical portion of the mandible.

r., meningeal. One of the primary branches of a spinal nerve that re-enters the vertebral foramen and supplies meninges and vertebral column.

r., posterior. One of the primary branches of a spinal nerve that supplies muscles and skin of the back.

rancid (răn'sĭd) [L. *rancidus,* stink]. Offensive; having a disagreeable smell or taste from partial decomposition, esp. of a fatty substance.

rancidify (răn-sĭd'ĭ-fī). To make rancid.

rancidity (răn-sĭd'ĭ-tē). Condition of being rancid.

random controlled trial. An experimental study for assessing the effects of a particular variable (such as a drug or treatment) in which subjects are assigned on a random basis to either of two groups, experimental or control. The experimental group receives the drug or procedure, while the control group does not. Laboratory tests or clinical evaluations are performed on both groups (usually using the double-blind technique, q.v.) to determine the effects of the drug or procedure.

randomization. In research, a method used to assign subjects to experimental groups. Prior to this step every attempt is made to ensure that the subjects are as equivalent as possible. Then by some random method, such as tossing a coin or using a list of numbers, each individual in the study is assigned to either a treatment or nontreatment group. Use of this technique helps to prevent inadvertent selection bias in the study. SEE: *clinical trial; double-blind technique.*

random sample. In experimental medicine and in epidemiology, the selection of samples from a population, or some other grouping, so that each individual or item in the group has the same opportunity of being selected in the sample.

range [ME., series]. The difference between the highest and lowest in a set of variables or in a series of values or observations.

range of accommodation. Difference between least and greatest distance of distinct vision. SEE: *accommodation.*

range of motion. ABBR: ROM. The range of movement of a joint. SEE: *goniometer.*

range-of-motion exercise. SEE: *exercise, range-of-motion.*

ranine (rā′nīn) [L. *rana*, a frog]. 1. Pert. to a ranula, or to the region beneath the tip of the tongue. 2. Branch of the lingual artery supplying that area. 3. Pert. to frogs.

ranula (răn′ū-lă) [L., little frog]. A large cystic tumor seen on underside of tongue on either side of the frenum; a retention cyst of the submandibular or sublingual ducts. The swelling may be small or large.

SYM: Semitranslucent; soft, large, dilated veins coursing over it. Fullness and discomfort. Usually no pain. Contains clear glairy fluid, due to dilatation of ducts of salivary glands and to obstruction of those of sublingual mucous glands.

TREAT: Periodic emptying of sac by careful needle aspiration will provide temporary relief. Surgical intervention is required for complete removal.

   r., pancreatic. Cystic disease of pancreas due to obstruction of its ducts.

Ranvier's nodes (rŏn-vē-āz′) [Louis A. Ranvier, Fr. pathologist, 1835–1922]. Constrictions in the medullary substance of a nerve fiber at more or less regular intervals. SEE: *nerve fiber.*

RAO. *right anterior oblique* position.

rape (rāp) [L. *rapere*, to seize]. Heterosexual or homosexual intercourse against the will of the victim. Complete penetration of the vagina (or other body orifice) by the penis or emission of seminal fluid is not necessary to constitute rape. Rape includes penetration of the vagina or other orifice by a penis, finger, or inanimate object. Most rapes include force or violence, but acquiescence due to verbal threats indicates lack of consent. It is an accepted fact that rape is a violent criminal act that happens to be associated with sexual activity. In many cases in which the male is the rapist, there is no evidence that orgasm occurred. SEE: *abused person; rape and sexual assault prevention; sexual abuse.*

NURSING IMPLICATIONS: Provide sensitive care, esp. psychological support. Remain with the patient and encourage verbalization. Follow state regulations regarding reporting the rape to police. Explain the need for and assist with the physical examination, pelvic and rectal examinations, and diagnostic tests. Follow directions exactly in assisting with collection of rape evidence for police investigation: obtain head and pubic hair combings, nail scrapings, etc. Allow the patient as much control as possible throughout examination, treatment, and interview procedures. Obtain a history of the assault and sexual history; discover whether or not the female rape victim was menstruating and, if so, the type of menstrual protection used.

Perform prescribed treatments on associated injuries. Administer prescribed prophylactic medications for venereal disease. Offer services of crisis intervention for emotional expression by the victim. Provide information concerning antipregnancy measures if indicated. Provide cleansing measures if patient desires. Assist patient in explaining situation to his or her family. Provide follow-up services and written and verbal instructions for prescribed medications, including drug actions and possible side effects. Arrange for escort home. SEE: *Nursing Diagnoses* in *Appendix.*

   r., date. Rape occurring while the individual raped was involved in a social relationship with the rapist. The individual may have been an intimate friend, but the sexual assault at that time was unsolicited and unwelcome.

   r., gang. An individual being forced against his or her will to have sexual intercourse or other sexual activity with several persons. SEE: *rape.*

   r., marital. Forcible sexual assault by a spouse at a time when the sexual encounter was neither solicited nor welcome.

   r., prison. Rape that occurs when the victim is assaulted by another prisoner or by a prison employee.

   r., statutory. Sexual intercourse with an individual younger than the legal age of consent.

rape and sexual assault prevention. A situation in which rape occurs usually means the victim is confronted by an irrational person; thus, rational behavior in attempting to prevent a potential rape may be of no avail, which is not to say that such behavior should not be considered. A rapist may fit any description, but many are neither "crazy" nor "macho" but, in fact, quite ordinary. Many of these individuals are persons with low self-esteem who do not have control over their lives. Most rapes are committed by persons known by the victim, and the act occurs in the home of either the victim or the attacker. Rape by a complete stranger does occur, but this is not the usual situation. Because alcohol consumption is a related factor in many rapes, it is advisable to keep alcohol intake to a minimum and do not allow a companion who is intoxicated into your home. In the following suggestions, it is assumed that the potential victim is a female who is being forced against her will to have sexual intercourse or participate in other sexual acts.

As much as possible, preventive measures should be directed at remaining in a well-secured area close to persons who can be called for assistance, either day or night. If the latter is not possible, emergency police and fire department phone numbers should be kept readily available. A call for help should be made without delay if it is suspected that one's apartment or home is being illegally entered.

When preparing to enter a car, be constantly alert for the presence of a stranger hidden either in the dark or behind, under, or within a car. Before leaving a well-lighted and populated area, have the car keys in hand and ready for quick use. Try to leave one arm free of packages, handbag, or other items. Placing individual keys firmly between the fingers like claws can prove a useful weapon. Walk quickly and with assurance to the car, and look under and inside it before unlocking the door. Once it has been ascertained that entrance is safe, enter quickly; do not fumble with keys. Immediately after entering, lock the car door(s) and close any windows that may be open.

When preparing to enter the home, be alert to any outward signs of danger; i.e., nonfunctioning hall light; unfamiliar noises or odors in the hallways; barking of a normally quiet resident dog; unlatched or ajar hall door that is normally secure; unfamiliar persons loitering outside or standing at or inside the hall door. Often, even the sense of danger can be a useful warning. If the situation does not "feel" familiarly safe, do not attempt to enter or brush by a stranger. Leave and go to a secure phone and call a neighbor who might assist in safe entry.

If possible, never enter an empty home or apartment dwelling alone. If this is unavoidable then, before closing the door, immediately turn on a light. Speak aloud as if a friend is present. Holding keys in hand and spread through the fingers, walk through the entire apartment, from front to back, checking closets, behind open doors, the shower, and any other places where an intruder might hide. Always leave at least one possible exit available before ascertaining safety of the apartment and closing the door.

Once safely inside, bolt the door securely. If a stranger comes to the door, keep a security chain on and preferably use a peephole through which to communicate until identification has been properly presented. If in doubt about the credentials or demeanor of a stranger at the door, refuse admission and phone for help immediately.

When on the street, avoid unlighted or dimly lighted streets, parks, and parking lots. Walk in the street if traffic permits. If walking on a sidewalk, stay on the middle or street side, avoiding dark alleyways or doors. Always try to walk with assurance and at a quick pace.

It is not possible to provide advice that would be applicable for all situations and which would guarantee that rape and injury would not occur. Even if it seems advisable to attempt to resist, the attacker usually has the advantage of being stronger than the victim. Nevertheless, if the victim is certain that persons are close by who could both hear a cry for help and would be willing to render assistance, a loud scream might be advisable. Even this approach could lead to injury or death if the attacker has a gun or other weapon ready to use at the first sign of resistance.

If raped, attempt to remember all details of the attacker: clothes; size; race; accent; hair color; identifying marks, scars, facial hair; vehicle; evidence of drug or alcohol use.

rape counseling. The emotional reaction and sequelae of rape may be devastating to the mental well-being of the victim. It is therefore important that the victim be reassured concerning what to expect both from internal feelings and potential reactions of society. Historically, law enforcement officers have been less than sympathetic to rape victims, but now most police departments have officers trained in investigating the crime of rape and they are sensitive to the emotional and physical trauma the victim has experienced. There are a variety of services available to the victim, including health care persons experienced in counseling victims of rape and various advocate groups.

rapeseed [L. *rapa,* turnip]. Seed of *Brassica campestris* and other Brassica species. Rape oil, which is used in foods and industry, is obtained from this seed.

raphania (ră-fā′nē-ă) [Gr. *rhaphanos,* radish]. A spasmodic disease caused by eating seeds of the wild radish; allied to ergotism, q.v. SYN: *rhaphania.*

raphe (rā′fē) [Gr. *rhaphe*]. [NA] A crease, ridge, or seam noting union of the halves of a part.

    r., abdominal. Linea alba.

r., buccal. Raphe on cheek indicating line of fusion of maxillary and mandibular processes.

r., lateral. A ridge along the lateral margin of the erector spinae muscles formed by the aponeurosis of the latissimus dorsi internal obliques and transversus abdominis and layers of the thoracolumbar fascia.

r. of penis. [NA] A median ridge on the posterior surface of the penis, a continuation of the raphe of the scrotum.

r. of scrotum. A ridge in the midline of the scrotum.

r. of tongue. A median groove on the dorsum of the tongue.

r., palatine. A line or ridge in the median line of the palate.

r., perineal. A line or ridge in the midline of the perineum.

r., pterygomandibular. A tendinous line of fusion between the buccinator and superior pharyngeal constrictor muscles that passes between the pterygoid process and the mandible, serving as an important landmark in dental anesthesia.

rapport (ră-por') [Fr. *rapporter*, to bring back]. A relationship of mutual trust and understanding, esp. between the patient and physician, nurse, or other health care provider.

rapture. A state of great joy, delight, or ecstasy.

raptus (răp'tŭs) [L.]. A sudden seizure or attack.

rarefaction (răr"ĕ-făk'shŭn) [L. *rarefacere*, to make thin]. Process of decreasing density and weight, as of air. The farther from the surface of the earth, the less dense the atmosphere becomes.

r. of bone. The process of making bone more porous because of absorption of mineral substances.

ETIOL: Disturbed calcium-phosphorus metabolism possibly resulting from excess parathyroid hormone. SEE: *osteoporosis; parathyroid.*

rarefy (răr'ĕ-fī). To make less dense, or to increase porosity of.

rarefying osteitis. Chronic bone inflammation marked by development of granulation tissue in marrow spaces with absorption of surrounding hard bone.

RAS. *reticular activating system.*

rash (răsh) [O. Fr. *rasche*]. General term applied to any eruption of the skin, esp. those associated with communicable diseases. Usually temporary. The rash usually is a shade of red, which varies with disease. SYN: *exanthema.* SEE: *eruption; lesion; roseola.*

NURSING IMPLICATIONS: Assess the location and characteristics of the lesions, such as color, size (height and diameter), pattern, whether discrete or coalesced, and any secondary changes (crusting, scaling, lichenification). Also assess for associated symptoms such as pruritus or discomfort, temporal elements, and history of known allergies, drugs used, and contacts with communicable diseases during preceding two-week period. Discontinue suspect drugs and isolate potential communicable disease patient until physician can be contacted. Apply cool compresses to relieve itching. As prescribed, apply topical preparations and dressings, and administer systemic medications. Instruct patient to keep hands clean and nails short and even, and to avoid touching rash. Teach patient about treatment regimen, its actions, and side effects, and evaluate for these responses.

r., butterfly. Skin rash of both cheeks joined by an extension across the bridge of the nose. Seen in systemic lupus erythematosus, esp. after the patient's face has been exposed to sunlight. Also seen in seborrheic dermatitis, tuberous sclerosis, q.v., and dermatomyositis, q.v. SEE: *lupus erythematosus.*

r., cable. An acneiform eruption caused by contact with chlorinated waxes, which are used to lubricate cables.

r., diaper. Irritant contact dermatitis as a reaction to friction, maceration, and prolonged contact with urine, feces, soap retained in diapers, and topical preparations.

TREAT: Symptomatic; change diapers frequently; if washable cloth diapers are used, be certain they are thoroughly washed and rinsed; do not use occlusive plastic pants over diaper; wash perianal and genital area with warm water and mild, nonperfumed soap. If these measures and application of a bland protective agent, e.g., zinc oxide paste, do not promote healing, apply a small amount of 0.5-1% topical hydrocortisone cream to the area after each diaper change. Do this for several days. SYN: *diaper dermatitis.*

r., drug. Rash caused by use of certain drugs, such as bromide or iodine. SYN: *dermatitis medicamentosa.* SEE: *drug rashes; idiosyncrasy.*

r., ecchymotic. R., hemorrhagic.

r., gum. A red, papular eruption of the chin and anterior chest area of children seen during teething. A form of miliaria due to excess saliva coming in contact with the skin. SYN: *r., red; strophulus.*

r., heat. Prickly heat, q.v.

r., hemorrhagic. Rash consisting chiefly of hemorrhages or ecchymoses.

r., macular. Rash in which the lesions are flat and level with the surrounding skin.

r., maculopapular. Rash in which there are discrete macular and papular lesions or a combination of these types of lesions.

r., mulberry. Rash seen in typhus fever; dusky in color.

r., nettle. Smooth, elevated, itchy, white patches. SYN: *hives; urticaria.*

r., red. R., gum.

r., rose. Any rose-colored rash. SYN: *roseola.*

r., serum. Rash accompanying serum sickness resulting from injection of a foreign serum. SEE: *serum sickness.*

r., sunburnlike. Macular rash resembling the reddened skin characteristic of a severe sunburn. It may be associated with circulating bacterial toxins. See: *toxic shock syndrome.*

r., tooth. R., gum, q.v.

r., wandering. Condition of tongue marked by numerous denuded patches on the dorsal surface coalescing into freeform shapes similar to geographic presentations on maps. SYN: *geographic tongue.*

rasion (rā′zhŭn) [L. *rasio*]. Grating of drugs by use of a file.

raspatory (răs′pă-tō″rē) [L. *raspatorium*]. File used in surgery, esp. for trimming surfaces of bone. SYN: *xyster.*

RAST. *radioallergosorbent test.*

Rastafarian cult. A religious cult that originated in Jamaica in the 1930s and has members in the Caribbean, Europe, Canada, and the U.S. It is of medical importance because cult members' dietary practices may lead to vitamin B_{12} deficiency with subsequent neurological disease or megaloblastic anemia or both.

rasura (ră-sū′ră) [L. *rasura*, a scraping]. 1. Process of scraping or shaving. 2. Scrapings or filings. SYN: *rasure.*

rat [ME]. A rodent of the genus *Rattus*, found in and around human habitations. In addition to causing economic loss due to crop destruction, rats are of primary importance in the spread of human and animal diseases. They serve as hosts of various protozoans, flukes, tapeworms, and threadworms; reservoirs of amebiasis, murine and scrub typhus, and plague (bubonic, septicemic, pneumonic). The plagues are transmitted to man principally through arthropods (rat flea). Rats also transmit rat-bite fever, q.v. SEE: *flea; vector.*

rat-bite fever. Either of two infectious diseases transmitted by the bite of a rat. One is caused by *Streptobacillus moniliformis,* characterized by skin inflammation, headache, vomiting, and back and joint pain; the other is caused by *Spirillum minus.* Associated with it are ulceration, rash, and recurrent fever. The latter disease is rare in the U.S.

rate (rāt) [L. *rata,* calculated]. The speed or frequency of occurrence of an event. Usually expressed with respect to time or some other known standard.

r., attack. Rate of occurrence of new cases of a disease.

r., basal metabolic. SEE: *basal metabolic rate.*

r., birth. The number of live births per 1000 in the population in a given year.

r., case. R., morbidity, q.v.

r., case fatality. The ratio of the number of deaths caused by a disease to the total number of people who contract the disease.

r., death. The number of deaths in a specified population. Usually expressed as number of deaths per 100,000 population. Also called *mortality rate.*

r., DMF. An expression concerning the dental caries experienced in school children in whom observations are made of the number of teeth that are: D, decayed; M, missing or requiring extraction; F, filled or with restorations. SEE: *DMF index.*

r., dose. The quantity of medicine administered per unit of time.

r., erythrocyte sedimentation. ABBR: ESR. SEE: *sedimentation rate.*

r., false-negative. Rate of occurrence of negative results of a test in individuals who actually have the attribute or disease being tested for.

r., false-positive. Rate of occurrence of positive results of a test in individuals who actually do not have the attribute or disease being tested for.

r., glomerular filtration. ABBR: GFR. Rate of filtrate formation as the blood passes through the glomeruli of the kidneys.

r., growth. Rate of growth of an individual, tissue, or organ. It may be expressed as rate per arbitrary unit of time such as hours, days, months, or years.

r., heart. The number of heart contractions per unit of time.

r., infant mortality. The number of deaths in a year of live-born infants less than one year of age divided by the number of live births in the same year. This value is usually expressed as deaths per 100,000 live births. SEE: *rate, perinatal; rate, neonatal.*

r., maternal mortality. The number of maternal deaths in one year from puerperal causes (i.e., associated with pregnancy, childbirth, and the puerperium) within 42 days after delivery divided by the number of live births in that same year. This value is usually expressed as deaths per 100,000 live births.

r., morbidity. The number of cases per year of certain diseases in relation to the population in which they occur.

r., mortality. The frequency of all deaths over a period of time, usually a year, in relation to the total population in which the deaths occur. SYN: *r., death*.

r., neonatal mortality. The number of deaths in one year of infants aged 0 to 28 days divided by the number of live births in that same year. SEE: *rate, maternal mortality; rate, perinatal mortality*.

r., perinatal mortality. The number of stillbirths (in which the gestation period was 28 weeks or more) in the first 7 days of life divided by the number of live births plus stillbirths in the same year. This value is usually expressed as deaths per 100,000 live births plus stillbirths. SEE: *rate, infant mortality; rate, neonatal mortality*.

r., periodontal disease. SEE: *periodontal index*.

r., pulse. The number of contractions of the heart per unit of time that can be detected by palpating a peripheral artery.

r., respiration. The number of breaths per unit of time.

r., sedimentation. Sedimentation rate, q.v.

Rathke's pouch (răth′kĕz) [Martin H. Rathke, Ger. anatomist, 1793–1860]. A depression in the mouth of the embryo. It is just anterior to the buccopharyngeal membrane. The anterior lobe of the pituitary arises from this structure.

ratio (rā′shē-ō) [L., computation]. Relationship in degree or number between two things.

r., A/G. R., albumin-globulin.

r., albumin-globulin. Ratio of albumin to globulin in blood plasma or serum. Normally 1.3 : 1 to 3.0 : 1.

r., arm. In chromosomes, the relation of the length of the long arm of the mitotic chromosome to the short arm.

r., body-weight. Body weight in grams divided by body height in centimeters.

r., cardiothoracic. The relation of the overall diameter of the heart to the widest part of the inside of the thoracic cavity. Usually the heart diameter is one-half or less than that of the thoracic cavity.

r., curative. R., therapeutic.

r., dextrose-nitrogen. Ratio of dextrose to nitrogen in urine.

r., lecithin-sphingomyelin. ABBR: L/S ratio. The ratio of lecithin in the amniotic fluid to sphingomyelin. This is used to determine fetal maturity. The ratio increases as the pregnancy approaches term, so that by the time of delivery, it is two or more to one.

r., odds. In epidemiological, case-control studies, a relative measure of disease occur-

rence. The odds in favor of a particular event occurring in an exposed group are divided by the odds in favor of the disease occurring in an unexposed group. If the condition being studied is rare, the odds ratio is a close approximation to the relative risk. SEE: *relative risk*.

r., sex. Ratio of males to females in a given population. Usually expressed as number of males per 100 females.

r., therapeutic. Ratio obtained by dividing effective therapeutic dose by minimum lethal dose. SYN: *r., curative*.

ration (rā′shŭn). Fixed allowance of food and drink for a certain period.

rational (răsh′ŭn-ăl) [L. *rationalis*, reason]. 1. Of sound mind. SYN: *sane*. 2. Reasonable or logical; employing treatments based on reasoning or general principles, opposed to empiric.

rationale (răsh″ŭn-ăl′) [L.]. The logical or fundamental reason for a course of action or procedure.

rationalization (răsh″ŭn-ăl-ĭ-zā′shŭn). In psychology, a justification for an unreasonable or illogical act or idea to make it appear reasonable.

rattle (răt′l) [ME. *ratelen*, to rattle]. A sound or rale heard on auscultation.

r., death. A gurgling sound or subcrepitant rale heard in the trachea of the dying.

rattlesnake. A poisonous snake of the genus *Crotalid*. It has articulated cuticular extensions at the tip of the tail. These produce a characteristic rattle. SEE: *snake*.

raucous (raw′kŭs) [L. *raucus, hoarse*]. Hoarse, harsh, as the sound of a voice.

Raudixin. Trade name for rauwolfia serpentina, USP.

Rauscher leukemia virus [Frank J. Rauscher, U.S. virologist, b. 1931]. Virus known to cause leukemia in mice.

Rauwiloid. Trade name for alseroxylon.

rauwolfia serpentina (raw-wŏlf′ē-ă) [Leonhard Rauwolf, Ger. botanist, 1535–1596]. USP. The dried roots of *Rauwolfia serpentina*. Extracts are potent hypotensive agents and sedatives with low toxicity. Derivatives are serpentine, serpentinine, and reserpine, q.v. Trade name is Raudixin.

rave (rāv) [ME. *raven*, to be delirious]. To talk irrationally, as in delirium.

raving. 1. Irrational utterance. 2. Talking irrationally.

raw egg. SEE: *eggs, raw*.

ray (rā) [L. *radius*, ray]. 1. One of a number of lines diverging from a common center. 2. Line of propagation of any form of radiant energy, esp. light or heat; loosely, any narrow beam of light.

RS: energy; energy, radiant; fluorescence; heat; radiation; "roentgen-" words; spectrum; x-ray.

r., actinic. A solar ray of the spectrum, capable of producing chemical changes. SYN: *r., chemical.*

r., alpha. Ray composed of positively charged particles of helium derived from atomic disintegration of radioactive elements. Velocity is one-tenth the speed of light. Alpha rays are completely absorbed by a thin sheet of paper and possess powerful fluorescent, photographic, and ionizing properties. They are less penetrative than beta rays.

r., antirachitic. Ultraviolet radiation from 2700 to 3020 A.U.

r., bactericidal. Ray between 1850 and 2600 A.U., which is strongly destructive to bacteria.

r.'s, Becquerel's. Rays emitted from radium, uranium, and other radioactive substances.

r.'s, beta. Negatively charged electrons expelled from atoms of disintegrating radioactive elements.

r.'s, border. R.'s, grenz.

r.'s, cathode. Negatively charged electrons discharged by the cathode through a vacuum, moving in a straight line and, upon hitting solid matter, producing roentgen rays.

r.'s, characteristic. Secondary roentgen rays, the wavelengths of which are determined by the chemical constitution of the object that emits, transmits, or scatters them.

r., chemical. R., actinic.

r.'s, cosmic. Electromagnetic waves (radiation) coming from sources in outer space. Cosmic rays have a short wavelength and exceptionally high velocity and penetrative power. SYN: *r.'s, Millikan.*

r.'s, delta. Highly penetrative waves given off by radioactive substances.

r., erythema-producing. Ray between 1800 and 4000 A.U., which produces erythema, with those around 2540 and between 2050 and 3100 A.U. being most effective.

r.'s, fluorescent roentgen. Secondary rays whose wavelengths are characteristic of the substance that emits them.

r.'s, gamma. Heterogeneous vibrations caused by electronic disturbance in atoms of radioactive elements during their disintegration. They appear identical with roentgen rays except that the wavelengths range from about 1.4 to 0.01 A.U. and they derive from the nucleus rather than from the orbit of the element. They have high velocity and penetrative power.

r.'s, grenz. Soft roentgen rays with an average wavelength of 2 A.U. (range from 1 to 3 A.U.); obtained with peak voltage of less

than 10 kilovolts. They lie between ultraviolet and roentgen rays.

r.'s, hard. Roentgen rays of short wavelength and great penetration.

r.'s, heat. Visible rays from 3900 to 7700 A.U. and infrared rays from 7700 to 14,000 A.U. The heating effect of visible rays on deeper tissue is proportionately stronger than that of infrared rays, because the visible rays have greater penetrating power. SEE: *heat.*

r.'s, hertzian. Electromagnetic waves used in radio communication.

r.'s, infrared. Radiations just beyond the red end of the spectrum. Their wavelengths range between 7700 and 500,000 A.U. The therapeutic range extends from about 7700 to about 14,000 A.U.

r., luminous. One of the visible rays of the spectrum.

r., medullary. In the kidney, one of many slender processes composed of straight tubules that project into the cortex from the bases of renal pyramids. SYN: *pars radiata lobuli corticalis renis.*

r.'s, Millikan. R.'s, cosmic.

r.'s, monochromatic. Rays characterized by a definite wavelength, as secondary rays.

r.'s, pigment-producing. Rays between 2540 and 3100 A.U. are most effective in stimulating the production of pigment in the skin. This is due to a local response to irritation of cutaneous prickle cells.

r.'s, positive. Rays of positively charged ions that, in a discharge tube, move from the anode toward the cathode.

r., primary. Ray discharged directly from a radioactive substance, as the alpha, beta, and gamma rays.

r.'s, roentgen. X-rays discovered by Wilhelm Konrad Roentgen. They have a penetrative power through opaque substances; used for photographing internal organs and parts, and for diagnostic and therapeutic purposes.

r.'s, scattered. Roentgen rays or gamma rays that, in their passage through a substance, have been deflected and changed by an increase in wavelength.

r.'s, Schumann. Rays in the region bounded between 1220 and 1850 A.U.

r.'s, secondary. Roentgen rays emitted in all directions by any matter irradiated with roentgen rays.

r.'s, ultraviolet. Invisible rays of the spectrum that are beyond the violet rays, and of varying wavelengths. They may be refracted, reflected, and polarized, but will not traverse many substances impervious to the rays of the visible spectrum. They rapidly destroy the vitality of bacteria. They produce photochemical and photographic effects.

r.'s, x-. R.'s, roentgen.

Raynaud's disease (rā-nōz') [Maurice Raynaud, Fr. physician, 1834–1881]. A peripheral vascular disorder found most frequently in females between the ages of 18 and 30. It is characterized by abnormal vasoconstriction of the extremities upon exposure to cold or emotional stress. A history of symptoms for at least 2 years is necessary for diagnosis.

SYM: Intermittent attacks of pallor or cyanosis of the digits (usually fingers) associated with cold or emotional disturbance, pallor or cyanosis that is bilateral or symmetrical, normal radial and ulnar pulse. No evidence of occlusive disease is present; gangrene may occur but is limited to the skin of the tips of the digits.

TREAT: Maintenance of warmth of extremities by wearing wool gloves, socks, avoidance of contact with cold materials, avoidance of use of tobacco. Vasodilators and tranquilizers may be helpful.

PROG: Attacks persist but can be controlled. No serious disability develops, but this condition is sometimes associated with the development of rheumatoid arthritis or scleroderma.

Raynaud's phenomenon. Intermittent attacks of pallor followed by cyanosis, then redness of digits, before return to normal. Initiated by exposure to cold or emotional disturbance. Numbness, tingling, and burning may occur during the attacks. Secondary to such conditions as occlusive arterial disease, systemic scleroderma, thoracic outlet syndrome, pulmonary hypertension, myxedema, or trauma. SEE: *Nursing Diagnoses in Appendix.*

TREAT: Based on recognition and treatment of the underlying condition.

rayon, purified. USP. A fibrous form of regenerated cellulose manufactured by the viscose process, desulfured, washed, and bleached. It is used in surgical dressings and bandages.

Rb. Chem. symb. for the element rubidium.

RBBB. *right bundle branch block.*

RBC, rbc. *red blood cell; red blood count.*

R.B.E. *relative biological effectiveness.*

RBRVS. *resource-based relative value scale.*

R.C.D. *relative cardiac dullness.*

R.C.P. *Royal College of Physicians.*

R.C.S. *Royal College of Surgeons.*

R.D.A. *right dorsoanterior,* presentation position of the fetus; *recommended dietary allowance.*

R.D.D.A. *recommended daily dietary allowance.*

RDMS. *registered diagnostic medical sonographer.*

R.D.P. *right dorsoposterior,* presentation position of the fetus.

RDS. *respiratory distress syndrome.*

R.E. *radium emanation; right eye; reticuloendothelium.*

Re. Chem. symb. for the element rhenium.

re- [L.]. Prefix meaning back or again.

reabsorb (rē″ăb-sorb'). To absorb again.

reabsorption (rē″ăb-sorp'shŭn). The process of absorbing again. It occurs in the kidney when some of the materials filtered out of the blood by the glomerulus are reabsorbed as the filtrate passes through the nephron.

reacher. A long grasping device for extending the reach of persons in wheelchairs or for those with limited strength or range of motion at the shoulder. SYN: *reaching tongs.*

react (rē-ăkt') [L. *re,* again, + *agere,* to act]. 1. To respond to a stimulus. 2. To participate in a chemical reaction.

reactant (rē-ăk'tănt). A chemical or substance taking part in a chemical reaction.

    r., acute phase. Any one of several serum proteins that increase or decrease in response to the progress or decline of inflammation.

reaction (rē-ăk'shŭn) [LL. *reactus,* reacted]. 1. Response of an organism, or part of it, to a stimulus. 2. In chemistry, a chemical process or change; transformation of one substance into another in response to a stimulus. 3. An opposing action or counteraction. 4. Emotional and mental state created by a situation.

    r., alarm. The first stage in the general adaptation syndrome, q.v., which includes changes occurring in the body when subjected to stressful stimuli. Physiological changes that occur are direct results of damage, shock, or both, or reactions of the body to defend itself against shock.

    r., allergic. Reaction resulting from hypersensitivity to an antigen.

    r., anamnestic. The reappearance of antibodies that may occur when an antigen is injected a considerable time after the first injection.

    r., anaphylactic. Reaction that follows injection or administration of a foreign substance to an animal that has been sensitized to it. SYN: *anaphylaxis.*

    r., antigen-antibody. The combination of molecules of an antigen with one or more molecules of its specific antibody.

    r., anxiety. In current psychiatric terminology, this condition is classed as an anxiety disorder, q.v.

    r., Arias-Stella. Decidual changes in the endometrial epithelium. These changes consist of hyperchromatic cells with large nuclei; they may be associated with ectopic pregnancy.

r., biuret. 1. A test for measuring proteins in serum. 2. A chemical test for urea.

r., chain. A self-renewing reaction in which the initial stage causes the next reaction, which in turn causes the next reaction, and so on.

r., complement-fixation. Reaction seen when the complement enters into combinations formed between soluble or particulate antigens and antibody. Used for diagnosis of certain diseases, esp. syphilis. SEE: *complement; fixation, complement.*

r., consensual. 1. An involuntary action. 2. A crossed reflex.

r., conversion. A conversion type of hysterical neurosis in which loss of or alteration in physical functioning suggests a physical disorder but instead represents the expression of a psychological conflict or need. The disturbance is not under voluntary control and cannot be explained by a disease process; it is not limited to pain or sexual dysfunction.

r., cross. Reaction between an antibody and an antigen that is not specific for the antibody but is closely allied to the one that is.

r., defense. A mental response the purpose of which is to protect the ego.

r., delayed. Reaction occurring a considerable time after a stimulus, esp. a reaction such as inflammation of the skin occurring hours or days after exposure to the allergen.

r., dissociative. A sudden, temporary alteration in the normal functions of consciousness, identity, or motor behavior. Thus the individuals may temporarily forget their identity; or important personal events cannot be recalled; or they may wander as if in a dream state.

r., false-negative. A test result that is inaccurate in that it was negative when in reality it should have been positive.

r., false-positive. A positive reaction in a test, esp. test for syphilis, that is due to faulty technique or to presence of another disease.

r., hemianopic. In some forms of homonymous hemianopia, the pupils of both eyes fail to react to a thin pencil of light from the blind side, but react normally to light from the normal side.

r., hemiopic pupillary. Reaction in certain cases of hemianopia in which light from one side will cause the iris to contract but light from the other side will not cause the contraction.

r., immune. Reaction that demonstrates the presence of antibodies in the blood. Indicative of a high degree of immunity.

r., leukemic or leukemoid. Changes in the blood smear of peripheral blood that are consistent with those present in leukemia. This may occur in patients with an infection or tumor but who do not have leukemia.

r., local. Reaction occurring at point of stimulation or injection of exciting substances.

r., myasthenic. Gradual decrease and eventual cessation of muscle contractions when a muscle is stimulated repeatedly by direct current.

r., neutral. In chemistry, a reaction indicating absence of acid or alkaline properties. Expressed as pH 7.0.

r. of degeneration. Change in muscle reactivity to electricity, seen in lower motor neuron paralysis.

r., ophthalmic. Local reaction of conjunctiva to introduction of toxins of tuberculosis and typhoid fever; more severe in those having the diseases.

r., Prausnitz-Küstner. SEE: *Prausnitz-Küstner reaction.*

r., quellung. The swelling of capsules of bacteria when mixed with their specific immune serum.

r., transfusion. Reaction that follows transfusion of incompatible blood, which causes agglutination and hemolysis of the recipient's or donor's red blood cells or both.

r., wheal and flare. The response within 10 to 15 minutes to an antigen injected into the skin. The area demonstrates an elevated blanched irregular wheal surrounded by erythema.

reaction time. The time required to respond to a stimulus.

reactivate. To make active again, esp. the process of returning activity to immune serum that has lost its potency by the addition of fresh normal serum, thus restoring the complement, which had become inactive through age, heat, or other factors.

reactive depression. In psychology, mental disorder resulting from bereavement, sadness, or a situation causing such emotions, lasting longer and more marked than the normal reaction.

reactivation (rē-ăk″tĭ-vā′shŭn). Process of making something active again.

reactivity (rē″ăk-tĭv′ĭ-tē). The action of reacting to a stimulus.

reading. Interpreting or perusing written or printed characters or material. Reading may or may not include comprehension of the material.

r., lip. Interpretation of what is being spoken by watching movements of the speaker's lips.

reading disorders. Conditions that interfere with or prevent comprehension of written or printed material. A term used esp. in reference to children. The condition seen in some adults may have developed due to injury to the brain or may have persisted from infancy. SEE: *dyslexia*.

reading machines for the blind. Electronic reading machines that convert printed matter into speech. Several machines for home use are available. For information, contact the Lighthouse National Center for Vision and Aging at (800) 334-5497 or the American Foundation for the Blind at (800) 232-5463.

read-only memory. ABBR: ROM. The portion of a computer's memory that contains permanent instructions as opposed to random access memory (RAM), which holds the temporary instructions (a program).

reagent (rē-ā′jĕnt) [L. *reagere*, to react]. 1. A substance involved in a chemical reaction. 2. A substance used to detect the presence of another substance. 3. Subject of a psychological experiment, esp. one reacting to a stimulus.

reagin (rē′ă-jĭn). A type of immunoglobulin gamma E (IgGE) present in the serum of atopic individuals. Reagin does not cross the placental barrier.

reaginic (rē-ă-jĭn′ĭk). Concerning reagin.

reality. The quality of being real.

reality orientation. A program intended to orient persons with dementia. It involves repetition of verbal and nonverbal information. The environment remains constant and the person is reminded and reviewed on names, dates, weather and other pertinent information.

reality principle (rē-ăl′ĭ-tē). Awareness of external demands and adjustment in a manner that meets these demands, yet assures continued self-gratification.

reality testing. The attempt by the individual to evaluate and understand the real world and his or her relation to it.

reality therapy. A psychiatric treatment based on the concept that some patients deny the reality of the world around them. Therapy is directed to assist such patients to recognize and accept the present situation. The main technique is confrontation; the therapist consistently confronts the client with the reality of the situation. Illness or pathology is viewed as a defense against the real world. The purpose of the confrontation is to minimize distortion.

reamer (rē′mĕr). A small instrument used in dentistry for enlarging the root canal of a tooth.

reanastomosis, surgical. The surgical procedure for rejoining structures, esp. vessels or tubes, that had been previously ligated.

reanimate (rē-ăn′ĭ-māt) [L. *re*, again, +

animare, fill with life]. To reactivate, restore to life, revive, resuscitate.

reapers' keratitis (rēp′ĕrs kĕr-ă-tī′tĭs). Inflammation of the cornea caused by dust from grain. SEE: *keratitis*.

reasonable care. Those acts performed or omitted that an ordinary prudent medical practitioner or health care professional would or would not have done. A measure against which a defendant's malpractice conduct is compared.

reasonable charge. The reimbursement for any service provided for health care. Under Medicare this is the lowest customary charge by a particular physician for a service or the prevailing charge of other physicians in that area for the same service.

reasonable cost. The amount a third party (usually the medical insurer) will actually reimburse for health care based on the cost to the provider for delivering that service.

reattachment (rē″ă-tăch′mĕnt). 1. Recementing a dental crown. 2. Re-embedding periodontal ligament fibers into the cementum of a tooth that has become dislodged. 3. Rejoining parts that have been separated, as a finger that has been traumatically detached.

rebase (rē-bās′). To refit a denture by replacing the base material without altering the occlusal characteristics.

rebound [ME. *rebounden*, to leap back]. Response even in reflexes in which sudden withdrawal of stimulus is followed by fresh activity, such as a strong contraction following a moderate one, marked relaxation following moderate relaxation, or contraction replacing inhibition.

rebound phenomenon. When a limb or a part is acting against a resistance and the resistance is suddenly removed, the limb will move forcibly in the direction toward which effort was being directed. This is indicative of a cerebellar lesion.

rebreathing. Inhalation of gases that had been previously exhaled.

Rebuck skin window test. An *in vivo* method of assessing inflammation. A superficial abrasion is made in the skin and a glass coverslip is applied to the area. Leukocytes accumulate at the site and adhere to the coverslip.

recalcification (rē″kăl-sĭ-fĭ-kā′shŭn) [L. *re*, again, + *calx*, lime, + *facere*, to make]. The restoration of calcium salts to tissues from which they have been withdrawn.

recall [″ + AS. *ceallian*, to call]. Act of bringing back to mind that which has been previously learned or experienced.

recanalization. Re-establishment of an opening through a vessel that had been previously occluded.

recapitulation theory (rē″kǎ-pĭt-ū-lā′shŭn) [″ + *capitulum*, a section]. The theory that an individual in its development from the ovum to maturity passes through successive stages that approximate the series of adult ancestors from which that organism has descended. Summarized in the statement "ontogeny recapitulates phylogeny."

receiver (rē-sēv′ĕr) [″ + *capere*, to take]. 1. Container for holding a gas or a distillate. 2. Apparatus for receiving electric waves or current, such as a radio receiver.

receptaculum (rē″sĕp-tăk′ū-lŭm) [L.] (pl. *receptacula*). A vessel or cavity in which a fluid is contained.

    r. chyli. Inferior, pear-shaped, expanded portion of the lower end of the thoracic duct, near 1st and 2nd lumbar vertebrae, into which the right and left lumbar trunks, an intestinal trunk, and some thoracic vessels empty. SYN: *cisterna chyli.*

receptor (rē-sĕp′tor) [L., a receiver]. 1. In pharmacology, a cell component that combines with a drug, hormone, or chemical mediator to alter the function of the cell. SEE: *Ehrlich's side-chain theory.* 2. Various sensory nerve endings.

    r., adrenergic. The area in certain cells that is thought to be the site of action of adrenergic stimulation whether produced by the body or drugs. There are two types of adrenergic receptors. Some act in response to sympathomimetic or adrenergic stimuli or drugs. These are called alpha-adrenergic receptors. Some react to inhibit the action of sympathomimetic or adrenergic stimuli, and these are called beta-adrenergic receptors. Epinephrine is a powerful activator of alpha-adrenergic receptors; and isoproterenol is a powerful activator of beta-adrenergic receptors.

    r., auditory. The hair cells in the organ of Corti in cochlea of the ear.

    r., cell. SEE: *r., drug.*

    r., cholinergic. Sites in nerve synapses or effector cells that respond to the effect of acetylcholine.

    r., contact. Receptor that gives rise to a sensation such as touch, temperature, or pain that can be localized in or on the surface of the body.

    r., cutaneous. Receptor located in the skin.

    r., distance. Receptor that responds to stimuli originating at a distance from the body. Includes visual, auditory, and olfactory sense organs. SYN: *teleceptor.*

    r.'s, drug. Cell constituents, including chemicals, protein, and portions of a membrane, that sense extracellular signals and translate them into intracellular physiological or metabolic events. In the case of drugs,

the receptors sense the presence of the pharmacologically active agent and produce the effects of the drug on the cell. There may be thousands of such receptors in *each* cell.

    r.'s, gravity. Macular hair cells of utricle and saccule, which respond to changes in position of the head and linear acceleration.

    r.'s, immunologic. Receptors on the surface of white blood cells that identify the type of cell and link with monokines, q.v., lymphokines, q.v., or other chemical mediators during the immune response.

    r.'s, olfactory. The olfactory cells, bipolar nerve cells, found in olfactory epithelium, whose axons form fibers of olfactory nerve.

    r.'s, optic. The rods and cones of the retina.

    r.'s, proprioceptive. Muscle and tendon spindles, the receptors of muscle or kinesthetic stimuli.

    r.'s, rotary. The hair cells in the cristae of the ampulla of semicircular ducts of the ear, which are stimulated by angular acceleration or rotation.

    r., sensory. A sensory nerve-ending, a cell or group of cells, or a sense organ that when stimulated gives rise to an afferent or sensory impulse.

    CLASSIF: Exteroreceptors: those located on or near the surface that respond to stimuli of the outside world. Include eye and ear (receptors for remote stimuli) and touch, temperature, and pain receptors (contact receptors). Interoceptors: those in mucous linings of alimentary and digestive tracts that respond to internal stimuli; also called visceroceptors. Proprioceptors: those responding to stimuli arising within body tissues.

    Receptors also are classified on the basis of nature of stimuli to which they respond: chemoreceptors, those that respond to chemical substances (taste buds, olfactory cells, receptors in aortic and carotid bodies); pressoreceptors, those that respond to pressure (receptors in aortic arch and carotid sinus); photoreceptors, those that respond to light (rods and cones); tangoreceptors, those that respond to touch (Meissner's corpuscle).

    r.'s, stretch. Neuromuscular and neurotendinar spindles and organs of Golgi, which are stimulated by stretch. SEE: *proprioceptor.*

    r.'s, taste. The gustatory cells of the taste buds.

    r.'s, temperature. Krause's end-bulbs (receptors of cold) and Ruffini's corpuscles (receptors for warmth).

    r.'s, touch. Merkel's disks, Meissner's corpuscles, and nerve plexus about the roots of hairs.

r., universal. SEE: *universal recipient.*

receptosome. SEE: *endosome.*

recess (rē'sĕs) [L. *recessus*, receded]. A small indentation, depression, or cavity. SYN: *recessus.*

    r., cochlear. A small concavity lying between the two limbs of the vestibular crest in vestibule of ear that lodges the beginning of the cochlear duct.

    r., elliptical. A small concavity lying superiorly and posteriorly on medial wall of vestibule that lodges the utricle of the ear.

    r., epitympanic. That portion of the tympanic cavity that lies above the level of tympanic membrane. It contains the head of the malleus and short limb of the incus. SYN: *attic.*

    r., infundibular. A small projection of the third ventricle that extends into the infundibular stalk of the hypophysis.

    r., lateral, of fourth ventricle. One of two lateral extensions of the 4th ventricle, forming narrow pockets on each side and around upper portions of the restiform bodies.

    r., nasopalatine. A small depression on the floor of the nasal cavity near the nasal septum. Lies immediately over the incisive foramen.

    r., omental. One of three pocketlike extensions of the omental bursa. The superior recess extends upward behind the caudate lobe of the liver; the inferior recess extends downward into the great omentum; and the lineal recess extends laterally to the hilus of the spleen.

    r., optic. A pocket of the 3rd ventricle lying anterior to the infundibular recess. It is bound inferiorly by the optic chiasma.

    r., pharyngeal. Recess in the lateral wall of the nasopharynx lying above and behind the opening to the auditory tube. SYN: *fossa, Rosenmüller's.*

    r., pineal. Recess of the roof of the 3rd ventricle extending into the stalk of the pineal body.

    r., piriform. A deep depression in the wall of the laryngeal pharynx lying lateral to the orifice of the larynx. It is bounded laterally by thyroid cartilage and medially by cricoid and arytenoid cartilages. It is a common site for lodgement of foreign objects.

    r., sphenoethmoidal. Small space in the nasal fossa lying above the superior concha. Lies between the ethmoid bone and the anterior surface of the body of the sphenoid bone and posteriorly receives the opening of the sphenoidal sinus.

    r., spherical. Recess on medial wall of the vestibule of the inner ear that accommodates the saccule.

    r., suprapineal. A posterior extension of roof of the 3rd ventricle forming a small cavity above the pineal body.

    r., tympanic membrane. One of two pouches of tympanic mucous membrane (anterior and posterior) lying between the tympanic membrane and anterior and posterior malleolar folds.

    r., umbilical. A dilatation on the left main branch of the portal vein that marks the position where the umbilical vein was originally attached.

recession (rē-sĕsh'ŭn) [L. *recessus*, recess]. 1. The withdrawal of a part from its normal position. 2. In dentistry, the shrinkage of gingival tissue in a direction toward the root of the tooth. This allows exposure of more of the tooth structure. SEE: *periodontitis.* SYN: *ulatrophia.*

recessive. Tending to recede or go back; lacking control; not dominant.

recessive gene. A gene that, in the presence of its dominant allele, does not express itself.

recessus (rē-sĕs'ŭs) [L.]. A small hollow or recess.

recidivation (rē-sĭd"ĭ-vā'shŭn) [L. *recidivus*, falling back]. 1. The relapse of a disease or recurrence of a symptom. 2. The return to criminal activity.

recidivism. Habitual criminality; repetition of antisocial acts.

recidivist. 1. A confirmed criminal. 2. A patient, esp. one with mental illness who has repeated relapses into behavior marked by antisocial acts.

recidivity. Tendency to relapse, or to return to a former condition.

recipe (rĕs'ĭ-pē) [L., take]. 1. Take, indicated by the sign ℞. 2. A prescription or formula for a medicine. SEE: *prescription.*

recipient (rĭ-sĭp'ē-ĕnt) [L. *recipiens*, receiving]. One who receives anything, esp. those who receive blood, tissues, or organs provided by a donor, as in a blood transfusion or kidney transplant. SEE: *donor.*

recipiomotor (rĭ-sĭp"ē-ō-mō'tor) [" + *motor*, mover]. Concerning the reception of motor stimuli.

reciprocal (rĭ-sĭp'rō-kăl) [L. *reciprocus*, alternate]. Interchangeable in character.

reciprocal inhibition. Inhibition of muscles antagonistic to those being facilitated; this is essential for coordinated movement.

reciprocation (rĭ-sĭp"rō-kā'shŭn) [L. *reciprocare*, to move backward and forward]. The condition of one action countering another reaction. In dentistry, the action of one part of a dental device to counter the effect of another part.

reciprocity. The recognition by one state of the license to practice granted to a health care professional by another state.

Recklinghausen, Friedrich D. von (rĕk' lĭng-how"zĕn). German pathologist, 1833–1910.

   R.'s canals. Rootlets of the lymphatics, minute spaces in connective tissue. SYN: *von Recklinghausen's canals.*

   R.'s disease. Multiple neurofibromata of nerve sheaths. They occur along peripheral nerves, where they are quite obvious, and on spinal and cranial nerve roots. Extremely variable in size, number, and shape. Area over tumor may be hyperpigmented. Symptoms may be completely absent or may be those of pain due to pressure on spinal cord or on the brain. SYN: *neurofibromatosis; von Recklinghausen's disease.*

   TREAT: Surgical as required to relieve symptoms.

   R.'s tumor. An adenoleiomyofibroma on wall of the fallopian tube or posterior uterine wall. SYN: *von Recklinghausen's tumor.*

reclination (rĕk"lĭ-nā'shŭn) [L. *reclinatio,* lean back]. The turning of a cataract-covered lens over into the vitreous to remove it from line of vision.

recline (rē-klīn') [L. *reclinare*]. To be in recumbent position; to lie down.

Reclus' disease (rā-klooz') [Paul Reclus, Fr. surgeon, 1847–1914]. Multiple benign cystic growths in the breast.

recombinant. In genetics and molecular biology, the result of combining genetic material from different sources.

recombinant DNA. Artificial manipulation of segments of DNA from one organism into the DNA of another organism. Using a technique known as gene splicing, it is possible to join genetic material of unrelated species. When the host's genetic material is reproduced, the transplanted genetic material is also copied. This technique permits isolating and examining the properties and action of specific genes. SEE: *plasmid; gene splicing.*

   Studies in this area must be done in a carefully controlled environment. Levels of need for containment have been defined and are designated as P-1 for the lowest level and P-4 for the highest. The P-4 level is for experiments involving animal virus DNA that contains potentially lethal genes. Experiments using DNA from pathogenic organisms, cancer-causing viruses, and viruses associated with certain toxins are prohibited in the U.S.

recombinant TPA. SEE: *tissue plasminogen inactivator.*

recombination (rē"kŏm-bĭ-nā'shŭn). 1. Joining together again. 2. In genetics, the joining together of gene combinations in the offspring that were not present in the par-

ents.

recomposition [L. *re,* again, + *composer,* to place together]. The recombining of constituents or parts.

recompression [" + LL. *compressare,* press together]. Resubjecting a person to increased atmospheric pressure, a procedure used in the treatment of caisson disease (bends).

reconstitution (rē"kŏn-stĭ-tū'shŭn). Returning a substance previously altered for preservation and storage to its approximate original state, as is done with dried blood plasma.

record (rĕk'ord). 1. A written account of something. SEE: *problem-oriented medical record.* 2. In dentistry, a registration of jaw relations in a malleable material or on a device.

   r., functional chew-in. Record of the natural chewing action of the mandible made on an occlusion rim by the teeth or scribing studs.

   r., interocclusal. Record of the positional relationship of teeth or jaws to each other. It is made by placing a plastic material that hardens between the teeth prior to biting down on the material.

recover (rĭ-kŭv'ĕr) [O. Fr. *recoverer*]. To regain health after illness; to regain a former state of health. To regain a normal state as to recover from fright.

recovery (rĭ-kŭv'ĕr-ē). The process or act of becoming well or returning to a state of health.

recovery room. Area provided with equipment and nurses needed to care for patients who have just come from surgery. Patients remain there until they regain consciousness and are no longer drowsy and stuporous from the effects of anesthesia. SEE: *postoperative care.*

recreation. Literally, to create anew. Participation in an endeavor that refreshes an individual and serves to provide mental or physical relaxation, or both. What would be considered work by one individual could very well be a form of recreation to another.

recreational drug. SEE: *drug, recreational.*

recrement (rĕk'rē-mĕnt) [L. *recrementum,* sifted again]. Secretion, such as the saliva or part of the bile, that is reabsorbed by the body.

recrudescence (rē"kroo-dĕs'ĕns) [L. *recrudescere,* to get worse]. Return of symptoms after a remission. SYN: *relapse.*

recrudescent (rē"kroo-dĕs'ĕnt). Assuming renewed activity after dormant or inactive period.

recruitment (rĭ-kroot'mĕnt) [O. Fr. *recrute,* new growth]. 1. Condition in which response in a reflex action increases to a maximum when a stimulus is prolonged, even though strength of stimulus is unchanged; due to activation of increasingly greater numbers of motor neurons. Ex.: If, while testing the patellar reflex, the normal patient clasps his or her hands together and attempts to pull them apart, the intensity of the reflex response will be increased. SEE: *Jendrassik's maneuver*. 2. In audiology, an increase in the perceived intensity of a sound out of proportion to the actual increase in the sound level.

recruitment of end organs. Increase in discharge from sensory end organs, resulting from increase in number of end organs discharging and increase in frequency in discharge from each.

rectal (rĕk'tăl) [L. *rectus*, straight]. Pert. to the rectum.

rectal alimentation. Rectal feeding.

rectal anesthesia. Introduction of anesthetic into rectum for local desensitization, used esp. in labor.

rectal crisis. Tenesmus and rectal pain in locomotor ataxia.

rectal feeding. The introduction of nutrients in fluid form into the colon through the rectum. SYN: *enema, nutrient; nutritive enema.*

rectalgia (rĕk-tăl'jē-ă) [L. *rectus*, straight, + Gr. *algos*, pain]. Pain in rectum.

rectal reflex. The normal desire to evacuate feces present in rectum.

rectectomy (rĕk-tĕk'tō-mē) [" + Gr. *ektome*, excision]. Excision of the rectum or anus. SYN: *proctectomy.*

rectification (rĕk"tĭ-fĭ-kā'shŭn) [" + *facere*, to make]. 1. Process of refining or purifying a substance. 2. Act of straightening or correcting. 3. Process of changing an alternating current into a pulsating direct current.

rectified (rĕk'tĭ-fīd). Made pure or straight. Set right.

rectifier (rĕk'tĭ-fī'ĕr) [L. *rectum*, straight, + *-ficare*, to make]. In electricity, a device for transforming an alternating current into a pulsating direct current.

rectitis (rĕk-tī'tĭs) [" + Gr. *itis*, inflammation]. Inflamed condition of the rectum. SYN: *proctitis.*

recto- [L. *rectus*, straight]. Combining form meaning straight or pert. to the rectum.

rectoabdominal (rĕk"tō-ăb-dŏm'ĭ-năl) [" + *abdomen*, belly]. Concerning the rectum and abdomen.

rectocele (rĕk'tō-sēl) [" + Gr. *kele*, tumor, swelling]. Protrusion or herniation of posterior vaginal wall with anterior wall of rectum through the vagina. SEE: *cystocele.*

rectoclysis (rĕk-tŏk'lĭ-sĭs) [" + Gr. *klysis*, a washing]. Slow introduction of fluid into rectum.

rectococcygeal (rĕk-tō-kŏk-sĭj'ē-ăl) [" + Gr. *kokkyx*, coccyx]. Concerning the rectum and coccyx.

rectococcypexia (rĕk"tō-kŏk-sĭ-pĕks'sē-ă) [" + " + *pexis*, fixation]. Fixation of rectum by suturing it to coccyx.

rectocolitis (rĕk"tō-kō-lī'tĭs) [" + Gr. *kolon*, colon, + *itis*, inflammation]. Inflamed condition of the rectum and colon. SYN: *proctocolitis.*

rectocystotomy (rĕk"tō-sĭs-tŏt'ō-mē) [" + Gr. *kystis*, bladder, + *tome*, incision]. Incision of the bladder through rectum, usually to remove a calculus.

rectolabial (rĕk"tō-lā'bē-ăl) [" + *labium*, lip]. Concerning the rectum and a labium of the vaginal introitus.

rectoperineorrhaphy (rĕk"tō-pĕr"ĭ-nē-or'ă-fē). Surgical repair of the anus and perineum. SYN: *proctoperineoplasty.*

rectopexy (rĕk'tō-pĕk-sē) [" + Gr. *pexis*, fixation]. Fixation of rectum by suturing to another part. SYN: *proctopexy.*

rectophobia (rĕk"tō-fō'bē-ă) [" + Gr. *phobos*, fear]. Acute anxiety concerning the possibility of having cancer in those patients with rectal disease.

rectoplasty (rĕk'tō-plăs"tē) [" + Gr. *plassein*, to form]. Plastic surgery on the anus and rectum. SYN: *proctoplasty.*

rectorrhaphy (rĕk-tor'ă-fē) [L. *rectus*, straight, + Gr. *rhaphe*, seam]. Suture of the rectum and anus. SYN: *proctorrhaphy.*

rectoscope (rĕk'tō-skōp) [" + Gr. *skopein*, to examine]. Proctoscope, q.v.

rectoscopy (rĕk-tŏs'kō-pē). Proctoscopy.

rectosigmoid (rĕk"tō-sĭg'moyd) [" + Gr. *sigma*, letter S, + *eidos*, form, shape]. Upper part of rectum and adjoining portion of the sigmoid colon.

rectosigmoidectomy (rĕk"tō-sĭg"moy-dĕk'tō-mē) [" + " + *ektome*, excision]. Surgical removal of the rectum and sigmoid colon.

rectostenosis (rĕk"tō-stĕn-ō'sĭs) [" + Gr. *stenos*, narrow]. Stricture of the rectum.

rectostomy (rĕk-tŏs'tō-mē) [" + Gr. *stoma*, mouth]. Creation of an artificial opening into the rectum to relieve stricture. SYN: *proctostomy.*

rectotomy (rĕk-tŏt'ō-mē) [" + Gr. *tome*, incision]. Incision for stricture of the rectum or other purposes. SYN: *proctotomy.*

rectourethral (rĕk"tō-ū-rē'thrăl) [" + Gr. *ourethra*, urethra]. Concerning the rectum and urethra.

rectouterine (rĕk"tō-ū'tĕr-ĭn) [" + *uterus*, womb]. Concerning the rectum and uterus.

rectovaginal (rĕk"tō-văj'ĭ-năl) [" + *vagina*, sheath]. Concerning the rectum and vagina.

rectovesical (rĕk"tō-vĕs'ĭ-kăl) [" + *ve-*

sica, bladder]. Concerning the rectum and bladder.

rectovestibular (rĕk″tō-vĕs-tĭb′ū-lăr) [″ + *vestibulum*, vestibule]. Concerning the rectum and vestibule of the vagina.

rectovulvar (rĕk″tō-vŭl′văr) [″ + *vulva*, covering]. Concerning the rectum and vulva.

rectum (rĕk′tŭm) [L., straight]. Lower part of large intestine, about 5 in. (12.7 cm) long, between sigmoid flexure and the anal canal. The centers for the defecation reflex are located in the medulla and 2nd, 3rd, and 4th sacral segments. SEE: *colon* for illus.

    PREPARATIONS   SOMETIMES GIVEN BY RECTUM: *Chloral Hydrate:* Prescribed dose dissolved in 3 oz (90 ml) of warm olive oil; 3 oz (90 ml) of very warm milk; or 3 oz (90 ml) of thin boiled cornstarch water. This makes a good preparation or base to hold the medicine in suspension. If adverse effects are noticed, as indicated by a sudden change in vital signs, action should be taken to prevent further absorption. A cleansing enema will accomplish this. SEE: *enema.*

    Sodium Bicarbonate: Four grams to 500 ml (or 1 pt) of water aids in the expulsion of the bowel content. The neutralizing action on the acidity of the bowel content brought about by the sodium bicarbonate solution serves to soothe the bowel.

    RS: anorectal; anus; archocele; archoptosis; archorrhagia; archostenosis; cloaca; colon; enema; feeding, rectal; hemorrhoid; sigmoid; "proct-" or "rect-" words.

rectus (rĕk′tŭs) [L.]. Straight; not crooked.

rectus muscles. 1. Two external abdominal muscles, one on each side, from pubic bone to the ensiform cartilage and 5th, 6th, and 7th ribs. 2. Four short muscles of the eye: exterior, interior, superior, and inferior.

recumbency (rĭ-kŭm′bĕn-sē) [L. *recumbens*, lying down]. State of leaning or reclining.

recumbent. 1. Lying down. SEE: *left lateral recumbent position; position, unilateral recumbent; prone.* 2. Inactive, idle.

    r., dorsal. Lying on one's back. SEE: *supine.*

    r., lateral. Lying on one's side.

    r., ventral. Lying with one's anterior side down. SEE: *prone.*

recuperation (rĭ-kū″pĕr-ā′shŭn) [L. *recuperare*, to recover]. Restoration to normal health.

recurrence (rĭ-kŭr′ĕns) [L. *re*, again, + *currere*, to run]. Return of symptoms after a period of quiescence, as in recurrent fever and in yellow fever. SYN: *relapse.*

recurrent (rĭ-kŭr′ĕnt) [L. *recurrens*, returning]. Returning at intervals, as a fever.

recurvation (rĭ″kŭr-vā′shŭn) [L. *recurvus*,

bent back]. The act of bending backward.

recurvatum. Backward bowing. At the knee, it is called genu recurvatum or back knee.

recurve (rē-kŭrv′). To bend backward.

red (rĕd) [AS. *read*]. A primary color of the spectrum.

    r., Congo. An odorless red-brown powder used as an indicator in testing for free hydrochloric acid in gastric fluids. Also used in testing for amyloid. In polarized light, amyloid treated with Congo red produces a green fluorescence.

    r., cresol. An indicator of pH. It is yellow below pH of 7.4 and red above 9.0.

    r., methyl. An indicator of pH. It is red at pH 4.4 and yellow at 6.2.

    r., neutral. An indicator of pH. It is red at pH 6.8 and yellow at 8.0.

    r., phenol. Phenolsulfonphthalein, a chemical used in testing renal function. It is also an indicator of pH. It is yellow at pH 6.8 and red at 8.4.

    r., scarlet. An azo dye used in staining tissues for microscopic examination.

    r., vital. A stain used in preparing tissues for microscopic examination.

red bag. Term used to describe infectious material or the placement of that material in a special container. SEE: *Universal Precautions* in *Appendix.*

red bag waste. Infectious material placed in a special container to prevent its being the source of infection to anyone exposed to it. SEE: *Universal Precautions* in *Appendix.*

red blindness. Inability to see red hues. The most frequent type of color blindness.

red blood cell. Blood corpuscle containing hemoglobin. SYN: *erythrocyte.*

    r.b.c., spiculed. Spiculed red cell, q.v.

red cross. A red cross on a white background is an internationally recognized sign of a medical installation or of medical personnel. It is also the emblem of the American Red Cross.

redia (rē′dē-ă) [Francesco Redi, It. naturalist, 1626–1698] (pl. *rediae*). Stage in life cycle of a trematode that follows the sporocyst stage. Rediae are saclike structures possessing an oral sucker and a blind gut. They arise parthenogenetically from germ masses within the sporocyst and in turn give rise to second- or third-generation rediae or to cercaria.

redifferentiation (rē″dĭf-ĕr-ĕn″shē-ā′shŭn). The resuming of the characteristics of mature cells by malignant cells.

red. in pulv. [L.] *reductus in pulverum*, let it be reduced to powder.

redintegration (rĕd-ĭn″tĕ-grā′shŭn) [L. *redintegratio*]. 1. Restitution of a part. 2. Restoration to health. 3. Recall by mental association.

Redisol. Trade name for cyanocobalamin.

redistribution. The matching of health care personnel resources to the population's site of care. Generally, the term is used in discussing the maldistribution of in-hospital personnel compared to in-community personnel.

red lead. Lead tetroxide, Pb_3O_4.

red-man (neck) syndrome. An adverse side effect of vancomycin therapy. Symptoms include one or more of the following: pruritus, erythema and flushing of the upper torso, angioedema and, rarely, cardiac depression. The reaction is probably due to an increase of histamine in plasma associated with the vancomycin.

red nucleus. Gray matter in the tegmentum of the midbrain. SYN: *nucleus ruber*, q.v.

red-out (rĕd'owt). A term used in aerospace medicine to describe what happens to the vision and central nervous system, i.e., seeing red and perhaps experiencing unconsciousness, when the aircraft is doing part or all of an outside loop at high speed, or any other maneuver that causes the pilot to experience a negative force of gravity. The condition is due to engorgement of the vessels of the head including those of the retina.

redox. Combined form indicating oxidation-reduction system or reaction.

red precipitate. Red mercuric oxide. Poisoning symptoms are similar to those of mercuric chloride, q.v.

redressement (rĕ-drĕs-mŏn') [Fr.]. 1. Correction of a deformity. 2. Dressing of a wound more than once.

reduce (rĭ-dūs') [L. *re*, again, + *ducere*, to lead]. 1. To restore to usual relationship, as the ends of a fractured bone. 2. To weaken, as a solution. 3. To diminish, as in bulk or weight.

reducible (rĭ-dūs'ĭ-bl). Capable of being replaced in a normal position, as a dislocated bone or a hernia.

reducing agent. A substance that loses electrons easily and therefore causes other substances to be reduced.

Ex.: hydrogen sulfide; sulfur dioxide.

reductant (rĭ-dŭk'tănt). The atom that is oxidized in an oxidation-reduction reaction.

reductase (rĭ-dŭk'tās) [" + *ducere*, to lead, + *ase*, enzyme]. An enzyme that accelerates the process of reduction of chemical compounds.

reduction (rĭ-dŭk'shŭn) [L. *reductio*, leading back]. 1. Restoration to normal position, as a fractured bone or a hernia. 2. In chemistry, a type of reaction in which a substance gains electrons and positive valence is decreased. SEE: *oxidation*.

r. of fractures, closed. Treatment of fractures of bones by placing the bones in proper position, i.e., reducing the fragments without the use of surgery.

r. of fractures, open. Treatment of fractures of bones by the use of surgery to place the bones in proper position, i.e., reducing the fragments.

reduction division. Cell division occurring in gametogenesis following synapsis in which diploid number of chromosomes is reduced to the haploid number (one-half the diploid number). SYN: *meiosis*.

redundant (rĭ-dŭn'dĕnt) [L. *redundare*, to overflow]. More than necessary.

reduplicated (rĭ-dū'plĭ-kā"tĕd) [L. *re*, again, + *duplicare*, to double]. 1. Doubled. 2. Bent backward upon itself, as a fold.

reduplication (rĭ-dū"plĭ-kā'shŭn). 1. A doubling, as of the heart sounds in some morbid conditions. 2. A fold.

Reduviidae (rē"dū-vī'ĭ-dē). A family of the order Hemiptera, including the assassin bugs.

Reduvius (rē-dū'vē-ŭs). A genus of true bugs belonging to the family Reduviidae.

R. personatus. A species that normally feeds on other insects, but sometimes attacks man, inflicting painful bites about the face. In some individuals, these bugs may cause severe allergic symptoms. SYN: *kissing bug*.

Reed-Sternberg cells [Dorothy Reed, U.S. pathologist, 1874–1964; Karl Sternberg, Aust. pathologist, 1872–1935]. Giant connective tissue cells with one or two large nuclei that are characteristic of Hodgkin's disease.

re-education (rē"ĕd-ū-kā'shŭn) [L. *re*, again, + *educare*, to educate]. 1. Training to partially restore lost competence to a disabled or mentally ill person. 2. Physical means for restoring muscular tone and activity.

reef (rēf). A fold or a tuck, usually taken in redundant tissue.

re-entry (rē-ĕn'trē). In cardiology, the diversion of a repolarization wave going in one direction where it is blocked to another where it is not blocked. The wave then goes back up the pathway that was blocked but is no longer blocked to produce a contraction. This leads to a continuing series of premature beats.

refection (rē-fĕk'shŭn) [L. *reficere*, to refresh]. 1. Act of restoring. 2. In the laboratory rat, recovery from symptoms of vitamin B–complex deficiency on a diet deficient in vitamin B. Thought to be due to bacterial synthesis of vitamins by intestinal bacteria.

reference man. Concept used in nutritional investigation and surveys. A man 22 years of age, weight 70 kg, living in an environment with a mean temperature of 20°C, wearing clothing compatible with thermal comfort, engaged in light physical activity, and with an estimated caloric intake of 2800 kcal/ day.

reference woman. A hypothetical model used in nutritional references, described the same as reference man, q.v., except in weight (58 kg) and caloric intake (2000 kcal/day).

referral. The practice of sending a patient to another practitioner or specialty program for consultation or service. Such referral involves a delegation of responsibility for patient care, which should be followed up to insure that satisfactory care has been delivered.

referred pain. Pain felt in a part removed from its point of origin. Referred pain may be the result of visceral pain or from proximal or deep musculoskeletal injury and is usually referred to areas distant from the source of the problem. Pain from the heart, angina pectoris, may be referred to either arm, but most commonly the left, or to the ear, jaw, back, or teeth.

refine (rē-fīn') [L. *re*, again, + ME. *fin*, finished]. To purify or render free from foreign material.

reflectance, diffuse. Reflectance of light from a rough or non-polished surface in which the radient energy tends to go in all directions. The angle of reflectance does not equal the angle of incidence.

reflectance, specular. Reflectance of light from a polished surface in which the angle of reflectance is equal to the angle of incidence.

reflectance photometer. An instrument used to measure reflectance. Clinically employed in chemical analyzers, glucometers and dip stick readers, such as the Ames serolyzer.

reflection (rĭ-flĕk'shŭn) [L. *reflexio*, a bending back]. 1. Condition of being turned back upon itself, as when the peritoneum passes from wall of a body cavity to and around an organ and back to the body wall. 2. The throwing back of a ray of radiant energy from a surface not penetrated. 3. Mental consideration of something previously considered.

reflector (rĭ-flĕk'tor) [L. *re*, again, + *flectere*, to bend]. Device or surface that reflects waves or radiant energy or sound.

reflex (rē'flĕks) [L. *reflexus*, bend back]. An involuntary response to a stimulus; a reflex action. Reflexes are specific and predictable and are usually purposeful and adaptive. They depend upon an intact neural pathway between point of stimulation and responding organ (muscle or gland). This pathway is called reflex arc. In a simple reflex this includes a sensory receptor, afferent or sensory neuron, reflex center in brain or spinal

cord, one or more efferent neurons, and an effector organ (muscle or gland). Most reflexes, however, are more complicated and include internuncial or associative neurons intercalated between afferent and efferent neurons. SEE: *arc, reflex,* for illus.

RS: Achilles jerk; areflexia; chemoreflex; chin jerk; conditioned reflex; consensual; intestinal reflex; jaw jerk reflex; jerk; reaction; reinforcement reflex; Setchenov's inhibitory centers; and reflexes under individual names.

r., abdominal. SEE: *abdominal reflexes.*

r., abdominocardiac. A change in heart rate, usually a slowing, resulting from mechanical stimulation of abdominal viscera.

r.'s, accommodation. The changes that take place when the eye adjusts to bring light rays from an object to focus on the retina. This involves change in the size of the pupil, convergence or divergence of the eyes, and either a decrease or increase in the convexity of the lens depending upon the previous condition of the lens.

r., Achilles. SEE: *Achilles tendon reflex.*

r., acquired. R., conditioned.

r., after-discharge of. Reflex activity that persists for a time after cessation of the stimulus.

r.'s, allied. Reflexes initiated by several stimuli originating in widely separated receptors whose impulses follow the final common path to effector organ and reinforce one another.

r., anal. SEE: *anal reflex.*

r., ankle. SEE: *ankle jerk.*

r.'s, antagonistic. Two or more reflexes initiated simultaneously in different receptors that involve the same motor center but produce opposite effects. The most important or adaptive response takes place.

r., auditory. SEE: *auditory reflex.*

r., autonomic. Any reflex involving the response of a visceral effector (cardiac muscle, smooth muscle, glands). Such reflexes always involve two efferent neurons (preganglionic and postganglionic).

r., autonomic, true. A visceral response in which afferent impulses do not pass through central nervous system, but instead enter prevertebral ganglia where connections are made with efferent neurons.

r., axon. A reflex that does not involve a complete reflex arc, hence is not a true reflex. The afferent and efferent limbs of the reflex are branches of a single nerve fiber, the axon (axonlike dendrite) of a sensory neuron. An example is vasodilation resulting from stimulation of skin.

r., Babinski's. SEE: *Babinski's reflex.*

r., Bainbridge. When an increase in blood pressure or distention of the heart occurs, the rate increases. SYN: *Bainbridge effect.*

r., biceps. Flexion of forearm upon percussion of tendon of biceps brachii.

r., Brain's. SEE: *Brain's reflex.*

r., carotid sinus. Pressure in the area of the neck over the carotid sinus causes reflex slowing of the heart.

r., cat's eye. In children, a pupillary flash or reflection from the eye that may be momentary, may be white, yellow, or pink, and is best seen under diminished natural illumination. This reflex, which may be noticed first by a child's parent, may be caused by a variety of conditions, the most important of which is retinoblastoma. Also observed in tuberous sclerosis, inflammatory diseases of the eye, and certain congenital malformations of the eye. SEE: *retinoblastoma.*

r.'s, Chaddock's. SEE: *Chaddock's reflexes.*

r., chain. Reflex initiated by several separate serial reflexes, each of which was activated by the preceding one.

r., chin. SEE: *chin reflex.*

r., ciliary. SEE: *ciliary reflex.*

r., ciliospinal. SEE: *ciliospinal reflex.*

r., clasp-knife. Quick inhibition of the stretch reflex when extensor muscles are forcibly stretched by flexing the limb. SYN: *reaction, lengthening.*

r., conditioned. Reflex acquired as a result of training in which the cerebral cortex is an essential part of the neural mechanism. Any reflex not inborn or inherited.

r., conjunctival. SEE: *conjunctival reflex.*

r., consensual. R., crossed.

r., convulsive. Condition in which a weak stimulus will induce a convulsion resulting in widespread uncoordinated and purposeless actions. Seen in strychnine poisoning.

r., corneal. SEE: *corneal reflex.*

r., cough. SEE: *cough reflex.*

r., cranial. Any reflex whose center lies in the brain.

r., cremasteric. SEE: *cremasteric reflex.*

r., crossed. Reflex in which stimulation of one side of the body results in response on the opposite side. SYN: *r., consensual; r., indirect.*

r., crossed extension. Extension of the opposite side lower extremity when a painful stimulus is applied to the skin.

r., deep. Reflex caused by stimulation of parts beneath skin, like tendons or bones, as the jaw, elbow, wrist, triceps, knee, and ankle jerk reflexes.

r., delayed. Reflex not taking place until some seconds after application of stimulus.

r., digital. SEE: *digital reflex.*

r., diving. Slowing of the heart rate when the head is immersed in water. This reflex helps to protect a person from drowning, esp. if immersed in cold water. SEE: *drowning.*

r., elbow. R., triceps.

r., elementary. A typical reflex common to all vertebrates. Includes postural, flexion, stretch, and extensor thrust reflexes.

r., embrace. SEE: *embrace reflex.*

r., extensor thrust. A quick and brief extension of a limb upon application of pressure to plantar surface.

r., flexor withdrawal. Flexion of the lower extremity when the foot receives a painful stimulus.

r., gag. SEE: *gag reflex.*

r., gastrocolic. SEE: *gastrocolic reflex.*

r., gastroileal. SEE: *gastroileal reflex.*

r., grasp. Grasping reaction of the fingers and toes when stimulated.

r., Grünfelder's. SEE: *Grünfelder's reflex.*

r., Hering-Breuer. SEE: *Hering-Breuer reflex.*

r., Hoffmann's. Flicking of the tip of the nail of the ring, middle, or index finger produces flexion of the terminal phalanx of the thumb and the second and third phalanges of another finger.

r., hung-up. Slowness of the relaxation phase of deep tendon reflexes. Present in hypothyroidism.

r., inborn. An unconditioned reflex; an innate or inherited reflex.

r., indirect. R., crossed.

r.'s, inhibition of. Prevention of a reflex action, as inhibiting a sneeze by pressure on facial nerve as it passes just under the upper lip.

r., intersegmental. Reflex in which several segments of spinal cord are involved.

r., intestinal. R., myenteric.

r., intrasegmental. Reflex that involves only a single segment of the spinal cord.

r.'s, irradiation of. The spreading of reflexes through the central nervous system whereby impulses entering the cord in one segment activate motor neurons located in many segments.

r., jaw. Chin reflex, q.v.

r., kinetic. R., labyrinthine.

r., knee-jerk. Extension of the leg resulting from percussion of patellar tendon. This is an example of a myotatic or stretch reflex of importance in the maintenance of posture. The reflex is diminished or abolished in lesions of the nerve supplying the muscle and tendon, lesions of posterior roots involving a sensory pathway as in tabes dorsalis, lesions of anterior root involving motor pathways, or lesions of lower motor neurons in anterior horns of gray matter of spinal cord, as in poliomyelitis. If, however, the upper motor neuron is destroyed, muscle tone and the motor response are greatly increased. So-called pathologic reflex under these conditions may appear. Reflexes are also modified by higher centers, e.g., emotional tension increases the knee jerk (and muscle tension generally). SEE: *Babinski's reflex; Jendrassik's maneuver.*

r., labyrinthine righting. Reflex, esp. a postural reflex, resulting from stimulation of receptors in semicircular ducts, utricle, and saccule of inner ear. This reflex provides orientation of the head in space and with the rest of the body. SYN: *r., kinetic; optical righting reflex.*

r., light. SEE: *light reflex.*

r., local. Reflex that does not involve the central nervous system.

Ex.: the myenteric reflex, which occurs even though extrinsic nerves to intestine have been cut.

r., long. Reflex involving many segments of the spinal cord.

r., lung. Dilatation of the lung tissue under the area of the skin that is irritated by percussion or cold.

r., Magnus-de Kleijn. In decerebrate rigidity, extension of the limbs on the side to which the chin is turned by rotating the head. There is flexion of the limbs of the opposite side.

r., mass. Condition following a section of spinal cord in which a weak stimulus through radiation brings about widespread responses due to release from inhibition of higher cortical centers.

r., Mayer's. Downward pressure on the index finger is followed by opposition and adduction of the thumb, flexion at the metacarpophalangeal joint, and extension at the interphalangeal joint.

r., Mendel-Bekhterev. Plantar flexion of the toes in response to percussion of the dorsum of the foot.

r., monosynaptic. Reflex involving only two neurons, an afferent and efferent.

r., Moro. SEE: *Moro reflex.*

r., myenteric. Reflex caused by distention of the intestine, resulting in contraction above the point of stimulation and relaxation below it. SYN: *r., intestinal.*

r., myotatic. R., stretch.

r., near. R., accommodation.

r., neck-righting. In the infant, rotation of the trunk in the same direction in response to the direction the head of the supine infant is turned. This reflex appears at age 4 to 6 months and is no longer obtainable

by age 2 years.

r., nociceptive. Reflex initiated by a painful stimulus.

r., optical righting. Use of visual stimuli to maintain the normal position of the body and head.

r., palatal. SEE: *palatal reflex.*

r., palmar grasp. The lightly stimulated palm grasps the stimulating object. This reflex is present at birth and is gone by the age of 6 months.

r., palm-chin. Vigorous stroking or scratching of the thenar eminence, producing contraction of the skin and lower lip muscles on the same side.

r. (response), parachute. Extension of the arms, hands, and fingers when the infant is suspended in the prone position and dropped a short distance onto a soft surface. This reaction appears at 9 months of age and persists. If the response is asymmetrical, a motor nerve abnormality is present.

r., paradoxical. Response to a stimulus that is unexpected and may be the opposite of what would be considered normal.

r., patellar. R., knee-jerk.

r., pathologic. Abnormal reflex due to disease; the reflex is seen as one of the symptoms of the disease.

r., pharyngeal. SEE: *pharyngeal reflex.*

r., pilomotor. SEE: *pilomotor reflex.*

r., placing. When an infant is held erect and the dorsum of one foot is dragged along the under-edge of a table top, the response is flexion of that leg and then extension. This reflex is present at birth and is no longer present by the age of 6 weeks.

r., plantar. SEE: *Babinski's reflex; plantar reflex.*

r., plantar grasp. Light stimulation of the sole of the foot produces a grasp reflex of the foot. This reflex is present at birth and is gone by the age of 10 months.

r., postural. Any reflex that is concerned with maintenance of posture.

r., pressor. Reflex that results in elevation of blood pressure brought about by constriction of arterioles.

r.'s, proprioceptive. Reflexes initiated by movement of the body to maintain the position of the moved part. Any reflex initiated by stimulation of a proprioceptor.

r., psychogalvanic. Decreased electric resistance of the skin in response to emotional stress or stimuli.

r., pupillary. Reflex that occurs when a beam of light strikes the retina, causing the pupil to contract (protective against excessive stimulation). The same effect results with accommodation to near objects.

r., quadriceps. R., knee-jerk, q.v.

r., quadrupedal extensor. Brain's reflex, q.v.

r., red. The red light reflection seen when examining the eye by use of the ophthalmoscope.

r., righting. Any of the reflexes that enable an animal to maintain the body in a definite relationship to the head and thus maintain its body right side up.

r., rooting. Stroking the cheek of the infant causes turning of the mouth toward the stimulus. This reflex is present at birth; by 7 months of age it is gone if done while the infant is asleep; it is gone by 4 months if done while the infant is awake.

r., Rossolimo's. SEE: *Rossolimo's reflex.*

r.´s, sexual. Reflexes concerned with sexual activities, esp. erection and ejaculation.

r., short. Reflex involving one or a few segments of spinal cord.

r., somatic. Reflex induced by stimulation of somatic sensory nerve endings.

r., spinal. Reflex whose center is in the spinal cord.

r., startle. Moro reflex, q.v.

r., static. Reflex concerned with establishment and maintenance of posture when body is at rest.

r.´s, statokinetic. Reflexes occurring when body is moving, e.g., walking or running.

r., stepping. Movements of progression elicited when the infant is held upright, inclined forward, as the soles of the feet are touching a flat surface. This reflex is present at birth and is gone by 6 weeks of age.

r., stretch. Contraction of a muscle as a result of quickly stretching the same muscle. SYN: *r., myotatic.*

r., sucking. Sucking movement of the infant produced by stroking the lips.

r., superficial. Cutaneous reflex caused by irritation of the skin or areas depending upon the spinal cord as a motor center, such as the scapular, epigastric, abdominal, cremasteric, gluteal, and plantar reflexes, or upon centers in the medulla, such as conjunctival, pupillary, and palatal reflexes.

r., swallowing. Production of the succession of reflexes and muscular activity concerned with swallowing when the palate is stimulated by food.

r., tendon. Deep reflex obtained by sharply tapping skin over tendon of a muscle. It is exaggerated in disease of an upper neuron and diminished or lost in disease of lower neuron.

r., tonic neck. A general term used to denote either the asymmetrical or symmetrical tonic neck reflexes seen in infants. Presence of the tonic neck reflexes suggests that head movements cause reflexive move-

ments of the upper extremities.

r., tonic neck, asymmetrical. In the infant, forcibly turning the head causes extension of one or both extremities on the side to which the head is turned. There is flexion of the extremities on the other side.

r., tonic neck, symmetrical. In infants, flexion of the neck causes flexion in the arms. Extension of the neck causes extension of the arms.

r., triceps. Sharp extension of forearm resulting from tapping of triceps tendon while arm is held loosely in bent position. SYN: *r., elbow.*

r., triceps surae. Achilles tendon reflex, q.v.

r., unconditioned. A natural or inherited reflex action; one not acquired.

r., vascular. R., vasomotor, q.v.

r., vasomotor. Constriction or dilatation of a blood vessel in response to a stimulus, as in becoming pale from fright. SYN: *r., vascular.*

r., visceral. Any reflex induced by stimulation of visceral nerves.

r., visceromotor. Contraction or tenseness of skeletal muscles resulting from painful stimuli originating in visceral organs.

reflex action. An involuntary response to a stimulus; a reflex.

reflex arc. The neural pathway or circuit between the point of stimulation and the responding organ in a reflex action. SEE: *arc, reflex,* for illus.

reflex center. A region, usually in the brain or spinal cord, where impulses from an afferent limb of a reflex arc initiate impulses in the efferent limb.

reflexogenic (rĭ-flĕks′ō-jĕn′ĭk) [L. *reflexus,* bend back, + Gr. *gennan,* to produce]. Causing a reflex action.

reflexogenous (rĭ″flĕks-ŏj′ĕ-nŭs). Reflexogenic, q.v.

reflexograph (rĭ-flĕks′ō-grăf) [″ + Gr. *graphein,* to write]. Device for recording and graphing a reflex, esp. one produced by muscular activity.

reflexology (rē″flĕk-sŏl′ō-jē) [″ + Gr. *logos,* word, reason]. 1. Study of the anatomy and physiology of reflexes. 2. A system of massage in which the feet and, sometimes, the hands are massaged for the purpose of attempting to favorably influence other body functions.

reflexometer (rē″flĕks-ŏm′ĕ-tĕr) [″ + Gr. *metron,* measure]. Instrument for measuring force of the tap required to produce a reflex.

reflexophil (rē-flĕks′ō-fĭl) [″ + Gr. *philein,* to love]. Characterized by activity of reflexes or by exaggerated reflexes.

reflexotherapy (rē-flĕks″ō-thĕr′ă-pē) ["
+ Gr. *therapeia*, treatment]. Treatment
by manipulation, anesthetizing, or cauterizing an area distant from seat of the disorder.
SEE: *spondylotherapy.*

reflex sympathetic dystrophy. A neurovascular complication of CVA characterized by
severe shoulder pain and stiffness, swelling
and pain in the hand. SYN: *shoulder-hand
syndrome.*

reflux (rē′flŭks) [L. *re*, back, + *fluxus*,
flow]. A return or backward flow. SEE: *regurgitation.*

    r., hepatojugular. Pressure on the liver
in patients with congestive heart failure
causes increased pressure in the cervical
venous pressure.

    r., vesicoureteral. Reflux of urine up the
ureter during micturition.

reflux disease. The illness produced when
gastric contents reflux into the esophagus.
The symptoms are heartburn, regurgitation
of acid, peptic ulcer-like pain, and difficulty
swallowing. If the symptoms are not controlled by medical therapy, surgery will be
needed.

refract (rĭ-frăkt′) [L. *refractus*, broken off]. 1.
To turn back; to deflect. 2. To detect errors
of refraction in the eyes and to correct them.

refracta dosi (rē-frăk′tă dō′sē) [L.]. In divided doses, denoting a definite amount of a
drug taken within a given time in a number
of fractional equal parts.

refraction (rĭ-frăk′shŭn) [LL. *refractio*, break
back]. 1. Deflection from a straight path, as
of light rays as they pass through media of
different densities; the change of direction
of a ray when it passes from one medium to
another of a different density. 2. Determination of amount of ocular refractive errors
and their correction.

    RS: ametropia; anisometropia; astigma-
tism; emmetropia; hypermetropia; myopia;
presbyopia.

    r., angle of. The angle formed by a re-
fracted ray of light with a line perpendicular
to surface at point of refraction.

    r., coefficient of. The quotient or sine of
angle of incidence divided by sine of angle of
refraction.

    r., double. Possessing more than one re-
fractive index, resulting in a double image.
SEE: *birefringent.*

    r., dynamic. Static refraction of the eye
plus that accomplished by accommodation;
the reciprocal of the near-point distance.

    r., errors of. Condition in which parallel
rays of light are not brought to a focus upon
the retina because of a defect in shape of the
eyeball or in refracting media of the eye.
SYN: *ametropia.*

    r., index of. 1. Ratio of angle made by in-
cident ray with the perpendicular (angle of
incidence) to that made by emergent ray
(angle of refraction). 2. The ratio of speed of
light in air to its speed in another medium.
The refractive index of water is 1.33; of crystalline lens of the eye it is 1.413.

    r., ocular. R. of eye.

    r. of eye. Ocular refraction brought
about by refractive media of the eye (cornea,
aqueous humor, crystalline lens, vitreous
body).

    r., static. Refraction of the eye when ac-
commodation is at rest or paralyzed.

refractionist (rĭ-frăk′shŭn-ĭst) [LL. *refractio*,
break back]. One skilled in determining and
correcting ocular refractive errors by use of
appropriate glass lenses.

refractive (rĭ-frăk′tĭv) [L. *refractus*, broken
off]. Concerning refraction.

refractive power. The degree to which a
transparent body deflects a ray of light from
a straight path. SEE: *diopter.*

refractivity (rē″frăk-tĭv′ĭ-tē). The quality of
being refractive; the ability to refract.

refractometer (rē-frăk-tŏm′ĕt-ĕr) [" +
Gr. *metron*, measure]. Device for measuring
refractive power, as of the eye.

refractometry (rē″frăk-tŏm′ĕ-trē). Measurement of refractive power of lenses.

refractory (rē-frăk′tō-rē) [L. *refractarius*]. 1.
Obstinate, stubborn. 2. Resistant to ordinary treatment. 3. Resistant to stimulation,
said of muscle or nerve.

refractory period, relative. Brief period of
relaxation of a muscle during which excitability is depressed. If stimulated, the muscle will respond, but a stronger stimulus is
required and response is less.

refracture (rē-frăk′chŭr) [L. *refractus*, broken off]. 1. To break again, as a bone set
wrongly. 2. Rebreaking of a fracture united
in a malaligned or incorrect position.

refrangible (rē-frăn′jĭ-bl) [L. *re*, again, +
ME. *frangible*, breakable]. Capable of being
refracted.

refresh (rĭ-frĕsh′) [O. Fr. *refreschir*, to renew].
1. To restore strength; to relieve from fatigue; to renew; to revive. 2. To scrape epithelial covering from two opposing surfaces
of a wound to facilitate the healing and joining together.

refrigerant (rĭ-frĭj′ĕr-ănt) [L. *refrigerans*,
making cold]. 1. Cooling. 2. Agent that produces coolness or reduces fever. SYN: *alge-
facient.*

refrigerant gases. A number of gases used in
ordinary household refrigerators; poisoning
due to leaks, faulty connections or breakage,
and gas dissipated into atmosphere may
occur.

refrigeration (rĭ-frĭj″ĕr-ā′shŭn) [L. *refrigera-
tio*, make cold]. Cooling; reduction of heat.

refrigeration anesthesia. Anesthesia resulting from cold, such as that produced in a limb by immersion in cold water.

refringent. Refractive.

Refsum's disease (rĕf'soomz) [Sigvald Bernhard Refsum, Norwegian physician, b. 1907]. An inherited metabolic disease due to inability to metabolize phytanic acid. Clinically there are visual disturbances, ataxia, and heart disease. Diets low in animal fat and milk products may relieve some of the symptoms.

refusion (rē-fū'zhŭn) [L. *refusus*, poured back]. The return of blood into the same circulatory system from which it was removed.

regainer (rē-gān'ĕr). 1. Device that ameliorates or restores that which was lost. 2. Device that applies pressure between teeth on either side of the space left by a missing tooth. This is done to push the teeth toward the edentulous space.

regel [Ger.]. Menstruation.

    r. kleine. Slight bloody discharge from the uterus at time of ovulation.

regeneration (rē-jĕn''ĕr-ā'shŭn) [L. *re*, again, + *generare*, to produce]. Repair, regrowth, or restoration of a part, such as tissues. Opposite of degeneration.

regimen (rĕj'ĭ-mĕn) [L., rule]. A systematic plan of activities and regulation of diet, sleep, and exercise designed to improve or maintain health or to keep a certain condition under control.

regio (rē'jē-ō) [L.]. Region.

region (rē'jŭn) [L. *regio*, boundary]. A portion of the body with natural or arbitrary boundaries.

    RS: abdomen; epigastrium; inguinal region; Kiesselbach's area; temple.

regional (rē'jŭn-ăl). Concerning a region.

register [LL. *regesta*, list]. 1. An official recording of names or facts. 2. The compass or range of a voice. 3. A series of tones of like quality or character, as low or high register, chest or head register.

registered nurse. A nurse who has graduated from a school of nursing, passed the State Board Examination administered by a State Board of Nursing Examiners, and is granted the right to practice for hire. The nurse is registered and licensed to practice.

registered record administrator. ABBR: R.R.A. A person who administers medical records and has been certified as an R.R.A. after passing the examination given by the American Medical Record Association.

registrant (rĕj'ĭs-trănt) [L. *registrans*, registering]. A nurse who is named on the books of a registry as being "on call" or available to be called for duty.

registrar (rĕj'ĭs-trăr) [O. Fr. *registreur*]. The official manager of a registry.

registration [L. *registratio*]. The act of recording information such as births or deaths; or the recording of those who are registered or licensed to practice within a state.

registry (rĕj'ĭs-trē) [LL. *regesta*, list]. An office or book where a list of nurses ready for duty is kept; a placement bureau for nurses.

Reglan. Trade name for metoclopramide hydrochloride.

Regonol. Trade name for pyridostigmine bromide.

regression (rĭ-grĕsh'ŭn) [L. *regressio*, go back]. 1. A turning back or return to a former state. 2. A return of symptoms. 3. Retrogression. 4. In psychology, an abnormal return to earlier reaction, characterized by mental state and behavior inappropriate to the situation. Regression may occur as a result of frustration or in states of fatigue, dreams, hypnosis, intoxication, illness, and in certain psychoses (schizophrenia). 5. In statistics, a procedure used to predict one variable on the basis of data about one or more other variables.

    r., filial. In biology, tendency of offspring to deviate less from the average of a population than their parents.

regressive (rĭ-grĕs'ĭv). Concerning or marked by regression.

regressive resistive exercise. ABBR: RRE. A form of active resistive exercise that advocates gradual reduction in the amount of resistance as muscles fatigue.

regular (rĕg'ū-lăr) [L. *regula*, rule]. 1. Conforming to rule or custom. 2. Methodical, steady in course, such as pulse. SYN: *normal; typical.*

regulation. 1. State of being controlled or directed. 2. The ability of an individual, such as a developing embryo, to develop normally in spite of experimental modifications.

regulation development. In embryology, condition in which a single blastomere, or a portion of an embryo, can give rise to a whole embryo. Opposite of mosaic development.

regulative. Pert. to regulation.

regulator. Device for adjusting or controlling the rate of flow or administration of fluids, oxygen, or blood.

regurgitant (rē-gŭr'jĭ-tănt) [L. *re*, again, + *gurgitare*, to flood]. Throwing back or flowing in a direction opposite to the normal.

regurgitation (rē-gŭr'jĭ-tā'shŭn). A backward flowing, as in the return of solids or fluids to the mouth from the stomach or the backward flow of blood through a defective heart valve.

    r., aortic. Backflow of blood into the left ventricle as a result of incompetent aortic valves.

r., cardiac. Backward flow of blood through the aortic, mitral, or tricuspid valves due to incomplete closure.

r., duodenal. Return flow of chyme from the duodenum to stomach.

r., functional. Regurgitation not due to valvular disorder but to dilatation of ventricles, the great vessels, or valve rings.

r., mitral. Backflow of blood from the left ventricle into the left atrium, resulting from imperfect closure of the mitral or bicuspid valve.

r., pulmonic. Backflow of blood from the pulmonary artery into the right ventricle.

r., tricuspid. Backflow of blood from the right ventricle into the right atrium.

r., valvular. Flow of blood back through a valve, esp. a heart valve, that is not completely closed as it would normally be.

REHABDATA. A computerized bibliographical database of rehabilitation information supplied by the National Rehabilitation Information Center (NARIC). For information, contact National Rehabilitation Information Center, 8455 Colesville Road, Suite 935, Silver Spring, MD 20910-3319. Telephone is (800) 34-NARIC.

rehabilitation (rē″hă-bĭl″ĭ-tā′shŭn) [L. *rehabilitare*]. 1. The processes of treatment and education that lead the disabled individual to attainment of maximum function, a sense of well-being, and a personally satisfying level of independence. The need for rehabilitation may be necessitated by any disease or injury that causes mental or physical impairment serious enough to result in disability. The post-coronary patient, the post-trauma patient, and the post-surgical patient need and can benefit from rehabilitation efforts. The individual who is recovering from a mental disorder is also in need of rehabilitative support. The combined efforts of the individual, family, friends, medical, nursing, and allied health personnel, and community resources are essential in order to make rehabilitation possible. 2. In dentistry, the methods used to restore dentition to its optimal functional condition. It may involve restoration of teeth by fillings, crowns, or bridgework; adjustment of occlusal surfaces by selective grinding; orthodontic realignment of teeth; or surgical correction of diseased or malaligned parts. It may be done to provide masticatory function; an acceptable aesthetic appearance of the face and teeth; improved phonetics; and preservation of the dentition and supporting tissues. Also called *occlusorehabilitation* and *mouth*, or *oral, rehabilitation.*

r., cardiac. A structured, interdisciplinary program of supervised activity, progressive exercise, psychological support, and patient education designed to enable attainment of maximum functional capacity by patients who have experienced a myocardial infarction.

rehabilitee (rē″hă-bĭl′ĭ-tē). A person rehabilitated.

rehalation (rē″hă-lā′shŭn) [L. *re*, again, + *halare*, to breathe]. Rebreathing process occasionally employed in anesthesia.

rehydration (rē″hī-drā′shŭn) [″ + Gr. *hydor*, water]. Restoration of fluid volume in a person who has been dehydrated. This may be done by use of fluids orally or parenterally.

Reichert's cartilage (rī′kĕrts) [Karl Bogislaus Reichert, Ger. anatomist, 1811–1883]. The second branchial arch of the embryo, which gives rise to stapes, styloid process, stylohyoid ligament, and lesser cornua to hyoid bone.

Reid's base line (rēdz) [Robert William Reid, Scottish anatomist, 1851–1939]. Line extending from lower edge of the orbit to center of aperture of external auditory canal backward to center of occipital bone.

Reil's island (rīlz) [Johann C. Reil, Ger. anatomist, 1759–1813]. Three or more small convolutions at bottom of fissure of Sylvius in the brain. SYN: *insula* [NA]; *island of Reil.*

reimplantation (rē″im-plăn-tā′shŭn) [L. *re*, again, + *in*, into, + *plantare*, to set]. Replacement of a part from where it has been taken out, as a tooth, finger, hand, or arm. Also called *replantation.*

reinfection (rē″in-fĕk′shŭn) [″ + ME. *infecten*, infect]. A second infection by the same organism. SEE: *superinfection.*

reinforcement (rē″in-fors′mĕnt) [″ + *inforce*, enforce]. Strengthening; augmentation of force. Part of the fundamental process of learning, along with motivation, stimulation, and action. The reward for the appropriate response in a learning situation.

reinforcement of reflex. Strengthening of the response to one stimulus by concurrent action of another; the exaggeration of a reflex by nervous activity elsewhere. Thus, during the raising of a heavy weight, the knee jerk is stronger. SEE: *Jendrassik's maneuver.*

reinforcer (rē″in-fors′ĕr). That which produces reinforcement.

reinfusion (rē″in-fū′zhŭn) [″ + *infusio*, to pour in]. The reinjection of blood serum or cerebrospinal fluid.

reinnervation (rē″in-ĕr-vā′shŭn) [″ + *in*, into, + *nervus*, nerve]. 1. Anastomosis of a paralyzed part with a living nerve. 2. Grafting of a fresh nerve for restoration of function in a paralyzed muscle.

reinoculation (rē″ĭn-ŏk″ū-lā′shŭn) [″ + *in*, into, + *oculus*, bud]. A second inoculation with the same virus or organism. SEE: *reinfection.*

reintegration. In psychology, the resumption of normal behavior and mental functioning following disintegration of personality in mental illness.

reinversion (rē″ĭn-vĕr′shŭn) [″ + *in*, into, + *versio*, turning]. Correction of an inverted organ, as of an inverted uterus by pressure on the fundus.

Reissner's membrane (rīs′nĕrz) [Ernst Reissner, Ger. anatomist, 1824–1878]. Delicate membrane separating the cochlear canal from the scala vestibuli.

Reiter's syndrome (rī′tĕrz) [Hans Conrad Julius Reiter, Ger. physician, 1881–1969]. ABBR: RS. Syndrome consisting of urethritis, arthritis, and conjunctivitis. Urethritis usually appears first. Occurs mainly in young men.

ETIOL: *Chlamydia* is the organism most frequently associated with RS.

TREAT: There is no specific therapy. Tetracycline or erythromycin is used for urethritis. The sexual partner should be treated if RS was sexually transmitted. Arthritis and conjunctivitis are treated symptomatically.

PROG: Generally good; however, recurrences are common.

rejection [L. *rejicere,* to throw back]. 1. Refusal to accept or to show affection for. In lower animals the young may be ignored or driven away by their mother. 2. In transplantation of tissues and organs, destruction of transplanted material at the cellular level by the host's immune mechanism. Transplant rejection is controlled primarily by T cells, but macrophages and B lymphocytes are also involved. Increased use of testing for HLA matching has lowered the incidence of organ transplant rejection. Immunosuppressant drugs, such as cyclosporine and corticosteroids, inhibit T cell function and reduce the possibility of rejection.

r., acute. Early destruction of grafted or transplanted material; usually begins a week after implantation. May be reversed by increased use of immunosuppressive agents.

r., chronic. Slow destruction of grafted or transplanted material. This may occur over a period of months or years.

r., hyperacute. Immediate, intense, and irreversible destruction of grafted material due to preformed antibodies.

r., parental. Refusal to accept or show affection for a son or daughter.

rejuvenation (rĭ-jū″vĕ-nā′shŭn) [L. *re*, again, + *juvenis*, young]. A return to youthful

conditions or to the normal.

rejuvenescence (rĭ-jū″vĕ-nĕs′ĕns) [″ + *juvenescere*, to become young]. The renewal of youth or return to earlier stage of existence.

Rela. Trade name for carisoprodol.

relapse (rē-lăps′) [L. *relapsus*]. Recurrence of a disease or symptoms after apparent recovery.

relapsing. Recurring after apparent recovery.

relapsing fever. An infectious disease marked by intermittent attacks of high fever.

ETIOL: Several species of spirochetes belonging to the genus *Borrelia* and transmitted by head lice, body lice, and ticks of the genus *Ornithodorus.*

TREAT: A single dose of either tetracycline, erythromycin, or procaine penicillin G and symptomatic treatment.

relation (rĭ-lā′shŭn) [L. *relatio,* a carrying back]. The condition, connection, or state of one thing compared to another.

r., jaw. Any relation of the position of the maxilla to the mandible.

r., occlusal jaw. Relation of the mandibular teeth to the maxillary teeth when the teeth are in contact.

r., unstrained jaw. Position of the jaw when normal tonus of all of the jaw muscles is present.

relative biological effect. Comparison of the effectiveness of types of radiation compared with that of x-rays or gamma rays.

relative risk. In epidemiological studies, a method of measuring the relative amount of disease occurring in different populations. The ratio of incidence rate in the exposed group to that in the unexposed group. SEE: *ratio, odds.*

relative value scale. ABBR: RVS. A proposal for setting the amount paid for medical services. It is based on the concept that payment rates for medical services should, as with other purchased services and goods, reflect the costs of producing those services.

relax [L. *relaxare,* to loosen]. To decrease tension or intensity, or to be rid of strain, anxiety, and nervousness.

relaxant (rĭ-lăk′sănt). 1. Rel. to or producing relaxation. 2. A drug that reduces tension. 3. A laxative.

r., muscle. A drug or therapeutic treatment that specifically relieves muscular tension.

r., neuromuscular. A drug, e.g., succinylcholine, that prevents transmission of stimuli to muscle tissue, esp. striated muscle.

r., smooth muscle. A drug that reduces the tension of smooth muscles such as those in the intestinal tract or bronchi.

relaxation (rē-lăk-sā′shŭn). 1. A lessening of tension or activity in a part. 2. Phase or period in a single muscle-twitch following contraction in which tension decreases, fibers lengthen, and muscle returns to resting position. 3. In magnetic resonance imaging, the return of an excited atom to alignment with the applied magnetic field.

 r., general. Relaxation of the entire body.

 r., local. Relaxation limited to a particular muscle group or to a certain part.

 r., pelvic. SEE: *pelvic relaxation.*

relaxation response. The physiological reaction that is sought and produced by sitting quietly and alone in a quiet place with eyes closed and arms and hands relaxed, paying careful attention to respiration, and repeating a brief word or phrase at each respiratory cycle. This is done for 15 to 30 minutes at a time, twice daily.

 This approach to quiet meditation is found in the practices of many religions and in Transcendental Meditation.

 It has been used by some physicians to produce therapeutic alteration in control of stress, as indicated by a reduction in blood pressure in hypertensive patients.

relaxed movement. Form of bodily movement that the operator carries through without the assistance or resistance of the patient. SYN: *passive exercise.*

relaxin (rĭ-lăk′sĭn). A polypeptide hormone secreted in the corpus luteum during pregnancy. Obtained commercially from ovaries of pregnant sows. In certain rodents, relaxin produces relaxation of the symphysis, inhibition of uterine contractions, and softening of the cervix.

relearning. Acquiring a skill or ability that had been previously present but was lost or removed due to physical damage to the muscles or brain.

release. A document which, if signed by the patient or the legal representative of the patient in the case of a minor, permits the treating physician to perform certain procedures, e.g., surgery, anesthesia, blood transfusion, removal of tissues or fluids for analysis. In addition to being signed by the patient, the release should also be signed by a witness. Most releases have a notation indicating the applicable time of the release.

releasing hormone. Hormone, releasing, q.v.

reliability. 1. Being dependable, accurate, and honest. 2. In statistics, the ability of the measuring method or device to produce reproducible data or information.

relief (rĭ-lēf′) [ME.]. Alleviation or removal of a distressing or painful symptom.

relieve [L. *relevare,* to raise]. To provide relief.

reline (rē-līn′). To replace or resurface the lining of a denture.

REM. *rapid eye movements.* Cyclic movement of the closed eyes observed or recorded during sleep. SEE: *sleep, stages of.*

rem. *roentgen equivalent* (in) *man.*

Remak's axis cylinder (rä′mäks) [Robert Remak, Ger. neurologist, 1815–1865]. The conducting part of a nerve.

Remak's band. The axis cylinder of a neuron.

Remak's fibers. The nonmedullated nerve fibers.

Remak's ganglion. A group of nerve cells in coronary sinus near its entry into the right atrium.

Remak's sign [Ernest Julius Remak, Ger. neurologist, 1849–1911]. A sign or symptom pertaining to perception of stimuli. It can be one of two types: one in which a single stimulus is perceived as if it were several stimuli applied in separate locations (polyesthesia) or one in which there is a delay in perception of stimuli. Both are seen in tabes dorsalis.

remedial (rĭ-mē′dē-ăl) [L. *remedialis*]. Curative; intended for a remedy.

remedy (rĕm′ĕd-ē) [L. *remedium,* medicine]. 1. To cure or relieve a disease. 2. Anything that relieves or cures a disease.

 r., local. Agent to relieve a local condition such as a sore.

 r., systemic. Agent to relieve or cure a disease affecting the entire organism.

remineralization (rē-mĭn″ĕr-ăl-ī-zā′shŭn). Therapeutic replacement of the mineral content of the body after it has been disrupted by disease or improper diet.

reminiscence therapy. A type of supportive talk therapy which is prescribed by health care professionals for patients who are aged and experiencing loss. Reminiscence therapy assists individuals to review and highlight the components of their past which have meaning. This is thought to increase self-esteem and life satisfaction. It can be conducted in groups or individually.

remission (rĭ-mĭsh′ŭn) [L. *remissio,* remit]. 1. Lessening of severity or abatement of symptoms. 2. The period during which symptoms abate.

remittance (rē-mĭt′ĕns). Temporary abatement of symptoms.

remittent (rē-mĭt′ĕnt) [L. *remittere,* to send back]. Alternately abating and returning at certain intervals. SEE: *fever.*

remittent fever. A fever alternately abating and returning, without intervals of afebrility. SEE: *malaria.*

remnant. That which remains or is left over.

remnant radiation. Ionizing radiation that passes through the part being examined to make the radiographic image.

remodeling. 1. The reshaping or reconstruction of a part or area. 2. Bone change or growth which is the net effect of all appositional growth and bone resorption and occurs continually in life to adapt the skeletal elements to the changing forces applied by growth, muscular activity, gravity, or mechanical pressures.

r., temporomandibular joint. The slow changes in the articular surfaces of the temporomandibular joint as it adapts to changing occlusal forces, resulting in shape changes or irregularities of the condyle or articular eminence.

Remsed. Trade name for promethazine hydrochloride.

ren (rĕn) [L.] (pl *renes*). [NA] The kidney.

r. amyloidens. Amyloid degeneration of the kidneys.

r. mobilis. Movable kidney.

r. unguliformis. Horseshoe kidney.

renal (rē′năl) [LL. *renalis*, kidney]. 1. Pert. to the kidney. SYN: *nephric.* SEE: *kidney* and *urinary tract* for illus. 2. Shaped like a kidney.

renal biopsy, percutaneous. Obtaining renal tissue for biopsy by use of a needle inserted through the skin. This is usually done after localizing the kidney by use of ultrasound, computed tomography, or angiography. The major complication is hematuria.

renal clearance test. One of several kidney function tests based on the ability of the kidney to eliminate a given substance in a standard time. Urea, phenolsulfonphthalein (PSP), iodopyracet, and other substances are employed.

renal failure, acute. Acute failure of the kidney to perform its essential functions. May be due to trauma; any condition that impairs the flow of blood to the kidneys; certain toxic substances such as compounds of mercury, carbon tetrachloride, or ethylene glycol; bacterial toxins; glomerulonephritis; acute obstruction of the urinary tract.

TREAT: Specific therapy for primary disease; either peritoneal dialysis or hemodialysis. SEE: *dialysis.*

NURSING IMPLICATIONS: Assist in identifying the cause and in its removal. Instruct patient regarding dietary restrictions, including fluid limitations; implement these restrictions. Promote prevention of infection. Instruct patient concerning activity restrictions due to metabolic alterations; implement dietary restrictions.

Prevent complications of immobility by respiratory toilet, position changes, and range-of-motion exercises. Assess neurologic status and provide appropriate safety measures. Monitor intake and output, acid-

base and electrolyte balance, particularly for signs and symptoms of hyperkalemia, and weigh daily. Assess the patient for GI and cutaneous bleeding and anemia, and replace blood components or administer erythropoietin therapy as prescribed. Record vital signs and assess for signs of pericarditis or hypotension.

If failure is not reversed but progresses to chronic (end-stage) renal failure, arrange for follow-up care and provide evaluation and appropriate patient and family teaching concerning dialysis if that is instituted. Establish learning plan for the patient and the family. Refer patient for vocational, sexual, or other counseling as needed. SEE: *Nursing Diagnoses* in *Appendix.*

renal insufficiency. The reduced capacity of the kidney to perform its functions.

renal papillary necrosis. Destruction of the papillae of the kidney. May be caused by a variety of conditions, including diabetes mellitus, acute pyelonephritis, urinary obstruction, sickle cell trait, and repeated use of phenacetin. Management consists of ureteral catheter irrigation of renal pelvis to remove obstruction; appropriate antibiotics; and adequate hydration.

renal pelvis. SEE: *pelvis, renal.*

renal scanning. Method of determining renal function and shape of the kidney. A radioactive substance that concentrates in the kidney is given intravenously. The irradiation emitted from the substance as it accumulates in the kidneys is recorded on a suitable photographic film.

renal transplantation. Surgical implantation of a donor kidney to replace one removed from a patient. SEE: *Nursing Diagnoses* in *Appendix.*

renal tubular acidosis. ABBR: RTA. A group of four disorders: Types I and II are hereditary; Type III, a combination of Types I and II, rarely occurs; Type IV is acquired. In all types the rate of excretion of acid by the kidneys is excessive. In addition, the kidneys resorb chloride in an excessive amount. This results in hyperchloremic acidosis.

Type I is characterized by hypercalciuria, calcium phosphate stones, and nephrocalcinosis. In children, rickets develops and growth is stunted. In adults there is osteomalacia.

TREAT: Sodium bicarbonate and Shohl's solution, q.v.

Type II may be a transient disorder of proximal tubular function; treatment, if required, consists of bicarbonate given in large amounts each day in combination with potassium supplements.

Type IV is usually associated with hypoaldosteronism due to diabetic nephropathy, or nephrosclerosis associated with hypertension, or chronic nephropathy. These patients have high serum potassium levels and low urine ammonia excretion. They do not have renal calculi.

TREAT: The hyperkalemia may be managed by administration of mineralocorticoids in combination with furosemide, q.v.

renal tubule. A nephron.

Rendu-Osler-Weber disease (rŏn-dū′ōs′lĕr-wĕb′ĕr). SEE: *Osler-Weber-Rendu disease.*

Renese. Trade name for polythiazide.

reniculus (rĕ-nĭk′ū-lŭs) [L.]. A lobule of the kidney.

renifleur (rā-nĭ-flŭr′) [Fr.]. One stimulated sexually by certain odors, esp. by the urine of others.

reniform (rĕn′ĭ-form) [L. *ren,* kidney, + *forma,* shape]. Shaped like a kidney. SYN: *nephroid.*

renin (rĕn′ĭn). An enzyme, produced by the kidney, that acts on angiotensin to form a pressor substance, angiotensin I. Renin is elevated in some forms of hypertension.

renin substrate. Alpha-2-globulin of the plasma. SYN: *hypertensinogen.*

renipelvic (rĕn″ĭ-pĕl′vĭk) [″ + *pelvis,* basin]. Concerning the pelvis of the kidney.

reniportal (rĕn″ĭ-por′tăl) [″ + *porta,* gate]. 1. Concerning the "hilum" of the kidney. 2. Concerning renal and portal circulations.

renipuncture (rĕn″ĭ-pŭnk′chūr) [″ + *punctura,* a piercing]. Surgical puncture of the capsule of the kidney.

rennet (rĕn′ĕt) [ME.]. 1. The lining of the fourth stomach of a calf. 2. A fluid containing rennin, a coagulating enzyme, used for making junket or cheese.

rennin (rĕn′ĭn). An enzyme that coagulates milk. Present in the gastric juice of ruminants but not in the human stomach.

renninogen (rĕn-ĭn′ō-jĕn) [ME. *rennet,* rennet, + Gr. *gennan,* to produce]. Antecedent or zymogen from which rennin is formed. The inactive form of rennin.

reno-. Combining form concerning the kidney.

renocutaneous (rē″nō-kū-tā′nē-ŭs) [″ + *cutis,* skin]. Concerning kidneys and skin.

renogastric (rē″nō-găs′trĭk) [L. *ren,* kidney, + Gr. *gaster,* belly]. Concerning the kidney and stomach.

renogram (rē′nō-grăm) [″ + Gr. *gramma,* something written]. Record of rate of removal from the blood by the kidneys of an intravenously injected dose of radioactive iodine (^{131}I).

renography (rē-nŏg′ră-fē) [″ + Gr. *graphein,* to write]. Radiography of the kidney.

renointestinal (rē″nō-ĭn-tĕs′tĭn-ăl) [″ +

intestinum, intestine]. Concerning the kidney and intestine.

renopathy (rē-nŏp′ă-thē) [″ + Gr. *pathos,* disease, suffering]. Any pathological condition of the kidneys.

renoprival (rē″nō-prī′văl). Related to loss of kidney function.

Renoquid. Trade name for sulfacytine.

renotrophic (rē″nō-trŏf′ĭk) [″ + Gr. *trophe,* nourishment]. Affecting the kidney. SYN: *nephrotrophic.*

renotropic (rē″nō-trŏp′ĭk) [″ + *trope,* a turn]. Renotrophic, q.v.

renovascular. Concerning the vascular supply of the kidney.

Renshaw cells (rĕn′shaw) [B. Renshaw, U.S. neurophysiologist, 1911–1948]. Small cells with short axons that serve to connect motor nerve axons with each other. The process functions to inhibit motor neurons.

reovirus (rē″ō-vī′rŭs) [*respiratory enteric orphan virus*]. One of the viruses found in the respiratory and digestive tracts of apparently healthy persons. Their exact importance in producing disease is not known. The group of viruses was formerly classed as ECHO virus, type 10.

rep. L. *repetatur,* let it be repeated.

repair (rĭ-păr′) [L. *reparare,* to prepare again]. To remedy, replace, or heal, as in a wound or a lost part.

   r., plastic. Utilization of plastic surgery to repair tissue.

   r., tooth. The state of recovery from pathological changes, involving the reduction of inflammation and the production of tertiary or reparative cementum. This is usually accompanied by improved health of the gingiva and the periodontal ligament.

repellent [L. *repellere,* to drive back]. An agent that repels noxious organisms such as insects, ticks, and mites. Repellents may be applied to surface of body as a liquid, spray, or dust, or they may be used to impregnate clothing.

repercolation (rē″pĕr-kō-lā′shŭn) [L. *re,* again, + *percolare,* to filter]. Repeated percolation using same materials.

repercussion (rē-pĕr-kŭsh′ŭn) [L. *repercussio,* rebound]. 1. Reciprocal action. 2. Action involved in causing subsidence of a swelling, tumor, or eruption. 3. In obstetrics, diagnosis of pregnancy by insertion of a finger into the vagina to push the uterus, causing embryo to rise and fall. SYN: *ballottement.*

repercussive (rē″pĕr-kŭs′ĭv). 1. Causing repercussion. 2. An agent that repels; a repellent.

reperfusion [L. *re,* back, + *perfundere,* to pour through]. 1. The reinstitution of blood flow to an area that was ischemic. In cardiology, the return of blood supply to a portion of the heart muscle that had become ischemic as the result of myocardial infarction, q.v. This is done by the use of thrombolytic agents such as streptokinase, q.v., or tissue plasminogen activator (tPA), q.v. The use of such agents has reduced in-hospital mortality for myocardial infarction by up to 50% when administered within the first hour of onset of symptoms. 2. Reperfusion of tissues that have been traumatized, esp. by a long period of crushing, may cause damage to other organs because of the material released from the traumatized tissues into the circulation. SEE: *crush syndrome; rhabdomyolysis.*

repetitive motion injury. Injury to tissues due to repeated trauma, usually associated with writing, painting, typing, or use of vibrating tools or hand tools. Almost any form of activity which produces repeated trauma to a particular area of soft tissue, including tendons and synovial sheaths, may cause this type of injury. Carpal tunnel syndrome, q.v., may be, but is not always, caused by repetitive motion of the wrist.

replacement. The act of replacing.

replantation [L. *re*, again, + *planto,* to plant]. Surgical reimplantation of that which has been removed from the body, esp. the surgical procedure of rejoining a hand, arm, or leg to the body after its having been removed as a result of an accident. In dentistry, replacement of a tooth that has been removed from its socket.

repletion (rē-plē'shŭn) [L. *repletio,* a filling up]. Condition of being full or satisfied.

replication (rĕp″lĭ-kā'shŭn). 1. A doubling back of tissue. 2. In medical investigations, the repetition of an experiment. 3. In genetics, the process of duplication of genetic material.

replicon (rĕp'lĭ-kŏn). Any genetic element that behaves as an autonomous unit of DNA replication. The element is able to replicate under its own control.

repolarization. Re-establishment of the electrical polarized state in a muscle or nerve fiber following contraction or conduction of a nerve impulse.

report. The account that the nursing staff going off duty gives to the oncoming staff. The purpose is to provide continuity of care despite the change in staff. The report is usually verbal. Obviously the information provided is of the utmost importance in caring for the critically ill.

reportable diseases. Diseases that must be reported by the physician to the health authorities. The communicable diseases required by International Health Regulations to be reported universally are the internationally quarantinable diseases: plague, cholera, and yellow fever. Other diseases that require such a report are those under surveillance by the World Health Organization. They are louse-borne typhus fever, relapsing fever, paralytic poliomyelitis, malaria, and influenza.

Special notification is required of all outbreaks or epidemics of diseases not listed above. Even a single case of a communicable disease long absent from a population or not previously recognized in that area is sufficient reason to require immediate reporting and institution of a full field investigation. SEE: *privacy.*

reposition (rē″pō-zĭsh'ŭn) [L. *repositio,* a replacing]. Restoration of an organ or tissue to its correct or original position.

repositioning (rē″pō-zĭsh'ŭn-ĭng). The placement of a part in its original place.

r., jaw. The changing of the position of the mandible in relation to the maxilla by altering occlusion of the teeth.

r., muscle. Surgical placement of a muscle to another attachment point in order to enhance function.

repositor. Instrument for restoring a tissue or an organ to its normal position.

r., inversion. Instrument for replacement of an inverted uterus.

r., uterine. Lever for replacement of the uterus when out of normal position.

repression (rē-prĕsh'ŭn) [L. *repressus,* press back]. In psychology, refusal to entertain distressing or painful ideas, thus submerging them in the unconscious, where they continue to exert their influence upon the individual. Psychoanalysis seeks to discover and to release repressions.

r., coordinate. Simultaneous reduction of the levels of enzymes of a metabolic pathway.

r., enzyme. An enzyme that interferes with a metabolic pathway, usually the same pathway that produced the enzyme.

repressor (rē-prĕs'or) [L. *repressus,* press back]. Something, esp. an enzyme, that inhibits or interferes with the initiation of protein synthesis by genetic material.

reproduction (rē-prō-dŭk'shŭn) [L. *re*, again, + *productio,* production]. 1. Process by which plants and animals give rise to offspring. SEE: *ovary* for illus. 2. The creation of a similar structure or situation; the act of duplicating.

r., asexual. Reproduction in which sex cells are not involved, as by fission or budding.

r., cytogenic. Reproduction by means of asexual single germ cells.

r., sexual. Reproduction by means of sexual or germ cells. Usually a male cell (spermatozoon) fuses with a female cell (egg or ovum). SYN: *syngamy.* SEE: *partheno-genesis.*

r., somatic. Asexual reproduction by budding of somatic cells.

reproductive (rē″prŏ-dŭk′tĭv). Concerning, or employed in, reproduction.

repullulation (rē-pŭl″ū-lā′shŭn) [″ + *pullulare,* to sprout]. Renewed growth by budding or sprouting.

repulsion (rĭ-pŭl′shŭn) [L. *repulsio,* a thrusting back]. 1. Act of driving back. 2. The force exerted by one body on another to cause separation. Opposite of attraction.

request for production of documents. In law, a written request for production of documents sent by plaintiff or defendant to discover additional information about a person, party, event, or subject at issue in a lawsuit.

In medical negligence cases, requests for medical records, office records, hospital policies and procedures can be made by using this discovery technique.

required services. Those services that must be included in a health program for it to qualify for federal funds.

RES. *reticuloendothelial system.*

rescinnamine (rē-sĭn′ă-mĭn). An antihypertensive drug derived from species of *Rauwolfia.* Trade name is Moderil.

rescue tools. Equipment used by rescuers in emergency medical service to free trapped victims. Rescue tools include a *come-a-long,* a hand-operated winch used to gain forceful entry during a rescue; *cutting tools,* used to cut open vehicles and metal to gain access to a patient; *jack,* a hand-operated jack used to lift objects away from patients; *power chisel,* a pressure-operated device used to cut into heavy metal. The trade name of one rescue tool is Jaws of Life.

research (rĭ-sĕrch′, rē′sĕrch) [O. Fr. *recerche,* research]. Scientific and diligent study, investigation, or experimentation in order to establish facts and analyze their significance. Inherent in such study is an orderly approach with accurate record-keeping. A hallmark of acceptable research is that it is conducted and described so that other scientists may read the report and have sufficient information concerning the design and methods to repeat it.

r., clinical. Research based mainly on bedside observation of the patient, rather than through laboratory work.

r., laboratory. Research done principally in the laboratory.

r., medical. Research concerned with any phase of medical science.

resect (rē-sĕkt′) [L. *resectus,* cut off]. To cut off, or to cut out, a portion of a structure or organ, as to cut off the end of a bone or to remove a segment of the intestine.

resectable (rē-sĕk′tă-bl). Able to be removed, esp. by surgical means. Usually used in reference to malignant growths that can be removed completely by use of surgery.

resection (rē-sĕk′shŭn) [L. *resectio,* a cutting off]. Partial excision of a bone or other structure.

r., gastric. Surgical resection of a part of the stomach.

r., transurethral. Surgical removal of the prostate by use of an instrument introduced through the urethra.

r., wedge. Surgical removal of a wedge-shaped piece of tissue, esp. from the ovary as a means of treating polycystic ovaries. SEE: *polycystic ovary syndrome.*

r., window. Resection of a portion of the nasal septum after reflection of a flap of mucous membrane.

resectoscope (rē-sĕk′tō-skōp) [L. *resectus,* cut off, + Gr. *skopein,* to examine]. Instrument for resection of the prostate gland through the urethra.

resectoscopy (rē″sĕk-tŏs′kō-pē). Resection of the prostate through the urethra.

reserpine (rĭ-sĕr′pĭn). USP. A chemically pure derivative of the plant *Rauwolfia serpentina.* A folk medicine used in India for centuries for snake bite, mental illness, and anxiety states. It lowers blood pressure and acts as a tranquilizer. Trade names are Sandril and Serpasil.

reserve (rē-zĕrv′) [L. *reservare,* to keep back]. 1. That which is held back for future use. 2. Self-control of one's feelings and thoughts.

r., alkali. Alkali content of body available for neutralization of acid.

r., cardiac. The ability of the heart to increase cardiac output to meet the needs of the body as energy output increases.

reserve air. Additional amount of air that can be expelled from the lungs over the normal quantity, which is 1200 to 1600 cc.

reservoir (rĕz′ĕr-vwor) [Fr.]. A place or cavity for storage of fluids.

reservoir of infectious agents. Any person, animal, arthropod, plant, soil, or substance in which an infectious agent normally lives and multiplies, on which it depends primarily for survival, and where it reproduces itself in such manner that it can be transmitted to a susceptible host.

residency. A period of at least one year and often 3 to 4 years of on-the-job training, usually postgraduate, that is part of the formal educational program for health care professionals.

resident. A physician who is obtaining further clinical training after internship. Usually this is done as a member of the house staff of a hospital.

residual (rĭ-zĭd′ū-ăl) [L. *residuum*, residue]. 1. Rel. to that which is left as a residue. 2. In psychology, any aftereffect of experience influencing later behavior.

residual function. The functional capacity remaining after an illness or injury.

residual urine. Urine left in bladder after urination. When this occurs, it is abnormal. May accompany enlargement of the prostate.

residue (rĕz′ĭ-dū). The remainder of something after a part is removed.

residue diet, high-. Diet with increased amounts of cellulose (fiber) and water.

residue diet, low-. Diet that includes solid food, but in which residue is reduced to a minimum. SEE: *nonlaxative diet.*

residue-free diet. Diet without cellulose or roughage. Semisolid and bland foods are included.

residuum (rē-zĭd′ū-ŭm) [L.] (pl. *residua*). Residue; the remainder.

resilience (rē-zĭl′ē-ĕns) [L. *resiliens,* leaping back]. The quality of coming back to normal shape after straining, as a stretched rubberband when released. SYN: *elasticity.*

resilient (rē-zĭl′ē-ĕnt). Elastic; coming back to normal shape after straining.

resin (rĕz′ĭn) [L. *resina,* fr. Gr. *rhetine,* resin of the pine]. 1. An amorphous, nonvolatile solid or soft-solid substance, a natural exudation from plants. It is practically insoluble in water, but soluble in alcohol. SEE: *rosin.* 2. Any of a class of solid or soft organic compounds of natural or synthetic origin. They are usually of high molecular weight, and most are polymers. Included are polyvinyl, polyethylene, and polystyrene. These are combined with chemicals such as epoxides, plasticizers, pigments, fillers, and stabilizers to form plastics.

   r., anion-exchange. SEE: *resin, ion-exchange.*

   r., cation-exchange. SEE: *resin, ion-exchange.*

   r., ion-exchange. Ionizable synthetic substances, which may be acid or basic, used accordingly to remove either acid or basic ions from solutions. Thus anionic-exchange resins may be used to absorb acid in the stomach. Cationic-exchange resins have the ability to remove basic (alkaline) ions from solutions.

   r., quick-cure. An autopolymer resin which can be polymerized by an activator and catalyst without the use of external heat. Used in many dental procedures. SYN: *cold-cure resin; self-curing resin.*

resinoid (rĕz′ĭ-noyd) [″ + Gr. *eidos,* form, shape]. Resembling a resin.

resinous (rĕz′ĭ-nŭs). Of the nature of, or pert. to, resin.

res ipsa loquitur [L.]. Literally, "the thing speaks for itself." In malpractice this concept is used for cases in which an injury occurs to the plaintiff in a situation solely under the control of the defendant. If the injury would not have occurred had the defendant exercised due care, the defendant is judged negligent. In medicine the classic example of this situation is when an object such as a sponge or clamp has been left in a patient's body after a surgical procedure or when a healthy organ has been removed.

resistance (rĭ-zĭs′tăns) [L. *resistens,* standing back]. 1. Opposition to, or the ability to oppose, anything, such as the power of a fluid to retard that which is passing through it; of the air; or opposition of the body to passage of an electric current. 2. The sum total of body mechanisms that interpose barriers to the progress of invasion, multiplication of infectious agents, or damage by their toxic products. Immunity is resistance associated with the presence of antibodies having a specific action on infectious microorganisms. Inherent resistance is the ability to resist disease independently of antibodies. 3. The force exerted to penetrate the unconscious or to submerge memories in the unconscious. 4. In psychoanalysis, condition in which the ego avoids bringing into consciousness conflicts and unpleasant events responsible for neurosis; reluctance of subject to give up old patterns of thought and behavior. It may take a variety of forms such as silence, failure to remember dreams, forgetfulness, and undue annoyance with trivial aspects of the treatment situation. 5. Force applied to a body part in the form of weights, machinery, or from another person to load muscles as an exercise to increase muscle strength.

   r., airway. The inherent resistance of the flow of air into the pulmonary tract.

   r., peripheral. The resistance of the arterial vascular system, esp. the arterioles and capillaries, to the flow of blood.

resistance exercise. Exercise in which an outside force is applied to a muscle, requiring it to develop greater tension. This is done to increase strength. If the resistance is applied by using weights, it is called mechanical resistance; if applied by a therapist, it is called manual resistance.

resistance transfer factor. A genetic factor in bacteria that controls resistance to certain antibiotic drugs. The factor is spread by bacteria to bacteria. This makes it possible for nonpathogenic bacteria to become resistant to antibiotics and to transfer that resistance to pathogens, thereby establishing a potential source for an epidemic.

resolution (rĕz-ō-lū′shŭn) [L. *resolutio,* a relaxing]. 1. Decomposition; absorption or breaking down of the products of inflammation. 2. Cessation of inflammation without suppuration. The return to normal. 3. The ability of the eye or series of lenses to distinguish fine detail.

resolve (rē-zŏlv') [L. *resolvere*, to release]. 1. To return to normal as after a pathological process. 2. To separate into component parts.

resolvent (rĭ-zŏl'vĕnt) [ME. *resolven*, releasing]. 1. Promoting disappearance of inflammation. 2. That which reduces inflammation or swelling.

resonance (rĕz'ō-nāns) [L. *resonantia*, resound]. 1. Quality or act of resounding. 2. Quality of the sound heard on percussion of a hollow structure such as the chest or abdomen. Absence of resonance is termed *flatness*; diminished resonance, *dullness*. 3. In physics, modification of sound due to vibrations of a body that are set up by waves of another vibrating body. 4. In electricity, state in which two electrical circuits are in tune with each other.

   r., amphoric. Sound similar to that produced when blowing across mouth of an empty bottle.

   r., bandbox. Pulmonary resonance heard in percussion of chests of patients with emphysema.

   r., bell-metal. Sound heard in pneumothorax in auscultation when coin is held against the chest wall and it is struck by another coin.

   r., cracked-pot. Sound having a peculiar clinking quality sometimes heard on percussion of chest in cases of advanced tuberculosis when cavities are present.

   r., normal. Normal pulmonary resonance.

   r., skodaic. Increased percussion sound over upper lung when there is pleural effusion in lower part.

   r., tympanic. Sound, low-pitched and drumlike, heard upon percussing over a large air-containing space.

   r., tympanitic. Resonance obtained by percussion of a hollow structure, such as the stomach or colon, when moderately distended with air.

   r., vesicular. Normal pulmonary resonance.

   r., vocal. In auscultation the vibrations of the voice transmitted to the ear, normally more marked over the right apex of the lung. Abnormally increased in pneumonic consolidation, in lungs infiltrated with tuberculosis, or in cavities that freely communicate with a bronchus.

Vocal resonance is diminished or absent in pleural effusion (air, pus, serum, lymph, or blood); emphysema; pulmonary collapse; pulmonary edema; egophony, a modified bronchophony characterized by a trembling, bleating sound usually heard above the upper border of dullness of pleural effusions and occasionally heard in beginning pneumonia.

   r., whispering. Auscultation sound heard when patient whispers.

resonant (rĕz'ō-nănt). Producing a vibrating sound on percussion.

resonating [L. *resonantia*, resound]. Vibrating sympathetically with a source of sound or electrical oscillations.

resonating cavities. The resonator of the human voice. Includes upper portion of the larynx, pharynx, nasal cavity, paranasal sinuses, and oral cavity.

resonator (rĕz'ō-nā"tĕr). 1. A structure that is capable of being set into sympathetic vibration when sound waves of the same frequency from another vibrating body strike it. 2. In electricity, an apparatus consisting of an electrical circuit in which oscillations of a certain frequency are set up by oscillations of the same frequency in another circuit.

resorb (rē-sorb', rē-zorb') [L. *resorbere*, to suck in]. 1. To undergo resorption. 2. To absorb again.

resorbent (rē-sor'bĕnt) [L. *resorbens*, sucking in]. An agent that promotes the absorption of abnormal matters, as exudates or blood clots.

   Ex.: potassium iodide, ammonium chloride.

resorcin (rē-zor'sĭn). Resorcinol.

resorcinol (rē-zor'sĭ-nŏl). USP. An agent with keratolytic, fungicidal, and bactericidal actions. It is used in treating certain skin diseases.

resorcinolphthalein (rē-zor"sĭ-nŏl-thăl'ē-ĭn). Fluorescein.

resorption (rē-sorp'shŭn) [L. *resorbere*, to suck in]. 1. Act of removal by absorption, as resorption of an exudate or pus. 2. Removal of enamel and other calcific portions of a tooth as a result of lysis and other pathological processes. 3. Often results from pressure or vascular changes as in root resorption of deciduous teeth prior to shedding, or bone resorption on the pressure side during tooth movement.

   r., bone. The removal of bone tissue by the process of resorption, q.v.

resource-based relative value scale. ABBR: RBRVS. The RBRVS was developed to increase payment to nonsurgeons for cognitive services, i.e., evaluation and management of patients. The scale is based on the total work required for a given service and on other considerations, including the cost of the physician's practice, the income lost during training, and the relative cost of liability insurance. This method of calculating medical care services was implemented by law in January 1992.

respirable (rĕ-spīr'ă-bl, rĕs'pĕr-ă-bl) [L. *respirare,* breathe again]. Fit or adapted for respiration.

respiration (rĕs-pĭr-ā'shŭn) [L. *respiratio,* breathing]. 1. The interchange of gases between an organism and the medium in which it lives. More specifically the taking in of oxygen, its utilization in the tissues, and the giving off of carbon dioxide. 2. The act of breathing, i.e., inhaling and exhaling, during which the lungs are provided with air, and the carbon dioxide is removed by exhaling. It is, of course, not possible to have normal respiratory exchange of oxygen and carbon dioxide in the lungs unless the pulmonary tissue is adequately perfused with blood. There are various abnormal forms of respiration: jerking, spasmodic, stertorous, stridulous, whistling, wavy, lack of evenness, abdominal, and thoracic. SEE: *lung; ventilation; diaphragm* for illus.

SOUNDS: *Friction:* These are produced by the rubbing together of roughened pleural surfaces; may be heard both in inspiration and expiration. Often resemble subcrepitant rales, but are more superficial and localized than the latter, and are not modified by cough or deep inspiration.

Metallic tinkling: Silvery bell-like sounds heard at intervals over a hydropneumothorax or large cavity. Speaking, coughing, and deep breathing usually induce them. Must not be confounded with similar sound produced by liquids in the stomach.

Rales: Abnormal bubbling sounds heard in air cells or bronchial tubes.

Succussion-splash or hippocratic succussion: A splashing sound produced by the presence of air and liquid in the chest, may be elicited by gently shaking the patient while auscultating. Nearly always indicates either a hydropneumothorax or a pyopneumothorax, although it has been detected over very large cavities. Air and liquid in stomach produce similar sounds.

AUSCULTATION: *Normal breath sounds:* In the normal person, breath sounds are low-pitched and have a frequency of 200 to 400 cycles per second (cps) and rarely greater than 500 cps. These are produced by air passing in and out of the alveoli, and are called vesicular breath sounds.

Bronchial and tracheal breath sounds: These are produced by the air passing over the walls of the bronchi and trachea. These sounds are normally heard only over the bronchi and trachea. The vesicular sounds

Rate of Respiration

Premature infant	.40–90/min
Newborn	30–80/min
1st year	20–40/min
2nd year	20–30/min
5th year	20–25/min
15th year	15–20/min
Adult	15–20/min

are heard over most of the lungs. These sounds are high-pitched and loud compared to vesicular sounds. Normally the inspiratory phase of respiration lasts longer than the expiratory.

Amphoric and cavernous breathing: These two are almost identical. Sounds are loud and the expiration is prolonged and hollow. Pitch of amphoric breathing is a little higher than cavernous type. May be imitated by blowing over the mouth of an empty jar. Heard in bronchiectatic cavities or pneumothorax when the opening to the lung is patulous; in the area of consolidation near a large bronchus; sometimes over a lung compressed by a moderate effusion.

METHOD OF COUNTING: With the hand in the same position as when taking the pulse, watch the patient's chest, without his or her knowledge if possible, because breathing is controlled by both the voluntary and involuntary muscles. Count each inspiration and expiration as one breath. Observe for one full minute by watching rise and fall of chest or upper abdomen. When the movements are scarcely perceptible, place the hand gently but firmly on chest or back and count in this manner. Note hour, frequency, and any abnormal condition, such as pain associated with breathing. SEE: table.

Total lung capacity (TLC): In normal adult males, depending upon their size, TLC range is 3.6 to 9.4 liters; in females, 2.5 to 6.9 liters.

    r., abdominal. Respiration in which chiefly the diaphragm exerts itself, while walls of chest are nearly at rest. Utilized in normal, quiet breathing, esp. by males, and in pathological conditions as in pleurisy, pericarditis, and fracture of ribs. SYN: *r., diaphragmatic.*

    r., absent. Respiration in which respiratory sounds are suppressed.

    r., accelerated. Respiration occurring at a rate that is faster than normal. Considered accelerated when it exceeds 25 per minute in the adult. Increased frequency may result from exercise, physical exertion, exposure to high altitudes, or mental disturbances, and frequently occurs in disease. It is present in many disorders of the lungs, such as pneumonia, bronchiectasis, advanced pulmonary tuberculosis, consolidation or compression of a lobe or of the entire lung, congestion, asthma, emphysema, abscess, tumors, aneurysms, diseases of the chest wall, hernia of the diaphragm, and partial obstruction to the entrance of air into the lungs. It may be seen in diseases of the blood, such as the anemias; in kidney disease; febrile disease; diseases of the heart; and as a result of drugs or nervous conditions such as anxiety, panic, and hysteria.

r., aerobic. Respiration in which air or free oxygen is utilized.

r., amphoric. Respiration having amphoric resonance. SEE: *resonance, amphoric.*

r., anaerobic. Respiration in which oxygen is obtained from chemical reactions not involving the liberation of free oxygen.

r., apneustic. Breathing characterized by prolonged inspiration unrelieved by attempts to exhale. Seen in patients who have had the upper part of the pons of the brain removed or damaged.

r., artificial. Artificial methods to restore respiration in cases of suspended breathing. For specific methods, SEE: *artificial respiration; cardiopulmonary resuscitation.*

r., Biot's. Breathing with irregularly alternating periods of apnea and hyperpnea. Occurs in meningitis and disorders of the brain that cause increased intracranial pressure.

r., cell. The combination of oxygen with various substances within cells resulting in formation of CO_2 and H_2O and release of energy. There are many intermediary reactions in which substances other than oxygen act as oxidizing agents, i.e., hydrogen or electron acceptors. Reactions are catalyzed by respiratory enzymes, which include the flavoproteins, cytochromes, and other enzymes. Certain vitamins (nicotinamide, riboflavin, thiamine, pyridoxine, and pantothenic acid) are essential in the formation of components of various intracellular enzyme systems.

r., Cheyne-Stokes. A common, usually abnormal, and bizarre breathing pattern characterized by a period of apnea lasting 10 to 60 seconds, followed by gradually increasing and then decreasing respirations. It accompanies depression of frontal lobe and diencephalic dysfunction. Postulated to be due to an abnormality in the respiratory center. May be normal in the elderly and present in premature infants. SEE: illus.

r., cogwheel. R., interrupted.

GRAPH OF RESPIRATORY MOVEMENTS IN CHEYNE-STOKES BREATHING

r., costal. Respiration in which the chest cavity is enlarged by raising the ribs.

r., decreased. Occurs in uremia, diabetic coma, most conditions that cause increased intracranial pressure, shock, hysteria, stenosis of the larynx, poisoning with opium or its derivatives, and approaching death.

r., diaphragmatic. R., abdominal.

r., direct. Respiration in which an organism, such as a one-celled ameba, secures its oxygen and gives up carbon dioxide directly to the surrounding medium.

r., electrophrenic. Application of intermittent electrical stimuli to cutaneous electrodes over the phrenic nerves in the neck to stimulate respiration rhythmically. Used in patients whose respiratory center has been damaged. SEE: *radiofrequency electrophrenic respiration.*

r., external. The processes involved in ventilating the lungs (breathing) and the exchange of gases (O_2 and CO_2) between the air in lungs and the blood within capillaries in the walls of alveoli.

Inspiration or drawing in of air is accomplished by expansion of the thoracic cavity. This is brought about by contraction of the diaphragm and raising the ribs and sternum. Expiration or the expulsion of air may be active or passive. In ordinary breathing it is passive, no muscular effort being needed to bring the chest wall back to normal position. In forced or labored respiration, muscular effort is involved.

If the aspiration of air is accomplished chiefly by contraction of the diaphragm, the abdomen will bulge with each inspiration because the diaphragm, forming at once the floor of the thorax and the roof of the abdominal cavity, is dome-shaped with its concavity downward. In contracting, it pushes the abdominal viscera down. This type of respiration is called diaphragmatic or abdominal. Its opposite is the thoracic type, in which the ribs and sternum must be raised. It is seen when the abdomen is confined by tight clothing.

r., fetal. Exchange of gases in the placenta between blood of fetus and maternal blood. SYN: *r., placental.*

r., forced. Voluntary hyperpnea (increase in rate and depth of breathing).

r., internal. The passage of oxygen from the blood into the cells, its utilization by the cells, and the passage of carbon dioxide from cells into the blood. Oxygen is carried in combination with hemoglobin. Oxyhemoglobin gives arterial blood its red color; reduced hemoglobin gives venous blood its dark red color. Carbon dioxide is carried in combination with metallic elements in the blood as bicarbonates and also as carbonic acid. Normally the partial pressure of oxygen in the blood is 75 to 100 mmHg, depending upon age; and for CO_2 it is 35 to 45 mm. SEE: *r., cell.*

r., interrupted. Respiration in which inspiratory or expiratory sounds are not continuous. SYN: *r., cogwheel.*

r., intrauterine. Respiration by fetus before birth. SEE: *r., fetal.*

r., Kussmaul's. Deep, gasping respiration characteristic of air hunger or diabetic coma.

r., labored. Dyspnea or difficult breathing; respiration that involves active participation of accessory inspiratory and expiratory muscles.

r., muscles of. *Inspiration:* diaphragm and external intercostals. *Forced inspiration:* (assist in elevating ribs and sternum) scaleni, levatores costorum, sternocleidomastoideus, pectoralis major, platysma myoides, and serratus posterior superior. *Expiration:* (voluntary deep breathing or forced expiration) rectus abdominis, external and internal oblique, transverse abdominis. SEE: *diaphragm; expiration; inspiration.*

The following accessory muscles may assist in depressing the ribs: internal intercostals, serratus posterior inferior, quadratus lumborum.

r., paradoxical. 1. A type of respiratory activity seen in pneumothorax. The affected side bulges out on expiration and caves in on inspiration. 2. Condition seen in paralysis of diaphragm in which diaphragm ascends during inspiration.

r., periodic. Breathing of uneven rhythm as in Cheyne-Stokes respiration, q.v.

r., placental. R., fetal.

r., slow. Breathing in which there are fewer than 12 respirations each minute. Generally the result of some structural or functional derangement of the nervous sys-

tem. Observed in apoplexy, increased intracranial pressure and hemorrhage, uremia, and in most of the circumstances that occasion coma. It may be induced by carbon monoxide, and opium or its derivatives.

r., stertorous. Respiration characterized by rattling or bubbling sounds.

r., stridulous. A high-pitched crowing or barking sound heard during inspiration caused by an obstruction in vicinity of glottis or in respiratory passageway.

r., thoracic. Respiration performed entirely by expansion of the chest when abdomen does not move. Observed when peritoneum or diaphragm is inflamed, when abdominal cavity is physically restricted by tight bandages or clothes, or during abdominal surgery.

r., tissue. R., internal, q.v.

respiration, words pert. to: air; anapnea; apnea; asphyxia; Biot's breathing; chest; Cheyne-Stokes respiration; diaphragm; dyspnea; eupnea; hyperpnea; hypopnea; infant; inspiration; lung; oligopnea; orthopnea; polypnea; respirator; respiratory; stridor; stridulous; tachypnea; thermometry.

respirator (rĕs′pĭ-rā″tor) [L. *respirare,* to breathe]. A machine for prolonged artificial respiration. Mechanical methods of assisting respiration usually include the capability of producing either intermittent or continuous positive pressure in the lungs. SEE: *Drinker respirator; ventilation, continuous positive-pressure; ventilation, intermittent positive-pressure.*

respiratory (rĕs-pīr′ă-tō-rē, rĕs′pĭ-ră-tō″rē) [L. *respiratio,* breathing]. Pert. to respiration.

respiratory anemometer. A form of respirometer used in investigating pulmonary function. The passage of air through the mask or mouthpiece drives a vane so that it rotates. This motion is recorded by use of a clockwise mechanism that permits measurement of the amount of air passed through the system.

respiratory arrest. Cessation of spontaneous respirations.

respiratory center. A region in the medulla oblongata of the brain stem that regulates movements of respiration. Consists of an inspiratory center, located in the rostral half of the reticular formation overlying the olivary nuclei, and an expiratory center, located dorsal to the inspiratory center. A pneumotaxic center, located in the pons, also is concerned with respiratory movements.

respiratory defense function. In addition to providing for the exchange of oxygen and carbon dioxide with the blood, the respiratory tract has other important functions such as: warming and humidifying the inspired air; providing the mucous secretions for protection of the epithelium of the airway; ciliated cells, each of which contains about 275 cilia that beat 1000 times a minute for moving the mucus toward the pharynx at the rate of 10 mm/minute in the trachea. Also, the lungs filter out inspired particles and the macrophages present in the alveolar and interstitial spaces can engulf and lyse inhaled bacteria. SEE: *lung; lung function.*

respiratory distress syndrome of the premature infant. ABBR: RDS. Severe impairment of the function of respiration in the premature newborn. This condition is rarely present in a newborn of greater than 37 weeks' gestation or in one weighing at least 2.2 kg (5 lb). RDS is the leading cause of death in prematurely born infants in the U.S. SYN: *hyaline membrane disease.* SEE: *adult respiratory distress syndrome.* SEE: *Nursing Diagnoses* in *Appendix.*

SYM: Shortly after birth the premature infant will have a low Apgar score, q.v., and develop signs of acute respiratory distress due to atelectasis of the lung, impaired blood perfusion of the lung, and reduced pulmonary compliance; tachypnea, tachycardia, retraction of the rib cage during inspiration, cyanosis, and grunting during expiration will be present. In addition to these symptoms, the blood gas studies will reflect the impaired ventilatory function; and x-ray of the lung will be typical for generalized atelectasis.

ETIOL: Delivery of an infant prior to maturation of the enzymatic system essential to the production of pulmonary surfactant.

TREAT: Premature infants with RDS require treatment in a specially staffed and equipped neonatal intensive care unit. Supportive therapy to assure adequate hydration and control of electrolytes. Every attempt should be made to reduce oxygen requirements by reducing fever if present and minimizing activity. Supplemental oxygen is used; and, if necessary, assisted ventilation is employed with great care to prevent the traumatic formation of pulmonary air leaks that could cause pulmonary emphysema and tension pneumothorax.

respiratory failure, acute. The clinical condition in which there is a marked drop in the patient's arterial oxygen concentration and an increase in the carbon dioxide concentration. In all cases, the diagnosis is made by comparing the previous "normal" base line for the blood gas values with those present in the acute situation. A drop in Pao_2 of 10 to 15 mmHg or more indicates acute failure. With respect to $Paco_2$, an acute rise in the arterial pH in the absence of metabolic acidemia to 7.3 or greater is diagnostic of hypercapnia and acute respiratory failure.

TREAT: If condition is due to obstruction, remove the cause. If condition is due to impaired gas exchange, positive-pressure ventilation is indicated. If the combination of ventilation and perfusion of the lung does not maintain the arterial oxygen concentration (Pao_2) of 50 to 55 mmHg or greater, supplemental oxygen will be required.

respiratory failure, chronic. Any disease process that interferes with ventilation and perfusion of the lungs will cause pulmonary insufficiency. The degree will depend on the severity and duration of the disease process. A great number of diseases can cause chronic pulmonary insufficiency. Examples are: airway obstruction due to asthma, emphysema, chronic bronchitis, or cystic fibrosis; chronic diseases of the pulmonary interstitial tissue such as sarcoidosis, pneumoconiosis, idiopathic pulmonary fibrosis, disseminated carcinoma, radiation sickness, and leukemia.

respiratory function monitoring. Use of various techniques to provide alarms that alert the patient's attendants to a change in the ability of the lungs to perform their functions. These include noninvasive devices for measuring the oxygen content of the blood, e.g., pulse oximetry; methods of monitoring respiratory muscle function; breathing pattern; device for monitoring carbon dioxide content of expired air, i.e., capnography. SEE: *apnea monitoring.*

respiratory insufficiency. Inability of the respiratory system to function adequately.

respiratory myoclonus. Leeuwenhoek's disease, q.v.

respiratory quotient. The relation of CO_2 produced and O_2 consumed. SEE: *quotient, respiratory.*

respiratory syncytial virus. A virus that induces formation of syncytial masses in infected cell cultures. It is a major cause of acute respiratory disease in children.

respiratory system. The organs involved in the interchange of gases between an organism and the atmosphere. In the human, it consists of the nose, pharynx, larynx, trachea, bronchi, and lungs. SEE: *lung* for illus.

respiratory therapist. Person who by training and background is qualified to provide respiratory therapy.

respiratory therapy. Treatment to preserve or improve pulmonary function.

respire. To breathe and to consume oxygen and release carbon dioxide.

respirometer (rĕs″pĭr-ŏm′ĕt-ĕr) [L. *respirare,* to breathe, + Gr. *metron,* a measure]. Instrument to ascertain character of respirations. Several devices are available for measuring specific respiratory qualities such as minute and tidal volume. SEE: *respiratory anemometer*.

response [L. *respondere*, to reply]. 1. A reaction, such as contraction of a muscle or secretion of a gland, resulting from a stimulus. SEE: *reaction*. 2. The sum total of reactions of an individual to specific conditions, e.g., the response (favorable or unfavorable) of a patient to a certain treatment or to a challenge to the immune system.

r., anamnestic. The rapid production of an antibody response after the injection of an antigen that had previously produced an immune response in the individual.

r., conditioned. SEE: *reflex, conditioned.*

r., galvanic skin. The measurement of the change in the electrical resistance of the skin in response to emotional stimuli.

r., immune. SEE: *immune response.*

r., inflammatory. A localized protective response elicited by the injury or destruction of tissue. Histologically, it involves the dilatation and increased permeability of small blood vessels, which result in migration and accumulation of leukocytes and exudation of plasma proteins into the area. The result serves to dilute, destroy, or wall off the injurious agent and injured tissue and is characterized by the classic signs of inflammation: pain (dolor), heat (color), redness (rubor), swelling (tumor), and loss of function (functio laesa). SEE: leukotrienes.

r., reticulocyte. The increase in reticulocyte production in response to administration of a hematinic agent.

r., triple. Three phases of vasomotor reactions occurring when a pointed instrument is drawn across the skin. Includes, in order of appearance, red reaction, flare or spreading flush, and wheal.

r., unconditioned. An inherent response rather than one that is learned. SEE: *r., conditioned.*

rest (rĕst) [AS. *raest*]. 1. Repose of body due to sleep. 2. Freedom from activity, as of mind or body. 3. To lie down; to cease voluntary motion. 4. A remnant of embryonic tissue that persists in the adult.

restenosis (rē″stĕ-nō′sĭs) [L. *re*, again, + Gr. *stenos*, narrow]. The recurrence of a stenosis condition as in a heart valve or vessel.

restiform (rĕs′tĭ-form) [L. *restis*, rope, + *forma*, shape]. Ropelike; rope-shaped.

restiform body. One of the inferior cerebellar peduncles of the brain. They are along the lateral border of the 4th ventricle. The nerve fibers contained in these bodies connect the medulla oblongata and spinal cord with the cerebellum.

resting. Inactive, motionless, at rest.

resting cell. 1. A cell not in the process of dividing. SEE: *interphase.* 2. A cell that is not performing its normal function, i.e., a nerve cell that is not conducting an impulse or a muscle cell that is not contracting.

resting pan splint. Splint designed to position fingers and stabilize hand in a functional position with the fingers held in opposition. Also called *resting hand splint.*

resting potential. The potential difference that exists across a cell membrane between the outside and the inside of a resting cell.

restitution ad integrum (rĕs″tĭ-tū′shē-ō ăd ĭn-tē′grŭm) [L.]. Complete restoration to health.

restitution (rĕs″tĭ-tū′shŭn) [L. *restitutio*]. 1. A return to a former status. 2. The act of making amends. 3. The turning of a fetal head to the right or left after it has completely emerged through the vagina.

restless legs syndrome. A condition of unknown etiology characterized by an intolerable creeping and internal itching sensation occurring in the lower extremities and causing an almost irresistible urge to move the legs. Symptoms are worse at the end of the day when patient is either seated or in bed. This symptom is sometimes associated with the onset of renal colic due to the attempt to pass or actual passage of a renal stone, and is sometimes seen as a side effect of psychotropic drugs. About 10% of pregnant women and 25% of people with iron-deficiency anemia will experience this condition. Also, the condition may be associated with intake of caffeine.

TREAT: Stop caffeine; clonazine or diazepam may be of benefit. SYN: *Ekbom's syndrome.*

restoration (rĕs″tō-rā′shŭn) [L. *restaurare*, to fix]. 1. To return anything to its previous state. 2. In dentistry, any treatment, material, or device that restores a tooth surface, or replaces a tooth or all of the teeth and adjacent tissues.

r., temporary. The use of zinc oxide and eugenol or some plastic material to provide a temporary filling of a tooth cavity.

restorative (rĭ-stor′ă-tĭv) [L. *restaurare*, to fix]. 1. Pert. to restoration. 2. An agent that is effective in the regaining of health and strength.

restraint (rĭ-strānt′) [O. Fr. *restrainte*]. 1. The process of refraining from any action, mental or physical. 2. State of being hindered. 3. That which hinders or restricts; device or method used to keep patients from injuring themselves. Various states have laws concerning methods to be used in restraining patients.

NURSING IMPLICATIONS: Use minimal restraint required to protect patient from injury (or from injuring others), obtaining physician's order prescribing specific restraints to be applied. Explain restraint to patient as "reminder" or "protection." Pad bony prominences in contact with restraining device, and secure snugly (to prevent escape) but not enough to interfere with blood flow to limb or trunk. Limit mobility only as much as is necessary to protect patient. Example: Applications of loose padded mitt may protect against removal of intravenous or other invasive tubing by limiting patient's ability to manipulate equipment with fingers and not cause the increase in restlessness and frustration that would occur if the patient's hands were tied down. Tie restraint to movable part of bed frame (but not to siderail) or to frame of chair, using a simple knot (half bow) that is easily untied when necessary. Assess patient and restraints every hour, and assess rationale for continued use. Examine neurovascular status distal to restraint. Remove restraints (one at a time only, if patient is unreliable) and assess skin under restraint and carry out range-of-motion exercise for joints that have been restricted. Document application of restraints and rationale, along with status of tissues affected by restraint prior to application. Also document interval assessment evaluations of patient and restraint sites, and measures taken to prevent problems. Periodically reevaluate need for continued restraint, reducing or discontinuing it as soon as patient's status permits.

r. in bed. If a proper bed is not available, the following may be used as a makeshift alternative. Move bed against wall, place straight-backed chairs along open side of bed. Tie them into place by interlacing with rope and then tying to foot and head of bed, or place a wide board the length of bed on either side and fasten through three or four holes bored near ends of the boards. Fold sheet lengthwise to width of one foot. Place under patient's back and cross in front below armpits. At sides secure hem ends to side bar or springs of bed. This allows some freedom for turning from side to side. The hands and feet may be restrained by a clove hitch of wide bandage around wrists and ankles and tied to side or foot of bed.

r., mechanical. Restraint by physical devices, esp. restraint of insane.

r., medicinal. Restraint of violent mentally ill patients through use of narcotics or sedatives.

r. of lower extremities. Tie a sheet across knees and tie feet together with a figure-of-eight bandage. Start loop under

ankles, cross between feet, bring ends around feet, and tie on top.

Caution: Restraint should not interfere with the circulation of blood to any extremity.

resuscitation (rĭ-sŭs″ĭ-tā′shŭn) [L. *resuscitatio*]. Revival after apparent death. SYN: *anabiosis.* SEE: *artificial respiration.*

r., cardiopulmonary. SEE: *cardiopulmonary resuscitation.*

r., heart-lung. SEE: *cardiopulmonary resuscitation.*

r., mouth-to-mouth. SEE: *cardiopulmonary resuscitation.*

r., oral. SEE: *artificial respiration.*

resuscitator (rĭ-sŭs′ĭ-tā″tor) [L. *resuscitare,* to revive]. An automatic breathing-assist machine that forces oxygen into the lungs under pressure of 4 oz per sq in. (1.4 mm Hg) when back pressure of 3 oz (about 1 mm Hg) trips the machine for exhalation.

r., manual. A device, usually a hand-held mask with bag attached, that permits air to be forced into the lungs each time it is squeezed. A patent airway is essential. The goal is to deliver at least 800 cc of air every 5 seconds. The device may or may not have provisions for adding supplemental oxygen to the bag.

ret. *roentgen equivalent therapy.* It is analogous to rem, q.v., used in describing radiation protection or exposure.

retainer (rĭ-tān′ĕr). 1. Any device or attachment for retaining or keeping something in place. 2. In dentistry, a device used in orthodontia for maintaining the teeth and jaws in position.

retardate (rĭ-tăr′dāt) [L. *retardare,* to delay]. One who is mentally retarded.

retardation (rē″tăr-dā′shŭn) [L. *retardare,* to delay]. 1. A holding back or slowing down; delay. 2. Delayed mental or physical response due to pathological conditions. SEE: *mental retardation.*

r., mental. SEE: *mental retardation.*

retarder. A substance used in dentistry to slow the hardening of a material.

retch (rĕch) [AS. *hraecan,* to cough up phlegm]. To make an involuntary attempt to vomit, q.v.

retching (rĕch′ĭng). Involuntary attempt to vomit.

rete (rē′tē) [L.] (pl. *retia*). [NA] A network. A plexus of nerves or blood vessels.

r., arterial; r. arteriosum. A vascular, arterial network just prior to the point where arteries become capillaries.

r., articular. Rete about a joint, esp. a deep anastomosis at knee joint.

r. cutaneum. A network of blood vessels at junction of the corium and superficial fascia.

r., malpighian. Stratum germinativum, q.v.

r. mirabile. [NA] A plexus formed by sudden division of a vessel into small twigs that unite again to form one vessel, as in the glomeruli of the kidneys.

r. olecrani. A network of vessels at back of elbow formed by divisions of the recurrent ulnar arteries.

r. ovarii. A layer of cells lying in the broad ligament and mesovarium of the ovary. They are homologous to rete testes in males.

r. patellae. [NA] A superficial network of vessels lying about the patella. Formed by branches of genicular arteries.

r. subpapillare. A network of vessels between papillary and reticular layers of the dermis.

r. testis. [NA] A network of tubules in mediastinum testis that receives sperm through the tubuli recti from the seminiferous tubules. From the rete testis, efferent ducts convey sperm to the epididymis.

r. venosum. Venous network.

r., vertebral. Two plexuses within the vertebral canal that extend from the foramen magnum to the coccyx. They lie posteriorly and laterally to the dura and between the dura and arches of the vertebrae.

retention (rĭ-těn'shŭn) [L. *retentio,* a holding back]. 1. The act or process of keeping in possession or of holding in place or position. 2. The persistent keeping within the body those materials normally excreted, such as urine, feces, or perspiration. 3. In dentistry, any of several procedures or materials used to keep a dental device or dentures in place.

retention cyst. Cyst caused by retention of a secretion in a gland, due to closure of the gland's duct.

retention defect. Inability to recall a name, number, or fact shortly after the subject was requested to remember it.

retention enema. Enema to be retained to provide nourishment, medicate the mucosa, or act as anesthetic. SEE: *enema.*

retention of urine. Inability to empty bladder. This may be due to a number of causes, such as loss of muscle tone of the bladder from anemia, old age, exposure to cold, or prolonged operation; lesions involving nervous pathways to and from the bladder; lesions involving reflex centers in brain and spinal cord; obstruction of the urethra, which may result from inflammation, stricture, stones, diverticula, cysts, tumors, or pressure from the outside as in cases of hypertrophy of the prostate; psychogenic factors; and medication such as morphine or certain antihistamines.

retention with overflow. Spasm of sphincter, causing failure to empty the bladder at one voiding, with only overflow dribbling away; due to same causes as urine retention.

rete ridges. The irregular internal surface of the epidermis in which downgrowths of epithelium surround the connective tissue papillae. Microscopic sections often appear as single downgrowths when in fact the epithelium is in a series of interconnecting ridges at the dermis/epidermis interface. SEE: *peg, rete.*

retia (rē'tē-ă) [L.]. Pl. of rete.

retial (rē'tē-ăl). Concerning a rete.

reticula (rē-tĭk'ū-lă) [L.]. Pl. of reticulum.

reticular (rĭ-tĭk'ū-lăr) [L. *reticula,* net]. Meshed, or in the form of a network.

reticular activating system. ABBR: RAS. The alerting system of the brain consisting of the reticular formation, subthalamus, hypothalamus, and medial thalamus. It extends from central core of the brain stem to all parts of the cerebral cortex. This system is essential in initiating and maintaining wakefulness and introspection, and in directing attention. Some of the tranquilizing drugs act to depress this system.

reticular cells. 1. Phagocytic cells present in lymphatic and myeloid tissues. 2. The cells of reticular connective tissue. SEE: *reticular tissue.*

reticular fibers. Extremely fine argyrophilic (i.e., silver-staining) fibers found in reticular tissue, q.v.

reticular formation. Groups of cells and fibers arranged in a diffuse network throughout the brain stem. These both fill the spaces and connect the tracts that ascend and descend through the area. They are important in controlling or influencing alertness, waking, sleeping, and various reflexes.

reticular layer. Layer of connective tissue forming deeper portion of dermis. Lies beneath papillary layer.

reticular membrane. Membrane formed by cuticular plates of distal ends of supporting cells in the organ of Corti of the ear.

reticular tissue. A form of connective tissue consisting of a network of reticular fibers and cells. Cells are stellate with protoplasmic processes anastomosing with adjacent cells. Protoplasm also encloses and extends along the fibers. Found principally in bone marrow and lymphatic organs (lymph nodes). Also found in various organs (liver, kidney), in tissue underlying mucous membranes, and in walls of blood vessels.

reticulate (rē-tĭk'ū-lāt). Of the nature of a network.

reticulated (rē-tĭk'ū-lā″těd) [L. *reticula,* net]. Netlike; pert. to a reticulum.

reticulate substance. Reticular formation.

reticulation (rē-tĭk″ū-lā′shŭn). The formation of a network mass.

reticulin (rē-tĭk′ū-lĭn) [L. *reticula*, net]. An albuminoid or scleroprotein substance in the connective tissue framework of reticular tissue.

reticulo-. Combining form concerning a reticulum.

reticulocyte (rē-tĭk′ū-lō-sīt) [″ + Gr. *kytos*, cell]. A red blood cell containing a network of granules or filaments representing an immature stage in development. Normally constitutes about 1% of circulating red blood cells.

reticulocytopenia (rē-tĭk″ū-lō-sī″tō-pē′nē-ă) [″ + ″ + *penia*, poverty]. Lowering of the number of the reticulocytes of the blood.

reticulocytosis (rē-tĭk″ū-lō-sī-tō′sĭs) [″ + ″ + *osis*, condition]. Increase in number of reticulocytes in circulating blood. Indicative of active erythropoiesis in red bone marrow. Occurs after hemorrhage, during acclimatization to high altitude, and following treatment for pernicious anemia.

reticuloendothelial (rē-tĭk″ū-lō-ĕn″dō-thē′lē-ăl) [″ + Gr. *endon*, within, + *thele*, nipple]. Pert. to the reticuloendothelial system.

reticuloendothelial cell. A phagocytic cell of the reticuloendothelial system. SYN: *histiocyte; macrophage.*

reticuloendothelial system. ABBR: RES. Term applied to the system on mononuclear phagocytes (monocytes and macrophages) located in the reticular connective tissue, q.v., of the body. These cells are responsible for phagocytosis of damaged or old cells, cellular debris, foreign substances, and pathogens, removing them from the circulation. Found in large concentrations in the spleen, liver (Kupffer's cells), lymph nodes, and alveoli, as well as other tissues such as the brain, blood vessels, and mucous membranes, they play a major role in the nonspecific immune response.

reticuloendothelioma (rē-tĭk″ū-lō-ĕn″dō-thē-lē-ō′mă) [″ + ″ + ″ + *oma*, tumor]. A neoplasm composed of reticuloendothelial tissue.

reticuloendotheliosis (rē-tĭk″ū-lō-ĕn″dō-thē-lē-ō′sĭs) [″ + ″ + *thele*, nipple, + *osis*, condition]. Hyperplasia of reticuloendothelium.

reticuloendothelium (rē-tĭk″ū-lō-ĕn″dō-thē′lē-ŭm). Tissue of the reticuloendothelial system, q.v. SEE: *reticuloendothelial system.*

reticulohistiocytoma (rē-tĭk″ū-lō-hĭs″tē-ō-sī-tō′mă) [L. *reticula*, net, + Gr. *histion*, little web, + *kytos*, cell, + *oma*, tumor]. A giant cell granulomacytosis involving the skin, mucous membranes, and synovial membranes of the long bones.

reticulohistiocytosis (rē-tĭk″ū-lō-hĭs″tē-ō-sī-tō′sĭs) [″ + ″ + *osis*, condition]. Reticuloendotheliosis, q.v.

reticuloid (rē-tĭk′ū-loyd) [″ + Gr. *eidos*, form, shape]. Resembling reticulosis.

reticuloma (rē-tĭk″ū-lō′mă) [″ + Gr. *oma*, tumor]. Neoplasm composed of reticuloendothelial cells.

reticulopenia (rē-tĭk″ū-lō-pē′nē-ă) [″ + Gr. *penia*, lack]. Decreased number of reticulocytes in the blood.

reticulopodium (rē-tĭk″ū-lō-pō′dē-ŭm). Rhizopodium, q.v.

reticulosarcoma (rē-tĭk″ū-lō-săr-kō′mă) [″ + Gr. *sarx*, flesh, + *oma*, tumor]. A neoplasm composed of large monocytic cells that originated in the reticuloendothelium of the lymph and other glands.

reticulosis (rē-tĭk-ū-lō′sĭs) [″ + Gr. *osis*, condition]. Reticulocytosis.

    r., familial histiocytic. A severe and fatal type of lymphoma characterized by anemia; granulocytopenia; enlargement of the spleen, liver, and the lymph nodes; and phagocytosis of red blood cells.

reticulum (rē-tĭk′ū-lŭm) [L., a little net] (pl. *reticula*). A network.

    r., endoplasmic. SEE: *endoplasmic reticulum.*

    r. of nucleus. A fine network of linin threads on which are arranged masses of chromatin.

    r., sarcoplasmic. The network of fine tubules, similar to endoplasmic reticulum, present in muscle tissues.

    r., stellate. The enamel pulp of a developing tooth, consisting of stellate cells lying between inner and outer epithelial layers of the enamel organ.

retiform (rĕt′ĭ-form) [L. *rete*, net, + *forma*, shape]. Resembling a network. SYN: *reticular.*

Retin-A. Trade name for tretinoin, USP.

retina (rĕt′ĭ-nă) [L.] (pl. *retinae*). [NA] Innermost layer of the eye, which receives image transmitted through the lens and is the immediate instrument of vision. SEE: illus.

    The retina is a light-sensitive structure upon which light rays come to a focus. It extends from the point of entrance of the optic nerve anteriorly to the margin of the pupil, completely lining the interior of the eye. It consists of three parts: pars optica, the nervous or sensory portion extending from the optic disk forward to the ora serrata, a wavy line immediately behind the ciliary process; pars ciliaris, the part lining the inner surface of the ciliary process; and pars iridica, the part forming the posterior surface of the

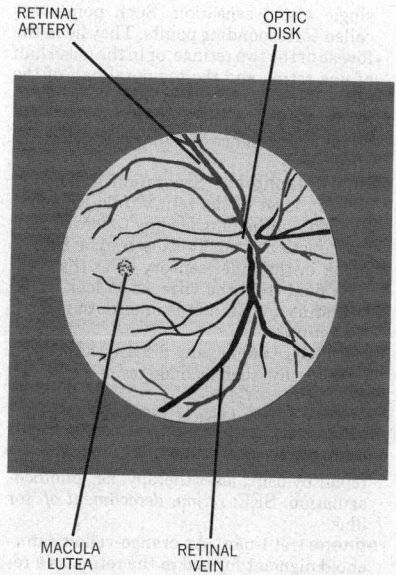

RETINAL ARTERY

OPTIC DISK

MACULA LUTEA

RETINAL VEIN

RETINA OF RIGHT EYE

iris. Slightly lateral to the posterior pole of the eye is a small, oval, yellowish spot, the macula lutea, in the center of which is a depression, the fovea centralis. This region contains only cones and is the region of most acute vision. About 3.5 mm nasally from the fovea is the optic papilla (optic disk), the point at which nerve fibers from the retina make their exit and form the optic nerve. This region is devoid of rods and cones and is insensitive to light, hence named the blind spot.

The retina, from without inward, consists of a layer of pigment epithelium, layer of rods and cones, external limiting membrane, external nuclear layer, external plexiform layer, internal nuclear layer, internal plexiform layer, layer of ganglion cells, layer of nerve fibers, and internal limiting membrane.

COLOR: Normally a purple-red tint, varying with complexion. It is colorless in severe anemia or in ischemia, and is reddened in hyperemia.

VESSELS: The arteries shown in the illustration are branches of a single central artery, a branch of the ophthalmic artery. The central artery enters at the center of the optic papilla, and it supplies the inner layers of retina. The outer layers, including rods and cones, are nourished by capillaries of

the choroid layer. The veins lack muscular coats. They parallel the arteries, blood leaving by a central vein that leads to the superior ophthalmic vein.

    r., coarctate. Condition in which there is an effusion of fluid between the retina and choroid, giving the retina a funnel shape.

    r., detachment of. Complete or partial separation of the retina from the choroid. May follow trauma, choroidal hemorrhages, or tumors. May also be associated with diabetes mellitus. SEE: illus. SEE: *Nursing Diagnoses in Appendix.*

    r., shot-silk. Retina having an opalescent appearance, sometimes seen in young persons.

    r., tigroid. Retina having a spotted or striped appearance seen in retinitis pigmentosa.

retinaculum (rĕt″ĭ-năk′ū-lŭm) [L., halter] (pl. *retinacula*). [NA] A band or membrane holding any organ or part in its place. Thickenings of the deep fascia in distal portions of limbs that hold tendons in position when muscles contract, called retinaculum tendinum.

    r. cutis. [NA] A fibrous band connecting the corium with underlying fascia.

    r., extensor, of ankle. 1. The superior extensor retinaculum, a band that crosses the

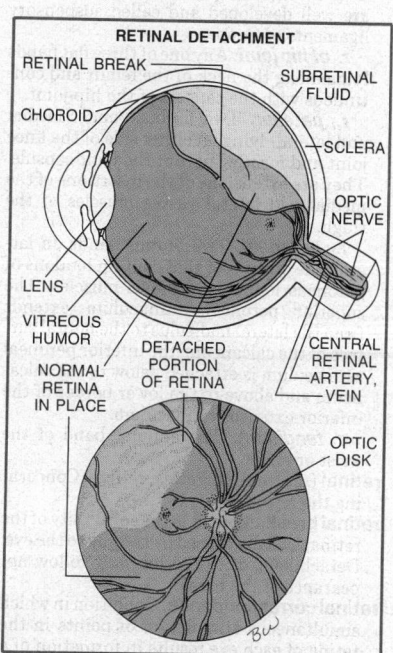

RETINAL DETACHMENT

RETINAL BREAK

SUBRETINAL FLUID

CHOROID

SCLERA

OPTIC NERVE

LENS

VITREOUS HUMOR

NORMAL RETINA IN PLACE

DETACHED PORTION OF RETINA

CENTRAL RETINAL ARTERY, VEIN

OPTIC DISK

extensor tendons of the foot and is attached to the lower portion of the tibia and fibula. 2. The inferior extensor retinaculum, a band located on dorsum of foot. Consists of two limbs having common origin on the lateral surface of the calcaneum. The upper limb is attached to the medial malleolus; the lower limb curves around the instep and is attached to the fascia of the abductor hallucis on the medial side of the foot.

    r., extensor, of wrist. An oblique band attached medially to the styloid process of the ulna, hammate bone, and medial ligament of the wrist joint. Laterally it is attached to the anterior border of the radius. Contains six separate compartments for passage of extensor tendons to hand.

    r., flexor, of ankle. Retinaculum extending from the medial malleolus to the medial tubercle of the calcaneum.

    r., flexor, of hand. The fascial band that holds down the flexor tendons of the digits.

    r., flexor, of wrist. Retinaculum extending from the trapezium and scaphoid bones laterally to the hammate and pisiform bones medially.

    r. mammae. Strands of connective tissue in the mammary gland extending from glandular tissue through fat toward the skin, where they are attached to deep fascia. Over the cephalic portion of mammae, they are well developed and called suspensory ligaments of Cooper.

    r. of hip joint. Any one of three flat bands lying along the neck of the femur and continuous with the capsule of the hip joint.

    r., patellar. Two fibrous bands (medial and lateral) lying on either side of the knee joint and forming part of the joint capsule. They are extensions of the insertions of the medial and lateral vastus muscles of the thigh.

    r., peroneal. Two fibrous bands on lateral side of the foot that contain tendons of peroneus longus and brevis muscles. The superior peroneal retinaculum extends from the lateral malleolus to the lateral surface of the calcaneum; the inferior peroneal retinaculum is attached below to the calcaneum and above to the lower border of the inferior extensor retinaculum.

    r. tendinum. The annular band of the wrist or ankle.

retinal (rĕt′ĭ-năl) [L. *retina*, retina]. Concerning the retina.

retinal break. A break in the continuity of the retina. Usually caused by trauma to the eye. Detachment of the retina may follow appearance of the break.

retinal correspondence. Condition in which simultaneous stimulation of points in the retina of each eye results in formation of a single visual sensation. Such points are called corresponding points. They lie in the foveae of the two retinae, or in the nasal half of one retina and the temporal half of the other. Abnormal correspondence results in double vision (diplopia) and usually is the result of imbalance of ocular muscles. SEE: *strabismus.*

retinal detachment. Separation of the inner sensory layer of the retina from the outer pigment epithelium, leading to loss of retinal function. Usually caused by a hole or break in the inner sensory layer that permits fluid from the vitreous to leak under the retina and lift off the innermost layer of the retina.

    ETIOL: trauma; any disease that causes retinopathy, such as diabetes or sickle cell disease.

    SYM: Blurred vision, flashes of light; vitreous floaters; and loss of visual acuity.

    TREAT: Determine location of holes and repair by using laser therapy, i.e., photocoagulation. SEE: *retina, detachment of,* for illus.

retinene (rĕt′ĭ-nēn). An orange-yellow carotenoid pigment formed in the retina as a result of the action of light on rhodopsin; an aldehyde of vitamin A. In dark adaptation, rhodopsin is regenerated from retinene. SYN: *xanthopsin.*

retinitis (rĕt-ĭ-nī′tĭs) [L. *retina*, retina, + Gr. *itis*, inflammation]. Inflamed condition of the retina.

    SYM: Diminished vision, contractions of fields or scotomata, alteration in size of objects, photophobia.

    TREAT: Absolute rest of eyes, protection from light, treatment of underlying cause.

    r., actinic. Retinitis due to exposure to intense light or other forms of radiant energy.

    r., albuminuric. Retinitis associated with chronic kidney disease and malignant hypertension. General signs of retinitis are present; it is distinguished by white patches in the fundus, esp. surrounding the papilla and in the macular region.

    r., apoplectic. Retinitis associated with hemorrhaging of retinal vessels.

    r., circinate. Retinitis in which there is a circle of white spots about the macula.

    r., circumpapillar. Retinitis in which there is a proliferation of outer layers of retina about the optic disk.

    r., diabetic. Retinitis occurring in diabetes, esp. that of long duration. Characterized by aneurysmal dilatation of blood vessels, hemorrhages, and waxy and cotton-wool exudates.

    r., disciform. Retinitis accompanied by degeneration of retina in region of macula.

r., exogenous purulent. Retinitis following introduction of infectious organisms into eye as a result of perforating wound or ulcer.

r., external exudative. Condition in which large masses of white and yellow crystals occur beneath retina as a result of organization of hemorrhages.

r., exudative. Chronic inflammation of the retina with elevated areas around the optic disk.

r., hemorrhagic. Retinitis with pronounced hemorrhage into the retina.

r., metastatic. Acute purulent retinitis resulting from presence of infective emboli in retinal vessels.

r. of prematurity. SEE: *retrolental fibroplasia.*

r. pigmentosa. A chronic progressive disease that has its onset in early childhood. It is characterized by degeneration of retinal epithelium, esp. rods; atrophy of the optic nerve; and widespread pigmentary changes in the retina. A degenerative condition without inflammation. An early event is defective night vision followed by constricted field of vision.

ETIOL: Unknown, but a hereditary tendency is suspected.

TREAT: No specific therapy, but professional and vocational guidance and genetic counseling can be provided. Family members should be examined to determine if their vision is affected.

r. proliferans. Vascularized masses of connective tissue that project from the retina into the vitreous. End result of recurrent hemorrhage from retina into the vitreous.

r. punctata albescens. A nonprogressive, degenerative, familial disease, characterized by presence of innumerable minute white spots scattered over entire retina, and without pigmentary changes. Usually starts early in life.

r., punctate. Retinitis characterized by numerous white or yellow spots in fundus of eye.

r., solar. Retinitis resulting from exposure of retina to rays of sun. SEE: scotoma, eclipse.

r., stellate. Retinitis characterized by presence of exudates, hemorrhages, blurring of optic disk, and formation of a star-shaped figure about macula.

r., suppurative. Retinitis associated with septicemia due to pyogenic organisms.

r., syphilitic. Retinitis resulting from, or associated with, syphilis. May also involve optic nerve (syphilitic neuroretinitis).

retinoblastoma (rĕt″ĭ-nō-blăs-tō′mă) [L. *retina*, retina, + Gr. *blastos*, germ, + *oma*, tumor]. A malignant glioma of the retina. Occurs in young children and shows a hereditary pattern. Usually unilateral. Initial diagnostic finding is usually a yellow or white light reflex seen at the pupil (cat's eye reflex).

retinochoroid (rĕt″ĭ-nō-kō′royd) [″ + Gr. *chorioeides*, skinlike]. Concerning the retina and the choroid of the eye.

retinochoroiditis (rĕt″ĭ-nō-kō-royd-ī′tĭs) [″ + ″ + *itis*, inflammation]. Inflamed condition of the retina and choroid.

r. juxtapapillaris. Retinochoroiditis close to the optic nerve.

retinocystoma (rĕt″ĭ-nō-sĭs-tō′mă) [″ + Gr. *kysis*, sac, + *oma*, tumor]. Glioma of the retina.

retinodialysis (rĕt″ĭ-nō-dī-ăl′ĭ-sĭs) [″ + Gr. *dialysis*, separation]. Detachment of the retina at its periphery. SYN: *disinsertion.*

retinoic acid. Metabolite of vitamin A used in the treatment of cystic acne.

retinoid (rĕt′ĭ-noyd). 1. [″ + Gr. *eidos*, form, shape] Like the retina. 2. [Gr. *rhetine*, resin, + *eidos*, form, shape] Resembling a resin; resinous.

retinol (rĕt′ĭ-nŏl). A form of vitamin A present in animal tissue.

retinopapillitis (rĕt″ĭ-nō-pă″pĭl-ī′tĭs) [L. *retina*, retina, + *papilla*, nipple, + Gr. *itis*, inflammation]. Inflamed condition of the retina and optic papilla. SYN: *papilloretinitis.*

retinopathy (rĕt″ĭn-ŏp′ă-thē) [″ + Gr. *pathos*, disease, suffering]. Any disorder of the retina.

r., arteriosclerotic. Retinopathy accompanying generalized arteriosclerosis and moderate hypertension.

r., circinate. A ring of degenerated white exudative area of the retina around the macula of the eye.

r., diabetic. Retinopathy occurring in diabetics.

r., hypertensive. Retinopathy associated with hypertension, toxemia of pregnancy, or glomerulonephritis.

r., solar. Pathological changes in the retina after looking directly at the sun. Seen frequently following an eclipse of the sun during which an individual looked directly at the sun. SEE: *scotoma, eclipse.*

r., syphilitic. Retinopathy occurring in later stages of syphilis.

retinopexy [″ + Gr. *pexis*, fixation]. In the treatment of retinal detachment, the formation of adhesions between the detached portion and the underlying tissue.

retinoschisis (rĕt″ĭ-nŏs′kĭ-sĭs) [″ + Gr. *schisis*, a splitting]. Splitting of the retina into two layers with cyst formation between the layers.

retinoscope (rĕt′ĭ-nō-skōp) [″ + Gr. *sko-*

pein, to examine]. An instrument used in performing retinoscopy.

retinoscopy (rĕt″ĭn-ŏs′kō-pē). Objective method of determining refractive errors of the eye. The examiner projects light into eyes and judges error of refraction by movement of reflected light rays. SYN: *skiascopy*.

retinosis (rĕt″ĭ-nō′sĭs) [″ + Gr. *osis*, condition]. Any degenerative process of the retina not associated with inflammation.

retire. 1. To discontinue formal employment or work at a specific place or task. In the past, in many industries, educational institutions, and public service, the age of retirement was mandated upon an employee's having attained a specified age. This practice has lost its attractiveness to a large segment of the work force, especially among those who enjoy work. SEE: *recreation*. 2. To go to bed.

retisolution (rĕt″ĭ-sō-lū′shŭn) [L. *rete*, net, + *solutio*, dissolution]. Dissolution of the Golgi structures.

retispersion (rĕt″ĭ-spĕr′zhŭn) [″ + *spersio*, a scattering]. Transference of Golgi structures to periphery of the cell.

retoperithelium (rē″tō-pĕr″ĭ-thē′lē-ŭm) [L. *rete*, net, + Gr. *peri*, around, + *thele*, nipple]. Epithelium covering a reticulum.

retort (rē-tort′) [L. *retortus*, bent back]. A flasklike, long-necked vessel used in distillation.

retothelium (rē″tō-thē′lē-ŭm) [L. *rete*, net, + Gr. *thele*, nipple]. Cellular layers covering reticular tissue. SYN: *reticuloendothelium*.

retract (rĭ-trăkt′) [L. *retractus*]. To draw back.

retractile (rĭ-trăkt′ĭl) [L. *retractilis*]. Capable of being drawn back or in.

retraction (rĭ-trăk′shŭn). A shortening; the act of drawing backward or state of being drawn back.

    r., clot. The shrinking of the clot that forms when blood is allowed to stand. The contraction is due to the fibrin network formed in the clot.

    r., uterine. The process by which muscular fibers of the uterus remain permanently shortened to a small degree following each contraction or labor pain.

retraction ring. A ridge sometimes felt on uterus above the pubes, marking line of separation between upper contractile and lower dilatable segments of the uterus. SEE: *Bandl's ring*.

retractor. 1. Instrument for holding back the margins of a wound. 2. Muscle that draws in any organ or part.

retrad (rē′trăd) [L. *retro*, backward]. Toward the posterior part of the body.

retrain. To instruct a person in a new skill or trade.

retreat (rĭ-trēt′) [ME. *retret*, draw back]. Act of retiring or withdrawing from difficult life situations. May be direct, as in physical flight, or indirect, as in malingering, illness, abnormal preoccupation, and self-deception.

retrenchment [Fr. *retrenchier*, to cut back]. Procedure used in plastic surgery to remove excess tissue.

retrieval (rĭ-trē′văl). In psychology, the process of bringing remembered information back to the conscious level.

retro- [L.]. Prefix meaning backward; back; situated behind.

retroaction (rĕt″rō-ăk′shŭn). Action in a reverse direction.

retroauricular (rĕt″rō-aw-rĭk′ū-lăr) [L. *retro*, behind, + *auricula*, ear]. Behind the auricle or ear.

retrobuccal (rĕt″rō-bŭk′ăl) [L. *retro*, back, +*bucca*, cheek]. Concerning the back part of the mouth or area behind the mouth.

retrobulbar (rĕt″rō-bŭl′băr) [L. *retro*, behind, + Gr. *bulbus*, bulb]. 1. Behind the eyeball. 2. Posterior to the medulla oblongata.

retrocecal (rĕt″rō-sē′kăl) [L. *retro*, back, + *caecum*, cecum]. Back of or pert. to the area posterior to the cecum.

retrocedent (rĕt″rō-sē′dĕnt) [L. *retrocedere*]. Going backward, returning.

retrocervical (rĕt″rō-sĕr′vĭ-kăl) [L. *retro*, back, + *cervix*, neck]. Back of the cervix uteri.

retrocession (rĕt″rō-sĕsh′ŭn) [L. *retrocessio*, going back]. 1. A going back; a relapse. 2. Metastasis of a condition from the surface to an internal organ. 3. An abnormal position of the uterus; backward displacement.

retroclusion (rĕt″rō-kloo′zhŭn) [″ + *claudere*, to close]. A method of stopping arterial bleeding. A needle is placed through the tissues over a severed artery and then turned around and down so that it is passed back through the tissues under the artery. This causes compression of the vessel.

retrocolic (rĕt″rō-kōl′ĭk) [L. *retro*, back, + Gr. *kolon*, colon]. Back of the colon.

retrocollic (rĕt″rō-kōl′ĭk) [″ + *collum*, neck]. Concerning the back of the neck.

retrocollic spasm. Wryneck with spasms affecting posterior muscles of neck.

retrocollis (rĕt″rō-kōl′ĭs). Spasm of posterior muscles of the neck with drawing of the head backward. SEE: *torticollis*.

retrocursive (rĕt″rō-kŭr′sĭv) [L. *retro*, back, + *curro*, to run]. Stepping or turning backward.

retrodeviation (rĕt″rō-dē″vē-ā′shŭn) [″ + *deviare*, to turn aside]. Backward displacement, as of an organ.

retrodisplacement (rĕt″rō-dĭs-plăs′mĕnt) [″

+ Fr. *desplacer,* displace]. Displacement backward of a part.

retroesophageal (rĕt″rō-ē-sŏf″ă-jē′ăl) [L. *retro,* behind, + Gr. *oisophagos,* gullet]. Located behind the esophagus.

retrofilling (rĕt″rō-fĭl′ĭng). Placement of filling material in a root canal by using an opening made in the apex of the tooth.

retroflexed (rĕt′rō-flĕkst″) [L. *retro,* backward, + *flexus,* bent]. Bent backward.

retroflexion (rĕt″rō-flĕk′shŭn). A bending or flexing backward.

retroflexion of uterus. Condition of the womb in which its body is bent backward at an angle with the cervix, whose position usually remains unchanged.

retrogasserian (rĕt″rō-găs-sē′rē-ăn). Referring to the posterior root of the gasserian ganglion.

retrognathia (rĕt″rō-năth′ē-ă) [L. *retro,* back, + Gr. *gnathos,* jaw]. Location of the mandible back of the frontal plane of the maxilla.

retrognathism (rĕt″rō-năth′ĭzm) [″ + Gr. *gnathos,* jaw]. Having retrognathia.

retrograde (rĕt′rō-grād) [L. *retro,* backward, + *gradi,* to step]. Moving backward; degenerating from better to worse state.

retrograde amnesia. Loss of memory for events and situations just preceding the time of patient's illness.

retrograde aortography. Roentgenography of the aorta by injecting a contrast medium into one of its branches, against the direction of blood flow.

retrograde flow. The flow of fluid in a direction opposite to that which is considered normal.

retrograde pyelography. Pyelography in which the radiopaque dye is injected into the kidneys from below, via the ureters.

retrography (rĕt″rŏg′ră-fē) [″ + Gr. *graphein,* to write]. Mirror writing, a symptom of certain brain diseases. Also may be present in persons with dyslexia.

retrogression (rĕt″rō-grĕsh′ŭn) [L. *retrogressus,* go backward]. A going backward as in the involution, degeneration, or atrophy of a tissue or structure.

retroinfection (rĕt″rō-ĭn-fĕk′shŭn) [L. *retro,* backward, + *infectio,* infection]. Infection communicated by the fetus in utero to the mother.

retroinsular (rĕt″rō-ĭn′sū-lăr) [″ + *insula,* island]. Situated behind the island of Reil in the brain.

retroiridian (rĕt″rō-ĭ-rĭd′ē-ăn) [L. *retro,* behind, + Gr. *iridos,* colored circle]. Posterior to the iris.

retrojection (rĕt″rō-jĕk′shŭn) [″ + *jacio,* throw]. Washing out a cavity from within by injection of a fluid.

retrolabyrinthine (rĕt″rō-lăb″ĭ-rĭn′thĭn) [L. *retro,* behind + Gr. *labyrinthos,* a maze]. Situated behind the labyrinth of the ear.

retrolental. Behind the crystalline lens.

retrolental fibroplasia. ABBR: RLF. A bilateral disease of the retinal vessels present in premature infants, some of whom were exposed to high postnatal oxygen concentrations. High oxygen concentration used in treating premature infants, esp. those weighing less than 1500 grams, causes vasoconstriction of the immature retinal vessels and eventually occlusion of the vessels. This may be followed by fibrous proliferation and invasion of the vitreous. Retinal detachment may occur at that time or many years later. Blindness develops within several weeks. Other factors can have an important role in the pathogenesis of RLF. Apnea, asphyxia, sepsis, nutritional deficiencies, and a large number of blood transfusions given over a short period of time have all been related to RLF.

In treating premature infants, it is possible to prevent RLF by using only the lowest possible effective oxygen concentration without endangering the life of the infant. Too severe restriction of oxygen will increase the likelihood of hyaline membrane disease and neurologic disorders. All premature infants treated with supplemental oxygen should have careful examination by an ophthalmologist prior to discharge from the hospital. Once blindness develops, there is no effective treatment. SYN: *retinopathy of prematurity.*

retrolenticular (rĕt″rō-lĕn-tĭk′ū-lăr) [″ + *lenticularis,* pert. to a lens]. Retrolental, q.v.

retrolingual (rĕt″rō-lĭng′gwăl) [L. *retro,* behind, + *lingua,* tongue]. Behind the tongue.

retromammary (rĕt″rō-măm′mă-rē) [″ + *mamma,* breast]. Located behind the mammary gland.

retromandibular (rĕt″rō-măn-dĭb′ū-lăr) [″ + *mandibulum,* jaw]. Located behind the lower jaw.

retromastoid (rĕt″rō-măs′toyd) [″ + Gr. *mastos,* breast, + *eidos,* form, shape]. Situated behind the mastoid process.

retromorphosis (rĕt″rō-mor′fō-sĭs) [″ + Gr. *morphe,* form, + *osis,* condition]. 1. Change in shape accompanying a transition from a higher to a lower type of structure. 2. Retrogressive changes within cells or tissues. SYN: *catabolism.*

retronasal (rĕt″rō-nā′zăl) [L. *retro,* back, + *nasus,* nose]. Rel. to, or situated at, the back part of the nose.

retroocular (rĕt″rō-ŏk′ū-lar) [L. *retro,* behind, + *oculus,* eye]. Located behind the eye.

retroparotid (rĕt″rō-pă-rŏt′ĭd) [″ + Gr. *para*, beside, + *ous*, ear]. Behind the parotid gland.

retroperitoneal (rĕt″rō-pĕr″ĭ-tō-nē′ăl) [″ + Gr. *peritonaion*, peritoneum]. Located behind the peritoneum and outside the peritoneal cavity, such as the kidneys.

retroperitoneal fibrosis. Development of a mass of fibrotic tissue in the retroperitoneal space. This may lead to physical compression of the ureters, and even the vena cava and aorta. This disease may be associated with taking methysergide for migraine, and with other drugs. SYN: *Ormond's syndrome.*

retroperitoneum (rĕt″rō-pĕr-ĭ-tō-nē′ŭm). The space behind the peritoneum.

retroperitonitis (rĕt″rō-pĕr″ĭ-tō-nī′tĭs). Inflammation behind the peritoneum.

retropharyngeal (rĕt″rō-făr-ĭn′jē-ăl) [L. *retro*, behind, + Gr. *pharynx*, throat]. Behind the pharynx.

retropharyngitis (rĕt″rō-făr″ĭn-jī′tĭs) [″ + ″ + *itis*, inflammation]. Inflammation of the retropharyngeal tissue.

retropharynx (rĕt″rō-făr′ĭnks) [″ + Gr. *pharynx*, throat]. Posterior portion of the pharynx.

retroplacental (rĕt″rō-plă-sĕn′tăl) [″ + *placenta*, a flat cake]. Behind the placenta, or behind both the placenta and the uterine wall.

retroplasia (rĕt″rō-plā′zē-ă) [″ + Gr. *plassein*, to form]. Degenerative change of a cell or tissue into a more primitive form.

retroposed (rĕt-rō-pōsd′) [L. *retro*, backward, + *positus*, placed]. Displaced backward.

retroposition (rĕt″rō-pō-zĭsh′ŭn). Backward displacement of a tissue or organ.

retropulsion (rĕt″rō-pŭl′shŭn) [″ + *pulsio*, a thrusting]. 1. Pushing back of any part, as of the fetal head in labor. 2. A walking or running backward involuntarily, seen in some of the nervous system disorders.

retrorunning. The practice of running backward. In addition to possibly being dangerous, this practice could cause muscle and joint pain.

retrospective study. A clinical study in which patients or their records are investigated after they have experienced the disease or condition. SEE: *prospective study.*

retrospondylolisthesis (rĕt″rō-spŏn″dĭ-lō-lĭs-thē′sĭs) [L. *retro*, behind + Gr. *spondylos*, vertebra, + *olisthesis*, a slipping]. Posterior displacement of a vertebra.

retrosternal (rĕt″rō-stĕr′năl) [″ + Gr. *sternon*, chest]. Behind the sternum.

retrosternal pulse. Venous pulse felt over the suprasternal notch.

retrotarsal (rĕt″rō-tăr′săl) [″ + Gr. *tarsos*, a broad, flat surface]. Located behind the tarsus of the eye.

retrouterine (rĕt″rō-ū′tĕr-ĭn) [L. *retro*, backward, + *uterus*, womb]. Located behind the uterus.

retroversioflexion (rĕt″rō-vĕr″sē-ō-flĕk′shŭn) [″ + *versio*, a turning, + *flexio*, flexion]. Retroversion and retroflexion of the uterus.

retroversion (rĕt″rō-vĕr′shŭn) [L. *retro*, back, + *versio*, a turning]. A turning, or state of being turned back, esp. an entire organ being tipped.

retroversion, femoral. A decrease in the head-neck angle of the femur, resulting in the shaft of the bone rotating outward when standing.

retroversion of uterus. Displacement of the uterus backward with the cervix pointing forward toward the symphysis pubis. Normally, the cervix points toward the lower end of the sacrum with the fundus toward the suprapubic region.

Retrovir. The previously accepted trade name for azidothymidine (AZT). The new trade name is Zidovudine.

retroviruses (rĕt″rō-vī′rŭs-ĕs). The common name for the family of Retroviridae; RNA-containing tumor viruses some of which are oncogenic and induce sarcomas, leukemias, lymphomas, and mammary carcinomas in lower animals. These viruses contain reverse transcriptase, which is essential for reverse transcription, i.e., the production of a molecule of DNA from an RNA model.

retrude (rī-trood′) [L. *re*, back, + *trudere*, to shove]. To force inward or backward.

retrusion (rī-troo′shŭn). 1. Process of forcing backward, esp. with reference to teeth. 2. Condition in which teeth are retroposed.

Retzius, lines of (rĕt′zē-ŭs) [Gustav Magnus Retzius, Swedish anatomist, 1842–1919]. Brownish incremental lines seen in microscopic sections of tooth enamel. They appear as concentric lines in transverse sections through the enamel crown.

Retzius, space of (rĕt′zē-ŭs) [Anders Adolf Retzius, Swedish anatomist, 1796–1860]. Space in lower portion of abdomen between bladder and pubic bones and bounded superiorly by peritoneum. Contains areolar tissue, fat, and a plexus of veins.

Retzius, veins of [A. A. Retzius]. Veins forming communications between the mesenteric veins and inferior vena cava.

reunient (rē-ūn′yĕnt) [L. *re*, again, + *unire*, to unite]. 1. Connecting or uniting tissues. 2. The ductus reuniens, q.v.

Reuss, August R. von (roys). Austrian ophthalmologist, 1841–1924.

    R.'s color charts. Colored letters that are printed on a colored background for use in testing color vision. To a color-blind person, the letters will appear to be the same color as the background.

revaccination (rē″văk-sĭ-nā′shŭn). Vaccination for a second time.

revascularization (rē-văs″kū-lăr-ĭ-zā′shŭn). Restoration of blood flow to a part. This may be done by using surgical means or by removing the obstruction from the original vessels.

revellent (rē-vĕl′ĕnt) [L. *re*, back, + *vellere*, to draw]. 1. Producing revulsion, the diversion of disease or blood from one part of the body to another. 2. Agent producing revulsion.

reverberation (rĭ″vĕr-bĕr-ā′shŭn) [L. *reverberare*, to cause to rebound]. 1. Process by which closed chains of neurons, when excited by a single impulse, will continue to discharge impulses from collaterals of their cells. 2. The repeated echoing of a sound.

Reverdin's needle (rā-vĕr-dănz′) [Jacques L. Reverdin, Swiss surgeon, 1842–1929]. A special needle with an eye at the tip that can be opened and closed by use of a lever.

reversal (rĭ-vĕr′săl) [L. *reversus*, revert]. 1. A change, or turning, in the opposite direction. 2. In psychology, a change in an instinct to its opposite, as from love to hate.

     r., sex. The process of changing an individual's sexual identity to that of the opposite sex. SEE: *sex reassignment.*

reversible (rĭ-vĕr′sĭ-bl). Able to change back and forth.

reversion (rĭ-vĕr′zhŭn). 1. Return to a previously existing condition. 2. In genetics, the appearance of traits possessed by a remote ancestor. SEE: *atavism.*

revertant. An organism that has reverted to a less advanced type by mutation.

review of systems. ABBR: ROS. In the process of examining and questioning a patient, esp. one not previously seen or examined, it is important to ask questions concerning each organ and region of the body. To fail to do this is to invite overlooking something in the history that is essential to the diagnosis of the disease process. This review is done in an orderly and systematic manner and is recorded. In general, it is true that if the examining person's findings are not recorded in the chart, they might as well have not been done—at least with respect to being available for others involved in the patient's care.

     In asking questions, keep in mind the possible differences between the examiner and the patient with respect to economic values, social and cultural mores, language, and life experiences. Thus questions concerning those areas generally considered to be personal, private, and confidential such as neuropsychiatric, sexual, and marital history must be tactful and done in a nonjudgmental manner. Also important is for the examiner to be aware constantly that the patient's vocabulary probably does not include complex or abstruse medical, anatomical, and chemical terms. Most individuals who know slang terms for urine, feces, and sexual intercourse are unaware of the usual medical terms. It is sometimes useful to do the ROS during the physical examination. The ROS outline that follows should not be used slavishly for each patient. Obviously the questions asked of an adolescent will reasonably be less detailed than those asked of an elderly patient.

     The systems and regions and questions include, but are not restricted to, the following.

     General. History of fatigue, weight loss, travel to other climates or countries, recent weight change, chills, fever, and lifestyle change. Has individual ever been refused for life insurance or military service? How many persons occupy the patient's dwelling? Patient's relationship to persons with whom he or she lives. Is it a happy home? Hobbies, outside interests. History of exercise and athletic activity. Religious activities, if any. History of exposure to animal pets and the health of those pets. Obtain history of military service and occupational record and in what locations, and sources of income. Health of spouse and sex partners. Highest level of education attained. Does the individual have a criminal record?

     Skin. Rash, itching, sunburn, change in size of moles, vesicles, hair loss.

     Head, face, and neck. Headache, migraine, vertigo, trauma, stiffness, pain, swelling.

     Eyes. Are glasses worn and when were eyes last examined concerning visual acuity and glaucoma? Pain, diplopia, scotomata, itch, discharge, redness, infection.

     Ears. Acute or chronic loss of hearing, pain, discharge, tinnitus, vertigo. Does ear wax collect and periodically need to be removed? History of failure to adjust to descent from altitude.

     Nose. Dryness, crust formation, bleeding, pain, discharge, obstruction, acuity of smell, malodor, sneezing. Do nose hairs have to be trimmed to prevent irritation?

     Mouth and teeth. Soreness, ulcers, pain, dryness, infection, hoarseness, bleeding gums, swallowing difficulty, condition of teeth either real or false, bruxism, temporomandibular syndrome.

     Breasts. Pain, swelling, tenderness, lumps, bleeding from nipple, infection, change in ability of nipples to become erect. Has plastic surgery been done and were implants used?

Respiratory. Cough, pain, sputum production, character of sputum, hemoptysis, exposure to persons with contagious diseases such as tuberculosis. History of occupational or other exposure to asbestos, silica, chickens, parrots, or dusty environment. Dyspnea, cyanosis, tuberculosis, pneumonia, pleurisy. If pulmonary function tests were done, the date(s). Extent and duration of use of tobacco.

Cardiac. Angina, dyspnea, orthopnea, palpitations, heart murmur, heart failure, cardiac infarction, surgical procedures on coronary arteries or heart valves, history of stress test results and how recently done, hypertension, rheumatic fever, cardiac arrhythmias, exercise tolerance, history of athletic participation (including jogging and running) and if these are current activities, the date(s) of ECG if ever taken.

Vascular. Claudication, history of cold intolerance (esp. of extremities), history of frostbite, phlebitis, ulcers (esp. of lower extremities).

Gastrointestinal. Appetite, history of recent gain or loss of weight, and has patient been on a particular diet for gaining or losing weight? Is patient a vegetarian? Difficulty in swallowing. Anorexia, nausea, vomiting and character of vomitus, diarrhea and possible explanation (such as foreign travel or food poisoning), belching, constipation, change in bowel habits, melena, hemorrhoids and history of surgery for this condition, use of laxatives or antacids, jaundice, hepatitis, other liver disease, use of injected "street" drugs.

Renal and urinary and genital tract. History of kidney or bladder stones and date of last occurrence, dysuria, hematuria, pyuria, nocturia, incontinence, urgency, history of antibiotics used for urinary tract infections, history of bedwetting, history of sexually transmitted diseases, libido, sexual preference, penile or urethral discharge, marital history, frequency of sexual activity.

In females, vulval pruritus, vaginal discharge, vaginal malodor, history of menarche, frequency and duration of menstrual periods, amount of flow, type of menstrual protection used, type(s) of contraception and douches used, total number of pregnancies, abortions, miscarriages, normal deliveries; number, sex, age, and health status of living children. Cause of death of children who died. Vaginal, cervical, uterine infections, pelvic inflammatory disease, tubal ligation, D & C, hysterectomy, dyspareunia. History of mother's use of diethylstilbestrol while pregnant with the patient.

In males, vasectomy, wet dreams, scrotal pain or swelling, prostate trouble.

Musculoskeletal. Muscle twitches, pain, heat, tenderness, swelling, loss of range of motion or strength, cramps, sprains, strains, trauma, fractures, stiffness, back pain, osteoporosis, and character with respect to time of day of onset and duration esp. with respect to effect of exercise, back pain, osteoporosis.

Hematological. Anemia, bleeding, bruising, hemarthrosis, history of hemophilia, sickle cell disease or trait, recent loss of blood, history of transfusions received and blood donation. Was transfusion received at a time when blood was not being screened for AIDS? Was patient ever turned down as a blood donor?

Endocrine. History of sexual maturation and development or lack of, weight change, tolerance to heat or cold esp. with respect to other persons in the same environment, dryness of hair and skin, hair loss, voice change. In men, change in rate of beard growth, development of facial hair in the female, increase in or loss of libido, polyuria, polydipsia, polyphagia, pruritus, diabetes, exophthalmos, goiter, unexplained flushing, and sweating.

Nervous system. Recent change in ability to control muscular activity, syncope, stroke ("shock"), seizures, tremor, coordination, sensory disturbance, falls, pain, change in memory, dizziness. History of trauma to head.

Emotional and psychological status. History of psychiatric illness, anxiety, depression, overactivity, mania, lassitude, change in sleep pattern, insomnia, hypersomnia, nightmares, sleepwalking, hallucinations, feeling of unreality, paranoia, phobias, obsessions, compulsions, criminal behavior, increase in or loss of libido, satyriasis, nymphomania, suicidal thoughts, satisfaction with occupation and life in general, marital and divorce record, family discord, employment history and recent job changes, educational history and achievement, self-image. History of drug abuse and sharing of needles. If appropriate, ask patient if he or she is happy and in love.

Révilliod sign [Leon Révilliod, Swiss physician, 1835–1919]. SEE: *wink.*

revised trauma score. ABBR: RTS. A method for scoring and quantifying the severity of trauma in pediatric patients. SYN: *pediatric trauma score.*

revivescence (rē″vī-vĕs′ĕns). Revivification, q.v.

revivification (rē-vĭv″ĭ-fĭ-kā′shŭn) [L. *re,* again, + *vivere,* to live, + *facere,* to make]. 1. Attempt to restore life to those apparently dead; restoration to life or consciousness. Also restoring life in local parts, as a limb after freezing. 2. Pairing of surfaces to facilitate healing, as in a wound.

revulsant (rĭ-vŭl'sănt) [L. *revulsio*, pulling back]. 1. Causing transfer of disease or blood from one part of the body to another. 2. Counterirritant that increases blood flow to an inflamed part.

revulsion (rĭ-vŭl'shŭn). 1. Act of driving backward, as diverting disease from one part to another by a quick withdrawal of the blood from that part. 2. In physical therapy, circulatory changes obtained by sudden and intense reactions to heat and cold. SEE: *counterirritation*.

revulsive (rĭ-vŭl'sĭv). 1. Causing revulsion. 2. A counterirritant.

reward. Something given to an individual as recognition of a good performance or of having achieved a certain level of competence in a field of endeavor.

rewarming. The process of warming the body of an individual whose body temperature has dropped to a subnormal level. It is usually accomplished by providing a warm environment; one way of doing this is to immerse the hypothermic individual in warm water.

Reye's syndrome (rīz) [R. D. K. Reye, Australian pathologist, 1912–1977]. A syndrome first recognized in 1963, characterized by acute encephalopathy and fatty infiltration of the liver and possibly of the pancreas, heart, kidney, spleen and lymph nodes. Seen in children under 15 years of age after an acute viral infection. The mortality rate is variable depending on severity, but may be as high as 80%.

SYM: Upper respiratory infection (viral) followed in about 6 days by pernicious nausea and vomiting and a change in mental status (disorientation, agitation, coma, seizures), hepatomegaly without jaundice in 40% of cases. The disease should be suspected in any child with acute onset of encephalopathy and altered liver function.

ETIOL: Unknown, but association with increased use of aspirin is evident from epidemiological studies.

Caution: Do not use aspirin as an antipyretic or for any reason in treating children with viral infections.

PROG: Outcome is related to severity of the central nervous system involvement.

TREAT: Supportive care including I.V. administration of fluids and electrolytes. Careful control of blood electrolytes.

NURSING IMPLICATIONS: Perform a neurological assessment at frequent intervals. Monitor temperature and perform prescribed measures to alleviate hyperthermia.

Implement seizure precautions. Monitor intake and output carefully. Observe for impaired hepatic function such as signs of bleeding. Instruct the parent or guardian not to administer aspirin to a child experiencing chicken pox or influenza, because use of aspirin in those conditions may induce Reye's syndrome.

RF, Rf. *rheumatoid factor*.

R.F.A. *right frontoanterior* fetal position.

R factor. Resistance transfer factor.

R.F.P. *right frontoposterior* fetal position.

R.F.T. *right frontotransverse* fetal position.

RH. *releasing hormone*.

Rh. 1. Chem. symb. for the element rhodium. 2. *Rhesus*, a monkey (*Macaca rhesus*) in which the Rh factor was first identified.

Rhabditis (răb-dī'tĭs) [Gr. *rhabdos*, rod]. A genus of small nematode worms, some of which are parasitic.

rhabdo- [Gr. *rhabdos*, rod]. Combining form meaning rod.

rhabdoid (răb'doyd) [″ + *eidos*, form, shape]. Resembling a rod.

rhabdomyoblastoma (răb″dō-mī″ō-blăs-tō'mă) [″ + *mys*, muscle, + *blastos*, germ, + *oma*, tumor]. Rhabdomyosarcoma.

rhabdomyolysis (răb″dō-mī-ŏl'ĭ-sĭs) [″ + ″ + *lysis*, dissolution]. An acute, sometimes fatal disease characterized by destruction of skeletal muscle. Rarely, this may occur following strenuous exercise and in association with use of drugs that can cause coma, such as alcohol, heroin, or cocaine.

Renal damage manifested by acute tubular necrosis may result if myoglobinuria is accompanied with acute dehydration or anoxia. SEE: *reperfusion*.

r., traumatic. SEE: *crush syndrome; reperfusion* (def. 2).

rhabdomyoma (răb″dō-mī-ō'mă) [″ + ″ + *oma*, tumor]. A striated muscular tissue tumor. SYN: *myoma striocellulare*.

rhabdomyosarcoma (răb″dō-mī″ō-săr-kō'mă) [″ + ″ + *sarx*, flesh, + *oma*, tumor]. An extremely malignant neoplasm originating in skeletal muscle.

rhabdophobia (răb-dō-fō'bē-ă) [″ + *phobos*, fear]. Abnormal fear of being hit or beaten with a stick or rod.

rhabdosarcoma (răb″dō-săr-kō'mă) [″ + *sarx*, flesh, + *oma*, tumor]. Rhabdomyosarcoma.

rhabdovirus (răb″dō-vī'rŭs) [″ + L. *virus*, poison]. Any of a group of rod-shaped RNA viruses with one important member, the rabies virus, pathogenic to man. The virus has a predilection for tissue of mucus-secreting glands and the central nervous system. All warm-blooded animals are susceptible to infection with these viruses.

rhachialgia (rā″kē-ăl′jē-ă) [Gr. *rhachis*, spine, + *algos*, pain]. Pain in the spine.

rhachiocampsis (rā″kē-ō-kămp′sĭs) [″ + *kampsis*, a bending]. Curvature of spine.

rhachioplegia (rā″kē-ō-plē′jē-ă) [″ + *plege*, stroke]. Spinal paralysis.

rhachioscoliosis (rā″kē-ō-skō″lē-ō′sĭs) [″ + *skoliosis*, curvature]. Curvature of the spine laterally.

rhachis (rā′kĭs) [Gr.]. Spinal column.

rhachischisis (ră-kĭs′kĭ-sĭs) [″ + *schisis*, a splitting]. A congenital cleft in the spinal column.

rhachitis (rā-kī′tĭs) [″ + *itis*, inflammation]. Constitutional disease of infancy marked by faulty nutrition and bone deformity. SYN: *rachitis; rickets.*

rhacoma (rā-kō′mă) [Gr. *rhakoma*, rags]. 1. Ragged, irregular abrasion, usually of the skin. 2. Relaxation of integument of scrotum.

rhagades (răg′ă-dēz) [Gr., tears]. Linear fissures appearing in skin, esp. at the corner of the mouth or anus, causing pain. If due to syphilis, they form a radiating scar on healing.

rhagadiform (rā-găd′ĭ-form) [Gr. *rhagas*, tear, + L. *forma*, shape]. Fissured; having cracks.

-rhage, -rhagia [Gr. *rhegnynai*, to burst forth]. Suffix meaning bleeding, profuse discharge.

Rh antiserum. Human serum that contains Rh antibodies.

rhaphania (ră-fā′nē-ă) [Gr. *raphanos*, radish]. Spasmodic disease caused by eating the seeds of wild radish; allied to ergotism. SYN: *raphania.*

rhaphe (rā′fē) [Gr.]. A seam or ridge. SYN: *raphe.*

-rhaphy [Gr. *rhaphe*]. Suffix meaning joining in a seam, or suturation.

Rh blood group. A blood group discovered on the surface of erythrocytes of the rhesus monkey. It is present to a variable degree in human populations. When the Rh blood group is present, an individual's blood type is designated Rh⁺ (Rh positive); when the Rh factor is absent, the blood type is Rh⁻ (Rh negative). If an individual with Rh⁻ blood receives a transfusion of Rh⁺ blood, it causes the formation of anti-Rh agglutinin. Subsequent transfusions of Rh⁺ blood may result in serious transfusion reactions (agglutination and hemolysis of red blood cells). A pregnant woman who is Rh⁻ may become sensitized by blood of an Rh⁺ fetus. In subsequent pregnancies, if the fetus is Rh⁺, Rh antibodies produced in maternal blood may cross the placenta and destroy fetal cells, giving rise to erythroblastosis fetalis, q.v.

-rhea [Gr. *rhoia*, flow]. Suffix meaning to flow.

rhegma (rĕg′mă) [Gr. *rhegma*, a tear]. Rupture, fracture, or rent.

rhegmatogenous (rĕg″mă-tŏj′ĕ-nŭs) [″ + *gennan*, to produce]. Originating or due to a rhegma.

rhenium (rē′nē-ŭm). SYMB: Re. At. wt. 186.2; at. no. 75. A metallic element similar to manganese.

rheo- [Gr. *rheos*, current]. Combining form indicating current, stream, or to flow.

rheobase (rē′ō-bās) [″ + *basis*, base]. In unipolar testing with the galvanic current using negative as active pole, the minimal voltage required to produce a stimulated response. This is the rheobase or threshold of excitation. SEE: *chronaxie.*

rheobasic (rē″ō-bā′sĭk). Concerning rheobase.

rheology (rē-ŏl′ō-jē) [″ + *logos*, word, reason]. Study of the deformation and flow of materials.

Rheomacrodex. Trade name for dextran 40.

rheometer (rē-ŏm′ĕt-ĕr) [″ + *metron*, measure]. 1. Instrument for qualitative determination of presence of an electric current. SYN: *galvanometer.* 2. Device for measuring velocity of the blood.

rheostat (rē′ō-stăt) [″ + *statos*, standing]. Device maintaining fixed or variable resistance for controlling the amount of electric current entering a circuit.

rheostosis (rē-ŏs-tō′sĭs) [″ + *osteon*, bone]. A hypertrophying and condensing osteitis occurring in streaks, involving long bones.

rheotachygraphy (rē″ō-tă-kĭg′ră-fē) [″ + *tachys*, swift, + *graphein*, to write]. Graphic recording of variation of electromotive force in a muscle.

rheotaxis (rē″ō-tăk′sĭs) [″ + *taxis*, arrangement]. Reaction to a current of fluid, causing the part acted upon to move against the current.

rheotropism (rē-ŏt′rō-pĭzm) [″ + *trope*, a turn, + *-ismos*, condition]. Rheotaxis, q.v.

rheum, rheuma (room, room′ă) [Gr. *rheuma*, discharge]. Any catarrhal or watery discharge.

rheumatic (roo-măt′ĭk) [Gr. *rheumatikos*]. Pert. to rheumatism.

rheumatic disease, functional class. The American Rheumatism Association has published the following classifications:

I. Complete functional capacity with ability to carry on all usual duties without handicaps.

II. Functional capacity adequate to conduct normal activities despite handicap or discomfort or limited mobility of one or more joints.

Jones Criteria for Diagnosis of Rheumatic Fever (revised)

Major Manifestations	Minor Manifestations
Carditis	Fever
Polyarthritis	Arthralgia
Chorea	Previous rheumatic fever or rheumatic heart disease
Erythema marginatum	Elevated ESR or positive CRP
Subcutaneous nodules	Prolonged P–R interval

Two major criteria or one major and two minor criteria indicate a high probability of the presence of rheumatic fever with supporting evidence of preceding streptococcal infection: history of recent scarlet fever; positive throat culture for group A streptococcus; increased ASO titer or other streptococcal antibodies.

Reprinted by permission of the American Heart Association.

III. Functional capacity adequate to perform only few or none of the duties of usual occupations or of self-care.

IV. Largely or wholly incapacitated with patient bedridden or confined to a wheelchair, permitting little or no self-care.

rheumatic fever. A systemic, febrile disease that is inflammatory and nonsuppurative in nature and variable in severity, duration, and sequelae. It is frequently followed by serious heart or kidney disease. SEE: table.

SYM: Following a streptococcal infection the patient will experience the sudden occurrence of fever and joint pain; this is the most common type of onset. Other symptoms include fever, migratory polyarthritis, pain upon motion, abdominal pain, chorea, cardiac involvement (pericarditis, myocarditis, and endocarditis). Later gives rise to precordial discomfort and development of heart murmurs. Skin manifestations include erythema marginatum or circinatum, and development of subcutaneous nodules. Epistaxis is common.

Rheumatic fever may occur without any sign or symptom of joint involvement. Two major manifestations (carditis, polyarthritis, chorea, erythema marginatum, subcutaneous nodules) or one major and two minor criteria (fever, arthralgia, previous rheumatic fever, elevated erythrocyte sedimentation rate or positive C-reactive protein, prolonged P-R interval) are required to establish the diagnosis of acute rheumatic fever. The Jones criteria for diagnosis of acute rheumatic fever, as revised, include the major and minor manifestations of this disease.

ETIOL: Unknown, but its onset follows a preceding infection with a strain of group A streptococci. Attacks usually occur in childhood; an individual is esp. susceptible to subsequent attacks.

PROPHYLAXIS: Prompt and adequate treatment of streptococcal infections with penicillin preferably, or erythromycin or clindamycin in appropriate dose, for a minimum of 10 days. Following an attack of rheumatic fever, an individual should receive continuous prophylaxis with penicillin G or V, amoxicillin, or sulfadiazene for an indefinite period.

Patients known to have carditis who must undergo dental or surgical procedures (especially those involving instrumentation of the urinary tract, rectum, or colon) should receive additional antibiotic coverage on the day of the treatment and for several days thereafter.

TREAT: Enforced bedrest until signs of active rheumatic fever have disappeared. Salicylates for symptomatic relief. Penicillin administered to eradicate streptococci. Complications, esp. those involving heart, require special treatment.

NURSING IMPLICATIONS: Ensure maintenance of bedrest by informing the patient of the significance of compliance. Monitor temperature frequently for elevation; institute appropriate nursing measures for fever reduction. Monitor pulse and notify the physician if an arrhythmia occurs. Instruct the patient concerning altered lifestyle and permitted activities. Instruct the patient concerning the prescribed bland, high-protein and high-carbohydrate diet. Force fluids unless the cardiac status contraindicates this, in which case the diet should also include salt restriction. Rheumatic fever is a known sequela of streptococcal pharyngitis. Instruct parents about the importance of prescribed prophylactic administration of penicillin for such infections. SEE: *Nursing Diagnoses* in *Appendix*.

rheumatid (roo'mă-tid). Skin lesion associated with rheumatic disease.

rheumatism (roo′mă-tĭzm) [Gr. *rheumatismos*]. A general term for acute and chronic conditions characterized by inflammation, soreness and stiffness of muscles, and pain in joints and associated structures. It includes arthritis (infectious, rheumatoid, gouty); arthritis due to rheumatic fever or trauma; degenerative joint disease; neurogenic arthropathy; hydroarthrosis; myositis; bursitis; fibromyositis; and many other conditions. SEE: *arthritis; rheumatic fever.*

    r., acute articular. Rheumatic fever.

    r., chronic. Rheumatism associated with a joint disorder, such as rheumatoid arthritis, gout, or degenerative joint disease, usually resulting in deformity of the joint.

    r., gonorrheal. Arthritis resulting from gonorrheal infection. SEE: *gonorrhea.*

    r., inflammatory. Rheumatism caused by rheumatic fever.

    r., muscular. Term applied to a number of muscular conditions characterized by tenderness, soreness, pain, and local spasm. Includes such conditions as fibromyositis, myositis, myalgia, and torticollis, q.v.

    r., palindromic. Intermittent joint pain with tenderness, heat, and swelling that lasts from a few hours to as long as a week. The knee is most often involved but the disease does not necessarily return to the same joint(s). Between attacks there is no evidence of the disease. The cause is unknown, and there is no specific treatment.

    r., psychogenic. Rheumatism of psychic origin, esp. that occurring under emotional stress.

    r., soft tissue. General term for a variety of localized and generalized conditions that cause pain around joints but are not related to or caused by joint disease. Included in this general classification are bursitis, tennis elbow, tendinitis, perichondritis, stiff man syndrome, and Tietze's disease.

rheumatismal (roo″mă-tĭz′măl). Concerning or related to rheumatism.

rheumatoid (roo′mă-toyd) [Gr. *rheuma*, discharge, + *eidos*, form, shape]. Of the nature of rheumatism; resembling rheumatism.

rheumatoid arthritis. Form of arthritis with inflammation of the joints, stiffness, swelling, cartilaginous hypertrophy, and pain. SEE: *arthritis, rheumatoid.*

rheumatoid factor. An immunoglobulin present in serum of 50% to 95% of adults with rheumatoid arthritis. This factor, although not specific for rheumatoid arthritis, is quite helpful in diagnosing and investigating the disease.

rheumatologist (roo″mă-tŏl′ō-jĭst). A physician who specializes in rheumatic diseases.

rheumatology (roo″mă-tŏl′ō-jē). The division of medicine concerned with rheumatic diseases.

rhexis (rĕk′sĭs) [Gr., rupture]. Rupture of any organ, blood vessel, or tissue.

Rh factor. SEE: *Rh blood group.*

Rh genes. A series of eight allelic genes that are responsible for the various Rh blood types and designated by A. S. Wiener as R^1, R^2, R^0, R^z, r, r', r'', and r_y. Genes represented by small r's are responsible for Rh-negative (Rh⁻) blood type; those by large R's for Rh-positive (Rh⁺) blood type.

rhigosis (rĭ-gō′sĭs) [Gr., shivering]. Perception of cold.

Rh immune globulin. A solution of gamma globulin containing anti-Rh. Given to an Rh-negative mother within 72 hours after delivery of an Rh-positive infant, it acts to prevent and suppress the Rh immune response. Also indicated in abortion done on an Rh-negative mother.

rhinal (rī′năl) [Gr. *rhis*, nose]. Concerning the nose. SYN: *nasal.*

rhinalgia (rī-năl′jē-ă) [″ + *algos*, pain]. Pain in the nose; nasal neuralgia.

rhinedema (rī″nĕ-dē′mă) [″ + *oidema*, swelling]. Edema of the nose.

rhinencephalon (rī-nĕn-sĕf′ă-lŏn) [″ + *enkephalos*, brain]. Portion of brain concerned with reception and integration of olfactory impulses. Includes olfactory bulb, olfactory tract and striae, intermediate olfactory area, piriform area, paraterminal area, hippocampal formation, and fornix. It constitutes the paleopallium and archipallium.

rhinencephalus (rī″nĕn-sĕf′ă-lŭs) [″ + *enkephalos*, brain]. Rhinocephalus.

rhinenchysis [″ + Gr. *enchein*, to pour in]. Nasal douche using medicated or nonmedicated solutions.

rhinesthesia (rī-nĕs-thē′zē-ă) [″ + *aisthesis*, sensation]. The sense of smell.

rhineurynter (rĭn″ū-rĭn′tĕr) [″ + *eurynein*, to dilate]. Elastic bag used for dilating the nostrils.

rhinion (rĭn′ē-ŏn) [Gr.]. Lower end of the suture between nasal bones; a craniometric point. SYN: *punctum nasale inferius.*

rhinism (rī′nĭzm) [Gr. *rhis*, nose, + *-ismos*, condition]. Nasal quality of the voice.

rhinitis (rī-nī′tĭs) [″ + *itis*, inflammation]. Inflammation of the nasal mucosa. Children with condition may have a characteristic way of rubbing their noses with an upward movement of their hands. This is called "allergic salute." SEE: *ozena.*

    r., acute. Acute congested condition of the nose with increased secretion of mucus. SYN: *coryza.*

    TREAT: No specific treatment is known. General measures include rest, adequate fluids, well-balanced diet. Analgesics and antipyretics may be used to make patient comfortable. Sulfonamides and other antibiotics are of no value and should not be administered. Antihistamines may relieve early symptoms but do not abort or alter course. Vasoconstrictors in form of inhalants, nasal sprays, or drops may give temporary relief. Their use helps prevent the development of middle ear infections by helping to maintain the patency of the eustachian tubes.

    r., allergic. Rhinitis due to sensitivity of nasal mucosa to an allergen. SYN: *hay fever; r., vasomotor.*

    TREAT: Same as for rhinitis in general, but intranasal corticosteroids are of benefit.

Caution: Overuse of corticosteroids may damage the nasal mucosa, and absorption of the drug can cause adverse side effects.

---

    r., atrophic. Chronic inflammation with marked atrophy of mucous membrane and with considerable dry crusting and disturbance in the sense of smell. Usually accompanied by ozena. The throat is dry and, as a rule, contains crusts. A husky voice or hoarseness often is common.

    SYM: Fetid odor from nose and throat with considerable crusting.

    TREAT: Irrigation of nose with warm alkalinized saline solution twice daily. General hygienic measures. Correction of any associated disorders. Surgical treatment seldom helpful.

    r. caseosa. Rhinitis characterized by accumulation of offensive cheeselike masses in nose and sinuses and accompanied by a seropurulent discharge.

    r., chronic hyperplastic. Chronic inflammation of mucous membrane accompanied by polypoid formation and underlying sinus pathology. SEE: *sinus.*

    r., chronic hypertrophic. Inflammation of the mucous membrane of the nose characterized by hypertrophy of the mucous membrane of the turbinates and the septum.

    SYM: Those of nasal obstruction, postnasal discharge, and recurrent head colds.

    TREAT: Consists in surgical removal of hypertrophic or mulberry ends of inferior turbinates and cauterization of mucosa of inferior turbinates and septum.

    r., fibrinous. Rhinitis characterized by formation of a false membrane in nasal cavities.

    r., hypertrophic. Rhinitis characterized by thickening and swelling of the nasal mucosa.

    r., membranous. Chronic rhinitis accompanied by a fibrinous exudate.

    r., perennial. Rhinitis that is nonseasonal, but continues indefinitely with variations in severity.

    r., periodic. R., allergic.

    r., pseudomembranous. R., fibrinous.

    r., purulent. Chronic rhinitis accompanied by pus formation.

    r., vasomotor. Rhinitis with rhinorrhea due to increased secretion of mucus from the nasal mucosa. May be caused by allergy or neurovascular imbalance.

rhino- [Gr. *rhis*]. Combining form indicating the nose.

rhinoanemometer (rī″nō-ăn″ĕ-mŏm′ĕ-tĕr). Device that determines the presence of nasal obstruction by measuring the rate of flow of air through the nasal passages.

rhinoantritis (rī″nō-ăn-trī′tĭs) [″ + *antron,* cavity, + *itis,* inflammation]. Inflamed condition of the nasal cavities and one or both maxillary antra.

rhinocanthectomy (rī″nō-kăn-thĕk′tō-mē) [Gr. *rhis,* nose, + *kanthos,* canthus, + *ektome,* excision]. Excision of inner corner of the eye. SYN: *rhinommectomy.*

rhinocele (rī′nō-sēl) [″ + *koilia,* cavity]. The ventricle or hollow of the olfactory lobe or rhinoencephalon.

rhinocephalus (rī″nō-sĕf′ă-lŭs) [″ + *kephale,* head]. An individual with rhinocephaly.

rhinocephaly (rī″nō-sĕf′ă-lē) [″ + *kephale,* head]. A congenital deformity in which the eyes are fused and the nose is present as a fleshy protuberance above the eyes.

rhinocheiloplasty (rī″nō-kī′lō-plăs″tē) [″ + *cheilos,* lip, + *plastos,* formed]. Plastic surgery of the nose and upper lip.

rhinocleisis (rī-nō-klī′sĭs) [Gr. *rhis,* nose, + *kleisis,* closure]. Nasal obstruction. SYN: *rhinostenosis.*

rhinodacryolith (rī″nō-dăk′rē-ō-lĭth) [″ + *dakryon,* tear, + *lithos,* stone]. A nasal calculus.

rhinodynia (rī″nō-dĭn′ē-ă) [″ + *odyne,* pain]. Nasal pain. SYN: *rhinalgia.*

Rhinoestrus (rī-nĕs′trŭs). A genus of flies belonging to the family Oestridae. Larvae may be deposited in eye, nasal, or buccal cavities of mammals.

    R. purpureus. Russian gadfly, whose larvae sometimes cause nasomyiasis and ophthalmomyiasis in humans.

rhinogenous (rī-nŏj′ĕn-ŭs) [″ + *gennan,* to produce]. Originating in the nose.

rhinokyphosis (rī″nō-kī-fō′sĭs) [″ + *kyphos,* hump, + *osis,* condition]. A deformity of the bridge of the nose.

rhinolalia (rī″nō-lā′lē-ă) [″ + *lalia,*

speech]. Nasal quality of the voice. SEE: *whinolalia.*

r. aperta. Rhinolalia caused by undue patency of posterior nares.

r. clausa. Rhinolalia caused by closure of nasal passages.

rhinolaryngitis (rī″nō-lăr″ĭn-jī′tĭs) [″ + *larynx,* larynx, + *itis,* inflammation]. Simultaneous inflammation of mucosa of nose and larynx.

rhinolith (rī′nō-lĭth) [″ + *lithos,* stone]. Nasal concretion.

rhinolithiasis (rī″nō-lĭth-ī′ă-sĭs). The formation of nasal calculi.

rhinologist (rī-nŏl′ō-jĭst) [″ + *logos,* word, reason]. A specialist in diseases of the nose.

rhinology (rī-nŏl′ō-jē). Science of the nose and its diseases.

rhinomanometer (rī″nō-măn-ŏm′ĕt-ĕr) [Gr. *rhis,* nose, + *manos,* thin, + *metron,* measure]. Device for measuring the amount of nasal obstruction.

rhinomanometry (rī″nō-mă-nŏm′ĕ-trē). Measurement of the air flow through and air pressure in the nose.

rhinometer (rī-nŏm′ĕt-ĕr). Device for measurement of the nose or its cavities.

rhinomiosis (rī″nō-mī-ō′sĭs) [″ + *meiosis,* a lessening]. Surgical reduction in size of the nose.

rhinommectomy (rī″nŏm-mĕk′tō-mē) [″ + *omma,* eye, + *ektome,* excision]. Surgical excision of the inner canthus of the eye. SYN: *rhinocanthectomy.*

rhinomycosis (rī″nō-mī-kō′sĭs) [″ + *mykes,* fungus, + *osis,* condition]. Fungi in mucous membranes and secretions of the nose.

rhinonecrosis (rī″nō-nē-krō′sĭs) [″ + *nekrosis,* state of death]. Necrosis of the nasal bones.

rhinopathy (rī-nŏp′ă-thē) [″ + *pathos,* disease]. Any nasal disease.

rhinopharyngeal (rī″nō-fă-rĭn′jē-ăl). Concerning the nasopharynx.

rhinopharyngitis (rī″nō-făr-ĭn-jī′tĭs) [″ + *pharynx,* throat, + *itis,* inflammation]. Inflamed condition of the nasopharynx.

rhinopharyngocele (rī″nō-făr-ĭn′gō-sēl) [″ + ″ + *kele,* tumor, swelling]. A nasopharyngeal tumor.

rhinopharyngolith (rī″nō-făr-ĭn′gō-lĭth) [″ + ″ + *lithos,* stone]. Concretion in the nasal pharynx.

rhinopharynx (rī″nō-făr′ĭnks). Upper portion of pharynx continuous with the nasal passages. SYN: *nasopharynx.*

rhinophonia (rī″nō-fō′nē-ă) [″ + *phone,* voice]. A nasal tone in speaking.

rhinophycomycosis (rī″nō-fī″kō-mī-kō′sĭs) [″ + *phykos,* seaweed, + *mykes,* fungus, + *osis,* condition]. A fungus infection that may occur in humans or animals. It affects the nasal and paranasal sinuses and may spread to the brain. It is caused by the phycomycete *Entomophthora coronata.*

rhinophyma (rī-nō-fī′mă) [″ + *phyma,* growth]. Lobular hypertrophy of nose, with red coloration, congestion, and retention of sebum. SYN: *acne rosacea.*

rhinoplasty (rī′nō-plăs″tē) [″ + *plastos,* formed]. Plastic surgery of the nose.

rhinopneumonitis (rī″nō-nū″mō-nī′tĭs) [Gr. *rhis,* nose, + *pneumon,* lung, + *itis,* inflammation]. Inflammation of the nasal and pulmonary mucous membranes.

rhinopolypus (rī″nō-pŏl′ĭ-pŭs) [″ + *polys,* many, + *pous,* foot]. Polypus of the nose.

rhinorrhagia (rī″nō-rā′jē-ă) [″ + *rhegnynai,* to burst forth]. Profuse hemorrhage from the nose. SYN: *epistaxis; nosebleed.*

rhinorrhea (rī″nō-rē′ă) [″ + *rhoia,* flow]. Thin watery discharge from the nose.

r., cerebrospinal. Discharge of spinal fluid from the nose due to a defect in or trauma to the cribriform plate.

r., gustatory. Flow of a thin watery material from the nose while one is eating.

rhinosalpingitis (rī″nō-săl″pĭn-jī′tĭs) [″ + *salpinx,* tube, + *itis,* inflammation]. Inflammation of the mucosa of the nose and eustachian tube.

rhinoscleroma (rī″nō-sklē-rō′mă) [″ + *skleros,* hard, + *oma,* tumor]. A chronic, infectious disease involving nose and upper portions of respiratory tract in which growths of almost stony hardness develop, sometimes leading to marked deformity.

SYM: The disease presents a hard, nodular growth, which usually begins at anterior end of nose and spreads to the lower respiratory tract. There usually is no pain and no tendency to ulceration.

ETIOL: *Klebsiella rhinoscleromatis,* a gram-negative encapsulated bacillus.

TREAT: Surgical, in combination with streptomycin.

rhinoscope (rī′nō-skōp) [″ + *skopein,* to examine]. Instrument for examination of the nose.

rhinoscopic (rī″nō-skŏp′ĭk). Concerning rhinoscopy.

rhinoscopy (rī-nŏs′kō-pē). Examination of nasal passages.

r., anterior. Examination through anterior nares.

r., posterior. Examination through posterior nares, usually with a small mirror in the nasopharynx.

rhinosporidiosis (rī″nō-spō-rĭd″ē-ō′sĭs) [″ + *sporidion,* little seed, + *osis,* condition]. Condition caused by a fungus, *Rhinosporidium seeberi,* characterized by development of pedunculated polyps on mucous membranes of nose, larynx, eyes, penis, vagina, and sometimes skin of various parts of body. Disease is contracted from cattle. Found in India, Sri Lanka, and other parts of the world.

Rhinosporidium (rī″nō-spō-rĭd′ē-ŭm). A genus of fungi that are pathogenic to man. *R. seeberi.* Causative agent of rhinosporidiosis.

rhinostenosis (rī″nō-stĕn-ō-′sĭs) [″ + *stenos*, narrow, + *osis*, condition]. Obstruction of the nasal passages. SYN: *rhinocleisis.*

rhinotomy (rī-nŏt′ō-mē) [″ + *tome*, incision]. Incision of the nose for drainage purposes.

rhinotracheitis (rī″nō-trā″kē-ī′tĭs) [″ + *tracheia*, rough, + *itis*, inflammation]. Inflammation of the nasal mucous membranes and the trachea.

rhinovaccination (rī″nō-văk-sĭn-ā′shŭn) [″ + L. *vaccinus*, pert. to cows]. Vaccine applied to the mucosa of the nose.

rhinovirus (rī″nō-vī′rŭs). One of a species of picornaviruses, q.v., that causes the common cold in man. There are probably more than 100 rhinoviruses and they occur worldwide. There is no specific therapy. Viruses other than rhinoviruses also cause the syndrome diagnosed as a cold. These include the A21 coxsackievirus and coronaviruses.

Rhipicephalus (rī″pĭ-sĕf′ă-lŭs) [Gr. *rhipis*, fan, + *kephale*, head]. A genus of ticks belonging to the family Ixodidae. Several species, esp. *R. sanguineus*, serve as vectors for the organisms of spotted fever, boutonneuse fever, and other rickettsial diseases.

rhitidectomy (rĭt″ĭ-dĕk′tō-mē) [Gr. *rhytis*, wrinkle, + *ektome*, excision]. Removal of wrinkles by plastic surgery. This is often referred to as a "face-lift." SYN: *rhytidectomy.*

rhitidosis (rĭt-ĭ-dō′sĭs) [Gr. *rhytidosis*]. Wrinkling of the cornea, indicating its disintegration. One of the signs of approaching death. SYN: *rhytidosis.*

rhizo- [Gr. *rhiza*]. Combining form meaning root.

rhizodontropy (rī″zō-dŏn′trō-pē) [Gr. *rhiza*, root, + *odous*, tooth, + *trope*, a turning]. Process of attaching an artificial crown upon the root of a tooth.

rhizodontrypy (rī″zō-dŏn′trī-pē) [″ + ″ + *trype*, a hole]. Puncture of root of a tooth.

rhizoid (rī′zoyd) [″ + *eidos*, form, shape]. 1. Rootlike. 2. A rootlike structure, usually one-celled, occurring in lower forms of plant life. 3. In bacteriology, term applied to a colony showing an irregular rootlike system of branching.

rhizome (rī′zōm) [Gr. *rhizoma*, mass of roots]. A rootlike stem growing horizontally along or below the ground and sending out roots and shoots.

rhizomelic (rī″zō-mĕl′ĭk) [Gr. *rhiza*, root, + *melos*, limb]. Concerning the hip joint and shoulder joint.

rhizomeningomyelitis (rī″zō-mē-nĭn″gō-mī″ē-lī′tĭs) [″ + *meninx*, membrane, + *myelos*, marrow, + *itis*, inflammation]. Radiculomeningomyelitis, q.v.

Rhizopoda (rī-zŏp′ō-dă) [″ + *pous*, foot]. A subclass of the class Sarcodina, phylum Protozoa, characterized by possession of lobose pseudopodia and lacking a central filament. Includes amebae and foraminifera.

rhizotomy (rī-zŏt′ō-mē) [″ + *tome*, incision]. Section of a root, as of a nerve or tooth. *r., anterior.* Section of the ventral root of the spinal nerve.
r., posterior. Section of the dorsal root of the spinal nerve for the relief of pain or the reduction of spasticity.

Rh$_o$(D) immune globulin. USP. Previously used name for immunoglobulin D.

rhodium (rō′dē-ŭm). SYMB: Rh. At. wt. 102.905; at. no. 45. A rare metallic element.

rhodo- (rō′dō) [Gr. *rhodon*, rose]. Combining form meaning red.

rhodogenesis (rō″dō-jĕn′ē-sĭs) [″ + *genesis*, generation, birth]. Regeneration of visual purple that has been bleached by light.

rhodophane (rō′dō-fān) [″ + *phainein*, to show]. A red pigment found in retinal cones of birds and fish.

rhodophylaxis (rō″dō-fī-lăk′sĭs) [″ + *phylaxis*, protection]. Ability of the retinal epithelium to regenerate visual purple that has been bleached by light.

rhodopsin (rō-dŏp′sĭn) [″ + *opsis*, vision]. Visual purple, a pigment in outer segment of retinal rods.

RhoGAM. Trade name for Rh$_o$(D) immune globulin.

rhombencephalon (rŏm″bĕn-sĕf′ă-lŏn) [Gr. *rhombos*, rhomb, + *enkephalos*, brain]. [NA] A primary division of the embryonic brain that gives rise to metencephalon and myelencephalon. Includes the pons, cerebellum, and medulla oblongata. SYN: *hindbrain.*

rhombocele (rŏm′bō-sēl) [″ + *koilos*, a hollow]. The cavity of the rhombencephalon.

rhomboid (rŏm′boyd) [″ + *eidos*, form, shape]. An oblique parallelogram.

rhomboideus (rŏm-bō-ĭd′ē-ŭs) [L.]. One of two muscles beneath the trapezius muscle. SEE: *Muscles* in *Appendix; muscle* for illus.

rhomboid fossa. The 4th ventricle of the brain.

rhombomere (rŏm′bō-mēr) [Gr. *rhombos*,

rhomb, + *meros,* a part]. Neuromere, q.v.

rhoncal, rhonchial (rŏng′kăl, rŏng′kē-ăl) [Gr. *rhonchos,* a snore]. Pert. to, or produced by, a rattle in the throat.

rhonchi. Plural of rhonchus.

rhonchus (rŏng′kŭs) (pl. *rhonchi*). A rale or rattling in the throat, esp. when it resembles snoring.

rhopheocytosis (rō″fē-ō-sī-tō′sĭs) [Gr. *rhophein,* gulp down, + *kytos,* cell, + *osis,* condition]. Mechanism of transfer of ferritin from one cell in the bone marrow to another. SEE: *pinocytosis.*

rhotacism (rō′tă-sĭzm) [Gr. *rhotakizein,* to overuse letter "r"]. Overuse or improper utterance of "r" sounds, with too much emphasis upon this letter.

rhubarb (roo′bărb) [ME. *rubarbe*]. Extract made from roots and rhizome of *Rheum officinale, R. palmatum,* and other species. Used as a cathartic and astringent. High in oxalic acid. The stems are used as food.

Rhus (rŭs) [L.]. A genus of trees and shrubs, some of which are poisonous and produce a severe dermatitis, e.g., poison ivy *(R. toxicodendron)* and poison sumac *(R. venenata).*

rhypophobia (rī″pō-fō′bē-ă) [Gr. *rhypos,* filth, + *phobos,* fear]. Abnormal disgust at the act of defecation, feces, or filth.

rhythm (rĭth′ŭm) [Gr. *rhythmos,* measured motion]. 1. A measured time or movement; regularity of occurrence of action or function. 2. In electroencephalography, the regular occurrence of an impulse.

   r., alpha. In electroencephalography, oscillations in electric potential occurring at a rate of 8½ to 12 per second.

   r., atrioventricular. Rhythmic discharges of impulses from atrioventricular (A-V) node that occur when activity of sinoatrial (S-A) node is depressed or abolished. SYN: *r., nodal.*

   r., beta. In electroencephalography, waves ranging in frequency from 15 to 30 per second and of lower voltage than alpha waves. More pronounced in frontomotor leads.

   r., bigeminal. The coupling of extrasystoles with previously normal beats of the heart. SEE: *bigeminal pulse.*

   r., biological. Regular occurrence of certain phenomena in living organisms. SEE: *circadian; clock, biological.*

   r., cantering. R., gallop.

   r., cardiac. The nature of the cyclical activity of the heart. It may be determined by obtaining the pulse rate or electronically by use of the electrocardiograph. SEE: *cardiac cycle; conduction system, cardiac; electrocardiogram.*

   r., circadian. The recurrence of certain biological activities approximately every 24 hours regardless of environmental influences.

   r., coupled. Rhythm in which every other heartbeat produces no pulse at the wrist.

   r., delta. In electroencephalography, slow waves with a frequency of 4 or fewer per second and of relatively high voltage (20 to 200 microvolts). May be found over the area of a gross lesion such as a tumor or hemorrhage.

   r., diurnal. Occurring during the day; a cycle of regular activities that occurs repetitively at approximately 24-hour intervals. Also called *circadian rhythm.*

   r., ectopic. A cardiac rhythm originating outside the sinoatrial node.

   r., escape. The heart rhythm when the supraventricular rate set by the sinoatrial node rhythm is completely blocked.

   r., gallop. Abnormal heart rhythm with three sounds in each cycle, resembling the gallop of a horse. SYN: *r., cantering.*

   r., gamma. The 50/second rhythm seen in the electroencephalogram.

   r., idioventricular. Rhythm of ventricles occurring in heart block resulting from establishment of a new center of rhythmicity in ventricular myocardium, usually in bundle of His.

   r., junctional. A cardiac rhythm originating within the A-V junction.

   r., nodal. R., atrioventricular.

   r., normal sinus. The normal cardiac rhythm. The stimulus arises in the sinoatrial node. It is characterized by a regular rhythm, ventricular rate of 60 to 100, upright P wave in lead II, P-R interval of 0.12 to 0.20 sec, and one P wave preceding each QRS complex.

   r., nyctohemeral. Day and night rhythm.

   r., pendulum. Rhythm with the two heart sounds alike, similar to the sound of a ticking clock.

   r., sinus. Normal cardiac rhythm proceeding from the sinoatrial node.

   r., theta. The 4 to 7/second rhythm seen in the electroencephalogram.

   r., tic-tac. A state of cardiac distress in which the first and second heart sounds are the same quality. SYN: *embryocardia.*

   r., ventricular. Very slow ventricular contractions in heart block.

rhythmic [Gr. *rhythmos*]. Pert. to, or marked by, rhythm.

rhythmicity (rĭth-mĭs′ĭ-tē). Characterized by rhythmic activity.

rhythm method of birth control. SEE: *contraception.*

rhytidectomy (rĭt″ĭ-dĕk′tō-mē) [Gr. *rhytis,*

wrinkle, + *ektome*, excision]. Excision of wrinkles by plastic surgery.

rhytidoplasty (rĭt″ĭ-dō-plăs″tē) [″ + *plassein*, to form]. Elimination of facial wrinkles by plastic surgery.

rhytidosis (rĭt″ĭ-dō′sĭs) [″ + *osis*, condition]. Wrinkling of cornea. Occurs in cases of great diminution in tension of eyeball, particularly after the escape of aqueous or vitreous humor, usually near death. SYN: *rhitidosis.*

RIA. *radioimmunoassay.*

rib (rĭb) [AS. *ribb*]. One of a series of 12 pairs of narrow, curved bones extending laterally and anteriorly from sides of thoracic vertebrae and forming a part of the skeletal thorax. With the exception of the floating ribs, they are connected to the sternum by means of costal cartilages.

   r., abdominal. False rib.

   r.'s, asternal. R.'s, false.

   r., bicipital. Irregular condition resulting from fusion of two ribs, usually involving the first rib.

   r., cervical. A supernumerary rib sometimes developing in connection with a cervical vertebra, usually the lowest.

   r.'s, false. Five ribs on each side that are not directly attached to the sternum. SYN: *r.'s, asternal.*

   r.'s, floating. Lower two ribs that are not attached to the sternum.

   r., lumbar. A rudimentary rib that develops in relation to a lumbar vertebra.

   r., slipping. Rib in which the costal cartilage is repeatedly dislocating.

   r.'s, sternal. R.'s, true.

   r.'s, true. The upper seven ribs on each side, which join the sternum by separate cartilages.

   r., vertebral. R., floating, q.v.

   r.'s, vertebrocostal. The upper three false ribs on each side.

   r., vertebrosternal. True rib.

ribbon (rĭb′ŭn). A ribbon or band-shaped structure.

riboflavin (rī″bō-flā′vĭn). USP. $C_{17}H_{20}N_4O_6$. A water-soluble vitamin of the B complex group. It is an orange-yellow crystalline powder comparatively stable to heat and air but unstable to light. SYN: *vitamin B₂.*

   FUNCT: It is a constituent of certain flavoproteins that function as coenzymes in cellular oxidations. Essential for tissue repair.

   SOURCES: Milk and milk products, leafy green vegetables, liver, beef, fish, dry yeast. Also synthesized by bacteria in body.

   DEFICIENCY SYM: Eye disorders, cheilosis, glossitis, seborrheic dermatitis, esp. of face and scalp.

   DAILY REQUIREMENT: Adults: 0.6

mg/1000 Cal of food intake. Infants, children, and pregnant and lactating women require increased amounts.

ribonuclease (rī″bō-nū′klē-ās). ABBR: RNase. An enzyme that catalyzes the depolymerization of ribonucleic acid (RNA) with formation of mononucleotides.

ribonucleic acid (rī″bō-nū″klē′ĭk). ABBR: RNA. A nucleic acid that controls protein synthesis in all living cells, and takes the place of DNA in certain viruses. It differs from DNA in that its sugar is ribose and the pyrimidine uracil rather than thymine is present. RNA occurs in several forms that are determined by the number of nucleotides. SEE: *deoxyribonucleic acid.*

   Messenger RNA (mRNA) carries the code for specific amino acid sequences from the DNA to the cytoplasm for protein synthesis.

   Transfer RNA (tRNA) carries the amino acid groups to the ribosome for protein synthesis.

   Ribosomal RNA exists within the ribosomes and is thought to assist in protein synthesis.

ribonucleoprotein (rī″bō-nū″klē-ō-prō′tē-ĭn). A compound containing both protein and ribonucleic acid.

ribonucleotide (rī″bō-nū′klē-ō-tīd). A nucleotide in which the sugar ribose is combined with the purine or pyrimidine base.

ribose (rī′bōs). $C_5H_{10}O_5$, a pentose sugar present in ribonucleic acids, riboflavin, and some nucleotides.

ribosome (rī′bō-sōm). An extremely small portion of the submicroscopic structure of a cell. It contains ribonucleoprotein and functions to synthesize protein. Ribosomes may be single units or in clusters called polyribosomes or polysomes. The ribosome functions to receive genetic information and translates those instructions into protein.

ribosyl (rī′bō-sĭl). The compound glycosyl, $C_5H_9O_4$, formed from ribose.

RICE. An acronym for *r*est, *i*ce, compression, and *e*levation, the elements of management of soft tissue stress or trauma, esp. sports injuries.

rice, polished. Rice that has been milled to produce the white product commercially available in Western countries. This treatment removes the hull, which contains the majority of the vitamin B₁.

rice water, boiled. The water remaining after rice has been cooked in it and removed. Useful as an oral rehydration agent esp. for children with diarrhea. SEE: *oral rehydration therapy.*

ricin (rī′sĭn). A white, amorphous, highly toxic protein (albumin) present in the seed of the castor bean, *Ricinus communis.*

ricinine (rĭs'ĭn-ēn, -ĭn). A poisonous alkaloid present in the leaves and seeds of castor bean plant, *Ricinus communis.*

ricinoleic acid. 12-hydroxy-9-octadecenoic acid. An unsaturated hydroxy acid comprising about 80% of fatty acids in the glycerides of castor oil. Has a strong laxative action.

rickets (rĭk'ĕts). A deficiency condition in children that results in inadequate deposition of lime salts in developing cartilage and newly formed bone, causing abnormalities in shape and structure of bones. SYN: *osteomalacia; rachitis.* SEE: *Nursing Diagnoses in Appendix.*

SYM: Restlessness and slight fever at night (101° to 102°F or 38.3° to 38.9°C); free perspiration about head; diffuse soreness and tenderness of body; pallor; slight diarrhea; enlargement of liver and spleen; delayed dentition and eruption of badly formed teeth; head large and more or less square in outline; craniotabes or skull bones often so thin they crackle like parchment.

Sides of thorax flattened; sternum prominent; nodules can be felt at sternal end of ribs, forming rachitic rosary. Deformity may be kyphosis, lordosis, or scoliosis. Liver and spleen may be considerably enlarged; long bones are curved and prominent at their extremities.

ETIOL: During childhood growth, any interference with the process of endochondral bone formation, i.e., the sequence of events that take place in the epiphyseal growth plates and result in the lengthening of long bones. Due primarily to vitamin D deficiency, which affects the absorption of calcium and phosphorus from the intestine and the reabsorption of phosphorus by the renal tubules. May also result from inadequate intake or excessive loss of calcium.

PREVENTION: Exposure to ultraviolet light (sunlight or artificial light) and administration of vitamin D in quantities to provide 400 I.U. of vitamin D activity per day.

TREAT: Careful regulation of diet to meet nutritive requirements of the child, plus administration of 2200 I.U. of vitamin D per day usually is effective. Some bone deformities may require surgery.

Caution: Excessive use of vitamin D (in infants, over 20,000 I.U. daily; in adults over 100,000 I.U. daily) is to be avoided because of danger of hypervitaminosis D.

PROG: Serum phosphatase studies are helpful in making diagnosis and prognosis. Usually favorable. Deformity disappears in 90% of cases treated early. SEE: *osteomala-*

cia.

   r., adult. Softening of bones, osteomalacia, occurring in adult life. It resembles rickets.

   r., late. Rickets that has its onset in older children.

   r., renal. A disturbance in epiphyseal growth during childhood due to severe chronic renal insufficiency resulting in persistent acidosis. Dwarfism and failure of gonadal development result. Prognosis is poor.

   TREAT: Diet low in meat, milk, cheese, and egg yolk. Administration of calcium lactate or calcium gluconate in large doses.

   r., vitamin D-resistant. Defect of renal tubular function that causes excessive loss of phosphorus and results in rickets poorly responsive to vitamin D therapy. SYN: *type II vitamin D-dependent rickets.*

Rickettsia (rĭ-kĕt'sē-ă) [Howard T. Ricketts, U.S. pathologist, 1871–1910]. A genus of microorganisms, family Rickettsiaceae, order Rickettsiales, that occupy a position intermediate between viruses and bacteria. They differ from bacteria in that they are obligate parasites requiring living cells for growth, and differ from viruses in that they are retained by the Berkefeld filter. They are the causative agents of many diseases and are usually transmitted by arthropods (lice, fleas, ticks, mites), which serve as vectors. SEE: *rickettsial disease; rickettsialpox; rickettsiosis.*

   R. typhi. The agent that causes fleaborne murine (endemic) typhus.

rickettsia (rĭ-kĕt'sē-ă) (pl. *rickettsiae*). Term applied to any of the microorganisms belonging to the genus *Rickettsia.*

rickettsial disease. A disease caused by an organism of the genus *Rickettsia.* The most common types are the spotted-fever group (Rocky Mountain spotted fever or rickettsialpox), epidemic typhus, endemic typhus, Brill's disease, human Ehrlichiosis, Q fever, scrub typhus, Sennetsu fever, and trench fever.

rickettsialpox (rĭ-kĕt'sē-ăl-pŏks″). An acute, febrile, self-limited disease caused by *Rickettsia akari.* It is transmitted from the house mouse to humans by a small colorless mite, *Allodermanyssus sanguineus.*

rickettsicidal (rĭ-kĕt″sĭ-sī'dăl). Lethal to rickettsiae.

rickettsiosis (rĭ-kĕt″sē-ō'sĭs). Infection with rickettsiae.

rickettsiostatic (rĭ-kĕt″sē-ō-stăt'ĭk). Preventing or slowing the growth of rickettsiae.

riders' bone. Bony formation in the adductor muscle of the leg. Seen in those who ride horses extensively. SYN: *cavalry bone.*

riders' sprain. Sprain of adductor muscles of

the thigh.

ridge (rĭj) [ME. *rigge*]. An elongated projecting structure or crest.

    r., alveolar. The bony process of the maxilla or mandible that contains the alveoli or tooth sockets; the alveolar process without teeth present.

    r., carotid. Sharp ridge between the carotid canal and the jugular fossa.

    r., dental. Any elevation on the crown of a tooth.

    r., dermal. One of the ridges on the surface of the fingers. These make up the fingerprints. SYN: *cristae cutis.*

    r., epicondylic. One of two ridges for muscular attachments on the humerus.

    r., gastrocnemial. Ridge on the posterior femoral surface for attachment of gastrocnemius muscles.

    r., genital. Ridge that develops on the ventromedial surface of the urogenital ridge and gives rise to gonads.

    r., gluteal. Ridge extending obliquely downward from the great trochanter of the femur for the attachment of the gluteus maximus muscle.

    r., interosseous. Ridge on the fibula for attachment of the interosseous membrane.

    r., interureteric. Ridge between the openings of the ureters in the bladder.

    r., mammary. In the embryo of mammals, a ridge extending from the axilla to the groin. The breasts arise from this ridge. In the human, only one breast normally remains on each side. SYN: *milk line.*

    r., mesonephric. Ridge that develops on the lateral surface of the urogenital ridge and gives rise to mesonephros. SYN: *r., wolffian.*

    r., mylohyoid. The line of attachment on the medial aspect of the body of the mandible for the mylohyoid muscle, which forms the floor of the mouth.

    r., pronator. Oblique ridge on the anterior surface of the ulna, providing attachment to the pronator quadratus.

    r., pterygoid. Ridge at angle of junction of temporal and infratemporal surface of great wing of the sphenoid bone.

    r., superciliary. Curved ridge of the frontal bone over supraorbital arch.

    r., supracondylar. One of two ridges (lateral and medial) on the distal end of the humerus, extending upward from the lateral to medial epicondyles.

    r., tentorial. Ridge on upper inner surface of the cranium to which is attached the tentorium.

    r., trapezoid. Oblique ridge on the upper surface of the clavicle giving attachment to the trapezoid ligament.

    r., urogenital. Ridge on dorsal wall of coelom that gives rise to genital and mesonephric ridges. SYN: *urogenital fold.* SEE: *r., genital; r., mesonephric.*

    r., wolffian. R., mesonephric.

ridgel (rĭj′ĕl). A male animal, esp. a horse, with only one testicle, or only one descended testicle.

Riedel's lobe (rē′dĕlz) [Bernhard M. C. L. Riedel, Ger. surgeon, 1846–1916]. A tongue-shaped process of liver, frequently found protruding over the gallbladder in cases of chronic cholecystitis.

Rifadin. Trade name for rifampin.

rifampin (rĭf′ăm-pĭn). USP. An antibiotic synthesized from rifamycin B, which in turn is produced by fermentation of *Streptomyces mediterranei.* It is used in treating *Mycobacterium tuberculosis* and carriers of *Neisseria meningitidis.* Trade names are Rimactane and Rifadin.

rifamycin (rĭf′ă-mī′sĭn). An antibiotic produced by certain strains of *Streptomyces mediterranei.*

Riga-Fede's disease (rē′gă fā′dāz) [Antonio Riga, It. physician, 1832–1919; Francesco Fede, It. physician, 1832–1913]. Ulceration of frenum of the tongue with membrane formation. Occurs after abrasion by the lower central incisors.

Riggs' disease [John M. Riggs, U.S. dentist, 1810–1885]. Periodontitis, q.v.

right (rīt) [AS. *riht*]. ABBR: R; rt. Pert. to the right side of the body; the side that on most persons is the stronger or preferred. SYN: *dexter.*

right-handedness. Condition of being more adept in use of the right hand. SYN: *dextrality.* SEE: *sinistrality.*

right to know law. Law that dictates that employers will inform their employees of the health effects and chemical hazards of the toxic substances used in each workplace. The employer must provide information concerning the generic and chemical names of the substances used; the level at which the exposure is hazardous; the effects of exposure at hazardous levels; the symptoms of such effects; the potential for flammability, explosion, and reactivity of the substances; the appropriate emergency treatment; proper conditions for safe use and exposure to the substances; and procedures for cleanup of leaks and spills. The law provides that an employee may refuse to work with a toxic substance until he or she has received information concerning its potential for being a hazardous substance. SEE: *hazardous material; health hazard; material safety data sheet; permissible exposure limits; toxic substance.*

rigid (rĭ′jĭd) [L. *rigidus*]. Stiff, hard, unyielding.

rigid cervical collar. Firm collar applied during extrication from any location of a traumatized person. This is done to patients with possible cervical spine injury to prevent neck movement.

rigidity (rĭ-jĭd'ĭ-tē). 1. Tenseness; immovability; stiffness; inability to bend or be bent. 2. In psychiatry, refers to one's excessive resistance to change.

    r., cadaveric. Rigor mortis.

    r., cerebellar. Stiffness of body and extremities resulting from lesion of middle lobe of cerebellum.

    r., clasp-knife. Passive flexion of the joint causes increased resistance of the extensors. This gives way abruptly if the pressure to produce flexion is continued.

    r., cogwheel. Condition noted upon passively stretching a hypertonic muscle in which resistance is jerky.

    r., decerebrate. Sustained contraction of extensor muscles of limbs resulting from a lesion in the brain stem between superior colliculi and vestibular nuclei.

    r., lead-pipe. Generalized muscular rigidity seen in parkinsonism.

rigor (rig'or) [L. *rigor*, stiffness]. 1. A sudden, paroxysmal chill with high temperature, called the cold stage, followed by a sense of heat and profuse perspiration, called the hot stage. 2. A state of hardness and stiffness, as in a muscle.

    r. mortis. The stiffness that occurs in dead bodies. SEE: *Nysten's law.*

rim. An edge or border.

    r., bite. R., occlusion, q.v.

    r., occlusion. Occluding surfaces built on denture bases in order to make maxillomandibular relation records and for arranging teeth.

rima (rī'mă) [L., a slit] (pl. *rimae*). [NA] A slit, fissure, or crack.

    r. cornealis. Groove in the sclera holding edge of the cornea.

    r. glottidis. [NA] An elongated slit between the vocal folds. SYN: *r. vocalis.*

    r. oris. [NA] Aperture of the mouth.

    r. palpebrarum. [NA] Slit between the eyelids.

    r. pudendi. [NA] Space between the labia majora, through which urethra and vagina open.

    r. respiratoria. Space behind the arytenoid cartilages.

    r. vestibuli. [NA] Space between the false vocal cords.

    r. vocalis. R. glottidis.

Rimactane. Trade name for rifampin.

rimose (rī'mōs, rī-mōs') [L. *rimosus*]. Fissured or marked by cracks.

rimula (rĭm'ū-lă) [L.] (pl. *rimulae*). A minute fissure or slit, esp. of the spinal cord or brain.

rind (rīnd) [AS.]. A thick or firm outer coating of an organ, plant, or animal.

ring (rĭng) [AS. *hring*]. 1. Any round area, organ, or band around a circular opening. SEE: *annulus.* 2. In chemistry, a collection of atoms chemically bound in a circular form.

    r.'s, abdominal. Apertures in the abdominal wall. SEE: *abdominal rings.*

    r., Albl's. A curved thin shadow seen on roentgenogram of an intracranial aneurysm.

    r., Bandl's. R., pathologic retraction, q.v.

    r., benzene. The closed ring of six carbon atoms.

    r., Cannon's. A contracted band of muscles in the transverse colon near the hepatic flexure.

    r., ciliary. Portion of the ciliary body consisting of a bandlike zone lying directly anterior to the ora serrata. SYN: *orbiculus ciliaris.*

    r., conjunctival. A narrow ring at the junction of the edge of the cornea with the conjunctiva. SYN: *anulus conjunctiva.*

    r., constriction. A stricture of the body of the uterus. A circular area of the uterus contracts around a part of the fetus.

    r., femoral. The superior aperture of the femoral canal.

    r., inguinal, abdominal. The internal opening of the inguinal canal. SEE: *abdominal rings.*

    r., inguinal, deep. The inguinal canal's opening deep inside the abdominal wall.

    r., inguinal, subcutaneous. The external opening of the inguinal canal. SEE: *abdominal rings.*

    r., inguinal, superficial. The opening of the superficial end of the inguinal canal.

    r., Kayser-Fleischer. SEE: *Kayser-Fleischer ring; Wilson's disease.*

    r., lymphoid. A ringlike arrangement of lymphoid tonsillar tissue around the oronasal region of the pharynx. It consists of the palatine, pharyngeal, and lingual tonsils, and provides protection against invading bacteria, viruses, and other foreign protein. Also called *Waldeyer's ring.*

    r., pathologic retraction. During delivery, a prolonged contraction of the ring formed by the junction of the body and isthmus of the uterus.

    r., physiologic retraction. A normal contraction of the ring formed by the junction of the body and isthmus of the uterus.

    r., Schatzki. SEE: *Schatzki ring.*

    r., Schwalbe's. The thickened peripheral margin of the Descemet's membrane of the cornea of the eye. It is formed by a circular bundle of connective tissue.

    r., tympanic. A band of bone formed by

three elements (squamous, petromastoid, and tympanic) that develop into the tympanic plate.

r., umbilical. The opening in the linea alba of the embryo. The umbilical vessels pass through this ring.

r., vascular. An anomalous ring of vascular structures around the trachea and esophagus.

r., Waldeyer's. SEE: *lymphoid ring.*

ring, removal from swollen finger. Technique for removal of ring from an injured or swollen finger. Pass one end of a length of string under the ring. Push the ring as far away from the swollen area toward the hand as is possible; wrap the string on the side of the swollen area around the finger for a dozen turns or so. Grasp the end of the string that extends under the ring and, while holding it firmly, unwind the string from the hand side of the ring. This will move the ring toward the free end of the finger. Continue this until the ring is free. If this technique fails, the ring will need to be cut from the finger.

Ringer, Sydney (ring'ĕr). British physiologist, 1835–1910.

R.'s injection, lactated. USP. A sterile solution of specified amounts of calcium chloride, potassium chloride, sodium chloride, and sodium lactate in water for injection. It is used intravenously to replace electrolytes.

R.'s irrigation. USP. A solution of recently boiled distilled water containing 8.6 gm sodium chloride, 0.3 gm potassium chloride, and 0.33 gm calcium chloride per liter. For topical use only. Previously used name was *Ringer's solution.*

ringworm (ring'wŭrm). Popular term for a dermatomycosis due to various species of fungi belonging to the genera *Microsporum* and *Trichophyton*. Ringworm of the scalp is called tinea capitis; of the body, tinea corporis; of the beard, tinea barbae; of the nails, tinea unguium; of the feet, athlete's foot. SEE: *tinea.* SEE: *Nursing Diagnoses in Appendix.*

SYM: Red-ringed patch of vesicles, itching, pain, scaling.

TREAT: Griseofulvin may be helpful in certain types. At the same time, treatment with topical fungistatic preparations is important.

Rinne test (rĭn'nē) [Heinrich Adolf Rinne, Ger. otologist, 1819–1868]. Use of tuning fork to compare bone conduction hearing with air conduction. The vibrating fork is held by its stem on the mastoid process of the ear until it is no longer heard by the patient. Then it is held close to the external auditory meatus. If the subject still hears

the vibrations, this is called a positive Rinne test. If the fork is not heard by air conduction the test is repeated; but first air conduction is tested until the sound is no longer heard, then the stem of the fork is placed on the mastoid process of the ear. If the sound is still heard, this is called a negative Rinne test. SEE: *Weber test.*

rinse. To wash lightly; a solution or water used to rinse.

r., mouth. A flavored, perhaps mildly antiseptic solution used to help cleanse the mouth or improve breath odor.

r., sodium fluoride. A 0.05% aqueous solution of sodium fluoride also containing coloring and flavoring agents used as a mouth rinse to help prevent dental caries.

Riolan's arch (rē″ō-länz′) [Jean Riolan, Fr. anatomist, 1577–1657]. Arch formed by the mesentery of the transverse colon.

Riolan's bouquet. Two ligaments and three muscles attached to styloid process of temporal bone.

Riolan's muscle. Ciliary portion of orbicularis oculi.

Riopan. Trade name for magaldrate.

ripa (rī′pă) [L., bank]. Any line of reflection of the ependyma of the brain from the ventricular wall to the choroid plexus.

Ripault's sign (rē-pōz′) [Louis H. A. Ripault, Fr. physician, 1807–1856]. Change in shape of pupil produced by unilateral (external) pressure upon eyeball.

ripening. 1. Softening and dilatation of the uterine cervix during labor. 2. Maturation of a cataract.

risk [origin obscure]. Exposure to the chance of developing a disease, or of experiencing an injury.

r., attributable. The portion of the risk of developing a condition that can be attributed to each of known risk factors, e.g., persons exposed to asbestos have a certain risk of developing lung cancer; and if they also smoke tobacco, they are also at risk from that factor. These risks may be estimated from cohort studies.

r., relative. The risk of developing a pathological condition because of being exposed to the entity as compared to what would have been the chance of developing the disease without the exposure.

risk-benefit analysis. In medical care and decision analysis, q.v., it is important that both the physician and the patient understand as precisely as possible the risk of undertaking a therapeutic course of action as well as the potential benefit of taking that action. An example would be the risk of dying from a surgical procedure versus the outcome if the procedure were successful and the course of the disease if the procedure were not done. SEE: *primum non nocere*.

risk factors. Factors in the environment, or chemical, psychological, physiological, or genetic elements, that are thought to predispose an individual to the development of a disease.

Ex.: Known risk factors for coronary artery disease include: hypertension, high circulating blood lipids and cholesterol, obesity, cigarette smoking, diabetes mellitus, inability to cope with stress, physical inactivity, and a family history of atherosclerosis. SEE: *odds ratio; relative risk*.

risk management. A subspecialty in the health care field which addresses the prevention and containment of liability by the careful and objective investigation and documentation of critical or unusual patient care incidents. In psychiatry, risk management deals with preventing suicide and patient-related violence and its associated liability.

risk-taker. An individual who willfully exposes himself or herself to a risk, e.g., a person who engages in activities that others regard as hazardous.

risorius (rĭ-sŏ′rē-ŭs) [L., laughing]. Muscular fibrous band arising over masseter muscle and inserted into tissues at the corner of the mouth. SEE: *Muscles in Appendix*.

ristocetin (rĭs″tō-sē′tĭn). An antibiotic obtained from cultures of *Nocardia lurida*.

risus (rī′sŭs) [L.]. Laughter; a laugh.

    r. sardonicus. A peculiar grin, as seen in tetanus, caused by acute spasm of facial muscles.

Ritalin Hydrochloride. Trade name for methylphenidate hydrochloride.

Ritter's disease (rĭt′ĕrz) [Gottfried Ritter von Rittershain, Ger. physician, 1820–1883]. A generalized form of impetigo of the newborn.

ritual (rĭch′ū-ăl). 1. A routine that the individual feels is essential and should not fail to be carried out. 2. In psychiatry, any activity that is performed compulsively in an attempt to relieve anxiety.

ritual circumcision. SEE: *circumcision, ritual*.

ritualistic surgery. Surgical procedures without scientific justification. Performed in primitive societies without the purpose of treatment or prevention of disease. Included in this are alterations of the skin, ears, lips, teeth, genitalia, and head. In some cases, even in nonprimitive societies, surgical procedures without rational justification are considered to be ritualistic. SEE: *circumcision*.

rivalry (rī′văl-rē). Competition between two individuals, groups, or systems seeking to attain the same goal.

    r., binocular. The continuous alternation in the conscious perception of visual stimuli to the two eyes.

    r., retinal. R., binocular, q.v.

    r., sibling. The competition between children for attention and affection of others, but esp. their parents.

rivalry strife. Alternate sensations of color and shape when the fields of vision of the two eyes cannot combine in one visual image.

Rivinus' canals (rē-vē′nŭs) [August Quirinus Rivinus, Ger. anatomist, 1652–1723]. Ducts of the sublingual glands.

Rivinus' gland. A sublingual gland.

Rivinus' incisure. The tympanic notch in the upper part of the tympanic portion of the temporal bone. It extends from the lesser to the greater tympanic spines and is occupied by the pars flaccida of the tympanic membrane.

Rivinus' ligament. Small portion of the tympanic membrane in the notch of Rivinus. SYN: *Shrapnell's membrane*.

rivus lacrimalis (rī′vŭs) [L. *rivus*, little stream, + *lacrima*, tear]. The pathway under the eyelids for the tears to travel from their source in the lacrimal glands to the punctum lacrimale.

riziform (rĭz′ĭ-form) [Fr. *riz*, rice, + L. *forma*, form]. Resembling rice grains.

R.L.E. *right lower extremity*.

RLF. *retrolental fibroplasia*.

R.L.L. *right lower lobe* of the lung.

RLQ. *right lower quadrant* (of abdomen).

R.M.A. *Registered Medical Assistant; right mentoanterior presentation* (of the fetal face).

RML. *right middle lobe* (of the lung).

R.M.P. *right mentoposterior presentation* (of the fetal face).

RMS. *rhabdomyosarcoma*.

R.M.T. *right mentotransverse* fetal position.

R.N. *registered nurse*.

Rn. Chem. symb. for the element radon.

RNA. *ribonucleic acid*.

RNase. *ribonuclease*.

R.O.A. *right occipitoanterior* fetal position.

Robaxin. Trade name for methocarbamol.

Robert's pelvis (rō′bärts) [Heinrich L. F. Robert, Ger. gynecologist, 1814–1874]. Transverse contraction of the pelvis due to osteoarthritis of the sacroiliac joints.

Robertson's pupil. Argyll Robertson pupil, q.v.

Robicillin VK. Trade name for penicillin V potassium.

Robimycin. Trade name for erythromycin.

Robinul. Trade name for glycopyrrolate.

Robitussin. Trade name for guaifenesin.

Rocaltrol. Trade name for calcitriol.

Rochalimaea quintana. The causative organism of the rickettsial disease trench fever.

Rochelle salt (rō-shĕl'). Potassium sodium tartrate; a colorless, transparent powder having a cooling and saline taste and used as a saline cathartic.

rocker knife. Adapted device for persons with limited upper extremity function. Allows one-handed stabilization and cutting of food.

rocking. A technique in neurodevelopmental rehabilitation designed to increase muscle tone in hypotonic patients through vestibular stimulation.

Rocky Mountain spotted fever. An infectious disease caused by the parasite *Rickettsia ricketsii* transmitted by the wood tick *Dermacentor andersoni* or *Dermacentor variabiles*. Originally thought to exist only in the western U.S., it can occur anywhere that the tick vector is present.

The organism causes vasculitis, giving rise to fever, headache, myalgia, and a characteristic rash. The rash appears several days after other symptoms, first erupting on the wrists and ankles, then on the palms and soles. It is nonpruritic and macular, and spreads to legs, arms, trunk, and face.

TREAT: Tetracycline is the drug of choice.

rod (rŏd) [AS. *rodd*, club]. 1. A slender, straight bar. 2. One of the slender, long, sensory bodies in the retina, which respond to faint light. 3. Bacterium shaped like a rod.

r., Corti's. Pillar cells, q.v.

r.'s, enamel. Minute calcareous rods or prisms laid down by ameloblasts and forming enamel of a tooth.

r., retinal. Visual cells in the eye that are the light-sensing elements of the retina, along with the cones.

rodent. Any mammal of the Rodentia order. Mice, rats, and squirrels are examples.

rodenticide (rō-dĕn'tĭ-sīd) [L. *rodens*, gnawing, + *caedere*, to kill]. An agent that kills rodents.

rodent ulcer [" + *ulcus*, ulcer]. A slowly growing, gnawing cancer that slowly destroys soft tissues and bones, causing great destruction. Usual sites are on outer angle of the eye, near side and on tip of nose, and on edges of the scalp. SYN: *Jacob's ulcer*.

rods and cones. The light-sensitive portions of rod and cone visual cells of the retina. They form the second layer lying between the external limiting membrane and the pigment epithelium. The rods contain visual purple (rhodopsin), which is essential for vision in dim light. SEE: *cone, ocular; night vision.*

Roentgen, Wilhelm Konrad (rĕnt'gĕn). German physicist, 1845–1923, who discovered roentgen rays in 1895 and won the Nobel Prize in physics in 1901.

roentgen (rĕnt'gĕn). ABBR: R. Unit for describing exposure dose of x- or γ-radiation. One unit is sufficient to liberate enough electrons and positrons to produce emissions of either charge of one electrostatic unit of electricity per 0.001293 gm of air. (One cc of dry air at 0°C and at 760 mmHg weighs 0.001293 gm.)

roentgenkymogram (rĕnt"gĕn-kī'mō-grăm) [*roentgen* + Gr. *kyme*, wave, + *gramma*, something written]. A record in the form of a tracing of the heart's action as determined by use of x-ray.

roentgenkymograph (rĕnt"gĕn-kī'mō-grăf) [" + " + *graphein*, to write]. Device for recording the movements of the heart and attached large vessels on a single x-ray film.

roentgenkymography (rĕnt"gĕn-kī-mŏg'ră-fē). Recording of heart movements by use of a roentgenkymograph.

roentgenocinematography (rĕnt"gĕn-ō-sīn"ĕ-mă-tŏg'ră-fē) [" + Gr. *kinema*, motion, + *graphein*, to write]. Moving picture photography of x-ray studies.

roentgenogram (rĕnt-gĕn'ō-grăm, rĕnt'gĕn-ō-grăm"). Film produced by roentgenography. SYN: *radiogram*. Preferred term is radiograph.

roentgenography (rĕnt"gĕn-ŏg'ră-fē) [*roentgen* + Gr. *graphein*, to write]. The process of obtaining pictures by use of roentgen rays. Preferred term is radiography.

r., body section. Tomography, q.v.

r., mucosal relief. X-ray of the intestinal mucosa after ingested barium has been removed and air under slight pressure has been injected. This leaves a light coat of barium on the mucosa and permits x-ray pictures of the fine detail of the mucosa.

r., serial. Taking repeated x-ray pictures of an area at defined but arbitrary intervals.

r., spot-film. X-ray picture taken of a small area during the course of fluoroscopy.

roentgenologist (rĕnt"gĕn-ŏl'ō-jĭst) [" + Gr. *logos*, word, reason]. A physician skilled in roentgen diagnosis, roentgenotherapy, or both. Preferred term is radiologist.

roentgenology (rĕnt"gĕn-ŏl'ō-jē). The science of applying roentgen rays for diagnostic and therapeutic purposes. Preferred term is radiology.

roentgenometer (rĕnt"gĕ-nŏm'ĕ-tĕr) [" + Gr. *metron*, measure]. Radiometer, q.v.

roentgenoscope (rĕnt-gĕn'ō-skōp) [" + Gr. *skopein*, to examine]. A fluoroscope, q.v.

roentgenoscopy (rĕnt"gĕ-nŏs'kō-pē). Fluoroscopy.

roentgenotherapy,   roentgentherapy (rĕnt"gĕn-ō-thĕr'ăp-ē) [*roentgen* + Gr. *therapeia*, treatment]. The treatment of disease by exposure of the patient to roentgen rays. Preferred term is radiotherapy.

roentgen ray. X-ray, q.v.

roeteln, roetheln (rĕt′ĕln) [Ger.]. German measles; rubella.

Roger's disease (rō-zhāz′) [Henri L. Roger, Fr. physician, 1809–1891]. Ventricular septal defect.

Rokitansky's disease (rō″kĭ-tăn′skēz) [Karl Freiherr von Rokitansky, Austrian pathologist, 1804–1878]. Acute yellow atrophy of the liver.

Rolaids. Trade name for dihydroxyaluminum sodium carbonate.

Rolando's area (rō-lăn′dōz) [Luigi Rolando, It. anatomist, 1773–1831]. Motor area in the cerebral cortex.

Rolando's fissure. Fissure between the parietal and frontal lobes. SYN: *sulcus centralis.*

role (rōl) [O. Fr. *rolle,* roll of paper on which a part is written]. The characteristic social behavior of an individual in relationship to the group.

    r., gender. SEE: *gender role.*

role model. The demonstration of the behavior associated with a particular position or profession that serves as an example for others.

role playing. The assignment and acting out of a role in a treatment setting to provide individuals the opportunity to see themselves as others do. Also used as a method of teaching such skills as interviewing, taking history, and doing a physical examination.

rolfing [Ida Rolf, U.S. physiotherapist, 1897–1979]. Deep massage of the tissues around muscles. The purpose is to increase the range of motion of the joints and to enhance suppleness.

rolitetracycline (rō″lē-tĕt″rä-sī′klēn). USP. An antibiotic drug. Trade name is Syntetrin.

roll. A usually solid, cylindrical structure.

    r., cotton. A cylindrical mass of purified and sterilized cotton used as packing or absorbent material in various dental procedures.

    r., ilial. A sausage-shaped mass in the left iliac fossa. It is due to a collection of feces in or induration of the walls of the sigmoid colon.

    r., scleral. Spur, scleral, q.v.

roller (rōl′ĕr) [O. Fr., roll]. 1. Strip of muslin or other cloth rolled up in cylinder form for surgeon's use. 2. A roller bandage. SEE: *bandage.*

ROM. *read-only memory; rupture of membranes.*

R.O.M. *range of motion.* SEE: *exercise, range of motion.*

roman numerals. Letters used by the ancient Romans for numeration in contradistinc-

tion to the arabic numerals that we now use. In roman notations, values are changed either by adding one or more symbols to the initial symbol or by subtracting a symbol from one or more to the right of it. Ex.: V is 5, IV is 4, and VI is 6. Thus, since X is 10, IX is 9 and XI is 11. SEE: *roman numerals* in *Appendix.*

romanopexy (rō-măn′ō-pĕk″sē) [L. *romanum,* the sigmoid, + Gr. *pexis,* fixation]. Fixation of the sigmoid flexure for prolapse of the rectum. SYN: *sigmoidopexy.*

romanoscope (rō-măn′ō-skōp) [″ + Gr. *skopein,* to examine]. Instrument for examining the sigmoid flexure.

rombergism (rŏm′bĕrg-ĭzm). While a patient is standing with feet close together, the tendency to fall when the eyes are closed. SEE: *Romberg's sign.*

Romberg's sign (rŏm′bĕrgs) [Moritz Heinrich Romberg, Ger. physician, 1795–1873]. Inability to maintain the body balance when the eyes are shut and the feet close together. The sign is positive if the patient sways and falls when the eyes are closed. Seen in sensory ataxia.

Rondomycin. Trade name for methacycline hydrochloride.

rongeur (rŏn-zhŭr′) [Fr., to gnaw]. An instrument for removing small amounts of tissue, particularly bone. A rongeur is a spring-loaded forceps with a sharp blade that may be either end cutting or side cutting. Also called *bone nippers.*

Roniacol. Trade name for nicotinyl alcohol.

roof nucleus. Small mass of gray matter in white substance of vermis of the cerebellum.

room [AS. *rum*]. An area or space in a building, partitioned off for occupancy or available for specific procedures.

    r., clean. Room, particularly one housing delicate electronic medical instruments, that is constructed so as to be isolated from the free entry of air. Air that enters is filtered, and personnel wear special clothing to prevent particles from their bodies from becoming freely dispersed in the room.

    r., dark-. SEE: *darkroom.*

    r., delivery. Room to which an obstetric patient is taken for childbirth.

    r., dust-free. A type of room designed to eliminate or reduce particulate matter, including airborne microorganisms, from circulating. This kind of room is useful in housing burn patients, in removing allergens from the air, in transplantation surgery, and in preparing drugs and solutions for intravenous use.

    r., intensive therapy. Intensive care room in which patients who need close medical attention and use of various medical devices such as resuscitation equipment are treated.

r., labor. Room in which an obstetric patient is placed during the first stage of labor, prior to being taken to the delivery room.

r., operating. A hospital room used for surgical procedures.

r., postdelivery. Room in which patients are kept following childbirth.

r., recovery. Recovery room, q.v.

rooming-in. The placing of infants in the same hospital room as their mothers, beginning immediately following birth.

root (rūt) [AS. *rot*]. 1. Underground part of a plant. 2. Proximal end of a nerve. 3. Portion of an organ implanted in tissues. SYN: *radix* [NA]. 4. Part of the human tooth covered by cementum, and designated by location, i.e., mesial, distal, buccal, lingual.

r., anterior. One of two roots by which a spinal nerve is attached to the spinal cord. Contains efferent nerve fibers.

r., dorsal. Radix dorsalis or sensory root of each spinal nerve.

r., motor. The anterior and motor division of a spinal nerve.

r., posterior. One of two roots by which a spinal nerve is attached to the spinal cord. Contains afferent nerve fibers.

r., sensory. R., dorsal, q.v.

r., ventral. R., motor, q.v.

root arteries. Arteries accompanying nerve roots into the spinal cord.

root canal. Pulp cavity of root of a tooth; colloquially, the procedure for preserving a tooth by removing its diseased pulp cavity.

root formation. The development of root of teeth by Hertwig's root sheath and the epithelial diaphragm. It involves the formation of root dentin with a covering of cementum essential for the attachment of the tooth to the surrounding bony tissues. Root formation or development continues for months or years after the tooth has erupted into the mouth.

rooting reflex. SEE: *reflex, rooting.*

root pick. A dental instrument for retrieving root fragments resulting from tooth extraction. SYN: *apical elevator.*

root planing. Deep scaling of tooth roots to remove calculus, diseased cementum or dentin, microbial flora and bacterial toxins. The smooth health root facilitates reattachment of the soft tissues of the periodontium.

root resorption of teeth. Condition of the roots of teeth caused by endocrine imbalance or excessive pressure of orthodontic appliances. X-ray photographs demonstrate roots that appear to be sawed off or shortened.

root sheath. 1. Epithelium covering the hair follicle. 2. The epithelial covering that induces root formation in teeth. Also: *Hert-*

wig's root sheath.

root zone. Burdach's column of the spinal cord. Outer tract of posterior funiculus or white column of the cord. SYN: *fasciculus cuneatus.*

R.O.P. *right occipitoposterior.* Fetal presentation, in which the occiput of the fetus is in relationship to the right sacroiliac joint of the mother.

Rorschach test (ror'shăk) [Hermann Rorschach, Swiss pyschiatrist, 1884–1922]. A psychological test consisting of 10 different inkblot designs. The subject is asked to interpret each design individually. This may reveal disturbances in personality.

rosa (rō'ză) [L.]. Rose.

rosacea (rō-zā'sē-ă) [L. *rosaceus,* rosy]. A chronic disease of the skin of the face in middle-aged and older persons. The cause is unknown. Characterized by varying degrees of papules, pustules, and hyperplasia (or rhinophyma) of the soft tissues of the nose. The onset is usually between 30 and 50 years of age, but may be as early as 10 or may occur first in old age. In adults, it occurs three times as often in females as in males.

TREAT: Symptomatic. Apply 15% precipitated sulfur to the lesions; give broad-spectrum antibiotics orally. Isotretinoin and topical metronidazole are also effective.

Rhinophyma may be treated surgically, but may recur.

rosaniline (rō-zăn'ĭ-lĭn). A basic dye used in preparing other dyes.

rosary (rō'ză-rē). Something that resembles a string of beads.

r., rachitic. Palpable areas at the site of joining of the ribs to their cartilages. This is seen in conjunction with rickets.

Rose, Frank A. (rōz). British surgeon.

R.'s position. The patient's head in a fully extended position is allowed to hang over the end of the operating room table. This prevents aspiration of blood during surgery on the mouth and lips.

rose bengal sodium I 131. USP. A standardized preparation of radioactive iodine and rose bengal used in photoscanning the liver and testing liver function.

rose fever. Summer or June cold; hay fever of early summer attributed to inhaling rose pollen. SEE: *hay fever.*

Rosenbach, Ottomar (rō'zĕn-bŏk). German physician, 1851–1907.

R.'s sign. 1. Fine rapid tremor of closed eyelids. Seen in hyperthyroidism. 2. In hysteria, inability to obey command to close eyes. 3. Absence of abdominal skin reflex in intestinal inflammation or hemiplegia.

R.'s test. A test for bile in the urine. Urine is passed several times through the same filter paper. After the paper has dried, a drop of nitric acid is added to it. If bile is present, a play of colors is produced.

Rosenmüller, Johann Christian (rō'zĕn-mil"ĕr). German anatomist, 1771–1820.

R.'s body. A rudimentary structure located in the mesosalpinx. Consisting of a longitudinal duct (duct of Gartner) and 10 to 15 transverse ducts, it is the remains of the upper portion of the mesonephros and is the homologue of the head of the epididymis in the male. SYN: *epoophoron; parovarium.*

R.'s cavity. Slitlike depression in the pharyngeal wall behind the opening of the eustachian tube.

roseo- [L. *roseus,* rosy]. 1. Combining form meaning rose-colored. 2. A prefix in chemical terms.

roseola (rō-zē'ō-lă, rō"zē-ō'lă) [L. *roseus,* rosy]. Skin condition marked by maculae or red spots of varying sizes on the skin; any rose-colored rash.

r. idiopathica. Macular eruptions not associated with any well-defined symptoms.

r. infantum. A noninfectious roseola occurring in infants. Characterized by high fever, splenomegaly, and a rash that appears just as the fever subsides. SYN: *exanthem subitum.*

r. symptomatica. Macular eruption occurring in well-defined disease.

roseolous (rō-zē'ō-lŭs) [L. *roseus,* rosy]. Resembling or pert. to roseola.

rosette [Fr., small rose]. 1. Something that resembles a rose. 2. A spherical group of fine red vacuoles surrounding cytocentrum of a monocyte.

rose water. Saturated aqueous solution of the oil of rose. Used to impart agreeable odor to lotions.

rose water ointment. USP. An emollient used to soften the skin. It contains waxes, almond oil, sodium borate, rose water, rose oil, and purified water.

rosin (rŏz'ĭn) [L. *resina*]. USP. Substance distilled from species of pine and used as a stiffening agent in preparing plasters.

Ross' bodies [Edward Halford Ross, Brit. pathologist, 1875–1928]. Copper-colored, round bodies showing dark granules. Found in blood and tissue fluids in syphilis. Sometimes they exhibit ameboid movements.

Rossolimo's reflex (rŏs"ō-lē'mōz) [Gregoriy I. Rossolimo, Russian neurologist, 1860–1928]. Plantar flexion of second to fifth toes in response to percussion of plantar surface of the toes.

rostellum (rŏs-tĕl'lŭm) [L., little beak] (pl. *rostella*). A fleshy protrusion on anterior end of scolex of tapeworms bearing one or more rows of spines or hooks.

rostral (rŏs'trăl) [L. *rostralis*]. 1. Resembling a beak. 2. Toward the front or cephalic end of the body.

rostrate (rŏs'trāt) [L. *rostratus,* beaked]. Having a beak or hook formation.

rostriform (rŏs'trĭ-form) [" + *forma,* shape]. Shaped like a beak.

rostrum (rŏs'trŭm) [L., beak] (pl. *rostrums, rostra*). Any hooked or beaked structure.

rosulate (rŏs'ū-lāt) [L. *rosulatus,* like a rose]. Shaped like a rosette.

R.O.T. *right occipitotransverse* fetal position.

rot (rŏt) [ME. *roten*]. To decay or decompose.

r., jungle. Common term for certain fungus diseases of the skin that occur in the tropics.

rotameter (rō-tăm'ē-tĕr). Device for measuring the flow of gas or a liquid.

rotate (rō-tāt) [L. *rotare,* to turn]. To twist or revolve.

rotating tourniquet. SEE: *tourniquet, rotating.*

rotation (rō-tā'shŭn) [L. *rotatio,* a turning]. Process of turning on an axis.

r., fetal. Twisting of the fetal head as it follows the curves of the birth canal downward.

r., optical. SEE: *optical activity.*

r., tooth. The process by which a tooth is repositioned by turning it on its long axis to a more normal occlusal position.

rotator (rō-tā'tor) (pl. *rotatores*). A muscle revolving a part on its axis.

rotaviruses (rō'tă-vī"rŭs-ĕs) [L. *rota,* wheel, + *virus,* poison]. A group of viruses that are a major cause of sporadic acute enteritis in infants and small children, and epidemic acute gastroenteritis.

röteln, rötheln (rĕt'ĕln) [Ger. *rot,* red]. German measles. SYN: *roeteln; rubella.*

rotenone (rō'tĕn-nōn). A poisonous chemical, $C_{23}H_{22}O_6$, used as an insecticide.

Roth's spots [Moritz Roth, Swiss physician and pathologist, 1839–1914]. Small white spots in the retina close to the optic disk. They are often surrounded by areas of hemorrhage.

ETIOL: Systemic infection, particularly cases of acute infective endocarditis.

rototome. Device for cutting tissue. Used in arthroscopic surgery.

rotoxamine tartrate (rō-tŏks'ă-mēn). An antihistamine drug.

Rouget's cells (roo-zhāz') [Charles M. B. Rouget, Fr. physiologist, 1824–1904]. Contractile cells that surround the capillaries. Observed in frogs and salamanders.

rough (rŭf). Not smooth.

roughage (rŭf'ĭj) [AS. *ruh,* rough]. Indigestible fiber of fruits, vegetables, and cereals that acts as a stimulant to aid intestinal peristalsis. Plenty of water should be added to consumption of roughage. Should not be used in colitis or in intestinal irritation.

SYN: *fiber, dietary.* SEE: *cellulose.*

rouleau (roo-lō′) [Fr., roll] (pl. *rouleaux*). A group of red blood corpuscles arranged like a roll of coins.

round (rownd) [O. Fr. *ronde*]. 1. Circular in shape. 2. Spherical, globular.

round ligament. 1. Curved fibrous cord attached to the center of articular surface of the head of the femur. 2. Two round cordlike structures passing from front of the body of the uterus in anterior wall of broad ligament, below the fallopian tubes, outward through the inguinal canals to soft tissues of the labia majora. 3. Fibrous cord that is the remnant of the umbilical vein.

roundworm. Any member of the phylum Nemathelminthes (Aschelminthes), esp. one belonging to the class Nematoda, q.v. SYN: *threadworm.*

Roux-en-Y. Anastomosis of the distal divided end of the small bowel to another organ such as the stomach or esophagus. The proximal end is anastomosed to the small bowel below the anastomosis.

Roven's IMDC [Milton D. Roven, contemporary U.S. podiatrist]. A new procedure for *intramedullary metatarsal decompression* performed through a small dorsal incision. It is less traumatic than previous procedures, allowing immediate ambulation and minimal postoperative pain and edema.

Royal Free disease [After Royal Free Hospital, London, from which cases were reported in 1955]. Postviral fatigue syndrome, q.v.

RPF. *renal plasma flow.*

rpm. *revolutions per minute.*

RPO. *right posterior oblique* position.

RPS. *renal pressor substance.* SEE: *renin.*

R.Q. *respiratory quotient.*

R.R.A. *registered record administrator.*

-rrhagia (rā′jē-ă) [Gr. *rhegnynai*, to burst forth]. Combining form indicating abnormal discharge, hemorrhage.

-rrhaphy [Gr. *raphe*, suture]. Suffix concerning sutures or surgical repair.

-rrhea [Gr. *rhoia*, flow]. Suffix concerning flow or discharge.

-rrhexis [Gr. *rhexis*, a breaking, bursting]. Suffix concerning rupture.

rRNA. *ribosomal RNA.*

R.S.A. *right sacroanterior* fetal position.

R.Sc.A. *right scapuloanterior* fetal position.

R.Sc.P. *right scapuloposterior* fetal position.

R.S.P. *right sacroposterior* fetal position.

R.S.T. *right sacrotransverse* fetal position.

R.S.V. *respiratory syncytial virus; Rous sarcoma virus.*

R.T. *radiation therapy; reading test; registered technologist.*

R.T.(N.) *registered technologist — nuclear medicine.*

R.T.(R.) *registered technologist radiographer.*

R.T.(T.). *registered technologist — radiation therapy.*

R.U. *rat unit.*

RU486. An abortifacient used in some countries. It is not used more than 47 days after the last menstrual period. A prostaglandin is administered by injection or as a suppository as an adjunct to RU486. One of its trade names is Mifepristone.

Ru. Chem. symbol for the element ruthenium.

rub. Friction of one surface moving over another. In auscultation, a roughened surface moving over another causes a characteristic sound.

    r., pericardial. The sound heard by use of auscultation with each heartbeat when the inflamed pericardial surface moves over the heart.

    r., pleural friction. Friction rub caused by inflammation of the pleural space.

rubber dam. Thin rubber tissue used by dentists to seal off the tooth from saliva in the mouth during dental treatment.

rubbing alcohol. USP. A preparation containing not less than 68.5% and not more than 71.5% by volume of dehydrated alcohol. The remainder consists of water and denaturants and may or may not contain color additives and perfume oils. Used as a rubefacient, q.v.

Caution: Because of the added denaturant, it is poisonous if taken internally.

---

rubedo [L. *ruber*, red]. Redness of the skin. May be temporary.

rubefacient (roo″bĕ-fā′shĕnt) [L. *rubefaciens*, making red]. 1. Causing redness, as of the skin. 2. Agent that reddens the skin, producing a local congestion, the vessels becoming dilated and the supply of blood increased. Rubefacients include mustard, turpentine, capsicum, flaxseed, arnica, rubbing alcohol, and liniments.

rubella (roo-bĕl′ă) [L. *rubellus*, reddish]. Acute infectious disease resembling both scarlet fever and measles, but differing from them in that it has a short course, causes a slight fever, and is free from sequelae. SYN: *German measles; roeteln; röteln.* SEE: *Nursing Diagnoses* in *Appendix.*

    SYM: Prodromes, slight or altogether absent. Drowsiness, slight fever, sore throat. Eruption first or second day. In some cases rash composed of pale red, scarcely elevated papules, more or less discrete rubella morbilliform; in others rash is bright red and diffuse like that of scarlet fever, rubella scarlatiniform. Rash begins on face, spreads rapidly over whole body, but fades so rapidly that face may be clear before extremities are affected. Slight desquamation frequently present, though not always. Superficial cervical and posterior auricular glands more swollen than in measles. Duration is 3 to 5 days.

INCUB: 14 to 21 days. Rubella produces a maculopapular rash that desquamates and vanishes in 2 to 3 days.

COMP: Rubella in pregnant women, esp. in first two or three months of gestation, is serious in that it may give rise to fetal anomalies, esp. congenital cataract.

TREAT: Nonspecific. Local antipruritics for itching; rest; liquid diet; sponging with tepid water.

PROG: Good.

rubella titer. Serology test to determine immune status to rubella.

rubella virus vaccine, live. USP. A standardized preparation of live rubella virus. Used to immunize against rubella. Trade name is Meruvax.

rubeola (roo-bē′ō-lă, roo″bē-ō′lă) [L. *rubeolus,* reddish]. 1. Acute contagious disease marked by fever, catarrhal symptoms, and a typical cutaneous eruption. SYN: *measles.* 2. Term occasionally applied to acute infectious disease with mild symptoms and rose-colored macular eruption.

rubeosis iridis. A condition in which new blood vessels form on the anterior surface of the iris. Associated with vascular disease that affects the retinal vein of the eye. Seen most frequently in diabetics, although it is not limited to these patients. Leads to painful, hemorrhagic glaucoma.

ruber (roo′bĕr) [L.]. Red.

rubescent (roo-bĕs′ĕnt) [L. *rubescere,* to grow red]. Growing red; flushing.

rubidium (roo-bĭd′ē-ŭm) [L. *rubidus,* red]. SYMB: Rb. At. wt. 85.47; at. no. 37. A soft, silvery metal that decomposes water with violence and bursts into flame spontaneously in air. Its salts are used medicinally.

rubiginous (roo-bĭj′ĭ-nŭs) [L. *rubiginosus*]. Rusty or rust-colored.

rubigo (roo-bī′gō) [L., rust]. Rust; mildew.

Rubin's test (roo′bĭns) [Isidor Clinton Rubin, U.S. physician, 1883–1958]. Transuterine insufflation of the fallopian tubes with carbon dioxide to test their patency. SEE: *sterility.*

Rubner's test (roob′nĕrz) [Max Rubner, Ger. physiologist, 1854–1932]. 1. A test for lactose or glucose in the urine. 2. A test for carbon monoxide in blood.

rubor (roo′bor) [L.]. Discoloration or redness caused by inflammation. It is one of the four classic symptoms of inflammation. The others are calor (heat), dolor (pain), and tumor (swelling).

Rubramin PC. Trade name for cyanocobalamin.

rubriblast (roo′brī-blăst) [L. *rubrica,* red, + Gr. *blastos,* germ]. Pronormoblast.

rubric (roo′brĭk) [L. *ruber,* red]. 1. Concerning or being red. 2. An established procedure or protocol.

rubricyte (roo′brī-sīt) [L. *ruber,* red, + Gr. *kytos,* cell]. Polychromatic normoblast.

rubrospinal (roo″brō-spī′năl) [″ + *spina,* thorn]. A descending tract consisting of a small bundle of nerve fibers in lateral funiculus of spinal cord. Fibers arise in cells of the red nucleus of midbrain and terminate in ventral horn of gray matter.

rubrothalamic (roo″brō-thăl-lăm′ĭk) [″ + Gr. *thalamos,* chamber]. Concerning the red nucleus of the brain and thalamus.

rubrum (roo′brŭm) [L., red]. Red nucleus of gray matter in crus cerebri near optic thalamus.

    r. scarlatinum. Scarlet red, a substance used as a healing agent and stain.

ructus (rŭk′tŭs) [L.]. Belching of air from stomach. SYN: *eructation.*

rudiment (roo′dĭ-mĕnt) [L. *rudimentum,* beginning]. 1. That which is undeveloped. 2. In biology, a part just beginning to develop. 3. Remains of a part functional at an earlier stage of one's development or in one's ancestors.

rudimentary (roo″dĭ-mĕn′tă-rē) 1. Elementary. 2. Undeveloped; not fully formed; remaining from an earlier stage. SYN: *vestigial.*

rudimentum (roo″dĭ-mĕn′tŭm) [L., beginning]. Rudiment.

Ruffini's corpuscles (roo-fē′nēz) [Angelo Ruffini, It. anatomist, 1864–1929]. Encapsulated sensory nerve endings found in subcutaneous tissue, thought to mediate sense of warmth. SYN: *organ of Ruffini.*

rufous (roo′fŭs) [L. *rufus,* red]. Ruddy; having a ruddy complexion and reddish hair.

ruga (roo′gă) [L.] (pl. *rugae*). A fold or crease, esp. one of the folds of mucous membrane seen on internal surface of the stomach.

    rugae of vagina. Small ridges on inner surface of the vagina extending laterally and upward from the columna rugarum (long ridges on anterior and posterior walls).

Ruggeri's reflex [Ruggero Ruggeri, It. physician, d. 1905]. Increase in pulse rate when eyes are strongly converged on a near object.

rugine (roo-zhēn′). 1. Periosteal elevator. 2. A raspatory.

rugose, rugous (roo′gōs, -gŭs) [L. *rugosus,* wrinkled]. Having many wrinkles or creases.

rugosity (rū-gŏs′ĭ-tē) [L. *rugositas*]. 1. Condition of being folded or wrinkled. 2. A ridge or wrinkle.

R.U.L. *right upper lobe* of lung.

rule (rool) [ME. *riule*]. A guide or principle based on experience or observation.

   r. of nines. Formula for estimating percentage of body surface areas. It is particularly helpful in judging the portion of skin that has been burned. The head represents 9%; each upper extremity 9%; the back of the trunk is 18%, and the front is 18%; each lower extremity represents 18%; and the perineum makes up the remaining 1%. SEE: *burn* for illus.

   r. of ten. Criteria used to judge the readiness of an infant for surgical repair of a cleft lip. The infant must weigh 10 pounds, be 10 weeks of age, have a hemoglobin of 10 grams, and a white blood cell count less than 10,000.

rum [origin obscure]. 1. An alcoholic beverage prepared from fermented sugar cane juice. 2. Colloquially, any alcoholic beverage.

rum fits. A type of convulsive seizure associated with withdrawal from the state of chronic inebriation due to abuse of alcohol. Most occur during the 7- to 48-hour period following abstinence. There may be a single seizure, but in most cases they occur in bursts of two to six. It is unlikely that this type of seizure represents a form of epilepsy.

ruminant (roo′mĭ-nănt). An animal that regurgitates food in order to chew it again. This is called chewing the cud.

rumination (roo″mĭ-nā′shŭn) [L. *ruminatio*]. 1. Regurgitation, esp. with rechewing, of previously swallowed food. This condition may be present in otherwise normal individuals, in emotionally deprived or mentally retarded infants, or mentally retarded adults. 2. In psychiatry, obsessional preoccupation of the mind by a single idea or a set of thoughts, and inability to dismiss or dislodge them. SYN: *merycism*.

rump (rŭmp) [ME. *rumpe*]. Posterior end of the back, the gluteal region, or buttocks.

Rumpf's symptom (roompfs) [Heinrich Theodor Rumpf, Ger. physician, 1851–1923]. 1. In neurasthenia, quickening of the pulse when pressure is exerted over a painful spot. 2. Twitching after strong faradization, in traumatic neuroses.

run [AS. *rinnan*, run]. To exude pus or mucus.

runaround, runround. Superficial infection encircling the fingernail. SYN: *whitlow*.

runners' high. Many persons who partake of an intensive exercise program, such as running, have found that after achieving a new level of physical fitness, they experience a feeling of elation and euphoria as they continue to run and at the completion of a running session. The relation of this to the stimulation of endorphin production by the exercise is unknown. SEE: *endorphins*.

rupia (roo′pē-ă) [Gr. *rhypos*, filth]. A cutaneous eruption, usually of tertiary syphilis, that first manifests itself by large elevations of the epidermis filled with a clear or blood-stained serum, soon becoming turbid and purulent. The bulla bursts and allows some fluid to escape. As it desiccates, it is covered with a crust that dries, accumulates new layers, and becomes covered with greenish-brown scales, sometimes to depth of ½ in. (13 mm). It is the thickest of all syphilides and presents the most extensive ulcerations.

   TREAT: Antisyphilitic antibiotics.

rupioid (roo′pē-oyd) [″ + *eidos*, form, shape]. Resembling rupia.

rupophobia (roo″pō-fō′bē-ă) [″ + *phobos*, fear]. Abnormal dislike for dirt or filth. SYN: *rhypophobia*.

rupture (rŭp′chŭr) [L. *ruptura*, breaking]. 1. A breaking apart of an organ or tissue. 2. Hernia.

   r. of membranes. Rupture of amniotic sac as normal result of dilation of the cervix uteri in labor.

   r. of perineum. Rupture of perineum in labor, a condition that can be prevented by episiotomy, q.v. More frequent in primiparas.

   r. of tubes. Rupture of a fallopian tube, a serious event in extrauterine pregnancy. May occur without the woman's knowledge of her pregnancy.

   r. of uterus. Rare rupture due to unrelieved obstructed labor.

RUQ. *right upper quadrant* of abdomen.

rush. 1. A strong contraction wave that moves down the small intestine. 2. The first surge of pleasure produced by a drug, esp. a narcotic drug.

Russell bodies (rŭs′ĕl) [William Russell, Scot. physician, 1852–1940]. Small spherical hyaline bodies in cancerous and simple inflammatory growths.

Russell's viper venom (rŭs′ĕlz) [Patrick Russell, Irish physician who worked in India, 1727–1805]. The venom from Russell's viper. It is used in investigating defective blood coagulation due to a deficiency of Factor X.

Russian bath. Hot vapor bath followed by friction and a plunge in cold water.

Rust's disease (rŭsts) [Johann N. Rust, Ger. surgeon, 1775–1840]. Tuberculosis of cervical vertebrae and their articulations.

rusts. Members of an order of parasitic fungi (Uredinales), all of which are parasitic on plants. Many are allergens.

rusty (rŭst′ē) [AS. *rustig*]. Reddish in color.

Resembling, or containing, rust. SYN: *rubiginous*.

rut (rŭt) [O. Fr. *ruit*, roaring of deer]. In lower male animals, seasonal period of sexual excitement during which mating usually takes place. SEE: *estrus; heat.*

rut-formation. In psychology, loss of interest in environment, fixation upon a single object, and concentration of emotional or other interests in a groove or rut.

ruthenium (roo-thē'nē-ŭm). SYMB: Ru. At. wt. 101.07; at. no. 44. A hard, brittle, metallic element of platinum group.

rutherford [Ernest Rutherford, Brit. physicist, 1871–1937]. ABBR: rd. A unit of radioactivity representing 10^6 disintegrations per second.

rutidosis (roo″tĭ-dō'sĭs) [Gr. *rhytis*, wrinkle].

Contraction or puckering of cornea just before death. SYN: *rhytidosis; rytidosis.*

rutilism (roo'tĭl-ĭzm) [L. *rutilis*, red, + Gr. *-ismos*, condition]. Having red or auburn-colored hair.

rutin (roo'tĭn). A crystalline glucoside of quercetin, closely related to hesperidin. Derived from buckwheat but present in many plants.

RV. *residual volume; right ventricle.*

rye (rī) [AS. *ryge*]. A cereal grass that produces a grain used in food and beverage production. When rye grain is infected with a certain fungus, ergot is produced.

rytidosis (rĭt″ĭ-dō'sĭs) [Gr. *rhytis*, a wrinkle, + *osis*, condition]. Wrinkling or contraction of cornea preceding death. SYN: *rhytidosis; rutidosis.*

S

σ. Sigma, the eighteenth letter of the Greek alphabet. In statistics, the symbol for standard deviation.

Σ. Capital of the Greek letter sigma. In statistics, the symbol for summation.

S. L. *signa*, mark, or let it be written — term used in prescription writing to indicate the instructions to the patient that the pharmacist will place on the dispensed medicine; *smooth*, description of bacterial colonies; *spherical* or *spherical lens; subject* (pl. *Ss*), participant in an experiment; chem. symb. for the element sulfur.

s. L. *semis*, half; *sinister*, left.

s̄, s. Symb. for [L.] *sine*, without; used as a form of shorthand in hospital charts and clinical records.

S1, S2, etc. *first sacral nerve, second sacral nerve.*

S_1, S_2. Normal first and second heart sounds.

S_3. Ventricular gallop.

S_4. Atrial gallop.

S-A, SA, S.A. *sinoatrial.*

saber shin. Anterior border of the tibia marked with sharp convexity, found in hereditary syphilis.

Sabin vaccine [Albert Bruce Sabin, Russ.-born U.S. virologist, b. 1906]. An oral vaccine for poliomyelitis. SYN: *live oral poliovirus vaccine.* SEE: *poliomyelitis.*

sabulous (săb'ū-lŭs) [L. *sabulosus*, sand]. Gritty; sandy.

saburra (să-bŭr'ră) [NL., sand]. Foulness of stomach or mouth due to decayed food. SYN: *sordes.*

sac (săk) [L. *saccus*, sack, bag]. A baglike part of an organ, a cavity or pouch, sometimes containing fluid. SYN: *saccus.* SEE: *cyst.*

    s., air. An alveolar cell in the lung. SEE: *s., alveolar.*

    s., allantoic. The expanded end of the allantois, well developed in birds and reptiles.

    s., alveolar. The terminal portion of an air passageway within the lung. Its wall contains pocketlike structures (alveoli), and each alveolar sac is connected to a respiratory bronchiole by an alveolar duct.

    s., amniotic. A thin membrane, containing a serous fluid, enclosing the embryo. SYN: *amnion.*

    s., chorionic. Saclike structure, consisting of chorion, that encloses the developing embryo.

    s., conjunctival. The cavity, lined with conjunctiva, that lies between the eyelids and anterior surface of the eye.

    s., dental. The mesenchymal tissue surrounding a developing tooth.

    s., endolymphatic. The expanded distal end of the endolymphatic duct.

    s., heart. Pericardium.

    s., hernial. Saclike protrusion of the peritoneum, containing a herniated organ. SEE: *hernia; hernial sac.*

    s., lacrimal. Upper dilated portion of the nasolacrimal duct.

    s., lesser peritoneal. A cavity within the layers of the peritoneum forming the great omentum. Its opening into the main peritoneal cavity is via the epiploic foramen. SYN: *omental bursa.*

    s., vitelline. S., yolk.

    s., yolk. An extra-embryonic membrane that encloses the yolk in reptiles, birds, and monotremes. It is formed of an inner layer of entoderm invested by splanchnic mesoderm. In marsupials and placental mammals that lack a yolk mass, the yolk sac is a rudimentary vesicle lying within the chorionic sac.

saccades (să-kāds') [Fr. *saccade*, jerk]. Fast, involuntary movements of the eyes as they change from one point of gaze to another.

saccadic (să-kăd'ĭk) [Fr. *saccade*, jerk]. Pert. to rapid intermittent movements, esp. of the eye. This type of eye movement is important when the fovea follows a moving target. SEE: *nystagmus; vergence.*

saccate (săk'āt) [NL. *saccatus*, baglike]. 1. Pert. to, like, or enclosed in a sac. SYN: *encysted.* 2. In bacteriology, marking a sac-shaped form, as in a type of liquefaction.

saccharase (săk'ă-rās) [Sanskrit *sarkara*, sugar]. An enzyme that catalyzes the breakdown of disaccharides to monosaccharides, esp. the hydrolysis of sucrose to dextrose. Ex.: sucrase, invertase.

saccharated (săk'ă-rāt"ĕd). Containing sugar.

saccharic acid. A dibasic acid, $C_6H_{20}O_8$, formed by the action of nitric acid on dextrose.

saccharide (săk'ă-rīd). A group of carbohydrates including sugars. It is divided into the following classifications: monosaccharides, disaccharides, trisaccharides, and polysaccharides.

sacchariferous (săk"ă-rĭf'ĕr-ŭs) [Sanskrit *sarkara*, sugar, + L. *ferre*, to carry]. Producing or containing sugar.

saccharification (săk"ăr-ĭ-fĭ-kā'shŭn) [" + L. *facere*, to make]. Conversion into sugar.

saccharin (săk′ă-rĭn). C₇H₅NO₃S. A sweet, white, powdered, synthetic product derived from coal tar, 300 to 500 times as sweet as sugar. Used as artificial sweetener. Its use is now restricted because of its ability to cause cancer in experimental animals.

saccharine (săk′ă-rĭn, -rīn) [L. *saccharum*, sugar]. Of the nature of, or having the quality of, sugar. SYN: *sweet*.

saccharo- [Sanskrit *sarkara*, sugar]. Combining form meaning sugar.

saccharogalactorrhea (săk″ă-rō-gă-lăk″tō-rē′ă) [″ + Gr. *gala*, milk, + *rhoia*, flow]. Excessive lactose secreted in milk.

saccharolytic (săk″ă-rō-lĭt′ĭk) [″ + Gr. *lysis*, dissolution]. Able to split up sugar.

Saccharomyces (săk″ă-rō-mī′sēz) [Sanskrit *sarkara*, sugar, + Gr. *mykes*, fungus] (pl. *saccharomycetes*). A genus of fungi, reproducing by budding. SYN: *yeasts*.

saccharomycosis (săk″ă-rō-mī-kō′sĭs) [″ + ″ + *osis*, condition]. Any disease or pathological condition due to yeasts or saccharomycetes.

saccharum (săk′ă-rŭm) [L.]. Sugar.
   s. album. White crystallized sugar.
   s. canadense. Maple sugar.
   s. candidum. Rock candy.
   s. lactis. Sugar of milk. SYN: *lactose*.
   s. ustum. Burnt sugar; caramel.

sacciform (săk′sĭ-form) [L. *saccus*, sack, bag, + *forma*, shape]. Bag-shaped or like a sac. SYN: *saccate*.

saccular (săk′ū-lăr) [NL. *sacculus*, small bag]. Having the shape of or resembling a sac.

sacculated (săk′ū-lāt″ĕd) [NL. *sacculus*, small bag]. Consisting of small sacs or saccules.

sacculation (săk″ū-lā′shŭn). 1. Formation into a sac or sacs. 2. Group of sacs, collectively.

saccule (săk′ūl) [NL. *sacculus*, small bag]. 1. A small sac. 2. The smaller of two sacs comprising the portion of the membranous labyrinth occupying the vestibule of the inner ear. It communicates with the utricle, cochlear duct, and endolymphatic duct, all of which are filled with endolymph. In its wall is the macula sacculi, a sensory area.
   s. laryngeal. A small diverticulum extending ventrally from the laryngeal ventricle lying between the ventricular fold and the thyroarytenoid muscle. SYN: *ventricular appendix*.

sacculocochlear (săk″ū-lō-kŏk′lē-ăr) [″ + Gr. *kokhlos*, land snail]. Concerning the saccule and cochlea of the ear.

sacculus (săk′ū-lŭs) [NL., small bag] (pl. *sacculi*). A saccule or little sac.
   s. laryngis. A blind sac extending up from the laryngeal ventricle to between the vestibular fold and the inner surface of the

thyroid cartilage.

saccus (săk′ŭs) [L., sack, bag] (pl. *sacci*). [NA] A sac or pouch.
   s. endolymphaticus. [NA] Dilated, blind end of the ductus endolymphaticus.
   s. lacrimalis. [NA] The lacrimal sac, into which empty the two lacrimal ducts.

SACH foot. Acronym for *solid ankle cushion heel foot*. A prosthetic (artificial) foot that has no definite ankle joint but is designed to absorb shock and allow movement of the shank over the foot during ambulation.

sacrad (sā′krăd) [L. *sacrum*, sacred, + *ad*, toward]. In the direction of the sacrum.

sacral (sā′krăl) [L. *sacralis*]. Rel. to the sacrum.

sacral bone. A triangular bone made up of five fused vertebrae just above the coccyx. SYN: *sacrum*.

sacral canal. Continuation of the vertebral canal in the sacrum.

sacral flexure. Rectal curve in front of the sacrum.

sacralgia (sā-krăl′jē-ă) [L. *sacrum*, sacred, + Gr. *algos*, pain]. Pain in the sacrum. SYN: *hieralgia*.

sacral index. Sacral breadth multiplied by 100 and divided by sacral length.

sacralization (sā″krăl-ĭ-zā′shŭn). Fusion of the sacrum and the 5th lumbar vertebra.

sacral nerves. Five pairs of spinal nerves, the upper four of which emerge through the posterior sacral foramina, the fifth pair through the sacral hiatus (termination of sacral canal). All are mixed nerves (motor and sensory).

sacral plexus. Plexus of sacral nerves from which sciatic nerve originates. It is a part of the lumbosacral plexus.

sacral vertebra. Fused vertebrae forming the sacrum.

sacrectomy (sā-krĕk′tō-mē) [L. *sacrum*, sacred, + Gr. *ektome*, excision]. Excision of part of the sacrum.

sacro- (sā′krō) [L. *sacrum*, sacred]. Prefix indicating relationship to the sacrum.

sacroanterior (sā″krō-ăn-tē′rē-or) [″ + *anterior*, before]. Denoting intrauterine fetal position in which the fetal sacrum is directed anteriorly.

sacrococcygeal (sā″krō-kŏk-sĭj′ē-ăl) [″ + Gr. *kokkyx*, coccyx]. Concerning the sacrum and coccyx.

sacrococcygeus (săk″rō-kŏk-sĭj′ē-ŭs). One of two small muscles (anterior and posterior) extending from the sacrum to coccyx.

sacrocoxalgia (sā″krō-kŏks-ăl′jē-ă) [″ + *coxa*, hip, + Gr. *algos*, pain]. Pain in the sacroiliac joint, usually due to inflammation. SEE: *sacrocoxitis*.

sacrocoxitis (sā″krō-kŏks-ī′tĭs) [″ + ″ + Gr. *itis*, inflammation]. Inflammation between the sacrum and coccyx.

sacrodynia (sā″krō-dĭn′ē-ă) [″ + *odyne*, pain]. Pain in the region of the sacrum.

sacroiliac (sā″krō-ĭl′ē-ăk) [″ + *iliacus*, hipbone]. Of, or pert. to, the sacrum and ilium.

sacroiliac joint. The articulation between the sacrum and the innominate bone of the pelvis. Joint movement is limited because of interlocking of the articular surfaces.

sacroiliitis (sā″krō-ĭl″ē-ī′tĭs) [″ + ″ + Gr. *itis*, inflammation]. Inflammation of the sacroiliac joint.

sacrolisthesis (sā″krō-lĭs-thē′sĭs) [″ + Gr. *olisthesis*, a slipping]. A deformity in which the sacrum is in front of the last lumbar vertebra. SEE: *spondylolisthesis*.

sacrolumbar (sā″krō-lŭm′băr) [″ + *lumbus*, loin]. Of, or concerning, the sacrum and lumbar area.

sacrolumbar angle. Angle formed by articulation of the last lumbar vertebra and the sacrum.

sacroposterior (sā″krō-pŏs-tē′rē-or) [″ + *posterus*, behind]. Denoting intrauterine fetal position in which the fetal sacrum is directed posteriorly.

sacrosciatic (sā″krō-sī-ăt′ĭk) [″ + *sciaticus*, hipjoint]. Concerning the sacrum and ischium.

sacrospinal (sā″krō-spī′năl) [″ + *spina*, thorn]. Concerning the sacrum and spine.

sacrospinalis [″ + *spina*, thorn]. A large muscle lying on either side of the vertebral column extending from the sacrum to the head. Its two chief components are the iliocostalis and longissimus muscles. SEE: *Muscles* in *Appendix*.

sacrotomy (sā-krŏt′ō-mē) [″ + Gr. *tome*, incision]. Surgical excision of the lower part of the sacrum.

sacrouterine (sā″krō-ū′tĕr-ĭn) [″ + *uterus*, womb]. Concerning the sacrum and uterus.

sacrovertebral (sā″krō-vĕr′tĕ-brăl) [″ + *vertebra*, vertebra]. Concerning the sacrum and spinal column.

sacrovertebral angle. Angle formed by the base of the sacrum and 5th lumbar vertebra.

sacrum (sā′krŭm) [L., sacred]. The triangular bone situated dorsal and caudal from the two ilia between the 5th lumbar vertebra and the coccyx. It is formed of five united vertebrae and is wedged between the two innominate bones, its articulations forming the sacroiliac joints. It forms the base of the vertebral column and, with the coccyx, forms the posterior boundary of the true pelvis. The sacrum in a male is narrower and more curved than in a female. SYN: *vertebra magnum*. SEE: illus.

sactosalpinx (săk″tō-săl′pĭnks) [Gr. *saktos*,

stuffed, + *salpinx*, tube]. Dilated fallopian tube due to retention of secretions, as in pyosalpinx or hydrosalpinx.

SAD. *seasonal affective disorder.*

saddle. A surface or structure that resembles a seat used to ride a horse. The base of artificial dentures is often referred to as a saddle.

saddle area. The portion of the buttocks, perineum, and thighs that would come in contact with the seat of the saddle when riding a horse.

saddle back. Term applied to an exaggerated curve of the lower back, lordosis, q.v.

saddle block anesthesia. Type of anesthesia produced by introducing the anesthetic agent into the 4th lumbar interspace. This anesthetizes the perineum and buttocks area.

saddle joint. Joint with articulating surfaces convex in one direction and concave in the other.

Ex.: carpometacarpal joint of the thumb.

saddle nose. A nose with a depressed bridge due to congenital absence of bony or cartilaginous support or due to a disease such as leprosy or congenital syphilis.

sadism (sā′dĭzm, săd′ĭzm) [Comte Donatien Alphonse François de Sade, Marquis de Sade, 1740–1814]. Conscious or unconscious sexual pleasure derived from inflicting mental or physical pain on others. SEE: *algolagnia; masochism*.

sadist (sā′dĭst, săd′ĭst). One who practices sadism.

sadness. A normal emotional feeling of dejection or melancholy. A result of an unhappy event or situation that warrants a change in the emotional state. Not to be confused with depression, in which the person is melancholic for no apparent reason or the degree of depression is out of proportion to the cause for sadness.

sadomasochism (sā″dō-măs′ĕ-kĭzm, săd″ō-măs′ĕ-kĭzm). Sexual pleasure related to both sadism and masochism.

sadomasochist (sā″dō-măs′ĕ-kĭst). One whose personality includes sadistic and masochistic elements.

Saemisch's ulcer (sā′mĭsh-ĕs) [Edwin Theodor Saemisch, Ger. ophthalmologist, 1833–1909]. Serpiginous infectious ulcer of the cornea.

safelight. Darkroom device that emits a light of a specified wavelength that is harmless to undeveloped film.

safe sex. With respect to protecting oneself from sexually transmitted diseases including AIDS, q.v., there are no absolutely safe sexual practices except celibacy and masturbation. Nevertheless, if both partners have no clinical or laboratory evidence of AIDS, then they could use condoms and en-

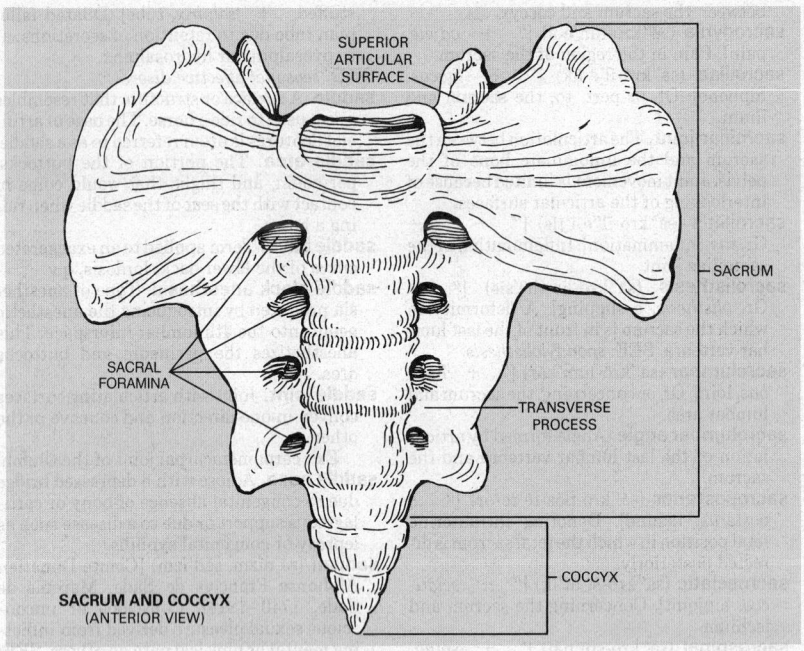

SUPERIOR
ARTICULAR
SURFACE

SACRUM

SACRAL
FORAMINA

TRANSVERSE
PROCESS

COCCYX

SACRUM AND COCCYX
(ANTERIOR VIEW)

gage in intimate sexual activities provided that neither partner has outside sexual partners or other risk factors for AIDS. Conversely, if both partners have evidence of infection with HIV (human immunodeficiency virus), then the main concern is that effective birth control measures be employed. Any heterosexual person having casual sexual contacts should avoid anal intercourse and should use condoms. Homosexuals engaging in casual sexual activity should avoid anal intercourse and should use condoms for all other sexual activity in which orgasm could lead to semen contacting the skin or mucosa of the partner. It is important to realize that a single negative laboratory test for AIDS may provide a false sense of security. Also, the time required for a test for AIDS to become positive after infection may be years. SEE: *AIDS; condom, instructions for use; sexually transmitted disease.*

safflower oil. Oil expressed from the seeds of the safflower plant, *Carthamus tinctorius.* It is high in linoleic acid and low in saturated fatty acids.

sagittal (săj′ĭ-tăl) [L. *sagittalis*]. Arrowlike; in an anteroposterior direction.

sagittalis (săj″ĭ-tā′lĭs) [L.]. Sagittal, q.v.

sagittal plane. A vertical plane through the longitudinal axis of the trunk dividing the body into two portions. If it is through the anterior-posterior midaxis and divides the body into right and left halves, it is called a median or midsagittal plane.

sagittal sinus. The superior longitudinal sinus.

sagittal sulcus. Groove on inner surface of parietal bones, forming a channel for the superior sagittal sinus.

sagittal suture. Suture between the two parietal bones.

sago (sā′gō) [Malay *sagu*]. A substance prepared from various palms, consisting principally of starches. Used as a demulcent and as a food with little residue.

St. Joseph's Cough Syrup for Children. Trade name for dextromethorphan hydrobromide.

Saint Vitus' dance. Nervous disease with involuntary jerking motions. SYN: *chorea, Sydenham's.*

sal (săl) [L.]. Salt; or a substance resembling salt.

    s. ammoniac. Chloride of ammonia.
    s. soda. Sodium carbonate.

salaam convulsion (sŭ-lŏm′) [Arabic *salam*, peace]. Clonic spasm of the sternomastoid muscles resulting in a bowing movement. SYN: *nodding spasm.*

salacious (sĕ-lā'shŭs) [L. *salax*, lustful]. Lustful or inciting to lust.

salicylamide (săl″ĭ-sĭl-ăm'ĭd). The amide of salicylic acid, $C_7H_7NO_2$. An analgesic drug.

salicylanilide (săl″ĭ-sĭl-ăn'ĭ-lĭd). An antifungal drug.

salicylate (săl″ĭ-sĭl'āt, săl-ĭs'ĭl-āt). Any salt of salicylic acid.

> **s., methyl.** The principal constituent of oil of wintergreen. It is applied externally as a counterirritant.

> **s., sodium.** White crystalline substance with disagreeable taste, in some cases even nauseating. Used to reduce pain and temperature. SEE: *acetylsalicylic acid.*

salicylated (săl-ĭs'ĭl-āt-ĕd). Impregnated with salicylic acid.

salicylate poisoning. SEE: *aspirin poisoning.*

salicylazosulfapyridine (săl″ĭ-sĭl″ă-zō-sŭl″fă-pĭr'ĭ-dēn). Previously used name for sulfasalazine, q.v.

salicylic acid (săl″ĭ-sĭl'ĭk). USP. $C_7H_6O_3$. A white crystalline acid derived from phenol.

> USES: In making aspirin; as a preservative and flavoring agent; and in external treatment of certain skin conditions.

salicylism (săl'ĭ-sĭl″ĭzm). Toxic condition caused by an overdose of salicylic acid or its derivatives.

salicylsulfonic acid test. Test for albumin in urine. SEE: *albumin.*

salicyluric acid (săl″ĭ-sĭ-lū'rĭk). Acid found in urine after an individual takes salicylic acid or its derivatives.

salient [L. *salio*, to spring, jump]. Prominent, conspicuous.

salifiable (săl″ĭ-fī′ă-bl) [L. *sal*, salt, + *fieri*, to be made]. Capable of forming a salt by combining with an acid.

salify (săl'ĭ-fī) [″ + *fieri*, to be made]. To convert to a salt.

salimeter (săl-ĭm'ĕ-ter) [″ + Gr. *metron*, a measure]. Device for testing strength of saline solutions.

saline (sā'līn, sā'lēn) [L. *salinus*, of salt]. Containing or pert. to salt; salty.

> **s., hypertonic.** Aqueous solution of sodium chloride of greater than 0.85%.

> **s., hypotonic.** Aqueous solution of sodium chloride of less than 0.85%.

saline cathartic. A salt, such as epsom salts, used to produce evacuation of the bowel.

saline enema. Enema consisting of a salt solution, used to induce peristalsis and evacuation. The salt solutions most frequently used are physiological saline; 1 teaspoonful (4 gm) table salt (sodium chloride) dissolved in 1 pint (500 ml) of warm water (115°F or 46.1°C); and epsom salts (magnesium sulfate) 15 to 113 gm in a sufficient quantity of warm water to dissolve the salt.

saline solution. A solution of sodium chloride and distilled water. A 0.9% solution of sodium chloride is considered isotonic to the body. A normal saline solution (one having an osmolality similar to blood serum) consists of 0.85% salt solution, which is necessary to maintain osmotic pressure and the stimulation and regulation of muscular activity. SEE: *physiological salt solution.*

salinometer (săl″ĭ-nŏm'ĕ-tĕr) [L. *salinus*, of salt, + *metron*, measure]. An instrument for determining the salt content of a solution.

saliva (să-lī'vă) [L., spittle]. Salivary gland and oral mucous gland fluid, the secretion that begins the process of digesting food.

> CHARACTER: It is normally tasteless, clear, odorless, viscid, and weakly alkaline, being neutralized after being acted upon by gastric acid in the stomach. Sp. gr. 1.002 to 1.006. The amount secreted in 24 hours is estimated to be 1500 ml. The flow varies from 0.2 ml per minute from resting glands to 4.0 ml per minute with maximum secretion.

> COMP: Inorganic substances: 99.5% water; salts (chlorides, carbonates, phosphates, sulfates); gases in solution; and sometimes abnormal substances being excreted from the body, e.g., acetone. Organic substances include enzymes (ptyalin, maltase, lysozyme); proteins (serum albumin and globulin, mucin); and small amounts of urea, uric acid, creatine, and amino acids. Cellular elements include epithelial cells and leukocytes.

> FUNCT: To moisten food, facilitating mastication and deglutition; to moisten and lubricate mouth parts; to act as a solvent for excretion of waste products; to initiate digestion of starches; to assist in regulation of water balance.

> RS: aptyalism; parotid; ptyalin; ptyalism; salivary digestion; salivary glands; sialagogue.

> **s., artificial.** A solution that is useful in treating excessive dryness of the mouth (xerostomia). One such formula is 20 ml of a 4% solution of methylcellulose, 10 ml of glycerin, sufficient normal saline to make 90 ml, and one drop of lemon oil.

saliva ejector. Device used during dental work to remove saliva.

salivant (săl'ĭ-vănt) [L. *saliva*, spittle]. Something that stimulates the flow of saliva.

salivary (săl'ĭ-vĕr-ē) [L. *salivarius*, slimy]. Pert. to, producing, or formed from saliva.

salivary corpuscles. Nucleated spherical bodies in saliva thought to be modified leukocytes from lymphatic tissue.

salivary digestion. Digestion occurring in the mouth resulting from action of salivary enzymes. Ptyalin, a salivary enzyme, is an amylase that initiates the breakdown of starch and glycogen to maltose and a small amount of glucose. Oral digestion is limited because of the short time food remains in the mouth, but digestion continues in the stomach until food becomes acidified by gastric juice. The optimum pH for ptyalin activity is 6.9. SEE: *digestion.*

salivary glands. The glands of the oral cavity that secrete saliva. The major glands are paired and include the parotid, below the ear and inside the ramus of the mandible; the sublingual, below the tongue in the anterior floor of the mouth; and the submandibular, below the posterior floor of the mouth, medial to the body of the mandible. Minor salivary glands are numerous in the oral cavity and are named according to their locations: lingual, sublingual, palatal, buccal, labial, and glossopharyngeal.

Salivary secretion is under nervous control, being reflexly initiated by mechanical, chemical, or radiant stimuli acting on taste buds (gustatory receptors) in the mouth, olfactory receptors, visual receptors (eyes), or other sense organs. Secretion may also occur as a result of conditioned reflexes, as when one thinks about food or hears a dinner bell.

NERVE SUPPLY: Facial and glossopharyngeal nerves and from the autonomic nervous system.

BLOOD SUPPLY: Branches from the external carotid artery.

salivation (săl″ĭ-vā′shŭn) [LL. *salivatio*, to spit out]. 1. The act of secreting saliva. 2. Excessive secretion of saliva. SYN: *ptyalism.*

salivatory (săl′ĭ-vă-tor″ē). Producing secretion of saliva.

salivolithiasis (să-lī″vō-lĭ-thī′ă-sĭs) [L. *saliva*, spittle, + Gr. *lithos*, stone, + *-iasis*, condition]. Sialolithiasis, q.v.

Salk vaccine (sŏlk) [Jonas E. Salk, U.S. microbiologist, b. 1914]. First successful poliomyelitis vaccine; it contains three types of formalin-inactivated poliomyelitis viruses. It induces immunity against the disease. SEE: *poliomyelitis.*

sallow (săl′ō) [AS. *salo*]. Of a sickly, yellow color, usually said of complexion or skin.

salmin(e) (săl′mēn, -mĭn) [L. *salmo*, salmon]. $C_{30}H_{57}N_{14}O_6$. A toxic protamine obtained from spermatozoa of salmon. SEE: *protamine; protein.*

Salmonella (săl″mō-nĕl′ă) [Daniel Elmer Salmon, U.S. veterinarian, 1850–1914]. A genus of bacteria belonging to the family Enterobacteriaceae. Salmonella are gram-negative, usually motile, rods. More than 1400 species have been classified. Several species are pathogenic, some producing mild gastroenteritis, others producing a severe and often fatal food poisoning. SEE: *egg, raw; salmonellosis.*

S. arizonae. Species that may be isolated from animals and humans. In humans, may cause gastroenteritis, urinary tract infection, bacteremia, meningitis, osteomyelitis, and brain abscess.

S. choleraesuis. Species often found to be the cause of septicemia.

S. enteritidis. Species causing gastroenteritis and food poisoning in humans.

S. paratyphi. A group of organisms of *Salmonella*, types A, B, and C, that cause paratyphoid fever.

S. typhi. Species causing typhoid fever, q.v., in humans.

S. typhimurium. Species frequently isolated from persons having acute gastroenteritis.

salmonellosis (săl-mō-nĕ-lō′sĭs). Infestation with bacteria of genus *Salmonella*. Three forms of salmonella infection occur in man: enteric fever (typhoid fever); septicemia, which usually is caused by *Salmonella choleraesuis;* and acute gastroenteritis, which can be caused by a variety of species of *Salmonella.* SEE: *egg, raw.*

salmon patch. Salmon-colored areas of the cornea in syphilitic keratitis. SYN: *Hutchinson's patch.*

salpingectomy (săl″pĭn-jĕk′tō-mē) [Gr. *salpinx*, tube, + *ektome*, excision]. Surgical removal of the fallopian tube.

salpingemphraxis (săl″pĭn-jĕm-frăk′sĭs) [″ + *emphraxis*, a stoppage]. Obstruction of the eustachian tube.

salpingian (săl-pĭn′jē-ăn). Concerning the eustachian tube or fallopian tube.

salpingion (săl-pĭn′jē-ŏn). A point at the inferior surface of the apex of the petrous portion of the temporal bone.

salpingitis (săl″pĭn-jī′tĭs) [Gr. *salpinx*, tube, + *itis*, inflammation]. Inflammation of the fallopian tube.

ETIOL: The condition may be acute, subacute, or chronic. The organisms most often associated with salpingitis are the gonococcus, staphylococcus, streptococcus, chlamydia, colon bacillus, and tubercle bacillus.

s., eustachian. Inflammation of the eustachian tube. SYN: *eustachitis.*

s., gonococcal. Salpingitis due to gonococci.

salpingo- [Gr. *salpinx*, tube]. Combining form concerning the auditory (eustachian) or fallopian tube.

salpingocatheterism (săl-pĭng″gō-kăth′ĕt-ĕr-ĭzm) [″ + *katheter*, something inserted, + *-ismos*, condition]. Catheterization of the eustachian tube.

salpingocele (săl-pĭng'gō-sēl) [″ + *kele*, tumor, swelling]. Hernial protrusion of a fallopian tube.

salpingocyesis (săl-pĭng″ō-sī-ē'sĭs) [″ + *kyesis*, pregnancy]. Pregnancy in which fetus begins to develop in a fallopian tube; tubal pregnancy.

salpingography (săl″pĭng-gŏg'ră-fē) [″ + *graphein*, to write]. Radiographic study of the fallopian tubes into which a radiopaque dye has been introduced. Used in testing for patency of the tubes in investigating infertility.

salpingolithiasis (săl-pĭng″gō-lĭ-thī'ă-sĭs) [″ + *lithos*, stone, + *iasis*, condition]. Presence of calculi in the fallopian tube.

salpingolysis (săl″pĭng-gŏl'ĭ-sĭs) [″ + *lysis*, dissolution]. Surgical disruption of adhesions in the fallopian tube.

salpingo-oophorectomy (săl-pĭng″gō-ō″ŏf-ō-rĕk'tō-mē) [″ + *oon*, egg, + *phoros*, a bearer, + *ektome*, excision]. Excision of an ovary and fallopian tube. SYN: *salpingo-ovariectomy*.

salpingo-oophoritis (săl-pĭng″ō-ō″ŏf-ō-rī'tĭs) [″ + ″ + ″ + *itis*, inflammation]. Inflammation of a fallopian tube and ovary. SYN: *salpingo-oothecitis*.

salpingo-oophorocele (săl-pĭng″gō-ō-ŏf'or-ō-sēl) [Gr. *salpinx*, tube, + *oon*, egg, + *phoros*, a bearer, + *kele*, tumor, swelling]. Hernia enclosing the ovary and fallopian tube.

salpingo-oothecitis (săl-pĭng″gō-ō″ō-thē-sī'tĭs) [″ + *ootheke*, ovary, + *itis*, inflammation]. Inflammation of a fallopian tube and ovary. SYN: *salpingo-oophoritis*.

salpingo-oothecocele (săl-pĭng″gō-ō″ō-thē'kō-sēl) [″ + ″ + *kele*, tumor, swelling]. Hernia of the ovary and fallopian tube.

salpingo-ovariectomy (săl-pĭng″gō-ō″văr-ē-ĕk'tō-mē) [″ + LL. *ovarium*, ovary, + Gr. *ektome*, excision]. Surgical removal of an ovary and fallopian tube. SYN: *salpingo-oophorectomy*.

salpingoperitonitis (săl-pĭng″gō-pĕr″ĭ-tō-nī'tĭs) [″ + *peritonaion*, peritoneum, + *itis*, inflammation]. Inflammation of the serosal covering of the fallopian tubes.

salpingopexy (săl-pĭng'ō-pĕk″sē) [″ + *pexis*, fixation]. Fixation of a fallopian tube.

salpingopharyngeal (săl-pĭng″gō-fă-rĭn'jē-ăl) [″ + *pharynx*, throat]. Concerning the eustachian tube of the ear and the pharynx.

salpingopharyngeus (săl-pĭng″gō-făr-ĭn'jē-ŭs) [″ + *pharynx*, throat]. The muscle arising near the opening of the eustachian tube. Raises the nasopharynx.

salpingoplasty (săl-pĭng'gō-plăs″tē) [″ + *plassein*, to form]. Plastic surgery of the fallopian tube. Used in treating female infertility. SYN: *tuboplasty*.

salpingorrhaphy (săl″pĭng-gor'ă-fē) [″ + *rhaphe*, seam, ridge]. Suture of a fallopian tube.

salpingosalpingostomy (săl-pĭng″gō-săl″pĭng-gŏs'tō-mē) [″ + *salpinx*, tube, + *stoma*, mouth]. The operation of attaching one fallopian tube to the other.

salpingoscope (săl-pĭng'gō-skōp″) [″ + *skopein*, to examine]. Device for examining the nasopharynx and eustachian tube.

salpingostenochoria (săl-pĭng″gō-stĕn″ō-kor'ē-ă) [″ + *stenos*, narrow, + *choreia*, dance]. Stenosis or stricture of the eustachian tube.

salpingostomatomy (săl-pĭng″gō-stō-măt'ō-mē) [″ + *stoma*, mouth, + *tome*, incision]. Creation of an artificial opening in a fallopian tube after it has been occluded as a result of inflammation and scarring.

salpingostomy (săl-pĭng-ŏs'tō-mē). Surgical opening of a fallopian tube that has been occluded, or for drainage purposes.

salpingotomy (săl-pĭng-ŏt'ō-mē) [″ + *tome*, incision]. Incision of a fallopian tube.

salpingo-ureterostomy (săl-pĭng″gō-ūr-ēt″ĕr-ŏs'tō-mē) [″ + *oureter*, ureter, + *stoma*, mouth]. Surgical connection of the ureter and the fallopian tube.

salpingysterocyesis (săl″pĭng-jĭs″tĕr-ō-sī-ē'sĭs) [″ + *hystera*, uterus, + *kyesis*, pregnancy]. Pregnancy in which the embryo is located at the entrance of the fallopian tube into the uterus; ectopic pregnancy.

salpinx (săl'pĭnks) [Gr., tube] (pl. *salpinges*). The fallopian or eustachian tube.

salt [AS. *sealt*]. 1. White crystalline compound occurring in nature, known chemically as sodium chloride, $NaCl$. 2. Containing, or treated with salt. 3. To treat with salt. 4. In the plural, any mineral salt or saline mixture used as an aperient or cathartic, esp. epsom salts or Glauber's salt. 5. In chemistry, a compound consisting of a positive ion other than hydrogen, and a negative ion other than hydroxyl. 6. A chemical compound resulting from the interaction of an acid and a base.

Salts and water are the inorganic or mineral constituents of the body. They play specific roles in the functions of cells and are indispensable for life. The principal salts are chlorides, carbonates, bicarbonates, sulfates, and phosphates, combined with sodium, potassium, calcium, or magnesium.

In general, salts serve the following roles in the body: maintenance of proper osmotic conditions; maintenance of water balance and regulation of blood volume; maintenance of proper acid-base balance; provision for essential constituents of tissue, esp.

bones and teeth; maintenance of normal irritability of muscle and nerve cells; maintenance of condition for coagulation of the blood; provision for essential components of certain enzyme systems, respiratory pigments, and hormones; regulation of cell membrane and capillary permeability. SEE: *sodium chloride.*

RS: chloride; low-salt diet; normal; sal; saline; salt-free diet; salt glow; secretion; sodium chloride.

s., acid. Salt in which one or more hydrogen atoms remain unreplaced by the hydroxyl (OH) radical.

s., basic. Salt in which the ability to react with an acid radical still remains.

s., bile. Salt of glycocholic and taurocholic acid present in bile.

s., buffer. Salt that fixes excess amounts of acid or alkali without a change in hydrogen-ion concentration.

s., double. Any salt formed from two other salts.

s., epsom. Magnesium sulfate.

s., Glauber's. Sodium sulfate.

s., haloid. Any salt of a halogen, i.e., chloride, iodide, bromide, or fluoride.

s., iodized. Salt containing 1 part sodium or potassium iodide to 10,000 parts of sodium chloride. An important source of iodine in the diet. Use of this form of salt will prevent goiter.

s., neutral. Any salt that contains no replaceable hydrogen or hydroxyl groups. SYN: *s., normal.*

s., Rochelle. Potassium sodium tartrate, used as a saline cathartic.

s., rock. Native sodium chloride.

s., smelling. Aromatized ammonium carbonate.

saltation (săl-tā′shŭn) [L. *saltatio*, leaping]. 1. Act of leaping or dancing, as in chorea. 2. Abrupt variation in character of a species. SYN: *mutation.*

saltatory (săl′tă-tō″rē). Marked by dancing or leaping.

saltatory conduction. Skipping from node to node, said of movement of the potential along myelinated neurons.

saltatory spasm. Tic of muscles of lower extremity, causing convulsive leaping upon attempt to stand. SEE: *Jumping Frenchmen of Maine; miryachit; palmus.*

salt-free diet. It is impractical to attempt to maintain a diet absolutely free of sodium chloride. Thus salt-free means a low-sodium diet that allows 500 mg (0.5 gm) or less of salt per day. On this diet, table salt should not be added to the food. Also, it is important to know the amount of salt in the drinking water and in commonly used beverages such as beer, because water in some

areas contains a large amount of sodium. Some medicines (for example, sodium salicylate) are quite high in sodium content. Exclusion of sodium-containing medicines is important in attempting to regulate the amount of sodium consumed. SEE: *salt.*

salt glow. Rubbing the entire body with moist salt for stimulation.

salting out. A method of separating a specific protein from a mixture of proteins by the addition of a salt, e.g., ammonium sulfate.

salt-losing syndrome. The condition of greatly increased loss of sodium from the body due to renal disease, adrenocortical insufficiency, or gastrointestinal disease.

saltpeter, saltpetre (sawlt-pē′těr) [L. *sal*, salt, + *petra*, rock]. A common name for potassium nitrate.

s., Chile. A common name for sodium nitrate, NaNO₃. Crystalline powder, saline in taste and soluble in water.

salt-poor diet. Diet in which all food is prepared and served without the addition of salt, including salt-free bread and butter. Milk intake is limited.

salts. Pl. of salt.

salt solution, normal. SEE: *salt solution, physiological.*

salt solution, physiological. A sterile solution containing 0.9% of sodium chloride in chemically pure distilled water (9 gm sodium chloride in 1000 ml or 1 liter of distilled water).

salt substitute. A substance intended for human consumption that has a flavor similar to salt, but is low in sodium content. Used by individuals whose medical condition requires limited salt intake.

salubrious (să-lū′brē-ŭs) [L. *salubris*, healthful]. Promoting or favorable to health; wholesome.

saluresis (săl″ū-rē′sĭs) [L. *sal*, salt, + Gr. *ouresis*, urination]. The excretion of sodium chloride in the urine.

saluretic (săl″ū-rĕt′ĭk). Something that promotes excretion of sodium chloride in the urine.

Saluron. Trade name for hydroflumethiazide.

salutary (săl′ū-tā″rē) [L. *salutaris*, health]. Healthful; promoting health; curative.

Salvarsan (săl′văr-săn) [L. *salvus*, safe, + Gr. *arsen*, arsenic]. An arsenical, yellow powder preparation developed by Paul Ehrlich for treatment of syphilis. Since the development of penicillin, there has been little need for Salvarsan. SYN: *arsphenamine.*

salve (săv) [AS. *sealf*]. 1. An ointment applied to wounds. 2. In pharmacology, any ointment or cerate made with a base of a fat, oil, petrolatum, or resin.

Samaritans. In England, a private organization providing 24-hour telephone service to befriend people passing through personal crises and in imminent danger of taking their own lives. In 1953, the founder, the Reverend Chad Varah, realized that persons in despair could be helped simply by talking with them. In 1985 the Samaritans received over 2 million telephone calls.

samarium (să-mā'rē-ŭm). SYMB: Sm. At. wt. 150.35; at. no. 62; sp. gr. approx. 7.50. A very rare metallic element.

sample. 1. A piece or portion of a whole that will demonstrate the characteristics or quality of the whole, such as a specimen of blood. 2. In research, a portion of a population selected to be representative of the entire population.

    s., biased. In epidemiology or medical research, a sample of a group of which each member did not have an equal opportunity of being selected in the sample.

sampling. The process of selecting a portion or part to represent the whole.

    s., random. One of several ways of selecting a sample of a population. This method involves using a listing of the entire population and a table of random numbers to select the sample.

sanative (săn'ă-tĭv) [L. *sanare*, to cure]. Of a healing nature. SYN: *curative.*

sanatorium (săn"ă-tō'rē-ŭm) [L. *sanatorius*, healing]. An establishment for preservation of health, or for the treatment of the chronically sick. SYN: *sanitarium.*

sanatory (săn'ă-tō"rē). Curative; conducive to health.

sand (sănd) [AS.]. Fine grains of disintegrated rock.

    s., auditory. Calcareous concretion in labyrinth of the ear. SYN: *ear dust; otoconium; otolith.*

    s., brain. Concretion of matter near base of the pineal gland. SYN: *acervulus cerebri.*

sandflies. Flies of the order Diptera belonging to the genus *Phlebotomus.* They transmit sandfly fever, Oroya fever, and various types of leishmaniasis.

sandfly fever. A mild virus disease that clinically resembles influenza, except for absence of respiratory symptoms. The causative organism, any one of three species of arboviruses, is transmitted by the common sandfly *Phlebotomus papatasii,* a small, hairy, blood-sucking midge that bites at night and has a limited flight range. The disease occurs in tropical and subtropical areas that experience long periods of hot, dry weather. There is no specific therapy. SYN: *pappataci fever; phlebotomus fever.*

Sandhoff's disease. A rare form of Tay-Sachs disease, q.v., in which two essential enzymes (hexosaminidase A and B) for metabolizing gangliosides are absent. In Tay-Sachs disease only one enzyme, hexosaminidase A, is absent.

Sandril. Trade name for reserpine, USP.

Sandwith's bald tongue (sănd'withs) [Fleming M. Sandwith, Br. physician, 1777–1843]. Abnormally clean tongue seen in late stages of pellagra.

sane (sān) [L. *sanus,* healthy]. Sound of mind; mentally normal.

Sanfilippo's disease [S. J. Sanfilippo, contemporary U.S. pediatrician]. A hereditary disease transmitted as an autosomal recessive. Characterized by severe progressive mental retardation and mild dwarfism, skeletal defects, and hepatosplenomegaly. SYN: *mucopolysaccharidosis III.*

sanguicolous (săng-gwĭk'ō-lŭs) [L. *sanguis,* blood, + *colere,* to dwell]. Inhabiting the blood, as a parasite.

sanguiferous (săng-gwĭf'ĕr-ŭs) [" + *ferre,* to carry]. Conducting or containing blood, as the circulatory organs.

sanguimotor, sanguimotory (săng"gwĭ-mō'tor, -tō-rē) [" + *motor,* a mover]. Pert. to blood circulation.

sanguine (săng'gwĭn) [L. *sanguineus,* bloody]. 1. Optimistic; cheerful. 2. Plethoric, bloody; marked by abundant and active blood circulation, particularly a ruddy complexion. 3. Pert. to, or consisting of, blood.

sanguineous (săng-gwĭn'ē-ŭs) [L. *sanguineus,* bloody]. 1. Bloody; rel. to blood. 2. Having an abundance of blood. SYN: *plethoric.*

sanguinolent (săng-gwĭn'ō-lĕnt) [L. *sanguinolentus,* bloody]. Containing, or tinged with, blood.

sanguinopoietic (săng"gwĭn-ō-poy-ĕt'ĭk) [L. *sanguis,* blood, + *poiein,* to form]. Forming or making blood. SYN: *hematopoietic; sanguifacient.*

sanguinopurulent (săng"gwĭ-nō-pū'rū-lĕnt) [" + *purulentus,* full of pus]. Concerning or containing blood and pus.

sanguinous (săng'gwĭ-nŭs) [L. *sanguineus,* bloody]. Sanguineous, q.v.

sanguirenal (săng"gwĭ-rē'năl) [L. *sanguis,* blood, + *ren,* kidney]. Pert. to the blood supply of the kidneys.

sanguis (săng'gwĭs) [L.] [NA] Blood.

sanguisuga (săng-gwĭ-sū'gă) [" + *sugere,* to suck]. A leech or bloodsucker. SEE: *Hirudo.*

sanguivorous (săng-gwĭv'ō-rŭs) [" + *vorare,* to eat]. Blood-eating.

sanies (sā'nē-ēz) [L., thin, fetid pus]. A thin, fetid, greenish discharge from a wound or ulcer, presenting appearance of pus tinged with blood.

saniopurulent (să"nē-ō-pū'roo-lĕnt) [L. *sanies,* thin, fetid pus, + *purulentus,* full of pus]. Having characteristics of sanies and pus; pert. to a fetid, serous, blood-tinged discharge containing pus.

sanioserous (să″nē-ō-sē′rŭs) [″ + *serum,* whey]. Composed of sanies and serum.

sanitarian (săn″ĭ-tā′rē-ăn) [L. *sanitas,* health]. A person who by training and experience is skilled in sanitation and public health.

sanitarium (săn-ĭ-tā′rē-ŭm) [L. *sanitas,* health]. Institution for treatment and recuperation of persons having physical or mental disorders; occasionally limited to place where conditions are prophylactic rather than therapeutic. SYN: *sanatorium.*

sanitary (săn′ĭ-tā″rē) [L. *sanitas,* health]. 1. Promoting or pertaining to conditions that are conducive to good health. 2. Clean, free of dirt.

sanitary napkin. Perineal pad, esp. one used for absorbing menstrual fluid. SEE: *tampon, menstrual.*

sanitation (săn″ĭ-tā′shŭn) [L. *sanitas,* health]. The formulation and application of measures to promote and establish conditions favorable to health, esp. public health. SEE: *hygiene.*

sanitization (săn″ĭ-tĭ-zā′shŭn) [L. *sanitas,* health]. The act of making sanitary.

sanitize (săn′ĭ-tīz). To make sanitary.

sanitizer. An agent that reduces the number of bacterial contaminants to safe levels as judged by public health requirements. Usually used to describe agents applied to eating and drinking utensils and dairy equipment.

sanity (săn′ĭ-tē). Soundness of health or mind; mentally normal.

San Joaquin valley fever. Coccidioidomycosis, q.v.

SA node. Sinoatrial node of the heart.

Sanorex. Trade name for mazindol.

Sansert. Trade name for methysergide maleate, USP.

santonin (săn′tō-nĭn). A colorless, crystalline substance obtained from the unexpanded flower heads of plants of the genus *Artemisia cina.*

ACTION/USES: A vermifuge against the roundworm. Because of its toxicity, it is not used.

sap (săp) [AS. *saep*]. 1. Any fluid essential to life and vitality of a living structure. 2. To cause gradual exhaustion or weakness, as to sap one's strength.

    s., cell. The fluid portion of protoplasm. SYN: *hyaloplasm.*

    s., nuclear. Liquid portion of a cell nucleus. SYN: *karyolymph.*

saphena (să-fē′nă) [Gr. *saphenes,* manifest] (pl. *saphenae*). Either of two large superficial veins of the leg. SEE: *saphenous veins.*

saphenectomy (săf″ē-něk′tō-mē) [″ + *ektome,* excision]. Surgical removal of the saphenous vein.

saphenous (să-fē′nŭs). Pert. to, or associated with, a saphenous vein or nerve in the leg.

saphenous nerve. A deep branch of the femoral nerve. In the lower leg, it follows the long saphenous vein that supplies the medial side of the leg, ankle, and foot.

saphenous opening. An aperture in the fascia, oval in shape, in inner and upper part of the thigh, transmitting the saphenous vein below Poupart's ligament. SYN: *fossa ovalis.*

saphenous veins. Two superficial veins, the great and small, passing up the leg. The great saphenous vein extends from the foot to the saphenous opening; the small vein runs behind the outer malleolus up the back of the leg, joining the popliteal vein. SYN: *saphenae.* SEE: *vein.*

sapid (săp′ĭd) [L. *sapidus,* tasty]. Savory; tasty; opposed to insipid.

sapo (să′pō) [L.]. Soap prepared from pure olive oil and sodium hydroxide.

saponaceous (să″pō-nā′shŭs) [NL. *saponaceus,* soapy]. Soapy; resembling soap in feel or quality.

saponatus (să″pō-nā′tŭs) [L.]. Mixed with soap.

saponification (să-pŏn″ĭ-fĭ-kā′shŭn) [L. *sapo,* soap, + *facere,* to make]. 1. Conversion into soap; chemically, the hydrolysis or the splitting of fat by an alkali yielding glycerol and three molecules of alkali salt of the fatty acid, the soap. 2. In chemistry, hydrolysis of an ester into corresponding alcohol and acid (free or in form of a salt).

saponification number. In analysis of fats, the number of milligrams of potassium hydroxide needed to saponify 1 gm of oil or fat.

saponify (să-pŏn′ĭ-fī). To convert into a soap, as when fats are treated with an alkali to produce a free alcohol plus the salt of the fatty acid. Thus, stearin, saponified with sodium hydroxide, yields the alcohol glycerol plus the soap sodium stearate.

saponin (săp′ō-nĭn) [Fr. *saponine,* soap]. Unabsorbable glucoside contained in the roots of some plants forming a lather in an aqueous solution. Saponins cause hemolysis of red blood cells even in high dilutions. When taken orally, they can produce diarrhea and vomiting.

sapophore (săp′ō-for) [L. *sapor,* taste, + Gr. *phoros,* bearing]. The component of a molecule that imparts taste to it.

saporific (săp″ō-rĭf′ĭk) [NL. *saporificus,* producing taste]. Imparting a taste or flavor.

sapphism (săf′ĭzm) [Sappho, Gr. poetess, 7th-century B.C.]. Female homosexuality. SYN: *lesbianism.*

sapro- [Gr. *sapros,* putrid]. Combining form meaning putrid or rotten.

saprobes (să′prŏbs) [Gr. *sapros,* putrid, +

bios, life]. Organisms that live as parasites because, as in the case of fungi, they do not possess photosynthetic pigments.

saprogen (săp'rō-jĕn) [" + *gennan*, to produce]. Any microorganism causing or produced by putrefaction.

saprogenic (săp"rō-jĕn'ĭk). Causing putrefaction, or resulting from it.

saprophilous (săp-rŏf'ĭl-ŭs) [Gr. *sapros*, putrid, + *philein*, to love]. Living on decaying or dead substances, as a microorganism. SYN: *saprophytic*.

saprophyte (săp'rō-fīt) [" + *phyton*, plant]. Any organism living on decaying or dead organic matter. Most of the higher fungi are saprophytes. SEE: *parasite*.

saprophytic (săp"rō-fĭt'ĭk). Living or growing in decaying or dead matter; characteristic of a saprophyte. SYN: *metatrophic; saprophilous*.

saprozoic (săp"rō-zō'ĭk) [" + *zoon*, animal]. Living on decaying or dead organic matter.

sarapus (săr'ă-pŭs) [Gr. *sarapous*]. A person having flat feet.

Sarcina (săr'sĭ-nă) [L., bundle]. A genus of spherical saprophytic bacteria of the family Micrococcaceae. The individual organisms remain adherent to each other after splitting in three planes. This process yields square tetrads or cubical packets.

sarcina (săr'sĭ-nă) (pl. *sarcinas* or *sarcinae*). Any organism of the genus *Sarcina*. SEE: *bacteria* for illus.

sarcitis (săr-sī'tĭs) [Gr. *sarx*, flesh, + *itis*, inflammation]. Inflammation of muscle tissue. SYN: *myositis*.

sarco- [Gr. *sarx*, flesh]. Combining form indicating flesh.

sarcoadenoma (săr"kō-ăd"ĕn-ō'mă) [" + *aden*, gland, + *oma*, tumor]. A fleshy tumor of a gland. SYN: *adenosarcoma*.

sarcobiont (săr"kō-bī'ŏnt) [" + *bioun*, to live]. A microorganism that lives on flesh.

sarcoblast (săr'kō-blăst) [" + *blastos*, a germ]. Embryonic cell that develops into a muscle cell. SYN: *myoblast*.

sarcocarcinoma (săr"kō-kăr"sĭn-ō'mă) [" + *karkinos*, crab, + *oma*, tumor]. A malignant tumor of sarcomatous and carcinomatous types.

sarcocele (săr'kō-sēl) [" + *kele*, tumor, swelling]. A fleshy tumor of the testicle.

sarcocyst (săr'kō-sĭst) [" + *kystis*, bladder]. An elongated tubular body produced by *Sarcocystis*.

Sarcocystis (săr"kō-sĭs'tĭs) [" + *kystis*, bladder]. A genus of sporozoa found in the muscles of higher vertebrates (reptiles, birds, and mammals).

   S. lindemanni. A species infesting the muscles of humans.

Sarcodina (săr-kō-dī'nă) [" + *eidos*, form, shape]. A class of protozoa characterized by absence of a thick pellicle and movement by pseudopodia. Sarcodines are typically holozoic and reproduce principally by asexual methods. Includes the families Amoebidae and Endamoebidae, the latter including many forms parasitic and pathogenic in humans.

sarcogenic (săr"kō-jĕn'ĭk) [" + *gennan*, to produce]. Producing flesh or muscle.

sarcoid (săr'koyd) [" + *eidos*, form, shape]. 1. Resembling flesh. 2. A small epithelioid tubercle-like lesion characteristic of sarcoidosis.

   s., Boeck's. SEE: *Boeck's sarcoid.*

sarcoidosis (săr"koyd-ō'sĭs) [" + " + *osis*, condition]. A disease of unknown etiology characterized by widespread granulomatous lesions that may affect any organ or tissue of the body. The liver is frequently affected, as are the skin, lungs, lymph nodes, spleen, eyes, and small bones of the hands and feet. Formerly called Boeck's sarcoid.

sarcolemma (săr"kō-lĕm'ă) [" + *lemma*, husk]. A delicate membrane surrounding each striated muscle fiber.

sarcology (săr-kŏl'ō-jē) [" + *logos*, word, reason]. Branch of medicine dealing with study of the soft tissues of the body.

sarcolysis (săr-kŏl'ĭ-sĭs) [" + *lysis*, dissolution]. Decomposition of the soft tissues or flesh.

sarcolytic (săr"kō-lĭt'ĭk). Decomposing flesh.

sarcoma (săr-kō'mă) [" + *oma*, tumor] (pl. *sarcomata*). Cancer arising from connective tissue such as muscle or bone. May affect the bones, bladder, kidneys, liver, lungs, parotids, and spleen.

   s., alveolar soft part. Malignant neoplasm composed of a reticular stroma of connective tissue surrounding clumps of large round cells.

   s., botryoid. Sarcoma of the uterus composed of a polypoid mass of soft edematous tissues. Most often seen in infants or children.

   s., chondro-. Sarcoma composed of masses of cartilage.

   s., endometrial. Malignant neoplasm of the endometrial stroma.

   s., Ewing's. A diffuse endothelioma or endothelial myeloma forming a fusiform swelling on a long bone.

   s., fibro-. Malignant tumor with fibrous tissue, many spindle cells, and dilated vessels.

   s., giant cell. Sarcoma from cancellous bone tissue with large cells with many nuclei. A special type called an epulis is seen in the jaw. SYN: *s., myeloid.*

s., Kaposi's. Kaposi's sarcoma, q.v. SEE: *AIDS.*

s., lipo-. A rare tumor of bone containing cells of various types with small vacuoles of fat.

s., lymphangio-. Sarcoma arising from endothelium of lymph vessels in a lymph gland.

s., myeloid. S., giant cell.

s., myxo-. Benign tumor of mucoid tissue, such as that of the umbilical cord. SYN: *myxoma.*

s., osteogenic. Sarcoma composed of osseous tissue containing variously shaped cells.

s., reticulum cell. A variety of malignant lymphoma involving the lymph nodes and other lymphatic tissue.

s., rhabdomyo-. An embryonal tumor of striated muscle containing multinucleated cells with a striated cytoplasm.

s., spindle cell. Sarcoma consisting of small and large spindle-shaped cells.

sarcomatoid (sar-kō'mă-toyd) [Gr. *sarx*, flesh, + *oma*, tumor, + *eidos*, form, shape]. Resembling a sarcoma.

sarcomatosis (săr″kō-mă-tō'sĭs) [" + " + *osis*, condition]. Condition marked by presence and spread of a sarcoma; sarcomatous degeneration.

sarcomatous (săr-kō'mă-tŭs). Of the nature of, or like, a sarcoma.

sarcomere (săr'kō-mēr) [" + *meros*, a part]. The portion of a striated muscle fibril lying between two adjacent dark lines called Krause's membranes.

sarcomphalocele (săr″kŏm-făl'ō-sēl) [" + *omphalos*, umbilicus, + *kele*, tumor, swelling]. Fleshy tumor of the umbilicus.

sarcomyces (săr″kō-mī'sēz) [" + *mykes*, fungus]. A fleshy growth having the appearance of a fungus.

Sarcophagidae (săr″kō-făj'ĭ-dē) [Gr. *sarx*, flesh, + *phagein*, to eat]. The family of the order Diptera that includes the flesh flies. Females deposit their eggs or larvae on decaying flesh of dead animals. Larvae of two genera, *Sarcophaga* and *Wohlfahrtia*, frequently infest open sores and wounds of humans, giving rise to cutaneous myiasis.

sarcophagy (săr-kŏf'ă-jē). Practice of eating flesh.

sarcoplasm (săr'kō-plăzm) [" + LL. *plasma*, form, mold]. Semifluid interfibrillary substance of striated muscle cells. The cytoplasm of muscle cells.

sarcoplasmic (săr″kō-plăz'mĭk). Concerning or containing sarcoplasm.

sarcopoietic (săr″kō-poy-ĕt'ĭk) [" + *poiein*, to form]. Forming muscle or flesh.

Sarcoptes (săr-kŏp'tēz). A genus of Acarina that includes the mites that infest humans

and animals. *Sarcoptes scabiei* causes scabies in humans.

Sarcoptidae (săr-kŏp'tĭ-dē). A family of mites of the order Acarina, class Arachnida, that includes *Sarcoptes scabiei*, the causative agent of scabies or itch in humans and mange and scab in other animals.

sarcosis (săr-kō'sĭs) [" + *osis*, condition]. 1. The development of multiple fleshy tumors. 2. Abnormal formation of flesh.

sarcosome (săr'kō-sōm) [" + *soma*, body]. Term previously used for mitochondria, particularly of muscle cells.

Sarcosporidia (săr″kō-spō-rĭd'ē-ă) [" + *sporos*, a seed]. An order of protozoa that belong to the class Sporozoa and are parasitic in the muscles of higher vertebrates. Includes the genus *Sarcocystis.*

sarcosporidiosis (săr″kō-spō-rĭd″ē-ō'sĭs) [" + " + *osis*, condition]. Infestation with organisms of the order Sarcosporidia or condition produced by them.

sarcostosis (săr″kŏs-tō'sĭs) [" + *osteon*, bone, + *osis*, condition]. Ossification of fleshy or muscular tissue.

sarcostyle (săr'kō-stīl) [" + *stylos*, a column]. Any one of the fine longitudinal fibrillae of a striated muscle fiber.

sarcotic (săr-kŏt'ĭk) [Gr. *sarx*, flesh]. 1. Producing or pert. to flesh formation. 2. Agent producing growth of flesh.

sarcotubules (săr″kō-tū'būlz). A continuous membranous tubule system present in striated muscle.

sarcous (săr'kŭs) [Gr. *sarko*, flesh]. Concerning flesh or muscle.

sardonic laugh. Old term for a spasmodic affection of facial muscles that gives the appearance of laughter. SYN: *risus sardonicus.*

sarin (GB). Isopropylmethylphosphonofluoridate. An extremely toxic "nerve gas."

sartorius (săr-tō'rē-ŭs) [L. *sartor*, tailor]. A long, ribbon-shaped muscle of the thigh. The longest muscle in the body, it functions to flex, abduct and laterally rotate the thigh, getting its name from its function in crossing the legs as tailors do. It also aids in flexing the knee. SEE: *Muscles* in *Appendix.*

SAS-500. Trade name for sulfasalazine.

sat. *saturated.*

satellite (săt'l-īt) [L. *satelles*, attendant]. A small structure attached to a larger one, esp. a minute body attached to a chromosome by a slender chromatin filament.

s., bacterial. A bacterial colony that grows best when close to a colony of another microorganism.

satellite cells. 1. Flat epithelium-like cells forming the inner portion of a double-layered capsule which covers a neuron. 2. Neuroglial cells enclosing the cell bodies of neurons in spinal ganglia.

satellitosis (săt″l-ĭ-tō′sĭs) [″ + Gr. *osis*, condition]. The accumulation of neuroglial cells about neurons of the central nervous system, seen in certain degenerative and inflammatory conditions.

satiety (să-tī′ĕt-ē) [L. *satietas*, enough]. Being full to satisfaction, esp. with food.

satiety center. An area in the hypothalamus that, following a meal, senses a feeling of satiety and thus inhibits the urge to eat by acting on the "feeding center," also located in the hypothalamus.

saturated (săt′ū-rā″tĕd) [L. *saturare*, to fill]. Holding all that can be absorbed, received, or combined, as a solution in which no more of a substance can be dissolved. Term is applied to hydrocarbons in which the maximum number of hydrogen atoms is present and there are no double or triple bonds between the carbon atoms.

saturated compound. An organic compound with all carbon bonds filled. It does not contain double or triple bonds. SEE: *unsaturated compound*.

saturated hydrocarbon. A carbon-hydrogen compound with all carbon bonds filled so there are no double or triple bonds. SEE: *polyunsaturated*.

saturated solution. Solution containing as much of the solid drug or other substance as can be dissolved.

saturation (săt″ū-rā′shŭn). 1. State in which all of a substance that can be dissolved in a solution is dissolved. Adding more of the substance will not increase the concentration. 2. In organic chemistry, to have all available carbon atom valences satisfied so that there are no double or triple bonds between the carbon atoms.

   s., oxygen. The ratio of amount of oxygen present in a known volume of blood to amount of oxygen that could be carried by that volume of blood.

saturation index. In hematology, the amount of hemoglobin present in a known volume of blood compared with the normal.

saturation time. Time required for arterial blood of a person inhaling pure oxygen to become saturated.

Saturday night paralysis. Paralysis, occurring often in alcoholics, from lying immobile with arm pressed against a projecting surface so that the musculospiral nerve is compressed. SYN: *paralysis, musculospiral.*

saturnine (săt′ŭr-nīn) [L. *saturnus*, lead]. Concerning or produced by lead.

saturnine breath. Sweet breath produced by lead poisoning.

saturnine gout. Goutlike symptoms produced by lead poisoning.

saturnism (săt′ŭr-nĭzm) [″ + Gr. *-ismos*, condition]. Lead poisoning. SYN: *plumbism.*

satyriasis (săt-ĭ-rī′ă-sĭs) [LL.]. Excessive, and often uncontrollable, sexual drive in men. SEE: *nymphomania.*

satyromania (săt″ĭ-rō-mā′nē-ă). Satyriasis, q.v.

saucerization (saw″sĕr-ĭ-zā′shŭn). Surgical creation of a shallow area in tissue; or the production of such a depression due to trauma.

sauna. An enclosure in which a person is exposed to high temperature and humidity, produced by pouring water on heated stones. This is done to produce moderate to very high temperatures and high humidity. After a stay in the enclosure, the person may bathe briefly in a cold lake or roll in snow.

   Sauna water is not sterile and may contain harmful microorganisms, including yeasts and molds.

   Even though the sauna has no proven benefit in preventing illnesses or promoting fitness, the regimen is beneficial in promoting relaxation, relieving aches and pains, and in helping to loosen stiff joints.

Caution: Saunas are not advised for those with fever, those who are dehydrated or are unable to sweat. Those who have recently used alcohol or have participated in strenuous exercise should not use a sauna. If soft tissue has been traumatized in the last 24 to 48 hours, the sauna should not be used. Prolonged exposure to the sauna may be dangerous due to induced hyperpyrexia, dehydration, and renal failure.

---

savory (sā′vō-rē) [O. Fr. *savoure*, tasty]. Having a pleasant or appetizing taste or odor.

saw [AS. *sagu*]. A cutting instrument with an edge of sharp toothlike projections; used esp. for cutting bone in surgery.

   s., Stryker's. An electric-powered oscillating saw that cuts through bone or dense tissue with minimal damage to the underlying soft tissues.

saxifragant (săks-ĭf′ră-gănt) [L. *saxum*, rock, + *frangere*, to break]. Dissolving or breaking calculi, esp. in the bladder.

saxitoxin (săk″sĭ-tŏk′sĭn). A toxin obtained from some forms of marine life, including mussels, clams, and plankton. It is the active ingredient in paralytic shellfish poisoning. If ingested, saxitoxin can produce death in a matter of hours; if inhaled, it can be lethal in minutes.

Sayre's jacket (sārz) [Lewis Albert Sayre, U.S. surgeon, 1820–1900]. A jacket of plaster of paris worn to support the spine in vertebral diseases.

Sb. Chem. symb. for the element antimony.

SbCl₃. Antimony trichloride.

**SCABIES ITCH MITE
(SARCOPTES SCABIEI)**

SBE. *subacute bacterial endocarditis.*

Sb$_2$O$_5$. Antimonic oxide; antimony pentoxide.

Sb$_4$O$_6$. Antimonious oxide.

Sc. Chem. symb. for the element scandium.

s.c. *subcutaneously.*

scab (skăb) [ME. *scabbe*]. 1. Crust of a cutaneous sore, wound, ulcer, or pustule formed by drying of the discharge. 2. To become covered with a crust.

scabicide (skă′bĭ-sīd). An agent that kills mites, esp. the causative agent of scabies.

scabies (skā′bē-ēz, -bēz) [L. *scabies*, itch]. A highly communicable skin disease caused by an arachnid, *Sarcoptes scabiei*, variety *hominis*, the itch mite. It is transmitted by direct contact with infected persons, and rarely by fomites. SYN: *itch* (def. 2). SEE: illus. SEE: *Nursing Diagnoses* in *Appendix.*

SYM: Papules, vesicles, pustules, burrows, and intense itching resulting in eczema. The impregnated females live in burrows that appear as slightly discolored lines several millimeters to several centimeters in length. Eggs deposited within the tunnel hatch within 3 to 5 days. The larvae molt into nymphs on the skin surface and mature in 2 to 3 weeks. Mature insects mate, and the gravid female invades the skin to begin a new cycle. Parts most commonly affected are hands, between fingers, wrists, axillae, genitalia, beneath the mammae, and inner aspect of the thighs.

DIAG: Identification of mites in tissue scraped from burrows, lesions, or fresh papules. Also, the clinical appearance is usually diagnostic.

TREAT: 1% gamma benzene hexachloride; 25% benzyl benzoate cream or lotion; lindane; or crotamiton applied to the entire body, except the eyes, nose, and mouth, after the patient has taken a prolonged hot bath or shower. The affected areas are scrubbed thoroughly, and then the medicine is applied. A second application is made the following morning.

A simpler, one-application treatment is possible with the use of permethrin. The 5% cream is applied and left overnight for 8 to 14 hours before being thoroughly washed off.

PROG: Favorable.

s., Norwegian. A rare form of scabies in which the mites are present in great number.

scabietic (skā″bē-ĕt′ĭk) [L. *scabies*, itch]. Concerning scabies.

scabieticide (skā″bē-ĕt′ĭ-sīd) [″ + *cidus*, killing]. Scabicide.

scabiphobia (skā″bĭ-fō′bē-ă) [″ + Gr. *phobos*, fear]. Abnormal fear of acquiring scabies.

scabrities (skā-brĭsh′ē-ēz) [L. *scaber*, rough]. 1. Scaly, roughened condition of the skin. 2. A morbid roughness of inner surface of eyelids causing sensation as if sand were in eyes.

s. unguium. Morbid degeneration of the nails making them rough, thick, distorted, and separated from the flesh at the root. Symptomatic of syphilis and leprosy.

scala (skā′lă) [L. *scala*, staircase]. Any one of the three spiral passages of the cochlea.

s. media. The cochlear duct that lies between the scala tympani and scala vestibuli. Its floor contains the spiral organ of Corti. It extends from the saccule to the tip of the cochlea and is filled with endolymph.

s. tympani. The cochlear duct filled with perilymph lying below the spiral lamina. Extends from tip of the cochlea to the round cochlear window.

s. vestibuli. The cochlear duct forming the upper portion of the osseous canal. It lies above the spiral lamina and extends from the floor of the vestibule to the tip of the cochlea, where it communicates with the scala tympani through an aperture, the helicotrema.

scald (skŏld) [ME. *scalden*, to burn with hot liquid]. 1. Burn to skin or flesh caused by moist heat and hot vapors, as steam. 2. To cause a burn with hot liquid or steam.

When the heat applied is approximately equivalent, a scald is deeper than a burn from dry heat and should be treated as a burn, q.v. Healing is slower and scar formation greater. Emergency treatment of a scalded area should be the immediate application of cold in the most readily available form, i.e., ice packs or immersion of the part in very cold water. This should be continued for at least an hour.

scalded skin syndrome, staphylococcal. Necrosis of the epidermal layer of the skin with very little damage to underlying dermis. Initially, there is an upper body and facial rash, fever, and extremely tender skin. Then bullae, filled with clear fluid, form. As much as 80% of the skin may be affected.

ETIOL: An exotoxin produced by one of several phage types of staphylococci.

TREAT: Beta-lactamase resistant synthetic penicillin; symptomatic therapy for bullae and denuded skin. Uncomplicated lesions heal without scarring.

scale (skāl). 1. [O. Fr. *escale*, husk] A small, thin, dry exfoliation shed from upper layers of skin. Shedding of scales from skin in small amounts is normal. More shedding is seen in cutaneous disorders such as squamous eczema, seborrhea sicca, psoriasis, ichthyosis, syphilis, lupus erythematosus, pityriasis rosea, and tinea tonsurans. SEE: *macule; rash.* 2. Film of tartar encrusting the teeth. 3. To remove a film of tartar from the teeth. 4. To form a scale on. 5. To shed scales. 6. [ME. *scole,* balance] An instrument for weighing. 7. [L. *scala,* staircase] A graduated or proportioned measure, a series of tests, or an instrument for measuring quantities or for rating, e.g., individual intelligence.

s., absolute. Scale used for indicating low temperatures based on absolute zero. SEE: *absolute temperature; absolute zero.*

s., Baumé. Scale for indicating the specific gravity of liquids.

s., Celsius. SEE: *Celsius scale.*

s., centigrade. Celsius scale.

s., Fahrenheit. Scale in which the freezing point of water is 32° and the boiling point is 212°. SEE: *Fahrenheit scale; thermometer* for table.

s., French. SEE: *French scale.*

s., Kelvin. SEE: *Kelvin scale.*

s. of contrast. The range of densities on a radiograph, the number of tonal grays that are visible.

scalene (skā-lēn') [Gr. *skalenos,* uneven]. 1. Having unequal sides and angles, said of a triangle. 2. Designating a scalenus muscle.

s. tubercle. Tubercle on upper surface of the first rib, the insertion of the scalenus anticus muscle. SYN: *tubercle, Lisfranc's.*

scalenectomy (skā″lĕ-nĕk′tŏ-mē) [″ + *ektome,* excision]. Resection of any of the scalenus muscles.

scaleniotomy (skā-lēn″ē-ŏt′ō-mē) [″ + *tome,* incision]. Incision of scalenus muscles near their insertion to check expansive movements in tuberculosis of the apex of the lung.

scalenotomy (skā″lē-nŏt′ō-mē) [″ + *tome,* incision]. Surgical division of one or more of the scalenus muscles.

scalenus (skā-lē′nŭs) [L., uneven]. One of three deeply situated muscles on each side of the neck, extending from the tubercles of the transverse processes of the 3rd through 6th cervical vertebrae to the 1st or 2nd rib. Known as scalenus anterior (anticus), medius, and posterior. SEE: *Muscles* in *Appendix.*

scalenus syndrome. A symptom complex characterized by brachial neuritis with or without vascular or vasomotor disturbance in the upper extremities. Also called *scalenus anticus syndrome.*

SYM: Not clearly defined but pain, tingling, and numbness may occur anywhere from shoulder to fingers. Atrophy of small muscles of the hand or even the deltoid or other muscles of arm.

TREAT: Correction of posture, and sometimes immobilization of arm and shoulder. When relief is not obtained, surgical correction may be required.

scaler (skā′lĕr) [O. Fr. *escale,* husk]. 1. A dental instrument used in the procedure of removing calculus from the teeth. 2. A device for counting pulses detected by a radiation detector.

s., ultrasonic. An instrument tip attached to a transducer through which a high frequency current causes ultrasonic vibrations (approx. 25,000 c.p.s.) These vibrations, usually accompanied by a stream of water, produce a turbulence which, in turn, removes stain and adherent deposits from teeth.

scaling (skā′lĭng) [O. Fr. *escale,* husk]. Removal of calculus from teeth.

scall (skawl) [Norse *skalli,* baldhead]. Dermatitis of the scalp producing a crusted scabby eruption.

scalp (skălp) [ME., sheath]. The hairy integument of the head. In anatomy, includes skin, dense subcutaneous tissue, occipitofrontalis muscle with the galea aponeurotica, loose subaponeurotic tissue, and the cranial periosteum.

scalpel (skăl′pĕl) [L. *scalpellum,* knife]. A small, straight surgical knife with a convex edge and thin keen blade. SEE: illus.

scalpriform (skăl′prī-form) [L. *scalprum,* knife, + *forma,* shape]. Shaped like a chisel.

scalprum (skăl′prŭm) [L., knife] (pl. *scalpra*). 1. A toothed instrument for removal of carious bone or for trephining. 2. A large scalpel. 3. Cutting edge of an incisor tooth.

scalp tourniquet. Tourniquet applied to the scalp during I.V. administration of antineoplastic drugs to restrict blood flow to the hair-bearing portion of the scalp. This procedure is helpful in preventing the cranial alopecia that may accompany chemother-

SCALPELS

BARD—PARKER HANDLE
WITH VARIOUS BLADES

GENERAL OPERATING

SINGLE—BLADE LISTON
AMPUTATING

LITTLE'S OPERATING

MAYO OPERATING

BISTOURY

DOUBLE—BLADE
AMPUTATING

apy used in treating certain types of cancer.

scaly (skā'lē) [O. Fr. *escale*, husk]. Resembling or characterized by scales.

scan. Short for scintiscan, q.v.

scandium [L. *Scandia*, Scandinavia]. SYMB: Sc. At. wt. 44.956; at. no. 21. A rare metal belonging to the aluminum group.

scanning. Recording, on a photographic plate, the emission of radioactive waves from a specific substance injected into the body. The radioactive agent selected is one that is concentrated in a specific tissue, such as thyroid, brain, or liver.

 s., radioisotope. Recording of radioisotope emanations from tissues into which the radioactive substances have been injected. The scanner can be moved around the site and a multiview picture obtained.

scanning electron microscope. ABBR: SEM. An electron microscope that scans an image point by point and displays the image on a photographic film or television screen. The SEM, unlike other types of microscopes, allows a three-dimensional view of the tissues, and tissues do not need to be extensively handled and prepared in order to be visualized. The magnification ranges from 20 to 100,000 times.

scanning speech. Pronunciation of words in syllables, or slowly and hesitatingly; a symptom of certain diseases of the cerebellum and advanced multiple sclerosis. SEE: *speech.*

scanty (skăn'tē) [ME. from O. Norse, *skamt*, short]. Not abundant; insufficient, as a secretion.

scapha (skā'fā) [NL., skiff]. [NA] Elongated depression of the ear between the helix and antihelix. SYN: *scaphoid fossa.*

scapho- [Gr. *skaphe*, skiff]. Combining form meaning boat.

scaphocephalic (skăf″ō-sěf-ăl'ĭk) [″ + *kephale*, head]. Having a deformed head, projecting like a boat's keel.

scaphocephalism (skăf″ō-sěf'ăl-ĭzm) [″ + ″ + *-ismos*, condition]. Condition of having a deformed head, projecting like the keel of a boat.

scaphocephalous (skăf″ō-sěf'ă-lŭs) [″ + *kephale*, head]. Scaphocephalic.

scaphocephaly (skăf″ō-sěf'ă-lē) [″ + *kephale*, head]. Scaphocephalism.

scaphohydrocephaly (skăf″ō-hī″drō-sěf'ă-lē) [″ + *hydor*, water, + *kephale*, head]. Hydrocephalus combined with scaphocephalism.

scaphoid (skăf'oyd) [″ + *eidos*, form, shape]. 1. Boat-shaped, navicular, hollowed.

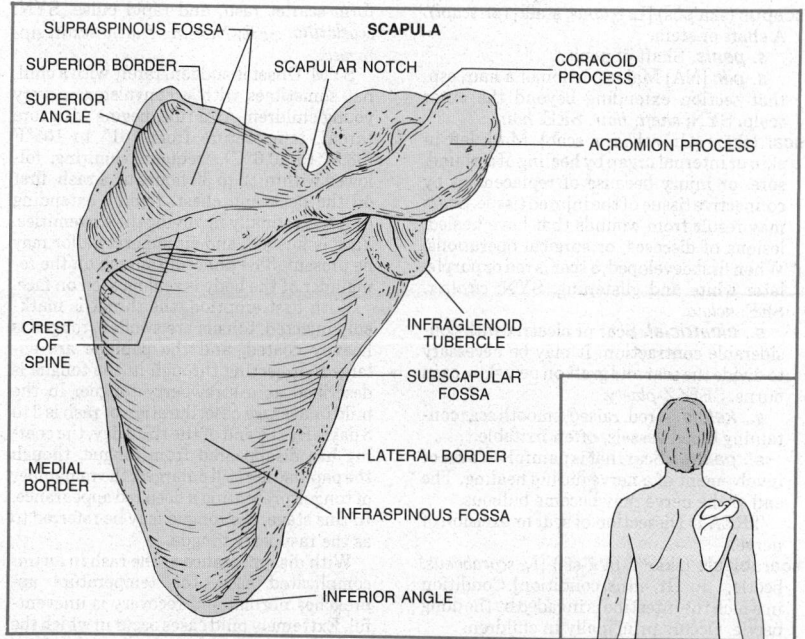

2. A proximal boat-shaped bone of the carpus or the tarsus. SYN: *os scaphoideum*.

scaphoid fossa. Scapha, q.v.

scaphoiditis (skăf″oyd-ī′tĭs) [″ + ″ + *itis*, inflammation]. Inflamed condition of the scaphoid bone.

scapula [L., shoulder blade] (pl. *scapulae*). [NA] The large, flat, triangular bone that forms the posterior part of the shoulder. It articulates with the clavicle and the humerus. SYN: *shoulder blade*. SEE: illus.; *triceps*.

    s., winged. Condition in which the medial border of the scapula is prominent, usually the result of paralysis of serratus anterior or trapezius muscles. SYN: *angel's wing*.

    RS: acromial; acromial angle; acromioclavicular joint; acromiocoracoid; acromion; glenoid cavity.

scapulalgia (skăp-ū-lăl′jē-ă) [L. *scapula*, shoulder blade, + Gr. *algos*, pain]. Pain in the region of the shoulder blade.

scapular (skăp′ū-lăr). Of, or pert. to, the shoulder blade.

scapular reflex. Muscular contraction following percussion or stimulus between the scapulae.

scapulary (skăp′ū-lă-rē). A shoulder bandage for keeping a body bandage in place. A broad roller bandage is split in half. The undivided section of the roller bandage is fastened in front with the two ends passing over the shoulders and attached to the back of the body bandage.

scapulectomy (skăp″ū-lĕk′tō-mē) [L. *scapula*, shoulder blade, + Gr. *ektome*, excision]. Surgical excision of the scapula.

scapulo- [L. *scapula*, shoulder blade]. Combining form meaning shoulder.

scapuloclavicular (skăp″ū-lō-klă-vĭk′ū-lar) [″ + *clavicula*, little key]. Concerning the scapula and clavicle.

scapulodynia (skăp″ū-lō-dĭn′ē-ă) [″ + *odyne*, pain]. Inflammation and pain in the shoulder muscles.

scapulohumeral (skăp″ū-lō-hū′mĕr-ăl) [″ + *humerus*, upper arm]. Concerning the scapula and humerus.

scapulohumeral reflex. Reflex in which the upper arm is adducted and rotated outward when vertebral border of scapula is percussed.

scapulopexy (skăp″ū-lō-pĕk′sē) [″ + Gr. *pexis*, fixation]. Fixation of the scapula to the ribs.

scapulothoracic (skăp″ū-lō-thō-răs′ĭk) [″ + Gr. *thorax*, chest]. Concerning the scapula and thorax.

scapus (skă′pŭs) [L. *scapus*, stalk] (pl. *scapi*). A shaft or stem.

    s. penis. Shaft of penis.

    s. pili. [NA] Major portion of a hair, esp. that section extending beyond the outer scalp. SYN: *shaft, hair.* SEE: *hair.*

scar (skăr) [Gr. *eskhara*, scab]. Mark left in skin or internal organ by healing of a wound, sore, or injury because of replacement by connective tissue of the injured tissue. Scars may result from wounds that have healed, lesions of diseases, or surgical operations. When first developed, a scar is red or purple, later white and glistening. SYN: *cicatrix.* SEE: *keloid.*

    s., cicatricial. Scar or cicatrix with considerable contraction. It may be necessary to divide the scar and graft on new skin, as in burns. SEE: *Z-plasty.*

    s., keloid. A red, raised, smooth scar containing blood vessels, often irritable.

    s., painful. Scar that is painful because of involvement of a nerve during healing. The end of the nerve may become bulbous.

    TREAT: Dissection of scar or excision of nerve.

scarabiasis (skăr″ă-bī′ă-sĭs) [L. *scarabaeus*, beetle, + Gr. -*iasis*, condition]. Condition in which the intestine is invaded by the dung beetle. Occurs principally in children.

scarification (skăr″ĭ-fĭ-kā′shŭn) [Gr. *skariphismos*, scratching up]. Making of numerous superficial incisions in the skin.

scarificator (skăr′ĭf-ĭ-kā″tor). Instrument for making small incisions in the skin. SYN: *scarifier.*

scarifier. Scarificator, q.v.

scarlatina (skăr″lă-tē′nă) [NL., red]. Scarlet fever.

    s. anginosa. A severe form of scarlatina with extensive necrosis and ulceration of the pharynx, and in some cases peritonsillar abscess.

    s. hemorrhagica. Scarlatina with hemorrhage into the skin and mucous membranes.

    s. maligna. A fulminant and usually lethal form of scarlatina.

scarlatinal (skăr″lă-tē′năl). Concerning or due to scarlatina.

scarlatinella (skăr-lăt″ĭ-nĕl′ă) [L.]. A mild disease resembling measles and scarlet fever.

scarlatiniform (skăr-lă-tĭn′ĭ-form) [L. *scarlatina*, red, + *forma*, shape]. Resembling scarlatina or its rash.

scarlatinoid (skăr-lăt′ĭ-noyd) [″ + Gr. *eidos*, form, shape]. Resembling scarlet fever.

scarlet fever [L. *scarlatum*, red]. An acute contagious disease characterized by sore throat, strawberry tongue, fever, puncti-form scarlet rash, and rapid pulse. SYN: *scarlatina.* SEE: *Nursing Diagnoses* in *Appendix.*

SYM: Onset is sudden, rarely with a chill, but sometimes with a convulsion in very young children. As a rule, begins with sore throat, temperature from 101° to 105°F (38.3° to 40.6°C), frequent vomiting; followed within 12 to 36 hours by a rash, first on the neck and chest, rapidly extending over body, finally involving the extremities. Face is flushed, and circumoral pallor may be present. The punctiform rash on the remainder of the body is seldom seen on face.

With first eruption, the throat is markedly injected, tonsils are swollen, tongue is heavily coated, and the papillae are enlarged, projecting through it; the tongue is described as a strawberry tongue. In the mild or average case, duration of rash is 2 to 3 days. By the end of the third day, the coating has disappeared from tongue, though the papillae are still enlarged, the remainder of tongue presenting a deep red appearance. In this stage, the tongue may be referred to as the raspberry tongue.

With disappearance of the rash in an uncomplicated case, the temperature approaches normal and recovery is uneventful. Extremely mild cases occur in which the rash is very faint and of very short duration, possibly not exceeding 24 hours. Scarlet fever may actually occur without any rash whatsoever. In any form, a leukocytosis is to be expected in the average case. Number of leukocytes may range from 10,000 to 20,000 with 75% to 90% neutrophils.

ETIOL: Many strains (over 40) of group A, β-hemolytic streptococci that elaborate an erythrogenic toxin. The toxin was discovered by Dick and Dick (1924–1925). SEE: *Dick method.*

INCUB: Probably never less than 24 hours. May be 1 to 3 days, rarely longer.

TREAT: Penicillin is the agent of choice. Penicillin should be given for a minimum of 10 days, no matter how mild the infection, in order to prevent the subsequent development of complications such as rheumatic fever, carditis, or acute glomerulonephritis.

Isolation from time of diagnosis until one day after beginning antibiotic therapy. Patients with uncomplicated scarlet fever should be kept in bed during the acute phase of the illness.

scarlet rash. A rose-colored rash, specifically that of German measles, q.v.

scarlet red. An azo dye, of the color its name suggests. Used to stimulate healing of indolent ulcers, burns, wounds, etc., or in histology, as a stain. SYN: *rubrum scarlatinum.*

Scarpa's fascia (skăr′păs) [Antonio Scarpa,

It. anatomist, 1752–1832]. Deep layer of superficial abdominal fascia around edge of the subcutaneous inguinal ring.

Scarpa's fluid. Fluid in membranous labyrinth of the ear. SYN: *endolymph*.

Scarpa's foramina. Bony passages opening into the incisor canal for passage of the nasopalatine nerves.

Scarpa's ganglion. The vestibular ganglion. SEE: *ganglion, vestibular*.

Scarpa's membrane. Membrane that closes the fenestra rotunda of the tympanic cavity.

Scarpa's triangle. Triangular space bounded laterally by the inner edge of the sartorius, above by Poupart's ligament, and medially by the adductor longus.

SCAT. *sheep cell agglutination test*.

scatemia (skă-tē′mē-ă) [Gr. *skato-*, dung, + *haima*, blood]. Toxemia from absorption of material present in the intestines. SYN: *scoretemia*.

scato- [Gr. *skato-*, dung]. Combining form denoting relationship to dung or fecal matter.

scatologic (skăt″ō-lŏj′ĭk). Concerning fecal matter.

scatology (skă-tŏl′ō-jē) [″ + *logos*, word, reason]. 1. Scientific study and analysis of the feces. SYN: *coprology*. 2. Interest in obscene things, esp. obscene literature.

scatoma (skă-tō′mă) [″ + *oma*, tumor]. Mass of inspissated feces in colon or rectum resembling an abdominal tumor. SYN: *fecaloma; stercoroma*.

scatophagy (skă-tŏf′ă-jē) [″ + *phagein*, to eat]. The eating of excrement. SYN: *coprophagy*.

scatoscopy (skă-tŏs′kō-pē) [″ + *skopein*, to examine]. Examination of excreta for diagnostic purposes.

scatter (skăt′ĕr). The diffusion of x-rays when they strike an object.

    s., back-. The scattering of x-rays back to the source after they have been reflected by striking an object.

scattered radiation. X-rays that have changed direction because of a collision with matter.

scattergram (skăt′ĕr-grăm). Display of data on a chart so that each value is indicated by a symbol. The symbols are not connected by a line.

scavenger cell (skăv′ĕn-jĕr) [ME. *skawager*, toll collector]. A phagocytic cell, such as a macrophage or a neutrophil leukocyte, that functions in the removal of disintegrating tissues.

Sc.D. *Doctor of Science* (degree).

scent (sĕnt). An emanation from living or dead tissues, or materials that stimulate the olfactory sense.

Schäffer's reflex (shā′fĕrs) [Max Schäffer, Ger. neurologist, 1852–1923]. Dorsiflexion

of toes and flexion of foot resulting when middle portion of Achilles tendon is pinched.

Schatzki ring [Richard Schatzki, U.S. radiologist, b. 1901]. A lower esophageal mucosal ring composed of an annular, thin, weblike tissue located at the squamocolumnar junction at or near the border of the lower esophageal sphincter. When the diameter of the ring is less than 1.3 cm, dysphagia is present.

    TREAT: Stretch the ring with rubber dilators.

schedule. A timetable, plan for action to achieve a certain goal. This is usually written.

Scheie's syndrome [Harold Glendon Scheie, U.S. ophthalmologist, 1909–1990]. SEE: *mucopolysaccharidosis*.

schema (skē′mă) [Gr., shape]. Shape, plan, or outline.

schematic (skē-măt′ĭk) [NL. *schematicus*, shape, figure]. Pert. to a diagram or model; showing part for part in a diagram.

scheroma (shē-rō′mă). A condition caused by lack of lacrimal fluid. SYN: *xerophthalmia*. SEE: *Schirmer's test*.

Schick test (shĭk) [Béla Schick, Hungarian-born U.S. pediatrician, 1877–1967]. Test to determine degree of immunity to diphtheria. Injection intradermally of 0.1 ml of dilute diphtheria toxin, 1⁄50 MLD. (MLD: minimum lethal dose, the amount of diphtheria toxin that would kill a small guinea pig in 4 days.)

    Results are obtained 3 to 4 days later. Susceptibility (positive test) is indicated by the development of a red inflamed area at point of injection, which slowly disappears after a few days. A negative test (little or no reaction) indicates the presence of antibodies sufficient to neutralize the toxin; hence the person is immune. SEE: *diphtheria*.

Schick test control. USP. Inactivated diphtheria toxin for Schick test. It is used in the Schick test as a control.

Schilder's disease (shĭl′dĕrs) [Paul Ferdinand Schilder, Austrian-U.S. neurologist, 1886–1940]. A rare but invariably fatal disease of the central nervous system characterized by adrenal atrophy and diffuse cerebral demyelination. This leads to mental deterioration and blindness. SYN: *adrenoleukodystrophy*.

Schiller's test (shĭl′ĕrs) [Walter Schiller, Austrian-U.S. pathologist, 1887–1960]. Test for superficial cancer, esp. of the cervix uteri. The tissue is painted with solution of iodine. Cells not containing glycogen fail to stain and their presence may indicate a malignant change.

Schilling's classification [Victor Schilling, Ger. hematologist, 1883–1960]. Method of classifying polymorphonuclear neutrophils into four categories according to number and arrangement of the nuclei in the cells.

Schilling test [Robert F. Schilling, U.S. hematologist, b. 1919]. A test, utilizing radioactive vitamin B_{12}, for gastrointestinal absorption of vitamin B_{12}. For diagnosis of primary pernicious anemia.

schindylesis (skĭn″dĭ-lē′sĭs) [Gr. *schindylesis*, a splitting]. A form of wedge and groove suture in which a crest of one bone fits into a groove of another.

Schiötz tonometer [Hjalamar Schiötz, Norwegian physician, 1850–1927]. Instrument for measuring intraocular pressure by the degree of indentation produced by pressure on the cornea.

Schirmer's test [Rudolph Schirmer, Ger. ophthalmologist, 1831–1896]. Use of a piece of absorbent paper placed so that it hangs out of the conjunctival sac of the eye. The rate and amount of wetting of the paper provide an estimate of tear production.

schisto- (skĭs′tō) [Gr. *schistos*, divided]. Combining form meaning split or cleft.

schistocelia (skĭs″tō-sē′lē-ă) [″ + *koilia*, belly]. Congenital abdominal fissure.

schistocephalus (skĭs″tō-sĕf′ă-lŭs) [″ + *kephale*, head]. Fetus with a cleft head.

schistocormia (skĭs″tō-kor′mē-ă) [″ + *kormos*, trunk]. Fetus with a cleft trunk.

schistocystis (skĭs″tō-sĭs′tĭs) [″ + *kystis*, bladder]. Fissure of the bladder.

schistocyte (skĭs′tō-sīt) [″ + *kytos*, cell]. Fragmented red blood cells that appear in a variety of shapes, from small triangular forms to round cells with irregular surfaces.

schistocytosis (skĭs″tō-sī-tō′sĭs) [″ + ″ + *osis*, condition]. Schistocytes in the blood.

schistoglossia (skĭs″tō-glŏs′ē-ă) [″ + *glossa*, tongue]. A cleft tongue.

schistomelus (skĭs-tŏm′ĕ-lŭs) [″ + *melos*, limb]. Fetus with a cleft in a limb.

schistoprosopia (skĭs″tō-prō-sō′pē-ă) [″ + *prosopon*, face]. Congenital fissure of the face.

schistorachis (skĭs-tor′ă-kĭs) [″ + *rhachis*, spine]. Protrusion of membranes through a congenital cleft in the lower vertebral column. SYN: *spina bifida cystica*.

Schistosoma (skĭs″tō-sō′mă) [″ + *soma*, body]. A genus of blood flukes belonging to the family Schistosomatidae, class Trematoda. Adults live in blood vessels of visceral organs. Eggs make their way into the bladder or intestine and are discharged in urine or feces. Eggs hatch into miracidia, which enter snails and transform into sporocysts. These develop daughter sporocysts, which give rise to fork-tailed cercariae. These leave the snail and enter the final host directly through the skin or through mucous membrane.

    S. haematobium. A species common in Africa and southwestern Asia. Adults infest pelvic veins of vesical plexus. Eggs work their way through the bladder wall and are discharged through urine. Cause of urinary schistosomiasis.

    S. japonicum. A species common in many parts of the Orient. Adults live principally in branches of the superior mesenteric vein. Eggs work their way through the intestinal wall into the lumen and are discharged with feces. Cause of Oriental schistosomiasis.

    S. mansoni. A species occurring in many parts of Africa and tropical America, including the West Indies. Adults live in branches of the inferior mesenteric veins. Eggs discharged through either the intestine or bladder. Cause of bilharzial dysentery or Manson's intestinal schistosomiasis.

schistosome dermatitis (skĭs′tō-sōm). Dermatitis resulting from penetration of skin of humans by cercariae of nonhuman blood flukes. Common in lake region of northern U.S. It is not associated with visceral schistosomiasis. SYN: *seabather's eruption; swimmer's itch.*

schistosomia (skĭs″tō-sō′mē-ă) [″ + *soma*, body]. Deformed fetus with a fissure in the abdomen; the limbs are rudimentary if present.

schistosomiasis (skĭs″tō-sō-mī′ăs-ĭs) [Gr. *schistos*, divided, + *soma*, body, + *-iasis*, infection]. A parasitic disease due to infestation with blood flukes belonging to the genus *Schistosoma*, q.v. The disease is endemic throughout Asia, Africa, and tropical America. Infestation occurs by wading or bathing in water containing cercariae that have issued from snails. SYN: *bilharziasis.*

schistosomicide (skĭs″tō-sō′mĭ-sīd) [″ + ″ + L. *cidus*, killing]. Something that destroys schistosomes.

schistosternia (skĭs″tō-stĕr′nē-ă) [″ + *sternon*, chest]. Schistothorax.

schistothorax (skĭs″tō-thō′răks) [″ + *thorax*, chest]. Fissure of the thorax.

schistotrachelus (skĭs″tō-tră-kē′lŭs). Fetus with a cleft in the neck.

schizamnion (skĭz-ăm′nē-ŏn) [Gr. *schizein*, to divide, + *amnion*, lamb]. An amnion formed by development of a cavity in the inner cell mass.

schizaxon (skĭz-ăk′sŏn) [″ + *axon*, axle]. An axon that divides in two equal, or nearly equal, branches.

schizencephaly (skĭz″ĕn-sĕf′ă-lē) [″ + *enkephalos*, brain]. Deformed fetus with a longitudinal cleft in the skull.

schizo- (skĭz′ō) [Gr. *schizein*, to split]. Combining form indicating division.

schizoblepharia (skĭz″ō-blĕf′ă-rē″ă) [″ + *blepharon*, eyelid]. Fissure of an eyelid.

schizocyte (skĭz′ō-sīt) [″ + *kytos,* cell]. Schistocyte, q.v.

schizocytosis (skĭz″ō-sī-tō′sĭs) [″ + ″ + *osis*, condition]. Schistocytosis.

schizogenesis (skĭz″ō-jĕn′ĕs-ĭs) [″ + *genesis*, generation, birth]. Reproduction by fission.

schizogony (skĭz-ŏg′ō-nē) [″ + *gone,* seed]. Reproduction by multiple asexual fission characteristic of sporozoa, esp. the life-cycle of the malarial parasite.

schizogyria (skĭz″ō-jī′rē-ă) [″ + *gyros,* a circle]. A cleft in the cerebral convolutions.

schizoid (skĭz′oyd) [″ + *eidos*, form, shape]. Resembling schizophrenia.

schizoid personality disorder. A disorder of the personality characterized by a persistent indifference to social interaction and a limited range of emotional experience and expression. It begins in early adulthood. These persons neither seek nor enjoy close relationships, nor do they want to be part of a family. They lead lonely lives and have no close friends or confidants; sexual interests and activity are almost nonexistent; rarely do they experience strong emotions such as anger and joy. They appear cold and aloof and rarely reciprocate gestures or facial expressions such as smiles or nods.

schizomycete (skĭz″ō-mī-sēt′) [″ + *mykes*, fungus]. Any organism belonging to the class Schizomycetes.

Schizomycetes (skĭz″ō-mī-sē′tēz) [″ + *mykes*, fungus]. Class of plant microorganisms or fungi that multiply by fission. Includes the bacteria.

schizont (skĭz′ŏnt) [″ + *ontos*, being]. 1. A stage appearing in the life cycle of a sporozoan protozoon resulting from multiple division or schizogony. 2. Stage in asexual phase of life cycle of *Plasmodium* organisms found in red blood cells. By schizogony, each gives rise to 12 to 24 or more merozoites. An early schizont is called a presegmenter; a mature schizont is called a rosette or segmenter.

schizonticide (skĭ-zŏn′tĭ-sīd) [″ + ″ + L. *cidus,* killing]. Something that destroys schizonts.

schizonychia (skĭz″ō-nĭk′ē-ă) [″ + *onyx,* nail]. Split condition of the nails.

schizophasia (skĭz″ō-fā′zē-ă) [″ + *phasis*, speech]. Muttered and incomprehensible speech of the schizophrenic.

schizophrenia (schizophrenic disorders). A group of related disorders of unknown etiology in which there is a special type of disordered thinking, affect, and behavior. Diagnosis is difficult to standardize because there are no specific physical findings or laboratory data. Because of this, the diagnosis of schizophrenia is imprecise. In addition, there may be a precise disease called schizophrenia, but at this time, it is virtually impossible to distinguish it from a disease that may only resemble schizophrenia. Clinically, patients exhibit disturbances of content of thought with delusions, such as the feeling that thoughts that have been inserted into their head are now being broadcast to the world. Speech may be coherent in actual words used but entirely unassociated with plausible thoughts or reality. Alternatively, the patient may be mute or completely incoherent. Perception is disordered by all forms of hallucinations. Affect may be flat or inappropriate to the situation. There is loss of a feeling of identity, and self-direction may be disturbed. All activity may be disturbed so that the ability to work or carry a task to completion is severely impaired. Interpersonal relations are abnormal and may manifest as social withdrawal and emotional detachment. The patient may be catatonic or otherwise unaware of his or her surroundings. In general, these disturbances are present for six months before the diagnosis of schizophrenia is accepted. Prognosis is usually poor, but, over a 25- to 30-year period, about one third of patients will show recovery or remission.

Schizophrenia occurs equally in males and females and at any age, but the usual age of admission to a hospital is 28 to 34. It occurs more frequently in the lowest socioeconomic groups. An estimated 100,000 to 200,000 new cases occur each year in the U.S. There is little doubt that genetic factors are important in schizophrenia, but the precise mode of inheritance has not been determined. SEE: *Nursing Diagnoses* in *Appendix.*

TREAT: Supportive psychotherapy for the patient and the family; antipsychotic drugs used in the lowest effective dose.

s., catatonic. A schizophrenic disorder dominated by any of the following: catatonic stupor or mutism; catatonic negativism; catatonic rigidity; catatonic excitement; catatonic posturing. The patients need careful attention to prevent hurting themselves or others, and to treat malnutrition, exhaustion, hyperpyrexia, or injury.

s., disorganized. Schizophrenia characterized by incoherence, grossly disorganized behavior, flat or inappropriate affect, fragmented (i.e., not systemized) delusions, stereotyped behavior with grimaces, mannerisms, and social withdrawal. SYN: *hebephrenic schizophrenia.*

s., paranoid. A type of schizophrenic disorder wherein there are delusions of persecution, grandiosity, jealousy, or hallucinations with persecutory or grandiose content.

s., undifferentiated. A type of schizophrenic disorder characterized by delusions, incoherence, or grossly disorganized behavior. It does not meet the criteria for some other type of schizophrenic disorder.

schizophrenic (skĭz″ō-frĕn′ĭk) [Gr. *schizein*, to divide, + *phren*, mind]. Afflicted with, or person afflicted with, schizophrenia.

schizoprosopia (skĭz″ō-prō-sō′pē-ă) [″ + *prosopon*, face]. Fissure of the face, such as harelip or cleft palate.

schizotonia (skĭz″ō-tō′nē-ă) [″ + *tonos*, tension]. Uneven tone of muscle groups.

schizotrichia (skĭz″ō-trĭk′ē-ă) [″ + *thrix*, hair]. Splitting of the tips of the hair.

schizozoite (skĭz″ō-zō′ĭt) [″ + *zoon*, animal]. Merozoite.

Schlatter-Osgood disease (shlăt′ĕr-ŏz′good). Osgood-Schlatter disease, q.v.

Schlemm, canal of (shlĕm) [Friedrich S. Schlemm, Ger. anatomist, 1795–1858]. Irregular space or spaces in the sclerocorneal region of the eye. It receives the aqueous humor from the anterior chamber of the eye.

Schmorl's disease [Christian G. Schmorl, Ger. pathologist, 1861–1932]. Herniation of the nucleus pulposus.

Schmorl's nodules. Schmorl's disease, q.v.

schneiderian membrane (shnī-dē′rē-ăn) [Conrad Viktor Schneider, Ger. anatomist, 1614–1680]. The nasal mucosa.

Schönlein's disease (shān′līnz) [Johann Lukas Schönlein, Ger. physician, 1793–1864]. An allergic or anaphylactic purpura occurring in individuals, esp. children, with drug sensitivities, serum sickness, and other allergic disorders. It is usually accompanied by pains in joints and abdomen. SYN: *purpura, idiopathic thrombocytopenic.*

Schönlein-Henoch purpura. SEE: *Henoch-Schönlein purpura.*

school phobia. A child's refusal to go to school because of fear.

Schüffner's dots (shĭf′nĕrz) [Wilhelm P. A. Schüffner, Ger. pathologist, 1867–1949]. Minute granules present in red blood cells infected by *Plasmodium vivax.*

Schüller's disease. SEE: *Hand-Schüller-Christian disease.*

Schultze's bundle (shooltz′ĕs) [Max Johann Schultze, Ger. biologist, 1825–1874]. Longitudinal mass of descending fibers, shaped like a comma, in the fasciculus cuneatus of spinal cord.

Schultze's cells. Olfactory cells.

Schultze's granule masses. Fine, granular masses formed by breaking up of plaques in the blood.

Schultz reaction [Werner Schultz, Ger. physician, 1878–1947]. A test that demonstrates the ability of muscle tissues from an animal that has been made anaphylactic to contract when re-exposed to the antigen. Either guinea pig uterine muscles or intestines are used. The test is very specific, as unrelated antigens will not cause the sensitized muscle to contract. Sir Henry Dale demonstrated the same phenomenon independent of Schultz's work. SYN: *Dale reaction.*

Schwabach test (shvă′băk) [Dagobert Schwabach, Ger. otologist, 1846–1920]. A test for hearing using five tuning forks, each of a different tone.

Schwalbe's ring (shvăl′bĕz) [Gustav Albert Schwalbe, Ger. anatomist, 1844–1916]. The peripheral edge of Descemet's membrane of the eye. Also called *Schwalbe's line.*

Schwann's cells (shvŏnz) [Theodor Schwann, Ger. anatomist, 1810–1882]. Cells of ectodermal origin that comprise the neurilemma.

schwannoma (shwŏn-nō′mă). A benign tumor of the neurilemma or sheath of Schwann of a nerve.

schwannosis (shwŏn-nō′sĭs). Hypertrophy of the sheath of Schwann of a nerve.

Schwann's sheath. The neurilemma of a nerve fiber. SYN: *neurilemma.*

Schwann's white substance. Myelin of a medullated nerve fiber.

sciage (sē-äzh′) [Fr., a sawing]. A movement of the hand in massage resembling that in sawing.

sciatic (sī-ăt′ĭk) [L. *sciaticus*]. 1. Pert. to the hip or ischium. 2. Pert. to, due to, or afflicted with sciatica. SYN: *ischiac; ischiatic.* SEE: *sciatica and low back pain.*

sciatica and low back pain (sī-ăt′ĭ-kă) [L.]. Severe pain in the leg along the course of the sciatic nerve felt at back of thigh running down the inside of the leg.

This symptom, which is usually self-limiting, costs patients at least 16 million dollars each year; low back pain will affect 60% to 90% of the population at some time in their lives. Annually, about 5% of the population will experience this type of pain. About 40% of the population will experience sciatica at some time during their lives. SEE: *meralgia; sciatic nerve.* SEE: *Nursing Diagnoses in Appendix.*

SYM: May begin abruptly or gradually and is characterized by a sharp shooting pain running down back of thigh. Movement of limb generally intensifies the suffering. Pain may be uniformly distributed along the limb, but frequently there are certain spots where it is more intense; numbness and tingling may be present; nerve may be extremely sensitive to touch.

ETIOL: 1. Compression or trauma of the sciatic nerve or its roots, esp. that resulting from ruptured intervertebral disk or osteoarthrosis of lumbosacral vertebrae. 2. Inflammation of sciatic nerve resulting from metabolic, toxic, or infectious disorders. 3. Pain referred to distribution of the sciatic nerve from other sources.

TREAT: If possible to determine the cause of the symptoms, the cause is treated with appropriate intervention. If the nerve is being compromised, surgery may be indicated. Because more than 50% of patients with sciatica recover in 6 weeks, surgical therapy should be delayed to provide time for recovery. In acute stage, rest is essential. Heat may give temporary relief from pain. Medication will depend on the diagnosis. Morphine or meperidine may be required to control pain, but the danger of habituation must be kept in mind. In arthritic patients, full doses of salicylates are useful. Early intervention with appropriate physical therapy may be indicated if mechanical positioning, traction, or stabilization decreases the symptoms. Ultimately, a therapeutic exercise program to develop stabilizing strength and endurance in the trunk musculature should be considered for functional recovery.

Because the illness is self-limiting in most patients, almost any form of noninvasive therapy will appear to be effective. This is true no matter what type of medical care practitioner is involved, i.e., physician, osteopath, or chiropractor.

PROG: Recovery follows in majority of cases.

sciatic nerve. Largest nerve in the body, arising from the sacral plexus on either side, passing from the pelvis through the greater sciatic foramen, down the back of the thigh, where it divides into tibial and peroneal nerves. Lesions cause paralysis of flexion and extension of toes, abduction and adduction of toes, rotation inward and adduction of foot, plantar flexion and lowering of ball of foot; anesthesia in cutaneous distribution (external popliteal nerve); paralysis of dorsiflexion and adduction of foot; paralysis of rotation of ball of foot outward and of raising external border of foot and of extension of toes; also anesthesia in cutaneous distribution. SEE: *Nerves* in *Appendix.*

sciatic nerve, small. The posterior femoral cutaneous nerve, a cutaneous nerve supplying skin of buttocks, perineum, popliteal region, and back of thigh and leg.

science (sī′ĕns) [L. *scientia,* knowledge]. The intellectual process for using all of the men-

tal and physical resources available in order to better understand, explain, quantitate, and predict normal as well as unusual natural phenomena. Thus, the scientific approach to understanding anything involves observation, measurement of entities that can be quantitated, the accumulation of data, and analysis of the findings as distinguished from an intuitive approach.

s.´s, life. SEE: *life sciences.*

Science of Unitary Human Beings. SEE: *Appendix 23.*

scieropia (sī-ĕr-ō′pē-ă) [Gr. *skieros,* shadow, + *opsis,* vision]. Abnormal vision in which things appear to be in a shadow.

scintigram (sĭn′tĭ-grăm). The record produced by a scintiscan, q.v.

scintillascope (sĭn-tĭl′ă-skōp) [L. *scintilla,* spark, + Gr. *skopein,* to examine]. Device for viewing the effect of ionizing radiation, alpha particles, on a fluorescent screen.

scintillation (sĭn″tĭ-lā′shŭn) [L. *scintillatio*]. 1. Sparkling; a subjective sensation, as of seeing sparks. 2. The emissions that come from radioactive substances.

scintiphotography (sĭn″tĭ-fō-tŏg′ră-fē). Photographing the scintillations emitted by radioactive substances injected into the body. Used to determine the outline and function of organs and tissues in which the radioactive substance collects or is secreted.

scintiscan (sĭn′tĭ-skăn). Use of scintiphotography to create a map of scintillations produced when a radioactive substance is introduced into the body. The intensity of the record indicates the differential accumulation of a substance in the various parts of the body.

scintiscanner (sĭn″tĭ-skăn′ĕr). The device used in doing a scintiscan.

scirrho- [Gr. *skirrhos,* hard]. Combining form meaning hard, or indicating relationship to a hard tumor or scirrhus.

scirrhoid (skĭr′oyd) [″ + *eidos,* form, shape]. Pert. to, or like, a hard carcinoma or scirrhus.

scirrhoma (skĭr-ō′mă) [″ + *oma,* tumor]. A hard carcinoma or scirrhus.

scirrhosarca (skĭr″ō-săr′kă) [″ + *sarx,* flesh]. Hardening of the flesh, esp. of the newly born. SYN: *sclerema neonatorum.*

scirrhous (skĭr′ŭs) [NL. *scirrhosus,* hard]. Hard, like a scirrhus.

scirrhus (skĭr′ŭs) [Gr. *skirrhos,* hard tumor]. A hard, cancerous tumor due to overgrowth of fibrous tissue.

scission (sĭzh′ŭn) [L. *scindere,* to split]. Dividing, cutting, or splitting.

scissor gait. Crossing the legs in walking. SEE: *gait.*

scissors (sĭz′ors) [LL. *cisorium*]. A cutting instrument composed of two opposed cutting blades with handles, held together by a central pin. This allows the cutting edge to be opened and closed.

scissura (sĭ-sū′rä) [L., to split] (pl. *scissurae*). A fissure or cleft; a splitting.

sclera (sklĕr′ä) [Gr. *skleros*, hard] (pl. *sclerae*). [NA] A tough white fibrous tissue that covers the so-called white of the eye. It extends from the optic nerve to the cornea. SYN: *sclerotica*.

    s., blue. Abnormal degree of blueness of the sclera. It may be a sign of osteogenesis imperfecta.

scleradenitis (sklĕ″răd-ĕn-ī′tĭs) [″ + *aden*, gland, + *itis*, inflammation]. Inflammation and induration of a gland.

scleral (sklĕr′ăl) [Gr. *skleros*, hard]. Concerning the sclera.

scleratogenous (sklĕ″rä-tŏj′ĕ-nŭs). Sclerogenous, q.v.

sclerectasia (sklĕ″rĕk-tā′zē-ä) [″ + *ektasis*, dilatation]. Protrusion of the sclera.

sclerectoiridectomy (sklĕ-rĕk″tō-ĭr″ĭ-dĕk′tō-mē) [″ + *iris*, colored circle, + *ektome*, excision]. Formation of a filtering cicatrix in glaucoma by combined sclerectomy and iridectomy.

sclerectoiridodialysis (sklĕ-rĕk″tō-ĭr″ĭd-ō-dī-ăl′ĭ-sĭs) [″ + ″ + *dialysis*, loosening]. Sclerectomy and iridodialysis for relief of glaucoma.

sclerectomy (sklĕ-rĕk′tō-mē) [″ + *ektome*, excision]. 1. Excision of a portion of the sclera. 2. Removal of adhesions in chronic otitis media.

scleredema (sklĕr″ē-dē′mä) [″ + *oidema*, swelling]. A condition usually following an acute infection characterized by edema and induration of the skin. It is a benign self-limited disease occurring more frequently in females than in males. It is often confused with scleroderma, q.v.

    s. adultorum. S., Buschke's, q.v.

    s., Buschke's. Generalized non-pitting edema that begins on the head or neck and spreads to the body. This lasts a year or less and leaves no sequelae. The cause is unknown.

    s. neonatorum. Sclerema, q.v.

sclerema (sklĕ-rē′mä) [Gr. *skleros*, hard]. Hardening of the skin. SYN: *scleroderma*.

    s. adiposum. S. neonatorum.

    s. adultorum. Scleroderma.

    s. neonatorum. Progressive hardening of the skin in the newborn; usually fatal.

sclerencephalia (sklĕ″rĕn-sē-fā′lē-ä) [″ + *enkephalos*, brain]. Sclerosis of the brain.

scleriasis (sklĕ-rī′ă-sĭs) [Gr. *skleriasis*]. 1. Progressive hardening of the skin. 2. Hardening of the eyelid.

scleriritomy (sklĕ-rĭ-rĭt′ō-mē) [″ + *iris*,

colored circle, + *tome*, incision]. Incision of the iris and sclera.

scleritis (sklĕ-rī′tĭs) [″ + *itis*, inflammation]. Superficial and deep inflammation of the sclera. SYN: *sclerotitis*. SEE: *episcleritis*.

    s., annular. Inflammation limited to the area surrounding the limbus of the cornea. A complete ring is formed.

    s., anterior. Scleritis of the area adjacent to the limbus of the cornea.

    s., posterior. Scleritis limited to the posterior half of the globe of the eye.

scleroblastema (sklĕ″rō-blăs-tē′mä) [Gr. *skleros*, hard, + *blastema*, sprout]. The embryonic tissue from which formation of bone takes place.

scleroblastemic (sklĕ″rō-blăs-tĕm′ĭk). Rel. to or derived from scleroblastema.

sclerocataracta (sklĕ″rō-kăt-ä-răk′tä) [″ + *katarrhaktes*, sheer, abrupt]. A hard cataract.

sclerochoroiditis (sklĕ″rō-kō″royd-ī′tĭs) [″ + *chorioeides*, skinlike, + *itis*, inflammation]. Inflammation of the sclera and choroid coat of the eye.

    s., posterior. Myopic choroiditis, posterior staphyloma.

scleroconjunctival (sklĕ″rō-kŏn″jŭnk-tī′văl) [″ + L. *conjunctivus*, to bind together]. Pertaining to the sclera and conjunctiva.

sclerocornea (sklĕ″rō-kor′nē-ä) [″ + L. *corneus*, horny]. The sclera and cornea together considered as one coat.

sclerodactylia (sklĕr″ō-dăk-tĭl′ē-ä) [″ + *daktylos*, a finger]. Induration of the skin of the fingers and toes. SYN: *acroscleroderma*.

scleroderma (sklĕr″ä-dĕr′mä) [Gr. *skleros*, hard, + *derma*, skin]. A chronic disease of unknown etiology that occurs four times as frequently in women as in men. It causes sclerosis of the skin and certain organs including the gastrointestinal tract, lungs, heart, and kidneys. The skin is taut, firm, and edematous and is firmly bound to subcutaneous tissue, which often causes limitation of range of motion; it feels tough and leathery, may itch, and later becomes hyperpigmented. The skin changes usually precede the development of signs of visceral involvement. For a limited period the only findings may be the CREST syndrome: calcinosis, Raynaud's phenomenon, esophageal dysfunction, sclerodactyly, and telangiectasia. SYN: *progressive systemic sclerosis*. SEE: *collagen diseases*. SEE: *Nursing Diagnoses* in *Appendix*.

    TREAT: There is no specific therapy. General supportive therapy is indicated. A great number of drugs including corticosteroids, vasodilators, D-penicillamine, and immunosuppressive agents have been tried. Physical therapy will help maintain range of motion and muscular strength but will not influence the course of joint disease.

PROG: Variable and unpredictable with respect to rate of pathological changes. Progression is worse in white males than in white females and is worse in black females than in black males. When the onset of the disease is later in life, the prognosis is poor.

s., circumscribed. Localized patches of linear sclerosis of the skin. There is no systemic involvement, and the course of the disease is usually benign.

s. neonatorum. Hardness and tightness of the skin in early infancy. SYN: *sclerema neonatorum.*

sclerodermatitis (sklĕ″rō-dĕr-mă-tī′tĭs) [Gr. *skleros,* hard, + *derma,* skin, + *itis,* inflammation]. Inflammation of the skin accompanied by thickening and hardening.

sclerodermatous (sklĕ″rō-dĕr′mă-tŭs) [″ + *derma,* skin]. Concerning scleroderma.

sclerogenic (sklĕ″rō-jĕn′ĭk) [″ + *gennan,* to produce]. Sclerogenous, q.v.

sclerogenous (sklĕ-rŏj′ĕ-nŭs) [″ + *gennan,* to produce]. Causing sclerosis or hardening of tissue.

scleroid (sklĕ′rŏyd) [″ + *eidos,* form, shape]. Having a hard or firm texture.

scleroiritis (sklĕ″rō-ī-rī′tĭs) [″ + *iris,* colored circle + *itis,* inflammation]. Inflammation of both the sclera and iris.

sclerokeratitis (sklĕr″ō-kĕr-ă-tī′tĭs) [″ + *keras,* horn, + *itis,* inflammation]. Cellular infiltration with inflammation of the sclera and cornea.

sclerokeratoiritis (sklĕ″rō-kĕr″ă-tō-ī-rī′tĭs) [″ + ″ + *iris,* colored circle, + *itis,* inflammation]. Inflamed condition of the sclera, cornea, and iris.

sclerokeratosis (sklĕr″ō-kĕr″ă-tō′sĭs) [″ + ″ + *osis,* condition]. Sclerokeratitis.

scleroma (sklĕ-rō′mă) [″ + *oma,* tumor]. Indurated, circumscribed area of granulation tissue in mucous membrane or skin. SEE: *sclerosis.*

scleromalacia (sklĕ″rō-mă-lā′sē-ă) [Gr. *skleros,* hard, + *malakia,* softening]. Softening of the sclera.

s. perforans. Scleromalacia accompanied by perforation.

scleromere (sklĕr′ō-mēr) [″ + *meros,* a part]. 1. Any segment of metamere of the skeleton. 2. The caudal half of a sclerotome, q.v.

scleromyxedema (sklĕr″ō-mĭk″sē-dē′mă) [″ + *myxa,* mucus, + *oidema,* swelling]. A type of lichen myxedematosus in which the skin under the papules is greatly thickened.

scleronychia (sklĕ″rō-nĭk′ē-ă) [″ + *onyx,* nail]. Thickening and hardening of the nails.

scleronyxis (sklĕ-rō-nĭk′sĭs) [Gr. *skleros,* hard, + *nyxis,* a piercing]. Surgical puncture of the sclera.

sclero-oophoritis (sklĕ″rō-ō-ŏf″ō-rī′tĭs) [″ + *oophoros,* bearing eggs, + *itis,* inflammation]. Induration and inflammation of the ovary.

sclerophthalmia (sklĕ″rŏf-thăl′mē-ă) [″ + *ophthalmos,* eye]. Congenital condition in which opacity of the sclera advances over the cornea.

scleroplasty (sklĕ′rō-plăs″tē) [″ + *plassein,* to form]. Plastic surgery of the sclera.

scleroprotein (sklĕ″rō-prō′tē-ĭn) [″ + *protos,* first]. A group of proteins noted for their insolubility in most chemicals. Found in skeletal tissue, cartilage, hair, nails, and in animal claws and horns.

sclerosal (sklĕ-rō′săl). Sclerous.

sclerosant (sklĕ-rō′sănt) [Gr. *skleros,* hard]. Something that produces sclerosis.

sclerose (sklĕ-rōs′) [Gr. *skleros,* hard]. To become hardened.

sclerosed (sklĕ-rōsd′, sklĕ′rōsd) [Gr. *skleros,* hard]. Having sclerosis; hardened. SYN: *indurated.*

sclerosing (sklĕ-rōs′ĭng). Causing or developing sclerosis.

sclerosing agent. A substance used to cause sclerosis, esp. in the lining of a vein. SEE: *varicose veins.*

sclerosis (sklĕ-rō′sĭs) [Gr. *sklerosis,* to harden]. 1. A hardening or induration of an organ or tissue, esp. that due to excessive growth of fibrous tissue. 2. Hardening within the nervous system, esp. of the brain and spinal cord, resulting from degeneration of nervous elements, as the myelin sheath. SYN: *cerebrosclerosis.* 3. Thickening and hardening of the layers in the wall of an artery. SEE: *arteriosclerosis; atherosclerosis.*

RS: cerebrosclerosis; Charcot-Marie-Tooth disease; scleritis.

s., Alzheimer's. Hyaline degeneration affecting small blood vessels of the brain.

s., amyotrophic lateral. Progressive muscular atrophy resulting from disease conditions, degenerative in nature, involving anterior horn cells and the pyramidal tracts. It is rapidly progressive, usually ending in bulbar paralysis.

s., annular. Sclerosis in which hardened substance forms a band about the spinal cord.

s., arterial. Hardening of the coats of the arteries. SYN: *arteriosclerosis.*

s., arteriolar. Sclerosis of arterioles.

s., diffuse. Sclerosis affecting large areas of the brain and spinal cord.

s., disseminated. S., multiple.

s., *hyperplastic.* S., medial.

s., *insular.* S., multiple.

s., *intimal.* Atherosclerosis.

s., *lateral.* Sclerosis of the lateral column of the spinal cord. SEE: *s., amyotrophic lateral.*

    s., *lobar.* Sclerosis of the cerebrum resulting in mental disturbances.

    s., *medial.* Sclerosis involving the tunica media of arteries, usually the result of involutional changes accompanying aging. SYN: *s., hyperplastic.*

    s., *multiple.* A chronic, slowly progressive disease of the central nervous system characterized by development of disseminated demyelinated glial patches called plaques. Symptoms and signs are numerous, but common early symptoms include paresthesias and visual disturbances, and in later stages, those of Charcot's triad (nystagmus, scanning speech, and intention tremor) are common. Occurs in the form of many clinical syndromes, the most common being the cerebral, brain stem-cerebellar, and spinal. A history of remissions and exacerbations is diagnostic. Etiological factors are unknown and there is no specific therapy. SYN: *s., disseminated.*

    s., *neural.* Sclerosis with chronic inflammation of a nerve trunk with branches.

    s., *renal.* Nephrosclerosis.

    s., *tuberous.* SEE: *tuberous sclerosis.*

    s., *vascular.* Sclerosis of the walls of blood vessels; arterial and venous sclerosis.

    s., *venous.* Phlebosclerosis.

scleroskeleton (sklĕr″ō-skĕl′ĕ-tŏn) [Gr. *skleros*, hard, + *skeleton*, a dried-up body]. Skeletal changes resulting from ossification of fibrous structures, such as ligaments, fasciae, and tendons.

sclerostenosis (sklĕr″ō-stĕ-nō′sĭs) [″ + *stenosis*, act of narrowing]. Contraction and induration of tissues, esp. those about an orifice.

    s. cutanea. Induration of the skin. SYN: *scleroderma.*

sclerostomy (sklĕ-rŏs′tō-mē) [″ + *stoma*, mouth]. Surgical formation of an opening in the sclera.

sclerotherapy (sklĕr″ō-thĕr′ă-pē) [″ + *therapeia*, treatment]. Use of sclerosing agents in treating diseases, esp. hemorrhoids.

sclerothrix (sklĕr′ō-thrĭks) [″ + *thrix*, hair]. Brittleness of the hair.

sclerotic (sklĕ-rŏt′ĭk) [L. *scleroticus*, hard]. Pert. to or affected with sclerosis.

sclerotica (sklĕ-rŏt′ĭ-kă) [L. *scleroticus*, hard]. The exterior white coat of the eye. SYN: *sclera.*

sclerotic acid. An amorphous, brown powder from ergot. A hemostatic and oxytocic.

sclerotic dentin. Areas of dentin where the tubules have been filled by mineralization, producing a more dense, radiopaque dentin; it is often produced in response to caries, attrition, and abrasion.

scleroticectomy (sklĕ-rŏt″ĭ-sĕk′tō-mē) [″ + Gr. *ektome*, excision]. Excision of a part of the sclera. SYN: *sclerectomy.*

scleroticochoroiditis (sklĕ-rŏt″ĭ-kō-kō″roy-dī′tĭs) [″ + Gr. *chorioeides*, skinlike, + *itis*, inflammation]. Inflammation of sclerotic and choroid coats of the eye. SYN: *scleroehoroiditis.*

scleroticonyxis (sklĕ-rŏt″ĭ-kō-nĭk′sĭs) [″ + Gr. *nyxis*, a piercing]. Surgical puncture of the sclera. SYN: *scleronyxis.*

scleroticopuncture (sklĕ-rŏt″ĭ-kō-pŭnk′tŭr) [″ + *punctura*, a piercing]. Surgical puncture of the sclera. SYN: *scleronyxis; scleroticonyxis.*

scleroticotomy (sklĕ-rŏt″ĭ-kŏt′ō-mē) [″ + Gr. *tome*, incision]. Incision of the sclerotic coat of the eye. SYN: *sclerotomy.*

sclerotic teeth. Teeth that are hard and highly resistant to caries.

sclerotitis (sklĕr-ō-tī′tĭs) [Gr. *skleros*, hard, + *itis*, inflammation]. Inflammation of the sclera. SYN: *scleritis.*

sclerotium (sklĕ-rō′shē-ŭm). Hardened mass formed by growth of certain fungi. That formed by ergot on rye is of medical importance.

sclerotome (sklĕr′ō-tōm) [″ + *tome*, incision]. 1. Knife used in incision of the sclera. 2. One of a series of segmentally arranged masses of mesenchymal tissue lying on either side of the notochord. They give rise to the vertebrae and ribs.

sclerotomy (sklĕ-rŏt′ō-mē). Surgical incision of sclera. SYN: *scleroticotomy.*

    s., *anterior.* Incision made at angle of the anterior chamber of the eye in glaucoma.

    s., *posterior.* Incision through the sclera into the vitreous for detached retina or removal of a foreign body.

sclerotrichia (sklĕ-rō-trĭk′ē-ă) [Gr. *sclerosis*, hard, + *thrix*, hair]. Hardness and brittleness of the hair.

sclerous (sklĕr′ŭs). Hard; indurated.

scobinate (skō′bĭn-āt) [L. *scobina*, rasp]. Having a rough, uneven, nodular surface.

scoleciasis (skō-lĕ-sī′ă-sĭs) [Gr. *skolex*, worm, + *-iasis*, condition]. Presence of larval forms of butterflies or moths in the body.

scoleciform (skō-lĕs′ĭ-form) [″ + L. *forma*, form]. Resembling a scolex.

scolecoid (skō′lĕ-koyd) [″ + *eidos*, form, shape]. Resembling a worm.

scolecology (skō″lĕ-kŏl′ō-jē) [″ + *logos*, word, reason]. Helminthology.

scolex (skō′lĕks) [Gr. *skolex*, worm] (pl. *sco-*

lices). The portion of a tapeworm, the so-called head, by which it attaches itself to the wall of the intestine. Scolices usually possess organs such as hooks, suckers, or grooves (bothria) for attachment.

scoliokyphosis (skō″lē-ō-kī-fō′sĭs) [Gr. *skolios*, twisted, + *kyphosis*, humpback]. Combined scoliosis and kyphosis.

scoliometer (skō″lē-ŏm′ĕt-ĕr) [″ + *metron*, measure]. Device for measuring curves, esp. lateral ones of the spine.

scoliorachitic (skō″lē-ō-ră-kĭt′ĭk) [″ + *rhachis*, spine]. Pert. to, or afflicted with, spinal curvature from rickets.

scoliosiometry (skō″lē-ō-sē-ŏm′ĕ-trē) [″ + *metron*, measure]. Measurement of degree of spinal curvature. SYN: *scoliosometry.*

scoliosis (skō″lē-ō′sĭs) [Gr. *skoliosis*, crookedness]. Lateral curvature of the spine. Usually consists of two curves, the original abnormal curve and a compensatory curve in the opposite direction.

NURSING IMPLICATIONS: Make provisions to assist the adolescent and family to meet the psychosocial needs associated with the illness. Teach the patient and family concerning treatment modality (cast, brace, traction, or electrical stimulation), exercises, activity level, skin care, prevention of complications, and breathing exercises. Provide preoperative teaching when necessary, including postanesthesia breathing exercises; explain apparatus that will be used postoperatively (such as a Stryker frame or Circ-O-Lectric bed); exercises and diet, as prescribed. Encourage socialization with peers and expend every effort to help the adolescent feel accepted and worthwhile. Provide patient and family with access to educational and support resources. SEE: *Nursing Diagnoses* in *Appendix.*

s., cicatricial. Scoliosis due to cicatricial contraction resulting from necrosis.

s., congenital. Scoliosis present at birth, usually the result of defective embryonic development of the spine.

s., coxitic. Scoliosis in the lumbar spine due to tilting of the pelvis in hip disease.

s., empyematic. Scoliosis following empyema and retraction of one side of the chest.

s., habit. Scoliosis due to habitually assumed improper posture or position.

s., idiopathic. Scoliosis due to unknown causes.

s., inflammatory. Scoliosis due to disease of the vertebrae.

s., ischiatic. Scoliosis due to hip disease.

s., myopathic. Scoliosis due to weakening of spinal muscles.

s., neuropathic. A structural scoliosis caused by congenital or acquired neurological disorders.

s., ocular. Scoliosis from tilting of the head because of visual defects or extraocular muscle imbalance.

s., osteopathic. Scoliosis caused by bony deformity of the spine.

s., paralytic. Scoliosis due to paralysis of muscles.

s., rachitic. Scoliosis due to rickets.

s., sciatic. Scoliosis due to sciatica.

s., static. Scoliosis due to difference in length of legs.

scoliosometry (skō″lē-ō-sŏm′ĕt-rē) [″ + *metron*, measure]. Determination of degree of spinal curvature. SYN: *scoliosiometry.*

scoliotic (skō-lē-ŏt′ĭk). Suffering from, or related to, scoliosis.

scoliotone (skō′lē-ō-tōn) [Gr. *skolios*, twisted, + *tonos*, tension]. An apparatus for correcting the curve in scoliosis by stretching the spine.

scombrine (skŏm′brĭn). A protamine present in mackerel sperm.

scombroid. Fish of the suborder Scombroidea. Included in this group are mackerels, tuna, bonitos, albacores, and skipjacks.

scombroid poisoning. Intoxication due to eating raw or inadequately cooked fish of the suborder Scombroidea. Certain bacteria act on the fish after they are caught to produce a histamine-like toxin.

Once the toxin forms, nothing can be done to destroy it, and there is usually no abnormal taste or smell to the fresh or cooked fish.

Fish known to have been associated with this type of toxin are tuna, mackerel of the Scombridae family, and amberjack, mahimahi, and bluefish, which are nonscombroid fish. These fish should be either eaten shortly after being caught or refrigerated immediately.

SYM: Nausea, vomiting, abdominal cramps, diarrhea, flushing, headache, urticaria, and a burning sensation and metallic taste in the mouth. The incubation period varies from 15 minutes to 3 hours and averages 45 minutes. Symptoms last less than one day.

TREAT: There is no specific therapy, but remove ingested fish by use of gastric lavage or emesis.

scoop (skoop) [ME., a ladle]. Spoon-shaped surgical instrument.

s., bone. Instrument for scraping or removing necrosed bone or contents of suppurative tracts.

s., bullet. Instrument for dislodging bullets.

s., cataract. Instrument for removing

fluids or foreign growths.

s., ear. Instrument for removing middle ear granulations.

s., lithotomy. Instrument for dislodging encysted calculi or removing stones, debris, etc.

s., mastoid. Instrument used in mastoid operations.

s., renal. Instrument to dislodge or remove small stones from pelvis of kidney.

scoparius (skō-pā'rē-ŭs). The fresh or dried tops of broom, *Cytisus scoparius*. It acts as a diuretic and emetic.

-scope [Gr. *skopein*, to examine]. Combining form meaning an instrument or device for viewing or examining.

scopolamine, transdermal. A method of delivering scopolamine by applying a patch containing the drug to the skin. The medicine is slowly absorbed over a period of several days. It is esp. useful in treating vertigo and motion sickness. In the latter condition, the medicine will be effective if applied several hours before the individual is exposed to the motion. The drug should be used cautiously in elderly patients because it may cause confusion, memory loss, and hallucinations.

scopolamine hydrobromide (skō-pŏl'ă-mēn hī''drō-brō'mīd). USP. The hydrobromide of alkaloids obtained from plants of the nightshade family.

ACTION/USES: As a sedative; locally as a mydriatic; and with morphine and pentobarbital in labor to produce "twilight" sleep. SYN: *hyoscine hydrobromide.*

scopometer (skō-pŏm'ē-tĕr) [Gr. *skopein*, to examine, + *metron*, measure]. Instrument for measuring the density of a suspension.

scopophilia (skō''pō-fil'ē-ă) [" + *philein*, to love]. Sexual pleasure derived from visual sources such as nudity and obscene pictures. SEE: *voyeur.*

scopophobia (skō''pō-fō'bē-ă) [" + *phobos*, fear]. Abnormal fear of being seen.

scopophobiac (skō''pō-fō'bē-ăk). One who is afraid of being seen.

-scopy [Gr. *skopein*, to examine]. Combining form meaning examination.

scoracratia (skor''ă-krā'shē-ă) [Gr. *skor*, dung, + *akratia*, lack of control]. Inability to retain the feces. SYN: *fecal incontinence.*

scorbutic (skor-bū'tĭk) [NL. *scorbuticus*, scurvy]. Concerning or affected with scurvy.

scorbutigenic (skor-bū''tĭ-jĕn'ĭk) [LL. *scorbutus*, scurvy, + Gr. *gennan*, to produce]. Something that causes scurvy.

scorbutus (skor-bū'tŭs) [LL., scurvy]. A deficiency disease due to lack of vitamin C in the diet. SYN: *scurvy.* SEE: *vitamin C.*

scordinema (skor-dĭ-nē'mă) [Gr. *skordinema*, yawning]. Yawning and stretching with fatigue and heaviness of the head, a prodromal symptom of an infectious disease.

score (skor). 1. A rating or grade as compared with a standard of other individuals, esp. in a competitive event. 2. To mark the skin with lines in order to have landmarks available, as in plastic surgery. 3. In dentistry, a rating that represents some assessment of the oral health or history of the individual. A DMF score or index represents decayed-missing-filled teeth; a periodontal score, or periodontal disease index, represents the relative health of the soft tissue of the mouth. SEE: *index, DMF; index, periodontal.*

s., Apgar. SEE: *Apgar score.*

scoretemia (skor-ē-tē'mē-ă) [Gr. *skor*, dung, + *haima*, blood]. Scatemia.

scorpion (skor'pē-ŏn) [Gr. *skorpios*, to cut off]. Insects of the class Arachnida and order Scorpionida. They vary in size from less than 2 in. (5 cm) in length for the small bark scorpions of Arizona to some African scorpions which may be 8 in. (20 cm) in length. The tail of the scorpion contains two venom glands connected to the tip of the stinger. Most scorpions are nocturnal and reclusive. Humans may encounter them by disturbing their daytime hiding places. They are most active during a time when the night temperatures remain above 70°F (21°C). The bites of most species in the U.S. seldom produce severe toxic reactions, but because of the difficulty of distinguishing one species of scorpion from another, each scorpion bite should be treated as if it had been inflicted by a species capable of delivering a very toxic dose of venom. SEE: *scorpion sting.*

scorpion sting. Scorpion bites may vary in severity from only a local tissue reaction consisting of swelling at the puncture site to a severe neurotoxic reaction which produces intense, aching pain and numbness radiating from the site of the bite, and paralysis and convulsions. Also present could be a rapid weak pulse, shock, excessive salivation, extreme thirst, and dysuria. The venom capable of causing the latter type reaction contains hemolysins, lytic enzymes, and neurotoxins. Death can occur, particularly in very young children.

TREAT: For mild reactions, application of cold compresses to the area will lessen the pain and may inhibit spread of the venom to the general circulation. In mild reactions, the symptoms usually subside within four hours. For the severe reactions use cold compresses to the area, treat the shock, and provide appropriate therapy for convulsions. Analgesics for pain.

Caution: Morphine and its derivatives are contraindicated because they act synergistically to increase the toxic effects of the venom.

Antivenins are available. Sources for those may be obtained by contacting the Information Officer, Centers for Disease Control, Atlanta, GA, 30333. Phone number is (404) 329-3311; or contact the nearest Poison Control Center. SEE: *Poison Control Centers in Appendix.*

scoto- (skō′tō) [Gr. *skotos,* darkness]. Combining form indicating a relation to darkness.

scotochromogen (skō″tō-krō′mō-jĕn) [″ + *chroma,* color, + *gennan,* to produce]. Any microorganism that produces a chromogen when grown in light or darkness.

scotodinia (skō″tō-dĭn′ē-ă) [″ + *dinos,* whirling]. Vertigo with black spots before the eyes and faintness of vision.

scotogram, scotograph (skō′tō-grăm, -grăf) [″ + *gramma,* something written; ″ + *graphein,* to write]. Any radiation effect recorded in the dark on a photographic plate.

scotoma (skō-tō′mă) [Gr. *skotoma,* to darken] (pl. *scotomata*). Islandlike blind gap in the visual field.

    s., absolute. An area in the visual field in which there is absolute blindness.

    s., annular. A scotomatous zone that encircles the point of fixation like a ring, not always completely closed, but leaving the fixation point intact.

    s., arcuate. Arc-shaped scotoma near the blind spot of the eye. It is caused by a nerve bundle defect on the temporal side of the optic disk.

    s., central. An area of depressed vision involving the point of fixation, seen in lesions of the macula.

    s., centrocecal. Defect in vision that is oval-shaped and includes the fixation point and the blind spot of the eye.

    s., color. Color blindness in a limited portion of the visual field.

    s., eclipse. An area of blindness in the visual field due to having looked directly at the sun during an eclipse.

    s., flittering. S., scintillating.

    s., negative. Scotoma not perceptible by the patient, being a blind spot in the visual field.

    s., peripheral. A defect in vision removed from the point of fixation of the vision.

    s., physiological. Blind spot due to absence of rods and cones where the optic nerve enters the retina.

    s., positive. Area that patient perceives in the visual field as a dark spot.

    s., relative. Scotoma in which perception of the object is impaired but not completely lost.

    s., ring. SEE: *s., annular.*

    s., scintillating. An irregular outline around a luminous patch in the visual field following mental or physical labor, following eyestrain, or in migraine. SYN: *s., flittering.*

scotomagraph (skō-tō′mă-grăf) [Gr. *skotoma,* to darken, + *graphein,* to write]. Device for recording scotomata.

scotomata (skō-tō′mă-tă) [Gr.]. Pl. of scotoma.

scotomatous (skō-tŏm′ă-tŭs) [Gr. *skotoma,* to darken]. Rel. to, of the nature of, or afflicted with scotoma.

scotometer (skō-tŏm′ĕt-ĕr) [″ + *metron,* a measure]. Device for detecting and measuring scotomata in the visual field.

scotometry (skō-tŏm′ĕ-trē). The locating and measurement of scotomata.

scotophilia (skō″tō-fĭl′ē-ă) [″ + *philein,* to love]. Preference for darkness or for the night. SYN: *nyctophilia.*

scotophobia (skō″tō-fō′bē-ă) [″ + *phobos,* fear]. Abnormal dread of darkness. SYN: *noctiphobia; nyctophobia.*

scotopia (skō-tō′pē-ă) [″ + *ops,* eye]. Adjustment of the eye for vision in dim light. Opposite of photopia.

scotopic (skō-tŏp′ĭk). Pert. to scotopia.

scotopic vision. Dark adaptation; the adjustment of the eyes for vision in dark or dim light. SYN: *night vision.*

scotopsin (skō-tŏp′sĭn). The protein portion of the rods of the retina of the eye. It combines with retinal to form rhodopsin.

scotoscopy (skō-tŏs′kō-pē) [Gr. *skotos,* darkness, + *skopein,* to examine]. Examination of internal organs by use of the fluoroscope. SYN: *skiascopy.*

scout film. In radiology, an x-ray, esp. of the abdomen, for detecting abnormalities. These films are of assistance in excluding or including certain diseases being considered as diagnostic possibilities.

scr. scruple.

scratch (skrăch) [ME. *cracchen,* to scratch]. 1. A mark or superficial injury produced by scraping with the nails on a rough surface. 2. To make a thin, shallow cut with a sharp instrument. 3. To rub the skin, esp. with fingernails, to relieve itching. Scratching temporarily relieves itching by soothing the cutaneous nerves, but in the long run, it may worsen the condition that caused the itching. SEE: *pruritus.*

scratch test. Placement of an appropriate dilution of a test material, suspected of being an allergen, in a lightly scratched area of the skin. If the material is an allergen, a wheal will develop within 15 minutes.

screatus (skrē-ā'tŭs) [L., a hawking]. A neurosis characterized by paroxysmal fits of hawking or snorting.

screen [O. Fr. *escren*]. 1. A flat area upon which movies or slides are viewed, or suitable for visualizing x-ray pictures. 2. To make a fluoroscopic examination. 3. To examine, using physical and mental examinations and laboratory tests to determine the presence of a certain disease or characteristics. 4. A structure or substance used to protect, guard, or shield from a damaging influence such as x-rays or sun rays. 5. A system used to select or reject personnel. 6. In psychiatry, the blocking of one memory with another.

   s., Bjerrum [Jannik P. Bjerrum, Danish ophthalmologist, 1827–1872]. A one-meter square planar surface viewed from a distance of one meter. It is used to plot the physiological blind spot, scotomata, and other visual field defects. SYN: *s., tangent.*

   s., fluorescent. A flat screen covered with a material that in a darkened room will light up when x-rays pass through it. Used in studying the image produced on the screen during fluoroscopy.

   s., intensifying. An apparatus that increases the brightness of the image being radiographed.

   s., tangent. SEE: *s., Bjerrum.*

screening. 1. The testing, usually using one diagnostic procedure including laboratory studies, of large groups of people to determine the presence of a particular disease or of certain risk factors known to be associated with that disease.

   Ex.: chest x-ray or tuberculin test for tuberculosis, urinalysis for diabetes, serum cholesterol for potential arteriosclerosis, intraocular pressure for glaucoma.

   2. In psychiatry, the initial examination to determine the mental status of an individual and the appropriate initial therapy.

   s., multiphasic. The use of many diagnostic tests to determine the presence of one or more diseases.

Scribner shunt [Belding Scribner, U.S. physician, b. 1921]. A tube usually made of synthetic material used to connect an artery to a vein. It is used in patients requiring frequent venipuncture, as in hemodialysis. This type of device and others have greatly simplified the care of patients requiring hemodialysis. Nevertheless, the shunts may develop complications such as infection, thrombosis, and release of septic emboli.

scrobiculate (skrō-bĭk'ū-lāt) [L. *scrobiculus*, little trench]. Having shallow depressions; pitted.

scrobiculus (skrō-bĭk'ū-lŭs) [L., little trench]. A small groove or pit.

   s. cordis. Pit of the stomach; precordial or epigastric depression.

scrofula (skrŏf'ū-lă) [L., breeding sow]. A variety of tuberculous adenitis that is most frequently encountered. It is thought to be a secondary involvement of cervical lymph nodes as a result of a localized hematogenous spread from a pulmonary lesion. Most common in childhood.

   TREAT: Responds to specific antituberculosis chemotherapy.

scrofulid(e) (skrŏf'ū-lĭd, -lĭd). Scrofuloderma.

scrofuloderma (skrŏf″ū-lō-dĕr'mă) [L. *scrofula*, breeding sow, + Gr. *derma*, skin]. A skin manifestation of tuberculous origin, usually secondary to scrofula. Marked by ulcers usually resulting from a tuberculous sinus. Occurs most commonly on chest, on neck, and in the axillae and groins, esp. in children and adolescents. Now very rare.

   TREAT: Responds to ultraviolet light treatments and specific chemotherapy for tuberculosis.

scrofulosis (skrŏf″ū-lō'sĭs) [″ + Gr. *osis*, condition]. Scrofula.

scrofulous (skrŏf'ū-lŭs) [L. *scrofula*, breeding sow]. Of the nature of, or afflicted with, scrofula.

scrotal (skrō'tăl) [L. *scrotum*, a bag]. Concerning the scrotum.

scrotal reflex. Slow vermicular contraction of scrotal muscle when perineum is stroked or cold applied.

scrotectomy (skrō-tĕk'tō-mē) [″ + Gr. *ektome*, excision]. Excision of part of the scrotum.

scrotitis [″ + Gr. *itis*, inflammation]. Inflamed condition of the scrotum.

scrotocele (skrō'tō-sēl) [″ + Gr. *kele*, tumor, swelling]. Hernia in the scrotum.

scrotoplasty (skrō'tō-plăs″tē) [″ + Gr. *plassein*, to form]. Plastic surgery on the scrotum.

scrotum (skrō'tŭm) [L., a bag] (pl. *scrota*, *-ums*). [NA] The double pouch of the male, which contains the testicles and part of the spermatic cord, found in most mammals. Constituent parts of the scrotum are skin; a network of nonstriated muscular fibers called dartos; cremasteric, spermatic, and infundibuliform fasciae; cremasteric muscle; and tunica vaginalis.

   RS: chimney-sweeps' cancer; chyloderma; dartos; oscheal; oscheitis; oscheoncus; rhacoma; urocele; varicocele.

scrubbing [MD. *schrubben*]. Term applied to washing the hands, fingernails, and lower arms in preparation for performing surgery.

The precise procedure to follow usually is posted in a special area where the washing is done.

METHOD: Scrubbing with soap and water and a nail brush, immersion in a mild germicidal solution, and the wearing of sterilized rubber gloves, cap, gown, and mask.

scrub nurse. Term applied to operating room nurse who hands instruments to the surgeon, and who has previously scrubbed his or her hands and wears a mask, sterile rubber gloves, and gown.

scrub typhus. An acute febrile illness caused by *Rickettsia tsutsugamushi* transmitted by several species of mites, including *Trombicula akamushi* and *T. deliensis*. Common in the Asiatic-Pacific area. If untreated, fever lasts for about 14 days. Fatality rate varies in untreated cases from 1% to 4%. SYN: *tsutsugamushi disease*.

TREAT: Tetracycline or chloramphenicol.

scruple (skrū′pl) [L. *scrupulus*, small, sharp stone]. ABBR: scr. SYMB: Ɔ Twenty grains in apothecaries' weight; 1.296 gm.

SCUBA. *self-contained underwater breathing apparatus.*

Scultetus bandage (skŭl-tē′tŭs) [Johann Schultes (Scultetus), Ger. surgeon, 1595–1645]. A many-tailed bandage or binder, applied around the abdomen so that the ends overlap each other as if they were roof shingles. The binder holds dressings in place and supports abdominal muscles postoperatively. SEE: *binder, Scultetus*, for illus.

Scultetus position. Position in which the head is low and the body is on an inclined plane.

scum (skŭm) [ME. *scume*]. Slimy floating islands of bacteria or impurities on the surface of a culture; an interrupted pellicle of bacterial growth.

scurf [AS. *scurf*]. A branny desquamation of the epidermis, esp. on the scalp. SEE: *dandruff*.

scurvy (skŭr′vē) [L. *scorbutus*]. A deficiency disease characterized by hemorrhagic manifestations and abnormal formation of bones and teeth.

SYM: Preceded by period of ill health characterized by sallow complexion; loss of energy; pains in legs, limbs, and joints. Anemia; great weakness; spongy, bleeding gums; fetor of breath; loosening of teeth; subcutaneous hemorrhages and hemorrhages from mucous membranes; painful, brawny indurations of muscles characterize overt symptoms.

ETIOL: Deficiency of vitamin C usually resulting from lack of fresh fruits and vegetables in diet.

TREAT: For infants, 300 mg of vitamin C

(ascorbic acid) daily for 1 week, then 150 mg daily for 1 month, or 4 to 8 oz (52 to 104 ml) of orange juice or 12 to 24 oz (155 to 311 ml) of tomato juice daily. For adults, 300 to 500 mg of ascorbic acid daily until symptoms have disappeared.

PROG: Favorable in early stages.

s., infantile. A form of scurvy that sometimes follows the prolonged use of condensed milk, sterilized milk, or proprietary foods that do not contain supplementary vitamin C. SYN: *Barlow's disease*.

SYM: Anemia, immobility of legs, pseudoparalysis, extreme tenderness, swelling without pitting, thickening of bones from subperiosteal hemorrhage, ecchymoses, and tendency toward fractures of epiphyses of bones.

scute (skūt) [L. *scutum*, shield]. 1. A thin plate or scale, esp. the horny plates found on the carapace of a turtle. 2. Term formerly applied to the tegmen tympani.

scutiform (skū′tĭ-form) [″ + *forma*, shape]. Shield-shaped.

scutular (skū′tū-lăr) [L. *scutulum*, a little shield]. Having small indented crusts of the skin.

scutulum (skū′tū-lŭm) [L., a little shield] (pl. *scutula*). Lesion of the scalp caused by the fungus *Trichophyton schoenleinii*. A yellow cup-shaped crust consisting of a dense mass of mycelia and epithelial debris. The cup faces up, and its center is pierced by the hair around which it has developed. SEE: *favus*.

scutum (skū′tŭm) [L., shield]. Plate of bone resembling a shield.

scybalous (sĭb′ă-lŭs) [Gr. *skybalon*, dung]. Of the nature of hard fecal matter.

scybalum (sĭb′ă-lŭm) (pl. *scybala*). A hard rounded mass of fecal matter.

scypho- [Gr. *skyphos*, cup]. Combining form meaning cup.

scyphoid (sī′foyd) [″ + *eidos*, form, shape]. Cup-shaped.

S.D. *skin dose; standard deviation.*

SDA. 1. *specific dynamic action.* 2. Abbreviation for Latin *sacrodextra anterior*. The right sacroanterior fetal position.

SDMS. *Society of Diagnostic Medical Sonographers.*

S.E. *standard error.*

Se. Chem. symb. for the element selenium.

seabather's eruption. Itching red papules that may appear on the skin within a few hours of swimming in the sea. The lesions progress to form crusted papules and disappear spontaneously in 7 to 10 days. Treatment is symptomatic. Caused by a form of schistosome found in coastal and inland waters of North America. SYN: *schistosome dermatitis; swimmer's itch*.

seal. 1. To close firmly. 2. A material such as

an adhesive or wax used to make an airtight closure.

s., border. Edge of a denture that contacts the tissues in order to close the area under the denture to entrance by food, air, or liquids.

s., posterior palatal. Seal at the posterior border of a denture.

s., velopharyngeal. Seal between the oral and nasopharyngeal cavities.

sealant. A substance applied to prevent leakage into or out of an area.

s., dental. Some type of resin that will bond to etched enamel of a tooth and form a protective coating resistant to chemical or physical breakdown.

s., pit and fissure. A method of helping to prevent dental caries by applying adhesive resins to teeth to fill the deep pits and fissures of the occlusal surfaces. This prevents accumulation of debris or decay-producing bacteria from entering these vulnerable areas.

seal finger. An infection of the finger due to the bite of a seal. The infectious agent has not been identified, but it is carried in the blood of the seal. It is sensitive to tetracycline.

searcher (sẽrch′ẽr) [ME. *serchen*]. Instrument for locating opening of ureter previous to inserting catheter or exploring sinuses, and esp. for detecting stones in the bladder. SYN: *sound.*

seasickness [AS. *sae*, sea, + *seocness*, illness]. Disorder due to motion of a boat, or riding in cars, trains, and elevators. A similar condition affects some air travelers. SYN: *motion sickness.*

SYM: Giddiness, vomiting, headache, nausea, and often extreme drowsiness, retching, prostration.

ETIOL: Motion affects the middle ear, and the vomiting center in the brain stem is stimulated. There is wide individual variation in susceptibility.

PREVENT: Select position in craft where up-and-down motion is least; avoid dietary and alcoholic excesses; avoid reading or unusual visual stimuli; assume a supine or recumbent position.

TREAT: 50 mg of Dramamine (dimenhydrinate) every four hours as necessary. This medicine causes some people to experience drowsiness; those individuals should not operate a motor vehicle or dangerous machinery when taking Dramamine. Sedatives and supportive therapy, such as intravenous fluids, may be required in severe and prolonged cases. Generally, antinausea pills should not be given to pregnant women during early pregnancy.

Transdermal scopolamine is effective in preventing seasickness if it is given several hours before the individual is exposed to the motion. The drug should be used cautiously in elderly patients because it may cause confusion, memory loss, and hallucinations.

seasonal affective disorder. ABBR: SAD. A disorder of mood characterized by mental depression related to a certain season of the year, esp. winter. Symptoms include daytime drowsiness, fatigue, and diminished concentration. Symptoms usually begin during adulthood. It is four times as common in women as in men. The part played by the decreased amount of sunlight during the winter is not clear. Nevertheless, the disorder is improved by exposure to bright light, esp. if it is used in the early morning.

seat. The structure upon which another structure rests or is supported.

s., basal. Tissues in the mouth that support a denture.

s., rest. An area upon which a denture or restoration rests.

Seattle foot [after the city Seattle, Washington, U.S., where it was developed]. An artificial foot that has a spring-back quality that makes it feel like a real foot. Use of this device allows single- or double-foot amputees to run and engage in other sports.

seatworm. A species of nematode worms, *Enterobius vermicularis*, which commonly infests humans. Adult worms inhabit large intestine in region of cecum and appendix. Gravid females migrate nightly to anus, where they deposit eggs in the perianal region. Movement of the worms about anus causes intense itching. SYN: *pinworm.*

sebaceous (sē-bā′shŭs) [L. *sebaceus*, made of tallow]. Containing, or pert. to, sebum, an oily, fatty matter secreted by the sebaceous glands.

sebaceous cyst. A cyst filled with sebum from a distended sebaceous gland. These cysts are sometimes known as wens. They frequently form on the scalp and consist of a small sac, containing sebaceous matter, that may grow to a large size. They may result from impairment of localized circulation and closure of sebaceous glands or ducts. Drainage does not remove them permanently because they will recur unless entirely extirpated. Extirpation, q.v., should be done with an electric current or cutting knife. One should never attempt to drain such a cyst without taking every precaution against infection.

sebaceous gland. Oil-secreting gland of the skin. The glands are simple or branched alveolar glands, most of which open into hair follicles. They are holocrine glands, their secretion, sebum, arising from disintegration of cells filling the alveoli. Most sebaceous glands have a hair follicle associated with them. Some aberrant glands are found in the cheeks or lips of the oral cavity, well separated from hair follicles. SEE: *Fordyce's spots.*

sebastomania (sē-băs″tō-mā′nē-ă) [Gr. *sebastos*, reverend, + *mania*, madness]. Religious insanity. SYN: *theomania.*

sebiferous (sē-bĭf′ĕr-ŭs) [L. *sebum*, tallow, + *ferre*, to carry]. Producing fatty or sebaceous matter. SYN: *sebiparous.*

sebiparous (sē-bĭp′ă-rŭs) [″ + *parere*, to produce]. Producing sebum or sebaceous matter. SYN: *sebiferous.*

sebo- [L. *sebum*, grease, tallow]. Combining form concerning the fatty substance secreted by sebaceous glands.

sebolite, sebolith (sĕb′ō-līt, -lĭth) [″ + Gr. *lithos*, a stone]. Concretion in a sebaceous gland. SYN: *sebolith.*

seborrhagia (sĕb″ō-rā′jē-ă) [″ + Gr. *rhegnynai*, to burst forth]. Excessive secretion of sebaceous glands. SYN: *seborrhea.*

seborrhea (sĕb-or-ē′ă) [″ + Gr. *rhoia*, flow]. Functional disease of the sebaceous glands marked by increase in the amount, and often alteration of the quality, of the sebaceous secretion.

TREAT: Mild dandruff may be treated with a shampoo containing selenium sulfide or sulfur. If severe, a lotion or cream containing corticosteroids, preferably in the form of hydrocortisone, is rubbed into the affected areas two or three times a day.

    s. capiti. Seborrhea of the scalp.

    s. congestiva. Facial form of seborrhea with elevated patches with red borders and covered with crusts and scars. SYN: *lupus erythematosus.*

    s. corporis. Seborrhea of the trunk.

    s. faciei. Seborrhea of the face.

    s. furfuracea. Dermatitis seborrheica.

    s. nigricans. Dark-colored crusts occurring in seborrhea.

    s. oleosa. Seborrhea in which fat elements predominate. Shows shiny skin with widely dilated follicular orifices, many of which contain comedones.

    s. sicca. Seborrhea with gray-brown or yellow scale and crust formation in addition to abnormal oiliness. Differentiation from seborrheic dermatitis is difficult. This form is most frequently observed on scalp and constitutes what is popularly called dandruff. Examination reveals an encrustation composed of thin yellowish-gray scales. In uncomplicated cases the skin is pale but often becomes hyperemic or inflamed from irritation. When allowed to continue, nutrition of hair is interfered with, and baldness results.

On the body, seborrhea sicca appears as

yellowish-gray, slightly elevated patches covered with greasy scales. Outlets of follicles are often dilated. There is generally more or less redness of the skin from hyperemia (seborrheal eczema).

seborrheic (sĕb″ō-rē′ĭk) [L. *sebum*, tallow, + Gr. *rhoia*, flow]. Afflicted with or like seborrhea.

seborrheid (sĕb″ō-rē′ĭd) [″ + Gr. *rhoia*, flow]. Seborrheic dermatitis.

seborrhoic (sĕb″ō-rō′ĭk). Suffering from or like seborrhea. SYN: *seborrheic.*

sebum (sē′bŭm) [L., tallow]. A fatty secretion of the sebaceous glands of the skin. It varies in different parts of the body. Sebum from the ears is called cerumen, q.v.; that from the foreskin is called smegma, q.v.

    s. palpebrale. Lema, q.v.

secernent (sē-sĕr′nĕnt) [L. *secernens*, secreting]. 1. Secreting. 2. A secreting organ.

seclusion of pupil. Shutting off of the pupil due to adherence of iris to the lenticular capsule. SYN: *synechia, annular.*

seclusio pupillae siderosis bulbi. Deposit of iron pigment within the eyeball. Seen in cases of iron foreign bodies retained in the eye.

secobarbital. USP. A barbiturate used for its sedative and hypnotic effects.

    s. sodium. USP. A hypnotic and sedative drug. Trade name is Seconal Sodium.

secodont (sē′kō-dŏnt) [L. *secare*, to cut, + Gr. *odous*, tooth]. Having molar teeth with cutting edges on the cusps.

Seconal. Trade name for secobarbital, USP.

Seconal Sodium. Trade name for secobarbital sodium.

secondary. 1. Next to or following; second in order. 2. Produced by a primary cause.

secondary areola. Pigmentation around the nipples during pregnancy. SEE: *areola.*

secondary care. Health care beyond the primary. Included are more sophisticated diagnostic methods and techniques, and laboratory facilities. This level of care is more nearly available in medical care institutions serving a large population. SEE: *primary care; tertiary care.*

secondary gain. SEE: *gain, secondary.*

secondary hemorrhage. 1. Hemorrhage appearing more than 24 hours after an injury or operation that is due to sepsis and septic ulceration into a blood vessel. 2. Uterine bleeding due to septic infection or from infant's umbilicus due to same cause.

secondary nursing care. Nursing care aimed at early recognition and treatment of disease. It includes general nursing intervention and teaching of early signs of disease conditions so that prompt medical care can be obtained.

secondary radiation. X-rays produced by

the interaction between primary radiation and the substance being examined.

second cranial nerve. A sensory nerve that conveys visual impulses from eye to thalamus. The two optic nerves undergo partial decussation at the optic chiasm. SEE: *cranial nerves; Cranial Nerves in Appendix.*

second intention. Healing by granulation or indirect union. Granulation tissue is formed to fill the gap between the edges of the wound with a thin layer of fibrinous exudate. It bars bacteria and aids in checking bleeding by the coagulation of the blood. Connective tissue cells support the new capillaries. This form of healing is slower than that by first intention, and its grayish-red surface may become pale and flabby if the healing is too long delayed. If the granulations show above the surface, they may have to be removed with caustics. If the granulations first form at the top instead of the bottom of the wound, the wound may have to be kept open with drainage. SEE: *intention; resolution.*

second sight. Alteration in refractive powers of the lens so that reading is possible again without glasses. This temporary condition occurs as a cataract develops over a period of years. SYN: *senopia.*

second stage of labor. Period in labor between complete dilation of the cervix and delivery of the child. During this stage involuntary contractions of the uterus become quite strong. This stage normally lasts 2 to 4 hours in primiparae and about 1 hour in multiparae. SEE: *labor.*

second wind. Condition occurring during strenuous exercise in which the feeling of subjective breathlessness subsides.

secreta (sē-krē′tă) [L.]. The products of secretion.

secretagogue (sē-krē′tă-gŏg) [L. *secretum,* secretion, + Gr. *agogos,* leading]. 1. That which stimulates secreting organs. 2. An agent that causes secretion. SYN: *secretogogue.*

secrete (sē-krēt′) [L. *secretio,* separation]. To separate from the blood, living organism, or gland; more specifically, to form a secretion.

secretin (sē-krē′tĭn). A hormone that stimulates pepsinogen secretion by the stomach and inhibits the secretion of acid by the stomach. It is also important in stimulating the secretion of bicarbonate (HCO_3) from both the pancreas and the liver. SEE: *cholecystokinin-pancreozymin.*

secretinase (sē-krē′tĭ-năs). An enzyme in blood that inactivates secretin.

secretion [L. *secretio,* separation]. 1. The process whereby cells of glandular organs produce certain materials from the blood. 2. The substance produced by glandular organs.

If the material flows out through a duct (e.g., saliva), it is called an external secretion; if it is returned to the blood or lymph (e.g., insulin), it is called an internal secretion.

FLUIDS OF BODY: *Blood:* Composed of 79% water, 21% solids, including the cellular elements of blood. *Bile:* Emulsifies fats and precipitates soluble peptones, 20 to 24 oz (259 to 311 ml) are produced daily. Sp. gr. 1.026 to 1.032. Reaction alkaline. *Chyle:* Absorbed by lacteals, the lymphatics of the small intestines. Contains fat absorbed from food. *Chyme:* Food that has undergone gastric digestion only. *Gastric juice:* Clear, acid, watery secretion of the glands of the stomach. Principal ingredients are hydrochloric acid, mucus, and pepsin. *Intestinal juice:* Has combined action of saliva and gastric and pancreatic juices. Starch and complex sugars are converted into monosaccharides. Reaction alkaline. *Lymph:* Characteristics vary with site of origin. If derived from a limb, it may be clear and have less than 1 gm of protein/100 ml. If derived from gut, protein is increased and fluid may have milky appearance. *Menstrual:* Menstrual flow. Average 60 ml during each period. Consists of blood, cellular tissue, and mucus. Blood clots are not usually abnormal. *Pancreatic juice:* Contains enzymes that act on fats, proteins or products of protein digestion, and carbohydrates. Approx. 2000 ml of a fluid of pH 7.5 to 8.0 secreted daily. *Perspiration:* The secretion of sweat glands. From 100 to 1000 ml/day under normal conditions. May be many times that amount in extremely hot and dry conditions. *Saliva:* Composition varies with particular glands, being watery if from parotid and viscous from submandibular glands. Approx. 1500 ml/day secreted. Serves to lubricate food and break down starch and glycogen. *Urine:* 1000 to 2500 ml/24 hours, but highly variable. Sp. gr. 1.003 to 1.025. Reaction acid. Contains 50 to 70 gm of solids, 12 to 20 gm/day of urea nitrogen, and chlorides 110 to 250 nmol/liter depending upon chloride intake. SEE: *urine.*

s., apocrine. Secretion in which the apical end of a secreting cell is broken off and its contents extruded, as in the mammary gland.

s., external. Secretion that passes through a duct and is discharged upon an epithelial surface, either internal or external. Also called *exocrine secretion.*

s., holocrine. Secretion in which the entire cell and its contents are extruded as a part of the secretory product, as in sebaceous glands.

s., internal. Secretion imparted to the blood instead of being eliminated by a duct. Also called *endocrine secretion.*

s., merocrine. Secretion in which the product is elaborated within cells and discharged through the cell membrane, the cell itself remaining intact.

s., paralytic. Continuous abundant watery secretion from a gland after section of its secretory nerves.

secretion, words pert. to: acrinia; amyxia; apolepsis; asteatosis; athyreosis; athyroidism; cerumen; ceruminal; ceruminosis; ceruminous; choleresis; chromocrinia; crinogenic; diacrisis; endocrine; errhine; exocrine; exsiccant; hormone; interstitial; saliva; sebum; secretagogue; secrete; secretin; semen; smegma; succorrhea.

secretogogue (sē-krē′tō-gŏg) [L. *secretio,* separation, + Gr. *agogos,* leading]. SEE: *secretagogue.*

secretoinhibitory (sē-krē″tō-ĭn-hĭb′ĭ-tō″rē). Inhibiting secretion.

secretomotor (sē-krē″tō-mō′tor). Something, esp. a nerve, that stimulates secretion.

secretor (sē-krē′tor) [L. *secretio,* separation]. A person who secretes ABO blood group substances into mucous secretions such as saliva or gastric juice.

secretory (sē-krē′tō-rē, sē′krē-tō″rē). Pert. to or promoting secretion; secreting.

secretory capillaries. Very small canaliculi receiving secretion discharged from gland cells.

secretory fibers. Centrifugal nerve fibers that excite secretion.

sectarian (sĕk-tā′rē-ăn) [L. *sectus,* having cut]. A medical practitioner who follows a dogma, tenet, or principle based on some unscientific belief.

sectile (sĕk′tĭl) [L. *sectilis*]. Capable of being cut.

sectio (sĕk′shē-ō) [L., a cutting]. Section or cut.

section [L. *sectio,* a cutting]. 1. Process of cutting. 2. A division or segment of a part. 3. A surface made by cutting.

s., abdominal. Any incision through the abdomen. SYN: *laparotomy.*

s., cesarean. Incision of the uterus for delivery of a fetus through the abdominal wall.

s., cesarean, postmortem. SEE: *cesarean section, postmortem.*

s., coronal. S., frontal.

s., frontal. Section dividing the body into two parts, dorsal and ventral. SYN: *s., coronal.*

s., frozen. A thin section of the body, an organ, or a piece of tissue that has been frozen before being sectioned and then studied microscopically.

s., midsagittal. Section that divides the body into right and left halves.

s., paraffin. Section of a tissue that has been infiltrated with paraffin.

s., perineal. External incision into the urethra to relieve stricture.

s., Pitres′. One of the series of sections made through the brain for postmortem examination.

s., sagittal. Section cut parallel to the median plane of the body.

s., serial. Microscopic sections made and arranged in consecutive order.

s., vaginal. Incision into the abdominal cavity through the vagina.

sectioning [L. *sectio,* a cutting]. The slicing of thin sections of tissue for examination under the microscope. SEE: *microtome.*

s., ultrathin. The cutting of sections extraordinarily thin (less than 1 micron in thickness), esp. for use in electron microscopy.

sector (sĕk′tor) [L., cutter]. The area of a circle included between two radii and an arc.

sectorial (sĕk-tō′rē-ăl). Having cutting edges, as teeth.

secundigravida (sē-kŭn″dĭ-grăv′ĭd-ă) [L. *secundus,* second, + *gravida,* pregnant]. A woman in her second pregnancy.

secundina (sē″kŭn-dī′nă) [L., from *secundinus,* following]. That which follows.

secundines (sĕk′ŭn-dīnz, sĭ-kŭn′dĭnz) [LL. *secundinae*]. The placenta, umbilical cord, and fetal membranes expelled during the third stage of labor. SYN: *afterbirth.*

secundipara (sē″kŭn-dĭp′ă-ră) [L. *secundus,* second, + *parere,* to bring forth, to bear]. A woman who has produced two infants at separate times that have weighed 500 grams or more, regardless of their viability. SEE: *gravida; para.*

secundiparity (sē-kŭn″dĭ-păr′ĭ-tē). The condition of being a secundipara.

secundum artem (sē-kŭn′dŭm ăr′tĕm) [L.]. In an approved manner; according to rule or science.

S.E.D. *skin erythema dose.*

sedation (sē-dā′shŭn) [L. *sedatio,* from *sedare,* to calm]. 1. Process of allaying nervous excitement. 2. State of being calmed.

sedative (sĕd′ă-tĭv) [L. *sedativus,* calming]. 1. Quieting. 2. An agent that exerts a soothing or tranquilizing effect. Sedatives may be general, local, nervous, or vascular.

s., cardiac. Sedative that decreases the heart's force.

s., nervous. Sedative affecting nervous system.

sedentary (sĕd′ĕn-tā″rē) [L. *sedentarius*]. 1. Sitting. 2. Pert. to an occupation or mode of living requiring minimal physical exercise.

sedentary living. A lifestyle involving little exercise, even of the least strenuous type. Increasing evidence indicates that this lifestyle is not conducive to maximum enjoyment of health or to longevity. SEE: *risk factors.*

sediment (sĕd'ĭ-mĕnt) [L. *sedimentum*, a settling]. The substance settling at bottom of a liquid. SYN: *hypostasis.* SEE: *precipitate.*

    s., urinary. Material that separates and accumulates at the bottom of a container of urine. This process may be accelerated by centrifuging the urine specimen. SEE: *urinary sediment.*

sedimentation (sĕd"ĭ-mĕn-tā'shŭn). Formation or depositing of sediment.

sedimentation rate. ABBR: ESR (erythrocyte sedimentation rate). A nonspecific laboratory test of speed at which erythrocytes settle. In this test, blood to which an anticoagulant has been added is placed in a long, narrow tube, and the distance the red cells fall in one hour is the rate, ESR. Normally, in males, it is less than 10 mm/hr; it is slightly higher in females.

    The speed at which the cells settle depends upon the size of the clumps into which the red cells aggregate, and the size of the clumps appears to depend upon the amount of fibrinogen in the blood. The sedimentation rate is a nonspecific indicator of disease, esp. inflammatory conditions. It is not a useful screening test. Some conditions retard sedimentation. These include polycythemia, congenital heart disease, and hypochromic microcytic anemia.

    An unexplained increase in the ESR is usally transitory and rarely due to serious disease.

seed (sēd) [AS. *saed*]. 1. The ripened ovule of a spermatophyte plant usually consisting of the embryo (germ) and a supply of nutrient material enclosed within the seed coats. It is a resting sporophyte. 2. Sperm; semen. 3. Capsule containing radon or radium for use in treatment of cancer. 4. Offspring. 5. To introduce microorganisms into a culture medium.

Seessel's pouch (zā'sĕlz) [Albert Seessel, U.S. embryologist and neurologist, 1850–1910]. In the embryo, a small ectodermal diverticulum of the foregut close to the buccopharyngeal membrane. It disappears in humans.

segment (sĕg'mĕnt) [L. *segmentum*, a portion]. 1. A part or section, esp. a natural one, of an organ or body. 2. One of the serial divisions of an animal.

    s., bronchopulmonary. A small subdivision of the lobes of the lung.

    s.'s, hepatic. Subdivision of the lobes of the liver.

    s., interannular. Portion of a neuron between two nodes of Ranvier.

    s., mesodermal. A somite.

    s.'s, uterine. Segments of the uterus during labor. The upper portion becomes thicker and the lower segment is thinned out.

segmental (sĕg-mĕn'tăl). Pert. to, resembling, or composed of segments.

segmental reflex. A reflex action in which afferent impulses enter the cord in the same segment or segments from which the efferent impulses emerge.

segmental static reactions. Postural reflexes in which movements of one extremity result in a movement in an opposite extremity.

segmentation (sĕg"mĕn-tā'shŭn) [L. *segmentum*, a portion]. 1. Division into similar parts. 2. Division of a fertilized egg into many smaller cells or blastomeres. SYN: *cleavage.* SEE: *blastomere; cleavage; embryo.*

    s., rhythmic. Division of the intestine and the chyme within it into segments by contraction of circular muscle fibers.

segmenter. Stage in development of the malarial organism (of the genus *Plasmodium*) in which the organism is undergoing schizogony. SYN: *rosette.* SEE: *schizont.*

segmentum (sĕg-mĕn'tŭm) [L.]. A portion or part of a structure.

segregation [L. *segregare*, to separate]. 1. Setting apart, separating. 2. In genetics, the process that takes place in the formation of germ cells (gametogenesis) in which each gamete (egg or sperm) receives only one of each pair of genes.

segregator. Instrument composed of two ureteral catheters for securing urine from each kidney separately.

Séguin's signal symptom (sā-gănz') [Edouard Séguin, Fr. psychiatrist in U.S., 1812–1880]. Involuntary contractions of muscles just before an epileptic attack.

SeHCAT. Selenium-75 labeled artificial bile salt; homologue to taurocholate.

Seidlitz powder (sĕd'lĭts, sīd'lĭtz) [Seidlitz, village in Bohemia]. Effervescent cathartic composed of tartaric acid, sodium bicarbonate, and sodium and potassium tartrate.

seismesthesia (sīz"mĕs-thē'zē-ă) [Gr. *seismos*, a shaking, + *aisthesis*, sensation]. Perception of vibrations.

seizure (sē'zhŭr) [O. Fr. *seisir*, to take possession of]. A sudden attack of pain, of a disease, or of certain symptoms.

    s., absence. SEE: *epilepsy.*

    s., convulsive. 1. A convulsion. 2. An attack of epilepsy. SEE: *epilepsy.*

    s., grand mal. SEE: *epilepsy.*

    s., jacksonian. SEE: *jacksonian epi-*

lepsy.

s., petit mal. SEE: *epilepsy.*

Seldinger technique. Method for introducing a catheter into a vein or artery. The vessel is located with a special needle that contains a wire; the needle is removed. The catheter is threaded into the vein while being guided by the wire over which it is moving. The wire is then removed from the catheter.

selection [L. *selectus,* having chosen]. 1. Choice; the process of choosing or selecting. 2. In biology, the factors that determine the reproductive ability of a certain genotype.

s., artificial. Process by which humans select desirable characteristics in animals and breed them for these phenotypes.

s., natural. Mechanism of evolution proposed by Darwin stating that the genotypes best adapted to their environment have a tendency to survive and reproduce.

s., sexual. Theory originated to account for differences in secondary sex characteristics between males and females. It assumes that individuals preferentially mate with individuals of the opposite sex who possess these characteristics.

selenium (sē-lē′nē-ŭm) [Gr. *selene,* moon]. SYMB: Se. At. wt. 78.96; at. no. 34. A chemical element resembling sulfur. It is poisonous to certain animals that feed on plants grown on soil that contains an excess of selenium.

s. sulfide. USP. A drug used in treating dandruff and tinea versicolor. Trade names for preparations including selenium sulfide are Exsel, Selsun, and Selsun Blue.

selenoid cells. SEE: *achromocytes.*

selenomethionine Se 75 injection (sĕl″ ĕn-ō-mĕ-thī′ō-nēn). USP. Radioactive L-selenomethionine in which the sulfur atom in the methionine has been replaced by selenium. The compound is used intravenously to investigate methionine metabolism.

self. In immunology, an individual's own antigenic make-up.

self-acceptance. Being realistic about oneself and at the same time comfortable with that personal assessment.

self-care. A concept central to Dorothea Orem's theory of nursing, self-care includes actions directed toward the self and toward the environment with the specific purpose of regulating one's functioning and wellbeing. The nurse's central function is to enhance the self-care of patients through the nursing process of assessment, planning, intervention, and evaluation.

self-care deficit. A deficit of thinking, action, emotion, or resources within a patient or his or her environment which impedes

successful self-care and necessitates the services of a nurse.

Self-Care Framework. SEE: *Appendix 23.*

self-concept. An individual's perception of self in relation to others and the environment.

self-conscious. Being aware of oneself, especially overly aware of appearance and actions, and thus being ill at ease.

self-contained underwater breathing apparatus. ABBR: SCUBA. A device used by free swimmers and divers. The mask worn is watertight and is connected to a tank of compressed air. Use of SCUBA permits great freedom for the swimmer as compared with the previously used diving suit that involved being enclosed in a watertight suit connected to a source of air on the surface of the water. SEE: *bends.*

self-defeating personality disorder. A behavior pattern involving not only self-defeat but, in many cases, avoidance of pleasurable situations. Socially this disorder manifests in persons who choose to relate to one who is abnormal, incompetent, or unavailable. The patient's response to positive personal events may be depression or guilt. Efforts to assist these individuals is rejected.

self-differentiation. The differentiation of tissues even though they are isolated.

self-digestion. Destruction or disintegration of a cell or tissue by its own juice, as that of the walls of the stomach by the gastric juice occurring in certain diseases of that organ. SYN: *autodigestion.*

self-esteem. One's personal evaluation or view of self, generally thought to influence feelings and behaviors. One's personal successes, expectations, and appraisals of the views others hold toward oneself are thought to influence this personal appraisal. SYN: *self-concept; self-worth.*

self-governance. A model of nursing management where the power base for decisions of patient care is decentralized. The responsibility and accountability for patient care rests directly with all levels of nurses through self-direction, self-regulation, and self-management. Advisory committees reflecting a cross section of nurses (new graduates, experienced nurses, faculty, and managers) maintain final decision-making authority within the work setting. SEE: *shared governance.*

self-hypnosis. Hypnotizing oneself.

self-limited disease. Disease that, without treatment, runs a definite course within a limited time.

self-ranging. Patient-administered passive range of motion following stroke. By using their unaffected arms and specific techniques, patients with hemiplegia can be taught to prevent contractures by moving their paralyzed extremities through full range of motion at the shoulder, elbow, wrist, and finger joints. Care should be exercised to prevent injury, especially at the shoulder.

self-tolerance. In immunology, tolerance to self-antigens.

sellar (sĕl'ăr). Concerning the sella turcica.

sella turcica (sĕl'ă tŭr'sĭ-kă) [NL., Turkish saddle]. [NA] A concavity on superior surface of body of sphenoid bone that houses the hypophysis cerebri (pituitary gland). SEE: *empty-sella syndrome.*

Sellick's maneuver. Application of digital pressure to cricoid cartilage in neck in an unconscious patient to prevent gastric regurgitation, and to permit visualization of glottic opening during endotracheal intubation.

Selsun. Trade name for selenium sulfide, USP.

Selsun Blue. Trade name for selenium sulfide, USP.

seltzer water. 1. Naturally occurring water with a high mineral and carbon dioxide content. 2. Water that has been artificially charged with carbon dioxide.

semantics (sē-măn'tĭks) [Gr. *semantikos*, significant]. The area of linguistics concerned with meaning.

semeiography (sē″mē-ŏg'ră-fē) [Gr. *semeion*, sign, + *graphein*, to write]. Description of the signs and symptoms of a disease.

semeiology (sē″mī-ŏl'ō-jē) [″ + *logos*, word, reason]. The branch of medicine dealing with the study of signs and symptoms. SYN: *symptomatology.*

semeiotics (sē″mī-ŏt'ĭks). 1. Branch of medicine concerned with signs and symptoms. SYN: *semiotics; symptomatology.* 2. Symptoms of a disease in a particular case considered as a whole.

semelincident (sĕm″ĕl-ĭn'sĭ-dĕnt) [L. *semel*, once, + *incidens*, falling upon]. Occurring only once in a person.

semen (sē'mĕn) [L., seed] (pl. *semina*). A thick, opalescent, viscid secretion discharged from the urethra of the male at the climax of sexual excitement (orgasm). Contains the spermatozoa. Semen is the mixed product of various glands (prostate and bulbourethral) plus the spermatozoa, which, having been produced in the testicles, are stored in the seminal vesicles.

Normal values for the seminal fluid ejaculate: volume, 2 to 5 ml; pH, 7.8 to 8.0; leukocytes, absent or only an occasional one seen per high-power field; sperm count, 60 to 150 million/ml; motility, 80% or more should be motile; morphology, 80% to 90% should be normal.

RS: aspermatism; azoospermia; bradyspermatism; coitus; copulation; ejaculation; emission; erection; fertilization; insemination; libido; orgasm; penis; prostate; semenarche; sexual intercourse; sperm; vesicle, seminal.

s., frozen. Semen stored in a bank for future use in insemination. It offers a supply of donors in small communities where it would be impossible to maintain anonymity of local donors. However, in artificial insemination the number of successful pregnancies is lower with frozen semen than with fresh.

semenarche (sē'mĕn-ăr″kē) [″ + *arche*, beginning]. During puberty, the beginning of production of semen. SEE: *pubarche; thelarche.*

semenuria (sē″mĕn-ū′rē-ă) [L. *semen*, seed, + Gr. *ouron*, urine]. Excretion of semen in the urine. SYN: *seminuria; spermaturia.*

semi- [L. *semis*, half]. Prefix meaning half.

semicanal (sĕm″ē-kăn-ăl′) [″ + *canalis*, channel]. A duct open on one side.

semicanalis (sĕm″ē-kă-nā'lĭs) [L., semicanal]. A channel open on one side.

 s. musculi tensoris tympani. Semicanal of tensor tympani muscle in the temporal bone.

 s. tubae auditivae. Semicanal of the auditory tube.

semicartilaginous (sĕm″ē-kăr″tĭ-lăj'ĭ-nŭs) [″ + *cartilago*, gristle]. Partially cartilaginous.

semicircular (sĕm″ē-sŭr′kū-lăr) [″ + *circulus*, a ring]. In the form of a half circle.

semicircular canals. Superior, posterior, and inferior passages forming part of inner ear.

semicoma (sĕm″ē-kō'mă) [″ + Gr. *koma*, a deep sleep]. Mild degree of impaired consciousness from which it is possible to arouse the patient.

semicomatose (sĕm″ē-kō'măt-ōs). In a condition of impaired consciousness from which patient may be aroused. SEE: *consciousness.*

semiconscious. Half-conscious or not fully conscious. SEE: *Glasgow coma scale.*

semicrista (sĕm″ē-krĭs'tă) [L.]. A small or rudimentary crest.

 s. incisiva. The nasal crest of the maxilla.

semidecussation (sĕm″ē-dē″kŭs-sā'shŭn) [″ + *decussare*, to make an X]. Incomplete crossing of nerve fibers.

semierection (sĕm″ē-ē-rĕk'shŭn) [″ + *erigere*, to erect]. An incomplete erection.

semiflexion (sĕm″ē-flĕk'shŭn) [″ + *flexio,*

bending]. Halfway between flexion and extension of a limb.

semi-Fowler's position. Semisitting position with knees flexed and supported by pillows on the bed.

semilunar (sĕm″ē-lū′năr) [L. *semis,* half, + *luna,* moon]. Shaped like a crescent.

semilunar bone. Half-moon-shaped bone of carpus. Also called the lunate bone.

semilunar cartilages. Two crescentic cartilages (medial and lateral) in the knee joint between the femur and tibia.

semilunar cusps. The three segments of the aortic valve between the left ventricle and the ascending aorta.

semilunare (sĕm″ē-lū-nā′rē) [L.]. The lunate bone of the wrist.

semilunar ganglion. The ganglion associated with the sensory root of the 5th cranial nerve. SYN: *gasserian ganglion; trigeminal ganglion.*

semilunar line. SEE: *line, semilunar.*

semilunar lobe. Lobe on upper surface of the cerebellum.

semilunar notch. Notch at the proximal end of the ulna for articulation with trochlea of the humerus.

semilunar valves. Heart valves between the ventricles and the vessels leaving the ventricles, i.e., the pulmonary artery and the aorta.

semiluxation (sĕm″ē-lŭk-sā′shŭn) [″ + *luxatio,* dislocation]. Subluxation.

semimembranosus (sĕm″ē-mĕm″brăn-ō′sŭs) [L.]. Large muscle of inner and back part of the thigh. SEE: *Muscles* in *Appendix.*

semimembranous (sĕm″ē-mĕm″bră-nŭs) [″ + L. *membrana,* membrane]. Composed partly of a membrane.

seminal (sĕm′ĭ-năl) [L. *seminalis*]. Concerning the semen or seed.

seminal duct. Any duct that conveys sperm, esp. the ductus deferens and the ejaculatory duct. SYN: *spermatic duct.*

seminal emission. Discharge of semen.

seminal fluid. Semen.

seminal vesicle. One of two saclike structures in the male, lying behind the bladder close to the prostate and connected to the ductus deferens on each side. They secrete a thick viscous fluid that forms a part of the semen.

semination (sĕm-ĭ-nā′shŭn) [L. *seminatio,* a begetting]. Introduction of semen into the female genital tract. Occurs during sexual intercourse or may be introduced artificially. SYN: *insemination.*

   s., artificial. Introduction of semen into the vagina or uterus by artificial means. SYN: *artificial insemination.*

seminiferous (sĕm-ĭn-ĭf′ĕr-ŭs) [L. *semen,* seed, + *ferre,* to produce]. Producing or

conducting semen, as the tubules of the testes.

seminoma (sĕm″ĭ-nō′mă) [″ + Gr. *oma,* tumor]. A tumor of the testis.

seminormal (sĕm″ē-nor′măl) [L. *semis,* half, + *norma,* rule]. One-half the normal standard.

seminal solution. Solution having half the quantity of the substance in the normal solution. Indicated thus: 0.5 N or N/2.

seminose (sĕm′ĭ-nōs). Mannose.

seminuria (sē″mĭn-ū′rē-ă) [L. *semen,* seed, + Gr. *ouron,* urine]. Semen in the urine. SYN: *semenuria; spermaturia.*

semiology (sē″mē-ŏl′ō-jē) [Gr. *semeion,* sign, + *logos,* word, reason]. Semeiology, q.v.

semiorbicular (sĕm″ē-or-bĭk′ū-lăr) [L. *semis,* half, + *orbiculus,* a small circle]. Semicircular.

semiotic (sē″mē-ŏt′ĭk) [Gr. *semeiotikos*]. Like or pert. to symptoms of disease. SYN: *semeiotic; symptomatic.*

semiotics (sē″mē-ŏt′ĭks). Scientific study of symptoms as a whole, or in one particular case. SYN: *semeiotics; symptomatology.*

semipenniform (sĕm″ē-pĕn′ĭ-form) [L. *semis,* half, + *penna,* feather, + *forma,* shape]. Penniform on one side.

semipermeable (sĕm″ē-per′mē-ă-bl) [″ + *per,* through, + *meare,* to pass]. Half-permeable; said of a membrane that will allow fluids, but not the dissolved substance, to pass through it. SEE: *membrane; osmosis.*

semipronation (sĕm″ē-prō-nā′shŭn) [″ + *pronus,* prone]. A semiprone position.

semiprone (sĕm-ē-prōn′) [″ + *pronus,* prone]. In a position on left side and chest, with both thighs flexed on abdomen, the right higher than the left, and left arm back. SYN: *Sims' position.*

semirecumbent (sĕm″ē-rē-kŭm′bĕnt) [″ + *recumbere,* to lie down]. Reclining, but not fully recumbent.

semis (sē′mĭs) [L.]. ABBR: ss. Half.

semisideratio, semisideration (sĕm″ē-sĭd-ĕr-ā′shē-ō, -ā′shŭn) [″ + *sideratio,* a blight]. Paralysis on one side of the body. SYN: *hemiplegia.*

semisopor (sĕm″ē-sō′por) [″ + *sopor,* deep sleep]. Light coma from which patient can be roused. SYN: *semicoma.*

semispinalis (sĕm″ē-spī-năl′ĭs) [L.]. Deep layer of muscle of back on either side of spinal column, divided into three parts. SEE: *Muscles* in *Appendix.*

semisulcus (sĕm″ē-sŭl′kŭs) [L. *semis,* half, + *sulcus,* groove]. A small sulcus or channel in a structure. It usually joins with another small channel to form a complete sulcus.

semisupination (sĕm″ē-sū-pĭn-ā′shŭn) [″

+ *supinus,* lying on the back]. A position halfway between supination and pronation.

semisupine (sĕm″ē-sū′pīn) [″ + *supinus,* lying on the back]. Not completely supine.

semisynthetic (sĕm″ē-sĭn-thĕt′ĭk) [″ + Gr. *synthetikos,* synthetic]. Chemical alteration of a portion of a natural substance.

semitendinosus (sĕm″ē-tĕn″dĭn-ō′sŭs) [L.]. Fusiform muscle of posterior and inner part of thigh. SEE: *Muscles* in *Appendix.*

semitendinous (sĕm″ē-tĕn″dĭ-nŭs) [L. *semis,* half, + *tendinosus,* tendinous]. Being partially tendinous.

senescence (sē-nĕs′ĕns) [L. *senescens,* growing old]. 1. The process of growing old. 2. The period of old age.

Sengstaken-Blakemore tube (sĕngz′tā-kĕn-blāk′mor) [Robert W. Sengstaken, U.S. neurosurgeon, b. 1923; Arthur H. Blakemore, U.S. surgeon, 1897–1970]. A three-lumen tube used to treat bleeding esophageal varices. One lumen leads to the stomach; another leads to a balloon at the gastric end — it is used to inflate the balloon after the tube is in place; the third lumen leads to an inflatable cuff around a portion of the entire tube. This third lumen allows the cuff to be inflated and provide pressure against the varices. The gastric balloon permits the cuff to resist being inadvertently removed and serves to keep the entire tube in place.

senile (sē′nīl, sĕn′īl) [L. *senilis,* old]. Pert. to growing old and the mental or physical weakness with which it is sometimes associated.

senilism (sē′nīl-ĭzm, -nīl-ĭzm) [″ + Gr. *ismos,* condition]. Old age, particularly when premature. SEE: *progeria.*

senility (sē-nĭl′ĭ-tē) [L. *senilis,* old]. Mental or physical weakness that may be associated with old age.

   s., premature. Onset of senile characteristics before old age, as early as 40 years.

   s., psychosis of. Mental disorder in old age.

senium (sē′nē-ŭm) [L.]. Old age, esp. its debility.

senna (sĕn′ă) [Arabic *sana*]. USP. The dried leaves of the plant *Cassia acutifolia* and *C. angustifolia.* Used as a cathartic.

sennosides (sĕn′ō-sīdz). USP. Anthraquinone glucosides present in senna that are used as cathartics. Trade name is Glysennid.

senology [Fr. *sein,* cavity, breast + Gr. *logos,* word, reason]. Study of the breast and breast disease.

senopia (sĕn-ō′pē-ă, sē-nō′-) [L. *senilis,* old, + Gr. *ops,* eye]. Improvement in near vision of old people. Usually precedes the development of nuclear cataract. SYN: *second sight.*

sensate. Perceived by the senses.

sensate focus. An area, such as an erogenous zone, q.v., that is particularly sensitive to tactile stimulation.

sensation (sĕn-sā′shŭn) [L. *sensatio*]. A feeling or awareness of conditions within or without the body resulting from the stimulation of sensory receptors.

   s., cincture. S., girdle.

   s., cutaneous. Sensation arising from receptors of the skin.

   s., delayed. Sensation not experienced immediately following a stimulus.

   s., epigastric. A sinking feeling in the stomach.

   s., external. Effect upon the mind of stimuli produced from a source outside the body.

   s., girdle. A painful sensation, as a bandage tightened about a limb or the trunk as in spinal disease. SYN: *zonesthesia.*

   s., gnostic. One of the more finely developed senses such as touch, tactile discrimination, position sense, and vibration.

   s., internal. S., subjective.

   s., palmesthetic. Sensation felt in the skin from vibration.

   s., primary. Sensation that results from a direct stimulus.

   s., proprioceptive. Proprioceptive sensation. This use is inappropriate because this sense rarely is at the conscious level.

   s., referred. Sensation that seems to arise from a source other than the actual one. SYN: *s., reflex.*

   s., reflex. S., referred.

   s., somesthetic. Sense, proprioception.

   s., subjective. Sensation that does not result from any external stimulus and is perceptible only by the subject. SYN: *s., internal.*

   s., tactile. Sensation produced through the sense of touch.

sense (sĕns) [L. *sensus,* a feeling]. 1. To perceive through a sense organ. 2. The general faculty by which conditions outside or inside the body are perceived. 3. Any special faculty of sensation connected with a particular organ. 4. Normal power of understanding.

   The most important of the senses are sight, hearing, smell, taste, touch and pressure, temperature, weight, resistance and tension (muscle sense), pain, position, proprioception, visceral and sexual sensations, equilibrium, and hunger and thirst.

   s., color. SEE: *color sense.*

   s., kinesthetic. S., muscular.

   s., light. SEE: *light sense.*

   s., muscular. Consciousness of muscular movement required in a given act. SYN:

s., kinesthetic.

s., posture. Ability through muscle sense to differentiate positions of the body or its structures. SYN: *proprioception.*

s., pressure. Faculty of feeling various degrees of pressure on the body surface. SYN: *baresthesia.*

s., proprioception. The correlation of unconscious sensations from the skin and joints that allows conscious appreciation of the position of the body.

s., sixth. General feeling of normal functioning of the body in general. SYN: *cenesthesia.*

s., space. Sense by which we recognize objects in space, their relationship, and dimensions.

s.'s, special. The five senses of sight, hearing, smell, touch, and taste.

s., static. Sense that makes it possible to maintain equilibrium.

s., stereognostic. Ability to judge consistency and shape of objects held in the fingers.

s., temperature. Ability to detect differences of temperature.

s., time. Ability to detect differences in time intervals.

s., tone. Ability to distinguish between different tones.

s., visceral. Subjective perception of the sensations of the internal organs.

sensibility (sĕn″sĭ-bĭl′ĭ-tē) [L. *sensibilitas*]. Capacity to receive and respond to stimuli.

s., deep. 1. Sensibility existing after an area of the skin is made anesthetic. 2. Sensation by which the position of a limb and estimation of difference in weight and tension are apparent.

s., mesoblastic. S., deep.

s., palmesthetic. The sensibility existing in the skin to vibration.

sensibilization (sĕn″sĭ-bĭl-ĭz-ā′shŭn). 1. The process of making sensitive; sensitization. 2. Production of hypersusceptibility to a foreign substance by injecting it into the body. SYN: *sensitization.*

sensible (sĕn′sĭ-bl) [L. *sensibilis*, capable of being perceived]. 1. Capable of being perceived by the senses; perceptible. 2. Capable of receiving sensations. SYN: *sensitive.* 3. Having reason.

sensiferous (sĕn-sĭf′ĕr-ŭs) [L. *sensus*, a feeling, + *ferre*, to bear]. Causing, conducting, or transmitting sensations.

sensimeter (sĕn-sĭm′ĕ-tĕr) [″ + Gr. *metron*, measure]. Machine for recording the degree of sensitiveness of various areas of the body.

sensitinogen (sĕn″sĭ-tĭn′ō-jĕn) [″ + Gr. *gennan*, to produce]. The collective of antigens which sensitize the body.

sensitive (sĕn′sĭ-tĭv) [L. *sensitivus*, of sensation]. 1. Capable of transmitting a sensation. 2. Able to feel a sensation. 3. Subject to destructive action of a complement. 4. Susceptible to suggestions, as a hypnotic. 5. Abnormally susceptible to a substance, as a drug or foreign protein. SEE: *allergy.*

sensitivity. A term used in assessing the value of a diagnostic test, procedure, or clinical observation. It is the proportion of people who truly have a specific disease and are so identified by the test. SEE: *specificity, diagnostic.*

sensitivity tests, antimicrobial. Laboratory method of determining the susceptibility of the patient's bacterial infection to antibiotics or antibacterials. The specimen obtained from the patient is cultured in various liquid dilutions of the drugs or on solid media containing various concentrations of the drugs in disks placed on the surface of the media. The disk-type test is not completely reliable.

sensitivity training. A form of group therapy in which individuals are given the opportunity to relate verbally and physically with complete candor and honesty with other members of the group. The goals of therapy are to increase self-awareness, learn constructive ways of dealing with conflicts, establish a better sense of inner direction, and relate to persons with warmth and affection.

sensitization (sĕn″sĭ-zā′shŭn). 1. A condition of being made sensitive to a specific substance (i.e., antigen) such as a protein or pollen. 2. Process of making a person susceptible to a substance by repeated injections of it.

s., active. Sensitization produced by injecting an antigen into a susceptible person.

s., autoerythrocyte. A syndrome characterized by spontaneous appearance of painful ecchymoses, usually at a site of a bruise. The areas itch and burn. The lesions may come and go, and in general, they are benign. The cause is assumed to be due to autosensitivity to a component of the red blood cell membrane. There is no specific therapy.

s., passive. The production of sensitization in a normal person by injecting the person with the serum from a sensitized animal or humans.

s., protein. Sensitization as a result of previous injection of a foreign protein into the body.

sensitized (sĕn′sĭ-tīzd). Made susceptible to a specific substance.

sensitized vaccine. A live culture that has been mixed with its antiserum before introduction.

sensitizer (sĕn′sĭ-tī″zĕr) [L. *sensitivus*, of

sensation]. In allergy and dermatology, a substance that makes the susceptible individual react to the same or other irritants.

sensomobile (sĕn″sō-mō′bĭl) [L. *sensus*, a feeling, + *mobilis*, mobile]. Movement in response to a stimulus.

sensomobility (sĕn″sō-mō-bĭl′ĭ-tē) [″ + *mobilitas*, mobility]. The capacity for movement in response to a stimulus.

sensomotor. Sensorimotor, q.v.

sensor. 1. A sense organ. 2. A device sensitive to light, heat, radiation, sound, or mechanical or other physical stimuli. These devices may be equipped to record the phenomena being detected and to sound an alarm if the value falls below a certain level or exceeds a specified limit.

sensorial (sĕn-sō′rē-ăl) [L. *sensorialis*]. Pert. to the sensorium, the seat of sensation.

sensoriglandular (sĕn″sō-rē-glănd′dū-lăr) [L. *sensus*, a feeling, + *glandula*, little acorn]. Concerning glandular excretion in response to stimulation of a nerve.

sensorimetabolism (sĕn″sō-rē-mĕ-tăb′ō-lĭzm) [″ + Gr. *metaballein*, to alter, + *-ismos*, condition]. Metabolic activity in response to sensory nerve stimulation.

sensorimotor (sĕn″sō-rē-mō′tor) [L. *sensus*, a feeling, + *motus*, moving]. Both sensory and motor. SYN: *sensomotor.*

sensorimuscular (sĕn″sō-rē-mŭs′kū-lăr) [″ + *muscularis*, muscular]. Muscular activity in response to a sensory stimulus.

sensorineural (sĕn″sō-rē-nū′răl) [″ + *neuralis*, neural]. Concerning a sensory nerve.

sensorium (sĕn-sor′ē-ŭm) [L., organ of sensation] (pl. *sensoriums, sensoria*). 1. That portion of the brain that functions as a center of sensations. 2. The sensory apparatus of the body taken as a whole.

sensorivasomotor (sĕn″sō-rē-văs″ō-mō′tor) [L. *sensus*, a feeling, + *vas*, vessel, + *motor*, a mover]. Vascular changes induced by sensory nerve stimulation.

sensory (sĕn′sō-rē) [L. *sensorius*]. 1. Conveying impulses from sense organs to the reflex or higher centers. SYN: *afferent*. 2. Pert. to sensation.

sensory amusia. Musical deafness; inability to comprehend music or musical sounds.

sensory aphasia. Inability to understand written or spoken words.

sensory area. Any area of the cerebral cortex in which sensations are perceived.

s.a., somesthetic. Area occupying the postcentral gyrus of the cerebral cortex and extending into adjacent areas in which sensations of general somatic sensibility are perceived.

sensory deprivation. Enforced absence of usual and accustomed sensory stimuli. Ex.: patients whose eyes are bandaged for extended periods following eye surgery, patients in respirators, astronauts, those who are isolated as would be the case of a sailor adrift alone following an accident, or those imprisoned in completely dark and soundproof cells. The absence of normal stimuli will, if continued, lead to severe mental changes including auditory and visual hallucinations, anxiety, depression, and insanity.

In psychological experimentation, sensory deprivation is achieved by confining a volunteer in a small soundproof room while wearing gloves, an eye mask, and ear muffs. Deprivation may also be produced by immersing an individual equipped for underwater breathing in a tank of water that is devoid of stimuli except for the sound of breathing.

NURSING IMPLICATIONS: Assess patient's usual response to prolonged quiet or isolation. Patients who require more environmental stimuli (radio, TV, noise, people) suffer more (and more quickly) in isolation than do those who prefer quiet. Provide stimulation to replace those stimuli that are deprived. Tell patient who cannot see, or whose visual field is limited by position or equipment, about weather, time of day, colors around him or her. Describe equipment, locations, food, anything the patient wishes to know about that cannot be visualized, allowing touch to help replace vision. For patient whose hearing is reduced by location or equipment (or by effects of drug therapy), use devices that assist hearing-impaired persons to understand speech. Encourage use of radio or TV as desired by any sensory deprived patient, and make frequent "stop-in" visits so patient knows he or she is not abandoned. Relate therapies to time of day (before breakfast, after dinner, at bedtime, etc.), and provide clock and calendar to assist with time orientation. If patient reports auditory or visual hallucinations, investigate thoroughly, seeking a source that could simulate sound or sight patient reported (linen cart may sound like truck going by, curtain moving may look like ghost). Validate reality for the patient, changing lighting or altering external noises as possible to eliminate confusion.

sensory ending. A termination of an afferent nerve fiber that upon stimulation gives rise to a sensation. SEE: *receptor, sensory.*

sensory epilepsy. Disturbances of sensation that replace epileptic convulsions.

sensory integration. Skill and performance required in the development and coordination of sensory input, motor output, and sensory feedback. Includes sensory awareness, visual spatial awareness, body integration, balance, bilateral motor coordination, visual-motor integration, praxis, and other components.

sensory nerve. An afferent nerve conveying sensory impulses to the sensorium, or one composed of sensory fibers.

sensory overload. The condition in which sensory stimuli are received at a rate and intensity beyond the level that the patient can handle. This stressful situation can lead to confusion, anxiety, mental distress, and panic.

sensory registration. The brain's ability to receive input and select that which will receive attention and that which will be inhibited from conscious attention.

sensory unit. A single sensory nerve fiber with all its branches and their terminal nerve endings.

sensual (sĕn'shū-ăl) [L. *sensus*, a feeling]. Concerning or consisting in the gratification of the senses; indulgence of the appetites; not spiritual or intellectual; carnal, worldly.

sensualism (sĕn'shū-ăl-ĭzm). State or condition of being sensual; condition in which one's actions are dominated by emotions.

sensuous (sĕn'shū-ŭs) [L. *sensus*, a feeling]. 1. Pert. to or affecting the senses. 2. Susceptible to influence through the senses.

sentient (sĕn'shē-ĕnt) [L. *sentiens*, perceive]. Capable of perceiving sensation. SYN: *sensitive.*

sentiment (sĕn'tĭ-mĕnt) [L. *sentio*, to feel]. Feeling, sensibility, esp. susceptibility to tender feelings; an emotional attitude toward an object or a group of objects.

sentinel gland. SEE: *sentinel node.*

sentinel node. An enlarged, superclavicular lymph node that is infiltrated with cancer cells that have metastasized from an obscurely located primary cancer.

separation. The process of disconnecting, disuniting, or severing.

separator [LL. *separator*]. 1. Anything that prevents two substances from mingling. 2. Any device or instrument used for separating two substances such as cream from milk.

separatorium (sĕp″ă-rā-tō′rē-ŭm) [L.]. Instrument for separating the pericranium from the skull.

sepsis (sĕp'sĭs) [Gr., putrefaction]. Pathologic state, usually febrile, resulting from the presence of microorganisms or their poisonous products in the bloodstream. May be manifested as cellulitis (local dissemination of infection), lymphangitis or lymphadenitis (dispersion along lymphatic channels), or bacteremia (widespread dissemination by way of the bloodstream). The latter is commonly called blood poisoning. SYN: *bacteremia; septicemia.*

s., puerperal. Infection of the genital tract following childbirth. The infection may occur through exogenous or endogenous means. Organisms most commonly associated with this type of infection are streptococci, staphylococci, and *Escherichia coli*. SYN: *childbed fever.* SEE: *Nursing Diagnoses* in *Appendix.*

SYM: Onset may be gradual or sudden. Patient begins to have general malaise, headache, chilly sensations or shaking chills, and rise in temperature. The uterus is tender, and there is some abdominal distention.

PATH: In minor cases of ulceration, the vaginal tract is covered by a dirty membrane. In streptococcal and staphylococcal infections, the endometrium is smooth and the lymphatics are congested with the invading organisms. As a rule, the uterine cavity is filled with very little lochia. The uterus shows poor involution. If the infection extends farther than the uterus, the parametrium or cellular tissues show edema, inflammation, and in some cases purulent infiltration. Extension of the process to the veins produces infectious thrombi, which in turn produce localized abscesses in other parts of the body.

COURSE: Early diagnosis and appropriate therapy will effectively control the course of the infection in most cases.

TREAT: Appropriate antibiotic and general measures include absolute bedrest, light or liquid diet, maintenance of fluid balance by parenteral injections if necessary, and analgesics for pain.

septa (sĕp'tă) [L. *saeptum*, a partition]. Pl. of septum.

septal (sĕp'tăl) [L. *saeptum*, a partition]. Concerning a septum.

septan (sĕp'tăn) [L. *septem*, seven]. Recurring every seventh day, as the paroxysms of malarial fever.

septate (sĕp'tāt) [L. *saeptum*, a partition]. Having a dividing wall.

septectomy (sĕp-tĕk'tō-mē) [″ + Gr. *ektome*, excision]. Excision of a septum, esp. the nasal septum or a part of it.

septemia (sĕp-tē'mē-ă). Septicemia.

septi- [L. *septem*, seven]. Combining form concerning seven.

septic (sĕp'tĭk) [Gr. *septikos*, putrefying]. 1. Pert. to sepsis. 2. Pert. to pathogenic organisms or their toxins.

septicemia (sĕp-tĭ-sē'mē-ă) [″ + *haima*, blood]. Presence of pathogenic bacteria in the blood. If allowed to progress, the organisms may multiply and cause an overwhelming infection and death. Symptoms and signs usually include chills and fever, petechiae, purpuric pustules, and abscesses. Shock may be present. SYN: *blood poisoning.* SEE: *Nursing Diagnoses in Appendix.*

   s., bronchopulmonary. Septicemia following entry, usually by aspiration, of infected material into the bronchi.

   s., cryptogenic. Septicemia in which no primary focus of infection can be found.

   s., fungal. Presence of pathogenic fungi in the blood. May be seen as a complication of parenteral hyperalimentation. SYN: *fungemia.*

   s., puerperal. Septicemia occurring following prolonged and difficult labor or incomplete abortion. SYN: *puerperal sepsis.*

septicemic (sĕp-tĭ-sē′mĭk). Relating to, resulting from, or of the nature of septicemia.

septic fever. Fever or infection due to presence of pathogenic organisms or their products in the blood. SYN: *septicemia.*

septicophlebitis (sĕp″tĭ-kō-flĕ-bī′tĭs) [Gr. *septikos,* putrefying, + *phleps,* vein, + *itis,* inflammation]. Septic inflammation of a vein.

septicopyemia (sĕp″tĭ-kō-pī-ē′mē-ă) [″ + *pyon,* pus, + *haima,* blood]. Septicemia and pyemia together.

septic shock. When fever, chills, tachycardia, tachypnea, and altered mental function, the signs of acute septicemia, are combined with hypotension and signs of inadequate organ perfusion, the condition of septic shock is present. Circulatory failure is manifest by decreased myocardial contractility, with pooling and altered distribution of blood in the microcirculation. This leads to widespread injury of tissues and eventually multiple organ failure and death.

   TREAT: Search for and reverse underlying disease. In immunosuppressed patients, treat the primary disease and, if on immunosupressing drugs, decrease the dose. Remove the source of infection. If an abscess is present, drain or remove it. All catheters should be removed and replaced. Vigorous support of pulmonary and cardiovascular function should be instituted without delay. This will require assisted respiration, I.V. fluids, pressor drugs such as dopamine. If acidosis develops, sodium bicarbonate solution is given I.V. The onset of disseminated intravascular coagulation (DIC) will necessitate replacement of clotting factors and administration of platelets. Antibiotics are given as soon as sepsis is diagnosed, but, if possible, not until material from all of the suspected sites and sources of infection is obtained. The value of glucocorticoids is controversial, and their use may be harmful. SEE: *toxic shock syndrome.*

septic sore throat. Streptococcal inflamma-

tion of the throat with fever and marked prostration.

septic tank. A tank for holding sewage. The material may be digested and biodegraded and the aqueous part allowed to drain into the ground, or the material may be periodically removed for disposal elsewhere. The colloquial terms for such a tank is *cesspool.*

septigravida (sĕp″tĭ-grăv′ĭ-dă) [L. *septem,* seven, + *gravida,* pregnant]. A woman pregnant for the seventh time.

septimetritis (sĕp″tĭ-mē-trī′tĭs) [Gr. *septos,* putrid, + *metra,* uterus, + *itis,* inflammation]. Inflammation of uterus due to sepsis.

septipara (sĕp-tĭp′ă-ră) [L. *septem,* seven, + *parere,* to bring forth]. A woman who has had seven pregnancies, each of which produced an infant, alive or dead, weighing 500 gm or more.

septivalent (sĕp-tĭ-vā′lĕnt, -tĭv′ă-lĕnt) [″ + *valere,* to be strong]. Having a valence of seven or combining with or replacing seven hydrogen atoms.

septomarginal (sĕp″tō-măr′jĭ-năl) [L. *saeptum,* a partition, + *marginalis,* border]. Pert. to the margin or the border of a septum.

septometer (sĕp-tŏm′ĕ-ter). 1. [L. *saeptum,* a partition, + Gr. *metron,* measure] Calipers for measuring the width of the nasal septum. 2. [Gr. *sepsis,* putrefaction, + *metron,* measure] Device for determining bacterial contamination of air.

septonasal (sĕp-tō-nā′zăl) [L. *saeptum,* a partition, + *nasus,* nose]. Concerning the nasal septum.

septoplasty (sĕp″tō-plăs′tē) [″ + Gr. *plassein,* to form]. Plastic surgery of the nasal septum.

septostomy (sĕp-tŏs′tō-mē) [″ + Gr. *stoma,* mouth]. Surgical formation of an opening in a septum.

   s., balloon. Procedure during cardiac catherization to enlarge the interatrial communication and thereby establish adequate mixing of oxygenated and unoxygenated blood.

septotome (sĕp′tō-tōm) [″ + Gr. *tome,* incision]. An instrument for cutting or removing a section of the nasal septum.

septotomy (sĕp-tŏt′ō-mē) [″ + Gr. *tome,* incision]. Incision of a septum, esp. the nasal septum.

septula (sĕp-tū′lă) [L.]. Pl. of septulum.

   s. testis. [NA] Thin partition extending inward from mediastinum testis and separating testis into the lobuli testis.

septulum (sĕp′tū-lŭm) [L.] (pl. *septula*). A small partition or septum.

septum (sĕp′tŭm) [L. *saeptum,* a partition] (pl. *septa*). A wall dividing two cavities.

s., atrial. A wall between the atria of the heart.

s. atriorum cordis. A wall between the atria of the heart. SYN: *s., interatrial.*

s., atrioventricular. Septum that separates the right and left atria of the heart from the respective ventricles.

s., crural. S., femoral.

s., femoral. Connective tissue that closes the femoral ring.

s., interatrial. S. atriorum cordis.

s., interdental. The bony partition across the alveolar process between adjacent teeth that contributes to the tooth sockets.

s., intermuscular. 1. A connective tissue septum that separates two muscles, esp. one from which muscles may take their origin. 2. One of two connective tissue septa that separate the muscles of the leg into anterior, posterior, and lateral groups.

s., interradicular. One of the thin bony partitions between the roots of a multi-rooted tooth which contribute to walls of the tooth socket.

s., interventricular. S., ventricular.

s., lingual. A sheet of connective tissue separating the halves of the tongue.

s. lucidum. 1. A translucent septum, the interior boundary of lateral ventricles of the brain. SYN: *s. pellucidum* [NA]. 2. The stratum corneum layer of the epidermis.

s., mediastinal. Mediastinum.

s., nasal. The partition that divides the nasal cavity into two nasal fossae. Bony portion formed by the perpendicular plate of ethmoid and the vomer bone; cartilaginous portion formed by septal and vomeronasal cartilages and medial crura of greater alar cartilages.

s., orbital. A fibrous sheet extending partially across the anterior opening of the orbit and partially closing it.

s. pectiniforme. Comblike partition that separates the corpora cavernosa.

s. pellucidum. [NA] A thin triangular sheet of nervous tissue consisting of two laminae attached to the corpus callosum above and the fornix below. It forms the medial wall of the lateral ventricles. SYN: *s. lucidum.*

s. primum. In the primitive, embryonic heart, a septum between the right and left chambers.

s., rectovaginal. Partition between the rectum and the vagina.

s., rectovesical. The membranous septum between the rectum and the urinary bladder.

s. scroti. [NA] Partition dividing the chambers of the scrotum.

s., ventricular. Partition between the ventricles of the heart. SYN: *s., interventricular.*

septuplet (sĕp'tŭ-plĕt) [L. *septuplus*, sevenfold]. One of seven children born from the same gestation.

sequel (sē'kwĕl) [L. *sequela*, sequel]. Sequela.

sequela (sē-kwē'lă) [L., sequel] (pl. *sequelae*). A condition following and resulting from a disease.

sequence (sē'kwĕns) [L.]. The order or occurrence of a series of related events.

sequential. Occurring in order, i.e., one after another.

sequester (sē-kwĕs'tĕr) [L. *sequestrare,* to separate]. 1. To isolate. 2. A piece of necrosed bone separated from surrounding tissue. SYN: *sequestrum.*

sequestra (sē-kwĕs'tră) [L.]. Pl. of sequestrum.

sequestral (sē-kwĕs'trăl). Concerning a sequestrum.

sequestration (sē"kwĕs-trā'shŭn) [L. *sequestratio,* a separation]. 1. The formation of sequestrum. 2. Isolation of a patient for treatment or quarantine. 3. Reduction of hemorrhage of head or trunk by temporarily stopping the return of blood from the extremities by applying tourniquets to the thighs and arms. 4. Fragment of nucleus pulposus of the intervertebral disk separating and freely floating in the spinal canal.

s., pulmonary. A nonfunctioning area of the lung that receives its blood supply from the systemic circulation.

sequestrectomy (sē"kwĕs-trĕk'tō-mē) [" + Gr. *ektome,* excision]. Excision of a necrosed piece of bone.

sequestrotomy (sē"kwĕs-trŏt'ō-mē) [" + Gr. *tome,* incision]. Operation for removal of a sequestrum, a fragment of necrosed bone. SYN: *sequestrectomy.*

sequestrum (sē-kwĕs'trŭm) [L., something set aside] (pl. *sequestra*). Fragment of a necrosed bone that has become separated from surrounding tissue. Designated primary if piece is entirely detached, secondary if still loosely attached, and tertiary if it is partially detached but still remaining in place.

sera (sē'ră) [L.]. Pl. of serum.

seralbumin (sĕr-ăl-bū'mĭn) [L. *serum,* whey, + *albumen,* white of egg]. Albumin of the blood.

Serax. Trade name for oxazepam.

serendipity (sĕr"ĕn-dĭp'ĭ-tē). The gift of finding, by chance and wisdom, valuable or agreeable things not sought for. In medical research an unexpected reaction or result may produce new insights into some area totally unrelated to that which prompted the investigation.

serial (sē'rē-ăl) [L. *series,* row, chain]. In numerical order, in continuity or sequence, as in a series.

serial sevens test. Test of mental status. The patient is asked to subtract seven from 100 and to take seven from that value and continue serially. The number of correct responses out of the 14 possible is the score.

series (sēr′ēz) [L. *series,* row, chain]. 1. Arrangement of objects in succession or in order. 2. In electricity, batteries or mode of arranging the parts of a circuit by connecting them successively end to end to form a single path for the current. The parts so arranged are said to be "in series."

s., aliphatic. Chemical compounds with a structure of an open chain of carbon atoms.

s., aromatic. Any series of organic compounds containing the benzene ring.

s., erythrocytic. The group of immature cells that develop into mature erythrocytes.

s., fatty. Aliphatic series, esp. those similar to methane.

s., granulocytic. The immature cells in the bone marrow that develop into mature granular leukocytes.

s., homologous. In chemistry, compounds that proceed from one to the next by some constant such as a CH_2 group.

s., leukocytic. S., granulocytic, q.v.

s., monocytic. The immature cells that proceed to develop into the mature monocyte.

s., thrombocytic. The immature cells that proceed to develop into platelets.

serine. 2-amino-3-hydroxypropionic acid. An amino acid present in many proteins including casein, vitellin, and others. Found in the urine of normal human beings.

seriscission (sĕr-ĭ-sĕsh′ŭn) [L. *sericum,* silk, + *scindere,* to cut]. Division of soft tissues, as a pedicle, by tying a silk ligature around it.

sero- [L.]. Combining form pert. to serum.

seroalbuminuria (sē″rō-ăl-bū″mĭn-ū′rē-ă) [L. *serum,* whey, + *albumen,* white of egg, + Gr. *ouron,* urine]. Serum albumin in the urine.

serocolitis (sē″rō-kō-lī′tĭs) [″ + Gr. *kolon,* colon, + *itis,* inflammation]. Inflammation of serous coat of the colon. SYN: *pericolitis.*

seroconversion. Development of evidence of antibody response to a disease or vaccine.

seroculture (sē′rō-kŭl-chŭr) [L. *serum,* whey, + *cultura,* tillage]. A bacterial culture on blood serum.

serocystic (sē″rō-sĭs′tĭk) [″ + Gr. *kystis,* bladder, sac]. Composed of cysts containing serous fluid.

serodermatosis (sē″rō-der-mă-tō′sĭs) [″ + Gr. *derma,* skin, + *osis,* condition]. Skin disease with serous effusion into tissues of the epidermis.

serodiagnosis (sē″rō-dī-ăg-nō′sĭs) [″ + Gr. *dia,* through, + *gnosis,* knowledge]. Diagnosis by observing the reactions of blood serum.

seroenteritis (sē″rō-ĕn-tĕr-ī′tĭs) [″ + Gr. *enteron,* intestine, + *itis,* inflammation]. Inflammation of serous covering of the intestine.

seroepidemiology (sē-rō-ĕp″ĭ-dē-mē-ŏl′ō-jē) [″ + *epi,* upon, + *demos,* people, + *logos,* word, reason]. Study of the epidemiology of a pathological condition by investigating the presence of a diagnostic characteristic in the serum.

serofast (sē′rō-făst″). Serum-fast, q.v.

serofibrinous (sē″rō-fī′brĭn-ŭs) [″ + *fibra,* fiber]. 1. Composed of both serum and fibrin. 2. Denoting a serofibrinous exudate.

serofibrous (sē″rō-fī′brŭs) [″ + *fibra,* fiber]. Concerning serous and fibrous surfaces.

seroflocculation (sē″rō-flŏk″ū-lā′shŭn) [″ + *flocculus,* little tuft]. Flocculation produced in serum by an antigen.

serohepatitis (sē″rō-hĕp-ă-tī′tĭs) [″ + Gr. *hepar,* liver, + *itis,* inflammation]. Inflammation of the peritoneal covering of the liver.

seroimmunity (sē″rō-ĭ-mū′nĭ-tē) [″ + *immunitas,* immunity]. Immunity produced by the administration of an antiserum.

serolipase (sē″rō-lĭp′ās) [″ + Gr. *lipos,* fat, + *ase,* enzyme]. Lipase found in blood serum.

serologic, serological (sē-rō-lŏj′ĭk, -ăl) [″ + Gr. *logos,* word, reason]. Pert. to or the study of sera.

serologist (sē-rŏl′ō-jĭst) [″ + Gr. *logos,* word, reason]. One who has special knowledge and ability in serology.

serology (sē-rŏl′ō-jē) [″ + Gr. *logos,* word, reason]. The scientific study of serum.

serolysin (sē-rŏl′ĭs-ĭn) [″ + Gr. *lysis,* dissolution]. A bactericidal substance or lysin found in the blood serum.

seroma (sĕr-ō′mă) [″ + Gr. *oma,* tumor]. A localized collection of serum that resembles a tumor.

seromembranous (sē″rō-mĕm′brăn-ŭs) [″ + *membrana,* membrane]. Both serous and membranous; rel. to a serous membrane.

seromucoid. Concerning a secretion that is part serous and part mucous.

seromucous (sē″rō-mū′kŭs) [″ + *mucus,* mucus]. Pert. to or composed of both serum and mucus.

seromuscular (sē″rō-mŭs′kū-lăr) [″ + *muscularis,* muscular]. Concerning the serous and muscular coats of the intestines.

seronegative (sē″rō-nĕg′ă-tĭv). Producing a negative reaction to serological tests.

seroperitoneum (sē″rō-pĕr″ĭ-tō-nē′ŭm) [″ + Gr. *peritonaion*, peritoneum]. Fluid in the peritoneum. SYN: *ascites; hydroperitoneum.*

seropositive (sē″rō-pŏz′ĭ-tĭv). Producing a positive reaction to serological tests.

seroprevention. Seroprophylaxis.

seroprognosis (sē″rō-prŏg-nō′sĭs) [″ + Gr. *pro*, before, + *gnosis*, knowledge]. Prognosis of disease determined by seroreactions.

seroprophylaxis (sē″rō-prō-fĭ-lăks′ĭs) [″ + Gr. *prophylatikos*, guarding]. Prevention of a disease by injection of serum. SYN: *seroprevention.*

seropurulent (sē″rō-pū′roo-lĕnt) [″ + *purulentus*, full of pus]. Composed of serum and pus, as an exudate.

seropus (sē″rō-pŭs′) [″ + *pus*, pus]. A collection of serum and pus.

seroreaction (sē″rō-rē-ăk′shŭn) [″ + *re*, back, + *actio*, action]. 1. Any reaction taking place in or involving serum. 2. Reaction to an injection of serum marked by rash, fever, pain, etc.

seroresistance (sē″rō-rē-zĭs′tăns). Failure of a serum reaction to become negative or be reduced in titer following treatment.

seroresistant (sē″rō-rē-zĭs′tănt). The serum becoming positive after exposure to a pathogen and after being treated.

serosa (sē-rō′să) [L. *serum*, whey]. A serous membrane. Examples are the peritoneum, pleura, and pericardium.

serosanguineous (sē″rō-săn-gwĭn′ē-ŭs) [L. *serum*, whey, + *sanguineus*, bloody]. Containing or of the nature of serum and blood.

seroserous (sē″rō-sē′rŭs) [L. *serosus*, serous, + *serum*, whey]. Pert. to two serous surfaces.

serositis (sē″rō-sī′tĭs) [″ + Gr. *itis*, inflammation] (pl. *serositides*). Inflamed condition of a serous membrane.

serosity (sē-rŏs′ĭ-tē) [Fr. *serosite*]. The quality of being serous.

serosynovial (sē″rō-sĭ-nō′vē-ăl) [L. *serum*, whey, + *synovia*, joint fluid]. Concerning serous and synovial material.

serosynovitis (sē″rō-sĭn″ō-vī′tĭs) [″ + *synovia*, joint fluid, + Gr. *itis*, inflammation]. Synovitis with increase of synovial fluid.

serotonergic neurons. Neural pathways that use serotonin as a neurotransmitter.

serotonin (sĕr″ō-tōn′ĭn). A chemical, 5-hydroxytryptamine (5-HT), present in platelets, gastrointestinal mucosa, mast cells, and in carcinoid tumors. Serotonin is a potent vasoconstrictor. It is thought to be involved in neural mechanisms important in sleep and sensory perception. SEE: *carci-*

noid syndrome.

serotype (sē′rō-tīp). In microbiology, a microorganism determined by the kinds and combinations of constituent antigens present in the cells.

serous (sēr′ŭs) [L. *serosus*]. 1. Having the nature of serum. 2. Producing a serous secretion, or containing serum or a serumlike substance.

serous cavity. Cavity lined by a serous membrane, specifically the pleural, peritoneal, and pericardial cavities.

serous cell. Cell that secretes a thin, watery, albuminous secretion.

serous effusion. Escape of serum into tissues or a body cavity.

serous exudate. Exudate consisting mostly of serum.

serous fluids. Liquids of the body, similar to blood serum, that are in part secreted by serous membranes.

serous glands. Glands secreting a watery, albuminous fluid, as the parotid gland.

serous inflammation. Inflammation of a part with serous exudate, or inflammation of a serous membrane.

serous membrane. Membrane lining a serous cavity.

serovaccination. A process with combined injection of serum, to secure immediate passive immunity, and bacterial vaccine, to acquire subsequent active immunity.

serovar [serological variation]. Variants within a species defined by variation in serological reactions. SEE: *biovar; morphovar.*

serozymogenic (sē″rō-zī″mō-jĕn′ĭk) [L. *serum*, whey, + Gr. *zyme*, ferment, + *gennan*, to produce]. Pert. to a serous fluid and enzymes.

serpiginous (sĕr-pĭj′ĭ-nŭs) [L. *serpere*, to creep]. Creeping from one part to another.

serrate (sĕr′āt) [L. *serratus*, toothed]. Notched; toothed. SYN: *dentate.*

Serratia (sĕr-ā′shē-ă) [Serafino Serrati, 18th-century It. physicist]. A genus of bacteria of the family Enterobacteriaceae. It is a gram-negative rod.

S. marcescens. Formerly called *Chromobacterium prodigiosum* and erroneously believed to be nonpathogenic to humans. Causes septicemia and pulmonary disease, esp. in immunocompromised patients. Found in water, soil, milk, and stools.

serration (sĕr-ā′shŭn) [L. *serratio*, a notching]. 1. Formation with sharp projections like the teeth of a saw. 2. A single tooth or notch in a serrated edge.

serratus muscle. Any of several muscles arising from the ribs or vertebrae by separate slips. SEE: *Muscles* in *Appendix.*

serrefine (sār-fēn′) [Fr.]. A small wire spring forceps for compressing bleeding vessels.

serrenoeud (sãr-nŭd') [Fr. *serrer*, to squeeze, + *noeud*, knot]. Device for tightening ligatures, esp. those placed on vessels in a deep cavity out of reach of fingers.

serrulate (sĕr'ū-lāt) [L. *serrulatus*]. Finely notched or serrated.

Sertoli's cells (sĕr-tō'lēz) [Enrico Sertoli, It. histologist, 1842–1910]. Supporting elongated cells of seminiferous tubules that nourish spermatids.

serum (sē'rŭm) [L., whey] (pl. *serums, sera*). 1. Any serous fluid, esp. the fluid that moistens the surfaces of serous membranes. 2. The watery portion of the blood after coagulation; a fluid found when clotted blood is left standing long enough for the clot to shrink. 3. Serum from an animal rendered immune against a pathogenic organism, to be injected into a patient with the disease resulting from the same organism. It consists of plasma minus fibrinogen.

    s. albumin. A protein found in blood serum. SEE: *blood; protein, simple.*

    s., anticrotalus. Serum used in treating rattlesnake poison.

    s., antidiphtheritic. Serum used to counteract the effects of diphtheria.

    s., antimeningococcal. Serum antagonistic to meningococcal infection.

    s., antipneumococcal. Serum used in treating pneumococcal infection.

    s., antitetanic. Serum given to counteract tetanus toxin.

    s., antitoxic. Serum containing antitoxin.

    s., antityphoid. Serum containing antibodies of the typhoid bacillus.

    s., bactericidal. Serum having no effect on toxins but destructive to bacteria.

    s., bacteriolytic. Serum containing a lysin that destroys certain bacteria.

    s., blood. The clear liquid portion of blood without its fibrin and corpuscles. SEE: *plasma.*

    s., convalescent. Blood serum from a person convalescing from an infection, the serum to be used in treating others having the same disease.

    s., foreign. Serum from one animal injected into one of another species, or into a human.

    s., immune. Serum containing antibodies for specific antigens.

    s., polyvalent. Serum containing antibodies to several types of the same bacterial species.

    s., pooled. Mixed blood serum from several persons.

    s., pregnancy. Blood serum from pregnant women.

    s., pregnant mare's. Serum derived from the blood of pregnant mares; source of hormones, esp. chorionic gonadotropin.

serum, words pert. to: agglutinin; agglutinogen; antigen; antitropin; antivenin; autoserodiagnosis; autoserotherapy; autoserous; autoserum; complement; icteric index; isohemagglutinin; opsonic index; opsonin; serology; serous.

serum bank. Place for long-term storage of samples of serum. Specimens are banked because of their potential future use in studying disease. Specimens are stored frozen or after lyophilization. Use of such specimens permits investigation of the presence of a newly discovered disease, e.g., AIDS, in persons whose serum was collected many years ago.

serum-fast. Capable of resisting the destructive forces present in serum.

serum glutamic-oxaloacetic transaminase. ABBR: SGOT. An intracellular enzyme involved in amino acid and carbohydrate metabolism. It is present in high concentrations in muscle, liver, and brain. An increased level of this enzyme in the blood indicates necrosis or disease in these tissues. SYN: *aspartate aminotransferase*, the preferred term.

serum glutamic pyruvic transaminase. ABBR: SGPT. An intracellular enzyme involved in amino acid and carbohydrate metabolism. It is present in high concentrations in muscle, liver, and brain. An increased level of this enzyme in the blood indicates necrosis or disease in these tissues. SYN: *alanine aminotransferase*, the preferred term.

serum protein. Any protein in blood serum. Serum protein forms weak acids mixed with alkali salts; this increases the buffer effects of the blood but to a lesser extent than cell protein.

serum rash. Rash first seen at site of an injection of serum. It remains thickest there, but may spread to other parts of the body. It resembles a combination of urticarial, morbilliform, and scarlatiniform rashes.

    SYM: Severe irritation; marked swelling of skin, esp. of the face; malaise; and constitutional symptoms.

serum sickness. An adverse (Type III hypersensitivity) immune response following administration of antitoxins derived from horses or other animals used for passive immunization against snake venom or rabies. Also occasionally occurs after the administration of penicillin or sulfonamides. The inflammatory response that results produces fever, myalgia, arthritis, urticaria, with an enlarged spleen and lymph nodes 7 to 14 days following exposure. SEE: *hypersensitivity.*

    TREAT: Symptomatic and adrenal cortical hormones if needed. SEE: *Nursing Diagnoses* in *Appendix.*

servomechanism (sŭr″vō-měk′ă-nĭzm). In biology and physiology, a control mechanism that operates by negative or positive feedback. For example, when in the normal person the blood glucose level rises, the pancreas responds by releasing insulin, which enables the glucose to be metabolized. The level of hormones is also regulated by this mechanism when the anterior pituitary responds to the levels of hormones circulating in the blood.

SES. *socioeconomic status.*

sesame oil. Oil obtained from the seeds of *Sesamum indicum.* It is used as a pharmaceutical aid and as a cooking oil.

sesamoid (sĕs′ă-moyd) [L. *sesamoides*]. Resembling a grain of sesame in size or shape.

sesamoid bone. An oval nodule of bone or fibrocartilage in a tendon playing over a bony surface. The patella is the largest one.

sesamoid cartilage. One or more small cartilage plates present in fibrous tissue between the lateral nasal and greater alar cartilages of the nose.

sesamoiditis (sĕs″ă-moy-dī′tĭs) [″ + Gr. *itis*, inflammation]. Inflammation of a sesamoid bone.

sesqui- [L.]. Prefix meaning one and one-half.

sesquihora (sĕs″kwĭ-hō′ră) [L.]. Every one and one-half hours.

sesquioxide (sĕs″kwē-ŏk′sĭd). Any oxide in which three parts of oxygen combine with two atoms of another element.

sessile (sĕs′l) [L. *sessilis*, low]. Having no peduncle but attached directly by a broad base.

set. 1. To fix firmly in place, as to set a bone in reduction of a fracture. 2. To allow an amalgam or plaster to harden. 3. In psychology, a group of conditions or attitudes that favor the occurrence of a certain response.

seta (sē′tă) [L., bristle] (pl. *setae*). A stiff, bristlelike structure. SEE: *vibrissae.*

setaceous (sē-tā′shŭs) [L. *setaceus*]. Bristly, hairy; resembling a bristle.

Setchenow's inhibitory centers (sĕtch′en-ŏfs) [Ivan M. Setchenow, Russian neurologist, 1829–1905]. Centers in the spinal cord and medulla oblongata involved in reflex inhibition of muscular and visceral activity.

setiferous (sē-tĭf′ĕr-ŭs) [L. *seta*, bristle, + *ferre*, to bear]. Having bristles.

setigerous (sē-tĭj′ĕr-ŭs) [″ + *gerere*, to carry]. Setiferous.

seton (sē″tŏn) [L. *seta*, bristle]. A thread or threads drawn through a fold of skin to act as a counterirritant or as a guide for instruments.

setose (sē′tōs). Having bristlelike appendages.

set point weight. SEE: *weight, set point.*

setup. The arrangement of teeth on a trial denture base.

seventh cranial nerve. Facial nerve; nervus facialis. SEE: *cranial nerves.*

seven-year itch. Scabies.

severe combined immunodeficiency disease. ABBR: SCID. An immunodeficiency disorder in which there are deficient T and B cell functions. Untreated, the disease may be quickly fatal. SCID occurs in less than one per million births.

    TREAT: Bone marrow transplant. If due to a deficiency of adenosine deaminase, that compound may be administered. The disease requires life-long therapy. SEE: *adenosine deaminase conjugated with polyethylene glycol.*

sevum (sē′vŭm) [L.]. Tallow or suet.

sewer gas. Gas produced by biodegradation of sewage. Contains methane and hydrogen sulfide. May be used for fuel. SEE: *carbon monoxide.*

sex [L. *sexus*]. 1. The characteristics that differentiate males and females in most plants and animals. 2. Motivation, both psychological and physiological, for behavior associated with procreation and erotic pleasure.

    s., chromosomal. Sex as determined by the presence of the female XX or male XY genotype in somatic cells.

    s., morphological. Sex of an individual as determined by the form of the external genitalia.

    s., nuclear. The genetic sex of an individual determined by the absence or presence of sex chromatin in the body cells, particularly blood cells.

    s., psychological. The individual's self-image of his or her gender. This may be at variance with the anatomical or morphological sex.

sex chromatin. Mass seen within the nuclei of normal female somatic cells. According to the Lyon hypothesis, one of the two X chromosomes in each somatic cell of the female is genetically inactivated. The sex chromatin represents the inactivated X chromosome. SYN: *Barr body.*

sex chromosomes. Chromosomes associated with determination of sex. In humans, these are the X (female) and Y (male) chromosomes. The normal female has two X chromosomes, and the normal male has one X and one Y chromosome. SEE: *Barr body.*

sex clinic. Clinic for diagnosis and treatment of an individual or couple with sexual problems.

sex determination. The concept that a couple may choose the sex of their offspring. To date, all efforts to make this a reality have been in vain. This concept should not be confused with determining the sexual identity of the fetus by analysis of cells obtained by amniocentesis or sampling of the chorionic villus.

sexdigital (sĕks-dĭj′ĭ-tăl) [L. *sex*, six, + *digitus*, digit]. Having six fingers and toes.

sexduction (sĕks-dŭk′shŭn). Process of transfer of bacterial genes from one cell to another by means of the sex factors within which they are incorporated.

sexism. All of the actions and attitudes that relegate individuals of either sex to a secondary and inferior status in society.

sexivalent (sĕks″ĭ-vă′lĕnt, -ĭv′ăl-ĕnt) [″ + *valere*, to be strong]. Capable of combining with six atoms of hydrogen.

sex-limited. Expression of a genetic character or trait in one sex only.

sex-linked. A character that is controlled by genes on the sex chromosomes.

sexology [L. *sexus*, sex, + Gr. *logos*, word, reason]. Scientific study of sexuality.

sex ratio. Ratio of females to males. Used in defining proportion of births of the two sexes or in the representation by sexual distribution in certain diseases.

sex surrogate. In sex therapy, a person serving as a surrogate sexual partner to assist in the therapeutic process.

sextan (sĕks′tăn) [L. *sextanus*, of the sixth]. Occurring every sixth day.

sextigravida (sĕks″tĭ-grăv′ĭd-ă) [L. *sextus*, six, + *gravida*, a pregnant woman]. A woman pregnant for the sixth time.

sextipara (sĕks-tĭp′ă-ră) [″ + *parere*, to bear a child]. A woman who has had six pregnancies that produced infants of 500 gm (or 20 weeks' gestation) regardless of their viability.

sextuplet (sĕks′tū-plĕt) [L. *sextus*, six]. One of six children born of a single gestation.

sexual (sĕks′ū-ăl) [L. *sexualis*]. 1. Pert. to sex. 2. Having sex.

sexual abuse. Rape, sexual assault, or sexual molestation. The active person in this may be male, female, adult, or child, and the abused person may be of the same or opposite sex of the abuser. Society gives much more publicity to the male abuser than it does to women who abuse adults and children, including their own sons and daughters. SEE: *incest; rape.*

sexual activity and aging. Medical studies of human sexual function and activity have provided no evidence that having attained a certain age is, of itself, reason to discontinue participating in and enjoying sexual intercourse.

sexual asphyxia. SEE: *asphyxia, sexual.*

sexual dysfunction. Inadequate enjoyment or failure to enjoy sexual activity. The areas of importance are desire, arousal, orgasm,

satisfaction, and pain. The dependence of most of these phases on the mental attitude of the partners is considerable, as is the hormonal balance of the patient(s). A careful history and physical examination will help to determine the possible pathological aspects of the various phases. Is desire absent, overactive, or is there aversion? Is arousal sufficient to maintain desire and, in the case of the male, to attain erection? Does orgasm occur, and if so, is it delayed or premature? Do the partners experience satisfaction at the completion of orgasm? Is pain present at any stage of the sexual activity?

ETIOL: A great number of physical and mental forces interact to culminate in enjoyable and fulfilling sexual activity. It is therefore important to keep this in mind in evaluating patients; and to realize that a great number of drugs have the undesired side effect of causing sexual dysfunction. Aging does not necessarily cause sexual dysfunction or obliteration of sexual capability.

Many commonly used drugs can cause sexual dysfunction in men and women; e.g., some antihypertensive agents; histamine-H_2-receptor antagonists; antipsychotic drugs; central nervous system depressants; and anticancer drugs.

TREAT: Treat the physical or mental factors that are involved, and attempt to use alternate drugs for those that appear to be the cause of the disorder.

sexual harassment. Especially between employers and employees, unsolicited and unprovoked sexual advances. In many instances, compliance with harasser's wishes is a condition of continued employment or advancement.

sexual health. The World Health Organization has defined three elements of sexual health: a capacity to enjoy and control sexual behavior in accordance with a social and personal ethic; freedom from fear, shame, guilt, false beliefs, and other psychological factors inhibiting sexual response and impairing sexual relationships; and freedom from organic disorder, disease, and deficiencies that interfere with sexual and reproductive functions. SEE: *AIDS.*

sexual intercourse. Sexual union between a male and a female. SYN: *coition; coitus; copulation.*

RS: clitoris; coitus interruptus; dyspareunia; ejaculation; emission; excitation; orgasm; penis; semen; vagina.

s.i., homosexual. Sexual union between persons of the same sex.

sexuality (sĕks-ū-ăl′ĭ-tē) [L. *sexus*, sex]. 1. State of having sex; the collective characteristics that mark the differences between the male and the female. 2. Constitution and life of individual as related to sex; all the dispositions related to the love life whether associated with the sex organs or not.

sexually transmitted disease. Disease acquired as a result of sexual intercourse with an infected individual. A more inclusive term than venereal disease, this term includes conditions such as syphilis, gonorrhea, AIDS, lymphogranuloma venereum, chancroid, granuloma inguinale, chlamydiosis, pelvic inflammatory disease, and other conditions such as trichomoniasis, genital candidiasis, genital herpes, genital warts, and bacterial vaginitis. For treatment of these diseases, see specific entries. SEE: *AIDS; Reiter's syndrome; venereal disease.* SEE: *Nursing Diagnoses* in *Appendix.*

sexual preference. The sexual orientation one prefers in choosing his or her sex partners.

sexual reassignment. Legal, surgical, or social action or decision to assign the appropriate sexuality to an individual who has been considered previously to be of the opposite sex.

sexual reflex. Erection and ejaculation resulting from direct genital stimulation or indirectly from emotion, whether asleep or awake.

Sézary cell [A. Sézary, Fr. dermatologist, 1880–1956]. A T cell lymphocyte, that contains an abundance of vacuoles filled with a mucopolysaccharide. Present in the blood of patients with Sézary syndrome.

Sézary syndrome. Skin disease characterized by infiltration with atypical Sézary cells. The exfoliative dermatitis is considered a variant form of mycosis fungoides, both of which are a form of cutaneous T cell lymphoma.

SGA. *small for gestational age.*

S.G.O. *Surgeon-General's Office.*

SGOT. *serum glutamic-oxaloacetic transaminase.* SEE: *transaminase, aspartate.*

SGPT. *serum glutamic pyruvic transaminase.* SEE: *transaminase, alanine.*

SH. *serum hepatitis.*

shadow [AS. *sceaduwe*]. A hemolyzed erythrocyte. SYN: *ghost corpuscle; phantom corpuscle.*

shadow-casting. A technique to increase the definition of the material being examined by use of electron microscopy. The object is sprayed from an oblique angle with a heavy metal.

shaft [AS. *sceaft*]. 1. The principal portion of any cylindrical body. 2. The diaphysis of a long bone.

    s., hair. The keratinized portion of a hair that extends from a hair follicle beyond the surface of the epidermis. SEE: *hair.*

shaken baby syndrome. A syndrome seen in abused infants and children. The patient has been subjected to violent, whiplash-type shaking injuries inflicted by the abusing individual. This may cause coma, convulsions, and increased intracranial pressure due to tearing of the cerebral veins with consequent bleeding into the subdural space. Retinal hemorrhages are usually present, and there may be bruises on the arms or trunk where the patient was forcefully grabbed. In domestic situations in which a child is abused, it is important to examine other children and infants living in the same home because about 20% of them will have signs of physical abuse. That examination should be done without delay in order to attempt to prevent further abuse of children in that home. SEE: *battered child syndrome; child abuse.*

shakes (shāks) [AS. *sceacen*]. 1. Shivering caused by a chill, esp. in intermittent fever. 2. Colloquial term for state of tremulousness and extreme irritability often seen in chronic alcoholics. SYN: *jitters.*

shaking. A passive movement in Swedish massage.

shaking palsy. A basal ganglion disease with progressive rigid tremulousness, peculiar gait, muscular contraction, and weakness. SYN: *paralysis agitans; Parkinson's disease.*

shaman (shā′mŭn, shŏ′-) [Russ., ascetic]. A traditional healer who, while in a trance, uses spirits, rather than techniques of Western medicine, to heal. Shamans have multifaceted holistic roles in their societies, which include judge, psychotherapist, magician, holder of the mores and traditions of the group, as well as medicine man or woman. SYN: *medicine man.* SEE: *shamanism.*

shamanism (shā′mŭn-ĭsm, shŏ′-). 1. Primitive religion of certain peoples of northern Asia who believe good and evil spirits pervade the world and can be influenced only by shamans acting as mediums. 2. Any similar form of primitive spiritualism, such as that practiced among American Indian tribes.

shank (shăngk) [AS. *sceanca*]. 1. The tibia or portion of leg from knee to ankle. SYN: *shin.* 2. The tapered portion of a dental hand instrument between the handle and the blade or nub. It may be straight or angled to provide better access or leverage in its use.

shape (shāp) [AS. *sceapan*]. 1. To mold to a particular form. 2. Outward form; contour.

    RS: aliform; arcate; arciform; arcuation; asteroid; bilateralism; bosselated; bosselation; bulbiform; calculus; caudate; circle; circumvallate.

shared decisions. The practice of the physician and patient discussing the approach to the medical care proposed for the patient.

The success of this sharing is, of course, dependent upon both the physician and patient being rational and competent.

shared governance. A model of nursing management in which the staff nurse shares responsibility and accountability for patient care with the hospital management. Shared governance assumes a participatory style of management and is aimed at quality patient care and a professional nursing practice. Shared governance is in contrast to self-governance and the traditional bureaucratic model of management. SEE: *self-governance.*

sharkskin. Condition seen in pellagra (nicotinic acid deficiency) in which openings of sebaceous glands become plugged with a dry yellowish material.

Sharpey's intercrossing fibers (shär′pēz) [William Sharpey, Scot. physiologist, 1802–1880]. Fibers forming the lamellae constituting the walls of the haversian canals in bone.

Sharpey's perforating fibers. 1. Fibers extending from the periosteum into the lamellae of bone. 2. Fibers extending from the periodontal membrane into the cementum of a tooth.

sharps. Medical articles that may cause punctures or cuts to those handling them. Included are all broken medical glassware, syringes, needles, scalpel blades, suture needles, and disposable razors. SEE: *AIDS; medical waste; Universal Precautions* in *Appendix.*

shear (shēr). A force applied parallel to the planes of an object but opposite in direction to whatever force was present.

sheath (shēth) [AS. *sceath*]. A covering structure of connective tissue, usually of an elongated part, such as the membrane covering a muscle.

    s., arachnoid. Delicate partition between pial sheath and dural sheath of the optic nerve.

    s., axon. The myelin sheath or neurilemma. SEE: *s., myelin.*

    s., carotid. Portion of cervical or pretracheal fascia enclosing the carotid artery, interior jugular vein, and vagus nerve.

    s., crural. Fascial covering of femoral vessels.

    s., dentinal. An obsolete term that was used when less complete microscopic information was available; no such sheath exists in dentin. It is an interface between peritubular and intertubular dentin that is apparent because of differing degrees of mineralization of the two areas, but it is of no significance and is not named. SYN: *s. of Neumann.*

    s., dural. A fibrous membrane or external investment of the optic nerve.

    s., femoral. The fascial covering of femoral vessels.

    s., lamellar. Connective tissue sheath covering a bundle of nerve fibers. SYN: *s., nerve; perineurium.*

    s., medullary. SEE: *s., myelin.*

    s., myelin. Layers of lipid and protein substances that form a semifluid covering of nerves. The layers are an extension of the plasma membrane of the Schwann cell. The sheath is relatively insensitive to the action of temperature and electrolytes. SEE: *nerve fiber; neuron.*

    s., nerve. S., lamellar.

    s. of Henle. Sheath of Key and Retzius.

    s. of Hertwig. SEE: *Hertwig's root sheath.*

    s. of Key and Retzius, connective tissue. Delicate reticular fibrils around individual nerve fibers.

    s. of Neumann. An obsolete term. SEE: *s., dentinal.*

    s. of Schwann. Membranous covering of myelin sheath of a nerve fiber.

    s. of Schweigger-Seidel. The thickened wall of a sheathed artery of the spleen.

    s., pial. Extension of the pia, closely investing surface of the optic nerve.

    s., root. The layers of a hair follicle derived from the epidermis. Includes the outer root sheath, which is a continuation of the stratum germinativum, and the inner root sheath, which consists of three layers of cells closely investing the root of the hair. SEE: *hair.*

    s., synovial. A double-walled tubelike bursa that encloses a tendon. Consists of an inner visceral layer lying upon and adhering to a tendon and an outer parietal layer, the two being separated by a space filled with synovial fluid. Found esp. in the hands and feet where tendons are confined to osteofibrous canals or pass over bony surfaces.

    s., tendon. A dense fibrous sheath that confines a tendon to an osseous groove, converting it into an osteofibrous canal. Found principally in the wrist and ankle. SEE: *s., synovial.*

shedding [ME. *sheden*, shed]. 1. The loss of deciduous teeth. 2. Casting off of surface layer of the epidermis. 3. Loss of bacteria from the skin.

Sheehan's syndrome. Hypopituitarism resulting from an infarct of the pituitary following postpartum shock or hemorrhage. Damage to the anterior pituitary gland causes partial to complete loss of thyroid, adrenocortical, and gonadal function.

sheep cell agglutination test. ABBR: SCAT. A test for rheumatoid factor in serum. Sheep erythrocytes sensitized with rabbit antisheep erythrocyte immune globulin will be agglutinated if serum containing the rheumatoid factor is added.

sheet (shēt) [AS. *sciete*, cloth]. Linen or cotton bedcovering next to the sleeper.

    s., draw. Sheet folded under a patient so that it may be withdrawn without lifting the patient. This is accomplished by turning the patient to the side of the bed to allow one side of the sheet to be removed and replaced with a clean one. The patient is then turned to the other side of the bed. The soiled sheet is removed and placement of the clean one is completed. SEE: *draw sheet*.

    s., lift. Sheet folded under a patient over the bottom sheet to assist with moving the patient up in bed.

shelf. Any shelflike structure.

    s., dental. SYN: *dental lamina*.

shelf-life. 1. The time a food may be kept on a store shelf and still be considered safe to eat. 2. The length of time a substance, preparation, or medication can be kept without separation or chemical changes of its component parts.

shell. A hard covering, as that for an egg or turtle.

shellac (shě-lăk'). A refined resinous substance obtained from plants that contain the secretions of certain insects. It is used in paints, varnishes, and as a coating for pills.

shellfish, paralytic poisoning from. Poisoning from eating fish which have ingested toxic dinoflaggelates, part of marine plankton. This causes paresthesias of the face and extremities, dysphonia, generalized muscle weakness, nausea, vomiting, and diarrhea. Sometimes paralysis and respiratory arrest are present.

    TREAT: Induce vomiting; give cathartic and whatever supportive therapy is needed.

shell shock. An obsolete term used during World War I to designate a wide variety of psychotic and neurotic disorders associated with the stress of combat. SEE: *hysteria*.

Shenton's line (shěn'tŏnz) [Thomas Shenton, Brit. radiologist, 1872–1955]. A radiographic line used to determine the relationship of the head of the femur to the acetabulum. The line follows the inferior border of the ramus of the pubic bone and continued outward follows the curve down the medial border of the neck of the femur.

shiatsu, shiatzu [Chinese, finger + pressure]. Japanese massage method used in treating disease. It incorporates acupressure.

shield (shēld) [AS. *scild*, shield]. 1. Any protecting device. 2. In biology, a protective plate or hard outer covering.

    s., embryonic. The two-layered blastoderm or blastodisk from which a mammalian embryo develops. SYN: *disk, embryonic*.

    s., gonadal. A lead device that is to be placed over the gonadal area to help reduce radiation exposure to this tissue.

    s., nipple. A cover to protect sore nipples of a nursing woman.

    s., phallic. An antiseptic covering for the male genitals during operations.

shift [AS. *sciftan*, to arrange]. A change in position or direction.

    s., antigenic. SEE: *antigenic drift*.

    s., chloride. The shift of chloride ions from the plasma into red blood cells upon the addition of carbon dioxide from the tissues and the reverse movement when carbon dioxide is released in the lungs. It is a mechanism for maintaining constant pH of the blood.

    s. to the left. Arneth's term for an increase in the number of young polymorphonuclear leukocytes in the blood. SEE: *Arneth's classification of neutrophils*.

    s. to the right. Arneth's term for an increase in the number of older polymorphonuclear leukocytes in the blood. SEE: *Arneth's classification of neutrophils*.

shift work. Work for a specific time period, esp. working a certain time of the day for a week or two and then shifting to a period either 8 hours prior to or after the original work period. This changing schedule every several weeks continues as long as one is on shift work rather than working the same period of time each day. SEE: *circadian; clock, biological; night work, maladaption to*.

Shiga's bacillus (shē'găs) [Kiyoshi Shiga, Japanese physician, 1870–1957]. The bacillus causing a form of dysentery. SYN: *Shigella dysenteriae*.

Shigella (shǐ-gěl'lä) [Kiyoshi Shiga]. A genus of non-lactose-fermenting, nonmotile, gram-negative rods belonging to the family Enterobacteriaceae. It contains a number of species that cause digestive disturbance ranging from mild diarrhea to a severe and often fatal dysentery. SEE: *dysentery, bacillary*.

    S. boydii. A species that causes acute diarrhea in humans. SYN: *Group C dysentery bacilli*.

    S. dysenteriae. Shiga's bacillus, a virulent strain isolated during a severe epidemic of dysentery in Japan in 1896.

    S. flexneri. A species that is a frequent cause of acute diarrhea in humans. SYN: *Group B dysentery bacilli*.

    S. sonnei. A species that is a frequent cause of bacillary dysentery. SYN: *Group D dysentery bacilli*.

shigellosis (shī"gěl-lō'sĭs) [*Shigella* + *osis*, condition]. The disease produced by infection with *Shigella* organisms.

shin (shĭn) [AS. *scinu*, shin]. Anterior edge of tibia, portion of leg between the ankle and knee. SYN: *shank*.

   s., saber. Condition seen in congenital syphilis in which anterior edge of tibia is extremely sharp.

shingles (shĭng'lz) [L. *cingulus*, a girdle]. Eruption of acute, inflammatory, herpetic vesicles on the trunk of the body along a peripheral nerve; occasionally elsewhere. SYN: *herpes zoster*, q.v.

   TREAT: Acyclovir.

shinsplints. Pain in the anterior compartment of the tibia. It usually follows strenuous exercise. The cause is ischemia of the muscles in the compartment and minute tears in the tissues. SYN: *medial tibial syndrome.*

shin spots. Hyperpigmented and retracted scars of the skin on the anterior lower legs. Condition is usually, but not always, associated with diabetes.

Shirodkar operation [Shirodkar, contemporary Indian physician]. Surgical placement of a purse-string suture around an incompetent cervical os to attempt to prevent premature onset of labor. The suture material used for this cerclage procedure is nonabsorbable and must be removed prior to delivery.

shiver (shĭv'ĕr) [ME. *chiveren*]. 1. Involuntary increased muscle activity in response to fear, onset of fever, or exposure to cold. The activity leads to increased heat production. 2. To tremble or shake.

shock (shŏk) [ME. *schokke*]. A clinical syndrome in which the peripheral blood flow is inadequate to return sufficient blood to the heart for normal function, particularly transport of oxygen to all organs and tissues. Shock may be caused by a variety of conditions including hemorrhage, infection, drug reaction, trauma, poisoning, myocardial infarction, and dehydration. Every injury is accompanied by some degree of shock and should be treated promptly. Syncope is caused by insufficient blood supply to the brain, and the clinical picture resembles shock. SEE: *catalepsy; insulin shock; s., septic; toxic shock syndrome*. SEE: *Nursing Diagnoses* in *Appendix.*

   SYM: The most outstanding symptoms are marked paleness of the skin; evidence of decreased oxygenation of the skin as shown by cyanosis as the process continues; the face is pinched and without expression; there may be a staring of the eyes, which often lose their characteristic luster, and the pupils may be dilated; the pulse is weak and rapid; the breathing rate is increased and is shallow; the blood pressure is decreased and may be unobtainable; there may be urinary retention and incontinence of feces; occasionally there is an unusual restlessness or excitement; and very often the patient expresses an extreme thirst. If conscious, the patient seems quite disinterested in the surroundings and complains little of pain even though he or she may be groaning.

   F.A.: Depends on diagnosis. In general, treat specific etiological factor and maintain body heat by warm but not hot blankets or water bottles. Keep body either flat or with head lower than feet. Do not move patient except to transport to a medical care facility. Give fluids sparingly but, in case of head injuries or suspected internal bleeding, do not give stimulants. Call a physician immediately.

   TREAT: Maintain circulation by keeping patient lying down with head lower than body. The lower extremities can be slightly elevated by placing the lower half of the body on pillows, or by elevating the foot of the bed.

   Patient should be kept comfortably warm, but application of external heat is not advisable. Avoid unnecessary questions and noises. Do not move patient unnecessarily.

   Even though thirst is present, give fluids by mouth sparingly in order to reduce the possibility of vomiting and aspirating vomitus. If bleeding is present, it should be controlled. If internal hemorrhage is suspected or head injuries are present, no stimulants are permissible.

   The use of intramuscular and intravenous injections such as norepinephrine, dopamine, or dobutamine may be recommended by the physician. Oxygen may be necessary. Blood transfusion or even artificial respiration may be required, depending on the seriousness of the condition.

   Relieve pain by splints, posture, supporting bandages, and drugs. Morphine is valuable. Blood transfusions may be lifesaving. If blood is not available, artificial substances for increasing plasma volume may be used.

   Respiration may be aided by administration of oxygen preferably mixed with 4% to 10% carbon dioxide as a respiratory stimulant. Constant, kindly, tactful encouragement and extreme gentleness in all procedures are of importance.

Caution: The shock syndrome is a serious life-endangering medical emergency and requires very careful therapy and monitoring. If the patient does not respond at once, it is essential that he be treated and monitored in the best facility available, such as an intensive care unit. It is important that the ECG, arterial and central venous blood pressures, blood gases, core and skin temperatures, pulse rate, blood volume, blood glucose, hematocrit, cardiac output, urine flow rate, changes in size, shape, and reaction of pupils, and mental state be monitored as frequently as needed. An electroencephalogram may be required.

Artificial blood has been used experimentally in treating shock due to blood loss.

s., anaphylactic. SEE: *anaphylactic shock.*

s., anesthesia. Shock due to an overdose of a general anesthetic. This calls for the immediate cessation of anesthesia. Artificial respiration, oxygen, and appropriate stimulants should be given at once. The condition is manifested by a weak rapid pulse, a fall or drop in blood pressure, cold clammy skin, and shallow respirations.

s., cardiogenic. Shock resulting from failure to maintain blood supply to the circulatory system and tissues because of inadequate cardiac output. SEE: *Nursing Diagnoses* in *Appendix.*

s., deferred. Late manifestation of shock following injury or burns. May appear in 3 to 30 hours and may be due to transportation, emotional stress, hemorrhage, dehydration, acidosis, or toxemia. SYN: *s., secondary.*

s., electric. Shock resulting from the passage of electric current through any part of the body.

s., endotoxin. Septic shock due to toxins from gram-negative bacteria. SEE: *septic shock.*

s., epigastric. Shock resulting from a blow or other trauma (surgery) in upper abdomen.

s., hemorrhagic. Shock due to loss of blood.

s., hypovolemic. Condition occurring when there is an insufficient amount of blood in the circulatory system. Usually, this is due to trauma that causes blood loss into a body cavity or frank external hemorrhage.

s., insulin. Shock resulting from an overdosage of insulin with subsequent hypoglycemia.

F.A.: Give orange juice, glucose, candy, lump of sugar. If unconscious, inject glucose intravenously. SEE: *insulin shock therapy.*

s., irreversible. Shock of such intensity that even heroic therapy cannot prevent death.

s., mental. Shock due to emotional stress or to seeing an injury or accident. SEE: *s., psychic.*

s., protein. Shock reaction resulting from parenteral administration of a protein.

s., psychic. Shock due to excessive fear, joy, anger, grief. SEE: *s., mental.*

s., secondary. S., deferred.

s., septic. SEE: *septic shock.*

s., serum. Shock occurring as part of a reaction to injection of serum.

s., spinal. Immediate flaccid paralysis and loss of all sensation and voluntary and involuntary reflex activity below the level of injury in acute transverse spinal cord injury.

s., surgical. Shock following operations and including traumatic shock. SEE: *s., traumatic.*

s. syndrome, toxic. SEE: *toxic shock syndrome.*

s., traumatic. Shock due to injury or surgery. May occur as the result of abdominal injury from any cause. Shock is proportional to the extent of injury. Esp. severe in upper abdomen and more marked when viscera are damaged. If prolonged, indicates hemorrhage or peritonitis, or both.

Cerebral injury: Concussion of brain or skull fracture. May come on immediately or later from edema or intracranial hemorrhage. *Chemical injury:* Shock due to pain from the effect of chemicals, esp. corrosives. *Crushing injury:* The greater the extent of injury, the more severe the degree of shock. *Fracture:* Esp. in compound fracture. Often extensive blood loss into tissues occurs, and hence circulation is impaired. *Heart damage:* As in angina pectoris, myocardial infarctions, pericarditis, or myocarditis. *Inflammation:* As acute general peritonitis or fulminating sepsis anywhere in the body. *Intestinal obstruction:* Shock is present when obstruction is acute. *Nerve injury:* Contusion of highly sensitive parts, as testicle, solar plexus, eye, urethra. *Operations:* May occur even after minor operations, as paracentesis and catheterization. *Perforation or rupture of viscera:* As in acute pneumothorax, ruptured aneurysm, perforated peptic ulcer, perforation in appendicitis, ectopic pregnancy. *Strangulation:* As in hernia, intussusception, volvulus. *Thermal injury:* As burns, frostbite, heat exhaustion. *Torsion of viscera:* As of an ovary, testicle.

shock-collapse. A shock-collapse or a hypotonic-hyporesponsive vascular collapse may be evidenced by signs or symptoms such as decrease in or loss of muscle tone, paralysis (partial or complete), hemiplegia, hemiparesis, skin pallor, unresponsiveness to environmental stimuli, depression of or loss of consciousness, prolonged sleeping with difficulty arousing or cardiovascular or respiratory arrest. SEE: *disseminated intravascular coagulation; septic shock.*

shock therapy. Form of treatment in mental illness. In electric shock therapy, convulsions are induced by passage of electric current through the brain, used chiefly in depression.

shoemakers' cramp. Spasm of muscles of hand and arm occurring in shoemakers.

short bowel syndrome. Inadequate absorption of ingested nutrients due to a surgical procedure in which a considerable length of the intestinal tract has been removed or bypassed. SEE: *total parenteral nutrition.*

shortsightedness (short-sīt'ĕd-nĕs). A condition of not being able to see very far, due to light rays coming to a focus in front of the retina. SYN: *myopia; nearsightedness.*

shot. A hypodermic injection.

shotgun prescription. Prescription containing many drugs given with hope that one of them may prove effective. Not a recommended approach to the treatment of disease.

shoulder (shōl'dĕr) [AS. *sculdor*]. The region of the proximal humerus, clavicle and scapula; a part of the shoulder girdle complex. SEE: *scapula.*

  s., dislocation of. Head of humerus is displaced beyond the boundaries of the glenoid fossa. Because dislocation of the shoulder is frequently accompanied by a fracture, surgeons advise making an x-ray examination of affected bones. Attempting to reduce dislocations without knowledge of the presence of fractures is very dangerous and sometimes results in serious paralysis of the entire upper extremity or grave damage to the large blood vessels in the armpit.

  ETIOL: The most common cause is from trauma with the arm in external rotation with abduction, causing the head of the humerus to sublux anteriorly; a posterior subluxation may occur from a fall on an outstretched arm. It is very common among athletes, esp. football and basketball players. A patient with a dislocated shoulder usually has a hollow in place of the normal bulge of the shoulder. There seems to be a slight depression at the outer end of the clavicle, and such patients cannot place their hand at their opposite shoulder while their elbow is on their chest. Always compare both sides. An inferior dislocation may occur from poor muscle tone as with hemiplegia and from the weight of the arm pulling the humerus downward.

  F.A.: Send for a physician as soon as possible. Lay the patient on the back, with a pillow (or folded pad) between the shoulders. Place a large, soft pad under the elbow on the affected side, then bind the forearm horizontally across the chest using an open sling that is reinforced by a broad cravat bandage, and apply cold applications to the affected shoulder. Treat for shock if present.

shoulder blade. The scapula.

shoulder girdle. The two scapulae and two clavicles attaching the bones of the upper extremities to the axial skeleton, i.e., the vertebrae of the backbone.

shoulder joint. Joint formed by humerus and glenoid cavity of the scapula. SYN: *glenohumeral joint.*

show (shō) [AS. *scewian*, to look at]. The sanguinoserous discharge from the vagina during the first stage of labor or just preceding menstruation.

Shrapnell's membrane (shrăp'nĕls) [Henry J. Shrapnell, Brit. anatomist, 1761–1841]. A small triangular portion of the tympanic membrane lying above the malleolar folds. It is thin and lax and attached directly to the petrous bone at the tympanic notch (notch of Rivinus). SYN: *pars flaccida.*

shreds (shrĕds) [AS. *screade*]. Slender strands of mucus seen in freshly voided urine, indicative of inflammation of the urinary tract or associated organs.

shrink. 1. To reduce in size. 2. Slang term for psychiatrist [from *headshrinker*].

shudder [ME. *shuddren*]. A temporary convulsive tremor resulting from fright, horror, or aversion.

shunt (shŭnt) [ME. *shunten*, to avoid]. 1. To turn away from; to divert. 2. Anomalous passage or one artificially constructed to divert flow from one main route to another. 3. Electric conductor connecting two points in a circuit to form a parallel circuit through which a portion of the current may pass.

  s., arteriovenous. An abnormal connection between an artery and the venous system.

  s., cardiovascular. An abnormal connection between the cavities of the heart or between the systemic and pulmonary vessels.

  s., dialysis. An arteriovenous shunt created for use during renal dialysis.

  s., left-to-right. Passage of blood from the left side of the heart to the right side through an abnormal opening, as in patent ductus arteriosus.

  s., LeVeen. SEE: *LeVeen shunt.*

  s., portacaval. Surgical creation of a connection between the portal vein and the vena cava.

  s., postcaval. S., portacaval.

  s., reversed. SEE: *s., right-to-left.*

  s., right-to-left. Passage of blood from the right to left side of the heart through some abnormal opening such as a septal defect. The shunted blood has no opportunity to become oxygenated because of having failed to pass through the lungs.

shy. The feeling of being timid, especially in

an unfamiliar setting or when encountering strangers. This feeling is so common that it cannot be classed as abnormal unless it interferes with activities essential to employment or interpersonal relations.

Shy-Drager syndrome [George Milton Shy, U.S. neurologist, 1919–1967; G. A. Drager, U.S. physician, 1917–1967]. Chronic orthostatic hypotension due to primary autonomic nervous system insufficiency.

SI. *Système International;* International System of Measurement. SEE: *SI Units* in *Appendix.*

Si. Chem. symb. for the element silicon.

SIADH. *syndrome of inappropriate antidiuretic hormone.*

siagonantritis (sī″ăg-ŏn-ăn-trī′tĭs) [Gr. *siagon,* jawbone, + *antron,* cavity, + *itis,* inflammation]. Inflammation of the maxillary sinus.

sial(o)- (sī′ă-lō) [Gr. *sialon,* saliva]. Combining form meaning saliva.

sialaden (sī-ăl′ă-dĕn) [″ + *aden,* gland]. A salivary gland.

sialadenitis (sī″ăl-ăd″ĕ-nī′tĭs) [″ + ″ + *itis,* inflammation]. Inflamed condition of a salivary gland.

sialadenoncus (sī″ăl-ăd″ĕ-nŏng′kŭs) [″ + ″ + *onkos,* tumor]. Tumor of salivary gland.

sialagogue (sī-ăl′ă-gŏg) [″ + *agogos,* leading]. Agent increasing flow of saliva. Also spelled sialogogue.

sialaporia (sī″ăl-ă-pō′rē-ă) [″ + *aporia,* lack]. Deficiency in secretion of saliva.

sialectasia, sialectasis (sī″ăl-ĕk-tā′sē-ă, sī″a-lĕk′tă-sĭs) [″ + *ektasis,* dilatation]. Hypertrophy or swelling of the salivary glands.

sialemesis (sī″ăl-ĕm′ĕs-ĭs) [″ + *emein,* to vomit]. Vomiting of saliva or vomiting caused by an excessive secretion of saliva.

sialic (sī-ăl′ĭk). Concerning or resembling saliva.

sialine (sī′ă-lĭn) [Gr. *sialon,* saliva]. Concerning saliva.

sialism, sialismus (sī′ăl-ĭzm, sī-ăl-ĭz′mŭs) [″ + *-ismos,* condition]. An excessive secretion of saliva. SYN: *ptyalism; salivation.*

sialitis (sī″ă-lī′tĭs) [″ + *itis,* inflammation]. Inflammation of a salivary gland.

sialoadenitis (sī″ă-lō-ăd″ĕ-nī′tĭs) [″ + *aden,* gland, + *itis,* inflammation]. Inflammation of a salivary gland. SYN: *sialadenitis.*

sialoadenotomy (sī″ă-lō-ăd″ĕ-nŏt′ō-mē) [″ + ″ + *tome,* incision]. Incision of a salivary gland.

sialoaerophagy (sī″ă-lō-ĕr″ŏf′ă-jē) [″ + *aer,* air, + *phagein,* to eat]. Constant swallowing, thus taking saliva and air into the stomach.

sialoangiectasis (sī″ă-lō-ăn″jē-ĕk′tă-sĭs) [Gr. *sialon,* saliva, + *angeion,* vessel, + *ektasis,* dilatation]. Dilation of a salivary gland duct.

sialoangiography (sī″ă-lō-ăn″jē-ŏg′ră-fē) [″ + ″ + *graphein,* to write]. Sialography.

sialoangitis, sialoangiitis (sī″ă-lō-ăn-jī′tĭs, -ăn″jē-ī′tĭs) [″ + ″ + *itis,* inflammation]. Inflamed condition of the salivary ducts.

sialocele (sī′ă-lō-sēl) [″ + *kele,* tumor, swelling]. Cyst or tumor of a salivary gland.

sialodochitis (sī″ă-lō-dō-kī′tĭs) [″ + *doche,* receptacle, + *itis,* inflammation]. Inflamed condition of salivary ducts.

s. fibrinosa. Sialodochitis with duct obstructed by a fibrinous exudate.

sialodochoplasty (sī″ă-lō-dō′kō-plăs″tē) [″ + ″ + *plassein,* to form]. Plastic surgery of a salivary gland.

sialoductitis (sī″ă-lō-dŭk-tī′tĭs) [″ + L. *ductus,* duct, + Gr. *itis,* inflammation]. Inflamed condition of Stensen's duct.

sialogenous (sī″ă-lŏj′ĕ-nŭs) [″ + *gennan,* to produce]. Forming saliva.

sialogogic (sī″ă-lō-gŏj′ĭk). Producing or promoting a secretion of saliva.

sialogogue (sī-ăl′ō-gŏg) [″ + *agogos,* leading]. 1. An agent that stimulates the secretion of saliva. 2. Producing or promoting the secretion of saliva. Also spelled sialagogue. SYN: *ptyalagogue.*

sialogram (sī-ăl′ō-grăm) [″ + *gramma,* something written]. A radiographic record of sialography, q.v.

sialography (sī″ă-lŏg′ră-fē) [″ + *graphein,* to write]. Examination of salivary ducts and glands with x-rays. SYN: *ptyalography.*

sialolith (sī-ăl′ō-lĭth) [″ + *lithos,* stone]. A salivary concretion or calculus.

sialolithiasis (sī″ă-lō-lĭ-thī′ă-sĭs). Presence of salivary calculi.

sialolithotomy (sī″ă-lō-lĭ-thŏt′ō-mē) [Gr. *sialon,* saliva, + *lithos,* stone, + *tome,* incision]. Removal of a calculus from a salivary gland or duct.

sialoncus (sī″ă-lŏng′kŭs) [″ + *onkos,* bulk, mass]. A tumor under the tongue caused by obstruction of a salivary gland or duct.

sialoporia (sī″ă-lō-pō′rē-ă) [″ + *aporia,* lack]. Deficient secretion of saliva.

sialorrhea (sī″ă-lō-rē′ă) [″ + *rhoia,* a flow]. Excessive flow of saliva. SYN: *sialism.* SEE: *transtympanic neurectomy.*

sialoschesis (sī″ă-lŏs′kĕ-sĭs) [″ + *schesis,* suppression]. Suppression or retention of saliva.

sialosemeiology (sī″ă-lō-sē″mī-ŏl′ō-jē) [″ + *semeion,* sign, + *logos,* word, reason]. Diagnosis based upon examination of saliva.

sialosis (sī-ă-lō′sĭs) [″ + *osis,* condition].

The flow of saliva.

sialostenosis (sī″ă-lō-stĕ-nō′sĭs) [″ + *stenosis*, act of narrowing]. Closure of a salivary duct.

sialosyrinx (sī″ă-lō-sī′rĭnks) [″ + *syrinx*, a pipe]. 1. Fistula into the salivary gland. 2. A syringe for washing out salivary ducts. 3. Drainage tube for a salivary duct.

sialotic (sī″ă-lŏt′ĭk) [Gr. *sialon*, saliva]. Concerning the flow of saliva.

Siamese twins (sī-ă-mēz′) [After Chang and Eng (1811–1874), joined Chinese twins born in Siam]. Congenitally united twins. In some cases the individuals are joined in a small area and are capable of activity, but the extent of union may be so great that survival is impossible. Nevertheless, modern surgical techniques have made it possible to separate infants who in the past would not have been expected to survive and have a good prognosis. SEE: *twin*.

sib [AS. *sibb*, kin]. 1. A brother or sister. SYN: *sibling*. 2. A blood relative.

sibilant (sĭb′ĭ-lănt) [L. *sibilans*, hissing]. Hissing or whistling, as a sound heard in a certain rale, q.v.

sibilation. Pronunciation in which the hissing sound is predominant.

sibilismus. A hissing sound.

   s. aurium. Tinnitus.

sibilus (sĭb′ĭ-lŭs) [L. *sibilans*, hissing]. A hissing rale.

sibling (sĭb′lĭng) [AS. *sibb*, kin, + *-ling*, having the quality of]. One of two or more children of same parents; a brother or sister.

   s., half. A half brother or sister.

sibship. Brothers and sisters of a single family.

siccant (sĭk′ănt) [L. *siccus*, dry]. Drying.

siccative (sĭk′ă-tĭv) [L. *siccativus*, drying]. Drying or that which dries. SYN: *siccant*.

siccolabile (sĭk″ō-lā′bĭl) [L. *siccus*, dry, + *labilis*, unstable]. Altered or destroyed by drying.

siccostabile (sĭk″ō-stā′bĭl) [″ + *stabilis*, stable]. Resistant to drying.

siccus (sĭk′ŭs) [L.]. Dry.

sick (sĭk) [AS *seoc*, ill]. 1. Not well. SYN: *ill*. 2. Mentally ill or disturbed. 3. Nauseated.

sickle cell. Abnormal red blood cell that has a crescent shape. SYN: *meniscocyte*.

sickle cell anemia. A hereditary chronic form of anemia in which abnormal sickle or crescent-shaped erythrocytes are present. Due to the presence of abnormal type of hemoglobin, hemoglobin S, in the red blood cells. The frequency of the gene that causes this disease is high in Mediterranean and African populations and in black populations.

   In addition to the hemolytic anemia, painful crises occur and multiple infarctions of most organ systems. This causes a great variety of signs and symptoms. The disease interferes with the development of infants and children. A common physical finding early in the history of the disease is the hand-foot syndrome. This form of inflammation of the small bones of the hands and feet occurs between ages of 3 and 20 months. The condition is characterized by fever, pallor, swelling of the hands and feet, and pain. It is usually reversible.

   DIAG: Observation of sickled red cells on blood smears; more than 80% of hemoglobin as shown by electrophoresis is hemoglobin S and not hemoglobin A.

   TREAT: Supportive, including supplemental iron and blood transfusion. A number of therapeutic approaches are being investigated. In the meantime, genetic counseling is indicated, and antenatal diagnosis by use of chorionic villus sampling is helpful.

   Because children with this disease under the age of 5 years are particularly prone to develop serious infections, it is of utmost importance to establish the diagnosis as early as possible in order to be prepared to institute therapy for infections without delay. SEE: *anemia; hemoglobin*.

sickle cell crisis. The sickled cells interfere with oxygen transport, obstruct capillary blood flow, and cause fever and severe pain in joints and the abdomen. The abdominal pain may simulate that caused by appendicitis or other indications for surgical intervention. The cause of the onset of symptoms is usually unknown, but a crisis may be precipitated by decreased ambient oxygen as can occur during flying at high altitude without use of supplemental oxygen. Also, acidosis and dehydration may precipitate a crisis.

sickle cell trait. The condition of having the heterozygous gene for sickle cell anemia, hemoglobin S. Thus each red cell has both normal hemoglobin A and abnormal hemoglobin S. These cells will not become sickled until extremely low concentrations of oxygen occur. SEE: *hemoglobin S*.

sicklemia (sĭk-lē′mē-ă) [AS. *sicol*, sickle, + Gr. *haima*, blood]. Sickle cells in the blood.

sickling. Tendency of red blood cells to be sickle-shaped. SEE: *sickle cell anemia*.

sickness [AS. *seoc*, ill]. State of being unwell. SYN: *illness*.

   s., balloon. Discomfort or illness due to ascent in a balloon to an altitude sufficient to cause symptoms of anoxia.

   s., bleeding. Abnormal tendency to bleed. SYN: *hemophilia*.

   s., car. Nausea and malaise from riding

in vehicles such as trains or automobiles. SYN: *motion sickness*.

s., falling. Epilepsy.

s., green. Form of anemia with greenish pallor. SYN: *chlorosis*.

s., morning. Nausea of early pregnancy.

s., motion. Nausea and vomiting caused by a variety of motions, such as those experienced on boats, airplanes, trains, automobiles, or rides in amusement parks.

s., mountain. Nausea and dyspnea caused by insufficient oxygen at high altitudes.

s., sea. Sickness caused by motion of a vessel while at sea.

s., serum. Sickness following injection of serum.

s., sleeping. 1. Infection with trypanosomes with involvement of central nervous system and ultimately continuous sleeping. The disease is transmitted by the bite of an infected tsetse fly, of the genus *Glossina*. The disease can be transmitted congenitally. SYN: *trypanosomiasis*. 2. Acute infectious disease with increasing lethargy. SYN: *encephalitis lethargica*.

sick sinus syndrome. ABBR: SSS. Several electrocardiographic abnormalities due to malfunction of the sinoatrial node of the heart. They may include persistent sinus bradycardia that may alternate with tachyarrhythmias; sinoatrial block; and sinus arrest for brief or prolonged periods. SEE: *Nursing Diagnoses* in *Appendix*.

SYM: Lightheadedness, dizziness, fainting, dyspnea, fatigue, and angina pectoris.

TREAT: Insertion of a pacemaker; anticoagulant therapy may be required to prevent thromboembolism.

SICU. *surgical intensive care unit*.

SID. *source-to-image receptor distance*.

S.I.D. *Society for Investigative Dermatology*.

side (sīd) [AS. *side*]. 1. Left or right part of trunk of the body. 2. An outer portion considered as facing in a particular direction.

side effect. The action or effect of a drug other than that desired. Commonly it is an undesirable effect such as nausea, headache, insomnia, acute toxic reaction, or drug interaction.

side-lyer. A device for positioning the patient with central nervous system dysfunction in the side-lying position in order to reduce decerebrate posturing and counteract the effects of the tonic labyrinthine (supine) reflex.

side-lying. A lateral recumbent position in which the individual rests on either the right or left side, usually with the knees slightly bent. This position is useful in persons with multiple disabilities resulting from damage to the central nervous system and allows re-

laxation while requiring minimal postural control.

side position. Position in which patient is lying on one side, thighs flexed, with underarm behind back. SYN: *Sims' position*. SEE: *position* for illus.

sideration (sĭd-ĕr-ā′shŭn) [L. *siderari*, to be struck by a star]. 1. Therapeutic application of electric sparks. 2. A sudden stroke, as in apoplexy. 3. Lightning stroke.

siderism, siderismus (sĭd′ĕr-ĭzm, sĭd-ĕr-ĭz′mŭs) [Gr. *sideros*, iron, + *-ismos*, condition]. Therapeutic application of metals to the skin. SYN: *metallotherapy*.

sidero- (sĭd′ĕr-ō) [Gr. *sideros*, iron]. Combining form meaning iron or steel.

sideroblast (sĭd′ĕr-ō-blăst″) [″ + *blastos*, germ]. A ferritin-containing normoblast in the bone marrow. They constitute from 20% to 90% of normoblasts in the marrow. The ferritin gives a positive Prussian-blue reaction, indicating the iron is ionized and not bound to the heme protein.

siderocyte (sĭd′ĕr-ō-sīt) [″ + *kytos*, cell]. A red blood cell containing iron in a form other than hematin.

sideroderma (sĭd′ĕr-ō-dĕr′mă) [″ + *derma*, skin]. Bronzed coloration of the skin from disordered hemoglobin disintegration.

siderodromophobia (sĭd″ĕr-ō-drō″mō-fō′bē-ă) [″ + *dromos*, a way, + *phobos*, fear]. Morbid fear of railway travel.

siderofibrosis (sĭd″ĕr-ō-fī-brō′sĭs) [″ + L. *fibra*, fiber, + Gr. *osis*, condition]. Fibrosis associated with deposits of iron.

siderogenous (sĭd″ĕr-ōj′ĕ-nŭs) [″ + *gennan*, to produce]. Producing or forming iron.

sideropenia (sĭd″ĕr-ō-pē′nē-ă) [″ + *penia*, poverty]. Iron deficiency; deficiency of iron in the blood.

sideropenic (sĭd″ĕr-ō-pē′nĭk). Characterized by deficiency of iron in the blood.

siderophil (sĭd′ĕr-ō-fĭl). A cell that has affinity for iron.

siderophilin (sī′dĭr-ŏf″ĭ-lĭn). Transferrin, q.v.

siderophilous (sĭd″ĕr-ŏf′ĭ-lŭs) [″ + *philein*, to love]. Having a tendency to absorb iron, as the red blood corpuscles.

siderophone (sĭd′ĕr-ō-fōn). A telephonelike device used to detect intraocular, iron-containing foreign bodies.

siderophore (sĭd′ĕr-ō-for) [″ + *phoros*, bearing]. A macrophage that contains hemosiderin.

sideroscope (sĭd′ĕr-ō-skōp) [″ + *skopein*, to examine]. Instrument for finding particles of iron in the eye.

siderosis (sĭd″ĕr-ō′sĭs) [″ + *osis*, condition]. A form of pneumoconiosis resulting from inhalation of dust or fumes containing iron particles. SYN: *arc-welder's disease*.

SEE: *hemosiderosis.*

  s., hepatic. Accumulation of an abnormal amount of iron in the liver.

  s., urinary. Hemosiderin granules in the urine.

siderosome (sĭd″ĕr-ō-sōm′) [″ + *soma,* body]. A reticulocyte in which iron-containing granules are present.

siderotic (sĭd″ĕr-ŏt′ĭk). Concerning siderosis.

SIDS. *sudden infant death syndrome.*

SIECUS. *Sex Information and Education Council of the U.S.*

siemens (sē′mĕnz). Unit of conductance derived from SI units. It is the reciprocal of the resistance in ohms. SYN: *mho* (ohm spelled backwards).

Siemens' syndrome [Hermann Werner Siemens, Ger. physician, 1891–1969]. Ichthyosis congenita.

sieve (sĭv). A device consisting of a mesh with holes of uniform size. Used to separate particles above a certain size from solutions or powders.

  s., molecular. A type of sieve in which the molecular material present in the gel or crystal will adsorb molecules of a certain size and let others pass.

sievert [Rolf Maximillian Sievert, Swedish radiologist, 1896–1966]. ABBR: Sv. A unit derived from the International System of Units (SI). A unit of absorbed radiation energy. One sievert is equal to one joule per kilogram or 100 rem.

sig. An abbreviation for the Latin *signa,* meaning in prescription writing to label it.

Sigault's operation (sē-gōz′) [Jean René Sigault, Fr. obstetrician, b. 1740]. Division of the symphysis pubis to facilitate childbirth by enlarging the pelvic outlet. SYN: *symphysiotomy.*

sigh [AS. *sican*]. A deep inspiration followed by a slow audible expiration.

sight (sīt) [AS. *sihth*]. 1. Power or faculty of seeing. 2. Range of sight. 3. A thing or view seen. SYN: *vision.*

  s., blind. SEE: *blind sight.*

  s., day. Night blindness. SYN: *nyctalopia.*

  s., far. Rays of light focusing behind the retina. SYN: *hypermetropia; hyperopia.*

  s., near. Rays of light focusing before the retina. SYN: *myopia.*

  s., night. Day blindness. SYN: *hemeralopia.*

  s., old. Loss of accommodation of near point. SYN: *presbyopia.*

  s., second. Alteration in refractive powers of the lens of the eye so that reading is again possible without glasses. May be caused by incipient cataract. SYN: *senopia.*

sight, words pert. to: achromatopsia; afterimage; alexia; amaurosis; amblyopia; ame-
tropia; aniseikonia; anisocoria; anisoiconia; anisometropia; anorthopia; aprosexia; asthenopia; astigmatism; blindness; brachymetropia; cataract; corneal transplant; glaucoma; hemeralopia; hypermetropia; hyperopia; lens, corneal contact; lens, implanted; Moore's lightning streaks; myopia; night blindness; nyctalopia; -phoria words; photophobia; presbyopia; squint.

sigma (sĭg′mă). The eighteenth letter, Σ or σ, in the Greek alphabet.

sigmatism (sĭg′mă-tĭzm) [Gr. *sigma,* letter S, + *-ismos,* condition]. Excessive or defective use of "s" sounds in speech.

sigmoid (sĭg′moyd) [Gr. *sigmoeides*]. 1. Shaped like the capital Greek letter sigma, Σ. 2. Pert. to the sigmoid flexure of the colon.

sigmoidectomy (sĭg″moyd-ĕk′tō-mē) [″ + *ektome,* excision]. Removal of all or part of the sigmoid flexure.

sigmoid flexure. The lower part of the descending colon, between the iliac crest and the rectum, shaped like the letter S. SEE: *cecosigmoidostomy; colon.*

sigmoiditis (sĭg″moyd-ī′tĭs) [″ + *itis,* inflammation]. Inflammation of the sigmoid flexure of the colon.

sigmoidopexy (sig-moy′dō-pĕk″sē) [″ + *pexis,* fixation]. Fixation of the sigmoid to an abdominal incision for prolapse of the rectum.

sigmoidoproctostomy (sĭg-moy″dō-prŏk-tŏs′tō-mē) [Gr. *sigmoeides,* shaped like Gr. letter S, + *proktos,* anus, + *stoma,* mouth]. Establishment of artificial passage by anastomosis of the sigmoid flexure with the rectum.

sigmoidorectostomy (sĭg-moy″dō-rĕk-tŏs′tō-mē) [″ + L. *rectus,* straight, + Gr. *stoma,* mouth]. Anastomosis of sigmoid flexure with the rectum to establish an artificial passage. SYN: *sigmoidoproctostomy.*

sigmoidoscope (sig-moy′dō-skōp) [″ + *skopein,* to examine]. Tubular speculum for examination of sigmoid flexure.

  s., flexible. Sigmoidoscope that utilizes fiberoptics. This permits the tubular extension to flex, enabling the examiner to visualize a greater portion of the colon than would be possible with a rigid sigmoidoscope.

sigmoidoscopy (sĭg″moy-dŏs′kō-pē) [″ + *skopein,* to examine]. Use of a sigmoidoscope to inspect the sigmoid colon.

sigmoidosigmoidostomy (sĭg-moy″dō-sĭg-moy-dŏs′tō-mē) [″ + *sigmoeides,* sigmoid, + *stoma,* mouth]. Surgical creation of a connection between two segments of the sigmoid colon.

sigmoidostomy (sĭg-moyd-ŏs′tō-mē) [″ + *stoma,* mouth]. Creation of an artificial anus in the sigmoid flexure.

sigmoidotomy (sĭg-moyd-ŏt′ō-mē) [″ +

tome, incision]. Incision of the sigmoid.

sigmoidovesical (sĭg-moy″dō-vĕs′ĭ-kăl) [″ + L. *vesica,* bladder]. Concerning a connection between the sigmoid colon and the urinary bladder.

sign (sīn) [L. *signum*]. 1. Symbol or abbreviation, esp. one used in pharmacy. 2. Any objective evidence or manifestation of an illness or disordered function of the body. Signs are more or less definitive and obvious, and apart from the patient's impressions, in contrast to symptoms, which are subjective. SEE: *symptom.* 3. To use sign language to communicate.

s., objective. In physical diagnosis, a sign that can be seen, heard, measured, or felt by the diagnostician. Finding of such sign(s) can be used to confirm or deny the diagnostician's impressions of the disease suspected of being present. SYN: *s., physical.*

s., physical. S., objective.

s.'s, vital. Those physical signs concerning functions essential to life, i.e., pulse, rate of respiration, blood pressure, and temperature.

signa (sĭg′nă) [L.]. ABBR: S or sig. A term used in writing prescriptions, q.v., meaning to label the subscription according to the dose and frequency of medication.

signal. Any form of communication that provides information. It is usually visual, verbal, or written, or it could be transmitted by electronic means, i.e., telephone, TV, radio, laser, or via optical fibers.

signature (sĭg′nă-tūr) [L. *signatura,* to mark]. The part of a prescription, q.v., giving instructions to the patient.

significance, statistical. SEE: *statistical significance.*

significant (sĭg-nĭf′ĭ-kănt). Important. In statistics, a difference is said to be statistically significant if the analysis indicates that the results have little probability of having occurred due to chance.

significant others. Persons with whom a patient or client has a close relationship. They may or may not include relatives or a spouse.

signing. The use of sign language to communicate with hearing-impaired persons.

sign language. Representing words by signs made with the position and movement of the fingers and hand. SEE: *American Sign Language; Manual Alphabet in Appendix.*

Silain. Trade name for simethicone.

Silastic. Trade name for a silicone material used in plastic surgery to help form body structures. SEE: *silicone, injectable.*

silent. Free from noise; mute; still.

silent disease. Disease that produces no clinically obvious symptoms or signs.

silent period. Period in a tendon reflex that immediately follows the contraction of the responding muscles during which the motor neurons do not respond to afferent impulses entering the reflex center.

silica (sĭl′ĭ-kă) [L. *silex,* flint]. SiO_2. Silicon dioxide.

silicate (sĭl′ĭ-kāt) [L. *silicus,* flintlike]. A salt of silicic acid.

siliceous, silicious (sĭ-lĭsh′ŭs). Containing silica.

silicic (sĭl-ĭs′ĭk). Pert. to silica or silicon.

silicoanthracosis (sĭl″ĭ-kō-ăn″thră-kō′sĭs) [L. *silex,* flint, + Gr. *anthrax,* coal, + *osis,* condition]. Silicosis combined with anthracosis, in coal miners.

silicofluoride (sĭl″ĭ-kō-floo′ō-rīd). A compound of silicon, fluorine, and the fluoride of a metal.

silicon (sĭl′ĭ-kŏn) [L. *silex,* flint]. SYMB: Si. At. wt. 28.086; at. no. 14; sp. gr. 2.33. A nonmetallic element found in the soil. Silicon makes up approximately 25% of the earth's crust, being exceeded only by oxygen. It occurs in traces in skeletal structures (bones and teeth). Silicon is commonly combined with oxygen to form silicon dioxide, SiO_2, which occurs in many forms, both crystalline and amorphous. In a pure state it forms quartz or rock crystal. It is present in many abrasive materials and is the principal constituent of glass.

silicone (sĭl′ĭ-kōn″). 1. An organic compound in which carbon has been replaced by silicon. 2. Any of a group of polymeric organic silicon compounds. Used in adhesives, lubricants, synthetic rubber, and prostheses.

s., injectable. Medical-grade silicone compounds suitable for implantation in the body. Used in plastic surgery. Use of non-medical-grade silicone for cosmetic breast augmentation has produced unfortunate results.

silicosiderosis (sĭl″ĭ-kō-sĭd″ĕr-ō′sĭs) [″ + Gr. *sideros,* iron, + *osis,* condition]. A type of pneumoconiosis in which the inhaled particles contain silicates and iron.

silicosis (sĭl-ĭ-kō′sĭs) [″ + Gr. *osis,* condition]. A form of pneumoconiosis resulting from inhalation of silica (quartz) dust, characterized by formation of small discrete nodules. In advanced cases, a dense fibrosis and emphysema with impairment of respiratory function may develop.

silicotic (sĭl-ĭ-kŏt′ĭk). 1. Relating to silicosis. 2. One affected with silicosis.

silicotuberculosis (sĭl″ĭ-kō-tū-bĕr-kū-lō′sĭs) [″ + *tuberculum,* a little swelling, + Gr. *osis,* condition]. Silicosis associated with pulmonary tuberculosis.

siliqua olivae (sĭl′ĭ-kwē ŏl′ĭ-vē) [L.]. Fibers that appear to encircle the olive of the brain.

siliquose (sĭl′ĭ-kwōs) [L. *siliqua,* pod]. Resembling a two-valve capsule or a pod.

siliquose cataract. Cataract with a dry, wrinkled capsule.

siliquose desquamation. Shedding of dried vesicles from the skin.

silo-filler's disease. Damage to the lungs produced in silo workers when they are exposed to nitrogen dioxide (NO_2), the highly toxic gas produced by the fermenting organic matter in the silo. If the concentration of NO_2 is high enough to cause immediate symptoms, i.e., irritation of eyes and pharynx, the person becomes unconscious. Unless the individual is removed from the site, death is the usual outcome. If the exposure is to low concentrations that do not cause immediate symptoms, delayed injury to the lungs may result.

PREVENTION: Allow no one to enter the silo until 7 to 10 days after it is filled; provide good ventilation above the base of the silo during the 7- to 10-day period; fence the area to prevent children or animals from straying into the space surrounding a silo; always activate the blower fan before entering a silo.

Silvadene. Trade name for silver sulfadiazine.

silver (sil'vĕr) [AS. *siolfor*]. SYMB: Ag. At. wt. 107.870; at. no. 47; sp. gr. 10.5. A white, soft, ductile malleable metal, its salts being widely used in medicine for their caustic, astringent, and antiseptic effects. In dentistry, silver is used in prosthetic devices, as an alloy with copper or mercury, as silver solder, and as tapering points to obliterate root canals in endodontic treatment of teeth. Silver nitrate has been used as a germicidal astringent with treatment of caries, root canal therapy, tooth sensitivity, and gingival diseases. SEE: *argyria.*

s. amalgam. An alloy of silver with varying amounts of tin or copper, using mercury as a major component to produce a silvery, malleable restorative material used in dentistry. It is mixed and condensed in place in a cavity preparation and hardens into a solid mass that can be shaped to the desired tooth form.

s. chloride. SYMB: AgCl. An insoluble salt of silver.

s., colloidal. Silver preparations in which the particles of silver or silver proteinate are suspended in the solution rather than being dissolved in it.

s. halide. The active ingredient in the radiographic film emulsion that, when exposed to radiant energy and developed, forms the image on the film.

s. nitrate. USP. $AgNO_3$. A toxic preparation made from silver. Most of its former uses have passed out of vogue, but it remains important as a germicide and local astringent.

INCOMPAT: Aspirin, sodium chloride. SEE: *silver nitrate poisoning.*

s. nitrate, toughened. USP. A mixture of silver nitrate and silver chloride used as a caustic on wounds and granulation tissue, and in treating warts.

s. picrate. A compound of silver and picric acid, containing 30% silver. Useful as an antiseptic, similar to other preparations of silver.

s. protein. A combination of silver and protein, containing from 7.5% to 8.5% (strong) silver.

s. sulfadiazine. A medicine used topically in treating burns of the skin. It is composed of silver and sulfadiazine. Trade name is Silvadene.

silverfish. An insect about one-half inch (13 mm) long that is fast, slick, and silver. It is carrot-shaped and has long antennae. The common variety, *Lepisma saccharina,* is not harmful, but it is destructive because it eats sugar, starch, glue, book bindings, and stamps. It will eat food-stained linen, rayon, and cotton. It may be controlled by use of insecticides.

silver fork deformity. Deformity in Colles' fracture of wrist and hand resembling curve on back of a fork.

silver nitrate poisoning. When taken by mouth, silver nitrate causes a grayish discoloration of mucous membranes.

SYM: Burning in throat and stomach; rather prompt vomiting. When small amounts of silver are taken over a long period, as in nose or eye drops, patient develops argyria, a peculiar bluish discoloration of all the exposed tissues of body, including the gingiva.

F.A.: Large volumes of ordinary table salt in water precipitate the silver as a slightly soluble chloride; follow with egg whites, oils, and other demulcents. SEE: *silver salts, nitrate, and other soluble salts* at *Poisons and Poisoning* in *Appendix.*

simesthesia (sĭm-ĕs-thē'zē-ă) [Gr. *aisthesis,* sensation]. Sensibility felt in a bone.

simethicone (sī-mĕth'ĭ-kōn). USP. A mixture of liquid demethylpolysiloxanes that because of its antifoaming properties is used in treating intestinal gas. Trade names are Mylicon and Silain.

simian crease. Crease on the palm of the hand, so termed because of its similarity to the transverse flexion crease found in some monkeys. Normally the palm of the hand at birth contains several flexion creases, two of which are separate and approx. transverse. When these two appear to fuse and thus form a single transverse crease, it is termed

SIMIAN AND NORMAL PALMAR CREASES

NORMAL   SIMIAN

simian crease. The crease may be present in a variety of developmental abnormalities including Down syndrome, rubella syndrome, Turner's syndrome, Klinefelter's syndrome, q.v., pseudohypoparathyroidism, q.v., and gonadal dysgenesis, q.v. SEE: illus.

similia similibus curantur (sĭ-mĭl′ē-ă sĭ-mĭl′ĭ-bŭs kū-răn′tūr) [L., likes are cured by likes]. The homeopathic doctrine that a drug producing pathological symptoms in those who are well will cure such symptoms in disease states.

similimum (sĭ-mĭl′ĭ-mŭm) [L., most like]. A medicine that causes a symptom quite similar to that produced by the disease. This therapeutic concept and practice is used in homeopathic medicine.

similitudes, doctrine of. In ancient times, the theory that an herb or plant root, because of its resemblance to the human form or some part of it, would be beneficial. Thus, roots such as those from ginseng or mandrake could act as tonics or aphrodisiacs.

Simmonds' disease (sĭm′mŏnds) [Morris Simmonds, Ger. physician, 1855–1925]. Condition in which complete atrophy of the pituitary body causes loss of function of the thyroid, adrenals, and gonads, premature senility, psychic symptoms, and cachexia. SYN: *cachexia, pituitary.*

Simon's position (zē′mŏns) [Gustav Simon, Ger. surgeon, 1824–1876]. An exaggerated lithotomy position in which the hips are somewhat elevated with thighs strongly abducted. Employed in operations on the vagina.

simple (sĭm′pl) [L. *simplex*]. 1. Not complex; not compound. 2. A medicinal plant.

simple fracture. Fracture without rupture of ligaments and skin.

simple inflammation. Inflammation without pus or other inflammatory exudates.

simple reflex. A reflex in which only two or

possibly three neurons are interposed between receptor and effector organs.

Simplesse. Trade name for a low-calorie fat replacement. SEE: *fat replacements.*

Sims' position (sĭmz) [James Marion Sims, U.S. gynecologist, 1813–1883]. A semiprone position with patient on left side, right knee and thigh drawn well up, left arm along patient's back, and chest inclined forward so patient rests upon it. It is the position of choice for administering enemas, because the sigmoid and descending colon are located on the left side of the body. Fluid is readily accepted in this position. Also employed in curettement of uterus, intrauterine irrigation after labor, and rectal examination.

simul (sĭ′mŭl, sĭm′ŭl) [L.]. At once or at the same time; term used in signature of prescription.

simulation (sĭm-ū-lā′shŭn) [L. *simulatio*, imitation]. 1. Pretense of having a disease; feigning of illness. SEE: *malingerer; Munchausen syndrome.* 2. Imitation of symptoms of one disease by another.

simulator (sĭm″ū-lā′tor). Any situation or device that creates a condition or situation similar to one that might be encountered. This technique is useful in teaching.

Simulium (sĭ-mū′lē-ŭm). A genus of insects of the order Diptera that includes the black flies (buffalo gnats), which are important annoyers of domestic animals and humans. The females are vicious blood suckers.

    S. damnosum. Species that serves as intermediate host of a filarial worm *Onchocerca volvulus.*

    S. venustum. A very annoying species common in North America.

simultanagnosia. Failure to perceive simultaneously all the elements of a scene.

Sinapis (sĭn-ā′pĭs) [Gr. *sinapi*, mustard]. A genus of plants, the mustard plant.

sinapism (sĭn′ă-pĭzm) [Gr. *sinapismos*]. A mustard plaster used to produce counterirritation by applying it to the skin. Enough water is added to flour to make a paste in these proportions: adult: 3 to 4 parts wheat flour to 1 of mustard flour; child: 8 to 10 parts wheat flour to 1 of mustard flour; and infant: 10 to 12 parts wheat flour to 1 of mustard flour.

sincipital (sĭn-sĭp′ĭ-tăl) [L. *sinciput*, half a head]. Concerning the sinciput.

sinciput (sĭn′sĭp-ŭt) [L., half a head]. [NA] 1. Fore and upper part of the cranium. 2. Upper half of the skull. SYN: *calvaria.*

Sinemet. Trade name for a combination of levodopa and carbidopa.

Sinequan. Trade name for doxepin hydrochloride.

sinew (sĭn′ū) [AS. *sinu*]. A tendon.

s., weeping. A ganglion cyst that contains synovial fluid.

sing. L. *singulorum*, of each. Used in writing prescriptions.

singer's node. A swelling between the arytenoid cartilages of singers. SYN: *chorditis nodosa.*

single-photon emission computed tomography. ABBR: SPECT. A medical imaging method for reconstructing cross-sectional images of radiotracer distributions. It is used in diagnosing and treating stroke, dementia, and epilepsy, and in diagnosing diseases of the heart and liver.

singleton. One of something described, esp. a single infant rather than a twin.

singultation (sĭng″gŭl-tā′shŭn) [L. *singultus*, a hiccup]. A hiccup.

singultus (sĭng-gŭl′tŭs) [L.]. Hiccup.

sinister (sĭn-ĭs′tĕr) [L.]. In anatomy, left; or present on the left side of the body.

sinistrad (sĭn′ĭs-trăd) [L. *sinister*, left, + *ad*, toward]. Toward the left.

sinistral (sĭn′ĭs-trăl) [L.]. 1. Pert. to or showing preference for the left hand, eye, or foot in certain actions. 2. On the left side.

sinistrality (sĭn″ĭs-trăl′ĭ-tē). Left-handedness.

sinistraural (sĭn-ĭs-traw′răl) [″ + *auris*, ear]. Having better hearing with the left ear.

sinistro- (sĭn′ĭs-trō) [L. *sinister*, left]. Combining form meaning left.

sinistrocardia (sĭn″ĭs-trō-kăr′dē-ă) [″ + Gr. *kardia*, heart]. Displacement of the heart to left of the medial line; opposed to dextrocardia.

sinistrocerebral (sĭn″ĭs-trō-sĕr′ē-brăl) [″ + *cerebrum*, brain]. Located in the left cerebral hemisphere.

sinistrocular (sĭn-ĭs-trŏk′ū-lar) [″ + *oculus*, eye]. Having stronger vision in the left eye.

sinistrocularity (sĭn″ĭs-trŏk″ū-lăr′ĭ-tē). Condition of having stronger vision in the left eye.

sinistrogyration (sĭn″ĭs-trō-jī-rā′shŭn) [″ + Gr. *gyros*, a circle]. Inclination to the left.

sinistromanual (sĭn″ĭs-trō-măn′ū-ăl) [″ + *manus*, hand]. Left-handed.

sinistropedal (sĭn-ĭs-trŏp′ĕd-ăl) [″ + *pes*, foot]. Left-footed.

sinistrotorsion (sĭn″ĭs-trō-tor′shŭn) [″ + *torsio*, a twisting]. A twisting or turning toward the left.

sinistrous (sĭn′ĭs-trŭs). Awkward, clumsy, unskilled; the opposite of dextrous.

sinoatrial (sĭn″ō-ā′trē-ăl). Pertaining to the sinus venosus and atrium. SYN: *sinoauricular.*

sinoatrial node. Node at junction of superior vena cava with right cardiac atrium, re-

garded as starting point of the heartbeat.

sinoauricular (sī″nō-aw-rĭk′ū-lar). Sinoatrial, which is the preferred term.

sinobronchitis (sī″nō-brŏng-kī′tĭs) [L. *sinus*, curve, + *bronchos*, windpipe, + Gr. *itis*, inflammation]. Paranasal sinusitis with bronchitis.

sinogram (sī′nō-grăm″) [L. *sinus*, curve, + Gr. *gramma*, something written]. Roentgenogram of a sinus injected with a radiopaque dye to determine the range and course of the sinus.

sinter (sĭn′tĕr). 1. The calcium or silica deposits formed from water obtained from mineral springs. 2. To reduce material to a solid form by heating without melting.

sinuous (sĭn′ū-ŭs) [L. *sinuosus*, winding]. Winding; wavy; tortuous.

sinus (sī′nŭs) [L., curve, hollow] (pl. *sinuses, sinus*). 1. A cavity within a bone. 2. Dilated channel for venous blood. 3. A canal or passage leading to an abscess. 4. Any cavity having a relatively narrow opening.

    RS: antritis; antronasal; antrotympanic; antrum; cephalhematocele; lateral sinus; sinusitis; transillumination.

s.'s, accessory nasal. The paranasal sinuses: frontal, maxillary, ethmoidal, and sphenoidal. Anterior group: frontal, maxillary, and anterior ethmoids. Posterior group: posterior ethmoids and sphenoid.

    Sinuses develop embryologically from nasal cavities, are lined with the same type of epithelium, are filled with air, and communicate with nasal cavities through their various ostia. Function of sinuses not definitely known. Various theories give them the same function as nasal cavities, namely, warming, moistening, and filtering the air.

s., anal. The saclike recesses behind the anal columns.

s., aortic. A dilatation of the aorta or pulmonary artery opposite the segment of the semilunar valve. SYN: *sinus of Valsalva.*

s., basilar. S., transverse.

s., carotid. SEE: *carotid sinus.*

s. cavernosus. [NA] A large sinus from the sphenoidal fissure to the apex of the petrous portion of the temporal bone.

s., cerebral. Any ventricle of the brain.

s., circular. A venous sinus around the pituitary body, communicating on each side with the cavernous sinus.

s., coccygeal. Sinus in the midline of the natal cleft just over the coccyx.

s., coronary, of heart. A vein in the transverse groove between the left cardiac atrium and ventricle.

s.'s, cranial. Venous canals between folds of the dura.

s., dermal. A congenital sinus tract connecting the surface of the body with the spinal canal.

s., draining. An abnormal passageway leading from inside the body to the outside. This is usually due to an infectious process.

s.'s, ethmoidal. Air cavities in the ethmoid bone.

s., frontal. An irregular cavity in the frontal bone on each side of the midline above the nasal bridge. One may be larger than the other. A duct carries secretions to the upper part of the nostrils.

s., genitourinary. S., urogenital.

s., hair. The sinus formed when hair is embedded in the skin and acts as a foreign body.

s., inferior longitudinal. A venous sinus along the posterior half of the lower border of the falx cerebri.

s., inferior petrosal. A large venous sinus from the cavernous sinus, running along the lower margin of the petrous portion of the temporal bone.

s., inferior sagittal. A venous sinus in the inferior margin of the falx cerebri.

s.'s, intercavernous. The anterior and posterior halves of the circular sinus.

s., lateral. One of two large venous sinuses in inner side of skull passing near the mastoid antrum and emptying into the jugular vein.

s.'s, lymph. Small spaces throughout the parenchyma of a lymphatic gland.

s., marginal. 1. A large venous sinus around part of the margin of the placenta. 2. Small bilateral venous sinuses of the dura mater at the edge of the foramen magnum. 3. A venous sinus around a portion of the white pulp of the spleen.

s., maxillary. A cavity in the maxillary bone communicating with the middle meatus of the nasal cavity. SYN: *antrum of Highmore.*

s., occipital. A small venous sinus in the attached margin of the falx cerebelli extending to the margin of the foramen magnum.

s. of the pulmonary trunk. One of the dilatations in the pulmonary trunk, across from a cusp of the pulmonary valve of the heart.

s. of spleen. A venous sinusoid in the reticulum of the spleen.

s. of Valsalva. A dilatation of the aorta or pulmonary artery opposite the segment of the semilunar valve. SYN: *s., aortic.*

s. of venal canal; s. venarum cavarum. The portion of the right atrium of the heart posterior to and to the left of the crista terminalis. The inferior and superior vena caval veins empty into it.

s.'s, paranasal. Accessory nasal sinuses.

s., pilonidal. SEE: *pilonidal fistula.*

s.'s, pleural. Spaces in the pleural sac along the lower and inferior portions of the lung that the lung does not occupy.

s. pocularis. Lacuna in prostatic part of the urethra. SYN: *s. prostaticus.*

s. prostaticus. S. pocularis.

s. rectus. Venous sinus at the junction of the falx cerebri and the cerebellar tentorium. SYN: *s. of the dura mater, straight; straight sinus.*

s., renal. The area in the kidney composed of the renal pelvis, renal calices, vessels, nerves, and fatty tissue.

s., rhomboid. The fourth cranial ventricle.

s., sigmoid. Continuation, on both sides, of the transverse sinuses down along the posterior border of the petrous part of the temporal bone to the jugular foramen and jugular veins.

s.'s, sphenoidal. Air sinuses that occupy the body of the sphenoid bone and connect with the nasal cavity.

s., sphenoparietal. 1. Venous sinus uniting the cavernous sinus and a meningeal vein. 2. The portion of the cavernous sinus below the ensiform process.

s., straight. SEE: *s. rectus.*

s., superior longitudinal. A triangular sinus along the upper edge of the falx cerebri.

s., superior petrosal. A venous canal running in a groove in the petrous portion of the temporal bone.

s., superior sagittal. Large venous sinus along the attached border of the falx cerebri from the crista galli to the internal occipital protuberance where it joins either the right or left transverse sinuses or both. SYN: *s. of the dura mater, superior sagittal.*

s., tarsal. A tunnel between the calcaneus and talus of the ankle.

s., tentorial. SEE: *s. rectus.*

s., terminal. A vein encircling the vascular area of the blastoderm.

s., transverse. 1. Sinus that unites the two inferior petrosal sinuses. 2. Venous network in the dura over the basilar process of the occipital bone. SYN: *s., basilar.*

s.'s, transverse, of the dura mater. Large, bilateral venous sinuses along the attached margin of the cerebellar tentorium. They receive the superior sagittal and straight sinuses and drain into the sigmoid sinuses and then into the jugular veins.

s., transverse, of the pericardium. A channel posterior to the aorta and the pulmonary trunk but in front of the atria.

s., tympanic. A deep recess in the labyrinthine wall of the tympanic cavity. It opens into the fenestra of the cochlea.

s., urogenital. 1. Duct into which, in the

embryo, the wolffian ducts and bladder empty; it opens into the cloaca. 2. The common receptacle of the genital and urinary ducts. SYN: *s., genitourinary.*

     s., uterine. Venous channels in the walls of the uterus during pregnancy.

     s.'s, uteroplacental. Slanting venous channels from the placenta serving to convey the maternal blood from the intervillous lacunae back into the uterine veins.

     s., venous. Sinus conveying venous blood.

     s.'s, venous, of the dura mater. Venous channels between the two layers of the dura mater. They drain the venous blood from the brain.

     s., venous, of sclera. A circular channel at the sclerocorneal junction in the sclera. It drains into the anterior ciliary vein. Aqueous humor leaves the eye via this sinus. SYN: *Schlemm's canal.*

sinus arrhythmia. Cardiac irregularity characterized by an increased heart rate during inspiration and decrease in heart rate on expiration. This arrhythmia has no clinical significance except in older patients, in whom it may occur in coronary artery disease.

sinusitis (sī-nŭs-ī'tĭs) [L. *sinus,* curve, hollow, + Gr. *itis,* inflammation]. Inflammation of a sinus, esp. a paranasal sinus. SYN: *sinuitis.*

     ETIOL: A number of causative agents, including viruses, bacteria, or allergy.

     PREDISPOSING FACTORS: Inadequate drainage, which may result from presence of polyps, enlarged turbinates, or deviated septum; chronic rhinitis; general debility; or dental abscess in maxillary bone.

     s., acute suppurative. Purulent inflammation with symptoms of pain over the sinus, fever, chills, and headache.

     TREAT: Conservative. Shrinkage in the nasal mucosa to facilitate ventilation and drainage of the sinus. Rest in bed, force fluids, decongestants, hot packs. If inflammation is due to bacterial infection, antibiotic therapy is indicated. Cefaclor, a cephalosporin, is effective against a great number of the organisms that can cause acute sinusitis.

     s., chronic hyperplastic. Polyps present in sinuses and nose and underlying osteitis of sinus walls.

     TREAT: Surgical. Conservative, removal of polyps and intranasal opening into sinuses for adequate ventilation and drainage, and radical, complete removal of sinus mucosa either through external or intranasal route.

sinusoid (sī'nŭs-oyd) [" + Gr. *eidos,* form, shape]. 1. Resembling a sinus. 2. A minute

blood vessel found in such organs as the liver, spleen, adrenal glands, and bone marrow. It is slightly larger than a capillary and has a lining of reticuloendothelium.

sinusoidal (sī-nŭs-oyd'ăl). Pert. to a sinusoid.

sinusoidal current. Alternating induced electric current, the two strokes of which are equal.

sinusoidalization (sī″nŭ-soy″dăl-ĭ-zā'shŭn) [L. *sinus,* hollow, curve, + Gr. *eidos,* form, shape]. Use of a sinusoidal current.

sinusotomy (sī-nŭs-ŏt'ō-mē) [" + Gr. *tome,* incision]. The operation of incising a sinus.

sinus rhythm. The normal cardiac rhythm commencing at the sinoatrial node.

SiO₂. Silicon dioxide.

si op sit. [L.] *si opus sit,* if needed. Used in writing prescriptions.

Sioux alarm. Long ago native American Indians of the Sioux tribe learned, after carefully controlled experiments, that they could use a full urinary bladder as a kind of alarm clock. By drinking a certain amount of fluids at bedtime, they found they would awaken in a specific number of hours. Were they to increase the amount of fluid taken, they would awaken earlier because of the urge to urinate; and if they took less, they would awaken later.

siphon (sī'fŭn) [Gr. *siphon,* tube]. A tube bent at an angle to form two unequal lengths for transferring liquids from one container to another by atmospheric pressure. One container must be higher than the other for this to work.

siphonage (sī'fŭn-ĭj). Use of a siphon to drain a body cavity such as the stomach or bladder.

Siphonaptera (sī″fō-năp'tĕr-ă) [" + *apteros,* wingless]. An order of insects commonly called fleas. They are wingless, undergo complete metamorphosis, and have piercing and sucking mouth parts, their food being the blood of birds and mammals. The body is compressed laterally, and the legs are adapted for leaping. In addition to being annoying pests, they transmit the causative organisms of several diseases (bubonic plague, endemic or murine typhus, and among rodents, tularemia). They also serve as intermediate hosts of certain tapeworms. SEE: *flea.*

siphonoma (sī-fŏn-ō'mă) [" + *oma,* tumor]. A tumor made up of fine tubes.

Sipple syndrome [John H. Sipple, U.S. physician, b. 1930]. Multiple endocrine neoplasia, type III, q.v.

sirenomelia (sī″rĕn-ŏm-ē'lē-ă) [Gr. *seiren,* mermaid, + *melos,* limb]. Congenital anomaly in which the lower extremities are fused.

siriasis (sĭ-rī′ă-sĭs) [Gr. *seirian*, to be hot].
Sunstroke, q.v.

-sis. Gr. suffix indicating condition or state.
Depending upon the preceding vowel, it may
appear in the form of -asis, -esis, -iasis, or
-osis.

sister. A term used by the British for nurse,
esp. a senior or head nurse.

Sister Mary Joseph nodule. SEE: *nodule,
Sister Mary Joseph.*

site [L. *situs*, place]. Position or location.

    s., active. The active portion of a chemi-
cal substance, esp. a catalyst or enzyme,
which binds to the material it is acting upon.

    s., binding. The particular location on a
cell surface or chemical to which other
chemical substances bind or attach.

    s., receptor. The particular component
of a cell surface that has the ability to react
with certain molecules such as proteins, or a
virus.

sitieirgia (sĭt-ē-ĭr′jē-ă) [Gr. *sition*, food, +
eirgein, to shut out]. Hysterical refusal to
take food.

sitio-, sito- [Gr. *sition, sitos*, food]. Combining
forms meaning bread or made from grain;
food.

sitophobia (sī″tō-fō′bē-ă) [″ + *phobos*,
fear]. Psychoneurotic abhorrence of food, or
morbid dread of or repugnance to food,
whether generally or only to specific dishes.

sitosterols (sī-tŏs′tĕr-ŏls). 1. A group of similar organic compounds that occur in plants.
They contain the steroid nucleus, perhydrocyclopentanophenanthrene, q.v. 2. A pharmaceutical compound that contains several
sitosterols. Used in treating hypercholesterolemia.

sitotaxis (sī″tō-tăk′sĭs) [″ + *taxis*, ar-
rangement]. Sitotropism, q.v.

sitotherapy (sī″tō-thĕr′ă-pē) [″ + *therapeia*, treatment]. The therapeutic use of
food.

sitotoxin (sī″tō-tŏk′sĭn) [″ + *toxikon*, poi-
son]. Any poison developed in food, esp. one
produced by bacteria growing in a cereal or
grain product.

sitotoxism (sī″tō-tŏks′ĭzm) [″ + ″ +
-ismos, condition]. Poisoning by vegetable
foods infested with molds or bacteria.

sitotropism (sī-tŏt′rō-pĭzm) [″ + *tropos*, a
turning, + *-ismos*, condition]. Response
of cells to the attraction or repulsion of food
elements.

situation. 1. A set of circumstances. 2. The location of an entity in relation to other objects, e.g., between a rock and a hard object.

situs (sī′tŭs) [L.]. A position.

    s. inversus viscerum. Abnormal rela-
tion and displacement of viscera to opposite
side of the body.

    s. perversus. Malposition of any vis-

ceral structure.

sitz bath (sĭtz). Bath to sit in with water above
and covering the hips. The water may be
warm and contain medication. The tub or
fixture is usually shaped to allow the legs to
be out of the water.

SI units. *International System of Units,* from
Fr. *Système International d'Unités.* ABBR:
SI. SEE: tables; *SI Units* in Appendix.

sixth cranial nerve. Abducens nerve that
supplies the external rectus of the eye. SEE:
cranial nerves.

Sjögren's syndrome. Syndrome occurring
in postmenopausal women including rheumatoid arthritis, xerostomia, and keratoconjunctivitis sicca. It is thought to be an
immunologic disorder.

SK-65. Trade name for propoxyphene hydrochloride.

SK-Apap. Trade name for acetaminophen
with codeine.

skateboard. A therapeutic device used for
upper or lower extremity rehabilitation. It
consists of a platform mounted on ball-
bearing rollers. It assists the patient in making coordinated movements.

skatol(e) (skăt′ōl) [Gr. *skatos*, dung]. C_9H_9N.
Beta-methyl indole, a malodorous, solid,
heterocyclic nitrogen compound found in
feces, formed by protein decomposition in
the intestines and giving them their odor.

skatoxyl (skă-tŏk′sĭl). A derivative of skatole.

SK-Bamate. Trade name for meprobamate.

SK-Chlorothiazide. Trade name for chlorothiazide.

SK-Dexamethasone. Trade name for dexamethasone.

skein (skān). A continuous tangled thread.
SYN: *spireme.*

skelalgia (skē-lăl′jē-ă) [Gr. *skelis*, leg, +
algos, pain]. Pain in the leg.

skeletal (skĕl′ĕ-tăl) [Gr. *skeleton*, a dried-up
body]. Pert. to the skeleton.

skeletal muscle. Muscle fibers that with few
exceptions are attached to parts of the skeleton and involved primarily in movements
of the parts of the body. SYN: *striated muscle; voluntary muscle.*

skeletal survey. Procedure in which entire
skeleton is radiographed to determine the
presence of pathology.

skeletal traction. Pulling force applied directly to the bone through surgically applied
pins and tongs.

    NURSING IMPLICATIONS: Place the
patient on a firm mattress and in prescribed
position while in traction. Daily assess
ropes, weights, and pulleys for wear, chafe,
and improper position. Care must be taken
to keep the insertion points of pins and
tongs on the skin clean and free of infection.
Infection at the insertion sites can lead to

Units of the International System of Units (SI units)

Basic Quantity	Basic Unit	Symbol
Length	meter	m
Mass	kilogram	kg
Time	second	s
Electric current	ampere	A
Thermodynamic temperature	kelvin	K
Luminous intensity	candela	cd
Amount of substance	mole	mol

osteomyelitis of the bone. Prevent such infection by assessing the area for odor and other signs of infection and cleansing the area utilizing aseptic technique, applying prescribed medication and a sterile dressing. Perform daily skin inspection for signs of pressure or friction, and institute appropriate nursing measures to alleviate any pressure or friction. Maintain proper traction alignment at all times; adjust as necessary. Establish exercise regimen for unaffected extremities. Assess any patient complaint without delay. Implement respiratory toilet regimen to prevent pulmonary complications. Administer analgesics as prescribed. Promote adequate nutrition and fluid intake for tissue healing and repair. Prevent constipation and fecal impaction by dietary and medical management. Assess affected extremity daily or more frequently if necessary for complications such as phlebitis, nerve or circulatory impairment, and, for lower extremity, examine for foot drop. Promote social and diversional activities. Teach the patient the use of a trapeze, exercises, and activity limitations. Establish discharge plan and follow-up.

skeletization (skĕl″ĕt-ĭ-zā′shŭn). Excessive emaciation.

skeleto- [Gr. *skeleton*, a dried-up body]. Combining form meaning skeleton.

skeletogenous (skĕl-ĕ-tŏj′ĕ-nŭs) [″ + *gennan*, to produce]. Forming skeletal structures or tissues.

skeletology (skĕl″ĕ-tŏl′ō-jē) [″ + *logos*, word, reason]. The special division of anatomy and biomechanics concerned with the skeleton.

skeleton (skĕl′ĕt-ŏn) [Gr., a dried-up body]. The bony framework of the body consisting of 206 bones: 80 axial or trunk and 126 of the limbs (appendicular). This number does not include teeth or sesamoid bones other than the patella. The various bones follow. SEE: illus.

```
AXIAL (80 Bones)
Head (29 Bones)
  Cranial (8)
    frontal — 1
    parietal — 2
    occipital — 1
```

Prefixes and Their Symbols Used to Designate Decimal Multiples and Submultiples in SI Units

Prefix	Symbol	Factor		
tera	T	10^{12}	=	1 000 000 000 000
giga	G	10^{9}	=	1 000 000 000
mega	M	10^{6}	=	1 000 000
kilo	k	10^{3}	=	1 000
hecto	h	10^{2}	=	100
deka	da	10^{1}	=	10
deci	d	10^{-1}	=	0.1
centi	c	10^{-2}	=	0.01
milli	m	10^{-3}	=	0.001
micro	μ	10^{-6}	=	0.000 001
nano	n	10^{-9}	=	0.000 000 001
pico	p	10^{-12}	=	0.000 000 000 001
femto	f	10^{-15}	=	0.000 000 000 000 001
atto	a	10^{-18}	=	0.000 000 000 000 000 001

SKELETON

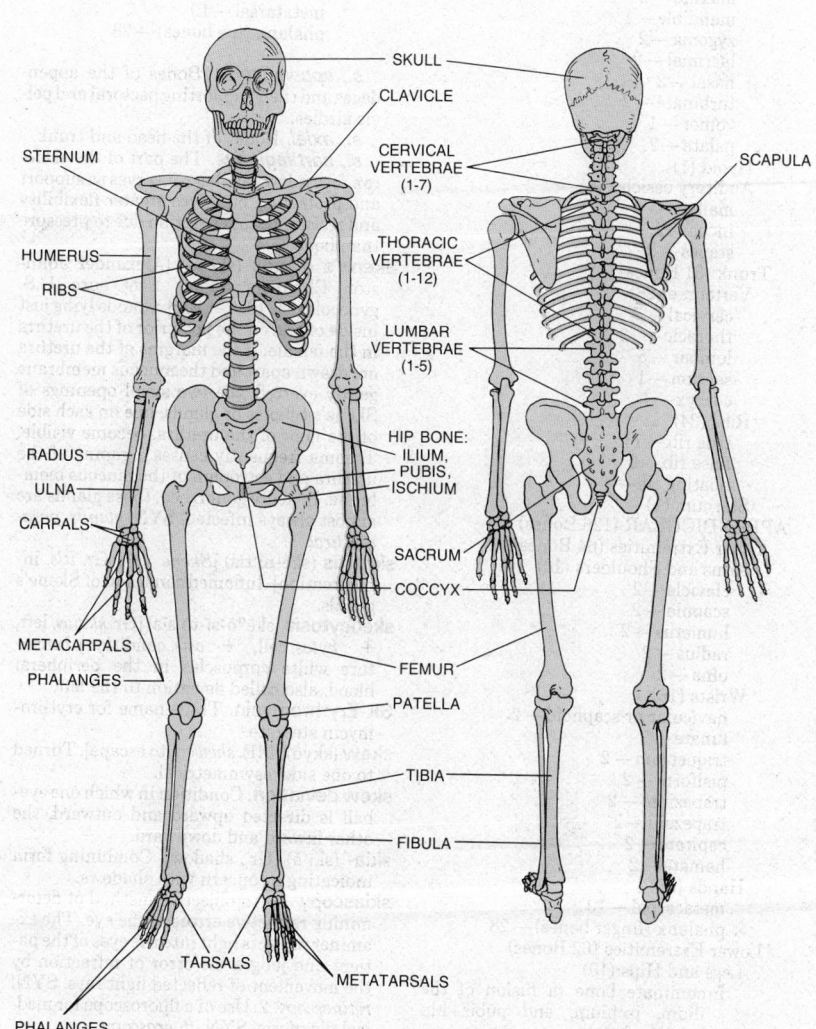

SKULL

CLAVICLE

CERVICAL
VERTEBRAE
(1-7)

SCAPULA

STERNUM

THORACIC
VERTEBRAE
(1-12)

HUMERUS

RIBS

LUMBAR
VERTEBRAE
(1-5)

RADIUS

ULNA

CARPALS

HIP BONE:
ILIUM,
PUBIS,
ISCHIUM

SACRUM

COCCYX

METACARPALS

PHALANGES

FEMUR

PATELLA

TIBIA

FIBULA

TARSALS

METATARSALS

PHALANGES

POSTERIOR VIEW

ANTERIOR VIEW

temporal — 2
sphenoid — 1
ethmoid — 1
Facial (14)
  maxilla — 2
  mandible — 1
  zygoma — 2
  lacrimal — 2
  nasal — 2
  turbinate — 2
  vomer — 1
  palate — 2
Hyoid (1)
Auditory ossicles (6)
  malleus — 2
  incus — 2
  stapes — 2
Trunk (51 Bones)
  Vertebrae (26)
    cervical — 7
    thoracic — 12
    lumbar — 5
    sacrum — 1
    coccyx — 1
  Ribs (24)
    true rib — 14
    false rib — 6
    floating rib — 4
  Sternum (1)
APPENDICULAR (126 Bones)
Upper Extremities (64 Bones)
  Arms and Shoulders (10)
    clavicle — 2
    scapula — 2
    humerus — 2
    radius — 2
    ulna — 2
  Wrists (16)
    navicular or scaphoid — 2
    lunate — 2
    triquetrum — 2
    pisiform — 2
    trapezium — 2
    trapezoid — 2
    capitate — 2
    hamate — 2
  Hands (38)
    metacarpal — 10
    phalanx (finger bones) — 28
Lower Extremities (62 Bones)
  Legs and Hips (10)
    innominate bone (a fusion of the ilium, ischium, and pubis – hip bone) — 2
    femur — 2
    tibia — 2
    fibula — 2
    patella (knee cap) — 2
  Ankles (14)
    astragaloid — 2
    calcaneus (heel bone) — 2
    scaphoid — 2

cuboid — 2
cuneiform, internal — 2
cuneiform, middle — 2
cuneiform, external — 2
Feet (38)
  metatarsal — 10
  phalanx (toe bones) — 28

s., appendicular. Bones of the appendages and their supporting pectoral and pelvic girdles.

  s., axial. Bones of the head and trunk.

  s., cartilaginous. The part of the skeleton formed by cartilage; it serves as support and protection but gives greater flexibility and resistance to resorption due to pressure than bone.

Skene's glands (skēns) [Alexander Johnston Chalmers Skene, Scot.-born U.S. gynecologist, 1837 – 1900]. Glands lying just inside of and on the posterior of the urethra in the female. If the margins of the urethra are drawn apart and the mucous membrane gently everted, the two small openings of Skene's tubules or glands, one on each side of the floor of the urethra, become visible. Trauma frequently causes a gaping of the urethra and ectropion of the mucous membrane. In acute gonorrhea, these glands are almost always infected. SYN: *glands, paraurethral.*

skenitis (skē-nī′tĭs) [*Skene* + Gr. *itis*, inflammation]. Inflamed condition of Skene's glands.

skeocytosis (skē″ō-sī-tō′sĭs) [Gr. *skaios*, left, + *kytos*, cell, + *osis*, condition]. Immature white corpuscles in the peripheral blood; also called deviation to the left.

SK-Erythromycin. Trade name for erythromycin stearate.

skew (skyū) [ME. *skewen*, to escape]. Turned to one side; asymmetrical.

skew deviation. Condition in which one eyeball is directed upward and outward, the other inward and downward.

skia- (skī′ă) [Gr., shadow]. Combining form indicating a concern with shadows.

skiascopy. 1. An objective method of determining refractive errors of the eye. The examiner projects light into the eyes of the patient and judges the error of refraction by the movement of reflected light rays. SYN: *retinoscopy.* 2. Use of a fluoroscope for medical diagnosis. SYN: *fluoroscopy.*

skill. One's level of proficiency in a specific task.

skimming. In health care, the practice of a for-profit corporation entering the market, attracting the business of those who can pay, and avoiding treating the indigent.

skin (skĭn) [Old Norse *skinn*]. The layer of tissue between the body and its environment.

A major organ of the body, skin is essential to life. It consists of two major divisions: the epidermis, which has four or five layers depending upon the type of skin present in specific locations, and the dermis. There is considerable variation in the thickness, strength, number of hairs, pigmentation, vascularization, nerve supply, keritinization, and types of glands present in skin depending upon the location of the skin. Skin may be classified as thin and hairy or thick and hairless (glabrous). The former covers most of the body and the latter covers the surface of the palms of the hands, soles of the feet, and flexor surfaces of the digits.

The outermost portion of skin, the epidermis, is a continually renewing, stratified, squamous epithelium that keratinizes and gives rise to structures called appendages, i.e., hair, nails, and sweat and sebaceous glands.

The innermost layer of the epidermis is the stratum germinativum, in which keratinocytes are formed. Above this lies the stratum spinosum (also known as stratum malpighii), in which progressive stages of keratinization occur. The keratinocytes in this layer have a well-developed capacity for phagocytosis. Melanin granules are present in the cytoplasm of some cells in the stratum spinosum. In the next layer, stratum granulosum, the cells making their way toward the surface become flattened and accumulate many large granules, termed keratohyalin. In this layer, the cells make the transition from a viable to a nonviable cell and become cornified. At that stage, the cells have lost their nucleus and the only material remaining is filaments of keratin. Above this layer is the stratum lucidum, which is found only in thick, glabrous skin and the cells of which closely resemble those of the next layer. The outermost layer, the stratum corneum, is composed of closely packed cornified, or horny, flattened cells that are the dead keratinocytes, called squames. This layer in the scalp may be only a few cells deep, but in thick skin may be 50 cells deep. Eventually, these cells separate from one another and become detached from the surface of the epidermis, a process called desquamation.

The time required for a newly formed keratinocyte to pass from the deepest layer to the surface and be shed has been estimated to be from 45 to 75 days. SEE: illus.; *hair* for illus; *melanin; nails; photoaging; tanning salon.*

DIFF. DIAGNOSIS: *Abnormal dryness:* May indicate abnormal deficiency of thyroid function, diabetes, and other conditions. *Ashy:* Malignant diseases, severe anemia, cancer, tuberculosis, chronic interstitial nephritis. *Bronzing:* Addison's disease, poisoning with certain dyes or metals, early stages of pellagra. *Brownish-yellow spots* (liver spots): May be due to aging; noted in pregnancy (chloasma uterinum), in exophthalmic goiter, and uterine and liver malignancies; also may be due to freckles, sunburn, cosmetics, mustard, turpentine, and other irritants.

Cherry red: Carbon monoxide poisoning. *Cold sweats:* Indicate great prostration, fear, anxiety, or depression.

Cyanosis: May be congenital; if acquired, may be due to asthma, pulmonary tuberculosis, whooping cough, advanced emphysema, croup, tracheal obstruction, aneurysm, goiter, flushing (hyperemia), emotion, febrile disorders, pulmonary tuberculosis, convulsions, large ovarian tumor, plethora, polycythemia. *Cyanosis alternating with pallor:* Cerebrospinal diseases, typhoid, vasomotor disturbances, menopause, argyria associated with ingestion of silver salts. May be noted in lips, mucous membranes, fingertips, and external ear. If extreme, entire body shows dusky, leaden tint. Indicates lack of oxygen and excess of carbon dioxide in blood. May be due to inflammation or abscess of pharynx and larynx, Ludwig's angina, croup, and disorders affecting respiration. Also to overdose of drugs or asphyxiation by gas.

Discolorations: Seen in icterus, chlorosis, leprosy, administration of silver nitrate, jaundice, carotenemia, vitiligo, albinism, malignant diseases, and asphyxia from gas. *Edema:* Seen in anemia, hydremia, obstruction, inflammation, and cardiac, circulatory and renal decompensation. If local, may be due to obstruction of return circulation or heart failure, in which case it will be evident in ankles and often legs, esp. at night. May also be due to renal diseases. *Emphysema:* Due to free air or gas in subcutaneous tissue. *Hot and dry:* Indicates fever, mental excitement, or excessive salt intake. *Moist:* Increased perspiration (hyperhidrosis) may be due to fevers, such as malarial, rheumatic, relapsing, or septic fever; pneumonic crisis; pulmonary tuberculosis; Graves' disease; neuralgia; migraine; drugs; hot drinks; exercise. Lack of moistness noted in dehydration and in ichthyosis.

Paleness: Nervous prostration, dropsy, paralysis, malnutrition. *Pallor:* Occurs in those living an indoor life, esp. in prisoners and night workers. May be due to anemia. Temporary pallor occurs in syncope, chills, shock, rigors, and some vasomotor instability. If sudden and persistent, may be sign of internal hemorrhage. Also seen in lead poi-

VIEW OF SKIN AND UNDERLYING TISSUES

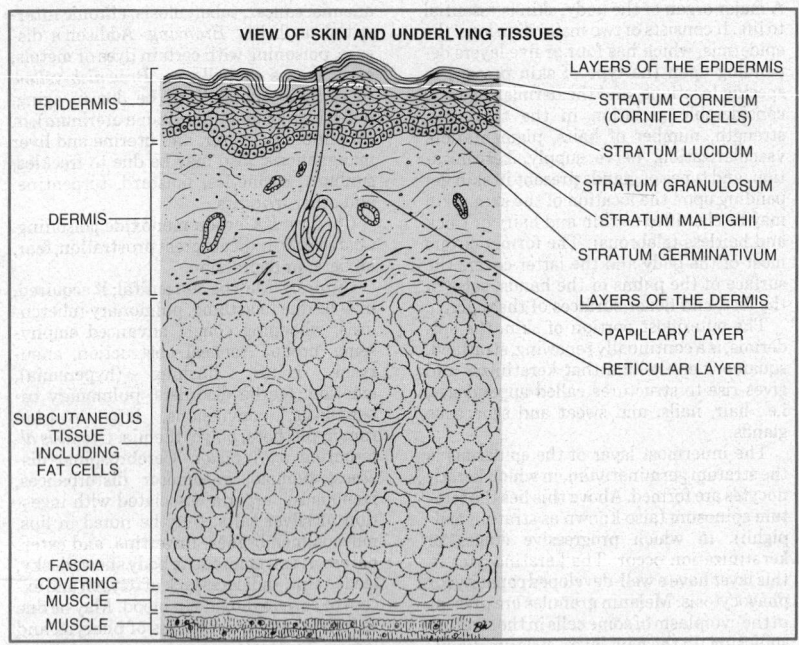

EPIDERMIS

DERMIS

SUBCUTANEOUS
TISSUE
INCLUDING
FAT CELLS

FASCIA
COVERING
MUSCLE

MUSCLE

LAYERS OF THE EPIDERMIS

STRATUM CORNEUM
(CORNIFIED CELLS)

STRATUM LUCIDUM

STRATUM GRANULOSUM

STRATUM MALPIGHII

STRATUM GERMINATIVUM

LAYERS OF THE DERMIS

PAPILLARY LAYER

RETICULAR LAYER

soning. If it gradually becomes permanent, may indicate chronic febrile disease, chronic gastrointestinal disease, cancer, arsenical poisoning, chronic suppuration, chronic mercurial poisoning, hemorrhages, leukemia, cachexia, nephrosis, nephritis, syphilis, parasitic diseases, tuberculosis, or malaria. *Purplish:* Interference of circulation common in asthma and typhus.

Rashes: SEE: *rash. Redness:* Local redness seen in inflammation, skin diseases, chronic alcoholism, vasomotor disturbances, and pyrexia. Local redness with pain indicates inflammation. Sunburn (actinic dermatitis). *Sallowness:* Cachexia, syphilis, chronic gallbladder disease, arthritis deformans, constipation, some anemias, gastric, pancreatic, enteric, or hepatic disorders.

Temperature: Usually correlates with internal temperature, unless raised by local applications of heat or exposure to cold. If generally cold, may be due to poor circulation or obstruction of same, vasomotor spasms, venous or arterial thrombosis, exposure to cold. General abnormal heat seen in febrile disorders, although in some of them a cold and clammy skin is present. *Wrinkling:* If permanent, may be due to

aging; temporary due to prolonged immersion in water or dehydration. *Yellow:* May be due to increased carotene intake; jaundice, liver disease. If jaundiced, plethoric, hyperemic, or pigmented, it should be noted.

Miscellaneous: Rashes, scars, and their causes are also diagnostic. Texture and temperature of skin are important signs. Undue moisture, cold or hot spots on body, dryness of skin are other points to look for in diagnosis. SEE: *anemia, pernicious; biliousness; endocarditis; face; liver.*

FUNCT: Protection against injuries and parasitic invasion; regulation of body temperature; aids in elimination; prevention of dehydration; reservoir for food and water; sense organ for the cutaneous senses; source of antirachitic vitamin (vitamin D) when the skin is exposed to sunlight.

s., alligator. Severe scaling of the skin with formation of thick plates resembling hide of an alligator. SEE: *ichthyosis.*

s., deciduous. Shedding of the epidermis. SYN: *keratolysis.*

s., elastic. Skin that has property of great elasticity.

s., glabrous. Skin which does not contain hair follicles, e.g., skin over the palms and soles.

s., glossy. Shining atrophy of the skin.

s., hidebound. Scleroderma.

s., loose. Hypertrophy of the skin.

s., parchment. Atrophy of the skin with stretching.

s., photoaged. SEE: *photoaged skin.*

s., piebald. Vitiligo.

s., scarf. Cuticle, epidermis, the outer layer of the skin.

s., true. Corium or inner layer of the skin.

skin, chemical peel of. SEE: *chemical peel of the skin.*

skin, tenting of. When normal skin and subcutaneous tissue are lightly pinched, raised up, and released, they return to their original position. Delay in the return is called tenting and is seen in dehydration. Delay becomes progressively slower as the skin ages and subcutaneous elastic tissue decreases. Thus, the test for tenting can be used as a rough index of the aging process. SEE: *dehydration.*

skin cancer. Cancer that may arise on the surface of the body and manifest as a small ulcer, pimple, or mole. It may be red, brown, black, or white, according to the type. It may be single or occur in a group, open or ulcerated. It may be localized or invade the blood vessels, lymph glands, and connecting ducts.

skinfold tenderness. Tenderness elicited by the examiner's rolling the skin and subcutaneous tissues over the upper border of the trapezius muscle. Normally, this produces minor discomfort, but in patients with nonarticular rheumatic disorders, this rolling of the skin consistently produces pain.

skinfold thickness. Measurement with calibrated calipers of thickness of a fold of skin at a selected body site. The sites usually are upper arm or triceps, subscapular region, and upper abdomen. The measurements are used in evaluating nutritional status by estimating the amount of subcutaneous fat.

skin graft. Using the skin from another part of the body, or from a donor, to repair a defect or trauma of the skin. SEE: *graft; Thiersch's graft.*

skin-marking. Application of nontoxic paints or dyes to the skin to provide landmarks during plastic surgery or to permit accurate alignment of the wound edges at the time the skin is closed.

Skinner box (skĭn′ĕr) [Burrhus Frederic Skinner, U.S. psychologist, 1904–1990]. A device used in experimental psychology. It is designed so that an animal presses a lever or button and is rewarded by receiving food. This is termed programmed learning.

skin rash. A usually temporary eruption of the skin covering a small area, a portion of the body, or the entire body. The rash may consist of macules, papules, vesicles, or pustules and is usually red or red-blue. It may be itchy. A rash is often indicative of a systemic disease such as measles or lupus, or it may indicate a local irritation such as contact dermatitis or diaper rash.

skin tag. SEE: *acrochordon.*

skin test. Any test in which a suspected allergen or sensitizer is applied to the skin.

skin tightening. Loss of normal skin folds and pliability due to various sclerosing disorders. This may be generalized or localized and may occur over any part of the body. The skin is taut, bound down to the underlying tissue, and may be thickened or indurated. In severe cases the skin may be so tight as to interfere with function of the fingers and toes. Flexion contractions of the mouth may decrease the patient's ability to open the mouth. Skin tightening due to edema is not included in this classification.

sklero- [Gr.]. SEE: words beginning with *sclero-.*

SK-Lygen. Trade name for chlordiazepoxide hydrochloride.

skodaic (skō-dā′ĭk). Concerning Josef Skoda. SEE: *Skoda's resonance.*

Skoda's rales (skō′dăs) [Josef Skoda, Austrian physician, 1805–1881]. Bronchial rales heard through consolidated tissue of the lungs in pneumonia.

Skoda's resonance. Tympanic resonance above the line of fluid in pleuritic effusion, or above consolidation in pneumonia.

SK-Penicillin VK. Trade name for penicillin V potassium.

SK-Phenobarbital. Trade name for phenobarbital.

SK-Potassium Chloride. Trade name for potassium chloride.

SK-Pramine. Trade name for imipramine hydrochloride.

SK-Prednisone. Trade name for prednisone.

SK-Probenecid. Trade name for probenecid.

SK-Quinidine Sulfate. Trade name for quinidine sulfate.

SK-Tetracycline. Trade name for tetracycline hydrochloride.

SK-Tolbutamide. Trade name for tolbutamide.

skull (skŭl) [ME. *skulle*, bowl]. The bony framework of the head, composed of eight cranial bones, the 14 bones of the face, and the teeth. SYN: *calvaria; cranium.* SEE: illus.; *skeleton.*

s., fracture of. Classified according to whether the fracture is in the vault or the base, but from the point of view of treatment, a more useful classification is as follows:

Simple uncomplicated fractures: Not

BONES OF SKULL

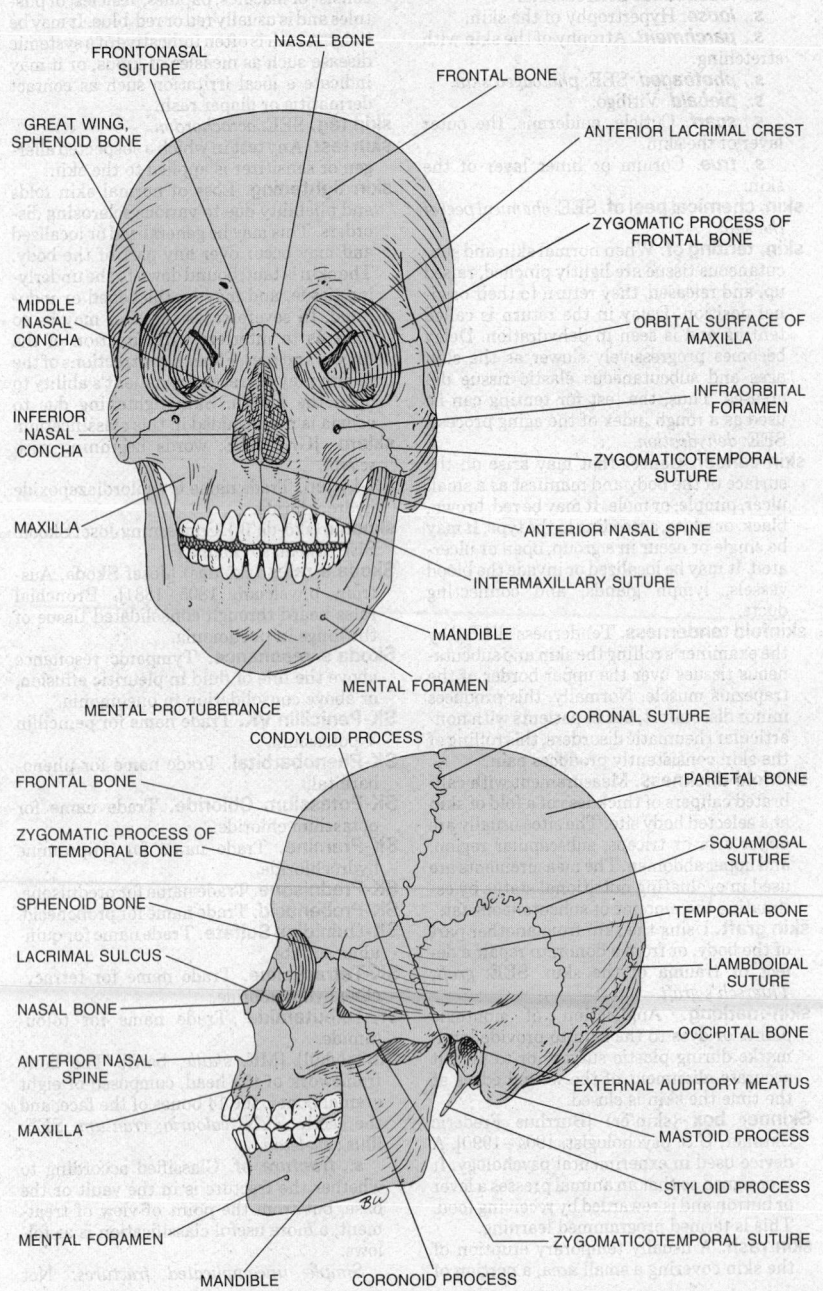

common.

Compound fractures: If in vault of skull, the bone is depressed and driven inward with possible damage to brain. Treatment is operative.

skullcap. Upper round portion of skull covering the brain. Also called calvaria.

slant. Tube of solid culture medium that is slanted to increase the surface area of the medium. Used in culturing bacteria.

slave. A device that allows the body movements to be transferred to a machine either directly or by remote control.

Ex.: apparatus for lifting, squeezing, and turning laboratory equipment containing radioactive materials. The remote "hands" are controlled by the operator from sufficient distance and proper shielding to prevent exposure to radiation or other highly toxic materials. Artificial arms and legs equipped to respond to physical or electrical stimulation have been developed.

SLE. *systemic lupus erythematosus.*

sleep (slēp) [AS. *slaep*]. A periodic state of rest accompanied by varying degrees of unconsciousness and relative inactivity. Although sleep is thought of as something that occurs once each 24-hour period, at least one-half the world's population has an afternoon nap or siesta as part of their lifelong sleep-wake pattern. The need for and value of sleep is obvious, yet the explanation of why it is so effective in providing a daily renewal of a feeling of health and well-being is lacking.

The sleep-wake cycle varies with age. The newborn may sleep as much as 20 hours each day; a child, 8 to 14 hours depending on age; adults, 3 to 12 hours with a mean of 7 to 8, and this may decrease to 6.5 hours in the elderly. Women past age 35 tend to sleep more than men. There is great individual variation in the amount and depth of sleep. Reports that some individuals never sleep are difficult to verify.

Attempts to generalize concerning the precise amount of sleep individuals need each night are not based on good evidence.

Investigators of sleep, using techniques involving recording of the electrical activity of the brain (electroencephalogram or EEG); muscles (electromyogram or EMG); eye movements; heart rate; respiratory rate; blood pressure; monitoring the state of the penis; and biochemical studies including analysis of hormone levels, have provided extensive information about the physiological changes that occur during sleep. There is a diurnal variation in body temperature, and the low point occurs during the night. It is erroneously thought that sleep is the cause of this decrease, but it is not.

Considerable research, in vain to date, has been done to attempt to isolate a chemical substance produced in animals or humans that induces sleep.

Sleep has been found to have two states: one with no rapid eye movements (NREM sleep) and one with rapid eye movements (REM sleep). In addition, four stages of sleep have been defined. During these stages, the person falling asleep passes from relaxed wakefulness to an early stage of light sleep and then to increasing degrees of deep sleep. Progression through these stages is discernible by alterations in the EEG, EMG, and eye movements.

The first four stages of sleep occur during a state of NREM. A period of REM sleep usually follows each period of NREM sleep. If sleep continues, these cycles repeat about 4 or 5 times during the sleep period. Most dream activity occurs during REM sleep, and the dream content is usually recallable if the subject is awakened at that time. A person may be easily awakened from REM sleep; but arousal from NREM sleep may require more than five minutes, and the person may be confused and disoriented during that arousal time. SEE: *sleep drunkenness.*

During normal sleep the body is not continually in one sleep state, but there is first a progression through the various stages of sleep; and, after more than one hour, REM sleep may occur. There is then a return to NREM sleep followed by REM sleep. This will be repeated several times during the sleep period. The time in each stage of the cycle will vary with age, and elderly persons may have little if any time in the deep sleep stages III and IV.

PHYSIOLOGIC CHANGES DURING SLEEP: A fall in body temperature; decreased secretion of urine; heart rate and respiration become slower and more regular during NREM sleep, then more rapid and less regular during REM sleep. Blood flow to the brain is increased during REM sleep; during REM sleep autonomic nervous functions tend to be activated, breathing is more irregular, heart rate and blood pressure vary, cerebral blood flow and metabolic rate increase; occurrence of penile erections, usually during REM sleep; increased secretion of growth hormone during the first two hours of sleep; surges of secretion of adrenocorticotropic hormone (ACTH) and cortisol occur in the last half of the sleep period; luteinizing hormone secretion is increased in both boys and girls during puberty; prolactin secretion is increased in both men and women during sleep, esp. immediately after onset of sleep.

In evaluating sleep, it is important to

know that hand waving, arm swinging, nose scratching, leg kicking, moaning, laughing, and flatus occur during normal sleep. Snoring may be clinically insignificant, but when accompanied by apnea, it can be harmful to the individual, and the sound aggravating to those close by.

s., hypnotic. 1. Sleep induced by hypnotic suggestion. 2. Sleep induced by the use of medicines classed as hypnotics.

s., NREM. Nonrapid eye movement sleep. SEE: *sleep.*

s., pathological. A term used in encephalitis lethargica (sleeping sickness). Here sleep is excessive. SEE: *encephalitis lethargica.*

s., REM. Rapid eye movement sleep. SEE: *sleep.*

s., twilight. A procedure of injection of scopolamine and morphine to abolish the subsequent memory of pain without completely abolishing pain at the time. At one time widely used during labor and delivery.

sleep, words pert. to: bruxism; dreams; hypnosis; hypnotic; hypnotism; insomnia; myoclonus; narcolepsy; noctambulism; sleep apnea; somnambulism; somnifacient; somniloquy; somnolence; somnolent; sopor; soporific.

sleep deprivation, effects of. Persons deprived of sleep for several days or more become irritable, fatigued, unable to concentrate, and usually disoriented. Performance of mental and physical tasks deteriorates. Some individuals will experience auditory, visual, and tactile illusions or hallucinations; and paranoid thoughts. Deprivation of REM sleep may cause anxiety, overeating, and hypersexuality. The effects of sleep deprivation are reversed when normal sleep-wake cycle is resumed.

sleep, disorders of. Any condition that interferes with sleep. This definition does not include the environmental factors that can disrupt sleep such as noise, excess heat or cold, or movement, as on a train, bus, or ship.

It is estimated that 20% to 40% of adults in the U.S. have difficulty sleeping, and about 5 million receive prescriptions for sleeping pills. SEE: various conditions below; *sleep-phase syndrome disorders.*

Cataplexy: The brief, sudden loss of muscle control brought on by strong emotion, such as a hearty laugh, excitement, surprise, or anger. Even though this may cause collapse, the patient remains fully conscious. The episode will last from seconds to minutes. Once the condition begins, it usually continues, but may be less severe with age. Most patients with narcolepsy (see below) will also have cataplexy.

TREAT: Imipramine hydrochloride (trade names are SK-Pramine and Tofranil) is of benefit.

Excessive somnolence: Condition in which the total time asleep is greatly increased during each 24-hour period. This may be associated with mental illness, drug or alcohol abuse, hypothyroidism, certain infectious diseases, and exposure to toxic chemicals.

Insomnia (disorders of initiating or maintaining sleep): Inability to sleep at a time when the person expected sleep to occur. The difficulty may be in either falling asleep or remaining asleep, or both. The disorder may be primary or secondary to some other illness, condition, or circumstance. Primary insomnia exists when there are no signs or symptoms of a mental or physical condition to account for the sleep disturbance. Secondary insomnia is usually readily explained by the existence of a condition that causes anxiety, stress, or pain; or by the use of a drug that interferes with sleep. The need for a careful sleep history is obvious. In addition to a careful search for mental or physical causes of insomnia, it is important that evidence of insomnia be obtained. It is also essential that the bed partner be questioned about the patient's sleep history.

TREAT: A great variety of drugs are available for insomnia. Their use on a short-term basis could be advisable, but all may have undesired side effects, such as overdose, habituation, tolerance, addiction, daytime drowsiness, lethargy, or amnesia. Insomnia requiring medication should be treated by a physician and the patient carefully advised of the possible undesired side effects. The use of drugs should be limited to short periods for primary insomnia. In secondary insomnia, the treatment consists of determining the condition causing the insomnia and then treating that disorder. If drugs are used, the benzodiazepines should be used only for short periods; insomnia should not be treated continuously with any drug. The benzodiazepines used for insomnia are triazolam, a drug with short duration of action (trade name is Halcion); temazepam, which has an intermediate duration of action (trade name is Restoril); and flurazepam with a long period of action (trade name is Dalmane). A great number of other medicines are available for treating insomnia, including over-the-counter preparations. In addition, some antihistamines promote drowsiness, but their use is not advised because they also cause diminished alertness during waking hours.

The insomniac should be advised that the body will eventually get as much sleep as is needed and that part of the treatment schedule should include not going to bed until drowsiness is present; and, if wakefulness occurs during the night, it would be appropriate to stay awake and do something pleasurable, such as read, work, or study. Other self-help measures include attempting to reduce the tension in one's lifestyle; establish a regular sleep routine; avoid anything that tends to excite just prior to attempting to sleep, such as horror movies, alcoholic beverages, coffee or tea, or strenuous exercise; a warm bath just prior to bed will relax tense muscles; avoid afternoon naps; sleep in a quiet, clean, cool, dark environment; orgasm may relax men but not women; a snack or glass of warm milk prior to going to bed will do no harm, but there is no evidence that this practice will help to induce sleep.

Caution: Some drugs used for treating insomnia are less rapidly biotransformed in elderly patients than in the young. Thus, these drugs have been associated with delirium, increased risk of falls and hip fractures, and excess sedation in elderly patients.

Narcolepsy: This disease of unknown etiology is not related to epilepsy or migraine. It is characterized by excessive daytime sleepiness and irresistible sleep attacks. These episodes may last from seconds to minutes and occur two to six times a day. In addition, the narcoleptic may have episodes of lapse of consciousness accompanied by automatic behavior, followed by amnesia. The diagnosis is confirmed by finding short-period REM sleep during the time the patient would normally be awake.

TREAT: The taking of naps prior to the time an attack might be expected may be beneficial; use of analeptic drugs or antidepressants is effective. It is important that patients be warned of the potential danger of the sleep attacks, and that they should avoid all activities in which a sleep attack could cause injury or death to themselves or others; thus, driving should be avoided. SEE: *cataplexy.*

Nightmares: These "bad dreams" occur in children and adults during REM sleep. The dream usually involves falling, death, or fear of attack. In the usual circumstance, nightmares are of no clinical importance, but they may be an indication of chronic alcohol or drug intoxication or withdrawal of drugs such as barbiturates.

Night Starts: Sudden "starts" or jerks that come during the transition between wakefulness and sleep. They may be intense enough to awaken the person. Even though these sudden movements may be of concern to the individual, he or she should be told that they are of no clinical importance. SYN: *hypnic jerks; somnolescent starts.*

Night Terrors: Shortly after falling asleep, the person awakens in fright, crying or screaming or moaning. There is tachycardia and hyperventilation. The episode lasts for only a few minutes, and it is not usually remembered the next morning. These usually begin in childhood but do occur in adults.

Sensory Paroxysms: At the onset of sleep, a sensation of hearing a sudden loud sound, a flash of light, or of being lifted and hurled to earth. Except for the disruption of sleep, these events are benign.

Shift work: A great number of persons work regularly at night, either on a permanent or rotating schedule. In most of those workers adaptation to the altered work schedule is inadequate. This leads to disturbed daytime sleep, decreased alertness and performance while at work, and an increased safety hazard. In addition, the general health of shift workers may be impaired.

TREAT: Shift changes should be clockwise; decrease frequency of shift changes so that they are done no more frequently than every two to three weeks; decrease the number of consecutive days worked at night to four or five.

Sleep Apnea: The symptom of a group of disorders characterized by cessation of breathing during sleep. In order to be so classified, the apnea lasts for at least 10 seconds and occurs 30 or more times during a seven-hour period of sleep. This strict definition may not apply to older persons in whom periods of sleep apnea are increased. The disorder is classified according to the mechanism involved: obstructive apnea, during which respiratory effort is present but is ineffective because of obstruction to the upper airway; central sleep apnea, which is associated with absence of respiratory muscle activity; and mixed apnea, when the apnea begins with absence of respiratory effort that is followed by upper airway obstruction.

Patients with obstructive sleep apnea are usually middle-aged, obese men with a history of excessive daytime sleepiness and sleep apnea associated with loud snorting, snoring, and gasping sounds.

The patient with central sleep apnea may present with excessive daytime sleepiness, but the snorting and gasping sounds during sleep are absent.

TREAT: Primary therapy is to assist breathing with continuous positive airway pressure. Correct the underlying disease; weight loss; surgical correction of palatal obstruction by uvulopalatopharyngoplasty, q.v. Medroxyprogesterone (trade name is Provera) may be of benefit.

Sleep Paralysis: Condition of being unable to speak or move even though fully aware of external events. Most commonly occurs upon falling asleep. The attack usually is of short duration, but, to the patient, the elapsed time may seem like hours. The exact cause or explanation of this condition is unknown.

Sleepwalking: This condition occurs mostly in children, and each episode usually lasts for less than 10 minutes. The patient appears to awaken, sits on the edge of the bed, and may walk. The eyes are open and the facial expression is blank. Even though their movements are clumsy, patients avoid obstructing objects. Night terrors (see above) may accompany sleepwalking. There is little if any memory of the event.

TREAT: The principal concern is to prevent injury by removing objects that could be dangerous and locking doors and windows, and to prevent from falling down stairs. Children usually outgrow this benign condition. SYN: *somnambulism.*

sleep drunkenness. The condition present in persons who require a great period of time to become fully alert upon awakening from deep sleep. During this transition period they may become ataxic, disoriented, or aggressive. Persons whose usual awakening sequence includes sleep drunkenness should not attempt to make decisions until they are fully alert and awake. SEE: *sleep, disorders of.*

sleep hygiene. Persons who have insomnia not caused by a known disease may find that attention to the following factors may assist in obtaining a good night's sleep: establishing a routine time to go to bed; avoiding trying to sleep; utilizing practices that assist in going to sleep such as reading, watching television, or listening to music; sleeping in a dark room, free of noise; avoiding caffeine prior to bedtime.

sleeping sickness. 1. Acute infectious disease marked by increasing lethargy, drowsiness, muscular weakness, and cerebral symptoms. SYN: *encephalitis lethargica.* 2. African trypanosomiasis caused by a protozoon introduced into the blood and cerebrospinal fluid by the bite of a tsetse fly; characterized by fever, protracted lethargy, weakness, tremors, and wasting.

sleep latency test. SEE: *Narcolepsy* in *sleep, disorders of.*

sleep-phase syndrome disorder. Persons who sleep well and for a normal amount of time, but not at the usual bedtime hours. Those with the delayed type of syndrome may function best if they go to sleep about the time most people are awakening. Those with the advanced type of syndrome do best when they go to sleep in late afternoon or early evening and arise about midnight.

When allowed to sleep at these hours, persons with this disease function normally.

sleep-wake cycle. The amount of time spent asleep and awake and the cycle of that schedule from day to day.

sleepwalking. SEE: *sleep, disorders of.*

slide. 1. A thin glass plate on which an object is placed for microscopic examination. 2. A photograph prepared so that it may be used in a film slide projector. 3. To move along a smooth surface in continuous contact, as the movement in dentistry of the mandibular teeth toward a centric position with the teeth in contact before closing completely in occlusion.

slime mold. A primitive mold that is not easily classified. It has been claimed by both the zoologists and the botanists.

slimy (slī′mē) [AS. *slim,* smooth]. Resembling slime or a viscid substance; of a growth, adhering to needle so it can be drawn out as a long thread.

sling (sling) [AS. *slingan,* to wind]. A support for an injured upper extremity. SEE: *bandage; triangular bandage* for illus.

    s., clove-hitch. Sling made as follows: Place a clove hitch in center of roller bandage. Fit to hand and carry ends over shoulder. Tie beside neck with square knot, making longer ends. They may be carried over and behind the shoulders, brought under each axilla, and tied over chest.

    s., counterbalanced. A rehabilitation device to assist upper extremity motion; it suspends the arm by way of an overhead frame and a pulley and weight system. SYN: *deltoid aid; suspension sling.*

    s., cravat. Sling made by placing the center of the cravat under wrist or forearm with ends tied around the neck.

    s., folded cravat. Lower-arm sling made by placing a broad fold of cloth in position on the chest with one end over affected shoulder and other hanging down in front of chest. Flex arm as desired across sling. Bring lower end up over sound shoulder, and secure with a knot located where it will not press on the affected shoulder.

    s., open. Sling made by placing the point of a triangular cloth at tip of elbow. The ends are brought around at back of neck and tied. The point should be brought forward and pinned or tied in a single knot, forming a cup to prevent elbow from slipping out.

    s., St. John's. Sling made by applying a

triangular bandage with point downward under elbow, upper end over sound shoulder. Flex arm acutely on chest. Bring lower end under affected arm and around back to knot with upper end on sound shoulder. Bring point up over elbow and fasten to base. Support is wholly for injured shoulder.

s., simple figure-of-eight roller arm. Sling made as follows: Flex arm on chest in desired position, then fix bandage with single turn toward uninjured side around arm and chest, crossing elbow just above external epicondyle of humerus. Make second turn overlapping two thirds of first, and bring bandage forward under tip of elbow, then upward along flexed forearm to root of neck of sound side. Then bring downward over scapula, cross chest and arm horizontally, overlapping, turn above, and continue as in progressive figure-of-eight.

s., swathe arm or cravat. Sling made as follows: Use folded cloth band. Place center under acutely flexed elbow, and carry to front and upward across the forearm and over affected shoulder. Proceed obliquely across back to sound axilla. Bring other end around front of arm and across body to sound axilla, where it is pinned to other end, continuing around back to part of sling surrounding affected elbow, where it is pinned again.

s., triangular. Sling made with suspension from uninjured side (brachioscapular sling). Place triangle on chest with one end over sound shoulder, the point under affected extremity, and fold the base. Flex injured arm outside of triangle. Carry lower end upward under axilla of injured side, back of shoulder, and tie with upper end behind back. Bring point of triangle anteriorly and medially around back of elbow, and fasten to body of bandage. This bandage changes point of carrying and also relieves the clavicle on injured side of the load. SEE: *triangular bandage* for illus.

s., triangular, reversed. Sling made as follows: Apply triangular bandage with one end over injured shoulder, point toward the sound side, base vertical under injured elbow. Flex arm acutely over triangle. Lower end is brought upward over front of arm and over sound shoulder. Pull ends taut and tie over sound shoulder. The point is pulled taut over forearm and fixed to anterior and posterior layers between forearm and arm. Holds elbow more acutely flexed—the weight is supported by the elbow.

slit [ME. *slitte*]. A narrow opening.

s., vestibular. The opening between left and right ventricular folds of the larynx.

slit lamp. SEE: *lamp, slit.*

slope. 1. An inclined plane or surface. 2. Tube

of solid culture medium that is slanted to increase the surface area of the medium. Used in culturing bacteria. SYN: *slant.*

s., lower ridge. The slope of the crest of the mandibular residual ridge from the third molar forward as viewed in profile.

Slo-Phyllin. Trade name for theophylline.

slough (slŭf) [ME. *slughe*, a skin]. 1. Dead matter or necrosed tissue separated from living tissue or an ulceration. 2. To separate in the form of dead or necrosed parts from living tissue. 3. To cast off, as dead tissue. SEE: *escharotic.*

sloughing (slŭf′ing). The formation of a slough; separation of dead from living tissue.

slow (slō) [AS. *slaw*, dull]. 1. Mentally dull. 2. Exhibiting retarded speed, as the pulse. 3. Said of a morbid condition or of a fever when it is not acute. SEE: words beginning with *brady-.*

Slow K. Trade name for potassium chloride.

slow-reacting substance of anaphylaxis. ABBR: SRS-A. A substance released by certain tissues, including the lungs, during anaphylaxis. It causes slow contraction of smooth muscle tissue and may be of major importance in allergic bronchospasm.

slows (slōz). A condition resulting from ingestion of plants such as snakeroot *(Eupatorium urticaefolium)* or jimmyweed *(Haplopappus heterophyllus).* Common in domestic animals and may occur in humans as a result of ingesting the plants or, more commonly, from drinking milk or eating the meat of poisoned animals. Symptoms are weakness; anorexia; nausea and vomiting; prostration; and possibly death. SYN: *trembles.*

slow virus infection. An infection caused by a virus that remains dormant in the body for a prolonged period prior to causing signs and symptoms of illness. Such viruses may require years to incubate prior to causing such diseases as scrapie in sheep or kuru in humans. Diseases of a chronic degenerative nature that are now suspected to be due to slow viruses include subacute sclerosing panencephalitis and progressive multifocal leukoencephalopathy.

sludge (slŭjh). Under the Resource Conservation and Recovery Act of 1976, sludge is defined as any solid, semisolid, or liquid waste generated from a municipal, commercial, or industrial wastewater treatment plant, or air pollution control facility, or any such waste having similar characteristics or effects.

sludged blood. Condition of the blood in certain abnormal states, such as tissue injury or shock, in which volume of plasma is reduced and the cells show a pronounced tendency to agglutinate and form large clumps or masses that move slowly through the vessels and sometimes clog the smaller vessels.

slurry (slŭr′ē) [ME. *slory*]. A thin, watery mixture.

Sm. Chem. symb. for the element samarium.

SMA-12. Trade name of device that does 12 blood chemistry tests on a single blood sample.

small-for-gestational age. ABBR: SGA. Term describing an infant whose birth weight is less than would be considered normal for the length of the calculated gestation period.

smallpox (smawl′pŏks) [AS. *smael*, tiny, + *poc*, pustule]. An acute, contagious, febrile disease, the constitutional symptoms of which are followed by the appearance of an eruption. SYN: *variola*. For complete description, SEE: *variola*.

NOTE: Smallpox is considered to have been eradicated.

smallpox vaccine. USP. A standardized preparation of the living virus of vaccinia. It was used in immunizing against smallpox, but its use is no longer thought to be necessary since smallpox is considered to have been eradicated worldwide.

smear (smēr) [AS. *smerian*, to anoint]. 1. In bacteriology, material spread on a surface, as a microscopic slide or a culture medium. 2. Material obtained from infected matter spread over solid culture media.

s., blood. A thin film of blood on a glass slide. Blood is prepared in this manner for staining and microscopic examination.

s., Pap; s., Papanicolaou. SEE: *Papanicolaou test.*

smegma (smĕg′mă) [Gr. *smegma*, soap]. Secretion of sebaceous glands, specifically, the thick, cheesy, odoriferous secretion found under the labia minora about the glans clitoridis or under the male prepuce from Tyson's glands.

s. clitoridis. Odoriferous secretion of the glands of the clitoris.

s. embryonum. Vernix caseosa.

s. praeputii. Cheesy odoriferous substance collecting under prepuce in the male.

smegmatic (smĕg-măt′ĭk). Pert. to or made up of smegma.

smegmolith (smĕg′mō-lĭth) [Gr. *smegma*, soap, + *lithos*, a stone]. Calcareous mass in the smegma.

smell (smĕl) [ME. *smellen*, to reek]. 1. To perceive by stimulation of the olfactory nerves. 2. To emit an odor, pleasant or offensive. In clinical medicine the smell arising from the patient's body, feces, breath, urine, vagina, and clothing may provide valuable information concerning the diagnosis. The smell on clothing may be due to a toxic chemical that

spilled on the clothes. Also, a patient may attempt to alter or mask the smell of alcohol on his breath by use of a medicated or flavored lozenge or mint. 3. A chemical sense dependent upon end organs on the surface of the upper part of the nasal septum and the superior nasal concha. These sensory cells live for an average of 30 days and are affected by a variety of factors including age, nutritional and hormonal states, drugs, and therapeutic radiation. 4. Property of a thing affecting the olfactory organs, pleasant or unpleasant. SYN: *odor.*

The sense of smell may be affected by many conditions, some of which are the following:

Anosmia: A loss of the sense of smell. It may be a local and a temporary condition resulting from acute and chronic rhinitis, mouth breathing, nasal polyps, dryness of the nasal mucous membrane, pollens, or very offensive odors. It may also result from disease or injury of the olfactory tract, bone disease near the olfactory nerve, disease of the nasal accessory sinuses, basal meningitis, or tumors or gumma affecting the olfactory nerve. It is sometimes found in locomotor ataxia, and frequently in hysteria and neurasthenia. Disease of one cranial hemisphere or of one nasal chamber may account for anosmia. SYN: *anodmia; anosphrasia.*

Hyperosmia: An increased sensitivity to odors.

Kakosmia: The perception of bad odors where none exist; it may be due to head injuries or occur in hallucinations in certain psychoses. SYN: *cacosmia.*

Parosmia: A perverted sense of smell. Odors that are considered agreeable are assumed to be offensive, and disagreeable odors may be found pleasant to those suffering from certain functional derangements and in some catarrhs. SYN: *parosphresia.* SEE: *cacosmia.*

smell, words pert. to: anosmia; anosphrasia; aroma; aromatic; cacosmia; dysosmia; hyperosmia; jumentous; kakosmia; odor; odoriferous; olfaction; olfactory; organoleptic tests; osmesthesia; osphresis; oxyosphresia.

smile. A facial expression that may represent pleasure, amusement, derision, or scorn. The corners of the mouth are turned up, and in expressions of pleasure or amusement, the eyes usually appear to be warm and friendly.

Smith's fracture [Robert W. Smith, Irish physician, 1807–1873]. Fracture of the lower end of the radius, with forward displacement of the lower fragment.

Smith-Magenis syndrome [Ann C. M. Smith, contemporary U.S. genetics counselor; Ellen Magenis, contemporary U.S.

physician]. A rare form of genetic mental retardation characterized by chronic ear infections, erratic sleep patterns, head banging, picking at skin, and pulling off fingernails and toenails. There is abnormality of chromosome 17. Treatment is symptomatic.

Smith-Petersen nail [Marius N. Smith-Petersen, U.S. orthopedic surgeon, 1886–1953]. A special nail that on cross-section has three flanges, used for stabilizing fractures of the neck of the femur.

Smith-Strang disease. An inherited disease due to malabsorption of methionine and in which the urine has a characteristic oasthouse odor. The patients have white hair, mental retardation, convulsions, diarrhea, and increased respiratory rate. SYN: *oasthouse urine disease.*

smog [blend of *smoke* and *fog*]. Dense fog combined with smoke and other forms of air pollution.

smoke inhalation. Persons exposed to gases produced by burning materials are at risk of developing acute injury to their lungs; and, depending upon the composition of the smoke and the duration of the exposure, the combination of heat and gases may be lethal. Firefighters are especially at risk from this kind of exposure. Modern construction and decorating materials produce a variety of volatile and irritating substances when burned. Repeated exposure to some of these gases may lead to chronic irritation of the respiratory tract. Firefighters should be aware that the "blackness" smoke produced by a fire may not be a true indicator of the amount of toxic substances, including carbon monoxide, in the smoke.

The normal half-life of carbon monoxide in the body is 4 hours. This can be reduced to 50 minutes by immediately inhaling 100% oxygen after exposure. Even more effective is the use of hyperbaric oxygen therapy. SEE: *smoke poisoning.*

smokeless tobacco. Tobacco used in the form of snuff, tobacco powder, or chewing tobacco. These products irritate the oral mucosa and gingiva, and their continued use results in an increased risk of cancer of the mouth, larynx, throat, and esophagus. Use of smokeless tobacco leads to addiction in the same manner as smoked tobacco products.

smoke poisoning. Toxicity produced by inhalation of gases and smoke produced by burning materials. The usual gas is carbon monoxide, but many combustion products will form corrosive acids or alkalies when they reach the moisture present in the upper respiratory tract. This will cause varying degrees of injury to the mucosa depending

upon the extent of exposure. This may lead to acute pulmonary edema, shock, and death.

TREAT: Administration of corticosteroids; oxygen; and therapy for pulmonary edema. SEE: *smoke inhalation.*

smoker's cancer. Cancer of the lip, throat, or lung caused by irritation from excessive smoking.

smoking, passive. The exposure of persons not smoking tobacco products to the smoke produced by other smokers. The extent and importance of such exposure in the workplace, the home, or in any other circumstance is directly related to the number of cigarettes and other tobacco products used by the smokers. It can lead to injury of the respiratory tract of the nonsmoker and to an increased incidence of all the other pathological conditions caused by smoking. Prevention of this type of exposure in a home in which smoking is allowed and where children have no alternative but to breathe the tobacco smoke is particularly important. SYN: *involuntary smoking.*

SMON. subacute myelo-optic neuropathy.

smooth muscle. SEE: *muscle, smooth.*

smudging (smŭj'ĭng). A speech defect in which difficult consonants are omitted.

Sn [L. *stannun*]. Chem. symb. for the element tin.

snail [ME.]. A small mollusk having a spiral shell and belonging to the class Gastropoda. Snails are important as intermediate hosts of many species of parasitic flukes.

snake [ME.]. A reptile possessing scales and lacking limbs, external ears, and functional eyelids.

  s., poisonous. A venom-producing snake. Venom is produced in a poison gland, which is connected by a tube or groove to a poison fang, one of two sharp elongated teeth present in the upper jaw. The following are poisonous snakes of the U.S.: coral snake, copperhead, water moccasin (cottonmouth), and rattlesnake, of which there are 15 species. All except the coral snake belong to a group known as pit vipers because of presence of a distinct pit between eye and nostril. SEE: illus.; *venom, snake.*

  A polyvalent antivenin serum for bites by pit vipers is prepared by Wyeth Lab. Inc., Radnor, PA. Antivenin for coral snake bite is also available from Wyeth.

  Information concerning the nearest source of antivenin may be obtained from the National Institutes of Health, Bethesda, MD; the Reptile Institute, Silver Springs, FL; or from large zoos.

  RS: antivenin; ophidism; ophiotoxemia; venenation; venene; veneniferous; venom.

snake bite. All snakes should be considered

SNAKES

BULL SNAKE
NONPOISONOUS
5' TO 7'
(152 TO 213 CM)

WATER SNAKE
NONPOISONOUS 3-½' TO 5'
(107 TO 152 CM)

EASTERN
DIAMONDBACK
RATTLESNAKE
POISONOUS
5'
(152 CM)

SCARLET KING SNAKE
NONPOISONOUS 18"
(40 CM)

GENERAL CHARACTERISTICS
OF POISONOUS SNAKES:
(PIT VIPERS)

ELLIPTICAL PUPIL — NOSTRIL

— PIT

— FANGS

— TONGUE

GENERAL CHARACTERISTICS
OF HARMLESS SNAKES:

ROUND PUPIL — NOSTRIL

— TONGUE

— TEETH

ANAL PLATE

RATTLESNAKE

RATTLES

SINGLE ROW
SUBCAUDAL PLATES

ANAL PLATE

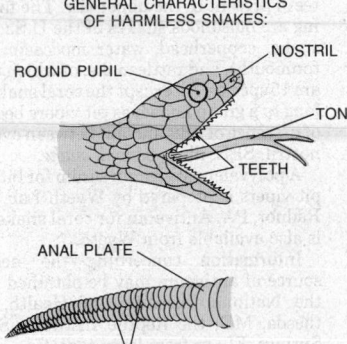

DOUBLE ROW SUBCAUDAL
PLATES

NO RATTLES

COPPERHEADS AND COTTONMOUTHS

poisonous, although only a few secrete an amount of venom sufficient to inoculate poison deeply into the tissues.

F.A.: Immediately transport patient to a medical facility equipped and staffed to handle snake bites. Do not apply tourniquet. Apply a band just above the bite. This should be tight enough to prevent lymph flow, but not tight enough to interfere with arterial flow or venous return. Do not apply cold to the area. If victim is more than several hours away from a hospital, attempt incision and suction only if this can be done by a qualified person.

In the hospital start intravenous infusion of Ringer's lactate or normal saline. If patient has actually received venom from the snake bite, and only about 50% of patients have, administer antivenin after first testing for sensitivity to horse serum. This should be done only if the equipment for treating anaphylaxis is available. Children require a larger dose of antivenin than adults.

If in doubt about the type of snake that bit the patient and the type of antivenin to use, call the nearest large zoo for emergency consultation, or call Poisindex central office in Denver, Colorado, at (800) 332-3037; or the Antivenin Index in Tucson, Arizona, at (602) 626-6016.

Caution: Alcoholic stimulants must not be taken, and nothing should be done to increase circulation. Do not cauterize with strong acids or depend upon home remedies. Antibiotics and tetanus prophylaxis are essential.

snap. A sharp cracking sound.

    s., closing. The intense first heart sound heard in mitral stenosis.

    s., opening. A sharp sound of increased pitch heard in early systole. It is associated with opening of the abnormal valve in mitral stenosis.

snapping finger. A snapping sound or feeling produced by bending the finger. In adults it is usually caused by tenosynovitis; in children by the sliding of tendons out of a cramped space when the finger is extended.

snapping hip. Slipping of the hip joint with a snap due to displacement over the great trochanter of a tendinous band.

snare (snār) [AS. *sneare*, noose]. Device for excision of polyps or tumors by tightening wire loops around them.

sneeze (snēz) [AS. *fneosan*, to pant]. 1. To expel air forcibly through the nose and mouth by spasmodic contraction of muscles of expiration due to irritation of nasal mucosa. The sneeze reflex may be produced by a great number of stimuli. Placing a foot on a

cold surface will provoke a sneeze in some people, while looking at a bright light or sunlight will cause it in others. Firm pressure applied to the middle of the upper lip and just under the nose will sometimes prevent a sneeze that is about to occur. SEE: *photic sneezing; ptarmus.* 2. The act of sneezing. SEE: *sternutation; sternutatory.*

sneeze reflex, solar. Sneeze that occurs following exposure to bright sunlight. This benign condition may affect a great number of normal persons, and it may also be associated with rhinitis. The mechanism of the cause of this type of sneeze reflex is unknown.

Snellen's chart (snĕl'ĕns) [Herman Snellen, Dutch ophthalmologist, 1834–1908]. Chart imprinted with lines of black letters graduating in size from smallest on the bottom to largest on top. Used for testing visual acuity.

Snellen's reflex. Congestion of ear on same side upon stimulation of the distal end of the divided auriculotemporal nerve. SYN: *auriculocervical nerve reflex.*

Snellen's test. Test for visual acuity where the patient reads Snellen's chart at a certain distance with one eye, then with the other eye, and then with both eyes.

sniff test. Test used to detect bacterial vaginosis. The discharge from the vaginal area is swabbed, placed on a slide, and 10% KON is added. The presence of a fishy odor is indicative of bacterial vaginosis.

snore (snor) [AS. *snora*]. During sleep, the noise produced while breathing through the mouth. The noise is caused by air passing through relaxed tissues in the pharynx. The majority of people snore to some extent. Snoring is of no clinical importance to the snorer unless it is prolonged and chronic, in which case it seems to be related to an increased risk of developing ischemic heart disease. Also, it is of importance if the snoring is so loud as to cause discomfort and lack of sleep in those sharing the sleeping space. Indeed, one man's snore was recorded at 88 decibels (equivalent to the sound produced by a loud motorcycle), and persons in the armed forces have had to be discharged because of their snoring interfering with the sleep of others.

    TREAT: In some cases, the snoring is of such clinical and social importance that plastic surgery, uvulopalatopharyngoplasty, q.v., for correcting the relaxed tissues in the pharynx is indicated. SYN: *stertor.*

snoring rale (snor'ĭng rāl). A sonorous rale, low in pitch, resembling a snore.

snow, carbon dioxide. SEE: *carbon dioxide solid therapy.*

snow blindness. Irritation of the conjunctiva caused by reflection of the sun on the snow. SEE: *Nursing Diagnoses* in *Appendix.*

SYM: Photophobia, blepharospasm, burning pain in the eyes, hyperemia, or temporary blindness.

SNS. *Society of Neurological Surgeons.*

snuff. 1. A medicinal powder inhaled through the nose. 2. A powdered form of tobacco inhaled through the nose, or placed in the posterior part of the buccal cavity on one side.

snuffbox, anatomical. Triangular area of the dorsum of the hand at the base of the thumb. When the thumb is extended, the tendons of the long and short extensor muscles of the thumb bound this area, which appears as a depression. When snuff was used, a small pinch could be placed in this "box" and snuffed up into the nose from that site. Tenderness in this area may be present when the navicular bone is fractured.

snuffles (snŭf'ls) [D. *snuffelen,* to snuff]. Obstructed nasal breathing with discharge from the nasal mucosa, esp. in infants, chiefly in congenital syphilis.

SOAP. Acronym for an organized structure for keeping progress notes in the chart. Each entry contains date, number, and title of the patient's particular problem, followed by the SOAP headings: Subjective findings; Objective findings; Assessment, the documented analysis and conclusions concerning the findings; and Plan for further diagnostic or therapeutic action. If the patient has multiple problems, a SOAP entry on the chart is made for each problem.

soap (sōp) [AS. *sape*]. A cleansing chemical compound formed by an alkali acting on a fatty acid, such as sodium stearate, NaC$_{18}$H$_{35}$O$_2$. Castile soap is made by saponifying olive oil with sodium hydroxide and contains mainly sodium oleate, NaC$_{18}$H$_{33}$O$_2$. SEE: *detergent; saponification.*

   s., green. S., soft medicinal.

   s., soft medicinal. A liquid soap made by saponification of vegetable oils excluding coconut oil and palm kernel oil and without removal of glycerin. Used in the treatment of skin diseases. SYN: *s., green.*

soap liniment. A solution of soap and camphor in alcohol and water. Used as a stimulant and rubefacient.

soapsuds enema. Enema given so that the irritating action of the soap will stimulate the bowel. Less harsh forms of enema are preferred. SEE: *enema, soapsuds.*

SOB. *short of breath.*

sob [ME. *sobben,* to catch breath]. 1. To weep with convulsive movements of the chest. 2. A cry or wail resulting from a sudden convulsive inspiration accompanied by spasmodic closure of the glottis. SEE: *sigh.*

socialization (sō″shǎ-lĭ-zā'shŭn). The process of adapting an individual to the social customs of society; in the process he or she becomes a useful member of the society.

social phobias. Persistent irrational fears and the need to avoid any situation in which one might be exposed to scrutiny by others and potentially embarrassed or humiliated. Even anticipating a phobia-producing situation, such as speaking in public, urinating in a restroom with others present, or eating in public, may cause extreme anxiety.

   TREAT: Relaxation therapy, desensitization, or use of beta blockers, such as propranolol, alprazolam, or atenolol, may be of benefit.

socioacusis (sō″sē-ō-ă-kū'sĭs) [L. *socius,* companion, + Gr. *akoustikos,* hearing]. The long-range ill effects of environmental noise on auditory acuity.

sociobiology (sō″sē-ō-bī-ŏl'ō-jē) [″ + Gr. *bios,* life, + *logos,* word, reason]. Analysis of social behavior in terms of modern evolutionary theory. It is the study of the social life of animals or humans on the assumption that populations evolve and adapt to their environments in different ways, through individual learning, cultural tradition, or genetic inheritance.

socioeconomic status. The combined social and economic level of individuals or groups. Such classification is useful in studying the relationship of income and living conditions to the prevalence and incidence of various diseases.

sociology (sō-sē-ŏl'ō-jē) [″ + *logos,* word, reason]. Study of human social behavior and the origins, institutions, and functions of human groups and societies.

sociomedical. Pert. to sociology and medicine, esp. the interrelationships between the two.

sociometry (sō″sē-ŏm'ĕ-trē) [″ + Gr. *metron,* measure]. The science concerned with measuring social behavior.

sociopath (sō'sē-ō-păth) [″ + Gr. *pathos,* suffering]. An individual with antisocial personality disorder. SEE: *personality, antisocial.*

sociopathic personality. SEE: *personality, antisocial.*

sociopathy (sō″sē-ŏp'ă-thē) [″ + Gr. *pathos,* disease, suffering]. The condition of being antisocial.

socket (sŏk'ĕt) [ME. *soket,* a spearhead]. 1. A hollow in a joint or part for another corresponding organ, as a bone socket or an eye socket. SEE: *acetabulum.* 2. The proximal portion of a prosthesis, into which the stump of an amputated extremity is fitted.

   s., alveolar. The bony space occupied by the tooth and periodontal ligament.

s., dry. Alveolitis following tooth extraction characterized by extreme pain but without suppuration.

s., tooth. A dental alveolus of the maxilla or mandible; a cavity that contains the root of a tooth.

soda (sō′dă) [Medieval L., barilla, from which soda is made]. 1. Term loosely applied to various salts of sodium, esp. to caustic soda (sodium hydroxide) and baking soda (sodium bicarbonate). SEE: *sodium.* 2. Short for soda water, which is water charged with carbon dioxide.

s., baking. Sodium bicarbonate.

s., caustic. Sodium hydroxide.

s. lime. A white granular substance consisting of a mixture of calcium hydroxide and sodium hydroxide or potassium hydroxide, or both. Used to absorb carbon dioxide.

Soda Mint. Trade name for sodium bicarbonate.

soda water. A solution of carbon dioxide under pressure; carbonic acid.

Sodestrin. Trade name for estrogens, conjugated.

sodic (sō′dĭk). Relating to or containing soda or sodium.

sodio-. Combining form denoting a compound containing sodium.

sodium (sō′dē-ŭm) [LL.]. SYMB: Na. At. wt. 22.9898; at. no. 11; sp. gr. 0.971. Sodium constitutes approximately 0.15% of elements of the body. Sodium (Na^+), K^+, Ca^{++}, and Mg^{++} constitute the principal cations of the body, their relative concentration determining the integrity of cell membranes and the bioelectric potentials of tissues. Na^+ is the principal cation found in extracellular fluids.

FUNCT: Sodium salts are found in the fluids of the body, serum, blood, and lymph, and in the tissues. They are necessary to preserve a balance between calcium and potassium to maintain normal heart action and the equilibrium of the body. They regulate osmotic pressure in the cells and fluids, act as an ion balance in tissues, produce a buffer action in the blood, and guard against an excessive loss of water from the tissues.

DEFICIENCY SYM: Weakness, nerve disorders, loss of weight, "salt hunger," miner's cramps, disturbed digestion.

s. acetate. USP. A chemical compound that is used to alkalize the urine, and is used in kidney dialysis solutions.

s. alginate. A purified carbohydrate product extracted from certain species of seaweed. It is used as a food additive and as a pharmaceutic aid.

s., amobarbital. The monosodium salt of isoamylethylbarbituric acid. Trade name

is Amytal Sodium.

ACTION/USES: Sedative and hypnotic in control of insomnia; preliminary to surgical anesthesia and in labor.

s. ascorbate. USP. The sodium salt of ascorbic acid, vitamin C. It may be used in a sterile solution when parenteral administration of vitamin C is required.

s. benzoate. A white, odorless powder with sweet taste. Used as a food preservative.

s. bicarbonate. USP. $NaHCO_3$. White odorless powder with saline taste. Used intravenously to treat acidosis, as in diabetic ketoacidosis or cardiopulmonary arrest.

ACTION/USES: Orally as an antacid. Effectiveness for this purpose is questionable. Externally, mild alkaline wash.

INCOMPAT: Acids, acid salts, ammonium chloride, lime water, ephedrine hydrochloride, iron chloride.

s. carbonate. Na_2CO_3. White crystalline powder (washing soda). Used as an alkali employed chiefly in alkaline baths.

s., carboxymethylcellulose. USP. The sodium salt of carboxymethylcellulose, q.v.

s. chloride. USP. NaCl. Common table salt.

ACTION/USES: In preparation of normal saline solution, emetic, and to add flavor to foods.

INCOMPAT: Silver nitrate.

In aqueous solution sodium chloride, a neutral salt, is a strong electrolyte, being almost completely ionized. The sodium and chlorine ions are important in maintaining the proper electrolyte balance in body fluids. The kidneys control excretion of sodium chloride in the urine. This control mechanism is complex, but the hormones vasopressin and aldosterone are essential to the process. Sodium chloride is also present in sweat, milk, and intestinal juices.

s. citrate. USP. White granular powder, saline in taste and soluble in water. Used as an anticoagulant for blood used for transfusion.

s. fluoride. USP. NaF. White crystalline powder, saline in taste, soluble in 25 parts of water.

ACTION/USES: In drinking water and in solution for local application to teeth for prevention of dental caries. Commercially, in etching glassware, for eradication of rats, insects, ants, and other pests. SEE: *fluoridation; sodium fluoride poisoning.*

s. hydroxide. NaOH. A whitish solid; soluble in water, making a clear solution. SYN: *soda, caustic; soda, lye.*

ACTION/USES: Antacid and caustic. In the laundry and in commercial compounds, in cleaning sink traps, toilets, etc., and in the preparation of soap.

Caution: Use great care in handling it, as it rapidly destroys organic tissues. Protective glasses should be worn while working with this chemical. If splashed in eye, may cause blindness.

s. hypochlorite [solution]. USP. An antiseptic used in root canal therapy.

Caution: This solution is not suitable for application to wounds.

s. iodide. USP. NaI. A salt resembling in appearance and action potassium iodide.

s. lactate [injection]. USP. Sodium salt of inactive lactic acid. In one-sixth or one-fourth molar solution, it is used I.V. to control electrolyte disturbances, esp. acidosis.

s. lauryl sulfate. An anionic surface-active agent that is used as a pharmaceutic acid.

s. monofluorophosphate. USP. An agent suitable for topical application to teeth to prevent dental caries.

s., morrhuate [injection]. USP. The sodium salt of the fatty acids, found in cod liver oil. Used as a sclerosing agent for the obliteration of varicose veins.

s. nitrite. USP. NaNO$_2$. White crystalline powder. Antidote for cyanide poisoning.

s. nitroprusside. USP. A powerful vasodilator used when rapid reduction in blood pressure is required.

s. phosphate, dibasic. USP. Chemical that is used as a cathartic.

s. phosphate P 32 [solution]. USP. A standardized preparation of radioactive phosphorus (^{32}P).

s. polystyrene sulfonate. USP. A cation-exchange resin used to lower the potassium in the body.

s. propionate. A pharmaceutic aid that also has antifungal action.

s. salicylate. USP. C$_7$H$_5$NaO$_3$. White powder or scales with sweet saline taste. Used as an analgesic and antipyretic.

INCOMPAT: Caffeine citrate, caffeine sodium benzoate.

s. sulfate. USP. A salt used as a saline cathartic and diuretic. Also has some uses in veterinary medicine. SYN: *Glauber's salt.*

s. thiosulfate. USP. White crystalline substance, having a cooling taste. Used externally to remove stains of iodine and intravenously an an antidote for cyanide poisoning.

sodium fluoride poisoning. Reaction to exposure to a toxic dose of sodium fluoride. This material is normally used in dentistry

or in fluoridating water supplies. Symptoms include conjunctivitis, retching, vomiting, nausea, eventual cardiac weakness, kidney disturbances, and interference with coagulation of blood.

F.A.: In addition to washing affected areas, precipitate by addition of soluble calcium salts such as lime water, calcium gluconate, or calcium lactate. Give emetics and soothing drinks such as milk, cream, or egg whites. SEE: *fluoride (salts, sodium)* at *Poisons and Poisoning* in *Appendix.*

sodium nitroprusside. ABBR: SNP. Antihypertensive. Trade names are Nipride and Nitropress.

Caution: Infusion of SNP at the maximum dose rate of 10 mcg/kg/min should never last for more than 10 minutes. For treatment of overdose, SEE: *cyanide poisoning.*

Sodium Versenate. Trade name for edetate disodium.

sodokosis (sŏd-ō-kō'sĭs) [Jap. *sodoku*, rat poison, + Gr. *osis*, condition]. Sodoku, q.v. SEE: *rat-bite fever.*

sodoku (sō-dō'koo). Infectious febrile disease due to *Spirillum minus* transmitted by rat bite. SEE: *rat-bite fever.* SYN: *rat-bite fever; sodokosis.*

sodomist, sodomite (sŏd'ō-mĭst, -mīt) [LL. *Sodoma,* Sodom]. A person who practices sodomy.

sodomy (sŏd'ō-mē) [LL. *Sodoma,* Sodom]. Anal intercourse, usually between males.

Soemmering's bone (sĕm'ĕr-ĭngz) [Samuel T. von Soemmering, German anatomist, 1755–1830]. Marginal process of malar (zygomatic) bone.

Soemmering's foramen. The fovea centralis retinae.

Soemmering's ring. Annular swelling of the periphery of the lens capsule.

Soemmering's spot. The macula lutea of the retina.

soft (sŏft) [AS. *softe*]. Not hard, firm, or solid.

soft diet. A diet consisting of nothing but soft or semi-solid foods or liquids. Includes fish, egg, and cheese dishes, chicken, cereals, bread, toast, and butter. Excluded are red meats, vegetables or fruits having seeds or thick skins, cellulose, raw fruits, and salads. SYN: *convalescent diet.*

softening (sŏf'ĕn-ing) [AS.]. Process of becoming soft. SYN: *malacia; mollities.*

s., anemic. White softening of the brain from lack of blood.

s., colliquative. The liquefying of tissues.

s., gray. Softening of the brain with absorption of fat following yellow softening.

s., hemorrhagic. S., red.

s., mucoid. Myxomatous degeneration.

s. of bones. Osteomalacia.

s. of brain. Paresis with progressive dementia. SYN: *encephalomalacia.*

s. of heart. Myomalacia cordis.

s. of stomach. Gastromalacia.

s., red. Softening of the brain with bleeding into necrosed portions. SYN: *s., hemorrhagic.*

s., white. S., anemic.

soft palate. The posterior portion of the roof of the mouth, partly separating the mouth and the pharynx. SYN: *velum palatinum.*

"soft sign." Any of a number of signs which, when considered collectively, are felt to indicate the presence of damage to the central nervous system. These signs include incoordination, visual motor difficulties, nystagmus, the presence of associated movements, and difficulties with motor control.

soft sore. A highly infectious nonsyphilitic venereal ulcer caused by Ducrey's bacillus. SYN: *chancroid, q.v.*

sol (sŏl, sōl) [Gr. *sole,* salt water]. State of a colloid system in which the dispersion medium or solvent forms a continuous phase in which the particles of the solute are dispersed, forming a fluid mass. It is called a hydrosol if dispersion medium is a liquid and aerosol if a gas. SEE: *gel.*

sol. Solution.

solace. An object or resource that does or seems to soothe pain or mental stress. In children a teddy bear or a "security" blanket may provide solace. In later life, one's spouse, a friend, or a hobby may be a source of comfort and security.

Solanaceae (sŏl″ă-nā′sē-ē). A family of herbs, shrubs, and trees from which several important drugs such as scopolamine and belladonna are derived. The potato is one of the species.

solanaceous (sŏl″ă-nā′shŭs). Concerning the family Solanaceae.

solanine (sō′lă-nēn). A poisonous narcotic alkaloid obtained from potato sprouts and tomatoes. SEE: *poisoning, potato.*

solar (sō′lăr) [L. *solaris*]. 1. Pert. to the sun or its rays. 2. The solar plexus.

solarium (sō-lā′rē-ŭm) [L. *solarium,* terrace]. 1. A room or porch exposed to the sun. 2. A room designed for heliotherapy or for the application of artificial light. 3. Day or recreational room for patients; often used as a waiting area for family or visitors.

solar plexus. The celiac plexus, behind the stomach and between the suprarenal glands and consisting of two large ganglia, the celiac and superior mesenteric ganglia, from which sympathetic fibers pass to visceral organs.

solar therapy. Treatment with the sun's rays.

SYN: *heliotherapy.*

solation (sō-lā′shŭn). In colloidal chemistry, the transformation of a gel into a sol.

solder (sŏd′ĕr). Any fusible alloy usually made of tin and lead but may be mostly silver or gold for use in dentistry. The alloy is applied in a melted state to build up or join metal parts.

s., building. An alloy of silver with large amounts of copper used to increase the height or bulk of contact areas of dental inlays or crowns. Also called sticky solder.

s., gold. A solder alloy with a high proportion of gold in it.

s., hard. A solder that is used in dentistry, has a high fusion point, and is stronger and more tarnish-resistant than softer, low-melting-point solders.

s., soft. A low-melting-point solder with less strength or tarnishing resistance than hard solder.

soldering. The joining of two pieces of metal by use of a lower melting-point alloy. When the melted solder cools and solidifies, it joins the parts together. Soldering is used to join many components of dental appliances or orthodontic bands and to add bulk or contours to crowns or inlays.

sole (sōl) [AS. *sole*]. 1. Underpart of the foot. SYN: *planta.* 2. The portion of a motor endplate at termination of a motor nerve fiber that is directly adjacent to the contractile substance of a muscle fiber. A large number of muscle nuclei are usually aggregated here. SEE: *antithenar; thenar.*

soleal line of tibia. A line on the posterior surface of the tibia extending diagonally from below the tibial condyle to the medial border of the tibia. The soleus muscle and fascia are attached to that line.

solenoid (sōl′lĕ-noyd). A coil of insulated wire in which a magnetic force is created in the long axis of the coil when an electric current flows through the wire. It may be used to activate switches.

sole reflex. Plantar flexion of the foot muscles when tickling the sole. SYN: *plantar reflex.*

soleus (sō′lĕ-ŭs) [L. *solea,* sole of foot]. A flat, broad muscle of the calf of the leg. SEE: *Muscles* in *Appendix.*

Solfoton. Trade name for phenobarbital, USP.

Solganal. Trade name for aurothioglucose, USP.

solid (sŏl′ĭd) [L. *solidus*]. 1. Not gaseous, hollow, or liquid. 2. A substance not gaseous, liquid, or hollow.

solipsism (sŏl′ĭp-sĭzm) [L. *solus,* alone, + *ipse,* self]. The theory that the self may know only its feelings and changes and there is then only subjective reality.

solitary (sŏl'ĭ-tăr-ē) [L. *solitarius,* aloneness]. Alone; single or existing separately.

solitary lymph nodules. Small spherical lymphatic nodules found in the lamina propria of the small and large intestine.

solo practitioner. A physician, dentist, or other practitioner who practices alone rather than with a group or partner.

solubility (sŏl″ū-bĭl'ĭ-tē) [LL. *solubilis,* to loosen, dissolve]. Capability of being dissolved.

soluble (sŏl'ū-bl). Able to be dissolved.

soluble immune response suppressor. ABBR: SIRS. A lymphokine, q.v., that suppresses antibody production.

Solu-Cortef. Trade name for hydrocortisone sodium succinate, USP.

Solu-Medrol. Trade name for methylprednisolone sodium succinate, USP.

solum tympani (sō'ŭm tĭm'pă-nē) [L.]. The floor of the tympanic cavity.

solute (sŏl'ūt) [L. *solutus,* to loosen, dissolve]. The substance that is dissolved in a solution.

solutio (sō-lū'shē-ō) [L. *solutus,* to loosen, dissolve]. Solution.

solution (sō-lū'shŭn) [L. *solutus,* to loosen, dissolve]. 1. Liquid containing dissolved substance. 2. Process by which a solid is homogeneously mixed with a fluid, solid, or gas so that the dissolved substances cannot be distinguished from the resultant fluid. 3. Mixture formed by dissolution of substances.

The liquid in which the substances are dissolved is called the solvent, q.v., and the substance dissolved, the solute, q.v.

s., aqueous. Solution containing water as the solvent.

s., buffer. Solution of a weak acid and its salt (e.g., carbonic acid, sodium bicarbonate) of importance in maintaining a constant pH, esp. of the blood.

s., colloidal. Solution in which the solute is suspended and not dissolved, such as gelatin or albumin.

s., contrast. Solution containing a radiopaque substance. These solutions are used to facilitate x-ray examination of body cavities.

s., hyperbaric. Solution with a specific gravity greater than one, or greater than the solution to which it is being compared. This is important in injecting medicines or anesthetic agents into the spinal fluid in the spinal canal.

s., hypertonic. Solution having a greater osmotic pressure than that of cells or body fluids; a solution that draws water out of cells, thus inducing plasmolysis.

Ex.: A concentrated solution of sodium chloride.

s., hypotonic. Solution having an osmotic pressure less than that of cells or body fluids; a solution that will cause water to enter cells, thus inducing turgor and possibly hemolysis.

Ex.: A sodium chloride solution containing less than 0.9 gm of NaCl in each 100 ml of water.

s., iodine. Solution of iodine and potassium iodine used as a source of iodine.

s., isobaric. Solution with a specific gravity equal to one or equal to the solution with which it is being compared. SEE: *s., hyperbaric.*

s., isohydric. Solution having the same hydrogen ion concentration or pH as another.

s., isosmotic. Solution with the same osmotic pressure as the solution with which it is being compared.

s., isotonic. Solution that has the same osmotic pressure as that of body cells or fluids.

Ex.: A sodium chloride solution containing 0.9 gm of NaCl in each 100 ml of water.

s., Locke-Ringer's. A buffered isotonic solution containing 9.0 gm sodium chloride, 0.42 gm potassium chloride, 0.24 gm calcium chloride, 0.5 gm sodium bicarbonate, 0.2 gm magnesium chloride, 0.5 gm dextrose, and distilled water to make 1000 ml.

s., molar. Solution containing a gram molecular weight or mole of the reagent dissolved in one liter (1000 ml) of solution. Designated 1M.

s., normal. Solution containing one gram equivalent weight of reagent in one liter (1000 ml) of solution. Designated 1N.

s., normal saline. An isotonic saline solution. SEE: *s., isotonic.*

s., ophthalmic. A sterile preparation suitable for instillation in the eye.

s., physiological saline. An isotonic solution of sodium chloride. SEE: *s., isotonic.*

s., repair. Any solution given intravenously to treat an electrolyte or metabolic disturbance.

s., Ringer's. Solution containing chlorides of sodium, calcium, and potassium. It contains 8.6 gm sodium chloride, 0.3 gm calcium chloride, 0.3 gm potassium chloride, and sufficient distilled water to make one liter (1000 ml).

s., saline. Solution of a salt, usually sodium chloride.

s., saturated. Solution containing all the solute it can dissolve. This limit is called the saturation point.

s., sclerosing. An irritating substance that produces sclerosis when applied to tissues or injected into a vein.

s., seminormal. ABBR: 0.5N or N/2. A

solution containing one-half of a gram equivalent weight of reagent in one liter (1000 ml) of solution.

   s., standard. Solution containing a definite amount of a substance as a normal solution. Used for comparison or analysis.

   s., supersaturation. Solution in which the saturation point is reached, but when heated, it is possible to dissolve more of the solute.

   s., test. A reagent solution, one used in performing a particular test.

   s., Tyrode's. A modified Ringer's solution containing, in addition, a small amount of magnesium chloride and acid and sodium phosphates.

   s., volumetric. A standard solution containing a definite amount of a substance in one liter (1000 ml) of solution. Used in volumetric analysis.

solv. L. *solve*, dissolve.

solvate (sŏl'vāt). A compound formed by reaction between solvent and solute.

solvation (sŏl-vā'shŭn). The formation of a solvate.

solvent (sŏl'vĕnt) [L. *solvens*]. 1. Producing a solution, dissolving. 2. A liquid holding another substance in solution. 3. A liquid that reacts with a solvent bringing it into solution.

solvent abuse. SEE: *glue sniffing.*

solvolysis (sŏl-vŏl'ĭ-sĭs). General term for reactions involving decomposition by hydrolysis, ammonolysis, and sulfolysis.

Soma. Trade name for carisoprodol.

soma (sō'mă) [Gr. *soma*, body]. 1. The body as distinct from the mind. 2. All of the body cells except the germ cells. 3. The body exclusive of the extremities.

soman. Pinacolyl methylphosphonofluoridate. An extremely toxic "nerve gas."

somasthenia (sōm″ăs-thē'nē-ă) [″ + *astheneia*, weakness]. A condition of chronic bodily weakness. SYN: *somatasthenia.*

somat(o)- (sō'mă-tō) [Gr. *soma*, body]. Combining form indicating a relationship to the body.

somatasthenia (sō″măt-ăs-thē'nē-ă). Chronic bodily weakness usually with low blood pressure, but not neurasthenia. SYN: *somasthenia.*

somatesthesia (sō″măt-ĕs-thē'zē-ă) [″ + *aisthesis*, sensation]. The consciousness of the body; bodily sensation.

somatic (sō-măt'ĭk) [Gr. *soma*, body]. 1. Pert. to nonreproductive cells or tissues. 2. Pert. to the body. 3. Pert. to structures of the body wall, e.g., skeletal muscles (somatic musculature) in contrast to structures associated with the viscera, e.g., visceral muscles (splanchnic musculature).

somaticosplanchnic (sō-măt″ĭ-kōsplănk′nĭk) [″ + *splanchnikos*, pert. to the viscera]. Somaticovisceral, q.v.

somaticovisceral (sō-măt″ĭ-kō-vĭs'ĕr-ăl) [″ + L. *viscera*, body organs]. Concerning the body and the viscera.

somatist (sō'mă-tĭst) [Gr. *soma*, body]. One who believes mental disorders have an organic basis.

somatization (sō″mă-tī-zā'shŭn). The process of expressing a mental condition as a disturbed bodily function.

somatization disorder. Condition of recurrent and multiple somatic complaints of several years' duration for which medical attention has been sought but no physical basis for the disorder has been found. The age of onset is usually prior to 30. The somatic complaints may be related to virtually any organ system.

somatoceptors (sō-măt″ō-sĕp'tors). Term applied to proprioceptors and exteroceptors collectively.

somatochrome (sō-măt'ō-krōm) [″ + *chroma*, color]. A nerve cell in which the nucleus is completely surrounded by cytoplasm.

somatocrinin. Growth hormone-releasing factor.

somatoform disorders. A group of disorders in which there are symptoms of a disease but no evidence of a physical disorder to explain the symptoms. Included are *body dysmorphic disorder*, in which there is preoccupation with some imagined defect in physical appearance; *conversion disorder*, in which psychological factors are thought to be related to an alteration in or loss of physical functioning due to a physical disorder; *hypochondriasis*, q.v.; and *psychogenic pain disorder*, characterized by preoccupation with pain that cannot be attributed to any other mental or physical disorder. Patients are noted for continually seeking another medical opinion for vague complaints. As a result, they may receive a great variety of medicines or have multiple surgical procedures, none of which affect the course of their disorder.

   TREAT: Repeated reassurance that the disorder is benign. Patient should be seen by as few health care professionals as possible in order to prevent needless repetition of tests and prescriptions for drugs.

somatogenic (sō″mă-tō-jĕn'ĭk) [″ + *gennan*, to produce]. Originating in the body. SEE: *psychogenic.*

somatology (sō″mă-tŏl'ō-jē) [″ + *logos*, word, reason]. Comparative study of structure, functions, and development of the human body.

somatome (sō'mă-tōm) [″ + *tome*, incision]. 1. A device for cutting the body of the fetus. 2. A somite.

somatomedin. ABBR: SM. *somatotropin-mediating.* A group of insulin-like growth factors, somatomedin C and somatomedin A, that require growth hormone in order to exert their function of stimulating growth. These proteins are produced in the liver and other tissues.

somatomegaly (sō″mă-tō-mĕg′ă-lē) [″ + *megas,* large]. Abnormally large size of the body.

somatometry (sō″mă-tŏm′ĕ-trē) [″ + *metron,* measure]. Measurement of the body.

somatopagus (sō″mă-tŏp′ă-gŭs) [″ + *pagos,* thing fixed]. A deformed twin fetus with the trunks merged.

somatopathic (sō″mă-tō-păth′ĭk) [″ + *pathos,* disease, suffering]. Organically ill, as distinguished from neuropathic or psychopathic diseases.

somatoplasm (sō-măt′ō-plăzm) [Gr. *soma,* body, + LL. *plasma,* form, mold]. The protoplasm of all the body cells as distinguished from that of the germ plasm.

somatopleural (sō″mă-tō-ploor′ăl). Concerning somatopleure.

somatopleure (sō-măt′ō-ploor) [″ + *pleura,* side]. The lateral and ventral body wall of an embryo, consisting of the outer ectoderm and a layer of somatic mesoderm underlying it. It continues beyond the embryo as the amnion and chorion.

somatopsychic (sō″măt-ō-sī′kĭk) [″ + *psyche,* mind]. Pert. to both body and mind.

somatopsychosis (sō″mă-tō-sī-kō′sĭs) [″ + ″ + *osis,* condition]. Any mental disorder that is a symptom of a bodily disease.

somatoschisis (sō″mă-tŏs′kĭ-sĭs) [″ + *schistos,* a splitting]. A deformed fetus with a cleft in the trunk.

somatoscopy (sō-mă-tŏs′kō-pē) [″ + *skopein,* to examine]. Physical examination of the body.

somatosensory evoked responses. ABBR: SER. Responses produced by small, painless electrical stimuli administered to large sensory fibers in mixed nerves of the hand or leg. The electroencephalographic record of the character of the subsequent waves produced help to determine the functional state of the nerves involved. SEE: *brain stem auditory evoked responses; evoked responses; visual evoked responses.*

somatosexual (sō″mă-tō-sĕks′ū-ăl) [″ + L. *sexus,* sex]. Concerning the body and sexual characteristics.

somatostatin (sō-măt′ō-stăt″ĭn). A hormone that inhibits the release of somatotropin. It is a hypothalamic peptide that also inhibits the secretion of insulin and gastrin. This hormone also inhibits the target tissues of

the hormones it inhibits. It has been used experimentally to inhibit hormone production by tumors. SYN: *somatotropin release-inhibitory factor (SRIF).*

somatotonia (sō″mă-tō-tō′nē-ă) [″ + L. *tonus,* a stretching]. A personality type, described by the anthropologist Sheldon, in which there is a predominance of physical assertiveness and activity.

somatotopic (sō″mă-tō-tŏp′ĭk) [″ + *topos,* place]. Concerning the correspondence between a particular part of the body and a particular area of the brain.

somatotrophic (sō″mă-tō-trŏf′ĭk) [″ + *tropos,* a turning]. 1. Having selective attraction for or influence on body cells. 2. Stimulating growth.

somatotrophin (sō″mă-tō-trō′fĭn) [″ + *trophe,* nourishment]. Growth hormone, somatotropin.

somatotropic (sō″mă-tō-trŏp′ĭk) [″ + *trope,* a turn]. Influencing the body or body cells.

somatotropin (sō″măt-ō-trō′pĭn) [″ + *tropos,* a turning]. The anterior pituitary lobe's growth-stimulating principle. In the human, this is called human growth hormone (HGH).

     s., bovine. A hormone used to increase milk production in cows. Its use is controversial.

somatotype (sō-măt′ō-tīp). A particular build or type of body, based on physical characteristics. SEE: *ectomorph; endomorph; mesomorph.*

Sombulex. Trade name for hexobarbital.

somesthesia (sŏm-ĕs-thē′sē-ă) [″ + *aisthesis,* sensation]. Awareness of bodily sensations. SYN: *somatesthesia.*

somesthetic (sō-mĕs-thĕt′ĭk). Pert. to sensations and sensory structures of the body.

somesthetic area. The region in the cortex in which the terminations of the axons of general sensory conduction paths.

somesthetic path. General sensory conduction path leading to the cortex.

somite (sō′mīt) [Gr. *soma,* body]. Embryonic blocklike segment formed on either side of the neural tube and its underlying notochord. Each somite gives rise to a muscle mass supplied by a spinal nerve and each pair gives rise to a vertebra.

somnambulance (sŏm-năm′bū-lăns) [L. *somnus,* sleep, + *ambulare,* to walk]. Somnambulism.

somnambule. A person who walks while asleep.

somnambulism (sŏm-năm′bū-lĭzm) [L. *somnus,* sleep, + *ambulare,* to walk]. Sleepwalking, an affection that prompts the sleeping person to perform, unconsciously, acts that naturally belong to the waking state.

somnambulist (sŏm-năm′bū-lĭst). One who is subject to sleepwalking.

somnifacient (sŏm-nĭ-fā′shĕnt) [″ + *facere*, to make]. 1. Producing sleep. SYN: *hypnotic*. 2. A medicine producing sleep. SYN: *soporific*.

somniferous (sŏm-nĭf′ĕr-ŭs) [″ + *ferre*, to bear]. Sleep-producing; pert. to that which promotes sleep.

somnific (sŏm-nĭf′ĭk). Producing sleep.

somniloquence (sŏm-nĭl′ō-kwĕns) [″ + *loqui*, to speak]. Somniloquism, q.v.

somniloquism (sŏm-nĭl′ō-kwĭzm) [″ + ″ + *-ismos*, condition]. Talking in one's sleep.

somniloquist (sŏm-nĭl′ō-kwĭst) [″ + *loqui*, to speak]. One who talks in his or her sleep.

somniloquy (sŏm-nĭl′ō-kwē) [″ + *loqui*, to speak]. Act of talking during sleep or in a hypnotic condition.

somnolence (sŏm′nō-lĕns) [L. *somnolentia*, sleepiness]. Prolonged drowsiness or a condition resembling trance that may continue for a number of days; sleepiness.

somnolent (sŏm″nō-lĕnt) [L. *somnolentus*]. Sleepy; drowsy.

somnolentia (sŏm″nō-lĕn′shē-ă) [L.]. 1. Drowsiness. 2. The sleep of drunkenness in which the faculties are only partially depressed.

somnolism (sŏm′nō-lĭzm) [″ + *-ismos*, condition]. Condition of being in a hypnotic trance.

Somogyi phenomenon [Michael Somogyi, U.S. biochemist, 1883–1971]. In diabetes mellitus, rebound hyperglycemia following an episode of hypoglycemia due to counter regulatory hormone release. Reduction of insulin dose will help control this condition. SEE: *dawn phenomenon; diabetes mellitus*.

Somophyllin-CRT. Trade name for theophylline.

sone (sōn) [L. *sonus*, sound]. A unit of loudness; the loudness of a pure tone of 1000 cycles per second, 40 decibels above the listener's threshold of audibility.

sonic [L. *sonus*, sound]. Pertaining to sound.

sonicate (sŏn′ĭ-kāt) [L. *sonus*, sound]. To expose to sound waves.

sonication (sŏn″ĭ-kā′shŭn). Exposure to high-frequency sound waves. Used to destroy bacteria.

sonic boom (sŏn′ĭk) [L. *sonus*, sound]. Noise caused by shock waves from an airborne object traveling at a speed in excess of the speed of sound. When the waves hit the ground, they may break windows and also affect the hearing.

sonogram (sō′nō-grăm) [L. *sonus*, sound, + Gr. *gramma*, something written]. The record obtained by use of ultrasonography.

sonographer. Technologist trained in the application of ultrasound for diagnostic and therapeutic purposes.

    s., diagnostic medical. One who provides patient services for those using diagnostic ultrasound under the supervision of a doctor of medicine or osteopathy.

sonography (sō-nŏg′ră-fē) [″ + Gr. *graphein*, to write]. Ultrasonography.

sonolucent (sō″nō-loo′sĕnt). In ultrasonography, the condition of not reflecting the ultrasound waves back to their source.

sonometer (sō-nŏm′ĕ-tĕr) [″ + Gr. *metron*, a measure]. Device to cause sound for production of anesthesia; used by dentists.

sonorous (sō-nō′rŭs) [L.]. Giving forth a loud and rounded sound.

sonorous rale. A dry or low-pitched rale often caused by vibration of mucous secretion in a bronchus.

sophistication (sō-fĭs″tĭ-kā′shŭn) [Gr. *sophistikos*, deceitful]. In medicine, the adulteration of any substance.

sophomania (sŏf″ō-mā′nē-ă) [Gr. *sophos*, wise, + *mania*, madness]. Unrealistic belief in one's own wisdom.

sopor (sō′por) [L.]. Deep, lethargic sleep. SYN: *stupor*.

soporiferous (sō″pō-rĭf′ĕr-ŭs) [″ + *ferre*, to bring]. Promoting sleep.

soporific (sō-pō-rĭf′ĭk) [″ + *facere*, to make]. 1. Inducing sleep. 2. Narcotic; a drug producing sleep.

soporose, soporous (sō′por-ōs, -ŭs) [L.]. Marked by or resembling sound sleep or coma.

sorbefacient (sor″bē-fā′shĕnt) [L. *sorbere*, to suck up, + *facere*, to make]. Causing or that which causes or promotes absorption.

sorbitol. $C_6H_{14}O_6$. A crystalline alcohol present in some berries and fruits. It is used as a sweetening agent and as an excipient in formulating tablets.

sorcery. The invoking of the force of evil spirits, magic, or witchcraft by a person to influence negatively the health and happiness of another person. The person against whom the force is directed may become seriously ill or even die even though there is no physical evidence of disease. SEE: *voodoo*.

sordes (sor′dēz) [L. *sordere*, to be dirty]. Foul brown crusts or accumulations on the teeth and about the lips from foul stomach or secretions of the mouth in mild fever.

    NURSING IMPLICATIONS: Prevent development with frequent oral hygiene for mouth breathers, patients who are unable to take or are not permitted oral fluids, and debilitated persons, evaluating patient response. A hydrogen peroxide mouthwash (one part hydrogen peroxide to three parts water) or glycerin applied with a soft brush or sponge stick (toothette) may be used to remove crusts. Always follow either treatment by rinsing with clear water (mouthwashes are astringent, and glycerin is drying to mucous membranes). Encourage oral intake if permitted, and position patient to discourage mouth-breathing. Provide water mist or spray for patient use in moistening membranes if fluids are restricted.

sore (sor) [AS. *sar*, sore]. 1. Tender; painful. 2. Any type of tender or painful ulcer or lesion of the skin or mucous membrane.

    s., bed. Gangrene of skin due to pressure. For detailed description, SEE: *bedsore*. SYN: *decubitus; pressure ulcer or sore.*

    s., canker. A small lesion of the mucous membrane of the mouth. Often accompanies a number of systemic conditions. Cause is unknown. SEE: *stomatitis, aphthous.*

    s., cold. Blister on the lips. SEE: *herpes simplex.*

    s., Delhi. Cutaneous leishmaniasis.

    s., desert. An ulcer of the skin associated with being in the desert.

    s., hard. Syphilitic chancre, q.v., primary lesion of syphilis.

    s., Oriental. Cutaneous leishmaniasis.

    s., pressure. A bedsore.

    s., soft venereal. Soft nonsyphilitic venereal sore occurring on the genitalia. SYN: *chancroid; s., venereal.*

    s., tropical. S., Oriental.

    s., venereal. S., soft venereal.

sore throat. Any inflammation of the tonsils, pharynx, or larynx.

    s.t., diphtheritic. Croupous tonsillitis.

    s.t., quinsy. Peritonsillar abscess. SEE: *quinsy.*

    s.t., septic. Severe, epidemic, pseudomembranous inflammation of fauces and tonsils caused by the hemolytic streptococcus.

    s.t., streptococcal. SEE: *scarlet fever.*

soroche (sō-rō'chā) [Sp.]. Mountain sickness, esp. that occurring in the Andes.

sororiation (sō-ror-ē-ā'shŭn) [L. *sororiare*, to increase together]. Growth of the breasts at puberty.

sorption (sorp'shŭn) [L. *sorbere*, to suck in]. The condition of being absorbed.

s.o.s. L. *si opus sit*, if necessary or required.

sotalol hydrochloride (sō'tă-lōl). An anti-adrenergic medicine.

soterenol hydrochloride (sō'tĕr'ĕ-nōl). An adrenergic medicine used as a bronchodilator.

souffle (soof'fl) [Fr. *souffler*, to puff]. A soft blowing sound heard in auscultation; a bruit; an auscultatory murmur.

    s., cardiac. Heart murmur.

    s., fetal. The soft blowing sound heard over the location of the umbilical cord of the fetus in utero and synchronous with the fetal heartbeat during late pregnancy. SYN: *s., funic.*

    s., funic. S., fetal.

    s., placental. SEE: *placental souffle.*

    s., splenic. Sound heard over spleen in malaria.

    s., uterine. Sound caused by blood entering dilated arteries of the uterus in last months of pregnancy; synchronous with maternal pulse. It is more frequent than the fetal souffle and is heard as a loud blowing murmur along left side of uterus, and frequently all over it. An enlarged uterus may cause it. That of pregnancy is variable, whereas other forms are constant.

sound (sownd) [L. *sonus*, sound]. 1. Auditory sensations produced by vibrations; noise. It is measured in decibels, which is the logarithm of the intensity of sound; thus 20 d. represents not twice 10 d., but ten times as much. Exposure to excessively loud noises, esp. in certain frequencies, if repeated will cause permanent injury to the hearing. SEE: *decibel; noise; sonic boom.* 2. A form of vibrational energy that gives rise to auditory sensations. SEE: *cochlea; ear; organ of Corti; sonic boom.* 3. Healthy, not diseased. 4. Heart sounds. SEE: *diastole; systole.* 5. [Fr. *sonder*, to probe] Instrument for introduction into a cavity or canal for exploration. SYN: *searcher.*

    s., anasarcous. Moist sound heard on auscultation when skin is edematous.

    s., blowing. Organic murmur as of air from an aperture expelled with moderate force.

    s., bottle. Noise as of fluid in a bottle. SEE: *amphoric.*

    s.'s, breath. Respiratory sounds heard on auscultation of the chest. In a normal chest, they are classified as vesicular, tracheal, and bronchovesicular.

    s., bronchial. Sound not heard in normal lung but occurring in pulmonary disease, indicating infiltration and solidification of lung.

    s.'s, bronchovesicular. A mixture of bronchial and vesicular sounds.

    s., cracked-pot. A tympanic resonance heard over pulmonary cavities.

    s., ejection. High-pitched clicking sound heard just after the first heart sound.

    s., fetal heart. Sound made by the fetal heart.

    s., friction. Sound produced by rubbing together two inflamed mucous surfaces.

    s.'s, heart. The two sounds "lubb" and "dupp" resulting from closure of atrial, pulmonic, mitral, and tricuspid valves. Third and fourth heart sounds may be present in some conditions. SEE: *heart.*

s.'s, Korotkoff's. SEE: *Korotkoff's sounds.*

s., percussion. SEE: *percussion.*

s.'s, physiological. Sound perceived when the auditory canals are closed. The sound is produced by the blood flowing through adjacent vessels.

s., respiratory. Any sound heard over the lungs, bronchi, or trachea.

s., succussion. Splashing sound heard over a cavity with fluid in it.

s., to-and-fro. Rasping friction sounds of pericarditis.

s., tracheal. Sound normally heard over the trachea or larynx.

s., tubular. Sound heard over the trachea or large bronchi.

s., urethral. A device suitable for use in exploring the urethra.

s., vesicular. Sound heard over the entire lung during inspiration resulting from distention of alveoli with air.

s., white. Sound made up of all audible frequencies.

sound, words pert. to: amphoric; aspirate; auscultation; capotement; clang; clapotage; heart; hyperacusis; murmur; rale; resonance; souffle; stridulous; succussion.

Souques' phenomenon [A. A. Souques, Fr. neurologist, 1860–1944]. Finger extension on the involved side of a hemiplegic patient when the extremity is raised to a position above 90° of shoulder flexion or abduction.

source-skin distance. In radiation therapy, the distance from the radiation source to the skin of the patient.

source-to-image receptor distance. ABBR: SID. In radiography, the distance from the x-ray tube to the radiographic film or the image digitizer.

soybean oil. USP. The refined oil obtained from seeds of the soya plant.

sp. L. *spiritus*, spirit; *species.*

spa (spä) [Spa, a Belgium resort town]. A mineral spring, esp. one allegedly having healing properties.

space (spās) [L. *spatium*, space]. 1. An area, region, or segment. 2. A cavity of the body. SYN: *spatium* [NA]. 3. The expanse in which the solar system, stars, and galaxies exist; outside the Earth's atmosphere.

s., anatomical dead. The area in the trachea, bronchi, and air passages containing air that does not reach the alveoli during respiration. Certain lung diseases, such as chronic obstructive pulmonary disease (emphysema), increase the amount of this dead space, thereby decreasing the effectiveness of respiration. SEE: *s., physiological dead.*

s., axillary. The axilla or space beneath the arm.

s., circumlental. Space between the equator of the lens and the ciliary body.

s., dead. 1. In respiratory physiology, the space between the nose and bronchioles that does not exchange oxygen and carbon dioxide. 2. Unobliterated space remaining after closure of a surgical wound. This space favors the accumulation of blood, and eventually infection.

s., epidural. Space between the dura mater and vertebral periosteum, or between the bones of the cranium and the dura mater, assumed to be lymph spaces.

s., extracellular. The space between cells. It contains fluid derived from plasma in the adjacent capillaries. The fluid flows back and forth from capillaries to cells. SEE: *extracellular fluid.*

s., intercostal. The interval between ribs.

s., interfascial. S., Tenon's.

s., interpleural. The mediastinum.

s., interproximal. Space between the surfaces of adjacent teeth in the dental arch; it is divided into the septal space, gingival to the contact point of the teeth and occupied normally by the interdental papilla of the gingiva, and the embrasure, the space occlusal to the contact point of the teeth.

s., interradicular. The area between the roots of a multirooted tooth, which contains an alveolar bony septum and the periodontal ligament.

s., intervillous. Space in the placenta that develops from early chorionic trophoblast. It forms a blood sinus in which chorionic villi of fetus are bathed in maternal blood received from uterine vessels.

s., lymph. Any space occupied by lymph tissue.

s., Meckel's. Cavum trigeminale, q.v.

s., mediastinal. The mediastinum.

s., medullary. The marrow-containing area of cancellous bone.

s., Nuel's. Space between outer hair cells and rods in the organ of Corti.

s.'s of Fontana. Spaces in scleral meshwork in angle of the iris through which aqueous humor passes from the anterior chamber to the canal of Schlemm.

s., palmar. The mid-palmar and thenar spaces of the hand.

s.'s, parasinoidal. Lateral spaces in the dura mater adjacent to the superior sagittal sinus that receive meningeal and diploic veins.

s., perforated. Space pierced by blood vessels at base of brain. SYN: *substantia perforata.*

s.'s, perivascular. Spaces within adventitia of larger blood vessels of the brain. They communicate with subarachnoid space.

s., personal. In psychiatry, an individual's personal area and the surrounding space. This space is important in interpersonal relations.

s., physiological dead. In the respiratory tract, the air in the alveoli not exposed to the capillary walls, plus the air in the anatomical dead space. SEE: *s., anatomical dead.*

s., plantar. One of four spaces between the fascial layers of the foot. When the foot is infected, pus may be found there.

s., pneumatic. Air-containing spaces in bone, esp. those in the paranasal sinuses.

s., popliteal. Space in back of the knee joint, containing the popliteal artery and vein and small sciatic and popliteal nerves.

s., prezonular. The anterior portion of the posterior chamber of the eye.

s., Prussak's. Space in tympanum behind Shrapnell's membrane.

s., retroperitoneal. The potential space outside the parietal peritoneum of the abdominal cavity.

s., retropharyngeal. Space behind pharynx separating prevertebral from visceral fascia. Important in dentistry as a possible path for the spread of infection from oral cavity trauma downward to visceral organs of the mediastinum. SYN: *retropharyngeal fascial cleft.*

s.'s, subarachnoid. Spaces between the pia mater and arachnoid containing the cerebrospinal fluid. The spaces, esp. in the cranium, are traversed by numerous trabeculae.

s., subdural. Narrow space between the dura and the arachnoid.

s., subphrenic. Space between the diaphragm and the abdominal organs.

s., suprasternal. Triangular space immediately above the sternum between layers of deep cervical fascia.

s., Tenon's. Lymph space between the sclera and Tenon's capsule. SYN: *s., interfascial.*

s., thenar. A deep fascial space in the hand lying anterior to the adductor pollicis muscle.

s., tissue. Any space within tissues not lined with epithelium and containing tissue fluid.

s.'s, zonular. Spaces within the zonule (suspensory ligament of lens).

space maintainer. An appliance placed within the dental arch to prevent adjacent teeth from moving into the space left by a missing tooth; it is a temporary placement until the permanent tooth erupts into the space, or until a bridge is placed to replace the missing permanent tooth.

space medicine. Branch of medical science concerned with the physiological and pathological problems encountered by humans who enter the area beyond the Earth's atmosphere. Included in space medicine are investigation of effects of weightlessness (zero gravity), sensory deprivation, motion sickness, enforced inactivity during lengthy travels in space, and the heat and decelerative forces encountered at the time of reentry into the Earth's atmosphere. SEE: *aerospace medicine.*

space sickness. A transient form of physiological vertigo encountered when the head is actively moved in a weightless environment. It may be accompanied by general malaise and nausea, with or without vomiting. The condition resembles seasickness but may or may not occur in individuals who normally experience that disorder and, conversely, may occur in persons known to be resistant to seasickness.

spallation (spawl-lā'shŭn). 1. The process of breaking into very small parts. The term may be applied to gross structures or to atomic particles. 2. The release of inert particles into the bloodstream. An example would be splintering of bits of plastic from the pump used in hemodialysis.

span. The distance from one fixed point to another, as the distance, when the hand is fully expanded, from the tip of the thumb to the tip of the little finger. Each individual should know that measurement of his or her own hand so that it may be used in estimating the length or size of objects.

Spanish fly. A strong rubefacient and blistering agent produced from these beetles. Believed by laymen to be an aphrodisiac, which it is not. SYN: *cantharides.*

sparer (spăr'ĕr) [AS. *sparian*, to refrain]. A substance destroyed by catabolism but that, nevertheless, decreases catabolic action upon other substances.

s.'s, protein. Carbohydrates and fats, so designated because their presence in diet prevents tissue proteins from being utilized as a source of energy.

sparganosis (spăr″gă-nō'sĭs). Infestation with a variety of Sparganum.

Sparganum (spăr'gă-nŭm) [Gr. *sparganon,* swathing band] (pl. *spargana*). The plerocercoid larva of tapeworms, esp. those of the genus *Diphyllobothrium.*

S. mansoni. An elongated plerocercoid species, 3 to 14 in. (7.6 to 35 cm) in length, found in muscles and connective tissue, esp. that around the eye. Common in the Far East.

S. mansonoides. Species occasionally occurring in U.S. The adult form is unknown.

S. proliferum. Minute species infesting

humans and producing acnelike nodules. It is thought to proliferate by means of budlike outgrowths.

sparge (spărj) [L. *spargere*, to scatter]. To introduce air or gas into a liquid.

spargosis (spär-gō'sĭs) [Gr. *spargosis*, swelling]. 1. Distention of the female breasts with milk. 2. Swelling or thickening of the skin. SYN: *elephantiasis.*

Sparine. Trade name for promazine hydrochloride.

spark coil. Coil consisting of primary and secondary coils with an interrupted current passing through them.

spark gap. 1. Arrangement of opposed points or surfaces between which an electric spark may jump. 2. An adjustable gap between needle points or between spheres used to measure high potentials.

> **s.g., quenched.** A multiple spark gap with numerous electrodes about 0.3 mm apart and equipped with a copper air-cooling device.

spasm (spăzm) [Gr. *spasmos*, convulsion]. An involuntary sudden movement or muscular contraction which occurs as a result of some irritant or trauma. Spasms may be clonic (characterized by alternate contraction and relaxation) or tonic (sustained). They may involve either visceral (smooth) muscle or skeletal (striated) muscle. When contractions are strong and painful, they are called cramps. The effect depends upon the part affected. Asthma is assumed to be due to spasm of muscular coats of smaller bronchi; renal colic to spasm of muscular coat of the ureter.

TREAT: General measures to reduce tension, induce muscle relaxation, and improve circulation. Specific measures include analgesics, massage, relaxation exercises, therapeutic modalities such as heat, cold, or electrotherapy, and, in some cases, gentle therapeutic exercises. Special orthopedic supports or braces are sometimes effective. For vascular spasm, chemical sympathectomy may give relief.

> **s., Bell's.** Convulsive tic of the face.
>
> **s., bronchial.** Contraction of the muscle fibers around bronchial tubes. This occurs in asthma.
>
> **s., choreiform.** Spasmodic movements resembling chorea.
>
> **s., clonic.** Intermittent contractions and relaxation of muscles.
>
> **s., diffuse.** Esophageal motor disorder characterized by dysphagia, odynophagia, and chest pain.
>
> **s., habit.** A habitual movement that some people develop. It may persist unchanged throughout life. Included are sniffing, clearing the throat, moving the neck as

if relieving collar tension, scratching or rubbing the skin in one place. These movements are voluntary but difficult for the individual to suppress. SEE: *peotillomania; trichotillomania.*

> **s., nodding.** A psychogenic condition in adults, causing nodding of the head from clonic spasms of the sternomastoid muscles. A similar nodding in babies with head turning from side to side.
>
> **s. of esophagus.** Paroxysmal dysphagia (inability to swallow), often associated with a sense of constriction in the chest. Characterized by intense dyspnea and occurs in spasmodic croup, true croup, ulceration of larynx, laryngismus stridulus, whooping cough, tetany, hysteria, hydrophobia, laryngeal crises of locomotor ataxia, when foreign bodies have lodged in larynx, and when aneurysms or mediastinal tumors press on the recurrent laryngeal nerve and irritate it.
>
> TREAT: Search for exciting cause and remove. Treatment largely dietetic, hygienic, and psychologic. Dilation by passage of a bougie may be of great value.
>
> PROG: Indefinite regarding duration, not threatening to life.
>
> **s., saltatory.** Term employed to designate a condition allied to hysteria in which a violent spasm seizes the muscles of the leg as soon as the feet touch the ground and, as a result, patient is thrown violently in the air.
>
> **s., tetanic.** Spasm in which contractions continue for a time without interruption.
>
> **s., tonic.** Continued involuntary contractions.
>
> **s., torsion.** Spasm characterized by a turning of a part, esp. the turning of the body at the pelvis.
>
> **s., toxic.** Convulsions due to poison.
>
> **s., winking.** Spasm of the muscles of the eyelids; may be unilateral. SYN: *blepharospasm.*

spasm, words pert. to: campospasm; cardiospasm; carpopedal; chirospasm; Chvostek's sign; clonic; clonospasm; clonus; face; habit; hypertonus; mobile; Raynaud's disease; spasticity; tetanus; tetany; tic douloureux; tonic spasm; torticollis; trismus; vaginismus.

spasmatic (spăz-măt'ĭk) [Gr. *spasmos*, convulsion]. Pert. to, like, or marked by spasm. SYN: *spasmodic.*

spasmatic asthma. Asthma caused by spasm of the bronchioles.

spasmatic croup. Laryngismus stridulus.

spasmatic stricture. Temporary narrowing of any canal, as the urethra, due to localized spasmodic muscular contraction of its coat.

spasmodic (spăz-mŏd'ĭk) [Gr. *spasmos*, convulsion]. Concerning spasms.

spasmogen (spăz'mō-jĕn) [" + *gennan*, to produce]. Something that causes spasms.

spasmology (spăz-mŏl'ō-jē) [" + *logos*, word, reason]. The study of spasms, their nature and cause.

spasmolygmus (spăz-mō-līg'mŭs) [" + *lygmos*, a sob]. 1. Spasmodic hiccup. 2. Spasmodic sobbing.

spasmolysin (spăz-mŏl'ĭ-sĭn). Something that abolishes spasms.

spasmolytic (spăz-mō-lĭt'ĭk) [" + *lysis*, dissolution]. Arresting spasms or that which acts as an antispasmodic.

spasmophemia (spăz-mō-fē'mē-ă) [" + *pheme*, speech]. A spasmodic disorder of speech. SYN: *stuttering.*

spasmophilia (spăz-mō-fĭl'ē-ă) [" + *philein*, to love]. A tendency to tetany and convulsions; almost always associated with rickets.

spasmous (spăz'mŭs) [Gr. *spasmos*, convulsion]. Of the nature of a spasm.

spasmus (spăz'mŭs) [Gr. *spasmos*, convulsion]. A spasm.

   s. agitans. Paralysis agitans.

   s. bronchialis. Bronchial asthma.

   s. caninus. Spasm of face causing a constant grin. SYN: *risus sardonicus.*

   s. coordinatus. Imitative or compulsive movements, as mimic tics or festination.

   s. cynicus. Spasmodic contraction of muscles on both sides of the mouth.

   s. Dubini. Rhythmic contractions, in rapid succession, of a group or groups of muscles, starting at an extremity or half of the face, and covering a large part or all of the body. Usually fatal.

   s. glottidis. Spasm of larynx. SYN: *laryngismus stridulus.*

   s. nictitans. A winking movement of the eyelid. SYM: *blepharospasm.*

   s. nutans. Nodding spasm in infants and young children. The eyes are also involved as manifested by rapid, pendular nystagmoid movements that may be observed in one eye. Spontaneous improvement always occurs.

spastic (spăs'tĭk) [Gr. *spastikos*, convulsive]. 1. Resembling or of the nature of spasms or convulsions. 2. Produced by spasms. 3. One afflicted with spasms.

spastic colon. A syndrome of disordered motility of the small and large intestines accompanied by pain, usually in the lower abdominal area, and constipation alternating with diarrhea. For complete description and treatment, SEE: *colon, irritable.*

spastic gait. A stiff movement of the legs while walking, usually the result of an upper motor neuron lesion and spasticity in the muscles of the lower extremity. There are several variations. Spasticity in the ankle

plantar flexors results in the toes dragging or walking on the toes; spasticity in the hip adductors results in a scissoring or crossing of the legs; spasticity in the quadriceps femoris results in the knee being held rigid. If the upper extremities are involved, the arms do not swing rhythmically but are usually held with the elbows and wrists flexed.

spastic hemiplegia. Spasticity occurring in one half of the body, usually due to a cardiovascular accident or cerebral palsy affecting only half of the brain.

spasticity (spăs-tĭs'ĭ-tē). Increased tone or contractions of muscles causing stiff and awkward movements: the result of upper motor neuron lesion.

spastic paralysis. Muscular rigidity accompanying partial paralysis. Usually due to a lesion involving upper motor neurons.

spastic paraplegia. Paraplegia due to transverse lesions of the cord or sclerosis. Both lower extremities exhibit spasticity.

spatial (spā'shăl). Pertaining to space.

spatial discrimination. Ability to perceive as separate points of contact the two blunt points of a compass when applied to the skin.

spatial localization disorder. Inability to describe or to find the way even though in familiar surroundings. A neurological condition usually due to bilateral occipitoparietal lesions of the brain.

spatial resolution. In radiology, the ability to distinguish two adjacent points of similar density as being separate.

spatium (spā'shē-ŭm) [L.] (pl. *spatia*). [NA] Space.

spatula (spăch'ū-lă) [L. *spatula*, blade]. Instrument for spreading or mixing semisolids. It is usually flat, thin, somewhat flexible, and shaped like a knife but without a cutting edge.

   s., eye. Blades for separating lips of corneal wounds, arresting hemorrhage, or for making pressure; made of sheet metal or rubber.

   s., nasal. Device for holding mucous flaps in place or to guard against burning from cautery.

spatulate (spăch'ū-lāt). To mix something by use of a spatula. In dentistry, to mix or manipulate certain dental materials with a spatula to achieve a uniform, homogenous mass.

spay, spaying (spā, spā'ĭng) [Gael. *spoth*, castrate]. Surgical removal of ovaries, usually said of animals. SEE: *castration.*

SPCA. *Society for the Prevention of Cruelty to Animals.*

specialist (spĕsh'ăl-ĭst) [L. *specialis*]. A dentist, nurse, physician, or other health professional who has advanced education and training in one clinical area of practice such as internal medicine, pediatrics, surgery, ophthalmology, neurology, maternal and child health, or cardiology. In most specialized areas of health care, there are organizations offering qualifying examinations. When an individual meets all of the criteria of such a board, he or she is called "board certified" in that area.

specialization (spĕsh″ăl-ĭ-zā′shŭn). The limitation of one's practice to a particular branch of medicine, surgery, dentistry, or nursing. This is customarily done after having received postgraduate training in the area of specialization.

specialty (spĕsh′ăl-tē). The branch of medicine, surgery, dentistry, or nursing in which a specialist practices.

speciation (spē″sē-ā′shŭn) [L. *species,* a kind]. The evolutionary process by which new species of living organisms are formed.

species (spē′shēz) [L. *species,* a kind]. In biology, a category of classification for living organisms. This group is just below genus and is usually capable of interbreeding.

species-specific. The characteristics of a species, esp. the immunological nature that differentiates that species from another.

species type. The original species that served as the basis for identifying a new genus or subgenus.

specific (spĕ-sĭf′ĭk) [L. *specificus,* pert. to a kind]. 1. A remedy having a curative effect on a particular disease or symptom. 2. Pert. to a species. 3. A disease always caused by the same organism. 4. Restricted, explicit; not generalized.

specific dynamic action. ABBR: SDA. The increase in metabolic rate resulting from absorption of food. For protein it amounts to about 30%, for carbohydrates, 7%, and for fats, 4%. After a general meal the increase would be 10% to 15%. This effect lasts for 4 to 6 hours.

specific gravity. Weight of a substance compared with an equal volume of water. For solid and liquid materials, water is used as a standard and considered to have a specific gravity of one (1.000). For gases, the weight per unit volume is compared with dry air at a specified temperature.

specificity (spĕ-sĭ-fĭs′ĭ-tē). State of being specific; having a relation to a definite result or to a particular cause.

   s., diagnostic. For a diagnostic or screening test, the proportion of people who are truly free of a specific disease and are so identified by the test. SEE: *sensitivity.*

specillum (spĕ-sĭl′lŭm) [L. *specere,* to look] (pl. *specilla*). 1. Lens. 2. Button-shaped silver probe.

specimen (spĕs′ĭ-mĕn) [L. *specere,* to look]. A part of a thing intended to show kind and quality of the whole, as a specimen of urine.

spectacles (spĕk′tăk-lz) [L. *spectare,* to see]. Two lenses supported by a nose bridge and side pieces passing over the ears. Used to aid vision or protect the eyes. SYN: *glasses.*

spectinomycin hydrochloride, sterile. USP. A sterile preparation of the antibiotic spectinomycin hydrochloride. When diluted with the appropriate amount of sterile water for injection, the medicine may be used intramuscularly.

spectral (spĕk′trăl) [L. *spectrum,* image]. Concerning a spectrum.

spectro- [L. *spectrum,* image]. Combining form meaning appearance, image, form, spectrum.

spectrocolorimeter (spĕk-trō-kŭl-or-ĭm′ĕ-tĕr) [″ + *color,* color, + Gr. *metron,* measure]. Device for detecting colorblindness by isolating a single spectral color.

spectrofluorometer (spĕk″trō-floo″or-ŏm′ĕ-tĕr). Instrument for measuring degree of fluorescence.

spectrograph (spĕk′trō-grăf) [″ + Gr. *graphein,* to write]. Instrument designed to photograph spectra on a sensitive photographic plate.

   s., mass. Device that separates ions of different masses by employing a magnetic field to deflect them as they travel along a given path.

spectrometer (spĕk-trŏm′ĕt-ĕr) [″ + Gr. *metron,* measure]. A spectroscope so constructed that angular deviation of a ray of light produced by a prism or by a diffraction grating thus indicates the wavelength.

spectrometry (spĕk-trŏm′ĕ-trē) [″ + Gr. *metron,* measure]. The process of determining the wavelength of light rays by use of a spectrometer.

spectrophotometer (spĕk″trō-fō-tŏm′ĕt-ĕr) [″ + Gr. *photos,* light, + *metron,* measure]. Device for measuring amount of color in a solution by comparison with the spectrum.

spectrophotometry (spĕk″trō-fō-tŏm′ĕt-rē). Estimation of coloring matter in a solution by use of the spectroscope or spectrophotometer.

spectropolarimeter (spĕk″trō-pō″lăr-ĭm′ĕ-tĕr) [″ + *polaris,* pole, + *metron,* measure]. Device for measuring the rotation of light rays of a specific wavelength by passage through a translucent solid.

spectropyrheliometer (spĕk″trō-pīr-hē-lē-ŏm′ĕ-tĕr) [″ + Gr. *pyr,* fire, + *helios,* sun, + *metron,* measure]. Instrument to measure solar radiation.

spectroscope (spĕk′trō-skōp) [″ + Gr. *skopein,* to examine]. An instrument for separating radiant energy into its component frequencies or wavelengths by means of a prism or grating to form a spectrum for inspection.

spectroscopic (spĕk"trō-skŏp'ĭk). Concerning a spectroscope.

spectroscopy (spĕk-trŏs'kō-pē). The branch of physical science that treats the phenomena observed with the spectroscope, or those principles on which the action is based; also, the art of using the spectroscope.

spectrum (spĕk'trŭm) [L., image] (pl. *spectra*). Charted band of wavelengths of electromagnetic vibrations obtained by refraction and diffraction of ray of white light.

  s., absorption. Spectrum recorded after light rays have passed through a substance that is capable of absorbing some of the wavelengths passing through. This spectrum is specific for various chemicals.

  s., broad. A term that refers to antibiotics effective against a variety of microorganisms.

  s., chromatic. That portion of the spectrum that produces visible light. Wavelengths of about 7700 to 3900 angstrom units are visible.

  s., invisible. Spectral portion either below the red (infrared) or above the violet (ultraviolet), which is invisible to the eye, the waves being too long or too short to affect the retina. The invisible spectrum includes rays less than 3900 angstrom units (A.U.) in length (ultraviolet, roentgen or x, gamma, and cosmic rays) and those exceeding 7700 A.U. in length (infrared, high-frequency oscillations used in short- and long-wave diathermy, radio, hertzian, and very long waves). These range in length from 7700 A.U. to 5,000,000 meters.

  s., visible. Portion of spectrum that is visible. The visible spectrum consists of the colors from red to violet with wavelengths of 3900 A.U. to 7700 A.U. When white light is passed through a prism, the various colors, because of different wavelengths, are refracted to various degrees, giving rise to the diverse colors of the rainbow. These are in order from the shortest wavelength to the longest violet, indigo, blue, green, yellow, orange, and red.

  s., visible electromagnetic. The complete range of wavelengths of electromagnetic radiation.

spectrum emission. In spectroscopy and fluorometry, the range of wavelengths emitted by a substance. In the case of atoms, the lines of emission.

speculum (spĕk'ū-lŭm) [L., a mirror] (pl. *specula*). 1. Instrument for examination of canals. 2. Membrane separating anterior cornua of lateral ventricles of brain. SYN: *septum pellucidum*.

  s., bivalve. A speculum with two opposed blades that can be separated or closed. SEE: *s., vaginal*.

  s., duck-bill. A bivalve speculum with wide blades.

  s., ear. Short, funnel-shaped tubes, tubular or bivalve; former preferable.

  s., eye. Device for separating eyelids. Plated steel wire, plain, Von Graefe's, Steven's, and Luer's are most common.

  s., Pedersen. A small vaginal speculum for examining prepubertal patients or others with quite small vaginal orifices.

  s., vaginal. A speculum, usually with two opposing portions that, after being inserted, can be pushed apart, for examining the vagina and cervix.

NOTE: A vaginal speculum should be warmed prior to use.

speech [AS. *spaec*]. 1. Verbal expression of one's thoughts. 2. The act of uttering articulate words or sounds. 3. Words that are spoken.

It is thought that certain crude sounds served as warnings or threats in much the same way as did facial and bodily expressions. As sounds became highly differentiated, each became associated and gradually identified with a certain idea. These word-symbols are a most valuable tool in ideation, and thinking is very largely dependent on this internal speech. Further identifications have made possible visual symbols (written language), though primitive written language was entirely unrelated—a series of pictures and crude representations.

External speech requires the coordination of larynx, mouth, lips, chest, and abdominal muscles. These have no special innervation for speech, but the upper neurons respond to complex motor pattern fields that convert the idea into suitable motor stimuli.

  s., aphonic. Whispering.

  s., ataxic. Defective speech resulting from muscular incoordination usually the result of cerebellar disorder.

  s., clipped. S., scamping.

  s., echo. Parrotlike repetition of words spoken by others. SYN: *echolalia*.

  s., esophageal. In persons who have had laryngectomies, the modulation of air expelled from the esophagus to produce sound that can be used in speech. The mouth, tongue, and pharynx participate in this.

  s., explosive. Sudden loud sounds produced by persons with organic brain disease or mental disorders.

  s., helium. The altered voice produced by inhaling helium and then speaking as the helium is exhaled. The very low density of the helium causes the alteration.

s., interjectional. Speech characterized by inarticulate sounds.

s., mirror. Speech characterized by reversing the order of syllables of a word.

s., scamping. Speech characterized by omission of consonants or syllables when unable to pronounce them. SYN: *s., clipped.*

s., scanning. A staccatolike speech with pauses between syllables.

s., slurring. Slovenly articulation of letters difficult to pronounce.

s., staccato. Slow and labored speech with each syllable pronounced separately, as in multiple sclerosis.

speech, words pert. to: alliteration; alogia; aphasia; aphonia; aphrasia; articulation; bradyarthria; bradylalia; Broca's area; deaf-mute; dyslalia; dyslexia; dysphasia; dysphonia; egophony; monophasia; mute; mutism; onomatomania; onomatopoiesis; perseveration; scanning speech; sign; stammering; stutter; tachyphasia; Wernicke's syndrome.

speech abnormalities. Speech failure results in motor aphasia, in which the patient is speechless but there is no paralysis of muscles of articulation. Although unable to express thoughts in words, the patient can still understand what he or she hears and reads.

Labialism is the excessive use of labial sounds.

Absence of speech or hoarseness may be part of a hysteria.

Word deafness is the condition in which a word is heard but the patient has no idea of its meaning. Similarly, word blindness means that the written symbol might as well be a foreign word. This is sometimes called alexia, q.v. Aphasia, q.v., in right-handed patients is classically referable to left-sided brain lesions, but the concept of centers for internal speech esp. is rather misleading. It is probably a diffuse cortical activity, and countless minor distortions occur in addition to those mentioned. Chief of those not enumerated is the slurring speech of paresis, q.v., in which letters and syllables are omitted without recognition of defect, and this further identifies the abnormality. Dysarthria, q.v., describes any defect of articulation; muscular tone disturbances as seen in cerebellar disease, chorea, paralysis agitans, lenticular degeneration, or multiple sclerosis, producing jerky, monotonous, or scanning speech.

Paralysis due to bilateral medullary pathology results in indistinct enunciation (mouthful speech) often entirely unintelligible. Pseudobulbar palsy (as in cases of double hemiplegia) adds a slow spastic characteristic. Peripheral nerve lesions, cleft palate, adenoids, and myasthenia gravis merely suggest the many possible modifications.

Stammering and stuttering are usually psychogenic.

Emotional values may be added to speech qualities; tremulousness and tension may render the voice high-pitched, irritating, or unsustained and broken. Emotional flattening may occur in the neuroses and psychoses. In the latter, diagnostic changes may occur in the stream of talk.

Slowing is common in all depressed states. When complete (mutism), it suggests the negativism esp. likely to occur in schizophrenia. Aphonic-like aphasia patients will find some means of communication.

Deaf persons may "speak" by using sign language at a slower rate if the normal speech is slow in their geographic area.

Excessive talk is generally seen in mania and excited states. When merely voluble but relevant, it constitutes circumstantiality. If the goal of the speech is lost, it may become a meaningless stream of words.

Neologisms are words created by the patient, often of no apparent significance.

Stereotyped speech is constant repetition of a word or phrase. It should be distinguished from perseveration in which the repetition is against the intention or wishes of the patient.

Amentia, q.v., invariably delays speech appearance and its faulty development is of diagnostic value. The delay or nonappearance of speech may be referable to deafness (deafmutism). Childish indistinctness (e.g., "r's" replaced by "w's") may persist in feeble-minded adults.

speech pathologist. An individual educated and trained to plan, direct, and conduct programs to improve communicative skills of children and adults with language and speech impairments arising from physiologic disturbances, defective articulation, or dialect. This individual can evaluate programs and may perform research related to speech and language problems.

speech synthesizer. An electronic device for producing speech. Activated by a keyboard, it permits persons lacking ability to speak to communicate.

speech therapy. The study, diagnosis, and treatment of defects and disorders of the voice and of spoken and written communication.

"speedballing". Among abusers of drugs, the use of cocaine and heroin combined and given I.V.

sperm (spĕrm) [Gr. *sperma*, seed]. 1. The ejaculate from the male; contains spermatozoa.

DOUBLE BODY

DOUBLE HEAD

ABERRANT IMPLANTATION
OF HEAD

CONE-SHAPED BODY

ABNORMAL CYTOPLASMIC
EXTRUSION OF HEAD

SWOLLEN POSTERIOR
PORTION OF HEAD

LEFT: TAIL CURLED AROUND BODY

RIGHT: INCOMPLETE
DEVELOPMENT OF TAIL

APLASTIC HEAD

IRREGULAR HEAD

ELONGATED HEAD

ROUGHENED HEAD
FORMATION

MEGALOSPERM

MICROSPERM

NORMAL

NORMAL AND ABNORMAL SPERM

SYN: *semen.* 2. Spermatozoa. SEE: illus.

sperma (spĕr'mă) [Gr.]. 1. Testicular secretion containing the male reproductive cells, spermatozoa. SYN: *semen.* 2. Individual male germ cell. 3. Also used as a combining form.

spermacrasia (spĕr″măk-rā'zē-ă) [Gr. *sperma*, seed, + *akrasia*, bad mixture]. Lack of spermatozoa in the semen. SYN: *aspermia.*

spermagglutination. Agglutination of spermatozoa.

spermatemphraxis (spĕr″măt-ĕm-frăk'sĭs) [" + *emphraxis*, stoppage]. An obstruction to emission of semen.

spermatic (spĕr-măt'ĭk) [Gr. *sperma*, seed]. Pert. to semen or sperm.

spermatic arteries. Two long slender vessels, branches of the abdominal aorta, following each spermatic cord to the testes.

spermatic cord. The cord suspending the testis composed of veins, arteries, lymphatics, nerves, and the ductus deferens. SEE: *cord, spermatic; infundibulum; varicocele.*

spermatic duct. Canal for passage of semen, esp. the ductus deferens and the ejaculatory duct. SYN: *seminal duct.*

spermaticidal (spĕrm″ăt-ĭ-sīd'ăl) [Gr. *sperma*, seed, + L. *cidus*, kill]. Destruc-

tive to or causing death of spermatozoa.

spermatic vein. One of two veins draining the testes. The right one empties into the inferior vena cava, the left into the left renal vein. In the spermatic cord, each forms a dilated pampiniform plexus.

spermatid (spĕr'mă-tĭd). A cell arising by division of the secondary spermatocyte to become a spermatozoon. SYN: *spermatoblast.*

spermatin (spĕr'mă-tĭn). A mucilaginous substance in the semen.

spermatism (spĕr'mă-tĭzm) [" + *-ismos*, condition]. Ejaculation of semen, voluntarily or otherwise.

spermatitis (spĕr″mă-tī'tĭs) [" + *itis*, inflammation]. Inflammation of the spermatic cord or of the ductus deferens. SYN: *deferentitis; funiculitis.*

spermato- [Gr. *sperma, spermatos*, seed]. Combining form meaning sperm, to sow seed.

spermatoblast (spĕr-măt'ō-blăst) [" + *blastos*, germ]. The rudimentary spermatozoon. SYN: *spermatid.*

spermatocele (spĕr-măt'ō-sēl) [" + *kele*, tumor, swelling]. A cystic tumor of the epididymis containing spermatozoa.

spermatocidal (spĕr″mă-tō-sī'dăl) [" + L. *cidus*, kill]. Destroying spermatozoa.

spermatocyst (spĕr-măt'ō-sĭst) [" + *kystis*, bladder]. 1. A seminal vesicle. 2. Tumor of epididymis containing semen. SYN: *spermatocele.*

spermatocystectomy (spĕr″măt-ō-sĭs-tĕk'tō-mē) [" + " + *ektome*, excision]. Removal of the seminal vesicles.

spermatocystitis (spĕr″măt-ō-sĭs-tī'tĭs) [" + " + *itis*, inflammation]. Inflammation of a seminal vesicle. SYN: *seminal vesiculitis.*

spermatocystotomy (spĕr″mă-tō-sĭs-tŏt'ō-mē) [" + " + *tome*, incision]. Drainage of the seminal vesicles by use of a surgical incision into the vesicle.

spermatocytal (spĕr″mă-tō-sī'tăl) [" + *kytos*, cell]. Concerning spermatocytes.

spermatocyte (spĕr-măt'ō-sīt) [" + *kytos*, cell]. A cell originating from a spermatogonium that forms by division the spermatids, which give rise to spermatozoa.

   s., primary. Cell arising by growth and development from a spermatogonium.

   s., secondary. Cell arising from primary spermatocyte by a meiotic division. It undergoes a second meiotic division, giving rise to two spermatids with haploid, q.v., number of chromosomes.

spermatocytogenesis (spĕr″mă-tō-sī″tō-jĕn'ĕ-sĭs) [" + " + *genesis*, generation, birth]. The initial stage of sperm formation.

spermatogenesis (spĕr″măt-ō-jĕn'ĕ-sĭs) [" + *genesis*, generation, birth]. The formation of mature functional spermatozoa. In the process, undifferentiated spermatogonia become primary spermatocytes, each of which divides to form two secondary spermatocytes. Each of these divides to form two spermatids, which transform into functional motile spermatozoa. In the process the chromosome number is reduced from the diploid to the haploid number. SEE: *gametogenesis; maturation; meiosis.*

spermatogenic, spermatogenous (spĕr″ mă-tō-jĕn′ĭk, spĕr″mă-tŏj′ĕ-nŭs). Producing sperm.

spermatogeny (spĕr″mă-tŏj′ĕ-nē). Spermatogenesis.

spermatogonium (spĕr″măt-ō-gō′nē-ŭm) [″ + *gone,* generation] (pl. *spermatogonia*). A large unspecialized germ cell that in spermatogenesis gives rise to a primary spermatocyte. SYN: *spermatospore.* SEE: *spermatogenesis.*

spermatoid (spĕr′mă-toyd) [″ + *eidos,* form, shape]. Resembling a spermatozoon.

spermatology (spĕr″mă-tŏl′ō-jē) [″ + *logos,* word, reason]. The study of the seminal fluid.

spermatolysin (spĕr″măt-ŏl′ĭ-sĭn) [″ + *lysis,* dissolution]. A lysin destroying spermatozoa.

spermatolysis (spĕr″măt-ŏl′ĭ-sĭs) [″ + *lysis,* dissolution]. Dissolution or destruction of spermatozoa.

spermatolytic (spĕr″măt-ō-lĭt′ĭk). Destroying spermatozoa.

spermatopathia, spermatopathy (spĕr″ mă-tō-păth′ē-ă, spĕr-mă-tŏp′ă-thē) [Gr. *spermatos,* seed, + *pathos,* disease]. Disease of sperm cells or their secreting glands or ducts.

spermatophobia (spĕr″mă-tō-fō′bē-ă) [″ + *phobos,* fear]. Abnormal fear of being afflicted with spermatorrhea, involuntary loss of semen.

spermatopoietic (spĕr″măt-ō-poy-ĕt′ĭk) [″ + *poiein,* to make]. Promoting the formation and secretion of semen.

spermatorrhea (spĕr″mă-tō-rē′ă) [″ + *rhoia,* flow]. Abnormally frequent involuntary loss of semen without orgasm.

spermatoschesis (spĕr″măt-ŏs′kĕ-sĭs) [″ + *schesis,* checking]. Suppression of the semen.

spermatospore (spĕr-măt′ō-spor) [″ + *sporos,* a seed]. A primitive cell from which spermatozoa arise. SYN: *spermatogonium.*

spermatotoxin (spĕr″mă-tō-tŏk′sĭn) [″ + *toxikon,* poison]. A toxin that destroys spermatozoa. SYN: *spermatoxin.*

spermatovum (spĕr″măt-ō′vŭm) [″ + L. *ovum,* egg]. A fecundated or impregnated ovum.

spermatoxin (spĕr″mă-tŏks′ĭn) [″ + *toxi-* *kon,* poison]. A toxin that causes destruction of spermatozoa. It is formed by injecting spermatozoa from an animal of another species.

spermatozoa (spĕr″măt-ō-zō′ă). Pl. of spermatozoon.

spermatozoal (spĕr″mă-tō-zō′ăl) [″ + *zoon,* life]. Concerning spermatozoa.

spermatozoicide (spĕr″mă-tō-zō′ĭ-sīd) [″ + ″ + L. *cidus,* kill]. Spermicide.

spermatozoon (spĕr″măt-ō-zō′ŏn) [″ + *zoon,* life] (pl. *spermatozoa*). The mature male sex or germ cell formed within the seminiferous tubules of the testes. The spermatozoon has a broad oval flattened head with a nucleus and a protoplasmic neck or middle piece and tail. It is about 51 microns long and resembles a tadpole. It has the power of self-propulsion by means of a flagellum. Develops after puberty from the spermatids in the testes in enormous quantities. The head pierces the envelope of the ovum and loses its tail when fusion of the two cells takes place. This process is called fertilization. SEE: *fertilization; sperm* for illus.

RS: acrosome; contraception; fertilization; gamete; ovum; semen; sperm; zygote.

spermaturia (spĕr″mă-tū′rē-ă) [″ + *ouron,* urine]. Semen discharged with the urine.

spermectomy (spĕr-mĕk′tō-mē) [″ + *ektome,* excision]. Resection of a portion of the spermatic cord and duct.

spermic (spĕr′mĭk). Concerning sperm, male reproductive cells.

spermicidal (spĕr″mĭ-sī′dăl) [″ + L. *cidus,* kill]. Killing spermatozoa.

spermicide (spĕr′mĭ-sīd). An agent that kills spermatozoa.

spermidine (spĕr′mĭ-dĭn). An amine present in semen.

spermiduct (spĕr′mĭ-dŭkt) [″ + L. *ductus,* a duct]. The ejaculatory duct and ductus deferens considered as one.

spermine (spĕr′mĭn). An amine present in semen and other animal tissues.

spermiogenesis (spĕr″mē-ō-jĕn′ĕ-sĭs). The processes involved in the transformation of a spermatid to a functional spermatozoon.

spermiogram (spĕr′mē-ō-grăm) [″ + *gramma,* something written]. Record of examining and classifying sperm in a semen sample.

spermoblast (spĕr′mō-blăst) [″ + *blastos,* a germ]. A cell developing into a spermatozoon. SYN: *spermatid; spermatoblast.*

spermolith (spĕr′mō-lĭth) [″ + *lithos,* stone]. A calculus in the seminal vesicle or spermatic duct.

spermolysin (spĕr′mŏl′ĭ-sĭn). A cytolysin formed following the inoculation of spermatozoa.

spermolytic (spĕr-mō-lĭt'ĭk) [" + *lysis*, dissolution]. Causing the destruction of spermatozoa.

spermoneuralgia (spĕr"mō-nū-răl'jē-ă) [" + *neuron*, nerve, + *algos*, pain]. Neuralgic pain in the testicles and spermatic cord.

spermophlebectasia (spĕr"mō-flē"bĕk-tā'zē-ă) [" + *phlebos*, vein, + *ektasis*, dilatation]. Varicosity of the spermatic veins.

spermoplasm (spĕr'mō-plăzm) [" + LL. *plasma*, form, mold]. The protoplasm of a male germ cell.

spermosphere (spĕr'mō-sfēr) [" + *sphaira*, a circle]. Mass of spermatoblasts derived from spermatogonia.

spermospore (spĕr'mō-spor) [" + *sporos*, seed]. A primitive cell from which spermatozoa originate. SYN: *spermatogonium*.

spermotoxin (spĕr"mō-tŏk'sĭn) [" + *toxikon*, poison]. Something that destroys sperm.

sp. gr. *specific gravity.*

sph. *spherical.*

sphacelate (sfăs'ĕl-āt) [Gr. *sphakelos*, gangrene]. 1. To affect with gangrene. 2. Gangrenous. SYN: *mortified; necrosed.*

sphacelation (sfăs"ĕl-ā'shŭn). Mortification; formation of a mass of gangrenous tissue. SYN: *gangrene; necrosis.*

sphacelism (sfăs'ĕl-ĭzm) [" + *-ismos*, condition]. Condition of being affected with sphacelus or gangrene. SYN: *necrosis.*

sphaceloderma (sfăs"ĕl-ō-dĕr'mă) [" + *derma*, skin]. Gangrene of the skin, esp. when symmetrical. SEE: *Raynaud's disease.*

sphacelotoxin (sfăs"ĕl-ō-tŏk'sĭn) [" + *toxikon*, poison]. Poisonous principle obtained from ergot used to produce abortion.

sphacelous (sfăs'ĕl-ŭs) [Gr. *sphakelos*, gangrene]. Pert. to a slough or patch of gangrene. SYN: *gangrenous; necrosed; necrotic.*

sphacelus (sfăs'ĕl-ŭs). 1. A necrosed mass of tissue. SYN: *slough.* 2. Process of becoming gangrenous. SYN: *gangrene; mortification; necrosis.*

sphenethmoid (sfĕn-ĕth'moyd) [Gr. *sphen*, wedge, + *ethmos*, sieve]. Sphenoethmoid, q.v.

sphenion (sfē'nē-ŏn) [Gr. *sphen*, wedge] (pl. *sphenia*). Point at apex of the sphenoidal angle of the parietal bone.

spheno- [Gr. *sphen*, wedge]. Combining form meaning a wedge; the sphenoid bone.

sphenobasilar (sfē"nō-băs'ĭ-lăr) [" + L. *basilaris*, basal]. Concerning the sphenoid bone and basilar portion of the occipital bone.

sphenoccipital (sfē"nŏk-sĭp'ĭ-tăl) [" + L. *occipitalis*, occipital]. Concerning the sphe-

noid and occipital bones.

sphenocephalus (sfē"nō-sĕf'ă-lŭs) [" + *kephale*, head]. A deformed fetus in which the head is wedge-shaped.

sphenoethmoid (sfē"nō-ĕth'moyd) [" + *ethmos*, sieve, + *eidos*, form, shape]. Pert. to the sphenoid and ethmoid bones.

sphenoethmoid recess. Groove back and above the superior concha, or turbinate bone.

sphenofrontal (sfē"nō-frŭn'tăl) [" + L. *frontalis*, frontal]. Concerning the sphenoid and frontal bones.

sphenoid (sfē'noyd) [" + *eidos*, form]. Cuneiform or wedge-shaped.

sphenoidal (sfē-noy'dăl). Concerning the sphenoid bone.

sphenoid bone. Large bone at base of the skull between the occipital and ethmoid in front, and the parietal and temporal bones at the side.

sphenoid fissure. Fissure in sphenoid and frontal bones for nerves and blood vessels.

sphenoiditis (sfē"noy-dī'tĭs) [" + " + *itis*, inflammation]. 1. Inflammation of the sphenoidal sinus. 2. Necrosis of the sphenoid bone.

sphenoidostomy (sfē"noy-dŏs'tō-mē) [" + " + *stoma*, mouth]. Surgically producing an opening into the sphenoid sinus.

sphenoidotomy (sfē"noyd-ŏt'ō-mē) [" + " + *tome*, incision]. Incision into the sphenoid bone.

sphenomalar (sfē"nō-mā'lăr) [" + L. *mala*, cheek]. Concerning the sphenoid and malar bones.

sphenomaxillary (sfē"nō-măk'sĭ-lā-rē) [" + L. *maxilla*, jawbone]. Concerning the sphenoid and maxilla.

spheno-occipital (sfē"nō-ŏk-sĭp'ĭ-tăl) [" + L. *occipitalis*, occipital]. Concerning the sphenoid and occipital bones.

sphenopalatine (sfē"nō-păl'ă-tēn) [" + L. *palatum*, palate]. Concerning the sphenoid and palatine bones.

sphenoparietal (sfē"nō-pă-rī'ē-tăl) [" + L. *paries*, a wall]. Concerning the sphenoid and parietal bones.

sphenorbital (sfē"nor'bĭ-tăl) [" + L. *orbita*, track]. Concerning the sphenoid bone and the orbits.

sphenosis [Gr., wedging]. Condition in which fetus becomes wedged in the pelvis.

sphenosquamosal (sfē"nō-skwă-mō'săl) [Gr. *sphen*, wedge, + L. *squamosa*, scaly]. Concerning the sphenoid bone and squamous portion of the temporal bone.

sphenotemporal (sfē"nō-tĕm'pō-răl) [" + L. *temporalis*, temporal]. Concerning the sphenoid and temporal bones.

sphenotic (sfē-nŏt'ĭk) [Gr. *sphen*, wedge, + *eidos*, form, shape]. A fetal bone that becomes part of the sphenoid bone.

sphenotresia (sfē″nō-trē′zē-ă) [Gr. *sphen,* wedge, + *tresis,* boring]. Perforating of the basal part of the fetal skull in craniotomy.

sphenotribe (sfē′nō-trīb) [″ + *tribein,* to crush]. Instrument for breaking up basal part of the fetal cranium.

sphenoturbinal (sfē″nō-tŭr′bĭ-năl) [″ + *turbo,* whirl]. A thin curved bone anterior to each of the lesser wings of the sphenoid.

sphenovomerine (sfē″nō-vō′mĕr-ĭn) [″ + L. *vomer,* plowshare]. Concerning the sphenoid and vomer bones.

sphenozygomatic (sfē″nō-zī″gō-măt′ĭk) [″ + *zygoma,* cheekbone]. Concerning the sphenoid and zygomatic bones.

sphere (sfēr) [Gr. *sphaira,* a globe]. 1. A ball or globelike structure. 2. The environment one controls or in which one lives and works.

    s., attraction. A clear region in cytoplasm close to nucleus and usually containing a centriole or diplosome (a divided centriole).

    s., segmentation. The segmented ovum or morula.

spheresthesia (sfēr″ĕs-thē′zē-ă) [″ + *aisthesis,* sensation]. A morbid sensation, as of a ball or lump ascending from stomach to throat. Seen in hysteria and other neuroses. SYN: *globus hystericus.*

spherical (sfēr′ĭ-kăl) [Gr. *sphairikos*]. Having the form of, or pert. to, a sphere. SYN: *globular.*

spherocylinder (sfē″rō-sĭl′ĭn-dĕr) [Gr. *sphaira,* globe, + *kylindros,* cylinder]. A lens with a spherical surface and a cylindrical surface.

spherocyte (sfē′rō-sīt) [″ + *kytos,* cell]. An erythrocyte that assumes a spheroid shape.

spherocytosis (sfē″rō-sī-tō′sĭs) [″ + ″ + *osis,* condition]. Condition in which erythrocytes assume a spheroid shape. Occurs in certain hemolytic anemias.

    s., hereditary. An inherited chronic disease characterized by hemolysis, anemia, spherocytosis, jaundice, and splenomegaly. The only effective treatment is splenectomy.

spheroid (sfē′royd) [″ + *eidos,* form, shape]. 1. A body shaped like a sphere. 2. Sphere-shaped.

spheroidal (sfē-roy′dăl). Shaped like a sphere.

spherolith (sfē′rō-lĭth) [″ + *lithos,* stone]. A minute concretion in the kidney of the newborn.

spheroma (sfē-rō′mă) [″ + *oma,* tumor]. A tumor of spherical form.

spherometer (sfē-rŏm′ĕt-ĕr) [″ + *metron,* measure]. Device to ascertain curvature of a surface.

spheroplast (sfēr′ō-plăst). In bacteriology, the cell wall remaining after gram-negative organisms have been lysed. Spheroplasts may be formed when synthesis of the cell wall is prevented by the action of certain chemicals while cells are growing. SEE: *protoplast.*

spherospermia (sfē″rō-spĕr′mē-ă) [″ + *sperma,* seed]. Round spermatozoa without tails.

spherule (sfēr′ūl) [LL. *sphaerula,* little globe]. 1. A very small sphere. 2. A minute granule found in the center of a centromere of a chromosome. 3. The structures present in tissues infected with *Coccidioides immitis.* These spherules contain up to hundreds of endospores.

sphincter (sfĭngk′tĕr) [Gr. *sphinkter,* band]. Circular muscle constricting an orifice. In normal tonic condition, it closes the orifice, i.e., the muscle must relax in order to allow the orifice to open.

    s. ampullae. Delicate network of fibers about papilla of Vater, occasionally present in adults, a part of sphincter of Oddi.

    s. ani. Sphincter that closes the anus, the external one being of striated muscle, the internal one, of plain muscle.

    s., bladder. Plain muscle about opening of bladder into the urethra.

    s., cardiac. Plain muscle about the esophagus at cardiac opening into the stomach.

    s. choledochus. Smooth muscle investing common bile duct just before its junction with pancreatic duct; a part of sphincter of Oddi.

    s., ileocecal. Plain muscle about the ileum at its opening into the cecum.

    s. of Oddi. Contracted region in common bile duct at papilla of Vater.

    s. pancreaticus. Smooth muscle encircling pancreatic duct just before it joins the ampulla.

    s., pyloric. A thickening of the muscular wall around the pyloric orifice.

sphincteral (sfĭngk′tĕr-ăl). Concerning a sphincter.

sphincteralgia (sfĭngk″tĕr-ăl′jē-ă) [Gr. *sphinkter,* band, + *algos,* pain]. Pain in the sphincter ani muscles.

sphincterectomy (sfĭngk″tĕr-ĕk′tō-mē) [″ + *ektome,* excision]. 1. Excision of any sphincter muscle. 2. Excision of part of the iris' pupillary border.

sphincteric (sfĭngk-tĕr′ĭk). Concerning a sphincter.

sphincterismus (sfĭngk″tĕr-ĭz′mŭs) [″ + *-ismos,* condition]. Spasm of sphincter ani muscles.

sphincteritis (sfĭngk″tĕr-ī′tĭs) [″ + *itis,* inflammation]. Inflammation of any sphincter muscle.

sphincterolysis (sfĭngk″tĕr-ŏl′ĭ-sĭs) [″ + *lysis*, dissolution]. Freeing of the iris from the cornea in anterior synechia affecting only the pupillary border.

sphincteroplasty (sfĭngk′tĕr-ō-plăs″tē) [″ + *plassein*, to form]. Plastic operation upon any sphincter muscle.

sphincteroscope (sfĭngk′tĕr-ō-skōp″) [″ + *skopein*, to examine]. Instrument for inspection of the anal sphincter.

sphincteroscopy (sfĭngk″tĕr-ŏs′kŏ-pē). Inspection of the internal anal sphincter.

sphincterotome (sfĭngk′tĕr-ō-tōm″) [″ + *tome*, incision]. Surgical instrument for cutting a sphincter.

sphincterotomy (sfĭngk″tĕr-ŏt′ō-mē) [″ + *tome*, incision]. Cutting of a sphincter muscle.

sphingolipid (sfĭng′gō-lĭp′ĭd) [Gr. *sphingein*, to bind, + *lipos*, fat]. Lipid containing one of several long-chain bases such as sphingosine, q.v., or dihydrosphingosine, q.v., or bases of similar chemical structure but containing longer chains.

sphingolipidosis [″ + ″ + *osis*, condition]. Any disease characterized by defective metabolism of sphingolipids. These genetically determined errors of metabolism include Sandhoff's disease, Fabry's disease, Tay-Sachs disease, Kufs' disease, Gaucher's disease, Krabbe's leukodystrophy, and Niemann-Pick disease. They are characterized by neurological deterioration, usually beginning a few months after birth, eventually leading to death except in the adult form of Gaucher's disease. These diseases can be detected by examining fluid obtained by amniocentesis.

sphingolipodystrophy (sfĭng′gō-lĭp″ō-dĭs′trō-fē) [″ + *dys*, bad, + *trophe*, nutrition]. A group of diseases caused by defective sphingolipid metabolism.

sphingomyelins (sfĭng′gō-mī′ĕl-ĭns). A major group of phosphorus-containing sphingolipids, q.v. They are found primarily in nervous tissue and in lipids in the blood. They are derived from choline phosphate and a ceramide.

sphingosine (sfĭng′gō-sĭn). A long-chain base, $C_{18}H_{37}O_2N$, present in sphingolipids. SEE: *dihydrosphingosine; sphingolipid.*

sphygmic (sfĭg′mĭk) [Gr. *sphygmikos*]. Rel. to the pulse.

sphygmo- [Gr. *sphygmos*, pulse]. Combining form indicating pulse.

sphygmobolometer (sfĭg″mō-bō-lŏm′ĕ-tĕr) [″ + *bolos*, mass, + *metron*, a measure]. Device to measure force of the pulse rather than the blood pressure.

sphygmocardiogram (sfĭg″mō-kăr′dē-ō-grăm) [″ + *kardia*, heart, + *gramma*, something written]. A tracing made by a sphygmocardiograph of the heartbeat and radial pulse.

sphygmocardiograph (sfĭg″mō-kăr′dē-ō-grăf) [″ + ″ + *graphein*, to write]. Device for simultaneous recording of the radial pulse and the heartbeat.

sphygmocardioscope (sfĭg″mō-kăr′dē-ō-skōp) [″ + ″ + *skopein*, to examine]. Device for recording the action of the pulse and heart. SYN: *sphygmocardiograph.*

sphygmochronograph (sfĭg″mō-krō′nō-grăf) [″ + *chronos*, time, + *graphein*, to write]. A sphygmograph graphically recording time between the heartbeat and the pulse.

sphygmogram (sfĭg′mō-grăm) [″ + *gramma*, something written]. A tracing of the pulse made by using the sphygmograph.

sphygmograph (sfĭg′mō-grăf) [″ + *graphein*, to write]. Instrument for recording the shape and force of the pulse wave. SYN: *polygraph.*

sphygmography (sfĭg-mŏg′rǎ-fē). Recording the arterial pulse by use of a sphygmograph.

sphygmoid (sfĭg′moyd) [Gr. *sphygmos*, pulse, + *eidos*, form, shape]. Resembling the pulse.

sphygmology (sfĭg-mŏl′ō-jē) [″ + *logos*, word, reason]. Scientific study of the pulse.

sphygmomanometer (sfĭg″mō-măn-ŏm′ĕt-ĕr) [″ + *manos*, thin, + *metron*, measure]. Instrument for determining arterial blood pressure indirectly. The two types are aneroid and mercury. SEE: *blood pressure.*

   s., random-zero. A special type of sphygmomanometer that allows the blood pressure to be taken without the observer's knowing where zero pressure is on the device. After the pressure is obtained, the mercury comes to rest at a point. The observed pressure is then corrected by subtracting the at-rest value on the device from the pressure obtained. Even though this device was developed to prevent subjective bias in determining blood pressure, it is not necessarily effective in achieving this goal.

sphygmometer (sfĭg-mŏm′ĕt-ĕr) [″ + *metron*, measure]. Instrument for measuring the pulse. SYN: *sphygmograph.*

sphygmopalpation (sfĭg″mō-păl-pā′shŭn) [″ + L. *palpatio*, palpation]. Palpating the pulse.

sphygmophone (sfĭg′mō-fōn) [Gr. *sphygmos*, pulse, + *phone*, voice]. Instrument for hearing the pulse beat.

sphygmoplethysmograph (sfĭg″mō-plĕth-ĭz′mō-grăf) [″ + *plethysmos*, to increase, + *graphein*, to write]. Device that traces the pulse with its curve of fluctuation in volume.

sphygmoscope (sfĭg′mō-skōp) [″ + *sko-*

pein, to examine]. Instrument for showing the heart's movements or pulsations of arteries and veins.

sphygmosystole (sfĭg″mō-sĭs′tō-lē) [Gr. *sphygmos,* pulse, + *systole,* contraction]. The segment of the sphygmogram that corresponds to the heart's systole.

sphygmotonograph (sfĭg″mō-tō′nō-grăf) [″ + *tonos,* tension, + *graphein,* to write]. Instrument for simultaneous recording and timing of arterial blood pressure, jugular or carotid pulse, and the brachial pulse.

sphygmotonometer (sfĭg″mō-tō-nŏm′ĕt-ĕr) [″ + ″ + *metron,* measure]. Instrument for ascertaining elasticity of walls of an artery.

sphygmus (sfĭg′mŭs) [Gr. *sphygmos,* pulse]. A pulse or pulsation.

sphyrectomy (sfī-rĕk′tō-mē) [Gr. *sphyra,* malleus, + *ektome,* excision]. Surgical excision of the malleus of the foot.

sphyrotomy (sfī-rŏt′ō-mē) [″ + *tome,* incision]. Surgical excision of a portion of the malleus of the foot.

spica (spī′kă) [L., ear of grain]. A reverse spiral bandage, the turn of which crosses like the letter V. SEE: *bandage, spica.*

spica hip cast. A cast containing the lower torso and extending to one or both lower extremities. If only one lower extremity is included, it is called a single hip spica; if two are included, it is called a double hip spica. These are used for treating pelvic and femoral fractures.

spicular (spīk′ū-lar) [L. *spiculum,* a dart]. Pert. to or resembling a spicule; dartlike.

spicule (spīk′ūl). A small, needle-shaped body.

  s., bony. A needle-shaped fragment of bone.

  s., cemental. An excementosis or pointed protuberance extending from the surface cementum of a tooth root.

spiculed red cell. Crenated red blood cells with surface projections. In most instances, this is a normal variation in red cell equilibrium, and is reversible.

spiculum (spīk′ū-lŭm) [L., a dart] (pl. *spicula*). A sharp, small spike. SYN: *spicule.*

spider (spī′dĕr). 1. An arachnid, belonging to the order Araneae, class Arachnida, phylum Arthropoda. The body is divided into cephalothorax and abdomen joined by a narrow waist. A spider usually possesses four pairs of legs as well as poison fangs. It often possesses spinnerets. 2. Anything resembling a spider in appearance.

  s., arterial. SEE: *spider nevus.*

  s., black widow. The female of *Latrodectus mactans.* It is glossy black in color with a brilliant red or yellow spot, usually shaped like an hourglass or two triangles, on

undersurface of the abdomen. Its bite causes excruciating pain and may prove fatal. SEE: *spider bites or poisoning.*

  s., brown recluse. *Loxosceles reclusa,* a small, three-eighth in. (10 mm) long spider native to North America. Its venom is quite toxic and is capable of causing death. The venom produces a large area of necrosis at the site of the bite. Treatment is symptomatic. SEE: *spider bites or poisoning.*

spider bites or poisoning. Not all spider bites are dangerous.

SYM: Local symptoms include slight burning followed in about one-half hour by severe radiating pains, often extending long distances from puncture. Sloughing at site and along lymphatics may occur. Collapse, unconsciousness, convulsions, and death sometimes follow.

  s.b. or poisoning, black widow. SYM: Initially the sensation resembles the prick of a pin. Pain usually lasts for a short period of time, subsides, and later the abdominal muscles become rigid. Within one-half hour severe abdominal cramps begin. The venom, which is neurotoxic, causes an ascending motor paralysis. Because of the extreme abdominal pain, the patient may be suspected of having an acute condition requiring abdominal surgery.

TREAT: Avoid all stimulants. Suction is of little value as the toxin is rapidly absorbed. Calcium gluconate intravenously often gives relief from pain. Large doses of morphine, repeated when necessary, given slowly by vein, also control pain. Apply heat either locally or by using a hot tub bath. Forcing fluids is also recommended. A specific antivenin, *Latrodectus mactans,* is available. This horse serum-containing preparation should be given intramuscularly as soon as the diagnosis is made, provided the patient is not sensitive to horse serum. SEE: *bites or stings.*

  s.b. or poisoning, brown recluse. SYM: The venom of the brown recluse spider may produce a large area of necrosis at the site of the bite. SEE: *spider, brown recluse.*

TREAT: Cleanse ulcers with solution of hydrogen peroxide suitable for topical applications; corticosteroids. Debridement if eschar develops. An antivenin is being investigated experimentally.

spider-burst. An area on the leg in which capillaries radiate from a central point. The veins, though dilated, are not varicosities.

spider cells. Branching cells in neuroglia. SYN: *cells, neuroglia,* q.v.; *Deiters' cells.*

spider fingers. Abnormally long phalanges of the hands. SYN: *arachnodactyly.* SEE: *Marfan's syndrome.*

spider nevus. A branched growth of dilated capillaries on the skin, resembling a spider. This abnormality may be associated with cirrhosis of the liver. SYN: *nevus araneus.*

Spielmeyer-Vogt disease [Walter Spielmeyer, Ger. neurologist, 1879–1935; Oskar Vogt, Ger. neurologist, 1870–1959]. Late juvenile cerebral sphingolipidosis. SYN: *Batten disease.*

spigelian line (spī-jē′lē-ăn) [Adriaan van den Spieghel, Flemish anatomist, 1578–1625]. Line on abdomen lying parallel to median line and marking edge of rectus abdominis muscle. SYN: *linea semilunaris; semilunar line.*

spigelian lobe. A small lobe behind right lobe of liver.

spike. The main peak in an oscillographic record of the action potential.

spikeboard. Adapted device for persons with limited upper extremity or one-handed function that allows for stabilization of food while it is being prepared.

spill (spĭl) [AS. *spillan,* to squander]. An overflow.

   s., cellular. Dissemination of cells through lymph or the blood resulting in metastasis.

   s., radioactive. Massive leak of radioactive materials from any source of those materials. SEE: *radiation accidents, emergency handling of.*

spillway (spĭl′wā). The contour of the teeth that allows food to escape from the cusps during mastication.

spiloma, spilus (spī-lō′mă, spī′lŭs) [Gr. *spiloma, spilos,* spot]. A mole or discoloration of skin. SYN: *nevus.*

spina (spī′nă) [L., thorn] (pl. *spinae*). [NA] 1. Any spinelike protuberance. 2. The spine.

   s. bifida cystica. Congenital defect in walls of the spinal canal caused by lack of union between the laminae of the vertebrae. Lumbar portion is section chiefly affected. SYN: *rachischisis.*

   SYM: As result of this deficiency, the membranes of the cord are pushed through the opening, forming a tumor known as *spina bifida cystica,* due to condition of spine that gives rise to the deformity, and *hydrorrhachis,* caused by the fluid contained in the tumor.

   s. bifida occulta. Failure of vertebrae to close without hernial protrusion.

   s. ventosa. Tuberculosis of the bone. The bone is expanded and the cortex thins.

spinal (spī′năl) [L. *spinalis*]. Pert. to the spine or spinal cord.

spinal accessory nerve. Accessory nerve, q.v.

spinal anesthesia. Anesthesia produced by an anesthetic injected into the spinal canal.

SYN: *narcosis, medullary.*

spinal canal. Canal of the vertebral column that contains the spinal cord.

spinal column. The vertebral column enclosing the spinal cord and consisting of 33 vertebrae: 7 cervical, 12 dorsal or thoracic, 5 lumbar, 5 sacral fused to form 1 bone, and 4 in the coccyx fused to form 1 bone. The number is sometimes increased by an additional vertebra in one region, and sometimes one may be absent in another. SEE: illus.

spinal cord. An ovoid column of nervous tissue averaging about 44 cm in length, flattened anteroposteriorly, extending from the medulla to the 2nd lumbar vertebra in the spinal canal. All nerves to the trunk and limbs are issued from the spinal cord, and it is the center of reflex action containing the conducting paths to and from the brain. In cross section, it does not fill the vertebral space, being surrounded by the pia mater, the cerebrospinal fluid, the arachnoid, and the dura mater, which fuses with the periosteum of the inner surfaces of the vertebrae.

   The gray substance approximates the shape of an "H," there being a posterior and anterior horn in either half. The anterior horn is composed of motor cells from which the fibers making up the motor portions of the peripheral nerves arise. Sensory neurons enter posteriorly. The "H" also divides the surrounding white matter into posterior, lateral, and anterior bundles. These serve to connect brain and cord in both directions (i.e., with efferent and afferent nerves) as well as various portions of the cord itself.

spinal cord injury, acute. Acute traumatic injury of the spinal cord. Traditionally, therapy for this condition has been ineffective with respect to neurologic outcome. Nevertheless, the use of intravenous methylprednisolone given as a bolus dose of 30 mg per kilogram and then a maintenance dose of 5.4 mg per kilogram per hour during the acute phase improved neurologic recovery.

spinal curvature. Abnormal curvature of the spine, frequently constitutional in children. It may be angular, lateral (scoliosis), or anteroposterior (kyphosis, q.v., lordosis, q.v.).

spinal curvature, angular. Caries of the spine. SYN: *Pott's disease.*

spinal curvature, lateral. Deviation of spine to one side or the other causing a twist of the spine.

spinal fluid. Cerebrospinal fluid. When normal, it contains 50 to 75 mg of sugar per 100 ml. The sugar content is lower than that in the blood.

CERVICAL CURVE

CERVICAL (SEVEN)

VERTEBRA SEEN FROM ABOVE

LAMINA

VERTEBRAL FORAMEN

ARTICULAR FACET

BODY

FOURTH CERVICAL VERTEBRA

THORACIC CURVE

THORACIC (TWELVE)

TRANSVERSE PROCESS

PEDICLE

SIXTH THORACIC VERTEBRA

LUMBAR CURVE

LUMBAR (FIVE)

THIRD LUMBAR VERTEBRA

SACRAL CURVE

SACRUM (ANTERIOR VIEW)

COCCYX

SPINAL COLUMN
INDICATING INDIVIDUAL VERTEBRAE
AT VARIOUS LEVELS

DIAG: *Cell count:* If normal, 0 to 5 mononuclear cells per ml. Increased in all diseased states, several hundred or thousands in meningitis, when fluid becomes opaque. *Lymphocytes:* Found in encephalitis and tuberculous meningitis; polymorphonuclears predominate in septic meningitis and epidemic meningitis. *Bloody fluid:* Brain hemorrhages due to arteriosclerosis, high blood pressure, tumors, and other causes. Spinal fluid may contain blood due to needle having punctured a small blood vessel. *Encephalitis:* Sugar content is increased, fluid clear, cell count 100 plus. *Globulin:* Its presence is abnormal.

Microorganisms: Meningococci, streptococci, pneumococci, tubercle bacilli, and influenza bacilli may be present, any of which may be indicative of meningitis. Epidemic meningitis indicated by gram-negative, intracellular diplococcus, biscuit-shaped microorganisms. Typhoid bacilli may produce meningeal symptoms in typhoid fever. Streptococci may enter the meninges through the ear; the invading point of pneumococci, influenza bacilli, and pneumobacilli is usually the lungs. All these may be found in smears or in culture of the spinal fluid. *Meningitis:* Lower spinal fluid sugar than sugar content of blood; 25 to 15 mg. If suppurative meningitis, spinal fluid is pus-like and turbid, but it is clear in tuberculous meningitis, encephalitis, and poliomyelitis. *Poliomyelitis:* Same as encephalitis.

RS: anhydromyelia; calcinorrhachia; cerebrospinal fluid; meningitis; poliomyelitis.

spinal fusion. Surgical immobilization of adjacent vertebrae. This procedure may be done for several conditions, including herniated disk.

spinal ganglion. Enlargement on dorsal or posterior root of a spinal nerve composed principally of cell bodies of somatic and visceral afferent neurons. Also called dorsal root ganglion.

spinalgia (spī-năl′jē-ă) [L. *spina,* thorn, + Gr. *algos,* pain]. Pain in a vertebra under pressure.

spinalis (spī-nā′lĭs) [L.]. A muscle attached to the spinal process of a vertebra. SEE: *Muscles* in *Appendix.*

spinal nerves. Nerves arising from the spinal cord: 31 pairs, consisting of 8 cervical, 12 thoracic, 5 lumbar, 5 sacral, and 1 coccygeal, corresponding with the spinal vertebrae. Each spinal nerve is attached to the spinal cord by two roots: a dorsal or posterior sensory root and a ventral or anterior root. The former consists of afferent fibers conveying impulses to the cord; the latter of efferent fibers conveying impulses from the cord. A typical spinal nerve, on passing through the intervertebral foramen, divides into four branches, a recurrent branch, a dorsal ramus or posterior primary division, a ventral ramus or anterior primary division, and two rami communicantes (white and gray), which pass to ganglia of the sympathethic trunk.

spinal puncture. Puncture of the spinal cavity with a needle to extract the spinal fluid for diagnostic purposes, to introduce anesthetic agents into the spinal canal, or to remove fluid so other fluids such as radiopaque substances may be injected.

The smallest needle possible should be used in order to decrease the chance of leakage of spinal fluid after the needle is withdrawn. This will help to prevent post-spinal puncture headache. SEE: *headache, postlumbar puncture; Queckenstedt's sign.*

SITE OF PUNCTURE: To prevent injury of the nerve fibers, the puncture is usually made at the juncture between the 3rd and 4th lumbar vertebrae. A line drawn posteriorly from the crest of one ilium over the crest of the other will usually pass over the tip of the spinous process of the 4th lumbar

vertebra. The point for the needle injection is directly above this line (i.e., toward the head).

NURSING IMPLICATIONS: Assess the patient's understanding of the procedure and correct any misinterpretations. Obtain permission or consent if necessary. Procure the equipment needed to perform the procedure. Have the patient void and defecate if possible. Provide privacy and position the patient properly. Assist as necessary during the procedure, and provide verbal and nonverbal reassurance to the patient. Send specimens to the laboratory as requested. Instruct patient concerning the need to remain flat, preferably in a prone position for the first several hours immediately following the procedure. This will help to prevent postspinal puncture headache. Document the specimens that were sent as well as the patient's response to the procedure.

Caution: If the cerebrospinal fluid pressure is elevated, it may be dangerous to perform spinal puncture.

---

spinal reflex. Any reflex centering in the spinal cord.

spinal shock. Effects resulting from transverse section of the spinal cord and occurring in segments below level of section. Principal effects are anesthesia, paralysis, loss of muscle tone, and suppression of reflexes, both visceral and somatic.

spinate (spī′nāt). Having spines or shaped like a thorn.

spindle (spĭn′dl) [AS. *spinel*]. 1. A fusiform-shaped body. 2. The portion of the achromatic apparatus seen in mitosis consisting of a bundle of delicate fibrils that connect the two centrosomes or asters. The chromosomes arrange themselves on the spindle in an equatorial plate.

s., aortic. A dilatation of the aorta following the aortic isthmus.

s., enamel. A tubular hypomineralized structure extending a short distance from the dentinoenamel junction into enamel, seen in ground sections of teeth.

s., muscle. A nerve receptor present in voluntary muscle tissues. This specialized tissue is involved in the stretch and myotatic reflexes.

s., neuromuscular. A complex sensory nerve ending consisting of muscle fibers enclosed within a capsule and supplied by an afferent nerve fiber. It mediates proprioceptive sensations and reflexes.

s., neurotendinous. A proprioceptive nerve ending found in a tendon, in muscle septa or sheaths, in a muscle tissue, or at junction of a muscle or tendon. SYN: *organ of Golgi.*

s., sleep. Specific waves that appear in the electroencephalogram during sleep.

spine (spīn). 1. A sharp process of bone. 2. The spinal column, consisting of 33 vertebrae: 7 cervical, 12 thoracic, 5 lumbar, 5 sacral, 4 coccygeal. The bones of the sacrum and coccyx are ankylosed in adult life and counted as one each. SYN: *backbone.*

RS: cephalorhachidian; cord, spinal; cramp; curvature; rachilysis, "rach-" words; scoliosis.

s., alar. Spinous process of the sphenoid bone.

s., anterior nasal. Projection formed by anterior prolongation of the inferior border of the nasal notch of the maxilla.

s., bifid. Spina bifida.

s., fracture of. A fractured spine often is treated in a plaster jacket with the spine hyperextended to reduce the fracture after essential treatment with skeletal traction. A window is cut over the abdomen. If the fracture is high, the neck is included. The jacket must be short enough to allow flexion of the thighs. The patient is allowed to walk in the jacket, which is left on for 3 or 4 months. A vest is put on under this plaster, and the prominences are padded with felt.

Traction and Balkan and Stryker frames are used if the fracture involves the cord with paralysis below the injury. Bedsores and cystitis must be prevented. An enema is given when needed.

s., frontal. Sharp-pointed medial process extending downward from nasal process of frontal bone. SYN: *s., nasal.*

s., hemal. That part of the hemal arch of a typical vertebra that closes it in.

s., Henle's. S., suprameatal.

s., iliac. One of four spines of the ilium, namely the anterior and posterior inferior spines and the anterior and posterior superior spines.

s., ischial. Spine of the ischium, a pointed eminence on its posterior border. SYN: *s., sciatic.*

s., mandibular. The small, tongue-shaped protuberance on the medial aspect of the mandibular ramus near the mandibular foramen, to which the sphenomandibular ligament is attached.

s., mental. Small process on the inner surface of mandible at back of the symphysis formed of one or more small projections (genial tubercles).

s., nasal. Sharp process descending in the middle line from the inferior surface of the frontal bone between the superior maxillae.

s., neural. Spinous process of a vertebra.

The posterior projection of the neural arch.

s. of pubis. A prominent tubercle on upper border of the pubis.

s. of scapula. An osseous plate projecting from the posterior surface of the scapula.

s. of sphenoid. Spinous process of the greater sphenoid wing.

s., pharyngeal. Ridge under the basilar process of the occipital bone.

s., posterior nasal. Spine formed by medial ends of the horizontal processes of the palatine bones.

s., sciatic. S., ischial.

s., suprameatal. A small spine at junction of superior and posterior walls of the external auditory meatus. SYN: *s., Henle's.*

s., typhoid. Acute arthritis due to infection causing spinal ankylosis during or following typhoid fever.

spinifugal (spī-nĭf'ū-găl) [L. *spina,* thorn, + *fugare,* to flee]. Moving away from the spinal cord.

spinipetal (spī-nĭp'ĕ-tăl) [" + *petere,* to seek]. Conducting nerve impulse toward the spinal cord.

spinnbarkeit (spĭn'băr-kīt) [Ger.]. The elasticity of cervical mucus. The cervical secretion is aspirated and placed on a slide. Spinnbarkeit (SBK) is measured by pulling upward on the secretion with a forceps. Before ovulation there is no elasticity. On the day of ovulation there is good elasticity, measuring 12 to 24 cm or more. The day after ovulation, elasticity diminishes.

Not all women have SBK changes that are clear-cut. Therefore, this test is used in conjunction with other signs of ovulation. SEE: *basal temperature chart; fern pattern; mittelschmerz; mucorrhea.*

spinobulbar (spī'nō-bŭl'băr) [" + Gr. *bulbos,* a bulb]. Concerning the spinal cord and medulla oblongata.

spinocellular (spī'nō-sĕl'ū-lăr) [" + *cellula,* little cell]. Pert. to or like prickle cells.

spinocerebellar (spī'nō-sĕr-ĕ-bĕl'ăr) [" + *cerebellum,* little brain]. Concerning the spinal cord and cerebellum.

spinocortical (spī'nō-kor'tĭ-kăl) [" + *cortex,* rind]. Pert. to the spinal cord and cerebral cortex. SYN: *corticospinal.*

spinocostalis (spī'nō-kŏs-tā'lĭs) [" + *costa,* rib]. The combination of the superior and inferior serratus muscles.

spinoglenoid (spī'nō-glĕn'oyd) [" + Gr. *glene,* socket, + *eidos,* form, shape]. Rel. to the spine of the scapula and the glenoid cavity.

spinoglenoid ligament. Ligament joining the spine of the scapula to the border of the glenoid cavity.

spinose (spī'nōs) [L. *spina,* thorn]. Spinous.

spinotectal (spī'nō-tĕk'tăl) [" + *tectum,*

roof]. Pert. to the spinal cord and the tectum, the dorsal portion (corpora quadrigemina) of the midbrain.

spinous (spī'nŭs) [L. *spina*, thorn]. Pert. to or resembling a spine.

spinous point. Spot over a spinous process very sensitive to pressure.

spinous process. Prominence at posterior part of each vertebra.

spintherism (spĭn'thĕr-ĭzm) [Gr. *spintherizein*, to emit sparks]. Sensation of sparks before the eyes.

spintheropia (spĭn"thĕr-ō'pē-ă) [Gr. *spinther*, spark, + *ops*, eye]. Subjective sensation of sparks before the eyes.

spiradenitis (spī"răd-ĕn-ī'tĭs) [Gr. *speira*, coil, + *aden*, gland, + *itis*, inflammation]. A funiculus beginning in coil of a sweat gland. SEE: *hidrosadenitis.*

spiradenoma (spī"răd-ĕn-ō'mă) [" + " + *oma*, tumor]. Benign tumor of the sweat glands.

spiral (spī'răl) [L. *spiralis*]. Coiling around a center like the thread of a screw.

   s., Curschmann's. SEE: *Curschmann's spirals.*

spiral bandage. Roller bandage to be applied spirally.

spiral canal of cochlea. The bony cochlea enclosing the scala tympani, scala vestibuli, and cochlear duct.

spiral canal of modiolus. Canal that runs spirally around the modiolus and contains the spiral ganglion.

spiral lamina. A thin, bony plate projecting from the modiolus into the cochlear canal, dividing it into two portions, the upper scala vestibuli and lower scala tympani. SYN: *lamina spiralis.*

spiral organ of Corti. Structure in floor of cochlear duct resting on basilar membrane. It contains hair cells, the receptors of stimuli produced by sound. SEE: *Corti, organ of.*

spirilla (spī-rĭl'ă) [L.]. Pl. of spirillum.

spirillicidal (spī-rĭl"ĭ-sīd'ăl) [L. *spirillum*, coil, + *cidus*, kill]. Destroying spirochetes or spirilla.

spirillicide (spī-rĭl'ĭ-sīd). Destructive to spirilla.

spirillolysis (spī"rĭ-lŏl'ĭ-sĭs) [" + Gr. *lysis*, dissolution]. The destruction of spirilla.

spirillosis (spī-rĭl-ō'sĭs) [" + Gr. *osis*, condition]. A disease caused by presence of spirilla in the blood.

spirillotropic (spī"rĭ-lō-trŏp'ĭk) [" + Gr. *trope*, a turning]. Having an attraction to spirilla.

spirillotropism (spī"rĭ-lŏt'rō-pĭzm) [" + " + *-ismos*, condition]. The ability to attract spirilla.

Spirillum (spī-rĭl'ŭm) [L., coil]. (pl. *Spirilla*) A genus of spiral-shaped motile microorganisms belonging to the family Pseudomonadaceae, tribe Spirilleae. Found in fresh water and salt water.

   S. minus. Species found in the blood of rats and mice. The causative agent of one form of rat-bite fever.

spirillum (pl. *spirilla*). A flagellated aerobic bacterium with an elongated spiral shape, of the genus *Spirillum.* SEE: *bacteria* for illus.

spirit (spĭr'ĭt) [L. *spiritus*, breath]. 1. A solution of essential or volatile liquid. 2. Any distilled or volatile liquid. 3. Alcoholic beverage.

   s. of ammonia. A pungent solution of approximately 4% ammonium carbonate in 70% alcohol flavored with lemon, lavender, and myristica oil. It is used to elicit reflex stimulation of respiration and as smelling salts to stimulate patients who have fainted.

   s. of bitter almond. A mixture of oil of bitter almond, almond, and distilled water, employed as a flavoring agent.

   s. of camphor. A mixture of camphor and alcohol, employed locally as a counterirritant.

   s. of juniper. A mixture of oil of juniper and alcohol.

   s. of lavender. A mixture of oil of lavender flowers and alcohol, employed as a flavoring agent.

   s. of mustard. A solution of volatile oil of mustard in alcohol, employed as a counterirritant.

   s. of peppermint. A mixture of oil of peppermint, peppermint, and alcohol, employed as a carminative.

spiritual therapy [L. *spiritus*, breath, + Gr. *therapeia*, treatment]. The application of spiritual knowledge in the treatment of mental and physical disorders. Based upon the assumption that man is a spiritual being living in a spiritual universe, that in proportion to his acceptance of this idea and in proportion to his success in using it, he may control his body and maintain the material elements in harmony with a divine plan.

spirituous (spĭr'ĭt-ū-ŭs") [L., *spiritus*, breath]. 1. Pert. to alcohol. 2. An alcoholic.

spiritus (spĭr'ĭ-tŭs) [L., breath]. Alcoholic solution of a volatile substance. Usually, 5% to 10% strength. SYN: *spirit.* SEE: *elixer.*

   s. frumenti. Whiskey.

   s. juniperi. Gin.

   s. myrciae. Bay rum.

   s. vini gallici. Brandy.

Spirochaeta (spī"rō-kē'tă) [Gr. *speira*, coil, + *chaite*, hair]. A genus of slender, spiral, motile microorganisms belonging to the family Spirochaetaceae, order Spirochaetales.

   S. icterohaemorrhagiae. Species found in Weil's disease or acute febrile jaundice.

SYN: *Leptospira interrogans icterohae-morrhagiae.*

S. pallida. The microorganism that causes syphilis. SYN: *Treponema pallidum.*

Spirochaetales (spī″rō-kē-tā′lēs). An order of slender spiral organisms belonging to the class Schizomycetes. It includes the families Spirochaetaceae and Treponemataceae.

spirochetal (spī″rō-kē′tăl) [″ + *chaite*, hair]. Pert. to spirochetes, esp. infections caused by them.

spirochetalytic (spī″rō-kē″tă-lĭt′ĭk) [″ + ″ + *lysis*, dissolution]. Destructive of spirochetes.

spirochete (spī′rō-kēt). Any member of the order Spirochaetales.

spirochetemia (spī″rō-kē-tē′mē-ă) [″ + *chaite*, hair, + *haima*, blood]. Spirochetes in the blood.

spirocheticidal (spī″rō-kē″tĭ-sī′dăl) [″ + ″ + L. *cidus*, kill]. Destructive to spirochetes.

spirocheticide (spī″rō-kē′tĭ-sīd). Anything that destroys spirochetes.

spirochetolysis (spī″rō-kē-tŏl′ĭ-sĭs) [″ + *chaite*, hair, + *lysis*, dissolution]. The destruction of spirochetes by specific antibodies, chemotherapy, or lysins.

spirochetosis (spī″rō-kē-tō′sĭs) [″ + ″ + *osis*, condition]. Any infection caused by spirochetes.

spirochetotic (spī″rō-kē-tŏt′ĭk). Pert. to or marked by spirochetosis.

spirocheturia (spī″rō-kē-tū′rē-ă) [Gr. *speira*, coil, + *chaite*, hair, + *ouron*, urine]. Spirochetes in the urine.

spirogram (spī′rō-grăm″) [L. *spirare*, to breathe, + Gr. *gramma*, something written]. A record made by a spirograph indicating respiratory movements.

spirograph (spī′rō-grăf) [″ + Gr. *graphein*, to write]. Graphic record of respiratory movements.

spiroid (spī′royd) [Gr. *speira*, coil, + *eidos*, form, shape]. Resembling a spiral.

spirokinesis (spī″rō-kĭn-ē′sĭs) [″ + *kinesis*, movement]. The tendency of motile organisms, including humans, to veer or move in a spiral direction when deprived of external reference points.

spiroma (spī-rō′mă) [″ + *oma*, tumor]. Multiple, benign, cystic epithelioma of the sweat glands. SYN: *spiradenoma.*

spirometer (spī-rŏm′ĕt-ĕr) [L. *spirare*, to breathe, + Gr. *metron*, measure]. An apparatus one form of which consists of a cylindrical bell immersed in water and so equipped with outlets that gases can be exhaled into it or inhaled out of it while measurements of volume are made. Less cumbersome forms are available. The following are typical measurements made on normal men by using the spirometer:

Complemental air (inspiratory reserve volume): 1600 cc, the amount that a subject can still inhale by special effort after a normal inspiration.

Dead space air: 150 cc, the air inhaled through the nose that gets only as far as nasopharynx, bronchi, bronchioles, and trachea and does not reach the lungs.

Functional residual air (functional residual capacity): About 2600 cc, the sum of the supplemental and residual air.

Minimal air: Less than 1000 cc, that which remains in the lungs after complete collapse, as in pneumothorax.

Reserve air: Supplemental air.

Residual air (residual volume): 1000 cc, the amount left in the lungs after a complete expiration.

Supplemental air (expiratory reserve volume): 1600 cc that can still be exhaled after a normal exhalation.

Tidal volume: 500 cc, the amount exhaled or inhaled during normal respiration.

spirometry (spī-rŏm′ĕ-trē) [L. *spirare*, to breathe, + Gr. *metron*, measure]. Measurement of air capacity of the lungs.

spironolactone (spī-rō″nō-lăk′tōn). USP. A diuretic drug that blocks the action of aldosterone on the renal tubules. It acts to decrease potassium loss in the urine. Trade name is Aldactone.

spissated (spĭs′āt-ĕd) [L. *spissatus*]. Thickened. SYN: *inspissated.*

spissitude (spĭs′ĭ-tūd) [L. *spissitudo*]. Condition of being inspissated, as a fluid thickened by evaporation almost to a solid; thickness.

spit (spĭt) [AS. *spittan*]. 1. Saliva. SYN: *expectoration; spittle; sputum.* 2. To expectorate spittle.

spittle [AS. *spatl*]. Saliva; spit.

splanchna (splăngk′nă) [Gr.]. The intestines or the viscera.

splanchnapophysis (splăngk″nă-pŏf′ĭ-sĭs) [Gr. *splanchnos*, viscus, + *apophysis*, offshoot]. 1. Any skeletal element involved with the function of the alimentary canal, as the lower jaw. 2. Outgrowth of a vertebra on opposite side of vertebral axis, enclosing some viscus.

splanchnectopia (splăngk″nĕk-tō′pē-ă) [″ + *ektopos*, out of place]. Dislocation of a viscus or of the viscera.

splanchnemphraxis (splăngk″nĕm-frăk′sĭs) [″ + *emphraxis*, stoppage]. Obstruction of any internal organ, particularly of the intestine.

splanchnesthesia (splăngk″nĕs-thē′zē-ă) [″ + *aisthesis*, sensation]. Visceral sensation.

splanchnesthetic (splăngk″nĕs-thĕt′ĭk).

Rel. to visceral consciousness or sensation.

splanchnic (splăngk′nĭk) [Gr. *splanchnikos*]. Pert. to the viscera.

splanchnicectomy (splăngk″nē-sĕk′tō-mē) [Gr. *splanchnos*, viscus, + *ektome*, excision]. Resection of the splanchnic nerves.

splanchnic nerves. Three nerves from the thoracic sympathetic ganglia distributed to the viscera.

splanchnicotomy (splăngk″nĭ-kŏt′ō-mē) [″ + *tome*, incision]. Section of a splanchnic nerve.

splanchnoblast (splăngk′nō-blăst) [″ + *blastos*, germ]. Incipient rudiment of a viscus. SEE: *anlage; proton*.

splanchnocele (splăngk′nō-sēl). 1. [″ + *koilos*, a cavity] That part of the coelom persisting in the adult, giving rise to the visceral cavities. SYN: *splanchnocoele*. 2. [″ + *kele*, tumor, swelling] Protrusion of any abdominal viscus.

splanchnocoele (splăngk′nō-sēl) [″ + *koilos*, a cavity]. Rudimentary embryonic cavity from which the visceral cavities arise.

splanchnocranium (splăngk″nō-krā′nē-ŭm) [″ + *kranion*, skull]. The portion of the skull derived from the visceral or branchial skeleton.

splanchnodiastasis (splăngk″nō-dī-ăs′tă-sĭs) [″ + *diastasis*, a separation]. Displacement or separation of any viscus.

splanchnodynia (splăngk-nō-dĭn′ē-ă) [Gr. *splanchnos*, viscus, + *odyne*, pain]. Pain in the abdominal region.

splanchnography (splăngk-nŏg′ră-fē) [″ + *graphein*, to write]. Descriptive treatise on anatomy of the viscera.

splanchnolith (splăngk′nō-lĭth) [″ + *lithos*, stone]. An intestinal calculus.

splanchnology (splăngk-nŏl′ō-jē) [″ + *logos*, word, reason]. The study of the viscera.

splanchnomegaly (splăngk″nō-mĕg′ă-lē) [″ + *megas*, large]. Visceromegaly, q.v.

splanchnomicria (splăngk″nō-mĭk′rē-ă) [″ + *mikros*, small]. The condition of having small splanchnic organs.

splanchnopathia (splăngk″nō-păth′ē-ă) [″ + *pathos*, disease, suffering]. Pathological conditions of the viscera.

splanchnopleural (splăngk″nō-ploor′ăl) [″ + *pleura*, side]. Concerning the splanchnopleure.

splanchnopleure (splăngk′nō-plūr) [″ + *pleura*, side]. The embryonic layer formed by the union of the visceral layer of the mesoderm with the entoderm. SEE: *somatopleure*.

splanchnoptosia,   splanchnoptosis (splăngk″nō-tō′sē-ă, -sĭs) [″ + *ptosis*, a dropping]. Prolapse of the viscera. SYN: *enteroptosis; ptosis, abdominal; visceroptosis*.

splanchnosclerosis (splăngk″nō-sklĕr-ō′sĭs) [″ + *sklerosis*, to harden]. Hardening of any of the viscera through overgrowth or infiltration of connective tissue.

splanchnoscopy (splăngk-nŏs′kō-pē) [″ + *skopein*, to examine]. Examination of the viscera with aid of roentgen rays or transillumination.

splanchnoskeleton (splăngk″nō-skĕl′ĕ-tŏn) [″ + *skeleton*, a dried-up body]. 1. In primitive vertebrates such as fishes, the cartilaginous or bony arches (branchial) that encircle pharyngeal portion of digestive tract. 2. In higher vertebrates, the bones derived from the branchial arches, which include the maxilla, mandible, malleus, incus, stapes, hyoid bone, and cartilages of the larynx.

splanchnosomatic (splăngk″nō-sō-măt′ĭk) [″ + *soma*, body]. Viscerosomatic, q.v.

splanchnotomy (splăngk-nŏt′ō-mē) [″ + *tome*, incision]. Dissection of the viscera.

splanchnotribe (splăngk′nō-trīb) [″ + *tribein*, to rub]. A crushing instrument for temporarily closing the lumen of the intestine prior to resection.

splayfoot [ME. *splayen*, to spread out, + AS. *fot*, foot]. A flatfoot or the deformity flatfoot. SYN: *pes planus; talipes valgus*.

spleen (splēn) [Gr. *splen*]. The largest collection of reticuloendothelial cells (monocytic phagocytes) in the body; an elongated, dark red, ovoid body lying in upper left quadrant of abdomen posterior and inferior to the stomach. It is composed of spongelike tissue (splenic pulp) consisting of lymphatic tissue differentiated into white pulp and pulp infiltrated with red blood cells (red pulp). It is enclosed by a dense capsule from which trabeculae extend into substance of the spleen. On one side is the hilus through which the splenic vessels and nerves enter and exit. SYN: *lien* [NA]. SEE: *abdominal quadrants* for illus.

FUNCT: *Blood formation:* In the embryo, all types of blood cells are formed by the spleen, but in the adult, only lymphocytes and monocytes. In the adult, if bone marrow is damaged, the spleen can function to produce various blood cells. *Blood storage:* Smooth muscle and elastic tissue fibers in the capsule and trabeculae enable the spleen to contract and discharge blood cells into circulation. *Blood filtration:* By which bacteria and particulate matter, esp. aged, nonfunctioning red blood cells, are removed from circulation. The spleen also removes inclusion bodies such as Heinz bodies and the nuclei of immature red blood cells from circulating red blood cells.

DISORDERS OF: Acute and chronic infections and certain infectionlike states, hypersplenism, primary splenic thrombocytopenia, primary splenic neutropenia, Felty's syndrome, Banti's disease, congestive splenomegaly, tumors. SEE: *asplenia syndrome; thrombosis.*

s., accessory. Splenic tissue nodules near the spleen.

s., floating. An enlarged movable spleen that is not protected by the ribs.

s., lardaceous. Enlargement of spleen due to fatty tissue. SEE: *degeneration, amyloid.*

s., sago. Spleen having appearance of grains of sago, q.v.

splenadenoma (splēn″ăd-ĕ-nō′mă) [Gr. *splen*, spleen, + *aden*, gland, + *oma*, tumor]. Enlargement of the spleen caused by hyperplasia of its pulp.

splenalgia (splē-năl′jē-ă) [″ + *algos*, pain]. Neuralgic pain in the spleen. SYN: *splenodynia.*

splenceratosis (splēn″sĕr-ă-tō′sĭs) [″ + *keras*, horn, + *osis*, condition]. Induration of the spleen.

splenectasia, splenectasis (splē″nĕk-tā′zē-ă, splē-nĕk′tă-sĭs) [″ + *ektasis*, dilatation]. Enlargement of the spleen.

splenectomy (splē-nĕk′tō-mē) [″ + *ektome*, excision]. Surgical excision of the spleen.

splenectomy, infections following. Because of the importance of the spleen in the control of bacteria in the bloodstream, its removal in young children has resulted in abnormal risk of their developing fulminant infections. Removal of the spleen in otherwise healthy adults causes only a slight alteration in their ability to resist infections.

splenectopia, splenectopy (splē″nĕk-tō′pē-ă, -nĕk′tō-pē) [″ + *ektopos*, out of place]. Displacement or mobility of the spleen. SYN: *spleen, floating.*

splenelcosis (splē″nĕl-kō′sĭs) [″ + *helkosis*, ulceration]. Ulceration or abscess of the spleen.

splenemia (splē-nē′mē-ă) [Gr. *splen*, spleen, + *haima*, blood]. 1. Splenic congestion with blood. 2. Leukemia with splenic hypertrophy.

splenemphraxis (splē″nĕm-frăk′sĭs) [″ + *emphraxis*, an obstruction]. Congested condition of the spleen.

spleneolus (splē-nē′ō-lŭs). Accessory spleen.

splenetic (splē-nĕt′ĭk). 1. Pert. to the spleen. 2. Suffering with chronic disease of the spleen. 3. Surly, fretful, impatient.

splenetic cords. Poorly defined cords of red pulp of the spleen.

splenetic nodule. A concentrated mass of white pulp in the spleen. SYN: *malpighian body* (def. 2).

splenetic sinus. One of a series of wide channels with thin walls forming an anastomosing plexus throughout red pulp of spleen. SYN: *terminal veins.*

splenetic vein. Vein carrying blood from spleen to the portal vein.

splenial (splē′nē-ăl) [Gr. *splen*, spleen]. Concerning the spleen.

splenic (splĕn′ĭk) [Gr. *splenikos*]. Splenetic.

splenic flexure. Junction of transverse and descending colon, making a bend on the left side near the spleen.

splenicterus (splē-nĭk′tĕr-ŭs) [Gr. *splen*, spleen, + *ikteros*, jaundice]. Inflammation of the spleen associated with jaundice.

splenification (splē″nĭ-fĭ-kā′shŭn) [″ + L. *facere*, to make]. Change in a structure whereby it resembles splenic tissue. SYN: *splenization.*

spleniform (splĕn′ĭ-form) [″ + L. *forma*, form]. Resembling the spleen.

splenitis (splē-nī′tĭs) [″ + *itis*, inflammation]. Inflamed condition of the spleen. Comprises acute and chronic hypertrophy, proliferative splenitis, and suppurative inflammation, the result of acute infectious disease.

SYM: Indefinite or absent. Usually little pain or tenderness unless perisplenitis exists. Considerable enlargement may be attended by sense of weight, tension, or distress in left hypochondrium, accompanied perhaps by slight dyspnea, sudden pain appearing in gastric region followed by vomiting of pus and blood in course of infectious disease, which may be due to abscess of spleen.

PROG: Depends upon systemic condition.

splenium (splē′nē-ŭm) [Gr. *splenion*, bandage]. 1. A compress or bandage. 2. A structure resembling a bandaged part.

s. corporis callosi. [NA] The thickened posterior end of the corpus callosum.

splenius (splē′nē-ŭs). A flat muscle on either side of back of neck and upper thoracic area. SEE: *muscle* for illus.; *Muscles* in Appendix.

splenization (splē″nĭ-zā′shŭn). The change in a tissue, as of the lung, when it resembles splenic tissue.

spleno-. Combining form concerning the spleen.

splenocele (splē′nō-sēl) [Gr. *splen*, spleen, + *kele*, tumor, swelling]. 1. A hernia of the spleen. 2. A splenic tumor.

splenoceratosis (splē″nō-sĕr″ă-tō′sĭs) [″ + *keras*, horn, + *osis*, condition]. Induration of the spleen.

splenocleisis (splē″nō-klī′sĭs) [″ + *kleisis*, closure]. Friction on the surface of the spleen or wrapping with gauze in order to induce the formation of fibrous tissue.

splenocolic (splē″nō-kŏl′ĭk) [″ + *kolon*,

colon]. Pert. to the spleen and colon or reference to a fold of peritoneum between the two viscera.

splenocyte (splē'nō-sīt) [" + *kytos,* cell]. A unicellular leukocyte or lymphocyte of the spleen. It probably originates elsewhere in the body.

splenodynia (splē"nō-dīn'ē-ă) [" + *odyne,* pain]. Pain in the spleen. SYN: *splenalgia.*

splenogenic, splenogenous (splē"nō-jĕn'ĭk, splē-nŏj'ĕn-ŭs) [" + *gennan,* to produce]. Originating in the spleen.

splenography (splē-nŏg'ră-fē) [" + *graphein,* to write]. A treatise on, or a description of, the spleen.

splenohepatomegaly (splē"nō-hĕp"ă-tō-mĕg'ă-lē) [Gr. *splen,* spleen, + *hepar,* liver, + *megas,* large]. Enlargement of the spleen and liver.

splenoid (splē'noyd) [" + *eidos,* form, shape]. Resembling the spleen.

splenokeratosis (splē"nō-kĕr"ă-tō'sĭs) [" + *keras,* horn, + *osis,* condition]. Induration of the spleen.

splenolaparotomy (splē"nō-lăp"ă-rŏt'ō-mē) [" + *lapara,* flank, + *tome,* incision]. Incision through the abdominal wall into the spleen.

splenology (splē-nŏl'ō-jē) [" + *logos,* word, reason]. The study of functions and diseases of the spleen.

splenolymphatic (splē"nō-lĭm-făt'ĭk) [" + L. *lympha,* lymph]. Concerning the spleen and lymph nodes.

splenolysin (splē-nŏl'ĭ-sĭn) [" + *lysis,* dissolution]. An antibody that destroys splenic tissue.

splenolysis (splē-nŏl'ĭ-sĭs). Destruction of splenic tissue.

splenoma (splē-nō'mă) [" + *oma,* tumor] (pl. *splenomas, -mata*). A tumor of the spleen. SYN: *splenocele.*

splenomalacia (splē"nō-mă-lā'shē-ă) [" + *malakia,* softening]. Softening of the spleen.

splenomedullary (splē"nō-mĕd'ū-lĕr"ē) [" + L. *medulla,* marrow]. Concerning the spleen and bone marrow, or originating in the spleen and bone marrow.

splenomegalia, splenomegaly (splē"nō-mē-gā'lē-ă, -mĕg'ă-lē) [" + *megas,* large]. Enlargement of the spleen.

    s., congestive. A syndrome consisting of anemia, splenic enlargement, hemorrhages, and ultimately cirrhosis of the liver. SYN: *Banti's syndrome.*

    s., hemolytic. Enlargement of the spleen in association with hemolytic disease of the blood.

splenometry (splē-nŏm'ĕ-trē) [" + *metron,* measure]. Determining the size of the spleen.

splenomyelogenous (splē-nō-mī"ĕ-lŏj'ĕ-nŭs) [" + *myelos,* marrow, + *gennan,* to produce]. Splenomedullary, q.v.

splenomyelomalacia (splē"nō-mī"ĕl-ō-mă-lā'shē-ă) [" + " + *malakia,* softening]. Abnormal softening of the spleen and bone marrow.

splenoncus (splē-nŏng'kŭs) [Gr. *splen,* spleen, + *onkos,* tumor]. Tumor of the spleen.

splenonephric (splē"nō-nĕf'rĭk) [" + *nephros,* kidney]. Rel. to the spleen and kidney. SYN: *lienorenal.*

splenonephroptosis (splē"nō-nĕf"rŏp-tō'sĭs) [" + " + *ptosis,* a dropping]. Downward displacement of the spleen and kidney.

splenopancreatic (splē"nō-păn"krē-ăt'ĭk) [" + *pankreas,* pancreas]. Rel. to the spleen and pancreas.

splenopathy (splē-nŏp'ă-thē) [" + *pathos,* disease, suffering]. Any disorder of the spleen.

splenopexy (splē'nō-pĕk"sē) [" + *pexis,* fixation]. Artificial fixation of a movable spleen.

splenophrenic (splĕn-ō-frĕn'ĭk) [" + *phren,* diaphragm]. Concerning the spleen and diaphragm.

splenopneumonia (splē"nō-nū-mō'nē-ă) [" + *pneumonia,* inflammation of lung]. Pneumonia with splenization, q.v., of the lung.

splenoportography (splē"nō-por-tŏg'ră-fē) [" + L. *porta,* gate, + Gr. *graphein,* to write]. X-ray study of the spleen and portal vein after injection of a radiopaque dye into the spleen.

splenoptosis (splē"nŏp-tō'sĭs) [" + *ptosis,* a dropping]. Downward displacement of the spleen.

splenorenal (splē"nō-rē'năl). Pert. to the spleen and kidney.

splenorenal shunt. Anastomosis of splenic vein to renal vein to enable blood from portal system to enter general venous circulation. Performed in cases of portal hypertension.

splenorrhagia (splē"nō-rā'jē-ă) [" + *rhegnynai,* to burst forth]. Hemorrhage from a ruptured spleen.

splenorrhaphy (splē-nor'ă-fē) [" + *rhaphe,* seam, ridge]. Suture of wound of the spleen.

splenotomy (splē-nŏt'ō-mē) [" + *tome,* incision]. Incision of the spleen.

splenotoxin (splē"nō-tŏks'ĭn) [" + *toxikon,* poison]. Cytotoxin having specific action on splenic cells. SYN: *lienotoxin.*

splenulus (splĕn'ū-lŭs) [L., a little spleen]. A rudimentary or accessory spleen.

splenunculus (splē-nŭng'kū-lŭs). Accessory

spleen.

splint (splĭnt) [MD. *splinte*, a wedge]. An appliance made of bone, wood, metal, or plaster of paris, used for the fixation, union, or protection of an injured part of the body. It may be movable or immovable.

s., acrylic resin bite-guard. Device fashioned to cover the incisal and occlusal surfaces of a dental arch for the purpose of stabilizing the teeth, treating bruxism, or facilitating proper occlusal positioning.

s., Agnew's. Splint used in fractures of the patella and metacarpus.

s., airplane. An appliance usually used on ambulatory patients in the treatment of fractures of the humerus. It takes its name from the elevated (abducted) position in which it holds the arm suspended away from the body.

s., anchor. Splint for fracture of the jaw, with metal loops fitting over the teeth and held together by a rod.

s., Ashhurst's. A bracketed splint of wire with a footpiece to cover the thigh and leg after excision of the knee joint.

s., Balkan. Splint used for continuous extension in fracture of the femur.

s., banjo traction. Splint made out of a steel rod bent to resemble the shape of a banjo. Used for the treatment of contractures and fractures of the fingers.

s., Bavarian. An immovable dressing in which the plaster is applied between two layers of flannel.

s., blow-up. Tubular material that fits around the injured extremity. It contains compartments that can be inflated. These immobilize the injured part when filled with air.

s., Bond's. Splint used for fracture of the lower end of the radius.

s., Bowlby's. Splint used for fracture of the shaft of the humerus.

s., bracketed. Splint composed of two pieces of metal or wood united by brackets.

s., Cabot's. Splint composed of a metal structure placed posterior to the thigh and leg.

s., Carter's intranasal. A steel bridge with wings connected by a hinge. Used for operation of depressed nasal bridge.

s., coaptation. Small splint adjusted about a fractured part to prevent overriding of the fragments of bones. Usually covered by a longer splint for fixation of entire section.

s., Denis Browne. Splint used to treat talipes equinovarus (clubfoot) and consisting of a curved bar attached to the soles of a pair of high-topped shoes. Often used in late infancy and applied at bedtime. Generally employed following casting and manipula-

tion which have reduced the deformity.

s., dental. A rigid or flexible device or compound used to support, protect, or immobilize teeth that have been loosened, replanted, fractured, or subjected to surgical procedures.

s., Dupuytren's. Splint used to prevent eversion in Pott's fracture, q.v.

s., dynamic. Splint that assists in movements initiated by the patient.

s., flail arm. SEE: *flail arm splint.*

s., Fox's. Splint used for fractured clavicle.

s., functional. S., dynamic, q.v.

s., Gibson walking. Splint that is a modification of Thomas splint.

s., Gordon's. A side splint used for the arm and hand in Colles' fracture, q.v.

s., inflatable. Inflatable device for immobilizing part or all of an extremity. The hollow tubular device is placed around the part and then inflated. SEE: *s., blow-up.*

Caution: Do not inflate tightly enough to prevent flow of blood to and from the extremity. If the patient is to be transported by air, an inflatable splint should not be used without carefully monitoring and adjusting the pressure during flight and at time of descent.

s., Jones' nasal. Splint used for fracture of nasal bones.

s., Kanavel. Splint used for stiffened hands.

s., Levis'. Splint of perforated metal extending from below the elbow to the end of the palm; shaped to fit the arm and hand.

s., McIntire's. Splint shaped like a double inclined plane, used as a posterior splint for leg and thigh.

s., permanent fixed. A nonremovable prosthesis firmly attached to an abutment used to stabilize or immobilize teeth. A fixed bridge may serve as a permanent fixed splint for such support.

s., Sayre's. One of three varieties of splint: ankle, knee, and hip joint disease.

s., Stromeyer's. Splint with two hinged sections that can be set at any angle, used esp. for the knee.

s., temporary removable. One of a variety of splints used for temporary or intermittent support and stabilization of teeth.

s., Thomas. A long wire splint with a proximal ring. The ring fits over the lower extremity and is placed as far as it will go toward the hip. Used in emergency treatment of femoral fracture.

s., Thomas' knee. A rigid metal used to remove pressure of body weight from a weak knee joint by transferring weight to the ischium and perineum.

s., Thomas' posterior. SEE: *Thomas splint.*

s., Volkmann's. Splint used for fracture of lower extremity, consisting of a footpiece and two lateral supports.

splinter (splĭn'tĕr) [MD. *splinte*, a wedge]. 1. A fragment from a fractured bone. 2. A slender, sharp piece of material piercing or imbedded in the skin.

splinter hemorrhage. Small linear hemorrhage under the fingernails or toenails. May be due to subacute bacterial endocarditis.

splinter skill. Any trained, developed, or learned skill that is acquired in an intermittent or inconsistent pattern and is unrelated to any variety or integration of previous skills. SEE: *cross-training.*

splinting. Fixation of a dislocation or fracture with a splint. Splints are also used to help support weak joints, to actively assist with functional movement, to immobilize to promote healing, and to protect from injury and deformity.

split (splĭt) [D. *splitten*, to divide]. 1. A longitudinal fissure. 2. Characterized by a deep fissure.

split foot. Congenital deformity, the division of the toes extending into the metatarsal region.

split hand. Congenital deformity, the division between the fingers extending into the metacarpal region. SYN: *cleft hand.*

split pelvis. Congenital failure of pubic bones to form a union at the symphysis.

splitting (splĭt'ĭng) [D. *splitten*, to divide]. In chemistry, the breaking up of complex molecules into two or more simpler compounds.

split tongue. A cleft or bifid tongue resulting from developmental arrest.

spodogenous (spō-dŏj'ĕn-ŭs) [Gr. *spodos*, ashes, + *gennan*, to produce]. Caused by waste material.

spodophagous (spō-dŏf'ă-gŭs) [" + *phagein*, to eat]. Destroying the waste matters in the body; said of scavenger cells.

spondee (spŏn-dē). Two-syllable words that receive equal stress on each syllable.

spondee threshold [Fr., a two-syllable word with equal stress on each syllable]. In audiometry, the intensity at which speech is recognized as a meaningful symbol. This is tested by presenting, through an audiometer, two-syllable words in which each symbol is accented equally. SEE: *audiometry.*

spondyl- (spŏn'dĭl) [Gr. *spondylos*, vertebra]. Combining form for vertebra.

spondylalgia (spŏn"dĭl-ăl'jē-ă) [" + *algos*, pain]. Painful condition of a vertebra.

spondylarthritis (spŏn"dĭl-ăr-thrī'tĭs) [" + *arthron*, joint, + *itis*, inflammation]. Inflammation of the joints of the vertebrae;

arthritis of the spine. SEE: *spondylitis.*

spondylarthrocace (splon"dĭl-ăr-thrŏk'ă-sē) [" + " + *kake*, badness]. Tuberculous condition of the vertebrae.

spondylexarthrosis (spŏn"dĭl-ĕks"ăr-thrō'sĭs) [" + *exarthrosis*, dislocation]. Dislocation of a vertebra.

spondylitic (spŏn"dĭ-lĭt'ĭk) [" + *itis*, inflammation]. 1. A person with spondylitis. 2. Concerning spondylitis.

spondylitis (spŏn-dĭl-ī'tĭs) [" + *itis*, inflammation]. Inflammation of one or more vertebrae, esp. tuberculous disease of the vertebrae, Pott's disease, q.v.

s., ankylosing. S., rheumatoid.

s. deformans. Inflammation of the vertebral joints resulting in the outgrowth of bonylike deposits on the vertebrae, which may fuse and cause rigid and distorted spine.

s., hypertrophic. Condition occurring in most people over 50 in which bodies of vertebrae hypertrophy. Bony changes such as slipping at bases and the development of bony outgrowths on articular processes occur.

s., Kümmell's. Traumatic spondylitis in which symptoms do not appear until some time after the injury.

s., Marie-Strümpell. S., rheumatoid.

s., rheumatoid. A chronic progressive disease involving the joints between articular processes, costovertebral joints, and sacroiliac joints. Bilateral sclerosis of sacroiliac joints is a diagnostic sign. Changes occurring in joints are similar to those seen in rheumatoid arthritis. Ankylosis may occur, giving rise to stiff back (poker spine). SYN: *s., ankylosing.*

s., tuberculous. SEE: *Pott's disease.*

spondylizema (spŏn"dĭl-ĭ-zē'mă) [Gr. *spondylos*, vertebra, + *izema*, depression]. Downward displacement of a vertebra caused by the disintegration of the one below it.

spondylo- [Gr. *spondylos*, vertebra]. Combining form meaning a vertebra.

spondylocace (spŏn"dĭ-lŏk'ă-sē) [" + *kake*, badness]. Tuberculosis of the vertebrae. SYN: *spondylarthrocace.*

spondylodiagnosis (spŏn"dĭ-lō-dī"ăg-nō'sĭs) [" + *dia*, through, + *gnosis*, knowledge]. Diagnosis by means of visceral reflexes obtained by percussion of the vertebrae.

spondylodymus (spŏn"dĭ-lŏd'ĭ-mŭs) [" + *didymos*, twin]. Twin fetuses joined at the vertebrae.

spondylodynia (spŏn"dĭ-lō-dĭn'ē-ă) [" + *odyne*, pain]. Pain in a vertebra.

spondylolisthesis (spŏn"dĭ-lō-lĭs"thē'sĭs) [" + *oblisthesis*, a slipping]. Any forward slipping of one vertebrae on the one below it. Predisposing factors include spondylolysis, degeneration, elongated pars, elongated pedicles, and birth defects in the spine such as spina bifida. SEE: *retrospondylolisthesis.*

spondylolisthetic (spŏn″dĭ-lō-lĭs-thĕt′ĭk). Concerning spondylolisthesis.

spondylolysis (spŏn″dĭ-lŏl′ĭ-sĭs) [″ + *lysis,* dissolution]. The breaking down of a vertebral structure.

spondylomalacia (spŏn″dĭ-lō-mă-lā′shē-ă) [″ + *malakia,* softening]. Softening of the vertebrae.

spondylopathy (spŏn″dĭl-ŏp′ă-thē) [″ + *pathos,* disease, suffering]. Any disorder of the vertebrae.

spondyloptosis (spŏn″dĭ-lō-tō′sĭs) [″ + *ptosis,* a dropping]. Spondylolisthesis, q.v.

spondylopyosis (spŏn″dĭ-lō″pī-ō′sĭs) [″ + *pyosis,* suppuration]. Suppuration with inflammation of a vertebra.

spondyloschisis (spŏn″dĭ-lŏs′kĭ-sĭs) [″ + *schisis,* a splitting]. Congenital fissure of one or more of the vertebral arches. SYN: *rhachioschisis.*

spondylosis (spŏn″dĭ-lō′sĭs) [Gr. *spondylos,* vertebra, + *osis,* condition]. Vertebral ankylosis.

   s., cervical or lumbar. Degenerative arthritis, osteoarthritis, of the cervical or lumbar vertebrae and related tissues. It may cause pressure on nerve roots with subsequent pain or paresthesia in the extremities.

   s., rhizomelic. Ankylosis interfering with movements of hips and shoulders.

spondylosyndesis (spŏn″dĭ-lō-sĭn′dĕ-sĭs) [″ + *syndesis,* a binding together]. Surgical formation of an ankylosis between vertebrae.

spondylotherapy (spŏn″dĭl-ō-thĕr′ă-pē) [″ + *therapeia,* treatment]. Spinal therapeutics; spinal manipulation in the treatment of disease.

spondylotomy (spŏn″dĭl-ŏt′ō-mē) [″ + *tome,* incision]. Removal of part of the vertebral column to correct a deformity or facilitate delivery of a fetus. SYN: *rachitomy.*

spondylous (spŏn′dĭ-lŭs) [Gr. *spondylos,* vertebra]. Concerning a vertebra.

sponge (spŭnj) [Gr. *sphongos,* sponge]. 1. Elastic, porous mass forming internal skeleton of certain marine animals; or rubber or synthetic substance that resembles sponge in properties and appearance. Used to hold liquids for washing or mopping up spillage. 2. An absorbent pad made of gauze and cotton used to absorb fluids and blood in surgery or to dress wounds. 3. Short term for sponge bath. 4. To moisten, clean, cool, or wipe with a sponge.

   s., abdominal. Flat sponges from ½ to 1 in. (1.27 to 2.54 cm) thick, 3 to 6 in. (7.62 to

15.24 cm) in diameter, used as packing, to prevent closing or obstruction by intrusion of viscera, as covering to prevent tissue injury, and as absorbents.

   s., contraceptive. A sponge impregnated with a spermicide. It is used intravaginally during sexual intercourse as a method of contraception. SYN: *spermicidal sponge.* SEE: *contraceptive.*

   s., gauze. A sterile pad made of absorbent material. It is used during surgery.

   s., gelatin. Spongy substance prepared from gelatin. It is a nonantigenic, readily absorbable material used esp. to stop internal bleeding. Sold under trade name of Gelfoam.

sponge graft. Sponge placed in an ulcer to cause granulation.

spongia (spŏn′jē-ă) [Gr. *sphongos,* sponge]. Sponge.

spongiform (spŭn′jĭ-form) [Gr. *sphongos,* sponge, + L. *forma,* shape]. Having the appearance or quality of a sponge.

spongio-. Combining form indicating sponge-like.

spongioblast (spŭn′jē-ō-blăst) [″ + *blastos,* germ]. Cell that develops from embryonic neural tube and serves as forerunner of ependymal cells and astrocytes.

spongioblastoma (spŭn″jē-ō-blăs-tō′mă) [″ + ″ + *oma,* tumor]. A glioma of the brain derived from spongioblasts.

spongiocyte (spŭn′jē-ō-sīt″) [″ + *kytos,* cell]. A neuroglial cell.

spongioid (spŭn′jē-oyd) [″ + *eidos,* form, shape]. Resembling a sponge. SYN: *spongiform.*

spongiosis (spŭn″jē-ō′sĭs) [Gr. *sphongos,* sponge, + *osis,* condition]. Intercellular edema of the spongy layer of the skin.

spongiositis (spŭn″jē-ō-sī′tĭs) [″ + *itis,* inflammation]. Inflammation of the corpus spongiosum of the urethra.

spongy (spŭn′jē). Resembling a sponge in texture.

spontaneous (spŏn-tā′nē-ŭs) [L.]. Occurring unaided or without apparent cause; voluntary.

spontaneous fracture. Fracture of a demineralized bone as in osteoporosis. This type of fracture may be painless.

   ETIOL: Fragilitas ossium; nerve conditions such as tabes; secondary malignant growths; osteoporosis of bones of the aged.

spontaneous version. The unaided conversion of a transverse presentation of a fetus into a vertex or breech presentation.

spoon [AS. *spon,* a chip]. Instrument consisting of a small bowl on a handle, used in scooping out tissues or tumors, or in measuring quantities.

spoon nail. A toenail or fingernail having a

concave outer surface.

sporadic (spō-răd′ĭk) [Gr. *sporadikos*]. Occurring occasionally or in scattered instances, as a disease. SEE: *endemic; epidemic; pandemic*.

sporangiophore (spō-răn′jē-ō-for) [Gr. *sporos*, seed, + *angeion*, vessel, + *phoros*, a bearer]. In bacteriology, the supporting stalk for a spore sac of certain fungi.

sporangium (spō-răn′jē-ŭm). A sac enclosing spores, seen in certain fungi.

spore (spor) [Gr. *sporos*, seed]. A reproductive cell, usually unicellular, produced by plants and some protozoa. Usually spores are asexual, but certain fungi form sexual spores (oospores, zygospores, or ascospores). Spores usually possess a thick wall enabling the cell to withstand unfavorable environmental conditions.

Sporing is an asexual method of reproduction in many unicellular animals and plants. Certain bacteria also form spores, but more in the nature of a defensive mechanism than for reproduction. The spores of bacteria are difficult to destroy because they are very resistant to heat and require prolonged exposure to high temperatures to destroy them.

sporicidal (spor-ĭ-sī′dăl) [″ + L. *cidus*, kill]. Destructive to spores.

sporicide (spor′ĭ-sīd). An agent that destroys bacterial and mold spores. Because spores are more difficult to kill than vegetative cells, a sporicide also acts as a sterilizing agent.

sporiferous (spor-ĭf′ĕr-ŭs) [″ + L. *ferre*, to bear]. Producing spores.

spork. Adapted utensil for persons with limited upper extremity function. Distal end may swivel to allow food to remain level due to gravitational force. The bowl end is shaped like a spoon but has modified tines, like a fork.

sporoblast (spor′ō-blăst) [″ + *blastos*, germ]. Structure within the oocyst of certain parasitic protozoa (*Eimeria* and *Isospora*) that gives rise to a sporocyst and eventually a spore.

sporocyst (spor′ō-sĭst) [″ + *kystis*, sac]. 1. Any sac containing spores or reproductive cells. 2. Sac secreted around a sporoblast by certain protozoa prior to spore production. 3. Stage in life cycle of a trematode worm usually found in tissues of first intermediate host, a mollusk. It develops from a miracidium and is essentially a germinal sac containing germ cells. It gives rise to daughter sporocysts or rediae.

sporogenesis (spor″ō-jĕn′ĕ-sĭs) [Gr. *sporos*, seed, + *genesis*, generation, birth]. The production or formation of spores.

sporogenic (spor″ō-jĕn′ĭk) [″ + *gennan*,

to produce]. Having the ability of developing into spores.

sporogenous (spor-ŏj′ĕ-nŭs) [″ + *gennan*, to produce]. Concerning sporogenesis.

sporogeny (spor-ŏj′ĕ-nē). Sporogenesis.

sporogony (spor-ŏg′ō-nē) [″ + *goneia*, generation]. Reproducing by development of spores. SYN: *sporogenesis*.

sporophore (spor′ō-for) [″ + *phoros*, bearing]. The spore-bearing portion of an organism.

sporophyte (spor′ō-fīt) [″ + *phyton*, plant]. The spore-bearing stage of a plant exhibiting alternation of generation.

sporoplasm (spor′ō-plăzm) [″ + LL. *plasma*, form, mold]. The cell protoplasm of spores.

Sporothrix (spor′ō-thrĭks). A genus of fungi of the family Moniliaceae.

   S. schenckii. Causative agent of sporotrichosis.

sporotrichin (spor-ŏ′trĭ-kĭn). Antigenic substance derived from *Sporothrix* organisms and used for diagnostic purposes.

sporotrichosis (spor″ō-trī-kō′sĭs) [″ + *thrix*, hair, + *osis*, condition]. A chronic granulomatous infection usually involving the skin and superficial lymph nodes; characterized by formation of abscesses, nodules, and ulcers. It is caused by the fungus *Sporothrix schenckii*, q.v.

Sporotrichum (spō-rŏt′rĭ-kŭm). Former name for *Sporothrix*, q.v.

   S. schenckii. Former name for *Sporothrix schenckii*, q.v.

Sporozoa (spor″ō-zō′ă) [″ + *zoon*, animal]. A subphylum of the phylum Protozoa that includes a miscellaneous assortment of organisms that are parasitic, usually with complicated life cycles, including sexual and asexual forms. Locomotor organs are not present in the adult forms. The medically important genera are *Isospora, Plasmodium*, and *Toxoplasma*.

sporozoan. 1. Pert. to the sporozoa. 2. Sporozoon.

sporozoite (spor″ō-zō′īt) [″ + *zoon*, animal]. 1. An animal spore. 2. An elongated sickle-shaped cell that develops from a sporoblast within the oocyst in the life cycle of the malaria organism. Upon bursting of oocyst, sporozoites are released into the body cavity and make their way to salivary gland. They are introduced into human blood by a mosquito and almost immediately enter tissue cells, where they go through two schizogonic divisions and then reenter bloodstream and infect erythrocytes.

sporozoon (pl. *sporozoa*). A protozoon belonging to the subphylum Sporozoa.

sport [ME. *sporten*, to divert]. A sudden permanent variation in a gene that is not characteristic of previous generations. SYN: *mutation.*

sporular (spor'ū-lăr) [L. *sporula*, little spore]. Concerning a spore.

sporulation (spor-ū-lā'shŭn) [L. *sporula*, little spore]. Production of spores, a method of reproduction of unicellular organisms.

spot (spŏt) [MD. *spotte*]. A small area of surface differing from surrounding parts in appearance. SYN: *loculus; macula; papule; pustule.*

   s., blind. The optic disk where the optic nerve enters the retina. SEE: *scotoma.*

   s., blue. S., mongolian.

   s., cherry-red. Red spot occurring on retina in cases of Tay-Sachs disease.

   s., cold. Area on surface of skin that, when stimulated, gives rise to sensation of coldness.

   s., corneal. An opaque area on the cornea. SYN: *leukoma.*

   s.'s, Fordyce's. Ectopic sebaceous glands seen frequently as yellow spots in oral mucosa of the cheek or lip.

   s., genital. Area on nasal mucosa that tends to bleed during menstruation. SEE: *menstruation, vicarious.*

   s., hot. S., warm.

   s., hypnogenic. A point on the body that, when pressed, will throw a susceptible person into hypnosis or sleep.

   s.'s, Koplik's. Minute white or bluish-white spots on mucous membrane of mouth before appearance of the rash of measles.

   s.'s, liver. Popular term for pigmentary skin discolorations, usually in yellow-brown patches. SEE: *chloasma; lentigo.*

   s., milk. 1. A thickened and opaque area seen on epicardium at autopsy. 2. A dense area of macrophages in the omentum.

   s., mongolian. One of the blue or mulberry-colored spots usually located in the sacral region. May be present at birth in Asian, American Indian, black, and Southern European infants. It usually disappears during childhood. SYN: *s., blue.*

   s.'s, rose. Rose-colored maculae occurring on abdomen or loins in eruption of typhoid fever.

   s., ruby. A tumor consisting of a compressible mass of blood vessels. SYN: *angioma, senile.*

   s., temperature. A cutaneous spot that responds to temperature changes. SEE: *s.,*

cold; *s., warm.*

   s.'s, warm. Areas on surface of skin that, when stimulated, give rise to sensation of warmth. SYN: *s., hot.*

   s.'s, white. Light-colored, elevated areas of various sizes occurring on ventricular surface of anterior leaflet of mitral valve.

   s., yellow. Area surrounding and including the fovea centralis in the retina. SYN: *macula lutea retinae.*

spotted fever. General and imprecise name for various eruptive fevers: typhus, tick fever, and rickettsial fevers. SEE: *Rocky Mountain spotted fever.*

spotting. Appearance of blood-tinged discharge from the vagina, usually between menstrual periods or at onset of labor.

spp. *species* (plural).

sprain (sprān) [O. Fr. *espraindre*, to wring]. Trauma to a joint that causes pain and disability depending upon degree of injury to ligaments. In severe sprain, ligaments may be completely torn. The ankle joint is the most often sprained. SEE: *fracture; strain.*

   SYM: The signs of a sprain are rapid swelling, heat, and disability; often discoloration and limitation of function. It is important to understand that the intensity of the symptoms and signs may not be accurate indicators of the difference between a sprain and a fracture.

   TREAT: During the first 24 to 48 hours, use cold compresses, bandage, and elevate the joint. After initial treatment with cold, apply heat. If recovery proves slow, immobilization of the joint is indicated, followed by careful massage.

   s. of ankle or foot. Trauma to the ankle or foot or both, with soft tissue and possibly ligament and tendon injury, but without fracture. SEE: *Nursing Diagnoses* in *Appendix.*

   SYM: Pain, tenderness, swelling, ecchymosis of area, and limitation of motion.

   TREAT: Treat as a fracture until the results of radiological studies of the ankle and foot are available. If there is no fracture, immobilize and elevate the lower extremity, apply cold for 24 hours (do not apply ice directly to the foot and ankle). Analgesics and nonsteroidal anti-inflammatory agents may be required. If a ligament is partially or completely torn, it may be necessary to immobilize the lower extremity by applying a cast.

   s. of back. Overstretching of muscles, ligaments, or other spinal structures, often associated with small fractures.

   SYM: Pain, esp. on extreme movements; tenderness; muscle spasm.

   TREAT: If patient is supine, keep him in that position; if not, have him lie down on rigid support; do not allow to sit up or walk until fracture is ruled out. Intermittent heat, rest, with adhesive strapping, and brace. After acute symptoms have subsided, physical therapy is prescribed.

s., riders'. Sprain of the adductor longus muscles of the thigh, resulting from strain in riding horseback.

sprain fracture. The separation of a tendon or ligament from its insertion, taking with it a piece of the bone.

spray (sprā) [MD. *spraeyen,* to sprinkle]. 1. A jet of fine medicated vapor applied to a diseased part or discharged into the air. 2. A pressurized container. SYN: *atomizer.* 3. To discharge fluid in a fine stream.

spreader (sprĕd'ĕr). 1. An instrument for distributing something evenly over a tissue or culture plate. 2. A bacterial culture that, as it grows, spreads over the surface of the culture medium.

s., bladder-neck. An instrument used to expose the bladder neck and prostatic cavity while doing a retropubic prostatectomy.

s., root canal. In dentistry, an instrument that is pointed and of variable diameter and taper. It is used to apply force to the material used in filling a root canal.

spreading (sprĕd'ĭng) [AS. *spraedan,* to strew]. Term indicating a growth on a bacterial culture, extending much (several millimeters or more) beyond the site of inoculation.

spring [AS. *springan,* to jump]. 1. The season of the year that comes after winter and before summer. SYN: *vernal season.* 2. A flying back of a body to its original position through its elasticity.

spring conjunctivitis. A form of conjunctivitis recurring each year in the spring but disappearing with the first frost. SYN: *vernal conjunctivitis.*

spring fever. A feeling of lassitude, rejuvenation, or increased sex drive that affects some people in the spring.

spring finger. Arrested movement of a finger in flexion or extension followed by a jerk. SYN: *trigger finger.*

spring ligament. Interior calcaneoscaphoid ligament of the sole of the foot. It joins the os calcis to the scaphoid bone.

sprue (sproo) [D. *sprouwe*]. In dentistry, the wax, metal, or plastic used to form the aperture(s) through which molten gold or resin will pass to make a casting; also, the part of the casting that later fills the sprue hole.

s., tropical. A disease endemic in many tropical regions. Characterized by weakness, anemia, loss of weight, steatorrhea, and malabsorption of essential nutrients; its cause is unknown, but thought to be due to a bacterial infection of the intestine. An-

other type, called nontropical sprue, is caused by intolerance to gluten. SEE: *gluten-induced enteropathy.*

TREAT: Folic acid and tetracyclines for about a month.

s., nontropical. Gluten-induced enteropathy, q.v.

spud (spŭd) [ME. *spudde,* short knife]. Short, flattened, spadelike blade to dislodge a foreign substance.

spur [AS. *spura,* a pointed instrument]. 1. A sharp or pointed projection. 2. A sharp horny outgrowth of the skin.

s., calcaneal. An exostosis of the heel, often painful and resulting in disability.

s., femoral. Spur sometimes present on medial and underside of neck of femur.

s., scleral. A pointed portion of sclera that projects into the deeper part of cornea immediately behind canal of Schlemm at angle of iris.

spurious (spū'rē-ŭs) [L. *spurius*]. Not true or genuine; adulterated; false.

sputum (spū'tŭm) [L.] (pl. *sputa*). Substance expelled by coughing or clearing the throat. It may contain a variety of material from the respiratory tract including one or more of the following: cellular debris, mucus, blood, pus, caseous material, and microorganisms. SEE: *Charcot-Leyden crystals.*

DIFF. DIAG: *Amount:* Copious; seen in chronic inflammations of lower respiratory tract. Scanty; in all pulmonary bronchial acute inflammations and the early stages of lobar pneumonia and beginning bronchopneumonia.

Color: This varies with the origin, cause, and amount of decomposition.

Conditions: Anthracosis (coal dust): sputum is black. *Bronchiectasis:* sputum is mucopurulent and foul if expectoration is infrequent. *Bronchial asthma:* scanty sputum and frothy, later becoming purulent and grayish, containing eosinophils. *Bronchitis:* sputum is mucous, later purulent, and in chronic cases, greenish-yellow and thick. *Bronchopneumonia:* frothy, mucoid, thin, mucopurulent, copious often with blood, or prune juice in color. *Calcinosis:* shows a sputum containing particles of lime or chalky deposits such as plaster of paris. *Empyema:* if accompanied by perforations, the sputum resembles that of pulmonary abscess. *Gangrene of lung and putrid bronchitis:* sputum has an obnoxious odor and is purulent, separates on standing into three layers containing pus cells, hematoidin crystals, and leukocytes. *Lobar pneumonia:* scanty and viscid, yellowish, and somewhat mucopurulent during early stages; in later stages, rusty, bloody, tenacious and viscid, esp. near or soon after crisis. *Pulmonary abscess:* usually purulent and fetid with many pus cells and pieces of lung tissue. *Pulmonary tuberculosis:* in early stages, scanty, whitish, or grayish-yellow, frothy, and expectorated in small quantities during coughing; later when consolidation takes place, it becomes more copious, tenacious, and yellowish-gray; and in the late stages, it becomes mucopurulent, musty and fetid, containing fibers and tubercle bacilli, sometimes blood-tinged or mixed with blood. *Pneumonoconiosis:* depends upon character of inhaled dust that produced the disease. *Siderosis:* contains particles of iron or other metals and resembles sputum of chronic bronchitis. It also contains alveolar cells. *Silicosis:* contains particles of silica or other stone dusts.

NURSING IMPLICATIONS: Inspect sputum for color, consistency, and odor. Question the patient about times when sputum is raised; changes in volume, color, consistency, odor; and presence of blood previously and currently, and whether this changes with coughing. Provide appropriate disposal equipment and hygienic instructions for proper use of the equipment to prevent contamination. Patient to wash hands after disposing of sputum. Instruct the patient in how to expectorate to prevent air contamination. The nurse should turn the patient's head away while coughing. Wash hands after handling items containing sputum. Wear a face mask if the patient is suspected of having a contagious disease that can be spread through the air. Explain postural drainage technique and its use to help promote sputum production.

Keep the patient clean and comfortable. Promote frequent mouth and nose care to minimize mouth odors and eliminate unpleasant taste. Hard candy may be sucked on to freshen mouth between meals. Administer prescribed medications to loosen secretions and alleviate irritation. Encourage cessation of smoking to increase ciliary action and decrease inflammation. Conduct physical examination of the chest, inspecting skin color and general appearance, respiratory rate, depth, and rhythm, and symmetry of chest wall movements. Palpate for thoracic excursions, areas of tenderness, and tactile fremitus. Percuss for dullness related to fluid or consolidation of lung fields. Auscultate for normal and adventitial breath sounds, noting timing and location. Promote adequate hydration of the patient to help liquefy secretions. Use disposable equipment whenever possible. SEE: *Universal Precautions* in *Appendix*.

s., bloody. Condition occurring most often in hemorrhages, although sputum can be blood-tinged from vigorous coughing. If the blood is mixed with the sputum, the hemorrhage is in the finer bronchioles. Large quantities of blood indicate rupture of a larger vessel. SYN: *hemoptysis*.

s., nummular. Round, coin-shaped, flat forms that sink in water; seen in bronchiectasis and advanced pulmonary tuberculosis.

s., prune juice. Thin, reddish, bloody sputum seen in gangrene, cancer of the lung, and certain pneumonias.

s., rusty. Sputum seen in lobar pneumonia.

s., septicemia. Sputum acquired from inoculation with organisms in saliva or sputum.

sputum specimen. A specimen of material expectorated from the mouth. If produced after a cough, it may contain, in addition to saliva, material from the throat and bronchi. The physical and bacterial characteristics of the sputum depend upon the disease process involved and the ability of the patient to cough up material. Some bronchial secretions are quite tenacious and difficult to cough up. SEE: *postural drainage*.

NURSING IMPLICATIONS: Explain the procedure to the patient. Have the patient rinse the mouth to remove food particles. Provide the appropriate collection container. Encourage deep coughing. Have the patient collect the specimen in the early morning prior to ingesting food or drink if possible. Examine the specimen to differentiate between sputum and saliva. Document characteristics (color, viscosity, odor) and volume, and record date and time the specimen was sent to the laboratory and reason for specimen. If the patient is unable to produce a specimen, heated aerosol may be prescribed to induce expectoration, or the airway may be suctioned using a sputum trap attached to the suction catheter to collect the specimen. Also, postural drainage, q.v., may help to produce a specimen. If the specimen is to be sterile, give the patient explicit instructions on the usage of the container. Send the specimen to the laboratory immediately or refrigerate. Treat all sputum specimens as infective until proved otherwise. Thus specimens are handled by using appropriate isolation procedures.

sq. *subcutaneous.*

squalene (skwāl'ēn). An unsaturated carbohydrate present in shark-liver oil and some vegetable oils. It is an intermediate in the biosynthesis of cholesterol.

squama (skwā'mă) [L.] (pl. *squamae*). 1. [NA] A thin plate of bone. 2. A scale from the epidermis.

squamate (skwā'māt) [L. *squama*, scale]. Scaly; squamous.

squamatization (skwă″mă-tĭ-zā′shŭn) [L. *squama*, scale]. The changing of cells into squamous cells.

squame (skwām) [L. *squama*, scale]. Squama.

squamocellular (skwā″mō-sĕl′ū-lăr) [L. *squama*, scale, + *cellula*, little cell]. Rel. to or having squamous cells.

squamofrontal (skwā″mō-frŏn′tăl) [″ + *frontalis*, frontal]. Concerning or belonging to the orbital palate.

squamomastoid (skwā″mō-măs′toyd) [″ + Gr. *mastos*, breast, + *eidos*, form, shape]. Concerning the squamous and mastoid portions of the temporal bone.

squamo-occipital (skwā″mō-ŏk-sĭp′ĭ-tăl) [″ + *occipitalis*, occipital]. Concerning the squamous portion of the occipital bone.

squamoparietal (skwā″mō-pă-rī′ĕ-tăl) [″ + *paries*, a wall]. Rel. to the squamous and parietal bones.

squamopetrosal (skwā″mō-pē-trŏ′săl) [″ + *petrosus*, stony]. Concerning the squamous and petrosal portions of the temporal bone.

squamosa (skwā-mō′săl) [L. scaly]. The squamous part of the temporal bone.

squamosal (skwā-mō″săl) [L. *squama*, scale]. Squamous.

squamosphenoid (skwā″mō-sfē′noyd) [″ + Gr. *sphen*, wedge, + *eidos*, form, shape]. Concerning the squamous portion of the temporal bone and the sphenoid bone.

squamous (skwā′mŭs) [L. *squamosus*]. Scale-like.

squamous bone. Upper anterior portion of temporal bone.

squamous cell. Flat, scaly, epithelial cell.

squamous epithelium. Flat form of epithelial cells.

squamous suture. Line uniting squamosa and parietal bone.

squamozygomatic (sqwā″mō-zī″gō-măt′ĭk) [″ + *zygoma*, cheekbone]. Concerning the squamous and zygomatic parts of the temporal bone.

square knot. Double knot in which ends and standing parts are together and parallel to each other. This knot is used universally because it holds well. It is quite easy to tie but may be very difficult to untie. SEE: *knot* for illus.

Hold one end in each hand, carry right end over left end, and make a simple knot. Now reverse by carrying left end over right end and again tying, thus forming a simple symmetrical knot. If this is not done correctly, a false or granny knot results, a type of knot that usually slips. To untie, steady the knot, take one end and draw it over knot, and then continue pulling in this direction until knot slips or jumps and forms two half hitches that may be slipped off.

square lobe. 1. The quadrate lobe of the liver. 2. A lobe on upper surface of the cerebellum.

squarrose, squarrous (skwăr′ōs, -ŭs) [L. *squarrosus*]. Scurfy or scaly; full of scabs or scales.

squatting position. Position in which person crouches with legs drawn up closely in front of, or beneath, body; sitting on one's haunches and heels.

squeeze-bottle. Bottle made of a flexible, semirigid material that can be deformed by applying hand pressure to it. Used to contain irrigating solutions, esp. those required in ophthalmology.

squill (skwĭl) [Gr. *skilla*, a sea onion]. A drug derived from a liliaceous plant. It was once popular as an expectorant and diuretic.

A form known as red squill has been used as a rat poison.

squint (skwĭnt) [ME. *asquint*, sidelong glance]. 1. Abnormality in which the right and left visual axes do not bear toward an objective point simultaneously. SYN: *strabismus*. 2. To close the eyes partly as in excess light. 3. To be unable to direct both eyes simultaneously toward a point.

   s., convergent. Condition existing when eyes are turned toward the medial line. SYN: *esotropia*.

   s., divergent. Condition existing when eyes are turned outward. SYN: *exotropia*.

   s., external. S., divergent.

   s., internal. S., convergent.

SR. *sedimentation rate.*

Sr. Chem. symb. for the element strontium.

SRF. *somatotropin releasing factor.*

sRNA. *soluble ribonucleic acid.*

SRS, SRS-A. *slow-reacting substance; slow-reacting substance of anaphylaxis.*

SS. *saliva sample; soapsuds; sterile solution.*

ss. [L. *semis*, half] One-half; *subjects*, as in ss of an experiment or clinical study.

SSD. *source-skin distance.*

SSE. *soapsuds enema.*

SSS. *sterile saline soak.*

SSSS. *Society for the Scientific Study of Sex.*

ST. *sedimentation time.*

S.T. 37. Proprietary germicide and disinfectant. SYN: *hexylresorcinol*.

stab (stăb) [ME. *stob*, stick]. 1. To pierce with a knife. 2. Wound produced by piercing with a knife or pointed instrument. 3. A stab culture.

stab culture. Bacterial culture in which organism is introduced into a solid gelatin medium with a wire or needle.

stabile (stā′bĭl) [L. *stabilis*, stable]. Not moving; fixed.

stability. Remaining unchanged, even in the presence of forces that would normally change the state or condition, e.g., a chemical compound that remains unchanged; or a mature mental state that resists change.

stabilization (stā″bĭl-ĭ-zā′shŭn) [L. *stabilis*, stable]. 1. Act of making something, such as a structure or chemical reaction, stable. 2. The fixation or seating of a fixed or partial denture so that it will not be displaced in function.

stable (stā′bl). 1. Firm; steady. 2. The structure of an atom that prevents spontaneous disintegration.

stable condition. Term used in describing a patient's condition. It indicates that the patient's disease process has not changed precipitously or significantly.

staccato speech (stă-kä′tō) [It. *staccare*, to detach]. Jerky pronunciation with words and syllables separated by pauses. SYN: *scanning speech*. SEE: *speech*.

stachyose. A nonabsorbable carbohydrate present in beans. Because the substance is not absorbed or metabolized in the small intestine, it passes into the colon where it is acted upon by bacteria to form gas. This may be related to the flatus produced by eating beans.

stactometer (stăk-tŏm′ĕt-ĕr) [Gr. *staktos*, dropping, + *metron*, measure]. Instrument for measuring fluid in drops.

stadium (stā′dē-ŭm) [Gr. *stadion*, alteration]. A stage or period in the progress of a disease. SEE: *fastigium*.

   s. acmes. The height of a disease.

   s. augmenti. Period of rising temperature or other symptoms.

   s. caloris. The hot stage in a fever or disease.

   s. decrementi. Period of defervescence or decrease of symptoms.

   s. fluorescentiae. Stage of eruption in an exanthematous disease.

   s. frigoris. Cold shivering stage in intermittent fevers, as malaria.

   s. incrementi. S. augmenti.

   s. invasionis. Incubation period of an infectious disease.

   s. sudoris. Sweating stage of a paroxysm of malaria.

Stadol. Trade name for butorphanol tartrate.

staff (stăf) [AS. *staef*, a stick]. 1. An instrument to be introduced into the urethra and bladder as a guide to a surgical knife. 2. The medical, nursing, and other personnel attached to a hospital.

   s., attending. The group of physicians and surgeons who are in regular attendance at a hospital.

   s., consulting. Physicians and surgeons attached to a hospital who may be consulted by members of the attending staff.

   s., house. SEE: *house staff*.

   s. of Wrisberg. Prominence of the cuneiform cartilage seen in the normal larynx

during examination.

stage (stāj) [O. Fr. *estage*]. 1. Period in the course of a disease or in the life history of an organism. SYN: *stadium*. 2. The platform of a microscope on which the slide is placed.

   s., algid. Period of chilliness at the beginning of a fever.

   s., amphibolic. Stage that intervenes between acme of a disease and its outcome, at a time when the outcome is unknown.

   s., asphyxial. Preliminary stage of Asiatic cholera.

   s., cold. Chill or rigor of a malarial paroxysm.

   s., defervescent. Period in which temperature is declining.

   s., end-. The final phase of a disease process.

   s., eruptive. 1. Period in which an exanthem appears. 2. The middle stage in the pre-eruptive, eruptive, or posteruptive categorization of tooth eruption. It is characterized by root elongation and movement of the tooth mesially and toward the occlusal plane.

   s., expulsive, of labor. Stage of dilatation of the cervix uteri during which the child is expelled from uterus; second stage of labor, q.v.

   s., first, of labor. Period when the fetal head is molded and the cervix is dilated.

   s., fourth, of labor. The postpartum period immediately following delivery of the placenta.

   s., hot. Febrile stage in a malarial paroxysm.

   s. of invasion. Period in which the causative agent is present in the body prior to the onset of a disease.

   s. of latency. The incubation period of an infectious disorder.

   s., placental, of labor. Period of labor during which placenta and fetal membranes are discharged; third stage of labor, q.v.

   s., pre-eruptive. Stage following infection and before appearance of eruption.

   s., pyrogenetic. Stage of onset in a febrile disease.

   s., resting. Stage of relative inactivity between periods of activity, as in a cell between mitotic divisions; a dormant stage.

   s., second, of labor. Expulsive stage of labor.

   s., sweating. The third or terminal stage of malaria during which sweating occurs.

   s., third, of labor. S., placental.

staggers (stăg′ĕrz). Vertigo and confusion that occur in decompression illness.

staging. Process of classifying tumors, esp. malignant tumors, with respect to their degree of differentiation, to their potential for responding to therapy, and to the patient's prognosis.

stagnation (stăg-nā'shŭn) [L. *stagnans,* stagnant]. 1. Cessation of motion. 2. In pathology, a stoppage of motion of any fluid in the body, as blood. SYN: *stasis.*

stain (stān) [O. Fr. *desteindre,* deprive of color]. 1. Any discoloration. SEE: *anti-stain formulary.* 2. A pigment or dye used in coloring microscopic objects and tissues. 3. To apply pigment to a tissue or microscopic object.

   s., acid. Stain in which the color-bearing ion (chromatophore) is the anion.

   Ex.: eosin, commonly used for staining the cytoplasmic or basic elements of cells.

   s., acid-fast. Stain used in bacteriology, esp. for staining *Mycobacterium tuberculosis.* A special solution of carbolfuchsin is used, which the organism retains in spite of washing with the decolorizing agent acid alcohol. SEE: *Ziehl-Neelsen method.*

   s., basic. Stain in which the color-bearing ion is the cation.

   Ex.: methylene blue, commonly used to stain the nucleic or acidic elements of cells.

   s., Commission Certified. Stain that has been certified by the Biological Stain Commission.

   s., contrast. Stain used to color one part of a tissue or cell unaffected when another part is stained by another color.

   s., counter. Stain, usually a contrast stain, used following the staining of specific elements of a tissue.

   s., dental. A discoloration accumulating on the surface of teeth, denture, or denture base material, most often attributed to use of tea, coffee, or tobacco. Many stains are due to inhalation through the mouth of metal-containing dust or orally administered drugs. Copper and nickel produce a green stain; manganese and silver produce a black stain; mercury produces a green-black stain; and iron produces a brown color. A green or green-yellow stain is often present on the gingival third of maxillary teeth of children and is thought to be caused by bacteria such as those of the genera *Penicillium* and *Aspergillus.* Both the metallic and bacterial stains are thought to be localized in the enamel cuticle remnants on the crown. Yellow, brown, or green fluorescent lines may be incorporated into the calcified structure of teeth due to medication with tetracyclines. Some orange dental stains seen on both labial and lingual surfaces of teeth are thought to be caused by chromogenic bacteria, e.g., *Serratia marcescens.*

   s., differential. In bacteriology, a stain such as Gram's stain that enables one to differentiate between different types of bacteria.

   s., double. A mixture of two contrasting dyes, usually an acid and a basic stain.

   s., Giemsa. Stain that contains azure II-eosin and azure II. It is used in staining tissues including blood cells, Negri bodies, and chromosomes.

   s., Gram's. SEE: *Gram's stain.*

   s., hematoxylin-eosin. A widely used method of staining tissues for microscopic examination. It stains nuclei deep blue-black and cytoplasm pink.

   s., intravital. A nontoxic dye that, when introduced into an organism, selectively stains certain cells or tissues. SYN: *s., vital.*

   s., inversion. A basic stain that, when under the influence of a mordant, acts as an acid stain.

   s., metachromatic. Stain with which the constituents of cells or tissues develop a color different from the stain itself.

   s., neutral. A combination of an acid and a basic stain.

   s., nuclear. A basic stain affecting nuclei.

   s., port-wine. Nevus flammeus, q.v.

   s., substantive. Stain that is directly absorbed by the tissues when they are immersed in the staining solution.

   s., supravital. Stain that will color living cells or tissues that have been removed from the body.

   s., tumor. In arteriography, an abnormally dense area in an x-ray image caused by the collection of contrast medium in the vessels. This may be a sign of neoplastic growth.

   s., vital. S., intravital.

   s., Wright's. A polychrome stain used for staining blood smears. SEE: *Wright's technique.*

staining (stān'ĭng) [O. Fr. *desteindre*]. Process of impregnating a substance, esp. a tissue, with pigments so that its component parts may be visible under a microscope. SEE: *Wright's technique.*

staircase breaths. In basic life support, q.v., the serial application of several small breaths rather than a single large volume breath. SEE: *cardiopulmonary resuscitation.*

staircase phenomenon. The effect exhibited by skeletal and heart muscle when subjected to rapidly repeated maximal stimuli following a period of rest. In the resulting series of contractions, each is greater than the preceding one until a state of maximum contraction is reached. SYN: *treppe.* SEE: *stress test.*

stalagmometer (stăl-ăg-mŏm'ĕ-tĕr) [Gr. *stalagmos,* dropping, + *metron,* a measure]. Instrument for measuring number of drops in a given amount of fluid.

stalk (stawk) [ME]. An elongated structure usually serving to attach or support an organ or structure.

   s., belly. Structure in embryo that develops into umbilical cord.

   s., body. A bridge of mesoderm that connects the caudal end of embryo with chorion. Into it grow the allantois and embryonic blood vessels, the latter forming the umbilical arteries and vein, which connect the embryo with the placenta.

   s., cerebellar. One of the cerebellar peduncles that connect the cerebellum with brain stem.

   s., infundibular. Stalk that connects the diencephalon with the neural lobe of the hypophysis. SYN: *infundibulum.*

   s., optic. Structure that connects the optic vesicle or cup to the forebrain.

   s., yolk. The narrow constricted portion by which the yolk sac is connected to the midgut of the embryo. SYN: *vitelline duct.*

stamina (stăm′ĭ-nă) [L., thread of the warp, thread of human life]. Inherent force, constitutional energy; strength; endurance.

stammering (stăm′ĕr-ĭng) [AS. *stamerian*]. Hesitant or faltering speech disorder. May be due to hesitation, mispronunciation, transposing the letters *l*, *r*, or *s*, or repetition. This condition may be made worse by anxiety and fear. Even though there is no known cause for this condition, it can be improved by speech therapy. SYN: *anarthria literalis; spasmophemia; stuttering.*

   s. of bladder. Interrupted and irregular flow of urine, the muscles which control micturition acting spasmodically.

standard [O. Fr. *estandard*, marking rallying place]. That which is established by custom or authority as a model, criterion, or rule for comparison of measurement.

   s., biological. The standardization of drugs or biological products (vitamins, hormones, antibiotics) by testing their effects upon animals. Utilized when chemical analysis is impossible or impracticable.

standard deviation. SYMB: σ. ABBR: S.D. In statistics, commonly used measure of dispersion or variability in a distribution. The square root of the variance, q.v.

standard error. ABBR: S.E. A measure of variability that could be expected of a statistical constant following the taking of random samples of a given size in a particular set of observations. An important standard error is that of the difference between the means of two samples.

standardization. The process of standardizing, esp. that of determining the strength or scale value of a substance or device by comparing with some standard, as standardization of solutions or thermometers.

standard of care. 1. In forensic medicine, a measure by which the defendant's conduct is compared to determine negligence or malpractice. 2. The acts of omission or commission that an ordinary prudent person would have done or not done if in the defendant's position.

standards of practice. The criteria against which one measures one's practice; for example, the American Nurses' Association Standards of Practice.

standing orders. Orders, rules, regulations, or procedures prepared by the professional staff of a hospital or clinic. Used as guidelines in preparation for and carrying out medical and surgical procedures. Standing orders serve to assure that such procedures are carried out correctly without being dependent upon an individual's fallible memory.

standstill. A cessation of activity.

   s., atrial. Cessation of atrial contractions.

   s., cardiac. Cessation of contractions of the heart.

   s., inspiratory. Temporary cessation of inspiration normally following each inspiration resulting from stimulation of proprioceptors in alveoli of lungs. SEE: *Hering-Breuer reflex.*

   s., respiratory. Cessation of respiratory movements.

   s., ventricular. Cessation of ventricular contractions.

stannic (stăn′ĭk) [L. *stannum*, tin]. 1. Resembling or containing tin. 2. In chemistry, containing tetravalent tin.

stannous (stăn′ŭs) [L. *stannum*, tin]. 1. Resembling or containing tin. 2. In chemistry, containing divalent tin.

stannous fluoride. USP. A fluoride compound used in toothpaste to prevent dental caries.

stannum (stăn′ŭm) [L.]. Tin.

stanolone (stăn′ō-lōn). An anabolic steroid drug.

stanozolol (stăn′ō-zō-lŏl″). USP. An anabolic steroid. Trade name is Winstrol.

Stanton's disease. Melioidosis, q.v.

stapedectomy (stā″pē-dĕk′tō-mē) [L. *stapes*, stirrup, + Gr. *ektome*, excision]. Excision of the stapes in order to improve hearing, esp. in cases of otosclerosis. The stapes is replaced by a prosthesis.

   During the first 24 hours following surgery, the patient remains flat in bed, head movements are kept to a minimum, and the patient is instructed to refrain from blowing his or her nose or sneezing (if possible). In the second 24 hours the patient moves or arises only if assisted. The patient should not allow the ear to get wet for at least 10 days postoperatively. For 30 days following surgery, the patient should not fly, climb to high altitudes, or be exposed to loud sounds such as those produced by jet aircraft. Sudden movements, even in elevators, should be avoided. SEE: *Nursing Diagnoses* in *Appendix.*

stapedial (stă-pē'dē-ăl). Rel. to the stapes.

stapediotenotomy (stă-pē"dē-ō-těn-ŏt'ō-mē) [" + Gr. *tenon*, tendon, + *tome,* incision]. Division of the tendon of the stapedius muscle.

stapediovestibular (stă-pē"dē-ō-věs-tĭb'ū-lar) [" + *vestibulum,* an antechamber]. Rel. to the stapes and vestibule of the ear.

stapedius (stă-pē'dē-ŭs) [L. *stapes,* stirrup]. A small muscle of the middle ear inserted in the stapes. SEE: *Muscles* in *Appendix.*

stapes (stā'pēz) [L., stirrup]. [NA] Ossicle in the middle ear that articulates with the incus. Commonly called stirrup. The footplate of the stapes fits into the oval window. SEE: *ear.*

Staphcillin. Trade name for methicillin sodium.

staphylectomy (stăf"ĭ-lĕk'tō-mē) [" + *ek-tome,* excision]. Amputation of the uvula. SYN: *staphylotomy* (def. 1); *uvulotomy.*

staphyledema (stăf"ĭl-ē-dē'mă) [" + *oi-dema,* swelling]. Swelling of the uvula.

staphyline (stăf'ĭ-lĭn) [Gr. *staphyle,* a bunch of grapes]. 1. Resembling a bunch of grapes. SYN: *botryoid.* 2. Rel. to the uvula. SYN: *uvular.*

staphylion (stăf-ĭl'ē-ŏn) [Gr., little grape]. 1. Craniometric point at median line of posterior border of hard palate. 2. Uvula. 3. A nipple or teat.

staphylitis (stăf"ĭl-ī'tĭs) [Gr. *staphyle,* a bunch of grapes, + *itis,* inflammation]. Inflammation of the uvula.

staphylo- [Gr. *staphyle,* a bunch of grapes]. Combining form indicating the uvula, pert. to or resembling a bunch of grapes, or pert. to *Staphylococcus.*

staphyloangina (stăf"ĭl-ō-ăn'jĭ-nă) [" + L. *angina,* sore throat]. Sore throat due to staphylococcus.

staphylococcal (stăf"ĭl-ō-kŏk'ăl) [" + *kokkos,* berry]. Pert. to or caused by staphylococci.

staphylococcal actinophytosis. Botryomycosis, a condition characterized by granulomatous lesions resembling those of actinomycoses; however, when organisms recovered from the lesions are cultured, they grow as staphylococci.

staphylococcal food poisoning. Poisoning by food containing any one of several heat-stable enterotoxins produced by certain strains of staphylococci. When ingested, the toxin causes nausea, vomiting, diarrhea, in-

testinal cramps, and in severe cases prostration and shock. Attack usually lasts three to six hours. Fatalities are rare.

staphylococcemia (stăf"ĭl-ō-kŏk-sē'mē-ă) [" + " + *haima,* blood]. The presence of staphylococcus in the blood.

staphylococci (stăf"ĭl-ō-kŏk'sē). Pl. of staphylococcus.

Staphylococcus (stăf"ĭl-ō-kŏk'ŭs) [Gr. *staphyle,* a bunch of grapes, + *kokkos,* berry]. A genus of micrococci belonging to the family Micrococcaceae, order Eubacteriales. They are gram-positive and when cultured on agar produce white, yellow, or orange-colored colonies. Some species are pathogenic, causing suppurative conditions and elaborating endotoxins destructive to tissue cells. Some produce enterotoxins and are the cause of a common type of food poisoning.

S. aureus. A species commonly present on skin and mucous membranes, esp. those of nose and mouth, characterized by production of a golden-yellow pigment. They are gram-positive, coagulase-positive anaerobes. A cause of suppurative conditions such as boils, carbuncles, and internal abscesses in humans. Various strains of this species produce toxins including those that cause food poisoning, staphylococcal scalded skin syndrome, and toxic shock syndrome. Some strains also produce hemolysins and staphylokinase.

S. aureus, **methicillin-resistant.** ABBR: MRSA. Staphylococci that produce β-lactamase and thus are resistant to the action of antibiotics that are destroyed or inactivated by that enzyme.

S. epidermidis. A species of low pathogenicity characterized by formation of white colonies. Previously termed *S. albus.*

S. saprophyticus. A newly classified species. It can cause urinary tract infections.

staphylococcus (stăf"ĭl-ō-kŏk'ŭs) (pl. *staphylococci*). Term applied loosely to any pathogenic micrococci. SEE: *bacteria* for illus.; *Staphylococcus.*

staphyloderma (stăf"ĭ-lō-děr'mă) [" + *derma,* skin]. Cutaneous infection with staphylococci.

staphylodermatitis (stăf"ĭl-ō-derm"ă-tī'tĭs) [" + " + *itis,* inflammation]. A dermatitis caused by staphylococci.

staphylodialysis (stăf"ĭ-lō-dī-ăl'ĭ-sĭs) [" + *dia,* through, + *lysis,* dissolution]. Relaxed and elongated condition of the uvula.

staphylohemia (stăf"ĭ-lō-hē'mē-ă) [" + *haima,* blood]. Staphylococci in the blood. SYN: *staphylococcemia.*

staphylokinase (stăf"ĭ-lō-kī'năs). Material

produced by some strains of *Staphylococcus aureus* that can convert plasminogen to plasmin.

staphylolysin (stăf″ĭ-lŏl′ĭ-sĭn) [″ + *lysis*, dissolution]. A hemolysin produced by staphylococci.

staphyloma (stăf″ĭl-ō′mă) [Gr.]. A protrusion of the cornea or sclera of the eye.

   s., anterior. Globular enlargement of anterior part of the eye. SYN: *keratoglobus.*

   s., ciliary. Staphyloma in region of the ciliary body.

   s. corneae. Thinning and bulging of the cornea.

   s., equatorial. Staphyloma in equatorial region of the eye.

   s., intercalary. Staphyloma in the region of union of the sclera with periphery of the iris.

   s., partial. Staphyloma that extends in one direction, displacing the pupil; the remainder of the cornea is clear.

   s., posterior. Bulging of sclera backward.

   s., total. Opaque, protuberant cicatrix found in place of the cornea.

   ETIOL: Perforation of cornea resulting in poor vision, increased tension, rupture of thin scar.

   TREAT: Incision, excision, ablation.

   s., uveal. Protrusion of any portion of the uvea through the sclera.

staphylomatous (stăf″ĭ-lŏm′ă-tŭs). Concerning or similar to a staphyloma.

staphyloncus (stăf″ĭ-lŏng′kŭs) [Gr. *staphyle,* a bunch of grapes, + *onkos,* bulk, mass]. A tumor or enlargement of the uvula.

staphylopharyngeus (stăf″ĭ-lō-făr-ĭn′jē-ŭs) [″ + *pharynx,* throat]. Muscle of soft palate narrowing fauces and occluding nasopharynx. SYN: *palatopharyngeus.*

staphylopharyngorrhaphy (stăf″ĭ-lō-făr″ĭn-gor′ă-fē) [″ + ″ + *rhaphe,* seam, ridge]. Term used to describe several different operations on the soft palate and uvula.

staphyloplasty (stăf′ĭ-lō-plăs″tē) [″ + *plassein,* to form]. Plastic surgery of the uvula or soft palate.

staphyloptosia, staphyloptosis (stăf″ĭ-lŏp-tō′sē-ă, -sĭs) [″ + *ptosis,* a dropping]. Relaxation or elongation of the uvula. SYN: *staphylodialysis.*

staphylorrhaphy (stăf″ĭl-or′ă-fē) [″ + *rhaphe,* seam, ridge]. Suture of a cleft palate.

staphyloschisis (stăf″ĭ-lŏs′kĭ-sĭs) [″ + *schisis,* a splitting]. Fissure of the uvula. SYN: *cleft palate.*

staphylotome (stăf′ĭ-lō-tōm) [″ + *tome,* incision]. Instrument for cutting the uvula.

staphylotomy (stăf″ĭ-lŏt′ō-mē). 1. [″ + *tome,* incision] Amputation or any incision

of the uvula. 2. [Gr. *staphyloma,* corneal protrusion, + *tome,* incision] Excision of a staphyloma.

staphylotoxin (stăf″ĭ-lō-tŏk′sĭn) [Gr. *staphyle,* a bunch of grapes, + *toxikon,* poison]. A toxin elaborated by one of the staphylococci, esp. *S. aureus.* Among some of the toxins produced are an enterotoxin, a cause of food poisoning, and exotoxins, including a hemotoxin that lyses red blood cells, a dermonecrotic toxin, toxic shock syndrome toxin-1, and leukocidins.

staple food. Any food that supplies a substantial part, at least 25% to 35%, of the caloric requirement and is regularly consumed by a certain population.

stapling. In surgery, a means of fastening tissues together by using special staples compatible with tissues. The staples are U-shaped lengths of wire that are pushed through the tissues. The ends are then bent over on an anvil.

star [AS. *steorra*]. Any structure resembling a star. SYN: *aster.*

   s., lens. A starlike structure developing in the lens of the eye as a result of unequal growth of lens fibers.

   s.'s of Verheyen. Star-shaped masses of veins on the surface of the kidney. SYN: *stellate veins; venulae stellatae.*

starch [AS. *stercan*]. Noncrystalline carbohydrate of the polysaccharide group found in plants. Included are vegetable starches, pectins, dextrins, and gums. All are rather easily decomposed, have high molecular weights, and yield monosaccharides on complete hydrolysis. Those that the body can hydrolyze into hexoses are useful as concentrated energy-giving foods. All are reduced to simple sugars before they are absorbed. When some fruits ripen, the starch is changed to sugar, while some vegetables (peas and corn) change sugar into starch as their seeds develop. SEE: table.

   The amylases of saliva and pancreatic juice hydrolyze starches to dextrins and maltose. These in turn are hydrolyzed to glucose, which is absorbed into the bloodstream. Glucose not immediately needed for energy is converted into glycogen, a form of starch that is stored in the liver or in muscle tissue.

   Pure starches, having the formula $(C_6H_{10}O_5)_n$, if normally metabolized, leave no residue and give rise only to carbon dioxide and water.

   s., animal. Glycogen.

   s., corn. Starch obtained from ordinary corn or maize *(Zea mays).* It is used as a dusting powder and an absorbent and is a constituent in many pastes and ointments. It is widely used in industry and as a food.

Classification of Starches

Groups	Examples
I. Potato Group	Canna, potato, arrowroot
II. Leguminous Group	Beans, peas, lentils
III. Wheat Group	Wheat, barley, rye
IV. Sago Group	Sago, cassava, arum
V. Rice Group	Rice, corn (maize), oats

Starches

Name	From
1. Cornflour	Maize or corn
2. Arrowroot	Maranta
3. Cassava	Brazilian arrowroot
4. Curcuma	East Indian arrowroot
5. Arum	Portland arrowroot
6. Tous-les-mois	Canna (West India)
7. Sago	Palm (East India)
8. Inulin	Dahlia tubers
9. Lichen	Iceland moss
10. Glycogen	Animal livers

NOTE: Starch is soluble at 150°F (65.5°C). Only slightly so in cold water.
IODINE acting on starch gives a deep blue color.
BROMINE acting on starch paste gives an orange-yellow color.

Percentage of Starch in Various Foods

Article	Percent	Article	Percent
Arrowroot	23	Oatmeal (uncooked), dry	68
Bananas	22	Peanuts, roasted and salted	19
Barley	79	Peas, dried	60
Beans, common	61	Peas, green, canned, drained	
Beans, green	26	solids	17
Bread fruit, raw	26	Potatoes (uncooked)	17
Buckwheat flour	72	Potatoes, sweet (uncooked)	26
Chestnuts, dried	79	Rice, white, uncooked	80
Corn grits (degermed, dry)	78	Rye flour, light	78
Corn meal (degermed, dry)	78	Soybeans (dry, uncooked)	34
Lentils, raw	60	Wheat flour, all purpose	76

starch glycerite. A combination of starch, benzoic acid, purified water, and glycerin. Used as an emollient in formulations for external use.

starch-iodine blue test. SEE: *test, starch-iodine.*

stare (stār) [AS. *starian*]. To gaze fixedly at anyone or anything.

Starling's law of heart [Ernest Henry Starling, Brit. physiologist, 1866–1927]. The force of the heartbeat is determined primarily by the length of the fibers constituting its muscular wall, i.e., an increase in diastolic filling increases force of heartbeat.

Starling's law of intestine. A stimulus within the intestine, i.e., the presence of food, initiating a band of constriction on proximal side and relaxation on distal side. This results in a peristaltic wave.

Star of Life symbol. Symbol approved by Department of Transportation to represent the emergency medical services and displayed on ambulances and outside of emergency departments. SEE: illus.

starter. A pure culture of bacteria or other microorganism used to initiate a particular fermentation, as in the making of cheese.

star test pattern. In radiography, a test to evaluate the resolution of the focal spot of the x-ray tube.

startle syndromes. The uncontrollable startle reaction that follows any stimulus for which there is usually no adaptation, such as a sudden noise, flash of light, or touching of a person. This causes a stiffening of the body, flexion of the arms, and sometimes a

STAR OF LIFE

EMERGENCY MEDICAL CARE SYMBOL

shout and fall to the ground. The verbal portion of the response may be related to what the individual is thinking or viewing at the time and may be a source of embarrassment. This syndrome was originally described as the Jumping Frenchmen of Maine, q.v., but it exists in other areas of the world. SYN: *hyperexplexias.*

TREAT: Clonazepam is beneficial.

starvation [AS. *steorfan,* to die]. 1. Condition of being without food for a long period of time. When everything but air and water is withheld, the sequence of events is as follows: (1) hunger, beginning about four hours after the last meal, accompanied by special activity of the stomach and general restlessness, becoming more acute periodically, esp. at times when meals were customarily taken; (2) loss of weight; (3) utilization of glycogen stored in liver and muscles; (4) utilization of stored fat; (5) spells of nausea and diminishing acuteness of the sensation of hunger; (6) destruction of body protein. The greatest loss of weight is in the fatty tissues, spleen, and liver. 2. Condition in which the supply of a specific food is below minimum bodily requirements, such as protein starvation. SEE: *kwashiorkor.* 3. Condition resulting from failure of the body to digest and ab-

sorb essential foodstuffs. SEE: *deficiency disease; diet; dietetics.*

stasibasiphobia (stā″sĭ-bā″sĭ-fō′bē-ă) [Gr. *stasis,* a standing, + *basis,* step, + *phobos,* fear]. Delusion of one's inability to stand or walk, or fear to make the attempt.

stasimorphia, stasimorphy (stā″sĭ-mor′fē-ă, -fē) [″ + *morphe,* form]. Deformity due to failure to develop and grow.

stasiphobia (stā″sĭ-fō′bē-ă) [″ + *phobos,* fear]. Delusion of one's inability to stand erect or hesitation to make the attempt.

stasis (stā′sĭs) [Gr. *stasis,* a standing]. Stagnation of normal flow of fluids, as of the blood or urine, or of the intestinal mechanism.

  s., diffusion. Stasis with diffusion of lymph or serum.

  s., intestinal. Condition in which peristaltic movements fail to move food along the intestine.

  s., venous. Stasis of blood caused by venous congestion.

stat. [L.] *statim,* immediately.

state [L. *status,* condition]. 1. A condition. 2. A mode or condition of being.

  s., anxiety. Condition characterized by more or less continuous anxiety and apprehension. SEE: *neurosis, anxiety.*

  s., central excitatory. ABBR: CES. Condition of increased excitability in the central nervous system, esp. in the spinal cord, following an excitatory stimulus.

  s., central inhibitory. ABBR: CIS. Condition of decreased excitability in the central nervous system, esp. in the spinal cord, resulting from an inhibitory stimulus.

  s., dream. State of diminished consciousness in which the surroundings are perceived as if in a dream.

  s., excited. The new state produced when energy is added to a nucleus, atom, or molecule. The energy is added by the absorption of photons or by collisions with other particles.

  s., fatigue. Nervous exhaustion, commonly following depressed states. SYN: *neurasthenia.*

  s., ground. State of the lowest energy of a system such as an atom or molecule.

  s., refractory. Condition of reduced ability to be excited just after a muscle and nerve have been stimulated.

  s., steady. In physiology, the condition of the metabolic needs of a system such as the muscles being supplied with nutrients at the same rate the energy is expended. Dynamic equilibrium.

static (stăt′ĭk) [Gr. *statikos,* causing to stand]. At rest; in equilibrium; not in motion.

static electricity. Electricity produced by friction.

static equilibrium. The ability to maintain a steady position of the head and body in relation to gravity. Opposite of dynamic equilibrium or dynamic balance. SYN: *static balance.*

static pressure. The pressure existing in all points in the circulation when the heart is stopped. It provides a measure of how well the circulatory bed is filled with blood.

static reactions. Postural reflex responses important to standing and walking. Included are local static reactions acting on individual limbs, segmental static reactions linking the extremities together, and general static reactions to the position of the head in space.

static reflex. A reflex action having to do with maintenance of posture or maintenance of muscle tone.

statics (stăt'ĭks). Study of matter at rest and forces bringing about equilibrium. SEE: *dynamics.*

static splint. Any orthosis that is without movable parts and is used for positioning, stability, protection, or support.

statim (stăt'ĭm) [L.]. ABBR: stat. Immediately; at once.

station (stā'shŭn) [L. *statio,* standing]. 1. The manner of standing. 2. A stopping place. 3. In obstetrics, the relationship in centimeters between the leading bony portion of the fetal head and the level of the ischial spines. This is useful in judging the level of application of forceps to aid in delivery. SEE: *forceps.*

   s., aid. Site in the army for collecting the wounded in battle.

   s., dressing. A temporary station for wounded soldiers in the field.

   s., rest. A temporary relief station for the sick on a military road or railway.

stationary (stā'shŭn-ĕr-ē) [L. *stationarius,* belonging to a station]. Remaining in a fixed condition.

statistical (stă-tĭs'tĭ-kăl). Pert. to statistics.

statistical significance. In statistics, after appropriate analysis of the data, the conclusion that the event being investigated had a certain probability of being due to chance, but the probability was so slight that it is presumed that the event did not occur due to mere chance. Probability is referred to as the *p value;* and, if the analysis indicated that there was only a one in 20 chance or less (i.e., *p* equal to or less than 0.05) that the observed results occurred due to chance, then the study results are arbitrarily considered to be statistically significant.

statistics (stă-tĭs'tĭks) [LL. *statisticus*]. The systematic collection, organization, analysis, and interpretation of numerical data pert. to any subject. SEE: *statistical signifi-*

cance.

   s., medical. Statistics pert. to medical sciences, esp. data pert. to human disease.

   s., morbidity. Statistics pert. to sickness.

   s., vital. Statistics dealing with births, deaths, and marriages.

statoacoustic (stăt″ō-ă-koo'stĭk) [Gr. *statos,* placed, + *akoustikos,* acoustic]. Concerning balance and hearing.

statoconia (stăt″ō-kō'nē-ă) [″ + *konos,* dust]. Minute bits of calcium adhering to the hair cells of the maculae of the utricle and saccule of the middle ear. These are important in sensing the orientation to gravity.

statokinetic (stăt″kō-kĭn-ĕt'ĭk) [″ + *kinetikos,* moving]. Pert. to reactions of the body produced by movement.

statokinetic reflexes. Reactions that are the result of movement of the body (positive or negative acceleration) or movements of the head. SYN: *accelerator reflexes; reflexes, kinetic.*

statolith (stăt'ō-lĭth) [″ + *lithos,* stone]. Statoconia, q.v.

statometer (stă-tŏm'ĕt-ĕr) [″ + *metron,* a measure]. Instrument for measuring amount of abnormal protrusion of eyeball.

statosphere (stăt'ō-sfēr) [″ + *sphaira,* a globe]. Centrosome.

stature (stăt'ūr) [L. *statura*]. Height of the body in a standing position.

   s., short. Body height below the level obtained at that age by 70% of the population. A number of disease states, including hormonal, nutritional, and intrauterine growth retardation, may cause this condition.

   TREAT: It is important to initiate therapy as soon as possible.

status (stā'tŭs) [L.] (pl. *statuses*). A state or condition.

   s. anginosus. A sustained attack of angina pectoris.

   s. arthriticus. Predisposition to having attacks of gout.

   s. asthmaticus. Persistent and intractable asthma.

   s. dysraphicus. Condition resulting from imperfect closure of neural tube of embryo.

   s. epilepticus. SEE: *epilepsy.*

   s. parathyreoprivus. Condition resulting from loss of parathyroid tissue.

   s. praesens. The state of a patient at time observed.

   s. raptus. A state of ecstasy.

   s. sternuens. Continual sneezing that may be caused by transient irritation of the nasal mucosa.

   TREAT: Application of topical anesthetic to the nasal mucosa.

   s. verrucosus. Defective development of

the cerebral gyri with many small gyri. This gives a warty appearance to the surface of the brain.

s. vertiginosus. Persistent condition of vertigo.

statute of limitations. A law that sets a legal time limit during which claims or lawsuits can be brought. If not brought during the time allowed by law, the person or party loses the right to file a claim or lawsuit. In medical negligence claims, the statute of limitations usually starts from the time the wrong occurred or was or should have been discovered.

staunch (stŏnch) [O. Fr. *estanche*, firm]. To stop the flow of blood from a wound. SYN: *stanch.*

staurion (staw'rē-ŏn) [Gr. *stauros*, little cross]. Craniometric point where transverse palatine suture crosses the median one.

stauroplegia (staw"rō-plē'jē-ă) [" + *plege*, stroke]. Alternate hemiplegia.

S.T.D. 1. *skin test dose.* SEE: *Dick test.* 2. *sexually transmitted disease.*

steal (stēl). The deviation of blood flow from its normal course or rate of flow.

s., subclavian. SEE: *subclavian steal syndrome.*

steam (stēm) [AS. *steam*, vapor]. 1. Invisible vapor into which water is converted at boiling point by heat. 2. Mist formed by condensation of water vapor. 3. Any vaporous exhalation.

steam tent. Device that permits inhalation of vapors. If no tent is available, a makeshift tent may be improvised. It is important that the method used does not burn the patient.

SOLUTIONS: Approx. 1 quart (or 1 liter) of boiling water to which is added a teaspoonful (5 ml) of compound tincture of benzoin or a teaspoonful (5 ml) of tincture of benzoin (this does not contain aloe), a few crystals of menthol or camphor, or a few drops of methyl salicylate. These ingredients are pleasant to smell but have relatively little therapeutic effect. Most of the value is in the water vapor.

steapsin (stē-ăp'sĭn) [Gr. *stear*, fat, + *pepsis*, digestion]. A lipolytic enzyme present in pancreatic juice that hydrolyzes fats to fatty acid and glycerine. The bile salts prepare the fats for the action of steapsin by emulsifying them. SYN: *lipase, pancreatic.* SEE: *enzyme; pancreas.*

stearate (stē'ă-rāt). An ester or salt of stearic acid.

stearic acid (stē-ăr'ĭk) [Gr. *stear*, fat]. A white, fatty acid found in solid animal fats and a few vegetable fats.

steariform (stē-ăr'ĭ-form) [" + *forma*, shape]. Resembling fat.

stearin (stē'ă-rĭn) [Gr. *stear*, fat]. A white

crystalline solid in animal and vegetable fats; $C_3H_5(C_{18}H_{35}O_2)_3$; any of the esters of glycerol and stearic acid, specifically glyceryl tristearate. One of the commonest fats in the body, esp. the solid ones. It breaks down into stearic acid and glycerol.

stearodermia (stē"ă-rō-dĕr'mē-ă) [" + *derma*, skin]. Disease of the sebaceous glands of the skin.

stearopten(e) (stē"ă-rŏp'tēn) [" + *ptenos*, volatile]. The more solid portion of a volatile oil as distinguished from the more fluid portion or eleoptene. Ex.: menthol, thymol.

stearrhea (stē"ă-rē'ă) [Gr. *stear*, fat, + *rhoia*, flow]. Excessive secretion of sebum or fat. SYN: *seborrhea oleosa.*

s. flavescens. Stearrhea with yellow sebaceous matter deposited on the skin.

s. nigricans. Stearrhea with black sweat due to presence of indican. SEE: *chromidrosis; chromodermatosis.*

s. simplex. Excessive discharge of sebum.

steatadenoma (stē-ăt"ăd-ĕ-nō'mă) [Gr. *steatos*, fat, + *aden*, gland, + *oma*, tumor]. Tumor of the sebaceous glands.

steatite (stē'ă-tīt). Talc.

steatitis (stē"ă-tī'tĭs) [" + *itis*, inflammation]. Inflammation of adipose tissue.

steato- [Gr. *steatos*, fat]. Prefix meaning fatty.

steatocele (stē-ăt'ō-sēl, stē'ăt-ō-sēl) [" + *kele*, tumor, swelling]. Fatty tumor within the scrotum.

steatocryptosis (stē"ă-tō-krĭp-tō'sĭs) [" + *krypte*, a sac, + *osis*, condition]. Any disease of sebaceous glands. SEE: *stearodermia.*

steatocystoma multiplex. A skin disorder characterized by development of many sebaceous cysts.

steatogenous (stē"ă-tŏj'ĕn-ŭs) [Gr. *steatos*, fat, + *gennan*, to produce]. 1. Causing fatty degeneration. 2. Producing any sebaceous gland disease.

steatolysis (stē"ă-tŏl'ĭ-sĭs) [" + *lysis*, dissolution]. 1. The process by which fats are first emulsified and then hydrolyzed to fatty acids and glycerine preparatory to absorption. 2. The decomposition of fat. SYN: *lipolysis.*

steatolytic (stē"ă-tō-lĭt'ĭk). Concerning steatolysis.

steatoma (stē"ă-tō'mă) [" + *oma*, tumor]. 1. Sebaceous cyst. SYN: *wen.* 2. Benign tumor composed of fat cells. SYN: *lipoma.*

Smooth, shiny, globular, cutaneous or subcutaneous tumor from pea to orange size arising from sebaceous glands, single or multiple, usually on neck, scalp, back, or scrotum.

ETIOL: Duct occlusion is causative in

some.

TREAT: Surgical excision by dissection without perforating sac. Packing in suppurative cases.

PROG: Prolonged irritation may cause suppuration.

steatomatous (stē″ă-tō′mă-tŭs). Presence of multiple sebaceous cysts.

steatonecrosis (stē″ă-tō-nē-krō′sĭs) [″ + *nekros*, corpse, + *osis*, condition]. Necrosis of fatty tissue in small patches.

steatopathy (stē-ă-tŏp′ă-thē) [″ + *pathos*, disease, suffering]. Disease of the sebaceous glands of the skin.

steatopygia (stē″ă-tō-pĭj′ē-ă) [″ + *pyge*, buttock]. Abnormal fatness of the buttocks occurring more frequently in women than in men. Seen in some tropical areas of Africa. Location of this excess fat accumulation in the buttocks may represent an adaptation to a very hot climate. It is thought that if this fat were evenly spread throughout the subcutaneous tissue, normal cooling of the skin would be severely limited.

steatopygous (stē″ă-tŏp′ĭ-gŭs) [″ + *pyge*, buttock]. Concerning or having steatopygia.

steatorrhea (stē″ă-tō-rē′ă) [Gr. *steatos*, fat, + *rhoia*, flow]. 1. Increased secretion of sebaceous glands. SYN: *seborrhea.* 2. Fatty stools, as seen in pancreatic diseases.

  s., idiopathic. Term applied to gastrointestinal disorders characterized by impaired absorption. SYN: *sprue.*

  s. simplex. Excessive secretion of sebaceous glands of the face.

steatosis (stē″ă-tō′sĭs) [″ + *osis*, condition]. 1. Fatty degeneration. 2. Disease of the sebaceous glands.

stegnosis (stĕg-nō′sĭs) [Gr. *stegnosis*, obstruction]. 1. Checking of a secretion or discharge. 2. Closing of a passage. SYN: *stenosis.* 3. Constipation. SYN: *costiveness.*

stegnotic (stĕg-nŏt′ĭk). Bringing about stegnosis. SYN: *astringent; constipating.*

Stegomyia (stĕg″ō-mĭ′ē-ă). A subgenus of mosquito of the genus *Aedes,* family Culicidae, suspected of transmitting the causative organism of yellow fever.

Steinert's disease (stīn′ĕrts) [Hans Steinert, Ger. physician, b. 1875]. A hereditary disease characterized by muscular wasting, myotonia, and cataract. SYN: *dystrophia myotonia.*

Stein-Leventhal syndrome (stīn-lĕv′ĕn-thäl) [Irving F. Stein, Sr., U.S. gynecologist, b. 1887; Michael L. Leventhal, U.S. obstetrician and gynecologist, 1901–1971]. The polycystic ovary syndrome characterized by normal growth and development with or without hirsutism. Menses may or may not be regular, but later oligomenorrhea develops and then amenorrhea, but infrequently ovulation will occur. Infertility is usually persistent but may be treated with clomiphene, gonadotropins, or wedge resection of the ovary. SYN: *polycystic ovary syndrome.*

Steinmann's extension (stīn′mănz) [Fritz Steinmann, Swiss surgeon, 1872–1932]. Traction applied to a limb by applying weight to a pin placed through the bone at right angles to the direction of pull of the traction force.

Steinmann pin. A sturdy pin placed in the distal end of a long bone so that a weight may be attached in order to apply traction.

Stelazine. Trade name for trifluoperazine hydrochloride.

stella [L.] (pl. *stellae*). Star.

  s. lentis hyaloidea. Posterior pole of the crystalline lens of the eye.

  s. lentis iridica. Anterior pole of the crystalline lens of the eye.

stellate [L. *stellatus*]. Star-shaped; arranged with parts radiating from a center.

stellate bandage. Bandage that is wrapped on the back, crossways.

stellate cell. Any cell that appears star-shaped.

  Ex.: neurons of molecular layer of cerebellum; Kupffer's cells of the liver sinusoids; astrocytes.

stellate fracture. Fracture with numerous fissures radiating from central point of injury.

stellate ganglion. A sympathetic ganglion formed by the fusion of inferior cervical and first thoracic ganglions.

stellate ligament. One of the anterior costovertebral ligaments.

stellate reticulum. The central cellular portion of the enamel organ, considered to be a nutritive store or protective covering of the developing enamel crown. SYN: *enamel pulp.*

stellate veins. Venous plexuses beneath the kidney's capsule. SYN: *stars of Verheyen.*

stellectomy (stĕl-lĕk′tō-mē) [″ + *ektome*, excision]. Surgical removal of the stellate ganglion.

Stellwag's sign (stĕl′văgs) [Carl Stellwag von Carion, Austrian oculist, 1823–1904]. Widening of palpebral aperture with absence or lessened frequency of winking, seen in Graves' disease.

stem. 1. [AS. *stemn,* tree trunk] Any stalklike structure. 2. To derive from or originate in. 3. [ME. *stemmen*] To check, stop, or hold back.

  s., brain. The lower portion of the brain excluding the cerebrum and cerebellum. Includes the medulla oblongata, pons, midbrain, and diencephalon.

stem cell. A cell that gives rise to a specific type of cell as in hematopoiesis.

stenion (stĕn'ē-ŏn) [Gr. *stenos,* narrow]. Craniometric point at extremities of the smallest transverse diameter in the temporal region.

steno- [Gr. *stenos,* narrow]. Combining form meaning narrow or short.

stenobregmatic (stĕn″ō-brĕg-măt'ĭk) [″ + *bregma,* front of head]. Term applied to a skull with narrowing of the upper and frontal portion.

stenocardia (stĕn″ō-kăr'dē-ă) [″ + *kardia,* heart]. Angina pectoris.

stenocephaly (stĕn″ō-sĕf'ă-lē) [″ + *kephale,* head]. Narrowness of the cranium in one or more diameters.

stenochoria (stĕn″ō-kō'rē-ă) [″ + *choros,* space]. Partial constriction, esp. of the lacrimal duct. SYN: *stenosis.*

stenocompressor (stĕn″ō-kŏm-prĕs'or) [″ + L. *compressor,* that which presses together]. An instrument for compressing Stensen's ducts to stop the flow of saliva.

stenocoriasis (stĕn″ō-kō-rī'ă-sĭs) [″ + *kore,* pupil, + -*iasis,* state]. Narrowing of pupil of the eye.

stenocrotaphia (stĕn″ō-krō-tă'fē-ă) [″ + *krotaphos,* the temple]. Abnormal narrowness of the temporal area of the head.

stenopaic, stenopeic (stĕn-ŏ-pā'ĭk, -pē'ĭk) [Gr. *stenos,* narrow, + *ope,* opening]. Provided with a narrow opening or slit, esp. denoting optical devices to protect against snow blindness.

stenosal (stē-nō'săl) [Gr. *stenos,* narrow]. Stenotic.

stenosed (stē-nōst', stĕn'ōzd). Characterized by stenosis; constricted.

stenosis (stē-nō'sĭs) [Gr., act of narrowing]. Constriction or narrowing of a passage or orifice. SYN: *stricture.*
  ETIOL: May result from embryonic maldevelopment, hypertrophy and thickening of a sphincter muscle, inflammatory disorders, or excessive development of fibrous tissue. It may involve almost any tube or duct.

  s., aortic. Constriction of the aortic orifice at cardiac base, or narrowing of the aorta.

  s., cardiac. A narrowing or constriction of any of the orifices leading into or from the heart or between chambers of the heart.

  s., cicatricial. Stenosis resulting from any contracted cicatrix.

  s., mitral. Stenosis of mitral valve or orifice of heart, or of both. Usually the result of rheumatic heart disease.

  s., pulmonary. SEE: *pulmonary stenosis.*

  s., pyloric. Obstruction caused by hypertrophy of walls of the pyloric orifice.

  s., subaortic. Congenital constriction of aortic tract below aortic valves.

  s., tricuspid. Narrowing of the opening to the tricuspid valve.

stenostomia (stĕn″ō-stō'mē-ă) [Gr. *stenos,* narrow, + *stoma,* mouth]. Narrowing of the mouth.

stenothermal (stĕn″ō-thĕr'măl) [″ + *therme,* heat]. Resisting only a small change of temperature.

stenothorax (stĕn″ō-thō'răks) [″ + *thorax,* chest]. An unusually narrow thorax.

stenotic [Gr. *stenosis,* act of narrowing]. Produced by or characterized by stenosis.

Stensen's duct (stĕn'sĕns) [Niels Stensen, Danish anatomist, 1638 – 1686]. The excretory duct of the parotid gland.

Stensen's foramina. Incisive foramina of the hard palate, transmitting anterior branches of the descending palatine vessels.

stent [Charles R. Stent, Brit. dentist, 1845 – 1901]. 1. Originally a compound used in making dental molds. 2. Any material used to hold tissue in place or to provide a support for a graft or anastomosis while healing is taking place.

  s., intraluminal coronary artery. A stent made of stainless steel with a self-expanding mesh introduced into the coronary artery. Used to prevent lumen closure (restenosis) following bypass surgery and to treat acute vessel closure after angioplasty.

step. A series of rests for the foot in ascending or descending.

  s., Rönne's. A steplike defect in the visual field.

stephanion (stē-fā'nē-ŏn) [Gr. *stephanos,* crown]. Point at intersection of the superior temporal ridge and coronal suture.

steppage gait. A high-stepping gait seen with paralysis of the dorsiflexors of the ankle; seen in diabetic neuropathy of the peroneal nerve. Patient lifts the foot very high in walking to raise the drooping toes from the ground or floor.

stepping reflex. SEE: *reflex, stepping.*

steradian (stē-rā'dē-ăn). The unit of measurement of solid angles. It encloses an area on the surface of a sphere equal to the square of the radius of the sphere.

Sterane. Trade name for prednisolone, USP.

sterco- [L. *stercus,* dung]. Combining form indicating a relationship to feces.

stercobilin (stĕr″kō-bī'lĭn) [″ + *bilis,* bile]. A brown pigment derived from the bile, giving the characteristic color to feces. SEE: *urobilin.*

stercobilinogen (stĕr″kō-bī-lĭn'ō-jĕn). A colorless substance derived from urobilinogen. It is present in the feces and turns brown on oxidation.

stercolith (stĕr'kō-lĭth) [″ + Gr. *lithos,* stone]. A fecal calculus.

stercoraceous (stĕr″kō-rā′shŭs) [L. *stercoraceus*]. Having the nature of, pert. to, or containing feces.

stercoral (stĕr′kō-răl) [L. *stercus*, dung]. Pert. to feces. SYN: *stercoraceous*.

stercorin (stĕr′kō-rĭn). A sterol, $C_{27}H_{47}OH$, in feces.

stercorolith (stĕr′kō-rō-lĭth) [″ + Gr. *lithos*, stone]. A fecal concretion. SYN: *coprolith; fecalith.*

stercoroma (stĕr″kō-rō′mă) [″ + Gr. *oma*, tumor]. A fecal tumorlike mass in the rectum. SYN: *fecaloma; scatoma.*

stercorous (stĕr′kō-rŭs) [L. *stercorosus*]. Resembling excrement. SYN: *stercoraceous; stercoral.*

stercus (stĕr′kŭs) [L.]. (pl. *stercora*) Feces. SYN: *excreta; excrement.*

stere (stĕr, stār) [Gr. *stereos*, solid]. Combining form meaning solid or indicating three-dimensional.

stereo-. Combining form concerning three dimensions, e.g., sound-producing devices in which the sound comes from several sources, such as speakers.

stereoagnosis (stĕr″ē-ō-ăg-nō′sĭs) [″ + *a-*, not, + *gnosis*, knowledge]. Astereognosis, q.v.

stereoanesthesia (stĕr″ē-ō-ăn″ĕs-thē′zē-ă) [″ + *an-*, not, + *aisthesis*, sensation]. Inability to recognize objects by feeling their form.

stereoarthrolysis (stĕr″ē-ō-ăr-thrŏl′ĭ-sĭs) [″ + *arthron*, joint, + *lysis*, dissolution]. Surgical formation of a movable new joint in bony ankylosis.

stereoauscultation (stĕr″ē-ō-aws″kŭl-tā′shŭn) [″ + L. *auscultare*, listen to]. Auscultation by use of a stethoscope with two ends on it so each may be placed on different parts of the chest. One tube of each instrument is inserted into an ear while the other is squeezed shut by the fingers.

stereocampimeter (stĕr″ē-ō-kăm-pĭm′ē-tĕr) [″ + L. *campus*, field, + Gr. *metron*, measure]. Device for measuring the visual field of both eyes simultaneously.

stereochemical (stĕr″ē-ō-kĕm′ĭ-kăl) [″ + *chemeia*, chemistry]. Concerning stereochemistry.

stereochemistry (stĕr″ē-ō-kĕm′ĭs-trē). That branch of chemistry dealing with atoms in their space relationship; and the effect of such relationship on the action and effects of the molecule.

stereocilia (stĕr″ē-ō-sĭl′ē-ă) (sing. *stereocilium*). Nonmotile protoplasmic projections from free surfaces of cells of ductus epididymis and ductus deferens.

stereocinefluorography (stĕr″ē-ō-sĭn″ē-flū″or-ŏg′ră-fē). Motion picture photography of the images produced by stereofluo-rography. This provides a three-dimensional visualization.

stereoencephalotomy (stĕr″ē-ō-ĕn-sĕf″ă-lŏt′ō-mē) [″ + *enkephalos*, brain, + *tome*, incision]. Surgical incision by use of stereotaxis.

stereognosis (stĕr″ē-ŏg-nō′sĭs) [″ + *gnosis*, knowledge]. Ability to recognize form of solid objects by touch.

stereogram (stĕr′ē-ō-grăm) [″ + *gramma*, something written]. Stereoscopic roentgenogram.

stereoisomer (stĕr″ē-ō-ī′sō-mĕr). A substance exhibiting stereoisomerism.

stereoisomerism (stĕr″ē-ō-ī-sō′mĕr-ĭzm). Condition in which two or more substances may have the same empirical formula, but a different structural formula, structural formulas being mirror images of each other.

Ex.: Dextrose and levulose differ in optical activity with regard to their effect on a plane of polarized light.

stereology (stĕr″ē-ŏl′ō-jē) [Gr. *stereos*, solid, + *logos*, word, reason]. Study of three-dimensional aspects of objects.

stereometer (stĕr″ē-ŏm′ē-tĕr) [″ + *metron*, measure]. An instrument used in stereometry.

stereometry (stĕr″ē-ŏm′ē-trē) [″ + *metron*, a measure]. The measurement of a solid body or the cubic contents of a hollow body.

stereo-ophthalmoscope (stĕr″ē-ō-ŏf-thăl′mō-skōp) [″ + *ophthalmos*, eye, + *skopein*, to examine]. An ophthalmoscope that is designed to permit the fundus to be seen simultaneously by both eyes of the examiner.

stereo-orthopter (stĕr″ē-ō-or-thŏp′tĕr) [″ + *orthos*, straight, + *opsis*, vision]. A mirror reflecting device for treatment of strabismus.

stereophantoscope (stĕr″ē-ō-făn′tō-skōp) [″ + *phantos*, visible, + *skopein*, to examine]. A stereoscopic device with rotating disks for testing vision.

stereophorometer (stĕr″ē-ō-for-ŏm′ē-tĕr) [″ + *phoros*, a bearer, + *metron*, measure]. A prism-refracting device for use in correcting extraocular eye muscle imbalance.

stereophotography (stĕr″ē-ō-fō-tŏg′ră-fē) [″ + *phos*, light, + *graphein*, to write]. Photography that produces effect of solidity or depth in the pictures.

stereophotomicrograph (stĕr″ē-ō-fō″tō-mī′krō-grăf) [″ + ″ + *mikros*, tiny, + *graphein*, to write]. A photograph showing solidity or depth of a microscopic subject.

stereopsis (stĕr″ē-ŏp′sĭs) [″ + *opsis*, vision]. Stereoscopic vision.

stereoradiography (stĕr″ē-ō-rā″dē-ŏg′rá-fē) [″ + L. *radius*, ray, + Gr. *graphein*, to write]. Taking roentgenograms from two slightly different angles so that when they are viewed through a stereoscope, there will be a stereoscopic effect.

stereoroentgenography (stĕr″ē-ō-rĕnt″gĕn-ŏg′rá-fē) [″ + *roentgen*, + Gr. *graphein*, to write]. Stereoradiography.

stereoscope (stĕr′ē-ō-skōp) [″ + *skopein*, to examine]. Instrument that creates an impression of solidity or depth of objects seen by combining images of two pictures.

stereoscopic, stereoscopical. Pert. to the stereoscope or its use.

stereoscopic vision. Vision in which things have the appearance of solidity and relief as though seen in three dimensions. Binocular vision produces this effect.

stereospecific (stĕr″ē-ō-spĕ-sĭf′ĭk). Specific for only one of the possible receptors on a cell.

stereotactic (stĕr″ē-ō-tăk′tĭk). Stereotaxic, q.v.

stereotaxic (stĕr″ē-ō-tăk′sĭk) [Gr. *stereos*, solid, + *taxis*, arrangement]. Concerning stereotaxis.

stereotaxis (stĕr″ē-ō-tăk′sĭs) [″ + *taxis*, arrangement]. A method of precisely locating areas in the brain; use of this technique is essential in certain neurosurgical procedures.

stereotropic (stĕr″ē-ō-trŏp′ĭk) [″ + *trope*, a turn]. Concerning stereotropism.

stereotropism (stĕr″ē-ŏt′rō-pĭzm) [″ + *tropos*, a turning, + *-ismos*, condition]. A response toward (positive stereotropism) or away from (negative stereotropism) a solid object. SYN: *thigmotropism.*

stereotypy (stĕr-ē-ō-tī′pē) [″ + *typos*, type]. Persistent repetition of words, posture, or movement without meaning; seen in catatonic partial stupors.

steric (stē′rĭk). Concerning the spatial arrangement of atoms in a chemical compound.

sterile (stĕr′ĭl) [L. *sterilis*, barren]. 1. Free from living microorganisms. Solutions that have passed through certain filters are called sterile solutions because bacteria, fungi, and their spores have been removed. However, viruses can pass through some filters, and the term sterile is incorrectly used in this context. 2. Not fertile; unable to reproduce young. SYN: *barren.* SEE: *sterility.*

sterility (stĕr-ĭl′ĭ-tē) [L. *sterilitas*, barrenness]. 1. Condition of being free from living microorganisms. 2. Inability of the female to become pregnant or for the male to impregnate a female.

Investigation into the cause of sterility includes investigation of both partners. A routine examination for sterility in the female includes a study of the vaginal secretions, a bimanual pelvic examination, visualization of the cervix, in some cases a test for patency of the fallopian tubes, and a record of basal body temperature. A history of pelvic disorder in the female is of great importance. The male should have the seminal fluid examined for the number, motility, viability, and normality of the spermatozoa.

TREAT: Treatment of sterility depends upon the finding and correction of any or all causes of the condition. A high percentage of couples who have an infertility problem in the first year of marriage will, without treatment, produce offspring within two to three years. SEE: *embryo transfer; gamete intrafallopian transfer; fertilization, in vitro.*

s., absolute. Complete and incurable inability to produce offspring as a result of anatomical or physiological factors that prevent production of functional germ cells, conception, or normal development of a zygote.

s., acquired. The failure of further conception after once having given birth to a child.

s., female. The inability of the woman to conceive.

ETIOL: *Congenital abnormalities:* Absence or maldevelopment of the uterus, tubes, or ovaries; infantile uterus. *Acquired local conditions: Vagina:* Inflammation. *Cervix:* Narrowing of the internal os; acute and chronic endocervicitis; polyps occluding the cervical canal; cervical mucus that, due to either its chemical or physical qualities, is hostile to sperm. *Body of the uterus:* Fibroids of the uterus that block the canal; diseased endometrium, particularly endometritis. *Fallopian tube:* Chronic salpingo-oophoritis with closure of the tubal ostium and where the ovary is embedded in adhesions. *Ovarian dysfunction:* Congenital conditions, or secondary to endocrine disorders, infections, trauma, neoplasms, x-ray or surgical castration, or effects of toxic agents. Psychological and emotional disturbances, coital difficulties, and dietary deficiencies may also result in sterility. SEE: *embryo transfer; gamete intrafallopian transfer; fertilization, in vitro.*

s., male. Inability of a male either to produce sperm or to produce viable sperm. This results in inability to fertilize the ovum.

ETIOL: May result from congenital factors such as cryptorchidism or maldevelopment of testicular ducts or testis; acquired factors; lack of libido or impotence.

s., primary. Sterility resulting from failure of the testis or ovary to produce functional germ cells.

s., relative. Sterility due to causes other than defect of sex organs.

sterilization (stĕr″ĭl-ĭ-zā′shŭn) [L. *sterilis*, barren]. 1. Process of completely removing or destroying all microorganisms on a substance by exposure to chemical or physical agents, exposure to ionizing radiation, or by filtering gas or liquids through porous materials that remove microorganisms. A substance cannot be properly described as being partially sterile. SEE: *sterile.* 2. Process of rendering barren. Can be accomplished by surgical removal of testes or ovaries (castration) or inactivation by irradiation, or by tying off or removing a portion of reproductive ducts (ductus deferens or uterine tubes). SEE: *salpingectomy; tubal ligation; vasectomy.*

s., dry heat. Sterilization of microorganisms accomplished by subjection to high heat (165° to 170°C) for 2 to 3 hours in ovens.

s., fractional. Sterilization of microorganisms in which heating is done at separated intervals, so that spores can develop into bacteria and be destroyed. Usually accomplished by subjecting organisms to free-flowing steam for 15 min. for three or four successive days. SYN: *s., intermittent.*

s., gas. Exposure to gases such as formaldehyde or ethylene oxide that destroy microorganisms.

s., intermittent. S., fractional.

s., laparoscopic. Sterilization by use of a laparoscope.

s., steam. Sterilization by exposure of microorganisms at 212°F (100°C) to flowing steam in an unsealed receptacle or by exposure of microorganisms to steam under pressure in an autoclave.

sterilize (stĕr′ĭ-līz) [L. *sterilis*, barren]. 1. To free from microorganisms. 2. To make incapable of reproduction.

sterilizer (stĕr′ĭ-lī″zĕr). Oven or appliance for sterilizing.

s., steam. An autoclave that sterilizes by steam under pressure at temperatures above 100°C.

sternad (stĕr′năd) [Gr. *sternon*, chest]. Toward the sternum.

sternal (stĕr′năl) [Gr. *sternalis*]. Rel. to the sternum or breastbone.

sternalgia (stĕr-năl′jē-ă) [Gr. *sternon*, chest, + *algos*, pain]. Pain in the sternum. SYN: *sternodynia.*

sternal puncture. Use of a large-bore needle to obtain a specimen of marrow from the sternum.

Sternberg-Reed cell. SEE: *Reed-Sternberg cell.*

sternebra (stĕr′nē-bră) [″ + L. *vertebra*, vertebra]. Parts of the sternum prior to fusion.

sternen (stĕr′nĕn) [Gr. *sternon*, chest]. Concerning the sternum and no other structures.

sterno- [Gr. *sternon*, chest]. Combining form meaning sternum.

sternoclavicular (stĕr″nō-klă-vĭk′ū-lăr) [″ + L. *clavicula*, little key]. Concerning the sternum and clavicle.

sternocleidal (stĕr″nō-klī″dăl) [″ + *clavis*, key]. Sternoclavicular.

sternocleidomastoid (stĕr″nō-klī″dō-măs′ toyd) [″ + *clavis*, key, + *mastos*, breast, + *eidos*, form, shape]. One of two muscles arising from the sternum and inner part of the clavicle. SEE: *Muscles* in *Appendix.*

sternocostal (stĕr″nō-kŏs′tăl) [″ + L. *costa*, rib]. Rel. to sternum and ribs.

sternodymia (stĕr″nō-dĭm′ē-ă) [″ + *didymos*, twin]. Condition in which deformed twin fetuses are joined at the sternum.

sternodynia (stĕr″nō-dīn′ē-ă) [″ + *odyne*, pain]. Pain in the sternum. SYN: *sternalgia.*

sternohyoid (stĕr″nō-hī′oyd) [″ + *hyoeides*, U-shaped]. Muscle from the medial end of the clavicle and sternum to the hyoid bone. SEE: *Muscles* in *Appendix.*

sternoid (stĕr′noyd) [″ + *eidos*, form, shape]. Resembling the breastbone.

sternomastoid (stĕr″nō-măs′toyd) [″ + *mastos*, breast, + *eidos*, form, shape]. Pert. to the sternum and mastoid process of the temporal bone.

sternomastoid region. Wide area on lateral region of the neck covered by sternocleidomastoid muscle.

sternopagia (stĕr″nō-pā′jē-ă) [″ + *pagos*, thing fixed]. Sternodymia, q.v.

sternopericardial (stĕr″nō-pĕr″ĭ-kăr′dē-ăl) [″ + *peri*, around, + *kardia*, heart]. Concerning the sternum and pericardium.

sternoschisis (stĕr-nŏs′kĭ-sĭs) [″ + *schisis*, a splitting]. A cleft or fissured sternum.

sternothyroid (stĕr″nō-thī′royd) [″ + *thyreos*, shield, + *eidos*, form, shape]. Muscle extending beneath the sternohyoid that depresses thyroid cartilage. SEE: *Muscles* in *Appendix.*

sternotomy (stĕr-nŏt′ō-mē) [″ + *tome*, incision]. The operation of cutting through the sternum.

sternotracheal (stĕr″nō-trā′kē-ăl) [″ + *tracheia*, trachea]. Concerning the sternum and trachea.

sternotrypesis (stĕr″nō-trī-pē′sĭs) [″ + *trypesis*, a boring]. Surgical perforation of the sternum.

sternovertebral (stĕr″nō-vĕr′tĕ-brăl) [″ + L. *vertebra*, vertebra]. Concerning the sternum and vertebrae.

sternum (stĕr'nŭm) [L.]. [NA] The narrow, flat bone in the median line of the thorax in front. It consists of three portions distinguished as the manubrium, the gladiolus, and the ensiform or xiphoid process. SEE: illus.

RS: breast, chicken; chondrosternal; cleft; ensiform; manubrium; xiphoid process.

s., cleft. Congenital fissure of the sternum.

sternutament (stĕr-nū'tăm-ĕnt) [L. *sternutare,* to sneeze]. A substance causing sneezing.

sternutatio (stĕr-nū-tā'shē-ō) [L.]. Sneezing.

s. convulsiva. Paroxysmal sneezing as in hay fever.

sternutation (stĕr-nū-tā'shŭn). Act of sneezing.

s., convulsive. Spasmodic or paroxysmal sneezing with profusion of watery secretion from the nose.

sternutator (stĕr'nū-tā″tor) [L. *sternutatorius,* causing sneezing]. An agent, such as a war gas, that induces sneezing.

sternutatory (stĕr-nū'tă-tō″rē). Causing sneezing.

steroid (stĕr'oyd). 1. An organic compound containing in its chemical nucleus the perhydrocyclopentanophenanthrene ring. SEE: *perhydrocyclopentanophenanthrene; steroid hormones* for illus. 2. Term applied to any one of a large group of substances chemically related to sterols. Includes sterols, D vitamins, bile acids, certain hormones, saponins, glucosides of digitalis, and certain carcinogenic substances.

steroidal withdrawal syndrome. The appearance of symptoms of adrenal insufficiency in persons who discontinue the use of corticosteroids after having been treated with them for a prolonged period. In those patients, adrenal function has been suppressed to such an extent that the adrenal glands do not provide an appropriate response when the patient has a serious infection, surgery, or an accident. This failure to respond to stress may be present for as long as a year after discontinuation of corticosteroid therapy. The syndrome may be prevented by gradual rather than abrupt withdrawal of corticosteroid therapy.

steroid hormones. The sex hormones and hormones of the adrenal cortex. SEE: illus.

steroid hormone therapy. Treatment with various steroid hormones, esp. those from the adrenal cortex. If therapy is continued for more than a few days, the following general precautions should be observed: low-salt diet; high-protein diet; control gastric acidity; adequate potassium intake; deter

STERNUM

JUGULAR NOTCH

MANUBRIUM

CLAVICULAR NOTCH

POINT OF ATTACHMENT OF FIRST RIB, SECOND RIB

BODY OF STERNUM

POINT OF ATTACHMENT OF THIRD RIB, FOURTH RIB, FIFTH RIB, SIXTH RIB, SEVENTH RIB

XIPHOID PROCESS

ANTERIOR VIEW

STEROID HORMONE NUCLEUS

PERHYDROCYCLOPENTANOPHENANTHRENE, THE BASIC STRUCTURE OR "BUILDING BLOCK" OF STEROID HORMONES. CARBON ATOMS ARE NUMBERED.

mine need for covering antibiotic such as isoniazid in sarcoidosis or in those who have a positive tuberculin test; nitrogen balance (androgen or estrogen therapy may be needed); observe for osteoporosis, particularly in postmenopausal women.

steroidogenesis (stē-roy″dō-jĕn′ē-sĭs). Production of steroids.

sterol (stēr′ŏl, stēr′ŏl) [Gr. *stereos*, solid, + L. *oleum*, oil]. One of a group of substances related to fats and belonging to the lipoids. They are alcohols with a cyclic nucleus (cyclopentanoperhydrophenanthrene) and are found free or esterified with fatty acids (cholesterides). They are found in animals (zoosterols) or in plants (phytosterols). Generally colorless, crystalline compounds, nonsaponifiable and soluble in certain organic solvents.
    Ex.: cholesterol.

stertor (stĕr′tor) [NL. *stertor*, to snore]. Snoring or laborious breathing due to obstruction of air passages in the head, seen in certain diseases such as apoplexy.

stertorous (stĕr′tō-rŭs). Pert. to laborious breathing provoking a snoring sound.

stethalgia (stĕth-ăl′jē-ă). Pain in the chest.

stetho- [Gr. *stethos*, chest]. Combining form indicating the chest.

stethocyrtograph (stĕth″ō-sĕr′tō-grăf) [″ + *kyrtos*, bent, + *graphein*, to write]. Stethokyrtograph, q.v.

stethogoniometer (stĕth″ō-gō″nē-ŏm′ĕt-ĕr) [″ + *gonia*, angle, + *metron*, measure]. Device for measuring the curvature of the chest.

stethogram (stĕth′ō-grăm) [″ + *gramma*, something written]. A record of heart sounds. The record may be stored for later comparison with subsequent heart sounds. SYN: *phonocardiogram*.

stethograph (stĕth′ō-grăf) [″ + *graphein*, to write]. Device to record chest movements in respiration.

stethokyrtograph (stĕth″ō-kĭr′tō-grăf) [″ + *kyrtos*, bent, + *graphein*, to write]. Device for measuring and recording the dimensions and amount of curves of the chest.

stethometer (stĕth-ŏm′ĕt-ĕr) [″ + *metron*, measure]. Device for measuring the chest's expansion during respiration.

stethomyitis, stethomyositis (stĕth″ō-mī-ī′tĭs, -mī″ō-sī′tĭs) [″ + *mys*, muscle, + *itis*, inflammation]. Inflammation of the muscles of the chest.

stethoparalysis (stĕth″ō-pă-răl′ĭ-sĭs) [″ + *paralyein*, to disable]. Paralysis of the muscles of the chest.

stethophonometer (stĕth″ō-fō-nŏm′ĕt-ĕr) [″ + *phone*, voice, + *metron*, measure]. Instrument for determining intensity of sound emitted in auscultation.

stethoscope (stĕth′ō-skōp) [″ + *skopein*, to examine]. Instrument used to mediate sounds produced in the body. Ordinarily consists of rubber tubing in a Y shape.
    s., binaural. Stethoscope designed for use with both ears.
    s., compound. Stethoscope in which more than one set is attached to the same fork and chest piece.
    s., double. Stethoscope with two earpieces and tubes.
    s., electronic. Stethoscope equipped to electronically amplify sounds from the body.
    s., single. Rigid or flexible stethoscope designed for one ear only.

stethoscopic (stĕth″ō-skŏp′ĭk). Concerning or done by use of a stethoscope.

stethoscopy (stĕth-ŏs′kō-pē) [″ + *skopein*, to examine]. Examination by means of the stethoscope.

stethospasm (stĕth′ō-spăzm) [″ + *spasmos*, convulsion]. Spasm of the pectoral or chest muscles.

Stevens-Johnson syndrome (stē′vĕnz-jŏn′sŏn) [Albert M. Stevens, 1884–1945, Frank C. Johnson, 1894–1934, U.S. pediatricians]. Erythema multiforme, q.v.

STH. *somatotropic hormone*; somatotropin, the growth hormone.

sthenia (sthē′nē-ă) [Gr. *sthenos*, strength]. Normal or unusual strength. Opposite of asthenia.

sthenic (sthĕn′ĭk). Active; strong.

sthenometer (sthĕn-ŏm′ĕ-tĕr) [Gr. *sthenos*, strength, + *metron*, measure]. Device for measuring muscular strength.

sthenometry (sthĕn-ŏm′ĕ-trē). Determination of bodily strength.

stibialism (stĭb′ē-ăl-ĭzm) [L. *stibium*, antimony, + Gr. *-ismos*, condition]. Antimony poisoning.

stibiated (stĭb′ē-āt″ĕd) [L. *stibium*, antimony]. Containing antimony.

stibium (stĭb'ē-ŭm) [L.]. Antimony.

stibophen (stĭb'ō-fĕn). A trivalent antimony compound, used in treating schistosomiasis and granuloma inguinale.

stiff [AS. *stif*]. Rigid, firm, inflexible.

stiff joint. Joint with reduced mobility.

stiff man syndrome. Intermittent aching, tightness, and stiffness of the muscles, which progresses to permanent stiffness to the extent of limiting voluntary movement. Etiology is unknown, but an autoimmune basis is suspected.

TREAT: Immunosuppressive therapy and exchange transfusion have been used. Diazepam is of benefit in some patients.

stiff neck. Rigidity of neck resulting from spasm of neck muscles. It is a symptom of many disorders. SYN: *torticollis; wryneck.*

stigma (stĭg'mă) [Gr., mark] (pl. *stigmata, -mas*). 1. A mark or spot on the skin; lesions or sores of hands and feet that resemble crucifixion wounds. 2. Spot on ovarian surface where rupture of a graafian follicle will occur. 3. Mental or physical mark characterizing a specific disease. There is often shame and embarrassment because of a stigmatizing condition; there is often some mental anguish because one has a condition that marks one as being different.

    s., hysterical. Any of the peculiar marks or symptoms of hysteria, such as spots on the skin or impairment of sensory functions.

    s. of degeneration. Any of the developmental variations from the normal. Formerly thought to be associated with mental degeneracy.

DEGENERATION CHANGES: *Face:* May be unusually hairy in the female and abnormally smooth in the male. *Fingers and toes:* May include an extra one, or may be adherent or webbed. *Forehead:* May be sloping and very low. *Eyes:* May be different in color or set at different levels. *Ears:* Unusual in many ways. *Jaws:* Either one may project unusually. *Head:* May be unusually large or small. *Teeth:* May be irregular or project. *Roof of mouth:* May be high and pointed or unusually narrow. Only several of these irregularities may be considered as indicative of defective mentality.

    s., psychic. Mental state characterized by susceptibility to suggestion.

stigmata. Marks on the body at the same locations as those on Christ's body caused by having been nailed to the cross. Allegedly, these are evidence of divine action, esp. on priests, nuns, and other members of religious orders.

stigmatic (stĭg-măt'ĭk) [Gr. *stigma,* mark]. Pert. to or marked with a stigma.

stigmatism. 1. Condition characterized by

possession of stigmata. 2. Condition in which the rays of light are accurately focused on the retina. SEE: *astigmatism.*

stigmatization (stĭg″mă-tĭ-zā'shŭn). The formation of stigmata, esp. hysterical stigmata on the skin.

stigmatometer (stĭg″mă-tŏm'ĕ-tĕr) [″ + *metron,* measure]. Device for testing eye refraction. SYN: *astigmatometer.*

stilbestrol (stĭl-bĕs'trŏl). Diethylstilbestrol, q.v.

stilet, stilette (stī-lĕt') [Fr. *stilette*]. 1. Small, sharp-pointed instrument for probing. 2. Wire used to pass through or stiffen a flexible catheter.

stillbirth [AS. *stille,* quiet, + Old Norse *burdhr,* birth]. Birth of a dead fetus.

stillborn [″ + *boren,* to bring forth]. Dead at birth.

Still's disease [Sir George F. Still, Brit. physician, 1868–1941]. Arthritis, juvenile rheumatoid, q.v.

stillicidium (stĭl″ĭ-sĭd'ē-ŭm) [L. *stilla,* drop, + *cadere,* to fall]. A dribbling or flowing, drop by drop.

    s. lacrimarum. Watering of the eye. SYN: *epiphora.*

    s. narium. Watery mucus discharged at onset of coryza.

    s. urinae. Urinary incontinence from a distended bladder. SYN: *strangury.*

Stilphostrol. Trade name for diethylstilbestrol diphosphate.

stimulant (stĭm'ū-lănt) [L. *stimulans,* goading]. Any agent temporarily increasing functional activity. Stimulants may be classified according to the organ upon which they act as follows: cardiac, bronchial, gastric, cerebral, intestinal, nervous, motor, vasomotor, respiratory, and secretory.

stimulate (stĭm'ū-lāt) [L. *stimulare,* to goad on]. To increase functional activity of an organ or structure.

stimulation (stĭm″ū-lā'shŭn). 1. Process of being stimulated. 2. Irritating action of agents on muscles, nerves, or sensory end organs by which activity in a part is evoked.

stimulator (stĭm″ū-lā'tor). Something that stimulates.

    s., long-acting thyroid. A substance present in the blood of persons with hyperthyroidism that stimulates the thyroid. It is an immune gamma globulin.

stimulus (stĭm'ū-lŭs) [L., a goad] (pl. *stimuli*). 1. Any agent or factor able to influence living protoplasm directly, as one capable of causing muscular contraction or secretion in a gland, or of initiating an impulse in a nerve. 2. A change of environment of sufficient intensity to evoke a response in an organism. 3. An excitant or irritant.

    s., adequate. 1. Any stimulus capable of

evoking a response, i.e., an environmental change possessing a certain intensity, acting for a certain length of time, and occurring at a certain rate. 2. A stimulus capable of initiating a nerve impulse in a specific type of receptor.

s., chemical. A chemical substance (liquid, gaseous, or solid) that is capable of evoking a response.

s., conditioned. Stimulus that gives rise to a conditioned response. SEE: *reflex, conditioned.*

s., electric. Stimulus resulting from initiation of or cessation of a flow of electrons as from a battery, induction coil, or generator.

s., homologous. Stimulus that acts only on specific sensory end organs.

s., iatrotropic. Stimulus or event that makes a person seek or receive medical attention; also called the sick person's chief complaint. However, medical care is voluntarily sought by apparently healthy people for many reasons, e.g., an Armed Forces draft examination, pre-employment or premarital examination, or in a health screening survey. Thus it is possible for disease to be discovered prior to the time when it would ordinarily make itself known to the individual.

s., liminal. S., threshold.

s., mechanical. Stimulus produced by a physical change such as contact with objects or changes in pressure.

s., minimal. S., threshold.

s., nociceptive. A painful and usually injurious stimulus.

s., subliminal. Stimulus that is weaker than a threshold stimulus.

s., thermal. Stimulus produced by a change in temperature of the skin, a rise giving sensations of warmth, a fall giving sensations of coldness.

s., threshold. The least or weakest stimulus that is capable of initiating a response or giving rise to a sensation. SYN: *s., liminal.*

s., unconditioned. Any stimulus that elicits an unconditioned response, i.e., a response that was inherently present rather than one that was learned.

sting [AS. *stingan*]. 1. Sharp, smarting sensation, as of a wound or astringent. 2. A puncture wound made by an insect. SEE: *bites or stings.*

stingray. A group of rays of the family Dasyatidae. A number of species are found in the coastal waters of the United States. It is flat with wide pectoral fins that resemble wings. A venomous spine runs along the top of its whiplike tail. It is used to inflict severe injuries.

TREAT: Pain relievers, debridement of

wound, irrigation with removal of foreign material and stinger if it is present, and injection of site with local anesthetic. Soak area in hot water (45° to 60°C) 30 to 60 min. to inactivate venom.

S-T interval. The interval in an electrocardiogram that represents the initial and final ventricular complexes. SEE: *QRST complex; electrocardiogram* for illus.

stippling (stĭp′lĭng) [Dutch *stippelen*, to spot]. A spotted condition, as in the retina in certain ocular diseases or in basophilic red corpuscles.

s., gingival. An orange-peel appearance of the attached gingiva in health, believed to be due to the enlargement of the underlying connective tissue papillae in response to massage and toothbrushing; the indent lies between the bulging papillae where the epithelia grow downward as rete ridges.

stirrup, stirrup bone (stĭr′ŭp) [AS. *stigrap*, a stirrup]. Stapes of the ear. SEE: *ear.*

stitch (stĭch) [AS. *stice*, a pricking]. 1. A local sharp, lancinating, or spasmodic pain. 2. A single loop of suture material passed through skin or flesh by a needle, to facilitate healing of a wound. 3. To unite skin or flesh with a needle and suture material. Stitches made of nonabsorbable materials are removed after a few days, and other types are absorbed by the body. SYN: *suture.*

stitch abscess. Abscess developing in a suture and due to infection.

stochastic model (stō-kăs′tĭk) [Gr. *stokastikos*, skillful in guessing]. A statistical model that attempts to reproduce the sequence of events that would be expected to occur in a real-life situation. This technique has some usefulness in predicting the importance and extent of disease in a specified population.

stock (stŏk) [AS. *stocc*, tree trunk]. The original individual, race, or tribe from which others have descended.

stock culture. Permanent culture of a microorganism reinforced from time to time by fresh media.

Stockholm syndrome [Named after the romantic involvement of a terrorist and a bank employee held hostage during a 1973 bank robbery in Stockholm]. The emotional involvement between a hostage and the person holding him or her captive. The hostage's action may be due to sympathy for the terrorist's "cause," stress, or the need to cooperate in order to survive.

stockinet. Tubular woven material of uniform size that is open at both ends. Used to hold bandages in place or to place uniform pressure on a leg, finger, arm, or other part of an extremity.

stocking. Snug covering for the foot and leg.

A stocking made of elastic material will place firm, even pressure on the extremity, which is useful in preventing thrombophlebitis of the leg in bedfast patients and in treating varicose veins.

stocking aid. A device for assisting persons with limited function to put on socks or stockings.

stoichiometry (stoy″kē-ŏm′ĕ-trē) [Gr. *stoicheion*, element, + *metron*, measure]. Study of the mathematics of chemistry and chemical reactions; chemical calculations.

stoke (stōk) [Sir George Stokes, Brit. physicist, 1819–1903]. A unit of viscosity equal to 10^{-4} square meters per second (10^{-4}m. s^{-1}).

Stokes-Adams syndrome (stōks-ăd′ăms) [William Stokes, Irish physician, 1804–1878; Robert Adams, Irish physician, 1791–1875]. Altered state of consciousness caused by decreased flow of blood to brain. Caused by any transient interference with cardiac output such as incomplete or complete heart block. The patient may be lightheaded or become completely unconscious and have convulsions.

TREAT: Intracardiac epinephrine, a sharp blow to the precordium, or use of an external electric pacemaker.

Stokes' disease (stōks) [William Stokes]. Exophthalmic goiter. SEE: *hyperthyroidism.*

Stokes' law (stōks) [William Stokes]. A muscle lying above an inflamed serous or mucous membrane may be paralyzed.

Stokes' lens [George Stokes]. Device used to diagnose astigmatism.

stoma (stō′mă) [Gr., mouth] (pl. *stomata, -mas*). 1. A mouth, small opening, or a pore. 2. Artificially created opening between two passages or body cavities or between a cavity or passage and the body's surface. 3. A minute opening between cells of certain epithelial membranes, esp. peritoneum and pleura.

stomach (stŭm′ăk) [Gr. *stomachos*, mouth]. A dilated, saclike, distensible portion of the alimentary canal below the esophagus and below the diaphragm to right of spleen, partly under the liver. It is composed of a fundus or round part, a body or middle portion, and pyloric portion, which is the small, distal end.

It has two openings: the upper cardiac orifice opens into the esophagus and the lower pyloric orifice opens into the duodenum. The stomach is composed of four layers. The outer serous coat covers almost all of the organ. The muscular layer just beneath is formed of three layers of smooth muscle fibers: an outer longitudinal layer, a medial circular layer, and an inner oblique layer. Submucous layer is a connecting medium

between the muscular and mucous layer, the inner lining of the stomach.

The cardiac, fundic (parietal or oxyntic), and pyloric glands of the stomach are composed of columnar and tubular cells that secrete gastric juice containing hydrochloric acid and pepsin. SEE: illus.

FUNCT: Although it has limited ability to absorb, the stomach secretes gastric juice and converts proteins into peptones. In addition to its basic function as an organ of digestion, the stomach serves in the following ways: regulation of passage of food to the remainder of the gut by reservoir action; stomach acid destroys a large proportion of microbes present in most food; actions involved in acid-base equilibrium of the body, particularly when electrolytes are removed from the body during vomiting; excretion of some parenterally administered drugs into the gastric juice; receptor for chemical and nervous mechanisms by which secretion and movement are stimulated in lower parts of the gastrointestinal tract; formation of hematinic principle (antianemic factor), effective in prevention of pernicious anemia, by the action of an intrinsic factor (present in gastric juice) on an extrinsic factor (vitamin B$_{12}$) present in foods.

DIET IN SOME DISORDERS: *Atony and hypomotility*: Food is retained longer than normal and decomposition may occur if hydrochloric acid is deficient. Liquids are retained longer than solids. Therefore, diet should consist of quickly and easily digested foods — soft-cooked vegetables, chicken, fish, strained beef, and moderate amount of skim milk. Avoid liquids, pastries, and rich gravies. *Hypermotility*: The stomach empties too rapidly; therefore, diet should be liquid, soft, in small amounts, and in frequent feedings. Fats delay the emptying of the stomach. *Hyperacidity*: Give protein to combine with acid. Frequent small feedings are advisable.

s., bilocular. S., hourglass.

s., cardiac. Fundus of the stomach.

s., cascade. A form of hourglass stomach in which there is a constriction between cardiac and pyloric portions. Cardiac portion fills first, and then contents cascade into pyloric portion.

s., cow horn. A high, transversely placed stomach.

s., foreign bodies in. In the average case foreign bodies pass through the alimentary tract without disturbance. However, these patients should be under a physician's care. Usually symptoms are absent, but the patient may be alarmed. Give nothing by mouth. Under no circumstances should salts, cathartics, and enemas be used, as

STOMACH

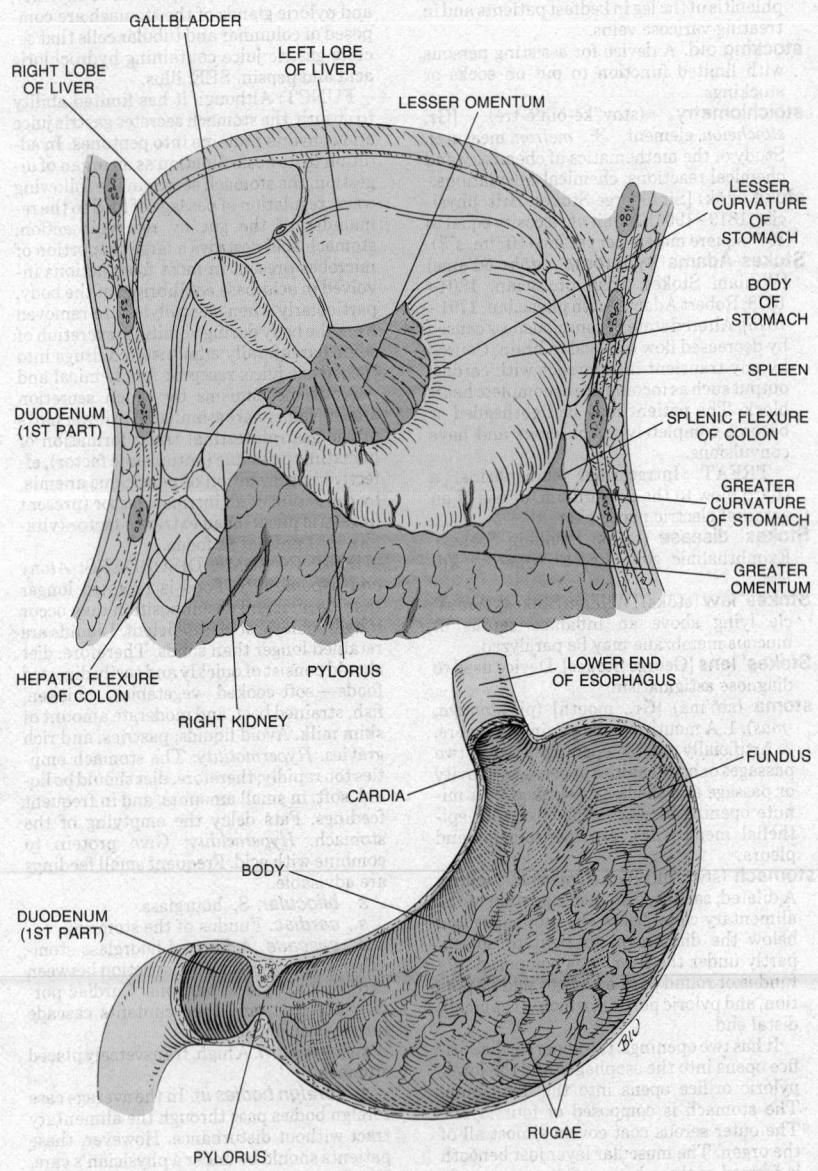

GALLBLADDER

LEFT LOBE
OF LIVER

RIGHT LOBE
OF LIVER

LESSER OMENTUM

LESSER
CURVATURE
OF
STOMACH

BODY
OF
STOMACH

SPLEEN

DUODENUM
(1ST PART)

SPLENIC FLEXURE
OF COLON

GREATER
CURVATURE
OF STOMACH

GREATER
OMENTUM

HEPATIC FLEXURE
OF COLON

PYLORUS

LOWER END
OF ESOPHAGUS

RIGHT KIDNEY

FUNDUS

CARDIA

DUODENUM
(1ST PART)

BODY

PYLORUS

RUGAE

INSIDE VIEW

they can make the condition worse.

s., hourglass. Stomach resembling an hourglass, caused by constriction from a band of fibrous tissue. SYN: *s., bilocular.*

s., leather-bottle. Condition of the stomach caused by hypertrophy of the stomach walls or their infiltration with malignant tissue.

s., thoracic. Condition in which stomach lies above the diaphragm. May result from an embryonic anomaly in which the stomach fails to descend, or from hernia of diaphragm. The latter results in so-called upside-down stomach.

s., water-trap. Stomach with the pylorus situated unusually high, causing slow emptying.

stomach, words pert. to: abdominal cavity; absorption; achylia gastrica; acidity; anachlorhydria; atony; cardialgia; cardiopyloric; cardiospasm; chlorhydria; cholangiogastrostomy; clapotage; digestion; ectasia; feeding, artificial; gastric digestion; gastric juice; gastric lavage; "gastr-" words; gastroesophageal reflux; gavage; hernia, hiatal; hourglass stomach; hunger; lavage; linitis; pylorus; secretagogue; ulcer; ventriculus.

stomach ache. Pain in the stomach. SYN: *gastralgia; gastrodynia.*

stomachal (stŭm′ă-kăl) [Gr. *stomachos*, mouth]. Rel. to the stomach.

stomachalgia [″ + *algos*, pain]. Pain in the stomach.

stomach cancer. May be carcinoma, lymphoma, or sarcoma.

SYM: General symptoms of dyspepsia with following characteristic symptoms: continued pain, often tenderness; vomiting of partially digested food; absence of free hydrochloric acid in gastric juice; hematemesis or blood in stools, slight in amount and blood-altered so it has a coffee-grounds appearance; presence of tumor; loss of weight and strength; extreme anemia; involvement of superficial lymph glands. When the pylorus is involved, symptoms of gastric dilatation will also be present.

TREAT: Early treatment. Surgery; liquid or semiliquid diet.

PROG: Very poor.

stomachic (stō-măk′ĭk) 1. Concerning the stomach. 2. Medicine that stimulates the action of the stomach.

stomach intubation. Passage of a tube into the stomach to obtain gastric contents for examination, for prophylaxis and treatment of ileus, or to remove ingested poisons.

stomachoscopy [″ + *skopein*, to examine]. Examination of the stomach. SYN: *gastroscopy.*

stomach pump. Device for removing contents of the stomach through a tube inserted through the mouth.

stomach tooth. A lower canine tooth during first dentition.

stomach tube. Tube used to wash out or to introduce fluid or liquids into the stomach.

stomal (stō′măl) [Gr. *stoma*, mouth]. Concerning a stoma.

stomata. Pl. of stoma.

stomatal (stō′mă-tăl) [Gr. *stoma*, mouth]. Concerning stomata.

stomatalgia (stō″mă-tăl′jē-ă) [Gr. *stoma*, mouth, + *algos*, pain]. Pain in the mouth. SYN: *stomatodynia.*

stomatic. Pert. to or rel. to the mouth.

stomatitis (stō-mă-tī′tĭs) [″ + *itis*, inflammation]. Inflammation of the mouth. SEE: *gangrene; noma; thrush.*

SYM: Heat, pain, increased flow of saliva, fetor of breath, restlessness, languor, disinclination to nurse in infants, sometimes fever.

ETIOL: Stomatitis may be caused by many factors or conditions. Among them are pathogenic organisms, including bacteria and viruses; mechanical trauma; irritants such as alcohol, tobacco, hot foods, spices; sensitization to chemical substances in toothpastes or mouthwashes; nutritional deficiencies, esp. avitaminoses; blood disorders; poisoning by drugs, esp. heavy metals; certain skin disorders; systemic infections such as measles, scarlet fever, syphilis. There are also several forms with unknown etiology.

s., aphthous. SEE: *aphthous ulcer.*

s., catarrhal. Simple stomatitis.

SYM: General symptoms of stomatitis with diffuse red swelling of mucous membrane.

TREAT: Good hygienic conditions; cleanse mouth with weak solution of boric acid as a wash.

s., corrosive. Stomatitis resulting from intentional or accidental exposure to corrosive substances.

s., diphtheritic. Diphtheria of mucous membranes of the gums or cheeks.

s., follicular. S., aphthous.

s., herpetic. Stomatitis characterized by cold sores (fever blisters).

s., membranous. Stomatitis accompanied by the formation of a false or adventitious membrane.

s., mercurial. A form of stomatitis seen in those who work with mercury; after the administration of very large doses of mercurials; and after small doses in individuals who have a high susceptibility to mercury.

SYM: Early symptoms are tenderness of gums, redness near insertion of teeth, metallic taste, and increase of saliva. Later symptoms include profuse salivation and fetor of breath; redness, swelling, and tenderness of gums. Tongue may be similarly affected and protrude from mouth. In severe cases, ulceration of mucous membrane, loss of teeth, and necrosis of jaw result.

TREAT: If due to acute poisoning, early administration of dimercaprol (British antilewisite) will be helpful. If chronic, remove patient from source of poison and treat symptomatically.

s., mycotic. Fungus infection of the mouth or throat, esp. in infants and young children. Characterized by formation of white patches and ulcers, frequently with fever and gastrointestinal inflammation. SYN: *thrush*.

s. parasitica. Stomatitis caused by a yeastlike fungus, *Candida albicans.* SEE: *thrush.*

SYM: Those of general stomatitis with milk-white elevations on tongue and mouth, which on removal leave a raw surface. Disease may extend to pharynx, esophagus, and larynx. Microscopic examination reveals fungus.

TREAT: Correct hygiene. Treat any gastric disturbance; locally, milk alkaline mouthwash. Diluted gentian violet mouthwash is effective also. Topical application of diluted nystatin solution may be necessary.

PROG: Good.

s., simple. Erythematous inflammation of the mouth occurring in patches on the mucous membranes.

s., traumatic. Stomatitis resulting from mechanical injury as from ill-fitting dentures, sharp jagged teeth, or biting cheek.

s., ulcerative. Thought by some to be an infectious disease, as it often occurs in epidemics and attacks both children and adults when congregated and unable to practice good oral hygiene. SYN: *trench mouth; Vincent's angina.*

SYM: Gums of lower jaw chiefly affected; are swollen, red, and spongy. Linear ulcers soon form and may extend to cheek; gland under jaw swollen. In severe cases, loosening of teeth and necrosis of jaw may follow.

TREAT: Debridement of ulceration, proper dental hygiene, rinsing of mouth with saline or suitable hydrogen peroxide solution. Avoid chemical or physical trauma to mucosa. Force fluids and provide proper nutrition. Systemic antibiotics are usually not required.

PROG: Guardedly favorable.

s., vesicular. S., aphthous.

s., Vincent's. S., ulcerative.

stomato- [Gr. *stoma,* mouth]. Combining form indicating mouth.

stomatodynia (stō″mă-tō-dĭn′ē-ă) [Gr. *stoma,* mouth, + *odyne,* pain]. Pain in the

mouth. SYN: *stomatalgia.*

stomatogastric (stō″mă-tō-găs′trĭk) [″ + *gaster,* belly]. Concerning the stomach and mouth.

stomatognathic (stō″mă-tŏg-năth′ĭk) [″ + *gnathos,* jaw]. Indicating the mouth and jaws together.

stomatologist (stō″mă-tŏl′ō-jĭst) [″ + *logos,* word, reason]. Specialist in treatment of diseases of the mouth.

stomatology (stō″mă-tŏl′ō-jē). Science of the mouth and teeth and their diseases.

stomatomalacia (stō″mă-tō-mă-lā′shē-ă) [″ + *malakia,* softening]. Pathological softening of any structures of the mouth.

stomatomenia (stō″mă-tō-mē′nē-ă) [″ + *meniaia,* menses]. Bleeding from the mouth at the time of menstruation.

stomatomy (stō-măt′ō-mē) [″ + *tome,* incision]. Surgical nicking of the edges of the os uteri to facilitate delivery.

stomatomycosis (stō″mă-tō-mī-kō′sĭs) [″ + *mykes,* fungus, + *osis,* condition]. Any disease of the mouth caused by fungi.

stomatopathy (stō″mă-tŏp′ă-thē) [″ + *pathos,* disease, suffering]. Any mouth disease.

stomatoplasty (stō′mă-tō-plăs″tē) [″ + *plassein,* to form]. Plastic surgery or repair of the mouth.

stomatorrhagia (stō″mă-tō-rā′jē-ă) [″ + *rhegnynai,* to burst forth]. Hemorrhage from the mouth or gums.

stomatoscope (stō-măt′ō-skōp) [″ + *skopein,* to examine]. Instrument for examining the mouth.

stomatosis (stō″mă-tō′sĭs) [″ + *osis,* condition]. Any disease of the mouth.

stomatotomy (stō″mă-tŏt′ō-mē) [″ + *tome,* incision]. Stomatomy, q.v.

stomion (stō′mē-ŏn) [Gr., dim. of *stoma,* mouth]. A landmark used in physical anthropology. It is the central point in the oral fissure when the lips are together.

stomocephalus (stō″mō-sĕf′ă-lŭs) [Gr. *stoma,* mouth, + *kephale,* head]. Deformed fetus with very small head and neck.

stomodeal (stō″mō-dē′ăl). Concerning the stomodeum.

stomodeum (stō″mō-dē′ŭm) [″ + *hodaios,* a way]. An external depression lined with ectoderm and bounded by frontonasal, mandibular, and maxillary processes of the embryo. It forms the anterior portion of the oral cavity. Its floor, the pharyngeal membrane, separates the stomodeum from the foregut.

stone [AS. *stan.*] 1. Hardened mineral matter, as a gallstone or a kidney stone. SYN: *calculus.* 2. In Britain, a unit of weight, 14 pounds avoirdupois.

s., dental. A hemihydrate of gypsum divided into four classes according to the qualities resulting from differing methods of preparation. It is used in dentistry in the preparation of models and study casts.

s., gray. A synthetic stone composed of carborundum and rubber used to polish dental restorations.

s., pulp. A calcified structure present in the pulp chamber of a tooth. SYN: *denticle.*

s., red. An abrasive stone with garnet as its main component for polishing dental restorations.

s., salivary. A calcified stone present in the ducts of salivary glands. Also called sialolith.

stool (stool) [AS. *stol*, a seat]. 1. Evacuation of the bowels. 2. Waste matter discharged from the bowels. SYN: *feces.*

COLOR: Iron and bismuth turn the stool black, and certain vegetables and berries darken it or produce a distinct color. Pathological stools are usually grayish or a whitish glistening color; and tarry in hemorrhage or show fresh blood.

CHARACTER: *Fatty stools:* These are observed in obstructive jaundice, cancer of the pancreas, pancreatic calculi, and in indigestion or overfeeding in infants.

Frothy, poorly formed stools: They may indicate a spastic colon, the presence of gas, or intestinal inflammation.

Lienteric stools: These contain much undigested food and are noted in inflammatory conditions of the stomach and upper bowel.

Tarry stools: They may indicate gastric hemorrhage, swallowed blood from the nose or lungs, bleeding ulcers of the gastrointestinal tract, hepatic cirrhosis, or cancer. If intestinal transport time is rapid, blood entering the upper gastrointestinal tract may not appear as tarry in the stool but may be bright red.

Membranous shreds: They may exist in cancer of the colon, dysentery, relapsing fever, acute proctitis, and in sloughing of intestinal mucosa.

Mucous stools: Exist in catarrhal or inflamed conditions of the intestines or rectum, in dysentery, enterocolitis, proctitis, impaction, and ulcerative colitis.

SHAPE: *Cylindrical:* If of small caliber, they may be indicative of prolapsus ani, annular rectal stricture, or intestinal spasms.

Ribbon-shaped: Indicative of stricture or cancer of the rectum; possibly enlargement of the prostate in males, hemorrhoids, spasm of the lower bowel and anus, prostatic abscess, and prolapse of the uterus.

Scybala: Rounded masses or balls of fecal matter or hardened feces, the result of habitual constipation, atony or sacculation (diverticulum) of the colon, gastric ulcer, di-

lation, rectal cancer, or dysentery.

s., bilious. Yellow or yellow-brown discharges in diarrhea becoming darker on exposure.

s., fatty. Fat in the feces, as in pancreatic disease.

s., lienteric. Stool containing undigested food.

s., pea soup. Liquid stools characteristic of typhoid.

s., rice water. Watery serum stools with detached epithelium, as in cholera.

stool softeners. Substances that act as wetting agents and thus promote soft malleable bowel movements. They are not laxatives and therefore are not indicated for constipation caused by decreased or absent peristaltic activity. Docusate sodium or docusate calcium may be used to soften stools.

stopcock (stŏp′kŏk). A valve, usually made of glass if used in chemistry, that regulates the flow of fluid from a container.

stop needle. A needle with an eye at the tip and a disk on the shaft to prevent penetration deeper than desired.

stoppage (stŏp′ăj) [AS. *stoppian*]. Obstruction of an organ. SEE: *cholestasia.*

storax (stō′răks). USP. A balsam obtained from the scarred trunk of *Liquidambar orientalis.* It has been used as an expectorant. It is a component of tincture of benzoin.

storm [AS.]. A sudden outburst or exacerbation of symptoms of a disease.

s., renal. A sudden attack of renal symptoms accompanying a neurosis sometimes occurring in patients suffering from aortic regurgitation.

s., thyroid. A complication of thyrotoxicosis that, if untreated, is almost always fatal. Consists of abrupt onset of fever, sweating, tachycardia, pulmonary edema or congestive heart failure, tremulousness, and restlessness. Occurs in patients with untreated or poorly treated thyrotoxicosis. Usually precipitated by infection, trauma, or a surgical emergency.

stout (stowt) [O. Fr. *estout*, bold]. 1. Having a bulky body. SYN: *corpulent.* 2. Strong, dark beer.

Stoxil. Trade name for idoxuridine.

STP. *standard temperature and pressure.*

STPD. *standard temperature and pressure, dry.* Gas volume at 0°C 760 mm of mercury total pressure and partial pressure of water of zero, i.e., dry.

Str. *Streptococcus.*

strabismal (stră-bĭz′măl) [Gr. *strabismos,* a squinting]. Strabismic, q.v.

strabismic (stră-bĭz′mĭk) [Gr. *strabismos,* a squinting]. Pert. to or afflicted with strabismus.

strabismometer (stră-bĭz-mŏm′ĕt-ĕr) ["

+ *metron,* a measure]. Instrument for determining amount of strabismus.

strabismus (strǎ-bǐz′mǔs) [Gr. *strabismos,* a squinting]. Disorder of eye in which optic axes cannot be directed to same object. The squinting eye always deviates to the same extent when the eyes are carried in different directions: *unilateral* when same eye always deviates; *alternating* when either deviates, the other being fixed; *constant* when the squint remains permanent; *periodic* when eyes are occasionally free from it. Strabismus can result from reduced visual acuity, unequal ocular muscle tone, or an oculomotor nerve lesion. SYN: *heterotropia; squint.* SEE: *microstrabismus.*

   s., accommodative. Strabismus due to disorder of ocular accommodation. SYN: *s., bilateral.*

   s., alternating. Strabismus affecting either eye alternately.

   s., bilateral. S., accommodative.

   s., concomitant. Strabismus in which both eyes move freely but retain unnatural relationship to each other.

   s., convergent. Strabismus in which the deviating eye turns inward.

   s. deorsum vergens. Vertical strabismus, the deviating eye turning downward. SYN: *hypotropia.*

   s., divergent. Strabismus in which the deviating eye turns outward.

   s., horizontal. Strabismus in which the deviation of the visual axis is in the horizontal plane.

   s., intermittent. Strabismus recurring at intervals.

   s., monocular. Strabismus in which the same eye habitually deviates.

   s., monolateral. Strabismus with the squinting eye always the same.

   s., nonconcomitant. Strabismus of an eye that varies in degree with the change in direction in which the eye moves.

   s., paralytic. Strabismus that is due to paralysis of a muscle. The deviation is present only in the sphere of action of the paralyzed muscle. In paralytic squint, the secondary deviation is greater than the primary. This condition is due to paralysis of one or more ocular muscles and may point to grave cerebral disease or to some constitutional disease. This form of strabismus is recognized by the fact that if a light or the finger of the examiner is carried from right to left before the face of the patient, the deviating eye fails to follow to its proper limit. This response leads the physician to look for lesions of the 6th nerve in failure of external rectus, of the 3rd nerve in failure of internal rectus of either side, and of the 4th nerve in impairment of superior oblique muscles. In

adults this usually is caused by syphilis involving the nerve centers or trunks.

   TREAT: Directed to the cause. Eyeglasses or contact lenses; miotics; corrective surgery.

   PROG: In general, guarded.

   s., spastic. Strabismus due to contraction of an ocular muscle.

   s. sursum vergens. Vertical upward squint. SYN: *hypertropia.*

   ETIOL: Defects of fusion faculty, errors of refraction, poor vision in one eye, anisometropia.

   TREAT: Refraction with prescribing of correcting lenses, orthoptic training (training of fusion), operative.

   s., vertical. Strabismus in which the eye turns upward. The vision is double (diplopia) unless there is unconscious suppression of the image in the squinting eye. Expression of face is bizarre. Vertical strabismus usually is the result of ametropia in childhood, or of central nervous system disease in adult life.

strabometer (strǎ-bŏm′ět-ěr) [Gr. *strabos,* squinting, + *metron,* a measure]. Instrument to ascertain the degree of strabismus.

strabotome (strǎ′bō-tōm) [″ + *tome,* incision]. A knife for performing strabotomy.

strabotomy (strǎ-bŏt′ō-mē) [″ + *tome,* incision]. Operation for strabismus.

strain (strān). 1. [AS. *streon,* offspring] A stock, said of bacteria or protozoa from a specific source and maintained in successive cultures or animal inoculation. 2. Hereditary streak or tendency. 3. [O. Fr. *estreindre,* to draw tight] To pass through, as a filter. 4. To injure by making too strong an effort or by excessive use. 5. Excessive use of a part of the body so that it is injured. 6. Trauma to the muscle or the musculotendinous unit from violent contraction or excessive forcible stretch. May be associated with failure of synergistic action of muscles. SEE: *sprain.* 7. To make a great effort as in straining to have a bowel movement. This is done by means of the Valsalva maneuver, which increases intra-abdominal pressure and helps to expel feces. 8. Force applied per unit area. Tension, compression or shear stress placed on tissue leads to distortion of the structure and release of energy.

strainer (strān′ěr). Device used for retaining solid pieces while liquid passes through. SYN: *filter.*

strain x-ray. Radiographic picture taken with the subject, usually a bone or joint, under static force or tension. Used to better demonstrate the pathological change, which might be inapparent if this technique were not employed.

strait (strāt) [O. Fr. *estreit,* narrow]. A constricted or narrow passage.

s., inferior. The lower outlet of the pelvic canal.

s.'s of pelvis. The inferior and superior openings of the true pelvis.

s., superior. The upper opening or inlet of the pelvic canal.

straitjacket. Shirt with long sleeves laced on patient and fastened to restrain the arms. SYN: *camisole.*

stramonium (stră-mō'nē-ŭm) [L.]. Jamestown weed, jimsonweed. The dried leaves of *Datura stramonium.*

USES: An ingredient in asthma powder used for its antispasmodic effect.

stramonium poisoning. Caused in children by accidental ingestion of medicine or by self-administered overdose. SEE: *atropine sulfate poisoning.*

SYM: Similar to those of atropine overdose.

strand. A single thread or fiber.

strangalesthesia (străng″găl-ĕs-thē'zē-ă) [L. *strangulare,* halter, + *aisthesis,* sensation]. A girdlelike sensation of constriction. SYN: *zonesthesia.*

strangle (străng'gl) [L. *strangulare,* halter]. To choke or suffocate or be choked from compression of the trachea.

strangulated (străng'gū-lā″tĕd). Constricted so that air or blood supply is cut off, as a strangulated hernia.

strangulation (străng″gū-lā'shŭn) [L. *strangulare,* halter]. Compression or constriction of a part, as the bowel or throat, causing suspension of breathing or of passage of contents; congestion accompanies condition.

s., internal. Slipping of a coil of the intestine through the diaphragm or an abnormal opening.

strangury (străng'gū-rē) [Gr. *stranx,* drop, squeezed out, + *ouron,* urine]. Painful and interrupted urination in drops produced by spasmodic muscular contraction of urethra and bladder.

strap (străp) [Gr. *strophos,* a cord]. 1. A band, as one of adhesive plaster, used to hold dressings in place or to approximate surfaces of a wound. 2. To bind with strips of adhesive plaster.

s., Montgomery. SEE: *Montgomery straps.*

strapping (străp'ĭng). 1. Adhesive plaster or other substance used to bind surfaces together or hold dressings in place. 2. Application of adhesive plaster strips on a part to give it support or compress it.

stratification (străt″ĭ-fĭ-kā'shŭn) [L. *stratificare,* to arrange in layers]. Act or process of arranging in layers.

stratified (străt'ĭ-fīd) [L. *stratificare,* to arrange in layers]. Arranged in the form of layers.

stratified epithelium. Epithelium in superimposed layers with differently shaped cells in the various layers.

stratiform (străt'ĭ-form) [L. *stratum,* layer, + *forma,* shape]. Arranged in layers, as manner of liquefaction of gelatin stab culture, in which there is liquefaction to the walls of the tube at the top and then downward horizontally.

stratum (strā'tŭm, străt'ŭm) [L.] (pl. *strata*). A layer.

s. basale. Innermost or deepest layer of the endometrium of the uterus. Also refers to the innermost layer of the epidermis and other stratified squamous epithelium. SYN: *malpighian layer; stratum germinativum.*

s. compactum. Superficial or outermost layer of the endometrium.

s. corneum. Outermost horny layer of the epidermis.

s. disjunction. Outermost layer of the stratum corneum, which is being shed constantly.

s. germinativum. Innermost layer of epidermis. A row of columnar cells that divide to replace the rest of the epidermis as it wears away. SYN: *s. malpighii.* SEE: *s. basale.*

s. granulosum. Layer of cells containing deeply staining granules of keratohyalin found in the epidermis of skin lying between stratum germinativum and stratum lucidum.

s. lucidum. Translucent layer of the epidermis lying between stratum corneum and stratum granulosum. It is frequently absent.

s. malpighii. The inner layer of epidermis. First seen with low magnification and described in the 1600s by Marcello Malpighi. It includes both stratum germinativum and stratum spinosum of today's nomenclature.

s. mucosum. S. malpighii.

s. papillare. Papillary layer of the corium lying adjacent to the epidermis.

s. reticulare. Recticular layer of the corium lying just beneath the papillary layer.

s. spinosum. Prickle cell layer, so called because of prominent intercellular attachments. Part of the stratum malpighii.

s. spongiosum. Middle layer of decidua of the endometrium.

s. submucosum. Layer of smooth muscle fibers of the myometrium lying contiguous with the endometrium.

s. subserosum. Layer of smooth muscle fibers of myometrium that lies immediately under the serous coat.

s. supravasculare. Layer of circular and longitudinal muscle fibers lying between stratum subserosum and stratum vasculare of the endometrium.

s. vasculare. Layer of smooth muscles in myometrium lying between stratum submucosum and stratum supravasculare of the endometrium.

strawberry mark. A soft, modular, vascular nevus usually present on face or neck, occurring at birth or shortly afterward. SEE: *nevus flammeus.*

strawberry tongue. The peculiar red, papillated tongue characteristic of scarlatina, q.v. SEE: *tongue.*

straw itch. A skin condition accompanied by itching due to working in straw or sleeping on a straw mattress. The straw contains a mite that causes the pruritic eruption. It is self-limiting.

streak (strēk) [AS. *strica*]. A line or stripe. SYN: *stria.*

s., angioid. A dark streak seen in the retinae of individuals with pseudoxanthoma elasticum and sickle cell anemia.

s., medullary. Deep longitudinal groove on dorsal surface of the embryo that becomes the medullary tube.

s., meningitic. A red line across the skin formed by drawing a pointed article across it; seen in meningitis and nerve center affections. SYN: *tache cérébrale.*

s., Moore's lightning. Subjective visual sensation of lightninglike flashes at time of eye movements. These are especially noticeable in dim or absent light. They are usually vertical and on the lateral part of the visual field. The flashes are accompanied by or followed by dark spots before the eyes. This condition is not related to significant eye disease.

s., primitive. SEE: *primitive streak.*

stream (strēm). A steady flow of a liquid.

strength. The quality of being strong or powerful as it relates to muscular activity; concentration of a solution or substance; intensity of light, color, or sound; ability to resist deformation, fracture, or abrasion. In research related to dental materials, several methods of testing strength are utilized.

s., breaking. The point at which applied force breaks a material. SYN: *tensile strength.*

s., compression. The point at which material loses shape when force is applied. SYN: *crushing strength.*

s., ego. SEE: *ego strength.*

s., impact. The force required to fracture a material.

s., shear. The resistance of a material to shear force.

strephosymbolia (strĕf″ō-sĭm-bō′lē-ă) [Gr. *strephein*, to twist, + *symbolon*, symbol]. 1. Difficulty in distinguishing between letters that are similar but face in opposite directions. Ex.: p-q, b-d. 2. Perception of objects reversed as in a mirror.

strepitus (strĕp′ĭ-tŭs) [L.]. A sound or noise, as that heard on auscultation.

Streptase. Trade name for streptokinase.

strepticemia (strĕp″ĭ-sē′mē-ă) [Gr. *streptos*, twisted, + *haima*, blood]. Streptococci present in the blood causing infection. SYN: *streptococcemia.*

strepto- [Gr. *streptos*, twisted]. Combining form meaning twisted.

streptoangina (strĕp″tō-ăn′jĭ-nă) [″ + L. *angina*, quinsy]. Sore throat with membranous formation due to streptococci.

streptobacillus moniliformis. A gram-negative bacillus present in the mouths of rats, mice, and cats. It is transmitted to humans through bites or by ingestion of milk contaminated by rats. It causes one form of ratbite fever, characterized by prolonged fever, skin rash, and generalized arthritis. SYN: *Haverhill fever.* SEE: *Spirillum minus.*

TREAT: Penicillin.

streptococcal (strĕp″tō-kŏk′ăl) [″ + *kokkos*, berry]. Caused by or pert. to streptococci.

streptococcemia (strĕp″tō-kŏk-sē′mē-ă) [″ + ″ + *haima*, blood]. Presence of streptococci in the blood causing infection. SYN: *strepticemia.*

streptococci (strĕp″tō-kŏk′sī). Pl. of streptococcus. SEE: *Streptococcus.*

streptococcic (strĕp″tō-kŏk′sĭk) [″ + *kokkos*, berry]. Resembling, produced by, or pert. to streptococci.

streptococcicosis (strĕp″tō-kŏk″sĭ-kō′sĭs) [″ + ″ + *osis*, condition]. Any streptococcal infection.

streptococcolysin (strĕp″tō-kŏk-kŏl′ĭ-sĭn) [″ + ″ + *lysis*, dissolution]. A lysin produced by streptococci.

Streptococcus (strĕp″tō-kŏk′ŭs) [″ + *kokkos*, berry]. ABBR: Str. A genus of bacteria belonging to the family Lactobacillaceae, tribe Streptococceae. They are grampositive cocci occurring in chains. Most species are harmless saprophytes, but some are among the most common and dangerous pathogens of humans. They are differentiated on the basis of their reactions on blood-agar plates into three types: alpha (α), beta (β), and gamma (γ). Those of the alpha type form a greenish coloration about colonies and partially hemolyze blood; those of the beta or hemolytic type form clear zones about colonies and completely hemolyze blood; those of the gamma type are non-hemolytic and produce a grayish coloration about colonies.

Streptococci were also classified into a number of immunologic groups designated by the letters A through H, and K through O.

Most human infections are caused by groups A, B, D, F, G, H, K, and O. More than 55 types of group A beta-hemolytic streptococci have been identified. SEE: *rheumatic fever; scarlet fever.*

Str. bovis. A species found in the alimentary tract of cattle. It may cause endocarditis in humans.

Str. equisimilis. An organism that has been isolated from the upper respiratory tract. May be associated with erysipelas, puerperal sepsis, pneumonia, osteomyelitis, bacteremia, and endocarditis.

Str. faecalis. A group D enterococcus that may or may not be hemolytic. It may be part of the normal flora of the intestinal tract, and it may be pathogenic.

Str. mutans. A species of streptococci that has been implicated in dental caries and endocarditis.

Str. pneumoniae. A species of bacteria, oval or spherical in shape, gram-positive, and nonmotile. It possesses a capsule. The species is made up of a number of distinct strains of which more than 84 serological types have been isolated. It is the causative agent of certain types of pneumonia, esp. lobar pneumonia, and is associated with other infectious diseases such as meningitis, conjunctivitis, endocarditis, peridontitis, septic arthritis, osteomyelitis, otitis media, septicemia, and, rarely, urinary tract infections.

Str. pyogenes. Any of the group A beta-hemolytic streptococci causing suppurative processes. The causative agent of scarlet fever, erysipelas, septic sore throat, puerperal sepsis, and various pyogenic infections.

Str. viridans. This is not the name of a particular species. A group of α-hemolytic streptococci that are normally present in the upper respiratory tract. Minor trauma such as vigorous chewing may result in their being admitted to the bloodstream. Thus when heart valves are damaged, these organisms are the ones that most frequently colonize on them. When this occurs, subacute bacterial endocarditis has an excellent chance of developing.

Streptococcus mitis and *salivarius* are members of the viridans group. These may be normal inhabitants of the respiratory tract or be pathogenic.

streptococcus (strĕp″tō-kŏk′ŭs) (pl. *streptococci*). An organism of the genus *Streptococcus.* SEE: *bacteria* for illus.

s., β-hemolytic. Streptococci that, when grown on blood-agar, produce hemolysis around each colony. The hemolysis is complete, and a clear zone is present at the site. Group A β-hemolytic streptococci are the type pathogenic for humans.

s., group B. Beta-hemolytic streptococci that are important in causing invasive infections in infants and pregnancy-related morbidity in women. In women, this is characterized by urinary tract infection, chorioamnionitis, postpartum endometritis, bacteremia, and wound infections complicating cesarean section. A vaccine for type III strains of group B streptococci is being investigated.

streptocolysin (strĕp″tō-kŏl′ĭ-sĭn) [″ + *lysis,* dissolution]. A hemolysin produced by streptococci. SYN: *streptococcolysin; streptolysin.*

streptodermatitis (strĕp″tō-dĕr″mă-tī′tĭs) [″ + *derma,* skin, + *itis,* inflammation]. Inflammation of the skin caused by streptococci.

streptodornase (strĕp″tō-dor′nās). One of the enzymes (streptokinase is another) produced by certain strains of hemolytic streptococci. It is capable of liquefying fibrinous and purulent exudates. SEE: *streptokinase.*

streptokinase (strĕp″tō-kĭ′nās). Enzyme produced by certain strains of streptococci that is capable of converting plasminogen to plasmin. SEE: *reperfusion* (def. 1); *streptodornase.*

streptokinase-streptodornase. A mixture of these two enzymes. They are produced by hemolytic streptococci, and are used topically and in body cavities to remove clotted blood and purulent material.

streptoleukocidin (strĕp″tō-lū″kō-sī′dĭn) [″ + *leukos,* white, + L. *caedere,* to kill]. A toxin produced by streptococci, destructive to leukocytes.

streptolysin (strĕp-tŏl′ĭ-sĭn). A hemolysin produced by streptococci. SYN: *streptococolysin; streptocolysin.*

s. O. Streptolysin that is inactivated by oxygen.

s. S. Streptolysin that is inactivated by heat or acid, but not by oxygen.

streptomycin sulfate (sterile) (strĕp″tō-mī′sĭn). USP. An antibiotic derived from a soil microbe, *Streptomyces griseus.* Trade name is Isoject-Streptomycin.

streptomycosis (strĕp″tō-mī-kō′sĭs) [″ + *mykes,* fungus, + *osis,* condition]. Infection caused by microorganisms of the genus *Streptomyces.*

streptosepticemia (strĕp″tō-sĕp″tĭ-sē′mē-ă) [″ + *septikos,* putrid, + *haima,* blood]. Septicemia resulting from streptococcus infection. SYN: *streptococcemia; streptomycosis.*

streptothricin (strĕp″tō-thrī′sĭn). An antibiotic biosynthesized by *Streptomyces lavendulae.* It is effective against both gram-negative and gram-positive bacteria and some fungi. Because of its toxicity, it is of limited usefulness.

streptothricosis (strĕp"tō-thrī-kō'sĭs) [Gr. *streptos,* twisted, + *thrix,* hair, + *osis,* condition]. Infection caused by a species of *Streptothrix.* Produces a chronic suppurative inflammation. SEE: *actinomycosis.*

stress (strĕs) [O. Fr. *estresse,* narrowness]. In medicine, the result produced when a structure, system, or organism is acted upon by forces that disrupt equilibrium or produce strain. In health care, the term denotes the physical (gravity, mechanical force, pathogen, injury) and psychological (fear, anxiety, crisis, joy) forces that are experienced by individuals. It is generally believed that biological organisms require a certain amount of stress in order to maintain their well-being. However, when stress occurs in quantities that the system cannot handle, it produces pathological changes. This biological concept of stress was developed by the late Hans Selye, who intended originally for stress to indicate cause rather than effect. But through a linguistic error, he gave the term *stress* to effect and later had to use the word *stressor* for the cause.

The amount of stress humans can withstand without having a pathological reaction to it varies from individual to individual and from situation to situation. From data obtained in World War II, it was determined that individuals exposed to the stress of combat would become nonfunctional at different levels of degree of stress experienced, but there were degrees of intensity and duration of stress that none of the soldiers could experience and remain functional.

In physical sciences, stress may be equated to certain types of forces (for example: impact, shear, torsion, compression, and tension) that result in deformation or fracture of the material being stressed or tested. In dentistry, the pressure of the upper teeth on the lower teeth in mastication produces stress. Mechanical forces of tension, compression, shear, or torsion may all be applied to teeth or dental prostheses during the movements of mastication and represent stress. SEE: *general adaptation syndrome.*

stress-breaker. Device incorporated into a removable denture. It is designed to relieve abutting teeth from excessive stress during chewing.

stress fracture. A fine hairline fracture that appears without evidence of soft tissue injury. This type of fracture is difficult to diagnose by roentgenographic examination and may not become visible until 3 to 4 weeks after the onset of symptoms. It occurs from repetitive microtraumas, as with run-

ning, aerobic dancing or marching, with improper shoes, on hard surfaces, or inadequate healing time after stress.

stressor. An agent or condition capable of producing stress.

    s., systemic. Stress that produces generalized systemic responses.

    s., topical. Stress that causes mild inflammation or local damage.

stress radiography. Strain x-ray, q.v. Stress is placed on the involved region while the radiograph is being taken to determine if a partial tear or rupture of the ligaments has occurred. Greater than normal gaping of the joint surfaces indicates a tear.

stress test. Method of evaluating cardiovascular fitness. While exercising, usually on a treadmill or a bicycle ergometer, the individual is subjected to steadily increasing levels of work. At the same time, the amount of oxygen consumed is being determined, and an electrocardiogram is being monitored. If certain abnormalities are noted in the ECG, the test is terminated.

stress ulcer. Peptic ulcer caused by acute or chronic stress such as cerebral trauma, burns, surgery, or acute infection.

stretch (strĕch) [AS. *streccan,* extend]. To draw out or extend to full length.

    s., static. A sustained, long-duration lengthening of soft tissue such as muscle or tendon applied to increase range of motion. The stretch force is usually applied at a low intensity and continuously for as little as 12-15 seconds or as long as several minutes.

stretcher (strĕch'er). A litter for carrying the sick, injured, or dead.

    s., basket (Stokes). Stretcher made of metal or strong synthetic material in which a patient is placed for removal from accident site. The stretcher may also be lifted by ropes.

    s., pole. Also known as the Army type, composed of folding cloth or canvas supported by poles.

    s., spineboard. Wooden board used to secure patients with spinal trauma to prevent movement.

    s., split-frame (scoop). Metal stretcher that can be split down the middle, slid under a patient, and reconnected.

stretching of contractures. Process performed to loosen contracted ligaments, muscles, and adhesions in stiff joints. There should be a slow, steady, and gradually increasing pull by the operator or with gradually increasing weights.

stretch marks. Striae, q.v.

stretch receptor. A proprioceptor located in a muscle or tendon that is stimulated by a stretch or pull.

stretch reflex. The contraction of a muscle as

a result of a pull exerted upon the tendon of the responding muscle. Stretch reflexes are of primary importance in maintenance of posture. SYN: *myotactic reflex.*

stria (strī′ă) [L., a channel] (pl. *striae*). [NA] A line or band elevated above or depressed below surrounding tissue, or differing in color and texture. SYN: *streak.*

striae acusticae. Horizontal white stripes on floor of the 4th ventricle of the brain. SYN: *striae medullares.*

s. atrophica. A fine pinkish-white or gray line, usually 14 cm long, seen in parts of body where skin has been stretched. Commonly seen on thighs, abdomen, and breasts of women who are or have been pregnant; in persons whose skin has been stretched by obesity, tumor, or edema; or in persons who have taken adrenocortical hormones for a prolonged period. SYN: *striae distensae; stria gravidarum.*

striae cerebellares. S. acusticae.

striae distensae. S. atrophica.

s. gravidarum. S. atrophica.

s. longitudinalis lateralis. One of the longitudinal bands of gray matter, slightly elevated on upper part of the corpus callosum.

striae medullares. S. acusticae.

striae of Retzius. The incremental lines seen periodically in calcified enamel of teeth. These are benign.

s. terminalis. A band of fibers in roof of inferior horn running to floor of body of the lateral ventricle.

striatal (strī-ā′tăl) [L. *striatus*, striped]. Concerning the corpus striatum.

striate, striated (strī′āt, strī′ā-tĕd) [L. *striatus*]. Striped; marked by streaks or striae.

striated arteries. Branches of the middle cerebral artery that supply basal nuclei of brain.

striated body. Mass of gray and white bands in each cerebral hemisphere. SYN: *corpus striatum.*

striated muscle. Skeletal muscle, consisting of fibers marked by cross striations. SEE: *muscle.*

striated veins, inferior. Branches of basal vein that drain corpus striatum.

striation (strī-ā′shŭn) [L. *striatus*, striped]. 1. State of being striped or streaked. 2. One of a series of streaks. SYN: *stria.*

striatum (strī-ā′tŭm) [L., grooved]. The caudate and lentiform nuclei of the brain considered as one. SYN: *corpus striatum.*

stricture (strĭk′chŭr) [LL. *strictura*, contraction]. A narrowing or constriction of the lumen of a tube, duct, or hollow organ such as the esophagus, ureter, or urethra. Strictures may be congenital or acquired. Acquired strictures may result from infection,

trauma, fibrosis resulting from mechanical or chemical irritation, muscular spasm, or pressure from adjacent structures or tumors. They may be temporary or permanent, depending on cause.

s., annular. Ringlike obstruction of an organ involving entire circumference of structure.

s., anorectal. Fibrotic narrowing of the anorectal canal.

s., bridle. Stricture caused by a band of membrane stretched across a tube, partially occluding it.

s., cicatricial. Stricture resulting from a scar or wound.

s., functional. Stricture due to muscular spasm. SYN: *s., spasmodic.*

s., impermeable. Stricture closing the lumen of a tube or canal so that an instrument cannot pass through it.

s., irritable. Stricture causing pain when an instrument is passed.

s. of urethra. Partial or complete narrowing of the urethra. Occurs most commonly in men.

SYM: Straining to pass urine, esp. at commencement of urination.

ETIOL: Spasm of urethral muscle, congestion of urethra, and fibrous formation.

s., spasmodic. S., functional.

stricturotome (strĭk′chŭr-ō-tōm) [L. *strictura*, contraction, + Gr. *tome*, incision]. Instrument for cutting strictures.

stricturotomy (strĭk″chŭr-ŏt′ō-mē). Operation of cutting strictures of the urethra.

stride length. The length of the stride. It is useful to measure the right and left leg stride lengths in attempting to determine a neuromuscular disease that affects only one leg.

strident (strī′dĕnt). Stridulous, q.v.

stridor (strī′dor) [L., a harsh sound]. Harsh sound during respiration, high pitched and resembling the blowing of wind, due to obstruction of air passages.

s., congenital laryngeal. Stridor present at birth or during first three weeks.

s. dentium. Noise from grinding of the teeth.

s. serraticus. Sound of respiration like that of sawing, produced by patient's tracheostomy tube.

stridulous (strĭd′ū-lŭs) [L. *stridulus*]. Making a shrill, grating sound.

string-of-pearls deformity. Fusiform enlargement of proximal and middle phalanges seen in rickets.

string sign. A greatly narrowed terminal ileum seen in roentgenological examination of abdomen in regional enteritis.

striocerebellar (strī″ō-sĕr′ĕ-bĕl′ăr) [L. *striatus*, striped, + *cerebellum*, little brain]. Concerning or affecting the corpus striatum and the cerebellum.

strip (strip) [AS. *striepan*, to plunder]. To remove all contents from, esp. by gentle pressure, as to strip the seminal vesicles.

stripper. Surgical instrument used to remove a vein.

strobila (strō-bī'lă) [Gr. *strobilos*, anything twisted up]. The adult form of a tapeworm.

strobiloid (strō'bĭ-loyd) [" + *eidos*, form]. Resembling a twisted chain. Tapeworm segments have this appearance.

stroboscope (strō'bō-skōp) [Gr. *strobos*, whirl, + *skopein*, to examine]. Device that produces an interrupted light. The light is shown on moving or vibrating objects. This makes the object appear to be stationary. A photograph taken at the precise time the light is flashed on the object will not be blurred.

stroke (strōk) [ME.]. 1. A sharp blow. 2. To rub gently in one direction, as in massage. 3. Gentle movement of the hand across a surface. 4. In dentistry, a complete simple movement that is often repeated with modifications of position, strength, or speed, perhaps as a part of a continuing activity; for example, the closing stroke in mastication when the jaw closes and the teeth come together. In scaling or planing the roots of teeth, the scaling instrument is introduced carefully into the subgingival area in what is called an exploratory stroke, perhaps followed by a power stroke designed to break or dislodge encrusted calculus. This is followed by a shaving stroke, intended to smooth or plane the root surface.

5. Sudden loss of consciousness followed by paralysis caused by one of several different mechanisms including hemorrhage into brain; formation of an embolus or thrombus that occludes an artery; or rupture of an extracerebral artery causing subarachnoid hemorrhage.

Stroke is one of the leading causes of death and disability among adults in the U.S. An estimated 150,000 persons die each year, and several hundred thousand are disabled. SYN: *apoplexy; cerebrovascular accident; a "shock."* SEE: *excitotoxin; transient ischemic attack.*

SYM: Onset acute. Unconsciousness. Stertorous breathing due to paralysis of portion of the soft palate; expiration puffs out the cheeks and mouth. Pupils sometimes unequal, the larger one being on the side of the hemorrhage. Paralysis usually involves one side of the face, arm and leg of one side, with eyeballs turned away from the side of the body paralysis; skin covered with clammy sweat, the surface temperature of which is often subnormal; speech disturbances. Onset more gradual if caused by a thrombosis, q.v.

F.A.: Keep patient quiet and sitting up or lying down with head and shoulders elevated. Do not give stimulants. Apply cooling applications to head and neck. Do not transport unless absolutely imperative, and then very carefully.

PROG: Depends upon symptoms. Often grave. The prognosis is directly related to the degree and length of time blood flow to the affected area of the brain is deficient or completely blocked. A regional cerebral blood flow of at least 15 to 18 mL/100 grams of brain tissue is necessary to maintain electrical activity in that part of the brain, but certain functions may remain viable until the flow rate falls to below 10 mL/100 grams of tissue. From animal studies, recovery of neuronal tissue is unlikely if occlusion continues longer than 4 to 6 hours. A treatment time beginning within 2 hours of the stroke is probably necessary to avoid or mitigate alterations in function. Thus, the immediate initiation of therapeutic measures is of the utmost importance if the extent of damaged cerebral tissue is to be kept to a minimum. SEE: *risk factors.*

NURSING IMPLICATIONS: Maintain a patent airway, assessing and promoting adequate ventilation and oxygenation. Suction pharynx or trachea gently, as necessary to remove obstructing secretions. Position patient in lateral or semiprone position, but with head elevated 15 to 30 degrees to decrease cerebral venous pressure. Monitor neurologic status (Glasgow coma scale, vital signs, pupillary responses, respiratory patterns, and sensory and motor responses to verbal, touch or painful stimulation), and document findings on a neurologic flow sheet, evaluating for deterioration or improvement. Obtain history of incident, time-frame, related past medical history (hypertension, use of anticoagulant drugs, cardiac dysrhythmias) and associated injuries. Prepare patient for prescribed diagnostic studies, including computed tomography, nuclear magnetic resonance imaging, x-rays of skull, cervical spine, and soft tissues of neck, arteriography, and lumbar puncture.

Orient patient frequently, and reassure with frequent verbal and tactile contacts. Assess aphasia type, if present, and support appropriately. Maintain normal body temperature, avoiding environmental heat or cold excesses. Assess bladder function, encouraging voiding with non-invasive measures in the presence of urinary retention, and attempting to discover voiding pattern; keep patient clean and dry in the presence of incontinence. Avoid use of indwelling catheters, as these promote urinary tract infections. Assess bowel function, and utilize dietary intervention, stool softeners, or laxatives as necessary to prevent constipation. Avoid straining at stool or use of enemas. Monitor and maintain fluid and electrolyte balance (intake, output, daily weight, laboratory values). Provide adequate enteral or parenteral nutrition, as appropriate. Initiate nursing measures to prevent complications of immobility: repositioning at least every 2 hours, maintaining correct body alignment, supporting joints to prevent flexion and rotation contractures, and providing range-of-motion exercises (passive to involved joints, active-assisted or active to uninvolved joints, as possible and appropriate). Prevent oral mucous membranes and eyes (cornea) from drying, using irrigation and lubrication. Administer prescribed therapy to decrease cerebral edema, and antihypertensives or anticoagulants as appropriate for etiology. Observe for seizure activity, and initiate drug therapy and safety precautions.

Begin rehabilitation after the acute phase has subsided. Collaborate with speech, physical and occupational therapists to develop with the patient and family a comprehensive care plan based on realistic goals. Provide positive reinforcement for all patient efforts. Make communication with patient and by patient a priority. Continue to prevent deformities through exercises, proper positioning, and supportive devices such as splints. Use of foot boards is controversial because they may facilitate spasticity. Provide quiet rest periods at appropriate intervals, based on evaluation of patient's response to activity. Encourage patient to participate in and perform own personal hygiene and to establish independence in activities of daily living. Evaluate patient's ability to feed himself or herself and continue to provide enteral feeding as necessary. Initiate a bowel and bladder retraining program, and instruct patient and support persons in its management. Teach patient and family about therapeutic regimen (activity and rest, diet, medications), including desired actions and side effects or concerns to report. Recognize and explain emotional lability, assisting patient in dealing with outbursts or inappropriate emotional affect. Assist with acceptance of deficits and disabilities, and in maintaining hope while establishing realistic expectations. Inform patient and others about social and financial support groups and services available to them, and encourage them to participate and avail themselves of these resources. Help them to accept residual deficits present after six months, as these may be permanent. Recognize that patient's recovery and survival expectations may be influenced by age and presence of other chronic illnesses, in addition to initial and later responses to stroke damage and therapies.

s., cryptogenic. An ischemic stroke that occurs in persons, esp. young patients, who have no known risk factors for that disease. One possible cause of this may be a clinically unapparent patent foramen ovale.

s., heat. An acute and dangerous reaction to heat exposure. The basic defect is failure of the heat-regulating mechanisms of the body. SEE: *heat; hyperpyrexia.*

s., ischemic. Stroke due to diminished blood supply to the brain or a particular area of the brain, e.g., the lodging of an embolus from the heart in an artery of the brain.

s., little. A pathologic change in the brain caused by diminished or lack of blood flow to a very small area of the brain. When this occurs, there may be no clinically detectable changes in the patient, or the changes may be subtle and unnoticed by the patient, but apparent to others. An example would include a person whose habits concerning personal neatness were well known, but after the little stroke the person no longer noticed that his or her clothes and appearance were no longer neat and clean. A group of little strokes may cause progressive dementia.

s., mini-. SEE: *mini-stroke.*

s., paralytic. Sudden onset of paralysis resulting from injury to brain or spinal cord. SEE: *stroke* (def. 5).

stroke volume. The amount of blood ejected by the left ventricle at each heartbeat. Amount varies with age, sex, and exercise. SYN: *systolic discharge.*

stroking. Technique of slow tactile stimulation over the posterior primary rami used to inhibit muscle responses and promote relaxation during neuromotor rehabilitation.

stroma (strō'mă) [Gr., bed covering] (pl. *stromata*). [NA] 1. Foundation-supporting tissues of an organ. Opposite of parenchyma. 2. Spongy, colorless framework of an erythrocyte.

stromal, stromatic (strō'măl, strō-măt'ĭk). Concerning or resembling the stroma of an organ.

stromatolysis (strō″mă-tŏl'ĭ-sĭs) [″ + *lysis,* dissolution]. Destruction of the stroma of a cell.

stromatosis (strō″mă-tō'sĭs) [″ + *osis,* condition]. Presence of mesenchyma-like tissue throughout the endometrium of the uterus.

Stromeyer's splint (strō'mī-ĕrz) [Georg F. L. Stromeyer, Ger. surgeon, 1804–1876]. A hinged splint for a joint, which can be fixed at an angle.

stromuhr (strō'moor) [Ger. *strom*, stream, + *uhr*, clock]. Device for measuring velocity of blood flow. SYN: *rheometer*. SEE: *flowmeter*.

Strongyloides (strŏn"jĭ-loy'dēz). A genus of roundworms that infect humans.

S. stercoralis. A roundworm that infrequently causes infection in humans, which may be fatal. In the U.S., *S. stercoralis* is found mainly in the rural South. The ova hatch in the intestines of the host, and rod-shaped larvae are passed in the stool. In the soil these may develop into adults and continue their life cycle or may metamorphose into filiform larvae that can infect humans. The filiform larvae enter the skin, pass through the venous system to the lungs, where they migrate upward and are swallowed. A rash or pneumonia may accompany their migration. The rod-shaped larvae have the ability to metamorphose into the filiform larvae in the human intestine. This form then enters the circulation, migrates to the lungs, and begins the cycle again.

This life cycle allows for a massive infection sufficient to cause overwhelming systemic infection with fever, severe abdominal pain, shock, and possibly death. Severe reactions are more likely to occur in immunosuppressed patients or patients with diseases that alter their immune status.

TREAT: Thiabendazole or mebendazole are the drugs of choice. Repeated courses of treatment may be required.

strongyloidosis (strŏn"jĭ-loy-dō'sĭs) [Gr. *strongylos*, compact, + *osis*, condition]. Infestation with organisms of the genus *Strongyloides*.

strongylosis (strŏn"jĭ-lō'sĭs). Infestation with organisms of the genus *Strongylus*.

Strongylus (strŏn'jĭ-lŭs). A genus of parasitic nematodes.

strontium (strŏn'shē-ŭm) [Strontian, mining village in Scotland]. SYMB: Sr. At. wt. 87.62; at. no. 38; sp. gr. 2.6. A dark yellow metal. Medically it is of interest because its radioactive isotope ^{90}Sr constitutes a radioactive hazard in fallout from atom bombs. The isotope has a half-life of 28 years and is stored in bone when ingested.

Strophanthus (strō-fǎn'thŭs) [Gr. *strophos*, twisted cord, + *anthos*, flower]. A genus of plants yielding a poisonous, white, crystalline glucoside, used chiefly in the form of alkaloid, strophanthin. Used as a heart stimulant.

strophocephaly (strŏf"ō-sĕf'ǎ-lē) [" + *kephale*, head]. Distortion of the head and face due to a developmental anomaly.

structural (strŭk'tū-rǎl) [L. *structura*, structure]. Pert. to organic structure.

structure (strŭk'shŭr). The arrangement of the component parts of an organism.

s., denture-supporting. The tissues that support a partial or complete denture.

struma (stroo'mǎ) [L. *struma*, a mass]. Enlargement of the thyroid gland. SYN: *goiter*.

s. aberranta. Struma of the accessory thyroid glands.

s., cast iron. Chronic thyroiditis accompanied by extreme development of fibrous tissue.

s. congenita. Goiter present at birth.

s. lingualis. Presence of thyroid tissue in tongue in region of foramen cecum.

s. lymphomatosa. Rare form involving a diffuse and extensive infiltration of the entire thyroid gland. SYN: *Hashimoto's struma.*

s. maligna. Carcinoma of the thyroid gland.

s. ovarii. Form of ovarian teratoma in which mass is composed of typical thyroid follicles filled with colloid.

s., Riedel's. Form of chronic thyroiditis in which the gland becomes enlarged, hard, and adherent to adjacent tissues. Follicles become atrophic and fibrosis occurs.

strumectomy (stroo-mĕk'tō-mē) [" + *ektome*, excision]. Removal of a goiter.

strumiprivous (stroo"mĭ-prī'vŭs) [" + *privus*, deprived]. Rel. to or caused by removal of the thyroid gland.

strumitis (stroo-mī'tĭs) [" + Gr. *itis*, inflammation]. Inflammation of a thyroid gland with goiter. SYN: *thyroiditis.*

strumous (stroo'mŭs) [L. *strumosus*]. 1. Affected with scrofula. SYN: *scrofulous.* 2. Affected with goiter.

Strümpell's disease (strĭm'pĕlz). Strümpell-Marie disease, q.v.

Strümpell-Marie disease [Adolf G. G. von Strümpell, Ger. physician, 1853–1925; Pierre Marie, Fr. neurologist, 1853–1940]. Ankylosing or rheumatoid spondylitis. SEE: *spondylitis, rheumatoid.*

Strümpell's sign (strĭm'pĕls). Dorsiflexion of foot when thigh is flexed on abdomen. May be associated with spastic paralysis of the leg.

struvite. Crystals of magnesium ammonium phosphate. Sometimes found as a harmless ingredient of canned food, where the crystals may be mistaken for glass. Struvite crystals will dissolve in vinegar. This simple test will distinguish struvite from glass. Struvite crystals are also present in some renal calculi. They are formed by the action of the bacterial enzyme urease.

strychnine (strĭk'nĭn, -nēn, -nĭn) [Gr. *strychnos*, nightshade]. A poisonous alkaloid ob-

STRYKER FRAME

tained from plants, as nux vomica. It has no therapeutic usefulness but has been used as an experimental tool in neuropharmacology.

strychnine poisoning. SEE: *Poisons and Poisoning* in *Appendix.*

strychninism (strik'nĭn-ĭzm) [" + *-ismos*, condition]. Chronic strychnine poisoning.

strychnism (strĭk'nĭzm). Poisoning from use of strychnine.

Stryker frame. Device that supports two rectangular pieces of lightweight but strong material so that one side is on the anterior surface of the patient and the other is on the posterior surface. The patient is held firmly between the pieces of material as if part of a sandwich. The device may be rotated around the patient's long axis. This permits turning the patient without his or her assistance. After a turn is completed, the uppermost portion of the frame can be moved away from the patient. SEE: illus.

STS. *serological test for syphilis.*

STU. *skin test unit.*

Stuart factor. The 10th factor (factor X) in blood coagulation. It is present in plasma and serum and is essential for blood coagulation. SYN: *thrombokinase.*

study, case-control. SEE: *case-control study.*

stump. The distal portion of an amputated extremity.

stump hallucination. Sensation of possessing a limb after its amputation. SYN: *phantom limb.*

stun (stŭn) [O. Fr. *estoner*, a blow]. To render unconscious or stupefied by a blow.

stupe (stūp) [L. *stupa*, tow]. A counterirritant for topical use. It is prepared by adding a small amount of an irritant such as turpentine to a hot liquid.

stupefacient (stū"pĕ-fā'shĕnt) [L. *stupefaciens*, stupefying]. Causing or that which causes stupor. SYN: *narcotic; soporific.*

stupefactive (stū"pĕ-făk'tĭv) [L. *stupefaciens*, stupefying]. Producing narcosis or stupor.

stupor (stū'por) [L., numbness]. 1. Condition of unconsciousness, torpor, or lethargy with suppression of sense or feeling. 2. In psychiatry, a state of lessened responsiveness. Stupor occurs in visceral and infectious diseases, melancholia, catatonia, epilepsy, paresis, poisonings, and hysteria. A benign form is seen in manic-depressive psychosis.

    RS: carotic; catatonia; collapse; coma; lethargy; syncope; unconsciousness.

    s., anergic. Stupor accompanied by immobility seen in certain psychoses.

s., delusional. Stupor accompanied by delusions.

s., epileptic. Stupor sometimes following an attack of epilepsy.

s., lethargic. Stupor accompanied by lethargy. SEE: *trance.*

s. melancholicus. Stupor associated with mental depression.

stuporous. Affected with stupor.

stuporous depression. An extremely depressed phase of manic-depressive psychosis typified by extreme psychomotor retardation and unresponsiveness to surrounding conditions.

Sturge-Weber syndrome [William Sturge, Brit. physician, 1850–1919; Frederick Parkes Weber, Brit. physician, 1863–1962]. Congenital syndrome characterized by port-wine nevi along the distribution of the trigeminal nerve, angiomas of leptomeninges and choroid, intracranial calcifications, mental retardation, epileptic seizures, and glaucoma. SYN: *amentia, nevoid.*

sturine (stū′rĭn) [NL. *sturio,* sturgeon]. Protamine obtained from sperm of sturgeon. SEE: *protamine; salmin(e).*

stutter (stŭt′ĕr) [ME. *stutten,* to stutter]. To hesitate and repeat or stumble spasmodically in speaking. Due to a variety of causes, among them difficulty in pronouncing initial consonants, caused by spasm of lingual and palatal muscles.

Understanding of the physiological and pathological aspects of stuttering is incomplete, e.g., some individuals who stutter in most situations will not stutter when alone, when singing, when ambient noise prevents their hearing the sound of their own voice, when talking to animals or reading to small children.

There is evidence that stuttering can be associated with an underlying neurologic dysfunction.

stuttering (stŭt′ĕr-ĭng). Defect in speech in which there is stumbling and spasmodic repetition of the same syllable. SYN: *anarthria literalis; stammering.* SEE: *lallation; speech.*

s., urinary. Irregular, spasmodic urination. SYN: *stammering of bladder.*

sty(e) (stī) [AS. *stigan,* to rise] (pl. *styes; sties*). A localized circumscribed inflammatory swelling of one of several sebaceous glands of the eyelid. Caused by a bacterial infection. External styes are superficial and affect Zeis' glands or glands of Moll at the edge of the lid. Internal styes concern the meibomian or tarsal glands under the eyelid and are more severe. SYN: *hordeolum.* SEE: *chalazion.*

SYM: General edema of lid, pain, local-

ized conjunctivitis. As the internal sty progresses, an abscess that can be seen through the conjunctiva will form.

TREAT: Frequent application of hot packs usually brings about drainage and resolution. Incision and drainage if not resolved. Topical antibiotics will prevent spread of infection.

s., meibomian. Inflammation of a meibomian gland.

s., zeisian. Inflammation of one of Zeis' glands.

style, stylet (stīl, stī′lĕt) [Gr. *stylos,* pillar]. 1. A slender, solid or hollow, plug of metal for making a canal permanent after operation or for stiffening or clearing a cannula or catheter. 2. A thin probe.

styliform (stī′lĭ-form) [″ + L. *forma,* form]. Long and pointed.

styliscus (stī-lĭs′kŭs) [Gr. *styliskos,* a pillar]. A slender, cylindrical plug for dilating a channel or for keeping a wound open.

styloglossus (stī-lō-glŏs′ŭs) [Gr. *stylos,* pillar, + *glossa,* tongue]. A muscle connecting the tongue and styloid process that raises and retracts the tongue. SEE: *Muscles* in *Appendix.*

stylohyal (stī′lō-hī′ăl) [″ + *hyoeides,* hyoid]. Stylohyoid, q.v.

stylohyoid (stī-lō-hī′oyd) [″ + *hyoeides,* hyoid]. Pert. to the styloid process of the temporal and hyoid bones.

stylohyoideus (stī″lō-hī-oyd′ē-ŭs). A muscle having its origin on the styloid process and its insertion on the hyoid bone. It draws the hyoid bone upward and backward. SEE: *Muscles* in *Appendix.*

styloid (stī′loyd) [″ + *eidos,* form, shape]. Resembling a stylus or pointed instrument.

styloiditis (stī″loyd-ī′tĭs) [″ + ″ + *itis,* inflammation]. Inflammation of a styloid process.

styloid process. 1. A pointed process of the temporal bone, projecting downward, and to which some of the muscles of the tongue are attached. 2. A pointed projection behind the head of the fibula. 3. A protuberance on the outer portion of the distal end of the radius. 4. An ulnar projection on the inner side of the distal end.

stylomandibular (stī″lō-măn-dĭb′ū-lar) [″ + L. *mandibula,* lower jawbone]. Concerning the styloid process of the temporal bone and mandible.

stylomastoid (stī″lō-măs′toyd) [″ + *mastos,* breast, + *eidos,* form, shape]. Concerning the styloid and mastoid processes of the temporal bone.

stylopharyngeus (stī″lō-făr-ĭn′jē-ŭs) [″ + *pharynx,* throat]. Muscle connecting the styloid process and pharynx that elevates and dilates the pharynx. SEE: *Muscles* in *Appendix*.

stylostaphyline (stī″lō-stăf′ĭ-lĭn) [″ + *staphyle*, bunch of grapes]. Concerning the styloid process of the temporal bone and uvula.

stylosteophyte (stī-lŏs′tē-ō-fīt). A peg-shaped outgrowth from bone.

stylus (stī′lŭs) [Gr. *stylos*, a pillar]. 1. A probe or slender wire for stiffening or clearing a canal or catheter. 2. Pointed medicinal preparation in stick form for external application.

stype (stīp) [Gr., tow]. A pledget or tampon of cotton or other material.

stypsis (stĭp′sĭs) [Gr., *styphein*, to contract]. Astringency or the use of an astringent.

styptic (stĭp′tĭk) [Gr. *styptikos*, contracting]. 1. Contracting a blood vessel; stopping a hemorrhage by astringent action. 2. Anything that stops a hemorrhage such as alum, ferrous sulfate, or tannic acid. SYN: *astringent; hemostat*.

sub- [L. *sub*, under, below]. Combining form meaning under, beneath, in small quantity, less than normal. SYN: [Gr.] *hypo-*.

subabdominal (sŭb″ăb-dŏm′ĭ-năl) [L. *sub*, under, below, + *abdomen*, abdomen]. Below the abdomen.

subabdominoperitoneal (sŭb″ăb-dŏm″ĭ-nō-pĕr″ĭ-tō-nē′ăl) [″ + ″ + Gr. *peritonaion*, peritoneum]. Deep to the abdominal peritoneum.

subacetate (sŭb-ăs′ĕ-tāt) [″ + *acetum*, vinegar]. A basic acetate.

subacid (sŭb-ăs′ĭd) [″ + *acidus*, sour]. Moderately acid.

subacromial (sŭb-ă-krō′mē-ăl) [″ + Gr. *akron*, point, + *osmos*, shoulder]. Under the acromial process.

subacute (sŭb″ă-kūt′) [″ + *acutus*, sharp]. Between acute and chronic, but with some acute features, said of the course of a disease or of the healing process following tissue injury.

subacute myelo-optic neuropathy. ABBR: SMON. Neurological disease that usually begins with abdominal pain or diarrhea followed by sensory and motor disturbances in the lower limbs, ataxia, impaired vision, and convulsions or coma. Reported mostly in Japan and Australia. Most patients survive but neurological disability remains. Many of those who have the disease have a history of taking drugs of the halogenated oxyquinoline group; e.g., clioquinol (previously called iodochlorhydroxyquin).

subacute sclerosing panencephalitis. ABBR: SSPE. A cerebral degenerative disease thought to be secondary to entrance of the measles virus into the brain. The first signs are due to a progressive decrease in higher cerebral functions, usually mani-

fested as failure to progress in school. There are personality changes, emotional instability, and generalized myoclonic jerks. In late stages dementia and generalized rigidity occur. There is no treatment and most patients die of the disease. SYN: *panencephalitis*.

subalimentation (sŭb″ăl-ĭ-mĕn-tā′shŭn) [″ + *alimentum*, nourishment]. A state of insufficient nourishment.

subanal (sŭb-ā′năl) [″ + *analis*, anal]. Below the anus.

subanconeus (sŭb″ăn-kō′nē-ŭs) [″ + Gr. *ankon*, elbow]. 1. Below the elbow. 2. Muscle beneath the elbow that contracts its posterior ligament. SEE: *Muscles* in *Appendix*.

subapical (sŭb-ăp′ĭ-kăl) [″ + *apex*, tip]. Below the apex.

subaponeurotic (sŭb″ăp-ō-nū-rŏt′ĭk) [″ + Gr. *apo*, from, + *neuron*, sinew]. Below an aponeurosis.

subarachnoid (sŭb″ă-răk′noyd) [″ + Gr. *arachne*, spider, + *eidos*, form, shape]. Below or under the arachnoid membrane and the pia mater of the covering of the brain.

subarachnoid cisternae. Spaces at the base of the brain where the arachnoid becomes widely separated from the pia, giving rise to large cavities.

subarachnoid space. Space between the pia proper and arachnoid containing the cerebrospinal fluid.

subarcuate (sŭb-ăr′kū-āt) [L. *sub*, under, below, + *arcuatus*, bowed]. Slightly arched.

subarcuate fossa. Depression that extends backward as a blind tunnel under the superior semicircular canal of the temporal bone.

subareolar (sŭb″ă-rē′ō-lăr) [″ + *areola*, a small space]. Below the areola.

subastragalar (sŭb-ăs-trăg′ă-lăr) [″ + Gr. *astragalos*, ball of the ankle joint]. Beneath the astragalus.

subastringent (sŭb″ăs-trĭn′jĕnt) [″ + *astringere*, to bind fast]. Mildly astringent.

subatomic (sŭb″ă-tŏm′ĭk) [″ + Gr. *atomos*, indivisible]. Less than the size of an atom.

subaural (sŭb-aw′răl) [″ + *auris*, ear]. Below the ear.

subauricular (sŭb″aw-rĭk′ū-lăr) [″ + *auricula*, little ear]. Below an auricle, esp. of the ear.

subaxial (sŭb-ăk′sē-ăl) [″ + *axis*, axis]. Below an axis.

subaxillary (sŭb-ăk′sĭ-lĕr″ē) [″ + *axilla*, armpit]. Below the axilla, or armpit.

subbrachycephalic (sŭb″brā-kē-sĕ-făl′ĭk) [″ + Gr. *brachys*, short, + *kephale*, head]. Having a cephalic index of 78 to 79.

subcalcarine (sŭb-kăl′kăr-īn) [″ + *calcar*,

spur]. Below the calcarine sulcus.

subcapsular (sŭb-kăp′sū-lăr) [″ + *capsula,* little box]. Below any capsule, esp. the capsule of the brain, or a capsular ligament.

subcarbonate (sŭb-kăr′bō-nāt) [″ + *carbo,* carbon]. A basic carbonate; one having proportion of carbonic acid radical less than the normal carbonate.

subcartilaginous (sŭb″kăr-tĭ-lăj′ĭn-ŭs) [″ + *cartilago,* gristle]. 1. Located beneath a cartilage. 2. Cartilaginous in part.

subception (sŭb-sĕp′shŭn). Subliminal perception.

subchondral (sŭb″kŏn′drăl) [″ + Gr. *chondros,* cartilage]. Below or under a cartilage.

subchoroidal (sŭb″kō-roy′dăl) [″ + Gr. *chorioeides,* skinlike]. Below the choroid.

subchronic (sŭb-krŏn′ĭk) [″ + Gr. *chronos,* time]. Noting a condition between subacute and chronic; almost chronic.

subclass (sŭb′klăs). In taxonomy, a category between class and an order.

subclavian (sŭb-klā′vē-ăn) [″ + *clavis,* key]. Under the clavicle or collarbone. SYN: *subclavicular.*

subclavian artery. Large artery at base of neck that supplies blood to the arm. The right subclavian artery branches from the innominate artery; the left subclavian artery branches from the aortic arch.

subclavian steal syndrome. Shunting of blood, which was destined for the brain, away from the cerebral circulation. This occurs when the subclavian artery is occluded. Blood then flows from the opposite vertebral artery across to and down the vertebral artery on the side of the occlusion.
SYM: Signs of insufficient blood flow to the brain. Symptoms are transient and are aggravated by exercise. Usually the blood pressure in the arm on the affected side will be significantly lower than in the other arm.

subclavian triangle. Triangle-shaped part of the neck formed by the clavicle and the omohyoid and sternomastoid muscles.

subclavian vein. Large vein draining arm. It unites with the interior jugular to form the innominate vein.

subclavicular (sŭb″klă-vĭk′ū-lăr) [L. *sub,* under, below, + *clavicula,* little key]. Beneath the clavicle. SYN: *subclavian.*

subclavius (sŭb-klā′vē-ŭs) [″ + *clavis,* key]. A tiny muscle from the first rib to the undersurface of the clavicle. SEE: *Muscles in Appendix.*

subclinical (sŭb-klĭn′ĭ-kăl) [″ + Gr. *klinikos,* pert. to a bed]. Pert. to a period before appearance of typical symptoms of a disease or to a disease or condition that does not present clinical symptoms. Some infections may not produce characteristic symptoms,

but can be demonstrated by antigenic reactions.

subcollateral (sŭb-kō-lăt′ĕr-ăl) [″ + *con,* together, + *lateralis,* pert. to a side]. Below the collateral fissure, indicating a cerebral convolution.

subconjunctival (sŭb″kŏn-jŭnk-tī′văl) [″ + *conjungere,* to join together]. Beneath the conjunctiva.

subconsciousness (sŭb-kŏn′shŭs-nĕs) [″ + *conscius,* aware]. 1. The state of being partially unconscious. 2. The condition in which mental processes take place without the individual's being aware of their occurrence. SEE: *subliminal.*

subcontinuous (sŭb″kŏn-tĭn′ū-ŭs) [″ + *continere,* to hold together]. Almost continuous; with periods of abatement.

subcontinuous fever. Fever with periods of remission and exacerbation. SYN: *remittent fever.*

subcoracoid (sŭb-kor′ă-koyd) [″ + Gr. *korakoeides,* like a crow's beak]. Beneath the coracoid process.

subcortex (sŭb-kor′tĕks) [″ + *cortex,* rind]. White substance of the brain underlying the cortex.

subcortical (sŭb-kor′tĭ-kăl). Pert. to the region beneath the cerebral cortex.

subcostal (sŭb-kŏs′tăl) [″ + *costa,* rib]. Beneath the ribs.

subcostalgia (sŭb″kŏs-tăl′jē-ă) [″ + ″ + Gr. *algos,* pain]. Pain in region over the subcostal nerve.

subcranial (sŭb-krā′nē-ăl) [″ + Gr. *kranion,* skull]. Beneath or below the cranium.

subcrepitant (sŭb-krĕp′ĭ-tănt) [″ + *crepitare,* to rattle]. Partially crepitant or crackling in character; noting a rale.

subcrureus (sŭb-kroo-rē′ŭs) [″ + *crus,* leg]. Small muscle between anterior surface of femoral shaft and synovial membrane of knee joint. SEE: *Muscles in Appendix.*

subculture (sŭb-kŭl′chŭr) [″ + *cultura,* tillage]. To make a culture of bacteria with material derived from another culture.

subcutaneous (sŭb″kū-tā′nē-ŭs) [″ + *cutis,* skin]. Beneath or to be introduced beneath the skin. SYN: *hypodermic.*

subcutaneous surgery. Operation performed through a small opening in the skin.

subcutaneous wound. A wound with only a small opening through the skin.

subcuticular (sŭb″kū-tĭk′ū-lăr) [L. *sub,* under, below, + *cuticula,* little skin]. Beneath the cuticle or epidermis. SYN: *subepidermal.*

subcutis (sŭb-kū′tĭs). The layer of connective tissue beneath the skin.

subdelirium (sŭb″dē-lĭr′ē-ŭm) [″ + *de,* away from, + *lira,* track]. A mild or partial state of delirium.

subdeltoid (sŭb-dĕl′toyd) [″ + Gr. *delta*, letter d, + *eidos*, form, shape]. Beneath the deltoid muscle.

subdental (sŭb-dĕn′tăl) [″ + *dens*, tooth]. Beneath the teeth or a tooth.

subdermal [″ + Gr. *derma*, skin]. Below the skin.

subdiaphragmatic (sŭb″dī-ă-frăg-măt′ĭk) [″ + Gr. *diaphragma*, a partition]. Beneath the diaphragm. SYN: *subphrenic.*

subdorsal (sŭb-dor′săl) [″ + *dorsum*, back]. Below the dorsal area.

subduct (sŭb-dŭkt′) [″ + *ducere*, to lead]. To draw down.

subdural (sŭb-dū′răl) [″ + *durus*, hard]. Beneath the dura mater.

subdural space. Space between the arachnoid and dura mater.

subendocardial (sŭb″ĕn-dō-kăr′dē-ăl) [″ + Gr. *endon*, within, + *kardia*, heart]. Below the endocardium.

subendothelial, subendothelium (sŭb″ĕn-dō-thē′lē-ăl, sŭb″ĕn-dō-thē′lē-ŭm) [″ + Gr. *endon*, within, + *thele*, nipple]. Beneath the endothelium.

subependymal (sŭb″ĕp-ĕn′dĭ-măl) [″ + Gr. *ependyma*, an upper garment, wrap]. Beneath the ependyma.

subepidermal (sŭb″ĕp-ĭ-dĕr′măl) [″ + Gr. *epi*, upon, + *derma*, skin]. Beneath the epidermis. SYN: *subcuticular.*

subepithelial (sŭb″ĕp-ĭ-thē′lē-ăl) [″ + ″ + *thele*, nipple]. Beneath the epithelium.

suberosis (sū″bĕr-ō′sĭs) [L. *suber*, cork, + Gr. *osis*, condition]. Pulmonary hypersensitivity reaction in workers exposed to cork. The antigen is present in a mold in the cork.

subfamily (sŭb-făm′ĭ-lē). In taxonomy, between a family and a tribe.

subfascial (sŭb-făsh′ē-ăl) [L. *sub*, under, below, + *fascia*, a band]. Beneath a fascia.

subfebrile (sŭb-fē′brĭl) [″ + *febris*, fever]. Mild fever, usually considered to be less than 101°F (38.3°C).

subfertility (sŭb″fĕr-tĭl′ĭ-tē) [″ + *fertilis*, fertile]. Not as fertile as would be considered normal.

subflavous (sŭb-flā′vŭs) [″ + *flavus*, yellow]. Yellowish.

subflavous ligament. Yellowish ligament connecting the laminae of the vertebrae.

subfolium (sŭb-fō′lē-ŭm) [″ + *folium*, leaf]. A leaflike division of the cerebellar folia.

subfrontal (sŭb-frŏn′tăl) [″ + *frontalis*, brow]. Below a frontal convolution or lobe of the brain.

subgenus (sŭb-jē′nŭs). In taxonomy, between a genus and species.

subgingival (sŭb-jĭn′jĭ-văl) [″ + *gingiva*, gum]. Beneath the gingiva. Related to a point or area apical to the margin of the free gingiva, usually within the confines of the gingival sulcus, e.g., subgingival calculus, or subgingival margin of a restoration.

subglenoid (sŭb-glē′noyd) [″ + Gr. *glene*, socket, + *eidos*, form, shape]. Below the glenoid fossa or glenoid cavity.

subglossal (sŭb-glŏs′ăl) [″ + Gr. *glossa*, tongue]. Under the tongue. SYN: *hypoglossal; sublingual.*

subglossitis (sŭb-glŏs-sī′tĭs) [″ + ″ + *itis*, inflammation]. Inflammation of the undersurface or tissues of the tongue.

subglottic (sŭb-glŏt′ĭk) [″ + Gr. *glottis*, back of tongue]. Beneath the glottis.

subgranular (sŭb-grăn′ū-lăr) [″ + *granulum*, little grain]. Not completely granular.

subgrondation, subgrundation (sŭb-grŏn-dă′shŭn, -grŭn-dă′shŭn) [Fr.]. Depression of one fragment of a broken bone beneath the other, as of the cranium.

subhepatic (sŭb″hĕ-păt′ĭk) [L. *sub*, under, below, + Gr. *hepatikos*, pert. to the liver]. Beneath the liver.

subhyaloid (sŭb-hī′ă-loyd) [″ + Gr. *hyalos*, glass, + *eidos*, form, shape]. Located beneath the hyaloid membrane.

subhyoid (sŭb-hī′oyd) [″ + Gr. *hyoeides*, U-shaped]. Beneath the hyoid bone.

subicteric (sŭb″ĭk-tĕr′ĭk) [″ + Gr. *ikteros*, jaundice]. Mildly jaundiced.

subicular (sŭ-bĭk′ū-lăr). Concerning the uncinate gyrus.

subiliac (sŭb-ĭl′ē-ăk) [″ + *iliacus*, pert. to the ilium]. 1. Below the ilium. 2. Pert. to the subilium.

subilium (sŭb-ĭl′ē-ŭm). The lowest part of the ilium.

subincision. Production of a fistula of the penile urethra. May interfere with conception. Used by some primitive groups, esp. Australian aborigines.

subintimal (sŭb-ĭn′tĭ-măl) [″ + *intima*, innermost]. Beneath the intima.

subintrant (sŭb-ĭn′trănt) [L. *subintrans*, stealing into]. Having cycles or paroxysms in such rapid succession that they intermingle and thus overlap. SYN: *proleptic.*

subintrant fever. Intermittent fever in which the paroxysms occur so rapidly that one comes on before the previous one has disappeared.

subinvolution (sŭb″ĭn-vō-lū′shŭn) [L. *sub*, under, below, + *involutio*, a turning into]. Imperfect involution; incomplete return of a part to normal dimensions after physiological hypertrophy, as when the uterus fails to reduce to normal size following childbirth. SEE: *uterus.*

subjacent (sŭb-jā′sĕnt) [″ + *jacere*, to lie]. Lying underneath.

subject (sŭb′jĕkt) [L. *subjectus*, brought

under]. 1. A patient undergoing treatment, observation, or investigation; a well person participating in a medical or scientific investigation. 2. A body used for dissection. 3. To have a liability to develop attacks of a particular disease. 4. To submit to a procedure or to the action of another.

subjective [L. *subjectivus*]. Arising from or concerned with the individual; not perceptible to an observer. Opposite of objective.

subjective sensation. A sensation occurring when stimuli due to internal causes excite the nervous system; one not of objective origin.

subjective symptoms. Symptoms of internal origin, evident only to the patient.

subjugal (sŭb-jū'găl) [L. *sub*, under, below, + *jugum*, yoke]. Below the malar bone or os zygomaticum.

sublatio (sŭb-lā'shē-ō) [L.]. Removal, elevation, or detachment of a part.

    s. retinae. Detachment of the retina.

sublation (sŭb-lā'shŭn) [L. *sublatio*, elevation]. The displacement, elevation, or removal of a part.

sublesional (sŭb-lē'shŭn-ăl) [L. *sub*, under, below, + *laesio*, wound]. Beneath a lesion.

sublethal (sŭb-lē'thăl) [" + Gr. *lethe*, oblivion]. Less than lethal; almost fatal.

sublethal dose. Dose containing not quite enough of a toxin or noxious substance to cause death.

sublimate (sŭb'lĭ-māt) [L. *sublimare*, to elevate]. 1. A substance obtained or prepared by sublimation. 2. To cause a solid or gas to change state without becoming a liquid during transition. Ex.: Ice may evaporate without first becoming a liquid. 3. An ego defense mechanism by which one diverts unwanted aggressive or sexual drives into socially acceptable activities.

sublimation (sŭb"lĭ-mā'shŭn) [L. *sublimatio*]. 1. Altering the state of a gas or solid without first changing it into a liquid. 2. Conversion of unwanted aggressive or sexual drives into socially accepted channels. A freudian term pert. to unconscious mental processes of ego defense whereby unwanted sexual or aggressive drives find an outlet through creative mental work.

Sublimaze. Trade name for fentanyl citrate.

sublime (sŭb-līm') [L. *sublimis*, to the limit]. To evaporate a substance directly from the solid into the vapor state and condense it again. Thus metallic iodine on heating does not liquefy, but forms directly a violet gas.

subliminal (sŭb-lĭm'ĭn-ăl) [L. *sub*, under, below, + *limen*, threshold]. 1. Below the threshold of sensation; too weak to arouse sensation or muscular contraction. 2. Below the normal consciousness.

subliminal self. In psychiatry, part of the normal individual's personality in which mental processes function without consciousness under normal waking conditions.

sublimis (sŭb-lī'mĭs) [L.]. Near the surface.

sublingual (sŭb-lĭng'gwăl) [L. *sub*, under, below, + *lingua*, tongue]. Beneath or concerning the area beneath the tongue.

sublingual gland. The smallest of the major salivary glands, located in the tissue in the floor of the mouth between the tongue and mandible on each side. It is a mixed seromucous gland whose main duct opens into or near the submandibular duct, but there may be several smaller ducts opening to the oral cavity independently along the sublingual fold. Numerous minor sublingual glands are scattered throughout the mucosa under the tongue, each with its own duct to the oral surface.

sublinguitis (sŭb"lĭng-gwī'tĭs) [" + " + Gr. *itis*, inflammation]. Inflammation of the sublingual gland.

sublobular (sŭb-lŏb'ū-lăr) [" + *lobulus*, small lobe]. Beneath a lobule.

sublumbar (sŭb-lŭm'băr) [" + *lumbus*, loin]. Below the lumbar region.

subluxation (sŭb"lŭks-ā'shŭn) [" + *luxatio*, dislocation]. 1. A partial or incomplete dislocation. 2. In dentistry, injury to supporting tissues that results in abnormal loosening of teeth without displacement, or when loosely applied to the temporomandibular joint, refers to the relaxation or stretching of the capsule and ligaments that results in popping noises during movement or partial dislocation of the mandible forward.

submammary (sŭb-măm'ă-rē) [" + *mamma*, breast]. Below the mammary gland.

submandibular [" + *mandibula*, lower jawbone]. Beneath the mandible or lower jaw.

submandibular gland. One of the salivary glands, a mixed tubuloalveolar gland about the size of a walnut that lies in digastric triangle beneath the mandible. Its main duct (Wharton's duct) opens at the side of the frenulum linguae.

submandibularitis. Inflammation of or mumps affecting the submandibular gland.

submarginal (sŭb-măr'jĭn-ăl) [" + *marginalis*, border]. Close to or next to a margin or border of a part. In dentistry, pert. to a deficiency in material or contour at the margin of a restoration in a tooth.

submaxillary. Below the maxilla or upper jaw.

submedial, submedian (sŭb-mē'dē-ăl, -ăn) [" + *medianus*, middle]. Below or close to the middle.

submembranous (sŭb-mĕm′bră-nŭs) [″ + membrana, membrane]. Containing partly membranous material.

submental [″ + mentum, chin]. Under the chin.

submerge (sŭb-mĕrj′) [″ + mergere, to immerse]. To place under water.

submerged tooth. A tooth which is below the plane of occlusion; usually a deciduous tooth retained as a result of ankylosis.

submetacentric (sŭb″mĕt-ā-sĕn′trĭk) [″ + Gr. meta, beyond, + kentron, center]. Concerning a chromosome in which the centromere is within the two central quarters but away from the middle.

submicron [″ + Gr. mikros, tiny]. A particle smaller than 10^{-5} cm in diameter. Visible only with an ultramicroscope. SEE: micron.

submicroscopic [″ + ″ + skopein, to examine]. Too minute to be seen through a microscope. SYN: amicroscopic.

submorphous (sŭb-mor′fŭs) [″ + Gr. morphe, form]. Neither completely amorphous nor crystalline, as some calculi.

submucosa (sŭb″mū-kō′să) [L. sub, under, below, + mucosus, mucus]. The layer of connective tissue below the mucosa. It may vary from areolar to quite dense irregular connective tissue and, in addition to the distributing vessels and nerves, may contain extensive deposits of fat, mucous glands, or muscle.

submucous (sŭb-mū′kŭs) [″ + mucus, mucus]. Beneath a mucous membrane.

submucous resection. Removal of tissue below the mucosa, esp. excision of cartilaginous tissue beneath the mucosal tissue of the nose.

subnarcotic (sŭb-năr-kŏt′ĭk) [″ + Gr. narkotikos, benumbing]. Mildly narcotic.

subnasal [″ + nasus, nose]. Under the nose.

subnasale (sŭb″nā-sā′lē) [″ + nasus, nose]. The base of the anterior nasal spine.

subnasal point. Craniometric point at base of the nasal spine.

subnasion (sŭb-nā′zē-ŏn) [″ + nasus, nose]. Subnasal.

subneural (sŭb-nū′răl) [″ + Gr. neuron, nerve]. Beneath the neural axis or the central nervous system.

subnormal (sŭb-nor′măl) [″ + normalis, accord. to pattern]. Less than normal or average.

subnucleus (sŭb-nū′klē-ŭs) [″ + nucleus, kernel]. One of the secondary nuclei into which a nucleus of the central nervous system may be divided.

suboccipital (sŭb″ŏk-sĭp′ĭ-tăl) [″ + occiput, back of head]. Situated below the occi-

put or occipital bone.

suboperculum (sŭb″ō-pĕr′kū-lŭm) [″ + operculum, a covering]. Portion of occipital convolution overlapping the insula. SEE: operculum.

suboptimal (sŭb-ŏp′tĭ-măl) [″ + optimus, best]. Less than optimum.

suborbital (sŭb-or′bĭ-tăl) [″ + orbita, track]. Beneath the orbit.

suborder (sŭb-or′dĕr). In taxonomy, a category below the grouping in the order.

suboxides (sŭb-ŏk′sīdz). In a series of oxides, ones that contain the smallest amount of oxygen.

subpapular (sŭb-păp′ū-lăr) [″ + papula, pimple]. Very slightly papular, as papules elevated being scarcely more than macules.

subparietal (sŭb″pă-rī′ĕ-tăl) [″ + paries, a wall]. Below the parietal bone or lobe.

subpatellar (sŭb″pă-tĕl′ăr) [″ + patella, a small pan]. Beneath the patella.

subpectoral (sŭb-pĕk′tor-ăl) [″ + pectus, chest]. Below the pectoral area; beneath the pectoral muscles.

subpeduncular (sŭb″pē-dŭn′kū-lăr) [″ + pedunculus, a little foot]. Below a peduncle.

subpeduncular lobe. Tiny lobe on undersurface of either cerebellar hemisphere. SYN: flocculus.

subpelviperitoneal (sŭb-pĕl″vē-pĕr″ĭ-tō-nē′ăl) [L. sub, under, below, + pelvis, basin, + Gr. peritonaion, peritoneum]. Beneath the pelvic peritoneum.

subpericardial (sŭb″pĕr-ĭ-kăr′dē-ăl) [″ + Gr. peri, around, + kardia, heart]. Beneath the pericardium.

subperiosteal (sŭb″pĕr-ē-ŏs′tē-ăl) [″ + ″ + osteon, bone]. Beneath the periosteum.

subperitoneal (sŭb″pĕr-ĭ-tō-nē′ăl) [″ + Gr. peritonaion, peritoneum]. Beneath the peritoneum.

subperitoneoabdominal (sŭb″pĕr-ĭ-tō-nē′ō-ăb-dŏm′ĭ-năl) [″ + ″ + L. abdomen, belly]. Subperitoneal.

subpharyngeal (sŭb″făr-ĭn′jē-ăl) [″ + Gr. pharynx, throat]. Beneath the pharynx.

subphrenic (sŭb-frĕn′ĭk) [″ + Gr. phren, diaphragm]. Beneath the diaphragm. SYN: subdiaphragmatic.

subphrenic abscess. Collection of pus beneath the diaphragm.

subphylum (sŭb-fī′lŭm). In taxonomy, between a phylum and a class.

subpial (sŭb-pī′ăl) [″ + pia, soft]. Beneath the pia.

subplacenta (sŭb″plă-sĕn′tă) [″ + placenta, a flat cake]. During pregnancy, the endometrium that lines the entire uterine cavity except at the site of the implanted blastocyst. SYN: decidua parietalis [NA].

subpleural (sŭb-plū′răl) [″ + Gr. pleura, side]. Beneath the pleura.

subpoena. A court document that requires a person to appear at a certain time and place to give testimony regarding a particular matter. Failure to appear can result in punishment by the court.

subpontine (sŭb-pŏn′tĭn, -tīn) [″ + *pons*, bridge]. Below the pons.

subpreputial (sŭb″prē-pū′shăl) [″ + *praeputium*, prepuce]. Under the prepuce.

subpubic (sŭb-pū′bĭk) [″ + *pubes*, pubic region]. Beneath the pubic arch, as a ligament, or performed beneath the pubic arch.

subpulmonary (sŭb-pŭl′mō-nā-rē) [″ + *pulmon*, lung]. Below the lung.

subpyramidal (sŭb″pī-răm′ĭ-dăl) [″ + Gr. *pyramis*, a pyramid]. Beneath a pyramid of the kidney.

subretinal (sŭb-rĕt′ĭ-năl) [″ + *rete*, a net]. Beneath the retina.

subscapular (sŭb-skăp′ū-lăr) [″ + *scapula*, shoulder blade]. Below the scapula.

subscleral (sŭb-sklē′răl) [″ + Gr. *skleros*, hard]. Beneath the sclera of the eye.

subsclerotic (sŭb-sklē′rŏt-ĭk) [″ + Gr. *skleros*, hard]. 1. Subscleral. 2. Not completely sclerosed.

subscription (sŭb-skrĭp′shŭn) [L. *subscriptas*, written under]. That part of a prescription that contains directions for compounding ingredients.

subserous (sŭb-sē′rŭs) [L. *sub*, under, below, + *serum*, whey]. Beneath a serous membrane.

subsibilant (sŭb-sĭb′ĭ-lănt) [″ + *sibilans*, hissing]. Having the sound of a muffled whistle.

subsidence (sŭb-sīd′ĕns) [L. *subsidere*, to sink down]. The gradual disappearance of symptoms or manifestations of a disease.

subsistence. The minimum amount of something essential for life, e.g., a subsistence diet.

subspecies (sŭb′spē-sēz) [L. *sub*, under, below, + *species*, a kind]. In taxonomy, subordinate to a species.

subspinale (sŭb″spī-nā′lē) [″ + *spina*, thorn]. The deepest point between the nasal spine and the crest of the maxilla.

subspinous (sŭb-spī′nŭs) [″ + *spina*, thorn]. 1. Beneath any spinous process. 2. Anterior to or beneath the spinal column.

subspinous dislocation. Dislocation with head of the humerus resting below spine of the scapula.

substage (sŭb′stāj) [″ + O. Fr. *estage*, position]. That part of the microscope below the stage by which attachments are held in place.

substance (sŭb′stăns) [L. *substantia*]. Material of which any organ or tissue is composed; matter.

   s., anterior perforated. Portion of rhin-encephalon lying immediately anterior to optic chiasm. It is perforated by numerous small arteries.

   s., anterior pituitary-like. Chorionic gonadotropin. SEE: *gonadotropin.*

   s., black. Substantia nigra.

   s., chromophilic. Substance found in the cytoplasm of certain cells that stains similar to chromatin with basic dyes. Includes Nissl bodies of neurons and granules in serozymogenic cells.

   s., colloid. Jellylike substance in colloid degeneration.

   s., gray. Gray matter of the brain and spinal cord.

   s., ground. The matrix or intercellular substance in which the cells of an organ or tissue are embedded.

   s., ketogenic. Substance that, in its metabolism, gives rise to ketone bodies.

   s., medullary. The soft inner material of any part such as a bone or organ.

   s., Nissl. Chromatophilic substance of nerve cells. SEE: *Nissl bodies.*

   s., posterior perforated. A triangular area forming floor of the interpeduncular fossa. It lies immediately behind the corpora mammillaria and contains numerous openings for blood vessels.

   s., pressor. Substance that elevates arterial blood pressure.

   s., reticular. The skein of threads present in some red blood cells. These are visible only when the cells are appropriately stained.

   s., slow-reacting. SEE: *slow-reacting substance of anaphylaxis.*

   s., specific soluble. ABBR: SSS. A polysaccharide hapten obtained from the capsules of pneumococci.

   s., threshold, high. Substance such as glucose or sodium chloride present in the blood and excreted by the kidney only when its concentration exceeds a certain level.

   s., threshold, low. Substance such as urea or uric acid that is excreted by the kidney from the blood almost in its entirety. It occurs in the urine in high concentrations.

   s., transmitter. Neurotransmitter.

   s., white. White matter of brain and spinal cord.

   s., white, of Schwann. A nerve fiber's medullary sheath.

substance abuse. Prolonged use of drugs that cause physical and mental impairment, including alcohol.

substance P. An 11-amino acid peptide that is believed to be important as a neurotransmitter in the pain fiber system. This substance may also be important in eliciting local tissue reactions resembling inflammation. SEE: *neurotransmitter; pain.*

substandard. Failing to meet the usual or accepted standard.

substantia (sŭb-stăn'shē-ă) [L.]. Material of which any organ or tissue is composed; matter. SYN: *substance*.

s. alba. [NA] White substance of the brain. SEE: *matter, white.*

s. cinerea. Gray substance of the brain and spinal cord.

s. ferruginea. [NA] Elongated mass of pigmented cells in the locus ceruleus.

s. gelatinosa. [NA] Gray matter of the cord surrounding central canal and capping head of posterior horns of spinal cord.

s. grisea. [NA] Gray matter of the spinal cord. SEE: *matter, gray.*

s. nigra. [NA] Black substance in a section of the crus cerebri. SYN: *locus niger.*

s. propria membranae tympani. Fibrous middle layer of drum membrane.

substernal (sŭb-stěr'năl) [L. *sub*, under, below, + Gr. *sternon*, chest]. Situated beneath the sternum.

substernal thrust. In children, a thrusting of the substernal area of the chest. This indicates right ventricular hypertrophy. SEE: *apical heave.*

substernomastoid (sŭb-stěr-nō-măs'toyd) [" + " + Gr. *mastos*, breast, + *eidos*, form, shape]. Beneath the sternomastoid muscle.

substituent. One part of a molecule substituted with another atom or group.

substitute (sŭb'stĭ-tūt). Something that may be used in place of another.

s., blood. A fluid used to expand the plasma volume, but not a true substitute for the blood. Artificial substances capable of functioning as blood are being investigated, but no completely satisfactory ones are available.

substitution (sŭb-stĭ-tū'shŭn) [L. *substitutio*, replacing]. 1. Displacing an atom (or more than one) of an element in a compound by atoms of another element of equal valence. 2. In psychiatry, the ego defense mechanism of turning from an obstructed desire to one whose gratification is socially acceptable. 3. The turning from an obstructed form of behavior to a more primitive one, as a substitution neurosis. 4. The replacement of a substance by another. 5. In pharmacy, the replacement of one drug by another drug in dispensing. Usually a generic drug is substituted for a proprietary one.

substitution products. Compounds formed by an element or a radical replacing another element or radical in a compound.

substitution therapy. The use in treatment of a substance such as a product of glandular secretion (hormone or enzyme) to replace natural substance in the body. This method is employed when glands fail to secrete properly or the substance secreted is unavailable to tissues.

substitutive (sŭb'stĭ-tū"tĭv) [L. *substitutivus*]. Causing a change or substitution of characteristics.

substitutive therapy. Treatment to overcome an inflammation of a specific character by exciting an acute nonspecific inflammation.

substrate, substratum (sŭb'strāt, sŭb-strā'tŭm) [L. *substratum*, to lie under]. 1. An underlying layer or foundation. 2. A base, as of a pigment. 3. The substance acted upon, as by an enzyme. SYN: *zymolyte.* SEE: *enzyme.*

substructure (sŭb'strŭk-chūr). The underlying structure of supporting material.

subsultus (sŭb-sŭl'tŭs) [L., to leap up]. Any tremor, twitching, or spasmodic movement.

s. tendinum. Involuntary twitchings of muscles, esp. of arms and feet, causing movement of tendons. Observed in certain febrile conditions.

subsylvian (sŭb-sĭl'vē-ăn). Below the fissure of Sylvius.

subtarsal (sŭb-tăr'săl) [L. *sub*, under, below, + Gr. *tarsos*, a broad, flat surface]. Below the tarsus.

subtentorial. Located beneath the tentorium.

subterminal (sŭb-těr'mĭ-năl) [" + *terminus*, a boundary]. Close to the end of an extremity.

subtetanic (sŭb"tē-tăn'ĭk) [" + Gr. *tetanikos*, suffering from tetanus]. Moderately tetanic.

subthalamic (sŭb"thă-lăm'ĭk) [" + Gr. *thalamos*, inner chamber]. Located below the thalamus.

subthalamic nucleus. An elliptical mass of gray matter lying in the ventral thalamus above the cerebral peduncle and rostral to substantia nigra. It receives fibers from the globus pallidus.

subthalamus. Portion of the diencephalon lying below the thalamus and above the hypothalamus. SEE: *thalamus.*

subtile, subtle (sŭb'tĭl, sŭt'l) [L. *subtilis*, fine]. 1. Very fine or delicate. 2. Very acute. 3. Mentally acute or crafty or piercing, as sharp. 4. Causing injury without attracting attention, as subtle poisons or early symptoms of a disease.

subtilin (sŭb'tĭl-ĭn). An antibiotic biosynthesized by *Bacillus subtilis.* It is of low toxicity and effective against gram-positive organisms.

subtotal (sŭb-tō'tăl) [L. *sub*, under, below, + *totus*, all]. Less than total, as partial removal of a gland.

subtraction. Process by which undesired,

overlying structures can be removed from a radiographic image.

subtrapezial (sŭb″tră-pē′zē-ăl) [″ + Gr. *trapezion*, a little table]. Beneath the trapezius muscle.

subtribe (sŭb′trīb). In taxonomy, between a genus and a tribe.

subtrochanteric (sŭb″trō-kăn-tĕr′ĭk) [″ + Gr. *trochanter*, to run]. Below a trochanter.

subtrochlear (sŭb-trŏk′lē-ăr) [″ + Gr. *trokhileia*, system of pulleys]. Beneath the trochlea.

subtuberal (sŭb-tū′bĕr-ăl) [″ + *tuber*, a swelling]. Located under a tuber.

subtympanic (sŭb-tĭm-păn′ĭk) [″ + Gr. *tympanon*, drum]. Below the tympanum.

subumbilical (sŭb″ŭm-bĭl′ĭ-kăl) [″ + *umbilicus*, navel]. Below the umbilicus.

subumbilical space. Space within the body cavity below the navel, resembling a triangle in shape.

subungual, subunguial (sŭb-ŭng′gwăl, -gwē-ăl) [″ + *unguis*, nail]. Situated beneath the nail of a finger or toe.

subungual hematoma. Collection of blood under the nail as a result of trauma. Condition may be treated by heating the end of a paper clip and then placing its point against the nail. This permits a small hole to be melted painlessly in the nail. The blood is then permitted to escape from under the nail.

subunit. In chemistry, a portion of a compound that represents smaller part of the molecule than the remainder of the substance. SEE: *beta subunit.*

suburethral (sŭb″ū-rē′thrăl) [″ + Gr. *ourethra*, urethra]. Below the urethra.

subvaginal (sŭb-văj′ĭn-ăl) [″ + *vagina*, sheath]. 1. Below the vagina. 2. On inner side of any tubular sheathing membrane.

subvertebral (sŭb-vĕr′tĕ-brăl) [″ + *vertebra*, vertebra]. Beneath, or on ventral side of, the vertebral column or a vertebra.

subvirile (sŭb-vĭr′ĭl, -vī′rĭl) [″ + *virilis*, masculine]. Deficient in, or lacking, virility.

subvitrinal (sŭb-vĭt′rĭn-ăl) [″ + *vitrina*, vitreous body]. Located beneath the vitreous body.

subvolution (sŭb″vō-lū′shŭn) [″ + *volutus*, turning]. Method of turning over a flap surgically to prevent adhesions.

subwaking (sŭb-wāk′ĭng). Between waking and sleeping.

subzonal (sŭb-zō′năl). Beneath a zone.

subzygomatic (sŭb″zī-gō-măt′ĭk) [″ + Gr. *zygoma*, cheekbone]. Beneath the zygomatic bone.

succagogue (sŭk′ă-gŏg) [L. *succus*, juice, + Gr. *agogos*, leading]. 1. To stimulate glandular secretion. 2. A substance that

stimulates glandular secretion.

succedaneous (sŭk″sē-dā′nē-ŭs) [L. *succedaneus*, substituting]. Acting as a substitute or relating to one. In dentistry, it refers to the secondary or permanent set of teeth, which follow an earlier deciduous set.

succedaneum (sŭk″sē-dā′nē-ŭm) [L. *succedaneus*, substituting]. Something that may be used as a substitute.

succenturiate (sŭk″sĕn-tū′rē-āt) [L. *succenturiare*, to substitute]. Acting as a substitute.

succi. Pl. of succus.

succinate (sŭk′sĭ-nāt). Any salt of succinic acid.

succinic acid. SEE: *acid, succinic.*

succinylcholine chloride (sŭk″sĭ-nĭl-kō′lēn). USP. A drug used for its neuromuscular blocking effect. It is used as an adjuvant in surgical anesthesia, and to prevent trauma in electroconvulsive shock therapy. Trade names are Anectine and Sucostrin.

Caution: This drug should be used only by physicians who have had extensive training in its use and in a setting where facilities for respiratory and cardiovascular resuscitation are immediately at hand.

succinylsulfathiazole (sŭk″sĭ-nĭl-sŭl″fă-thī′ă-zōl). 2-(N^4-succinylsulfanilamido) thiazole. Because of lack of evidence of its clinical efficacy, the drug is no longer used.

succorrhea (sŭk-kō-rē′ă) [L. *succus*, juice, + Gr. *rhoia*, flow]. Unnatural increase in secretion of any juice, esp. of a digestive fluid.

succubus (sŭk′ū-bŭs) [L.]. 1. A nightmare. 2. An evil demon thought to have sexual intercourse with men during sleep.

succus (sŭk′kŭs) [L. *succus*, juice] (pl. *succi*). A juice or fluid secretion.

   s. entericus. The intestinal juice. It is alkaline. The secretion of the minute glands lining the small intestine.

   s. gastricus. The gastric juice.

   s. pyloricus. An alkaline secretion by the pyloric end of the stomach.

succussion (sŭ-kŭsh′ŭn) [L. *succussio*, a shaking]. Shaking of a person to detect the presence of fluid in the body cavity by listening for a splashing sound, esp. in the thorax.

suck [AS. *sucan*, to suck]. 1. To draw fluid into the mouth, as from the breast. 2. To exhaust air from a tube and thus siphon fluid from a container. 3. That which is drawn into the mouth by sucking.

sucking pad. Mass of fat in cheeks, esp. well developed in an infant, aiding it to suck. SEE: *buccal fat pad.*

suckle. To nurse at the breast.

Sucostrin Chloride. Trade name for succinylcholine chloride.

sucralfate. A medicine consisting of a complex formed from sucrose octasulfate and polyaluminum hydroxide. It is effective in treating peptic ulcer by forming a coating over the ulcer crater. The coating will stay in place for over 8 hours. The dose is one gram 1 hour before each meal and at bedtime. Trade name is Carafate. SEE: *peptic ulcer.*

sucrase (sū'krās) [Fr. *sucre*, sugar]. An enzyme in the intestinal juice that splits cane sugar into glucose and fructose, the two being absorbed into the portal circulation. SYN: *invertase.*

sucrose (sū'krōs) [Fr. *sucre*, sugar]. NF. A saccharose, $C_{12}H_{22}O_{11}$, obtained from sugar cane, sugar beet, and other sources. It is hydrolyzed in the intestine to glucose and fructose by sucrase present in intestinal juice.

ACTION/USES: Only a little is retained by the stomach, and it is all absorbed in the intestines. The lack of residue tends to cause constipation. Sucrose is stored by the hepatic cells of the liver after it is made into glycogen, for future use.

RS: carbohydrates; disaccharose; fructose; galactose; glucose; lactose; levulose; maltose.

sucrosemia (sū"krō-sē'mē-ă) [" + Gr. *haima*, blood]. Sucrose in the blood.

sucrose polyester. A nonabsorbable synthetic fat. It has been used experimentally as a fat substitute in treating obesity.

sucrosuria (sū"krō-sū'rē-ă) [" + Gr. *ouron*, urine]. Sucrose in the urine.

suction [LL. *suctio*, sucking]. The act of, or capacity for, sucking up by reduction of air pressure over part of the surface of a substance. SEE: *aspiration.*

　　s., nasogastric. Suction of gas, fluid and solid material from the gastrointestinal tract by use of a tube extending from the suction device to the stomach or intestines via the nasal passage. SEE: *Wangensteen tube.*

　　s., post-tussive. Suction sound over a lung cavity heard on auscultation after a cough.

suction abortion. Removing the products of conception from the uterus by using a device that sucks the tissues away from the lining of the uterus.

suction biopsy. Obtaining tissue by use of a device that applies suction to the area from which tissue is desired. This technique is used in obtaining tissue from the mucosa of the stomach and intestines.

suction lipectomy. SEE: *lipectomy, suction.*

suctorial (sŭk-tō'rē-ăl) [LL. *suctio*, sucking]. 1. Concerning sucking. 2. Equipped for

sucking.

Sudafed. Trade name for pseudephedrine hydrochloride.

sudamen (sū-dā'měn) [L., sweat] (pl. *sudamina*). Noninflammatory eruption from sweat glands characterized by whitish vesicles caused by the retention of sweat in corneous layer of the skin, appearing after profuse sweating or in certain febrile diseases, disappearing by absorption.

sudamina (sū-dăm'ĭn-ă). Pl. of sudamen.

sudaminal (sū-dăm'ĭ-năl) [L. *sudamen*, sweat]. Concerning sudamina, q.v.

Sudan (sū-dăn'). One of a number of related biological stains for which fats have a special affinity. Includes Sudan II, Sudan III (G), Sudan IV, and Sudan R.

sudanophil (sū-dăn'ō-fĭl) [*sudan* + Gr. *philein*, to love]. A leukocyte that stains readily with Sudan III, indicative of fatty degeneration.

sudanophilia (sū-dăn"ō-fĭl'ē-ă). Affinity for Sudan stains.

sudanophilic (sū-dăn"ō-fĭl'ĭk). Staining easily with Sudan stain.

sudation (sū-dā'shŭn) [L. *sudatio*]. 1. The act of sweating. 2. Excessive perspiration.

sudatoria (sū"dă-tō'rē-ă) [L.] (sing. *sudatorium*). Excessive sweating. SYN: *ephidrosis; hyperhidrosis.*

sudatorium (sū"dă-tō'rē-ŭm) [L. *sudatorium*, a sweating room] (pl. *sudatoria*). 1. A hot air bath or any bath to induce perspiration. 2. A room used to induce sweat baths.

sudden death. Death occurring unexpectedly and instantaneously or within one hour of onset of symptoms in a patient with or without known preexisting heart disease. Sudden death due to cardiac conditions occurs in the U.S. at the rate of one each minute.

ETIOL: A number of cardiovascular conditions, including ischemic heart disease, aortic stenosis, coronary embolism, myocarditis, ruptured or dissecting aortic aneurysm, Stokes-Adams syndrome, cerebrovascular accident, pulmonary thromboembolism, and other noncardiovascular-related disorders, such as disturbances of electrolyte balance, drug toxicity, or idiosyncrasy.

sudden infant death syndrome. ABBR: SIDS. The completely unexpected and unexplained death of an apparently well, or virtually well, infant. The most common cause of death between the second week and first year of life. In the U.S. SIDS is responsible for the deaths of approximately 7000 infants each year. This worldwide syndrome has been of a constant rate over the years. Occurs more frequently in the third and fourth months of life, in premature infants, in males, and in infants living in poverty. The deaths usually occur during sleep and are more likely to happen in winter than in summer. SYN: *crib death.* SEE: *apnea; apnea alarm mattress.*

ETIOL: The cause is uncertain at this time. SIDS cannot be predicted or prevented.

NOTE: Loss of an infant because of SIDS may produce a severe grief and guilt reaction. Thus, the family needs expert counseling in the several months after the death.

Further information can be obtained from the National SIDS Foundation, 2 Metro Plaza, Suite 104, 8200 Professional Pl., Landover, MD 20785.

Sudeck's disease or atrophy (soo'dĕks) [Paul Herman Martin Sudeck, Ger. surgeon, 1866–1938]. Acute atrophy of the bone at the site of an injury. SYN: *traumatic osteoporosis.*

sudokeratosis (sū"dō-kĕr"ă-tō'sĭs) [L. *sudor,* sweat, + Gr. *keras,* horn, + *osis,* condition]. Circumscribed horny overgrowths that obstruct the sweat ducts.

sudomotor (sū"dō-mō'tor) [" + *motor,* a mover]. Pert. to stimulating the secretion of sweat; noting certain nerves.

sudor (sū'dor) [L.]. Secretion from the sweat glands. SYN: *perspiration; sweat.*

RS: anhidrosis; bromidrosis; chromidrosis; hematidrosis; hydrosis; perspiration; pore; skin; sudorific; sweat; uridrosis.

s. cruentus. Blood-tinged sweat. SYN: *hematidrosis.*

sudoral (sū'dor-ăl). Pert. to, caused by, or marked by perspiration.

sudoresis (sū"dō-rē'sĭs) [L.]. Profuse sweating. SYN: *diaphoresis.*

sudoriferous (sū-dor-ĭf'ĕr-ŭs) [" + *ferre,* to bear]. Conveying or producing sweat.

sudoriferous glands. Sweat-secreting glands of the skin.

sudorific (sū"dor-ĭf'ĭk) [L. *sudorificus*]. 1. Secreting or promoting the secretion of sweat. 2. Agent that produces sweating. SYN: *diaphoretic.*

sudoriparous (sū"dor-ĭp'ă-rŭs) [L. *sudor,* sweat, + *parere,* to produce]. Secreting sweat. SYN: *sudoriferous.*

suet (sū'ĕt) [Fr. *sewet,* suet]. Hard fat from cattle or sheep kidneys and loins. Used as the base of certain ointments and as an emollient.

suffocate (sŭf'ō-kāt) [L. *suffocare*]. To impair respiration; to smother, asphyxiate.

suffocation (sŭf"ō-kā'shŭn). 1. State of being choked by obstruction of air passages by drowning, smothering, throttling, or inhalation of noxious gases. SYN: *asphyxiation.* SEE: *asphyxia; resuscitation; unconsciousness.* 2. Act of obstructing the air passages.

SYM: Insensibility, breathing slight, face purple and swollen, livid lips. Symptoms not always present.

TREAT: Dash cold water in face. Slap chest. Apply aromatic spirits of ammonia to nostrils. Artificial respiration. Tracheotomy may be required.

suffusion (sŭ-fū'zhŭn) [L. *suffusio,* a pouring over]. 1. Spreading of a bodily fluid into surrounding tissues. SYN: *extravasation.* 2. Pouring of a fluid over the body as treatment.

sugar [O. Fr. *zuchre*]. A sweet-tasting carbohydrate belonging to the monosaccharose and disaccharose groups. Crystalline carbohydrates of comparatively low molecular weight and generally having a sweet taste. Sugar has been used as a thin paste applied to the area to treat infected wounds and ulcers. SEE: *bedsore; carbohydrates.*

CLASSIF: They are classified in two ways: the number of atoms of simple sugars yielded on hydrolysis by a molecule of the given sugar and the number of carbon atoms in the molecules of the simple sugars so obtained. Thus, dextrose, q.v., is a monosaccharide because it cannot be hydrolyzed to a simpler sugar; it is a hexose because it contains six carbon atoms per molecule. Sucrose is a disaccharide because on hydrolysis it yields two molecules, one of dextrose and one of levulose.

s., beet. Sucrose obtained from sugar beets.

s., blood. The carbohydrate present in the blood, principally glucose.

s., brain. Galactose.

s., cane. Sucrose obtained from sugar cane.

s., diabetic. Glucose in the urine of diabetics.

s., fruit. Levulose or fructose.

s., grape. Glucose.

s., invert. Mixture consisting of one molecule of glucose and one of fructose resulting from the hydrolysis of sucrose.

s., liver. Glycogen.

s., malt. Maltose.

s., milk. Lactose.

s., muscle. Inositol; it is not a true sugar.

s., starch. Dextrin, a carbohydrate but not a true sugar.

s., wood. Xylose.

sugar, words pert. to: aglycosuric; blood; carbohydrates; dextrose; disaccharide; fructose; galactose; glucide; hypoglycemia; invert; invertase; lactose; levulose; mannitol; melitemia; monosaccharide; pentose; pentosuria; polysaccharide; sucrose; xylose; words beginning with "gluco-," "glyco-," and "sacchar-."

sugar as a therapeutic agent. Sugar has

been applied directly to decubitus ulcers to aid the healing process. Also, sugar taken orally or in appropriate I.V. solution is quite beneficial in preventing the hypoglycemia caused by excess insulin dose.

suggestibility (sŭg-jĕs″tĭ-bĭl′ĭ-tē) [L. *suggestus,* suggested]. A condition in which a person responds readily to suggestions or opinions of another. SYN: *sympathism.*

suggestible (sŭg-jĕs′tĭ-bl). Very susceptible to the opinions or suggestions of others.

suggestion (sŭg-jĕs′chŭn) [L. *suggestio*]. 1. Imparting of an idea indirectly; act of implying. 2. The idea so conveyed. 3. The psychological process of having an individual adopt or accept an idea without argument or persuasion.

   s., auto-. Self-suggestion as distinguished from that coming from another person, esp. in hypnotic state.

   s., hypnotic. Suggestion placed in the mind of a person while under the influence of hypnosis.

   s., posthypnotic. Suggestion made to a subject while under hypnosis. After emerging from the hypnotic state, the person usually performs the suggested act.

suggestive (sŭg-jĕs′tĭv). Stimulating or pert. to suggestion.

suggestive medicine. Therapy by suggestion during either consciousness or hypnosis.

suggestive therapeutics. The practice of treating disease by hypnotic suggestions.

suicide (sū′ĭ-sīd) [L. *sui,* of oneself, + *caedere,* to kill]. Intentionally and voluntarily taking one's own life. In the U.S., approximately 30,000 people commit suicide each year. This is equivalent to one suicide every 20 minutes. Most of these persons have consulted with a physician in the six months prior to death, and 10% have seen a physician during the week preceding suicide.

During the last 30 years, the rate of suicide in persons 15 to 24 years of age, particularly in young men, has tripled. From this information it is obvious that physicians and other health care workers have great potential for recognizing and treating individuals at risk of taking their own lives.

Persons at high risk of suicide include older white males without a spouse, unemployed, and in poor health; depressed patients; alcoholics; drug addicts; and those with clinical conditions, including spinal cord injuries, cancer (particularly in male patients shortly after diagnosis), schizophrenia, or seizure disorders. Suicide occurs in hospitalized patients at 3½ times the rate of the general population.

Patients admitted for accidents are believed to be at high risk because the "accident" was in fact a suicide attempt. Health care professionals should be alert to warning signs of suicide, such as statements indicating a desire to die or prediction that suicide will occur. Persons contemplating suicide may be depressed, act to get their lives in order, may give away possessions, have failing grades or poor work performance, take risks, or have a history of alcoholism or drug abuse.

Management of persons who are contemplating or have attempted suicide includes removal of lethal means from them and the provision of professional, social, and family support. If the patient is being treated as an outpatient, then he or she should be scheduled for specific future appointments and informed of a telephone number where help or assistance will be immediately available on a 24-hour basis. During a crisis, the patient should not be left alone even for a few minutes. For medicolegal reasons, careful and complete medical records should be kept concerning the plans and actions for management of the patient. SEE: *Samaritans.*

suicide, assisted. SEE: *assisted suicide.*

suicide clusters. A cluster, q.v., of suicides within a defined location and time.

suicidology (soo″ĭ-sīd-ŏl′ō-jē) [″ + ″ + Gr. *logos,* word, reason]. The science of suicide including its cause, prediction of those susceptible, and prevention.

suint (swĭnt). The crude oily substance containing potassium obtained from lamb's wool. Lanolin is obtained from this substance.

suit. 1. Lawsuit; legal action; court proceeding by one party against another for damages or other legal remedies. 2. An outer garment.

   s., anti-G. SEE: *anti-G suit.*

sulcal (sŭl′kăl) [L.]. Pert. to a sulcus.

sulcal artery. A tiny branch of the anterior spinal artery.

sulcate, sulcated (sŭl′kāt, -ĕd) [L. *sulcatus*]. Furrowed or grooved.

sulciform (sŭl′sĭ-form) [L. *sulcus,* groove, + *forma,* form]. Resembling a sulcus.

sulculus (sŭl′kū-lŭs) [L.]. A small sulcus.

sulcus (sŭl′kŭs) [L., groove] (pl. *sulci*). A furrow, groove, slight depression, or fissure, esp. of the brain.

   s., alveololingual. The space in the floor of the mouth between the base of the tongue and the alveolar ridge, on each side extending from the frenum of the tongue back to the retromolar wall.

   s., calcarine. A deep horizontal fissure on the medial surface of the occipital lobe of the brain.

   s. centralis. Fissure dividing the frontal and parietal lobes of each cerebral hemisphere. SYN: *fissure, Rolando's.*

s., collateral. Sulcus on the tentorial surface of the brain. It bounds the inferior lingual gyrus and is parallel to the calcarine and postcalcarine sulci.

sulci cutis. The ridges on the skin of the palmar surface of the fingers and toes. These comprise the fingerprints.

s., gingival. The space or crevice between the free gingiva and the tooth surface; the depth of the sulcus varies according to the state of oral hygiene, deepening to become a periodontal pocket.

s., hippocampal. Sulcus on the medial side of the hippocampal gyrus.

s., intraparietal. Groove that separates the inferior from the superior parietal bones and lobes.

s. precentralis. [NA] An interrupted sulcus generally parallel with the fissure of Rolando and anterior to it.

s. pulmonalis. [NA] Depression on either side of the vertebral column.

s. spiralis cochleae. Groove between the labium tympanicum and labium vestibulare.

Sulf-10. Trade name for sulfacetamide sodium, 10%.

sulfacetamide (sŭl″fă-sĕt′ă-mīd). An antibacterial sulfonamide that is highly soluble. It is particularly useful for topical application to the eye.

s., sodium. USP. A very soluble sulfonamide used in solution to treat infections of the cornea and conjunctiva. Trade names are Belph-10 Liquifilm, Sulamyd Sodium, and Isopto Cetamide.

sulfadiazine (sŭl″fă-dī′ă-zēn). USP. One of a group of diazine derivatives of sulfanilamide. Because it readily penetrates the blood-brain barrier, it has been used extensively in treating meningococcal meningitis. Some strains of meningococci have become resistant to sulfadiazine.

s., silver. USP. SEE: *silver sulfadiazine.*

sulfa drugs. Drugs of the sulfonamide group possessing bacteriostatic properties. SEE: *sulfonamides.*

sulfamerazine (sŭl″fă-mĕr′ă-zēn). USP. An antibacterial sulfonamide that is more readily absorbed than sulfadiazine, from which it is derived. SEE: *sulfadiazine.*

sulfamethazine (sŭl″fă-mĕth′ă-zēn). USP. An antibacterial sulfonamide similar to sulfadiazine.

sulfamethizole (sŭl″fă-mĕth′ĭ-zōl). USP. A sulfonamide used in treating urinary tract infections. Trade names are Proklar and Thiosulfil.

sulfamethoxazole (sŭl″fă-mĕth-ŏks′ă-zōl). USP. A sulfonamide used in treating urinary tract infections. Usually used in com-

bination with trimethoprim. Trade name is Gantanol. SEE: *trimethoprim.*

Sulfamylon. Trade name for mafenide.

sulfanilamide (sŭl″făn-ĭl′ă-mīd). Para-aminobenzenesulfonamide. White, slightly bitter crystalline substance from coal tar, the parent of the azo dyes. Formerly it was widely used in the treatment of a number of infections, but because of its toxic reactions it has been superseded by more effective and less toxic sulfonamides.

sulfapyridine (sŭl″fă-pĭr′ĭ-dēn). USP. A sulfonamide that is used only in treating dermatitis herpetiformis.

s., sodium monohydrate. A soluble salt of sulfapyridine for intravenous use only.

sulfarsphenamine (sŭlf″ăr-sfĕn′ă-mēn). A sulfur compound, containing 19% arsenic; effective in treating syphilis.

sulfasalazine (sŭl″fă-săl′ă-zēn). USP. A sulfonamide that is poorly absorbed from the gastrointestinal tract. It is used in treating ulcerative colitis. Trade names are Azulfidine and SAS-500.

sulfatase (sŭl′fă-tās). An enzyme that hydrolyzes sulfuric acid esters.

sulfate (sŭl′fāt) [L. *sulphas*]. A salt or ester of sulfuric acid.

s., cupric. USP. The penta hydrate salt of copper, $CuSO_4 .5H_2O$, used as an antidote in treating phosphorus poisoning.

s., ferrous. USP. An iron compound used in treating iron-deficiency anemia.

s., iron. Green vitriol; copperas. Fatal in large dosage. SEE: *ferrous sulfate; copper salts* in *Poisons and Poisoning* in *Appendix.*

s., magnesium. Magnesium sulfate.

sulfathiazole (sŭl″fă-thī′ă-zōl). A rapidly absorbed and excreted sulfanilamide compound. Largely replaced by less toxic sulfonamides.

sulfatide (sŭl′fă-tīd). Any cerebroside with a sulfate radical esterified to the galactose.

sulfhemoglobin (sŭlf″hēm-ō-glō′bĭn). Substance formed by action of hydrogen sulfide on blood. SYN: *sulfmethemoglobin.*

sulfhemoglobinemia (sŭlf″hēm-ō-glō″bĭn-ē′mē-ă). Persistent cyanotic condition due to sulfhemoglobin in blood.

sulfhydryl (sŭlf-hī′drĭl). The univalent radical, SH, of sulfur and hydrogen.

sulfide (sŭl′fīd). Any compound of sulfur with an element or base.

sulfinpyrazone (sŭl″fĭn-pī′ră-zōn). USP. A drug used to promote excretion of uric acid in the urine. Trade name is Anturane.

sulfisoxazole (sŭl″fĭ-sŏk′să-zōl). USP. A sulfonamide used for treating certain bacterial infections, esp. certain urinary tract infections. Trade names are SK-Soxazole and Gantrisin.

sulfmethemoglobin (sŭlf″mĕt-hē″mō-glō′

bĭn). The greenish hemoglobin compound formed when hemoglobin and hydrogen sulfide are combined. SYN: *sulfhemoglobin*.

sulfo-. A combining form usually indicating the presence of the sulfo- group, $-SO_3OH$.

sulfobromophthalein (sŭl″fō-brō″mō-thăl′ē-ĭn). USP. A drug administered intravenously in testing liver function.

sulfonamides. A group of compounds consisting of amides of sulfanilic acid derived from their parent compound sulfanilamide. They are bacteriostatic, their action on bacteria resulting from interference with functioning of enzyme systems necessary for normal metabolism, growth, and multiplication.

sulfone (sŭl′fōn). An oxidation product of sulfur compound in which the $=SO_2$ is united to two hydrocarbon radicals.

sulfourea (sŭl″fō-ū-rē′ă). Urea with oxygen replaced by sulfur. SYN: *thiourea*.

sulfoxide (sŭl-fŏk′sīd). The divalent radical $=SO$.

sulfoxone sodium (sŭl-fŏks′ŏn). USP. A drug used in treating leprosy and dermatitis herpetiformis. The leprosy bacillus has, in some areas, become resistant to this drug.

sulfur (sŭl′fŭr) [L.]. SYMB: S. At. wt. 32.06, at. no. 16; sp. gr. 2.07. A pale yellow, crystalline element that burns with a blue flame, producing sulfur dioxide.

The amount of sulfur excreted in urine varies with amount of protein in diet but more or less parallels the amount of nitrogen excreted, as both are derived from protein catabolism. The S:N ratio is approx. 1:14, i.e., for each gm of sulfur excreted, 14 gm of nitrogen are excreted. The amount of sulfur excreted daily is about 1 gm. It is oxidized to sulfate and required for the synthesis of body proteins as cystine, cysteine, or their combination.

DEFICIENCY SYM: Dermatitis, imperfect development of hair and nails. Deficiency of cystine or cysteine proteins in diet restricts growth and may be fatal. Tissue oxidation of cystine forms inorganic sulfate if the protein intake is sufficient.

   s. dioxide. An irritating gas used in industry to manufacture acids. Also used in mechanical refrigerators. A bactericide and important disinfectant.

   s., precipitated. USP. A form of sulfur used in various skin diseases, including scabies. Its keratolytic effect helps to make it effective in those disorders.

   s., sublimed. USP. A form of sulfur used in various skin diseases. Its keratolytic effect helps to make it effective in those disorders. It is a scabicide.

sulfurated, sulfureted (sŭl′fū-rā″tĕd, -rĕt″ĕd). Combined or impregnated with sulfur.

sulfurated hydrogen. H_2S. A colorless, inflammable gas of disagreeable odor resulting from decomposition of organic matter containing sulfur; used as a chemical reagent. SYN: *hydrogen sulfide*.

sulfuric acid (sŭl-fū′rĭk). A colorless, odorless liquid of heavy, oily consistency. It is extremely caustic and corrosive. It is widely used in manufacturing. SYN: *vitriol, oil of*.

   s.a., dilute. An aqueous 10% solution of H_2SO_4. Used as an astringent and for gastric hypoacidity.

sulfuric acid poisoning. Sulfuric acid is sometimes accidentally taken by mouth, as it resembles syrup or glycerin.

SYM: Local effects. Burning, with destruction of skin. If it strikes eye, it may result in blindness. If taken by mouth, intense injury to mucosa extending from mouth to esophagus and down to stomach, causing marked, excruciating pain, swelling of affected tissues; salivation; painful swallowing; often gasping for breath, and hoarse voice. Mucous membrane has a grayish-white coating. There is persistent, painful vomiting. Patient quickly goes into shock.

TREAT: Dilute acid with large volumes of water. Neutralize acid with milk of magnesia, baking soda, or other well-diluted alkalies. Follow by soothing substances, as raw eggs. SEE: *acids* at *Poisons and Poisoning* in *Appendix*.

Caution: Do not attempt gastric lavage by using a stomach tube if poisoning has occurred more than an hour previously.

---

sumac (soo′măk). General term applied to several species of *Rhus*.

   s., poison. A type of sumac that causes a contact dermatitis. SEE: *poison sumac*.

summation (sŭm-ā′shŭn) [L. *summatio*, adding]. Cumulative action or effect, as of stimuli. Thus an organ reacts to two or more weak stimuli as if they were a single strong one.

summer (sŭm′ĕr) [AS. *sumer*]. The warmest season of the year, occurring between spring and autumn.

Sumycin. Trade name for tetracycline hydrochloride.

sunburn [AS. *sunne*, sun, + *bernan*, to burn]. Dermatitis due to excessive exposure to the actinic rays of the sun. The rays that produce the characteristic changes in the skin are ultraviolet, between 290 and 320 nanometers (sunburn rays). Some people are more resistant to these rays than others, but the skin will be damaged in anyone who has sufficient exposure.

PREVENTION: Avoid direct exposure of the skin to sunlight between 10 a.m. and 3 p.m., when sunburn rays are generally present. Wear clothing to cover the skin, or use a sun-blocking agent with a sun protective factor (SPF) of 15. This should be reapplied each hour if the person is sweating heavily.

TREAT: Cool, wet dressings applied to burned area if reaction is moderate. For severe sunburn, use lukewarm baths with oatmeal or cornstarch and baking soda. Aspirin or other nonsteroidal anti-inflammatory agents may reduce inflammation and pain.

Sunday morning paralysis. Radial nerve palsy, sometimes the indirect result of acute alcoholism resulting from stuporous patient lying immobile with arm pressed over a projecting surface. SYN: *Saturday night paralysis.*

sunflower eyes. Slang term for the appearance of the eyes of patients with Wilson's disease. Deposits of copper around the edge of the cornea (Kayser-Fleischer rings) cause this condition.

sunglasses. Eyeglasses that protect the eyes from exposure to visible as well as ultraviolet rays. Because of the great variability of sunglasses to perform this function, it is advisable for the potential user to consult an ophthalmologist or optometrist concerning the need for sunglasses and the type needed. SEE: *glasses, sun-.*

sunscreen. Substance used to protect the skin from ultraviolet radiation of the sun. Usually applied as an ointment or cream. SEE: *ultraviolet radiation.*

sunscreen protective factor index. In preparations (sunscreens) for protecting the skin from the sun, the ratio of the amount of exposure needed to produce a minimal erythema response with the sunscreen in place divided by the amount of exposure required to produce the same reaction without the sunscreen.

sunstroke (sŭn′strōk) [AS. *sunne*, sun, + *strake*, a blow]. An acute and dangerous reaction to heat exposure. Characterized by high body temperature, usually above 105°F (40.6°C); cessation of sweating; headache; numbness; tingling and confusion prior to sudden delirium or coma; fast pulse; rapid respiratory rate; usually elevated blood pressure. The basic defect is failure of the heat-regulating mechanisms of the body. SYN: *heatstroke.*

TREAT: Effective therapy may save the patient's life. Without delay, the nude patient should be placed in a bathtub filled with ice water. This will not cause pain, shock, or cutaneous vasoconstriction. The patient's temperature will need to be monitored carefully. Remove from bath when body temperature falls to 103°F (39.4°C). If ice water and a bathtub are not available, place wet sheets on nude body, fan vigorously, and massage the skin. The use of sedatives may be required to control convulsions. Careful observation of patient for signs of fluid imbalance and renal failure will be required for several days.

suntan. Darkening of the skin due to exposure to the sun. SEE: *photoaging; tanning salon; sunburn; sunscreen.*

super- [L., over, above]. Combining form meaning above, beyond, superior.

superabduction (soo″pĕr-ăb-dŭk′shŭn) [L. *super*, over, above, + *abducens*, drawing away]. Pronounced or extreme abduction.

superacidity (soo″pĕr-ă-sĭd′ĭ-tē). Excess acidity.

superacromial (soo″pĕr-ă-krō′mē-ăl). Supra-acromial.

superactivity (soo″pĕr-ăk-tĭv′ĭ-tē). Hyperactivity.

superacute (soo″pĕr-ă-kūt′) [″ + *acutus*, sharp]. Markedly acute.

superalimentation (soo″pĕr-ăl″ĭ-mĕn-tā′shŭn) [″ + *alimentum*, nourishment]. Therapeutic administration of food in excess of body needs or appetite. SYN: *hyperalimentation.*

superalkalinity (soo″pĕr-ăl″kă-lĭn′ĭ-tē) [″ + *alkalinus*, alkaline]. Excessive alkalinity.

superciliary (soo″pĕr-sĭl′ē-ă-rē) [L. *supercilium*, eyebrow]. Pert. to or in the region of an eyebrow.

supercilium (soo″pĕr-sĭl′ē-ŭm) [L.]. (pl. *supercilia*) 1. [NA] Eyebrow. 2. A hair of the eyebrow.

superclass (soo′pĕr-klăs). In taxonomy, between a phylum and a class.

superduct (soo″pĕr-dŭkt′) [L. *super*, over, above, + *ducere*, to lead]. To elevate.

superego (soo″pĕr-ē′gō) [″ + *ego*, I; later translators of Freud's writings feel the word *uber-ich* should have been translated to over-I or upper-I and not to superego]. In freudian psychoanalytical theory, the portion of the personality associated with ethics, self-criticism, and the moral standard of the community. It is formed in infancy by the individual's adopting as his or her personal standards the values of the significant persons with whom he or she identifies. This serves to help form the conscience. The superego functions to protect and to reward when the ego-ideal of behavior or thought is satisfied; and to criticize, punish, and evoke a sense of guilt when the reverse is true. In neuroses, symptoms develop when instinctual drives conflict with those dictated by the superego. SEE: *ego.*

superexcitation (soo″pĕr-ĕk″sī-tā′shŭn) [″ + *excitatio*, excitation]. Excess excitement.

superextension (soo″pĕr-ĕks-tĕn′shŭn) [″ + *extensio*, extension]. Excess extension.

superfamily (soo″pĕr-făm′ĭ-lē). In taxonomy, between an order and a family.

superfecundation (soo″pĕr-fē″kŭn-dā′shŭn) [″ + *fecundare*, to fertilize]. Successive fertilization by two or more separate instances of sexual intercourse of two or more ova formed during the same menstrual cycle. Fertilization may be by the same male or by two different males.

superfemale. A female having three X chromosomes.

superfetation (soo″pĕr-fē-tā′shŭn) [″ + *fetus*, fetus]. Fertilization of two ova in the same uterus at different menstrual periods within a short interval. SYN: *hypercyesis*.

superficial (soo″pĕr-fish′ăl) [L. *superficialis*]. 1. Confined to the surface. 2. Not thorough; cursory.

superficialis (soo″pĕr-fĭsh-ē-ā′lĭs) [L.]. Superficial; noting a structure such as an artery, vein, or nerve that is near the surface.

superficial reflex. Reflex induced by very light stimulus, such as stroking skin lightly with soft cotton wad.

superficies (soo″pĕr-fĭsh′ē-ēz) [L.]. An outer surface.

superflexion (soo″pĕr-flĕk′shŭn) [L. *super*, over, above, + *flexio*, flexion]. Excess flexion.

supergenual (soo″pĕr-jĕn′ū-ăl) [″ + *genu*, knee]. Above the knee.

superglue. An extremely strong adhesive made of cyanoacrylate.

Caution: This glue is quite effective in gluing skin to skin. Thus, avoid contact with it, esp. on the eyelids.

superimpregnation (soo″pĕr-ĭm″prĕg-nā′shŭn) [″ + *impregnare*, to make pregnant]. Conception during pregnancy; fertilization from two different ovulations. SEE: *superfecundation; superfetation.*

superinduce (soo″pĕr-ĭn-dūs′) [″ + *in*, into, + *ducere*, to lead]. To bring on, over, or above an already existing condition or situation.

superinfection (soo″pĕr-ĭn-fĕk′shŭn) [″ + *infectio*, a putting into]. A new infection caused by an organism different from that which caused the initial infection. The microbe responsible is usually resistant to the treatment given for the initial infection.

superinvolution (soo″pĕr-ĭn-vō-lū′shŭn) [″ + *involutus*, a turning]. Excessive reduction of the uterus to less than its normal size following childbirth. SYN: *hyperinvolution.*

superior (soo-pē′rē-or) [L. *superus*, upper]. 1. [NA] Higher than; situated above something else. 2. Better than. 3. One in charge of others.

superiority complex. An exaggerated conviction of one's own superiority; a pretense of superiority in order to compensate for one's feeling of inferiority.

superior vena cava syndrome. Partial occlusion of the superior vena cava with resulting interference of venous blood flow from the head and neck to the heart. This is usually due to some form of cancer.

SYM: Venous engorgement and edema of the head and neck.

superjacent (soo″pĕr-jā′sĕnt). Immediately above.

superlactation (soo″pĕr-lăk-tā′shŭn) [L. *super*, over, above, + *lactatio*, a sucking]. Oversecretion of milk, or continuance of lactation beyond normal time.

superlethal (soo″pĕr-lē′thăl) [″ + Gr. *lethe*, oblivion]. A dose of a drug, or exposure to trauma, greater than that required to produce death.

supermedial (soo″pĕr-mē′dē-ăl) [″ + *medium*, middle]. Above the middle.

supermoron (soo″pĕr-mō′rŏn) [″ + Gr. *moros*, stupid]. One only slightly mentally deficient.

supermotility (soo″pĕr-mō-tĭl′ĭ-tē) [″ + *motilis*, moving]. Excessive motility in any part. SYN: *hyperkinesia.*

supernatant (soo″pĕr-nā′tănt) [″ + *natare*, to float]. 1. Floating on surface, as oil on water. 2. The clear liquid remaining at the top after a precipitate settles. 3. The cell-derived fluids containing chemical mediators that develop in a laboratory culture of leukocytes mixed with an antigen or mitogen, q.v., stimulus. Supernatants can be assessed for the presence of monokines or lymphokines by adding them to other white blood cell cultures and measuring cell proliferation and activity.

supernate (soo′pĕr-nāt). A supernatant fluid.

supernumerary (soo″pĕr-nū′mĕr-ăr″ē) [L. *supernumerarius*]. Exceeding the regular number.

supernumerary teeth. More than the usual number of teeth. Extra teeth develop in approx. 2% of the population, with almost all of them being maxillary incisors or mesiodens, q.v. Cleft palate or other developmental disturbances disrupt the dental lamina and often result in palatal supernumerary teeth.

supernutrition (soo″pĕr-nū-trĭ′shŭn) [L. *super*, over, above, + *nutritio*, nourish]. More than normal nutrition. SEE: *hyperalimentation.*

superolateral (soo″pĕr-ō-lăt′ĕr-ăl) [″ + *latus*, side]. Above and to the side.

superovulation (soo″pĕr-ŏv″ū-lā′shŭn) [″ + *ovulum*, little egg]. Increased frequency of ovulation or production of a greater number of ova at one time. This is usually caused by the administration of gonadotropins.

superoxide. A highly reactive form of oxygen ($\overline{O}_2$), the superoxide anion, produced when oxygen is reduced by a single electron. Superoxide is produced during the normal catalytic function of certain enzymes, by the oxidation of hemoglobin to methemoglobin, and when ionizing radiation passes through water. It is also produced when granulocytes phagocytose bacteria. Superoxide is destroyed by the enzyme superoxide dismutase, which catalyzes the conversion of two molecules of superoxide anion to one molecule of oxygen and one of hydrogen peroxide: $\overline{O}_2 + \overline{O}_2 + 2H^+ \leftrightarrow H_2O_2 + O_2$.

superoxide dismutase. Enzyme that destroys superoxide. One form of the enzyme contains manganese and another contains copper and zinc.

superparasite (soo″pĕr-păr′ă-sīt) [″ + Gr. *para*, beside, + *sitos*, food]. 1. A parasite that lives upon another parasite. 2. A parasite involved in superparasitism.

superparasitism (soo″pĕr-păr′ă-sī″tĭzm) [″ + ″ + *-ismos*, condition]. Condition in which the host is infested or infected with a greater number of parasites than can be supported.

superphosphate (soo″pĕr-fŏs′fāt). Acid phosphate.

supersaturate. To add more of a substance to a solution than can be dissolved permanently.

superscription (soo″pĕr-skrĭp′shŭn) [L. *super*, over, above, + *scriptio*, a writing]. The beginning of a prescription noted by the sign ℞, signifying (L.) *recipe*, take.

supersecretion (soo″pĕr-sē-krē′shŭn) [″ + *secretio*, separation]. An excess of any secretion.

supersensitiveness (soo″pĕr-sĕn′sĭ-tĭv″nĕs) [″ + *sensitivus*, feeling]. Excessive susceptibility to a foreign protein or other antigenic substance. SYN: *hypersensitiveness*.

supersoft (soo″pĕr-sŏft′) [″ + AS. *softe*, soft]. Exceptionally soft; noting roentgen rays of extremely long wavelength and low penetrating power.

supersonic (soo″pĕr-sŏn′ĭk) [″ + *sonus*, sound]. 1. Pert. to vibrations of sound space waves of frequencies above 20,000 cycles per second, which are inaudible to the human ear. SYN: *ultrasonic*. 2. Used to describe speeds greater than that of sound. At sea level, in air at 0°C, the speed of sound is about 331 meters, or 1087 feet per second (741 miles per hour).

superstructure (soo″pĕr-strŭk′chŭr). The visible portion of a structure, esp. those parts external to the main structure.

supertension (soo″pĕr-tĕn′shŭn) [″ + *tensio*, a stretching]. Extremely high tension.

supervenosity (soo″pĕr-vē-nŏs′ĭ-tē). Abnormally decreased oxygen in the venous blood.

supervention (soo″pĕr-vĕn′shŭn) [L. *superventio*, a coming over]. The development of an additional condition as a complication to an existing disease.

supervirulent (soo″pĕr-vĭr′ū-lĕnt) [L. *super*, over, above, + *virulentus*, full of poison]. More virulent than usual.

supervisor (soo′pĕr-vīz″ĕr) [L. *supervisus*, having looked over]. One who directs and evaluates the performance of others. In a health care setting, the supervisor has the knowledge and skills to provide the same service as those being directed, e.g., the supervisor of the pharmacy, physical therapy, or maternity nursing.

supervitaminosis. Excess accumulation of vitamins in the body due to administration of an excess dose. SYN: *hypervitaminosis*.

supervoltage (soo′pĕr-vŏl″tĭj). A term applied to x-rays produced by very high voltage.

supinate (sū′pĭ-nāt) [L. *supinatus*, bent backward]. 1. To turn the forearm or hand so that the palm faces upward. 2. To rotate the foot and leg outward. 3. A triplanar motion of the foot involving the accessory motions of inversion, plantarflexion and adduction so that the sole of the foot rotates inward and upward. If the foot is fixed on the ground when the hind foot supinates, the arch of the foot increases. Opposite of pronate.

supination (sū″pĭn-ā′shŭn) [L. *supinatio*]. 1. Turning of the palm or the hand anteriorly or the foot inward and upward. 2. Act of lying flat upon the back. 3. Condition of being on the back or having the palm of the hand facing upward or the foot turned inward and upward.

supinator (sū″pĭn-ā′tor) [L.]. A muscle producing the motion of supination of the forearm. SEE: *Muscles* in *Appendix*.

supinator longus reflex. Flexion of the forearm caused by tapping of the tendon of the supinator longus. SYN: *brachioradial reflex*.

supine (sū-pīn′) [L. *supinus*, lying on the back]. 1. Lying on the back with the face upward. 2. Noting position of the hand or foot with the palm or foot facing upward. Opposite of prone.

suppedania (sŭp″ĕ-dā′nē-ă) [L. *sub*, under, + *pes*, foot]. Applications to the soles of the feet.

supplemental (sŭp″lĕ-mĕn′tăl) [L. *supple-*

mentum, an addition]. Referring to something added to supply a need or to reinforce.

supplemental air. The air that by the most forcible effort can be expelled after an ordinary expiration that has followed a normal inspiration. In adult males, it averages about 1500 cc. SYN: *reserve air.*

support (sŭp-port'). 1. That which assists in maintaining something in place. 2. In dentistry, the abutting teeth, alveolar ridge, and mucosal tissues upon which the denture rests.

suppository (sŭ-pŏz'ĭ-tō-rē) [L. *suppositorium*, something placed underneath] (pl. *suppositories*). A semisolid substance for introduction into the rectum, vagina, or urethra, where it dissolves. It often serves as a vehicle for medicines to be absorbed. Commonly shaped like cylinder or cone and made of soap, glycerinated gelatin, or cocoa butter (oil of theobroma).

NURSING IMPLICATIONS: Provide privacy. Instruct the patient to retain suppository for approximately 20 minutes for effectiveness. Position the patient appropriately. Lubricate suppository prior to insertion, and be certain it is inserted into the appropriate orifice. For neurological rehabilitation, a rectal suppository may be utilized by the patient after the patient has been taught bowel management. Check with the patient for effectiveness and note in chart.

suppression (sŭ-prĕsh'ŭn) [L. *suppressio*, a pressing under]. 1.Repression of the external manifestation of a morbid condition. 2. Complete failure of natural production of a secretion or excretion, as distinguished from retention, in which normal secretion occurs but the discharge is retained within the organ or body. 3. In psychoanalysis, the freudian ego defense mechanism of conscious inhibition of an idea or desire, as distinguished from repression, which is considered an unconscious process.

suppression of menses. 1. Amenorrhea in which menstruation ceases after once being established and from some cause other than hysterectomy, pregnancy, or menopause. 2. Any suppression of the menses.

suppressor T cells. Term used for a subpopulation of T lymphocytes that slow and stop the specific immune response, q.v.

suppurant (sŭp'ū-rănt) [L. *suppurans*]. 1. Producing, tending to produce, or characterized by pus formation. 2. Agent causing pus formation. SYN: *suppurative.*

suppurate (sŭp'ū-rāt) [L. *suppurare*]. To form or generate pus.

suppuration (sŭp-ū-rā'shŭn) [L. *suppuratio*]. 1. The process of pus formation. SYN: *pyogenesis; pyopoiesis.* 2. The discharge pro-

duced by suppuration. SYN: *purulence; pus.*

Inflammation is caused by the presence of certain microorganisms called pyogenic (pus-forming) bacteria. Suppuration does not always develop even though microorganisms are present in the affected part, as may be the case in erysipelas and acute joint affections where exudate is serous. Liquefaction of tissues and formation of pus will continue while the microorganisms are alive. They cause the death of the leukocytes (white cells) and the cells of the part, liquefying the tissue so that the area becomes filled with a liquid containing the dead and dying cells. This fluid is called pus. An abscess may form because of the accumulation of this liquid. The abscess is indicated by redness, swelling, heat, and pain. It will show fluctuation, which may be felt by palpating it with two fingers. When the abscess reaches the surface, it will burst and discharge its contents. In most cases it is advisable to surgically incise the abscess rather than to wait for it to burst spontaneously.

RS: abscess; gangrene; infection; inflammation; purulent; pus; pustulant; pustule; pyogenic.

suppurative (sŭp'ū-rā″tĭv, -rā-tĭv) [L. *suppuratus*]. 1. Producing or associated with generation of pus. 2. Agent producing pus formation.

supra- [L.]. Combining form meaning above, beyond, or on the top side.

supra-acromial (soo″pră-ă-krō'mē-ăl) [L. *supra*, above, on top, beyond, + Gr. *akron*, extremity, + *omos*, shoulder]. Located above the acromion.

supra-anal (soo-pră-ā'năl) [″ + *analis*, anal]. Located above the anus.

supra-auricular (soo″pră-ŏ-rĭk'ū-lăr) [″ + *auricula*, little ear]. Located above the auricle.

supra-axillary (soo″pră-ăk'sĭ-lĕr″ē) [″ + *axilla*,underarm]. Located above the axilla.

suprabuccal (soo″pră-bŭk'ăl) [″ + *bucca*, cheek]. Located above the buccal area.

suprabulge (soo′pră-bŭlj). The part of the crown of a tooth that curves toward the occlusal surface.

supracerebellar (soo″pră-sĕr″ĕ-bĕl′ăr) [″ + *cerebellum*, little brain]. On or above the upper surface of the cerebellum.

suprachoroid (soo″pră-kō'royd) [″ + Gr. *chorioeides*, skinlike]. Situated upon or above the choroid layer of the eyeball.

suprachoroidea (soo″pră-kō-roy'dē-ă). Outermost layer of the choroid. SYN: *suprachoroid lamina.*

suprachoroid lamina. Superficial layer of the choroid consisting of thin transparent layers, the outermost adhering to the sclera. SYN: *lamina suprachoroidea.*

supraciliary (soo″pră-sĭl′ē-ĕr″ē) [L. *supra,* above, on top, beyond, + *cilia,* eyelid]. Superciliary, q.v.

supraclavicular (soo″pră-klă-vĭk′ū-lar) [″ + *clavicula,* little key]. Located above the clavicle.

supraclavicular fossa. Depression on either side of the neck extending down behind the clavicle.

supraclavicular point. A stimulation point over the clavicle at which contraction of arm muscles may be produced.

supracondylar (soo″pră-kŏn′dĭ-lar) [″ + Gr. *kondylos,* knuckle]. Above a condyle.

supracostal (soo″pră-kŏs′tăl) [″ + *costa,* rib]. Above the ribs.

supracotyloid (soo″pră-kŏt′ĭ-loyd) [″ + Gr. *kotyloeides,*cup-shaped]. Above the acetabulum.

supradiaphragmatic (soo″pră-dī″ă-frăg-măt′ĭk) [″ + Gr. *dia,* across, + *phragma,* wall]. Above the diaphragm.

supraduction (soo″pră-dŭk′shŭn) [″ + *ducere,* to lead]. Turning upwards of the eye.

supraepicondylar (soo″pră-ĕp″ĭ-kŏn′dĭ-lar) [″ + Gr. *epi,* upon, + *kondylos,* condyle]. Located above an epicondyle.

supragingival. A dental term referring to the location of dental restorations, bacterial plaque, or calculus on the tooth. It is often contrasted with subgingival, the gingival margin being the point of reference.

supraglenoid (soo″pră-glē′noyd) [″ + Gr. *glene,* socket, + *eidos,* form, shape]. Above the glenoid cavity or fossa.

supraglenoid tuberosity. A rough surface of the scapula above the glenoid cavity to which is attached the long head of the biceps muscle.

supraglottic (soo″pră-glŏt′ĭk). Located above the glottis.

supraglottitis. Inflammation of the epiglottis.

suprahepatic (soo″pră-hē-păt′ĭk) [″ + Gr. *hepar,* liver]. Located above the liver.

suprahyoid (soo″pră-hī′oyd) [″ + *hyoeides,* U-shaped]. Located above the hyoid bone; denoting accessory thyroid glands within the geniohyoid muscle.

suprahyoid muscles. The digastric, geniohyoid, mylohyoid, and stylohyoid muscles.

suprainguinal (soo″pră-ĭn′gwĭn-ăl) [″ + *inguinalis,* pert. to the groin]. Above the groin.

supraintestinal (soo″pră-ĭn-tĕs′tĭ-năl) [″ + *intestinum,* intestine]. Overlying the intestine.

supraliminal (soo″pră-lĭm′ĭ-năl) [L. *supra,* above, on top, beyond, + *limen,* threshold]. 1. Above the threshold of consciousness; conscious. 2. Exceeding the stimulus threshold. SEE: *subliminal.*

supralumbar (soo″pră-lŭm′băr) [″ + *lumbus,* loin]. Above the lumbar region.

supramalleolar (soo″pră-mă-lē′ŏ-lăr) [″ + *malleolus,* little hammer]. Located above either malleolus.

supramammary (soo″pră-măm′ă-rē) [″ + *mamma,* breast]. Located above the breast.

supramandibular (soo″pră-măn-dĭb′ū-lăr) [″ + *mandibula,* lower jawbone]. Located above the mandible.

supramarginal (soo″pră-măr′jĭn-ăl) [″ + *marginalis,* border]. Above any border.

supramarginal convolution. A cerebral convolution on lateral surface of the parietal lobe above the posterior part of the sylvian fissure.

supramastoid (soo″pră-măs′toyd) [″ + *mastos,* breast, + *eidos,* form, shape]. Above the mastoid process of the temporal bone.

supramastoid crest. A ridge on the temporal bone. SYN: *temporal line.*

supramaxilla (soo″pră-măk-sĭl′ă) [″ + Gr. *maxilla,* jawbone]. The upper jawbone. SYN: *maxilla.*

supramaxillary (soo″pră-măk′sĭ-lĕr-ē). 1. Rel. to the upper jaw. 2. Located above the upper jaw.

suprameatal (soo″pră-mē-ā′tăl) [″ + *meatus,* passage]. Above a meatus, esp. the exterior auditory meatus, noting the spine of Henle, a small bony projection at the posterosuperior margin of the external auditory meatus.

suprameatal spine. Small bony projection at the posterosuperior margin of the external auditory meatus marking the anterosuperior apex of the suprameatal triangle, q.v. SYN: *spine, Henle's.*

suprameatal triangle. Triangular space bordered by the posterior wall of the external auditory meatus and the posterior root of the zygomatic process of the temporal bone.

supramental (soo″pră-mĕn′tăl) [L. *supra,* above, on top, beyond, + *mentum,* chin]. Located above the chin.

supranasal (soo″pră-nā′zăl) [″ + *nasus,* nose]. Located above the nose.

supranuclear (soo″pră-nū′klē-lăr) [″ + *nucleus,* little kernel]. Concerning nerve fibers located above a nucleus in the brain.

supraoccipital (soo″pră-ŏk-sĭp′ĭ-tăl) [″ + *occiput,* back of head]. Lying above or in upper portion of the occiput.

supraocclusion (soo″pră-ŏ-kloo′zhŭn) [″ + *occlusio,* occlusion]. The condition of teeth that are beyond the occlusal plane.

supraorbital (soo″pră-or′bĭ-tăl) [″ + *orbita,* track]. Located above the orbit.

supraorbital neuralgia. Neuralgia of the supraorbital nerve. SYN: *hemicrania* (def. 1).

supraorbital notch. A notch in the superior margin arch of the orbit for transmitting supraorbital vessels and nerve.

supraorbital reflex. Contraction of orbicularis oculi muscle with closure of lids resulting from percussion above the supraorbital nerve.

suprapatellar (soo″pră-pă-tĕl′ăr) [″ + *patella*, a small pan]. Above the patella.

suprapelvic (soo″pră-pĕl′vĭk) [″ + *pelvis*, basin]. Located above the pelvis.

suprapontine (soo″pră-pŏn′tīn) [″ + *pons*, bridge]. Located above the pons varolii.

suprapubic (soo″pră-pū′bĭk) [″ + NL. *(os) pubis*, bone of the groin]. Above the pubic arch.

suprapubic aspiration of urine. Use of a sterile needle and syringe to obtain urine from the bladder. There is less chance of introducing bacteria into the bladder with this method than during routine catheterization.

TECHNIQUE: Patient is instructed to drink fluids and not to urinate. When the bladder is palpable, the suprapubic area is cleaned with alcohol and a 21-gauge sterile needle is inserted through the skin into the bladder. Urine is then aspirated. Local anesthetic may not be required.

Caution: The needle may pierce a loop of bowel that is lying over the anterior surface of the bladder.

---

suprapubic catheter. Catheter inserted through a suprapubic incision into the bladder to drain urine. Generally used when unable to insert through the urethra due to obstruction or there is a need to allow the urethra and bladder sphincter to heal. SEE: *suprapubic aspiration of urine.*

NURSING IMPLICATIONS: Observe for hemorrhage or prolonged hematuria. Utilize aseptic technique during dressing and equipment changes. Perform bladder irrigation only as prescribed. Observe patient for signs of local or systemic infection. Administer prescribed medications such as analgesics, antispasmodics, and bowel stimulants. Evaluate the patient's ability to micturate. Monitor and record intake and output. Force fluids unless otherwise restricted to insure passage of dilute urine.

suprapubic cystostomy. Surgical opening of the bladder from just above the symphysis pubis.

suprapubic reflex. Deflection of linea alba toward stroked side when abdomen is stroked above Poupart's ligament.

suprarenal (soo″pră-rē′năl) [L. *supra*, above, on top, beyond, + *ren*, kidney]. 1. Above

the kidney. 2. Pert. to the tiny gland above each kidney. SEE: *adrenal gland.*

suprarenalectomy (soo″pră-rē″năl-ĕk′tō-mē) [″ + ″ + Gr. *ektome*, excision]. Adrenalectomy.

suprarenal gland. An endocrine gland lying adjacent to and in a superior and medial position to the kidney. SYN: adrenal gland. SEE: *ACTH; adrenalin; corticosterone; cortisone; endocrine gland; epinephrine; norepinephrine.*

suprarenalopathy (soo″pră-rē-năl-ŏp′ă-thē) [″ + ″ + Gr. *pathos*, disease, suffering]. A disorder due to abnormal functioning of the adrenal glands.

suprascapular (soo″pră-skăp′ū-lăr) [″ + *scapula*, shoulder blade]. Located above the scapula.

suprascleral (soo″pră-sklē′răl) [″ + Gr. *skleros*, hard]. On the surface of the sclera.

suprasegmental [″ + *segmentum*, segment]. Above the segmented portion.

suprasegmental brain. The cerebrum, midbrain, and cerebellum as distinguished from the segmental portion (pons and medulla oblongata).

suprasellar (soo″pră-sĕl′ăr) [″ + *sella*, saddle]. Above or over the sella turcica.

suprasonic, supersonic (soo″pră-sŏn′ĭk) [″ + *sonus*, sound]. Noting sound with frequencies of vibration above 20,000 cycles per second. SEE: *supersonic.*

supraspinal (soo″pră-spī′năl) [″ + *spina*, thorn]. Above a spine.

supraspinous. Above any spinous process.

supraspinous fossa. A groove above the spine of the scapula.

suprastapedial (soo″pră-stă-pē′dē-ăl) [″ + *stapes*, stirrup]. Above the stapes of the inner ear.

suprasternal (soo″pră-stĕr′năl) [L. *supra*, above, on top, beyond, + Gr. *sternon*, chest]. Above the sternum. SYN: *episternal.*

suprasterol (soo″pră-stĕr′ŏl). Substance related to ergosterol produced by excessive irradiation of vitamin D.

suprasylvian (soo″pră-sil′vē-ăn). Above the sylvian fissure of the brain.

supratemporal (soo″pră-tĕm′pō-răl) [″ + *temporalis*, temporal]. Above the temporal bone or fossa.

supratentorial (soo″pră-tĕn-tō′rē-ăl). Located above the tentorium.

suprathoracic (soo″pră-thō-răs′ĭk) [″ + Gr. *thorax*, chest]. Above the thorax.

supratonsillar (soo″pră-tŏn′sĭ-lăr) [″ + *tonsilla*, almond]. Above the tonsil.

supratrochlear (soo″pră-trŏk′lē-ăr) [″ + *trochlea*, pulley]. Above a trochlea, esp. that of the humerus.

supratympanic (soo″pră-tĭm-păn′ĭk) [″ + *tympanon*, drum]. Above the tympanic membrane of the ear.

supravaginal (soo″pră-văj′ĭ-năl) [″ + *vagina*, sheath]. Above the vagina or any sheathing membrane.

supraventricular (soo″pră-věn-trĭk′ū-lăr) [″ + *ventriculus*, a little belly]. Above the ventricle, esp. the heart ventricles.

supravergence (soo″pră-věr′jĕns) [″ + *vergere*, to be inclined]. Condition in which one eye moves upward in the vertical plane while the other does not.

supraversion (soo″pră-věr′zhŭn) [″ + *versio*, a turning]. 1. A turning upward. 2. In dentistry, a tooth out of occlusal line.

sura (sū′ră) [L.]. [NA] Calf of the leg; muscular posterior portion of lower leg.

sural (sū′răl). Rel. to the calf of the leg.

suralimentation (sŭr″ăl-ĭ-měn-tā′shŭn) [Fr. *sur*, above, + L. *alimentum*, nourishment]. Treatment by overfeeding. SYN: *hyperalimentation; superalimentation.*

suramin sodium (soo′ră-mĭn). A urea derivative used in treating African trypanosomiasis (sleeping sickness). It is available only from the Parasitic Disease Division of the Centers for Disease Control (CDC), Atlanta, Georgia 30333, U.S.A.

surditas (sŭr′dĭ-tăs) [L.]. Deafness.

surdity (sŭr′dĭ-tē) [L. *surditas*, deafness]. Inability to hear. SYN: *deafness.*

surdomute (sŭr′dō-mūt″) [L. *surdus*, deaf, + *mutus*, dumb]. 1. A deaf-mute. 2. Deaf and dumb.

surefooted. Being able to walk or run without stumbling or falling.

surface (sŭr′fĕs) [Fr. *sur*, above, + L. *facies*, face]. 1. The exterior boundary of an object. 2. The external or internal exposed portions of a hollow structure, as the outer or inner surfaces of the cranium or stomach. 3. The face or faces of a body such as a bone. 4. The side of a tooth or the dental arch; is usually named for the adjacent tissue or space. The outer or facial surface is called the labial surface of the incisors or canines, and the buccal surface for the premolars and molars. The facial surface may also be called the vestibular surface. The inner surface of each tooth is called the lingual or oral surface. Within the arch, each tooth is said to have a mesial surface, the side toward the midpoint in the front of the dental arch, and a distal surface, the side of the tooth furthest from the midpoint in the front of the dental arch.

   s., body. SEE: *body surface area.*

surface tension. Condition at the surface of a liquid in contact with a gas or another liquid that causes its surface to act as a stretched rubber membrane. It is the result of mutual attraction of the molecules to each other, thus producing a cohesive state that causes

liquids to assume a shape presenting the smallest surface area to the surrounding medium. This accounts for the spherical shape assumed by fluids, such as drops of oil or water.

surfactant (sŭr-făk′tănt). An agent that lowers surface tension.

   Ex.: oils and various forms of detergents.

   s., pulmonary. A phospholipid substance important in controlling the surface tension of air-liquid emulsion that is present in the lungs. Abnormalities in this surfactant have been noted in prematurity, hyaline membrane disease, and pulmonary edema.

Surfak. Trade name for docusate calcium.

surfer's ear. Growth of a bony area in the subcutaneous area of the ear due to prolonged exposure to cold as may occur in persons who participate in surfing.

surfer's knots. Nodular swelling and possibly bone changes of area of lower leg and foot exposed to pressure and trauma while on a surfboard. Nodules may be painful.

surgeon (sŭr′jŭn) [L. *chirurgia*]. A medical practitioner who specializes in surgery.

   s., dental. A dentist whose training and skills are in the area of surgery of the mouth and teeth. SYN: *stomatologist.*

surgeon general. The chief medical officer in one of the armed forces of the U.S. or the U.S. Public Health Service.

surgery (sŭr′jĕr-ē) [L. *chirurgia*]. 1. Branch of medicine dealing with manual and operative procedures for correction of deformities and defects, repair of injuries, and diagnosis and cure of certain diseases. 2. Surgeon's operating room. 3. Treatment or work performed by a surgeon. SYN: *operation.* SEE: *Nursing Diagnoses* in *Appendix.*

   s., ambulatory. Surgery done between the time the patient is admitted in the morning and the time the patient is discharged the same day.

   s., aseptic. Operative procedures carried on under aseptic conditions or in the absence of pathogenic organisms.

   s., aural. Surgery of the ear.

   s., conservative. Surgery in which as much as possible of a part or structure is retained. Opposite of radical surgery.

   s., cosmetic. Surgery done to revise or change the texture, configuration, or relationship of contiguous structures of any feature of the human body that would be considered by the average observer to be within the broad range of normal and acceptable variation for age and ethnic origin. In addition, the procedure is performed for a condition that is judged by competent medical opinion to be without potential for jeopardy to physical or mental health. (Adapted from official A.M.A. definition, 1974.) SEE: *s., plastic.*

s., major. Important and serious operations involving a risk to life.

s., maxillofacial. The branch of dental practice that deals with the diagnosis and the surgical and adjunctive treatment of diseases, injuries, and defects of the human mouth and dental structures. Formerly called oral surgery and dental surgery.

s., minor. Simple operations not considered to involve a risk to life.

s., mucogingival. A plastic surgical method for correcting disease conditions relating to the gingiva and adjacent mucosa of the mouth.

s., oral. Operative procedures pert. to the mouth and associated structures, esp. the teeth and jaws. SEE: *surgery, maxillofacial.*

s., orthopedic. Surgery for correction of deformities and treatment of chronic joint diseases.

s., plastic. Surgery concerned with the repair or restoration of defective or missing structures, frequently involving the transference of tissue from a part or person to another part or person. SEE: *s., cosmetic; tissue expansion, soft.*

s., radical. Surgery involving extensive extirpation to remove diseased tissues or adjoining areas of lymphatic drainage in an attempt to obtain complete cure. Opposite of conservative surgery.

surgery, antimicrobial prophylaxis in. Use of antibiotics prior to a surgical procedure. Even though this may decrease the incidence of infection in certain procedures the benefit must be considered with respect to the potential side effects. This practice is more nearly suited to procedures involving contaminated areas or those involving implantation of prosthetic material.

surgical (sŭr'jĭ-kăl). Of the nature of or pert. to surgery.

surgical diathermy. The use of high-frequency electrical oscillations in such a way that animal tissues are destroyed.

surgical dressing. Sterile protective covering of gauze or other substance applied to an operative wound.

surgical fever. Fever following an operation or injury.

surgical neck. Constricted part of shaft of humerus below the tuberosities; commonly the seat of fracture.

surgical resident. A physician who has graduated from medical school and is enrolled in a hospital-based training program to complete the requirements for certification as a board-qualified surgeon.

surgical suture, absorbable. Suture, absorbable surgical, q.v.

surgical suture, nonabsorbable. Suture, nonabsorbable surgical, q.v.

Surgicel. Trade name for oxidized cellulose.

surimi. Foods made from fish paste. These preparations may be flavored and formed into realistic replications of various foods, including crab meat, shrimp, lobster, and scallops.

Surital. Trade name for thiamylal sodium.

Surmontil. Trade name for trimipramine.

surname. The family name, as distinguished from the individual's given or Christian name.

In some societies, the surname is written first.

surrogate (sŭr'ō-gāt) [L. *surrogatus,* substituted]. 1. Something or someone replacing another; a substitute, esp. an emotional substitute for another. 2. In psychoanalysis, the respresentation of one whose identity is concealed from conscious recognition as in a dream; a figure of importance may represent one's loved one.

s., sex. SEE: *sex surrogate.*

surrogate father. An individual who stands in for the natural father. SEE: *surrogate mother; surrogate parenting.*

surrogate mother. An individual who is not the biological mother but stands in for her. SEE: *surrogate parenting.*

surrogate parenting. An alternative method of parenting in cases in which a wife is infertile. The surrogate mother-to-be is artificially inseminated with the husband's sperm, and if pregnancy is achieved, she carries the child to term and agrees to relinquish all parental rights to the child. The individual bearing the child is, of course, the biological mother. SEE: *fertilization, in vitro; GIFT; parenting, surrogate.*

sursumduction (sŭr"sŭm-dŭk'shŭn) [L. *sursum,* upward, + *ducere,* to lead]. Elevation, as the power or act of turning an eye upward independently of the other one.

sursumvergence (sŭr"sŭm-vĕr'jĕns) [" + *vergere,* to turn]. An upward turning, as of the eyeballs.

sursumversion (sŭr"sŭm-vĕr'zhŭn) [" + *versio,* turning]. Process of turning upward; simultaneous movement of both eyes upward.

surveillance (sŭr-vāl'ăns). The monitoring or controlling of something.

s., immunological. The idea that the body defenses recognize alien materials or malignant cells and destroy them when they appear.

survey. 1. To comprehensively appraise an area of study or research. 2. To conduct a study of a particular disease or condition, esp. its epidemiological aspects.

survival. Continuing to live, esp. under conditions in which death would be the expected outcome.

survivor guilt. The feeling of guilt present in some persons who have survived an event in which others have lost their lives, e.g., a war, ship sinking, holocaust, or prison camp.

susceptibility (sŭs-sĕp″tĭ-bĭl′ĭ-tē). Being susceptible.

susceptible (sŭ-sĕp′tĭ-bl) [L. *susceptibilis*, capable of receiving]. 1. Having little resistance to a disease or foreign protein. 2. An individual with little resistance to an infectious disease or who is not known to have become immune to one. 3. Easily impressed or influenced.

sushi (soo′shē). A general term for a food made of raw fish, usually wrapped in a soft rice shell. Some raw fish contain adults of the larvae of the nematodes of the family Anisakidae. In order to prevent these organisms from infecting persons who eat raw fish, the U.S. Food and Drug Administration has directed that prior to serving, the fish must be suddenly frozen to −31°F (−34.4°C) or below for 15 hours, or held in a commercial freezer at −4°F (−20°C) for 24 hours. After that period, the fish may be thawed and served. SYN: *sashimi.* SEE: *anisakiasis.*

suspended (sŭs-pĕnd′ĕd) [L. *suspendere,* to hang up]. 1. Hanging. 2. Temporarily inactive.

suspension (sŭs-pĕn′shŭn) [L. *suspensio,* a hanging]. 1. A condition of temporary cessation, as of any vital process. 2. Treatment by immobilization of a part or whole by hanging from a suspension in desired position. 3. State of a solid when its particles are mixed with, but not dissolved in, a fluid or another solid; also a substance in this state.

   s., cephalic. Supported suspension of a patient by the head to extend the vertebral column.

   s., colloid. A colloidal solution in which particles of the dispersed phase are relatively large.

   s., tendon. Fixation of a tendon. SYN: *tenodesis.*

suspensoid (sŭs-pĕn′soyd) [″ + Gr. *eidos,* form, shape]. A colloid solution in which the dispersed particles are solid, as distinguished from emulsoid. SYN: *colloid suspension.*

suspensory (sŭs-pĕn′sō-rē) [L. *suspensorius,* hanging]. 1. Supporting a part, as a muscle, ligament, or bone. 2. A structure of the body that supports a part. 3. Bandage or sac for supporting or compressing a part, esp. the scrotum.

suspensory bandage. A sling for support of the testicles.

suspensory ligament. Any one of a number

of ligaments that support a specific organ or structure. SEE: *ligament.*

Sus-Phrine. Trade name for epinephrine hydrochloride.

suspiration (sŭs″pĭr-ā′shŭn) [L. *suspiratio*]. A sigh or the act of sighing.

suspirious (sŭs-pī′rē-ŭs) [L. *suspirare,* to sigh]. Breathing with apparent effort; sighing.

sustentacular (sŭs″tĕn-tăk′ū-lăr) [L. *sustentaculum,* support]. Supporting; upholding.

sustentacular cell. A supporting cell such as those found in the acoustic macula, organ of Corti, olfactory epithelium, taste buds, or testes. SEE: *Sertoli's cells.*

sustentacular fibers of Müller [Friedrich von Müller, Ger. physician, 1858–1941]. Fibers forming the supporting framework of the retina.

sustentaculum (sŭs″tĕn-tăk′ū-lŭm) [L.] (pl. *sustentacula*). A supporting structure.

   s. hepatis. A fold of peritoneum upon which rests the right margin of the liver.

   s. lienis. Phrenocolic ligament that apparently supports the spleen.

   s. tali. [NA] A process of the calcaneum that supports part of the astragalus or talus.

susurrus (sū-sŭr′ŭs) [L., a whisper]. A murmur.

sutilains (soo′tĭ-lāns). USP. Proteolytic enzymes derived from the bacterium *Bacillus subtilis.* Calculated on the dry basis, it contains not less than 2,500,000 USP casein units. It is used in ointment form to debride necrotic lesions. Trade name is Travase.

Caution: Keep away from the eyes.

Sutton's disease (sŭt′ŏnz). 1. [Richard L. Sutton, Sr., U.S. dermatologist, 1878–1952] A halo nevus. 2. [Richard L. Sutton, Jr., U.S. dermatologist, b. 1908] Granuloma fissuratum.

Sutton's law [Named for Willie Sutton, a U.S. bank robber]. Originally, the concept that a bank robber robs banks because "that is where the money is." (A reporter coined the phrase and attributed it to Sutton.) Applied to medicine, the law indicates one should look for diseases where they are most likely to be. Ex.: malaria in tropical areas that harbor *Anopheles* mosquitoes; atherosclerosis in patients who are middle-aged or older.

sutura (sū-tū′ră) [L., a seam] (pl. *suturae*). 1. [NA] A kind of fibrous union found only in the skull; one in which bony surfaces are closely united by a thin fibrous membrane that does not permit movement. SYN: *synarthrosis.* 2. Suture of any kind.

   s. dentata. Sutura with interlocking of

bony processes resembling the teeth of a saw.

s. harmonia. Simple apposition of two contiguous bones.

s. limbosa. Beveled suture in which opposing margins fit in parallel ridges as between parietal and frontal bones.

s. notha. A false suture with ill-defined projections.

s. serrata. [NA] Suture with deeper and more irregular indentations than a dental suture.

s. squamosa. [NA] Suture formed by overlapping of contiguous bones by broad beveled edges as in suture between squamous portion of temporal and parietal bones.

s. vera. A true suture in which no movement of united bones can occur.

sutural (sū′tū-răl) [L. *sutura*, a seam]. Rel. to a suture.

sutural joint. Articulation between two bones.

sutural ligament. Fibers uniting opposed bones forming a cranial suture.

suturation (sū″tū-rā′shŭn). Application of sutures; stitching.

suture (sū′chŭr) [L. *sutura*, a seam]. 1. Line of union in an immovable articulation, as those between the skull bones; also such an articulation itself. SYN: *sutura; synarthrosis*. SEE: *raphe*. 2. Operation of uniting parts by stitching them together. 3. The thread or wire or other material used in the operation of stitching parts of the body together. 4. The seam or line of union formed by surgical stitches. 5. To unite by stitching.

s., absorbable surgical. USP. A sterile strand prepared from collagen derived from healthy mammals or from synthetic polymer. This type of suture is absorbed and thus does not need to be removed.

s., apposition. Suture in the superficial layers of the skin in order to produce precise apposition of the edges.

s., approximation. A deep suture for joining the deep tissues of a wound.

s., basilar. Suture between the occipital bone and sphenoid bone which persists until the 16th to 18th year as the anteroposterior growth center of the base of the skull. Also known as spheno-occipital synchondrosis.

s., bifrontal. Suture between the frontal and parietal bones.

s., biparietal. Suture between the two parietal bones.

s.'s, buried. Sutures placed so that they are completely covered by skin.

s., button. Suture in which the threads are passed through buttons on the surface and tied to prevent the suture material from cutting into the skin. SEE: *s., quilled*.

s., catgut. Material used in suturing, made from a portion of the small intestine of sheep. It can be sterilized. Eventually it is absorbed by body fluids.

s., coaptation. Superficial suture for cutaneous wounds.

s., cobbler's. Suture in which the thread has a needle at each end.

s., continuous. The closure of a wound by means of one continuous thread, usually by transfixing one edge of the wound and then the other alternately from within outward. SYN: *s., uninterrupted.*

s., coronal. Suture between the frontal and parietal bones. SYN: *s., frontoparietal.*

s.'s, cranial. Sutures between the bones of the skull.

s., dentate. Suture consisting of long and toothlike processes.

s., ethmoidofrontal. Suture between the ethmoid and frontal bones.

s., ethmoidolacrimal. Suture between the ethmoid and lacrimal bones.

s., ethmosphenoid. Suture between the ethmoid and sphenoid bones.

s., false. Any form of suture in which one surface is smooth.

s., figure-of-eight. Suture that has shape of the figure eight.

s., frontal. An occasional suture in the frontal bone from the sagittal suture to root of the nose. SYN: *s., mediofrontal; s., metopic.*

s., frontolacrimal. Suture between the frontal and lacrimal bones.

s., frontomalar. Suture between the frontal and malar bones.

s., frontomaxillary. Suture between the frontal bone and superior maxilla.

s., frontonasal. Suture between the frontal bone and the alae of the sphenoid bone.

s., frontoparietal. S., coronal.

s., frontotemporal. Suture between the frontal and temporal bones.

s., glover's. A continuous suture in which the needle is passed through the loop of the preceding stitch.

s., harmonic. Suture in which there is simple apposition of bone.

s., implanted. Suture formed by placing pins opposite each other on the two sides of a wound, and approximating the lips by winding thread or other similar material about the pins.

s., intermaxillary. Suture between the superior maxillae.

s., internasal. Suture between the nasal bones.

s., interparietal. S., sagittal.

s., interrupted. Suture formed by single stitches inserted separately, the needle usually being passed through one lip from without inward, and through the other from within outward.

s., lambdoid. Suture between the parietal bones and the two superior borders of the occipital bone. SYN: *s., occipital; s., occipitoparietal.*

s., longitudinal. S., sagittal.

s., maxillolacrimal. Suture between the maxilla and lacrimal bone.

s., mediofrontal. S., frontal.

s., metopic. S., frontal.

s., nasomaxillary. Suture between the nasal bone and superior maxilla.

s., nonabsorbable. Suture made from a material that is not absorbed by the body, such as silk, silkworm gut, horsehair, certain synthetic materials, and wire.

s., nonabsorbable surgical. USP. A sterile or nonsterile strand of material that is suitably resistant to the action of living mammalian fluids and tissue. This suture should be used only in those applications in which it may eventually be removed or its staying in the tissues will cause no harm.

s., occipital. S., lambdoid.

s., occipitomastoid. Suture between the occipital bone and mastoid portion of temporal bone. SYN: *s., temporo-occipital.*

s., occipitoparietal. S., lambdoid.

s., palatine. Suture between the palatine bones.

s., palatine transverse. Suture between the palatine processes and superior maxilla.

s., parietal. S., sagittal.

s., parietomastoid. Suture between the parietal bone and mastoid portion of the temporal bone.

s., petro-occipital. Suture between the petrous portion of the temporal bone and occipital bone.

s., petrosphenoidal. Suture between the petrous portion of the temporal bone and ala magna of the sphenoid bone.

s., purse-string. Suture entering and exiting around the periphery of a circular opening, closing when drawn taut.

s., quilled. An interrupted suture in which a double thread is passed deep into the tissues below the bottom of the wound, needle being so withdrawn as to leave a loop hanging from one lip and the two free ends of the thread from the other. A quill, or more commonly a piece of bougie, is passed through the loops, which are tightened upon it, and the free ends of each separate thread are tied together over a second quill. Purpose of quilled suture is prevention of tearing when tension becomes greater. SEE: *s., button.*

s., relaxation. Suture that may be loosened to relieve excessive tension.

s., relief. A row of supplementary sutures including the tissues to the extent of 1 to 1½ in. (2.5 to 3.8 cm) on each side of a fistula or a deep wound, for the purpose of lessening the strain on the coaptation sutures.

s., right-angled. A suture used in sewing intestine. The needle is passed in the same direction as the long axis of the incision, and the process is repeated on the opposite side of the incision, the suture being continuous.

s., sagittal. Suture between the two parietal bones. SYN: *s., interparietal; s., longitudinal; s., parietal.*

s., serrated. An articulation by suture in which there is an interlocking of bones by small, fine, and delicate projections and indentations.

s., shotted. Suture in which both ends of a wire or silkworm gut are passed through a perforated shot that is then compressed tightly over them.

s., silk. Type of suture made of silk. May be twisted, braided, or floss.

s., silkworm gut. Type of suture that causes little friction, is pliable, does not curl or twist, and is less liable to produce irritation.

s., sphenoparietal. Suture between the parietal bone and ala magna of the sphenoid bone.

s., sphenosquamous. Articulation of the great wing of the sphenoid with squamous portion of the temporal bone.

s., sphenotemporal. Suture between the sphenoid and temporal bones.

s., squamoparietal. Suture between the parietal and squamous portions of the temporal bone.

s., squamosphenoidal. Suture between the squamous portion of the temporal bone and great wing of the sphenoid.

s., squamous. Suture between flat overlapping bones.

s., subcuticular. A buried continuous suture in which the needle is passed horizontally under the epidermis into the cutis vera, emerging at the edge of the wound but beneath the skin, then in a similar manner passed through the cutis vera of the opposite side of the wound, and so on until the other angle of the wound is reached.

s., temporo-occipital. S., occipitomastoid.

s., temporoparietal. Suture between the temporal and parietal bones.

s., twisted. Suture in which pins are passed through the opposite lips of a wound and material is wound about the pins, crossing them first at one end and then at the other in a figure-of-eight fashion, thus holding the lips of the wound firmly together.

s., uninterrupted. S., continuous.

s., vertical mattress. An interrupted suture in which a deep stitch is taken and the needle inserted upon the same side as that from which it emerged, and passed back through both lips of the wound. The suture is then tied to the free end on the side the needle originally entered. This suture is particularly useful in holding together thick fragile tissues.

s., wire. Type of suture adapted for cases in which there is tension or resection, or for uniting ends of bones. Usually stainless steel or silver wire is used.

suxamethonium chloride (sŭk″să-mĕ-thō′nē-ŭm). Succinylcholine chloride, USP.

Sv. *sievert.*

SV 40 virus. Simian virus 40, which is a member of the papovavirus family. The virus will produce sarcomas after subcutaneous inoculation into newborn hamsters.

swab (swăb) [Dutch *swabbe*, mop]. 1. Cotton or gauze on end of slender stick used for cleansing cavities, applying remedies, or for obtaining a piece of tissue or secretion for bacteriological examination. 2. To wipe with a swab.

s., test tube. Swab for cleansing tubes.

s., urethral. A slender rod for holding cotton used in examinations with the speculum, in treating ulcers or removing secretions. The male urethral swab is a rod about 7 in. (17.8 cm) long.

s., uterine. A slender flattened wire, plain rod, or one with coarse thread on the distal end for absorbing or wiping away discharges.

swaddling. Restraining an infant by wrapping with strips of cloth. This practice has almost disappeared, but is still done in Turkey and China. The restraining procedure may interfere with respiratory function which, in turn, can lead to an increased risk of the infant's developing acute respiratory infections.

swage (swāj). 1. To shape metal, esp. around something in order to make a close fit. 2. Fusing a suture to a needle.

swager. A dental tool or device used to shape silver amalgam or gold by applying pressure from different directions simultaneously.

swallow (swăl′ō) [AS. *swelgan*]. To cause or enable the passage of something from the mouth through the throat and esophagus into the stomach by muscular action. SYN: *deglutition.*

swallowed blood syndrome. Passage of blood in an infant's stool. This may be confused with bleeding from the infant's gastrointestinal tract when in fact it is due to ingested blood from a bleeding nipple. It is important to determine whether or not the blood originated from the infant or from the breast of the person who is nursing the infant. SEE: *APT test.*

swallowing (swăl′ō-ĭng). A complicated act, usually initiated voluntarily but always completed reflexively, whereby food is moved from the mouth through the pharynx and esophagus to the stomach. It occurs in the following three stages.

In the *first stage,* food is placed on the surface of the tongue. The tip of the tongue is placed against the hard palate; then elevation of the larynx and backward movement of the tongue forces food through the isthmus of the fauces in the pharynx.

In the *second stage,* the food passes through the pharynx. This involves constriction of the walls of the pharynx, backward bending of the epiglottis, and an upward and forward movement of the larynx and trachea. This may be observed externally with the bobbing of the Adam's apple. Food is kept from entering the nasal cavity by elevation of the soft palate and from entering the larynx by closure of the glottis and backward inclination of the epiglottis. During this stage, respiratory movements are inhibited by reflex.

In the *third stage,* food moves down the esophagus and into the stomach. This movement is accomplished by momentum from the second stage, peristaltic contractions, and gravity. With the body in upright position, liquids pass rapidly and do not require assistance from the esophagus. However, second stage momentum and peristaltic contractions are sufficient to allow liquids to be drunk even when the head is lower than the stomach.

Difficulty in swallowing is called dysphagia, q.v. It may be caused by congenital defects such as cleft palate or esophageal obstruction; neural and psychogenic disturbances; muscular dysfunction; or local conditions such as presence of tumors, abscesses, and inflammation. SYN: *deglutition.*

RS: aglutition; aphagia; choking; Heimlich maneuver.

s., air. Introduction of air into the stomach or intestines while eating, drinking, chewing gum, or smoking. May be habitual on part of the patient or brought on by hysteria. SYN: *aerophagia.*

s., tongue. Condition in which the tongue has a tendency to fall backward and obstruct the openings to the larynx and esophagus. The tongue is not swallowed and the term is inaccurate; nevertheless, it is commonly used. The condition is due to excessive flaccidity of tongue during unconsciousness. Control of this requires forceful elevation of the chin and extension of the head during artificial respiration in order to help provide an airway. The tongue may also be pulled forward to clear the airway.

swallow's nest. Cerebral depression between the uvula and the posterior velum. SYN: *nidus hirundinis.*

Swan-Ganz catheter [Harold James Swan, U.S. physician, b. 1922; Willian Ganz, U.S. physician, b. 1919]. A soft, flexible catheter that contains a balloon near its tip. The sterile catheter is passed through the vein to the right heart, being carried along by the blood returning to the heart. The balloon then helps, without the use of fluoroscopy, to guide the catheter to the pulmonary artery. Once in the pulmonary artery, the balloon is inflated sufficiently to block the flow of blood from the right heart to the lung. This allows the back pressure in the pulmonary artery distal to the balloon to be recorded. This pressure reflects the pressure transmitted back from the left atrial chamber of the heart.

A catheter similar to the Swan-Ganz was originally developed in 1953 and used in dogs by the U.S. physiologists Michael Lategola and Hermann Rahn.

swan-neck deformity. Finger deformity frequently seen in rheumatoid arthritis characterized by flexion of the distal interphalangeal joints and hyperextension of the proximal interphalangeal joints due to hypermobility in the proximal interphalangeal joint and slipping of the link ligament posteriorly. The interossei muscles may become tight as a result of the position.

swarming (sworm′ing). The spread of bacteria over a culture medium.

sway-back (swā′băk). Lordosis.

sweat (swĕt) [AS. *sweatan*]. 1. The secretion of the sudoriparous glands of the skin. SYN: *perspiration; sudor.* SEE: *glands, Moll's.* 2. Condition of perspiring or of being made to perspire freely, as to order a sweat for a patient. 3. To emit moisture through the skin's pores. SYN: *perspire.* 4. To cause to emit moisture through the pores.

Perspiration is a colorless, slightly turbid, salty, aqueous fluid, although that from the sweat glands in the axillae, around the anus, and of the ceruminous glands has an oil consistency. It contains urea, fatty substances, and sodium chloride. This salty, watery fluid is difficult to collect without contamination with sebum, q.v.

Ingestion of spicy foods such as those flavored with chili peppers may cause sweating. Capsaicin, a chemical in chili that activates nerve endings in the mouth and tongue, causes sweating of the face. SEE: *perspiration, insensible; perspiration, sensi-*

ble.

FUNCT: To cool the body by evaporation and to rid it of what waste may be expressed through the pores of the skin. The amount per day is about a liter; this figure is subject to extreme variation according to physical activity and atmospheric conditions, and in extreme conditions may be as much as 10 to 15 liters in 24 hours.

PHYS: Perspiration is controlled by the sympathetic nervous system through true secretory fibers supplying sweat glands.

   s., bloody. Sweat tinged with blood. SYN: *hematidrosis.*

   s., colliquative. Profuse, clammy sweat.

   s., colored. Sweat tinged with a pigment. SYN: *chromidrosis.*

   s., fetid. Sweat with a foul odor. SYN: *bromidrosis.*

   s., night. Sweating during the night; may be a symptom of pulmonary tuberculosis.

   s., profuse. Excessive perspiration. SYN: *hyperhidrosis.*

   s., scanty. Abnormally small amount of or lack of sweat. SYN: *anhidrosis.*

sweat, words pert. to: bromidrosis; chromidrosis; diaphoresis; diaphoretic; dyshidria; dysidrosis; hidradenitis; hidrorrhea; hidrosis; hydradenitis; hydradenoma; hyperhidrosis, hyphidrosis; melanidrosis; perspiration; sudor; sudorific; sudoriparous; uridrosis.

sweat centers. Principal centers controlling perspiration located in the hypothalamus; secondary centers are present in the spinal cord.

sweat glands. Simple, coiled, tubular glands found on all body surfaces except margin of lips, glans penis, and inner surface of prepuce. The coiled secreting portion lies in the corium or subcutaneous portion of skin; the excretory duct follows a straight or oblique course through the dermis, but becomes spiral in passing through the epidermis to its opening, a sweat pore.

Most sweat glands are merocrine; those of the axilla, areola, mammary gland, labia majora, and circumanal region are apocrine. Sweat glands are most numerous on the palms of the hands and soles of the feet. SEE: illus.; *gland, eccrine; gland, apocrine.*

sweating (swĕt′ing) [AS. *swat*, sweat]. 1. Act of exuding sweat. 2. Emitting sweat. 3. Causing profuse sweat.

To induce sweat in a localized area, paint 2 in. (5.1 cm) square of skin under each axilla with mixture of equal parts of olive oil and guaiacol solution. Cover with several layers of gauze, then flannel, and hold with adhesive tape. Wrap patient in warm blankets.

   s., deficiency of. Diminished or com-

ECCRINE AND APOCRINE SWEAT GLANDS

PORE OF SKIN

SHAFT OF HAIR

CONNECTS WITH DUCT OF SEBACEOUS GLAND

SEBACEOUS GLAND

ELASTIC TISSUE SURROUNDING THE DUCT

BLOOD VESSELS

SUBCUTANEOUS TISSUE

DERMAL PAPILLA

APOCRINE TYPE OF SWEAT GLAND

SECRETORY PORTION OF ECCRINE TYPE SWEAT GLAND

BULB OF HAIR FOLLICLE

plete absence of secretion of sweat. Seen in profuse diarrhea, polyuria, vomiting, hemorrhage, diabetes insipidus, myxedema, general anasarca, ichthyosis, and in high temperature. SYN: *anhidrosis*.

s., excessive. Overabundance of secretion of sweat. Seen in rheumatic, malarial, and relapsing fever, septic fevers, pneumonia at crisis, pulmonary tuberculosis, hyperthyroidism, migraine, neuralgia. Locally of hands and feet in hysteria, neurasthenia, vagotonia, nervous irritability, exophthalmic goiter, fright, and other emotions. SYN: *hyperhidrosis*.

s., insensible. Evaporation of water from the skin without the production of visible sweat. This is done by the water vapor diffusing through the skin rather than being secreted by the sweat glands.

s., sensible. Production of moisture on the skin by means of the secretions of the sweat glands.

s., urinous. Presence of urea in the sweat. Often found in uremia. SYN: *uridrosis*.

RS: anhidrosis; bromidrosis; chromidrosis; hidrosis; perspiration; pores; skin; sudor; sudorific; sweat; uridrosis.

Swedish gymnastics. System of active and

passive exercise of the various muscles and joints of the body without using apparatus.

Swedish massage. Massage combined with Swedish gymnastics.

sweet [AS. *swete*, sweet]. 1. Pleasing to the taste or smell. SEE: *taste*. 2. Containing or derived from sugar. 3. Free from excess of acid, sulfur, or corrosive salts.

Sweet's procedure. A radiographic procedure used to locate foreign objects in the eye.

Sweet's syndrome [R. D. Sweet, contemporary Brit. physician]. A condition characterized by fever; raised painful plaques on the limbs, face, and neck; neutrophil leukocytosis; and dense dermal infiltration with mature neutrophil polymorphs. The cause is unknown, but treatment with adrenal cortical hormone is usually effective.

swelling (swĕl'ing) [AS. *swellan*, swollen]. An abnormal transient enlargement, esp. one appearing on the surface of the body. SEE: *edema*.

TREAT: Ice water applied to area helps to reduce swelling.

RS: detumescence; node; nodule; turgescence; turgid.

s., albuminous. S., cloudy.

s., Calabar. Swelling occurring in infestations by the nematode *Loa loa*. Temporary and painless, the swelling is thought to be the result of temporary sensitization.

s., cloudy. Degeneration of tissues marked by cloudy appearance, swelling, and appearance of tiny albuminoid granules in the cells as observed with the microscope. SYN: *s., albuminous.*

s., fugitive. Temporary swellings such as those occurring in infestations of *Loa loa,* which appear at one place, persist for two or three days, then disappear, possibly to recur at another position.

s., glassy. Swelling occurring in amyloid degeneration of tissues. SEE: *amyloid degeneration; erythredema.*

s., white. Swelling seen in tuberculous arthritis, esp. of the knee.

Swift's disease. Acrodynia.

swimmer's ear. A type of external otitis seen in persons who swim for a considerable period of time or fail to completely dry their ear canals after swimming. If excess cerumen is not present, the condition can be prevented by placing a few drops of 70% alcohol in the ear canals at the end of each swimming session.

swimmer's itch. Appearance of papules resembling insect bites on the skin of persons who swim in water containing the cercariae of certain schistosomes. Usually present only on exposed surfaces of the skin. The papules appear from 4 to 13 days after exposure. Disease is self-limited; thus treatment is symptomatic. SYN: *dermatitis, cercarial.* SEE: *schistosome dermatitis; seabather's eruption.*

swimming pool granuloma. A chronic skin granuloma caused by *Mycobacterium marinum.* The lesion may develop in those who experience an abrasion of the skin while working in a home aquarium or in a marine environment.

TREAT: Tetracycline to begin with; then, if lesions do not heal, prolonged therapy with rifampin and ethambutol will be required.

switch (swĭch) [MD. *swijch,* bough]. In physical therapy, device used to break or open an electrical circuit or to divert current from one conductor to another.

s., foot. A foot-activated switch that enables the operator to use both hands in application of surgical high-frequency currents, at the same time activating the current with his or her foot.

s., pole-changing. A switch by which the polarity of a circuit may be reversed.

swoon [AS. *swogan,* to suffocate]. 1. A fainting spell. SYN: *syncope.* 2. To faint.

sycoma (sī-kō′mă) [Gr. *sykoma*]. A large soft wart. SYN: *condyloma.*

sycophant (sĭk′ō-fănt). One who seeks to incur favor or advance oneself by flattery and praise of persons of influence.

sycosiform (sī-kō′sĭ-form) [Gr. *sykosis,* figlike disease, + L. *forma,* shape]. Resembling sycosis.

sycosis (sī-kō′sĭs) [Gr. *sykosos,* figlike disease]. Chronic inflammation of hair follicles.

SYM: Inflammation of hairy areas of the body characterized by an aggregation of papules and pustules, each of which is pierced by a hair. Pustules show no disposition to rupture but dry to yellow-brown crusts. Itching and burning. If disease persists, may lead to extreme destruction of hair follicles and permanent alopecia.

ETIOL: *Staphylococcus aureus* and *epidermidis* entering through hair follicles. Trauma and disability are predisposing factors.

TREAT: Organism should be cultured and tested to determine systemic and topical antibiotic of choice.

PROG: Disease is curable under prolonged treatment; relapses occur.

s. barbae. Sycosis of the beard marked by papules and pustules perforated by hairs and surrounded by infiltrated skin.

s., lupoid. Pustular lesions of the hair follicles of the beard.

s. vulgaris. S. barbae, q.v.

Sydenham's chorea (sĭd′ĕn-hămz) [Thomas Sydenham, Brit. physician, 1624–1689]. A disease of childhood commonly occurring between 5 and 15 years of age; more females than males are affected. Usually associated with rheumatic fever. Characterized by involuntary purposeless contractions of the muscles of the trunk and extremities; anxiety; impairment of memory and sometimes of speech.

TREAT: Rest; remove child from school. Protection against injury if chorea is severe. Sedation is indicated in some cases.

PROG: Recovery usually in course of 6 to 10 weeks. Relapses not infrequent, esp. in pregnancy. A possible sequel is chronic chorea. Rare complication is death from heart disease.

syllabic utterance (sĭ-lăb′ĭk) [Gr. *syllabikos*]. A staccato accentuation of syllables, slowly but separately, observed in multiple sclerosis. SYN: *scanning speech.*

syllable stumbling (sĭl′ă-bl) [Gr. *syllabe,* syllable]. Hesitating utterance (dysphasia) with difficulty in pronouncing certain syllables.

syllabus (sĭl′ă-bŭs) [Gr. *syllabos,* table of contents]. Abstract of a lecture or outline of a course of study or of a book.

sylvatic plague. Bubonic plague that is endemic among wild rodents. The causative organism is transmitted by fleas. SEE: *plague.*

sylvian aqueduct (sĭl'vē-ăn). A narrow canal from 3rd to 4th ventricle.

sylvian artery [François (Franciscus de la Boë) Sylvius, Dutch anatomist, 1614–1672]. Middle cerebral artery in the fissure of Sylvius.

sylvian fissure [François Sylvius]. The fissure separating the temporal lobe from the frontal and parietal lobes.

sylvian line [François Sylvius]. Line on exterior of the cranium, marking direction of the sylvian fissure.

sym- [Gr. *syn,* together]. Combining form meaning with, along, together with, beside.

symballophone (sĭm-băl'ō-fōn) [" + *ballein,* to throw, + *phone,* sound]. A special stethoscope with two chest pieces. Its use assists in locating a lesion in the chest by comparing the different sounds detected by the two chest pieces.

symbion, symbiont (sĭm'bē-ŏn, -bē-ŏnt) [Gr. *syn,* together, + *bios,* life]. An organism that lives with another in a state of symbiosis, q.v. SYN: *commensal.*

symbiosis (sĭm"bē-ō'sĭs) [Gr.]. 1. The living together in close association of two organisms of different species. If neither organism is harmed, such is referred to as commensalism; if the association is beneficial to both, it is mutualism; if one is harmed and the other benefited, it constitutes parasitism. 2. In psychiatry, a dependent, mutually reinforcing relationship between two persons. In a health context, it is characteristic of the infant-mother relationship. In an unhealthy context, it may reinforce the psychopathology present in close associates.

symbiote (sĭm'bī-ōt) [Gr. *syn,* together, + *bios,* life]. An organism symbiotic with another.

symbiotic (sĭm"bī-ŏt'ĭk). Concerning symbiosis.

symblepharon (sĭm-blĕf'ă-rŏn) [" + *blepharon,* eyelid]. Adhesion between conjunctivae of lid and eyeball due to injuries, esp. burns from lime or acids. Also seen in trachoma, in pemphigus, and following operations.

    SYM: Interference with movement of eyeball, conjunctival irritation.

    TREAT: Division of cicatricial bands and keeping raw surfaces separated. Mucous membrane grafts.

symblepharopterygium (sĭm-blĕf"ă-rō-tĕr-ĭj'ē-ŭm) [" + " + *pterygion,* wing]. Abnormal joining of the eyelid to the eyeball.

symbol (sĭm'bŏl) [Gr. *symbolon,* a sign]. 1. An object or sign that represents an idea or quality by association, resemblance, or convention. SEE: *Prescription Writing* and *Symbols* in *Appendix.* 2. In psychology, an object used as an unconscious substitute that is not connected consciously with the libido, but into which the libido is concentrated. 3. A mark or letter representing an atom or an element in chemistry. SEE: *Physical Constants of Elements* in *Appendix.*

    s., phallic. An object that bears some resemblance to the penis.

symbolia (sĭm-bō'lē-ă). Ability to identify or recognize an object by the sense of touch.

symbolism (sĭm'bŏl-ĭzm) [" + *-ismos,* condition]. 1. Unconscious substitutive expression of subconscious thoughts of sexual significance in terms recognized by the objective consciousness. 2. An abnormal condition in which everything that occurs is interpreted as a symbol of the patient's own thoughts.

symbolization. An unconscious process by which an object or idea comes to represent another object or idea on the basis of similarity or association.

symbolophobia (sĭm"bŏl-ō-fō'bē-ă) [" + *phobos,* fear]. Hesitancy in expressing oneself in words or action for fear that it may be interpreted as possessing a symbolic meaning.

symbrachydactyly (sĭm-brăk"ē-dăk'tĭ-lē) [" + *brachys,* short, + *daktylos,* finger]. Webbing of fingers that are abnormally short.

Syme's operation (sīmz) [James Syme, Scottish surgeon, 1799–1870]. 1. Amputation of the foot at the ankle joint with removal of the malleoli. 2. Excision of the tongue. 3. External urethrotomy.

symmelia (sĭm-mē'lē-ă) [Gr. *syn,* together, + *melos,* limb]. Fusion of limbs.

symmelus, symelus (sĭm'ĕ-lŭs, -ē-lŭs) [" + *melos,* limb]. Sirenomelia, q.v.

Symmetrel. Trade name for amantadine hydrochloride.

symmetromania (sĭm"ĕ-trō-mā'nē-ă) [Gr. *symmetria,* symmetry, + *mania,* madness]. A compulsive impulse to make symmetrical motions such as moving both arms instead of one.

symmetry (sĭm'ĕt-rē). Correspondence in shape, size, and relative position of parts on opposite sides of a body.

    s., bilateral. Symmetry of an organism or body whose right and left halves are mirror images of each other or in which a median longitudinal section divides the organism or body into equivalent right and left halves.

    s., radial. Symmetry of an organism whose parts radiate from a central axis.

sympathectomize (sĭm"pă-thĕk'tō-mīz). To perform a sympathectomy.

sympathectomy (sĭm″pă-thĕk′tō-mē) [Gr. *sympathetikos*, sympathy, + *ektome*, excision]. Excision of a portion of the sympathetic division of the autonomic nervous system. It may include a nerve, plexus, ganglion, or a series of ganglia of the sympathetic trunk.

s., chemical. The use of chemicals to destroy or temporarily inactivate part of the sympathetic nervous system.

s., periarterial. Removal of sheath of an artery in which sympathetic nerve fibers are located; used in trophic disturbances.

sympatheoneuritis (sĭm-păth″ē-ō-nū-rī′tĭs) [″ + *neuron*, nerve, + *itis*, inflammation]. Inflammation of the sympathetic nerve.

sympathetic (sĭm″pă-thĕt′ĭk). 1. Pert. to sympathetic nervous system. 2. Caused by or pert. to sympathy.

sympatheticalgia (sĭm″pă-thĕt″ĭ-kăl′jē-ă) [″ + *algos*, pain]. Pain in the cervical sympathetic ganglion.

sympathetic irritation. Irritation of one structure caused by irritation of a related one.

sympathetic nervous system. A large part of the autonomic nervous system. It consists of ganglia, nerves, and plexuses that supply the involuntary muscles. Most of the nerves of the system are motor, but some are sensory. SEE: *nervous system; parasympathetic nervous system; autonomic nervous system* for illus.

sympatheticoparalytic (sĭm″pă-thĕt″ĭ-kō-păr″ă-lĭt′ĭk) [″ + *paralysis*, a loosening at the sides]. Resulting from paralysis of the sympathetic nervous system.

sympatheticopathy (sĭm″pă-thĕt″ĭ-kŏp′ă-thē) [″ + *pathos*, disease, suffering]. Any condition resulting from disorder of the sympathetic nervous system.

sympathetic ophthalmia. Inflammation of the uveal tract in one eye due to similar inflammation in the other eye.

sympatheticotonia (sĭm″pă-thĕt″ĭ-kō-tō′nē-ă) [″ + *tonos*, act of stretching, tension]. Condition characterized by excessive tone of the sympathetic nervous system with unusually high blood pressure, fine tremor of hands, and insomnia. May be present in thyrotoxic patients. SYN: *sympathicotonia*.

sympatheticotonic (sĭm″pă-thĕt″ĭ-kō-tŏn′ĭk). Marked by increased arterial tone or vasoconstriction due to overaction of the sympathetic nervous system.

sympatheticotripsy. Sympathicotripsy, q.v.

sympathetic plexuses. Plexuses formed at intervals by the sympathetic nerves and ganglia.

sympathetoblast (sĭm″pă-thĕt′ō-blăst) [Gr. *sympathetikos*, sympathy, + *blastos*, germ]. Sympathoblast, q.v.

sympathic (sĭm-păth′ĭk) [Gr. *sympathetikos*, sympathy]. Sympathetic.

sympathicectomy (sĭm-păth″ĭ-sĕk′tō-mē) [″ + *ektome*, excision]. Excision of part of the sympathetic nervous pathways. SYN: *sympathectomy*.

sympathicoblast (sĭm-păth′ĭ-kō-blăst) [″ + *blastos*, a germ]. A primitive sympathetic nerve cell. SEE: *sympathoblast*.

sympathicoblastoma (sĭm-păth″ĭ-kō-blăs-tō′mă) [″ + *oma*, tumor]. A tumor consisting of sympathicoblasts.

sympathicolytic (sĭm-păth″ĭ-kō-lĭt′ĭk) [″ + *lytikos*, dissolving]. Interfering with, opposing, inhibiting, or destroying impulses from the sympathetic nervous system. SYN: *sympatholytic*.

sympathicomimetic (sĭm-păth″ĭ-kō-mĭm-ĕt′ĭk) [″ + *mimetikos*, imitating]. Adrenergic. Producing effects resembling those resulting from stimulation of the sympathetic nervous system, such as effects following the injection of epinephrine.

sympathiconeuritis (sĭm-păth″ĭ-kō-nū-rī′tĭs) [″ + *neuron*, nerve, + *itis*, inflammation]. Inflammation of the sympathetic nerves.

sympathicopathy (sĭm-păth″ĭ-kŏp′ă-thē) [″ + *pathos*, disease, suffering]. Disease or disordered function due to malfunction of the autonomic nervous system.

sympathicotonia (sĭm-păth″ĭ-kō-tō′nē-ă) [″ + *tonos*, act of stretching, tension]. Increased tonus of the sympathetic system with marked tendency to vascular spasm and heightened blood pressure. Opposite of vagotonia. SYN: *sympatheticotonia*.

sympathicotripsy (sĭm-păth″ĭ-kō-trĭp′sē) [″ + *tripsis*, a crushing]. Crushing of a sympathetic ganglion. SYN: *sympatheticotripsy*.

sympathicotropic (sĭm-păth″ĭ-kō-trŏp′ĭk) [″ + *tropos*, a turning]. Having a special affinity for the sympathetic nerve.

sympathicus (sĭm-păth′ĭ-kŭs). The sympathetic nervous system.

sympathism (sĭm′pă-thĭzm) [″ + *-ismos*, condition]. Condition of susceptibility to the suggestions and opinions of others. SYN: *suggestibility*.

sympathist (sĭm′pă-thĭst) [″ + *-ismos*, condition]. One susceptible to sympathism.

sympathoadrenal (sĭm″păth-ō-ă-drē′năl) [″ + L. *ad*, to, + *ren*, kidney]. Concerning the sympathetic part of the autonomic nervous system and the adrenal medulla.

sympathoblast (sĭm-păth′ō-blăst) [″ + *blastos*, germ]. A primitive cell from which arises a sympathetic ganglion cell. SYN: *sympathicoblast*.

sympathoblastoma (sĭm″păth-ō-blăs-tō′mă) [″ + ″ + *oma*, tumor]. A malignant tumor made up of sympathetic nerve cells.

sympathoglioblastoma (sĭm″păth-ō-glī″ō-blăs-tō′mă) [Gr. *sympathetikos*, sympathy, + *glia*, glue, + *blastos*, germ, + *oma*, tumor]. A tumor made up primarily of sympathoblasts with scattered neuroblasts and spongioblasts.

sympathogonia (sĭm″pă-thō-gō′nē-ă) [″ + *gone*, seed]. Primitive cells from which sympathetic nervous system cells are derived.

sympathogonioma (sĭm″pă-thō-gō″nē-ō′mă) [″ + ″ + *oma*, tumor]. A tumor containing sympathogonia.

sympatholytic. Opposing or inhibiting adrenergic nerve function.

sympathoma [″ + *oma*, tumor]. A tumor composed of tissue similar to that of the sympathetic nervous system.

sympathomimetic (sĭm″pă-thō-mĭm-ĕt′ĭk) [″ + *mimetikos*, imitating]. Adrenergic. SYN: *sympathicomimetic*.

sympathy (sĭm′pă-thē) [Gr. *sympatheia*]. 1. An association or feeling of closeness between individuals such that something that affects one affects the other. SEE: *empathy*. 2. In biology, something that affects one of a paired organ may also influence the other. There may be no clear understanding of the mechanism of this interaction.

sympexion (sĭm-pĕks′ē-ŏn) [Gr. *sympexis*, concretion]. A concretion in certain sites such as the prostate or seminal vesicles.

sympexis (sĭm-pĕks′ĭs). Arrangement of red blood cells due to the effect of surface tension.

symphalangism (sĭm-făl′ăn-jĭzm) [Gr. *syn*, together, + *phalanx*, closely knit row]. 1. Ankylosis of joints of the fingers or toes. 2. Web-fingered or web-toed condition.

symphyogenetic (sĭm″fē-ō-jĕ-nĕt′ĭk) [Gr. *syn*, together, + *phyein*, to grow, + *gennan*, to produce]. Concerning the combined effect of heredity and environment upon the development and function of an organism.

symphyseal (sĭm-fĭz′ē-ăl) [Gr. *symphysis*, growing together]. Pert. to symphysis.

symphyseotomy (sĭm-fĭz″ē-ŏt′ō-mē) [″ + *tome*, incision]. Section of symphysis pubis to enlarge the pelvic diameters during delivery. SYN: *hebosteotomy; hebotomy; pelvioplasty; pubiotomy; symphysiectomy; symphysiotomy*.

symphysiectomy (sĭm-fĭz″ē-ĕk′tō-mē) [″ + *ektome*, excision]. Resection of the symphysis pubis to facilitate delivery.

symphysion (sĭm-fĭz′ē-ŏn) [Gr. *symphysis*, growing together]. Most anterior point of the alveolar process of the lower jaw.

symphysiorrhaphy (sĭm-fĭz″ē-or′ă-fē) [″ + *rhaphe*, seam, ridge]. Surgical repair of a divided symphysis.

symphysiotome (sĭm-fĭz′ē-ō-tōm) [″ + *tome*, incision]. An instrument for dividing a symphysis.

symphysiotomy (sĭm-fĭz″ē-ŏt′ō-mē) [″ + *tome*, incision]. Section of the symphysis pubis to facilitate childbirth by enlarging the pelvic outlet.

symphysis (sĭm′fĭ-sĭs) [Gr., growing together] (pl. *symphyses*). 1. A line of fusion between two bones that are separate in early development, as symphysis of mandible. 2. [NA] A form of synchondrosis in which the bones are separated by a disk of fibrocartilage, as in joints between bodies of vertebrae or between pubic bones. SEE: *intervertebral disk*.

   s. **cartilaginosa.** Synchondroses.

   s. **ligamentosa.** Syndesmoses.

   s. **mandibulae.** S. menti.

   s. **menti.** The symphysis of the chin or the ridge marking the line of union of the two halves of the mandible. SYN: *symphysis mandibulae.*

   s. **of jaw.** An anterior, median, vertical ridge upon outer surface of lower jaw representing line of union of its halves.

   s. **pubis.** The junction of the pubic bones on midline in front; the bony eminence under the pubic hair.

symphysodactyly (sĭm″fĭ-sō-dăk′tĭ-lē) [″ + *daktylos*, finger]. Fusion of the fingers or toes. SYN: *syndactylism*.

symplasm (sĭm′plăzm) [Gr. *syn*, together, + LL. *plasma*, form, mold]. Living nucleated material lacking in cellular structure. SYN: *syncytium*.

sympodia (sĭm-pō′dē-ă) [″ + *pous*, foot]. Condition in which lower extremities are united.

symporter (sĭm-por′tĕr). Mechanism for carrying two different molecules or ions in the same direction through a membrane.

symptom (sĭm′tŭm, sĭmp-) [Gr. *symptoma*, occurrence]. Any perceptible change in the body or its functions that indicates disease or the kind or phases of disease. Symptoms may be classified as objective, subjective, cardinal, and sometimes as constitutional. However, another classification considers all symptoms as being subjective, with objective indications being called signs, q.v.

   Aspects of general symptom analysis include the following. *Onset:* date, manner (gradual or sudden), precipitating factors. *Characteristics:* character, location, radiation, severity, timing, aggravating or relieving factors, associated symptoms. *Course since onset:* incidence, progress, effects of therapy.

ABDOMEN: May be distended, rigid, flat, flabby, adipose, tympanitic, shiny, enlarged, or bulging in certain areas, certain discolorations, stripings, or markings. Muscles may be tensed and little affected by pressure. Cold areas may be noted. Various sounds may be heard such as splashings, roarings, and rumblings (borborygmus, also known as intestinal flatus).

Pain is closely associated with abdominal symptoms. Locate exact area affected, and note nature, duration, time when it arises, and any causes that might be responsible. Also the effect of movement or pressure on the pain; and the alteration in the pain if pressure applied to the area is suddenly released. SEE: *tenderness, rebound.*

Emesis is another condition associated with symptoms pert. to the abdominal region. It may consist of simple regurgitation of stomach contents or be extremely forcible. In the latter case, it is called projectile vomiting. Emesis may be watery, clear, or contain mucus or undigested food; may be stertorous, bilious, frothy, profuse, purulent, colored from food or medication, and contain blood (hematemesis). If blood is present in large quantity and has been acted on by gastric juices, it may resemble coffee grounds. Emesis may be sour, have odor of feces or garlic, may be ammoniacal, or have odor characteristic of some food or drug.

The patient may complain of abdominal distention, gas, and pain caused by gas, crowding in the region of the heart, and interference with respiration. Heartburn may be present, or gastritis and regurgitation. Pain may be felt when food enters the stomach, or relieved by eating or shortly after eating or by changing body position. Distention after eating as well as desire to eructate or to expel flatus should be noted. Colicky pains in the abdomen may be accompanied by pain in the shoulder. Pain at pit of stomach and in lower right quadrant may indicate appendicitis. When pains are over the lower right ribs or a little below, disease of the gallbladder may be suspected. SEE: *abdomen; emesis.*

BACK: The dorsal side of the body may reveal edema, deformities, irregularities of the spine, discolorations, eruptions, impaired motion, decubitus, or any condition affecting the skin. SEE: *back pain.*

BREATH: May have a fecal odor, a sweet (acetone) odor, one of wet hay, an odor of fish, ammonia, urine, blood, or pus. Respiration may be abdominal or thoracic and show dyspnea, orthopnea, apnea, or it may be normal (eupnea). SEE: *apnea; breath; dyspnea; orthopnea.*

CHEST: The chest may show abnormalities and deformities. It may move asymmetrically with one lung being inflated much less than the other. Coughing may be whooping, hacking, crowing, hoarse, dry, rasping, or hysterical. There may or may not be expectoration. A cough may be spasmodic or occur on awakening; during sleep it may awaken patient; it may or may not produce sputum; it may occur when swallowing food; when in a horizontal position, or when subjected to change of temperatures. If hiccupping is present, note when it occurs. Sputum may be mucoid, yellowish, thick, tenacious, ropy, gelatinous, dark green, offensive in odor, copious, streaked with bright (brick red) or dark blood (hemoptysis), or it may resemble cheesy lumps. It may be clear and watery, scanty, or profuse.

Frequency of coughing and clearing throat should be noted. Patient's respirations may be shallow; dyspnea may be present, or inability to expand the lungs, complaints of irritation, sticking pains, or catchy pains on inspiration. There may be an accumulation of phlegm in the air passages or a tickling in the throat. Patient may not be able to take deep inspirations or may be constantly yawning. There may be migrating knifelike pains in region of heart or throughout chest. Heart-consciousness may be present, or a fluttering feeling about the heart, or cardiac pain. Queer sensations, the loud beating of the heart, and heaviness in cardiac region are other symptoms. SEE: *apnea; chest; cough; dyspnea; hiccough; sputum.*

DEFECATION: Symptoms to observe are the frequency of defecation; the presence of constipation; hemorrhoids; the nature of the feces such as formation (ribbon-shaped, soft, semiformed, hard or scybalous, cylindrical) and whether watery, liquid, or semiliquid; the color, whether dark brown, light brown, clay-colored, green, yellowish, black, bloody; and whether lienteric, serous, mucous, purulent, tarry, or containing membranous shreds, calculi, or foreign substances. The amount should be noted, as small, medium, large, or copious. The odor may be characteristic of various conditions: sour, putrid, offensive, or fetid. The nature of the evacuation should be noted, as natural, difficult, involuntary, or painful. SEE: *feces; stool.*

DENTITION: Teeth may be irregular, missing, misshapen, or affected by caries. There may be a partial or complete denture. Dental hygiene may be good or poor. There may be a loosening of teeth, a film over them, or they may show the presence of sordes.

EARS: Tinnitus aurium, q.v., (ringing in the ears) occurs in certain diseases. Pain in or about ears, or swelling under either or both, should be noted. Impacted cerumen, foreign bodies, or insects may be present in auditory canals. SEE: *ear*.

EYES: May be staring, have an excited look, or be expressionless. Nystagmus, strabismus, and coma vigil, q.v., may be present. Pupils may be contracted or dilated, or one pupil may be affected. Patient may keep eyes closed constantly, or keep one open and the other closed. Eyes may be sunken or protruding. Lacrimation may be present. Eyelids may be edematous, and eyeball soft to the touch; or the eyeball may be extremely hard. Accommodation may be faulty. Nictitation, squinting, or tremor of the eyelids should always be recorded. Blurring of vision usually is associated with other symptoms. Patient may complain of specks dancing before the eyes (muscae volitantes). These may be colorless or colored. SEE: *eye*.

GAIT: May be faltering, scissors, festinating, unsteady, staggering, weakened, swaying, or movements may be stiff, awkward, or unusual. There may be total disability or immobility. SEE: *gait*.

GENERAL APPEARANCE: The face may show an expression of anxiety or have a pinched look or a drawn expression. Patient may have air of apathy, a distorted or a blank look, an emotional expression, a risus sardonicus, or lack of all expression (mask-like).

GENERAL SYM: Burning sensations may be complained of in various parts of the body, as in the head, throat, arms, chest, or abdomen. They may or may not be accompanied by tenderness. The complaint may be of feeling too hot or too cold without apparent cause, or of having a general feeling of distress.

Anorexia and nausea upon taking food, at the thought of food, or with no reference to food are significant and should be noted; also when nausea occurs: on awakening, when taking fluids, after eating, when changing a position, when taking medication, or in the presence of odors. There always should be an explanation for nausea, either somatic or psychiatric.

Fear of death (angor animi), anxiety, agitation, or panic may be present.

LIMBS: The symptoms pert. to the skin, of course, apply to skin of the limbs. Note if there are deformities, abnormalities, impaired motion, discolorations, sensitivity, varicosities.

LIPS: May be pale, dry, cyanotic, edematous, drawn, deformed, out of proportion, motionless and expressionless, flushed, fissured, or show other lesions or growths. SEE: *lip*.

MOUTH AND GUMS: May be pale or ulcerated, highly inflamed and red, infected, discolored, edematous, or abnormally shaped. Pyorrhea or edema may be present. Patient may complain of bitter, sweet, salty, sour, fishy, or flat tastes, or an absence of taste. Medication may have much to do with temporary disorders of taste. SEE: *gum; mouth*.

NOSE: May appear deformed, discolored, edematous, or enlarged. Nostrils may discharge or show obstruction. There may be inability to breathe through one or both nostrils. Patient may complain of odors not usually manifested as objective symptoms, or for which there is no known cause. SEE: *nose*.

PAIN: Determine if the patient's perception of pain is local or referred so that the exact area affected can be ascertained. The wording of the patient's complaint of pain must be charted or reported. Note if pain is in nature of a cramp or spasm; if it is dull, superficial, deep, remittent, shifting, shooting, lancinating, gnawing, fixed, sharp; or if there is an absence of pain, esp. in conditions in which pain usually occurs. Note whether pain is relieved or increased by pressure, heat, cold, change of body position or environment, or other conditions. When is pain experienced, how often does the same type of pain recur, and does it awaken the patient from sleep, esp. at night? Observe the facial expression during an attack of pain and listen carefully to the patient's description.

The patient may locate a *headache* around the eyes and nose, in the center of the forehead, above the nose, in one or both temples accompanied by throbbing, at the top of the head, or at the base of the brain. It may be felt as a tight, bandlike sensation around the head above the eyes. It may be in the center of the forehead above the eyebrow line, in the upper region of the center forehead, all over the top of the head, over one or both ears, or back of both ears. Pain may be sharp, dull, or shifting. It may accompany head noises, or a roaring in the head may be experienced without pain. Vertigo or a sensation of fainting may be present. Pulsations may be felt in the occiput or in the temporal region. A patient may be very sensitive to light and sound, and headaches may be accompanied by nausea, vomiting, the sensation of flashing lights, and chills. Tenderness or soreness may be associated with rigidity. SEE: *headache; pain*.

POSITIONS AND POSTURES: An inability to lie down; to arise; or to lie on one side, on the back, or in any special position reveals much to the physician. Whether lying on the affected or unaffected side is also important to observe. Left or right legs, or both, may be flexed, or there may be an inclination to lie with the arms above the head. The legs may be restless. SEE: *posture.*

SKIN: May appear pale, flushed all over or in spots; may be cyanotic, jaundiced, shiny, erupted, burned, blistered, sunburned, wrinkled, lacerated, nodular, bruised; or may exhibit dermographia, lesions, growth, or deformities; or may be puffy and edematous, ashy, gray, wet with perspiration, or discolored. SEE: *skin.*

THROAT: May show abnormalities, discoloration, swelling, inflammation, diseased tonsils, and presence of adenoids. Dysphagia and hoarseness or aphonia and other conditions affecting the voice may be present. A lump in the throat (globus hystericus), or a dry, scratchy irritation or fullness or pulsations may be present.

TONGUE: May be coated, clean, smooth, atrophic, shiny, dry on top and moist on the sides or dry all over; may look like raw beef or appear furry, glossy, tremulous, or sharp-pointed. It may be edematous or abnormal in size; there may be fissures; the papillae may have disappeared; there may be a strawberry tongue, or it may have various colors. SEE: *tongue.*

URINE: May be blue, milky, pale, lemon, smoky, brick-colored, clear, amber, straw-colored, orange, or almost any other color. Hematuria may be present. Polyuria or oliguria may be indicated, or there may be frequent urination of small amounts. The odors may be ammoniacal, aromatic, stercorous, or like that of new-mown hay, ripe apples, or violets. There may be retention, suppression, or dribbling, and urination may be painful. SEE: *urine.*

s., accessory. A minor symptom, or one that is not pathognomonic.

s., accidental. Symptom occurring incidentally during course of a disease, but having no relationship to the disease.

s., assident. S., accessory.

s., cardinal. A principal symptom in the diagnosis of a disease.

s., concomitant. Symptom occurring along with the essential symptoms of a disease.

s., constitutional. Symptom caused by or indicating disease of the whole body. SYN: *s., general.*

s., delayed. Symptom appearing sometime after the precipitating cause.

s., direct. Symptom resulting from direct effects of the disease.

s., dissociation. Anesthesia to heat, cold, and pain without loss of tactile sensibility. Seen in syringomyelia.

s., equivocal. Symptom that may occur in several diseases.

s., focal. Symptom at a specific location.

s., general. S., constitutional.

s., indirect. Symptom occurring secondarily as a result of a disease.

s., labyrinthine. A group of symptoms, such as tinnitus, vertigo, or nausea, indicating a disease or lesion of the inner ear.

s., local. Symptom indicating the specific location of the pathological process.

s., negative pathognomonic. Symptom that never occurs in a certain disease or condition; hence its occurrence rules out the existence of that disease.

s., objective. Symptom apparent to the observer. SEE: *sign.*

s., passive. S., static.

s., pathognomonic. Symptom that is unmistakably associated with a particular disease.

s., presenting. Symptom that led the patient to seek medical care.

s.´s, prodromal. Symptoms that indicate an approaching disease. SYN: *prodrome.*

s., rational. Symptom apparent only to the patient. SYN: *s., subjective.*

s., signal. Symptom that is premonitory of an impending condition such as the aura that precedes an attack of epilepsy or migraine.

s., static. Symptom pert. to the condition of a single organ or structure without reference to remainder of body. SYN: *s., passive.*

s., subjective. Symptom apparent only to the patient. SYN: *s., rational.*

s., sympathetic. Symptom for which there is no specific inciting cause and usually occurring at a point more or less remote from the point of disturbance. SEE: *sympathy* (def. 1).

s.´s, withdrawal. Those symptoms following sudden withdrawal of a substance to which a person has become addicted.

symptomatic (sĭmp″tō-măt′ĭk) [Gr. *symptomatikos*]. Of the nature of or concerning a symptom.

symptomatology (sĭmp″tō-mă-tŏl′ō-jē) [Gr. *symptoma*, symptom, + *logos*, word, reason]. 1. Science of symptoms and indications. SYN: *semeiology.* 2. All of the symptoms of a given disease as a whole.

symptomatolytic (sĭmp″tō-măt″ō-lĭt′ĭk) [″ + *lysis*, dissolution]. Causing the removal of symptoms.

symptom complex. A group of symptoms

that occur together and thus characterize a specific disease. SYN: *syndrome*.

symptom magnification syndrome. Term used in conjunction with the rehabilitation of persons with work-related injuries to refer to behaviors which exaggerated pain or functional limitation.

symptomolytic (sĭmp″tō-mō-lĭt′ĭk) [″ + *lysis*, dissolution]. Pert. to the removal of symptoms. SYN: *symptomatolytic*.

symptosis (sĭmp-tō′sĭs) [Gr. *syn*, together, + *ptosis*, a dropping]. Emaciation; wasting away of the body or an organ.

sympus (sĭm′pŭs) [″ + *pous*, foot]. A deformed fetus fused at the lower limbs.

syn- [Gr., together]. Prefix meaning joined, together. SEE: words beginning with *con-*.

synache. Inflammation of the throat that obstructs the airway.

synactosis (sĭn″ăk-tō′sĭs) [Gr. *syn*, together, + L. *actio*, function, + Gr. *osis*, condition]. Malformation resulting from the abnormal fusion of parts.

synadelphus (sĭn″ă-dĕl′fŭs) [″ + *adelphos*, brother]. A deformed fetus with eight limbs.

Synalar. Trade name for fluocinolone acetonide, USP.

synalgia (sĭn-ăl′jē-ă) [″ + *algos*, pain]. Referred or reflex pain felt in a part distant from the site of its origin.

synalgic (sĭn-ăl′jĭk) [. Pert. to or characterized by referred pain.

synapse (sĭn′ăps) [Gr. *synapsis*, point of contact]. The point of junction between two neurons in a neural pathway, where the termination of the axon of one neuron comes into close proximity with the cell body or dendrites of another. At this point, where the relationship of the two neurons is one of contact only, the impulse traveling in the first neuron initiates an impulse in the second neuron. Synapses are polarized, i.e., the impulses pass in one direction only. They are susceptible to fatigue, offer a resistance to the passage of impulses, and are markedly susceptible to the effects of oxygen deficiency, anesthetics, and other agents, including therapeutic drugs and toxic chemicals.

s., axodendritic. Connection between an axon of one neuron and the dendrites of another.

s., axodendrosomatic. Connection between the axon of one neuron and the dendrites and body of another.

s., axosomatic. Connection between the axon of one neuron and the body of another.

synapsis (sĭn-ăp′sĭs) [Gr., point of contact]. 1. Synapse. 2. The process of first maturation division in gametogenesis, in which there is

conjugation of pairs of homologous chromosomes forming double or bivalent chromosomes. In the resulting meiotic division, the chromosome number is reduced from the diploid to the haploid number. It is at this stage that crossing over occurs.

RS: crossing over; meiosis; oogenesis; spermatogenesis.

synaptic. Pert. to a synapse or synapsis.

synaptic field. A field in the cerebral cortex, cerebellar cortex, and retina where large numbers of contacts between neurons can take place.

synaptolemma (sĭn-ăp″tō-lĕm′ă). The membrane at a synapse separating two neurons.

synaptology (sĭn″ăp-tŏl′ō-jē) [″ + *logos*, word, reason]. Study of the synapse.

synarthrodia (sĭn″ăr-thrō′dē-ă) [Gr. *syn*, together, + *arthron*, joint, + *eidos*, form, shape]. Type of immovable cartilaginous joint without a joint cavity in which bones are separated by only a connective tissue membrane; a fixed articulation. SYN: *synarthrosis*. SEE: *joint*.

synarthrodial. Pert. to a synarthrosis.

synarthrophysis (sĭn″ăr-thrō-fĭ′sĭs) [″ + *arthron*, joint, + *physis*, growth]. Progressive ankylosis of joints.

synarthrosis [″ + *arthron*, joint, + *osis*, condition] (pl. *synarthroses*). A type of joint in which the skeletal elements are united by a continuous intervening substance (cartilage, fibrous tissue, or bone). Movement is absent or limited, and a joint cavity is lacking. It includes the synchondrosis, suture, and syndesmosis types of joints. SYN: *synarthrodia*.

syncanthus (sĭn-kăn′thŭs) [″ + *kanthos*, angle]. Adhesion of the eyeball to the structures of the orbit.

syncaryon (sĭn-kăr′ē-ŏn). Synkaryon, q.v.

syncephalus (sĭn-sĕf′ă-lŭs) [″ + *kephale*, head]. A deformed fetus with one head, one face, and four ears.

synchilia (sĭn-kī′lē-ă) [″ + *cheilos*, lip]. Congenital adhesions of the lips or atresia of the mouth.

synchiria (sĭn-kī′rē-ă) [″ + *cheir*, hand]. Disorder of sensibility in which stimulus applied to one side of the body is felt on both sides. SEE: *achiria; allochiria; dyschiria*.

synchondroseotomy (sĭn″kŏn-drŏ″sē-ŏt′ō-mē) [″ + *chondros*, cartilage, + *tome*, incision]. An operation of cutting through the sacroiliac ligaments and closing the arch of the pubes in congenital absence of the anterior wall of the bladder (exstrophy).

synchondrosis (sĭn″kŏn-drŏ′sĭs) [″ + ″ + *osis*, condition]. An immovable joint having surfaces between the bones connected by cartilages. This may be temporary, in which case the cartilage eventually becomes ossified, or permanent.

synchondrotomy (sĭn-kŏn-drŏt'ō-mē) [" + " + *tome*, incision]. 1. Division of articulating cartilage of a synchondrosis. 2. Section of the symphysis pubis to facilitate childbirth. SEE: *symphyseotomy.*

synchorial (sĭn-kō'rē-ăl) [" + *chorion*, chorion]. Pert. to multiple fetuses that share a single placenta.

synchronism (sĭn'krō-nĭzm) [" + *chronos*, time, + *-ismos*, condition]. Simultaneous occurrence of acts or events.

synchronous (sĭn'krō-nŭs). Occurring simultaneously.

synchrony. Simultaneous occurrence of separate events.

synchrotron (sĭn'krō-trŏn). An apparatus that accelerates atomic particles around a circular path by use of electrostatic forces.

synchysis (sĭn'kĭs-ĭs) [Gr., confound]. Fluid state of vitreous of the eye.

  s. scintillans. Bright flashes of light resulting from presence of crystals of cholesterol or fat substances in vitreous body.

syncinesis (sĭn″sĭn-ē'sĭs) [" + *kinesis*, movement]. An involuntary movement produced in association with a voluntary one. SYN: *synkinesis.*

  s., imitative. Involuntary movement occurring on sound side when movement is attempted on paralyzed side.

  s., spasmodic. Syncinesis occurring on paralyzed side when muscles of opposite side are voluntarily moved.

synciput (sĭn'sĭ-pŭt). Anterior upper half of the cranium. SYN: *sinciput.*

synclinal (sĭn-klī'năl) [Gr. *synklinein*, to lean together]. Inclined in the same direction toward a point.

synclitism (sĭn'klĭt-ĭzm) [Gr. *synklinein*, to lean together, + *-ismos*, condition]. Parallelism between the planes of the fetal head and those of the maternal pelvis.

synclonus (sĭn'klō-nŭs) [" + *klonos*, turmoil]. 1. Clonic contraction of several muscles together. 2. A disease marked by muscular spasms.

  s. ballismus. Paralysis agitans.

  s. tremens. Generalized tremor.

syncopal (sĭn'kō-păl) [Gr. *synkope*, fainting]. Rel. to or marked by syncope.

syncope (sĭn'kō-pē) [Gr. *synkope*, fainting]. A transient loss of consciousness due to inadequate blood flow to the brain. SYN: *fainting; swoon.* SEE: *coma; transient ischemic attack; unconsciousness.*

  ETIOL: Syncope or fainting may be due to deficient blood flow resulting from peripheral circulatory failure, cerebral vascular accident (stroke), cardiac arrhythmia or transient cardiac standstill in Stokes-

Adams syndrome, q.v., or altered blood chemistry as in hyperventilation or hypoglycemia. Predisposing factors include fatigue, prolonged standing, nausea, pain, emotional disturbances, anemia, dehydration, poor ventilation, and many others.

  F.A.: Place the person in a horizontal position, preferably with the head low in order to facilitate blood flow to the brain. At the same time, be certain there is a clear airway. The clothing must be loose, esp. if a tight collar was being worn. Fainting usually is of short duration and is counteracted by the individual's being in a supine position. Nevertheless it is important to attempt to establish the cause of the faint prior to dismissing the episode as being of no consequence. If recovery from fainting is not prompt, move the person to a hospital.

  s. anginosa. Syncope occurring with anginal pain.

  s., cardiac. Syncope of cardiac origin as in Stokes-Adams syndrome, aortic stenosis, tachycardia, bradycardia, or myocardial infarction.

  s., carotid sinus. Syncope resulting from pressure on, or hypersensitivity of, carotid sinus. May result from turning head to one side or from too tight a collar.

  s., cough. Syncope occurring during a coughing spell.

  s., defecation. SEE: *defecation syncope.*

  s., hysterical. Syncope resulting from anxiety.

  s., laryngeal. Brief unconsciousness following coughing and tickling in the throat. SYN: *vertigo, laryngeal.*

  s., local. Numbness of a part with sudden blanching, as of the fingers; a symptom of Raynaud's disease or of local asphyxia.

  s., micturition. SEE: *micturition syncope.*

  s., swallow. Fainting that occurs in relation to swallowing. This may be related to an abnormality of the esophagus or heart; but may also occur in normal persons.

  s., vasovagal. Syncope resulting from fall in blood pressure due to failure of peripheral resistance with concomitant reduced venous return, or due to slowing of the heart. May be caused by emotional stress, pain, acute loss of blood, fear, or by assuming an upright position after having been in bed for a prolonged period.

syncopic (sĭn-kŏp'ĭk) [Gr. *synkope*, fainting]. Syncopal.

syncretio (sĭn-krē'shē-ō) [L.]. Development of adhesions between opposing inflamed surfaces.

syncytial (sĭn-sĭ'shăl). Of the nature of a syncytium.

syncytiolysin (sĭn″sĭt-ē-ŏl'ĭ-sĭn) [Gr. *syn*, together, + *kytos*, cell, + *lysis*, dissolution]. A cytolysin that is formed from injections of emulsions of placental tissue.

syncytioma (sĭn″sĭt-ē-ō′mă) [″ + ″ + *oma*, tumor]. A tumor of the chorion. SYN: *chorioma; deciduoma.*

  s. benignum. A mole.

  s. malignum. A tumor formed of cells from the syncytium and chorion, occurring frequently after abortion or during puerperium at site of placenta.

syncytiotrophoblast (sĭn-sĭt″ē-ō-trō′fō-blăst) [″ + ″ + *trophe*, nourishment, + *blastos*, germ]. The outer layer of cells covering the chorionic villi of the placenta. These cells are in contact with the maternal blood or decidua. SYN: *syntrophoblast.*

syncytium (sĭn-sĭt′ē-ŭm) [″ + *kytos*, cell]. 1. A multinucleated mass of protoplasm such as a striated muscle fiber. 2. A group of cells in which the protoplasm of one cell is continuous with that of adjoining cells such as the mesenchyme cells of the embryo. SYN: *coenocyte.*

syndactylism (sĭn-dăk′tĭl-ĭzm) [″ + *daktylos*, finger, + *-ismos*, condition]. A fusion of two or more toes or fingers.

syndactylous (sĭn-dăk′tĭ-lŭs) [″ + *daktylos*, finger]. Concerning syndactylism.

syndectomy (sĭn-dĕk′tō-mē) [″ + *dein*, to bind, + *ektome*, excision]. Excision of a circular strip of the conjunctiva around the cornea to relieve pannus. SYN: *peritomy* (def. 1).

syndesis (sĭn-dē′sĭs) [″ + *desis*, binding]. 1. Condition of being bound together. 2. Surgical fixation or ankylosis of a joint.

syndesmectomy (sĭn″dĕs-mĕk′tō-mē) [Gr. *syndesmos*, ligament, + *ektome*, excision]. Excision of a section of a ligament.

syndesmectopia (sĭn″dĕs-mĕk-tō′pē-ă) [″ + *ektopos*, out of place]. Abnormal position of a ligament.

syndesmitis (sĭn″dĕs-mī′tĭs) [″ + *itis*, inflammation]. 1. Inflammation of a ligament or ligaments. 2. Inflammation of the conjunctiva.

syndesmochorial (sĭn″dĕs″mō-kor′ē-ăl). Pert. to a type of placenta found in ungulates (e.g., sheep and goats) in which there is destruction of surface layer of uterine mucosa, thus allowing chorionic villi to come into direct contact with maternal blood vessels.

syndesmography (sĭn-dĕs-mŏg′ră-fē) [Gr. *syndesmos*, ligament, + *graphein*, to write]. Treatise on the ligaments.

syndesmologia (sĭn″dĕs-mō-lō′jē-ă) [″ + *logos*, word, reason]. A term concerned with the articulations of joints and their related ligaments.

syndesmology (sĭn″dĕs-mŏl′ō-jē) [″ + *logos*, word, reason]. Study of the ligaments, joints, their movements, and their disorders.

syndesmoma (sĭn″dĕs-mō′mă) [″ + *oma*, tumor]. A connective tissue tumor.

syndesmopexy (sĭn″dĕs′mō-pĕk″sē) [″ + *pexis*, fixation]. Joining of two ligaments or fixation of a ligament in a new place, used in correction of a dislocation.

syndesmophyte (sĭn-dĕs′mō-fīt) [″ + *phyton*, plant]. 1. A bony bridge formed between adjacent vertebrae. 2. A bony outgrowth from a ligament.

syndesmoplasty (sĭn-dĕs′mō-plăs″tē) [″ + *plassein*, to form]. Plastic surgery on a ligament.

syndesmorrhaphy (sĭn″dĕs-mor′ă-fē) [″ + *rhaphe*, seam, ridge]. Repair or suture of a ligament.

syndesmosis (sĭn″dĕs-mō′sĭs) [Gr. *syndesmos*, ligament, + *osis*, condition) (pl. *syndesmoses*). [NA] Articulation in which the bones are united by ligaments. Ex.: the distal tibiofibular articulation.

syndesmotomy (sĭn″dĕs-mŏt′ō-mē) [″ + *tome*, incision]. Surgical section of ligaments.

syndrome (sĭn′drōm) [Gr., a running together]. A group of symptoms and signs of disordered function related to one another by means of some anatomic, physiologic, or biochemical peculiarity. This definition does not include a precise cause of an illness but does provide a framework of reference for investigating it.

  s., Adair-Dighton. A familial condition characterized by fragility of bones, deafness, and blue sclerae. SEE: *osteogenesis imperfecta.*

  s., adiposogenital. S., Fröhlich's.

  s., adrenogenital. Syndrome characterized by abnormally early puberty in children, overmasculinization in adults, virilism, and hirsutism, due to excess production of adrenocortical hormones. SEE: *Cushing's syndrome.*

  s., Angelman. A rare genetic condition characterized by severe mental retardation, microcephaly, and paroxysms of laughter. Due to an abnormal chromosome 15 of maternal origin. SEE: *s., Prader-Willi.*

  s., Angelucci's. Palpitation, excitable temperament, and vasomotor disturbance in some individuals who experience spring conjunctivitis.

  s., congenital rubella. Infection of the fetus from maternal rubella. The newborn may have severe central nervous system impairment, including deafness and mental retardation. SEE: *vaccine, rubella.*

  s., dumping. Symptom complex that may follow partial or complete gastrectomy.

Appears to be related to rapid emptying of the gastric pouch. Occurs immediately after eating. Consists of weakness, varying degrees of syncope, nausea, sweating, and palpitation, and sometimes diarrhea and sensation of warmth. Usually lying down affords some relief.

s., Fröhlich's. Syndrome characterized by increase in fat, atrophy of the genitals, transition to feminine type due to lesions of the pituitary and hypothalamus. SYN: *dystrophy, adiposogenital.*

s., Gilles de la Tourette's. SEE: *Gilles de la Tourette's syndrome.*

s., Gradenigo's. Paralysis of the external rectus muscle with severe temporoparietal pain and suppurative otitis media on affected side. Caused by infection in petrous portion of the temporal bone involving the 6th nerve.

s., Horner's. Contracted pupil, ptosis, enophthalmos, and dry, cool face on affected side produced by paralysis of sympathetic nerves. Caused by tumors in neck, trauma, apical tuberculosis, tabes, syringomyelia, and neuritis of cervical plexus.

s., Korsakoff's. A pyschosis, ordinarily due to chronic alcoholism, with polyneuritis, disorientation, insomnia, muttering delirium, hallucinations, and a bilateral wrist or foot drop.

s., Marfan's. A hereditary syndrome characterized by disorders of connective tissue, bones, eyes, muscles, ligaments, and skeletal structures.

s. of inappropriate antidiuretic hormone. ABBR: SIADH. Increased ADH activity in spite of reduced plasma osmolarity. Often first recognized by a relative hyponatremia, it is most commonly associated with CNS disorders, various tumors, and drugs.

s., Prader-Willi [Andrea Prader and Heinrich Willi, 20th century Swiss pediatricians]. A rare congenital condition characterized by genetic obesity, mental retardation, short stature, sexual infantilism, and hypotonia. Due to an abnormal chromosome 15 of maternal origin. SEE: *s., Angelman.*

s., shoulder-hand. A reflex neurovascular problem in the upper extremity caused by trauma in the shoulder region, involving the wrist and hand with edema, vasomotor instability and trophic changes in the skin.

s., sick sinus. SEE: *sick sinus syndrome.*

s., skin-eye. Syndrome consisting of deposits on the anterior surface of the lens and posterior cornea, and skin pigmentation. Due to extensive medication with some of the phenothiazine-type tranquilizers. SEE: *iatrogenic disorder.*

s., Stokes-Adams. Syndrome of brady-

cardia and intermittent convulsive seizures with loss of consciousness due to decreased flow of blood to the brain. Caused by partial or complete heart block.

s., toxic shock. SEE: *toxic shock syndrome.*

s., Weber's. Paralysis of hypoglossal nerve on one side and of oculomotor nerve on other with paralysis of limbs due to lesion of a cerebral peduncle.

syndromic (sĭn-drŏm'ĭk) [Gr. *syndrome,* a running together]. Pert. to or occurring as a syndrome.

synechia (sĭn-ĕk'ē-ă) [Gr. *synecheia,* continuity] (pl. *synechiae*). Adhesions of parts, esp. adhesion of iris to lens and cornea.

s., annular. Adhesion of iris to lens throughout its entire pupillary margin.

s., anterior. Adhesion of iris to cornea.

s., posterior. Adhesion of iris to capsule of lens.

s., total. Adhesion of entire surface of iris to lens.

s. vulvae. Fusion of the vulvae, usually congenital.

synechotome (sĭn-ĕk'ō-tōm) [″ + *tome,* incision]. An instrument for cutting synechia.

synechotomy (sĭn″ĕk-ŏt'ō-mē) [″ + *tome,* incision]. Division of a synechia or adhesion.

synechtenterotomy (sĭn″ĕk-tĕn″tĕr-ŏt'ō-mē) [″ + *enteron,* intestine, + *tome,* incision]. Division of an intestinal adhesion.

synecology (sĭn″ē-kŏl'ō-jē) [Gr. *syn,* together, + *oikos,* house, + *logos,* word, reason]. The study of organisms in relationship to their environment in group form.

Synemol. Trade name for fluocinolone acetonide, USP.

synencephalocele (sĭn″ĕn-sĕf'ă-lō-sēl″) [″ + *enkephalos,* brain, + *kele,* tumor, swelling]. Encephalocele with adhesions to adjacent structures.

syneresis (sĭn-ĕr'ĕ-sĭs) [Gr. *synairesis,* drawing together]. Contraction of a gel resulting in its separation from the liquid, as a shrinkage of fibrin when blood clots.

synergetic (sĭn″ĕr-jĕt'ĭk) [Gr. *syn,* together, + *ergon,* work]. Exhibiting cooperative action, said of certain muscles; working together. SYN: *synergic.*

synergia (sĭn-ĕr'jē-ă). The association and correlation of the activity of synergetic muscle groups.

synergic (sĭn-ĕr'jĭk) [″ + *ergon,* work]. Rel. to or exhibiting cooperation, as certain muscles. SYN: *synergetic.*

synergism (sĭn'ĕr-jĭzm) [″ + ″ + *-ismos,* condition]. The harmonious action of two agents, such as drugs or organs, producing an effect that neither could produce alone or one that is greater than the total effects of each agent operating by itself.

synergist (sĭn′ĕr-jĭst). 1. A remedy that acts to enhance the action of another. SYN: *adjuvant.* 2. A muscle or organ functioning in cooperation with another, as the flexor muscles. Opposite of antagonist.

synergistic (sĭn″ĕr-jĭs′tĭk). 1. Concerning synergy. 2. Acting together.

synergy (sĭn′ĕr-jē) [Gr. *synergia*]. Action of two or more agents or organs working with each other; cooperation. Combined action; coordinated action. SEE: *synergism.*

synesthesia (sĭn″ĕs-thē′zē-ă) [Gr. *syn*, together, + *aisthesis*, sensation]. 1. A sensation in one area from a stimulus applied to another part. 2. A subjective sensation of a sense other than the one being stimulated. Hearing a sound may also produce the sensation of smell. SEE: *phonism.*

   s. algica. Painful synesthesia.

synesthesialgia (sĭn″ĕs-thē-zē-ăl′jē-ă) [″ + ″ + *algos*, pain]. A painful sensation giving rise to a subjective one of different character. SEE: *synesthesia.*

synezesis (sĭn″ē-zē′sĭs) [Gr. *synizesis*, a sitting together]. Closure of the pupil.

Syngamus (sĭn′gă-mŭs). A genus of nematode worms parasitic in the respiratory tract of birds and mammals.

   S. laryngeus. Species normally parasitic in ruminants, but sometimes accidentally infesting humans.

syngamy (sĭn′gă-mē) [Gr. *syn*, together, + *gamos*, marriage]. 1. Sexual reproduction. 2. Cell union as of gametes in fertilization.

syngeneic. Term used to describe individuals or cells without detectable tissue incompatibility. Strains of mice that are inbred for a great number of generations become syngeneic. Identical twins may be syngeneic.

syngenesioplasty (sĭn″jĕ-nē″zē-ō-plăs′tē) [″ + *genesis*, generation, birth, + *plassein*, to form]. Indicating transplantation of tissue from one individual to one related and of the same species.

syngenesious (sĭn″jĕ-nē′shŭs) [″ + *genesis*, generation, birth]. Derived from an individual of the same species, said of tissue transplants.

syngenesis (sĭn-jĕn′ē-sĭs) [″ + *genesis*, generation, birth]. Arising from the germ cells derived from both parents, rather than from a single cell from one parent.

syngnathia (sĭn-nā′thē-ă) [″ + *gnathos*, jaw]. Congenital adhesions between the jaws.

synhidrosis (sĭn″hī-drō′sĭs) [″ + *hidrosis*, sweat]. Sweating, esp. excessive sweating associated with another condition.

synizesis (sĭn″ĭ-zē′sĭs) [Gr. *synizesis*]. 1. An occlusion, or shutting. 2. Clumping of nu-

clear chromatin during prophase of mitosis.

   s. pupillae. Closure of the pupil of the eye with loss of vision.

synkaryon (sĭn-kăr′ē-ŏn) [Gr. *syn*, together, + *karyon*, kernel]. A nucleus resulting from fusion of two pronuclei.

synkinesis (sĭn″kĭ-nē′sĭs) [″ + *kinesis*, movement]. An involuntary movement of one part occurring simultaneously with reflex or voluntary movement of another part.

   s., imitative. An involuntary movement in a healthy or normal muscle accompanying an attempted movement of a paralyzed muscle on the opposite side.

synnecrosis (sĭn″nĕ-krō′sĭs) [″ + *nekrosis*, state of death]. The condition of association between groups or individuals that causes mutual inhibition or death.

synonym (sĭn′ō-nĭm) [Gr. *synonymon*]. ABBR: syn. One of two words that have the same or very similar meaning; an additional or substitute name for the same disease, sign, symptom, or anatomical structure.

synophrys (sĭn-ŏf′rĭs) [Gr. *syn*, together, + *ophrys*, eyebrow]. Condition in which the eyebrows grow across the midline.

synophthalmus (sĭn″ŏf-thăl′mŭs) [″ + *ophthalmos*, eye]. Cyclops.

synopsia (sĭn″ŏp-sē-ă) [″ + *opsis*, vision]. Condition in which there is a congenital fusion of the eyes.

synopsis (sĭn-ŏp′sĭs) [Gr.]. A summary; a general review of the whole.

synoptophore (sĭn-ŏp′tō-for) [″ + *ops*, sight, + *phoros*, bearing]. Apparatus for diagnosis and treatment of strabismus.

synoptoscope (sĭn-ŏp′tō-skōp) [″ + ″ + *skopein*, to examine]. An instrument for diagnosis and treatment of strabismus. SYN: *synoptophore.*

synorchidism, synorchism (sĭn-or′kĭd-ĭzm, -kĭzm) [″ + *orchis*, testicle, + *-ismos*, condition]. Union or partial fusion of the testicles.

synoscheos (sĭn-ŏs′kē-ŏs) [″ + *oscheon*, scrotum]. Adhesions between the penis and scrotum.

synosteology (sĭn″ŏs-tē-ŏl′ō-jē) [″ + ″ + *logos*, word, reason]. The branch of medical science concerned with joints and articulations.

synosteosis (sĭn″ŏs-tē-ō′sĭs). Synostosis.

synosteotomy (sĭn″ŏs-tē-ŏt′ō-mē) [″ + *osteon*, bone, + *tome*, incision]. Dissection of joints.

synostosis (sĭn″ŏs-tō′sĭs) [″ + ″ + *osis*, condition] (pl. *synostoses*). 1. [NA] Articulation by osseous tissue of adjacent bones. 2. Union of separate bones by osseous tissue.

synostotic (sĭn″ŏs-tŏt′ĭk) [″ + ″ + *osis*, condition]. Concerning synostosis.

synotia (sĭn-ō′shē-ă) [″ + *ous*, ear]. The

union of, or approximation of, the ears occurring in embryonic development, usually associated with absence of, or incomplete development of, the lower jaw.

synotus (sĭ-nō'tŭs) [" + *ous*, ear]. A fetus with synotia.

synovectomy (sĭn″ō-vĕk′tō-mē) [L. *synovia*, joint fluid, + Gr. *ektome*, excision]. Excision of synovial membrane.

synovia (sĭn-ō′vē-ă) [L.]. [NA] A colorless viscid, lubricating fluid of joints, bursae, and tendon sheaths secreted within synovial membranes. It contains mucin, albumin, fat, and mineral salts. SYN: *synovial fluid*. SEE: *asynovia; joint, synovial* for illus.

synovial (sĭn-ō′vē-ăl). Pert. to synovia, the lubricating fluid of the joints.

synovial bursa. A cavity in connective tissue between muscles, tendons, ligaments, and bones lined by a synovial membrane and containing synovia. SYN: *bursa*.

synovial crypt. Diverticulum of a synovial membrane of a joint.

synovial cyst. Accumulation of synovia in a bursa, synovial crypt, or sac of a synovial hernia, causing a tumor.

synovial fluid. Clear lubricating fluid secreted by the synovial membrane of a joint. SYN: *synovia*. SEE: *joint, synovial* for illus.

synovial folds. Smooth folds of synovial membrane on inner surface of the joint capsule. SYN: *plica synovialis* [NA].

synovial hernia. Protrusion of a portion of synovial membrane through a tear in the stratum fibrosum of a joint capsule.

synovialis (sĭ-nō″vē-ā′lĭs) [L.]. Synovial.

synovial membrane. Membrane lining the capsule of a joint. SYN: *synovium*.

synovialoma (sĭ-nō″vē-ă-lō′mă) [L. *synovia*, joint fluid, + Gr. *oma*, tumor]. Synovioma.

synovial tendon sheaths. Sheaths that develop in osteofibrous canals through which tendons pass. Each is a double-layered tube, the space between the two layers being occupied by synovial fluid. SYN: *vagina mucosa tendinis*.

synovial villi. Slender avascular processes on the free surface of a synovial membrane projecting into the joint cavity.

synovioma (sĭn″ō-vē-ō′mă) [L. *synovia*, joint fluid, + Gr. *oma*, tumor]. A tumor arising from a synovial membrane.

synoviparous (sĭn″ō-vĭp′ă-rŭs) [" + *parere*, to produce]. Forming synovia.

synovitis (sĭn″ō-vī′tĭs) [" + Gr. *itis*, inflammation]. Inflammation of a synovial membrane. SEE: *Nursing Diagnoses in Appendix.*

SYM: The joint is painful, much more so on motion, esp. at night. Swollen, tense; may be fluctuating. In synovitis of the knee, patella is floated up from condyles, and it can be readily depressed, to rise again when pressure is taken off. The part is never in full extension, as this increases the pain. Skin, which is very sensitive to pressure only at certain points, is neither thickened nor reddened. After a few days, when pain lessens and swelling diminishes as the effusion and extravasated blood are absorbed, the limb takes its natural position, and recovery follows.

ETIOL: Simple inflammation may be the result of an aseptic wound, a subcutaneous injury (contusion or sprain), irritation produced by damaged cartilage, or exposure to cold and dampness.

s., chronic. Synovitis in which active congestion appears but an undue amount of fluid remains in the cavity, and the membrane itself is edematous. Later if disease does not subside, membrane and articular structures become irregularly thickened by plastic exudation and formation of fibrous tissue. Joint is weak but not esp. painful, except on pressure and sometimes not even then. Movements, esp. in extension, are restricted, and generally attended by some grating or creaking. Symptoms are well marked when there is great accumulation of liquid. Fluid, which is straw-colored, somewhat viscid, sometimes flocculent, and may or may not be bloodstained, can be drawn off with the hypodermic needle.

s., dendritic. Synovitis with villous growths developing in the sac.

s., dry. Synovitis with little or no effusion. SYN: *s. sicca*.

s., purulent. Synovitis with purulent effusion within the sac. SYN: *arthritis, suppurative*.

s., serous. Synovitis with nonpurulent, copious effusion.

s. sicca. S., dry.

s., simple. Synovitis with effusion only slightly turbid, if not clear.

s., tendinous. Inflammation of a tendon sheath.

s., vaginal. S., tendinous.

s., vibration. Synovitis resulting from a wound near a joint.

synovium (sĭn-ō′vē-ŭm) [L. *synovia*, joint fluid]. A synovial membrane.

syntactic (sĭn-tăk′tĭk). Concerning or affecting syntax.

syntasis (sĭn-tā′sĭs) [Gr. *syn*, together, + *teinein*, to stretch]. Stretching.

syntaxis (sĭn-tăk′sĭs) [" + *taxis*, arrangement]. A junction between two bones. SYN: *articulation*.

syntectic (sĭn-tĕk′tĭk). Concerning syntexis.

syntexis (sĭn-tĕk′sĭs) [Gr.]. Wasting or cachexia.

synthase. Any enzyme that acts as a catalyst for synthesizing high-energy phosphate bonds. SEE: *synthetase.*

synthermal (sĭn-thĕr'măl) [" + *therme,* heat]. Having the same temperature.

synthesis (sĭn'thĕs-ĭs) [Gr.]. In chemistry, the union of elements to produce compounds; the process of building up. In general, the process or processes involved in the formation of a complex substance from simpler elements or compounds, as the synthesis of proteins from amino acids. Opposite of decomposition.

synthesize (sĭn"thĕ-sīz'). To produce by synthesis.

synthetase (sĭn'thĕ-tās). An enzyme that acts as a catalyst for joining two molecules with the loss or splitting off of a high-energy phosphate group. SYN: *ligase.*

synthetic (sĭn-thĕt'ĭk) [Gr. *synthetikos*]. Rel. to or made by synthesis; artificially prepared.

synthetic blood. SEE: *blood, synthetic.*

synthorax (sĭn-thō'răks) [Gr. *syn,* together, + *thorax,* chest]. Thoracopagus, q.v.

Synthroid. Trade name for levothyroxine sodium.

Syntocinon. Trade name for oxytocin injection.

syntone (sĭn'tōn) [" + *tonos,* act of stretching, tension]. An individual whose personality indicates a stable responsiveness to the environment and its social demands. SEE: *syntonic.*

syntonic (sĭn-tŏn'ĭk). Pert. to a personality characterized by an even temperament, a normal emotional responsiveness to life situations. Opposite of schizoid. Syntonic type is exaggerated in manic states or in depression. SEE: *syntone.*

syntonin (sĭn'tō-nĭn). An acid albumin formed by the action of dilute hydrochloric acid on muscle during gastric digestion.

syntoxoid (sĭn-tŏk'soyd) [Gr. *syn,* together, + *toxikon,* poison, + *eidos,* form, shape]. A toxoid having the same degree of affinity for an antitoxin as that possessed by the toxin.

syntripsis (sĭn-trĭp'sĭs) [Gr., destruction]. A comminuted fracture or act causing it.

syntrophism (sĭn'trŏf-ĭzm) [" + *trophe,* nourishment, + *-ismos,* condition]. Stimulation of an organism to grow by mixing with or closeness of another strain.

syntrophoblast (sĭn-trŏf'ō-blăst) [" + " + *blastos,* germ]. The outer syncytial layer of the trophoblast. SEE: *trophoblast.*

syntropic (sĭn-trŏp'ĭk) [" + *trope,* a turn]. Concerning syntropy.

syntropy (sĭn'trō-pē) [" + *trope,* a turn]. Turning or pointing in the same direction.

synulosis (sĭn"ū-lō'sĭs) [Gr. *synoulosis*]. Formulation of scar tissue.

synulotic (sĭn"ū-lŏt'ĭk). 1. Promoting cicatrization. 2. An agent stimulating cicatrization.

syphilelcosis (sĭf-ĭl-ĕl-kō'sĭs) [*syphilis* + Gr. *helkosis,* ulceration]. Syphilitic ulceration.

syphilelcus (sĭf"ĭl-ĕl'kŭs) [" + Gr. *helkos,* ulcer]. A syphilitic ulcer or chancre.

syphilid(e) (sĭf"ĭl-ĭd) [Fr.] (pl. *syphilides*). Skin eruption caused by secondary syphilis.

syphilionthus (sĭf"ĭl-ē-ŏn'thŭs) [" + Gr. *ionthos,* eruption]. A copper-colored, branny-scaled syphilide.

syphiliphobia (sĭf"ĭl-ĭ-fō'bē-ă) [" + Gr. *phobos,* fear]. Morbid fear of syphilis. SYN: *syphilophobia.*

syphilis (sĭf'ĭ-lĭs) [*Syphilis,* shepherd having the disease in a Latin poem]. An infectious, chronic, venereal disease characterized by lesions that may involve any organ or tissue. It usually exhibits cutaneous manifestations, relapses are frequent, and it may exist without symptoms for years. SYN: *lues.*

SYM: *Primary stage:* Initial lesion appears 2 to 4 weeks after inoculation, changing from a small red papule to a small ulcer to a hard chancre. Usually upon prepuce or vulva but may be on any skin or mucous membrane site. Lymph nodes enlarge about 2 weeks after appearance of lesion.

Secondary stage: Symptoms appear about 6 weeks after appearance of primary lesion, principally in the form of lesions of the skin and mucous membranes. The character of the skin lesions is protean, syphilis often being called the "great imitator." Systemic symptoms such as headache, fever, and malaise are common but may be absent. Enlargement and induration of regional lymph nodes occur. Eruptions of skin, maculae (roseola), syphilide, reddish-brown coppery spots continuing for a week or two and possibly recurring later.

Tertiary stage: The heart and blood vessels (cardiovascular syphilis) and the central nervous system (neurosyphilis) are frequently involved. Tabes dorsalis, paresis (general paralysis of the insane), and various types of psychoses may result.

ETIOL: *Treponema pallidum,* a spirochete that is transmitted by direct contact between humans, contact with freshly contaminated material, transfusion of infected blood or plasma, or in utero by passage of the organism from mother to fetus. The organism may enter through skin or any mucous membrane.

DIAG: Laboratory tests for syphilis are based on three procedures: *microscopic,* dark-field demonstration of spirochetes in material taken from a chancre or other early lesion; *biopsy,* examination of cerebrospinal fluid; *serologic tests for syphilis* (S.T.S.), done on blood and spinal fluid. The VDRL (Venereal Disease Research Laboratory), *Treponema pallidum* immobilization (TPI), and fluorescent treponemal antibody (FTA) tests also are useful in diagnosing syphilis and distinguishing it from biological false-positive serologic reactions. Serologic tests for syphilis are negative during the primary and early secondary stages of the disease.

Caution: A person who contracts gonorrhea also may have been exposed to syphilis at the same time. Because the clinical signs and symptoms of gonorrhea develop several weeks prior to those of syphilis, the patient may be treated for that disease. The treatment for gonorrhea may be sufficient to mask or delay the signs of syphilis, but insufficient to rid the patient of the spirochetes. When this occurs, syphilis will develop and may be unnoticed by the patient. It is therefore of vital importance either to treat each case of gonorrhea as if syphilis had also been contracted, or to test the patient for serologic evidence of syphilis each month for at least four months following the treatment for gonorrhea.

TREAT: Penicillin is the treatment of choice for all types and stages. A dose that assures an adequate blood level for more than 7 days is needed. Benzathine penicillin in a dose of 2.4 million units given over 2 to 3 days will suffice. Should allergic reactions occur, other antibiotics (doxycycline, tetracycline, or erythromycin) may be substituted.

NURSING IMPLICATIONS: Teach the patient about the illness and the importance of locating all contacts, treatment, and the significance of follow-up care. Administer penicillin as prescribed or alternative antibiotic if patient is allergic to penicillin. Encourage follow-up care. Refer to public health agency to assist in identification of contacts. Teach methods of prevention. Provide supportive counseling. Report disease to infection control authorities as prescribed by local health agency. Utilize caution when handling laboratory specimens. Instruct patient to avoid sexual contact with anyone until he or she has completed therapy; and to avoid sexual contact with previous partners who have not received adequate investigation for the possible presence of syphilis, and treatment if indicated. Employ secretory precautions from the time the disease is suspected until 24 hours after

the initiation of proper antibiotic therapy. SEE: *Universal Precautions* in *Appendix.*

s., cardiovascular. Syphilis involving the heart and great blood vessels, esp. the aorta. Saccular aneurysms of the aorta and aortic insufficiency frequently result.

s., congenital. Syphilis transmitted from the mother to the fetus in utero. SYN: *s., prenatal.* SEE: *Nursing Diagnoses* in *Appendix.*

s., endemic. Chronic, nonvenereal syphilis infection of childhood. It is characterized in its early stages by mucocutaneous or membrane lesions. Later, gummas of bone and skin occur.

ETIOL: The causative organism is *T. pallidum.*

TREAT: Penicillin.

s., extragenital. Syphilis in which the primary chancre is located elsewhere than on genital organs.

s., latent. Phase of syphilis in which symptoms are absent and the disease can be diagnosed only by serological tests.

s., meningovascular. A form of neurosyphilis in which the meninges and vascular structures of the brain and spinal cord are involved. May be localized or general.

s., neuro-. Involvement of the nervous system by syphilis.

s., prenatal. S., congenital.

s., visceral. Syphilis in which visceral organs are involved.

syphilitic (sĭf″ĭ-lĭt′ĭk) [L. *syphiliticus*]. Rel. to, caused by, or affected with syphilis.

syphilitic fever. Rise in temperature in early stage of secondary syphilis.

syphilitic macules. Small red eruptions manifested in secondary syphilis, often covering the entire body.

SYM: Associated with chancre or scar, alopecia, pain in bones, swollen glands, and sore throat.

syphiloderm, syphiloderma (sĭf″ĭl-ō-dĕrm″, sĭf″ĭl-ō-dĕr′mă) [″ + Gr. *derma*, skin]. A syphilitic cutaneous disorder.

syphilogenesis, syphilogeny (sĭf″ĭl-ō-jĕn′ĕ-sĭs, sĭf″ĭl-ōj′ĕn-ē) [″ + Gr. *genesis*, generation, birth]. The development or origin of syphilis.

syphilography (sĭf″ĭl-ŏg′ră-fē). A treatise on syphilis.

syphiloid (sĭf′ĭ-loyd) [″ + Gr. *eidos*, form, shape]. Resembling syphilis.

syphilology (sĭf″ĭl-ŏl′ō-jē). The study of syphilis and its treatment.

syphiloma (sĭf″ĭl-ō′mă) [″ + Gr. *oma*, tumor]. A syphilitic tumor; a gumma, q.v.

syphilomania (sĭf″ĭl-ō-mā′nē-ă) [″ + Gr. *mania*, madness]. Morbid fear of syphilis or inference that one is suffering with it. SYN:

syphilophobia.

syphilopathy (sĭf″ĭ-lŏp′ă-thē) [″ + Gr. *pathos*, disease, suffering]. Any syphilitic disorder.

syphilophobia (sĭf″ĭl-ō-fō′bē-ă) [″ + Gr. *phobos*, fear]. 1. Morbid fear of syphilis. 2. Delusion of having syphilis.

syphilophobic (sĭf″ĭl-ō-fō′bĭk). Pert. to or affected with syphilophobia.

syphilophyma (sĭf″ĭl-ō-fī′mă) [″ + Gr. *phyma*, a growth]. 1. Any growth or excrescence due to syphilis. 2. Syphiloma of the epidermis.

syphilosis (sĭf″ĭ-lō′sĭs) [″ + Gr. *osis*, disease]. Generalized syphilitic disease.

syphilotherapy (sĭf″ĭl-ō-thĕr′ă-pē) [″ + Gr. *therapeia*, treatment]. Treatment of syphilis.

syphionthus (sĭf″ē-ŏn′thŭs) [″ + Gr. *ionthos*, eruption]. Copper-colored patches of the skin seen in syphilis.

syr. L. *syrupus*, syrup.

syrigmophonia (sĭr″ĭg-mō-fō′nē-ă) [Gr. *syrigmos*, a whistle, + *phone*, voice]. 1. A sibilant rale. 2. A whistling sound in pronunciation of "s" due to a denture peculiarity.

syrigmus (sĭr-ĭg′mŭs) [Gr. *syrigmos*, a whistle]. A subjective sound such as a hissing or ringing heard in the ears.

syringadenoma (sĭr-ĭng″ă-dē-nō′mă) [Gr. *syrinx*, pipe, + *aden*, gland, + *oma*, tumor]. Tumor of a sweat gland.

syringe (sĭr-ĭnj′, sĭr′ĭng) [Gr. *syrinx*, pipe]. 1. Instrument for injecting fluids into cavities or vessels. 2. To wash out or introduce fluid with a syringe.

   s., hypodermic. Syringe, fitted with a needle, used to administer drugs by injecting them into the subcutaneous tissue.

   s., oral. Syringe made of plastic or glass. It is not fitted with a needle. It is graduated and is used to dispense liquid medication to children. The tip is constructed to prevent its breaking in the child's mouth.

syringectomy (sĭr″ĭn-jĕk′tō-mē) [″ + *ektome*, excision]. Removal of the walls of a fistula.

syringitis (sĭr″ĭn-jī′tĭs) [″ + *itis*, inflammation]. Inflammation of eustachian tube.

syringoadenoma (sĭ-rĭng″gō-ăd″ĕ-nō′mă) [″ + *aden*, gland, + *oma*, tumor]. Syringocystadenoma, q.v.

syringobulbia (sĭr-ĭn″gō-bŭl′bē-ă) [″ + *bulbos*, a bulb]. A chronic progressive disease characterized by development of cavities in the medulla oblongata. SEE: *syringomyelia.*

syringocarcinoma (sĭ-rĭng″gō-kăr″sĭ-nō′mă) [″ + *karkinos*, crab, + *oma*, tumor]. Carcinoma of the sweat gland.

syringocele (sĭr-ĭn′gō-sēl) [″ + *koilia*, cav-

ity]. 1. The central canal of the myelon or spinal cord. 2. A form of meningomyelocele that contains a cavity in the ectopic spinal cord.

syringocystadenoma (sĭr-ĭn″gō-sĭs″tă-dĕ-nō′mă) [″ + *kystis*, bladder, sac, + *aden*, gland, + *oma*, tumor]. Adenoma of sweat glands characterized by tiny, hard, papular formations.

syringocystoma (sĭr-ĭn″gō-sĭs-tō′mă) [″ + ″ + *oma*, tumor]. Cystic tumor having its origin in ducts of the sweat gland.

syringoencephalomyelia (sĭ-rĭng″gō-ĕn-sĕf″ă-lō-mī-ē′lē-ă) [″ + *enkephalos*, brain, + *myelos*, marrow]. Condition of cavities in the brain and spinal cord.

syringoid (sĭr-ĭn′goyd) [Gr. *syrinx*, pipe, + *eidos*, form, shape]. Resembling a tube; fistulous.

syringoma (sĭr″ĭn-gō′mă) [″ + *oma*, tumor]. Tumor of the sweat glands.

syringomeningocele (sĭr-ĭn″gō-mĕn-ĭn′gō-sēl) [″ + *meninx*, membrane, + *kele*, tumor, swelling]. Meningocele that is similar to a syringomyelocele.

syringomyelia (sĭr-ĭn″gō-mī-ē′lē-ă) [″ + *myelos*, marrow]. A chronic progressive disease of the spinal cord characterized by the development of cavities and gliosis of surrounding tissue. Usually begins before age of 30 and is more common among males than among females. Its cause is unknown. SEE: *Nursing Diagnoses in Appendix.*

   SYM: Cavitation occurs in cervical and lumbar regions and soon involves pathways of the cord that carry impulses of pain and temperature sensations, resulting in dissociated sensory loss. Destruction of lateral and anterior gray matter causes muscular atrophy and weakness.

   TREAT: There is no satisfactory treatment. Sudden enlargement of cavity may warrant surgical intervention with decompression of cavity. Persistent pain may necessitate chordotomy or medullary tractotomy for relief.

syringomyelitis (sĭr-ĭn″gō-mī″ē-lī′tĭs) [″ + *myelos*, marrow, + *itis*, inflammation]. Inflammation coincident with abnormal dilation of the central canal of the spinal cord.

syringomyelocele (sĭr-ĭn″gō-mī″ĕl-ō-sēl) [″ + ″ + *kele*, tumor, swelling]. A form of spina bifida in which the cavity of the projecting portion communicates with the central canal of the spinal cord.

syringomyelus (sĭr-ĭn″gō-mī′ĕl-ŭs). Abnormal dilatation of the central canal of the spinal cord.

syringopontia (sĭr-ĭn″gō-pŏn′shē-ă) [″ + L. *pons*, bridge]. Cavity formation in the pons varolii similar to syringomyelia.

syringosystrophy (sĭr-ĭn″gō-sĭs′trō-fē) [″ + *systrophe*, a twist]. Twisting of the oviduct.

syringotome (sĭr-ĭn′gō-tōm) [″ + *tome*, incision]. Instrument for incision of a fistula.

syringotomy (sĭr″ĭn-gŏt′ō-mē). Operation for incision of a fistula.

syrinx (sĭr′ĭnks) [Gr., pipe]. 1. The eustachian tube. 2. Pathological cavity in the spinal cord or brain. 3. A fistula.

syrup (sĭr′ŭp) [L. *syrupus*]. ABBR: syr. Concentrated solution of sugar in water. Usually specific medicinal substances are added. Syrup usually does not represent a very high percentage of the active drug. Some syrups are used principally to give a pleasant odor and taste to solutions.

    s., simple. A combination of purified water and sucrose.

syssarcosis (sĭs″ăr-kō′sĭs) [Gr. *syn*, together, + *sarkosis*, fleshy growth]. The union of bones by muscles; a muscular articulation such as the hyoid and patella.

systaltic (sĭs-tăl′tĭk) [Gr. *systaltikos*, contracting]. Contracting and dilating alternately; having a systole. SYN: *pulsating.*

system (sĭs′tĕm) [Gr. *systema*, a composite whole]. 1. An organized grouping of related structures or parts. 2. A group of structures or organs related to each other and performing certain functions together, e.g., the digestive system. 3. A group of cells or aggregations of cells that perform a particular function such as the mononuclear phagocyte, cardiovascular, respiratory, and central nervous systems.

    s., alimentary. S., digestive, q.v.

    s., autonomic nervous. That portion of the peripheral nervous system that innervates all smooth muscle, cardiac muscle, and glands, the activities of which are involuntary. It includes the craniosacral (parasympathetic) and thoracolumbar (sympathetic) divisions, each of which provides fibers for most of the visceral structures or organs. SYN: *system, vegetative nervous.*

    s., cardiovascular. The heart and blood vessels (aorta, arteries, arterioles, capillaries, venules, veins, venae cavae).

    s., centimeter-gram-second. ABBR: CGS. System of measurement in units of length, mass, and time. SYN: *metric system.*

    s., central nervous. That portion of the nervous system consisting of the brain and spinal cord.

    s., chromaffin. The mass of tissue forming paraganglia and medulla of suprarenal glands, which secretes epinephrine and stains readily with chromium salts. Similar tissue is found in the organs of Zuckerkandl,

and in the liver, testes, ovary, and heart.

    s., circulatory. System concerned with circulation of body fluids. It includes the cardiovascular and lymphatic systems. SYN: *s., vascular.*

    s., conduction, of the heart. SEE: *heart, conduction system of.*

    s., cytochrome. Cytochrome oxidase and three hemochromogen-like pigments (cytochromes a, b, and c) that make molecular oxygen available for the oxidation of hydrogen liberated from cellular metabolites.

    s., digestive. The alimentary canal (mouth, teeth, tongue, pharynx, esophagus, stomach, small and large intestines) and accessory glands (salivary glands, liver, pancreas). SEE: *digestion; digestive system* for illus.

    s., endocrine. The ductless glands or the glands of internal secretion, which include the pineal body, pancreas, and paraganglia and pituitary, thyroid, parathyroid, and adrenal glands. SEE: *endocrine gland.*

    s., extrapyramidal motor. Functional system including all descending fibers arising in cortical and subcortical motor centers that reach the medulla and spinal cord by pathways other than recognized pyramidal tracts. The system is important in maintenance of equilibrium and muscle tone.

    s., genital. S., reproductive.

    s., genitourinary. The organs of reproduction combined with the urinary organs. SEE: *genitalia* for illus.

    s., haversian. Architectural unit of bone consisting of a central tube (haversian canal) with alternate layers of intercellular material (matrix) surrounding it in concentric cylinders. Alternating layers of matrix and cells are called haversian lamellae.

    s., hematopoietic. The blood-forming tissues and organs of the body. Includes the bone marrow, spleen, and lymphatic tissue.

    s., heterogeneous. Any system the components of which may be separated by mechanical means.

    s., homogeneous. Any system the components of which cannot be separated by mechanical means.

    s., hypophyseoportal. The series of vessels that lead from the hypothalamus to the anterior lobe of the pituitary. The releasing factors are carried to the pituitary through this system.

    s., impulse-conducting. System of atypical muscle fibers (Purkinje fibers) within the heart that conduct impulses regulating contractions of the atria and ventricles. Includes S-A and A-V nodes and bundle of His.

    s., integumentary. The skin and its derivatives (hair, nails).

s., lymphatic. System concerned with the circulation of lymph. Includes lymph vessels and ducts and lymphatic organs (lymph nodes, tonsils, thymus, spleen). SEE: *lymph; lymphatic.*

s., metric. A system of weights and measures based on the meter (39.37 in.) as the unit of linear measure; the gram (15.432 gr) as the unit of weight; the liter (1.057 qt.) as the unit of volume. SEE: *Metric System* and *SI Units* in *Appendix.*

s., muscular. System that includes all the muscles (smooth, cardiac, striated, or skeletal) of the body. SEE: *muscle.*

s., nervous. System that includes the brain, spinal cord, ganglia, and nerves.

S. of Units, International. ABBR: SI. The modern version of the metric system. SEE: *SI Units* in *Appendix.*

s., osseous. The bony structures of the body; the skeleton. SEE: *skeleton.*

s., parasympathetic nervous. SEE: *parasympathetic nervous system.*

s., peripheral nervous. That part of the nervous system outside the central nervous system.

s., portal. System of vessels in which blood passes through a capillary network, a large vessel, and then another capillary network before returning to the systemic circulation, as the circulation of blood through the liver.

s., reproductive. The gonads and their associated structures and ducts. In the female this system includes the ovaries, uterine tubes (oviducts), uterus, vagina, and vulva. In the male it includes the testes, efferent ducts, epididymis, ductus deferens, ejaculatory duct, urethra and accessory glands (bulbourethral, prostate, seminal vesicles), and penis. SYN: *s., genital.* SEE: *genitalia* for illus.

s., respiratory. The air passageways and organs (nasal cavities, oral cavity, pharynx, larynx, trachea, and lungs, including bronchi, bronchioles, alveolar ducts, and alveoli). SEE: *lung* for illus.

s., reticuloendothelial. ABBR: RES. Collectively, all the phagocytic cells of the body excepting the leukocytes. Includes macrophages, histiocytes, Kupffer's cells of the liver, reticular cells of lymphatic organs, microglia of the brain, and many others. NOTE: This system is also called the mononuclear phagocyte system.

s., skeletal. The bony framework of the body. SEE: *skeleton.*

s., sympathetic nervous. The thoracolumbar or sympathetic division of the autonomic nervous system.

s., urinary. The kidneys, ureters, bladder, and urethra.

s., urogenital. The urinary and reproductive systems combined. SEE: *genitalia* for illus.

s., vascular. System of all vessels of the body (heart, blood vessels, and lymphatics). SYN: *s., circulatory.*

s., vasomotor. The part of the nervous system that controls the size of the vascular system vessels.

s., vegetative nervous. S., autonomic nervous.

s., visceral efferent. System that includes all efferent nerve fibers conveying impulses to the visceral organs; the autonomic nervous system, q.v.

systema (sĭs-tē″mă) [Gr., a composite whole]. System.

systematic (sĭs″tĕ-măt′ĭk). Concerning a system or organized according to a system.

systematization (sĭs-tĕm″ă-tī-zā′shŭn). The process of organizing something according to a plan.

systemic (sĭs-tĕm′ĭk). Pert. to a whole body rather than to one of its parts; somatic.

systemic circulation. The blood flow from the left ventricle through the aorta and all its branches (arteries) to the capillaries of the tissues and its return to the heart through veins and the venae cavae, which empty into the right atrium.

systemic lupus erythematosus. SEE: *lupus erythematosus.*

systemic remedies. Remedies that will act on the body as a whole.

systemoid (sĭs′tĕ-moyd) [″ + *eidos,* form, shape]. 1. Resembling a system. 2. Pert. to tumors made up of several types of tissues.

Systems Model. SEE: *Appendix 23.*

systems theory. As used in clinical medicine, an approach that considers the human being as a whole as opposed to his parts. Human beings are considered open systems constantly exchanging information, matter, and energy with the environment. There are three levels of reference for systems; the system-level on which one is focusing, such as man; the suprasystems-level above the focal system, such as man's family, the community, and the culture; and subsystem, the level below the focal system, such as the bodily systems and the cell. Those involved in health care must view persons as being affected constantly by supra- and subsystems. Health care, in the systems approach, transcends the idea of treating illness and addresses the larger issue of attaining and maintaining health through assessment and treatment of the total person. SYN: *general systems theory.* SEE: *holism; holistic medicine.*

systole (sĭs′tō-lē) [Gr., contraction]. That

part of the heart cycle in which the heart is in contraction, i.e., the myocardial fibers are tightening and shortening. Occurs in the interval between first and second heart sounds during which blood is surged through the aorta and pulmonary artery. SEE: *diastole; murmur; presystole.*

s., aborted. A premature cardiac systole in which arterial pressure is increased little if at all because of inadequate filling of ventricles due to shortening of preceding diastole.

s., anticipated. Systole that is aborted because it occurs before the ventricle is filled.

s., arterial. The rebound or recoil of the stretched elastic walls of the arteries following ventricular systole.

s., atrial. The contraction of the atria. Precedes the ventricular systole.

s., electrical. The total duration of the QRST complex in an electrocardiogram. Approximately the same as that of the mechanical systole.

s., extra-. A premature systole occurring in addition to the fundamental rhythm.

s., premature. Systole slightly preceding a normal systole. SYN: *extrasystole.*

s., ventricular. Ventricular contraction.

systolic (sĭs-tŏl'ĭk) [Gr. *systole,* contraction]. Pert. to the systole.

systolic discharge. The amount of blood ejected by the heart at each systole.

systolic murmur. A cardiac murmur during systole.

systolic pressure. Maximum blood pressure. This occurs during contraction of the ventricle. SEE: *blood pressure; diastolic pressure; pulse; pulse pressure.*

systremma (sĭs-trĕm'ă) [Gr. *systremma,* anything twisted together]. Cramp in calf of the leg, the muscles assuming form of a hard knot.

Sytobex. Trade name for cyanocobalamin.

syzygial (sĭ-zĭj'ē-ăl) [Gr. *syzygia,* conjunction]. Pert. to a syzygium.

syzygiology (sĭ-zĭj"ē-ŏl'ō-jē) [" + *logos,* word, reason]. Study of interdependence or interrelationship of the whole as opposed to that of isolated functions or separate parts. SEE: *holism.*

syzygium (sĭ-zĭj'ē-ŭm) [Gr. *syzygia,* conjunction]. Fusion of two parts or structures without loss of identity of the parts.

syzygy (sĭz'ĭ-jē). Fusion of organs, each remaining distinct.

T

T. *temperature; time; intraocular tension.*

t. *temporal;* L. *ter,* three times.

t$_{1/2}$ T$_{1/2}$. In nuclear medicine, the symbol of half-life of a radioactive substance.

T$_3$. Triiodothyronine. SEE: *thyroid function tests.*

T$_4$. Tetraiodothyronine. SEE: *thyroid function tests.*

T-1824. Evans blue dye.

T.A. *toxin-antitoxin.*

Ta. Chem. symb. for the element tantalum.

tabacism (tăb″ă-sĭzm) [L. *tabacum,* tobacco, + Gr. *-ismos,* condition]. Chronic tobacco poisoning. SYN: *tabacosis.* SEE: *tobacco.*

tabacosis (tăb″ă-kŏ′sĭs) [″ + Gr. *osis,* condition]. Chronic tobacco poisoning or pneumoconiosis from inhaling tobacco dust.

tabacum (tă-bā′kum, tăb′ă-kum) [L.]. Tobacco.

tabagism (tăb′ă-jĭzm) [″ + Gr. *-ismos,* condition]. Poisoning from excessive use of tobacco or nicotine. SYN: *nicotinism.*

tabanid (tăb′ă-nĭd) [L. *tabanus,* horsefly]. A member of the dipterous family Tabanidae, q.v.

Tabanidae (tă-băn′ĭ-dē) [L. *tabanus,* horsefly]. A family of insects belonging to the order Diptera. It includes horseflies, gadflies, deer flies, and mango flies, all bloodsucking insects that attack man and other warm-blooded animals. Tabanidae is of medical importance because flies serve in the transmission of the filaria worm, *Loa loa,* tularemia, anthrax, and other diseases. Their bites are extremely painful and heal with difficulty.

Tabanus (tă-bā′nŭs) [L., horsefly]. A genus of flies of the family Tabanidae, q.v.

tabardillo (tăb″ăr-dē′lyō) [Sp.]. Spanish term for epidemic louse-borne typhus fever that occurs in parts of Mexico. SEE: *typhus.*

tabatière anatomique (tă-bă″tē-ăr′ ă-nă″tō-mēk′) [Fr., anatomical snuffbox]. Depression at base of thumb in back when thumb is extended. Triangular area of the dorsum of the hand at the base of the thumb. When the thumb is extended, the tendons of the long and short extensor muscles of the thumb bound this area, which appears as a depression. When snuff was used, a small pinch could be placed in this box and snuffed up into the nose from that site. SYN: *snuffbox, anatomical.*

tabella (tă-bĕl′ă) [L., tablet] (pl. *tabellae*). A medicated mass of material formed into a small disk. SEE: *lozenge; tablet; troche.*

tabes (tā′bēz) [L., wasting disease]. A gradual, progressive wasting in any chronic disease.

t., diabetic. Peripheral neuritis affecting diabetics. May affect spinal cord and simulate tabes caused by syphilis.

t. dorsalis. Sclerosis of the posterior columns of the spinal cord. SYN: *ataxia, locomotor.* SEE: *syphilis.*

SYM: Postural instability, esp. when eyes are closed, and a staggering wide-base gait are characteristic; hence the name locomotor ataxia. Pain and paresthesias are common, esp. lightning pains, described as sharp, stabbing, and paroxysmal. Ankle and knee reflexes are diminished or lost. Many symptoms characteristic of syphilis such as pupillary changes, optic atrophy, bladder disturbances, and development of trophic ulcers, esp. on feet, make diagnosis certain.

ETIOL: Infection of central nervous system with *Treponema pallidum,* the causative agent of syphilis.

TREAT: Treat for syphilis. Special measures should be taken to relieve severe pains. Rehabilitation measures are often essential for those with disturbed gait. SEE: *syphilis.*

t. ergotica. Tabes resulting from the use of ergot.

t. mesenterica. Emaciation and general disorder of the functions of nutrition due to engorgement and tubercular degeneration of the mesenteric glands.

tabescent (tă-bĕs′ĕnt) [L. *tabes,* wasting disease]. Progressive withering or wasting away.

tabetic (tă-bĕt′ĭk) [L. *tabes,* wasting disease]. Pert. to or afflicted with tabes.

tabetic crises. Paroxysms of pain or other acute manifestations of episodic character in tabes due to syphilis.

tabetic foot. Twisted foot in locomotor ataxia.

tabetiform (tă-bĕt′ĭ-form) [″ + *forma,* shape]. Resembling or characteristic of tabes.

tabic, tabid (tăb′ĭk, tăb′ĭd). Tabetic.

tablature (tăb′lă-chūr). The formation of the cranial bones into two outer hard layers and a spongy center, the diploë.

table (tā′bl) [L. *tabula,* board]. 1. A flat-topped structure, as an operating table. 2. A thin flat plate, as of bone.

t.'s of skull. Inner and outer condensed layers of the cranial bone separated by diploë (cancellous bony tissue).

t., periodic. SEE: *periodic table.*

t., tilt. Table that may be tilted. A person is secured to it, and the circulatory response to various angles of tilt from flat to perpendicular is observed and recorded. It is useful in studying postural hypotension.

t., vitreous. The inner cranial table.

t., water. The level at which rock or any underground stratum is saturated with water. This overlies an impervious stratum. SYN: *groundwater level.*

tablespoon (tā′bl-spoon). ABBR: Tbs. A rough measure utilizing a household spoon. When instructed to administer a tablespoon of medicine, give 15 ml of the substance.

tablet (tăb′lĕt) [O. Fr. *tablete,* a small table]. A small, disklike mass of medicinal powder.

t., buccal. Tablet designed to be placed in the mouth and held between the cheek and gum until dissolved and absorbed through the buccal mucosa.

t., coated. Type of tablet usually made by coating compressed tablets with sugar or chocolate.

t., compressed. Tablet made by forcibly compressing the powdered substances into the desired shape; usually made to contain from 65 to 650 mg of the active drug. Frequently they are very hard and not readily soluble.

t., dispensing. Tablet that contains a comparatively large amount of the active drug. Used by pharmacists and dispensing physicians to avoid the necessity of weighing small amounts of a potent drug in filling prescriptions.

t., enteric-coated. Tablet with an outer layer that is resistant to dissolution by gastric juices.

t., fluoride. Tablet of sodium fluoride taken for dental caries prevention.

t., hypodermic. Tablet that frequently contains, in addition to the active drug, some agents that produce chemical action when water is added, thus causing a rapid disintegration of the mass. Used to form injectable solutions.

t., sublingual. Small, flat, oval tablet placed beneath the tongue to permit direct absorption of the active substance.

t. triturate. Tablet made by moistening the medication mixed with a powdered lactose or sucrose, and then molding into shape and allowing the liquid to evaporate. Such tablets seldom contain more than 65 mg of the active agent. They usually disintegrate readily and are a very desirable form for administering certain drugs.

tablier (tă-blyā′) [Fr., apron]. Pudendal apron; enlarged vulvae. SEE: *Hottentot apron.*

taboo [Polynesian *tabu, tapu,* inviolable]. An act, object, or social custom separated or set aside as being sacred or profane, thus forbidden for general use.

taboparalysis (tă″bō-păr-ăl′ĭ-sĭs) [L. *tabes,* wasting disease, + Gr. *paralyein,* to disable]. Tabes associated concurrently with general paralysis. SYN: *taboparesis.*

taboparesis (tă″bō-păr-ē′sĭs, -păr′ē-sĭs) [″ + Gr. *paresis,* relaxation]. General paralysis in combination with tabes. SYN: *taboparalysis.*

tabophobia (tă″bō-fō′bē-ă) [″ + Gr. *phobos,* fear]. A morbid fear of being afflicted with tabes, a common symptom of neurasthenia.

tabular (tăb′ū-lăr) [L. *tabula,* board]. 1. Resembling a table. 2. Set up in columns, as a tabulation.

tabular bone. A flat bone, or one with two compact bonelike parts with cancellous tissue between them.

tabun. Ethyl N-dimethylphosphoramidocyanidate. An extremely toxic "nerve gas."

Tacaryl Hydrochloride. Trade name for methdilazine hydrochloride.

TACE. Trade name for chlorotrianisene.

tache (tŏsh) [Fr., spot]. A colored spot or macule on the skin, as a freckle.

t. blanche. A white spot on the liver in some infectious diseases.

t. bleuâtre. A blue spot on the skin, usually due to bite of cutaneous parasites. SYN: *macula caerulea.*

t. cérébrale. The red line that occurs in meningitis and other nervous disorders when the fingernail is drawn across the skin.

t. motrice. The motor endplate of a striated muscle fiber.

t. noire. A small round or oval ulcer covered by a black scab; the primary lesion of boutonneuse fever and rickettsialpox.

tachetic (tăk-ĕt′ĭk) [Fr. *tache,* spot]. Marked by purple or reddish blue patches (taches).

tachistoscope (tă-kis′tō-skōp) [Gr. *tachistos,* swiftest, + *skopein,* to view]. Device used to determine the speed of visual perception. The time of exposure can be adjusted so that the length of time needed for detection of the viewed object can be measured.

tachogram (tăk′ō-grăm) [Gr. *tachos,* speed, + *gramma,* something written]. A graphic tracing of rate of flow of blood.

tachography (tăk-ŏg′ră-fē) [″ + *graphein,* to write]. The recording of the speed of the blood circulation.

tachy- [Gr. *tachys,* swift. Combining form meaning swift.

tachyarrhythmia (tăk″ē-ă-rĭth′mē-ă) [″ + *a,* not, + *rhythmos,* rhythm]. Irregularity of heartbeat combined with rapid rate.

tachyauxesis (tăk″ē-awk-sē′sĭs) [″ + *auxesis,* increase]. Condition in which a part of an organism grows more rapidly than the whole.

tachycardia (tăk″ē-kăr′dē-ă) [″ + *kardia*, heart]. Abnormal rapidity of heart action, usually defined as a heart rate over 100 beats per minute in adults.

    t., atrial. Rapid heart rate usually less than 200 beats per minute. The beats arise from an atrial focus.

    t., ectopic. Rapid heartbeat due to stimuli arising from outside the sinoatrial node.

    t., essential. Rapid persistent heart action due to functional disturbance.

    t., nodal. Tachycardia resulting from an increase in rhythmicity of A-V node over the S-A node. May be the result of digitalis therapy.

    t., paroxysmal atrial. Atrial tachycardia beginning and ending suddenly. Rate is usually from 150 to 240 beats per minute.

    t., paroxysmal nodal. Tachycardia due to increased activity of the A-V junctional focus. Rate is usually 120 to 180 beats per minute.

    t., paroxysmal supraventricular. Rapid ectopic atrial arrhythmia originating proximal to the His bundle bifurcation. A re-entry impulse occurs in the atrial, A-V node, or His bundle.

    t., paroxysmal ventricular. Ventricular tachycardia beginning and ending suddenly.

    t., polymorphic ventricular. Very rapid ventricular tachycardia characterized by a gradually changing QRS complex in the ECG. It is usually self-limiting but may change into ventricular fibrillation. SYN: *torsade de pointes.*

    t., reflex. Tachycardia resulting from stimuli outside the heart, reflexly accelerating heart rate or depressing vagal tone.

    t., sinus. Uncomplicated tachycardia when sinus rhythm is faster than 100 beats per minute, as that due to exercise. Causes other than exercise include hyperthermia, thyrotoxicosis, hemorrhage, anoxia, infections, cardiac failure, and certain drugs such as atropine, epinephrine, and nicotine.

    TREAT: Tachycardia sometimes ceases following procedures that cause vagal stimulation. Among these are pressure on one or both carotid sinuses, pressure on eyeballs, induction of gagging or vomiting, attempted expiration with glottis closed, lying down with feet in air, and bending over. If these procedures when employed singly are unsuccessful, two or more combined may produce desirable results. If these general measures are ineffective, specific therapy based on etiological factors will be required.

    t. strumosa exophthalmica. Tachycardia occurring as a symptom of exophthalmic goiter.

    t., ventricular. A series of beats arising from a ventricular focus at a rate greater than 100 beats per minute. The beats usually arise from a single focus and are at a rate of 150 to 200 beats per minute.

tachycardia-bradycardia syndrome. A form of sick sinus syndrome. A group of arrhythmias produced by a defect in the sinus node impulse generation or conduction. Arrhythmias associated may include supraventricular tachycardias, atrial fibrillation, atrial flutter that alternates with sinus arrest, and sinus bradycardia.

tachycardiac (tăk″ē-kăr′dē-ăk) [Gr. *tachys*, swift, + *kardia*, heart]. Pert. to or afflicted with tachycardia.

tachygastria. Increased rate of contractions of the stomach.

tachylalia (tăk″ē-lā′lē-ă) [″ + *lalein*, to speak]. Rapid speech.

tachymeter (tăk-ĭm′ĕ-tĕr) [″ + *metron*, measure]. Instrument for estimating the speed of any body in motion.

tachyphagia (tăk″ē-fā′jē-ă) [″ + *phagein*, to eat]. Rapid eating.

tachyphasia (tăk″ē-fā′zē-ă) [″ + *phasis*, speech]. Very rapid or voluble speech. SYN: *tachyphrasia.*

tachyphemia (tăk″ē-fē′mē-ă) [″ + *pheme*, speech]. Tachyphrasia, q.v.

tachyphrasia (tăk″ē-frā′zē-ă) [″ + *phrasis*, speech]. Excessive volubility or rapidity of speech, as seen in mental disorders. SYN: *tachyphasia.*

tachyphrenia (tăk″ē-frē′nē-ă) [″ + *phren*, mind]. Abnormally rapid mental activity.

tachyphylaxis (tăk″ē-fĭ-lăk′sĭs) [″ + *phylaxis*, protection]. Rapid immunization to a toxic dose of a substance by previously injecting tiny doses of the same substance.

tachypnea (tăk″ĭp-nē′ă) [″ + *pnoia*, breath]. Abnormal rapidity of respiration.

    t., nervous. Respiratory rate of 40 or more per minute. It occurs in hysteria and neurasthenia. If prolonged, it will cause excess loss of CO_2 and the hyperventilation syndrome will develop. SEE: *alkalosis, respiratory; hyperventilation.*

tachyrhythmia (tăk″ē-rĭth′mē-ă) [″ + *rhythmos*, rhythm]. 1. Rapid heart action. SYN: *tachycardia.* 2. Increase in frequency of brain waves in electroencephalography up to 12 to 50/sec.

tachysterol (tă-kĭs′tĕ-rŏl). One of the isomers of ergosterol, q.v., obtained by irradiation.

tachytrophism (tăk″ē-trō′fĭzm) [″ + *trophe*, nourishment, + *-ismos*, condition]. Accelerated metabolism.

tactile (tăk′tĭl) [L. *tactilis*]. Perceptible to the touch.

tactile corpuscles. Minute elongated bodies

enclosing the endings of several afferent nerve fibers and serving as the receptor for slight pressure or touch. They are located in dermal papillae just beneath the epidermis and are most numerous on fingertips, toes, soles, palms, lips, nipples, and tip of tongue. SYN: *Meissner's corpuscles.*

tactile defensiveness. A defense reaction due to sensitivity to being touched.

tactile discrimination. The ability to localize two points of pressure on the surface of the skin and to identify them as discrete sensations.

tactile disk. Tiny expanded end of a sensory nerve fiber found in epidermis and in epithelial root sheath of a hair.

tactile localization. An individual's ability to accurately identify the site of tactile stimulation (touch, pressure, or pain). Tactile localization is often tested in sensory evaluations following disease or trauma of the nervous system.

tactile system. That portion of the nervous system concerned with the sensation of touch. Includes sensory nerve endings (Meissner's corpuscles, Merkel's tactile disks, hair-root endings), afferent nerve fibers, conducting pathways in the cord and brain, and sensory (somesthetic) area of cerebral cortex.

taction (tăk′shŭn) [L. *tactio*]. 1. Sense of touch. 2. Touching.

tactometer (tăk-tŏm′ĕt-ĕr) [L. *tactus*, touch, + Gr. *metron*, measure]. Instrument for determining acuity of tactile sensitiveness.

tactor (tăk′tor). Any tactile organ.

tactual (tăk′tū-ăl) [L. *tactus*, touch]. Rel. to the sense of touch. SYN: *tactile.*

tactus (tăk′tŭs) [L.]. Touch.

   t. eruditus. Sensitiveness of touch acquired by long practice.

taedium vitae (tē′dē-ŭm vē″tī) [L.]. Weariness of life with suicidal inclination.

Taenia (tē′nē-ă) [L., tape]. A genus of parasitic flatworms belonging to the class Cestoda, phylum Platyhelminthes. They are elongated ribbonlike worms consisting of a scolex, usually armed, and a chain of segments (proglottids). Adults live as intestinal parasites of vertebrates; larvae parasitize both vertebrates and invertebrates, which serve as intermediate hosts. SEE: *taeniasis; tapeworm.*

   T. echinococcus. *Echinococcus granulosus,* q.v.

   T. lata. Diphyllobothrium latum, q.v. SYN: *tapeworm, fish.*

   TREAT: Niclosamide or praziquantel.

   T. saginata. Tapeworm whose larvae live in cattle. The adult worm lives in the intestines of humans, who acquire it by eating insufficiently cooked beef infested with the encysted larval form (cysticercus or bladderworm). Adult worms may reach a length of 15 to 20 feet (4.6 to 6.1 meters) or longer. SYN: *tapeworm, beef.*

   T. solium. Tapeworm whose larvae live in hogs. The adult worm lives in the intestines of humans, who acquire it by eating insufficiently cooked pork infested with the larval form. Infected pork containing the bladderworm *(Cysticercus cellulosae)* is called measly pork. The cysticerci may also develop in humans, infection occurring from self-infection with eggs from contaminated hands or by hatching of eggs liberated in the intestine. SYN: *tapeworm, pork.*

   TREAT: Niclosamide or praziquantel.

taenia (tē′nē-ă) [L., tape]. 1. Any bandlike structure. SYN: *tenia* [NA]. 2. A tapeworm.

   t. coli. One of three bands of the large intestines into which muscular fibers are collected. They are taenia mesocolica (mesenteric insertion), taenia libera (opposite mesocolic band), and taenia omentalis (at place of attachment of omentum to transverse colon).

   t. fimbriae. The folded or recurved lateral edge of the fimbria to which the epithelium covering the choroid plexus of the inferior horn of the lateral ventricle is attached.

   t. pontis. One or two small transverse bands of fiber at rostral border of the pons.

   t. semicircularis. Stria terminalis.

   t. thalami. Structure separating the superior surface from the lateral surface of the thalamus, its lateral portion containing the stria medullaris.

   t. ventriculi tertii. The taenia of the third ventricle.

taeniacide (tē′nē-ă-sīd) [L. *taenia*, tapeworm, + *cidus*, kill]. An agent that kills tapeworms.

taeniafuge (tē′nē-ă-fūj″) [″ + *fugere*, to put to flight]. Anything that expels tapeworms.

taeniasis (tē-nī′ă-sĭs) [″ + Gr. *-iasis*, condition]. Condition of being infested with tapeworms of the genus *Taenia.* SEE: *tapeworm.*

taeniform (tē′nĭ-form) [″ + *forma*, shape]. Having the structure of, or resembling, a tapeworm.

taenifuge (tē′nĭ-fūj) [″ + *fuga*, flight]. An agent that expels tapeworms.

taeniophobia (tē″nē-ō-fō′bē-ă) [″ + Gr. *phobos*, fear]. Morbid fear of becoming infested with tapeworms.

tag. 1. A small polyp or growth. 2. A label or tracer; or application of a label or tracer.

   t., hemorrhoidal. The remaining anal skin tag from an old external hemorrhoid.

   t., radioactive. A radioactive isotope that is incorporated into a chemical or organic material to allow its detection in metabolic or chemical processes.

t., skin. A small outgrowth of skin, usually occurring on the neck, axilla, and groin. SEE: *acrochordon.*

Tagamet. Trade name for cimetidine.

tagging. Introduction of a radioactive isotope into a molecule in order to distinguish the molecule from others without that "tag." SYN: *labeling.*

tagliacotian operation (tă-lē-ă-kō′shē-ăn) [Gasparo Tagliacozzi, It. surgeon, 1546–1599]. Plastic operation on the nose in which skin is used from another part of the body.

tail (tāl) [AS. *taegel*]. Posterior, long, flexible terminus, as the extremity of the spinal column. SEE: *cauda* [NA].

tailgut (tāl′gŭt). A transient diverticulum of the entodermal cloaca of the embryo. It extends into the tail.

tailor's cramp. An occupational syndrome characterized by spasm of the muscles of the arms and hands.

taint (tānt) [O. Fr. *teint,* color, tint]. To spoil or cause putrefaction, as in tainted meat.

Takayasu's arteritis (pulseless disease) [Michishige Takayasu, Japanese physician, b. 1872]. An inflammatory disease of the aorta that occludes one or more of the large branches of the aortic arch. This decreases the flow of blood to the areas supplied by these branches, which in turn leads to a lack of pulse in those areas. Dr. Takayasu noted the lack of pulse in the arteries of the eye, thus the name pulseless disease. The etiology is unknown and the only effective treatment is to implant vascular grafts to bypass the occluded vessels.

take. To be effective, as in administering a vaccine; or to be successful in grafting skin or transplanting an organ.

talalgia (tăl-ăl′jē-ă) [L. *talus,* heel, + Gr. *algos,* pain]. Pain in the heel or ankle.

talar (tā′lăr) [L. *talaris,* of the ankle]. Pert. to the talus, the ankle.

talbutal (tăl′bū-tăl). USP. A barbiturate that acts as a hypnotic and sedative. Trade name is Lotusate.

talc (tălk) [Persian *talk*]. Powdered soapstone; a soft, soapy powder; native hydrous magnesium silicate, $Mg_3Si_4O_{10}(OH)_2$, used as a dusting powder.

Caution: Talc used either for industrial, cosmetic, or health products should not contain asbestos fibers.

talcosis (tăl-kō′sĭs) [Persian *talk,* talc, + Gr. *osis,* condition]. Disease due to inhalation or implantation of talc in the body.

talcum (tălk′ŭm) [L.]. Talc.

tali (tā′lī). Pl. of talus.

talipedic (tăl″ĭ-pē′dĭk) [L. *talus,* ankle, + *pes,* foot]. Clubfooted. SEE: *talipes.*

talipes (tăl′ĭ-pēz) [L. *talus,* ankle, + *pes,* foot]. Any of a number of deformities of the foot, esp. those occurring congenitally; a nontraumatic deviation of the foot in the direction of one or the other of the four lines of movement, or of two of these combined. SYN: *clubfoot.*

t. arcuatus. Talipes in which there is an exaggerated normal arch of the foot. SYN: *talipes cavus.*

t. calcaneus. Talipes in which the foot is flexed and the heel alone touches the ground, causing the patient to walk on the inner side of the heel. Often follows infantile paralysis of the muscle of Achilles tendon.

t. cavus. T. arcuatus.

t. equinus. Talipes in which the foot is extended and the person walks on the toes.

t. percavus. Talipes in which there is excessive plantar curvature.

t. valgus. Talipes in which the heel and foot are turned outward.

t. varus. Talipes in which the heel is turned inward, away from the midline.

talipomanus (tăl″ĭp-ŏm′ăn-ŭs) [L. *talus,* ankle, + *pes,* foot, + *manus,* hand]. Deformity of the hand in which it is twisted out of position. SYN: *clubhand.*

tallow (tăl′ō). Fat obtained from suet, the solid fat of certain ruminants.

talocalcaneal (tā″lō-kăl-kā′nē-ăl) [″ + *calcaneus,* heel bone]. Pert. to the talus and calcaneus, bones of the tarsus.

talocrural (tā″lō-kroo′răl) [″ + *crus,* leg]. Pert. to the talus and leg bones.

talocrural articulation. The ankle joint, a ginglymus or hinge joint.

talofibular (tā″lō-fĭb′ū-lăr) [″ + *fibula,* pin]. Concerning the talus and fibula.

talon (tăl′ōn) [L.]. The portion of the claw of a bird, esp. a bird of prey, that projects posteriorly.

t. noir. Minute intracutaneous black areas of the heels, toes, or hands. They are thought to be areas of hemorrhage caused by trauma.

talonavicular (tā″lō-nă-vĭk′ū-lăr) [L. *talus,* ankle, + *navicula,* boat]. Concerning the talus and navicular bones.

talonid (tăl′ō-nĭd) [ME. *talon,* heel]. The crushing region, the posterior or heel part, of a lower molar tooth.

taloscaphoid (tā″lō-skăf′oyd) [L. *talus,* ankle, + Gr. *skaphe,* skiff, + *eidos,* form, shape]. Talonavicular.

talotibial (tā″lō-tĭb′ē-ăl) [″ + *tibia,* shinbone]. Concerning the talus and tibial bones.

talus (tā′lŭs) [L., ankle] (pl. *tali*). [NA] The

ankle bone articulating with the tibia, fibula, calcaneus, and navicular bone. Formerly called astragalus.

Talwin (tăl'wĭn). Trade name for pentazocine.

tambour (tăm-boor') [Fr., drum]. A shallow, drum-shaped appliance used in transmitting and registering arterial pulsations, blood pressure, respiratory movements, peristaltic contractions, and other slight movements.

Tamm-Horsfall mucoprotein. SEE: *mucoprotein, Tamm-Horsfall.*

tamoxifen citrate (tă-mŏks'ĭ-fĕn). An antiestrogen drug used in treating carcinoma of the breast. Trade name is Nolvadex.

tampon (tăm'pŏn) [Fr., plug]. A roll or pack made of various absorbent substances, such as cotton, rayon, wool, and gauze, used to arrest hemorrhage or absorb secretions from a wound or body cavity.

   t., menstrual. An absorbent material suitably shaped and prepared to provide a hygienic means of absorbing menstrual fluid in the vagina. A cord is attached and remains outside the vagina to facilitate removal. These tampons are made for self-insertion. SEE: *sanitary napkin.*

   t., Mikulicz's. A large-scale capillary drain. It consists of a square piece of iodoform gauze of requisite size, placed in a cavity and filled with narrow strips of plain gauze until the necessary degree of compression is secured. Used if there is parenchymatous oozing. Serves as a tampon to arrest bleeding and also acts as a capillary drain. SYN: *Mikulicz's drain.*

   t., nasal. Soft rubber bulb dilated with compressed air, used in plugging nostrils to stop hemorrhage from the nose.

tamponade (tăm″pŏn-ād') [Fr., plug]. 1. Act of using a tampon. SYN: *tamponage.* 2. Pathologic compression of a part.

   t., balloon. Producing pressure against some object by use of a catheter surrounded by an elongated balloon. Often used in the esophagus to arrest bleeding from varices. The Sengstaken-Blakemore tube is most frequently used. This is a three-lumen tube: one is used to administer fluids to the patient or to provide gastric suction, another goes to a balloon inserted in the stomach to hold the tube in place, and the third is attached to the balloon for application of pressure to the esophageal walls. SEE: *epistaxis; varicose veins.*

   NURSING IMPLICATIONS: After balloon insertion, monitor vital signs, electrolyte status, and changes in the hematocrit. Because the balloon prevents swallowing, administer fluids and tube feedings as prescribed. Instruct the patient to expectorate

saliva, and provide emesis basin for oral secretions. Aspiration of secretions is necessary. If patient is comatose, continuous drainage of the esophagus above the balloon will be required.

   t., cardiac. Pathological condition resulting from accumulation of excess fluid in the pericardium. May result from pericarditis or injuries to the heart or great blood vessels, with accumulation of blood.

   NURSING IMPLICATIONS: Question patient for history of trauma. Perform physical assessment, including measurement of arterial pressure, if possible. Administer oxygen as prescribed. Explain cardiac pericardiocentesis to the patient. Obtain the necessary supplies and equipment and place them at bedside. Assist the physician with the procedure. Administer blood and intravenous fluids as prescribed. Maintain and care for thoracotomy tubes if they are inserted.

   t., nasal. SEE: *epistaxis; nosebleed* for illus.

tamponage (tăm'pŏn-ōj) [Fr., plug]. Tamponade.

tamponing, tamponment (tăm'pŏn-ĭng, tăm-pŏn'mĕnt). Tamponade, q.v.

Tandearil. Trade name for oxyphenbutazone.

tang. 1. A strong taste or flavor. 2. A long slender projection or prong forming a part of a chisel, file, or knife. 3. In dentistry, an apparatus for joining the rests and retainers to palatal or lingual bars of a denture.

Tangier disease (tăn-jēr') [Tangier Island, in Chesapeake Bay, where the disease was first discovered]. A rare disease caused by familial high-density lipoprotein deficiency. Symptoms and signs include polyneuropathy, lymphadenopathy, orange-yellow discoloration of enlarged tonsillar tissue, hepatosplenomegaly, and a marked decrease in high-density lipoproteins. Cholesterol esters accumulate in various organs. There is no specific therapy.

tank, Hubbard. SEE: *Hubbard tank.*

tannase (tăn'ās). An enzyme that is capable of hydrolyzing tannins. It is present in certain plants and is produced by cultures of various microorganisms, esp. molds.

tannate (tăn'āt). Any salt or ester of tannic acid.

tannic acid. SEE: *acid, tannic.*

tannin (tăn'ĭn) [Fr. *tanin*]. 1. Acid substance found in bark of certain plants and trees or their products, usually from nutgall. Found in coffee and to a greater extent in tea. 2. Any of several substances containing tannin.

   ACTION/USES: Astringent, antidote for various poisons, and as a topical hemostatic. It is constipating. It is partly eliminated in the urine as gallic acid.

tanning salon. A place equipped to provide exposure to artificial light in order to produce a "suntan." The ultraviolet radiation emitted by the units is different from that in natural sunlight. If this type of tan is obtained and the individual is then exposed to sunlight, the skin damage may be greater than that induced by sunlight alone.

tantalum (tăn′tă-lŭm). SYMB: Ta. At. wt. 180.947; at. no. 73. A rare metallic element derived from tantalite. Because it is non-corrosive and malleable, it has been used to repair cranial defects, as a wire suture, and in prostheses.

tantrum (tăn′trŭm). Display of great anger, which may or may not include violent action. SEE: *temper tantrums.*

Tanyoz's sign. In ascites the umbilicus is displaced downward and in pregnancy it is displaced upward.

TAO. Trade name for troleandomycin.

tap (tăp). 1. [AS. *taeppa*]. To puncture or to empty a cavity of fluid. SEE: *lumbar puncture; paracentesis; thoracentesis.* 2. [O. Fr. *taper*]. A light blow.

    t., spinal. SEE: *spinal puncture.*

Tapar. Trade name for acetaminophen.

Tapazole (tăp′ă-zōl). Trade name for methimazole, USP.

tape (tāp) [AS. *taeppe*]. 1. A long, flexible, narrow strip of linen, cotton, paper, or plastic such as adhesive tape. 2. To wrap a part with a long bandage made of adhesive or other type of material.

    t., adhesive. USP. A fabric, film, or paper, one side of which is coated with an adhesive substance, that adheres to the skin. SYN: *plaster, adhesive.*

tapeinocephalic (tăp″ī-nō-sĕ-făl′ĭk) [Gr. *tapeinos*, low-lying, + *kephale*, head]. Pert. to tapeinocephaly.

tapeinocephaly (tăp″ī-nō-sĕf′ă-lē). A flattened head in which the vertical index of the skull is less than 72.

tapetum (tă-pē′tŭm) [NL., a carpet]. A layer of fibers from the corpus callosum forming roof and lateral walls of inferior and posterior horns of lateral ventricles of the brain. Fibers pass to temporal and occipital lobes.

    t. choroideae. T. lucidum, q.v.

    t. lucidum. A layer of tissue in the choroid of the eye between the vascular and capillary layers in some animals, but not in humans. This membrane reflects light shown into the animal's eyes. It produces a green reflex, readily seen in cats. SYN: *t. choroideae.*

tapeworm [AS. *taeppe*, a narrow band, + *wyrm*, worm]. Any of the species of parasitic worms belonging to the class Cestoda, phylum Platyhelminthes. A typical tapeworm consists of a scolex with hooks and suckers for attachment, and a series of segments or proglottids that vary in number from a few to several thousand. New proglottids are budded off of the scolex, so that a worm is actually a linear colony consisting of immature, mature, and ripe or gravid proglottids. Adults live as endoparasites in the intestine. The terminal ripe proglottids containing the ova break off and pass out with the feces. The eggs develop into minute six-hooked oncospheres, which when ingested by the proper intermediate host (usually another vertebrate) develop in muscle tissues into an encysted larva known as a cysticercus. Infestation occurs when uncooked meat containing encysted larvae is eaten. These larvae develop into the mature adult in the primary host.

    Species of medical importance are *Diphyllobothrium latum, Echinococcus granulosus, Hymenolepis nana, H. diminuta, Taenia saginata,* and *T. solium,* q.v. SEE: *cysticercosis; cysticercus; hydatid; taeniasis.*

    SYM: Often absent. If numerous, may cause intestinal obstruction. Occasionally mild systemic symptoms may occur from absorption of metabolic wastes. Sometimes there are dyspeptic symptoms.

    t., armed. Taenia solium, the pork tapeworm, whose scolex possesses a row of hooks about the rostellum.

    t., beef. Taenia saginata.

    t., broad. Diphyllobothrium latum, q.v.

    t., dog. Dipylidium caninum.

    t., dwarf. Hymenolepis nana.

    t., fish. Diphyllobothrium latum.

    t., hydatid. Echinococcus granulosus, q.v.

    t., mouse. Hymenolepis nana.

    t., pork. Taenia solium.

    t., rat. Hymenolepis nana.

    t., unarmed. Taenia saginata.

taphephobia (tăf″ē-fō′bē-ă) [Gr. *taphos*, grave, + *phobos*, fear]. Abnormal fear of being buried alive.

taphophilia (tăf″ō-fīl′ē-ă) [″ + *philos*, love]. Abnormal attraction for graves.

Tapia syndrome (tă′pē-ă) [Antonio García Tapia, Sp. physician, 1875–1950]. Paralysis of the pharynx and larynx on one side and atrophy of the tongue on the opposite side. Caused by a lesion affecting the vagus (tenth) and hypoglossal (twelfth) cranial nerves on the side in which the pharynx is affected.

tapinocephalic (tăp″ĭn-ō-sĕf-ăl′ĭk) [Gr. *tapeinos*, lying low, + *kephale*, head]. Pert. to flatness of top of cranium.

tapinocephaly (tăp″ĭn-ō-sĕf′ă-lē). Flatness of top of the skull.

tapioca. An edible starch obtained from cassava. It may be prepared in several forms, including flakes, flour, or pellets.

tapiroid (tă'pĭr-oyd) [Amerind. *tapira*, tapir, + Gr. *eidos*, form, shape]. Resembling a tapir's snout; said of an elongated cervix uteri.

tapotement (tă-pōt-mŏn') [Fr.]. Percussion in massage. Techniques include beating with the clinched hand, clapping performed with the palm of the hand, hacking with the ulnar border of the hand, and punctuation with the tips of the fingers.

The strength of the manipulations is an essential factor in the massage treatment, and care must be taken not to bruise the patient. As a rule, begin with moderate pressure, ascertaining from the patient the sensation. A lubricating lotion or cream should be used to avoid abrading the skin. SEE: *massage*.

tapping (tăp'ĭng). 1. [O. Fr. *taper*, of imitative origin]. Percussion in massage. SYN: *tapotement*. 2. [AS. *taeppa*, tap]. Removal of fluid from a cavity. SYN: *paracentesis*.

tar. A term applied to a dark, viscid mass of complex chemicals obtained by destructive distillation of coal, shale, and organic matter, esp. wood from pine and juniper trees.

t., coal. Coal tar, USP, q.v.

t., juniper. USP. Material obtained from destructive distillation of oil obtained from the wood of the juniper tree, *Juniperus oxycedrus*. It is used in certain medicines applied topically in treating certain skin diseases.

t., pine. Pine tar, USP, q.v.

Taractan. Trade name for chlorprothixene.

tarantism (tăr'ăn-tĭzm) [*Taranto*, seaport in southern Italy, + Gr. *-ismos*, condition]. A nervous affection marked by stupor, melancholy, and uncontrollable dancing mania. Popularly attributed to bite of the tarantula.

tarantula (tă-răn'tū-lă). A large venomous spider feared by many people; however, its bite is comparable in severity to a bee sting. SEE: *spider bites or poisoning*.

Tardieu's spots (tăr-dyŭz') [Auguste A. Tardieu, Fr. physician, 1818–1879]. Subpleural spots of ecchymosis following death by strangulation.

tardive (tăr'dĭv) [Fr., tardy]. Characterized by lateness, esp. pert. to a disease in which the characteristic sign or symptom appears late in the course of the disease.

tardive dyskinesia. SEE: *dyskinesia, tardive*.

tare (tăr). The weight of an empty container. That weight is subtracted from the total weight of the vessel and substance added to it in order to determine the precise weight of the material added to the container.

tared. A container of known and predetermined tare, q.v.

tarentism (tăr'ĕn-tĭzm). Tarantism.

target (tăr'gĕt) [O. Fr. *targette*, light shield]. 1. A structure or organ that something is directed to. SEE: *target organ*. 2. The electrode on which cathode rays within an x-ray tube are focused and from which roentgen rays are emitted; usually of a heavy metal such as tungsten.

target cell. An abnormal erythrocyte with a rounded central area, which stains deeply, surrounded by a lightly staining area, which in turn is surrounded by denser cytoplasm at the periphery of the cell, the whole somewhat resembling a target with a bull's eye. Found in certain types of anemia and after splenectomy.

target organ. The organ or structure toward which the effects of a drug, hormone, or therapeutic agent are primarily directed.

tarichatoxin (tăr''ĭk-ă-tŏk'sĭn). A neurotoxin from the *Taricha* newt.

Tarnier's sign (tăr-nē-āz') [Etienne Stéphene Tarnier, Fr. obstetrician, 1828–1897]. A sign of impending miscarriage; the disappearance of the angle between upper and lower uterine segments in pregnancy.

tarnish. Surface discoloration or reduced luster of metals due to the effect of corrosive substances or galvanic action. In dental restorations such action may be enhanced by accumulation of bacterial plaque.

tarsadenitis (tăr''săd-ĕn-ī'tĭs) [Gr. *tarsos*, a broad, flat surface, + *aden*, gland, + *itis*, inflammation]. Inflammation of the tarsal or meibomian glands of the eyelid.

tarsal (tăr'săl) [Gr. *tarsalis*]. 1. Pert. to the tarsus or supporting plate of the eyelid. 2. Pert. to the ankle or tarsus.

tarsal arches. Two branches, superior and inferior, of the median palpebral artery supplying the eyelid.

tarsal bones. The seven bones of the ankle, hind foot and midfoot, consisting of the talus, calcaneus, navicular, cuboid and three cuneiform bones.

tarsal cartilages. The dense connective tissue of the tarsus of the eyelid. It is not true cartilage.

tarsalgia (tăr-săl'jē-ă) [Gr. *tarsos*, a broad, flat surface, + *algos*, pain]. Pain in tarsus or ankle. May be due to flatfoot, shortening of Achilles tendon, or other causes.

tarsal glands. Branched sebaceous alveolar glands embedded in the tarsus and opening on the margin of the eyelid. SYN: *meibomian glands*.

tarsalia (tăr-sā'lē-ă) [L.] (sing. *tarsale*). The tarsal bones.

tarsalis (tăr-sā'lĭs) [L.]. One of the tarsal muscles. SEE: *Muscles* in *Appendix*.

tarsal lacrimal glands. Accessory lacrimal glands located on the inner surface of the eyelids, esp. the upper lid.

tarsal tunnel. In the ankle, the bony-fibrous passage for the posterior tibial vessels, tibial nerve, and flexor tendons.

tarsal tunnel syndrome. Neuropathy of the distal portion of the tibial nerve at the ankle due to chronic pressure on the nerve at the point it passes through the tarsal tunnel. It causes pain in and numbness of the sole of the foot and weakness of plantar flexion of the toes.

tarsectomy (tar-sĕk′tō-mē) [″ + *ektome,* excision]. 1. Excision of tarsus or a tarsal bone. 2. Removal of tarsal plate of an eyelid.

tarsectopia (tăr″sĕk-tō′pē-ă). Dislocation of the tarsus.

tarsi. Pl. of tarsus.

tarsitis (tăr-sī′tĭs) [″ + *itis,* inflammation]. 1. Inflammation of tarsus of the foot. 2. Inflammation of the margin of an eyelid. SYN: *blepharitis.*

tarso- [Gr. *tarsos,* a broad, flat surface]. Combining form meaning the flat of the foot or the edge of the eyelid.

tarsocheiloplasty (tăr″sō-kī′lō-plăs″tē) [″ + *cheilos,* lip, + *plassein,* to form]. Plastic surgery of borders of the eyelid.

tarsoclasia, tarsoclasis (tăr″sō-klă′sē-ă, tăr-sŏk′lăs-ĭs) [″ + *klasis,* a breaking]. Surgical fracture of the tarsus for correction of clubfoot.

tarsomalacia (tăr″sō-mă-lā′sē-ă) [″ + *malakia,* a softening]. Softening of the tarsal cartilages of the eyes.

tarsomegaly (tăr″sō-mĕg′ă-lē) [″ + *megas,* large]. Enlargement of the heel bone, calcaneus.

tarsometatarsal (tăr″sō-mĕt″ă-tăr′săl) [″ + *meta,* between, + *tarsos,* a broad, flat surface]. Pert. to the tarsus and the metatarsus.

tarso-orbital (tăr″sō-or′bĭ-tăl) [″ + L. *orbita,* track]. Concerning the tarsus of the eyelid and the orbit.

tarsophalangeal (tăr″sō-fă-lăn′jē-ăl) [″ + *phalanx,* closely knit row]. Concerning the tarsus of the foot and the phalanges of the toes.

tarsophyma (tăr″sō-fī′mă) [″ + *phyma,* a growth]. Any tarsal tumor of the eyelid. SYN: *hordeolum; sty.*

tarsoplasia, tarsoplasty (tăr″sō-plā′zē-ă, tăr′sō-plăs″tē) [″ + *plassein,* to form]. Plastic surgery of margin of the eyelid. SYN: *blepharoplasty.*

tarsoptosis (tăr″sŏp-tō′sĭs) [″ + *ptosis,* falling]. Flat foot; fallen arch of the foot.

tarsorrhaphy (tăr-sor′ă-fē) [″ + *rhaphe,* seam, ridge]. The operation of uniting the edges of the lids at the outer commissure for the purpose of reducing the width of the palpebral fissure.

tarsotarsal (tăr″sō-tăr′săl) [″ + *tarsos,* a broad, flat surface]. Concerning the articulation between two rows of tarsal bones.

tarsotibial (tăr″sō-tĭb′ē-ăl) [″ + L. *tibia,* shinbone]. Concerning the tarsus and the tibia of the foot.

tarsotomy (tăr-sŏt′ō-mē) [″ + *tome,* incision]. 1. Incision of tarsal cartilage of an eyelid. 2. Any surgical incision of the tarsus of the foot.

tarsus (tăr′sŭs) [Gr. *tarsos,* a broad, flat surface] (pl. *tarsi*). 1. The ankle with its seven bones located between bones of the lower leg and metatarsus. It forms the proximal portion of the foot. It consists of the following bones: calcaneus (os calcis), talus (astragalus), cuboid (os cuboideum), navicular (scaphoid), and first, second, and third cuneiform bones. The talus articulates with the tibia and fibula, the cuboid and cuneiform bones with the metatarsals. SEE: *foot; skeleton;* names of individual bones. 2. A curved plate of dense white fibrous tissue forming the supporting structure of the eyelid. Also called *tarsal plate.*

   t. inferior palpebrae. The firm layer of connective tissue that provides internal support for the lower eyelid.

   t. superior palpebrae. The firm layer of connective tissue that provides internal support for the upper eyelid.

tartar [Gr. *tartaron,* dregs]. 1. An acid compound found in the juice of grapes and deposited on the sides of casks during winemaking. 2. Calcareous matter deposited upon the teeth. SYN: *calculus; plaque, dental.*

   t., cream of. Potassium bitartrate.

   t. emetic. Antimony potassium tartrate. Used as an emetic.

tartaric acid (tăr-tăr′ĭk). Any one of four isomers of an organic compound, $C_4H_6O_6$. Used in making potassium bitartrate, which is cream of tartar.

tart cells. Certain cells containing altered nuclear material appearing along with L.E. cells in suspensions of leukocytes or bone marrow cells.

tartrate. A salt of tartaric acid.

tartrazine. A pyrazole aniline dye widely used to color foods, cosmetics, drugs, and textiles.

taste (tāst) [O. Fr. *taster,* to feel, to taste]. 1. To attempt to determine the flavor of a substance by touching it with the mouth. 2. A chemical sense dependent upon sense organs on the surface of the tongue. These organs, called taste buds, when appropriately stimulated, produce one or a combination of the four fundamental taste sensations: sweet, bitter, sour, and salty. The nervous impulses are carried to the brain by the lingual (from the anterior two-thirds of the surface) and the glossopharyngeal (from the posterior third) nerves. Loss of taste may be due to bilateral disease of chorda tympani nerve and of gustatory fibers of the glossopharyngeal nerve or to cytotoxic drugs used therapeutically.

The cells of the taste buds have an average life span of 10 to 10½ days; thus, they are constantly being renewed. If a cytotoxic agent used in cancer therapy destroys the cells, taste will return in a minimum of 10 days but usually over a much longer period.

RS: ageusia; agnosia; appetite; degustation; dysgeusia; gustation; gustatory; hypogeusia.

t., after-. The persistence of a taste sensation after removal of original stimulus.

taste area. Area in cerebral cortex at lower end of somesthetic area.

taste blindness. Inability to taste certain substances such as phenylthiocarbamide (PTC). This inability is due to a hereditary factor that is transmitted as an autosomal recessive trait.

taste buds. Sensory end-organs that mediate the sensation of taste. They are oval structures located on the surface of the tongue, esp. the sides of the circumvallate papillae, on soft palate, epiglottis, and portions of the pharynx. Each contains sensory and gustatory (taste) cells and supporting (sustentacular) cells. When stimulated by chemical stimuli, they give rise to sense of taste. SEE: *chemoreceptor; taste cells.*

taste cells. Neuroepithelial cells within a taste bud that serve as receptors for the sense of taste. Each possesses on the free surface a short taste hair that projects through the inner taste pore. SYN: *cell, gustatory.*

taster (tās′tĕr). 1. A person capable of detecting a particular substance by using the taste sense. SEE: *phenylthiocarbamide.* 2. An individual who tastes food prior to its being approved for ingestion by a person whom others might wish to poison.

TAT. *thematic apperception test.*

T.A.T. *tetanus antitoxin; toxin-antitoxin.*

tattooing (tă-too′ĭng) [Tahitian *tatau*]. Indelible marking of the skin produced by introducing minute amounts of pigments into the skin. Tattooing is usually done to produce a certain design, picture, or name. When it is done commercially, sterile procedures are rarely used and infectious hepatitis or AIDS virus or both may be transmitted to the customer. The technique may also be used to conceal a corneal leukoma, to mask pigmented areas of skin, or to color skin to look like the areola in mammoplasty.

t., removal of. The pigment in a tattoo may be "erased" by use of a ruby laser. This usually causes no permanent skin changes.

t., traumatic. Following abrasion of the skin, embedding of fine dirt particles under the superficial layers of the skin; or as a result of forceful deposit of gunpowder granules. This can be prevented by immediate removal of the particles.

taurine (taw′rĭn). A derivative of cysteine. It is present in bile, as taurocholic acid, in combination with bile acid.

taurocholate (taw″rō-kō′lāt). A salt of taurocholic acid.

taurocholemia (taw″rō-kō-lē′mē-ă) [Gr. *tauros*, a bull, + *chole*, bile, + *haima*, blood]. Taurocholic acid in the blood.

taurocholic acid. A substance occurring in bile and yielding cholic acid and taurine on hydrolysis.

taurodontism (taw″rō-dŏn′tĭzm) [″ + *odous*, tooth, + *-ismos*, condition]. Condition in which teeth have greatly enlarged pulp chambers that are deepened. In that shape, the pulp chamber encroaches on the roots of the teeth.

Taussig-Bing syndrome (taw′sĭg-bĭng) [Helen B. Taussig, U.S. pediatrician, b. 1898; Richard J. Bing, U.S. surgeon, b. 1909]. Congenital deformity of the heart in which the aorta arises from the right ventricle and the pulmonary artery arises from both ventricles. An intraventricular septal defect is present.

tauto- [Gr. *tautos*, identical]. Prefix meaning the same.

tautomenial (taw″tō-mē′nē-ăl) [″ + *meniaia*, menses]. Concerning the same menstrual period.

tautomer (taw′tō-mĕr) [″ + *meros*, a part]. A chemical that is capable of tautomerism.

tautomeral, tautomeric (taw-tŏm′ĕr-ăl, -tō-mĕr′ĭk) [″ + *meros*, a part]. Noting certain neurons that send processes to the white matter on the same side of the spinal cord.

tautomerase (taw-tŏm′ĕr-ās) [″ + ″ + *-ase*, enzyme]. An enzyme that catalyzes tautomeric reactions.

tautomerism (taw-tŏm′ĕr-ĭzm) [″ + ″ + *-ismos*, condition]. Phenomenon in which two formulae are possible and exist in dynamic equilibrium so that as the amount of one substance is altered, the second is changed into the other form in order to maintain the equilibrium. SEE: *isomerism.*

tautorotation (taw″tō-rō-tā′shŭn) [″ + L. *rotare*, to turn round]. A change in specific rotation that occurs when a solution of certain sugars stands for a while.

Tavist. Trade name for clemastine fumarate.

taxis (tăk′sĭs) [Gr., arrangement]. 1. Manual replacement or reduction of a hernia or dislocation. 2. The response of an organism to its environment; a turning toward (positive taxis) or away from (negative taxis) a particular stimulus. SEE: *chemotaxis.*

t., bipolar. Replacing of a retroverted uterus by applying traction on the cervix while the uterus is pushed upward by manipulating it through the rectum.

taxol. A chemical obtained from the bark of the yew tree, *Taxus brevifolia.* In clinical trials taxol has shown great promise in treating certain advanced cancers of the ovary and the breast. Like all drugs, taxol has the potential for causing undesired side effects.

taxon (tăk'sŏn) [Gr. *taxis,* arrangement]. A taxonomic group.

taxonomic (tăk″sō-nŏm'ĭk). Concerning taxonomy.

taxonomy (tăks-ŏn'ō-mē) [″ + *nomos,* law]. Laws and principles of classification of animals and plants. Also used for classification of learning objectives.

Taylor brace (tā'lĕr) [Charles Fayette Taylor, U.S. surgeon, 1827–1899]. Brace with two rigid posterior oblique portions and soft straps crossed anteriorly over the chest.

Tay-Sachs disease [Warren Tay, Brit. physician, 1843–1927; Bernard Sachs, U.S. neurologist, 1858–1944]. An inherited disease transmitted as an autosomal recessive trait. The rate of occurrence in Ashkenazi Jews in the U.S. is estimated to be 400 per 1 million births. SYN: G_{M2} *gangliosidosis.* SEE: *Nursing Diagnoses in Appendix.*

SYM: Neurological deterioration characterized by mental and physical retardation, blindness, cherry-red spots on the macula, an exaggerated startle response, spasticity, convulsions, and enlargement of the head. Carriers of the trait can be accurately detected by assay of hexosaminidase A. It is possible to detect affected embryos by measurement of hexosaminidase A in amniotic fluid.

ETIOL: Because of the lack of the enzyme hexosaminidase A, which is important in sphingolipid metabolism, sphingolipids accumulate in the cells, esp. those of nerves and the brain.

PROG: Death usually occurs prior to the age of 4.

TREAT: There is no specific therapy.

Tay's spot. Spot, cherry-red, q.v.

TB. Colloquialism for *tuberculosis.*

Tb. Chem. symb. for the element terbium.

T.b. *tubercle bacillus; tuberculosis.*

T bandage. Bandage resembling the letter T, used for the head and the perineum.

T-bar. T-shaped tubing connected to an endotracheal tube in situ. Used to deliver O_2 therapy to an intubated patient who does not require mechanical ventilation.

TBI. *total body irradiation.*

TBP. *thyroxine-binding protein.*

Tbs. *tablespoon.*

TBSA. *total body surface area.*

Tc. Chem. symb. for the element technetium.

T cell mediated immunity. One part of the specific immune response during which T lymphocytes act to destroy or neutralize organisms that have invaded the body.

Physiologic Actions: Unlike B cells, T cells are unable to recognize foreign antigens on their own. A foreign antigen is recognized by a macrophage that engulfs it and displays part of the antigen on its surface next to a histocompatibility, q.v., or "self" antigen (macrophage processing), q.v. The presence of these two markers plus the secretion of a chemical monokine, interleukin-1 (IL-1), activates one type of T cell, the helper/T4 cell, which controls the activities of other T cells.

T4 cells secrete interleukin-2 (IL-2), q.v., which stimulates the activity of natural killer cells, cytotoxic T cells, and B cells. Gamma interferon is also secreted by T4 cells to inhibit the growth of viruses and to stimulate macrophages' cytotoxicity and processing of antigens. T4 cells also activate suppressor or T8 cells that inhibit the responses of T4 cells and B cells after several days, providing a protective feedback mechanism that prevents excessive lymphocyte activity. SEE: *B cells; interleukin-1; interleukin-2; interferon; macrophage; T cells.*

T cell receptors. ABBR: TCR. Molecules on the surface of T cells that are specific for an antigen. Thus, for each of the great number of antigens to which the human may be exposed, there is a specific TCR for each one. SEE: *immune response; T cells.*

T cell replacing factor. ABBR: TRF. A lymphokine, q.v., that induces differentiation of B cell lymphocytes into antibody-secreting plasma cells.

T cells. Lymphoid cells from the bone marrow that migrate to the thymus gland, where they develop into mature differentiated lymphocytes that circulate between blood and lymph. Immature T cells are called thymocytes. Mature T cells are "antigen specific," meaning that each one responds to only one antigen. Different T cells have effector or regulator functions, or both. Effector activities are the secretion of chemicals called lymphokines and the ability to kill cells (cytotoxicity). Regulator functions include modulating the activities of other lymphocytes, including B cells.

T cells cannot recognize foreign antigens without the help of macrophage processing. However, once the macrophage has helped them identify an antigen as "non-self," T cells dominate the specific immune response, q.v., directing macrophages, B cells and other T cells in the body's defense. T cells also are responsible for tumor immunity, graft rejection, and hypersensitivity reactions.

Subpopulations of T lymphocytes include T4 (CD4) or helper cells, which are the major regulatory cells. These cells secrete interleukin-2 (IL-2), which stimulates the activity of B cells and other T lymphocytes. They also secrete gamma interferon, q.v., which inhibits viruses. T4 cells are the primary cells attacked by the human immunodeficiency virus (HIV) in AIDS. T8 (CD8) or supressor cells stop the specific immune response after several days and create memory cells. At least two classes of T lymphocytes directly kill other cells: cytotoxic T cells and natural killer cells. SEE: *antigen; B cells; immune response; immune surveillance; immunity, cell-mediated; immunity, humoral; lymphocytes; macrophage processing; plasma cells; rejection; T cell receptors.*

TCID$_{50}$. *Tissue culture infective dose* that will produce a cytopathic effect in 50% of the cultures inoculated.

t.d.s. L. *ter die sumendum,* to be taken three times a day.

Te. Chem. symb. for the element tellurium.

tea (tē). 1. An infusion of a medicinal plant. 2. Leaves of the plant *Thea chinensis*, from which a beverage is made by steeping the leaves in boiling hot water.

COMP: The principal ingredients are caffeine, tannin, and a volatile oil that gives the beverage prepared from tea leaves its characteristic taste and aroma. Caffeine, which constitutes 1% to 4% of tea leaves, is one of the medically important ingredients in tea. Fluoride is present in green tea at about twice the amount in black tea, but in both teas the concentration is sufficient to help prevent tooth decay. The caloric content is negligible until sugar and milk are added to the beverage. SEE: *caffeine.*

t., black. Tea made from leaves that have been fermented before they are dried.

t., green. Tea prepared by heating leaves in open trays.

t., herb. Tea made of a variety of plants, including leaves of certain flowers, herbs, barks, and grasses. Some herbs used in these teas are known to be harmful.

t., Paraguay copper. Tea made from the leaves and stems of *Ilex paraguayensis*. It is a stimulating drink and contains volatile oil, tannin, and caffeine.

TEAB. *tetraethylammonium bromide.*

TEAC. *tetraethylammonium chloride.*

tear (tār) [AS. *taer*]. 1. To separate or pull apart by force. 2. (tēr) The liquid excreted

into the eyes by the lacrimal glands.

t., bucket handle. A longitudinal tear, usually beginning in the middle of the semilunar cartilage of the knee.

tear duct, test of patency of. This can be easily done by placing several drops of a weak solution of sugar in the eye. If the person detects a sweet taste in the mouth, then the duct is patent.

tears (tērs) [AS. *tear*]. The watery saline solution secreted continuously by the lacrimal glands, q.v. They lubricate the surfaces between the eyeball and eyelids, i.e., the conjunctiva. These are called continuous tears. Irritant tears are produced when a foreign object or substance is in the eye. SEE: *Schirmer's test.*

t.'s, artificial. Solution of materials used to lubricate the conjunctivae.

t.'s, crocodile. Crocodile tears, q.v.

tease (tēz) [AS. *taesan,* to pluck]. To separate a tissue into minute parts with a needle to prepare it for the microscope.

teaspoon (tē'spoon). ABBR: tsp. A household measure equal to approximately 5 ml. Teaspoons used in the home vary from 3 to 6 ml. Because household measures are not accurate, when a teaspoon dose is prescribed or ordered, give 5 ml of the substance.

teat (tēt) [ME. *tete,* from AS. *tit,* teat]. 1. The nipple of the mammary gland. SYN: *papilla mammae.* SEE: *nipple; breast.* 2. Any protuberance resembling a nipple.

teatulation (tēt″ū-lā'shŭn) [AS. *tit,* teat]. The development of a nipplelike elevation.

technetium (těk-nē'shē-ŭm). SYMB: Tc. At. wt. is 98.9062; at. no. 43. A synthetic metallic chemical element.

technetium-99m. SYMB: ^{99m}Tc. An isomer of technetium that emits gamma rays. It has a half-life of six hours.

technetium Tc 99m albumin aggregated injection. USP. A radioactive isotope of technetium-99m. It is used intravenously for scanning the lung.

technic (těk'nĭk) [Gr. *techne,* art]. SEE: *technique.*

technical (těk'nĭ-kăl) [Gr. *tekhnikos,* skilled]. Requiring technique or special skill.

technician (těk-nĭsh'ăn) An individual who has the knowledge and skill required to carry out specific technical procedures. This individual usually has a diploma from a specialized school or an associate degree from college or has received training through preceptorship.

t., biomedical engineering. Technician who assembles, repairs, and adapts medical equipment used for the delivery of health care and assists in the development and maintenance of these systems.

t., dental. Technician who constructs

complete and partial dentures, makes orthodontic appliances, and fixes bridgework, crowns, and other dental restorations as authorized by dentists.

t., dialysis. Technician who operates and maintains an artificial kidney machine following approved methods to provide dialysis treatment for patients with kidney disorders.

t., dietetic. Technician who works with the food service manager and dietitian in a health care facility assisting with planning, implementing, and evaluating food programs, and may train and supervise dietary aides.

t., electrocardiographic. Technician who operates and maintains electrocardiographic machines, records the heart's electrical activity, and provides data for diagnosis and treatment of heart ailments by physicians.

t., electromyographic. Technician who assists the physician in recording and analyzing bioelectric potentials that originate in muscle tissue. This includes the operation of various electronic devices, maintenance of electronic equipment, assisting with patient care during testing, and record keeping.

t., emergency medical, -paramedic. Technician who responds to medical emergency calls, evaluates the nature of the emergency, and carries out specific diagnostic measures and emergency treatment procedures under the standing orders or specific directions of a physician.

t., environmental health. Technician who assists in the survey of environmental hazards and performs technical duties under professional supervision in areas such as pollution control, radiation protection, and sanitation.

t., histologic. Technician who works under the supervision of a pathologist in sectioning, staining, and mounting human and animal tissue and fluid for microscopic study.

t., medical laboratory. Technician who performs biological and chemical tests requiring limited independent judgment or correlation competency under the supervision of a medical technologist, pathologist, or physician.

t., medical record. Technician who assists the medical record administrator by coding, analyzing, and preserving patients' medical records and compiling reports, disease indices, and statistics in health care institutions.

t., orthopedic. Technician who is trained in maintaining traction devices, applies all types of traction, makes casts, and applies splints.

t., pharmacy. Technician who assists the pharmacist in certain activities such as medication profile reviews for drug incompatibilities, typing prescription labels, prescription packaging, handling purchase records, inventory control, and may, where state law and hospital policy permit, dispense drugs to patients under the supervision of a registered pharmacist.

t., psychiatric. Technician who works under the supervision of a professional in the care of mentally ill patients in a psychiatric care facility; assists in carrying out the prescribed treatment plan and assigned individual and group activities with patients.

t., respiratory therapy. Technician who routinely treats patients requiring noncritical respiratory care and who recognizes and responds to a limited number of specified respiratory emergencies.

technique (těk-nēk') [Fr., Gr. *technikos*]. 1. Systematic procedure or methods by which an involved or scientific task is completed. 2. The skill in performing details of a procedure or operation. 3. In radiology, the various technical factors that must be determined in order to produce a diagnostic radiograph, such as kilovoltage, milliamperage, time of exposure, and focal-film distance.

techno- [Gr. *techne*, art]. Combining form meaning art or skill.

technologist (těk″nŏl′ō-jĭst). Technologist specializing in the application of scientific knowledge in solving practical or theoretical problems. The knowledge and skills required for performing these functions are achieved through formal education and a period of supervised clinical practice.

t., blood bank. Technologist trained to assist in all of the routine and special functions and tasks concerned with blood bank and transfusion services.

t., cardiovascular. Technologist who performs a wide range of tests related to the functions and therapeutic care of the heart and lung system. These include operating and maintaining a heart-lung machine, assisting in cardiac catheterization, cardiac resuscitation, postoperative monitoring, and in care and treatment of patients who have undergone heart or lung surgery.

t., cyto-. Medical laboratory technologist who works under the supervision of a pathologist to examine cells in order to diagnose cancer or other diseases.

t., electroencephalographic. Technologist who operates and maintains electroencephalographic machines.

t., histologic. Technologist who performs all the functions of the histologic technician as well as more complex procedures for processing tissues, such as identifying tissue structures, cell components, and their staining characteristics, and relates them to physiological functions; may also implement and test new techniques and procedures.

t., medical. A technologist who works in conjunction with pathologists, physicians, and scientists in all general areas of the clinical laboratory. Independent and correlational judgments are made in a wide range of complex procedures. A medical technologist may teach and supervise laboratory personnel.

t., nuclear medicine. Technologist who assists in caring for patients receiving radioactive materials for diagnostic or therapeutic purposes. The nuclear medicine technologist prepares and administers these materials and is skilled in the use of radiation detection devices.

t., radiation therapy. Nuclear medicine technologist, q.v.

t., radiologic. Technologist trained in the safe application of ionizing radiation to portions of the body to assist the physician in the diagnosis of injuries and disease.

t., surgical. Technologist who assists in providing a safe environment for surgical care and assists surgeon, nurses, and other operating room staff.

technology (těk-nŏl′ō-jē) [″ + *logos*, word, reason]. 1. The application of scientific knowledge. 2. The entire scientific knowledge used in solving or approaching problems and situations. 3. The entire body of knowledge available to a civilization.

tectocephalic (těk″tō-sě-făl′ĭk) [L. *tectum*, roof, + Gr. *kephale*, head]. Concerning tectocephaly.

tectocephaly (těk-tō-sěf′ăl-ē). Possession of a boat-shaped cranium. SYN: *scaphocephalism.*

tectorial (těk-tō′rē-ăl) [L. *tectum*, roof]. Pert. to a roof or covering. SYN: *tegmental.*

tectorium (těk-tō′rē-ŭm) [L. *tectorium*, a covering] (pl. *tectoria*). 1. Any rooflike structure. SYN: *tectum; tegmentum; tegument.* 2. Corti's membrane.

tectospinal (těk″tō-spī′năl) [L. *tectum*, roof, + *spina*, thorn]. From the tectum mesencephali to the spinal cord.

tectospinal tract. A tract of white fibers of the spinal cord passing from the tectum of the midbrain and going down through the medulla to the spinal cord. It begins on one side and crosses to the other.

tectum (těk′tŭm) [L., roof]. 1. Any structure serving as, or resembling, a roof. 2. The dorsal portion of the midbrain consisting of the superior and inferior colliculi (corpora

quadrigemina). SYN: *tegmentum.*

t. mesencephali. Roof of the midbrain, including the corpora quadrigemina.

T.E.D. *threshold erythema dose.*

teenage. Pert. to those who are 13 through 19 years of age. SYN: *adolescent.*

teeth (tēth) [AS. *toth*, tooth] (sing. *tooth*). Hard bony projections in jaws serving as organs of mastication, there being 32 permanent teeth, 16 in each jaw. They include the following types: incisors, canines (cuspids), premolars (bicuspids), and molars. An average child should have 6 teeth at 1 year, 12 at 18 months, 16 at 2 years, and 20 at 2½ years. A child may be born with teeth, and in other cases the teeth may not appear until 16 months. SEE: *dentition* for illus.; *tooth; toothbrush and toothbrushing; plaque, dental; periodontal disease.*

t., anterior. Teeth located close to the midline of the dental arch on either side of the jaw, including the incisors and canine.

t., auditory. Minute toothlike projections along the free margin of the labium vestibulare of the cochlea. SYN: *Huschke's auditory teeth.*

t., charting and numbering. The various systems developed for designating teeth in a chart system include numbers, letters, or symbols and are not uniformly accepted; widely used are the two-digit system of Federation Dentaire Internationale (FDI system) and the American system, which numbers the permanent teeth consecutively from upper right third molar as #1, through the maxillary teeth to #16, and then to left mandibular third molar as #17 and through the mandibular teeth to the right third molar as #32.

t., deciduous. Teeth making up the first dentition, which are shed and replaced by the permanent teeth. SYN: *teeth, milk; teeth, temporary.* SEE: illus.

t., Hutchinson's. Condition in which lateral incisors of the upper jaw are pegged and central incisors of same jaw have convex sides and crescentic notches on their cutting edges; noted only on permanent teeth, sometimes indicating hereditary syphilis.

t., malacotic. Teeth that are esp. prone to decay, soft in structure and white in color.

t., milk. T., deciduous.

t., permanent. Teeth of the second dentition, replacing the deciduous teeth. SEE: illus.

t., reimplantation or repair of. F.A.: If a tooth is completely knocked out of its socket by trauma or fracture, the tooth or fragment should be gently cleaned (do not scrub tooth), placed in clean water, and taken with the patient without delay to a dentist. For an

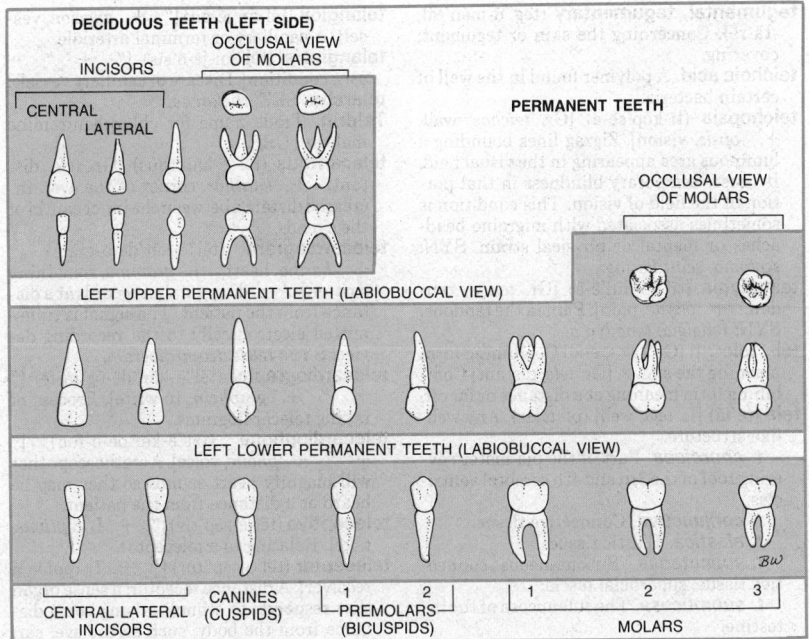

DECIDUOUS TEETH (LEFT SIDE)

OCCLUSAL VIEW OF MOLARS

INCISORS

CENTRAL

LATERAL

PERMANENT TEETH

OCCLUSAL VIEW OF MOLARS

LEFT UPPER PERMANENT TEETH (LABIOBUCCAL VIEW)

LEFT LOWER PERMANENT TEETH (LABIOBUCCAL VIEW)

CENTRAL LATERAL INCISORS   CANINES (CUSPIDS)   1 2 PREMOLARS (BICUSPIDS)   1 2 3 MOLARS

adult who is conscious, the tooth may be replaced in the socket while it is being transported to the dentist. The dentist may be able to save the tooth; and for fragments, to glue them to the remaining part of the tooth.

t., sclerotic. Yellowish teeth that are naturally hard and not subject to ready decay.

t., secondary. T., permanent.

t., stained. Deep or superficial discoloration of teeth. There are a number of conditions that will cause staining of teeth, e.g., exposure of the fetus to tetracycline the mother took during pregnancy or mottling due to exposure to high levels of fluoride in drinking water. No matter what the cause, the stains may be covered up by applying a plastic resin or porcelain laminate coating over them, a process called bonding. This same technique may be used to rebuild or repair chipped or cracked teeth.

t., temporary. T., deciduous.

t., twinning of. A dental anomaly in which two teeth are joined together.

t., wisdom. The third molar teeth of the permanent dentition, which are the last to erupt.

teething (tēth'ĭng) [AS. *toth*, tooth]. Eruption of the teeth. SEE: *dentition*.

Teflon. Trade name for polytetrafluorethylene.

tegmen (tĕg'mĕn) [L. *tegmen*, covering] (pl. *tegmina*). A structure that covers a part.

   t. mastoideum. Bony roof of mastoid cells.

   t. tympani. [NA] Roof of tympanum separating middle ear from cranial cavity.

   t. ventriculi quarti. [NA] The roof of the 4th ventricle.

tegmental (tĕg-mĕn'tăl) [L. *tegmentum*, covering]. Relating to a tegument or tegmentum; a covering. SYN: *tentorial*.

tegmental nuclei. Several masses of gray matter lying in the tegmentum of the midbrain and upper portion of the pons. Include the dorsal, pedunculopontile, reticular, and ventral nuclei.

tegmentum (tĕg-mĕn'tŭm) [L. *tegmentum*, covering]. 1. A roof or covering. SYN: *tectorium; tegument.* 2. The dorsal portion of the cruri cerebri of the midbrain. It contains the red nucleus and nuclei and roots of the oculomotor nerve. SYN: *tectum.*

Tegopen (tĕg'ō-pĕn). Trade name for cloxacillin sodium, USP.

tegument (tĕg'ū-mĕnt). 1. The skin; the covering of the body. SYN: *integument.* 2. A covering structure.

tegumental, tegumentary (tĕg"ū-mĕn'tăl, -tă-rē). Concerning the skin or tegument; covering.

teichoic acid. A polymer found in the wall of certain bacteria.

teichopsia (tī-kŏp'sē-ă) [Gr. *teichos*, wall, + *opsis*, vision]. Zigzag lines bounding a luminous area appearing in the visual field. It causes temporary blindness in that portion of the field of vision. This condition is sometimes associated with migraine headaches or mental or physical strain. SYN: *scotoma, scintillating.*

teinodynia (tī"nō-dĭn'ē-ă) [Gr. *tenon*, tendon, + *odyne*, pain]. Pain in the tendons. SYN: *tenalgia; tenodynia.*

tel-, tele-. 1. [Gr. *telos*, end] Combining form meaning the end. 2. [Gr. *tele*, distant] Combining form meaning at a distance or far off.

tela (tē'lă) [L. *tela*, web] (pl. *telae*). Any weblike structure.

    t. choroidea. Part of the pia mater covering roof of the 3rd and 4th cerebral ventricles.

    t. conjunctiva. Connective tissue.

    t. elastica. Elastic tissue.

    t. subcutanea. Subcutaneous connective tissue; superficial fascia.

    t. submucosa. The submucosa of the intestine.

telalgia (tĕl-ăl'jē-ă) [Gr. *tele*, distant, + *algos*, pain]. Pain felt at a distance from its stimulus. SYN: *referred pain.*

telangiectasia, telangiectasis (tĕl-ăn"jē-ĕk-tā'zē-ă, -ĕk'tă-sĭs) [Gr. *telos*, end, + *angeion*, vessel, + *ektasis*, dilatation]. A vascular lesion formed by dilatation of a group of small blood vessels. It may appear as a birthmark or become apparent in young children. May occur anywhere on the skin but is seen most frequently on the face and thighs.

    t., hereditary hemorrhagic. A hereditary disease characterized by thinness of walls of blood vessels of nose, skin, and digestive tract and tendency to hemorrhage. SYN: *Osler-Weber-Rendu disease.*

    t. lymphatica. Tumor composed of dilated lymph vessels.

    t., spider. A stellate angioma (nevus araneus).

telangiectatic (tĕl-ăn"jē-ĕk-tăt'ĭk). Concerning telangiectasia.

telangiectodes (tĕl-ăn"jē-ĕk-tō'dēz). Tumors that have telangiectasia.

telangiitis (tĕl-ăn"jē-ī'tĭs) [" + " + *itis*, inflammation]. Inflammation of the capillaries.

telangioma (tĕl-ăn"jē-ō'mă) [Gr. *telos*, end, + *angeion*, vessel, + *oma*, tumor]. A tumor made up of dilated capillaries or arterioles.

telangion (tĕl-ăn'jē-ŏn) [" + *angeion*, vessel]. A capillary or terminal arteriole.

telangiosis (tĕl"ăn-jē-ō'sĭs) [" + " + *osis*, condition]. Disease of capillary vessels.

telarche. SEE: *thelarche.*

Teldrin. Trade name for chlorpheniramine maleate, USP.

telecanthus (tĕl"ē-kăn'thŭs) [Gr. *tele*, distant, + *kanthos*, corner of the eye]. Increased distance between the inner canthi of the eyelids.

telecardiogram (tĕl"ē-kăr'dē-ō-grăm) [" + *kardia*, heart, + *gramma*, something written]. A cardiogram that records at a distance from the patient. The signal is transmitted electronically to the recording device. SYN: *telelectrocardiogram.*

telecardiography (tĕl"ē-kăr"dē-ŏg'ră-fē) [" + " + *graphein*, to write]. Process of taking telecardiograms.

telecardiophone (tĕl"ē-kăr'dē-ō-fōn) [" + *phone*, voice]. A stethoscope that will magnify heart sounds so they may be heard at a distance from the patient.

teleceptive (tĕl-ē-sĕp'tĭv) [" + L. *ceptivus*, take]. Relating to a teleceptor.

teleceptor (tĕl'ē-sĕp"tor) [" + L. *ceptor*, a receiver]. A distance receptor; a sense organ that responds to stimuli arising some distance from the body, such as the eye, ear, and nose. SYN: *teloceptor.*

telecinesia (tĕl"ē-sĭn-ē'zē-ă) [" + *kinesis*, movement]. Apparent automatic movement of an object produced without contact with any stimulus or power.

telecurietherapy (tĕl-ē-kū"rē-thĕr'ă-pē) [" + *curie*, + Gr. *therapeia*, treatment]. Application of radiation therapy from a source distant from the lesion or patient.

teledendrite, teledendron (tĕl-ē-dĕn'drīt, -dĕn'drŏn) [Gr. *telos*, end, + *dendron*, a tree]. The terminal processes of an axon. SYN: *telodendron.*

telediagnosis (tĕl"ē-dī"ăg-nō'sĭs) [Gr. *tele*, distant, + *diagignoskein*, to discern]. Diagnosis made on the basis of data transmitted electronically to the physician's location.

telediastolic (tĕl"ē-dī-ă-stŏl'ĭk) [Gr. *telos*, end, + *diastole*, a dilatation]. Concerning the last phase of the diastole.

telefluoroscopy (tĕl"ē-floo"or-ŏs'kō-pē). Transmission of fluoroscopic images by electronic means.

telekinesis (tĕl"ē-kĭ-nē'sĭs) [" + *kinesis*, movement]. Willful movement of articles without touching them. Some practitioners of the occult claim to have this ability. Be skeptical.

telelectrocardiogram (tĕl"ē-lĕk"trō-kăr'dē-ō-grăm) [Gr. *tele*, distant, + *elektron*, amber, + *kardia*, heart, + *gramma*, something written]. An electrocardiogram taken with a galvanometer attached to the patient by a wire some distance from the instrument. SYN: *telecardiogram*.

telemeter (tĕl'ĕ-mē"tĕr) [" + *metron*, measure]. To transmit information to a distant point by using electronic devices.

telemetry (tĕ-lĕm'ĕ-trē). The transmission of data electronically to a distant location.

telencephalic (tĕl"ĕn-sĕf-ăl'ĭk) [Gr. *telos*, end, + *enkephalos*, brain]. Pert. to the endbrain (telencephalon).

telencephalization (tĕl"ĕn-sĕf"ăl-ĭ-zā'shŭn). The evolutionary degree of control over functions previously mediated by lower nerve centers.

telencephalon (tĕl-ĕn-sĕf'ă-lŏn) [" + *enkephalos*, brain]. The embryonic endbrain or posterior division of the prosencephalon from which the cerebral hemispheres, corpora striata, and rhinencephalon develop.

teleneurite (tĕl"ĕ-nū'rīt) [" + *neuron*, nerve]. The branching end of an axon.

teleneuron (tĕl"ĕ-nū'rŏn) [" + *neuron*, nerve]. A nerve ending.

teleo- [Gr. *teleos*, complete]. Combining form meaning perfect or complete.

teleological (tē"lē-ō-lŏj'ĭ-kăl). Concerning teleology.

teleology (tĕl-ē-ŏl'ō-jē) [" + *logos*, word, reason]. The belief that everything is directed toward some final purpose. The doctrine of final causes.

teleomitosis (tĕl"ē-ō-mī-tō'sĭs) [" + *mitos*, thread, + *osis*, condition]. Mitosis that is complete.

teleonomic (tĕl"ē-ō-nŏm'ĭk). Concerning teleonomy.

teleonomy (tĕl"ē-ŏn'ō-mē) [" + *nomos*, law]. The concept that, in an organism or animal, the existence of a structure, capability, or function indicates that it had a survival function.

teleoperators. A machine or device operated by a person at a distance. The location of the device could be in an adjacent room or on another planet. Use of such a machine allows tasks to be done deep in the ocean or on orbiting satellites, or in closer conditions where the goal is to manipulate radioactive materials without danger of exposure to the radioactivity.

teleopsia (tĕl-ē-ŏp'sē-ă) [Gr. *tele*, distant, + *ops*, eye]. A visual disorder in which objects perceived in space have excessive depth or in which close objects appear far away.

teleorganic (tĕl"ē-or-găn'ĭk) [Gr. *teleos*, complete, + *organon*, organ]. Necessary to organic life. SYN: *vital*.

teleotherapeutics (tĕl"ē-ō-thĕr-ă-pū'tĭks) [Gr. *tele*, distant, + *therapeutikos*, treat-

ing]. The use of hypnotic suggestion in the treatment of disease. SYN: *suggestive therapeutics*.

Telepaque (tĕl'ĕ-pāk). Trade name for iopanoic acid.

telepathist (tĕ-lĕp'ă-thĭst) [" + *pathos*, disease, suffering]. One who claims the ability to read the mind of others.

telepathy (tĕ-lĕp'ă-thē). Supposed communication of one mind with another at a distance without any physical or psychological explanation. SYN: *telesthesia*.

teleradiography (tĕl"ĕ-rā-dē-ŏg'ră-fē) [Gr. *tele*, distant, + L. *radius*, ray, + Gr. *graphein*, to write]. Radiography with the radiation source about 2 meters (6½ ft) from the body. Done to minimize distortion by having rays virtually parallel at that distance. SYN: *teleroentgenography*.

teleradiology. Transmission of an x-ray image to a distant center where it may be interpreted by a radiologist.

teleradium (tĕl"ĕ-rā'dē-ŭm). A radium source distant from the area being treated.

teleroentgenogram (tĕl"ĕ-rĕnt-gĕn'ō-grăm) [" + *roentgen* + Gr. *gramma*, something written]. An x-ray picture obtained by teleroentgenography.

teleroentgenography (tĕl"ĕ-rĕnt"gĕn-ŏg'ră-fē) [" + " + Gr. *graphein*, to write]. Radiography in which the radiation source is about 2 meters (6½ ft) from the body. SYN: *teleradiography*.

telesthesia (tĕl-ĕs-thē'zē-ă) [" + *aisthesis*, sensation]. 1. An impression received at a distance without normal operation of organs of sense. 2. Distance perception. SYN: *telepathy*. SEE: *paranormal*.

telesystolic (tĕl"ĕ-sĭs-tŏl'ĭk) [Gr. *telos*, end, + *systole*, contraction]. Pert. to the termination of the cardiac systole.

teletactor (tĕl"ĕ-tăk'tor) [" + L. *tactus*, touch]. A device used by the deaf to receive vibrations through the skin.

teletherapy (tĕl-ĕ-thĕr'ă-pē) [Gr. *tele*, distant, + *therapeia*, treatment]. 1. Treatment of disease by telepathy. 2. Cancer treatment in which the radiation source is placed outside the body.

teletypewriter. ABBR: TTY. A typewriter that may be connected to a telephone. Use of this device permits deaf persons to communicate by sending and receiving type-written messages.

telluric (tĕ-lūr'ĭk) [L. *tellus*, earth]. Of or rel. to the earth.

tellurism (tĕl'ū-rĭzm) [" + Gr. *-ismos*, condition]. The concept that emanations from the earth cause disease.

tellurium (tĕl-ū're-ŭm) [L. *tellus*, earth]. SYMB: Te. At. wt. 127.60; at. no. 52; sp. gr. 6.24. A nonmetallic element used as an electric rectifier and in coloring glass.

tellurium poisoning. Characterized by a garlic odor of all secretions and excretions and a disagreeable odor to the breath. Perspiration and saliva are suppressed, resulting in dry skin and mouth. Anorexia, nausea, drowsiness, and weakness.

TREAT: Give saline cathartics; increase fluid intake; induce perspiration; otherwise treatment is symptomatic.

telocentric (tĕl″ō-sĕn′trĭk) [Gr. *telos*, end, + *kentron*, center]. Location of the centromere in the extreme end of the replicating chromosome so that there is only one arm on the chromosome.

teloceptor. Teleceptor.

telodendron (tĕl-ō-dĕn′drŏn) [Gr. *telos*, end, + *dendron*, tree]. The more or less diffuse arborizations at the end of an axon or its collaterals. SYN: *teledendrite.*

telogen (tĕl′ō-jĕn) [″ + *genesis*, generation, birth]. Resting stage of hair growth cycle. SEE: *anagen; catagen.*

telogloia (tĕl-ŏg′lē-ă). Cells that cover the outer surface of the motor endplate.

telolecithal. Concerning an egg in which the large yolk mass is concentrated at one pole.

telolemma (tĕl″ō-lĕm′mă) [″ + *lemma*, rind]. The membrane covering the motor endplate in a striated muscle fiber.

telomere (tĕl′ō-mēr) [″ + *meros*, part]. The end of an arm of a chromosome.

telophase (tĕl′ō-fāz) [″ + *phasis*, an appearance]. The final phase or stage of mitosis (karyokinesis) during which reconstruction of the daughter nuclei takes place and the cytoplasm of the cell divides, giving rise to two daughter cells.

telophragma (tĕl″ō-frăg′mă) [″ + *phragmos*, a fencing in]. The Z line or disk in striated muscle. SEE: *Z disk.*

telosynapsis (tĕl″ō-sĭ-năp′sĭs) [″ + *synapsis*, point of contact]. End-to-end union of pairs of homologous chromosomes during gametogenesis.

telotism (tĕl′ō-tĭzm) [″ + *-ismos*, condition]. The entire performance of a function, as that of one of the senses.

TEM. *triethylene melamine.* SEE: *nitrogen mustards.*

Temaril (tĕm′ă-rĭl). Trade name for trimeprazine tartrate.

tempeh. A wheat-soybean food developed as an excellent inexpensive source of protein for children. It is used in economically depressed countries. Quality of protein in tempeh is almost equal to casein.

temper [AS. *temprian*, to mingle]. State of an individual's mood, disposition, or mind, e.g., even-tempered or foul-tempered.

temperament (tĕm′pĕr-ă-mĕnt) [L. *temperamentum*, mixture]. The combination of intellectual, emotional, ethical, and physical characteristics of a specific individual.

temperance. Moderation in one's thoughts and actions, especially with respect to use of alcoholic beverages.

temperate (tĕm′pĕr-ĭt). Moderate; not excessive.

temperature (tĕm′pĕr-ă-tūr) [L. *temperatura*, proportion]. 1. Degree of heat of a living body. 2. Degree of hotness or coldness of a substance.

Body temperature varies with the body area in which it is measured and with the time of day. The temperature in the liver may be 105°F (40.6°C), while that under the tongue is 98.6°F (37°C); the rectal temperature is likely to be 0.5° to 1.0°F (0.28° to 0.56°C) above the oral.

Muscular work (as in shivering) is a mechanism for raising body temperature; sweating lowers it.

Body temperature may be measured by a clinical thermometer placed in the mouth, in the rectum, or under the arm. Rectal temperature usually is from 0.5° to 1.0°F (0.28° to 0.56°C) higher than by mouth; axillary temperature is about 0.5°F (0.28°C) lower than by mouth. Oral temperature may be inaccurate if taken just after the patient has ingested cold substances or has been breathing with the mouth open.

Body temperature is the result of the balance between heat production and heat loss. Eighty-five percent of body heat is lost through the skin, the remainder through lungs and fecal and urinary excretions. Regulation of body temperature is accomplished principally through thermoregulatory centers located in the hypothalamus. Elevation of temperature above normal is designated fever (pyrexia), and subnormal temperature is hypothermia. SEE: *ear thermometry.*

t., absolute. Temperature measured from absolute zero, which is −273.15°C.

t., ambient. The surrounding temperature or that present in the place, site, or location indicated.

t., axillary. Temperature obtained by placing thermometer in apex of the axilla with arm pressed closely to side of body. Temperature obtained by this method is usually 0.5° to 1.0°F (0.28° to 0.56°C) lower than oral.

t., body. Temperature of the body.

t. chart, basal. SEE: *basal temperature chart.*

t., core. Core temperature, q.v.

t., critical. Temperature below which a gas may be converted to liquid form by pressure.

t., inverse. Condition in which body

temperature is higher in the morning than in the evening.

t., maximum. Temperature above which bacterial growth will not take place.

t., mean. The average temperature for a stated period in a given locality.

t., minimum. In bacteriology, temperature below which bacterial growth will not take place.

t., normal. Temperature of the body, taken orally, in a healthy individual; 98.6°F (37°C) in humans.

t., optimum. Temperature at which a procedure is best carried out, such as the culture of a given organism or the action of an enzyme.

t., oral. Temperature obtained by placing a thermometer under the patient's tongue with lips closed for 3 minutes. It should not be taken for at least 10 minutes after ingestion of hot or cold liquids. It is not advisable for infants, mouth-breathers, comatose patients, or those extremely ill.

t., rectal. Temperature obtained by inserting the thermometer into the anal canal to a depth of at least 1½ in. (3.8 cm) and allowing it to remain there for 3 to 5 minutes. Do not take following a rectal operation or if rectum is diseased. Rectal temperature is more accurate than either oral or axillary temperature. It averages about 1°F (0.56°C) higher than the oral temperature.

t., room. Temperature between 65° and 80°F (18.3° and 26.7°C).

t., subnormal. Temperature below the normal of 98.6°F (37°C).

t., tympanic. Temperature obtained by placing an electronic probe in the ear canal. SEE: *ear thermometry; thermometer, tympanic.*

temperature, words pert. to: algid; algid stage; algogenic; chauffage; cold; frigid; frigidity; frigorific; hardening; heat; infant; myothermic; pseudocrisis; respiration; temperature scale; "therm-" words.

temperature senses. The sensations of warmth resulting from raising the temperature of the skin and that of cold aroused by lowering it. The sensation of warmth is mediated by Ruffini's corpuscles; that of cold, by end-bulbs of Krause. These receptors are distributed so as to form cold and warm sensing spots on the skin. Afferent impulses from receptors, on reaching the thalamus, may give rise to crude uncritical temperature sensations; on being relayed to the somesthetic area of the cortex, they result in discrete and fairly well localized sensations of heat and cold. Adaptation is rapid.

temper tantrums. A stage of anger and reaction in which the individuals, esp. children, are no longer in control of themselves and they are unaware of how their condition appears to others. The parents or associates need to realize that it is not possible to talk the child out of this behavior or reaction. The child needs to be separated, at that time, from the person who the child thinks caused the incident. The parents or those involved should not demean the child or make fun of him or her during the episode. The child will eventually learn that control of anger is important and that, at times, controlled anger is an appropriate response to certain situations.

template (těm′plāt). A pattern, mold, or form used as a guide in duplicating a shape, structure, or device.

t., occlusal. Stone or metal base made from a wax occlusal registration against which artificial teeth are set in the preparation of a denture.

t., wax. Wax impression of the occlusion of teeth made by closing the jaw until the teeth are embedded in the wax plate.

temple (těm′pl) [O. Fr. from L. *tempora*, pl. of *tempus*, temple]. The region of the head in front of the ear and over the zygomatic arch.

tempolabile (těm″pō-lā′bl) [L. *tempus*, period of time, + *labi*, to slip]. Becoming altered spontaneously within a definite time.

tempora (těm′pō-ră) [L. pl. of *tempus*, period of time]. The temples.

temporal (těm′por-ăl) [L. *temporalis*, period of time]. 1. Pert. to or limited in time. 2. Rel. to the temples.

temporal bone. A bone on both sides of the skull at its base. Composed of squamous, mastoid, and petrous portions, the latter enclosing the organ of hearing. SYN: *os temporale.* SEE: *Arnold's canal; mastoid; petrosa; styloid process.*

temporalis (těm″pō-rā′lĭs) [L.]. Muscle in temporal fossa that elevates the mandible. SEE: *Muscles* in *Appendix.*

temporal line. One of two lines on lateral surface of the frontal and parietal bones that mark upper limit of temporal fossa.

temporal lobe. Lobe of the cerebrum located laterally and below the frontal and occipital lobes. Contains auditory receptive areas.

temporal-sequential organization. The ability of a child to develop concepts of time and sequence. This function is localized in the left hemisphere of the brain. This ability is essential to the function of a child in daily activities concerned with routines such as telling time or following multistep directions. Skill in this function increases with age. SEE: *digit span test.*

temporo- [L. *tempora*]. Combining form meaning temples of the head.

temporoauricular (těm″pō-rō-aw-rĭk′ū-lăr) [″ + *auricula*, little ear]. Concerning the temples and auricular areas.

temporohyoid (tĕm″pō-rō-hī′oyd) [″ + Gr. *hyoeides*, U-shaped]. Concerning the temporal and hyoid bones.

temporomalar (tĕm″pō-rō-mā′lăr) [″ + *mala*, cheek]. Temporozygomatic, q.v.

temporomandibular (tĕm″pō-rō-măn-dĭb′ū-lăr) [″ + *mandibula*, lower jawbone]. Pert. to the temporal and mandible bones; esp. important in dentistry because of the articulation of the bones of the temporomandibular joint.

temporomandibular joint(s). The encapsulated, double, synovial joints between the condyles of the mandible and the temporal bones of the skull. SYN: *craniomandibular joints.*

temporomandibular joint syndrome. ABBR: TMJ syndrome. Severe aching pain in and about the temporomandibular joint, made worse by chewing. There are limited movement of the joint and clicking sounds during chewing. Tinnitus, pain, and deafness may be present. SYN: *Costen's syndrome.*

ETIOL: A variety of conditions, including malocclusion, ill-fitting dentures, rheumatoid arthritis, and neoplastic diseases.

TREAT: Definitive therapy for the primary disease or condition.

temporomaxillary (tĕm″pō-rō-măk′sĭ-lĕr-ē) [″ + *maxilla*, jawbone]. Pert. to the temporal and maxillary bones.

temporo-occipital (tĕm″pō-rō-ŏk-sĭp′ĭ-tăl) [″ + *occipitalis*, pert. to the occiput]. Pert. to the temporal and occipital bones or their regions.

temporoparietal (tĕm″pō-rō-pă-rī′ĕ-tăl) [″ + *paries*, wall]. Concerning the temporal bone and parietal bones.

temporopontine [″ + *pons*, bridge]. Concerning or situated between the temporal lobe of the brain and the pons.

temporosphenoid (tĕm″pō-rō-sfē′noyd) [″ + Gr. *sphen*, wedge, + *eidos*, form, shape]. Pert. to the temporal and sphenoid bones.

temporozygomatic (tĕm″pō-rō-zī″gō-măt′ĭk) [″ + Gr. *zygoma*, cheekbone]. Concerning the temporal and zygomatic bones.

tempostabile (tĕm″pō-stā′bĭl) [L. *tempus*, time, + *stabilis*, stable]. Descriptive of something, esp. a chemical compound, that remains stable with the passage of time.

Tempra. Trade name for acetaminophen.

tenacious (tĕ-nā′shŭs) [L. *tenax*]. Adhering to; adhesive; retentive.

tenacity (tĕ-năs′ĭ-tē). Condition of being tough, stubborn, or obstinate.

tenaculum (tĕn-ăk′ū-lŭm) [L., a holder]. Sharp, hooklike, pointed instrument with slender shank for grasping and holding a part, as an artery.

tenalgia (tĕn-ăl′jē-ă) [Gr. *tenon*, tendon, + *algos*, pain]. Pain in a tendon. SYN: *tenodynia.*

   t. crepitans. Inflammation of a tendon sheath that on movement results in a crackling sound. SYN: *tendosynovitis crepitans; tenosynovitis crepitans.*

Tenckhoff peritoneal catheter. SEE: *catheter, Tenckhoff peritoneal.*

tenderizers. Preparations containing proteolytic enzymes such as papain or bromelin that are used to make meat more tender.

tender loving care. ABBR: TLC. The concept of administering medical and nursing care and attention to a patient in a kindly, compassionate, and humane manner as distinguished from a cold technical approach. This is particularly important in intensive care units, where patients are connected to electronic monitors and devices.

tenderness (tĕn′dĕr-nĕs). Sensitiveness to pain upon pressure.

   t., rebound. Production of or intensification of pain when pressure is released.

tendinitis (tĕn″dĭn-ī′tĭs) [L. *tendo*, tendon, + Gr. *itis*, inflammation]. Inflammation of a tendon. SYN: *tenonitis; tenontitis.*

tendinoplasty (tĕn′dĭ-nō-plăs″tē) [″ + Gr. *plassein*, to form]. Plastic surgery of tendons. SYN: *tendoplasty; tenontoplasty; tenoplasty.*

tendinosuture (tĕn″dĭn-ō-sū′tŭr) [″ + *sutura*, a seam]. The suturing of a divided tendon. SYN: *tenorrhaphy.*

tendinous (tĕn′dĭ-nŭs) [L. *tendinosus*]. Pert. to, composed of, or resembling tendons.

tendinous synovitis. Inflammation of a tendon's synovial sheath.

tendo [L.] (pl. *tendines*). [NA] A tendon.

tendolysis (tĕn-dŏl′ĭ-sĭs) [″ + Gr. *lysis*, dissolution]. The process of freeing a tendon from adhesions.

tendon (tĕn′dŭn) [L. *tendo*, tendon]. Fibrous connective tissue serving for the attachment of muscles to bones and other parts. SYN: *sinew.*

   t., Achilles. The large tendon at lower end of the gastrocnemius muscle, inserted into the os calcis. It is the strongest and thickest tendon in the body.

   t., calcaneal. T., Achilles.

   t., central. The central portion of the diaphragm, consisting of a flat aponeurosis into which the muscle fibers of the diaphragm are inserted.

   t. of Zinn. Portion of the fibrous ring (annulus tendineus communis) from which inferior rectus muscle of eye originates.

   t., superior, of Lockwood. Portion of fibrous ring from which the superior oblique muscle of the eye originates.

tendon action. Passive movement of a joint when a two- or multi-joint muscle is stretched across it.

tendon cells. Fibroblasts of white fibrous connective tissue of tendons arranged in parallel rows.

tendonitis [″ + Gr. *itis*, inflammation]. Inflammation of a tendon.

tendon reflex. Reflex act in which a muscle contracts when its tendon is percussed.

   t.r., patellar. Slight extension of the leg when tendon of quadriceps muscle is tapped immediately below the patella. Tested with leg slightly bent at the knee if patient is in bed. May be tested while leg hangs free when patient is sitting on edge of bed. SYN: *knee jerk; patellar reflex.* SEE: *Jendrassik's maneuver.*

tendon spindle. Fusiform nerve ending in a tendon.

tendoplasty (těn′dō-plăs″tē) [″ + Gr. *plassein*, to mold]. Reparative surgery of an injured tendon. SYN: *tendinoplasty; tenontoplasty; tenoplasty.*

tendosynovitis (těn″dō-sĭn″ō-vī′tĭs) [″ + *synovia*, joint fluid, + Gr. *itis*, inflammation]. Inflammation of a tendon or of a sheath of a tendon. SYN: *tendovaginitis; tenosynovitis.*

   t. crepitans. Tendosynovitis accompanied by a crackling sound on movement. SYN: *tenalgia crepitans; tenosynovitis crepitans.*

tendotome (těn′dō-tōm) [″ + Gr. *tome*, incision]. Instrument for severing a tendon. SYN: *tenotome.*

tendotomy (těn-dŏt′ō-mē). Division of a tendon. SYN: *tenotomy.*

tendovaginal (těn″dō-văj′ĭ-năl) [L. *tendo*, tendon, + *vagina*, sheath]. Rel. to a tendon and its sheath.

tendovaginitis (těn″dō-văj″ĭn-ī′tĭs) [″ + ″ + Gr. *itis*, inflammation]. Inflamed condition of a tendon and its sheath. SYN: *tenosynovitis.*

Tenebrio (tě-něb′rē-ō). A genus of beetles including the species of *T. molitor*, which serves as intermediate host of helminth parasites of vertebrates.

tenectomy [″ + *ektome*, excision]. Excision of a lesion of a tendon or tendon sheath; removal of a ganglion or xanthoma.

   t., graduated. Partial division of a tendon.

tenesmic (těn-ěz′mĭk). Pert. to or like tenesmus.

tenesmus (tě-něz′mŭs) [Gr. *teinesmos*, a stretching]. Spasmodic contraction of anal or vesical sphincter with pain and persistent desire to empty the bowel or bladder, with involuntary ineffectual straining efforts.

teni-. SEE: words beginning with *taeni-.*

tenia (tē′nē-ă) [L. *taenia*, tape]. A flat band or strip of soft tissue.

teniasis (tē-nī′ă-sĭs) [L. *taenia*, tapeworm, + Gr. *-iasis*, a condition]. Presence of tapeworms in the body.

tenicide (těn′ĭ-sīd) [″ + *cidus*, killing]. Taeniacide, q.v.

tenifuge (těn′ĭ-fūj) [″ + *fuga*, flight]. Causing or that which causes expulsion of tapeworms.

tennis elbow. Condition characterized by pain over lateral epicondyle of humerus radiating to outer side of arm and forearm and aggravated by dorsiflexion and supination of wrist. Present are weakness of wrist and difficulty in grasping objects. A reliable diagnostic sign is increased pain when the middle finger is extended against resistance. Usually caused by strain or overuse, as may occur in playing tennis. SYN: *lateral epicondylitis.*

   TREAT: In mild cases, immobilization by a splint or adhesive strapping, supplemented by application of cold, use of nonsteroidal anti-inflammatory agents, and muscle relaxants. Also, it may be possible to decrease the pain and inflammation by applying a wide strap just below the elbow. This will alter the action of the stressed muscles in the forearm and splint the area. This strap should be worn during exercise. Injection of cortisone and local anesthetic into the painful area may be of assistance in cases that have not been helped by conservative therapy. In long continued cases, surgical intervention may be indicated.

teno- [Gr. *tenon*]. Combining form indicating tendon.

tenodesis (těn-ŏd′ě-sĭs) [″ + *desis*, a binding]. 1. Surgical fixation of a tendon. Usually a tendon is transferred from its initial point of origin to a new origin in order to restore muscle balance to a joint, to restore lost function, or to increase active power of joint motion. 2. Closing of the fingers through tendon action of the extrinsic finger flexor muscles when they are stretched across the wrist joint during wrist extension. This mechanism is used for functional grip in the quadriplegic individual when paralysis is due to loss below the sixth cervical vertebra. SEE: *tendon action.*

tenodesis splint. Orthosis fabricated to allow pinch and grasp movements through use of wrist extensors. Also called *wrist-driven flexor hinge hand splint.*

tenodynia (těn″ō-dĭn′ē-ă) [″ + *odyne*, pain]. Pain in a tendon. SYN: *tenalgia.*

tenofibril (těn′ō-fī″brĭl) [″ + *fibrilla*, little fiber]. A fine thread present in the cytoplasm of epithelial cells.

tenolysis (tĕn-ŏl'ĭ-sĭs) [″ + *lysis,* dissolution]. Tendolysis, q.v.

tenomyoplasty (tĕn″ō-mī'ō-plăs″tē) [″ + *mys,* muscle, + *plassein,* to form]. Reparative operation upon a tendon and muscle. SYN: *tenontomyoplasty.*

tenomyotomy (tĕn″ō-mī-ŏt'ō-mē) [″ + ″ + *tome,* incision]. Excision of lateral portion of a tendon or muscle.

Tenon's capsule (tē'nŏns) [Jacques R. Tenon, Fr. surgeon, 1724–1816]. A thin connective tissue envelope of the eyeball behind the conjunctiva.

tenonectomy (tĕn″ō-nĕk'tō-mē) [″ + *ektome,* excision]. Excision of a portion of a tendon.

tenonitis (tĕn″ō-nī'tĭs) [″ + *itis,* inflammation]. 1. Inflammation of a tendon. SYN: *tenontitis.* 2. Inflammation of Tenon's capsule.

tenonometer (tĕn″ō-nŏm'ĕ-tĕr) [Gr. *teinein,* to stretch, + *metron,* measure]. Device for measuring degree of intraocular tension. SYN: *tonometer.*

Tenon's space. Space between the posterior surface of the eyeball and Tenon's capsule, q.v.

tenontitis (tĕn″ŏn-tī'tĭs) [Gr. *tenontos,* tendon, + *itis,* inflammation]. Inflammation of a tendon. SYN: *tendinitis; tenositis.*

tenontodynia (tĕn″ŏn-tō-dīn'ē-ă) [″ + *odyne,* pain]. Pain in a tendon. SYN: *tenalgia; tenodynia.*

tenontography (tĕn″ŏn-tŏg'ră-fē) [″ + *graphein,* to write]. A treatise on the tendons.

tenontolemmitis (tĕn-ŏn″tō-lĕm-mī'tĭs) [″ + *lemma,* rind, + *itis,* inflammation]. Tenosynovitis, q.v.

tenontology (tĕn″ŏn-tŏl'ō-jē) [″ + *logos,* word, reason]. Study of tendons.

tenontomyoplasty (tĕn-ŏn″tō-mī'ō-plăs″tē) [″ + *mys,* muscle, + *plassein,* to form]. Plastic surgery, including muscle and tendon repair in treatment of hernia. SYN: *myotenontoplasty; tenomyoplasty.*

tenontomyotomy (tĕn-ŏn″tō-mī-ŏt'ō-mē) [″ + ″ + *tome,* incision]. Cutting of the principal tendon of a muscle with excision of the muscle in part or in whole. SYN: *myotenotomy.*

tenontoplasty (tĕn-ŏn″tō-plăs″tē) [″ + *plassein,* to form]. Plastic surgery of defective or injured tendons. SYN: *tenoplasty.*

tenontothecitis (tĕn-ŏn″tō-thē-sī'tĭs) [″ + *theke,* sheath, + *itis,* inflammation]. Inflammation of a tendon and its sheath. SYN: *tendosynovitis; tendovaginitis; tenosynovitis.*

    t. stenosans. A chronic form of tenontothecitis with narrowing of the sheath.

tenophyte (tĕn'ō-fīt) [″ + *phyton,* a growth]. A cartilaginous or osseous growth on a tendon.

tenoplastic (tĕn″ō-plăs'tĭk). Concerning tenoplasty.

tenoplasty (tĕn'ō-plăs″tē) [″ + *plassein,* to form]. Reparative surgery of tendons. SYN: *tendinoplasty; tenontoplasty.*

tenoreceptor (tĕn″ō-rē-sĕp'tor) [″ + L. *receptor,* receiver]. Proprioceptive nerve ending in a tendon.

tenorrhaphy (tĕn-or'ă-fē) [″ + *rhaphe,* seam, ridge]. Suturing of a tendon.

tenositis (tĕn″ō-sī'tĭs) [″ + *itis,* inflammation]. Inflammation of a tendon. SYN: *tenontitis.*

tenostosis (tĕn″ŏs-tō'sĭs) [Gr. *tenon,* tendon, + *osteon,* bone, + *osis,* condition]. Calcification of a tendon.

tenosuspension (tĕn″ō-sŭs-pĕn'shŭn) [″ + L. *suspensio,* a hanging under]. In surgery, use of a tendon to support a structure.

tenosuture (tĕn″ō-sū'chŭr) [″ + L. *sutura,* a seam]. Suture of a partially or completely divided tendon. SYN: *tenorrhaphy.*

tenosynovectomy (tĕn″ō-sĭn″ō-vĕk'tō-mē) [″ + *synovia,* joint fluid, + Gr. *ektome,* excision]. Excision of a tendon sheath.

tenosynovitis (tĕn″ō-sĭn″ō-vī'tĭs) [″ + ″ + Gr. *itis,* inflammation]. Inflammation of a tendon sheath.

    t. crepitans. Inflammation of a tendon sheath in which a crackling sound is heard on motion. Most commonly affects flexor tendons.

    SYM: Pain, excessive tenderness.

    ETIOL: May follow puncture wounds, contusions, and lacerations or be caused by lymphatic extension of inflammation.

    TREAT: Early drainage, rest, heat, and appropriate antibiotics.

    t. hyperplastica. Painless swelling of extensor tendons over the wrist joint.

tenotome (tĕn'ō-tōm) [″ + *tome,* incision]. Instrument for section of a tendon.

tenotomist (tĕ-nŏt'ō-mĭst). Specialist in tenotomy.

tenotomy (tĕ-nŏt'ō-mē). Surgical section of a tendon.

tenovaginitis (tĕn″ō-văj″ĭn-ī'tĭs) [″ + L. *vagina,* sheath, + Gr. *itis,* inflammation]. Inflammation of a tendon sheath. SYN: *tendosynovitis; tenontothecitis; tenosynovitis.*

TENS. *transcutaneous electrical nerve stimulation,* q.v.

tense (tĕns). Tight, rigid, anxious, under mental stress.

Tensilon. Trade name for edrophonium chloride.

Tensilon test. Diagnostic test for juvenile myasthenia gravis. Tensilon is injected I.V. with an improvement of muscle strength that lasts for 5 minutes.

tensiometer (těn″sē-ŏm′ē-tĕr) [L. *tensio,* a stretching, + Gr. *metron,* measure]. 1. A device for determining the surface tension of liquids. 2. A device used to measure the amount of force a muscle can produce. Also called *cable tensiometer.*

tension (těn′shŭn) [L. *tensio,* a stretching]. 1. Process or act of stretching; state of being strained or stretched. 2. Pressure, as arterial tension. 3. Expansive force of a gas or vapor. 4. Mental, emotional, or nervous strain.

　　t., arterial. Tension resulting from the force exerted by the blood pressure on the walls of arteries.

　　t., intraocular. The pressure of the fluid within the eyeball. SEE: *tonometry.*

　　t., intravenous. Force exerted by the blood pressure on the walls of a vein.

　　t., muscular. Condition of a muscle in which fibers tend to shorten and thus perform work or liberate heat.

　　t., premenstrual. Condition occurring periodically in some individuals a few days before menstruation; characterized by varying degrees of nervousness and irritability, emotional instability, headaches, and sometimes depression. Usually disappears a short time after onset of menstrual flow. SEE: *premenstrual syndrome.*

　　t., surface. Molecular property of film on surface of a liquid to resist rupture, the particles tending to pull inward.

　　t., tissue. The theoretical state of equilibrium between the cells of a tissue.

tension headache. Headache caused by sustained tension of muscles of the face, neck, and scalp.

tension myalgia. SEE: *fibromyalgia.*

tension of gases. Gas pressure usually measured in millimeters of mercury (mmHg).

tension pneumothorax. Pneumothorax, valvular, q.v.

tension suture. Suture used to reduce pull of the edges of a wound.

tensometer (těn-sŏm′ē-tĕr) [L. *tensio,* a stretching, + Gr. *metron,* measure]. Device for testing the tensile strength of materials.

tensor (těn′sor) [L., a stretcher]. Any muscle that makes a part tense. SEE: *Muscles* in *Appendix.*

tent (těnt) [O. Fr. *tente,* from L. *tenta,* stretched out]. 1. A plug of soft material used to maintain or dilate the opening to a sinus, canal, or body cavity. A variety of cylindrically shaped materials may be used. 2. A portable covering or shelter composed of fabric.

　　t., laminaria. A plug made of *Laminaria digitata,* q.v., that is placed in the cervical canal to dilate it.

　　t., oxygen. Tent that can be placed over a bed for the continuous administration of oxygen.

　　t., sponge. A plug made of compressed sponge that is placed in the cervical canal to dilate it.

tentacle (těn′tă-k'l). A slender projection of invertebrates. It is used for prehension, tactile purposes, or feeding.

tentative (těn′tă-tǐv) [L. *tentativus,* feel, try]. 1. Noting a diagnosis subject to change because of insufficient data. 2. Indecisive.

tenth cranial nerve. Nerve supplying most of the abdominal viscera, the heart, lungs, and esophagus. SYN: *vagus nerve.* SEE: *cranial nerves.*

tentorial (těn-tō′rē-ăl). Pertaining to a tentorium.

tentorial notch. An arched cavity formed by the anterior and inner border of the tentorium cerebelli.

tentorial pressure cone. Projection of a portion of the temporal lobe of the cerebrum through the incisure of the tentorium due to increased intracranial pressure.

tentorium (těn-tō′rē-ŭm) [L., tent] (pl. *tentoria*). A tentlike structure or part.

　　t. cerebelli. [NA] The process of the dura mater between the cerebrum and cerebellum supporting the occipital lobes.

Tenuate. Trade name for diethylpropion hydrochloride.

Tepanil. Trade name for diethylpropion hydrochloride.

tephromyelitis (těf″rō-mī″ěl-ī′tǐs) [″ + *myelos,* marrow, + *itis,* inflammation]. Inflammation of the gray matter of the spinal cord.

tephrosis (těf-rō′sǐs) [″ + *osis,* condition]. Incineration; cremation.

tephrylometer (těf″rǐ-lŏm′ē-tĕr) [″ + *hyle,* matter, + *metron,* measure]. Device for measuring the thickness of the cerebral cortex, the gray matter of brain.

tepid (těp′ǐd) [L. *tepidus,* lukewarm]. Slightly warm; lukewarm.

tepidarium (těp″ǐd-ā′rē-ŭm) [L.]. A place for a warm bath.

tepor (tē′por) [L., lukewarmness]. Moderate heat.

TEPP. tetraethylpyrophosphate.

ter- [L., thrice]. Combining form meaning three times.

teracurie (těr″ă-kū′rē). A unit of radioactivity, 10^{12} curies.

teramorphous (těr-ă-mor′fŭs) [Gr. *teras,* monster, + *morphe,* form]. Similar to, or of the nature of, a congenitally deformed fetus, infant, or child.

teras (těr′ăs) [Gr.] (pl. *terata*). A severely deformed fetus.

teratic (těr-ăt′ǐk) [Gr. *teratikos,* monstrous].

Pert. to a severely malformed fetus.

teratism (tĕr′ă-tĭzm) [Gr. *teratisma*]. An anomaly or structural abnormality either inherited or acquired.

t., acquired. Abnormality resulting from a prenatal environmental influence.

t., atresic. Teratism in which natural openings such as the mouth or anus fail to form.

t., ceasmic. Teratism in which a normal union of parts fails to occur, e.g., as in spina bifida or cleft palate.

t., ectogenic. Condition in which parts are absent or defective.

t., ectopic. Abnormality in which a part becomes displaced.

t., hypergenic. Teratism in which a part is duplicated, e.g., polydactylism.

t., symphysic. Teratism in which parts that are normally separate are fused.

terato- [Gr. *teratos*, monster]. Combining form indicating a severely malformed fetus.

teratoblastoma (tĕr″ă-tō-blăs-tō′mă) [″ + *blastos*, germ, + *oma*, tumor]. A tumor that contains embryonic material but that is not representative of all three germinal layers. SEE: *teratoma*.

teratocarcinoma (tĕr″ă-tō-kăr″sĭ-nō′mă) [″ + *karkinos*, cancer, + *oma*, tumor]. A carcinoma that has developed from the epithelial cells of a teratoma.

teratogen (tĕr-ăt′ō-jĕn) [″ + *gennan*, to produce]. Anything that causes teratogenesis. SEE: table.

teratogenesis (tĕr″ă-tō-gĕn′ĕ-sĭs) [″ + *genesis*, generation, birth]. The development of abnormal structures in an embryo resulting in a severely deformed fetus.

teratogenetic (tĕr″ă-tō-jĕ-nĕt′ĭk) [″ + *genesis*, generation, birth]. Concerning teratogenesis.

teratogenic (tĕr″ă-tō-gĕn′ĭk). Causing abnormal development of the embryo.

teratogenous (tĕr″ă-tŏj′ĕ-nŭs) [″ + *gennan*, to produce]. Developed from severely deformed fetal parts.

teratogeny (tĕr″ă-tŏj′ĕ-nē). Teratogenesis.

teratoid (tĕr′ă-toyd) [Gr. *teratos*, monster, + *eidos*, form, shape]. Resembling a severely malformed fetus.

teratoid tumor. Tumor of embryonic remains from all germinal layers. SYN: *teratoma*.

teratologic (tĕr″ă-tō-lŏj′ĭk). Concerning teratology.

teratology (tĕr-ă-tŏl′ō-jē) [″ + *logos*, word, reason]. Branch of science dealing with the study of congenitally deformed fetuses.

teratoma (tĕr-ă-tō′mă) [″ + *oma*, tumor]. Congenital tumor containing one or more of the three primary embryonic germ layers. Thus, hair and teeth as well as endodermal elements may be present. SYN: *dermoid cyst.* SEE: *fetus in fetu.*

teratomatous (tĕr″ă-tō′mă-tŭs). Pert. to or resembling a teratoma.

teratophobia (tĕr″ă-tō-fō′bē-ă) [″ + *phobos*, fear]. Abnormal fear of giving birth to a malformed fetus or being in contact with one.

teratosis (tĕr″ă-tō′sĭs) [″ + *osis*, condition]. A deformed fetus.

teratospermia (tĕr″ă-tō-spĕr′mē-ă) [″ + *sperma*, seed]. Malformed sperm in semen.

terazosin hydrochloride. A hypertensive agent. Trade name is Hytrin.

terbium (tĕr′bē-ŭm). SYMB: Tb. At. wt. 158.9254; at. no. 65; sp. gr. 8.272. A metal of the rare earths.

terbutaline sulfate. USP. A synthetic sympathomimetic amine used in treating asthma. It is an effective bronchodilator. Trade names are Brethine and Bricanyl.

terchloride (tĕr-klō′rīd). Trichloride.

terebrant (tĕr′ē-brănt). Piercing pain.

terebration (tĕr″ē-brā′shŭn) [L. *terebratio*]. 1. Boring, trephination. 2. A boring pain.

teres (tē′rēz) [L., round]. Round and smooth; cylindrical. Used to describe certain muscles and ligaments.

tergal (tĕr′găl) [L. *tergum*, back]. Concerning the back or dorsal surface.

tergum (tĕr′gŭm) [L.]. The back.

ter in die (tĕr ĭn dē′ă) [L.]. Three times a day. ABBR: t.i.d.

term [L. *terminus*, a boundary]. 1. A limit or boundary. 2. A definite period of duration such as the normal period of pregnancy, approx. nine calendar months.

terminal (tĕr′mĭ-năl) [L. *terminalis*]. Pert. to or placed at the end.

terminal arteriole. Arteriole that has no branches, but it splits into capillaries.

terminal bars. Minute bars of dense intercellular cement that occupy and close spaces between epithelial cells and bind them together.

terminal cancer. Term used to describe the condition of having advanced cancer. Previously the use of this description may have been applicable; but with the therapeutic techniques now available, its use may not be warranted.

terminal device. Component of an upper extremity prosthesis that substitutes for the functions of the hand. There are many types of terminal devices, some of which are designed for use with specific tools and implements. These devices are classified basically by whether or not the action of the prosthesis wearer results in opening the device (voluntary opening) or closing it (voluntary closing). SYN: *hook.*

terminal ganglia. Ganglia of the parasympa-

Teratogenic and Fetotoxic Drugs

Maternal Medication	Fetal or Neonatal Effect
Established Teratogenic Agents	
Antineoplastic agents	Multiple anomalies, abortion
Antimetabolites (amethopterin, fluorouracil, diazo-oxonorleucine, 6-azauridine, etc.)	
Alkylating agents (cyclophosphamide, etc.)	
Antibiotics (amphotericin B, mitomycin, etc.)	
Estrogens	Vaginal adenocarcinoma in daughter in later years*
Other sex hormones (androgens, progestogens)	Masculinization, advanced bone age
Thalidomide	Fetal death or phocomelia; deafness; cardiovascular, gastrointestinal, or genitourinary abnormalities
Organic mercury	Cerebral palsy
Polychlorinated biphenyls (PCBs) (contaminants in manufacture of rice, cooking oil)	"Cola"-colored neonates with other developmental defects
Possible Teratogens	
Insulin (shock or hypoglycemia)	Anomalies
LSD	"Fractured chromosomes," anomalies
Sulfonylurea derivatives	Anomalies
Vitamin D	Cardiopathies
Fetotoxic Drugs	
Analgesics, narcotics	
Heroin, morphine	Neonatal death or convulsions, tremors
Salicylates (excessive)	Neonatal bleeding
Cardiovascular drugs	
Ammonium chloride	Acidosis
Hexamethonium	Neonatal ileus
Reserpine	Nasal congestion, drowsiness
Coumarin anticoagulants	Fetal death or hemorrhage
Poliomyelitis immunization (Sabin)	Death or neurologic damage
Sedatives, hypnotics, tranquilizers	
Meprobamate	Retarded development
Phenobarbital (excessive)	Neonatal bleeding
Phenothiazines	Hyperbilirubinemia
Smallpox vaccination	Death or fetal vaccinia
Tetracyclines	Dental discoloration and abnormalities
Thiazides	Thrombocytopenia
Tobacco smoking	Undersized babies
Vitamin K (excessive)	Hyperbilirubinemia

Source: Krupp, MA and Chatton, MJ (eds): Current Medical Diagnosis and Treatment. Appleton & Lange, Los Altos, CA, 1982.
* FDA Drug Bulletin (Nov) 1971: Diethylstilbestrol contraindicated in pregnancy.

thetic division of the autonomic nervous system that are located in or close to walls or visceral structures such as heart or intestines.

terminal illness. Illness that because of its nature can be expected to cause the patient to die. Usually a chronic disease for which there is no known cure.

NURSING IMPLICATIONS: Support patient and family by anticipating their loss and grief. Help patient to deal with major concerns: pain, fear, hopelessness, dependency, disability, loss of self-esteem, loss of pleasure. Provide hospice care if desired and available. Provide caring comfort and help patient to adjust to the lack of quality of life; attempt to ensure that death is with dignity.

terminal infection. Infection appearing in the late stage of another disease; often fatal.

terminal veins. One of two veins (anterior and posterior) draining portions of the brain and emptying into interior cerebral veins.

terminatio (tĕr″mĭ-nā′shē-ō) [L.]. The termination or ending.

termination [L. *terminatio*, limiting]. 1. The distal end of a part. 2. The cessation of anything.

terminology (tĕr-mĭ-nŏl′ō-jē) [L. *terminus*, a boundary, + Gr. *logos*, word]. The vocabulary of scientific and technical terms used in specific arts, trades, or professions. SYN: *nomenclature.*

terminus (tĕr′mĭ-nŭs) [L.]. An ending; a boundary.

ternary (tĕr′nă-rē) [L. *ternarius*, triple]. 1. Threefold; triple; third. 2. Chemical substance containing three different elements or radicals.

terpene (tĕr′pēn). Any member of the family of hydrocarbons of the formula $C_{10}H_{16}$.

terpin hydrate (tĕr′pĭn hī′drāt). White crystalline substance with a turpentine taste; made by the interaction of rectified spirits of turpentine, alcohol, and nitric acid.

ACTION/USES: In the form of an elixir; used as an expectorant.

terra (tĕr′ă) [L.]. Earth; soil.

   t. alba. White clay.

   t. fullonica. Fuller's earth.

terracing (tĕr′ăs-ĭng) [O. Fr. *terrasse*]. Suturing in several rows through thick tissues in closing a wound.

Terramycin (tĕr″ă-mī′sĭn). A trade name for oxytetracycline. An antibiotic biosynthesized by *Streptomyces rimosus.* It is a broadspectrum antibiotic effective against both gram-negative and gram-positive bacteria, rickettsias, and some viruses.

territoriality (tĕr″ĭ-tor″ē-ăl′ĭ-tē). The tendency of animals and human groups to defend a particular area or region.

terror [L. *terrere*, to frighten]. Very great fear.

   t., night. Nightmare, esp. of children.

tertian (tĕr′shŭn) [L. *tertianus*, the third]. Occurring every third day. Usually pertaining to a form of malarial fever.

tertiary (tĕr′shē-ār-ē) [L. *tertiarius*]. Third in order or stage.

tertiary alcohol. Alcohol containing the trivalent group ≡COH.

tertiary care. A level of medical care that would be available only in large medical care institutions. Included would be techniques and methods of therapy and diagnosis involving equipment and personnel that would not be economically feasible to have in a smaller institution because of the lack of utilization. SEE: *primary care; secondary care.*

tertiary syphilis. Third and most advanced stage of syphilis.

tertigravida (tĕr″shē-grăv′ĭ-dă) [″ + *gravida*, pregnant]. A woman pregnant for the third time.

tertipara (tĕr-shĭp′ă-ră) [L. *tertius*, third, + *parere*, to bring forth]. A woman who has had three pregnancies terminating after the twentieth week of gestation or has produced three infants of at least 500 grams of weight, regardless of their viability.

tesla [Nikola Tesla, U.S. physicist, 1856–1943]. ABBR: T. In the SI system, a measure of magnetic strength. One tesla equals 10,000 gauss or one newton/amp-m.

Teslac. Trade name for testolactone.

Tessalon. Trade name for benzonatate.

tessellated (tĕs′ĕ-lā″tĕd) [L. *tessella*, a square]. Composed of little squares.

test [L. *testum*, earthen vessel]. 1. An examination. 2. Method to determine the presence or nature of a substance or the presence of a disease. 3. A chemical reaction. 4. A reagent or substance used in making a test.

   t., acetic acid. Test for albumin in urine. Adding a few drops of acetic acid to urine that has been boiled causes a white precipitate if albumin is present.

   t., acetone. Test for presence of acetone in the urine; made by adding a few drops of sodium nitroprusside to the urine along with strong ammonia water. Presence of acetone causes formation of a magenta ring at outline of contacts.

   t., agglutination. A widely used test in which adding an antiserum containing antibodies to cells or bacteria causes them to agglutinate.

   t., alkali denaturation. Test for hemoglobin F (fetal hemoglobin) in the blood. Spectrophotometry is used in this test.

   t., Allen-Doisy. Test to determine amount of estrogen content in female blood serum by its reaction on secretions of mice.

   t., aptitude. Test used to determine an

t., Aschheim-Zondek. Test for pregnancy by injecting the patient's urine subcutaneously into immature female mice. If the patient is pregnant, the ovaries of the mouse begin to mature prematurely.

t., association. Test used to determine an individual's response to word stimuli. The nature of the response and time required may provide insight into the subject's personality and previous experiences.

t., autohemolysis. Test of the rate of hemolysis of sterile defibrinated whole blood incubated at 37°C. Normal cells hemolyze at a certain rate and blood cells from persons with certain types of disease hemolyze at a faster rate.

t., biuret. Test to determine the presence of proteins or urea.

t., challenge. Administering a substance in order to determine its ability to cause a response, esp. the giving of an antigen and observing or testing for the antibody response.

t., chromatin. Test for genetic sex in which blood or tissue cells are examined for presence or absence of Barr bodies, q.v.

t., coin. Test for pneumothorax. A metal coin is placed flat on the chest and struck with another coin. The chest is auscultated at the same time. If a pneumothorax is present, a sharp, metallic ringing sound is heard.

t., complement-fixation. SEE: *complement fixation.*

t., concentration. A kidney function test based on the ability of the person to produce concentrated urine under conditions that would normally cause such production, as in intentional dehydration.

t., conjunctival. An allergy test in which the suspected antigen is placed in the conjunctival sac; if it is allergenic for that patient, the conjunctiva becomes red, itches, and lacrimates.

t., cover. Test for strabismus, q.v. The eyes are observed and the patient is asked to focus on an object. A cover is placed first over one eye and then the other. If either eye moves, strabismus is present.

t., creatinine clearance. Test of glomerular function of the kidney. The amount of creatinine present in a timed volume of urine is compared with the plasma creatinine value.

t., double-blind. SEE: *double-blind technique.*

t., finger-nose. Test of cerebellar function wherein the patient is asked to, while keeping the eyes open, touch the nose with the finger and remove the finger, and repeat this rapidly. The test is done by using a finger of each hand successively or in concert. How fast and well this is done is recorded.

t., finger-to-finger. A test for coordination of the movements of the upper extremities. The patient is asked to touch the tips of the fingers of one hand to the opposite finger tips.

t., Friedman. Test for pregnancy by injecting urine of the patient into unmated mature female rabbits, a positive reaction being indicated by formation of corpora lutea and corpora haemorrhagica.

t., galactose tolerance. Test of the ability of the liver to metabolize galactose. A standard dose of galactose is administered to the fasting patient, and the amount of galactose excreted in the urine in the next five hours is determined. If the liver is damaged, the galactose is not metabolized to glycogen, but is instead excreted in the urine.

t., glucose tolerance. SEE: *glucose tolerance test.*

t., guaiac. Test for occult blood in the feces. An alcoholic solution of guaiac resin and hydrogen peroxide is mixed with the specimen. The appearance of a blue color indicates a positive test.

t., hardness. Test designed to determine the relative hardness of materials by correlating the size or depth of an indent produced by a particular instrument with known amount of compressive force. SEE: *hardness number.*

t., histamine. 1. Injection of histamine subcutaneously in order to stimulate gastric secretion of hydrochloric acid. 2. Test for vasomotor headache; a histamine injection precipitates the onset of a headache in persons with this disease.

t., Huhner. Aspiration of vagina within an hour after coitus, to investigate sperm activity.

t., human repeated patch insult. The test material is applied fresh to the same skin site every other day for 10 applications. Each application remains on for 48 hours. After a rest period of about two weeks, the test material is applied again for 48 hours to a different skin site than that originally used. This area is examined daily for the next four days for evidence of irritation. The test measures the ability of the test substance to cause sensitization or irritation reactions or both.

t., intracutaneous. Injection of an antigen intracutaneously and observing the response.

t., Kahn. Precipitation test for syphilis.

t., McMurray. Test for torn meniscus of the knee. The supine patient flexes the knees completely. One foot is slowly rotated outward by the examiner as the knee is slowly extended. If a painful click occurs, the medial meniscus of that knee is torn; if as the foot is rotated inward a click is felt, then the lateral meniscus is torn.

t., multiple-puncture. Any skin test, but esp. a tuberculin test, in which the material is placed on the skin and multiple superficial punctures are produced under the material, thus allowing the material to enter the skin.

t., neutralization. Test of the ability of an antibody to neutralize the toxic effects of an antigen.

t., patch. A skin test in which a low concentration of a substance is applied to the skin under an occlusive dressing for 48 hours to assess for hypersensitivity to a suspected allergen, q.v. If the concentration of the agent is too high or an allergy exists to the material used in the dressing, false positive reactions can occur due to local irritation. False negative reactions may result if the concentration of the suspected allergen is too low. Intradermal injection may be used instead of patch testing as another form of delayed hypersensitivity skin testing.

t., precipitin. An antigen-antibody test in which a specific antigen is added to a solution. If the solution contains the antibody to that antigen, a precipitate is formed.

t., pregnancy. SEE: *pregnancy test.*

t., prothrombin consumption. Test for amount of thromboplastin present in the plasma that reacts with prothrombin. This is determined by quantitating the prothrombin that remains in the serum after coagulation is complete.

t., pulp vitality. A determination of the vitality of a tooth pulp by the application of hot, cold, or electrical stimuli. Also called *vitalometry.*

t., Rubin. Test for patency of the fallopian tubes by insufflation with carbon dioxide; used in investigating the cause of sterility.

t., Schiller's. Test for detection of cancer of the cervix by painting the tissue with iodine solution; areas that contain glycogen are stained by the iodine. Those sites that do not stain, but become white or yellow, are assumed to be abnormal. Tissue is taken from those areas for microscopic examination.

t., Schwabach. Test for hearing using tuning forks.

t., scratch. An allergy test in which the antigen is applied to skin that has been lightly scratched.

t., serial sevens. SEE: *serial sevens test.*

t., serologic. Any test done on serum.

t., sickling. Test for the ability of red cells to sickle. The red cells are placed in an atmosphere of reduced oxygen tension. If they contain hemoglobin S, they will sickle.

t., standardized. Test that has been developed empirically, has adequate norms, definite instructions for administration, and evidence of reliability and validity.

t., starch-iodine. A test for presence of starch. When an iodine solution is applied to a substance or material that contains starch, a dark blue color appears.

t., thematic apperception. A projective test in which the subject is shown life situations in pictures that could be interpreted in several ways. The subject is asked to provide a story of what the picture represents. The results may provide insights into the subject's personality.

t., three-glass. Upon awakening, the patient urinates sequentially into three glasses. The amount of cellular debris visible to the naked eye in the glasses helps to locate the site of urinary tract infection, i.e., whether it is in the anterior urethra, posterior urethra, or prostate. If the first glass is turbid and the other two are clear, the anterior urethra is inflamed but the rest of the urinary tract is clear. If the initial specimen is clear and the second and third ones are turbid, the posterior urethra or prostate is inflamed. If only the third specimen is turbid, then only the prostate is inflamed.

t., tine. SEE: *tine test.*

t., tolerance. Test of the ability of the patient or subject to endure the medicine given or exercise taken.

t., tourniquet. Test for capillary fragility. A blood pressure cuff is inflated sufficiently to occlude venous return from the arm. It is kept in place for a set time. After the cuff is removed, the skin distal to the cuff is examined for petechiae.

t., tuberculin. SEE: *tuberculin test.*

t., urea balance. Test of kidney function by measuring intake and output of urea.

t., Wassermann. Previously used diagnostic test for syphilis based on principle of fixation of complement.

testa (tĕs'tä) [L.]. A shell.

testalgia (tĕs-tăl'jē-ă) [L. *testis*, testicle, + Gr. *algos*, pain]. Pain in the testicle.

testectomy (tĕs-tĕk'tō-mē) [" + Gr. *ektome*, excision]. 1. Removal of a testicle. SYN: *castration.* 2. Removal of a corpus quadrigeminum.

testes (tĕs'tēs) [L.]. Pl. of testis.

testicle (tĕs'tĭ-kl) [L. *testiculus*, a little testis]. A testis.

t., self-examination of. Each testicle is examined. The best time to perform the test is just after a warm bath or shower. The scrotal tissue will be more nearly relaxed at that time. While standing, place the thumbs on the anterior surface of the testicle and support the testicle by the index and middle fingers of both hands. The testicle is gently rolled between the fingers and thumbs. Carefully feel for lumps, hardness or thickening, esp. as compared with the other testicle. The epididymis is a soft, slightly tender, tubelike body behind the testicle. Masses outside the testicle are not tumors of the testes.

testicond (tĕs′tĭ-kŏnd) [L. *testis,* testicle, + *condere,* to hide]. The condition of having the testicles remain undescended. It is abnormal in man and in many animals.

testicular (tĕs-tĭk′ū-lăr). Rel. to a testicle.

testicular cancer, germ-cell. A particular type of testicular cancer. Metastatic cancer of this type is treated with ifosfamide, q.v., and mesna, q.v.

testis (tĕs′tĭs) [L.] (pl. *testes*). [NA] The male gonad. One of two reproductive glands located in the scrotum that produce the male reproductive cells or spermatozoa and the male hormone, testosterone. Each is an ovoid body about 4 cm long and 2 to 2.5 cm in width and thickness enclosed within a dense inelastic fibrous tunica albuginea. The testis is divided into numerous lobules separated by septa, each lobule containing one to three seminiferous tubules within which the spermatozoa arise. The lobules lead to straight ducts that join a plexus, the rete testis, from which 15 to 20 efferent ducts lead to the epididymis. The epididymis leads to the ductus deferens, through which sperm are conveyed to the urethra. Between the seminiferous tubules are located the interstitial cells (cells of Leydig), which are considered to be the source of the male hormone.

The testes are suspended from the body by the spermatic cord, a structure extending from the inguinal ring to the testis. It contains the ductus deferens, testicular vessels (spermatic artery, vein, lymph vessels), and nerves. SYN: *testicle.*

Hyperfunction (hypergonadism) may cause early maturity such as dentition, large sexual organs with early functional activity, and increased growth of hair.

Hypofunction (hypogonadism) is indicated by undeveloped testes, absence of body hair, high-pitched voice, sterility, smooth skin, loss of sexual desire, low metabolism, and eunuchoid or eunuch body type.

   t., descent of. Change in position of the testis from abdominal cavity to scrotum during fetal life.

   t., displaced. Testis located abnormally within the inguinal canal or pelvis.

   t., femoral. An inguinal testis near or over the femoral ring.

   t., inverted. Testis reversed in the scrotum so that the epididymis attaches to the anterior instead of the posterior part of the gland.

   t., perineal. Testis located in the perineal region outside the scrotum.

   t., undescended. Testis remaining in the inguinal canal or abdominal cavity. This may be present at birth or develop later.

testis compression reflex. Contraction of abdominal muscles following moderate compression of testis.

testitis (tĕs-tī′tĭs) [L. *testis,* testicle, + Gr. *itis,* inflammation]. Inflammation of a testis. SEE: *orchitis.*

testitoxicosis (tĕs″tĭ-tŏk-sĭ-kō′sĭs) [″ + Gr. *toxikon,* poison, + *osis,* condition]. A toxic state sometimes following ligation of the ductus deferens.

test meal. A meal usually small and of definite quality and composition, given to aid in chemical analysis of the stomach contents or x-ray diagnosis of the stomach.

testoid (tĕs′toyd). Resembling a testis.

testolactone (tĕs-tō-lăk′tōn). USP. An anabolic steroid used in treating carcinoma of the breast. Trade name is Teslac.

testopathy (tĕs-tŏp′ă-thē) [″ + Gr. *pathos,* disease, suffering]. Any disease of the testes.

testosterone (tĕs-tŏs′tĕr-ōn) [L. *testis,* testicle]. USP. An androgen isolated from the testes of a number of animals including man and considered to be the principal testicular hormone produced in man. It is a steroid produced by the interstitial cells of Leydig of the testicles. This hormone is also normally produced by the adrenal cortex of both human males and females. It has been prepared synthetically by conversion of other sterols, esp. cholesterol.

   ACTION: It accelerates growth in tissues upon which it acts and stimulates blood flow. It stimulates and promotes the growth of secondary sexual characteristics and is essential for normal sexual behavior and the occurrence of erections. It is essential for normal growth and development of the male accessory sexual organs. It is responsible for deepening of the male voice at puberty, greater muscular development in men, development of beard and pubic hair, and distribution of fat in adult men. It also affects many metabolic activities.

Testred. Trade name for methyltestosterone.

test tube baby. A baby born to a mother whose ovum was removed, fertilized outside her body, and then implanted in her uterus.

SEE: *gamete intrafallopian transfer; in vitro fertilization.*

test type. Letters or figures of various size printed on paper. These are used in testing visual acuity.

tetanic (tĕ-tăn'ĭk) [Gr. *tetanikos*]. 1. Pert. to or producing tetanus. 2. Any agent producing tetanic spasms.

tetanic convulsion. A tonic convulsion with constant muscular contraction.

tetaniform (tĕ-tăn'ĭ-form) [Gr. *tetanos*, stretched, + L. *forma*, shape]. Resembling tetanus.

tetanigenous (tĕt"ă-nĭj'ĕ-nŭs) [" + *gennan*, to produce]. Causing tetanus or tetanic spasms.

tetanism (tĕt'ă-nĭzm) [" + *-ismos*, condition]. Persistent muscular hypertonicity resembling tetanus, esp. in infants.

tetanization (tĕt"nĭ-zā'shŭn) [Gr. *tetanos*, stretched]. 1. Production of tetanus or tetanic spasms by induction of the disease. 2. Induction of tetanic contractions in a muscle by electrical stimuli.

tetanize (tĕt'ă-nīz). To induce tonic muscular spasms.

tetanode (tĕt'ă-nōd) [" + *eidos*, form, shape]. In tetany the quiet period between spasms.

tetanoid (tĕt'ă-noyd) [" + *eidos*, form, shape]. Resembling tetanus. SYN: *tetaniform.*

tetanoid paraplegia. Paralysis of lower extremities due to lateral sclerosis of the spinal cord. SYN: *paraplegia, spastic.*

tetanolysin (tĕt"ă-nŏl'ĭ-sĭn). A hemolytic component of the toxin produced by *Clostridium tetani,* causative organism of tetanus. It does not cause the clinical signs and symptoms of this disease.

tetanomotor (tĕt"ăn-ō-mō'tor) [" + L. *motor,* a mover]. Appliance for the production of tetanic motor spasms mechanically by electrical stimulation of a nerve.

tetanophil,   tetanophilic (tĕt'ăn-ō-fĭl, tĕt"ăn-ō-fĭl'ĭk) [" + *philein,* to love]. Possessing an affinity for tetanus toxin.

tetanospasmin (tĕt"ă-nō-spăs'mĭn) [" + *spasmos,* a convulsion]. A component of the toxin produced by tetanus bacillus that is responsible for tetanic convulsions and the clinical disease state.

tetanus (tĕt'ă-nŭs) [Gr. *tetanos,* stretched]. 1. An acute infectious disease due to the toxin of tetanus bacillus, *Clostridium tetani,* growing anaerobically at the site of injury. There is a state of more or less persistent painful tonic spasm of some of the voluntary muscles. SEE: *tetanolysin; tetanospasmin.* 2. A state of sustained contraction of a muscle, esp. that induced by stimulation.

Tetanus usually begins gradually but may begin suddenly, may be of brief duration, or last some weeks. The first sign is stiffness of the jaw, esophageal muscles, and some of the muscles of the neck. Soon the jaws become rigidly fixed (trismus or lockjaw), the voice is altered, and muscles of the face contract, producing a wild excited expression, a compound of bitter laughter and crying (risus sardonicus). The muscles of the back and extremities become tetanic.

If the patient is bent back in a bow, the condition is termed opisthotonos; if bent to the side, pleurothotonos; if bent forward, emprosthotonos.

The paroxysms are reflex and are excited by noises, currents of air, and irritation of bedclothes. The temperature usually rises and may become extremely high. The pain is great; the patient also suffers from hunger, thirst, and want of sleep. The mind is clear. This disease is usually, but not always, fatal, the patient expiring from asphyxia or exhaustion.

TREAT: The patient is treated in an intensive care unit. Debride the wound and give penicillin if wound is infected. Give tetanus immune globulin intramuscularly. If this is unavailable, give 10,000 units of tetanus antitoxin intravenously after testing for horse serum sensitivity. Antiserum does not neutralize toxin fixed to central nervous system cells and is of little use in patients with symptoms present at time of hospitalization. It is esp. beneficial if administered early in mild to moderately severe cases. Patients should receive antibiotics to treat infection and to stop toxin production. The muscle spasms are treated with sedatives, muscle relaxants, or neuromuscular blocking agents. Airway management is of utmost importance, esp. in patients with diffuse rigidity. Tracheostomy is an important treatment and reduces the risk of aspiration when laryngospasm prevents respiration. Establish intravenous access. Insert a foley catheter to prevent urinary retention.

NOTE: Recovery from tetanus does not guarantee natural immunity. Therefore, the patient should begin an immunization series before leaving the hospital.

RS: emprosthotonos; lockjaw; opisthotonos; pleurothotonos; posture; risus sardonicus.

   t. anticus. Form of tetanus in which the body is bowed forward.

   t., artificial. Tetanus produced by a drug such as strychnine.

   t., ascending. Tetanus in which muscle spasms occur first in lower part of body and then spread upward, finally involving muscles of head and neck.

   t., cephalic. Form of tetanus due to a

wound of the head, esp. one near the eyebrow. It is marked by trismus, facial paralysis on one side, and pronounced dysphagia; resembles rabies; often fatal. SYN: *t., hydrophobic.*

t., cerebral. Form of tetanus produced by inoculating the brain of animals with tetanus antitoxin, marked by epileptiform convulsions and excitement.

t., chronic. 1. A latent infection in a healed wound, reactivated upon opening the wound. 2. Form of tetanus in which onset and progress of the disease are slower and more prolonged and symptoms less severe.

t., cryptogenic. Tetanus in which the site of entry of the organism is not known.

t., descending. Tetanus in which muscle spasms occur first in head and neck and later are manifested in other muscles of the body.

t. dorsalis. Tetanus in which the body is bent backward.

t., extensor. Tetanus that affects the extensor muscles especially.

t., hydrophobic. T., cephalic.

t., idiopathic. Tetanus that occurs without any visible lesion.

t., imitative. Hysteria that simulates tetanus.

t. infantum. T. neonatorum.

t. lateralis. Form of tetanus in which the body is bent sideways.

t., local. Tetanus characterized by spasticity of a group of muscles near the wound. Trismus, tonic contraction of jaw muscles, is usually absent.

t. neonatorum. Tetanus of very young infants, usually due to infection of the navel caused by using nonsterile technique in ligating the umbilical cord.

t. paradoxus. Cephalic tetanus in which condition is combined with paralysis of the facial or other cranial nerve.

t., postoperative. Tetanus that follows an operation.

t., puerperal. Tetanus that occurs following childbirth.

t., toxic. Tetanus produced by overdose of strychnine.

tetanus antitoxin. 1. An antibody that develops in the blood of man or other animals (horses) as a result of infection by the tetanus organism *(Clostridium tetani)* or inoculation with tetanus toxin or toxoid. 2. An antitoxin derived from the blood of horses or cattle immunized against tetanus toxin. It is used to produce passive immunity to prevent the development of tetanus and in the treatment of active tetanus. Prophylactic dose is 1500 units injected subcutaneously; for active tetanus, 5000 to 20,000 units injected intravenously or subcutaneously.

tetanus immune globulin. USP. Immune globulin from human blood for use in persons not previously immunized against tetanus whose wound would indicate the need for tetanus prophylaxis. Tetanus immune globulin (human) will produce fewer side effects than will tetanus antitoxin produced from horse serum.

tetanus toxoid. Tetanus toxin modified so that its toxicity is greatly reduced, but its capacity to promote active immunity has been retained.

tetany (tĕt′ă-nē) [Gr. *tetanos*, stretched]. A nervous affection characterized by intermittent tonic spasms that are usually paroxysmal and involve the extremities; most frequent in the young; frequently associated with pregnancy or lactation.

SYM: Characterized by nervousness, irritability and apprehension, numbness and tingling of the extremities, cramps of the various muscles (particularly those of the hands, producing a typical accoucheur type of hand, such as carpopedal spasm) and extreme extension of the feet. Bilateral tonic spasms in arms and legs with jaws rarely involved. Contractions are usually paroxysmal and are attended with pain. May be slight edema. Sensation not disturbed; mind clear; fever slight or absent.

SIGNS: Characteristic diagnostic signs are Trousseau's sign, Chvostek's sign, and the peroneal sign. Prolongation of the isoelectric phase of the S–T segment of the ECG usually is indicative of low calcium. SEE: *Chvostek's sign; hyperventilation; Trousseau's sign.*

ETIOL: Tetany is induced by changes in pH and extracellular calcium that increase nervous and muscular excitability. Causative factors are parathyroid deficiency or inadvertent operative removal of parathyroids during thyroidectomy, alkalosis, vitamin D deficiency, or hyperventilation.

PROG: Usually favorable. Attacks following thyroidectomy sometimes fatal.

t., alkalotic. Tetany resulting from respiratory alkalosis, as in hyperventilation, or from metabolic alkalosis induced by excessive intake of sodium bicarbonate or excessive loss of chlorides by vomiting, gastric lavage, or suction.

t., duration. Continuous contraction, esp. in degenerated muscles, in response to a continuous electric current.

t., epidemic. A form of tetany occurring in Europe, esp. in the winter season. It is of short duration and seldom fatal.

t., gastric. Severe tetany from stomach disorders accompanied by tonic, painful spasms of the extremities.

t., hyperventilation. Tetany caused by

continued hyperventilation.

t., hypocalcemic. Tetany due to low serum calcium and high serum phosphate levels. May be due to lack of vitamin D, factors that interfere with calcium absorption such as steatorrhea or infantile diarrhea, or defective renal excretion of phosphorus.

t., latent. Tetany that requires mechanical or electrical stimulation of nerves to show characteristic signs of excitability.

t., manifest. Tetany in which the characteristic symptoms such as carpopedal spasm, laryngospasm, and convulsions are present. Opposite of latent tetany.

t., parathyroid. Tetany resulting from excision of the parathyroid gland or from hyposecretion of the parathyroid gland as a result of disease or disorders of the gland. SEE: *hypoparathyroidism.*

t., rachitic. Tetany due to hypocalcemia accompanying vitamin D deficiency.

t., thyreoprival. Tetany resulting from removal of the thyroid gland accompanied by removal of parathyroid glands.

tetarcone (tĕt′är-kōn) [Gr. *tetartos*, fourth, + *konos*, cone]. Fourth or distolingual cusp of an upper premolar tooth. SYN: *tetartocone.*

tetartanopia, tetartanopsia (tĕt″är-tăn-ō′pē-ă, -ŏp′sē-ă) [″ + *opsis*, vision]. Symmetrical blindness in the same quadrant of each visual field. SYN: *quadrantanopsia.*

tetartocone (tĕt-är′tō-kōn) [″ + *konos*, cone]. The distolingual cusp of an upper premolar tooth. SYN: *tetarcone.*

tetra-, tetr- [Gr. *tetras*, four]. Combining forms meaning four.

tetrabasic (tĕt″ră-bā′sĭk) [″ + *basis*, base]. Having four replaceable hydrogen atoms, said of an acid or acid salt.

tetrablastic (tĕt″ră-blăs′tĭk) [″ + *blastos*, germ]. Having four germinal layers: the ectoderm, endoderm, and two mesodermic layers.

tetrabrachius (tĕt″ră-brā′kē-ŭs) [″ + *brachion*, arm]. A deformed fetus with four arms.

tetrabromofluorescein (tĕt″ră-brōm″ō-flū-or-ĕs′ĭn, -ē-ĭn). A dye, $C_{20}H_8Br_4O_5$, obtained from action of bromine on fluorescein, used as a stain in microscopy. SYN: *eosin.*

tetracaine hydrochloride. USP. A local anesthetic agent used topically, and by infiltration. Trade name is Pontocaine Hydrochloride.

tetrachirus (tĕt″ră-kī′rŭs) [″ + *cheir*, hand]. A deformed fetus with four hands.

tetrachlorethylene (tĕt″ră-klor-ĕth′ĭ-lēn). USP. A clear, colorless liquid with a characteristic odor, used as a solvent.

tetrachloride (tĕt″ră-klō′rĭd). A radical with four atoms of chlorine.

tetracid (tĕ-trăs′ĭd) [″ + L. *acidus*, sour]. 1. Able to react with four molecules of a monoacid or two of a diacid to form a salt or ester, said of a base or alcohol; term disapproved by some authorities. 2. Having four hydrogen atoms replaceable by basic atoms or radicals, said of acids.

Tetracoccus (tĕt″ră-kŏk′ŭs) [″ + *kokkos*, berry]. Genus of micrococcus arranged in groups of four by division into two planes.

tetracrotic (tĕt″ră-krŏt′ĭk) [″ + *krotos*, beat]. Noting a pulse or pulse tracing with four upward strokes in the descending limb of the wave.

tetracycline (tĕt″ră-sī′klēn). USP. A member of the tetracycline group of broad-spectrum antibiotics having similar pharmacological activity (i.e., tetracycline, chlortetracycline, oxytetracycline). Adverse effects may include hypersensitivity, burning of the eyes, glossitis, gastrointestinal disorders, various leukocyte changes, liver and kidney disorders, and staining of the teeth of a child whose mother took tetracycline during pregnancy. There are a great number of trade names for this antibiotic. SEE: *teeth, staining of.*

tetrad (tĕt′răd) [Gr. *tetras*, four]. 1. A group of four things with something in common. 2. An element having a valence or combining power of four. 3. A group of four similar bodies. 4. A group of four parts, said of cells produced by division in two planes, or of a chromosome in four parts in preparation for two mitotic divisions in maturation.

tetradactyly (tĕt″ră-dăk′tĭ-lē) [″ + *daktylos*, finger]. Having four digits on a hand or foot.

tetraethylammonium chloride (tĕt-ră-ĕth-ĭl-ăm-ō′nē-ŭm klō′rĭd). ABBR: TEAC. A quaternary ammonium compound used as a ganglionic blocking agent in diagnosis and treatment of circulatory diseases.

tetraethylpyrophosphate (tĕt-ră-ĕth″ĭl-pī-rō-fōs′făt). ABBR: TEPP. A powerful cholinesterase inhibitor used as an insecticide; poisonous to man. Has had some use in treatment of myasthenia gravis. The antidote is atropine.

tetragenous (tĕt-răj′ĕn-ŭs) [Gr. *tetras*, four, + *gennan*, to produce]. Pert. to organisms, esp. bacteria, that divide into groups of four.

tetrahydrocannabinol (tĕt″ră-hī″drō-kă-năb′ĭ-nŏl). A chemical, $C_{21}H_{30}O_2$, that is the principal active component in cannabis, or marijuana.

tetrahydrozoline hydrochloride (tĕt″ră-hī-drō′zō-lēn). USP. A vasoconstrictor agent used as a nasal decongestant and ophthalmic vasoconstrictor. Trade name is Tyzine.

tetraiodothyronine (tĕt″ră-ī″ō-dō-thī′rō-nēn). ABBR: T_4. One of the principal hormones secreted by the thyroid gland. Chemically it is 3,5,3′,5′-tetraiodothyronine. SEE: *thyroid; thyroid function tests; triiodothyronine.* SYN: *thyroxine.*

tetralogy. The combination of four symptoms or elements.

t. of Fallot. An anomaly of the heart consisting of pulmonary stenosis, interventricular septal defect, dextroposed aorta that receives blood from both ventricles, and hypertrophy of the right ventricle.

tetramastia, tetramazia (tĕt″ră-măs′tē-ă, tĕt″ră-mā′zē-ă) [″ + *mastos, mazos,* breast]. Condition characterized by presence of four breasts.

tetramastigote (tĕt″ră-măs′tĭ-gōt) [″ + *mastix,* lash]. Having four flagella.

tetrameric, tetramerous (tĕt″ră-mĕr′ĭk, tĕt-răm′ĕr-ŭs) [″ + *meros,* a part]. Having four parts.

tetranopsia (tĕt″ră-nŏp′sē-ă) [″ + *an-,* not, + *opsis,* vision]. Obliteration of one-quarter of the visual field.

tetraotus (tĕt″ră-ō′tŭs) [Gr. *tetras,* four, + *otos,* ear]. Tetrotus, q.v.

tetraparesis (tĕt″ră-păr′ĕ-sĭs) [″ + *parienai,* to let fall]. Muscular weakness of all four extremities.

tetrapeptide (tĕt″ră-pĕp′tīd). A peptide that yields four amino acids when it is hydrolyzed.

tetraplegia (tĕt″ră-plē′jē-ă) [″ + *plege,* a stroke]. Paralysis of both arms and legs. SYN: *quadriplegia.*

tetraploid (tĕt′ră-ployd) [″ + *ploos,* a fold, + *eidos,* form, shape]. 1. Concerning tetraploidy. 2. Having four sets of chromosomes.

tetrapus (tĕt′ră-pŭs) [″ + *pous,* foot]. A deformed fetus having four feet.

tetrasaccharide (tĕt″ră-săk′ă-rīd). A carbohydrate composed of four monosaccharides.

tetrascelus (tĕt-răs′ē-lŭs) [″ + *skelos,* leg]. A deformed fetus having four legs.

tetrasomic (tĕt-ră-sō′mĭk) [″ + *soma,* body]. Possessing four instead of the usual pair of chromosomes in an otherwise diploid cell, that is, having a chromosome number of 2n + 2.

tetraster (tĕt-răs′tĕr) [″ + *aster,* star]. A mitotic figure in which there are four asters instead of the usual two; occurring abnormally in mitosis.

tetrastichiasis (tĕt″ră-stĭ-kī′ă-sĭs) [″ + *stichos,* row, + *-iasis,* condition]. A deformed fetus having four rows of eyelashes.

tetratomic (tĕt″ră-tŏm′ĭk) [″ + *atomos,* indivisible]. Having four atoms.

tetravalent (tĕt″ră-vā′lĕnt). Having a valence or combining power of four. SYN: *quadrivalent.*

Tetrex. Trade name for tetracycline phosphate complex.

tetrodotoxin (tĕt″rō-dō-tŏks′ĭn). A powerful nerve poison found in the eggs of the California newt and in certain puffer fish in Japan. In concentrated form it is more toxic than cyanide.

tetrotus (tĕt-rō′tŭs) [″ + *otos,* ear]. A deformed fetus with two faces, four eyes, and four ears.

tetroxide (tĕ-trŏk′sīd). A chemical compound containing four oxygen atoms.

textiform (tĕks′tĭ-form) [L. *textum,* something woven, + *forma,* shape]. Resembling a network, web, or mesh.

textoblastic (tĕks″tō-blăs′tĭk) [L. *textus,* tissue, + Gr. *blastos,* germ]. Forming adult tissue; regenerative.

textural (tĕks′tū-răl) [L. *textura,* weaving]. Concerning the texture or constitution of a tissue.

texture (tĕks′tūr) [L. *textura*]. The organization of a tissue or structure.

textus (tĕks′tŭs) [L.]. Tissue.

T fracture. Fracture in which bone splits both longitudinally and transversely.

T-group. Group of individuals who meet in sensitivity training sessions in order to become more sensitive to themselves and others.

Th. Chem. symbol for the element thorium.

thalamencephalon (thăl″ă-mĕn-sĕf′ă-lŏn) [Gr. *thalamos,* inner chamber, + *enkephalos,* brain]. [NA] The part of the diencephalon that includes the thalamus, pineal body, and geniculate bodies. SYN: *diencephalon.*

thalamic (thăl-ăm′ĭk) [Gr. *thalamos,* inner chamber]. Pert. to the thalamus.

thalamic syndrome. Vascular lesions of the thalamus, causing disturbances of sensation and partial or complete paralysis of one side of the body. An extremely severe, sharp, boring-type pain may occur spontaneously. There also is a tendency to over-respond to a sensory stimulus and to be aware of the stimulus long after it has ceased.

    ETIOL: Optic thalamus lesion.

thalamo- [Gr. *thalamos,* inner chamber]. 1. Combining form meaning chamber, part of brain at which a nerve originates. 2. Pert. to the thalamus.

thalamocele, thalamocoele (thăl′ăm-ō-sēl) [″ + *koilia,* a hollow]. The 3rd ventricle of the brain.

thalamocortical (thăl″ăm-ō-kor′tĭ-kăl) [″ + L. *cortex,* rind]. Pert. to the optic thalamus and the cerebral cortex.

thalamolenticular (thăl′ăm-ō-lĕn-tĭk′ū-lăr) [″ + L. *lenticula,* lentil]. Concerning the optic thalamus and the lenticular nucleus.

thalamotomy (thăl-ă-mŏt′ō-mē) [″ + *tome,* incision]. Destruction by one of several methods of a portion of the thalamus in order to treat psychosis or intractable pain.

thalamus (thăl′ă-mŭs) [L.] (pl *thalami*). [NA] The largest subdivision of the diencephalon on either side, consisting chiefly of an ovoid gray nuclear mass in the lateral wall of the 3rd ventricle. Each consists of a number of nuclei (anterior, medial, lateral, and ventral), the medial and lateral geniculate bodies, and the pulvinar.

FUNCT: All sensory stimuli, with the exception of olfactory, are received by the thalamus. These are associated, synthesized, and then relayed through thalamocortical radiations to specific cortical areas. Impulses are also received from the cortex, hypothalamus, and corpus striatum and relayed to visceral and somatic effectors. The thalamus is also the center for appreciation of primitive uncritical sensations of pain, crude touch, and temperature.

thalassemia (thăl-ă-sē′mē-ă) [Gr. *thalassa*, sea, + *haima*, blood]. A group of hereditary anemias occurring in populations bordering the Mediterranean and in Southeast Asia. Anemia is produced by either a defective production rate of the alpha or beta hemoglobin polypeptide chain or a decreased synthesis of the beta chain. Heterozygotes are usually asymptomatic. The severity in homozygotes varies according to the complexity of the inheritance pattern, but thalassemia may be fatal. SEE: *anemia, sickle cell.*

   t. major. The homozygous form of deficient beta chain synthesis, which is very severe and presents during childhood. Characterized by fatigue, splenomegaly, severe anemia, enlargement of the heart, slight jaundice, leg ulcers, and cholelithiasis. Increased bone marrow activity causes thickening of the cranial bones and increased malar eminences. Prognosis varies; however, the younger the child when the disease appears, the more unfavorable the outcome. SYN: *Cooley's anemia.*

   t. minor. Heterozygosity for either β or α chain produces a mild disease that may be completely asymptomatic. Usually revealed by chance or as a result of study of the family of an individual having thalassemia major. Prognosis is excellent.

thalassophobia (thăl-ăs″ō-fō′bē-ă) [Gr. *thalassa*, sea, + *phobos*, fear]. Abnormal fear of the sea.

thalassoposia (thăl-lăs″sō-pō′zē-ă) [″ + *posis*, drinking]. Ingestion of sea water.

thalassotherapy (thăl-ăs″sō-thĕr′ă-pē) [″ + *therapeia*, treatment]. Treatment of disease by living at the seaside, by sea bathing, or by sea voyages.

thalidomide (thă-lĭd′ō-mīd). A chemical substance α (N-phthalimido) glutarimide, used extensively as a sedative and sleeping pill in Europe in the early 1960s. Its use was discontinued when it was discovered to cause severe malformation in limbs of developing fetuses exposed to the drug in their very early intrauterine life. SEE: *phocomelia.*

thallinization (thăl″ĭn-ĭ-zā′shŭn). Treatment with doses of thalline or its salts.

thallitoxicosis (thăl″ĭ-tŏk″sĭ-kō′sĭs). Poisoning by accidental ingestion of thallium sulfate-containing pesticides. SEE: *thallium* in *Poisons and Poisoning* in *Appendix.*

thallium (thăl′ē-ŭm) [Gr. *thallos*, a young shoot]. SYMB: Tl. At. wt. 204.37; at. no. 81; sp. gr. 11.85. A metallic element. Its salts are poisonous.

   t. sulfate. A chemical used as a rodenticide. It is also quite toxic to humans.

thallium poisoning. Characterized by severe abdominal pain, vomiting, diarrhea, tremors, delirium, convulsions, paralysis, coma, and death. SEE: *Poisons and Poisoning* in *Appendix.*

thallotoxicosis (thăl″ō-tŏk″sĭ-kō′sĭs). Thallitoxicosis, q.v.

THAM. Trade name for tromethamine.

thanato- [Gr. *thanatos*, death]. Combining form meaning death.

thanatobiological (thăn″ă-tō-bī-ō-lŏj′ĭ-kăl) [Gr. *thanatos*, death, + *bios*, life, + *logos*, word, reason]. Rel. to the processes of life and death.

thanatognomonic (thăn″ăt-ŏg-nō-mŏn′ĭk) [″ + *gnomonikos*, knowing]. Indicative of the approach of death.

thanatoid (thăn′ă-toyd) [″ + *eidos*, form, shape]. Resembling death.

thanatology (thăn″ă-tŏl′ō-jē) [Gr. *thanatos*, death, + *logos*, word, reason]. The study of death.

thanatomania (thăn″ă-tō-mā′nē-ă) [″ + *mania*, madness]. Condition of homicidal or suicidal mania.

thanatophidia (thăn″ă-tō-fĭd′ē-ă) [″ + *ophis*, snake]. Venomous snakes.

thanatophobia (thăn″ă-tō-fō′bē-ă) [″ + *phobos*, fear]. Morbid fear of death. SYN: *necrophobia.*

thanatophoric (thăn″ă-tō-for′ĭk) [″ + *pherein*, to bear]. Lethal.

thanatophoric dwarfism. Dwarfism caused by generalized failure of endochondral bone formation. Characterized by large head, prominent forehead, hypertelorism, saddle nose, and short limbs extending straight out from the trunk. Most of these infants die soon after birth. SEE: *dwarf, micromelic.*

thaumato- [Gr. *thauma*, wonder]. Combining form meaning wonder, marvel.

thaumaturgic [″ + *ergon*, work]. To work miracles or magic.

Thayer-Martin medium. A special medium used for growing the causative organism of gonorrhea, *Neisseria gonorrhoeae.*

theaism (thē'ă-ĭzm) [L. *thea,* tea, + Gr. *-ismos,* condition]. Chronic poisoning from excessive tea drinking.

thebaic (thē-bā'ĭk) [L. *Thebaicus,* Theban, from Thebes, where opium was once prepared]. Concerning opium.

thebaine (thē-bā'ĭn). An alkaloid present in opium.

thebesian foramina (thē-bē'zē-ăn) [Adam Christian Thebesius, Ger. physician, 1686–1732]. Orifices of the thebesian veins, opening into the right auricle of the heart.

thebesian valve. An endocardial fold at entrance of the coronary sinus into right auricle.

thebesian veins. Venules conveying blood from the myocardium to the atria or ventricles.

theca (thē'kă) [Gr. *theke,* sheath] (pl. *thecae*). A sheath of investing membrane.

  t. cordis. Pericardium that sheaths the heart.

  t. folliculi. [NA] Outer wall of a graafian follicle, consisting of an inner vascular layer (theca interna) and outer fibrous layer (theca externa).

thecal (thē'kăl) [Gr. *theke,* sheath]. Pert. to a sheath.

thecitis (thē-sī'tĭs) [″ + *itis,* inflammation]. Inflammation of the sheath of a tendon.

theco- [Gr. *theke,* sheath]. Combining form meaning sheath, case, or receptacle.

thecodont (thē'kō-dŏnt) [″ + *odous,* tooth]. Having teeth that are inserted in sockets.

thecoma (thē-kō'mă) [″ + *oma,* tumor]. A tumor of the ovary usually occurring during or following menopause. It is usually benign.

thecomatosis (thē″kō-mă-tō'sĭs) [″ + ″ + *osis,* condition]. Increased connective tissue in the ovary.

thecostegnosia, thecostegnosis (thē″kō-stĕg-nō'sē-ă, -nō'sĭs) [″ + *stegnosis,* a narrowing]. Constriction of a tendon sheath.

Theelin. Trade name for estrone.

thelalgia (thē-lăl'jē-ă) [Gr. *thele,* nipple, + *algos,* pain]. Pain in the nipples.

thelarche (thē-lăr'kē) [″ + *arche,* beginning]. The beginning of breast development at puberty. SEE: *pubarche; semenarche.*

thelasis (thē-lăs'ĭs) [″ + *-iasis,* condition]. The act of sucking.

Thelazia (thē-lā'zē-ă) [Gr. *thelazo,* to suck]. A genus of nematodes that inhabit the conjunctival sac and lacrimal ducts of various species of vertebrates. Occasionally species of *Thelazia* are found in humans.

thelaziasis (thē″lā-zī'ă-sĭs) [″ + *-iasis,* condition]. Condition of being infested by worms of the genus *Thelazia.*

theleplasty (thē'lē-plăs″tē) [Gr. *thele,* nipple, + *plassein,* to form]. Plastic surgery of the nipple. SYN: *mammilliplasty.*

thelerethism (thĕl-ĕr'ĕ-thĭzm) [″ + *erethisma,* stimulation]. Erection of the nipple.

thelitis (thē-lī'tĭs) [″ + *itis,* inflammation]. Inflammation of the nipples. SYN: *acromastitis.*

thelium (thē'lē-ŭm) [L.] (pl. *thelia*). 1. A papilla. 2. A nipple. 3. A cellular layer.

theloncus (thē-lŏn'kŭs) [″ + *onkus,* bulk, mass]. A tumor of a nipple.

thelophlebostemma (thē″lō-flĕb″ō-stĕm'mă) [″ + *phelps,* vein, + *stemma,* wreath]. A dark or venous circle of veins about the nipple.

thelorrhagia (thē″lō-rā'jē-ă) [″ + *rhegnynai,* to burst forth]. Hemorrhage from a nipple.

thelothism (thē'lō-thĭzm) [″ + *erethisma,* stimulation]. Erection of a nipple brought about by contraction of smooth muscle fibers. SEE: *thelerethism.*

thelygenic (thē″lē-jĕn'ĭk) [Gr. *thelys,* female, + *gennan,* to produce]. Producing only female children.

thenad (thē'năd) [Gr. *thenar,* palm, + L. *ad,* toward]. Toward the palm or thenar eminence.

thenal (thē'năl) [Gr. *thenar,* palm]. Pert. to the palm or thenar eminence.

thenal aspect. Outer side of the palm.

thenar (thē'năr) [Gr. *thenar,* palm]. 1. Palm of hand or sole of foot. 2. Fleshy eminence at base of thumb. 3. Concerning the palm.

thenar cleft. A fascial cleft of the palm overlying volar surface of adductor pollicis muscle.

thenar eminence. A prominence at the base of the thumb.

thenar fascia. A thin membrane covering the short muscles of the thumb.

thenar muscles. Abductor and flexor muscles of the thumb.

theobromine (thē-ō-brō'mēn) [Gr. *theos,* god, + *broma,* food]. A white powder obtained from *Theobroma cacao,* the plant from which chocolate is obtained.

  ACTION/USES: Dilates blood vessels in the heart and peripherally. Used as a mild stimulant and as a diuretic.

theomania (thē-ō-mā'nē-ă) [Gr. *theos,* god, + *mania,* madness]. Religious insanity; esp. that in which the patient thinks he or she is a deity or has devine inspiration.

theophobia (thē″ō-fō'bē-ă) [″ + *phobos,* fear]. Abnormal fear of the wrath of God.

theophylline (thē″ŏ-fĭl′ēn, -ĭn) [L. *thea*, tea, + Gr. *phyllon*, plant]. USP. A white crystalline powder with action resembling caffeine and theobromine. Trade names include Elixophyllin and Slo-Phyllin.

    t. ethylenediamine. Previously used name for aminophylline.

    t. olamine. A smooth-muscle relaxant. A theophylline preparation available only as a solution for rectal administration.

    t. sodium glycinate. USP. A smooth-muscle relaxant.

theorem (thē′ŏ-rĕm) [Gr. *theorema*, principle arrived at by speculation]. A proposition that can be proved by use of logic, or by argument, from information previously accepted as being valid.

    t., Bayes. SEE: *Bayes theorem.*

theory (thē′ŏ-rē) [Gr. *theoria*, speculation as opposed to practice]. A supposition or an assumption based on certain evidence or observations but lacking scientific proof. When a theory becomes generally accepted and firmly established, it is called a doctrine or principle.

    t., cell. The proposition that living things are composed of cells capable of life.

    t., clonal selection, of immunity. Theory formulated by the Australian Nobel prize winner F. M. Burnett, in 1959, that mesenchymal cells, precursors of the cells that form antibodies, are made up of innumerable clones. The clones capable of reacting with "self" components, i.e., the individual's own cells, are eliminated or suppressed in the prenatal period. Those clones not eliminated or suppressed that are specific for foreign substances react with the antigen fitting to the receptor, and this leads to the proliferation of that clone.

    t., germ. The proposition that infectious diseases are due to microorganisms.

    t., quantum. The proposition that energy can be emitted in discrete quantities (quanta) and that atomic particles can exist only in certain energy states. Quanta are measured by multiplying the frequency of the radiation, v, by h, Planck's constant. SYN: *Planck's theory.*

    t., recapitulation. Theory that during development an individual organism goes through the same progressive stages as did the species in developing from lower to higher forms of life. The theory that ontogeny recapitulates phylogeny.

Theory of Clinical Nursing. SEE: *Appendix 23.*

Theory of Cultural Care Diversity and Universality. SEE: *Appendix 23.*

Theory of Health as Expanding Consciousness. SEE: *Appendix 23.*

Theory of Human Becoming. SEE: *Appendix 23.*

Theory of Human Caring. SEE: *Appendix 23.*

Theory of Interpersonal Relations in Nursing. SEE: *Appendix 23.*

Theory of the Nursing Process Discipline. SEE: *Appendix 23.*

theotherapy (thē″ŏ-thĕr′ă-pē) [Gr. *theos*, god, + *therapeia*, treatment]. Treatment of disease by spiritual and religious methods.

thèque (tĕk) [Fr., a box]. A nest of nevus cells or other cells close to the basal layer of the epidermis.

Theralax. Trade name for bisacodyl, USP.

therapeusis (thĕr″ă-pū′sĭs). Therapeutics.

therapeutic (thĕr-ă-pū′tĭk) [Gr. *therapeutikos*, treating]. 1. Pert. to results obtained from treatment. 2. Having medicinal or healing properties. 3. A healing agent.

therapeutic exercise. Scientific supervision of exercise for the purpose of preventing muscular atrophy, restoring joint and muscle function, increasing muscular strength, and improving efficiency of cardiovascular and pulmonary function.

therapeutic recreation. A specialized field within recreation whose specialists plan and direct recreational activities for patients recovering from physical or mental illness or who are attempting to cope with a permanent or temporary disability.

therapeutics (thĕr″ă-pū′tĭks) [Gr. *therapeutike*, treatment]. That branch of medicine concerned with the application of remedies and the treatment of disease. SYN: *therapy.*

therapia sterilisans magna (thĕr″ă-pē′ă stē-rĭl′ĭ-săns măg′nă) [L.]. Ehrlich's method of administering a chemical agent that would destroy in one large dose all the parasites in a patient without causing serious injury to the patient.

therapist (thĕr′ă-pĭst) [Gr. *therapeia*, treatment]. A person skilled in giving therapy, usually in a specific field of health care.

    t., occupational. Therapist skilled in using environmental or task modification to assist persons unable to accomplish usual tasks because of disability.

    t., physical. A person educated to evaluate, establish, and administer a program of physical therapy using rehabilitative and therapeutic exercise techniques and physical modalities.

    t., radiation. Therapist trained to use ionizing radiation for the treatment of diseases.

    t., respiratory. A person skilled in managing the techniques and equipment used in treating those with acute and chronic respiratory diseases.

t., speech. A person skilled in assisting patients who have speech and language difficulties.

therapy (thĕr'ă-pē) [Gr. *therapeia*, treatment]. Treatment of a disease or pathological condition. SEE: *treatment.*

t., adjuvant. SEE: *adjuvant therapy.*

t., anticoagulant. Use of anticoagulants to decrease the tendency of the blood to coagulate and cause thrombosis.

t., aversion. Aversion therapy, q.v.

t., behavior. In psychiatry, the use of conditioning techniques to directly modify behavior. Even though the technique may be of benefit, the basic cause of the difficulty is not abolished.

t., collapse. Production of a pneumothorax on one side in order to treat pulmonary tuberculosis. It allows the lung on that side to be at rest.

t., electroconvulsive. SEE: *electroconvulsive therapy.*

t., fever. Therapy involving artificially produced fever. This is accomplished by exposure to high environmental temperature or by the injection of foreign proteins.

t., group. SEE: *group therapy.*

t., immunosuppressive. SEE: *immunosuppressive agent.*

t., inhalation. Administration of medicines, water vapor, gases (such as oxygen, carbon dioxide, or helium), or anesthetics by inhalation. The medicines usually are nebulized by using an aerosol or spray apparatus. SEE: *intermittent positive-pressure breathing.*

t., insulin shock. SEE: *insulin shock therapy.*

t., light. Treatment with radiation from the visible spectrum.

t., milieu. Treatment of mental illness by altering the patient's immediate social and environmental circumstances in order to facilitate whatever other therapy is being used.

t., neoadjuvant. SEE: *neoadjuvant therapy.*

t., nonspecific. Use of injections of foreign proteins or bacterial vaccines in treatment of infection to stimulate general cellular activity. SEE: *t., specific.*

t., occupational. SEE: *occupational therapy.*

t., opsonic. Use of bacterial vaccines to elevate the opsonic index of the blood. SYN: *t., vaccine.*

t., parenteral. A medicine or solution administered via a route other than ingestion.

t., photodynamic. Method of treating cancer by using light-absorbing chemicals

that are selectively retained by malignant cells. When these cells are exposed to light in the visible range, the cancer cells are killed.

t., physical. Appropriate use of therapeutic exercise, rehabilitative programs, and physical agents such as massage, heat, hydrotherapy, radiation, and electricity, under the direction of a licensed physical therapist.

t., play. The use of play, esp. with dolls and toys, to allow children to express their feelings. This may permit insight into their thought processes that could not be obtained through verbal communication.

t., radiation. Treatment of diseases by the use of ionizing radiation.

t., replacement. The therapeutic use of a medicine to substitute for a natural substance that is either absent or diminished, e.g., insulin or thyroid hormone.

t., serum. Use of injections of blood serum from immunized animals or persons in the treatment of disease. SYN: *serotherapy.*

t., shock. SEE: *shock therapy.*

t., specific. Administration of a remedy acting directly against the cause of a disease, as arsphenamine or mercury for syphilis, or quinine for malaria.

t., speech. SEE: *speech therapy.*

t., spiritual. SEE: *spiritual therapy.*

t., substitution. Administration of a substance that the body normally produces, such as a hormone.

t., vaccine. Injection of bacteria or their products to produce active immunization against a disease.

therapy putty. Generic name for malleable plastic material used as a therapeutic modality to provide resistance in various hand exercises. One brand is available under the trade name Theraplast.

therm [Gr. *therme*, heat]. Term used to indicate a variety of quantities of heat. SEE: MET.

thermacogenesis (thĕr"mă-kō-jĕn'ĕs-ĭs) [Gr. *therme*, heat, + *genesis*, generation, birth]. Production of an increase of body temperature by drug therapy.

thermaerotherapy (thĕr-mā"ĕr-ō-thĕr'ă-pē) [" + *aer*, air, + *therapeia*, treatment]. Therapeutic application of hot air.

thermal (thĕr'măl) [Gr. *therme*, heat]. Pert. to heat.

thermal death point. In bacteriology, the degree of heat that will kill organisms in a fluid culture in 10 minutes.

thermalgesia (thĕr"măl-jē'zē-ă) [" + *algesis*, sense of pain]. Pain caused by heat.

thermalgia (thĕr-măl'jē-ă) [" + *algos*, pain]. Neuralgia accompanied by intense burning sensation, pain, redness, and sweating of the area involved. SYN: *causalgia.*

thermal radiation. Heat radiation.

thermal sense. Capacity for recognition of heat. SYN: *thermesthesia.*

thermanalgesia (thĕrm″ăn-ăl-jē′zē-ă) [″ + *an-,* not, + *algesis,* sense of pain]. Inability to experience sensation of heat because of a cerebral lesion.

thermanesthesia (thĕrm″ăn-ĕs-thē′zē-ă) [″ + ″ + *aisthesis,* sensation]. Inability to recognize sensations of heat and cold; insensibility to heat changes. It sometimes occurs in syringomyelia. SYN: *thermoanesthesia.*

thermatology (thĕr-mă-tŏl′ō-jē) [Gr. *therme,* heat, + *logos,* word, reason]. The study of heat in treatment of disease.

thermelometer (thĕr″mĕl-ŏm′ĕ-tĕr) [″ + *elektron,* amber, + Gr. *metron,* a measure]. An electric thermometer used to indicate temperature changes too slight to be measured on an ordinary thermometer.

thermesthesia (thĕr″mĕs-thē′zē-ă) [″ + *aisthesis,* sensation]. Capability of perceiving heat and cold; temperature sense. SYN: *thermoesthesia.*

thermesthesiometer (thĕrm″ĕs-thē-zē-ŏm′ĕt-ĕr) [″ + *aisthesis,* sensation, + *metron,* a measure]. Device for determining sensibility to heat.

thermhyperesthesia (thĕrm″hī-pĕr-ĕs-thē′zē-ă) [″ + Gr. *hyper,* over, above, excessive, + *aisthesis,* sensation]. Excessive sensitivity to heat.

thermhypesthesia (thĕrm″hī-pĕs-thē′zē-ă) [″ + *hypo,* under, below, + *aisthesis,* sensation]. Lessened sensibility of the temperature sense. SYN: *thermohypesthesia.*

thermic (thĕr′mĭk) [Gr. *therme,* heat]. Pert. to heat.

thermic sense. The temperature sense; ability to react to heat stimuli.

thermistor (thĕr-mĭs′tor). An apparatus for quickly determining very small changes in temperature. Materials that alter their resistance to the flow of electricity as the temperature changes are used in these devices.

thermo- [Gr. *therme,* heat]. Combining form indicating hot or heat.

thermoalgesia (thĕr″mō-ăl-jē′zē-ă) [Gr. *therme,* heat, + *algesis,* sense of pain]. Condition in which pain is caused by application of moderate heat. SYN: *thermalgesia.*

thermoanalgesia (thĕr″mō-ăn″ăl-jē′zē-ă) [″ + *an,* not, + *algesis,* sense of pain]. Loss of heat sensation. SYN: *thermanalgesia.*

thermoanesthesia (thĕr″mō-ăn″ĕs-thē′zē-ă) [″ + ″ + *aisthesis,* sensation]. 1. Inability to distinguish between heat and cold. 2. Insensibility to heat or temperature changes.

thermobiosis (thĕr″mō-bī-ō′sĭs) [″ + *biosis,* way of life]. Ability to withstand high temperature.

thermobiotic (thĕr″mō-bī-ŏt′ĭk) [″ + *bios,* life]. Able to exist at high temperature.

thermocauterectomy (thĕr″mō-kaw-tĕr-ĕk′tō-mē) [″ + *kauterion,* branding iron, + *ektome,* excision]. Excision by thermocautery.

thermocautery (thĕr″mō-kaw′tĕr-ē). 1. Cautery by application of heat. 2. Cauterizing iron.

thermochemistry (thĕr″mō-kĕm′ĭs-trē). The branch of science concerned with the interrelationship of heat and chemical reactions.

thermochroic (thĕr″mō-krō′ĭk) [″ + *chroa,* color]. Concerning thermochroism.

thermochroism (thĕr-mŏk′rō-ĭzm) [″ + *chroa,* color]. Property of a substance reflecting or transmitting portions of thermal radiation and absorbing or altering others.

thermocoagulation (thĕr″mō-kō-ăg-ū-lā′shŭn) [″ + L. *coagulatio,* clotting]. The use of high-frequency currents to produce coagulation to destroy tissue.

thermocouple (thĕr′mō-kŭ″pl) [″ + L. *copula,* a bond]. Device for measuring slight temperature changes. SYN: *thermopile.*

thermocurrent (thĕr″mō-kŭr′ĕnt). An electric current produced by thermoelectric means.

thermode. Device for heating or cooling a part of the body. Thermodes have been used in studying the effect on body function when temperature of some organ or tissue is changed.

thermodiffusion (thĕr″mō-dĭ-fū′zhŭn). Increased diffusion of a substance as a result of increased heat.

thermodilution (thĕr″mō-dī-lū′shŭn). Use of an injected cold liquid such as sterile saline into the bloodstream and measuring the temperature change downstream. This has been used in determining cardiac output.

thermoduric (thĕr″mō-dū′rĭk) [″ + L. *durus,* resistant]. Able to live in high temperatures. SEE: *thermophylic.*

thermodynamics (thĕr″mō-dī-năm′ĭks) [″ + *dynamis,* power]. The branch of physics concerned with laws that govern heat production, changes, and conversion into other forms of energy.

thermoelectric (thĕr″mō-ē-lĕk′trĭk). Concerning thermoelectricity.

thermoelectricity (thĕr″mō-ē-lĕk-trĭs′ĭ-tē). Electricity generated by heat.

thermoesthesia (thĕr″mō-ĕs-thē′zē-ă). [Gr. *therme,* heat, + *aisthesis,* sensation]. Ability to recognize temperature differences. SYN: *thermesthesia.*

thermoexcitatory (thĕr″mō-ĕk-sī′tă-tor-ē) [″ + L. *excitare,* to irritate]. Stimulating the production of heat in the body.

thermogenesis (thĕr″mō-jĕn′ĕ-sĭs) [″ + *genesis,* generation, birth]. The production of heat, esp. in the body.

thermogenics (thĕr″mō-jĕn′ĭks). The study and science of heat production.

thermogram (thĕr′mō-grăm). A graphic record of variation in heat.

thermograph (thĕr′mō-grăf) [″ + *graphein,* to write]. Device for registering variations of heat.

thermography. In medicine, the use of a device that detects and records the heat present in very small areas of the part being studied. When these multiple readings are accumulated, the relatively hot and cold spots on the body surface are revealed. The technique has been used to study blood flow to limbs and to detect cancer of the breast.

thermohyperalgesia (thĕr″mō-hī″pĕr-ăl-jē′zē-ă) [″ + *hyper,* excessive, + *algesis,* sense of pain]. Unbearable pain upon the application of heat.

thermohyperesthesia (thĕr″mō-hī″pĕr-ĕs-thē′zē-ă) [″ + *hyper,* excessive, + *aisthesis,* sensation]. Exceptional sensitiveness to heat.

thermohypesthesia (thĕr″mō-hī″pĕs-thē′zē-ă) [″ + *hypo,* below, + *aisthesis,* sensation]. Diminished perception of heat.

thermohypoesthesia (thĕr″mō-hī″pō-ĕs-thē′zē-ă) [″ + ″ + *aisthesis,* sensation]. Thermohypesthesia, q.v.

thermoinhibitory (thĕr″mō-ĭn-hĭb′ĭ-tor″ē) [″ + L. *inhibere,* to restrain]. Arresting or impeding the generation of body heat.

thermolabile (thĕr″mō-lā′bĭl) [″ + *labilis,* unstable]. Destroyed or changed easily by heat; unstable. SEE: *heat; heat, latent.*

thermolamp (thĕr′mō-lămp) [″ + *lampe,* torch]. Lamp used for providing heat.

thermology (thĕr-mŏl′ō-jē) [″ + *logos,* word, reason]. The science of heat.

thermoluminescent dosimeter. A monitoring device consisting of a small crystal in a container that can be attached to a patient or to a health care worker. It stores energy when struck by ionizing radiation. When heated, it will emit light proportional to the amount of radiation to which it has been exposed.

thermolysis (thĕr-mŏl′ĭ-sĭs) [″ + *lysis,* dissolution]. 1. Loss of heat from the body, as by evaporation. 2. Chemical decomposition by heat.

thermolytic (thĕr″mō-lĭt′ĭk) [″ + *lytikos,* dissolving]. Promoting thermolysis.

thermomassage (thĕr″mō-mă-săzh′). Massage by use of heat.

Comparative Thermometric Scale

	Celsius*	Fahrenheit
Boiling point	100°	212°
of water	90	194
	80	176
	70	158
	60	140
	50	122
	40	104
Body temperature	37°	98.6°
	30	86
	20	68
	10	50
Freezing point	0°	32°
of water	−10	14
	−20	−4

CONVERSION: *Fahrenheit to Celsius:* Subtract 32 and multiply by 5/9. *Celsius to Fahrenheit:* Multiply by 9/5 and add 32.
* Also called Centigrade.

thermometer (thĕr-mŏm′ĕ-tĕr) [″ + *metron,* measure]. An instrument for indicating the degree of heat or cold. First mention of a thermometer in diagnosis of disease was given by It. physician Sanctorius in 1626. The glass clinical thermometer used today is little different from the one he used.

   t., alcohol. Thermometer containing alcohol.

   t., Celsius. Thermometric scale generally used in scientific notation. Temperature of boiling water at sea level 100°C and freezing point 0°C, with 100° between. SEE: tables.

   t., centigrade. T., Celsius.

   t., clinical. Thermometer for measuring temperature of the body; one in which the mercury remains stationary at the registration point until shaken down. SEE: *clinical thermometer.*

   t., differential. Thermometer recording slight variations of temperature.

   t., Fahrenheit. Thermometric scale used in English-speaking countries. Boiling point 212°F, freezing point 32°F. SEE: tables.

   t., gas. Thermometer filled with gas, such as air, helium, or oxygen. SEE: *t., air.*

   t., Kelvin. Thermometric scale in which absolute zero is zero degrees Kelvin; the freezing point of water is 273.15°; the boiling point of water is 373.15°. Thus one degree on the Kelvin scale is exactly equivalent to one degree on the Celsius scale.

   t., mercury. Thermometer containing

Thermometric Equivalents (Celsius and Fahrenheit)

C°	F°	C°	F°	C°	F°	C°	F°
0	32	27	80.6	54	129.2	81	177.8
1	33.8	28	82.4	55	131	82	179.6
2	35.6	29	84.2	56	132.8	83	181.4
3	37.4	30	86.0	57	134.6	84	183.2
4	39.2	31	87.8	58	136.4	85	185
5	41	32	89.6	59	138.2	86	186.8
6	42.8	33	91.4	60	140	87	188.6
7	44.6	34	93.2	61	141.8	88	190.4
8	46.4	35	95	62	143.6	89	192.2
9	48.2	36	96.8	63	145.4	90	194
10	50	37	98.6	64	147.2	91	195.8
11	51.8	38	100.4	65	149	92	197.6
12	53.6	39	102.2	66	150.8	93	199.4
13	55.4	40	104	67	152.6	94	201.2
14	57.2	41	105.8	68	154.4	95	203
15	59	42	107.6	69	156.2	96	204.8
16	60.8	43	109.4	70	158	97	206.6
17	62.6	44	111.2	71	159.8	98	208.4
18	64.4	45	113	72	161.6	99	210.2
19	66.2	46	114.8	73	163.4	100	212
20	68	47	116.6	74	165.2		
21	69.8	48	118.4	75	167		
22	71.6	49	120.2	76	168.8		
23	73.4	50	122	77	170.6		
24	75.2	51	123.8	78	172.4		
25	77	52	125.6	79	174.2		
26	78.8	53	127.4	80	176		

mercury for measurement of temperature.

t., recording. Device with a suitable sensor that continuously monitors and records temperature.

t., rectal. Thermometer that is inserted into the rectum for determining body temperature.

t., self-registering. Thermometer recording variations of temperature.

t., spirit. Thermometer filled with alcohol instead of mercury for registering low temperatures.

t., surface. Thermometer for indicating temperature of the body's surface.

t., tympanic. Thermometer which determines the temperature electronically by measuring it from the tympanic membrane. SEE: *ear thermometry; temperature, tympanic.*

t., wet-and-dry-bulb. Device for determining relative humidity consisting of two thermometers, the bulb of one being kept saturated with water vapor. The difference in temperatures between the two is dependent upon relative humidity.

thermometer, disinfection of. Disinfection of a thermometer with a substance that is able to kill ordinary bacteria and *Mycobac-*

terium tuberculosis as well as viruses. A variety of chemical solutions are used, but the effectiveness of these agents can be greatly diminished if the thermometer is not washed thoroughly prior to being disinfected.

thermometric (thĕr″mō-mĕt′rĭk) [Gr. *therme*, heat, + *metron*, measure]. Pert. to heat measurement or a thermometer.

thermometry (thĕr-mŏm′ĕ-trē). Measurement of temperature.

t., clinical. Oral temperature of the healthy body ranges between 96.6° and 100°F (35.9° and 37.8°C). During a 24-hour period, a person's body temperature may vary from 0.5° to 2.0°F (0.28° to 1.1°C). It is highest in late afternoon and lowest during sleep in early hours of the morning. Slightly increased by eating, exercising, and external heat; reduced about 1.5°F (0.8°C) during sleep. In disease the temperature of the body deviates several degrees above or below that considered the average in healthy persons.

In acute infections such as meningitis, pneumonia, scarlatina, typhoid, typhus, smallpox, and intermittent fever, body temperature sometimes rises as high as 106° to

107°F (41.1° to 41.7°C). In other febrile diseases, it rarely reaches 104°F (40°C). However, temperature may reach as high as 110°F (43.3°C) in sunstroke. The lowest extreme of temperature is found sometimes in the cold stage of cholera, when temperature may be very low (85° to 90°F or 29.4° to 32.2°C) for several days.

Subnormal temperatures, below 98°F (36.7°C), are observed in the following conditions: during convalescence from certain febrile conditions; after pneumonia and typhoid fever; in collapse resulting from shock, hemorrhage, or rupture of a viscus, as the bowel in typhoid or the stomach in perforating ulcer.

In general, for every degree of fever the pulse rises 10 beats per minute, but elevation of temperature to 99.5°F (37.5°C) provides greater evidence of disease than a pulse rate increase from 70 to 90 beats per minute. If temperature remains above normal after general symptoms subside during convalescence, the patient is in danger of a relapse or the supervention of some other disease. The range of the increase of heat in different febrile diseases extends to 110°F (43.3°C) or more and as a rule the amount of increase is a criterion of the intensity of the disease.

Artificial fever induced through diathermy, continuous hot bath, or malarial injections was formerly utilized in treating some diseases but is seldom used in modern medicine.

thermoneurosis (thĕr″mō-nū-rō′sĭs) [Gr. *therme*, heat, + *neuron*, nerve, + *osis*, condition]. Elevation of body temperature in hysteria and other nervous conditions.

thermonuclear (thĕr″mō-nū′klē-ăr). Concerning thermonuclear reactions.

thermopenetration (thĕr″mō-pĕn-ĕ-trā′shŭn) [″ + L. *penetrare*, to go within]. Application of heat to the deeper tissues of the body by diathermy. SYN: *thermoradiotherapy.*

thermoperiodicity (thĕr″mō-pĕr-ē-ō-dĭs′ĭ-tē). Condition in which an organism grows better when exposed to alternating high and low temperatures.

thermophagy (thĕr-mŏf′ă-jē) [″ + *phagein*, to eat]. Eating of extremely hot food.

thermophilic (thĕr″mō-fĭl′ĭk) [″ + *philein*, to love]. Preferring or thriving best at high temperatures, said of bacteria that thrive best at temperatures between 40° and 70°C (104° and 158°F).

thermophils (thĕr′mō-fĭlz). Organisms that grow best at elevated temperatures, i.e., 40° to 70°C.

thermophobia (thĕr″mō-fō′bē-ă) [″ + *phobos*, fear]. Abnormal dread of heat.

thermophore (thĕr′mō-for) [″ + *phoros*, a bearer]. Apparatus for applying heat to a part, consisting of water heater and tubes conveying water to a coil and returning to heater, or salts that produce heat when moistened.

thermophylic (thĕr″mō-fĭ′lĭk) [″ + *phylake*, guard]. Resistant to destruction by heat, characteristic of certain bacteria.

thermopile (thĕr′mō-pīl) [″ + L. *pila*, pile]. In physical therapy, a thermoelectric battery used in measuring small variations in the degree of heat. It consists of a number of connected dissimilar metallic plates. Under the influence of heat, these produce an electric current.

thermoplacentography (thĕr″mō-plăs″ĕn-tŏg′ră-fē) [″ + L. *placenta*, a flat cake, + Gr. *graphein*, to write]. Use of thermography for determining the location of placental attachment.

thermoplastic (thĕr″mō-plăs′tĭk). Concerning or being softened or made malleable by heat.

thermoplegia (thĕr″mō-plē′jē-ă) [″ + *plege*, a stroke]. Heatstroke.

thermopolypnea (thĕr″mō-pŏl-ĭp-nē′ă) [″ + *polys*, many, + *pnoia*, breath]. Quickened breathing caused by high fever or great heat.

thermoradiotherapy (thĕr″mō-rā″dē-ō-thĕr′ă-pē) [″ + L. *radius*, ray, + Gr. *therapeia*, treatment]. Application of heat to deep tissues by diathermy. SYN: *thermopenetration.*

thermoreceptor (thĕr″mō-rē-sĕp′tor) [″ + L. *receptor*, a receiver]. A sensory receptor that is stimulated by a rise of body temperature.

thermoregulation (thĕr″mō-rĕg″ū-lā′shŭn). Heat regulation.

thermoregulatory (thĕr″mō-rĕg″ū-lă-tor′ē). Pert. to the regulation of temperature, esp. body temperature.

thermoregulatory centers. Centers in the hypothalamus that regulate heat production and heat loss, esp. the latter, so that a normal body temperature is maintained. They are influenced by nervous impulses from cutaneous receptors and by the temperature of the blood flowing through them.

thermoresistant (thĕr″mō-rē-zĭs′tănt) [″ + L. *resistentia*, resistance]. Ability to survive in relatively high temperature. Characteristic of some types of bacteria.

thermostabile (thĕr″mō-stā′bl) [″ + L. *stabilis*, stable]. Not changed or destroyed by heat.

thermostasis (thĕr″mō-stā′sĭs) [″ + *stasis*, standing still]. The maintenance of body temperature.

thermostat (thĕr′mō-stăt) [″ + *statikos*,

standing]. An automatic device for regulating the temperature.

thermosteresis (thĕr″mō-stĕ-rē′sĭs) [″ + steresis, deprivation]. The deprivation of or loss of heat.

thermosterilization. Bacterial sterilization by use of heat.

thermosystaltic (thĕr″mō-sĭs-tăl′tĭk) [Gr. therme, heat, + systellein, to contract]. Pert. to contraction of the muscles under stimulus of heat.

thermotactic, thermotaxic (thĕr″mō-tăk′tĭk, -tăks′ĭk) [″ + taktikos, regulating]. Rel. to regulation of the body temperature.

thermotaxis (thĕr″mō-tăks′ĭs) [″ + taxis, arrangement]. 1. Regulation of bodily temperature. 2. Reaction of organisms or of protoplasm in the living body to heat. 3. The movement of certain organisms or cells toward (positive thermotaxis) or away from (negative thermotaxis) heat. SYN: thermotropism.

thermotherapeutics (thĕr″mō-thĕr-ă-pū′tĭks) [″ + therapeutike, treatment]. Use of heat in treatment of disease. SYN: thermotherapy.

thermotherapy (thĕr″mō-thĕr′ă-pē) [″ + therapeia, treatment]. The therapeutic application of heat. Heat may be applied locally by radiant heating devices that give off infrared rays and by conductive heating that utilizes hot water bottles, paraffin baths, and hot packs. The temperature of the body may be increased by artificial fever, by raising environmental temperature, or by preventing heat loss from the body. SEE: heat; hyperthermia.

thermotics (thĕr-mŏt′ĭks). The science of heat.

thermotolerant (thĕr″mō-tŏl′ĕr-ănt) [″ + L. tolerare, to tolerate]. Able to live normally in high temperature.

thermotonometer (thĕr″mō-tō-nŏm′ĕ-tĕr) [″ + tonos, tension, + metron, measure]. Device for measuring muscle contraction caused by heat stimuli.

thermotoxin (thĕr″mō-tŏks′ĭn) [″ + toxikon, poison]. A poison formed in the tissues as a result of excessive heat.

thermotropism (thĕr-mŏt′rō-pĭzm) [″ + trope, turning, + -ismos, condition]. Thermotaxis.

theroid (thē′royd) [Gr. theriodes, beastlike]. Having animal instincts and characteristics.

thiabendazole (thī″ă-bĕn′dă-zōl). USP. An antihelmintic drug used in treating cutaneous larva migrans and strongyloidiasis. Trade name is Mintezol.

thiaminase (thī-ăm′ĭ-nās). An enzyme that hydrolyzes thiamine.

thiamine hydrochloride. $C_{12}H_{17}ClN_4OS \cdot HCl$. A white crystalline compound occurring naturally and produced synthetically. It is widely distributed in various animal and plant foods, dry yeast and wheat germ being the richest natural sources. It is present in the outer layers of seeds and in nuts, legumes, most vegetables, and in some meats (pork, muscle, liver, heart, and kidneys). SYN: vitamin B_1.

FUNCT: It is essential for the normal metabolism of carbohydrates and fats. It acts as a coenzyme of carboxylases in the carboxylation of pyruvic acid, hence is essential for the liberation of energy and disposal of pyruvic acid.

DEFICIENCY SYM: Moderate deficiency results in impaired functioning of nervous, circulatory, digestive, and endocrine systems. Neurasthenia, neurological disorders, and cardiac and gastrointestinal symptoms may result. Loss of appetite, fatigue, muscle tenderness, and increased irritability are symptoms. Severe and prolonged deficiency results in beriberi, q.v.

DAILY REQUIREMENTS: For children and adults 0.5 mg per 1000 Cal of food intake.

thiamine monohitrate. USP. Thiamine in which the chloride has been replaced by nitrate.

thiamine pyrophosphate. An enzyme important in carbohydrate metabolism. It is the active form of thiamine. SYN: cocarboxylase.

thiamylal sodium for injection (thī-ăm′ĭ-lăl). USP. An ultra-short-acting barbiturate. Trade name is Surital.

thiemia (thī-ē′mē-ă) [Gr. theion, sulfur, + haima, blood]. An excess of sulfur in the blood.

Thiersch's graft (tērsh′ĕz) [Karl Thiersch, Ger. surgeon, 1822–1895]. A method of skin grafting using epidermis and a portion of the dermis.

thiethylperazine malate (thī-ĕth″ĭl-pĕr′ă-zēn). USP. An antiemetic drug.

thigh (thī) [AS. theoh]. The proximal portion of the lower extremity; the portion lying between the hip joint and the knee. SEE: femur; hip; pectineus; sartorius.

thigmesthesia (thĭg″mĕs-thē′zē-ă) [Gr. thigma, touch, + aisthesis, sensation]. Sensitivity to touch.

thigmotaxis (thĭg″mō-tăks′ĭs) [″ + taxis, arrangement]. The negative or positive response of certain motile cells to touch.

thigmotropism (thĭg-mŏt′rō-pĭzm) [″ + tropos, a turning, + -ismos, condition]. The response of certain motile cells to move toward something that touches them.

thimerosal (thī-měr′ō-săl). USP. An organic mercurial antiseptic used topically and as a preservative in pharmaceutical preparations. Trade name is Merthiolate.

thinking. The highest order of intellectual activity, but it is difficult to describe and analyze. Involved in thinking are the interpretation and ordering of symbols for learning, for organizing information, and for problem solving. The logical progression of this process would be to have and develop the capacity to reason and form sound judgments.

thin-layer chromatography. ABBR: TLC. Chromatography involving the adsorption and partitioning of compounds on a thin porous solid applied as a thin layer on a glass plate.

thinning hair. Colloquialism for loss of hair from the scalp, i.e., as in becoming bald.

thio- [Gr. *theion*, sulfur]. Prefix denoting the presence of sulfur replacing oxygen.

thiocyanate (thī″ō-sī′ă-nāt). Any compound containing the radical —SCN.

thiogenic (thī″ō-jěn′ĭk) [Gr. *theion*, sulfur, + *gennan*, to produce]. Able to convert hydrogen sulfide into higher sulfur compounds, said of bacteria in the water of some mineral springs.

thioglucosidase (thī″ō-glū-kō′sĭ-dās). An enzyme that catalyzes the hydrolysis of thioglycoside to a thiol and a sugar.

thioguanine (thī″ō-gwă′nēn). USP. An antimetabolite used in treating certain types of leukemia. It also acts as an immunosuppressant.

thioneine (thī′ō-nēn) [″ + *neos*, new]. Thiolhistidine-betaine, a compound containing crystalline sulfur. Found in ergot and red blood cells. Also: *ergothioneine.*

thionic (thī′ō-nĭk). Concerning sulfur.

thiopectic, thiopexic (thī-ō-pĕk′tĭk, -pĕks′ ĭk) [″ + *pexis*, fixation]. Pert. to the fixation of sulfur.

thiopental sodium (thī″ō-pĕn′tăl). USP. An ultra-short-acting barbiturate used as an adjuvant in surgical anesthesia. Trade name is Pentothal Sodium.

thiopexy (thī″ō-pĕks′ē). The fixation of sulfur.

thiophil, thiophilic (thī″ō-fĭl, thī″ō-fĭl′ĭk) [Gr. *theion*, sulfur, + *philein*, to love]. Thriving in the presence of sulfur or its compounds, which is true of some bacteria.

thioridazine hydrochloride (thī″ō-rĭd′ă-zēn). USP. An antipsychotic drug. Trade name is Mellaril.

thiosulfate (thī″ō-sŭl′fāt). Any salt of thiosulfuric acid.

Thiosulfil. Trade name for sulfamethizole.

thiotepa (thī″ō-tē′pă). USP. An alkylating agent that is cytotoxic. It is used in treating certain types of neoplasms.

Caution: Great care should be taken to prevent inhaling particles of thiotepa or exposing the skin to it.

---

thiothixene (thī″ō-thĭks′ēn). USP. An antipsychotic drug. Trade name is Navane.

thiouracil (thī″ō-ū′ră-sĭl). An antithyroid drug that is little used now. SEE: *propylthiouracil.*

thiourea (thī″ō-ūr-ē′ă) [Gr. *theion*, sulfur, + *ouron*, urine]. Colorless crystalline compound of urea in which sulfur replaces the oxygen. SYN: *sulfourea.*

thiram (thī′răm). An antifungal agent.

thiram poisoning. Toxic exposure may occur in those engaged either in manufacturing or applying this compound in agricultural work.

third cranial nerve. Oculomotor nerve. SEE: *cranial nerves.*

third intention. Healing of a wound by filling with granulations. SEE: *healing.*

third ventricle. Third ventricle of the brain, a narrow cavity between the two optic thalami. It communicates anteriorly with the lateral ventricles and posteriorly, via the cerebral aqueduct of Sylvius, with the 4th ventricle. SYN: *ventriculus tertius.*

thirst [AS. *thurst*]. 1. Desire for fluid, esp. for water. It may occur in fevers and certain other maladies, or it may be entirely lacking in some conditions. The nurse should note whether the intake of fluids allays the patient's thirst. 2. The sensation resulting from the lack of or the need for water. Thirst may result from drying of mucous membranes, esp. those of the pharynx, or from reduced salivary secretion. It also results from general dehydration, as may occur following hemorrhage, profuse sweating, vomiting, or excessive loss of urine as in diabetes mellitus or insipidus. SEE: *adipsia; anadipsia; aposia.*

Thiry's fistula (tē′rēz) [Ludwig Thiry, Austrian physiologist, 1817–1897]. An artificial fistula placed in a dog's intestines for obtaining intestinal juices for experimental purposes.

Thiuretic. Trade name for hydrochlorothiazide.

thixolabile (thĭk″sō-lā′bĭl). Especially susceptible to being changed by shaking.

thixotropy (thĭks-ŏt′rō-pē) [Gr. *thixis*, a touching, + *trope*, turning]. The property of certain gels in which they liquefy when agitated and revert to a gel upon standing.

thlipsencephalus (thlĭp″sĕn-sĕf′ă-lŭs) [Gr. *thlipsis*, pressure, + *enkephalos*, brain].

A deformed fetus with a malformed or absent skull.

Thomas splint [Hugh Owen Thomas, Brit. orthopedic surgeon, 1834–1891]. A splint originally developed to treat hip-joint disease. It is now used mainly to place traction on the leg in its long axis. It is used in treating fractures of the upper leg. It consists of a proximal ring that fits around the upper leg and to which two long rigid slender steel rods are attached. These extend down to another smaller ring distal to the foot.

Thomas-White hypothesis [Clayton Thomas, b. 1921, U.S. physician; Arthur White, b. 1925, U.S. physician]. The hypothesis that there will eventually be reported a congenital abnormality in which a fetus has two umbilici.

Thomsen's disease (tŏm′sĕnz) [Asmus Julius Thomsen, Danish physician, 1815–1896]. Myotonia congenita, q.v.

thoracalgia (thō″răk-ăl′jē-ă) [Gr. *thorakos*, chest, + *algos*, pain]. Pain in the chest wall. SYN: *pleurodynia*.

thoracectomy (thō″ră-sĕk′tō-mē) [″ + *ektome*, excision]. Incision of the chest wall with resection of a portion of rib.

thoracentesis (thō″ră-sĕn-tē′sĭs) [″ + *kentesis*, a puncture]. Surgical puncture of the chest wall for removal of fluids. Usually done by using a large-bore needle. SYN: *pleurocentesis; thoracocentesis*.

NURSING IMPLICATIONS: Before procedure obtain chest x-ray report if available. Explain procedure to patient and verify signed consent. Prepare patient for sensations that may be experienced and emphasize importance of remaining still during the procedure. Obtain baseline vital signs. Identify allergies and administer sedative if prescribed. Position the patient comfortably. Assist physician and support patient throughout procedure. Check the patient's vital signs frequently throughout the procedure and assess for dizziness, faintness, tachycardia, dyspnea, chest pain, nausea, pallor or cyanosis, weakness, diaphoresis, and cough or expectoration of blood. Apply occlusive dressing to puncture wound as needle or cannula is removed. Send specimen for desired diagnostic testing and document procedure and patient response. Arrange for postprocedure chest x-ray to detect pneumothorax, and evaluate results. Continue to monitor vital signs and dressing status and assess patient for coughing or expectoration of blood.

thoracic (thō-răs′ĭk) [Gr. *thorax*, chest]. Pert. to the chest or thorax.

thoracic cage. The bony structure surrounding the thorax, consisting of the 12 paired ribs, the thoracic vertebrae, and the sternum.

thoracic cavity. The space lying above the diaphragm and enclosed within the walls of the thorax; the space occupied by the thoracic viscera. It includes the pleural cavities occupied by the lungs and the mediastinum, the space between the lungs (which is occupied by the heart, lying within the pericardium), the thoracic aorta, pulmonary artery and veins, vena cava, thymus gland, lymph nodes, trachea, bronchi, esophagus, and thoracic duct. It is separated from the abdominal cavity by the diaphragm. SEE: *lymphatic system* for illus.

RS: chyle; cisterna chyli; lacteal; lymphatic; lymphatic system.

thoracic duct. The main lymph duct of the body, having its origin at the cisterna chyli on the abdomen. It passes upward through the diaphragm into the thorax, continuing upward alongside the aorta and esophagus to the neck, where it turns to the left and enters the left subclavian vein near its junction with the left internal jugular vein. It receives lymph from all parts of the body except the right side of the head, neck, and thorax and right upper extremity.

thoracic limbs. Upper extremities.

thoracicoabdominal (thō-răs″ĭ-kō-ăb-dŏm′ĭ-năl). Concerning the thorax and abdomen.

thoracicohumeral (thō-răs″ĭ-kō-hū′mĕr-ăl). Concerning the thorax and humerus bone.

thoracic outlet compression syndrome. A symptom complex caused by conditions in which nerves or vessels are compressed in the neck or axilla. Anatomically, the cause is compression by structures, such as the first rib pressing against the clavicle. Also, the condition may be associated with a cervical rib or scalenus anticus syndrome. It is characterized by brachial neuritis with or without vascular or vasomotor disturbance in the upper extremities. The condition may be confused with cervical disk lesions; osteoarthritis affecting cervical vertebrae; bursitis; brachial plexus injury; angina; and cancer of the lung.

thoracic squeeze. A rare occurrence in divers who are skilled enough to go approx. 80 to 100 feet (24.4 to 30.5 meters) deep while holding their breath. The lungs become compressed sufficiently to cause rupture of alveolar capillaries.

TREAT: Immediate removal from the water; artificial respiration preferably with an apparatus that will deliver increased oxygen concentration rather than just air.

thoracic surgery. Surgery involving the rib cage and structures contained within the thoracic cage.

NURSING IMPLICATIONS: *Preop:* Preparation involves the usual preop teaching, with special emphasis on breathing and coughing, incisional splinting, pain evaluation, invasive and noninvasive relief measures that will be available, and basic information about the chest drainage tube and system that will be required in most such surgeries. Encourage patient to voice fears and concerns, allay misapprehensions, and correct misconceptions. *Postop:* Monitor vital signs and breath sounds. Maintain water-seal chest drainage as prescribed, and monitor volume and characteristics of drainage. Maintain sterile impervious wound dressings. Provide analgesia and comfort measures to insure patient cooperation with respiratory toilet, exercises, and rest and activity. Provide emotional support and encouragement. Provide instructions to be followed by patient and family after discharge, and follow-up care.

thoraco- [Gr. *thorakos,* chest]. Combining form meaning chest or chest wall.

thoracoacromial (thō″ră-kō-ă-krō′mē-ăl). Concerning the thorax and acromion.

thoracobronchotomy (thō″răk-ō-brŏn-kŏt′ō-mē) [″ + *bronchos,* windpipe, + *tome,* incision]. Incision through the thoracic wall into the bronchus.

thoracocautery (thō″răk-ō-kaw′tĕr-ē) [″ + *kauterion,* branding iron]. The use of cautery in breaking up pulmonary adhesions to collapse the lung.

thoracoceloschisis (thō″răk-ō-sē-lŏs′kĭ-sĭs) [Gr. *thorakos,* chest, + *koilia,* belly, + *schisis,* a splitting]. Congenital fissure of the thoracic and abdominal cavities.

thoracocentesis (thō″răk-ō-sĕn-tē′sĭs) [″ + *kentesis,* a puncture]. Surgical entry into the thoracic cavity in order to remove fluid. Usually done by using a needle. SYN: *thoracentesis.*

thoracodelphus (thō″ră-kō-dĕl′fŭs) [″ + *adelphos,* brother]. A deformed fetus with a single head and thorax, but four legs.

thoracodidymus (thō″ră-kō-dĭd′ĭ-mŭs) [″ + *didymos,* twin]. Conjoined twins united at the thorax.

thoracodynia (thō″răk-ō-dĭn′ē-ă) [″ + *odyne,* pain]. Pain in the thorax.

thoracogastroschisis (thō″răk-ō-găs-trŏs′kĭ-sĭs) [″ + *gaster,* belly, + *schisis,* a splitting]. Congenital fissure of abdomen and thorax.

thoracograph (thō-răk′ō-grăf) [″ + *graphein,* to write]. Device for plotting and recording the contour of the thorax and its change during inspiration and expiration.

thoracolaparotomy (thō″ră-kō-lăp″ă-rŏt′ō-mē) [″ + *lapara,* loin, + *tome,* incision]. Surgical incision of the thoracic wall and the diaphragm in order to gain access to adjacent areas.

thoracolumbar (thō″răk-ō-lŭm′bar) [″ + L. *lumbus,* loin]. Pert. to the thoracic and lumbar parts of the spine; noting their ganglia and the fibers of the sympathetic nervous system.

thoracolysis (thō″răk-ŏl′ĭ-sĭs) [″ + *lysis,* dissolution]. The freeing of a lung that is attached to the chest wall. SYN: *pneumonolysis.*

thoracomelus (thō″ră-kŏm′ē-lŭs) [″ + *melos,* limb]. A deformed fetus with an extra leg attached to the thorax.

thoracometer (thō″ră-kŏm′ē-tĕr) [Gr. *thorakos,* chest, + *metron,* measure]. Device for measuring the expansion of the chest.

thoracometry (thō″ră-kŏm′ĕt-rē) [″ + *metron,* measure]. The measurement of the thorax.

thoracomyodynia (thō″ră-kō-mī″ō-dĭn′ē-ă) [″ + *mys,* muscle, + *odyne,* pain]. Pain in chest muscles.

thoracopagus (thō″ră-kŏp′ă-gŭs) [″ + *pagos,* fixed]. Two malformed fetuses joined at the thorax.

thoracoparacephalus (thō″ră-kō-păr″ă-sĕf′ă-lŭs) [″ + *para,* beside, + *kephale,* head]. Thoracopagus twins in which a rudimentary head is attached to the smaller twin.

thoracopathy (thō″răk-ŏp′ă-thē) [″ + *pathos,* disease, suffering]. Any disease of the thorax, thoracic organs, or tissues.

thoracoplasty (thō″ră-kō-plăs″tē, thō-rā′kō-plăs″tē) [″ + *plassein,* to form]. A plastic operation upon the thorax; removal of portions of the ribs in stages to collapse diseased areas of the lung. SEE: *empyema.*

thoracopneumoplasty (thō″ră-kō-nū′mō-plăs-tē) [″ + *pneumon,* lung, + *plassein,* to form]. Plastic surgery involving the chest and lung.

thoracoschisis (thō″ră-kŏs′kĭ-sĭs) [″ + *schisis,* a splitting]. Congenital fissure of the chest wall.

thoracoscope (thō-rā′kō-skōp, -răk′ō-skōp) [″ + *skopein,* to examine]. 1. Instrument for inspection of the thoracic cavity. It has an electric light and is inserted through an intercostal space. 2. Instrument used in auscultation to convey the sounds of the chest to the ear. SYN: *stethoscope.*

thoracoscopy (thō″ră-kŏs′kō-pē). Diagnostic examination of the pleural cavity with an endoscope.

thoracostenosis (thō″ră-kō-stĕn-ō′sĭs) [″ + *stenosis,* act of narrowing]. Narrowness of the thorax due to atrophy of trunk muscles. SYN: *wasp waist.*

thoracostomy (thō″răk-ŏs′tō-mē) [″ + *stoma,* mouth]. Resection of chest wall to allow drainage of the chest cavity.

thoracotomy (thō″răk-ŏt′ō-mē) [″ +

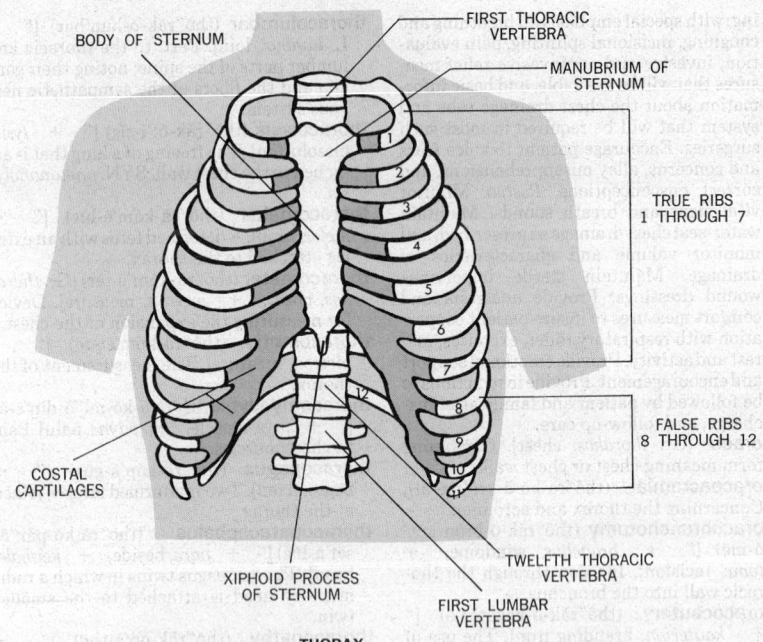

THORAX

tome, incision]. Surgical incision of the chest wall.

thorax (thō′răks) [Gr., chest] (pl. *thoraces*, *thoraxes*). [NA] That part of the body between the base of the neck superiorly and the diaphragm inferiorly.

The surface of the thorax is divided into regions as follows: *Anterior surface:* supraclavicular, above the clavicles; suprasternal, above the sternum; clavicular, over the clavicles; sternal, over the sternum; mammary, the space between the 3rd and 6th ribs on either side; inframammary, below the lower border of the mamma and above the lower border of the 12th rib on either side. *Posterior surface:* scapular, over the scapulae; interscapular, between the scapulae; infrascapular, below the scapulae. *On sides:* axillary, above the 6th rib. SYN: *chest.* SEE: illus.

RS: acromiothoracic; cholohemothorax; "thorac-" words.

t., barrel-shaped. A malformed chest rounded like a barrel seen in advanced pulmonary emphysema.

t., bony. The part of the skeleton that is made up of the thoracic vertebrae, 12 pairs of ribs and the sternum.

t. paralyticus. The long, flat chest of patients with constitutional visceroptosis.

t., Peyrot′s. A chest that has an obliquely oval deformed shape, seen with large pleural effusions.

Thorazine. Trade name for chlorpromazine hydrochloride. It is an antipsychotic agent useful in controlling excited psychotic behavior. It is also valuable as an antiemetic. Use with caution when administering concomitantly with sedatives and general anesthetics, as it potentiates their actions.

Thorel′s bundle (tō′rĕlz) [Christen Thorel, Ger. physician, 1880–1935]. A muscle bundle in the heart that connects the sinoatrial and atrioventricular nodes and passes medial to the orifice of the inferior vena cava.

thorium (thō′rē-ŭm). SYMB: Th. At. wt. 232.038; at. no. 90. A metallic element that is radioactive. At one time it was used to outline blood vessels in roentgenography.

Thorn test [George W. Thorn, U.S. physician, b. 1906]. Administration of corticotrophin, which causes a decrease in circulating eosinophils of a normal person, but does not cause a decrease if given to patients with adrenal insufficiency.

thoron (thō′rŏn). SYMB: Tn. At. wt. 220; at. no. 86. A radioactive isotope of radon. It has a half-life of 51.5 seconds.

thread (thrĕd). 1. Any thin filamentous structure, e.g., a stringy substance present in the urine in some infectious diseases of the urinary tract. 2. Suture material.

threadworm. Common name applied to the pinworm, *Enterobius vermicularis.*

three-day fever. A viral disease transmitted by the sandfly, *Phlebotomus papatasii.* The disease resembles dengue but is less severe. SYN: *sandfly fever.*

thremmatology (thrĕm″ă-tŏl′ō-jē) [Gr. *thremma,* nursling, + *logos,* word, reason]. Scientific breeding of plants and animals.

threonine (thrē′ō-nīn). Alpha-amino-beta-hydroxy butyric acid. One of the essential amino acids.

threshold (thrĕsh′ōld) [AS. *therscold*]. 1. Point at which a psychological or physiological effect begins to be produced. 2. A measure of the sensitivity of an organ or function that is obtained by finding the lowest value of the appropriate stimulus that will give the response.

 t., absolute. The lowest amount or intensity of a stimulus that will give rise to a sensation or a response.

 t., acoustic reflex. SEE: *acoustic reflex threshold.*

 t., auditory. Minimum audible sound perceived.

 t., differential. The lowest limit at which two stimuli can be differentiated from each other.

 t., erythema. Stage in which erythema of the skin due to radiation just begins.

 t., ketosis. The lower limit at which ketone bodies (acetoacetic acid, hydroxybutyric acid, and acetone), upon their accumulation in the blood, are excreted by the kidney. At that point ketone bodies are being produced faster by the liver than the body can oxidize them.

 t. of consciousness. In psychoanalysis, point at which a stimulus is just barely perceived.

 t., renal. The concentration at which a substance in the blood normally not excreted by the kidney begins to appear in the urine. The renal threshold for glucose is 160 to 180 mg/dl.

 t., sensory. The minimal stimulus for any sensory receptor that will give rise to a sensation.

 t. stimulus. The least or minimal stimulus that will give rise to a sensation or bring about a response such as a muscle contraction. SYN: *liminal stimulus.* SEE: *rheobase.*

threshold dose. Minimum dose that will produce an effect on the patient.

threshold substance. A substance present in the blood that, on being filtered through glomeruli of the kidney, is reabsorbed by the tubules up to a certain limit, that being the upper limit of the concentration of the substance in normal plasma. High-threshold substances are those that are entirely or almost entirely reabsorbed. Ex.: chlorides; glucose. Low-threshold substances are those that are reabsorbed in limited quantities. Ex.: phosphates; urea. No-threshold substances are those excreted in their entirety. Ex.: creatinine sulfate.

thrifty. Thriving, growing vigorously, and being healthy, esp. when assessing the health status of animals or plants. SEE: *unthrifty.*

thrill (thrĭl) [ME. *thrillen,* to pierce]. 1. Abnormal tremor accompanying a vascular or cardiac murmur felt on palpation. SYN: *fremitus.* 2. A tingling or shivering sensation of tremulous excitement as from pain, pleasure, or horror.

 t., aneurysmal. Thrill felt on palpation of an aneurysm.

 t., aortic. Thrill heard over aortic aperture on lesions of valves.

 t., arterial. Thrill heard over an artery.

 t., diastolic. Thrill felt over the heart during diastole of the ventricle.

 t., hydatid. Peculiar tremor felt on palpation of a hydatid cyst.

 t., presystolic. Thrill sometimes felt over apex of the heart preceding ventricular contraction.

 t., systolic. Thrill felt during systole over the precordium. It may be associated with aortic or pulmonary stenosis, or interventricular septal defect.

thrix. Hair.

 t. annulata. Hair with light and dark segments alternating along the shaft.

-thrix [Gr. *thrix,* hair]. A word ending indicating hair.

throat (thrōt) [AS. *throte*]. 1. The pharynx and fauces. 2. Cavity from the arch of the palate to the glottis and superior opening of the esophagus. 3. The anterior portion of the neck. 4. Any narrow orifice.

throat, foreign bodies in. Symptoms depend somewhat on the location and size of the foreign body, and vary from simple discomfort to distressing coughing, difficulty in breathing, retching, and cyanosis. If not relieved, suffocation results in unconsciousness.

 If the symptoms are relieved but it is not known whether the foreign body has been removed, it is important to seek medical attention in case the object has moved farther down the respiratory tract.

 F.A.: If complete airway obstruction is present as evidenced by inability to speak or absence of intake of air, the Heimlich maneuver should be performed. It consists of

(1) wrapping your arms around victim's waist from behind; (2) making a fist with one hand and placing it against the victim's abdomen between the navel and rib cage; (3) clasping your fist with your free hand and pressing in with a quick, forceful upward thrust. Repeat several times if necessary. If the airway remains obstructed, tracheostomy will be required to save the patient's life. SEE: *Heimlich maneuver* for illus.

Caution: Do not perform the Heimlich maneuver unless complete airway obstruction is present. If the patient is able to cough, do not perform the Heimlich maneuver. In children and infants, place in head-down position to facilitate removal of obstruction.

throb (thrŏb) [ME. *throbben,* of imitative origin]. 1. A beat or pulsation, as of the heart. 2. To pulsate.

throbbing (thrŏb'ĭng). Pulsation; a beating rhythmic movement.

Throckmorton's reflex (thrŏk'mor"tŭnz) [Thomas Bentley Throckmorton, U.S. neurologist, 1885–1961]. Extension of great toe and flexion of others when dorsum of foot is percussed in metatarsophalangeal region.

throe (thrō) [AS. *thruve,* paroxysm]. A severe spasm of pain.

thrombase (thrŏm'bās). Thrombin.

thrombasthenia (thrŏm"băs-thē'nē-ă) [Gr. *thrombos,* clot, + *astheneia,* weakness]. A hemorrhagic disorder due to abnormal platelet function characterized by abnormal clot retraction, prolonged bleeding time, and lack of aggregation of the platelets on a blood smear.

thrombectomy (thrŏm-bĕk'tō-mē) [" + *ektome,* excision]. Excision of a thrombus.

thrombi (thrŏm'bī). Pl. of thrombus.

thrombin (thrŏm'bĭn) [Gr. *thrombos,* clot]. 1. An enzyme formed in shed blood from prothrombin, which reacts with soluble fibrinogen converting it to fibrin, which forms the basis of a blood clot. SEE: *coagulation, blood.* 2. USP. A sterile plasma protein substance prepared from prothrombin of bovine origin. Used topically to control capillary oozing during surgical procedures. Used alone, it is not capable of controlling arterial bleeding.

thrombinogen (thrŏm-bĭn'ō-jĕn). An obsolete term for prothrombin.

thrombo- [Gr.]. Combining form meaning clot of blood; a thrombus.

thromboangiitis (thrŏm"bō-ăn"jē-ī'tĭs) [Gr. *thrombos,* clot, + *angeion,* vessel, + *itis,* inflammation]. Inflammation of inner coat of a blood vessel with clot formation. SEE: *thrombosis.*

   t. obliterans. A chronic, recurring, inflammatory, vascular occlusive disease, chiefly of the peripheral arteries and veins of the extremities. The disease is seen most commonly in males 20 to 40 years of age who smoke cigarettes. SYN: *Buerger's disease.*

   SYM: Occlusion; thrombosis; excruciating pain in leg or foot that is worse at night; cyanotic, clammy, cold extremity; diminished sense of heat and cold; gangrene of toes or foot may develop.

thromboarteritis (thrŏm"bō-ăr-tĕ-rī'tĭs) [" + *arteria,* artery, + *itis,* inflammation]. Inflammation of an artery in connection with thrombosis.

thromboclasis (thrŏm-bŏk'lă-sĭs) [" + *klasis,* a breaking]. The breaking up or lysis of a thrombus. SYN: *thrombolysis.*

thromboclastic (thrŏm"bō-klăs'tĭk). Pert. to or producing the dissolution of a thrombus. SYN: *thrombolytic.*

thrombocyst (thrŏm'bō-sĭst) [Gr. *thrombos,* clot, + *kystis,* a sac]. A membranous sac enveloping a thrombus. Also: *thrombocystis.*

thrombocyte (thrŏm'bō-sīt) [" + *kytos,* cell]. An old term for a blood platelet.

thrombocythemia (thrŏm"bō-sī-thē'mē-ă) [" + " + *haima,* blood]. An absolute increase in the number of platelets in the blood.

thrombocytocrit (thrŏm"bō-sī'tō-krĭt) [" + " + *krinein,* to separate]. Device for estimating the platelet content of the blood.

thrombocytolysis (thrŏm"bō-sī-tŏl'ĭ-sĭs) [" + " + *lysis,* dissolution]. Dissolution of thrombocytes.

thrombocytopathy (thrŏm"bō-sī-tŏp'ă-thē) [" + " + *pathos,* disease, suffering]. Deficient function of platelets.

thrombocytopenia (thrŏm"bō-sī"tō-pē'nē-ă) [" + " + *penia,* lack]. Abnormal decrease in number of the blood platelets. SYN: *thrombopenia.*

   NURSING IMPLICATIONS: Watch for signs of internal hemorrhage, esp. intracranial, and handle the patient gently to prevent trauma and hemorrhage. Observe carefully for signs of hemorrhage such as hematuria, hematemesis, bleeding gums, abdominal distention, melena, prolonged menstruation, epistaxis, ecchymosis, petechiae, or purpura. Evaluate emesis, urine, and stools for evidence of occult bleeding. Control bleeding by applying pressure to bleeding sites. Promote bedrest to prevent excessive activity and exhaustion. Advise the patient to avoid constipation and straining and to avoid exposure to upper respiratory infections, which may cause sneezing and coughing. Instruct the patient to prevent injury by using a soft toothbrush. If the patient shaves, an electric razor should be used. Administer platelet transfusions as prescribed and observe for chills, fever, or allergic reactions. Avoid aspirin and other nonsteroidal anti-inflammatory agents, as platelet function may be inhibited by these drugs. Administer platelet transfusions as prescribed, assessing for chills, fever, or allergic reactions. If splenectomy is performed, provide required preoperative and postoperative nursing care. Allow for time to talk with patient and for expression of patient's feelings.

thrombocytopoiesis (thrŏm″bō-sī″tō-poy-ē′sĭs) [″ + ″ + poiesis, production]. The formation of blood platelets.

thrombocytosis (thrŏm″bō-sī-tō′sĭs) [″ + kytos, cell]. Increase in number of blood platelets.

thromboembolism (thrŏm″bō-ĕm′bō-lĭzm) [″ + embolos, thrown in, + -ismos, condition]. An embolism; the blocking of a blood vessel by a thrombus that has become detached from its site of formation.

thromboendarterectomy (thrŏm″bō-ĕnd″ăr-tĕr-ĕk′tō-mē) [″ + endon, within, + arteria, artery, + ektome, excision]. Surgical removal of a thrombus from an artery, and removal of the diseased intima of the artery.

thromboendarteritis (thrŏm″bō-ĕnd-ăr″tĕr-ī′tĭs) [″ + ″ + ″ + itis, inflammation]. Thromboarteritis.

thromboendocarditis (thrŏm″bō-ĕn″dō-kăr-dī′tĭs) [″ + endon, within, + kardia, heart, + itis, inflammation]. Formation of a clot on inflamed surface of a heart valve.

thrombogenesis (thrŏm″bō-jĕn′ē-sĭs) [″ + genesis, generation, birth]. The formation of a blood clot.

thrombogenic (thrŏm″bō-jĕn′ĭk) [″ + gennan, to produce]. Producing or tending to produce a clot.

thromboid (thrŏm′boyd) [″ + eidos, form, shape]. Resembling a thrombus or clot.

thrombokinase (thrŏm″bō-kĭn′ās) [″ + kinesis, movement]. Obsolete term for the tenth blood coagulation factor (factor X) or Stuart factor, q.v.

thrombokinesis (thrŏm″bō-kĭ-nē′sĭs) [″ + kinesis, movement]. The coagulation of the blood.

thrombolymphangitis (thrŏm″bō-lĭm″făn-jī′tĭs) [″ + L. lympha, lymph, + Gr. angeion, vessel, + itis, inflammation]. Inflammation of a lymphatic vessel due to obstruction by thrombus formation.

thrombolysis (thrŏm-bŏl′ĭ-sĭs) [″ + lysis, dissolution]. The breaking up of a thrombus. SYN: thromboclasis.

thrombolytic (thrŏm-bō-lĭt′ĭk). Pert. to or causing the breaking up of a thrombus.

thrombon (thrŏm′bŏn) [Gr. thrombos, clot].

The portion of the hematopoietic system concerned with platelet formation.

thrombopathy (thrŏm-bŏp′ă-thē) [″ + pathos, disease, suffering]. A defect in the coagulation apparatus of the blood.

thrombopenia (thrŏm-bō-pē′nē-ă) [″ + penia, lack]. Abnormal decrease in the number of blood platelets.

thrombophilia (thrŏm-bō-fĭl′ē-ă) [″ + philein, to love]. A tendency to the occurrence of clot formation.

thrombophlebitis (thrŏm″bō-flē-bī′tĭs) [″ + phleps, vein, + itis, inflammation]. Inflammation of a vein in conjunction with the formation of a thrombus. Usually occurs in an extremity, most frequently a leg. SEE: phlebitis; phlegmasia alba dolens.

TREAT: The therapeutic goal is to prevent a thrombus from becoming an embolus that may reach the lung. The anticoagulant heparin is used but requires careful monitoring of the patient's response. Therapy may also include ligation of the vein proximal to the thrombus to prevent pulmonary embolism.

NURSING IMPLICATIONS: Prevent by identifying patients at risk and encouraging leg exercises, use of antiembolic stockings, and early ambulation to prevent venous stasis. Avoid prolonged pressure on the popliteal areas. Assess patient at regular intervals for signs of inflammation, tenderness, aching, positive Homans' sign, and differences in calf circumference measurements. If condition is present, follow physician's prescribed regimen regarding elevation of leg or keeping it flat and intermittent or continuous application of warm, moist heat. Administer anticoagulants as prescribed, evaluating patient for signs of bleeding, and monitor coagulation results. Instruct patient to avoid rubbing or massaging extremities. Assess patient every two hours for signs of pulmonary emboli, dyspnea, tachypnea, chest pain, changes of level of consciousness, arterial blood gas abnormalities, or ECG changes. Prepare the patient for diagnostic procedures, medical or surgical interventions prescribed. SEE: Nursing Diagnoses in Appendix.

t. migrans. Recurring attacks of thrombophlebitis in various sites.

t., postpartum, iliofemoral. Thrombophlebitis of the iliofemoral artery that occurs during the postpartum period.

thromboplastic (thrŏm″bō-plăs′tĭk) [″ + plassein, to form]. Pert. to or causing acceleration of clot formation in the blood.

thromboplastid (thrŏm″bō-plăs′tĭd). A blood platelet.

thromboplastin (thrŏm″bō-plăs′tĭn) [″ + plassein, to form]. The third blood coagulation factor (factor III), a substance found in both blood and tissues. Tissue thromboplastin is found in most parts of the body as an intracellular substance. A substance with thromboplastic activity is also present in red blood cells. Even though these two substances are separate and act in different manners, both are able to accelerate the clotting of blood.

thromboplastinogen (thrŏm″bō-plăs-tĭn′ō-jĕn). Blood clotting factor VIII. SEE: *coagulation factors.*

thrombopoiesis (thrŏm″bō-poy-ē′sĭs) [″ + *poiesis,* production]. The formation of blood platelets.

thrombosed (thrŏm′bōzd) [Gr. *thrombos,* a clot]. 1. Coagulated; clotted. 2. Denoting a vessel containing a thrombus.

thrombosinusitis (thrŏm″bō-sī-nŭs-ī′tĭs) [″ + L. *sinus,* a curve, hollow, + Gr. *itis,* inflammation]. Thrombus formation of a dural sinus.

thrombosis (thrŏm-bō′sĭs) [″ + *osis,* condition]. The formation, development, or existence of a blood clot or thrombus within the vascular system. This is a life-saving process when it occurs during hemorrhage. It is a life-threatening event when it occurs at any other time because the clot can occlude a vessel and stop the blood supply to an organ or a part. The thrombus, if detached, becomes an embolus and occludes a vessel at a distance from the original site; for example, a clot in the leg may break off and cause a pulmonary embolus.

ETIOL: Trauma, esp. following an operation and parturition; cardiac and vascular disorders, obesity, heredity, increasing age, an excess of erythrocytes and of platelets, an overproduction of fibrinogen, and sepsis are predisposing causes.

SYM: Lungs: Obstruction of smaller vessels in the lungs causes an infarct manifested by sudden pain in the side of the chest, similar to pleurisy; also the spitting of blood, a pleural friction rub, and signs of consolidation. Kidneys: Blood appears in the urine, and in small hemorrhagic spots in the skin. Spleen: Pain is felt in the left upper abdomen. Extremities: If a large artery in one of the extremities, such as the arm, is suddenly obstructed, the part becomes cold, pale, bluish, and the pulse disappears below the obstructed site. Gangrene of the digits or of the whole limb may ensue. Same symptoms may be present with an embolism, q.v.

If the limb is swollen, watch for pressure sores. Guard against burning with hot water bottle or electric pad. Prolonged bedrest may be necessary, depending on the condition of the patient.

TREAT: Anticoagulant therapy is neces-

sary. When a thrombus or embolus is large, surgical removal may be necessary.

RS: angina pectoris; embolus; "thromb-" words.

t., cardiac. Thrombosis of an artery supplying the heart muscle (myocardium).

t., coagulation. Thrombosis due to coagulation of fibrin in a blood vessel.

t., coronary. Thrombosis of a coronary artery. A common cause of myocardial infarction.

SYM: Sudden onset of severe and prolonged substernal oppression and pain, the pain arising over the precordium and being referred to the upper and middle sternum and often radiating to the left and sometimes right arm and into the neck or back. Blood pressure usually falls, pulse becomes rapid, fever and leukocytosis are usually observed within 24 hours. Erythrocyte sedimentation rate becomes elevated and electrocardiographic changes occur.

Certain enzyme tests are very helpful in diagnosing myocardial infarction. The serum level of creatine phosphokinase (CPK) is elevated in the first 24 hours following the infarction; the degree of elevation is proportional to the amount of cardiac muscle damaged. The CPK level may also be elevated if skeletal muscle damage is present. In that case other enzyme tests such as aspartate aminotransferase or lactic dehydrogenase (LDH) will be helpful in diagnosis.

TREAT: Complete physical and mental rest for a variable length of time depending upon severity. This is sometimes best accomplished by allowing the patient to rest in a reclining chair rather than a bed and to use a bedside toilet instead of having to strain to use a bedpan. Special nursing care is desirable. Prompt and complete relief from pain by use of intravenous morphine sulfate; oxygen administration sometimes necessary. Vasopressor drugs to elevate blood pressure; digitalis when there is evidence of congestive heart failure; treatment of cardiac arrhythmias, esp. tachycardia; anticoagulants. Treatment in coronary care unit is usually mandatory.

If given within the first several hours after the acute thrombosis, medicines such as streptokinase or tissue plasminogen activator (tPA) given to lyse the thrombus have greatly improved the prognosis in these patients. SEE: *streptokinase; tissue plasminogen activator.*

DIET: As requested by patient but restrict caloric intake to 1000 to 1500 Cal. Restrict salt intake and maintain record of fluid intake and output.

COMPLICATIONS: Shock; acute pulmonary edema; pulmonary embolism; paroxysmal ventricular tachycardia; congestive heart failure; aneurysm of the ventricle.

Most patients will develop some form of cardiac arrhythmia. This can be simple sinus tachycardia, bradycardia, atrial fibrillation, ventricular tachycardia, ventricular fibrillation, or cardiac arrest. The latter two are life-threatening and require prompt and diligent therapeutic intervention. Depending on the cause, the arrhythmia will be treated with one or more of the following: atropine, lidocaine, digitalis, defibrillation, or a pacemaker.

t., deep vein. Thrombosis of a vein or veins in the deep venous system of the upper or lower extremities. This may occur without obvious cause but is more likely to occur as a result of any condition that involves venous stasis or damage to the endothelial area of a vein, or as a result of conditions associated with certain surgical procedures and the accompanying inactivity of the patient. In many cases the result of this is that the thrombus will form and a portion of it will travel to the lung and create pulmonary embolism. To prevent this, anticoagulants, elastic stockings, operative thrombectomy, or vena caval interruption may be utilized. Also, a vena caval filter may be inserted to prevent emboli from entering the lung. SEE: *embolism, pulmonary.*

t., embolic. Thrombosis caused by an embolus obstructing a vessel.

t., infective. Thrombosis in which there is bacterial infection.

t., marasmic. Thrombosis due to wasting diseases of infancy and old age.

t., placental. Thrombi in the placenta and veins of the uterus.

t., plate. Thrombus formed from an accumulation of blood platelets.

t., puerperal. Coagulation in veins following labor.

t., sinus. Formation of a blood clot in a venous sinus.

t., traumatic. Thrombosis due to a wound or injury of a part.

t., venous. Thrombosis of a vein. SEE: *Nursing Diagnoses* in *Appendix.*

thrombostasis (thrŏm-bŏs′tă-sĭs) [″ + *stasis,* standing still]. Stasis of blood in a part causing or due to formation of thrombus.

thrombosthenin (thrŏm″bō-sthē′nĭn) [″ + *sthenos,* strength]. A contractile protein present in the platelets. Because of this protein that is active in clot retraction, the platelets have been characterized as being a form of muscle cell.

thrombotic (thrŏm-bŏt′ĭk) [Gr. *thrombos,* clot]. Related to, caused by, or of the nature

of a thrombus.

thromboxane A₂. ABBR: TXA₂. An unstable compound synthesized in platelets and other cells from a prostaglandin, PGH₂. It acts to aggregate platelets. In addition, it is a potent vasoconstrictor. SEE: *eicosanoids; prostaglandins; prostanoids.*

thrombus (thrŏm′bŭs) [Gr. *thrombos*]. A blood clot that obstructs a blood vessel or a cavity of the heart. Anticoagulants are used in prevention and treatment of this condition.

t., agonal. Blood clot formed in the heart just at the time of death.

t., annular. Thrombus whose circumference is attached to the walls of a vessel, an opening still remaining in the center.

t., antemortem. A clot formed in the heart or large vessels before death.

t., ball. A round clot in the heart, esp. in the atria.

t., hyaline. Thrombus having a glassy appearance usually occurring in smaller blood vessels.

t., Laennec's. A globular thrombus that forms in the heart, usually in cases of fatty degeneration.

t., lateral. T., mural.

t., milk. A curdled milk tumor in the female breast due to obstruction in a lactiferous duct.

t., mural. Thrombus attached to the wall of a vessel or the heart. SYN: *t., parietal.*

t., obstructing. Thrombus completely occluding the lumen of a vessel.

t., occluding. Thrombus that completely closes the vessel.

t., parietal. Thrombus attached to the wall of a vessel.

t., postmortem. Blood clot formed in the heart or a large blood vessel after death.

t., progressive. Thrombus that increases in size.

t., stratified. Thrombus composed of layers.

t., white. A pale thrombus in any site. Made up principally of platelets.

through-and-through drainage. Irrigation and drainage of a cavity or an organ such as the bladder by placing two perforated tubes, drains, or catheters in the area. A solution is instilled through one tube, usually by continuous drip, and the other tube is attached to either straight or gravity drainage or to a suction machine.

through illumination. Passage of light through the walls of an organ or cavity for medical examination. SYN: *transillumination.*

throwback. SEE: *atavism.*

thrush (thrŭsh) [D. *troske,* rotten wood]. Infection of mouth or throat, esp. in infants and young children, caused by *Candida albicans*. Characterized by formation of white patches and ulcers and frequently by fever and gastrointestinal inflammation. SEE: *aphtha; sprue; stomatitis.*

thrust. To move forward suddenly and forcibly, as in tongue thrust when the tongue is pushed against the teeth or alveolar ridge at the beginning of deglutition. This may cause open bite or malformed jaws.

thrypsis (thrĭp'sĭs) [Gr., breaking in pieces]. A fracture in which the bone is splintered or crushed.

thulium (thū'lē-ŭm). SYMB: Tm. At. wt. 168.934; at. no. 69. A rare metallic element found in combination with minerals.

thumb (thŭm) [AS. *thuma*, thumb]. The short thick first finger on the radial side of the hand, having two phalanges and being opposable to the other four digits. SYN: *pollex* [NA]. SEE: *hand* for illus.

   t., tennis. Calcification and inflammation of the tendon of the flexor pollicis longus muscle due to repeated irritation and stress while playing tennis.

thumb sign. Protrusion of the thumb across the palm and beyond the clenched fist. Seen in children with Marfan's syndrome.

thumb sucking. The habit of sucking one's thumb. Intermittent thumb sucking is not abnormal, but prolonged and intensive thumb sucking past the time the first permanent teeth erupt at five or six years of age can lead to a misshapen mouth and displaced teeth. If the habit persists, combined dental and psychological therapy should be instituted.

thus (thŭs) [L.]. Frankincense, the oleoresin obtained as an exudate from trees of the *Pinus* genus. Genuine frankincense is obtained from the bark of trees of the genus *Boswellia*.

thylacitis (thī"lă-sī'tĭs) [Gr. *thylax*, pouch, + *itis*, inflammation]. Inflammation of the sebaceous glands of the skin.

thylakoid (thī'lă-koyd) [Gr. *thylakon*, a small sac, + *eidos*, form]. Part of the lamellae of chloroplasts. Thylakoids contain photosynthetic pigments and catalytic enzymes for light-dependent reactions.

thymectomize (thī-mĕk'tō-mīz). Surgical removal of the thymus gland.

thymectomy (thī-mĕk'tō-mē) [Gr. *thymos*, mind, + *ektome*, excision]. Surgical removal of the thymus gland.

thymelcosis (thī"mĕl-kō'sĭs) [" + *helkosis*, ulceration]. Ulceration of the thymus gland.

-thymia [Gr. *thymos*, mind]. A word ending indicating a state of the mind.

thymic (thī'mĭk) [L. *thymicus*]. Rel. to the thymus gland.

thymicolymphatic (thī"mĭ-kō-lĭm-făt'ĭk). Rel. to the thymus and lymph glands.

thymidine (thī'mĭ-dēn). A nucleoside present in deoxyribonucleotide. It is formed from the condensation product of thymine and deoxyribase.

thymine (thī'mĭn). A base 5-methyl uracil present in deoxyribonucleic acid.

thymion (thĭm'ē-ŏn) [Gr.]. A wart on the skin.

thymitis (thī-mī'tĭs) [Gr. *thymos*, mind, + *itis*, inflammation]. Inflammation of the thymus gland.

thymo-. 1. [Gr. *thymos*, mind] Combining form indicating relationship to the thymus. 2. [Gr. *thymos*, mind, spirit] Combining form indicating relationship with the soul or emotions.

thymocyte (thī'mō-sīt) [Gr. *thymos*, mind, + *kytos*, cell]. A cell in the thymus that migrated there as a prothymocyte from the bone marrow. Thymocytes mature as they develop, and some of them leave the thymus to become various types of T lymphocytes.

thymokesis (thī"mō-kē'sĭs). Abnormal enlargement of the thymus in the adult.

thymokinetic (thī"mō-kĭ-nĕt'ĭk) [" + *kinesis*, movement]. Stimulating the thymus gland.

thymol (thī'mōl) [Gr. *thumon*, thyme, + L. *oleum*, oil]. White crystals obtained from oil of thyme. Formerly used in treatment of hookworm.

   t. iodide. An antifungal and antibacterial agent.

thymolysis (thī-mŏl'ĭ-sĭs) [Gr. *thymos*, mind, + *lysis*, dissolution]. Dissolution of thymus tissue.

thymolytic (thī-mō-lĭt'ĭk). Destructive to thymus tissue.

thymoma (thī-mō'mă) [" + *oma*, tumor]. A tumor originating in epithelial tissues of the thymus gland.

thymopathy (thī-mŏp'ă-thē). Disease of the thymus.

thymopexy (thī"mō-pĕks'ē) [" + *pexis*, fixation]. Fixation of an enlarged thymus in a new position.

thymopoietin (thī"mō-poy'ĕ-tĭn). A substance produced by the thymus that stimulates differentiation of thymocytes.

thymoprivic (thī"mō-prĭv'ĭk) [" + L. *privus*, deprived of]. Concerning or caused by removal of the thymus.

thymotoxic (thī"mō-tŏks'ĭk) [" + *toxikon*, poison]. Poisonous to thymic tissue.

thymus (thī'mŭs) [Gr. *thymos*]. An unpaired organ located in the mediastinal cavity anterior to and above the heart. It consists of two flattened symmetrical lobes, each enclosed in a capsule, from which trabeculae extend into the gland and divide each lobe into many lobules. These contain a cortex and medulla. The cortex is composed of dense lymphoid tissue containing many cells (thymocytes) closely packed together. The medulla also contains thymocytes but they are less numerous. It also contains characteristic thymic (Hassall's) corpuscles.

At birth, the average weight of the thymus is 10 to 15 gm. Growth is rapid during the first two years, then slow; the thymus attains a weight of about 40 gm at puberty, after which it begins to undergo involution and the thymic tissue is replaced with adipose and connective tissue.

FUNCT: Important in development of immune response in newborn. Its removal during early childhood has been associated with an increased susceptibility to acute infectious diseases at a later time.

The thymus is essential to the maturation of the thymic lymphoid cells, called T cells. When the T cells enter the circulation they are the small and medium-sized lymphocytes; they may survive for up to 5 years. These cells are important in the body's cellular immune response.

PATH: Sometimes it is much larger than it should be and is then known as an enlarged thymus. Children having these enlarged structures were routinely irradiated in the past. This practice has been discontinued because of the high incidence of cancer of the thyroid in these individuals when they reached adulthood. It is recommended that anyone who has undergone thymus irradiation be examined for possible thyroid cancer. SEE: *asthma, thymic.*

t., accessory. A lobule isolated from the mass of the thymus gland.

t. persistens hyperplastica. Thymus persisting into adulthood, sometimes hypertrophying.

thymus dependent antigens. Foreign antigens that require B lymphocyte stimulation by T cells before production of antibodies and memory cells can occur.

thymus independent antigens. Foreign antigens that are capable of stimulating B cell activation and the production of antibodies without T cell interaction. Most of these antibodies fall into the IgM, q.v., class. A few memory cells are created.

thymusectomy (thī″mŭs-ĕk′tō-mē) [Gr. *thymos,* mind, + *ektome,* excision]. Surgical excision of the thymus.

thyreo-, thyro- [Gr. *thyreos,* shield]. Combining forms meaning oblong, shield, or thyroid.

thyreoplasia. Defective functioning of the thyroid gland due to abnormal development.

thyroadenitis (thī″rō-ăd-ĕ-nī′tĭs) [″ +

aden, gland, + *itis,* inflammation]. Inflammation of the thyroid gland.

thyroaplasia (thī″rō-ă-plā′zē-ă) [″ + *a-,* not, + *plasis,* a molding]. Imperfect development of the thyroid gland.

thyroarytenoid (thī″rō-ă-rĭt′ĕn-oyd) [″ + *arytaina,* ladle, + *eidos,* form, shape]. Rel. to the thyroid and arytenoid cartilages.

thyrocalcitonin (thī″rō-kăl″sĭ-tō′nĭn). Calcitonin, q.v.

thyrocardiac (thī″rō-kăr′dē-ăk) [″ + *kardia,* heart]. 1. Pert. to the heart and thyroid gland. 2. A person suffering from thyroid disease complicated by heart disorder.

thyrocele (thī′rō-sēl) [″ + *kele,* tumor, swelling]. Enlarged condition of the thyroid gland. SYN: *goiter.*

thyrochondrotomy (thī″rō-kŏn-drŏt′ō-mē) [″ + *chondros,* cartilage, + *tome,* incision]. Surgical incision of thyroid cartilage.

thyrocolloid (thī″rō-kŏl′oyd). Colloid contained in the thyroid gland.

thyrocricotomy (thī″rō-krī-kŏt′ō-mē) [″ + *krikos,* ring, + *tome,* incision]. Division of the cricothyroid membrane.

thyroepiglottic (thī″rō-ĕp″ĭ-glŏt′ĭk) [″ + *epi,* upon, + *glottis,* back of tongue]. Rel. to the thyroid and epiglottis.

thyroepiglottic muscle. Muscle arising on inner surface of thyroid cartilage. It extends upward and backward and is inserted on the epiglottis. It depresses the epiglottis.

thyroepiglottideus (thī″rō-ĕp″ĭ-glŏt-ĭd′ē-ŭs). Muscle in the thyroid cartilage that depresses the epiglottis.

thyrofissure (thī″rō-fĭsh′ŭr). Surgical creation of an opening through the thyroid cartilage in order to expose the inside of the larynx.

thyrogenic, thyrogenous (thī-rō-jĕn′ĭk, thī-rŏj′ĕ-nŭs) [″ + *gennan,* to produce]. Having its origin in the thyroid.

thyroglobulin (thī″rō-glŏb′ū-lĭn) [″ + L. *globulus,* globule]. 1. An iodine-containing protein secreted by the thyroid gland and stored within its colloid substance. 2. USP. A substance obtained by the fractionation of thyroid glands from the hog, *Sus scrofa.* Trade name is Proloid.

thyroglossal (thī″rō-glŏs′săl) [″ + *glossa,* tongue]. Pert. to the thyroid gland and the tongue.

thyroglossal duct. A duct that in the embryo connects the thyroid diverticulum with the tongue. It eventually disappears, its point of origin being indicated as a pit, the foramen cecum. It sometimes persists as an anomaly.

thyrohyal (thī″rō-hī′ăl). Concerning the thyroid cartilage and the hyoid bone.

thyrohyoid (thī″rō-hī′oyd) [″ + *hyoeides,* U-shaped]. Rel. to thyroid cartilage and hyoid bone.

thyroid (thī′royd) [″ + *eidos*, form, shape].
1. A gland of internal secretion in the neck, anterior to and partially surrounding the thyroid cartilage and upper rings of the trachea. SEE: *thyroid gland*. 2. USP. The cleaned, dried, and powdered thyroid gland of animals, usually pigs, slaughtered for food. The preparation is free of fat and connective tissue.

ACTION/USES: Used in cases of deficient action of the gland (hypothyroidism) or following thyroidectomy.

ADM: Tablet form by mouth. The maximum effect will not be obtained for at least 7 to 10 days. It is advisable to start with a small dose and increase it gradually until the proper dose is determined.

thyroid cachexia. Exophthalmic goiter. SEE: *hyperthyroidism.*

thyroid cartilage. The principal cartilage of the larynx, consisting of two broad laminae united anteriorly to form a V-shaped structure. It forms a subcutaneous projection called the laryngeal prominence or Adam's apple. SEE: *thyroid gland* for illus.

thyroid crisis. Thyroid storm.

thyroidea accessoria; thyroidea ima (thī-roy′dē-ă). Accessory thyroid.

thyroidectomized (thī″roy-dĕk′tō-mīzd) [″ + *eidos*, form, shape, + *ektome*, excision]. With the thyroid gland removed.

thyroidectomy (thī″royd-ĕk′tō-mē). Excision of the thyroid gland.

NURSING IMPLICATIONS: *Preop:* Provide a calm atmosphere and a diet high in carbohydrates, protein, and supplemental vitamins to restore a positive nitrogen balance. Administer prescribed antithyroid drugs to establish euthyroid state. Evaluate patient response and report side effects. Carry out usual preoperative teaching plus special considerations related to moving the head and voice rest. *Postop:* Assess vital signs and intake and output, provide emotional support, and administer analgesics as prescribed. Assess patient frequently during initial 48 hours for signs of tracheal compression with acute airway obstruction (choking, irregular respirations, or stridor). Have oxygen, suction, and tracheostomy equipment available at the bedside. Observe incisional area for swelling or bleeding, assessing dressings at back of neck where blood would accumulate. Maintain the patient in a semi-Fowler's position as tolerated, immobilizing the head with sandbags or pillows and supporting the head during moving or turning. Assess for signs of damage to the recurrent laryngeal nerve (hoarseness, weak whispery voice persisting for more than four days). Encourage voice rest by asking questions that can be an-

swered with hand signals, and assist patient in using a "magic slate" or other written communication tool. Assess for signs of tetany (tingling of toes, fingers, circumoral area, positive Chvostek's and Trousseau's signs) leading to seizure activity, and have calcium chloride available for emergency I.V. administration. Watch for signs of thyroid storm (hyperpyrexia, tachydysrhythmias, profuse diaphoresis, hypotension, and diarrhea), which can progress to delirium, coma, cardiovascular collapse, and death. *Discharge planning:* Teach patient to observe for and report signs of hypo- or hyperthyroid function. Encourage neck exercise regimen for optimal range of motion post suture removal. Instruct the patient about prescribed medications and counsel about rest, relaxation, and nutrition. SEE: *Nursing Diagnoses* in *Appendix.*

t., subtotal. Surgical excision of most of the thyroid to relieve hyperthyroidism.

thyroid function tests. Tests for evidence of increased or decreased thyroid function, including clinical physical examination, which is usually reliable, and a variety of reliable laboratory tests. Some of the more common tests are based on direct or indirect determination of the two thyroid hormones, triiodothyronine (T_3) and tetraiodothyronine (T_4). Also frequently used are tests on radioactive iodine uptake by the thyroid.

Most thyroid function tests are unreliable in certain circumstances. They may be influenced by the patient's having been exposed to organic or inorganic iodides or to drugs that interfere with the binding capacity of serum proteins.

Hypothyroidism is confirmed by finding a subnormal level of free serum thyroxine (T_4) in the serum.

In 95% of patients with hyperthyroidism, the level of free serum thyroxine (T_4) is increased. It is also helpful to obtain the serum thyroid stimulating hormone level (TSH), which is decreased in hyperthyroidism. SEE: *goiter, exophthalmic; hyperthyroidism.*

thyroid gland. A gland of internal secretion located in the base of the neck on both sides of the lower part of the larynx and upper part of trachea. It consists of two lateral lobes connected by an isthmus. Sometimes a third medial or pyramidal lobe extends upward from the isthmus. Histologically it consists of a large number of closed vesicles called follicles that contain a homogeneous substance called colloid, which contains the thyroglobulin. It in turn contains various active substances such as thyroxine. The thyroid gland is enlarged in goiter and it may pulsate. SEE: illus.

THYROID GLAND AND RELATED STRUCTURES

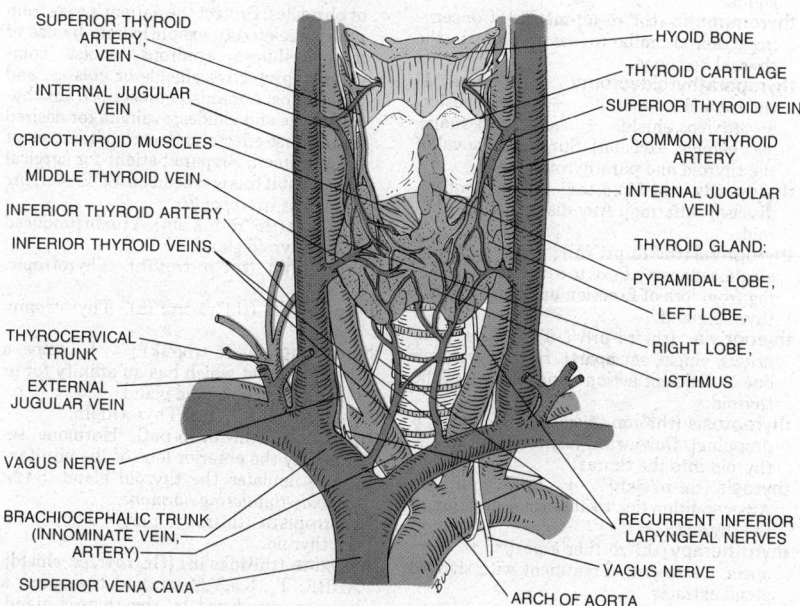

RS: endocrine gland; hormone; hyperthyroidism; hypothyroidism; iodine; struma; thyrotropic hormone; thyroxine.

thyroidism (thī'royd-izm). Disease caused by hyperactivity of the thyroid gland.

thyroiditis (thī"royd-ī'tĭs) [" + *eidos*, form, shape, + *itis*, inflammation]. Inflammation of the thyroid gland. SEE: *struma, Riedel's*.

  t., giant cell. Thyroiditis characterized by presence of giant cells, round-cell infiltration, fibrosis, and destruction of follicles.

  t., Hashimoto's. A form of autoimmune thyroiditis that affects women eight times more often than men. Clinically there is an enlarged thyroid and hypothyroidism. The treatment is life-long replacement therapy with thyroid hormone.

  t., Reidel's. A rare form of thyroiditis characterized by fibrotic destruction of the thyroid gland. The fibrotic tissue extends beyond the capsule of the gland into the surrounding structures of the neck and may develop sufficiently to compress the trachea. The etiology is unknown.

thyroidomania (thī"royd-ō-mā'nē-ă) [" + " + *mania*, frenzy]. Mental disorder associated with hyperthyroidism.

thyroidotomy (thī"royd-ŏt'ō-mē) [" + "

+ *tome*, incision]. Incision of the thyroid gland.

thyroidotoxin (thī"royd-ō-tŏk'sĭn). A substance that is specifically toxic for cells of the thyroid gland.

thyroid-stimulating hormone. ABBR: TSH. Hormone secreted by the anterior lobe of the pituitary that stimulates the thyroid gland. SYN: *thyrotropin*.

thyroid storm. A complication of thyrotoxicosis that if untreated is almost uniformly fatal. Consists of abrupt onset of fever, sweating, tachycardia, pulmonary edema or congestive heart failure, tremulousness, and restlessness. Occurs in a patient in whom existing thyrotoxicosis has been treated poorly or not at all. It usually is precipitated by infection, trauma, or a surgical emergency. SYN: *thyrotoxic crisis*.

  TREAT: Catecholamine inhibitors. Both guanethidine and propranolol have been reported to be quite effective.

Thyrolar. Trade name for liotrix.

thyrolysin (thī-rŏl'ĭ-sĭn). Anything that destroys thyroid tissue.

thyrolytic (thī"rō-lĭt'ĭk) [Gr. *thyreos*, shield, + *lysis*, dissolution]. Causing destruction of thyroid tissue.

thyromegaly (thī"rō-mĕg'ă-lē) [" +

megas, large]. Enlargement of the thyroid gland.

thyromimetic (thī″rō-mī-mĕt′ĭk). Concerning action(s) similar to that produced by the thyroid hormone.

thyroparathyroidectomy (thī″rō-păr″ă-thī″royd-ĕk′tō-mē) [″ + *para,* beside, + *thyreos,* shield, + *eidos,* form, shape, + *ektome,* excision]. Surgical removal of the thyroid and parathyroid glands.

thyropathy (thī-rŏp′ă-thē) [″ + *pathos,* disease, suffering]. Any disease of the thyroid.

thyroprival (thī″rō-prī′văl) [″ + L. *privus,* single, set apart]. Pert. to a condition resulting from loss of function or removal of the thyroid gland.

thyroprivia (thī″rō-prĭv′ē-ă) [″ + L. *privus,* single, set apart]. Hypothyroidism due to deficient action of or removal of the thyroid.

thyroptosis (thī″rŏp-tō′sĭs) [″ + *ptosis,* a dropping]. Downward displacement of the thyroid into the thorax.

thyrosis (thī-rō′sĭs) [″ + *osis,* condition]. Any condition due to abnormal function of the thyroid.

thyrotherapy (thī″rō-thĕr′ă-pē) [″ + *therapeia,* treatment]. Treatment with thyroid gland extracts.

thyrotome (thī′rō-tōm) [″ + *tome,* incision]. Knife for cutting the thyroid cartilage.

thyrotomy (thī-rŏt′ō-mē). 1. The splitting of the thyroid cartilage anteriorly in midline in order to expose laryngeal structures. 2. Surgery on the thyroid gland.

thyrotoxic (thī″rō-tŏks′ĭk) [″ + *toxikon,* poison]. Pert. to, affected by, or marked by toxic activity of the thyroid gland.

thyrotoxic crisis. SEE: *thyroid storm.*

thyrotoxicosis (thī″rō-tŏks″ĭ-kō′sĭs) [″ + ″ + *osis,* condition]. Toxic condition due to hyperactivity of the thyroid gland. SYN: *goiter, exophthalmic.*

SYM: Rapid heart action; tremors; elevated basal metabolism; enlarged gland; exophthalmos; nervous symptoms; and loss of weight.

NURSING IMPLICATIONS: Assist the patient in coping with the anxiety and irritability related to this condition by providing a restful atmosphere, encouraging expression of feelings, and avoiding known stressors and stimulants. Promote nutritional intake high in carbohydrates, proteins, and vitamins to maintain an anabolic state and prevent muscle weakness and wasting. Provide comfort measures to reduce effects of pyrexia, diaphoresis, abdominal cramping, and diarrhea. As ordered, replace fluids and electrolytes lost by diaphoresis or diarrhea. Prevent accidental injury by removing environmental hazards or obstacles. Protect the patient's eyes from injuries related to exophthalmia by use of methylcellulose eyedrops, moist compresses, protective shields or glasses, and positioning. Administer prescribed antithyroid drugs and iodides; evaluate for desired and adverse effects, and teach patient about drug regimen. Prepare patient for surgical treatment if this is scheduled. SEE: *Nursing Diagnoses* in *Appendix.*

thyrotoxin (thī″rō-tŏk′sīn). A toxin produced in the thyroid gland.

thyrotrophic (thī″rō-trōf′ĭk). Thyrotropic, q.v.

thyrotrophin (thī″rō-trōf′ĭn). Thyrotropin, q.v.

thyrotropic (thī″rō-trŏp′ĭk) [″ + *trope,* a turning]. That which has an affinity for or stimulates the thyroid gland.

thyrotropic hormone. Thyrotropin.

thyrotropin (thī-rŏt′rō-pĭn). Hormone secreted by the anterior lobe of the pituitary that stimulates the thyroid gland. SYN: *thyroid-stimulating hormone.*

thyrotropism (thī-rŏt′rō-pĭzm). Affinity for the thyroid.

thyroxine (thī-rŏks′ĭn) [Gr. *thyreos,* shield]. ABBR: T_4. 3,5,3′,5′-tetraiodothyronine, a hormone produced by the thyroid gland. Used in the treatment of hypothyroidism.

Ti. Chem. symb. for titanium.

TIA. *transient ischemic attack.*

tibia (tĭb′ē-ă) [L., *tibia,* shinbone]. The inner and larger bone of the leg between the knee and the ankle; it articulates with the femur above and with the talus below.

   t., saber-shaped. A deformity of the tibia due to gummatous periostitis (syphilitic) in which it curves outward.

   t. valga. A bulging of the lower legs in which the convexity is inward. SYN: *genu valgum.*

   t. vara. A bowing of the lower legs in which the convexity is outward. SYN: *genu varum.*

tibiad (tĭb′ē-ăd) [″ + *ad,* to]. Toward the tibia.

tibial (tĭb′ē-ăl) [L. *tibialis*]. Concerning the tibia.

tibialgia (tĭb″ē-ăl′jē-ă) [″ + Gr. *algos,* pain]. Pain in the tibia.

tibialis (tĭb″ē-ā′lĭs) [L.]. [NA] Pert. to the tibia.

tibioadductor reflex (tĭb″ē-ō-ăd-dŭk′tor) [L. *tibia,* shinbone, + *adducere,* to lead to]. Adduction of either the stimulated leg or the opposite one when the tibia is percussed on the inner side.

tibiocalcanean (tĭb″ē-ō-kăl-kā′nē-ăn). Concerning the tibia and calcaneus bones.

tibiofemoral (tĭb″ē-ō-fĕm′or-ăl) [″ + L. *femur*, thigh]. Rel. to the tibia and femur.

tibiofibular (tĭb″ē-ō-fĭb′ū-lăr) [″ + L. *fibula*, pin]. Rel. to the tibia and fibula.

tibionavicular (tĭb″ē-ō-nă-vĭk′ū-lăr). Concerning the tibia and navicular bones.

tibioperoneal (tĭb″ē-ō-pĕr″ō-nē′ăl). Tibiofibular.

tibioscaphoid (tĭb″ē-ō-skăf′oyd). Tibionavicular.

tibiotarsal (tĭb″ē-ō-tăr′săl) [″ + Gr. *tarsos*, broad, flat surface]. Rel. to the tibia and tarsus.

tic (tĭk) [Fr.]. A spasmodic muscular contraction, most commonly involving the face, mouth, eyes, head, neck, or shoulder muscles. The spasms may be tonic, q.v., or clonic, q.v. The movement appears purposeful, is often repeated, is involuntary, and can be inhibited for a short time only to burst forth with increased severity.

Children between the ages of 5 and 10 years are especially likely to develop tics or habit spasms. These tend to cease in a few weeks if they are ignored. SYN: *habit spasm.* SEE: *Gilles de la Tourette's syndrome; neuralgia.*

ETIOL: In most cases the cause is unknown. In some individuals they are related to anxiety and nervous tension.

t., convulsive. Spasm of muscles of face supplied by the seventh cranial nerve.

t. douloureux. Degeneration of or pressure on the trigeminal nerve, resulting in neuralgia of that nerve. The pain comes on in severe lightning-like stabs and radiates from the angle of the jaw along one of the involved branches. If it is the first branch, a shocklike pain is felt along the eye and back over the forehead. If it is the middle fiber, the upper lip, nose, and cheek under the eye are affected. If it is the third branch, pain is in the lower lip and outer border of the tongue on the affected side. Pain is momentary but may occur repetitively for as long as 20 seconds. Paroxysms may last for hours and then subside for weeks or months. SYN: *prosopalgia; neuralgia, trigeminal.* SEE: *Nursing Diagnoses* in *Appendix.*

TREAT: Injection of the nerve with alcohol. Anticonvulsants may be helpful to shorten attacks or cause remission. Surgical therapy may be required.

t., facial. Tic of the facial muscles.

t., habit. Habitual repetition of a grimace or muscular action.

t. rotatoire. Spasmodic torticollis in which head and neck are forcibly rotated or turned from one side to the other.

t., spasmodic. Tonic contractions and paralysis of muscles of one or both sides of the face.

t.'s, vocal. Grunts and barking sounds that may be made by persons with Tourette's syndrome, q.v.

Ticar. Trade name for ticarcillin disodium.

ticarcillin disodium, sterile (tī″kăr-sĭl′ĭn). USP. A semisynthetic penicillin esp. effective against *Pseudomonas aeruginosa.* Trade name is Ticar.

tick (tĭk) [ME. *tyke*]. Any of the numerous bloodsucking acarids of the order Acarida. Ixodidae is the hard tick family and Argasidae the soft. They transmit specific diseases to humans and lower animals.

tick bite. Ticks can be vectors for several diseases, including Rocky Mountain spotted fever, Q fever, tularemia, borreliosis, human babesiosis, and Lyme disease, but the bite itself usually produces a mildly itching papule. If the tick is incompletely removed, the retained mouth parts may cause a pruritic nodule. The nodule should be surgically excised. Removal of a tick should not be done by crushing but by either gentle traction or application of petroleum jelly, oil, or nail polish to the tick, which will facilitate removal.

tick-borne rickettsiosis. A variety of tick-borne rickettsial diseases similar to Rocky Mountain spotted fever. They are caused by a rickettsial organism *(Rickettsia rickettsii)* transmitted by Ixodid ticks.

tickle (tĭk′l) [ME. *tikelen*]. 1. Peculiar sensation caused by titillation or touching, esp. in certain areas of the body, resulting in reflex muscular movements, laughter, or hysteria. 2. To arouse such a sensation by touching a surface lightly.

tickling (tĭk′lĭng). Gentle stimulation of a sensitive surface and its reflex effect, such as involuntary laughter. SYN: *titillation.*

t.i.d. L. *ter in die,* three times a day.

tidal (tī′dăl). Periodically rising and falling, increasing and decreasing.

tidal air. Air that is inhaled and exhaled during normal quiet breathing. SEE: *air; respiration.*

tidal drainage. The drainage of a paralyzed bladder by use of an automatic irrigation apparatus.

tide [AS. *tid,* time]. Alternate rise and fall; a space of time.

t., acid. Temporary increase in acidity of urine due to increased secretion of alkaline substances into the duodenum or after fasting.

t., alkaline. Temporary decrease in acidity of urine following awakening and after meals. The former results from an increased rate of breathing, in which excess CO_2 is eliminated; the latter results from increase of base in the blood following the secretion of HCl into gastric juice.

t., fat. Increased fat in the lymph and blood after a fatty meal.

Tietze's syndrome (tēt'sĕz) [Alexander Tietze, Ger. surgeon, 1864–1927]. Inflammation of the costochondral cartilages. A self-limiting disease of unknown etiology. Pain may be confused with that of myocardial infarction. There is no specific therapy, but some relief will be provided by injecting the area with procaine and corticosteroids.

Tigan. Trade name for trimethobenzamide hydrochloride.

tigering [Gr. *tigris*, tiger]. Tigerlike striped appearance of heart muscle due to irregular areas of fatty degeneration. Seen in conditions that cause severe anoxemia, such as anemia.

tigretier (tē-grĕt"ē-ā') [Fr.]. A dancing mania or form of tarantism due to bite of a poisonous spider, occurring in Tigré, Abyssinia.

tigroid (tī'groyd) [Gr. *tigroeides*, tiger-spotted]. Striped, spotted, or marked like a tiger.

tigroid bodies. Masses of chromophil substance present in the cell bodies of neurons. SYN: *Nissl bodies.*

tigrolysis (tīg"rŏl'ĭ-sĭs). Dissolution and disappearance of chromophil substance of a nerve cell. May occur following injury to an axon (retrograde degeneration) or subsequent to direct injury to a nerve cell. SYN: *chromatolysis.*

tilmus (tĭl'mŭs) [Gr. *tilmos*, a plucking]. Delirious picking at the bedclothes by the patient. SYN: *carphology.*

tiltometer (tĭl-tŏm'ē-tĕr). A device for measuring the degree of tilt of a bed or operating table. Used when spinal anesthesia has been given in order to know which end of the spinal canal is lower.

timbre (tĭm'bĕr, tăm'br) [Fr., a bell to be struck with a hammer]. Resonance quality of a sound by which it is distinguished, other than pitch or intensity, depending upon the number and character of vibrating body's overtones.

time (tīm) [AS. *tima*, time]. Interval between beginning and ending; measured duration.

t., bleeding. Time required for bleeding from a small wound to cease. Usually tested by puncturing the lobe of the ear. Normal time is 1 to 3 minutes. SEE: *bleeding time.*

t., clot retraction. Time required following withdrawal of blood for a clot to completely contract and express the serum entrapped within the fibrin net. Normal time is about 1 hour. Clot retraction is dependent upon the number of platelets in the specimen.

t., coagulation. Time required for clotting to occur in whole blood that has been placed in tubes coated with silicone. Time required is somewhat different for each lab-

oratory but will usually vary from 20 to 60 minutes.

t., doubling. Length of time needed for a malignant tumor cell population to double in size.

t., median lethal. Time required for the death of 50% of the individuals of an organism group that were given an exposure to ionizing radiation.

t., prothrombin. Time needed for oxalated plasma to clot, measured in seconds, after adding thromboplastin and recalcifying.

t., reaction. Period between application of a stimulus and the response.

t., setting. Time required for a material to polymerize or harden, as in dental amalgam, cement, plaster, resin, or stone.

t., thermal death. Time required to kill a bacterium at a certain temperature.

time frame. The limits of time for any event or occurrence.

time inventory. An assessment approach used by occupational therapists to determine a patient's perception of the value of time and its organization.

time-out. Alternative method of discipline that involves removing the child from social interaction and placing him or her in a nonstimulating location (i.e., in a chair facing a corner) for a few minutes after an unacceptable behavior has occurred.

timer (tīm'ĕr). Device for measuring, signaling, recording, or otherwise indicating elapsed time. Various forms of timers are used in x-ray, surgical, and laboratory work.

Timoptic Solution. Trade name for timolol maleate.

tin (tĭn) [AS.]. SYMB: Sn. At. wt. 118.69; at. no. 50. A metallic element used in various industries, and in making certain tissue stains. SEE: *tin poisoning.*

Tinactin. Trade name for tolnaftate.

tinct. *tincture.*

tinctable (tĭnk'tă-bl). Stainable.

tinction (tĭnk'shŭn) [L. *tingere*, to dye]. 1. The process of staining. 2. A stain.

tinctorial (tĭnk-tō'rē-ăl) [L. *tinctorius*, dyeing]. Rel. to staining or color.

tinctura (tĭnk-tū'ră) [L., a dyeing] (pl. *tincturae*). Tincture.

tincturation (tĭnk"tū-rā'shŭn). Making a tincture from an appropriate drug.

tincture (tĭnk'chūr) [L. *tincture*, a dyeing]. An alcoholic extract of vegetable or animal substances. Simple alcoholic solutions of pure substances such as iodine and quinine are no longer called tinctures. The name of material contained in the tincture other than alcohol is added to the name of the tincture.

This class of preparations usually contains tannic acid, so, in most instances, cannot be employed with agents that are incompatible with that drug. Those tinctures that contain much resinous matter or oils will precipitate with water. Some examples are tinctures of belladonna, ginger, benzoin, and guaiac. Tinctures of the most potent drugs usually contain 10% of the crude drug, as tinctures of opium and digitalis. When more than a teaspoon of a 10% tincture would have to be taken to get a dose of the drug, the tincture is usually made to contain 20%, or more, of the agent.

tincture of iodine. Obsolete term for simple alcoholic solution of iodine.

tincture of iodine poisoning. This commonly used antiseptic is sometimes taken by mouth either accidentally or for the purpose of suicide.

SYM: Very strong irritation of mouth, esophagus, and stomach. Stains membranes dark brown or black. Pain is intense and leads to early vomiting and purging; extreme thirst; often collapse.

TREAT: Give large amounts of water, milk and starchy paste; gruels, as boiled rice or cream of wheat. Gastric lavage with either one to 10% starch solution, or sodium thiosulfite or protein solution such as egg white or milk. Control pain, circulatory collapse, and fluid and electrolyte balance with appropriate therapy. Tracheotomy may be required. SEE: *iodine* at *Poisons and Poisoning* in *Appendix.*

Tindal. Trade name for acetophenazine maleate.

tine. A sharp, pointed prong.

tinea (tǐn′ē-ă) [L., worm]. Any fungus skin disease occurring on various parts of the body, the name indicating the part affected. Ex.: tinea barbae (beard), tinea corporis (body). Commonly called ringworm. SEE: *dermatomycosis.*

SYM: Of two types. Superficial symptoms are marking by scaling; slight itching; reddish or grayish patches; dry, brittle hair that is easily extracted with hair shaft. The deep type is characterized by flat, reddish, kerion-like tumors, the surface studded with dead or broken hairs or by gaping follicular orifices. Nodules may be broken down in center, discharging pus through dilated follicular openings.

TREAT: Griseofulvin, given orally for all types of true trichophyton infections. Local treatment alone is of little benefit in ringworm of the scalp, nails, and in most cases the feet. Topical preparations containing fungicidal agents are useful in treatment of tinea cruris and tinea pedis.

Personal hygiene is important in controlling these two common diseases. The use of antiseptic foot baths to control tinea pedis does not prevent spread of the infection from one person to another. Persons affected should not allow their personal items, such as clothes, towels, and sports equipment, to be used by others.

Tinea of the scalp, tinea capitis, is particularly resistant if due to *Microsporum audouini.* Do not treat topically. Systemic griseofulvin is quite effective.

t. amiantacea. Sticky scaling of the scalp following infection or trauma.

t. barbae. A fungus skin disease of the bearded portions of neck and face. SYN: *barber's itch.*

t. capitis. A fungal infection of the scalp. May be due to one of several types of *Microsporum* or *Trichophyton tonsurans.* SEE: *kerion.*

t. corporis. Tinea of the body. Begins with red, slightly elevated scaly patches that on examination reveal minute vesicles or papules. New patches spring from the periphery while central portion clears up. Often considerable itching.

t. cruris. A fungus skin disease of surfaces of contact in the scrotal, crural, anal, and genital areas. SYN: *dhobie itch.*

t. imbricata. Chronic tinea caused by *Trichophyton concentricum.* It is present in tropical regions. The annular lesions have scales at their periphery.

t. kerion. Kerion, q.v.

t. nigra. An asymptomatic superficial fungal infection that affects the skin of the palms. Characterized by deeply pigmented, macular, non-scaly patches. SYN: *pityriasis nigra.*

ETIOL: *Cladosporium werneckii* or *C. mansonii.*

t. nodosa. Sheathlike nodular masses in hair of beard and mustache from growth of either *Piedraia hortai,* which causes black piedra, or *Trichosporon beigelii,* which causes white piedra. The masses surround the hairs, which become brittle; hairs may be penetrated by fungus and thus split. SYN: *piedra.*

t. pedis. A fungus skin infection of the foot. SYN: *athlete's foot; dermatophytosis.*

t. profunda. A rare type of tinea characterized by indolent nodules and plaques. These skin lesions may ulcerate.

t. sycosis. T. barbae, q.v.

t. tonsurans. T. capitis, q.v.

t. unguium. Onychomycosis.

t. versicolor. Fungus infection of skin producing branny patches that are yellow or fawn-colored. Topically applied acrisorcin cream is effective in treating the causative agent, the fungus *Malassezia furfur.* SYN: *pityriasis versicolor.*

Tinel's sign (tǐn-ĕlz′) [Jules Tinel, Fr. neurologist, 1879–1952]. Cutaneous tingling sensation produced by pressing on or tapping the nerve trunk that has been damaged or is regenerating following trauma.

tine test. A skin test for tuberculosis. The tuberculin is on metal tines that are barely pressed into the skin. The test is read in 48 and 72 hours. The unit is sterile and disposable and therefore is very useful in mass surveys. Several multiple puncture tests are available including Mantoux, Aplitest, and Heaf test. SEE: *tuberculin test.*

tingibility (tĭn″jī-bĭl′ĭ-tē). The property of being stainable.

tingible (tĭn′jī-bl) [L. *tingere*, to stain]. Capable of being stained by a dye.

tingle (tĭng′gl). A prickling or stinging sensation. May be caused by cold or nerve injury.

tinnitus (tĭn-ī′tŭs) [L., a jingling]. A subjective ringing or tinkling sound in the ear.

    t. aurium. Ringing, tinkling, buzzing, or other sounds in the ear. Found in certain diseases of the exterior, middle, or inner ear.

    ETIOL: Impacted cerumen; myringitis; otitis media; labyrinthitis; Ménière's symptom complex; otosclerosis; hysteria. Also follows prolonged therapy with drugs such as quinine and salicylates, including aspirin.

tin poisoning. Tin in soldered containers has occasionally been responsible for poisoning. This is exceedingly rare.

    SYM: Metallic taste in mouth, gastrointestinal irritation, nausea, vomiting, cramping, and diarrhea.

    TREAT: Wash out stomach and administer bland or soothing drinks.

tint. A variety of color or hue.

tintometer (tĭn-tŏm′ĕ-ter) [L. *tinctus*, a dyeing, + Gr. *metron*, a measure]. A scale of different shades of color to determine by comparison the intensity of color of the blood or other fluid.

tintometric (tĭn″tō-mĕt′rĭk). Rel. to tintometry.

tintometry (tĭn-tŏm′ĕ-trē). Estimation of color by comparison with a scale of colors.

tip (tĭp) [ME]. A point or apex of a part.

tipped uterus. In the past, malposition of the uterus has been invoked as the cause of numerous conditions, including pelvic pain, back pain, abnormal uterine bleeding, infertility, and emotional difficulties. Simple malposition of the uterus without evidence of a specific disease condition that accounts for the malposition is felt to be harmless and virtually symptomless. It is essential therefore that individuals who have been told that a tipped uterus is the cause of their symptoms be carefully examined in order to attempt to find a specific organic cause for the symptoms. If in the absence of other findings a vaginal pessary relieves symptoms associated with a retrodisplaced uterus and these symptoms return when the pessary is removed, then surgical suspension of the uterus is indicated. If surgery is not acceptable to the patient, the pessary may be worn intermittently. Evidence that a tipped uterus is an important cause of pelvic pain and discomfort is lacking.

tipping (tĭp′ĭng). Angulation of a tooth about its long axis.

tiqueur (tĭ-kĕr′) [Fr.]. One afflicted with a tic.

tire (tīr) [AS. *teorian*, to tire]. 1. To become fatigued. 2. To exhaust or fatigue.

tirefond (tēr-fōn′) [Fr.]. Appliance like a corkscrew for raising depressed portions of bone or for removing foreign bodies.

tires (tīrz). Condition marked by constipation, vomiting, muscular tremors, and pain. SYN: *trembles.*

tiring (tīr′ĭng). Fastening wire around the fragments of a bone.

tissue (tĭsh′ū) [O. Fr. *tissu*, from L. *texere*, to weave]. A group or collection of similar cells and their intercellular substance that act together in the performance of a particular function. The primary tissues are epithelial, connective, skeletal, muscular, glandular, and nervous.

    t., adenoid. Lymphoid tissue.

    t., adipose. Areolar tissue containing aggregations of densely packed fat cells. SYN: *fat.*

    t., areolar. A form of loose connective tissue consisting of interlacing collagenous and elastic fibers embedded in a semifluid matrix together with fibroblasts, histiocytes, mast cells, plasma cells, and other cellular elements. It is widely distributed, forming the interstitial tissue of most organs, the membranes surrounding blood vessels and nerves, and the principal portion of fascia.

    t., bony, bone. Bone in its usual or abnormal site, i.e., in calcified tissue.

    t., brown adipose, brown fat. A special type of fat in which brown pigment and small fat droplets are present. It is in some mammals, esp. between the scapulae of hibernating animals.

    t., cancellous. Spongy bone with many marrow cavities. It is present at the ends of long articular bones and in the interior of most flat bones.

    t., cartilage. The dense connective tissue of cartilage consisting of cells embedded in a matrix.

    t., chondroid. Embryonic cartilage.

    t., chordal. Tissue of the notochord or derived therefrom. The nucleus pulposus is derived from the notochord.

    t.'s, chromaffin. Tissues containing

cells that give the chromaffin reaction. Found in the adrenal medulla and ganglia of the parasympathetic nervous system. SEE: *chromaffin system.*

t., cicatricial. The thick fibrous tissue formed as part of the healing process in soft tissue wounds.

t., connective. Tissue that supports and connects other tissues and parts of the body. The cells of connective tissue are comparatively few in number, the bulk of the tissue consisting of intercellular substance or matrix, the nature of which gives each type of connective tissue its particular properties. Connective tissues are highly vascular with the exception of cartilage. Connective tissue proper includes the following types: mucous, fibrous (areolar, white fibrous, yellow fibrous, or elastic), reticular, and adipose. Dense connective tissue includes cartilage and bone (osseous tissue).

t., elastic. A form of connective tissue in which yellow elastic fibers predominate. Found in certain ligaments and the walls of blood vessels, esp. the larger arteries.

t., embryonic. T., mucous.

t., endothelial. Endothelium, q.v.

t., epithelial. A form of tissue composed of cells arranged in a continuous sheet consisting of one or several layers. It forms the epidermis of skin, covers surfaces of organs, lines cavities and canals, and forms tubes and ducts and secreting portions of glands. SYN: *epithelium.*

t., erectile. Spongy tissue, the spaces of which fill with blood, causing it to harden and expand. Found in the penis, clitoris, and nipples.

t., extracellular. All of the tissue and fluids outside of the cells of the body. Included are plasma, serum, lymph, aqueous and vitreous humors, and connective tissue such as collagen, cartilage, and some bone.

t., fatty. T., adipose.

t., fibrous. Connective tissue consisting principally of fibers. Includes three types: areolar or loose connective, white fibrous, and yellow fibrous or elastic.

t., gelatiginous. Tissue from which gelatin may be obtained by treating it with hot water.

t., glandular. A group of epithelial cells capable of producing secretions.

t., granulation. The newly formed vascular and cellular tissue produced in the early stages of wound healing.

t., hard. In dentistry, term used to denote any of the three calcified tissue components of the tooth: enamel, dentin, and cementum.

t., indifferent. Tissue composed of undifferentiated cells as in embryonic tissue.

t., interstitial. Connective tissue that forms a network with the cellular elements of an organ.

t., lymphadenoid. Lymphoid tissue present in various sites, including the liver, spleen, and bone marrow.

t., lymphoid. A collection of developing and mature lymphocytes mingled with a supporting lattice of connective tissue. Such collections are present in the adenoids, tonsils, and in Peyer's patches in the intestines.

t., mesenchymal. The embryonic mesenchyme.

t., mucous. Jellylike tissue from which connective tissue is derived. SYN: *t., embryonic.*

t., muscular. The material composing the muscles. *Voluntary:* Striped or striated tissue principally connected with the bony framework. In animals it is known as lean meat or flesh. It is a cross-striped muscular tissue, the fibers like a long cylinder with flattened sides and conical ends, enveloped in a delicate sheath, the sarcolemma. *Involuntary:* Smooth or unstriped, or nonstriated, not under control of the will. Principally found in walls of hollow organs, tubes, arteries, and veins. SEE: *muscle.*

t., myeloid. The red bone marrow in which most blood cells are formed.

t., nerve, nervous. All of the tissue of the central and peripheral nervous systems.

t., osseous. Connective tissue with intercellular substance impregnated with phosphate and carbonate of calcium, the mineral substances being two thirds of the bone's dry weight. SYN: *bony tissue.*

t., reticular. A type of connective tissue consisting of delicate fibers forming interlacing networks. Fibers stain selectively with silver stains and are called argyrophil fibers. Reticular tissue supports lymph nodes and is found in muscular tissue and bone marrow, the spleen, liver, lungs, kidneys, and mucous membranes of the gastrointestinal tract.

t., scar. T., cicatricial, q.v.

t., sclerous. Firm connective tissues such as bone and cartilage.

t., skeletal. The bones, cartilages, and connective tissues that make up the skeleton.

t., splenic. The highly vascular splenic pulp.

t., subcutaneous. Areolar tissue under and becoming part of the corium.

t., subcutaneous adipose. Adipose tissue within subcutaneous tissue.

t., white fibrous. Connective tissue with white inelastic fibers, forming tendons, ligaments, and resistant membranes.

t., white nervous. Nervous tissue of medullated nerve fibers.

tissue bank. A facility for collecting, processing, and storing tissue for later transplantation. Tissue stored includes bone, skin, nerve, fascial, tendon, heart valve, dura mater, cornea, and bone marrow. These are tested for microbial pathogens and stored either in a freeze-dried or frozen state.

tissue culture. Growth of tissue in vitro on artificial media for experimental research.

tissue expansion, soft. A technique used in plastic surgery to expand skin in order to remove an area for cosmetic reasons. One or more expander balloons are inserted under the skin. The balloon(s) is then expanded by progressively increasing the amount of saline solution in it. This is done on a weekly basis for whatever time is required to sufficiently stretch the overlying skin. Once the expansion is completed the plastic surgical procedure is done. This permits removal of skin without having to cover the area by use of a skin graft. SEE: *surgery, plastic; W-plasty; Z-plasty.*

tissue factor. ABBR: TF. A protein on the surface of all cells outside the bloodstream, combines with factor 7 and forms TF-7 that combines with factor 10 to form 10 molecules of 10a; these molecules combine with factor 5a which bind to the protein prothrombin and in so doing create 2 million thrombin molecules. This creates 160 billion molecules of fibrin. The fibrin polymer is the major component of a blood clot.

tissue plasminogen activator. ABBR: TPA. A drug used to dissolve the blood clots (thrombolysis) that cause occlusion of the arteries in myocardial infarction. It is administered within the first six hours of the attack. It has been shown to reduce the chances of dying following a heart attack by over 50%. The undesired side effect of causing intracranial bleeding as a result of the therapy has not been a problem when the correct dose is given; and the drug may have a place in the treatment of stroke due to intravascular clots in the arteries of the central nervous system. Patients over 75 years of age or any patient with a history of stroke or history of potential bleeding sites should not be given the drug. In addition, it should be used cautiously in pregnant women. This drug has a half life of about 5 minutes. It is metabolized in the liver and excreted in the urine. Within 10 minutes of its administration, about 80% of a dose has been cleared from the blood. SYN: *recombinant TPA.* SEE: *streptokinase; reperfusion.*

NURSING IMPLICATIONS: Maintain patient on strict bedrest throughout infusion. Initiate additional IV access site(s) for adjuvant therapies or required blood studies prior to initiating TPA. No further needle sticks should occur during therapy. Inspect intravenous access site for bleeding throughout therapy, and assess patient for indications of intracerebral or gastric bleeding. Administer heparin with or following therapy as prescribed to maintain activated partial thromboplastin time (APTT) at 2 times patient's normal baseline. Evaluate for indications of reperfusion: sudden cessation of chest pain, early peak of creatine phosphokinase-MB (CPK-MB) enzyme (at 12 hours post injury), resolution of EKG injury current patterns, and "reperfusion dysrhythmias," including accelerated idioventricular rhythm, ventricular tachycardia, sinus bradycardia, and atrioventricular (AV) block with hypotension. Assess for, document, and treat mild allergic responses to therapy (pruritus, urticaria, flushing, fever, headache, nausea and malaise); also assess for more acute allergic manifestations (bronchospasm, angioedema), immediately initiating emergency treatment to protect airway and prevent circulatory collapse.

tissue reaction. The response of living tissues to altered conditions or types of restorative materials, metals, cements.

tissue typing. Techniques utilized in determining the histocompatibility of tissues to be used in grafts and transplants with the recipient's tissues and cells. SEE: *transplantation.*

tissular (tǐsh′ū-lăr). Concerning living tissues.

titanium (tī-tā′nē-ŭm) [L. *titan,* the sun]. SYMB: Ti. At. wt. 47.90; at. no. 22; sp. gr. 4.54. A metallic element found in combination with minerals. In dentistry, it is used as an alloy chiefly for appliances and implants because of its biological acceptance and resistance to corrosion.

    t. dioxide. USP. A chemical used to protect the skin from the sun. It is also used in industrial applications to produce a white color in paints and plastics.

titer (tī′tĕr) [F. *titre,* standard]. Standard of strength per volume of a volumetric test solution.

    t., agglutination. The highest dilution of a serum that will cause clumping or agglutination of the bacteria being tested.

    t., antibody. A measure of the amount of antibody against a particular antigen present in the blood. One use is in detection of antibodies against herpes simplex virus and Epstein Barr virus. Researchers believe that any elevated antibody titers may indicate a decrease in lymphocyte activity as the result of the stress response or other condition since these viruses are generally controlled by T lymphocytes. This titer is also useful in following the course of many acute infectious diseases. A rising titer usually indicates the disease is present and the body is reacting to the specific antigen.

titillation (tĭt″ĭl-ā′shŭn) [L. *titillatio*, a tickling]. 1. Act of tickling, as in the throat. 2. State of being tickled. 3. Sensation produced by tickling.

titrate (tī′trāt). To determine or estimate by titration.

titration (tī-trā′shŭn) [Fr. *titre*, a standard]. 1. Estimation of the concentration of a chemical solution by adding known amounts of standard reagents until alteration in color or electrical state occurs. 2. Determination of quantity of antibody in an antiserum.

titre. Titer.

titrimetric (tī″trī-mĕt′rĭk) [″ + Gr. *metron*, measure]. Employing the process of titration.

titrimetry (tī-trĭm′ĕ-trē) [*titration* + Gr. *metron*, measure]. To analyze something by using titration.

titubation (tĭt″ū-bā′shŭn) [L. *titubatio*, a staggering]. A staggering gait, seen in diseases of the cerebellum.

t., lingual. Stuttering, stammering.

Tl. Chem. symb. for the element thallium.

TLC. 1. *tender loving care.* The concept of administering medical and nursing care and attention to a patient in a kindly, compassionate, and humane manner as distinguished from a cold technical approach. This is particularly important in intensive care units, where patients are connected to electronic monitors and devices. 2. *total lung capacity. 3. thin-layer chromatography.* SEE: *chromatography, thin-layer.*

T.L.R. *tonic labyrinthine reflex.*

Tm. 1. Chem. symb. for the element thulium. 2. Symb. for maximal tubular excretory capacity of the kidneys.

TMJ. *temporomandibular joint.*

Tn. Symb. for normal intraocular tension.

TNF. *tumor necrosis factor.*

TNM classification. Method of classifying malignant tumors with respect to primary tumor, involvement of regional lymph nodes, and presence or absence of metastases. SEE: *cancer.*

TNT. *trinitrotoluene.*

TO. *old tuberculin* (also abbr. OT).

toadskin (tōd′skin). Condition characterized by excessive dryness, wrinkling, and scaling of skin sometimes seen in vitamin deficiencies. SEE: *phrynoderma.*

toadstool (tōd′stool). Any of various fungi with an umbrella-shaped cap; popularly a poisonous mushroom.

toadstool poisoning. The toxicity experienced from ingestion of a poisonous mushroom.

SYM: Symptoms appear from a few minutes to 15 hours after ingestion, characterized by marked abdominal pain, vomiting, and intense diarrhea. Profound weakness comes early and remains. Sometimes perspiration and lacrimation are present and occasionally convulsions or coma.

F.A.: Absolute bedrest. Empty stomach and bowels promptly and completely with gastric lavage and quick-acting cathartic and enemas. Atropine is especially helpful and may be given by any route. Fluid, sodium chloride, and high carbohydrate intake should be maintained intravenously if required. Excitement, hypotension, convulsions, pain, and fever are treated symptomatically. Dialysis has been used in treating poisoning due to *Amanita phalloides.* SEE: *amanita* at *Poisons and Poisoning* in *Appendix.*

tobacco (tō-băk′ō) [Sp. *tabaco*]. Dried leaves of *Nicotiana tabacum* and other species. It contains nicotine, pyridine, picoline, and collidin. Widely used in forms of cigars, cigarettes, pipe tobacco, snuff, and chewing tobacco. During its combustion, various products are given off, the most important being nicotine, q.v., and certain compounds that have an adverse effect on the lungs. For this reason, the use of tobacco products has proved injurious to health.

Even though chewing tobacco and snuff are not smoked, they, too, are harmful. SEE: *risk factors; smokeless tobacco; smoking, passive.*

tobramycin (tō″bră-mī′sĭn). USP. An antibiotic drug.

tocainide (tō-kāy′nīd). A lidocaine analogue used in treating ventricular arrhythmias. Trade name is Tonocard.

toco- [Gr. *tokos*, birth]. Prefix indicating a relationship to childbirth.

tocodynagraph (tō″kō-dī′nă-grăf) [″ + *dynamis*, power, + *graphein*, to write]. A device for measuring the intensity of uterine contractions.

tocodynamometer (tō″kō-dī″năm-ŏm′ĕ-tĕr) [″ + *dynamis*, power, + *metron*, a measure]. Device for estimating force of uterine contractions in childbirth. SYN: *tocometer.*

tocograph (tŏk′ō-grăf) [″ + *graphein*, to write]. A device for estimating and recording the force of uterine contractions.

tocography (tō″kŏg′ră-fē). Recording the intensity of uterine contractions.

tocology (tō-kŏl′ō-jē) [″ + *logos*, word, reason]. Science of parturition and obstetrics.

tocolysis (tō″kō-lĭ′sĭs) [″ + *lysis*, dissolution]. Inhibition of uterine contractions.

Drugs used for this include adrenergic agonists, magnesium sulfate, and ethanol.

tocometer (tō-kŏm′ĕt-ĕr) [″ + *metron*, a measure]. Device for estimating force of contractions of the uterus during labor. SYN: *tocodynamometer.*

tocopherol (tō-kŏf′ĕr-ŏl) [″ + *pherein*, to carry, + L. *oleum*, oil]. Generic term for vitamin E (alpha tocopherol) and a number of chemically related compounds, most of which have the biological activity of vitamin E.

tocophobia (tō″kō-fō′bē-ă) [″ + *phobos*, fear]. Abnormal fear of childbirth.

tocus (tō′kŭs) [L.]. Parturition; childbirth.

toe (tō) [AS. *ta*]. A digit of the foot. SYN: *digit.* SEE: *foot* for illus.

RS: acroataxia; acrodynia; bunion; camptodactylia; clavus; corn; dactylus; gout; hallux; metatarsus.

   t., claw. Hammertoe.

   t., dislocations of. Treated essentially same as dislocations of the fingers. SEE: *finger, dislocation of.*

   t.'s., fanning of. Spreading of toes, esp. when sole is stroked.

   t., hammer-. Condition of dorsal flexion of the first phalanx and plantar flexion of the second and third phalanges.

   t., Morton's. Metatarsalgia.

   t., pigeon. Walking with the toes turned inward.

   t.'s, webbed. Toes joined by webs of skin.

toe clonus. Contraction of the big toe due to sudden extension of the first phalanx.

toe drop. Inability to lift the toes.

toenail (tō′nāl). Unguis. SEE: *nail.*

toe reflex. Reflex in which strong flexion of the great toe flexes all muscles below the knee.

Tofranil. Trade name for imipramine hydrochloride.

Togaviridae [L. *toga,* coat, + *virus,* poison]. A family of arthropod-borne viruses including the genera *Alphavirus* and *Rubivirus* (rubella virus; german measles virus), which affect humans, and *Pestivirus,* a genus that affects only animals.

In humans, the two genera cause a great number of diseases characterized by symptoms such as encephalitis, headache, and arthritis. These diseases are controlled by eradicating the arthropod vectors.

toilet (toy′lĕt) [Fr. *toilette,* a little cloth]. 1. Cleansing of a wound after operation, or cleansing of an obstetrical patient. 2. An apparatus for use during defecation and urination to collect and dispose of these waste products. The disposal may be immediate by flushing with water, by chemical digestion, or by incineration.

toilet training. Teaching the child to control urination and defecation until placed on a toilet. The bowel movements of an infant may habitually occur at the same time each day very early in life, but it is not advisable to begin to train the child until the end of the second year. Close to that time, placing the child on a small potty chair for a short period of time at regular intervals may allow the child to stay dry. First the diapers are removed while the child is awake. Later they are removed during naps and the child is told he or she should be able to stay dry. This schedule may need to be interrupted for a period if the child does not remain dry. Later on there will be no need for diapers during the day or night. To protect the bed a rubber sheet should be used during the training period. Children who are unsuccessful in remaining dry or training their bowel habits should not be punished. To do so may promote the later development of enuresis or constipation.

toko-. Toco-, q.v.

tokodynagraph (tō″kō-dī′nă-grăf) [Gr. *tokos,* birth, + *dynamis,* power, + *graphein,* to write]. Tocodynagraph, q.v.

tolazamide (tŏl-ăz′ă-mīd). USP. An oral hypoglycemia agent of the sulfonylurea class. Trade name is Tolinase.

Caution: This drug should be used only in patients with diabetes of the insulin-independent type who cannot be treated with diet alone and who are unwilling or unable to take insulin if weight reduction and dietary control fail.

---

tolazoline hydrochloride (tŏl-ăz′ō-lēn). USP. An α-adrenergic blocking agent used to produce peripheral vasodilation. Trade name is Priscoline Hydrochloride.

tolbutamide (tŏl-bū′tă-mīd). USP. An oral hypoglycemic agent of the sulfonylurea class. Trade name is Orinase.

Caution: This drug should be used only in patients with diabetes of the insulin-independent type who cannot be treated with diet alone and who are unwilling or unable to take insulin if weight reduction and dietary control fail.

Tolectin. Trade name for tolmetin sodium.

tolerance (tŏl′ĕr-ăns) [L. *tolerantia,* tolerance]. Capacity for enduring a large amount of a substance (food, drug, or poison) without an adverse effect and showing a decreased sensitivity to subsequent doses of the same substance.

   t., drug. Progressive decrease in effectiveness of a drug.

t., exercise. The amount of physical activity that can be done under supervision before exhaustion.

t., glucose. The ability of the body to absorb and utilize glucose. SEE: *glucose tolerance test.*

t., immunologic. A state of immunologic inactivity or diminution so that an antigen that would ordinarily induce an immune response does not.

t., pain. The degree of pain an individual can withstand.

tolerant. Capable of enduring or withstanding drugs without experiencing ill effects.

tolerogen (tŏl'ĕr-ō-jĕn). That which causes immunological tolerance or failure of the body to react to an antigen by forming an antibody. The mechanism of formation of this specific unresponsive state is poorly understood.

tolerogenic (tŏl"ĕr-ō-jĕn'ĭk). Producing immunological tolerance.

Toleron. Trade name for ferrous fumarate.

Tolinase. Trade name for tolazamide, USP.

tollwut (tŏl-voot') [Ger.]. Rabies.

tolnaftate (tŏl-năf'tāt). USP. A synthetic antifungal agent used topically in treating various forms of tinea. Trade name is Tinactin.

tolu balsam. USP. A balsam obtained from *Myroxylon balsamum*. It is used as an expectorant.

toluene. A hydrocarbon derived from coal tar.

toluene poisoning. SEE: *benzene* in *Poisons and Poisoning* in *Appendix.*

toluidine (tŏl-ū'ĭ-dĭn). C_7H_9N. Aminotoluene, a derivative of toluene.

tomaculous neuropathy (tŏ-mā'cū-lŭs) [L. *tomaculum*, a kind of sausage]. The presence of sausage-shaped areas of thickened myelin with secondary axon constriction in some cases of familial recurrent brachial neuropathy.

tomatine (tō'mă-tēn). A substance derived from tomato plants affected by wilt. It has antifungal action.

-tome [Gr. *tome*, incision]. Combining form meaning cutting, or cutting instrument.

tomo- [Gr. *tome*, incision]. Combining form indicating a section or layer.

tomogram (tō'mō-grăm) [" + *gramma*, something written]. The x-ray picture obtained by use of tomography.

tomograph (tō'mō-grăf) [" + *graphein*, to write]. A special type of x-ray apparatus that demonstrates the organ or tissue at a particular depth.

tomography (tō-mŏg'ră-fē). Any of several noninvasive special techniques of roentgenography designed to show detailed images of structures in a selected plane of tissue by blurring images of structures in all other planes.

t., computerized. ABBR: CT. Tomography in which transverse planes of tissue are swept by a pinpoint radiographic beam and a computerized analysis of the variance in absorption produces a precise reconstructed image of that area. This technique has a greater sensitivity in showing the relationship of structures than conventional radiography and has been used most successfully in diagnostic studies of the brain.

t., computerized axial. ABBR: CAT. SEE: *tomography, computerized; magnetic resonance imaging.*

t., positron emission. ABBR: PET. SEE: *positron emission tomography.*

-tomy. A word ending indicating a cutting or an incision.

tonaphasia (tō"nă-fā'sē-ă) [L. *tonus*, a stretching, + *a-*, not, + *phasis*, speech]. Inability to remember a tune due to cerebral lesion.

tone (tōn) [L. *tonus*, a stretching]. 1. That state of a body or any of its organs or parts in which the functions are healthy and normal. In a more restricted sense, the resistance of muscles to passive elongation or stretch. 2. Normal tension or responsiveness to stimuli, as of arteries or muscles, seen particularly in involuntary muscle (such as the sphincter of the urinary bladder). SYN: *tonicity.* 3. A musical or vocal sound.

t., muscular. Condition in which a muscle is in a steady state of contraction; the ability of a muscle to resist a force for a considerable period of time without change in length.

tone deafness. Inability to detect differences in musical sounds. SYN: *amusia.*

tongs, Crutchfield. SEE: *Crutchfield tongs.*

tongue (tŭng) [AS. *tunge*]. A freely movable muscular organ lying partly in the floor of the mouth and partly in the pharynx. Its function is manipulation of food in mastication and deglutition, speech production, and taste. Its surface is covered with mucous membrane. SYN: *lingua.* SEE: illus.

ANAT: The tongue consists of a body and root and is attached by muscles to the hyoid bone below, the mandible in front, the styloid process behind, and the palate above, and by mucous membrane to the floor of the mouth, the lateral walls of the pharynx, and the epiglottis. A median fold, the frenulum linguae, connects the tongue to the floor of the mouth. The surface of the tongue bears numerous papillae of three types: filiform, fungiform, and vallate. Taste buds are present on the surfaces of many of the papillae, esp. the vallate papillae. Mucous and serous glands (lingual glands) are present, their ducts opening on the surface. Lym-

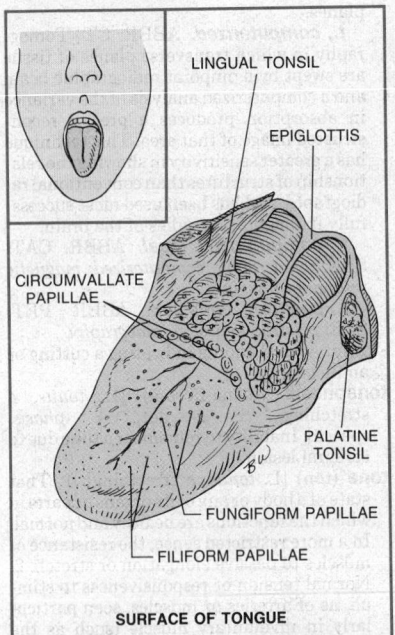

LINGUAL TONSIL

EPIGLOTTIS

CIRCUMVALLATE PAPILLAE

PALATINE TONSIL

FUNGIFORM PAPILLAE

FILIFORM PAPILLAE

SURFACE OF TONGUE

phoid tissue composing the lingual tonsils is present in the posterior third of the tongue. A median fibrous septum extends the entire length of the tongue.

Arteries: Lingual, exterior maxillary, and ascending pharyngeal. *Muscles:* Extrinsic muscles include genioglossus, hypoglossus, and styloglossus. Intrinsic muscles consist of four groups: superior, inferior, transverse and vertical lingualis muscles. *Nerves:* Lingual nerve (containing fibers from trigeminal and facial nerves), glossopharyngeal, vagus, and hypoglossal.

DIFF. DIAG: *Pain:* Occurs in local lesions; fissures; glossitis; malignancies; and pernicious anemia. *Protrusion and movement:* This occurs with very sick patients, as in advanced typhoid fever and toxemia. The tongue is tremulous in early typhoid and in meningitis. In chorea it is thrust out suddenly and at once withdrawn. If it is protruded very slowly or if left exposed after being shown, it is a sign of great exhaustion, vascular congestion, or disorder of the nerve supply. If the tongue when protruded points to the right or left involuntarily, a central or peripheral lesion of the nerve supply is present. Some persons have the ability to curl the tongue along its long axis. This abil-

ity is genetically determined. *Thrust to one side:* Indicates hemiplegia if continually held in this position. *Scars:* These may be the result of injury or bulbar palsy causing ulceration and resulting in scars. *Spasm:* Occurs in multiple sclerosis, general paresis, melancholia, and stuttering. *Tremors:* Noted in asthenia, alcoholism, bulbar palsy, and Graves' disorder. In hemiplegia it is turned toward the paralyzed side if the face is affected. If turned toward the unaffected side, it denotes a lesion of the medulla. *Tremulousness:* In all acute diseases but no particular significance in chronic nervous disorders.

Color: The tongue may be temporarily discolored by a variety of colored medicines, foods, and liquids. *Black coating:* Glossophytia; may be due to stain or presence of microphytes. In dysentery, indicates impending death. Onset of jaundice is usually first detectable in the yellowish discoloration of the area seen under the tongue when its tip is placed against the roof of the mouth. *Bluish:* Denotes impaired circulation, interference with respiration, heart disease, asthma, cyanosis. *Black hairy:* SEE: t., black hairy. *Pale:* Indicates severe anemia; the tongue appears smaller than normal. *Red:* An early sign in typhoid fever. *Bright red:* Indicates glossitis or stomatitis. *Clean red:* With papillae prominent, or a white-coated tongue with papillae projecting through the fur, indicates scarlatina. *Red tip and edges,* or having red dry streak in center, typical of typhoid. *Strawberry:* White fur through which project bright red and prominent papillae. Seen in early stage of scarlet fever. *Yellow:* With thick fur covering the tongue, indicates jaundice.

Macroglossia: Large tongue, generally congenital, or may result from inflammation, Ludwig's angina, glossitis, actinomycosis, acromegaly, myxedema. If localized, may be due to gumma, carcinoma, or local trauma. *Microglossia:* Small tongue, observed in anemia, emaciation, convalescence from typhoid. These conditions are temporary.

t., bifid. Tongue with a cleft at its anterior end. SYN: *t., forked.*

t., black hairy. Condition in which tongue possesses a brown furlike area on its dorsum. The area is composed of hypertrophied filiform papillae pigment and possibly microorganisms. Sometimes results from excessive use of oxygen-liberating mouthwashes or antibiotic therapy. SYN: *lingua nigra.*

t., burning. Burning sensation of the tongue. SYN: *glossopyrosis.*

t., cleft. T., bifid.

t., coated. Tongue covered with layer of whitish or yellowish material consisting of desquamated epithelium, bacteria, or food debris. Significance is difficult to interpret. May mean only that patient slept with mouth open or has not eaten because of loss of appetite. If darkly coated, it may indicate a fungus infection.

t., deviation of. Marked turning of tongue from the midline when protruded. Indicative of lesions of the hypoglossal nerve.

t., dry. Tongue that is dry and shriveled, usually indicative of dehydration. May also be the result of mouth breathing.

t., fern-leaf. Tongue possessing a prominent central furrow and lateral branches.

t., filmy. Tongue possessing symmetrical whitish patches.

t., fissured. Tongue bearing deep furrows in its epithelium. May be normal. Causes are obscure. If deep and inflamed, may be due to syphilitic infection, dissecting glossitis, a broken tooth, chronic dysentery, hepatic disease, or diabetes mellitus.

t., forked. T., bifid.

t., furred. Coated tongue on which surface epithelium appears as a coat of white fur. Seen in nearly all fevers. Unilateral furring may result from disturbed innervation, as in condition affecting 2nd and 3rd branches of the 5th nerve. Has been noted in neuralgia of those branches and in fractures of the skull involving the foramen rotundum. Yellow fur indicates jaundice.

t., geographic. Tongue possessing white raised areas resembling mountain ranges on a relief map. Areas consist of heaped-up epithelium surrounding areas of atrophy.

t., magenta. Magenta-colored tongue seen in cases of riboflavin deficiency.

t., parrot. A dry shriveled tongue, seen in typhus.

t., raspberry. T., strawberry, q.v.

t., scrotal. Furrowed and fissured tongue, resembling skin of scrotum. SEE: *t., fissured.*

t., smoker's. Condition of tongue characterized by white opaque patches of thickened epithelium later thickening and becoming fissured. SYN: *leukoplakia.*

t., smooth. Condition of tongue resulting from atrophy of papillae. Characteristic of many conditions, such as anemia and malnutrition.

t., strawberry. Tongue that first has a white coat except at tip and along edges, with enlarged papillae standing out distinctly against white surface. Later white coat disappears, leaving a bright red surface. Characteristic of scarlet fever.

t., trifid. Tongue in which anterior end is divided into three parts.

t., trombone. Rapid involuntary movement of the tongue in and out.

tongue, words pert. to: circumvallate papillae; cleft; frenulum linguae; "gloss-" words; hypoglossal; hypoglottis; lingua; macroglossia; ranula; sublingual gland.

tongue-swallowing. In an unconscious person lying on the back, the tendency for the relaxed tongue to slip back into the pharynx. Although the tongue is not actually swallowed, the airway becomes blocked and respiration is seriously impeded. To correct, elevate the shoulders and extend the head; this maneuver will open the airway. Also a mechanical airway device may be used to hold or push the tongue forward.

tongue thrust. In the infant, the habit of extending the tongue from the mouth during sucking and swallowing.

tongue-tie. Lay term for ankyloglossia, congenital shortness of the frenum of the tongue.

    SYM: Interference in sucking and in articulation.

    TREAT: Surgical freeing of the frenum.

tonic (tŏn′ĭk) [Gr. *tonikos,* from *tonos,* tone]. 1. Pert. to or characterized by tension or contraction, esp. muscular tension. 2. Restoring tone. 3. A medicine that increases strength and tone. Tonics are subdivided according to action such as cardiac or general. Ex.: iron; digitalis.

tonicity (tō-nĭs′ĭ-tē) [Gr. *tonos,* act of stretching]. 1. Property of possessing tone, esp. muscular tone. 2. State of normal tension or partial contracion of muscle fibers while at rest. SYN: *tone.*

tonic labyrinthine reflex. In animals, the postural reflex. In decerebrate humans, this reflex manifests as extension of the four extremities when the person is in a supine position with the head in midline.

tonic neck reflex. Reflex, tonic neck, q.v.

tonicoclonic (tŏn″ĭ-kō-klŏn′ĭk). Tonoclonic.

tonic spasm. A persistent, involuntary, firm or violent muscular contraction. SEE: *clonic spasm.*

tonoclonic (tŏn″ō-klŏn′ĭk) [″ + *klonos,* tumult]. Both tonic and clonic, said of muscular spasms.

tonofibril (tŏn′ō-fī″brĭl). Tenofibril, q.v.

tonofilament (tŏn″ō-fĭl′ă-mĕnt). A filament of a tonofibril.

tonogram (tō′nō-grăm) [″ + *gramma,* something written]. The record produced by a tonograph.

tonograph (tō′nō-grăf) [″ + *graphein,* to write]. A recording tonometer.

tonography (tō-nŏg′ră-fē). The recording of changes in intraocular pressure.

tonometer (tŏn-ŏm′ĕ-tĕr) [″ + *metron,*

measure]. Instrument for measuring tension or pressure, esp. intraocular pressure.

tonometer, Schiötz [Hjalmar Schiötz, Norwegian physician, 1850–1927]. Instrument for measuring intraocular pressure by the degree of indentation produced by pressure on the cornea.

tonometry (tŏn-ŏm′ĕ-trē). The measurement of tension of a part, as intraocular tension. This test is extremely useful in detecting glaucoma.

   t., digital. Determining intraocular pressure by use of the fingers.

   t., non-contact. The intraocular pressure is determined by measuring the alteration in the cornea produced by a puff of air.

tonoplast (tŏn′ō-plăst) [″ + *plassein,* to form]. The membrane surrounding an intracellular vacuole.

tonsil (tŏn′sĭl) [L. *tonsilla,* almond]. 1. A mass of lymphatic tissue located in depressions of the mucous membrane of fauces and pharynx. 2. A rounded mass on the inferior surface of the cerebellum lying lateral to the uvula.
FUNCT: Acts as a filter to protect body from invasion of bacteria, and aids in the formation of white cells.

   t., cerebellar. One of a pair of cerebellar lobules on either side of the uvula, q.v., projecting from the inferior surface of the cerebellum.

   t., faucial T., palatine.

   t., lingual. A mass of lymphoid tissue located in the root of the tongue.

   t., Luschka's. T., pharyngeal.

   t., nasal. Lymphoid tissue on the nasal septum.

   t., palatine. A mass of lymphoid tissue that lies in tonsillar fossa on each side of oral pharynx between glossopalatine and pharyngopalatine arches. The free surface of each tonsil is covered with stratified squamous epithelium that forms deep indentations or crypts extending into the substance of the tonsil. The lateral surface of each tonsil is covered with a firm fibrous capsule. Efferent lymph vessels convey lymph from the tonsil.

   t., pharyngeal. Lymphoid tissue on the roof of the posterior wall of the pharynx. SYN: *t., Luschka's.* SEE: *adenoid.*

   t., tubal. Lymphatic tissue present in mucous membrane of the auditory tube near its opening into the pharynx.

tonsilla (tŏn-sĭl′ă) [L.]. General anatomic term for a small, discrete, rounded mass of tissue.

tonsillar (tŏn′sĭ-lăr). Pert. to a tonsil, esp. the faucial or palatine tonsil.

tonsillar area. Area composed of the palatine arch, tonsillar fossa, glossopalatine sulcus,

and posterior faucial pillar.

tonsillar crypt. A deep indentation into the pharyngeal surface of a tonsil. It is lined with stratified epithelium.

tonsillar fossa. Depression between the glossopalatine and pharyngopalatine arches in which the palatine tonsil is situated.

tonsillar ring. The almost complete ring of tonsillar tissue encircling the pharynx. Includes the palatine, lingual, and pharyngeal tonsils. SEE: *Waldeyer's ring.*

tonsillar sinus. Space lying between the plica triangularis and the anterior surface of the palatine tonsil.

tonsillectomy (tŏn-sĭl-ĕk′tō-mē) [L. *tonsilla,* almond + Gr. *ektome,* excision]. Surgical removal of the tonsils.
NURSING IMPLICATIONS: *Preop:* Explain to adults the anesthetic method to be used and expected sensations. Offer child a simple, nonthreatening explanation, explain hospital routines, permit child to try on operating room garb, and show the operating room and recovery areas as appropriate to age. Encourage parent to remain with child.
   Postop: Maintain a patent airway and prevent aspiration by positioning patient semiprone or on side until fully reactive from anesthesia. Monitor vital signs and assess for bleeding (excessive swallowing in semiconscious child), restlessness, tachycardia, and pallor. After patient's gag reflex has returned, allow water by mouth and encourage intake of nonirritating fluids. Also encourage deep breathing and turning to prevent pulmonary complications. Administer ice packs and analgesics as prescribed. Encourage voice rest and instruct patient not to clear throat or cough, as this may precipitate bleeding. Provide written discharge instructions for patient and family, including use of fluids and soft diet as tolerated and avoidance of overactivity. Inform them that a white scab may form in throat within 5 to 10 days postoperatively and instruct to report bleeding, ear discomfort, or persistent fever. SEE: *Nursing Diagnoses* in *Appendix.*

tonsillith (tŏn′sĭ-lĭth) [″ + Gr. *lithos,* stone]. Tonsillolith.

tonsillitis (tŏn-sĭl-ī′tĭs) [″ + Gr. *itis,* inflammation]. Inflammation of a tonsil, esp. the faucial tonsil. SEE: *Nursing Diagnoses* in *Appendix.*

   t., acute. Inflammation of the lymphatic tissue of the pharynx, esp. the palatine or faucial tonsils. May occur sporadically or in epidemic form. SEE: *rheumatic fever.*
   SYM: Onset is sudden, usually accompanied by chills. Temperature may reach 105°F (40.6°C). Malaise; headache; pains

and aches in back and extremities; pain in tonsils, esp. when swallowing, may be present. Tonsils appear enlarged and red with yellowish exudate projecting from crypts.

ETIOL: May be caused by a variety of organisms. If due to group A beta-hemolytic streptococci, sequelae such as rheumatic fever, carditis, and nephritis must be considered.

PROG: Usually self-limited but serious complications, such as sinusitis, otitis media, mastoiditis, or peritonsillar abscess, may occur.

TREAT: *General:* Bedrest; liquid diet; antipyretics; hot saline or 30% glucose gargles or throat irrigations. *Specific:* Procaine penicillin or tetracycline drugs.

If the disease is thought to be due to group A beta-hemolytic streptococci, the throat should be cultured and then penicillin therapy instituted for a full 10-day course. If therapy was instituted prior to the report of the culture and the report is negative for these organisms, the penicillin therapy may be discontinued when clinical signs of infection have subsided.

If throat culture technique is not available and infection with group A beta-hemolytic streptococci is suspected, then a full 10-day course of penicillin should be given. This regimen will prevent the streptococci from elaborating the toxic substances that cause rheumatic fever, rheumatic heart disease, and certain kidney diseases. Administration of penicillin for less than 10 days when tonsillitis is due to group A beta-hemolytic streptococci is not advisable, even though clinical signs of infection may disappear within the first several days of treatment.

t., follicular. Tonsillitis in which the crypts are affected.

t., parenchymatous, acute. Tonsillitis in which the entire tonsil is affected.

tonsilloadenoidectomy (tŏn″sĭl-ō-ăd″ĕ-noy-dĕk′tō-mē). Excision of the tonsils and adenoids of the pharynx.

tonsillolith (tŏn′sĭl-ō-lĭth) [″ + Gr. *lithos*, stone]. A concretion within a tonsil. SYN: *amygdalolith*.

tonsillopathy (tŏn″sĭ-lŏp′ă-thē). Any disease of the tonsil.

tonsilloscopy (tŏn″sĭl-lŏs′kō-pē) [″ + Gr. *skopein*, to examine]. Inspection of the tonsils.

tonsillotome (tŏn-sĭl′ō-tōm). Surgical instrument used in tonsillectomy.

tonsillotomy (tŏn″sĭl-ŏt′ō-mē) [″ + Gr. *tome*, incision]. Incision of the tonsils.

tonus (tō′nŭs) [L., tension]. That partial steady contraction of muscle which deter-

mines tonicity or firmness. Opposite of clonus. SYN: *tone, tonicity.*

tooth [AS. *toth*] (pl. *teeth*). One of the conical hard structures of the upper and lower jaws used for mastication. A tooth consists of a crown or portion above the gum, a root portion embedded in a socket (alveolus) of the jaw bone, and a neck or cervical constricted region between the crown and root. The soft tissue gingiva covers the neck and root to a variable extent, depending on age and oral hygiene. The major portion of a tooth consists of dentin, which surrounds the pulp chamber in the crown and root of the tooth. Ivory is an example of dentin, which is harder than bone. Enamel is the hardest tissue of the body and covers the crown. Cementum is similar to bone and covers the root, attaching the tooth to the surrounding bony socket by the periodontal ligament fibers embedded in both bone and cementum. The pulp cavity contains the dental pulp, a loose connective tissue containing many cells, nerves, and blood or lymph vessels. SEE: illus.; *dentition; periodontal disease; plaque, dental; teeth; teeth, reimplantation or repair of; teeth, stained;* words beginning with *odonto-*.

t., accessional. The permanent molar teeth which arise without deciduous predecessors in the dental arch.

t., baby. Deciduous tooth.

t., impacted. A tooth that is unable to erupt due to adjacent teeth or malposition of the tooth.

t., implanted. An artificial tooth implanted permanently into the jaw.

toothache. Pain in a tooth or the region about a tooth. SYN: *odontalgia; odontodynia.*

tooth bleaching. Application of chemical bleaching agents to teeth to make them whiter.

toothbrush and toothbrushing. The teeth can be cleansed by using a soft brush specifically designed for cleaning teeth; it consists of tufts of soft, synthetic fibers or natural bristles mounted in a handle that may be straight or angled for better access or brushing action. It is usually used with fluoride toothpaste (a mildly abrasive, flavored dentifrice) in a manner suggested by dentists and dental hygienists as being a suitable method for cleaning. Proper use of a toothbrush stimulates periodontal tissue.

Good oral hygiene, consisting of proper brushing of the teeth with a soft bristle brush, use of a fluoride containing toothpaste, and daily use of dental floss will help to prevent dental plaque. If brushing or flossing causes bleeding, pain, or irritation, see your dentist without delay.

Some people with conditions that limit

STRUCTURE OF TOOTH

CROWN

ENAMEL

DENTIN

GINGIVAL SULCUS

GINGIVA

NECK

PULP CHAMBER

PERIODONTAL LIGAMENT

PERIODONTAL MEMBRANE

ROOT

ROOT CANALS WITH VESSELS AND NERVES

BONE

APICAL FORAMEN

INFERIOR ALVEOLAR NERVE, ARTERY AND VEIN

motion of their hands may have difficulty holding and using a toothbrush. This may be overcome by attaching the brush handle to the hand with a wide elastic band, or the handle may be enlarged by attaching a rubber or foam ball to it. Those with limited shoulder or elbow movement may find that lengthening the handle by attaching it to a long piece of wood or plastic is beneficial. In addition, an electric toothbrush may be of benefit. SEE: *periodontal disease; plaque, dental; teeth; tooth.*

Caution: If the toothbrush used has hard bristles or if any toothbrush is used too forcibly, gingival tissue may be eroded and damaged.

tooth migration, pathologic. Drifting or movement of teeth due to the pathological changes in areas adjacent to the moving teeth. SEE: *mesial drift; tooth movement.*

tooth migration, physiologic. The natural and expected movement of teeth as growth and development occur. SYN: *physiologic drift.* SEE: *mesial drift; tooth migration, pathologic; tooth movement.*

tooth movement. Change in position of a tooth or teeth in the dental arch. This may occur due to abnormal pressure from the tongue, pathological changes in tooth-supporting structures, malocclusion, missing teeth, or may be due to a therapeutic orthodontic procedure. Thumb sucking, q.v., if prolonged, may cause malocclusion and, eventually, displacement of teeth. SEE: *tooth migration, pathologic.*

toothpaste. A dentifrice used with a toothbrush to clean the exposed surfaces of teeth. It may contain mild abrasives, whiteners, deodorants, or caries-preventing agents. SEE: *toothbrush and toothbrushing.*

toothpick. Any small tapering sliver of wood or other materials used to remove food debris from between the teeth. Early examples were made of gold, carved bone or ivory.

top-, topo-. Combining form meaning place or locale.

topagnosis (tŏp″ăg-nō′sĭs) [Gr. *topos*, place, + *a*, not, + *gnosis*, knowledge]. Loss of ability to localize site of tactile sensations.

topalgia (tō-păl′jē-ă) [″ + *algos*, pain]. Pain in a localized site.

topectomy (tō-pĕk′tō-mē) [″ + *ektome*, excision]. A modified form of frontal lobotomy in which small incisions are made through the thalamofrontal tracts. A psychosurgical procedure used in the treatment of certain mental diseases.

topesthesia (tŏp″ĕs-thē′zē-ă) [″ + *aisthesis*, sensation]. Ability through tactile sense to determine that skin is touched. SYN: *topognosia*.

tophaceous (tō-fā′shŭs) [L. *tophaceus*, sandy]. 1. Relating to a tophus. 2. Sandy or gritty.

tophus (tō′fŭs) [L., porous stone] (pl. *tophi*). 1. Deposit of sodium biurate in tissues near a joint, in the ear, or in bone in gout. 2. A salivary calculus. 3. Tartar on the teeth.

tophyperidrosis (tŏf″ĭ-pĕr″ĭ-drō′sĭs) [Gr. *topos*, place, + *hyper*, above, + *hidros*, sweat]. Excessive sweating in local areas.

topical [Gr. *topos*, place]. Pert. to a definite area; local.

Topicort. Trade name for desoximetasone.

Topicycline. Trade name for tetracycline hydrochloride.

topoalgia (tō″pō-ăl′jē-ă) [″ + *algos*, pain]. Localized pain; common in neurasthenia following emotional upsets.

topoanesthesia (tō″pō-ăn″ĕs-thē′zē-ă) [″ + *an-*, not, + *aisthesis*, sensation]. Loss of ability to recognize the location of a tactile sensation.

topognosia, topognosis (tō″pŏg-nō′sē-ă, -sĭs) [″ + *gnosis*, knowledge]. Recognition of the location of a tactile sensation. SYN: *topesthesia*.

topographic (tŏp″ō-grăf′ĭk) [″ + *graphein*, to write]. Pert. to description of special regions.

topographic anatomy. A study of all the structures and their relationships in a given region, for example, the axilla.

topography (tō-pŏg′ră-fē). Description of a part of the body.

topology (tō-pŏl′ō-jē). 1. Topographic anatomy, q.v. 2. In obstetrics, the relationship of the presenting fetal part to the pelvic outlet. 3. In mathematics, the study of the properties of geographic configurations, both solid and plane.

toponarcosis (tō″pō-năr-kō′sĭs) [″ + *narkosis*, a benumbing]. Local anesthesia.

toponeurosis (tō″pō-nū-rō′sĭs) [″ + *neuron*, nerve, + *osis*, condition]. Neurosis of a limited area.

toponym (tŏp′ō-nĭm). The name of a region.

toponymy (tō-pŏn′ĭ-mē) [″ + *onoma*, name]. Nomenclature of the regions of the body.

topophobia (tō″pō-fō′bē-ă) [″ + *phobos*, fear]. A neurotic fear of being in certain areas.

topothermesthesiometer (tŏp″ō-thĕr″mĕs-thē-zē-ŏm′ĕ-ter) [″ + *therme*, heat, + *aisthesis*, sensation, + *metron*, measure]. Device for measuring local temperature sense.

TOPS. Acronym for an organization that assists obese persons to *Take Off Pounds Sensibly*.

Topsyn. Trade name for fluocinonide.

TOPV. *trivalent oral polio vaccine*. SEE: *poliovirus vaccine, trivalent oral*.

torcular Herophili (tor′kū-lăr). The confluence of sinuses at the internal occipital protuberance of the skull.

toric (tō′rĭk). Concerning a torus.

tormina (tor′mĭn-ă) [L., twistings] (sing. *tormen*). Intestinal colic with griping pains.

torose, torous (tō′rōs, -rŭs) [L. *torosus*, full of muscle]. Knobby or bulging; tubercular.

torpent (tor′pĕnt) [L. *torpens*, numbing]. 1. Medicine that modifies irritation. 2. Not capable of functioning; dormant, apathetic, torpid.

torpid (tor′pĭd) [L. *torpidus*, numb]. Not acting vigorously; sluggish.

torpidity (tor-pĭd′ĭ-tē). Sluggishness; inactivity.

torpor [L. *torpor*, numbness]. Abnormal inactivity; dormancy; numbness; apathy.

   t. retinae. Reduced sensitivity of retina to light stimuli.

torque (tork) [L. *torquere*, to twist]. A force producing rotary motion. In dentistry, applying force to rotate a tooth around its long axis.

torr (tor). The pressure of 1/760 of the standard atmospheric pressure. This is virtually equivalent to the pressure of 1 mm of mercury.

torrefaction (tor″ĕ-făk′shŭn) [L. *torrefactio*]. Roasting or parching something, esp. drugs, in order to dry it.

torrefy (tor′ĕ-fī) [L. *torrefacere*]. To parch or roast.

torsade de pointes. Very rapid ventricular tachycardia characterized by a gradually changing QRS complex in the ECG. It is usually self-limiting but may change into ventricular fibrillation. SYN: *tachycardia, polymorphic ventricular.*

torsiometer (tor″sē-ŏm′ĕ-tĕr). Device for measuring the rotation of the eyeball around the visual axis, i.e., its anterior-posterior axis.

torsion (tor′shŭn) [L. *torsio*, a twisting]. 1. Act of twisting or condition of being twisted. In dentistry, the state of a tooth when rotated around its long axis. 2. Rotation of the vertical meridians of the eye.

torsionometer (tor″shŭn-ŏm′ĕ-tĕr) [″ + Gr. *metron*, measure]. Device for measuring the rotation of the vertebral column around the long axis.

torsive (tor′sĭv). Twisted, as in a spiral.

torsiversion (tor″sĭ-vĕr′zhŭn). Rotating a tooth around its long axis.

torso (tor′sō) [It.]. The trunk of the body.

torsoclusion (tor″sō-kloo′zhŭn) [″ + L.

occlusio, to occlude]. 1. Acupressure in combination with torsion to stop a bleeding vessel. 2. Malocclusion characterized by rotation of a tooth on its long axis.

torticollar (tor"tĭ-kŏl'ăr). Concerning torticollis.

torticollis (tor"tĭ-kŏl'ĭs) [L. *tortus,* twisted, + *collum,* neck]. A deformity of the neck secondary to shortening of neck muscles which tilts the head to affected side with chin pointing to the other side. Congenital or acquired. The muscles affected are principally those supplied by the spinal accessory nerve. SYN: *wryneck.*

    ETIOL: Results of scars; disease of cervical vertebrae; adenitis; tonsillitis; rheumatism; enlarged cervical glands; retropharyngeal abscess; cerebellar tumors. It may be spasmodic (clonic) or permanent (tonic). The latter type may be due to Pott's disease (tuberculosis of the spine).

    t., fixed. Abnormal position of head due to organic shortening of the muscles.

    t., intermittent. T., spasmodic.

    t., ocular. Torticollis from inequality in sight of the two eyes.

    t., rheumatic. T., symptomatic.

    t., spasmodic. Torticollis with recurrent but transient contractions of muscles of the neck and esp. of the sternocleidomastoid. SYN: *t., intermittent.*

    TREAT: Botulinus toxin has been used experimentally with good results. The toxin acts to inhibit the spastic contractions of the affected muscles. SEE: *toxin, botulinus.*

    t., spurious. Torticollis from caries of the cervical vertebrae.

    t., symptomatic. Rheumatic stiff neck. SYN: *t., rheumatic.*

tortipelvis (tor"tĭ-pĕl'vĭs) [" + *pelvis,* basin]. Muscular spasms that distort the spine and hip. SYN: *dystonia musculorum deformans.*

tortuous (tor'choo-ŭs) [L. *tortuosus,* fr. *torqueo,* to twist]. Having many twists or turns.

torture (tor'chūr) [LL. *tortura,* a twisting]. Infliction of severe mental or physical pain by various methods, usually for the purpose of coercion.

Torula (tor'ū-lă). Former name of a genus of yeastlike organism, now called *Cryptococcus.*

toruloid (tor'ū-loyd) [L. *torulus,* a little bulge, + Gr. *eidos,* form, shape]. Beaded; noting an aggregate of colonies like those seen in the budding of yeast.

toruloma (tor-ū-lō'mă) [*Torula,* old name for Cryptococcus, + *oma,* tumor]. The nodular lesion of cryptococcosis (torulosis).

Torulopsis glabrata. A yeast of the family Cryptococcaceae. It is closely related to the *Candida* species. Usually nonpathogenic for humans but may cause serious illness in immunocompromised patients no matter what the cause, and in patients receiving immunosuppressive drugs, antibiotics, or corticosteroids.

torulosis (tor-ū-lō'sĭs). Infestation with *Torula* or yeast cells. *Cryptococcosis* is the preferable term.

torulus (tor'ū-lŭs) [L. *torulus,* a little elevation]. A very small nipplelike elevation. SYN: *papilla.*

    t. tactiles. A tactile cutaneous elevation on palms and soles.

torus (tō'rŭs) [L., swelling] (pl. *tori*). A rounded elevation or swelling.

    t. mandibularis. An exostosis that develops on the lingual aspect of the body of the mandible, perhaps transmitted as a genetic trait.

    t. palatinus. A benign exostosis located in the midline of the hard palate. SYN: *palatine protuberance.*

Totacillin. Trade name for ampicillin.

total allergy syndrome. The mistaken belief of some patients, and occasionally their medical advisers, that they are allergic to everything in their environment. Even though their symptoms resemble an allergic condition, the difficulty is most probably due to acute or chronic emotional stress. These individuals may go to great lengths to isolate themselves from environmental materials. Treatment is difficult, but psychotherapy should be tried. This condition has been termed "20th Century syndrome."

total hip replacement. Surgical procedure used in treating severe arthritis of the hip. Both the head of the femur and the acetabulum are replaced with synthetic components. SEE: *arthroplasty.*

    NURSING IMPLICATIONS: *Preop:* Ascertain patient's knowledge of surgery, care, and expected outcome; provide necessary information and correct misconceptions. Teach patient about postoperative limitations, hip abduction methods, use of trapeze and mobility regimen. Teach gluteal and quadriceps setting and triceps exercises. Explain importance of and teach technique for respiratory toilet. Teach patient how to evaluate pain and explain analgesic availability. Administer prescribed antibiotic or other drugs. Review reports of laboratory and radiologic studies, and notify physician if abnormal. Perform prescribed preoperative preparations (skin, GI tract, urinary bladder, pre-medication), explaining significance to patient. Encourage patient to express and discuss feelings and concerns.

    Postop: Monitor dressings and drainage

devices for excessive bleeding, inspecting beneath the buttocks for gravity pooling of drainage. Reinforce or replace dressings according to surgeon's protocol, using aseptic technique. Monitor vital signs, and perform frequent neurovascular checks of affected extremity. Administer analgesia as prescribed and required, and evaluate response. Reposition patient frequently, using prescribed positions and maintaining integrity of all supportive equipment (splints, pillows, traction devices). Teach patient to avoid leg crossing and internal rotation, which enhance potential for prosthesis dislocation and interfere with venous return. Assess respiratory status, and encourage deep breathing and coughing to prevent pulmonary complications. Initiate exercise program and ambulation when prescribed by surgeon (regarding type and extent of weight-bearing on affected limb), collaborating with physical therapist. Avoid hip flexion by use of raised toilet seats and semireclining chairs. Provide diet high in protein and vitamin C, assess wound healing, and prevent skin breakdown. Apply antiembolic stockings if prescribed, and assess for complications such as thrombophlebitis, embolism, and dislocation. Provide discharge teaching regarding exercise regimen and activity limitations, stressing the importance of swimming and walking programs. Arrange for outpatient orthopedic follow-up care and physical therapy as required. Involve patient in weight reduction program if pertinent.

total parenteral nutrition. ABBR: TPN. Provision of the total caloric needs by intravenous route for a patient who is unable to take food orally. Although this is extremely difficult, patients have been maintained in a healthy state for prolonged periods with nutrients through a catheter extending through the subclavian vein to the superior vena cava.

The daily feeding of 2500 to 3000 kcal for an adult includes 2500 to 3000 ml of water; 100 to 130 gm protein hydrolysate (amino acids); 12 to 18 gm nitrogen; 525 to 625 gm dextrose; 125 to 150 mEq sodium; 75 to 120 mEq potassium; 4 to 8 mEq magnesium; vitamins A, D, E, C, thiamine, riboflavin, niacin, and pantothenic acid. Calcium, phosphorus, and iron given as required; vitamin B_{12}, folic acid, and vitamin K given intramuscularly as needed. Trace elements required after one month of continuous feeding.

NURSING IMPLICATIONS: Explain procedure to patient. Obtain a nutritional assessment of the patient. Monitor and record intake and output. Assist with the catheter insertion. Observe for adverse effects. Document procedure and initial fluid administration, and continue to monitor fluid intake. Inspect and redress catheter site every 25 to 48 hours using strict aseptic technique. Document condition of site and position of catheter. Evaluate for catheter leakage and, if present, report to physician immediately. Monitor electrolytes. Administer vitamin supplements as prescribed. Observe for presence of edema or dehydration. If diarrhea or nausea occurs, slow the infusion rate. Perform urine sugar and acetone tests every six hours. Monitor blood sugar levels as ordered. Weigh patient daily. Never discontinue solution abruptly, and taper off with isotonic glucose administered for several hours. In the event of catheter blockage or removal, notify physician immediately. Provide instructions for patient and those in the household who will care for the patient at home.

totem [American Indian]. An object representing a tribe and often serving as a distinctive and venerated symbol.

totipotency (tō″tē-pō′tĕn-sē). The ability of a cell to develop into a great number of different tissues.

totipotent (tō-tĭp′ō-tĕnt) [L. *totus*, all, + *potentia*, power]. A cell capable of differentiating into a large variety of cells. The fertilized ovum has this ability.

touch (tŭch) [O. Fr. *tochier*]. 1. To perceive by the tactile sense; to feel with the hands, to palpate. 2. The sense by which pressure on the skin or mucosa is perceived; the tactile sense. 3. Examination with the hand. SYN: *palpation.*

Various disorders may disturb or impair the tactile sense or the ability to feel normally. There are a number of words and suffixes pert. to sensation and its modifications. A few of the more important ones are as follows: algesia; -algia; anesthesia; dysesthesia; -dynia; esthesia; esthesioneurosis; hyperesthesia; paresthesia; synesthesia.

   t., abdominal. Palpation of the abdomen. SEE: *abdominal examination.*

   t., after-. Persistence of the sensation of touch after contact with stimulus has ceased.

   t., double. Vaginal and rectal examination made at the same time.

   t., rectal. Digital examination of the rectum.

   t., vaginal. Digital examination of the vagina.

   t., vesical. Digital examination of the bladder.

touch, words pert. to: astereognosis; atopognosis; delire de toucher; hallucination; haptic; polyesthesia; stereognosis; tactile.

tour de maître (toor" dĕ mā-tr') [Fr., the master's turn]. A method of introducing a catheter or sound into the male bladder or into the uterus. This involves very carefully turning and angulating the device so as to follow the curvature of the canal.

Tourette's syndrome, disorder. SEE: *Gilles de la Tourette's syndrome.*

Tournay's sign (tūr-nāz') [Auguste Tournay, Fr. ophthalmologist, 1878–1969]. Dilatation of the pupil of the eye on unusually strong lateral fixation.

tourniquet (toor'nĭ-kĕt) [Fr., a turning instrument]. Any constrictor used on an extremity to apply pressure over an artery and thereby control bleeding; also used to distend veins to facilitate venipuncture or intravenous injections.

Arterial hemorrhage: Apply tourniquet between the wound and the heart, close to the wound, placing a hard pad over point of pressure. Should be discontinued as soon as possible and a tight bandage substituted under the loosened tourniquet. SEE: *bleeding, arterial,* for Arrest of Arterial Bleeding table.

Venous hemorrhage: Place tourniquet below bleeding point, but close to the wound. The tourniquet should remain in place with periodic momentary loosening until released by a physician.

Caution: Tourniquet should never be left in place too long. Ordinarily, it should be released from 12 to 18 minutes after application to determine whether bleeding has ceased. If it has, leave tourniquet loosely in place so that it may be retightened if necessary. If bleeding has not ceased, retighten at once. In general, a tourniquet should not be used if steady firm pressure over the bleeding site will stop the flow.

---

t., rotating. In certain types of medical emergencies such as acute pulmonary edema, it is essential to reduce the return of blood to the heart. This is accomplished by applying blood pressure cuffs to three extremities; the patient is placed in a head-high position (Fowler's). The pressure is kept midway between systolic and diastolic. Every 10 minutes the cuffs are deflated and when inflated, the previously free extremity is now used. This allows each extremity to be free of a tourniquet for 10 minutes out of each 40-minute cycle. Obviously, a cuff would not be applied to an extremity into which an intravenous infusion is running.

tourniquet paralysis. Injury to a nerve due to a tourniquet's having been applied for too long a period or too tightly.

tourniquet test. Test for determining the ability of capillaries to withstand increased pressure.

Touton cells (toot'ŏn) [Karl Touton, Ger. dermatologist, 1858–1934]. Giant multinucleated cells found in lesions of xanthomatosis.

towelette (tow"ĕl-ĕt') [ME. *towelle,* towel]. A small towel for surgical or obstetrical use.

tox-, toxi-, toxo-. Combining forms indicating toxic, poison.

toxanemia (tŏks"ă-nē'mē-ă) [Gr. *toxikon,* poison, + *an-,* not, + *haima,* blood]. Anemia due to a hemolytic toxin.

toxemia (tŏks-ē'mē-ă) [" + Gr. *haima,* blood]. Distribution throughout the body of poisonous products of bacteria growing in a focal or local site, thus producing generalized symptoms.

SYM: Fever; diarrhea; vomiting; pulse and respiration quickened or depressed; shock. In tetanus, the nervous system is esp. affected; in diphtheria, nerves and muscles.

t. alimentary. Illness due to absorption of bacterial or other toxins from the gastrointestinal tract.

t., eclamptogenic. Toxemia of pregnancy. SEE: *eclampsia.*

t. of pregnancy. Previously used term for pregnancy-induced hypertension. SEE: *eclampsia; pre-eclampsia.* SEE: *Nursing Diagnoses* in Appendix.

toxenzyme (tŏks-ĕn'zĭm) [" + Gr. *en,* in, + *zyme,* leaven]. A poisonous enzyme.

toxic (tŏks'ĭk) [Gr. *toxikon,* poison]. Pert. to, resembling, or caused by poison. SYN: *poisonous.*

toxic-allergic syndrome. A disease characterized by toxic-allergic pneumonopathy, with respiratory distress, fever, headache, nausea, myalgia, abdominal pains, rash, hepatosplenomegaly, and eosinophilia.

ETIOL: Ingestion of rapeseed oil adulterated with aniline and containing acetanilide.

TREAT: There is no specific therapy, but mechanically assisted respiratory therapy and corticosteroids are helpful.

toxicant (tŏks'ĭ-kănt) [L. *toxicans,* poisoning]. 1. Poisonous; toxic. 2. Any poison.

toxicemic. Toxemic.

toxic erythema. Redness of skin or a rash resulting from toxic agents such as drugs.

toxicide (tŏks'ĭ-sīd) [Gr. *toxikon,* poison, + L. *cidus,* kill]. 1. Destructive to toxins. 2. A chemical antidote for poisons.

toxicity (tŏks-ĭs'ĭ-tē). The extent, quality, or degree of being poisonous.

toxic-nutritional optic neuropathy. Onset of bilateral visual impairment with central scotomas, occurring over a period of days or weeks. This is usually associated with a toxic or nutritional disorder. An example is the optical nerve pathology caused by ingestion of methyl alcohol, q.v.

toxico- [Gr. *toxikon*, poison]. Combining form meaning poisonous.

Toxicodendron (tŏk″sĭ-kō-dĕn′drŏn). A genus of plants that includes poison ivy and poison oak.

toxicoderma (tŏks″ĭ-kō-dĕr′mă) [″ + *derma*, skin]. Any skin disease resulting from a poison.

toxicodermatitis (tŏks″ĭ-kō-dĕrm-ă-tī′tĭs) [″ + ″ + *itis*, inflammation]. Inflammation of the skin due to a poison.

toxicodermatosis (tŏks″ĭ-kō-dĕrm-ă-tō′sĭs) [″ + ″ + *osis*, condition]. Toxicoderma.

toxicogenic (tŏks″ĭ-kō-jĕn′ĭk) [″ + *gennan*, to produce]. Caused by, or producing, a poison.

toxicoid (tŏks′ĭ-koyd) [″ + *eidos*, form, shape]. Of the nature of a poison.

toxicologist (tŏks″ĭ-kŏl′ō-jĭst) [″ + *logos*, word, reason]. A specialist in the field of poisons or toxins.

toxicology (tŏks″ĭ-kŏl′ō-jē). Division of medical and biological science concerned with toxic substances, detecting them, studying their chemistry and pharmacological actions, and establishing antidotes and treatment of toxic manifestations, prevention of poisoning, and methods for controlling exposure to harmful substances.

toxicomania (tŏks″ĭ-kō-mā′nē-ă) [″ + *mania*, madness]. Abnormal craving for narcotics, intoxicants, or poisons.

toxicopathic (tŏks″ĭ-kō-păth′ĭk) [″ + *pathos*, disease, suffering]. Pert. to any condition caused by a poison.

toxicopathy (tŏks″ĭ-kŏp′ă-thē) [″ + *pathos*, disease, suffering]. Any disease caused by a poison.

toxicopexy (tŏk′sĭ-kō-pĕk″sē) [″ + Gr. *pexis*, fixation]. Neutralization of a toxin or poison in the body.

toxicophidia (tŏk″sĭ-kō-fĭd′ē-ă) [″ + Gr. *ophis*, snake]. Poisonous snakes. SYN: *thanatophidia.*

toxicophobia (tŏks″ĭ-kō-fō′bē-ă) [″ + *phobos*, fear]. Abnormal fear of being poisoned by any medium: food, gas, water or drugs.

toxicosis (tŏks″ĭ-kō′sĭs) [″ + *osis*, condition]. A diseased condition resulting from poisoning.

    t., endogenic. Disease due to poisons generated within the body. SYN: *autointoxication.*

    t., exogenic. Any toxic condition resulting from a poison not generated in the body.

    t., retention. Toxicosis from retained products that normally are excreted shortly after formation.

toxic shock syndrome. ABBR: TSS. A rare and sometimes fatal disease caused by a toxin or toxins produced by certain strains of the bacterium *Staphylococcus aureus*. The diagnosis is made when the following criteria are met: fever of 102°F (38.9°C) or greater; diffuse macular erythematous rash followed in one or two weeks by desquamation, particularly of the palms and soles; hypotension or orthostatic syncope; and involvement of three or more of the following organ systems: gastrointestinal (vomiting or diarrhea at onset of illness); muscular (severe myalgia); mucous membrane (vaginal, oropharyngeal, or conjunctival hyperemia); renal; hepatic; hematologic (platelets less than 100,000/cubic millimeter); central nervous system (disorientation or alteration in consciousness without focal neurologic signs when fever and hypotension are absent). In addition, negative results on the following tests if obtained: blood, throat, or cerebrospinal fluid culture, but blood culture may be positive for *Staphylococcus aureus;* and no rise in titer to tests for Rocky Mountain spotted fever, leptospirosis, or rubeola.

The disease has occurred in young menstruating women, most of whom were using vaginal tampons for menstrual protection. About one-half of the total cases reported occur in males, menstruating women who are not using tampons, and women who do not menstruate. TSS has occurred in patients with streptococcal infections. SEE: *Nursing Diagnoses* in *Appendix.*

Caution: Anyone who develops these symptoms and signs should seek medical attention immediately. If a tampon is being used, it should be removed at once.

TREAT: Beta-lactamase-resistant antimicrobials and immediate therapy to combat shock and renal failure if present.

toxic substance. Any substance that can cause acute or chronic injury to the human body, or is suspected of being able to cause disease or injury under some conditions. In the U.S., the National Institute of Occupational Safety and Health (NIOSH) publishes a registry of toxic chemicals. SEE: *hazardous material; health hazard; permissible exposure limits; right to know law.*

toxidermitis (tŏks″ĭ-dĕr-mī′tĭs) [″ + *derma*, skin, + *itis*, inflammation]. Any inflammatory skin disease due to poisoning. SYN: *toxicodermatitis.*

toxiferous (tŏks-ĭf′ĕr-ŭs) [″ + L. *ferre*, to carry]. Containing a poison. SYN: *poisonous.*

toxigenic (tŏks″ĭ-jĕn′ĭk) [″ + *gennan*, to produce]. Producing toxins or poisons.

toxigenicity (tŏks″ĭ-jĕn-ĭs′ĭ-tē). The virulence of a toxin-producing pathogenic organism.

toxignomic (tŏks″ĭg-nŏm′ĭk) [″ + *gnomikos*, knowing]. Having the toxic action peculiar to a poison.

toxin (tŏks′ĭn) [Gr. *toxikon*, poison]. A poisonous substance of animal or plant origin. SEE: *antitoxin; phytotoxin; toxoid.*

   t., bacterial. Toxin produced by bacteria. Includes exotoxins, which diffuse from bacterial cells into surrounding medium, and endotoxins, which are liberated only when the bacterial cell is destroyed. SEE: *bacteria.*

   t., botulinus. Toxin produced by *Clostridium botulinum*, the causative organism for botulism. Seven types of the toxin have been identified.

   t., dermonecrotic. Any one of a group of different toxins that can cause necrosis of the skin. Coagulase-positive *Staphylococcus aureus* produce several such toxins. SEE: *Kawasaki disease; scalded skin syndrome, staphylococcal; toxic shock syndrome.*

   t., Dick. An erythrogenic toxin produced by some streptococci.

   t., diphtheria. The specific toxin produced by *Corynebacterium diphtheriae.*

   t., dysentery. The exotoxin of various species of *Shigella.*

   t., erythrogenic. T., Dick, q.v.

   t., extracellular. Toxin produced and excreted by microorganisms; an exotoxin, q.v.

   t., fatigue. An alleged toxin present in the body due to muscular fatigue.

   t., intracellular. Toxin produced in the bacterial cell, but retained therein; an endotoxin, q.v.

   t., plant. Any toxin produced by a plant; a phytotoxin.

toxin-antitoxin (tŏks′ĭn-ăn″tĭ-tŏks′ĭn) [Gr. *toxikon*, poison, + *anti*, against, + *toxikon*, poison]. ABBR: T.A.T. Diphtheria toxin with its antitoxin in a nearly neutral mixture, the diphtheria toxin being about 85% neutralized. Used for immunization against diphtheria.

toxinicide (tŏks-ĭn′ĭs-īd) [″ + *cidus*, kill]. That which is destructive to toxins.

toxinology (tŏk″sĭn-ŏl′ō-jē) [″ + Gr. *logos*, word, reason]. The branch of science concerned with toxins.

toxinosis (tŏk″sĭ-nō′sĭs) [″ + Gr. *osis*, condition]. Any disease or condition caused by a toxin.

toxipathic. Concerning toxipathy.

toxipathy (tŏks-ĭp′ă-thē) [″ + Gr. *pathos*, disease, suffering]. Any disease due to poison.

toxiphobia (tŏks″ĭ-fō′bē-ă) [″ + Gr.

phobos, fear]. Abnormal fear of being poisoned.

toxisterol (tŏk-sĭs′tĕr-ŏl). Toxic derivative obtained by radiating ergosterol.

toxitherapy (tŏks″ĭ-thĕr′ă-pē) [″ + Gr. *therapeia*, treatment]. Use of toxins in treatment of disease; e.g., the use of botulinum toxin injected locally to treat certain eye muscle imbalance conditions and to treat spasmodic torticollis.

toxituberculid (tŏks″ĭ-tū-bĕr′kū-lĭd). A skin lesion resulting from action of toxin of tuberculosis organism.

toxocariasis (tŏks″ō-kār-ī′ă-sĭs) [″ + *kara*, head, + *-iasis*, condition]. A self-limiting disease due to infection with nematode worms *Toxocara canis* or *T. cati.* In humans, the eggs penetrate the bowel wall and enter the circulation. Larvae may be carried to any part of the body where the blood vessel is large enough to accommodate them. They may end up in the brain, retinal vessels, liver, lung, or heart. The larvae cause hemorrhage, inflammation, and necrosis in these tissues. Thus the patient may have myocarditis, endophthalmitis, epilepsy, or encephalitis. Diagnosis is made by immunological tests and by presence of larvae in tissue obtained by liver biopsy. It is important that toxocariasis be considered in cases diagnosed as retinoblastoma. SYN: *larva migrans, visceral.*

toxogenin (tŏks-ŏj′ĕn-ĭn) [Gr. *toxikon*, poison, + *gennan*, to produce]. Hypothetical substance in the blood caused by injection of antigens, innocuous in itself, but causing anaphylaxis upon addition of fresh antigen.

toxoid (tŏks′oyd) [″ + *eidos*, form, shape]. A toxin that has been treated to destroy its toxicity, but is still capable of inducing formation of antibodies on injection. SYN: *anatoxin.*

   t., alum-precipitated. Toxoid of diphtheria or tetanus precipitated with alum.

   t., diphtheria. Diphtheria toxin detoxified by formaldehyde treatment.

   t., tetanus. Tetanus toxoid, q.v.

toxolecithin (tŏks″ō-lĕs′ĭ-thĭn) [″ + *lekithos*, egg yolk]. A compound of lecithin with a toxin such as certain snake venoms.

toxolysin (tŏks-ŏl′ĭ-sĭn) [″ + *lysis*, dissolution]. Substance destroying toxins. SYN: *antitoxin; toxicide.*

toxomucin (tŏks″ō-mū′sĭn) [″ + L. *mucus*, mucus]. Specific toxic albuminoid from cultures of tubercle bacilli.

toxonosis (tŏks″ō-nō′sĭs) [″ + *osis*, condition]. A disease caused by poisoning. SYN: *toxicosis.*

toxopeptone (tŏks″ō-pĕp′tōn) [″ + *pepton*, digesting]. A protein derivative produced by action of a toxin on peptones.

toxophil(e) (tŏks′ō-fĭl, -fīl) [″ + *philein*, to love]. Having a special affinity for toxins.

toxophilic (tŏk″sō-fĭl′ĭk) [″ + *philein*, to love]. Concerning a toxophile.

toxophore (tŏks′ō-for) [″ + *phoros*, a bearer]. That portion of a toxin which gives to a toxin its poisonous qualities.

toxophorous (tŏk-sŏf′ō-rŭs). Concerning a toxophore.

toxophylaxin (tŏks″ō-fĭ-lăks′ĭn) [″ + *phylax*, guard]. A substance that neutralizes bacterial toxins.

Toxoplasma (tŏks″ō-plăs′mă). A genus of protozoa.

   T. gondii. The causative agent of toxoplasmosis.

toxoplasmin (tŏk″sō-plăs′mĭn). An antigen obtained from mouse peritoneal fluid infected with *Toxoplasma gondii.*

toxoplasmosis (tŏks-ō-plăs-mō′sĭs). A disease due to infection with the protozoa *Toxoplasma gondii.* The organism is found in many mammals and birds. Symptoms may be so mild as to be barely noticeable or may be more severe with lymphadenopathy, malaise, muscle pain, and little if any fever. In the severe disseminated form, there are pneumonitis, hepatitis, and encephalitis. In the congenital form, destructive lesions of the central nervous system, jaundice, anemia, and generalized lymphadenopathy usually are present.

   DIAG: By identification of culture of the organism and by serologic test.

   TREAT: Even though treatment is not entirely satisfactory, trisulfapyrimidines or pyrimethamine and sulfadiazine are indicated. The latter combination is less toxic if folinic acid is given with each dose.

Toynbee maneuver [Joseph Toynbee, Brit. physician, 1815–1866]. Changing the pressure within the middle ear by swallowing or blowing while the nose is pinched closed and the mouth is tightly shut. This maneuver is used to "clear the ears" when quickly changing altitude, as in an airplane flight.

   In some cases the effect of this maneuver may be enhanced by tilting the head backward while it is done. This places tension on the tensor tympani muscle and helps to open the eustachian tubes. SEE: *Valsalva's maneuver.*

T.P.I. test. *Treponema pallidum immobilizing test* (for syphilis).

TPN. *triphosphopyridine nucleotide; total parenteral nutrition.*

TPR. *temperature, pulse, respiration.*

tr. L. *tinctura,* tincture.

trabecula (tră-bĕk′ū-lă) [L., a little beam] (pl. *trabeculae*). [NA] 1. Fibrous cord of connective tissue that serves as supporting fiber by forming a septum that extends into an organ from its wall or capsule. 2. The network of osseous tissue which makes up the cancellous structure of a bone.

trabeculae carneae cordis. [NA] Thick muscular tissue bands attached to inner walls of the ventricles of the heart.

trabecular (tră-bĕk′ū-lăr). Concerning a trabecula.

trabecularism (tră-bĕk′ū-lăr-ĭzm). Condition of having a trabecular structure.

trabeculate (tră-bĕk′ū-lāt). Having trabeculae.

trabeculoplasty. Surgical procedure on the trabecular meshwork of the eye. This procedure is used to allow escape of aqueous humor in the treatment of glaucoma. SEE: *glaucoma.*

trabs (trăbz) [L., a beam] (pl. *trabes*). A supporting band.

   t. cerebri. Arched band of white fibers connecting the cerebral hemispheres. SYN: *corpus callosum* [NA].

trace (trās) [O. Fr. *tracier*]. 1. A very small quantity. 2. A visible mark or sign.

   t., primitive. Pale white streak in germinal area indicating beginning of development of the blastoderm. SYN: *primitive streak.*

trace elements. Organic elements normally found in minute quantities in foods and tissues.

   Ex.: aluminum, bromine, chromium, cobalt, copper, fluorine, iron, iodine, manganese, nickel, silicon, zinc, and other rare minerals.

tracer. A radioactive isotope, capable of being incorporated into compounds, that when introduced into the body "tags" a specific portion of the molecule so that its course may be traced. Used in absorption and excretion studies, in identification of intermediary products of metabolism, and in determination of distribution of various substances in the body. Radioactive carbon (^{14}C), calcium (^{42}Ca), and iodine (^{131}I) are examples of tracers commonly used. SEE: *label.*

trachea (tră′kē-ă) [Gr. *tracheia*, rough] (pl. *tracheae*). [NA] A cylindrical cartilaginous tube, 4½ in. (11.3 cm) long, from the larynx to the bronchial tubes. It extends from the 6th cervical to the 5th dorsal vertebra, where it divides at a point called the carina into two bronchi, one leading to each lung. It is lined with mucous membrane and its inner surface is lined with ciliated epithelium. SYN: *windpipe.* SEE: *bronchi.*

tracheaectasy (tră″kē-ă-ĕk′tă-sē) [Gr. *tracheia*, rough, + *ektasis*, dilatation]. Dilatation of the trachea.

tracheal (tră′kē-ăl). Pert. to the trachea.

trachealgia (tră″kē-ăl′jē-ă) [″ + *algos,*

pain]. Pain in the trachea.

trachealis (trā″kē-ā′lĭs) [L.]. A muscle composed of smooth muscle fibers that extends between the ends of the tracheal rings. Its contraction reduces the size of the lumen.

tracheal tickle. A maneuver designed to elicit a reflex cough.

tracheal tugging. Pulsation of the larynx or downward pull of the trachea, symptomatic of thoracic aneurysm.

tracheitis (trā″kē-ī′tĭs) [Gr. *tracheia*, rough, + *itis*, inflammation]. An inflammation of the trachea. It may be acute or chronic and may be associated with bronchitis and laryngitis.

    NURSING IMPLICATIONS: Monitor vital signs and assess for fever and acute airway obstruction (croupy cough, stridor) due to presence of copious, thick, and purulent secretions. Administer humidified oxygen as prescribed and suction as necessary to remove secretions. Administer prescribed antibiotic therapy. Be prepared for emergency endotracheal intubation or tracheostomy if airway obstruction persists. Provide comfort to child and parents to reduce anxiety.

trachelectomopexy (trā″kĕ-lĕk′tŏm-ō-pĕk″sē) [″ + *ektome*, excision, + *pexis*, fixation]. Fixation of uterine neck with partial excision.

trachelectomy (trā″kĕl-ĕk′tō-mē) [″ + *ektome*, excision]. Amputation of the cervix uteri.

trachelematoma (trā″kĕl-ĕm″ā-tō′mă) [″ + *haima*, blood, + *oma*, tumor]. A hematoma situated on the neck.

trachelism, trachelismus (trā″kĕ-lĭzm, trā-kĕ-lĭz′mŭs) [″ + *-ismos*, condition]. Backward spasm of the neck, sometimes preceding an epileptic attack.

trachelitis (trā-kĕ-lī′tĭs) [″ + *itis*, inflammation]. Inflammation of mucous membrane of the cervix uteri. SYN: *cervicitis*.

trachelo- [Gr. *trachelos*, neck]. Combining form meaning neck.

trachelobregmatic (trā″kĕ-lō-brĕg-măt′ĭk) [″ + *bregma*, front of the head]. Pert. to the neck and the bregma.

trachelocele (trăk′ĕ-lō-sēl) [″ + *kele*, tumor, swelling]. Tracheocele.

trachelocyrtosis (trā″kĕ-lō-sĭr-tō′sĭs) [″ + *kyrtos*, curved, + *osis*, condition]. Trachelokyphosis.

trachelocystitis (trā″kĕl-ō-sĭs-tī′tĭs) [″ + *kystis*, bladder, + *itis*, inflammation]. Inflammation of the neck of the bladder.

trachelodynia (trā″kĕ-lō-dĭn′ē-ă) [″ + *odyne*, pain]. Pain in the neck.

trachelokyphosis (trā″kĕl-ō-kī-fō′sĭs) [″ + *kyphosis*, humpback]. Excessive anterior curvature of cervical portion of spine.

trachelology (trā″kĕ-lŏl′ō-jē) [″ + *logos*,

word, reason]. Scientific study of the neck, its diseases and injuries.

trachelomastoid (trā″kĕ-lō-măs′toyd) [″ + *mastos*, breast, + *eidos*, form, shape]. A muscle of the neck. SEE: *Muscles* in *Appendix.*

trachelomyitis (trā″kĕ-lō-mī-ī′tĭs) [″ + *mys*, muscle, + *itis*, inflammation]. Inflammation of muscles of the neck.

trachelopexy (trā″kĕl-ō-pĕks″ē) [″ + *pexis*, fixation]. Surgical fixation of the cervix uteri to an adjacent part.

tracheloplasty (trā″kĕl-ō-plăs″tē) [″ + *plassein*, to form]. Surgical repair or plastic surgery of the neck of the uterus.

trachelorrhaphy (trā″kĕl-or′ă-fē) [″ + *rhaphe*, seam, ridge]. Suturing of a torn cervix uteri.

tracheloschisis (trā″kĕ-lŏs′kĭ-sĭs) [″ + *schisis*, a splitting]. Congenital opening or fissure in the neck.

trachelotomy (trā″kĕl-ŏt′ō-mē) [″ + *tome*, incision]. Incision of the cervix of the uterus.

tracheo- [Gr. *tracheia*, rough]. Combining form meaning trachea or windpipe.

tracheoaerocele (trā″kĕ-ō-ĕr′-ō-sēl) [Gr. *tracheia*, rough, + *aer*, air, + *kele*, tumor, swelling]. Hernia or cyst of trachea containing air.

tracheobronchial (trā″kē-ō-brŏng′kē-ăl). Concerning the trachea and bronchus.

tracheobronchomegaly (trā″kē-ō-brŏng″kō-mĕg′ă-lē). Congenitally enlarged size of the trachea and bronchi.

tracheobronchoscopy (trā″kē-ō-brŏng-kŏs′kō-pē) [″ + *bronchos*, windpipe, + *skopein*, to examine]. Inspection of the trachea and bronchi through a bronchoscope.

tracheocele (trā′kē-ō-sēl) [″ + *kele*, hernia]. Protrusion of mucous membrane through the wall of the trachea.

tracheoesophageal (trā″kē-ō-ē-sŏf″ă-jē′ăl) [″ + *oisophagos*, esophagus]. Pert. to the trachea and esophagus.

tracheolaryngeal (trā″kē-ō-lăr-rĭn′jē-ăl). Concerning the trachea and larynx.

tracheolaryngotomy (trā″kē-ō-lăr″ĭn-gŏt′ō-mē) [″ + *larynx*, larynx, + *tome*, incision]. Incision into larynx and trachea.

tracheomalacia. Softening of the cartilage of the trachea.

tracheopathia, tracheopathy (trā″kē-ō-păth′ē-ă, -ŏp′ă-thē) [″ + *pathos*, disease, suffering]. Diseased condition of the trachea.

tracheopharyngeal (trā″kē-ō-făr-ĭn′jē-ăl) [″ + *pharynx*, throat]. Pert. to both the trachea and pharynx.

tracheophony (trā″kē-ŏf′ō-nē) [″ + *phone*, a sound]. Sound heard over the trachea in auscultation.

tracheoplasty (trā′kē-ō-plăs″tē) [″ + *plassein*, to form]. Plastic operation on the trachea.

tracheopyosis (trā″kē-ō-pī-ō′sĭs) [″ + *pyon*, pus, + *osis*, condition]. Tracheitis with suppuration.

tracheorrhagia (trā″kē-ō-rā′jē-ă) [Gr. *tracheia*, rough, + *rhegnynai*, to burst forth]. Tracheal hemorrhage.

tracheoschisis (trā″kē-ŏs′kĭs-ĭs) [″ + *schisis*, a splitting]. Fissure of the trachea.

tracheoscopy (trā″kē-ŏs′kō-pē) [″ + *skopein*, to examine]. Inspection of interior of trachea by means of reflected light.

tracheostenosis (trā″kē-ō-stĕn-ō′sĭs) [″ + *stenosis*, act of narrowing]. Contraction or narrowing of lumen of the trachea.

tracheostoma (trā″kē-ŏs′tō-mă). Opening into the trachea, via the neck.

tracheostomize (trā″kē-ŏs′tō-mīz). To perform a tracheostomy.

tracheostomy (trā″kē-ŏs′tō-mē) [″ + *stoma*, mouth]. Operation of incising the skin over the trachea and making a surgical wound in the trachea in order to permit an airway during tracheal obstruction. This technique is used to provide an airway in emergency situations and to replace the airway provided by an endotracheal tube that has been in place for more than several weeks. The latter indication is necessary to prevent permanent damage of the larynx. SEE: *tube, endotracheal.*

Caution: Tracheostomy should be done by someone who is thoroughly trained in performing this surgical procedure.

NURSING IMPLICATIONS: Monitor vital signs frequently after surgery. Administer warmed, humidified oxygen. Place patient in semi-Fowler's position to enhance drainage and promote ease of breathing. Provide a restful environment. Establish communication via questions with yes and no answers, hand signals, and simple sign language, and the use of a "magic slate" for writing, or an alphabet board. (Written communication requires vision, hand strength, and dexterity and is often difficult or impossible for acutely ill patients.) Later, as appropriate, teach patient how to cover tracheostomy to permit vocalization. Be alert to patient's unmet needs and assist with these to prevent increased anxiety. Establish range-of-motion exercises and physical therapy of the chest to promote aeration of the lung. Administer analgesics, antibiotics, and other prescribed medications. Monitor and record intake and output; provide adequate fluids and nutrition. Perform suctioning of secretions and tra-

cheostomy care, q.v., as necessary. Change the dressing frequently during the first 24 hours postoperative, and observe for excessive bleeding. Encourage coughing and deep breathing at regular intervals. Establish a learning plan for the patient; this should include stoma care, consisting of cleansing, removing crusts, and filtering air with a suitable filter. Be alert for signs of infection. Instruct the patient to avoid crowds, to continue coughing and deep-breathing regimen, to take adequate fluids and nutrition, and to avoid smoking. Activities may gradually be increased to include non-contact sports, but should not include swimming. Showering may be permitted if the patient wears a protective plastic bib or uses the hand to cover the stoma. Reassure the patient that secretions will decrease and that taste and smell will gradually return. Stress the importance of follow-up care.

t., mini-. Placement of a small, 4 mm (about 1/6th of an inch) cannula through an incision made through the cricothyroid membrane into the trachea. This is done using local anesthesia. This type of tracheostomy is especially useful in removing sputum retained in the tracheobronchial tree.

tracheostomy care. Suction as often as necessary to remove secretions. Before suctioning, aerate the patient well; this can be accomplished by using an Ambu bag attached to a source of oxygen. Maintain sterile technique throughout the procedure. Before suctioning, test the patency of the suction catheter by aspirating sterile normal saline through it. Insert the catheter without applying suction until the patient coughs. Apply suction intermittently and withdraw the catheter in a rotating motion. Assess the airway by auscultating the lungs; repeat suctioning procedure until the airway is clear. Each suctioning episode should take no longer than 15 seconds, and the patient should be allowed to rest and breathe between suctioning episodes. Cleanse the suction catheter with sterile normal saline solution and cleanse the oral cavity if necessary. The inner cannula should be cleansed or replaced after each aspiration. Metal cannulas should be cleansed with sterile water.

Keep an emergency tracheotomy set at the bedside at all times. Also keep a Kelly clamp at the bedside to hold open the tracheostomy site in an emergency. Cuffed tracheostomy tubes must be inflated if the patient is on positive-pressure ventilation unless ordered otherwise. In other cases, keep the cuff deflated if the patient has problems with aspiration. Using aseptic technique, change dressing and tape every 8 hours. Tracheostomies should always be covered with a dressing to prevent skin breakdown. To apply neck tapes, obtain two lengths of twill tape approx. 10 in. (25 cm) long; fold the end of each and make a slit ½ in. (1.3 cm) long about 1 in. (2.5 cm) from the fold; slip the slit end under the neck plate, and pull the other end of the tape through the slit; repeat for the other side; wrap the tape around the neck and secure it with a square knot on the side. Neck tapes should be left in place until new tapes are attached. Culture tracheal secretions as ordered; observe and record their color, viscosity, amount, and abnormal odor, if any. Inspect site daily for bleeding, hematoma formation, subcutaneous emphysema, and signs of infection. Provide appropriate skin care. Help to alleviate the patient's anxiety and apprehension, and provide a communication process. Document patient response.

tracheotome (trā′kē-ō-tōm) [″ + *tome,* incision]. Instrument used in opening of the trachea.

tracheotomy (trā″kē-ŏt′ō-mē). Incision of the trachea through the skin and muscles of the neck overlying the trachea. SEE: *tracheostomy.*

trachitis (trā-kī′tĭs) [″ + *itis,* inflammation]. Inflammation of the trachea. SYN: *tracheitis.*

trachoma (trā-kō′mă) [Gr., roughness]. A chronic contagious form of conjunctivitis, noted by hypertrophy of conjunctiva and formation of follicles with subsequent cicatricial changes. The disease affects 400,000,000 people, mostly in Asia and Africa, but is also seen in the southwestern part of the United States. Approximately 20,000,000 persons have been blinded by this disease. SYN: *ophthalmia, Egyptian; conjunctivitis, granular.*

ETIOL: The causative agent is a strain of *Chlamydia trachomatis.* Chlamydial organisms are responsible for psittacosis, inclusion conjunctivitis, lymphogranuloma venereum, genital tract infections, neonatal infections, and pneumonia. The disease is readily transmitted, esp. in early stages. Transmission occurs by direct contact with trachomatous material or indirectly through contaminated articles such as towels or handkerchiefs. SEE: *Universal Precautions* in *Appendix.*

COMPLICATIONS: Pannus, ptosis, corneal ulcers.

SEQUELAE: Blindness; corneal opacities; ectropion; entropion; staphyloma; symblepharon; trichiasis.

TREAT: Tetracycline or erythromycin used topically and systemic tetracycline are effective. Surgery may be necessary when lid deformities occur.

   t., brawny. Trachoma with general lymphoid infiltration without granulation of the conjunctiva.

   t. deformans. Trachoma with cicatricial contractions.

   t., diffuse. Trachoma with large granulations.

trachomatous (tră-kō′mă-tŭs). Concerning trachoma.

trachychromatic (trā″kĭ-krō-măt′ĭk) [Gr. *trachys,* rough, + *chroma,* color]. Pert. to a nucleus with very deeply staining chromatin.

trachyphonia (trā″kĭ-fō′nē-ă) [″ + *phone,* voice]. Roughness or hoarseness of the voice.

tracing (trā′sĭng). 1. A graphic record of some event that changes with time such as respiratory movements or electrical activity of the heart or brain. 2. In dentistry, a graphic display of movements of the mandible.

tract (trăkt) [L. *tractus,* extent]. 1. A course or pathway. 2. A group or bundle of nerve fibers within the spinal cord or brain that constitutes an anatomical and functional unit. SEE: *fasciculus.* 3. A group of organs or parts forming a continuous pathway.

   t., afferent. T., ascending.

   t., alimentary. The canal or passage from the mouth to the anus. SYN: *t., digestive.*

   t., ascending. White fibers in the spinal cord that carry nerve impulses toward the brain. SYN: *t., afferent.*

   t., biliary. SEE: *biliary tract.*

   t., descending. Fibers in the spinal cord that carry nerve impulses from the brain.

   t., digestive. T., alimentary.

   t., dorsolateral. A spinal cord tract superficial to the tip of the dorsal horn. It is made up of short pain and temperature fibers that are processes of neurons having their cell bodies in the dorsal root ganglion. SYN: *Lissauer's tract.*

   t., extrapyramidal. SEE: *system, extrapyramidal.*

   t., gastrointestinal. The stomach and intestines.

   t., genitourinary. The genital and urinary pathways.

   t., iliotibial. A thickened area of fascia lata extending from the lateral condyle of the tibia to the iliac crest.

   t., intestinal. The small and large intestines.

   t., motor. Descending pathway that conveys motor impulses from the brain to lower portions of the spinal cord.

   t., olfactory. A narrow white band that entends from the olfactory bulb to the anterior perforated substance of the brain.

t., optic. A band of fibers that extends from the optic chiasma to the lateral geniculate body of the thalamus. Some fibers of the tract continue on to the midbrain and hypothalamus.

t., pyramidal. Any of the columns of "motor" fibers in the spinal cord that are continuations of pyramids in the medulla.

t., respiratory. The respiratory organs in continuity.

t., rubrospinal. A descending tract of fibers arising from cell bodies located in red nucleus of the midbrain. Fibers terminate in gray matter of the spinal cord.

t., supraopticohypophyseal. A tract consisting of fibers arising from cell bodies located in supraoptic and paraventricular nuclei of the hypothalamus and terminating in the posterior lobe of the hypophysis.

t., urinary. The urinary passageway from kidney to the outside of the body. Includes the pelvis of the kidney, ureter, bladder, and urethra.

t., uveal. The vascular and pigmented tissues that constitute the middle coat of the eye. Included are the iris, ciliary body, and choroid.

tractellum (trăk-tĕl´ŭm) [L.]. An anterior flagellum of a protozoan. It propels the body by traction.

traction (trăk´shŭn) [L. *tractio*]. Process of drawing or pulling. SEE: *Nursing Diagnoses in Appendix.*

t., axis. Traction in line with the long axis of a course through which a body (fetus) is to be drawn.

t., cervical. Traction applied to the cervical spine by applying a force to lift the head or a mobilization technique to distract individual joints of the vertebrae. SEE: *Crutchfield tongs.*

t., elastic. Traction exerted by elastic devices such as rubber bands.

t., external. Traction applied to any fracture, e.g., compression fractures of the face using metal or plaster headgear for anchorage.

t., head. Traction applied to the head as in the treatment of injuries to cervical vertebrae.

t., intermittent. The force of traction alternately applied and released at specified intervals.

t., lumbar. Traction applied to the lumbar spine usually by applying a force to pull on the pelvis, or by using a mobilization technique to distract individual joints of the lumbar vertebrae.

t., manual. The application of traction to the joints of the spine or extremities by a therapist trained to know appropriate posi-

tions and intensities for the force.

t., maxillomandibular. Traction applied to the maxilla and mandible by means of elastic or wire ligatures and interdental wiring or splints.

t., mechanical. The use of a device or mechanical linkage, i.e., pulleys and weights, to apply a traction force.

t., sustained. Application of a constant traction force up to one-half hour.

t., weight. Traction exerted by means of weights.

tractor (trăk´tor) [L., drawer]. Any device or instrument for applying traction.

tractotomy (trăk-tŏt´ō-mē). Surgical section of a fiber tract of the central nervous system. Sometimes resorted to for relief of intractable pain.

tractus (trăk´tŭs) [L.] (pl. *tractus*). A tract, q.v., or path.

tragacanth (trăg´ă-kănth) [Gr. *tragakantha,* a goat thorn]. The dried gummy exudation from the plant *Astragalus gummifer* and related species, grown in Asia. Used in the form of mucilage as a greaseless lubricant and as an application for chapped skin.

tragal (trā´găl) [Gr. *tragos,* goat]. Relating to the tragus.

tragi (trā´jī). Pl. of tragus.

tragicus (trăj´ĭk-ŭs) [L.]. Muscle on the outer surface of the tragus. SEE: *Muscles in Appendix.*

tragion (trăj´ē-ŏn). An anthropometric point at the upper margin of the tragus of the ear.

tragomaschalia (trăg″ō-măs-kăl´ē-ă) [Gr. *tragos,* goat, + *maschale,* the armpit]. Odorous perspiration (bromidrosis) of the axilla.

tragophonia, tragophony (trăg″ō-fō´nē-ă, -ŏf´ō-nē) [″ + *phone,* voice]. A bleating sound heard in auscultation at level of fluid in hydrothorax. SYN: *egophony.*

tragopodia (trăg″ō-pō´dē-ă) [″ + *pous,* foot]. Knock-knee.

tragus (trā´gŭs) [Gr. *tragos,* goat] (pl. *tragi*). [NA] Cartilaginous projection in front of the exterior meatus of the ear. SYN: *antilobium.*

train (trān). To participate in a special program of instruction in order to attain competence in a certain occupation or profession.

trainable (trān´ă-bl). 1. A mentally deficient individual who is capable of being trained. 2. To have the ability to be instructed and to learn from being taught. In classifying severity of mental retardation or brain damage it is important to know to what extent individuals may be trainable in various areas such as safety, personal care, or self-feeding.

training. An organized system of instruction.

t., assertiveness. A type of behavior

therapy in which the patient is taught to respond in a more positive and assertive manner to the normal stimuli encountered in daily activities. The goal is to be able to express one's true feelings, whether positive or negative. Role playing in group therapy may be used to teach this to patients.

t., athletic. 1. The physical and mental conditioning program used by athletes in order to increase their proficiency in sports endeavors. 2. Performing the tasks that an athletic trainer, q.v., is prepared to do.

t., aversive. SEE: *aversion therapy.*

trait (trāt). A distinguishing feature; a characteristic or property of an individual.

t., acquired. Trait that is not inherited; one resulting from effects of environment.

t., inherited. Trait due to genes transmitted through germ cells.

trajector (tră-jĕk'tor) [L. *trajectus,* thrown across]. Device for determining approximate location of a bullet in a wound.

Tral. Trade name for hexocyclium methylsulfate.

tramazoline hydrochloride (tră-măz'ō-lēn). An adrenergic drug.

trance (trăns) [L. *transitus,* a passing over]. A sleeplike state, as in deep hypnosis, appearing also in hysteria and in some spiritualistic mediums, with limited sensory and motor contact with the ordinary surroundings, and with subsequent amnesia of what has occurred during the state.

t., death. Trance simulating death.

t., induced. Trance caused by some external event such as hypnosis.

Trancopal. Trade name for chlormezanone.

tranquilizer (trăn"kwī-līz'ĕr) [L. *tranquillus,* calm]. A drug that acts to reduce mental tension and anxiety without interfering with normal mental activity. This ideal state of tranquilization is difficult to attain. Thus, patients taking these medicines may find that their reactions are slowed. The use of tranquilizers has facilitated the treatment of severely disturbed psychiatric patients. Among the drugs in use are chlordiazepoxide (Librium), chlorpromazine (Thorazine), diazepam (Valium), meprobamate (Miltown, Equanil), alprazolam (Xanax), and reserpine (Serpasil).

Side effects, particularly from chlorpromazine and reserpine, have included jaundice, nausea, rashes, and in some instances severe mental depression. The U.S. Public Health Service has warned of "a significant incidence of severe depression, with suicidal tendencies in some instances," in persons under heavy reserpine dosage.

Persons taking tranquilizers regularly should not discontinue their use suddenly. To prevent withdrawal signs, which include convulsions, muscle cramps, sweating, and vomiting, reduce the dose slowly.

Caution: Some tranquilizers may be injurious to the developing embryo. Therefore, prior to prescribing one, it is important to know whether it is approved for use during pregnancy, esp. during early pregnancy.

---

trans- [L.]. Prefix meaning across, over, beyond, through.

transabdominal (trăns"ăb-dŏm'ĭ-năl). Through or across the abdomen or abdominal wall.

transacetylation (trăns-ăs"ē-tĭl-ā'shŭn). Transfer of an acetyl group,

$$CH_3 - \overset{\displaystyle \underset{\|}{}}{C} -$$
$$\underset{O}{\|}$$

in a chemical reaction.

transaction. The interaction of a person with others.

transactional analysis. Psychotherapy involving role playing in an attempt to understand the relation between patient and therapist and eventually the relation of the patient to reality.

transamidination (trăns-ăm"ĭ-dĭn-ā'shŭn). The transfer of an amidine group from one amino acid to another.

transaminase (trăns-ăm'ĭn-ās). An enzyme that catalyzes transamination.

t., glutamic-oxaloacetic. ABBR: GOT, or SGOT for serum GOT. Enzyme present in the serum and body tissue; the highest concentration being in the heart and the liver. Tissue injury stimulates its release in the bloodstream and measurement of serum levels can indicate myocardial infarction or hepatic cell damage. Previously used name for aspartate aminotransferase, q.v.

t., glutamic-pyruvic. ABBR: GPT, or SGPT for serum GPT. Enzyme present in the serum and many tissues; the highest concentration is found in the liver. Injury of hepatic cells liberates the enzyme into the bloodstream. Thus measurement of the level in the serum (SGPT) provides a valuable test for hepatic cell injury. Previously used name for alanine aminotransferase, q.v.

transamination (trăns"ăm-ĭ-nā'shŭn). The transfer of an amino group from one compound to another or the transposition of an amino group within a single compound.

transaortic (trăns"ā-or'tĭk). Done through the aorta, e.g., a surgical procedure.

transatrial (trăns-ā'trē-ăl). Done through the atrium, e.g., a surgical procedure.

transaudient (trăns-aw'dē-ĕnt) [" + *audire,* to hear]. Permeable to sound waves.

transaxial (trăns-ăk′sē-ăl). Across the long axis of a structure or part.

transcalent (trăns-kā′lĕnt) [″ + *calere*, to be hot]. Permeable by heat rays. SYN: *diathermal*.

transcapillary (trăns″kăp′ĭl-lă-rē) [″ + *capillaris*, relating to hair]. Across the endothelial wall of a capillary.

transcapillary exchange. The passage of substances between blood and tissue (interstitial) fluid.

transcervical (trăns-sĕr′vĭ-kăl). Done through the cervical os of the uterus.

transcervical balloon tuboplasty. SEE: *tuboplasty, transcervical balloon.*

transcortical (trăns-kor′tĭ-kăl). Joining two parts of the cerebral cortex.

transcortin (trăns-kor′tĭn). A corticosteroid-binding globulin.

transcriptase (trăns-krĭp′tās). A polymerase that performs transcription by converting a DNA base sequence into its complementary RNA base sequence.

transcription (trăn-skrĭp′shŭn). In synthesizing genes and proteins, the necessary process of duplication or copying of information from certain aspects of the chemical compound deoxyribonucleic acid (DNA). Messenger ribonucleic acid (mRNA) is synthesized by copying information from DNA and bringing that information to ribosomes, which are particles containing RNA.

transcutaneous. Percutaneous.

transcutaneous electrical nerve stimulation. ABBR: TENS. Application of mild electrical stimulation to skin electrodes placed over a painful area. It causes interference with transmission of painful stimuli.

transdermal infusion system. A method of delivering medicine by placing it in a special gel-like matrix that is applied to the skin. The medicine is absorbed through the skin at a fixed rate. Each application will provide medicine for from one to several days. Nitroglycerin and scopolamine are examples of medicines that have been prepared for use in this type of system. SYN: *transdermal drug-delivery system.*

transducer (trăns-dū′sĕr) [L. *trans*, across, + *ducere*, to lead]. Device that converts one form of energy to another. Used in medical electronics to receive the energy produced by sound or pressure and relay it as an electrical impulse to another transducer, which can either convert the energy back into its original form or make a record of it on a recording device. The telephone is an example.

    t., ultrasonic. Device used in ultrasound that sends and receives the sound wave signal.

transduction (trăns-dŭk′shŭn). A phenomenon causing genetic recombination in bacteria in which DNA is carried from one bacterium to another by bacteriophage. SEE: *transformation.*

transection (trăn-sĕk′shŭn) [″ + *sectio*, cutting]. A cutting made across a long axis; a cross section.

transfection (trans-fĕk′shŭn). The infection of bacteria by purified phage DNA after pretreatment with calcium ions or conversion to spheroplasts.

transfer, transference (trăns′fer, trăns-fĕr′ĕns) [″ + *ferre*, to bear]. 1. The mental process whereby a person transfers patterns of feelings and behavior that had previously been experienced with important figures such as parents or siblings to another person. Quite often these feelings are shifted to the caregiver. 2. State in which the symptoms of one area are transmitted to a similar area.

transferase (trăns′fĕr-ās). An enzyme that catalyzes the transfer of atoms or groups of atoms from one chemical compound to another.

transfer board. Device used to bridge the space between a wheelchair and a bed, toilet, or carseat. Used to facilitate independent or assisted transferring of the patient from one of these sites to another. Also called sliding board.

transfer factor. In immunology, a factor present in lymphocytes that have been sensitized to antigens, which can, in humans, be transferred to a nonsensitized recipient. Thus the recipient will react to the same antigen that was originally used to sensitize the lymphocytes of the donor. In humans the factor can be transferred by injecting the recipient with either intact lymphocytes or extracts of disrupted cells.

transferrin (trăns-fĕr′rĭn). A globulin in the blood that binds and transports iron.

transferring. The act of moving a person with limited function from one location to another. May be accomplished by the patient or with assistance.

transfix (trăns-fĭks′) [″ + *figere*, to fix]. To pierce through or impale with a sharp instrument.

transfixion (trăns-fĭk′shŭn). Maneuver in performing an amputation in which a knife is passed into the soft parts and cutting is from within outward.

transforation (trăns″for-ā′shŭn) [″ + *forare*, to pierce]. The perforation of the fetal skull at the base in craniotomy.

transforator (trăns′for-ā″tor). Instrument for perforating fetal skull.

transformation (trăns″for-mā′shŭn) [″ + *formatio*, a forming]. 1. Change of shape or form. SYN: *metamorphosis.* 2. In oncology, the change of one tissue into another. SEE: *metastasis.* 3. A type of mutation occurring in bacteria. It results from DNA of a bacterial cell penetrating the host cell and becoming incorporated into the genotype of the host.

transformer (trăns-form′er) [″ + *formare,* to form]. A stationary induction apparatus to change electrical energy at one voltage and current to electrical energy at another voltage and current through the medium of magnetic energy, without mechanical motion.

    t., step-down. Transformer that changes electricity to a lower voltage.

    t., step-up. Transformer that changes electricity to a higher voltage.

transfuse. The act of transfusion.

transfusion (trăns-fū′zhŭn) [″ + *fusio,* a pouring]. 1. The injection of blood or a blood component into the bloodstream. SEE: *blood transfusion; interosseous infusion.* 2. Injection of saline or other solutions into a vein for a therapeutic purpose.

    t., autologous. Procedure for collecting and storing patient's own blood several weeks prior to its anticipated need by the patient. Alternatively, blood lost during a surgical procedure can be recovered from the operation site and processed for transfusion.

    This method of providing blood for an individual is to prevent transmission of disease by using blood obtained from donors. SEE: *blood doping.*

    t., cadaver blood. Transfusion using blood obtained from a cadaver within a short time after death.

    t., direct. Transfer of blood directly from one person to another.

    t., exchange. Transfusion and withdrawal of small amounts of blood repeated until blood volume is almost entirely exchanged. Used in infants born with hemolytic disease and in patients with uremia.

    t., indirect. Transfusion of blood from a donor to a suitable storage container and then to the patient.

    t., replacement. T., exchange.

    t., single unit. SEE: *blood, transfusion of a single unit.*

transfusion reactions. A variety of reactions can occur as a result of blood transfusions. The most serious is the response of the recipient when incompatible blood is administered. In that case, massive intravascular clumping and lysis of red cells occur. Other causes of hemolytic reactions are administering hemolyzed or fragile red blood cells due to the age of the blood or to its having been stored at an inappropriate tempera-

ture or having come in contact with incompatible I.V. solutions. If the reaction is severe, the patient will experience a bursting feeling in the head, face flushing, pain in the neck and lumbar area, vomiting, and shock. If the blood contains something to which the patient is allergic, the symptoms of urticaria, edema, wheezing, and headache will be present. Infrequently, anaphylactic shock will occur. Some patients with compromised cardiovascular systems will experience heart failure, shock, pulmonary edema, and cyanosis if too much blood is administered. The transfusion must be stopped when these symptoms and signs appear. Such patients should not receive whole blood.

    Prevention of these types of reactions is dependent upon meticulous attention to detail and accuracy in labeling the patient's blood sample for typing and cross-matching, double checking this at the time of transfusion, and starting the blood flow very slowly during the first 15 minutes and observing carefully for reactions. To prevent allergic reactions in persons with a history of allergies, an antihistamine may be administered orally or intramuscularly just before the transfusion is started.

transfusion syndrome, multiple. Development of hemorrhagic tendency caused by multiple transfusions with blood low in platelets and by increased fibrinolytic activity in the blood. SEE: *post-transfusion syndrome.*

    TREAT: Transfuse with blood that is only a few hours old and give fibrinogen.

transgenic. An organism into which hereditary (i.e., genetic) material from another organism has been introduced.

Transgrow. Proprietary name of a special medium for culturing *Neisseria gonorrhoeae.* The specimen may be placed in the medium and then shipped to the laboratory. The bacteria will remain viable even though they were not incubated while being transported.

transient [L. *transi,* to go by]. Not lasting; of brief duration.

transient ischemic attack. ABBR: TIA. Temporary interference with blood supply to the brain. The symptoms of neurological deficit may last for only a few moments or several hours. After the attack no evidence of residual brain damage or neurological damage remains. It is not necessarily true that individuals who have experienced transient ischemic attacks will within the predictable future develop a full vascular occlusion and have a stroke. SEE: *bruit, carotid; stroke.*

    SYM: Usually abrupt onset of giddiness

or light-headed sensation. The specific signs and symptoms will depend upon the portion of the brain affected. Thus, any one or a combination of several of the following may be present: fleeting monocular blindness, hemiparesis, hemiplegia, aphasia, astereognosis, dizziness, staggering, numbness, difficulty in swallowing, or paresthesias.

ETIOL: Insufficient blood flow to the brain due to decreased cardiac output, hypotension, overmedication with antihypertensive agents, or cerebrovascular spasm. Intravascular microembolization is suspected of causing some cases.

NURSING IMPLICATIONS: Support patient and family during diagnostic procedures, offering procedural and sensation information, and encourage them to ventilate concerns and fears. Provide planned therapeutic interventions and teach patient about actions and side effects of prescribed drugs. Teach patient safety measures to prevent injury related to uncoordinated gait or weakness in subsequent attacks.

transiliac (trăns-ĭl′ē-ăk) [L. *trans*, across, + *iliacus*, pert. to ilium]. Extending between the two ilia.

transilient (trăns-sĭl′ē-ĕnt). Jumping across or passing over as occurs when nerve fibers in the brain link nonadjacent convolutions.

transillumination (trăns″ĭl-lū″mĭ-nā′shŭn) [″ + *illuminare*, to light up]. Inspection of a cavity or organ by passing a light through its walls. When pus or lesion is present, the transmission of light is diminished or absent.

transinsular (trăns-ĭn′sū-lăr). Across the insula of the brain.

transischiac (trăns-ĭs′kē-ăk). Across or between the ischia of the pelvis.

transisthmian (trăns-ĭs′mē-ăn). Across an isthmus.

transition (trăn-zĭ′shŭn) [L. *transitio*, a going across]. Passage from one state or position to another, or from one part to another part.

transitional (trăn-zĭsh′ŭn-ăl). Marked by or relating to change.

translation (trăns-lā′shŭn) [L. *trans*, across, + *latus*, borne]. 1. The synthesis of proteins under the direction of ribonucleic acid. 2. To change to another place or to convert into another form.

translocation (trăns″lō-kā′shŭn) [″ + *locus*, place]. 1. The alteration of a chromosome either by transfer of a portion of it to another chromosome or to another portion of the same chromosome. The latter is called shift or intrachange. When two chromosomes interchange material, it is called reciprocal translocation. 2. Movement of bacteria across the intestinal wall to invade the body.

translucent (trăns-lū′sĕnt) [″ + *lucens*, shining]. Not transparent but permitting passage of light.

transmethylase (trăns-mĕth′ĭ-lās). Methyltransferase.

transmethylation (trăns″mĕth-ĭ-lā′shŭn). Process in the metabolism of amino acids in which a methyl group is transferred from one compound to another; for example, the conversion in the body of homocysteine to methionine. In this case the methyl group is furnished by choline or betaine.

transmigration (trănz″mī-grā′shŭn) [″ + *migrare*, to move from place to place]. Wandering across or through, especially the passage of white blood cells through capillary membranes into the tissues.

    t., external. Transfer of an ovum from an ovary to an opposite tube through the pelvic cavity.

    t., internal. Transfer of an ovum through the uterus to the opposite oviduct.

transmissible (trăns-mĭs′ă-bl) [L. *transmissio*, a sending across]. Capable of being carried from one person to another, as an infectious disease.

transmission (trăns-mĭsh′ŭn). Transfer of anything, as a disease or hereditary characteristics.

    t., biological. Condition in which the organism that transmits the causative agent of a disease plays an essential role in the life history of a parasite or germ.

    t., duplex. Passage of impulses through a nerve trunk in both directions.

    t., mechanical. The passive transfer of causative agents of disease, esp. by arthropods. May be indirect, as when flies pick up organisms from excreta of humans or animals and deposit them on food, or direct, as when they pick up organisms from body of a diseased individual and directly inoculate them into body of another individual by bites or through open sores. SEE: *vector.*

    t., neuromyal. Transmission of excitation from a motor neuron to a muscle fiber at a neuromyal (myoneural) junction.

    t., placental. Transmission of substances in the mother's blood to the blood of the fetus by way of the placenta.

    t., synaptic. The mechanism by which an impulse in one neuron gives rise to an impulse in another neuron.

    t., transovarial. Transmission of causative agents of disease to offspring following invasion of ovary and infection of eggs. Occurs in ticks and mites.

transmogrify. Transform. To change in appearance, esp. to a grotesque shape or form.

transmural (trăns-mū′răl) [L. *trans*, across, + *murus*, a wall]. Across the wall of an organ or structure, as in transmural myocardial thrombosis, in which the tissue in the entire thickness of a portion of the cardiac wall is affected.

transmutation (trăns″mū-tā′shŭn) [L. *transmutatio*, a changing across]. A transformation or change, as the evolutionary change of one species into another.

transocular (trăns-ŏk′ū-lăr) [″ + *oculus*, eye]. Across the eye.

transonance (trăns′ō-năns) [L. *trans*, across + *sonans*, sounding]. Transmission of sounds through an organ, as heart sounds through the lungs and chest wall.

transorbital (trăns-or′bĭ-tăl) [″ + *orbita*, track]. Passing through the orbit of the eye.

transovarial passage (trăns-ō-vā′rē-ăl). The passage of infectious or toxic agents into the ovary. A process that might invade and infect the oocytes.

transparent (trăns-păr′ĕnt) [″ + *parere*, to appear]. 1. Transmitting light rays so that objects are visible through the substance. 2. Pervious to radiant energy. SEE: *clearing agent*.

transparietal (trăns″pă-rī′ĕ-tăl) [″ + *paries*, a wall]. Through a parietal region or wall.

transpeptidase (trăns-pĕp′tĭ-dās). An enzyme that catalyzes the transfer of a peptide from one compound to another.

transperitoneal (trăns″pĕr-ĭ-tō-nē′ăl). Across or through the peritoneum.

transphosphorylase (trăns-fŏs-for′ĭ-lās). An enzyme that catalyzes the transfer of a phosphate group from one compound to another.

transphosphorylation (trăns-fŏs″for-ĭ-lā′shŭn). The exchange of phosphate groups from one compound to another.

transpirable (trăns-pī′ră-bl) [″ + *spirare*, to breathe]. Permitting excretion through the skin or membranes, as perspiration.

transpiration (trăns″pī-rā′shŭn) [″ + *spirare*, to breathe]. 1. Act of exhaling water, gas, or vapor through the skin or a membrane. SEE: *perspiration*. 2. Substance exhaled.

   t., cutaneous. Giving off sweat from pores of the skin. SYN: *perspiration*.

   t., pulmonary. Escape of watery vapor from the blood to the air in the lungs.

transpire. To emit vapor through the skin or other tissues. SEE: *perspire*.

transplacental (trăns″plă-sĕn′tăl). Through the placenta, esp. penetration of the placenta by a toxin, chemical, or organism that would affect the fetus.

transplant [″ + *plantare*, to plant]. 1. (trăns-plănt′) To transfer tissue or an organ from one part to another as in grafting or plastic surgery. 2. (trăns′plănt) A piece of

tissue or organ used in transplantation, q.v.

transplantar (trăns-plăn′tăr) [″ + *planta*, sole]. Across the sole of the foot.

transplantation (trăns″plăn-tā′shŭn). 1. The grafting of living tissue from its normal position to another site or the transplantation of an organ or tissue from one person to another. Organs and tissues that have been successfully transplanted include the heart, lung, kidney, liver, pancreas, cornea, large blood vessels, tendon, cartilage, skin, bone, and bone marrow. Brain tissue has been implanted experimentally in treating parkinsonism. The most important factor in successful transplantation is the matching of histocompatibility antigens that differentiate one individual's cells from another's. Cyclosporine has been used to attempt to prevent rejection of the transplant. SEE: *autotransplantation; graft; heart transplantation; organ donation; renal transplantation; replantation.* 2. In dentistry, the transfer of a tooth from one alveolus to another.

   t., autoplastic. Transplantation of tissue from one part to another part of the same body. SYN: *t., homoplastic.*

   t., bone marrow. ABBR: BMT. Infusion of bone marrow cells into a patient. These cells may have been previously obtained from the patient, i.e., autologous cells, or from a donor, i.e., allogeneic cells. This procedure is used in treating various life-threatening diseases including some types of leukemia, aplastic anemia, and severe immunodeficiency state. SEE: *National Marrow Donor Program.*

   t., heteroplastic. Transplantation of a part from one individual to another individual of the same or a closely related species.

   t., heterotopic. Transplantation in which transplant is placed in a different location in host than it had in donor.

   t., homoplastic. T., autoplastic.

   t., homotopic. Transplantation in which transplant occupies the same location in the host as it had in the donor.

   t., tenoplastic. Transplantation of tissue between individuals belonging to different genera.

transplantation antigens. The commonly used term for histocompatibility antigens that cause the immune system of one individual to reject transplanted tissue.

transpleural (trăns-ploor′răl). Through the pleura.

transport. Movement or transfer of substances in a biological system, esp. movement of electrolytes, nutrients, and liquids across cell membranes. Transport may occur actively, passively, or with the assistance of a carrier.

t., active. Transfer of a substance across a membrane even though its concentration may be higher on the side toward which the movement is taking place.

transportation of the injured. *Carrying in arms:* Patient is picked up in both arms, as a child.

One-arm assist: Patient's arm is placed about neck of bearer and bearer's arm is placed about waist, thus assisting patient to walk.

Chair carry, chair stretcher: Any ordinary firm chair may be used. Patient is seated upon the tilted-back chair. One bearer grasps back of the chair and the other the legs of the chair (either the front or rear, depending on the construction of the chair). Both bearers face in the same direction.

Fireman's drag: Patient's wrists are crossed and tied with a belt or rope. Bearer kneels astride patient, with head under patient's wrists, and walks on all fours, dragging patient underneath.

Fireman's lift: Bearer grasps patient's left wrist with right hand; bearer's head is placed under patient's left armpit, drawing patient's body over bearer's left shoulder. Bearer's left arm should encircle both thighs, then lift patient. Patient's wrist is transferred to bearer's left hand, thus leaving one hand free to remove obstacles or to open doors.

Four-handed basket seat: Each of two bearers grasps own wrist and then grasps partner's free wrist. Patient sits upon this support.

Pack-strap carry: Patient is supported along bearer's back. Patient's right arm is brought over bearer's right shoulder and held by bearer's left hand. Left arm is brought over left shoulder and held by bearer's right hand. Patient is thus carried on the back, with arms resembling pack straps.

Piggyback carry: Patient is supported along bearer's back with knees raised to sides of bearer's torso. This leaves patient practically in a sitting position astride bearer's back, with arms around the bearer's neck or trunk.

Six- or eight-person carry: This is done as the three-person carry, q.v., except three or four bearers are on each side of patient, thus dividing weight more uniformly.

Three-handed basket seat: Bearer grasps own wrist, partner grasps the free wrist and leaves one arm free for supporting patient.

Three- or four-person carry: The litter-type carry used by emergency squads. Three persons kneel on one side of patient, place their hands under patient and lift up. The head bearer supports the patient's head and shoulders, center bearer lifts waist and hips, and third bearer lifts both lower extremities. A fourth person, if available, should help steady patient while patient is being lifted.

Two-handed seat: Bearers kneel on either side of patient. Each passes one arm around back (under armpits) and other arm under knees and lifts patient carefully in a sitting position.

Wheel chair, improvised: Fasten the legs of a chair, preferably one with arms, to parallel boards and attach skates or casters to the bottom of the boards. A footrest can be made by attaching a broom handle or stick across the parallel boards in front of the chair.

Vehicles: If an ambulance is not available, stretchers can be improvised with ropes and chairs, ladders, or poles. The patient should always be tied to the stretcher during transportation. Several bearers will be necessary to assist entering and leaving the vehicle.

transport proteins. Proteins important to transporting materials such as hormones from their site of origin to the site of cellular action and metabolism.

transpose. To change places, e.g., moving the insertion of a muscle or ligament to another site.

transposition (trănz″pō-zi′shŭn) [L. *trans*, across, + *positio*, a placing]. 1. A transfer of position from one spot to another. SYN: *metathesis.* 2. Displacement of an organ, esp. a viscus, to the opposite side. 3. Transplantation of a flap of tissue without severing it entirely from its original position until it has united in the new position.

transposition of great vessels. A fetal deformity of the heart in which the aorta arises from the right ventricle and the pulmonary artery arises from the left ventricle.

transposon (trănz-pō′zŏn). A genetic unit such as a DNA sequence that is transferred from one cell's genetic material to another.

transrectal ultrasonography of the prostate. SEE: *prostate, transrectal ultrasonography of the.*

transsection (trăns-sĕk′shŭn). Transection.

transsegmental (trăns″sĕg-mĕn′tăl) [″ + *segmentum*, a cutting]. Extending across or beyond a segment, as of a limb.

transseptal (trăns-sĕp′tăl) [″ + *saeptum*, partition]. Across a septum.

transsexual (trăns-sĕks′ū-ăl) [″ + *sexus*, sex]. 1. An individual who has an overwhelming desire to be of the opposite sex. 2. An individual who has had his or her external sex changed by surgery.

transsexualism (trăns-sĕks′ū-ă-lĭzm). The condition of being of a certain definite sex, i.e., male or female, but feeling and acting as if a member of the opposite sex. In some instances the desire to alter this situation leads individuals to seek medical and surgical assistance in order to alter anatomical characteristics so that their anatomy would more nearly match their feelings about their true sexuality. The success of this therapy is controversial.

transsexual surgery. Surgical therapy for alteration of the anatomical sex of an individual whose psychological gender is not consistent with the anatomical sexual characteristics.

transsphenoidal (trăns″sfē-noy′dăl). Done through the sphenoid bone.

transtemporal (trăns-tĕm′pō-răl) [″ + temporalis, pert. to a temple]. Crossing the temporal lobe of the cerebrum.

transthalamic (trăns″thăl-ăm′ĭk) [″ + Gr. thalamos, chamber]. Passing across the optic thalamus.

transthermia (trăns-thĕr′mē-ă) [″ + Gr. therme, heat]. Production of heat in the deep tissues by electric currents. SYN: diathermy; thermopenetration.

transthoracic (trăns″thō-răs′ĭk) [″ + Gr. thorax, chest]. Across the thorax.

transthoracotomy (trăns″thō-ră-kŏt′ō-mē) [″ + Gr. thorax, chest, + tome, incision]. The operation of incising across the thorax.

transtracheal. Across or through the trachea.

transtracheal jet insufflation. Life-saving technique of ventilating a patient with a complete airway obstruction. A small catheter is placed via a cricothyroid puncture and attached to a pressure-controlled oxygen outlet via a one-way valve.

transtympanic neurectomy. Surgical interruption of the parasympathetic nerve supply to the parotid and submandibular glands by bilateral sectioning of the tympanic and chorda tympani nerves. The technique is used in treating sialorrhea in mentally retarded children.

transubstantiation (trăn″sŭb-stăn″shē-ā′shŭn) [″ + substantia, substance]. The process of replacing one tissue by another.

transudate (trăns′ū-dāt) [″ + sudare, to sweat]. The fluid that passes through a membrane, esp. that which passes through capillary walls. Compared to an exudate, q.v., a transudate has fewer cellular elements and is of a lower specific gravity.

transudation (trăns-ū-dā′shŭn). Oozing of a fluid through pores or interstices, as of a membrane.

transureteroureterostomy (trăns″ū-rē″tĕr-ō-ū-rē″tĕr-ŏs′tō-mē). Section of one ureter and joining both ends to the opposite ureter.

transurethral (trăns″ū-rē′thrăl) [″ + Gr. ourethra, urethra]. Pert. to an operation performed through the urethra.

transurethral resection of the prostate. ABBR: TUR. Removal of prostatic tissue by use of a device inserted through the urethra. SEE: prostate.

transvaginal (trăns-văj′ĭn-ăl) [″ + vagina, sheath]. Through the vagina or across its wall as in a surgical procedure.

transvector (trăns-vĕk′tor). An animal that transmits a toxin that it does not produce and by which it is itself unaffected, as when a bivalve mollusc, such as the oyster, filters viruses out of the water and transmits them to those who ingest the mollusc.

transversalis (trăns″vĕr-să′lĭs) [″ + vertere, to turn]. A structure occurring at right angles to the long axis of the body.

transversalis fascia. A thin membrane forming the peritoneal surface of the transversus muscle and its aponeurosis.

transverse (trăns-vĕrs′) [L. transversus]. Lying at right angles to the long axis of the body; crosswise.

transversectomy (trăns″vĕr-sĕk′tō-mē) [″ + Gr. ektome, excision]. Excision of a transverse vertebral process.

transverse foramen. Canal through the transverse processes of the cervical vertebrae for passage of the vertebral arteries.

transverse plane. Plane that divides the body into a top and bottom portion.

transversion (trăns-vĕr′zhŭn). The eruption of a tooth at an abnormal site.

transversocostal (trăns-vĕr″sō-kŏs′tăl). Costotransverse, q.v.

transversospinalis (trăns-vĕr″sō-spī-nā′lĭs) [L. transversus, turned across, + spina, thorn]. Semispinalis capitis, semispinalis cervicis. SEE: Muscles in Appendix.

transversourethralis (trăns-vĕr″sō-ū″rē-thră′lĭs). The transverse fibers of the sphincter urethrae muscle.

transversus (trăns-vĕr′sŭs) [L.]. 1. Any of several muscles. SEE: Muscles in Appendix. 2. Lying across the long axis of a part or organ.

transvesical (trăns-vĕs′ĭ-kăl). Across or through the bladder.

transvestism, transvestitism (trăns-vĕst′ĭzm, -ĭ-tĭzm) [L. trans, across, + vestitus, clothed, + Gr. -ismos, condition]. The desire to dress in the clothes of and be accepted as a member of the opposite sex. SEE: eonism.

transvestite (trăns-vĕs′tīt). An individual who practices transvestism.

Trantas' dots (trăn′tăs) [Alexios Trantas, Gr. ophthalmologist, 1867–1960]. Chalky concretions of the conjunctiva around the limbus. These are associated with vernal conjunctivitis.

Tranxene. Trade name for chlorazepate dipotassium.

tranylcypromine (trăn″ĭl-sĭ′prō-mēn). USP. An antidepressant drug. Trade name is Parnate.

trap, food. A space or area in or between teeth where particles of food can and do become trapped.

trapeze bar. Triangular device suspended above a bed to facilitate transferring and positioning the patient. Also called *swivel trapeze bar.*

trapezial (tră-pē′zē-ăl). Concerning the trapezium.

trapeziform (tră-pē′zĭ-form). Shaped like a trapezoid.

trapezii. The trapezium and trapezoid carpal bones once they have fused. They function as one bone in the mechanics of the wrist.

trapeziometacarpal (tră-pē″zē-ō-mĕt″ă-kăr′păl). Concerning or connecting the trapezium and the metacarpus of the thumb.

trapezium (tră-pē′zē-ŭm) [Gr. *trapezion*, a little table]. 1. A four-sided, single-plane geometric figure in which none of the sides are parallel. 2. The os trapezium, the first bone on the radial side of the distal row of the bones of the wrist. It articulates with the base of the metacarpal bone of the thumb. SYN: *multangular bone, greater.*

trapezius (tră-pē′zē-ŭs). A flat, triangular muscle covering posterior surface of neck and shoulder. SEE: *Muscles* in *Appendix.*

trapezoid (trăp′ē-zoyd) [Gr. *trapezoeides*, table-shaped]. A four-sided figure having two parallel sides and two divergent sides.

trapezoid body. A bundle of transverse fibers in the ventral portion of tegmentum of pons. SYN: *corpus trapezoideum* [NA].

trapezoid bone. The second bone in the distal row of carpal bones. It lies between the greater multangular and capitate bones. SYN: *multangular bone, lesser.*

trapezoid ligament. The lateral portion of the coracoclavicular ligament.

trauma (traw′mă) [Gr. *trauma*, wound] (pl. *traumata* or *traumas*). 1. A physical injury or wound caused by external force or violence. It may be self-inflicted. In the U.S. trauma is the principal cause of death between the ages of one and 38 years. In addition to each death from trauma, there were at least two cases of permanent disability due to trauma. The principal types of trauma involved include motor vehicle accidents, suicide, homicide, falls, burns, and drowning. The majority of deaths occur in the first several hours after the event. 2. An emotional or psychological shock that may produce disordered feelings or behavior.

   t., birth. Injury to the fetus during the birthing process.

   t., occlusal. Any injury to part of the masticatory system as a result of malocclusion or occlusal dysfunction. It may be abrupt in its development in response to a restoration or ill-fitting prosthetic device, or result from years of tooth wear, drift, or faulty oral habits. It may produce adverse periodontal changes, tooth mobility, or excessive wear, pain in the temporomandibular joints, or spasms and pain in the muscles of mastication.

   t., psychic. A painful emotional experience that may cause anxiety.

   t., toothbrush. Abrasion or grooving of teeth and gingival injury or recession as a result of improper brushing with a stiff-textured brush.

trauma center. A regional hospital capable of providing care for critically injured patients. Available on a 24-hour basis are a surgical team, operating suite, surgical subspecialties, intensive care unit, and specialized nursing team.

Trauma Score. Numerical grading system that combines the Glasgow Coma Scale, q.v., and measurements of cardiopulmonary function as a gauge of severity of injury and predictor of survival after blunt trauma to the head. Each parameter is given a number (high for normal and low for impaired function). Severity of injury is estimated by summing the numbers. The lowest score is 1, and the highest score is 16. SEE: table.

traumatic (traw-măt′ĭk) [Gr. *traumatikos*]. Caused by or relating to an injury.

traumatic psychosis. Psychosis resulting from physical injuries or emotional shock.

traumatic rhabdomyolysis. SEE: *fibromyalgia.*

traumatism (traw′mă-tĭzm) [Gr. *traumatismos*]. Morbid condition of system due to an injury or wound.

traumato-. A combining form indicating a relationship to trauma.

traumatology (traw-mă-tŏl′ō-jē) [Gr. *trauma*, wound, + *logos*, word, reason]. The branch of surgery dealing with wounds and their care.

traumatopathy (traw″mă-tŏp′ă-thē) [″ + *pathos*, disease, suffering]. Pathological state caused by trauma.

traumatophilia (traw″mă-tō-fĭl′ē-ă) [″ + *philein*, to love]. The enjoyment of or unconscious desire to be traumatized, either mentally or physically. SEE: *masochism.*

traumatopnea (traw″mă-tŏp-nē′ă) [″ + *pnoia*, breath]. Passage of air in and out of a wound in the chest wall.

traumatopyra (traw″mă-tō-pī′ră) [″ + *pyr*, fever]. Fever caused by trauma.

traumatotherapy (traw″mă-tō-thĕr′ă-pē). Treatment of injury.

Trauma Score

Cardiopulmonary*			Neurologic† (Glasgow Coma Scale)		
Respiratory Rate	10–24/min	4	Eye Opening	Spontaneous	4
	24–35/min	3		To Voice	3
	36/min or greater	2		To Pain	2
	1–9/min	1		None	1
	None	0	Verbal Response	Oriented	5
Respiratory Expansion	Normal	1		Confused	4
				Inappropriate Speech	3
	Retractive	0		Incomprehensible Sounds	2
				None	1
Systolic Blood Pressure	90 mmHg or greater	4	Motor Response	Obeys Command	6
				Localizes Pain	5
	70–89 mmHg	3		Withdraws (pain)	4
	50–69 mmHg	2		Flexion (pain)	3
				Extension (pain)	2
	0–49 mmHg	1		None	1
	No Pulse	0	Glasgow Coma Score Total		
Capillary Refill	Normal	2	**Total Glasgow Coma Scale Points**		
	Delayed	1	14–15 = 5 11–13 = 4 8–10 = 3 5– 7 = 2 3– 4 = 1	CONVERSION = APPROXIMATELY ONE THIRD TOTAL VALUE	
	None	0			
Cardiopulmonary Assessment			Neurologic Assessment		
Total Trauma Score = Cardiopulmonary + Neurologic					

* Adapted from Champion, HR, Sacco, WJ, Carnazzo, AJ, et al: Trauma score. Crit Care Med 9(9):672–676, 1981.

† Adapted from Teasdale, G, and Jennett, B: Lancet II, 1974, p. 81, and Teasdale, G, et al: Acta Neurochirurgica Suppl. 28, 1979, pp 13–16.

travail (trắ-vāl′). The labor during childbirth.

Travase. Trade name for sutilains.

travelers' diarrhea. SEE: *diarrhea, travelers'*.

travel, medical preparation for. For travel in the U.S., no particular medical provisions need be made other than the usual ones concerning a spare pair of glasses, provisions for any medicines taken regularly, and suitable clothing. International travel requires more planning with respect to required immunizations, knowledge of climatic conditions that will be encountered, and the availabil-

ity of medical care in the places that will be visited. Knowledge of the altitude of the area to be visited is particularly important if the traveler has chronic diseases of the heart or lungs. Persons who use wheelchairs will need to know how well suited the places to be visited are for wheelchair access. It is also important to know whether your medical insurance will cover medical expenses incurred abroad. SEE: *diarrhea, travelers'*.

tray (trā). A flat surface with raised edges.

    t., impression. In dentistry, a U-shaped receptacle with raised edges made of metal or acrylic resin used to carry impression material and support it in contact with the surfaces to be recorded until the impression material is set or firm.

Treacher Collins syndrome [Edward Treacher Collins, Brit. ophthalmologist, 1862–1919]. Mandibulofacial dysostosis.

treacle (trē′kl) [Gr. *theriaka*]. A thick molasses-like residue that remains when sugar is refined.

treatment (trēt′ment) [ME. *treten*, to handle]. 1. Medical, surgical, dental, or psychiatric management of a patient. 2. Any specific procedure used for the cure or the amelioration of a disease or pathological condition. SEE: *therapy.*

t., active. Treatment directed specifically toward cure of a disease.

t., causal. Treatment directed toward removal of the cause of the disease.

t., conservative. 1. The withholding of administration of medicine or utilization of operative procedures until such procedures are clearly indicated. 2. In surgical cases, the preservation of the organ or part if at all possible with the least possible mutilation.

t., dental. Any of a variety of treatments of the teeth and adjacent tissues to restore or maintain normal oral health and function.

t., dietetic. Treatment of disease based on regulation of diet.

t., electric shock. Electroshock therapy, shock therapy, q.v.

t., empiric. Treatment based on observation and experience rather than having a scientific basis.

t., expectant. Relief of symptoms as they arise, i.e., not directed at the specific cause.

t., Kenny. Treatment of acute poliomyelitis by use of wet hot pack applications to the affected muscles. SEE: *Kenny treatment.*

t., palliative. Treatment designed for the relief of symptoms of the disease rather than curing the disease.

t., preventive. Treatment directed to prevention of disease.

t., rational. Treatment based on scientific principles.

t., shock. Shock therapy.

t., specific. Treatment directed to the cause of a disease.

t., starvation. Treatment in which food is withheld, as in cases of bacillary dysentery following hemorrhage.

t., supportive. Special measures employed to supplement specific therapy.

t., surgical. Treatment by means of operation.

t., symptomatic. Treatment directed toward constitutional symptoms, such as pyrexia, shock, and pain.

treatment plan. The projected series and sequence of treatment procedures based on an individualized evaluation of what is needed to restore or improve the health and function of a patient.

Trecator SC. Trade name for ethionamide.

tree. A structure that resembles a tree.

t., bronchial. The right or left bronchus with its branches and their terminal arborizations.

t., tracheobronchial. The trachea, bronchi, and their branches.

trehala (trē-hā′lă). A sweet substance secreted by the insect *Larinus maculatus.*

trehalase (trē-hā′lās). An enzyme that hydrolyzes trehalose to form two molecules; D-glucose.

trehalose (trē-hā′lōs). A disaccharide of trehala, q.v. It is also present in certain fungi.

Trematoda (trĕm″ă-tō′dă) [Gr. *trematodes,* pierced]. A class of flatworms commonly called flukes belonging to the phylum Platyhelminthes. It includes two orders: Monogenea, which are external or semi-external parasites having direct development with no asexual multiplication, and Digenea, internal parasites with asexual generation in their life cycle. The Digenea usually require two or more hosts, the hosts alternating. SEE: *fluke.*

trematode (trĕm′ă-tōd). A fluke, a parasitic flatworm belonging to the class Trematoda. SEE: *cercaria; fluke.*

trematodiasis (trĕm″ă-tō-dī′ă-sĭs). Infestation with a trematode.

tremble (trĕm′bl) [O. Fr. *trembler*]. 1. An involuntary quivering or shaking. 2. To shiver, quiver, or shake.

trembles (trĕm′blz). A condition resulting from ingestion of plants such as snakeroot (*Eupatorium urticaefolium*) or jimmyweed (*Haplopappus heterophyllus*). Common in domestic animals and may occur in humans as a result of ingesting the plants or more commonly from drinking milk or eating the meat of poisoned animals. Symptoms are weakness; anorexia; nausea and vomiting; prostration; and possibly death. In humans, the illness is called milk sickness.

tremelloid, tremellose (trĕm′ĕ-loyd, -lōs). Jellylike.

tremetol (trĕm′ĕ-tŏl). A poisonous substance occurring in snakeroot, rayless goldenrod, and other plants that may cause trembles in animals or humans. SEE: *trembles.*

Tremin. Trade name for trihexyphenidyl hydrochloride.

tremogram (trĕm′ō-grăm) [L. *tremere,* to shake, + Gr. *gramma,* something written]. Graphic representation made by a tremograph.

tremograph (trĕm′ō-grăf) [″ + Gr. *graphein*, to write]. Device for recording tremors.

tremolabile (trē″mō-lā′bl) [″ + *labi*, to slip]. Easily destroyed or inactivated by shaking; said of a ferment.

tremophobia (trĕ″mō-fō′bē-ă) [″ + Gr. *phobos*, fear]. Abnormal fear of trembling.

tremor (trĕm′or, trē′mor) [L. *tremor*, a shaking]. 1. A quivering, esp. continuous quivering of a convulsive nature. 2. An involuntary movement of a part or parts of the body resulting from alternate contractions of opposing muscles.

Tremors may be classified as involuntary, static, dynamic, kinetic, hereditary, and hysteric. Pathologic tremors are independent of the will. The trembling may be fine or coarse, rapid or slow, and may appear on movement (intention tremor) or improve when the part is employed. Often due to organic disease; trembling may express an emotion (e.g., fear). All abnormal tremors except palatal and ocular myoclonus disappear during sleep. SEE: *subsultus*.

    t., action. T., intention.

    t., alcoholic. The visible tremor exhibited by alcoholics.

    t., cerebellar. An intention tremor of 3 to 5 Hz frequency, associated with cerebellar disease.

    t., coarse. Tremor in which oscillations are relatively slow.

    t., continuous. Tremor that resembles tremors of paralysis agitans.

    t., enhanced physiologic. An action tremor associated with catecholamine excess, e.g., in association with anxiety, thyrotoxicosis, hypoglycemia, or alcohol withdrawal. It may occur as a side effect of drugs, such as epinephrine, caffeine, theophylline, amphetamines, levodopa, tricyclic antidepressants, lithium, and corticosteroids.

    t., essential. A benign tremor, usually of the head, chin, outstretched hands, and occasionally in the voice, that needs to be differentiated from the tremor of parkinsonism. Essential tremor, which is made worse by anxiety or action, is usually eight to ten cycles per second and that of parkinsonism four to five. There is usually a family history of essential tremor but not in parkinsonism. The medicines that are effective in treating parkinsonism have no effect on essential tremor.

    t., fibrillary. Tremor caused by consecutive contractions of separate muscular fibrillae rather than of a muscle or muscles.

    t., fine. A rapid tremor.

    t., flapping. Coarse tremor of a muscle group. The supported part momentarily loses its support and there is an attempt to regain the support. When seen in the outstretched arm and hand, the part flaps like a wing. Seen in hepatic coma and other diseases that cause encephalopathy. SYN: *asterixis*.

    t., forced. Tremor continuing after voluntary motion has ceased.

    t., Hunt's. Tremor associated with all voluntary movements. It is present in certain cerebellar lesions.

    t., hysterical. A fine tremor occurring in hysteria. May be limited to one extremity or generalized.

    t., intention. Tremor when voluntary motion is attempted.

    t., intermittent. Tremor common to paralyzed muscles in hemoplegia when attempting voluntary movement.

    t., muscular. Slight oscillating muscular contractions in rhythmical order.

    t., parkinsonian. A rest tremor that is suppressed briefly during voluntary activity. Parkinson's disease can occur without tremor. The tremor disappears during all but the lightest phases of sleep.

    t., physiologic. A tremor occurring in normal individuals. It may be transient and occur in association with excessive physical exertion, excitement, hunger, fatigue, or other causes. SEE: *tremor, enhanced physiologic*.

    t., rest. Tremor present when the involved part is at rest but absent or diminished when active movements are attempted. SYN: *t., static*.

    t., senile. Tremor occurring in old age.

    t., static. T., rest.

    t., volitional. Trembling of limbs or of body when making a voluntary effort. Seen in multiple sclerosis and other nervous diseases.

tremorgram (trĕm′or-grăm). Tremogram.

tremulor (trĕm′ū-lor). Device for administering vibratory massage.

tremulous (trĕm′ū-lŭs) [L. *tremulus*]. Trembling or shaking.

trench fever. A nonfatal, febrile disease of diverse signs, symptoms, and severity. Usually present are headache, malaise, pain, tenderness esp. in the shins, splenomegaly, and sometimes a transient macular rash. The causative Rickettsial organism, *Rochalimaea quintana,* may be cultured from the blood. Even though humans are the hosts for the organism, the disease is not directly transmitted from person to person. The body louse, *Pediculus humanus humanus*, is the intermediate host. It begins to excrete infectious feces five to twelve days after ingesting blood from an infected human.

    TREAT: The causative organism is sensitive *in vitro* to antibiotics such as tetracyclines and chloramphenicol, but there is no evidence that they are clinically effective.

trench foot. A condition resembling frostbite affecting feet of soldiers who are obliged to keep their feet in wet socks and shoes for long periods of time.

trench mouth. Painful pseudomembranous ulceration of the mucous membranes of the mouth and pharynx. SYN: *gingivitis, necrotizing ulcerative.*

trend [ME. *trenden,* to revolve]. The inclination to proceed in a certain direction or at a certain rate. Used to describe the prognosis or course of a symptom or disease.

Trendelenburg position (trĕn-dĕl'ĕn-bŭrg) [Friedrich Trendelenburg, Ger. surgeon, 1844–1924]. Position in which the patient's head is low and the body and legs are on an elevated and inclined plane. This may be accomplished by having the patient flat on a bed and elevating the foot of the bed. In this position, the abdominal organs are pushed up toward the chest by gravity. The foot of the bed may be elevated by resting it upon blocks. This position is used in abdominal surgery. In treating shock, this position is usually used, but if there is an associated head injury, the head should not be kept lower than the trunk.

Trental. Trade name for pentoxifylline.

trepan (trē-păn') [Gr. *trypanon,* a borer]. 1. To perforate the skull with a trepan to relieve the brain from pressure. 2. An instrument resembling a carpenter's bit for incision of the skull. SYN: *trephine.*

trepanation (trĕp"ă-nā'shŭn) [L. *trepanatio*]. Surgery utilizing a trepan.

   t., corneal. Keratoplasty.

trephination (trĕf"ĭn-ā'shŭn) [Fr. *trephine,* a bore]. Process of cutting out a piece of bone with the trephine.

trephine (trē-fīn'). 1. To perforate with a trephine. 2. A cylindrical saw for cutting circular piece of bone out of skull. SYN: *trepan.*

trephining. 1. The process of cutting bone with a trephine. 2. The removal of a piece of cornea for the relief of glaucoma.

trephocyte (trĕf'ō-sīt) [Gr. *trephein,* to feed, + *kytos,* cell]. Trophocyte, q.v.

trepidant (trĕp'ĭ-dănt) [L. *trepidans,* trembling]. Marked by tremor.

trepidatio (trĕp"ĭ-dā'shē-ō) [L.]. Trepidation.

   t. cordis. Palpitation of the heart.

trepidation (trĕp"ĭ-dā'shŭn) [L. *trepidatio,* a trembling]. 1. Fear, anxiety. 2. Trembling movement, esp. when involuntary.

Treponema (trĕp"ō-nē'mă) [Gr. *trepein,* to turn, + *nema,* thread]. A genus of spirochetes, parasitic in humans, which belongs to the family Treponemataceae. They move by flexing, snapping, and bending. SEE: *bacteria* for illus.

   T. carateum. The causative agent of pinta, an infectious disease of the skin.

   T. pallidum. Causative organism of syphilis. SYN: *Spirochaeta pallida.*

   T. pertenue. Causative organisms of yaws (frambesia).

Treponemataceae (trĕp"ō-nē"mă-tā'sē-ē). A family of spiral organisms belonging to the order Spirochaetales. Includes the genera *Borrelia, Leptospira,* and *Treponema.*

treponematosis (trĕp"ō-nē-mă-tō'sĭs). Infection with *Treponema.*

treponeme (trĕp'ō-nēm). Any organism of the genus *Treponema.*

treponemiasis (trĕp"ō-nē-mī'ă-sĭs) [" + *nema,* thread, + *-iasis,* condition]. Infestation with Treponema.

treponemicidal (trĕp"ō-nē"mĭ-sī'dăl) [" + " + L. *cidus,* to kill]. Destructive to Treponema.

trepopnea (trĕp-ŏp'nē-ă) [" + *pnoia,* breath]. Condition of being able to breathe with less difficulty when in a certain position.

tretinoin (trĕt'ĭ-noyn). USP. All-transretinoic acid. It is a keratolytic agent used topically in treating acne. Trade name is Retin-A.

TRF. *thyrotropin releasing factor.*

TRH. *thyrotropin releasing hormone.*

tri- [Gr. *treis,* three]. Combining form meaning three.

triacetate (trī-ăs'ē-tāt). Any acetate that contains three acetic acid groups.

triacetin (trī-ăs'ē-tĭn). USP. An antifungal agent used topically. Trade name is Enzactin. Previously used name was glyceryl triacetate.

triacetyloleandomycin (trī-ăs"ē-tĭl-ō"lē-ăn"dō-mī'sĭn). Previously used name for troleandomycin.

triacylglycerols. Combination of glycerol and three fatty acids. The fatty acids may be of a single kind or different. They are the major components of storage (or deposit) fat in plant and animal cells. These substances are referred to as fats, neutral fats, or triglycerides. These fats provide the major source of stored energy in the body. SEE: *fat.*

triad (trī'ăd) [Gr. *trias,* group of three]. 1. Any three things having something in common. 2. A trivalent element. 3. Trivalent.

   t., Hutchinson's. Syndrome characteristic of prenatal syphilis consisting of notched teeth, interstitial keratitis, and eighth-nerve deafness due to meningeal involvement.

triage (trē-äzh') [Fr., sorting]. The screening and classification of sick, wounded, or injured persons during war or other disasters to determine priority needs for efficient use of medical and nursing manpower, equipment, and facilities. It is also done in emergency rooms and in acute care clinics to determine priority of treatment. Use of triage is essential if the maximum number of lives is to be saved during an emergency situation that produces many more sick and wounded than the available medical care facilities and personnel can possibly handle.

NURSING IMPLICATIONS: For each patient, the emergency room staff must obtain a brief history, perform a rapid physical assessment including vital signs, perform first aid if necessary, assist in determining the severity of illness, and transfer the patient to the appropriate place of care. In order of diagnosis and treatment, bleeding with subsequent shock is the second priority after establishment of an airway and basic life support measures. Arterial bleeding, whether internal or external, needs immediate care. Next, the neurological status and attention to traumatized bones and tissues receives attention. After the emergency conditions have been diagnosed and treated, the staff should perform an orderly and complete physical examination to be certain no life-threatening condition is neglected. Reassess patient frequently and alter prescribed care as necessary.

triakaidekaphobia (trī″ă-kī″děk-ă-fō′bē-ă) [Gr. *treis*, three, + *kai*, and, + *deka*, ten, + *phobos*, fear]. Superstition regarding the number 13. SYN: *triskaidekaphobia*.

triamcinolone (trī″ăm-sĭn′ō-lōn). USP. A synthetic glucosteroid drug. Trade names are Aristocort, Kenacort, and SK-Triamcinolone.

triamterene (trī-ăm′tĕr-ēn). USP. A diuretic drug of the potassium-sparing type. Trade name is Dyrenium.

triangle (trī′ăng-gl) [L. *triangulum*]. A figure or area formed by three angles and three sides.

    t., anal. Triangle with its base between the two ischial tuberosities and its apex at the coccyx.

    t., anterior, of neck. The space bounded by the middle line of the neck, the anterior border of the sternocleidomastoid muscle, and a line running along the lower border of the mandible and continued to the mastoid process of the occipital bone.

    t., carotid, inferior. The space bounded by the middle line of the neck, the sternomastoid muscle, and the anterior belly of the omohyoid muscle. SYN: *t., muscular.*

    t., carotid, superior. The space bounded by the anterior belly of the omohyoid muscle, the posterior belly of the digastricus muscle, and the sternomastoid muscle. SYN: *t., omohyoid.*

    t., cephalic. Triangle on the anteroposterior plane of the skull formed by lines joining the occiput and forehead and chin, and a line uniting the occiput and the chin.

    t., digastric. Triangular region of the neck. Its borders are the mandible, stylohyoid muscle, and the anterior belly of the digastric muscle. SYN: *trigonum submandibulare.*

    t., facial. Triangle bounded by lines uniting the basion and the alveolar and nasal points, and one uniting the nasal and basion.

    t., femoral. Triangle on the inner part of the thigh, bounded by sartorius and adductor longus muscles and above by the inguinal ligament. SYN: *t., inguinal; t., Scarpa's.*

    t., frontal. Triangle bounded by the maximum frontal diameter and lines joining its extremities and the glabella.

    t., Hesselbach's. The interval in the groin bounded by Poupart's ligament, the edge of the rectus muscle, and the deep epigastric artery.

    t., inferior occipital. Area having the bimastoid diameter for its base and the inion for its apex.

    t., inguinal. T., femoral.

    t., Lesser's. Triangle bounded below by anterior and posterior bellies of the digastric muscle and above by the hypogastric nerve.

    t., lumbocostoabdominal. Triangle bounded in front by the obliquus abdominis externus, above by the lower border of the serratus posticus inferior and the point of the 12th rib, behind by the outer edge of the erector spinae, and below by the obliquus abdominis internus.

    t., muscular. T., carotid, inferior.

    t., mylohyoid. The triangular space formed by the mylohyoid muscle and the two bellies of the digastric muscle.

    t., occipital, of the neck. Triangle bounded by the sternocleidomastoid, the trapezius, and the omohyoid muscles.

    t. of elbow. The area in front of the elbow bounded by the brachioradialis and the pronator teres muscles on the sides, and with the base toward the humerus.

    t. of necessity. T., carotid, inferior, q.v.

    t. of Petit. The space above the hip bone between the exterior oblique muscle, the latissimus dorsi, and the interior oblique muscle.

    t., omoclavicular. T., subclavian.

    t., omohyoid. T., carotid, superior.

    t., posterior cervical. Triangle bounded by the upper border of the clavicle, the posterior border of the sternocleidomastoid muscle, and the anterior border of the trapezius muscle.

t., pubourethral. A triangular space in the perineum bounded externally by the ischiocavernous muscle, internally by the bulbocavernous muscle, and posteriorly by the transversus perinei muscle.

t., Scarpa's. T., femoral.

t., subclavian. A triangular space bounded by the posterior belly of the omohyoid, the upper border of the clavicle, and the posterior margin of the sternocleidomastoid. SYN: *t., omoclavicular; t., supraclavicular.*

t., submandibular. The triangular region of the neck, bounded by the inferior border of the mandible, the stylohyoid muscle and the posterior belly of the digastric muscle, and the anterior belly of the digastric muscle; it is one of three triangles included in the anterior triangle of the neck. Formerly called submaxillary triangle.

t., suboccipital. Triangle bounded by the obliquus inferior and superior muscles on two sides and the rectus capitis posterior major muscle on the third side. The floor contains the posterior arch of the atlas bone and the vertebral artery. It is covered by the semispinalis capitis muscle.

t., supraclavicular. T., subclavian.

t., suprameatal. Triangle slightly above and behind the exterior auditory meatus. It is bounded above by the root of the zygoma and anteriorly by the posterior wall of the exterior auditory meatus.

t., urogenital. Triangle with its base formed by a line between the two ischial tuberosities and its apex just below the symphysis pubis.

t., vesical. The triangular space at the base of the bladder. SYN: *trigone.*

triangular. Having three sides; shaped like a triangle.

triangular bandage. A square bandage folded diagonally. When folded, the several thicknesses can be applied to afford support. SEE: illus.; *bandage.*

triangularis (trī-ăng″gū-lā′ris) [L.]. A muscle of the chin. SEE: *Muscles* in *Appendix.*

triangular ligament. One of two ligaments, right and left, connecting posterior portions of the right and left lobes of the liver with corresponding portions of the diaphragm.

triangular nucleus of Schwalbe. The chief or dorsal nucleus of the vestibular division of the 8th cranial nerve. Located in the pons and occupying most of the acoustic area of the rhomboid fossa.

Triatoma (trī-ăt′ō-mă). A genus of bloodsucking bugs belonging to the order Hemiptera, family Reduviidae. Commonly called cone-nosed bugs or assassin bugs. It includes the species *T. braziliensis, T. dimi-*

diata, T. infestans, T. protracta, T. recurva, T. rubida, and others. They are house-infesting pests and some species, especially *T. infestans,* serve to transmit *Trypanosoma cruzi,* causative agent of Chagas' disease.

triatomic (trī″ă-tŏm′ĭk). Composed of three atoms.

tribade. A lesbian.

tribadism (trĭb′ăd-ĭzm) [Gr. *tribein,* to rub, + *-ismos,* condition]. A relationship in which women attempt to imitate heterosexual intercourse with each other.

tribasic (trī-bā′sĭk) [Gr. *treis,* three, + L. *basis,* base]. Composed of three replaceable hydrogen atoms.

tribasilar (trī-băs′ĭl-ăr) [″ + L. *basilaris,* base]. Having three bases.

tribasilar synostosis. Condition resulting from premature fusion of three skull bones —the occipital, sphenoid, and temporal. Results in arrested cerebral development and mental deficiency.

tribe (trīb) [L. *tribus,* division of the Roman people]. In taxonomy, an occasional subdivision of a family; often equal to or below subfamily and superior to genus.

tribology (trī-bŏl′ō-jē). Study of the effect of friction on the body, esp. the articulating joints.

triboluminescence (trī″bō-lū″mĭ-nĕs′ĕns) [Gr. *tribein,* to rub, + L. *lumen,* light, + O. Fr. *escence,* continuing]. Luminescence or sparks produced by friction or mechanical force applied to certain chemicals. Has been observed when wintergreen mints are broken by the teeth in the dark.

tribrachia (trī-brā′kē-ă). Condition of having three arms.

tribrachius (trī-brā′kē-ŭs). Deformed fetus, usually conjoined twins, exhibiting three arms.

tribromide (trī-brō′mīd) [Gr. *treis,* three, + *bromos,* stench]. A compound having three atoms of bromine in the molecule.

tribromoethanol (trī-brō″mō-ĕth′ă-nŏl). A white crystalline substance that is used in anesthesia.

TRIC agents. Acronym for *tra*choma and *i*nclusion conjunctivitis. SEE: *Chlamydia trachomatis.*

tricarboxylic acid cycle. A complicated series of reactions in the body involving the oxidative metabolism of pyruvic acid and liberation of energy. It is the main pathway of terminal oxidation in the utilization of carbohydrates, fats, and proteins. SYN: *citric acid cycle; Krebs cycle.* SEE: *Krebs cycle* for illus.

tricellular (trī-sĕl′ū-lăr). Three-celled.

tricephalus (trī-sĕf′ă-lŭs) [Gr. *treis,* three, + *kephale,* head]. A deformed fetus having three heads.

TRIANGULAR BANDAGE

STEPS IN MAKING SLING FOR ARM

triceps (trī′sĕps) [″ + L. *caput*, head]. A muscle arising by three heads with a single insertion. SEE: *Muscles* in *Appendix*.

triceps reflex. Sharp extension of forearm resulting from tapping of triceps tendon while arm is held loosely in bent position.

Tricercomonas (trī″sĕr-cŏm-ō′năs). Genus of very small protozoa considered identical to *Enteromonas*. SEE: *Enteromonas hominis*.

trichalgia. Pain caused by touching or moving the hair.

trichangiectasia, trichangiectasis (trĭk″ăn-jē-ĕk-tā′zē-ă, -ĕk′tă-sĭs) [Gr. *thrix*, hair, + *angeion*, vessel, + *ektasis*, dilatation]. Dilatation of capillaries. SYN: *telangiectasia*.

trichatrophia (trĭk″ă-trō′fē-ă) [″ + *atrophia*, atrophy]. Brittleness of hair resulting from atrophy of the root.

trichauxe, trichauxis (trĭk-awk′sē, -sĭs) [″ + *auxe*, increase]. Excessive growth of hair. SYN: *hypertrichosis*.

trichi-, tricho- [Gr. *thrix*]. Combining forms meaning hair.

trichiasis (trĭk-ī′ă-sĭs) [Gr. *thrix*, hair, + *-iasis*, condition]. Inversion of eyelashes so that they rub against the cornea, causing a continual irritation of the eyeball.

SYM: Photophobia, lacrimation, and feeling of foreign body in the eye.

TREAT: Epilation, electrolysis, and operation, such as correcting the underlying entropion with which this condition is usually associated.

trichilemma cyst. SEE: *cyst, pilar*.

trichilemmoma (trĭk″ī-lĕm-ō′mă). A benign tumor of the outer root sheath epithelium of a hair follicle.

Trichina (trĭk-ī′nă) [Gr. *trichinos*, of hair]. *Trichinella*, q.v.

trichina (trī-kī′nă) (pl. *trichinae*). A larval worm of the genus *Trichinella*.

Trichinella (trĭk″ī-nĕl′lă). A genus of nematode worms belonging to the suborder Trichurata. They are parasitic in humans, hogs, rats, and many other mammals.

    T. spiralis. The species of *Trichinella* that commonly infests humans, causing trichinosis. Infection occurs when raw or improperly cooked meat, particularly pork, containing cysts is eaten. Larvae encyst in the duodenum and invade mucosa of small intestine, becoming adults in five to seven days. After fertilization, each female deposits 1000 to 2000 living larvae, which enter blood or lymph vessels and circulate to various parts of the body where they encyst

HEAD

EYE

TEMPLE

OPEN HAND

HIP

GROIN

STUMP

FOOT

FIST

PALM

TRIANGULAR BANDAGES

in various areas, esp. in striated muscle.
SEE: *trichinosis.*

trichinelliasis (trĭk″ĭ-nĕl-lī′ă-sĭs). Trichinosis.

trichinellosis (trĭk″ĭ-nĕl-lō′sĭs) [Gr. *trichinos,* of hair, + *osis,* condition]. Disease caused by *Trichinella spiralis.* SYN: *trichinosis.*

trichiniasis (trĭk″ĭ-nī′ă-sĭs). Trichinosis.

trichiniferous (trĭk″ĭ-nĭf′ĕr-ŭs) [″ + L. *ferre,* to bear]. Containing trichinae.

trichinization (trĭk″ĭn-ĭ-zā′shŭn). Infestation with trichinae.

trichinophobia (trĭk″ĭn-ō-fō′bē-ă) [Gr. *trichinos,* of hair, + *phobos,* fear]. Abnormal fear of developing trichinosis.

trichinosis (trĭk″ĭn-ō′sĭs) [″ + *osis,* condition]. Disease caused by the ingestion of *Trichinella spiralis* when raw or insufficiently cooked infected pork is eaten. SEE: *Nursing Diagnoses* in *Appendix.*

SYM: Sometimes lacking. When large numbers have been ingested, gastrointestinal symptoms develop in a few days. These are pain, nausea, vomiting, and serous diarrhea. In one to two weeks muscular symptoms develop. Muscles become swollen, firm, and extremely painful. Movement is inhibited and dyspnea results from involvement of respiratory muscles. Edema, esp. of the face, is a prominent symptom. Profuse sweating is observed sometimes and high fever is usually present, as is eosinophilia.

In the third to sixth week of the disease, signs and symptoms of encephalitis and meningitis with visual and auditory symptoms may develop.

TREAT: For acute stage, thiabendazole may be helpful. In later stages, after worms have involved muscles, muscle pains should be relieved by analgesics. Corticosteroids are indicated for allergic reaction or central nervous system involvement. Treatment is in general symptomatic and supportive to enable patient to survive the acute toxemia following invasion of muscles. After encystment, the only symptom is vague muscular pains, which may persist for weeks.

PROG: Depends on number of worms ingested. Majority of patients recover.

trichinous (trĭk′ĭn-ŭs) [Gr. *trichinos,* of hair]. Infested with trichinae.

trichinous myositis. Myositis trichinosa, q.v.

trichion (trĭk′ē-ŏn) [Gr.]. The anthropometric point at which the midsagittal plane of the head intersects the hairline.

trichitis (trĭk-ī′tĭs) [Gr. *thrix,* hair, + *itis,* inflammation]. Inflammation of hair bulbs.

trichloride (trī-klō′rīd). A compound containing three atoms of chlorine.

trichlormethiazide (trī-klor″mĕ-thī′ă-zīd). USP. A diuretic drug of the thiazide type. Trade names are Metahydrin and Naqua.

trichloroacetic acid. USP. A drug used as a caustic to destroy certain types of warts, condylomata, keratoses, and hyperplastic tissue.

trichloroethylene (trī″klor-ō-ĕth′ĭl-ēn). A colorless clear volatile liquid with a specific gravity of 1.47 at 59°F (15°C). It is inhaled and used as an analgesic and anesthetic agent to supplement the action of nitrous oxide. It is a halogenated hydrocarbon having the chemical formula $CCl_2{=}CHCl$. Marketed under the trade names Triline and Trimar. It should not be used with epinephrine.

Caution: Should never be used in a system that requires soda lime. The heat generated in this type of system by the action of CO_2 and the lime will break down trichloroethylene to form the toxic gas phosgene and hydrochloric acid. Also in the presence of alkali the toxic and flammable substance dichloroacetylene is formed.

2,4,5-trichlorophenoxyacetic acid. ABBR: 2,4,5-T. A widely used herbicide that contains dioxin, q.v., a toxic, unwanted, and undesirable contaminant.

tricho- [Gr. *thrix, trichos,* hair]. A prefix denoting a relationship to hair.

trichoanesthesia (trĭk″ō-ăn″ĕs-thē′zē-ă). Loss of ability to sense stimulation of the hair.

trichobacteria (trĭk″ō-băk-tē′rē-ă) [″ + *bakterion,* rod]. 1. Filamentous bacteria. 2. Bacteria possessing flagella.

trichobezoar (trĭk″ō-bē′zor) [″ + Arabic *bazahr,* protecting against poison]. A hair ball or concretion in the intestine or stomach.

trichocardia (trĭk-ō-kăr′dē-ă) [″ + *kardia,* heart]. Pericardial inflammation with elevations resembling hair. SYN: *heart, hairy; pericardium, shaggy.*

trichoclasia, trichoclasis (trĭk″ō-klā′zē-ă, -ŏk′lăs-ĭs) [″ + *klasis,* a breaking]. Brittleness of the hair. SYN: *trichorrhexis.*

trichocryptosis (trĭk″ō-krĭp-tō′sĭs) [″ + *kryptos,* concealed]. Any disease of the hair follicles.

trichocyst (trĭk′ō-sĭst) [″ + *kystis,* bladder]. 1. A cell structure derived from cytoplasm. 2. In some single-celled organisms, a vesicle equipped with a thread that can be thrust out for the purposes of defense or attack.

Trichodectes (trĭk″ō-dĕk′tēz) [″ + *dektes,* biter]. A genus of lice of the suborder Mallophaga. It does not bite humans.

trichoepithelioma (trĭk″ō-ĕp″ĭ-thē-lē-ō″mă) [″ + *epi,* upon, + *thele,* nipple, + *oma,* tumor]. A benign skin tumor originating in the hair follicles.

trichoesthesia (trĭk″ō-ĕs-thē′zē-ă) [″ + *aisthesis,* sensation]. 1. Sensation felt when a hair is touched. 2. A paresthesia causing a sensation of the presence of a hair on a mucous membrane or on the skin.

trichogen (trĭk′ō-jĕn) [″ + *gennan,* to produce]. An agent stimulating growth of hair.

trichogenous (trĭk-ŏj′ĕn-ŭs). Promoting hair growth.

trichoglossia (trĭk″ō-glŏs′ē-ă) [″ + *glossa,* tongue]. Hairy condition of the tongue.

trichohyalin (trĭk″ō-hī′ă-lĭn) [″ + *hyalos,* glass]. The hyaline of the hair.

trichoid (trĭk′oyd) [″ + *eidos,* form, shape]. Hairlike.

trichokryptomania (trĭk″ō-krĭp″tō-mā′nēă) [″ + *kryptos,* hidden, + *mania,* madness]. Abnormal desire to break off the hair or beard with the fingernail. SYN: *trichorrhexomania.*

tricholith (trĭk′ō-lĭth) [″ + *lithos,* stone]. 1. A hairy nodule on the hair. Seen in piedra. 2. A calcified intestinal bezoar that contains hair.

trichology (trĭk-ŏl′ō-jē) [″ + *logos,* word, reason]. Study of the hair and its care and treatment.

trichoma (trĭk-ō′mă) [Gr., hairiness]. 1. Inversion of one or more eyelashes. SYN: *entropion.* 2. Matted, verminous, encrusted state of the hair. SYN: *plica polonica.*

trichomatosis (trĭk″ō-mă-tō′sĭs) [″ + *osis,* condition]. Entangled matted hair due to fungus disease of the scalp and lack of cleanliness. SYN: *plica polonica.*

trichomatous (trī-kŏm′ă-tŭs). Of the nature of or affected with trichoma.

trichome (trī′kōm) [Gr. *trichoma,* a growth of hair]. 1. A hair or other appendage of the skin. 2. A colony of blue-green algae that grows end-to-end in chainlike fashion.

trichomegaly (trĭk″ō-mĕg′ă-lē) [Gr. *trichos,* hair, + *megas,* large]. Long, coarse eyebrows.

trichomonacide (trĭk″ō-mō′nă-sīd). Anything that is lethal to trichomonads.

trichomonad (trĭk″ō-mō′năd). Related to or resembling the genus of flagellate *Trichomonas.*

Trichomonas (trĭk″ō′mō′năs) [″ + *monas,* unit]. Genus of flagellate parasitic protozoa.

T. hominis. Species in human intestines sometimes causing diarrhea and bacillary dysentery.

T. tenax. A benign trichomonas that may be present in the mouth. SYN: *T. buccalis.*

T. vaginalis. Species found in the vagina that produces discharge. A fairly common condition in women, esp. during pregnancy or following vaginal surgery. It is sometimes found in the male urethra and may be transmitted through sexual intercourse.

SYM: Persistent burning, redness, and itching of the vulvar tissue associated with a profuse vaginal discharge that may be frothy or malodorous or both. Occasionally *T. vaginalis* is present but asymptomatic.

TREAT: Metronidazole (Flagyl) taken orally by the female and her partner. Alcohol should not be consumed during metronidazole therapy. SEE: *colpitis macularis.*

trichomoniasis (trĭk″ō-mō-nī′ă-sĭs) [″ + ″ *-iasis,* infection]. Infestation with a parasite of genus *Trichomonas.*

trichomycosis (trĭk″ō-mī-kō′sĭs) [″ + *mykes,* fungus, + *osis,* condition]. Any disease of the hair due to a fungus.

t. axillaris. An affection of the axillary region and sometimes pubic hairs caused by *Nocardia tenuis.*

t. nodosa. Disease marked by nodule formations on the hair shafts. SYN: *piedra.*

trichonodosis (trĭk″ō-nō-dō′sĭs). Trichorrhexis nodosa, q.v.

trichonosis, trichonosus (trĭk-ō-nō′sĭs, -ŏn′ō-sŭs) [Gr. *trichos,* hair, + *nosos,* disease]. Any diseased condition of the hair.

trichopathic (trĭk″ō-păth′ĭk). Concerning disease of the hair.

trichopathophobia (trĭk″ō-păth″ō-fō′bē-ă) [″ + *pathos,* disease, suffering, + *phobos,* fear]. Morbid fear of hair on the face experienced by women, or any abnormal anxiety regarding hair.

trichopathy (trĭk-ŏp′ă-thē) [″ + *pathos,* disease, suffering]. Any disease of the hair.

trichophagia, trichophagy (trĭk-ō-fā′jē-ă, -ŏf′ă-jē) [″ + *phagein,* to eat]. The habit of eating hair.

trichophobia (trĭk″ō-fō′bē-ă) [″ + *phobos,* fear]. Abnormal dread of hair or of touching it.

trichophytic (trĭk″ō-fĭt′ĭk) [″ + *phyton,* plant]. 1. Relating to *Trichophyton.* 2. Promoting hair growth.

trichophytic granulosa (trĭk″ō-fĭt′ĭk) Tinea profunda, q.v.

trichophytid (trī-kŏf′ĭ-tĭd). A skin disorder considered to be an allergic reaction to fungi of the genus *Trichophyton.*

trichophytin (trī-kŏf′ĭ-tĭn). An extract prepared from cultures of the fungi of the genus *Trichophyton.* Used as an antigen for skin tests and for the treatment of certain trichophytid infections.

trichophytobezoar (trĭk-ō-fī″tō-bē′zor) [″ + *phyton,* plant, + Arabic *bazahr,* protecting against poison]. A hair ball found in the stomach or intestine composed of hair, vegetable fibers, and miscellaneous debris.

Trichophyton (trĭ-kŏf'ĭt-ŏn). A genus of parasitic fungi that lives in or on the skin or its appendages (hair and nails) and is the cause of various dermatomycoses and ringworm infections. Species that produce spores arranged in rows on the outside of the hair are designated ectothrix; if spores are within the hair, endothrix.

　　T. mentagrophytes. Species, one form of which, called granulare, is parasitic on several mammals including horses, dogs, and rodents and can also affect humans; another variety, called interdigitale, is associated with tinea pedis.

　　T. schoenleinii. Causative agent of favus of the scalp. SEE: *favus.*

　　T. tonsurans. The most frequent cause of ringworm of the scalp. SEE: *tinea capitis.*

　　T. violaceum. Causative agent of some forms of ringworm of the scalp, beard, or nails.

trichophytosis (trĭk″ō-fī-tō'sĭs) [″ + *phyton,* plant, + *osis,* condition]. Infestation with *Trichophyton* fungi.

trichoptilosis (trĭk″ŏp-til-ō'sĭs) [″ + *ptilon,* feather, + *osis,* condition]. 1. The splitting of hairs at their ends, giving them a featherlike appearance. 2. Disease of hair marked by development of nodules along the hair shaft, at which point it splits off. SYN: *trichorrhexis nodosa.*

trichorrhea (trĭk-or-ē'ă) [″ + *rhoia,* a flow]. Rapid loss of hair.

trichorrhexis (trĭk″ō-rĕks'ĭs) [″ + *rhexis,* a breaking]. Condition in which the hair splits. SYN: *trichoschisis.*

　　t. nodosa. Sparse, brittle hairs with bamboolike nodes. These apparent nodes are actually partial fractures of the hair shaft. This is caused by an atrophic condition of the hair. SYN: *hair, bamboo.*

trichorrhexomania (trĭk″ō-rĕks″ō-mā'nē-ă) [″ + ″ + *mania,* madness]. The abnormal habit of breaking off the hair with the fingernails.

trichoschisis (trĭ-kŏs'kĭs-ĭs) [″ + *schisis,* a splitting]. Splitting of the hairs.

trichoscopy (trĭk-ŏs'kō-pē) [″ + *skopein,* to examine]. Inspection of the hair.

trichosiderin (trĭk″ō-sĭd'ĕr-ĭn) [″ + *sideros,* iron]. An iron-containing pigment normally present in red hair.

trichosis (trĭ-kō'sĭs) [″ + *osis,* condition]. Any disease of the hair or its abnormal growth or development in an abnormal place.

　　t. decolor. Any abnormal coloring or lack of coloring of the hair. SYN: *canities.*

　　t. setosa. Coarse hair.

Trichosporon (trĭ-kŏs'pō-rŏn) [″ + *sporos,* a seed]. A genus of fungi that grows on hair and causes piedra.

　　T. beigelii. The causative agent of white piedra. SEE: *piedra.*

trichosporosis (trĭk″ō-spō-rō'sĭs) [″ + ″ + *osis,* condition]. Infestation of the hair with *Trichosporon.*

trichostasis spinulosa (trĭ-kŏs'tă-sĭs spĭn″ū-lō'să) [″ + *stasis,* a standing]. A congenital condition in which the hair follicle is plugged with keratin and fine, lanugo hairs.

trichostrongyliasis (trĭk″ō-strŏn-jī-lī'ă-sĭs). Infestation with the intestinal parasite *Trichostrongylus.* A rare disease in the U.S.

trichostrongylosis (trĭk″ō-strŏn″jī-lō'sĭs). Infestation with *Trichostrongylus.*

Trichostrongylus (trĭk″ō-strŏn'jī-lŭs). A genus of nematode worms of the family Trichostrongylidae. These worms are of economic importance because of the damage they cause to domestic animals and birds.

Trichothecium (trĭk″ō-thē'sē-ŭm) [″ + *theke,* a box]. A genus of mold fungi causing disease of the hair.

　　T. roseum. A species of mold fungus found in certain cases of inflammation of the eardrum (mycomyringitis).

trichotillomania (trĭk″ō-tĭl″ō-mā'nē-ă) [″ + *tillein,* to pull, + *mania,* madness]. The unnatural and irresistible urge to pull out one's own hair. It is estimated that 8 million Americans are affected by this compulsive action. Clomipramine has been effective in treating this condition.

trichotomous (trī-kŏt'ō-mŭs) [Gr. *tricha,* threefold, + *tome,* incision]. Divided into three.

trichotomy (trī-kŏt'ō-mē). Division into three parts.

trichotoxin (trĭk″ō-tŏks'ĭn) [Gr. *trichos,* hair, + *toxikon,* poison]. An antibody or cytotoxin that destroys ciliated epithelial cells.

trichotrophy (trī-kŏt'rō-fē) [″ + *trophe,* nourishment]. Nutrition of the hair.

trichroic (trī-krō'ĭk) [Gr. *treis,* three, + *chroa,* color]. Presenting three different colors when viewed along each of three different axes.

trichroism (trī'krō-ĭzm) [″ + ″ + *-ismos,* condition]. Quality of showing a different color when viewed along each of three axes.

trichromatic (trī″krō-măt'ĭk) [″ + *chroma,* color]. Rel. to or able to see the three primary colors; denoting normal color vision. SYN: *trichromic.*

trichromatism (trī-krō'mă-tĭzm). Trichroism.

trichromatopsia (trī″krō-mă-tŏp'sē-ă). Normal color vision.

trichromic (trī-krō'mĭk). Pert. to normal color vision or ability to see the three primary colors. SYN: *trichromatic.*

trichterbrust (trĭch'tĕr-broost) [Ger.]. Funnel chest.

trichuriasis (trĭk″ū-rī'ă-sĭs) [Gr. *trichos,* hair, + *oura,* tail + *-iasis,* condition]. Presence of worms of genus *Trichuris* in the colon or in the ileum.

Trichuris (trĭ-kū'rĭs). Parasitic nematode worms that belong to the class Nematoda.

T. trichiura. Species of *Trichuris* that infects humans when the ova that have undergone incubation in the soil are ingested. The larvae develop into adults, which inhabit the large intestine. If the infection is heavy, the patient will develop diarrhea and abdominal pain. Rectal prolapse may occur if a great number of worms are present. It is not definitely known that infection with *Trichuris* causes intestinal blood loss. SYN: *whipworm.*
   TREAT: Mebendazole is the drug of choice.

tricipital (trī-sĭp'ĭ-tăl) [Gr. *treis,* three, + L. *caput,* head]. Three-headed, as the triceps muscle.

tricitrates oral solution. A solution of sodium citrate, potassium citrate, and citric acid in a suitable aqueous medium. The sodium and potassium ion contents of the solution are approximately one mEq per ml.

triclofos sodium (trī'klō-fōs). A sedative-hypnotic drug. Trade name is Triclos.

tricornic (trī-kor'nĭk) [″ + L. *cornu,* horn]. Having three horns or cornua. SYN: *tricornute.*

tricornute (trī-kor'nūt) [″ + L. *cornutus,* horned]. Having three horns.

tricrotic (trī-krŏt'ĭk) [Gr. *trikrotos,* rowed with a triple stroke]. Condition in which three accentuated waves or notches occur on a sphygmograph tracing from one beat of the pulse.

tricrotism (trī'krŏt-ĭzm) [″ + *-ismos,* condition]. Condition of being tricrotic.

tricuspid (trī-kŭs'pĭd) [Gr. *treis,* three, + L. *cuspis,* point]. 1. Pert. to the tricuspid valve. 2. Having three points or cusps.

tricuspid area. Lower portion of the body of the sternum where sounds of the right atrioventricular orifice are best heard.

tricuspid atresia. Stenosis of the tricuspid valve. A fairly uncommon congenital malformation that causes cyanosis and clubbing.
   SYM: Paroxysmal dyspnea; difficulty in feeding.

tricuspid murmur. Murmur caused by stenosis of the tricuspid valve or by its incompetency.

tricuspid orifice. Right atrioventricular cardiac aperture.

tricuspid tooth. Tooth with a crown that has three cusps.

tricuspid valve. Right atrioventricular valve. SYN: *valvula tricuspidalis.*

trident, tridentate (trī'dĕnt, trī-dĕn'tāt) [L. *tres, tria,* three, + *dens,* tooth]. Having three prongs.

tridermic (trī-dĕr'mĭk) [Gr. *treis,* three, + *derma,* skin]. Developed from the ectoderm, endoderm, and mesoderm.

tridermoma (trī″dĕr-mō'mă) [″ + ″ + *oma,* tumor]. A teratoid growth containing all three germ layers.

Tridesilon. Trade name for desonide.

tridihexethyl chloride (trī″dī-hĕks-ĕth'ĭl). USP. An anticholinergic drug that acts similarly to belladonna. Trade name is Pathilon.

Tridione. Trade name for trimethadione.

tridymite (trĭd'ĭ-mīt). A crystalline form of silica, SiO_2, that may be obtained by heating quartz.

trielcon (trī-ĕl'kŏn) [″ + *helkein,* to draw]. Instrument with three branches for removing bullets or other foreign bodies from wounds.

triencephalus (trī″ĕn-sĕf'ă-lŭs) [″ + *enkephalos,* brain]. A deformed fetus lacking organs of sight, hearing, and smell.

triethanolamine (trī″ĕth-ă-nōl'ă-mēn). Previously used name for trolamine, q.v.

triethylenemelamine (trī-ĕth″ĭ-lēn-mēl'ă-mēn). ABBR: TEM. One of the nitrogen mustard compounds. SEE: *nitrogen mustards.*

triethylenethiophosphoramide (trī-ĕth″ĭ-lēn-thī″ō-fŏs-for'ă-mīd). An alkylating agent used in treating certain types of malignancies. SYN: *thiotepa.*

trifacial (trī-fā'shăl) [L. *trifacialis*]. Pert. to the fifth cranial nerve. SYN: *trigeminal.*

trifacial neuralgia. Neuralgia of one of the branches of the fifth cranial nerve; often severe. SYN: *tic douloureux.*

trifid (trī-fĭd) [L. *trifidus,* split thrice]. Split into three; having three clefts.

trifluoperazine hydrochloride (trī″floo-ō-pār'ă-zēn). USP. An antipsychotic drug. Trade name is Stelazine.

triflupromazine (trī″floo-prō'mă-zēn). USP. An antipsychotic drug that is also used in treating nausea and vomiting.

trifurcation (trī″fŭr-kā'shŭn) [Gr. *treis,* three, + L. *furca,* fork]. Division into three branches.

trigastric (trī-găs'trĭk) [Gr. *treis,* three, + *gaster,* belly]. Having three bellies, as certain muscles.

trigeminal (trī-jĕm'ĭn-ăl) [L. *tres, tria,* three, + *geminus,* twin]. Pert. to the trigeminus or fifth cranial nerve.

trigeminal cough. A reflex cough from irritation of the trigeminal terminations in respiratory upper passages.

trigeminal nerve. A large mixed nerve arising superficially from the side of the pons near its superior border. It is attached to the brain stem by two roots: a large sensory root and a small motor root. The sensory root bears an enlargement, the semilunar gasserian ganglion, from which three large branches arise. These are *ophthalmic*, purely sensory, from skin of upper part of head, mucous membranes of nasal cavity and sinuses, cornea and conjunctiva; *maxillary*, purely sensory, from dura mater, gums and teeth of upper jaw, upper lip, and orbit; *mandibular*, the largest division, containing sensory fibers from tongue, gums and teeth of lower jaw, skin of cheek, lower jaw and lip, and motor fibers supplying principally muscles of mastication. SYN: *fifth cranial nerve; nervus trigeminus.*

trigeminal neuralgia. Facial neuralgia. SYN: *tic douloureux*. SEE: *neuralgia, trigeminal.*

NURSING IMPLICATIONS: Observe and record characteristics of attack. Encourage the patient to maintain independence and social activities. Administer analeptic drugs as prescribed and observe for side effects. Inform the patient receiving alcohol injections that pain will return with nerve regeneration and to notify physician of pain recurrence. Before surgery, eliminate causative factors such as extreme temperatures of foods and jarring of the bed. Instruct the patient to use a cotton pad to cleanse the face and a blunt-toothed comb to comb the hair.

After surgery, assess sensory deficits to prevent trauma to the face and affected areas. Instruct the patient who has had an ophthalmic branch resection to examine the eye with a hand mirror every hour for foreign substances, as they cannot be felt, and to wear protective glasses to minimize entry of foreign substances into the eye. Instruct the patient who has had a mandibular or maxillary branch resection to be careful when eating. Teach the patient to chew food on the unaffected side so as to be aware of inner cheek injury. Tell the patient to have frequent dental examinations to detect any abnormalities that the patient cannot feel. Care for the patient who undergoes an intracranial surgical approach is similar to that for any patient undergoing intracranial surgery. Provide emotional support.

trigeminal pulse. Pulse with longer or shorter interval after each three beats because the third beat is an extrasystole.

trigeminus (trī-jĕm'ĭ-nŭs). The fifth cranial nerve. SYN: *trigeminal nerve*. SEE: *Cranial Nerves* in *Appendix*.

trigeminy (trī-jĕm'ĭ-nē). Occurring in threes, esp. three pulse beats in rapid succession.

trigenic (trī-jĕn'ĭk) [Gr. *treis*, three, + *gennan*, to produce]. In genetics, condition in which three alleles are present at any particular locus on the chromosome.

trigger (trĭg'ĕr) [D. *trekker*, something pulled]. 1. An event or impulse that initiates other actions or events. SYN: *stimulus*. 2. To initiate or start with suddenness.

trigger action. A physiological process or a pathological change initiated by a sudden stimulus.

trigger finger. State in which flexion or extension of a digit is arrested temporarily but finally completed with a jerk. Any finger may be involved, but the ring or middle fingers are most often affected.

TREAT: A finger splint or cortisone injection may be used. Surgery may be required.

trigger point or zone. Any place on the body that when stimulated causes a sudden pain in a specific area, esp. a type of pain previously felt spontaneously at the same location.

trigger substance. A chemical substance that initiates a function or action.

trigger zone. 1. An area that when stimulated will initiate an attack of neuralgia. 2. An area of cerebral cortex that when stimulated produces abnormal reactions similar to those in acquired epilepsy. SEE: *epileptogenic zone.*

triglycerides (trī-glĭs'ĕr-īds). Combinations of glycerol with three of five different fatty acids. These substances, triacylglycerols, are also called neutral fats. A large portion of the fatty substances, i.e., lipids, in the blood is triglycerides. Because these lipids are insoluble in water, they are transported in combination with proteins (lipoproteins). About one or two grams of triglycerides per kilogram of body weight are ingested daily in the usual diet in the U.S. In addition, they are produced in the liver from carbohydrates. SEE: *hyperlipoproteinemia.*

trigonal (trĭg'ō-năl) [Gr. *trigonon*, a three-cornered figure]. Triangular; pert. to a trigone.

trigone (trī'gōn). A triangular space, esp. one at the base of the bladder. SYN: *trigonum; triangle, vesical.*

    t., carotid. The triangular area in the neck bounded by the posterior belly of the digastric muscle, the sternocleidomastoid muscle, and the midline of the neck.

    t. of bladder. A triangular area at the base of the bladder. It is between the two openings of the ureters and the urethra.

    t., olfactory. A small triangular eminence at the root of the olfactory peduncle and anterior to the anterior perforated space of the base of the brain.

t., vesical. T. of bladder.

trigonectomy (trī″gŏn-ĕk′tō-mē) [″ + *ektome*, excision]. Excision of the base of the bladder.

trigonid (trī-gō′nĭd). The first three cusps of a lower molar tooth.

trigonitis (trĭg″ō-nī′tĭs) [″ + *itis*, inflammation]. Inflammation confined to mucous membrane of the trigone of the bladder.

trigonocephalic (trī″gō-nō-sĕ-făl′ĭk) [″ + *kephale*, head]. Having a head shaped like a triangle.

trigonocephalus (trĭg″ō-nō-sĕf′ă-lŭs). A fetus exhibiting trigonocephaly.

trigonocephaly (trī-gō″nō-sĕf′ă-lē). The condition of the head of the fetus being shaped like a triangle.

trigonum (trī-gō′nŭm) [L.] (pl. *trigona*). Any triangular area. SYN: *trigone*.

t. lumbale. Petit's triangle, q.v.

trihexyphenidyl hydrochloride (trī-hĕk″sē-fĕn′ĭ-dĭl). USP. An anticholinergic drug used in treating parkinsonism. Trade names are Antitrem, Artane, Pipanol, and Tremin.

trihybrid (trī-hī′brĭd) [Gr. *treis*, three, + L. *hybrida*, mongrel]. In genetics, the offspring of a cross between two individuals differing in three unit characters.

tri-iniodymus (trī″ĭn-ē-ŏd′ĭ-mŭs) [″ + *inion*, nape of the neck, + *didymos*, twin]. A deformed fetus with a single body and three heads joined at the occiput.

triiodothyronine (trī″ī-ō″dō-thī′rō-nēn). ABBR: T₃. One of two forms of the principal hormone secreted by the thyroid gland. Chemically it is 3,5,3′-triiodothyronine (liothyronine). SEE: *tetraiodothyronine; thyroid-function tests.*

trikates. USP. A solution of potassium acetate, potassium bicarbonate, and potassium citrate. Used in treating electrolyte deficiencies.

trilabe (trī′lāb) [Gr. *treis*, three, + *labe*, a handle]. Three-pronged forceps for removing foreign substances from the bladder. SEE: *lithotrite.*

Trilafon. Trade name for perphenazine.

trilaminar (trī-lăm′ĭ-năr). Composed of three layers.

trilateral (trī-lăt′ĕr-ăl) [″ + L. *latus*, side]. Concerning three sides.

trill (trĭl) [It. *trillare*, probably imitative]. A tremulous sound, esp. in vocal music.

trilobate (trī-lō′bāt) [″ + *lobos*, lobe]. Having three lobes.

trilocular (trī-lŏk′ū-lăr) [″ + L. *loculus*, cell]. Having three compartments.

trilogy (trĭl′ō-jē). A series of three events.

trimanual (trī-măn′ū-ăl) [″ + *manualis*, by

hand]. Performed with three hands, as an obstetrical maneuver.

trimensual (trī-mĕn′shū-ăl) [″ + *mensualis*, monthly]. Occurring every three months.

trimeprazine tartrate (trī-mĕp′ră-zēn). USP. A drug used for its antipruritic action. Trade name is Temaril.

trimester (trī-mĕs′tĕr). A three-month period.

t., first. The first three months of pregnancy.

t., second. The middle three months of pregnancy.

t., third. The third and final three months of pregnancy.

trimethadione (trī″mĕth-ă-dī′ōn). USP. An anticonvulsive agent used in treating certain forms of epilepsy. Trade name is Tridione.

trimethaphan camsylate (trī-mĕth′ă-făn). USP. A ganglionic blocking agent used to diminish blood pressure in acute hypertensive crisis. Trade name is Arfonad.

trimethidinium methosulfate (trī-mĕth″ĭ-dĭn′ē-ŭm). An antihypertensive drug.

trimethobenzamide hydrochloride (trī-mĕth″ō-bĕn′ză-mīd). USP. An antiemetic drug. Trade name is Tigan.

trimethoprim (trī-mĕth′ō-prĭm). USP. An antibacterial drug usually used in combination with sulfamethoxazole because they act to interfere with two sequential steps in the metabolism of certain bacteria. The combination is useful in treating various bacterial infections. Trade names are Proloprim and Trimpex. SEE: *sulfamethoxazole.*

trimethylene (trī-mĕth′ĭ-lēn). Cyclopropane, q.v.

trimmer. Device or instrument used to shape something by cutting off the material along its margin.

t., gingival margin. A cutting instrument for shaping gingival contours. It has a curved and angled shaft for use either on the right or left sides and on the mesial or distal surfaces.

t., model. A rotary flat grinder used to trim dental plaster or stone casts. Water keeps the cutting surface clean and obviates any dust problem as the casts are squared into proper study models.

trimorphous (trī-mor′fŭs) [″ + *morphe*, form]. 1. Having three different forms as the larva, pupa, and adult of certain insects. 2. Having three different forms of crystals.

Trimox. Trade name for amoxicillin trihydrate.

Trimpex. Trade name for trimethoprim.

Trinitroglycerol (trī-nī″trō-glĭs′ĕr-ŏl). Nitroglycerin.

trinitrophenol (trī″nī-trō-fē′nŏl). A yellow

crystalline powder that precipitates proteins. Used as a dye and as a reagent. SYN: *acid, picric.*

trinitrotoluene (trī″nĭ-trō-tŏl′ū-ēn). An explosive compound. SYN: *TNT.*

triocephalus (trī″ō-sĕf′ă-lŭs) [″ + *kephale,* head]. A deformed fetus with a rudimentary head without eyes, nose, or mouth.

triolein. Olein, q.v.

triolism (trī′ō-lĭzm). A sexual activity involving two persons of one sex and the other of the opposite sex.

triophthalmos (trī″ŏf-thăl′mōs) [″ + *ophthalmos,* eye]. A deformed fetus with three eyes.

triopodymus (trī″ō-pŏd′ĭ-mŭs) [″ + *ops,* face, + *didymos,* twin]. A deformed fetus with three fused heads and three faces.

triorchid, triorchis (trī-or′kĭd, -kĭs) [″ + *orchis,* testicle]. Person who has three testicles.

triorchidism (trī-or′kĭd-ĭzm) [″ + ″ + *-ismos,* condition]. The condition of having three testicles.

triose (trī′ōs). A monosaccharide having three carbon atoms in its molecule.

triotus (trī-ō′tŭs) [″ + *ous,* ear]. A person with a third ear.

trioxsalen (trī-ŏk′să-lĕn). USP. An agent used to promote repigmentation in vitiligo. Trade name is Trisoralen. SEE: *psoralen; vitiligo.*

trip (trĭp). A slang term used to refer to hallucinations produced by various drugs, including LSD, mescaline, and some narcotics.

tripara (trĭp′ă-ră) [L. *tres, tria,* three, + *parere,* to bear]. A woman who has had three pregnancies that have lasted beyond 20 weeks or have produced an infant of 500 grams. Designated Para III. SYN: *tertipara.*

tripelennamine citrate (trī″pĕ-lĕn′ă-mĭn). USP. An antihistamine drug. Trade name is Pyribenzamine Citrate.

tripeptide (trī-pĕp′tĭd) [Gr. *treis,* three, + *pepton,* digested]. Product of combination of three amino acids formed during proteolytic digestion.

triphalangia (trī″fă-lăn′jē-ă) [″ + *phalanx,* closely knit row]. Deformity marked by presence of three phalanges in a thumb or great toe.

triphasic (trī-fā′sĭk) [″ + *phasis,* phase]. Consisting of three phases or stages, said of electric currents.

triphenylmethane (trī-fĕn″ĭl-mĕth′ān). A coal tar-derived chemical that serves as the basis of some dyes and stains.

Tripier's amputation (trĭp-ē-āz′) [Léon Tripier, Fr. surgeon, 1842–1891]. Amputation of a foot with part of the calcaneus removed.

triple (trĭp′l) [L. *triplus,* threefold]. Consisting of three; threefold; treble.

triplegia (trī-plē′jē-ă) [″ + *plege,* stroke]. Hemiplegia with paralysis of one limb on the other side of the body.

triple response. The three reactions of the skin to injury: a red reaction along line of injury; a red area (flare or erythema) about injury; and an elevated area (welt or wheal) resulting from localized edema.

triplet (trĭp′lĕt) [L. *triplus,* threefold]. 1. One of three children produced in one gestation and one birth. SEE: *Hellin's law.* 2. A combination of three of a kind.

triplex (trī′plĕks, trĭp′lĕks) [Gr. *triploos,* triple]. Triple; threefold.

triploblastic (trĭp″lō-blăst′ĭk) [″ + *blastos,* germ]. Consisting of three germ layers: ectoderm, entoderm, and mesoderm.

triploid (trĭp′loyd). Concerning triploidy.

triploidy (trĭp′loy-dē). In the human, having three sets of chromosomes.

triplokoria (trĭp″lō-kor′ē-ă) [″ + *kore,* pupil]. Possessing three pupillary openings in one eye.

triplopia (trĭp-lō′pē-ă) [″ + *ope,* vision]. Condition in which three images of the same object are seen.

tripod (trī′pŏd) [Gr. *treis,* three, + *pous,* foot]. A stand having three supports, usually legs.

   t., Haller's. Truncus celiacus, q.v.

   t., vital. The three essentials for life-support: brain, lungs, and heart.

tripodia (trī-pō′dē-ă). Having three feet.

tripoding (trī′pŏd-ĭng). Use of three bases for support, e.g., two legs and a cane, or one leg and two crutches.

triprolidine hydrochloride (trī-prō′lĭ-dēn). USP. An antihistamine drug. Trade name is Actidil.

triprosopus (trī″prō-sō′pŭs) [″ + *prosopon,* face]. A deformed fetus with three faces.

tripsis (trĭp′sĭs) [Gr. *tripsis,* friction]. 1. The process of trituration. 2. Massage.

-tripsy (trĭp′sē) [Gr. *tripsis,* friction]. A word ending indicating intentional crushing of something.

triquetral (trī-kwē′trăl) [L. *triquetrus*]. Triangular.

triquetral bone. 1. The third carpal bone in the proximal row, enumerated from radial side. 2. Any wormian bone. SYN: *cuneiform bone.*

triquetrous (trī-kwē′trŭs) [L. *triquetrus,* triangular]. Triangular.

triquetrum (trī-kwē′trŭm) [L.]. Three-cornered.

triradial, triradiate (trī-rā′dē-ăl, -ăt) [Gr. *treis,* three, + L. *radiatus,* rayed]. Having three rays; radiating in three directions.

triradius (trī-rā′dē-ŭs). In classifying fingerprints, the point of convergence of dermal ridges coming from three directions.

trisaccharide (trī-săk'ă-rĭd). A carbohydrate that upon hydrolysis yields three molecules of simple sugars (monosaccharides).

triskaidekaphobia (trĭs-skī-dĕk-ă-fō'bē-ă) [Gr. *triskaideka,* thirteen, + *phobos,* fear]. Superstition concerning the number 13. SYN: *triakaidekaphobia.*

trismic (trĭz'mĭk). Concerning trismus.

trismoid (trĭz'moyd) [Gr. *trismos,* grating, + *eidos,* form, shape]. 1. Of the nature of trismus. 2. A form of trismus nascentium; once thought to be due to pressure on occiput during delivery.

trismus (trĭz'mŭs) [Gr. *trismos,* grating]. Tonic contraction of the muscles of mastication. May occur in mouth infections, encephalitis, inflammation of salivary glands, and tetanus. SYN: *ankylostoma; lockjaw.*

  t. nascentium. In the newborn, inability to open the mouth.

trisomic (trī-sōm'ĭk). In genetics, an individual possessing 2n + 1 chromosomes, that is, one set of chromosomes contains an extra (third) chromosome. SEE: *chromosome; karyotype.*

trisomy (trī'sō-mē). In genetics, having three homologous chromosomes per cell instead of two.

  t. 13. Trisomy of chromosome 13, which causes severe congenital deformation and mental retardation. These children usually do not survive past the first year of life. They have a large broad nose, widely spaced small eyes (hypertelorism), low-set ears, and poorly formed lower jaw.

  t. 18. Trisomy of chromosome 18, which causes severe deformity and mental retardation. These children usually do not survive beyond the first year of life. Characterized by prominent occiput, overlapping of index finger over third finger, frequent facial abnormalities, straight nose coming off sharply from the forehead, low-set ears, and cleft palate and lip.

  t. 21. A variety of congenital moderate-to-severe mental retardation. Marked by sloping forehead, presence of epicanthal folds causing an Oriental appearance of eyes, gray or very light yellow spots at periphery of iris (Brushfield's spots), short broad hand with a single palmar crease (simian crease), a flat nose or absent bridge, low-set ears, and generally dwarfed physique. SYN: *Down syndrome.*

trisplanchnic (trī-splănk'nĭk) [Gr. *treis,* three, + *splanchna,* viscera]. Pert. to the three large body cavities: the skull, thorax, and abdomen.

tristichia (trī-stĭk'ē-ă) [" + *stichos,* row]. The presence of three rows of eyelashes.

tristimania (trĭs"tĭ-mā'nē-ă) [L. *tristis,* sad, + Gr. *mania,* madness]. Melancholia.

trisulcate (trī-sŭl'kāt) [L. *tres, tria,* three, + *sulcus,* groove]. Having three grooves or furrows.

trisulfapyrimidines oral suspension (trī-sŭl"fă-pī-rĭm'ĭ-dēnz). USP. A combination of sulfadiazene, sulfamerazine, and sulfamethazine. This antimicrobial combination was developed in order to reduce the precipitation of crystals of the sulfonamides in the urinary tract. Trade names are Neotrizine and Terfonyl.

trisulfate (trī-sŭl'fāt). A chemical compound containing three sulfate, SO_4, groups.

trisulfide (trī-sŭl'fĭd). A chemical compound containing three sulfur atoms.

tritanomalopia (trī"tă-nŏm'ă-lō-pē-ă) [Gr. *tritos,* third, + *anomalos,* irregular, + *ope,* sight]. Color vision defect similar to tritanopia, q.v., but the defect is less pronounced.

tritanomaly (trī"tă-nŏm'ă-lē). Tritanomalopia.

tritanopia (trī"tă-nō'pē-ă) [Gr. *tritos,* third, + *an-,* not, + *ope,* vision]. Blue blindness; color blindness in which there is a defect in the perception of blue. SEE: *color blindness.*

Triten. Trade name for dimethindene maleate.

tritiate (trĭt'ē-āt). To treat with tritium.

tritiated thymidine. ^{3}H-Tdr. A radioactively labeled nucleoside used to measure T lymphocyte proliferation in vitro. Thymidine is essential for DNA synthesis, thus the amount of ^{3}H-Tdr taken up is a general measure of the number of new lymphocytes produced.

triticeous (trĭt-ĭsh'ŭs) [L. *triticeus,* of wheat]. Shaped like a grain of wheat.

  t. cartilage. A cartilaginous nodule in the thyrohyoid ligament.

tritium (trĭt'ē-ŭm, trĭsh'ē-ŭm) [Gr. *tritos,* third]. The mass three isotope of hydrogen; triple-weight hydrogen.

triturable (trĭt'ū-ră-bl) [L. *triturare,* to pulverize]. Capable of being powdered.

triturate (trĭt'ū-rāt). 1. To reduce to a fine powder by rubbing. 2. A finely divided substance made by rubbing.

trituration (trĭt-ū-rā'shŭn) [LL. *triturare,* to pulverize]. 1. The act of reducing to a powder. 2. A finely ground and easily mixed powder. 3. The creation of a homogenous mixture of metal alloy particles and mercury to form dental amalgam. SYN: *amalgamation.*

trivalence (trĭv'ă-lĕns). Condition of being trivalent.

trivalent (trī-vā'lĕnt, trĭv'ăl-ĕnt) [Gr. *treis,* three, + L. *valens,* powerful]. Combining with or replacing three hydrogen atoms.

trivalve (trī'vălv). Having three valves.

trivial name. A nonsystematic or semisystematic name and qualifying term used to name drugs. These names do not provide assistance in determining biological function of the drug. Examples are aspirin, caffeine, and belladonna.

trizonal (trī-zō'năl). Having three zones or layers.

tRNA. *transfer RNA.*

Trobicin. Trade name for spectinomycin hydrochloride.

trocar (trō'kăr) [Fr. *trois quarts,* three quarters]. A sharply pointed surgical instrument contained in a cannula. Used for aspiration or removal of fluids from cavities.

troch. Troche.

trochanter (trō-kăn'tĕr) [Gr. *trokhanter,* to run]. Either of the two bony processes below the neck of the femur.

   t., greater. T. major.

   t., lesser. T. minor.

   t. major. [NA] A thick process at upper end of the femur projecting upward externally to union of neck and shaft. SYN: *t., greater.*

   t. minor. [NA] A conical tuberosity upon inner and posterior surface of upper end of femur, at junction of shaft and neck. SYN: *t., lesser.*

   t. tertius. [NA] The gluteal ridge of the femur when it is unusually prominent.

   t., third. T. tertius.

trochanterian, trochanteric (trō″kăn-tē'rē-ăn, trō-kăn-tĕr'ĭk). Rel. to a trochanter.

trochanterplasty (trō-kăn'tĕr-plăs″tē). Plastic surgery of the neck of the femur.

trochantin (trō-kăn'tĭn). Trochanter minor.

trochantinian (trō″kăn-tĭn'ē-ăn). Concerning the lesser trochanter of the femur.

troche (trō'kē, trōk') [Gr. *trokhiskos,* a small wheel]. Solid, discoid, or cylindrical mass consisting chiefly of medicinal powder, sugar, and mucilage. Troches are intended to be used by placing them in the mouth and allowing them to remain until, through slow solution or disintegration, their purpose of mild medication is effected. SYN: *lozenge.*

trochiscus (trō-kĭs'kŭs) [L., Gr. *trochiskos,* a small disk]. A medicated tablet or troche.

trochlea (trŏk'lē-ă) [Gr. *trokhileia,* system of pulleys] (pl. *trochleae*). 1. A structure having the function of a pulley; a ring or hook through which a tendon or muscle projects. 2. The articular smooth surface of a bone upon which glides another bone.

trochlea of the elbow. A surface on the distal humerus that articulates with the ulna.

trochlear (trŏk'lē-ăr). 1. Of the nature of a pulley. 2. Pert. to a trochlea.

trochlear fovea. A depression on the orbital plate of the frontal bone for attachment of the cartilaginous pulley of the superior oblique muscle.

trochleariform (trŏk″lē-ăr'ĭ-form). Pulley-shaped.

trochlearis (trŏk″lē-ā'rĭs) [L.]. Superior oblique muscle of the eye. SEE: *Muscles* in *Appendix.*

trochlear nerve. A small mixed nerve exiting from the dorsal surface of the midbrain. It contains efferent motor fibers to the superior oblique muscle of the eye and afferent sensory fibers conveying proprioceptive impulses from the same muscle. SYN: *nerve trochlearis; fourth cranial nerve.* SEE: *Cranial Nerves* in *Appendix.*

trochocardia (trō″kō-kăr'dē-ă) [Gr. *trokhos,* a wheel, + *kardia,* heart]. Rotary displacement of the heart on its axis.

trochocephalia, trochocephaly (trō″kō-sē-fā'lē-ă, -sĕf'ă-lē) [″ + *kephale,* head]. Roundheadedness, a deformity due to premature union of the frontal and parietal bones.

trochoid (trō'koyd) [Gr. *trokhos,* a wheel, + *eidos,* form, shape]. Rotating or revolving, noting an articulation resembling a pivot or pulley. SEE: *joint, pivot.*

trochoides (trō-koy'dēz). A pivot or rotary joint.

Troglotrematidae (trŏg″lō-trē-măt'ĭ-dē). A family of flukes that includes *Paragonimus* (human lung fluke).

Troisier's node (trwă-zē-āz') [Charles E. Troisier, Fr. physician, 1844–1919]. Sentinel node, q.v.

trolamine (trō'lă-mēn). An alkalizing agent. Previously used name is triethanolamine.

troland (trō'lănd). A unit of visual stimulation to the retina of the eye. It is one equal to the illumination received per square millimeter of pupil from a source of one lux brightness.

troleandomycin (trō″lē-ăn-dō-mī'sĭn). An antibacterial drug. Previously used name is triacetyloleandomycin.

trolnitrate phosphate (trŏl-nī'trāt). A vasodilator drug. Trade name is Metamine.

Trombicula (trŏm-bĭk'ū-lă). A genus of mites belonging to the Trombiculidae. The larvae, called redbugs or chiggers, are annoying pests causing an irritating dermatitis and rash. They may serve as vectors of various diseases.

   T. akamushi. Species of mites that transmits the causative agent of scrub typhus.

trombiculiasis (trŏm-bĭk″ū-lī'ă-sĭs). Infestation with Trombiculidae.

Trombiculidae (trŏm-bĭk'ū-lī″dē). A family of mites; only the genus *Trombicula* is of medical significance.

tromethamine (trō-mĕth′ă-mēn). USP. A drug used intravenously to correct acidosis. It should not be used longer than one day. Trade name is THAM.

Tronothane Hydrochloride. Trade name for pramoxine hydrochloride.

troph-, tropho- [Gr. *trophe*]. Combining forms meaning nourishment.

trophectoderm (trŏf-ĕk′tō-dĕrm) [Gr. *trophe,* nourishment, + *ectoderm*]. Trophoblast.

trophedema (trŏf″ĕ-dē′mă) [Gr. *trophe,* nourishment, + *oidema,* a swelling]. Localized edema due to congenital hypoplasia of lymphatic vessels or resulting secondarily from obstruction to lymph flow by external pressure. Repeated low-grade infection may also obstruct the flow of lymph.

trophic (trŏf′ĭk) [Gr. *trophikos*]. Concerned with nourishment. Applied particularly to a type of efferent nerves believed to control the growth and nourishment of the parts they innervate. SEE: *autotrophic; center, trophic.*

trophism (trŏf′ĭzm). Nutrition.

trophoblast (trŏf′ō-blăst) [Gr. *trophe,* nourishment, + *blastos,* germ]. The outermost layer of the developing blastocyst (blastodermic vesicle) of a mammal. It differentiates into two layers, the cytotrophoblast and syntrophoblast, the latter coming into intimate relationship with the uterine endometrium, with which it establishes nutrient relationships. SEE: *fertilization* for illus.

trophoblastic (trŏf′ō-blăs′tĭk). Concerning trophoblasts.

trophoblastoma (trŏf″ō-blăs-tō′mă) [″ + ″ + *oma,* tumor]. A neoplasm due to excessive proliferation of chorionic epithelium. SYN: *chorioepithelioma.*

trophocyte (trŏf′ō-sīt). A cell, Sertoli cell, of the testicle, that supports and nourishes the developing spermatozoa.

trophoderm (trŏf′ō-dĕrm) [Gr. *trophe,* nourishment, + *derma,* skin]. Term applied to the trophoblast and its underlying layer of mesoderm. It is homologous to the serosa of birds, reptiles, and lower mammals.

trophodynamics (trŏf″ō-dī-năm′ĭks). Study of the forces and factors concerned with nutrition.

trophology (trō-fŏl′ō-jē) [″ + *logos,* word, reason]. The science of nutrition.

trophoneurosis (trŏf″ō-nū-rō′sĭs) [″ + *neuron,* nerve, + *osis,* condition]. Any trophic disorder due to defective function of the nerves concerned with nutrition of the part.

t., disseminated. Thickening and hardening of the skin. SYN: *sclerema; scleroderma.*

t., facial. Progressive facial atrophy.

t., muscular. Muscular changes in connection with nervous disorders.

trophoneurotic (trŏf″ō-nū-rŏt′ĭk). Rel. to a trophoneurosis.

trophonosis (trŏf″ō-nō′sĭs) [″ + *nosos,* disease]. Trophopathia.

trophonucleus (trŏf″ō-nū′klē-ŭs) [″ + *nucleus,* kernel]. Protozoan nucleus concerned with vegetative functions in metabolism and not reproduction.

trophopathia (trŏf″ō-păth′ē-ă) [″ + *pathos,* disease, suffering]. 1. Any disorder of nutrition. 2. A trophic disease.

trophopathy (trŏf-ŏp′ă-thē). Trophopathia.

trophotaxis (trŏf″ō-tăks′ĭs) [″ + *taxis,* arrangement]. The movement of cells away from or toward nutrients. SYN: *trophotropism.*

trophotherapy (trŏf″ō-thĕr′ă-pē). Nutritional therapy of disease.

trophotonus (trŏf-ŏt′ŏn-ŭs) [″ + *tonos,* tension]. A rigid state of contractile tissue resulting from trophic disorder.

trophotropism (trŏf-ŏt′rō-pĭzm) [″ + *tropos,* a turning, + *-ismos,* condition]. Attraction and repulsion of cells to nutritive substances; positive and negative trophotropism respectively. SYN: *trophotaxis.*

trophozoite (trŏf″ō-zō′īt) [″ + *zoon,* animal]. A sporozoan nourished by its hosts during its growth stage.

tropia (trō′pē-ă) [Gr. *trope,* turn]. Deviation of the eye or eyes away from the visual axis. Observed with the eyes open and uncovered. Esotropia indicates inward or nasal deviation; exotropia, outward; hypertropia, upward; hypotropia, downward. SYN: *manifest squint; strabismus.* SEE: *phoria.*

tropical (trŏp′ĭ-kal) [Gr. *tropikos,* turning]. Pert. to the tropics.

tropical immersion foot. Syndrome with severe wrinkling and maceration of the soles of the feet and marked lowering of the threshold of pain. Due to prolonged exposure of the feet to warm water as would occur in the tropics. May be prevented by allowing feet to dry thoroughly each night, use of dry socks and shoes the next day, and protecting the feet with silicone grease.

tropical lichen. Acute inflammation of the sweat glands. SYN: *prickly heat.*

tropical sprue. Sprue, q.v.

tropicamide (trō-pĭk′ă-mīd). USP. An anticholinergic drug used to produce mydriasis and cycloplegia in treating eye conditions. Trade name is Mydriacyl.

-tropin [Gr. *tropos,* a turn]. Suffix indicating the stimulating effect of a substance, esp. a hormone, on its target organ.

tropine (trō′pĭn). An alkaloid, $C_8H_{15}NO$, that smells like tobacco. It is present in certain plants.

tropism (trō'pĭzm) [Gr. *trope*, turn, + *-ismos*, condition]. 1. Reaction of living organisms involuntarily toward or away from light, darkness, heat, cold, or other stimuli. 2. The involuntary response of an organism as a bending, turning, or movement toward (positive tropism) or away from (negative tropism) an external stimulus. SYN: *taxis*. SEE: *chemotropism; galvanotropism; phototropism*.

-tropism. Combining form meaning a response to or a turning toward or away from an external stimulus.

tropocollagen (trō″pō-kŏl′ă-jĕn) [″ + *collagen*]. The basic molecular unit of collagen fibrils, composed of three polypeptide chains.

tropometer (trŏp-ŏm′ĕ-ter) [″ + *metron*, measure]. 1. Device for measuring the rotation of the eyeballs. 2. Instrument for measuring torsion in long bones.

tropomyosin (trō″pō-mī′ō-sĭn). A muscle protein that is involved in the formation of cross-bridges during muscle contraction.

troponin (trō′pō-nĭn). A muscle protein that attaches to both actin and tropomyosin. It is concerned with calcium binding and inhibiting cross-bridge formation.

trough (trŏf). A groove or channel.

   t., gingival. Gingival sulcus, q.v.

   t., synaptic. The depression in a muscle fiber that is occupied by the axon termination in a motor endplate.

Trousseau's sign (troo-sōz′) [Armand Trousseau, Fr. physician, 1801–1867]. Muscular spasm resulting from pressure applied to nerves and vessels of the upper arm. It is indicative of latent tetany. Also occurs in osteomalacia. SEE: *tetany*.

Trousseau's spots. Streaking of the skin with the fingernail, seen in meningitis and other cerebral diseases.

Trousseau's symptom. Spasmodic muscular contractions produced by pressing the principal vessel and nerve of the limb. Presence of this symptom is a sign of tetany.

troxidone (trŏk′sĭ-dōn). Trimethadione.

troy weight. A system of weighing gold, silver, precious metals, and jewels in which 5760 grains equal 1 pound; one grain equals 0.0648 grams. SEE: *Weights and Measures* in *Appendix*.

true (troo) [AS. *treowe*, faithful]. Not false; real; genuine.

true conjugate diameter of pelvic inlet. The distance from the posterior surface of the symphysis pubis to the promontory of the sacrum (about 11 cm in female).

true pelvis. Portion of the pelvis that falls below the iliopectineal line.

true ribs. The seven upper ribs on each side

with cartilages articulating directly with the sternum. SYN: *costa vera*. SEE: *rib*.

truncal (trŭng′kăl) [L. *truncus*, trunk]. Rel. to the trunk.

truncate (trŭng′kāt) [L. *truncare*, to cut off]. 1. Having a square end as if it were cut off; lacking an apex. 2. To shorten by amputation of a part of the entity.

truncus (trŭng′kŭs). Trunk.

   t. arteriosus. The arterial trunk from the embryonic heart.

   t. brachiocephalicus. Initial branch of the arch of the aorta.

   t. celiacus. Trunk arising from the abdominal artery. Most of the blood supply for the liver, stomach, spleen, gallbladder, pancreas, and duodenum comes from this trunk.

   t. pulmonalis. The vessel arising from the right ventricle. It transports venous blood to the lungs.

trunk (trŭnk) [L. *truncus*, trunk]. 1. The body exclusive of the head and limbs. SYN: *torso*. 2. Main stem of a lymphatic vessel, nerve, or blood vessel.

   t., celiac. Truncus celiacus, q.v.

   t., lumbosacral. Truncus pulmonalis, q.v.

   t., pulmonary. The great vessel that arises from the right ventricle of the heart and gives rise to the right and left pulmonary arteries to the lungs.

   t., sympathetic. The two long chains of ganglia, connected by sympathetic nerve fibers, that extend along the vertebral column from the skull to the coccyx.

trusion (troo′zhŭn) [L. *trudere*, to show]. Malposition of a tooth or teeth.

truss (trŭs) [ME. *trusse*, a bundle]. 1. A restraining device for pushing a hernia, esp. an inguinal or abdominal wall hernia, back in place. 2. To tie or bind as with a cord or string.

trust. In the relations between health care providers and patients, reliance by both parties on the integrity and sincerity of each other, and the patient's confidence in the ability of the care provider or confidence that the provider would be willing to seek assistance when his or her ability is lacking. Trust is essential in the relationship between patients and those who provide medical care for them.

truth serum. One of several hypnotic drugs supposedly having the effect of causing a person upon questioning to talk freely and without inhibition. In actual practice, serum is not given, but a short-acting barbiturate or Pentothal Sodium is given intravenously. The reliability of information obtained is questionable.

trybutyrase. An enzyme present in the stomach that digests the short chain diglycerides of butter. SEE: *digestion.*

try-in. The temporary placement of a dental restoration or device to determine its fit and comfortableness.

trypanocide, trypanocidal (trĭp-ăn′ō-sīd, trĭp″ăn-ō-sī′dăl) [Gr. *trypanon,* a borer, + L. *cide,* kill]. 1. Destructive to trypanosomes. 2. An agent that kills trypanosomes. SYN: *trypanosomicide.*

trypanolysis (trĭp-ăn-ōl′ĭ-sĭs) [″ + *lysis,* dissolution]. The dissolution of trypanosomes.

Trypanoplasma (trī″păn-ō-plăz′mă) [″ + LL. *plasma,* form, mold]. A genus of protozoan parasites resembling trypanosomes.

Trypanosoma (trī″păn-ō-sō′mă) [″ + *soma,* a body]. A genus of parasitic, flagellate protozoa found in the blood of many vertebrates, including humans. They are transmitted by insect vectors.

   T. brucei. The causative agent of trypanosomiasis in horses and other domestic animals. Nonpathogenic in man.

   T. cruzi. The causative agent of American trypanosomiasis in many animals and specifically Chagas' disease in humans. It is transmitted by blood-sucking insects (triatomids) belonging to the family Reduviidae.

   T. gambiense. The causative agent of African sleeping sickness. It is transmitted by the tsetse fly.

   T. rhodesiense. An organism parasitic in wild game and domestic animals of portions of Africa. May cause East African sleeping sickness in humans.

trypanosomal (trī-păn-ō-sō′măl). Pert. to trypanosomata.

trypanosome (trī′păn-ō-sōm). Any protozoan belonging to the genus Trypanosoma.

trypanosomiasis (trī-păn″ō-sō-mī′ă-sĭs) [″ + *soma,* body, + *-iasis,* infection]. Any of the several diseases occurring in humans and domestic animals caused by a species of *Trypanosoma.* SEE: *sleeping sickness.*

   t., African. African sleeping sickness, caused by *Trypanosoma gambiense.* SEE: *eflornithine.*

   t., South American. Disease caused by *Trypanosoma cruzi* and transmitted by the biting reduviid bug. It is characterized by fever, lymphadenopathy, hepatosplenomegaly, and facial edema. Chronic cases may be mild or asymptomatic, or may be accompanied by myocardiopathy, megaesophagus, and megacolon, with fatal outcome. In Brazil and Argentina, the disease is often severe; in Chile, the disease is mild. SYN: *Chagas' disease.*

   TREAT: Treat acute phase with nifurtimox, which is available in the U.S. only from the Parasitic Disease Drug Service, Centers for Disease Control, Atlanta, GA 30333.

   Nifurtimox is not effective in treating the chronic disease.

trypanosomic (trī-păn″ō-sō′mĭk). Concerning trypanosomes.

trypanosomicide. Trypanocide, q.v.

trypanosomid (trī-păn′ō-sō-mĭd). A skin eruption in any disease caused by a trypanosome.

tryparsamide (trĭp-ărs′ă-mĭd, -mĭd). An arsenic compound containing about 25% arsenic. Used chiefly in sleeping sickness.

trypsin (trĭp′sĭn) [Gr. *tripsis,* friction]. 1. A proteolytic enzyme formed in the intestine from the action of enterokinase of the intestinal juice (succus entericus) on trypsinogen secreted by the pancreas and present in pancreatic juice. It catalyzes the hydrolysis of peptide bonds in partly digested proteins and some native proteins, the final products being amino acids and various polypeptides. 2. USP. Proteolytic enzyme crystallized from an extract of the pancreas gland of an ox. SEE: *chymotrypsin; digestion; enzyme; pancreas.*

   t., crystallized. USP. A standardized preparation of the proteolytic enzyme trypsin. It is extracted from the pancreas of the ox, *Bos taurus.*

trypsinized (trĭp′sĭ-nīzd). Subjected to action of trypsin, thus having antitryptic power abolished.

trypsinogen (trĭp-sĭn′ō-jĕn) [″ + *gennan,* to produce]. The proenzyme, or inactive form of trypsin found in pancreatic juice. Activated when mixed in the intestine with the enterokinase of the succus entericus.

tryptic (trĭp′tĭk). Rel. to trypsin.

tryptolysis (trĭp-tŏl′ĭ-sĭs) [″ + *lysis,* dissolution]. The hydrolysis of proteins or their derivatives by trypsin.

tryptone (trĭp′tōn). A peptide produced by the action of trypsin on a protein.

tryptophan (trĭp′tō-făn). USP. An essential amino acid present in high concentrations in animal and fish protein. It is necessary for normal growth and development. Tryptophan is a precursor of serotonin, a chemical important in the transmission of nerve impulses across nerve cell connections. In high doses it may cause nausea and vomiting.

tryptophanase (trĭp′tō-făn-ās). An enzyme that catalyzes the splitting of tryptophan into indole, pyruvic acid, and ammonia.

tryptophan-induced eosinophilia-myalgia syndrome. SEE: *eosinophilia-myalgia syndrome, tryptophan-induced.*

tryptophanuria (trĭp″tō-fă-nū′rē-ă) [*tryptophan* + Gr. *ouron,* urine]. Tryptophan in the urine.

T/S. *thyroid:serum* (thyroid to serum iodine

ratio).

T.S. *test solution; triple strength.*

TSD. *target skin distance.*

tsetse fly (tsĕt′sē) [S. African]. One of several species of blood-sucking flies belonging to the genus *Glossina*, order Diptera, confined to Africa south of the Sahara Desert. It is an important transmitter of trypanosomes, the causative agents of African sleeping sicknesses in humans and nagana and other diseases of cattle and game animals. SEE: *Trypanosoma; trypanosomiasis.*

TSH. *thyroid-stimulating hormone.*

TSH-RF. *thyroid-stimulating hormone releasing factor.*

tsp. *teaspoon.*

TSTA. *tumor-specific transplantation antigen.*

tsutsugamushi disease (soot″soo-gă-moo′ shĭ) [Japanese, dangerous bug]. Scrub typhus.

TT. *transit time* of blood through heart and lungs.

T-tube. Device inserted into the biliary duct after removal of the gallbladder. It allows for drainage of the gallbladder and introduction of contrast medium for postoperative cholangiography.

T.U. *toxic unit; toxin unit.*

tuaminoheptane sulfate (too-ăm″ĭ-nō-hĕp′tān). USP. A sympathomimetic drug used to produce vasoconstriction of the nasal mucosa or the conjunctiva. It is prepared in an appropriate solution and applied topically.

tub (tŭb) [ME. *tubbe*]. 1. A receptacle for bathing. 2. The use of the cold bath. 3. To treat by using a cold bath.

tuba (too′bă) [L. *tubus,* tube]. Tube.

tubal (tū′băl) [L. *tubus,* tube]. Pert. to a tube, esp. the fallopian tube.

tubal nephritis. Inflammation of kidney tubules.

tubal pregnancy. SEE: *pregnancy, tubal.*

tubatorsion (tū″bă-tor′shŭn) [″ + *torsio,* a twisting]. The twisting of an oviduct.

tubba, tubboe (tŭb′ă, -ō). Yaws that attacks the palms and soles.

tube (tūb) [L. *tubus,* a tube]. A long, hollow, cylindrical structure.

    t., auditory. Eustachian tube, q.v.

    t., Cantor. T., intestinal decompression.

    t., cathode ray. Vacuum tube with a thin window at the end opposite the cathode to allow the cathode rays to pass outside. More generally, any discharge tube in which the vacuum is fairly high.

    t., Coolidge. A kind of hot cathode tube that is so highly exhausted that the residual gas plays no part in the production of the cathode stream, and that is regulated by variable heating of the cathode filament.

    t., Crookes′. Vacuum tube used in producing roentgen rays.

    t., drainage. Glass or rubber tube that, when inserted into a cavity, drains away its fluid contents.

    t., endobronchial. Double-lumen tube used in anesthesia. One tube may be used to aerate a portion of the lung, while the other is occluded in order to deflate the other lung or a portion of it. SYN: *Carlen's catheter.*

    t., endotracheal. A catheter inserted into the trachea for the purpose of providing an airway.

    t., esophageal. T., stomach.

    t., eustachian. Tube passing from the throat to the middle ear.

    t., fallopian. One of two oviducts leading from the peritoneal cavity into the uterine cavity.

    t., fermentation. U-shaped tube open only at one end. If they produce gas, bacteria cultured in media in the upright tubes will cause the level of fluid to decrease in the tube with the closed end.

    t., hot-cathode. Vacuum tube in which the cathode is electrically heated to incandescence and in which the supply of electrons depends on the temperature of the cathode.

    t., hot cathode roentgen-ray. Vacuum roentgen-ray tube in which the electron stream is supplied by a heated cathode. The cathode stream may be regulated by varying the current through the cathode filament.

    t., intestinal decompression. Tube placed in the intestinal tract, usually via the nose and esophagus, in order to relieve gas pressure produced when paralytic ileus or intestinal obstruction is present. Tubes may be plain; made of rubber, plastic, or silicone; or they may be equipped with a mercury-filled tip to facilitate passage into the intestinal tract. The latter is called a Cantor tube. The tubes are impregnated with a radiopaque substance in order to allow x-ray visualization of their location.

    t., intubation. Tube for passing into the larynx to facilitate breathing. SEE: *intubation.*

    t., Levin. Tube passed via the nose into the gastrointestinal tract.

    t., Miller-Abbott. Double-channel intestinal tube used to relieve intestinal distention. Inserted through a nostril, the tube is passed through the stomach into the small intestine.

    t., nasogastric. Tube passed via the nose into the gastrointestinal tract for the purpose of instilling liquid foods into the stomach.

    t., neural. SEE: *neural tube.*

    t., otopharyngeal. Eustachian tube, q.v.

t., Sengstaken-Blakemore. Three-element nasogastric tube used in treating esophageal bleeding. One tube is for aspiration, another is for feeding, and the third is attached to an elongated balloon that surrounds the tubes. The balloon is inflated after the tube is inserted. The goal is to compress the bleeding areas.

t., Southey's. Very small tube pushed into tissue to help drain edema fluid. Used in severe congestive heart failure to relieve edema of the legs.

t., stomach. Rubber tube for introducing food into the stomach or for washing out the stomach. SYN: *t., esophageal.*

t., test. Glass tube closed at one end. It is used in chemistry to hold chemicals and materials being tested.

t., thoracostomy. Tube inserted into the pleural space via the chest wall in order to remove air or fluid present in the space.

t., tracheotomy. Tube for inserting into the trachea.

t., uterine. Fallopian tube, q.v.

t., ventilation. SEE: *grommets.*

t., Wangensteen. Tube used in Wangensteen method, q.v.

tubectomy (too-bĕk′tō-mē). Surgical removal of all or part of a tube, esp. the fallopian tube.

tube feeding. Providing the patient's fluids and nutritional requirements by instilling foods into the stomach via a nasogastric tube.

An alternative method utilizes a gastrostomy tube inserted into the stomach via the abdominal wall. This can be done under local anesthesia.

This method of providing food for comatose patients who have no hope of recovery is controversial.

tuber (tū′bĕr) [L., a swelling] (pl. *tubera*). A swelling or enlargement.

t. cinereum. A part of the base of the hypothalamus bordered by mammillary bodies, the optic chiasma, and on either side by the optic tract. It is connected by the infundibulum with the posterior lobe of the pituitary.

tubercle (tū′bĕr-kl) [L. *tuberculum*, a little swelling]. 1. A small rounded elevation or eminence on a bone. 2. A small nodule, esp. a circumscribed solid elevation of the skin or mucous membrane. 3. The characteristic lesion resulting from infection by tubercle bacilli. It consists typically of three parts: a central giant cell, a midzone of epithelioid cells, and a peripheral zone of nonspecific structure. SYN: *tuberculum.* SEE: *tuberculosis.*

t., adductor. Tubercle of the femur to which is attached the tendon of the adductor

magnus.

t., articular. Tubercle at the base of the zygomatic arch to which is attached the temporomandibular ligament; lateral to the articular eminence of the glenoid fossa, with which it is often confused. SYN: *t., zygomatic.*

t., condyloid. An eminence on the mandibular condyle for the attachment of the lateral ligament of the temporomandibular joint.

t., deltoid. Tubercle on the clavicle for attachment of the deltoid muscle.

t., dental. A small elevation of variable size on the crown of a tooth representing a thickened area of enamel or an accessory cusp.

t., fibrous. Fibrous tissue that has replaced a previously inflamed area.

t., genial. Tubercle on either side of the lower jawbone.

t., genital. The embryonic structure that becomes the clitoris or the penis.

t., lacrimal. A small tubercle between the lacrimal crest and the frontal process of the maxilla.

t., laminated. The cerebellar nodule.

t., Lisfranc's. Tubercle on the first rib for attachment of the scalenus anticus muscle.

t., mental. A small tubercle on either side of the midline of the chin.

t., miliary. A small tubercle resembling a millet seed; the lesion of tuberculosis.

t. of the upper lip. The prominence of the upper part of the vermilion border that represents the distal termination of the philtrum of the upper lip.

t., pharyngeal. The point of attachment of the superior pharyngeal constrictor and its fibrous raphe on the inferior surface of the basilar part of the occipital bone.

t., pubic. A small projection at the crest at the lateral end of the crest of the pubic bone. The inguinal ligament attaches to it.

t., supraglenoid. A rough, elevated area just above the glenoid cavity of the clavicle. The long head of the biceps muscle of the arm attaches to this tubercle.

t., zygomatic. Tubercle on the zygoma at the junction of the anterior root.

tubercula (tū-bĕr′kū-lă). Pl. of tuberculum.

tubercular (tū-bĕr′kū-lăr) [L. *tuberculum,* a little swelling]. Relating to or marked by nodules. SYN: *torose.*

tuberculate, tuberculated (tū-bĕr′kū-lāt, -lāt″ĕd) [L. *tuberculum,* a small swelling]. Covered with nodules. SYN: *tubercular.*

tuberculation (tū-bĕr″kū-lā′shŭn). The formation of tubercles.

tuberculid(e) (tū-bĕr′kū-lĭd, -līd) [L. *tuberculum,* a little swelling]. A tuberculous cutaneous eruption due to toxins of tuberculosis. SYN: *tuberculoderma.*

t., follicular. A cutaneous eruption characterized by presence of groups of follicular lesions, esp. on the trunk.

t., papulonecrotic. Form of tuberculid characterized by symmetrically distributed bluish papules, esp. on extremities. These undergo central necrosis and, on healing, leave deep scars.

tuberculigenous (tū-bĕr-kū-lĭj′ĕn-ŭs) [″ + Gr. *gennan,* to produce]. Causing or predisposing to tuberculosis.

tuberculin (tū-bĕr′kū-lĭn) [L. *tuberculum, a little swelling*]. 1. A soluble cell substance prepared from the tubercle bacillus, usually the human type, which is used to determine the presence of a tuberculosis infection. Among the types of tuberculin used are Koch's original or old tuberculin (ABBR: OT or TO) and tuberculin purified protein derivative (ABBR: PPD). 2. USP. The tuberculin used for diagnostic tests of the ability of the skin to react to the intradermal injection of tuberculin. Trade names are Aplisol and Aplitest.

t., new. A suspension of tubercle bacilli fragments from which the soluble materials have been removed and to which glycerine has been added. Tuberculin, USP, is now used in place of this preparation.

t., old. Tuberculin originally prepared by Koch from cultures of *Mycobacterium tuberculosis.*

t., purified protein derivative. A purified tuberculin obtained by the same technique as that used for old tuberculin except a synthetic broth is used to culture the *Mycobacterium tuberculosis.*

tuberculin test. A test to determine the presence of a tuberculosis infection based on positive reaction of subject to tuberculin. Tests commonly used are Mantoux test, involving intradermal injection of tuberculin, and other multiple-puncture tests. In all tests a local inflammatory reaction is observed in infected persons after 48 to 96 hours. Tests do not reveal whether infection is active or inactive. SEE: *tine test.*

tuberculin tine test. Tuberculin test performed by using a special disposable instrument that contains multiple sharp points or prongs for piercing the skin. These tines penetrate the skin and introduce the tuberculin that has been applied to them. The test is read in 48 to 72 hours.

tuberculitis (tū″bĕr-kū-lī′tĭs). Inflammation of a tubercle.

tuberculocele (tū-bĕr′kū-lō-sēl″) [″ + *kele,* tumor]. Tuberculosis of the testis.

tuberculocidal (tū-bĕr″kū-lō-sī′dăl). Anything that destroys *Mycobacterium tubercu-*

losis.

tuberculoderma (tū-bĕr″kū-lō-dĕr′mă) [″ + Gr. *derma,* skin]. A tuberculous lesion of the skin. SYN: *tuberculide.*

tuberculofibroid (tū-bĕr″kū-lō-fī′broyd) [″ + *fibra,* fiber, + Gr. *eidos,* form, shape]. Denoting fibroid degeneration of tubercles.

tuberculofibrosis (tū-bĕr″kū-lō-fī-brō′sĭs) [″ + ″ + Gr. *osis,* condition]. 1. Chronic pulmonary inflammation with formation of fibrous tissue. 2. Interstitial pneumonia.

tuberculoid (tū-bĕr′kū-loyd) [L. *tuberculum,* a little swelling, + Gr. *eidos,* form, shape]. Resembling tuberculosis or a tubercle.

tuberculoma (tū-bĕr″kū-lō′mă) [″ + Gr. *oma,* tumor]. 1. A tuberculous abscess. 2. Any tuberculous neoplasm.

tuberculophobia (tū-bĕr″kū-lō-fō′bē-ă) [″ + Gr. *phobos,* fear]. An abnormal fear of being infected with tuberculosis.

tuberculoprotein (tū-bĕr″kū-lō-prō′tē-ĭn). A protein derived from tubercle bacilli.

tuberculosilicosis (tū-bĕr″kū-lō-sĭl″ĭ-kō′sĭs). Silicosis and pulmonary tuberculosis at the same time.

tuberculosis (tū-bĕr″kū-lō′sĭs) [″ + Gr. *osis,* condition]. ABBR: TB. An infectious disease caused by the tubercle bacillus, *Mycobacterium tuberculosis,* and characterized pathologically by inflammatory infiltrations, formation of tubercles, caseation, necrosis, abscesses, fibrosis, and calcification. It most commonly affects the respiratory system, but other parts of the body such as gastrointestinal and genitourinary tracts, bones, joints, nervous system, lymph nodes, and skin may become infected. Fish, amphibians, birds, and mammals (esp. cattle) are subject to the disease. Three types of the tubercle bacillus exist: human, bovine, and avian. Humans may become infected by any of the three types, but in the U.S. the human type predominates. Infection usually is acquired from contact with an infected person or an infected cow or through drinking contaminated milk.

Tuberculosis may occur in an acute generalized form (miliary tuberculosis) or in a chronic localized form. In humans, the primary infection usually consists of a localized lesion and regional adenitis, these constituting the primary complex. From this state, lesions may heal by fibrosis and calcification and the disease may exist in an arrested or inactive stage. Reactivation or exacerbation of the disease or reinfection gives rise to the chronic progressive form.

In the last several decades tuberculosis decreased in incidence. But a great number of new cases have been reported in patients with AIDS. In many cases of tuberculosis, the cause is a drug-resistant strain of the bacillus. For these reasons individuals with AIDS and others who have risk factors for AIDS should be screened for TB; if they test positive, the tubercle bacillus will need to be tested for sensitivity to antituberculous agents.

Other factors that increase the risk of developing TB include: silicosis; gastrectomy; jejunoileal bypass; weight of 10% or more below ideal weight of an infant; chronic renal failure; diabetes mellitus; conditions requiring prolonged high-dose corticosteroid therapy and immunosuppressive therapy; and malignancies. People with those conditions should be tested for tuberculosis. SEE: *tuberculin test; tine test.* SEE: *Nursing Diagnoses* in *Appendix.*

NOTE: Many varieties of *Mycobacterium* that previously were thought to be nonpathogenic for humans have been found to cause chronic progressive pulmonary disease closely resembling pulmonary tuberculosis. These organisms have been termed anonymous or atypical *Mycobacterium.* They have been classified into four groups: photochromogens, scotochromogens, nonphotochromogens, and rapid growers.

TREAT: For treating uncomplicated tuberculosis, daily isoniazid (INH), pyrazinamide (PZA), and rifampin (RMP) for 2 months followed by 4 months of daily rifampin and isoniazid is effective. In this regimen the medicines are self-administered. To ensure compliance and to help prevent the development of drug-resistant strains of the tubercle bacillus, it may be necessary for the health care worker to watch the patient take the medicine.

RS: mycobacterium; tubercle; tubercle bacillus; tuberculin; tuberculin test; tuberculin tine test.

t., avian. Tuberculosis of birds, due to *Mycobacterium avium.*

t., bovine. Tuberculosis of cattle due to *Mycobacterium tuberculosis.*

t., endogenous. Tuberculosis originating in a tubercle in another body site.

t., exogenous. Tuberculosis originating from a source outside the body.

t., hematogenous. Spread of tuberculosis from a primary site to another site via the bloodstream.

t., miliary. Tuberculosis that spreads throughout the body via the bloodstream. It may be fatal.

t., open. Tuberculosis in which the tubercle bacilli are present in bodily secretions that leave the body.

t. verrucosa. Tuberculosis of the skin or mucous membranes characterized by formation of warty lesions.

tuberculostatic (tū-bĕr″kū-lō-stăt′ĭk). Arresting the growth of the tubercle bacillus.

tuberculotic (tū-bĕr″kū-lŏt′ĭk). Concerning tuberculosis.

tuberculous (tū-bĕr′kū-lŭs) [L. *tuberculum,* a little swelling]. Relating to or affected with tuberculosis, or conditions marked by infiltration of a specific tubercle, as opposed to the term tubercular, referring to nonspecific tubercle.

tuberculum (tū-bĕr′kū-lŭm) [L. *tuberculum,* a little swelling] (pl. *tubercula*). A small knot or nodule; a tubercle.

   t. acusticum. Dorsal nucleus of the cochlear nerve.

   t. majus humeri. [NA] Larger tuberosity of the humerus at upper end of its lateral surface, giving attachment to infraspinatus, supraspinatus, and teres minor muscles.

   t. minus humeri. [NA] The projection at the proximal end of the anterior humerus, providing attachment to the subscapularis muscle.

tuberin (tū′bĕr-ĭn) [L. *tuber,* a swelling]. A simple protein; a globulin in potatoes.

tuberosis (tū″bĕr-ō′sĭs). A condition in which nodules develop; a nonspecific term that indicates no specific disease process.

tuberositas (tū-bĕr-ŏs′ĭt-ăs) [L.] (pl. *tuberositates*). A projection, nodule, or prominence.

tuberosity (tū-bĕr-ŏs′ĭ-tē) [L. *tuberositas,* tuberosity]. 1. An elevated round process of a bone. 2. A tubercle or nodule.

   t., ischial. A palpable prominence on the inferior margin of the ischium which supports a person's weight when sitting.

   t., maxillary. A rounded eminence on the posteroinferior surface of the maxilla that enlarges with the development and eruption of the third molar. It articulates medially with the palatine bone and laterally with the lateral pterygoid process of the sphenoid. It forms the anterior surface of the pterygopalatine fossa, including a groove for the passage of the maxillary nerve which is anesthetized in this region for a maxillary or second-division block.

tuberous (tū′bĕr-ŭs). Pert. to tubers.

tuberous sclerosis. ABBR: TS. A syndrome manifested by convulsive seizures, progressive mental disorder, adenoma sebaceum, and tumors of the kidneys and brain with projections into the cerebral ventricles.

tubo- [L. *tubus*]. Combining form meaning tube.

tuboabdominal (tū″bō-ăb-dŏm′ĭn-ăl) [L. *tubus,* tube, + *abdominalis,* pert. to the abdomen]. Pert. to the fallopian tubes and the abdomen.

tuboabdominal pregnancy. Ectopic gestation with embryo partly in tube and partly in the abdominal cavity.

tubocurarine chloride (tū″bō-kū-rä′rĭn klō′rīd). USP. Drug used to produce skeletal muscle relaxation during anesthesia and convulsive states and to treat poisoning due to black widow spider bites. Tubocurarine was originally obtained from the Indian arrow poison, curare, q.v.

Caution: Tubocurarine should be administered only by those who have the proper equipment and are fully capable of providing artificial ventilation, tracheal intubation, appropriate antidotes, and additional therapy in case of overdose.

---

tuboligamentous (tū″bō-lĭg-ă-mĕn′tŭs) [″ + *ligamentum,* a band]. Pert. to the fallopian tube and broad ligament of the uterus.

tubo-ovarian (tū″bō-ō-vā′rē-ăn) [″ + LL. *ovarium,* ovary]. Pert. to the fallopian tube and the ovary.

tubo-ovariotomy (tū″bō-ō-vā-rē-ŏt′ō-mē) [″ + LL. *ovarium,* ovary, + Gr. *tome,* incision]. Excision of ovaries and oviducts. SYN: *salpingo-oothecotomy.*

tubo-ovaritis (tū″bō-ō″vă-rī′tĭs) [″ + ″ + Gr. *itis,* inflammation]. Inflammation of the ovary and fallopian tube.

tuboperitoneal (tū″bō-pĕr-ĭ-tō-nē′ăl) [″ + Gr. *peritonaion,* peritoneum]. Rel. to the oviduct and peritoneum.

tuboplasty (tū′bō-plăs″tē). 1. Plastic repair of any tube. 2. Plastic repair of fallopian tube or tubes in an attempt to restore patency so that fertilization of the ovum may occur.

tuboplasty, transcervical balloon. An experimental procedure for treating occlusion of the fallopian tubes. The procedure does not involve surgery. A balloon catheter is inserted through the cervical os of the uterus and into the fallopian tube to the point of occlusion in the tube. The balloon is then expanded by filling it with sterile saline. This dilation of the tube may restore tubal patency. This technique is used to help individuals with bilateral occlusion of the fallopian tubes to conceive. SEE: *infertility; catheter, balloon.*

tuborrhea (tū-bor-rē′ă) [″ + Gr. *rhoia,* flow]. Discharge from the eustachian tube.

tubotorsion (tū″bō-tor′shŭn). The act of twisting a tube.

tubotympanal (tū″bō-tĭm′pă-năl) [″ + Gr. *tympanon,* a drum]. Rel. to the tympanum of the ear and the eustachian tube.

tubouterine (tū″bō-ū′tĕr-ĭn) [″ + *uterinus,* pert. to the uterus]. Rel. to the oviduct and the uterus.

tubovaginal (tū″bō-văj′ĭ-năl). Concerning the fallopian tube and vagina.

tubular (tū′bū-lăr) [L. *tubularis,* like a tube]. Rel. to or having the form of a tube or tubule.

tubule (tū′būl) [L. *tubulus,* a tubule]. A small tube or canal.

   t., collecting. Tubule in the renal medulla that is part of the discharging tubule.

   t.'s, convoluted, of kidney. The convoluted tubules of the nephron unit of the kidney that, along with the loop of Henle, the distal convoluted tubule, and the collecting tubule, provide a passageway for the glomerular filtrate to reach the renal pelvis. SEE: *kidney; nephron.*

   t.'s, convoluted seminiferous. Tubules present in each lobe of the testes.

   t.'s, dentinal. Very small canals in the dentin. They extend from the pulp cavity of the tooth to the enamel and are occupied by odontoblastic processes and occasional nerve filaments.

   t.'s, excretory. The uriniferous tubules in medullary portion of the kidneys.

   t.'s, galactophorous. The lactiferous ducts of the breast. They provide a channel for the milk formed in the lobes of the breast to pass to the nipple.

   t., Henle's. Henle's loop, q.v.

   t., junctional. Short part of a uriniferous tubule connecting with a collecting tubule.

   t.'s, lactiferous. T.'s, galactophorous, q.v.

   t.'s, mesonephric. Tubes that make up the temporary kidney of amniotes (animals that form amnions).

   t.'s, metanephric. Tubes that make up the permanent kidneys of amniotes.

   t.'s, renal. Tubules that connect the glomeruli to the renal pelvis. Included, in order, are the proximal convoluted tubules, loop of Henle, distal convoluted tubules, and the collecting tubules. SEE: *kidney; nephron.*

   t.'s, seminiferous. Very small channels of the testes in which spermatozoa develop and through which they leave the testes.

   t.'s, uriniferous. Minute canals forming the glandular substance of the kidney, originating in Bowman's capsules and emptying into the pelvis of the kidney.

tubulin (tū′bū-lĭn). A protein present in the microtubules of cells.

tubulization (too″bū-lĭ-zā′shŭn). A method of repairing severed nerves in which the nerve ends are placed in a tube of absorbable material.

tubuloalveolar. Consisting of tubes and alveoli, as in a tubuloalveolar salivary gland.

tubulocyst (too′bū-lō-sĭst). The cystic dilatation of a functionless duct or canal.

tubulodermoid (tū″bū-lō-dĕr′moyd) [″ +

Gr. *derma,* skin, + *eidos,* form, shape]. A dermoid tumor due to the persistent embryonic tubular structure.

tubuloracemose (too″bū-lō-răs′ē-mōs). Pert. to a gland that has tubular and racemose characteristics.

tubulorrhexis (too″bū-lō-rĕk′sĭs) [″ + *rhexis,* a breaking]. Focal ruptures of renal tubules.

tubulous (too′bū-lŭs). Containing tubules.

tubulus (tū′bū-lŭs) [L.] (pl. *tubuli*). [NA] A tubule; a small tube.

tubus (too′bŭs) [L.]. Tube.

    t. digestorius. The alimentary canal.

tuft. A small clump, cluster, or coiled mass.

    t., enamel. Abnormal structure formed in development of enamel consisting of poorly calcified twisted rods.

    t., malpighian. The renal glomerulus.

tugging. A dragging or pulling.

    t., tracheal. An indication of thoracic aneurysm.

    SYM: A sense of downward pulling of larynx with cardiac systole when thyroid cartilage is gently raised between the finger and thumb.

tularemia (tū-lăr-ē′mē-ă) [*Tulare,* part of California where disease was first discovered]. An acute plaguelike infectious disease caused by *Francisella tularensis* (formerly classed as *Pasteurella tularensis*). Transmitted to humans by the bite of an infected tick or other bloodsucking insect; by direct contact with infected animals; by eating inadequately cooked meat or by drinking water that contains the organism. SYN: *deer fly fever; rabbit fever.*

    SYM: May appear from 1 to 10 days but averaging 3 days after infection, headache, chilliness, vomiting, aching pains, and fever develop. Site of infection develops into an ulcer. Glands at elbow or in armpit become enlarged, tender, and painful; later may develop into an abscess. Sweating, loss of weight, and debility.

    TREAT: Streptomycin or gentamicin is effective.

tumbu fly. Species of fly belonging to the genus *Cordylobia* in Africa and the genus *Dermatobia* in tropical America. Their larvae develop in the skin of wild domesticated animals, and humans are frequently attacked.

tumefacient (tū-mĕ-fā′shĕnt) [L. *tumefaciens,* producing swelling]. Producing or tending to produce swelling; swollen.

tumefaction (tū″mĕ-făk′shŭn) [L. *tumefactio,* a swelling]. 1. A swelling. 2. Act of swelling or the state of being swollen. SYN: *intumescence.*

tumentia (tū-mĕn′shē-ă). [L.]. Swelling.

    t., vasomotor. Irregular swellings in lower extremities associated with vasomotor disturbances.

tumescence (tū-mĕs′ĕns). 1. Condition of being swollen or tumid. 2. A swelling.

tumid (tū′mĭd) [L. *tumidus*]. Swollen.

tumor (tū′mor) [L. *tumor,* a swelling]. 1. A swelling or enlargement. 2. Swelling, one of the four classical signs of inflammation. The others are calor (heat), dolor (pain), and rubor (redness). 3. A spontaneous new growth of tissue forming an abnormal mass. It is with few exceptions of unknown cause, noninflammatory, and develops independent of and unrestrained by normal laws of growth and morphogenesis. SYN: *neoplasm.* SEE: *cancer.*

    TYPES: *Myeloid sarcomata* or *giant-celled sarcomata:* Consist of elements formed chiefly of protoplasm containing two or more nuclei, up to 20 or even 50; with a varying number of round, spindle, or mixed cells. Vary in consistency from that of jelly to that of muscle. More frequently occur on lower jaw, femur, and tibia. *Round-celled sarcomata:* Usually soft, vascular, rapidly growing, become large, and give rise to metastatic deposits in distant parts and in viscera. Occur in periosteum, bone, lymphatic glands, subcutaneous tissue, testicle, eye, ovary, uterus, lung, and kidneys, although they may occur wherever fibrous tissue exists. *Glioma:* Grows from the connective tissue of nerve centers and its basic substance resembles that structure. Occurs in retina and brain. *Melanotic sarcoma:* In cells may be of either round or spindle variety. This type of tumor is extremely malignant. *Spindle-cell sarcoma:* Cells vary much in size, from small oat-shaped cells to greatly elongated bodies with long, fine, tapering extremities. Chiefly in bones. *Endotheliomata:* Occur, in different forms, in the testicle, pia mater, pleura, and peritoneum.

    Acinous or *spheroidal-celled carcinoma:* Occurs in two forms: (1) hard, spheroidal-celled (scirrhus or chronic carcinoma) and (2) soft, spheroidal-celled (encephaloid or acute carcinoma). It resembles brain tissue in appearance and consistency. Occurs in testicle, liver, bladder, kidney, ovary, fundus oculi, and more rarely in the breast. SEE: *scirrhus. Colloid carcinoma:* One of preceding varieties that has undergone mucoid degeneration and so distended the alveoli that they may be seen by the naked eye. Occurs in stomach, intestine, omentum, and ovary. *Epithelial carcinoma:* (1) The squamous-celled epitheliomata that always spring from skin or mucous membranes or their glands, esp. at junctions of mucous and cutaneous surfaces. Are not encapsulated. Commence as wartlike growth, flattened tubercle, or fissure, ulceration in all these forms setting in early. (2) Cylindrical or columnar-celled. Less common form of carcinoma. Originates from either the cylindrical surface epithelium of a mucous membrane or its glands, closely imitating these structures in microscopic appearance. These growths form indurated infiltrating masses in the walls of organs attacked, producing considerable stenosis of lumen of hollow viscera; as rectum and small intestinal obstruction. Occur in uterus and intestinal tract.

Warty or villous growth (papillomata): Resemble in their structure hypertrophied papillae of skin or mucous membrane. These include condylomata and mucous tubercles. Occur about the anus and genitals or in the mouth and throat. Warts and warty growths on skin of hands and genitalia and mucous surface of larynx. Villous growths, bladder, rectum, and larynx. *Teratoma:* tumors containing bone, hair, or teeth, usually situated in ovaries or testicles but may also be present in other tissues.

t., carotid body. Benign tumor of the carotid body, q.v.

t., connective tissue. Any tumor of connective tissue such as fibroma, lipoma, chondroma, or sarcoma.

t., desmoid. Tumor of the fibrous connective tissue.

t., erectile. Tumor composed of erectile tissue.

t., Ewing's. Malignant tumor of bone.

t., false. An enlargement due to hemorrhage into tissue or extravasation of fluid into a space but not due to a neoplastic growth.

t., fibroid. Benign fibrous tissue tumor of the myometrium.

t., giant cell, of bone. Benign or malignant tumor of bone in which the cells are multinucleated and surrounded by cellular spindle cell stroma.

t., giant cell, of tendon sheath. Localized nodular tenosynovitis.

t., granulosa, granulosa cell. An estrin-secreting tumor of the granulosa cells of the ovary.

t., granulosa-theca cell. An estrogen-secreting tumor of the ovary made up of either granulosa or theca cells.

t., heterologous. Tumor the tissue of which differs from the tissue in which it is growing.

t., homoiotypic, homologous. Tumor the tissue of which resembles the tissue in which it is growing.

t., Hürthle cell. Benign or malignant tumor of the thyroid gland. The cells are large and acidophilic.

t., islet cell. Tumor of the islets of Langerhans of the pancreas.

t., Krukenberg's. Tumor of the ovary due to metastases from a tumor in the gastrointestinal tract.

t., lipoid cell, of the ovary. A masculinizing tumor of the ovary. It may be malignant.

t., mast cell. A benign nodular accumulation of mast cells.

t., melanotic neuroectodermal. Benign tumor of the jaw. It occurs mostly during the first year of life.

t., mesenchymal mixed. Tumor composed of tissue that resembles mesenchymal cells.

t. of pregnancy. The abdominal swelling produced by the growing conceptus of pregnancy.

t., phantom. Gaseous distention of the intestinal tract.

t., sand. Psammoma, q.v.

t., turban. Multiple cutaneous cylindromata that cover the scalp like a turban.

t., Wilms'. SEE: *Wilms' tumor.*

tumoraffin (tū'mor-ăf-ĭn) [L. *tumor,* a swelling, + *affinis,* related]. Having an affinity for tumor cells. SYN: *oncotropic.*

tumor angiogenesis factor. ABBR: TAF. A protein present in animal and human cancer tissue that in experimental studies appears to be essential to growth of the cancer. The substance is thought to act by stimulating the growth of new blood capillaries for supplying the tumor with nutrients and removing waste products.

tumor burden. The sum of cancer cells present in the body.

tumoricidal (too″mor-ĭ-sī'dăl). Lethal to neoplastic cells.

tumorigenesis (too″mor-ĭ-jĕn'ĕ-sĭs). Production of tumors.

tumorigenic (tū″mor-ĭ-jĕn'ĭk) [″ + Gr. *genesis,* generation, birth]. Producing tumors, esp. malignancies. SYN: *oncogenic.* SEE: *carcinogenic.*

tumor markers, serum. Certain substances in blood serum that serve as biochemical indicators for the possible presence of a malignancy. The substances produced may be normal materials present in abnormal amounts or chemicals not normally present. None of these is perfectly reliable, but they do serve the purpose of monitoring response to therapy and estimating prognosis. Examples of the markers and the malignancies concerned are carcinoembryonic antigen (ABBR: CEA) for tumors of the colon, lung, breast, and ovary; beta subunit of chorionic gonadotropin for trophoblastic and testicular tumors; alpha-fetoprotein for testicular teratocarcinoma and primary hepatocellular carcinoma; and prostatic acid phosphatase and prostate-specific antigen for malignancy of prostate.

tumor necrosis factor. ABBR: TNF. A monokine produced in various parts of the body by activated phagocytes, including monocytes. TNF is important in stimulating leukocytosis, fever, and necrosis of some tumors; and induces acute phase reactions, q.v. TNF is also essential to the mediation of the toxic effects of endotoxin and other bacterial products. SYN: *cachectin*. SEE: *acute phase reactions; cytokines; monokines; shock, septic.*

tumorous (too′mor-ŭs). Tumorlike.

tumor viruses. Viruses that cause malignant neoplasms. This is known to occur in a variety of species, including some primates, but conclusive proof that any human tumor is virus-induced is lacking. Viruses that are suspected of being oncogenic, i.e., tumor-inducing, in humans are Epstein-Barr virus linked to African Burkitt's lymphoma; hepatitis B virus with primary hepatocellular carcinoma; herpes simplex type 2 with carcinoma of the cervix; and cytomegalovirus with Kaposi's sarcoma.

tumultus (tū-mŭl′tŭs) [L.]. Excessive or agitated activity.

   t. cordis. Irregular heart action with palpitation.

   t. sermonis. Extreme stuttering due to pathologic cause.

Tunga (tŭng′ă). A genus of fleas of the family Hectopsyllidae.

   T. penetrans. A small flea common in tropical regions. It infests humans, cats, dogs, rats, pigs, and other animals and produces a severe local inflammation frequently liable to secondary infection.

tungiasis (tŭng-gī′ă-sĭs). Infestation of the skin with *Tunga penetrans.*

tungsten (tŭng′stĕn). SYMB: W (for wolfram). At. wt. 183.85; at. no. 74. A metallic element.

tunic (tū′nĭk) [L. *tunica,* a sheath]. An investing membrane.

   t., Bichat's. Tunica intima, q.v.

tunica (tū′nĭ-kă) [L. *tunica,* a sheath] (pl. *tunicae*). A coat or covering; in anatomy, the term defines a covering or lining layer of connective tissue or epithelium respectively.

   t. adventitia. [NA] The outermost fibroelastic layer of a blood vessel or other tubular structure.

   t. albuginea. The white fibrous coat of the eye, testicle, ovary, or spleen.

   t. conjunctiva. Conjunctiva, q.v.

   t. dartos. [NA] The muscular, contractile tissue beneath the skin of the scrotum.

   t. externa. SYN: *t. adventitia.*

   t. interna. SEE: *t. intima.*

   t. intima. The internal lining of blood vessels composed of an epithelial (endothelium) layer and the basement membrane, a subendothelial connective tissue layer, and usually an internal elastic lamina.

   t. media. The middle layer in the wall of a blood vessel composed of circular or spiraling smooth muscle and some elastic fibers.

   t. mucosa. Mucous membrane lining of various structures.

   t. muscularis. The muscular tissue around structures such as the bronchi, intestines, and blood vessels.

   t. propria. The subepithelial component of a mucosal layer containing loose connective tissue and small blood vessels, nerves, and glands. It is similar to the papillary layer of dermis of the skin except for hair follicles and the differing types of glands.

   t. serosa. The mesothelial lining of the external walls of the body cavities such as the pleural, peritoneal, and pericardial.

   t. vaginalis. Serous membrane surrounding the front and sides of the testicle.

   t. vasculosa. Any vascular layer.

tunicin (too′nĭ-sĭn). A celluloselike substance found in the covering of some lower vertebrates.

tuning fork. Device that when struck at the forked end vibrates and thus can be heard and felt. It is used in testing the sensations of hearing, including bone conduction and vibration. A fork that vibrates at 256 cycles per second is suitable for use in these tests.

tunnel (tŭn′ĕl). A narrow channel or passageway.

   t., carpal. The canal in the wrist bounded by osteofibrous material through which the flexor tendons and the median nerve pass.

   t., flexor. T., carpal, q.v.

   t., inner. Triangular canal lying between the inner and outer pillars of Corti in the organ of Corti of inner ear.

   t., tarsal. The osteofibrous canal in the tarsal area bounded by the flexor retinaculum and tarsal bones. The posterior tibial vessels, tibial nerve, and flexor tendons pass through this tunnel.

tunnel vision. 1. A condition seen in hysteria in which the field of vision is the same regardless of distance from the visual screen. 2. Severe constriction of the visual field due to advanced chronic glaucoma. 3. A figure of speech indicating an individual's very narrow view or perspective of a situation or condition.

TUR. *transurethral resection* (of prostate).

turbid (tŭr′bĭd) [L. *turba,* a tumult]. Cloudy;

not clear. SEE: *turbidity*.

turbidimeter (tŭr-bĭ-dĭm′ĕ-ter) [L. *turbidus,* disturbed, + Gr. *metron,* measure]. Device for estimating degree of turbidity of a fluid.

turbidimetry (tŭr-bĭ-dĭm′ĕ-trē) [″ + Gr. *metron,* measure]. Estimation of the turbidity of a liquid.

turbidity (tŭr-bĭd′ĭ-tē) [L. *turbiditas,* turbidity]. 1. Quality of not having translucent appearance of liquid due to growth of microorganisms. 2. Having flaky or granular particles suspended in a clear liquid, giving it a cloudy appearance. SEE: *clarificant.*

turbinal, tubinate (tŭr′bĭ-năl, -nāt) [L. *turbinalis,* fr. *turbo,* a child's top]. Shaped like an inverted cone.

turbinated (tŭr′bĭ-nā″tĕd) [L. *turbo,* whirl]. Top- or cone-shaped. SEE: *concha.*

turbinectomy (tŭr-bĭn-ĕk′tō-mē) [″ + Gr. *ektome,* excision.] Excision of a turbinated bone.

turbinotome (tŭr-bĭn′ō-tōm) [″ + Gr. *tome,* incision]. Instrument for excision of a turbinated bone.

turbinotomy (tŭr-bĭn-ŏt′ō-mē) [″ + Gr. *tome,* incision]. Surgical incision of a turbinated bone.

turgescence (tŭr-jĕs′ĕns) [L. *turgescens,* swelling]. Swelling or enlargement of a part.

turgescent (tŭr-jĕs′ĕnt) [L. *turgescens,* swelling]. Swollen; inflated.

turgid (tŭr′jĭd) [L. *turgidus,* swollen]. Swollen; bloated.

turgometer (tŭr-gŏm′ĕ-tĕr) [L. *turgor,* swelling, + Gr. *metron,* measure]. Device for measuring turgescence.

turgor [L., a swelling]. 1. Normal tension in a cell. 2. Distention, swelling.

    t., skin. The resistance of the skin to deformation, esp. to being grasped between the fingers. The skin of the healthy person may, on the back of the hand, be grasped between the fingers and upon release either reform immediately to its normal appearance or it may gently and relatively slowly settle back into its normal appearance. Which of these reactions occurs depends on several factors, including state of hydration of the skin, but age is the most important factor. In the skin of the older person, the skin returns much more slowly to its normal position after having been pinched between the fingers of the examiner.

    t. vitalis. Normal fullness of the capillaries and blood vessels.

Turing test [Alan M. Turing, Brit. mathematician, 1912–1954]. A test of the degree of artificial intelligence of a computer. A human being "talks" to a computer for 30 minutes and if, after that time, the human is unable to tell whether or not the respondent

was a machine or a human, then the machine, according to this test, has human intelligence. SEE: *artificial intelligence.*

turista (tū-rēs′tä) [Sp.]. One of the many names applied to travelers' diarrhea, q.v., esp. that which occurs in tourists in Mexico.

Turner's syndrome [Henry Hubert Turner, U.S. physician, 1892–1970]. Congenital endocrine disorder caused by failure of the ovaries to respond to pituitary hormone stimulation. Clinically there is amenorrhea, failure of sexual maturation, and usually short stature. About one-third of these patients have webbing of the neck and may have marked cubitus valgus. Intelligence may be impaired. These patients usually have only 45 chromosomes, the second X chromosome being absent. SYN: *gonadal dysgenesis.* SEE: *karyotype.*

turning [AS. *turnian,* to turn]. Process of manually changing position of fetus in utero to permit normal delivery. SYN: *version.*

turpentine (tŭr′pĕn-tīn) [Gr. *terebinthos,* turpentine tree]. Oleoresin obtained from various species of pine trees. A mixture of terpenes and other hydrocarbons obtained from pine trees. It was previously used in liniments and counterirritants, applied topically. It is the source of oil of turpentine or spirits of turpentine.

turpentine poisoning. Usually contracted by inhalation. SEE: *Poisons and Poisoning* in *Appendix.*

    SYM: Warm or burning sensation in the esophagus and stomach, followed by cramping, vomiting, and diarrhea. Pulse and respiration become weak, slow, and irregular; irritation of urinary tract and central nervous system resembling alcoholic intoxication.

    F.A.: Gastric lavage, soothing drinks, and stimulants. Increase fluid intake.

turricephaly (tŭr″ĭ-sĕf′ă-lē). Oxycephaly.

turunda (tū-rŭn′dă) [L.]. 1. A surgical tent, drain, or tampon. 2. A suppository.

tussal (tŭs′ăl) [L. *tussis,* cough]. Rel. to a cough. SYN: *tussive.*

tussicular (tŭ-sĭk′ū-lăr) [L. *tussis,* cough]. Pertaining to a cough.

tussiculation (tŭ-sĭk″ū-lā′shŭn). A short, dry cough.

tussis (tŭs′ĭs) [L.]. A cough.

    t. convulsiva. Pertussis or whooping cough.

    t. stomachalis. Reflex cough from irritation of the mucosa forming the lining of the stomach.

tussive (tŭs′ĭv) [L. *tussis,* cough]. Relating to a cough. SYN: *tussal.*

tussive syncope. SEE: *laryngeal vertigo.*

tutamen (tū-tā′mĕn) [L.] (pl. *tutamina*). Any tissue that has a protective action.

tutamina oculi. The structures around the eye that protect it: the eyebrows, eyelids, and eyelashes.

tutin (too′tĭn). A highly poisonous glycoside present in the New Zealand toot plant.

T.V.R. *tonic vibration reflex.* A polysynaptic reflex believed to depend on spinal and supraspinal pathways.

T wave. Portion of the electrocardiogram that is due to repolarization of the ventricles. The wave may be positive or negative depending upon the lead involved in recording the ECG and whether or not the electrical activity of the heart is within normal limits. SEE: *electrocardiogram; QRST complex.*

twelfth cranial nerve. One of a pair of cranial nerves distributing to the base of the tongue. SEE: *cranial nerves; hypoglossal nerve; Nerves in Appendix.*

twig. The final branch of a structure such as a nerve or vessel.

twilight sleep. A state of partial anesthesia and hypoconsciousness in which pain sense has been greatly reduced by the injection of morphine and scopolamine. Patient responds to pain, but afterward memory of pain is dulled or effaced. SEE: *labor.*

twilight state. State in which consciousness is disordered, making possible actions subsequently forgotten. May occur in hysteria and epilepsy.

twin (twĭn) [AS. *twinn*]. One of two children developed within the uterus at the same time from the same impregnation. Identical and fraternal twins provide a unique resource for investigating the origin and natural history of various diseases and in attempts to discover the differential importance of environmental and hereditary factors in causing physical and mental disorders. The latter type of investigation is esp. important in following the course of identical twins who were separated shortly after birth and grew up in different social, economic, educational, and environmental conditions. SEE: illus.; *fetus papyraceus; Hellin's law.*

 t.'s, biovular. Dizygotic twins.

 t.'s, conjoined. Twins that are united. SEE: *Siamese twins.*

 t.'s, dizygotic. Twins from two separate ova fertilized at the same time. SYN: *t.'s, biovular; t.'s, fraternal.* SEE: *t.'s, monozygotic.*

 t.'s, enzygotic. T.'s, monozygotic.

 t.'s, fraternal. T.'s, dizygotic.

 t.'s, identical. T.'s, monozygotic.

 t.'s, impacted. Twins so entwined in utero as to prevent normal delivery.

 t.'s, interlocked. Twins in which the neck of one becomes interlocked with the head of the other, making vaginal delivery impossible.

 t.'s, monozygotic. Twins that develop from a single fertilized ovum. Monozygotic twins have the same genetic makeup and, consequently, are of the same sex and resemble each other strikingly in physical, physiological, and mental traits. They develop within a common chorionic sac and have a common placenta. Each usually develops its own amnion and umbilical cord. Such twins may result from development of two inner cell masses within a blastocyst, development of two embryonic axes on a single blastoderm, or the division of a single embryonic axis into two centers. SYN: *t.'s, enzygotic; t.'s, identical; t.'s, true; t.'s, uniovular.*

 t., parasitic. The smaller of a pair of conjoined twins, when there is a marked disparity in size.

 t.'s, Siamese. Symmetrically conjoined twins. SEE: *Siamese twins.*

 t.'s, true. T.'s, monozygotic.

 t.'s, unequal. Twins, one of which is underdeveloped.

 t.'s, uniovular. T.'s, monozygotic.

 t., vanishing. SEE: *gestation, multiple.*

twinge (twĭnj) [AS. *twengan*, to pinch]. A sudden keen pain.

twinning (twĭn′ĭng). Delivery of or producing twins.

twitch (twĭch) [ME. *twicchen*]. 1. A simple, quick, spasmodic contraction of a muscle. SEE: *myokymia; myopalmus.* 2. To jerk convulsively.

twitching (twĭtch′ĭng). Repeated contractions of portions of muscles.

two-point discrimination test. Test of cutaneous sensation involving determination of the ability of the patient to detect that the skin is being touched by two pointed objects at once. It is used to determine the degree of sensory loss following disease or trauma affecting the nervous system.

TXA₂. *thromboxane A_2.*

tybamate (tī′bă-māt). A minor tranquilizer. Trade name is Tybatran.

tylectomy (tī-lĕk′tŏ-mē) [Gr. *tylos*, knot, + *ektome*, excision]. Local removal of a lesion. SYN: *lumpectomy.*

tylion (tĭl′ē-ŏn) [Gr. *tyleion*, knot]. Point at middle of anterior edge of the optic groove.

tyloma (tī-lō′mă) [Gr. *tylos*, knot, + *oma*, tumor]. A callosity.

tylosis (tī-lō′sĭs) [″ + *osis*, condition]. Formation of a callus.

tyloxapol (tī-lŏks′ă-pōl). USP. A nonionic liquid polymer of the alkyl aryl polyether alcohol type. It is a detergent used to reduce the viscosity of bronchopulmonary secretions. Trade name is Superinone.

POSSIBLE RELATIONS OF FETAL MEMBRANES IN TWIN PREGNANCIES

SEPARATE PLACENTAS

CHORION   AMNION

SEPARATE PLACENTAS

CHORION   AMNION

SINGLE PLACENTA

CHORION   AMNION

TWO PLACENTAS, TWO AMNIONS,
TWO CHORIONS

ONE PLACENTA, ONE AMNION,
ONE CHORION

TWO PLACENTAS, TWO AMNIONS,
SINGLE CHORION

tympanal (tĭm′păn-ăl) [Gr. *tympanon*, drum].
Rel. to the tympanum. SYN: *tympanic*.

tympanectomy (tĭm″păn-ĕk′tō-mē) [″ +
ektome, excision]. Excision of the tympanic
membrane.

tympania (tĭm-păn′ē-ă). Tympanites.

tympanic (tĭm-păn′ĭk) [Gr. *tympanon*,
drum]. 1. Pert. to the tympanum. SYN: *tympanal*. 2. Resonant.

tympanicity (tĭm″pă-nĭs′ĭ-tē). The condition
of having a tympanic quality.

tympanic membrane. Membrane serving as
the lateral wall of the tympanic cavity and
separating it from the external acoustic
meatus. SYN: *eardrum*. SEE: *ear thermometry; tympanum*.

tympanism (tĭm′păn-ĭzm) [Gr. *tympanon*,
drum, + *-ismos*, condition]. Abdominal
inflation from gas. SYN: *tympanites*.

tympanites (tĭm-păn-ī′tēz) [Gr., distention].
Distention of the abdomen or intestines by
gas.

tympanitic (tĭm-păn-ĭt′ĭk). 1. Pert. to or
characterized by tympanites. 2. Resonant.
SYN: *tympanic*.

tympanitic resonance. A sound produced by
percussion over an air- or gas-filled cavity.

tympanitis (tĭm-păn-ī′tĭs) [Gr. *tympanon*,
drum, + *itis*, inflammation]. Inflammation of the middle ear. SYN: *otitis media*.

tympano- [Gr. *tympanon*, drum]. Combining
form meaning eardrum, tympanum of the
ear.

tympanoeustachian (tĭm″pă-nō-ū-stā′kē-
ăn). Concerning the tympanic cavity and
eustachian tube.

tympanography. Radiographic examination
of the eustachian tubes and middle ear after
introduction of a contrast medium.

tympanohyal (tĭm″pă-nō-hī′ăl). Concerning
the tympanic cavity and hyoid arch.

tympanomalleal (tĭm″pă-nō-măl′ē-ăl). Concerning the tympanic membrane and malleus.

tympanomandibular (tĭm″pă-nō-măn-dĭb′
ū-lăr). Concerning the middle ear and mandible.

tympanomastoiditis (tĭm″păn-ō-măs″toy-
dī′tĭs) [″ + *mastos*, breast, + *eidos*,
form, shape, + *itis*, inflammation]. Inflammation of the tympanum and mastoid
cells.

tympanometry (tĭm″pă-nŏm′ĕ-trē). Procedure for objective evaluation of the mobility
and patency of the eardrum and for detection of middle-ear disorders and patency of
the eustachian tubes. SEE: *audiometry*.

tympanoplasty (tĭm″păn-ō-plăs′tē) [″ +

plassein, to form]. Any one of several surgical procedures designed either to cure a chronic inflammatory process in the middle ear or to restore function to the sound-transmitting mechanism of the middle ear. SEE: *Nursing Diagnoses* in *Appendix*.

tympanosclerosis (tĭm″pă-nō-sklĕ-rō′sĭs). Infiltration by hard fibrous tissue around the ossicles of the middle ear.

tympanosis (tĭm-pă-nō′sĭs) [″ + *osis,* condition]. Tympanites.

tympanosquamosal (tĭm″pă-nō-skwă-mō′săl). Concerning the pars tympanica and pars squamosa of the temporal bone.

tympanostapedial (tĭm″pă-nō-stă-pē′dē-ăl). Concerning the tympanic cavity and stapes.

tympanostomy. Myringotomy, q.v.

tympanostomy tubes. Tubes placed through the tympanic membrane of the ear in order to allow ventilation of the middle ear as part of the treatment of otitis media with effusion, q.v. SYN: *ventilation tubes.* SEE: *otitis media with effusion, Type A.*

tympanotemporal (tĭm″pă-nō-tĕm′pō-răl). Concerning the tympanic cavity and area of the temporal bone.

tympanotomy (tĭm″păn-ŏt′ō-mē) [″ + *tome,* incision]. Incision of the membrana tympani. SYN: *myringotomy.*

tympanous (tĭm′păn-ŭs) [Gr. *tympanon,* a drum]. Marked by abdominal distention with gas.

tympanum (tĭm′păn-ŭm) [L.; Gr. *tympanon*]. The middle ear or tympanic cavity. SYN: *cavum tympani; eardrum.* SEE: *ear, middle.*

tympany (tĭm′pă-nē). 1. Abdominal distention with gas. 2. Tympanic resonance on percussion. It is a clear hollow note like that of a drum having no vesicular quality. It indicates a pathological condition of the lung or of a cavity.

type (tīp) [Gr. *typos,* mark]. The general character of a person, disease, or substance.

   t., asthenic. Having a thin, flat, long-chested body build with poor muscular development.

   t., athletic. Having broad shoulders, deep chest, flat abdomen, thick neck, and excellent muscular development.

   t., blood. SEE: *blood groups.*

   t., phage. Distinguishing subgroups of bacteria by the type of bacteriophage associated with that specific bacterium.

   t., pyknic. Having a rounded body, large chest, thick shoulders, broad head, thick neck, and usually short stature.

type A personality. SEE: *behavior patterns, types A and B.*

type B personality. SEE: *behavior patterns, types A and B.*

typhlectasis (tĭf-lĕk′tă-sĭs) [Gr. *typhlon,*

cecum, + *ektasis,* dilatation]. Cecal distention.

typhlectomy (tĭf-lĕk′tō-mē) [″ + *ektome,* excision]. Excision of the cecum. SYN: *cecectomy.*

typhlenteritis (tĭf″lĕn-tĕr-ī′tĭs) [″ + *enteron,* intestine, + *itis,* inflammation]. Inflammation of the cecum. SYN: *typhlitis.*

typhlitis (tĭf-lī′tĭs) [″ + *itis,* inflammation]. Inflammation of the cecum.

typhlo-. 1. Combining form indicating a relationship to the cecum. 2. Combining form indicating a relationship to blindness.

typhlodicliditis (tĭf″lō-dĭk-lĭ-dī′tĭs) [″ + *diklis,* door, + *itis,* inflammation]. Inflammation of the ileocecal valve.

typhloempyema (tĭf″lō-ĕm-pī-ē′mă) [″ + *en,* in, + *pyon,* pus, + *haima,* blood]. An abdominal abscess following appendicitis.

typhloenteritis (tĭf″lō-ĕn-tĕr-ī′tĭs) [″ + *enteron,* intestine, + *itis,* inflammation]. Inflammation of the cecum. SYN: *typhlenteritis; typhlitis.*

typhlolexia (tĭf″lō-lĕk′sē-ă) [Gr. *typhlos,* blind, + *lexis,* speech]. Alexia.

typhlolithiasis (tĭf″lō-lĭ-thī′ă-sĭs) [Gr. *typhlon,* cecum, + *lithos,* stone, + *-iasis,* condition]. Formation of a concretion in the cecum.

typhlology (tĭf-lŏl′ō-jē) [Gr. *typhlos,* blind, + *logos,* word, reason]. Study of blindness, its causes and effects.

typhlomegaly (tĭf″lō-mĕg′ă-lē) [Gr. *typhlon,* cecum, + *megas,* large]. Abnormally large cecum.

typhlon (tĭf′lŏn) [Gr.]. The cecum.

typhlopexy (tĭf′lō-pĕks″ē) [Gr. *typhlon,* cecum, + *pexis,* fixation]. Suturing of a movable cecum to the abdominal wall.

typhlorrhaphy (tĭf-lor′ă-fē). Surgical repair of the cecum.

typhlosis (tĭf-lō′sĭs) [Gr. *typhlos,* blind, + *osis,* condition]. Blindness.

typhlospasm (tĭf′lō-spăsm). Spasm of the cecum.

typhlostenosis (tĭf″lō-stĕn-ō′sĭs) [Gr. *typhlon,* cecum, + *stenosis,* act of narrowing]. Stenosis or stricture of the cecum.

typhlostomy (tĭf-lŏs′tō-mē) [″ + *stoma,* mouth]. Establishment of a permanent cecal fistula.

typhlotomy (tĭf-lŏt′ō-mē) [Gr. *typhlon,* cecum, + *tome,* incision]. Incision of the cecum.

typhloureterostomy (tĭf″lō-ū-rĕ″tĕr-ŏs′tō-mē) [″ + *oureter,* ureter, + *stoma,* mouth]. Implantation of a ureter in the cecum.

typho- [Gr. *typhos,* fever]. Combining form pert. to fever or to typhoid.

typhohemia (tī″fō-hē′mē-ă) [″ + *haima,*

blood]. Degeneration of the blood due to presence of bacilli.

typhoid (tī'foyd) [Gr. *typhos,* fever, + *eidos,* form, shape]. Resembling typhus.

typhoidal (tī-foy'dăl). Resembling typhoid.

typhoid carrier. An individual who has recovered from typhoid fever but who harbors the bacteria, usually in the gallbladder, and who excretes the organism in urine and feces.

typhoid fever. An acute infectious disease characterized by definite lesions in Peyer's patches, mesenteric glands, and spleen accompanied by fever, headache, and abdominal pain.

SYM: Early symptoms are headache, general weakness, indefinite pains, and nosebleed. Constipation may occur. Within a few days to a week the temperature may reach a maximum of 104° to 105°F (40° to 40.6°C) and during this time, or up to the 10th day, rose spots can usually be seen, particularly on the abdomen, though they may be observed on the chest and back. They usually come out in crops during a period of several days. They will blanch upon pressure. Abdominal tenderness develops and with it, generally, distention. Splenomegaly will be found in more than half of the cases by the end of the first week.

During following weeks, fever is characterized by marked daily remissions, evening temperature being from 1° to 3°F (0.56° to 1.7°C) higher than that in the morning. In the young, the temperature often rises very abruptly. When the diurnal remissions are slight, a protracted case is forecast. As defervescence advances, the temperature becomes more irregular. Remissions are more decided, and not infrequently a higher temperature is recorded in the morning. Rapid respiratory rate, slight cough, and bronchial rales are common. Pulse is usually slow in comparison with the temperature rise and is dicrotic. Heart sounds are often feeble, expression dull and heavy, cheeks somewhat flushed, conjunctivae clear, pupils dilated.

Tongue tremulous; at first red at tip and edges, and covered posteriorly with a whitish furlike material. In severe cases, tongue becomes dry, brown and fissured, and sordes collect on teeth. Gastric symptoms not common but when present they are obstinate. Vomiting sometimes develops and becomes a serious complication. Abdomen is tympanitic and there is tenderness on palpation, esp. in the iliac fossa. Diarrhea generally present but not a constant symptom. Bowel movements vary from three to six or more a day; thin, offensive, yellowish. Stupor, muttering, delirium, twitching of the muscles, carphologia, and coma vigil may be

present. Proteinuria and retention of urine are common. White blood count demonstrates a leukopenia. Convalescence marked by anemia, loss of hair, often desquamation. The patient gives evidence of having suffered from a protracted illness that has produced general mental and physical debilitation.

ETIOL: Causative organism is *Salmonella typhi,* a gram-negative, motile bacillus. It may be transmitted by infected water or milk supplies. Human carriers, particularly food handlers, may be responsible for spread of infection. Body discharges from active or convalescent cases may be the means of infecting others.

DIFF. DIAG: Paratyphoid, pneumonia, dysentery, meningitis, smallpox, appendicitis. Diagnostic points of value will be the presence of rose spots, splenomegaly, leukopenia, the Widal serological test, blood culture, and examination of feces for presence of causative organism.

PROPHYLAXIS: Immunity can ordinarily be established by administering two injections of vaccine several weeks apart. SEE: *typhoid vaccine.*

INCUBATION: Average of two weeks; varies from one to three weeks.

TREAT: General care, isolation of patient, and disinfection of all discharges are of primary importance. Those caring for the typhoid patient should be immunized against the disease. All precautions applicable to such infections must be adopted. Articles in contact with the patient must be sterilized or disinfected before being handled by persons other than the immediate attendant. It is necessary to guard against development of bedsores. Because delirium is not infrequent, patient may require constant watching to prevent his or her leaving the bed. The mouth should be kept as clean as possible to prevent development of sordes. Chloramphenicol is the drug of choice, but ampicillin is given if chloramphenicol-resistant strains are present.

Ice bags and cold sponging are little used at the present time. On the other hand, sponging with tepid water, or with alcohol, is sometimes used when the temperature has reached unusual heights. Surgical intervention will be necessary if antibiotics and bowel decompression fail to control severe hemorrhage or if intestinal perforation occurs.

COMPLICATIONS: These occur in approximately 25% of untreated cases and account for the majority of deaths. The most frequent and dangerous complications are intestinal hemorrhage and intestinal perforation. An abrupt fall of several degrees in temperature is suggestive of intestinal hemorrhage or perforation. Usually occurs during 3rd or 4th week.

PROG: Should always be guarded, no matter how mild the case appears to be. Fatality rate varies in different epidemics. Hemorrhages in any form, together with excessive diarrhea, are unfavorable signs. SEE: *Universal Precautions* in *Appendix.*

NURSING IMPLICATIONS: Follow enteric precautions (handwashing, patient handwashing, glove and gown for disposal of feces or fecally contaminated objects) until three consecutive stool cultures at 24-hour intervals are negative. Administer drugs as prescribed, and observe for signs and symptoms of complications, such as bacteremia, intestinal bleeding, and bowel perforation. During the acute phase, monitor temperature and administer prescribed antipyretics; tepid sponge baths to promote vasodilation without shivering. Cleanse the incontinent patient and encourage high fluid intake by mouth or I.V. to maintain adequate hydration. Provide frequent oral hygiene and skin care. Reposition the patient and carry out passive to active range-of-motion exercises. Watch for bladder distention and monitor intake and output. Maintain adequate nutrition. Inform the patient of the importance of follow-up care and examination to be certain of being or not being a carrier.

Charting: A four-hour chart should be kept of temperature, pulse, and respiration, although the pulse should be taken much more frequently than this. In the 3rd week, the temperature should be taken every two hours. A sudden drop in temperature indicates hemorrhage.

Disinfection: The usual methods of disinfection should be observed in handling all excreta and secretions, linens, and utensils. Disinfection for the nurse is also very important. SEE: *Universal Precautions* in *Appendix.*

typhoid vaccine. A vaccine containing killed *Salmonella typhi.* Even though its effectiveness in preventing typhoid fever is limited to protecting only those who have experienced a small infecting dose of *Salmonella typhi,* its use is advisable in persons who will be exposed to typhoid bacilli.

typholysin (tī-fŏl′ĭ-sĭn) [″ + *lysis,* dissolution]. A lysin destructive to typhoid bacilli.

typhomalarial (tī″fō-mă-lā′rē-ăl) [″ + It. *malaria,* bad air]. Having symptoms of both typhoid and malarial fever.

typhomania (tī-fō-mā′nē-ă) [″ + *mania,* madness]. Muttering delirium characteristic of typhoid fever and typhus.

typhopneumonia (tī″fō-nū-mō′nē-ă) [″ +

pneumon, lung, + *-ia,* condition, abnormal state]. 1. Pneumonia occurring in typhoid fever. 2. Pneumonia with typhoid symptoms.

typhous (tī′fŭs) [Gr. *typhos,* fever]. Pert. to typhus fever.

typhus (tī′fŭs) [Gr. *typhos,* fever]. Any of a group of acute infectious diseases characterized by great prostration, severe headache, generalized maculopapular rash, sustained high fever, and usually progressive neurologic involvement, ending in a crisis in 10 to 14 days.

Three diseases are included in the group: epidemic (louse-borne) typhus, caused by *Rickettsia prowazekii;* Brill-Zinsser disease (recrudescent typhus), caused by *Rickettsia prowazekii;* and murine (flea-borne) typhus, caused by *Rickettsia typhi.* Although clinically and pathologically similar, they differ in intensity of symptoms, severity, and mortality rate.

Epidemic typhus is particularly prevalent amid unsanitary conditions. It often develops on shipboard, in army camps, and where living conditions are unfavorable and congestion is marked. The disease is rare in the U.S. SEE: *Nursing Diagnoses* in *Appendix.*

SYM: Onset sudden. Severe headache, pain in back and limbs, extreme prostration. Fever rises rapidly, often reaching 104° to 105°F (40° to 40.6°C) in two to three days; remains high for about 10 days, then falls by crisis. Pulse rapid, weak, often dicrotic. Tongue tremulous, may be covered with whitish fur; in severe cases becomes black and rolled up like a ball in back of mouth. Face dusky, conjunctivae injected, pupil contracted, headache, stupor, delirium, muscle twitching, picking at the bedclothes (carphologia).

From 4th to 5th day, bluish spots appear over body, esp. on abdomen. These are petechial in character and do not disappear on pressure. The extent of eruption is indicative of severity of attack. Sometimes there is a diffuse, dark red, subcuticular mottling. Bowels are constipated; urine is scanty, pigmented and often albuminous.

DIFF. DIAG.: Typhoid fever, hemorrhagic smallpox, Henoch's purpura, epidemic meningitis of fulminating type, and ulcerative endocarditis may have to be considered.

INCUBATION: One to two weeks except for Brill-Zinsser disease, which may recur years after the initial attack.

TREAT: *Preventive:* Absolute cleanliness, sterilization of clothing, and the use of apparel to prevent infestation by the body louse. Patient must be isolated. Absolute rest necessary, and liquid diet. *Specific:*

Broad-spectrum antibiotics, such as the tetracyclines and chloramphenicol, give excellent results. SEE: *Universal Precautions* in *Appendix.*

COMPLICATIONS: Bronchopneumonia occurs more frequently than lobar. Hypostatic congestion of lungs, nephritis, and parotid abscess.

PROG: Variable. Mortality may be quite high in epidemic typhus and almost nonexistent in murine typhus. Broad-spectrum antibiotics will be life-saving if given early enough.

t., classic. T., epidemic.

t., endemic. T., murine.

t., epidemic. An infectious disease caused by *Rickettsia prowazekii* and transmitted by human body louse *(Pediculus humanus humanus).* SYN: *t., classic.*

t., flea-borne. T., murine.

t., Mexican. A louse-borne epidemic typhus present in certain portions of Mexico. SYN: *tabardillo.*

t., mite-borne. Tsutsugamushi disease or scrub typhus.

t., murine. A disease caused by *Rickettsia mooseri* and occurring in nature as a mild infection of rats and transmitted from rat to rat by the rat-louse or flea. Humans may acquire it by being bitten by infected rat fleas or ingesting food contaminated by rat urine or flea feces. SYN: *t., endemic; t., flea-borne; t., shop.*

t., recrudescent. A recurrence or recrudescence of a preceding attack of epidemic typhus after initial attack.

t., rural. T., scrub.

t., scrub. A self-limited febrile disease of two weeks' duration caused by *Rickettsia tsutsugamushi* and transmitted by two species of mites (chiggers) of the genus *Thrombicula.* Occurs principally in Pacific-Asiatic area. SYN: *t., mite-borne; t., rural; tsutsugamushi disease.*

t., shop. T., murine.

t., urban. T., epidemic.

typhus vaccine. USP. A sterile suspension of the killed rickettsial organism of a strain or strains of epidemic typhus rickettsiae.

typical (tĭp'ĭ-kăl) [Gr. *typikos*, pert. to type]. Having the characteristics of, pert. to, or conforming to, a type or condition or group.

typing (tīp'ĭng). Identification of type.

t., bacteriophage. Determination of the subdivision of a bacterial species using a type-specific bacteriophage.

t., blood. Determination of the specific blood group of an individual. SEE: *blood transfusion.*

t., tissue. Determination of the histocompatibility of tissues to be used in grafts and transplants. SEE: *transplantation.*

typo- [Gr. *typos*]. Combining form meaning a type.

typoscope (tī'pō-skōp) [" + *skopein*, to examine]. A reading aid device for patients with amblyopia or cataract.

typus (tī'pŭs) [L.]. Type.

tyramine (tī'ră-mēn). Intermediate product in the conversion of tyrosine to epinephrine. Tyramine is found in most cheeses and in beer, broad bean pods, yeast, wine, and chicken liver. When persons taking certain types of antidepressant monoamine oxidase inhibitors also eat these foods, they may experience severe hypertension, headache, palpitation, neck pain, and perhaps intracranial hemorrhage. This is due to the tyramine's not being inactivated by monoamine oxidation. This has been called the "cheese reaction."

tyrannism (tĭr'ăn-ĭzm) [Gr. *tyrannos*, tyrant, + *-ismos*, condition]. Abnormal tendency to exercise cruelty. SYN: *sadism.*

tyrogenous (tī-rŏj'ĕn-ŭs) [Gr. *tyros*, cheese, + *gennan*, to produce]. Having origin in or produced by cheese.

Tyroglyphus (tī-rŏg'lĭ-fŭs) [Gr. *tyros*, cheese, + *glyphein*, to carve]. A genus of sarcoptoid mites commonly known as cheese mites. They infest cheese and dried vegetable food products and occasionally infest humans, causing a pruritus. Contains species causing grocer's itch, vanillism, and copra itch.

tyroid (tī'royd) [" + *eidos*, form, shape]. Caseous; cheesy.

tyroma (tī-rō'mă). A tumor that contains cheeselike material.

tyromatosis (tī″rō-mă-tō'sĭs) [" + *oma*, tumor, + *osis*, condition]. Conversion of necrotic tissue into a granular amorphous mass resembling cheese. SYN: *caseation.*

tyrosinase (tī-rō'sĭn-ās) [Gr. *tyros*, cheese]. An enzyme that acts on tyrosine to produce melanin.

tyrosine (tī'rō-sĭn). USP. An amino acid present in many proteins, esp. casein. It serves as a precursor of epinephrine, thyroxine, and melanin. Two vitamins, ascorbic acid and folic acid, are essential for its metabolism.

tyrosinemia (tī″rō-sĭ-nē'mē-ă). A disease of tyrosine metabolism due to a deficiency of the enzyme tyrosine aminotransferase. In addition to an accumulation of tyrosine in the blood, mental retardation, keratitis, and dermatitis are present. Treatment consists of controlling the phenylalanine and tyrosine intake.

tyrosinosis (tī″rō-sĭn-ō'sĭs) [" + *osis*, condition]. Condition resulting from faulty metabolism of tyrosine, whereby its oxidation products appear in the urine.

tyrosinuria (tī″rō-sĭn-ū′rē-ă) [″ + *ouron,* urine]. Tyrosine in the urine.

tyrosis (tī-rō′sĭs) [″ + *osis,* condition]. 1. Curdling of milk. 2. Vomiting of cheesy substance by infants. 3. Cheesy degeneration. SYN: *tyromatosis.*

tyrosyluria (tī″rō-sĭl-ū′rē-ă). Increased tyrosine-derived products in the urine.

tyrothricin (tī″rō-thrī′sĭn). An antibacterial drug.

tyrotoxism (tī″rō-tŏks′ĭzm) [″ + *toxikon,* a poison, + *-ismos,* condition]. Poisoning produced by a milk product or by cheese.

Tyrrell's fascia (tĭr′rĕlz) [Frederick Tyrrell, Brit. anatomist, 1797–1843]. An ill-defined fibromuscular layer from the middle aponeurosis of the perineum, behind the prostate gland.

Tyson's glands (tī′sŭnz) [Edward Tyson, Brit. physician and anatomist, 1650–1708]. Modified sebaceous glands located on neck of penis and inner surface of prepuce. Their secretion is one of the components of smegma. SYN: *preputial glands.*

tysonitis (tī″sŏn-ī′tĭs). Inflammation of Tyson's glands.

tyvelose (tī′vĕl-ōs). A carbohydrate, 3-6-di-deoxy-D-mannose, derived from certain strains of *Salmonella.* It is a somatic antigen.

Tyzine Trade name for tetrahydrozoline hydrochloride.

Tzanck test (tsănk) [Arnault Tzanck, Russ. dermatologist in Paris, 1886–1954]. Examination of tissue from the lower surface of a lesion in vesicular disease to determine the cell type.

tzetze (sĕt′sē). Tsetse.

U

U. 1. *unit.* 2. Chem. symb. for the element uranium.

²³⁵U. Isotope of uranium with mass number 235.

UAO. *upper airway obstruction.*

uberous (ū'bĕr-ŭs) [L. *uber*, udder]. Prolific; fruitful; fertile.

uberty (ū'bĕr-tē) [L. *uber*, udder]. Fruitfulness; fertility.

ubiquinol (ū-bĭk'wĭ-nŏl). Coenzyme QH₂, the reduced form of ubiquinone, q.v.

ubiquinone (ū-bĭk'wĭ-nōn) [*ubi*quitous + coenzyme *quinone*]. Coenzyme Q, a lipid-soluble quinone present in virtually all cells. It is a collector of reducing equivalents during intracellular respiration. It is converted to its reduced form, ubiquinol, while involved in this process.

ubiquitin. A small protein present in eukaryotic cells that combines with other proteins and makes these proteins susceptible to destruction. This protein is also important in promoting the functions of proteins that make up ribosomes.

udder (ŭd'ĕr). The mammary gland of animals such as cows and goats.

UDP. *uridine diphosphate.*

Uffelmann's test (oof'ĕl-mänz) [Jules Uffelmann, Ger. physician, 1837–1894]. Test for determination of lactic acid in gastric juice.

U-Gencin. Trade name for gentamicin sulfate.

Uhthoff's sign (oot'hŏfs) [Wilhelm Uhthoff, Ger. ophthalmologist, 1853–1927]. The nystagmus that occurs in multiple disseminated sclerosis.

ulalgia (ū-lăl'jē-ă) [Gr. *oulon*, gum, + *algos*, pain]. Pain in the gums.

ulcer (ŭl'sĕr) [L. *ulcus*, ulcer]. An open sore or lesion of the skin or mucous membrane accompanied by sloughing of inflamed necrotic tissue. If the sore becomes infected, pus is discharged. Simple ulcers may result from trauma, caustics, intense heat or cold, or arterial or venous stasis. They may occur as a complication of varicose veins due to stasis of blood leading to inflammation, necrosis, and sloughing of tissue. Ulcers of the mucous membrane of the stomach or duodenum are caused by the effect of gastric acid and pepsin. The sores of acquired syphilis are caused by blockage of small vessels. The secretion from these sores contains the causative agent *Treponema pallidum.*

RS: abscission; anthracosis; aphtha; argema; carcinomelcosis; dieresis; phagedena; slough; stomach.

u., amputating. Ulcer that destroys tissue to the bone by encircling the part.

u., aphthous. SEE: *aphthous ulcer.*

u., atonic. A chronic ulcer.

u., callous. A chronic ulcer with indurated, elevated edges and no granulations, which does not heal.

u., chronic leg. Any long-standing slow-to-heal ulcer of the lower extremity, esp. one due to occlusive disease of the arteries or veins, or varicose veins.

u., Curling's. Peptic ulcer that sometimes occurs following severe burns to the body. A form of stress ulcer.

u., decubitus. Ischemic necrosis and ulceration of tissue, esp. over a bony prominence. Due to pressure from prolonged confinement in bed or from a cast or splint. SYN: *bedsore.* SEE: *decubitus ulcer.* SEE: *Nursing Diagnoses* in *Appendix.*

u., duodenal. Ulcer on the mucosa of the duodenum, due to the action of the gastric juice. SEE: *peptic ulcer.*

u., follicular. A tiny ulcer having its origin in a lymph follicle and affecting a mucous membrane.

u., fungus. Ulcer in which the granulations protrude above edges of the wound and bleed easily.

u., gastric. Ulcer of the gastric mucosa. SEE: *peptic ulcer.*

u., Hunner's. A painful, slow-to-heal ulcer of the urinary bladder.

u., indolent. Nearly painless ulcer usually found on the leg, characterized by an indurated and elevated edge and a nongranulating base.

u., peptic. Ulcer of the mucosa of the duodenum or stomach. SEE: *peptic ulcer.* SEE: *Nursing Diagnoses* in *Appendix.*

u., perforating. Ulcer that permeates the entire thickness of the part, as the foot or intestine.

u., phagedenic. Ulcer that spreads rapidly and disintegrates the tissues, producing a slough and discharge.

u., rodent. A deeply infiltrating ulcer that slowly destroys bones and soft tissues; commonly affects the upper part of the face. SYN: *Jacob's ulcer.*

u., serpiginous. A creeping ulcer that heals in one part and extends to another.

u., simple. A local ulcer with no severe inflammation or pain.

u., specific. Ulcer caused by a specific disease, as syphilis or lupus.

u., stasis. SEE: *decubitus ulcer.*

u., stercoral. 1. Ulcer caused by pressure from impacted feces. 2. Ulcer through which feces escape.

u., stress. Peptic ulcer due to acute or chronic stress such as may be present with cerebral trauma, burns, surgery, acute infection, prolonged adrenal corticosteroid therapy, or central nervous system disease.

u., trophic. Ulcer due to failure of supply of nutrients to a part.

u., tropical. 1. An indolent ulcer, usually of the lower extremity, that occurs in persons living in hot, humid areas. The etiology may or may not be known, and it may be due to a combination of bacterial, environmental, and nutritional factors. 2. The tropical sore caused by leishmaniasis.

u., varicose. Ulcer, esp. of the lower extremity, associated with varicose veins.

u., venereal. Ulcer caused by a venereal disease, i.e., chancre, or chancroid.

ulcera. Pl. of ulcus.

ulcerate (ŭl′sĕr-āt) [L. *ulcerare,* to form ulcers]. To produce or become affected with an ulcer.

ulcerated (ŭl′sĕr-ā″tĕd). Of the nature of an ulcer or affected with one.

ulcerated tooth. Suppuration of the alveolar periosteum with ulceration of gum surrounding the decaying root of a tooth.

ulceration (ŭl″sĕr-ā′shŭn). Suppuration occurring on a free surface, as on the skin or on a mucous membrane, to form an ulcer. SEE: *eye, trophic ulceration of.*

ulcerative (ŭl′sĕr-ā-tĭv) [L. *ulcerare,* to form ulcers]. Pert. to or causing ulceration.

ulcerogangrenous (ŭl″sĕr-ō-găng′grĕ-nŭs). An ulcer that contains gangrenous tissue.

ulcerogenic drugs. Medicines that, because of their systemic rather than local effects, may cause peptic ulcers.

ulceromembranous (ŭl″sĕr-ō-mĕm′brăn-ŭs) [″ + *membrana,* membrane]. Pert. to ulceration and formation of a fibrous pseudomembrane.

ulceromembranous tonsillitis. Tonsillitis that ulcerates and develops a membranous film.

ulcerous (ŭl′sĕr-ŭs). Pert. to or affected with an ulcer.

ulcus (ŭl′kŭs) [L.] (pl. *ulcera*). Ulcer.

u. cancrosum. Cancerous ulcer that eats away the tissues. SYN: *rodent ulcer.*

u. induratum. A chancre, q.v.

u. vulvae acutum. An acute erosive ulcer on the female external genitalia. The cause is unknown but the ulcers may appear in association with acute infectious diseases such as typhoid fever, viral pneumonia, or brucellosis, or may appear as a variant of Behçet's syndrome, q.v. The disease may be confused with herpes simplex and ulcers caused by trauma.

ulegyria (ū″lĕ-jī′rē-ă) [Gr. *oule,* scar, + *gyros,* ring]. Condition in which gyri of the cerebral cortex are abnormal due to scar tissue from injuries usually occurring in early development.

ulerythema (ū-lĕr-ĭ-thē′mă) [Gr. *oule,* scar, + *erythema,* redness]. An erythematous disorder with atrophic scar formation.

u. ophryogenes. Folliculitis of eyebrows characterized by falling out of hair and scarring.

u. sycosiforme. Inflammation of the hair follicles of the beard with alopecia in the affected area.

uletic (ū-lĕt′ĭk) [Gr. *oulon,* gum]. Pert. to the gums.

uletomy (ū-lĕt′ō-mē) [Gr. *oule,* scar, + *tome,* incision]. Incision of a scar to relieve tension. SYN: *cicatricotomy.*

uliginous (ū-lĭj′ĭ-nŭs) [L. *uliginosus,* wet]. Muddy; slimy.

ulna (ŭl′nă) [L., elbow]. The inner and larger bone of the forearm, between the wrist and the elbow, on the side opposite that of the thumb. It articulates with the head of the radius and humerus above and with the radius below.

RS: coronoid process; cubital; cubitus; elbow; olecranon; skeleton.

ulnad (ŭl′năd) [″ + *ad,* to]. In the direction of the ulna.

ulnar (ŭl′năr) [L. *ulna,* elbow]. 1. Rel. to the ulna, or to nerve or artery named from it. 2. Cuneiform carpal bone.

ulnar drift. A joint change at the metacarpophalangeal joints frequently seen in rheumatoid arthritis, resulting from chronic synovitis. In this condition the long axis of the fingers deviate in an ulnar direction with respect to the metacarpals.

ulnaris (ŭl-nā′rĭs). 1. Ulnar. 2. Concerning the ulna.

ulnocarpal (ŭl″nō-kăr′păl) [″ + Gr. *karpos,* wrist]. Relating to the carpus and ulna, or to the ulnar side of the wrist.

ulnoradial (ŭl″nō-rā′dē-ăl) [″ + *radius,* spoke of a wheel]. Rel. to the ulna and radius, as their ligaments and articulations.

Ulo. Trade name for chlophedianol hydrochloride.

ulo- [Gr. *oule,* scar]. Combining form concerning a scar.

ulodermatitis (ū″lō-dĕrm-ă-tī′tĭs) [Gr. *oule,* scar, + *derma,* skin, + *itis,* inflammation]. Dermatitis with scar tissue formation.

uloid (ū′loyd) [Gr. *oule,* scar, + *eidos,* form, shape]. 1. Scarlike. 2. A scarlike lesion caused by subcutaneous degeneration.

ulosis (ū-lō′sĭs) [Gr. *oule,* scar, + *osis,* condition]. Formation of scar tissue. SYN: *cica-*

trization.

ulotic (ū-lŏt′ĭk) [Gr. *oule,* scar]. Causing cicatrization. SYN: *cicatricial.*

ulotrichous (ū-lŏt′rĭk-ŭs) [Gr. *oulos,* woolly, + *thrix,* hair]. Having short woolly hair, characteristic of some races.

ultimate (ŭl′tĭm-ĭt) [L. *ultimus,* last]. Final or last.

ultimobranchial bodies (ŭl″tĭ-mō-brăng′kē-ăl). Two embryonic pharyngeal pouches usually considered as rudimentary fifth pouches. They become separated from the pharynx and incorporated into substance of the thyroid gland, where they give rise to parafollicular cells that secrete calcitonin, a hormone used to regulate blood calcium level.

ultra- [L.]. Prefix meaning beyond, excess.

ultrabrachycephalic (ŭl″tră-brăk″ĭ-sē-făl′ĭk) [L. *ultra,* beyond, + Gr. *brachys,* short, + *kephale,* head]. Having a cephalic index of 90 or more.

ultracentrifugation (ŭl″tră-sĕn-trĭf″ū-gā′shŭn). Treatment or preparation of substances by use of the ultracentrifuge.

ultracentrifuge (ŭl-tră-sĕn′trĭ-fūj) [″ + *centrum,* center, + *fugere,* to flee]. A high-speed centrifuge capable of producing centrifugal forces more than 100,000 times gravity. Used in the study of proteins, viruses, etc.

ultradian (ŭl-trā′dē-ăn) [″ + *dies,* day]. Concerning biologic rhythms that occur less frequently than every 24 hours.

ultrafilter (ŭl-tră-fĭl′tĕr). A filter by which colloidal particles may be separated from their dispersion medium or from crystalloids.

ultrafiltration (ŭl″tră-fĭl-trā′shŭn) [″ + *filtrum,* a filter]. Filtration of a colloidal substance in which the dispersed particles, but not the liquid, are held back.

ultraligation (ŭl″tră-lĭ-gā′shŭn) [″ + *ligare,* to bind]. Ligation of a blood vessel beyond the origin of a branch.

ultramicrobe (ŭl″tră-mī′krōb) [″ + Gr. *mikros,* small, + *bios,* life]. A microorganism too small to be visible by the ordinary microscope.

ultramicroscope (ŭl″tră-mī′krō-skōp) [″ + ″ + *skopein,* to examine]. Microscope by which objects invisible through an ordinary microscope may be seen by means of powerful side illumination. SYN: *microscope, darkfield.*

ultramicroscopy (ŭl″tră-mī-krŏs′kō-pē). The use of the ultramicroscope.

ultramicrotome (ŭl″tră-mī′krŏ-tōm). A microtome that makes extremely thin slices of tissue.

ultrasonic (ŭl-tră-sŏn′ĭk) [″ + *sonus,* sound]. Pertaining to sounds of frequencies

above approx. 20,000 cycles per second. They are inaudible to the human ear. SEE: *supersonic; ultrasound; ultrasonography.*

ultrasonic cleaning. Use of ultrasonic energy to clean objects, including medical and surgical instruments.

ultrasonics (ŭl-tră-sŏn′ĭks). The division of acoustics that studies inaudible sounds with frequencies greater than 20,000 cycles per second. Biological effects may result depending on intensity of beams. Heating effects are produced by beams of low intensity, paralytic effects by those of moderate intensity, and lethal effects by those of high intensity. The lethal action of ultrasonics is primarily the result, either directly or indirectly, of cavitation of tissues. Ultrasonics are utilized clinically for therapeutic and diagnostic purposes. In dentistry, instruments are used which produce 29,000 vibrations/sec in periodontal surgery, curettage, and root planing. SEE: *ultrasound.*

ultrasonogram (ŭl″tră-sŏn′ō-grăm). The image produced by use of ultrasonography.

ultrasonography (ŭl-tră-sŏn-ŏg′ră-fē). Use of ultrasound to produce an image or photograph of an organ or tissue. Ultrasonic echoes are recorded as they strike tissues of different densities.

ultrasound. Inaudible sound in the frequency range of approx. 20,000 to 10 billion (10^9) cycles per second. Ultrasound has different velocities in tissues that differ in density and elasticity from others. This property permits the use of ultrasound in outlining the shape of various tissues and organs in the body. Use of ultrasound for diagnostic and therapeutic purposes requires special equipment. SEE: *ultrasonography.*

u., A-mode. Sonographic information presented as a single line representing the time it takes for the ultrasound wave to reach the interface of a structure and reflect back to the transducer.

u., real-time. Sonographic procedure which provides rapid, multiple images of an anatomical structure in the form of motion.

ultrastructure (ŭl′tră-strŭk″chŭr). The fine structure of tissues. It is visible only by use of electron microscopy.

ultraviolet (ŭl″tră-vī′ō-lĕt) [″ + *viola,* violet]. Beyond the visible spectrum at its violet end, said of rays between the violet rays and roentgen rays. SEE: *infrared rays.*

ultraviolet radiation. ABBR: UVR. Rays emitted by natural and artificial sources, including very hot bodies, the sun, and by ionized gases with wavelengths between 290 and 400 nanometers (nm). From a therapeutic standpoint, physiological effects include erythema production, pigmentation of skin, antirachitic effect through production of vitamin D, bactericidal effects, and various effects on metabolism. In clinical practice, dosage is measured in terms of minimum erythema dose (M.E.D.).

In addition to erythema UVR can cause degenerative and neoplastic changes in skin, retinal damage, cataracts, and modification of the immunological system of the skin.

The UVR spectrum has been described and categorized as follows:

UV-A which includes wavelengths of 320 to 400 nm. UV-A can produce skin erythema but a 1000 time dose is required as compared to UV-B.

UV-B with the included wavelength of 290 to 320 nm is the principal portion of the UVR spectrum that is important in causing sunburn. A large portion of the UV-B emitted by the sun is absorbed by the ozone layer in the earth's atmosphere.

UV-C includes those wavelengths below 280 nm. These rays are completely absorbed by the ozone layer and have no role in causing pathological changes caused by exposure to sunlight.

UVR in combination with various chemical compounds may cause phototoxic or photoallergic reactions. SEE: *photoaging; sun screen; tanning salon.*

ultraviolet therapy. Treatment with ultraviolet radiation. SEE: *heliotherapy; light therapy.*

ululation (ŭl″ū-lā′shŭn) [L. *ululare*, to howl]. The crying and screaming of mentally ill persons.

umbilical (ŭm-bĭl′ĭ-kăl) [L. *umbilicus*, navel]. Pert. to the umbilicus.

umbilical artery catheter. Catheter placed in the umbilical artery of an infant in order to facilitate administration of medicines parenterally or to do an exchange transfusion.

umbilical cord. The attachment connecting the fetus with the placenta. It contains two arteries and one vein surrounded by a gelatinous substance, Wharton's jelly, q.v. The embryo receives nourishment from the blood supplied by the arteries of the umbilical cord, which go from the placenta to the fetus. SEE: illus.

The umbilical cord is surgically severed after the birth of the child. In order to give the infant a better blood supply, the cord should not be cut or tied until umbilical vessels have ceased pulsating. The stump of severed cord atrophies and leaves a depression on the abdomen of the child, called a navel or umbilicus.

umbilical fissure. Portion of hepatic longitudinal fissure in which the umbilical vein is lodged.

umbilical hernia. Hernia in the region of the umbilicus.

umbilical souffle. A hissing sound said to arise from the umbilical cord.

umbilical vesicle. That part of the embryonic yolk sac leading from the umbilicus.

umbilicate (ŭm-bĭl′ĭ-kāt) [L. *umbilicatus*, dimpled]. Pert. to or shaped like the navel, noting a bacterial colony with a central depression resembling an umbilicus.

umbilication (ŭm-bĭl-ĭ-kā′shŭn) [L. *umbilicatus*, dimpled]. 1. A depression resembling a navel. 2. Formation at apex of a pustule or vesicle of a pit or depression.

umbilicus (ŭm-bĭ-lī′kŭs, -bĭl′ī-kŭs) [L., a pit] (pl. *umbilici*). [NA] A depressed point in the middle of the abdomen; the scar that marks the former attachment of the umbilical cord to the fetus. SEE: *Cullen's sign; nodule, Sister Mary Joseph; Tanyoz's sign; Thomas-White hypothesis.*

RS: funic souffle; funiculus; funis; hydromphalus; mesogastrium; navel; "omphal-" words; umbilical cord; varicomphalus.

umbo (ŭm′bō) [L., boss of a shield]. Projecting center of a round surface.

u. of tympanic membrane. The central depressed portion of the concavity on the lateral surface of the tympanic membrane. It marks the point where the handle (manubrium of malleus) is attached to the inner surface.

umbra (ŭm′bră) [L., shade, shadow]. The edge of the radiographic image proper.

umbrella filter. Filter placed in a blood vessel in order to prevent emboli from passing that point. Has been used in the vena cava to prevent emboli in the veins from reaching the lungs.

UMP. *uridine monophosphate.*

un- [AS. *un-*, against]. Prefix meaning back, reversal, annulment of, and not.

uncal (ŭng′kăl). Concerning the uncus of the brain.

uncal herniation. Herniation, transtentorial, q.v.

unciform (ŭn′sĭ-form) [L. *uncus*, hook, + *forma*, shape]. Hook-shaped.

unciform bone. Hook-shaped bone on ulnar side of distal row of the carpus. SYN: *os hamatum* [NA].

unciforme (ŭn″sĭ-for′mē) [L.]. Uncinate, q.v.

unciform fasciculus. Bundle of fibers connecting frontal cerebral lobes with the temporosphenoid lobes.

unciform process. 1. Long thin lamina of bone from orbital plate of the ethmoid articulating with the inferior turbinate. 2. Hook at anterior end of the hippocampal gyrus. 3. Hooked end of unciform bone.

uncinariasis (ŭn″sĭn-ă-rī′ă-sĭs). Condition of

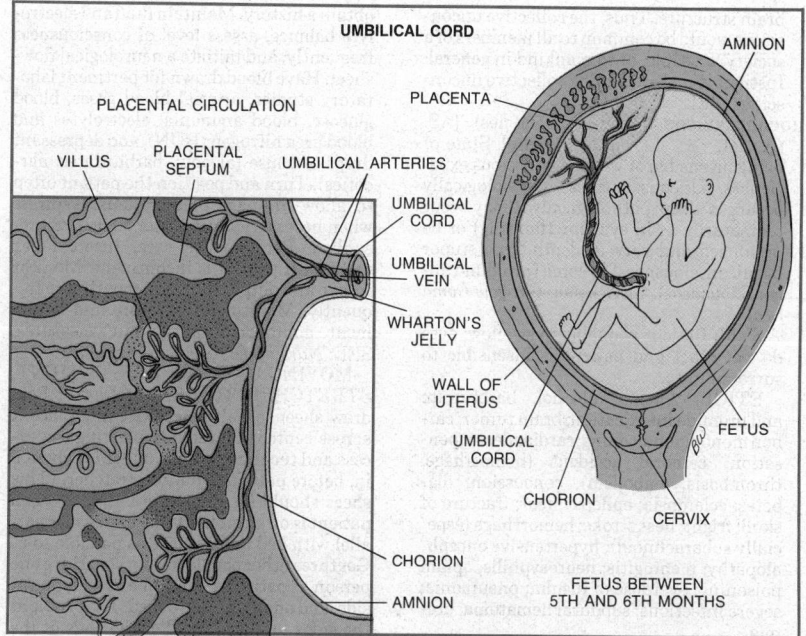

UMBILICAL CORD

AMNION

PLACENTA

PLACENTAL CIRCULATION

VILLUS   PLACENTAL SEPTUM   UMBILICAL ARTERIES

UMBILICAL CORD

UMBILICAL VEIN

WHARTON'S JELLY

WALL OF UTERUS

UMBILICAL CORD

CHORION

AMNION

FETUS

CERVIX

FETUS BETWEEN 5TH AND 6TH MONTHS

being infested with hookworms, i.e., worms of the genus *Uncinaria.*

uncinate (ŭn′sĭn-āt) [L. *uncinatus,* hooked]. Hook-shaped; hooked.

uncinate bundle of Russell [James S. Risien Russell, Brit. physician, 1863–1939]. Fibers that arise in the fastigial superior cerebellar peduncle and pass inferiorly to the vestibular nuclei and reticular formation by which impulses are carried to muscles, esp. those of the neck and body.

uncinate convolution. Uncinate gyrus.

uncinate epilepsy. Form of epilepsy occurring in disease of uncinate area of the temporal lobe.

uncinate fasciculus. Bundle of fibers connecting orbital gyri of frontal lobe with rostral portion of temporal lobe. They curve sharply as they pass over lateral fissure of cerebrum.

uncinate fits. Episodic attacks characterized by olfactory and gustatory hallucinations, usually disagreeable, a sense of unreality, and sometimes convulsions and temporary loss of senses of taste and smell. Associated with lesions of uncinate gyrus.

uncinate gyrus. Gyrus of the temporal lobe of the brain consisting of recurved rostral portion of hippocampal gyrus. SYN: *uncinate*

convolution; uncus.

uncinatum (ŭn″sĭ-nā′tŭm) [L.]. Hooked.

uncipressure (ŭn′sĭ-prĕsh″ŭr) [L. *uncus,* hook, + *pressura,* pressure]. Pressure applied with the use of a blunt hook to arrest bleeding.

uncomplemented (ŭn-kŏm′plē-mĕnt″ĕd). Not joined or associated with complement and thus inactive.

unconditioned reflex. An inborn or natural reflex; one not dependent upon previous experience or training.

unconscious (ŭn-kŏn′shŭs) [AS. *un,* not, + L. *conscius,* aware]. 1. Insensible; lacking in awareness of the environment. State in which a person experiences no sensory impressions and has no subjective experiences. SEE: *unconsciousness.* 2. In freudian psychiatry, that part of our personality consisting of a complex of feelings and drives of which we are unaware and that are not available to our consciousness.

   u., collective. Carl Jung divided the unconscious into personal and collective. Personal unconscious included all of the material stored in the unconscious that was acquired through personal experience. The collective unconscious is made up of material that the species inherits as part of the brain structure. Thus, the collective unconscious would be common to all members of a society, a people, or to mankind in general. Instinct is included in the collective unconscious. SEE: *sociobiology.*

unconsciousness (ŭn-kŏn'shŭs-nĕs) [AS. *un,* not, + L. *conscius,* aware]. State of being insensible or without conscious experiences. Unconsciousness physiologically occurs in sleep; pathologically it may occur temporarily as in syncope (fainting) or be prolonged and vary in depth from stupor (semiconsciousness) to coma (profound unconsciousness). SEE: *coma; Glasgow Coma Scale.*

SYM: Patient is unable to swallow; eyes do not react and patient is insensible to surroundings.

ETIOL: Anoxia; alcohol, barbiturate and bromide intoxication; brain tumor; carbon monoxide poisoning; cardiac decompensation; cerebral accident (hemorrhage, thrombosis, embolism), concussion; diabetes; eclampsia; epilepsy; fear; fracture of skull; fright; heat stroke; hemorrhage (especially subarachnoid); hypertensive encephalopathy; meningitis; neurosyphilis; opium poisoning; overdose of insulin; pneumonia; severe infections; subdural hematoma; uremia.

TREAT: If the face is flushed or if hemorrhage is present or suspected, do not lower head and do not give stimulants. In other instances, it is desirable to lower head and shoulders, loosen clothing, and keep patient comfortably warm but not hot. Remove false teeth if present. Turn head to one side to prevent vomitus, if any, from being inhaled. Provide artificial respiration, if necessary. Look for evidence of blows to the head, and for fractures and paralysis. Test pulse, respiration, odor of breath, condition of skin, and pupils of eyes. It is important to diagnose the cause of unconsciousness prior to instituting specific therapy.

Caution: The patient should be examined for a Medic Alert bracelet or pendant or a medical record card indicating chronic illness, critical medications, or allergy to drugs.

NURSING IMPLICATIONS: In the initial approach, follow the ABCs of emergency care, i.e., airway, bleeding, consciousness, digestive organs, excretory organs, and fractures. Establish adequate circulation and ventilation. Remove false teeth if present. Assess the patient for other health problems and treat them if they are of immediate concern. Implement safety measures to prevent further trauma. Re-examine the patient, and if he or she is conscious,

obtain a history. Maintain fluid and electrolyte balance, assess level of consciousness frequently, and initiate a neurological flowsheet. Have blood drawn for pertinent laboratory studies: arterial blood gases, blood glucose, blood ammonia, electrolytes and blood urea nitrogen (BUN), and depressant drugs of abuse (alcohol, barbiturates, narcotics). Turn and position the patient often to allow drainage of secretions. Aspirate when necessary. Administer oxygen as prescribed. Perform eye care. Insert Foley catheter if patient is incontinent. Monitor intake and output. Perform mouth care frequently. Monitor temperature and implement appropriate antipyretic measures. SEE: *Nursing Diagnoses* in *Appendix.*

MOVING UNCONSCIOUS PATIENT, STRETCHER TO BED: *Method I:* Fold draw sheet in half lengthwise and place it across center of stretcher, pleating the excess and tucking the ends under for about 6 in. before patient is put on stretcher. (This sheet should be under the buttocks when patient is on stretcher.) Place stretcher parallel with bed and as close as possible to it. Get three other people to help you. Have one person at patient's head, one at feet, one at side, and one at far side of bed. The people at the sides take firm hold of the ends of the draw sheet and all four lift together, the person at the far side pulling the draw sheet toward the bed.

Method II: This movement requires three people. Place stretcher at right angles to the foot of the bed with patient's head at end of bed nearest stretcher. Standing side by side the three people put their arms under the patient and lift and swing the patient around onto the bed.

unconsciousness, words pert. to: apoplexy; asphyctic; asphyxial; asphyxia; cataplexy; collapse; coma; epilepsy; fainting; Glasgow Coma Scale; shock; sleep; stroke; stupor; syncope; trance; twilight sleep.

unco-ossified (ŭn″kō-ŏs'ĭ-fĭd). Not ossified into one bone.

uncovertebral (ŭn″kō-vĕr'tĕ-brăl). Concerning the uncinate process of a vertebra.

unction (ŭnk'shŭn) [L. *unctio,* ointment]. 1. The application of an ointment. 2. Substance used for anointing. SYN: *unguent.*

unctuous (ŭnk'chū-ŭs) [L. *unctus,* an ointment]. Oily; greasy.

uncus (ŭn'kŭs) [L. *uncus,* hook]. 1. Any structure that is hook-shaped. 2. Hooked anterior end of hippocampal gyrus.

undecylenic acid. USP. An antifungal drug used topically to treat tinea pedis.

underachiever. A person whose achievements are less than what is predicted to be possible.

undercut (ŭn'dĕr-kŭt). A condition of having overhanging tissue as could be the case in preparing a dental cavity for restoration. Undercutting helps to keep the filling material in place.

undernutrition (ŭn"dĕr-nū-trĭsh'ŭn) [AS. *under*, beneath, + LL. *nutritio*, nourish]. Inadequate nutrition from any cause.

SYM: Loss of body weight representing at first mostly loss of body fat; then loss of protein manifested by atrophy of muscles, weakness, and edema.

undertoe (ŭn'dĕr-tō) [" + *ta*, toe]. Condition of displacement of the great toe underneath the others.

underweight (ŭn'dĕr-wāt"). Condition in which body weight is at least 10% less than what would be considered within normal limits for a particular individual. It is an imprecise term.

undifferentiation (ŭn-dĭf"ĕr-ĕn-shē-ā'shŭn) [AS. *un*, not, + L. *differens*, bearing apart]. Alteration in cell character to a more embryonic type or toward a malignant state. SYN: *anaplasia*.

undine (ŭn'dĭn) [L. *unda*, wave]. A small glass flask used for irrigating the eye.

undinism (ŭn'dĭn-ĭzm). Awakening of the libido by running water, as by urination or at sight of urine. SEE: *urolagnia*.

undulant (ŭn'dū-lănt). [L. *undulatio*, wavy]. Rising and falling like waves, or moving like them.

undulant fever (ŭn'dū-lănt). Brucellosis, q.v.

undulate (ŭn'dū-lāt) [L. *undulatio*, wavy]. Wavy; having a wavy border with shallow sinuses, said of bacterial colonies.

undulation (ŭn-dū-lā'shŭn). A continuous wavelike motion or pulsation.

  u., jugular. A venous pulse.

  u., respiratory. Fluctuation in blood pressure due to respiratory movements.

unemployment. Condition of being unemployed, esp. involuntary idleness due to not having a job. Medically, this is important because it is known that being unemployed is not conducive to mental health, and only in rare cases does the experience of being unemployed prove to be a positive experience. Also, it is known that one's work provides a tie to reality.

ung. [L.]. *unguentum*, ointment.

ungual (ŭng'gwăl) [L. *unguis*, nail]. Pert. to or resembling the nails. SYN: *unguinal*.

ungual phalanx. Terminal phalanx of each finger and toe.

ungual tuberosity. Spatula-shaped extremity of the terminal phalanx that supports the nails of fingers and toes.

unguent (ŭng'gwĕnt) [L. *unguentum*, ointment]. A lubricant or salve for sores or burns. SYN: *ointment*.

unguentum (ŭn-gwĕn'tŭm) [L., ointment]. 1. Fatty, soft, solid preparation intended to be applied to the skin by inunction. 2. Simple ointment. SYN: *ointment*.

unguiculate (ŭng-gwĭk'ū-lāt). Having nails or claws rather than hooves.

unguinal. Ungual, q.v.

unguis (ŭng'gwĭs) [L., nail] (pl. *ungues*). 1. [NA] A fingernail or toenail. SYN: *onyx*. 2. The lacrimal bone. 3. A white prominence on floor of the posterior horn of the lateral ventricle. SYN: *hippocampus minor.*

  u. incarnatus. An ingrowing nail, esp. a toenail.

ungula (ŭn'gū-lă) [L., claw]. Instrument for removal of dead fetus from the uterus.

ungulate. Having hooves.

uni- [L. *unus*]. Combining form meaning one.

uniarticular (ū"nē-ăr-tĭk'ū-lăr) [L. *unus*, one, + *articulus*, joint]. Pertaining to a single joint.

uniaxial (ū"nē-ăk'sē-ăl) [" + *axis*, axis]. Having a single axis.

unibasal (ū"nē-bā'săl) [" + *basis*, base]. Having a single base.

unicameral (ū"nĭ-kăm'ĕr-ăl) [" + *camera*, vault]. Having a single cavity.

unicellular (ū"nĭ-sĕl'ū-lăr) [" + *cellula*, a little box]. Having only one cell.

unicentral (ū"nĭ-sĕn'trăl) [" + *centrum*, center]. Having a single center.

uniceps (ū'nĭ-sĕps) [" + *caput*, head]. Having a single head or origin, as in muscles.

unicorn, unicornous (ū'nĭ-korn, ū-nĭ-kor'nŭs) [" + *cornu*, horn]. Having a single cornu or horn.

unicuspid (ū"nĭ-kŭs'pĭd). Having a single cusp.

uniflagellate (ū"nĭ-flăj'ĕ-lāt). Having a single flagellum.

uniforate (ū"nĭ-fō'rāt) [" + *foratus*, pierced]. Having a single opening.

uniform. Having the identical shape or form of other objects of the same class.

unigerminal (ū"nĭ-jĕr'mĭ-năl). Concerning a single ovum or germ.

uniglandular (ū"nĭ-glăn'dū-lăr). Concerning one gland.

unigravida (ū"nĭ-grăv'ĭ-dă) [" + *gravida*, pregnant]. Woman who is pregnant for the first time. SEE: *primigravida.*

unilaminar (ū"nĭ-lăm'ĭ-năr). Having a single layer.

unilateral (ū"nĭ-lăt'ĕr-ăl) [" + *latus*, side]. Affecting or occurring on only one side. SEE: *contralateral; homolateral; ipsilateral.*

unilobar (ū"nĭ-lō'băr). Having a single lobe.

unilocular (ū"nĭ-lŏk'ū-lăr) [" + *loculus*, a small space]. Having only one cavity.

uninuclear (ū"nĭ-nū'klē-ăr) [" + *nucleus*, a kernel]. Having only one nucleus.

uninucleated (ū"nĭ-nū'klē-āt"ĕd). Having a

single nucleus.

uniocular (ū″nē-ŏk′ū-lăr) [″ + *oculus*, eye]. Pert. to or having only one eye.

union (ūn′yŭn) [L. *unio*]. 1. Act of joining two or more things into one part, or the state of being so united. 2. Growing together of severed or broken parts, as of bones or lips of a wound. SEE: *healing*.

    u., non-. Failure to unite, as a fractured bone that fails to heal completely.

    u., secondary. A healing by second intention with adhesion of granulating surfaces. SEE: *healing*.

    u., vicious. Union of ends of a broken bone in such a way as to cause deformity.

unioval (ū″nē-ō′văl) [L. *unus*, one, + *ovum*, egg]. Developed from one ovum, as identical twins.

uniovular (ū″nē-ŏv′ū-lăr) [″ + *ovum*, egg]. Monozygotic, as in the case of twins that develop from a single ovum.

unipara (ū-nĭp′ă-ră) [″ + *parere*, to bring forth, to bear]. A woman who has had one pregnancy over 20 weeks or has produced a fetus of 500 grams, regardless of the viability of the fetus. SEE: *primipara*.

uniparous (ū-nĭp′ă-rŭs) [″ + *parere*, to bring forth, to bear]. 1. Giving birth to one offspring at a time. 2. Having produced one child of 500 grams or having a pregnancy lasting 20 weeks, regardless of the viability of the fetus.

Unipen. Trade name for nafcillin sodium.

unipolar (ū″nĭ-pō′lăr) [″ + *polus*, pole]. 1. Having or pert. to one pole. 2. Having a single process, as a unipolar neuron.

unipotent, unipotential (ū-nĭp′ō-tĕnt, ū″nĭ-pō-tĕn′shăl). Concerning a cell that can only develop in a specific way to produce a certain end-result.

uniseptate (ū″nē-sĕp′tāt). Having only one septum.

unisex. 1. Lack of gender distinction by external appearance, esp. with respect to hair style or clothing. 2. Suitable for use by either sex.

Unisom. Trade name for doxylamine succinate.

unit (ū′nĭt) [L. *unus*, one]. 1. One of anything. 2. ABBR: u. A determined amount adopted as a standard of measurement.

    u., amboceptor. The smallest amount of amboceptor required in the presence of which a given quantity of red blood corpuscles will be hemolyzed by an excess of complement.

    u., angström. ABBR: Å or A.U. An internationally adopted unit of measurement of wavelength, 1/10,000,000 of a millimeter, or 1/254,000,000 of an inch.

    u., antigen. Smallest quantity of antigen required to fix one unit of complement.

    u., antitoxin. Unit for expressing the strength of an antitoxin. Originally the various units were defined biologically but now are compared to a weighed standard specified by the U.S. Public Health Service and the World Health Organization. SYN: *immunizing unit.*

    u., atomic mass. ABBR: AMU. One-twelfth of the mass of a neutral carbon atom. This is equal to 1.657×10^{-24} gram.

    u., Bodansky. In clinical chemistry, a unit of alkaline phosphatase equal to that which will liberate 1 mg of phosphorus as inorganic phosphate after one hour of incubation with a buffered substrate containing sodium β-glycerophosphate. SEE: *phosphatase, alkaline.*

    u., British thermal. ABBR: BTU. The amount of heat necessary to raise the temperature of one pound of water from 39°F to 40°F.

    u., cat. The amount of drug per kg of body weight just sufficient to kill a cat when injected intravenously slowly and continuously.

    u., complement. Smallest quantity of complement required for hemolysis of a given amount of red blood corpuscles with one amboceptor unit present.

    u., dental. 1. A masticatory unit consisting of a single tooth and its adnexa. 2. A mobile or fixed piece of equipment, usually complete with chair, light, engine, and other accessories or utilities necessary for dental examinations or operations.

    u., electrostatic. ABBR: ESU or ESE (from the German *elektrostatische Einheit*). Any static electricity unit based on the unit electrostatic charge expressed in the centimeter-gram-second system of measurement.

    u., hemolytic. The amount of inactivated immune serum that causes complete hemolysis of 1 ml of a 5% emulsion of washed red blood corpuscles in the presence of complement.

    u., international. Unit defined and adopted by the International Conference for Unification of Formulae. Used for measurement of hormones, enzymes, and some vitamins.

    u., light. A foot-candle, or the amount of light one ft from a standard candle. SEE: *candela; lumen.*

    u., Mache. ABBR: M.u. Unit of measurement of radium emanation.

    u., motor. Unit that provides motor activity. It consists of a somatic neuron cell and the muscles innervated by it.

    u., mouse. Least amount of estrogen that induces, in a spayed mouse, a characteristic desquamation of the vaginal epithelium.

u. of capacity. Capacity of a condenser that gives a difference of potential of one volt when charged with one coulomb. SYN: *curie; farad.*

u., rat. Greatest dilution of estrogen that will cause desquamation and cornification of vaginal epithelium during first day, if given to a mature spayed rat in three injections, every four hours.

u., SI. Any of the units specified by the International System of Units adopted by an International Conference of Weights and Measures in 1960. SEE: *SI Units* for tables; *SI Units* in *Appendix.*

u., Todd. In a test of inhibition hemolysis by enzymes such as antistreptolysin O, the reciprocal of the highest dilution that inhibits hemolysis.

u., USP. Any unit specified in the U.S. Pharmacopeia.

unitarian (ū-nĭ-tār′ē-ăn) [L. *unitarius*]. Composed of a single unit.

unitary (ū′nĭ-tĕr-ē). Rel. to a single unit.

unit dose. A dose form in which individual doses of medicine are prepared in each packet. This saves time in dispensing medicines, esp. to hospitalized patients.

United Network for Organ Sharing. ABBR: UNOS. An organization established in 1984 to facilitate donation of organs for possible transplantation. All hospitals are required by law to inform relatives of potential donors about UNOS. SEE: *death; dying; do not resuscitate; organ donation; transplantation.*

United States Adopted Names. ABBR: USAN. Dictionary of nonproprietary names, brand names, code designations, and Chemical Abstracts Service registry numbers for drugs published by the U.S. Pharmacopeial Convention, Inc. The purpose is to have nonproprietary names assigned to new drugs in accordance with established principles. SEE: *USAN and the USP Dictionary of Drug Names.*

United States Pharmacopeia. ABBR: USP followed by the edition number expressed in Roman numerals. USP XXII was published in 1985. The official pharmacopeia of the United States. SEE: *pharmacopeia, United States.*

United States Public Health Service. ABBR: USPHS. An agency of the U.S. Department of Health and Human Services (HHS). Broadly, its function is to assess needs and promote national and international health. Included in the organization are the Centers for Disease Control (CDC), Food and Drug Administration (FDA), Alcohol, Drug Abuse and Mental Health Administration, Agency for Toxic Substances

and Disease Registry, and various USPHS Regional Offices.

uniterminal (ū″nĭ-tĕr′mĭn-ăl) [L. *unus*, one, + *terminus*, end]. Having only one terminal. SEE: *monoterminal.*

univalence (ū″nĭ-vā′lĕns). The condition of having but one valence.

univalent (ū″nĭ-vā′lĕnt, ū-nĭv′ă-lĕnt) [″ + *valens*, to be powerful]. 1. Possessing the power of combining or replacing one atom of hydrogen. SYN: *monovalent.* 2. Single, noting a chromosome that lacks or fails to unite with a synaptic mate.

universal (ū″nĭ-vĕr′săl) [L. *universalis*, combined into one whole]. General or applicable or common to all situations or conditions.

universal antidote. Antidote used in poisoning where specific antidote is unknown or not available. Two parts activated charcoal; one part tannic acid; one part magnesium oxide. Give orally a paste of 5 heaping tsp of the mixture dissolved in a glass of water. After the patient has swallowed the antidote, the stomach contents should be removed by gastric lavage. In general, there is no universal antidote. The preferred general antidote is activated charcoal alone.

Caution: Do not use gastric lavage in patients who have ingested caustics. The stomach or esophagus may be ruptured by introduction of the tube.

---

universal cuff. An adapted device fitted around the palm of the hand to permit attachment of self-care tools when normal grasp is absent. SYN: *palmar cuff.*

universal donor. A person whose blood type is O, Rh negative. As a rule, blood from a universal donor may be transfused without danger of untoward reactions into persons belonging to any of the other ABO blood groups.

NOTE: Because there are multiple blood type factors in addition to those of ABO, it would be dangerous to assume that type O, Rh-negative blood could, without further tests for compatibility, be given to persons of different blood type.

universal dressing. A large flat bandage that may be folded several times to make a relatively large dressing or folded several more times to make a smaller and thicker bandage. This process can be continued until the unit is suitable for use as a cervical collar. SEE: *dressing, universal,* for illus.

universal recipient. A person belonging to blood type AB, Rh positive, whose serum will not agglutinate the cells of the other ABO blood. Nevertheless, the recipient's blood must be tested by cross-matching prior to the transfusion.

unmedullated (ŭn-mĕd′ū-lāt″ĕd). A nerve that does not contain a myelin sheath.

unmyelinated (ŭn-mī′ĕ-lĭ-nāt″ĕd). A nerve that does not contain a myelin sheath.

Unna's paste (oo′năz) [Paul G. Unna, Ger. dermatologist, 1850–1929]. A combination of 15% zinc oxide in a glycogelatin base. Trade name is Dome paste.

Unna's (paste) boot. A bootlike dressing of the lower extremity made of layers of gauze and Unna's paste. It is used in treating chronic ulcers, usually due to varicosities, of the leg.

unofficial (ŭn-ō-fĭsh′ăl) [AS. *un*, not, + L. *officialis*, doing work]. Indicates a drug not listed by the U.S. Pharmacopeia or National Formulary.

unorganized (ŭn-or′găn-īzd) [″ + L. *organizare*, to form a structure]. 1. Not organized into an organic structure. 2. Without characteristics of a living organism; inorganic.

UNOS. *United Network for Organ Sharing.*

unphysiological (ŭn-fĭz-ē-ō-lŏj′ĭk-ăl). Contrary to physiological principles.

unrest. Turbulence, instability, or irregularity.

unsaturated (ŭn-săt′ū-rāt″ĕd) [″ + L. *saturare*, to fill]. 1. Capable of dissolving or absorbing to a greater degree. 2. Not combined to the greatest possible extent.

unsaturated compound. An organic compound having double or triple bonds between the carbon atoms.

unsex (ŭn-sĕks′) [″ + L. *sexus*, sex]. 1. To castrate; to spay or excise the ovaries. 2. To deprive of sexual character.

unstriated (ŭn-strī′ăt-ĕd) [″ + *striatus*, striped]. Unstriped, as smooth muscle fiber.

unthrifty. Not healthy or robust, esp. when describing plants or animals.

Unverricht's disease, syndrome (oon′fĕr-ĭkts) [Heinrich Unverricht, Ger. physician, 1853–1912]. A rare, fatal disease inherited as an autosomal recessive trait. It is characterized by the onset in later childhood of progressive myoclonic epilepsy, tetraplegia, and dementia. Also: *Unverricht-Lafora disease.*

unwell [″ + *wel*, well]. Sick; ill; indisposed.

upper airway obstruction. ABBR: UAO. Condition of the respiratory system in which it has the capability of functioning but is prevented from doing so by an obstruction in the upper portion of the airway, such as the main bronchus, larynx, mouth, or nose. SEE: *cardiopulmonary resuscitation; tracheostomy.*

upper GI. *upper gastrointestinal.* Radiographic and fluoroscopic examinations of the stomach and duodenum after the ingestion of a contrast medium.

upper motor neuron lesion. Neurological condition resulting from damage to corticospinal or pyramidal tract in the brain or spinal cord. Results in hemiplegia, paraplegia, or quadriplegia, depending upon the location and extent of the lesion. Clinical signs include loss of voluntary movement, spasticity, sensory loss, and pathological reflexes.

upper respiratory infection. ABBR: URI. An imprecise term for almost any kind of infectious disease process involving the nasal passages, pharynx, and bronchi. The etiological agent may be bacterial or viral.

upsiloid (ŭp′sĭ-loyd) [Gr. *upsilon*, letter U, + *eidos*, form, shape]. Shaped like the letter U or V.

uptake (ŭp′tāk). The absorption of nutrients, chemicals (including radioactive materials), and medicines by tissues or by an entire organism.

urachal (ū′ră-kăl) [Gr. *ourachos*, fetal urinary canal]. Rel. to the urachus.

urachus (ū′ră-kŭs) [Gr. *ourachos*, fetal urinary canal]. An epithelioid cord surrounded by fibrous tissue extending from the apex of the bladder to the umbilicus. In the embryo it is continuous with the allantoic stalk; postnatally it forms the middle umbilical ligament of the bladder.

   u., patent. Condition in which the urachus remains as a hollow tube that connects the vertex of the bladder with the umbilicus, resulting in an umbilical urinary fistula.

uracil (ū′ră-sĭl). $C_4H_4N_2O_2$. A pyrimidine base found in ribonucleic acids.

uracil mustard. USP. An alkylating type of cytotoxic drug used in treating certain types of malignant tumors.

Caution: Handle this drug with exceptional care. It must be handled in a well-ventilated hood, using a protective mask, protective glasses, and gloves. Thoroughly clean the work area afterward, and rinse hands in water for several minutes; then wash with soap and water.

---

uracrasia (ū-ră-krā′sē-ă) [Gr. *ouron*, urine, + *akrasia*, bad mixture]. Inability to retain urine. SEE: *enuresis; incontinence, urinary stress.*

uracratia (ū-ră-krā′shē-ă) [″ + *akratia*, incontinence]. Incontinence of the urine.

uragogue (ū′ră-gŏg) [″ + *agogos*, leading]. Increasing the secretion of urine. SYN: *diuretic.*

uranisconitis (ū-răn-ĭs″kŏn-ī′tĭs) [Gr. *ouraniskos*, palate, + *itis*, inflammation]. Inflammation of the palate.

uraniscoplasty (ū-răn-ĭs′kō-plăs″tē) [″ + *plassein*, to form]. Operation for repair of cleft palate. SYN: *uranoplasty; uranorrhaphy.*

uraniscorrhaphy (ū″răn-ĭs-kor′ră-fē) [″ + *rhaphe*, seam, ridge]. Operation for suturing of a cleft palate. SYN: *uraniscoplasty.*

uraniscus (ū-răn-ĭs′kŭs) [Gr. *ouraniskos*, palate]. Palate, or roof of mouth.

uranium (ū-rā′nē-ŭm) [LL., planet Uranus]. SYMB: U. At. wt. 238.029; at. no. 92. A radioactive element, the parent of radium and other radioelements. Uranium ore contains the isotopes ^{238}U, ^{235}U, and ^{234}U.

uranoplasty (ū′răn-ō-plăs″tē) [Gr. *ouranos*, palate, + *plassein*, to form]. Operation for cleft palate. SYN: *uraniscoplasty.*

uranoplegia (ū″ră-nō-plē′jē-ă) [″ + *plege*, stroke]. Paralysis of muscles of the soft palate.

uranorrhaphy (ū-răn-or′ră-fē) [″ + *rhaphe*, seam, ridge]. Operation for suture of a cleft palate. SYN: *uraniscorrhaphy.*

uranoschisis (ū-răn-ŏs′kĭs-ĭs) [″ + *schisis*, a splitting]. Cleft palate.

uranostaphyloplasty (ū″răn-ō-stăf″ĭl-ō-plăs″tē) [″ + *staphyle*, uvula, + *plassein*, to form]. Operation for correction of a defect of the soft and hard palates.

uranostaphylorrhaphy (ū″răn-ō-stăf-ĭl-or′ă-fē) [″ + ″ + *rhaphe*, seam, ridge]. Operation for repair of cleft of hard and soft palates.

uranostaphyloschisis (ū″ră-nō-stăf″ĭ-lŏs′kĭ-sĭs). Cleft of the hard and soft palate.

uranyl (ū′ră-nĭl). The bivalent uranium radical UO^{++}. It forms salts with many acids. An example is uranyl nitrate, UO_2 $(NO_3)_2$.

urapostema (ū″ră-pŏs-tē′mă) [Gr. *ouron*, urine, + *apostema*, abscess]. An abscess containing urine.

uraroma (ū-ră-rō′mă) [″ + *aroma*, spice]. Aromatic spicy odor of the urine.

urarthritis (ū″răr-thrī′tĭs). Arthritis due to gout.

urase (ū′rās). Urease.

urate (ū′rāt) [Gr. *ouron*, urine]. Combination of uric acid with a base; a salt of uric acid. Urates are normally present in urine.

uratemia (ū″ră-tē′mē-ă) [″ + *haima*, blood]. Urates, esp. sodium urate, in the blood.

uratic (ū-răt′ĭk). Concerning urates or gout.

uratoma (ū″ră-tō′mă). Concretions of urates around joints caused by gout; a tophus.

uratosis (ū″ră-tō′sĭs). Any condition leading to deposition of urates in tissues.

uraturia (ū″ră-tū′rē-ă) [Gr. *ouron*, urine]. Excess of urates in the urine. SYN: *lithuria.*

urceiform (ŭr-sē′ĭ-form) [L. *urceus*, pitcher, + *forma*, shape]. Pitcher-shaped.

urceolate (ŭr-sē′ō-lāt). Urceiform, q.v.

ur-defense(s) (ŭr″dē-fēns′) [Ger. *ur*, ultimate, + *defense*]. Basic beliefs, such as

religious or scientific ones, that are thought by the individual to be essential to man's emotional well-being. These beliefs may include faith in a personal or universal God or the fundamental goodness of mankind.

urea (ū-rē′ă) [Gr. *ouron*, urine]. 1. The diamide of carbonic acid, a crystalline solid having the formula CH_4N_2O; found in blood, lymph, and urine. It is formed in the liver from ammonia derived from amino acids by deamination. It may also be formed directly from arginine.

Urea is the chief nitrogenous constituent of urine and, along with CO_2, is the final product of protein metabolism in the body. In normal conditions, urea represents 80% to 90% of the total urinary nitrogen. It is odorless and colorless, appearing as white prismatic crystals, and forming salts with acids. Its excess is one of the signs of uremia, q.v. The amount of urea excreted varies directly with the amount of protein in the diet. Excretion is increased in fever, diabetes, or increased activity of the adrenal gland.

USES: As a diuretic.

2. USP. A standardized preparation of urea used as a diuretic. Trade name is Ureaphil.

urea cycle. The complex cyclic chemical reactions in some (ureotelic) animals, including man, that produce urea from the metabolism of nitrogen-containing foods. This cycle provides a method of excreting the nitrogen produced by the metabolism of amino acids as urea. The cycle was first described by Sir Hans Krebs [1900–1981].

urea frost. White flaky deposits of urea seen on skin in patients with advanced uremia.

ureagenesis. Ureapoiesis, q.v.

ureagenetic (ū-rē″ă-jĕn-ĕt′ĭk) [″ + *genesis*, generation, birth]. Pert. to or producing urea.

ureal (ū-rē′ăl). Rel. to or containing urea.

ureametry (ū-rē-ăm′ĕt-rē). Determination of amount of urea in urine.

urea nitrogen. ABBR: BUN. The nitrogen of urea as distinguished from nitrogen in blood proteins.

Ureaphil. Trade name for urea.

Ureaplasma urealyticum. A microorganism of the genus Mycoplasma. It is usually sexually transmitted. It may cause inflammation of the urogenital tract in males and females.

urease (ū′rē-ās) [Gr. *ouron*, urine]. An enzyme that accelerates hydrolysis of urea into ammonium carbonate and hippuric acid into glycocoll and benzoic acid. It is found in alkaline fermentation of urine, is produced by many microorganisms, and is also found in jack beans and soybeans. It is used in determining the amount of urea in blood or in urine.

urecchysis (ū-rĕk'ĭs-ĭs) [" + *ekchysis,* a pouring out]. Effusion of urine into tissues.

Urecholine. Trade name for bethanechol chloride.

uredema (ū-rĕ-dē'mă) [" + *oidema,* swelling]. Urine in the subcutaneous tissues, thus distending them.

ureide (ū'rē-īd) [Gr. *ouron,* urine]. Any compound of urea in which acid radicals have taken the place of one or more of its hydrogen atoms.

urelcosis (ū-rĕl-kō'sĭs) [" + *helkosis,* ulceration]. Ulceration of the urinary tract.

uremia (ū-rē'mē-ă) [" + *haima,* blood]. Toxic condition associated with renal insufficiency produced by the retention in the blood of nitrogenous substances normally excreted by the kidney. SEE: *azotemia; coma, uremic.*

SYM: Nausea, vomiting, headache, dizziness, dimness of vision, coma or convulsions, urinous odor of breath and perspiration. Stupor, stertorous respiration. No change in pupillary reaction; dry skin; hard rapid pulse; elevated blood pressure; scanty urine containing casts and albumin. There is a reduction of urea in the urine, and tube casts are present. Urea retention is 150 to 500 mg or more per decaliter of blood.

ETIOL: Result of disturbed kidney function seen in nephritis and due to suppression or deficient secretion of urine from any cause.

TREAT: Dialysis.

u., extrarenal. U., prerenal.

u., prerenal. Uremia occurring not as a result of primary renal disease but due to other conditions such as disturbances in circulation, fluid balance, or metabolism arising in other parts of the body.

uremic (ū-rē'mĭk). Pert. to or caused by uremia.

uremigenic (ū-rē'mĭ-jĕn'ĭk) [Gr. *ouron,* urine, + *haima,* blood, + *gennan,* to produce]. Caused by or producing uremia.

ureogenesis (ūr''ē-ō-jĕn'ē-sĭs) [" + *genesis,* generation, birth]. Formation of urea.

ureotelic (ū''rē-ō-tĕl'ĭk) [*urea* + Gr. *telikos,* belonging to the completion]. Concerning animals that excrete amino nitrogen in the form of urea. Included in this group are mammals, including most terrestrial vertebrates. SEE: *ammonotelic; urea cycle; uricotelic.*

uresiesthesia, uresiesthesis (ū-rē''sē-ĕs-thē'zē-ă, -sĭs) [Gr. *ouresis,* urination, + *aisthesis,* sensation]. The normal inclination to void urine.

uresis (ū-rē'sĭs) [Gr. *ouresis*]. The passage of urine. SYN: *urination.*

ureter (ū'rĕ-ter, ū-rē'tĕr) [Gr. *oureter*]. The tube that carries urine from the kidney to the bladder. It originates in the pelvis of the kidney and terminates in the base of the bladder. Each kidney has one ureter measuring from 28 to 34 cm long, the right being slightly shorter than the left. The diameter varies from 1 mm to 1 cm. The wall consists of three layers: the mucosal, muscular, and fibrous coats. SEE: *kidney; urethra.*

ureteral (ū-rē'tĕr-ăl). Concerning the ureter.

ureteralgia (ū''rē-tĕr-ăl'jē-ă) [" + *algos,* pain]. Pain in the ureter.

uretercystoscope (ū-rē''tĕr-sĭs'tō-skōp) [" + *kystis,* bladder, + *skopein,* to examine]. A cystoscope combined with a ureteral catheter.

ureterectasis (ū-rē''tĕr-ĕk'tă-sĭs) [" + *ektasis,* dilatation]. Dilatation of the ureter.

ureterectomy (ū-rē''tĕr-ĕk'tō-mē) [" + *ektome,* excision]. Excision of a ureter.

ureteric (ū''rĕ-tĕr'ĭk). Ureteral, q.v.

ureteritis (ū-rē''tĕr-ī'tĭs) [" + *itis,* inflammation]. Inflammation of the ureters.

uretero-. Combining form concerning the ureter.

ureterocele (ū-rē'tĕr-ō-sēl) [" + *kele,* tumor, swelling]. Cystlike dilatation of the ureter near its opening into the bladder. Usually a result of congenital stenosis of ureteral orifice.

ureterocelectomy (ū-rē''tĕr-ō-sē-lĕk'tō-mē) [" + " + *ektome,* excision]. Surgical removal of a ureterocele.

ureterocervical (ū-rē''tĕr-ō-sĕr'vĭ-kăl) [" + L. *cervicalis,* pert. to cervix]. Concerning the ureter and the cervix uteri.

ureterocolostomy (ū-rē''tĕr-ō-kō-lŏs'tō-mē) [" + *kolon,* colon, + *stoma,* mouth]. The implantation of the ureter into the colon.

ureterocystanastomosis (ū-rē''tĕr-ō-sĭs''tă-năs''tō-mō'sĭs) [Gr. *oureter,* ureter, + *kystis,* bladder, + *anastomosis,* opening]. Ureteroneocystostomy, q.v.

ureterocystoneostomy (ū-rē''tĕr-ō-sĭst''ō-nē-ŏs'tō-mē) [" + *kystis,* bladder, + *neos,* new, + *stoma,* mouth]. Ureteroneocystostomy.

ureterocystoscope (ū-rē''tĕr-ō-sĭs'tō-skōp) [" + " + *skopein,* to view]. Uretercystoscope, q.v.

ureterocystostomy (ū-rē''tĕr-ō-sĭs-tŏs'tō-mē) [" + " + *stoma,* mouth]. Ureteroneocystostomy.

ureterodialysis (ū-rē''tĕr-ō-dī-ăl'ĭ-sĭs) [" + *dialysis,* a separation]. Rupture of a ureter. SYN: *ureterolysis.*

ureteroenterostomy (ū-rē''tĕr-ō-ĕn-tĕr-ŏs'tō-mē) [" + *enteron,* intestine, + *stoma,* mouth]. Formation of a passage between a ureter and the intestine.

ureterography (ū-rē''tĕr-ŏg'ră-fē) [" +

graphein, to write]. Radiography of the ureter after injection of a radiopaque substance into it.

ureteroheminephrectomy (ū-rē″tĕr-ō-hĕm″ĭ-nĕ-frĕk′tō-mē) [″ + *hemi-*, half, + *nephros*, kidney, + *ektome*, excision]. In cases of reduplication of the upper urinary tract on one side, surgical removal of the reduplicated portion.

ureterohydronephrosis (ū-rē″tĕr-ō-hī″drō-nĕ-frō′sĭs) [″ + *hydor*, water, + *nephros*, kidney, + *osis*, condition]. Dilatation of ureter and pelvis of the kidney resulting from a mechanical or inflammatory obstruction in the urinary tract.

ureteroileostomy (ū-rē″tĕr-ō-ĭl″ē-ŏs′tō-mē) [″ + *ileum*, ileum, + *stoma*, mouth]. Surgical anastomosis of a ureter to an isolated segment of the ileum. The ileum is connected to an abdominal stoma so that urine leaves the body via that opening.

ureterolith (ū-rē′tĕr-ō-lĭth) [″ + *lithos*, stone]. A stone or calculus in the ureter.

ureterolithiasis (ū-rē″tĕr-ō-lĭth-ī′ăs-ĭs) [″ + ″ + *iasis*, condition]. Development of a calculus in the ureter.

ureterolithotomy (ū-rē″tĕr-ō-lĭth-ŏt′ō-mē) [″ + ″ + *tome*, incision]. Surgical incision for removal of a calculus from the ureter.

ureterolysis (ū-rē″tĕr-ŏl′ĭ-sĭs) [″ + *lysis*, dissolution]. 1. Rupture of the ureter. 2. Paralysis of the ureter. 3. The process of loosening adhesions around the ureter.

ureteroneocystostomy (ū-rē″tĕr-ō-nē″ō-sĭs-tŏs′tō-mē) [″ + *neos*, new, + *kystis*, bladder, + *stoma*, mouth]. Surgical formation of a new passage between a ureter and the bladder. SYN:*ureterocystoneostomy; ureterocystostomy.*

ureteroneopyelostomy (ū-rē″tĕr-ō-nē″ō-pī-ĕ-lŏs′tō-mē) [″ + ″ + *pyelos*, pelvis, + *stoma*, mouth]. Excision of a portion of the ureter with attachment of the severed end of the lower portion to a new aperture in the renal pelvis. SYN: *ureteropyeloneostomy.*

ureteronephrectomy (ū-rē″tĕr-ō-nĕf-rĕk′tō-mē) [″ + *nephros*, kidney, + *ektome*, excision]. Removal of a kidney and its ureter.

ureteropathy (ū-rē″tĕr-ŏp′ă-thē) [″ + *pathos*, disease]. Any diseased condition of the ureter.

ureteropelvioplasty (ū-rē″tĕr-ō-pĕl′vē-ō-plăs″tē) [Gr. *oureter*, ureter, + L. *pelvis*, basin, + Gr. *plassein*, to mold]. Plastic surgery of the junction of the ureter and the pelvis of the kidney.

ureterophlegma (ū-rē″tĕr-ō-flĕg′mă) [″ + *phlegma*, phlegm]. Accumulation of mucus in the ureter.

ureteroplasty (ū-rē′tĕr-ō-plăs″tē) [″ + *plassein*, to form]. Plastic surgery of the ureter.

ureteroproctostomy (ū-rē″tĕr-ō-prŏk-tŏs′tō-mē) [″ + *proktos*, anus, + *stoma*, mouth]. Formation of a passage from the ureter to the lower rectum.

ureteropyelitis (ū-rē″tĕr-ō-pī-ĕl-ī′tĭs) [″ + *pyelos*, pelvis, + *itis*, inflammation]. Inflammation of the pelvis of the kidney and a ureter.

ureteropyeloneostomy (ū-rē″tĕr-ō-pī″ĕl-ō-nē-ŏs′tō-mē) [″ + ″ + *neos*, new, + *stoma*, mouth]. Ureteroneopyelostomy.

ureteropyelonephritis (ū-rē″tĕr-ō-pī″ĕl-ō-nĕf-rī′tĭs) [″ + ″ + *nephros*, kidney, + *itis*, inflammation]. Inflammation of the renal pelvis and the ureter.

ureteropyeloplasty (ū-rē″tĕr-ō-pī′ĕl-ō-plăs″tē) [″ + ″ + *plassein*, to mold]. Plastic surgery of the ureter and renal pelvis.

ureteropyelostomy (ū-rē″tĕr-ō-pī″ĕ-lŏs′tō-mē) [″ + ″ + *stoma*, mouth]. Ureteropyeloneostomy.

ureteropyosis (ū-rē″tĕr-ō-pī-ō′sĭs) [″ + *pyon*, pus, + *osis*, condition]. Suppurative inflammation within a ureter.

ureterorectostomy (ū-rē″tĕr-ō-rĕk-tŏs′tō-mē) [″ + L. *rectum*, straight, + Gr. *stoma*, mouth]. Ureteroproctostomy.

ureterorrhagia (ū-rē″tĕr-or-ră′jē-ă) [″ + *rhegnynai*, to burst forth]. Hemorrhage from the ureter.

ureterorrhaphy (ū-rē″tĕr-or′ră-fē) [″ + *rhaphe*, seam, ridge]. Suture of the ureter, as for fistula.

ureterosigmoidostomy (ū-rē″tĕr-ō-sĭg-moyd-ŏs′tō-mē) [″ + *sigma*, letter S, + *eidos*, shape, + *stoma*, mouth]. Surgical implantation of the ureter into the sigmoid flexure.

ureterostegnosis (ū-rē″tĕr-ō-stĕg-nō′sĭs). Ureterostenosis.

ureterostenosis (ū-rē″tĕr-ō-stĕn-ō′sĭs) [″ + *stenosis*, a narrowing]. Stricture of a ureter.

ureterostoma (ū″rē-tĕr-ō-stō′mă) [Gr. *oureter*, ureter, + *stoma*, mouth]. The orifice through which the ureter enters the urinary bladder.

ureterostomy (ū-rē″tĕr-ŏs′tō-mē) [″ + *stoma*, mouth]. Formation of a permanent fistula for drainage of a ureter.

   u., cutaneous. Surgical implantation of the ureter into the skin. This allows urine to drain via the ureter to the outside of the body by going through the stoma.

ureterotomy (ū-rē″tĕr-ŏt′ō-mē) [″ + *tome*, incision]. Incision or surgery of the ureter.

ureterotrigonoenterostomy (ū-rē″tĕr-ō-trī-gŏ"nō-ĕn"tĕr-ŏs'tō-mē) [" + *tri-gonon*, three-sided figure, + *enteron*, intestine, + *stoma*, mouth]. Surgical removal of the trigone of the bladder with one or both of the ureteral openings and implanting it into the intestine.

ureteroureteral (ū-rē"tĕr-ō-ū-rē'tĕr-ăl) [" + *oureter*, ureter]. Concerning two parts of the same ureter or the union of one ureter with the other.

ureteroureterostomy (ū-rē"tĕr-ō-ū-rē"tĕr-ŏs'tō-mē) [" + " + *stoma*, mouth]. 1. Formation of a connection from one ureter to the other. 2. Re-establishment of a passage between the ends of a divided ureter.

ureterouterine (ū-rē"tĕr-ō-ū'tĕr-ĭn) [" + L. *uterus*, womb]. Concerning the ureter and uterus or a fistula between them.

ureterovaginal (ū-rē"tĕr-ō-văj'ĭ-năl) [" + L. *vagina*, sheath]. Relating to a ureter and the vagina, noting a fistula connecting them.

ureterovesical (ū-rē"tĕr-ō-vĕs'ĭ-kăl) [" + L. *vesica*, bladder]. Pert. to a connection between the ureter and bladder.

ureterovesicostomy (ū-rē"tĕr-ō-vĕs"ĭ-kŏs'tō-mē) [" + " + Gr. *stoma*, mouth]. Reimplantation of a ureter into the bladder.

urethra (ū-rē'thră) [Gr. *ourethra*]. A canal for the discharge of urine extending from the bladder to the outside. In the female its orifice lies in the vestibule between the vagina and clitoris; in the male the urethra traverses the penis, opening at the tip of the glans penis. In the male it serves as the passage for semen as well as urine. Its inner lining, the mucosa, is thrown into folds and contains openings of lacunae into which the glands of Littre open. Surrounding the mucosa is a lamina propria containing many elastic fibers and blood vessels, outside of which is an indefinite muscular layer. SEE: *penis*.

    u. muliebris. The female urethra.

    u. virilis. The male urethra.

urethra, words pert. to: aerourethroscopy; anaspadias; ankylurethria; atreturethria; bulb; bulbourethral glands; corpus spongiosum; gleet; habenula urethralis; hypospadias; meatus urinarius; Skene's glands; urelcosis; "urethr-" words.

urethral (ū-rē'thrăl) [Gr. *ourethra*, urethra]. Relating to the urethra.

urethralgia (ū-rē-thrăl'jē-ă) [" + *algos*, pain]. Pain in the urethra.

urethral syndrome. SEE: *acute urethral syndrome.*

urethrascope (ū-rē'thră-skōp). Urethroscope.

urethratresia (ū-rē"thră-trē'zē-ă) [" + *a-*, not, + *tresis*, a perforation]. Occlusion, or

imperforation of the urethra.

urethrectomy (ū-rē-thrĕk'tō-mē) [" + *ektome*, excision]. Surgical excision of the urethra or part of it.

urethremphraxis (ū"rē-thrĕm-frăk'sĭs) [" + *emphraxis*, an obstruction]. Urethral obstruction. SYN: *urethrophraxis.*

urethreurynter (ū-rĕth"rūr-ĭn'tĕr) [" + *eurynein*, to dilate]. Appliance for dilating the urethra.

urethrism, urethrismus (ū'rē-thrĭzm, ū"rē-thrĭz'mŭs) [" + *-ismos*, condition]. Irritability or spasm of the urethra.

urethritis (ū"rē-thrī'tĭs) [" + *itis*, inflammation]. Inflammation of the urethra.

    u., anterior. Inflammation of that portion of the urethra anterior to the anterior layer of the triangular ligament.

    u., gonococcal. Urethritis caused by gonococcus.

    u., nongonococcal. ABBR: NGU. U., nonspecific, q.v.

    u., nonspecific. ABBR: NSU. Inflammation and irritation of the urethra that in the past was not directly attributable to a specific organism. About half of the cases are due to *Chlamydia trachomatis.*

    TREAT: Both tetracyclines and erythromycin are of benefit. The latter drug should be used if the patient is pregnant. Test for syphilis before and after initiating therapy. Patient should abstain from sexual intercourse until cured.

    u., posterior. Inflammation of membranous and prostatic portions of the urethra.

    u., specific. Urethritis due to a specific organism, usually gonococcus.

urethro- [Gr. *ourethra*]. Combining form meaning urethra.

urethrobulbar (ū-rē"thrō-bŭl'băr). Concerning the urethra and the bulbar penis.

urethrocele (ū-rē'thrō-sēl) [" + *kele*, tumor, swelling]. 1. Pouchlike protrusion of the urethral wall in the female. 2. Thickening of connective tissue around the urethra in the female.

urethrocystitis (ū-rē"thrō-sĭs-tī'tĭs) [" + *kystis*, bladder, + *itis*, inflammation]. Inflammation of the urethra and bladder.

urethrocystopexy (ū-rē"thrō-sĭs'tō-pĕk"sē) [" + *kystis*, bladder, + *pexis*, fixation]. Plastic surgery of the urethral-bladder junction in order to relieve urinary stress incontinence.

urethrodynia (ū-rē"thrō-dĭn'ē-ă) [" + *odyne*, pain]. Urethralgia.

urethrograph (ū-rē'thrō-grăf). Device for recording the caliber of the urethra.

urethrography (ū-rē-thrŏg'ră-fē) [" + *graphein*, to write]. Roentgenography of the urethra after the injection of a radiopaque substance into it.

u., voiding. Radiographic examination of the urethra during micturition after the introduction of a contrast medium.

urethrometer (ū-rē-thrŏm'ĕt-ĕr) [Gr. *ourethra,* urethra, + *metron,* measure]. Instrument for measuring diameter of the urethra or lumen of a stricture.

urethropenile (ū-rē″thrō-pē'nīl) [″ + L. *penis,* penis]. Relating to the urethra and penis.

urethroperineal (ū-rē″thrō-pĕr-ĭ-nē'ăl) [″ + *perinaion,* perineum]. Rel. to the urethra and perineum.

urethroperineoscrotal (ū-rē″thrō-pĕr-ĭ-nē″ō-skrō'tăl) [″ + ″ + L. *scrotum,* a bag]. Relating to the urethra, perineum, and scrotum.

urethropexy (ū-rē'thrō-pĕks-ē) [″ + Gr. *pexis,* fixation]. Surgical fixation of the urethra.

urethrophraxis (ū-rē-thrō-frăks'ĭs) [″ + *phrassein,* to obstruct]. Urethral obstruction. SYN: *urethremphraxis.*

urethrophyma (ū-rē-thrō-fī'mă) [″ + *phyma,* growth]. A neoplasm in the urethra.

urethroplasty (ū-rē'thrō-plăs″tē) [″ + *plassein,* to mold]. Reparative surgery of the urethra.

urethroprostatic (ū-rē″thrō-prŏs-tăt'ĭk). Concerning the urethra and prostate.

urethrorectal (ū-rē″thrō-rĕk'tăl) [Gr. *ourethra,* urethra, + L. *rectus,* straight]. Rel. to the urethra and rectum.

urethrorrhagia (ū-rē″thror-ā'jē-ă) [″ + *rhegnynai,* to burst forth]. Hemorrhage from the urethra.

urethrorrhaphy (ū-rē-thror'ăf-ē) [″ + *rhaphe,* seam, ridge]. Suture of the urethra or of a urethral fistula.

urethrorrhea (ū-rē″thror-ē'ă) [″ + *rhoia,* flow]. Abnormal discharge from the urethra.

u. ex libidine. The discharge of normal glandular secretions resulting from sexual stimulation, esp. that preceding sexual intercourse. SEE: *Cowper's glands.*

urethroscope (ū-rē'thrō-skōp) [″ + *skopein,* to examine]. Device for examining the interior of the urethra.

urethroscopic (ū-rē″thrō-skŏp'ĭk). Relating to the urethroscope or urethroscopy.

urethroscopy (ū-rē-thrŏs'kō-pē). An examination of the mucous membrane of the urethra with a urethroscope.

urethrospasm (ū-rē'thrō-spăzm) [″ + *spasmos,* a convulsion]. Spasmodic stricture of the urethra.

urethrostaxis (ū-rē″thrō-stăks'ĭs) [″ + *staxis,* a dropping]. Oozing of blood from the urethral mucous membrane.

urethrostenosis (ū-rē″thrō-stĕn-ō'sĭs) [″ + *stenosis,* act of narrowing]. Stricture of

the urethra.

urethrostomy (ū-rē-thrŏs'tō-mē) [″ + *stoma,* mouth]. Formation of a permanent fistula opening into the urethra by perineal section and fixation of membranous urethra in the perineum.

urethrotome (ū-rē'thrō-tōm) [″ + *tome,* incision]. An instrument for incision of urethral stricture.

urethrotomy (ū-rē-thrŏt'ō-mē). Incision of a urethral stricture.

urethrotrigonitis (ū-rē″thrō-trī″gō-nī'tĭs) [″ + *trigonon,* three-sided figure, + *itis,* inflammation]. Inflammation of the urethra and the trigone of the bladder.

urethrovaginal (ū-rē″thrō-văj'ĭ-năl) [″ + L. *vagina,* sheath]. Pert. to the urethra and vagina.

urethrovesical (ū-rē″thrō-vĕs'ĭ-kăl) [″ + L. *vesicula,* little bladder]. Concerning the urethra and the bladder.

uretic. Concerning urine.

urhydrosis (ūr″hī-drō'sĭs) [Gr. *ouron,* urine, + *hidros,* sweat]. Excretion of urea in sweat.

URI. *upper respiratory infection.*

uric (ū'rĭk) [Gr. *ourikos,* urine]. Of or pert. to urine.

uric acid. $C_5H_4N_4O_3$. A crystalline acid occurring as an end product of purine metabolism. It is formed from purine bases derived from nucleoproteins. It is a common constituent of urinary and renal calculi and of gouty concretions.

OUTPUT: Between 0.5 and 1 gm per day if patient is on ordinary mixed diet. Uric acid must be excreted because it cannot be destroyed within the body.

Increased elimination is observed in ingestion of proteins and nitrogenous foods, after exercise, and in gout, leukemia, and acute articular rheumatism. Decreased elimination is observed in nephritis, chlorosis, lead poisoning, and protein-free diet.

u.a., endogenous. Uric acid derived from purines undergoing metabolism from the nucleoprotein of body tissues.

u.a., exogenous. Uric acid derived from those purines from food made up of free purines and nucleoproteins. SEE: *urate; uraturia.*

uricacidemia (ū″rĭk-ăs-ĭd-ē'mē-ă) [Gr. *ourikos,* urine, + L. *acidus,* sour, + Gr. *haima,* blood]. Excess uric acid in the blood.

uricaciduria (ū″rĭk-ăs-ĭd-ū'rē-ă) [″ + ″ + Gr. *ouron,* urine]. Excessive amount of uric acid in the urine.

uricase (ū'rĭ-kāz) [″ + *-ase,* enzyme]. An enzyme present in the liver and kidneys of most mammals, but not humans. This enzyme is capable of oxidizing uric acid into allantoin and carbon dioxide.

uricemia (ū-rĭ-sē'mē-ă) [" + *haima*, blood]. Excess uric acid in the blood. SYN: *uricacidemia.*

uricocholia (ū″rĭ-kō-kō'lē-ă) [" + *chole*, bile]. Uric acid in the bile.

uricolysis (ū-rĭ-kŏl'ĭ-sĭs) [" + *lysis*, dissolution]. The decomposition of uric acid.

uricolytic (ū″rĭ-kō-lĭt'ĭk). Decomposing uric acid.

uricometer (ū″rĭk-ŏm'ĕ-ter) [" + *metron*, measure]. Apparatus for quantitative estimation of uric acid in the urine.

uricopoiesis (ū″rĭ-kō-poy-ē'sĭs) [" + *poiesis*, formation]. Producing uric acid.

uricosuria (ū″rĭ-kō-sū'rē-ă) [" + *ouron*, urine]. The excessive excretion of uric acid in the urine.

uricosuric (ū″rĭ-kō-sū'rĭk). Potentiating the excretion of uric acid in the urine.

uricosuric agent. A drug (such as probenecid) that increases the urinary excretion of uric acid, thereby reducing the concentration of uric acid in the blood. Used in treatment of gout.

   NURSING IMPLICATIONS: Assess patient for history of gastrointestinal complaints or ulceration. Assess for drug sensitivities and drug regimens to prevent interactions. Advise patient to take drugs with milk or food. Advise fluid intake of at least 3000 ml/day (unless contraindicated), and alkalinization of urine with sodium bicarbonate and alkaline ash diet to prevent uric acid crystallization until serum urate levels return to normal. Instruct patient to avoid use of salicylates while probenecid is being taken; acetaminophen may be used for analgesia. Instruct patient to report gastrointestinal side effects.

uricotelic (ū″rĭ-kō-tĕl'ĭk) [" + *telikos*, belonging to the completion]. Concerning animals that excrete amino nitrogen in the form of uric acid. Included in this group are birds, snakes, and lizards. SEE: *ammonotelic; urea cycle; ureotelic.*

uricoxidase (ū″rĭk-ŏks'ĭ-dās) [" + *oxys*, sharp, + *-ase*, enzyme]. An enzyme capable of oxidizing uric acid.

uridine (ūr'ĭ-dĭn). A nucleoside that is one of the four main riboside components of ribonucleic acid. It consists of uracil and D-ribose.

   u. diphosphate. A uridine-containing nucleotide important in certain metabolic reactions, in which it transports sugars such as glucose and galactose.

uridrosis (ū-rĭ-drō'sĭs) [" + *hidrosis*, a sweating]. The presence of urea in the sweat. Evaporation may show white scales, the crystals of urea.

   u. crystallina. White powder of uric acid deposited on the skin. SYN: *urea frost.*

uriesthesis (ū-rē-ĕs-thē'sĭs) [" + *aisthesis*, sensation]. Normal desire to void urine.

urinaccelerator (ū″rĭn-ăk-sĕl'ĕr-ā″tor). Musculus bulbospongiosus.

urinal (ū'rĭn-ăl) [L. *urina*, urine]. A container into which one urinates. Also a toilet or bathroom fixture for receiving urine and flushing it away.

   u. condom. Catheter, condom, q.v.

urinalysis (ū″rĭ-năl'ĭ-sĭs) [" + Gr. *ana*, apart, + *lysis*, a loosening]. Analysis of the urine. SEE: *urine.*

urinary (ū'rĭ-năr″ē) [L. *urina*, urine]. Pert. to, secreting, or containing urine.

urinary bladder. Receptacle for urine excreted by the kidneys. SEE: *bladder.*

urinary calculi. Concretions formed in the urinary passages. They vary in composition but may contain urates, calcium, oxalate, calcium carbonate, phosphates, and cystine. SEE: *calculus, renal; lithotriptor.*

   NURSING IMPLICATIONS: Allow the patient to verbalize anxieties and concern related to severe pain. Administer pain relief measures as prescribed, such as analgesics and antispasmodics, and warm, moist heat. Strain all urine, watch for stone passage, and send calculus for analysis. If a lithotriptor is to be used, carefully explain procedure with respect to duration and follow-up care. Offer procedural explanation concerning diagnostic studies and therapeutic interventions, and encourage patient to voice fears and concerns. Observe for hematuria. Test for specific gravity of voided specimens. Monitor vital signs; if temperature is elevated, institute appropriate antipyretic measures as ordered. Force fluids to enhance dilution of urine, and monitor intake and output. Be alert for complications such as infection, stasis, and retention. Catheterize as ordered. Monitor renal function studies. Dietary management is based on the composition of the stone. If calcium stones are present, dietary calcium generally should be reduced and foods that acidify the urine, such as cereals and cranberry and grape juices, should be encouraged. If phosphate stones are present, acid-ash foods such as cereals, eggs, meat, and cranberry and grape juices should be given. Persons prone to uric acid stones are advised to consume an alkaline-ash diet of green vegetables and fruits. To minimize urinary tract infection, esp. for female patient, teach the patient adequate perineal hygiene, and emphasize that increased fluid intake is essential.

urinary casts. Casts of kidney tubules passed in the urine.

urinary director appliance. A hand-held, hollow, plastic device that fits over the vulva, enabling a woman to urinate while standing. The device collects urine and allows it to be directed away from the user through an outlet spout. Intended use is for women who are active outdoors and need to urinate without partially disrobing. Medically, the appliance has been found to be useful in patients who have had a radical vulvectomy. Trade name is Sani-Fem Urinary Director and it is available from Sani-Fem, Downey, California.

Other devices for use by women in collecting urine are available. Some of these have the capacity to contain the specimen for later disposal rather than merely redirecting the flow.

urinary incontinence. SEE: *incontinence; incontinence, urinary stress.*

urinary organs. The structures concerned with the secretion and excretion of urinary products, consisting of the two kidneys, two ureters, the bladder, and the urethra.

urinary pigments. Urochrome, urobilin, uroerythrin, and hematoporphyrin.

urinary reflex. Desire to void resulting from accumulation of urine in the bladder.

urinary sediment. Substances present in urine, i.e., bacteria, mucus, phosphates, uric acid, calcium oxalate, calcium carbonate, calcium phosphate, magnesium and ammonium phosphate; more rarely, cystine, tyrosine, xanthine, hippuric acid, hematoidin. SEE: *sediment, urinary.*

urinary stammering. Temporary interruptions in voiding urine.

urinary system. Kidneys, ureters, bladder, and urethra.

urinary tract. Organs and ducts participating in secretion and elimination of urine. SEE: illus.

urinary tract infection. ABBR: UTI. Infection of the urinary tract with microorganisms. SEE: *clean-catch method; urinary tract infection, risk factors for.*

NURSING IMPLICATIONS: Administer the prescribed antimicrobial specific for the causative organism. Obtain serial urine culture to validate the effectiveness of drug therapy. Administer antispasmodics as prescribed to relieve bladder irritation. Force fluids to 3 liters (approx. 3 quarts) a day to dilute the bacterial concentration. Monitor and record intake and output. Encourage the patient to void every 2 hours to empty the bladder and excrete the bacteria. Measure specific gravity of voided specimens. Provide relief from urgency by administering analgesics, sitz baths, and warm tub baths. Monitor vital signs every 4 hours; if temperature is elevated, administer prescribed antipyretic medications. Because urinary tract infections recur frequently in females, teach the patient the following: wear cotton pants; drink large amounts of fluids; avoid bubble baths; cleanse the perineum from front to back after elimination; take a shower rather than a bath; void immediately after sexual intercourse and take prescribed single dose of antimicrobial after intercourse. If symptoms persist after taking prescribed course of antibiotics, notify the physician.

urinary tract infection, risk factors for. In sexually active women, certain conditions predispose an individual to development of urinary tract infection. They are: use of a contraceptive diaphragm; method of sexual intercourse, i.e., greatly prolonged or cunnilingus; failure to void immediately following intercourse.

urinate (ū′rĭ-nāt) [L. *urinare*, to discharge urine]. To pass urine from the bladder. SYN: *micturate.*

urination (ū″rĭ-nā′shŭn) [L. *urinatio*, a discharging of urine]. The act of voiding urine. Although this act is somewhat under voluntary control, it is accomplished chiefly by the action of involuntary muscles. The musculus sphincter vesicae relaxes, while the general musculature of the wall of the urinary bladder contracts to force out its contents. SYN: *micturition; uresis.*

DIFF. DIAG: Increased frequency is seen in polyuria; nervous excitement; irritation of bladder, urethra, or urinary meatus; disease of spinal cord; enlarged prostate in male; pregnancy in female; beer drinking; interstitial nephritis; diabetes; phimosis. Decreased frequency occurs after sweating, diarrhea, or bleeding; in anuria, oliguria, uremia, brain disease, drug poisoning, coma, and parenchymatous nephritis. SEE: *urine.*

urination, words pert. to: anisuria; bacilluria; bladder; bradyuria; catheterization; clean-catch method; diuresis; diuretic; dysuria; enuresis; kidney; melanuria; micturate; micturition; nocturia; nycturia; oliguria; polyuria; strangury; uracratia; urea; "uret-" words; uric acid; "urin-" words; void.

urine (ū′rĭn) [L. *urina;* Gr. *ouron,* urine]. The fluid excreted by the kidneys, stored in the bladder, and discharged, usually voluntarily, through the urethra. It is conveyed to the bladder by two ureters, one from each of the kidneys. SEE: table.

In healthy persons, urine is of amber color with a slightly acid reaction, has a peculiar odor with a bitter saline taste, frequently deposits a precipitate of phosphates when fresh, but esp. on standing. Its specific gravity varies from 1.005 to 1.030.

The greater the amount of urine excreted, the lower the specific gravity. The normal amount of nonprotein nitrogen is from 25 to

URINARY TRACT AND ADJACENT ARTERIAL STRUCTURES — FEMALE

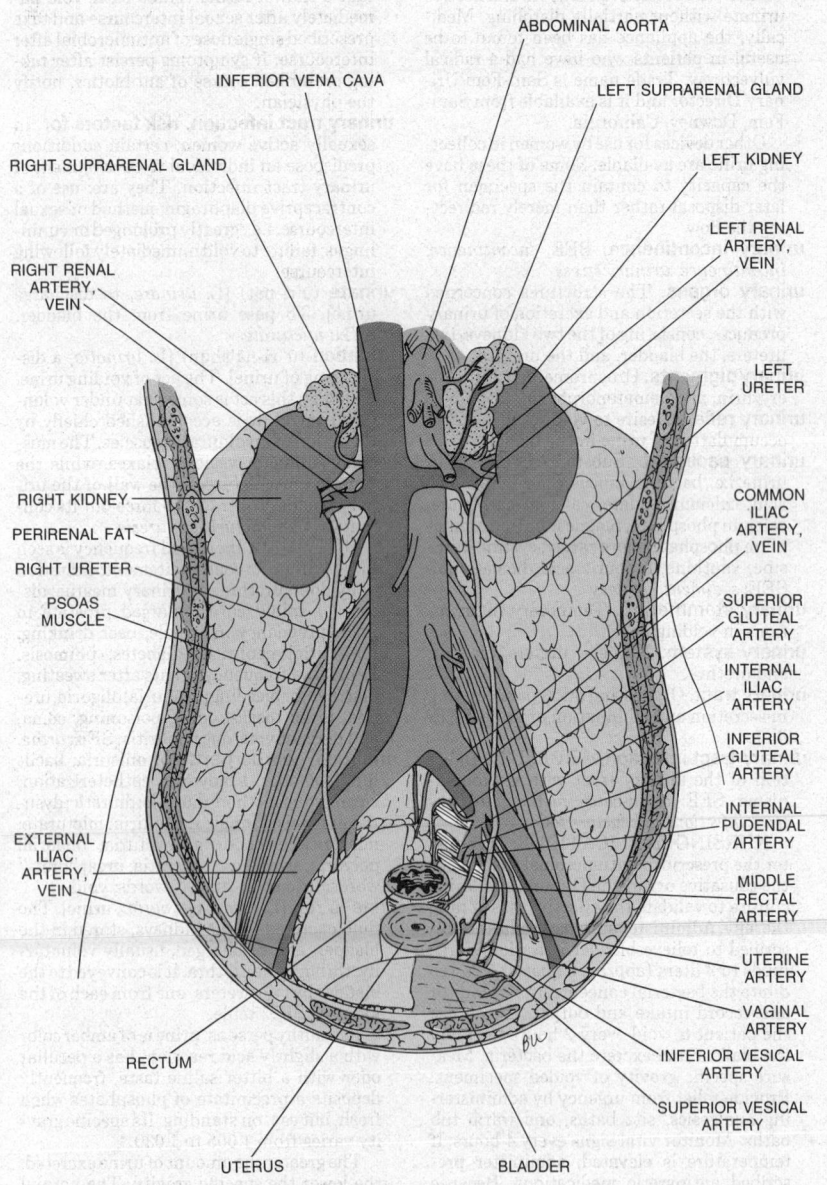

ABDOMINAL AORTA

INFERIOR VENA CAVA

LEFT SUPRARENAL GLAND

LEFT KIDNEY

RIGHT SUPRARENAL GLAND

LEFT RENAL ARTERY, VEIN

RIGHT RENAL ARTERY, VEIN

LEFT URETER

RIGHT KIDNEY

COMMON ILIAC ARTERY, VEIN

PERIRENAL FAT

RIGHT URETER

SUPERIOR GLUTEAL ARTERY

PSOAS MUSCLE

INTERNAL ILIAC ARTERY

INFERIOR GLUTEAL ARTERY

INTERNAL PUDENDAL ARTERY

EXTERNAL ILIAC ARTERY, VEIN

MIDDLE RECTAL ARTERY

UTERINE ARTERY

VAGINAL ARTERY

RECTUM

INFERIOR VESICAL ARTERY

SUPERIOR VESICAL ARTERY

UTERUS

BLADDER

Significance of Changes in Urine

QUANTITY

Normal	Abnormal	Significance
1000–1500 ml (approx. 95% H_2O)		Depends upon water and fluid, foods consumed, exercise, temperature, kidney function
	High (polyuria)	Diabetes mellitus, diabetes insipidus, nervous diseases, certain types of chronic nephritis (kidney disorder), diuretics (drugs as caffeine, digitalis, causing increased urinary excretion)
	Low (oliguria)	Acute nephritis, heart disease, fevers, eclampsia, diarrhea, vomiting, inadequate fluid intake
	None (anuria)	Uremia (urinary substances in blood), acute nephritis, metal poisoning, e.g., due to bichloride of mercury, complete obstruction of biliary tract

COLOR

Normal	Abnormal	Significance
Yellow to amber		Depends upon concentration of pigment (urochrome)
	Pale	Diabetes insipidus, due to a very dilute urine
	Milky	Fat globules, pus in genitourinary infections
	Reddish	Blood pigments, drugs, or food pigments
	Greenish	Bile pigment, associated with jaundice
	Brown-black	Poisoning (mercury, lead, phenol), hemorrhage

TRANSPARENCY

Normal	Abnormal	Significance
Clear		No significance
Cloudy on standing		Precipitation of mucin from urinary tract; not pathological
Turbid		Precipitation of calcium phosphate; not pathological
	Milky	Presence of fat globules; pathological
	Turbid	Presence of pus as result of inflammation of urinary tract; pathological

ODOR

Normal	Abnormal	Significance
Faintly aromatic		No significance
	Pleasant (sweet)	Acetone, associated with diabetes mellitus
	Unpleasant	Decomposition or ingestion of certain drugs or foods
Peppermint		Menthol ingestion
Acrid		Asparagus in diet
Spicy		Ingestion of sandalwood oil or saffron

Significance of Changes in Urine (Continued)

PROTEINURIA

Normal	Abnormal	Significance
Albumin and globulin		
	Albumin	Excretion of 10–100 mg each 24 hr is normal but this amount is not detected by usual tests
	Albumin	Evidence of altered renal function, which may be due to renal pathology or a systemic disease such as diabetes mellitus
	Globulin	Bence Jones proteins are associated with multiple myeloma and diseases of globulin metabolism. Other types of globulins may be present in acute and chronic pyelonephritis

SPECIFIC GRAVITY

Normal	Abnormal	Significance
1.010–1.025 sp. gr.		Ordinary, sp. gr. inversely proportional to volume
	Low	Dilution if volume is large; otherwise nephritis
	High	Acute nephritis; concentrated if volume is small; otherwise, if volume is large and light colored, diabetes mellitus

ACIDITY

Normal	Abnormal	Significance
Acid (slight)		Diet of acid-forming foods (meats, eggs, prunes, wheat) overbalancing the base-forming foods (vegetables and fruits)
	High acidity	Acidosis, diabetes mellitus, many pathological disorders (fevers, starvation)
	Alkaline	Putrefying bacteria change urea into ammonium carbonate; infection or ingestion of alkaline compounds

35 mg per 100 ml of blood. The amount of this substance present in the blood is related to how well the kidneys are functioning. The daily output is equally variable, being adapted to the amount of water taken in and to the amount lost by evaporation from the skin in expired air.

COMP: Urine consists of approx. 95% water and 5% solids. Solids amount to 30 to 70 gm per liter and include the following (values are in grams per 24 hours unless otherwise noted): *Organic substances:* urea, uric acid (20 to 40), creatine (0 to 40 mg/d. in men and 0 to 80 in women), creatinine (15 to 25 mg/kg of body weight/day), ammonia (0.5 to 1.3). *Inorganic substances:* chlorides (110 to 250 nmol/liter depending upon chloride intake), calcium (0.1 to 0.2), magnesium (3 to 5 nmol/d.), phosphorus (0.4 to 1.3).

In addition to the above, many other substances may be present depending on the diet and state of health of the individual. Among component substances indicating pathological states are abnormal amounts of albumin, glucose, ketone bodies, blood, pus, casts, and bacteria.

COLLECTION OF URINE: For a routine urinalysis, a voided specimen of urine in a clean container is usually sufficient. For culture, either a clean-catch or a catheterized specimen is required. For a clean-catch specimen the individual cleanses the perineum or glans penis with soap and water or an antiseptic solution such as benzalkonium chloride prior to voiding. A midstream specimen of urine is then collected in a sterilized container. A catheterized specimen is obtained by passing a catheter into the bladder, using sterile technique. SEE: *suprapubic catheter.*

NOTE: A urine specimen may be obtained in order to test for excretion of drugs of abuse. In such cases, care must be taken to be sure that the specimen was produced by the individual and that there was no opportunity for the specimen to be diluted with water or someone else's urine.

DIAG: *Color:* Normal urine is amber in color, resulting from the presence of urobilin, q.v., a pigment mainly derived from bilirubin, q.v., in the bile. This pigment is found in excessive quantities in fever, and it may indicate excess destruction of red blood cells. The effect of food and medication must be considered before concluding that the color of the urine is abnormal. *Black:* Melanuria, malignant pigmented tumor, melanotic cancer, or carbolic acid poisoning. *Bile-colored:* Seen in jaundice. *Blue:* May result from methylene blue or the presence of indigo. *Colorless:* This is known as achromaturia and is usually due to the urine's being extremely dilute. *Lime green:* Presence of a blue-colored substance such as methylene blue, or indican and yellow urochrome to produce a bright green color. *Milky:* May be due to chyluria, lipuria, or pus. *Orange-red:* May indicate the presence of pyridine dyes. *Pale:* Indicates an excess of water; it is found in conditions causing polyuria. *Red or reddish color:* May be due to the presence of blood in the urine, hematuria, phenolsulfonphthalein, the laxative danthron, or to senna or rhubarb, which may color the urine either brown or orange. Psychopathic or malingering patients have added ketchup or tomato juice to their urine specimen to make it appear to be blood-stained.

Odor: Ammoniacal: May result from decomposition products. *Aromatic:* This is the odor of normal urine. *Fecal:* Due to fistulous communications between the intestinal and urinary tracts. *Fishy:* Cystitis. *New-mown hay:* Indicative of diabetes. *Overripe apple:* Indicative of acetonuria or the presence of acetone bodies in the urine. *Violet:* May be caused by turpentine.

NOTE: Some foods but esp. asparagus may cause the urine to have a characteristic odor. This is a transient phenomenon.

PRODUCTS IN DISEASE: *Acidic:* May be found in acidosis and pyelonephritis. *Alkaline:* May show a white sediment. *Albumin:* Due to nephritis and inflammation of mucous membrane of any portion of the urinary apparatus. *Acetone:* Represents the by-products of excessive fat metabolism excreted by the kidneys and known as ketonuria. *Animal parasites:* Rare, found as result of contamination. *Bacteria:* Usually regarded as being of little importance if fewer than 100,000 can be cultured from each ml of urine. Appears cloudy. *Bile:* Bile in the urine indicates abnormal retention of bile. *Blood:* Shows a smoky sediment and is reddish-brown. Indicates hemorrhagic nephritis, calculi, congestion of a kidney, renal carcinoma, tuberculosis of kidney, chronic infections, or trauma. *Casts:* These indicate renal disease. A few hyaline casts in the aged denote slight damage to kidneys. Casts are found in large numbers in nephritis. The less acute the disease, the finer are the granular casts. *Crystals:* Calcium oxalate and uric acid crystals will be present in acid urine; crystals of ammonium biurate and phosphates will be present in alkaline urine. Crystals have little significance except leucine and tyrosine crystals, which may indicate liver disease. *Cylindroids:* No special significance. *Acetoacetic acid:* Deficient carbohydrate metabolism of an advanced stage; it is preceded by the presence of acetone. *Epithelial cells* (squamous): If in large numbers from urinary bladder and ureters, they indicate inflammation of these parts; renal epithelial cells of kidney indicate serious damage to the same. *Fat droplets:* Fatty degeneration of kidneys and lipemia. *Froth:* Indicates presence of bile. *Indican:* Small significance but is seen in intestinal putrefaction. *Mucus:* If visible and in quantity, urethritis is indicated. No special significance in women if the quantity is small. *Mucous threads:* Mucoid ribbonlike structures of no great significance. *Pus:* This is mucoid and shows a white sediment. It is found in bacterial infections of the urinary tract. The presence of the occasional pus cell may be normal per high-power field; if accompanied by red cells, pus cells indicate inflammation. *Red blood cells:* Stones or inflammation of kidney or urinary tract. No significance if due to contamination by menstrual fluid. *Sediment:* Pinkish due to excess of urates; white, caused by phosphates. In order to obtain sediment, the examination should be made quickly by centrifuging for 3 min. after urine is voided. *Sugar* (glucose): Denotes faulty carbohydrate metabolism as seen in diabetes mellitus. *Urea:* Principal end product of protein metabolism. *Yeasts and molds:* Result of contamination.

CONDITIONS: *Difficult urination* (dysuria): Found in urethral stricture, enlarged prostate, atony and impairment of the bladder's muscular power, and in gonorrhea and other inflammatory conditions involving the urethra, bladder, or lower ureter. *Diminished* (oliguria): Diminished in disease of the liver and in low protein intake. Scanty in all fevers unless fluid intake is increased. Accompanies cardiac failure; acute, chronic, and parenchymatous nephritis; obstruction of return venous circulation of kidney; thrombosis of renal vein or inferior vena cava; loss of fluids through hemorrhages, vomiting, or diarrhea; inadequate fluid intake; obstruction or pressure upon ureter; lead poisoning.

Incontinence (enuresis, q.v.): Inability to retain urine because of paralysis or relaxation of sphincters or contraction of longitudinal muscular layer of bladder; incontinence and dribbling are results. This can occur in all forms of coma, during an epileptic seizure, shock, typhoid, and typhus. It may also occur in conjunction with injuries to or tumors of the spinal cord; transverse myelitis, spinal meningitis, locomotor ataxia, paralysis, and reflex excitability of nervous system. Other causes include local irritation of the bladder, cystitis, phimosis, vesical calculus, contracted meatus, ascarides, and very concentrated urine. SEE: *incontinence, urinary stress.*

Increased (polyuria): In fevers, esp. if weight is lost: after pregnancy; during parturition; after the intake of large quantities of liquid. May be indicative of chronic interstitial nephritis; diabetes mellitus or insipidus; amyloid disease of kidney; reabsorption of effusions; functional disease of nervous system, as in hysteria and neurasthenia. Persistent in bulbar, cerebellar, and spinal tumors, locomotor ataxia, and meningitis. *Obstructive:* Result of occlusion of one or both ureters; or occlusion of urethra. *Painful:* Dysuria, q.v., vesical tenesmus. There is a persistent desire to urinate. *Residual:* That remaining in bladder after urination; usually indicative of a pathological condition such as prostatic hypertrophy or disease or cystocele. *Retention* (ischuria): Inability to urinate; almost same diseases and injuries of cord that produce incontinence. All forms of coma; typhoid; peritonitis; hysteria; atony; prostatic enlargement; urethral stricture; urethritis, cystitis; tumors of bladder; calculus in urethra. *Strangury:* Painful and spasmodic. May be indicative of cystitis; neuralgia; acute nephritis; tuberculosis; cancer or ulceration of

bladder; urethritis; urethral stricture; hypertrophied, cancerous, or inflamed prostate; prolapsus uteri; pelvic peritonitis and abscess; vesical tenesmus. Pain and burning often caused by concentrated or acid urine. *Suppression:* Failure of kidneys to secrete urine. May be complete (anuria) or partial (oliguria). Failure of kidneys to secrete the urine or failure of urine to reach the bladder if secreted may be found in acute nephritis or congestion, renal abscess, last stages of chronic nephritis. Renal damage caused by patient's having received a blood transfusion with incompatible blood.

    u., double-voided. SEE: *double-voided urine.*

    u., residual. Residual urine, q.v.

urine, words pert. to: acetoacetic acid; acetone; acetone bodies; acetone in urine, tests for; acetonuria; achromaturia; acidaminuria; albuminuria; alkalinuria; alkaptone; alkaptonuria; allantoinuria; alloxuria; aminuria; ammoniuria; amylosuria; amyluria; anisuria; antidiuretic; anuria; arabinosuria; azoturia; Bence Jones albumose; Benedict's test for sugar; bilirubinuria; bladder, stammering of; bladder, urinary; calcariuria; calculi; cast; ceramuria; cerebrosuria; chloride, test for, in urine; chloriduria; chondroituria; chromaturia; chyluria; enuresis; epithelium; galactosuria; galacturia; glucose; glycosuria; Heller's test; hemoglobinuria; hippuria; hyaline casts; hydruria; incontinence; ischuria; ketonuria; ketosis; kidney; lactosuria; lipuria; lithotripsy; lithuria; melanuria; mucus; myosinuria; nocturia; oliguresis; oxaluria; pentosuria; pus; pyuria; residual urine; retention of urine; secretion; tyrosinuria; uraturia; urea; uredema; uremia; ureter; uric acid; uricosuria; urinalysis; urolagnia; "uro-" words.

urinemia (ūʺrĭ-nēʹmē-ă) [L. *urina,* urine, + Gr. *haima,* blood]. Accumulation in the blood of substances such as urea, which are normally excreted in the urine. SYN: *uremia.*

uriniferous (ū-rĭ-nĭfʹĕr-ŭs) [ʺ + *ferre,* to bear]. Carrying urine.

urinific (ūʺrĭ-nĭfʹĭk). Uriniparous.

uriniparous (ū-rĭ-nĭpʹă-rŭs) [ʺ + *parere,* to bring forth, to bear]. Producing or secreting urine.

urino-. Combining form concerning urine.

urinogenital (ūʺrĭ-nō-jĕnʹĭ-tăl) [ʺ + *genitalia,* genitals]. Pert. to the genital and urinary organs. SYN: *urogenital.*

urinogenous (ūʺrĭ-nŏjʹĭ-nŭs) [ʺ + Gr. *gennan,* to produce]. 1. Producing urine. 2. Originating in urine. SYN: *urogenous.*

urinology (ūʺrĭ-nŏlʹō-jē). Urology.

urinoma (ūʺrĭ-nōʹmă) [ʺ + Gr. *oma,* mass]. A cyst containing urine.

urinometer (ū″rĭ-nŏm′ĕ-tĕr) [″ + Gr. *metron*, measure]. Device for determining specific gravity of urine.

urinometry (ū″rĭ-nŏm′ĕ-trē). Determination of specific gravity of the urine.

urinophil (ū′rĭ-nō-fĭl) [″ + Gr. *philein*, to love]. Capable of existing in the urine, such as bacteria that grow best in urine.

urinoscopy (ū″rĭ-nŏs′kō-pē). Uroscopy.

urinose, urinous (ū′rĭ-nōs, ū′rĭ-nŭs) [L. *urina*, urine]. Having the characteristics of or containing urine.

urinosexual (ū″rĭ-nō-sĕks′ū-ăl). Urogenital.

uriposia (ū″rĭ-pō′zē-ă) [″ + *posis*, drinking]. Drinking of urine.

urisolvent (ū″rĭ-sŏl′vĕnt) [″ + *solvens*, dissolving]. Dissolving uric acid or causing it to be dissolved.

Urispas. Trade name for flavoxate hydrochloride.

uro- [Gr. *ouron*]. Combining form meaning pert. to urine.

uroammoniac (ū″rō-ă-mō′nē-ăk). Containing urine and ammonia.

uroanthelone (ū″rō-ăn′thĕ-lōn). Urogastrone.

urobilin (ū″rō-bī′lĭn) [″ + L. *bilis*, bile]. A brown pigment formed by the oxidation of urobilinogen, a decomposition product of bilirubin. Urobilin may be formed from the urobilinogen in stools or in urine after exposure to air.

urobilinemia (ū″rō-bī″lĭn-ē′mē-ă) [″ + ″ + Gr. *haima*, blood]. Urobilin in blood.

urobilinicterus (ū″rō-bī-lĭn-ĭk′tĕr-ŭs) [″ + L. *bilis*, bile, + Gr. *ikteros*, jaundice]. Jaundice resulting from urobilinemia.

urobilinogen (ū″rō-bī-lĭn′ō-jĕn) [″ + ″ + Gr. *gennan*, to produce]. A colorless derivative of bilirubin, from which it is formed by the action of intestinal bacteria.

urobilinogenemia (ū″rō-bī″lĭn-ō-jĕn-ē′mē-ă) [″ + ″ + ″ + *haima*, blood]. Urobilinogen in the blood.

urobilinuria (ū″rō-bī″lĭn-ū′rē-ă) [″ + ″ + Gr. *ouron*, urine]. Excess of urobilin in the urine.

urocele (ū′rō-sēl) [″ + *kele*, tumor, swelling]. Escape of urine into the scrotum.

urocheras (ū-rŏk′ĕr-ăs) [″ + *cheras*, gravel]. Gravel of calcareous sediment in the urine.

urochesia (ū-rō-kē′zē-ă) [″ + *chezein*, to defecate]. A discharge of urine in the feces.

urochrome (ū′rō-krōm) [″ + *chroma*, color]. The pigment that gives urine its characteristic color. It is derived from urobilin.

uroclepsia (ū-rō-klĕp′sē-ă) [″ + *kleptein*, judge]. Involuntary urination without being aware of it.

urocrisia (ū″rō-krĭz′ē-ă) [″ + *krinein*, to

judge]. Diagnosis by examining the urine.

urocyanin (ū-rō-sī′ă-nĭn) [″ + *kyanos*, blue]. A blue pigment present in the urine in certain diseases, esp. scarlet fever.

urocyanogen (ū″rō-sī-ăn′ō-jĕn) [″ + ″ + *gennan*, to produce]. A blue pigment in urine, esp. in cholera patients.

urocyanosis (ū″rō-sī-ăn-ō′sĭs) [″ + ″ + *osis*, condition]. Blue discoloration of the urine. May be due to presence of indigo blue from oxidation of indican, or from ingestion of drugs such as methylene blue. SYN: *indicanuria.*

urocyst (ū′rō-sĭst) [Gr. *ouron*, urine, + *kystis*, bladder]. The urinary bladder.

urocystic (ū″rō-sĭs′tĭk). Concerning the urinary bladder.

urocystis (ū″rō-sĭs′tĭs). The urinary bladder.

urocystitis (ū″rō-sĭs-tī′tĭs). Inflammation of the urinary bladder.

urodynamics (ū″rō-dī-năm′ĭks). Study of the holding or storage of urine in the bladder; the facility with which it empties; and the rate of movement of urine out of the bladder during micturition.

urodynia (ū″rō-dĭn′ē-ă) [″ + *odyne*, pain]. Pain associated with urination.

uroedema (ū″rō-ĕ-dē′mă) [″ + *oidema*, swelling]. Extravasation of urine distending the tissues. SYN: *uredema.*

uroenterone (ū″rō-ĕn′tĕr-ōn). Urogastrone.

uroerythrin (ū″rō-ĕr′ĭth-rĭn) [″ + *erythros*, red]. A reddish pigment sometimes present in urine. SYN: *purpurin.*

uroflavin (ū″rō-flā′vĭn). A fluorescent compound present in the urine of persons taking riboflavin.

uroflowmeter. Device for recording urine flow. Used to quantitate obstruction to urine flowing from the bladder.

urofuscin (ū″rō-fūs′ĭn) [″ + L. *fuscus*, dark brown]. A red-brown pigment sometimes found in samples of urine, esp. in cases of porphyrinuria.

urofuscohematin (ū″rō-fūs″kō-hĕm′ăt-ĭn) [″ + ″ + Gr. *haima*, blood]. A reddish-brown pigment in urine in some diseases.

urogastrone (ū″rō-găs′trōn) [″ + *gaster*, belly]. A polypeptide present in urine that has an inhibitory effect on gastric secretion.

urogenital (ū″rō-jĕn′ĭ-tăl) [″ + L. *genitalia*, genitals]. Pert. to the urinary and reproductive organs. SYN: *urinogenital.*

urogenital fold. Ridge, urogenital, q.v.

urogenous (ū-rŏj′ĕn-ŭs) [″ + *gennan*, to produce]. 1. Producing urine. 2. Originating in urine. SYN: *urinogenous.*

uroglaucin (ū″rō-glaw′sĭn) [″ + *glaukos*, green]. Urocyanin.

urogram (ū′rō-grăm) [″ + *gramma*, something written]. A roentgenogram of any part of the urinary tract.

urography (ū′rŏg′ră-fē) [Gr. *ouron*, urine, + *graphein*, to write]. Roentgenography of any part of the urinary tract after introduction of a radiopaque substance.

    u., ascending; u., cystoscopic. Urography in which the radiopaque dye is injected into the bladder during cystoscopy.

    u., descending; u., excretion; u., excretory; u., intravenous. Urography in which an injected dye is excreted by the kidney and studied by x-ray during excretion.

    u., retrograde. U., ascending, q.v.

urohematin (ū″rō-hĕm′ăt-ĭn) [″ + *haima*, blood]. Pigment in urine, considered as identical with hematin, q.v., that alters color of urine in proportion to degree of oxidation.

urohematonephrosis (ū″rō-hĕm″ă-tō-nē-frō′sĭs) [″ + ″ + *nephros*, kidney]. Pathological condition of the kidney in which the pelvis is distended with blood and urine.

urohematoporphyrin (ū″rō-hĕm″ă-tō-por′fĭr-ĭn) [″ + ″ + *porphyra*, purple]. Iron-free hematin in urine when hemolysis occurs.

urokinase (ū-rō-kī′nās). An enzyme obtained from human urine. Used experimentally for dissolving venous thrombi and pulmonary emboli. It is administered intravenously.

urokinetic (ū″rō-kĭ-nĕt′ĭk) [″ + *kinesis*, movement]. Resulting reflexly from stimulation of the urinary organs.

urolagnia (ū-rō-lăg′nē-ă) [″ + *lagneia*, lust]. Sexual excitation associated with urine or urination. This may include watching others urinate or having someone urinate on their body. SEE: *undinism.*

urolith (ū′rō-lĭth) [″ + *lithos*, stone]. A concretion in the urine.

urolithiasis (ū″rō-lĭ-thī′ă-sĭs) [″ + ″ + *-iasis*, condition]. Formation of urinary calculi and the illness associated with the presence of calculi in the urinary tract. SEE: *calculus, renal.* SEE: *Nursing Diagnoses in Appendix.*

urolithic (ū″rō-lĭth′ĭk). Concerning urinary calculi.

urolithology (ū″rō-lĭ-thŏl′ō-jē) [″ + ″ + *logos*, word, reason]. Science dealing with urinary calculi.

urologic (ū-rō-lŏj′ĭk) [″ + *logos*, word, reason]. Pert. to urology.

urologist (ū-rŏl′ō-jĭst). A physician who specializes in the practice of urology.

urology (ū-rŏl′ō-jē) [″ + *logos*, word, reason]. The branch of medicine concerned with the urinary tract in both sexes and the genital tract in the male. SYN: *uronology.*

urolutein (ū-rō-lū′tē-ĭn) [″ + L. *luteus*, yellow]. A yellow pigment seen in the urine.

uromancy (ūr′ō-măn″sē) [″ + *manteia*, a divination]. Use of urinalysis for diagnosis of disease.

uromedulin, human. The most abundant protein of renal origin in normal urine. This glycoprotein is the same protein termed Tamm-Horsfall mucoprotein. SEE: *mucoprotein, Tamm-Horsfall.*

uromelanin (ū-rō-mĕl′ăn-ĭn) [″ + *melas*, black]. A black pigment occurring in urine resulting from the decomposition of urochrome.

uromelus (ū-rŏm′ē-lŭs) [Gr. *oura*, tail, + *melos*, limb]. Congenitally deformed fetus in which the lower extremities are fused. SYN: *sirenomelus.*

urometer (ū-rŏm′ĕt-ĕr) [Gr. *ouron*, urine, + *metron*, measure]. Instrument for determining specific gravity of urine. SYN: *urinometer.*

uroncus (ū-rŏn′kŭs) [″ + *onkos*, bulk, mass]. A swelling or cyst containing urine.

uronephrosis (ū″rō-nĕf-rō′sĭs) [″ + *nephros*, kidney, + *osis*, condition]. Dilatation of renal structures from obstruction of urinary flow. Distention of renal pelvis and tubules with urine. SYN: *hydronephrosis.*

uronology (ū-rō-nŏl′ō-jē) [″ + *logos*, word, reason]. The science of urine and genitourinary diseases. SYN: *urology.*

uronophile (ū-rŏn′ō-fīl) [″ + *philein*, to love]. A microorganism that grows best in a culture containing urine.

uropathogen (ū″rō-păth′ō-jĕn) [″ + *pathos*, disease, suffering, + *gennan*, to produce]. A microorganism capable of causing disease of the urinary tract.

uropathy (ū-rŏp′ă-thē). Any disease affecting the urinary tract.

    u., obstructive. Any disease resulting from obstruction of the urinary tract.

uropenia (ū-rō-pē′nē-ă) [″ + *penia*, a lack]. Lack of urinary secretion.

uropepsin (ū″rō-pĕp′sĭn). The end product of pepsin metabolism. It is excreted in the urine.

urophanic (ū-rō-făn′ĭk) [″ + *phainein*, to appear]. Appearing in the urine.

urophein (ū″rō-fē′ĭn) [″ + *phaios*, gray]. Gray pigment in urine said to cause its characteristic odor. Also spelled *urophaein.*

urophosphometer (ū″rō-fŏs-fŏm′ē-tĕr) [″ + L. *phosphas*, phosphorus]. Device for estimating amount of phosphorus in the urine.

uroplania (ū″rō-plā′nē-ă) [″ + *plane*, a wandering]. Condition in which urine is present or discharged from parts other than the urinary organs.

uropoiesis (ū″rō-poy-ē′sĭs) [Gr. *ouron*, urine, + *poiesis*, production]. Formation of urine by the kidneys.

uropoietic (ū″rō-poy-ĕt′ĭk) [″ + *poiein*, to form]. Pert. to the formation of urine.

uroporphyria (ū″rō-por-fîr′ē-ă). Porphyria in which an excess amount of uroporphyrin is excreted in the urine.

uroporphyrin (ū″rō-por′fĭ-rĭn). A red pigment present in the urine and feces in cases of porphyria. May also be present in the urine of persons taking certain drugs.

uroporphyrinogen (ū″rō-por″fĭ-rĭn′ō-jĕn). Any one of several porphyrins that are the precursors of uroporphyrins.

    u. l. An abnormal isomer of a precursor of protoporphyrin, which accumulates in one form of porphyria. It causes the urine to be red, the teeth to fluoresce brightly in ultraviolet light, and the skin to be abnormally sensitive to sunlight. This is observed in congenital erythropoietic porphyria.

uropsammus (ū″rō-săm′ŭs) [″ + *psammos*, sand]. Gravel or calcareous sediment in the urine.

uropyonephrosis (ū″rō-pī-ō-nĕf-rō′sĭs) [″ + *pyon*, pus, + *nephros*, kidney, + *osis*, condition]. Urine and pus in the renal pelvis.

uropyoureter (ū″rō-pī″ō-ū-rē′tĕr) [″ + + *oureter*, ureter]. Accumulation of urine and pus in the ureter.

urorosein (ū″rō-rō′zē-ĭn) [″ + L. *roseus*, rosy]. A rose-colored pigment in urine, which is increased in certain diseases. SYN: *urorrhodin.*

urorrhagia (ū-rō-rǎ′jē-ă) [″ + *rhegnynai*, to burst forth]. Excessive secretion of urine. SYN: *polyuria.*

urorrhea (ū-rō-rē′ă) [″ + *rhoia*, a flow]. Involuntary flow of urine. SYN: *enuresis.*

urorrhodin (ū-rō-rō′dĭn) [″ + *rhodon*, rose]. A rose-colored pigment in the urine in certain infectious diseases such as typhoid fever and tuberculosis.

urorrhodinogen (ū″rō-rō-dĭn′ō-jĕn) [Gr. *ouron*, urine, + *rhodon*, rose, + *gennan*, to produce]. A chromogen of the urine that, when decomposed, forms urorrhodin.

urorubin (ū-rō-roo′bĭn) [″ + L. *ruber*, red]. A red pigment obtained from urine by treatment with hydrochloric acid.

urorubrohematin (ū″rō-rū″brō-hĕm′ă-tĭn) [″ + + Gr. *haima*, blood]. A red pigment occasionally found in the urine in some chronic diseases.

urosacin (ū-rō′sā-sĭn). A red pigment in the urine. SYN: *urorrhodin.*

uroscheocele (ū-rŏs′kē-ō-sēl) [″ + *oscheon*, scrotum, + *kele*, tumor, swelling]. Swelling of the scrotum from extravasation of urine into the scrotal sac. SYN: *urocele.*

uroschesis (ū-rŏs′kĕs-ĭs) [″ + *schesis*, a holding]. 1. Suppression of urine. 2. Retention of the urine.

uroscopy (ū-rŏs′kō-pē) [″ + *skopein*, to examine]. 1. Examination of the urine. 2. Diagnosis by examination of the urine.

urosepsis (ū-rō-sĕp′sĭs). Sepsis due to retention and absorption of urinary products in the tissues.

urospectrin (ū-rō-spĕk′trĭn) [″ + L. *spectrum*, image]. A pigment derived from normal urine; seen when urine is shaken with acetic ether.

urostealith (ū″rō-stē′ă-lĭth) [″ + *stear*, fat, + *lithos*, stone]. A fatty substance in some urinary calculi.

urotoxicity (ū″rō-tŏks-ĭs′ĭ-tē) [″ + *toxikon*, poison]. The toxic character of the urine.

urotoxin (ū″rō-tŏk′sĭn). Toxic substances in the urine.

uroureter (ū″rō-ū′rĕ-tĕr, ū″rō-ū-rē′tĕr) [″ + *oureter*, ureter]. Distention of the ureter with urine due to stricture or obstruction.

urous (ū′rŭs) [Gr. *ouron*, urine]. Having the nature of urine.

uroxanthin (ū″rō-zăn′thĭn) [″ + *xanthos*, yellow]. Yellow pigment of the urine; an indigo-forming substance.

uroxin (ū-rŏk′sĭn) [″ + *oxys*, sharp]. Alloxantin, a derivative of alloxan.

urtica (ŭr-tī′kă) [L., nettle] (pl. *urticae*). A wheal.

urticant (ŭr′tĭ-kănt). That which causes an urticarial reaction in the skin.

urticaria (ŭr-tĭ-kā′rē-ă) [L. *urtica*, nettle]. A vascular reaction of the skin characterized by the eruption of pale evanescent wheals, which are associated with severe itching. SYN: *hives; nettle rash*. SEE: *allergy; angioneurotic edema.*

    SYM: Sudden general eruption of papules or wheals associated with intense itching.

    ETIOL: Contact with an external irritant such as the nettle, physical agents, foods, insect bites, serum sickness, pollens, drugs, or neurogenic factors.

    TREAT: *General measures:* Because the skin manifestation is an allergic reaction, identify and remove the antigenic offender if possible. Check diet for common offenders such as wheat, milk, eggs, shellfish, and other suspected food allergens. Avoid unnecessary medications, as drugs are often causative factors. *Specific measures:* Antihistaminic drugs often give quick relief. Injection of epinephrine (subcutaneous). Ephedrine may be used. In severe cases ACTH or cortisone used with caution has proved effective. Locally, antipruritic lotions and baths are frequently beneficial. If dietary cause is suspected, use elimination diet to attempt to determine the identity of the food(s).

    u., aquagenic. Urticaria caused by exposure of the skin to ordinary water.

u. bullosa. Eruption of temporary vesicles with infusion of fluid under the epidermis.

u., cold. Cold-induced urticarial eruption that may progress to angioedema.

u. factitia. Urticaria following slight irritation of the skin. SYN: *dermatographia.*

u. gigantea. Angioneurotic edema.

u. haemorrhagica. Urticaria with lesions infiltrated with blood.

u. maculosa. A chronic form of urticaria with red-colored lesions.

u. maritima. Urticaria due to salt water bathing.

u. medicamentosa. Urticaria due to certain drugs.

u. papulosa. In this form of urticaria, the wheal is followed by a lingering papule that is attended by considerable itching. Most commonly observed in debilitated children. SYN: *lichen urticatus; prurigo simplex.*

u. pigmentosa juvenilis. A form of urticaria pigmentosa that begins in infancy.

u. solaris. Urticaria occurring in certain individuals following exposure to sunlight.

urticarial (ŭr″tĭ-kā′rē-ăl) [L. *urtica,* nettle]. Pert. to urticaria. SYN: *urticarious.*

urticate (ŭr′tĭ-kāt). 1. To produce urticaria. 2. Marked by the appearance of wheals.

urtication (ŭr-tĭ-kā′shŭn). 1. Flogging of a part with nettles to induce counterirritation. 2. Burning or itching sensation. 3. Eruption of itching wheals. SYN: *urticaria.*

urushiol (ū-roo′shē-ŏl″) [Japanese *urushi,* lac, + L. *oleum,* oil]. The principal toxic irritant substance of plants such as poison ivy, which produces characteristic severe dermatitis upon contact.

U.S. AEC. *U.S. Atomic Energy Commission.*

USAN. *United States Adopted Names* (for drugs), q.v.

USAN and the USP Dictionary of Drug Names. A dictionary of nonproprietary names, brand names, code designations, and Chemical Abstracts Service registry numbers for drugs. The 1993 edition is cumulative for U.S. adopted names (USAN) from June 15, 1961, through June 15, 1992.

Usher's syndrome [Charles Howard Usher, Brit. ophthalmologist, 1865–1942]. A hereditary disorder characterized by a combination of congenital deafness and retinitis pigmentosa that results in a gradual loss of vision.

USP, U.S. Phar. *United States Pharmacopeia.*

U.S.P.H.S. *United States Public Health Service.*

USP-PRN. *United States Pharmacopeia-Practitioners' Reporting Network.*

ustilaginism (ŭs-tĭl-ăj′ĭn-ĭzm) [L. *ustulatus,*

scorched, + Gr. *-ismos,* condition]. Poisoning resulting from eating corn infected with smut fungus, *Ustilago maydis.*

Ustilago (ŭs-tĭl-ā′gō). A moldlike fungus, *Ustilago maydis,* commonly called smut.

ustion (ŭs′chŭn) [L. *ustio,* a burning]. Cauterization with actual cautery.

ustulation (ŭs-tū-lā′shŭn) [L. *ustulare,* to scorch]. Roasting, parching, or drying of a moist drug.

ustus (ŭs′tŭs) [L.]. Burned. SEE: *calcination.*

uta (ū′tă). Infection with *Leishmania braziliensis* involving the nasopharyngeal and mucocutaneous membranes. Common in Central and South America. SYN: *leishmaniasis, American.*

ut dict. L. *ut dictum,* as directed.

utend. L. *utendus,* to be used.

uter-, utero- [L. *uterus,* womb]. Combining forms denoting relationship to the uterus.

uteralgia (ū″tĕr-ăl′jē-ă) [L. *uterus,* womb, + Gr. *algos,* pain]. Uterine pain.

uterectomy (ū″tĕr-ĕk′tō-mē) [″ + Gr. *ektome,* excision]. Removal of uterus through the abdomen or vagina. SYN: *hysterectomy.*

uterine (ū′tĕr-ĭn, -īn) [L. *uterinus*]. Pert. to the uterus.

uterine artery Doppler velocimetry. SEE: *Doppler echocardiography.*

uterine bleeding. Bleeding from the uterus. Physiologic bleeding via the vagina occurs in normal menstruation. Abnormal forms include excessive menstrual flow (hypermenorrhea, menorrhagia) or too frequent menstruation (polymenorrhea). Nonmenstrual bleeding is called metrorrhagia. Pseudomenstrual or withdrawal bleeding may occur following estrogenic therapy. Breakthrough bleeding is the term used for intermenstrual bleeding that sometimes occurs in women who take progestational agents such as birth control pills. SEE: *amenorrhea; menstruation; tampon, menstrual.* SEE: *Nursing Diagnoses* in Appendix.

uterine glands. The tubular glands in the endometrium.

uterine milk. A milky white substance between the gravid uterus and placental villi.

uterine souffle. A vascular sound that may be heard in the pregnant uterus by using a stethoscope.

uterine subinvolution. Failure of the uterus to return to normal size after childbirth. A uterus that weighs more than 100 gm is considered to be enlarged.

uterine tube. One of two small tubes attached to either side of the uterus and leading from the region of the ovary. SYN: *fallopian tube.*

uteroabdominal (ū″tĕr-ō-ăb-dŏm′ĭ-năl) [L. *uterus,* womb, + *abdomen,* belly]. Pert. to both the uterus and abdomen.

uterocele (ū-tĕr′ō-sēl) [″ + Gr. *kele*, tumor, swelling]. Hernia containing the uterus.

uterocervical (ū″tĕr-ō-sĕr′vĭ-kăl) [″ + *cervix*, neck]. Rel. to the uterus and cervix.

uterocystostomy (ū″tĕr-ō-sĭs-tŏs′tō-mē) [″ + Gr. *kystis*, bladder, + *stoma*, mouth]. Formation of a passage between the uterine cervix and the bladder.

uterofixation (ū″tĕr-ō-fĭks-ā′shŭn) [″ + *fixatio*, a fixing]. Fixation of a displaced uterus. SYN: *hysteropexy*.

uterogenic (ū″tĕr-ō-jĕn′ĭk). Formed in the uterus.

uterogestation (ū″tĕr-ō-jĕs-tā′shŭn) [″ + *gestare*, to bear]. Pregnancy in the uterus; normal pregnancy.

uterography (ū″tĕr-ŏg′ră-fē) [″ + Gr. *graphein*, to write]. Roentgenography of the uterus.

uterolith (ū′tĕr-ō-lĭth) [″ + Gr. *lithos*, stone]. A uterine concretion.

uterometer (ū″tĕr-ŏm′ĕt-er) [″ + Gr. *metron*, measure]. Device for measuring the uterus and for determining its position.

uteroovarian (ū″tĕr-ō-ō-vā′rē-ăn) [″ + LL. *ovarium*, ovary]. Rel. to the uterus and ovary.

uteropexia, uteropexy (ū″tĕr-ō-pĕks′ē-ă, ū′tĕr-ō-pĕks″ē) [″ + Gr. *pexis*, fixation]. Fixation of the uterus to the abdominal wall. SYN: *hysteropexy*.

uteroplacental (ū″tĕr-ō-plă-sĕn′tăl) [″ + *placenta*, a flat cake]. Rel. to the placenta and uterus.

uteroplasty (ū″tĕr-ō-plăs′tē) [″ + Gr. *plassein*, to form]. Plastic surgery of the uterus.

uterorectal (ū″tĕr-ō-rĕk′tăl). Concerning the uterus and rectum.

uterosacral (ū″tĕr-ō-sā′krăl) [″ + *sacralis*, pert. to the sacrum]. Rel. to the uterus and sacrum.

uterosalpingography (ū″tĕr-ō-săl-pĭng-ŏg′ră-fē) [″ + Gr. *salpinx*, tube, + *graphein*, to write]. Visualization of the interior of the uterus and fallopian tubes by roentgenography.

uteroscope (ū′tĕr-ō-skōp) [″ + Gr. *skopein*, to examine]. Device for viewing the uterine cavity.

uterotome (ū′tĕr-ō-tŏm) [″ + Gr. *tome*, incision]. An instrument used for uterotomy.

uterotomy (ū-tĕr-ŏt′ō-mē). Incision of the uterus.

uterotonic (ū″tĕr-ō-tŏn′ĭk) [L. *uterus*, womb, + Gr. *tonos*, act of stretching, tension]. Giving muscular tone to the uterus.

uterotractor (ū″tĕr-ō-trăk′tor) [″ + *tractor*, drawer]. An instrument for applying traction to the cervix uteri.

uterotubal (ū″tĕr-ō-tū′băl) [″ + *tuba*, tube]. Relating to the uterus and oviducts.

uterotubography (ū″tĕr-ō-tū-bŏg′ră-fē) [″ + ″ + Gr. *graphein*, to write]. Hysterosalpingography.

uterovaginal (ū″tĕr-ō-văj′ĭ-năl) [″ + *vagina*, sheath]. Rel. to the uterus and vagina.

uteroventral(ū″tĕr-ō-vĕn′trăl).Uteroabdominal, q.v.

uterovesical (ū″tĕr-ō-vĕs′ĭ-kăl) [″ + *vesica*, bladder]. Rel. to the uterus and bladder.

uterus (ū′tĕr-ŭs) [L.]. [NA] An organ of the female reproductive system for containing and nourishing the embryo and fetus from the time the fertilized egg is implanted to the time of birth of the fetus. SYN: *womb*. SEE: *genitalia, female*, for illus.; *pregnancy test*.

ANAT: A muscular, hollow, pear-shaped structure. It is partly covered by peritoneum and the cavity is lined by a mucous membrane, the endometrium.

The uterus consists of three areas: the body or expanded upper portion, the isthmus or constricted central area, and the cervix, the lowermost cylindrical portion that joins the uterus to the upper end of the vagina. The rounded portion of the body lying above the openings of the two uterine tubes is the fundus.

The uterus is situated in the midpelvis, approximately halfway between the sacrum and the symphysis pubis. It is supported in this position by the pelvic diaphragm, supplemented by two broad ligaments, two round ligaments, and two uterosacral ligaments, as well as other lesser ligaments. The upper part of the body is called the fundus, and the lateral borders of the fundus to which the tubes are attached are called the cornual ends. The fallopian tubes communicate with the peritoneal cavity and provide the pathway for the ova to go from the ovary to the cavity of the uterus. The cavity of the uterus, a potential space, is triangular in shape with the base of the triangle in the fundal portion. The canal of the cervix is long and narrow and is constricted at the upper end by the internal os and at the lower end by the external os.

The largest portion of the uterus is made up of musculature that is longitudinal and circular. The outer covering of the uterus is peritoneum, with the exception of that part upon which the bladder rests and the vaginal portion of the cervix. The inner lining of the body of the uterus varies in form and histological structure with the period of life in which it is studied, the prepuberty stage, the actively menstruating stage, and the menopausal stage, each having its own characteristics. The uterus is normally anteflexed. Its blood supply is derived from the uterine and ovarian arteries.

POSITIONS: Anteflexion: bending forward. Anteversion: forward displacement of fundus toward pubis, while cervix is tilted up toward sacrum. Retroflexion: bending backward at junction of body and cervix. Retroversion: inclination backward with retention of normal curve; opposite of anteversion.

AUSCULTATION: After the fourth month of gestation, if the uterus contains a living fetus, three distinct sounds may be heard. *Fetal heart sounds*: Consist of a succession of short, rapid, double pulsations varying in frequency from 120 to 140 per minute. First sound is short, feeble, and obscure, while the second, the one usually heard, is loud and distinct; sounds like ticking of a watch wrapped in a napkin. Sound is usually transmitted over a space of 3 or 4 in. (7.6 to 10.2 cm) square. Location is determined by the position of the fetus. Generally, when maximum intensity is on the level of or above the umbilicus, it is a breech presentation. During labor, examinations, if made, should be between uterine contractions. In protracted labors the fetal heart sound is of value in indicating the time for manual or instrumental interference to save life of child. Irregularity and feebleness of sound are indicative of a life-threatening situation for the fetus.

Funic souffle: The soft blowing sound heard over the location of the umbilical cord of the fetus in utero and synchronous with the fetal heartbeat during late pregnancy.

Uterine bruit: This sound is single, intermittent in character, and a combination of blowing and hissing sounds. Increases in intensity up to the period of labor. Believed to depend upon rapid passage of blood from the arteries into the distended venous sinuses of the uterus. Synchronous with maternal pulse, subject to same variations, and is always heard before the pulsations of the fetal heart. The area over which it is audible varies, with the greatest point of intensity in a median line a little above the pubes.

PALPATION: During the third month of pregnancy, if walls of abdomen are not too thick, palpate by placing patient upon her back with head raised and thighs flexed, and pressing points of fingers gently downward and backward above the pubes. A hard round mass will be found beneath the median line, rising out of the pelvis. Two or four weeks later the increase is marked. As pregnancy advances, the mass loses its hardness and becomes more elastic, like a cyst filled with water. In doubtful cases in which decided enlargement of abdomen is present, a standard hormonal test for pregnancy should be done.

By vaginal examination one may be able to diagnose the stage of gestation, stage of parturition, or if the woman is near term, the progress of labor, the presentation and position of the child, and the position of the uterus. The sensation of the tip of the cervix of an unimpregnated uterus to the touch is like that imparted to the finger by touching the tip of the nose, i.e., firm and cartilaginous; of the impregnated, like that of touching the lips and is soft like velvet, but deeper, beyond the softness, is a hardness, as of board.

PERCUSSION: The nonpregnant uterus is inaccessible to touch externally or to percussion. In pregnancy at end of second month a dull sound on percussion just above the pubes indicates the enlarging uterus; later, as uterus increases in volume and rises into abdomen, one is able, by oval tumor felt in hypogastrium and by circumscribed area of dullness corresponding to situation of the tumor, to establish strong presumptive evidence of pregnancy. This presumption becomes strengthened if the area of dullness increases as gestation progresses. Palpation and percussion, however, are not sufficient to determine whether the enlargement is due to pregnancy or to some other form of new growth. After the fifth month, both these methods are inferior to auscultation.

u. acollis. Uterus without a cervix.

u. arcuatus. Uterus with a depressed arched fundus.

u. bicornis. Uterus in which the fundus is divided into two parts.

u. biforis. Uterus in which the external os is divided into two parts by a septum.

u. bilocularis. Uterus in which the cavity is divided into two parts by a partition. SYN: *uterus septus.*

u., bipartite. Uterus in which the body is partially divided by a median septum.

u., cancer of. Malignant neoplasm of the uterus. Detected by size, intermittent bleeding, purulent discharge, vaginal or Papanicolau smear, or cervical or endometrial biopsy. May produce sterility, abortion, hemorrhage, sepis. Extremely rare in pregnancy; however, if present, a tumor will usually increase in size during pregnancy.

u. cordiformis. Heart-shaped uterus.

u., Couvelaire. SEE: *Couvelaire uterus.*

u. didelphys. Double uterus.

u. duplex. Double uterus resulting from failure of union of müllerian ducts.

u., fetal. Uterus that is retarded in development and possesses an extremely long cervical canal.

u., fibroids of. SEE: *fibroma, uterine.*

u., gravid. Pregnant uterus.

u. masculinus. The prostatic utricle. SEE: *utricle, prostatic.*

u. parvicollis. Normal uterus with disproportionately small vaginal portion.

u., prolapse of. Defective pelvic floor allowing the uterus or part of it to protrude out of the vagina. SYN: *descensus uteri; procidentia.*

VARIETIES: First degree: where the cervix uteri reaches down to the vaginal introitus. Second degree: where the cervix uteri protrudes out of the vagina. Third degree: where the entire uterus lies outside of the vagina.

SYM: The condition is most often seen following instrumental deliveries or when the patient has been allowed to bear down before the cervix is fully dilated. Frequently associated with this is a prolapse of the anterior and posterior vaginal walls, as seen in cystocele and rectocele. In the early stages there are dragging sensations in the lower abdomen, back pain while standing and on exertion, sensation of weight and bearing down in the perineum, frequency of urination and incontinence of urine in cases associated with cystocele. In the later stages a protrusion or swelling at the vulva is noticed on standing or straining, and leukorrhea is present. In procidentia, q.v., there is frequently pain on walking, inability to urinate unless the mass is reduced, and cystitis.

ETIOL: This condition may be congenital or acquired; most often it is acquired. The etiological factors are congenital weakness of the uterine supports and injury to the pelvic floor or uterine supports during childbirth.

TREAT: The treatment depends upon the age of the patient, the degree of prolapse, and the associated pathology. Abdominal surgery with fixation of the uterus will be required if the prolapse is complete.

u., pubescent. Adult uterus that resembles a uterus of a prepubertal female.

u., rupture of, in pregnancy. Rare but serious. May be spontaneous or traumatic. Fetus and amniotic sac may be expelled into peritoneal cavity. SEE: *Nursing Diagnoses* in *Appendix.*

SYM: Obstruction usually precedes symptoms. Abdominal pains, shock, hemorrhage. Fetus easily palpated. However, spontaneous rupture may occur without warning.

ETIOL: Obstruction, weakness of uterine wall. Scars may cause weakness.

TREAT: Combat shock and hemorrhage, and surgically remove products of conception from peritoneal cavity.

u. septus. U. bilocularis.

u., subinvolution of. The lack of involution of the uterus following childbirth. It is manifested by a large uterus and a continuation of lochia rubra beyond the usual time. The factors in its causation are usually puerperal infection, multiparity, overdistention of the uterus by multiple pregnancy or polyhydramnios, lack of lactation, malposition of the uterus, and retained secundines. Involution is aided by certainty that the placenta is intact at the time of delivery, and the use of ecbolics, q.v., to cause contraction of the uterus.

u., tipped. SEE: *tipped uterus.*

u., tumors of. May cause sterility or abortion or obstruct labor; may become infected or twisted on their attachments. Myomata (fibroids) are possible but not common in young women; fibroids are more common beyond age 30 and in black women. Subserous tumors do not affect pregnancy, may impede labor, or may disappear following labor. Interstitial and submucous type may interfere with pregnancy and produce abortion.

EFFECTS UPON LABOR: Tumors usually have no effect. If low, may cause malpresentation or impossible labor; labor pains may be weak and inefficient. Often there will be severe pains and rupture of uterus. Submucous tumors may protrude before or after birth. Placenta may be retained. Tumor may be infected postpartum. Knee-chest position helps patient if tumor is in pelvis. If in fundus, delivery is through vagina; if not, cesarean section may be needed. Control hemorrhage by packing.

u. unicornis. Uterus possessing only one lateral half and usually having only one uterine tube.

Uticillin VK. Trade name for penicillin V potassium.

Uticort. Trade name for betamethasone benzoate.

utilization review. Evaluation of the necessity, quality, effectiveness, or efficiency of medical services, procedures, and facilities. In regard to a hospital, the review includes appropriateness of admission, services ordered and provided, length of stay, and discharge practices.

Utimox. Trade name for amoxicillin.

utricle (ū′trĭk′l) [L. *utriculus*, a little bag]. 1. One of two sacs of the membranous labyrinth in the bony vestibule of the inner ear. It communicates with the semicircular ducts by five openings on posterior wall and with the sacculus and endolymphatic duct by an opening on anterior wall. On its inner surface is an area of sensory epithelium, the macula utriculi, containing cells that respond to movement of otoliths due to changes in position. 2. Any small sac.

u. of urethra. The prostatic vesicle of the male.

u. of vestibule. Vestibular cavity connecting with the semicircular canals.

u., prostatic. A small blind pouch of the urethra extending into substance of prostate gland. It is a remnant of the embryonic mullerian duct. SYN: *uterus masculinus.*

utricular (ū-trĭk′ū-lăr) [L. *utriculus*, a little bag]. 1. Pert. to the utricle. 2. Like a bladder.

utriculitis (ū-trĭk-ū-lī′tĭs) [″ + Gr. *itis*, inflammation]. Inflammation of the utricle, either that of the vestibule or the prostatic utricle.

utriculoplasty (ū-trĭk′ū-lō-plăs″tē) [″ + Gr. *plassein*, to form]. Surgical reduction of the size of the uterus by excision of a longitudinal wedge-shaped section.

utriculosaccular (ū-trĭk″ū-lō-săk′ū-lăr) [″ + *sacculus*, a small bag]. Pert. to the utricle and saccule of the labyrinth.

utriculosaccular duct. Duct uniting the utricle and saccule.

utriculus (ū-trĭk′ū-lŭs) [L., a little bag]. A utricle.

u. masculinus. Utricle, prostatic.

u. prostaticus. Utricle, prostatic.

utriform (ū′trĭ-form) [L. *uter*, a skin bag, + *forma*, shape]. Having a shape like a bottle.

uva (ū′vă) [L., grape]. The dried fruit of the grapevine; the raisin.

uvea (ū′vē-ă) [L. *uva*, grape]. The second or vascular coat of the eye lying immediately beneath the sclera. It consists of the iris, ciliary body, and choroid, and forms the pigmented layer.

uveal (ū′vē-ăl). Pert. to the middle coat of the eye, or uvea.

uveitic (ū-vē-ĭt′ĭk) [″ + Gr. *itis*, inflammation]. Marked by or pert. to uveitis.

uveitis (ū-vē-ī′tĭs). A nonspecific term for any intraocular inflammatory disorder. The uveal tract structures — iris, ciliary body, and choroid — are usually involved, but other nonuveal parts of the eye, including the retina and cornea, may be involved.

Uveitis that is not associated with known infections or that is associated with diseases of unknown cause is termed endogenous uveitis. This is thought to be due to an autoimmune phenomenon.

TREAT: Corticosteroids and other immunosuppressive agents, including cyclosporine, are used in treating some causes of uveitis, but their use may make some types of uveitus worse.

Short-acting cycloplegic agents such as hematropine, scopolamine, or cyclopentolate are used during therapy to prevent inflammatory adhesions (posterior synechiae) between the iris and lens.

u., sympathetic. Severe, bilateral uveitis that started as inflammation of the uveal tract of one eye resulting from a puncture wound. The injured eye is termed the "exciting eye." If the affected eye is not removed within 10 days of the accident that caused the wound, blindness will be the outcome. SEE: *ophthalmia, sympathetic.*

uveoparotitis (ū″vē-ō-păr-ō-tī′tĭs) [″ + Gr. *para*, beside, + *ous*, ear, + *itis*, inflammation]. Inflammation of the parotid gland and uveitis.

uveoplasty (ū′vē-ō-plăs″tē) [″ + Gr. *plassein*, to form]. Reparative operation of the uvea.

uveoscleritis (ū″vē-ō-sklĕr-ī′tĭs). Inflammation of the sclera in which the infection has spread from the uvea.

uviform (ū′vĭ-form) [″ + *forma*, form]. Shaped like a grape.

uviofast (ū′vē-ō-făst). Unaffected by ultraviolet radiation.

uviol (ū′vē-ŏl). Glass that is unusually transparent to ultraviolet rays.

uviolize (ū′vē-ō-līz). To use ultraviolet radiation therapeutically.

uviometer (ū″vē-ŏm′ĕ-tĕr). An instrument for measuring the intensity of ultraviolet light.

uvioresistant (ū″vē-ō-rē-zĭs′tănt). Resistant to effects of ultraviolet radiation. SYN: *uviofast.*

uviosensitive (ū″vē-ō-sĕn′sĭ-tĭv). Sensitive to effects of ultraviolet radiation.

uvula (ū′vū-lă) [L. *uvula*, a little grape]. Small, soft structure hanging from free edge of soft palate in midline above the root of the tongue. It is composed of muscle, connective tissue, and mucous membrane. SYN: *cion; staphyle.*

u. fissa. A cleft uvula.

u. of cerebellum. A small lobule of the cerebellum lying on inferior surface of inferior vermis, anterior to the pyramis.

u. vermis. A small, triangular elevation on the vermis of the cerebellum of the brain.

u. vesicae. A median projection of mucous membrane of the urinary bladder located immediately anterior to the orifice of the urethra.

uvulaptosis (ū″vū-lăp-tō′sĭs) [″ + Gr. *ptosis*, a dropping]. A relaxed condition of the uvula. SYN: *uvuloptosis.*

uvular (ū′vū-lăr) [L. *uvula*, little grape]. Pert. to the uvula.

uvularis (ū-vū-lā′rĭs) [L.]. The azygos uvulae muscle. SEE: *Muscles* in *Appendix.*

uvulatome (ū′vū-lă-tōm) [″ + Gr. *tome*, incision]. Instrument for removal of the uvula.

uvulatomy (ū-vū-lăt′ō-mē). Excision of the uvula.

uvulectomy (ū″vū-lĕk′tō-mē) [″ + Gr. *ek-*

tome, excision]. Surgical removal of the uvula.

uvulitis (ū″vū-lī′tĭs) [″ + Gr. *itis*, inflammation]. Inflammation of the uvula.

uvulopalatopharyngoplasty. ABBR: UPPP. Plastic surgery of the oropharynx in which redundant soft palate, uvula, pillars, fauces, and sometimes posterior pharyngeal wall mucosa are removed. This procedure is usually done to correct intractable snoring or sleep apnea. SEE: *sleep, disorders of; snore.*

uvuloptosis (ū″vū-lŏp-tō′sĭs) [″ + Gr. *ptosis*, a dropping]. Relaxed and pendulous condition of the palate.

uvulotome (ū′vū-lō-tōm) [L. *uvula*, little grape, + Gr. *tome*, incision]. Instrument for performing uvulotomy. SYN: *uvulatome.*

uvulotomy (ū-vū-lōt′ō-mē). Amputation of the uvula.

U wave. In the electrocardiogram, a low-amplitude deflection that follows the T wave. Its significance is unknown, and its absence does not indicate abnormality. SEE: *QRST complex; electrocardiogram.*

V

V. 1. *Vibrio; vision; visual acuity.* 2. Chem. symb. for the element vanadium.

V. 1. Symbol for gas flow. 2. Symbol for ventilation.

v. L. *vena*, vein; *volt*.

vaccigenous (văk-sĭj′ĕn-ŭs) [L. *vaccinus*, pert. to cows, + Gr. *gennan*, to produce]. Producing vaccine. SYN: *vaccinogenous*.

vaccina (văk-sī′nă). Vaccinia, q.v.

vaccinable (văk-sĭn′ă-b′l). Capable of being successfully vaccinated.

vaccinal (văk′sĭn-ăl). Rel. to vaccine or to vaccination.

vaccinate (văk′sĭn-āt) [L. *vaccinus*, pert. to cows]. To inoculate with vaccine to produce immunity against disease.

vaccination (văk″sĭ-nā′shŭn) [L. *vaccinus*, pert. to cows]. 1. Inoculation with any vaccine or toxoid to establish resistance to a specific infectious disease. SEE: *immunization*. 2. A scar left on the skin by inoculation of a vaccine.

vaccinator (văk′sĭ-nā″tor). One who vaccinates.

vaccine (văk′sēn, văk-sēn′) [L. *vaccinus*, pert. to cows]. A suspension of infectious agents, or some part of them, given for the purpose of establishing resistance to an infectious disease. SEE: table.

Vaccines are of four general classes:

(1) Those containing living attenuated infectious organisms. Ex.: vaccine for poliomyelitis.

(2) Those containing infectious agents killed by physical or chemical means. Ex.: vaccines used to protect human beings against typhoid fever, rabies, and whooping cough.

(3) Those containing soluble toxins of microorganisms, sometimes used as such, but generally forming toxoids. Ex.: toxoid used in the prevention of diphtheria and tetanus.

(4) Those containing substances extracted from infectious agents. Ex.: capsular polysaccharides extracted from pneumococci.

FUNCT: To stimulate an immune response in the body by creating antibodies or activated T lymphocytes capable of controlling the organism. The result is more or less permanent protection against a disease. An attack of smallpox or diphtheria, for example, usually leaves the recovered patient permanently immune to those diseases. As a result of infection, the body succeeds in building up its own defenses, so that a new infection causes no illness. A successful vaccine does the same thing without risk of illness. SEE: *immune response; immunity; immunization; immunobiologics.*

v., autogenous. Bacterial vaccine prepared from lesions of the individual to be inoculated. SYN: *v., homologous.*

v., bacterial. A suspension of bacteria, killed or attenuated, in saline solution. Used for injection into body to induce development of active immunity to the same organism.

v., BCG. USP. Bacille Calmette-Guérin, a preparation of a dried, living culture of *Mycobacterium tuberculosis.* In areas with a high incidence of tuberculosis, it is used in prophylactic vaccination of infants against tuberculosis. It is also used in adults who are at high and unavoidable risk of becoming infected with tuberculosis. Virulence of the bacillus has been reduced by repeated cultures on glycerinated ox bile.

v., cholera. Vaccine prepared from killed *Vibrio cholerae.* It is effective for only a few months.

v., diphtheria. SEE: *v., DTP.*

v., DTP. A preparation of diphtheria and tetanus toxoids and killed pertussis vaccine that is used in active immunization. It is administered intramuscularly.

v., Haemophilus influenza type b. Vaccine prepared from the bacterial polysaccharide (HbPV) or polysaccharide converted to protein (HbCV).

v., hepatitis B. Vaccine prepared from inactivated hepatitis B viral antigen.

v., heterologous. Vaccine derived from an organism different from the organism against which the vaccine is used.

v., human diploid cell rabies (HDCV). An inactivated virus vaccine prepared from fixed rabies virus grown in human diploid cell tissue culture.

v., influenza. A polyvalent vaccine containing inactivated antigenic variants of the influenza virus for use in areas expected to have epidemics. Its use is particularly helpful to the aged and chronically ill.

v., killed. Vaccine prepared from dead microorganisms. This type of vaccine is used for strains that have a high virulence.

v., measles virus, live attenuated. Vaccine prepared from live strains of measles virus. It is the preferred form except in patients who have one of the following: lymphoma, leukemia, or other generalized malignancy; radiation therapy; pregnancy; active tuberculosis; egg sensitivity; pro-

Vaccines

Name	Age Administered	Booster Schedule	Comments
BCG (bacillus of Calmette and Guerin)	In epidemic conditions, administer to infants as soon as possible after birth.	None	The only contraindications are symptomatic human immunodeficiency virus (HIV) infection or other illnesses known to cause suppression of immunity.
Cholera	See Comments	Every 3 to 6 mo. for those who remain in epidemic areas.	Only those traveling to countries where cholera is present need to be vaccinated. Whole cell vaccines provide partial protection for 3 to 6 mo.
DPT (diphtheria, pertussis, tetanus)	Given routinely beginning as early as 2 mo., a total of 3 inoculations at 4–6 wk intervals. A 4th dose is given a yr later. Administered I.M.	Repeat inoculation at time of entering school. After that children need only tetanus and diphtheria immunization every 10 yr.	Tetanus booster may be required following a wound even though all routine and booster immunizations have been received. Booster of diphtheria toxoid should be given if child under six is exposed to diphtheria.
Haemophilus influenza b (Polysaccharide or conjugate)	Between 18 months and 2 years.	None	SEE: *Haemophilus influenza b infections.*
Hepatitis B	All ages of persons at risk of contracting the virus, e.g., dialysis patients.	Every 6 to 12 mo.	The vaccine is expensive and should be given only to those at high risk of developing the disease who do not show evidence of immunity to the virus. Immune globulin or hepatitis B globulin may be given to produce passive immunity in exposed contacts.
Influenza (flu)	All ages.	Annually, given prior to time influenza is expected.	Recommended for those who may become seriously ill if they develop flu, i.e., the elderly and those of any age who have chronic diseases of the heart or lungs or metabolic diseases such as diabetes.
Measles (live attenuated rubeola)	At or after 15 mo.	If vaccinated before 10 mo of age, should be revaccinated within a year.	Vaccine will usually prevent measles if given within 2 days after a child has been exposed to the disease. Not given to adults.

Vaccines (Continued)

Name	Age Administered	Booster Schedule	Comments
Mumps	Any age after 15 mo.	Not indicated.	Particularly valuable for children approaching puberty, adolescents, and adults who have never had mumps. Contraindicated in those known to be hypersensitive to eggs, chicken, chicken feathers, or neomycin.
Plague	See Comments	See Comments	Recommended for those traveling to Southeast Asia, persons who work closely with wild rodents in plague areas, and laboratory personnel working with *Yersinia pestis* organisms.
Pneumococcal vaccine, polyvalent	Do not give to children under age 2 or to pregnant women.	None	Vaccine is effective against the 23 most prevalent types of pneumococci. Administered to those who have an increased risk of developing pneumococcal pneumonia. Included are those who have chronic diseases, are recovering from an acute illness, are in chronic care facilities, or are 65 years of age or older.
Polio (live oral trivalent vaccine)	Three doses, first at 2 mo, then at 4 mo, and at 18 mo.	At time of entering school.	Administration is postponed in those with persistent vomiting, diarrhea, or acute illness.
Rabies	See Comments	See Comments	Each exposure to rabies needs to be evaluated on an individual basis by the physician. The use of human diploid cell rabies vaccine is the treatment of choice for those never previously immunized against rabies. SEE: *rabies*.
Rh immune globulin	1 dose 72 hr after delivery, abortion, or accidental transfusion of Rh-positive blood to Rh-negative patient.	None	Should be given to Rh-negative women who give birth to Rh-positive infants and to Rh-negative women who have abortions.

Vaccines (Continued)

Name	Age Administered	Booster Schedule	Comments
Rubella (German measles)	No earlier than 1 yr of age.	Not indicated.	Object is to prevent infection of the fetus. Because the major source of virus dissemination is from children in elementary school, all children regardless of their previous experience with rubella should be vaccinated. CAUTION: Pregnant women should not be given rubella vaccine. Vaccine should not be given to persons with defective or compromised immune systems.
Smallpox	See Comments	See Comments	Because smallpox is considered to have been eradicated worldwide, the vaccine is no longer administered.
Typhoid	See Comments	See Comments	Immunization is indicated when a person has come into contact with a known typhoid carrier, if there is an outbreak of typhoid fever, or prior to traveling to an area where typhoid is endemic.
Yellow fever	See Comments	Every 10 years.	Vaccine should be given to all persons traveling in or living in areas where yellow fever is present.

longed treatment with drugs that suppress the immune response, i.e., corticosteroids or antimetabolites; administration of gamma globulin, blood, or plasma. Those persons should be given immune globulin immediately following exposure. SEE: *vaccine, measles virus, inactivated.*

v., meningococcal. Vaccine prepared from bacterial polysaccharides from certain types of meningococci.

v., MMR. A vaccine prepared from the live viruses of measles, mumps, and rubella.

v., mumps. A live attenuated vaccine used to prevent mumps. Its use should be governed by the same restrictions listed for live attenuated measles virus vaccine.

v., pertussis. SEE: *v., DTP.*

v., plague. Vaccine made from a crude fraction of killed plague bacilli for immunizing against plague.

v., pneumococcal, polyvalent. A vac-

cine effective against the 23 most prevalent types of pneumococci. Do not give to children under two years of age or to pregnant women.

v., poliovirus, inactivated. USP. Oral vaccine prepared from three types of inactivated polioviruses. Previously used name: poliomyelitis vaccine.

v., poliovirus, live oral. USP. Vaccine prepared from three types of live poliovirus.

v., rabies. Vaccine prepared from killed, fixed virus of rabies, used prophylactically following bite by a rabid animal. SEE: *v., human diploid cell rabies (HDCV); rabies.*

v., rubella. A live virus vaccine used to prevent rubella (German measles). All nonpregnant susceptible women of childbearing age should be provided with this vaccine in order to prevent fetal infection and the congenital rubella syndrome, i.e., possible fetal death, prematurity, impaired hearing, cataract, mental retardation, and other serious conditions.

v., Sabin. V., poliovirus, live oral. USP. SEE: *poliomyelitis.*

v., Salk. V., poliovirus inactivated.

v., sensitized. Vaccine prepared from bacteria treated with their specific immune serum.

v., smallpox. Vaccine made from lymph of cowpox vesicles obtained from healthy vaccinated bovine animals. NOTE: This vaccine is no longer used because smallpox has been eradicated world-wide.

v., tetanus. SEE: *v., DTP.*

v., typhoid. Vaccine made of killed *Salmonella typhii* organisms for immunizing against typhoid. May not be effective if person receives unusually large doses of the live organism at time of exposure. An orally administered vaccine is available.

v., varicella. Although there is no vaccine for varicella (chickenpox), varicella-zoster immune globulin is available. SEE: *varicella* (prevention).

v., yellow fever. Vaccine made from a live attenuated strain of yellow fever virus.

vaccinia (văk-sĭn′ē-ă) [L. *vaccinus,* pert. to cows]. A contagious disease of cattle, produced in humans by inoculation with cowpox virus to confer immunity against smallpox. Papules form about third day after vaccination, changing to umbilicated vesicles about the fifth day, and at end of first week becoming umbilicated pustules surrounded by red areolae. They dry and form scabs, which fall off about the second week, leaving a white pitted depression. SYN: *cowpox.* SEE: *vaccination; varicella; variola.*

v. necrosum. Spreading necrosis at the site of smallpox vaccination. May be accompanied by similar necrotic areas elsewhere on the body.

vaccinia immune globulin. USP. Hyperimmune gamma globulin. The therapeutic agent of choice for dermal complications of vaccination for smallpox, i.e., eczema vaccinatum and progressive vaccinia. May be obtained commercially or by contacting one of the designated consultants listed by the Regional Blood Centers of the American Red Cross.

NOTE: There is no longer a need for this material because smallpox has been eradicated world-wide.

vaccinial (văk-sĭn′ē-ăl). Resembling vaccinia.

vacciniform (văk-sĭn′ĭ-form) [L. *vaccinus,* pert. to cows, + *forma,* shape]. Of the nature of vaccinia or cowpox.

vacciniola (văk″sĭn-ē-ō′lă) [L., little cows].

Secondary general eruption after local eruption from vaccine.

vaccinogen (văk-sĭn′ō-jĕn). A source of vaccine.

vaccinogenous (văk″sĭn-ŏj′ĕn-ŭs) [L. *vaccinus,* pert. to cows, + Gr. *gennan,* to produce]. Producing vaccine or pert. to its production.

vaccinoid (văk′sĭn-oyd) [″ + Gr. *eidos,* form, shape]. 1. Resembling vaccinia. 2. Modified or spurious vaccinia.

vaccinostyle (văk-sĭn′ō-stīl). A pointed stylus used in vaccination.

vaccinotherapeutics (văk″sĭn-ō-thĕr″ă-pū′tĭks). Treatment by injection of bacterial vaccines.

vaccinum (văk-sī′nŭm) [L.]. Vaccine.

vacuolar (văk′ū-ō-lăr) [L. *vacuum,* empty]. Pert. to or possessing vacuoles.

vacuolar degeneration. Swelling of cells with increase in number and size of vacuoles. SYN: *cloudy swelling.*

vacuolated (văk′ū-ō-lāt″ĕd). Possessing or containing vacuoles.

vacuolation (văk″ū-ō-lā′shŭn). Formation of vacuoles. SYN: *vacuolization.*

vacuole (văk′ū-ōl) [L. *vacuum,* empty]. A clear space in cell protoplasm filled with fluid or air.

v., autophagic. Vacuole that contains recognizable fragments of the ribosomes or mitochondria.

v., contractile. A cavity filled with fluid in the cytoplasm of a protozoan. The cavity is emptied by sudden contraction of its walls.

v., heterophagous. Vacuole that contains substances that come from outside the cell.

v., plasmocrine. Vacuole present in cytoplasm of secretory cell that is filled with crystalloid material.

v., rhagiocrine. Vacuole present in cytoplasm of secretory cell that is filled with colloid material.

vacuolization (văk″ū-ō-lĭ-zā′shŭn) [L. *vacuum,* empty]. Vacuolation.

vacuome (văk′ū-ōm). A system of vacuoles in cells that stain in the living cell with neutral red.

vacuum (văk′ū-ŭm) [L., empty]. A space exhausted of its air content.

vacuum aspiration. Removal of uterine contents by using a hollow curet or catheter to which a suction apparatus is attached. Used prior to 12th week of pregnancy.

vacuum extractor. Device, using a suction cup attached to the fetal head, for applying traction to the fetus during delivery. Its use may be hazardous except in the hands of experts.

vacuum tube. A vessel of insulating material (usually glass) that is sealed and has a vacuum sufficiently high to permit the free flow of electrons between the electrodes that extend into the tube from the outside. In England, it is called a vacuum valve.

vade mecum (vā″dē mē′kŭm) [L., go with me]. A useful object that a person has available at all times. A dictionary or handbook.

vagabond's disease. Discoloration of skin caused by exposure and scratching due to presence of lice. SEE: *pediculosis corporis.*

vagal (vā′găl) [L. *vagus,* wandering]. Pert. to the vagus nerve.

vagal attack. Condition of dyspnea with cardiac distress and a fear of impending death. A sinking sensation assumed to be the result of vasomotor spasm.

vagal escape. Condition in which one or more beats of the heart occur even though the vagus nerve is being continuously stimulated. Stimulation of the vagus normally inhibits heartbeat.

vagal tone. Condition in which impulses over the vagus nerve exert a continuous inhibitory effect upon the heart.

vagi (vā′gī). Pl. of vagus.

vagina (vă-jī′nă) [L., sheath] (pl. *vaginae, vaginas*). 1. A sheathlike part. 2. [NA] A musculomembranous tube that forms the passageway between the cervix uteri and the vulva.

ANAT: In the uppermost part, the cervix divides the vagina into four fornices: the two lateral, the anterior, and the posterior. The bladder is situated adjacent to the anterior wall of the vagina, and the rectum is behind the posterior wall. The vagina represents a potential space, the walls of which are in contact with each other. Close to the cervix uteri the walls form a horizontal crescent shape, at the midpoint an H shape, and close to the vulva the shape of a vertical slit. The vagina is lined by mucous membrane made up of squamous epithelium. It is surrounded by fasciae that allow for easy distensibility. The blood supply of the vagina is furnished from the inferior vesical, inferior hemorrhoidal, and uterine arteries. Except for the area close to the entrance, the vaginal tissue and mucosa contain few, if any, sensory nerve endings.

PHYS: A passage for the intromission of the penis, for the reception of semen, and for the discharge of the menstrual flow; and the passageway through which the fetus is delivered.

v., artificial. A plastic surgery procedure in which an artificial vagina is constructed. This is done for a patient whose vagina was removed for treatment of carcinoma.

v., bulb of. Small erectile body on each side of the vestibule. SYN: *Bartholin's*

glands; bulbi vestibuli.

v. fibrosa tendinis. A fibrous sheath surrounding a tendon that usually confines it to an osseous groove.

v., foreign bodies in. SEE: *foreign bodies.*

v. masculina. The prostatic utricle. SEE: *utricle, prostatic.*

v. mucosa tendinis. A synovial sheath that develops about a tendon.

v., septate. Congenital condition in which the vagina is divided longitudinally into two parts. Division may be partial or complete.

vagina, words pert. to: bulbus vestibuli; coitus; "colp-" words; cystocele; "elytr-" words; endocolpitis; enterocele; fistula; fornix; fourchette; gynatresia; hematocolpometra; hydrocolpos; hymen; leukorrhea; paravaginal; pronaus; rectocele; supravaginal; transvaginal; "vagin-" words.

vaginal (văj′ĭn-ăl) [L. *vagina,* sheath]. Pert. to the vagina or to any enveloping sheath.

vaginal atrophy, postmenopausal. Atrophy of the vagina and vaginal mucosa that may occur following menopause. Hormonal changes occur following menopause. These changes are believed to influence the onset of vaginal atrophy. Menopausal women who continue to engage in sexual intercourse during menopause have less vaginal atrophy than do those women who become sexually inactive.

vaginalectomy (văj″ĭn-ăl-ĕk′tō-mē) [″ + Gr. *ektome,* excision]. Excision of the tunica vaginalis. SYN: *vaginectomy* (def. 1).

vaginal hysterectomy. Surgical removal of uterus through the vagina.

vaginitis (văj-ĭn-ăl-ī′tĭs) [″ + Gr. *itis,* inflammation]. Inflammation of tunica vaginalis testis.

vaginal lubricant. A substance, usually a water-soluble ointment or cream, used to lubricate the vagina. Vaseline has little if any benefit when used as a vaginal lubricant. A natural and effective lubricant is human saliva.

vaginal vibrator. A device used intravaginally to produce vibrations. May be used for erotic stimulation.

vaginapexy (văj″ĭn-ă-pĕk′sē) [″ + Gr. *pexis,* fixation]. Repair of a relaxed and prolapsed vagina. SYN: *colpopexy; vaginofixation.*

vaginate (văj′ĭn-āt) [L. *vaginatus*]. Forming or enclosed in a sheath.

vaginectomy (văj-ĭn-ĕk′tō-mē) [L. *vagina,* sheath, + Gr. *ektome,* excision]. 1. Resection of tunica vaginalis. 2. Excision of the vagina or a part of it.

vaginismus (văj″ĭn-ĭz′mŭs) [L.]. Painful spasm of vagina from contraction of the muscles surrounding the vagina. May interfere with coitus. This is usually the result of real, imagined, or anticipated attempts at vaginal penetration. There may be a physical condition, i.e., an anatomical abnormality to account for the condition, but this is not the usual case. The patient and her sex partner should be seen together by the physician. If there are no anatomical causes, the following therapy may help: The patient may be desensitized by teaching her relaxation techniques; then self-insertion of a small vaginal dilator. Over time, the dilator size is increased and, eventually, when both the patient and her sex partner are agreeable, female-superior intercourse may be tried while he is passive. Later, male-superior intercourse is prescribed. SEE: *Nursing Diagnoses* in Appendix.

vaginitis (văj-ĭn-ī′tĭs) [L. *vagina*, sheath, + Gr. *itis*, inflammation]. 1. Inflammation of a sheath. 2. Inflammation of the vagina. SYN: *colpitis*.

SYM: Free purulent vaginal discharge, sometimes malodorous and occasionally stained with blood. There is irritation and itching of the vulvae and perineum, increased frequency of micturition, and smarting pain on the passage of urine. The vaginal mucous membrane is reddened and there may be superficial ulceration.

ETIOL: May be caused by microorganisms such as gonococci, chlamydiae, *Gardnerella vaginalis*, staphylococci, streptococci, spirochetes; viruses; irritation from use of strong chemicals in douching; fungus infection (candidiasis) caused by *Candida albicans*; protozoal infection (*Trichomonas vaginalis*); neoplasms of cervix or vagina; irritation from foreign bodies (pessaries), retained tampon; vitamin deficiency as in pellagra; conditions involving vulva and surrounding area, such as uncleanliness or intestinal parasites.

TREAT: Specific therapy as indicated. Improve perineal hygiene by instructing in proper method of cleaning anus after a bowel movement, proper use of menstrual protection materials, and necessity of drying vulva following urination.

NURSING IMPLICATIONS: Use aseptic technique in collecting specimens. Support patient throughout diagnostic and therapeutic interventions, providing warning concerning procedures and possible discomfort. If vaginitis is due to a sexually transmitted disease, see that sexual partner is treated along with patient to prevent reinfection. Certain sexually transmitted vaginal infections are reported to the local Public Health Service officials along with patient's known sexual contacts. SEE: *Nursing Diagnoses* in Appendix.

v. adhaesiva. Inflammation of the vagina causing adhesions between its walls.

v., atrophic. Vaginitis following the menopause. SYN: *v., postmenopausal; v., senile.*

v., candidal. Vaginitis due to infection with *Candida albicans.* SYN: *candidal vulvovaginitis.*

TREAT: Specific therapy with intravaginal miconazole cream, clotrimazole, or butoconazole are effective, as is ketoconazole administered orally. Also, the ingestion of yogurt containing *Lactobacillus acidophilus* is effective in decreasing colonization of the vagina by candida.

NOTE: Even though some manufacturers claim their yogurt contains lactobacilli, the yogurt may not contain the microorganism.

v., diphtheritic. Vaginitis with membranous exudate caused by infection with *Corynebacterium diphtheriae.*

v., emphysematous. Vaginitis with gas-bubble formation in connective tissues.

v., Gardnerella vaginalis. SEE: *Gardnerella vaginalis vaginitis; vaginosis, bacterial.*

v., granular. Vaginitis with cellular infiltration and enlargement of papillae.

v., nonspecific. In the past, a term used to describe virtually all cases of vaginitis in which no specific etiological agent could be identified. It is now known that the majority of cases are caused by either *Gardnerella vaginalis* or *Trichomonas vaginalis* organisms.

DIAG: A fresh specimen diluted with normal saline will upon microscopic examination reveal *Trichomonas* organisms; if short motile rods are seen to cover vaginal epithelial cells (so-called "clue" cells), then *Gardnerella* organisms are the cause. The vaginal aspirate is usually acid and, when mixed with a 10% potassium hydroxide solution, emits a characteristic offensive (fishy) odor.

TREAT: For *Trichomonas* or *Gardnerella* use metronidazole. SEE: *vaginosis, bacterial.*

v., postmenopausal. V., atrophic.

v., senile. V., atrophic.

v. testis. Inflammation of the tunica vaginalis of the testis.

v., Trichomonas vaginalis. Vaginitis associated with or caused by infection by *Trichomonas vaginalis,* a flagellate protozoon. *T. vaginalis* may be present in the vagina without causing disease in the host. Because the causative organism may be spread by direct contact during sexual intercourse, *T. vaginalis* vaginitis is classified as a sexually transmitted disease.

vaginoabdominal (văj″ĭn-ō-ăb-dŏm′ĭn-ăl) [L. *vagina*, sheath, + *abdominalis*, abdominal]. Rel. to the vagina and abdomen.

vaginocele (văj′ĭn-ō-sēl) [″ + Gr. *kele*, tumor, swelling]. Vaginal hernia. SYN: *colpocele*.

vaginodynia (văj″ĭn-ō-dĭn′ē-ă) [″ + Gr. *odyne*, pain]. Pain in the vagina.

vaginofixation (văj″ĭn-ō-fĭks-ā′shŭn) [″ + *fixatio*, a fixing]. 1. Process of rendering the vagina immovable. 2. Attachment of the uterus to vaginal peritoneum.

vaginogenic (văj″ĭn-ō-jěn′ĭk) [″ + Gr. *gennan*, to produce]. Developed from or originating in the vagina.

vaginogram (văj′ĭn-ō-grăm) [″ + *gramma*, something written]. Radiographic study of the vagina by use of a solution of radiopaque material into the vagina. This technique is useful in diagnosing ureterovaginal fistula.

vaginography (văj-ĭn-ŏg′ră-fē) [″ + Gr. *graphein*, to write]. Roentgenography of the vagina.

vaginolabial (văj″ĭn-ō-lā′bē-ăl) [″ + *labium*, lip]. Rel. to the vagina and labia. SYN: *vaginovulvar; vulvovaginal*.

vaginometer (văj-ĭn-ŏm′ĕ-tĕr) [″ + Gr. *metron*, measure]. Device for measuring the length and expansion of the vagina.

vaginomycosis (văj″ĭn-ō-mī-kō′sĭs) [″ + Gr. *mykes*, fungus, + *osis*, condition]. A fungus infection (mycosis) of the vagina.

vaginopathy (văj″ĭ-nŏp′ă-thē) [″ + Gr. *pathos*, disease, suffering]. Any disease of the vagina.

vaginoperineal (văj″ĭn-ō-pĕr-ĭ-nē′ăl) [″ + Gr. *perinaion*, perineum]. Rel. to the vagina and perineum.

vaginoperineoplasty. Plastic surgery procedure involving the vagina and perineum.

vaginoperineorrhaphy (văj″ĭn-ō-pĕr″ĭ-nē-or′ăf-ē) [″ + ″ + *rhaphe*, seam, ridge]. Repair of a laceration involving both the perineum and vagina. SYN: *colpoperineorrhaphy*.

vaginoperineotomy (văj″ĭn-ō-pĕr″ĭn-ē-ŏt′ō-mē) [″ + ″ + *tome*, incision]. Surgical incision of the vagina and perineum. Usually done in order to facilitate childbirth. SEE: *episiotomy*.

vaginoperitoneal (văj″ĭn-ō-pĕr″ĭ-tō-nē′ăl). Rel. to the vagina and peritoneum.

vaginopexy (vă-jĭ′nō-pĕk″sē) [″ + Gr. *pexis*, fixation]. Fixation of the vagina. SYN: *colpopexy*.

vaginoplasty (vă-jĭ′nō-plăs″tē) [″ + Gr. *plassein*, to form]. Plastic surgery on the vagina.

vaginoscope (văj′ĭn-ō-skōp) [″ + Gr. *skopein*, to examine]. Instrument for inspection of the vagina. May be a speculum or an optical instrument.

vaginoscopy (văj′ĭn-ŏs′kō-pē). Visual examination of the vagina.

vaginosis, bacterial. Inflammation of the vagina due to *Gardnerella vaginalis*. Prior to identification of this organism, this form of vaginitis was classed as nonspecific. The diagnosis is confirmed when *Candida* and trichomonal vaginitis are excluded, the characteristic clue cells are found in vaginal secretions, and the characteristic fishy odor is produced when the vaginal discharge is mixed with 10% potassium hydroxide.
    SEE: *Gardnerella vaginalis vaginitis*.

vaginotome (vă-jĭ′nō-tōm) [″ + Gr. *tome*, incision]. An instrument for making an incision in the vaginal walls.

vaginotomy (văj″ĭ-nŏt′ō-mē) [″ + Gr. *tome*, incision]. Incision of the vagina.

vaginovesical (văj″ĭ-nō-vĕs′ĭ-kăl) [″ + *vesica*, bladder]. Rel. to the vagina and bladder. SYN: *vesicovaginal*.

vaginovulvar (văj″ĭn-ō-vŭl′văr) [″ + *vulva*, covering]. Pert. to the vulva and vagina. SYN: *vaginolabial; vulvovaginal*.

vagitis (vă-jī′tĭs) [L. *vagus*, wandering, + Gr. *itis*, inflammation]. Inflammation of the vagal nerve.

vagitus (vă-jī′tŭs) [L. *vagire*, to squall]. First cry of newly born infant.
    v. uterinus. Crying of the fetus before birth while still in the uterus.
    v. vaginalis. Cry of an infant with head still in the vagina.

vagolysis (vă-gŏl′ĭ-sĭs) [L. *vagus*, wandering, + Gr. *lysis*, dissolution]. Surgical destruction of the vagus nerve.

vagolytic (vă″gō-lĭt′ĭk). 1. Concerning vagolysis. 2. An agent, surgical or chemical, that prevents function of the vagus nerve.

vagomimetic (vă″gō-mĭ-mĕt′ĭk) [″ + Gr. *mimetikos*, imitating]. Resembling action caused by stimulation of the vagus nerve.

vagosympathetic (vă″gō-sĭm-pă-thĕt′ĭk) [″ + Gr. *sympathetikos*, suffering with]. The cervical sympathetic and the vagus nerves considered together.

vagotomy (vă-gŏt′ō-mē) [″ + Gr. *tome*, incision]. Section of the vagus nerve.
    v., medical. Administration of drugs to prevent function of the vagus nerve.

vagotonia (vă″gō-tō′nē-ă) [″ + Gr. *tonos*, tension]. Hyperirritability of the parasympathetic nervous system. SEE: *sympatheticotonia*.

vagotonic (vă″gō-tŏn′ĭk). Pert. to vagotonia.

vagotropic (vă″gō-trŏp′ĭk) [″ + Gr. *tropos*, a turning]. Acting upon the vagus nerve.

vagotropism (vă-gŏt′rō-pĭzm) [″ + ″ + *-ismos*, condition]. Affinity for the vagus nerve, as a drug.

vagovagal (vă″gō-vā′găl). Reflex activity

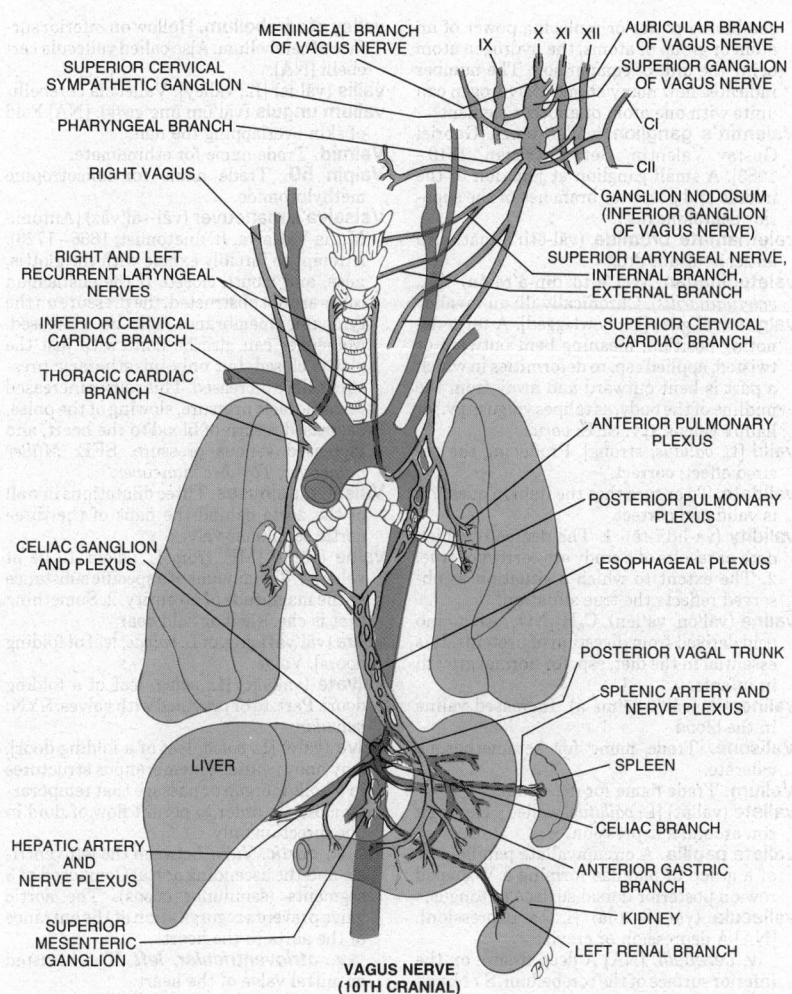

SUPERIOR CERVICAL
SYMPATHETIC GANGLION

MENINGEAL BRANCH
OF VAGUS NERVE

PHARYNGEAL BRANCH

RIGHT VAGUS

RIGHT AND LEFT
RECURRENT LARYNGEAL
NERVES

INFERIOR CERVICAL
CARDIAC BRANCH

THORACIC CARDIAC
BRANCH

CELIAC GANGLION
AND PLEXUS

LIVER

HEPATIC ARTERY
AND
NERVE PLEXUS

SUPERIOR
MESENTERIC
GANGLION

X XI XII

IX

AURICULAR BRANCH
OF VAGUS NERVE

SUPERIOR GANGLION
OF VAGUS NERVE

CI

CII

GANGLION NODOSUM
(INFERIOR GANGLION
OF VAGUS NERVE)

SUPERIOR LARYNGEAL NERVE,
INTERNAL BRANCH,
EXTERNAL BRANCH

SUPERIOR CERVICAL
CARDIAC BRANCH

ANTERIOR PULMONARY
PLEXUS

POSTERIOR PULMONARY
PLEXUS

ESOPHAGEAL PLEXUS

POSTERIOR VAGAL TRUNK

SPLENIC ARTERY AND
NERVE PLEXUS

SPLEEN

CELIAC BRANCH

ANTERIOR GASTRIC
BRANCH

KIDNEY

LEFT RENAL BRANCH

VAGUS NERVE
(10TH CRANIAL)

mediated entirely through the vagus nerve,
i.e., via efferent and afferent impulses
transmitted through the vagus nerve.

vagrant (vā′grănt) [L. *vagrans*]. 1. Wandering
from place to place without a fixed home. 2.
A homeless person who wanders from place
to place.

vagus (vā′gŭs) [L., wandering] (pl. *vagi*). The
pneumogastric or 10th cranial nerve. It is a
mixed nerve, having motor and sensory
functions and a wider distribution than any
of the other cranial nerves. SEE: illus.; *cranial nerves.*

vagus pulse. Decreased heart rate due to the
slowing action of stimuli from the vagus
nerve. SEE: *vagotomy; vagotonia.*

vagusstoff (vā′gŭs-stŏf) [″ + Ger. *Stoff*,
substance]. Acetylcholine.

Valadol. Trade name for acetaminophen.

valence, valency (vā′lĕns, -lĕn-sē) [L. *valens*,
powerful]. 1. Property of an atom or group of
atoms causing them to combine in definite
proportion with other atoms or groups of
atoms. Valency may be as high as 8 and is
determined by the number of electrons in
the outer orbit of the atom. 2. Degree of the

combining power or replacing power of an atom or group of atoms, the hydrogen atom being the unit of comparison. The number indicates how many atoms of hydrogen can unite with one atom of another element.

Valentin's ganglion (văl'ĕn-tēnz) [Gabriel Gustav Valentin, Ger. physician, 1810–1883]. A small ganglion at junction of the middle and posterior branches of the superior dental plexus.

valethamate bromide (văl-ĕth'ă-māt). An anticonvulsant drug.

valetudinarian (văl''ē-tū''dĭn-ā'rē-ăn) [L., *valetudinarius*]. Chronically ill; an invalid.

valgus (văl'gŭs) [L., bowlegged]. A term denoting position, meaning bent outward or twisted, applied esp. to deformities in which a part is bent outward and away from the midline of the body, as talipes valgus, q.v., or hallux valgus, q.v. SEE: *varus.*

valid [L. *validus*, strong]. Producing the desired effect; correct.

validate. To ensure that the item in question is valid and correct.

validity (vă-lĭd'ĭ-tē). 1. The degree to which data or results of a study are correct or true. 2. The extent to which a situation as observed reflects the true situation.

valine (văl'ēn, vā'lēn). $C_5H_{11}NO_2$. An amino acid derived from digestion of proteins. It is essential in the diet, esp. for normal growth in infants.

valinemia (văl''ĭ-nē'mē-ă). Increased valine in the blood.

Valisone. Trade name for betamethasone valerate.

Valium. Trade name for diazepam.

vallate (văl'āt) [L. *vallatus*, walled]. Having a rim around a depression.

vallate papilla. A circumvallate papilla; one of a group of papillae forming a V-shaped row on posterior dorsal surface of tongue.

vallecula (văl-lĕk'ū-lă) [L., a depression]. [NA] A depression or crevice.

   v. cerebelli. [NA] A deep fissure on the inferior surface of the cerebellum. SYN: *valley of cerebellum.*

   v. epiglottica. [NA] Depression lying lateral to the median epiglottic fold and separating it from the pharyngoepiglottic fold.

   v. ovata. Depression in the liver in which rests the gallbladder.

   v. sylvii. Depression marking beginning of the fissure of Sylvius.

   v. unguis. Fold of skin in which the proximal and lateral edges of the nails are embedded.

Valleix's points (văl-lāz') [François L. I. Valleix, Fr. physician, 1807–1855]. In neuralgia, distinct painful points along the course of the affected nerve.

valley fever. Coccidioidomycosis, q.v.

valley of cerebellum. Hollow on inferior surface of cerebellum. Also called vallecula cerebelli [NA].

vallis (văl'ĭs) [L., valley]. Vallecula cerebelli.

vallum unguis (văl'ŭm ŭng'gwĭs). [NA] Fold of skin overlapping the nail.

Valmid. Trade name for ethinamate.

Valpin 50. Trade name for anisotropine methylbromide.

Valsalva's maneuver (văl-săl'văz) [Antonio Maria Valsalva, It. anatomist, 1666–1723]. Attempt to forcibly exhale with the glottis, nose, and mouth closed. If the eustachian tubes are not obstructed, the pressure on the tympanic membranes will be increased. Maneuver can also be done with just the glottis closed, but only intrathoracic pressure will be increased. This causes increased intrathoracic pressure, slowing of the pulse, decreased return of blood to the heart, and increased venous pressure. SEE: *Müller maneuver; Toynbee maneuver.*

Valsalva's sinuses. Three dilatations in wall of the aorta behind the flaps of the three aortic semilunar valves.

value (văl'ū) [ME. from L. *valere*, to be of value]. 1. The amount of a specific substance or the magnitude of an entity. 2. Something that is cherished or held dear.

valva (văl'vă) [sing. of L. *valvae*, leaf of folding doors]. Valve.

valvate (văl'vāt) [L. *valva*, leaf of a folding door]. Pert. to or provided with valves. SYN: *valvular.*

valve (vălv) [L. *valva*, leaf of a folding door]. Any one of various membranous structures in a hollow organ or passage that temporarily closes in order to permit flow of fluid in one direction only.

   v., aortic. Valve between the left ventricle and the ascending aorta. Composed of 3 segments (semilunar cusps). The aortic valve prevents regurgitation at the entrance of the aorta to the heart.

   v., atrioventricular, left. The bicuspid or mitral valve of the heart.

   v., atrioventricular, right. The tricuspid valve of the heart.

   v., bicuspid. Valve that closes the orifice between the left cardiac atrium and the left ventricle. SYN: *v., mitral.*

   v., Bjork-Shiley concavo-convex heart. A synthetic, artificial heart valve that is no longer commercially available, but is still implanted in thousands of patients. The valve has been known to fracture in use. When that occurs, death results in the majority of cases.

   v.'s, cardiac. The four valves that control the flow of blood into, through, and out of the heart. In order of the entry of the venous blood into the right atrium, they are right atrioventricular, pulmonary, left atrioventricular, and aortic.

v., coronary. The coronary sinus valve at the entrance of the coronary sinus into the right atrium.

v.'s, Houston's. Mucosal folds of the rectum. SYN: *plicae transversales recti.*

v., ileocecal. Valve between the ileum and large intestine that prevents regurgitation of intestinal contents. It is composed of two membranous folds. SYN: *v. of Varolius; valvula coli.*

v., mitral. V., bicuspid.

v. of Varolius. V., ileocecal.

v., pulmonary. Valve composed of three cusps, separating the pulmonary artery and right ventricle.

v., pyloric. Prominent circular membranous fold at pyloric orifice of the stomach.

v., semilunar. Valve between heart and the aorta and valve between the heart and the pulmonary artery.

v., thebesian. V., coronary, q.v.

v., tricuspid. Valve between the right cardiac atrium and right ventricle.

valvectomy. Surgical excision of a valve, esp. a heart valve. SEE: *valvuloplasty.*

valvotomy (văl-vŏt'ō-mē) [" + Gr. *tome,* incision]. Incision into a valve.

valvula (văl'vū-lă) [L., a small fold] (pl. *valvulae*). [NA] A valve, specifically a small valve.

v. bicuspidalis. Valve between the left cardiac atrium and left ventricle. SYN: *valve, bicuspid.*

v. coli. Valve between ileum and large intestine. SYN: *valve, ileocecal.*

v. pylori. Prominent mucosal fold at pyloric entrance of the stomach. SYN: *valve, pyloric.*

v. semilunaris. [NA] Valve separating heart and aorta and heart and pulmonary artery. SYN: *valve, semilunar.*

v. tricuspidalis. Valve between the right atrium and right ventricle of the heart. SYN: *valve, tricuspid.*

valvulae (văl'vū-lē). Pl. of valvula.

v. conniventes. Circular membranous folds that project into the lumen of the small intestine; they do not disappear on distention of the bowel. They act by retarding passage of food along the bowel and provide a greater absorbing area. SYN: *plicae circulares.*

valvular (văl'vū-lăr) [L. *valvula,* a small fold]. Rel. to or having a valve. SYN: *valvate.*

valvulitis (văl"vū-lī'tĭs) [" + Gr. *itis,* inflammation]. Inflammation of a valve, esp. a cardiac valve.

valvuloplasty (văl'vū-lō-plăs"tē). Plastic or restorative surgery on a valve, esp. a cardiac valve.

valvulotome (văl'vū-lō-tōm) [" + Gr. *tome,* incision]. An instrument for incising a valve.

valvulotomy (văl"vū-lŏt'ō-mē). Process of cutting through a valve, as a rectal fold that is too rigid. SYN: *valvotomy.*

vanadium (vă-nā'dē-ŭm) [*Vanadis,* a Scandinavian goddess]. SYMB: V. At. wt. 50.941; at. no. 23. A light gray metallic element.

vanadiumism (vă-nā'dē-ŭm-ĭzm). Toxicity due to chronic exposure to vanadium. The symptoms include bronchitis, pneumonitis, conjunctivitis, and anemia.

van Buren's disease (văn bū'rĕnz) [William Holme van Buren, U.S. surgeon, 1819–1883]. Induration of the corpora cavernosa of the penis. SYN: *Peyronie's disease.*

Vanceril. Trade name for beclomethasone dipropionate.

Vancocin Hydrochloride. Trade name for vancomycin hydrochloride.

vancomycin hydrochloride (văn'kō-mī"sĭn). USP. An antibacterial drug. Trade name is Vancocin Hydrochloride.

van den Bergh's test (văn"dĕn bŭrgz') [A. A. Hijmans van den Bergh, Dutch physician, 1869–1943]. A test to detect the presence of bilirubin in blood serum or plasma.

van der Hoeve's syndrome [Jan van der Hoeve, Dutch ophthalmologist, 1878–1952]. Conductive deafness due to otosclerosis-like changes in the temporal bone. Blue sclerae and osteogenesis imperfecta are also present.

van der Waals forces [Johannes D. van der Waals, Dutch physicist, 1837–1923]. The definite but weak forces of attraction between the nuclei of atoms of compounds. These forces do not exist on the basis of ionic attraction, hydrogen bonding, or sharing of electrons.

vanilla (vă-nĭl'ă) [Sp. *vainilla,* little sheath]. Any one of a group of tropical orchids. The cured seed pods of *Vanilla planifolia* contain an aromatic substance, also called vanilla, that is used for flavoring.

vanillin. A crystalline compound found in vanilla pods or produced synthetically used for flavoring foods and in pharmaceuticals.

vanillism (vă-nĭl'ĭzm). Irritation of the skin, mucous membranes, and conjunctiva sometimes experienced by workers handling raw vanilla. It is caused by a mite.

vanillylmandelic acid. ABBR: VMA. 3-methoxy-4-hydroxymandelic acid. Approx. 90% of the catecholamines epinephrine and norepinephrine are metabolized to VMA and are secreted in the urine. Persons with pheochromocytoma produce excess amounts of catecholamines; thus VMA is present in their urine in increased amount.

vanishing twin. SEE: *gestation, multiple.*

van't Hoff's rule [Jacobus Henricus van't Hoff, Dutch chemist, 1852–1911]. The speed of chemical reactions is doubled, at least, for each 10°C rise in temperature.

Vapo-Iso. Trade name for isoproterenol hydrochloride.

vapor (vā'por) [L., steam]. 1. Gaseous state of any substance. 2. Medicinal substance for administration by inhalation.

vaporium (vā-pō'rē-ŭm) [L.]. Apparatus for applying hot, cold, or medicated vapors.

vaporization (vā"por-ĭ-zā'shŭn) [L. *vapor*, steam]. 1. The conversion of a liquid or solid into vapor. 2. Therapeutic use of a vapor.

vaporize (vā'por-īz). To change a material to a vapor form.

vaporizer (vā'por-ī"zer). Device for converting liquids into a vapor spray.

vaporous (vā'por-ŭs) [L. *vapor*, steam]. Consisting of, pert. to, or producing vapors.

vapor permeable membrane. A membrane, usually transparent, that is permeable to oxygen and water vapor. It may be prepared with an adhesive backing that will stick only to dry skin. This type of membrane has been used in treating wounds. The membrane must be applied properly without wrinkles and changed as often as necessary in order to prevent excess accumulation of fluid and bacteria under it.

vapotherapy (vā"pō-thĕr'ă-pē). Therapeutic use of vapors.

Vaquez's disease (vă-kāz') [Louis Henri Vaquez, Fr. physician, 1860–1936]. Polycythemia vera.

variability (văr"ē-ă-bĭl'ĭ-tē). Condition of being variable.

variable (vā'rē-ă-b'l) [L. *variare*, to vary]. 1. Anything that is not constant but can and does change in different circumstances. In statistics, it is often possible to graph the relationship of one variable to another, e.g., the increase in height and weight in the growing child. 2. Changing form, or structure, behavior, or physiology.

    v., dependent. In research studies, a variable influenced by the independent variable.

    v., independent. In research studies, a variable controlled by the investigator.

variance (văr'ē-ăns) [L. *variare*, to vary]. A statistical index of the degree to which measurements in a data set are different from each other or deviate from the mean; the square of the standard deviation.

variant (văr'ē-ănt). That which is different from the characteristics of the other organisms or entities in a particular classification, esp. a disease, species, or physical appearance.

variate (vā'rē-āt). Variable.

variation (vā"rē-ā'shŭn). Differences between individuals of a certain species or class.

    v., continuous. Variation in which the difference between successive groups or individuals is quite small.

    v., meristic. Variation in number as opposed to kind.

varication (văr"ĭ-kā'shŭn). 1. Formation of a varix. 2. The condition of a varicosity.

variced. Concerning a varix.

varicella (văr"ĭ-sĕl'ă) [L., a tiny spot]. An acute, highly contagious viral disease characterized by an eruption that makes its appearance in successive crops, and passes through stages of macules, papules, vesicles, and crusts. SYN: *chickenpox.*

SYM: There may be a slight elevation of temperature at onset, followed within 24 hr by appearance of the eruption, after which time temperature usually rises still further. Eruption first appears on back and chest, crops continuing to make their appearance for a period of 2 to 3 days on an average. Each crop requires about 36 hr to pass through the several stages. Because of this, macules, papules, vesicles, and crusts may be found side by side in the same general locality. Lesions are superficial and rupture very easily. They tend to be ovoid. On the chest their distribution is often particularly marked along the course of the intercostal nerves. Some, though possibly few, scars nearly always remain as evidence of a varicella attack. The extremities are relatively free as compared with the trunk.

ETIOL: Varicella-zoster virus, which also is the causative agent of herpes zoster. May occur at any age, though far less common in adults than in children. Epidemics most frequent in winter and spring and in temperate zones. Approx. 75% of all children will contract varicella by age 15.

DIFF. DIAG: Confusion between this disease and smallpox is responsible for the chief importance given varicella. Impetigo, dermatitis herpetiformis, herpes zoster, and furunculosis may require consideration.

COMPLICATIONS: Secondary infections due to scratching, which may result in abscess formation; at times development of erysipelas or even septicemia. Occasionally lesions in the vicinity of the larynx may cause edema of the glottis and threaten the life of the patient. Encephalitis is a rare complication. Varicella may be fatal in children with leukemia or who are taking adrenocorticosteroids.

PREVENTION: Administration of varicella-zoster immune globulin (VZIg) within 72 hr of exposure will prevent clinical varicella in susceptible, normal children. The following conditions should alert one to the possible need for use of VZIg: immunocompromised children; newborns of mothers who develop varicella in the period 5 days before to 48 hr after delivery; postnatal exposure of newborn infants (esp. those who are premature) to varicella; normal adults who are susceptible to varicella and who have been exposed; pregnant women who have no history of having had varicella and who have had significant exposure. Use of VZIg in pregnant women will not prevent fetal infection or congenital varicella syndrome. Live, attenuated vaccine is being investigated but is not available for general use.

Caution: Severe illness and death have resulted from varicella in children being treated with corticosteroids. Children being treated with corticosteroids should avoid exposure to varicella.

INCUB: From 2 to 3 weeks; usually 13 to 17 days.

TREAT: Isolation. Restrain the hands in the case of infants or young children so that the lesions may not be scratched. Use of calamine lotion locally may alleviate irritation. Keep the skin, bedclothes, and sheets clean to help prevent skin infections. Also keep patient's fingernails well trimmed. The usual duration of the disease is from 2 to 3 weeks. Cases usually classed as contagious from 5 days prior to the skin eruption until not more than 6 days after the first crop of vesicles.

PROG: Always favorable except in a very severe type, which is described as varicella gangrenosa. In this variety, gangrene may develop about the site of the lesions.

v. gangrenosa. Varicella in which necrosis occurs around the vesicles, resulting in gangrenous ulceration.

varicella-zoster immune globulin. ABBR: VZIg. An immune globulin obtained from the blood of normal persons found to have high antibody titers to varicella-zoster. For indications for its use, SEE: PREVENTION under _varicella._

varicelliform (văr″ĭ-sĕl′ĭ-form). Resembling varicella.

varicelloid (văr′ĭ-sĕl′oyd) [″ + Gr. _eidos,_ form, shape]. Resembling varicella.

varices (văr′ĭ-sēz) [L.]. Pl. of varix.

variciform (văr-ĭs′ĭ-form) [L. _varix,_ twisted vein, + _forma,_ shape]. Resembling a varix. SYN: _varicose._

varicoblepharon (văr″ĭ-kō-blĕf′ă-rŏn) [″ + Gr. _blepharon,_ eyelid]. Varicose tumor of the eyelid.

varicocele (văr′ĭ-kō-sēl) [″ + Gr. _kele,_ tumor, swelling]. Enlargement of the veins of the spermatic cord (pampiniform plexus), commonly occurring on the left side in adolescent males; these seldom require treatment.

SYM: Vessels on affected side of scrotum are full, feeling like a bundle of worms, sometimes purplish in color. Dull ache along the cord. Slight dragging sensation in groin.

TREAT: Dragging sensation from exceptionally large varicocele may be relieved by a suspensory. Surgery is required for persistent symptomatic varicocele.

v., ovarian. Varicosity of veins of the ovarian or pampiniform plexus of the broad ligament.

v., utero-ovarian. Varicosity of the veins of the ovarian (pampiniform) plexus and uterine plexus of the broad ligament.

varicocelectomy (văr″ĭ-kō-sē-lĕk′tō-mē) [L. _varix,_ twisted vein, + Gr. _kele,_ tumor, swelling, + _ektome,_ excision]. Excision of portion of scrotal sac with ligation of the dilated veins to relieve varicocele.

varicography (văr″ĭ-kŏg′ră-fē) [″ + Gr. _graphein,_ to write]. Roentgenography of varicose veins.

varicoid (văr′ĭ-koyd) [″ + Gr. _eidos,_ form, shape]. Resembling a varix.

varicole (văr′ĭ-kōl). Varicocele.

varicomphalus (văr″ĭ-kŏm′fă-lŭs) [″ + Gr. _omphalos,_ navel]. Varicose tumor of the navel.

varicophlebitis (văr″ĭ-kō-flē-bī′tĭs) [″ + Gr. _phleps,_ vein, + _itis,_ inflammation]. Phlebitis combined with varicose veins.

varicose (văr′ĭ-kōs) [L. _varicosus,_ full of dilated veins]. Pert. to varices; distended, swollen, knotted veins.

varicose ulcers. Ulcers that form as a result of varicose veins. When thrombophlebitis develops in varicose veins, this leads to venous stasis and eventually edema and ulcer formation.

NURSING IMPLICATIONS: Maintain patient on bedrest. Continuously apply warm, moist compresses to relieve discomfort and infection. Use aseptic technique when applying dressings and therapeutic agents.

varicose veins. Enlarged, twisted superficial veins. May occur in almost any part of the body but are most commonly observed in the lower extremities and in the esophagus.

SYM: Pain in feet and ankles, swelling, ulcers on skin. Severe bleeding if a vein is injured.

ETIOL: Incompetent venous valves that may be acquired or congenital. The development of varicose veins is promoted and aggravated by pregnancy, obesity, and occupations that require prolonged standing. Esophageal varices are caused by portal hypertension that accompanies cirrhosis of the liver.

F.A.: In hemorrhage, elevation of extremity and gentle but firm pressure over wound will stop bleeding. The use of a tourniquet is undesirable. Sterile dressing should be held in place with a firm bandage. Patient should not be permitted to walk for some time. The Sengstaken-Blakemore tube may be used to control bleeding due to hemorrhage from esophageal varices. SEE: *tamponade, balloon.*

TREAT: In general, consists of rest, elevation of extremity, and use of an external support. The use of elastic stockings is much preferred to elastic bandages. Unna's paste boots recommended for elderly or debilitated persons with cutaneous ulcers. Injection of sclerosing solutions may be utilized for small varicosities. High ligation and removal of vein by stripping may be necessary for major varicosities.

NURSING IMPLICATIONS: Teach the patient to avoid anything that impedes venous return, such as wearing garters and tight girdles, crossing the legs at the knees, and prolonged sitting. Apply support hose after the legs have been elevated for 10 to 15 minutes. Instruct the patient not to sit in a chair for longer than 1 hour at a time. Encourage ambulation for at least 5 minutes every hour. Elevate legs whenever possible, but no less than twice a day for 30 minutes each time. Instruct the patient to avoid prolonged standing. Teach the patient the signs of thrombophlebitis, a common complication of varicose veins; these are heat, local pain, and a positive Homans' sign, q.v. If surgery is performed, postoperatively apply elastic stockings and elevate the foot of the bed above the level of the heart. Encourage the overweight patient to lose weight. SEE: *Nursing Diagnoses* in *Appendix.*

varicosis (văr″ĭ-kō′sĭs) [L.]. Varicose condition of veins.

varicosity (văr″ĭ-kŏs′ĭ-tē) [L. *varix*, twisted vein]. 1. Condition of being varicose. 2. A swollen, twisted vein. SYN: *varix.*

varicotomy (văr″ĭ-kŏt′ō-mē) [″ + Gr. *tome*, incision]. Excision of a varicose vein.

varicula (văr-ĭk′ū-lă) [L., a tiny dilated vein]. A small varix, esp. of the conjunctiva.

variety (vă-rī′ĕ-tē) [L., *varietas*, variety]. A term used in classifying individuals in a subpopulation of a species.

variola (vă-rī′ō-lă) [L., pustule]. An acute, contagious, systemic, viral disease characterized by a prodromal stage during which the constitutional symptoms usually are severe, followed by an eruption that passes through the successive stages of macules,

papules, vesicles, pustules, and crusts. SYN: *smallpox.*

NOTE: This disease is considered to have been completely eradicated world-wide. Cultures of the virus are kept in only one or two research laboratories.

v. minor. Mild form of smallpox with sparse rash and low-grade fever.

variolar (văr-ī′ō-lăr) [L. *variola*, pustule]. Pert. to smallpox.

variolate (văr″ē-ō-lāt). 1. To vaccinate with smallpox virus. 2. Having lesions like those of smallpox.

variolation, variolization (văr″ē-ō-lā′shŭn, văr″ē-ō-lĭ-zā′shŭn) [L. *variola*, pustule]. Inoculation with smallpox.

variolic (văr″ē-ŏl′ĭk). Variolar.

varioliform (vă″rē-ŏl′ĭ-form). Resembling smallpox.

varioloid (văr′ē-ō-loyd) [″ + Gr. *eidos*, form, shape]. 1. Resembling smallpox. 2. Pert. to varioloid. 3. A mild but contagious type of smallpox in those who have had smallpox or have been vaccinated.

variolous (vă-rī′ō-lŭs). Rel. to smallpox.

varix (vā′rĭks) [L., twisted vein] (pl. *varices*). 1. A tortuous dilatation of a vein. SEE: *varicose veins.* 2. Less commonly, dilatation of an artery or lymph vessel.

v., aneurysmal. A direct communication between an artery and a varicose vein without an intervening sac.

v., arterial. A varicosity or dilation of an artery.

v., chyle. Varix of a lymphatic vessel that conveys chyle.

varices, esophageal. SEE: *esophageal varices.* SEE: *Nursing Diagnoses* in *Appendix.*

v. lymphaticus. Dilatation of a lymphatic vessel.

v., turbinal. Permanent dilatation of veins of turbinate bodies.

varnish (văr′nĭsh). A solution of gums and resins in a solvent. When these are applied to a surface, the solvent evaporates and leaves a hard, more or less flexible film. In dentistry, varnishes are used to protect sensitive tooth areas such as the pulp.

v., cavity. The material applied to the walls and floor of a tooth cavity preparation to protect against acidic cements or metallic restorations. It reduces microleakage and seals the dentinal tubules, thereby reducing pulp irritation.

v., periodontal. A protective coating applied to the outer tooth surface to alleviate pain and promote healing after deep scaling or curettage.

varolian (vă-rō′lē-ăn) [Costanzo Varolio (Varolius), It. anatomist, 1543–1575]. Rel.

to the pons varolii.

varolian bend. Anterior extension of hindgut on its ventral surface in the fetus.

varus (vā′rŭs) [L.]. 1. Turned inward. 2. A condition in which a clubfooted person walks on outer border of the foot. SYN: *talipes varus.* SEE: *valgus.*

vas (văs) [L., vessel] (pl. *vasa*). [NA] A vessel or duct.

    v. aberrans. 1. A narrow tube varying in length from 1½ to 14 in. (3.8 to 35.6 cm), occasionally found connected with the lower part of the canal of the epididymis or with the commencement of the vas deferens. 2. Vestige of the biliary ducts sometimes found in the liver.

    v. afferens. [NA] An afferent vessel of a lymph node.

    v. afferens glomeruli. [NA] The afferent arteriole that conveys blood to the glomerulus of a renal corpuscle.

    v. capillare. [NA] A capillary blood vessel.

    v. deferens. The excretory duct of the testis, the continuation of the canal of the epididymis. This slim, muscular tube, approximately 18 in. (45.7 cm) long, transports the sperm from each testis to the prostatic urethra. SYN: *ductus deferens* [NA]. SEE: *genitalia* for illus.
    RS: ampullitis; cord; deferentitis; spermatic.

    v. lymphaticum. [NA] One of the vessels carrying the lymph.

    v. prominens. [NA] Blood vessel on the cochlea's accessory spiral ligament.

    v. spirale. A large blood vessel beneath the tunnel of Corti in the basilar membrane.

vasa (vā′să) [L. *vas*, vessel]. Pl. of vas.

    v. afferentia. [NA] The lymphatic vessels entering a lymph node.

    v. brevia. Branches of the splenic artery going to greater curvature of the stomach.

    v. efferentia. 1. Lymphatics that leave a lymph node. 2. Excretory ducts of the testis to the head of the epididymis.

    v. praevia. The blood vessels of the umbilical cord presenting before the fetus.

    v. recta. 1. Tubules that become straight prior to entering the mediastinum testis. 2. Straight collecting tubules of the kidney.

    v. vasorum. [NA] Tiny blood vessels that are distributed to the walls of the larger veins and arteries.

    v. vorticosa. Stellate veins of the choroid, carrying blood to the superior ophthalmic vein.

vasal (vā′săl) [L. *vas*, vessel]. Rel. to a vas or vessel.

vasalgia (vă-săl′jē-ă). Pain in a vessel of any kind.

vascular (văs′kū-lăr) [L. *vasculum*, a small vessel]. Pert. to or composed of blood vessels.

vascular endothelium. The cellular tissue lining the blood vessels. In addition to serving as a semipermeable barrier between the blood and the vascular smooth muscle, the endothelium is highly active as a metabolic and endocrine organ. The cells may function to inactivate vasoactive substances and, in turn, produce vasodilator substances. Damage to the endothelium leads to increased production of prostaglandins.

vascularity (văs″kū-lăr′ĭ-tē). State of being vascular.

vascularization (văs″kū-lăr-ĭ-zā′shŭn) [L. *vasculum*, a small vessel]. Development of new blood vessels in a structure.

vascularize (văs′kū-lăr″īz) [L. *vasculum*, a small vessel]. To become vascular by development of new blood vessels.

vascular ring. Congenital abnormality in which an arterial ring encircles the trachea and esophagus. This causes signs of compression of their structures. Surgery may be required to relieve the symptoms.

vascular system. The heart, blood vessels, lymphatics, and their parts considered collectively. It includes the pulmonary and portal systems.

vascular tuft. One of the vascular processes on the chorion in the fetus at an early stage of development. SYN: *chorionic villi.*

vascular tumor. Tumor containing dilated blood vessels. SYN: *angioma; telangioma.*

vasculature (văs′kū-lă-tūr″). The arrangement of blood vessels in the body or any part of it, including their relationship and functions.

vasculitis (văs″kū-lī′tĭs) [″ + *itis*, inflammation]. Inflammation of a blood or lymph vessel. SYN: *angiitis.*

vasculogenesis (văs″kū-lō-jĕn′ĕ-sĭs) [″ + Gr. *genesis*, generation, birth]. Development of the vascular system.

vasculomotor (văs″kū-lō-mō′tor). Vasomotor.

vasculopathy (văs″kū-lŏp′ă-thē). Any disease of blood vessels.

vasculum (văs′kū-lŭm) [L.]. A tiny vessel.

vasectomy (văs-ĕk′tō-mē) [L. *vas*, vessel, + Gr. *ektome*, excision]. Removal of all or a segment of the vas deferens. Usually done bilaterally to produce sterility in the male.
    NOTE: Persons who have had this surgical procedure ejaculate in a normal manner but the ejaculate does not contain sperm. There are no anatomical or physiological reasons for sterilization by this method to alter the sex drive or libido. Nevertheless, hematomas may occur postoperatively, and

granulomas in response to leakage of sperm may occur.

Caution: The patient should have about two dozen ejaculations to help insure that sterility has been accomplished. Sterility is not considered to have been achieved until two ejaculates have been found to be free of sperm. Spontaneous reanastomosis has been reported.

---

vasectomy reversal. Surgical procedure for the rejoining of the previously severed vas deferens. Even though this procedure may be successful, the chance of success varies in published reports.

Vaseline. Trade name for petrolatum.

vasifactive (văs″ĭ-făk′tĭv) [″ + *facere*, to make]. Forming new vessels. SYN: *vasofactive; vasoformative.*

vasiform (văs′ĭ-form) [″ + *forma*, shape]. Resembling a tubular structure or vas.

vasitis (vă-sī′tĭs). Inflammation of the ductus deferens of the testicle.

vaso- [L. *vas*, vessel]. Combining form meaning a vessel, as a blood vessel.

vasoactive (văs″ō-ăk′tĭv). Affecting blood vessels.

vasoactive intestinal polypeptide. ABBR: VIP. A peptide present in the mucosa of the gastrointestinal tract. One of its principal actions is to inhibit gastric function including gastric acid secretion. VIP is also present in nerve fibers of the female genital tract.

vasoconstriction (văs″ō-kŏn-strĭk′shŭn). Decrease in the caliber of blood vessels.

vasoconstrictive (văs″ō-kŏn-strĭk′tĭv) [″ + *constrictus*, bound]. Causing constriction of the blood vessels.

vasoconstrictor (văs″ō-kŏn-strĭk′tor) [″ + *constrictor*, a binder]. 1. Causing constriction of blood vessels. 2. That which constricts or narrows the caliber of blood vessels, as a drug or a nerve.

vasodentin (văs″ō-děn′tĭn) [″ + *dens*, tooth]. Modified dentin provided with blood capillaries. Present in fish but seldom seen in other animals.

vasodepression (văs″ō-dē-prĕsh′ŭn) [″ + *depressio*, a pressing down]. Vasomotor depression or collapse.

vasodepressor (văs″ō-dē-prĕs′or) [″ + *depressor*, that which presses down]. 1. Having a depressing influence on the circulation, lowering blood pressure by dilatation of blood vessels. 2. An agent that decreases circulation.

Vasodilan. Trade name for isoxsuprine hydrochloride.

vasodilatation (văs″ō-dĭl-ă-tā′shŭn) [″ + *dilatare*, to enlarge]. Dilatation of blood vessels, esp. small arteries and arterioles.

v., antidromic. Vasodilatation resulting from stimulation of dorsal root of a spinal nerve.

v., reflex. Blood vessel dilation due to stimulation of its dilator nerves or inhibition of its constrictor substance or nerves. This can be done by stimulating the sensory reflex arc.

vasodilation (văs″ō-dī-lā′shŭn). Increase in the caliber of blood vessels.

vasodilative (văs″ō-dī′lā-tĭv). Causing dilation of the blood vessels.

vasodilator (văs″ō-dī-lā′tor) [″ + *dilatare*, to enlarge]. 1. Causing relaxation of the blood vessels. 2. A nerve or drug that dilates the blood vessels.

vasoepididymostomy (văs″ō-ĕp″ĭ-dĭd-ĭ-mŏs′tō-mē) [″ + Gr. *epi*, upon, + *didymos*, testicle, + *stoma*, mouth]. Formation of a passage between the vas deferens and the epididymis.

vasofactive (văs″ō-făk′tĭv) [″ + *facere*, to make]. Forming new blood vessels. SYN: *vasifactive; vasoformative.*

vasoformative (văs″ō-for′mă-tĭv) [″ + *formare*, to form]. Forming new blood vessels. SYN: *vasifactive; vasofactive.*

vasoganglion (văs″ō-găng′glē-ŏn). Any mass of blood vessels.

vasography (văs-ŏg′ră-fē) [″ + Gr. *graphein*, to write]. Roentgenography of the blood vessels.

vasohypertonic (văs″ō-hī″pĕr-tŏn′ĭk) [″ + Gr. *hyper*, over, above, excessive, + *tonikos*, pert. to tension]. Causing or that which causes constriction of blood vessels. SYN: *vasoconstrictor.*

vasohypotonic (văs″ō-hī″pō-tŏn′ĭk) [″ + Gr. *hypo*, under, beneath, below, + *tonikos*, pert. to tension]. Relaxing or that which relaxes blood vessels. SYN: *vasodilator.*

vasoinhibitor (văs″ō-ĭn-hĭb′ĭ-tor) [″ + *inhibere*, to restrain]. An agent that decreases the action of vasomotor nerves.

vasoinhibitory (văs″ō-ĭn-hĭb′ĭ-tor-ē). Restricting vasomotor activity.

vasoligation (văs″ō-lī-gā′shŭn) [″ + *ligare*, to bind]. Ligation of a vessel, specifically the vas deferens.

vasomotion (văs″ō-mō′shŭn) [″ + *motio*, movement]. Change in caliber of a blood vessel.

vasomotor (văs″ō-mō′tor) [″ + *motor*, a mover]. Pert. to the nerves having muscular control of the blood vessel walls. The circularly arranged fibers of the muscles of arteries and veins can contract or relax; the affected region is accordingly either blanched or flushed. The former effect can commonly be produced by stimulating sympathetic fibers, and is consequently called vasoconstrictor; certain other nerves on stimulation cause vasodilation, examples being the nervus chorda tympani and the nervi erigentes. A vasomotor reflex is one in which the stimulus, such as a horrifying sight, results in a change in vasomotor tone, e.g., pallor. SEE: *vasoconstrictor; vasodilator.*

vasomotor epilepsy. Epilepsy with vasomotor changes in the skin.

vasomotor reflex. Constriction of cutaneous blood vessels in response to a stimulus to the skin.

vasomotor spasm. Spasm of smaller arteries.

vasoneuropathy (văs″ō-nū-rŏp′ă-thē). Disease due to the combined effect of vascular and neurologic effects.

vasoneurosis (văs″ō-nū-rō′sĭs) [L. *vas,* vessel, + Gr. *neuron,* nerve, + *osis,* condition]. A neurosis affecting blood vessels; a disorder of the vasomotor system. SEE: *angioneurosis.*

vaso-orchidostomy (văs″ō-or″kĭd-ŏs′tō-mē) [″ + Gr. *orchis,* testicle, + *stoma,* mouth]. Surgical connection of the epididymis to the severed end of the vas deferens.

vasoparesis (văs″ō-păr-ē′sĭs) [″ + Gr. *parienai,* to let fall]. Partial paralysis or weakness of the vasomotor nerves.

vasopressin (văs″ō-prĕs′ĭn). A hormone formed in supraoptic and paraventricular nuclei of hypothalamus and transported to posterior lobe of hypophysis through the hypothalamohypophyseal tract. It has an antidiuretic effect and a pressor effect that elevates blood pressure. This drug should not be used as an agent to increase blood pressure because of its effect of reducing coronary artery blood flow. Trade name is Pitressin. SYN: *antidiuretic hormone.* SEE: *oxytocin.*

vasopressin injection. USP. A sterile solution, in a suitable diluent, of material containing the polypeptide hormone having the properties of causing the contraction of vascular and other smooth muscle, and of diuresis. Trade name is Pitressin.

vasopressor (văs″ō-prĕs′or). 1. Causing contraction of the muscles of capillaries and arteries. This increases resistance to the flow of blood and thus elevates blood pressure. 2. Agent that stimulates contraction of muscles of capillaries and arteries.

vasopuncture (văs′ō-pŭnk″chūr) [″ + *punctura,* prick]. Puncture of the vas deferens.

vasoreflex (văs″ō-rē′flĕx). A reflex that alters the caliber of blood vessels.

vasorelaxation (văs″ō-rē-lăks-ā′shŭn) [″ + *relaxare,* to loosen]. Lessening of vascular pressure.

vasorrhaphy (văs-or′ă-fē) [″ + Gr. *rhaphe,* seam, ridge]. Surgical suture of the

vas deferens.

vasosection (văs″ō-sĕk′shŭn) [″ + *sectio,* a cutting]. Surgical division of the vasa deferentia.

vasosensory (văs″ō-sĕn′sō-rē) [″ + *sensorius,* pert. to sensation]. Rel. to sensation in the blood vessels.

vasospasm (văs′ō-spăzm) [″ + Gr. *spasmos,* a convulsion]. Spasm of a blood vessel. SYN: *angiohypotonia; angiospasm; vasoconstriction.*

vasospastic (văs″ō-spăs′tĭk). Concerning or characterized by vasospasm.

vasostimulant (văs″ō-stĭm′ū-lănt) [L. *vas,* vessel, + *stimulans,* goading]. Exciting vasomotor action.

vasostomy (va-sŏs′tō-mē) [″ + Gr. *stoma,* mouth]. Surgical procedure of making an opening into the vas deferens.

vasotomy (văs-ŏt′ō-mē) [″ + Gr. *tome,* incision]. Incision of the vas deferens.

vasotonia (văs″ō-tō′nē-ă) [″ + Gr. *tonos,* act of stretching, tension]. The tone of blood vessels.

vasotonic (văs″ō-tŏn′ĭk) [″ + Gr. *tonikos,* pert. to tone]. 1. Pert. to the tone of a vessel. 2. Causing vasotonia.

vasotribe (văs′ō-trīb) [″ + Gr. *tribein,* to rub]. Pressure forceps used for controlling hemorrhages. SYN: *angiotribe.*

vasotripsy (văs′ō-trĭp″sē) [″ + Gr. *tripsis,* a crushing]. Arrest of hemorrhages with a strong forceps by crushing an artery. SYN: *angiotripsy.*

vasotrophic (văs″ō-trŏf′ĭk) [″ + Gr. *trophe,* nourishment]. Concerned with the nutrition of blood vessels.

vasotropic (văs″ō-trŏp′ĭk). Affecting blood vessels.

vasovagal (văs″ō-vā′găl). Concerning the action of stimuli from the vagus nerve on blood vessels.

vasovagal syncope. Sudden faint due to hypotension induced by the response of the nervous system to abrupt emotional stress, pain, or trauma. This is accompanied by pallor, sweating, hyperventilation, and bradycardia. Vagal stimulation causes this reaction. Treatment consists of having the patient lie flat and being certain that there is a clear airway; treat the underlying condition if indicated. Anticholinergic agents, such as propantheline bromide, may be helpful. Vomiting does not usually occur, but if it does, position patient to prevent aspiration of vomitus.

vasovasostomy (văs″ō-vă-sŏs′tō-mē) [″ + *vas,* vessel, + *stoma,* mouth]. Rejoining of the previously severed ductus deferens of the testicle.

vasovesiculectomy (văs″o-vĕ-sĭk″ū-lĕk′tō-mē) [″ + *vesicula,* tiny sac, + Gr. *ek-*

tome, excision]. Excision of the vas deferens and seminal vesicles.

vasovesiculitis (văs″ō-vĕ-sĭk″ū-lī′tĭs) [″ + *vesicula*, a tiny bladder, + Gr. *itis*, inflammation]. Inflammation of the vas deferens and seminal vesicles.

Vasoxyl. Trade name for methoxamine hydrochloride.

vastus (văs′tŭs) [L., vast]. 1. Great, large, extensive. 2. One of three muscles of the thigh. SEE: *Muscles* in *Appendix*.

Vater's ampulla (fä′tĕrz) [Abraham Vater, Ger. anatomist, 1684–1751]. Former name for papilla of Vater.

Vater's corpuscles. Ovoid end organs of nerves supplying the skin. SYN: *pacinian corpuscles*.

Vater's papilla. The duodenal end of the drainage systems of the pancreatic and common bile ducts. Formerly called ampulla of Vater.

vault (vawlt). A part or structure resembling a dome or arched roof.

VC. *vital capacity*.

V-Cillin. Trade name for penicillin V.

V-Cillin K. Trade name for penicillin V potassium, USP.

V̇CO₂. Symbol for carbon dioxide output per unit of time.

VD. *venereal disease*.

VDH. *valvular disease of the heart*.

VDRL. *Venereal Disease Research Laboratories*.

vection (vĕk′shŭn) [L. *vectio*, a carrying]. 1. Transfer of disease agents by a vector from the sick to the well. 2. Illusion of self-motion. This may be produced experimentally by having the subject seated within a drum that rotates while the subject remains stationary.

vectis (vĕk′tĭs) [L., pole]. A curved lever for making traction on presenting part of fetus.

vector (vĕk′tor) [L., a carrier]. 1. Any force or influence that is a quantity completely specified by magnitude, direction, and sense, which can be represented by a straight line of appropriate length and direction. 2. A carrier, usually an arthropod or insect that transmits the causative organisms of disease from infected to noninfected individuals, esp. one in which the organism goes through one or more stages in its life cycle.

    v., biological. An animal vector in which the disease-causing organism multiplies or develops prior to becoming infective for a susceptible individual.

    v., mechanical. A vector in or upon which growth and development of the infective agent do not occur.

vectorcardiogram (vĕk″tor-kăr′dē-ō-grăm) [″ + Gr. *kardia*, heart, + *gramma*,

something written]. A graphic record of the direction and magnitude of the electrical forces of the heart's action by means of a continuous series of vector loops. Analysis of the configuration of these loops permits certain statements to be made about the state of health or diseased condition of the myocardium. At any moment the electrical activity of the heart can be represented as an electrical vector with a specific direction and magnitude. This is called the instantaneous cardiac vector. A series of these vectors may be established for the entire cardiac cycle. By joining the tips of these vectors with a continuous line, the vectorcardiogram loop is formed. The configuration so obtained may be projected on the frontal plane or viewed as a three-dimensional loop. Three vectorcardiogram loops are formed during each cardiac cycle — one for the electrical activity of the atrium; one for ventricular depolarization; one for ventricular repolarization.

    v., spatial. Depiction of the vectorcardiogram in three planes, i.e., frontal, sagittal, and horizontal.

vectorcardiography. Analysis of the direction and magnitude of the electrical forces of the heart's action by a continuous series of loops (vectors) that represent the cardiac cycle.

vectorial (vĕk-tō′rē-ăl) [L. *vector*, a carrier]. Rel. to a vector.

VEE. *Venezuelan equine encephalitis*.

vegan (vēj′ăn). An extreme vegetarian who omits all animal protein from the diet.

veganism (vēj′ă-nĭzm). Strict vegetarianism in which one eats no food, including milk or cheese products, from an animal source.

vegetable (vĕj′ĕ-tă-bl). 1. Pert. to, of the nature of, or derived from plants. 2. A herbaceous plant, esp. one cultivated for food. 3. The edible part or parts of plants that are used as food, including the leaves, stems, seeds and seed pods, flowers, roots, tubers, and fruits.

    Vegetables are important sources of minerals and vitamins; provide bulk, which stimulates intestinal motility; and are sources of energy. Caloric value is indirectly proportional to water content. Vegetables in general are valuable for their mineral content and for their fiber content. Copper is estimated at 1.2 mg/kg for leafy vegetables, and 0.7 mg/kg for nonleafy ones.

    Plant and vegetable proteins are nutritionally inferior to those from animal sources, but by combining certain vegetables in the diet, a completely adequate and balanced mixture of essential amino acids can be provided. Corn is low in lysine but has adequate amounts of tryptophan; beans are adequate in lysine but low in tryptophan. While neither of these two foods contains adequate amounts of essential amino acids, they are adequate when eaten in combination. Similarly, rice and soybeans eaten together provide adequate essential amino acids even though each is lacking in essential amino acids. SEE: *incaparina.*

All starches in vegetables must be changed to sugars before they can be absorbed. Dry heat changes starch to dextrin; heat and acid or an enzyme change dextrin to dextrose. In germinating grain, starch is changed to dextrin and dextrose. Dextrose in fermentation turns to alcohol and carbon dioxide.

vegetal (vĕj'ĕ-tăl). 1. Pertaining to plants. 2. Tropic or nutritional, esp. with reference to that part of an ovum which contains the yolk. SEE: *pole, vegetal.*

vegetarian (vĕj-ĕ-tā'rē-ăn) [from *vegetable,* coined 1847 by Vegetarian Society]. One whose diet consists mainly of vegetables, sometimes also excluding dairy products. A carefully planned vegetarian diet, even if devoid of dairy products, may provide adequate nutrition; but if the diet is limited to fats, oils, refined carbohydrates, starches, or alcohol, it may not be nutritionally adequate.

vegetarianism (vĕj-ĕ-tā'rē-ăn-īzm) [" + Gr. *-ismos,* condition]. The belief and practice of eating vegetables and fruits only; may or may not exclude dairy products.

vegetate (vĕj'ĕ-tāt) [LL. *vegetare,* to grow]. 1. To grow luxuriantly with the production of fleshy or warty outgrowths such as a polyp. 2. To lead a passive existence mentally or physically, or both; to do little more than eat and maintain autonomic body functions.

vegetation (vĕj-ĕ-tā'shŭn). A morbid luxurious outgrowth on any part, esp. wartlike projections made up of collections of fibrin in which are enmeshed white and red blood cells; sometimes seen on denuded areas of the endocardium covering the valves of the heart.

  v., adenoid. Funguslike masses of lymphoid tissue in nasopharynx.

vegetative (vĕj'ĕ-tā"tĭv). 1. Having the power to grow, as plants. 2. Functioning involuntarily. 3. Quiescent, passive, noting a stage of development.

vegetative state. An imprecise term indicating a patient who was previously comatose, but whose eyes are now open and give the appearance that he or she is awake. It is properly characterized as a severe dementia due to global damage to the cerebral cortex. There is complete inability to respond to stimuli or to communicate.

vegetoanimal (vĕj"ĕ-tō-ăn'ĭ-măl). Concerning plants and animals.

vehicle (vē'ĭ-kl) [L. *vehiculum,* that which carries]. A substance, usually inactive therapeutically, used in a medicinal preparation as the agent for carrying the active ingredient.

  Ex.: a syrup in liquid preparations.

veil (vāl) [L. *velum,* a covering]. 1. Any veillike structure. 2. A piece of the amniotic sac occasionally covering the face of a newborn infant. SYN: *caul.* 3. Slight alteration in the voice in order to disguise it.

vein (vān) [L. *vena,* vein]. Vessel carrying dark red (unaerated) blood to the heart, except for the pulmonary vein, which carries oxygenated blood. Veins have three coats: inner, middle, and outer. They differ from arteries in their larger capacity and greater number; also in their thinner walls, larger and more frequent anastomoses, and presence of valves that prevent backward circulation. They consist of two sets, superficial or subcutaneous, and the deep veins, with frequent communications between the two. The former do not usually accompany an artery, as do the latter. The systemic veins consist of three groups — those entering the heart through the superior vena cava, those through the inferior vena cava, and those through the coronary sinus. Blood from the capillary plexuses enters the right atrium of the heart. SEE: *circulation; vena; Veins* in *Appendix.*

vein, words pert. to: basilic vein; cephalic vein; innominate veins; intravenous; jugular veins; phlebectomy; phlebitis; phlebogram; phlebotomy; phlegmasia alba dolens; portal vein; thrombophlebitis; thrombus; "varic-" words; varix; vascular; vasoconstrictor; vasodilator; vasomotor; vasoparesis; vena; vena cava; venesection; venosity; venotomy; venous; venule.

velamen (vē-lā'mĕn) [L., veil] (pl. *velamina*). Any covering membrane.

  v. nativum. The skin covering the body.

  v. vulvae. Abnormal elongation of the nymphae. SEE: *Hottentot apron.*

velamentous (vĕl"ă-mĕn'tŭs). Expanding like a veil, or sheet.

velamentum (vĕl"ă-mĕn'tŭm) [L., a cover] (pl. *velamenta*). A membranous covering.

velar (vē'lăr) [L. *velum,* a veil]. Pert. to a velum or veil-like structure.

Velban. Trade name for vinblastine sulfate.

Velcro. Trade name for fabric tape closures frequently used in orthotic fabrication and in adapting garments and devices for use by disabled persons with limited upper extremity function. The material contains a hooked side that adheres to the opposite side, which contains loops when the two are pressed together. The material may be applied and removed many times without losing its ability to adhere.

veliform (vĕl′ĭ-form). Velamentous.

vellication (vĕl-ĭk-ā′shŭn) [L. *vellicare*, to twitch]. Spasmodic twitching of muscular fibers.

vellus (vĕl′ŭs) [L., fleece]. The fine hair present on the body after the lanugo hair of the newborn is gone.

velopharyngeal (vĕl″ō-fă-rĭn′jē-ăl) [L. *velum*, veil, + Gr. *pharynx*, throat]. Concerning the soft palate and the pharynx.

velosynthesis (vĕl″ō-sĭn′thĕs-ĭs) [″ + Gr. *synthesis*, a placing together]. Suture of a cleft palate, particularly the soft palate. SYN: *staphylorrhaphy*.

Velpeau's bandage (vĕl-pōz′) [Alfred Velpeau, Fr. surgeon, 1795–1867]. A special immobilizing roller bandage that incorporates the shoulder, forearm, and arm. SEE: *bandage* for illus.

Velpeau's deformity. Deformity seen in Colles' fracture, q.v., in which lower fragment is displaced backward.

velum (vē′lŭm) [L., veil]. [NA] Any veil-like structure.

   v. palatinum. [NA] The soft palate.

vena (vē′nă) [L.] (pl. *venae*). A vein. SEE: *Veins* in *Appendix*.

   v. cava inferior. [NA] The principal vein draining the lower portion of the body. It is formed by junction of the two common iliac veins and terminates in the right atrium of the heart. SEE: *heart*.

   v. cava superior. [NA] The principal vein draining the upper portion of the body. It is formed by the junction of the right and left innominate veins and empties into the right atrium of the heart. SEE: *heart*.

venacavography (vē″nă-kā-vŏg′ră-fē). Radiography of the vena cava during the injection of a contrast media.

venae comitantes [L.]. Two or more veins accompanying an artery. They are usually present with the deep arteries of the extremities.

venation. The distribution of veins to an organ or structure.

venectasia (vē″nĕk-tā′zē-ă) [L. *vena*, a vein, + Gr. *ektasis*, dilation]. Dilation of a vein. SYN: *phlebectasia*.

venectomy (vē-nĕk′tō-mē) [″ + Gr. *ektome*, excision]. Phlebectomy.

veneer. In dentistry, a manmade material, such as an acrylic resin, that can be bonded to the surface of a tooth. Sometimes used for cosmetic reasons.

venenation (vĕn″ē-nā′shŭn) [L. *venenum*, poison]. 1. Condition of being poisoned. 2. Act of poisoning.

venene (vē-nēn′). A mixture of venoms from poisonous snakes.

veneniferous (vĕn″ē-nĭf′ĕr-ŭs) [″ + *ferre*, to carry]. Transmitting or carrying poison.

venenific (vĕn″ē-nĭf′ĭk) [″ + *facere*, to make]. Producing poison.

venenosalivary (vĕn″ē-nō-săl′ĭ-vĕr″ē). Venomosalivary, q.v.

venenosity (vĕn″ē-nŏs′ĭ-tē). State of being venomous.

venenous (vĕn′ĕn-ŭs) [L. *venenum*, poison]. Poisonous.

venepuncture (vĕn′ē-pŭnk″chŭr) [L. *vena*, vein, + *punctura*, a point]. Venipuncture.

venereal (vē-nē′rē-ăl) [L. *venereus*]. Pert. to or resulting from intercourse.

venereal bubo. Enlarged lymph node in the groin, the result of a venereal disease.

venereal collar. Mottled condition of the neck seen occasionally in syphilis.

venereal disease. Disease acquired ordinarily as a result of heterosexual or homosexual intercourse with an individual who is afflicted. The diseases so classified include gonorrhea, nonspecific urethritis, chlamydiosis, syphilis, AIDS, and chancroid. *Trichomonas vaginalis* vaginitis can be, but is not always, contracted through sexual intercourse. Genital candidiasis, lymphogranuloma venereum, granuloma inguinale, genital herpes, genital warts, balanoposthitis, and proctitis are also included in this classification. Bacterial pathogens, such as those of the genera *Salmonella*, *Shigella*, *Campylobacter*, and parasitic organisms including those of the genera *Giardia* and *Amoeba* may be transmitted by sexual activity involving anal-oral contact. SYN: *sexually transmitted disease*. SEE: *AIDS*. SEE: *Nursing Diagnoses* in *Appendix*.

venereal sore. Chancroid.

venereal urethritis. Urethritis occurring in gonorrhea.

venereal wart. Moist reddish elevation on genitals and anus. SYN: *condyloma; verruca acuminata*.

venereologist (vē-nēr″ē-ŏl′ō-jĭst) [″ + Gr. *logos*, word, reason]. A doctor who specializes in the treatment of venereal diseases.

venereology (vē-nēr″ē-ŏl′ō-jē). The scientific study and treatment of venereal diseases.

venereophobia (vē-nēr″ē-ŏ-fō′bē-ă) [L. *venereus*, pert. to sexual intercourse, + Gr. *phobos*, fear]. Abnormal fear of venereal disease. SYN: *cypridophobia*.

venery (vĕn′ĕr-ē) [L. *venerus*, pert. to Venus]. Archaic term for indulgence in sexual activity.

venesection (vĕn″ē-sĕk′shŭn) [L. *vena*, vein, + *sectio*, a cutting]. Surgical opening of a vein for withdrawal of blood. SYN: *phlebotomy; venisection*.

venin(e) (věn′ĭn) [L. *venenum*, poison]. Toxic substance in snake venom. SYN: *venene*.

venipuncture (věn′ĭ-pŭnk″chūr) [L. *vena*, vein, + *punctura*, a point]. Puncture of a vein for any purpose. The pain of venipuncture may be diminished by several methods, including application of cold to the area just prior to the puncture; injection of sterile, normal saline intracutaneously to produce blanching of the site; and use of a local anesthetic to produce a wheal at the site. SEE: *intravenous infusion* for illus.

venisection (věn″ĭ-sĕk′shŭn). Venesection.

venisuture (věn′ĭ-sū″chūr) [″ + *sutura*, a seam]. Suture of a vein. SYN: *phleborrhaphy*.

veno-. Combining form concerning veins.

venoatrial (vē″nō-āt′rē-ăl) [″ + *atrium*, corridor]. Rel. to the vena cava and the atrium. SYN: *venoauricular*.

venoauricular (vē″nō-aw-rĭk′ū-lăr) [″ + *auricula*, little ear]. Venoatrial.

venoclysis (vē-nŏk′lĭ-sĭs) [″ + Gr. *klysis*, a washing]. The continuous injection of medicinal or nutrient fluid intravenously. SYN: *phleboclysis*.

venofibrosis (vē″nō-fī-brō′sĭs). Phlebosclerosis.

venogram (vē′nō-grăm) [″ + Gr. *gramma*, something written]. 1. A roentgenogram of the veins. SYN: *phlebogram*. 2. A tracing of the venous pulse.

venography (vē-nŏg′ră-fē) [″ + Gr. *graphein*, to write]. 1. Roentgenography of veins. 2. The making of a tracing of the venous pulse.

venom (věn′ŏm) [L. *venenum*, poison]. A poison excreted by some animals, such as insects or snakes, and transmitted by bites or stings.

   v., ***Russell's viper***. SEE: *Russell's viper venom*.

   v., ***snake***. The poisonous secretion of the labial glands of certain snakes. Venoms contain proteins, chiefly toxins and enzymes, which are responsible for their toxicity. They are classified as neurocytolysins, hemolysins, hemocoagulins, proteolysins, and cytolysins on the basis of the effects produced. SEE: *snake, poisonous*.

venomization (věn″ŭm-ĭ-zā′shŭn). Treatment of a material with snake venom.

venomosalivary (věn″ō-mō-săl′ĭ-věr″ē). Secreting saliva with venom in it.

venomotor (vē″nō-mō′tor) [L. *vena*, vein, + *motus*, moving]. Pert. to constriction or dilatation of veins.

venomous (věn′ō-mŭs). 1. Poisonous. 2. Pert. to animals or insects that have venomsecreting glands.

venomous snake. In the U.S., the coral snakes and pit vipers (copperhead, cotton-mouth moccasin, and rattlesnake). SEE: *snake, poisonous*.

veno-occlusive (vē″nō-ō-kloo′sĭv). Concerning obstruction of veins.

venoperitoneostomy (vē″nō-pěr″ĭ-tō″nē-ŏs′tō-mē) [L. *vena*, vein, + Gr. *peritonaion*, peritoneum, + *stoma*, mouth]. Surgically inserting the cut end of the saphenous vein into the cavity of the peritoneum. This is done to allow ascitic fluid from the peritoneal cavity to drain into the vein.

venopressor (vē′nō-prěs″or) [″ + *pressor*, that which squeezes]. Pert. to venous blood pressure.

venosclerosis (vē″nō-sklě-rō′sĭs) [″ + Gr. *sklerosis*, to harden]. Sclerosis of veins. SYN: *phlebosclerosis*.

venose (vē′nōs). Having veins.

venosinal (vē″nō-sī′năl). Concerning the vena cava and the right atrium of the heart.

venosity (vē-nŏs′ĭ-tē) [L. *vena*, vein]. 1. Condition in which there is an excess of venous blood in a part, causing venous congestion. 2. Deficient aeration of venous blood.

venospasm (vē′nō-spăzm) [″ + Gr. *spasmos*, a convulsion]. Contraction of a vein. May follow infusion of cold or irritating substance into the vein.

venostasis (vē″nō-stā′sĭs) [″ + Gr. *stasis*, standing still]. The trapping of blood in an extremity by compression of veins, a method sometimes employed for reducing the amount of blood in circulation.

venostat (vē′nō-stăt) [″ + Gr. *statikos*, standing]. Appliance for performing venous compression.

venothrombotic (vē″nō-thrŏm-bŏt′ĭk). Having the property of inducing the formation of thrombi in veins.

venotomy (vē-nŏt′ō-mē) [″ + Gr. *tome*, incision]. Incision of a vein.

venous (vē′nŭs) [L. *vena*, vein]. Pert. to the veins or blood passing through them.

venous access devices. Specially designed catheters for use in gaining and maintaining access to the venous system. These devices are for use in providing access for patients who require intravenous fluids or medications for several days or more, e.g., patients having a bone marrow transplant or who are receiving long-term total parenteral nutrition.

venous blood. The dark blood in the veins.

venous cutdown. Surgical incision in a vein to permit intravenous administration of fluids or drugs. Required in patients with vascular collapse due to shock or other causes. SEE: illus.

venous hum. Murmur heard upon auscultation over larger veins of the neck.

venous hyperemia. Excess of venous blood

VENOUS CUTDOWN

CEPHALIC VEIN

SAPHENOUS VEIN

INFILTRATE INCISION AREA WITH LOCAL ANAESTHETIC

TOURNIQUET

BASILIC VEIN

CEPHALIC VEIN

INCISION SITE

A

LEFT ARM

LIGATURE TO ELEVATE VEIN

B

HEMOSTAT

DISTAL SUTURE

BASILIC VEIN

LIGATURE

VEIN

HANDLE VEIN GENTLY

USE SHARP POINTED SCISSORS TO CUT HALF OF CIRCUMFERENCE OF THE VEIN

C

45°

DIRECTION OF FLOW OF BLOOD PRIOR TO CUTDOWN

TOURNIQUET REMOVED AFTER PROXIMAL SUTURE IS TIED AROUND VEIN AND CATHETER. THEN ATTACH IV TUBING AND START FLUID

D

CATHETER INTRODUCER PLACED UNDER FLAP

CATHETER IS PLACED IN VEIN

DISTAL SUTURE

CATHETER

CUTDOWN SITE IS SUTURED

CATHETER SUTURED TO SKIN

E

FLUID TUBING

in a part. SYN: *venosity*.

venous return. The amount of blood returning to the atria of the heart.

venous sinus. A channel that carries venous blood. Important venous sinuses are those of the dura mater draining the brain and those of the spleen.

venous sinus of sclera. The canal of Schlemm. SEE: *canal, Schlemm's*.

venous thrombosis. SEE: *thrombosis, venous*.

venovenostomy (vē″nō-vē-nŏs′tō-mē) [″ + ″ + Gr. *stoma*, mouth]. Formation of an anastomosis of a vein joined to a vein.

vent (vĕnt) [O. Fr. *fente*, slit]. An opening in any cavity, esp. one for excretion.

    v., alveolar. An opening between adjacent alveoli of the lung.

venter (vĕn′tĕr) [L., belly]. 1. A belly-shaped part. 2. The cavity of the abdomen. 3. [NA] The wide swelling part or belly of a muscle.

ventilation (vĕn″tĭ-lā′shŭn) [L. *ventilare*, to air]. 1. Circulation of fresh air in a room and withdrawal of foul air. 2. Oxygenation of blood. 3. In physiology, the amount of air inhaled per day. This can be estimated by spirometry, multiplying the tidal air by the number of respirations per day. An average figure is 10,000 liters. This must not be confused with the total amount of oxygen consumed, which is on the average only 360 liters per day. These volumes are more than doubled during hard physical labor.

    v., continuous positive-pressure. Method of mechanically assisted pulmonary ventilation. A device administers air or oxygen to the lungs under a continuous pressure that never returns to zero.

    v., high frequency jet. A type of ventilation which provides continuous ventilation delivered at 100 to 150 cycles per minute. Used in respiratory failure to provide continuous ventilation without the side effects of positive pressure ventilation.

    v., intermittent positive-pressure. Mechanical method for assisting pulmonary ventilation employing a device that administers air or oxygen for the inflation of the lungs under positive pressure. Exhalation is usually passive. SYN: *breathing, intermittent positive-pressure*.

    v., pulmonary. The inspiration and expiration of air from the lungs.

ventilation coefficient. The amount of air that must be respired for each liter of oxygen to be absorbed.

ventilation rate. ABBR: VR. The amount of air breathed in one minute.

ventilation tube. SEE: *grommet*.

ventilator. A mechanical device for artificial ventilation of the lungs. The mechanism may be hand operated or machine driven,

and in the latter case may be automatic and very sophisticated with respect to being able to control and monitor flow of air to the lungs.

ventouse (vĕn-toos′) [Fr.]. A glass or glass-shaped vessel used in cupping, q.v.

ventrad (vĕn′trăd) [L. *venter*, belly, + *ad*, to]. Toward the ventral aspect. Opposite of dorsad.

ventral (vĕn′trăl) [L. *ventralis*, pert. to the belly]. Pert. to the belly. Hence, in quadrupeds, pertaining to the lower or underneath side of the body; in humans, pertaining to the anterior portion or the front side of the body. Opposite of dorsal.

ventral hernia. Hernia through the abdominal wall, esp. at points other than the umbilicus and groin.

ventralis (vĕn-trā′lĭs) [L.]. Anterior, or closer to the front.

ventricle (vĕn′trĭk-l) [L. *ventriculus*, a little belly]. 1. A small cavity. 2. Either of two lower chambers of the heart that when filled with blood contract to propel it into the arteries. The right ventricle forces blood into the pulmonary artery and thence into the lungs; the left pumps blood through the aorta into the arteries. 3. One of the cavities of the brain. SEE: illus.; *Arantius' body*.

    v., aortic. Left ventricle of the heart.

    v., fifth. Cavity of the septum lucidum of the brain. It is between the two laminae of the septum lucidum.

    v., fourth. The cavity above the pons and medulla of the brain. It extends from the central canal of the upper end of the spinal cord to the aqueduct of the midbrain. Its roof is the cerebellum and the superior and inferior medullary vela. Its floor is the rhomboid fossa.

    v., lateral. The cavity in each cerebral hemisphere that communicates with the third ventricle through the interventricular foramen. It consists of a triangular central body; and four horns, two inferior and two posterior.

    v., left. The cavity of the heart that receives blood from the left atrium and pumps it out into the general circulation through the aortic valve.

    v., Morgagni's. The recess in the lateral wall on each side of the larynx between the vestibular and vocal folds.

    v. of Arantius. The terminal depression of the median sulcus of the fourth ventricle of the brain.

    v. of larynx. The space between the true and false vocal cords.

    v., pineal. The pineal recess of the third ventricle of the brain.

    v., right. The cavity of the heart that receives blood from the right atrium and

VENTRICLES OF THE BRAIN

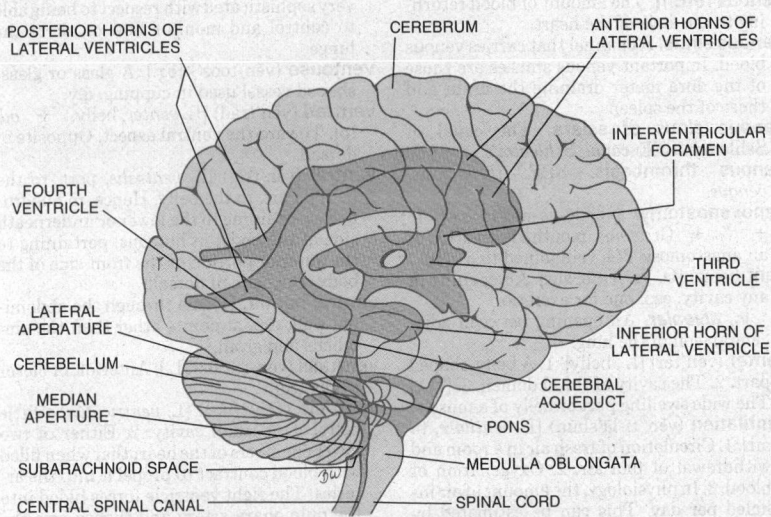

POSTERIOR HORNS OF LATERAL VENTRICLES

CEREBRUM

ANTERIOR HORNS OF LATERAL VENTRICLES

INTERVENTRICULAR FORAMEN

FOURTH VENTRICLE

THIRD VENTRICLE

LATERAL APERTURE

INFERIOR HORN OF LATERAL VENTRICLE

CEREBELLUM

CEREBRAL AQUEDUCT

MEDIAN APERTURE

PONS

SUBARACHNOID SPACE

MEDULLA OBLONGATA

CENTRAL SPINAL CANAL

SPINAL CORD

RIGHT LATERAL VIEW

pumps it into the lungs via the pulmonary veins.

v., third. The median cavity in the brain bounded by the thalamus and hypothalamus on either side, anteriorly by the optic chiasm; the floor is made up of the tuber cinereum, mammillary body, the posterior perforated substance and tegmentum of the cerebral peduncle; the roof is the ependyma. Anteriorly, it communicates with the lateral ventricles, and posteriorly, with the aqueduct of the midbrain.

ventricornu (věn″trĭ-kor′nū) [L. *venter,* belly, + *cornu,* horn]. The anterior ventral horn of gray matter of the spinal cord.

ventricose (věn′trĭ-kōs) [L. *ventricosus,* bigbellied]. 1. Inflated or distended. 2. Corpulent.

ventricular (věn-trĭk′ū-lăr) [L. *ventriculus,* a little belly]. Pert. to a ventricle.

ventricular assist pumping. Use of a device to replace the pumping action of a diseased or nonfunctioning heart. These devices are for temporary use.

ventricular compliance. Distensibility or stiffness of the relaxed ventricle of the heart.

ventricular folds. The false vocal cords or folds of mucous membrane parallel or above the true vocal cords.

ventricular ligament. A narrow band of fibrous tissue lying within each ventricular fold.

ventricular septal defect. Defect in the septum between the left and right ventricles of the heart. This permits blood to be shunted between the ventricles.

ventriculitis (věn-trĭk″ū-lī′tĭs) [″ + Gr. *itis,* inflammation]. Inflammation of a ventricle.

ventriculoatriostomy (věn-trĭk″ū-lō-ā″trē-ŏs′tō-mē) [″ + *atrium,* corridor, + Gr. *stoma,* mouth]. Plastic surgery for the relief of hydrocephalus. Subcutaneous catheters are placed to connect a cerebral ventricle to the right atrium via the jugular vein. The catheters contain one-way valves so that cerebral spinal fluid can flow into the catheters but blood may not be pumped into the cerebral ventricle.

ventriculocisternostomy (věn-trĭk″ū-lō-sĭs″těr-nŏs′tō-mē) [″ + *cisterna,* box, chest, + Gr. *stoma,* mouth]. Plastic surgery to create an opening between the ventricles of the brain and the cisterna magna.

ventriculocordectomy (věn-trĭk″ū-lō-kor-dĕk′tō-mē) [″ + Gr. *khorde,* cord, + *ektome,* excision]. Surgery for relief of laryngeal stenosis. The ventricular floor is removed, but the buccal processes are left in place.

ventriculogram (věn-trĭk′ū-lō-grăm) [″ + Gr. *gramma,* something written]. Roentgenogram of the cerebral ventricles.

ventriculography (věn-trĭk″ū-lŏg′ră-fē) [″ + Gr. *graphein*, to write]. 1. An x-ray process used for visualizing the size and shape of the cerebral ventricles by injecting air to display the cerebrospinal fluid that normally fills these cavities. 2. Visualization of ventricles of the heart by x-ray after injection of a contrast material.

ventriculometry (věn-trĭk″ū-lŏm′ĕ-trē) [″ + Gr. *metron*, measure]. The measurement of the intraventricular cerebral pressure.

ventriculonector (věn-trĭk″ū-lō-něk′tor) [L. *ventriculus*, a little belly, + *nector*, a joiner]. The atrioventricular bundle.

ventriculopuncture (věn-trĭk′ū-lō-pǔnk″tūr) [″ + *punctura*, a point]. Use of a needle to puncture a lateral ventricle of the brain.

ventriculoscopy (věn-trĭk″ū-lŏs′kō-pē) [″ + Gr. *skopein*, to examine]. Examination of the ventricles of the brain with an endoscope.

ventriculostomy (věn-trĭk″ū-lŏs′tō-mē) [″ + Gr. *stoma*, mouth]. Plastic surgery in order to establish communication between the floor of the third ventricle of the brain and the cisterna interpeduncularis. This is done to treat hydrocephalus.

ventriculosubarachnoid (věn-trĭk″ū-lō-sǔb″ă-răk′noyd). Concerning the cerebral ventricles and the subarachnoid spaces.

ventriculotomy (věn-trĭk″ū-lŏt′ō-mē) [″ + Gr. *tome*, incision]. Surgical incision of a ventricle.

ventriculus (věn-trĭk′ū-lǔs) [L., a little belly]. [NA] 1. Ventricle. 2. The stomach. 3. A ventricle of the brain or heart.

v. tertius. Third ventricle, q.v.

ventricumbent (věn″trĭ-kǔm′běnt) [L. *venter*, belly, + *cumbere*, to lie]. Lying on the belly. SYN: *prone.*

ventriduct (věn′trĭ-dǔkt) [″ + *ducere*, to lead]. To draw toward the abdomen.

ventriduction (věn″trĭ-dǔk′shǔn). Pulling or placing a part ventrad.

ventrimeson (věn″trĭ-měs′ŏn) [″ + Gr. *mesos*, middle]. The median line on the ventral surface of the body.

ventripyramid (věn″trĭ-pĭr′ă-mĭd) [″ + Gr. *pyramis*, a pyramid]. An anterior pyramid of the medulla oblongata.

ventro- [L. *venter*, belly]. Combining form denoting the abdomen or ventral (anterior) surface of the body.

ventrocystorrhaphy (věn″trō-sĭs-tor′ă-fē) [″ + Gr. *kystis*, sac, + *rhaphe*, seam, ridge]. Suture of a cyst or the bladder to the abdominal wall.

ventrodorsal (věn″trō-dor′săl) [″ + *dorsum*, back]. In a direction from the front to the back.

ventrofixation (věn″trō-fĭks-ā′shǔn) [″ + *fixatio*, to fix]. The suture of a displaced viscus to the abdominal wall.

ventrohysteropexy (věn″trō-hĭs′těr-ō-pěks″ē) [″ + Gr. *hystera*, womb, + *pexis*, fixation]. Attachment of the uterus to the abdominal wall.

ventroinguinal (věn″trō-ĭng′gwĭ-năl) [″ + *inguen*, groin]. Concerning the ventral and inguinal regions.

ventrolateral (věn″trō-lăt′ĕr-ăl) [″ + *latus*, side]. Both ventral and lateral.

ventromedial (věn″trō-mē′dē-ăl) [″ + *medianus*, median]. Both ventral and medial.

ventroptosia, ventroptosis (věn″trŏp-tō′sē-ă, -sĭs) [″ + Gr. *ptosis*, a dropping]. Downward displacement of the stomach. SYN: *gastroptosis.*

ventroscopy (věn-trŏs′kō-pē) [L. *venter*, belly, + Gr. *skopein*, to examine]. Examination of the abdominal cavity by illumination. SYN: *celioscopy.*

ventrose (věn′trōs). Having a swelling like a belly.

ventrosity (věn-trŏs′ĭ-tē). Having an enlarged belly; corpulence.

ventrosuspension (věn″trō-sǔs-pěn′shǔn) [″ + *suspensio*, a hanging]. Fixation of displaced uterus to abdominal wall.

ventrotomy (věn-trŏt′ō-mē) [″ + Gr. *tome*, incision]. Incision into abdominal cavity. SYN: *celiotomy; laparotomy.*

ventrovesicofixation (věn″trō-věs″ĭ-kō-fĭks-ā′shǔn) [″ + L. *vesica*, bladder, + *fixare*, to fix]. Suture of uterus to abdominal wall and bladder. SYN: *hysterocystopexy.*

Venturi mask [Giovanni Battista Venturi, It. scientist, 1746–1822]. A special mask for administering a controlled concentration of oxygen to a patient.

venturimeter (věn″tūr-ĭm′ě-těr). Device for measuring flow of fluids through vessels.

venula (věn′ū-lă) [L., little vein]. Venule.

venule (věn′ūl) [L., *venula*, little vein]. A tiny vein continuous with a capillary.

Venus, crown of. An eruption around the hairline caused by syphilis.

Venus, mount of. The mons pubis or mons veneris, q.v.

Venus's collar (vē′nǔs) [L., the Roman goddess of love]. Pigmentation around the neck in eruption due to syphilis.

verbigeration (věr-bĭj″ěr-ā′shǔn) [L. *verbigerare*, to chatter]. Repetition of words that are either meaningless or have no significance.

verbomania (věr″bō-mā′nē-ă) [L. *verba*, word, + Gr. *mania*, madness]. The flow of talk in some forms of psychosis.

Vercyte. Trade name for pipobroman.

verdigris (věr′dĭ-grĭs) [O. Fr. *vert de Grece*,

green of Greece]. 1. Mixture of basic copper acetates. 2. Deposit of copper carbonate upon copper and bronze vessels. It is a green-gray color.

verdigris poisoning. Same as for copper sulfate. SEE: *copper salts* in *Poisons and Poisoning* in *Appendix.*

verdohemoglobin (vĕr″dō-hēm′ō-glōb″ĭn). A greenish pigment occurring as an intermediate product in the formation of bilirubin from hemoglobin.

Verga's ventricle (vĕr′găz) [Andrea Verga, It. neurologist, 1811–1895]. Cleftlike space between the corpus callosum and the body of the fornix of the brain.

verge (vĕrj). An edge or margin.

    v., anal. The transitional area between the smooth perianal area and the hairy skin.

vergence (vĕr′jĕns) [L. *vergere,* to bend]. A turning of one eye with reference to the other. May be horizontal (convergence or divergence) or vertical (intravergence or supravergence). SEE: *phoria.*

Verheyen's stars (fĕr-hī′ĕns) [Philippe Verheyen, Flemish anatomist, 1648–1710]. Starlike venous plexuses on surface of the kidney below its capsule.

vermicidal (vĕr″mĭ-sī′dăl) [L. *vermis,* worm, + *cidus,* kill]. Destroying worms parasitic in the intestines.

vermicide (vĕr′mĭ-sīd). 1. Destroying worms. 2. An agent that will kill intestinal worms.

vermicular (vĕr-mĭk′ū-lăr) [L. *vermicularis*]. Resembling a worm.

vermicular movements. The wormlike movements of peristalsis.

vermicular pulse. Small rapid pulse resulting in wormlike feeling in the fingers.

vermiculation (vĕr″mĭk″ū-lā′shŭn) [L. *vermiculare,* to wriggle]. A wormlike motion, as in the intestines. SEE: *peristalsis.*

vermicule (vĕr′mĭ-kūl) [L. *vermiculus,* a small worm]. A small worm, or having a wormlike shape.

vermiculose, vermiculous (vĕr-mĭk′ū-lōs, vĕr-mĭk′ū-lŭs) [L. *vermicularis,* wormlike]. 1. Infested with worms or larvae. 2. Wormlike.

vermiform (vĕr′mĭ-form) [L. *vermis,* worm, + *forma,* shape]. Contoured like a worm.

vermiform appendix. A long, narrow, worm-shaped tube connected to the cecum. It varies in length from less than 1 to more than 8 in. (2.5 to 20.3 cm) with an average of about 3 in. (7.6 cm). Its distal end is closed. It is lined with mucosa similar to that of the large intestine. Inflammation of it is called appendicitis, q.v. SEE: illus.

vermifugal (vĕr-mĭf′ū-găl) [″ + *fugare,* to put to flight]. Expelling worms from the intestines.

vermifuge (vĕr′mĭ-fūj). Agent for expelling

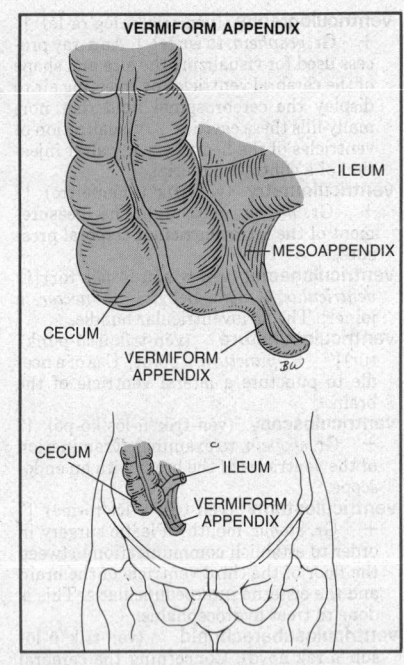

VERMIFORM APPENDIX

ILEUM

MESOAPPENDIX

CECUM

VERMIFORM APPENDIX

CECUM

ILEUM

VERMIFORM APPENDIX

intestinal worms. SYN: *anthelmintic; vermicide.*

vermilion border (vĕr-mĭl″yŏn) [ME. *vermilioun,* bright red]. The red boundary of the lips which represents the highly vascular, hyalinized epithelial covering between the outer skin and moist oral mucosa of the mouth.

vermilionectomy (vĕr-mĭl″yŏn-ĕk′tō-mē) [″ + Gr. *ektome,* excision]. Surgical removal of the vermilion border of the lip.

vermin (vĕr′mĭn) [L. *vermis,* worm]. Small insects and animals such as mice, lice, or bedbugs that are annoying or cause destruction or disease.

verminal (vĕr′mĭ-năl). Concerning or caused by worms.

vermination (vĕr″mĭn-ā′shŭn). Vermin or worm infestation.

verminosis (vĕr″mĭn-ō′sĭs) [″ + Gr. *osis,* condition]. Infestation with vermin.

verminous (vĕr′mĭn-ŭs). Pert. to or infested with worms.

vermiphobia (vĕr″mĭ-fō′bē-ă) [″ + Gr. *phobos,* fear]. An abnormal fear of being infested with worms.

vermis (vĕr′mĭs) [L. worm]. 1. A worm. 2. Vermis cerebelli.

    v. cerebelli. [NA] Median connecting

lobe of the cerebellum.

v., inferior. The anteroinferior portion of the vermis of the cerebellum. Includes the nodule, uvula, pyramis, and tuber.

v., superior. The posterior dorsal portion of the vermis. Includes the folium, declive, culmen, and central lobule.

Vermox. Trade name for mebendazole.

vernal (vĕr′năl) [L. *vernalis*, pert. to spring]. Occurring in or pert. to the spring.

Vernet's syndrome (vĕr-nāz′) [Maurice Vernet, Fr. physician, b. 1887]. Paralysis of glossopharyngeal, vagus, and spinal accessory nerves on the opposite side of a lesion involving the jugular foramen.

vernix (vĕr′nĭks) [L.]. Varnish.

v. caseosa. A sebaceous deposit covering the fetus. It is protective during intrauterine life. Most abundant in creases and flexor surfaces. Consists of exfoliations of outer skin layer, lanugo, and secretions of sebaceous glands. It is not necessary to remove this after the fetus is delivered. SEE: *sebum.*

verruca (vĕr-roo′kă) [L., wart] (pl. *verrucae*). Tumor of the epidermis of the skin. Produces a circumscribed elevated area of hypertrophy of the papillae. SYN: *wart.*

ETIOL: Caused by a papillomavirus.

TREAT: Removal with sharp spoon curet under local anesthesia. If elevated, clip off with sharp scissors and touch with iodine. Freezing with carbon dioxide snow or fulguration.

PROG: Essentially benign and may disappear spontaneously, particularly in children and young adults. In elderly with long-standing dry seborrhea, lesions are potentially malignant.

v. acuminata. A pointed, reddish, moist wart about the genitals and the anus. Develops near mucocutaneous junctures, forming pointed, tufted, or pedunculated pinkish or purplish projections of varying lengths and consistency. Venereal warts should be treated with topically applied podophyllum resin. SYN: *venereal wart.*

v. digitata. Form of verruca seen on face and scalp, possibly serving as starting point of cutaneous warts. Several filiform projections with horny caps are formed, closely grouped on a comparatively narrow base that in turn may be separated from skin surface by slightly contracted neck.

v. filiformis. A small threadlike growth on the neck and eyelids covered with smooth and apparently normal epidermis.

v. gyri hippocampi. One of the small wartlike protuberances on the convex surface of the gyrus hippocampi.

v. plana. A flat or slightly raised wart.

v. plantaris. Wart on the sole of the foot.

SYN: *plantar wart.*

v. vulgaris. The common wart, usually on backs of hands and fingers, but may occur anywhere on the skin.

verruciform (vĕ-roo′sĭ-form) [L. *verruca*, wart, + *forma*, shape]. Wartlike.

verrucose, verrucous (vĕr′roo-kōs, vĕr-roo′kŭs) [L. *verrucosus*, wartlike]. Wartlike, with raised portions.

verrucosis (vĕr″oo-kō′sĭs) [L. *verruca*, wart, + Gr. *osis*, condition]. The condition of having multiple warts.

verruga peruana (vĕ-roo′gă pĕr-wăn′ă) [Sp., Peruvian wart]. The eruptive second clinical stage of bartonellosis, q.v. Oroya fever is the first or febrile stage.

Versapen. Trade name for hetacillin.

Versapen K. Trade name for hetacillin potassium.

Versed. Trade name for midazolam hydrochloride, q.v.

Versene. Ethylenediaminetetraacetic acid, q.v.

versicolor (vĕr′sĭ-kŏl″or) [L., of changing colors]. 1. Having many shades or colors. 2. Changeable in color. SEE: *tinea versicolor.*

version (vĕr′zhŭn) [L. *versio*, a turning]. 1. Altering of position of the fetus in the uterus. May occur naturally or may be done mechanically by the physician in order to facilitate delivery. 2. Deflection of an organ such as the uterus from its normal position.

v., bipolar. Changing the position of the fetus by combined internal and external manipulation.

v., cephalic. Turning of fetus so that the head presents.

v., combined. Mechanical version by combined internal and external manipulation.

v., external. Version of the fetus through the abdominal wall.

v., internal. Version of the fetus with one hand inserted through the vagina.

v., pelvic. Version of a cross-presentation until it is changed to a pelvic presentation.

v., podalic. Version of fetus by the feet so that the breech presents.

v., spontaneous. Version of fetus by uterine muscular contraction without artificial assistance.

vertebra (vĕr′tĕ-bră) [L.] (pl. *vertebrae*). [NA] Any one of the 33 bony segments of the spinal column. The spinal vertebrae contain 7 cervical, 12 thoracic (dorsal), 5 lumbar, 5 sacral, and 4 coccygeal vertebrae. In adults, the five sacral vertebrae fuse to form a single bone, the sacrum, and the four rudimentary coccygeal vertebrae fuse to form the coccyx.

A typical vertebra consists of a ventral body and a dorsal or neural arch. In the thoracic region, the body bears on each side two costal pits for reception of the head of the rib. The arch that encloses the vertebral foramen is formed of two roots or pedicles and two laminae. The arch bears seven processes: a dorsal spinous process, two lateral transverse processes, and four articular processes (two superior and two inferior). A deep concavity, inferior vertebral notch, on the inferior border of the arch provides a passageway for a spinal nerve. The successive vertebral foramina surround the spinal cord.

The bodies of successive vertebrae articulate with one another and are separated by intervertebral disks, disks of fibrous cartilage enclosing a central mass, the nucleus pulposus. The inferior articular processes articulate with the superior articular processes of the next succeeding vertebra in the caudal direction. Several ligaments (supraspinous, interspinous, anterior and posterior longitudinal, and the ligamenta flava) hold the vertebrae in position, yet permit a limited degree of movement. SEE: *sacrum* for illus.

RS: acantha; anapophysis; anticlinal; atlas; axis; lamina; "spondyl-" words.

   v., basilar. The lowest of the lumbar vertebrae.

   v., cervical. The seven vertebrae of the neck.

   v., coccygeal. The rudimentary vertebrae of the coccyx.

   v. dentata. The second cervical vertebra. SYN: *axis* [NA]; *v., odontoid.*

   v., false. The sacral and coccygeal vertebrae that fuse. SYN: *v., fixed.*

   v., fixed. V., false.

   v., flexion. Forward bending of one vertebra on the one below it.

   v., lumbar. The five vertebrae between the thoracic vertebrae and the sacrum.

   v. magnum. The sacrum.

   v., odontoid. V. dentata.

   v. prominens. [NA] The seventh cervical vertebra.

   v., rotation. The direction the anterior part of the body of the more superior vertebra moves on the vertebra below it.

   v., sacral. The five fused vertebrae forming the sacrum. SEE: *sacrum* for illus.

   v., sternal. The segments of the sternum.

   v., thoracic. The 12 vertebrae that connect the ribs and form part of the posterior wall of the thorax. SEE: *spinal column* for illus.

   v., true. The vertebrae that remain unfused through life: the cervical, thoracic, and lumbar.

vertebral (vĕr′tĕ-brăl) [L. *vertebra*, vertebra].

Pertaining to a vertebra or the vertebral column.

vertebral arch. The thoracic portion of a vertebra that encloses a vertebral foramen.

vertebral canal. Cavity of the spinal column that contains the spinal cord. SYN: *spinal canal.*

vertebral column. Spinal column.

vertebral foramen. The hollow space enclosed by a vertebral arch.

vertebral groove. Groove lying on either side of the spinous processes of the vertebrae.

vertebral notch. Notch on inferior surface of vertebral arch for transmission of a spinal nerve.

vertebral ribs. The lower two, or floating, ribs.

vertebrarium (vĕr′tĕ-brā′rē-ŭm) [L.]. The vertebral column.

Vertebrata (vĕr′tĕ-brā′tă). A subphylum of the phylum Chordata characterized by possession of segmented backbone or spinal column. They possess an axial notochord at some period of their existence. Includes the following classes: Agnatha (cyclostomes); Chondrichthyes (cartilaginous fishes); Osteichthyes (bony fishes); Amphibia; Reptilia; Aves; and Mammalia.

vertebrate (vĕr′tĕ-brāt) [L. *vertebra*, vertebra]. Having or resembling a vertebral column.

vertebrated (vĕr′tĕ-brāt″ĕd). Composed of jointed segments.

vertebrectomy (vĕr′tĕ-brĕk′tō-mē) [″ + Gr. *ektome*, excision]. Excision of a vertebra or part of one.

vertebro-. Combining form concerning a vertebra or vertebrae.

vertebroarterial (vĕr″tĕ-brō-ăr-tē′rē-ăl) [″ + Gr. *arteria*, artery]. Concerning the vertebral artery.

vertebrobasilar (vĕr″tĕ-brō-băs′ĭ-lăr) [″ + *basilaris*, basilar]. Concerning the vertebral and basilar arteries.

vertebrochondral (vĕr″tĕ-brō-kŏn′drăl) [″ + Gr. *chondros*, cartilage]. Denoting the vertebra and the costal cartilages.

vertebrocostal (vĕr″tĕ-brō-kŏs′tăl) [″ + *costa*, rib]. Pert. to a vertebra and a rib. SYN: *costovertebral.*

vertebrofemoral (vĕr″tĕ-brō-fĕm′or-ăl) [″ + *femur*, thigh]. Concerning the vertebrae and femur.

vertebroiliac (vĕr″tĕ-brō-ĭl′ē-ăk) [″ + *iliacus*, pert. to ilium]. Concerning the vertebrae and ilium.

vertebromammary (vĕr″tĕ-brō-măm′mă-rē) [″ + *mamma*, breast]. Pert. to the vertebral and mammary areas.

vertebrosacral (vĕr″tĕ-brō-sā′krăl) [″ + *sacrum*, sacred]. Concerning the vertebrae and sacrum.

vertebrosternal (věr″tě-brō-stěr′năl) [″ + Gr. *sternon*, chest]. Pert. to a vertebra and the sternum.

vertex (věr′těks) [L., summit]. [NA] The top of the head. SYN: *corona capitis; crown*.
  v. cordis. Apex of the heart.

vertical (věr′tǐ-kăl) [L. *verticalis*, summit]. 1. Pert. to or situated at the vertex. 2. Perpendicular to the plane of the horizon of the earth; upright.

verticalis (věr″tǐ-kā′lǐs) [L.]. Vertical. Indicating any plane that passes through the body parallel to the long axis of the body.

verticality. The ability to accurately perceive the vertical position in the absence of environmental cues.

verticillate (věr-tǐs′ǐl-āt, -tǐs-ǐl′āt) [L. *verticillus*, a little whirl]. Arranged like the spokes of a wheel or a whorl.

verticomental (věr″tǐ-kō-měn′tăl) [L. *vertex*, summit, + *mentum*, chin]. Concerning the crown of the head and the chin.

vertiginous (věr-tǐj′ǐ-nŭs) [L. *vertiginosus*, one suffering from dizziness]. Pert. to or afflicted with vertigo.

vertigo (věr′tǐ-gō, věr-tī′gō) [L. *vertigo*, a turning round]. True vertigo is the sensation of moving around in space (subjective vertigo) or of having objects move about the person (objective vertigo) and is a result of a disturbance of equilibratory apparatus. Sometimes used as a synonym for dizziness, lightheadedness, and giddiness. SEE: *vection* (def. 2).

ETIOL: May be caused by a variety of entities, including middle ear disease; toxic conditions such as those caused by salicylates, alcohol, or streptomycin; sunstroke; postural hypotension; or toxemia due to food poisoning or infectious diseases.

NURSING IMPLICATIONS: Assessment should include whether or not the patient feels that he or she, or the environment, is turning or whirling; direction of the sensation of motion; whether it is intermittent or constant; time of day it occurs; whether or not it is related to position, drugs, occupation, or menses; whether it is associated with nausea and vomiting or with nystagmus and migraine. Implement safety measures such as use of siderails while in bed. Ambulate gradually after a slow, assisted move from a sitting position. Have the call bell available at all times; make sure tissues, water, and other needed supplies are within easy reach and that furniture and other obstacles are removed from the path of ambulation. The patient who received a fenestration operation on the ear and is experiencing severe vertigo should be confined to bed for several days and then begin a gradual increase in activity.

  v., alternobaric. Vertigo associated with sudden decrease in the pressure to which the inner ear is exposed. This could occur when a SCUBA diver ascends quickly or when an aircraft ascends quickly. SEE: *bends*.

  v., auditory. Vertigo due to disease of the ear.

  v., benign positional. A benign disorder of the labyrinth of the inner ear characterized by paroxysmal vertigo and nystagmus only when the head is in a certain position or moves in a certain direction. The diagnosis is made at the bedside by moving the patient from the sitting position to recumbency with the head tilted down 30° over the end of the table and 30° to one side. This causes a paroxysm of vertigo. This test is called the Hallpike maneuver. The episodes may last less than a minute, but may recur for months. SYN: *positional vertigo of Báránay*.

  v., central. Vertigo caused by disease of the central nervous system.

  v., cerebral. Vertigo due to brain disease.

  v., epidemic. Vertigo that may occur in epidemic form. It is believed to be due to vestibular neuronitis.

  v., epileptic. Vertigo attending an epileptic attack or following it.

  v., essential. Vertigo from an unknown cause.

  v., gastric. Vertigo associated with gastric disturbance.

  v., horizontal. Vertigo that occurs while the patient is supine.

  v., hysterical. Vertigo accompanying hysteria.

  v., labyrinthine. Vertigo due to disease of labyrinth of the ear. SYN: *Ménière's disease*.

  v., laryngeal. Vertigo accompanying laryngeal spasm.

  v., objective. Vertigo in which stationary objects appear to be moving.

  v., ocular. Vertigo caused by disease of the eye.

  v., organic. Vertigo due to a brain lesion.

  v., peripheral. Vertigo due to disturbances in the peripheral areas of the central nervous system.

  v., positional; v., postural. Vertigo that occurs when the head is in a specific position.

  v., rotary. Vertigo in which the sensation is that of rotation.

  v., subjective. Vertigo in which the patient has the sensation of turning or rotating.

  v., toxic. Vertigo from presence of a toxin in the body.

  v., vertical. Vertigo upon standing; or produced by looking up or down.

  v., vestibular. Vertigo due to disease or

malfunction of the vestibular apparatus.

verumontanitis (věr″ū-mŏn″tăn-ī′tĭs) [L. *veru*, spit, dart, + *montanus*, mountainous, + Gr. *itis*, inflammation]. Inflammation of the verumontanum. SYN: *colliculitis*.

verumontanum (věr″ū-mŏn-tā′nŭm) [L. *veru*, spit, dart, + *montanus*, mountainous]. An elevation on the floor of the prostatic portion of the urethra where the seminal ducts enter.

very low density lipoproteins. ABBR: VLDL. Plasma lipids bound to albumin consisting of chylomicrons and prelipoproteins. This class contains a greater ratio of lipid than low-density lipoproteins and are the least dense. SEE: *lipoprotein.*

vesalianum (věs-ā″lē-ā′nŭm) [Andreas Vesalius, Flemish anatomist and physician, 1514–1564]. One of the sesamoid bones in the tendon of origin of the gastrocnemius muscle, and another on outer border of foot in the angle between the cuboid and fifth metatarsal.

Vesalius, foramen of (věs-ā′lē-ŭs) [Andreas Vesalius]. Opening in base of the skull transmitting an emissary vein.

Vesalius, vein of. Small emissary vein from cavernous sinus passing through foramen of Vesalius and conveying blood to the pterygoid plexus.

vesica (vě-sī′kă) [L.]. [NA] A bladder.

    v. fellea. [NA] The gallbladder.

    v. prostatica. A minute pouch in the prostatic urethra, remnant of the müllerian duct. SYN: *utriculus prostaticus.*

    v. urinaria. [NA] The urinary bladder.

vesical (věs′ĭ-kăl). Pert. to or shaped like a bladder.

vesical reflex. Inclination to urinate caused by moderate bladder distention.

vesicant (věs′ĭ-kănt) [L. *vesicare*, to blister]. 1. Blistering; causing or forming blisters. 2. Agent used to produce blisters. It is much less severe in its effects than are escharotics. 3. A blistering gas used in chemical warfare. SEE: *gas, vesicant.*

vesication (věs″ĭ-kā′shŭn). 1. Process of blistering. 2. A blister.

vesicatory (věs′ĭ-kă-tor″ē). 1. Causing or pert. to blisters. 2. Agent causing blisters. SYN: *vesicant.*

vesicle (věs′ĭ-kl) [L. *vesicula*, a little bladder]. 1. A small sac or bladder containing fluid. 2. A blisterlike small elevation on the skin containing serous fluid.

    Vesicles may vary in diameter from a few millimeters to a centimeter. They may be round, transparent, opaque, or dark elevations of the skin, sometimes containing seropurulent or bloody fluid. They are seen in sudamina as the result of sweat that cannot

escape from the skin; in herpes, mounted on an inflammatory base, having no tendency to rupture but associated with burning pain. In herpes zoster they follow the line of the nerve trunks. They are seen in dermatitis venenata as the result of contact with poison ivy or oak and accompanied by great itching; they are also seen in dermatitis herpetiformis or multiformis. In impetigo contagiosa they occur, especially in children, in discrete form, flat and umbilicated, filled with straw-colored fluid, with no tendency to break. They dry up, forming yellow crusts with little itching. They are also seen in vesicular eczema, molluscum contagiosum, miliaria (prickly heat or heat rash), chickenpox, smallpox, and scabies. SEE: *herpes; miliaria.*

    v., allantoic. The hollow, enlarged part of the allantois, esp. in birds and reptiles.

    v., auditory. That portion of the cerebral vesicle from which the exterior ear is formed.

    v., blastodermic. Sac developed from the blastoderm.

    v.'s, brain. The five embryonic subdivisions of the brain.

    v.'s, brain, primary. The three earliest subdivisions of the embryonic neural tube.

    v.'s, cerebral. Expansion of neural embryonic canal from which the brain develops.

    v., chorionic. The outer villus-covered layer of the early embryo. It encloses the embryo, amnion, umbilical cord, and yolk stalk.

    v., compound. Multilocular vesicles.

    v.'s, encephalic. V.'s, brain.

    v., lens. The embryonic vesicle formed from the lens pit. It develops into the lens of the eye.

    v.'s, multilocular. Vesicles that contain multiple chambers.

    v.'s, optic. Hollow outgrowths from the lateral aspects of the embryonic brain. The retinae and optic nerves develop from these paired vesicles.

    v., otic. V., auditory, q.v.

    v., seminal. One of the two membranous sacculated tubes situated at the base of the bladder, between it and the rectum, serving as a reservoir for the semen and having a secretion of its own.

    v., umbilical. Portion of embryonic yolk sac outside the body cavity.

vesico- (věs′ĭ-kō) [L. *vesica*, bladder]. Combining form meaning bladder.

vesicoabdominal (věs″ĭ-kō-ăb-dŏm′ĭ-năl) [″ + *abdomen*, belly]. Concerning the urinary bladder and the abdomen.

vesicocele (věs′ĭ-kō-sēl″) [L. *vesica*, bladder, + Gr. *kele*, tumor, swelling]. Hernia of the bladder into the vagina. SYN: *cystocele.*

vesicocervical (věs″ĭ-kō-sĕr′vĭ-kăl) [″ + *cervix,* neck]. Rel. to the urinary bladder and cervix uteri.

vesicoclysis (věs″ĭ-kŏk′lĭ-sĭs) [″ + Gr. *klysis,* a washing]. Injection of fluid into the bladder.

vesicoenteric (věs″ĭ-kō-ĕn-tĕr′ĭk) [″ + Gr. *enteron,* intestine]. Concerning the urinary bladder and intestine.

vesicofixation (věs″ĭ-kō-fĭks-ā′shŭn) [L. *vesica,* bladder, + *fixatio,* a fixing]. Attachment of the uterus to the bladder or the bladder to the abdominal wall.

vesicointestinal (věs″ĭ-kō-ĭn-tĕs′tĭ-năl). Vesicoenteric.

vesicoprostatic (věs″ĭ-kō-prŏs-tăt′ĭk) [″ + Gr. *prostates,* prostate]. Relating to the bladder and prostate.

vesicopubic (věs″ĭ-kō-pū′bĭk) [″ + NL. *(os) pubis,* bone of the groin]. Pert. to the bladder and os pubis.

vesicopustule (věs″ĭ-kō-pŭs′tūl) [″ + *pustula,* blister]. A vesicle in which pus has developed.

vesicosigmoid (věs″ĭ-kō-sĭg′moyd) [″ + Gr. *sigmoid,* shaped like Gr. letter S]. Concerning the urinary bladder and sigmoid colon.

vesicosigmoidostomy (věs″ĭ-kō-sĭg″moy-dŏs′tō-mē) [″ + ″ + *stoma,* mouth]. Surgical creation of an anastomosis between the urinary bladder and sigmoid colon.

vesicospinal (věs″ĭ-kō-spī′năl) [″ + *spina,* thorn]. Relating to the urinary bladder and spinal cord.

vesicostomy (věs″ĭ-kŏs′tō-mē) [″ + Gr. *stoma,* mouth]. Surgical production of an opening into the bladder.

vesicotomy (věs″ĭ-kŏt′ō-mē) [″ + Gr. *tome,* incision]. Incision of the bladder.

vesicoumbilical (věs″ĭ-kō-ŭm-bĭl′ĭ-kăl) [″ + *umbilicus,* navel]. Concerning the urinary bladder and umbilicus.

vesicoureteral (věs″ĭ-kō-ū-rē′tĕr-ăl) [″ + Gr. *oureter,* ureter]. Concerning the urinary bladder and a ureter.

vesicouterine (věs″ĭ-kō-ū′tĕr-ĭn) [″ + *uterinus,* pert. to the womb]. Pert. to the urinary bladder and uterus.

vesicouterine pouch. Downward extension of the peritoneal cavity located between bladder and uterus.

vesicouterovaginal (věs″ĭ-kō-ū″tĕr-ō-văj′ĭ-năl) [″ + *uterus,* womb, + *vagina,* sheath]. Concerning the urinary bladder, the uterus, and the vagina.

vesicovaginal (věs″ĭ-kō-văj′ĭ-năl) [″ + *vagina,* sheath]. Pert. to the urinary bladder and vagina.

vesicovaginorectal (věs″ĭ-kō-văj″ĭ-nō-rĕk′tăl) [″ + *vagina,* sheath, + *rectum,* straight]. Concerning the urinary bladder, vagina, and rectum.

vesicula (vĕ-sĭk′ū-lă) [L.] (pl. *vesiculae*). [NA] A small bladder or vesicle.

   v. seminalis. [NA] Tiny reservoir of semen at base of the bladder. SYN: *seminal vesicle.*

vesicular (vĕ-sĭk′ū-lăr). Pert. to vesicles or small blisters.

vesicular breathing. Murmur heard in normal breathing. SYN: *vesicular murmur.*

vesicular eczema. Eczema accompanied by formation of vesicles.

vesicular murmur. The normal sound of respiration heard on auscultation. SYN: *vesicular breathing.*

vesicular rale. The crepitant rale, a crackling sound heard at end of inspiration.

vesicular resonance. Percussion sound heard over the normal lung.

vesiculase (vĕ-sĭk′ū-lās). An enzyme in prostatic fluid said to coagulate semen.

vesiculated (vĕ-sĭk′ū-lāt″ĕd). Having vesicles present.

vesiculation (vĕ-sĭk′ū-lā′shŭn) [L. *vesicula,* a tiny bladder]. Formation of vesicles or state of having or forming them.

vesiculectomy (vĕ-sĭk″ū-lĕk′tō-mē) [″ + Gr. *ektome,* excision]. Partial or complete excision of a vesicle, particularly a seminal vesicle.

vesiculiform (vĕ-sĭk′ū-lĭ-form) [″ + *forma,* shape]. Having the shape of a vesicle.

vesiculitis (vĕ-sĭk″ū-lī′tĭs) [″ + Gr. *itis,* inflammation]. Inflammation of a vesicle, particularly the seminal vesicle.

vesiculobronchial (vĕ-sĭk″ū-lō-brŏng′kē-ăl) [″ + Gr. *bronchos,* windpipe]. Both vesicular and bronchial.

vesiculocavernous (vĕ-sĭk″ū-lō-kăv′ĕr-nŭs) [″ + *caverna,* a hollow]. Vesicular and cavernous.

vesiculogram (vĕ-sĭk″ū-lō-grăm) [″ + Gr. *gramma,* something written]. Radiograph of the seminal vesicles.

vesiculography (vĕ-sĭk″ū-lŏg′ră-fē) [″ + Gr. *graphein,* to write]. Roentgenography of the seminal vesicles.

vesiculopapular (vĕ-sĭk″ū-lō-păp′ū-lăr) [″ + *papula,* pimple]. Composed of vesicles and papules.

vesiculopustular (vĕ-sĭk″ū-lō-pŭs′tū-lăr) [″ + *pustula,* blister]. Having both vesicles and pustules.

vesiculotomy (vĕ-sĭk″ū-lŏt′ō-mē) [″ + Gr. *tome,* incision]. Surgical incision into a vesicle, as a seminal vesicle.

vesiculotubular (vĕ-sĭk″ū-lō-tū′bū-lăr) [″ + *tubularis,* like a tube]. Sounds from auscultation of the chest that have both vesicular and tubular qualities.

vesiculotympanic (vĕ-sĭk″ū-lō-tĭm-păn′ĭk) [″ + Gr. *tympanon,* drum]. Having both vesicular and tympanic qualities.

Vespidae [L. *vespa,* wasp]. Family of wasps, including paper wasps, hornets, and yellow jackets.

Vesprin. Trade name for triflupromazine hydrochloride.

vessel (vĕs′ĕl) [O. Fr. from L. *vascellum,* a little vessel]. A tube, duct, or canal to convey the fluids of the body. SYN: *vas* [NA].

RS: anastomose; anastomosis; angiitis; angiodystrophia; arrosion; endothelial; intima; rhegma; vas; vascular.

v.'s, absorbent. The lacteals, lymphatics, and capillaries of the intestines.

v., blood. Any of the vessels carrying blood, i.e., arteries, veins, and capillaries.

v.'s, chyliferous. Vessels arising in the villi of the intestinal walls carrying chyle and terminating in the thoracic duct.

v., collateral. Vessel parallel to the vessel from which it arose.

v.'s, great. The large blood vessels entering and leaving the heart.

v., lacteal. A lymph vessel that collects chyle from the intestinal villi.

v.'s, lymphatic. Vessels conveying lymph.

v.'s, nutrient. Vessels supplying specific areas such as the interior of bones.

v., radicular. Branch of a vertebral artery supplying cerebral nerve root.

vestibular (vĕs-tĭb′ū-lăr) [L. *vestibulum,* vestibule]. Pert. to a vestibule.

vestibular bulbs. Two sacculated collections of veins, lying on either side of the vagina beneath the bulbocavernosus muscle, connected anteriorly by the pars intermedia, and through this strip of cavernous tissue communicating with the erectile tissue of the clitoris. The vestibular bulbs are the homologues of the male corpus spongiosum. Injury during labor may give rise to troublesome bleeding. SEE: *Bartholin's glands; vagina; vestibule of vagina.*

vestibular nerve. A main division of the auditory nerve. Arises in the vestibular ganglion and is concerned with equilibrium.

vestibule (vĕs′tĭ-būl). A small space or cavity at the beginning of a canal, such as the aortic vestibule.

v., aortic; v. of aorta. The part of the left ventricle of the heart just below the aortic valve.

v. of ear. The middle part of the inner ear, behind the cochlea, and in front of the semicircular canals; it contains the utriculus and sacculus.

v. of larynx. The portion of the larynx above the vocal cords.

v. of mouth. The part of the oral cavity

between the lips and the cheeks and between the teeth and the gums.

v. of nose. The anterior part of the nostrils, containing the vibrissae.

v. of pharynx. The space surrounded by the soft palate, base of the tongue, and the palatoglossal and palatopharyngeal arches.

v. of vagina. An almond-shaped space between the lines of attachment of the labia minora. At the anterior angle the clitoris is situated; the posterior boundary is the fourchette. The vestibule is approx. 4 to 5 cm long and 2 cm in greatest width when the labia minora are separated. Four major structures open into the vestibule: the urethra anteriorly, the vagina posteriorly, and the two excretory ducts of the glands of Bartholin laterally. The covering membranes are pink in color and constructed of delicate stratified squamous epithelium. Collections of cavernous tissue are disposed beneath the integument. SEE: *Bartholin's glands; vagina; vestibular bulbs.*

vestibulocochlear nerve (vĕs-tĭb″ū-lō-kŏk′lē-ăr) [L. *vestibulum,* vestibule, + Gr. *kokhlos,* land snail]. The 8th cranial nerve, which emerges from the brain behind the facial nerve between the pons and medulla oblongata. SYN: *acoustic nerve.* SEE: illus.

vestibuloplasty (vĕs-tĭb′ū-lō-plăs″tē) [″ + Gr. *plassein,* to mold]. Plastic surgery of the vestibule of the mouth.

vestibulotomy (vĕs-tĭb″ū-lŏt′ō-mē) [″ + Gr. *tome,* incision]. Surgical incision into the vestibule of the inner ear.

vestibulourethral (vĕs-tĭb″ū-lō-ū-rē′thrăl) [″ + Gr. *ourethra,* urethra]. Rel. to the vestibule of the vagina and urethra.

vestibulum (vĕs-tĭb′ū-lŭm) [L.] (pl. *vestibula*). [NA] Vestibule.

vestige (vĕs′tĭj) [L. *vestigium,* footstep]. A small degenerate or incompletely developed structure that has been more fully developed in the embryo or in a previous stage of species.

vestigial (vĕs-tĭj′ē-ăl). Of the nature of a vestige. SYN: *rudimentary.*

vestigium (vĕs-tĭj′ē-ŭm) [L., a footstep] (pl. *vestigia*). Vestige.

veta (vā′tă) [Sp.]. Mountain sickness, esp. that which occurs in the Andes.

veterinarian (vĕt″ĕr-ĭ-nār′ē-ăn). One who is trained and licensed to practice veterinary medicine and surgery.

veterinary (vĕt′ĕr-ĭ-nār″ē). 1. Pert. to animals, their diseases and treatment. 2. A veterinarian.

veterinary medicine. That which deals with diseases of animals and their treatment.

VF. *ventricular fibrillation; vocal fremitus.*

V.H. *viral hepatitis.*

VESTIBULOCOCHLEAR NERVE
(8TH CRANIAL)

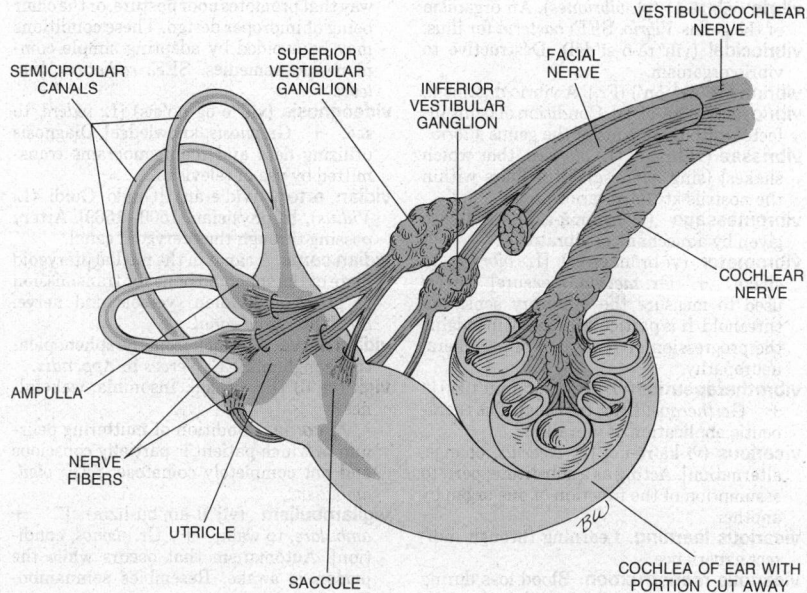

SEMICIRCULAR
CANALS

SUPERIOR
VESTIBULAR
GANGLION

INFERIOR
VESTIBULAR
GANGLION

FACIAL
NERVE

VESTIBULOCOCHLEAR
NERVE

COCHLEAR
NERVE

AMPULLA

NERVE
FIBERS

UTRICLE

SACCULE

COCHLEA OF EAR WITH
PORTION CUT AWAY

via (vē′ă, vī′ă) [L.] (pl. *viae*). Any passage in the body such as nasal, intestinal, or vaginal.

viability (vī″ă-bǐl′ĭ-tē) [L. *vita*, life, + *habilis*, fit]. Ability to live, grow, and develop.

viable (vī′ă-bl) [L. *vita*, life, + *habilis*, fit]. Capable of living, as a newborn or a fetus that has reached a stage, usually 24 weeks or greater than 500 gm, that will permit it to live outside the uterus.

vial (vī′ăl) [Gr. *phiale*, a drinking cup]. A small glass bottle for medicines or chemicals.

vibex (vī′běks) [L. *vibix*, mark of a blow] (pl. *vibices*). Narrow linear mark of hemorrhage into the skin.

Vibramycin. Trade name for doxycycline.

vibrapuncture (vī″bră-pŭnk′tūr). Medical use of tattoo technique to introduce medicine into skin lesions. Multiple punctures are made into the skin by a needle that has passed through a small amount of the solution of medicine placed on the site.

Vibra-Tabs. Trade name for doxycycline hyclate.

vibratile (vī′bră-tĭl) [L. *vibrare*, to shake]. Adapted to or used in vibratory motion; moving to and fro. SEE: *vibratory*.

vibration (vī-brā′shŭn). 1. A to-and-fro movement. SYN: *oscillation*. 2. Therapeutic shaking of the body, a form of massage. Consists of a quick motion of the fingers or the hand vertical to the body or use of a mechanical vibrator.

vibrative (vīb′ră-tĭv). 1. Vibratory. 2. Indicating sound produced by vibration of parts of the respiratory tract as air passes through.

vibrator (vī′bră-tor) [L. *vibrator*, a shaker]. Device for causing artificial vibration of body or its parts.

   v., vaginal. SEE: *vaginal vibrator.*

   v., whole body. Exposure of the entire body as would occur in occupations such as truck and tractor drivers, jackhammer operators, helicopter pilots, and construction workers using various vibration-producing tools. There is evidence that such exposure may produce diseases of the peripheral nerves, prostatitis, and back disorders.

vibratory (vī′bră-tō″rē) [L. *vibrator*, a shaker]. Having a vibrating or oscillatory movement.

vibratory sense. The ability to perceive vibrations transmitted through the skin to deep tissues. Usually tested by placing a vibrating tuning fork over bony prominences.

Vibrio (vĭb′rē-ō). A genus of curved, motile, gram-negative bacilli, several of which may be pathogenic for humans. Included are V.

cholerae, the comma-shaped organism that causes cholera, and *V. vulnificus.*

vibrio (vĭb′rē-ō) (pl. *vibriones*). An organism of the genus *Vibrio.* SEE: *bacteria* for illus.

vibriocidal (vĭb″rē-ō-sī′dăl). Destructive to vibrio organism.

vibrion (vē″brē-ŏn′) [Fr.]. A vibrio organism.

vibriosis (vĭb″rē-ō′sĭs). Condition of being infected with organisms of the genus *Vibrio.*

vibrissae (vī-brĭs′ē) [L. *vibrissa,* that which shakes] (sing. *vibrissa*). Stiff hairs within the nostrils at the anterior nares.

vibromassage (vī″brō-mă-săj′). Massage given by a mechanical vibrator.

vibrometer (vī-brŏm′ĕt-ĕr) [L. *vibrare,* to shake, + Gr. *metron,* measure]. Device used to measure the vibratory sensation threshold. It is particularly useful in judging the progression or remission of peripheral neuropathy.

vibrotherapeutics (vī″brō-thĕr″ă-pū′tĭks) [" + Gr. *therapeutikos,* treating]. The therapeutic application of vibration.

vicarious (vī-kā′rē-ŭs) [L. *vicarius,* change, alternation]. Acting as a substitute; pert. to assumption of the function of one organ by another.

vicarious learning. Learning through indirect experience.

vicarious menstruation. Blood loss during menstruation at some site other than the vagina, as hemorrhage from the nose, the breast, or eyes. SEE: *stigmata.*

vicarious respiration. Increased respiration in one lung when respiration in the other is lessened or abolished.

Vicq d′Azyr′s tract (vĭk dă-zērz′) [Felix Vicq d′Azyr, Fr. anatomist, 1748–1794]. A large myelinated bundle arising in mammillary nuclei and terminating in anterior thalamic nuclei of the brain.

vidarabine (vī-dār′ă-bēn). USP. An antiviral agent effective against the herpes simplex and herpes zoster-varicella viruses. It has been successfully used in treating encephalitis due to herpes simplex. Trade name is Vira-A. SYN: *ara-A.*

video display terminal. ABBR: VDT. Terminals used in information processing (computer terminals) and entertainment (TV picture tubes) that produce an image on a screen (target) by bombarding it with electrons. This causes the fluorescent material that coats the screen to emit light. The effects on workers involved with the use of VDTs have been investigated with respect to a variety of factors. There is no evidence that reproductive or visual health is impaired by working with VDTs.

Those who work with VDTs may experience musculoskeletal difficulties if the workplaces are poorly designed. This may be due to the screen being positioned in a way that promotes poor posture, or the chair being of improper design. These conditions may be avoided by adapting simple commonsense remedies. SEE: *radiation, low-level.*

videognosis (vĭd″ē-ŏg-nō′sĭs) [L. *videre,* to see, + Gr. *gnosis,* knowledge]. Diagnosis utilizing data and roentgenograms transmitted by use of television.

vidian artery (vĭd′ē-ăn) [Guido Guidi (L. *Vidius*), It. physician, 1500–1569]. Artery passing through the pterygoid canal.

vidian canal. A canal in the medial pterygoid plate of the sphenoid bone for transmission of pterygoid (vidian) vessels and nerve. SYN: *pterygoid canal.*

vidian nerve. A branch from the sphenopalatine ganglion. SEE: *Nerves* in *Appendix.*

vigil (vĭj′ĭl) [L., awake]. Insomnia, wakefulness.

    v., coma. Condition of muttering delirium in which patient is partially conscious and not completely comatose. SEE: *vigilambulism.*

vigilambulism (vĭj″ĭl-ăm′bū-lĭzm) [" + *ambulare,* to walk, + Gr. *-ismos,* condition]. Automatism that occurs while the person is awake. Resembles somnambulism.

vigilance (vĭj′ĭ-lăns) [L. *vigilantia,* wastefulness]. Being attentive, alert, and watchful.

vigintinormal (vī-jĭn″tĭ-nor′măl) [L. *viginti,* twenty, + *normal,* rule]. Consisting of one-twentieth of what is normal, as a solution.

vigor (vĭg′or) [L.]. Active force or strength of body or mind.

Villaret′s syndrome (vē-lär-āz′) [Maurice Villaret, Fr. neurologist, 1877–1946]. Ipsilateral paralysis of the ninth, tenth, eleventh, twelfth, and sometimes the seventh cranial nerves and the cervical sympathetic fibers. It is caused by a lesion in the posterior retroparotid space. The signs and symptoms include paralysis and anesthesia of the pharyngeal area with difficulty swallowing; loss of taste sensation in the posterior third of the tongue; paralysis of the vocal cords, sternocleidomastoid and trapezius muscles; and Horner′s syndrome, q.v.

villi (vĭl′ī) [L.]. Pl. of villus.

    v., chorionic. Tiny branching processes of the surface of chorion that become vascular and help to form the placenta.

villiferous (vĭl-ĭf′ĕr-ŭs) [" + *ferre,* to bear]. Having villi or tufts of hair.

villoma (vĭ-lō′mă) [L. *villus,* tuft of hair, + Gr. *oma,* tumor]. A villous tumor.

villose, villous (vĭl′ōs, vĭl′ŭs) [L. *villus,* tuft of

VILLI OF THE SMALL INTESTINE

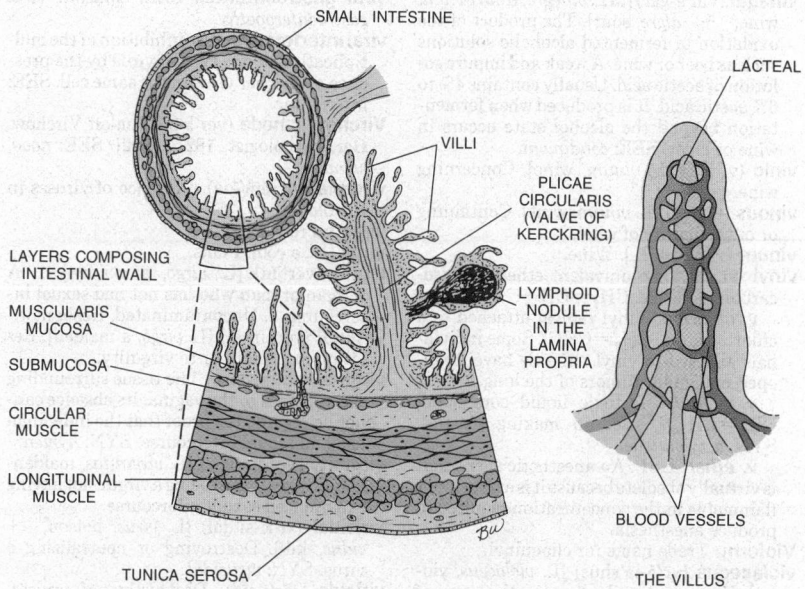

hair]. Pert. to or furnished with villi or with fine hairlike extensions.

villositis (vĭl″ōs-ī′tĭs) [″ + Gr. *itis*, inflammation]. Inflammation of the placental villi.

villosity (vĭ-lŏs′ĭ-tē). Condition of being covered with villi.

villus (vĭl′ŭs) [L., tuft of hair] (pl. *villi*). The short filamentous processes found on certain membranous surfaces.

   v., arachnoid. A protrusion of the cerebral arachnoid into the dural wall of a venous sinus or its lacuna.

   v., chorionic. Tiny vascular projections of the chorionic surface that help to form the placenta. SEE: *chorion.*

   v., intestinal. Multiple, minute projections of the intestinal mucosa into the lumen of the small intestines. These serve to absorb fluids and nutrients. SEE: illus.

   v., synovial. Thin projections of synovial membrane into the joint cavity.

villusectomy (vĭl″ŭs-ĕk′tō-mē) [″ + Gr. *ektome*, excision]. Surgical removal of a synovial villus.

vinblastine sulfate (vĭn-blăs′tēn). USP. A fraction of an extract obtained from the periwinkle plant, *Vinca rosea*, a species of myrtle. It is a cytotoxic agent used in treating

certain types of malignant tumors. Trade name is Velban.

Caution: Handle vinblastine sulfate with great care, since it is a potent cytotoxic agent.

Vinca (vĭn′kă). A genus of herbs including periwinkles, from which vincristine and vinblastine are obtained.

Vincent's angina (vĭn′sĕnts ăn-jī′nă) [Henri Vincent, Fr. physician, 1862–1950]. SYN: *trench mouth.* SEE: *gingivitis; gingivitis, acute necrotizing.*

vincristine sulfate (vĭn-krĭs′tēn). USP. A fraction of an extract obtained from the periwinkle plant, *Vinca rosea*, a species of myrtle. It is a cytotoxic agent used in treating certain types of malignant tumors. Trade name is Oncovin.

Caution: Handle vincristine sulfate with great care, since it is a potent cytotoxic agent.

---

vinculum (vĭn′kū-lŭm) [L., to bind, tie] (pl. *vincula*). A uniting band or bundle. SYN: *frenulum; frenum; ligament.*

   v. tendinum. 1. Slender tendinous filaments connecting the phalanges with the

Labels on figure:
SMALL INTESTINE
LACTEAL
VILLI
PLICAE CIRCULARIS (VALVE OF KERCKRING)
LAYERS COMPOSING INTESTINAL WALL
LYMPHOID NODULE IN THE LAMINA PROPRIA
MUSCULARIS MUCOSA
SUBMUCOSA
CIRCULAR MUSCLE
LONGITUDINAL MUSCLE
BLOOD VESSELS
THE VILLUS
TUNICA SEROSA

flexor tendons. 2. The ringlike ligament of the ankle or wrist.

vinegar (vĭn'ĕ-găr) [ME. *vinegre,* from Fr. *vin,* wine, + *aigre,* sour]. The product of the oxidation of fermented alcoholic solutions such as beer or wine. A weak and impure solution of acetic acid. Usually contains 4% to 6% acetic acid. It is produced when fermentation beyond the alcohol state occurs in wine or cider. SEE: *condiment.*

vinic (vī'nĭk) [L. *vinum,* wine]. Concerning wine.

vinous (vī'nŭs) [L. *vinum,* wine]. Containing or of the nature of wine.

vinum (vī'nŭm) [L.]. Wine.

vinyl (vī'nĭl). The univalent ethenyl hydrocarbon molecule, $CH_2=CH-$.

   v. chloride. Vinyl radical attached to a chlorine atom, $CH_2=CHCl$. Some individuals exposed to vinyl chloride have developed malignant tumors of the lung.

   v. cyanide. A toxic liquid compound, $CH_2=CHCN$, used in making plastics. SYN: *acrylonitrile.*

   v. ether. USP. An anesthetic agent that is virtually obsolete because it is explosive or flammable in the concentration required to produce anesthesia.

Vioform. Trade name for clioquinol.

violaceous (vī"ĕ-lā'shŭs) [L. *violaceus,* violet]. Having a purple discoloration, esp. of the skin.

violate (vī'ĕ-lāt") [L. *violare,* to injure]. To harm or injure a person, especially to rape a female.

violence (vī'ō-lĕnts) [L. *violentia*]. 1. The use of force or physical compulsion to abuse or damage. 2. The act of violent behavior.

violet (vī'ō-lĕt) [ME. *violett,* from L. *viola,* violet]. One of the colors of the spectrum; similar to purple.

   v., gentian. SEE: *gentian violet.*

violet blindness. Inability to see violet tints.

viomycin (vī-ō-mī'sĭn). An antibiotic produced by strains of *Streptomyces griseus.*

viosterol (vī-ŏs'tĕr-ōl). A solution of irradiated ergosterol in vegetable oil. SYN: *calciferol.*

viper (vī'pĕr). Any venomous snake of the family Viperidae.

vipoma [*vasoactive intestinal polypeptide* + *oma,* tumor]. ABBR: VIP. A rare form of islet cell tumor of the pancreas that is characterized by watery diarrhea, hypokalemia, and achlorhydria. This is caused by the release of vasoactive intestinal peptide (VIP) from the tumor.

Vira-A. Trade name for vidarabine.

viraginity (vĭr"ă-jĭn'ĭ-tē) [L. *virago,* an amazon or manlike woman]. A condition in which a woman believes that she should be a male even though she is aware that her body is female. SEE: *transsexual.*

viral. Pert. to or caused by a virus.

viral gastroenteritis. SEE: *epidemic viral gastroenteropathy.*

viral interference. The inhibition of the multiplication of one type of virus by the presence of another virus in the same cell. SEE: *interferon.*

Virchow's node (vĕr'kōz) [Rudolf Virchow, Ger. pathologist, 1821–1902]. SEE: *node, signal.*

viremia (vī"rĕm'ē-ă). Presence of viruses in the blood.

vires (vī'rēs). Pl. of vis.

virga [L., a rod]. Penis.

virgin (vĕr'jĭn) [L. *virgo,* a maiden]. 1. A woman or man who has not had sexual intercourse. 2. Uncontaminated; fresh; new.

virginal (vĕr'jĭn-ăl) [L. *virgo,* a maiden]. Relating to a virgin or to virginity.

virginal membrane. The tissue surrounding the entrance to the vagina. Its absence cannot be regarded as proof that the individual has had sexual intercourse. SYN: *hymen.*

virginity (vĕr-jĭn'ĭt-ē) [L. *virginitas,* maidenhood]. The state of being a virgin; not having experienced sexual intercourse.

viricidal (vĭ-rĭ-sī'dăl) [L. *virus,* poison, + *cidus,* kill]. Destroying or neutralizing a virus. SYN: *virucidal.*

viricide (vĭr'ĭ-sīd). Destructive of viruses. SYN: *virucide.*

virile (vĭr'ĭl) [L. *virilis,* masculine]. Having characteristics of a mature male. SYN: *masculine.*

virile reflex. 1. Sudden downward movement of penis when the prepuce or gland of a completely relaxed penis is pulled upward. SYN: *bulbocavernosus reflex.* 2. Contraction of bulbocavernous muscle on percussing dorsum of penis. 3. Contraction of bulbocavernous muscle resulting from compression of glans penis.

virilescence (vĭr-ĭl-ĕs'ĕns) [L. *virilis,* masculine]. The acquisition of secondary masculine characteristics in the female.

virilia (vĭr-ĭl'ē-ă) [L.]. The male sexual organs.

virilism (vĭr'ĭl-ĭzm) [" + Gr. *-ismos,* condition]. Presence or development of male secondary characteristics in a woman.

virility (vĭr-ĭl'ĭ-tē) [L. *virilitas,* masculinity]. 1. The state of possessing masculine qualities. 2. Sexual potency in the male.

virilization (vĭr"ĭ-lĭ-zā'shŭn). Production of masculine secondary sex changes in the female. Included would be voice change, development of male-type baldness, clitoral enlargement, and increased growth of facial and body hair. Virilization may be caused by one of several endocrine diseases that lead to excess production of testosterone, or by the female's taking anabolic steroids. In the latter case, this if often done in order to attempt to enhance muscular development.

virion (vī'rē-ŏn, vĭ'rē-ŏn). A complete virus particle; a unit of genetic material, the genome, surrounded by a protective protein coat, the capsid. Sometimes the capsid is surrounded by an envelope. SEE: *capsid.*

viripotent (vī-rĭp'ō-těnt) [L. *viripotens*]. 1. Sexually mature, as applied to a male. 2. Marriageable, as applied to a female.

viroids. Small, naked, infectious molecules of RNA. Viroids differ from viruses by the absence of a dormant phase and by genomes that are much smaller than those of known viruses.

virology (vī-rŏl'ō-jē) [L. *virus,* poison, + Gr. *logos,* word, reason]. The study of viruses and viral diseases.

viropexis (vī"rō-pĕk'sĭs) [" + Gr. *pexis,* fixation]. The fixation of a virus particle to a cell. This leads to the inclusion of the virus inside the cell.

Viroptic. Trade name for trifluridine.

virose, virous (vī'rōs, vī'rŭs) [L. *virus,* poison]. Having poisonous qualities or effects. SYN: *poisonous.*

virtual (věr'tū-ăl) [L. *virtus,* capacity]. Appearing to exist but not in actual fact or form.

virucidal (vĭr-ū-sī'dăl) [L. *virus,* poison, + *cidus,* to kill]. Destructive of a virus. SYN: *viricidal.*

virucide. An agent that destroys or inactivates a virus, esp. a chemical substance used on living tissue.

virulence (vĭr'ū-lĕns) [LL. *virulentia,* stench]. 1. Relative power and degree of pathogenicity possessed by organisms to produce disease. Whether or not a microorganism will cause disease in the host is dependent upon a number of factors other than its virulence, e.g., the inherent resistance of the host and the actual dose of organisms that have gained access to the host. SEE: *immunocompetent; immunocompromised.* 2. Property of being virulent; venomousness, as of a disease. SEE: *attenuation.*

virulent (vĭr'ū-lĕnt) [L. *virulentus,* poison]. 1. Very poisonous. 2. Infectious; able to overcome the host's defensive mechanism.

viruliferous (vĭr-ū-lĭf'ĕr-ŭs) [L. *virus,* poison, + *ferre,* to bear]. Conveying or producing a virus.

viruria (vī-rū-rē'ă) [" + Gr. *ouron,* urine]. Presence of viruses in the urine.

virus (vī'rŭs) [L., poison]. A minute organism not visible with ordinary light microscope. It is parasitic in that it is entirely dependent on nutrients inside cells for its metabolic and reproductive needs. Some bacteria share these properties but not the distinctive features of viruses such as their simple organization and composition and their mechanism of replication. Viruses can be seen by use of electron microscopy. They consist of a strand of either deoxyribonucleic acid (DNA) or ribonucleic acid (RNA), but not both, and are surrounded by a capsid, a covering of protein. There is no cell wall.

More than 300 viruses have been isolated from animals; some of these appear to be harmless to humans. However, viruses cause a variety of important infectious diseases, among them the common cold, AIDS, smallpox, yellow fever, many childhood diseases, and the majority of infections of the upper respiratory passages. Certain viruses cause cancer in laboratory animals. Evidence that they cause cancer in humans is inconclusive, but there is evidence that some lymphomas and leukemias are caused by a virus. Infection with a virus induces an antibody response in the host.

A virus was first synthesized in the laboratory in 1967. This was done by using natural virus DNA as a template for forming the synthetic virus DNA.

CLASSIF: There are a variety of ways to classify viruses. Not all will be given here, but the more generally accepted types of classification follow. They may be broken down into two groups according to whether they contain DNA or RNA, with these groups further classified. They may be classed as to the host they dominate: bacteria (bacteriophages), animal, or plant.

They are also classified as to origin (reoviruses), mode of transportation (arboviruses), manifestation they produce in the host (polioviruses), and geographical site first located (coxsackievirus).

RS: adenovirus; AIDS; arboviruses; capsid; coxsackievirus; deoxyribonucleic acid; ECHO virus; enterovirus; herpesvirus; immunocompromised; microscope, electron; myxoviruses; papovaviruses; paramyxoviruses; picornaviruses; poliovirus; poxvirus; reovirus; retrovirus; rhabdovirus; rhinovirus; ribonucleic acid.

v., arbor. Former name for arboviruses, q.v.

v., attenuated. Virus with reduced pathogenicity due to treatment or repeated passage through hosts.

v., bacterial. Virus capable of inducing lysis or dissolution of certain bacterial cells. SYN: *bacteriophage.*

v., chikungunya. SEE: *chikungunya virus.*

v., coxsackie. SEE: *coxsackievirus.*

v., cytomegalic. ABBR: CMV. A member of herpesvirus family that is widely distributed and causes clinically detectable disease in infants. It is transmitted either transplacentally or at the time of birth to the fetus from a mother with a latent infection. The virus may also be transmitted by blood transfusion. SYN: *cytomegalovirus*.

v., defective. A virus particle that, because of lack of certain essential factors, is unable to replicate. Sometimes this can be overcome by the presence of a helper virus that provides the missing factor or factors.

v., EB. Epstein-Barr virus, q.v.

v., ECHO. *enteric cytopathogenic human orphan.* Virus that was accidentally discovered in human feces and not known to be associated with a disease, thus the name "orphan." Initially 33 ECHO virus serotypes were designated, but numbers 10 and 28 have been reclassified. Various serotypes have been associated with aseptic meningitis, encephalitis, acute upper respiratory infection, enteritis, pleurodynia, and myocarditis.

v., enteric. Enterovirus, q.v.

v., enteric orphan. SEE: *v., ECHO.*

v., filtrable. Virus causing infectious disease, the essential elements of which are so tiny that they retain infectivity after passing through a filter of the Berkefeld type. SEE: *filter, Berkefeld.*

v. fixé, v., fixed. Rabies virus that was stabilized and modified but only partially attenuated by serial passage through rabbits.

v., helper. Virus that permits a defective virus present in the same cell to replicate. SEE: *v., defective.*

v., hepadna-. A family of hepatotropic DNA viruses that infect the liver of certain animal species.

v., herpes. SEE: *herpesvirus.*

v., human immunodeficiency. ABBR: HIV. The virus that causes AIDS, q.v.

v., latent. Some viruses have the ability to infect the host, initially causing little or no signs of illness but persisting for the lifetime of the infected individual. Later on, a specific triggering mechanism may cause the virus to produce a clinically apparent disease. This occurs with herpes simplex virus that remains latent in sensory ganglia and is reactivated by trauma to the skin supplied by the distal sensory nerves associated with these ganglia. After reactivation, the virus may cause localized or generalized lesions in the affected area and the central nervous system.

v., lytic. Any virus that, after infecting a cell, lyses it.

v., masked. Virus that ordinarily occurs in the host in a noninfective state but is activated and demonstrated by indirect methods.

v.'s, neurotropic. Viruses that reproduce in nerve tissue.

v.'s, orphan. Viruses that initially were thought not to be associated with pathogenicity. However, since then, a number of them have been shown to be associated with disease. Includes enteroviruses and rhinoviruses.

v., parainfluenza. One of a group of viruses that affect infants and young children. Causes respiratory infections that may be mild or may progress to pneumonia. Most infections are so mild as to be clinically inapparent.

v., plant. Any virus that is pathogenic for plants.

v., pox. Poxvirus, q.v.

v., respiratory syncytial. Virus that is a major cause of lower respiratory tract disease during infancy and early childhood. It induces formation of large syncytial masses in cell cultures, and this led to its being so named. Attempts to develop an effective and safe vaccine have been in vain. Because it is difficult to recognize the disease early and inapparent cases are frequent, isolation and public health measures are not adequate to control the spread of the disease.

v., slow. SEE: *slow virus infection.*

v., street. Rabies virus obtained from an infected animal rather than from a laboratory strain.

v., tumor. Tumor viruses, q.v.

virusemia (vī″rŭs-ēm′ē-ă) [″ + Gr. *haima*, blood]. Virus in the blood. SYN: *viremia.*

virus shedding. Release of virus from the host.

virustatic (vīr″ŭ-stăt′ĭk) [″ + Gr. *statikos*, bringing to a standstill]. Stopping the growth of viruses.

vis (vĭs) [L., strength] (pl. *vires*). Force, strength, energy, power.

v. medicatrix naturae. The healing power of nature.

viscera (vĭs′ĕr-ă) [L.] (sing. *viscus*). Internal organs enclosed within a cavity, esp. the abdominal organs. SEE: *celosomia; evisceration; splanchnic.*

viscerad (vĭs′ĕr-ăd) [″ + *ad*, toward]. Toward the viscera.

visceral (vĭs′ĕr-ăl) [L. *viscera*, body organs]. 1. Pert. to viscera. 2. Pert. to or derived from the gill arches of vertebrates.

visceral arches. Branchial arches.

visceral cavity. Body cavity containing the viscera.

visceral clefts. The fissures separating the visceral arches.

visceralgia (vĭs″ĕr-ăl′jē-ă) [″ + Gr. *algos*, pain]. Neuralgia of any of the viscera.

visceral skeleton. The pelvis, ribs, and sternum enclosing the viscera.

viscerimotor (vĭs″ĕr-ĭ-mō′tor) [″ + *motor*, mover]. A nerve supplying motor stimuli to a viscus. SYN: *visceromotor*.

viscero- (vĭs′ĕr-ō) [L. *viscera*, body organs]. Combining form meaning pertaining to the viscera.

viscerocranium (vĭs″ĕr-ō-krā′nē-ŭm). That portion of the skull derived from the pharyngeal arches.

viscerogenic (vĭs″ĕr-ō-jĕn′ĭk) [″ + Gr. *gennan*, to produce]. Originating in the viscera.

visceroinhibitory (vĭs″ĕr-ō-ĭn-hĭb′ĭ-tō-rē) [″ + *inhibere*, to restrain]. Checking the action of the viscera.

visceromegaly (vĭs″ĕr-ō-mĕg′ă-lē) [″ + Gr. *megalos*, great]. Generalized enlargement of the abdominal visceral organs.

visceromotor (vĭs″ĕr-ō-mō′tor) [L. *viscera*, body organs, + *motor*, a mover]. Conveying motor impulses to the viscera.

visceromotor reflex. Increase in tonus of abdominal muscles resulting from painful stimuli originating in a viscus.

visceroparietal (vĭs″ĕr-ō-pă-rī′ĕ-tăl) [″ + *paries*, wall]. Rel. to the viscera and abdominal wall.

visceroperitoneal (vĭs″ĕr-ō-pĕr″ĭ-tō-nē′ăl) [″ + Gr. *peritonaion*, peritoneum]. Rel. to the abdominal viscera and peritoneum.

visceropleural (vĭs″ĕr-ō-ploo′răl) [″ + Gr. *pleura*, a side]. Rel. to the thoracic viscera and pleura. SYN: *pleurovisceral.*

visceroptosis (vĭs″ĕr-ŏp-tō′sĭs) [″ + Gr. *ptosis*, a dropping]. Downward displacement of a viscus.

visceroreceptors (vĭs″ĕr-ō-rē-sĕp′torz). A group of receptors that includes those located in visceral organs. Their stimulation gives rise to poorly localized and ill-defined sensations. In hollow visceral organs they are stimulated principally by excessive contraction or by distention.

viscerosensory (vĭs″ĕr-ō-sĕn′sō-rē) [″ + *sensorius*, sensory]. Pert. to sensations aroused by stimulation of visceroreceptors.

viscerosensory reflex. Pain or tenderness elicited in somatic structures (skin and muscle) due to visceral disorder. SEE: *referred pain.*

visceroskeletal (vĭs″ĕr-ō-skĕl′ĕt-ăl) [″ + Gr. *skeleton*, a dried-up body]. Rel. to the visceral skeleton.

viscerosomatic (vĭs″ĕr-ō-sō-măt′ĭk) [″ + Gr. *soma*, body]. Rel. to the viscera and the body.

viscerosomatic reaction. A reaction occurring in muscles of the body wall as a result of stimulation of visceroreceptors.

viscerotome (vĭs″ĕr-ō-tōm) [″ + Gr. *tome*, incision]. That part of an abdominal organ that is supplied with afferent nerves from a single posterior root.

viscerotonia (vĭs″ĕr-ō-tōn′ē-ă) [″ + Gr. *tonos*, tension]. Personality traits characterized by predominance of social over intellectual and physical traits. Individual is sociable and convivial, exhibits gluttony for food, and loves company, affection, and social support.

viscerotrophic (vĭs″ĕr-ō-trŏf′ĭk) [″ + Gr. *trophe*, nourishment]. Pertaining to trophic conditions related to or associated with visceral conditions.

viscerotropic (vĭs″ĕr-ō-trŏp′ĭk) [″ + Gr. *tropos*, a turn]. Primarily affecting the viscera.

viscerovisceral reaction (vĭs″ĕr-ō-vĭs″ĕr-ăl). A reaction taking place in the viscera as a result of stimulation of visceral receptors. Such reactions are usually below the level of consciousness.

viscid (vĭs′ĭd) [L. *viscum*, mistletoe, birdlime]. Adhering, glutinous, sticky. In bacteriology, said of a colony that strings out by clinging to a needle when it is touched to the culture and withdrawn. The sediment rises in a coherent whirl when the liquid culture is shaken.

viscidity (vĭ-sĭd′ĭ-tē). The property of being viscid or sticky. SYN: *viscosity.*

viscoelasticity. The property of being viscous and elastic.

viscometer (vĭs-kŏm′ĕ-tĕr). Viscosimeter.

viscosimeter (vĭs″kŏs-ĭm′ĕ-tĕr) [LL. *viscosus*, viscous, + Gr. *metron*, measure]. Device for estimating the viscosity of a fluid, esp. of blood.

viscosimetry (vĭs″kō-sĭm′ĕ-trē). Measurement of the viscosity of a substance.

viscosity (vĭs″kŏs′ĭ-tē) [LL. *viscosus*, viscous]. 1. State of being sticky or gummy. 2. Resistance offered by a fluid to change of form or relative position of its particles due to attraction of molecules to each other.

   v., specific. The internal friction of a fluid, measured by comparing the rate of flow of the liquid through a tube with that of some standard liquid, or by measuring the resistance to rotating paddles.

viscous (vĭs′kŭs). Sticky, gummy, gelatinous, with high viscosity.

viscus (vĭs′kŭs) [L., body organ] (pl. *viscera*). Any internal organ enclosed within a cavity, such as the thorax or abdomen.

visibility (vĭz″ĭ-bĭl′ĭ-tē) [L. *visibilitas*]. Quality of being visible.

visible (vĭz′ĭ-bl) [L. *visibilis*]. Capable of being seen.

visile (vĭz′ĭl) [L. *visum*, seeing]. 1. Pert. to vision. 2. Readily recalling what is seen, more than that which is audible or motile.

vision (vĭzh′ŭn) [L. *visio*, a seeing]. 1. Act of viewing external objects. SYN: *sight*. SEE:

reading machines for the blind. 2. Sense by which light and color are apprehended. 3. An imaginary sight.

v., achromatic. Complete color blindness.

v., artificial. A technique, still in experimental stage, designed to make it possible for some blind persons to see. SEE: *Optacon.*

v., binocular. Visual sensation that is produced when the images perceived by each eye are fused to appear as one.

v., central. Vision resulting from rays falling on the fovea centralis.

v., day. Condition in which patient sees better during the day than at night, found in peripheral lesions of the retina such as retinitis pigmentosa.

v., dichromatic. A form of defective color vision in which only two of the primary colors are perceived.

v., double. Seeing of one object as two. SYN: *diplopia.*

v., field of. The space within which an object can be seen while the eye remains fixed on one point.

v., half. Blindness in one or both eyes for half of the visual field. SYN: *hemianopia.*

v., indirect. V., peripheral, q.v.

v., monocular. Vision utilizing only one eye.

v., multiple. Seeing of one object as two or more. SYN: *polyopia.*

v., night. Ability to see when illumination is reduced.

v., oscillating. Oscillopsia, q.v.

v., peripheral. Vision resulting from rays falling on the retina outside of the macular field.

v., phantom. An experience of visual sensations following surgical removal of an eye. Usually a transient condition.

v., tunnel. Tunnel vision, q.v.

vision, words pert. to: aberration; accommodation; aftercataract; afterimage; amblyopia; ametropia; anopsia; anotropia; asthenope; asthenopia; astigmatic; astigmatism; bifocal; blind; cataract; chloropsia; chromatic; chromatopsia; chromopsia; contact lens; convergence; cyclophoria; depth perception; diplopia; emmetropia; erythropsia; farpoint; farsightedness; glare; glaucoma; halation; hypermetropia; hypometropia; image; macropsia; metamorphosis; micropsia; Moore's lightning streaks; muscae volitantes; myope; myopia; night blindness; night vision; nyctalopia; nyctamblyopia; nyctotyphlosis; ocular; oculist; Optacon; reading machines for the blind; retina; retinal detachment; scintillation; scotoma; second sight; strabismus; vergence; visile; visual; xanthopsia; words ending in "-phoria."

visit. An encounter between a patient and a health professional that requires either the patient to travel from his or her home to the professional's usual place of practice (office visit) or vice versa (home visit).

Visiting Nurse Association. A voluntary health agency that provides nursing services in the home, including health supervision, education and counseling, and maintenance of the medical regimen. Nurses and other personnel such as home health aides who are specifically trained for tasks of personal bedside care provide the services offered by the agency. These agencies originated in the visiting or district nurse service provided to the poor in their homes by voluntary agencies such as the New York City Mission, which existed in the 1870s. The first visiting nurse associations were established in Buffalo, Boston, and Philadelphia between 1886 and 1887.

Vistaril Pamoate. Trade name for hydroxyzine pamoate.

Vistaril Parenteral. Trade name for hydroxyzine hydrochloride.

visual (vĭzh′ū-ăl) [L. *visio,* a seeing]. 1. Pert. to vision. 2. One whose learning and memorizing processes are largely of a visual nature.

visual acuity. A measure of the resolving power of the eye. Usually determined by having the subject read letters of various sizes at a standard distance from the test chart. The result is expressed as a fraction. For example, 20/20 is normal vision. This means the subject's eye has the ability to see from a distance of 20 feet (6.1 meters) what the normal eye would see at that distance. 20/40 means that a person sees at 20 feet (6.1 meters) what the normal eye could see at 40 feet (12.2 meters).

visual angle. Angle between line of sight and the extremities of object seen.

visual axis. The line of vision from object seen through the pupil's center to macula lutea.

visual cone. The cone whose vertex is at the eye and whose generating lines touch the boundary of a visible object.

visual evoked responses. ABBR: VER. While the patient is watching a pattern projected on a screen, the electroencephalogram is recorded. The characteristics of the wave form, its latency, and the amplitude of the wave can be compared with the normal, and important information concerning the function of the visual apparatus in transmitting stimuli to the brain can be obtained. SEE: *brain stem auditory evoked responses; evoked responses; somatosensory evoked responses.*

visual field. The area within which objects may be seen when the eye is fixed. SEE: *pe-*

rimetry.

visual function. The process of receiving stimuli transmitted to the eye and then to the brain and translating those stimuli into images. There are three aspects of visual function: form sense, color sense, and light sense. Form sense is tested by determining visual acuity; color sense by having the patient distinguish colors depicted in standard charts; and light sense is evaluated by testing peripheral vision.

There is evidence that the human eye must see an object twice in order to form an image of an object in the brain. This is done when the eye fixes on an object and then almost instantaneously and imperceptibly shifts to look at the object from a slightly different angle.

visualization (vĭzh″ū-ăl-ĭ-zā′shŭn). The act of viewing or sensing a picture of an object, esp. the picture of a body structure as obtained by x-ray study.

visualize (vĭzh′ū-ăl-īz). 1. To make visible. 2. To imagine or picture something in one's mind.

visual object agnosia. Loss of the ability to visually recognize objects presented, even though some degree of ability to see is intact.

visual plane. The plane in which both optic axes lie.

visual point. Center of vision.

visual yellow. A pigment formed in the retina by the action of light on rhodopsin.

visuoauditory (vĭzh″ū-ō-aw′dĭ-tor″ē) [L. *visio,* a seeing, + *auditorius,* pert. to hearing]. Rel. to sight and hearing, as connecting nerve fibers between auditory and visual centers.

visuognosis (vĭzh″ū-ŏg-nō′sĭs) [″ + Gr. *gnosis,* knowledge]. The recognition and appreciation of what is seen.

visuopsychic (vĭzh″ū-ō-sī′kĭk) [″ + Gr. *psyche,* soul, mind]. Both visual and psychic, applied to cerebral area involved in apprehension of visual sensations.

visuosensory (vĭzh″ū-ō-sĕn′sō-rē) [L. *visio,* a seeing, + *sensorius,* sensory]. Rel. to the recognition of visual impressions.

visuospatial. Concerning the ability to discern spatial relationships from visual presentations.

vita glass (vī′tă-glăs) [L. *vita,* life, + AS. *glaes,* glass]. Window glass containing quartz for transmitting the ultraviolet rays of sunlight.

vital (vī′tăl) [L. *vitalis,* pert. to life]. 1. Pert. to or characteristic of life. 2. Contributing to or essential for life.

vital capacity. Volume of air that can be expelled following full inspiration.

vital capacity, timed. Test of vital capacity of the lungs expressed with respect to the volume of air that can be quickly and forcibly breathed out in a certain amount of time. SEE: *FEV₁.*

vital center. Respiratory center in the medulla.

vitalism (vī′tăl-ĭzm) [″ + Gr. *-ismos,* condition]. The opinion that a force neither chemical nor mechanical is responsible for some phenomena.

vitalist (vī′tăl-ĭst) [L. *vitalis,* pert. to life]. One who believes in vitalism.

vitalistic (vī-tăl-ĭs′tĭk). Relating to vitalism.

vitality (vī-tăl′ĭ-tē). 1. That which distinguishes living things from the nonliving. 2. Animation, action. 3. State of being alive.

vitalize (vī′tăl-īz). To instill life or force in anything.

vital signs. The traditional signs of life, i.e., heartbeat, body temperature, respiration, and blood pressure.

vital statistics. Statistics relating to births (natality), deaths (mortality), marriages, health, and disease (morbidity). Vital statistics for the U.S. are published annually by the National Center for Health Statistics of the Department of Health and Human Services.

vitamer (vī′tă-mĕr). Any one of a number of compounds that have specific vitamin activity.

vitamin (vī′tă-mĭn) [L. *vita,* life, + *amine*]. Any of a group of organic substances other than proteins, carbohydrates, fats, minerals, and organic salts which are essential for normal metabolism, growth, and development of the body. Vitamins are not sources of energy, nor do they contribute significantly to the substance of the body. They are indispensable for the maintenance of health. They are effective in minute quantities. They act principally as regulators of metabolic processes and play a role in energy transformations, usually acting as coenzymes in enzymatic systems.

Vitamins are extremely complex chemical substances, but the nature, chemical structure, and composition of most of them are known. Most have been isolated and some have been synthesized. In general, none of the vitamins can be formed in the body but must be obtained preformed from animal or plant sources. Exceptions to the above are the formation of vitamin A from its precursor, carotene, the formation of vitamin D by the action of ultraviolet light on the skin, and the formation of vitamin K by symbiotic bacteria of the intestines. Some vitamins are unstable, being readily destroyed by oxidation, heat, esp. in an alkaline medium, strong acids, light, and aging. SEE: *Vitamins* in *Appendix.*

There are several broad classifications of

vitamins, for example, the fat-soluble vitamins (A, D, E, and K) and the water-soluble (B and C). This is of clinical importance in patients with diseases that interfere with digestion of fat, because they will eventually develop deficiencies of the fat-soluble vitamins, which are essential to body growth, development, and function. Certain vitamins cannot be manufactured by certain species. Humans belong to one of the few species that cannot manufacture vitamin C.

A variety of conditions increase the need for vitamins above the usual recommended dose. These include lactation, pregnancy, use of certain drugs, excess use of alcohol or tobacco, and certain illnesses.

RS: avitaminosis; deficiency disease.

v., antiberiberi. Thiamine; vitamin B_1.

v., antidermatitis. Vitamin B_6.

v., antihemorrhagic. Vitamin K.

v., anti-infective. Vitamin A.

v., antineuritic. Thiamine (B_1).

v., antipellagra. Nicotinamide.

v., antirachitic. The vitamin D group.

v., antiscorbutic. Vitamin C.

v., antixerophthalmic. Vitamin A.

v., coagulation. Vitamin K.

vitamin A. USP. A fat-soluble vitamin formed in the body from precursors, yellow pigments of plants (alpha, beta, and gamma carotene). It is essential for normal growth and development, the integrity of epithelial tissues, and for normal tooth and bone development. It is stored in the liver. Trade names are Alphalin, and Aquasol-A. Recommended daily requirement for the adult female is 800 μg and 1000 μg for the adult male. SYN: *retinol; vitamin, anti-infective.* SEE: *Vitamins* in *Appendix.*

SOURCES: Butter, butterfat in milk, egg yolks, and cod liver oil are rich sources. Liver; green leafy and yellow vegetables and some fruits: prunes, pineapples, oranges, limes, and cantaloupes.

TOXICITY: Excess intake of vitamin A may cause acute or chronic effects. SEE: *hypervitaminosis.*

ACTION/USES: Essential to the normal function of epithelial cells and the formation of visual purple.

STABILITY: Resists boiling for some time if not exposed to oxidation. Quite stable to brief exposure to heat but not to continued high temperatures (above 100°C or 212°F). Vitamin A is present in fish liver oils, egg yolks, liver, butter, cream, green leafy vegetables, and yellow vegetables such as carrots.

DEFICIENCY DISORDERS: Interference with growth, reduced resistance to infections, interference with nutrition of cornea, conjunctiva, trachea, hair follicles, and renal pelvis. Thus these tissues have an increased susceptibility to infections. Interference with ability of eyes to adapt to darkness (night blindness). Visual acuity will also be impaired. Children will experience impaired growth and development. SEE: *Bitot's spots.*

vitamin A_1. Form of vitamin A found in fish liver oils.

vitamin A_2. A compound found in the livers of freshwater fish. Similar in properties to vitamin A but with different ultraviolet absorption spectra.

vitamin B complex. A group of water-soluble vitamins isolated from liver, yeast, and other sources. Only grain-made yeast that is dried at once preserves its potency. Among vitamins included are thiamine (B_1), riboflavin (B_2), niacin (nicotinic acid), pyridoxine (B_6), biotin, folic acid, and cyanocobalamin (B_{12}).

SOURCES: *Thiamine:* Whole grains, wheat embryo, brewer's yeast, legumes, nuts, egg yolk, fruits, and vegetables. *Riboflavin:* Brewer's yeast, liver, meat, esp. pork and fish, poultry, eggs, milk, and green vegetables. *Nicotinic acid:* Brewer's yeast, liver, meat, poultry, and green vegetables. *Pyridoxine:* Rice, bran, yeast. *Folic acid:* Leafy green vegetables, organ meats, lean beef and veal, wheat cereals.

ACTION/USES: Affects growth, appetite, lactation, and the gastrointestinal, nervous, and endocrine systems; aids in marasmus; stimulates appetite; important in metabolism of carbohydrates, including sugar; stimulates biliary action; and is used as an adjunct when some antituberculosis drugs are used.

B_1, thiamine, affects growth and nutrition and carbohydrate metabolism. B_2, riboflavin, affects growth and cellular metabolism. Nicotinic acid prevents pellagra.

Although not destroyed by ordinary cooking, B complex vitamins may be destroyed by excessive heating for 2 to 4 hours. Bicarbonate of soda used in cooking aids destruction. Riboflavin and nicotinic acid, more stable than thiamine, are not destroyed by heat or oxidation.

NOTE: Prolonged use of antibiotics may destroy the intestinal bacteria that normally produce some of the B vitamins. In those cases supplemental vitamins will be required.

STABILITY: Long-continued cooking or high-temperature cooking destroys vitamin B; bicarbonate of soda used in cooking aids its destruction. Ordinary cooking or heat does not destroy it.

DEFICIENCY DISORDERS: Beriberi, pellagra, digestive disturbances, enlargement of liver, disturbance of the thyroid, degeneration of sex glands, disturbance of the nervous system. Deficiency induces edema, affects the heart, liver, spleen, and kidneys, enlarges the adrenals, and causes dysfunction of the pituitary and salivary glands.

vitamin B₁. Thiamine, or thiamine hydrochloride. Recommended daily allowance: approx. 1.5 mg for the adult male and 1.1 mg for the adult female. SEE: *Vitamins in Appendix.*

vitamin B₂. Riboflavin. SEE: *Vitamins in Appendix.*

vitamin B₆. Pyridoxine. Found in rice, bran, and yeast. Excess doses (2 to 5 gm/day for months) has caused impairment of central nervous system function. SEE: *Vitamins in Appendix.*

vitamin B₁₂. A red crystalline substance, a cobamide, extracted from liver that is essential for the formation of red blood cells. Its deficiency results in pernicious anemia. It is used for prophylaxis and treatment of these and other diseases in which there is defective red cell formation. Recommended daily requirement: 2 μg per day for adults. The terms vitamin B₁₂ and cyanocobalamin are used interchangeably as the generic term for all of the cobamides active in humans. SYN: *cyanocobalamin.* SEE: *Vitamins in Appendix.*

vitamin C. Ascorbic acid, a factor necessary for formation of intercellular substance of connective tissue and essential in maintenance of integrity of intercellular cement in many tissues, especially capillary walls. Deficiency leads to scurvy. SYN: *ascorbic acid.* SEE: *Vitamins in Appendix.*

NOTE: Recommended daily allowance for adults is 60 mg. Large daily doses of vitamin C have been recommended for prevention and treatment of the common cold. Although the effectiveness of vitamin C for this purpose has not been established, it is felt that the vitamin may at least decrease the severity of symptoms of a cold. Excess doses of vitamin C for an extended period can interfere with absorption of vitamin B₁₂, cause uricosuria, and promote formation of oxalate kidney stones.

SOURCES: Raw cabbage, young carrots, orange juice, lettuce, celery, onions, tomatoes, radishes, and green peppers. Citrus fruits are especially rich in this vitamin. Strawberries are about as rich a source as tomatoes. Apples, pears, apricots, plums, peaches, and pineapples. Rutabagas are also rich in this vitamin.

STABILITY: Destroyed easily by heat in the presence of oxygen, as in open-kettle boiling. Less affected by heat in an acid medium; otherwise stable.

DEFICIENCY DISORDERS: Scurvy, imperfect prenatal skeletal formation, defective teeth, pyorrhea, anorexia, anemia, undernutrition injury to bone, cells, and blood vessels.

vitamin D. One of several vitamins having antirachitic activity. The vitamin D group, which is fat-soluble, includes D₂ (calciferol), D₃ (irradiated 7-dehydrocholesterol), D₄ (irradiated 22-dihydroergosterol), and D₅ (irradiated dehydrositosterol). It is essential in calcium and phosphorus metabolism; consequently it is required for normal development of bones and teeth. Recommended daily allowance is 10 μg. SEE: *Vitamins in Appendix.*

SOURCES: Milk; cod liver oil; salmon and cod livers; egg yolk; butter fat. Ergosterol in the skin activated by sunlight or ultraviolet radiation possesses vitamin D potency.

ACTION/USES: Related to utilization of calcium and phosphorus in blood and bone building. It is called the antirachitic vitamin because deficiency of it interferes with calcium and phosphorus utilization, which in turn causes rickets, q.v. Exposure to the sun or ultraviolet radiation synthesizes this vitamin in the body. Necessary for most efficient absorption of calcium and phosphorus. A specific in treatment of infantile rickets, spasmophilia (infantile tetany), and softening of bone; valuable also in prevention of these conditions. Important in normal growth and mineralization of skeleton and teeth.

Excess doses of vitamin D (100,000 I.V. daily) for a prolonged period will cause hypercalcemia with anorexia, nausea, vomiting, polyuria, polydipsia, weakness, anxiety, pruritus, and altered renal function.

STABILITY: Not affected by oxidation or by heat unless over 100°C (212°F) or long-continued cooking.

DEFICIENCY DISORDERS: Imperfect skeletal formation; bone diseases; rickets; caries.

vitamin E. USP. An essential nutrient for humans, although the exact biochemical mechanism whereby vitamin E functions in the body is unknown. Because of the amount of vitamin E present in foods, its deficiency is absent in the general population. Excess doses (100 mg/kg/day) in low-birth-weight neonates has been implicated in the development of necrotizing enterocolitis and sepsis. Recommended daily allowance is 10 mg for the adult male and 8 mg for the adult female. SYN: *alpha-tocopherol.* SEE: *Vitamins in Appendix.*

vitamin K. An antihemorrhagic factor whose activity is associated with compounds derived from naphthoquinone. Vitamin K, which is fat-soluble, is present in alfalfa; vitamin K_2 in fishmeal; vitamin K_3 is synthesized as menadione sodium bisulfite. Vitamin K aids blood coagulation and is necessary for formation of prothrombin. Its deficiency prolongs blood-clotting time and causes hemorrhages. Vitamin K is not present in the digestive tract of newborn infants until food is ingested and bacteria produced in the intestines to synthesize vitamin K. Thus an intramuscular injection of 1 mg of water-soluble vitamin K_1 (phytonadione) is recommended for all infants.

Large doses may cause hemolysis in persons with G6PD deficiency and in some normal individuals. Large doses in the newborn may lead to anemia and kernicterus. Recommended daily allowance is 65 μg for the adult female and 80 μg for the adult male. SEE: *Vitamins* in *Appendix.*

SOURCES: Found in fats, fishmeal, oats, wheat, rye, and alfalfa.

ACTION/USES: Helps to eliminate prolonged bleeding in operations and in biliary tract of jaundiced patients. Bile salts necessary for its absorption.

vitamin loss. Loss of vitamin content in food products because of vitamin instability, esp. in oxidation and during heating. Methods of preserving foods add to the loss of vitamins. Pickling, salting, curing, or fermenting processes usually cause complete loss of vitamin C. Commercial canning destroys from 50% to 85% of vitamin C contained in peas, lima beans, spinach, and asparagus. Pasteurization, unless special precautions are observed, causes a loss of from 30% to 60% of vitamin C. Apple pie and freshly prepared applesauce retain only from 20% to 30% of the vitamin C value of the apple. Vitamin B_1 in wheat is lost through milling because the wheat embryo, rich in vitamin B_1, is removed in milling.

vitaminoid (vī'tă-mĭn-oyd) [*vitamin* + Gr. *eidos,* form, shape]. Of the nature of vitamins.

vitaminology (vī''tă-mĭn-ŏl'ō-jē). Study of vitamins.

vitamin supplements. Any vitamin tablet or capsule containing one or more vitamins. Thus, a tablet or capsule may contain a single vitamin or many, and in some instances, a preparation will contain more than a dozen vitamins and an even greater number of minerals. The rationale for daily use of this latter type of vitamin and mineral supplement has not been established. In general, healthy adult men and healthy non-pregnant, non-lactating women consuming a normal, varied diet do not need vitamin supplements.

The difficulty of individuals choosing to treat themselves with vitamin supplements are: 1. People who take the supplements are usually already consuming an adequate diet. 2. The vitamins chosen are often not the ones inadequate in their diet. 3. The dose may be many times greater than the daily needs.

Also, if too large a dose of pyridoxine (vitamin B-6) or vitamins A and D are ingested, toxic symptoms can develop. SEE: *vitamin C.*

vitellary (vĭt'ĕl-ā-rē) [L. *vitellus,* yolk of an egg]. Pert. to the vitellus. SYN: *vitelline.*

vitellin (vī-tĕl'ĭn). A protein that can be extracted from egg yolk and contains lecithin. SEE: *nucleoprotein; ovovitellin.*

vitelline (vī-tĕl'ēn). Pert. to the yolk of an egg or the ovum.

vitelline circulation. The embryonic circulation of blood to the yolk sac via vitelline arteries and its return to general circulation through the vitelline veins.

vitelline duct. The narrow duct connecting the yolk sac with the embryonic gut.

vitelline membrane. 1. The membrane forming the surface layer of an ovum. 2. In a chicken egg, the membrane forming the surface layer of the vitellus or yolk.

vitelline veins. Two veins conveying blood from the yolk sac.

vitellogenesis (vī''tĕl-ō-jĕn'ĕ-sĭs). Production of yolk.

vitellointestinal (vī'tĕl-ō-ĭn-tĕs''tĭn-ăl). Concerning the embryonic yolk sac and the intestinal tract.

vitellolutein (vī''tĕl-ō-lū'tē-ĭn) [L. *vitellus,* yolk, + *luteus,* yellow]. Yellow pigment present in lutein.

vitellorubin (vī''tĕl-ō-rū'bĭn) [" + *ruber,* red]. Red pigment present in lutein.

vitellose (vī-tĕl'ōs). A proteose present in vitellin.

vitellus (vī-tĕl'ŭs) [L.]. The yolk of an ovum, esp. the yolk of a hen's egg.

vitiation (vish''ē-ā'shŭn) [L. *vitiare,* to corrupt]. Injury, contamination, impairment of use or efficiency.

vitiligines (vĭt''ĭ-lĭj'ĭ-nēz). Depigmented areas of skin. SEE: *vitiligo.*

vitiliginous (vĭt''ĭ-lĭj'ĭ-nŭs). Concerning vitiligo.

vitiligo (vĭt-ĭl-ī'gō) [L.]. An acquired cutaneous affection characterized by milk-white patches, surrounded by areas of normal pigmentation. More common in the tropics and in blacks. Cause unknown. SYN: *leukoderma; piebald skin.*

ETIOL: Unknown, but it may be associated with systemic diseases such as hypothyroidism or hyperthyroidism, diabetes mellitus, Addison's disease, pernicious anemia, leprosy, or chronic mucocutaneous candidiasis syndrome.

TREAT: Oral and topical synthetic trioxsalen, USP, and a natural psoralen, methoxsalen, USP, are used with exposure to long-wave ultraviolet light, but the efficacy is doubtful. The lesions may be masked by use of cosmetic preparations. Vitiliginous areas should be protected from sunburn by applying a 5% aminobenzoic acid solution or gel to the affected areas. The use of 5% fluorouracil cream applied under an occlusive dressing to the depigmented areas may cause erosion of the dermis and, after re-epithelialization, pigment may reappear.

v. capitis. Vitiligo of the scalp with depigmentation of the hairs of the affected area.

v., perinevic. Vitiligo surrounding a nevus.

vitiligoidea (vĭt″ĭl-ĭg-oy′dē-ă) [″ + Gr. eidos, form, shape]. Disease marked by formation of tiny yellow patches or nodules on the skin, as on the eyelids. SYN: xanthoma.

vitium (vĭsh′ē-ŭm) [L., fault] (pl. vitia). A fault, defect, or vice.

v. cordis. An organic heart lesion.

vitrectomy (vĭ-trĕk′tō-mē) [L. vitreus, glassy, + Gr. ektome, excision]. Use of a special instrument in order to remove the contents of the vitreous chamber, and replacing them with a sterile physiological saline solution.

vitreocapsulitis (vĭt″rē-ō-kăp″sū-lī′tĭs) [L. vitreus, glassy, + capsula, capsule, + Gr. itis, inflammation]. Inflammation of the vitreous humor. SYN: hyalitis.

vitreodentin (vĭt″rē-ō-dĕn′tĭn). A particularly hard and brittle form of dentin.

vitreoretinal (vĭt″rē-ō-rĕt′ĭ-năl). Concerning the vitreous and the retina.

vitreous (vĭt′rē-ŭs) [L. vitreus, glassy]. 1. Glassy. 2. Pertaining to the vitreous body of the eye. 3. The vitreous body.

vitreous body. A transparent jellylike mass composed of collagen fibrils and a gel (vitreous humor). It fills the cavity of the eyeball, behind the lens and in front of the retina.

vitreous chamber. The portion of the cavity of the eyeball behind the lens.

vitreous degeneration. Retrogressive change of a part into a translucent shining substance, esp. of a blood vessel wall. SEE: degeneration, hyaline.

vitreous humor. The clear watery gel filling the interstices of the stroma of the vitreous body, q.v.

vitreous membrane. 1. Inner membrane of the choroid. 2. The innermost layer of the connective tissue sheath surrounding a hair follicle.

vitreous table. The inner layer of compact tissue characteristic of most of the bones of the cranium.

vitrescence (vĭ-trĕs′ĕns). Becoming hard and transparent like glass.

vitreum (vĭt′rē-ŭm). The vitreous body of the eye.

vitrification. The process of converting a silicate material into a smooth, viscous substance by heat. It hardens on cooling and possesses a smooth, glossy surface, preserving its liquid properties in a solidified form as glass. In dentistry, it is related to the extensive use of ceramics, cements, and porcelains. These vary by the additive components which determine the density and refractive qualities.

vitriol (vĭt′rē-ōl) [L. vitriolum]. A sulfate of any of various metals.

v., blue. Copper sulfate.

v., green. Ferrous sulfate.

v., oil of. Sulfuric acid.

v., white. Zinc sulfate.

vitropression (vĭt″rō-prĕsh′ŭn) [L. vitrum, glass, + pressio, a squeezing]. Method of temporarily eliminating redness of the skin caused by hyperemia by pressure with a glass slide on the skin for purpose of studying any lesions or discolorations.

vitrum (vĭt′rŭm) [L.]. Glass.

Vivactil. Trade name for protriptyline hydrochloride.

vivi- (vĭv′ĭ) [L. vivus]. Combining form meaning alive.

vividialysis (vĭv″ĭ-dī-ăl′ĭ-sĭs). Dialysis through a living membrane.

vividiffusion (vĭv″ĭ-dĭf-ū′zhŭn) [L. vivus, alive, + dis, apart, + fundere, to pour]. The process of removing diffusible substances from blood of a living animal by allowing it to flow through dialyzing membranes immersed in saline solution.

vivification (vĭv″ĭ-fĭ-kā′shŭn) [″ + facere, to make]. 1. Trimming of the surface layer of a wound to aid union of tissues. 2. Transformation of protein food through assimilation into the living matter of cellular organisms.

viviparity (vĭv″ĭ-păr′ĭ-tē). The ability to produce living young rather than producing young by laying an egg and then having it hatch.

viviparous (vĭv-ĭp′ăr-ŭs) [″ + parere, to bring forth, to bear]. Developing young within the body, the young being expelled and born alive, the opposite of oviparous.

vivisect (vĭv′ĭ-sĕkt) [L. vivus, alive, + sectio, a cutting]. To dissect a living animal for experimental purposes.

vivisection (vĭv″ĭ-sĕk′shŭn) [″ + sectio, a cutting]. Cutting of or operation upon a living animal for physiological investigation and the study of disease. The operations are usually performed upon an anesthetized animal under conditions similar to those encountered in an operating room of a hospital.

vivisectionist (vĭv″ĭ-sĕk′shŭn-ĭst). One who practices or believes in vivisection. SEE: *antivivisection.*

vivisector (vĭv-ĭs-ĕk′tor) [″ + *sector,* a cutting]. One who practices vivisection.

vivisepulture (vĭv″ĭ-sĕp′ŭl-tūr) [″ + *sepultura,* buried]. The practice or act of burying an individual alive.

VLDL. *very low density lipoprotein.*

Vleminckx's solution (flĕm′ĭnks) [Jean François Vleminckx, Belgian physician, 1800–1876]. A solution of sulfurated lime used in various skin diseases.

VMA. *vanillylmandelic acid.*

V$_{max}$. *maximum velocity.*

V.N.A. *Visiting Nurse Association.*

Vo$_2$. Symbol for oxygen consumption per unit of time.

vocal (vō′kăl) [L. *vocalis,* talking]. Pert. to the voice.

vocal cord. Two thin, reedlike folds of tissue within the larynx that vibrate as air passes between them, producing sounds that are the basis of speech.

vocal cords, false. The ventricular folds of the larynx.

vocal cords, true. Vocal folds.

vocal folds. The thin edges of the vocal lips of the larynx, each of which encloses the vocal ligament. They form the edges of the rima glottidis, and are involved in the production of sound. SYN: *vocal cords.*

vocal fremitus. Chest-wall vibration felt on palpation while patient is speaking.

vocal ligament. A strong band of elastic tissue lying within the vocal fold.

vocal lips. Two shelflike projections of the lateral walls of the larynx. Their edges bear the vocal folds, q.v.

vocal muscle. The inner portion of the thyroarytenoid muscle, which lies in the vocal lip lateral to and in contact with the vocal ligament.

vocal process. The area of the arytenoid cartilage to which are attached the vocal cords.

vocal resonance. Sound heard in auscultation of lung while patient is speaking.

vocal signs. Indication of disease by changes in the voice.

voces (vō′sēz) [L.]. Pl. of vox.

voice (voys) [L. *vox*]. Sound uttered by human beings produced by vibration of the vocal cords.

    v., amphoric. V., cavernous, q.v.

    v., cavernous. The quality of the voice as heard during auscultation of the chest over an area underneath that is a cavity. SEE: *amphoric.*

    v., eunuchoid. The characteristic high-pitched voice of a male in whom the normal sexual development has not occurred or in a male who was castrated prior to puberty.

voice, words pert. to: amphoriloquy; arytenoid; heterophonia; hoarseness; phonation; resonance; rhinolalia; rhinophonia; trachyphonia.

voiceprint. Technique for depicting graphically the characteristics of an individual's speech pattern. Because voiceprints, like fingerprints, can be used to distinguish one person from another, the technique is useful in medicine and in identifying the voices of criminal suspects.

voices (voys′ēz). In psychiatry, verbal-auditory hallucinations expressed as being heard by the patient.

void (voyd) [O. Fr. *voider,* to empty]. To evacuate the bowels or bladder.

vol. *volume.*

vol.%. *volume percent.*

vola, volar (vō′lă, vō′lăr) [L.]. Terms originally used to refer to the palm of the hand or sole of the foot. The preferred terms for reference to the palm of the hand are palmar and palmaris.

vola manus (vō′lă). Palm, q.v.

vola pedis. The sole of the foot.

volaris (vō-lā′rĭs). Volar.

volatile (vŏl′ă-tĭl) [L. *volatilis,* flying]. Easily vaporized or evaporated. Examples of volatile liquids are ether (boiling point, 34.5°C) and ethyl chloride (boiling point, 12.2°C).

volatilization (vŏl″ă-tĭl-ĭ-zā′shŭn). Conversion of a solid or liquid into a vapor.

volatilize (vŏl′ă-tĭl-īz). To vaporize a liquid or solid.

vole (vōl). A mouselike rodent of the genus *Clethrionomys* or *Microtus.*

volition (vō-lĭsh′ŭn) [L. *volitio,* will]. The act or power of willing or choosing.

volitional (vō-lĭsh′ŭn-ăl). Performed by volition.

Volkmann's canals (fōlk′mänz) [Alfred Wilhelm Volkmann, Ger. physiologist, 1800–1877]. Vascular channels in compact bone. They are not surrounded by concentric lamellae as are the haversian canals.

Volkmann's contracture (fōlk′mänz) [Richard von Volkmann, Ger. surgeon, 1830–1889]. Degeneration, contracture, fibrosis, and atrophy of a muscle resulting from injury to its blood supply. Usually seen in the hand. SYN: *paralysis, ischemic.*

volley (vŏl′ē) [L. *volare,* to fly]. The simultaneous or nearly simultaneous discharge of a number of nerve impulses from a center within the brain or spinal cord.

volsella (vŏl-sĕl′ă) [L., tweezers]. Forceps with sharp, pointed hooks at end of each blade.

volt (vōlt) [Count Alessandro Volta, It. physicist, 1745–1827]. An electrical unit of pressure, the electromotive force required to produce one ampere of current through a resistance of one ohm.

voltage (vōl′tĭj). Electromotive force or difference in potential expressed in volts.

voltaic (vŏl-tā′ĭk). Concerning electricity produced by a battery.

voltaism (vŏl′tă-ĭzm). Galvanism, q.v.

voltammeter (vōlt-ăm′mē-tĕr). A device for measuring both volts and amperes.

voltampere (vōlt-ăm′pēr). The value obtained by multiplying volts times amperes.

voltmeter. A device for measuring the potential, i.e., electrical, between two positions.

volubility (vŏl″ū-bĭl′ĭ-tē) [L. *volubilitas,* flow of discourse]. Excessive speech.

volume (vŏl′ūm). The space occupied by a substance, usually a gas or liquid. Liquid volume is expressed in liters or milliliters; gas volume is expressed in cubic centimeters.

    v., expiratory reserve. The maximal amount of air that can be forced from the lungs after normal expiration.

    v., inspiratory reserve. The maximal amount of air that can be inspired after the end of a normal inspiration.

    v., mean corpuscular. ABBR: MCV. The mean volume of an average erythrocyte. Normal values range from 82 to 92 cubic microns.

    v., minute. The amount of blood discharged from one ventricle in one minute.

    v., packed cell. The volume of packed erythrocytes in a sample of centrifuged blood. Average volume equals 47% of blood volume in men, 42% in women. SYN: *hematocrit.*

    v., residual. Volume of air remaining in the lungs after maximal expiration.

    v., stroke. The amount of blood discharged by a ventricle in one contraction. Determined by dividing the minute volume by the number of heartbeats occurring in one minute.

    v., tidal. Volume of air inspired and expired in one normal respiratory cycle.

volumenometer (vŏl″ūm-nŏm′ĕ-tĕr). Volumometer.

volume percent. The number of cubic centimeters (milliliters) of a substance (usually O_2 or CO_2) contained in 100 cc (or ml) of another substance, e.g., blood. ABBR: vol.%.

volumetric (vŏl″ū-mĕt′rĭk) [L. *volumen,* a volume, + Gr. *metron,* measure]. Pert. to measurement of volume.

volumometer (vŏl″ū-mŏm′ĕ-tĕr). A device for measuring volume.

voluntary (vŏl′ŭn-tĕr″ē) [L. *voluntas,* will].

Pert. to or under control of the will.

voluntary health agency. Any nonprofit, nongovernmental agency, governed by lay or professional individuals, organized on a national, state, or local level, whose primary purpose is health related. This term applies to agencies supported mainly by voluntary public contributions. They are usually engaged in programs of service, education, and research related to a particular disability or group of diseases and disabilities; for example, the American Heart Association, American Cancer Society, National Foundation, National Lung Institute, and their state and local affiliates. The term can also be applied to such agencies as nonprofit hospitals, visiting nurse associations, and other local service organizations that have both lay and professional governing boards and are supported by both voluntary contributions and charges and fees for service provided.

voluntary muscle. Any muscle that is normally controlled by the will. They are generally attached to the skeleton and are innervated by myelinated nerves coming directly from the brain or spinal cord. Microscopically they consist of long cylindrical fibers bearing crosswise striations. The terms voluntary, striped, striated, cross-striated, and skeletal are practically synonymous when applied to muscle.

voluptuous (vō-lŭp′tū-ŭs) [L. *voluptas,* pleasure]. 1. Pert. to, arising from, or provoking, consciously or otherwise, sensual desire, usually applied to the female sex. 2. Given to sensualism.

volupty (vŏl′ŭp-tē) [O. Fr. *volupte,* pleasure]. Sexual pleasure.

volute (vō-lūt′) [L. *volutus,* rolled]. Spiral, rolled up. SYN: *convoluted.*

volvulosis (vŏl″vū-lō′sĭs). Onchocerciasis, q.v.

volvulus (vŏl′vū-lŭs) [L. *volvere,* to roll]. A twisting of the bowel upon itself causing obstruction. A prolapsed mesentery is the predisposing cause. Usually occurs at sigmoid and ileocecal areas of intestines.

vomer (vō′mĕr) [L., plowshare]. The plowshaped bone that forms the lower and posterior portion of the nasal septum, articulating with the ethmoid, sphenoid, the two palate bones, and two superior maxillary bones.

vomerine (vō′mĕr-ĭn). Pert. to the vomer.

vomerobasilar (vō″mĕr-ō-băs′ĭ-lăr). Concerning the vomer and base of the skull.

vomeronasal (vō″mĕr-ō-nā′săl). Pert. to the vomer and nasal bones.

vomeronasal cartilages. Two narrow strips of cartilage lying along the anterior portion of the inferior border of the septal cartilage of the nose.

vomeronasal organ. A small tubular epithelial sac lying on the anteroinferior surface of the nasal septum. Rudimentary in humans. SYN: *Jacobson's organ.*

vomica (vŏm'ĭ-kă) [L., ulcer] (pl. *vomicae*). 1. A cavity in the lungs, as from suppuration. 2. Sudden and profuse expectoration of putrid purulent matter.

vomicose (vŏm'ĭ-kōs). Marked by many ulcers; ulcerous; purulent.

vomit (vŏm'ĭt) [L. *vomere*, to vomit]. 1. Material that is ejected from the stomach through the mouth. 2. To eject stomach contents through the mouth. SEE: *melena; nausea; vomitus.*

PHYS: The act is usually reflex involving coordinated activity of both voluntary and involuntary muscles. A certain position is assumed, the glottis is closed, the diaphragm and abdominal muscles contract, and the cardiac sphincter of the stomach relaxes while antiperistaltic waves course over the duodenum, stomach, and esophagus.

v., bilious. Bile forced back into the stomach and ejected with vomited matter.

v., black. Vomit containing blood acted on by the gastric juice. Seen in worst form of yellow fever.

v., coffee-ground. Vomit having the appearance and consistency of coffee grounds because of blood mixed with gastric contents. Occurs in any condition associated with hemorrhage into the stomach.

vomiting (vŏm'ĭt-ing) [L. *vomere*, to vomit]. Ejection through the mouth of the gastric contents, and, in cases of bowel obstruction, intestinal contents. It may result from toxins from ptomaines, drugs, uremia, and specific fevers; cerebral tumors and meningitis (often unaccompanied by nausea and does not relieve associated headache); diseases of the stomach such as ulcer, cancer, dilatation, dyspepsia; reflex from pregnancy, uterine or ovarian disease, irritation of the fauces, worms, biliary colic; intestinal obstruction; motion sickness; nervous affections such as hysteria and migraine. Vomiting may result from taking poisons such as arsenic, aconite, antimony, barium, colchicum, cantharides, copper, corrosive alkalis, acids, digitalis, iodine, mercury, phenol, phosphorus, veratrum, wood alcohol (methanol), food toxins or poisons, and zinc. Periodic vomiting may be in itself a neurosis or associated with the gastric crises of locomotor ataxia. Esophageal vomiting results from obstruction, and the vomitus, q.v., is alkaline in reaction. SYN: *emesis.* SEE: *anorexia nervosa.*

TREAT: Antinausea medicines by mouth

if possible, otherwise intramuscularly or intravenously. Fluids may be given by mouth if patient will accept them. If vomiting continues, fluids and electrolytes intravenously will be required to replace those lost in the vomitus.

In pregnancy (hyperemesis gravidarum, q.v.): If severe, fluid intake by mouth should be restricted but maintained by intravenous route. In less severe cases, frequent small feedings of more or less dry foods are advisable.

Caution: It is of utmost importance not to use medicines during pregnancy unless there is evidence that the drug being prescribed has been investigated and found to be harmless to the embryo and its development.

NURSING IMPLICATIONS: Assess causative factors such as drugs, food, disease entities, and psychological factors. Remove causative factor if possible. Assess frequency of vomiting, amount, time of occurrence, and characteristics of fluid. Provide an emesis basin and empty it as often as needed. Position patient to prevent aspiration, and have suction equipment available. Administer antiemetics as prescribed. Withhold food and fluids for several hours, and offer frequent mouth care. If surgery during pregnancy is required, prevent vomiting by restricting foods and fluids for approximately 8 hours before surgery. Use comfort measures such as a cool cloth to the face. Monitor serum electrolytes, and keep accurate intake and output records to ensure proper fluid replacement. Monitor vital signs and institute antipyretic measures if temperature is elevated. To prevent vomiting, encourage the patient to take deep breaths or to swallow. Promote a calm environment and provide distraction.

RS: anorexia nervosa; antiemetic; emesis; emetic; hyperemesis; vomit; vomitus.

v., cyclic. Periodic and recurring attacks of vomiting occurring in patients with a nervous temperament. The condition is associated with acidosis.

v., dry. Nausea without vomitus.

v., epidemic. Sudden unexplained attacks of gastroenteritis characterized by nausea, vomiting, and sometimes diarrhea. Though not proven, the symptoms are believed to be due to a virus. Treatment is symptomatic.

v., incoercible. Uncontrollable vomiting.

v., induced. Production of vomiting by administering certain types of emetics, e.g., syrup of ipecac or amorphine; or by physical stimulation of the posterior pharynx.

Caution: In the past, salt solutions were used to induce vomiting. Because sodium chloride in high doses is toxic and may be lethal, it should not be used.

---

v. of pregnancy. Vomiting of pregnancy, esp. morning sickness.

v., pernicious. Severe vomiting of pregnancy.

v., projectile. Ejection of vomitus with great force.

v., psychogenic. SEE: *psychogenic vomiting.*

v., stercoraceous. Vomiting of fecal matter.

vomitive (vŏm′ĭ-tĭv). Emetic.

vomitory (vŏm′ĭ-tō-rē) [L. *vomitorius,* pert. to vomit]. 1. Causing vomiting. 2. An agent inducing emesis. 3. A vessel to receive vomitus.

vomiturition (vŏm″ĭ-tū-rĭsh′ŭn) [L. *vomitus,* vomit]. Repeated involuntary and ineffective efforts to vomit. SYN: *retching.*

vomitus (vŏm′ĭ-tŭs). 1. Act of ejecting matter from the stomach through the mouth. 2. Material ejected from the stomach by vomiting.

    CHARACTER: *Ammoniacal odor:* Indicates uremia. *Bilious:* Green or greenish-yellow, containing bile, appears after frequent and violent vomiting. *Fecal:* Indicative of intestinal obstruction, general peritonitis, and abnormal communication between the intestines and stomach. *Garlic odor:* Denotes phosphorus poisoning.

    Hematemesis: The vomiting of blood. If bright and fluid, it has not been long in the stomach; otherwise, it has the appearance of coffee grounds, reddish-brown, or it forms in clots. Also, this may indicate rupture of an aneurysm into the stomach or esophagus or rupture of esophageal varicose veins; gastric ulcer; cirrhosis of liver; enlarged spleen; or carcinoma of the stomach. It is not necessarily fatal. Hematemesis may result from swallowed blood. It may occur in vicarious menstruation, gastritis, corrosive poisoning, or after ingestion of strong alkalies or acids, or it may result from anemia, leukemia, or Hodgkin's disease. Sometimes it is present in chronic nephritis, scurvy, purpura hemorrhagica, acute yellow atrophy of the liver, and in malaria.

    Profuse: The ejection of large quantities of frothy fermented material is highly significant of gastric dilatation. *Purulent:* This may result from the rupture of an abscess into the esophagus or stomach. *Without nausea, distress, or other phenomena:* This may occur in certain neuroses, in hysteria,

uremia, central nervous system disease as from a tumor, or as a precursor of apoplexy. The vomitus may be colored by certain fruits, by wine, coffee, cocoa, soups, and bile.

v., coffee-ground. Vomitus of dark red or black granular material (resembling coffee grounds), which is blood. The blood has been in the stomach or intestinal tract long enough to be changed from red to black by the action of gastric and intestinal juices. Occurs in conditions associated with hemorrhage into the stomach.

v. cruentus. Bloody vomit.

v. marinus. Seasickness.

v. matutinus. The vomiting of morning sickness.

von Gierke's disease (fŏn gēr′kĕz) [Edgar von Gierke, Ger. pathologist, 1877–1945]. Glycogen storage disease, type 1a. SYN: *glycogenosis; glycogen storage disease.*

von Graefe's sign (fŏn grā′fēz) [Albrecht von Graefe, Ger. ophthalmologist, 1828–1870]. Failure of lid to move downward promptly with eyeball, the lid moving tardily and jerkily; seen in exophthalmic goiter.

von Hippel's disease. Hippel's disease, q.v.

von Jaksch's disease [Rudolf von Jaksch-Wartenhorst, Austrian physician, 1855–1947]. A symptom complex consisting of anemia, hepatosplenomegaly, and infections that are associated with a number of chronic diseases such as tuberculosis and malnutrition.

von Pirquet's test (fŏn pēr′kāz) [Clemens Peter Johann von Pirquet, Austrian pediatrician, 1874–1929]. A diagnostic test for tuberculosis in which a small amount of tuberculin is applied to a scarified area of the skin of the arm. A positive reaction is seen if a red papillar eruption appears several days later at the site of inoculation.

von Recklinghausen's canals. Recklinghausen's canals, q.v.

von Recklinghausen's disease. Recklinghausen's disease, q.v.

von Recklinghausen's tumor. Recklinghausen's tumor, q.v.

Vontrol. Trade name for diphenidol.

von Willebrand's disease [Erik Adolph von Willebrand, Finnish physician, 1870–1949]. A congenital bleeding disorder. The bleeding tendency manifests at an early age, usually as epistaxis and easy bruising but petechiae are rare. Bleeding in the intestinal tract during surgery and excess loss of blood during menstruation are common. The symptoms decrease in severity with age and during pregnancy.

    ETIOL: Deficiency of coagulation factor VIII.

    DIAG: Prolonged bleeding time and factor VIII deficiency.

TREAT: Administer factor VIII 24 to 48 hours prior to surgery or during attacks of bleeding.

voodoo [Creole Fr., *voudou*, a good or bad spirit or demon]. A religious cult of African origin. It is practiced in the Caribbean by some Haitians. Practitioners believe in sorcery, fetishes, and rituals for communicating with ancestors or saints. Some persons believe in the power of a "hex" being placed on someone in order to cause death. There seems to be good evidence that otherwise normal persons have had a hex put upon them and they later experienced an otherwise unexplained death. SEE: *hex; miracle, medical; zombie.*

Voorhees' bag (voor'ēz) [James Ditmors Voorhees, U.S. obstetrician, 1869–1929]. An inflatable rubber bag for dilating the cervix uteri to induce and facilitate labor.

voracious (vō-rā'shŭs) [L. *vorare*, to devour]. Having an insatiable or ravenous appetite.

vortex (vor'tĕks) [L., a whirlpool] (pl. *vortices*). A structure having a spiral or whorled appearance.

    v., coccygeal. The region over the coccyx where lanugo hairs of the embryo come to a point.

    v. lentis. Spiral patterns on the surface of the lens due to concentric pattern of fiber growth.

    v. of heart. Region at apex of heart where muscle fibers of the ventricles make a tight spiral and turn inward.

vortices (vor'tĭ-sēz) [L.]. Pl. of vortex.

    v. pilorum. Hair whorls as in arrangement of hairs on the scalp.

vorticose (vor'tĭk-ōs) [L. *vortices*, whirlpools]. Whirling or having a whorled arrangement.

vorticose veins. Four veins (two superior and two inferior) that receive blood from all parts of the choroid of the eye. They empty into posterior ciliary and superior ophthalmic veins.

vox (vŏks) [L.] (pl. *voces*). Voice.

    v. abscissa. Loss of voice.

    v. capitus. Falsetto voice or a voice in the upper register.

    v. cholerica. The suppressed voice in last stages of cholera.

    v. rauca. A hoarse voice.

voxel. Volume element. In magnetic resonance imaging, a three-dimensional area in the structure being examined, which is represented as a pixel (picture element) on the matrix of the final digital image.

voyeur (voy-yĕr') [Fr., one who sees]. One who derives sexual pleasure from observing nude persons or the sexual activity of others.

voyeurism (voy'yĕr-ĭzm). The experiencing of sexual gratification by observing nude persons or the sexual activity of others.

V.R. *right vision; ventilation rate; vocal resonance.*

V.S. *vesicular sound; vital signs; volumetric solution.*

VSD. *ventricular septal defect.*

vuerometer (vū"ĕr-ŏm'ĕ-tĕr) [Fr. *vue*, sight, + Gr. *metron*, measure]. Apparatus for measuring interpupillary distance of the eyes.

vulgaris (vŭl-gā'rĭs) [L.]. Ordinary, common.

vulnerable (vŭl'nĕr-ă-bl) [L. *vulnerare*, to wound]. Easily injured or wounded.

vulnerant (vŭl'nĕr-ănt). 1. Something that wounds or injures. 2. To inflict injury.

vulnerary (vŭl'nĕr-ār"ē). 1. Pert. to wounds. 2. An agent, esp. a folk remedy or herb, used to promote wound healing.

vulnerate (vŭl'nĕr-āt). To wound.

vulnus (vŭl'nŭs) [L.] (pl. *vulnera*). A wound or injury.

Vulpian-Heidenhain-Sherrington phenomenon [Edme-Felix Alfred Vulpian, French physician, 1826–1887; Rudolph Peter Heinrich Heidenhain, Ger. physiologist, 1834–1897; Sir Charles Scott Sherrington, Brit. physiologist, 1857–1952]. Contraction of denervated skeletal muscle by stimulating autonomic cholinergic fibers innervating its blood vessels.

vulsella, vulsellum (vŭl-sĕl'ă, vŭl-sĕl'ŭm) [L. *vulsella*, tweezers]. A forceps with a hook on each blade. SYN: *volsella.*

vulva (vŭl'vă) [L., covering] (pl. *vulvae*). That portion of the female external genitalia lying posterior to the mons veneris, consisting of the labia majora, labia minora, clitoris, vestibule of the vagina, vaginal opening, and bulbs of the vestibule. SYN: *pudendum femininum* [NA].

    v. connivens. Vulva in which the labia majora are in apposition.

    v. hians. Vulva in which labia majora are gaping.

    v., velamen. Abnormally elongated clitoris.

vulval, vulvar [L. *vulva*, covering]. Relating to the vulva.

vulvar dystrophies. Non-neoplastic epithelial disorders of the vulvar skin and mucosa. These conditions may be associated with squamous cell hyperplasia, lichen sclerosus, or other dermatoses.

vulvar leukoplakia. Condition characterized by diffuse or focal translucent thickening of the vulva. Often gives rise to carcinoma.

vulvar vestibulitis syndrome. Presence of severe pain upon pressing or touching the vestibule of the vagina or attempted vaginal entry. Physical findings of a mild degree of localized erythema are limited to the mucosa of the vestibule. The etiology of this distressing syndrome is unknown, and therapy, including vestibulectomy, has not been 100% effective.

vulvectomy (vŭl-vĕk′tō-mē) [″ + Gr. *ektome*, excision]. Excision of the vulva.

vulvismus (vŭl-vĭz′mŭs) [″ + Gr. *-ismos*, condition]. Painful spasm of the vagina. SYN: *vaginismus*.

vulvitis (vŭl-vī′tĭs) [L. *vulva*, covering, + Gr. *itis*, inflammation]. Inflammation of the vulva.

v., acute nongonorrheal. Vulvitis resulting from chafing of opposed lips of vulva or from accumulated sebaceous material around the clitoris.

v., follicular. Inflammation of hair follicles of the vulva.

v., gangrenous. Necrosis and sloughing of areas of vulva, often a complication of infectious diseases such as diphtheria, scarlatina, herpes genitalis, or typhoid fever.

v., leukoplakic. A chronic atrophic vulvitis. SEE: *kraurosis vulvae.*

v., mycotic. Vulvitis caused by various fungi, most commonly by *Candida albicans.*

vulvo- [L. *vulva*, covering]. Combining form meaning a covering, or the vulva.

vulvocrural (vŭl″vō-kroo′răl) [″ + *cruralis*, pert. to the leg]. Rel. to the vulva and thigh.

vulvodynia [″ + *dynia*, pain]. A nonspecific syndrome that has no known cause. It is characterized by pain, especially during sexual intercourse, itching, and discomfort.

vulvopathy (vŭl-vŏp′ă-thē) [″ + Gr. *pathos*, disease, suffering]. Any disorder of the vulva.

vulvouterine (vŭl″vō-ū′tĕr-ĭn) [″ + *uterinus*, pert. to the uterus]. Rel. to the vulva and uterus.

vulvovaginal (vŭl″vō-văj′ĭ-năl) [″ + *vagina*, a sheath]. Pert. to the vulva and vagina. SYN: *vaginolabial; vaginovulvar.*

vulvovaginal glands. Small glands on either side of the vulvar orifice. SYN: *Bartholin's glands.*

vulvovaginitis (vŭl″vō-văj″ĭ-nī′tĭs) [″ + ″ + Gr. *itis*, inflammation]. Inflammation of both the vulva and vagina at the same time, or of the vulvovaginal glands. The condition may be due to chemical irritation produced by materials present in medications, tight-fitting underclothes, inadequate perineal hygiene, allergic conditions, or a variety of infectious agents including bacteria, yeasts, viruses, and parasites.

v., diabetic. Mycotic vulvar infection commonly occurring with diabetes.

vv. *veins.*

v/v. Volume of dissolved substance per volume of solvent.

V.W. *vessel wall.*

v/w. Volume of a substance per unit of weight of another component.

V-Y-plasty. A method used in plastic surgery to repair a skin defect. A V-shaped incision is made, and the tissue at the top of the V is pulled toward that position. The edges of the new wound are then sutured so that a Y-shaped scar is now produced.

W

W. Chem. symbol for the element tungsten (wolfram).

w. *watt*, a unit of electric energy; *week; wife; with.*

Waardenburg syndrome [Petrus Johannes Waardenburg, Dutch ophthalmologist, 1886–1979]. A congenital defect involving pigmentation. It consists of a white forelock, vitiligo, heterochromic irides, broad nasal root, dystopia canthorum (lateral displacement of the inner canthi), deficient pigmentation of the fundus, synophrys (growing together of the two sets of eyebrows), and cutaneous hypopigmentation. Congenital deafness may or may not be present. The condition is inherited as an autosomal dominant.

Wachendorf's membrane (vŏk'ĕn-dorfs) [Eberhard J. Wachendorf, Dutch physician, 1703–1758]. 1. A thin membrane occluding the pupil of the embryo. SYN: *membrana pupillaris.* 2. The outer membrane ensheathing a cell.

wafer (wā'fĕr) [Ger. *wafel*]. 1. A thin sheet of flour paste used to enclose a medicinal dose of powder. 2. A flat vaginal suppository.

Wagstaffe's fracture (wăg'stăfs) [William Warwick Wagstaffe, Brit. surgeon, 1843–1910]. Fracture with separation of the internal malleolus of the ankle.

waist (wāst) [ME. *wast*, growth]. Small part of the human trunk between thorax and hips. SEE: *cincture sensation.*

wakeful (wāk'fŭl) [AS. *wacian*, to be awake, + *full*, complete]. Not able to sleep; sleepless.

Walcher's position (vŏl'kĕrz) [Gustav Adolf Walcher, Ger. gynecologist, 1856–1935]. Position in which the patient assumes dorsal recumbent posture with hips at the edge of the bed and legs hanging down.

Wald, Lillian (wăld). U.S. nurse, 1867–1940, who founded the Henry Street Settlement in New York City, and one of the world's first visiting nurse associations.

Wald cycle. The transformations involved in the breakdown of resynthesis of rhodopsin.

Waldenström's disease (văl'dĕn-strĕmz) [Johann Henning Waldenström, Swedish surgeon, b. 1877]. Osteochondritis deformans juvenilis, q.v.

Waldeyer's gland (vŏl'dī-ĕrz) [Wilhelm von Waldeyer, Ger. anatomist, 1836–1921]. Sweat glands of the eyelids. Usually most prominent in the lower lid margin.

Waldeyer's neuron. The nerve cell and its processes.

Waldeyer's ring. The ring of tonsillar (lymphatic) tissue that encircles the nasopharynx and oropharynx. Consists of the two palatine tonsils, lingual and pharyngeal tonsils.

walk. 1. Method of locomotion of upright bipeds such as humans. 2. The particular way an individual moves. SEE: *gait.*

walker. A mobile device used to assist a person in walking. It consists of a stable platform made of metal tubing that the patient grasps while taking a step. The walker is then moved forward and another step is taken. SEE: *crutch.*

walking [AS. *wealcan*, to roll]. Act of moving on foot; advancing by steps.
RS: abasia; acathisia; astasia; atremia; basophobia; claudication; dysbasia; gait.
w., sleep-. Somnambulism.

walking cast. A cast that allows the patient to be ambulatory.

walking system. A complex device that enables patients with spinal injuries resulting in paralysis of the legs to walk. The device uses computer-controlled electrical stimulation to muscles so that walking may be accomplished. Each of these devices is made especially for each patient, and their use is experimental.

walking typhoid. Typhoid fever in which the symptoms are mild so that the patient is ambulatory.

walking well. Persons who are indeed ill, but still able to walk.

walking wounded. In military medicine, an ambulatory case.

wall [AS. *weall*]. The limiting or surrounding substance or material of a cell, vessel, or cavity such as an artery, vein, chest, or bladder. In dentistry, it may refer to specific boundaries of a cavity preparation or its location within the tooth, e.g., cavity walls: buccal, lingual, mesial, distal, pulpal, coronal, axial, cervical, facial, incisal, gingival, enamel.

Wallenberg's syndrome (vŏl'ĕn-bĕrgz) [Adolf Wallenberg, Ger. physician, 1862–1949]. A complex of symptoms resulting from occlusion of the posteroinferior cerebellar artery or one of its branches supplying the lower portion of the brain stem. Dysphagia, muscular weakness or paralysis, impairment of pain and temperature senses, and cerebellar dysfunction are characteristic.

wallerian degeneration (wŏl-ē'rē-ăn) [Augustus Volney Waller, Brit. physician,

1816–1870]. Degeneration of a nerve fiber (axon) that has been severed from its cell body. The myelin sheath also degenerates and is transformed into a chain of lipoid droplets that stains by the Marchi method, which is utilized in tracing the course of injured nerve fibers. The neurilemma does not degenerate but forms a tube that directs the growth of the regenerating axon.

walleye [ME. *wawil-eghed*]. 1. Eye in which iris is light-colored or white. 2. Leukoma or dense opacity of cornea. 3. Squint in which both visual axes diverge. SYN: *strabismus, divergent.*

Walthard's islets or inclusions [Max Walthard, Swiss gynecologist, 1867–1933]. Nests or small cysts of embryological squamous epithelium-like cells in the superficial parts of the ovary, tubes, and uterine ligaments. They are thought to represent the beginning Brenner tumor.

wandering (wăn′dĕr-ing) [AS. *wandrian*]. Moving about; not fixed.

wandering abscess. Abscess that burrows and comes to the surface at a point distant from its origin.

wandering kidney. Dislocated floating kidney.

wandering mind. Daydream or reverie.

wandering spleen. Dislocated floating spleen.

Wangensteen tube (wăn′gĕn-stēn) [Owen H. Wangensteen, U.S. surgeon, 1898–1981]. Tube used for relieving postoperative abdominal distention, nausea, vomiting, and certain cases of mechanical bowel obstruction. It is used as an intranasal catheter in combination with a suction siphonage apparatus. SEE: *decompression.*

Warburg apparatus [Otto H. Warburg, Ger. biochemist, 1883–1970]. A capillary manometer used for determining oxygen consumption and carbon dioxide production of small bits of cellular tissue. Widely used in metabolism studies.

ward [AS. *weard*, watching over]. A large room in a hospital for the care of several patients, usually more than four.

    w., accident. Ward reserved for accident cases.

    w., psychiatric. Ward in a general hospital for mentally ill patients.

Wardrop's disease (wăr′drŏps) [James Wardrop, Brit. surgeon, 1782–1869]. Acute inflammation of the nailbed with fetid ulceration and loss of the nail. SYN: *onychia maligna.*

Wardrop's operation. Ligation of an artery for aneurysm at a distance beyond the sac.

warehousemen's itch. Eczema of hands from touching irritating substances.

warfarin poisoning. Caused by accidental administration of an overdose of the drug, or by the cumulative effect of repeated administration of the drug. Warfarin is also used as a rodenticide. Repeated ingestion of those materials by children may cause poisoning. SEE: *Poisons and Poisoning* in *Appendix.*

warfarin potassium. USP. An anticoagulant drug. Trade name is Athrombin-K.

warfarin sodium [name derived from initials of Wisconsin Alumni Research Foundation]. An anticoagulant drug. Coumadin and Panwarfin are trade names.

NURSING IMPLICATIONS: Instruct the patient to observe for signs of bleeding such as epistaxis, bleeding gums, hematuria, melena, and skin trauma (ecchymosis, purpura, or petechia). Preventive measures should include gentle blowing of the nose, use of an electric razor and a soft-bristled toothbrush, gentle cleaning of the anal area, and avoidance of tight, constrictive clothing. Stress the importance of having blood studies as prescribed by the physician and the significance of regular medical follow-up. Provide the patient with an identification card listing the prescribed drug, dosage, frequency of administration, and physician's name and phone number. It is important for the patient to consult with the physician before taking any over-the-counter medications. This is necessary because many drugs interact with anticoagulants to interfere with their action.

war gases. Any chemical substances, whether solid, liquid, or vapor, used to produce poisonous or irritant effects. SEE: *gas, war.*

wart (wort) [AS. *wearte*]. A circumscribed cutaneous elevation resulting from hypertrophy of the papillae and epidermis. It is caused by a papillomavirus. Also applied to benign conditions, such as verruca, that resemble warts.

    RS: condyloma; keratosis, seborrheic; sycoma; venereal wart; verrucose.

    w., fig. Growth of filiform projections usually occurring on genitalia. Frequently they are covered with a foul-smelling secretion. SYN: *venereal wart; verruca acuminata.*

    w., genital. Wart of the genitalia. It is caused by human papillomavirus (HPV). In the female, there is a question of the association of these warts with cancer of the cervix. It is estimated that as many as 1 million new cases of genital warts occur each year in the U.S.

    A variety of therapies, including topically applied chemicals such as podophyllin, laser therapy, surgery, and recombinant interferon alfa-2a, have been used with varying degrees of success. Nevertheless, there is no completely safe and effective therapy available for genital warts.

w., plantar. Wart on pressure-bearing areas, esp. the sole of the foot. SYN: *verruca plantaris.*

w., seborrheic. Patch of corneous hypertrophy on face of the aged.

w., senile. W., seborrheic.

w., venereal. Vegetating growth upon skin, esp. on the mucocutaneous juncture of the genitals, having an offensive discharge. SYN: *verruca acuminata.*

wash (wăsh) [AS. *wacsan*]. 1. Act of cleaning, esp. a part or all of the body. 2. A medicinal preparation used in washing or coating.

w., eye. A lotion for the eyes. SYN: *collyrium.*

washerwoman's itch. Eczema of the hands of laundry workers.

washout, nitrogen. Removal of nitrogen from the body by breathing either 100% oxygen or a combination of oxygen and helium. Even though complete removal of nitrogen will require 12 hours of breathing nitrogen-free air, 2 hours may be sufficient to prevent the development of bends, q.v., in aviators preparing to ascend to high altitudes.

wasp [AS. *waesp*]. Term sometimes applied to all insects belonging to the suborder Apocrita, order Hymenoptera (except the Formicidae or ants), but more generally restricted to the superfamilies Scolioidea, Vespoidea, and Specoidea. Members have the base of the abdomen constricted, and females have a piercing ovipositor, which in many species is modified into a sting. Many are social, living in large colonies. Common representatives are yellow jackets and hornets.

wasp sting. The injection of wasp venom into the skin, resulting in a painful wound and sometimes a mild systemic reaction. Multiple stings may be dangerous, esp. to sensitized individuals.

TREAT: Apply bicarbonate of soda paste, strong epsom salt, or household ammonia solution locally. If pain is severe, infiltrate area with 2% procaine solution. Severe allergic reaction may require injection of epinephrine and cortisone. Application of cold to a large area around bite will slow absorption of the venom.

waste (wāst) [L. *vastus*, empty]. 1. To shrink in physical bulk or strength, as from disease. SYN: *cachexia.* 2. Loss by breaking down of bodily tissue. 3. Excreted material no longer useful to an organism.

waste products. Carbon dioxide, organic and inorganic salts, urine, dead skin, hair, nails, undigested foods.

w.p., metabolic. Soluble salts in the form of nitrogenous salts (urea) and inorganic salts (sodium chloride), gas in form of carbon dioxide, and liquid in the form of water. They are excreta, removed by the process of elimination, q.v.

wasting (wāst'ĭng) [L. *vastare*, to devastate]. Enfeebling; causing loss of strength or size; emaciating. SEE: *marasmus.*

wasting palsy. Chronic disease marked by gradual atrophy of muscular tissue with paralysis. SYN: *progressive muscular atrophy.* SEE: *atrophy, muscular.*

water (wă'tĕr) [AS. *waeter*]. 1. H_2O, hydrogen combined with oxygen, forming a tasteless, clear, odorless fluid. 2. A lay term used to refer to urine or urinating.

Water freezes at 32°F (0°C) and boils at 212°F (100°C). It is the principal chemical constituent of the body, composing approx. 65% of the body weight of an adult male and 55% of the adult female. It is distributed within the intracellular fluid and outside of the cells in the extracellular fluid. Water is indispensable for metabolic activities within cells, as it is the medium in which chemical reactions can take place. Outside of cells, it is the principal transporting agent of the body. The following properties of water are important to living organisms: it is almost a universal solvent; it is a medium in which acids, bases, and salts ionize, and the concentrations of these substances (electrolytes) must be and are normally regulated quite precisely by the body; it possesses a high specific heat and has a high latent heat of vaporization, of importance in regulation and maintenance of a constant body temperature; it possesses a high surface tension; it is an important reacting agent and essential in all hydrolytic reactions.

Water is the principal constituent of all body fluids (blood, lymph, tissue fluid), secretions (salivary juice, gastric juice, bile, sweat), and excretory fluid (urine). Intake of water is determined principally by the sense of thirst. Excessive intake may lead to water intoxication; excessive loss to dehydration. Humans can survive for only a short time without water intake. The exact length of survival time varies with ambient temperature, moisture in available food, and amount of physical activity.

w., bound. Water that in protoplasm is attached to organic substances. It is not available for metabolic processes.

w., deionized. Water that has been passed through a substance that removes cations and anions present as contaminants.

w., distilled. Water that has been purified by distillation, q.v. Used for pharmaceutical purposes.

w., emergency preparation of safe drinking. Water must be purified when only unclean water is available or if there is reason to believe that available drinking water has become contaminated. One of the following methods may be used: (1) Strain water through a clean cloth and boil water vigorously for 30 minutes. (2) Add 3 drops of alcoholic solution of iodine to each quart (approx. 1 liter) of water. Mix well and let it stand for 30 minutes prior to using. (3) Add either 10 drops of 1% chlorine bleach, or 2 drops of 4% to 6% chlorine bleach, or 1 drop of 7% to 10% chlorine bleach to each quart (liter) of water. Mix well and let stand for 30 minutes. If water is cloudy to begin with, use double the amount of chlorine.

If *Giardia* organisms are contaminating the water, heating to 55°C (131°F) will kill the protozoa. Methods (2) and (3) will also kill the cysts, but more time will be required. Vegetative bacteria and viruses are killed by water kept at 60°C (140°F) for 30 minutes.

NOTE: If traveling in an area where the potability of water is questionable and there is no easy method of purification available, using water from the hot water tap may help to decrease the possibility of ingesting live pathogenic microorganisms. The water is allowed to cool to drinking temperature.

w., hard. Water that contains dissolved salts of magnesium or calcium.

w., heavy. D₂O. An isotopic variety of water, esp. deuterium oxide, in which hydrogen has been displaced by its isotope, deuterium. Its properties differ from ordinary water in that heavy water has a higher freezing and boiling point and is incapable of supporting life.

w., lime. Calcium hydroxide solution.

w., potable. Water suitable for drinking both from the hygienic point as well as being free of odor and objectionable minerals.

w., purified. USP. Water that is mineral free. Obtained by distillation, q.v., or deionization, q.v.

w., pyrogen-free. Water that has been rendered free of fever-producing proteins (bacteria and their metabolic products). SEE: *water for injection.*

w., soft. Water that contains very little, if any, dissolved salts of magnesium or calcium.

water bed. A rubber mattress partially filled with warm water (100°F or 37.8°C). If too full, the mattress will be hard. Used in preventing and treating bedsores.

water brash. Reflex salivary hypersecretion in response to peptic esophagitis.

water cure. Use of water in treatment of a condition. SYN: *hydrotherapy.*

water for injection. Water for parenteral use that has been distilled and sterilized. Distilled, sterilized water that is stored in sealed containers will remain free of pyrogens and may be used after longer periods of storage.

waterhammer pulse. Pulse marked by a quick, powerful beat, collapsing suddenly. SYN: *pulse, Corrigan's.*

Waterhouse-Friderichsen syndrome [Rupert Waterhouse, Brit. physician, 1873–1958; Carl Friderichsen, Danish physician, b. 1886]. Acute adrenal insufficiency due to hemorrhage into the adrenal gland caused by meningococcal infection. SEE: *adrenal gland; meningitis, acute meningococcal.*

water intoxication. Excess water and sodium retention. Clinically, abdominal cramps, dizziness, lethargy, nausea, vomiting, convulsions, and coma may be present.

ETIOL: Excess ingestion of water, I.V. administration of hypotonic solutions, excess tap water enemas, hypothalamic tumors, cerebral concussion, or excess secretion of antidiuretic hormone. SEE: *brain edema.*

water on brain. Disease marked by abnormal increase in cerebrospinal fluid. SYN: *hydrocephalus.*

waters. Common term for the amniotic fluid surrounding the fetus.

water syringe. In dentistry, a syringe for delivering water spray to a localized area. The flow, pressure, and temperature may be controlled.

Watson-Crick helix [James Dewey Watson, U.S. biochemist, b. 1928; Francis Harry Compton Crick, Brit. biochemist, b. 1916]. A double helix named after the scientists who established its structure. Each half of the helix contains chemical compounds arranged in a specific sequence. Variation in the sequence of these compounds enables genetic information to be transmitted. The double helix is the structure of DNA (deoxyribonucleic acid).

Watson-Schwartz test (wŏt′sŏn-shwärts) [Cecil J. Watson, U.S. physician, 1901–1983; Samuel Schwartz, U.S. physician, b. 1916]. A test used in acute porphyria to differentiate porphobilinogen from urobilinogen.

watt [James Watt, Scottish engineer, 1736–1819]. Unit of electrical power. May be expressed as work at the rate of one joule per second. One watt is the power produced by one ampere of current flowing with a force or pressure, i.e., electromotive force, of one volt. In SI units, one watt equals one joule/second. And in other units, one watt equals one newton meter/second. This is also equal

COMPONENTS OF WAVES

to 0.7376 foot pounds/second. SEE: *electromotive force.*

wattage (wŏt'ij). The electrical energy produced or consumed by an electrical device, expressed in watts.

wave (wāv) [ME. *wave*]. 1. A disturbance, usually orderly and predictable, observed as a moving ridge on the surface of a liquid. 2. An undulating or vibrating motion. 3. An oscillation seen in the recording of an electrocardiogram, electroencephalogram, or other graphic record of physiological activity. SEE: illus.

    w., a. Venous neck wave produced by atrial contraction. Also, component of right atrial and pulmonary artery wedge pressure tracings produced by atrial contraction. The a wave just precedes the first heart sound. Absent in atrial fibrillation. Larger in A-V dissociation and in conditions causing dilation of the right atrium.

    w., alpha. SEE: *rhythm, alpha.*

    w., beta. SEE: *rhythm, beta.*

    w., brain. The fluctuation, usually rhythmic, of electrical impulses produced by the brain. SEE: *electroencephalography.*

    w., c. Component of right atrial and pulmonary capillary wedge pressure waves. Reflects the closing of the tricuspid valve at the beginning of ventricular systole. An abnormal configuration is seen in increased right heart pressure and with abnormalities of the tricuspid valve.

    w., delta. SEE: *rhythm, delta.*

    w., electromagnetic. A wave-form produced by simultaneous oscillation of electric and magnetic fields perpendicular to each other. The direction of propagation of the wave is perpendicular to the oscillations. The following waves are electromagnetic. They are listed in order of increasing frequency and decreasing wavelength: radio, television, microwave, infrared, visible light, ultraviolet, x-rays, and gamma rays. SEE: *electromagnetic spectrum* for table.

    w., excitation. The excitatory impulse(s) that originate in the sinoatrial node of the heart and sweep through the musculature of the atria, stimulating the atrioventricular node and then continuing through the conductile tissue of the ventricles. They bring about the contraction of the chambers of the heart.

    w.'s, hertzian. Electromagnetic radiations used in radio and wireless transmission.

    w.'s, light. Electromagnetic waves that produce the sensation of visible light on the retina.

    w., P. SEE: *electrocardiogram.*

    w., pulse. The pressure wave originated by the systolic discharge of blood into the aorta. It is not due to the passage of the ejected blood but is the result of the impact being transmitted through the arterial walls. Its speed of transmission varies with the nature of the arterial wall, increasing with age as the arteries become less resilient. Thus in arteriosclerosis, the velocity is increased over normal.

    w., Q. SEE: *electrocardiogram.*

    w., R. SEE: *electrocardiogram.*

    w.'s, radio. Electromagnetic waves between the frequencies of 10^{11} and 10^4 hertz.

    w., S. SEE: *electrocardiogram.*

    w.'s, sound. Vibrations of a vibrating medium that, upon stimulating sensory receptors of the cochlea, are capable of giving rise to sensations of sound. Velocity: in dry air, 1087 ft (331.6 meters) per sec at 0°C; in water, approx. 4 times faster than in air.

    w., T. SEE: *electrocardiogram.*

    w.'s, theta. Brain waves present in the electroencephalogram. They have a frequency of about 4 to 7 hertz.

    w., ultrashort. Arbitrary designation of radio waves of a wavelength of less than 1 meter.

    w., ultrasonic. A sound wave of greater frequency than 20 kilohertz. These waves do not produce sound audible to the human ear.

wavelength (wāv'lĕngth). The distance between the beginning and end of a single wave cycle, usually measured from the top of one wave to the top of the next one.

wax [AS. *weax*]. 1. Beeswax, secreted by bees; a substance that is solid at room temperature. In medicine, a purified form, white wax, is used in making ointments and to stop bleeding from bones during surgery. 2. Any substance with the consistency of beeswax. 3. Earwax. SYN: *cerumen.*

    w., dental. A variety of waxes compounded for their specific properties desired for dental procedures, e.g., baseplate wax, bone wax, boxing wax, burnout wax, casting wax, inlay wax, and pattern wax.

waxing-up. In dentistry, the shaping of wax around the contours of a trial denture.

waxy (wăks'ē) [AS. *weax*, wax]. Resembling or pert. to wax.

waxy cast. Dense, highly refractile urinary

cast. Such casts have clean-cut contours; sometimes irregular curves and notches. Occurs in severe chronic renal disease.

waxy degeneration. Amyloid degeneration seen in wasting diseases.

WBC. *white blood cells; white blood count.*

weak (wĕk) [Old Norse *veikr*, flexible]. 1. Lacking physical strength or vigor; infirm, esp. as compared with what would be the normal or usual for that individual.

RS: asthenia; atony; cardiasthenia; enervation; ergasthenia; fatigue; lassitude.

2. Dilute, as in a weak solution; or weak tea.

weakness. A precise but subjective term used by a patient to indicate a lack of strength as compared with what he or she feels is normal. The cause may be organic or a combination of an organic and a mental state. In either event, the symptom, if it is unremitting, requires careful investigation with special attention being given to determining potentially lethal causes that may be curable, e.g., cancer, anemia, certain parasitic or infectious diseases, or neurologic conditions.

wean (wēn) [AS. *wenian*]. 1. To accustom an infant to discontinuation of breast milk by substitution of other nourishment. 2. The slow discontinuation of ventilatory support therapy.

weanling. A young child or infant recently changed from breast to formula feeding.

weanling diarrhea. Severe gastroenteritis that sometimes occurs in infants who recently have been weaned.

web. A tissue or membrane extending across a space.

    w., esophageal. A tissue in the form of a web that extends across the esophageal lumen and thus interferes with the swallowing of food.

    w., terminal. A weblike network, microscopic in size, that is beneath the microvilli of absorption cells of the intestines, and beneath the hair cells of the inner ear.

webbed (wĕbd) [AS. *webb*, a fabric]. Having a membrane or tissue connecting adjacent structures, as the toes of a duck's feet.

Weber-Christian disease (wĕb′ĕr-krĭs′ chĕn) [Fredrick Parkes Weber, Brit. physician, 1863–1962; Henry A. Christian, U.S. physician, 1876–1951]. Relapsing, febrile, nodular, nonsuppurative panniculitis, a generalized disorder of fat metabolism characterized by recurring episodes of fever and development of crops of subcutaneous fatty nodules.

Weber's glands (vā′bĕrz) [Moritz I. Weber, Ger. anatomist, 1795–1875]. Mucous glands on the lateral borders of the lateral edges of the tongue.

Weber's paralysis (wĕb′ĕrz) [Sir Hermann David Weber, Brit. physician, 1823–1918]. Paralysis of oculomotor nerve on one side with contralateral spastic hemiplegia.

    ETIOL: Lesion of the crus cerebri.

Weber test [Friedrich Eugen Weber, Ger. otologist, 1823–1891]. Test for unilateral deafness. A vibrating tuning fork held against the midline of the top of the head is perceived as being so located by those with equal hearing ability in the ears; to persons with unilateral conductive-type deafness, the sound will be perceived as being more pronounced on the diseased side; in persons with unilateral nerve-type deafness, the sound will be perceived as being louder in the good ear.

Wechsler Intelligence Scale for Children. ABBR: WISC. A widely used intelligence test for children aged 5 to 16.

wedge. A solid object with a broad base and two sides arising from the base to intersect each other and to form an acute angle opposite the base.

wedge pressure. Pulmonary artery wedge pressure, q.v.

WEE. *western equine encephalomyelitis.*

weeping [AS. *wepan*, to lament]. 1. Shedding tears. 2. Moist, dripping.

weeping eczema. Dermatitis with eruption of vesicles exuding serum.

weeping sinew. Circumscribed cystic swelling of a tendon sheath.

Wegener's granulomatosis or syndrome [F. Wegener, 20th century Ger. pathologist]. A rare condition characterized by vasculitis, granulomatous lesions of the entire respiratory tract, and glomerulonephritis. The symptoms are fever, weakness, malaise, weight loss, purulent rhinitis, sinusitis, polyarthralgia, ulcerations of the nasal septum, and signs of severe progressive renal disease. The prognosis is very good if it is diagnosed early and treated initially with cyclophosphamide and corticosteroids and then with cyclophosphamide alone. If undesired side effects occur due to cyclophosphamide, azathioprine may be used in place of it. If it is not treated early, death is the outcome, usually within one year.

Weidel reaction (vī′dĕl) [Hugo Weidel, Austrian chemist, 1849–1899]. Test for presence of xanthine bodies or uric acid.

Weigert's law (vī′gĕrts) [Carl Weigert, Ger. pathologist, 1845–1904]. An observation that states that loss or destruction of tissue results in an excess of new tissue during repair.

weight (wāt) [AS. *gewiht*]. The gravitational force exerted on an object, usually by the earth. The unit of weight is the newton. One newton equals 0.225 pounds. The difference

1983 Metropolitan Height and Weight Tables for Men and Women According to Frame, Ages 25–59

	Men				Women		
Height (In Shoes)*	**Weight in Pounds (In Indoor Clothing)†**			**Height (In Shoes)***	**Weight in Pounds (In Indoor Clothing)†**		
Ft. In.	Small Frame	Medium Frame	Large Frame	Ft. In.	Small Frame	Medium Frame	Large Frame
5 2	128–134	131–141	138–150	4 10	102–111	109–121	118–131
5 3	130–136	133–143	140–153	4 11	103–113	111–123	120–134
5 4	132–138	135–145	142–156	5 0	104–115	113–126	122–137
5 5	134–140	137–148	144–160	5 1	106–118	115–129	125–140
5 6	136–142	139–151	146–164	5 2	108–121	118–132	128–143
5 7	138–145	142–154	149–168	5 3	111–124	121–135	131–147
5 8	140–148	145–157	152–172	5 4	114–127	124–138	134–151
5 9	142–151	148–160	155–176	5 5	117–130	127–141	137–155
5 10	144–154	151–163	158–180	5 6	120–133	130–144	140–159
5 11	146–157	154–166	161–184	5 7	123–136	133–147	143–163
6 0	149–160	157–170	164–188	5 8	126–139	136–150	146–167
6 1	152–164	160–174	168–192	5 9	129–142	139–153	149–170
6 2	155–168	164–178	172–197	5 10	132–145	142–156	152–173
6 3	158–172	167–182	176–202	5 11	135–148	145–159	155–176
6 4	162–176	171–187	181–207	6 0	138–151	148–162	158–179

* Shoes with 1-inch heels.
† Indoor clothing weighing 5 pounds for men and 3 pounds for women.
Source of basic data: Build Study, 1979, Society of Actuaries and Association of Life Insurance Medical Directors of America, 1980.
Copyright 1983 Metropolitan Life Insurance Company.

between weight and mass is that the weight of an object varies with the force of gravity, but the mass remains the same; e.g., an object will weigh less on the moon than on earth because the force of gravity is less on the moon; but the mass of the object would be the same in both places. SEE: *mass* (def. 3).

Weight of the body increases in pathological obesity and decreases in Addison's disease, AIDS, cancer, chronic diarrhea, chronic suppurations, untreated Type I diabetes mellitus, hysteria, anorexia, fevers, lactation when prolonged, marasmus, obstruction of pylorus or thoracic duct, starvation, tuberculosis, and ulcer of the stomach.

Normal weight depends upon the frame of the individual. SEE: table.

w., apothecaries'. SEE: *apothecaries' weights and measures.*

w., atomic. ABBR: at. wt. Weight of an atom of an element compared with that of oxygen which is taken as 16; the mean value of the isotopic weights of an element.

w., avoirdupois. SEE: *avoirdupois measure.*

w., equivalent. Weight of a chemical element that is equivalent to and will replace a hydrogen atom (1.008 grams) in a chemical reaction.

w., molecular. ABBR: mol. wt. The sum of all the atomic weights of all the elements in one molecule of a compound.

w., set point. The concept that body weight is controlled by the central nervous system and set at a certain value; the value is more or less stable until something occurs to alter it. An example of resetting of the set point occurs in persons with a disturbance of hypothalamic function that interferes with the satiety center, q.v., and the feeding center, q.v.

weightlessness. Condition of not being acted upon by the force of gravity. It is present when astronauts travel in areas so distant from the earth, moon, or planets that the force of gravity is virtually absent.

weights and measures. SEE: *Weights and Measures* in *Appendix.*

Weil's disease (vīlz) [Adolf Weil, Ger. physician, 1848–1916]. Severe leptospirosis caused by any one of several serotypes of *Leptospira interrogans* such as *L. icterohemorrhagica* in rats, *L. pomona* in swine, or *L. canicola* in dogs. All of these may be pathogenic for humans.

ETIOL: An organism found in rat urine and feces, and acquired by humans through contaminated food or water or by contact of broken skin with an infected rat or its feces or urine. It is a specific infection accompanied by muscular pains, fever, jaundice, and enlargement of liver and spleen.

TREAT: Symptomatic; also, if given very early in the disease, large doses of penicillin G or tetracycline I.V. may be of benefit.

Weil-Felix reaction, test (vīl-fā'līks) [Edmund Weil, Austrian bacteriologist, 1880–1922; Arthur Felix, Ger. bacteriologist, 1887–1956]. The agglutination of certain *Proteus* organisms due to the development of *Proteus* antibodies in certain rickettsial diseases.

Weir Mitchell's treatment (wēr mĭt'chĕlz) [Silas Weir Mitchell, U.S. neurologist, 1829–1914]. Treatment for hysteria and neurasthenia that consists of rest in bed, massage, nourishing diet, and isolation.

weismannism (wīs'măn-ĭzm) [August F. L. Weismann, Ger. biologist, 1834–1914]. The theory that acquired characteristics are not inherited.

Weitbrecht's foramen (vīt'brĕkts) [Josias Weitbrecht, Ger.-born Russian anatomist, 1702–1747]. An opening in the articular cartilage of the shoulder joint.

Weitbrecht's ligament. The oblique cord connecting the ulna and radius.

Welch's bacillus (wĕlsh'ĕz) [William Henry Welch, U.S. pathologist, 1850–1934]. *Clostridium perfringens,* the causative organism of gas gangrene. SEE: *gangrene, gas.*

welding. The joining of separate pieces of metal by compression and fusion with heat but without solder. Different names are applied designating the energy source or type of welding, such as arc w., fusion w., gas w., laser w., pressure w., and spot w.

welt [ME. *welte*]. An elevation on the skin produced by a lash, blow, or allergic stimulus. The skin is unbroken and the mark is reversible.

wen (wĕn) [AS.]. A cyst resulting from the retention of secretion in a sebaceous gland. SYN: *sebaceous cyst; steatoma.* SEE: *Fordyce's disease.*

SYM: One or more rounded or oval elevations, varying in size from a few millimeters to about 10 centimeters, slowly appear on scalp, face, or back; painless, rather soft, containing a yellow-white caseous mass.

TREAT: Sac and contents should be carefully dissected in order to prevent its recurrence.

Wenckebach's period, pauses, or phenomenon (vĕn'kĕ-bäks) [Karel F. Wenckebach, Dutch-born Aust. internist, 1864–1940]. A form of incomplete heart block in which, as detected by electrocardiography, there is progressive lengthening of the P-R interval until there is not a ventricular response; and then the cycle of increasing P-R intervals begins again.

Werdnig-Hoffmann disease (vĕrd'nĭg-hŏf'măn) [Guido Werdnig, Austrian neurologist, 1844–1919; Johann Hoffmann, Ger. neurologist, 1857–1919]. A hereditary, progressive, infantile form of muscular atrophy resulting from degeneration of anterior horn cells of the spinal cord. Characterized by early onset, hypotonia and wasting of muscles, complete flaccid paralysis, and death.

Werdnig-Hoffmann paralysis. Infantile muscular atrophy, considered by some to be identical with amyotonia congenita. SEE: *Hoffmann's syndrome.*

Werdnig-Hoffmann syndrome. SEE: *Hoffmann's syndrome.*

Werlhof's disease (vĕrl'hŏfs) [Paul G. Werlhof, Ger. physician, 1699–1767]. Idiopathic thrombocytopenic purpura. SEE: *purpura, idiopathic thrombocytopenic.*

Wermer's syndrome [Paul Wermer, U.S. physician, d. 1975]. Multiple endocrine neoplasia, q.v.

Wernicke's encephalopathy (vĕr'nĭ-kēz) [Karl Wernicke, Ger. neurologist, 1848–1905]. Encephalopathy associated with thiamine deficiency. Usually associated with chronic alcoholism, gastric carcinoma, or hyperemesis gravidarum.

Wernicke's syndrome. Frequent condition of old age marked by loss of memory and disorientation with confabulation. SYN: *presbyophrenia.* SEE: *polioencephalitis, anterior superior.*

western blotting. A technique for analyzing protein antigens. Initially, the antigens are separated by electrophoresis and transferred to a solid membrane by blotting. The membrane is incubated with antibodies; and then the bound antibodies are detected by enzymatic or radioactive methods. This method is used to detect small amounts of antibodies.

Westphal-Edinger nucleus [Karl Westphal, Ger. neurologist, 1833–1890; Ludwig Edinger, Ger. neurologist, 1855–1918]. Small group of nerve cells in rostral portion of nucleus of oculomotor nerve. Efferent fibers pass to ciliary ganglion conveying impulses destined for intrinsic muscles of the eye.

Westphal-Strümpell pseudosclerosis (vĕst'fäl-strĭm'p'l) [K. Westphal; Adolf G. G. von Strümpell, Ger. physician, 1853–1925]. 1. Hepatolenticular degeneration. SEE: *Wilson's disease.* 2. Hysteria with symptoms of disseminated sclerosis but no pathological changes in the nervous system.

wet (wĕt) [AS. *waet*]. Soaked with moisture, usually water.

wet brain. Increased amount of cerebrospinal fluid with edema of the meninges. May be associated with alcoholism.

wet cup. A cupping glass used after scarification.

wet dream. Nocturnal seminal emission.

wet-dry dressing or pack. SEE: *pack, wet-dry.*

wet nurse. A woman who breastfeeds another's child.

wet nurse phenomenon. The production of milk in response to repeated stimulation of the nipples in women who have previously been pregnant.

wet pack. A form of bath given by wrapping patient in hot or cold wet sheets, covered with a blanket, used esp. to reduce fever.

Wetzel grid (wĕt′sĕl) [Norman C. Wetzel, U.S. pediatrician, b. 1897]. A graph for use in evaluating growth and development in children aged 5 to 18 years.

Wharton's duct (hwăr′tŏnz) [Thomas Wharton, Brit. anatomist, 1614–1673]. Duct of the submandibular salivary gland opening into the mouth at side of the frenulum linguae.

Wharton's jelly. A gelatinous intercellular substance consisting of primitive connective tissue of the umbilical cord. It is rich in hyaluronic acid.

wheal (hwēl). 1. [AS. *hwele*] More or less round and evanescent elevation of the skin, white in center with pale red periphery, accompanied by itching. Seen in urticaria, insect bites, anaphylaxis, angioneurotic edema. SYN: *pomphus.* 2. [ME. *wale,* a stripe] An elongated mark or ridge. Such a ridge produced for intradermal injection or caused by injection or tests.

wheat (hwēt) [AS. *hwaete*]. Any of various cereal grasses, widely cultivated for its important edible grain used in making flour. Boiled whole wheat is an excellent food. SEE: *bread.*

STRUCTURE: Husk or outer coat, removed before grinding; bran coats, removed in making white flour and containing the mineral substances; gluten, contains the fat and protein; starch, center of the kernel.

Refined wheat products do not include the bran and germ, which contain B complex vitamins, phosphorus, and iron.

WHEAT PREPARATIONS AND PASTAS: Macaroni, vermicelli, and noodles are made from flour and water, molded, dried, and slightly baked. They are easy to digest, and not over 10% of nitrogen content is lost.

wheat germ oil. The oil expressed from the germ of the wheat seed.

wheatstone bridge. An electric circuit with two branches each containing two resistors. These branches are joined to complete the circuit. If the resistance in three resistors is known, the resistance of the fourth and unknown one can be calculated.

wheel. A disc attached through its middle to an axle that rotates. In dentistry, small wheels are attached to a handpiece and used for polishing and shaping teeth and restorations.

    w., carborundum. A cutting wheel containing silicon carbide. Variable grit sizes are available.

    w., diamond. In dentistry, a wheel that contains diamond chips.

    w., polishing. In dentistry, a wheel made of soft material suitable for polishing teeth or restorations.

    w., wire. A wheel containing pieces of wire. It is used for cleaning metal surfaces.

wheelchair. A special chair equipped with usually two large and two small wheels for transporting patients. Especially useful in enabling partially paralyzed individuals to be mobile and to have occupations that might otherwise be impossible.

Wheelchairs are made in a variety of sizes and weights to accommodate the patient and the type of injury. The universal wheelchair has larger wheels in the back and may be used indoors or outdoors. A wheelchair for amputees is available with rear wheels that are set farther back to compensate for the loss of weight of the amputated limbs. Power-driven wheelchairs are especially useful for patients who cannot propel themselves.

A tread-equipped wheelchair capable of negotiating curbs, rough terrain, and stairs has been used experimentally.

wheeze (hwēz) [ME. *whesen*]. A whistling or sighing sound resulting from narrowing of the lumen of a respiratory passageway. Often only noted by use of stethoscope. Occurs in asthma, croup, hay fever, mitral stenosis, and pleural effusion. May result from presence of tumors, foreign obstructions, bronchial spasm, tuberculosis, obstructive emphysema, or edema.

wheezing. Production of whistling sounds during difficult breathing such as occurs in asthma, coryza, croup, and other respiratory disorders. SEE: *wheeze.*

whelk (hwĕlk) [AS. *hwylca*]. A wheal; a protuberance on the face as a nodule or tubercle.

whey. The watery material separated from the curd of milk that has coagulated.

whiff. 1. A slight gust or puff of air, esp. one conveying an odor. 2. A quick inhalation or exhalation, as of tobacco smoke.

whinolalia (wĭn"ō-lā′lē-ă) [AS. *whinan,* whine, + Gr. *lalein,* to talk]. Hypernasality and distortion of speech. Occurs in incompetent palate syndrome.

whiplash injury. Imprecise term for injury to the cervical vertebrae and adjacent soft tissues. Produced by a sudden jerking or relative backward or forward acceleration of the head with respect to the vertebral column. Injury may occur to those in a vehicle that is suddenly and forcibly struck from the rear.

Whipple's disease (hwĭp′ĕlz) [George Hoyt Whipple, U.S. pathologist, 1878–1976]. Intestinal lipodystrophy, characterized by abnormal skin pigmentation, fatty stools, loss of weight and strength, chronic arthritis, a distinctive lesion of the mucosa of the jejunum and ileum, and other signs of a malabsorption syndrome. This rare disease resembles idiopathic steatorrhea. SYN: *intestinal lipodystrophy.*

TREAT: Intensive antibiotic therapy with procaine penicillin followed by maintenance therapy with tetracycline provides good results.

whipworm. Common name for a roundworm often parasitic in the human intestines. SYN: *Trichuris trichiura.*

whirl (hwŭrl) [Old Norse *hvirfla*]. 1. To revolve rapidly. 2. To feel giddiness.

whirlbone. 1. The kneecap. SYN: *patella.* 2. The head of the femur.

whirlpool bath. SEE: *bath, whirlpool.*

whiskey, whisky (hwĭs′kē). A distilled alcoholic liquor made from grain. The alcohol present is ethyl alcohol.

Caution: Wood or methyl alcohol should never be used in alcoholic beverages intended for human consumption. It is extremely toxic and may cause death. In those who survive, blindness is a common occurrence.

---

whisper (hwĭs′pĕr) [AS. *hwisprian*]. 1. Speech with a low, soft voice; a low, sibilant sound. 2. To utter in a low sound.

w., cavernous. Direct transmission of a whisper through a cavity in auscultation.

whistle (hwĭs′ĕl). 1. A sound produced by pursing one's lips and blowing. 2. A tubular device driven by wind that produces a loud and usually shrill sound.

whistling face syndrome. A congenital malformation with muscle dysfunction that produces a masklike "whistling face." Also present are hypoplastic nasal bones and clubfeet. The genetic transmission may be autosomal recessive.

white (hwīt) [AS. *hwit*]. 1. The achromatic color of maximum lightness that reflects all rays of the spectrum. 2. The color of milk or fresh snow; opposite of black.

white cell. The leukocyte.

white gangrene. Gangrene due to local anemia.

whitehead (hwĭt′hĕd). Milium, q.v.

white leg. Phlebitis of femoral vein marked by white swelling of the leg. SYN: *phlegmasia alba dolens.*

white line. White tendinous attachment of abdominal oblique and transverse muscles. Visible in the midline of the skin covering the anterior wall of the abdomen. SYN: *linea alba.*

white lotion. USP. A combination of zinc sulfate, and sulfurated potassium diluted in purified water, used in treating certain skin diseases.

white matter. Any nervous structure composed of white medullated nerve fibers.

white of egg. The albumin of an egg.

white of eye. Conjunctiva.

white ointment. USP. Ointment containing white wax and white petrolatum.

whitepox (hwĭt′pŏks). Variola minor.

white precipitate. A white amorphous powder used principally in ointments for external treatment of some skin diseases. SYN: *ammoniated mercury.*

whites. Slang for leukorrhea, q.v.

white softening. Stage of softening of any substance in which the affected area has become white and anemic.

whitlow (hwĭt′lō) [ME. *whitflawe,* white flow]. Suppurative inflammation at the end of a finger or toe. It may be deep seated, involving the bone and its periosteum, or superficial, affecting parts of the nail. SYN: *felon; panaris; paronychia; runaround.*

w., herpetic. Whitlow due to herpes simplex virus. It is painful and accompanied by lymphadenopathy.

Whitmore's disease [Alfred Whitmore, Brit. surgeon, 1876–1946]. Melioidosis, q.v.

W.H.O. *World Health Organization.*

whole body counter. Instrument that detects the radiation present in the entire body.

whole bowel irrigation. Decontamination technique to mechanically cleanse the entire gastrointestinal tract in cases of poisoning in which emesis is dangerous because aspiration may occur and in cases where ingested pills are too big to be evacuated via gastric lavage. Involves oral administration of several liters of isotonic, isosmotic polyethylene glycol in a balanced salt solution. Trade name is Go-Lytely.

wholism. Holism, q.v.

wholistic health. SEE: *holistic medicine.*

whoop (hoop) [AS. *hwopan,* to threaten]. The sonorous and convulsive inspiratory crow following a paroxysm of whooping cough.

whooping cough. An acute infectious disease caused by *Bordetella pertussis* with re-current spasms of coughing ending in a whooping inspiration. SYN: *pertussis*.

whorl (hwŭrl) [ME. *whorle*]. 1. Spiral arrangement of cardiac muscular fibers. SYN: *vortex.* 2. A type of fingerprint in which the central papillary ridges turn through at least one complete circle. SEE: *fingerprint* for illus.

Widal's reaction or test (vē-dŏlz') [Georges Fernand Isidore Widal, Fr. physician, 1862–1929]. An agglutination test for typhoid fever.

wig. A covering for the head either to simulate hair if the individual is bald or partially bald, or to cover one's own hair as part of a ceremony or costume.

Wigs are especially beneficial for use by patients who have lost their hair due to natural causes or as a result of therapy with certain types of cytotoxic agents used in cancer chemotherapy.

Wigs may be made of hair or synthetic fibers such as acrylic.

wild cherry. The dried bark of *Prunus sero-tina*, used principally in the form of syrup as a flavored vehicle for cough medicine.

will [AS.]. 1. The mental faculty used in choosing or deciding upon an act or thought. 2. Power of controlling one's actions or emotions.

Willis' circle (wĭl'ĭs) [Thomas Willis, Brit. anatomist, 1621–1675]. An intercommunicating set of arteries that encircles the optic chiasm and hypophysis, from which the principal arteries supplying the brain are derived. It receives blood from the two internal carotid arteries and the basilar artery formed by union of the two vertebral arteries. SEE: illus.

Willis' cords. Cords crossing the superior longitudinal sinus transversely.

Wilms' tumor (vĭlmz) [Max Wilms, Ger. surgeon, 1867–1918]. Rapidly developing tumor of the kidney that usually occurs in children. In the past, the mortality from this cancer was extremely high. Newer approaches to therapy have been very effective in controlling the tumor. SYN: *embryonal carcinosarcoma; nephroblastoma.* SEE: *Nursing Diagnoses* in *Appendix*.

Wilson's disease (wĭl'sŭnz) [Samuel Alexander Kinnier Wilson, Brit. internist, 1877–1937]. A hereditary syndrome transmitted as an autosomal recessive trait in which a decrease of ceruloplasmin, q.v., permits accumulation of copper in various organs (brain, liver, kidney, and cornea) associated with increased intestinal absorption of copper. A pigmented ring (Kayser-Fleischer ring) at the outer margin of the cornea is pathognomonic. Syndrome is characterized by degenerative changes in the brain, cirrhosis of the liver, splenomegaly, tremor, muscular rigidity, involuntary movements, spastic contractures, psychic disturbances, dysphagia, and progressive weakness and emaciation. SYN: *degeneration, hepatolenticular.*

TREAT: The untreated disease is fatal. The goal is to prevent further buildup of copper accumulation in tissues. This is done by avoiding foods high in copper. Also to reduce the copper in the tissues by giving the copper binder, D-penicillamine, until serum copper level returns to normal.

Caution: The copper binder, D-penicillamine, may cause pyridoxine and iron deficiency.

Wilson-Mikity syndrome [Miriam G. Wilson, U.S. pediatrician, b. 1922; Victor G. Mikity, U.S. radiologist, b. 1919]. A so-called pulmonary dysmaturity syndrome seen in premature infants. The symptoms are insidious onset of dyspnea, tachypnea, and cyanosis in the first month of life. Roentgenograms of the lungs reveal evidence of emphysema that develops into multicysts. Therapy is directed to the pulmonary insufficiency and cardiac failure. The death rate is about 25%.

Winckel's disease (vĭng'kĕlz) [Franz von Winckel, Ger. gynecologist, 1837–1911]. A fatal disease of the newborn characterized by profuse hemorrhages, hematuria, jaundice, enlarged spleen, collapse, and convulsions.

windburn. Erythema, and irritation of the skin due to exposure to wind. Simultaneous exposure to the sun, moisture, wind, and cold may cause a severe dermatitis.

windchill. The cooling effect wind has on exposed human skin.

windchill factor. Loss of heat from exposure of skin to wind. Heat loss is proportional to the speed of the wind. Thus, skin exposed to a wind velocity of 20 miles per hour (mph) (32 kilometers per hour) when the temperature is 0°F (−17.8°C) will be cooled at the same rate it would be in still air at −46°F (−43.3°C). Similarly when the temperature is 20°F (−6.7°C) and the wind is 10, 20, or 35 mph (16.1, 32.2, or 56.3 kilometers per hour), the equivalent skin temperature would be −4°, −18°, or −28°F (−20°, −27.8°, or −33.3°C), respectively.

Windchill factor is calculated for dry skin. Skin that is wet from any cause and exposed to wind will lose heat at a much higher rate than dry skin. Wind blowing over wet skin can cause frostbite, even on a comfortably warm day as judged by the thermome-

ARTERIES OF THE CIRCLE OF WILLIS OF THE BRAIN

POSTERIOR COMMUNICATING ARTERY

POSTERIOR CEREBRAL ARTERY

SUPERIOR CEREBELLAR ARTERY

PONTINE ARTERIES

ANTERIOR COMMUNICATING ARTERY

INTERNAL CAROTID ARTERY

BASILAR ARTERY

INTERNAL AUDITORY ARTERY

ANTERIOR INFERIOR CEREBELLAR ARTERY

VERTEBRAL ARTERIES

ter.

windchill index. A table listing the windchill factor for various combinations of temperature and wind velocity.

winding sheet. Sheet used to wrap a dead body. SYN: *shroud*.

window [Old Norse *vindauga*]. 1. An aperture for the admission of light or air or both. 2. A small aperture into a cavity, esp. that of the inner ear. SEE: *fenestra*.

   w., aortic. In radiology, in a left anterior oblique or lateral view of the chest, a clear area bounded by the aortic arch, the bifurcation of the trachea, and the pericardial border.

   w., cochlear. The fenestra cochleae. SYN: *fenestra rotunda*.

   w., oval. The fenestra vestibuli.

   w., round. The fenestra cochleae. SYN: *fenestra rotunda*.

   w., vestibular. The oval window. SYN: *fenestra vestibuli*.

windowing. Cutting a hole in anything, esp. a plaster cast. Use to relieve pressure on skin or bony area.

windpipe. The tubular structure through which air passes from the larynx to the lungs. SYN: *trachea*.

wine (wīn) [L. *vinum*, wine]. 1. Fermented juice of any fruit, usually made from grapes and containing 10% to 15% alcohol. 2. Solution of a medicinal substance in wine. SYN: *vinum*.

wineglass. A fluid measure of approx. 2 fl. oz (60 ml).

wine sores. Slang term for superficial infected areas of the skin seen in alcoholics with poor personal hygiene. Erroneously thought to be due to specific action of the wine.

wing [Old Norse *vaengi*]. A structure resembling the wing of a bird, esp. the great and small wings of the sphenoid bone, q.v. SEE: *ala*.

wink [AS. *wincian*]. Brief, voluntary closure of one eye. In hemiplegia, the patient may not be able to blink or close the eye on the paralyzed side without at the same time closing the other eye. This is called *Revilliod sign* or *orbicularis sign*. SEE: *blink; Marcus Gunn syndrome*.

winking. SEE: *wink*.

   w., jaw. Involuntary simultaneous closing of the eyelid as the jaw is moved.

   w., jaw-, syndrome. Unilateral ptosis of the eye at rest; and rapid exaggerating elevation of the lid when the mandible is either depressed or moved to the opposite side of the ptosed lid. SYN: *Marcus Gunn syndrome.*

Winslow, foramen of (wĭnz′lō) [Jacob Benignus Winslow, Danish-born Fr. anatomist, 1669–1760]. The epiploic foramen.

Winslow, ligament of. The oblique popliteal ligament located at back of knee.

Winslow, pancreas of. The processus uncinatus of the pancreas.

Winstrol. Trade name for stanozolol.

wintergreen oil. Methyl salicylate, a colorless, yellowish, or reddish liquid that has a characteristic taste and odor. It is used as a flavoring substance and as a counterirritant applied topically in the form of salves, lotions, and ointments. Trade name is Wintergreen Oil. SYN: *methyl salicylate; sweet birch oil.*

winter itch. Itching occurring only in cold weather. Probably due to drying of skin that is deficient in natural lubrication. SYN: *pruritus hiemalis.*

wire (wīr). 1. Metal drawn out into threads of varying thickness. 2. To join fracture fragments together by use of wire.

w., arch. In dentistry, application of wire around the dental arch in order to correct irregularities of position of the teeth.

w., Kirschner. Steel wire placed through a long bone in order to apply traction to the bone.

w., ligature. Soft, thin wire used in orthodontics to anchor other dental devices to an arch wire.

w., separating. Soft wire used in dentistry to separate teeth prior to banding them.

wired. Slang for describing a person who is tense and anxious, esp. when the condition is caused by the effect of a psychoactive drug.

wiring (wīr′ĭng). Fastening bone fragments together by use of wire.

w., circumferential. Method of treating a fractured mandible by passing wires around the bone and a splint in the oral cavity.

w., continuous loop. Forming wire loops on both mandibular and maxillary teeth in order to provide attachment sites for rubber bands. This is used in treating fractures of the mandible.

w., craniofacial suspension. Use of bones not contiguous with the oral cavity for attachment of wires that lead from those bones to the fractured jaw segments.

w., Gilmer. Wiring of single opposed teeth by use of wire passed circumferentially around the two teeth and the ends twisted

together. Used to produce intermaxillary fixation.

w., Ivy loop. Placement of wire around adjacent teeth in order to provide an attachment of elastics.

w., perialveolar. Use of wires to fix a splint to the mandible. The wires are passed through the alveolar process from the buccal plate to the palate.

w., pyriform. Use of the nasal bones for stabilizing a fracture of the jaw. The wires are passed through the pyriform aperture of the nasal bone and then to the segment.

w., Stout's. W., continuous loop.

Wirsung, duct of (vēr′soong) [Johann Georg Wirsung, Ger. physician, 1600–1643]. Excretory duct of the pancreas. SYN: *duct, pancreatic.*

wisdom tooth (wĭz′dŏm). The last molar tooth on each side of the jaw. These four molars may appear as late as the 25th year or may never erupt.

Wiskott-Aldrich syndrome [Alfred Wiskott, Ger. pediatrician, b. 1898; Robert A. Aldrich, U.S. pediatrician, b. 1917]. A sex-linked, recessive disorder with a defect in both T and B cell function. It is characterized by eczema, thrombocytopenia with bleeding tendency, and infections, esp. of the ears. Treatment consists of antibiotics, but the possibility of superinfection by viruses, fungi, and *Pneumocystis carinii* must be watched for. The use of transfer factor obtained from activated lymphocytes has been effective in about half of the cases. Because of the variable severity of the disease, some patients have lived into their teens, but death may occur at an earlier age.

witch doctors. An imprecise term for native healers in some countries who attempt to treat illnesses by use of magic or use of bizarre combinations of materials such as baked insects, dried reptiles, and shrivelled flesh from a white man.

In some cultures the witch doctor may provide health-giving spells cast by marking the body of the patient with charcoal or razor blades.

In the Zulu culture, the witch doctor is known as isangoma, who serves as a link between spirits and their descendants. SEE: *voodoo.*

witches' milk. Milk secreted by the newly born infant's breast, stimulated by the lactating hormone circulating in the mother.

withdrawal. Cessation of administration of a drug, esp. a narcotic, or alcohol to which the individual has become either physiologically or psychologically addicted. Withdrawal symptoms vary with the type of drug used. Neonates may exhibit withdrawal symptoms from drugs or alcohol ingested by the mother during pregnancy. SEE: *drug addiction.*

withdrawal syndrome. Partial collapse resulting from withdrawal of alcohol, stimulants, or some opiates. SYN: *abstinence syndrome.*

witkop (wĭt'kŏp) [Afrikaans, white scalp]. Matted crusts in the hair producing a scalplike structure. Seen in South African natives. SYN: *dikwakwadi; white head.*

witness. A person having knowledge or information about a particular subject or event.

    w., expert. A person having superior knowledge, skills, education, experience, and training concerning a relevant subject. In litigation, expert witnesses are used to testify about liability, damage, and injury issues.

    w., fact. A person having personal knowledge about circumstances surrounding an event or transaction.

witzelsucht (vĭt'sĕl-zookt) [M. Jastrowitz, Ger. physician, b. 1839]. Condition produced by frontal lobe lesions characterized by self-amusement from poor jokes and puns. SEE: *moria.*

    w., primary affective. A peculiar variety of witzelsucht characterized by teutonization of nomenclature.

Wohlfahrtia (vōl-fär'tē-ä). A genus of flies parasitic in animal tissue, belonging to the family Sarcophagidae, order Diptera.

    W. magnifica. Species found in southeast Europe. The larvae may occur in human and animal wounds.

    W. opaca. Species occurring in Canada, a common parasite of wild animals. Human infants may become infested.

    W. vigil. Species found in Canada and northern United States.

wolffian body (wool'fē-ăn) [Kaspar Friedrich Wolff, Ger. anatomist, 1733–1794]. An embryonic organ on each side of the vertebral column. SYN: *mesonephros.* SEE: *archinephron; embryo; paroophoron; parovarium.*

wolffian cyst. One of the broad ligaments of the uterus.

wolffian duct. Duct in the embryo leading from the mesonephros to cloaca. From it develop the ductus epididymis, ductus deferens, seminal vesicle, ejaculatory duct, ureter, and pelvis of kidney. SYN: *mesonephric duct.*

wolffian tubules. One of 30 to 34 tubules that develop within the mesonephros and empty into the mesonephric duct. Most are transitional, persisting for only a short time. Some persist in adult males as the efferent ductules of the testis; others persist only as vestigial structures. SYN: *mesonephric tubules.* SEE: *epoophoron; paradidymis; paroophoron.*

Wolff-Parkinson-White syndrome [Louis Wolff, U.S. cardiologist, 1898–1972; Sir John Parkinson, Brit. physician b. 1885; Paul Dudley White, U.S. cardiologist, 1886–1973]. ABBR: WPW. Abnormality of cardiac rhythm that manifests as supraventricular tachycardia. The diagnosis is made by use of electrocardiography. The P-R interval is less than 0.12 second and the QRS complex contains an initial slur, called the delta wave, that broadens the complex. SEE: *pre-excitation, ventricular.*

Wolfina 100. Trade name for rauwolfia serpentina.

wolfram (wool'frăm). Tungsten.

wolfsbane (wŏlfs'bān). Old name for aconite root.

Wolhynia fever. Trench fever, q.v.

Wolman's disease [M. Wolman, Israeli physician, b. 1914]. An inherited metabolic disorder in which infants develop hepatosplenomegaly, calcification of the adrenal glands, and foam cells in the bone marrow and other tissues.

woman. An adult human female. SEE: *man.*

womb (woom) [AS. *wamb*]. Female organ for containing, protecting, and nourishing the fetus. SYN: *uterus.* SEE: *placenta.*

wood alcohol. CH_3OH. Alcohol obtained by distillation from wood. It is a poisonous substance; its ingestion may cause death, and in those who survive, loss of eyesight. SEE: *methanol; methyl alcohol.*

Wood's rays [Robert Williams Wood, U.S. physicist, 1868–1955]. Ultraviolet rays. Used to detect fluorescent materials in the skin and hair in certain disease states such as tinea capitis. The terms Wood's light and Wood's lamp have become synonymous for Wood's rays, even though these are misnomers.

wood tick. *Dermacentor andersoni,* an important North American species of tick, which causes tick paralysis and transmits causative organisms of Rocky Mountain spotted fever and tularemia.

wool. The curly hair that composes the fleece of sheep and other animals. Lanolin is obtained from sheep wool.

wool fat. Anhydrous lanolin, a fatty substance obtained from sheep's wool. Used as a base for ointments.

woolsorter's disease. A pulmonary form of anthrax that develops in those who handle wool contaminated with *Bacillus anthracis.*

word blindness. Inability to comprehend written words; a form of aphasia, q.v. SYN: *alexia.*

word salad. The use of words with no apparent meaning attached to them or to their relationship with one another. Usually found in schizophrenia.

work [Ger. *wirken*]. A force moving a resistance. The amount of work done is the product of the force in the direction of movement times the distance the resisting object is moved. Regardless of the force applied, if the resisting object is not moved, then no work has been done. This is not to say that energy has not been expended. Work is measured in units of force times distance, or newton meters. SEE: *calorie; erg.*

work, shift. SEE: *shift work.*

work and mental health. Though little studied, work is one of the major forces in promoting mental health. Freud noted, "Work has a greater effect than any other technique of living in binding the individual more closely to reality; in his work, at least, he is securely attached to a part of reality, his community." Goethe said, "Employment is nature's physician and is essential to human happiness." Assuming the truth of their statements, it is essential that one's work be meaningful, challenging, and worthy of human effort in order to be satisfying and effective in promoting mental health.

work hardening. A series of conditioning exercises that an injured worker performs in a rehabilitation program. These are designed to simulate the functional tasks encountered on the job to which the individual will return.

working through. In psychiatry, the combined endeavor of the patient and the therapist to understand the unconscious genesis of a symptom or mental illness.

workout. In athletics, a practice or training session.

work-up. The process of obtaining all of the necessary data for diagnosing and treating a patient. It should be done in an orderly manner so that essential elements will not be overlooked. Included are retrieval of all previous medical and dental records, the patient's family and personal medical history, social and occupational history, physical examination, laboratory studies, x-rays, and indicated diagnostic surgical procedures. The patient's work-up is an ongoing process wherein all hospital personnel involved cooperate in attempting to determine the correct diagnosis and effective therapy. SEE: *medical record, problem-oriented; nursing histories* for table.

World Health Organization. ABBR: W.H.O. The United Nations agency concerned with health. Its definition of health is as follows.

"Health is a state of complete physical and social well being, and not merely the absence of disease or infirmity. The enjoyment of the highest attainable standards of health is one of the fundamental rights of every human being without distinction of race, religion, political belief, economic or social condition. The health of all peoples is fundamental to the attainment of peace and security and is dependent upon the fullest cooperation of individuals and States. The achievement of any State in the promotion and protection of health is of value to all."

worm (wŭrm) [AS. *wyrm*]. 1. An elongated invertebrate belonging to one of the following phyla: Platyhelminthes (flatworms); Nemathelminthes or Aschelminthes (roundworms or threadworms); Acanthocephala (spinyheaded worms); and Annelida (Annulata) (segmented worms). SYN: *helminth.* SEE: individual worms by name. 2. Any small, limbless, creeping animal. 3. Median portion of the cerebellum. 4. Any wormlike structure.

wormian bones (wŭr′mē-ăn) [Ole Worm, Danish physician, 1588–1654]. Small, irregular bones in the course of the cranial sutures.

wormseed (wĕrm′sēd). The dried, unexpanded capitula of several ragweeds, such as *Artemisia santonica, A. maritima,* or *A. pauciflora,* from which the vermifuge santonin is obtained.

    w., American. *Chenopodium ambrosioides.*

wormwood (wĕrm′wood). A toxic substance, absinthium, obtained from *Artemisia absinthium.* It was used in certain alcoholic beverages (absinthe), but because of its toxicity, such use is prohibited in most countries.

worried well. Persons who are indeed well, but because of their anxiety or imagined illness, they frequent medical care facilities seeking reassurances concerning their health status.

wound (woond) [AS. *wund*]. Break in the continuity of soft parts of body structures caused by violence or trauma to tissues. In treating any wound, give the previously immunized patient a tetanus toxoid booster injection. If not previously immunized, the patient should be given tetanus immune globulin. If tetanus immune globulin is not available, the equine form may be used, but the patient must be tested for hypersensitivity prior to administering the full dose.

    w., abdominal. Frequently sustained and ordinarily involves structure of the abdominal wall. In such instances, the wound may be treated as an ordinary one. Where a cavity has been opened, and esp. if viscera have been exposed, attempt to keep the area sterile and moist. This will help to prevent infection.

w., bullet. A puncture wound from a bullet. Usually there is a small point of entrance. If the bullet left the body, there is a larger point of exit; it is associated with injuries of bone, tendon, or blood vessels. SEE: *Nursing Diagnoses* in *Appendix.*

SYM: Depend on site, speed, and character of bullet.

TREAT: Tetanus booster injection or tetanus immune globulin. Apply appropriate bandage. Antibiotics if indicated. Treat complications, including hemorrhage and shock.

w., cellulitis of. Local inflammation of a wound, occurring when wound has been closed without drainage, esp. in appendicitis.

SYM: Elevation of temperature from 4th to 7th day with an accompanying tenderness. Inspect dressing and chart findings.

TREAT: Evacuation of the abscess; hot, wet dressings; antibiotics.

w., contused. A bruise in which the skin is not broken. It may be caused by a blunt instrument. Injury of the tissues under the skin, leaving the skin unbroken, traumatizes the soft tissue. The blood vessels ruptured underneath the skin cause discoloration. If extravasated blood becomes encapsulated, it is termed hematoma; if it is diffused, ecchymosis. SEE: *ecchymosis; hematoma.*

TREAT: Cold compresses, pressure, and rest. Elevation of injured area will help prevent or reduce swelling. When acute stage is over (24 to 48 hr), continued rest, heat, and elevation are prescribed. Aseptic drainage may be indicated.

w., crushing. Trauma due to force applied to tissues so they are mashed or compressed, but with minimal or no lacerations. If wound is bleeding, apply cold cloths; if not, apply dressing and treat as an ordinary wound until patient can be given definitive surgical treatment. If bone is fractured, apply splint.

w., fishhook. Injury caused by fishhook becoming embedded in soft tissue. Deeply embedded fishhooks are difficult to remove. Push the hook through, then cut off barb with an instrument, and pull the remainder of the fishhook out by the route it entered. Antitetanus treatment as indicated. Frequently these injuries become infected, so prophylactic use of a broad-spectrum antibiotic is indicated.

w., incised. Any sharp cut in which the tissues are not severed; a clean cut caused by a keen cutting instrument. The wound may be either aseptic or infected, depending on

circumstances that caused it.

An aseptic wound, one occurring under surgical conditions, should heal if conditions are favorable and no contaminations due to pathogenic organisms or foreign material enter into it. During the healing process, the area of the wound must be kept aseptic. The skin must be cleansed with plain soap and water, rinsed thoroughly, and covered securely with sterile dressings to keep the wound clean. A clean wound should be left alone. The dressings should be changed only often enough to keep the wound clean. There should be no squeezing or pulling of its edges.

w., lacerated. A torn wound with ragged edges; not a clean wound. It is a type of wound that provides many avenues for infection. May be caused by many kinds of implements that may be covered with any kind of pathogenic bacteria. Thus a variety of types of wound infections may be expected. Antitetanus and gas gangrene prophylaxis may be needed.

TREAT: The wound should be cleansed with mild soap and water and rinsed thoroughly. If wound edges are ragged, they will need to be trimmed and dead tissue removed. The patient should be given tetanus antitoxin or tetanus booster, depending on previous history. The wound should never be sealed. It is best to hold the wound open with some form of drain.

w., nonpenetrating. Wound in which the surface of the skin remains intact.

w., open. Contusion in which skin is also broken, such as a gunshot, incised, or lacerated wound.

w., penetrating. Wound in which the skin is broken and the agent causing the wound enters subcutaneous tissue or a deeply lying structure or cavity.

w., perforating. Wound in which the object that caused it, such as a bullet, projectile, or knife, entered the body and emerged.

w., puncture. Wound made by a sharp-pointed instrument such as a dagger, ice pick, or needle. The chief danger is from thrombosis and possible release of emboli. A puncture wound usually is collapsed. This provides ideal conditions for infection. Placement of a drain, antitetanus therapy or prophylaxis, and gas gangrene prophylaxis may be required. This will depend on the nature of the instrument that caused the injury.

w., subcutaneous. All wounds, such as contusions, that are unaccompanied by a break in skin.

w., tunnel. Wound having a small entrance and exit of uniform diameter.

wound ballistics. Study of the effects on the

body produced by penetrating projectiles.

wound healing. SEE: *inflammation.*

W-plasty. Technique used in plastic surgery to prevent contractures in straight-line scars. Each side of the edges of a wound is cut in the form of connected W's, and the edges are sutured together in a zig-zag fashion. SEE: *tissue expansion; Z-plasty.*

wreath (rēth). A structure that encircles something so that it resembles a circlet of leaves and branches (laurel) worn around the head.

Wright's stain [James H. Wright, U.S. pathologist, 1871–1928]. A combination of eosin and methylene blue used in staining blood cells to reveal malarial parasites. SEE: *Wright's technique.*

Wright's technique. Method of staining blood smears. Cover the dried blood smear with 5 to 10 drops of Wright's stain. Let stand 1 min. Add an equal amount of neutral distilled water to the stain. Let diluted stain stand for 3 to 10 min. A metallic sheen should appear. Remove stain by gently washing with distilled water. Stand slide on end and allow to dry. Mount in balsam or methacrylate. If staining results are good, red cells will have a pink or copper color, white cells will have densely stained blue nuclei, and the cytoplasmic granules will stain variously in the different types of leukocytes. SEE: *leukocyte.*

wrinkle (rĭng'kl) [AS. *gewrinclian,* to wind]. 1. A crevice, furrow, or ridge in the skin. 2. To make creases or furrows, as in the skin by habitual frowning.

Wrisberg's cardiac ganglion (rĭs'bŭrgz) [Heinrich August Wrisberg, Ger. anatomist, 1739–1808]. Wrisberg's ganglion, q.v.

Wrisberg's cartilages. The cuneiform cartilages of the larynx.

Wrisberg's ganglion. Ganglion of the superficial cardiac plexus. It is between the aortic arch and the pulmonary artery. SYN: *Wrisberg's cardiac ganglion.* SEE: *ganglion, cardiac.*

Wrisberg's nerve. 1. The medial brachial cutaneous nerve, a branch of the medial cord of the brachial plexus. 2. The nervus intermedius (pars intermedia), a branch of the facial nerve lying between the motor root and the acoustic nerve.

wrist (rĭst) [AS]. The joint or region lying between the hand and the forearm.

wrist bones. The carpus, consisting of eight bones. SEE: *skeleton; hand* for illus.

wrist drop. Condition in which hand is flexed at wrist and cannot be extended; due to injury of radial nerve or paralysis of extensor muscles of wrist and hand.

wrist unit. A component of an upper extremity prosthesis that attaches the terminal device to the forearm section and provides for pronation or supination.

writer's cramp. A cramp affecting muscles of the thumb and two adjacent fingers after prolonged writing.

writing. The act of placing characters, letters, or words on a surface, usually paper, for the purpose of communicating ideas.

   w., dextrad. Writing that progresses from left to right.

   w., mirror. Writing so that letters and words are reversed and appear as in a mirror.

writing hand. Position of hand seen in paralysis agitans, marked by contraction of muscles of the hand. The fingers assume a position similar to that used in holding a pen.

wrongful birth or wrongful life. The concept that a birth or life would not have occurred if the parents had been adequately informed of the possibility that the mother would give birth to a physically or mentally defective child.

wryneck (rī'nĕk). Contracted state of one or more muscles of the neck, producing an abnormal position of the head. Occasionally it is acute, due to cold or trauma; more commonly it is chronic, spastic in character, and dependent upon nerve irritation. Has been produced by habitual malposition of the head assumed because of existing ocular defect. May be congenital. When acute, it generally passes away under influence of rest, heat, and time. Chronic wryneck may require surgical therapy. SYN: *loxia; torticollis.* SEE: *torticollis.*

w.s. *water-soluble.*

wt. *weight.*

Wuchereria (voo″kĕr-ē'rē-ă) [Otto Wucherer, Ger. physician, 1820–1873]. A genus of filarial worms belonging to the superfamily Filarioidea, class Nematoda. Common in warm regions of the world.

   W. bancrofti. The causative agent of elephantiasis. Adults of the species live in lymph nodes and ducts of humans. Females give birth to sheathed microfilariae, which remain in internal organs during the day but at night are in circulating blood, where they are sucked up by night-biting mosquitoes, in which they continue their development, becoming infective larvae in about two weeks. They are then passed on to the human when the mosquito bites. SYN: *Filaria bancrofti.*

   W. malayi. Species occurring in Southeast Asia and largely responsible for lymphangitis and elephantiasis in that region. Closely resembles *W. bancrofti.*

wuchereriasis (voo″kĕr-ē-rī'ă-sĭs). Infestation with filarial worms of the genus *Wuchereria.* SYN: *elephantiasis; filariasis.*

w/v. *weight in volume.* It indicates the amount

by weight of a solid substance dissolved in a measured quantity of liquid. Percent w/v expresses number of grams of an ingredient in 100 ml of solution.

w/w. *weight in weight.* It indicates the amount by weight of a solid substance dissolved in a known amount (by weight) of liquid. Percent w/w expresses the number of grams of one ingredient in 100 grams of solution.

Wyamine Sulfate. Trade name for mephentermine sulfate.

Wyamycin Liquid. Trade name for erythromycin ethylsuccinate.

Wyamycin S. Trade name for erythromycin stearate.

Wycillin. Trade name for penicillin G procaine.

Wydase. Trade name for hyaluronidase (injection).

X

X. Symbol for Kienböck's unit of x-ray dose; symbol for xanthine.

Xanax. Trade name for alprazolam, a triazolo-benzodiazepine antianxiety agent.

xanchromatic (zăn″krō-măt′ĭk). Xanthochromic.

xanthelasma (zăn″thĕl-ăz′mă) [Gr. *xanthos,* yellow, + *elasma,* plate]. 1. Yellow. 2. Flat or slightly raised yellowish tumor occurring in elderly persons, found most frequently on the upper and lower lids, esp. near the inner canthus. SYN: *xanthoma.*

xanthelasmoidea (zăn″thĕl-ăz-moy′dē-ă) [″ + ″. + *eidos,* form, shape]. Chronic disease of childhood marked by wheals and followed by yellow-brown patches. SYN: *urticaria pigmentosa.*

xanthematin (zăn-thĕm′ă-tĭn). A yellow substance produced by the action of nitric acid on hematin.

xanthemia (zăn-thē′mē-ă) [″ + *haima,* blood]. Occurrence of yellow pigment in the blood. SYN: *carotenemia.*

xanthene (zăn′thēn). A crystalline compound, $O=(C_6H_4)_2=CH_2$, from which various dyes are formed, including rhodamine and fluorescein.

xanthic (zăn′thĭk) [Gr. *xanthos,* yellow]. 1. Yellow. 2. Pert. to xanthine.

xanthic calculus. A urinary concretion containing xanthine.

xanthine (zăn′thĭn, -thēn). A nitrogenous compound present in muscle tissue, liver, spleen, pancreas, and other organs, and in the urine. It is formed during the metabolism of nucleoproteins.

    x., dimethyl-. Theobromine.

xanthine base. A group of chemical compounds including xanthine, hypoxanthine, uric acid, and theobromine, which have a purine as their base. SYN: *purine base.*

xanthinuria (zăn″thĭn-ū′rē-ă) [″ + *ouron,* urine]. Excretion of large amounts of xanthine in the urine.

xanthiuria (zăn″thē-ū′rē-ă). Xanthinuria.

xanthochroia (zan″thō-krō′ē-ă) [″ + *chroia,* skin]. Yellowish discoloration of the skin.

xanthochromatic (zăn″thō-krō-măt′ĭk). Xanthochromic.

xanthochromia (zăn″thō-krō′mē-ă) [″ + *chroma,* color]. Yellow discoloration, as of the skin in patches or of the cerebrospinal fluid, resembling jaundice.

xanthochromic (zăn″thō-krō′mĭk). 1. Pert. to anything that is yellow. 2. Pert. to xanthochromia.

xanthochroous (zăn-thŏk′rō-ŭs) [Gr. *xanthochroos*]. Having a yellowish or light complexion.

xanthocyanopia, xanthocyanopsia (zăn″thō-sī-ăn-ŏ′pē-ă, -ŏp′sē-ă) [Gr. *xanthos,* yellow, + *kyanos,* blue, + *opsis,* sight]. A form of color blindness in which yellow and blue are distinguishable, but not red and green. SYN: *xanthokyanopy.*

xanthocyte (zăn′thō-sīt) [″ + *kytos,* cell]. A cell containing yellow pigment.

xanthoderma (zăn″thō-dĕr′mă) [″ + *derma,* skin]. Yellowness of the skin.

xanthodont (zăn′thō-dŏnt) [″ + *odous,* tooth]. One who has yellow teeth.

xanthoerythrodermia perstans (zăn″thōĕrĭth″rō-dĕr′mē-ă). A rare symptomless disease requiring no treatment. It consists of persistent patches of erythema covered with fine scales, mostly on the trunk and limbs. SYN: *parapsoriasis.*

xanthogranuloma (zăn″thō-grăn″ū-lō′mă) [″ + L. *granulum,* grain, + *oma,* tumor]. A tumor having characteristics of both an infectious granuloma and a xanthoma.

    x., juvenile. A skin disease that may be present at birth or develop in the first months of life. The firm dome-shaped yellow, pink, or orange papules, ranging from a few mm to 4 cm in diameter, are usually present on the scalp, face, and upper trunk. Biopsy of these lesions reveals lipid-filled histiocytes, inflammatory cells, and Touton giant cells (multinucleated vacuolated cells with a wreath of nuclei and peripheral rim of foamy cytoplasm). Even though this illness is distressing, there is no need to attempt to treat the lesions because they regress spontaneously during the first years of life.

xanthokyanopy (zăn″thō-kī-ăn′ō-pē) [″ + *kyanos,* blue, + *opsis,* sight]. Partial blindness for color, only yellow and blue being discerned. SEE: *xanthocyanopia.*

xanthoma (zăn-thō′mă) [Gr. *xanthos,* yellow, + *oma,* tumor]. Flat, slightly elevated, soft rounded plaque or nodule, usually on the eyelids. May occur in patches of yellowish macule on orbital regions, confined to middle life or later. Consists of a degenerative process involving fibers of the orbicularis muscle.

    x., diabetic. Cutaneous disease associated with uncontrolled diabetes mellitus.

    x. disseminatum. Condition characterized by presence of xanthomata throughout the body, esp. on the face, in tendon sheaths, and in mucous membranes. SYN: *Hand-Schüller-Christian disease.*

   x. multiplex. Xanthomata all over the body.

   x. palpebrarum. Xanthoma affecting the eyelids.

   x. tuberosum. A form of xanthoma that may appear on the neck, shoulders, trunk, or extremities, consisting of small elastic and yellowish-colored nodules.

xanthomatosis (zăn"thō-mă-tō'sĭs) [" + " + *osis,* condition]. Condition in which there is a deposition of lipid in tissues usually accompanied by hyperlipemia. Cholesterol may accumulate in tumor nodules (xanthoma) or in individual cells, esp. histiocytes and reticuloendothelial cells.

xanthomatous (zăn-thō'mă-tŭs). Concerning xanthoma.

xanthophose (zăn'thō-fōz) [" + *phos,* light]. Any yellow phose. SEE: *phose.*

xanthophyll (zăn'thō-fĭl) [" + *phyllon,* leaf]. A yellow pigment derived from carotene. It is present in some plants and egg yolk.

xanthoprotein (zăn"thō-prō'tē-ĭn). Yellow substance produced by heating proteins with nitric acid.

xanthopsia (zăn-thŏp'sē-ă) [" + *opsis,* sight]. Condition in which objects appear to be yellow.

xanthopsin (zăn-thŏp'sĭn). The visual purple produced by light acting on rhodopsin.

xanthopsis (zăn-thŏp'sĭs). Yellow pigmentation seen in certain cancers and degenerating tissue.

xanthorrhea (zăn"thō-rē'ă) [" + *rhoia,* to flow]. Discharge of a yellow purulent substance from the vagina.

xanthosine (zăn'thō-sēn). 7-xanthine-D-ribose, a nucleoside formed by the deamination of guanosine.

xanthosis (zăn-thō'sĭs) [" + *osis,* condition]. A yellowing of the skin seen in carotenemia resulting from ingestion of excessive quantities of carrots, squash, egg yolk, and other foods containing carotenoids. Condition usually harmless, but it may indicate increase of lipochromes in blood due to other conditions such as hypothyroidism or diabetes.

xanthous (zăn'thŭs) [Gr. *xanthos,* yellow]. Yellow.

xanthurenic acid. $C_{10}H_7NO_4$. 4,8-dihydroxyquinaldic acid. Acid excreted in the urine of pyridoxine-deficient animals after they are fed tryptophan.

xanthuria (zăn-thū'rē-ă) [" + *ouron,* urine]. Excretion of an excess of xanthine in the urine. SYN: *xanthinuria.*

X chromosome. Chromosome that determines female sex characteristics. In the normal female there are two X chromosomes, and in the male one X chromosome and one Y chromosome. SEE: *chromosome.*

x-disease. Poisoning caused by ingestion of peanuts or peanut products contaminated with *Aspergillus flavus* or other *Aspergillus* strains that produce aflatoxin, q.v. Farm animals and humans are susceptible to this toxicosis. SYN: *aflatoxicosis.*

Xe. Chem. symbol for the element xenon.

xeno- [Gr. *xenos,* stranger]. Combining form indicating strange or a foreign material.

xenobiotic (zĕn"ō-bī-ŏt'ĭk). An antibiotic chemical substance not produced by the body, and thus foreign to it.

xenogeneic (zĕn"ō-jĕn-ā'ĭk) [" + *gennan,* to produce]. Tissues used for transplantation that are obtained from a species different from that of the recipient. SEE: *heterologous.*

xenogenesis (zĕn"ō-jĕn'ĕ-sĭs). Heterogenesis, q.v.

xenogenous (zĕn-ŏj'ĕn-ŭs) [Gr. *xenos,* stranger, + *gennan,* to produce]. 1. Caused by a foreign body. 2. Originating in the host, as a toxin resulting from stimuli applied to cells of the host.

xenograft (zĕn'ō-grăft) [" + L. *graphium,* stylus]. Surgical graft of tissue from one species to an individual of a different species. SYN: *heterograft.*

xenology (zĕn-ŏl'ō-jē) [" + *logos,* word, reason]. The study of parasites and their relationships to one another, and their hosts.

xenomenia (zĕn-ō-mē'nē-ă) [" + *meniaia,* menses]. Menstruation from a part of the body other than the normal one. SYN: *menstruation, vicarious; stigmata.*

xenon (zē'nŏn) [Gr. *xenos,* stranger]. SYMB: Xe. At. wt. 131.29; at. no. 54. A gaseous element in the atmosphere.

xenon-133. USP. A radioactive isotope of xenon used in photoscanning studies of the lung. SYN: $^{133}Xe.$

xenoparasite (zĕn"ō-păr'ă-sīt). An ectoparasite of a weakened animal, one that would not normally serve as a host.

xenophobia (zĕn"ō-fō'bē-ă) [" + *phobos,* fear]. Abnormal dread of strangers.

xenophonia (zĕn"ō-fō'nē-ă) [" + *phone,* voice]. Alteration in accent and intonation of a person's voice due to defect of speech.

xenophthalmia (zĕn"ŏf-thăl'mē-ă) [" + *ophthalmia,* eye inflammation]. Inflammation of the eye caused by a foreign body.

Xenopsylla (zĕn"ŏp-sĭl'ă) [" + *psylla,* flea]. A genus of fleas belonging to the family Pulicidae, order Siphonaptera.

   X. cheopis. The rat flea, but other hosts include humans and various animals. It is a vector for a number of pathogens including *Hymenolepis nana,* the dwarf tapeworm;

Salmonella organisms; and causative organisms of bubonic and sylvatic plague, and endemic typhus.

xenorexia (zĕn″ō-rĕk′sē-ă) [″ + *orexis*, appetite]. An abnormality of appetite marked by persistent swallowing of foreign objects.

xerantic (zē-răn′tĭk) [Gr. *xeros*, dry]. Causing dryness. SYN: *siccant; siccative.*

xerasia (zē-rā′sē-ă) [Gr. *xeros*, dry]. Disease of the hair in which there is abnormal dryness, brittleness, and eventual loss of hair.

xero- [Gr. *xeros*]. Prefix meaning dry.

xerocheilia (zē″rō-kī′lē-ă) [″ + *cheilos*, lip]. Dryness of the lips; a type of cheilitis.

xeroderma (zē″rō-dĕr′mă) [″ + *derma*, skin]. Roughness and dryness of the skin; mild ichthyosis.

x. pigmentosum. A rare disease of the skin starting in childhood and marked by disseminated pigment discolorations, ulcers, cutaneous and muscular atrophy, and death. SYN: *Kaposi's disease; melanosis lenticularis.*

xerography (zē-rŏg′ră-fē). Xeroradiography, q.v.

xeroma (zē-rō′mă) [″ + *oma*, tumor]. An abnormally dry state of the conjunctiva. SYN: *xerophthalmia.*

xeromammography (zē″rō-măm-mŏg′ră-fē). Xeroradiography of the breast.

xeromenia (zē″rō-mē′nē-ă) [″ + *meniaia*, menses]. The occurrence of the symptoms of menstruation without menstrual flow.

xeromycteria (zē″rō-mĭk-tē′rē-ă) [″ + *mykter*, nose]. Dryness of the nasal passages.

xeronosus (zē-rŏn′ō-sŭs) [″ + *nosos*, disease]. Dryness of the skin.

xerophagia (zē″rō-fā′jē-ă) [″ + *phagein*, to eat]. The eating of dry food only.

xerophagy (zē-rŏf′ă-jē). Xerophagia, q.v.

xerophthalmia (zē-rŏf-thăl′mē-ă) [″ + *ophthalmos*, eye]. Conjunctival dryness with keratinization of epithelium following chronic conjunctivitis and in disease due to deficiency of vitamin A. SEE: *Schirmer's test.*

xerophthalmus (zē″rŏf-thăl′mŭs). Xerophthalmia.

xeroradiography (zē″rō-rā″dē-ŏg′ră-fē). Method of photoreproduction used in radiography. It is a dry process involving the use of plates covered with a powdered substance, such as selenium, electrically and evenly charged. This is held between metal plates. The x-rays alter the charge or the substance to varying degrees dependent upon the tissues they have traversed. This produces the image.

xerosis (zē-rō′sĭs) [Gr.]. 1. Abnormal dryness of skin, mucous membranes, or the conjunctiva. 2. Normal sclerosis of tissues in the aged.

xerostomia (zē″rō-stō′mē-ă) [″ + *stoma*, mouth]. Dryness of the mouth caused by abnormal reduction in the amount of salivary secretion. It may occur in diabetes, hysteria, paralysis of facial nerve involving chorda tympani, acute infections, and some types of neuroses. It is induced by certain drugs such as nicotine and atropine. SEE: *ptyalism.*

xerotes (zē′rō-tēz) [Gr.]. Dryness.

xerotic (zē-rŏt′ĭk) [Gr. *xeros*, dry]. Dry; characterized by dryness.

xerotocia (zē″rō-tō′sē-ă) [″ + *tokos*, birth]. Dry labor due to diminished amount of amniotic fluid.

xerotripsis (zē″rō-trĭp′sĭs) [″ + *tripsis*, friction]. Dry friction.

xiphi-, xipho- [Gr. *xiphos*, sword]. Prefixes pert. to the xiphoid cartilage.

xiphisternum (zĭf″ĭ-stĕr′nŭm) [Gr. *xiphos*, sword, + *sternon*, chest]. The pointed process of the lower end of the sternum. SYN: *xiphoid process.*

xiphocostal (zĭf″ō-kŏs′tăl) [″ + L. *costa*, rib]. Rel. to the xiphoid cartilage and ribs.

xiphocostal ligament. Ligament connecting the xiphoid cartilage to the cartilage of the 8th rib.

xiphodynia (zĭf″ō-dĭn′ē-ă) [″ + *odyne*, pain]. Pain in the ensiform cartilage.

xiphoid (zĭf′oyd) [Gr. *xiphos*, sword, + *eidos*, form, shape]. Sword-shaped, ensiform.

xiphoiditis (zĭf″oyd-ī′tĭs) [″ + ″ + *itis*, inflammation]. Inflammation of the ensiform or xiphoid cartilage.

xiphoid process. The lowest portion of the sternum; sword-shaped cartilaginous process supported by bone. It has no ribs attached to it, but some of the abdominal muscles are attached to it. It ossifies in the aged. SEE: *sternum* for illus.

xiphopagotomy (zī-fŏp″ă-gŏt′ō-mē). Surgical separation of twins joined at the xiphoid process.

xiphopagus (zī-fŏp′ă-gŭs) [″ + *pagos*, thing fixed]. Symmetrical twins joined at the xiphoid process.

X-linked. Denoting characters that are transmitted by genes on the X chromosome. SEE: *choroideremia; hemophilia.*

X-linked disorders. Diseases due to genes located on the X chromosome.

x radiation. 1. Electromagnetic waves or energy composed of x-rays. 2. Treatment with or exposure to x-rays.

X-rated. 1. A motion picture considered to have obscene sections, thus making it suitable for showing to adults only. This rating terminology has been superseded. 2. Obscene, sexually explicit, or vulgar.

x-ray. A high-energy electromagnetic wave

varying in length from 0.05 to 100 angstrom units. X-rays are produced by bombarding a target in a vacuum tube with high-velocity electrons. Because of their ability to penetrate most solid matter to some extent and to act on photographic film, they are used both in diagnosis and therapy. SYN: *roentgen ray*. SEE: *roentgenogram*.

NURSING IMPLICATIONS: Explain diagnostic or therapeutic rationale to patient, and advise concerning procedures and possible discomfort. Prepare the patient according to protocol. Following procedure, recognize that most patients are fatigued and require a period of rest. Insure nutrition and hydration in patients who were kept n.p.o. prior to the procedure, esp. elderly or debilitated patients.

    x-r., bitewing. Roentgenogram taken with the film holder held between the teeth and the film parallel to the teeth. This technique permits film to be taken of several upper and lower teeth at the same time.

    x-r., strain. Roentgenogram taken with the part, usually a bone or joint, under static force or tension. Used to better demonstrate the pathological change that might be inapparent if this technique were not employed.

x-ray dermatitis. Cutaneous inflammation due to exposure to x-rays.

xylene (zī'lēn, zī-lēn'). A mixture of isomeric dimethylbenzenes used in making lacquers and rubber cement.

xylene poisoning. SEE: *benzene* in *Poisons and Poisoning* in *Appendix*.

xylenin (zī'lē-nĭn) [Gr. *xylon*, wood]. A toxic

substance extracted by xylene from tubercle bacilli.

xylenol (zī'lē-nŏl). General name for a series of dimethylphenols found in the pine-type coal tar disinfectants.

xylitol. A five-carbon sugar alcohol that has a sweet taste and has similar chemical properties to sucrose. It may be used in place of sucrose as a sweetener. Use of xylitol in the diet might reduce tooth decay in children.

xylo- [Gr. *xylon*, wood]. Prefix pert. to wood.

Xylocaine. Trade name for lidocaine hydrochloride.

xylol (zī'lŏl). Xylene.

xylometazoline hydrochloride (zī"lō-mĕt"ă-zō'lēn). USP. A vasoconstrictor drug used as a nasal decongestant. Trade name is Otrivin Hydrochloride.

xylose (zī'lōs) [Gr. *xylon*, wood]. USP. Wood sugar, a crystalline, nonfermentable pentose.

xylulose (zī'lū-lōs). A pentose sugar present in nature as L-xylulose. It appears in the urine in essential pentosuria; and in the form of D-xylulose.

xylyl (zī'lĭl). A radical, $CH_3C_6H_4CH_2$—, derived by the removal of a hydrogen atom from xylene.

xyrospasm (zī'rō-spăzm) [Gr. *xyron*, razor, + *spasmos*, a convulsion]. Occupational spasm or neurosis involving the fingers and arms. Seen in barbers.

xysma (zĭz'mă) [Gr. *zysma*, filings]. Shreds of tissue sometimes seen in diarrhea stools.

xyster (zĭs'tĕr) [Gr., scraper]. File or rasp used in surgery. SYN: *raspatory*.

Y

Y. Chem. symb. for the element yttrium.

yard [AS. *gerd*, a rod]. A measure of 3 feet or 36 inches. Equal to 0.9144 meter. SEE: *Weights and Measures* in *Appendix.*

yaw (yaw). The primary lesion of yaws, q.v.

   y., mother. The initial lesion of yaws, q.v., occurring at site of inoculation 3 to 4 weeks after infection. SYN: *frambesioma.*

yawn (yawn) [AS. *geonian*]. 1. To open the mouth involuntarily and usually take a deep breath as in drowsiness or fatigue; yawning may also be an expression of boredom. Yawning may stimulate observers to yawn. 2. Involuntary act of gaping, accompanied by attempts at inspiration, excited by drowsiness.

yawning (yawn'ĭng). Deep inspiration with mouth wide open; induced by drowsiness, boredom, or fatigue. SYN: *oscitation.* SEE: *pandiculation.*

yaws (yawz). An infectious nonvenereal disease caused by a spirochete, *Treponema pertenue.* Mainly found in humid, equatorial regions. SYN: *bouba; frambesia; tropica; parangi; pian.*

   SYM: Febrile disturbances, rheumatism, eruption of tubercles with a caseous crust on hands, feet, face, and external genitals.

   TREAT: Penicillin.

Yb. Chem. symb. for the element ytterbium.

Y cartilage. The cartilage that connects the pubis, ilium, and ischium and extends into the acetabulum.

Y chromosome. The chromosome that determines the male sex. Normal males possess one Y chromosome and one X chromosome; normal females possess two X chromosomes. SEE: *chromosome; Lyon hypothesis.*

years of life lost. The number of years a person is estimated to have remained alive if the disease experienced had not happened.

yeast (yēst) [AS. *gist*]. 1. Any of several unicellular fungi of the genus *Saccharomyces,* which reproduce by budding. They are capable of fermenting carbohydrates.

   Yeasts, esp. *Candida albicans,* may cause systemic infections as well as vaginitis. Yeast infections are frequently present in patients with malignant lymphomas, severe diabetic mellitus, AIDS, or other immuno-compromised individuals. SEE: *candida; candidiasis; fungi.*

   2. A commercial product composed of meal impregnated with living yeast.

   y., brewer's. Yeast obtained during the brewing of beer. May be used in the dried

form as a good source of vitamin B.

   y., dried. Dried yeast cells from strains of *Saccharomyces cerevisiae.* It is used as a source of proteins and vitamins, esp. B complex.

yellow (yĕl'ō) [AS. *geolu*]. 1. One of the primary colors resembling that of a ripe lemon. 2. Colored yellow, as the skin in disease.

   y., visual. SEE: *visual yellow.*

yellow body. The corpus luteum.

yellow fever. An acute infectious disease characterized by jaundice, epigastric tenderness, vomiting, hemorrhages, and a febrile course consisting of two paroxysms.

   There are two forms of yellow fever: urban, in which the transmission cycle is mosquito to human to mosquito; and sylvan, in which the reservoir is wild primates. Also, in sylvan yellow fever, the mosquito will remain infected for life.

   Except for a few cases in Trinidad in 1954, urban yellow fever has not been reported in North or South America since 1942. Outbreaks do occur in Africa adjacent to rain forests. Yellow fever has not been reported in Asia or the eastern coast of Africa. Sylvan yellow fever is enzootic in South America and parts of Africa.

   In general, the disease is erroneously thought to be minor with respect to the number of annual cases. Further study has revealed that the true incidence is generally underestimated.

   SYM: *First Stage:* Disease begins with sudden onset of fever, sometimes accompanied by a chill, followed by pain in head, back, and limbs. Temperature rises rapidly till it reaches its maximum 103° to 105°F (39.4° to 40.6°C). Face flushed, conjunctivae injected, pupils small, gastroenteritis, urine scanty and albuminous. This stage lasts from a few hours to several days. It is followed by a marked fall in temperature and an improvement in general symptoms. At this time convalescence may begin or patient may pass into second febrile paroxysm. Jaundice rarely appears before the third day.

   Second Stage, Period of Intoxication: Three to nine days. Fever rises to its original height, skin becomes yellow, vomiting persistent; vomitus may contain dark blood. Sometimes hemorrhages occur from other mucous membranes. Pulse rapid but not in proportion to the fever. Urine becomes very scanty and contains albumin and casts. Death frequently results from exhaustion or uremia, though recovery may follow the gravest symptoms.

ETIOL: The virus of yellow fever, a *flavivirus,* subgroup III of the Togaviridae family, is transmitted by the bite of a female mosquito, *Aedes aegypti.* The incubation period is 3 to 6 days.

DIAG: Diagnosis on clinical grounds alone is almost impossible during the period of infection or in atypical mild forms. Yellow fever viral antigen or antibodies may be detected during the acute phase of the illness.

PROPH: Preventive measures include mosquito control by screening, spraying with nontoxic insecticides, and destruction of breeding areas. Yellow fever vaccine prepared from the 17D strain is available for those who plan to travel or live in areas where the disease is endemic.

TREAT: There is no specific therapy. Absolute rest; cool, well-ventilated room; liquid diet; vitamin K and calcium gluconate for hemorrhagic tendency. Dehydration and electrolyte balance must be controlled by appropriate I.V. fluid replacement therapy. Parenteral fluids containing 10% to 20% glucose should be given to prevent fluid overload. Transfusion may be required. Heparin may be required if there is evidence of disseminated intravascular coagulation. Dopamine may be required to maintain blood pressure in cases that do not respond to fluid administration. Control fever by cool applications. Analgesics for pain.

PROG: Always grave. Mortality is 5% for natives of an area where the disease is endemic.

yellow ointment. An ointment containing yellow wax and petrolatum.

yellow spot. 1. Yellow nodule of anterior end of vocal cord. SYN: *macula flava laryngis.* 2. Center of the retina, the point of clearest vision. SYN: *macula lutea retinae.*

yellow vision. Condition in which objects seem yellow in color. SYN: *xanthopsia.*

yerba (yěr′bä) [Sp.]. An herb.

    y. maté. Herbal tea made from the dried leaves of maté, an evergreen tree. Popular in South America.

Yersinia (yěr-sĭn′ē-ä) [Yersin]. A genus of gram-negative bacteria.

    Y. enterocolitica. Species of large coccobacilli that are pathogenic for humans. Clinical infections may be characterized by acute mesenteric lymphadenitis or enterocolitis. The disease may progress to a septicemic form in children, and mortality may be as high as 50%. Therapy with trimethoprim-sulfamethoxazole, aminoglycosides, tetracycline, third-generation cephalosporin, or quinolones is effective.

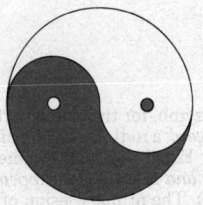

YIN-YANG

    Y. pestis. Causative organism of plague, q.v. Formerly termed *Pasteurella pestis.*

    Y. pseudotuberculosis. A gram-negative coccoid or ovoid organism that produces pseudotuberculosis in humans.

yersiniosis (yěr-sĭn″ē-ō′sĭs). Infection with *Yersinia* organisms.

Yersin's serum (yěr′sĭnz) [Alexandre Emil Jean Yersin, Swiss bacteriologist who worked in Paris, 1863–1943]. An antitoxic serum for the plague.

yin-yang. The Chinese symbol of opposing but complementary entities or concepts such as light-dark; male-female; sun-moon. In Chinese philosophy and medicine, the goal is to have a proper balance of such biological forces. Applied to contemporary biology, this would embody a feedback type of control of physiological phenomena. SEE: illus.

-yl [Gr. *hyle,* matter, substance]. Suffix signifying a radical in chemistry.

-ylene. Suffix denoting a bivalent hydrocarbon radical in chemistry.

Y ligament. A Y-shaped band covering the upper and anterior portions of the hip joint.

Yodoxin. Trade name for iodoquinol.

yoga [Sanskrit, union]. A system of beliefs and practices, the goal of which is to attain a union of the individual self with Supreme Reality or the Universal Self. The term yoga, as used in the Western world, has been associated almost exclusively with physical postures and regulation of breathing. These are yoga exercises but not yoga in the spiritual sense.

yogurt, yoghurt (yōg′hŭrt) [Turkish]. A form of curdled milk, curdling caused by action of *Lactobacillus bulgaricus.* Extensive claims have been made concerning the therapeutic value of yogurt for various ailments. These have not been substantiated. Yogurt may be of benefit in persons with lactase deficiency. In those persons, the absorption of lactose is probably the result of intraintestinal digestion of lactose by the lactase released from the yogurt organisms. SEE: *milk.*

yohimbine (yō-hĭm′bĕn). A poisonous alkaloid derived from the bark of the tree *Corynanthe yohimbi*. It is an α-adrenergic blocking agent and causes antidiuresis, increased blood pressure, tachycardia, irritability, tremor, sweating, nausea, and vomiting.

yoke (yōk). A tissue connecting two structures.

yolk (yōk) [AS. *geolca*]. The contents of the ovum; sometimes only the nutritive portion. SYN: *vitellus*. SEE: *zona pellucida*.

    y. sac. Membranous sac surrounding food yolk in the embryo.

    y. stalk. The umbilical duct connecting the yolk sac with the embryo.

Young-Helmholtz theory (yŭng-hĕlm′hōlts) [Thomas Young, Brit. physician, 1773–1829; Hermann Ludwig Ferdinand von Helmholtz, Ger. physician, 1821–1894]. Theory that color vision depends on three different sets of retinal fibers responsible for perception of red, green, and violet. The loss of either red, green, or violet as color perceptive elements in the retina causes an inability to perceive a primary color or any color of which it forms a part.

Young's rule (yŭngz) [Thomas Young]. A method for calculating the dose of medicine a child should receive. Divide the age by the age plus 12. The result represents the fraction of the adult dose suitable for the child.

    Ex.: a child of 4 years of age requires the following fraction of the adult dose:

$$\frac{4}{4+12} = \frac{1}{4}$$

youth (yooth) [AS. geoguth]. Period between childhood and maturity.

    In some modern societies there is a fascination with being young, or avoiding being old. Thus, a large industry has developed to provide potions, pills, and devices promoted to prevent aging. Jonathan Swift summarized this quest for youth: "Every man desires to live long, but no man would be old."

ypsiliform (ĭp-sĭl′ĭ-form). Y-shaped.

y.s. *yellow spot* of the retina.

ytterbium (ĭ-tŭr′bē-ŭm). SYMB: Yb. At. wt. 173.04; at. no. 70. A rare metallic element; a rare earth substance used in screens in radiography.

yttrium (ĭt′rē-ŭm). SYMB: Y. At. wt. 88.905; at. no. 39. A metallic element.

yushi. Minamata disease, q.v.

Yutopar. Trade name for ritodrine hydrochloride.

Z

Z. 1. Ger. *Zuckung,* contraction. 2. Symb. for atomic number.

z. *zero; zone.*

Zaglas' ligament (ză'glŭs). The part of the posterior sacroiliac ligament from the posterosuperior spinous process of the ilium to the side of the sacrum.

Zahn's lines (zŏnz) [Frederick W. Zahn, Ger. pathologist, 1845–1904]. Transverse whitish marks on the free surface of a thrombus made by the edges of the lamellae of blood platelets.

Zanelli maneuver. In obstetrics, the manual return of the head of a partially born fetus with intractable shoulder dystocia to the vagina. This is followed by cesarean section.

Zang's space (zăngz) [Christoph B. Zang, Ger. surgeon, 1772–1835]. Space between the two lower tendons of the sternomastoid muscle in the supraclavicular fossa.

Zaroxolyn. Trade name for metolazone.

Z disk. A thin, dark disk that transversely crosses through and bisects the clear zone of a striated muscle and bisects the clear zone (isotropic disk) of a striated muscle fiber. The portion between two disks constitutes a sarcomere. SYN: *Krause's membrane.*

zea. Maize or corn.

zeatin (zē'ă-tĭn). A cytotoxin that can be isolated from sweet corn.

zeaxanthin (zē"ă-zăn'thĭn). A carotenoid that is an isomer of xanthophyll. It is present in a great number of plants and animals.

zein (zē'ĭn) [Gr. *zeia,* a kind of grain]. A protein obtained from maize. It is deficient in tryptophan and lysine.

Zeis' glands [Eduard Zeis, Ger. ophthalmologist, 1807–1868]. Sebaceous glands of the eyelid, close to the free edge of the lid. Each gland is associated with an eyelash. SEE: *Moll's glands.*

zeisian (zī'sē-ăn). Pert. to something originally described by Edvard Zeis.

zeitgeist [German]. The spirit of the people, or trend of thought at a particular time.

zelotypia (zē"lō-tĭp'ē-ă) [Gr. *zelos,* zeal, + *typtein,* to strike]. 1. Morbid or monomaniacal zeal in the interest of any project or cause. 2. Insane jealousy.

Zenker, Friedrich Albert von (zĕng'kĕr). German pathologist, 1825–1898.

   Z.'s degeneration. A glassy or waxy hyaline degeneration of skeletal muscles in acute infectious diseases, esp. in typhoid. SYN: *zenkerism.*

   Z.'s diverticulum. Herniation of the mucous membrane of the esophagus through a defect in the wall of the esophagus. The location is usually in the posterior hypopharyngeal wall. Small ones are asymptomatic, but larger ones may collect food and cause esophageal obstruction. Treatment is surgical. SYN: *hypopharyngeal diverticulum.*

zenkerism (zĕng'kĕr-ĭzm). Zenker's degeneration, q.v.

Zephiran chloride. Trade name for benzalkonium chloride.

zero (zē'rō) [It.]. 1. Corresponding to nothing. SYMB: 0. 2. The point from which the graduation figures of a scale commence.

On the Celsius scale, zero (0°) is the temperature of melting ice, equivalent to 32° on the Fahrenheit scale. To obtain this fixed point, the thermometer is immersed in melting ice, and when the mercury column ceases to fall, the level at which it remains is fixed as 0° on the C and as 32° on the F scale. SEE: *thermometer.*

   z., absolute. The temperature at which all atoms and molecules cease movement or at which all gases liquefy: $-273.15°C$ or $-459.67°F$.

   z., limes. SYMB: L0. The greatest amount of toxin that, when mixed with one unit of antitoxin and injected into a guinea pig weighing 250 gm, will cause no local edema.

zero population growth. ABBR: ZPG. The demographic condition when in a given period of time the population neither increases nor decreases.

zero-sum game. A game in which the sum of the wins is equal to the sum of the losses.

zestocausis (zĕs"tō-kŏw'sĭs) [Gr. *zestos,* boiling hot, + *kausis,* burning]. Cauterization with a tube containing heated steam.

Zide. Trade name for hydrochlorothiazide.

zidovudine. An antiviral medicine which has been used in treating AIDS. Trade name is Retrovir.

Ziehl-Neelsen method (zēl-nēl'sĕn) [Franz Ziehl, Ger. bacteriologist, 1857–1926; Friedrich Karl Adolf Neelsen, Ger. pathologist, 1854–1894]. Method for staining *Mycobacterium tuberculosis.* A solution of carbolfuchsin is applied, which the organism retains after rinsing with acid alcohol.

Zieve's syndrome [L. Zieve, U.S. physician, b. 1915]. Hyperlipidemia, jaundice, hemolytic anemia, and abdominal pain following intake of a large amount of alcoholic beverages.

Zim jar opener. Trademarked name for a variety of devices allowing one-handed opening of bottles and jars for persons with disability.

zinc (zĭnk) [L. *zincum*]. SYMB: Zn. At. wt. 65.37; at. no. 30; sp. gr. 7.13. A bluish-white, crystalline metallic element that boils at 906°C. It is found as a carbonate and silicate, known as calamine, and as a sulfide (blende).

    z. acetate. USP. White, pearly crystals.
ACTION/USES: Astringent and antiseptic. Used chiefly in eye solutions, in a 0.1% to 0.5% solution.

    z. bacitracin. SEE: *bacitracin zinc.*

    z. cadmium sulfide. Fluorescent material used in radiographic screens.

    z. carbonate. A mild astringent used topically in dusting powders.

    z. chloride. USP. White granular powder used as an antiseptic.

    z. gelatin. USP. A combination of zinc oxide, glycerin, and purified water. This smooth jelly is placed between layers of gauze dressing to serve as a protective dressing and to support varicosities. It is removed by soaking in warm water.

    z. oxide. USP. Very fine white powder of zinc.
ACTION/USES: Slightly antiseptic and astringent. Used chiefly in the form of ointment, 20%.

    z. oxide and eugenol. Two substances that react together to produce a relatively hard mass, used in dentistry for impression material, cavity liners, temporary restorations, and cementing layers.

    z. peroxide. A topical anti-infective agent, used in powder form.

    z. salts. A bluish-white metal used to make various containers and also to galvanize iron to prevent rust. The most commonly used compounds are zinc oxide as a pigment for paints, in ointments, and in chloride and sulfate, which resemble epsom salts and have been administered accidentally. The salts also are used as a wood preservative, in soldering, in medicine to neutralize tissue, and in dilute solutions as an astringent and emetic. SEE: *zinc salts poisoning.*

    z. stearate. USP. A very fine smooth powder used as a nonirritating antiseptic and astringent for burns, scalds, and abrasions.

    z. sulfate. USP. Transparent white crystals used externally as an ophthalmic astringent. Trade names are Op-Thal-Zin and Verazinc.

    z. undecylenate. USP. An antifungal agent used in treating fungal infection of the skin. It is a component of Desenex ointment.

    z., white. Z. oxide.

zinc-eugenol cement. USP. A cement and protectant used in dentistry. SEE: *zinc oxide and eugenol.*

zinciferous (zĭng-kĭf′ĕr-ŭs). Containing zinc.

zincoid (zĭng′koyd) [L. *zincum*, zinc, + Gr. *eidos*, form, shape]. Resembling or concerning zinc.

zinc ointment. An ointment consisting of 20% zinc oxide mixed with petrolatum and white ointment. Used topically in treating skin diseases.

zinc salts poisoning. Characterized by metallic taste with prompt burning of mouth, throat, esophagus, and stomach. Violent vomiting, often bloody; increased salivation; painful diarrhea; coma. If patient recovers, nervous complications are frequent. SEE: *Poisons and Poisoning* in *Appendix.*
    F.A. Wash out stomach and treat as for sulfuric acid ingestion.

Zinn's ligament (zĭnz) [Johann G. Zinn, Ger. anatomist, 1727–1759]. Connective tissue giving attachment to the rectus muscles of the eyeball. SEE: *zonule of Zinn.*

zipper pull. An adaptive device allowing persons with limited function to fasten zippers on clothing, especially those in back.

zirconium (zir-kō′nē-ŭm). SYMB: Zr. At. wt. 91.22; at. no. 40. A metallic element found only in combination. Used in corrosion-resistant alloys and as a white pigment in dental porcelain and other ceramics.

Zn. Chem. symb. for the element zinc.

zoacanthosis (zō″ăk-ăn-thō′sĭs). Dermatitis due to foreign bodies such as bristles, hairs, or stingers from animals.

zoanthropy (zō-ăn′thrŏ-pē) [Gr. *zoon*, animal, + *anthropos*, man]. Delusion that one is an animal.

zoescope (zō′ĕ-skōp) [Gr. *zoe*, life, + *skopein*, to view]. Stroboscope.

zoetic (zō-ĕt′ĭk) [Gr. *zoe*, life]. Pert. to life. SYN: *vital.*

zoic (zō′ĭk). Concerning animal life.

Zollinger-Ellison syndrome [Robert M. Zollinger, b. 1903, and Edwin H. Ellison, 1918–1970, U.S. surgeons]. Condition caused by non-insulin-secreting tumors of the pancreas, which secrete excess amounts of gastrin. This stimulates the stomach to secrete great amounts of hydrochloric acid and pepsin, which in turn leads to peptic ulceration of the stomach and small intestines. About 60% of the tumors are malignant.
    TREAT: Total gastrectomy and local excision of pancreatic tumor if metastases have not appeared.

Zolyse. Trade name for chymotrypsin.

Zomax. Trade name for zomepirac sodium.

zombie [African *nzambi*, god]. In voodoo, the

apparent giving of life to a dead person. One investigator determined that the exhumed "body" is given a hallucinogen, datura, and the nerve toxin tetrodotoxin, derived from roasted puffer fish; however, this alone did not completely explain the phenomenon of zombiism. SEE: *hex; voodoo.*

zona (zō'nä) [L., a girdle] (pl. *zonae*). 1. A band or girdle. 2. An acute inflammatory disease, characterized by groups of small vesicles mounted on inflammatory bases, associated with neuralgic pain and following the distribution of certain nerve trunks. SYN: *herpes zoster.*

z. ciliaris. Ciliary processes combined.

z. facialis. Herpes zoster of the face.

z. fasciculata. The adrenal cortex.

z. glomerulosa. The outer layer of the adrenal cortex just inside the capsule.

z. ophthalmica. Old name for herpes zoster of the area supplied by the ophthalmic nerve.

z. pellucida. Inner, solid, thick, membranous envelope of the ovum. It is pierced by many radiating canals, giving it a striated appearance. SYN: *vitelline membrane; z. radiata.*

z. radiata. Z. pellucida, q.v.

z. reticularis. The inner layer of the cortex of the adrenal gland.

z. striata. Z. pellucida, q.v.

zonae. Pl. of zona.

zonal (zō'năl) [L. *zonalis*]. Pert. to a zone.

zonary (zō'năr-ē) [L. *zona*, a girdle]. Pert. to or shaped like a zone.

zonary placenta. Placenta arranged in the form of a broad ring around the chorion.

Zondek-Aschheim test (zŏn'dĕk-ăsh'hīm) [Bernhardt Zondek, Ger.-born Israeli obstetrician-gynecologist, 1891–1966; Selmar Aschheim, Ger. gynecologist, 1878–1965]. A test for pregnancy by injecting the patient's urine subcutaneously into immature female mice.

zone (zōn) [L. *zona*, a girdle]. An area or belt.

z., cell-free. In dentistry, a cellular area below the odontoblastic layer of the dental pulp. Also called zone of Weil.

z., cell-rich. Area of increased cell frequency between the cell-free zone and the central pulp of the tooth.

z., ciliary. The peripheral part of the anterior surface of the iris of the eye.

z., comfort. The range of temperature, humidity, and, when applicable, solar radiation and wind in which an individual doing work at a specified rate and in a certain specified garment is comfortable.

z., epileptogenic. Any area of the brain that after stimulation produces an epileptic seizure.

z., erogenous. An area of the body that may produce erotic desires when stimulated. These areas include, but are not limited to, the breasts, lips, genital and anal regions, buttocks, and sometimes the special senses that cause sexual excitation, such as the sense of smell or taste.

z., hypnogenic, hypnogenous. Any area of the body that when pressed on induces a hypnotic state.

z., transitional. The area of the lens of the eye where the epithelial capsule cells change into lens fibers.

zonesthesia (zōn"ĕs-thē'zē-ă) [" + *aisthesis*, sensation]. A sensation, as a cord constricting the body. SYN: *cincture sensation; girdle pain.*

zonifugal (zō-nĭf'ū-găl) [" + *fugere*, to flee]. Passing outward from within any zone or area.

zoning. The occurrence of a stronger fixation of complement in a lesser amount of suspected serum; a phenomenon occasionally observed in diagnosing syphilis by complement-fixation method.

zonipetal (zō-nĭp'ĕt-ăl) [" + *petere*, to seek]. Passing from without into a zone or area of the body.

zonoskeleton (zōn"ō-skĕl'ĕ-tŏn). Proximal bones to which limbs attach, such as the hip bone, scapula, and clavicle.

zonula (zōn'ū-lä) [L.]. A small zone. SYN: *zonule.*

z. adherens. The portion of the junctional complex between columnar epithelial cells below the zonula occludens where there is an intercellular space of about 200 angstroms and the cellular membranes are supported by filamentous material.

z. ciliaris. [NA] Suspensory ligament of the crystalline lens. SYN: *zonule of Zinn.*

z. occludens. The portion of the junctional complex between columnar epithelial cells just below the free surface where the intercellular space is obliterated. Also called tight junction.

zonular (zōn'ū-lăr). Pert. to a zonula.

zonular cataract. Cataract with opacity limited to certain layers of the lens.

zonular fibers. Interlacing fibers of the zonula ciliaris.

zonular spaces. Spaces between fibers of ligaments of the lens.

zonule (zōn'ūl) [L. *zonula*, small zone]. A small band or area. SYN: *zonula.*

z. of Zinn. Suspensory ligament of the crystalline lens. SYN: *zonula ciliaris* [NA].

zonulitis (zōn-ū-lī'tĭs) [" + Gr. *itis*, inflammation]. Inflammation of zonule of Zinn.

zonulolysis (zōn"ū-lŏl'ĭ-sĭs) [" + Gr. *lysis*, dissolution]. Use of enzymes to dissolve the zonula ciliaris of the eye.

zonulotomy (zōn"ū-lŏt'ō-mē) [" + Gr.

tome, incision]. Surgical incision of the ciliary zonule.

zonulysis (zŏn″ū-lī′sĭs). Zonulolysis.

zoo-. Combining form concerning an animal.

zoobiology (zō″ō-bī-ŏl′ō-jē) [Gr. *zoon,* animal, + *bios,* life, + *logos,* word, reason]. The biology of animals.

zooblast (zō′ō-blăst) [″ + *blastos,* germ]. An animal cell, esp. an immature form.

zoochemistry (zō″ō-kĕm′ĭs-trē). Biochemistry of animals.

zoodermic (zō″ō-dĕr′mĭk) [″ + *derma,* skin]. Performed with the skin of an animal, said of a method of skin grafting.

zoodynamics (zō″ō-dī-năm′ĭks) [″ + *dynamis,* power]. Physiology of animals.

zooerasty (zō″ō-ē′răs-tē). Sexual intercourse with an animal. SYN: *bestiality.*

zoofulvin (zō″ō-fŭl′vĭn). A yellow pigment derived from certain animal feathers.

zoogenesis (zō″ō-jĕn′ĕ-sĭs). Zoogeny, q.v.

zoogenous (zō-ŏj′ĕn-ŭs) [″ + *gennan,* to produce]. Derived or acquired from animals.

zoogeny (zō″ŏj′ĕ-nē) [″ + *gennan,* to produce]. The development and evolution of animals.

zoogeography (zō″ō-jē-ŏg′ră-fē). Study of the distribution of animals on the earth.

zooglea (zō″ō-glē′ă) [″ + *gloios,* sticky]. A stage in development of certain organisms in which colonies of microbes are embedded in a gelatinous matrix.

zoogonous (zō-ŏg′ō-nŭs). Viviparous, q.v.

zoogony (zō-ŏg′ō-nē) [″ + *gone,* offspring]. 1. Production of living young from within the body. 2. Breeding of animals.

zoograft (zō′ō-grăft) [″ + L. *graphium,* stylus]. A graft of tissue obtained from an animal.

zoografting (zō″ō-grăft′ĭng). Use of animal tissue in grafting on a human body.

zooid (zō′oyd) [″ + *eidos,* form, shape]. 1. Resembling an animal. 2. A form resembling an animal; an organism produced by fission. 3. An animal cell that can move or exist independently.

zoolagnia (zō″ō-lăg′nē-ă) [″ + *lagneia,* lust]. Sexual desire for animals.

zoologist (zō-ŏl′ō-jĭst) [″ + *logos,* word, reason]. A biologist who specializes in the study of animal life.

zoology (zō-ŏl′ō-jē). The science of animal life.

zoom. A type of lens that can be adjusted to focus on near or distant objects.

zoomania (zō″ō-mā′nē-ă) [Gr. *zoon,* animal, + *mania,* madness]. A morbid and excessive affection for animals.

zoonoses (zō-ō-nō′sēz) [″ + *nosos,* disease]. Diseases communicable from animals to humans under natural conditions.

zoonotic (zō″ō-nŏt′ĭk). Concerning zoonoses.

zooparasite (zō″ō-păr′ă-sīt) [″ + *para,* beside, + *sitos,* food]. An animal parasite.

zoopathology (zō″ō-păth-ŏl′ō-jē) [″ + *pathos,* disease, + *logos,* word, reason]. Science of the diseases of animals.

zoophagous (zō-ŏf′ă-gŭs) [″ + *phagein,* to eat]. Living upon animal food.

zoophilia. The preference for obtaining sexual gratification by having intercourse with or other sexual activity with animals.

zoophile (zō′ō-fīl) [″ + *philein,* to love]. 1. One who likes animals. 2. An antivivisectionist.

zoophilism (zō-ŏf′ĭl-ĭzm) [″ + ″ + *-ismos,* condition]. Abnormal love of animals.

zoophobia (zō″ō-fō′bē-ă) [″ + *phobos,* fear]. Abnormal fear of animals.

zoophyte (zō′ō-fīt) [″ + *phyton,* plant]. A plantlike animal; any of numerous invertebrate animals resembling plants in appearance or mode of growth.

zooplankton (zō″ō-plănk′tŏn) [″ + *planktos,* wandering]. Small animal organism present in natural waters. SEE: *phytoplankton.*

zooplasty (zō′ō-plăs″tē) [″ + *plassein,* to form]. Transplantation of animal tissue to humans.

zoopsia (zō-ŏp′sē-ă) [″ + *opsis,* vision]. Hallucinations involving animals.

zoopsychology (zō″ō-sī-kŏl′ō-jē). Animal psychology.

zoosadism (zō″ō-sā′dĭzm). Being sadistic to animals.

zooscopy (zō-ŏs′kō-pē) [″ + *skopein,* to examine]. 1. Zoopsia. 2. Scientific observation of animals.

zoosmosis (zō″ōs-mō′sĭs) [Gr. *zoe,* life, + *osmos,* impulsion]. Process of passage of living protoplasm into the tissues from blood vessels.

zoospore (zō′ō-spor) [″ + *sporos,* seed]. A motile asexual spore that moves by means of one or more flagella.

zoosterol (zō″ō-stē′rŏl). Any sterol derived from animals.

zootechnics (zō″ō-tĕk′nĭks) [Gr. *zoon,* animal, + *techne,* art]. The complete care, management, and breeding of domestic animals.

zootic (zō-ŏt′ĭk). Concerning animals.

zootomy (zō-ŏt′ō-mē) [″ + *tome,* incision]. Dissection of animals.

zootoxin (zō″ō-tŏks′ĭn) [″ + *toxikon,* poison]. Any toxin or poison produced by an animal, as snake venom.

zootrophic (zō″ō-trŏf′ĭk) [″ + *trophe,* nutrition]. Concerning animal nutrition.

zoster (zŏs′tĕr) [Gr. *zoster,* girdle]. Acute inflammatory disease with vesicles grouped in the course of cutaneous nerves. SYN: *herpes*

Z-PLASTY METHOD OF CORRECTING A DEFORMING SCAR

SCAR TISSUE AND INCISION LINES

zoster; zona.

   z. auricularis. Herpes zoster of the ear.
   z. ophthalmicus. Herpes zoster affecting the ophthalmic nerve.
zosteriform (zŏs-tĕr′ĭ-form) [″ + L. *forma,* shape]. Resembling herpes zoster. SYN: *zosteroid.*
zosteroid (zŏs′tĕr-oyd) [″ + *eidos,* form, shape]. Resembling herpes zoster. SYN: *zosteriform.*
ZPG. *zero population growth.*
Z-plasty. A technique with a Z-shaped incision used in plastic surgery to relieve tension in scar tissue. The area under tension is lengthened at the expense of the surrounding elastic tissue. SEE: illus.; *tissue expansion; W-plasty.*
Zr. Chem. symb. for the element zirconium.
Z-track. An injection technique in which the surface (skin and subcutaneous) tissues are pulled and held to one side prior to insertion of the needle deep into the muscle in the identified site. The medication is injected slowly, followed by a 10-second delay; then the needle is removed, and the tissues are quickly permitted to resume their normal position. This provides a Z-shaped track, which makes it difficult for the injected irri-

tating drug to seep back into subcutaneous tissues.
zwitterions (tsvĭt′ĕr-ī′ŏns). Dipolar ions that contain positive and negative charges of equal strength. They are therefore not attracted to either an anode or cathode. In a neutral solution, amino acids function as zwitterions.
zygal (zī′găl) [Gr. *zygon,* yoke]. Concerning or shaped like a yoke.
zygapophyseal (zī″gă-pō-fĭz′ē-ăl). Concerning zygapophysis.
zygapophysis (zī″gă-pŏf′ĭ-sĭs) [″ + *apo,* from, + *physis,* growth]. One of the articular processes of the neural arch of a vertebra.
zygion (zĭj′ē-ŏn) [Gr. *zygon,* yoke] (pl. *zygia*). Craniometrical point on the zygoma at either end of the bizygomatic diameter.
zygocyte. Zygote, q.v.
zygodactyly (zī″gō-dăk′tĭl-ē) [″ + *daktylos,* digit]. Fusion of two or more fingers or toes. SYN: *syndactylism.*
zygoma (zī-gō′mă) [Gr., cheekbone]. 1. The long arch that joins zygomatic processes of the temporal and malar bones on the sides of the skull. 2. The malar bone.
zygomatic (zī″gō-măt′ĭk). Pert. to the zygoma.
zygomatic arch. The formation on each side of the cheeks of the zygomatic process of each malar bone articulating with the zygomatic process of the temporal bone.
zygomatic bone. Bone on either side of the face below the eye. SYN: *malar bone.*
zygomaticoauricularis (zī″gō-măt″ĭ-kō-ăw-rĭk″ū-lā′rĭs) [L.]. Muscle that draws the pinna of the ear forward. SEE: *Muscles* in *Appendix.*
zygomaticofacial (zī″gō-măt″ĭ-kō-fā′shăl). Concerning the zygoma and face.
zygomaticofrontal (zī″gō-măt″ĭ-kō-frŏn′tăl). Concerning the zygoma and frontal bone of the face.
zygomaticomaxillary (zī″gō-măt″ĭ-kō-măk′sĭ-lĕr″ē). Concerning the zygoma and maxilla.
zygomatico-orbital (zī″gō-măt″ĭ-kō-or′bĭtăl). Concerning the zygoma and orbit of the eye.
zygomaticosphenoid (zī″gō-măt″ĭ-kō-sfē′noyd). Concerning the zygoma and sphenoid bone.
zygomaticotemporal (zī″gō-măt″ĭ-kō-tĕm′por-ăl). Concerning the zygoma and temporal bone.
zygomatic process. 1. A thin projection from the temporal bone bounding its squamous portion. 2. A part of the malar bone helping to form the zygoma.
zygomatic reflex. Movement of lower jaw toward percussed side when zygoma is per-

cussed.

zygomaticum (zī″gō-măt′ĭ-kŭm) [L.]. The zygomatic bone.

zygomaticus (zī″gō-măt′ĭk-ŭs) [L.]. A muscle that draws the upper lip upward and outward. SEE: *Muscles* in *Appendix*.

zygomaxillary (zī″gō-măks′ĭl-ār-ē) [Gr. *zygoma*, cheekbone, + L. *maxilla*, jawbone]. Pert. to the cheekbone and upper jaw.

zygomaxillary point. A craniometrical point marked at the lower end of the zygomatic suture.

zygomycosis. Mucormycosis, q.v.

zygon (zī′gŏn) [Gr.]. The short crossbar connecting the parallel limbs of a cerebral fissure.

zygopodium (zī″gō-pō′dē-ŭm). The intermediate-distal portion of a limb, i.e., the ulna and radius, and the tibia and fibula.

zygosis (zī-gō′sĭs) [Gr. *zygosis*, a balancing]. Sexual union of two unicellular animals.

zygosity (zī-gŏs′ĭ-tē) [Gr. *zygon*, yoke]. Concerning zygosis.

zygosperm (zī′gō-spĕrm). Zygospore.

zygospore (zī′gō-spor). A spore formed by fusion of morphologically identical structures.

zygote (zī′gōt) [Gr. *zygotos*, yoked]. Cell produced by union of two gametes. The fertilized ovum. SYN: *oosperm; zygocyte*.

zygotene (zī′gō-tēn) [Gr. *zygotos*, yoked]. The second stage of the prophase of the first meiotic division. During this stage, the homologous chromosomes pair side by side. SEE: *cell division*.

zygotic (zī-gŏt′ĭk). Concerning a zygote.

zygotoblast (zī-gō′tō-blăst) [″ + *blastos*, germ]. Sporozoite, q.v.

zygotomere (zī-gō′tō-mēr) [″ + *meros*, part]. Sporoblast, q.v.

Zyloprim. Trade name for allopurinol.

zymase (zī′mās) [Gr. *zyme*, leaven, + -*ase*, enzyme]. Any of a group of enzymes that, in the presence of oxygen, convert certain carbohydrates into carbon dioxide and water or, in absence of oxygen, into alcohol and carbon dioxide or lactic acid. It is found in yeast, bacteria, and higher plants and animals. SEE: *enzyme, fermenting*.

zyme (zīm) [Gr. *zyme*, leaven]. 1. An enzyme or ferment. 2. An agent that produces an infectious disease.

zymic (zī′mĭk). Concerning enzymes.

zymogen (zī′mō-jĕn) [″ + *gennan*, to produce]. A substance that develops into a chemical ferment or enzyme. It exists in an inactive form antecedent to the active enzyme. SYN: *proenzyme*. SEE: *pepsinogen; trypsinogen*.

zymogene (zī′mō-jēn). Microbe causing fermentation.

zymogen granules. Secretory granules of a pre-enzyme substance seen in cells of synthetic organs such as salivary glands or pancreas.

zymogenic (zī″mō-jĕn′ĭk). 1. Causing a fermentation. 2. Pert. to or producing a zymogen.

zymogenous (zī-mŏj′ē-nŭs). Zymogenic.

zymogram (zī′mō-grăm). Electrophoretic graph of the separation of the enzymes in a solution.

zymohexase (zī″mō-hĕk′sās). The enzyme that is involved in splitting fructose 1,6-diphosphate into dihydroxyacetone phosphate and phosphoglyceric aldehyde.

zymohydrolysis (zī″mō-hī-drŏl′ĭ-sĭs) [″ + *hydor*, water, + *lysis*, dissolution]. Decomposition brought about by a ferment. SYN: *zymosis*.

zymoid (zī′moyd) [″ + *eidos*, form, shape]. Resembling an enzyme.

zymologic (zī″mō-lŏ′jĭk) [″ + *logos*, word, reason]. Rel. to zymology.

zymologist (zī-mŏl′ō-jĭst). One who specializes in study of ferments.

zymology (zī-mŏl′ō-jē). The science of fermentation.

zymolysis (zī-mŏl′ĭ-sĭs) [Gr. *zyme*, leaven, + *lysis*, dissolution]. Changes produced by an enzyme; action of enzymes. SYN: *fermentation; zymosis*.

zymolyte (zī′mō-līt″). Substance upon which a ferment acts. SYN: *substrate*.

zymolytic (zī″mō-lĭt′ĭk) [″ + *lytikos*, dissolved]. Causing fermentation; fermentative.

zymometer (zī-mŏm′ĕ-tĕr) [″ + *metron*, measure]. Device for measuring fermentation.

Zymonema (zī″mō-nē′mă) [″ + *nema*, thread]. A genus of fungi.

zymophore (zī′mō-for) [″ + *phoros*, a bearer]. Noting the atomic group bearing the ferment.

zymophoric, zymophorous (zī″mō-for′ĭk, zī-mŏf′or-ŭs). Having fermentative properties.

zymophyte (zī′mō-fīt) [″ + *phyton*, growth]. A microorganism causing fermentation.

zymoplastic (zī″mō-plăs′tĭk) [″ + *plassein*, to form]. Producing a ferment.

zymoprotein (zī″mō-prō′tē-ĭn). Any protein that also functions as an enzyme.

zymosan (zī′mō-săn). An anticomplement obtained from the walls of great cells.

zymoscope (zī′mō-skōp) [″ + *skopein*, to examine]. Device for determining zymotic power of yeast.

zymose (zī′mōs). An enzyme that changes a disaccharide into a monosaccharide, such as cane sugar into invert sugar. SYN: *invertin.*

zymosis (zī-mō'sĭs) [Gr. *zymosis,* fermentation]. 1. Fermentation. 2. Process by which an infectious disease is supposed to develop. 3. An infectious disease.

  z. gastrica. Organic acid in the stomach due to action of yeasts.

zymosterol (zī-mŏs'tĕr-ŏl). A sterol obtained from yeast.

zymosthenic (zī-mŏs-thĕn'ĭk) [Gr. *zyme,* leaven, + *sthenos,* strength]. Increasing the power and activity of an enzyme.

zymotic (zī-mŏt'ĭk). Rel. to or produced by fermentation.

Z.Z.'Z.". Symb. for increasing strengths of contraction.

Appendix

Table of Contents
for Appendix

Index to Appendix

App. 1: Normal Ranges of Laboratory Values

Body Fluids, Tissues, and Excreta
Including SI Unit Conversion Table*

The normal ranges listed are suggested ones and are included as a helpful guide. Different laboratories use a variety of analytical methods and are likely to have normal ranges different from the ones included in this table. For many constituents in the table, there are several different normal ranges for pediatric patients (e.g., newborns, infants, and adolescents), many of which are different from those for adults. The conversion factors are not affected by this difference. Therefore, although the conversion factors are suitable for pediatric patients, the normal ranges in the table should be used for adult patients only (with a few clearly noted exceptions). For pediatric normal ranges, see *Nelson: Textbook of Pediatrics* by R.E. Behrman and V.C. Vaughan III.

To obtain a consensus on whether plasma, serum, or whole blood are suitable samples for analysis of blood-borne compounds, the author reviewed published tables from articles listed in the Massachusetts General Hospital Clinical Laboratory Handbook and laboratory handbooks from several large commercial laboratories. It is understood that plasma specimens may be suitable only if collected in a specific anticoagulant (e.g., heparin may be acceptable, but not citrate). It is also understood that the normal range for a given compound may not be identical for serum and for plasma. However, since the suggested normal range is only an approximation of the normal range for a given laboratory, and the difference in normal values between serum and plasma is usually small, there variations are not taken into account. It is further recognized that certain compounds listed as being measured only in plasma or only in serum may in fact be accurately measured in both. Whole blood is listed in the table as the sample fluid for determining RBC number and mean RBC corpuscular volume because anticoagulated whole blood is aspirated into an automated cell counter.

Abbreviations found in the table include multiples and submultiples of the gram (g), the mole (mol), the liter (L), the meter (m), the equivalent (Eq), the International enzyme unit (U or IU), the katal (kat), the pascal (Pa), and the osmole (Osm). The units of time — the second (s), the minute (min), the hour (hr), and the day (d) are also found in the table.

To convert a value from the traditional to the SI unit, multiply the conversion factor times the traditional value. Similarly, to convert the SI unit to traditional, divide the SI value by the conversion factor.

---

* Adapted from Laposato, Michael. New England Journal of Medicine SI Unit Conversion Guide. Boston: NEJM Books, 1992.

CONSTITUENT	FLUID	TRADITIONAL APPROXIMATE NORMAL RANGE	TRADITIONAL UNITS	CONVERSION FACTOR MULT → / DIV ←	SI APPROXIMATE NORMAL RANGE	SI UNITS
Acetaminophen						
Therapeutic	plasma, serum	0.2 - 0.6	mg/dL	66.16	13 - 40	µmol/L
Toxic	plasma, serum	> 5.0	mg/dL	66.16	>330	µmol/L
Acetoacetate	plasma, serum	0.3 - 3.0	mg/dL	97.95	30 - 300	µmol/L
Acetone	plasma, serum	0	mg/dL	172.2	0	µmol/L
Acid Phosphatase (prostatic)	serum	0 - 0.8 (37°C)	Units/L	1	0 - 0.8	U/L
	serum	0 - 0.8 (37°C)	Units/L	16.67	0 - 13.3	nkat/L
ACTH (adrenocorticotropin)	plasma	20 - 100	pg/mL	0.2202	4 - 22	pmol/L
Adrenocorticotropin (ACTH)	plasma	20 - 100	pg/mL	0.2202	4 - 22	pmol/L
Alanine Aminotransferase (ALT, SGPT)	serum	0 - 35 (37°C)	Units/L	1	0 - 35	U/L
	serum	0 - 35 (37°C)	Units/L	0.01667	0 - 0.58	µkat/L
Alanine, amino acid fractionation	plasma, serum	2.2 - 4.5	mg/dL	112.20	245 - 500	µmol/L
Albumin	serum	4.0 - 6.0	g/dL	10	40 - 60	g/L
Aldolase	serum	0 - 6 (37°C)	Units/L	1	0 - 6	U/L
	serum	0 - 6 (37°C)	Units/L	16.67	0 - 100	nkat/L
Aldosterone						
Normal Salt Diet	serum	8.1 - 15.5	ng/dL	27.74	220 - 430	pmol/L
Restricted Salt Diet	serum	20.8 - 44.4	ng/dL	27.74	580 - 1240	pmol/L
Aldosterone, sodium excretion						
= 25 mmol/24 hr	urine	18 - 85	µg/24 hr	2.774	50 - 235	nmol/d
= 75 - 125 mmol/24 hr	urine	5 - 26	µg/24 hr	2.774	15 - 70	nmol/d
= 200 mmol/24 hr	urine	1.5 - 12.5	µg/24 hr	2.774	5 - 35	nmol/d
Alkaline phosphatase	serum	30 - 120 (37°C)	Units/L	1	30 - 120	U/L
	serum	30 - 120 (37°C)	Units/L	0.01667	0.5 - 2.0	µkat/L
ALT (alanine aminotransferase, SGPT)	serum	0 - 35 (37°C)	Units/L	1	0 - 35	U/L
	serum	0 - 35 (37°C)	Units/L	0.01667	0 - 0.58	µkat/L
Aluminum	serum	0 - 15	µg/L	37.06	0 - 560	nmol/L
Alpha-Aminobutyric acid, amino acid fractionation	plasma, serum	0.1 - 0.2	mg/dL	96.97	10 - 20	µmol/L
Alpha-1-Antitrypsin	serum	150 - 350	mg/dL	0.01	1.5 - 3.5	g/L
Alpha-Fetoprotein	amniotic fluid	gestation dependent	mg/dL	10	gestation dependent	mg/L
Alpha-Fetoprotein	serum	0 - 20	ng/mL	1	0 - 20	µg/L
17-alpha-Hydroxyprogesterone						
Children	plasma, serum	0.2 - 1.4	µg/L	3.026	0.5 - 4.5	nmol/L
Male	plasma, serum	0.5 - 2.5	µg/L	3.026	1.5 - 7.5	nmol/L
Female	plasma, serum	0.3 - 4.2	µg/L	3.026	1.0 - 13.0	nmol/L
Female, postmenopausal	plasma, serum	0.3 - 1.7	µg/L	3.026	1.0 - 5.0	nmol/L
Alpha-2-Macroglobulin	serum	145 - 410	mg/dL	0.01	1.5 - 4.1	g/L
Alpha-Tocopherol (vitamin E)	plasma, serum	0.78 - 1.25	mg/dL	23.22	18 - 29	µmol/L
Amikacin, therapeutic (peak)	serum	15 - 25	µg/mL	1.71	25.6 - 42.7	µmol/L

CONSTITUENT	FLUID	TRADITIONAL APPROXIMATE NORMAL RANGE	UNITS	CONVERSION FACTOR MULT ⟶ / DIV ⟵	SI APPROXIMATE NORMAL RANGE	UNITS
Amino Acid fractionation						
Alanine	plasma, serum	2.2 - 4.5	mg/dL	112.20	245 - 500	µmol/L
Alpha-Aminobutyric acid	plasma, serum	0.1 - 0.2	mg/dL	96.97	10 - 20	µmol/L
Arginine	plasma, serum	0.5 - 2.5	mg/dL	57.40	30 - 145	µmol/L
Asparagine	plasma, serum	0.5 - 0.6	mg/dL	75.69	35 - 45	µmol/L
Aspartic acid	plasma, serum	0.0 - 0.3	mg/dL	75.13	0 - 20	µmol/L
Citrulline	plasma, serum	0.2 - 1.0	mg/dL	57.08	15 - 55	µmol/L
Cystine	plasma, serum	0.2 - 2.2	mg/dL	41.61	10 - 90	µmol/L
Glutamic acid	plasma, serum	0.2 - 2.8	mg/dL	67.97	15 - 190	µmol/L
Glutamine	plasma, serum	6.1 - 10.2	mg/dL	68.42	420 - 700	µmol/L
Glycine	plasma, serum	0.9 - 4.2	mg/dL	133.20	120 - 560	µmol/L
Histidine	plasma, serum	0.5 - 1.7	mg/dL	64.45	30 - 110	µmol/L
Hydroxyproline	plasma, serum	0 - trace	mg/dL	76.26	0 - trace	µmol/L
Isoleucine	plasma, serum	0.5 - 1.3	mg/dL	76.24	40 - 100	µmol/L
Leucine	plasma, serum	1.0 - 2.3	mg/dL	76.24	76 - 176	µmol/L
Lysine	plasma, serum	1.2 - 3.5	mg/dL	68.40	80 - 240	µmol/L
Methionine	plasma, serum	0.1 - 0.6	mg/dL	67.02	5 - 40	µmol/L
Ornithine	plasma, serum	0.4 - 1.4	mg/dL	75.67	30 - 400	µmol/L
Phenylalanine	plasma, serum	0.6 - 1.5	mg/dL	60.54	35 - 90	µmol/L
Proline	plasma, serum	1.2 - 3.9	mg/dL	86.86	105 - 340	µmol/L
Serine	plasma, serum	0.8 - 1.8	mg/dL	95.16	75 - 170	µmol/L
Taurine	plasma, serum	0.3 - 2.1	mg/dL	79.91	25 - 170	µmol/L
Threonine	plasma, serum	0.9 - 2.5	mg/dL	83.95	75 - 210	µmol/L
Tryptophan	plasma, serum	0.5 - 2.5	mg/dL	48.97	25 - 125	µmol/L
Tyrosine	plasma, serum	0.4 - 1.6	mg/dL	55.19	20 - 90	µmol/L
Valine	plasma, serum	1.7 - 3.7	mg/dL	85.36	145 - 315	µmol/L
Amino Acid Nitrogen	plasma	4.0 - 6.0	mg/dL	0.7139	2.9 - 4.3	mmol/L
Amino Acid Nitrogen	urine	50 - 200	mg/24 hr	0.07139	3.6 - 14.3	mmol/d
delta-Aminolevulinate (as aminolevulinic acid)	urine	1.0 - 7.0	mg/24 hr	7.626	8 - 53	µmol/d
Amitriptyline, therapeutic	serum	50 - 200	ng/mL	3.605	180 - 720	nmol/L
Ammonia						
as ammonia (NH3)	plasma	10 - 80	µg/dL	0.5872	5 - 50	µmol/L
as ammonium (NH4+)	plasma	10 - 85	µg/dL	0.5543	5 - 50	µmol/L
as nitrogen (N)	plasma	10 - 65	µg/dL	0.7139	5 - 50	µmol/L
Amylase	serum	0 - 130 (37°C)	Units/L	1	0 - 130	U/L
	serum	0 - 130 (37°C)	Units/L	0.01667	0 - 2.17	µkat/L
ANA (Antinuclear Antibodies)	serum	negative at 1:10 dil	highest pos. dil	1	negative at 1:10 dil	highest pos. dil
Androstenedione						
Male > 18 yrs	serum	0.2 - 3.0	µg/L	3.492	0.5 - 10.5	nmol/L
Female >18 yrs	serum	0.8 - 3.0	µg/L	3.492	3.0 - 10.5	nmol/L

CONSTITUENT	FLUID	TRADITIONAL APPROXIMATE NORMAL RANGE	UNITS	CONVERSION FACTOR MULT → / DIV ←	SI APPROXIMATE NORMAL RANGE	UNITS
Androsterone (ketosteroid fractions)						
Female	urine	0.5 - 3.0	mg/24 hr	3.443	1 - 10	µmol/d
Male	urine	2.0 - 5.0	mg/24 hr	3.443	7 - 17	µmol/d
Angiotensin converting enzyme	serum	< 40 (37°C)	U/L	1	<40	U/L
	serum	< 40 (37°C)	U/L	16.67	<670	nkat/L
Antibodies:						
Antibody to Centromeres	serum	negative at 1:40 dil.	highest pos. dil	1	negative at 1:40 dil.	highest pos. dil.
Antibody to delta Hepatitis Virus	serum	negative	highest pos. dil	1	negative	highest pos. dil.
Antibody to Hepatitis A Virus (IgG, IgM)	serum	negative	highest pos. dil	1	negative	highest pos. dil.
Antibody to Hepatitis B core antigen	serum	negative	highest pos. dil	1	negative	highest pos. dil.
Antibody to Hepatitis B surface antigen	serum	negative	highest pos. dil	1	negative	highest pos. dil.
Antibody to Hepatitis C Virus	serum	negative	highest pos. dil	1	negative	highest pos. dil.
Antibody to SS-A (Ro)	serum	negative	highest pos. dil	1	negative	highest pos. dil.
Antibody to SS-B (La)	serum	negative	highest pos. dil.	1	negative	highest pos. dil.
Anti-DNA (native or double stranded)	serum	negative at 1:10 dil.	highest pos. dil.	1	negative at 1:10 dil.	highest pos. dil.
	serum	0 - 15	%	0.01	0 - 0.15	fraction of 1.00
Anti-gastric Parietal Cell antibody	serum	negative at 1:20 dil.	highest pos. dil	1	negative at 1:20 dil.	highest pos. dil.
Anti-glomerular Basement Membrane antibody	serum	negative	highest pos. dil	1	negative	highest pos. dil.
Anti-HIV antibody	serum	negative	highest pos. dil	1	negative	highest pos. dil.
Anti-mitochondrial antibody (AMA)	serum	negative at 1:20 dil.	highest pos. dil	1	negative at 1:20 dil.	highest pos. dil.
Anti-neutrophil antibodies	serum	negative	highest pos. dil	1	negative	highest pos. dil.
Anti-RNP antibodies	serum	negative	highest pos. dil.	1	negative	highest pos. dil.
Anti-Smith (Sm) antibody	serum	negative	highest pos. dil.	1	negative	highest pos. dil.
Anti-smooth Muscle antibody	serum	negative at 1:20 dil.	highest pos. dil.	1	negative at 1:20 dil.	highest pos. dil.
Anti-thyroid Colloid antibody	serum	negative at 1:10 dil.	highest pos. dil.	1	negative at 1:10 dil.	highest pos. dil.
Anti-thyroid Microsomal antibody	serum	negative at 1:10 dil.	highest pos. dil.	1	negative at 1:10 dil.	highest pos. dil.
Antihemophilic globulin (Coagulation Factor VIII)	plasma	50-200	%	0.01	0.50-2.00	fraction of 1.00
Antinuclear Antibodies (ANA)	serum	negative at 1:10 dil.	highest pos. dil.	1	negative at 1:10 dil.	highest pos. dil.
Alpha-1-Antitrypsin	serum	150 - 350	mg/dL	0.01	1.5 - 3.5	g/L
Arginine, amino acid fractionation	plasma, serum	0.5 - 2.5	mg/dL	57.40	30 - 145	µmol/L
Arsenic						
as As	hair	<1	µg/g (ppm)	13.35	<13.0	nmol/g
as As	urine	0 - 5	µg/24 hr	13.35	0 - 67	nmol/d
as As203	urine	<25	µg/dL	0.05055	<1.3	µmol/L
Ascorbate (as ascorbic acid)(Vitamin C)	plasma, serum	0.6 - 2.0	mg/dL	56.78	30 - 110	µmol/L
Asparagine, amino acid fractionation	plasma, serum	0.5 - 0.6	mg/dL	75.69	35 - 45	µmol/L
Aspartate Aminotransferase (AST, SGOT)	serum	0 - 35 (37°C)	Units/L	1	0 - 35	U/L
	serum	0 - 35 (37°C)	Units/L	0.01667	0 - 0.58	µkat/L
Aspartic acid, amino acid fractionation	plasma, serum	0.0 - 0.3	mg/dL	75.13	0 - 20	µmol/L

CONSTITUENT	FLUID	TRADITIONAL APPROXIMATE NORMAL RANGE	UNITS	CONVERSION FACTOR → MULT / ← DIV	SI APPROXIMATE NORMAL RANGE	UNITS
AST (aspartate aminotransferase, SGOT)	serum	0 - 35 (37°C)	Units/L	1	0 - 35	U/L
	serum	0 - 35 (37°C)	Units/L	0.01667	0 - 0.58	μkat/L
Barbiturate - overdose, total expressed as:						
phenobarbital	serum	Depends on	mg/dL	43.06	Depends on	μmol/L
sodium phenobarbital	serum	composition	mg/dL	39.34	composition	μmol/L
barbitone	serum	of mixture	mg/dL	54.29	of mixture	μmol/L
Barbiturate - therapeutic						
phenobarbital	plasma, serum	2 - 5	mg/dL	43.06	85 - 215	μmol/L
pentobarbital	plasma, serum	20 - 40	mg/L	4.419	90 - 170	μmol/L
thiopental	plasma, serum	individual	mg/L	4.126	individual	μmol/L
Bence-Jones protein	urine	0	absent/present	1	0	absent/present
Beta-Carotenes	serum	50 - 250	μg/dL	0.01863	0.9 - 4.6	μmol/L
Beta-Hydroxybutyrate (as beta-hydroxybutyric acid)	serum	<1.0	mg/dL	96.05	<100	μmol/L
Beta-2-Microglobulin <50 yrs	serum	0.80 - 2.40	mg/L	84.750	68 - 204	nmol/L
Beta-2-Microglobulin <50 yrs	urine	<140	μg/24 hr	0.08475	<12	nmol/d
Bicarbonate + CO2 (carbon dioxide content)	wh bld, plasma, serum	22 - 28	mEq/L	1	22 - 28	mmol/L
Bile Acids						
Total	serum	trace - 3.3	μg/mL	2.547	trace - 8.4	μmol/L
Chenodeoxycholic acid	serum	trace - 1.3	μg/mL	2.547	trace - 3.4	μmol/L
Cholic acid	serum	trace - 1.0	μg/mL	2.448	trace - 2.4	μmol/L
Deoxycholic acid	serum	trace - 1.0	μg/mL	2.547	trace - 2.6	μmol/L
Lithocholic Acid	serum	trace	μg/mL	2.656	trace	μmol/L
Bile Acids (after cholecystokinin stimulation)						
Total	duodenal fluid	14.0 - 58.0	mg/mL	2.547	35.0 - 148.0	mmol/L
Chenodeoxycholic acid	duodenal fluid	4.0 - 24.0	mg/mL	2.547	10.0 - 61.4	mmol/L
Cholic acid	duodenal fluid	2.4 - 33.0	mg/mL	2.448	6.8 - 81.0	mmol/L
Deoxycholic acid	duodenal fluid	0.8 - 6.9	mg/mL	2.547	2.0 - 18.0	mmol/L
Lithocholic Acid	duodenal fluid	0.3 - 0.8	mg/mL	2.656	0.8 - 2.0	mmol/L
Bilirubin						
Total	serum	0.1 - 1.0	mg/dL	17.1	2 - 18	μmol/L
Conjugated	serum	0 - 0.2	mg/dL	17.1	0 - 4	μmol/L
Blood Gases						
pCO2	art whole blood	35 - 45	mm Hg	0.1333	4.7 - 6.0	kPa
pH	art whole blood	7.35 - 7.45	pH units	1	7.35 - 7.45	pH units
pO2	art whole blood	75 - 100	mm Hg	0.1333	10.0 - 13.3	kPa
Blood Urea Nitrogen (BUN, urea nitrogen)	plasma, serum	8 - 18	mg/dL	0.357	3.0 - 6.5	mmol/L of urea
Blood volume	patient	8.5 - 9.0	% body weight	9.4	80-85	mL/kg

CONSTITUENT	FLUID	TRADITIONAL APPROXIMATE NORMAL RANGE	UNITS	CONVERSION FACTOR MULT → / DIV ←	SI APPROXIMATE NORMAL RANGE	UNITS
Bromide, toxic						
as bromide ion	serum	> 120	mg/dL	0.1252	> 15	mmol/L
as sodium bromide	serum	> 150	mg/dL	0.09719	> 15	mmol/L
as sodium bromide	serum	> 15	mEq/L	1	> 15	mmol/L
BUN (blood urea nitrogen, urea nitrogen)	plasma, serum	8 - 18	mg/dL	0.357	3.0 - 6.5	mmol/L of urea
C1 Esterase Inhibitor	serum	12 - 30	mg/dL	0.01	12 - 30	g/L
C3 (complement, C3)	serum	70 - 160	mg/dL	0.01	0.7 - 1.6	g/L
C4 (complement, C4)	serum	20 - 40	mg/dL	0.01	0.2 - 0.4	g/L
Cadmium	serum	< 3	µg/dL	0.08897	< 0.27	µmol/L
Calcitonin	serum	<100	pg/mL	1	<100	ng/L
Calcium						
Male	serum	8.8 - 10.3	mg/dL	0.250	2.20 - 2.58	mmol/L
Female <50 yr	serum	8.8 - 10.0	mg/dL	0.250	2.20 - 2.50	mmol/L
Female >50 yr	serum	8.8 - 10.2	mg/dL	0.250	2.20 - 2.56	mmol/L
All populations	serum	4.4 - 5.1	mEq/L	0.500	2.20 - 2.56	mmol/L
Calcium, ionized						
All populations	wh bld, plsm, ser	2.00 - 2.30	mEq/L	0.500	1.00 - 1.15	mmol/L
All populations	wh bld, plsm, ser	4.00 - 4.60	mg/dL	0.250	1.00 - 1.15	mmol/L
Calcium, normal diet	urine	<250	mg/24 hr	0.02495	<6.2	mmol/d
cAMP (cyclic adenosine monophosphate)	plasma, serum	2.6 - 6.6	µg/L	3.038	8 - 20	nmol/L
cAMP (cyclic adenosine monophosphate)						
Total Urinary	urine	2.9 - 5.6	µmol/g of creatinine	113.1	330 - 630	nmol/mmol of creatinine
Renal Tubular	urine	<2.5	µmol/g of creatinine	113.1	<280	nmol/mmol of creatinine
Carbamazepine, therapeutic	plasma, serum	4 - 12	mg/L	4.233	17 - 51	µmol/L
Carbon Dioxide Content [bicarb. + CO2]	wh bld, plasma, serum	22 - 28	mEq/L	1	22 - 28	mmol/L
Carbon monoxide (proportion of Hb that is COHb)	plasma	<15	% saturation	0.01	< 0.15	fraction of 1.00
Carcinoembryonic Antigen (CEA)	serum	<3.0	ng/mL	1	<3.0	µg/L
Carotenes, beta	serum	50 - 250	µg/dL	0.01863	0.9 - 4.6	µmol/L
Catecholamines, total (as norepinephrine)	urine	< 100	µg/24 hr	5.911	< 590	nmol/d
CBC (Complete Blood Count)						
Hematocrit						
Female	whole blood	33 - 43	%	0.01	0.33 - 0.43	1
Male	whole blood	39 - 49	%	0.01	0.39 - 0.49	1
Hemoglobin						
Mass Concentration						
Female	whole blood	14.0 - 18.0	g/dL	10.0	140 - 180	g/L
Male	whole blood	11.5 - 15.5	g/dL	10.0	115 - 155	g/L

CONSTITUENT	FLUID	TRADITIONAL APPROXIMATE NORMAL RANGE	UNITS	CONVERSION FACTOR MULT ⟶ / DIV ⟵	SI APPROXIMATE NORMAL RANGE	UNITS
CBC (Complete Blood Count) (continued)						
Hemoglobin						
Substance Concentration Hb [Fe]						
Female	whole blood	12.0 - 15.0	g/dL	0.6206	7.45 - 9.30	mmol/L
Male	whole blood	13.6 - 17.2	g/dL	0.6206	8.45 - 10.65	mmol/L
Mean Corpuscular Hemoglobin (MCH)						
Mass	whole blood	27 - 33	pg		27 - 33	pg
Amount of substance Hb [Fe]	whole blood	27 - 33	pg	0.06206	1.70 - 2.05	fmol
Mean Corpuscular Hemoglobin Conc. (MCHC)						
Mass Concentration	whole blood	33 - 37	g/dL	1.0	330 - 370	g/L
	whole blood	33 - 37	%	0.01	0.33 - 0.37	fraction of 1.00
Amount of substance Hb[Fe]	whole blood	33 - 37	g/dL	0.6206	20 - 23	mmol/L
Mean Corpuscular Volume (MCV)	whole blood	76 - 100	μm^3	1	76 - 100	fL
Platelet count	whole blood	130 - 400	$10^3/mm^3$	1	130 - 400	$10^9/L$
RBC Count (erythrocyte count)						
Female	whole blood	3.5 - 5.0	$10^6/mm^3$	1	3.5 - 5.0	$10^{12}/L$
Male	whole blood	4.3 - 5.9	$10^6/mm^3$	1	4.3 - 5.9	$10^{12}/L$
WBC Count	whole blood	3.2 - 9.8	$10^3/mm^3$	0.001	3.2 - 9.8	$10^9/L$
WBC Differential						
Bands	whole blood	3 - 5	%	0.01	0.03 - 0.05	fraction of 1.00
Neutrophils	whole blood	54 - 62	%	0.01	0.54 - 0.62	fraction of 1.00
Lymphocytes	whole blood	25 - 33	%	0.01	0.25 - 0.33	fraction of 1.00
Monocytes	whole blood	3 - 7	%	0.01	0.03 - 0.07	fraction of 1.00
Eosinophils	whole blood	1 - 3	%	0.01	0.01 - 0.03	fraction of 1.00
Basophils	whole blood	0 - 0.75	%	0.01	0 - 0.0075	fraction of 1.00
Bands	whole blood	150 - 400	cells/mm³ (μL)	1	150 - 400	10^6 cells / L
Neutrophils	whole blood	3000 - 5800	cells/mm³ (μL)	1	3000 - 5800	10^6 cells / L
Lymphocytes	whole blood	1500 - 3000	cells/mm³ (μL)	1	1500 - 3000	10^6 cells / L
Monocytes	whole blood	285 - 500	cells/mm³ (μL)	1	285 - 500	10^6 cells / L
Eosinophils	whole blood	50 - 250	cells/mm³ (μL)	1	50 - 250	10^6 cells / L
Basophils	whole blood	15 - 50	cells/mm³ (μL)	1	15 - 50	10^6 cells / L
CEA (Carcinoembryonic Antigen)	serum	< 3.0	ng/mL	1	< 3.0	μg/L
Ceruloplasmin	serum	20 - 25	mg/dL	10	200 - 350	mg/L
cGMP (cyclic guanine monophosphate)	plasma	0.6 - 3.5	μg/L	2.897	1.7 - 10.1	nmol/L
cGMP (cyclic guanine monophosphate)	urine	0.3 - 1.8	μmol/g of creatinine	113.1	30 - 200	nmol/mmol of creatinine
CH50 (Hemolytic Complement, Total)	serum	150-250	units/mL	1	150-250	arb unit
Chloramphenicol, therapeutic	serum	10 - 20	μg/mL	3.1	31.0 - 62.0	μmol/L
Chlordiazepoxide						
Therapeutic	plasma, serum	0.5 - 5.0	mg/L	3.336	2 - 17	μmol/L
Toxic	plasma, serum	>10.0	mg/L	3.336	>33	μmol/L

| CONSTITUENT | FLUID | TRADITIONAL | | CONVERSION FACTOR | SI | |
		APPROXIMATE NORMAL RANGE	UNITS	MULT ⟶ / DIV ⟵	APPROXIMATE NORMAL RANGE	UNITS
Chloride	plasma, serum	95 - 105	mEq/L	1	95 - 105	mmol/L
Chloride	CSF	120 - 130	mEq/L	1	120 - 130	mmol/L
Chlorimipramine (includes desmethyl metabolite), therapeutic	plasma, serum	50 - 400	ng/mL	3.76	150 - 1270	nmol/L
Chlorpromazine, therapeutic	plasma, serum	50 - 300	ng/mL	3.136	150 - 950	nmol/L
Chlorpropamide, therapeutic	plasma, serum	75 - 250	mg/L	3.613	270 - 900	µmol/L
Cholecalciferol (vitamin D3)	serum	24 - 40	ng/mL	2.599	60 - 105	nmol/L
25-OH-cholecalciferol	serum	18 - 36	ng/mL	2.496	45 - 90	nmol/L
Cholestanol (as a fraction of total cholesterol)	plasma, serum	1 - 3	%	0.01	0.01 - 0.03	fraction of 1.00
Cholesterol, HDL (high density lipoproteins)						
Male	plasma, serum	30 - 70	mg/dL	0.02586	0.80 - 1.80	mmol/L
Female	plasma, serum	30 - 90	mg/dL	0.02586	0.80 - 2.35	mmol/L
Cholesterol, LDL (low density lipoproteins)	plasma, serum	50 - 190	mg/dL	0.02586	1.30 - 4.90	mmol/L
Cholesterol, total						
<29 yr	plasma, serum	<200	mg/dL	0.02586	<5.20	mmol/L
30 - 39 yr	plasma, serum	<225	mg/dL	0.02586	<5.85	mmol/L
40 - 49 yr	plasma, serum	<245	mg/dL	0.02586	<6.35	mmol/L
>50 yr	plasma, serum	<265	mg/dL	0.02586	<6.85	mmol/L
Cholesterol esters (as a fraction of total cholesterol)	plasma, serum	60-75	%	0.01	0.60-0.75	fraction of 1.00
Cholinesterase	plasma, serum	620-1370 (25°C)	Units/L	1	620-1370	U/L
	plasma, serum	620-1370 (25°C)	Units/L	0.01667	10.3 - 22.8	µkat/L
Chorionic gonadotropin (HCG)	serum	< 10 if not pregnant	mIU/mL	1	< 10 if not pregnant	IU/L
Chorionic gonadotropin (HCG)	urine	negative	neg/pos	1	negative	neg/pos
Citrate (as citric acid)	serum	1.2 - 3.0	mg/dL	52.05	60 - 160	µmol/L
Citrulline, amino acid fractionation	plasma, serum	0.2 - 1.0	mg/dL	57.08	15 - 55	µmol/L
CK, (Creatine phosphokinase, creatine kinase)	serum	0 - 150 (37°C)	Units/L	1	0 - 150	U/L
	serum	0 - 150 (37°C)	Units/L	0.01667	0 - 2.50	µkat/L
CK (Creatine kinase) isoenzymes, MB fraction	serum	> 5 % in myocardial infarction	%	0.01	>0.05	fraction of 1.00
CO2 (carbon dioxide content, bicarb. + CO2)	wh bld, plasma, serum	22 - 28	mEq/L	1	22 - 28	mmol/L
Clot retraction	plasma	50-100	% @ 2 hour	1	0.50 - 1.00	fraction of 1.00
Coagulation Factor I (fibrinogen)	plasma	0.15 - 0.35	g/dL	29.41	4.4 - 10.3	µmol/L
	plasma	150 - 350	mg/dL	0.01	1.5 - 3.5	g/L
Coagulation Factor II (prothrombin)	plasma	70 -130	%	0.01	0.70-1.30	fraction of 1.00
Coagulation Factor V	plasma	70 -130	%	0.01	0.70-1.30	fraction of 1.00
Coagulation Factor VII	plasma	60 - 140	%	0.01	0.60 - 1.40	fraction of 1.00
Coagulation Factor VIII C	plasma	50 - 200	%	0.01	0.50 - 2.00	fraction of 1.00
Coagulation Factor VIII VW (RCoF. Ristocetin Cofactor, von Willebrand Factor)	plasma	50 - 150	%	0.01	0.50 - 1.50	fraction of 1.00

CONSTITUENT	FLUID	TRADITIONAL			CONVERSION FACTOR		SI	
		APPROXIMATE NORMAL RANGE	UNITS		→ MULT DIV ←		APPROXIMATE NORMAL RANGE	UNITS
Coagulation Factor IX	plasma	70 -130	%		0.01		0.70-1.30	fraction of 1.00
Coagulation Factor X	plasma	70 -130	%		0.01		0.70-1.30	fraction of 1.00
Coagulation Factor XI	plasma	70 -130	%		0.01		0.70-1.30	fraction of 1.00
Coagulation Factor XII	plasma	70 -130	%		0.01		0.70-1.30	fraction of 1.00
Complement - hemolytic total (CH50)	serum	150 - 250	units/mL		1		150-250	arb unit
Complement Component 3	serum	70 - 160	mg/dL		0.01		0.7 - 1.6	g/L
Complement Component 4	serum	20 - 40	mg/dL		0.01		0.2 - 0.4	g/L
Complete Blood Count (CBC)								
Hematocrit								
Female	whole blood	33 - 43	%		0.01		0.33 - 0.43	1
Male	whole blood	39 - 49	%		0.01		0.39 - 0.49	1
Hemoglobin								
Mass Concentration								
Female	whole blood	14.0 - 18.0	g/dL		10.0		140 - 180	g/L
Male	whole blood	11.5 - 15.5	g/dL		10.0		115 - 155	g/L
Substance Concentration Hb [Fe]								
Female	whole blood	12.0 -15.0	g/dL		0.6206		7.45 - 9.30	mmol/L
Male	whole blood	13.6 - 17.2	g/dL		0.6206		8.45 - 10.65	mmol/L
Mean Corpuscular Hemoglobin (MCH)								
Mass	whole blood	27 - 33	pg		1		27 - 33	pg
Amount of substance Hb [Fe]	whole blood	27 - 33	pg		0.06206		1.70 - 2.05	fmol)
Mean Corpuscular Hemoglobin Conc. (MCHC)								
Mass Concentration	whole blood	33 - 37	g/dL		10		330 - 370	g/L
	whole blood	33 - 37	%		0.01		0.33 - 0.37	fraction of 1.00
Amount of substance Hb[Fe]	whole blood	33 - 37	g/dL		0.6206		20 - 23	mmol/L
Mean Corpuscular Volume (MCV)	whole blood	76 - 100	μm³		1		76 - 100	fL
Platelet count	whole blood	130 - 400	10³/mm³		1		130 - 400	10⁹/L
RBC Count (erythrocyte count)								
Female	whole blood	3.5 - 5.0	10⁶/mm³		1		3.5 - 5.0	10¹²/L
Male	whole blood	4.3 - 5.9	10⁶/mm³		1		4.3 - 5.9	10¹²/L
WBC Count.	whole blood	3.2 - 9.8	10³ / mm³		0.001		3.2 - 9.8	10⁹/L
WBC Differential								
Bands	whole blood	3 - 5	%		0.01		0.03 - 0.05	fraction of 1.00
Neutrophils	whole blood	54 - 62	%		0.01		0.54 - 0.62	fraction of 1.00
Lymphocytes	whole blood	25 - 33	%		0.01		0.25 - 0.33	fraction of 1.00
Monocytes	whole blood	3 - 7	%		0.01		0.03 - 0.07	fraction of 1.00
Eosinophils	whole blood	1 - 3	%		0.01		0.01 - 0.03	fraction of 1.00
Basophils	whole blood	0 - 0.75	%		0.01		0 - 0.0075	fraction of 1.00
Bands	whole blood	150 - 400	cells/mm³ (μL)		1		150 - 400	10⁶ cells / L
Neutrophils	whole blood	3000 - 5800	cells/mm³ (μL)		1		3000 - 5800	10⁶ cells / L
Lymphocytes	whole blood	1500 - 3000	cells/mm³ (μL)		1		1500 - 3000	10⁶ cells / L

CONSTITUENT	FLUID	APPROXIMATE NORMAL RANGE (Traditional)	UNITS (Traditional)	CONVERSION FACTOR MULT → DIV ←	APPROXIMATE NORMAL RANGE (SI)	UNITS (SI)
Complete Blood Count (CBC) (continued)						
WBC Differential						
Monocytes	whole blood	285 - 500	cells/mm³ (µL)	1	285 - 500	10⁶ cells / L
Eosinophils	whole blood	50 - 250	cells/mm³ (µL)	1	50 - 250	10⁶ cells / L
Basophils	whole blood	15 - 50	cells/mm³ (µL)	1	15 - 50	10⁶ cells / L
Copper (Copper (II), Cu)	serum	70 - 140	µg/dL	0.1574	11.0 - 22.0	µmol/L
Copper (Copper (II), Cu)	urine	<40	µg/24 hr	0.01574	<0.6	µmol/d
Coproporphyrin	urine	<200	µg/24 hr	1.527	<300	nmol/d
Corticotropin (ACTH)	plasma	20 - 100	pg/mL	0.2202	4 - 22	pmol/L
Cortisol						
0800 hr	plasma, serum	4 - 19	µg/dL	27.59	110 - 520	nmol/L
1800 hr	plasma, serum	2 - 15	µg/dL	27.59	50 - 410	nmol/L
2400 hr	plasma, serum	<5	µg/dL	27.59	<140	nmol/L
Cortisol, free	urine	10 - 110	µg/24 hr	2.759	30 - 300	nmol/d
Creatine						
Male	serum	0.17 - 0.50	mg/dL	76.25	10 - 40	µmol/L
Female	serum	0.35 - 0.93	mg/dL	76.25	30 - 70	µmol/L
Creatine						
Male	urine	0 - 40	mg/24 hr	7.625	0 - 300	µmol/d
Female	urine	0 - 80	mg/24 hr	7.625	0 - 600	µmol/d
Creatine kinase (CK, creatine phosphokinase)	serum	0 - 150 (37°C)	Units/L	1	0 - 150	U/L
	serum	0 - 150 (37°C)	Units/L	0.01667	0 - 2.50	µkat/L
Creatine kinase isoenzymes, MB fraction	plasma, serum	> 5 % in myocardial infarction	%	0.01	>0.05	fraction of 1.00
Creatinine	plasma, serum	0.6 - 1.2	mg/dL	88.4	50 - 110	µmol/L
Creatinine						
Male	urine	20 - 26	mg/kg/24hr	0.0088	0.18 - 0.23	mmol/kg/d
	urine	1.0 - 2.0	g/24hr	8.8	8.8 - 17.6	mmol/d
Female	urine	14 - 22	mg/kg/24hr	0.0088	0.12 - 0.19	mmol/kg/d
	urine	0.8 - 1.8	g/24hr	8.8	7.0 - 15.8	mmol/d
Creatinine clearance	plsm, ser. & urine	75 - 125	mL/min	0.01667	1.24 - 2.08	mL/s
creatinine clearance µmol/L (urine creatinine) · mL/s corrected for body µmol/L (serum creatinine) surface area		$\dfrac{1.73}{A}$ (where A is the body surface area in square meters)				
Cryoglobulins	serum	0	neg/pos	1	0	neg/pos
Cyanide, lethal	plasma	>0.10	mg/dL	384.3	>40	µmol/L
Cyanocobalamin (vitamin B12)	serum	200 - 1000	pg/mL	0.7378	150 - 750	pmol/L
	serum	20 - 100	ng/dL	7.378	150 - 750	pmol/L
Cyclic adenosine monophosphate (cAMP)	plasma	2.6 - 6.6	µg/L	3.038	8 - 20	nmol/L

CONSTITUENT	FLUID	TRADITIONAL APPROXIMATE NORMAL RANGE	UNITS	CONVERSION FACTOR → MULT ← DIV	SI APPROXIMATE NORMAL RANGE	UNITS
Cyclic adenosine monophosphate (cAMP)						
Total Urinary	urine	2.9 - 5.6	μmol/g of creatinine	113.1	330 - 630	nmol/mmol of creatinine
Renal Tubular	urine	<2.5	μmol/g of creatinine	113.1	<280	nmol/mmol of creatinine
Cyclic guanine monophosphate (cGMP)	plasma, serum	0.6 - 3.5	μg/L	2.897	1.7 - 10.1	nmol/L
Cyclic guanine monophosphate (cGMP)	urine	0.3 - 1.8	μmol/g of creatinine	113.1	30 - 200	nmol/mmol of creatinine
Cystine, amino acid fractionation	plasma, serum	0.2 - 2.2	mg/dL	41.61	10 - 90	μmol/L
Cystine	urine	10 - 100		4.161	40 - 420	μmol/d
Dehydroepiandrosterone (DHEA)						
1 - 4 years	plasma, serum	0.2 - 0.4	μg/L	3.467	0.6 - 1.4	nmol/L
4 - 8 years	plasma, serum	0.1 - 1.9	μg/L	3.467	0.4 - 6.6	nmol/L
8 - 10 years	plasma, serum	0.2 - 2.9	μg/L	3.467	0.6 - 10.0	nmol/L
10 - 12 years	plasma, serum	0.5 - 9.2	μg/L	3.467	1.8 - 31.8	nmol/L
12 - 14 years	plasma, serum	0.9 - 20.0	μg/L	3.467	3.2 - 69.4	nmol/L
14 - 16 years	plasma, serum	2.5 - 20.0	μg/L	3.467	8.6 - 69.4	nmol/L
Premenopausal female	plasma, serum	2.0 - 15.0	μg/L	3.467	7.0 - 52.0	nmol/L
Male	plasma, serum	0.8 - 10.0	μg/L	3.467	2.8 - 34.6	nmol/L
Dehydroepiandrosterone (ketosteroid fractions)						
Female	urine	0.2 - 1.8	mg/24 hr	3.467	1 - 6	μmol/d
Male	urine	0.2 - 2.0	mg/24 hr	3.467	1 - 7	μmol/d
Dehydroepiandrosterone sulphate (DHEA-S)						
newborn	plasma, serum	1670 - 3640	ng/mL	0.002714	4.5 - 9.9	μmol/L
pre-pubertal children	plasma, serum	100 - 600	ng/mL	0.002714	0.3 - 1.6	μmol/L
male	plasma, serum	2000 - 3350	ng/mL	0.002714	5.4 - 9.1	μmol/L
female [premenopausal]	plasma, serum	820 - 3380	ng/mL	0.002714	2.2 - 9.2	μmol/L
female [post-menopausal]	plasma, serum	110 - 610	ng/mL	0.002714	0.3 - 1.7	μmol/L
pregnancy [term]	plasma, serum	230 - 1170	ng/mL	0.002714	0.6 - 3.2	μmol/L
Delta-Aminolevulinate (as aminolevulinic acid)	urine	1.0 - 7.0	mg/24 hr	7.626	8 - 53	μmol/d
11-Deoxycortisol	plasma	0 - 2	μg/dL	28.86	0 - 60	nmol/L
Desipramine, therapeutic	plasma, serum	50 - 200	ng/mL	3.754	170 - 700	nmol/L
Desmethylsuximide, therapeutic	plasma, serum	10 - 40	μg/L	5.285	50 - 210	μmol/L
Diazepam						
Therapeutic	plasma, serum	0.1 - 0.25	mg/L	3512	350 - 900	nmol/L
Toxic	plasma, serum	>1.0	mg/L	3512	>3510	nmol/L
Dicoumarol, therapeutic	plasma, serum	8 - 30	mg/L	2.974	25 - 90	μmol/L
Dilantin, (Diphenylhydantoin, Phenytoin)						
Therapeutic	plasma, serum	10 - 20	mg/L	3.964	40 - 80	μmol/L
Toxic	plasma, serum	>30	mg/L	3.964	>120	μmol/L

CONSTITUENT	FLUID	TRADITIONAL APPROXIMATE NORMAL RANGE	UNITS	CONVERSION FACTOR MULT ⟶ DIV ⟵	SI APPROXIMATE NORMAL RANGE	UNITS
Digoxin						
Therapeutic	plasma, serum	0.5 - 2.2	ng/mL	1.281	0.6 - 2.8	nmol/L
Therapeutic	plasma, serum	0.5 - 2.2	µg/L	1.281	0.6 - 2.8	nmol/L
Toxic	plasma, serum	>2.5	ng/mL	1.281	>3.2	nmol/L
Dimethadione, therapeutic	plasma, serum	<1	g/L	7.745	<7.7	mmol/L
Diphenylhydantoin (phenytoin)						
Therapeutic	plasma, serum	10 - 20	mg/L	3.964	40 - 80	µmol/L
Toxic	plasma, serum	>30	mg/L	3.964	>120	µmol/L
Disopyramide, therapeutic	plasma, serum	2.0 - 6.0	mg/L	2.946	6 - 18	µmol/L
Doxepin, therapeutic	plasma, serum	50 - 200	ng/mL	3.579	180 - 720	nmol/L
D-Xylose (25 g dose)	plasma, serum	30 - 40 (30-60 min)	mg/dL	0.06661	2.0 - 2.7 (30-60 min)	mmol/L
D-Xylose excretion (25 g dose)	urine (excreted in 5 hr)	21 - 31	%	0.01	0.21 - 0.31 (excreted in 5 hr)	fraction of 1.00
Electrolytes						
Chloride	plasma, serum	95 - 105	mEq/L	1	95 - 105	mmol/L
CO2	wh bld, plsm, ser	22 - 28	mEq/L	1	22 - 28	mmol/L
Potassium	plasma, serum	3.5-5.0	mEq/L	1	3.5 - 5.0	mmol/L
Sodium	plasma, serum	135 - 147	mEq/L	1	135 - 147	mmol/L
Electrophoresis, protein						
Albumin	serum	60 - 65	%	0.01	0.60 - 0.65	fraction of 1.00
Alpha 1 Globulin	serum	1.7 - 5.0	%	0.01	0.02 - 0.05	fraction of 1.00
Alpha 2 Globulin	serum	6.7 - 12.5	%	0.01	0.07 - 0.13	fraction of 1.00
Beta Globulin	serum	8.3 - 16.3	%	0.01	0.08 - 0.16	fraction of 1.00
Gamma Globulin	serum	10.7 - 20.0	%	0.01	0.11 - 0.20	fraction of 1.00
Albumin	serum	3.6 - 5.2	g/dL	10.0	36 - 52	g/L
Alpha 1 Globulin	serum	0.1 - 0.4	g/dL	10.0	1 - 4	g/L
Alpha 2 Globulin	serum	0.4 - 1.0	g/dL	10.0	4 - 10	g/L
Beta Globulin	serum	0.5 - 1.2	g/dL	10.0	5 - 12	g/L
Gamma Globulin	serum	0.6 - 1.6	g/dL	10.0	6 - 16	g/L
Electrophoresis, Protein	urine	no monoclonal paraproteins	neg/pos	1	no monoclonal paraproteins	neg/pos
Epinephrine	plasma	31 - 95 (at rest for 15 min)	pg/mL	5.458	170 - 520 (at rest for 15 min)	pmol/L
Epinephrine	urine	<10	µg/24 hr	5.458	<55	nmol/d
Erythrocyte count (RBC count)						
Female	whole blood	3.5 - 5.0	10⁶/mm³	1	3.5 - 5.0	10¹²/L
Male	whole blood	4.3 - 5.9	10⁶/mm³	1	4.3 - 5.9	10¹²/L
Erythrocyte count (RBC count)	CSF	0	per mm³	1	0	10⁶/L
Erythrocyte Sedimentation Rate (ESR)						
Female	whole blood	0 - 30	mm/hr	1	0 - 30	mm/hr

CONSTITUENT	FLUID	TRADITIONAL APPROXIMATE NORMAL RANGE	UNITS	CONVERSION FACTOR MULT →/ DIV ←	SI APPROXIMATE NORMAL RANGE	UNITS
Erythrocyte Sedimentation Rate (ESR) (continued)						
Male	whole blood	0 - 20	mm/hr	1	0 - 20	mm/hr
Estradiol, (as estrogens)						
Female	plasma, serum	20 - 300	pg/mL	3.671	70 - 1100	pmol/L
Peak production	plasma, serum	200 - 800	pg/mL	3.671	750 - 2900	pmol/L
Male	plasma, serum	<50	pg/mL	3.671	<180	pmol/L
Estriol (nonpregnant)						
Onset of menstruation	urine	4 - 25	µg/24 hr	3.468	15 - 85	nmol/d
Ovulation peak	urine	28 - 99	µg/24 hr	3.468	95 - 345	nmol/d
Luteal peak	urine	22 - 105	µg/24 hr	3.468	75 - 365	nmol/d
Menopausal women	urine	1.4 - 19.6	µg/24 hr	3.468	5 - 70	nmol/d
Male	urine	5 - 18	µg/24 hr	3.468	15 - 60	nmol/d
Estrogens (as estradiol)						
Female	plasma, serum	20 - 300	pg/mL	3.671	70 - 1100	pmol/L
Peak production	plasma, serum	200 - 800	pg/mL	3.671	750 - 2900	pmol/L
Male	plasma, serum	<50	pg/mL	3.671	<180	pmol/L
Estrogens, placental (as estriol)	urine	gestation dependent	mg/24 hr	3.468	gestation dependent	µmol/d
Estrogen receptors						
Negative Result	tissue	0 - 3	fmol of estradiol bound/mg of cytosol protein	1	0 - 3	fmol of estradiol bound/mg of cytosol protein
Doubtful Result	tissue	4 - 10	fmol of estradiol bound/mg of cytosol protein	1	4 - 10	fmol of estradiol bound/mg of cytosol protein
Positive Result	tissue	>10	fmol of estradiol bound/mg of cytosol protein	1	>10	fmol of estradiol bound/mg of cytosol protein
Estrone						
Female, 1-10 days of cycle	plasma, serum	43 - 180	pg/mL	3.699	160 - 665	pmol/L
Female, 11-20 days of cycle	plasma, serum	75 - 196	pg/mL	3.699	275 - 725	pmol/L
Female, 20-29 days of cycle	plasma, serum	131 - 201	pg/mL	3.699	485 - 745	pmol/L
Male	plasma, serum	29 - 75	pg/mL	3.699	105 - 275	pmol/L
Estrone, female	urine	2 - 25	µg/24 hr	3.699	5 - 90	nmol/d
Ethanol, toxic (ethyl alcohol)	plasma, serum	>100	mg/dL	0.2171	>22	mmol/L
Ethchlorvynol, therapeutic	plasma, serum	< 40	mg/L	6.915	< 280	µmol/L
Ethyl Alcohol, toxic (ethanol)	plasma, serum	>100	mg/dL	0.2171	>22	mmol/L
Etiocholanolone						
Female	urine	0.8 - 4.0	mg/24 hr	3.443	2 - 14	µmol/d
Male	urine	1.4 - 5.0	mg/24 hr	3.443	4 - 17	µmol/d
Ethosuximide, therapeutic	plasma, serum	40 - 110	mg/L	7.084	280 - 780	µmol/L

CONSTITUENT	FLUID	TRADITIONAL APPROXIMATE NORMAL RANGE	UNITS	CONVERSION FACTOR → MULT ← DIV	SI APPROXIMATE NORMAL RANGE	UNITS
Ethylene glycol, toxic	plasma, serum	>30	mg/dL	0.1611	>5	mmol/L
Factor I (fibrinogen)	plasma	0.15-0.35	g/dL	29.41	4.4 - 10.3	µmol/L
	plasma	150 - 350	mg/dL	0.01	1.5 - 3.5	g/L
Factor II (prothrombin)	plasma	70 -130	%	0.01	0.70 -1.30	fraction of 1.00
Factor V	plasma	70 -130	%	0.01	0.70 -1.30	fraction of 1.00
Factor VII	plasma	60 - 140	%	0.01	0.60 - 1.40	fraction of 1.00
Factor VIII C	plasma	50 - 200	%	0.01	0.50 - 2.00	fraction of 1.00
Factor VIII VW (Ristocetin Cofactor, von Willebrand Factor)	plasma	50 - 150	%	0.01	0.50 - 1.50	fraction of 1.00
Factor IX	plasma	70 -130	%	0.01	0.70 -1.30	fraction of 1.00
Factor X	plasma	70 -130	%	0.01	0.70 -1.30	fraction of 1.00
Factor XI	plasma	70 -130	%	0.01	0.70 -1.30	fraction of 1.00
Factor XII	plasma	70 -130	%	0.01	0.70 -1.30	fraction of 1.00
Fatty Acids, nonesterified	plasma	8 - 20	mg/dL	10	80 - 200	mg/L
	plasma	8 - 20	mg/dL	0.01	0.08 - 0.20	g/L
Fecal fat (as stearic acid)	feces	2.0 - 6.0	g/24 hr	3.515	7 - 21	mmol/d
Ferritin	plasma, serum	18 - 300	ng/mL	1	18 - 300	µg/L
Fetal hemoglobin (Hemoglobin F)	whole blood	<2	%	0.01	<0.02	fraction of 1.00
alpha-Fetoprotein	amniotic fluid	gestation dependent	mg/dL	10	gestation dependent	mg/L
alpha-Fetoprotein	serum	0 - 20	ng/mL	1	0 - 20	µg/L
Fibrinogen (coagulation factor I)	plasma	0.15-0.35	g/dL	29.41	4.4 - 10.3	µmol/L
	plasma	150 - 350	mg/dL	0.01	1.5 - 3.5	g/L
Fibrin(ogen) Split Products	serum	<10	µg/mL	1	<10	mg/L
5'Nucleotidase	plasma, serum	2 - 17 (37°C)	U/L	1	2 - 17	U/L
	plasma, serum	2 - 17 (37°C)	U/L	0.01667	0.03 - 0.28	µkat/L
Fluoride	urine	<1.0	mg/24 hr	52.63	<50	µmol/d
Folate (folic acid, pteroylglutamic acid)	serum	2 - 10	ng/mL	2.266	4 - 22	nmol/L
Folate	serum	0.2 - 1.0	µg/dL	22.66	4 - 22	nmol/L
Folate	RBC	140 - 960	ng/mL	2.266	550 - 2200	nmol/L
Follicle Stimulating Hormone (FSH)						
Female	plasma, serum	2.0 - 15.0	mIU/mL	1	2 - 15	IU/L
Peak Production - Female	plasma, serum	20 - 50	mIU/mL	1	20 - 50	IU/L
Male	plasma, serum	1.0 - 10.0	mIU/mL	1	1 - 10	IU/L
Follicle Stimulating Hormone (FSH)						
Follicular phase	urine	2 - 15	IU/24 hr	1	2 - 15	IU/d
Midcycle	urine	8 - 40	IU/24 hr	1	8 - 40	IU/d
Luteal phase	urine	2 - 10	IU/24 hr	1	2 - 10	IU/d
Menopausal women	urine	35 - 100	IU/24 hr	1	35 - 100	IU/d
Male	urine	2 - 15	IU/24 hr	1	2 - 15	IU/d
Fructose	plasma	<10	mg/dL	0.05551	<0.55	mmol/L
Galactose (children)	plasma	<20	mg/dL	0.05551	<1.10	mmol/L

CONSTITUENT	FLUID	TRADITIONAL APPROXIMATE NORMAL RANGE	UNITS	CONVERSION FACTOR MULT → / DIV ←	SI APPROXIMATE NORMAL RANGE	UNITS
Gamma Glutamyl Transferase (GGT)	serum	0 - 30 (30°C)	Units/L	1	0 - 30	U/L
	serum	0 - 30 (30°C)	Units/L	0.01667	0 - 0.50	µkat/L
Gases (arterial)						
pCO2	art whole blood	35 - 45	mm Hg	0.1333	4.7 - 6.0	kPa
pH	art whole blood	7.35 - 7.45	pH units	1	7.35 - 7.45	pH units
pO2	art whole blood	75 - 100	mm Hg	0.1333	10.0 - 13.3	kPa
Gastrin	plasma, serum	0 - 180	pg/mL	1	0 - 180	ng/L
GGT (Gamma Glutamyl Transferase)	serum	0 - 30 (30°C)	Units/L	1	0 - 30	U/L
	serum	0 - 30 (30°C)	Units/L	0.01667	0 - 0.50	µkat/L
Globulins, as immunoglobulins						
IgG	serum	500 - 1200	mg/dL	0.01	5.00 - 12.00	g/L
IgA	serum	50 - 350	mg/dL	0.01	0.50 - 3.50	g/L
IgM	serum	30 - 230	mg/dL	0.01	0.30 - 2.30	g/L
IgD	serum	<6	mg/dL	10	<60	mg/L
IgE						
0 - 3 years	serum	0.5 - 10	IU/mL	2.40	1 - 24	µg/L
> 3 years	serum	5 - 100	IU/mL	2.40	12 - 240	µg/L
Glucagon	plasma, serum	50 - 100	pg/mL	1	50 - 100	ng/L
Glucose (fasting)	plasma, serum	70 - 110	mg/dL	0.05551	3.9 - 6.1	mmol/L
Glucose	CSF	50 - 80	mg/dL	0.05551	2.8 - 4.4	mmol/L
Glutamic acid, amino acid fractionation	plasma, serum	0.2 - 2.8	mg/dL	67.97	15 - 190	µmol/L
Glutamine, amino acid fractionation	plasma, serum	6.1 - 10.2	mg/dL	68.42	420 - 700	µmol/L
Glutethimide						
Therapeutic	plasma, serum	<10	mg/L	4.603	<46	µmol/L
Toxic	plasma, serum	>20	mg/L	4.603	>92	µmol/L
Glycerol (free)	serum	<1.5	mg/dL	0.1086	<0.16	mmol/L
Glycine, amino acid fractionation	plasma, serum	0.9 - 4.2	mg/dL	133.20	120 - 560	µmol/L
Gold, therapeutic	serum	300 - 800	µg/dL	0.05077	15.0 - 40.0	µmol/L
Gold	urine	<500	µg/24 hr	0.005077	<2.5	µmol/d
Growth hormone						
Male (fasting)	plasma, serum	0 - 5	ng/mL	1	0 - 5	µg/L
Female (fasting)	plasma, serum	0 - 10	ng/mL	1	0 - 10	µg/L
Haptoglobin	serum	50 - 220	mg/dL	0.01	0.50 - 2.20	g/L
HCG (human chorionic gonadotropin)	serum	< 10 if not pregnant	mIU/mL	1	< 10 if not pregnant	IU/L
HCG (human chorionic gonadotropin)	urine	negative	neg/pos	1	negative	neg/pos
HDL (high density lipoproteins)						
Male	plasma, serum	30 - 70	mg/dL	0.02586	0.80 - 1.80	mmol/L
Female	plasma, serum	30 - 90	mg/dL	0.02586	0.80 - 2.35	mmol/L
Hematocrit						
Female	whole blood	33 - 43	%	0.01	0.33 - 0.43	fraction of 1.00
Male	whole blood	39 - 49	%	0.01	0.39 - 0.49	fraction of 1.00

CONSTITUENT	FLUID	APPROXIMATE NORMAL RANGE	UNITS	CONVERSION FACTOR MULT ---> / DIV <---	APPROXIMATE NORMAL RANGE	UNITS
Hemoglobin						
Mass Concentration						
Female	whole blood	14.0 - 18.0	g/dL	10.0	140 - 180	g/L
Male	whole blood	11.5 - 15.5	g/dL	10.0	115 - 155	g/L
Substance Concentration Hb [Fe]						
Female	whole blood	12.0 -15.0	g/dL	0.6206	7.45 - 9.30	mmol/L
Male	whole blood	13.6 - 17.2	g/dL	0.6206	8.45 - 10.65	mmol/L
Hemoglobin, methemoglobin and sulfhemoglobin	whole blood	absent/present		1.0	0	absent/present
Hemoglobin A1C	whole blood	3.8 - 6.4	%	0.01	0.038 - 0.064	fraction of 1.00
Hemoglobin A2	whole blood	2.0-3.0	%	0.01	0.02-0.03	fraction of 1.00
Hemoglobin F (fetal hemoglobin)	whole blood	<2	%	0.01	< 0.02	fraction of 1.00
Hemolytic Complement, Total (CH50)	serum	150-250	units/mL	1	150-250	arb unit
Hgb-oxyhemoglobin, substance fraction Oxygen saturation	art whole blood	96-100	%	0.01	0.96-1.00	fraction of 1.00
Hepatitis Tests						
Antibodies						
Antibody to delta Hepatitis Virus	serum	negative	highest pos. dil.	1	negative	highest pos. dil.
Antibody to Hepatitis A Virus	serum	negative	highest pos. dil.	1	negative	highest pos. dil.
Antibody to Hepatitis B Core Antigen	serum	negative	highest pos. dil.	1	negative	highest pos. dil.
Antibody to Hepatitis B Surface Antigen	serum	negative	highest pos. dil.	1	negative	highest pos. dil.
Antibody to Hepatitis C Virus	serum	negative	highest pos. dil.	1	negative	highest pos. dil.
Hepatitis Be Antibody	serum	negative	highest pos. dil.	1	negative	highest pos. dil.
Antigens						
Hepatitis B Surface Antigen	serum	negative	highest pos. dil.	1	negative	highest pos. dil.
Hepatitis Be Antigen	serum	negative	highest pos. dil.	1	negative	highest pos. dil.
5-HIAA (5-Hydroxyindoleacetate, 5-hydroxy-indoleacetic acid)	urine	2 - 8	mg/24 hr	5.230	10 - 40	μmol/d
High Density Lipoproteins (HDL)						
Male	plasma, serum	30 - 70	mg/dL	0.02586	0.80 - 1.80	mmol/L
Female	plasma, serum	30 - 90	mg/dL	0.02586	0.80 - 2.35	mmol/L
Histidine, amino acid fractionation	plasma, serum	0.5 - 1.7	mg/dL	64.45	30 - 110	μmol/L
Homogentisate (homogentisic acid)	urine	0	mg/24 hr	5.947	0	μmol/d
Homovanillate (homovanillic acid)	urine	<8	mg/24 hr	5.489	<45	μmol/d
HPL (human placental lactogen)	plasma, serum	> 4, after 30 wk gestation	μg/mL	46.3	>180	nmol/L
	plasma, serum	> 4, after 30 wk gestation	mg/mL	46.3	>180	nmol/L
Human chorionic gonadotropin (HCG)	serum	< 10 if not pregnant	mIU/mL	1	< 10 if not pregnant	IU/L
Human chorionic gonadotropin (HCG)	urine	negative	neg/pos	1	negative	neg/pos
beta-Hydroxybutyrate (beta-hydroxybutyric acid)	serum	<1.0	mg/dL	96.05	<100	μmol/L

2203

CONSTITUENT	FLUID	TRADITIONAL APPROXIMATE NORMAL RANGE	UNITS	CONVERSION FACTOR MULT → / DIV ←	SI APPROXIMATE NORMAL RANGE	UNITS
Hydroxycorticosteroids (as cortisol)						
Female	urine	2.0 - 8.0	mg/24 hr	2.759	5 - 25	µmol/d
Male	urine	3.0 - 10.0	mg/24 hr	2.759	10 - 30	µmol/d
5-Hydroxyindoleacetate (5-hydroxyindoleacetic acid; 5-HIAA)	urine	2 - 8	mg/24 hr	5.230	10 - 40	µmol/d
4-Hydroxy-3-methoxymandelic acid (vanillylmandelic acid, VMA)	urine	<6.8	mg/24 hr	5.046	<35	µmol/d
17-alpha-Hydroxyprogesterone						
Children	plasma, serum	0.2 - 1.4	µg/L	3.026	0.5 - 4.5	nmol/L
Male	plasma, serum	0.5 - 2.5	µg/L	3.026	1.5 - 7.5	nmol/L
Female	plasma, serum	0.3 - 4.2	µg/L	3.026	1.0 - 13.0	nmol/L
Female, postmenopausal	plasma, serum	0.3 - 1.7	µg/L	3.026	1.0 - 5.0	nmol/L
Hydroxyproline						
1 week - 1 yr	urine	55 - 220	mg/24 hr/m²	7.626	420 - 1680	µmol/(d·m²)
1 - 13 yr	urine	25 - 80	mg/24 hr/m²	7.626	190 - 610	µmol/(d·m²)
22 - 65 yr	urine	6 - 22	mg/24 hr/m²	7.626	40 - 170	µmol/(d·m²)
>65 yr	urine	5 - 17	mg/24 hr/m²	7.626	40 - 130	µmol/(d·m²)
Hydroxyproline, amino acid fractionation	plasma, serum	0 - trace	mg/dL	76.26	0 - trace	µmol/L
5-hydroxytryptamine (serotonin)	plasma	8 - 21	µg/dL	0.05675	0.45 - 1.20	µmol/L
Imipramine, therapeutic	plasma, serum	50 - 200	ng/mL	3.566	180 - 710	nmol/L
Immunoglobulins						
IgG	serum	500 - 1200	mg/dL	0.01	5.00 - 12.00	g/L
IgA	serum	50 - 350	mg/dL	0.01	0.50 - 3.50	g/L
IgM	serum	30 - 230	mg/dL	0.01	0.30 - 2.30	g/L
IgD	serum	<6	mg/dL	10	<60	mg/L
IgE						
0 - 3 years	serum	0.5 - 10	IU/mL	2.40	1 - 24	µg/L
> 3 years	serum	5 - 100	IU/mL	2.40	12 - 240	µg/L
Inderal (propranolol hydrochloride), therapeutic	serum	50 - 200	ng/mL	3.856	190 - 770	nmol/L
Insulin						
	plasma, serum	5 - 20	µU/mL	7.175	35 - 145	pmol/L
	plasma, serum	5 - 20	mU/L	7.175	35 - 145	pmol/L
	plasma, serum	0.20 - 0.84	µg/L	172.2	35 - 145	pmol/L
Ionized Calcium						
All populations	wh bld, plsm, ser	2.00 - 2.30	mEq/L	0.500	1.00 - 1.15	mmol/L
All populations	wh bld, plsm, ser	4.00 - 4.60	mg/dL	0.250	1.00 - 1.15	mmol/L
Iron						
Male	serum	80 - 180	µg/dL	0.1791	14 - 32	µmol/L
Female	serum	60 - 160	µg/dL	0.1791	11 - 29	µmol/L
Iron-binding capacity	serum	250 - 460	µg/dL	0.1791	45 - 82	µmol/L
Isoleucine, amino acid fractionation	plasma, serum	0.5 - 1.3	mg/dL	76.24	40 - 100	µmol/L

| CONSTITUENT | FLUID | TRADITIONAL | | CONVERSION FACTOR | | SI | |
		APPROXIMATE NORMAL RANGE	UNITS	→ MULT	DIV ←	APPROXIMATE NORMAL RANGE	UNITS
Isoniazid							
Therapeutic	serum	<2.0	mg/L	7.291		<15	µmol/L
Toxic	serum	>3.0	mg/L	7.291		>22	µmol/L
Isopropanol	plasma, serum	0	mg/dL	0.1664		0	mmol/L
17-Ketogenic steroids (as dehydroepiandrosterone)							
Female	urine	7.0 - 12.0	mg/24 hr	3.467		25 - 40	µmol/d
Male	urine	9.0 - 17.0	mg/24 hr	3.467		30 - 60	µmol/d
17-Ketosteroids (as dehydroepiandrosterone)							
Female	urine	6.0 - 17.0	mg/24 hr	3.467		20 - 60	µmol/d
Male	urine	6.0 - 20.0	mg/24 hr	3.467		20 - 70	µmol/d
Ketosteroid fractions							
Androsterone							
Female	urine	0.5 - 3.0	mg/24 hr	3.443		1 - 10	µmol/d
Male	urine	2.0 - 5.0	mg/24 hr	3.443		7 - 17	µmol/d
Dehydroepiandrosterone							
Female	urine	0.2 - 1.8	mg/24 hr	3.467		1 - 6	µmol/d
Male	urine	0.2 - 2.0	mg/24 hr	3.467		1 - 7	µmol/d
Etiocholanolone							
Female	urine	0.8 - 4.0	mg/24 hr	3.443		2 - 14	µmol/d
Male	urine	1.4 - 5.0	mg/24 hr	3.443		4 - 17	µmol/d
Lactate (lactic acid)	plasma	0.5 - 2.0	mEq/L	1		0.5 - 2.0	mmol/L
	plasma	5 - 20	mg/dL	0.1110		0.5 - 2.0	mmol/L
Lactate dehydrogenase	serum	50 -150 (37°C)	Units/L	1		50 - 150	U/L
	serum	50 -150 (37°C)	Units/L	0.01667		0.82 - 2.66	µkat/L
Lactate dehydrogenase isoenzymes							
LD1	serum	15 - 40	%	0.01		0.15 - 0.40	fraction of 1.00
LD2	serum	20 - 45	%	0.01		0.20 - 0.45	fraction of 1.00
LD3	serum	15 - 30	%	0.01		0.15 - 0.30	fraction of 1.00
LD4	serum	5 - 20	%	0.01		0.05 - 0.20	fraction of 1.00
LD5	serum	5 - 20	%	0.01		0.05 - 0.20	fraction of 1.00
LD1	serum	10 - 60	Units/L	0.01667		0.16 - 1.00	µkat/L
	serum	10 - 60	Units/L	1		10 - 60	U/L
LD2	serum	20 - 70	Units/L	0.01667		0.32 - 1.16	µkat/L
	serum	20 - 70	Units/L	1		20 - 70	U/L
LD3	serum	20 - 70	Units/L	1		20 - 70	U/L
	serum	10 - 45	Units/L	0.01667		0.17 - 0.76	µkat/L
LD4	serum	10 - 45	Units/L	1		10 - 45	U/L
	serum	5 - 30	Units/L	0.01667		0.08 - 0.50	µkat/L
LD5	serum	5 - 30	Units/L	1		5 - 30	U/L
	serum	5 - 30	Units/L	0.01667		0.08 - 0.50	µkat/L
	serum	5 - 30	Units/L	1		5 - 30	U/L

CONSTITUENT	FLUID	TRADITIONAL APPROXIMATE NORMAL RANGE	UNITS	CONVERSION FACTOR →MULT / DIV←	SI APPROXIMATE NORMAL RANGE	UNITS
Lead (Lead (II), Pb) - toxic	plasma	>60	μg/dL	0.04826	>2.90	μmol/L
Lead (Lead (II), Pb) - toxic	plasma	>0.06	mg/dL	48.26	>2.90	μmol/L
Lead (Lead (II), Pb) - toxic	urine	>80	μg/24 hr	0.004826	>0.40	μmol/d
LDL (low density lipoproteins)	plasma, serum	50 - 190	mg/dL	0.02586	1.30 - 4.90	mmol/L
Leucine, amino acid fractionation	plasma, serum	1.0 - 2.3	mg/dL	76.24	76 - 176	μmol/L
Leukocyte count	whole blood	3.2 - 9.8	10³/mm³	0.001	3.2 - 9.8	10⁹/L
Number Fraction "Differential"						
Bands	whole blood	3 - 5	%	0.01	0.03 - 0.05	fraction of 1.00
Neutrophils	whole blood	54 - 62	%	0.01	0.54 - 0.62	fraction of 1.00
Lymphocytes	whole blood	25 - 33	%	0.01	0.25 - 0.33	fraction of 1.00
Monocytes	whole blood	3 - 7	%	0.01	0.03 - 0.07	fraction of 1.00
Eosinophils	whole blood	1 - 3	%	0.01	0.01 - 0.03	fraction of 1.00
Basophils	whole blood	0 - 0.75	%	0.01	0 - 0.0075	fraction of 1.00
Bands	whole blood	150 - 400	cells/mm³ (μL)	1	150 - 400	10⁶ cells / L
Neutrophils	whole blood	3000 - 5800	cells/mm³ (μL)	1	3000 - 5800	10⁶ cells / L
Lymphocytes	whole blood	1500 - 3000	cells/mm³ (μL)	1	1500 - 3000	10⁶ cells / L
Monocytes	whole blood	285 - 500	cells/mm³ (μL)	1	285 - 500	10⁶ cells / L
Eosinophils	whole blood	50 - 250	cells/mm³ (μL)	1	50 - 250	10⁶ cells / L
Basophils	whole blood	15 - 50	cells/mm³ (μL)	1	15 - 50	10⁶ cells / L
Leukocyte count	CSF	0 - 5	per mm³	1	0 - 5	10⁹/L
Lidocaine (Xylocaine)	plasma, serum	1.0 - 5.0	mg/L	4.267	4.5 - 21.5	μmol/L
Lipase	serum	0 - 160 (30°C)	Units/L	1	0 - 160	U/L
Lipase	serum	0 - 160 (30°C)	Units/L	0.01667	0 - 2.66	μkat/L
Lipids, total	plasma	400 - 850	mg/dL	0.01	4.0 - 8.5	g/L
Lipoproteins						
Low density (LDL) cholesterol	plasma, serum	50 - 190	mg/dL	0.02586	1.30 - 4.90	mmol/L
High-density (HDL) cholesterol						
Male	plasma, serum	30 - 70	mg/dL	0.02586	0.80 - 1.80	mmol/L
Female	plasma, serum	30 - 90	mg/dL	0.02586	0.80 - 2.35	mmol/L
Lithium, therapeutic	serum	0.50 - 1.50	mEq/L	1	0.50 - 1.50	mmol/L
Lithium, therapeutic	serum	347 - 1041	μg/dL	0.001441	0.50 - 1.50	mmol/L
Lithium, therapeutic	serum	0.35 - 1.04	mg/dL	1.441	0.50 - 1.50	mmol/L
Low Density Lipoproteins (LDL)	plasma, serum	50 - 190	mg/dL	0.02586	1.30 - 4.90	mmol/L
Luteinizing hormone, (LH)						
Male	plasma, serum	3 - 25	mIU/mL	1	3 - 25	IU/L
Female	plasma, serum	2 - 20	mIU/mL	1	2 - 20	IU/L
Peak Production - Female	plasma, serum	30 - 140	mIU/mL	1	30 - 140	IU/L
Lysine, amino acid fractionation	plasma, serum	1.2 - 3.5	mg/dL	68.40	80 - 240	μmol/L
Lysozyme (muramidase)	serum	1 - 15	μg/mL	1	1 - 15	mg/L
Lysozyme (muramidase)	urine	<2	μg/mL	1	<2	mg/L
alpha-2-Macroglobulin	serum	145 - 410	mg/dL	0.01	1.5 - 4.1	g/L

CONSTITUENT	FLUID	TRADITIONAL APPROXIMATE NORMAL RANGE	UNITS	CONVERSION FACTOR ---> MULT DIV <---	SI APPROXIMATE NORMAL RANGE	UNITS
Magnesium (Mg)	plasma, serum	1.8 - 3.0	mg/dL	0.4114	0.80 - 1.20	mmol/L
	plasma, serum	1.6 - 2.4	mEq/L	0.500	0.80 - 1.20	mmol/L
Maprotiline, therapeutic	plasma	50 - 200	ng/mL	3.605	180 - 720	nmol/L
MCH (Mean Corpuscular Hemoglobin)						
Mass	whole blood	27 - 33	pg	1	27 - 33	pg
Amount of substance Hb [Fe]	whole blood	27 - 33	pg	0.06206	1.70 - 2.05	fmol
MCHC (Mean Corpuscular Hemoglobin Conc.)						
Mass Concentration	whole blood	33 - 37	g/dL	10	330 - 370	g/L
	whole blood	33 - 37	%	0.01	0.33 - 0.37	fraction of 1.00
Amount of substance Hb[Fe]	whole blood	33 - 37	g/dL	0.6206	20 - 23	mmol/L
MCV (Mean Corpuscular Volume)	whole blood	76 - 100	μm³	1	76 - 100	fL
Mean Corpuscular Hemoglobin (MCH)						
Mass	whole blood	27 - 33	pg	1	27 - 33	pg
Amount of substance Hb [Fe]	whole blood	27 - 33	pg	0.06206	1.70 - 2.05	fmol
Mean Corpuscular Hemoglobin Conc.(MCHC)						
Mass Concentration	whole blood	33 - 37	g/dL	10	330 - 370	g/L
	whole blood	33 - 37	%	0.01	0.33 - 0.37	fraction of 1.00
Amount of substance Hb[Fe]	whole blood	33 - 37	g/dL	0.6206	20 - 23	mmol/L
Mean Corpuscular Volume (MCV)	whole blood	76 - 100	μm³	1	76 - 100	fL
Meprobamate						
Therapeutic	plasma, serum	<20	mg/L	4.582	<90	μmol/L
Toxic	plasma, serum	>40	mg/L	4.582	>180	μmol/L
Mercury						
Normal	whole blood	<1.0	μg/dL	49.85	<50	nmol/L
Chronic	whole blood	>20	μg/dL	0.04985	>1.00	μmol/L
Mercury						
Normal	urine	<30	μg/24 hr	4.985	<150	nmol/d
Exposure						
Organic	urine	>45	μg/24 hr	4.985	>220	nmol/d
Inorganic	urine	>450	μg/24 hr	0.004985	>2.20	μmol/d
Metanephrines (as normetanephrine)	urine	0 - 2.0	mg/24 hr	5.458	0 - 11.0	μmol/d
Methanol	plasma, serum	0	mg/dL	0.3121	0	mmol/L
Methaqualone						
Therapeutic	plasma, serum	<10	mg/L	3.995	<40	μmol/L
Toxic	plasma, serum	>30	mg/L	3.995	>120	μmol/L
Methionine, amino acid fractionation	plasma, serum	0.1 - 0.6	mg/dL	67.02	5 - 40	μmol/L
Methotrexate, toxic	plasma, serum	>2.3	mg/L	2.20	>5.0	μmol/L
Methsuximide (as desmethylsuximide), therapeutic	plasma, serum	10 - 40	mg/L	5.285	50 - 210	μmol/L
Methyprylon						
Therapeutic	plasma	<10	mg/L	5.457	<50	μmol/L
Toxic	plasma	>40	mg/L	5.457	>220	μmol/L

CONSTITUENT	FLUID	TRADITIONAL APPROXIMATE NORMAL RANGE	UNITS	CONVERSION FACTOR ⟶ MULT / DIV ⟵	SI APPROXIMATE NORMAL RANGE	UNITS
beta-2-Microglobulin, <50 yrs	serum	0.80 - 2.40	mg/L	84.750	68 - 204	nmol/L
beta-2-Microglobulin, <50 yrs	urine	<140	μg/24 hr	0.08475	<12	nmol/d
Muramidase (lysozyme)	serum	1 - 15	μg/mL	1	1 - 15	mg/L
Muramidase (lysozyme)	urine	<2	μg/mL	1	<2	mg/L
N-acetylprocainamide, therapeutic	plasma, serum	4.0 - 8.0	mg/L	3.606	14 - 29	μmol/L
Nitrogen, amino acid	plasma	4.0 - 6.0	mg/dL	0.7139	2.9 - 4.3	mmol/L
Nitrogen, amino acid	urine	50 - 200	mg/24 hr	0.07139	3.6 - 14.3	mmol/d
Nitrogen, total	urine	diet dependent		0.07139	diet dependent	mmol/d
Nitroprusside toxicity (thiocyanate)	plasma	>10.0	g/24 hr	0.1722	>1.75	mmol/L
Norepinephrine	plasma	215 - 475 (at rest for 15 min)	pg/mL	0.005911	1.27 - 2.81 (at rest for 15 min)	nmol/L
Norepinephrine	urine	<100	μg/24 hr	5.911	<590	nmol/d
Nortriptyline, therapeutic	plasma, serum	25 - 200	ng/mL	3.797	90 - 760	nmol/L
5'Nucleotidase	plasma, serum	2 - 17 (37°C)	U/L	1	2 - 17	U/L
	plasma, serum	2 - 17 (37°C)	U/L	0.01667	0.03 - 0.28	μkat/L
Ornithine, amino acid fractionation	plasma, serum	0.4 - 1.4	mg/dL	75.67	30 - 400	μmol/L
Osmolality	plasma, serum	280 - 300	mOsm/kg	1	280 - 300	mmol/kg
	urine	50 - 1200	mOsm/kg	1	50 - 1200	mmol/kg
Oxalate (as anhydrous oxalic acid)	urine	10 - 40	mg/24 hr	11.11	110 - 440	μmol/d
Oxygen saturation (Hgb-oxyhemoglobin, substance fraction)	art whole blood	96-100	%	0.01	0.96-1.00	fraction of 1.00
Palmic acid	amniotic fluid	gestation dependent		1000	gestation dependent	μmol/L
Partial Thromboplastin Time (PTT) - activated	plasma	22-37	seconds	1	22-37	seconds
pCO2	art whole blood	35 - 45	mm Hg	0.1333	4.7 - 6.0	kPa
Pentobarbital, therapeutic	plasma, serum	20 - 40	mg/L	4.419	90 - 170	μmol/L
pH	art whole blood	7.35 - 7.45	pH units	1	7.35 - 7.45	pH units
Phenobarbital, therapeutic	plasma, serum	2 - 5	mg/dL	43.06	85 - 215	μmol/L
Phensuximide	plasma, serum	4 - 8	mg/L	5.285	20 - 40	μmol/L
Phenylalanine, amino acid fractionation	plasma, serum	0.6 - 1.5	mg/dL	60.54	35 - 90	μmol/L
Phenylbutazone, therapeutic	plasma	<100	mg/L	3.243	<320	μmol/L
Phenytoin (Dilantin, Diphenylhydantoin) Therapeutic	plasma, serum	10 - 20	mg/L	3.964	40 - 80	μmol/L
Toxic	plasma, serum	>30	mg/L	3.964	>120	μmol/L
Phosphatase, acid (prostatic)	serum	0 - 0.8 (37°C)	Units/L	1	0 - 0.8	U/L
	serum	0 - 0.8 (37°C)	Units/L	16.67	0 - 13.3	nkat/L
Phosphatase, alkaline	serum	30 - 120 (37°C)	Units/L	1	30 - 120	U/L
	serum	30 - 120 (37°C)	Units/L	0.01667	0.5 - 2.0	μkat/L
Phosphate (as phosphorus, inorganic)	serum	2.5 - 5.0	mg/dL	0.3229	0.80 - 1.60	mmol/L
Phosphate (as phosphorus, inorganic)	urine	diet dependent	g/24 hr	32.29	diet dependent	mmol/d
Phospholipid phosphorus	plasma, serum	5 - 12	mg/dL	0.3229	1.60 - 3.90	mmol/L
Phospholipid phosphorus, total	RBC	1.2 - 12.0	mg/dL	0.3229	0.40 - 3.90	mmol/L

CONSTITUENT	FLUID	TRADITIONAL APPROXIMATE NORMAL RANGE	UNITS	CONVERSION FACTOR ---> MULT DIV <---	SI APPROXIMATE NORMAL RANGE	UNITS
Phospholipids, substance fraction of total phospholipid						
Phosphatidylcholine	plasma, serum	65 - 70	%	0.01	0.65 - 0.70	fraction of 1.00
Phosphatidylethanolamine	plasma, serum	4 - 5	%	0.01	0.04 - 0.05	fraction of 1.00
Sphingomyelin	plasma, serum	15 - 20	%	0.01	0.15 - 0.20	fraction of 1.00
Lysophosphatidylcholine	plasma, serum	3 - 5	%	0.01	0.03 - 0.05	fraction of 1.00
Phospholipids, substance fraction of total phospholipid						
Phosphatidylcholine	RBC	28 - 33	%	0.01	0.28 - 0.33	fraction of 1.00
Phosphatidylethanolamine	RBC	24 - 31	%	0.01	0.24 - 0.31	fraction of 1.00
Sphingomyelin	RBC	22 - 39	%	0.01	0.22 - 0.29	fraction of 1.00
Phosphatidylserine and Phosphatidylinositol	RBC	12 - 20	%	0.01	0.12 - 0.20	fraction of 1.00
Lysophosphatidylcholine	RBC	1 - 2	%	0.01	0.01 - 0.02	fraction of 1.00
Phosphorus, inorganic (phosphate)	serum	2.5 - 5.0	mg/dL	0.3229	0.80 - 1.60	mmol/L
Phosphorus, inorganic (phosphate)	urine	diet dependent	g/24 hr	32.29	diet dependent	mmol/d
Phytanic acid	plasma	trace - 0.3	mg/dL	32.00	<10	µmol/L
Placental lactogen, human (HPL)	plasma, serum	> 4, after 30 wk gestation	µg/mL	46.3	>180	nmol/L
		> 4, after 30 wk gestation	mg/L	46.3	>180	nmol/L
Plasminogen	plasma	90 - 136	%	0.01	0.90 - 1.36	fraction of 1.00
Platelet count	whole blood	130 - 400	$10^3/mm^3$	1	130 - 400	10^9/L
pO2	art whole blood	75 - 100	mm Hg	0.1333	10.0 - 13.3	kPa
Porphobilinogen	urine	0.0 - 2.0	mg/24 hr	4.420	0 - 9.0	µmol/d
Porphyrins						
Coproporphyrin	urine	45 - 180	µg/24 hr	1.527	68 - 276	nmol/d
Protoporphyrin	RBC	15 - 50	µg/dL	0.0177	0.28 - 0.90	µmol/L
Uroporphyrin	urine	5 - 20	µg/24 hr	1.204	6 - 24	nmol/d
Potassium	plasma, serum	3.5-5.0	mEq/L	1	3.5-5.0	mmol/L
	plasma, serum	13.7 - 19.5	mg/dL	0.2558	3.5-5.0	mmol/L
Potassium (diet dependent)	urine	25 - 100	mEq/24 hr	1	25 - 100	mmol/d
Pregnanediol						
Normal	urine	1.0 - 6.0	mg/24 hr	3.120	3.0 - 18.5	µmol/d
Pregnancy	urine	gestation dependent	mg/24 hr	3.120	gestation dependent	µmol/d
Pregnanetriol	urine	0.5 - 2.0	mg/24 hr	2.972	1.5 - 6.0	µmol/d
Primidone						
Therapeutic	plasma, serum	6.0 - 10.0	mg/L	4.582	25 - 46	µmol/L
Toxic	plasma, serum	>10.0	mg/L	4.582	>46	µmol/L
Procainamide						
Therapeutic	plasma, serum	4.0 - 8.0	mg/L	4.249	17 - 34	µmol/L
Toxic	plasma, serum	>12	mg/L	4.249	>50	µmol/L
N-acetylprocainamide, therapeutic	plasma, serum	4.0 - 8.0	mg/L	3.606	14 - 29	µmol/L

CONSTITUENT	FLUID	TRADITIONAL APPROXIMATE NORMAL RANGE	UNITS	CONVERSION FACTOR MULT → / DIV ←	SI APPROXIMATE NORMAL RANGE	UNITS
Progesterone						
Follicular phase	plasma, serum	<2	ng/mL	3.180	<6	nmol/L
Luteal phase	plasma, serum	2 - 20	ng/mL	3.180	6 - 64	nmol/L
Progesterone Receptors						
Negative Result	tissue	0 - 3	fmol of progesterone bound/mg of cytosol protein	1	0 - 3	fmol of progesterone bound/mg of cytosol protein
Doubtful Result	tissue	4 - 10	fmol of progesterone bound/mg of cytosol protein		4 - 10	fmol of progesterone bound/mg of cytosol protein
Positive Result	tissue	>10	fmol of progesterone bound/mg of cytosol protein	1	>10	fmol of progesterone bound/mg of cytosol protein
Prolactin	plasma, serum	<20	ng/mL	1	<20	µg/L
Proline, amino acid fractionation	plasma, serum	1.2 - 3.9	mg/dL	86.86	105 - 340	µmol/L
Propoxyphene, toxic	plasma, serum	>2.0	mg/L	2.946	>5.9	µmol/L
Propranolol hydrochloride (Inderal), therapeutic	serum	50 - 200	ng/mL	3.856	190 - 770	nmol/L
Protein, electrophoresis						
Albumin	serum	60 - 65	%	0.01	0.60 - 0.65	fraction of 1.00
Alpha 1 Globulin	serum	1.7 - 5.0	%	0.01	0.02 - 0.05	fraction of 1.00
Alpha 2 Globulin	serum	6.7 - 12.5	%	0.01	0.07 - 0.13	fraction of 1.00
Beta Globulin	serum	8.3 - 16.3	%	0.01	0.08 - 0.16	fraction of 1.00
Gamma Globulin	serum	10.7 - 20.0	%	0.01	0.11 - 0.20	fraction of 1.00
Albumin	serum	3.6 - 5.2	g/dL	10	36 - 52	g/L
Alpha 1 Globulin	serum	0.1 - 0.4	g/dL	10	1 - 4	g/L
Alpha 2 Globulin	serum	0.4 - 1.0	g/dL	10	4 - 10	g/L
Beta Globulin	serum	0.5 - 1.2	g/dL	10	5 - 12	g/L
Gamma Globulin	serum	0.6 - 1.6	g/dL	10	6 - 16	g/L
Protein, electrophoresis	urine	no monoclonal paraproteins	neg/pos	1	no monoclonal paraproteins	neg/pos
Protein, total	plasma, serum	6.0 - 8.0	g/dL	10	60-80	g/L
Protein	CSF	<40	mg/dL	0.01	<0.40	g/L
Protein (quantitative)	urine	<150	mg/24 hr	0.001	<0.15	g/d
Prothrombin (coagulation factor II)	plasma	70-130	%	0.01	0.70-1.30	fraction of 1.00
Prothrombin Time (as PT)	plasma	9 - 12	seconds	1	9 - 12	seconds
Protoporphyrin	RBC	15 - 50	µg/dL	0.0177	0.28 - 0.90	µmol/L
Protriptyline	plasma, serum	100 - 300	ng/mL	3.797	380 - 1140	nmol/L
Pteroylglutamic acid (folate, folic acid)	serum	2 - 10	ng/mL	2.266	4 - 22	nmol/L
	serum	2 - 10	µg/dL	22.66	4 - 22	nmol/L
PT (Prothrombin Time)	plasma	9 - 12	seconds	1	9 - 12	seconds
PTT (Partial Thromboplastin Time) - activated	plasma	22-37	seconds	1	22-37	seconds

CONSTITUENT	FLUID	TRADITIONAL APPROXIMATE NORMAL RANGE	UNITS	CONVERSION FACTOR → MULT ← DIV		SI APPROXIMATE NORMAL RANGE	UNITS
Pyridoxal (vitamin B6)	plasma	20 - 90	ng/mL	5.982		120-540	nmol/L
Pyruvate (pyruvic acid)	plasma	0.30 - 0.90	mg/dL	113.6		35 - 100	µmol/L
Quinidine							
Therapeutic	plasma, serum	1.5 - 3.0	mg/L	3.082		4.6 - 9.2	µmol/L
Toxic	plasma, serum	>6.0	mg/L	3.082		>18.5	µmol/L
RBC Count (erythrocyte count)							
Female	whole blood	3.5 - 5.0	$10^6/mm^3$	1		3.5 - 5.0	$10^{12}/L$
Male	whole blood	4.3 - 5.9	$10^6/mm^3$	1		4.3 - 5.9	$10^{12}/L$
RBC Count (erythrocyte count)	CSF	0	per mm^3	1		0	$10^6/L$
RCoF (Coagulation Factor VIII VW, Histocetin Cofactor, von Willebrand Factor)	plasma	50 - 150	%	0.01		0.50 - 1.50	fraction of 1.00
Renin							
Normal sodium diet	plasma	1.1 - 4.1	ng/mL/hr	0.2778		0.30 - 1.14	ng/(L·s)
Restricted sodium diet	plasma	6.2 - 12.4	ng/mL/hr	0.2778		1.72 - 3.44	ng/(L·s)
Reticulocyte count - adults							
Number fraction	whole blood	10 - 75	$10^3/mm^3$	0.001		10 - 75	$10^9/L$
	whole blood	1 - 24	number per 1,000 RBC	0.001		0.001 - 0.024	fraction of 1.00
Number fraction	whole blood	0.1 - 2.4	%	0.01		0.001 - 0.024	fraction of 1.00
Retinol (vitamin A)	plasma, serum	10 - 50	µg/dL	0.03491		0.35 - 1.75	µmol/L
Rheumatoid Factor	serum	< 80	IU/mL	1		< 80	kIU/L
	serum	neg at < 1:80 dil	highest pos. dil	1		neg at < 1:80 dil	highest pos. dil
Rheumatoid Factor	synovial fluid	< 80	IU/mL	1		< 80	kIU/L
	synovial fluid	neg at < 1:80 dil	highest pos. dil	1		neg at < 1:80 dil	highest pos. dil
Riboflavin (vitamin B2)	serum	2.6 - 3.7	µg/dL	26.57		70-100	nmol/L
Ristocetin Cofactor (Coagulation Factor VIII VW, RCoF, von Willebrand Factor)	plasma	50 - 150	%	0.01		0.50 - 1.50	fraction of 1.00
Salicylate, toxic	plasma, serum	>20	mg/dL	0.07240		>1.45	mmol/L
Sedimentation Rate (RBC)							
Female	whole blood	0 - 30	mm/hr	1		0 - 30	mm/hr
Male	whole blood	0 - 20	mm/hr	1		0 - 20	mm/hr
Serine, amino acid fractionation	plasma, serum	0.8 - 1.8	mg/dL	95.16		75 - 170	µmol/L
Serotonin (5-hydroxytryptamine)	plasma	8 - 21	µg/dL	0.05675		0.45 - 1.20	µmol/L
Serum Protein Electrophoresis							
Albumin	serum	60 - 65	%	0.01		0.60 - 0.65	fraction of 1.00
Alpha 1 Globulin	serum	1.7 - 5.0	%	0.01		0.02 - 0.05	fraction of 1.00
Alpha 2 Globulin	serum	6.7 - 12.5	%	0.01		0.07 - 0.13	fraction of 1.00
Beta Globulin	serum	8.3 - 16.3	%	0.01		0.08 - 0.16	fraction of 1.00
Gamma Globulin	serum	10.7 - 20.0	%	0.01		0.11 - 0.20	fraction of 1.00
Albumin	serum	3.6 - 5.2	g/dL	10		36 - 52	g/L
Alpha 1 Globulin	serum	0.1 - 0.4	g/dL	10		1 - 4	g/L
Alpha 2 Globulin	serum	0.4 - 1.0	g/dL	10		4 - 10	g/L

CONSTITUENT	FLUID	APPROXIMATE NORMAL RANGE (TRADITIONAL)	UNITS	CONVERSION FACTOR MULT → / DIV ←	APPROXIMATE NORMAL RANGE (SI)	UNITS
Serum Protein Electrophoresis (continued)						
Beta Globulin	serum	0.5 - 1.2	g/dL	10	5 - 12	g/L
Gamma Globulin	serum	0.6 - 1.6	g/dL	10	6 - 16	g/L
Serum Viscosity	serum	1.4 - 2.0 times that of water		1	1.4 - 2.0 times that of water	
SGOT (aspartate aminotransferase, AST)	serum	0 - 35 (37°C)	Units/L	1	0 - 35	U/L
	serum	0 - 35 (37°C)	Units/L	0.01667	0 - 0.58	µkat/L
SGPT (alanine aminotransferase, ALT)	serum	0 - 35 (37°C)	Units/L	1	0 - 35	U/L
	serum	0 - 35 (37°C)	Units/L	0.01667	0 - 0.58	µkat/L
Sodium	plasma, serum	135 - 147	mEq/L	1	135 - 147	mmol/L
Sodium	urine	diet dependent		1	diet dependent	mmol/d
Stearic acid (as fecal fat)	feces	2.0 - 6.0	g/24 hr	3.515	7 - 21	mmol/d
Steroids						
Hydroxycorticosteroids (as cortisol)						
Female	urine	2.0 - 8.0	mg/24 hr	2.759	5 - 25	µmol/d
Male	urine	3.0 - 10.0	mg/24 hr	2.759	10 - 30	µmol/d
17-Ketogenic steroids (as dehydroepiandrosterone)						
Female	urine	7.0 - 12.0	mg/24 hr	3.467	25 - 40	µmol/d
Male	urine	9.0 - 17.0	mg/24 hr	3.467	30 - 60	µmol/d
17-Ketosteroids (as dehydroepiandrosterone)						
Female	urine	6.0 - 17.0	mg/24 hr	3.467	20 - 60	µmol/d
Male	urine	6.0 - 20.0	mg/24 hr	3.467	20 - 70	µmol/d
Ketosteroid fractions						
Androsterone						
Female	urine	0.5 - 3.0	mg/24 hr	3.443	1 - 10	µmol/d
Male	urine	2.0 - 5.0	mg/24 hr	3.443	7 - 17	µmol/d
Dehydroepiandrosterone						
Female	urine	0.2 - 1.8	mg/24 hr	3.467	1 - 6	µmol/d
Male	urine	0.2 - 2.0	mg/24 hr	3.467	1 - 7	µmol/d
Etiocholanolone						
Female	urine	0.8 - 4.0	mg/24 hr	3.443	2 - 14	µmol/d
Male	urine	1.4 - 5.0	mg/24 hr	3.443	4 - 17	µmol/d
Androstenedione						
Male > 18 yrs	serum	0.2 - 3.0	µg/L	3.492	0.5 - 10.5	nmol/L
Female >18 yrs	serum	0.8 - 3.0	µg/L	3.492	3.0 - 10.5	nmol/L
Sulfonamides (as sulfanilamide), therapeutic	plasma	10.0 - 15.0	mg/dL	58.07	580 - 870	µmol/L
T3 uptake, thyroid test	serum	25 - 35	%	0.01	0.25 - 0.35	fraction of 1.00
T3 (triiodothyronine)	serum	75 - 220	ng/dL	0.01536	1.2 - 3.4	nmol/L
T4 (thyroxine)	serum	4.0 - 11.0	µg/dL	12.87	51 - 142	nmol/L
Taurine, amino acid fractionation	plasma, serum	0.3 - 2.1	mg/dL	79.91	25 - 170	µmol/L

CONSTITUENT	FLUID	TRADITIONAL APPROXIMATE NORMAL RANGE	UNITS	CONVERSION FACTOR --> MULT <-- DIV	SI APPROXIMATE NORMAL RANGE	UNITS
TBG (thyroxine-binding globulin), thyroid test for thyroxine	serum	12.0 - 28.0	µg/dL	12.87	150 - 360	nmol/L
Testosterone						
Female	plasma, serum	<0.6	ng/mL	3.467	<2.0	nmol/L
Male	plasma, serum	4.0 - 8.0	ng/mL	3.467	14.0 - 28.0	nmol/L
Theophylline, therapeutic	plasma, serum	10.0 - 20.0	mg/L	5.550	55 - 110	µmol/L
Thiamine hydrochloride (vitamin B1)	urine	60 - 500	µg/24 hr	0.002965	0.18 - 1.48	µmol/d
Thiocyanate (nitroprusside toxicity)	plasma	> 10.0	mg/dL	0.1722	> 1.75	mmol/L
Thiopental, therapeutic	plasma, serum	individual	mg/L	4.126	individual	µmol/L
Threonine, amino acid fractionation	plasma, serum	0.9 - 2.5	mg/dL	83.95	75 - 210	µmol/L
Thrombin time	plasma	<17	seconds	1	<17	seconds
Thyroid tests						
Thyroid-stimulating hormone (TSH)	serum	2 - 11	µU/mL	1	2 - 11	mU/L
Thyroid Hormone Binding Index (THBI)	serum	0.83 - 1.17	unitless ratio	1	0.83 - 1.17	unitless ratio
Thyroxine (T4)	serum	4.0 - 11.0	µg/dL	12.87	51 - 142	nmol/L
Thyroxine-binding globulin (TBG), for thyroxine	serum	12.0 - 28.0	µg/dL	12.87	150 - 360	nmol/L
Thyroxine, free	serum	0.8 - 2.8	ng/dL	12.87	10 - 36	pmol/L
Triiodothyronine (T3)	serum	75 - 220	ng/dL	0.01536	1.2 - 3.4	nmol/L
T3 uptake	serum	25 - 35	%	0.01	0.25 - 0.35	fraction of 1.00
Tobramycin, therapeutic (peak)	serum	4 - 8	µg/mL	2.1	8.4 - 16.8	µmol/L
alpha-Tocopherol (vitamin E)	plasma, serum	0.78 - 1.25	mg/dL	23.22	18 - 29	µmol/L
Total Hemolytic Complement (CH50)	serum	150-250	units/mL	1	150-250	arb unit
Total Lipids	plasma	400 - 850	mg/dL	0.01	4.0 - 8.5	g/L
Total Protein	plasma, serum	6.0-8.0	g/dL	10	60-80	g/L
	CSF	<40	mg/dL	0.01	<0.40	g/L
	urine	<150	mg/24 hr	0.001	<0.15	g/d
Transferrin	serum	170 - 370	mg/dL	0.01	1.70 - 3.70	g/L
Triglycerides (as triolein)	plasma, serum	<160	mg/dL	0.01129	<1.80	mmol/L
Triiodothyronine (T3)	serum	75 - 220	ng/dL	0.01536	1.2 - 3.4	nmol/L
Trimethadione, therapeutic	plasma	<50	mg/L	6.986	<350	µmol/L
Trimipramine, therapeutic	plasma	50 - 200	ng/mL	3.397	170 - 680	nmol/L
Tryptophan, amino acid fractionation	plasma, serum	0.5 - 2.5	mg/dL	48.97	25 - 125	µmol/L
TSH (thyroid-stimulating hormone)	serum	2 - 11	µU/mL	1	2 - 11	mU/L
Tyrosine, amino acid fractionation	plasma, serum	0.4 - 1.6	mg/dL	55.19	20 - 90	µmol/L
Urate (as uric acid)	serum	2.0 - 7.0	mg/dL	59.48	120 - 420	µmol/L
Urate (as uric acid)	urine	diet dependent	g/24 hr	5.948	diet dependent	mmol/d
Urea nitrogen (BUN)	plasma, serum	8 - 18	mg/dL	0.357	3.0 - 6.5	mmol/L of urea
Urea nitrogen (BUN)	urine	12 - 20 (diet dep)	g/24 hr	35.70	450 - 700	mmol/d of urea
Uric Acid (Urate)	serum	2.0 - 7.0	mg/dL	59.48	120 - 420	µmol/L
Uric Acid (Urate)	urine	diet dependent	g/24 hr	5.948	diet dependent	mmol/d
Urine Protein Electrophoresis	urine	no monoclonal paraproteins	neg/pos	1	no monoclonal paraproteins	neg/pos

CONSTITUENT	FLUID	TRADITIONAL APPROXIMATE NORMAL RANGE	UNITS	CONVERSION FACTOR MULT → / DIV ←	SI APPROXIMATE NORMAL RANGE	UNITS
Urobilinogen	urine	0 - 4.0	mg/24 hr	1.693	0.0 - 6.8	μmol/d
Uroporphyrin	urine	5 - 20	μg/24 hr	1.204	6 - 24	nmol/d
Valine, amino acid fractionation	plasma, serum	1.7 - 3.7	mg/dL	85.36	145 - 315	μmol/L
Valproic acid, therapeutic	plasma, serum	50 - 100	mg/L	6.934	350 - 700	μmol/L
Vanillylmandelic acid (VMA, 4-hydroxy-3-methoxymandelic acid)	urine	<6.8	mg/24 hr	5.046	<35	μmol/d
Viscosity	serum	1.4 - 2.0 times that of water		1	1.4 - 2.0 times that of water	
Vitamin A (retinol)	plasma, serum	10 - 50	μg/dL	0.03491	0.35 - 1.75	μmol/L
Vitamin B1 (thiamine hydrochloride)	urine	60 - 500	μg/24 hr	0.002965	0.18 - 1.48	μmol/d
Vitamin B2 (riboflavin)	serum	2.6 - 3.7	μg/dL	26.57	70 - 100	nmol/L
Vitamin B6 (pyridoxal)	plasma	20 - 90	ng/mL	5.982	120 - 540	nmol/L
Vitamin B12 (cyanocobalamin)	serum	200 - 1000	pg/mL	0.7378	150 - 750	pmol/L
Vitamin B12 (cyanocobalamin)	serum	20 - 100	ng/dL	7.378	150 - 750	pmol/L
Vitamin C (ascorbate)	plasma, serum	0.6 - 2.0	mg/dL	56.78	30 - 110	μmol/L
Vitamin D3 (cholecalciferol)	serum	24 - 40	ng/mL	2.599	60 - 105	nmol/L
25-OH-cholecalciferol	serum	18 - 36	ng/mL	2.496	45 - 90	nmol/L
Vitamin E (alpha-tocopherol)	plasma, serum	0.78 - 1.25	mg/dL	23.22	18 - 29	μmol/L
VMA (vanillylmandelic acid, 4-hydroxy-3-methoxymandelic acid)	urine	<6.8	mg/24 hr	5.046	<35	μmol/d
von Willebrand Factor (Coagulation Factor VIII VW, RCoF, Ristocetin Cofactor)	plasma	50 - 150	%	0.01	0.50 - 1.50	fraction of 1.00
Warfarin sodium, therapeutic	plasma	1.0 - 3.0	mg/L	3.243	3.3 - 9.8	μmol/L
WBC Differential	whole blood				3.2 - 9.8	10⁹/L
Bands	whole blood	3 - 5	%	0.01	0.03 - 0.05	fraction of 1.00
Neutrophils	whole blood	54 - 62	%	0.01	0.54 - 0.62	fraction of 1.00
Lymphocytes	whole blood	25 - 33	%	0.01	0.25 - 0.33	fraction of 1.00
Monocytes	whole blood	3 - 7	%	0.01	0.03 - 0.07	fraction of 1.00
Eosinophils	whole blood	1 - 3	%	0.01	0.01 - 0.03	fraction of 1.00
Basophils	whole blood	0 - 0.75	%	0.01	0 - 0.0075	fraction of 1.00
Bands	whole blood	150 - 400	cells/mm³ (μL)	1	150 - 400	10⁶ cells/L
Neutrophils	whole blood	3000 - 5800	cells/mm³ (μL)	1	3000 - 5800	10⁶ cells/L
Lymphocytes	whole blood	1500 - 3000	cells/mm³ (μL)	1	1500 - 3000	10⁶ cells/L
Monocytes	whole blood	285 - 500	cells/mm³ (μL)	1	285 - 500	10⁶ cells/L
Eosinophils	whole blood	50 - 250	cells/mm³ (μL)	1	50 - 250	10⁶ cells/L
Basophils	whole blood	15 - 50	cells/mm³ (μL)	1	15 - 50	10⁶ cells/L
Xylocaine (Lidocaine)	plasma, serum	1.0 - 5.0	mg/L	4.267	4.5 - 21.5	μmol/L
D-Xylose (25 g dose)	plasma, serum	30 - 40 (30 - 60 min)	mg/dL	0.06661	2.0 - 2.7 (30-60 min)	mmol/L
D-Xylose excretion (25 g dose)	urine	21 - 31 (excreted in 5 hr)	%	0.01	0.21 - 0.31 (excreted in 5 hr)	fraction of 1.00
Zinc	serum	75 - 120	μg/dL	0.1530	11.5 - 18.5	μmol/L
Zinc	urine	150 - 1200	μg/24 hr	0.01530	2.3 - 18.3	μmol/d

App. 2: Units of Measurement

Scientific Notation

Sometimes it is necessary to use very large and very small numbers. These can best be indicated and handled in calculations by use of scientific notation, which is to say by use of exponents. Use of scientific notation requires writing the number so that it is the result of multiplying some whole number power of 10 by a number between 1 and 10. Examples are:

$$1234 = 1.234 \times 10^3 \qquad\qquad 0.01234 = 1.234 \times \frac{1}{100} = 1.234 \times 10^{-2}$$

$$0.001234 = 1.234 \times \frac{1}{1000} = 1.234 \times 10^{-3}$$

To convert a number to its equivalent in scientific notation:

Place the decimal point to the right of the first non-zero digit. This will now be a number between 1 and 9.

Multiply this number by a power of 10, the exponent of which is equal to the number of places the decimal point was moved. The exponent is positive if the decimal point was moved to the left, and negative if it was moved to the right. For example:

$$\frac{1,234,000.0 \times 0.000072}{6000.0} = \frac{1.234 \times 10^6 \times 7.2 \times 10^{-5}}{6.0 \times 10^3}$$

Now, by simply adding or subtracting the exponents of ten, and remembering that moving an exponent from the denominator of the fraction to the numerator changes its sign,

$$= \frac{1.234 \times 10^6 \times 10^{-5} \times 10^{-3} \times 7.2}{6} = \frac{1.234 \times 10^{-2} \times 7.2}{6}$$

Now, dividing by 6,

$$= 1.234 \times 10^{-2} \times 1.2 = 1.4808 \times 10^{-2} = \frac{1.4808}{100} = 0.014808$$

The last operation changed 1.4808×10^{-2} into the final value, 0.014808, which is not expressed in scientific notation.

Metric System

Masses

Scale	Table	Grams	Grains
Kilo	1 Kilogram =	1000.0	= 15,432.35
Hecto	1 Hectogram =	100.0	= 1,543.23
Deca	1 Decagram =	10.0	= 154.323
Unit	1 Gram =	1.0	= 15.432
Deci	1 Decigram =	0.1	= 1.5432
Centi	1 Centigram =	0.01	= 0.15432
Milli	1 Milligram =	0.001	= 0.01543
Micro	1 Microgram =	10^{-6}	= 15.432×10^{-6}
Nano	1 Nanogram =	10^{-9}	= 15.432×10^{-9}
Pico	1 Picogram =	10^{-12}	= 15.432×10^{-12}
Femto	1 Femtogram =	10^{-15}	= 15.432×10^{-15}
Atto	1 Attogram =	10^{-18}	= 15.432×10^{-18}

Arabic numbers are used with masses and measures, as 10 gm, or 3 ml, etc. Portions of masses and measures are usually expressed decimally. 10^{-1} indicates 0.1; $10^{-6} = 0.000001$; etc. SEE: *Scientific Notation* above.

SI Units (Système International d'Unités) or International System of Units

This system includes two types of units important in clinical medicine. The *base units* are shown in the first table, derived units in the second table, and derived units with special names in the third table.

SI Base Units

Quantity	Name	Symbol
Length	meter	m
Mass	kilogram	kg
Time	second	s
Electric current	ampere	A
Temperature	kelvin	K
Luminous intensity	candela	cd
Amount of a substance	mole	mol

Some SI Derived Units

Quantity	Name of Derived Unit	Symbol
Area	square meter	m^2
Volume	cubic meter	m^3
Speed, velocity	meter per second	m/s
Acceleration	meter per second squared	m/s^2
Mass density	kilogram per cubic meter	kg/m^3
Concentration of a substance	mole per cubic meter	mol/m^3
Specific volume	cubic meter per kilogram	m^3/kg
Luminescence	candela per square meter	cd/m^2

SI Derived Names With Special Names

Quantity	Name	Symbol	Expressed in Terms of Other Units
Frequency	hertz	Hz	s^{-1}
Force	newton	N	$kg \cdot m \cdot s^{-2}$ or $kg \cdot m/s^2$
Pressure	pascal	Pa	$N \cdot m^{-2}$ or N/m^2
Energy, work, amount of heat	joule	J	$kg \cdot m^2 \cdot s^{-2}$ or $N \cdot m$
Power	watt	W	$J \cdot s$ or J/s
Quantity of electricity	coulomb	C	$A \cdot s$
Electromotive force	volt	V	W/A
Capacitance	farad	F	C/V
Electrical resistance	ohm	Ω	V/a
Conductance	siemens	S	A/V
Inductance	henry	H	$W\phi/A$
Illuminance	lux	lx	ln/m^2
Absorbed (radiation) dose	gray	Gy	J/kg
Dose equivalent (radiation)	sievert	Sv	J/kg
Activity (radiation)	becquerel	Bq	s^{-1}

Prefixes and Multiples Used in SI

Prefix	Symbol	Power	Multiple or Portion of a Multiple
tera	T	10^{12}	1,000,000,000,000
giga	G	10^9	1,000,000,000
mega	M	10^6	1,000,000
kilo	k	10^3	1,000
hecto	h	10^2	100
deca	da	10^1	10
unity			1
deci	d	10^{-1}	0.1
centi	c	10^{-2}	0.01
milli	m	10^{-3}	0.001
micro	μ	10^{-6}	0.000001
nano	n	10^{-9}	0.000000001
pico	p	10^{-12}	0.000000000001
femto	f	10^{-15}	0.000000000000001
atto	a	10^{-18}	0.000000000000000001

Tables of Data

Arabic numerals are used with masses and measures, as 10 gm, or 3 ml, etc. Portions of masses and measures are usually expressed decimally. For practical purposes, 1 cm³ (cubic centimeter) is equivalent to 1 ml (milliliter) and 1 drop (gtt.) of water is equivalent to a minim (m).

Units of Length

Millimeters	Centimeters	Inches	Feet	Yards	Meters
1 mm = 1.0	0.1	0.03937	0.00328	0.0011	0.001
1 cm = 10.0	1.0	0.3937	0.03281	0.0109	0.01
1 in. = 25.4	2.54	1.0	0.0833	0.0278	0.0254
1 ft. = 304.8	30.48	12.0	1.0	0.333	0.3048
1 yd = 914.40	91.44	36.0	3.0	1.0	0.9144
1 m = 1000.0	100.0	39.37	3.2808	1.0936	1.0

1 μm = 1 micrometer = 0.001 millimeter. 1 mm = 1000 μm

1 km = 1 kilometer = 1000 meters = 0.62137 statute mile.

1 statute mile = 5280 feet = 1.609 kilometers.

1 nautical mile = 6076.042 feet = 1852.276 meters

Units of Volume (fluid or liquid)

	Milliliters	U.S. Fluid Drams	Cubic Inches	U.S. Fluid Ounces	U.S. Fluid Quarts	Liters
1 ml =	1.0	0.2705	0.061	0.03381	0.00106	0.001
1 fl. ℨ =	3.697	1.0	0.226	0.125	0.00391	0.00369
1 cu. in. =	16.3866	4.4329	1.0	0.5541	0.0173	0.01639
1 fl. ℥ =	29.573	8.0	1.8047	1.0	0.03125	0.02957
1 qt. =	946.332	256.0	57.75	32.0	1.0	0.9463
1 L =	1000.0	270.52	61.025	33.815	1.0567	1.0

1 gallon = 4 quarts = 8 pints = 3.785 liters.

1 pint = 473.16 ml

Units of Weight

	Grains	Grams	Apothecaries' Ounces	Avoirdupois Pounds	Kilograms
1 gr =	1.0	0.0648	0.00208	0.0001429	0.000065
1 gm =	15.432	1.0	0.03215	0.002205	0.001
1 ℥ =	480.0	31.1	1.0	0.06855	0.0311
1 lb =	7000.0	453.5924	14.583	1.0	0.45354
1 kg =	15432.358	1000.0	32.15	2.2046	1.0

1 microgram (μg) = 0.001 milligram

1 mg = 1 milligram = 0.001 gm; 1000 mg = 1 gm

1 grain = 64.8 mg; 1 mg = 0.0154 grain.

Weights* and Measures

Apothecaries' Weight

20 grains = 1 scruple	3 scruples = 1 dram
8 drams = 1 ounce	12 ounces = 1 pound

Avoirdupois Weight

27.343 grains = 1 dram	16 drams = 1 ounce
16 ounces = 1 pound	100 pounds = 1 hundredweight
2000 pounds = 1 short ton	2240 pounds = 1 long ton
1 oz troy = 480 grains	1 oz avoirdupois = 437.5 grains
1 lb troy = 5760 grains	1 lb avoirdupois = 7000 grains

Circular Measure

60 seconds = 1 minute	60 minutes = 1 degree
90 degrees = 1 quadrant	4 quadrants = 360 degrees = circle

Cubic Measure

1728 cubic inches = 1 cubic foot	27 cubic feet = 1 cubic yard
2150.42 cubic inches = 1 standard bushel	268.8 cubic inches = 1 dry (U.S.) gallon
1 cubic foot = about four-fifths of a bushel	128 cubic feet = 1 cord (wood)

Dry Measure

2 pints = 1 quart	8 quarts = 1 peck	4 pecks = 1 bushel

Liquid Measure

16 ounces = 1 pint	4 quarts = 1 gallon	2 barrels = 1 hogshead (U.S.)
1000 milliliters = 1 liter	31.5 gallons = 1 barrel (U.S.)	1 quart = 946.35 milliliters
4 gills = 1 pint	2 pints = 1 quart	1 liter = 1.0566 quart

Barrels and hogsheads vary in size. A U.S. gallon is equal to 0.8327 British gallon; therefore, a British gallon is equal to 1.201 U.S. gallons.

1 liter is equal to 1.0567 quarts.

Linear Measure

1 inch = 2.54 centimeters	40 rods = 1 furlong	8 furlongs = 1 statute mile
12 inches = 1 foot	3 feet = 1 yard	5.5 yards = 1 rod
1 statute mile = 5280 feet	3 statute miles = 1 statute league	1 nautical mile = 6076.042 feet

Troy Weight

24 grains = 1 pennyweight	20 pennyweights = 1 ounce	12 ounces = 1 pound

Used for weighing gold, silver, and jewels.

Household Measures** and Weights

Approximate Equivalents: 60 gtt. = 1 teaspoonful = 5 ml = 60 minims = 60 grains = 1 dram = ⅛ ounce

1 teaspoon = ⅙ fl. oz; 1 dram	16 teaspoons (liquid) = 1 cup
3 teaspoons = 1 tablespoon	12 tablespoons (dry) = 1 cup
1 tablespoon = ½ fl. oz; 4 drams	1 cup = 8 fl. oz

1 tumbler or glass = 8 fl. oz; ½ pint

---

* For abbreviations and symbols of these weights, see *Symbols* in *Appendix*.

** Household measures are not precise. For instance, household tsp will hold from 3 to 5 ml of liquid substances. Therefore, do not substitute household equivalents for medication prescribed by the physician.

Note: Traditionally, the word "weights" is used in these tables, but "masses" is the correct term.

Conversion Rules

To convert units of one system into the other, multiply the number of units in column I by the equivalent factor opposite that unit in column II.

Weight*

I		II
1 milligram	=	0.015432 grain
1 gram	=	15.432 grains
1 gram	=	0.25720 apothecaries' dram
1 gram	=	0.03527 avoirdupois ounce
1 gram	=	0.03215 apothecaries' or troy ounce
1 kilogram	=	35.274 avoirdupois ounces
1 kilogram	=	32.151 apothecaries' or troy ounces
1 kilogram	=	2.2046 avoirdupois pounds
1 grain	=	64.7989 milligrams
1 grain	=	0.0648 gram
1 apothecaries' dram	=	3.8879 gram
1 avoirdupois ounce	=	28.3495 grams
1 apothecaries' or troy ounce	=	31.1035 grams
1 avoirdupois pound	=	453.5924 grams

Volume (air or gas)

I		II
1 cubic centimeter (cm³)	=	0.06102 cubic inch
1 cubic meter (m³)	=	35.314 cubic feet
1 cubic meter	=	1.3079 cubic yard
1 cubic inch (in³)	=	16.3872 cubic centimeters
1 cubic foot (ft³)	=	0.02832 cubic meter

Capacity (fluid or liquid)

I		II
1 milliliter	=	16.23 minims
1 milliliter	=	0.2705 fluidram
1 milliliter	=	0.0338 fluidounce
1 liter	=	33.8148 fluidounces
1 liter	=	2.1134 pints
1 liter	=	1.0567 quart
1 liter	=	0.2642 gallon
1 fluidram	=	3.697 milliliters
1 fluidounce	=	29.573 milliliters
1 pint	=	473.1765 milliliters
1 quart	=	946.353 milliliters
1 gallon	=	3.785 liters

To Convert Degrees Celsius (Centigrade) to Degrees Fahrenheit**

Multiply the number of degrees Celsius by ⅘ and add 32 to the result.

Example: $55°C \times ⅘ = 99 + 32 = 131°F$

To convert degrees Fahrenheit to degrees Celsius: Subtract 32 from the number of degrees Fahrenheit and multiply the difference by ⅘.

Example: $243°F - 32 = 211 \times ⅘ = 117.2°C$

---

* Traditionally, the word "weight" is used in these tables, but "mass" is the correct term.

** See: thermometer for table.

Miscellaneous Conversion Factors

Pressure

To obtain	multiply	by
lb/sq. in.	atmospheres	14.696
lb/sq. in.	in. of water	0.03609
lb/sq. in.	ft. of water	0.4335
lb/sq. in.	in. of mercury	0.4912
lb/sq. in.	kg/sq. meter	0.00142
lb/sq. in.	kg/sq. cm	14.22
lb/sq. in.	cm of mercury	0.1934
lb/sq. ft.	atmospheres	2116.8
lb/sq. ft.	in. of water	5.204
lb/sq. ft.	ft. of water	62.48
lb/sq. ft.	in. of mercury	70.727
lb/sq. ft.	cm of mercury	27.845
lb/sq. ft.	kg/sq. meter	0.20482
lb/cu. in.	gm/ml	0.03613
lb/cu. ft.	lb/cu. in.	1728.0
lb/cu. ft.	gm/ml	62.428
lb/U.S. gal	gm/L	8.345
in. of water	in. of mercury	13.60
in. of water	cm of mercury	5.3543
ft. of water	atmospheres	33.95
ft. of water	lb/sq. in.	2.307
ft. of water	kg/sq. meter	0.00328
ft. of water	in. of mercury	1.133
ft. of water	cm of mercury	0.4461
atmospheres	ft. of water	0.02947
atmospheres	in. of mercury	0.03342
atmospheres	kg/sq. cm	0.9678
bars	atmospheres	1.0133
in. of mercury	atmospheres	29.921
in. of mercury	lb/sq. in.	2.036
mm of mercury	atmospheres	760.0
gm/ml	lb/cu. in.	27.68
gm/sq. cm	kg/sq. meter	0.1
kg/sq. meter	lb/sq. in.	703.1
kg/sq. meter	in. of water	25.40
kg/sq. meter	in. of mercury	345.32
kg/sq. meter	cm of mercury	135.95
kg/sq. meter	atmospheres	10332.0
kg/sq. cm	atmospheres	1.0332

Flow Rate

To obtain	multiply	by
cu. ft./hr	cc/min.	0.00212
cu. ft./hr	L/min.	2.12
L/min.	cu. ft./hr	0.472

Parts Per Million

Conversion of parts per million (ppm) to percent: 1 ppm = 0.0001%, 10 ppm = 0.001%, 100 ppm = 0.01%, 1000 ppm = 0.1%, 10,000 ppm = 1%, etc.

Miscellaneous Units of Measurement

Units of Time

1 millisecond = one thousandth (0.001) of a second
1 second = 1/60 of a minute

1 minute = 1/60 of an hour
1 hour = 1/24 of a day

Units of Temperature

Given a temperature on the Fahrenheit scale; to convert it to degrees Celsius, subtract 32 and multiply by 5/9. Given a temperature on the Celsius scale; to convert it to degrees Fahrenheit, multiply by 9/5 and add 32. Degrees celsius are equivalent to degrees Centigrade.

Units of Energy

1 foot pound = 1.35582 joule
1 joule = 0.2389 Calorie (kilocalorie)
1 Calorie (kilocalorie) = 1000 calories = 4184 joules
A large Calorie, or kilocalorie, is always written with a capital C.

---

pH Table

The pH scale is simply a series of numbers stating where a given solution would stand in a series of solutions arranged according to acidity or alkalinity. At one extreme (i.e., high pH) lies a highly alkaline solution which may be made by dissolving 4 gm of sodium hydroxide in water to make a liter of solution; at the other extreme (i.e., low pH) is an acid solution containing 3.65 gm of hydrogen chloride per liter of water. Halfway between lies purified water, which is neutral. All other solutions can be arranged on this scale, and their acidity or alkalinity can be stated by giving the numbers that indicate their relative positions.

Tenth-normal HCl	−1.00	Litmus is red in this acid range.
Gastric juice	*1.4	
Urine	*6.0	
Water	7.00-Neutral	
Blood	7.35 – 7.45	
Bile	*7.5	Litmus is blue in this alkaline range
Pancreatic juice	8.5	
Tenth-normal NaOH	13.00	

If one is told that the pH of a certain solution is 5.3, one knows at once that it falls between gastric juice and urine on the above scale, is moderately acid, and will turn litmus red.

---

* These body fluids vary rather widely in pH; typical figures have been used for simplicity. Urine samples obtained from healthy individuals may have pH's anywhere between 4.7 and 8.0.

App. 3: Physical Constants of the Elements

Element	Symbol	Atomic Number	Approx. Relative Atomic Weight
Actinium	Ac	89	(227)
Aluminum	Al	13	27.0
Americium	Am	95	(243)
Antimony	Sb	51	122
Argon	Ar	18	39.9
Arsenic	As	33	74.9
Astatine	At	85	(210)
Barium	Ba	56	137
Berkelium	Bk	97	(249)
Beryllium	Be	4	9.01
Bismuth	Bi	83	209
Boron	B	5	10.8
Bromine	Br	35	79.9
Cadmium	Cd	48	112
Calcium	Ca	20	40.1
Californium	Cf	98	(251)
Carbon	C	6	12.0
Cerium	Ce	58	140
Cesium	Cs	55	133
Chlorine	Cl	17	35.5
Chromium	Cr	24	52.0
Cobalt	Co	27	58.9
Copper	Cu	29	63.5
Curium	Cm	96	(247)
Dysprosium	Dy	66	162
Einsteinium	Es	99	(254)
Erbium	Er	68	167
Europium	Eu	63	152
Fermium	Fm	100	(253)
Fluorine	F	9	19.0
Francium	Fr	87	(223)
Gadolinium	Gd	64	157
Gallium	Ga	31	69.7
Germanium	Ge	32	72.6
Gold	Au	79	197
Hafnium	Hf	72	178
Helium	He	2	4.00
Holmium	Ho	67	165
Hydrogen	H	1	1.01
Indium	In	49	115
Iodine	I	53	127
Iridium	Ir	77	192
Iron	Fe	26	55.8
Krypton	Kr	36	83.8
Lanthanum	La	57	139
Lawrencium	Lr	103	(257)
Lead	Pb	82	207
Lithium	Li	3	6.94
Lutetium	Lu	71	175
Magnesium	Mg	12	24.3
Manganese	Mn	25	54.9
Mendelevium	Md	101	(256)
Mercury	Hg	80	201
Molybdenum	Mo	42	95.9
Neodymium	Nd	60	144

Physical Constants of the Elements *(Continued)*

Element	Symbol	Atomic Number	Approx. Relative Atomic Weight
Neon	Ne	10	20.2
Neptunium	Np	93	(237)
Nickel	Ni	28	58.7
Niobium	Nb	41	92.9
Nitrogen	N	7	14.0
Nobelium	No	102	(253)
Osmium	Os	76	190
Oxygen	O	8	16.0
Palladium	Pd	46	106
Phosphorus	P	15	31.0
Platinum	Pt	78	195
Plutonium	Pu	94	(242)
Polonium	Po	84	(210)
Potassium	K	19	39.1
Praseodymium	Pr	59	141
Promethium	Pm	61	(147)
Protactinium	Pa	91	231
Radium	Ra	88	(226)
Radon	Rn	86	(222)
Rhenium	Re	75	186
Rhodium	Rh	45	103
Rubidium	Rb	37	85.5
Ruthenium	Ru	44	101
Samarium	Sm	62	150
Scandium	Sc	21	45.0
Selenium	Se	34	79.0
Silicon	Si	14	28.1
Silver	Ag	47	108
Sodium	Na	11	23.0
Strontium	Sr	38	87.6
Sulfur	S	16	32.1
Tantalum	Ta	73	181
Technetium	Tc	43	(98.9)
Tellurium	Te	52	128
Terbium	Tb	65	159
Thallium	Tl	81	204
Thorium	Th	90	232
Thulium	Tm	69	169
Tin	Sn	50	119
Titanium	Ti	22	47.9
Tungsten	W	74	184
Unnilhexium	Uah	106	(263)
Unnilpentium	Unp	105	(262)
Unnilquadium	Unq	104	(264)
Unnilseptium	Uns	107	(262)
Uranium	U	92	238
Vanadium	V	23	50.9
Xenon	Xe	54	131
Ytterbium	Yb	70	173
Yttrium	Y	39	88.9
Zinc	Zn	30	65.4
Zirconium	Zr	40	91.2

* The relative atomic mass values have been rounded off to three significant figures. Values for elements with no stable isotope are shown in parentheses and represent the most stable known isotopes.

SOURCE: Adapted from the 1989 Table of Atomic Weights from the International Union of Pure and Applied Chemistry.

App. 4: Anatomy

Muscles with Their Action, Origin, Insertion, and Innervation

The muscles in the body number over 650, the total varying according to the authority, as some list as separate muscles what others regard as portions of adjacent muscles. Most of the muscles occur in pairs; five are single muscles.

HEAD AND FACE

auricularis anterior (aw-rĭk″ū-lā′rĭs ăn-tē′rĭ-or). ACTION: Draws pinna of ear forward and upward. ORIGIN: Superficial temporal fascia. INSERTION: Helix of ear anteriorly. INNERVATION: Facial.

auricularis posterior (aw-rĭk″ū-lā′rĭs pŏs-tē′rē-or). ACTION: Draws pinna of ear backward. ORIGIN: Mastoid process. INSERTION: Root of auricle. INNERVATION: Facial.

auricularis superior (aw-rĭk″ū-lā′rĭs sū-pē′rē-or). ACTION: Elevates pinna of ear. ORIGIN: Galea aponeurotica. INSERTION: Upper portion of pinna of ear. INNERVATION: Facial.

buccinator (bŭk″sĭn-ā′tor). ACTION: Compresses cheek, retracts angle of mouth. ORIGIN: Alveolar process of maxilla, pterygomandibular ligament, buccinator ridge of mandible. INSERTION: Orbicularis oris. INNERVATION: Facial.

ciliaris (sĭl-ĭ-ā′rĭs). ACTION: Alters shape of crystalline lens in accommodation. ORIGIN: (1) Meridional: Junctions of cornea and sclera. (2) Circular: Fibers forming a circle close to iris. INSERTION: (1) External layers of choroid. (2) Ciliary process. INNERVATION: Short ciliary.

corrugator supercilii (kōr′ū-gā′tor sū-pĕr-sĭl′ĭ-ī). ACTION: Draws eyebrows down and in. ORIGIN: Inner end of supercilliary arch. INSERTION: Skin above orbital arch. INNERVATION: Facial.

depressor anguli oris (dē-prĕs′or ăng′ū-lī ō′rĭs). ACTION: Depresses angle of mouth. ORIGIN: External oblique line of mandible. INSERTION: Angle of mouth. INNERVATION: Facial.

depressor labii inferioris (dē-prĕs′or lā′bĭ-ī ĭn-fē″rĭ-ō′rĭs). ACTION: Draws lower lip down. ORIGIN: External oblique line of the mandible. INSERTION: Lower lip and orbicularis oris. INNERVATION: Facial.

depressor septi nasi (dē-prĕs′or sĕp′tī nā′sī). ACTION: Draws outer wall of nostril downward. ORIGIN: Incisive fossa of superior maxillary bone. INSERTION: Septum and ala of nose. INNERVATION: Facial.

dilator naris anterior (dĭl′ă-tā-tor nā′rĭs ăn-tē′rĭ-or). ACTION: Dilates apertures of nostril. ORIGIN: Cartilage of ala of nose. INSERTION: Border of ala. INNERVATION: Facial.

dilator naris posterior (dĭl′ă-tā-tor nā′rĭs pŏs-tē′rē-or). ACTION: Dilates apertures of nostril. ORIGIN: Nasal notch of superior maxilla and the sesamoid cartilages. INSERTION: Integument of margin of nostril. INNERVATION: Facial.

levator anguli oris (lē-vā′tor ăng′ū-lī ō′rĭs). ACTION: Elevates angle of mouth. ORIGIN: Canine fossa of maxilla. INSERTION: Angle of mouth and orbicularis oris. INNERVATION: Facial.

levator labii superioris (lē-vā′tor lā′bĭ-ī sū-pē″rē-ō′rĭs). ACTION: Elevates and extends upper lip. ORIGIN: Lower margin of orbit, malar bone. INSERTION: Upper lip. INNERVATION: Infraorbital branch of facial.

levator labii superioris alaeque nasi (lē-vā′tor lā′bĭ-ī sū-pē″rē-ō′rĭs ā-lē′kwĕ nā′sī). ACTION: Elevates upper lip, dilates nostril. ORIGIN: Nasal process of maxilla. INSERTION: Cartilage of ala of nose and upper lip. INNERVATION: Infraorbital branch of facial.

levator palpebrae superioris (lē-vā′tor păl′pē-brē sū-pē″rē-ō′rĭs). ACTION: Raises upper eyelid. ORIGIN: Lesser wing of the sphenoid bone. INSERTION: Upper tarsal cartilage. INNERVATION: Oculomotor.

masseter (mă-sē′tĕr). ACTION: Mastication. ORIGIN: Zygomatic arch and malar process of superior maxilla. INSERTION: Angle ramus and coronoid process of mandible. INNERVATION: Mandibular division of trigeminal.

mentalis (mĕn-tā′lĭs). ACTION: Elevates and protrudes lower lip, wrinkles skin of chin. ORIGIN: Incisive fossa of mandible. INSERTION: Integument of chin. INNERVATION: Facial.

nasalis (nā-sā′lĭs). Consists of transverse and alar parts. ACTION: Depresses cartilaginous part of nose and draws the alae medially. ORIGIN: Maxilla. INSERTION: Bridge of nose. INNERVATION: Buccal branches of facial.

obliquus inferior oculi (ŏb-lī′kwŭs ĭn-fē′rĭ-or ŏk′ū-lī). ACTION: Rotates eyeball up and out. ORIGIN: Orbital plate of superior maxillary bone. INSERTION: Sclerotic coat at right angles to insertion of rectus externus just below it. INNERVATION: Oculomotor.

obliquus superior oculi (ŏb-lī′kwŭs sū-pē′rē-or ŏk′ū-lī). ACTION: Rotates eyeball down and out. ORIGIN: Above optic foramen. IN-

SERTION: By a tendon through trochlea to the sclerotic coat. INNERVATION: Trochlear.

occipitofrontalis (ŏk-sĭp'ĭ-tō-frŏn-tā'lĭs). Consists of (1) occipitalis and (2) frontalis bellies. ACTION: (1) Draws scalp back. (2) Draws scalp forward, raises eyebrows. ORIGIN: (1) Occipital and temporal bones. (2) Procerus, corrugator, and orbicularis oris muscles. INSERTION: Galea aponeurotica. INNERVATION: Facial.

orbicularis oculi (or-bĭk"ū-lā'rĭs ŏk'ū-lī). ACTION: Closes eyelid, wrinkles forehead vertically, compresses lacrimal sac. ORIGIN: (1) *(Pars lacrimalis)* Lacrimal bone. (2) *(Pars orbitalis)* Frontal processes of maxilla and frontal bone. (3) *(Pars palpebralis)* Inner canthus. INSERTION: (1) Joins palpebral portion. (2) Encircles orbit to orbit. (3) Outer canthus. INNERVATION: Facial.

orbicularis oris (or-bĭk"ū-lā'rĭs ō'rĭs). ACTION: Closes lips. ORIGIN: Nasal septum and canine fossa of mandible by accessory fibers. INSERTION: Buccinator and adjacent muscles surrounding mouth. INNERVATION: Facial.

procerus (prō-sē'rŭs). ACTION: Draws skin of forehead down. ORIGIN: Bridge of nose. INSERTION: Skin over root of nose. INNERVATION: Facial.

pterygoideus lateralis (tĕr-ĭ-goyd'ē-ŭs lăt"ĕr-ā'lĭs). ACTION: Brings jaw forward, moves jaw from side to side, opens jaws. ORIGIN: (1) Outer plate of pterygoid process. (2) Great wing of sphenoid and infratemporal ridge. INSERTION: Neck of condyle of mandible. INNERVATION: Lateral pterygoid from trigeminal nerve.

pterygoideus medialis (tĕr-ĭ-goyd'ē-ŭs mē-dĭ-ā'lĭs). ACTION: Closes jaw by raising and advancing it. ORIGIN: Pterygoid fossa of sphenoid bone. INSERTION: Inner surface of angle of mandible. INNERVATION: Medial pterygoid from trigeminal nerve.

rectus externus or lateralis (rĕk'tŭs ĕks-tĕr'nŭs, lăt"ĕr-ā'lĭs). ACTION: Rotates eyeball outward. ORIGIN: Margin of sphenoidal fissure and outer margin of optic foramen. INSERTION: Sclerotic coat. INNERVATION: Abducent.

rectus inferior (rĕk'tŭs ĭn-fē'rĭ-or). ACTION: Rotates eyeball downward. ORIGIN: Lower margin of optic foramen. INSERTION: Sclerotic coat. INNERVATION: Oculomotor.

rectus internus or medialis (rĕk'tŭs ĭn-tĕr'nŭs, mē-dĭ-ā'lĭs). ACTION: Rotates eyeball inward. ORIGIN: Lower margin of optic foramen. INSERTION: Sclerotic coat. INNERVATION: Oculomotor.

rectus superior (rĕk'tŭs sū-pē'rē-or). ACTION: Rotates eyeball upward. ORIGIN: Upper margin of optic foramen. INSERTION: Sclerotic coat. INNERVATION: Oculomotor.

risorius (rī-sō'rī-ŭs). ACTION: Draws angle of mouth outward ("laughing muscle"). ORIGIN: Fascia over masseter muscle. INSERTION: Angle of mouth. INNERVATION: Facial, buccal branch.

temporalis (tĕm-pō-rā'lĭs). ACTION: Closes jaws. ORIGIN: Temporal fossa and temporal fascia. INSERTION: Coronoid process of lower jaw. INNERVATION: Trigeminal, mandibular division.

zygomaticus major (zī-gō-măt'ĭ-kŭs mā'jor). ACTION: Draws upper lip backward, upward, and outward. ORIGIN: Malar bone, zygomatic arch. INSERTION: Angle of mouth. INNERVATION: Facial.

zygomaticus minor (zī-gō-măt'ĭ-kŭs mī'nor). ACTION: Draws the upper lip up and out. ORIGIN: Malar bone behind the maxillary arch. INSERTION: Angle of mouth, orbicularis oris. INNERVATION: Facial.

EAR

antitragicus (an-tī-trā'jī-kŭs). ORIGIN: Anterior part of antitragus. INSERTION: Opposite side at larger auricular fissure. INNERVATION: Posterior auricular branch of facial.

helicis major and minor (hĕl'ĭ-sĭs mā'jor, mī'nor). ACTION: Tighten the skin of auditory canal. ORIGIN: Tuberosity on helix. INSERTION: Rim of helix. INNERVATION: Auriculotemporal and posterior auricular.

obliquus auriculae (ŏb-lī'kwŭs aw-rĭk'ū-lē). ORIGIN: Concha of the ear. INSERTION: Fossa of antihelix. INNERVATION: Posterior auricular branch of facial.

stapedius (stă-pē'dĭ-ŭs). ACTION: Depresses base of the stapes. ORIGIN: Interior of pyramid. INSERTION: Neck of stapes. INNERVATION: Tympanic branch of facial.

tensor tympani (tĕn'sor tĭm'păn-ī). ACTION: Draws the membrana tympani tense. ORIGIN: Temporal tube, eustachian tube and canal. INSERTION: Handle of malleus. INNERVATION: Branch of mandibular through otic ganglion.

tragicus (tră'jī-kŭs). ORIGIN and INSERTION: Outer part of tragus. INNERVATION: Temporal branch of facial.

transversus auriculae (trăns-vĕr'sŭs aw-rĭk'ū-lē). ACTION: Retracts helix. ORIGIN: Cranial surface of pinna. INSERTION: Circumference of pinna. INNERVATION: Posterior auricular branch of facial.

NECK

constrictor pharyngis inferior (kŏn-strĭk'tor făr-ĭn'jĭs ĭn-fē'rĭ-or). ACTION: Narrows pharynx, as in swallowing. ORIGIN: Sides of cricoid and thyroid cartilage. INSERTION: Posterior raphe of pharyngeal wall. INNERVATION: Pharyngeal plexus.

constrictor pharyngis medius (kŏn-strĭk'tor fär-ĭn'jĭs mē'dē-ŭs). ACTION: Narrows pharynx, as in swallowing. ORIGIN: Both cornua of hyoid bone and stylohyoid ligament. INSERTION: Middle of posterior pharyngeal wall. INNERVATION: Pharyngeal plexus.

constrictor pharyngis superior (kŏn-strĭk'tor fär-ĭn'jĭs sū-pē'rē-or). ACTION: Narrows pharynx, as in swallowing. ORIGIN: Internal pterygoid plate, pterygomandibular ligament, jaw, side of tongue. INSERTION: Posterior pharyngeal wall. INNERVATION: Pharyngeal plexus.

digastricus (dī-găs'trĭ-kŭs). Consists of (1) anterior and (2) posterior bellies. ACTION: (1) Draws hyoid bone forward. (2) Draws hyoid bone backward. ORIGIN: (1) Lower border of lower jaw. (2) Mastoid groove of temporal bone. INSERTION: Intermediate tendon between both bellies. INNERVATION: (1) Mylohyoid. (2) Facial.

genioglossus (jē-nē″ō-glŏs'ŭs). ACTION: Protrudes and retracts tongue, elevates hyoid. ORIGIN: Inner surface of symphysis of mandible. INSERTION: Hyoid and bottom of tongue. INNERVATION: Hypoglossal.

geniohyoideus (jē-nē″ō-hī-oyd'ē-ŭs). ACTION: Elevates and advances hyoid and helps to depress jaw. ORIGIN: Mental spine of inferior maxilla. INSERTION: Hyoid. INNERVATION: Hypoglossal.

glossopalatinus (glŏs″ō-păl-ă-tī'nŭs). ACTION: Elevates back of tongue and constricts fauces. ORIGIN: Undersurface of soft palate. INSERTION: Side of tongue. INNERVATION: Pharyngeal plexus.

hyoglossus (hī″ō-glŏs'ŭs). ACTION: Depresses side of tongue and retracts tongue. ORIGIN: Cornua and body of hyoid. INSERTION: Side of tongue. INNERVATION: Hypoglossal.

levator veli palatini (lē-vā'tor vē'lī păl″ă-tī'nī). ACTION: Elevates soft palate. ORIGIN: Petrous portion of temporal bone and cartilaginous eustacian tube. INSERTION: Aponeurosis of soft palate. INNERVATION: Pharyngeal plexus.

linguae (ling-gwē). ACTION: Elevates sides and center of tongue. ORIGIN: Undersurface of tongue. INSERTION: Edge of tongue. INNERVATION: Hypoglossal.

longus capitis (lŏng'ŭs kăp'ĭ-tĭs). ACTION: Flexes head. ORIGIN: Transverse processes of 3rd to 6th cervical vertebrae. INSERTION: Occipital bone, basilar process. INNERVATION: Branches of 1st to 3rd cervical nerves.

longus colli (lŏng'ŭs kŏl'ī). Consists of three parts: (1) superior oblique, (2) inferior oblique, and (3) vertical. ACTION: Twists and bends neck forward. ORIGIN: (1) Trans-

verse processes of 3rd to 5th cervical vertebrae. (2) Bodies of 1st to 3rd thoracic vertebrae. (3) Bodies of three upper thoracic and three lower cervical vertebrae. INSERTION: (1) Anterior tubercle of atlas. (2) Transverse processes of 5th and 6th cervical vertebrae. (3) Bodies of 2nd to 4th cervical vertebrae. INNERVATION: Branches of 2nd to 7th cervical.

mylohyoideus (mī″lō-hī-oyd'ē-ŭs). ACTION: Elevates floor of mouth and hyoid, depresses jaw. ORIGIN: Mylohyoid line of mandible. INSERTION: Body of hyoid and median raphe. INNERVATION: Mylohyoid.

omohyoideus (ō″mō-hī-oyd'ē-ŭs). ACTION: Depresses hyoid. ORIGIN: Upper border of scapula. INSERTION: Hyoid bone. INNERVATION: Upper cervical through ansa hypoglossi.

pharyngopalatinus (fär-ĭn″gō-păl-ă-tī'nŭs). ACTION: Narrows fauces and shuts off nasopharynx. ORIGIN: Soft palate. INSERTION: Thyroid cartilage and aponeurosis of the pharynx. INNERVATION: Pharyngeal plexus.

platysma (plă-tĭz'mă). ACTION: Wrinkles skin of neck and chest, depresses jaw and lower lip. ORIGIN: Clavicle, acromion and fascia over deltoid, and pectoralis major. INSERTION: Lower border of mandible, risorius, and opposite platysma. INNERVATION: Cervical branch of facial.

rectus capitis anterior (rĕk'tŭs kăp'ĭ-tĭs ăn-tē'rĭ-or). ACTION: Turns and inclines the head. ORIGIN: Base of atlas. INSERTION: Occipital bone, basilar process. INNERVATION: Between 1st and 2nd cervical.

rectus capitis lateralis (rĕk'tŭs kăp'ĭ-tĭs lăt″ĕr-ā'lĭs). ACTION: Inclines head laterally and supports it. ORIGIN: Transverse process of atlas. INSERTION: Jugular process of occipital bone. INNERVATION: Between 1st and 2nd cervical nerves.

salpingopharyngeus (săl-pĭn″gō-fär-ĭn'jē-ŭs). ACTION: Elevates nasopharynx. ORIGIN: Eustachian tube close to nasopharynx. INSERTION: Posterior portion of the pharyngopalatinus. INNERVATION: Plexus.

scalenus anterior (skā-lē'nŭs ăn-tē'rĭ-or). ACTION: Elevates 1st rib and flexes neck. ORIGIN: Transverse processes of 3rd to 6th cervical vertebrae. INSERTION: Tubercle of 1st rib. INNERVATION: Cervical plexus.

scalenus medius (skā-lē'nŭs mē'dē-ŭs). ACTION: Elevates 1st rib and flexes neck. ORIGIN: Transverse processes of 2nd to 6th cervical vertebrae. INSERTION: First rib. INNERVATION: Cervical plexus.

scalenus posterior (skā-lē'nŭs pŏs-tē'rē-or). ACTION: Elevates 2nd rib and flexes neck. ORIGIN: Transverse processes of 4th to 6th cervical vertebrae. INSERTION: Second rib. INNERVATION: Cervical and brachial plexus.

Muscles *(Continued)*

sternocleidomastoideus (stĕr″nō-klī-dō-măs-toyd′ē-ŭs). ACTION: Rotates and laterally flexes neck. ORIGIN: By two heads, from sternum and clavicle. INSERTION: Mastoid process and outer part of superior curved line of occipital bone. INNERVATION: Spinal accessory.

sternohyoideus (stĕr″nō-hī-oyd′ē-ŭs). ACTION: Depresses hyoid bone. ORIGIN: Manubrium sterni and 1st costal cartilage. INSERTION: Body of hyoid bone. INNERVATION: Upper cervical through ansa hypoglossi.

sternothyroideus (stĕr″nō-thī-rē-oyd′ē-ŭs). ACTION: Depresses thyroid cartilage. ORIGIN: Sternum and 1st costal cartilage. INSERTION: Side of thyroid cartilage. INNERVATION: Upper cervical through ansa hypoglossi.

styloglossus (stī″lō-glŏs′ŭs). ACTION: Retracts and elevates tongue. ORIGIN: Styloid process. INSERTION: Side of tongue. INNERVATION: Hypoglossal.

stylohyoideus (stī″lō-hī-oyd′ē-ŭs). ACTION: Fixes hyoid, drawing it up and back. ORIGIN: Styloid process. INSERTION: Body of hyoid bone. INNERVATION: Facial.

stylopharyngeus (stī″lō-făr-ĭn′jē-ŭs). ACTION: Elevates and dilates pharynx. ORIGIN: Styloid process. INSERTION: Thyroid cartilage and side of pharynx. INNERVATION: Glossopharyngeal.

tensor veli palatini (tĕn′sŏr vē′lī păl″ă-tī′nī). ACTION: Stretches soft palate. ORIGIN: Spine of sphenoid, scaphoid fossa of internal pterygoid process and eustachian tube. INSERTION: Posterior border of hard palate and aponeurosis of soft palate. INNERVATION: Otic ganglion, trigeminal nerve.

thyrohyoideus (thī-rō-hī-oyd′ē-ŭs). ACTION: Depresses hyoid bone; elevates thyroid cartilage if hyoid bone is fixed. ORIGIN: Side of thyroid cartilage. INSERTION: Cornu and body of hyoid bone. INNERVATION: Hypoglossal.

uvulae (ū′vū-lē). ACTION: Elevates the uvula. ORIGIN: Posterior nasal spine. INSERTION: Forms large part of uvula. INNERVATION: Pharyngeal plexus.

LARYNX AND EPIGLOTTIS

aryepiglotticus (ăr″ē-ĕp″ĭ-glŏt′ĭk-ŭs). ACTION: Closes glottic opening. ORIGIN: Arytenoid cartilage. INSERTION: Epiglottis. INNERVATION: Laryngeal, recurrent.

arytenoideus (ăr″ē-tē-noyd′ē-ŭs). Consists of (1) arytenoideus obliquus and (2) arytenoideus transversus. ACTION: Closes glottic opening. ORIGIN: Arytenoid cartilage. INSERTION: (1) Aryepiglottic fold. (2) Crosses between the two cartilages of the obliquus

portion. INNERVATION: Laryngeal, recurrent.

cricoarytenoideus lateralis (krī″kō-ăr″ē-tē-noyd′ē-ŭs lăt″ĕr-ā′lĭs). ACTION: Narrows glottis. ORIGIN: Upper border of arch of cricoid cartilage. INSERTION: Muscular process of arytenoid cartilage. INNERVATION: Laryngeal, recurrent.

cricoarytenoideus posterior (krī″kō-ăr″ē-tē-noyd′ē-ŭs pŏs-tē′rē-or). ACTION: Opens glottis. ORIGIN: Back of cricoid cartilage. INSERTION: Muscular process of arytenoid cartilage. INNERVATION: Laryngeal, recurrent.

cricothyroideus (krī″kō-thī-royd′ē-ŭs). ACTION: Tightens vocal cords. ORIGIN: Anterior surface of cricoid cartilage. INSERTION: Thyroid cartilage. INNERVATION: Laryngeal, superior.

thyroarytenoideus (thī″rō-ăr″ē-tē-noyd′ē-ŭs). ACTION: Relaxes vocal cords. ORIGIN: Thyroid cartilage. INSERTION: Arytenoid cartilage. INNERVATION: Laryngeal, recurrent.

thyroepiglotticus (thī″rō-ĕp″ĭ-glŏt′ĭk-ŭs). ACTION: Depresses epiglottis. ORIGIN: Thyroid cartilage. INSERTION: Epiglottis and sacculus laryngis. INNERVATION: Laryngeal, recurrent.

BACK

iliocostalis cervicis (ĭl″ē-ō-kŏs-tă′lĭs sĕr′vĭ-sĭs). ACTION: Extends cervical spine. ORIGIN: Angles of 3rd to 6th ribs. INSERTION: Transverse processes of 4th to 6th cervical vertebrae. INNERVATION: Branches of cervical.

iliocostalis lumborum (ĭl″ē-ō-kŏs-tă′lĭs lŭm-bō′rŭm). ACTION: Extends lumbar spine. ORIGIN: With sacrospinalis. INSERTION: In angles of 5th to 12th ribs. INNERVATION: Branches of dorsal and lumbar.

iliocostalis thoracis (ĭl″ē-ō-kŏs-tă′lĭs thō-rā′sĭs). ACTION: Keeps dorsal spine erect. ORIGIN: Angles of 12th to 7th ribs. INSERTION: Sixth to 1st ribs and 7th cervical vertebra. INNERVATION: Branches of dorsal.

interspinales (ĭn-tĕr-spī-nă′lēz). A series. ACTION: Supports and extends vertebral column. ORIGIN: Undersurface of spine of one vertebra. INSERTION: Spine of vertebra above. INNERVATION: Branches of spinal.

intertransversarii (ĭn-tĕr-trăns-vĕr-sā′rī-ī). ACTION: Flexes vertebral column. ORIGIN: Between transverse processes of contiguous vertebrae. INNERVATION: Branches of ventral and dorsal divisions of spinal.

latissimus dorsi (lă-tĭs′ĭ-mŭs dŏr′sī). ACTION: Adducts, extends, and rotates arm. ORIGIN: Lower thoracic and lumbar vertebrae, sacrum, and tip of iliac crest. INSERTION: Intertubercular groove of humerus.

Muscles *(Continued)*

INNERVATION: Brachial plexus.

levator scapulae (lē-vā′tor skăp′ū-lē). ACTION: Elevates posterior angle of scapula. ORIGIN: Transverse process of four upper cervical vertebrae. INSERTION: Superior edge of scapula. INNERVATION: Dorsal scapular from 5th cervical and branches of 3rd and 4th cervical.

longissimus capitis (lŏn-jĭs′ĭ-mŭs kăp′ĭ-tĭs). ACTION: Keeps head erect, draws it backward or to one side. ORIGIN: Upper thoracic and lower and middle cervical vertebrae. INSERTION: Mastoid process. INNERVATION: Branches of cervical.

longissimus cervicis (lŏn-jĭs′ĭ-mŭs sĕr′vĭ-sĭs). ACTION: Extends cervical spine. ORIGIN: Upper thoracic vertebrae. INSERTION: Ribs and upper lumbar and thoracic vertebrae. INNERVATION: Branches of dorsal divisions of spinal.

longissimus thoracis (lŏn-jĭs′ĭ-mŭs thō-rā′sĭs). ACTION: Extends spinal column. ORIGIN: Transverse processes of lumbar and dorsal vertebrae. INSERTION: Lowest ribs and lumbar and dorsal vertebrae. INNERVATION: Lumbar and dorsal divisions of spinal.

multifidus (mŭl-tĭf′ĭ-dŭs). ACTION: Rotates spinal column. ORIGIN: Sacrum, iliac spine, lumbar, cervical, and dorsal vertebrae. INSERTION: Laminae and spinous processes of next four vertebrae above. INNERVATION: Branches of dorsal divisions of spinal.

obliquus capitis inferior (ŏb-lī′kwŭs kăp′ĭ-tĭs ĭn-fē′rĭ-or). ACTION: Rotates head. ORIGIN: Spine of axis. INSERTION: Transverse process of atlas. INNERVATION: Suboccipital.

obliquus capitis superior (ŏb-lī′kwŭs kăp′ĭ-tĭs sū-pē′rē-or). ACTION: Rotates head. ORIGIN: Transverse process of axis. INSERTION: Occipital bone. INNERVATION: Suboccipital.

rectus capitis posterior major (rĕk′tŭs kăp′ĭ-tĭs pŏs-tē′rē-or mā′jor). ACTION: Rotates and draws head backward. ORIGIN: Spine of axis. INSERTION: Inferior curved line of occipital bone. INNERVATION: Suboccipital.

rectus capitis posterior minor (rĕk′tŭs kăp′ĭ-tĭs pŏs-tē′rē-or mī′nor). ACTION: Rotates and draws head backward. ORIGIN: Posterior tubercle of atlas. INSERTION: Inferior curved line of occipital bone. INNERVATION: Suboccipital.

rhomboideus major (rŏm-boy′dē-ŭs mā′jor). ACTION: Retracts, elevates, and downwardly rotates scapula. ORIGIN: Spinous processes of 2nd to 5th thoracic vertebrae. INSERTION: Vertebral border of scapula below spine. INNERVATION: Dorsal scapular from brachial plexus.

rhomboideus minor (rŏm-boy′dē-ŭs mī′nor). ACTION: Retracts and elevates scapula. ORIGIN: Spinous processes of 7th cervical vertebra and 1st thoracic vertebra. INSERTION: Border of scapula above spine. INNERVATION: Dorsal scapular from brachial plexus.

rotatores (rō-tā-tō′rēz). ACTION: Extends and rotates the vertebral column. ORIGIN: Transverse processes of 2nd to 12th dorsal vertebrae. INSERTION: Lamina of next vertebra above. INNERVATION: Branches of dorsal divisions of spinal.

sacrospinalis (sā″krō-spī-nā′lĭs). ACTION: Extends vertebral column. ORIGIN: Sacrum, lumbar vertebrae, iliac crest. INSERTION: Iliocostalis and longissimus dorsi. INNERVATION: Posterior branches of spinal.

semispinalis capitis (sĕm″ē-spī-nā′lĭs kăp′ĭ-tĭs). ACTION: Rotates and draws head backward. ORIGIN: Transverse processes of upper six or seven thoracic and lower four cervical vertebrae. INSERTION: Occipital bone, between inferior and superior curved line. INNERVATION: Branches of dorsal division of cervical.

semispinalis cervicis (sĕm″ē-spī-nā′lĭs sĕr′vĭ-sĭs). ACTION: Extends the vertebral column and rotates it toward the opposite side. ORIGIN: Transverse processes of upper five or six thoracic vertebrae. INSERTION: Spines from axis to 5th cervical vertebra. INNERVATION: Branches of dorsal divisions of spinal.

semispinalis thoracis (sĕm″ē-spī-nā′lĭs thō-rā′sĭs). ACTION: Extends the vertebral column and rotates it toward the opposite side. ORIGIN: Transverse processes of 6th to 10th thoracic vertebrae. INSERTION: Spines of upper four thoracic and lower two cervical vertebrae. INNERVATION: Branches of dorsal divisions of spinal.

serratus posterior inferior (sĕr-ā′tŭs pŏs-tē′rē-or ĭn-fē′rĭ-or). ACTION: Draws ribs back and downward. ORIGIN: Spines of lower two thoracic and upper two lumbar vertebrae. INSERTION: Lower four ribs. INNERVATION: Branches of ventral divisions of 9th to 12th thoracic.

serratus posterior superior (sĕr-ā′tŭs pŏs-tē′rē-or sū-pē′rē-or). ACTION: Elevates the ribs. ORIGIN: Spines of 7th cervical and two upper thoracic vertebrae. INSERTION: Angles of 2nd to 5th ribs. INNERVATION: Branches of ventral divisions of thoracic.

spinalis capitis (spī-nā′lĭs kăp′ĭ-tĭs). ORIGIN: Inconstant; from spines of upper dorsal and lower cervical vertebrae. INSERTION: Blends with the semispinalis capitis.

spinalis cervicis (spī-nā′lĭs sĕr′vĭ-sĭs). ACTION: Extends cervical spine. ORIGIN: Spines of 5th, 6th, and 7th cervical vertebrae. INSERTION: Axis and, occasionally, the two vertebrae below. INNERVATION: Branches of cervical.

Muscles *(Continued)*

spinalis thoracis (spī-nā′lĭs thō-rǎ′sĭs). AC-
TION: Erects spinal column. ORIGIN: Spines
of first two lumbar and last two thoracic
vertebrae. INSERTION: Spines of middle and
upper thoracic vertebrae. INNERVATION:
Dorsal branches of spinal.

splenius capitis (splē′nē-ŭs kǎp′ĭ-tĭs). AC-
TION: Rotates and extends head. ORIGIN:
Ligamentum nuchae, 7th cervical and first
three thoracic vertebrae. INSERTION: Mastoid process and superior curved line of occiput. INNERVATION: Branches of dorsal divisions of cervical.

splenius cervicis (splē′nē-ŭs sĕr′vĭ-sĭs). AC-
TION: Rotates and flexes head and neck. OR-
IGIN: Spines of 3rd to 6th thoracic vertebrae.
INSERTION: Transverse processes of 1st and
2nd cervical vertebrae. INNERVATION:
Branches of dorsal divisions of cervical.

suspensorius duodeni (sŭs-pĕn-sō′rē-ŭs
doo″ō-dē′nē). ACTION: Acts as a suspensory
ligament. ORIGIN: Wide, flat band of tissue
and unstriped muscle attached to the left
crus of diaphragm and continuous with the
muscular coat of the duodenum at its line of
junction with the jejunum. INNERVATION:
Celiac plexus.

trapezius (trǎ-pē′zē-ŭs). ACTION: Draws head
back and to the side, rotates scapula. ORI-
GIN: Superior curved line of occipital, spinous processes of 7th cervical and all thoracic vertebrae. INSERTION: Clavicle,
acromion, base of spine of scapula. INNER-
VATION: Spinal accessory and cervical
plexus.

ABDOMEN

cremaster (krē-mǎs′tĕr). ACTION: Raises testicle. ORIGIN: Midportion of inguinal ligament. INSERTION: Cremasteric fascia and
pubic bone. INNERVATION: Genitofemoral.

obliquus externus abdominis (ŏb-lī′kwŭs
ĕks-tĕr′nŭs ăb-dŏm′ĭ-nĭs). ACTION: Contracts abdomen and viscera. ORIGIN: Lower
8 ribs. INSERTION: Iliac crest, Poupart's ligament, linea alba, pubic crest. INNERVATION:
Iliohypogastric, ilioinguinal, and branches
of intercostal.

obliquus internus abdominis (ŏb-lī′kwŭs
ĭn-tĕr′nŭs ăb-dŏm′ĭ-nĭs). ACTION: Compresses viscera, flexes thorax forward. ORI-
GIN: Iliac crest, inguinal ligament, lumbar
fascia. INSERTION: Few lowest ribs, linea
alba, pubic crest. INNERVATION: Iliohypogastric, ilioinguinal, and branches of intercostal.

pyramidalis (pĭ-răm″ĭ-dǎ′lĭs). ACTION:
Tightens linea alba. ORIGIN: Pubic crest. IN-
SERTION: Linea alba. INNERVATION: Branch
of 12th thoracic.

quadratus lumborum (kwǎd-rǎ′tŭs lŭm-

bō′rŭm). ACTION: Flexes trunk laterally and
assists lumbar vertebral extension. ORIGIN:
Iliac crest, iliolumbar ligament, lower lumbar vertebrae. INSERTION: Twelfth rib and
the upper lumbar vertebrae. INNERVATION:
Branches of 1st lumbar and 12th thoracic.

rectus abdominis (rĕk′tŭs ăb-dŏm′ĭ-nĭs).
ACTION: Compresses or flattens abdomen.
ORIGIN: Pubis. INSERTION: Cartilage of 5th
to 7th ribs. INNERVATION: Branches of 7th to
12th intercostal.

transversus abdominis (trăns-vĕr′sŭs ăb-
dŏm′ĭ-nĭs). ACTION: Compresses abdomen,
flexes thorax. ORIGIN: Lumbar fascia, 7th to
12th costal cartilages, inguinal ligament,
iliac crest. INSERTION: Xiphoid cartilage,
linea alba, pubic crest, and iliopectineal line.
INNERVATION: Iliohypogastric, ilioinguinal,
branches of intercostal.

PERINEUM

bulbospongiosus (bŭl″bō-spŏn″jē-ō′sŭs).
ACTION: Constricts bulbous urethra in male;
constricts urethra in female. ORIGIN: Central point of perineum and medial raphe. IN-
SERTION: Undersurface of bulb, spongy and
cavernous part of penis; root of clitoris. IN-
NERVATION: Perineal branch of pudendal.

coccygeus (kŏk-sĭj′ē-ŭs). ACTION: Supports
coccyx, closes pelvic outlet. ORIGIN: Ischial
spine and sacrospinous ligament. INSER-
TION: Coccyx and lowest portion of sacrum.
INNERVATION: Third and 4th sacral.

corrugator cutis ani (kŏr′ū-gā′tŏr kū′tĭs
ā′nī). ACTION: Wrinkles skin of anus. ORI-
GIN: Submucous tissue, interior of anus. IN-
SERTION: Subcutaneous tissue on opposite
side of anus. INNERVATION: Sympathetic.

depressor urethrae (dē-prĕs′or ū-rē′thrē).
ACTION: Depresses urethra. ORIGIN: Ramus
of ischium near the transversus perinei profundus. INSERTION: Fibers of constrictor vaginae.

ischiocavernosus (ĭs″kē-ō-kǎ″vĕr-nō′sŭs).
ACTION: Maintains erection of penis or clitoris. ORIGIN: Tuberosity of ischium and great
sacrosciatic ligament. INSERTION: Corpora
cavernosum of clitoris or penis. INNERVA-
TION: Perineal branch of pudendal.

levator ani (lē-vā′tor ā′nī). ACTION: Supports
rectum and pelvic floor, aids in defecation.
ORIGIN: Pubis, pelvic fascia, ischial spine.
INSERTION: Rectum, coccyx, and fibrous
raphe of perineum. INNERVATION: Sacral and
perineal.

sphincter ani externus (sfĭngk′tĕr ā′nī ĕks-
tĕr′nŭs). ACTION: Closes anus. ORIGIN: Ring
of fibers surrounding anus. INSERTION: Coccyx and central point of perineum. INNERVA-
TION: Hemorrhoidal branch of pudendal.

sphincter ani internus (sfĭngk′tĕr ā′nī ĭn-

Muscles *(Continued)*

tĕr'nŭs). ACTION: Contracts rectum and anus, but not voluntarily. ORIGIN: Muscular ring of rectal fibers above canal.

sphincter urethrae membranaceae (sfĭngk'tĕr ū-rē'thrē mĕm-bră-nā'sē-ē). ACTION: Constricts membranous urethra. ORIGIN: Ramus of pubis. INSERTION: Behind and in front of urethra. INNERVATION: Perineal branch of pudendal.

sphincter vesicae (sfĭngk'tĕr vĕs'ĭ-kē). ACTION: Shuts off internal orifice of urethra. ORIGIN: Near urethral orifice of bladder. INNERVATION: Sacral and hypogastric.

transversus perinei profundus (trăns-vĕr'sŭs pĕr-ĭ-nē'ĭ prō-fŭn'dŭs). ACTION: Assists compressor urethrae. ORIGIN: Ramus of ischium. INSERTION: Central tendon. INNERVATION: Perineal branch of pudendal.

transversus perinei superficialis (trăns-vĕr'sŭs pĕr-ĭ-nē'ĭ soo″pĕr-fĭsh-ē-ā'lĭs). ACTION: Tenses central tendon. ORIGIN: Ramus of ischium. INSERTION: Central point of perineum. INNERVATION: Perineal branch of pudendal.

THORAX

diaphragma (dī″ă-frăg'mă). ACTION: Increases chest capacity and decreases pressure within the thoracic cavity. ORIGIN: Ensiform cartilage, 7th to 12th ribs, arcuate ligaments, and lumbar vertebrae. INSERTION: Central tendon. INNERVATION: Phrenic.

intercostalis externus (ĭn″tĕr-kŏs-tă'lĭs ĕks-tĕr'nŭs). ACTION: Draws ribs together and raises ribs. ORIGIN: Lower border of rib. INSERTION: Upper border of rib below. INNERVATION: Intercostal.

intercostalis internus (ĭn″tĕr-kŏs-tă'lĭs ĭn-tĕr'nŭs). ACTION: Draws ribs together and lowers ribs. ORIGIN: Lower border of rib. INSERTION: Upper border of rib below. INNERVATION: Intercostal.

levatores costarum (lē-vā-tō'rez kŏs-tă'rŭm). ACTION: Raises ribs, flexes vertebral column. ORIGIN: Transverse process of 7th cervical and upper 11 thoracic vertebrae. INSERTION: Rib next below. INNERVATION: Branches of intercostal.

subcostales (sŭb-kŏs-tă'lēz). ACTION: Draws ribs together and lowers ribs. ORIGIN: Inconstant; inner surface of the ribs. INSERTION: Inner surface of one of the ribs just below. INNERVATION: Intercostal.

transversus thoracis (trăns-vĕr'sŭs thō-rā'sĭs). ACTION: Narrows the chest. ORIGIN: Xiphoid cartilage and sternum. INSERTION: Costal cartilages, 2nd to 6th ribs. INNERVATION: Branches of intercostal.

SHOULDER

deltoideus (dĕl-toy'dē-ŭs). ACTION: Raises and rotates arm. ORIGIN: Clavicle, acromion process, and spine of scapula. INSERTION: Shaft of humerus. INNERVATION: Axillary (circumflex) from brachial plexus.

infraspinatus (ĭn″fră-spī-nā'tŭs). ACTION: Rotates arm back and out. ORIGIN: Infraspinous fossa of scapula. INSERTION: Great tuberosity of humerus. INNERVATION: Suprascapular from brachial plexus.

pectoralis major (pĕk″tō-rā'lĭs mā'jor). ACTION: Flexes, adducts, and rotates arm. ORIGIN: Sternum, clavicle, and cartilages of 1st to 6th ribs. INSERTION: Bicipital ridge of humerus. INNERVATION: Anterior thoracic from brachial plexus.

pectoralis minor (pĕk″tō-rā'lĭs mī'nor). ACTION: Draws down scapula and point to shoulder, raises ribs. ORIGIN: Third to 5th ribs. INSERTION: Coracoid process of scapula. INNERVATION: Anterior thoracic from brachial plexus.

serratus anterior (sĕr-ā'tŭs ăn-tē'rĭ-or). ACTION: Elevates ribs, rotates scapula. ORIGIN: Upper eight or nine ribs. INSERTION: Angles and vertebral border of scapula. INNERVATION: Long thoracic from brachial plexus.

subclavius (sŭb-klā'vē-ŭs). ACTION: Draws clavicle down and forward or elevates the 1st rib. ORIGIN: First rib and cartilage. INSERTION: Undersurface of clavicle. INNERVATION: Special nerve with fibers from 5th and 6th cervical.

subscapularis (sŭb-skăp-ū-lā'rĭs). ACTION: Rotates humerus inward and lowers it. ORIGIN: Subscapular fossa. INSERTION: Lesser tubercle of humerus. INNERVATION: Subscapular.

supraspinatus (soo″pră-spī-nā'tŭs). ACTION: Abducts and raises arm. ORIGIN: Supraspinous fossa of scapula. INSERTION: Greater tubercle of humerus. INNERVATION: Branches of suprascapular.

teres major (tē'rēz mā'jor). ACTION: Inwardly rotates, adducts, and extends arm. ORIGIN: Axillary border of scapula. INSERTION: Lesser tubercle of humerus. INNERVATION: Branch of lower subscapular.

teres minor (tē'rēz mī'nor). ACTION: Rotates arm outward. ORIGIN: Axillary border of scapula. INSERTION: Greater tubercle of humerus. INNERVATION: Branch of axillary (circumflex).

ARM AND FOREARM

anconeus (ăn-kō'nē-ŭs). ACTION: Extends forearm. ORIGIN: Lateral epicondyle of humerus. INSERTION: Olecranon and posterior surface of ulna. INNERVATION: Branch of radial.

biceps brachii (bī'sĕps brā'kē-ī). ACTION: Flexes arm and forearm and supinates forearm. ORIGIN: (1) Short head from coracoid process. (2) Long head from the supraglenoid tuberosity at the margin of the glenoid cavity. INSERTION: Bicipital tuberosity of radius. INNERVATION: Musculocutaneous.

brachialis (brā"kē-ăl'ĭs). ACTION: Flexes forearm. ORIGIN: Lower half of anterior surface of humerus. INSERTION: Coronoid process of ulna. INNERVATION: Musculocutaneous and radial.

brachioradialis (brā"kē-ō-rā"dē-ā'lĭs). ACTION: Flexes and supinates forearm. ORIGIN: Supracondylar ridge of humerus. INSERTION: Styloid process of radius. INNERVATION: Branch of radial. SYN: *supinator longus.*

coracobrachialis (kor"ă-kō-brā"kē-ăl'ĭs). ACTION: Raises and adducts arm. ORIGIN: Coracoid process of scapula. INSERTION: Middle of inner border of humerus. INNERVATION: Musculocutaneous.

extensor carpi radialis brevis (ĕks-tĕn'sŏr kar'pī rā"dē-ā'lĭs brē'vĭs). ACTION: Extends and abducts wrist. ORIGIN: External condyloid ridge of humerus. INSERTION: Base of 3rd metacarpal. INNERVATION: Branch of radial.

extensor carpi radialis longus (ĕks-tĕn'sŏr kar'pī rā"dē-ā'lĭs lŏng'ŭs). ACTION: Extends and abducts wrist. ORIGIN: External condyloid ridge of humerus. INSERTION: Base of 2nd metacarpal. INNERVATION: Branch of radial.

extensor carpi ulnaris (ĕks-tĕn'sŏr kar'pī ŭlnā'rĭs). ACTION: Extends and adducts hand and wrist. ORIGIN: Lateral epicondyle of humerus. INSERTION: Base of 5th metacarpal. INNERVATION: Branch of radial.

extensor digiti minimi (ĕks-tĕn'sŏr dĭj'ĭ-tī mĭn'ĭm-ī). ACTION: Extends little finger. ORIGIN: External epicondyle of humerus. INSERTION: Dorsum of 1st phalanx of little finger. INNERVATION: Branch of radial.

extensor digitorum communis (ĕks-tĕn'sŏr dĭj-ĭ-tō'rŭm kŏm-mū'nĭs). ACTION: Extends fingers and wrist. ORIGIN: External epicondyle of humerus. INSERTION: Second and 3rd phalanges. INNERVATION: Branch of radial.

extensor indicis proprius (ĕks-tĕn'sŏr ĭn'dĭsĭs prō'prē-ŭs). ACTION: Extends index finger. ORIGIN: Dorsal surface of ulna and interosseous membrane. INSERTION: First tendon of extensor digitorum communis. INNERVATION: Branch of radial.

extensor pollicis brevis (ĕks-tĕn'sŏr pŏl'ĭsĭs brē'vĭs). ACTION: Extends thumb and abducts 1st metacarpal. ORIGIN: Dorsal surface of radius. INSERTION: Base of 1st phalanx of thumb. INNERVATION: Branch of radial.

extensor pollicis longus (ĕks-tĕn'sŏr pŏl'ĭsĭs lŏng'ŭs). ACTION: Extends terminal phalanx of thumb and abducts hand. ORIGIN: Dorsal surface of ulna. INSERTION: Base of 2nd phalanx of thumb. INNERVATION: Branch of radial.

flexor carpi radialis (flĕks'or kar'pī rā"dēā'lĭs). ACTION: Flexes and abducts wrist. ORIGIN: Medial epicondyle of humerus. INSERTION: Base of 2nd metacarpal. INNERVATION: Branch of median.

flexor carpi ulnaris (flĕks'or kar'pī ŭl-nā'rĭs). Consists of (1) humeral head and (2) ulnar head. ACTION: Flexes and adducts wrist. ORIGIN: (1) Medial epicondyle of humerus. (2) Olecranon process and posterior border of ulna. INSERTION: Pisiform bone and 5th metacarpal. INNERVATION: Branch of ulnar.

flexor digitorum profundus (flĕks'or dĭj-ĭtō'rŭm prō-fŭn'dŭs). ACTION: Flexes the distal interphalangeal joints of the fingers. ORIGIN: Upper three-fourths of shaft of ulna. INSERTION: Terminal phalanges of fingers. INNERVATION: Branch of ulnar and branch of median.

flexor digitorum sublimis (flĕks'or dĭj-ĭtō'rŭm sŭb-lī'mĭs). SAME AS: *flexor digitorum superficialis*

flexor digitorum superficialis (flĕks'or dĭj-ĭtō'rŭm soo"pĕr-fĭsh-ē-ā'lĭs). Consists of three heads (1) humeral, (2) ulnar, and (3) radial. ACTION: Flexes the middle and proximal phalanges, carpal flexion of hand. ORIGIN: (1) Medial epicondyle of humerus. (2) Medial side of coronoid process. (3) Outer border of radius. INSERTION: Second phalanx of each finger. INNERVATION: Branches of median. SYN: *flexor digitorum sublimis.*

flexor pollicis longus (flĕks'or pŏl'ĭ-sĭs lŏng'ŭs). ACTION: Flexes thumb. ORIGIN: Anterior surface of middle third of radius. INSERTION: Terminal phalanx of thumb. INNERVATION: Branch of median.

palmaris longus (păl-mā'rĭs lŏng'ŭs). ACTION: Tightens palmar fascia, flexes wrist. ORIGIN: Medial epicondyle of humerus. INSERTION: Transverse carpal ligament and palmar fascia. INNERVATION: Branch of median.

pronator quadratus (prō-nā'tor kwădrā'tŭs). ACTION: Pronates forearm. ORIGIN: Lower fourth of ulna. INSERTION: Lower fourth of radius. INNERVATION: Volar interosseous.

pronator teres (prō-nā'tor tĕ'rēz). Consists of (1) humeral head and (2) ulnar head. ACTION: Pronates hand. ORIGIN: (1) Medial epicondyle of humerus. (2) Coronoid process of ulna. INSERTION: Lateral surface of shaft of radius. INNERVATION: Branch of median.

supinator (soo″pĭ-nā′tor). ACTION: Supinates forearm. ORIGIN: Lateral epicondyle of humerus, oblique line of ulna, elbow joint. INSERTION: Outer surface of radius. INNERVATION: Branch of radial.

supinator longus (soo″pĭ-nā′tor lŏng′ŭs). SAME AS: *brachioradialis.*

triceps brachii (trī′sĕps brā′kē-ī). Consists of three heads: (1) long, (2) lateral, and (3) medial. ACTION: Extends forearm and arm. ORIGIN: (1) Infraglenoid tubercle of scapula. (2) Posterior surface of humerus below great tubercle. (3) Humerus below radial groove. INSERTION: Olecranon process of ulna. INNERVATION: Branches of radial.

HAND

abductor digiti minimi manus (ăb-dŭk′tor dĭj-ĭ-tī mĭn′ĭ-mī mă′nŭs). ACTION: Abducts little finger. ORIGIN: Pisiform bone and ligaments. INSERTION: Inner side of 1st phalanx of little finger. INNERVATION: Ulnar, palmar branch.

abductor pollicis brevis (ăb-dŭk′tor pŏl′ĭ-sĭs brē′vĭs). ACTION: Abducts thumb. ORIGIN: Ridge of trapezius and transverse carpal ligament. INSERTION: Outer side of 1st phalanx of thumb. INNERVATION: Branch of median.

abductor pollicis longus (ăb-dŭk′tor pŏl′ĭ-sĭs lŏng′ŭs). ACTION: Abducts and assists in extending thumb. ORIGIN: Posterior surface of radius and ulna. INSERTION: Outer side of base of 1st metacarpal. INNERVATION: Branch of radial.

adductor pollicis (ăd-dŭk′tor pŏl′ĭ-sĭs). ACTION: Adducts thumb. ORIGIN: Third metacarpal bone. INSERTION: Inner side of base of 1st phalanx of thumb. INNERVATION: Ulnar.

flexor digiti quinti brevis manus (flĕks′or dĭj-ĭ-tī kwĭn′tī brē′vĭs mă′nŭs). ACTION: Flexes 1st phalanx of little finger. ORIGIN: Unciform bone. INSERTION: First phalanx of little finger. INNERVATION: Branch of ulnar.

flexor pollicis brevis (flĕks′or pŏl′ĭ-sĭs brē′vĭs). ACTION: Flexes 1st phalanx of thumb. ORIGIN: Transverse carpal ligament, metacarpal bone. INSERTION: Base of 1st phalanx of thumb. INNERVATION: Branch of median and ulnar.

interossei dorsales manus (ĭn″tĕr-ŏs′ē-ī dŏr-sā′lēz mă′nŭs). Four. ACTION: Abducts and adducts fingers. ORIGIN: Sides of metacarpal bones. INSERTION: First phalanges. INNERVATION: Branch of ulnar.

interossei volares (ĭn″tĕr-ŏs′ē-ī vō-lā′rēz). Three. ACTION: Adducts index finger, abducts ring and little fingers. ORIGIN: Metacarpal bones laterally. INSERTION: Ulnar side of index finger, and radial sides of ring and little fingers. INNERVATION: Branch of ulnar.

lumbricales manus (lŭm-brĭ-kā′lēz mă′nŭs). Four. ACTION: Flexes 1st and extends 2nd and 3rd phalanges. ORIGIN: Tendon of flexor digitorum profundus. INSERTION: First phalanx and extensor tendon. INNERVATION: Median and ulnar.

opponens digiti quinti (ŏp-pō′nĕns dĭj-ĭ-tī kwĭn′tī). ACTION: Flexes and adducts little finger. ORIGIN: Unciform bone, transverse carpal ligament. INSERTION: Fifth metacarpal bone. INNERVATION: Branch of ulnar.

opponens pollicis (ŏp-pō′nĕns pŏl′ĭ-sĭs). ACTION: Flexes and adducts thumb. ORIGIN: Trapezium and transverse carpal ligament. INSERTION: First metacarpal bone. INNERVATION: Median.

palmaris brevis (păl-mā′rĭs brē′vĭs). ACTION: Wrinkles skin on inner side of hand. ORIGIN: Central portion of palmar aponeurosis and transverse carpal ligament. INSERTION: Skin of ulnar side of hand. INNERVATION: Branch of ulnar.

HIP, THIGH, LOWER EXTREMITY

adductor brevis (ăd-dŭk′tor brē′vĭs). ACTION: Flexes, adducts, and tends to rotate thigh medially. ORIGIN: Ramus of pubis. INSERTION: Upper portion of linea aspera of femur. INNERVATION: Branch of obturator.

adductor longus (ăd-dŭk′tor lŏng′ŭs). ACTION: Adducts, flexes and tends to rotate thigh medially. ORIGIN: Pubic crest and symphysis. INSERTION: Middle of linea aspera of femur. INNERVATION: Branch of obturator.

adductor magnus (ăd-dŭk′tor măg′nŭs). ACTION: Adducts thigh and rotates it outward. ORIGIN: Ramus of ischium and pubis. INSERTION: Linea aspera of femur and medial condyle. INNERVATION: Branch of sciatic and obturator.

articularis genus (ăr-tĭk″ū-lā′rĭs jē′nŭs). ACTION: Elevates capsule of knee joint. ORIGIN: Lower quarter of anterior surface of femoral shaft. INSERTION: Synovial membrane of knee joint. INNERVATION: Branch of femoral.

biceps femoris (bī′sĕps fĕm′ō-rĭs). ACTION: Flexes knee and rotates it outward. ORIGIN: (1) Short head from linea aspera. (2) Long head from ischial tuberosity. INSERTION: Head of fibula; lateral condyle of tibia. INNERVATION: (1) Peroneal, and (2) tibial portions of sciatic.

gemellus inferior (jĕ-mĕl′ŭs ĭn-fē′rĭ-or). ACTION: Rotates thigh outward. ORIGIN: Ischial tuberosity. INSERTION: Medial surface of greater trochanter. INNERVATION: Sacral.

gemellus superior (jĕ-mĕl′ŭs sū-pē′rē-or). ACTION: Rotates thigh outward. ORIGIN: Spine of ischium. INSERTION: Medial surface of greater trochanter. INNERVATION: Sacral plexus.

gluteus maximus (gloo′tē-ŭs măk′sē-mŭs). ACTION: Extends and rotates thigh. ORIGIN: Superior curved iliac line and crest, coccyx, and sacrum. INSERTION: Fascia lata and femur below greater trochanter. INNERVATION: Inferior gluteal.

gluteus medius (gloo′tē-ŭs mē′dē-ŭs). ACTION: Abducts and rotates thigh. ORIGIN: Lateral surface of ilium. INSERTION: Greater trochanter. INNERVATION: Branches of superior gluteal.

gluteus minimus (gloo′tē-ŭs mĭn′ĭ-mŭs). ACTION: Abducts and extends thigh. ORIGIN: Lateral surface of ilium. INSERTION: Greater trochanter. INNERVATION: Branch of superior gluteal.

gracilis (grăs′ĭ-lĭs). ACTION: Flexes and adducts leg, adducts thigh. ORIGIN: Symphysis pubis and pubic arch. INSERTION: Medial surface of shaft of tibia. INNERVATION: Branch of obturator.

iliacus (ĭ-lī′ă-kŭs). ACTION: Flexes and rotates thigh. ORIGIN: Margin of iliac fossa. INSERTION: Lesser trochanter. INNERVATION: Branches of femoral.

obturator internus (ŏb′tū-rā″tor ĭn-tĕr′nŭs). ACTION: Rotates thigh outward. ORIGIN: Pubes, ischium, obturator foramen. INSERTION: Inner surface of greater trochanter. INNERVATION: Branch of obturator.

pectineus (pĕk-tĭn′ē-ŭs). ACTION: Flexes and adducts thigh. ORIGIN: Pubic spine, iliopectineal line. INSERTION: Pectineal line of femur. INNERVATION: Branch of obturator and femoral.

piriformis (pĭ-rĭ-for′mĭs). ACTION: Abducts and rotates thigh outward. ORIGIN: Margins of anterior sacral foramina and sacrosciatic notch of ilium. INSERTION: Upper margin of greater trochanter. INNERVATION: Branch of sacral.

psoas major (sō′ăs mā′jor). ACTION: Flexes thigh, adducts and rotates it medially. ORIGIN: Last thoracic and all of the lumbar vertebrae. INSERTION: Lesser trochanter of femur. INNERVATION: Lumbar plexus.

psoas minor (sō′ăs mī′nor). ACTION: Tenses iliac fascia. ORIGIN: Twelfth thoracic and 1st lumbar vertebrae. INSERTION: Iliac fascia and iliopectineal tuberosity. INNERVATION: Branch of lumbar.

quadratus femoris (kwăd-rā′tŭs fĕm′ō-rĭs). ACTION: Rotates thigh outward. ORIGIN: Ischial tuberosity. INSERTION: Intertrochanteric ridge. INNERVATION: Sciatic.

quadriceps femoris (kwăd′rĭ-sĕps fĕm′ō-rĭs). ACTION: Extends leg. ORIGIN: By four heads: rectus femoris, vastus medialis, vastus lateralis, and vastus intermedius. INSERTION: Patella and tibial tuberosity. INNERVATION: Branches of femoral.

rectus femoris (rĕk′tŭs fĕm′ō-rĭs). ACTION: Extends leg and assists flexion of thigh. ORIGIN: Iliac spine, upper margin of acetabulum. INSERTION: Base of patella. INNERVATION: Femoral.

sartorius (săr-tō′rē-ŭs). ACTION: Flexes and rotates thigh and leg. ORIGIN: Anterior superior iliac spine. INSERTION: Tibial tuberosity. INNERVATION: Branches of femoral.

semimembranosus (sĕm″ē-mĕm″brăn-ō′sŭs). ACTION: Flexes and rotates leg, extends thigh. ORIGIN: Ischial tuberosity. INSERTION: Medial condyle of tibia. INNERVATION: Tibial portion of sciatic.

semitendinosus (sĕm″ē-tĕn″dĭn-ō′sŭs). ACTION: Flexes and rotates leg, extends thigh. ORIGIN: Ischial tuberosity. INSERTION: Shaft of tibia below internal tuberosity. INNERVATION: Tibial portion of sciatic.

tensor fasciae latae (fĕm′ō-rĭs făsh′ē-ē lā′tē). ACTION: Flexes and rotates thigh. ORIGIN: Iliac crest, iliac spine, fascia lata. INSERTION: Iliotibial band of fascia lata. INNERVATION: Branch of superior gluteal.

vastus intermedius (văs′tŭs ĭn″tĕr-mē′dē-ŭs). ORIGIN: Upper part of anterior surface of shaft of femur. INSERTION: Common tendon of quadriceps femoris. INNERVATION: Branches of femoral.

vastus lateralis (văs′tŭs lăt″ĕr-ā′lĭs). ACTION: Extends knee. ORIGIN: Linea aspera to greater trochanter. INSERTION: Common tendon of quadriceps femoris. INNERVATION: Branches of femoral.

vastus medialis (văs′tŭs mē-dĭ-ā′lĭs). ACTION: Extends leg, draws patella in. ORIGIN: Linea aspera of femur. INSERTION: Common tendon of quadriceps femoris. INNERVATION: Branches of femoral.

LEG

extensor digitorum longus (ĕks-tĕn′sōr dĭj-ĭ-tō′rŭm lŏng′ŭs). ACTION: Extends toes, dorsiflexes foot. ORIGIN: External tuberosity of tibia; body of fibula. INSERTION: Second and 3rd phalanges of toes. INNERVATION: Branches of peroneal.

extensor hallucis longus (ĕks-tĕn′sōr hăl-oo′sĭs lŏng′ŭs). ACTION: Extends great toe, flexes foot. ORIGIN: Front of fibula and interosseous membrane. INSERTION: Terminal phalanx of great toe. INNERVATION: Branch of peroneal.

flexor digitorum longus (flĕks′or dĭj-ĭ-tō′rŭm lŏng′ŭs). ACTION: Flexes the toes. ORIGIN: Posterior surface of tibia. INSERTION: Terminal phalanges of lesser toes. INNERVATION: Branch of tibial.

flexor hallucis longus (flĕks′or hăl-oo′sĭs lŏng′ŭs). ACTION: Flexes phalanges, primarily the distal phalanges, and plantar flexes the foot. ORIGIN: Lower portion of shaft of fibula. INSERTION: Distal phalanx of great toe. INNERVATION: Posterior tibial.

gastrocnemius (găs″trŏk-nē′mē-ŭs). ACTION: Plantar flexes foot and flexes knee. ORIGIN: External and internal femoral condyles. INSERTION: By tendo calcaneus into os calcis. INNERVATION: Branches of tibial.

peroneus brevis (pĕr-ō-nē′ŭs brĕ′vĭs). ACTION: Extends and abducts foot. ORIGIN: Midportion of shaft of fibula. INSERTION: Base of 5th metatarsal bone. INNERVATION: Branch of peroneal.

peroneus longus (pĕr-ō-nē′ŭs lŏng′ŭs). ACTION: Extends, abducts, and everts foot. ORIGIN: Upper fibula and external condyle of tibia. INSERTION: By tendon to internal cuneiform and 1st metatarsal bone. INNERVATION: Branch of peroneal.

peroneus tertius (pĕr-ō-nē′ŭs tĕr′shē-ŭs). ACTION: Flexes foot. ORIGIN: Lower part of fibula. INSERTION: Fifth metatarsal bone. INNERVATION: Branch of peroneal.

plantaris (plăn-tăr′ĭs). ACTION: Extends foot. ORIGIN: External supracondyloid ridge of femur. INSERTION: Inner border of tendo calcaneus. INNERVATION: Branch of tibial.

popliteus (pŏp-lĭt′ē-ŭs, -lĭt-ē′ŭs). ACTION: Flexes leg and rotates it inward. ORIGIN: External condyle of femur. INSERTION: Posterior surface of tibia. INNERVATION: Branch of tibial.

soleus (sō′lē-ŭs). ACTION: Plantar flexes foot. ORIGIN: Upper shaft of fibula, oblique line of tibia. INSERTION: By tendo calcaneus to os calcis. INNERVATION: Tibial.

tibialis anterior (tĭb″ē-ā′lĭs ăn-tē′rĭ-or). ACTION: Dorsiflexes foot and increases the arch in the takeoff of walking. ORIGIN: Upper tibia, interosseus membrane, and intermuscular septum. INSERTION: Internal cuneiform and 1st metatarsal. INNERVATION: Branch of peroneal.

tibialis posterior (tĭb″ē-ā′lĭs pŏs-tē′rē-or). ACTION: Plantar flexes foot. ORIGIN: Shaft of fibula and tibia. INSERTION: Tuberosity of scaphoid, 2nd to 4th metatarsal, internal cuneiform. INNERVATION: Branch of tibial.

FOOT

abductor digiti minimi pedis (ăb-dŭk′tor dĭj-ĭ-tī mĭn′ĭ-mī pē′dĭs). ACTION: Abducts little toe. ORIGIN: Outer tuberosity of calcaneus, plantar fascia, and intermuscular septum. INSERTION: External side of 1st phalanx of little toe. INNERVATION: Lateral plantar.

abductor hallucis (ăb-dŭk′tor hăl-oo′sĭs). ACTION: Abducts great toe. ORIGIN: Inner tuberosity of os calcis, plantar fascia. INSERTION: Inner side, 1st phalanx of great toe. IN-

NERVATION: Medial plantar.

adductor hallucis (ăd-dŭk′tor hăl-oo′sĭs). ACTION: Adducts great toe. ORIGIN: Tarsal terminations of the three middle metatarsal bones. INSERTION: Lateral side of base of 1st phalanx of great toe. INNERVATION: Branch of lateral plantar.

extensor digitorum brevis (ĕks-tĕn′sŏr dĭj-ĭ-tō′rŭm brĕ′vĭs). ACTION: Extends toes. ORIGIN: Dorsal surface of os calcis. INSERTION: To 1st phalanx of great toe and the tendons of extensor digitorum longus. INNERVATION: Branch of peroneal.

flexor accessorius (flĕks′or ăk-sĕ-sō′rē-ŭs). SAME AS: *quadratus plantae*

flexor digiti quinti brevis pedis (flĕks′or dĭj-ĭ-tī kwĭn′tī brĕ′vĭs pē′dĭs). ACTION: Flexes the little toe. ORIGIN: Base of metatarsal of little toe and sheath of peroneus longus. INSERTION: Outer side of base of 1st phalanx of little toe. INNERVATION: External plantar.

flexor digitorum brevis (flĕks′or dĭj-ĭ-tō′rŭm brĕ′vĭs). ACTION: Flexes toe. ORIGIN: Os calcis and plantar fascia. INSERTION: Second phalanges of lesser toes. INNERVATION: Internal plantar.

flexor hallucis brevis (flĕks′or hăl-oo′sĭs brĕ′vĭs). ACTION: Flexes great toe. ORIGIN: Internal surface of cuboid and middle and external cuneiform bones. INSERTION: Sides of base of 1st phalanx of great toe. INNERVATION: Internal and external plantar.

interossei dorsales pedis (ĭn″tĕr-ŏs′ē-ī dōr-sā′lēz pē′dĭs). Four. ACTION: Adducts 2nd toe, abducts 2nd, 3rd, and 4th toes. ORIGIN: Shafts of adjacent metatarsal bones. INSERTION: First phalanges of lesser toes. INNERVATION: External plantar.

interossei plantares (ĭn″tĕr-ŏs′ē-ī plăn-tăr′ĭs). Three. ACTION: Adducts three outer toes. ORIGIN: 3rd, 4th, and 5th metatarsals. INSERTION: First phalanx of corresponding toe. INNERVATION: External plantar.

lumbricales plantar (lŭm-brĭ-kā′lēz plăn′tăr). Four. ACTION: Flexes 1st and extends 2nd and 3rd phalanges. ORIGIN: Tendons of flexor digitorum longus. INSERTION: First phalanx and extensor tendon. INNERVATION: External and internal plantar.

quadratus plantae (kwăd-rā′tŭs plăn′tē). ACTION: Assists flexion of toes. ORIGIN: Inferior surface of os calcis by two heads from outer and inner borders. INSERTION: Tendons of flexor digitorum longus. INNERVATION: Branch of lateral plantar.

GENERAL

arrectores pilorum (ă″rĕk-tō′rĕz pĭl-ō′rŭm). ACTION: Elevates hairs of skin. ORIGIN: Papillary layer of skin. INSERTION: Hair follicles. INNERVATION: Sympathetic.

Principal Joints

Name	Type	Ligaments
Acromioclavicular	Arthrodial	Capsular; superior and inferior acromioclavicular; articular disk; coracoclavicular (trapezoid and conoid)
Ankle	Ginglymus (hinge)	Capsular; deltoid; anterior and posterior talofibular; calcaneofibular
Atlas	Trochoid (pivot); arthrodial	Capsular; anterior and posterior atlantoaxial; transverse
Calcaneocuboid	Arthrodial	Capsular; dorsal calcaneocuboid; bifurcated; long plantar; plantar calcaneocuboid
Carpometacarpal	Arthrodial	Dorsal; volar; interosseous
Elbow	Ginglymus (hinge)	Capsular; ulnar and radial collateral
Hip	Enarthrodial	Capsular; iliofemoral; pubocapsular; ischiofemoral; round ligament of femur; transverse acetabular
Intercarpal Carpal, proximal Carpal, distal Carpal bones, two rows with each other	 Arthrodial Arthrodial 	 Dorsal; volar; interosseous Dorsal; volar; interosseous Volar; dorsal; collateral
Intermetacarpal		Dorsal; volar; interosseous; transverse metacarpal
Intermetatarsal	Arthrodial	Dorsal; plantar; interosseous
Interphalangeal	Ginglymus (hinge)	Collateral; volar in fingers and plantar in toes
Knee	Condyloid and arthrodial	Capsular; patellar; oblique and arcuate popliteal; tibial and fibular collateral; anterior and posterior cruciate; medial and lateral menisci; transverse; coronary
Mandible (Jaw)	Ginglymus (hinge); arthrodial	Capsular; temporomandibular; sphenomandibular; articular disk; stylomandibular
Metacarpophalangeal	Condyloid	Volar; collateral
Metatarsophalangeal	Condyloid	Plantar; collateral
Pubic	Amphiarthrodial	Superior and arcuate pubic; interpubic fibrocartilaginous layer
Radioulnar, distal	Trochoid (pivot)	Ulnar collateral; articular disk

Principal Joints *(Continued)*

Name	Type	Ligaments
Radioulnar, middle	Trochoid (pivot)	Oblique; interosseous
Radioulnar, proximal	Trochoid (pivot)	Annular
Ribs, heads of	Arthrodial	Capsular; radiate; intra-articular
Ribs, tubercles and necks of	Arthrodial	Capsular; anterior and posterior costotransverse; neck of rib; tubercle of rib
Sacrococcygeal	Amphiarthrodial	Anterior, posterior, and lateral sacrococcygeal; interposed fibrocartilaginous; interarticular
Sacroiliac		Anterior and posterior sacroiliac; interosseous
Sacrum and ischium		Sacrotuberous; sacrospinous
Shoulder	Enarthrodial (ball-and-socket)	Capsular; coracohumeral; glenohumeral; transverse humeral; glenoid of humerus
Sternoclavicular	Double arthrodial	Capsular; anterior and posterior sternoclavicular; inter- and costoclavicular; articular disk
Sternocostal	Arthrodial	Capsular; radiate and intra-articular sternocostal; costoxiphoid
Subtalar	Arthrodial	Capsular; anterior, posterior, lateral, medial, and interosseous; talocalcaneal
Talocalcaneonavicular	Arthrodial	Capsular; dorsal talonavicular
Tarsometatarsal	Arthrodial	Dorsal; plantar; interosseous
Tibiofibular	Arthrodial	Capsular; anterior; posterior
Tibiofibular syndesmosis	Arthrodial	Anterior and posterior tibiofibular; inferior transverse; interosseous
Vertebral arches	Arthrodial	Capsular; flaval; supraspinal; nuchal; interspinal; intertransverse
Vertebral bodies	Amphiarthrodial	Anterior and posterior longitudinal; intervertebral fibrocartilaginous
Vertebral column with cranium	Condyloid	Capsular; anterior and posterior atlanto-occipital membrane; lateral; tectorial membrane; alar; apical odontoid
Wrist	Condyloid	Volar and dorsal radiocarpal; ulnar and radial collateral

Nerves

Name	NA Term*	Origin	Function	Distribution
Abducent (6th cranial n.)	N. abducens	Pons	Motor	Lateral rectus muscle of eye.
Accessory (11th cranial n.)	N. accessorius	Medulla oblongata and spinal cord	Motor	Sternomastoid and trapezius muscles.
Auditory (8th cranial n.)	N. vestibulocochlearis	Cochlea	Special sense of hearing	Internal auditory meatus.
Auricular, great	N. auricularis magnus	Second and third cervical through cervical plexus	Sensory	Side of neck; skin of ear and cheek.
Auricular, posterior	N. auricularis posterior	Facial	Motor	Posterior auricular muscle.
Auriculotemporal	N. auriculotemporalis	Mandibular div. of trigeminal	Sensory	Side of scalp.
Buccal	N. buccalis	Mandibular div. of trigeminal	Sensory	Skin and mucous membrane of cheek.
Cervical n., superficial (cutaneous cervical n.; transverse n. of neck)	N. transversus colli	Second and third cervical through cervical plexus	Sensory	Skin of front of neck.
Chorda tympani		Facial	Motor	Sublingual and submaxillary glands.
Ciliary, long	Nn. ciliares longi	Nasal	Sensory and motor	Cornea, iris, and ciliary body.
Ciliary, short	Nn. ciliares breves	Ciliary ganglion	Sensory and motor	Cornea, iris, and ciliary body.
Circumflex (Axillary)	N. axillaris	Posterior cord of brachial plexus	Motor and sensory	Deltoid, teres minor, shoulder joint, and overlying skin.
Coccygeal	N. coccygeus	Spinal cord	Motor and sensory	Coccygeus muscle and skin over coccyx.
Cochlear. SEE: *Vestibulocochlear n.*		Auditory	Special sense of hearing	Cochlea.
Cutaneous, medial	N. cutaneus antebrachii medialis	Inner cord of brachial plexus	Sensory	Skin of inner aspect of forearm.
Cutaneous, lesser medial	N. cutaneus brachii medialis	Inner cord of brachial plexus	Sensory	Skin of inner aspect of upper arm.

		Mandibular div. of trigeminal	Sensory and motor	Teeth of lower jaw, mylohyoid muscle, and skin of chin.
Dental, inferior	N. alveolaris inferior	Mandibular div. of trigeminal	Sensory and motor	Teeth of lower jaw, mylohyoid muscle, and skin of chin.
Dental, superior	Nn. alveolares superiores	Maxillary div. of trigeminal	Sensory	Upper teeth and gums.
Digastric		Facial	Motor	Stylohyoid and posterior belly of digastric muscle.
Facial (7th cranial n.)	N. facialis	Pons	Motor	Muscles of expression.
Femoral (anterior crural n.)	N. femoralis	2nd, 3rd, and 4th lumbar	Motor and sensory	Muscles and skin of thigh.
Frontal	N. frontalis	Ophthalmic div. of trigeminal	Sensory	Skin of forehead.
Genitofemoral (genitocrural n.)	N. genitofemoralis	1st and 2nd lumbar	Sensory and motor	Cremaster muscle and skin of groin and upper part of thigh.
Glossopharyngeal (9th cranial n.)	N. glossopharyngeus	Medulla oblongata	Motor and sensory	Muscles and mucous membrane of pharynx, fauces, and posterior third of tongue.
Gluteal, inferior	N. gluteus inferior	5th lumbar and 1st and 2nd sacral	Motor	Gluteus maximus.
Gluteal, superior	N. gluteus superior	4th and 5th lumbar and 1st sacral	Motor	Gluteus medius and minimus, tensor fasciae femoris.
Hypogastric	N. hypogastricus	Iliohypogastric	Motor and sensory	Muscles and skin of abdominal wall.
Hypoglossal (12th cranial n.)	N. hypoglossus	Hypoglossal nucleus in medulla oblongata	Motor	Intrinsic muscles of tongue.
Iliohypogastric	N. iliohypogastricus	1st lumbar	Sensory and motor	Muscles and skin of hypogastrium.
Ilioinguinal	N. ilioinguinalis	1st lumbar	Sensory and motor	Muscles of abdominal wall, skin of upper thigh, skin of root of penis and scrotum (in male), and skin of mons pubis and labium majus (in female).

* Nomina Anatomica

Nerves (Continued)

Name	NA Term*	Origin	Function	Distribution
Infraorbital	N. infraorbitalis	Maxillary div. of trigeminal	Sensory	Skin of cheek and all upper teeth except molars.
Infratrochlear	N. infratrochlearis	Nasociliary	Sensory	Skin of lower eyelid and root of nose, conjunctiva, and lacrimal sac and caruncle.
Intercostal	Nn. intercostales	Thoracic	Sensory and motor	Muscles and skin of back, thorax, and upper abdomen.
Intercostobrachial	Nn. intercostobrachiales	2nd intercostal	Sensory	Skin of axilla and medial side of arm.
Interosseous anterior (volar interosseous n.)	N. interosseus anterior	Median	Motor	Deep flexor and pronator muscles of forearm.
Interosseous, posterior	N. interosseus posterior	Musculospiral (radial)	Motor and sensory	Muscles and skin of back of forearm and wrist.
Lacrimal	N. lacrimalis	Ophthalmic div. of trigeminal	Sensory	Lacrimal gland, conjunctiva, and skin of upper eyelid.
Laryngeal, inferior	N. laryngeus inferior	Branch of recurrent laryngeal	Motor	Muscles of larynx except cricothyroid.
Laryngeal, recurrent	N. laryngeus recurrens	Vagus	Motor	Muscles of larynx except cricothyroid.
Laryngeal, superior	N. laryngeus superior	Vagus	Motor and sensory	Mucous membrane of larynx; arytenoid and cricothyroid muscles.
Lingual	N. lingualis	Mandibular div. of trigeminal	Sensory	Mucous membrane of anterior two-thirds of tongue and floor and outer wall of mouth.
Lumbar	Nn. lumbales	Spinal cord	Motor and sensory	Loins and front of lower abdomen and thigh to help in forming lumbar and sacral plexuses.

Mandibular	N. mandibularis	Trigeminal	Motor and sensory	Teeth, gums, and skin of lower jaw and cheek; muscles of mastication; mucous membrane of anterior two-thirds of tongue.
Masseteric	N. massetericus	Mandibular div. of trigeminal	Motor	Masseter muscle.
Maxillary	N. maxillaris	Trigeminal	Sensory	Nasal pharynx, palate, teeth of upper jaw and skin of cheek.
Median	N. medianus	Internal and external cords of brachial plexus	Motor and sensory	Pronators and flexors of forearm, two external lumbricales, thenar muscles, skin of palm and first four fingers.
Mental	N. mentalis	Inferior dental	Sensory	Skin and mucous membrane of lower lip and chin.
Musculocutaneous	N. musculocutaneous	External cord of brachial plexus	Motor and sensory	Flexors of upper arm and skin of external aspect of forearm.
Mylohyoid	N. mylohyoideus	Inferior dental	Motor	Mylohyoid muscle and anterior belly of digastric muscle.
Nasal (nasociliary n.)	N. nasociliaris	Ophthalmic div. of trigeminal	Sensory	Ciliary ganglion, iris, conjunctiva, ethmoid cells, mucous membrane and skin of nose.
Nasopalatine	N. nasopalatinus	Meckel's ganglion (sphenopalatine ganglion)	Sensory	Mucous membrane of nose and palate.
Obturator	N. obturatorius	2nd, 3rd, and 4th lumbar through lumbar plexus	Motor and sensory	Adductors of thigh, hip, and knee joints; skin of inner aspect of thigh.
Occipital, greater	N. occipitalis major	2nd cervical	Motor and sensory	Muscles of back of neck; skin over occiput.
Occipital, lesser	N. occipitalis minor	2nd and 3rd cervical	Sensory	Skin behind ear and on back of scalp.

* Nomina Anatomica

Nerves (Continued)

Name	NA Term*	Origin	Function	Distribution
Occipital, third	N. occipitalis tertius	3rd cervical	Sensory	Skin of back of head and nape of neck
Oculomotor (3rd cranial n.)	N. oculomotorius	Floor of aqueduct of Sylvius	Motor	All ocular muscles except lateral rectus and superior oblique.
Olfactory (1st cranial n.)	Nn. olfactorii	Olfactory lobe	Special sense of smell	Nasal mucous membranes in olfactory region.
Ophthalmic	N. ophthalmicus	1st div. of trigeminal	Sensory	Lacrimal gland, conjunctiva, skin of forehead, skin and mucous membrane of nose.
Optic (2nd cranial n.)	N. opticus	Corpora quadrigemina	Special sense of sight	Retina.
Palatine, anterior, middle, and posterior	Nn. palatini	Meckel's ganglion	Motor	Mucous membrane of palate.
Perineal	N. perineales	Pudendal	Motor and sensory	Muscles and skin of perineum.
Peroneal, common (lateral popliteal n.)	N. peroneus communis	Sciatic	Motor and sensory	Extensor muscles of lower leg and foot and overlying skin.
Phrenic	N. phrenicus	3rd, 4th, and 5th cervical	Motor and sensory	Diaphragm.
Pneumogastric. SEE: *Vagus n.*				
Popliteal, lateral. SEE: *Peroneal n., common.*				
Pterygoid	N. pterygoideus	Mandibular div. of trigeminal	Motor	Lateral and medial pterygoid muscles.
Pterygoid canal, n. of. SEE: *Vidian n.*				
Pudendal	N. pudendus	2nd, 3rd, and 4th sacral	Sensory	Skin and muscles of perineum and genitalia.

Radial (musculospiral n.)	N. radialis	Brachial plexus	Motor and sensory	Skin of back of entire arm and hand; extensor muscles of entire arm and hand.
Sacral	Nn. sacrales	Spinal cord	Motor and sensory	Muscles and skin of loins and lower extremities.
Saphenous, external or short. SEE: *Sural n.*				
Saphenous, internal or long	N. saphenus	Femoral	Sensory	Skin of inner aspect of knee, leg, ankle, and dorsum of foot.
Sciatic (great sciatic n.)	N. ischiadicus	Sacral plexus	Motor and sensory	Muscles of calf and back of thigh; skin of lower calf and upper surface of foot.
Sphenopalatine	N. pterygopalatini	Maxillary div. of trigeminal	Sensory	Meckel's ganglion.
Spinal accessory (accessory n.; 11th cranial n.)	N. accessorius	Floor of 4th ventricle and cervical cord	Motor	Sternomastoid and trapezius muscles.
Stapedial	N. stapedius	Facial	Motor	Stapedius muscle.
Stylohyoid	N. stylohyoid	Facial	Motor	Stylohyoid muscle.
Suboccipital	N. suboccipitalis	Posterior div. of 1st cervical	Motor	Complexus oblique and rectus muscles of back of neck.
Subscapular	N. subscapularis	Posterior cord of brachial plexus	Motor	Teres major and subscapularis muscles.
Supraclavicular, intermediate (supraclavicular n., middle; supraclavicular n.)	Nn. supraclaviculares intermedii	3rd and 4th cervical	Sensory	Skin of fossa below collarbone.
Supraclavicular, lateral (supraclavicular n., posterior; supra-acromial n.)	Nn. supraclaviculares laterales	3rd and 4th cervical	Sensory	Skin of shoulder.
Supraclavicular, medial (supraclavicular n., anterior; suprasternal n.)	Nn. supraclaviculares mediales	3rd and 4th cervical	Sensory	Skin over upper part of thorax.

* *Nomina Anatomica*

Nerves (Continued)

Name	NA Term*	Origin	Function	Distribution
Supraorbital	N. supraorbitalis	Frontal	Sensory	Forehead, upper eyelid, scalp, and frontal sinus.
Suprascapular	N. suprascapularis	5th and 6th cervical	Motor	Supraspinatus and infraspinatus muscles and the shoulder joint.
Supratrochlear	N. supratrochlearis	Frontal	Sensory	Skin of upper eyelid and root of nose.
Sural	N. suralis	Common peroneal and tibial n.'s	Sensory	Skin of calf and medial side of foot to great toe.
Temporal, deep	Nn. temporales profundi	Mandibular div. of trigeminal	Motor	Temporal muscle.
Thoracic	Nn. thoracici	Spinal cord	Motor and sensory	Muscles and skin of thorax.
Thoracic, anterior		Brachial plexus	Motor	Pectoralis minor and major muscles.
Thoracic, long (posterior thoracic n.; external respiratory n. of Bell).	N. thoracicus longus	5th, 6th, and 7th cervical	Motor	Serratus anterior muscle.
Tibial	N. tibialis	Sciatic	Motor and sensory	Flexor muscles of back of knee joint and calf; skin of lower leg.
Trigeminal (5th cranial n.; trifacial n.)	N. trigeminus	Midbrain and pons	Motor and sensory	Skin of face, tongue, teeth; muscles of mastication.
Trochlear (4th cranial n.; pathetic n.)	N. trochlearis	Floor of aqueduct of Sylvius	Motor	Superior oblique muscle of eye.
Tympanic (Jacobson's n.)	N. tympanicus	Glossopharyngeal	Sensory	Tympanum, eustachian tube, and structures of middle ear.
Ulnar	N. ulnaris	Medial cord of brachial plexus	Motor and sensory	Muscles and skin of forearm and hand.

Vagus (10th cranial n.; pneumogastric n.)	N. vagus	Medulla oblongata	Motor and sensory	Pharynx, larynx, heart, lungs, stomach.
Vestibulocochlear (8th cranial n.; acoustic n.; auditory n.)	N. vestibulocochlearis	Ganglion of Scarpa and ganglion of Corti	Sense of hearing	Internal auditory meatus.
Vidian	N. canalis pterygoidei	Facial	Sensory	Meckel's ganglion (sphenopalatine ganglion).
Zygomatic	N. zygomaticus	Maxillary div. of trigeminal	Sensory	Skin of temple and cheekbone.
*Nomina Anatomica				

aortic (ā-or′tĭk). *(Abdominal).* ORIGIN: Semilunar, lumbar ganglia, renal and solar plexuses. LOCATION: Sides and front of aorta. DISTRIBUTION: Inferior mesenteric, spermatic and hypogastric plexus. Filaments to inferior vena cava. *(Thoracic).* ORIGIN: Thoracic ganglia of sympathetic nerve, cardiac plexus. LOCATION: Surrounding the thoracic aorta. DISTRIBUTION: Solar plexus, aorta.

brachial (brā′kē-ăl). ORIGIN: Anterior branches of 5th, 6th, 7th, 8th cervical and greater part of 1st dorsal nerves. LOCATION: Lower part of neck to axilla. DISTRIBUTION: Sixteen branches of suprascapular, subscapular, rhomboid, median, ulnar, musculospiral, posterior thoracic, musculothoracic, circumflex, musculocutaneous nerves.

cardiac (kär′dē-ăk). *(Great or Deep).* ORIGIN: Cardiac nerves of cervical ganglion of sympathetic and vagus. LOCATION: In front of bifurcation of trachea. DISTRIBUTION: Pulmonary, coronary and cardiac plexuses. *(Superficial or Anterior).* ORIGIN: Left superior cardiac nerve, branch of vagus and filaments of deep cardiac plexus. LOCATION: Beneath arch of aorta. Front of right pulmonary artery. DISTRIBUTION: Coronary and pulmonary plexuses.

carotid (kă-rŏt′ĭd). *(External).* ORIGIN: Pharyngeal plexus, superior cardiac nerve, and superior cervical ganglion. LOCATION: Around external carotid artery. DISTRIBUTION: External carotid artery and its branches. *(Internal).* ORIGIN: Postganglionic sympathetic fibers. LOCATION: Surrounding internal carotid artery. DISTRIBUTION: Tympanic plexus, sphenopalatine ganglion, abducens and oculomotor nerves, the cerebral vessels, and the ciliary ganglion.

cavernous (kăv′ĕr-nŭs). ORIGIN: 3rd to 6th cranial nerves and ophthalmic ganglion. LOCATION: Cavernous sinus. DISTRIBUTION: Wall of internal carotid artery.

celiac (sē′lē-ăk). ORIGIN: Solar plexus, branches from lesser splanchnic and vagus nerves. LOCATION: Behind stomach, in front of aorta at level of origin of celiac artery. DISTRIBUTION: Coronary, hepatic, pyloric, gastroduodenal, gastroepiploic and splenic plexuses. SYN: *solar plexus.*

cervical (ser′vĭ-kăl). ORIGIN: Anterior branches of first four cervical nerves. LOCATION: Beneath sternocleidomastoid muscle opposite first four cervical vertebrae. DISTRIBUTION: Cutaneous, muscular, and communicating rami.

coccygeal (kŏk-sĭj′ē-ăl). ORIGIN: Fourth and 5th sacral and the coccygeal nerves. LOCATION: Dorsal surface of coccyx and caudal end of sacrum. DISTRIBUTION: Anococcygeal nerves.

cystic (sĭs′tĭk). ORIGIN: Hepatic plexus. LOCATION: At gallbladder. DISTRIBUTION: Gallbladder.

esophageal (ē-sŏf″ă-jē′ăl). ORIGIN: Vagus nerve, thoracic sympathetic ganglia. LOCATION: Around the esophagus. DISTRIBUTION: Esophagus.

gastric (găs′trĭk). ORIGIN: Celiac plexus and continuations of esophageal plexuses. LOCATION: Gastric artery. DISTRIBUTION: Stomach.

hemorrhoidal (hĕm-ō-roy′dăl). ORIGIN: Pelvic and inferior mesenteric plexuses. LOCATION: Rectum and sides of rectum. DISTRIBUTION: Rectum.

hepatic (hē-păt′ĭk). ORIGIN: Celiac plexus, left vagus, right phrenic. LOCATION: Accompanies hepatic artery. DISTRIBUTION: Liver.

hypogastric (hī″pō-găs′trĭk). ORIGIN: Aortic plexus and lumbar ganglia. LOCATION: Promontory of sacrum. DISTRIBUTION: Pelvic plexus.

lumbar (lŭm′băr). ORIGIN: First four lumbar nerves. LOCATION: Psoas muscle. DISTRIBUTION: Iliohypogastric, ilioinguinal, genitocrural, external cutaneous, obturator, accessory, and anterior crural nerves.

Meissner's (mīs′nĕrz). ORIGIN: Superior mesenteric plexus (controls secretions of the bowels). LOCATION: Submucous coat of small intestines. DISTRIBUTION: Intestinal walls.

mesenteric (mĕs″ĕn-tĕr′ĭk). ORIGIN: Celiac plexus and left side of aortic plexus. LOCATION: Surrounding the inferior and superior mesenteric arteries. DISTRIBUTION: Descending colon, sigmoid, rectum, intestines.

myenteric (mī″ĕn-tĕr′ĭk). ORIGIN: Sympathetic system (controls peristalsis). LOCATION: Between the circular and longitudinal coats of small intestines. DISTRIBUTION: Intestinal walls.

ophthalmic (ŏf-thăl′mĭk). ORIGIN: Internal carotid plexus. LOCATION: Around ophthalmic artery and optic nerve. DISTRIBUTION: Optic region.

pancreatic (păn″krē-ăt′ĭk). ORIGIN: Splenic plexus. LOCATION: Near pancreas. DISTRIBUTION: Filaments to pancreas.

pancreaticoduodenal (păn″krē-ăt″ĭ-kō-dū-ō-dē′năl). ORIGIN: Hepatic plexus. LOCATION: Near head of pancreas. DISTRIBUTION: Filaments to pancreas and duodenum.

pelvic (pĕl′vĭk). ORIGIN: Hypogastric plexus, 2nd to 4th sacral nerves, 1st and 2nd sacral ganglia (pelvic brain). LOCATION: Side of rectum and bladder. DISTRIBUTION: Viscera of pelvis, pelvic plexus.

phrenic (frĕn′ĭk). ORIGIN: Solar plexus, semilunar ganglia. LOCATION: Accompanies phrenic artery to diaphragm. DISTRIBUTION: Diaphragm and suprarenal capsules.

prostatic (prŏs-tăt′ĭk). ORIGIN: Hypogastric plexus. LOCATION: Vesical arteries. DISTRIBUTION: Bladder.

pulmonary (pŭl′mō-nĕ-rē). ORIGIN: Anterior and posterior pulmonary branches of vagus and sympathetic nerves. LOCATION: Root of lungs, front and back. DISTRIBUTION: Root of lungs.

pyloric (pī-lor′ĭk). ORIGIN: Hepatic plexus. LOCATION: Near pylorus. DISTRIBUTION: Filaments to pylorus.

renal (rē′năl). ORIGIN: Solar and aortic plexuses and semilunar ganglia. LOCATION: Renal artery. DISTRIBUTION: Kidneys, posterior vena cava, spermatic plexus.

sacral (sā′krăl). ORIGIN: Anterior branch of 4th and 5th lumbar and 1st, 2nd, 3rd, and 4th sacral nerves. LOCATION: Front of sacrum on piriformis muscle. DISTRIBUTION: Muscular, pudic, superior gluteal, great and small sciatic nerves.

solar (sō′lăr). *(Epigastric).* ORIGIN: Splanchnics and right vagus. LOCATION: Back of stomach. DISTRIBUTION: Semilunar ganglia, phrenic, suprarenal, renal, spermatic, celiac, superior mesenteric, and aortic plexuses. Called *abdominal brain.* SYN: *celiac plexus.*

spermatic (spĕr-măt′ĭk). *(Ovarian).* ORIGIN: Aortic plexus. LOCATION: Accompanies spermatic vessels to testes or ovaries. DISTRIBUTION: Testes or ovaries.

splenic (splĕn′ĭk). ORIGIN: Celiac plexus, left semilunar ganglion, right vagus nerve. LOCATION: Accompanies splenic artery. DISTRIBUTION: Spleen, pancreatic plexus, left gastroepiploic plexus.

suprarenal (soo″prä-rē′năl). ORIGIN: Diaphragmatic, solar, and renal plexuses. LOCATION: Around suprarenal capsules. DISTRIBUTION: Filaments to medulla of suprarenal capsules.

thyroid (thī′royd). *(Inferior).* ORIGIN: Middle cervical ganglion. LOCATION: Around external carotid and inferior thyroid arteries. DISTRIBUTION: Larynx, pharynx, thyroid gland. *(Superior).* ORIGIN: Superior laryngeal and cardiac nerves. LOCATION: Around the thyroid gland. DISTRIBUTION: Thyroid region.

uterine (ū′tĕr-ĭn). ORIGIN: Pelvic plexus. LOCATION: Accompanies uterine arteries. DISTRIBUTION: Cervix and lower part of uterus.

vaginal (văj′ĭn-ăl). ORIGIN: Pelvic plexus. LOCATION: Vaginal walls. DISTRIBUTION: Vagina.

vertebral (vĕr′tĕ-brăl). ORIGIN: First part thoracic ganglion, upper cervical nerves. LOCATION: Surrounding basilar and vertebral arteries. DISTRIBUTION: Vertebral and cerebellar regions.

vesical (vĕs′ĭ-kăl). ORIGIN: Pelvic plexus. LOCATION: Accompanies vesical arteries. DISTRIBUTION: Vesicula seminalis, vas deferens.

Cranial Nerves

No.	Name	NA Term*	Origin	Function	Distribution
1st	Olfactory	Nn. olfactorii	Olfactory lobe	Smell	Nasal mucous membrane
2nd	Optic	N. opticus	Retina	Sight	Retina
3rd	Oculomotor	N. oculomotorius	Floor of aqueduct of Sylvius	Motor	All ocular muscles except lateral rectus and superior oblique
4th	Trochlear	N. trochlearis	Floor of aqueduct of Sylvius	Motor	Superior oblique muscle of eye
5th	Trigeminal	N. trigeminus	Midbrain and pons	Motor and chief sensory n. of face	Skin of face; tongue; teeth; muscles of mastication
6th	Abducent	N. abducens	Pons	Motor	Lateral rectus muscle of eye
7th	Facial	N. facialis	Pons	Motor	Muscles of expression
8th	Auditory	N. vestibulocochlearis	Brain	Hearing	Internal auditory meatus
9th	Glossopharyngeal	N. glossopharyngeus	Medulla oblongata	Motor and sensory	Sensation of pharynx and posterior third of tongue; paroid gland
10th	Vagus	N. vagus	Medulla oblongata	Motor and sensory	Pharynx; larynx; heart; lungs; esophagus; stomach; abdominal viscera
11th	Accessory	N. accessorius	Medulla oblongata and spinal cord	Motor	Sternomastoid and trapezius muscles
12th	Hypoglossal	N. hypoglossus	Medulla oblongata	Motor	Intrinsic muscles of tongue

Arteries

Name	NA*	Origin	Distribution	Branches
Alveolar, inferior	A. alveolaris inferior	Maxillary	Lower anterior skull	Dental; mylohyoid; mental
Angular	A. angularis	Terminal branch of external maxillary	Neck and face	
Aorta	SEE: *aorta* in vocabulary			

Arcuate (Metatarsal a.)	A. arcuata pedis	Dorsal a. of foot	Foot and toes	Deep plantar; dorsal metatarsal; dorsal digital
Auditory, internal	A. labyrinthi	Middle of basilar or anterior inferior cerebellar	Internal ear	
Auricular, deep	A. auricularis profunda	Maxillary	Skin of auditory canal, tympanic membrane, and temporomandibular joint	
Auricular, posterior	A. auricularis posterior	External carotid	Middle ear; mastoid cells; auricle; parotid gland	Stylomastoid; auricular; occipital
Axillary	A. axillaris	Subclavian	Forms brachial and seven branches	Superior; thoracic; thoracoacromial; lateral thoracic; subscapular; anterior and posterior humeral; thoracodorsal; brachial
Basilar	A. basilaris	Vertebral	Pons	Posterior cerebral; pontine; internal auditory; anterior inferior cerebellar; superior cerebellar
Brachial	A. brachialis	Axillary	Upper arm	Deep brachial; nutrient; superior and inferior collateral; muscular
Brachial, deep	A. profunda brachii	Brachial	Accompanies radial nerve	
Bronchial	Rr. bronchiales	Thoracic aorta	Bronchi; lower trachea; pulmonary vessels; pericardium; part of esophagus	Left and right bronchial
Buccal (Buccinator a.)	A. buccalis	Maxillary	Buccinator muscle; mucous membrane of mouth	
Capsular, middle SEE: *Suprarenal a., middle.*				
Carotid, common	A. carotis communis	Brachiocephalic trunk (right); aortic arch (left)	Neck and thyroid	External and internal carotid

* Nomina Anatomica

Arteries (Continued)

Name	NA*	Origin	Distribution	Branches
Carotid, external	A. carotis externa	Common carotid	Neck; face; skull	Superior thyroid; ascending pharyngeal; lingual; facial; occipital; posterior auricular; superficial temporal; maxillary
Carotid, internal	A. carotis interna	Common carotid	Anterior brain; eyes; forehead; nose	Caroticotympanic; vidian; cavernous; hypophyseal; semilunar; anterior meningeal; ophthalmic; anterior and middle cerebral; posterior communicating; choroidal
Celiac	Truncus celiacus	Abdominal aorta	Stomach; liver; pancreas; duodenum; spleen	Left gastric; common hepatic; splenic
Cerebellar, anterior inferior	A. cerebelli inferior anterior	Basilar	Anterior undersurface of cerebellum	
Cerebellar, posterior inferior	A. cerebelli inferior posterior	Vertebral	Cerebellum	
Cerebellar, superior	A. cerebelli superior	Near termination of basilar	Upper cerebellum; midbrain; pineal body	
Cerebral, anterior	A. cerebri anterior	Internal carotid	Cerebrum	Cortical; central; anterior communicating
Cerebral, posterior	A. cerebri posterior	Basilar	Cerebrum	Central; posterior choroidal; cortical temporal; calcarine; parieto-occipital
Cervical, ascending	A. cervicalis ascendens	Inferior thyroid	Muscles of neck and spinal cord	
Cervical, superficial		Thyroid axis	Muscles of shoulder	
Cervical, transverse	A. transversa colli	Thyroid axis	Muscles and glands of neck	Deep and superficial rami
Choroidal, anterior (Choroid)	A. choroidea anterior	Internal carotid	Internal capsule	

	Aa. ciliares anteriores[*]	Ophthalmic and lacrimal	Iris; conjunctiva	
Ciliary, anterior	Aa. ciliares anteriores	Ophthalmic and lacrimal	Iris; conjunctiva	
Ciliary, long posterior	Aa. ciliares posteriores longae	Ophthalmic	Iris and ciliary process	
Ciliary, short posterior	Aa. ciliares posteriores breves	Ophthalmic	Choroid coat of eye	
Circumflex, anterior humeral	A. circumflexa humeri anterior	Lateral side of axillary	Shoulder joint and upper arm	
Circumflex, posterior humeral	A. circumflexa humeri posterior	Axillary	Deltoid and shoulder joint; upper arm	
Colic, left	A. colica sinistra	Inferior mesenteric	Descending and transverse colon	Ascending and descending colic
Colic, middle	A. colica media	Superior mesenteric	Transverse colon	Right and left colic
Colic, right	A. colica dextra	Superior mesenteric	Ascending colon	Ascending and descending colic
Collateral, inferior ulnar	A. collateralis ulnaris inferior	Brachial	Muscles at back of elbow	
Collateral, superior ulnar	A. collateralis ulnaris superior	Brachial	Elbow joint and triceps muscles	
Communicating, posterior	A. communicans posterior	Internal carotid	Hippocampus; thalamus	
Coronary, left	A. coronaria sinistra	Ascending aorta	Left ventricle and atrium	Anterior descending coronary; circumflex
Coronary, right	A. coronaria dextra	Ascending aorta	Right ventricle and atrium	Posterior descending; marginal
Cystic	A. cystica	Proper hepatic	Gallbladder; liver	
Digital, common palmar	Aa. digitales palmares communes	Palmar arch	Fingers	Proper palmar digital
Digital, proper palmar (collateral digital a.)	Aa. digitales palmares propriae	Common palmar digital	Fingers	
Dorsal, of foot	A. dorsalis pedis	Continuation of anterior tibial	Foot	Lateral and medial tarsal; deep plantar; arcuate; first dorsal metatarsal
Epigastric, inferior	A. epigastrica inferior	External iliac	Abdominal muscles; peritoneum	Cremasteric
Epigastric, superficial	A. epigastrica superficialis	Femoral	Skin of abdomen; superficial fascia; inguinal lymph nodes	

* Nomina Anatomica

Arteries (Continued)

Name	NA*	Origin	Distribution	Branches
Epigastric, superior	A. epigastrica superior	Internal thoracic	Abdominal muscles and skin; diaphragm	
Esophageal		In front of aorta	Esophagus	
Ethmoidal, anterior	A. ethmoidalis anterior	Ophthalmic	Ethmoidal cells and frontal sinus; dura mater; nasal cavity	Anterior meningeal
Ethmoidal, posterior	A. ethmoidalis posterior	Ophthalmic	Ethmoidal cells; dura mater; nasal cavity	Posterior meningeal
Facial (External maxillary a.)	A. facialis	Carotid triangle	Face; tonsil; palate; submandibular gland	Ascending palatine; tonsillar; submental; inferior and superior labial; angular; glandular; lateral nasal; muscular
Facial, transverse	A. transversa faciei	Superficial temporal	Parotid gland; skin of face; masseter muscle	
Femoral	A. femoralis	Continuation of external iliac	Lower abdominal wall; external genitalia; lower extremity	Superficial epigastric; superficial circumflex iliac; external pudendal; deep femoral; descending genicular
Femoral, deep	A. profunda femoris	Femoral	Thigh muscles; hip joint; gluteal muscles; femur	Perforating; medial and lateral circumflex
Femoral, lateral circumflex	A. circumflexa femoris lateralis	Deep femoral a.	Hip joint; thigh muscles	Ascending; descending; transverse
Femoral, medial circumflex	A. circumflexa femoris medialis	Medial aspect of deep femoral a.	Hip joint; thigh muscles	Deep; acetabular; transverse; superficial
Fibular SEE: *Peroneal a.*				
Frontal	A. supratrochlearis	Ophthalmic	Forehead muscles; cranium	
Gastric, left	A. gastrica sinistra	Celiac trunk	Abdominal section of esophagus; stomach; left lobe of liver	Anterior and posterior gastric; cardioesophageal

Gastric, right	A. gastrica dextra	Common hepatic	Lesser curvature of stomach	
Gastric, short	Aa. gastricae breves	End of splenic	Greater curvature of stomach	
Gastroduodenal	A. gastroduodenalis	Common hepatic trunk	Stomach; duodenum; pancreas; greater omentum	Superior pancreaticoduodenal; right gastroepiploic; retroduodenal
Gastroepiploic, left	A. gastroepiploica sinistra	Splenic	Stomach; greater omentum	
Gastroepiploic, right	A. gastroepiploica dextra	Gastroduodenal	Stomach; greater omentum	Ascending pyloric and ascending branches to stomach.
Genicular, descending	A. genus descendens	Femoral	Knee joint; skin of upper and medial section of leg	Saphenous; musculo-articular
Genicular, inferior	A. genus inferior	Popliteal	Knee joint; skin of upper and middle leg	
Genicular, middle	A. genus media	Popliteal	Knee joint, ligaments and synovial membrane of knee	
Genicular, superior	A. genus superior	On either side of popliteal	Knee joint; femur; patella	
Gluteal, inferior (Sciatic a.)	A. glutea inferior	Internal iliac	Buttocks and back of thigh	Muscular; coccygeal; anastomotic; articular; cutaneous, comitans nervi; ishiadici
Gluteal, superior	A. glutea superior	Internal iliac	Gluteal region	Superficial and deep gluteal
Hemorrhoidal, middle	A. rectalis media	Internal iliac	Rectum; prostate; seminal vesicles	
Hemorrhoidal, superior	A. rectalis superior	Inferior mesenteric	Rectum	
Hepatic common	A. hepatica communis	Celiac trunk	Stomach; pancreas; duodenum; liver; gallbladder; greater omentum	Right gastric; gastroduodenal; proper hepatic
Hepatic, proper	A. hepatica propria	Common hepatic	Liver and gallbladder	Cystic

* Nomina Anatomica

Arteries (Continued)

Name	NA*	Origin	Distribution	Branches
Ileocolic	A. ileocolica	Superior mesenteric	Ileum; cecum; appendix; ascending colon	Superior and inferior ileocolic; appendicular
Iliac, common	A. iliaca communis	End of abdominal aorta	Pelvis; abdominal wall; lower limbs	External and internal iliac
Iliac, deep circumflex	A. circumflexa ilium profunda	External iliac	Muscles of skin and lower abdomen	
Iliac, external	A. iliaca externa	Common iliac	Abdominal wall; external genitalia; lower limb	Inferior epigastric; deep circumflex iliac
Iliac, internal	A. iliaca interna	Common iliac	Walls and viscera of pelvis, buttocks, reproductive organs; medial side of thighs	Superior, middle, and inferior vesical; middle hemorrhoidal; obturator; internal pudendal; inferior gluteal; uterine; vaginal; iliolumbar; lateral sacral; superior gluteal
Iliac, superficial circumflex	A. circumflexa ilium superficialis	Femoral	Inguinal glands; skin of thigh and abdomen	
Infraorbital	A. infraorbitalis	Maxillary	Maxillary sinus; center face	Anterior superior alveolar; orbital
Innominate	Truncus brachiocephalicus	Arch of aorta	Right side of head, neck, and arm	Right subclavian; right common carotid
Intercostal	Aa. intercostales posteriores	Thoracic aorta	Intercostal spaces; back muscles; vertebral column; thoracic wall	Anterior and posterior rami
Interosseous, anterior (Volar interosseous a.)	A. interossea anterior	Common interosseous	Deep structures of anterior forearm	Median; nutrient; muscular
Interosseous, common	A. interossea communis	Ulnar	Deep structure of forearm	Anterior and posterior interosseous
Interosseous, posterior	A. interossea posterior	Common interosseous	Muscles of posterior forearm	Recurrent interosseous
Intestinal		Superior mesenteric	Jejunum and ileum	

Labial, inferior	A. labialis inferior	Near angle of mouth	Lower lip
Labial, superior	A. labialis superior	Near angle of mouth	Upper lip
Lacrimal	A. lacrimalis	Ophthalmic	Lacrimal gland; eyelid; conjunctiva	Lateral palpebral; zygomatic; recurrent
Laryngeal, inferior	A. laryngea inferior	Inferior thyroid	Muscles and mucous membrane of trachea and larynx
Laryngeal, superior	A. laryngea superior	Superior thyroid	Muscles, mucous membrane, and glands of larynx
Lingual	A. lingualis	External carotid	Undersurface of tongue; tonsil; epiglottis	Suprahyoid; dorsal and deep lingual; sublingual
Lingual, deep	A. profunda linguae	End of lingual	Undersurface of tongue
Lingual, dorsal	Rr. dorsales linguae	Lingual	Mucous membrane on dorsum of tongue; glossopalatine arch; tonsil; soft palate; epiglottis
Lumbar	Aa. lumbales	Abdominal aorta	Abdominal wall; vertebrae; lumbar muscles; renal capsule	Posterior lumbar; muscular
Malleolar, lateral anterior	A. malleolaris anterior lateralis	Anterior tibial	Ankle joint
Malleolar, medial anterior	A. malleolaris anterior medialis	Anterior tibial	Ankle joint
Malleolar, medial posterior	Rr. malleolares mediales arteriae tibialis posterioris	Peroneal	Tibial malleolus
Masseteric	A. masseterica	Maxillary	Masseter muscle
Maxillary (Internal maxillary a.)	A. maxillaris	External carotid	Jaws and teeth; muscles of mastication; ear; meninges; nose; nasal sinus; palate	Anterior tympanic; deep auricular; middle and accessory meningeal; inferior and posterior superior alveolar; deep temporal; pterygoid; masseteric; buccal; infraorbital; greater palatine; pharyngeal; sphenopalatine

Nomina Anatomica

2255

Arteries (Continued)

Name	NA*	Origin	Distribution	Branches
Maxillary, external	SEE: *Facial a.*			
Mediastinal, anterior	Rr. mediastinales arteriae thoracicae internae	Internal thoracic	Anterior mediastinal cavity; portion of thymus	
Medullary (Bulbar a.)		Vertebral	Medulla oblongata	
Meningeal, middle	A. meningea media	Maxillary	Dura mater; cranial bones	Superficial; petrosal; superior tympanic; orbital; temporal; and numerous small vessels
Mesenteric, inferior	A. mesenterica inferior	Abdominal aorta	Left half of transverse colon; descending, iliac, and sigmoid colon; part of rectum	Left colic; sigmoid; superior hemorrhoidal
Mesenteric; superior	A. mesenterica superior	Abdominal aorta	Small intestine; cecum; ascending colon; part of transverse colon	Inferior pancreaticoduodenal; jejunal; ileal; ileocolic; right and middle colon
Metacarpal, palmar	Aa. metacarpales palmares	Deep palmar arch	Interosseous muscles and bones	
Metatarsal, first dorsal		Dorsal a. of foot	Medial border of foot	
Musculophrenic	A. musculophrenica	Internal thoracic	Diaphragm; abdominal and thoracic walls	
Nasal, dorsal	A. dorsalis nasi	Ophthalmic	Lacrimal sac; integuments of nose	Lacrimal
Obturator	A. obturatoria	Internal iliac	Pelvis and thigh	Iliac; vesical; pubic; anterior and posterior obturator
Occipital	A. occipitalis	Posterior part of external carotid	Muscles of neck and scalp; meninges; mastoid	Muscular; meningeal; sternomastoid; descending occipital; auricular
Ophthalmic	A. ophthalmica	Internal carotid	Eye and adjacent structures of face	Lacrimal; supraorbital; posterior and anterior ethmoidal; medial palpebral; frontal; dorsal nasal; central a. of retina; short posterior,

				long posterior, and anterior ciliary; muscular
Ovarian	A. ovarica	Abdominal aorta	Ovaries; uterine tubes; ureter	Ureteral
Palatine, ascending	A. palatina ascendens	Facial	Base of skull; palate; auditory tube	
Palatine, greater	A. palatina major	Maxillary	Palate and tonsils	Greater and lesser palatine
Palpebral, medial (Internal Palpebral a.)	Aa. palpebrales mediales	Ophthalmic	Upper and lower eyelids	Superior and inferior palpebral
Pancreaticoduodenal, inferior	Aa. pancreaticoduodenales inferiores	Superior mesenteric	Pancreas; duodenum	
Pancreaticoduodenal, superior	Aa. supraduodenales superiores	Gastroduodenal	Pancreas; duodenum	
Perforating	Aa. perforantes	Deep femoral	Back of thigh	
Pericardiacophrenic	A. pericardiacophrenica	Internal thoracic	Diaphragm; pericardium; pleura	
Peroneal	A. peronea	Posterior tibial	Ankle; deep calf muscles	Perforating; communicating; calcaneal; tibial and fibular nutrient; lateral and medial malleolar
Pharyngeal, ascending	A. pharyngea ascendens	Posterior part of external carotid	Pharynx; soft palate; ear; meninges; cranial nerves; capitis muscles	Pharyngeal; palatine; posterior meningeal; prevertebral; inferior tympanic
Phrenic	Aa. phrenicae inferiores and Aa. phrenicae superiores	Aorta, abdominal and thoracic	Diaphragm; adrenal glands	Medial, lateral, and superior adrenal
Plantar, deep	R. plantaris profunda	Dorsal a. of foot	Sole of foot	First plantar metatarsal
Plantar, lateral	A. plantaris lateralis	Posterior tibial	Toes and sole of foot	Plantar arch and plantar metatarsal
Plantar, medial	A. plantaris medialis	Posterior tibial	Muscles and skin of sole of foot and toes	Superficial digital

* Nomina Anatomica

Name	NA*	Origin	Distribution	Branches
Popliteal	A. poplitea	Continuation of femoral	Knee and calf	Anterior and posterior tibial; lateral and medial superior genicular; middle, sural, lateral, and medial inferior genicular; genicular articular
Pudendal, external	Aa. pudendae externae	Femoral	External genitalia; medial thigh	
Pudendal, internal	A. pudenda interna	Internal iliac	External genitalia	Posterior scrotal or posterior labial; inferior hemorrhoidal; perineal; urethral; a. of bulb of penis or vestibule; deep a. of penis or clitoris; dorsal a. of penis or clitoris
Pulmonary	Truncus pulmonalis	Right ventricle	Lungs	Right and left pulmonary
Pulmonary, left	A. pulmonalis sinistra	Pulmonary trunk	Left lung	Numerous branches
Pulmonary, right	A. pulmonalis dextra	Pulmonary trunk	Right lung	Numerous branches
Radial	A. radialis	Brachial	Forearm; wrist; hand	Recurrent radial; muscular; palmar and dorsal carpal; superficial palmar; first dorsal metacarpal; principal a. of thumb; perforating; recurrent; palmar
Radial, of index finger	A. radialis indicis	Principal a. of thumb	Index finger	
Recurrent, anterior tibial	A. recurrens tibialis anterior	Anterior tibial	Knee joint	
Recurrent, posterior tibial	A. recurrens tibialis posterior	Anterior tibial	Knee joint	
Recurrent, radial	A. recurrens radialis	Below elbow from radial	Elbow joint; muscles of forearm	
Recurrent, ulnar	A. recurrens ulnaris	Ulnar	Elbow joint; skin and muscles of elbow	Anterior and posterior recurrent
Renal	A. renalis	Abdominal aorta	Kidney; suprarenal gland; ureter	Inferior suprarenal

Retroduodenal		Gastroduodenal	Head of pancreas; duodenum; bile duct	
Sacral, lateral	Aa. sacrales laterales	Internal iliac	Coccyx and sacrum	
Sacral, middle	A. sacralis mediana	Abdominal aorta	Sacrum; coccyx; rectum	Lowest lumbar
Scapular, circumflex	A. circumflexa scapulae	Subscapular	Lateral border of scapula; infraspinous fossa; muscles of upper arm	
Scapular, descending (Dorsal scapular a.)	A. scapularis descendens	Subclavian	Medial border of scapula	
Sciatic SEE: *Gluteal a., inferior.*				
Sigmoid	Aa. sigmoideae	Inferior mesenteric	Iliac, sigmoid, and pelvic colon	
Spermatic, internal SEE: *Testicular a.*				
Sphenopalatine (Nasopalatine a.)	A. sphenopalatina	Maxillary	Nose	Posterior lateral nasal; posterior septal
Spinal, anterior (Ventral spinal a.)	A. spinalis anterior	Vertebral	Anterior spinal cord	
Spinal, posterior (Dorsal spinal a.)	A. spinalis posterior	Vertebral	Posterior spinal cord	
Splenic (Lienal a.)	A. lienalis	Celiac trunk	Pancreas; spleen; stomach; greater omentum	Pancreatic; left gastroepiploic; short gastric; splenic
Sternomastoid	Rr. sternocleidomastoidei arteriae occipitalis	Occipital or external carotid	Sternocleidomastoid muscles	
Stylomastoid	A. stylomastoidea	Posterior auricular	Mastoid; tympanic cavity; stapedius muscle	
Subclavian	A. subclavia	Innominate (right); arch of aorta (left)	Brain; meninges; spinal cord; neck; thoracic walls; upper limbs	Vertebral; internal thoracic; thyrocervical; costocervical; transverse cervical
Subcostal	A. subcostalis	Thoracic aorta	Upper abdominal wall	Dorsal and spinal

* *Nomina Anatomica*

Arteries (Continued)

Name	NA*	Origin	Distribution	Branches
Sublingual	A. sublingualis	Anterior margin of hypoglossus	Sublingual gland and mucous membrane of mouth and gums	
Submental	A. submentalis	Facial	Mylohyoid muscle; submandibular and sublingual glands; lower lip	
Subscapular	A. subscapularis	Axillary	Shoulder	Scapular circumflex and thoracodorsal
Supraorbital	A. supraorbitalis	Ophthalmic	Forehead; frontal sinus; upper eyelid; upper muscles of orbit	
Suprarenal, middle (Middle capsular a.)	A. suprarenalis media	Abdominal aorta	Suprarenal gland	
Suprascapular (Transverse scapular a.)	A. suprascapularis	Thyroid axis	Scapular; clavicle; shoulder joint	Acromial; suprasternal
Sural	Aa. surales	Popliteal opposite knee joint	Calf	
Tarsal, lateral	A. tarsea lateralis	Dorsal a. of foot	Muscles and joints of tarsus	
Tarsal, medial	Aa. tarseae mediales	Dorsal a. of foot	Middle portion of foot	
Temporal, middle	A. temporalis media	Above zygomatic arch	Temporal muscle	
Temporal, superficial	A. temporalis superficialis	End of external carotid	Parotid gland; auricle; scalp; skin of face; masseter muscle	Transverse facial; middle temporal; anterior auricular; frontal; parietal
Testicular (Internal spermatic a.)		Abdominal aorta	Ureter; epididymis; testes	Ureteral
Thoracic, internal (Internal mammary a.)	A. thoracica interna	Subclavian	Anterior thoracic wall; mediastinal structures; diaphragm	Pericardiacophrenic; anterior mediastinal; pericardial; sternal; intercostal; perforating; musculophrenic; superior epigastric

			Shoulder muscles and axillary glands	In the female, external mammary
Thoracic, lateral	A. thoracica lateralis	Axillary		
Thoracic, superior	A. thoracica suprema	Thoracoacromial	Muscles of chest	
Thoracoacromial	A. thoracoacromialis	Axillary	Muscles and skin of upper arm, shoulder, and chest	Pectoral; acromial; clavicular; deltoid
Thoracodorsal	A. thoracodorsalis	Subscapular	Posterior portion of axillary	
Thumb, principal a. of	a. princeps pollicis	Radial	Sides and palmar aspect of thumb	Radial a. of index finger
Thyroid, inferior	A. thyroidea inferior	Thyroid axis	Thyroid gland; esophagus	Inferior laryngeal; tracheal; muscular; esophageal; ascending cervical
Thyroid, superior	A. thyroidea superior	External carotid	Hyoid muscles; larynx; thyroid gland; pharynx	Hyoid; sternomastoid; superior laryngeal; cricothyroid
Tibial, anterior	A. tibialis anterior	Popliteal	Leg; ankle; foot	Anterior and posterior tibial recurrent; fibular; lateral and medial anterior malleolar
Tibial, posterior	A. tibialis posterior	Lower end of popliteal	Leg; foot; heel	Peroneal; lateral and medial posterior malleolar; communicating; plantar; tibial and fibular nutrient
Tympanic, anterior	A. tyrpanica anterior	Maxillary	Lining of tympanic arch	
Tympanic, inferior	A. tympanica inferior	Ascending pharyngeal	Tympanic cavity	
Ulnar	A. ulnaris	Brachial	Forearm; wrist and hand	Anterior and posterior recurrent; common interosseous; muscular; palmar and dorsal carpal; deep palmar; superficial palmar arch
Uterine	A. uterina	Internal iliac	Uterus; uterine tubes; ovary; vagina	Vaginal; ovarian; tubal

* Nomina Anatomica

Arteries (Continued)

Name	NA*	Origin	Distribution	Branches
Vaginal	A. vaginalis	Uterine	Vagina; bladder	
Vertebral	A. vertebralis	Subclavian	Muscles of neck; vertebrae; spinal cord; cerebellum; interior or cerebrum	Spinal; muscular; anterior and posterior spinal; posterior inferior cerebellar; medullary
Vesical, inferior	A. vesicalis inferior	Internal iliac	Bladder; prostate; seminal vesicles	
Vesical, superior	Aa. vesicales superiores	Internal iliac	Upper part of bladder	A. to the ductus deferens
Vidian (A. of the pterygoid canal)	A. canalis pterygoidei		Roof of pharynx; auditory (eustachian) tube	

Veins

Name	NA*	Origin	Distribution	Description
Angular	V. angularis	Union of supratrochlear and supraorbital veins	Continues inferiorly as facial v.	Short superficial v. in nasal region
Antebrachial, median	V. mediana antebrachii	Base of dorsum of thumb	Ascends forearm between cephalic and basilic veins to elbow where it joins these veins	Superficial v. forearm
Auricular, posterior	V. auricularis posterior	Plexus on side of head	From side of head it descends behind the pinna where it unites with retromandibular v. to form the external jugular v.	Superficial v. which drains parietal and posterior part of temporal region
Axillary	V. axillaris	Junction of basilic and brachial veins	Lower border of teres major muscles to lateral border of first rib where it becomes the subclavian v.	Portion of venous trunk of upper extremity
Azygos	V. azygos	Arises from ascending lumbar v.	From level of diaphragm up posterior thoracic wall on	Trunk which connects superior and inferior vena cavae

				right of vertebral bodies to superior vena cava
Basilic	V. basilica	Ulnar side of dorsal rete of hand	Ascends posteriorly on the forearm. Below the elbow it moves to exterior surface where it joins axillary v.	Superficial v. of hand and forearm
Brachial	Vv. brachiales	Tributaries from structures in upper arm	Follows course of brachial artery and joins axillary v.	Each v. drains an arm
Brachiocephalic (Innominate v.)	Vv. brachiocephalicae (dextra et sinistra)	Union of internal jugular and subclavian veins	From sternal end of clavicle it ascends vertically to untie below the cartilage of first rib to form superior vena cava	Paired veins which drain blood from heed, neck, and upper extremities. They unite to form superior vena cava
Bronchial	Vv. bronchiales	Capillaries of bronchi and roots of lungs	Empties into azygos v. on the right and into hemiazygos or superior intercostal veins on left	Several veins which return blood from larger bronchi and roots of lungs
Cardiac	Vv. cordis	Capillaries of tissues of heart	Circulates throughout heart, usually emptying into coronary sinus	Drain blood from tissues of heart
Cardinal		Each v. receives a v. from caudal and cephalic portions of embryo	Include precardinal and postcardinal veins	First veins to appear in body of embryo
Cephalic	V. cephalic	Radial border of dorsal rete of hand	Winds anteriorly up arm and empties into axillary v.	Superficial v. of arm and forearm
Cerebellar, inferior	Vv. cerebelli inferiores	Undersurface of cerebellum	Empty into transverse, superior, petrosal, and occipital sinuses	Large veins of undersurface of cerebellum
Cerebellar, superior	Vv. cerebelli superiores	Upper surface of cerebellum	Empty into straight sinus or transverse sinus	Veins from upper surface of cerebellum

* Nomina Anatomica

Veins (Continued)

Name	NA*	Origin	Distribution	Description
Cerebral, great	V. cerebri magna	Formed by union of two internal cerebral veins	Curves backward and upward around the splenium of the corpus callosum and continues as a straight sinus	Short median trunk
Cerebral, inferior	Vv. cerebri inferiores	Tributaries in lobes of cerebrum	From various lobes they empty into cavernous and transverse sinuses	Small-sized veins which drain undersurfaces of hemispheres
Cerebral, internal	Vv. cerebri internae	Formed near interventricular foramen by union of terminal and choroid veins	Run backward parallel to one another and unite at the splenium of the corpus callosum to form great cerebral v.	Two veins which drain deep parts of hemisphere
Cerebral, superficial middle	V. cerebri media superficialis	Lateral surface of cerebral hemisphere	Follows lateral cerebral fissure and empties into cavernous sinus	Drains lateral surface of cerebral hemisphere
Cerebral, superior	Vv. cerebri superiores	Capillaries of cerebrum	From cerebrum to longitudinal cerebral fissure, opening into superior sagittal sinus	Eight to twelve veins which drain the surface of the cerebral hemisphere
Cervical, deep	V. cervicalis profunda	Plexus in suboccipital triangle	Follows deep cervical artery down neck and empties into vertebral or brachiocephalic v.	Deep v. of neck
Cervical, transverse	Vv. transversae cervicis	Capillaries of supraspinous region of scapula and neck	From supraspinous region of scapula diagonally across shoulder to subclavian or external jugular v.	Drain blood from supraspinous region of scapula and neck
Cystic	V. cystica	Capillaries of gallbladder	From gallbladder along cystic duct to enter right branch of portal v. just below liver	Drains gallbladder
Deep		Extremities	Throughout the body	Accompany homonymous arteries and usually are enclosed in sheaths with those vessels

2264

Digital, palmar	Vv. digitales palmares	Capillaries of superficial tissues of palmar surface of fingers	Along proper and common digital arteries	Superficial veins of palmar surface of fingers
Digital, plantar	Vv. digitales plantares	Capillaries of toes	Along plantar surface of toes to foot to form four metatarsal veins	Veins of plantar surface of toes
Diploic	Vv. diploicae	Bony tissue between internal and external skull surface	Connect with meningeal veins, sinuses of the dura mater, and veins of the pericranium	Large veins of the skull. Main veins are frontal, anterior and posterior temporal, and occipital
Emissary	V. emissaria	Cerebral sinuses	Pass through foramina of skull	One of the small valveless veins which establish communication between sinuses inside the skull and veins external to it
Epigastric, inferior	V. epigastrica inferior	Capillaries of internal surface of lower anterior abdominal walls	Internal surface of abdominal wall diagonally across wall to flow into external iliac v.	V. of lower anterior abdominal wall
Epigastric, superficial	V. epigastrica superficialis	Superficial tissues of lower portion of anterior abdominal wall	Follows superficial epigastric artery and opens into great saphenous v.	Drains lower and medial portion of abdominal wall
Esophageal	Vv. esophageae	Capillaries of esophagus	From esophagus empties into inferior thyroid, hemiazygos, azygos, or left brachiocephalicus v.	One of several small trunks which drain esophagus
Facial	V. facialis	Continuation of angular v.	From inner angle of orbit it passes diagonally downward and outward to lower jaw	Deep v. of face. Branches drain deep structures of face
Femoral	V. femoralis	Continuation of popliteal v.	From posterior region of knee it follows course of femoral artery, becoming external iliac v. at inguinal ligament	Large v. of thigh

* Nomina Anatomica

Veins (Continued)

Name	NA*	Origin	Distribution	Description
Femoral, deep	V. profunda femoris	Tributaries from posterior region of thigh	Accompanies deep femoral artery to femoral triangle where it joins femoral v.	Deep v. of thigh
Gastric, left	V. gastrica sinistra	Gastrohepatic omentum	Right to left along lesser curvature of stomach to enter portal v.	Drains both surfaces of stomach
Gastric, right (Pyloric)	V. gastrica dextra	Small v. from upper portion of stomach	From upper stomach runs left to right along pyloric portion of lesser curvature of stomach to end in portal v.	Drains upper portion of stomach
Gastric, short	Vv. gastricae breves	Capillaries of fundus of stomach	From wall of stomach empty into splenic v.	Drain wall of stomach
Gastroepiploic, left	V. gastroepiploica sinistra	Branches from stomach and greater omentum	Right to left on greater curvature of stomach to empty into splenic v.	V. of upper stomach
Gastroepiploic, right	V. gastroepiploica dextra	Branches from greater omentum and lower surfaces of stomach	Left to right on greater curvature of stomach to empty into superior mesenteric v.	V. of lower stomach
Gluteal, inferior (Sciatic v.)	Vv. gluteae inferiores	Capillaries of upper part of back of thigh	Upper back thigh through lower sciatic foramen where they unite into a single v. and empty into internal iliac v.	V. of lower region of hip
Gluteal, superior	Vv. gluteae superiores	Capillaries of gluteal and adjacent muscles	From tissues of hip they pass through sciatic foramen to empty into internal iliac v.	Drain muscles of buttocks
Hemiazygos	V. hemiazygos	Left ascending lumbar v.	Lumbar region through diaphragm, crossing in front of spine and emptying into azygos v.	Single v. of lower left thoracic wall
Hemiazygos, accessory	V. hemiazygos accessoria	Capillaries of upper intercostal	From left side of vertebra	Drains blood from intercostal

2266

	Nomina Anatomica*	spaces		
			crosses over spine to enter azygos v.	spaces above level of sixth to seventh
Hemorrhoidal plexus	Plexus venous rectalis	Muscular wall and submucosa of rectum	Tissues of rectum via hemorrhoidal veins to internal pudendal v. to hypogastric v. to commencement of inferior mesenteric v.	Surround the rectum
Hepatic	Vv. hepaticae	Tissues of liver	From liver empty into inferior vena cava	Drain the liver
Ileocoli	V. ilecolica	Capillaries of organs in area of ileum and colon	From lower portion of ascending colon runs parallel with ileocolic artery and empties into superior mesenteric v.	Large tributary of mesenteric v. which drains the ileum, appendix, cecum, and lower part of ascending colon
Iliac, common	V. iliaca communis	Union of internal and external iliac veins	Diagonally across pelvis	Large v. which drains blood from pelvis and leg. One on each side meets to form inferior vena cava
Iliac, deep circumflex	V. circumflexa iliaca profunda	Capillaries of deep muscles of upper portion of thigh and lower portion of abdomen	Deep tissues of anterior superior spine along inner surface of pelvic brim to external iliac v.	V. of deep structures of iliac region
Iliac, external	V. iliaca externa	Begins behind inguinal ligament as continuation of external iliac v.	Behind inguinal ligament to sacroiliac articulation where it unites with internal iliac v. to form common iliac v.	Upward continuation of external iliac v.
Iliac, internal (Hypogastric v.)	V. iliaca interna	Near upper part of greater sciatic foramen	Upper part of greater sciatic foramen	Short v. which draws blood from pelvis
Intercostal		Tributaries of other veins of intercostal spaces	Intercostal spaces to region of lower ribs	One of a number of veins (anterior, posterior, right, left, superior, and highest) which drain blood from intercostal spaces

* Nomina Anatomica

Veins (Continued)

Name	NA*	Origin	Distribution	Description
Intervertebral	V. intervertebralis	Vertebral plexuses	Vertebral plexuses through intervertebral foramina where they empty into regional veins	One of numerous veins which drain vertebral plexuses and accompany spinal nerves
Jugular, anterior	V. jugularis anterior	From veins of region of lower lip	From lower jaw descends neck anteriorly and enters external jugular v.	Superficial v. of anterior region of neck
Jugular, external	V. jugularis externa	Formed at parotid gland by union of posterior auricular and retromandibular veins	From parotid gland descends perpendicularly in neck to empty into subclavian, internal jugular, or brachiocephalic v.	A large superficial v. which receives greater part of blood from exterior of cranium and deep parts of face
Jugular, internal	V. jugularis interna	Continuous from transverse sinus at base of skull	Runs vertically in neck and unites with subclavian v. at root of neck to form the brachiocephalic v.	Largest v. of head and neck. Collects blood from brain, superficial parts of face, and neck
Lingual	V. lingualis	Capillaries of tongue and sublingual areas	Follows distribution of lingual artery	Deep v. of tongue
Lumbar	Vv. lumbales	Capillaries of abdominal walls	Abdominal walls to ascending lumbar v., inferior vena cava, and iliolumbar v.	Four or five veins of abdominal walls
Lumbar, ascending	V. lumbalis ascendens	Lateral sacral veins	Lateral sacral v. along lateral border of spinal column to first lumbar vertebra where it becomes azygos v. on right side and hemiazygos v. on left side	Longitudinal v. which connects lumbar veins
Meningeal	Vv. meningeae	Meninges of brain	Accompany meningeal arteries from meninges and empty into regional sinuses and veins	Multiple veins of dura mater of brain
Mesenteric, superior	V. mesenterica superior	Capillaries of small intestine	From ileum in right iliac fossa	Large v. from small intestine

Name	NA*	Receives	Location / Course	Drains
			it follows distribution of its artery and unites with splenic v. behind pancreas to form portal v.	
Mesenteric, inferior	V. mesenterica inferior	Capillaries of colon and rectum	As a continuation of superior rectal v. ascends behind peritoneum and enters splenic v.	Drains blood from rectum and sigmoid and descending parts of colon
Metacarpal, dorsal	Vv. metacarpaea dorsales	Capillaries of hand	From digital venous arches join to form dorsal venous rete of hand	Superficial veins of back of hand
Metacarpal, palmar	Vv. metacarpeae palmares	Capillaries of palm	Deep tissues of palm along metacarpal bone to deep venous arches	Deep veins on both sides of hand
Metatarsal, dorsal	Vv. metatarsales dorsales pedis	Dorsal digital veins of toes	Through metatarsal spaces to unite to form dorsal venous arch	Deep veins of back of foot
Metatarsal, plantar	Vv. metatarsales plantares	Plantar digital veins	From toes to ankles and open into plantar venous arch	Deep veins of solar aspect of foot
Musculophrenic	Vv. musculophrenicae	Capillaries of upper abdominal wall, lower intercostal spaces, and diaphragm	Along thoracic surface of diaphragm upward lateral to sternum to unite with superior epigastric v. to form internal thoracic v.	Drains blood from thoracic surface of diaphragm and from walls of thorax and abdomen
Obturator	Vv. obturatoriae	Union of tributaries of hip and muscle of upper posterior thigh	From upper portion of adductor region of thigh run through upper part of obturator foramen and run back to empty into internal iliac v.	Drains blood from obturator foramen
Occipital	V. occipitalis	Plexus at back part of vertex of skull	From plexus of occipital region, occasionally following course of occipital artery, extends to internal or external jugular v.	Superficial v. which drains occipital region

* Nomina Anatomica

Veins (Continued)

Name	NA*	Origin	Distribution	Description
Ophthalmic, inferior	V. ophthalmica inferior	Venous network at forepart of orbit	Runs backward in lower orbit and divides into two branches. One passes through inferior orbital fissure and joins pterygoid venous plexus; the second enters cranium through superior orbital fissure and ends in cavernous sinus	Ophthalmic v. which divides into two terminal branches
Ophthalmic, superior	V. ophthalmica superior	Inner angle of orbit	Follows course of ophthalmic artery into cavernous sinus	Paired veins of orbital cavity
Ovarian, right and left	V. ovarica dextra and V. ovarica sinistra	Capillaries of ovaries, uterine tubes, and adjacent structures	Pampiniform plexus of broad ligament into inferior vena cava on right and left renal v. on left	Drains ovaries
Palatine, external	V. palatina externa	Capillaries of deep tissues of neck	Palatine regions into facial v.	Drains blood from tonsils and soft palate
Pancreatic	Vv. pancreaticae	Capillaries of pancreas	From pancreas into splenic and superior mesenteric veins	V. of pancreas
Parietal emissary	V. emissaria parietalis	Upper skull	Connects superior sagittal sinus with extra cranial veins	Small v. which passes through the parietal foramen of the skull
Parumbilical	Vv. parumbilicales	Cutaneous veins in region of umbilicus	From region of umbilicus run backward and upward to left portal v.	Small important veins which establish communication between portal v. and superior and inferior epigastric veins
Penis, dorsal v. of	V. dorsalis profunda penis	Capillaries of skin or tissue of penis	Runs length of penis between two dorsal arteries	Two (deep and superficial) veins of penis
Peroneal (Fibular v.)	Vv. peroneae (fibulares)	Veins of ankle and capillaries of tissues of leg	From venous plexus in region of heel upward along lateral	Deep v. of leg

Pharyngeal	Vv. pharyngeae	Pharyngeal plexus	Empty from pharyngeal plexus into internal jugular v.	Drain pharyngeal plexus
Phrenic, inferior	Vv. phrenicae inferiores	Tissues of diaphragm	From diaphragm flow to inferior vena cava on right side and left suprarenal v. on left side	Drain abdominal surface of diaphragm
Popliteal	V. poplitea	Union of tibial veins at lower border of popliteus muscle	From tibial veins upward to adductor hiatus to become femoral v.	Large v. in posterior region of knee
Portal	V. portae hepatis	Union of superior mesenteric and splenic veins	Abdominal cavity	Subdivision of systemic venous system. Collects blood from digestive tract and conveys it to the liver
Pudendal, external	Vv. pudendae externae	Capillaries of superficial tissues of lower abdomen, scrotum, or labia	From lower abdomen transversely across upper region of thigh to great saphenous or femoral v.	Drain blood from superficial regions of medial aspect of upper thigh and receive subcutaneous dorsal veins of external genitals
Pudendal, internal	V. pudenda interna	Deep veins of penis or clitoris	Follows course of internal pudendal artery and opens into internal iliac v.	Drains the perineum and external genitals
Pulmonary	Vv. pulmonales	Capillaries upon walls of air sacs of lungs	Lungs to left atrium	Four veins which return oxygenated blood from lungs to left atrium of heart
Radial	Vv. radiales	Palmar arches of hand	From palmar arches of hand accompany radial artery along lateral side of forearm in deep tissues to unite with ulnar v. to form brachial v.	Large deep veins on radial side of forearm

region of deep tissue to flow into posterior tibial v. below knee

* Nomina Anatomica

2271

Veins (Continued)

Name	NA*	Origin	Distribution	Description
Rectal, inferior	Vv. rectales inferiores	Venous plexus of anal canal	Anal canal to internal pudendal v.	Drain the rectal plexus
Rectal, middle	Vv. rectales mediae	Rectal plexus with tributaries from bladder, prostate, and seminal vesicles	Run laterally from rectal plexus to internal iliac v.	Drain the rectal plexus
Rectal, superior	V. rectalis superior	Capillaries of rectum	Ascends from rectal plexus to brim of pelvis into inferior mesenteric v.	Drains upper part of rectal plexus
Renal	Vv. renales	Capillaries of kidneys. The left v. receives the left suprarenal v. and left gonadal v.	From kidneys transversely across posterior abdominal wall to inferior vena cava	Short thick trunks which drain the kidneys. The left is longer than the right
Sacral, lateral	Vv. sacrales laterales	Tissues of posterior pelvic wall	Posterior pelvic wall upward along sacrum to empty into internal iliac v.	Large v. of posterior pelvic wall veins
Sacral, middle	V. sacralis mediana	Capillaries of tissues of posterior pelvic wall	From pelvic wall in sacral region follows middle sacral artery to empty into common iliac v.	Large v. of posterior pelvic wall
Saphenous, great	V. saphena magna	Medial marginal v. of dorsum of foot	Dorsum of foot to femoral v. just below the inguinal ligament	Longest v. in body
Saphenous, small	V. saphena parva	Continuation of marginal v.	From behind malleolus ascends back of leg to knee joint where it opens into popliteal v.	Large superficial. v. of back of leg
Sciatic SEE: *Gluteal v., inferior.*				
Spinal, anterior and posterior	Vv. spinales anteriores and Vv. superiores	Spinal cord and its pia mater	Spinal cord through roots to internal vertebral venous plexuses	Network of veins draining blood from spinal cord
Splenic	V. splenica	Union of several small veins at the hilus of the spleen	From spleen transversely across abdomen to head of pancreas	Large v. which drains blood from spleen and part of

Name	Latin	Receives	Course / Termination	Description
			where it forms portal v. by joining the superior mesenteric v.	stomach
Subcardinal				Paired vessels in embryo which replace postcardinal veins. SEE: Cardinal v.
Subclavian	V. subclavia	Continuation of axillary v.	Outer border of first rib to sternal end of clavicle where it joins the internal jugular v. to form the brachiocephalic v.	Main venous trunk of upper extremity
Superficial (Cutaneous v.)	V. cutanea	Capillaries of superficial tissues of body wall	Throughout subcutaneous tissue of body wall	Veins located beneath layers of superficial fascia immediately beneath the skin
Supraorbital	V. supraorbitalis	Capillaries and superficial tissues of region of eye	From region of eye along lateral wall of orbital cavity to root of nose where it unites with supratrochlear v. to form angular v.	Drains upper portion of orbital cavity
Suprarenal, left	V. suprarenalis sinistra	Capillaries of left adrenal gland	Hilum of left suprarenal gland, ascending to left renal v.	V. of left adrenal gland
Suprarenal, right	V. suprarenalis dextra	Capillaries of right adrenal gland	Hilum of right adrenal gland to inferior vena cava	V. of right adrenal gland
Supratrochlear (Frontal v.)	Vv. supratrochleares	Capillaries of anterior region of scalp	From venous plexuses in forehead diagonally to left of root of nose where they unite with supraorbital v. to form angular v.	Drain the anterior scalp
Temporal, middle	V. temporalis media	Substance of temporal muscle	From lateral superficial plexus of skull it passes to zygoma where it joins superficial temporal v. to form retromandibular v.	Superficial v. of lateral portion of stomach

* Nomina Anatomica

Veins (Continued)

Name	NA*	Origin	Distribution	Description
Temporal, superficial	Vv. temporales superficiales	Lateral scalp in parietal and frontal region	Temporal region of scalp diagonally to ear and downward to mandible where they unite with maxillary v. to form retromandibular v.	Veins of superficial tissues of skull
Testicular	V. testicularis dextra and sinistra	Testicular v. in male and ovarian v. in female	From brim of pelvis upward along posterior abdominal wall to inferior vena cava on right and renal v. on left	Receives blood from testis and epididymis
Thoracic, internal	Vv. thoracicae internae	Tributaries from tissues of intercostal spaces	Tributaries form a single trunk which runs up medial side of internal thoracic artery and ends in brachiocephalic v.	Deep v. of chest draining intercostal spaces
Thoracic, lateral (Long thoracic v.)	V. thoracica lateralis	Capillaries of muscles and glands of anterior chest	Tissues of anterior chest muscles to axillary v.	A large tributary v. of the axillary v. which drains the lateral thoracic wall
Thoracoepigastric	Vv. thoracoepigastricae	Region of superficial epigastric v.	Run laterally along trunk from superficial epigastric v. to lateral thoracic v.	Superficial v. of trunk which establishes an important communication between the femoral and axillary veins
Thyroid, inferior	V. thyroidea inferior	Veins from thyroid glands	Downward to brachiocephalic v.	Two or more veins which arise in venous plexuses on thyroid gland
Thyroid, superior	V. thyroidea superior	Substance and surface of thyroid gland	Accompanies superior thyroid artery and empties into internal jugular v.	One v. from either side of thyroid
Tibial, anterior	Vv. tibiales anteriores	Capillaries of leg tissue and dorsal metatarsal v.	Accompany anterior tibial artery, ascending between tibia and fibula and uniting with posterior tibial v. to form popliteal v.	Deep veins of anterior aspect of leg

Tibial, posterior	Vv. tibiales posteriores	Capillaries of deep tissues of leg	From ankle upward posterior aspect of leg to unite with anterior tibial v. to form popliteal v. just below knee	Deep veins of back of leg
Ulnar	Vv. ulnares	Palmar arches of hand	Palmar arches of hand upward in deep tissues along ulnar side of forearm to form brachial v. with radial v. at elbow	Large deep veins of medial aspect of forearm
Umbilical	V. umbilicalis sinistra	Placental tissues	Along umbilical cord through umbilicus to liver upward through inferior vena cava to heart	V. which carries blood from placenta to fetus
Uterine	Vv. uterinae	Tissues of uterus	Uterine plexus through part of the broad ligament to empty into internal iliac v.	Veins carrying blood from uterus
Vena cava inferior	V. cava inferior	Right and left iliac veins	From union of iliac veins at level of fifth lumbar vertebra to right atrium of heart	Returns blood from lower half of body
Vena cava superior	V. cava superior	Two innominate veins	From below right costal cartilage to right atrium of heart.	Drains blood from upper half of body
Vertebral	V. vertebralis	Numerous small tributaries in the suboccipital triangle	Base of skull down neck, opening into brachiocephalic v.	Drains blood from internal vertebral venous plexuses
Vertebral, anterior	V. vertebralis anterior	Plexus around transverse process of upper cervical vertebrae	Descends from region of upper cervical vertebrae with ascending cervical artery and opens into terminal part of vertebral v.	Small v.

* Nomina Anatomica

App. 5: Recommended Daily Dietary Allowances[a] (Revised 1989)

Category	Age (years) or Condition	Weight[b] (kg)	Weight[b] (lb)	Height[b] (cm)	Height[b] (in)	Protein (g)	Vit. A (μg RE)[c]	Vit. D (μg)[d]	Vit. E (mg α-TE)[e]	Vit. K (μg)	Vit. C (mg)	Thiamin (mg)	Riboflavin (mg)	Niacin (mg NE)[f]	Vit. B6 (mg)	Folate (μg)	Vit. B12 (μg)	Calcium (mg)	Phosphorus (mg)	Magnesium (mg)	Iron (mg)	Zinc (mg)	Iodine (μg)	Selenium (μg)
Infants	0.0–0.5	6	13	60	24	13	375	7.5	3	5	30	0.3	0.4	5	0.3	25	0.3	400	300	40	6	5	40	10
	0.5–1.0	9	20	71	28	14	375	10	4	10	35	0.4	0.5	6	0.6	35	0.5	600	500	60	10	5	50	15
Children	1–3	13	29	90	35	16	400	10	6	15	40	0.7	0.8	9	1.0	50	0.7	800	800	80	10	10	70	20
	4–6	20	44	112	44	24	500	10	7	20	45	0.9	1.1	12	1.1	75	1.0	800	800	120	10	10	90	20
	7–10	28	62	132	52	28	700	10	7	30	45	1.0	1.2	13	1.4	100	1.4	800	800	170	10	10	120	30
Males	11–14	45	99	157	62	45	1000	10	10	45	50	1.3	1.5	17	1.7	150	2.0	1200	1200	270	12	15	150	40
	15–18	66	145	176	69	59	1000	10	10	65	60	1.5	1.8	20	2.0	200	2.0	1200	1200	400	12	15	150	50
	19–24	72	160	177	70	58	1000	10	10	70	60	1.5	1.7	19	2.0	200	2.0	1200	1200	350	10	15	150	70
	25–50	79	174	176	70	63	1000	5	10	80	60	1.5	1.7	19	2.0	200	2.0	800	800	350	10	15	150	70
	51+	77	170	173	68	63	1000	5	10	80	60	1.2	1.4	15	2.0	200	2.0	800	800	350	10	15	150	70
Females	11–14	46	101	157	62	46	800	10	8	45	50	1.1	1.3	15	1.4	150	2.0	1200	1200	280	15	12	150	45
	15–18	55	120	163	64	44	800	10	8	55	60	1.1	1.3	15	1.5	180	2.0	1200	1200	300	15	12	150	50
	19–24	58	128	164	65	46	800	10	8	60	60	1.1	1.3	15	1.6	180	2.0	1200	1200	280	15	12	150	55
	25–50	63	138	163	64	50	800	5	8	65	60	1.1	1.3	15	1.6	180	2.0	800	800	280	15	12	150	55
	51+	65	143	160	63	50	800	5	8	65	60	1.0	1.2	13	1.6	180	2.0	800	800	280	10	12	150	55
Pregnant						60	800	10	10	65	70	1.5	1.6	17	2.2	400	2.2	1200	1200	300	30	15	175	65
Lactating	1st 6 months					65	1300	10	12	65	95	1.6	1.8	20	2.1	280	2.6	1200	1200	355	15	19	200	75
	2nd 6 months					62	1200	10	11	65	90	1.6	1.7	20	2.1	260	2.6	1200	1200	340	15	16	200	75

a The allowances, expressed as average daily intakes over time, are intended to provide for individual variations among most normal persons as they live in the United States under usual environmental stresses. Diets should be based on a variety of common foods in order to provide other nutrients for which human requirements have been less well defined.

b Weights and heights of Reference Adults are actual medians for the U.S. population of the designated age, as reported by NHANES II [second National Health and Nutrition Examination Survey]. The median weights and heights of those under 19 years of age were taken from Hamill et al. [Physical Growth: National Center for Health Statistics percentiles. Am J Clin Nutr 32:607, 1979]. The use of these figures does not imply that the height-to-weight ratios are ideal.

c Retinol equivalents. 1 RE = 1 μg retinol or 6 μg β-carotene.

d As cholecalciferol. 10 μg cholecalciferol = 400 IU (International Units) of vitamin D.

e α-tocopherol equivalents. 1 mg d-α tocopherol = 1 α-TE.

f 1 NE (niacin equivalent) = 1 mg of niacin or 60 mg of dietary tryptophan.

g Those who smoke cigarettes regularly should take at least 100 mg of vitamin C daily.

SOURCE: National Research Council (Food and Nutrition Board): Recommended Dietary Allowances, ed 10. National Academy Press, Washington, DC, 1989.

Estimated Safe and Adequate Daily Dietary Intakes of Selected Vitamins and Minerals[a]

Category	Age (years)	Vitamins		Trace Elements[b]				
		Biotin (µg)	Pantothenic Acid (mg)	Copper (mg)	Manganese (mg)	Fluoride (mg)	Chromium (µg)	Molybdenum (µg)
Infants	0.0–0.5	10	2	0.4–0.6	0.3–0.6	0.1–0.5	10–40	15–30
	0.5–1.0	15	3	0.6–0.7	0.6–1.0	0.2–1.0	20–60	20–40
Children and Adolescents	1–3	20	3	0.7–1.0	1.0–1.5	0.5–1.5	20–80	25–50
	4–6	25	3–4	1.0–1.5	1.5–2.0	1.0–2.5	30–120	30–75
	7–10	30	4–5	1.0–2.0	2.0–3.0	1.5–2.5	50–200	50–150
	11+	30–100	4–7	1.5–2.5	2.0–5.0	1.5–2.5	50–200	75–250
Adults		30–100	4–7	1.5–3.0	2.0–5.0	1.5–4.0	50–200	75–250

[a] Because there is less information on which to base allowances, these figures are not given in the main table of RDA and are provided here in the form of ranges of recommended intakes.

[b] Since the toxic levels for many trace elements may be only several times usual intakes, the upper levels for the trace elements given in this table should not be habitually exceeded.

SOURCE: National Research Council (Food and Nutrition Board): Recommended Dietary Allowances, ed 10. National Academy Press, Washington, DC, 1989, p 284.

App. 6: Vitamins*

(Summary of Vitamins Significant in Human Diet)

Vitamin	Chief Functions	Results of Deficiency	Characteristics	Good Sources
VITAMIN A Provitamin, carotene	Essential for maintaining the integrity of epithelial membranes. Helps maintain resistance to infections. Necessary for the formation of rhodopsin and prevention of night blindness.	*Mild:* Retarded growth. Increased susceptibility to infection. Abnormal function of gastrointestinal, genitourinary and respiratory tracts due to altered epithelial membranes. Skin dries, shrivels, thickens; sometimes pustule formation. Night blindness. *Severe:* Xerophthalmia, a characteristic eye disease, and other local infections.	Fat soluble. Not destroyed by ordinary cooking temperatures. Is destroyed by high temperatures when oxygen is present. Marked capacity for storage in the liver. NOTE: Excessive intake of carotene, from which vitamin A is formed, may produce yellow discoloration of the skin (carotenemia).	Animal fats butter cheese cream egg yolk whole milk. Fish liver oil. Liver. Vegetables 1. green leafy, esp. escarole, kale, parsley 2. yellow, esp. carrots. *Artificial:* Concentrates in several forms. Irradiated fish oils.
THIAMINE Vitamin B$_1$	Important role in carbohydrate metabolism. Essential for maintenance of normal digestion and appetite. Essential for normal functioning of nervous tissue.	*Mild:* Loss of appetite. Impaired digestion of starches and sugars. Colitis, constipation, or diarrhea. Emaciation. *Severe:* Nervous disorders of various types. Loss of coordinating power of muscles. Beriberi. Paralysis in man.	Water soluble. Not readily destroyed by ordinary cooking temperature. Destroyed by exposure to heat, alkali, or sulfites. Is not stored in body.	Widely distributed in plant and animal tissues but seldom occurs in high concentration, except in brewer's yeast. Other good sources are: Whole grain cereals Peas, beans Peanuts Oranges Glandular — heart, liver, kidney Many vegetables and fruits Nuts.

	Functions	Deficiency	Properties	Sources
				Artificial: Concentrates from yeast. Rice polishings. Wheat germ.
RIBOFLAVIN Vitamin B$_2$	Important in formation of certain enzymes and in cellular oxidation. Normal growth. Prevention of cheilosis and glossitis. Participates in light adaptation.	Impaired growth. Lassitude and weakness. Cheilosis. Glossitis. Atrophy of skin. Anemia. Photophobia. Cataracts.	Water soluble. Alcohol soluble. Not destroyed by heat in cooking unless with alkali. Unstable in light, esp. in presence of alkali.	Eggs Green vegetables Liver Kidney Lean meat Milk Wheat germ Yeast, dried Enriched foods.
NIACIN Nicotinic acid Nicotinamide Antipellagra vitamin	As the component of two important enzymes, it is important in glycolysis, tissue respiration, and fat synthesis. Nicotinic acid, but not nicotinamide, causes vasodilation and flushing. Prevents pellagra.	Pellagra. Gastrointestinal disturbances. Mental disturbances.	Soluble in hot water and alcohol. Not destroyed by heat, light, air, or alkali. Not destroyed in ordinary cooking.	Yeast Lean meat Fish Legumes Whole grain cereals and peanuts Enriched foods.
VITAMIN B$_{12}$ Cyanocobalamin	Produces remission in pernicious anemia. Essential for normal development of red blood cells.	Pernicious anemia.	Soluble in water or alcohol. Unstable in hot alkaline or acid solutions.	Liver Kidney Dairy products. Most of vitamin required by humans is synthesized by intestinal bacteria.

* See App. 5 for daily allowances recommended.

Vitamin (Continued)

Vitamins (Continued)

Vitamin	Chief Functions	Results of Deficiency	Characteristics	Good Sources
VITAMIN C Ascorbic acid	Essential to formation of intracellular cement substances in a variety of tissues including skin, dentin, cartilage, and bone matrix. Important in healing of wounds and fractures of bones. Prevents scurvy. Facilitates absorption of iron.	*Mild:* Lowered resistance to infections. Joint tenderness. Susceptibility to dental caries, pyorrhea, and bleeding gums. *Severe:* Hemorrhage. Anemia. Scurvy.	Soluble in water. Easily destroyed by oxidation; heat hastens the process. Lost in cooking, particularly if water in which food was cooked is discarded. Also loss is greater if cooked in iron or copper utensils. Quick-frozen foods lose little of their vitamin C. Stored in the body to a limited extent.	Abundant in most fresh fruits and vegetables, esp. citrus fruit and juices, tomato and orange. *Artificial:* Ascorbic acid. Cevitamic acid.
VITAMIN D	Regulates absorption of calcium and phosphorus from the intestinal tract. Antirachitic.	*Mild:* Interferes with utilization of calcium and phosphorus in bone and tooth formation. Irritability. Weakness. *Severe:* Rickets, may be common in young children. Osteomalacia in adults.	Soluble in fats and organic solvents. Relatively stable under refrigeration. Stored in liver. Often associated with vitamin A.	Butter Egg yolk Fish liver oils Fish having fat distributed through the flesh, salmon, tuna fish, herring, sardines Liver Oysters Yeast and foods irradiated with ultraviolet light. Formed in the skin by exposure to sunlight. Artificially prepared forms.
VITAMIN E Alpha tocopherol	Normal reproduction in rats. Prevention of muscular dystrophy in rats.	Red blood cell resistance to rupture is decreased.	Fat soluble. Stable to heat in absence of oxygen.	Lettuce and other green, leafy vegetables. Wheat germ oil Margarine Rice.

VITAMIN B₆ Pyridoxine	Essential for metabolism of tryptophan. Needed for utilization of certain other amino acids.	Dermatitis around eyes and mouth. Neuritis. Anorexia, nausea, and vomiting.	Soluble in water and alcohol. Rapidly inactivated in presence of heat, sunlight, or air.	Blackstrap molasses Meat Cereal grains Wheat germ.
FOLACIN	Essential for normal functioning of hematopoietic system.	Anemia.	Slightly soluble in water. Easily destroyed by heat in presence of acid. Decreases when food is stored at room temperature. NOTE: A large dose may prevent appearance of anemia in a case of pernicious anemia but still permit neurological symptoms to develop.	Glandular meats Yeast Green, leafy vegetables.

App. 7: Nutritive Value of Foods

QUICK VIEW OF FOOD CATEGORIES

Nutritive Value of Foods *(Continued)*

Foods, approximate measures, units, and weight (weight of edible portion only)			Water	Food energy	Protein	Fat	Saturated	Monounsaturated	Polyunsaturated
								Fatty Acids	
		Grams	*Percent*	*Calories*	*Grams*	*Grams*	*Grams*	*Grams*	*Grams*
BEVERAGES									
Alcoholic:									
Beer:									
Regular-----------	12 fl oz--------	360	92	150	1	0	0.0	0.0	0
Light-------------	12 fl oz--------	355	95	95	1	0	0.0	0.0	0.0
Gin, rum, vodka, whiskey:									
86-proof----------	1½ fl oz--------	42	64	105	0	0	0.0	0.0	0.0
Wines:									
Dessert-----------	3½ fl oz--------	103	77	140	Tr	0	0.0	0.0	0.0
Table:									
Red--------------	3½ fl oz--------	102	88	75	Tr	0	0.0	0.0	0.0
White-----------	3½ fl oz--------	102	87	80	Tr	0	0.0	0.0	0.0
Carbonated:[2]									
Club soda-----------	12 fl oz--------	355	100	0	0	0	0.0	0.0	0.0
Cola type:									
Regular-----------	12 fl oz--------	369	89	160	0	0	0.0	0.0	0.0
Diet, artificially sweetened-----------	12 fl oz--------	355	100	Tr	0	0	0.0	0.0	0.0
Ginger ale-----------	12 fl oz--------	366	91	125	0	0	0.0	0.0	0.0
Root beer-----------	12 fl oz--------	370	89	165	0	0	0.0	0.0	0.0
Coffee:									
Brewed-------------	6 fl oz---------	180	100	Tr	Tr	Tr	Tr	Tr	Tr
Instant, prepared (2 tsp powder plus 6 fl oz water)-------------	6 fl oz---------	182	99	Tr	Tr	Tr	Tr	Tr	Tr
Fruit drinks, noncarbonated:									
Canned:									
Fruit punch drink-----	6 fl oz---------	190	88	85	Tr	0	0.0	0.0	0.0
Grape drink--------	6 fl oz---------	187	86	100	Tr	0	0.0	0.0	0.0
Pineapple-grapefruit juice drink-------	6 fl oz---------	187	87	90	Tr	Tr	Tr	Tr	Tr
Fruit juices. See type under Fruits and Fruit Juices.									
Milk beverages. See Dairy Products									
Tea:									
Brewed-------------	8 fl oz---------	240	100	Tr	Tr	Tr	Tr	Tr	Tr
Instant, powder, prepared:									
Unsweetened (1 tsp powder plus 8 fl oz water)-----------	8 fl oz---------	241	100	Tr	Tr	Tr	Tr	Tr	Tr
Sweetened (3 tsp powder plus 8 fl oz water)---	8 fl oz---------	262	91	85	Tr	Tr	Tr	Tr	Tr
DAIRY PRODUCTS									
Cheese:									
Natural:									
Blue-------------	1 oz----------	28	42	100	6	8	5.3	2.2	0.2

(Tr indicates nutrient present in trace amounts.)

Nutrients in Indicated Quantity

Cho-les-terol	Carbo-hydrate	Calcium	Phos-phorus	Iron	Potas-sium	Sodium	Vitamin A value		Thiamin	Ribo-flavin	Niacin	Ascorbic acid
							(IU)	(RE)				
Milli-grams	Grams	Milli-grams	Milli-grams	Milli-grams	Milli-grams	Milli-grams	Inter-national units	Retinol equiva-lents	Milli-grams	Milli-grams	Milli-grams	Milli-grams
0	13	14	50	0.1	115	18	0	0	0.02	0.09	1.8	0
0	5	14	43	0.1	64	11	0	0	0.03	0.11	1.4	0
0	Tr	Tr	Tr	Tr	1	Tr	0	0	Tr	Tr	Tr	0
0	8	8	9	0.2	95	9	(1)	(1)	0.01	0.02	0.2	0
0	3	8	18	0.4	113	5	(1)	(1)	0.00	0.03	0.1	0
0	3	9	14	0.3	83	5	(1)	(1)	0.00	0.01	0.1	0
0	0	18	0	Tr	0	78	0	0	0.00	0.00	0.0	0
0	41	11	52	0.2	7	18	0	0	0.00	0.00	0.0	0
0	Tr	14	39	0.2	7	[3]32	0	0	0.00	0.00	0.0	0
0	32	11	0	0.1	4	29	0	0	0.00	0.00	0.0	0
0	42	15	0	0.2	4	48	0	0	0.00	0.00	0.0	0
0	Tr	4	2	Tr	124	2	0	0	0.00	0.02	0.4	0
0	1	2	6	0.1	71	Tr	0	0	0.00	0.03	0.6	0
0	22	15	2	0.4	48	15	20	2	0.03	0.04	Tr	[4]61
0	26	2	2	0.3	9	11	Tr	Tr	0.01	0.01	Tr	[4]64
0	23	13	7	0.9	97	24	60	6	0.06	0.04	0.5	[4]110
0	Tr	0	2	Tr	36	1	0	0	0.00	0.03	Tr	0
0	1	1	4	Tr	61	1	0	0	0.00	0.02	0.1	0
0	22	1	3	Tr	49	Tr	0	0	0.00	0.04	0.1	0
21	1	150	110	0.1	73	396	200	65	0.01	0.11	0.3	0

[1] indicates nutrient present in trace amounts.

Nutritive Value of Foods *(Continued)*

Foods, approximate measures, units, and weight (weight of edible portion only)		Water	Food energy	Protein	Fat	Fatty Acids Saturated	Monounsaturated	Polyunsaturated
		Grams	*Percent*	*Calories*	*Grams*	*Grams*	*Grams*	*Grams*

Foods, approximate measures, units, and weight (weight of edible portion only)		Water	Food energy	Protein	Fat	Saturated	Monounsaturated	Polyunsaturated
		Grams	*Percent*	*Calories*	*Grams*	*Grams*	*Grams*	*Grams*
DAIRY PRODUCTS—Con.								
Camembert (3 wedges per 4-oz container)- - - - -	1 wedge- - - - - - - -	38	52	115	8	9	5.8	2.7	0.3
Cheddar:								
Cut pieces- - - - - - - -	1 oz- - - - - - - - -	28	37	115	7	9	6.0	2.7	0.3
	1 in³- - - - - - - - -	17	37	70	4	6	3.6	1.6	0.2
Shredded- - - - - - - -	1 cup- - - - - - - - -	113	37	455	28	37	23.8	10.6	1.1
Cottage (curd not pressed down):								
Lowfat (2%)- - - - - - -	1 cup- - - - - - - - -	226	79	205	31	4	2.8	1.2	0.1
Uncreamed (cottage cheese dry curd, less than ½% fat)- - - - -	1 cup- - - - - - - - -	145	80	125	25	1	0.4	0.2	Tr
Cream- - - - - - - - - - - - -	1 oz- - - - - - - - -	28	54	100	2	10	6.2	2.8	0.4
Feta- - - - - - - - - - - - - -	1 oz- - - - - - - - -	28	55	75	4	6	4.2	1.3	0.2
Mozzarella, made with:								
Whole milk- - - - - - - -	1 oz- - - - - - - - - -	28	54	80	6	6	3.7	1.9	0.2
Parmesan, grated:								
Tablespoon- - - - - - - -	1 tbsp- - - - - - - -	5	18	25	2	2	1.0	0.4	Tr
Ounce- - - - - - - - - - -	1 oz- - - - - - - - - -	28	18	130	12	9	5.4	2.5	0.2
Provolone- - - - - - - - - -	1 oz- - - - - - - - - -	28	41	100	7	8	4.8	2.1	0.2
Ricotta, made with:								
Whole milk- - - - - - - -	1 cup- - - - - - - - -	246	72	430	28	32	20.4	8.9	0.9
Part skim milk- - - - -	1 cup- - - - - - - - -	246	74	340	28	19	12.1	5.7	0.6
Swiss- - - - - - - - - - - - -	1 oz- - - - - - - - - -	28	37	105	8	8	5.0	2.1	0.3
Pasteurized process cheese:								
American- - - - - - - - - -	1 oz- - - - - - - - - -	28	39	105	6	9	5.6	2.5	0.3
Swiss- - - - - - - - - - - - -	1 oz- - - - - - - - - -	28	42	95	7	7	4.5	2.0	0.2
Pasteurized process cheese food, American- - - - -	1 oz- - - - - - - - - -	28	43	95	6	7	4.4	2.0	0.2
Cream, sweet:								
Half-and-half (cream and milk)- - - - - - - - - - - - -	1 cup- - - - - - - - -	242	81	315	7	28	17.3	8.0	1.0
	1 tbsp- - - - - - - - -	15	81	20	Tr	2	1.1	0.5	0.1
Light, coffee, or table- - - -	1 cup- - - - - - - - -	240	74	470	6	46	28.8	13.4	1.7
	1 tbsp- - - - - - - - -	15	74	30	Tr	3	1.8	0.8	0.1
Whipping, unwhipped (volume about double when whipped):								
Light- - - - - - - - - - - - -	1 tbsp- - - - - - - - -	15	64	45	Tr	5	2.9	1.4	0.1
Heavy- - - - - - - - - - - - -	1 tbsp- - - - - - - - -	15	58	50	Tr	6	3.5	1.6	0.2
Whipped topping, (pressurized)- - - - - - - - - - - - -	1 tbsp- - - - - - - - -	3	61	10	Tr	1	0.4	0.2	Tr
Cream, sour- - - - - - - - - -	1 tbsp- - - - - - - - -	12	71	25	Tr	3	1.6	0.7	0.1
Cream products, imitation (made with vegetable fat):								

(Tr indicates nutrient present in trace amounts.)

2286

Cho-les-terol	Carbo-hydrate	Calcium	Phos-phorus	Iron	Potas-sium	Sodium	Vitamin A value		Thiamin	Ribo-flavin	Niacin	Ascorbic acid
							(IU)	(RE)				
Milli-grams	Grams	Milli-grams	Milli-grams	Milli-grams	Milli-grams	Milli-grams	Inter-national units	Retinol equiva-lents	Milli-grams	Milli-grams	Milli-grams	Milli-grams
27	Tr	147	132	0.1	71	320	350	96	0.01	0.19	0.2	0
30	Tr	204	145	0.2	28	176	300	86	0.01	0.11	Tr	0
18	Tr	123	87	0.1	17	105	180	52	Tr	0.06	Tr	0
119	1	815	579	0.8	111	701	1,200	342	0.03	0.42	0.1	0
19	8	155	340	0.4	217	918	160	45	0.05	0.42	0.3	Tr
10	3	46	151	0.3	47	19	40	12	0.04	0.21	0.2	0
31	1	23	30	0.3	34	84	400	124	Tr	0.06	Tr	0
25	1	140	96	0.2	18	316	130	36	0.04	0.24	0.3	0
22	1	147	105	0.1	19	106	220	68	Tr	0.07	Tr	0
4	Tr	69	40	Tr	5	93	40	9	Tr	0.02	Tr	0
22	1	390	229	0.3	30	528	200	49	0.01	0.11	0.1	0
20	1	214	141	0.1	39	248	230	75	0.01	0.09	Tr	0
124	7	509	389	0.9	257	207	1,210	330	0.03	0.48	0.3	0
76	13	669	449	1.1	307	307	1,060	278	0.05	0.46	0.2	0
26	1	272	171	Tr	31	74	240	72	0.01	0.10	Tr	0
27	Tr	174	211	0.1	46	406	340	82	0.01	0.10	Tr	0
24	1	219	216	0.2	61	388	230	65	Tr	0.08	Tr	0
18	2	163	130	0.2	79	337	260	62	0.01	0.13	Tr	0
89	10	254	230	0.2	314	98	1,050	259	0.08	0.36	0.2	2
6	1	16	14	Tr	19	6	70	16	0.01	0.02	Tr	Tr
159	9	231	192	0.1	292	95	1,730	437	0.08	0.36	0.1	2
10	1	14	12	Tr	18	6	110	27	Tr	0.02	Tr	Tr
17	Tr	10	9	Tr	15	5	170	44	Tr	0.02	Tr	Tr
21	Tr	10	9	Tr	11	6	220	63	Tr	0.02	Tr	Tr
2	Tr	3	3	Tr	4	4	30	6	Tr	Tr	Tr	0
5	1	14	10	Tr	17	6	90	23	Tr	0.02	Tr	Tr

Nutritive Value of Foods *(Continued)*

Foods, approximate measures, units, and weight (weight of edible portion only)		Water	Food energy	Pro- tein	Fat	Fatty Acids		
						Satu- rated	Mono- unsatu- rated	Poly- unsatu- rated
		Per- cent	Cal- ories	Grams	Grams	Grams	Grams	Grams
DAIRY PRODUCTS — Con.	Grams							
Sweet:								
Creamers:								
Powdered - - - - - - - - 1 tsp - - - - - - - - - -	2	2	10	Tr	1	0.7	Tr	Tr
Whipped topping:								
Frozen - - - - - - - - - - - 1 cup - - - - - - - -	75	50	240	1	19	16.3	1.2	0.4
1 tbsp - - - - - - - - -	4	50	15	Tr	1	0.9	0.1	Tr
1 tbsp - - - - - - - - -	12	75	20	Tr	2	1.6	0.2	0.1
Ice cream. See Milk desserts, frozen.								
Ice milk. See Milk desserts, frozen.								
Milk:								
Fluid:								
Whole (3.3% fat) - - - - - 1 cup - - - - - - - - -	244	88	150	8	8	5.1	2.4	0.3
Lowfat (2%):								
No milk solids added - 1 cup - - - - - - - - -	244	89	120	8	5	2.9	1.4	0.2
Lowfat (1%):								
No milk solids added - 1 cup - - - - - - - -	244	90	100	8	3	1.6	0.7	0.1
Nonfat (skim):								
No milk solids added - 1 cup - - - - - - - -	245	91	85	8	Tr	0.3	0.1	Tr
Buttermilk - - - - - - - - - 1 cup - - - - - - - -	245	90	100	8	2	1.3	0.6	0.1
Canned:								
Evaporated:								
Whole milk - - - - - - - 1 cup - - - - - - - -	252	74	340	17	19	11.6	5.9	0.6
Skim milk - - - - - - - 1 cup - - - - - - - -	255	79	200	19	1	0.3	0.2	Tr
Dried:								
Nonfat, instantized:								
Envelope, 3.2 oz, net wt.[6] - - - - - - - - - - - 1 envelope - - - - - -	91	4	325	32	1	0.4	0.2	Tr
Milk beverages:								
Chocolate milk (commer- cial):								
Regular - - - - - - - - - 1 cup - - - - - - - - -	250	82	210	8	8	5.3	2.5	0.3
Lowfat (2%) - - - - - - - 1 cup - - - - - - - - -	250	84	180	8	5	3.1	1.5	0.2
Cocoa and chocolate-flavored beverages:								
Eggnog (commercial) - - - - 1 cup - - - - - - - -	254	74	340	10	19	11.3	5.7	0.9
Malted milk:								
Chocolate:								
Powder								
Prepared (8 oz whole milk plus ¾ powder) - - - - - - - 1 serving - - - - - -	265	81	235	9	9	5.5	2.7	0.4
Shakes, thick:								
Chocolate - - - - - - - - - - 10-oz container - -	283	72	335	9	8	4.8	2.2	0.3
Vanilla - - - - - - - - - - - - 10-oz container - -	283	74	315	11	9	5.3	2.5	0.3

(Tr indicates nutrient present in trace amounts.)

Cholesterol	Carbohydrate	Calcium	Phosphorus	Iron	Potassium	Sodium	Vitamin A value		Thiamin	Riboflavin	Niacin	Ascorbic acid
							(IU)	(RE)				
Milligrams	Grams	Milligrams	Milligrams	Milligrams	Milligrams	Milligrams	International units	Retinol equivalents	Milligrams	Milligrams	Milligrams	Milligrams
0	1	Tr	8	Tr	16	4	Tr	Tr	0.00	Tr	0.0	0
0	17	5	6	0.1	14	19	[5]650	[5]65	0.00	0.00	0.0	0
0	1	Tr	Tr	Tr	1	1	[5]30	[5]3	0.00	0.00	0.0	0
1	1	14	10	Tr	19	6	Tr	Tr	Tr	0.02	Tr	Tr
33	11	291	228	0.1	370	120	310	76	0.09	0.40	0.2	2
18	12	297	232	0.1	377	122	500	139	0.10	0.40	0.2	2
10	12	300	235	0.1	381	123	500	144	0.10	0.41	0.2	2
4	12	302	247	0.1	406	126	500	149	0.09	0.34	0.2	2
9	12	285	219	0.1	371	257	80	20	0.08	0.38	0.1	2
74	25	657	510	0.5	764	267	610	136	0.12	0.80	0.5	5
9	29	738	497	0.7	845	293	1,000	298	0.11	0.79	0.4	3
17	47	1,120	896	0.3	1,552	499	[7]2,160	[7]646	0.38	1.59	0.8	5
31	26	280	251	0.6	417	149	300	73	0.09	0.41	0.3	2
17	26	284	254	0.6	422	151	500	143	0.09	0.41	0.3	2
149	34	330	278	0.5	420	138	890	203	0.09	0.48	0.3	4
34	29	304	265	0.5	500	168	330	80	0.14	0.43	0.7	2
30	60	374	357	0.9	634	314	240	59	0.13	0.63	0.4	0
33	50	413	326	0.3	517	270	320	79	0.08	0.55	0.4	0

Nutritive Value of Foods *(Continued)*

Foods, approximate measures, units, and weight (weight of edible portion only)		Water	Food energy	Pro-tein	Fat	Satu-rated	Mono-unsatu-rated	Poly-unsatu-rated
							Fatty Acids	
		Percent	*Cal-ories*	*Grams*	*Grams*	*Grams*	*Grams*	*Grams*
DAIRY PRODUCTS—Con.	*Grams*							
Milk desserts, frozen:								
Ice cream, vanilla:								
Regular (about 11% fat):								
Hardened--------- 1 cup --------	133	61	270	5	14	8.9	4.1	0.5
3 fl oz --------	50	61	100	2	5	3.4	1.6	0.2
Soft serve (frozen cus-								
tard)----------- 1 cup --------	173	60	375	7	23	13.5	6.7	1.0
Rich (about 16% fat),								
hardened-------- 1 cup --------	148	59	350	4	24	14.7	6.8	0.9
Ice milk, vanilla:								
Hardened (about								
4% fat)--------- 1 cup --------	131	69	185	5	6	3.5	1.6	0.2
Soft serve (about								
3% fat)--------- 1 cup --------	175	70	225	8	5	2.9	1.3	0.2
Sherbert (about 2% fat)-- 1 cup --------	193	66	270	2	4	2.4	1.1	0.1
Yogurt:								
With added milk solids:								
Made with lowfat milk:								
Fruit-flavored[8]----- 8-oz container---	227	74	230	10	2	1.6	0.7	0.1
Plain----------- 8-oz container---	227	85	145	12	4	2.3	1.0	0.1
Made with nonfat milk- 8-oz container--	227	85	125	13	Tr	0.3	0.1	Tr
EGGS								
Eggs, large (24 oz per dozen):								
Raw:								
Whole, without shell--- 1 egg ---------	50	75	80	6	6	1.7	2.2	0.7
White------------- 1 white--------	33	88	15	3	Tr	0.0	0.0	0.0
Yolk-------------- 1 yolk---------	17	49	65	3	6	1.7	2.2	0.7
Cooked:								
Fried in butter------- 1 egg---------	46	68	95	6	7	2.7	2.7	0.8
Hard-cooked, shell								
removed--------- 1 egg---------	50	75	80	6	6	1.7	2.2	0.7
Poached---------- 1 egg---------	50	74	80	6	6	1.7	2.2	0.7
Scrambled (milk added)								
in butter. Also omelet- 1 egg---------	64	73	110	7	8	3.2	2.9	0.8
FATS AND OILS								
Butter (4 sticks per lb):								
Tablespoon (⅛ stick)---- 1 tbsp---------	14	16	100	Tr	11	7.1	3.3	0.4
Pat (1 in square, ⅓ in high;								
90 per lb)----------- 1 pat---------	5	16	35	Tr	4	2.5	1.2	0.2
Fats, cooking (vegetable								
shortenings)--------- 1 tbsp---------	13	0	115	0	13	3.3	5.8	3.4
Lard----------------- 1 tbsp---------	13	0	115	0	13	5.1	5.9	1.5
Margarine:								
Imitation (about 40% fat),								
soft----------- 1 tbsp---------	14	58	50	Tr	5	1.1	2.2	1.9

(Tr indicates nutrient present in trace amounts.)

Nutrients in Indicated Quantity

Cholesterol	Carbohydrate	Calcium	Phosphorus	Iron	Potassium	Sodium	Vitamin A value (IU)	(RE)	Thiamin	Riboflavin	Niacin	Ascorbic acid
Milligrams	Grams	Milligrams	Milligrams	Milligrams	Milligrams	Milligrams	International units	Retinol equivalents	Milligrams	Milligrams	Milligrams	Milligrams
59	32	176	134	0.1	257	116	540	133	0.05	0.33	0.1	1
22	12	66	51	Tr	96	44	200	50	0.02	0.12	0.1	Tr
153	38	236	199	0.4	338	153	790	199	0.08	0.45	0.2	1
88	32	151	115	0.1	221	108	900	219	0.04	0.28	0.1	1
18	29	176	129	0.2	265	105	210	52	0.08	0.35	0.1	1
13	38	274	202	0.3	412	163	175	44	0.12	0.54	0.2	1
14	59	103	74	0.3	198	88	190	39	0.03	0.09	0.1	4
10	43	345	271	0.2	442	133	100	25	0.08	0.40	0.2	1
14	16	415	326	0.2	531	159	150	36	0.10	0.49	0.3	2
4	17	452	355	0.2	579	174	20	5	0.11	0.53	0.3	2
274	1	28	90	1.0	65	69	260	78	0.04	0.15	Tr	0
0	Tr	4	4	Tr	45	50	0	0	Tr	0.09	Tr	0
272	Tr	26	86	0.9	15	8	310	94	0.04	0.07	Tr	0
278	1	29	91	1.1	66	162	320	94	0.04	0.14	Tr	0
274	1	28	90	1.0	65	69	260	78	0.04	0.14	Tr	0
273	1	28	90	1.0	65	146	260	78	0.03	0.13	Tr	0
282	2	54	109	1.0	97	176	350	102	0.04	0.18	Tr	Tr
31	Tr	3	3	Tr	4	[9]116	[10]430	[10]106	Tr	Tr	Tr	0
11	Tr	1	1	Tr	1	[9]41	[10]150	[10]38	Tr	Tr	Tr	0
0	0	0	0	0.0	0	0	0	0	0.00	0.00	0.0	0
12	0	0	0	0.0	0	0	0	0	0.00	0.00	0.0	0
0	Tr	2	2	0.0	4	[11]134	[12]460	[12]139	Tr	Tr	Tr	Tr

Nutritive Value of Foods (Continued)

Foods, approximate measures, units, and weight (weight of edible portion only)			Water	Food energy	Pro-tein	Fat	Satu-rated	*Fatty Acids* Mono-unsatu-rated	Poly-unsatu-rated
		Grams	*Per-cent*	*Cal-ories*	*Grams*	*Grams*	*Grams*	*Grams*	*Grams*
FATS AND OILS—Con.									
Regular (about 80% fat):									
Hard (4 sticks per lb):									
Tablespoon (⅛ stick)-	1 tbsp- - - - - - - - -	14	16	100	Tr	11	2.2	5.0	3.6
Pat (1 in square, ⅓ in high; 90 per lb)- - - -	1 pat- - - - - - - - -	5	16	35	Tr	4	0.8	1.8	1.3
Soft- - - - - - - - - - - - - -	1 tbsp- - - - - - - - -	14	16	100	Tr	11	1.9	4.0	4.8
Spread (about 60% fat):									
Hard (4 sticks per lb):									
Tablespoon (⅛ stick)-	1 tbsp- - - - - - - - -	14	37	75	Tr	9	2.0	3.6	2.5
Pat (1 in square, ⅓ in high; 90 per lb)- - - -	1 pat- - - - - - - - -	5	37	25	Tr	3	0.7	1.3	0.9
Soft- - - - - - - - - - - - - -	8-oz container- - -	227	37	1,225	1	138	29.1	71.5	31.3
	1 tbsp- - - - - - - - -	14	37	75	Tr	9	1.8	4.4	1.9
Oils, salad or cooking:									
Corn- - - - - - - - - - - - - -	1 tbsp- - - - - - - - -	14	0	125	0	14	1.8	3.4	8.2
Olive- - - - - - - - - - - - - -	1 tbsp- - - - - - - - -	14	0	125	0	14	1.9	10.3	1.2
Peanut- - - - - - - - - - - - -	1 tbsp- - - - - - - - -	14	0	125	0	14	2.4	6.5	4.5
Safflower- - - - - - - - - - - -	1 tbsp- - - - - - - - -	14	0	125	0	14	1.3	1.7	10.4
Soybean oil, hydrogenated (partially hardened)- - -	1 tbsp- - - - - - - - -	14	0	125	0	14	2.1	6.0	5.3
Soybean-cottonseed oil blend, hydrogenated- - -	1 tbsp- - - - - - - - -	14	0	125	0	14	2.5	4.1	6.7
Sunflower- - - - - - - - - - - -	1 tbsp- - - - - - - - -	14	0	125	0	14	1.4	2.7	9.2
Salad dressings:									
Commercial:									
Blue cheese- - - - - - - - -	1 tbsp- - - - - - - - -	15	32	75	1	8	1.5	1.8	4.2
French:									
Regular- - - - - - - - - -	1 tbsp- - - - - - - - -	16	35	85	Tr	9	1.4	4.0	3.5
Low calorie- - - - - - - -	1 tbsp- - - - - - - - -	16	75	25	Tr	2	0.2	0.3	1.0
Italian:									
Regular- - - - - - - - - -	1 tbsp- - - - - - - - -	15	34	80	Tr	9	1.3	3.7	3.2
Low calorie- - - - - - - -	1 tbsp- - - - - - - - -	15	86	5	Tr	Tr	Tr	Tr	Tr
Mayonnaise:									
Regular- - - - - - - - - -	1 tbsp- - - - - - - - -	14	15	100	Tr	11	1.7	3.2	5.8
Imitation- - - - - - - - - -	1 tbsp- - - - - - - - -	15	63	35	Tr	3	0.5	0.7	1.6
Mayonnaise type- - - - -	1 tbsp- - - - - - - - -	15	40	60	Tr	5	0.7	1.4	2.7
Tartar sauce- - - - - - - -	1 tbsp- - - - - - - - -	14	34	75	Tr	8	1.2	2.6	3.9
Thousand island:									
Regular- - - - - - - - - -	1 tbsp- - - - - - - - -	16	46	60	Tr	6	1.0	1.3	3.2
Low calorie- - - - - - - -	1 tbsp- - - - - - - - -	15	69	25	Tr	2	0.2	0.4	0.9
Prepared from home recipe:									
Cooked type[13]- - - - - - -	1 tbsp- - - - - - - - -	16	69	25	1	2	0.5	0.6	0.3
FISH AND SHELLFISH									
Clams:									
Raw, meat only- - - - - - - -	3 oz- - - - - - - - - -	85	82	65	11	1	0.3	0.3	0.3
Canned, drained solids- - -	3 oz- - - - - - - - - -	85	77	85	13	2	0.5	0.5	0.4
Crabmeat, canned- - - - - - -	1 cup- - - - - - - - -	135	77	135	23	3	0.5	0.8	1.4

(Tr indicates nutrient present in trace amounts.)

Nutrients in Indicated Quantity

Cholesterol	Carbohydrate	Calcium	Phosphorus	Iron	Potassium	Sodium	Vitamin A value		Thiamin	Riboflavin	Niacin	Ascorbic acid
							(IU)	(RE)				
Milligrams	Grams	Milligrams	Milligrams	Milligrams	Milligrams	Milligrams	International units	Retinol equivalents	Milligrams	Milligrams	Milligrams	Milligrams
0	Tr	4	3	Tr	6	[11]132	[12]460	[12]139	Tr	0.01	Tr	Tr
0	Tr	1	1	Tr	2	[11]47	[12]170	[12]50	Tr	Tr	Tr	Tr
0	Tr	4	3	0.0	5	[11]151	[12]460	[12]139	Tr	Tr	Tr	Tr
0	0	3	2	0.0	4	[11]139	[12]460	[12]139	Tr	Tr	Tr	Tr
0	0	1	1	0.0	1	[11]50	[12]170	[12]50	Tr	Tr	Tr	Tr
0	0	47	37	0.0	68	[11]2,256	[12]7,510	[12]2,254	0.02	0.06	Tr	Tr
0	0	3	2	0.0	4	[11]139	[12]460	[12]139	Tr	Tr	Tr	Tr
0	0	0	0	0.0	0	0	0	0	0.00	0.00	0.0	0
0	0	0	0	0.0	0	0	0	0	0.00	0.00	0.0	0
0	0	0	0	0.0	0	0	0	0	0.00	0.00	0.0	0
0	0	0	0	0.0	0	0	0	0	0.00	0.00	0.0	0
0	0	0	0	0.0	0	0	0	0	0.00	0.00	0.0	0
0	0	0	0	0.0	0	0	0	0	0.00	0.00	0.0	0
0	0	0	0	0.0	0	0	0	0	0.00	0.00	0.0	0
3	1	12	11	Tr	6	164	30	10	Tr	0.02	Tr	Tr
0	1	2	1	Tr	2	188	Tr	Tr	Tr	Tr	Tr	Tr
0	2	6	5	Tr	3	306	Tr	Tr	Tr	Tr	Tr	Tr
0	1	1	1	Tr	5	162	30	3	Tr	Tr	Tr	Tr
0	2	1	1	Tr	4	136	Tr	Tr	Tr	Tr	Tr	Tr
8	Tr	3	4	0.1	5	80	40	12	0.00	0.00	Tr	0
4	2	Tr	Tr	0.0	2	75	0	0	0.00	0.00	Tr	0
4	4	2	4	Tr	1	107	30	13	Tr	Tr	Tr	0
4	1	3	4	0.1	11	182	30	9	Tr	Tr	0.0	Tr
4	2	2	3	0.1	18	112	50	15	Tr	Tr	Tr	Tr
2	2	2	3	0.1	17	150	50	14	Tr	Tr	Tr	0
9	2	13	14	0.1	19	117	70	20	0.01	0.02	Tr	Tr
43	2	59	138	2.6	154	102	90	26	0.09	0.15	1.1	9
54	2	47	116	3.5	119	102	90	26	0.01	0.09	0.9	3
135	1	61	246	1.1	149	1,350	50	14	0.11	0.11	2.6	0

Foods, approximate measures, units, and weight (weight of edible portion only)		Water	Food energy	Pro- tein	Fat	Fatty Acids		
						Satu- rated	Mono- unsatu- rated	Poly- unsatu- rated
FISH AND SHELLFISH—Con.	Grams	Per- cent	Cal- ories	Grams	Grams	Grams	Grams	Grams
Fish sticks, frozen, reheated, (stick, 4 by 1 by ½ in)- -	1 fish stick- - - - -	28	52	70	6	3	0.8	1.4	0.8
Flounder or Sole, baked, with lemon juice:									
With butter- - - - - - - - -	3 oz- - - - - - - - - -	85	73	120	16	6	3.2	1.5	0.5
With margarine- - - - - - - -	3 oz- - - - - - - - - -	85	73	120	16	6	1.2	2.3	1.9
Without added fat- - - - - -	3 oz- - - - - - - - - -	85	78	80	17	1	0.3	0.2	0.4
Haddock, breaded, fried[14]- - -	3 oz- - - - - - - - - -	85	61	175	17	9	2.4	3.9	2.4
Halibut, broiled, with butter and lemon juice- - - - - -	3 oz- - - - - - - - - -	85	67	140	20	6	3.3	1.6	0.7
Herring, pickled- - - - - - - - -	3 oz- - - - - - - - - -	85	59	190	17	13	4.3	4.6	3.1
Ocean perch, breaded, fried[14]	1 fillet - - - - - - - -	85	59	185	16	11	2.6	4.6	2.8
Oysters:									
Raw, meat only (13–19 me- dium Selects)- - - - - - - -	1 cup- - - - - - - - -	240	85	160	20	4	1.4	0.5	1.4
Breaded, fried[14]- - - - - - - -	1 oyster- - - - - -	45	65	90	5	5	1.4	2.1	1.4
Salmon:									
Canned (pink), solids and liquid- - - - - - - - - - - - -	3 oz- - - - - - - - - -	85	71	120	17	5	0.9	1.5	2.1
Baked (red)- - - - - - - - - - -	3 oz- - - - - - - - - -	85	67	140	21	5	1.2	2.4	1.4
Smoked- - - - - - - - - - - - -	3 oz- - - - - - - - - -	85	59	150	18	8	2.6	3.9	0.7
Sardines, Atlantic, canned in oil, drained solids- - - - -	3 oz- - - - - - - - - -	85	62	175	20	9	2.1	3.7	2.9
Scallops, breaded, frozen, re- heated- - - - - - - - - - - - -	6 scallops- - - - - -	90	59	195	15	10	2.5	4.1	2.5
Shrimp:									
Canned, drained solids- - -	3 oz- - - - - - - - - -	85	70	100	21	1	0.2	0.2	0.4
French fried (7 medium)[16]-	3 oz- - - - - - - - - -	85	55	200	16	10	2.5	4.1	2.6
Trout, broiled, with butter and lemon juice- - - - - - - -	3 oz- - - - - - - - - -	85	63	175	21	9	4.1	2.9	1.6
Tuna, canned, drained solids:									
Oil pack, chunk light- - - -	3 oz- - - - - - - - - -	85	61	165	24	7	1.4	1.9	3.1
Water pack, solid white- -	3 oz- - - - - - - - - -	85	63	135	30	1	0.3	0.2	0.3
Tuna salad[17]- - - - - - - - - - -	1 cup- - - - - - - - -	205	63	375	33	19	3.3	4.9	9.2
FRUITS AND FRUIT JUICES									
Apples:									
Raw:									
Unpeeled, without cores:									
2¾-in diam. (about 3 per lb with cores)- -	1 apple- - - - - - -	138	84	80	Tr	Tr	0.1	Tr	0.1
3¼-in diam. (about 2 per lb with cores)- -	1 apple- - - - - - -	212	84	125	Tr	1	0.1	Tr	0.2
Dried, sulfured- - - - - - - -	10 rings- - - - - -	64	32	155	1	Tr	Tr	Tr	0.1
Apple juice, bottled or canned[19]- - - - - - - - - - -	1 cup- - - - - - - - -	248	88	115	Tr	Tr	Tr	Tr	0.1
Applesauce, canned:									
Sweetened- - - - - - - - - - -	1 cup- - - - - - - - -	255	80	195	Tr	Tr	0.1	Tr	0.1

(Tr indicates nutrient present in trace amounts.)

Nutrients in Indicated Quantity

Cho-les-terol	Carbo-hydrate	Calcium	Phos-phorus	Iron	Potas-sium	Sodium	Vitamin A value		Thiamin	Ribo-flavin	Niacin	Ascorbic acid
							(IU)	(RE)				
Milli-grams	Grams	Milli-grams	Milli-grams	Milli-grams	Milli-grams	Milli-grams	Inter-national units	Retinol equiva-lents	Milli-grams	Milli-grams	Milli-grams	Milli-grams
26	4	11	58	0.3	94	53	20	5	0.03	0.05	0.6	0
68	Tr	13	187	0.3	272	145	210	54	0.05	0.08	1.6	1
55	Tr	14	187	0.3	273	151	230	69	0.05	0.08	1.6	1
59	Tr	13	197	0.3	286	101	30	10	0.05	0.08	1.7	1
75	7	34	183	1.0	270	123	70	20	0.06	0.10	2.9	0
62	Tr	14	206	0.7	441	103	610	174	0.06	0.07	7.7	1
85	0	29	128	0.9	85	850	110	33	0.04	0.18	2.8	0
66	7	31	191	1.2	241	138	70	20	0.10	0.11	2.0	0
120	8	226	343	15.6	290	175	740	223	0.34	0.43	6.0	24
35	5	49	73	3.0	64	70	150	44	0.07	0.10	1.3	4
34	0	[15]167	243	0.7	307	443	60	18	0.03	0.15	6.8	0
60	0	26	269	0.5	305	55	290	87	0.18	0.14	5.5	0
51	0	12	208	0.8	327	1,700	260	77	0.17	0.17	6.8	0
85	0	[15]371	424	2.6	349	425	190	56	0.03	0.17	4.6	0
70	10	39	203	2.0	369	298	70	21	0.11	0.11	1.6	0
128	1	98	224	1.4	104	1,955	50	15	0.01	0.03	1.5	0
168	11	61	154	2.0	189	384	90	26	0.06	0.09	2.8	0
71	Tr	26	259	1.0	297	122	230	60	0.07	0.07	2.3	1
55	0	7	199	1.6	298	303	70	20	0.04	0.09	10.1	0
48	0	17	202	0.6	255	468	110	32	0.03	0.10	13.4	0
80	19	31	281	2.5	531	877	230	53	0.06	0.14	13.3	6
0	21	10	10	0.2	159	Tr	70	7	0.02	0.02	0.1	8
0	32	15	15	0.4	244	Tr	110	11	0.04	0.03	0.2	12
0	42	9	24	0.9	288	[18]56	0	0	0.00	0.10	0.6	2
0	29	17	17	0.9	295	7	Tr	Tr	0.05	0.04	0.2	[20]2
0	51	10	18	0.9	156	8	30	3	0.03	0.07	0.5	[20]4

Nutritive Value of Foods (Continued)

Foods, approximate measures, units, and weight (weight of edible portion only)			Water	Food energy	Pro-tein	Fat	Satu-rated	Mono-unsatu-rated	Poly-unsatu-rated
								Fatty Acids	
		Grams	Per-cent	Cal-ories	Grams	Grams	Grams	Grams	Grams

FRUITS AND FRUIT JUICES—Con.									
Unsweetened	1 cup	244	88	105	Tr	Tr	Tr	Tr	Tr
Apricots:									
Raw, without pits (about 12 per lb with pits)	3 apricots	106	86	50	1	Tr	Tr	0.2	0.1
Canned (fruit and liquid):									
Heavy syrup pack	3 halves	85	78	70	Tr	Tr	Tr	Tr	Tr
Juice pack	3 halves	84	87	40	1	Tr	Tr	Tr	Tr
Dried:									
Uncooked (28 large or 37 medium halves per cup)	1 cup	130	31	310	5	1	Tr	0.3	0.1
Cooked, unsweetened, fruit and liquid	1 cup	250	76	210	3	Tr	Tr	0.2	0.1
Apricot nectar, canned	1 cup	251	85	140	1	Tr	Tr	0.1	Tr
Avocados, raw, whole, without skin and seed:									
California (about 2 per lb with skin and seed)	1 avocado	173	73	305	4	30	4.5	19.4	3.5
Florida (about 1 per lb with skin and seed)	1 avocado	304	80	340	5	27	5.3	14.8	4.5
Bananas, raw, without peel:									
Whole (about 2½ per lb with peel)	1 banana	114	74	105	1	1	0.2	Tr	0.1
Sliced	1 cup	150	74	140	2	1	0.3	0.1	0.1
Blackberries, raw	1 cup	144	86	75	1	1	0.2	0.1	0.1
Blueberries:									
Raw	1 cup	145	85	80	1	1	Tr	0.1	0.3
Frozen, sweetened	10-oz container	284	77	230	1	Tr	Tr	0.1	0.2
	1 cup	230	77	185	1	Tr	Tr	Tr	0.1
Cantaloup. See Melons.									
Cherries:									
Sour, red, pitted, canned, water pack	1 cup	244	90	90	2	Tr	0.1	0.1	0.1
Sweet, raw, without pits and stems	10 cherries	68	81	50	1	1	0.1	0.2	0.2
Cranberry juice cocktail, bottled, sweetened	1 cup	253	85	145	Tr	Tr	Tr	Tr	0.1
Cranberry sauce, sweetened, canned, strained	1 cup	277	61	420	1	Tr	Tr	0.1	0.2
Dates:									
Whole, without pits	10 dates	83	23	230	2	Tr	0.1	0.1	Tr
Figs, dried	10 figs	187	28	475	6	2	0.4	0.5	1.0
Fruit cocktail, canned, fruit and liquid:									
Heavy syrup pack	1 cup	255	80	185	1	Tr	Tr	Tr	0.1
Juice pack	1 cup	248	87	115	1	Tr	Tr	Tr	Tr

(Tr indicates nutrient present in trace amounts.)

Cho-les-terol	Carbo-hydrate	Calcium	Phos-phorus	Iron	Potas-sium	Sodium	Vitamin A value		Thiamin	Ribo-flavin	Niacin	Ascorbic acid
							(IU)	(RE)				
Milli-grams	Grams	Milli-grams	Milli-grams	Milli-grams	Milli-grams	Milli-grams	Inter-national units	Retinol equiva-lents	Milli-grams	Milli-grams	Milli-grams	Milli-grams
0	28	7	17	0.3	183	5	70	7	0.03	0.06	0.5	[20]3
0	12	15	20	0.6	314	1	2,770	277	0.03	0.04	0.6	11
0	18	8	10	0.3	119	3	1,050	105	0.02	0.02	0.3	3
0	10	10	17	0.3	139	3	1,420	142	0.02	0.02	0.3	4
0	80	59	152	6.1	1,791	13	9,410	941	0.01	0.20	3.9	3
0	55	40	103	4.2	1,222	8	5,910	591	0.02	0.08	2.4	4
0	36	18	23	1.0	286	8	3,300	330	0.02	0.04	0.7	[20]2
0	12	19	73	2.0	1,097	21	1,060	106	0.19	0.21	3.3	14
0	27	33	119	1.6	1,484	15	1,860	186	0.33	0.37	5.8	24
0	27	7	23	0.4	451	1	90	9	0.05	0.11	0.6	10
0	35	9	30	0.5	594	2	120	12	0.07	0.15	0.8	14
0	18	46	30	0.8	282	Tr	240	24	0.04	0.06	0.6	30
0	20	9	15	0.2	129	9	150	15	0.07	0.07	0.5	19
0	62	17	20	1.1	170	3	120	12	0.06	0.15	0.7	3
0	50	14	16	0.9	138	2	100	10	0.05	0.12	0.6	2
0	22	27	24	3.3	239	17	1,840	184	0.04	0.10	0.4	5
0	11	10	13	0.3	152	Tr	150	15	0.03	0.04	0.3	5
0	38	8	3	0.4	61	10	10	1	0.01	0.04	0.1	[21]108
0	108	11	17	0.6	72	80	60	6	0.04	0.06	0.3	6
0	61	27	33	1.0	541	2	40	4	0.07	0.08	1.8	0
0	122	269	127	4.2	1,331	21	250	25	0.13	0.16	1.3	1
0	48	15	28	0.7	224	15	520	52	0.05	0.05	1.0	5
0	29	20	35	0.5	236	10	760	76	0.03	0.04	1.0	7

Nutritive Value of Foods *(Continued)*

Foods, approximate measures, units, and weight (weight of edible portion only)		Water	Food energy	Protein	Fat	Fatty Acids		
						Saturated	Mono-unsaturated	Poly-unsaturated
	Grams	Per cent	Calories	Grams	Grams	Grams	Grams	Grams
FRUITS AND FRUIT JUICES—Con.								
Grapefruit:								
Raw, without peel, membrane and seeds (3¾-in diam., 1 lb 1 oz, whole, with refuse)- - - - - - - - ½ grapefruit- - - -	120	91	40	1	Tr	Tr	Tr	Tr
Canned, sections with syrup)- - - - - - - - - - - - 1 cup- - - - - - - - -	254	84	150	1	Tr	Tr	Tr	0.1
Grapefruit juice:								
Raw- - - - - - - - - - - - - - - - 1 cup- - - - - - - - -	247	90	95	1	Tr	Tr	Tr	0.1
Canned:								
Unsweetened- - - - - - - - 1 cup- - - - - - - - -	247	90	95	1	Tr	Tr	Tr	0.1
Frozen concentrate, unsweetened								
Diluted with 3 parts water by volume- - - - - - - - - 1 cup- - - - - - - - -	247	89	100	1	Tr	Tr	Tr	0.1
Grapes, European type (adherent skin), raw:								
Thompson Seedless- - - - - 10 grapes- - - - - - -	50	81	35	Tr	Tr	0.1	Tr	0.1
Tokay and Emperor, seeded types- - - - - - - - - - - - - - 10 grapes- - - - - - -	57	81	40	Tr	Tr	0.1	Tr	0.1
Grape juice:								
Canned or bottled- - - - - - 1 cup- - - - - - - - -	253	84	155	1	Tr	0.1	Tr	0.1
Kiwifruit, raw, without skin (about 5 per lb with skin)- 1 kiwifruit- - - - -	76	83	45	1	Tr	Tr	0.1	0.1
Lemons, raw, without peel and seeds (about 4 per lb with peel and seeds)- - - - - - - - 1 lemon- - - - - - -	58	89	15	1	Tr	Tr	Tr	0.1
Lemon juice:								
Raw- - - - - - - - - - - - - - - - 1 cup- - - - - - - - -	244	91	60	1	Tr	Tr	Tr	Tr
Canned or bottled, unsweetened- - - - - - - - - - - - - - 1 cup- - - - - - - - -	244	92	50	1	1	0.1	Tr	0.2
1 tbsp- - - - - - - - -	15	92	5	Tr	Tr	Tr	Tr	Tr
Lime juice:								
Raw- - - - - - - - - - - - - - - - 1 cup- - - - - - - - -	246	90	65	1	Tr	Tr	Tr	0.1
Canned, unsweetened- - - - 1 cup- - - - - - - - -	246	93	50	1	1	0.1	0.1	0.2
Mangos, raw, without skin and seed (about 1½ per lb with skin and seed)- - - - 1 mango- - - - - - -	207	82	135	1	1	0.1	0.2	0.1
Melons, raw, without rind and cavity contents:								
Cantaloup, orange-fleshed (5-in diam., 2⅓ lb, whole, with rind and cavity contents)- - - - - - - - - - - - - ½ melon- - - - - - -	267	90	95	2	1	0.1	0.1	0.3
Honeydew (6½-in diam., 5¼ lb, whole, with rind and cavity contents)- - - - - - ⅒ melon- - - - - - -	129	90	45	1	Tr	Tr	Tr	0.1

(Tr indicates nutrient present in trace amounts.)

Nutrients in Indicated Quantity

Cholesterol	Carbohydrate	Calcium	Phosphorus	Iron	Potassium	Sodium	Vitamin A value		Thiamin	Riboflavin	Niacin	Ascorbic acid
							(IU)	(RE)				
Milligrams	Grams	Milligrams	Milligrams	Milligrams	Milligrams	Milligrams	International units	Retinol equivalents	Milligrams	Milligrams	Milligrams	Milligrams
0	10	14	10	0.1	167	Tr	[22]10	[22]1	0.04	0.02	0.3	41
0	39	36	25	1.0	328	5	Tr	Tr	0.10	0.05	0.6	54
0	23	22	37	0.5	400	2	20	2	0.10	0.05	0.5	94
0	22	17	27	0.5	378	2	20	2	0.10	0.05	0.6	72
0	24	20	35	0.3	336	2	20	2	0.10	0.05	0.5	83
0	9	6	7	0.1	93	1	40	4	0.05	0.03	0.2	5
0	10	6	7	0.1	105	1	40	4	0.05	0.03	0.2	6
0	38	23	28	0.6	334	8	20	2	0.07	0.09	0.7	[20]Tr
0	11	20	30	0.3	252	4	130	13	0.02	0.04	0.4	74
0	5	15	9	0.3	80	1	20	2	0.02	0.01	0.1	31
0	21	17	15	0.1	303	2	50	5	0.07	0.02	0.2	112
0	16	27	22	0.3	249	[23]51	40	4	0.10	0.02	0.5	61
0	1	2	1	Tr	15	[23]3	Tr	Tr	0.01	Tr	Tr	4
0	22	22	17	0.1	268	2	20	2	0.05	0.02	0.2	72
0	16	30	25	0.6	185	[23]39	40	4	0.08	0.01	0.4	16
0	35	21	23	0.3	323	4	8,060	806	0.12	0.12	1.2	57
0	22	29	45	0.6	825	24	8,610	861	0.10	0.06	1.5	113
0	12	8	13	0.1	350	13	50	5	0.10	0.02	0.8	32

Nutritive Value of Foods *(Continued)*

Foods, approximate measures, units, and weight (weight of edible portion only)		Water	Food energy	Pro-tein	Fat	Fatty Acids		
						Satu-rated	Mono-unsatu-rated	Poly-unsatu-rated
FRUITS AND FRUIT JUICES—Con.		*Grams*	*Per-cent*	*Cal-ories*	*Grams*	*Grams*	*Grams*	*Grams*
Nectarines, raw, without pits (about 3 per lb with pits)	1 nectarine-----	136	86	65	1	1	0.1	0.2	0.3
Oranges, raw:									
Whole, without peel and seeds (2⅝-in diam., about 2½ per lb, with peel and seeds)------------	1 orange-------	131	87	60	1	Tr	Tr	Tr	Tr
Orange juice:									
Raw, all varieties-------	1 cup--------	248	88	110	2	Tr	0.1	0.1	0.1
Canned, unsweetened----	1 cup--------	249	89	105	1	Tr	Tr	0.1	0.1
Chilled-------------	1 cup--------	249	88	110	2	1	0.1	0.1	0.2
Frozen concentrate:									
Diluted with 3 parts water by volume--------	1 cup--------	249	88	110	2	Tr	Tr	Tr	Tr
Orange and grapefruit juice, canned-------------	1 cup--------	247	89	105	1	Tr	Tr	Tr	Tr
Papayas, raw, ½-in cubes---	1 cup--------	140	86	65	1	Tr	0.1	0.1	Tr
Peaches:									
Raw: Whole, 2½-in diam., peeled, pitted (about 4 per lb with peels and pits)-----------	1 peach--------	87	88	35	1	Tr	Tr	Tr	Tr
Canned, fruit and liquid:									
Heavy syrup pack-----	1 half---------	81	79	60	Tr	Tr	Tr	Tr	Tr
Juice pack----------	1 half---------	77	87	35	Tr	Tr	Tr	Tr	Tr
Dried:									
Uncooked----------	1 cup--------	160	32	380	6	1	0.1	0.4	0.6
Cooked, unsweetened, fruit and liquid-----	1 cup--------	258	78	200	3	1	0.1	0.2	0.3
Frozen, sliced, sweetened-	10-oz container--	284	75	265	2	Tr	Tr	0.1	0.2
	1 cup--------	250	75	235	2	Tr	Tr	0.1	0.2
Pears:									
Raw, with skin, cored:									
Bartlett, 2½-in diam. (about 2½ per lb with cores and stems)----	1 pear---------	166	84	100	1	1	Tr	0.1	0.2
Bosc, 2½-in diam. (about 3 per lb with cores and stems)-----------	1 pear---------	141	84	85	1	1	Tr	0.1	0.1
D'Anjou, 3-in diam. (about 2 per lb with cores and stems)----	1 pear---------	200	84	120	1	1	Tr	0.2	0.2
Canned, fruit and liquid:									
Heavy syrup pack-----	1 half---------	79	80	60	Tr	Tr	Tr	Tr	Tr
Juice pack----------	1 half---------	77	86	40	Tr	Tr	Tr	Tr	Tr
Pineapple:									
Raw, diced----------	1 cup--------	155	87	75	1	1	Tr	0.1	0.2

(Tr indicates nutrient present in trace amounts.)

Nutrients in Indicated Quantity

Cho-les-terol	Carbo-hydrate	Calcium	Phos-phorus	Iron	Potas-sium	Sodium	Vitamin A value		Thiamin	Ribo-flavin	Niacin	Ascorbic acid
							(IU)	(RE)				
Milli-grams	Grams	Milli-grams	Milli-grams	Milli-grams	Milli-grams	Milli-grams	Inter-national units	Retinol equiva-lents	Milli-grams	Milli-grams	Milli-grams	Milli-grams
0	16	7	22	0.2	288	Tr	1,000	100	0.02	0.06	1.3	7
0	15	52	18	0.1	237	Tr	270	27	0.11	0.05	0.4	70
0	26	27	42	0.5	496	2	500	50	0.22	0.07	1.0	124
0	25	20	35	1.1	436	5	440	44	0.15	0.07	0.8	86
0	25	25	27	0.4	473	2	190	19	0.28	0.05	0.7	82
0	27	22	40	0.2	473	2	190	19	0.20	0.04	0.5	97
0	25	20	35	1.1	390	7	290	29	0.14	0.07	0.8	72
0	17	35	12	0.3	247	9	400	40	0.04	0.04	0.5	92
0	10	4	10	0.1	171	Tr	470	47	0.01	0.04	0.9	6
0	16	2	9	0.2	75	5	270	27	0.01	0.02	0.5	2
0	9	5	13	0.2	99	3	290	29	0.01	0.01	0.4	3
0	98	45	190	6.5	1,594	11	3,460	346	Tr	0.34	7.0	8
0	51	23	98	3.4	826	5	510	51	0.01	0.05	3.9	10
0	68	9	31	1.1	369	17	810	81	0.04	0.10	1.9	[21]268
0	60	8	28	0.9	325	15	710	71	0.03	0.09	1.6	[21]236
0	25	18	18	0.4	208	Tr	30	3	0.03	0.07	0.2	7
0	21	16	16	0.4	176	Tr	30	3	0.03	0.06	0.1	6
0	30	22	22	0.5	250	Tr	40	4	0.04	0.08	0.2	8
0	15	4	6	0.2	51	4	Tr	Tr	0.01	0.02	0.2	1
0	10	7	9	0.2	74	3	Tr	Tr	0.01	0.01	0.2	1
0	19	11	11	0.6	175	2	40	4	0.14	0.06	0.7	24

Foods, approximate measures, units, and weight (weight of edible portion only)		Water	Food energy	Pro-tein	Fat	Fatty Acids		
						Satu-rated	Mono-unsatu-rated	Poly-unsatu-rated
		Per-cent	*Cal-ories*	*Grams*	*Grams*	*Grams*	*Grams*	*Grams*
FRUITS AND FRUIT JUICES—Con.	*Grams*							
Canned, fruit and liquid:								
Heavy syrup pack:								
Slices- - - - - - - - - - - -	1 slice- - - - - - - - -	58	79	45	Tr	Tr	Tr	Tr	Tr
Juice pack:								
Slices- - - - - - - - - - - -	1 slice- - - - - - - - -	58	84	35	Tr	Tr	Tr	Tr	Tr
Pineapple juice, unsweetened, canned- - - - - - - - - - - - - -	1 cup- - - - - - - - -	250	86	140	1	Tr	Tr	Tr	0.1
Plantains, without peel:								
Cooked, boiled, sliced- - - -	1 cup- - - - - - - - -	154	67	180	1	Tr	0.1	Tr	0.1
Plums, without pits:								
Raw:								
2⅛-in diam. (about 6½ per lb with pits)- - - - - - -	1 plum- - - - - - - -	66	85	35	1	Tr	Tr	0.3	0.1
1½-in diam. (about 15 per lb with pits)- - - - - - -	1 plum- - - - - - - -	28	85	15	Tr	Tr	Tr	0.1	Tr
Canned, purple, fruit and liquid:								
Heavy syrup pack- - - - -	3 plums- - - - - - - -	133	76	120	Tr	Tr	Tr	0.1	Tr
Juice pack- - - - - - - - - -	3 plums- - - - - - - -	95	84	55	Tr	Tr	Tr	Tr	Tr
Prunes, dried:								
Uncooked- - - - - - - - - - - -	4 extra large or 5 large prunes- - -	49	32	115	1	Tr	Tr	0.2	0.1
Cooked, unsweetened, fruit and liquid- - - - - - - - - -	1 cup- - - - - - - - -	212	70	225	2	Tr	Tr	0.3	0.1
Prune juice, canned or bottled- - - - - - - - - - -	1 cup- - - - - - - - -	256	81	180	2	Tr	Tr	0.1	0.1
Raisins, seedless:								
Cup, not pressed down- - -	1 cup- - - - - - - - -	145	15	435	5	1	0.2	Tr	0.2
Packet, ½ oz (1½ tbsp)- - -	1 packet- - - - - - -	14	15	40	Tr	Tr	Tr	Tr	Tr
Raspberries:								
Raw- - - - - - - - - - - - - - -	1 cup- - - - - - - - -	123	87	60	1	1	Tr	0.1	0.4
Frozen, sweetened- - - - - -	10-oz container- -	284	73	295	2	Tr	Tr	Tr	0.3
Rhubarb, cooked, added sugar- - - - - - - - -	1 cup- - - - - - - - -	240	68	280	1	Tr	Tr	Tr	0.1
Strawberries:								
Raw, capped, whole- - - - -	1 cup- - - - - - - - -	149	92	45	1	1	Tr	0.1	0.3
Frozen, sweetened, sliced-	10-oz container- -	284	73	275	2	Tr	Tr	0.1	0.2
	1 cup- - - - - - - - -	255	73	245	1	Tr	Tr	Tr	0.2
Tangerines:								
Raw, without peel and seeds (2⅜-in diam., about 4 per lb, with peel and seeds)-	1 tangerine- - - - -	84	88	35	1	Tr	Tr	Tr	Tr
Watermelon, raw, without rind and seeds:								
Piece (4 by 8 in wedge with rind and seeds; 1/16 of 32⅜-lb melon, 10 by 16 in)- -	1 piece- - - - - - - -	482	92	155	3	2	0.3	0.2	1.0

(Tr indicates nutrient present in trace amounts.)

Nutrients in Indicated Quantity

Cho-les-terol	Carbo-hydrate	Calcium	Phos-phorus	Iron	Potas-sium	Sodium	Vitamin A value (IU)	(RE)	Thiamin	Ribo-flavin	Niacin	Ascorbic acid
Milli-grams	Grams	Milli-grams	Milli-grams	Milli-grams	Milli-grams	Milli-grams	Inter-national units	Retinol equiva-lents	Milli-grams	Milli-grams	Milli-grams	Milli-grams
0	12	8	4	0.2	60	1	10	1	0.05	0.01	0.2	4
0	9	8	3	0.2	71	1	20	2	0.06	0.01	0.2	6
0	34	43	20	0.7	335	3	10	1	0.14	0.06	0.6	27
0	48	3	43	0.9	716	8	1,400	140	0.07	0.08	1.2	17
0	9	3	7	0.1	114	Tr	210	21	0.03	0.06	0.3	6
0	4	1	3	Tr	48	Tr	90	9	0.01	0.03	0.1	3
0	31	12	17	1.1	121	25	340	34	0.02	0.05	0.4	1
0	14	10	14	0.3	146	1	960	96	0.02	0.06	0.4	3
0	31	25	39	1.2	365	2	970	97	0.04	0.08	1.0	2
0	60	49	74	2.4	708	4	650	65	0.05	0.21	1.5	6
0	45	31	64	3.0	707	10	10	1	0.04	0.18	2.0	10
0	115	71	141	3.0	1,089	17	10	1	0.23	0.13	1.2	5
0	11	7	14	0.3	105	2	Tr	Tr	0.02	0.01	0.1	Tr
0	14	27	15	0.7	187	Tr	160	16	0.04	0.11	1.1	31
0	74	43	48	1.8	324	3	170	17	0.05	0.13	0.7	47
0	75	348	19	0.5	230	2	170	17	0.04	0.06	0.5	8
0	10	21	28	0.6	247	1	40	4	0.03	0.10	0.3	84
0	74	31	37	1.7	278	9	70	7	0.05	0.14	1.1	118
0	66	28	33	1.5	250	8	60	6	0.04	0.13	1.0	106
0	9	12	8	0.1	132	1	770	77	0.09	0.02	0.1	26
0	35	39	43	0.8	559	10	1,760	176	0.39	0.10	1.0	46

Nutritive Value of Foods *(Continued)*

Foods, approximate measures, units, and weight (weight of edible portion only)		Water	Food energy	Pro-tein	Fat	Fatty Acids		
						Satu-rated	Mono-unsatu-rated	Poly-unsatu-rated
		Grams	Per-cent	Cal-ories	Grams	Grams	Grams	Grams	Grams

		Grams	*Per-cent*	*Cal-ories*	*Grams*	*Grams*	*Grams*	*Grams*	*Grams*
GRAIN PRODUCTS									
Bagels, plain or water, enriched, 3½-in diam.[24]	1 bagel	68	29	200	7	2	0.3	0.5	0.7
Barley, pearled, light, uncooked	1 cup	200	11	700	16	2	0.3	0.2	0.9
Biscuits, baking powder, 2-in diam. (enriched flour, vegetable shortening):									
From home recipe	1 biscuit	28	28	100	2	5	1.2	2.0	1.3
Breadcrumbs, enriched: Soft. See White bread.									
Breads:									
Boston brown bread, canned, slice, 3¼ in by ½ in[25]	1 slice	45	45	95	2	1	0.3	0.1	0.1
Cracked-wheat bread (¾ enriched wheat flour, ¼ cracked wheat flour):[25]									
Slice (18 per loaf)	1 slice	25	35	65	2	1	0.2	0.2	0.3
French or vienna bread, enriched:[25] Slice:									
French, 5 by 2½ by 1 in	1 slice	35	34	100	3	1	0.3	0.4	0.5
Vienna, 4¾ by 4 by ½ in	1 slice	25	34	70	2	1	0.2	0.3	0.3
Italian bread, enriched:									
Slice, 4½ by 3¼ by ¾ in	1 slice	30	32	85	3	Tr	Tr	Tr	0.1
Mixed grain bread, enriched:[25]									
Slice (18 per loaf)	1 slice	25	37	65	2	1	0.2	0.2	0.4
Oatmeal bread, enriched:[25]									
Slice (18 per loaf)	1 slice	25	37	65	2	1	0.2	0.4	0.5
Pita bread, enriched, white, 6½-in diam.	1 pita	60	31	165	6	1	0.1	0.1	0.4
Pumpernickel (⅔ rye flour, ⅓ enriched wheat flour):[25]									
Slice, 5 by 4 by ⅜ in	1 slice	32	37	80	3	1	0.2	0.3	0.5
Raisin bread, enriched:[25]									
Slice (18 per loaf)	1 slice	25	33	65	2	1	0.2	0.3	0.4
Rye bread, light (⅔ enriched wheat flour, ⅓ rye flour):[25]									
Slice, 4¾ by 3¾ by ⁷⁄₁₆ in	1 slice	25	37	65	2	1	0.2	0.3	0.3
Wheat bread, enriched:[25]									
Slice (18 per loaf)	1 slice	25	37	65	2	1	0.2	0.4	0.3

(Tr indicates nutrient present in trace amounts.)

Nutrients in Indicated Quantity

Cho-les-terol	Carbo-hydrate	Calcium	Phos-phorus	Iron	Potas-sium	Sodium	Vitamin A value		Thiamin	Ribo-flavin	Niacin	Ascorbic acid
							(IU)	(RE)				
Milli-grams	Grams	Milli-grams	Milli-grams	Milli-grams	Milli-grams	Milli-grams	Inter-national units	Retinol equiva-lents	Milli-grams	Milli-grams	Milli-grams	Milli-grams
0	38	29	46	1.8	50	245	0	0	0.26	0.20	2.4	0
0	158	32	378	4.2	320	6	0	0	0.24	0.10	6.2	0
Tr	13	47	36	0.7	32	195	10	3	0.08	0.08	0.8	Tr
3	21	41	72	0.9	131	113	[26]0	[26]0	0.06	0.04	0.7	0
0	12	16	32	0.7	34	106	Tr	Tr	0.10	0.09	0.8	Tr
0	18	39	30	1.1	32	203	Tr	Tr	0.16	0.12	1.4	Tr
0	13	28	21	0.8	23	145	Tr	Tr	0.12	0.09	1.0	Tr
0	17	5	23	0.8	22	176	0	0	0.12	0.07	1.0	0
0	12	27	55	0.8	56	106	Tr	Tr	0.10	0.10	1.1	Tr
0	12	15	31	0.7	39	124	0	0	0.12	0.07	0.9	0
0	33	49	60	1.4	71	339	0	0	0.27	0.12	2.2	0
0	16	23	71	0.9	141	177	0	0	0.11	0.17	1.1	0
0	13	25	22	0.8	59	92	Tr	Tr	0.08	0.15	1.0	Tr
0	12	20	36	0.7	51	175	0	0	0.10	0.08	0.8	0
0	12	32	47	0.9	35	138	Tr	Tr	0.12	0.08	1.2	Tr

Nutritive Value of Foods *(Continued)*

Foods, approximate measures, units, and weight (weight of edible portion only)		Water	Food energy	Pro-tein	Fat	Fatty Acids		
						Satu-rated	Mono-unsatu-rated	Poly-unsatu-rated
		Per-cent	Cal-ories	Grams	Grams	Grams	Grams	Grams
GRAIN PRODUCTS—Con.	Grams							
Wheat bread, enriched:[25]								
Slice (18 per loaf)- - - - - 1 slice- - - - - - - - -	25	37	65	2	1	0.3	0.4	0.2
Whole-wheat bread:[25]								
Slice (16 per loaf)- - - - - 1 slice- - - - - - - - -	28	38	70	3	1	0.4	0.4	0.3
Breakfast cereals:								
Hot type, cooked:								
Corn, (hominy) grits:								
Regular and quick,								
enriched- - - - - - - - 1 cup- - - - - - - - -	242	85	145	3	Tr	Tr	0.1	0.2
Instant, plain- - - - - - 1 pkt- - - - - - - - -	137	85	80	2	Tr	Tr	Tr	0.1
Cream of Wheat®:								
Regular, quick,								
instant- - - - - - - - - 1 cup- - - - - - - - -	244	86	140	4	Tr	0.1	Tr	0.2
Mix'n Eat, plain- - - - 1 pkt- - - - - - - - -	142	82	100	3	Tr	Tr	Tr	0.1
Malt-O-Meal®- - - - - - - 1 cup- - - - - - - - -	240	88	120	4	Tr	Tr	Tr	0.1
Oatmeal or rolled oats:								
Regular, quick, instant,								
nonfortified- - - - - - 1 cup- - - - - - - - -	234	85	145	6	2	0.4	0.8	1.0
Ready to eat:								
All-Bran® (about								
⅓ cup)- - - - - - - - 1 oz- - - - - - - - -	28	3	70	4	1	0.1	0.1	0.3
Cap'n Crunch® (about ¾								
cup)- - - - - - - - - - - 1 oz- - - - - - - - -	28	3	120	1	3	1.7	0.3	0.4
Cheerios® (about 1¼								
cup)- - - - - - - - - - - 1 oz- - - - - - - - -	28	5	110	4	2	0.3	0.6	0.7
Corn Flakes (about 1¼								
cup):								
Kellogg's®- - - - - - - - 1 oz- - - - - - - - - -	28	3	110	2	Tr	Tr	Tr	Tr
40% Bran Flakes:								
Kellogg's® (about ¾								
cup)- - - - - - - - - - - 1 oz- - - - - - - - -	28	3	90	4	1	0.1	0.1	0.3
Post® (about ⅔ cup)- 1 oz- - - - - - - - -	28	3	90	3	Tr	0.1	0.1	0.2
Froot Loops® (about 1								
cup)- - - - - - - - - - - 1 oz- - - - - - - - -	28	3	110	2	1	0.2	0.1	0.1
Golden Grahams®								
(about ¾ cup)- - - - - 1 oz- - - - - - - - -	28	2	110	2	1	0.7	0.1	0.2
Grape-Nuts® (about ¼								
cup)- - - - - - - - - - - 1 oz- - - - - - - - -	28	3	100	3	Tr	Tr	Tr	0.1
Honey Nut Cheerios®								
(about ¾ cup)- - - - - 1 oz- - - - - - - - -	28	3	105	3	1	0.1	0.3	0.3
Lucky Charms® (about 1								
cup)- - - - - - - - - - - 1 oz- - - - - - - - -	28	3	110	3	1	0.2	0.4	0.4
Nature Valley® Granola								
(about ⅓ cup)- - - - - 1 oz- - - - - - - - -	28	4	125	3	5	3.3	0.7	0.7
100% Natural Cereal								
(about ¼ cup)- - - - - 1 oz- - - - - - - - -	28	2	135	3	6	4.1	1.2	0.5

(Tr indicates nutrient present in trace amounts.)

Cholesterol	Carbohydrate	Calcium	Phosphorus	Iron	Potassium	Sodium	Vitamin A value (IU)	Vitamin A value (RE)	Thiamin	Riboflavin	Niacin	Ascorbic acid
Milligrams	Grams	Milligrams	Milligrams	Milligrams	Milligrams	Milligrams	International units	Retinol equivalents	Milligrams	Milligrams	Milligrams	Milligrams
0	12	32	27	0.7	28	129	Tr	Tr	0.12	0.08	0.9	Tr
0	13	20	74	1.0	50	180	Tr	Tr	0.10	0.06	1.1	Tr
0	31	0	29	[27]1.5	53	[28]0	[29]0	[29]0	[27]0.24	[27]0.15	[27]2.0	0
0	18	7	16	[27]1.0	29	343	0	0	[27]0.18	[27]0.08	[27]1.3	0
0	29	[30]54	[31]43	[30]10.9	46	[31,32]5	0	0	[30]0.24	[30]0.07	[30]1.5	0
0	21	[30]20	[30]20	[30]8.1	38	241	[301]1,250	[30]376	[30]0.43	[30]0.28	[30]5.0	0
0	26	5	[30]24	[309]9.6	31	[33]2	0	0	[30]0.48	[30]0.24	[30]5.8	0
0	19	178		1.6	131	[34]2	40	4	0.26	0.05	0.3	0
0	21	23	264	[304]4.5	350	320	[301]1,250	[30]375	[30]0.37	[30]0.43	[305]5.0	[30]15
0	23	5	36	[277]7.5	37	213	40	4	[27]0.50	[27]0.55	[276]6.6	0
0	20	48	134	[304]4.5	101	307	[301]1,250	[30]375	[30]0.37	[30]0.43	[305]5.0	[30]15
0	24	1	18	[301]1.8	26	351	[301]1,250	[30]375	[30]0.37	[30]0.43	[305]5.0	[30]15
0	22	14	139	[308]8.1	180	264	[301]1,250	[30]375	[30]0.37	[30]0.43	[305]5.0	0
0	22	12	179	[304]4.5	151	260	[301]1,250	[30]375	[30]0.37	[30]0.43	[305]5.0	0
0	25	3	24	[304]4.5	26	145	[301]1,250	[30]375	[30]0.37	[30]0.43	[305]5.0	[30]15
Tr	24	17	41	[304]4.5	63	346	[301]1,250	[30]375	[30]0.37	[30]0.43	[305]5.0	[30]15
0	23	11	71	1.2	95	197	[301]1,250	[30]375	[30]0.37	[30]0.43	[305]5.0	0
0	23	20	105	[304]4.5	99	257	[301]1,250	[30]375	[30]0.37	[30]0.43	[305]5.0	[30]15
0	23	32	79	[304]4.5	59	201	[301]1,250	[30]375	[30]0.37	[30]0.43	[305]5.0	[30]15
0	19	18	89	0.9	98	58	20	2	0.10	0.05	0.2	0
Tr	18	49	104	0.8	140	12	20	2	0.09	0.15	0.6	0

Nutritive Value of Foods *(Continued)*

Foods, approximate measures, units, and weight (weight of edible portion only)			Water	Food energy	Pro-tein	Fat	Satu-rated	Mono-unsatu-rated	Poly-unsatu-rated
								Fatty Acids	
		Grams	*Per-cent*	*Cal-ories*	*Grams*	*Grams*	*Grams*	*Grams*	*Grams*

Foods	measure	Grams	Water (%)	Food energy (Cal)	Protein (Grams)	Fat (Grams)	Saturated (Grams)	Mono-unsat (Grams)	Poly-unsat (Grams)
GRAIN PRODUCTS — Con.									
Product 19® (about ¾ cup)- - - - - - - -	1 oz- - - - - - - - -	28	3	110	3	Tr	Tr	Tr	0.1
Raisin Bran:									
Kellogg's® (about ¾ cup)- - - - - - - - - -	1 oz- - - - - - - - -	28	8	90	3	1	0.1	0.1	0.3
Post® (about ½ cup)-	1 oz- - - - - - - - -	28	9	85	3	1	0.1	0.1	0.3
Rice Krispies® (about 1 cup)- - - - - - - - - -	1 oz- - - - - - - - -	28	2	110	2	Tr	Tr	Tr	0.1
Shredded Wheat (about ⅔ cup)- - - - - - - - -	1 oz- - - - - - - - -	28	5	100	3	1	0.1	0.1	0.3
Special K® (about 1⅓ cup)- - - - - - - - - -	1 oz- - - - - - - - -	28	2	110	6	Tr	Tr	Tr	Tr
Super Sugar Crisp® (about ⅞ cup)- - - - -	1 oz- - - - - - - - -	28	2	105	2	Tr	Tr	Tr	0.1
Sugar Frosted Flakes, Kellogg's® (about ¾ cup)- - - - - - - - - -	1 oz- - - - - - - - -	28	3	110	1	Tr	Tr	Tr	Tr
Sugar Smacks® (about ¾ cup)- - - - - - - - - -	1 oz- - - - - - - - -	28	3	105	2	1	0.1	0.1	0.2
Total® (about 1 cup)- -	1 oz- - - - - - - - -	28	4	100	3	1	0.1	0.1	0.3
Trix® (about 1 cup)- - -	1 oz- - - - - - - - -	28	3	110	2	Tr	0.2	0.1	0.1
Wheaties® (about 1 cup)- - - - - - - - - -	1 oz- - - - - - - - -	28	5	100	3	Tr	0.1	Tr	0.2
Buckwheat flour, light, sifted	1 cup - - - - - - - -	98	12	340	6	1	0.2	0.4	0.4
Bulgur, uncooked- - - - - - - -	1 cup - - - - - - - -	170	10	600	19	3	1.2	0.3	1.2
Cakes prepared from cake mixes with enriched flour:[35]									
Angelfood:									
Piece, 1/12 of cake- - - - -	1 piece- - - - - - - -	53	38	125	3	Tr	Tr	Tr	0.1
Coffeecake, crumb:									
Piece, ⅙ of cake- - - - -	1 piece- - - - - - - -	72	30	230	5	7	2.0	2.8	1.6
Devil's food with chocolate frosting:									
Piece, 1/16 of cake- - - - -	1 piece- - - - - - - -	69	24	235	3	8	3.5	3.2	1.2
Cupcake, 2½-in diam.- -	1 cupcake- - - - - -	35	24	120	2	4	1.8	1.6	0.6
Gingerbread:									
Piece, ⅑ of cake- - - - -	1 piece- - - - - - - -	63	37	175	2	4	1.1	1.8	1.2
Yellow with chocolate frosting:									
Piece, 1/16 of cake- - - - -	1 piece- - - - - - - -	69	26	235	3	8	3.0	3.0	1.4
Cakes prepared from home recipes using enriched flour:									
Carrot, with cream cheese frosting:[36]									
Piece, 1/16 of cake- - - - -	1 piece- - - - - - - -	96	23	385	4	21	4.1	8.4	6.7

(Tr indicates nutrient present in trace amounts.)

Cholesterol	Carbohydrate	Calcium	Phosphorus	Iron	Potassium	Sodium	Vitamin A value (IU)	Vitamin A value (RE)	Thiamin	Riboflavin	Niacin	Ascorbic acid
Milligrams	Grams	Milligrams	Milligrams	Milligrams	Milligrams	Milligrams	International units	Retinol equivalents	Milligrams	Milligrams	Milligrams	Milligrams
0	24	3	40	[30]18.0	44	325	[30]5,000	[30]1,501	[30]1.50	[30]1.70	[30]20.0	[30]60
0	21	10	105	[30]3.5	147	207	[30]960	[30]288	[30]0.28	[30]0.34	[30]3.9	0
0	21	13	119	[30]4.5	175	185	[30]1,250	[30]375	[30]0.37	[30]0.43	[30]5.0	0
0	25	4	34	[30]1.8	29	340	[30]1,250	[30]375	[30]0.37	[30]0.43	[30]5.0	[30]15
0	23	11	100	1.2	102	3	0	0	0.07	0.08	1.5	0
Tr	21	8	55	[30]4.5	49	265	[30]1,250	[30]375	[30]0.37	[30]0.43	[30]5.0	[30]15
0	26	6	52	[30]1.8	105	25	[30]1,250	[30]375	[30]0.37	[30]0.43	[30]5.0	0
0	26	1	21	[30]1.8	18	230	[30]1,250	[30]375	[30]0.37	[30]0.43	[30]5.0	[30]15
0	25	3	31	[30]1.8	42	75	[30]1,250	[30]375	[30]0.37	[30]0.43	[30]5.0	[30]15
0	22	48	118	[30]18.0	106	352	[30]5,000	[30]1,501	[30]1.50	[30]1.70	[30]20.0	[30]60
0	25	6	19	[30]4.5	27	181	[30]1,250	[30]375	[30]0.37	[30]0.43	[30]5.0	[30]15
0	23	43	98	[30]4.5	106	354	[30]1,250	[30]375	[30]0.37	[30]0.43	[30]5.0	[30]15
0	78	11	86	1.0	314	2	0	0	0.08	0.04	0.4	0
0	129	49	575	9.5	389	7	0	0	0.48	0.24	7.7	0
0	29	44	91	0.2	71	269	0	0	0.03	0.11	0.1	0
47	38	44	125	1.2	78	310	120	32	0.14	0.15	1.3	Tr
37	40	41	72	1.4	90	181	100	31	0.07	0.10	0.6	Tr
19	20	21	37	0.7	46	92	50	16	0.04	0.05	0.3	Tr
1	32	57	63	1.2	173	192	0	0	0.09	0.11	0.8	Tr
36	40	63	126	1.0	75	157	100	29	0.08	0.10	0.7	Tr
74	48	44	62	1.3	108	279	140	15	0.11	0.12	0.9	1

Foods, approximate measures, units, and weight (weight of edible portion only)		Water	Food energy	Pro-tein	Fat	Fatty Acids		
						Satu-rated	Mono-unsatu-rated	Poly-unsatu-rated
GRAIN PRODUCTS—Con.	*Grams*	*Per-cent*	*Cal-ories*	*Grams*	*Grams*	*Grams*	*Grams*	*Grams*
Fruitcake, dark:[36]								
Piece, 1/32 of cake,								
2/3-in arc · · · · · · · · · · 1 piece · · · · · · · ·	43	18	165	2	7	1.5	3.6	1.6
Plain sheet cake:[37]								
Without frosting:								
Piece, 1/9 of cake · · · · · 1 piece · · · · · · · ·	86	25	315	4	12	3.3	5.0	2.8
With uncooked white frosting:								
Piece, 1/9 of cake · · · · · 1 piece · · · · · · · ·	121	21	445	4	14	4.6	5.6	2.9
Pound:[38]								
Slice, 1/17 of loaf · · · · · · · 1 slice · · · · · · · · ·	30	22	120	2	5	1.2	2.4	1.6
Cakes, commercial, made with enriched flour:								
Pound:								
Slice, 1/17 of loaf · · · · · · · 1 slice · · · · · · · · ·	29	24	110	2	5	3.0	1.7	0.2
Snack cakes:								
Devil's food with creme filling (2 small cakes per pkg) · · · · · · · · · · 1 small cake · · · ·	28	20	105	1	4	1.7	1.5	0.6
Sponge with creme filling (2 small cakes per pkg) 1 small cake · · · · ·	42	19	155	1	5	2.3	2.1	0.5
White with white frosting:								
Piece, 1/16 of cake · · · · · · 1 piece · · · · · · · ·	71	24	260	3	9	2.1	3.8	2.6
Yellow with chocolate frost-ing:								
Piece, 1/16 of cake · · · · · · 1 piece · · · · · · · ·	69	23	245	2	11	5.7	3.7	0.6
Cheesecake:								
Piece, 1/12 of cake · · · · · · · 1 piece · · · · · · · ·	92	46	280	5	18	9.9	5.4	1.2
Cookies made with enriched flour:								
Brownies with nuts:								
Commercial, with frost-ing, 1½ by 1¾ by ⅞ in- 1 brownie · · · · · ·	25	13	100	1	4	1.6	2.0	0.6
From home recipe, 1¾ by ⅞ in[36] · · · · · · · 1 brownie · · · · · ·	20	10	95	1	6	1.4	2.8	1.2
Chocolate chip:								
Commercial, 2¼-in diam., ⅜ in thick · · · · 4 cookies · · · · · · ·	42	4	180	2	9	2.9	3.1	2.6
From home recipe, 2⅓-in diam.[25] · · · · · · · · · · 4 cookies · · · · · · ·	40	3	185	2	11	3.9	4.3	2.0
From refrigerated dough, 2¼-in diam., ⅜ in thick 4 cookies · · · · · · ·	48	5	225	2	11	4.0	4.4	2.0
Oatmeal with raisins, 2⅝-in diam., ¼ in thick · · · · 4 cookies · · · · · · ·	52	4	245	3	10	2.5	4.5	2.8
Peanut butter cookie, from home recipe, 2⅝-in diam.[25] · · · · · · · · · · · 4 cookies · · · · · · ·	48	3	245	4	14	4.0	5.8	2.8

(Tr indicates nutrient present in trace amounts.)

Nutrients in Indicated Quantity

Cholesterol	Carbohydrate	Calcium	Phosphorus	Iron	Potassium	Sodium	Vitamin A value		Thiamin	Riboflavin	Niacin	Ascorbic acid
							(IU)	(RE)				
Milligrams	Grams	Milligrams	Milligrams	Milligrams	Milligrams	Milligrams	International units	Retinol equivalents	Milligrams	Milligrams	Milligrams	Milligrams
20	25	41	50	1.2	194	67	50	13	0.08	0.08	0.5	16
61	48	55	88	1.3	68	258	150	41	0.14	0.15	1.1	Tr
70	77	61	91	1.2	74	275	240	71	0.13	0.16	1.1	Tr
32	15	20	28	0.5	28	96	200	60	0.05	0.06	0.5	Tr
64	15	8	30	0.5	26	108	160	41	0.06	0.06	0.5	0
15	17	21	26	1.0	34	105	20	4	0.06	0.09	0.7	0
7	27	14	44	0.6	37	155	30	9	0.07	0.06	0.6	0
3	42	33	99	1.0	52	176	40	12	0.20	0.13	1.7	0
38	39	23	117	1.2	123	192	120	30	0.05	0.14	0.6	0
170	26	52	81	0.4	90	204	230	69	0.03	0.12	0.4	5
14	16	13	26	0.6	50	59	70	18	0.08	0.07	0.3	Tr
18	11	9	26	0.4	35	51	20	6	0.05	0.05	0.3	Tr
5	28	13	41	0.8	68	140	50	15	0.10	0.23	1.0	Tr
18	26	13	34	1.0	82	82	20	5	0.06	0.06	0.6	0
22	32	13	34	1.0	62	173	30	8	0.06	0.10	0.9	0
2	36	18	58	1.1	90	148	40	12	0.09	0.08	1.0	0
22	28	21	60	1.1	110	142	20	5	0.07	0.07	1.9	0

Nutritive Value of Foods *(Continued)*

<table>
<tr><th rowspan="3">Foods, approximate measures, units, and weight
(weight of edible portion only)</th><th rowspan="3"></th><th rowspan="3">Water</th><th rowspan="3">Food
energy</th><th rowspan="3">Pro-
tein</th><th rowspan="3">Fat</th><th colspan="3">Fatty Acids</th></tr>
<tr><th>Satu-
rated</th><th>Mono-
unsatu-
rated</th><th>Poly-
unsatu-
rated</th></tr>
<tr></tr>
<tr><th>GRAIN PRODUCTS—Con.</th><th></th><th>Grams</th><th>Per-
cent</th><th>Cal-
ories</th><th>Grams</th><th>Grams</th><th>Grams</th><th>Grams</th><th>Grams</th></tr>
<tr><td>Sandwich type (chocolate
or vanilla), 1¾-in
diam., ⅜ in thick----</td><td>4 cookies-------</td><td>40</td><td>2</td><td>195</td><td>2</td><td>8</td><td>2.0</td><td>3.6</td><td>2.2</td></tr>
<tr><td>Shortbread:</td><td></td><td></td><td></td><td></td><td></td><td></td><td></td><td></td><td></td></tr>
<tr><td>Commercial---------</td><td>4 small cookies---</td><td>32</td><td>6</td><td>155</td><td>2</td><td>8</td><td>2.9</td><td>3.0</td><td>1.1</td></tr>
<tr><td>Sugar cookie, from refriger-
ated dough, 2½-in
diam., ¼ in thick----</td><td>4 cookies-------</td><td>48</td><td>4</td><td>235</td><td>2</td><td>12</td><td>2.3</td><td>5.0</td><td>3.6</td></tr>
<tr><td>Vanilla wafers, 1¾-in diam.,
¼ in thick--------</td><td>10 cookies------</td><td>40</td><td>4</td><td>185</td><td>2</td><td>7</td><td>1.8</td><td>3.0</td><td>1.8</td></tr>
<tr><td>Corn chips------------</td><td>1-oz package----</td><td>28</td><td>1</td><td>155</td><td>2</td><td>9</td><td>1.4</td><td>2.4</td><td>3.7</td></tr>
<tr><td>Cornmeal:</td><td></td><td></td><td></td><td></td><td></td><td></td><td></td><td></td><td></td></tr>
<tr><td>Whole-ground, unbolted,
dry form----------</td><td>1 cup---------</td><td>122</td><td>12</td><td>435</td><td>11</td><td>5</td><td>0.5</td><td>1.1</td><td>2.5</td></tr>
<tr><td>Bolted (nearly whole-
grain), dry form-----</td><td>1 cup---------</td><td>122</td><td>12</td><td>440</td><td>11</td><td>4</td><td>0.5</td><td>0.9</td><td>2.2</td></tr>
<tr><td>Degermed, enriched:</td><td></td><td></td><td></td><td></td><td></td><td></td><td></td><td></td><td></td></tr>
<tr><td>Dry form-----------</td><td>1 cup---------</td><td>138</td><td>12</td><td>500</td><td>11</td><td>2</td><td>0.2</td><td>0.4</td><td>0.9</td></tr>
<tr><td>Crackers:[39]</td><td></td><td></td><td></td><td></td><td></td><td></td><td></td><td></td><td></td></tr>
<tr><td>Cheese:</td><td></td><td></td><td></td><td></td><td></td><td></td><td></td><td></td><td></td></tr>
<tr><td>Plain, 1 in square-----</td><td>10 crackers-----</td><td>10</td><td>4</td><td>50</td><td>1</td><td>3</td><td>0.9</td><td>1.2</td><td>0.3</td></tr>
<tr><td>Sandwich type (peanut
butter)-----------</td><td>1 sandwich-----</td><td>8</td><td>3</td><td>40</td><td>1</td><td>2</td><td>0.4</td><td>0.8</td><td>0.3</td></tr>
<tr><td>Graham, plain,
2½ in square-------</td><td>2 crackers------</td><td>14</td><td>5</td><td>60</td><td>1</td><td>1</td><td>0.4</td><td>0.6</td><td>0.4</td></tr>
<tr><td>Melba toast, plain------</td><td>1 piece--------</td><td>5</td><td>4</td><td>20</td><td>1</td><td>Tr</td><td>0.1</td><td>0.1</td><td>0.1</td></tr>
<tr><td>Rye wafers, whole-grain, 1⅞
by 3½ in----------</td><td>2 wafers-------</td><td>14</td><td>5</td><td>55</td><td>1</td><td>1</td><td>0.3</td><td>0.4</td><td>0.3</td></tr>
<tr><td>Saltines[40]-----------</td><td>4 crackers------</td><td>12</td><td>4</td><td>50</td><td>1</td><td>1</td><td>0.5</td><td>0.4</td><td>0.2</td></tr>
<tr><td>Snack-type, standard----</td><td>1 round cracker--</td><td>3</td><td>3</td><td>15</td><td>Tr</td><td>1</td><td>0.2</td><td>0.4</td><td>0.1</td></tr>
<tr><td>Wheat, thin----------</td><td>4 crackers------</td><td>8</td><td>3</td><td>35</td><td>1</td><td>1</td><td>0.5</td><td>0.5</td><td>0.4</td></tr>
<tr><td>Whole-wheat wafers-----</td><td>2 crackers------</td><td>8</td><td>4</td><td>35</td><td>1</td><td>2</td><td>0.5</td><td>0.6</td><td>0.4</td></tr>
<tr><td>Croissants, made with
enriched flour, 4½ by 4 by
1¾ in---------------</td><td>1 croissant-----</td><td>57</td><td>22</td><td>235</td><td>5</td><td>12</td><td>3.5</td><td>6.7</td><td>1.4</td></tr>
<tr><td>Danish pastry, made with
enriched flour:</td><td></td><td></td><td></td><td></td><td></td><td></td><td></td><td></td><td></td></tr>
<tr><td>Plain without fruit or nuts:</td><td></td><td></td><td></td><td></td><td></td><td></td><td></td><td></td><td></td></tr>
<tr><td>Round piece, about 4¼-in
diam., 1 in high-----</td><td>1 pastry-------</td><td>57</td><td>27</td><td>220</td><td>4</td><td>12</td><td>3.6</td><td>4.8</td><td>2.6</td></tr>
<tr><td>Fruit, round piece------</td><td>1 pastry-------</td><td>65</td><td>30</td><td>235</td><td>4</td><td>13</td><td>3.9</td><td>5.2</td><td>2.9</td></tr>
<tr><td>Doughnuts, made with
enriched flour:</td><td></td><td></td><td></td><td></td><td></td><td></td><td></td><td></td><td></td></tr>
<tr><td>Cake type, plain, 3¼-in
diam., 1 in high------</td><td>1 doughnut-----</td><td>50</td><td>21</td><td>210</td><td>3</td><td>12</td><td>2.8</td><td>5.0</td><td>3.0</td></tr>
<tr><td>Yeast-leavened, glazed, 3¾-
in diam., 1¼ in high---</td><td>1 doughnut-----</td><td>60</td><td>27</td><td>235</td><td>4</td><td>13</td><td>5.2</td><td>5.5</td><td>0.9</td></tr>
</table>

(Tr indicates nutrient present in trace amounts.)

Cholesterol	Carbohydrate	Calcium	Phosphorus	Iron	Potassium	Sodium	Vitamin A value		Thiamin	Riboflavin	Niacin	Ascorbic acid
							(IU)	(RE)				
Milligrams	Grams	Milligrams	Milligrams	Milligrams	Milligrams	Milligrams	International units	Retinol equivalents	Milligrams	Milligrams	Milligrams	Milligrams
0	29	12	40	1.4	66	189	0	0	0.09	0.07	0.8	0
27	20	13	39	0.8	38	123	30	8	0.10	0.09	0.9	0
29	31	50	91	0.9	33	261	40	11	0.09	0.06	1.1	0
25	29	16	36	0.8	50	150	50	14	0.07	0.10	1.0	0
0	16	35	52	0.5	52	233	110	11	0.04	0.05	0.4	1
0	90	24	312	2.2	346	1	620	62	0.46	0.13	2.4	0
0	91	21	272	2.2	303	1	590	59	0.37	0.10	2.3	0
0	108	8	137	5.9	166	1	610	61	0.61	0.36	4.8	0
6	6	11	17	0.3	17	112	20	5	0.05	0.04	0.4	0
1	5	7	25	0.3	17	90	Tr	Tr	0.04	0.03	0.6	0
0	11	6	20	0.4	36	86	0	0	0.02	0.03	0.6	0
0	4	6	10	0.1	11	44	0	0	0.01	0.01	0.1	0
0	10	7	44	0.5	65	115	0	0	0.06	0.03	0.5	0
4	9	3	12	0.5	17	165	0	0	0.06	0.05	0.6	0
0	2	3	6	0.1	4	30	Tr	Tr	0.01	0.01	0.1	0
0	5	3	15	0.3	17	69	Tr	Tr	0.04	0.03	0.4	0
0	5	3	22	0.2	31	59	0	0	0.02	0.03	0.4	0
13	27	20	64	2.1	68	452	50	13	0.17	0.13	1.3	0
49	26	60	58	1.1	53	218	60	17	0.16	0.17	1.4	Tr
56	28	17	80	1.3	57	233	40	11	0.16	0.14	1.4	Tr
20	24	22	111	1.0	58	192	20	5	0.12	0.12	1.1	Tr
21	26	17	55	1.4	64	222	Tr	Tr	0.28	0.12	1.8	0

Nutritive Value of Foods *(Continued)*

Foods, approximate measures, units, and weight (weight of edible portion only)		Water	Food energy	Pro-tein	Fat	Satu-rated	Mono-unsatu-rated	Poly-unsatu-rated
							Fatty Acids	
	Grams	*Per-cent*	*Cal-ories*	*Grams*	*Grams*	*Grams*	*Grams*	*Grams*
GRAIN PRODUCTS—Con.								
English muffins, plain, enriched	1 muffin	57	42	140	5	1	0.3	0.2	0.3
Toasted	1 muffin	50	29	140	5	1	0.3	0.2	0.3
French toast, from home recipe	1 slice	65	53	155	6	7	1.6	2.0	1.6
Macaroni, enriched, cooked (cut lengths, elbows, shells):									
Firm stage (hot)	1 cup	130	64	190	7	1	0.1	0.1	0.3
Tender stage:									
Cold	1 cup	105	72	115	4	Tr	0.1	0.1	0.2
Hot	1 cup	140	72	155	5	1	0.1	0.1	0.2
Muffins made with enriched flour, 2½-in diam., 1½ in high:									
From home recipe:									
Blueberry[25]	1 muffin	45	37	135	3	5	1.5	2.1	1.2
Bran[36]	1 muffin	45	35	125	3	6	1.4	1.6	2.3
Corn (enriched, de-germed cornmeal and flour)[25]	1 muffin	45	33	145	3	5	1.5	2.2	1.4
From commercial mix (egg and water added):									
Blueberry	1 muffin	45	33	140	3	5	1.4	2.0	1.2
Bran	1 muffin	45	28	140	3	4	1.3	1.6	1.0
Corn	1 muffin	45	30	145	3	6	1.7	2.3	1.4
Noodles (egg noodles), enriched, cooked	1 cup	160	70	200	7	2	0.5	0.6	0.6
Noodles, chow mein, canned	1 cup	45	11	220	6	11	2.1	7.3	0.4
Pancakes, 4-in diam.:									
Buckwheat, from mix (with buckwheat and enriched flours), egg and milk added	1 pancake	27	58	55	2	2	0.9	0.9	0.5
Plain:									
From home recipe using enriched flour	1 pancake	27	50	60	2	2	0.5	0.8	0.5
From mix (with enriched flour), egg, milk, and oil added	1 pancake	27	54	60	2	2	0.5	0.9	0.5
Piecrust, made with enriched flour and vegetable short-ening, baked:									
From home recipe, 9-in diam.	1 pie shell	180	15	900	11	60	14.8	25.9	15.7
From mix, 9-in diam.	Piecrust for 2-crust pie	320	19	1,485	20	93	22.7	41.0	25.0

(Tr indicates nutrient present in trace amounts.)

Nutrients in Indicated Quantity

Cholesterol	Carbohydrate	Calcium	Phosphorus	Iron	Potassium	Sodium	Vitamin A value		Thiamin	Riboflavin	Niacin	Ascorbic acid
							(IU)	(RE)				
Milligrams	Grams	Milligrams	Milligrams	Milligrams	Milligrams	Milligrams	International units	Retinol equivalents	Milligrams	Milligrams	Milligrams	Milligrams
0	27	96	67	1.7	331	378	0	0	0.26	0.19	2.2	0
0	27	96	67	1.7	331	378	0	0	0.23	0.19	2.2	0
112	17	72	85	1.3	86	257	110	32	0.12	0.16	1.0	Tr
0	39	14	85	2.1	103	1	0	0	0.23	0.13	1.8	0
0	24	8	53	1.3	64	1	0	0	0.15	0.08	1.2	0
0	32	11	70	1.7	85	1	0	0	0.20	0.11	1.5	0
19	20	54	46	0.9	47	198	40	9	0.10	0.11	0.9	1
24	19	60	125	1.4	99	189	230	30	0.11	0.13	1.3	3
23	21	66	59	0.9	57	169	80	15	0.11	0.11	0.9	Tr
45	22	15	90	0.9	54	225	50	11	0.10	0.17	1.1	Tr
28	24	27	182	1.7	50	385	100	14	0.08	0.12	1.9	0
42	22	30	128	1.3	31	291	90	16	0.09	0.09	0.8	Tr
50	37	16	94	2.6	70	3	110	34	0.22	0.13	1.9	0
5	26	14	41	0.4	33	450	0	0	0.05	0.03	0.6	0
20	6	59	91	0.4	66	125	60	17	0.04	0.05	0.2	Tr
16	9	27	38	0.5	33	115	30	10	0.06	0.07	0.5	Tr
16	8	36	71	0.7	43	160	30	7	0.09	0.12	0.8	Tr
0	79	25	90	4.5	90	1,100	0	0	0.54	0.40	5.0	0
0	141	131	272	9.3	179	2,602	0	0	1.06	0.80	9.9	0

Nutritive Value of Foods *(Continued)*

Foods, approximate measures, units, and weight (weight of edible portion only)		Water	Food energy	Pro-tein	Fat	Satu-rated	Mono-unsatu-rated	Poly-unsatu-rated
							Fatty Acids	
		Per-cent	*Cal-ories*	*Grams*	*Grams*	*Grams*	*Grams*	*Grams*
GRAIN PRODUCTS—Con.	*Grams*							
Pies, piecrust made with enriched flour, vegetable shortening, 9-in diam.:								
Apple:								
Piece, ⅙ of pie - - - - - -	1 piece - - - - - - - -	158	48	405	3	18	4.6	7.4	4.4
Blueberry:								
Piece, ⅙ of pie - - - - - -	1 piece - - - - - - - -	158	51	380	4	17	4.3	7.4	4.6
Cherry:								
Piece, ⅙ of pie - - - - - -	1 piece - - - - - - - -	158	47	410	4	18	4.7	7.7	4.6
Creme:								
Piece, ⅙ of pie - - - - - -	1 piece - - - - - - - -	152	43	455	3	23	15.0	4.0	1.1
Custard:								
Piece, ⅙ of pie - - - - - -	1 piece - - - - - - - -	152	58	330	9	17	5.6	6.7	3.2
Lemon meringue:								
Piece, ⅙ of pie - - - - - -	1 piece - - - - - - - -	140	47	355	5	14	4.3	5.7	2.9
Peach:								
Piece, ⅙ of pie - - - - - -	1 piece - - - - - - - -	158	48	405	4	17	4.1	7.3	4.4
Pecan:								
Piece, ⅙ of pie - - - - - -	1 piece - - - - - - - -	138	20	575	7	32	4.7	17.0	7.9
Pumpkin:								
Piece, ⅙ of pie - - - - - -	1 piece - - - - - - - -	152	59	320	6	17	6.4	6.7	3.0
Pies, fried:								
Apple - - - - - - - - - - - -	1 pie - - - - - - - - -	85	43	255	2	14	5.8	6.6	0.6
Cherry - - - - - - - - - - - -	1 pie - - - - - - - - -	85	42	250	2	14	5.8	6.7	0.6
Popcorn, popped:								
Air-popped, unsalted - - - -	1 cup - - - - - - - - -	8	4	30	1	Tr	Tr	0.1	0.2
Popped in vegetable oil, salted - - - - - - - - - - - -	1 cup - - - - - - - - -	11	3	55	1	3	0.5	1.4	1.2
Sugar syrup coated - - - - - -	1 cup - - - - - - - - -	35	4	135	2	1	0.1	0.3	0.6
Pretzels, made with enriched flour:								
Stick 2¼ in long - - - - - - -	10 pretzels - - - - - -	3	3	10	Tr	Tr	Tr	Tr	Tr
Twisted, dutch 2¾ by 2⅝ in - - - - - - - - -	1 pretzel - - - - - - -	16	3	65	2	1	0.1	0.2	0.2
Twisted, thin, 3¼ by 2¼ by ¼ in - - - - - - - - - - - -	10 pretzels - - - - - -	60	3	240	6	2	0.4	0.8	0.6
Rice:								
Brown, cooked, served hot-	1 cup - - - - - - - - -	195	70	230	5	1	0.3	0.3	0.4
White enriched:								
Commercial varieties, all types:								
Cooked, served hot - - -	1 cup - - - - - - - - -	205	73	225	4	Tr	0.1	0.1	0.1
Instant, ready-to-serve, hot - - - - - - - - - - - - -	1 cup - - - - - - - - -	165	73	180	4	0	0.1	0.1	0.1
Parboiled:								
Cooked, served hot - - -	1 cup - - - - - - - - -	175	73	185	4	Tr	Tr	Tr	0.1

(Tr indicates nutrient present in trace amounts.)

Nutrients in Indicated Quantity

Cho-lesterol	Carbo-hydrate	Calcium	Phos-phorus	Iron	Potas-sium	Sodium	Vitamin A value (IU)	Vitamin A value (RE)	Thiamin	Ribo-flavin	Niacin	Ascorbic acid
Milli-grams	Grams	Milli-grams	Milli-grams	Milli-grams	Milli-grams	Milli-grams	Inter-national units	Retinol equiva-lents	Milli-grams	Milli-grams	Milli-grams	Milli-grams
0	60	13	35	1.6	126	476	50	5	0.17	0.13	1.6	2
0	55	17	36	2.1	158	423	140	14	0.17	0.14	1.7	6
0	61	22	40	1.6	166	480	700	70	0.19	0.14	1.6	0
8	59	46	154	1.1	133	369	210	65	0.06	0.15	1.1	0
169	36	146	172	1.5	208	436	350	96	0.14	0.32	0.9	0
143	53	20	69	1.4	70	395	240	66	0.10	0.14	0.8	4
0	60	16	46	1.9	235	423	1,150	115	0.17	0.16	2.4	5
95	71	65	142	4.6	170	305	220	54	0.30	0.17	1.1	0
109	37	78	105	1.4	243	325	3,750	416	0.14	0.21	1.2	0
14	31	12	34	0.9	42	326	30	3	0.09	0.06	1.0	1
13	32	11	41	0.7	61	371	190	19	0.06	0.06	0.6	1
0	6	1	22	0.2	20	Tr	10	1	0.03	0.01	0.2	0
0	6	3	31	0.3	19	86	20	2	0.01	0.02	0.1	0
0	30	2	47	0.5	90	Tr	30	3	0.13	0.02	0.4	0
0	2	1	3	0.1	3	48	0	0	0.01	0.01	0.1	0
0	13	4	15	0.3	16	258	0	0	0.05	0.04	0.7	0
0	48	16	55	1.2	61	966	0	0	0.19	0.15	2.6	0
0	50	23	142	1.0	137	0	0	0	0.18	0.04	2.7	0
0	50	21	57	1.8	57	0	0	0	0.23	0.02	2.1	0
0	40	5	31	1.3	0	0	0	0	0.21	0.02	1.7	0
0	41	33	100	1.4	75	0	0	0	0.19	0.02	2.1	0

Nutritive Value of Foods (Continued)

Foods, approximate measures, units, and weight (weight of edible portion only)		Water	Food energy	Pro-tein	Fat	Fatty Acids		
						Satu-rated	Mono-unsatu-rated	Poly-unsatu-rated
		Per-cent	Cal-ories	Grams	Grams	Grams	Grams	Grams
GRAIN PRODUCTS—Con.		*Grams*						
Rolls, enriched:								
Commercial:								
Dinner, 2½-in diam., 2 in high	1 roll	28	32	85	2	2	0.5	0.8	0.6
Frankfurter and ham-burger (8 per 11½-oz pkg.)	1 roll	40	34	115	3	2	0.5	0.8	0.6
Hard, 3¾-in diam., 2 in high	1 roll	50	25	155	5	2	0.4	0.5	0.6
Hoagie or submarine, 11½ by 3 by 2½ in	1 roll	135	31	400	11	8	1.8	3.0	2.2
From home recipe:								
Dinner, 2½-in diam., 2 in high	1 roll	35	26	120	3	3	0.8	1.2	0.9
Spaghetti, enriched, cooked:								
Firm stage, "al dente," served hot	1 cup	130	64	190	7	1	0.1	0.1	0.3
Tortillas, corn	1 tortilla	30	45	65	2	1	0.1	0.3	0.6
Waffles, made with enriched flour, 7-in diam.:								
From home recipe	1 waffle	75	37	245	7	13	4.0	4.9	2.6
From mix, egg and milk added	1 waffle	75	42	205	7	8	2.7	2.9	1.5
Wheat flours:								
All-purpose or family flour, enriched:								
Sifted, spooned	1 cup	115	12	420	12	1	0.2	0.1	0.5
Cake or pastry flour, enriched, sifted, spooned	1 cup	96	12	350	7	1	0.1	0.1	0.3
Self-rising, enriched, unsifted, spooned	1 cup	125	12	440	12	1	0.2	0.1	0.5
Whole-wheat, from hard wheats, stirred	1 cup	120	12	400	16	2	0.3	0.3	1.1
LEGUMES, NUTS, AND SEEDS								
Almonds, shelled:								
Slivered, packed	1 cup	135	4	795	27	70	6.7	45.8	14.8
Whole	1 oz	28	4	165	6	15	1.4	9.6	3.1
Beans, dry:								
Cooked, drained:								
Black	1 cup	171	66	225	15	1	0.1	0.1	0.5
Great Northern	1 cup	180	69	210	14	1	0.1	0.1	0.6
Lima	1 cup	190	64	260	16	1	0.2	0.1	0.5
Pea (navy)	1 cup	190	69	225	15	1	0.1	0.1	0.7
Pinto	1 cup	180	65	265	15	1	0.1	0.1	0.5

(Tr indicates nutrient present in trace amounts.)

Nutrients in Indicated Quantity

Cholesterol	Carbohydrate	Calcium	Phosphorus	Iron	Potassium	Sodium	Vitamin A value		Thiamin	Riboflavin	Niacin	Ascorbic acid
							(IU)	(RE)				
Milligrams	Grams	Milligrams	Milligrams	Milligrams	Milligrams	Milligrams	International units	Retinol equivalents	Milligrams	Milligrams	Milligrams	Milligrams
Tr	14	33	44	0.8	36	155	Tr	Tr	0.14	0.09	1.1	Tr
Tr	20	54	44	1.2	56	241	Tr	Tr	0.20	0.13	1.6	Tr
Tr	30	24	46	1.4	49	313	0	0	0.20	0.12	1.7	0
Tr	72	100	115	3.8	128	683	0	0	0.54	0.33	4.5	0
12	20	16	36	1.1	41	98	30	8	0.12	0.12	1.2	0
0	39	14	85	2.0	103	1	0	0	0.23	0.13	1.8	0
0	13	42	55	0.6	43	1	80	8	0.05	0.03	0.4	0
102	26	154	135	1.5	129	445	140	39	0.18	0.24	1.5	Tr
59	27	179	257	1.2	146	515	170	49	0.14	0.23	0.9	Tr
0	88	18	100	5.1	109	2	0	0	0.73	0.46	6.1	0
0	76	16	70	4.2	91	2	0	0	0.58	0.38	5.1	0
0	93	331	583	5.5	113	1,349	0	0	0.80	0.50	6.6	0
0	85	49	446	5.2	444	4	0	0	0.66	0.14	5.2	0
0	28	359	702	4.9	988	15	0	0	0.28	1.05	4.5	1
0	6	75	147	1.0	208	3	0	0	0.06	0.22	1.0	Tr
0	41	47	239	2.9	608	1	Tr	Tr	0.43	0.05	0.9	0
0	38	90	266	4.9	749	13	0	0	0.25	0.13	1.3	0
0	49	55	293	5.9	1,163	4	0	0	0.25	0.11	1.3	0
0	40	95	281	5.1	790	13	0	0	0.27	0.13	1.3	0
0	49	86	296	5.4	882	3	Tr	Tr	0.33	0.16	0.7	0

Nutritive Value of Foods *(Continued)*

Foods, approximate measures, units, and weight (weight of edible portion only)		Water	Food energy	Protein	Fat	Fatty Acids Saturated	Mono-unsaturated	Poly-unsaturated
		Grams	Per-cent	Cal-ories	Grams	Grams	Grams	Grams
LEGUMES, NUTS, AND SEEDS—Con.		Grams						
Canned, solids and liquid:								
White with:								
Frankfurters (sliced)-	1 cup	255	71	365	19	18	7.4	8.8	0.7
Pork and tomato								
sauce-	1 cup	255	71	310	16	7	2.4	2.7	0.7
Pork and sweet sauce-	1 cup	255	66	385	16	12	4.3	4.9	1.2
Red kidney-	1 cup	255	76	230	15	1	0.1	0.1	0.6
Black-eyed peas, dry, cooked (with residual cooking								
liquid)-	1 cup	250	80	190	13	1	0.2	Tr	0.3
Brazil nuts, shelled-	1 oz	28	3	185	4	19	4.6	6.5	6.8
Carob flour-	1 cup	140	3	255	6	Tr	Tr	0.1	0.1
Cashew nuts, salted:								
Dry roasted-	1 oz	28	2	165	4	13	2.6	7.7	2.2
Roasted in oil-	1 oz	28	4	165	5	14	2.7	8.1	2.3
Chestnuts, European (Italian), roasted,								
shelled-	1 cup	143	40	350	5	3	0.6	1.1	1.2
Chickpeas, cooked, drained-	1 cup	163	60	270	15	4	0.4	0.9	1.9
Coconut:								
Raw:								
Piece, about 2 by 2 by ½ in-	1 piece	45	47	160	1	15	13.4	0.6	0.2
Dried, sweetened, shredded-	1 cup	93	13	470	3	33	29.3	1.4	0.4
Filberts (hazelnuts), chopped-	1 oz	28	5	180	4	18	1.3	13.9	1.7
Lentils, dry, cooked-	1 cup	200	72	215	16	1	0.1	0.2	0.5
Macadamia nuts, roasted in oil, salted-	1 oz	28	2	205	2	22	3.2	17.1	0.4
Mixed nuts, with peanuts, salted:								
Dry roasted-	1 oz	28	2	170	5	15	2.0	8.9	3.1
Roasted in oil-	1 oz	28	2	175	5	16	2.5	9.0	3.8
Peanuts, roasted in oil, salted-	1 oz	28	2	165	8	14	1.9	6.9	4.4
Peanut butter-	1 tbsp	16	1	95	5	8	1.4	4.0	2.5
Peas, split, dry, cooked-	1 cup	200	70	230	16	1	0.1	0.1	0.3
Pecans, halves-	1 oz	28	5	190	2	19	1.5	12.0	4.7
Pine nuts (pinyons), shelled-	1 oz	28	6	160	3	17	2.7	6.5	7.3
Pistachio nuts, dried, shelled	1 oz	28	4	165	6	14	1.7	9.3	2.1
Pumpkin and squash kernels, dry, hulled-	1 oz	28	7	155	7	13	2.5	4.0	5.9
Refried beans, canned-	1 cup	290	72	295	18	3	0.4	0.6	1.4
Sesame seeds, dry, hulled-	1 tbsp	8	5	45	2	4	0.6	1.7	1.9
Soybeans, dry, cooked, drained-	1 cup	180	71	235	20	10	1.3	1.9	5.3

(Tr indicates nutrient present in trace amounts.)

Nutrients in Indicated Quantity

Cholesterol	Carbohydrate	Calcium	Phosphorus	Iron	Potassium	Sodium	Vitamin A value (IU)	Vitamin A value (RE)	Thiamin	Riboflavin	Niacin	Ascorbic acid
Milligrams	Grams	Milligrams	Milligrams	Milligrams	Milligrams	Milligrams	International units	Retinol equivalents	Milligrams	Milligrams	Milligrams	Milligrams
30	32	94	303	4.8	668	1,374	330	33	0.18	0.15	3.3	Tr
10	48	138	235	4.6	536	1,181	330	33	0.20	0.08	1.5	5
10	54	161	291	5.9	536	969	330	33	0.15	0.10	1.3	5
0	42	74	278	4.6	673	968	10	1	0.13	0.10	1.5	0
0	35	43	238	3.3	573	20	30	3	0.40	0.10	1.0	0
0	4	50	170	1.0	170	1	Tr	Tr	0.28	0.03	0.5	Tr
0	126	390	102	5.7	1,275	24	Tr	Tr	0.07	0.07	2.2	Tr
0	9	13	139	1.7	160	[41]181	0	0	0.06	0.06	0.4	0
0	8	12	121	1.2	150	[42]177	0	0	0.12	0.05	0.5	0
0	76	41	153	1.3	847	3	30	3	0.35	0.25	1.9	37
0	45	80	273	4.9	475	11	Tr	Tr	0.18	0.09	0.9	0
0	7	6	51	1.1	160	9	0	0	0.03	0.01	0.2	1
0	44	14	99	1.8	313	244	0	0	0.03	0.02	0.4	1
0	4	53	88	0.9	126	1	20	2	0.14	0.03	0.3	Tr
0	38	50	238	4.2	498	26	40	4	0.14	0.12	1.2	0
0	4	13	57	0.5	93	[43]74	Tr	Tr	0.06	0.03	0.6	0
0	7	20	123	1.0	169	[44]190	Tr	Tr	0.06	0.06	1.3	0
0	6	31	131	0.9	165	[44]185	10	1	0.14	0.06	1.4	Tr
0	5	24	143	0.5	199	[45]122	0	0	0.08	0.03	4.2	0
0	3	5	60	0.3	110	75	0	0	0.02	0.02	2.2	0
0	42	22	178	3.4	592	26	80	8	0.30	0.18	1.8	0
0	5	10	83	0.6	111	Tr	40	4	0.24	0.04	0.3	1
0	5	2	10	0.9	178	20	10	1	0.35	0.06	1.2	1
0	7	38	143	1.9	310	2	70	7	0.23	0.05	0.3	Tr
0	5	12	333	4.2	229	5	110	11	0.06	0.09	0.5	Tr
0	51	141	245	5.1	1,141	1,228	0	0	0.14	0.16	1.4	17
0	1	11	62	0.6	33	3	10	1	0.06	0.01	0.4	0
0	19	131	322	4.9	972	4	50	5	0.38	0.16	1.1	0

Nutritive Value of Foods *(Continued)*

Foods, approximate measures, units, and weight (weight of edible portion only)		Water	Food energy	Pro-tein	Fat	Fatty Acids Satu-rated	Mono-unsatu-rated	Poly-unsatu-rated
		Percent	Calories	Grams	Grams	Grams	Grams	Grams
LEGUMES, NUTS, AND SEEDS—Con.	Grams							
Soy products:								
Miso- - - - - - - - - - - - - - - -	1 cup - - - - - - - - -	276	53	470	29	13	1.8	2.6	7.3
Tofu, piece 2½ by 2¾								
by 1 in- - - - - - - - - - - -	1 piece - - - - - - - -	120	85	85	9	5	0.7	1.0	2.9
Sunflower seeds, dry, hulled-	1 oz - - - - - - - - -	28	5	160	6	14	1.5	2.7	9.3
Tahini - - - - - - - - - - - - - - -	1 tbsp - - - - - - - -	15	3	90	3	8	1.1	3.0	3.5
Walnuts:								
Black, chopped- - - - - - - -	1 oz - - - - - - - - - -	28	4	170	7	16	1.0	3.6	10.6
English or Persian, pieces or chips- - - - - - - - - - - -	1 oz - - - - - - - - - -	28	4	180	4	18	1.6	4.0	11.1
MEAT AND MEAT PRODUCTS								
Beef, cooked:[46]								
Cuts braised, simmered, or pot roasted:								
Relatively fat such as chuck blade:								
Lean and fat, piece, 2½ by 2½ by ¾ in - - - -	3 oz - - - - - - - - - -	85	43	325	22	26	10.8	11.7	0.9
Lean only- - - - - - - -	2.2 oz - - - - - - - -	62	53	170	19	9	3.9	4.2	0.3
Relatively lean, such as bottom round:								
Lean and fat, piece, 4⅛ by 2¼ by ½ in- - - -	3 oz - - - - - - - - -	85	54	220	25	13	4.8	5.7	0.5
Lean only- - - - - - - -	2.8 oz - - - - - - - -	78	57	175	25	8	2.7	3.4	0.3
Ground beef, broiled, patty, 3 by ⅝ in:								
Lean- - - - - - - - - - - - - -	3 oz - - - - - - - - - -	85	56	230	21	16	6.2	6.9	0.6
Regular- - - - - - - - - - -	3 oz - - - - - - - - - -	85	54	245	20	18	6.9	7.7	0.7
Liver, fried, slice, 6½ by 2⅜ by ⅜ in[47]- - - - - - - -	3 oz - - - - - - - - - -	85	56	185	23	7	2.5	3.6	1.3
Roast, oven cooked, no liquid added:								
Relatively fat, such as rib:								
Lean and fat, 2 pieces, 4⅛ by 2¼ by ¼ in - -	3 oz - - - - - - - - - -	85	46	315	19	26	10.8	11.4	0.9
Lean only- - - - - - - -	2.2 oz - - - - - - - -	61	57	150	17	9	3.6	3.7	0.3
Relatively lean, such as eye of round:								
Lean and fat, 2 pieces, 2½ by 2½ by ⅜ in- -	3 oz - - - - - - - - - -	85	57	205	23	12	4.9	5.4	0.5
Lean only- - - - - - - -	2.6 oz - - - - - - - -	75	63	135	22	5	1.9	2.1	0.2
Steak:								
Sirloin, broiled:								
Lean and fat, piece, 2½ by 2½ by ¾ in - - - -	3 oz - - - - - - - - - -	85	53	240	23	15	6.4	6.9	0.6
Lean only- - - - - - - -	2.5 oz - - - - - - - -	72	59	150	22	6	2.6	2.8	0.3
Beef, canned, corned- - - - - -	3 oz - - - - - - - - - -	85	59	185	22	10	4.2	4.9	0.4

(Tr indicates nutrient present in trace amounts.)

Nutrients in Indicated Quantity

Cholesterol	Carbohydrate	Calcium	Phosphorus	Iron	Potassium	Sodium	Vitamin A value		Thiamin	Riboflavin	Niacin	Ascorbic acid
							(IU)	(RE)				
Milligrams	Grams	Milligrams	Milligrams	Milligrams	Milligrams	Milligrams	International units	Retinol equivalents	Milligrams	Milligrams	Milligrams	Milligrams
0	65	188	853	4.7	922	8,142	110	11	0.17	0.28	0.8	0
0	3	108	151	2.3	50	8	0	0	0.07	0.04	0.1	0
0	5	33	200	1.9	195	1	10	1	0.65	0.07	1.3	Tr
0	3	21	119	0.7	69	5	10	1	0.24	0.02	0.8	1
0	3	16	132	0.9	149	Tr	80	8	0.06	0.03	0.2	Tr
0	5	27	90	0.7	142	3	40	4	0.11	0.04	0.3	1
87	0	11	163	2.5	163	53	Tr	Tr	0.06	0.19	2.0	0
66	0	8	146	2.3	163	44	Tr	Tr	0.05	0.17	1.7	0
81	0	5	217	2.8	248	43	Tr	Tr	0.06	0.21	3.3	0
75	0	4	212	2.7	240	40	Tr	Tr	0.06	0.20	3.0	0
74	0	9	134	1.8	256	65	Tr	Tr	0.04	0.18	4.4	0
76	0	9	144	2.1	248	70	Tr	Tr	0.03	0.16	4.9	0
410	7	9	392	5.3	309	90	[48]30,690	[48]9,120	0.18	3.52	12.3	23
72	0	8	145	2.0	246	54	Tr	Tr	0.06	0.16	3.1	0
49	0	5	127	1.7	218	45	Tr	Tr	0.05	0.13	2.7	0
62	0	5	177	1.6	308	50	Tr	Tr	0.07	0.14	3.0	0
52	0	3	170	1.5	297	46	Tr	Tr	0.07	0.13	2.8	0
77	0	9	186	2.6	306	53	Tr	Tr	0.10	0.23	3.3	0
64	0	8	176	2.4	290	48	Tr	Tr	0.09	0.22	3.1	0
80	0	17	90	3.7	51	802	Tr	Tr	0.02	0.20	2.9	0

Nutritive Value of Foods *(Continued)*

Foods, approximate measures, units, and weight (weight of edible portion only)		Water	Food energy	Pro-tein	Fat	Satu-rated	Mono-unsatu-rated	Poly-unsatu-rated
							Fatty Acids	
	Grams	*Per-cent*	*Cal-ories*	*Grams*	*Grams*	*Grams*	*Grams*	*Grams*
MEAT AND MEAT PRODUCTS—Con.								
Beef, dried, chipped- - - - - - - 2.5 oz - - - - - - - - -	72	48	145	24	4	1.8	2.0	0.2
Lamb, cooked:								
Chops, (3 per lb with bone):								
Arm, braised:								
Lean and fat- - - - - - - 2.2 oz - - - - - - - - -	63	44	220	20	15	6.9	6.0	0.9
Lean only- - - - - - - - - 1.7 oz - - - - - - - - -	48	49	135	17	7	2.9	2.6	0.4
Loin, broiled:								
Lean and fat- - - - - - - 2.8 oz - - - - - - - - -	80	54	235	22	16	7.3	6.4	1.0
Lean only- - - - - - - - - 2.3 oz - - - - - - - - -	64	61	140	19	6	2.6	2.4	0.4
Leg, roasted:								
Lean and fat, 2 pieces, 4⅛								
by 2¼ by ¼ in- - - - 3 oz - - - - - - - - - -	85	59	205	22	13	5.6	4.9	0.8
Lean only- - - - - - - - - 2.6 oz - - - - - - - - -	73	64	140	20	6	2.4	2.2	0.4
Rib, roasted:								
Lean and fat, 3 pieces, 2½								
by 2½ by ¼ in- - - - - 3 oz - - - - - - - - - -	85	47	315	18	26	12.1	10.6	1.5
Lean only- - - - - - - - - 2 oz - - - - - - - - - -	57	60	130	15	7	3.2	3.0	0.5
Pork, cured, cooked:								
Bacon:								
Regular- - - - - - - - - - - - 3 medium slices- -	19	13	110	6	9	3.3	4.5	1.1
Canadian-style- - - - - - - 2 slices- - - - - - - -	46	62	85	11	4	1.3	1.9	0.4
Ham, light cure, roasted:								
Lean and fat, 2 pieces, 4⅛								
by 2¼ by ¼ in- - - - - - 3 oz - - - - - - - - - -	85	58	205	18	14	5.1	6.7	1.5
Lean only- - - - - - - - - 2.4 oz - - - - - - - - -	68	66	105	17	4	1.3	1.7	0.4
Luncheon meat:								
Canned, spiced or un-spiced, slice, 3 by 2 by ½								
in- - - - - - - - - - - - - - 2 slices- - - - - - - -	42	52	140	5	13	4.5	6.0	1.5
Cooked ham (8 slices per 8-oz pkg):								
Regular- - - - - - - - - - 2 slices- - - - - - - -	57	65	105	10	6	1.9	2.8	0.7
Extra lean- - - - - - - - 2 slices- - - - - - - -	57	71	75	11	3	0.9	1.3	0.3
Pork, fresh, cooked:								
Chop, loin (cut 3 per lb with bone):								
Broiled:								
Lean and fat- - - - - - - 3.1 oz - - - - - - - - -	87	50	275	24	19	7.0	8.8	2.2
Lean only- - - - - - - - - 2.5 oz - - - - - - - - -	72	57	165	23	8	2.6	3.4	0.9
Pan fried:								
Lean and fat- - - - - - - 3.1 oz - - - - - - - - -	89	45	335	21	27	9.8	12.5	3.1
Lean only- - - - - - - - - 2.4 oz - - - - - - - - -	67	54	180	19	11	3.7	4.8	1.3
Ham (leg), roasted:								
Lean and fat, piece, 2½ by								
2½ by ¾ in- - - - - - - 3 oz - - - - - - - - - -	85	53	250	21	18	6.4	8.1	2.0
Lean only- - - - - - - - - 2.5 oz - - - - - - - - -	72	60	160	20	8	2.7	3.6	1.0

(Tr indicates nutrient present in trace amounts.)

Nutrients in Indicated Quantity

Cholesterol	Carbohydrate	Calcium	Phosphorus	Iron	Potassium	Sodium	Vitamin A Value		Thiamin	Riboflavin	Niacin	Ascorbic acid
							(IU)	(RE)				
Milligrams	Grams	Milligrams	Milligrams	Milligrams	Milligrams	Milligrams	International units	Retinol equivalents	Milligrams	Milligrams	Milligrams	Milligrams
46	0	14	287	2.3	142	3,053	Tr	Tr	0.05	0.23	2.7	0
77	0	16	132	1.5	195	46	Tr	Tr	0.04	0.16	4.4	0
59	0	12	111	1.3	162	36	Tr	Tr	0.03	0.13	3.0	0
78	0	16	162	1.4	272	62	Tr	Tr	0.09	0.21	5.5	0
60	0	12	145	1.3	241	54	Tr	Tr	0.08	0.18	4.4	0
78	0	8	162	1.7	273	57	Tr	Tr	0.09	0.24	5.5	0
65	0	6	150	1.5	247	50	Tr	Tr	0.08	0.20	4.6	0
77	0	19	139	1.4	224	60	Tr	Tr	0.08	0.18	5.5	0
50	0	12	111	1.0	179	46	Tr	Tr	0.05	0.13	3.5	0
16	Tr	2	64	0.3	92	303	0	0	0.13	0.05	1.4	6
27	1	5	136	0.4	179	711	0	0	0.38	0.09	3.2	10
53	0	6	182	0.7	243	1,009	0	0	0.51	0.19	3.8	0
37	0	5	154	0.6	215	902	0	0	0.46	0.17	3.4	0
26	1	3	34	0.3	90	541	0	0	0.15	0.08	1.3	Tr
32	2	4	141	0.6	189	751	0	0	0.49	0.14	3.0	[49]16
27	1	4	124	0.4	200	815	0	0	0.53	0.13	2.8	[49]15
84	0	3	184	0.7	312	61	10	3	0.87	0.24	4.3	Tr
71	0	4	176	0.7	302	56	10	1	0.83	0.22	4.0	Tr
92	0	4	190	0.7	323	64	10	3	0.91	0.24	4.6	Tr
72	0	3	178	0.7	305	57	10	1	0.84	0.22	4.0	Tr
79	0	5	210	0.9	280	50	10	2	0.54	0.27	3.9	Tr
68	0	5	202	0.8	269	46	10	1	0.50	0.25	3.6	Tr

Nutritive Value of Foods *(Continued)*

Foods, approximate measures, units, and weight (weight of edible portion only)		Water	Food energy	Pro-tein	Fat	Satu-rated	Fatty Acids Mono-unsatu-rated	Poly-unsatu-rated
		Per-cent	*Cal-ories*	*Grams*	*Grams*	*Grams*	*Grams*	*Grams*
		Grams						
MEAT AND MEAT PRODUCTS—Con.								
Rib, roasted:								
Lean and fat, piece, 2½ by ¾ in	3 oz	85	51	270	21	20	7.2	9.2	2.3
Lean only	2.5 oz	71	57	175	20	10	3.4	4.4	1.2
Shoulder cut, braised:								
Lean and fat, 3 pieces, 2½ by 2½ by ¼ in	3 oz	85	47	295	23	22	7.9	10.0	2.4
Lean only	2.4 oz	67	54	165	22	8	2.8	3.7	1.0
Sausages (See also Luncheon meats):								
Bologna, slice (8 per 8-oz pkg)	2 slices	57	54	180	7	16	6.1	7.6	1.4
Braunschweiger, slice (6 per 6-oz pkg)	2 slices	57	48	205	8	18	6.2	8.5	2.1
Brown and serve (10–11 per 8-oz pkg), browned	1 link	13	45	50	2	5	1.7	2.2	0.5
Frankfurter (10 per 1-lb pkg), cooked (reheated)	1 frankfurter	45	54	145	5	13	4.8	6.2	1.2
Pork link (16 per 1-lb pkg), cooked[50]	1 link	13	45	50	3	4	1.4	1.8	0.5
Salami:								
Cooked type, slice (8 per 8-oz pkg)	2 slices	57	60	145	8	11	4.6	5.2	1.2
Dry type, slice (12 per 4-oz pkg)	2 slices	20	35	85	5	7	2.4	3.4	0.6
Sandwich spread (pork, beef)	1 tbsp	15	60	35	1	3	0.9	1.1	0.4
Vienna sausage (7 per 4-oz can)	1 sausage	16	60	45	2	4	1.5	2.0	0.3
Veal, medium fat, cooked, bone removed:								
Cutlet, 4⅛ by 2¼ by ½ in, braised or broiled	3 oz	85	60	185	23	9	4.1	4.1	0.6
Rib, 2 pieces, 4⅛ by 2¼ by ¼ in, roasted	3 oz	85	55	230	23	14	6.0	6.0	1.0
MIXED DISHES AND FAST FOODS								
Mixed dishes:								
Chicken potpie, from home recipe, baked, piece, ⅓ of 9-in diam. pie[51]	1 piece	232	57	545	23	31	10.3	15.5	6.6
Chili con carne with beans, canned	1 cup	255	72	340	19	16	5.8	7.2	1.0
Chop suey with beef and pork, from home recipe	1 cup	250	75	300	26	17	4.3	7.4	4.2

(Tr indicates nutrient present in trace amounts.)

Cholesterol	Carbohydrate	Calcium	Phosphorus	Iron	Potassium	Sodium	Vitamin A value		Thiamin	Riboflavin	Niacin	Ascorbic acid
							(IU)	(RE)				
Milligrams	Grams	Milligrams	Milligrams	Milligrams	Milligrams	Milligrams	International units	Retinol equivalents	Milligrams	Milligrams	Milligrams	Milligrams
69	0	9	190	0.8	313	37	10	3	0.50	0.24	4.2	Tr
56	0	8	182	0.7	300	33	10	2	0.45	0.22	3.8	Tr
93	0	6	162	1.4	286	75	10	3	0.46	0.26	4.4	Tr
76	0	5	151	1.3	271	68	10	1	0.40	0.24	4.0	Tr
31	2	7	52	0.9	103	581	0	0	0.10	0.08	1.5	[40]12
89	2	5	96	5.3	113	652	8,010	2,405	0.14	0.87	4.8	[40]6
9	Tr	1	14	0.1	25	105	0	0	0.05	0.02	0.4	0
23	1	5	39	0.5	75	504	0	0	0.09	0.05	1.2	[40]12
11	Tr	4	24	0.2	47	168	0	0	0.10	0.03	0.6	Tr
37	1	7	66	1.5	113	607	0	0	0.14	0.21	2.0	[40]7
16	1	2	28	0.3	76	372	0	0	0.12	0.06	1.0	[40]5
6	2	2	9	0.1	17	152	10	1	0.03	0.02	0.3	0
8	Tr	2	8	0.1	16	152	0	0	0.01	0.02	0.3	0
109	0	9	196	0.8	258	56	Tr	Tr	0.06	0.21	4.6	0
109	0	10	211	0.7	259	57	Tr	Tr	0.11	0.26	6.6	0
56	42	70	232	3.0	343	594	7,220	735	0.32	0.32	4.9	5
28	31	82	321	4.3	594	1,354	150	15	0.08	0.18	3.3	8
68	13	60	248	4.8	425	1,053	600	60	0.28	0.38	5.0	33

Nutritive Value of Foods *(Continued)*

Foods, approximate measures, units, and weight (weight of edible portion only)		Water	Food energy	Pro-tein	Fat	Fatty Acids Satu-rated	Mono-unsatu-rated	Poly-unsatu-rated
		Per-cent	*Cal-ories*	*Grams*	*Grams*	*Grams*	*Grams*	*Grams*
MIXED DISHES AND FAST FOODS—Con.	*Grams*							
Macaroni (enriched) and cheese:								
Canned[52] - - - - - - - - - 1 cup - - - - - - - -	240	80	230	9	10	4.7	2.9	1.3
Quiche Lorraine, ⅛ of 8-in diam. quiche[51] - - - - - 1 slice - - - - - - - -	176	47	600	13	48	23.2	17.8	4.1
Spaghetti (enriched) in to-mato sauce with cheese:								
Canned - - - - - - - - - - - 1 cup - - - - - - - -	250	80	190	6	2	0.4	0.4	0.5
From home recipe - - - - - 1 cup - - - - - - - -	250	77	260	9	9	3.0	3.6	1.2
Spaghetti (enriched) with meatballs and tomato sauce:								
From home recipe - - - - - 1 cup - - - - - - - -	248	70	330	19	12	3.9	4.4	2.2
Fast food entrees:								
Cheeseburger:								
Regular - - - - - - - - - - - 1 sandwich - - - - -	112	46	300	15	15	7.3	5.6	1.0
4 oz patty - - - - - - - - - 1 sandwich - - - - -	194	46	525	30	31	15.1	12.2	1.4
Chicken, fried. See Poultry and Poultry Products.								
Enchilada - - - - - - - - - - 1 enchilada - - - - -	230	72	235	20	16	7.7	6.7	0.6
English muffin, egg, cheese, and bacon - - - - - - - - - 1 sandwich - - - - -	138	49	360	18	18	8.0	8.0	0.7
Fish sandwich:								
Regular, with cheese - - - 1 sandwich - - - - -	140	43	420	16	23	6.3	6.9	7.7
Large, without cheese - - 1 sandwich - - - - -	170	48	470	18	27	6.3	8.7	9.5
Hamburger:								
Regular - - - - - - - - - - - 1 sandwich - - - - -	98	46	245	12	11	4.4	5.3	0.5
4 oz patty - - - - - - - - - 1 sandwich - - - - -	174	50	445	25	21	7.1	11.7	0.6
Pizza, cheese, ⅛ of 15-in diam. pizza[51] - - - - - - 1 slice - - - - - - - -	120	46	290	15	9	4.1	2.6	1.3
Roast beef sandwich - - - - - 1 sandwich - - - - -	150	52	345	22	13	3.5	6.9	1.8
Taco - - - - - - - - - - - - - - 1 taco - - - - - - - - -	81	55	195	9	11	4.1	5.5	0.8
POULTRY AND POULTRY PRODUCTS								
Chicken:								
Fried, flesh, with skin:[53]								
Batter dipped:								
Breast, ½ breast (5.6 oz with bones) - - - - - - 4.9 oz - - - - - - - - -	140	52	365	35	18	4.9	7.6	4.3
Drumstick (3.4 oz with bones) - - - - - - - - - 2.5 oz - - - - - - - - -	72	53	195	16	11	3.0	4.6	2.7
Flour coated:								
Breast, ½ breast (4.2 oz with bones) - - - - - - 3.5 oz - - - - - - - - -	98	57	220	31	9	2.4	3.4	1.9
Drumstick (2.6 oz with bones) - - - - - - - - - 1.7 oz - - - - - - - - -	49	57	120	13	7	1.8	2.7	1.6

(Tr indicates nutrient present in trace amounts.)

Nutrients in Indicated Quantity

Cholesterol	Carbohydrate	Calcium	Phosphorus	Iron	Potassium	Sodium	Vitamin A value		Thiamin	Riboflavin	Niacin	Ascorbic acid
							(IU)	(RE)				
Milligrams	Grams	Milligrams	Milligrams	Milligrams	Milligrams	Milligrams	International units	Retinol equivalents	Milligrams	Milligrams	Milligrams	Milligrams
24	26	199	182	1.0	139	730	260	72	0.12	0.24	1.0	Tr
285	29	211	276	1.0	283	653	1,640	454	0.11	0.32	Tr	Tr
3	39	40	88	2.8	303	955	930	120	0.35	0.28	4.5	10
8	37	80	135	2.3	408	955	1,080	140	0.25	0.18	2.3	13
89	39	124	236	3.7	665	1,009	1,590	159	0.25	0.30	4.0	22
44	28	135	174	2.3	219	672	340	65	0.26	0.24	3.7	1
104	40	236	320	4.5	407	1,224	670	128	0.33	0.48	7.4	3
19	24	97	198	3.3	653	1,332	2,720	352	0.18	0.26	Tr	Tr
213	31	197	290	3.1	201	832	650	160	0.46	0.50	3.7	1
56	39	132	223	1.8	274	667	160	25	0.32	0.26	3.3	2
91	41	61	246	2.2	375	621	110	15	0.35	0.23	3.5	1
32	28	56	107	2.2	202	463	80	14	0.23	0.24	3.8	1
71	38	75	225	4.8	404	763	160	28	0.38	0.38	7.8	1
56	39	220	216	1.6	230	699	750	106	0.34	0.29	4.2	2
55	34	60	222	4.0	338	757	240	32	0.40	0.33	6.0	2
21	15	109	134	1.2	263	456	420	57	0.09	0.07	1.4	1
119	13	28	259	1.8	281	385	90	28	0.16	0.20	14.7	0
62	6	12	106	1.0	134	194	60	19	0.08	0.15	3.7	0
87	2	16	228	1.2	254	74	50	15	0.08	0.13	13.5	0
44	1	6	86	0.7	112	44	40	12	0.04	0.11	3.0	0

Foods, approximate measures, units, and weight (weight of edible portion only)		Water	Food energy	Pro-tein	Fat	Fatty Acids Saturated	Mono-unsatu-rated	Poly-unsatu-rated
		Per-cent	Cal-ories	Grams	Grams	Grams	Grams	Grams
POULTRY AND POULTRY PRODUCTS—Con.		Grams						
Roasted, flesh only:								
Breast, ½ breast (4.2 oz with bones and skin)- - - - - - -	3.0 oz - - - - - - - - -	86	65	140	27	3	0.9	1.1	0.7
Drumstick, (2.9 oz with bones and skin)- - -	1.6 oz - - - - - - - - -	44	67	75	12	2	0.7	0.8	0.6
Stewed, flesh only, light and dark meat, chopped or diced- - - - - - - - -	1 cup - - - - - - - - -	140	67	250	38	9	2.6	3.3	2.2
Chicken liver, cooked- - - - -	1 liver - - -¦- - - - - -	20	68	30	5	1	0.4	0.3	0.2
Duck, roasted, flesh only- - -	½ duck - - - - - - - -	221	64	445	52	25	9.2	8.2	3.2
Turkey, roasted, flesh only:								
Dark meat, piece, 2½ by 1⅝ by ¼ in - - - - - - - - - - -	4 pieces - - - - - - - -	85	63	160	24	6	2.1	1.4	1.8
Light meat, piece, 4 by 2 by ¼ in- - - - - - - - - - - - -	2 pieces- - - - - - - - -	85	66	135	25	3	0.9	0.5	0.7
Poultry food products:								
Turkey:								
Loaf, breast meat (8 slices per 6-oz pkg)- - - - - -	2 slices - - - - - - - -	42	72	45	10	1	0.2	0.2	0.1
Roast, boneless, frozen, seasoned, light and dark meat, cooked- - -	3 oz - - - - - - - - - -	85	68	130	18	5	1.6	1.0	1.4
SOUPS, SAUCES, AND GRAVIES								
Soups:								
Canned, condensed:								
Prepared with equal volume of milk:								
Clam chowder, New England - - - - - - - -	1 cup - - - - - - - - -	248	85	165	9	7	3.0	2.3	1.1
Cream of chicken- - - -	1 cup - - - - - - - - -	248	85	190	7	11	4.6	4.5	1.6
Cream of mushroom- - -	1 cup - - - - - - - - -	248	85	205	6	14	5.1	3.0	4.6
Tomato- - - - - - - -	1 cup - - - - - - - - -	248	85	160	6	6	2.9	1.6	1.1
Prepared with equal volume of water:								
Bean with bacon- - - -	1 cup - - - - - - - - -	253	84	170	8	6	1.5	2.2	1.8
Beef broth, bouillon, consomme- - - - - - -	1 cup - - - - - - - - -	240	98	15	3	1	0.3	0.2	Tr
Beef noodle- - - - - - -	1 cup - - - - - - - - -	244	92	85	5	3	1.1	1.2	0.5
Chicken noodle- - - - -	1 cup - - - - - - - - -	241	92	75	4	2	0.7	1.1	0.6
Chicken rice- - - - - - -	1 cup - - - - - - - - -	241	94	60	4	2	0.5	0.9	0.4
Clam chowder, Man-hattan- - - - - - - - -	1 cup - - - - - - - - -	244	90	80	4	2	0.4	0.4	1.3
Cream of chicken- - - -	1 cup - - - - - - - - -	244	91	115	3	7	2.1	3.3	1.5
Cream of mushroom- -	1 cup - - - - - - - - -	244	90	130	2	9	2.4	1.7	4.2
Minestrone- - - - - - - -	1 cup - - - - - - - - -	241	91	80	4	3	0.6	0.7	1.1
Pea, green- - - - - - - -	1 cup - - - - - - - - -	250	83	165	9	3	1.4	1.0	0.4

(Tr indicates nutrient present in trace amounts.)

Nutrients in Indicated Quantity

Cho-les-terol	Carbo-hydrate	Calcium	Phos-phorus	Iron	Potas-sium	Sodium	Vitamin A value		Thiamin	Ribo-flavin	Niacin	Ascorbic acid
							(IU)	(RE)				
Milli-grams	Grams	Milli-grams	Milli-grams	Milli-grams	Milli-grams	Milli-grams	Inter-national units	Retinol equiva-lents	Milli-grams	Milli-grams	Milli-grams	Milli-grams
73	0	13	196	0.9	220	64	20	5	0.06	0.10	11.8	0
41	0	5	81	0.6	108	42	30	8	0.03	0.10	2.7	0
116	0	20	210	1.6	252	98	70	21	0.07	0.23	8.6	0
126	Tr	3	62	1.7	28	10	3,270	983	0.03	0.35	0.9	3
197	0	27	449	6.0	557	144	170	51	0.57	1.04	11.3	0
72	0	27	173	2.0	246	67	0	0	0.05	0.21	3.1	0
59	0	16	186	1.1	259	54	0	0	0.05	0.11	5.8	0
17	0	3	97	0.2	118	608	0	0	0.02	0.05	3.5	[54]0
45	3	4	207	1.4	253	578	0	0	0.04	0.14	5.3	0
22	17	186	156	1.5	300	992	160	40	0.07	0.24	1.0	3
27	15	181	151	0.7	273	1,047	710	94	0.07	0.26	0.9	1
20	15	179	156	0.6	270	1,076	150	37	0.08	0.28	0.9	2
17	22	159	149	1.8	449	932	850	109	0.13	0.25	1.5	68
3	23	81	132	2.0	402	951	890	89	0.09	0.03	0.6	2
Tr	Tr	14	31	0.4	130	782	0	0	Tr	0.05	1.9	0
5	9	15	46	1.1	100	952	630	63	0.07	0.06	1.1	Tr
7	9	17	36	0.8	55	1,106	710	71	0.05	0.06	1.4	Tr
7	7	17	22	0.7	101	815	660	66	0.02	0.02	1.1	Tr
2	12	34	59	1.9	261	1,808	920	92	0.06	0.05	1.3	3
10	9	34	37	0.6	88	986	560	56	0.03	0.06	0.8	Tr
2	9	46	49	0.5	100	1,032	0	0	0.05	0.09	0.7	1
2	11	34	55	0.9	313	911	2,340	234	0.05	0.04	0.9	1
0	27	28	125	2.0	190	988	200	20	0.11	0.07	1.2	2

Nutritive Value of Foods *(Continued)*

Foods, approximate measures, units, and weight (weight of edible portion only)		Water	Food energy	Pro-tein	Fat	Satu-rated	Mono-unsatu-rated	Poly-unsatu-rated
							Fatty Acids	
		Per-cent	*Cal-ories*	*Grams*	*Grams*	*Grams*	*Grams*	*Grams*
SOUPS, SAUCES, AND GRAVIES—Con.	*Grams*							
Tomato- - - - - - - - - - 1 cup - - - - - - - - -	244	90	85	2	2	0.4	0.4	1.0
Vegetable beef - - - - - - 1 cup - - - - - - - - -	244	92	80	6	2	0.9	0.8	0.1
Vegetarian - - - - - - - - 1 cup - - - - - - - - -	241	92	70	2	2	0.3	0.8	0.7
Dehydrated:								
Prepared with water:								
Chicken noodle - - - - - 1 pkt (6-fl-oz) - - -	188	94	40	2	1	0.2	0.4	0.3
Onion - - - - - - - - - - - 1 pkt (6-fl-oz) - - -	184	96	20	1	Tr	0.1	0.2	0.1
Tomato vegetable - - - 1 pkt (6-fl-oz) - - -	189	94	40	1	1	0.3	0.2	0.1
Sauces:								
From dry mix:								
Hollandaise, prepared								
with water - - - - - - - 1 cup - - - - - - - - -	259	84	240	5	20	11.6	5.9	0.9
White sauce, prepared								
with milk - - - - - - - - 1 cup - - - - - - - - -	264	81	240	10	13	6.4	4.7	1.7
From home recipe:								
White sauce, medium[55] - 1 cup - - - - - - - - -	250	73	395	10	30	9.1	11.9	7.2
Ready to serve:								
Barbecue - - - - - - - - - 1 tbsp - - - - - - - - -	16	81	10	Tr	Tr	Tr	0.1	0.1
Soy - - - - - - - - - - - - 1 tbsp - - - - - - - - -	18	68	10	2	0	0.0	0.0	0.0
SUGARS AND SWEETS								
Candy:								
Caramels, plain or choco-								
late - - - - - - - - - - - - - 1 oz - - - - - - - - -	28	8	115	1	3	2.2	0.3	0.1
Chocolate:								
Milk, plain - - - - - - - - 1 oz - - - - - - - - -	28	1	145	2	9	5.4	3.0	0.3
Milk, with almonds - - - 1 oz - - - - - - - - -	28	2	150	3	10	4.8	4.1	0.7
Milk, with peanuts - - - 1 oz - - - - - - - - -	28	1	155	4	11	4.2	3.5	1.5
Milk, with rice cereal - - 1 oz - - - - - - - - -	28	2	140	2	7	4.4	2.5	0.2
Semisweet, small pieces								
(60 per oz) - - - - - - - - 1 cup or 6 oz - - - -	170	1	860	7	61	36.2	19.9	1.9
Sweet (dark) - - - - - - - 1 oz - - - - - - - - -	28	1	150	1	10	5.9	3.3	0.3
Fudge, chocolate, plain - - 1 oz - - - - - - - - -	28	8	115	1	3	2.1	1.0	0.1
Gum drops - - - - - - - - - 1 oz - - - - - - - - -	28	12	100	Tr	Tr	Tr	Tr	0.1
Hard - - - - - - - - - - - - - 1 oz - - - - - - - - -	28	1	110	0	0	0.0	0.0	0.0
Jelly beans - - - - - - - - - 1 oz - - - - - - - - -	28	6	105	Tr	Tr	Tr	Tr	0.1
Marshmallows - - - - - - - 1 oz - - - - - - - - -	28	17	90	1	0	0.0	0.0	0.0
Custard, baked - - - - - - - 1 cup - - - - - - - - -	265	77	305	14	15	6.8	5.4	0.7
Gelatin dessert prepared with								
gelatin dessert powder and								
water - - - - - - - - - - - - - ½ cup - - - - - - - - -	120	84	70	2	0	0.0	0.0	0.0
Honey, strained or extracted 1 cup - - - - - - - - -	339	17	1,030	1	0	0.0	0.0	0.0
1 tbsp - - - - - - - - -	21	17	65	Tr	0	0.0	0.0	0.0
Jams and preserves - - - - - 1 tbsp - - - - - - - - -	20	29	55	Tr	Tr	0.0	Tr	Tr
1 packet - - - - - - -	14	29	40	Tr	Tr	0.0	Tr	Tr
Jellies - - - - - - - - - - - - - 1 tbsp - - - - - - - - -	18	28	50	Tr	Tr	Tr	Tr	Tr
1 packet - - - - - - -	14	28	40	Tr	Tr	Tr	Tr	Tr
Popsicle, 3-fl-oz size - - - - 1 popsicle - - - - - -	95	80	70	0	0	0.0	0.0	0.0

(Tr indicates nutrient present in trace amounts.)

Nutrients in Indicated Quantity

Cholesterol	Carbohydrate	Calcium	Phosphorus	Iron	Potassium	Sodium	Vitamin A value		Thiamin	Riboflavin	Niacin	Ascorbic acid
							(IU)	(RE)				
Milligrams	Grams	Milligrams	Milligrams	Milligrams	Milligrams	Milligrams	International units	Retinol equivalents	Milligrams	Milligrams	Milligrams	Milligrams
0	17	12	34	1.8	264	871	690	69	0.09	0.05	1.4	66
5	10	17	41	1.1	173	956	1,890	189	0.04	0.05	1.0	2
0	12	22	34	1.1	210	822	3,010	301	0.05	0.05	0.9	1
2	6	24	24	0.4	23	957	50	5	0.05	0.04	0.7	Tr
0	4	9	22	0.1	48	635	Tr	Tr	0.02	0.04	0.4	Tr
0	8	6	23	0.5	78	856	140	14	0.04	0.03	0.6	5
52	14	124	127	0.9	124	1,564	730	220	0.05	0.18	0.1	Tr
34	21	425	256	0.3	444	797	310	92	0.08	0.45	0.2	3
32	24	292	238	0.9	381	888	1,190	340	0.15	0.43	0.8	2
0	2	3	3	0.1	28	130	140	14	Tr	Tr	0.1	1
0	2	3	38	0.5	64	1,029	0	0	0.01	0.02	0.6	0
1	22	42	35	0.4	54	64	Tr	Tr	0.01	0.05	0.1	Tr
6	16	50	61	0.4	96	23	30	10	0.02	0.10	0.1	Tr
5	15	65	77	0.5	125	23	30	8	0.02	0.12	0.2	Tr
5	13	49	83	0.4	138	19	30	8	0.07	0.07	1.4	Tr
6	18	48	57	0.2	100	46	30	8	0.01	0.08	0.1	Tr
0	97	51	178	5.8	593	24	30	3	0.10	0.14	0.9	Tr
0	16	7	41	0.6	86	5	10	1	0.01	0.04	0.1	Tr
1	21	22	24	0.3	42	54	Tr	Tr	0.01	0.03	0.1	Tr
0	25	2	Tr	0.1	1	10	0	0	0.00	Tr	0.0	0
0	28	Tr	2	0.1	1	7	0	0	0.10	0.00	0.0	0
0	26	1	1	0.3	11	7	0	0	0.00	Tr	Tr	0
0	23	1	2	0.5	2	25	0	0	0.00	Tr	Tr	0
278	29	297	310	1.1	387	209	530	146	0.11	0.50	0.3	1
0	17	2	23	Tr	Tr	55	0	0	0.00	0.00	0.0	0
0	279	17	20	1.7	173	17	0	0	0.02	0.14	1.0	3
0	17	1	1	0.1	11	1	0	0	Tr	0.01	0.1	Tr
0	14	4	2	0.2	18	2	Tr	Tr	Tr	0.01	Tr	Tr
0	10	3	1	0.1	12	2	Tr	Tr	Tr	Tr	Tr	Tr
0	13	2	Tr	0.1	16	5	Tr	Tr	Tr	0.01	Tr	Tr
0	10	1	Tr	Tr	13	4	Tr	Tr	Tr	Tr	Tr	Tr
0	18	0	0	Tr	4	11	0	0	0.00	0.00	0.0	0

Foods, approximate measures, units, and weight (weight of edible portion only)		Water	Food energy	Pro- tein	Fat	Fatty Acids		
						Satu- rated	Mono- unsatu- rated	Poly- unsatu- rated
	Grams	Per- cent	Cal- ories	Grams	Grams	Grams	Grams	Grams
SUGARS AND SWEETS— Con.								
Puddings:								
Canned:								
Vanilla- - - - - - - - - - - - 5-oz can- - - - - -	142	69	220	2	10	9.5	0.2	0.1
Dry mix, prepared with whole milk:								
Chocolate:								
Instant- - - - - - - - - - ½ cup- - - - - - - - -	130	71	155	4	4	2.3	1.1	0.2
Regular (cooked)- - - - ½ cup- - - - - - - - -	130	73	150	4	4	2.4	1.1	0.1
Rice- - - - - - - - - - - - - ½ cup- - - - - - - - -	132	73	155	4	4	2.3	1.1	0.1
Tapioca- - - - - - - - - - - ½ cup- - - - - - - - -	130	75	145	4	4	2.3	1.1	0.1
Vanilla:								
Instant- - - - - - - - - - ½ cup- - - - - - - - -	130	73	150	4	4	2.2	1.1	0.2
Sugars:								
Brown, pressed down- - - - 1 cup- - - - - - - - -	220	2	820	0	0	0.0	0.0	0.0
White:								
Granulated- - - - - - - - - 1 cup- - - - - - - - -	200	1	770	0	0	0.0	0.0	0.0
	1 tbsp- - - - - - - - -	12	1	45	0	0	0.0	0.0	0.0
	1 packet- - - - - - -	6	1	25	0	0	0.0	0.0	0.0
Powdered, sifted, spooned into cup- - - - 1 cup- - - - - - - - -	100	1	385	0	0	0.0	0.0	0.0
Syrups:								
Chocolate-flavored syrup or topping:								
Thin type- - - - - - - - - 2 tbsp- - - - - - - - -	38	37	85	1	Tr	0.2	0.1	0.1
Fudge type- - - - - - - - - 2 tbsp- - - - - - - - -	38	25	125	2	5	3.1	1.7	0.2
Molasses, cane, blackstrap 2 tbsp- - - - - - - - -	40	24	85	0	0	0.0	0.0	0.0
Table syrup (corn and maple)- - - - - - - - - - 2 tbsp- - - - - - - - -	42	25	122	0	0	0.0	0.0	0.0
VEGETABLES AND VEGETABLE PRODUCTS								
Alfalfa seeds, sprouted, raw- 1 cup- - - - - - - - -	33	91	10	1	Tr	Tr	Tr	0.1
Artichokes, globe or French, cooked, drained- - - - - - - - 1 artichoke- - - - -	120	87	55	3	Tr	Tr	Tr	0.1
Asparagus, green:								
Cooked, drained:								
From raw:								
Cuts and tips- - - - - - 1 cup- - - - - - - - -	180	92	45	5	1	0.1	Tr	0.2
Spears, ½-in diam. at base- - - - - - - - - - 4 spears- - - - - - -	60	92	15	2	Tr	Tr	Tr	0.1
From frozen:								
Cuts and tips- - - - - - 1 cup- - - - - - - - -	180	91	50	5	1	0.2	Tr	0.3
Spears, ½-in diam. at base- - - - - - - - - - 4 spears- - - - - - -	60	91	15	2	Tr	0.1	Tr	0.1
Canned, spears, ½-in diam. at base- - - - - - - - - - 4 spears- - - - - - -	80	95	10	1	Tr	Tr	Tr	0.1
Bamboo shoots, canned, drained- - - - - - - - - - - - 1 cup- - - - - - - - -	131	94	25	2	1	0.1	Tr	0.2

(Tr indicates nutrient present in trace amounts.)

Cho-les-terol	Carbo-hydrate	Calcium	Phos-phorus	Iron	Potas-sium	Sodium	Vitamin A value		Thiamin	Ribo-flavin	Niacin	Ascorbic acid
							(IU)	(RE)				
Milli-grams	Grams	Milli-grams	Milli-grams	Milli-grams	Milli-grams	Milli-grams	Inter-national units	Retinol equiva-lents	Milli-grams	Milli-grams	Milli-grams	Milli-grams
1	33	79	94	0.2	155	305	Tr	Tr	0.03	0.12	0.6	Tr
14	27	130	329	0.3	176	440	130	33	0.04	0.18	0.1	1
15	25	146	120	0.2	190	167	140	34	0.05	0.20	0.1	1
15	27	133	110	0.5	165	140	140	33	0.10	0.18	0.6	1
15	25	131	103	0.1	167	152	140	34	0.04	0.18	0.1	1
15	27	129	273	0.1	164	375	140	33	0.04	0.17	0.1	1
0	212	187	56	4.8	757	97	0	0	0.02	0.07	0.1	0
0	199	3	Tr	0.1	7	5	0	0	0.00	0.00	0.0	0
0	12	Tr	Tr	Tr	Tr	Tr	0	0	0.00	0.00	0.0	0
0	6	Tr	Tr	Tr	Tr	Tr	0	0	0.00	0.00	0.0	0
0	100	1	Tr	Tr	4	2	0	0	0.00	0.00	0.0	0
0	22	6	49	0.8	85	36	Tr	Tr	Tr	0.02	0.1	0
0	21	38	60	0.5	82	42	40	13	0.02	0.08	0.1	0
0	22	274	34	10.1	1,171	38	0	0	0.04	0.08	0.8	0
0	32	1	4	Tr	7	19	0	0	0.00	0.00	0.0	0
0	1	11	23	0.3	26	2	50	5	0.03	0.04	0.2	3
0	12	47	72	1.6	316	79	170	17	0.07	0.06	0.7	9
0	8	43	110	1.2	558	7	1,490	149	0.18	0.22	1.9	49
0	3	14	37	0.4	186	2	500	50	0.06	0.07	0.6	16
0	9	41	99	1.2	392	7	1,470	147	0.12	0.19	1.9	44
0	3	14	33	0.4	131	2	490	49	0.04	0.06	0.6	15
0	2	11	30	0.5	122	[56]278	380	38	0.04	0.07	0.7	13
0	4	10	33	0.4	105	9	10	1	0.03	0.03	0.2	1

Nutritive Value of Foods *(Continued)*

Foods, approximate measures, units, and weight (weight of edible portion only)			Water	Food energy	Pro-tein	Fat	Fatty Acids Saturated	Mono-unsatu-rated	Poly-unsatu-rated
		Grams	Per-cent	Cal-ories	Grams	Grams	Grams	Grams	Grams
VEGETABLES AND VEGETABLE PRODUCTS—Con.									
Beans:									
Lima, immature seeds, frozen, cooked, drained:									
Thick-seeded types (Fordhooks)	1 cup	170	74	170	10	1	0.1	Tr	0.3
Thin-seeded types (baby limas)	1 cup	180	72	190	12	1	0.1	Tr	0.3
Snap:									
Cooked, drained:									
From raw (cut and French style)	1 cup	125	89	45	2	Tr	0.1	Tr	0.2
From frozen (cut)	1 cup	135	92	35	2	Tr	Tr	Tr	0.1
Canned, drained solids (cut)	1 cup	135	93	25	2	Tr	Tr	Tr	0.1
Beans, mature. See Beans, dry and Black-eyed peas, dry.									
Bean sprouts (mung):									
Raw	1 cup	104	90	30	3	Tr	Tr	Tr	0.1
Beets:									
Cooked, drained:									
Diced or sliced	1 cup	170	91	55	2	Tr	Tr	Tr	Tr
Canned, drained solids, diced or sliced	1 cup	170	91	55	2	Tr	Tr	Tr	0.1
Beet greens, leaves and stems, cooked, drained	1 cup	144	89	40	4	Tr	Tr	0.1	0.1
Black-eyed peas, immature seeds, cooked and drained:									
From raw	1 cup	165	72	180	13	1	0.3	0.1	0.6
From frozen	1 cup	170	66	225	14	1	0.3	0.1	0.5
Broccoli:									
Raw	1 spear	151	91	40	4	1	0.1	Tr	0.3
Cooked, drained:									
From raw:									
Spear, medium	1 spear	180	90	50	5	1	0.1	Tr	0.2
Spears, cut into ½-in pieces	1 cup	155	90	45	5	Tr	0.1	Tr	0.2
Brussels sprouts, cooked, drained:									
From frozen	1 cup	155	87	65	6	1	0.1	Tr	0.3
Cabbage, common varieties:									
Raw, coarsely shredded or sliced	1 cup	70	93	15	1	Tr	Tr	Tr	0.1
Cooked, drained	1 cup	150	94	30	1	Tr	Tr	Tr	0.2
Cabbage, Chinese:									
Pak-choi, cooked, drained	1 cup	170	96	20	3	Tr	Tr	Tr	0.1
Pe-tsai, raw, 1-in pieces	1 cup	76	94	10	1	Tr	Tr	Tr	0.1

(Tr indicates nutrient present in trace amounts.)

Nutrients in Indicated Quantity

| Cho-les-terol | Carbo-hydrate | Calcium | Phos-phorus | Iron | Potas-sium | Sodium | Vitamin A value | | Thiamin | Ribo-flavin | Niacin | Ascorbic acid |
							(IU)	(RE)				
Milli-grams	Grams	Milli-grams	Milli-grams	Milli-grams	Milli-grams	Milli-grams	Inter-national units	Retinol equiva-lents	Milli-grams	Milli-grams	Milli-grams	Milli-grams
0	32	37	107	2.3	694	90	320	32	0.13	0.10	1.8	22
0	35	50	202	3.5	740	52	300	30	0.13	0.10	1.4	10
0	10	58	49	1.6	374	4	[57]830	[57]83	0.09	0.12	0.8	12
0	8	61	32	1.1	151	18	[58]710	[58]71	0.06	0.10	0.6	11
0	6	35	26	1.2	147	[59]339	[60]470	[60]47	0.02	0.08	0.3	6
0	6	14	56	0.9	155	6	20	2	0.09	0.13	0.8	14
0	11	19	53	1.1	530	83	20	2	0.05	0.02	0.5	9
0	12	26	29	3.1	252	[61]466	20	2	0.02	0.07	0.3	7
0	8	164	59	2.7	1,309	347	7,340	734	0.17	0.42	0.7	36
0	30	46	196	2.4	693	7	1,050	105	0.11	0.18	1.8	3
0	40	39	207	3.6	638	9	130	13	0.44	0.11	1.2	4
0	8	72	100	1.3	491	41	2,330	233	0.10	0.18	1.0	141
0	10	205	86	2.1	293	20	2,540	254	0.15	0.37	1.4	113
0	9	177	74	1.8	253	17	2,180	218	0.13	0.32	1.2	97
0	13	37	84	1.1	504	36	910	91	0.16	0.18	0.8	71
0	4	33	16	0.4	172	13	90	9	0.04	0.02	0.2	33
0	7	50	38	0.6	308	29	130	13	0.09	0.08	0.3	36
0	3	158	49	1.8	631	58	4,370	437	0.05	0.11	0.7	44
0	2	59	22	0.2	181	7	910	91	0.03	0.04	0.3	21

Foods, approximate measures, units, and weight (weight of edible portion only)		Water	Food energy	Pro-tein	Fat	Satu-rated	Mono-unsatu-rated	Poly-unsatu-rated
							Fatty Acids	
		Grams	Per-cent	Cal-ories	Grams	Grams	Grams	Grams

VEGETABLES AND VEGETABLE PRODUCTS—Con.

Foods, approximate measures, units, and weight		Water	Food energy	Pro-tein	Fat	Satu-rated	Mono-unsatu-rated	Poly-unsatu-rated
Cabbage, red, raw, coarsely shredded or sliced- - - - -	1 cup- - - - - - - - -	70	92	20	1	Tr	Tr	Tr	0.1
Cabbage, savoy, raw, coarsely shredded or sliced- - - - - -	1 cup- - - - - - - - -	70	91	20	1	Tr	Tr	Tr	Tr
Carrots:								
Raw, without crowns and tips, scraped:								
Whole, 7½ by 1⅛ in, or strips, 2½ to 3 in long-	1 carrot or 18 strips- - - - - - - -	72	88	30	1	Tr	Tr	Tr	0.1
Cooked, sliced, drained:								
From frozen- - - - - - - - -	1 cup- - - - - - - - -	146	90	55	2	Tr	Tr	Tr	0.1
Canned, sliced, drained solids- - - - - - - - - - - -	1 cup- - - - - - - - -	146	93	35	1	Tr	0.1	Tr	0.1
Cauliflower:								
Cooked, drained:								
From raw (flowerets)- - -	1 cup- - - - - - - - -	125	93	30	2	Tr	Tr	Tr	0.1
From frozen (flowerets)-	1 cup- - - - - - - - -	180	94	35	3	Tr	0.1	Tr	0.2
Celery, pascal type, raw:								
Stalk, large outer, 8 by 1½ in (at root end)- - - - - - - -	1 stalk- - - - - - - -	40	95	5	Tr	Tr	Tr	Tr	Tr
Collards, cooked, drained:								
From raw (leaves without stems)- - - - - - - - - - - - -	1 cup- - - - - - - - -	190	96	25	2	Tr	0.1	Tr	0.2
Corn, sweet:								
Cooked, drained:								
From raw, ear 5 by 1¾ in- - - - - - - - - - - -	1 ear- - - - - - - - -	77	70	85	3	1	0.2	0.3	0.5
From frozen:								
Kernels- - - - - - - - - -	1 cup- - - - - - - - -	165	76	135	5	Tr	Tr	Tr	0.1
Canned:								
Cream style- - - - - - - -	1 cup- - - - - - - - -	256	79	185	4	1	0.2	0.3	0.5
Whole kernel, vacuum pack- - - - - - - - - - -	1 cup- - - - - - - - -	210	77	165	5	1	0.2	0.3	0.5
Cowpeas. See Black-eyed peas.								
Cucumber, with peel, slices, ⅛ in thick (large, 2⅛-in diam.; small, 1¾-in diam.)- - - - -	6 large or 8 small slices- - - - - - - -	28	96	5	Tr	Tr	Tr	Tr	Tr
Dandelion greens, cooked, drained- - - - - - - - - - - - -	1 cup- - - - - - - - -	105	90	35	2	1	0.1	Tr	0.3
Eggplant, cooked, steamed- -	1 cup- - - - - - - - -	96	92	25	1	Tr	Tr	Tr	0.1
Endive, curly (including escarole), raw, small pieces- - - - - - - - - - - - - -	1 cup- - - - - - - - -	50	94	10	1	Tr	Tr	Tr	Tr
Jerusalem-artichoke, raw, sliced- - - - - - - - - - - - - -	1 cup- - - - - - - - -	150	78	115	3	Tr	0.0	Tr	Tr

(Tr indicates nutrient present in trace amounts.)

Nutrients in Indicated Quantity

Cholesterol	Carbohydrate	Calcium	Phosphorus	Iron	Potassium	Sodium	Vitamin A value		Thiamin	Riboflavin	Niacin	Ascorbic acid
							(IU)	(RE)				
Milligrams	Grams	Milligrams	Milligrams	Milligrams	Milligrams	Milligrams	International units	Retinol equivalents	Milligrams	Milligrams	Milligrams	Milligrams
0	4	36	29	0.3	144	8	30	3	0.04	0.02	0.2	40
0	4	25	29	0.3	161	20	700	70	0.05	0.02	0.2	22
0	7	19	32	0.4	233	25	20,250	2,025	0.07	0.04	0.7	7
0	12	41	38	0.7	231	86	25,850	2,585	0.04	0.05	0.6	4
0	8	37	35	0.9	261	[62]352	20,110	2,011	0.03	0.04	0.8	4
0	6	34	44	0.5	404	8	20	2	0.08	0.07	0.7	69
0	7	31	43	0.7	250	32	40	4	0.07	0.10	0.6	56
0	1	14	10	0.2	114	35	50	5	0.01	0.01	0.1	3
0	5	148	19	0.8	177	36	4,220	422	0.03	0.08	0.4	19
0	19	2	79	0.5	192	13	[63]170	[63]17	0.17	0.06	1.2	5
0	34	3	78	0.5	229	8	[63]410	[63]41	0.11	0.12	2.1	4
0	46	8	131	1.0	343	[64]730	[63]250	[63]25	0.06	0.14	2.5	12
0	41	11	134	0.9	391	[65]571	[63]510	[63]51	0.09	0.15	2.5	17
0	1	4	5	0.1	42	1	10	1	0.01	0.01	0.1	1
0	7	147	44	1.9	244	46	12,290	1,229	0.14	0.18	0.5	19
0	6	6	21	0.3	238	3	60	6	0.07	0.02	0.6	1
0	2	26	14	0.4	157	11	1,030	103	0.04	0.04	0.2	3
0	26	21	117	5.1	644	6	30	3	0.30	0.09	2.0	6

Nutritive Value of Foods *(Continued)*

Foods, approximate measures, units, and weight (weight of edible portion only)			Water	Food energy	Pro-tein	Fat	Fatty Acids		
							Satu-rated	Mono-unsatu-rated	Poly-unsatu-rated
VEGETABLES AND VEGETABLE PRODUCTS—Con.		*Grams*	*Per-cent*	*Cal-ories*	*Grams*	*Grams*	*Grams*	*Grams*	*Grams*
Kale, cooked, drained:									
From raw, chopped- - - - -	1 cup- - - - - - - - -	130	91	40	2	1	0.1	Tr	0.3
From frozen, chopped- - - -	1 cup- - - - - - - - -	130	91	40	4	1	0.1	Tr	0.3
Kohlrabi, thickened bulb-like stems, cooked, drained, diced- - - - - - - - - - - - - - -	1 cup- - - - - - - - -	165	90	50	3	Tr	Tr	Tr	0.1
Lettuce, raw:									
Butterhead, as Boston types:									
Head, 5-in diam- - - - - -	1 head- - - - - - - -	163	96	20	2	Tr	Tr	Tr	0.2
Leaves- - - - - - - - - - - -	1 outer or 2 inner leaves- - - - - - -	15	96	Tr	Tr	Tr	Tr	Tr	Tr
Crisphead, as iceberg:									
Head, 6-in diam- - - - - -	1 head- - - - - - - -	539	96	70	5	1	0.1	Tr	0.5
Looseleaf (bunching varie-ties including romaine or cos), chopped or shredded pieces- - - - -	1 cup- - - - - - - - -	56	94	10	1	Tr	Tr	Tr	0.1
Mushrooms:									
Raw, sliced or chopped- - -	1 cup- - - - - - - - -	70	92	20	1	Tr	Tr	Tr	0.1
Cooked, drained- - - - - - -	1 cup- - - - - - - - -	156	91	40	3	1	0.1	Tr	0.3
Canned, drained solids- - -	1 cup- - - - - - - - -	156	91	35	3	Tr	0.1	Tr	0.2
Mustard greens, without stems and midribs, cooked, drained- - - - - - - - - - - - -	1 cup- - - - - - - - -	140	94	20	3	Tr	Tr	0.2	0.1
Okra pods, 3 by ⅝ in, cooked	8 pods- - - - - - - - -	85	90	25	2	Tr	Tr	Tr	Tr
Onions:									
Raw:									
Sliced- - - - - - - - - - - - -	1 cup- - - - - - - - -	115	91	40	1	Tr	0.1	Tr	0.1
Cooked (whole or sliced), drained- - - - - - - - - - -	1 cup- - - - - - - - -	210	92	60	2	Tr	0.1	Tr	0.1
Onions, spring, raw, bulb (⅜-in diam.) and white portion of top- - - - - - - - - - - - - - -	6 onions- - - - - - -	30	92	10	1	Tr	Tr	Tr	Tr
Onion rings, breaded, par-fried, frozen, prepared- - -	2 rings- - - - - - - -	20	29	80	1	5	1.7	2.2	1.0
Parsley:									
Raw- - - - - - - - - - - - - - -	10 sprigs- - - - - - -	10	88	5	Tr	Tr	Tr	Tr	Tr
Parsnips, cooked (diced or 2 in lengths), drained- - - - - - -	1 cup- - - - - - - - -	156	78	125	2	Tr	0.1	0.2	0.1
Peas, edible pod, cooked, drained- - - - - - - - - - - - -	1 cup- - - - - - - - -	160	89	65	5	Tr	0.1	Tr	0.2
Peas, green:									
Canned, drained solids- - -	1 cup- - - - - - - - -	170	82	115	8	1	0.1	0.1	0.3
Frozen, cooked, drained- -	1 cup- - - - - - - - -	160	80	125	8	Tr	0.1	Tr	0.2
Peppers:									
Hot chili, raw- - - - - - - - -	1 pepper- - - - - - -	45	88	20	1	Tr	Tr	Tr	Tr

(Tr indicates nutrient present in trace amounts.)

Nutrients in Indicated Quantity

Cho-les-terol	Carbo-hydrate	Calcium	Phos-phorus	Iron	Potas-sium	Sodium	Vitamin A value		Thiamin	Ribo-flavin	Niacin	Ascorbic acid
							(IU)	(RE)				
Milli-grams	Grams	Milli-grams	Milli-grams	Milli-grams	Milli-grams	Milli-grams	Inter-national units	Retinol equiva-lents	Milli-grams	Milli-grams	Milli-grams	Milli-grams
0	7	94	36	1.2	296	30	9,620	962	0.07	0.09	0.7	53
0	7	179	36	1.2	417	20	8,260	826	0.06	0.15	0.9	33
0	11	41	74	0.7	561	35	60	6	0.07	0.03	0.6	89
0	4	52	38	0.5	419	8	1,580	158	0.10	0.10	0.5	13
0	Tr	5	3	Tr	39	1	150	15	0.01	0.01	Tr	1
0	11	102	108	2.7	852	49	1,780	178	0.25	0.16	1.0	21
0	2	38	14	0.8	148	5	1,060	106	0.03	0.04	0.2	10
0	3	4	73	0.9	259	3	0	0	0.07	0.31	2.9	2
0	8	9	136	2.7	555	3	0	0	0.11	0.47	7.0	6
0	8	17	103	1.2	201	663	0	0	0.13	0.03	2.5	0
0	3	104	57	1.0	283	22	4,240	424	0.06	0.09	0.6	35
0	6	54	48	0.4	274	4	490	49	0.11	0.05	0.7	14
0	8	29	33	0.4	178	2	0	0	0.07	0.01	0.1	10
0	13	57	48	0.4	319	17	0	0	0.09	0.02	0.2	12
0	2	18	10	0.6	77	1	1,500	150	0.02	0.04	0.1	14
0	8	6	16	0.3	26	75	50	5	0.06	0.03	0.7	Tr
0	1	13	4	0.6	54	4	520	52	0.01	0.01	0.1	9
0	30	58	108	0.9	573	16	0	0	0.13	0.08	1.1	20
0	11	67	88	3.2	384	6	210	21	0.20	0.12	0.9	77
0	21	34	114	1.6	294	[66]372	1,310	131	0.21	0.13	1.2	16
0	23	38	144	2.5	269	139	1,070	107	0.45	0.16	2.4	16
0	4	8	21	0.5	153	3	[67]4,840	[67]484	0.04	0.04	0.4	109

Foods, approximate measures, units, and weight (weight of edible portion only)		Water	Food energy	Pro-tein	Fat	Fatty Acids		
						Satu-rated	Mono-unsatu-rated	Poly-unsatu-rated
		Per-cent	*Cal-ories*	*Grams*	*Grams*	*Grams*	*Grams*	*Grams*
VEGETABLES AND VEGETABLE PRODUCTS—Con.	*Grams*							
Sweet (about 5 per lb, whole), stem and seeds removed:								
Raw- - - - - - - - - - - - -	1 pepper- - - - - - -	74	93	20	1	Tr	Tr	Tr	0.2
Cooked, drained- - - - - -	1 pepper- - - - - - -	73	95	15	Tr	Tr	Tr	Tr	0.1
Potatoes, cooked:								
Baked (about 2 per lb, raw):								
With skin- - - - - - - - - -	1 potato- - - - - - -	202	71	220	5	Tr	0.1	Tr	0.1
Flesh only- - - - - - - - - -	1 potato- - - - - - -	156	75	145	3	Tr	Tr	Tr	0.1
Boiled (about 3 per lb, raw):								
Peeled after boiling- - - -	1 potato- - - - - - -	136	77	120	3	Tr	Tr	Tr	0.1
Peeled before boiling- - -	1 potato- - - - - - -	135	77	115	2	Tr	Tr	Tr	0.1
French fried, strip, 2 to 3½ in long, frozen:								
Oven heated- - - - - - - - -	10 strips- - - - - - -	50	53	110	2	4	2.1	1.8	0.3
Fried in vegetable oil- - -	10 strips- - - - - - -	50	38	160	2	8	2.5	1.6	3.8
Potato products, prepared:								
Hashed brown, from frozen	1 cup - - - - - - - - -	156	56	340	5	18	7.0	8.0	2.1
Mashed:								
From home recipe:								
Milk added- - - - - - - -	1 cup - - - - - - - - -	210	78	160	4	1	0.7	0.3	0.1
Milk and margarine added- - - - - - - - - -	1 cup - - - - - - - - -	210	76	225	4	9	2.2	3.7	2.5
Potato salad, made with mayonnaise- - - - - -	1 cup - - - - - - - - -	250	76	360	7	21	3.6	6.2	9.3
Scalloped:								
From dry mix- - - - - - -	1 cup - - - - - - - - -	245	79	230	5	11	6.5	3.0	0.5
Potato chips- - - - - - - - - - -	10 chips- - - - - - -	20	3	105	1	7	1.8	1.2	3.6
Pumpkin:								
Cooked from raw, mashed-	1 cup - - - - - - - - -	245	94	50	2	Tr	0.1	Tr	Tr
Canned- - - - - - - - - - - - -	1 cup - - - - - - - - -	245	90	85	3	1	0.4	0.1	Tr
Radishes, raw, stem ends, rootlets cut off- - - - - - - -	4 radishes- - - - - -	18	95	5	Tr	Tr	Tr	Tr	Tr
Sauerkraut, canned, solids and liquid- - - - - - - - - - -	1 cup - - - - - - - - -	236	93	45	2	Tr	0.1	Tr	0.1
Seaweed:								
Kelp, raw- - - - - - - - - - - -	1 oz- - - - - - - - - -	28	82	10	Tr	Tr	0.1	Tr	Tr
Southern peas. See Black-eyed peas.								
Spinach:								
Raw, chopped- - - - - - - - -	1 cup - - - - - - - - -	55	92	10	2	Tr	Tr	Tr	0.1
Cooked, drained:								
From raw- - - - - - - - - -	1 cup - - - - - - - - -	180	91	40	5	Tr	0.1	Tr	0.2
Canned, drained solids- - -	1 cup - - - - - - - - -	214	92	50	6	1	0.2	Tr	0.4
Squash, cooked:								
Summer (all varieties), sliced, drained- - - - - -	1 cup - - - - - - - - -	180	94	35	2	1	0.1	Tr	0.2

(Tr indicates nutrient present in trace amounts.)

Cholesterol	Carbohydrate	Calcium	Phosphorus	Iron	Potassium	Sodium	Vitamin A value		Thiamin	Riboflavin	Niacin	Ascorbic acid
							(IU)	(RE)				
Milligrams	Grams	Milligrams	Milligrams	Milligrams	Milligrams	Milligrams	International units	Retinol equivalents	Milligrams	Milligrams	Milligrams	Milligrams
0	4	4	16	0.9	144	2	[68]390	[68]39	0.06	0.04	0.4	[68]95
0	3	3	11	0.6	94	1	[70]280	[70]28	0.04	0.03	0.3	[71]81
0	51	20	115	2.7	844	16	0	0	0.22	0.07	3.3	26
0	34	8	78	0.5	610	8	0	0	0.16	0.03	2.2	20
0	27	7	60	0.4	515	5	0	0	0.14	0.03	2.0	18
0	27	11	54	0.4	443	7	0	0	0.13	0.03	1.8	10
0	17	5	43	0.7	229	16	0	0	0.06	0.02	1.2	5
0	20	10	47	0.4	366	108	0	0	0.09	0.01	1.6	5
0	44	23	112	2.4	680	53	0	0	0.17	0.03	3.8	10
4	37	55	101	0.6	628	636	40	12	0.18	0.08	2.3	14
4	35	55	97	0.5	607	620	360	42	0.18	0.08	2.3	13
170	28	48	130	1.6	635	1,323	520	83	0.19	0.15	2.2	25
27	31	88	137	0.9	497	835	360	51	0.05	0.14	2.5	8
0	10	5	31	0.2	260	94	0	0	0.03	Tr	0.8	8
0	12	37	74	1.4	564	2	2,650	265	0.08	0.19	1.0	12
0	20	64	86	3.4	505	12	54,040	5,404	0.06	0.13	0.9	10
0	1	4	3	0.1	42	4	Tr	Tr	Tr	0.01	0.1	4
0	10	71	47	3.5	401	1,560	40	4	0.05	0.05	0.3	35
0	3	48	12	0.8	25	66	30	3	0.01	0.04	0.1	(¹)
0	2	54	27	1.5	307	43	3,690	369	0.04	0.10	0.4	15
0	7	245	101	6.4	839	126	14,740	1,474	0.17	0.42	0.9	18
0	7	272	94	4.9	740	[72]683	18,780	1,878	0.03	0.30	0.8	31
0	8	49	70	0.6	346	2	520	52	0.08	0.07	0.9	10

Foods, approximate measures, units, and weight (weight of edible portion only)		Water	Food energy	Pro-tein	Fat	Fatty Acids		
						Satu-rated	Mono-unsatu-rated	Poly-unsatu-rated
		Per-cent	*Cal-ories*	*Grams*	*Grams*	*Grams*	*Grams*	*Grams*
VEGETABLES AND VEGETABLE PRODUCTS—Con.								
	Grams							
Winter (all varieties), baked, cubes	1 cup	205	89	80	2	1	0.3	0.1	0.5
Sunchoke. See Jerusalem-artichoke.									
Sweet potatoes:									
Cooked (raw, 5 by 2 in; about 2½ per lb):									
Baked in skin, peeled	1 potato	114	73	115	2	Tr	Tr	Tr	0.1
Boiled, without skin	1 potato	151	73	160	2	Tr	0.1	Tr	0.2
Candied, 2½ by 2-in piece	1 piece	105	67	145	1	3	1.4	0.7	0.2
Canned:									
Solid pack (mashed)	1 cup	255	74	260	5	1	0.1	Tr	0.2
Vacuum pack, piece 2¾ by 1 in	1 piece	40	76	35	1	Tr	Tr	Tr	Tr
Tomatoes:									
Raw, 2⅗-in diam. (3 per 12 oz pkg.)	1 tomato	123	94	25	1	Tr	Tr	Tr	0.1
Canned, solids and liquid	1 cup	240	94	50	2	1	0.1	0.1	0.2
Tomato juice, canned	1 cup	244	94	40	2	Tr	Tr	Tr	0.1
Tomato products, canned:									
Paste	1 cup	262	74	220	10	2	0.3	0.4	0.9
Puree	1 cup	250	87	105	4	Tr	Tr	Tr	0.1
Sauce	1 cup	245	89	75	3	Tr	0.1	0.1	0.2
Turnips, cooked, diced	1 cup	156	94	30	1	Tr	Tr	Tr	0.1
Turnip greens, cooked, drained:									
From raw (leaves and stems)	1 cup	144	93	30	2	Tr	0.1	Tr	0.1
From frozen (chopped)	1 cup	164	90	50	5	1	0.2	Tr	0.3
Vegetable juice cocktail, canned	1 cup	242	94	45	2	Tr	Tr	Tr	0.1
Vegetables, mixed:									
Frozen, cooked, drained	1 cup	182	83	105	5	Tr	0.1	Tr	0.1
Water chestnuts, canned	1 cup	140	86	70	1	Tr	Tr	Tr	Tr
MISCELLANEOUS ITEMS									
Baking powders for home use:									
Sodium aluminum sulfate:									
With monocalcium phos-phate monohydrate	1 tsp	3	2	5	Tr	0	0.0	0.0	0.0
Catsup	1 cup	273	69	290	5	1	0.2	0.2	0.4
	1 tbsp	15	69	15	Tr	Tr	Tr	Tr	Tr
Chili powder	1 tsp	2.6	8	10	Tr	Tr	0.1	0.1	0.2
Chocolate:									
Bitter or baking	1 oz	28	2	145	3	15	9.0	4.9	0.5
Semisweet, see Candy									
Cinnamon	1 tsp	2.3	10	5	Tr	Tr	Tr	Tr	Tr
Curry powder	1 tsp	2	10	5	Tr	Tr	(¹)	(¹)	(¹)

(Tr indicates nutrient present in trace amounts.)

Nutrients in Indicated Quantity

Cholesterol	Carbohydrate	Calcium	Phosphorus	Iron	Potassium	Sodium	Vitamin A value		Thiamin	Riboflavin	Niacin	Ascorbic acid
							(IU)	(RE)				
Milligrams	Grams	Milligrams	Milligrams	Milligrams	Milligrams	Milligrams	International units	Retinol equivalents	Milligrams	Milligrams	Milligrams	Milligrams
0	18	29	41	0.7	896	2	7,290	729	0.17	0.05	1.4	20
0	28	32	63	0.5	397	11	24,880	2,488	0.08	0.14	0.7	28
0	37	32	41	0.8	278	20	25,750	2,575	0.08	0.21	1.0	26
8	29	27	27	1.2	198	74	4,400	440	0.02	0.04	0.4	7
0	59	77	133	3.4	536	191	38,570	3,857	0.07	0.23	2.4	13
0	8	9	20	0.4	125	21	3,190	319	0.01	0.02	0.3	11
0	5	9	28	0.6	255	10	1,390	139	0.07	0.06	0.7	22
0	10	62	46	1.5	530	[73]391	1,450	145	0.11	0.07	1.8	36
0	10	22	46	1.4	537	[74]881	1,360	136	0.11	0.08	1.6	45
0	49	92	207	7.8	2,442	[75]170	6,470	647	0.41	0.50	8.4	111
0	25	38	100	2.3	1,050	[76]50	3,400	340	0.18	0.14	4.3	88
0	18	34	78	1.9	909	[77]1,482	2,400	240	0.16	0.14	2.8	32
0	8	34	30	0.3	211	78	0	0	0.04	0.04	0.5	18
0	6	197	42	1.2	292	42	7,920	792	0.06	0.10	0.6	39
0	8	249	56	3.2	367	25	13,080	1,308	0.09	0.12	0.8	36
0	11	27	41	1.0	467	883	2,830	283	0.10	0.07	1.8	67
0	24	46	93	1.5	308	64	7,780	778	0.13	0.22	1.5	6
0	17	6	27	1.2	165	11	10	1	0.02	0.03	0.5	2
0	1	58	87	0.0	5	329	0	0	0.00	0.00	0.0	0
0	69	60	137	2.2	991	2,845	3,820	382	0.25	0.19	4.4	41
0	4	3	8	0.1	54	156	210	21	0.01	0.01	0.2	2
0	1	7	8	0.4	50	26	910	91	0.01	0.02	0.2	2
0	8	22	109	1.9	235	1	10	1	0.01	0.07	0.4	0
0	2	28	1	0.9	12	1	10	1	Tr	Tr	Tr	1
0	1	10	7	0.6	31	1	20	2	0.01	0.01	0.1	Tr

Foods, approximate measures, units, and weight (weight of edible portion only)		Water	Food energy	Pro-tein	Fat	Satu-rated	Fatty Acids Mono-unsatu-rated	Poly-unsatu-rated
MISCELLANEOUS ITEMS—Con.	Grams	Per-cent	Cal-ories	Grams	Grams	Grams	Grams	Grams
Garlic powder	1 tsp	2.8	6	10	Tr	Tr	Tr	Tr	Tr
Gelatin, dry	1 envelope	7	13	25	6	Tr	Tr	Tr	Tr
Mustard, prepared, yellow	1 tsp or individual packet	5	80	5	Tr	Tr	Tr	0.2	Tr
Olives, canned:									
Green	4 medium or 3 extra large	13	78	15	Tr	2	0.2	1.2	0.1
Ripe, Mission, pitted	3 small or 2 large	9	73	15	Tr	2	0.3	1.3	0.2
Oregano	1 tsp	1.5	7	5	Tr	Tr	Tr	Tr	0.1
Paprika	1 tsp	2.1	10	5	Tr	Tr	Tr	Tr	0.2
Pepper, black	1 tsp	2.1	11	5	Tr	Tr	Tr	Tr	Tr
Pickles, cucumber:									
Dill, medium, whole, 3¾ in long, 1¼-in diam.	1 pickle	65	93	5	Tr	Tr	Tr	Tr	0.1
Fresh-pack, slices 1½-in diam., ¼ in thick	2 slices	15	79	10	Tr	Tr	Tr	Tr	Tr
Sweet, gherkin, small, whole, about 2½ in long, ¾-in diam.	1 pickle	15	61	20	Tr	Tr	Tr	Tr	Tr
Popcorn. See Grain Products									
Salt	1 tsp	5.5	0	0	0	0	0.0	0.0	0.0
Vinegar, cider	1 tbsp	15	94	Tr	Tr	0	0.0	0.0	0.0
Yeast:									
Baker's, dry, active	1 pkg	7	5	20	3	Tr	Tr	0.1	Tr

(Tr indicates nutrient present in trace amounts.)

[1] Value not determined.

[2] Mineral content varies depending on water source.

[3] Blend of aspartame and saccharin; if only sodium saccharin is used, sodium is 75 mg; if only aspartame is used, sodium is 23 mg.

[4] With added ascorbic acid.

[5] Vitamin A value is largely from beta-carotene used for coloring.

[6] Yields 1 qt of fluid milk when reconstituted according to package directions.

[7] With added vitamin A.

[8] Carbohydrate content varies widely because of amount of sugar added and amount and solids content of added flavoring. Consult the label if more precise values for carbohydrate and calories are needed.

[9] For salted butter; unsalted butter contains 12 mg sodium per stick, 2 mg per tbsp, or 1 mg per pat.

[10] Values for vitamin are year-round average.

[11] For salted margarine.

[12] Based on average vitamin A content of fortified margarine. Federal specifications for fortified margarine require a minimum of 15,000 IU per pound.

[13] Fatty acid values apply to product made with regular margarine.

[14] Dipped in egg, milk, and breadcrumbs; fried in vegetable shortening.

[15] If bones are discarded, value for calcium will be greatly reduced.

[16] Dipped in egg, breadcrumbs, and flour; fried in vegetable shortening.

[17] Made with drained chunk light tuna, celery, onion, pickle relish, and mayonnaise-type salad dressing.

Cholesterol	Carbohydrate	Calcium	Phosphorus	Iron	Potassium	Sodium	Vitamin A value		Thiamin	Riboflavin	Niacin	Ascorbic acid
							(IU)	(RE)				
Milligrams	Grams	Milligrams	Milligrams	Milligrams	Milligrams	Milligrams	International units	Retinol equivalents	Milligrams	Milligrams	Milligrams	Milligrams
0	2	2	12	0.1	31	1	0	0	0.01	Tr	Tr	Tr
0	0	1	0	0.0	2	6	0	0	0.00	0.00	0.0	0
0	Tr	4	4	0.1	7	63	0	0	Tr	0.01	Tr	Tr
0	Tr	8	2	0.2	7	312	40	4	Tr	Tr	Tr	Tr
0	Tr	10	2	0.2	2	68	10	1	Tr	Tr	Tr	0
0	1	24	3	0.7	25	Tr	100	10	0.01	Tr	0.1	1
0	1	4	7	0.5	49	1	1,270	127	0.01	0.04	0.3	1
0	1	9	4	0.6	26	1	Tr	Tr	Tr	0.01	Tr	0
0	1	17	14	0.7	130	928	70	7	Tr	0.01	Tr	4
0	3	5	4	0.3	30	101	20	2	Tr	Tr	Tr	1
0	5	2	2	0.2	30	107	10	1	Tr	Tr	Tr	1
0	0	14	3	Tr	Tr	2,132	0	0	0.00	0.00	0.0	0
0	1	1	1	0.1	15	Tr	0	0	0.00	0.00	0.0	0
0	3	3	90	1.1	140	4	Tr	Tr	0.16	0.38	2.6	Tr

[18] Sodium bisulfite used to preserve color; unsulfited product would contain less sodium.

[19] Also applies to pasteurized apple cider.

[20] Without added ascorbic acid. For value with added ascorbic acid, refer to label.

[21] With added ascorbic acid.

[22] For white grapefruit; pink grapefruit have about 310 IU or 31 RE.

[23] Sodium benzoate and sodium bisulfite added as preservatives.

[24] Egg bagels have 44 mg cholesterol and 22 IU or 7 RE vitamin A per bagel.

[25] Made with vegetable shortening.

[26] Made with white cornmeal. If made with yellow cornmeal, value is 32 IU or 3 RE.

[27] Nutrient added.

[28] Cooked without salt. If salt is added according to label recommendations, sodium content is 540 mg.

[29] For white corn grits. Cooked yellow grits contain 145 IU or 14 RE.

[30] Value based on label declaration for added nutrients.

[31] For regular and instant cereal. For quick cereal, phosphorus is 102 mg and sodium is 142 mg.

[32] Cooked without salt. If salt is added according to label recommendations, sodium content is 390 mg.

[33] Cooked without salt. If salt is added according to label recommendations, sodium content is 324 mg.

[34] Cooked without salt. If salt is added according to label recommendations, sodium content is 374 mg.

[35] Excepting angelfood cake, cakes were made from mixes containing vegetable shortening and frostings were made with margarine.

[36] Made with vegetable oil.

(Footnotes continue on next page.)

[37] Cake made with vegetable shortening; frosting with margarine.

[38] Made with margarine.

[39] Crackers made with enriched flour except for rye wafers and whole-wheat wafers.

[40] Made with lard.

[41] Cashews without salt contain 21 mg sodium per cup or 4 mg per oz.

[42] Cashews without salt contain 22 mg sodium per cup or 5 mg per oz.

[43] Macadamia nuts without salt contain 9 mg sodium per cup or 2 mg per oz.

[44] Mixed nuts without salt contain 3 mg sodium per oz.

[45] Peanuts without salt contain 22 mg sodium per cup or 4 mg per oz.

[46] Outer layer of fat was removed to within approximately ½ inch of the lean. Deposits of fat within the cut were not removed.

[47] Fried in vegetable shortening.

[48] Value varies widely.

[49] Contains added sodium ascorbate. If sodium ascorbate is not added, ascorbic acid content is negligible.

[50] One patty (8 per pound) of bulk sausage is equivalent to 2 links.

[51] Crust made with vegetable shortening and enriched flour.

[52] Made with corn oil.

[53] Fried in vegetable shortening.

[54] If sodium ascorbate is added, product contains 11 mg ascorbic acid.

[55] Made with enriched flour, margarine, and whole milk.

[56] For regular pack; special dietary pack contains 3 mg sodium.

[57] For green varieties; yellow varieties contain 101 IU or 10 RE.

[58] For green varieties; yellow varieties contain 151 IU or 15 RE.

[59] For regular pack; special dietary pack contains 3 mg sodium.

[60] For green varieties; yellow varieties contain 142 IU or 14 RE.

[61] For regular pack; special dietary pack contains 78 mg sodium.

[62] For regular pack; special dietary pack contains 61 mg sodium.

[63] For yellow varieties; white varieties contain only a trace of vitamin A.

[64] For regular pack; special dietary pack contains 8 mg sodium.

[65] For regular pack; special dietary pack contains 6 mg sodium.

[66] For regular pack; special dietary pack contains 3 mg sodium.

[67] For red peppers; green peppers contain 350 IU or 35 RE.

[68] For green peppers; red peppers contain 4220 IU or 422 RE.

[69] For green peppers; red peppers contain 141 mg ascorbic acid.

[70] For green peppers; red peppers contain 2740 IU or 274 RE.

[71] For green peppers; red peppers contain 121 mg ascorbic acid.

[72] With added salt; if none is added, sodium content is 58 mg.

[73] For regular pack; special dietary pack contains 31 mg sodium.

[74] With added salt; if none is added, sodium content is 24 mg.

[75] With no added salt; if salt is added, sodium content is 2070 mg.

[76] With no added salt; if salt is added, sodium content is 998 mg.

[77] With salt added.

Adapted from Nutritive Value of Foods, Home and Garden Bulletin, No. 72, U.S. Dept. of Agriculture.

App. 8: Phobias

Fear of	Condition	Fear of	Condition
air	aerophobia	fire	pyrophobia
animals	zoophobia	fish	ichthyophobia
anything new	neophobia	floods	antlophobia
bacilli	bacillophobia	fog	homichlophobia
bearing a deformed child	teratophobia	food	cibophobia, sitophobia
bees	apiphobia, melissophobia	forest	hylophobia
being buried alive	taphephobia	frogs	batrachophobia
birds	ornithophobia	ghosts	phasmophobia
blood	hematophobia,	girls	parthenophobia
	hemophobia	glare of light	photaugiaphobia
blushing	ereuthrophobia	glass	crystallophobia,
brain disease	meningitophobia		hyalophobia
bridges (crossing of)	gephyrophobia	God	theophobia
cats	ailurophobia, galeophobia	gravity	barophobia
change or novelty	kainophobia	hair	trichopathophobia
childbirth	tocophobia	heat	thermophobia
choking	pnigophobia	height	acrophobia
cold or something cold	psychrophobia	hell	hadephobia, stygiophobia
color(s)	chromatophobia,	heredity and hereditary	patroiophobia
	chromophobia	disease	
confinement	claustrophobia	high objects or being on	batophobia
contamination or	molysmophobia	tall buildings	
infection		house, being in a	domatophobia,
corpses	necrophobia		oikophobia
crowds	ochlophobia	ideas	ideophobia
dampness	hygrophobia	injury	traumatophobia
darkness	nyctophobia, scotophobia	innovation	neophobia
dawn	eosophobia	insane, becoming	maniaphobia
daylight	phengophobia	insects	acarophobia,
death	thanatophobia		entomophobia
definite, specific disease	monopathophobia	jealousy	zelophobia
deformity	dysmorphophobia	justice	dikephobia
depth	bathophobia	knife or pointed objects	aichmophobia
developing a phobia	phobophobia	large objects	megalophobia
dirt	mysophobia, rupophobia	left	levophobia
disease	nosophobia, pathophobia	light	photophobia
dogs	cynophobia	lightning	astraphobia,
dolls	pediophobia		astrapophobia,
drafts	anemophobia		keraunophobia
dust	amathophobia	locked in, being	clithrophobia
eating	phagophobia	looked at, being	scopophobia
electricity	electrophobia	machinery	mechanophobia
emptiness	kenophobia, cenophobia	men	androphobia
error	hamartophobia	many things	polyphobia
everything	panphobia, panophobia,	marriage	gamophobia
	pantophobia	medicine	pharmacophobia
excrement	coprophobia	metals	metallophobia
eyes	ommatophobia	mice	musophobia
failure	kakorrhaphiophobia	mirror and seeing	eisoptrophobia,
fatigue	kopophobia	oneself in	spectrophobia
feathers	pteronophobia	missiles	ballistophobia
fever	pyrexeophobia	moisture	hygrophobia
filth	mysophobia	money	chrematophobia
filth or odor, personal	automysophobia	motion	kinesophobia

Phobias (Continued)

Fear of	Condition	Fear of	Condition
myths	mythophobia	skin lesion	dermatophobia
naked body	gymnophobia	skin of animals	doraphobia
name, hearing a certain	onomatophobia	sleep	hypnophobia
needles	belonephobia	small objects	microphobia,
neglect or omission of duty	paralipophobia		microbiophobia
night	noctiphobia, nyctophobia	smothering	pnigerophobia
northern lights	auroraphobia	snake	ophidiophobia
novelty	kainophobia	snow	chionphobia
odor	olfactophobia,	solitude or being alone	eremophobia
	osmophobia,	sounds	acousticophobia
	osphresiophobia	sourness	acerophobia
odor, personal	bromidrosiphobia	speaking, talking	lalophobia
open space	agoraphobia	spider	arachnophobia
overwork	ponophobia	stairs	climacophobia
pain	algophobia, odynophobia	standing up	stasiphobia
parasites	parasitophobia	standing or walking	stasibasiphobia
people	anthropophobia	stars	siderophobia
place	topophobia	stealing	kleptophobia
pleasure	hedonophobia	stories	mythophobia
pointed objects	aichmophobia	strangers	xenophobia
poison	iophobia, toxicophobia	street	agyiophobia
poverty	peniaphobia	string	linonophobia
precipices	cremnophobia	sunlight	heliophobia
punishment	poinephobia	symbolism	symbolophobia
rabies	cynophobia, lyssophobia	syphilis	syphilophobia
railroad or train	siderodromophobia	tapeworms	taeniophobia
rain or rain storm	ombrophobia	taste	geumaphobia
rectum	proctophobia	teeth	odontophobia
red	erythrophobia	thinking	phronemophobia
responsibility	hypengyophobia	thunder	astraphobia,
returning home	nostophobia		brontophobia
right	dextrophobia	time	chronophobia
river	potamophobia	touched, being	haphephobia,
robbers	harpaxophobia		haptephobia
rod or instrument of	rhabdophobia	travel	hodophobia
punishment		trembling	tremophobia
ruin	atephobia	trichinosis	trichinophobia
sacred things	hierophobia	tuberculosis	phthisiophobia,
scabies	scabiphobia		tuberculophobia
school	school phobia	vaccination	vaccinophobia
scratches or being	amychophobia	vehicle, being in	amaxophobia
scratched		venereal disease	cypridophobia
sea	thalassophobia	voice, one's own	phonophobia
self	autophobia	void	kenophobia
semen, loss of	spermatophobia	vomiting	emetophobia
sex	genophobia	walking	basiphobia
sexual intercourse	coitophobia	water	hydrophobia
shock	hormephobia	weakness	asthenophobia
sin	hamartophobia	wind	anemophobia
sinning	peccatiphobia	women	gynephobia
sitting	thaasophobia	words, hearing certain	onomatophobia
sitting down	kathisophobia	work	ergasiophobia
skin disease	dermatosiophobia	writing	graphophobia

Adapted from Campbell, R.J.: Psychiatric Dictionary, ed 5. Oxford University Press, N.Y., 1981.

App. 9: Symbols

Symbol	Meaning	Symbol	Meaning
♍	Minim.	+	Plus; excess; acid reaction; positive.
℈	Scruple.	−	Minus; deficiency; alkaline reaction; negative.
ʒ	Dram.		
fʒ	Fluidram.	±	Plus or minus; either positive or negative; indefinite.
℥	Ounce.		
f℥	Fluidounce.	♯	Number; following a number, pounds.
O	Pint.	÷	Divided by.
℔	Pound.	×	Multiplied by; magnification.
℞	Recipe (L. take)	/	Divided by.
M	Misce (L. mix)	=	Equals.
a͞a	Of each.	≈	Approximately equal.
A, Å	angström unit.	>	Greater than; from which is derived.
C-1, C-2, etc.	Complement.	<	Less than; derived from.
c, c̄	cum (L. with).	≮	Not less than.
Δ	Change; heat	≯	Not greater than.
E₀	Electroaffinity.	≦	Equal to or less than.
F₁	First filial generation.	≧	Equal to or greater than.
F₂	Second filial generation.	≠	Not equal to.
mμ	Millimicron, nanometer.	√	Root; square root; radical.
μg	Microgram.	²√	Square root.
mEq	Milliequivalent.	³√	Cube root.
mg	Milligram.	∞	Infinity.
mg%	Milligrams percent; milligrams per 100 ml.	:	Ratio; "is to."
		::	Equality between ratios, "as."
Qo₂	Oxygen consumption.	∴	Therefore.
m-	Meta-.	°	Degree.
o-	Ortho-.	%	Percent.
p-	Para-.	π	3.1416 — ratio of circumference of a circle to its diameter.
p̄	After.		
Po₂	Partial pressure of oxygen.	□, ♂	Male.
Pco₂	Partial pressure of carbon dioxide.	○, ♀	Female.
s̄	Without	⇌	Denotes a reversible reaction.
ss, ss	[L. semis]. One-half.	n	Subscripted n indicates the number of the molecules can vary from two to greater.
μm	Micrometer.		
μ	Micron (former term for micrometer).	↑	Increase.
μμ	Micromicron.	↓	Decrease.

2351

App. 10: Abbreviations*

Principal Medical Abbreviations†

Abbreviation	Latin (unless indicated)	English Definition
ad	ad	to; up to
ad lib.	ad libitum	freely; at pleasure
ALT		alanine aminotransferase (formerly SGPT)
AQ	aqua	water
AST		aspartate aminotransferase (formerly SGOT)
AV		atrioventricular
av.	(French)	avoirdupois
		average
B.P.		British Pharmacopeia
BUN		blood urea nitrogen
C		Calorie (kilocalorie)
		Celsius
		centigrade
C	congius	gallon
ca.	circa	about
CBC		complete blood count
cc.	(French)	cubic centimeter
CDC		Centers for Disease Control
cg	(French)	centigram
cm	(French)	centimeter
comp.	compositus	compound
CNS		central nervous system
cong.	congius	gallon
CSF		cerebrospinal fluid
CV		cardiovascular
d	dexter	right
	dies	day (24 hours)
/d		per day
D&C		dilatation and curettage
DPT		diphtheria-pertussis-tetanus
dr.	drachma	dram
ECG		electrocardiogram
ECT		electroconvulsive therapy
EEG		electroencephalogram
elix.	(Arabic)	elixir
EMG		electromyogram
emp.	emplastrum	a plaster
ENT		ear, nose, and throat
ESR		erythrocyte sedimentation rate
F	(proper name)	Fahrenheit
f		female
FDA		Food and Drug Administration
FEV		forced expiratory volume
Fld	fluidus	fluid
fl. dr.	fluidrachma	fluidram
fl. oz.	fluidus uncia	fluidounce
FSH		follicle-stimulating hormone
GI		gastrointestinal
Gm; gm	gramme (French)	gram
gr	granum	grain
Gtt, gtt	guttae	drops

* For other abbreviations used in the book, see page xli in the front of the book.
† See also *Charting* and *Prescription Writing* on following pages and *Elements* and *Symbols* in *Appendix*.

Abbreviation	Latin (unless indicated)	English Definition
h.	hora	hour
hgb		hemoglobin
I.M.		intramuscular
inf.	infusum	infusion
inhal.	inhalatio	inhalation
inj.	injectio	injection
instill.		instillation
IQ		intelligence quotient
I.U.		international unit
IUD		intrauterine device
I.V.		intravenously
kg	(French)	kilogram
l	litre (French)	liter
lab.		laboratory
lb.	libra	pound
LD$_{50}$		lethal dose, median
liq.	liquor	liquid; fluid
m		male
	(French)	meter
	minimum	minim
MED		minimum effective dose
mEq		milliequivalent
mg		milligram
ml		milliliter
mM		millimole
mm	(French)	millimeter
mol. wt.		molecular weight
mph		miles per hour
MPN		most probable number
μEq		microequivalent
μg		microgram
no.	numerus	number
NPN		nonprotein nitrogen
O	octarius	pint
OC		oral contraceptive
O.D.	oculus dexter	right eye
O.L.	oculus laevus	left eye
O.S.	oculus sinister	left eye
oz.	uncia	ounce
paren.		parenterally
PBI		protein-bound iodine
pH		hydrogen ion concentration
ppm		parts per million
pt	pinte (French)	pint
qt	quartina	quart
rad		radiation absorbed dose
s	sans	without
s̄	sine	without
S	signa	mark
s.c.	sub cutis	subcutaneously
s.cut.		subcutaneously
SGOT		serum glutamic oxaloacetic transaminase (see AST)
SGPT		serum glutamic pyruvic transaminase (see ALT)
sp. gr.	gravitus	specific gravity
spt.	spiritus	spirit
s.q.		subcutaneously
stat.	statim	immediately

Principal Medical Abbreviations *(Continued)*

Abbreviation	Latin (unless indicated)	English Definition
syr.	syrupus	syrup
top.		topically
tr., tinct.	tinctura	tincture
UHF		ultrahigh frequency
ung.	unguentum	ointment
UV		ultraviolet
vin.	vinum	wine
Vo$_2$		maximum oxygen consumption
vol. %		volume per cent
WBC		white blood count
Wt.	wiht (Old English)	weight
w/v.		weight in volume
x		multiplied by

Charting: Abbreviations and Their Meanings

Some of these abbreviations are used rarely if at all. They are recorded for their historical interest. See also *Principal Medical Abbreviations* and *Prescription Writing* in *Appendix*.

Abbreviation	Latin Phrase	English Definition
ā	ante	before
abs. feb.	absente febre	without fever
a.c.	ante cibum	before a meal
ad effect.	ad effectum	to effect
adhib.	adhibendus	to be administered
ad lib.	ad libitum	at pleasure
ad part. dolent.	ad partes dolentes	to the aching parts
adst. feb.	adstante febre	when fever is present
ad us.	ad usum	according to custom
ad us. ext.	ad usum externum	for external use
ag. feb.	aggrediente febre	when the fever increases
alt. dieb.	alternis diebus	every other day
alt. hor.	alternis horis	every other hour
alt. noc.	alterna nocte	every other night
aq.	aqua	water
bal.	balneum	bath
bal. sin.	balneum sinapis	mustard bath
bis in 7d.	bis in septem diebus	twice a week
BM		bowel movement
BP		blood pressure
c̄	cum	with
cat.	cataplasma	a poultice
CC		chief complaint
cito disp.	cito dispensetur	let it be dispensed quickly
c.m.	cras mane	tomorrow morning
c.m.s.	cras mane sumendus	to be taken tomorrow morning
c.n.	cras nocte	tomorrow night
cont. rem.	continuentur remedia	let the medicine be continued
c.v.	cras vespere	tomorrow evening
cyath.	cyathus	ladle (wineglass)
cyath. vinos.	cyathus vinosus	wineglassful
d	da	give
d	dies	day
/d		per day
DC		discharge
dc		discontinue
DDX		differential diagnosis
decub.	decubitus	lying down

Abbreviation	Latin Phrase	English Definition
DNA		does not apply
donec. alv. sol. ft.	donec alvus soluta fuerit	until the bowels are open
dur. dolor.	durante dolore	while pain lasts
Dx		diagnosis
en., enem.		enema
exhib.	exhibeatur	let it be displayed
h.n.	hoc nocte	tonight
hor. som, h.s.	hora somni	bedtime
in d.	in dies	daily
lmp		last menstrual period
mod. praesc.	modo praescripto	as prescribed
mor. dict.	more dicto	in the manner directed
mor. sol.	more solito	in the usual manner
n.b.	nota bene	note well
noct.	nocte	of the night
n.p.o.		nothing by mouth
p̄	post	after
p.a.a.	parti affectae applicetur	let it be applied to the affected region
PERRL		Pupils equal, regular, react to light
PI		present illness
post. cib. or p. c.	post cibos	after meals
p.r.	per rectum	through the rectum
p.r.n.	pro re nata	as needed
p.v.	per vaginam	through the vagina
Q.h.	quaque hora	every hour
Q. 2h.		every two hours
Q. 3h.		every three hours
q.i.d.	quater in die	four times a day
q.l.	quantum libet	as much as wanted
q.p.	quantum placeat	as much as desired
q.s.	quantum sufficiat	as much as may be needed
quotid.	quotidie	daily
s̄	sine	without
s.a. or sec. a.	secundum artem	by skill
semih.	semihora	half an hour
SOB		shortness of breath
s.o.s.	si opus sit	if necessary
S/P	status post	no change after
st.	stet, stent	let it (them) stand
sum.	sumat, sumendum	let him take; to be taken
s.v.	spiritus vini	alcoholic spirit
s.v.v.	spiritus vini vitus	brandy
T		temperature
ter.	tere	rub
t.i.d.	ter in die	three times a day
t.i.n.	ter in nocte	three times a night
ur.		urine
WDWN		well developed, well nourished
WF/BF		white female/black female
WM/BM		white male/black male

Prescription Writing: Abbreviations and Their Meanings

Some of these abbreviations are used rarely if at all. They are recorded for their historical interest. See also *Principal Medical Abbreviations* and *Charting* on previous pages.

Abbreviation	Latin (unless indicated)	English Definition
aa or ā	ana (Greek)	of each
add.	adde	add
adhib.	adhibendus	to be administered
admov.	admove	apply
ad sat.	ad saturandum	to saturation
aeq.	aequales	equals
agit.	agita	shake; stir
agit. ante sum.	agita ante sumendum	shake before taking
alb.	albus	white
aq. bull.	aqua bulliens	boiling water
aq. cal.	aqua calida	hot water
aq. dest.	aqua destillata	distilled water
aq. ferv.	aqua fervens	boiling water
aq. font.	aqua fontis	spring water
aq. frig.	aqua frigida	cold water
aq. menth. pip.	aqua menthae piperitae	peppermint water
aq. pur.	aqua pura	pure water
bib.	bibe	drink
b.i.d.	bis in die	twice daily
b.i.n.	bis in noctus	twice a night
bol.	bolus	a pill
bull.	bulliat	let it boil
c̄	cum	with
cap.	capsula	a capsule
chart. or cht.	chartula	a small medicated paper
coch. mag.	cochleare magnum	a large spoonful
coch. med	cochleare medium	a half spoonful
coch. parv.	cochleare parvum	a teaspoonful
collyr.	collyrium	an eyewash
comp.	compositus	compounded of
cuj. lib.	cujus libet	of any you please
D	dosis	dose
d.	da	give
d.d. in d.	de die in diem	from day to day
dec.	decanta	pour off
dent. tal. dos.	dentur tales doses	give of such doses
det.	detur	let it be given
dieb. alt.	diebus alternis	every other day
dieb. tert.	diebus tertiis	every 3rd day
dil.	dilue, dilutus	dilute, diluted
dim.	dimidius	halved
div.	dividatur	divide
div. in p. aeq.	dividatur in partes aequales	let it be divided into equal parts
donec. alv. sol. ft.	donec alvus soluta fuerit	until the bowels are open
dos.	dosis	dose
dur. dolor.	durante dolore	while pain lasts
e.m.p.	ex modo praescripto	as directed
emp.	emplastrum	a plaster
emuls.	emulsio	an emulsion
epistom.	epistomium	a stopper
ext.	extendere	to spread
	extractum	extract
ferv.	fervens	boiling
f.h.	fiat hastus	let a draught be made
filt.	filtra	filter

2356

Prescription Writing: Abbreviations
and Their Meanings *(Continued)*

Abbreviation	Latin (unless indicated)	English Definition
f.m.	fiat mistura	let a mixture be made
f.p.	fiat potio	let a potion be made
f. pil.	fiat pilula	let a pill be made
ft.	fiat	let it be made
garg.	gargarisma	a gargle
grad.	gradatim	by degrees
gtt	guttae	drops
guttat.	guttatim	drop by drop
haust.	haustus	a draught
hor. decub.	hora decubitus	at bedtime
hor. som. or h. s.	hora somni	at bedtime
hor. 1 spat.	horae unis spatio	one hour's time
inf.	infusum	an infusion
int.	intime	to the innermost
int. cib	inter cibos	between meals
lin.	linimentum	a liniment
liq.	liquor	a solution
lot.	lotio	a lotion
M	misce	mix
mac.	macera	soften
man. prim.	mane primo	first thing in the morning
mas.	massa	a mass
med.	medicamentum	a medicine
m. et n.	mane et nocte	morning and night
mist.	mistura	a mixture
mitt.	mitte	let go
mitt. x tal.	mitte decem tales	send 10 like this
mod.	modicus	moderate-sized
mod. praesc.	modo praescripto	in the manner prescribed
moll.	mollis	soft
mor. dict.	more dicto	in the manner directed
mor. sol.	more solito	as accustomed
ne tr. s. num.	ne tradas sine nummo	deliver not without the money
no.	numerus	number
noct. maneq.	nocte maneque	night and morning
non. rep., n. r.	non repetatur	do not repeat
omn. bid.	omni bidendis	every 2 days
omn. bih.	omni bihoris	every 2 hours
omn. hor.	omni hora	every hour
omn. noct.	omni nocte	every night
om. ¼ h.	omni quadranta hora	every 15 minutes
om. mane vel. noc.	omni mane vel nocte	every morning or night
part. aeq.	partes aequales	equal parts
part. vic.	partitis vicibus	in divided doses
p.c.	post cibos	after meals
pil.	pilula	a pill
p.o.	per os	by mouth
p. p. a.	phiala prius agitata	the bottle having first been shaken
pro. rat. aet.	pro ratione aetatis	according to patient's age
pulv.	pulvis	powder
red. in pulv.	redactus in pulverem	reduced to powder
repetat., rep.	repetatur	let it be repeated
rub.	ruber	red
sig.	signa	write
	signetur	let it be labeled
sing.	singulorum	of each
sol.	solutio	a solution
solv.	solve	dissolve
ss.	semi- or semisse	a half

Prescription Writing: Abbreviations
and Their Meanings *(Continued)*

Abbreviation	Latin (unless indicated)	English Definition
subind.	subinde	immediately after
sum.	sume	take
sum. tal.	sumat talem	take 1 like this
suppos.	suppositorium	a suppository
s.v.r.	spiritus vini rectificatus	rectified spirit of wine
tab.	tabella	a medicated tablet
tinct.	tinctura	a tincture
trit.	tritura	triturate or grind
ult. praes.	ultimus praescriptus	the last ordered
ung.	unguentum	ointment
ut dict.	ut dictum	as directed
vitel.	vitellus	yolk of an egg

App. 11: Documentation Terms

ALERT. A charting system used primarily in long-term care in which the patient's chart is tagged to indicate that special charting procedures/precautions need to be initiated and followed for a specified time.

CBE. Acronym for *Charting By Exception*, a system for documentation which eliminates the need to chart repetitious findings and tasks. The nurse uses specially designed admission history and flow sheets which highlight important findings and trends. Only significant findings or exceptions to established standards of care and protocols are documented in the progress notes.

CORE. Documentation system designed to support nursing process. Key elements include data base, care plans, flow sheets, progress notes, and discharge summaries. Progress notes use a three-column format and are organized using (D) patient *Database*; (A) *Action* of the health care worker; and (E) *Evaluation* of patient outcome.

DAR. Acronym for the organizing structure for writing progress notes using Focus Charting®. Each Focus entry includes (D) *Database* describing the current patient condition; (A) *Action* taken by the health care worker; and (R) patient *Response* or outcome to the intervention.

FACT. Acronym for documentation system including these key elements: *F*lowsheets for specific patient populations; standardized *A*ssessment parameters printed on the chart form; *C*oncise integrated progress notes; and *T*imely entries by nurses at the time care is given.

FOCUS CHARTING®. Trademark title for three-column format for organizing the progress notes in the patient record. The FOCUS column serves as an index. The body of the note is organized by identifying the DATAbase describing the current patient condition; ACTION taken by the health care worker; and patient RESPONSE to or outcome of the intervention.

PIE. Acronym for a process-oriented documentation system. The progress notes in the patient record use (P) to define the particular problem; (I) to document intervention; and (E) to evaluate the patient outcome. PIE charting integrates care planning with progress notes.

POMR. Acronym for *Problem-Oriented Medical Record*, a method of establishing and maintaining the patient's medical record so that problems are clearly stated. These data are kept in the front of the chart and are evaluated as frequently as indicated with respect to recording changes in the patient's problems as well as progress made in solving the problems. Use of this system may bring a degree of comprehensiveness to total patient care that might not be possible with conventional medical records.

SOAP. Acronym for an organized structure for keeping progess notes in the chart. Each entry contains date, number, and title of the patient's particular problem, followed by the SOAP headings, *S*ubjective findings; *O*bjective findings; *A*ssessment, the documented analysis and conclusions concerning the fndings; and *P*lan for further diagnostic or therapeutic action. If the patient has multiple problems, a SOAP entry on the chart is made for each problem.

SOAPIER. Adds to the SOAP headings listed above: documentation of *I*ntervention implemented to solve the identified problem; the *E*valuation of the effectiveness of the intervention; and care plan *R*evisions indicated.

App. 12: Prefixes and Suffixes

a-, an-. Negative.

a-, ab-, abs-. Away from.

ad-, -ad. Toward.

-aemia. Blood.

aer-. Air.

-aesthesia. Sensation.

-algesia, -algia. Suffering; pain.

algi-. Pain.

all-. Other.

amb-. Both; on both sides.

amph-. Around; on both sides.

ana-, an-. Up.

angio-. Relating to blood or lymph vessels.

ante-. Before.

anti-. Against.

apo-. From; opposed.

-ase. Enzyme.

aut-, auto-. Self.

bi-, bis-. Twice; double.

brachy-. Short.

brady-. Slow.

cac-, caco-. Bad; evil.

cat-, cata-, cath-. Down.

-cele. A tumor; a cyst; a hernia.

cent-. Hundred.

cephal-. Relating to a head.

chrom-, chromo-. Color.

-cide. Causing death.

circum-. Around.

co-, com-, con-. Together.

contra-. Against.

cyst-, -cyst. Bag; bladder.

-cyte. A cell.

dacry-. Tears.

dactyl-. Fingers.

de-. From; not.

deca-. Ten.

deci-. Tenth.

demi-. Half.

dent-. Relating to the teeth.

derma-. The skin.

di-. Double; apart from.

dia-. Through; between; asunder.

dipla-, diplo-. Double.

dis-. Negative; double; apart; absence of.

-dynia. Pain.

dys-. Difficult; bad.

ec-, ecto-. Out; on the outside.

-ectomy. A cutting out.

ef-, es-, ex-, exo-. Out.

-emesis. Vomiting.

-emia. Blood.

en-. In; into.

endo-. Within.

entero-. Relating to the intestine.

ento-. Within.

epi-. Upon.

-esthesia. Sensation.

eu-. Well.

ex-, exo-. Out.

extra-. On the outside; beyond.

fore-. Before; in front of.

-form. Form.

-fuge. To drive away.

galact-, galacto-. Milk.

gaster-, gastro-. The stomach; the belly.

-gene, -genesis, -genetic, -genic. Production; origin; formation.

glosso-. Relating to the tongue.

-gog, -gogue. To make flow.

-gram. A tracing; a mark.

-graphy. A writing; a record.

hem-, hemato-. Relating to the blood.

hemi-. Half.

hepa-, hepar-, hepato-. Liver.

hetero-. Other; indicating dissimilarity.

holo-. All.

homo-, homeo-. Same; similar.

hydra-, hydro-. Relating to water.

hyp-, hyph-, hypo-. Under.

hyper-. Over; above; beyond.

hypo-. Under.

-iasis. Condition; pathological state.

idio-. Peculiar to the individual or organ.

ileo-. Relating to the ileum.

in-. In; into; not.

infra-. Beneath.

inter-. Between.

intra-, intro-. Within.

-ism. Condition; theory.

iso-. Equal.

-itis. Inflammation.

-ize. To treat by special method.

juxta-. Near.

karyo-. Nucleus; nut.

kata-, kath-. Down.

kera-. Horn; indicates hardness.

kinesi-. Movement.

-kinesis. Motion.

lact-. Milk.

laparo-. The loin; relating to the loin or abdomen.

laryng-, laryngo-. The larynx.

latero-. Side.

lepto-. Small; soft.

leuko-. White.

-lite, -lith. A stone; a calculus.

lith-. A stone.

-logia, -logy. Science of; study of.

-lysis. Setting free; disintegration.

macro-. Large; long; big.

mal-. Bad; poor; evil.

med-, medi-. Middle.

mega-, megal-. Large; great.

-megalia, -megaly. Large; great; extreme.

melan-, melano-. Black.

mes-, meso-. Middle.

meta-. Beyond; over; between; change, or transposition.

-meter. Measure.

metra-, metro-. The uterus.

micro-. Small.

mio-. Less; smaller.

mono-. Single.

multi-. Many.

my-, myo-. Muscle.

myel-, myelo-. Marrow.

myxa-, myxo-. Mucus.

neo-. New.

nephr-, nephra-, nephro-. Kidney.

neu-, neuro-. Nerve.

niter-, nitro-. Nitrogen.

non-, not-. No.

nucleo-. Nucleus.

ob-. Against.

oculo-. The eye.

-ode, -oid. Form; shape; resemblance.

odont-. A tooth.

oligo-. Few.

-oma. A tumor.

omo-. Shoulder.

o-. An egg; ovum.

oophoron-. Ovary.

opisth-. Backward.

orchid-. Testicle.

ortho-. Straight; normal.

os-. A mouth; a bone.

-osis. Condition; disease; intensive.

oste-, osteo-. A bone.

-ostomosis, -ostomy. To furnish with a mouth or an outlet.

-otomy. Cutting.

oxy-. Sharp; acid.

pachy-. Thick.

pan-. All; entire.

para-. Alongside of.

path-, -path, -pathy. Disease; suffering.

-penia. Lack.

per-. Excessive; through.

peri-. Around.

-phobia. Fear.

-phylaxis. Protection.

-plasm. To mold.

-plastic. Molded; indicates restoration of lost or badly formed features.

-plegia. A stroke.

plur-. More.

pneu-. Relating to the air or lungs.

poly-. Much; many.

post-. After.

pre-. Before.

pro-. Before; in behalf of.

proto-. First.

pseud-, pseudo-. False.

psych-. The soul; the mind.

py-, pyo-. Pus.

re-. Back; again.

retro-. Backward.

-rhage, -rhagia. Hemorrhage; flow.

-rhaphy. A suturing or stitching.

-rhea. To flow; indicates discharge.

sacchar-. Sugar.

sacro-. Sacrum.

salping-, salpingo-. A tube; relating to a fallopian tube.

sarco-. Flesh.

sclero-. Hard; relating to the sclera.

-sclerosis. Dryness; hardness.

-scopy. To see.

semi-. Half.

-stomosis, -stomy. To furnish with a mouth or outlet.

sub-. Under.

super-, supra-. Above.

syn-. With; together.

tele-. Distant; far.

tetra-. Four.

thio-. Sulfur.

thyro-. Thyroid gland.

-tomy. Cutting.

trans-. Across.

tri-. Three.

-trophic. Relating to nourishment.

tropho-. Relating to nutrition.

uni-. One.

-uria. Relating to the urine.

urino-, uro-. Relating to the urine or urinary organs.

vaso-. A vessel.

venter-, ventro-. The abdomen.

xanth-. Yellow.

App. 13: Latin and Greek Nomenclature

Greek Alphabet

Name of Letter	Capital	Lower Case	Trans-literation	Name of Letter	Capital	Lower Case	Trans-literation
alpha	A	α	a	nu	N	ν	n
beta	B	6 or β	b	xi	Ξ	ζ	x
gamma	Γ	γ	g	omicron	O	o	o short
delta	Δ	δ	d	pi	Π	π	p
epsilon	E	ϵ	e short	rho	P	ρ	r
zeta	Z	ζ	z	sigma	Σ	σ or s	s
eta	H	η	e long	tau	T	τ	t
theta	Θ	θ	th	upsilon	Y	υ	y
iota	I	ι	i	phi	Φ	ϕ or φ	f
kappa	K	κ	k, c	chi	X	χ	ch as in German echt
lambda	Λ	λ	l	psi	Ψ	ψ	ps
mu	M	μ	m	omega	Ω	ω	o long

English with Latin and Greek Equivalents

acid. Acidum.
ague. Febris.
and. Et.
arm. Brachium. Gr., brachion.
artery. Arteria.
attachment. Adhesio.
back. Tergum; dorsum.
backbone. Spina.
backward. Retro.
bath. Balneum.
beef. Bubula.
belly. Venter; abdomen.
bend. Flexus.
bile. Bilis. Gr., chole
bladder. Vesica.
bleed. Fluere.
blind. Obscurus.
blister. Pustulo; vesicatorium.
bloat. Tumeo.
blood. Sanguis. Gr., haima.
blood vessel. Vena.
body. Corpus. Gr., soma.
boiling up. Effervescens.
bone. Os. Gr., osteon.
bony. Osseus.
bowels. Intestina; viscera.
bowlegged. Valgus.
brain. Cerebrum. Gr., enkephalos.
breach. Ruptura.
breast. Mamma. Gr., mastos.
breath. Halitus.
bubble. Pustula.
bulb. Bulbus.
buttock. Clunis. Gr., gloutos.
calcareous. Calci similis.
canal. Canalis.
cartilage. Cartilago. Gr., chondros.
catarrh. Coryza.
cavity. Caverna.

change. Mutatio.
chest. Thorax. Gr., thorax.
chin. Mentum. Gr., geneion.
choke. Strangulo.
clavicle. Clavicula.
confinement. Puerperium.
congestion. Conglobatio.
consumption. Phthisis, pulmonaria.
convulsion. Convulsio.
cord. Corda.
corn. Callus-clavus.
cornea. Cornu. Gr., keras.
costive. Astrictus.
cough. Tussio.
countenance. Vultus.
cramp. Spasmus.
crisis. Dies crisimus.
cup. Poculum.
cure. Sano.
curvature. Curvatura.
cuticle. Cuticula.
daily. Diurnus.
dandruff. Furfures capitas.
day. Dies.
dead. Mortuus; defunctus.
deadly. Lethalis.
deafness. Surditas.
decompose. Dissolvo.
dental. Dentalis.
depression. Depressio.
digestive. Digestorius; pepticus.
dilute. Dilutus.
discharge. Eluvies; effluens.
disease. Morbus.
dorsal. Dorsalis.
dose. Potio.
dram. Drachma.
drink. Bibo; potis.
dropsy. Hydrops; opis.

drug. Medicamentum.
duct. Ductus.
dysentery. Dysenteria.
ear. Auris, Gr., ous.
eat. Edo. Gr., phagos.
egg. Ovum.
elbow. Cubitum. Gr., ankon.
embryo. Partus immaturus.
emission. Emissio.
entrails. Viscera.
epidemic. Epidemus.
epilepsy. Morbus comitalis; epilepsia.
epileptic. Epilepticus.
erection. Erectio.
erotic. Amatorius.
eunuch. Eunuchus.
every. Omnis.
excrement. Excrementum.
excretion. Excrementum; excretio.
exhalation. Exhalatio.
exhale. Exhalo.
expel. Expello.
expire. Expiro.
external. Externus.
extract. Extractum.
eye. Oculus. Gr., ophthalmos.
eyeball. Pupula.
eyebrow. Supercilium.
eyelid. Palpebra.
eyetooth. Dens caninus.
face. Facies.
faculty. Facultas.
faint. Collabor.
fat. Adeps. Gr., lipos.
feature. Lineomentum.
febrile. Febriculosus.
fecundity. Fecunditas.
feel. Tactus.
fever. Febris.
film. Membranula.
filter. Percolo.
finger. Digitus. Gr., daktylos.
fistula. Fistula putris.
fit. Accessus.
flesh. Carnis, Gr., sarx.
fluid. Fluidus.
food. Cibus.
foot. Pes, pedis. Gr., pous.
forearm. Brachium.
forehead. Frons.
freckle. Lentigo.
gall. Bilis.
gangrene. Gangraena.
gargle. Gargarizo.
gland. Glandula.
gleet. Ichor.
gout. Morbus articularis; (in feet) podagra.
grain. Granum.
gravel. Calculus.
grinder tooth. Dens maxillaris.

gullet. Gula.
gum. Gingiva.
gut. Intestinum.
hair. Capillus. Gr., thrix.
half. Dimidius.
hand. Manus. Gr., cheir.
harelip. Labrum fissum.
haunch. Clunis.
head. Caput. Gr., kephale.
heal. Sano.
healer. Medicus.
healing. Salutaris.
health. Sanitas.
healthful. Salutaris; saluber.
healthy. Sanus.
hear. Audio.
hearing. Auditio; (sense of) auditus.
heart. Cor. Gr., kardia.
heartburn. Redundatio stomachi.
heat. Calor.
hectic. Hecticus.
heel. Calx, talus.
hirsute. Hirsutus.
homeopathic. Homeopathicus.
hysterics. Hysteria.
illness. Morbus.
incisor. Dens acutus.
infant. Infans; puerilis.
infect. Inficio.
infectious. Contagiosus.
infirm. Infirmus; debilis.
inflammation. Inflammatio; (of lungs)
    inflammatio pulmonaria.
injection. Injectio.
insane. Insanus.
intellect. Intellectus.
intercourse. Congressus.
internal. Intestinus.
intestine. Intestinum. Gr., enteron.
itch. Scabies.
itching. Pruritus.
jaw. Maxilla.
joint. Artus. Gr., arthron.
jugular vein. Vena jugularis.
kidney. Ren. Gr., nephros.
knee. Genu. Gr., gonu.
kneepan. Patella.
knuckle. Condylus.
labor. Partus.
labyrinth. Labyrinthus.
lacerate. Lacero.
larynx. Guttur.
lateral. Lateralis.
leech. Sanguisuga.
leg. Tibia.
leprosy. Leprosus.
ligament. Ligamentum. Gr., syndesmos.
ligature. Ligatura.
limb. Membrum.
lime. Calx.

listen. Ausculto.
liver. Jecur. Gr., hepar.
livid. Lividus.
loin. Lumbus. Gr., lapara.
looseness. Laxitas.
lotion. Lotio.
lukewarm. Tepidus.
lung. Pulmo. Gr., pneumon.
lymph. Lympha.
mad. Insanus.
malady. Morbus.
male. Masculinus.
malignant. Malignus.
maternity. Conditio matris.
medicated. Medicatus.
medicine. (Remedy) Medicamentum.
milk. Lac.
mind. Animus.
mix. Misceo.
mixture. Mistura.
moist. Humidus.
molar. Dens molaris.
month. Mensis.
monthly. Menstruus.
morbid. Morbidus.
mouth. Os. Gr., stoma.
mucous. Mucosus.
muscle. Musculus. Gr., mys.
mustard. Sinapis.
nail. Unguis.
navel. Umbilicus. Gr., omphalos.
neck. Cervix; collum. Gr., trachelos.
nerve. Nervus. Gr., neuron.
nipple. Papilla.
no, none. Nullus.
normal. Normalis.
nose. Nasus. Gr., rhis.
nostril. Naris.
not. Non.
nourish. Nutrio.
nourishment. Alimentus.
now. Nunc.
nudity. Nudatio.
nurse. Nutrix.
obesity. Obesitas.
ocular. Ocularis.
oculist. Ocularis medicus.
oil. Oleum.
ointment. Unguentum.
operator. Manus curatio.
opiate. Medicamentum somnificum.
optics. Optice.
orifice. Foramen.
pain. Dolor.
palate. Palatum.
palm. Palma.
parasite. Parasitus.
part. Pars.
patient. Patiens.
pectoral. Pectoralis.

pedal. Pedale.
phlegm. Pituita.
pill. Pilus.
pimple. Pustula.
plaster. Emplastrum.
poison. Venenum.
poultice. Cataplasma.
powder. Pulvis.
pregnant. Gravida.
prepare. Paro.
prescribe. Praescribo.
prescription. Praescriptum.
puberty. Pubertas.
pubic bone. Os pubis. Gr., pecten.
pulverize. Pulvero.
pupil. Pupilla.
purgative. Purgativus.
putrid. Putridus.
quinsy. Cynanche; angina.
rash. Exanthema.
recover. Convalesco.
recumbent. Recumbens.
recur. Recurro.
redness. Rubor.
remedy. Remedium.
respiration. Respiratio.
rheum. Fluxio.
rib. Costa.
rigid. Rigidus.
ringing. Tinnitus.
rupture. Hernia.
saliva. Sputum.
sallow. Salix.
salt. Sal.
salve. Unguentum.
sane. Sanus.
scab. Scabies.
scalp. Pericranium.
scaly. Squamosus.
scar. Cicatrix.
sciatica. Ischias.
scruple. Scrupulum.
seed. Semen.
senile. Senilis.
serum. Sanguinis pars equosa.
sheath. Vagina.
shin. Tibia.
shock. Concussio; (of electricity) ictus electricus.
short. Brevis.
shoulder. Humerus. Gr., omos.
shoulder blade. Scapula.
shudder. Tremor.
sick. Aegrotus.
side. Latus.
sinew. Nervus.
skeleton. Gr., skeleton.
skin. Cutis. Gr., derma.
skull. Cranium. Gr., kranion.
sleep. Somnus.
smallpox. Variola.

smell. Odoratus.
soap. Sapo.
socket. Cavum.
soft. Mollis.
solid. Solidus.
solution. Dilutum.
soporific. Soporus.
sore. Ulcus.
spasm. Spasmus.
spinal. Dorsalis; spinalis.
spine. Spina.
spirit. Spiritus.
spittle. Sputum.
spleen. Lien.
spoon. Cochleare.
sprain. Luxatio.
stomach. Stomachus. Gr., gaster.
stone. Calculus.
stricture. Strictura.
sugar. Saccharum.
suture. Sutura.
swallow. Glutio.
sweat. Sudor. Gr., hidros.
symptom. Symptoma.
system. Systema.
tail. Cauda.
take. Sumo.
tapeworm. Taenia.
taste. Gustatus.
tear. Lacrima.
teeth. Dentes.
tendon. Tendo. Gr., tenon.
testicle. Testis. Gr., orchis.
thigh. Femur.

throat. Fauces. Gr., pharynx.
throb. Palpito.
thumb. Pollex.
tongue. Lingua. Gr., glossa.
tonsil. Tonsilla.
tooth. Dens. Gr., odous.
troche. Trochiscus.
tube. Tuba.
twin. Geminus.
twitching. Subsultus.
ulcer. Ulcus.
unless. Nisi.
urine. Urina.
uterine. Uterinus.
vaccine. Vaccinum.
vagina. Vagina. Gr., kolpos.
valve. Valvula.
vein. Vena. Gr., phleps.
vertebra. Vertebra. Gr., spondylos.
vessel. Vas.
wash. Lavo.
water. Aqua.
wax. Cera.
waxed dressing. Ceratum.
weary. Lassus.
wet. Humidus.
windpipe. Arteria aspera.
wine. Vinum.
woman. Femina.
womb. Uterus. Gr., hystera.
worm. Vermis.
wound. Vulnus.
wrist. Carpus. Gr., karpos.
yolk. Luteum.

COLORS

black. Niger; nigra; nigrum.
blue. Caeruleus; cyaneus; lividus.
brown. Fulvus.
crimson. Coccum; coccineus.
gray. Cinereus.
green. Viridis.
lemon. Citreum.
pink. Rosaceus.
purple. Purpura; purpureus.
red. Ruber.
scarlet. Coccineus.
violet. Violaceus.
white. Albus.
yellow. Flavus; luteus; croceus.

heavy. Gravis; ponderosus.
hot. Calidus; fervens; candens.
light. Levis.
liquid. Liquidus.
moist. Humidus; uvidus.
sharp. Acutus.
short. Brevis.
sour. Acidus.
sweet. Dulcis.
tall. Longus; celsus; procerus.
thick. Densus.
thin. Tenuis; macer.
warm. Calidus.
warmth. Calor.
weary. Lassus; languidus; fatigatus.
wet. Humidus.

QUALITIES

bitter. Acerbus.
chill. Friguscolum.
cold. Frigidus.
dry. Aridus.
dull. Stupidus; hebes.
faintness. Languor.
fat. Obesus; pinguis.
heat. Calor; ardor; fervor.

METALS

copper. Cuprum; cuprinus.
gold. Aurum; aureus.
iron. Ferrum; ferreus.
silver. Argentum; argenteus.
tin. Stannum; plumbum album.

TIME

afternoon. Post meridiem.
age. Aetas; maturas; adultus; impubis.
autumn. Autumnus.
birth. Partus; natales.
breakfast. Prandium.
child. Infans; puer; filius.
daily. Diurnus.
date. Status dies.
dawn. Prima lux.
day. Dies.
death. Mors.
dinner. Cena.
evening. Vesper.
hour. Hora.
infant. Infans.
maturity. Maturitas; aetas matura.
meal. Epulae.
midnight. Media nox.
midsummer. Media aestas.
moment. Punctum.

month. Mens.
monthly. Menstruus.
morning. Matutinum.
night. Nox, noctis.
noon. Meridies.
old. Antiquus.
puberty. Pubertas.
second. Secundum.
spring. Ver; veris.
summer. Aestas.
sunrise. Solis ortus.
sunset. Solis occasus.
supper. Cena.
time. Tempus.
winter. Hiems, hiemis.
year. Annus.
young. Parvus; infans.
youth. Adolescentia.

NUMERALS (ROMAN)

SEE: *Roman Numerals* in *Appendix.*

Latin Numerals

	Cardinals			Ordinals
1	unus		1st	primus
2	duo		2nd	secundus
3	tres		3rd	tertius
4	quattuor		4th	quartus
5	quinque		5th	quintus
6	sex		6th	sextus
7	septem		7th	septimus
8	octō		8th	octāvus
9	novem		9th	nōnus
10	decem		10th	decimus
11	ūndecim		11th	ūndecimus
12	duodecim		12th	duodecimus
13	tredecim		13th	tertius decimus
14	quattuordecim		14th	quartus decimus
15	quīndecim		15th	quīntus decimus
16	sēdecim		16th	septus decimus
17	septendecim		17th	septimus decimus
18	duodēvīgintī		18th	duodēvīcēsimus
19	ūndēvīgintī		19th	ūndēvīcēsimus
20	vīgintī		20th	vīcēsimus
21	vīgintī ūnus,		21st	vīcēsimus primus,
	or ūnus et vīgintī			*or* prīmus et vīcēsimus
22	vīgintī duo,		22nd	vīcēsimus secundus,
	or duo et vīgintī			*or* duo et vīcēsimus
28	duodētrīgintā		28th	duodētrīcēsimus
29	ūndētrīgintā		29th	ūndētrīcēsimus
30	trīgintā		30th	trīcēsimus
40	quadrāgintā		40th	quadrāgēsimus
50	quīnquāgintā		50th	quīnquāgēsimus
60	sexāgintā		60th	sexāgēsimus
70	septuāgintā		70th	septuāgēsimus
80	octōgintā		80th	octōgēsimus
90	nōnāgintā		90th	nōnāgēsimus
100	centum		100th	centēsimus

101	centum ūnus, *or*	101st	centēsimus prīmus,
	centum et ūnus		*or* centēsimus et prīmus
102	centum duo, *or*	102nd	centēsimus secundus, *or*
	centum et duo		centēsimus et secundus
200	ducentī	200th	ducentēsimus
300	trecentī	300th	trecentēsimus
400	quadringentī	400th	quadringentēsimus
500	quīngentī	500th	quīngentēsimus
600	sēscentī, *or* sexcenti	600th	sēscentēsimus
700	septingentī	700th	septingentēsimus
800	octingentī	800th	octingentēsimus
900	nōngentī	900th	nōngentēsimus
1,000	mīlle	1,000th	mīllēsimus
2,000	duo mīllia	2,000th	bis mīllēsimus
10,000	decem mīllia	10,000th	decies mīllēsimus
100,000	centum mīllia	100,000th	centiēs mīllēsimus

Roman Numerals

A line placed over a letter increases its value one thousand times.

1	I	6	VI	11	XI	40	XL	90	XC	5000	$\overline{\text{V}}$
2	II	7	VII	12	XII	50	L	100	C	10,000	$\overline{\text{X}}$
3	III	8	VIII	15	XV	60	LX	500	D	100,000	$\overline{\text{C}}$
4	IV	9	IX	20	XX	70	LXX	1000	M	1,000,000	$\overline{\text{M}}$
5	V	10	X	30	XXX	80	LXXX	2000	MM		

App. 14: Braille Alphabet and Numerals

	Braille		Braille		Braille		Braille
A	●	J	● ● ●	S	● ●	2	● ●
B	● ●	K	● ● ●	T	● ● ●	3	● ●
C	● ●	L	● ● ●	U	● ● ●	4	● ● ●
D	● ● ●	M	● ● ●	V	● ● ● ●	5	● ●
E	● ●	N	● ● ●	W	● ● ● ●	6	● ●
F	● ● ●	O	● ● ●	X	● ● ● ●	7	● ● ● ●
G	● ● ● ●	P	● ● ● ●	Y	● ● ● ● ●	8	● ● ●
H	● ● ●	Q	● ● ● ● ●	Z	● ● ● ●	9	● ●
I	● ●	R	● ● ● ●	1	●	0	● ● ●

App. 15: Manual Alphabet

App. 16: The Interpreter

Basic Medical Diagnosis and Treatment
English, Spanish, Italian, French, German

Table of Contents

Introduction

When attempting to communicate with a patient whose language is foreign to you, it is important to establish that while you may be able to say a few words in his or her language you will not be able to understand the patient's replies. The patient may need to use signs in replying. The following paragraphs are given for your convenience in explaining your language difficulty to the patient.

English

Hello. I want to help you. I do not speak (English) but will use this book to ask you some questions. I will not be able to understand your spoken answers. Please respond by shaking your head or raising one finger to indicate "no"; nod your head or raise two fingers to indicate "yes."

Spanish

(Translation)

Saludos. Quiero ayudarlo. Yo no hablo español, pero voy a usar este libro para hacerle algunas preguntas. No voy a poder entender sus respuestas; por eso haga el favor de contestar, negando con la cabeza o levantando un dedo para indicar "no" y afirmando con la cabeza o levantando dos dedos para indicar "sí."

(Phonetic)

Sah-loo'dohs. Ki-air'oh ah-joo-dar'loh. Joh noh ah'bloh es'panyohl, pair'oh voy ah oo-sawr' es'tay lee'broh pahr'ah ah-sair'lay ahl-goo'nahs pray-goon'tahs. Noh voy ah poh-dair' en-ten-dair' soos res-poo-es'rahs; pore es-soh ah'gah el fah-vohr' day kohn-tes-tahr', nay-gahn'doh kohn lah kah-bay'thah oh lay-vahn-tahn'doh oon day'doh pahr'ah een-dee-kahr' noh ee ah-feer-mahn'doh kohn lah kah-bay'thah oh lay-vahn-tahn'doh dohs day'dohs pahr'a een-dee-kahr' see.

Italian

(Translation)

Buon giorno. La voglio aiutare. Io non parlo italiano, ma userò questo libro per farle qualche domanda. Non potrò comprendere le Sue domande. Per favore risponda con un cenno di testa. Alzi un dito per indicare 'no'; muova la Sua testa su e giu o alzi due dita per indicare 'si.'

(Phonetic)

Bwon jih-or'noh. Lah vol'yoh ah-yoo-tar'day. Ee'oh nohn par'loh ee-towl-ee-ah'noh mah oo-say'roh kwes'toh lee'broh pehr fahr'lay kwall'kay doh-mahn'dah. Non poh'throh kohm-prehn'deh-ray lay soo'ee doh-mahn'day. Pehr fah-vohr'ay ray-spohn'dah kohn oon chay'noh dee tes'tah. Ahlt'zih oon dee'toh pehr in-dee-kar'ay noh; moo-eh'vah lah soo'ah tes'tah soo eh joo oh alht'zih doo'ay dee'tay pehr in-dee-kar'ay see.

French

(Translation)

Bonjour. Je veux bien vous aider. Je ne parle pas français mais tout en me servant de ce livre je vais vous poser des questions. Je ne comprendrai pas ce que vous dites en français. Je vous en prie, pour répondre: pour indiquer "non", secouez la tête ou levez un seul doigt; pour indiquer "oui", faites un signe de tête ou levez deux doigts.

(Phonetic)

Bon-zhoor'. Zheh voo bih-ehn' voo ay-day'. Zheh neh parl pah frahn-say' may too ahn meh sehr-vahn' d' seh lee'vrah zheh vay voo poh-say' day kehs-tih-on'. Zheh neh kahm-prahn'dry pah seh keh voo deet ahn frahn-say'. Zheh voo ahn pree, por ray-pahn'drah; por ahn-dee-kay nohn, seh-kway' lah teht oo leh-vay' oon sool dwoit; por ahn-dee-kay wee', fayt oon seen deh teht oo leh-vay' duh dwoit.

German

(Translation)

Hallo! Ich mochte Ihnen helfen. Ich spreche kein Deutsch, aber ich werde dieses Buch benützten um Sie einiges zu fragen. Ich werde Ihre Antworten nicht verstehen. Deshalb antworten Sie mir indem Sie Ihren Kopf schütteln oder heben Sie Ihren Finger um "nein" auszudrücken; nicken Sie mit dem Kopf oder heben Sie zwei Finger um "ja" auszudrücken.

(Phonetic)

Ha-loh! Ich möhh'tuh ee'nuhn hel'fuhn. Ich shpre'huh kīn doitsh, ah'buhr ich ver'duh dee'zuhs bookh bā-nüt'zuhn um zee ī'ni-guhs tsoo frah'guhn. Ich ver'duh ee'ruh ant'vor-tuhn nihht fer-shtay'uhn. Dās'halb' ant'vor-tuhn zee meer in-dām' zee ee'ruhn kopf shü'tln ō'der hāb'uhn zee ee'ruhn fing'uhr um nīn ows'tsoo-drük-uhn; nick'uhn zee mit dām kopf ō'der hāb'uhn zee tsvī fing'uhr um ya ows'tsoo-drük-uhn.

The Interpreter in Five Languages
GENERAL
Basic Questions and Replies

English	Spanish	Italian	French	German
Good morning.	Buenos días.	Buon giorno.	Bonjour.	Guten Morgen.
What is your name?	¿Cómo se llama?	Come si chiama Lei?	Quel est votre nom?	Wie heissen Sie?
How old are you?	¿Cuántos años tiene?	Quanti anni ha?	Quel âge avez-vous?	Wie alt sind Sie?
Do you understand me?	¿Me entiende?	Mi capisce?	Me comprenez-vous?	Verstehen Sie mich?
Answer only . . .	Conteste solamente . . .	Risponda solamente . . .	Répondez seulement . . .	Antworten Sie nur . . .
Yes No	Sí No	Sì No	Oui Non	Ja Nein
What do you say?	¿Qué dice?	Cosa dice?	Que dites-vous?	Was sagen Sie?
Speak slower.	Hable más despacio.	Parli più adagio.	Parlez plus lentement.	Sprechen Sie langsamer.
Say it once again.	Repítalo, por favor.	Lo dica ancora una volta.	Répétez ça.	Wiederholen Sie das.
Don't be afraid.	No tenga miedo.	Non abbia paura.	N'ayez pas peur.	Haben Sie keine Angst.
Try to recollect.	Trate de recordar.	Cerchi di ricordarsi.	Cherchez à vous en rappeler.	Versuchen Sie sich zu erinnern.
You cannot remember?	¿No recuerda?	Non si ricorda?	Ne vous en souvenez pas?	Können Sie sich nicht erinnern?
Come to my office.	Venga a mi oficina.	Venga al mio ufficio.	Venez à mon bureau.	Kommen Sie in mein sprechzimmer
Please remove all your clothes.	Por favor, desvístase completamente.	Per cortesia, si spogli.	Veuillex-vous déshabiller.	Ziehen Sie sich bitte ganz aus.
You will?	¿Ud. quiere?*	Desidera?	Vous voulez bien?	Sie wollen?
You will not?	¿No quiere Ud.?	Non desidera?	Vous ne voulez pas?	Sie wollen nicht?
You don't know?	¿No sabe?	Non sa?	Vous ne savez pas?	Wissen Sie nicht?

* Ud.—Usted.

English	Spanish	Italian	French	German
Is it impossible?	¿Es imposible?	È impossible?	C'est impossible?	Ist es unmöglich?
It is necessary.	Es necesario.	È necessario.	C'est necéssaire.	Es ist unbedingt nötig.
That is right.	Está bien.	Va bene.	C'est bien.	Das ist richtig.
Show me . . .	Enséñeme . . .	Mi faccia vedere . . .	Montrez-moi . . .	Zeigen Sie mir . . .
Here There	Aquí Allí	Qui Qua	Ici Là	Hier Da
Which side?	¿En qué lado?	Quale lato?	Quel côté?	Auf welcher Seite?
Since when?	¿Desde cuándo?	Da quando?	Depuis quand?	Seit wann?
Right	Derecha	A destra	A droit	Rechts
Left	Izquierda	A sinistra	A gauche	Links
More or less	Más o menos	Più o meno	Plus ou moins	Mehr oder weniger
How long?	¿Cuánto tiempo?	Da quanto tempo?	Combien de temps?	Wie lange?
Not much	No mucho	Non molto	Pas beaucoup	Nicht viel
Try again.	Trate otra vez.	Provi di nuovo.	Essayez encore une fois.	Versuchen Sie es noch ein mal.
Never	Nunca	Mai	Jamais	Niemals
Never mind.	Olvídelo.	Non importa.	Ça ne fait rien.	Lassen Sie es gut sein.
That will do.	Suficiente.	Basta così.	Ça suffit.	Das ist genug.
About how much daily?	¿Más o menos qué cantidad diaramente?	Circa quanto al giorno?	A peu près combien par jour?	Ungefähr wie viel täglich?
So much?	¿Tanto?	Tanto?	Autant?	So viel?
You must be very careful.	Tiene que tener mucho cuidado.	Deve usare molte precauzioni.	Vous devez prendre garde.	Sie müssen sehr vorsichtig sein.

Seasons

English	Spanish	Italian	French	German
In the spring.	En la primavera.	Nella primavera.	Au printemps.	Im Frühjahr.
In summer.	En el verano.	Nell' estate.	En été	Im Sommer.

The Interpreter in Five Languages (Continued)

English	Spanish	Italian	French	German
In autumn.	En el otoño.	Nell' autunno.	En automne.	Im Herbst.
In winter.	En el invierno.	Nell' inverno.	En hiver.	Im Winter.

Months

English	Spanish	Italian	French	German
The months	Los meses	I mesi	Les mois	Die Monate
January	enero	gennaio	janvier	Januar
February	febrero	febbraio	février	Februar
March	marzo	marzo	mars	März
April	abril	aprile	avril	April
May	mayo	maggio	mai	Mai
June	junio	giugno	juin	Juni
July	julio	luglio	juillet	Juli
August	agosto	agosto	août	August
September	septiembre	settembre	septembre	September
October	octubre	ottobre	octobre	Oktober
November	noviembre	novembre	novembre	November
December	diciembre	dicembre	décembre	Dezember

Days of the Week

English	Spanish	Italian	French	German
Sunday	domingo	domenica	dimanche	Sonntag
Monday	lunes	lunedì	lundi	Montag
Tuesday	martes	martedì	mardi	Dienstag
Wednesday	miércoles	mercoledì	mercredi	Mittwoch
Thursday	jueves	giovedì	jeudi	Donnerstag

Numbers and Time of Day
(office hours, age, diagnosis, treatment)

	viernes	venerdì	vendredi	Freitag
Friday	sábado	sabato	samedi	Sonnabend
Saturday				
One	Uno	Uno	Un	Eins
Two	Dos	Due	Deux	Zwei
Three	Tres	Tre	Trois	Drei
Four	Cuatro	Quattro	Quatre	Vier
Five	Cinco	Cinque	Cinq	Fünf
Six	Seis	Sei	Six	Sechs
Seven	Siete	Sette	Sept	Sieben
Eight	Ocho	Otto	Huit	Acht
Nine	Nueve	Nove	Neuf	Neun
Ten	Diez	Dieci	Dix	Zehn
Twenty	Veinte	Venti	Vingt	Zwanzig
Thirty	Treinta	Trenta	Trente	Dreissig
Forty	Cuarenta	Quaranta	Quarante	Vierzig
Fifty	Cincuenta	Cinquanta	Cinquante	Fünfzig
Sixty	Sesenta	Sessanta	Soixante	Sechzig
Seventy	Setenta	Settanta	Soixante-dix	Siebzig
At 10:00	A las diez	Alle dieci	A dix heures	Um zehn Uhr
At 2:30	A las dos y media	Alle due e mezzo	A deux heures et demie	Um halb drei
Early in the morning	Temprano por la mañana	Di buon mattino	De bon matin	Frühmorgens
In the daytime	En el día	Durante il giorno	Pendant la journée	Bei Tag
At noon	A mediodía	A mezzo giorno	A midi	Mittags
At bedtime	Al acostarse	All' ora di coricarsi	A l'heure de se coucher	Vor dem Schlafengehen
At night	Por la noche	Alla sera	Le soir	Abends

The Interpreter in Five Languages (Continued)

English	Spanish	Italian	French	German
Before meals	Antes de las comidas	Prima del pasto	Avant les repas	Vor den Mahlzeiten
After meals	Después de las comidas	Dopo il pasto	Après les repas	Nach den Mahlzeiten
Today	Hoy	Oggi	Aujourd'hui	Heute
Tomorrow	Mañana	Domani	Demain	Morgen
Every day	Todos los días	Ogni giorno	Chaque jour	Jeden Tag
Every hour	Cada hora	Ogni ora	Chaque heure	Jede Stunde
How long have you felt this way?	¿Desde cuándo se siente así?	Da quanto tempo si sente così?	Depuis quand vous sentez-vous comme ça?	Seit wann fühlen Sie sich so?
It came all of a sudden?	¿Vino de repente?	Venne tutto ad un tratto?	Ça vous est arrivé tout à coup?	Ist es ganz plötzlich gekommen?
For how many days or weeks?	¿Cuántos días o semanas?	Da quanti giorni o settimane?	Depuis combien de jours ou semaines?	Seit wievielen Tagen oder Wochen?
Do they come every day?	¿Los tiene todos los días?	Le vengono tutti i giorni?	Ça vous gêne tous le jours?	Kommt es jeden Tag?
At the same hour?	¿A la misma hora?	Alla stessa ora?	A la même heure?	Zur selben Stunde?
At intervals?	¿De vez en cuando?	Ad intervalli?	De temps à autre?	Dann und wann?
It will be too late.	Será demasiado tarde.	Sarà troppo tardi.	Ce sera trop tard.	Es wird zu spät sein.

Colors

English	Spanish	Italian	French	German
Black	Negro	Nero	Noir	Schwarz
Blue	Azul	Blu	Bleu	Blau
Green	Verde	Verde	Vert	Grün
Pink	Rosado	Rosa	Rose	Rosa
Red	Rojo	Rosso	Rouge	Rot
White	Blanco	Bianco	Blanc	Weiss
Yellow	Amarillo	Giallo	Jaune	Gelb

Parts of Body

English	Spanish	Italian	French	German
In the abdomen?	¿En el vientre?	Nel ventre?	Dans le abdomen?	Im Leib?
The ankle	El tobillo	La caviglia	La cheville	Das Fussgelenk
The arm	El brazo	Il braccio	Le bras	Der Arm
The back	La espalda	Il dorso	Le dos	Der Rücken
The bones	Los huesos	La ossa	Le os	Die Knochen
The chest	El pecho	Il petto	La poitrine	Die Brust
The ears	Los oídos	Le orecchie	Les oreilles	Die Ohren
The elbow	El codo	Il gomito	Le coude	Der Ellenbogen
The eye	El ojo	L'occhio	L'oeil	Das Auge
The foot	El pie	Il piede	Le pied	Der Fuss
The gums	Las encías	Le gengive	Les gengives	Das Zahnfleisch
The hand	La mano	La mano	La main	Die Hand
The head	La cabeza	La testa	La tête	Der Kopf
The heart	El corazón	Il cuore	Le coeur	Das Herz
The leg	La pierna	La gamba	La jambe	Das Bein
The liver	El hígado	Il fegato	Le foie	Die Leber
The lungs	Los pulmones	I polmoni	Les poumons	Die Lungen
The mouth	La boca	La bocca	La bouche	Der Mund
The muscles	Los músculos	I muscoli	Les muscles	Die Muskeln
The neck	El cuello	Il collo	Le cou	Der Nacken
The nerves	Los nervios	I nervi	Les nerfs	Die Nerven
The nose	La nariz	Il naso	Le nez	Die Nase
The ribs	Las costillas	Le costole	Les côtes	Die Rippen
The shoulder blades	Las paletillas	Le scapole	Les omoplates	Die Schulterblätter
The side	El flanco	Il fianco	Le côté	Die Seite
The skin	La piel	La pelle	La peau	Die Haut

The Interpreter in Five Languages (Continued)

English	Spanish	Italian	French	German
The skull	El cráneo	Il cranio	Le crâne	Der Schädel
The stomach	El estómago	Lo stomaco	L'estomac	Der Magen
The teeth	Los dientes	I denti	Les dents	Die Zähne
The temples	Las sienes	Le tempie	Les tempes	Die Schläfen
The thigh	El muslo	La coscia	La cuisse	Der Oberschenkel
The throat	La garganta	La gola	La gorge	Der Hals
The thumb	El dedo pulgar	Il pollice	Le pouce	Der Daumen
The tongue	La lengua	La lingua	La langue	Die Zunge
The wrist	La muñeca	Il polso	Le poignet	Das Handgelenk

Work History

English	Spanish	Italian	French	German
What work do you do?	¿Cuál es su ocupación?	Che lavoro fa?	Quelle est votre profession?	Was ist Ihr Beruf?
Is it heavy physical work?	¿Es un trabajo corporal pesado?	È un pesante lavoro manuale?	Est-ce que c'est un travail physiquement fatigant?	Ist es eine schwere körperliche Arbeit?
What work have you done?	¿Qué trabajo ha hecho?	Che lavoro ha fatto?	A quoi avez-vous travaillé?	Welche Arbeit haben Sie getan?

HISTORY
Family

English	Spanish	Italian	French	German
Are you married?	¿Es Ud. casado?	È sposato?	Etes-vous marié?	Sind Sie verheiratet?
A widower?	¿Viudo?	È vedovo?	Veuf?	Ein Witwer?
A widow?	¿Viuda?	È vedova?	Veuve?	Eine Witwe?
Do you have children?	¿Tiene Ud. hijos?	Ha bambini?	Avez-vous des enfants?	Haben Sie Kinder?
Are they still living?	¿Viven todavía?	Vivono ancora?	Sont-ils encore vivants?	Leben sie noch?
Do you have any sisters?	¿Tiene hermanas?	Ha sorelle?	Avez-vous des soeurs?	Haben Sie Schwestern?

English	Spanish	Italian	French	German
Do you have any brothers?	¿Tiene hermanos?	Ha fratelli?	Avez-vous des frères?	Haben Sie Brüder?
Of what did your mother die?	¿De qué murió su madre?	Di checosa è morta Sua mamma?	De quoi est morte votre mère?	Woran ist Ihre Mutter gestorben?
And your father?	¿Y su padre?	E Suo padre?	Et votre père?	Und Ihr Vater?
Your grandfather?	¿Su abuelo?	Suo nonno?	Votre grand-père?	Ihr Grossvater?
Your grandmother?	¿Su abuela?	Sua nonna?	Votre grand-mère?	Ihre Grossmutter?

General

English	Spanish	Italian	French	German
Do you have . . . ?	¿Tiene . . . ?	Ha Lei . . . ?	Avez-vous . . . ?	Haben Sie . . . ?
Have you ever had . . . ?	¿Ha tenido . . . ?	Ha mai avuto . . . ?	Avez-vous jamais eu . . . ?	Haben Sie je . . . gehabt?
Chills	Escalofríos	I brividi	Les frissons	Ein Fieberfrösteln
An attack of fever	Un ataque de calentura	Un attacco di febbre	Une attaque de fièvre	Ein Fieberanfall
Toothache	Dolor de muelas	Mal di denti	Le mal aux dents	Zahnschmerzen
Hemorrhage	Hemorragia	Emorragia	De hémorragie	Die Blutergüsse
Nosebleeds	Hemorragia por la nariz	Emorragia nasale	Saignements de nez	Das Nasenbluten
Unusual vaginal bleeding	Hemorragia vaginal fuera de los periodos	Perdite di sangue irregulari dalla vagina	Du saignement vaginal anormal	Jemals unregelmässiges bluten aus der Scheide
When did you last have a period?	¿Cuándo tuvo Ud. su última menstruación?	Quando ha avuto l'ultima volta le mestruazione?	Quand avez-vous eu vos règles pour la dernière fois?	Wann war die letze Menstruation?
Do you take birth control pills?	¿Toma. Ud. píldoras anticonceptivas	Prende pillole contro la gravibanza	Est-ce que vous prenez des médicaments anti-conceptionnels?	Nehmen Sie Geburtskontroll-pillen?
Hoarseness	Ronquera	Raucedine	Enrouement	Heiserkeit

Diseases

English	Spanish	Italian	French	German
What diseases have you had?	¿Qué enfermedades ha tenido?	Che malattie ha avuto?	Quelles maladies avez-vous eues?	Welche Krankheiten haben Sie gehabt?
Allergy	Alergia	Allergie	Une maladie allergique	Überempfindlichkeiten

The Interpreter in Five Languages (Continued)

English	Spanish	Italian	French	German
Anemia	Anemia	Anemia	L'anémie	Blutarmut
Bleeding tendency	Tendencia a sangrar	Tendenza alle emorragie	Une tendance à saigner	Neigung zum Bluten
Cancer	Cáncer	Cancro	Le cancer	Krebs
Chicken pox	Varicela	Varicella	La varicelle	Windpocken
Diabetes	Diabetes	Diabete	Le diabète	Zuckerkrankheit
Diphtheria	Difteria	Difterite	La diphthérie	Diphtherie
German measles	Rubéola	Rosolia	Rubéole	Röteln
Gonorrhea	Gonorrea	Gonorrea	La gonorrhée	Gonorrhöe, Tripper
Heart disease	Enfermedad del corazón	Malattia di cuore	Une maladie de coeur	Herzkrankheit
High blood pressure	Presion sanguinea elevada	Pressione alta del sangue	La tension arterielle trop élevée	Hohen Blutdruck
Influenza	Gripe (influenza)	Influenza	La grippe	Grippe
Lead poisoning	Envenenamiento con plomo	Avvelenamento da piombo	Empoisonnement causé par le plomb	Bleivergiftung
Liver disease	Enfermedad del hígado	Una malattia del fegato	Une maladie de foie	Eine Leberkrankheit
Malaria	Malaria (paludismo)	Malaria	La malaria	Malaria
Measles	Sarampión	Morbillo	La rougeole	Die Masern
Mental disease	Enfermedades mentales	Malattie mentali	Une maladie mentale	Geisteskrankheit
Mumps	Paperas	Orecchioni	Les oreillons	Mumps
Nervous disease	Enfermedades nerviosas	Malattie nervose	Une maladie nerveuse	Nervenkrankheit
Pleurisy	Pleuresía	Pleurite	Une pleurésie	Rippenfellentzündung
Pneumonia	Pulmonía	Polmonite	Pneumonie	Die Lungenentzündung
Rheumatic fever	Reumatismo (fiebre reumática)	Febbre reumatica	La fièvre rhumatismale	Rheumatisches Fieber

Rheumatism	Reumatismo	Reumatismo	Le rhumatisme	Der Rheumatismus
Scarlet fever	Escarlatina	Febre scarlattina	La fièvre scarlatine	Das Scharlachfieber
Smallpox	Viruela	Vaiolo	La variole	Pocken
Syphilis	Sífilis	Sifilide (lue)	La syphilis	Syphilis
Tuberculosis	Tuberculosis	Tubercolosi	Tuberculose	Die Tuberkulose
Typhoid fever	Tifoidea	Febre il tifo	La fièvre typhoide	Der Typhus

EXAMINATION
General

How do you feel?	¿Cómo se siente?	Come stà?	Comment vous sentez-vous?	Wie fühlen Sie sich?
Good	Bien	Bene	Bien	Gut
Bad	Mal	Male	Mal	Schlecht
Let me see . . .	Déjeme ver . . .	Mi lasci vedere . . .	Permettez-moi de voir . . .	Lassen Sie mich sehen . . .
Let me feel your pulse.	Déjeme tomarle el pulso.	Mi lasci sentire il polso.	Permettez-moi de vous tâter le pouls.	Lassen Sie mich Ihren Puls fühlen.
Whisper: one, two, three.	Repita en voz baja: uno, dos, tres.	Dica piano: uno, due, tre.	Dites tout bas: un, deux, trois.	Flüstern Sie: eins, zwei, drei.
Say it out loud.	Dígalo en voz alta.	Lo dica ad alta voce.	Dites-le à voix haute.	Sagen Sie es laut.
Sit down.	Siéntese.	Si sieda.	Asseyez-vous.	Setzen Sie sich.
Stand up.	Levántese.	Si alzi.	Levez-vous.	Stehen Sie auf.
Can you not rise quicker?	¿No puede levantarse más rápidamente?	Non si può alzare un po' più presto?	Vous ne pouvez pas vous lever plus vite?	Können Sie sich nicht schneller erheben?
Walk a little way.	Ande algunos pasos.	Cammini un po'.	Faites quelques pas.	Gehen Sie einige Schritte.
Return; go backwards.	Vuelva; ande para atrás.	Ritorni; cammini all' indietro.	Revenez; allez à retours.	Kommen Sie zurück; gehen Sie rückwärts.
Do you feel like falling?	¿Le parece que se va a caer?	Si sente come se dovesse cadere?	Vous sentez vous comme si vous allez tomber?	Ist es Ihnen als ob Sie fallen werden?
Do you feel dizzy?	¿Tiene Ud. vértigo?	Ha delle vertigini?	Avez-vous le vertige?	Ist Ihnen schwindlig?
Are you tired?	¿Está Ud. cansado?	Si sente molto stanco?	Êtes vous fatigué?	Sind Sie müde?

The Interpreter in Five Languages (Continued)

English	Spanish	Italian	French	German
Have you slept well?	¿Ha dormido bien?	Ha dormito bene?	Avez-vous bien dormi?	Haben Sie gut geschlafen?
Have you any difficulty in breathing?	¿Tiene dificultad al respirar?	Ha difficoltà di respirare?	C'est difficile à respirer?	Fällt Ihnen das Atemholen schwer?
Have you lost weight?	¿Ha perdido Ud. peso?	É dimagrito?	Avez-vous maigri?	Haben Sie abgenommen?
Since when have you had this eruption?	¿Desde cuándo tiene esta erupción?	Da quanto ha questa eruzione?	Depuis quand avez-vous cette éruption?	Seit wann haben Sie diesen Ausschlag?
Do you sweat much at night?	¿Suda mucho por la noche?	Suda molto alla notte?	Transpirez-vous beaucoup pendant la nuit?	Schwitzen Sie viel in der Nacht?
Are you warm?	¿Tiene calor?	Ha caldo?	Avez-vous chaud?	Ist Ihnen heiss?
Are you cold?	¿Tiene frío?	Ha freddo?	Avez-vous froid?	Ist Ihnen kalt?
Have you been exposed much to the wet weather?	¿Ha estado expuesto a la intemperie?	Si è mai esposto all' umidità?	Avez-vous été longtemp sous la pluie?	Sind Sie dem feuchten Wetter ausgesetzt gewesen?
Can you eat?	¿Puede comer?	Può mangiare?	Pouvez-vous manger?	Können Sie essen?
Have you a good appetite?	¿Tiene Ud. buen apetito?	Ha buon appetito?	Avez-vous un bon appétit?	Haben Sie guten Appetit?
Are you thirsty?	¿Tiene sed?	Ha sete?	Avez-vous soif?	Haben Sie Durst?
Do you still feel very weak?	¿Se siente muy débil todavía?	Si sente ancora molto debole?	Vous sentez-vous encore très faible?	Fühlen Sie sich noch sehr schwach?
Had you been drinking?	¿Había tomado alguna bebida alcohólica?	Ha bevúto?	Est-ce que vous-aviez bu quelque chose d'alcoolique?	Waren Sie angetrunken?
Are you a drinking man?	¿Toma Ud. bebidas alcohólicas habitualmente?	Ha l'abitudine di bere?	Buvez-vous des choses alcooliques d'habitude?	Sind Sie em Trinker?
Are you nervous?	¿Está Ud. nervioso?	É nervoso?	Etes-vous nerveux?	Sind Sie nervös?
When were you first taken sick?	¿Cuándo le empezó esta enfermedad?	Quando si è ammalato la prima volta?	Quand êtes-vous tombé malade d'abord?	Wann hat diese Krankheit begonnen?
How did this illness begin?	¿Cómo empezó esta enfermedad?	Come ha incominciato questa malattia?	Comment cette maladie a-t-elle commencé?	Wie hat diese Krankheit begonnen?

English	Spanish	Italian	French	German
Did you take anything for it?	¿Tomó algo para mejorarla?	Ha preso qual cosa per curarsi?	Avez-vous pris quelque chose pour cela?	Haben Sie etwas dafür genommen?
Have you taken the medicine?	¿Ha tomado Ud. la medicina?	Ha preso la medicina?	Avez-vous pris la medicament?	Haben Sie die Medizin genommen?
A wound	Una herida	Una piaga	Une plaie	Eine Wunde
Are you subject to them?	¿Lo sucede a menudo?	Ne è soggetto?	Ça vous gêne souvent?	Haben Sie dieselben häufig?
Did a dog bite you?	¿Lo mordió un perro?	L'ha morsicato un cane?	Est-ce qu'un chien vous a mordu?	Hat Sie eine Hund gebissen?
Did a fly sting you?	¿Lo picó una mosca?	L'ha punto una mosca?	Est-ce qu'une mouche vous a piqué?	Hat Sie eine Fliege gestochen?
Did you prick yourself with a pin?	¿Se ha pinchado con un alfiler?	Si è punto con una spilla?	Vous êtes-vous piqué avec une épingle?	Haben Sie sich mit einer Stecknadel gestochen?
Did you burn yourself?	¿Se quemó?	Si è bruciato?	Vous êtes-vous brulé?	Haben Sie sich verbrannt?
Did you sprain your foot?	¿Se torció el pie?	Si ha dislocato un piede?	Vous êtes-vous fait une entorse au pied?	Haben Sie Ihren Fuss verstaucht?

Pain

English	Spanish	Italian	French	German
Have you any pain?	¿Tiene dolor?	Ha dolori?	Avez-vous mal quelque?	Haben Sie Schmerzen?
Where does it hurt?	¿Dónde le duele?	Dove le duele?	Où avez-vous mal?	Wo haben Sie Schmerzen?
Do you have pain here?	¿Le duele aquí?	Ha dolori qui?	Avez-vous mal par ici?	Haben Sie Schmerzen hier?
Do you have a pain in your side?	¿Le duele el costado?	Avete dolori al fianco?	Avez-vous mal au côté?	Haben Sie Seitenstechen?
Show me where.	Enséñeme dónde.	Mi mostri dove.	Montrez-moi où.	Zeigen Sie mir wo.
What did you feel in the beginning?	¿Qué sentía cuando empezó?	Che sentiva al principio?	Qu'avez-vous senti au commencement?	Was haben Sie anfangs gespürt?
Shooting pains?	¿Dolores agudos?	Dei dolori acuti?	Des elancements?	Stechende Schmerzen?
As if one were pricking you with pins?	¿Como si estuvieran pinchándole con alfileres?	Come se fossero delle spille?	Comme si l'on vous piquâit avec des épingles?	Als ob man Sie mit Stecknadeln stäche?
Did you feel much pain at the time?	¿Sintió mucho dolor entonces?	Avete sentito molto dolore allora?	Est-ce que ça vous a fait beaucoup de mal alors?	Haben Sie gleich damals arge Schmerzen gespürt?

The Interpreter in Five Languages (Continued)

English	Spanish	Italian	French	German
Is it worse now?	¿Está peor ahora?	È peggio ora?	Est-ce que c'est encore pire maintenant?	Ist es jetzt schlimmer?
Does it still pain you?	¿Le duele todavía?	Fa male ancora?	Est-ce que ça vous fait mal toujours?	Schmerzt er noch?
Do you still have that heavy pain?	¿Le duele mucho todavía?	Ha ancora quel dolore pesante?	Avez-vous toujours la douleur pesante?	Haben Sie noch den drückenden Schmerz?
Does it pain you to breathe?	¿Le duele al respirar?	Le fa male respirare?	Votre respiration est-elle douloureuse?	Spüren Sie Schmerzen beim Atmen?

Head

English	Spanish	Italian	French	German
How does your head feel?	¿Cómo siente la cabeza?	Come si sente la testa?	Comment va votre tête?	Wie geht es Ihrem Kopf?
Your memory	Su memoria	La sua memoria	Votre mémoire	Ihr Gedächtnis
Is it good?	¿Es buena?	È buona?	Est-elle bonne?	Ist es gut?
Have you any pain in the head?	¿Le duele la cabeza?	Ha dolor di testa?	Avez-vous mal à la tête?	Haben Sie Kopfschmerzen?
Did you fall and how did you fall?	¿Se cayó, y cómo se cayó?	È caduto, e come è caduto?	Etes-vous tombé et comment êtes-vous tombé?	Sind Sie gefallen und wie sind Sie gefallen?
Did you faint?	¿Se desmayó?	È svenuto?	Vous êtes-vous évanoui?	Sind Sie ohnmächtig geworden?
Have you ever had fainting spells?	¿Ha tenido desmayos alguna vez?	È mai svenuto regolarmente?	Avez-vous jamais eu des évanouissements?	Haben Sie jemals Ohmachtsanfälle gehabt?

Ears

English	Spanish	Italian	French	German
Do you have ringing in the ears?	¿Le pitan los oídos?	Le tentennano le orecchie?	Avez-vous des bourdonnements d'oreilles?	Haben Sie Ohrenbrausen?
Do you have discharge from the ears?	¿Le supuran los oídos?	Le esce materia dalle orecchie?	Est-ce que vous avez un écoulement des oreilles?	Eitern Ihre Ohren?

English	El oído	L'udito	L'ouïe	Das Gehör
The hearing				
Is it affected?	¿Está afectado?	È compromesso?	Est-elle changée?	Ist es angegriffen?

Eyes

English	El oído	L'udito	L'ouïe	Das Gehör
Look up.	Mire para arriba.	Guardi sù.	Regardez en haut.	Schauen Sie hinauf.
Look down.	Mire para abajo.	Guardi giu.	Regardez en bas.	Schauen Sie hinunter.
Look toward your nose.	Mire la nariz.	Si guardi il naso.	Regardez le nez.	Schauen Sie auf Ihre Nase.
Look at me.	Míreme.	Mi guardi.	Regardez-moi.	Sehen Sie mich an.
Can you see what is on the wall?	¿Puede ver lo que está en la pared?	Può vedere cosa c'è sui muro?	Pouvez-vous voir ce qu'il y a contre le mur?	Können Sie sehen was hier an der Wand ist?
You cannot?	¿No puede?	Non può?	Vous ne pouvez pas?	Können Sie es nicht erkennen?
Can you see it now?	¿Puede verlo ahora?	Può vederlo adesso?	Le voyez-vous maintenant?	Können Sie es jetzt sehen?
And now?	¿Y ahora?	Ed ora?	Et maintenant?	Und nun?
What is it?	¿Qué es ésto?	Che cosa è?	Qu'est-ce que c'est?	Was ist es?
Tell me what number it is?	Dígame qué número es éste.	Mi dica che numero è.	Dites-moi quel est le numéro.	Sagen Sie mir welche Nummer es ist.
Tell me what letter it is.	Dígame qué letra es ésta.	Mi dica che lettera è.	Dites-moi quelle est la lettre.	Nennen Sir mir diesen Buchstaben.
Do you see things through a mist?	¿Ve las cosas a traves de una niebla?	Vede le cose come se fossero fra la nebbia?	Voyez-vous les choses à travers d'un brouillard?	Sehen Sie alles durch einen Nebel?
Can you see clearly?	¿Puede ver claramente?	Può vedere chiaro?	Pouvez-vous voir clairement?	Sehen Sie deutlich?
Better at a distance?	¿Mejor a cierta distancia?	Meglio a distanza?	Mieux à distance?	Besser aus der Entfernung?
Do your eyes water a good deal?	¿Le lagrimean mucho los ojos?	Le lacrimano molto gli occhi?	Est-ce que les yeux vous coulent beaucoup?	Tränen Ihre Augen stark?
Can't you open your eye?	¿No puede abrir el ojo?	Non puo aprire l'occhio?	Ne pouvez-vous pas ouvrir l'oeil?	Können Sie Ihr Auge nicht öffnen?
Do not try to open it when you awaken.	No trate de abrirlo al despertarse.	Quando si sveglia si forzi ad aprirlo.	N'essayez pas de l'ouvrir en vous réveillent.	Versuchen Sie nicht, es beim Aufwachen zu öffnen.

The Interpreter in Five Languages (Continued)

English	Spanish	Italian	French	German
Did anything get into your eye?	¿Le entró algo en el ojo?	Le è entrata qualche cosa nell'occhio?	Est-ce que quelque chose est entré dans l'oeil?	Ist Ihnen etwas ins Auge geflogen?
Do you sometimes see things double?	¿Ve las cosas doble algunas veces.	Vede qualche volta le cose doppie?	Est-ce que la vue est double parfois?	Sehen Sie manchmal doppelt?
Does the eyeball feel as if it were swollen?	¿Le parece que el ojo está hinchado?	Le sembra che l'occhio sia gonfio?	L'oeil vous semble-t-il gonflé?	Fühlt sich das Auge wie geschwollan?
You must be careful not to go out yet.	Tenga cuidado de no salir todavía.	Deve aver cura a non andar fuori.	Gardez vous de sortir maintenant.	Sie dürfen durchaus noch nicht ausgehen.
It would harm your eyes.	Le haría daño a los ojos.	Le farà male agli occhi.	Cela vous abimerait les yeux.	Es wurde Ihren Augen schaden.
Since when has your eyesight failed you?	¿Desde cuando ha disminuido su vista?	Da quanto tempo la sua vista E diminuita?	Depuis quand votre vue s'est-elle diminuée?	Seit wann hat Ihre Sehkraft nachgelassen?

Throat and Mouth

English	Spanish	Italian	French	German
Cough.	Tosa.	Tossisca.	Toussez.	Husten Sie.
Cough again.	Tosa otra vez.	Tossisca ancora.	Toussez encore une fois.	Husten Sie noch einmal.
Open your mouth.	Abra la boca.	Apra la bocca.	Ouvrez la bouche.	Öffnen Sie den Mund.
Does it hurt you to open your mouth?	¿Le duele al abrir la boca?	Le fa male aprir la bocca?	Ouvrir la bouche vous fait-il mal?	Spüren Sie Schmerzen wenn Sie den Mund offnen?
Since when do you cough?	¿Desde cuándo tose Ud?	Da quando ha la tosse?	Depuis quand avez-vous la toux?	Seit wann husten Sie?
You cough a little?	¿Tose poco?	Tossisca poco?	Toussez-vous un peu?	Husten Sie manchmal?
Take a deep breath.	Respire profundamente.	Prenda un gran respiro.	Respirez profondement.	Atmen Sie tief.
Do you expectorate much?	¿Escupe mucho?	Sputa molto?	Crachez-vous beaucoup?	Spucken Sie viel aus?
What is the color of your expectorations?	¿De qué color es el esputo?	Di che color lo sputo?	De quelle sont vos crachats?	Welche Farbe hat der Speichel?

English	Italian	Spanish	French	German
Does your tongue feel swollen?	Ha la lingua gonfia?	¿Siente Ud. la lengua hinchada?	Est-ce que la langue vous paraît gonflée?	Fühlt sich Ihre Zunge wie geschwollen an?
Do you have a sore throat?	Ha mal di gola?	¿Le duele la garganta?	Avez-vous mal à la gorge?	Haben Sie Halsschmerzen?
Does it hurt to swallow?	Quando ingoia le fa male?	¿Le duele al tragar?	Ça vous fait mal à avaler?	Spüren Sie Schmerzen beim Schlucken?

Arms and Hands

English	Italian	Spanish	French	German
Let me see your hand.	Mi faccia vedere la sua mano.	Enséñeme la mano.	Montrez-moi la main.	Zeigen Sie mir Ihre Hand.
Have you no power in it?	Non ha forza nella mano?	¿No tiene fuerza en la mano?	Est-elle complètement inerte?	Ist sie ganz kraftlos?
Grasp my hand.	Mi stringa la mano.	Apriete mi mano.	Serrez-moi la main.	Drücken Sie mir die Hand.
Can you not do it better than that?	Non può far meglio?	¿No puede hacerlo más fuerte?	Vous ne pouvez-pas serrer plus fort que cela?	Können Sie nicht fester greifen?
Your arm feels paralyzed?	Si sente il braccio paralizzato?	¿Parece que el brazo está paralizado?	Est-ce que le bras vous paraît paralysé?	Ihr Arm erscheint Ihnen gelähmt?
Raise your arm.	Alzi il braccio.	Levante el brazo.	Levez le bras.	Heben Sie den Arm.
Raise it more.	Ancora di più.	Más alto.	Plus haut.	Höher.
Now the other.	Adesso l'altro.	Ahora el otro.	Maintenant l'autre.	Jetzt den andern.
Since when is your arm so powerless?	Da quando il suo braccio è senza forza?	Desde cuándo no tiene fuerza en el brazo?	Depuis quand votre bras a-t-il perdu la force?	Seit wann ist Ihr Arm so kraftlos?
Had you been sleeping on your arm?	Ha dormito col braccio sotto la testa?	¿Ha dormido encima del brazo?	Vous êtes-vous endormi sur le bras?	Sind Sie auf Ihrem Arm eingeschlafen?

Gastrointestinal

English	Italian	Spanish	French	German
Do you have stomach cramps?	Ha dei dolori acuti allo stomaco?	¿Tiene calambres en el estómago?	Avez-vous des crampes de l'estomac?	Haben Sie Magenkrämpfe?
Since when is your tongue that color?	Da quando la sua lingua è di questo colore?	¿Desde cuándo tiene la lengua de ese color?	Depuis quand votre langue a-t-elle cette couleur?	Seit wann hat Ihre Zunge diese Farbe?
Have you a pain in the pit of your stomach?	Ha dei dolori alla bocca dello stomaco?	¿Tiene dolor en la boca del estómago?	Est-ce que ça vous fait mal dans le creux de l'estomac?	Haben Sie Schmerzen in der Magengrube?

The Interpreter in Five Languages (Continued)

English	Spanish	Italian	French	German
Nausea	Náusea	La nausea	La nausée	Die Übelkeit
Does eating make you vomit?	¿El comer le hace vomitar?	Vomita dopo aver manginto?	Rendez-vous ce que vous mangez?	Erbrechen Sie nachdem Sie gegessen haben?
How are your stools?	¿Cómo son sus defecaciones?	Come va di corpo?	Comment allez-vous à la selle?	Wie ist der Stuhlgang?
Are they regular?	¿Son regulares?	Va regolarmente?	Allez-vous à la selle régulièrment?	Ist er regelmässig?
Have you noticed their color?	¿Se ha fijado en el color?	Si è accorto di che colore?	Avez-vous remarqué la couleur de vos selles?	Haben Sie auf die Farbe geachtet?
Are you constipated?	¿Está estreñido?	È stitico?	Etes-vous constipé?	Leiden Sie an Verstopfung?
Do you have diarrhea?	¿Tiene diarrea?	Ha diarrea?	Avez-vous la diarrhée?	Haben Sie Durchfall?
Do you pass any blood?	¿Con sangre?	Passa sangue?	Y-a-t-il du sang?	Ist Blut im Stuhl?
Have you vomited?	¿Ha vomitado?	Ha vomitato?	Avez-vous vomi?	Haben Sie erbrochen?
Do you still vomit?	¿Vomita todavía?	Vomita ancora?	Vomissez-vous encore?	Erbrechen Sie noch immer?
Do you vomit blood?	¿Vomita sangre?	Vomita sangue?	Vomissez-vous du sang?	Erbrechen Sie Blut?
Is it of a dark or bright red color?	¿Es de color rojo oscuro o claro?	È di colore rosso chiaro o rosso scuro?	La couleur du sang est elle foncée ou claire?	Ist es dunkel oder hellrot?

Kidneys

English	Spanish	Italian	French	German
Have you any difficulty passing water?	¿Tiene dificultad en orinar?	Ha della difficoltà nell' urinare?	Avez-vous de la difficulté à uriner?	Haben Sie Schwierigkeiten beim Wasserlassen?
Do you pass water involuntarily?	¿Orina sin querer?	Urina involontariamente?	Urinez-vous involontaire-ment?	Lassen Sie den Harm ohne es zu wollen?
Are any of your limbs swollen?	¿Están hinchados alguno de sus miembros?	Si sente gonfio in qualche parte?	Avez-vous des membres gonflés?	Ist irgendeines Ihrer Glieder geschwollen?
How long have they been swollen like this?	¿Desde cuándo estan hinchados asi?	Da quanto tempo che li ha cosi gonfi?	Depuis quand sont-ils gonflés comme ça?	Seit wann sind sie so angeschwollen?

2388

English	Spanish	Italian	French	German
Were they ever swollen before?	¿Han estado hinchados alguna vez antes?	Sono stati mai gonfi prima?	Ont-ils jamais été gonflés autrefois?	Sind sie je früher so angeschwollen gewesen?

TREATMENT
General

English	Spanish	Italian	French	German
It is nothing serious.	No es nada grave.	Non è nulla.	Ce n'est rien de grave.	Es ist nichts ernstliches.
You will get better.	Ud. se mejorará.	Si sentirà meglio.	Vous vous remettrez.	Es wird besser werden.
Do exactly as I tell you.	Haga exactamente lo que le digo.	Faccia estattamente ciò che Le dico.	Faites exactement ce que je vous dis.	Tun Sie genau was ich Ihnen sage.
Take a bath.	Tome un baño.	Si faccia un bagno.	Prenez un bain.	Nehmen Sie ein bad
A sponge bath	Un baño de esponja	Un bagno con la spugna	Un bain à l'éponge	Ein Schwamm bad
A bran bath	Un baño de salvado	Un bagno con crusca	Un bain au son	Ein Kleie bad
A soda bath	Un baño de soda	Un bagno con soda	Un bain à la soude	Ein Soda bad
Bathe with hot water.	Báñese con agua caliente.	Faccia il bagno con acqua calda.	Baignez-vous dans de l'eau chaude.	Baden Sie mit heissem Wasser.
Bathe with cold water.	Báñese con agua fría.	Si faccia il bagno con acqua fredda.	Baignez-vous dans de l'eau froide.	Baden Sie mit kaltem Wasser.
Bathe with alcohol.	Báñese con alcohol.	Si bagni con alcool.	Baignez-vous avec de l'alcool.	Reiben Sie sich alkoholab.
Paint the swelling with this.	Pinte la hinchazón con esto.	Deve pitturare il gonfiore con questo.	Badigeonnez l'enflure avecececi.	Pinseln Sie die Geschwulst damit.
I will use electricity.	Usaré electricidad.	Userò dell'elettricità.	Je ferai un traitment a la electricité.	Ich werde elektrischen Strom anwenden.
Apply bandage to . . .	Ponga un vendaje a . . .	Si metta una fasciatura	Mettez un bandage à . . .	Verbinden Sie . . .
Apply ointment	Aplíquese ungüento.	Applichi un unguento.	Appliquez un onguent.	Verwenden Sie Salbe.
Keep very quiet.	Estése muy quieto.	Sia tranquillo.	Restez tranquille.	Verhalten Sie sich sehr ruhig.
You must not speak.	No debe hablar.	Non deve parlare.	Vous ne devez pas parler.	Sie dürfen nicht sprechen.
Swallow small pieces of ice.	Trague pedacitos de hielo.	Ingoi dei pezzettini di ghiaccio.	Avalez de petits morceaux de glace.	Schlucken Sie kleine Eisstücke.

The Interpreter in Five Languages (*Continued*)

English	Spanish	Italian	French	German
		Diet		
In a few days you may eat food.	Dentro de algunos días podrá comer.	Fra pochi giorni potrà mangiare.	Après quelques jours vous pouvez prendre de la nourriture.	In einigen Tagen dürfen Sie essen.
And remain on a diet.	Y estar a dieta.	E rimanga a dieta.	Et suivez un régime.	Und Diät halten.
You may eat . . .	Puede comer . . .	Potrà mangiare . . .	Vous pouvez manger . . .	Sie dürfen essen . . .
Two eggs	Dos huevos	Due d'uova	Deux oeufs	Zwei Eier
Toast	Pan tostado	Pane tostato	Du pain grillé	Geröstetes Brot
Bread	Pan	Pane	Du pain	Das Brot
Oysters	Ostras	Delle óstriche	Des huîtres	Die Austern
Chicken	Pollo	Pollo	Du poulet	Das Huhn
You may drink icewater.	Puede tomar agua con hielo.	Lei può bere acqua ghiacciata.	Vous pouvez boir de l'eau glacée.	Sie dürfen Eiswasser trinken.
Milk	Leche	Latte	Du lait	Die Milch
Tea	Té	Il té	Du thé	Der Tee
Coffee	Café	Il caffè	Du café	Der Kaffee
Chocolate	Chocolate	La cioccolatta	Du chocolat	Die Schokolade
Beef bouillon	Caldo de carne	Brodo	Le bouillon	Die Bouillon
		Operation		
An operation will be necessary.	Tendrá que operarse.	Una operazione è necessaria.	Il faut que l'on fasse une operation.	Eine Operation ist notwendig.
We will operate . . .	Lo operaremos . . .	Opereremo . . .	Nous opérerons . . .	Wir werden operieren . . .

Medication
(use with numbers and time of day)

English	Spanish	Italian	German
I will give you something for that.	Le daré algo para eso.	Le darò qualche cosa per questo.	Ich werde Ihnen etwas dafür geben.
I will leave a prescription.	Le dejaré una receta.	Lascerò una ricetta.	Ich werde Ihnen ein Rezept hierlassen.
Use it regularly.	Tómelo con regularidad.	Lo usi regolarmente.	Gebrauchen Sie es regelmässig.
Take one teaspoonful three times daily (in water).	Tome una cucharadita tres veces al día, con agua.	Ne beva un cucchiaio tre volte al giorno (con acqua).	Nehmen Sie einen Teelöffel voll dreimal täglich (mit Wasser).
Gargle.	Haga gárgaras.	Faccia gargarismi.	Gurgeln Sie.
Use injection.	Use una inyección.	Si faccia un iniezione.	Injizieren Sie.
Take a purgative.	Tome una purga.	Un purgante	Nehmen Sie ein Abführmittel.
A pill	Una píldora	Una pillola	Eine Pille
A powder	Un polvo	Una polverina	Ein Pulver
Drop into one eye.	Vierta gotas en un ojo.	Metta delle gocce nell'occhio	Träufeln Sie in das eine Auge.
Drop into each eye.	Vierta gotas en cada ojo.	Metta delle gocce in ciascun occhio.	Träufeln Sie in beide Augen.

App. 17: Universal Precautions

Part I—Guidelines for Prevention of Transmission of Human Immunodeficiency Virus (HIV) and Hepatitis B Virus (HBV) to Health-Care and Public-Safety Workers

In 1985, the Centers for Disease Control (CDC) developed the strategy of "universal blood and body fluid precautions" to address concerns regarding transmission of HIV in the health-care setting. The concept, now referred to simply as "universal precautions," stresses that *all patients should be assumed to be infectious for HIV and other blood-borne pathogens.* In the hospital and other health-care settings, universal precautions should be followed when workers are exposed to blood, certain other body fluids (amniotic fluid, pericardial fluid, peritoneal fluid, pleural fluid, synovial fluid, cerebrospinal fluid, semen, and vaginal secretions), or any body fluid visibly contaminated with blood. Since HIV and HBV transmission has not been documented from exposure to feces, nasal secretions, sputum, sweat, tears, urine, and vomitus, universal precautions do not apply to these fluids, or to saliva, except in the dental setting, where saliva is likely to be contaminated with blood.

For the purpose of this document, human "exposure" is defined as contact with blood or other body fluids to which universal precautions apply through percutaneous inoculation or contact with an open wound, nonintact skin, or mucous membrane during the performance of normal job duties.

The unpredictable and emergent nature of exposures encountered by emergency and public-safety workers may make differentiation between hazardous body fluids and those which are not hazardous very difficult and often impossible. Therefore, *when emergency medical and public-safety workers encounter body fluids under uncontrolled, emergency circumstances in which differentiation between fluid types is difficult, if not impossible, they should treat all body fluids as potentially hazardous.*

Disinfection, Decontamination, and Disposal

1. **Needle and sharps disposal.** All workers should take precautions to prevent injuries caused by needles, scalpel blades, and other sharp instruments or devices during procedures; when cleaning used instruments; during disposal of used needles; and when handling sharp instruments after procedures. To prevent needle-stick injuries, needles should not be recapped, purposely bent or broken by hand, removed from disposable syringes, or otherwise manipulated by hand. After they are used, disposable syringes and needles, scalpel blades, and other sharp items should be placed in puncture-resistant containers for disposal; the puncture-resistant containers should be located as close as practical to the use area (e.g., in the ambulance or, if sharps are carried to the scene of victim assistance from the ambulance, a small puncture-resistant container should be carried to the scene, as well). Reusable needles should be left on the syringe body and should be placed in a puncture-resistant container for transport to the reprocessing area.

2. **Hand washing.** Hands and other skin surfaces should be washed immediately and thoroughly if contaminated with blood, other body fluids to which universal precautions apply, or potentially contaminated articles. Hands should always be washed after gloves are removed, even if the gloves appear to be intact. Hand washing should be completed using appropriate facilities, such as utility or restroom sinks. Waterless antiseptic hand cleanser should be provided on responding units to use when hand-washing facilities are not available. When hand-washing facilities are available, wash hands with warm water and soap. When hand-washing facilities are not available, use a waterless antiseptic hand cleanser. The manufacturer's recommendations for the product should be followed.

3. **Cleaning, disinfecting, and sterilizing.** The following table presents the methods and applications for cleaning, disinfecting, and sterilizing equipment and surfaces in the prehospital setting. These methods also apply to housekeeping and other cleaning tasks.

Reprocessing Methods for Equipment

Sterilization

Destroys: All forms of microbial life including high numbers of bacterial spores.

Methods: Steam under pressure (autoclave), gas (ethylene oxide), dry heat, or immersion in EPA-approved chemical "sterilant" for prolonged period of time, e.g., 6–10 hours or according to manufacturers' instructions. Note: liquid chemical "sterilants" should be used only on those instruments that are impossible to sterilize or disinfect with heat.

Use: For those instruments or devices that penetrate skin or contact normally sterile areas of the body, e.g., scalpels, needles, etc. Disposable invasive equipment eliminates the need to reprocess these types of items. When indicated, however, arrangements should be made with a health-care facility for reprocessing of reusable invasive instruments.

High-Level Disinfection

Destroys: All forms of microbial life except high numbers of bacterial spores.

Methods: Hot water pasteurization (80–100 C, 30 minutes) or exposure to an EPA-registered "sterilant" chemical as above, except for a short exposure time (10–45 minutes or as directed by manufacturer).

Use: For reusable instruments or devices that come into contact with mucous membranes (e.g., laryngoscope blades, endotracheal tubes, etc.).

Intermediate-Level Disinfection

Destroys: *Mycobacterium tuberculosis,* vegetative bacteria, most viruses, and most fungi, but does not kill bacterial spores.

Methods: EPA-registered "hospital disinfectant" chemical germicides that have a label claim for tuberculocidal activity; commercially available hard-surface germicides or solutions containing at least 500 ppm free available chlorine (a 1:100 dilution of common household bleach — approximately 1/4 cup bleach per gallon of tap water).

Use: For those surfaces that come into contact only with intact skin, e.g., stethoscopes, blood pressure cuffs, splints, etc., and have been visibly contaminated with blood or bloody body fluids. Surfaces must be precleaned of visible material before the germicidal chemical is applied for disinfection.

Low-Level Disinfection

Destroys: Most bacteria, some viruses, some fungi, but not *Mycobacterium tuberculosis* or bacterial spores.

Methods: EPA-registered "hospital disinfectants" (no label claim for tuberculocidal activity).

Use: These agents are excellent cleaners and can be used for routine housekeeping or removal of soiling in the absence of visible blood contamination.

Environmental Disinfection

Environmental surfaces which have become soiled should be cleaned and disinfected using any cleaner or disinfectant agent which is intended for environmental use. Such surfaces include floors, woodwork, ambulance seats, countertops, etc.

IMPORTANT: To assure the effectiveness of any sterilization or disinfection process, equipment and instruments must first be thoroughly cleaned of all visible soil.

Universal Precautions (*Continued*)

4. **Cleaning and decontaminating spills of blood.** All spills of blood and blood-contaminated fluids should be promptly cleaned up using an EPA-approved germicide or a 1:100 solution of household bleach in the following manner *while wearing gloves.* Visible material should first be removed with disposable towels or other appropriate means that will ensure against direct contact with blood. If splashing is anticipated, protective eyewear should be worn along with an impervious gown or apron which provides an effective barrier to splashes. The area should then be decontaminated with an appropriate germicide. Hands should be washed following removal of gloves. Soiled cleaning equipment should be cleaned and decontaminated or placed in an appropriate container and disposed of according to agency policy. Plastic bags should be available for removal of contaminated items from the site of the spill.

    Shoes and boots can become contaminated with blood in certain instances. Where there is massive blood contamination on floors, the use of disposable impervious shoe coverings should be considered. Protective gloves should be worn to remove contaminated shoe coverings. The coverings and gloves should be disposed of in plastic bags.

5. **Laundry.** Although soiled linen may be contaminated with pathogenic microorganisms, the risk of actual disease transmission is negligible. Rather than rigid procedures and specifications, hygienic storage and processing of clean and soiled linen are recommended. Soiled linen should be handled as little as possible and with minimum agitation to prevent gross microbial contamination of the air and of persons handling the linen. All soiled linen should be bagged at the location where it was used. Linen soiled with blood should be placed and transported in bags that prevent leakage. Normal laundry cycles should be used according to the washer and detergent manufacturers' recommendations.

6. **Decontamination and laundering of protective clothing.** Protective work clothing contaminated with blood or other body fluids to which universal precautions apply should be placed and transported in bags or containers that prevent leakage. Personnel involved in the bagging, transport, and laundering of contaminated clothing should wear gloves.

7. **Infective waste.** The selection of procedures for disposal of infective waste is determined by the relative risk of disease transmission and application of local regulations, which vary widely. In all cases, local regulations should be consulted prior to disposal procedures and followed. Infective waste, in general, should either be incinerated or be decontaminated before disposal in a sanitary landfill. Bulk blood, suctioned fluids, excretions, and secretions may be carefully poured down a drain connected to a sanitary sewer, where permitted. Sanitary sewers may also be used to dispose of other infectious wastes capable of being ground and flushed into the sewer, where permitted. Sharp items should be placed in puncture-proof containers and other blood-contaminated items should be placed in leak-proof plastic bags for transport to an appropriate disposal location.

    Prior to the removal of protective equipment, personnel remaining on the scene after the patient has been cared for should carefully search for and remove contaminated materials. Debris should be disposed of as noted above.

Fire and Emergency Medical Services

Fire and emergency medical service personnel are engaged in delivery of medical care in the prehospital setting. The following guidelines are intended to assist these personnel in making decisions concerning use of personal protective equipment and resuscitation equipment, as well as for decontamination, disinfection, and disposal procedures.

1. **Gloves.** Disposable gloves should be a standard component of emergency response equipment, and should be donned by all personnel prior to initiating any emergency patient care tasks involving exposure to blood or other body fluids to which universal precautions apply. Extra pairs should always be available. Considerations in the choice of disposable gloves should include dexterity, durability, fit, and the task being performed. Thus, there is no single type or thickness of glove appropriate for protection in all situations. For situations where large amounts of blood are likely to be encountered, it is important that gloves fit tightly at the wrist to prevent blood contamination of hands around the cuff. For multiple trauma victims, gloves should be changed between patient contacts, if the emergency situation allows.

    While wearing gloves, avoid handling personal items, such as combs and pens, that could become soiled or contaminated. Gloves that have become contaminated with blood or other body fluids to which universal precautions apply should be removed as soon as possible, taking care to avoid skin contact with the exterior surface. Contaminated gloves should be placed and transported in bags that prevent leakage and should be disposed of or, in the case of reusable gloves, cleaned and disinfected properly.

2. **Masks, eyewear, and gowns.** Masks, eyewear, and gowns should be present on all emergency vehicles that respond to medical emergencies or victim rescues. These protective barriers should be

used in accordance with the level of exposure encountered. Minor lacerations or small amounts of blood do not merit the same extent of barrier use as required for exsanguinating victims or massive arterial bleeding. Management of the patient who is not bleeding, and who has no bloody body fluids present, should not routinely require use of barrier precautions. Masks and eyewear (e.g., safety glasses) should be worn together, or a face shield should be used by all personnel prior to any situation where splashes of blood or other body fluids to which universal precautions apply are likely to occur. Gowns or aprons should be worn to protect clothing from splashes with blood. If large splashes or quantities of blood are present or anticipated, impervious gowns or aprons should be worn. An extra change of work clothing should be available at all times.

3. **Resuscitation equipment.** No transmission of HBV or HIV infection during mouth-to-mouth resuscitation has been documented. However, because of the risk of salivary transmission of other infectious diseases (e.g., herpes simplex and *Neisseria meningitidis*) and the theoretical risk of HIV and HBV transmission during artificial ventilation of trauma victims, disposable airway equipment or resuscitation bags should be used. Disposable resuscitation equipment and devices should be used once and disposed of or, if reusable, thoroughly cleaned and disinfected after each use according to the manufacturer's recommendations.

Mechanical respiratory assist devices (e.g., bag-valve-masks, oxygen demand valve resuscitators) should be available on all emergency vehicles and to all emergency response personnel that respond or potentially respond to medical emergencies or victim rescues.

Pocket mouth-to-mouth resuscitation masks designed to isolate emergency response personnel (i.e., double lumen systems) from contact with victims' blood and blood-contaminated saliva, respiratory secretions, and vomitus should be provided to all personnel who provide or potentially provide emergency treatment.

Other Considerations

1. **Handling deceased persons and body removal.** For any personnel who may have to touch or remove a body, the response should be the same as for situations requiring CPR or first aid: wear gloves and cover all cuts and abrasions to create a barrier and carefully wash all exposed areas after any contact with blood. The precautions to be used with blood and deceased persons should also be used when handling amputated limbs, hands, or other body parts. Such procedures should be followed after contact with the blood of *anyone*, regardless of whether they are known or suspected to be infected with HIV or HBV.

2. **Autopsies.** Protective masks and eyewear (or face shields), laboratory coats, gloves, and waterproof aprons should be worn when performing or attending all autopsies. All autopsy material should be considered infectious for both HIV and HBV. Onlookers with an opportunity for exposure to blood splashes should be similarly protected. Instruments and surfaces contaminated during postmortem procedures should be decontaminated with an appropriate chemical germicide.

3. **Forensic laboratories.** Blood from *all* individuals should be considered infective. To supplement other worksite precautions, the following precautions are recommended for workers in forensic laboratories.

   a. All specimens of blood should be put in a well-constructed, appropriately labelled container with a secure lid to prevent leaking during transport. Care should be taken when collecting each specimen to avoid contaminating the outside of the container and of the laboratory form accompanying the specimen.

   b. All persons processing blood specimens should wear gloves. Masks and protective eyewear or face shield should be worn if mucous-membrane contact with blood is anticipated (e.g., removing tops from vacuum tubes). Hands should be washed after completion of specimen processing.

   c. For routine procedures, such as histologic and pathologic studies or microbiological culturing, a biological safety cabinet is not necessary. However, biological safety cabinets (Class I or II) should be used whenever procedures are conducted that have a high potential for generating droplets. These include activities such as blending, sonicating, and vigorous mixing.

   d. Mechanical pipetting devices should be used for manipulating all liquids in the laboratory. Mouth pipetting must not be done.

   e. Use of needles and syringes should be limited to situations in which there is no alternative, and the recommendations for preventing injuries with needles should be followed.

   f. Laboratory work surfaces should be cleaned of visible materials and then decontaminated with an appropriate chemical germicide after a spill of blood, semen, or blood-contaminated body fluid and when work activities are completed.

   g. Contaminated materials used in laboratory tests should be decontaminated before reprocessing or be placed in bags and disposed of in accordance with institutional and local regulatory policies for disposal of infective waste.

  h. Scientific equipment that has been contaminated with blood should be cleaned and then decontaminated before being repaired in the laboratory or transported to the manufacturer.

  i. All persons should wash their hands after completing laboratory activities and should remove protective clothing before leaving the laboratory.

  j. Area posting of warning signs should be considered to remind employees of continuing hazard of infectious disease transmission in the laboratory setting.

Part II — Recommendations for Preventing Transmission of Human Immunodeficiency Virus (HIV) and Hepatitis B Virus (HBV) to Patients During Exposure-Prone Invasive Procedures

Infection Control Practices

Previous recommendations have specified that infection-control programs should incorporate principles of universal precautions (i.e., appropriate use of hand washing, protective barriers, and care in the use and disposal of needles and other sharp instruments) and should maintain these precautions rigorously in all health-care settings. Proper application of these principles will assist in minimizing the risk of transmission of HIV or HBV from patient to health-care worker, health-care worker to patient, or patient to patient.

As part of standard infection control practice, instruments and other reusable equipment used in performing invasive procedures should be appropriately disinfected and sterilized as follows:

1. Equipment and devices that enter the patient's vascular system or other normally sterile areas of the body should be sterilized before being used for each patient.
2. Equipment and devices that touch intact mucous membranes but do not penetrate the patient's body surfaces should be sterilized when possible or under high-level disinfection if they cannot be sterilized before being used for each patient.
3. Equipment and devices that do not touch the patient or that only touch intact skin of the patient need only be cleaned with a detergent or as indicated by the manufacturer.

Compliance with universal precautions and recommendations for disinfection and sterilization of medical devices should be scrupulously monitored in all health-care settings. Training of health-care workers in proper infection control technique should begin in professional and vocational schools and continue as an ongoing process. Institutions should provide all health-care workers with appropriate inservice education regarding infection control and safety and should establish procedures for monitoring compliance with infection control policies.

All health-care workers who might be exposed to blood in an occupational setting should receive hepatitis B vaccine, preferably during their period of professional training and before any occupational exposures could occur.

Exposure-Prone Procedures

Despite adherence to the principles of universal precautions, certain invasive surgical and dental procedures have been implicated in the transmission of HBV from infected health-care workers to patients, and should be considered exposure-prone. Reported examples include certain oral, cardiothoracic, colorectal, and obstetric/gynecologic procedures.

Certain other invasive procedures should also be considered exposure-prone. In a prospective study CDC conducted in four hospitals, one or more percutaneous injuries occurred among surgical personnel during 96 (6.9%) of 1,382 operative procedures on the general surgery, gynecology, orthopedic, cardiac, and trauma services. Percutaneous exposure of the patient to the health-care worker's blood may have occurred when the sharp object causing the injury recontacted the patient's open wound in 28 (32%) of the 88 observed injuries to surgeons.

Characteristics of exposure-prone procedures include digital palpation of a needle tip in a body cavity or the simultaneous presence of the health-care worker's fingers and a needle or other sharp instrument or object in a poorly visualized or highly confined anatomic site. Performance of exposure-prone procedures presents a recognized risk of percutaneous injury to the health-care worker, and — if such injury occurs — the health-care worker's blood is likely to contact the patient's body cavity, subcutaneous tissues, and/or mucous membranes.

Experience with HBV indicates that invasive procedures that do not have the above characteristics would be expected to pose substantially lower risk, if any, of transmission of HIV and other blood-borne pathogens from an infected health-care worker to patients.

Recommendations

Investigations of HIV and HBV transmission from health-care workers to patients indicate that, when health-care workers adhere to recommended infection control procedures, the risk of transmitting HBV from an infected health-care worker to a patient is small, and the risk of transmitting HIV is likely to be even smaller. However, the likelihood of exposure of the patient to a health-care worker's blood is greater for certain procedures designated as exposure-prone. To minimize the risk of HIV or HBV transmission, the following measures are recommended:

1. All health-care workers should adhere to universal precautions, including the appropriate use of hand washing, protective barriers, and care in the use and disposal of needles and other sharp instruments. Health-care workers who have exudative lesions or weeping dermatitis should refrain from all direct patient care and from handling patient-care equipment and devices used in performing invasive procedures until the condition resolves. Health-care workers should also comply with current guidelines for disinfection and sterilization of reusable devices used in invasive procedures.

2. Currently available data provide no basis for recommendations to restrict the practice of health-care workers infected with HIV or HBV who perform invasive procedures not identified as exposure-prone, provided the infected health-care workers practice recommended surgical or dental technique and comply with universal precautions and current recommendations for sterilization/ disinfection.

3. Exposure-prone procedures should be identified by medical/surgical/dental organizations and institutions at which the procedures are performed.

4. Health-care workers who perform exposure-prone procedures should know their HIV antibody status. Health-care workers who perform exposure-prone procedures and who do not have serologic evidence of immunity to HBV from vaccination or from previous infection should know their HbsAg status and, if that is positive, should also know their HbeAg status.

5. Health-care workers who are infected with HIV or HBV (and are HBeAg positive) should not perform exposure-prone procedures unless they have sought counsel from an expert review panel and been advised under what circumstances, if any, they may continue to perform these procedures. Such circumstances should include notifying prospective patients of the health-care worker's seropositivity before they undergo exposure-prone invasive procedures.

   The review panel should include experts who represent a balanced perspective. Such experts might include all of the following: a) the health-care worker's personal physician(s), b) an infectious disease specialist with expertise in the epidemiology of HIV and HBV transmission, c) a health professional with expertise in the procedures performed by the health-care worker, and d) state or local public health official(s). If the health-care worker's practice is institutionally based, the expert review panel might also include a member of the infection-control committee, preferably a hospital epidemiologist. Health-care workers who perform exposure-prone procedures outside the hospital/ institutional setting should seek advice from appropriate state and local public health officials regarding the review process. Panels must recognize the importance of confidentiality and the privacy rights of infected health-care workers.

6. Mandatory testing of health-care workers for HIV antibody, HBsAg, or HBeAg is not recommended. The current assessment of the risk that infected health-care workers will transmit HIV or HBV to patients during exposure-prone procedures does not support the diversion of resources that would be required to implement mandatory testing programs. Compliance by health-care workers with recommendations can be increased through education, training, and appropriate confidentiality safeguards.

SOURCES: Adapted from Centers for Disease Control: Guidelines for prevention of transmission of human immunodeficiency virus and hepatitis B virus to health-care and public-safety workers. MMWR 38 (no. S-6), 1989. Recommendations for preventing transmission of human immunodeficiency virus and hepatitis B virus to patients during exposure-prone invasive procedures. MMWR 40 (no. RR-8), 1991.

App. 18: Poisons, Drug Abuse, and Medical Emergencies

Poisons and Poisoning

(Note: See Poison Control Centers, United States and Canada, in Appendix.)

Toxic Substances	Symptoms of Poisoning	Emergency Measures	Supportive and Follow-up Treatment	Pathology
Acetaminophen	Early: may be asymptomatic. Nausea and vomiting, pallor, diaphoresis, early signs of liver damage. Late: In 24 to 48 hours nausea and vomiting, jaundice, blood coagulation defects, hypoglycemia, hepatic and renal failure.	Emesis or gastric lavage. N-acetylcysteine should be given as soon as possible, with the first dose being 140 mg/kg and then 70 mg/kg every 4 hours for 3 days. Instillation of activated charcoal in stomach should not be used at the same time as the N-acetylcysteine because it interferes with absorption of the antidote.	If liver and renal failure develop, treat accordingly.	Liver and kidney damage.
Acetophenetidin, acetanilid and aniline inks and oils	Sweating; nausea; vomiting; chills; ringing in ears; fall in blood pressure; circulatory collapse; cyanosis; coma; convulsions; death from respiratory failure.	Gastric lavage or induce emesis. Instill sodium bicarbonate into stomach. Whole blood or plasma. Artificial respiration or oxygen. Analeptics.	Keep patient warm and quiet. If cyanosis becomes severe, 1–2 mg/kg of 1% methylene blue.	Methemoglobinemia, CNS stimulation, kidney and liver injury.
Acetylsalicylic acid — SEE: Salicylates.				
Acids (acetic, hydrochloric, nitric, phosphoric, sulfuric, etc.)	Immediate pain and corrosion of mucous membranes of mouth, throat, and esophagus; difficulty in swallowing; stomach pain; nausea; coffee-ground vomitus; thirst; shock syndrome; death in circulatory collapse.	Give orally magnesium oxide, milk of magnesia, lime water, or aluminum hydroxide gel. Avoid carbonates as neutralizers. Give large amounts of water or milk immediately. Demulcents and morphine for pain.	Correct shock with fluids, plasma, or whole blood. Tracheotomy or gastrectomy may become necessary.	Asphyxia from glottic edema, gastric and pyloric strictures, and stenosis or perforation.

2398

Amanita muscaria mushroom	Parasympathetic stimulation: lacrimation, sweating, salivation, vomiting, abdominal cramps, diarrhea, vertigo, coma, and convulsions may occur within a few minutes or up to 2 hours after eating.	For signs of parasympathetic stimulation, give atropine, 1-2 mg I.M. and repeat dose every 4 hours until symptoms are alleviated. Remove mushrooms from stomach by inducing emesis and by gastric lavage.	Fluid therapy as indicated.	With appropriate therapy, complete recovery within 24 hours.
Amanita phalloides mushroom	After 6 to 15 hours, abdominal pain, nausea, vomiting, purging, weakness, thirst, shock syndrome, restlessness, delirium, hallucinations, coma, late jaundice, acute renal failure. Death may be from cardiac, kidney, liver, or CNS lesions.	Induce vomiting immediately. Slurry of activated charcoal as lavage fluid, leaving some in stomach along with saline cathartic. Meperidine for pain. I.V. 10% dextrose and sodium chloride to treat hypoglycemia.	Correct fluid and electrolyte balance. Prepare to treat renal or hepatic failure. Treatment with artificial kidney may be required.	Acute yellow atrophy of the liver, acute renal failure, cardiac damage.
Aminophylline (theophylline ethylenediamine) or caffeine	Restlessness; excitement alternating with drowsiness; ringing in ears; fast pulse; nausea; vomiting; fever; diuresis; dehydration; thirst; tremor; delirium; convulsions; coma; death in cardiovascular and respiratory collapse.	Lavage, induce emesis with saline cathartic unless vomiting and purging have already begun. Treat CNS excitation with phenobarbital or diazepam.	Oxygen and artificial respiration. Treat shock. Maintain fluid and electrolyte balance. Dialysis or charcoal hemoperfusion may be required.	CNS stimulation and gastric ulceration.
Ammonia and ammonium hydroxide	Irritation of eyes and respiratory tract (sometimes pulmonary edema, glottic spasm, or laryngeal edema). Other symptoms are like lye poisoning (SEE: *Lye* in table).	Give large amounts of diluted vinegar, lemon juice, or orange juice. Demulcents and morphine for pain. Oxygen under pressure to help prevent pulmonary edema.	Treat for shock. Tracheotomy may be needed. NOTE: Do not give drugs such as narcotics which would depress respiration.	Corrosive esophagitis and gastritis, laryngeal edema, pulmonary edema.
d-Amphetamine	Excitement; talkativeness; restlessness; tremors; dizziness; hyperactive reflexes; dry mouth; nausea; vomiting; diarrhea; palpitations; fever; dehydration; mydriasis;	Gastric lavage with tap water and activated charcoal, or induce emesis. Artificial respiration and administration of oxygen.	Isolate patient and avoid sensory stimuli. Ice packs and sponge baths for hyperpyrexia. Chlorpromazine, 1-2 mg/kg I.M., may be required. Peritoneal dialysis may be	CNS and peripheral sympathetic stimulation; petechial hemorrhages in the brain.

Poisons and Poisoning (Continued)

Toxic Substances	Symptoms of Poisoning	Emergency Measures	Supportive and Follow-up Treatment	Pathology
	tachycardia; hallucinations; delirium; mania; convulsions; coma; death in circulatory collapse.	indicated.		
Aniline — SEE: *Acetanilid.*				
Antabuse — SEE: *disulfram.*				
Antihistamines (tripelennamine, diphenhydramine, chlorphenidramine, etc.)	Drowsiness or excitement; lethargy; fatigue; ataxia; dryness of mouth; fixed dilated pupils; coma. Sometimes, however, only excitement is seen with tremors, anxiety, delirium, convulsions, hyperpyrexia, nausea, vomiting, diarrhea, death in cardiovascular collapse or respiratory arrest.	Lavage or induce emesis. Cautious use of sedatives if excited. Oxygen and artificial respiration.	Ice packs and alcohol sponges for hyperpyrexia.	Mechanism of death not precisely known. Cerebral edema has been described.
Arsenic	Symptoms may be delayed several hours. Metallic taste and odor of garlic on breath; burning pain throughout gastrointestinal tract; vomiting and purging; dehydration; shock syndrome; coma; convulsions; paralysis; severe diarrhea which becomes bloody. Death may occur.	Induce emesis, gastric lavage. Leave demulcent in stomach. Chelation therapy with penicillamine. Administer dimercaprol (BAL) in accordance with supplier's dosage schedule.	Maintain fluid and electrolyte balance. Morphine for pain. Treat for shock. Treat anemia and renal failure if either is present. Administer saline cathartic.	Shock secondary to hemorrhagic gastroenteritis. Skin eruptions are of no toxicological significance.

Aspirin — SEE: *salicylates*.

Atropine	Dryness of mouth and burning pain in throat; thirst; mydriasis; blurring of vision; skin is dry, hot, and flushed; hyperpyrexia; tachycardia; palpitations; restlessness; excitement; convulsions; confusion; mania; delirium. Death is rare.	Induce emesis. Lavage with slurry of activated charcoal or 10% tannic acid. Physostigmine salicylate I.V., given slowly, may reverse effects. CAUTION: Atropine, 1 mg, should be available for immediate injection if physostigmine causes bradycardia, convulsions or bronchoconstriction.	Intense CNS excitation and parasympathetic paralysis.
		Oxygen and artificial respiration. Maintain airway. Ice packs for hyperpyrexia. Catheterize if necessary.	
Barbiturates	Confusion; drowsiness; ataxia; vertigo; slurred speech; shallow respiration and pulse; mental confusion; headache; stupor; coma; areflexia; cyanosis; hypotension; hypothermia or hyperthermia; cardiovascular collapse; death in respiratory arrest.	Establish airway; gastric lavage; artificial respiration; oxygen; maintain fluid and electrolyte balance. Hemodialysis to remove barbiturate may be helpful but is rarely required. Treat hypothermia or hyperthermia if either is present.	CNS depression with respiratory arrest. Pulmonary edema occurs in prolonged coma.
		Gastric lavage will be of benefit up to 24 hours after last dose of barbiturate. Record vital signs frequently. Correct airway obstruction. Oxygen and artificial respiration as needed. When vital signs have stabilized and kidney function is ensured, induce diuresis with urea, and alkalinize urine. Antibiotic therapy if aspiration of vomitus has occurred.	
Barium salts, absorbable (barium carbonate, barium hydroxide, barium chloride)	Salivation; nausea; vomiting; abdominal cramps; violent and bloody diarrhea; slow and irregular pulse; ringing in ears; dizziness; twitching; convulsions or paralysis; death from respiratory failure and cardiac arrest.	Give sodium sulfate rapidly by mouth. Lavage or induce emesis. Diazepam for convulsions. Morphine may relieve abdominal pain. Artificial respiration and oxygen.	Violent peristalsis, atrial hypertension, cardiac disturbances, late kidney damage.
		Intravenous saline for dehydration. Potassium I.V. if hypokalemia is present. Treat for shock.	Barium stimulates contraction of all muscle cells.

Toxic Substances	Symptoms of Poisoning	Emergency Measures	Supportive and Follow-up Treatment	Pathology
Benzene, xylene, toluene	Burning sensation in mouth and stomach; nausea; vomiting; chest pains; cough; headache; giddiness; vertigo; ataxia; confusion; stupor; convulsions and coma; late severe anemia due to aplasia of bone marrow. Death from respiratory failure or ventricular fibrillation.	Cautious lavage with tap water, leave saline cathartic in the stomach. Diazepam for convulsions.	Oxygen, artificial respiration, parenteral fluids. *Avoid* epinephrine and ephedrine.	Respiratory failure from CNS depression or ventricular fibrillation. Severe and possibly fatal bone marrow damage.
Benzene hexachloride	Irritability; vomiting; diarrhea; restlessness; ataxia; spasms; convulsions; coma; respiratory failure.	Cautious lavage with tap water and activated charcoal, then instill saline cathartic into the stomach. Control convulsions with diazepam.	Rest and quiet. *Avoid* fats, oils, epinephrine and ephedrine.	Liver function may be impaired.
Bleach, household — SEE: *Hypochlorite salts.*				
Boric acid and borate salts	Headache; nausea; vomiting; fever; oliguria or anuria; diarrhea; stomach pain; weakness and lethargy; restlessness; tremor; convulsions; coma; cyanosis. Distinctive, fine, bright red rash. Shock with death in vascular collapse.	Induce emesis. Establish airway and maintain respiration. Lavage stomach with 1% sodium bicarbonate solution and instill activated charcoal. Control convulsions with diazepam.	Fluids and electrolytes for replacement therapy. Maintain urinary output.	In fatal cases, liver and kidney damage are found along with cerebral edema.
Botulinum toxin	In adults, symptoms begin as early as 8 hours and as late as a week after ingestion: nausea,	Lavage with tap water or a slurry of activated charcoal if within a few hours postingestion.	Oxygen and artificial respiration. Tracheotomy and assisted respiration if needed. Patient	Blocks transmission of nerve impulses at motor end plate. Congestion and hemorrhage

	Symptoms	Treatment	Pathology
(continued)	vomiting, occasionally diarrhea, difficulties swallowing, double vision, loss of visual acuity and pupillary reflexes, weakness and paralysis of respiratory muscles. Profuse sweating, and pulse is rapid and weak.	Instill saline cathartic. Give specific or polyvalent botulinus antitoxin. NOTE: The antitoxin is available from the state or local health department or the Bacterial Diseaese Division, Centers for Disease Control, Atlanta, GA 30333, (404) 639-3670 during the day or (404) 639-2888 at night. Test for hypersensitivity to horse serum prior to administering.	should be in intensive care unit. CNS.
Bromides (sodium, potassium, ammonium, etc.)	Prompt vomiting; drowsiness; irritability; abdominal pain; ataxia; vertigo; confusion; mania; hallucinations; coma; skin rashes; neurological signs; sensory disturbances; increased spinal fluid pressure. Death is rare.	Induce emesis. Give sodium chloride, one gram in water, orally every hour. Continue sodium chloride until blood bromide is reduced to below 50 mg/dl.	Maintain hydration and mild diuresis. Restrain delirious patient.	Acne-like skin eruption, inflammation of mucous membranes, CNS depression.
Cadmium salts	Nausea; vomiting; diarrhea; salivation; abdominal cramps; headache; vertigo; exhaustion; collapse; shock and immediate death or delayed death from acute renal failure. Inhaling dusts and fumes very hazardous, producing pulmonary edema.	Demulcents; lavage with milk or water if vomiting is not prompt. Give saline cathartic. If pulmonary edema develops, treat with positive pressure oxygen administration. Use of EDTA will hasten removal of cadmium.	Maintain fluid and electrolyte balance. Prophylactic and supportive measures for liver injury or acute renal failure.	Severe gastroenteritis, mild liver damage, and acute renal failure. Inhalation as a dust or fume produces pulmonary edema.
Camphor	Nausea; vomiting; feeling of warmth; headache; confusion; vertigo; excitement; restlessness; delirium; hallucinations; tremor; convulsions; depression; coma; death from respiratory failure.	Diazepam to prevent or stop convulsions. Gastric lavage with tap water.	Protect the patient from all possible sensory stimuli. Oxygen and artificial respiration as needed. Avoid fats, oils, alcohol, and opiates.	Intense CNS excitation.

Toxic Substances	Symptoms of Poisoning	Emergency Measures	Supportive and Follow-up Treatment	Pathology
Carbon disulfide	Irritation of skin, eyes, and mucous membranes; headache; nausea; vomiting; diarrhea; weak pulse; palpitations; fatigue; ataxia; vertigo; mania; hallucinations; CNS depression with respiratory paralysis.	Induce emesis. Provide artificial respiration and oxygen. Lavage with tap water.	Treat pulmonary edema. Bed rest for several days.	CNS depression sometimes with permanent neurological sequelae.
Carbon monoxide	Mild headache, breathlessness on moderate exertion; irritability; fatigue; nausea; vomiting; confusion; ataxia; syncope with periods of convulsions; incontinence of urine and feces; death from respiratory arrest. In some cases the skin will be bright red, and blistering may occur.	Artificial respiration and 100% oxygen by mask. Treatment in a hyperbaric chamber may be life-saving. Treat cerebral edema with diuretics and prednisone 1 mg/kg every 4 hours if needed. Stimulants are contraindicated.	Keep patient warm. Strict bedrest for 24 hours. Assisted ventilation if needed.	High concentrations of carboxyhemoglobin in circulating erythrocytes lead to an asphyxial death.
Carbon tetrachloride	Nausea; vomiting; intense abdominal pain; headache; confusion; drowsiness; CNS depression; coma; late kidney and liver injury with possible acute renal failure. Death from respiratory arrest, circulatory collapse, or ventricular fibrillation.	If swallowed: Gastric lavage or emetic. If inhaled: Artificial respiration, oxygen, stimulants but avoid alcohol. Remove clothes contaminated with carbon tetrachloride; and wash from skin.	No specific therapy but be prepared to treat renal and hepatic failure. Do not give stimulants. Maintain urinary output.	CNS depression, hepatic central lobular necrosis, necrosis of renal tubular epithelium.
Chloral hydrate	CNS alteration with confusion, drowsiness, respiratory depression; shock; liver and	Induce emesis, gastric lavage, if drug administered per rectum, give enema.	Support ventilation; if kidney function is intact, force fluids	Acute renal and hepatic failure.

kidney may be injured.

Chlorate salts	Vomiting; diarrhea; abdominal pain; methemoglobinemia; intravascular hemolysis; delirium; coma; convulsions; cyanosis; jaundice; death in acute renal failure.	Induce emesis. Gastric lavage followed by instillation of activated charcoal. Protect airway. Administer sodium thiosulfate 2-5 gm in 200 ml of 5% sodium bicarbonate orally.	Methemoglobinemia, intravascular hemolysis, liver damage, acute renal failure.
Chlordane, heptachlor	Irritability; hyperexcitability; convulsions and tremors punctuated by periods of depression; late liver damage.	Gastric lavage with activated charcoal in 2-4 L of tap water, saline cathartic. Diazepam or ultrashort-acting barbiturates for convulsions.	Liver and kidney damage.
Chlorpromazine and other drugs derived from phenothiazine	Drowsiness; somnolence; stupor; coma; areflexia; hypotension; ventricular arrhythmias; hypothermia; restlessness; tremor; spasm; rigidity; convulsions; respiratory or vasomotor collapse; jaundice.	Induce emesis. Lavage with tap water. Diphenhydramine for ataxia and muscle spasms. Phenytoin for ventricular arrhythmias. A cardiac pacemaker may be needed.	Fluids and electrolytes to treat hypotension. Oxygen or artificial respiration. *Avoid* use of norepinephrine for treatment of hypotension.	CNS depression, extrapyramidal seizures, liver damage, aplastic anemia.
Cocaine	Initially stimulation with euphoria, restlessness, anxiety, hallucinations, convulsions, and then depression, convulsions with loss of reflexes, coma, and death.	Administer oxygen and provide respiratory and circulatory support. Gastric lavage with activated charcoal in tap water. Attempts to remove drug more than 30 minutes after ingestion or injection may be ineffective. Monitor core temperature for sign of onset of hyperthermia. Diazepam for convulsions.	Therapy for circulatory collapse. Do not use vasopressors. If malignant hyperthermia is present, use aggressive cooling procedures. If hypertension develops, administer nitroprusside.	CNS stimulation and then depression.
Copper salts, sulfate	Pain in mouth, esophagus, and stomach; vomiting; diarrhea with abdominal pain; metallic taste; shock; convulsions; paralysis; coma; death.	Induce emesis; gastric lavage; chelation therapy with calcium disodium edetate, penicillamine.	Respiratory and circulatory support.	Widespread capillary damage, hemorrhagic gastroenteritis, kidney injury, liver damage.

Poisons and Poisoning *(Continued)*

Toxic Substances	Symptoms of Poisoning	Emergency Measures	Supportive and Follow-up Treatment	Pathology
Cyanide (sodium, potassium, hydrogen, etc.)	Large doses produce immediate death. In smaller doses, an acrid taste is noted preceding numbness in the throat, anxiety, confusion, vertigo, hyperpnea followed by dyspnea; pulmonary edema may cause death within minutes; odor of bitter almonds on breath, unconsciousness followed by convulsions and death from respiratory arrest.	Start artificial respiration with 100% oxygen immediately, keeping airway clear. Give inhalations from amyl nitrite perles for 15-20 seconds each time. Inject 10 ml of freshly prepared 3% sodium nitrite I.V. over a 2- to 4-minute period. Do not remove needle. Urgency may necessitate use of nonsterile solutions. Through the same needle give 50 ml of 25% sodium thiosulfate over a 10-minute period. Repeat this regimen if symptoms recur.	If cyanide has been swallowed, gastric lavage should *follow* specific therapy.	Cyanide combines with enzymes which are essential in transfer of oxygen to the cells. Death is due to tissue anoxia.
DDT (chlorophenothane) and halogenated organic insecticides	Vomiting (may be delayed); numbness and tickling of lips, tongue, and face; headache; sore throat; fatigue; tremors; ataxia; weakness; confusion; convulsions; coma.	Induce emesis; if convulsions are not present, instill activated charcoal in stomach. Do not give stimulants.	Diazepam for convulsions. Parenteral fluids.	No pathological changes from DDT ingestion. Changes seen in experimental animals have not been found in humans.
2,4-Dichlorophen-oxyacetic acid (2,4-D)	Weakness; hypotension; lethargy; diarrhea; spastic myotonia; ventricular fibrillation and cardiac arrest. Possibly hypermetabolism and hyperpyrexia with convulsions and coma.	Induce emesis or lavage with activated charcoal in tap water. Lidocaine may be of value for cardiac symptoms.	If fever occurs, treat vigorously with cold packs, alcohol sponges, and other means for promoting heat loss.	Mechanism of death not known; abnormal EEGs have been recorded and severe protracted peripheral neuropathy has occurred.

Dieldrin or aldrin — SEE: *DDT*.

Digitalis and digoxin	Nausea; salivation; vomiting; diarrhea; headache; fatigue; weakness; drowsiness; confusion; disorientation; delirium; hallucinations; visual disturbances; death from ventricular fibrillation.	Slurry of activated charcoal followed by gastric lavage. Disturbances in cardiac rate and rhythm may be controlled by appropriate therapy. Do not use potassium if atrioventricular block or hyperkalemia is present. Propranolol should not be used if severe heart failure is present. Electroconversion may be required for ventricular fibrillation.	Preserve water and electrolyte balance. Specific fragment antigen binding (Fab) is used in severe cases. SEE: *digoxin immune Fab (ovine) for injection.*	Produces cardiac arrhythmia and all grades of impaired conduction. Striking lack of human pathological changes in comparison with those seen in experimentally poisoned animals.
2,4-Dinitrophenol	Fatigue; insatiable thirst; sweating; flushing; nausea; vomiting; abdominal pain; restlessness; excitement; severe hyperpyrexia; tachycardia; hyperpnea; dyspnea; cyanosis; coma; death in respiratory or circulatory collapse.	Gastric lavage with 5% sodium bicarbonate solution and instill saline cathartic. Ice packs, alcohol sponges, or cold water enemas to reduce body temperature.	Appropriate fluid therapy for dehydration or acidosis, mild stimulants, oxygen, artificial respiration.	Tremendously increased BMR through uncoupling of oxidative phosphorylation.
Disulfiram (Antabuse)	Nausea; vomiting; diarrhea; ataxia; hyperexcitability; hypothermia; flaccid paralysis. If patient has also ingested ethyl alcohol in even trivial amounts, symptoms are quite different and include flushing, fall in blood pressure, hyperventilation, palpitations, sweating, vertigo, confusion, circulatory collapse, coma, and death.	Lavage with tap water. Strictly prohibit alcohol in all forms. Also avoid fats, oils, and oil solvents. Artificial respiration and oxygen.	Symptomatic and supportive care for gastrointestinal symptoms and neurological complications. In case complicated by alcohol, parenteral glucose, ascorbic acid, ephedrine, and diphenhydramine may be beneficial. Wash skin if contaminated and remove clothing.	Altered liver function tests.

Poisons and Poisoning (Continued)

Toxic Substances	Symptoms of Poisoning	Emergency Measures	Supportive and Follow-up Treatment	Pathology
Ergot and ergotamine	Vomiting; diarrhea; dizziness; weak pulse; thirst; tingling in feet; numbness and coldness of extremities; variable effects on blood pressure; dyspnea; convulsions; loss of consciousness.	Slurry of activated charcoal by mouth followed by emesis or lavage. Atropine sulfate for spasm; diazepam for convulsions. Artificial respiration and oxygen if necessary. Treat hypotension but do not use vasopressors.	Keep patient warm and quiet; massage extremities; treat for shock. Treat hypercoagulability with heparin. Blood clotting time should be kept at about 3 times normal.	Congestion and inflammatory changes in gastrointestinal tract and kidneys. Gangrene of fingers and toes from persistent peripheral vasoconstriction.
Ethyl alcohol	Emotional instability and moods depending on personality, circumstances, and surroundings. Impaired motor coordination; slurred speech; ataxia; peripheral vasodilation with flushing, rapid pulse, and sweating, nausea and vomiting; drowsiness; stupor and coma; peripheral vascular collapse; hypotension; tachycardia; hypothermia; death from respiratory or circulatory failure.	Lavage with tap water or 3% sodium bicarbonate, mild stimulants, oxygen and artificial respiration. Dialysis may be required for blood levels above 300 mg/dl.	Intravenous saline or lactate and dextrose for circulatory collapse, and prevention of hypoglycemia. Mild external heat. Avoid aspiration of vomitus. Hypertonic glucose or urea for cerebral edema.	Irregularly descending CNS depression leading to respiratory or circulatory failure. In death from an acute overdose, pathological changes in liver, kidneys, heart, and brain.
Ethylene glycol	Transient excitement; nausea; vomiting, hypotension; abdominal cramps; weakness; muscle cramps; ataxia; vertigo; stupor; coma; death from respiratory paralysis or delayed acute renal failure with uremia.	Induce emesis and then gastric lavage; I.V. infusion of ethanol sufficient to maintain a blood level of 100 mg/dl to prevent conversion of glycol to toxic metabolites. Treat acidosis and hypocalcemia without delay. Diazepam for convulsions.	Mild stimulants, oxygen and artificial respiration. Immediate use of artificial kidney.	Edema of brain and hydropic degeneration of the liver and kidneys.

Ferrous or ferric salts — SEE: *Iron salts.*

Fluoride (salts, sodium)	Peculiar taste with salivation and thirst; nausea; abdominal pain; vomiting; diarrhea; muscle weakness; tremors; central depression; death due to vascular collapse and shock.	Give 10 ml of 10% calcium gluconate I.V. Repeat at signs of tetany. Dextrose in saline I.V. Lavage with milk or solution of lime water or calcium chloride, leaving some solution in the stomach. If a fluoride is inhaled, oxygen therapy plus prednisone to treat chemical pneumonitis.	Treat shock and acidosis vigorously. Maintain urine output. Calcium gluconate I.V. if hypocalcemia is present.	Hemorrhagic gastroenteritis, inhibition of cellular glycolysis, hypocalcemia.
Fluoroacetate (salts, sodium)	Vomiting; paresthesias of face; CNS excitation progressing to convulsions, punctuated by periods of severe CNS depression; disturbances in heartbeat; ventricular fibrillation; death.	Induce vomiting or lavage. Leave 15-30 gm sodium or magnesium sulfate in stomach. Glycerol monoacetate has been effective in treating experimental animals.	Oxygen, artificial respiration, short-acting barbiturates for convulsions.	Cardiac disturbances leading to fatal ventricular fibrillation.
Formaldehyde	Pain in epigastrium; nausea; vomiting; anxiety; weak and rapid pulse; coma; anuria; collapse; death in respiratory failure.	Give milk, tap water, or solution of activated charcoal by mouth. *Do not* give emetic or use gastric lavage. If eyes have been exposed, flush with saline. If skin is exposed, wash thoroughly.	Treat for shock; morphine for pain; antibiotics at the first signs of infection; sodium bicarbonate or lactate for acidosis.	Inflammation and ulceration of mucous membranes, acidosis, kidney damage, circulatory collapse.
Hydrogen sulfide	Sudden collapse and unconsciousness in acute poisoning with death from respiratory paralysis. Subacutely, gas is an irritant to eyes, respiratory tract, and skin.	Terminate exposure immediately; artificial respiration; oxygen with 5% CO_2; bedrest for 3-4 days; treat pulmonary edema. Treat as for cyanide poisoning but do not use thiosulfate.	Antibiotics at first signs of infection.	No significant pathological changes except in chronic poisoning in which pulmonary edema may be seen.
Hypochlorite salts or solutions (liquid household bleach)	Pain and inflammation of mouth, pharynx, esophagus, and stomach; coffee-ground vomitus; circulatory collapse;	Dilute bleach in stomach by giving milk, beaten eggs, melted ice cream, starch paste, or antacids such as milk of	Treat shock with intravenous fluids. Tracheotomy or gastrectomy may be indicated.	Edema of pharynx, glottis, or larynx. Perforation of stomach or esophagus. Fumes may produce pulmonary edema.

Poisons and Poisoning (Continued)

Toxic Substances	Symptoms of Poisoning	Emergency Measures	Supportive and Follow-up Treatment	Pathology
	confusion; delirium; coma; edema of glottis. All systemic symptoms are secondary to local injury and shock.	magnesia or aluminum hydroxide gel.		
Iodine	Burning pain in mouth, throat, and stomach; lips and mouth are stained brown; thirst; vomiting (blue vomitus if stomach contained starches); bloody diarrhea; anuria or strangury, urine containing albumin or blood. Death from circulatory collapse, asphyxia from glottic edema or aspiration pneumonia.	Immediately give milk, oral cornstarch or flour solution, 15 gm in 500 ml (2 cups) water. Morphine for pain and mild stimulants as indicated, but do not use if esophagus is injured. Epinephrine, diphenhydramine (Benadryl), or hydrocortisone for anaphylaxis.	Give fluids and electrolytes, supportive therapy for circulatory collapse, antibiotics for secondary infections, prepare for emergency tracheotomy.	Irritation and swelling within throat (glottic edema), esophagus, and stomach. Shock secondary to fluid and electrolyte loss. More rarely, late esophageal stenosis.
Ipecac syrup or fluidextract	Nausea; vomiting; diarrhea; abdominal albuminuria; abdominal cramps; bloody vomitus and feces; dehydration; myocarditis; myocardial infarction; cardiac arrest or shock secondary to cardiac depression and fluid loss.	Lavage with activated charcoal solution or induce emesis if spontaneous vomiting has not occurred. Do not give additional emetic agents. Saline cathartic if purging has not occurred.	General supportive and symptomatic measures for impending shock.	Intractable vomiting and diarrhea due to intense irritation of entire gastrointestinal tract leading to shock. Pathological changes in kidneys, heart, and liver.
Iron salts	Severe gastroenteritis; abdominal pain; vomiting and diarrhea which eventually becomes bloody; dehydration; pallor; cyanosis; shock leading to death in 3 to 4 hours.	Milk by mouth and induce vomiting if not already spontaneous. Gastric lavage with 5% sodium bicarbonate. The specific antidote deferoxamine should be given orally and intravenously in	Intravenous fluids for dehydration and whole blood or plasma for shock.	Pulmonary edema, cardiac dilatation, severe gastroenteritis. Pathological changes in liver and kidneys.

appropriate dose.

	Signs and Symptoms	Treatment	Notes
Isopropyl alcohol	Dizziness, incoordination, headache, confusion, stupor, coma, nausea, vomiting, respiratory depression, and oliguria, followed by diuresis. Symptoms closely resemble ethyl alcohol intoxication. Death from circulatory collapse or respiratory failure.	Intravenous dextrose and saline, and correct electrolyte imbalance. Anticipate liver or kidney injury.	Acetonuria without glycosuria is pathognomonic. Severe CNS depression. Aspiration pneumonitis.
Kerosene (coal oil), diesel oil, gasoline, naphtha, and petroleum distillates	Burning sensation in mouth, throat, and stomach; nausea with vomiting and diarrhea; drowsiness; restlessness; disorientation; coma. Signs of pulmonary involvement indicate grave prognosis of impending fulminating hemorrhagic bronchopneumonia.	If risks of lavage and emetics are undertaken, an endotracheal tube with inflatable cuff should be employed. This is done to prevent inhalation of gastric contents. Dilute sodium bicarbonate is satisfactory lavage fluid.	Severe chemical pneumonitis. Pathological changes in liver, kidneys, and if inhalation of high concentrations, depression of bone marrow may occur.
		Antibiotics for secondary infection. Support respiration with oxygen. Observe patient in hospital for at least 24 hours.	
Lead or its salts	Metallic taste in mouth; burning pain in stomach and abdomen; constipation followed by diarrhea; convulsions; muscular weakness; paralysis of extremities; skin cold and cyanotic; delayed severe anemia; death is due to peripheral vascular collapse or encephalopathy. In children, the lead also interferes with the development of the central nervous system.	Gastric lavage with magnesium sulfate or sodium sulfate. Analgesics for pain. Diazepam I.V. for convulsions. Intravenous calcium disodium edetate in accordance with supplier's directions. Dimercaprol is also used. Treat cerebral edema with corticosteroids and mannitol.	Gastrointestinal inflammation, liver and kidney injury when sufficient lead has been absorbed. Encephalopathy is frequent in children.
		Keep patient quiet. Maintain fluid and electrolyte balance. Long-term therapy (1 to 2 months for adults and 3 to 6 months for children) with penicillamine to decrease the blood lead level to 60 μg/dl.	
Lye, sodium and potassium hydroxides and carbonates	Severe pain in mouth and difficulty in swallowing; gastrointestinal pain and	Do not induce vomiting. Large amounts of water or milk by mouth; avoid emetics and	Laryngeal or glottic edema; corrosion and possible perforation of upper
		Morphine for pain; fluids and electrolytes; cortisone. Use of bougies to prevent esophageal	

Poisons and Poisoning (Continued)

Toxic Substances	Symptoms of Poisoning	Emergency Measures	Supportive and Follow-up Treatment	Pathology
	vascular collapse; death in shock or asphyxia from glottic edema.	lavage. For hypocalcemia, slowly administer 5 ml of 10% calcium gluconate I.V. Tracheotomy may be required.	stricture. Broad-spectrum antibiotics.	gastrointestinal tract; late esophageal stenosis.
Meprobamate (Equanil, Miltown)	Drowsiness; relaxation; stupor; sleep; chills; fever; coma; areflexia; muscular flaccidity; severe and persistent hypotension; pulmonary edema.	Lavage or induce emesis; plasma or pressor agents for hypotension; mild stimulants. Artificial respiration and oxygen. Hemoperfusion if brain stem function is impaired.	Symptomatic and supportive care with frequent recording of vital signs.	In fatal cases, pulmonary edema, cerebral edema, and pneumonia.
Mercuric chloride or other soluble salts	Metallic taste and burning in mouth and throat; thirst; abdominal pain and cramps with nausea and vomiting; diarrhea and bloody stools; scanty urine containing albumin; collapse in shock with weak, rapid pulse, slow and shallow respirations, and cold and clammy skin. If patient survives acute episode, death from renal failure may occur after several days. Chronic mercury poisoning is also common with primarily neurological symptoms.	Egg white, milk, or flour by mouth. Lavage with activated charcoal. Dimercaprol (BAL) I.M. in accordance with supplier's directions. Penicillamine.	Saline cathartic if purging has not already occurred. Demulcents and analgesics. Treat for shock. Prepare for management of acute renal failure. Hemodialysis may be required.	Ulceration of gums and mouth, loosening of teeth, progressive peripheral neuritis are all seen in chronic poisonings or cases in which death is delayed. In acute cases, usual cause of death due to peripheral vascular collapse secondary to fluid or electrolyte loss, or acute renal failure.
Methyl alcohol (wood alcohol)	Fatigue, headache, muscular weakness, nausea, dizziness, vomiting, and abdominal pain; delirium with visual	If patient is seen within 2 hours of ingesting methanol use gastric lavage with 5% sodium bicarbonate, leaving some	To prevent formation of formic acid, give 10 ml of ethyl alcohol orally. If poisoning is severe, give ethyl alcohol I.V.	Intense metabolic acidosis. Partial to complete blindness due to atrophy of the ganglion cells of the retina if patient

Poison	Symptoms	Treatment		Remarks
	disturbances which may progress to blindness; weak and rapid pulse; shallow respirations; cyanosis; coma; death from respiratory failure, metabolic acidosis.	in 10% solution with 5% dextrose. Maintain blood level of 100 mg/ml. Bedrest, treat shock with respiratory and cardiovascular support, mild external heat, stimulants as indicated, protect patient's eyes from light. Oxygen.		survives. Pathological changes in heart, liver, lungs, and kidneys.
Morphine	Gross overdosages produce prompt depression, but smaller doses may cause transient period of excitement before drowsiness. Weariness; loss of pain sensation; nausea; vomiting; pinpoint pupils; coma with muscular relaxation and slowing of respiratory rate; cyanosis; slow pulse; fall in blood pressure; death in respiratory arrest.	Gastric lavage, even if several hours after ingestion. Naloxone is specific antagonist given I.V. 5 μg/kg may be repeated 10 to 20 times. Artificial respiration. Inhalation of oxygen with 5% CO_2.	Keep patient awake with mild stimulation. Maintain airway. Maintain fluid and electrolyte balance. Keep patient warm.	Pulmonary congestion. Death is from respiratory failure due to central depression.
Mushrooms — SEE: *Amanita.*				
Naphthalene (mothballs)	Abdominal pain; nausea; vomiting, diarrhea; headache; diaphoresis; coma with or without convulsions. Certain individuals exhibit intense intravascular hemolysis accompanied by anemia, jaundice, hematuria, and renal insufficiency.	Induce emesis or lavage with tap water, saline cathartic, demulcents, and mild stimulants. Sodium bicarbonate every 4 hours to maintain alkaline urine in order to prevent renal blockage with acid hematin crystals.	Anemia from hemolysis may require whole blood transfusions. Supportive measures for acute renal failure. Give oral fluids in large quantities along with a diuretic (furosemide) to produce diuresis. Avoid use of milk, oils, or fatty foods. Diazepam for convulsions.	Various states of central excitement or depression. Rarely, liver necrosis. Acute hemolytic anemia.
Nicotine	Burning sensation in mouth and throat; salivation; vomiting; diarrhea; hypertension; headache; sweating; dizziness; weakness; pupils contracted	Slurry of activated charcoal as lavage fluid with additional portion left in stomach. Artificial respiration and oxygen.	Diazepam for convulsions. Relief for symptoms of parasympathetic or sympathetic stimulation is obtained with atropine or	Transient stimulation and then depression of CNS, all autonomic ganglia and nerve endings in skeletal muscle.

Poisons and Poisoning *(Continued)*

Toxic Substances	Symptoms of Poisoning	Emergency Measures	Supportive and Follow-up Treatment	Pathology
	at first then dilated; pulse slow at first then rapid; respirations deep and rapid at first then dyspneic; death from paralysis of respiratory musculature.		phentolamine.	
Nitroglycerin, nitrites, and nitrates	Prompt fall in blood pressure; intense throbbing in head; dizziness; faintness; excessive muscular relaxation; tremors; nausea; vomiting; skin flushed, then cold and cyanotic; methemoglobinemia; postural hypotension; respiratory paralysis; convulsions; death.	Gastric lavage or administer emetic. Mild stimulants as indicated. Oxygen and artificial respiration. Methylene blue, 1% solution I.V., slowly for methemoglobinemia.	Keep patient in reclining position and comfortably warm. Transfusions, if needed, with whole blood or plasma.	Anoxia due to methemoglobinemia aggravated by stagnation of blood in capillaries, venules, and veins from peripheral vasodilatation.
Oxalic acid and oxalate salts	Severe gastrointestinal irritation and intense pain in upper gastrointestinal tract; vomiting and intense thirst; pulse weak and thready; skin cold and cyanotic; twitching of facial musculature; convulsions; coma; collapse; death, which may occur immediately.	In order to precipitate oxalate, immediately give large amounts of calcium lactate, lime water, magnesia, or chalk orally, or lavage cautiously with any of these. Calcium gluconate I.V.	Keep patient quiet and in recumbent position. Morphine for pain; demulcents. Treat shock. If renal function remains normal, give 4 liters of fluid daily.	Severe gastroenteritis and secondary shock, hypocalcemia and kidney injury. Calcium oxalate crystals in kidneys and other tissues.
Parathion and other organophosphorus insecticides (cholinesterase inhibitors)	Nausea; vomiting; diarrhea; abdominal cramps; salivation; headache; vertigo; runny nose; pinpoint pupils; generalized and profound muscular weakness; confusion; jerky movements; convulsions;	Give atropine 1 to 4 mg I.M. immediately and repeat every 3–8 minutes until parasympathetic symptoms are controlled. Give oxygen and artificial respiration. If available, valuable adjunct is	Endotracheal intubation or tracheotomy may be necessary. Treat dehydration. Keep patient under constant observation.	All signs and symptoms are referable to the inhibition of the enzyme acetycholinesterase and consequent accumulation of acetylcholine at all nervous junctions where it is the

coma; death in respiratory failure.	pralidoxime chloride in accordance with manufacturer's directions.	chemical mediator. Pulmonary edema; hyperemia of lungs and brain.
Petroleum distillates — SEE: *Kerosene.*		
Phenol Corrosive burns in mouth, esophagus, and stomach; abdominal pain; bloody diarrhea; pallor; sweating; weakness; headache; dizziness; ringing in ears; shock with weak pulse; fall in blood pressure and body temperature; shallow respiration; cyanosis; coma; death from respiratory failure. Skin contact produces pain followed by numbness and corrosive burn.	NOTE: If stomach wall is severely corroded, passage of a tube into it may cause rupture. If there is no corrosive damage to esophagus, cautious gastric lavage with activated charcoal. Instill 240 ml of milk into stomach. Avoid mineral oils and alcohol. Demulcents, morphine, mild respiratory stimulants, as needed. Wash skin thoroughly with water and activated charcoal; avoid use of alcohol or castor oil. Diazepam for convulsions.	Corrosive burns of skin and mucous membranes; gastric perforation. More rarely, esophageal stricture and renal failure.
Phosphorus Skin contact produces painful penetrating burns. Ingestion leads to burning pain in throat or abdomen with intense thirst followed by nausea, vomiting, diarrhea, odor of garlic on breath, luminescent vomitus and feces. Patient often appears to recover for several days, then suddenly relapses with severe liver, kidney, and cardiac damage.	Repeated lavage of the stomach with tap water. Give morphine for pain. Calcium gluconate I.V. to maintain serum calcium level.	Fatty degeneration of liver, kidneys, and heart; pulmonary edema.
Salicylates (sodium, methyl, acetylsalicylic acid, aspirin) Stimulation of the CNS including the respiratory center. The resulting hyperpnea leads to CO_2 loss, respiratory alkalosis,	Protect airway while giving gastric lavage with activated charcoal. Administer saline cathartic. Artificial respiration with oxygen. Diazepam for	Disturbed acid-base balance. Children often exhibit metabolic acidosis while adults more commonly show respiratory alkalosis. Intense

Poisons and Poisoning (Continued)

Toxic Substances	Symptoms of Poisoning	Emergency Measures	Supportive and Follow-up Treatment	Pathology
	hyperthermia, convulsions and shock, hypokalemia, and dehydration.	convulsions.	requires vigorous therapy. Attempt to keep urine at pH 8 or above, but do this with minimal increase in urinary output.	CNS stimulation followed by depression.
Silver salts, nitrate, and other soluble salts	Intense pain in mouth, throat, and gastrointestinal tract; bloody stools; vertigo; coma; convulsions; death.	Gastric lavage with several liters of saline solution. Saline cathartic. Treat shock. Diazepam for convulsions. Meperidine (Demerol) or codeine for pain.	Give milk, stimulants as indicated; treat for shock; maintain fluid and electrolyte balance.	Severe corrosion of gastrointestinal tract. Deposits of metallic silver occur under skin in chronic poisoning, but these are of minor cosmetic concern.
Strychnine	Apprehension; stiffness of muscles; twitching of face and arms; sweating; sudden tetanic convulsions of entire body; cyanosis of face and lips; pulse slow and strong; death in 1-3 hours with face fixed in a grin and body arched in hyperextension.	Slurry of activated charcoal by mouth is not administered until convulsions are controlled with diazepam I.V. Use muscle-relaxing drugs for tetany.	Place patient in a quiet, dark room. Avoid drafts. Artificial respiration may be needed. Constant nursing care. Treat acidosis and hypokalemia.	Stimulation of spinal cord leading to contraction of respiratory musculature and death from anoxia.
Thallium and salts, sulfate	Severe abdominal pain; bilateral ptosis; ataxia; fever; vomiting; diarrhea; tremors; delirium; convulsions; paralysis; coma; death. Loss of hair is peculiar to chronic poisoning.	Induce emesis and gastric lavage with activated charcoal. Give saline cathartic, demulcents. Diazepam for convulsions. Hemoperfusion may be of help.	Treat for shock; maintain fluid and electrolyte balance; calcium salts or milk; symptomatic and supportive therapy for CNS disorders. Antibiotics for pneumonia.	Hemorrhagic gastroenteritis and encephalopathy.
Turpentine	Sensation of warmth or pain in mouth, throat, and stomach followed by abdominal pain,	If patient is alert, put 240 ml of milk in stomach and induce gastric lavage. Give	Force fluids.	Irritation of kidneys; hematuria, albuminuria, and sometimes acute renal failure.

Drug	Symptoms and Signs	Treatment		
	vomiting and diarrhea. Aspiration into lungs may cause pneumonitis. Excitement, ataxia, delirium, and stupor, followed by convulsions, coma, and death from respiratory failure.	demulcents and saline cathartic. Atropine to decrease bronchial secretions.		Capillary dilatation and increased fragility with hypoprothrombinemia leading to internal hemorrhage.
Warfarin and anticoagulants	After few days of repeated ingestions; nosebleed; bleeding gums; pallor; hemorrhagic areas in skin, especially knees and buttocks; blood in urine or feces; death in hemorrhagic shock.	Gastric lavage with tap water in case of large single dose. Vitamin K is specific antidote and should be given until prothrombin levels return to normal.	Transfuse with fresh blood or plasma if hemorrhage is severe.	
Zinc salts (chloride, sulfate, acetate, etc.)	Increased salivation; fever; muscular aches; violent vomiting and purging, followed by prostration.	Lavage with milk or lime water. Follow with egg white and other demulcents. Aspirin for fever and pain. Treat pulmonary edema. If zinc fumes inhaled, give corticosteroids.	Recumbent position, external heat to body; treat for shock; maintain fluid and electrolyte balances.	Stricture of esophagus, pylorus, and destruction of glandular structure of stomach. Ulceration or perforation of the stomach.

Toxicity Rating Chart*

Toxicity Rating or Class	Probable Oral LETHAL Dose (Human)	
	Dose	For 70 kg person (150 lb)
6 Super toxic	less than 5 mg/kg	A taste (less than 7 drops)
5 Extremely toxic	5–50 mg/kg	Between 7 drops and 1 teaspoonful
4 Very toxic	50–500 mg/kg	Between 1 tsp and 1 ounce
3 Moderately toxic	0.5–5 gm/kg	Between 1 oz and 1 pint (or 1 lb)
2 Slightly toxic	5–15 gm/kg	Between 1 pt and 1 quart
1 Practically nontoxic	above 15 gm/kg	More than 1 quart (2.2 lb)

*From Gosselin, R. E., Smith, R. P., and Hodge, H. C.: Clinical Toxicology of Commercial Products, ed. 5. The Williams & Wilkins Co., Baltimore, 1984

Symptoms and Signs of Drug Abuse*

Drug	Acute Intoxication and Overdose	Withdrawal Syndrome

CNS Stimulants

Cocaine; amphetamine; dextroamphetamine; methylphenidate; phenmetrazine; phenylpropanolamine; STP[1]; MDMA[2]; Bromo-DMA[3]; diethylpropion; most amphetaminelike anti-obesity drugs

Vital Signs: temperature elevated; heart rate increased; respirations shallow; BP elevated. *Mental Status:* sensorium hyperacute or confused; paranoid ideation; hallucinations; delirium; impulsivity; agitation; hyperactivity; sterotypy. *Physical Exam:* pupils dilated and reactive; tendon reflexes hyperactive; cardiac arrhythmias; dry mouth; sweating; tremors; convulsions; coma; stroke.

Muscular aches; abdominal pain; chills, tremors; voracious hunger; anxiety; prolonged sleep; lack of energy; profound depression, sometimes suicidal; exhaustion

Opioids

Heroin; morphine; codeine; meperidine; methadone; hydromorphone; opium; pentazocine; propoxyphene; fentanyl; sufentanil

Vital Signs: temperature decreased; respiration depressed; BP decreased, sometimes shock. *Mental Status:* euphoria; stupor. *Physical Exam:* pupils constricted (may be dilated with meperidine or extreme hypoxia); reflexes diminished to absent; pulmonary edema; constipation; convulsions with propoxyphene or meperidine; cardiac arrhythmias with propoxyphene; coma.

Pupils dilated; *pulse* rapid; gooseflesh; lacrimation; abdominal cramps; muscle jerks; "flu" syndrome; vomiting; diarrhea; tremulousness; yawning; anxiety

CNS Depressants

Barbiturates; benzodiazepines; glutethimide; meprobamate; methaqualone; ethchlorvynol; chloral hydrate; methyprylon; paraldehyde

Vital Signs: respiration depressed; BP decreased, sometimes shock. *Mental Status:* drowsiness or coma; confusion; delirium. *Physical Exam:* pupils dilated with glutethimide or in severe poisoning; tendon reflexes depressed; ataxia; slurred speech; nystagmus; convulsions or hyperirritability with methaqualone; signs of anticholinergic poisoning with glutethimide; cardiac arrhythmias with chloral hydrate.

Tremulousness; insomnia; sweating; fever; clonic blink reflex; anxiety; cardiovascular collapse; agitation; delirium; hallucinations; disorientation; convulsions; shock

Symptoms and Signs of Drug Abuse *(Continued)*

Drug	Acute Intoxication and Overdose	Withdrawal Syndrome
Hallucinogens LSD[4]; psilocybin; mescaline; PCP[5]	*Vital Signs:* temperature elevated; heart rate increased; BP elevated. *Mental Status:* euphoria; anxiety or panic; paranoia; sensorium often clear; affect inappropriate; illusions; time and visual distortions; visual hallucinations; depersonalization; with PCP hypertensive encephalopathy. *Physical Exam:* pupils dilated (normal or small with PCP); tendon reflexes hyperactive; with PCP: cyclic coma or extreme hyperactivity, drooling, blank stare, mutism, amnesia, analgesia, nystagmus (sometimes vertical), gait ataxia, muscle rigidity, impulsive or violent behavior; violent, scatological, pressured speech.	None
Cannabis Group Marijuana; hashish; THC[6]; hash oil; sinsemilla	*Vital Signs:* heart rate increased; BP decreased on standing. *Mental Status:* anorexia, then increased appetite; euphoria; anxiety; sensorium often clear; dreamy, fantasy state; time-space distortions; hallucinations may be rare. *Physical Exam:* pupils unchanged; conjunctiva injected; tachycardia, ataxia, and pallor in children.	Nonspecific symptoms including anorexia, nausea, insomnia, restlessness, irritability, anxiety, depression
Anticholinergics Atropine; belladonna; henbane; scopolamine; trihexyphenidyl; benztropine mesylate; procyclidine; propantheline bromide; jimson weed seed	*Vital Signs:* temperature elevated; heart rate increased; possibly decreased BP. *Mental Status:* drowsiness or coma; sensorium clouded; amnesia; disorientation; visual hallucinations; body image alterations; confusion; with propantheline restlessness, excitement. *Physical Exam:* pupils dilated and fixed; decreased bowel sounds; flushed, dry skin and mucous membranes; violent behavior; convulsions; with propantheline circulatory failure, respiratory failure, paralysis, coma.	Gastrointestinal and musculoskeletal symptoms

*Mixed intoxications produce complex combinations of signs and symptoms.

1. STP (2,5-dimethoxy-4-methylamphetamine)
2. MDMA (3,4-methylenedioxymethamphetamine)
3. Bromo-DMA (4-Bromo-2,5-dimethoxyamphetamine)
4. LSD (D-lysergic acid diethylamide)
5. PCP (phencyclidine)
6. THC (delta-9-tetrahydrocannabinol)

From The Medical Letter, Vol. 29, Sept. 11, 1987, with permission.

Substances Generally Nontoxic When Ingested*

Ball-point inks (amt. in 1 pen)
Barium sulfate
Bathtub toys (floating)
Blackboard chalk (calcium carbonate)
Candles (insect-repellent type may be toxic)
Carbowax (polyethylene glycol)
Carboxymethylcellulose (dehydrating material
   packed with drugs, film, etc.)
Castor oil
Cetyl alcohol
Crayons (children's: marked A.P., C.P., or C.S.
   130–46)
Detergents, anionic and nonionic
Dichloral (herbicide)
Dry cell battery
Glycerol
Glyceryl monostearate
Graphite
Gums (acacia, agar, ghatti, etc.)
Hormones
Kaolin
Lanolin
Lauric acid
Linoleic acid
Linseed oil (not boiled)

Lipstick
Magnesium silicate (antacid)
Matches
Methylcellulose
Modeling clay
Paraffin, chlorinated
Pencil lead (graphite)
Pepper, black (except inhaled in mass)
Petrolatum
Polyethylene glycols
Polyethylene glycol stearate
Polysorbate (Tweens®)
Putty
Red oil (turkey-red oil, sulfated castor oil)
Silica (silicon dioxide)
Spermaceti
Stearic acid
Sweetening agents
Talc
Tallow
Thermometer fluid or mercury
Titanium oxide
Triacetin (glyceryl triacetate)
Vitamins, multiple without iron

*Substances listed here may, however, be present in combination with phenol, petroleum distillate vehicles, or other toxic chemicals. Since manufactured products may be changed in their composition, this table is intended only as a guide, and prudence requires that a poison center be consulted for up-to-date information.

From The Merck Manual, Ed. 15, Merck Sharp and Dohme, 1987, with permission.

Suffocation, Asphyxiation, Drowning

Type	History	Pathology	Symptoms and Color	Pulse	Breathing	Muscles	Pupils	Complications	Treatment
Choking	Edema of larynx; diseases of larynx. Foreign bodies aspirated into the larynx.	Trauma of larynx.	Patient in a state of apprehension. Color is cyanotic.	Rapid due to exertion.	Respirations are very rapid or patient may gasp occasionally.	May be voluntarily contracted.	Dilated.	Pneumonia; sinusitis; complete obstruction of the bronchi; lung abscess.	Manual removal of foreign object or perform Heimlich maneuver. Tracheotomy may be required.
Drowning	Body discovered in water.	Waterlogging of lungs and asphyxia.	Patient is unconscious. Color is gray and changing to blue (cyanosis).	If perceptible, it is rapid and may be shallow.	If respirations are present, the patient may gasp occasionally or very irregularly.	Muscles are relaxed and body is very limp.	May be dilated.	Fracture of neck; heart failure; suffocation, shock, and collapse.	Artificial respiration (mouth to mouth); external cardiac massage if needed; oxygen; treat for shock; heart stimulants.
Gas Poisoning	Victim rescued from room with escaping gas from open jet or victim overcome in closed garage.	Changes in the blood chemistry and then anemia. Respiratory paralysis which leads to death.	Patient unconscious. Color typical cherry red, or pallor and cyanosis, carbon monoxide in poisoning.	Rapid, may be irregular.	Respirations are usually slow but may be rapid and shallow very early after the exposure to gas.	Muscles are relaxed and body is limp.	Varies with the type of gas poisoning.	Respiratory failure; depletion of O_2 supply in the blood.	Artificial respiration; oxygen; shock treatment.

2421

Suffocation, Asphyxiation, Drowning (Continued)

Type	History	Pathology	Symptoms and Color	Pulse	Breathing	Muscles	Pupils	Complications	Treatment
Strangulation and Hanging	Patient found during or after the act. Very definite signs of violence.	Fracture of cervical vertebrae; suffocation; trauma of medulla by odontoid process of axis.	If living, may be unconscious or in a state of excitement or desperation. Cyanotic if death occurred sometime previous to discovery.	May be perceptible or absent.	No respirations, or respirations are very rapid, or patient may gasp occasionally.	May be voluntarily contracted.	Dilated. Unequal if there is cerebral injury.	Fracture of neck; suffocation; contusions on neck.	Release pull of rope by placing chair under patient's feet and cutting rope. Oxygen therapy; artificial respiration; treat for shock; treat fractures.

Unconsciousness

Type	History	Skin and Color	Pupils	Muscles	Pulse	Breathing	Reflexes	Complications	Treatment
Acid and Alkali Poisoning	Accidental or intentional poisoning.	Clammy skin. Skin pale; face cyanotic.	Dilated. Eyes sunken, staring.	Tense. Patient in convulsion.	Rapid, feeble pulse.	Shallow, rapid, labored, irregular.	Increased.	Corrosion of mucous membranes; ulcers of stomach; gastritis; jaundice.	Acids: Milk of magnesia, egg albumin, lime water, no chalk or alkaline carbonate. Alkalies: Neutralize with acetic acid (vinegar). In both cases careful gastric lavage.

		Skin	Pupils	Muscles	Pulse	Respiration	Reflexes	Complications	Treatment
Bleeding	Trauma causing bright red spurting or welling bleeding. Bleeding after an operation.	Skin shows pallor which progresses to a yellow or greenish tinge.	Dilated.	Relaxed.	Rapid, becoming thready.	Respirations are rapid and shallow. Air hunger is evident.	Diminished.	Shock; anemia; heart failure; death.	Digital pressure and tourniquet; pad in joint. Keep patient quiet; treat for shock; transfusion if necessary.
Concussion	Head injury caused by fall or blow upon the head.	Skin pale, cold, and clammy. Varies with degree of pathology.	Dilated. Varies with degree and area of injury.	May be spastic.	Pulse rate usually shows a slight increase. May be weak and rapid.	Respirations are usually deep.	Deep tendon reflexes may be increased.	Shock in severe cases; paralysis of limbs may occur.	Bedrest; keep patient flat and warm.
Drowning	Victim is found unconscious in body of water. May have a fractured neck or skull.	Skin is cold, clammy, and cyanotic.	Dilated.	Relaxed if victim is living. Rigor mortis if dead.	If perceptible, it is rapid and weak, or very irregular.	No respirations. Occasional gasp if living.	None.	Heart failure; pneumonia; shock; aspiration of foreign material.	Resuscitation (Mouth-to-mouth is most effective method if a manual positive pressure type of device is not available). Keep body warm but not hot. Stimulating drinks when conscious.
Drunkenness	Victim is unable to cope with the amount of intoxicants taken. Be	Color varies. Face may be flushed; skin is moist, relaxed, and cool.	Usually dilated but equal.	Relaxed. Body and limbs are limp.	Strong and slow.	Respirations are slow, deep, stertorous, accompanied by character-	Involuntary reflexes usually increased.	Pneumonia.	Keep the body warm. If conscious give emetic. Gastric lavage. Give hot cof-

2423

Unconsciousness (Continued)

Type	History	Skin and Color	Pupils	Muscles	Pulse	Breathing	Reflexes	Complications	Treatment
	certain the physical condition is not due to cerebral concussion.					istic "lip blowing" and Cheyne-Stokes type of breathing.			fee or aromatic spirits of ammonia.
Electric Shock	Victim is found after coming in contact with a live wire.	Skin is pale, cold, and clammy.	Pupils may be unequal.	Tense.	Weak and imperceptible.	Respirations cease suddenly.	Deep tendon reflexes usually are increased.	Low voltage affects heart action, makes resuscitation impossible. High voltage affects the respiratory center in medulla and patient may be resuscitated.	Carefully release the patient from current. Artificial respiration by prone pressure; electrical defibrillation may be required. If heart fails to resume contraction, use of an external cardiac pacemaker is indicated. Each moment of delay increases the chances of death.
Epilepsy	Previous occurrence of fits or spells	Pallor to flush followed by cyanosis—	Pupils are unequal, eyes rolling.	May be spastic. Tonic type of convulsion	Usually rapid.	Respirations are deep and stertorous.	May be increased.	Injuries in falling or biting the tongue.	Bedrest. Prevent falling or biting

Condition	Cause	Skin	Pupils	Muscles	Pulse	Respiration	Temperature	Complications	Treatment
	with or without aura.	may be slight and gradually increased to marked cyanosis.		is followed by the clonic type.				Patient may react violently (fighting others).	tongue. Sedative.
Fainting	Fatigue, lightheadedness, shock, or horrifying experience.	Face and lips are blanched. Body is cold and clammy.	Normal.	Completely relaxed.	Rapid and thready.	Respirations are rapid and shallow.	Slightly increased.	Shock usually a serious complication. Body injury and fracture if patient falls.	Apply cold water to face, head, and chest. Place head in low position. Have patient inhale aromatic spirits of ammonia.
Freezing	Exposure to intense cold or prolonged period of exposure to cold.	Frostbite: Skin is cold, pale, and blanched. Frozen: Skin is livid and later cyanotic, then turns to purplish or greenish black.	Dilated.	Tense and becoming very rigid.	Rapid and weak.	Breathing is slower and deeper. Patient falls into very deep slumber.	Not discernible.	Pneumonia; certain damage due to mechanical destruction of the cells' sloughing and gangrene of the part previously frozen.	Gradual warming of the parts; slight massage of extremities for better circulation; elevation of parts; treatment of dry gangrene.
Gases	Victim rescued from a mine, burning building, or room with open gas jet. Overcome in garage or car.	In carbon monoxide poisoning, skin is cyanotic and changing to cherry red color.	Eyes fixed. Pupils are usually fully dilated. Varies with type of gas.	Relaxed if victim is living. Rigor mortis if dead.	Weak, slow, and irregular.	Respirations irregular and jerky to only an occasional gasp.	None.	Respiratory failure; asphyxia; collapse.	Place the patient in the open air; give oxygen and resuscitation (mouth-to-mouth). Treat for shock.

Unconsciousness (Continued)

Type	History	Skin and Color	Pupils	Muscles	Pulse	Breathing	Reflexes	Complications	Treatment
Hanging	Victim is found hanging with a rope, wire, or other flexible material around the neck.	Skin is pale and face is cyanotic.	Dilated and unequal if cerebral injury.	Relaxed. Varies with the level of tenure.	Pulse is rapid, weak, and irregular if strangulation is incomplete. If complete, pulse is absent.	Respirations have ceased or an occasional gasp is observed.	None.	Respiratory and circulatory failure; fracture of neck.	Release the patient and cut the rope. Artificial respiration; treat for shock and possible fracture of neck.
Heat Exhaustion	Victim is overcome by the degree of heat and loss of sodium chloride through perspiration.	Skin may be pale and cool. Temperature is usually normal.	Moderately contracted.	Tense with muscle cramps.	Rapid and may become weak.	Respirations shallow with rigidity of the chest muscles.	Increased.	Shock.	Treat for shock; keep body warm. Give salt by mouth and I.V.
Heatstroke (sunstroke, heat hyperpyrexia)	Exposure to intense degree, or prolonged period, of heat from environment.	Skin is flushed and hot when touched. Body temperature may be 106°F (41°C) or higher.	Dilated.	Relaxed.	Rapid and weak.	Respirations may be shallow and gasping or deep and slow.	Increased.	Suppressed sweating for prolonged period. Paralysis of vasomotor centers within medulla. Paralysis of heart, collapse, and death.	Place patient in cool area. Cold application to head and body. Wrap in cold, wet sheet. Continue to lower body temperature. No stimulants or sedatives unless required to treat convulsions. Judge

2426

Condition	History / Cause	Skin	Pupils (Eyes)	Muscles	Pulse	Respiration	Temperature	Complications	Treatment ... effectiveness of therapy by continual monitoring of rectal temperature.
Mineral Poisoning	Accidental or suicidal poisoning.	Skin is cold and clammy. Pallor.	Dilated. Eyes fixed, staring.	Tense, convulsive to relaxed when in stupor.	Rapid, feeble to imperceptible.	Respirations are shallow, rapid, labored.	Increased.	Nephritis; liver degeneration; colitis.	Gastric lavage; emetics.
Narcotic Poisoning	History of addiction or allergic reaction to the drug.	Skin is ashen, cyanotic, and cold.	Pupils are contracted to pinpoint if due to opiate derivative.	Relaxed.	Usually slow but varies with type of drug poisoning.	Respirations slow, irregular, stertorous.	Diminished.	Addiction to drug or production of a marked sensitivity to a drug.	Removal of the drug by emetics or lavage; use of antidotes; specific counteractives.
Obstruction in throat	Aspiration of a foreign body or respiratory tract is obstructed by edema or disease.	Skin is cyanotic.	Dilated.	Sternal retraction. Muscles are tense with efforts of trying to breathe and remove obstruction.	Rapid and very weak.	Respirations are deep and labored.	Increased.	Asphyxia; pulmonary infection; shock.	Remove obstruction. Use Heimlich maneuver. Institute basic life support procedures. Tracheotomy if indicated.
Stroke (Apoplectic)	Patient may have history of hypertension and arteriosclerosis. Usually past 40 years of age.	Skin is injected. May be cyanotic or ashen. Hot and dry to flushed. Elevation of temperature.	Pupils vary. May be dilated, often unequal. Inactive in deep coma.	Muscles of the involved side (hemiplegia) are usually spastic with a facial palsy.	Slow, full with increased tension.	Respirations are slow, loud, usually deep.	Diminished on one side. May be hyperactive on the other side.	Pneumonia; injury from falling.	Rest and absolute quiet with head of bed elevated and feet lowered. Ice cap to head; no stimulants.

App. 19: Burn Care Resources
And Skin Banks

The first part of this appendix lists the addresses and phone numbers of 166 hospitals at which burn care physicians in the United States and Canada reported the presence of beds designated for burn care in 1991. The list includes 148 burn care facilities in the United States and 18 in Canada. The second part of the appendix lists 36 active skin banks in the United States and Canada.

The information in this appendix was adapted from the American Burn Association's Directory of Burn Care Resources in North America (1991–92). Besides the information reported here, the ABA directory provides the names of key contact personnel at the burn centers listed as well as a separate list of burn care fellowship programs. It also provides detailed information regarding the ability of skin banks to supply tissue to other institutions upon request, the preservation techniques they use, and the quality assurance tests performed by each skin bank. For a copy of the directory, contact the ABA at (800) 548–2876.

BURN CARE SERVICES
United States

ALABAMA

Birmingham
Children's Hospital of Alabama
1600 7th Ave., South (Zip: 35233)
(205) 939-9398

University of Alabama Hospital
619 South 19th St. (Zip: 35233)
(205) 934-7250

Mobile
University of South Alabama Burn Center
2451 Fillingrim St. (Zip: 36617)
(205) 471-7520

ALASKA

Anchorage
Providence Hospital
3200 Providence Drive, Pouch 6604 (Zip: 99519-6604)
(907) 261-3651

Fairbanks
Fairbanks Memorial Hospital
1650 Cowles St. (Zip: 99701)
(907) 452-8181

ARIZONA

Phoenix
Maricopa Medical Center
2601 East Roosevelt St. (Zip: 85008)
(602) 267-5726

Tucson
Carondelet St. Mary's Hospital
1601 W. St. Mary's Rd. (Zip: 85745)
(602) 622-5833

ARKANSAS

Little Rock
Arkansas Children's Hospital
800 Marshall St. (Zip: 72205-3591)
(501) 320-1323

CALIFORNIA

Berkeley
Alta-Bates-Herrick Hospital
3001 Colby St. (Zip: 94705)
(415) ICU-BURN (428-2876)

Castro Valley
Eden Hospital Medical Center
20103 Lake Chabot Rd. (Zip: 94546)
(415) 537-1234, ext. 5066

Chico
Chico Community Hospital
560 Cohasset Ave. (Zip: 95926)
(916) 896-5085

Downey
Rancho Los Amigos Medical Center
7601 East Imperial Hwy. (Zip: 90242)
(213) 940-7454

Fresno
Valley Medical Center
445 South Cedar Ave. (Zip: 93702)
(209) 453-4220

Los Angeles
Children's Hospital of Los Angeles
4650 Sunset Blvd. (Zip: 90027-0700)
(213) 669-2154 (days); 669-2120 (24 hr)

Los Angeles County – University of Southern California
  Medical Center
1200 N. State St. (Zip: 90033)
(213) 226-7991

Oakland
Children's Hospital of Oakland
51st and Martin Luther King (Zip: 94609)
(415) ICU-BURN (428-2876)

Orange
UCI Medical Center
101 The City Drive (Zip: 92668)
(714) 634-5304

Sacramento
University of California Davis Medical Center
2315 Stockton Blvd. (Zip: 95817)
(916) 734-3636

San Bernardino
San Bernardino County Medical Center
780 E. Gilbert St. (Zip: 92404)
(714) 387-8028

San Diego
University of California San Diego Medical Center
225 Dickinson St. (Zip: 92103)
(619) 294-2833

San Francisco
Saint Francis Memorial Hospital
900 Hyde St. (Zip: 94109)
(415) 923-4759

San Francisco General Hospital
1001 Potrero Ave. (Zip: 94110)
(415) 821-8201

San Jose
Santa Clara Valley Medical Center
751 S. Bascom Ave. (Zip: 95128)
(408) 299-5242

San Pablo
Brookside Hospital
2000 Vale Rd. (Zip: 94806)
(415) 235-7000

Sherman Oaks
Sherman Oaks Community Hospital
4929 Van Nuys Blvd. (Zip: 91403)
(818) 981-7111

Stockton
Dameron Hospital
525 W. Acacia St. (Zip: 95203)
(209) 944-5550

Torrance
Torrance Memorial Medical Center
3330 Lomita Blvd. (Zip: 90505)
(213) 517-4622

COLORADO

Colorado Springs
Penrose Hospital
2215 N. Cascade Ave. (Zip: 80907)
(719) 630-5770

Denver
Children's Hospital
1056 East 19th Ave. (Zip: 80218)
(303) 861-6516

University Hospital, University of Colorado
4200 East Ninth Ave. (Zip: 80262)
(303) 270-8052

Grand Junction
St. Mary's Hospital and Medical Center
7th St. and Patterson Rd. (Zip: 81501)
(303) 244-2273

Greeley
North Colorado Medical Center
16th St. and 17th Ave. (Zip: 80631)
(303) 350-6570

CONNECTICUT

Hartford
Hartford Hospital
80 Seymour St. (Zip: 06115)
(203) 524-3112

New Haven
Yale University School of Medicine
333 Cedar St. (Zip: 06510)
(203) 785-2876

DISTRICT OF COLUMBIA

Washington
Children's Hospital National Medical Center
111 Michigan Ave. NW (Zip: 20010)
(202) 745-5116

Washington Hospital Center
110 Irving St. NW (Zip: 20010)
(202) 877-7241

FLORIDA

Gainesville
University of Florida Medical Center
1600 Archer Rd. (Zip: 32601)
(904) 395-0200

Miami
University of Miami–Jackson Memorial Medical Center
1611 NW 12th Ave. (Zip: 33136)
(305) 549-7085

Orlando
Orlando Regional Medical Center
1414 S. Kuhl Ave. (Zip: 32806-2093)
(407) 841-5176

Tampa
Tampa General Hospital
Davis Island (Zip: 33606)
(813) 253-0711

GEORGIA

Atlanta
Grady Memorial Hospital
80 Butler St. SE (Zip: 30335)
(404) 589-4307

Augusta
Humana Hospital–Augusta Burn Center
3651 Wheeler Rd. (Zip: 30910)
(404) 863-3232

Medical College of Georgia
1120 15th St. (Zip: 30912)
(404) 721-4721

HAWAII

Honolulu
Straub Hospital
888 S. King St. (Zip: 96813)
(808) 522-4000

ILLINOIS

Chicago
Cook County Hospital
700 S. Wood St. (Zip: 60612)
(312) 633-6565

Burn Center, University of Chicago
5841 S. Maryland (Zip: 60637)
(312) 702-6302

Maywood
Foster G. McGaw Hospital/Loyola University Medical
  Center
2160 S. First Ave. (Zip: 60153)
(708) 216-3988

Rock Island
Franciscan Medical Center
2701 17th St. (Zip: 61201)
(309) 793-3173

Rockford
St. Anthony Medical Center
5666 E. State St. (Zip: 61108)
(815) 395-5313

Springfield
Memorial Medical Center
800 N. Rutledge St. (Zip: 62781)
(217) 788-3325

INDIANA

Fort Wayne
St. Joseph's Medical Center
700 Broadway (Zip: 46802)
(219) 424-BURN (-2876)

Indianapolis
Indiana University Medical Center
Wishard Memorial Hospital (adults)
1001 W. Tenth St. (Zip: 46202)
(317) 630-6471

James Whitcomb Riley Hospital (children)
702 Barnhill Dr. (Zip: 46202-5124)
(317) 274-3927

IOWA

Des Moines
Iowa Methodist Medical Center
1200 Pleasant St. (Zip: 50309)
(515) 283-5042

Iowa City
University of Iowa Burn Treatment Center
8322 John Colloton Pavilion (Zip: 52242)
(319) 356-2496

Sioux City
St. Luke's Regional Medical Center
2720 Stone Park Blvd. (Zip: 51104)
(712) 279-3440

KANSAS

Kansas City
University of Kansas Medical Center
39th and Rainbow Blvd. (Zip: 66103)
(913) 588-6540

Wichita
St. Francis Regional Medical Center
929 N. St. Francis Ave. (Zip: 67214-3882)
(316) 268-5388

KENTUCKY

Lexington
Chandler Medical Center
800 Rose St. (Zip: 40536)
(606) 233-5260

Louisville
Kosair-Children's Hospital
P.O. Box 35070 (Zip: 40232-5070)
(502) 895-5466

Humana Hospital-University of Louisville
530 S. Jackson St. (Zip: 40202)
(502) 562-3983

LOUISIANA

Baton Rouge
Baton Rouge General Medical Center
3600 Florida St. (Zip: 70821)
(504) 387-7716

Shreveport
LSU Medical Center
1501 Kings Hwy. (Zip: 71130)
(318) 674-6850)

MAINE

Portland
Maine Medical Center
22 Bramhall St. (Zip: 04102)
(207) 871-2176

MARYLAND

Baltimore
Francis Scott Key Medical Center
4940 Eastern Ave. (Zip: 21224)
(301) 550-0890

MASSACHUSETTS

Boston
Boston City Hospital
818 Harrison Ave. (Zip: 02118)
(617) 434-5689

Brigham and Women's Hospital
75 Francis St. (Zip: 02115)
(617) 732-7715

Shriners Burns Institute
51 Blossom St. (Zip: 02114)
(617) 722-3000

Springfield
Baystate Medical Center
759 Chestnut (Zip: 01199)
(413) 784-4800

MICHIGAN

Ann Arbor
University of Michigan Medical Center
1500 E. Medical Center Drive (Zip: 48109-0033)
(313) 936-9666

Detroit
Children's Hospital of Michigan
3901 Beaubien Blvd. (Zip: 48201)
(313) 745-BURN (-2876)

Detroit Receiving Hospital
4201 St. Antoine (Zip: 48201)
(313) 745-3078

Flint
Hurley Medical Center
1 Hurley Plaza (Zip: 48502)
(313) 257-9188

Grand Rapids
West Michigan Burn Unit
1840 Wealthy St. SE (Zip: 49506)
(616) 774-7670

Kalamazoo
Bronson Methodist Hospital Burn Center
252 Lovell St. (Zip: 49009)
(616) 341-6485

Lansing
E. W. Sparrow Hospital
1215 E. Michigan Ave. (Zip: 48909-7980)
(517) 483-2647

MINNESOTA

Duluth
Miller-Dwan Medical Center
502 E. Second St. (Zip: 55805)
(218) 720-1215

Minneapolis
Hennepin County Medical Center
(Zip: 55415)
(800) 321-BURN (-2876)

St. Paul
St. Paul-Ramsey Medical Center
640 Jackson St. (Zip: 55101)
(612) 221-3351

MISSISSIPPI

Greenville
Mississippi Firefighters Memorial Burn Center
1400 E. Union Ave. (Zip: 38703)
(601) 378-3783

MISSOURI

Columbia
University of Missouri-Columbia Hospital and Clinics
One Hospital Dr. (Zip: 65212)
(314) 882-7994

Burn Care Resources (*Continued*)

Kansas City
Children's Mercy Hospital
24th at Gilham Rd. (Zip: 64108)
(816) 234-3520

St. Louis
Barnes Hospital Burn Center
One Barnes Hospital Plaza (Zip: 63110)
(314) 362-4060

St. John's Mercy Medical Center
615 S. New Ballas Rd. (Zip: 63141)
(314) 569-6055

Springfield
St. John's Regional Burn Unit
1235 E. Cherokee St. (Zip: 65804-2263)
(417) 885-2876

MONTANA

Billings
St. Vincent Hospital and Health Center
Box 35200 (Zip: 59107-5200)
(406) 657-7067

NEBRASKA

Lincoln
St. Elizabeth Community Health Center
500 S. 70th St. (Zip: 68510)
(402) 486-7680

NEVADA

Las Vegas
University Medical Center of Southern Nevada
1800 W. Charleston Blvd. (Zip: 89102)
(702) 383-2268

NEW JERSEY

Livingston
Saint Barnabas Medical Center
Old Short Hills Rd. (Zip: 07039)
(201) 533-5920

NEW MEXICO

Albuquerque
University of New Mexico Regional Burn Center
2211 Lomas Blvd. NE (Zip: 87106)
(505) 843-2715

NEW YORK

Buffalo
Erie County Medical Center
462 Grider St. (Zip: 14215)
(716) 898-LIFE (-5433)

East Meadow
Nassau County Medical Center
2201 Hempstead Turnpike (Zip: 11554)
(516) 542-3207

Elmira
St. Joseph's Hospital
555 E. Market St. (Zip: 14902)
(607) 737-7882

New York (Manhattan)
New York Hospital
525 E. 68th St. (Zip: 10021)
(212) 746-5317

Rochester
Strong Memorial Hospital
601 Elmwood Ave. (Zip: 14642)
(716) 275-2222

Stony Brook
University Hospital – SUNY at Stony Brook
(Zip: 11794)
(516) 444-2270

Syracuse
SUNY Health Science Center
750 E. Adams St. (Zip: 13210)
(315) 464-6083

Valhalla
Westchester County Medical Center
(Zip: 10595)
(914) 285-8677

West Islip
Good Samaritan Hospital
800 Montauk Highway (Zip: 11795)
(516) 587-7800

NORTH CAROLINA

Chapel Hill
The Hospitals at the University of North Carolina
(Zip: 27514)
(919) 966-3693

Durham
Duke University Hospital
Box 3708 (Zip: 27710)
(919) 681-2404

Winston-Salem
North Carolina Baptist Hospital
300 S. Hawthorne Rd. (Zip: 27103)
(919) 748-7766

Burn Care Resources (*Continued*)

NORTH DAKOTA

Fargo
St. Luke's Hospitals-Meritcare
720 Fourth St., S. (Zip: 58122)
(701) 234-5222

OHIO

Akron
Children's Hospital Medical Center of Akron
281 Locust St. (Zip: 44308)
(216) 379-8224

Cincinnati
Shriners Burns Institute
202 Goodman St. (Zip: 45219)
(513) 872-6000

University of Cincinnati Hospital
234 Goodman St. (Zip: 45219)
(513) 558-8199

Cleveland
MetroHealth Medical Center
3395 Scranton Rd. (Zip: 44109)
(216) 398-6000

Columbus
Children's Hospital
700 Children's Dr. (Zip: 43205)
(614) 461-2560

Ohio State University Hospitals
410 W. Tenth Ave. (Zip: 43210)
(614) 293-8744

Dayton
Miami Valley Hospital
One Wyoming St. (Zip: 45409)
(513) 220-2126

OKLAHOMA

Oklahoma City
Baptist Medical Center
3300 Northwest Expressway (Zip: 73112)
(405) 949-3345

Tulsa
Hillcrest Medical Center
1120 S. Utica (Zip: 74104)
(918) 560-5745

OREGON

Portland
Emanuel Hospital
2801 N. Gantenbein Ave. (Zip: 97227)
(503) 280-4232

PENNSYLVANIA

Allentown
Lehigh Valley Hospital Center
1200 S. Cedar Crest Blvd. (Zip: 18103)
(215) 776-8734

Erie
Hamot Medical Center
201 State St. (Zip: 16550)
(814) 870-6130

Philadelphia
Saint Agnes Medical Center
1900 S. Broad St. (Zip: 19145)
(215) 339-4341

St. Christopher's Hospital for Children
Erie Ave. at Front St. (Zip: 19134-1095)
(215) 427-5323

Pittsburgh
Mercy Hospital of Pittsburgh
1400 Locust St. (Zip: 15219)
(412) 232-8225

Western Pennsylvania Hospital
4800 Friendship Ave. (Zip: 15224)
(412) 578-5274

Upland
Crozer-Chester Medical Center
One Medical Center Blvd. (Zip: 19013)
(215) 447-2800

RHODE ISLAND

Providence
Rhode Island Hospital
593 Eddy St. (Zip: 02903)
(401) 277-5753; 277-5754

SOUTH CAROLINA

Charleston
Medical University of South Carolina
171 Ashley Ave. (Zip: 29425)
(803) 792-3681 (adults); 792-2123 (children)

SOUTH DAKOTA

Sioux Falls
McKennan Hospital
800 E. 21st St. (Zip: 57117-5045)
(605) 339-8000

TENNESSEE

Chattanooga
Erlanger Medical Center
975 E. Third St. (Zip: 37403)
(615) 778-7881

Memphis
Regional Burn Center at Memphis
877 Jefferson Ave. (Zip: 38103)
(901) 575-8090

Nashville
Vanderbilt University Hospital
S-4400 RW
Medical Center North (Zip: 37232-2165)
(615) 322-4590

TEXAS

Dallas
Parkland Memorial Hospital
5301 Harry Hines Blvd. (Zip: 75235)
(214) 590-7650

El Paso
Sun Towers Hospital
1801 N. Oregon St. (Zip: 79902)
(915) 521-1780

Fort Sam Houston
U.S. Army Institute of Surgical Research
(Zip: 78234-5012)
(512) 222-BURN (-2876); 221-6604; 221-6943

Galveston
Shriners Burns Institute
610 Texas Ave. (Zip: 77550)
(409) 770-6600

University of Texas Medical Branch
Eighth and Mechanic Sts. (Zip: 77550)
(409) 761-2023

Houston
Hermann Hospital
6411 Fannin St. (Zip: 77030-1501)
(713) 797-4350

Lubbock
University Medical Center
602 Indiana Ave. (Zip: 79417)
(806) 743-3406

San Antonio
St. Luke's Lutheran Hospital
P.O. Box 29100 (Zip: 78229-0100)
(512) 692-8768

UTAH

Salt Lake City
University of Utah Medical Center
50 N. Medical Dr. (Zip: 84132)
(801) 581-2700

VERMONT

Burlington
Medical Center Hospital of Vermont
Colchester Ave. (Zip: 05404)
(802) 656-5555

VIRGINIA

Charlottesville
University of Virginia Health Sciences Center
(Zip: 22908)
(804) 924-BURN (-2876)

Norfolk
Sentara Norfolk General Hospital
600 Gresham Dr. (Zip: 23507)
(804) 628-3117

Richmond
Medical College of Virginia/Virginia Commonwealth
    University
Box 7, MCV Station (Zip: 23298)
(804) 786-9240

St. Mary's Hospital
5801 Bremo Rd. (Zip: 23226)
(804) 285-2011 Pager 486

WASHINGTON

Seattle
Harborview Medical Center
325 Ninth Ave. (Zip: 98104)
(206) 284-BURN (-2876)

Spokane
Sacred Heart Medical Center
W. 101 8th Ave. TAF C9 (Zip: 99204)
(509) 455-4644

Tacoma
St. Joseph Hospital and Health Care Center
1718 So I St. (Zip: 98405)
(206) 591-6677

WEST VIRGINIA

Huntington
Cabell Huntington Hospital
1340 Hal Greer Blvd. (Zip: 25701)
(304) 526-2390

WISCONSIN

Madison
University of Wisconsin Hospital and Clinics
600 Highland Ave. (Zip: 53792)
(608) 263-1490

Milwaukee
St. Mary's Regional Burn Center
2323 N. Lake Dr. (Zip: 53201)
(414) 225-8000

Canada

ALBERTA

Calgary
Foothills Hospital
1403 29 St. NW (Code: T2N 2T9)
(403) 270-4922

Edmonton
University of Alberta Hospital
8440 112th St. (Code: T6G 2B7)
(403) 492-6149

BRITISH COLUMBIA

Vancouver
Vancouver General Hospital
855 W. 12th Ave. (Code: V5Z 1M9)
(604) 875-4030

MANITOBA

Winnipeg
Health Sciences Center
820 Sherbrook St. (Code: R3A 1R9)
(204) 787-3775

Winnipeg Children's Hospital
840 Sherbrook St. (Code: R3A 1S1)
(204) 787-4785

NEW BRUNSWICK

Moncton
The Moncton Hospital
135 MacBeath Ave. (Code: E1C 6Z8)
(506) 857-5227

NOVA SCOTIA

Halifax
Victoria General Hospital
1278 Tower Rd. (Code: B3H 2Y9)
(902) 428-2527

Izaak Walton Killam Children's Hospital
P.O. Box 3070 (Code: B3J 3G9)
(902) 428-8352

ONTARIO

Hamilton
Hamilton General Hospital
237 Barton St. East (Code: L8I 2X2)
(416) 527-0271, ext. 6350

Kingston
Hotel Dieu Hospital (Code: K7L 5G2)
(613) 544-3310, ext. 2461

London
Victoria Hospital
375 South St. (Code: N6A 4G5)
(519) 685-8500, ext. 5735

Ottawa
Children's Hospital of Eastern Ontario
401 Smyth Rd. (Code: K1H 8L1)
(613) 737-7600

Scarborough
Scarborough General Hospital
(Code: M1P 2V5)
(416) 438-2911

Toronto
The Hospital for Sick Children
555 University Ave. (Code M5G 1X8)
(416) 598-6932

Wellesley Hospital
160 Wellesley St. East (Code: M4Y 1J3)
(416) 926-7021

Windsor
Metropolitan General Hospital
1995 Lens Ave. (Code: N8W 1L9)
(519) 254-1661

QUEBEC

Montreal
Montreal Children's Hospital
2300 Tupper St. (Code: H3H 1P3)
(514) 934-4400

SASKATCHEWAN

Saskatoon
Royal University Hospital
(Code: S7N 0X0)
(306) 966-1957

SKIN BANKS
United States

ARIZONA

Phoenix
Maricopa Medical Center
2601 E. Roosevelt St. (Zip: 85008)
(602) 267-5637

CALIFORNIA

San Diego
San Diego Regional Tissue Bank
7606 Miramar Rd., #7400 (Zip: 92126)
(619) 578-8010

UCSD Regional Tissue Bank
225 Dickinson St. (Zip: 92103)
(619) 294-6034

Torrance
Southern California Tissue Bank
381 Van Ness Ave., Suite 1502-03 (Zip: 90501)
(213) 548-5935

COLORADO

Denver
University of Colorado Health Sciences
   Center Skin Bank
4200 E. Ninth Ave., Box B211 (Zip: 80262)
(303) 270-4505

CONNECTICUT

New Haven
Yale University Skin Bank
333 Cedar St. (Zip: 06510)
(203) 785-2575

FLORIDA

Miami
University of Miami Tissue Bank
P.O. Box 16960 (Zip: 33101)
(305) 547-6786

ILLINOIS

Chicago
Cook County Hospital Skin Bank
700 S. Wood St. (Zip: 60612)
(312) 633-6570

University of Chicago Skin Bank
5841 S. Maryland Ave. (Zip: 60637)
(312) 702-6302

INDIANA

Fort Wayne
American Red Cross
1212 E. California Rd. (Zip: 46825)
(219) 480-8267

Indianapolis
Central Indiana Regional Blood Center and Tissue Bank
3450 N. Meridian St. (Zip: 46208)
(317) 927-1692

IOWA

Iowa City
University of Iowa Burn Center
8322 John Colloton Pavilion (Zip: 52242)
(319) 356-3221

KANSAS

Kansas City
University of Kansas Medical Center
39th St. and Rainbow Blvd. (Zip: 66103)
(913) 588-6540

KENTUCKY

Louisville
University of Louisville Skin Bank
305 W. Broadway (Zip: 40202)
(800) 525-3456

MARYLAND

Baltimore
Maryland Tissue Bank
Hospital Box 98
22 S. Greene St. (Zip: 21201)
(301) 328-3626

MASSACHUSETTS

Boston
Skin Bank, Shriners Burns Institute
51 Blossom St. (Zip: 02114)
(617) 722-3000

MICHIGAN

Ann Arbor
University of Michigan Hospitals' Skin Bank
1500 E. Medical Center Dr. (Zip: 48109-0033)
(313) 936-9673

MINNESOTA

Minneapolis
Hennepin County Medical Center Regional Tissue Bank
701 Park Ave. (Zip: 55415)
(612) 347-2810

St. Paul
American Red Cross Transplantation Services
100 S. Robert St. (Zip: 55107)
(800) 247-4273

NEW YORK

New York
New York Firefighters Skin Bank at New York Hospital
525 E. 68th St. (Zip: 10021)
(212) 746-5010

NORTH CAROLINA

Winston-Salem
North Carolina Baptist Hospital Skin Bank
300 S. Hawthorne Rd. (Zip: 27103)
(919) 748-4541

OHIO

Akron
Children's Hospital Medical Center Skin Bank
281 Locust St., Room 560 (Zip: 44308)
(216) 379-8200

Cincinnati
Ohio Valley Tissue and Skin Center
2939 Vernon Place (Zip: 45219)
(513) 558-4361

Dayton
Dayton Regional Tissue Bank
349 S. Main St. (Zip: 45402)
(513) 223-6192, ext. 3588

OREGON

Portland
Oregon Tissue Bank
Emanuel Hospital and Health Center
2801 N. Gantenbein Ave. (Zip: 97227)
(503) 280-4932

PENNSYLVANIA

Exton
Keystone Skin Bank
71 W. Uwchlan Ave., Suite 120 (Zip: 19341)
(215) 594-2172

TENNESSEE

Memphis
Regional Skin Bank
877 Jefferson Ave. (Zip: 38104)
(901) 575-8313

TEXAS

Dallas
Transplant Services
University of Texas Southwestern Medical Center
5323 Harry Hines Blvd. (Zip: 75218)
(214) 688-2609

Fort Sam Houston
U.S. Army Institute of Surgical Research
(Zip: 78234-5012)
(512) 221-2720

Galveston
Galveston Burn Services Skin Bank
610 Texas Ave. (Zip: 77550)
(409) 770-6731

UTAH

Salt Lake City
Intermountain Skin Bank
University of Utah Health Sciences Center
Dept. of Surgery, 3B-306 (Zip: 84132)
(801) 581-3595

VIRGINIA

Virginia Beach
LifeNet Tissue Services
5809 Ward Court (Zip: 23455)
(800) 847-7831

WASHINGTON

Seattle
Northwest Tissue Center
921 Terry Ave (Zip: 98104)
(206) 292-1879 (9 a.m.-5 p.m.)
(206) 292-6525 (after 5 p.m.)

Canada

ALBERTA

Calgary
Foothills Hospital
1403 29th St. NW (Code: T2N 2T8)
(403) 283-3853

Edmonton
Firefighters Burn Unit Skin Bank
Canadian Red Cross Bldg.
University of Alberta (Code: T6G 2B7)
(403) 431-0202, ext. 260

BRITISH COLUMBIA

Vancouver
Vancouver General Hospital Tissue Bank
855 W. 12th Ave. (Code: V5Z 1M9)
(604) 873-9333

NOVA SCOTIA

Halifax
Nova Scotia Firefighters Burn Treatment
  Society Skin Bank
Victoria General Hospital
1278 Tower Rd. (Code: B3H 2Y9)
(904) 428-2525

App. 20: Poison Control Centers

Centers in boldface have a 24-hour separate staff, and those that also have an asterisk (*) meet the American Association of Poison Control Centers' criteria for certification. Centers in lightface lack those qualifications but handle a minimum of 2000 information calls and 500 actual human exposures annually, except in areas where the population is too small to produce that number of calls.

United States

ALABAMA

Birmingham
The Children's Hospital of Alabama Regional Poison Control Center*
(800) 292-6678 (Alabama only); (205) 933-4050; (205) 939-9201; (205) 939-9202

Tuscaloosa
Alabama Poison Control System, Inc.*
(800) 462-0800 (Alabama only); (205) 345-0600

ALASKA

Anchorage
Anchorage Poison Center, Providence Hospital
(800) 478-3193 (Alaska only); (907) 261-3193

ARIZONA

Phoenix
Samaritan Regional Poison Center*, Good Samaritan Medical Center
(602) 253-3334

Tucson
Arizona Poison and Drug Information Center*, University of Arizona, Arizona Health Sciences Center
(800) 362-0101 (Arizona only); (602) 626-6016

ARKANSAS

Little Rock
Arkansas Poison and Drug Information Center, University of Arkansas for Medical Sciences, College of Pharmacy
(800) 482-8948 (MDs and hospitals, Arkansas only); (501) 661-6161; (501) 666-5532 (MDs and hospitals)

CALIFORNIA

Fresno
Fresno Regional Poison Control Center*, Fresno Community Hospital and Medical Center
(800) 346-5922 (Fresno, Kern, Kings, Madera, Mariposa, Merced, and Tulare counties only); (209) 445-1222

Los Angeles
Los Angeles County Regional Poison Control Center*
(800) 777-6476 (Los Angeles, Santa Barbara, and Ventura counties only); (800) 825-2722 (MDs and hospitals; California only); (213) 484-5151; (213) 664-2121 (MDs and hospitals)

Orange
UC Irvine Regional Poison Center*, University of California, Irvine, Medical Center
(800) 544-4404 (Inyo, Mono, Orange, Riverside, and San Bernardino counties only); (714) 634-5988; (714) 634-6665 (hazardous materials hotline)

Sacramento
UC Davis Medical Center Regional Poison Control Center*
(800) 342-9293 (northern California only); (916) 734-3692

San Diego
San Diego Regional Poison Center*, University of California, San Diego, Medical Center
(800) 876-4766 (Imperial and San Diego counties only); (619) 543-6000

San Francisco
San Francisco Bay Area Regional Poison Control Center*, San Francisco General Hospital
(800) 523-2222 (Alameda, Contra Costa, Del Norte, Humboldt, Marin, Mendocino, Napa, San Francisco, San Mateo, and Sonoma counties only); (415) 476-6600

San Jose
Santa Clara Valley Medical Center, Regional Poison Control Center
(800) 662-9886 (Monterey, San Benito, San Luis Obispo, Santa Clara, and Santa Cruz counties only); (408) 299-5112

COLORADO

Denver
Rocky Mountain Poison and Drug Center*
(800) 332-3073 (Colorado only); (800) 525-5042 (Montana only); (800) 446-6179 (Las Vegas, Nev., only); (303) 629-1123

CONNECTICUT

Farmington
Connecticut Poison Control Center, University of Connecticut Health Center
(800) 343-2722 (Connecticut only); (203) 679-3473 (administration); (203) 679-4346 (TDD)

DELAWARE

Wilmington
Poison Information Center, Medical Center of Delaware, Wilmington Hospital
(302) 655-3389

DISTRICT OF COLUMBIA

Washington
National Capital Poison Center*, Georgetown
University Hospital
(202) 625-3333; (202) 784-4660 (TTY)

FLORIDA

Jacksonville
St. Vincent's Medical Center, Poison Control Center
(904) 387-7500; (904) 387-7499 (TDD)

Tallahassee
Tallahassee Memorial Regional Medical Center
(904) 681-5411

Tampa
**Florida Poison Information Center at Tampa
General Hospital***
(800) 282-3171 (Florida only); (813) 253-4444

GEORGIA

Atlanta
Georgia Regional Poison Control Center*, Grady
Memorial Hospital
(800) 282-5846 (Georgia only); (404) 589-4400; (404)
525-3323 (TTY)

Macon
Medical Center of Central Georgia Poison Control Center
(912) 744-1427; 744-1146; 744-1000

Savannah
Savannah Regional Poison Control Center, Dept. of
Emergency Medicine, Memorial Medical Center
(912) 355-5228 (southeastern Georgia and
southwestern South Carolina only)

Interstate Centers
Palmetto Poison Center, Columbia, S.C.
(800) 922-1117 (central Savannah River area of
Georgia only)

HAWAII

Honolulu
Hawaii Poison Center, Kapiolani Medical Center for
Women and Children
(800) 362-3585 (outer islands of Hawaii only); (800)
362-3586; (808) 941-4411

IDAHO

Boise
Idaho Poison Center, St. Alphonsus Regional
Medical Center
(800) 632-8000 (Idaho only); (208) 378-2707

Interstate Centers
Spokane Poison Center, Spokane, Wash.
(800) 572-5842 (northern Idaho only)

ILLINOIS

Chicago
**Chicago & Northeastern Illinois Regional Poison
Control Center,** Rush-Presbyterian-St. Luke's
Medical Center
(800) 942-5969 (northeastern Illinois only); (312) 942-
5969

Springfield
**Central and Southern Illinois Regional Poison
Resource Center,** St. John's Hospital
(800) 252-2022 (Illinois only); (217) 753-3330

Interstate Centers
**Cardinal Glennon Children's Hospital Regional
Poison Center*,** St. Louis, Mo.
(800) 366-8888 (western Illinois only)

INDIANA

Indianapolis
Indiana Poison Center*, Methodist Hospital of
Indiana
(800) 382-9097 (Indiana only); (317) 929-2323; (317)
929-2336 (TTY)

Interstate Centers
**Kentucky Regional Poison Center of Kosair
Children's Hospital*,** Louisville, Ky.
(502) 589-8222 (southern Indiana only)

IOWA

Des Moines
Variety Club Poison and Drug Information Center,
Iowa Methodist Medical Center
(800) 362-2327 (Iowa only); (515) 283-6254

Iowa City
Poison Control Center, University of Iowa Hospitals
and Clinics
(800) 272-6477 (Iowa only); (319) 356-2922

Interstate Centers
McKennan Hospital Poison Center, Sioux Falls, S.D.
(800) 843-0505

The Poison Control Center*, Omaha, Neb.
(800) 955-9119

KANSAS

Kansas City
Mid-America Poison Control Center, University of
Kansas Medical Center
(800) 332-6633 (Kansas only); (913) 588-6633

Wichita
HCA Wesley Medical Center
(316) 688-2277

Interstate Centers
Cardinal Glennon Children's Hospital Regional Poison Center*, St. Louis, Mo.
(800) 366–8888 (Topeka only)

KENTUCKY

Louisville
Kentucky Regional Poison Center of Kosair Children's Hospital*
(800) 722–5725 (Kentucky only); (502) 589–8222 (metropolitan Louisville and southern Indiana only)

Interstate Centers
Knoxville Poison Control Center, Knoxville, Tenn.
(615) 544–9400 (southern Kentucky only)

MAINE

Portland
Maine Poison Control Center at Maine Medical Center
(800) 442–6305 (Maine only); (207) 871–2381 (Emergency Room)

MARYLAND

Baltimore
Maryland Poison Center*, University of Maryland School of Pharmacy
(800) 492–2414 (Maryland only); (301) 528–7701

MASSACHUSETTS

Boston
Massachusetts Poison Control System*
(800) 682–9211 (Massachusetts only); (617) 232–2120

MICHIGAN

Detroit
Poison Control Center*, Children's Hospital of Michigan
(313) 745–5711

Grand Rapids
Blodgett Regional Poison Center*, Blodgett Memorial Medical Center
(800) 632–2727 (517, 616, and 906 area codes only); (800) 356–3232 (TTY); (616) 774–2963

Kalamazoo
Bronson Poison Center, Bronson Methodist Hospital
(800) 442–4112 (Michigan only); (616) 341–6409

Interstate Centers
Poison Information Center of Northwest Ohio, Toledo, Ohio
(800) 589–3897 (southeastern Michigan only)

MINNESOTA

Minneapolis
Hennepin Regional Poison Center*, Hennepin County Medical Center
(612) 347–3141; 337–7474 (TTY)

St. Paul
Minnesota Regional Poison Center*, St. Paul-Ramsey Medical Center
(800) 222–1222 (Minnesota only); (612) 221–2113

Interstate Centers
McKennan Hospital Poison Center, Sioux Falls, S.D.
(800) 843–0505

North Dakota Poison Information Center, Fargo, N.D.
(701) 234–5575 (northwestern Minnesota only–call collect)

St. Luke's Midland Regional Medical Center, Poison Control Center, Aberdeen, S.D.
(800) 592–1889

MISSISSIPPI

Jackson
Mississippi Regional Poison Control Center, University Medical Center
(601) 354–7660

MISSOURI

Kansas City
Children's Mercy Hospital
(816) 234–3000

St. Louis
Cardinal Glennon Children's Hospital Regional Poison Center*
(800) 366–8888 (Missouri, western Illinois, and Topeka, Kan.); (800) 392–9111 (Missouri only); (314) 772–5200; (314) 577–5336 (TTY)

Interstate Centers
The Poison Control Center*, Omaha, Neb.
(800) 955–9119

MONTANA

Interstate Centers
Rocky Mountain Poison and Drug Center*, Denver, Colo.
(800) 525–5042

Spokane Poison Center, Spokane, Wash.
(800) 572–5842 (western Montana only)

NEBRASKA

Omaha
The Poison Center*, Children's Memorial Hospital
(800) 955–9119 (Nebraska, Iowa, Missouri, South Dakota, and Wyoming); (402) 390–5555

Interstate Centers
McKennan Hospital Poison Center, Sioux Falls, S.D.
(800) 843–0505

Poison Control Centers *(Continued)*

NEVADA

Interstate Centers
Rocky Mountain Poison and Drug Center*,
Denver, Colo.
(800) 446-6179 (Las Vegas only)

NEW HAMPSHIRE

Lebanon
New Hampshire Poison Information Center,
Dartmouth Hitchcock Memorial Hospital
(800) 562-8236 (New Hampshire only); (603) 650-5000

NEW JERSEY

Newark
**New Jersey Poison Information and Education
System*,** Newark Beth Israel Medical Center
(800) 962-1253 (New Jersey only); (201) 923-0764;
(201) 926-8008 (TTY)

NEW MEXICO

Albuquerque
**New Mexico Poison and Drug Information
Center*,** University of New Mexico
(800) 432-6866 (New Mexico only); (505) 843-2551

Interstate Centers
El Paso Poison Control Center, El Paso, Tex.
(915) 533-1244 (southern New Mexico only)

NEW YORK

Buffalo
Western New York Regional Poison Control Center at
Children's Hospital of Buffalo
(800) 888-7655 (New York only); (716) 878-7654;
878-7655

East Meadow
Long Island Regional Poison Control Center*,
Nassau County Medical Center
(516) 542-2323; 542-2324; 542-2325; 542-3813; 747-
3323 (TTY)

New York
New York City Poison Control Center*
(212) 340-4494; 764-7667

Nyack
Hudson Valley Regional Poison Center, Nyack
Hospital
(800) 336-6997 (New York only); (914) 353-1000

Rochester
**Life Line/Finger Lakes Regional Poison Control
Center,** University of Rochester Medical Center
(800) 333-0542 (Ontario and Wayne counties only);
(716) 275-5151; 275-2700 (TTY)

Syracuse
Central New York Poison Control Center,
University Hospital at Syracuse
(800) 252-5655 (New York only); (315) 476-4766

Interstate Centers
Northwest Regional Poison Center, Erie, Pa.
(800) 822-3232 (southwestern New York only)

Vermont Poison Center, Burlington, Vt.
(802) 658-3456 (bordering Vermont only)

NORTH CAROLINA

Asheville
Western N.C. Poison Control Center, Memorial
Mission Hospital
(800) 542-4225 (North Carolina only); (704) 255-4490

Charlotte
Mercy Hospital Poison Control Center
(704) 379-5827

Durham
**Duke University Regional Poison Control
Center,** Duke University Medical Center
(800) 672-1697 (North Carolina only); (919) 684-8111

Greensboro
**Triad Poison Center at Moses H. Cone Memorial
Hospital**
(800) 722-2222 (Alamance, Forsyth, Guilford,
Rockingham, and Randolph counties only); (919)
379-4105

Hickory
Catawba Memorial Hospital, Poison Control Center
(704) 322-6649

NORTH DAKOTA

Fargo
North Dakota Poison Information Center, St. Luke's
Hospitals
(800) 732-2200 (North Dakota only); (701) 234-5575
(local northwestern Minnesota only-call collect)

Interstate Centers
St. Luke's Midland Regional Medical Center, Poison
Control Center, Aberdeen, S.D.
(800) 592-1889

OHIO

Akron
Akron Regional Poison Control Center, Children's
Hospital Medical Center of Akron
(800) 362-9922 (Ohio only); (216) 379-8562; (216)
379-8446 (TTY)

2441

Cincinnati
**Regional Poison Control System and Drug &
Poison Information Center***, University of
Cincinnati College of Medicine
(800) 872–5111 (Ohio only); (513) 558–5111

Cleveland
Greater Cleveland Poison Control Center
(216) 231–4455

Columbus
Central Ohio Poison Center*, Children's Hospital
(800) 682–7625 (Ohio only); (614) 228–1323; (614)
228–2272 (TTY)

Dayton
Western Ohio Poison and Drug Information Center,
Children's Medical Center
(800) 762–0727 (Ohio only); (513) 222–2227

Lorain
Poison Control Center of Lorain County, Lorain
Community Hospital
(800) 821–8972 (Ohio only); (216) 282–2220

Toledo
Poison Information Center of Northwest Ohio,
Medical College of Ohio Hospital
(800) 589–3897 (northwestern Ohio and southeastern
Michigan only); (419) 381–3897

Youngstown
Mahoning Valley Poison Center, St. Elizabeth
Hospital Medical Center
(800) 426–2348 (Ohio, and Mercer and Lawrence
counties in Pennsylvania, only); (216) 746–2222;
(216) 746–5510 (TTY)

Interstate Centers
Northwest Regional Poison Center, Erie, Pa.
(800) 822–3232 (northeastern Ohio only)

OKLAHOMA

Oklahoma City
Oklahoma Poison Control Center, Children's Hospital
of Oklahoma
(800) 522–4611 (Oklahoma only); (405) 271–5454

OREGON

Portland
Oregon Poison Center*, Oregon Health Sciences
University
(800) 452–7165 (Oregon only); (503) 494–8968

Interstate Centers
Spokane Poison Center, Spokane, Wash.
(800) 572–5842 (northwestern Oregon only)

PENNSYLVANIA

Allentown
Lehigh Valley Poison Center, Allentown Hospital
(215) 433–2311

Danville
Susquehanna Poison Center, Geisinger Medical
Center
(800) 352–7001 (Pennsylvania only)

Erie
Northwest Regional Poison Center, Saint Vincent
Health Center
(800) 822–3232 (northwestern Pennsylvania,
northeastern Ohio, and southwestern New York
only); (814) 452–3232

Hershey
Central Pennsylvania Poison Center, University
Hospital, Milton S. Hershey Medical Center
(800) 521–6110; (717) 531–6111; (717) 531–6039

Philadelphia
**The Poison Control Center (Serving the Greater
Philadelphia Metropolitan Area)***
(215) 386–2100; (215) 590–2003

Pittsburgh
Pittsburgh Poison Center*, Children's Hospital of
Pittsburgh
(412) 681–6669

Interstate Centers
Mahoning Valley Poison Center, Youngstown, Ohio
(800) 426–2348 (Lawrence and Mercer counties only)

RHODE ISLAND

Providence
Rhode Island Poison Center*, Rhode Island Hospital
(401) 277–5727

SOUTH CAROLINA

Columbia
Palmetto Poison Center, University of South Carolina,
College of Pharmacy
(800) 922–1117 (South Carolina and central Savannah
River area of Georgia only); (803) 765–7359

Interstate Centers
Savannah Regional Poison Control Center, Savannah,
Ga.
(912) 355–5228 (southwestern South Carolina only)

SOUTH DAKOTA

Aberdeen
St. Luke's Midland Regional Medical Center, Poison
Control Center
(800) 592–1889 (South Dakota, Minnesota, North
Dakota, and Wyoming only); (605) 622–5678

Sioux Falls
McKennan Hospital Poison Center
(800) 952–0123 (South Dakota only); (800) 843–0505
  (Iowa, Minnesota, and Nebraska only); (605) 336–3894

Interstate Centers
The Poison Control Center*, Omaha, Neb.
(800) 955–9119

TENNESSEE

Knoxville
Knoxville Poison Control Center, University of
  Tennessee Memorial Research Center and Hospital
(615) 544–9400 (eastern Tennessee and southern
  Kentucky only)

Memphis
Southern Poison Center, Inc.
(901) 528–6048; (901) 522–5985 (administration)

Nashville
**Middle Tennessee Regional Poison/Clinical
  Toxicology Center**
(800) 288–9999 (mid-Tennessee only); (615) 322–6435
  (Nashville and adjacent counties only)

TEXAS

Dallas
North Texas Poison Center*, Parkland Hospital
(800) 441–0040 (Texas only); (214) 590–5000

El Paso
El Paso Poison Control Center, R.E. Thomason
  General Hospital
(915) 533–1244 (southwestern Texas and southern
  New Mexico only)

Galveston
Texas State Poison Control Center*, University of
  Texas Medical Branch
(800) 392–8548 (MDs and ambulance personnel; Texas
  only); (409) 772–1420; (713) 654–1701 (Houston only)

UTAH

Salt Lake City
Intermountain Regional Poison Control Center*
(800) 456–7707 (Utah only); (801) 581–2151

VERMONT

Burlington
Vermont Poison Center, Medical Center Hospital of
  Vermont
(802) 658–3456 (Vermont and bordering New York
  only); 656–2721 (education programs)

VIRGINIA

Charlottesville
Blue Ridge Poison Center*, University of Virginia
  Health Sciences Center, Blue Ridge Hospital
(800) 451–1428 (Virginia, West Virginia, North
  Carolina, District of Columbia, Tennessee, and
  Maryland); (804) 924–5543

Richmond
Virginia Poison Center, Virginia Commonwealth
  University
(800) 552–6337 (Virginia only); (804) 786–9123

WASHINGTON

Seattle
Seattle Poison Center, Children's Hospital and
  Medical Center
(800) 732–6985 (Washington only); (206) 526–2121;
  (206) 526–2223 (TTY)

Spokane
Spokane Poison Center, St. Luke's Hospital
(800) 572–5842 (eastern Washington, northern Idaho,
  western Montana, and northwestern Oregon only);
  (509) 747–1077

Tacoma
Mary Bridge Poison Center, Mary Bridge
  Children's Hospital
(800) 542–6319 (Washington only); (206) 594–1414

Yakima
Central Washington Poison Center, Yakima Valley
  Memorial Hospital
(800 572-9176 (Washington only); (509) 248–4400

WEST VIRGINIA

Charleston
West Virginia Poison Center*, West Virginia
  University Health Sciences Center, Charleston
  Division
(800) 642–3625 (West Virginia only); (304) 348–4211

WISCONSIN

Green Bay
Green Bay Poison Control Center, St. Vincent Hospital
(414) 433–8100

Madison
**University of Wisconsin Hospital Regional
  Poison Control Center**
(608) 262–3702

Milwaukee
The Poison Center, Children's Hospital of Wisconsin
(414) 266–2222

WYOMING

Interstate Centers
The Poison Control Center*, Omaha, Neb.
(800) 955-9119

St. Luke's Midland Regional Medical Center, Poison
Control Center, Aberdeen, S.D.
(800) 592-1889

Canada

ALBERTA

Poison treatment centres are found in every active
treatment hospital.

Poison Information Centres
Calgary
Calgary General Hospital
(403) 262-5982

Foothills General Hospital, Poison and Drug
Information Services
(800) 332-1414 (Alberta only); (403) 670-1414

Edmonton
Royal Alexandra Hospital
(403) 477-4444

University of Alberta Hospital
(403) 432-8432

BRITISH COLUMBIA

Poisoning treatment available in every active treatment
hospital emergency service.

Vancouver
B.C. Drug and Poison Information Centre, St. Paul's
Hospital
(604) 682-5050

Victoria
Emergency Department, Royal Jubilee Hospital
(604) 595-9212

MANITOBA

Poisoning treatment available in every active treatment
hospital emergency service.

Winnipeg
Provincial Poison Information Centre, Children's
Hospital Health Sciences Centre
(204) 787-2591

NEW BRUNSWICK

Poison treatment centres are found in most active
treatment hospital emergency services.

Bathurst
Chaleur General Hospital
(906) 546-4666

Campbellton
Hôtel-Dieu St. Joseph
(506) 753-5212

Edmundston
Hôtel-Dieu St. Joseph
(506) 735-7384

Fredericton
Dr. Everett Chalmers Hospital
(506) 452-5400

Moncton
Moncton City Hospital
(506) 388-3005

Saint John
Saint John General Hospital, Central Division
(506) 648-7111

NEWFOUNDLAND AND LABRADOR

St. John's
Provincial Poison Control Centre, Dr. Charles A.
Janeway Child Health Centre
(709) 722-1110

Corner Brook
Western Memorial Hospital
(709) 634-7121

Gander
James Paton Memorial Hospital
(709) 651-2500

Grand Falls
Central Newfoundland Hospital
(709) 489-6661

Labrador City
Capt. Wm. Jackman Memorial Hospital
(709) 944-2632

St. Anthony
Charles S. Curtis Memorial Hospital (International
Grenfell Association)
(709) 454-3333

NORTHWEST TERRITORIES

Fort Smith
Fort Smith Health Centre
(403) 872-2713

Frobisher Bay
Baffin Regional Hospital
(819) 979-5231

Poison Control Centers *(Continued)*

Hay River
H. H. Williams Memorial Hospital
(403) 874-6512

Inuvik
Inuvik General Hospital
(403) 979-2955

Yellowknife
Stanton Yellowknife Hospital
(403) 920-4111

NOVA SCOTIA

Main Centre
Halifax
Izaak Walton Killam Hospital for Children, Poison
  Control Centre
(902) 428-8161

Satellite Centres
Amherst
Highland View Regional Hospital
(902) 667-3361, ext. 145

Antigonish
St. Martha's Hospital
(902) 863-2830, ext. 122

Bridgewater
Dawson Memorial Hospital
(902) 543-4603

Dartmouth
Dartmouth General Hospital
(902) 469-9520, ext. 238

Halifax
Victoria General Hospital
(902) 428-2043

Kentville
Valley Health Services Association
(902) 678-7381, ext. 215

New Glasgow
Aberdeen Hospital
(902) 752-8311

Sydney
Sydney City Hospital
(902) 539-6400, ext. 118

Yarmouth
Yarmouth Regional Hospital
(902) 742-3541, ext. 111

ONTARIO

Main Centres
Ottawa
Children's Hospital of Eastern Ontario
(800) 267-1373 (area code 807, call collect); (613) 737-
  1100

Toronto
Hospital for Sick Children
(800) 268-9017 (area code 807, call collect); (416) 598-
  5900

Other Centres
Brantford
Brantford General Hospital
(519) 752-7871

Guelph
St. Joseph's Hospital Emergency Department
(519) 824-2620, ext. 208

Kingston
Kingston General Hospital
(613) 547-2001

Kirkland Lake
Kirkland and District Hospital
(705) 567-5251

Kitchener
Kitchener-Waterloo Hospital
(519) 749-4220

St. Mary's General Hospital
(519) 744-3311

London
Victoria Hospital, South St. Campus
(519) 432-5241

St. Catharines
St. Catharines General Hospital
(416) 684-7271, ext. 461

Sarnia
Sarnia General Hospital
(519) 336-6311

St. Joseph's Hospital
(519) 336-3111

Sault Ste. Marie
Plummer Memorial Public Hospital
(705) 254-5161

Simcoe
Norfolk General Hospital
(519) 426-0750

Poison Control Centers *(Continued)*

Sudbury
Sudbury General Hospital
(705) 674-3636

Thunder Bay
McKellar General Hospital
(807) 623-5561

Port Arthur General Hospital
(807) 344-6621

Toronto
East General and Orthopaedic Hospital
(416) 461-8272, ext. 200

Windsor
Hôtel-Dieu de St. Joseph
(519) 973-4400

PRINCE EDWARD ISLAND

Charlottetown
Queen Elizabeth Hospital
(902) 566-6250

Summerside
Prince County Hospital
(902) 436-9131

QUEBEC

Poison treatment centres are found in every active
treatment hospital emergency service or Centre Local
de Santé Communautaire.

Main Centres
Montreal
Hôpital Sainte-Justine
(514) 731-4931

Montreal Children's Hospital
(514) 937-8511

Québec City
Centre Hospitalier de l'Université Laval
(800) 463-5090; (418) 656-8090

Provincial Poison Control Program
Québec City
Centre de Toxicologie de Québec
Centre Hospitalier de l'Université Laval
(418) 656-8326

SASKATCHEWAN

Poison treatment centres are found in most active
treatment hospital emergency services.

Main Centres
Regina
Regina General Hospital, Poison Control Centre
(306) 359-4545

Saskatoon
Saskatoon University Hospital, Poison Control Center
(306) 343-3323

YUKON TERRITORY

Whitehorse
Whitehorse General Hospital, Emergency Department
(403) 668-9444

SOURCES: U.S. information provided courtesy of Emergency Medicine magazine, Cahners Publishing Co., New
York. Canadian information provided courtesy of Childrens' Hospital of Eastern Ontario, Ottawa, Ontario, and
Health and Welfare Canada, Health Protection Branch, Ottawa, Ontario.

App. 21: AIDS-Related Organizations And Hotlines

United States

AIDS Action Council
2033 M St. NW, Suite 802, Washington, DC 20036; (202) 293-2886

American Association for Marriage and Family Therapy
1717 K St. NW, Suite 407, Washington, DC 20006; (202) 429-1825

American Association of Physicians for Human Rights
2940 16th St., #105, San Francisco, CA 94103; (415) 255-4547

American Civil Liberties Union Foundation, AIDS and Civil Liberties Project
132 W. 43rd St., New York, NY 10036; (212) 944-9800

American Foundation for AIDS Research
733 3rd Ave., 12th fl., New York, NY 10017-3204; (212) 682-7440

American Red Cross
HIV/AIDS Education Program
1709 New York Ave. NW, #208, Washington, DC 20006; (202) 639-3223

Association for Retarded Citizens of the United States
HIV Prevention Project
500 E. Border St., Suite 300, Arlington, TX 76010; (800) 433-5255; (817) 261-6003; (817) 277-0553 (TTY/TDD)

Center for Attitudinal Healing
19 Main St., Tiburon, CA 94920; (415) 435-5022

Computerized AIDS Information Network
1213 N. Highland Ave., Los Angeles, CA 90038; (213) 464-7400

Gay Men's Health Crisis
129 W. 20th St., New York, NY 10011; (212) 807-6655

Lambda Legal Defense and Education Fund
666 Broadway, New York, NY 10012; (212) 995-8585

Mothers of AIDS Patients
P.O. Box 1763, Lomita, CA 90717; (213) 542-3019; 541-3134

National AIDS Minority Information and Education Program
Howard University, College of Allied Health Sciences
2139 Georgia Ave. NW, Suite 313, Washington, DC 20001; (202) 865-3720

National AIDS Support Center
1915 Rosina St., Santa Fe, NM 87501; (505) 986-8337

National Association of People With AIDS
1413 K St. NW, 10th fl., Washington, DC 20005; (800) 898-0414; (202) 898-0414

National Council of Churches AIDS Task Force
475 Riverside Dr., Room 350, New York, NY 10115; (212) 870-3871

National Foundation for Infectious Diseases
4733 Bethesda Ave., Suite 750, Bethesda, MD 20815; (301) 656-0003

National Gay and Lesbian Task Force
1734 14th St. NW, Washington, DC 20009-4309; (202) 332-6483

National Hemophilia Foundation
110 Greene St., New York, NY 10012; (800) 42-HANDI; (212) 219-8180

National Hospice Organization
1901 N. Moore St., Suite 901, Arlington, VA 22209; (800) 658-8898; (703) 243-5900

National Leadership Coalition on AIDS
1730 M St. NW, Suite 905, Washington, DC 20036; (202) 429-0930

National Lesbian and Gay Health Foundation
P.O. Box 65472, Washington, DC 20035; (202) 797-3578

National Native American AIDS Prevention Center
3515 Grand Ave., Suite 100, Oakland, CA 94610; (800) 283-2437; (415) 444-2051

New York Department of Health
AIDS Institute
Corning Tower, Room 359, 1315 Empire State Plaza, Albany, NY 12237-0684; (518) 473-7238; 486-1595

Pan American Health Organization
AIDS Program
525 23rd St. NW, Washington, DC 20037; (202) 861-4346

Project Inform
347 Delores St., #301, San Francisco, CA 94110; (800) 334-7422 — California only; (800) 822-7422; (415) 558-8669

San Francisco AIDS Foundation
25 Van Ness Ave., 6th fl., San Francisco, CA 94101-6182; (415) 864-5855; 861-3397

Sex Information and Education Council of the U.S.
130 W. 42nd St., Suite 2500, New York, NY 10036; (212) 819-9770

U.S. Conference of Mayors AIDS Program
1620 I St. NW, Washington, DC 20006; (202) 293-7330

U.S. Department of Health and Human Services
Public Health Service

CDC National AIDS Clearinghouse
P.O. Box 6003, Rockville, MD 20849-6003; (800) 458-5231

National AIDS Information and Education Program
Centers for Disease Control, 1600 Clifton Rd. NE, Atlanta, GA 30333; (404) 639-3311

AIDSLINE — National Library of Medicine
8600 Rockville Pike, Bethesda, MD 20894; (800) 638-8480; (301) 999-9999

National AIDS Demonstration Research Project
National Institute on Drug Abuse, 5600 Fishers Lane, Room 10-46, Rockville, MD 20857; (301) 443-3783

Canada

National AIDS Clearinghouse
Canadian Public Health Association, 400-1565 Carling Ave., Ottawa, ON K1Z 8R1; (613) 725-3769

ALBERTA

AIDS Calgary Awareness Association
300-1021 10th Ave. SW, Calgary, AB T2R 0B7; (403) 228-0198

Calgary Council on AIDS
c/o Calgary Health Services, P.O. Box 4016, Postal Station C, 320-17th Ave. SW, Calgary, AB T2T 5T1; (403) 228-7430

South Peace AIDS Council
Box 902, Grande Prairie, AB T8V 3Y1; (403) 538-3388

AIDS: A Positive Co-ordinated Response Society of Jasper
Box 1090, Jasper, AB T0E 1E0; (403) 852-3381

Lethbridge AIDS Connection Society
421, 515-7 St South, Lethbridge, AB T1J 2G8; (403) 328-8186

Central Alberta AIDS Network Society
4935-51 St., Red Deer, AB T4N 2A8; (403) 346-8858

AIDS Network of Edmonton Society
10704-108th St., 2nd fl., Edmonton, AB T5H 3A3; (403) 424-4767

Foothills AIDS Awareness Association
P.O. Box 758, Okotoks, AB T0L 1T0; (403) 938-4911

BRITISH COLUMBIA

Mid-Island AIDS Network
311 Fitzwilliam St., Room 4, Nanaimo, BC V9R 3A6; (604) 755-1034

AIDS Vancouver Island
304-733 Johnson St., Victoria, BC V8W 3C7; (604) 384-2366

AIDS Vancouver
Box 4991, Vancouver Main Post Office, Vancouver, BC V6B 4A6; (604) 687-5220

Vancouver PWA Society
1447 Hornby St., Vancouver, BC V6Z 1W8; (604) 683-3381

MANITOBA

Village Clinic
668 Corydon Ave., Winnipeg, MB R3M 0X7; (204) 453-0045

Body Positive Coalition of Manitoba
c/o Village Clinic, 668 Corydon Ave., Winnipeg, MB R3M 0X7; (204) 452-7704

NEW BRUNSWICK

SIDA Nouveau-Brunswick/AIDS New-Brunswick
65 Brunswick St., Fredericton, NB E3B 1G5; (506) 459-7518

SIDA-AIDS Moncton
427-100 Arden St., Moncton, NB E1C 4B7; (506) 859-9616

AIDS Saint John
116 Cobourg St., Saint John, NB E2L 3K1; (506) 652-AIDS

NEWFOUNDLAND

Newfoundland and Labrador AIDS Committee
Box 626, Station "C," St. John's, NF A1C 5K8; (709) 579-8656

AIDS-Related Organizations (*Continued*)

NOVA SCOTIA

AIDS Nova Scotia
206–5224 Blowers St., Halifax, NS B3J 1J7; (902) 425-4882

Nova Scotia PWA Coalition
2093 Gottingen St., Halifax, NS B3K 3B1; (902) 429-7922

ONTARIO

AIDS Committee of Thunder Bay
Box 3586, Thunder Bay, ON P7B 6E2; (807) 345-1516

ACCESS (AIDS Committee of Sudbury/Comité du SIDA de Sudbury)
23 Durham St., Sudbury, ON P3C 5E2; (705) 688-0505

AIDS Committee of Windsor
Box 7186, Windsor, ON N9C 3Z1; (519) 973-0222

AIDS Committee of London
343 Richmond St., Suite 301, London, ON N6A 3C2; (519) 434-1601

AIDS Committee of Cambridge Kitchener/Waterloo and Area
13–1601 River Rd. East, Kitchener, ON N2A 3Y4; (519) 748-5556

AIDS Committee of Guelph and Wellington County
202–73 Delhi St., Guelph, ON N1E 6L9; (519) 763-2255

AIDS Committee of Niagara
Box 158, 541 Glenridge Ave., St. Catharines, ON L2R 6S5; (416) 984-8684

Hamilton AIDS Network for Dialogue and Support (HANDS)
900–143 James St. South, Hamilton, ON L8P 3A1; (416) 528-0854

Kingston AIDS Project
Box 120, Kingston, ON K7L 4V6; (613) 545-3698

AIDS Committee of Ottawa/Comité du SIDA d'Ottawa
201–267 Dalhousie St., Ottawa, ON K1N 7E3; (613) 238-5014

AIDS Housing Group of Ottawa
101–44 Bayswater Ave., Ottawa, ON K1Y 4K3; (613) 729-3822

AIDS Committee of North Bay and Area
Box 494, North Bay, ON P1B 8J1; (705) 497-3560

Peterborough AIDS Resource Network
P.O. Box 1582, Peterborough, ON K9J 7H7; (705) 749-9110

AIDS Committee of Durham Region
22 Simcoe St. North, Oshawa, ON L1G 4R8; (416) 723-8201

AIDS Network of Superior Waters East Region (ANSWER)
P.O. Box 98, Wawa, ON P0S 1K0; (705) 856-1960

TORONTO AREA

AIDS Committee of Toronto
202–464 Yonge St., Toronto, ON M4Y 1W9; (416) 926-0063

Prostitute's Safe Sex Project
Box 1143, Station "F," Toronto, ON M4Y 2T8; (416) 964-0150

Casey House Hospice Inc.
9 Huntley St., Toronto, ON M4Y 2K8; (416) 962-7600

Toronto PWA Foundation
201B–464 Yonge St., Toronto, ON M4Y 1W9; (416) 925-7112

St. Stephen's Community House AIDS Education Program
91 Bellevue Ave., Toronto, ON M5T 2N8; (416) 323-1498

AIDS Action Now!
321–517 College St., Toronto, ON M6G 1A8; (416) 928-2206

Street Health AIDS Project
323 Dundas St. East, Toronto, ON M5A 2A2; (416) 863-1610

Anishnawbe Health Toronto
225 Queen St. East, Toronto, ON M5A 1S4; (416) 360-0486

Black Coalition for AIDS Prevention
103–597 Parliament St., Toronto, ON M4X 1W3; (416) 926-0122

Gay Asian AIDS Project
17 St. Joseph St., Suite 214, Toronto, ON M4Y 1S8; (416) 963-4300

The Works
277 Victoria St., 1st fl., Toronto, ON M5B 1W1; (416) 392-0520

Alliance for South Asian AIDS Prevention
320½ Bloor St. West, Toronto, ON M5S 1W1; (416) 966-2727

Community AIDS Treatment Information Exchange (CATIE)
324–517 College St., Toronto, ON M6G 1A8; (416) 944-1916

Youthlink-Inner City
151 Gerrard St. East, Toronto, ON M5A 2E4; (416) 922-3335

Gays and Lesbians of the First Nations (GLFN)
201 Church St., 2nd fl., Toronto, ON M5B 1Y7; (416) 324-8279

PRINCE EDWARD ISLAND

AIDS PEI
199 Grafton St., Suite 103, Charlottetown, PEI C1A 1L2; (902) 566-2437

QUEBEC

Comité SIDA aide Montréal (C-SAM)
3600, rue Hôtel-de-Ville, Montréal (QC) H2X 3B6; (514) 282-9888

Comité des personnes atteintes du VIH (CPAVIH)
3600, rue Hôtel-de-Ville, Montréal (QC) H2X 3B6; (514) 282-6673

CHRISCOQ
8170 blvd Gouin est, Montréal (QC) H1E 1B7

Bureau régional d'action SIDA
811 blvd St-Réné ouest, Pièce 700, Gatineau (QC) J8R 2S4; (819) 568-2727

Groupe d'action pour la prévention du SIDA dans la communauté haitienne (GAP-SIDA)
2577-A rue Jean-Talon est, Bureau 101, Montréal (QC) H2A 1T8; (514) 722-5655

Chez Ma Cousine
P.O. Box 325, Place du Parc, Montréal (QC) H2W 2N8; (514) 523-4457

Centre Pierre Hénault Inc.
1732, rue Orléans, Montréal (QC) H1W 3R3; (514) 522-3339

Mouvement d'information, d'éducation et d'entraide dans la lutte contre le SIDA (MIENS)
CP 723, Chicoutimi (QC) G7H 5E1; (418) 693-8983

Bureau local d'intervention traitant du SIDA (BLITS)
55, rue Monfette, Local 110, Victoriaville (QC) G6P 1J8; (819) 758-2662

Mouvement d'information et d'entraide dans la lutte contre le SIDA à Québec (MIELS-Québec)
575, boulevard St-Cyrille ouest, Québec (QC) G1S 1S6; (418) 687-4310

Intervention régionale et information sur le SIDA, (IRIS/Estrie)
CP 1766, Sherbrooke (QC) J1H 5N8; (819) 823-6704

SASKATCHEWAN

AIDS Saskatoon
Box 4062, Saskatoon, SK S7K 4E3; (306) 242-5005

PLWA Network of Saskatchewan
Box 7123, Saskatoon, SK S7K 4J1

AIDS Regina, Inc.
Box 432, Regina, SK S4P 3A2; (306) 525-0902

U.S. Hotlines

CDC National AIDS Hotline
(800) 342-AIDS

Alabama
Alabama AIDS Hotline, Montgomery
(800) 228-0469

Alaska
Alaska AIDS Hotline, Juneau
(800) 478-2437

Arizona
Arizona AIDS Hotline, Phoenix
(800) 334-1540

California
Southern California AIDS Hotline, Los Angeles
(800) 922-2437; (800) 553-2437 (TTY/TDD)

Northern California AIDS Hotline, San Francisco
(800) FOR-AIDS; (415) 864-6606 (TTY/TDD)

Colorado
Colorado Dept. of Health, Denver
(800) 252-2437

Connecticut
Connecticut AIDS Hotline, Hartford
(203) 566-1157

Delaware
Delaware AIDS Hotline, Wilmington
(800) 422-0429

District of Columbia
District of Columbia AIDS Hotline, Washington
(202) 332-2437

Florida
Florida AIDS Hotline, Tallahassee
(800) 545-SIDA; (800) 352-2437 (English Hotline); (800) AID-S101 (Haitian Creole Hotline)

Georgia
Georgia AIDS Hotline
(800) 551-2728; (404) 876-9944; (404) 876-9950 (TTY/
TDD)

Hawaii
Hawaii AIDS Hotline, Honolulu
(808) 922-1313

Idaho
Idaho AIDS Hotline, Boise
(800) 677-2437

Illinois
Illinois AIDS Hotline, Chicago
(800) 243-2437; (800) 782-0423 (TTY/TDD)

Indiana
Indiana AIDS Hotline, Indianapolis
(800) 848-2437

Iowa
Iowa AIDS Hotline, Des Moines
(800) 445-2437

Kentucky
Kentucky AIDS Information Service, Frankfort
(800) 654-2437

Louisiana
Louisiana AIDS Hotline, New Orleans
(800) 992-4379

Maine
Maine AIDS Hotline, Portland
(800) 851-2437

Maryland
Maryland AIDS Hotline, Baltimore
(800) 638-6252; (800) 553-3140 (TTY/TDD)

Massachusetts
Massachusetts AIDS Hotline, Boston
(800) 235-2331; (800) 235-2331 (TTY/TDD); (617) 262-
7248 (Spanish Hotline)

Michigan
Michigan AIDS Hotline, Royal Oak
(800) 872-2437; (800) 332-0849 (TTY/TDD)

Minnesota
Minnesota AIDSline, Minneapolis
(800) 248-2437

Mississippi
Mississippi AIDS Hotline, Jackson
(800) 537-0851

Missouri
Missouri AIDS Hotline, Jefferson City
(800) 533-2437

Montana
Montana AIDS Hotline, Helena
(800) 233-6668

Nebraska
Nebraska AIDS Hotline, Omaha
(800) 782-2437

Nevada
Nevada AIDS Hotline, Carson City
(800) 842-2437

New Hampshire
New Hampshire AIDS Information Line, Concord
(800) 872-8909

New Jersey
New Jersey AIDS Hotline, Trenton
(800) 624-2377

New Mexico
New Mexico AIDS Hotline, Santa Fe
(800) 545-2437

New York
New York AIDS Hotline, Buffalo
(800) 541-2437; (800) 233-SIDA

North Dakota
North Dakota AIDS Hotline, Bismarck
(800) 472-2180

Ohio
Ohio AIDS Hotline, Columbus
(800) 332-2437; (800) DEA-FTTY (TTY/TDD)

Oklahoma
Oklahoma AIDS Hotline, Oklahoma City
(800) 522-9054; (800) 522-9054 (TTY/TDD)

Oregon
Oregon AIDS Hotline, Portland
(800) 777-2437

Pennsylvania
Pennsylvania AIDS Hotline, Harrisburg
(800) 445-7720

Puerto Rico
Linea de Auxilio SIDA y Enfermedades de Transmision
Sexual, Rio Piedras
(809) 765-1010

Rhode Island
Rhode Island AIDS Hotline, Providence
(800) 726-3010

South Carolina
South Carolina AIDS Hotline, Columbia
(800) 322-2437

South Dakota
South Dakota AIDS Hotline, Sioux Falls
(800) 592-1861

Tennessee
Tennessee AIDS Hotline, Nashville
(800) 525-2437

Texas
Texas AIDSLINE, Austin
(800) 299-2437; (800) 252-8012 (TTY/TDD)

Utah
Utah AIDS Hotline, Salt Lake City
(801) 538-6094

Vermont
Vermont AIDS Hotline, Burlington
(800) 882-AIDS

Virginia
Virginia AIDS Hotline, Richmond
(800) 533-4148; (800) 533-4148 (TTY/TDD)

Virgin Islands
Virgin Islands AIDS Hotline, Christiansted
(809) 773-1311

Washington
Washington AIDS Hotline, Olympia
(800) 272-AIDS

West Virginia
West Virginia AIDS Hotline, Charleston
(800) 642-8244

Wisconsin
Wisconsin AIDSline, Milwaukee
(800) 334-2437

Wyoming
Wyoming AIDS Hotline, Cheyenne
(800) 327-3577

Canadian Hotlines

Alberta
Alberta Health — STD Control
(403) 427-2830 (Edmonton)
(800) 772-AIDS (throughout Alberta)

British Columbia
British Columbia Ministry of Health
(604) 872-6652 (Vancouver)
(800) 972-2437 (throughout BC)

Manitoba
AIDS Infoline — Manitoba Dept. of Health
(204) 945-AIDS (Winnipeg)
(800) 782-AIDS (throughout Manitoba)

Newfoundland
Newfoundland Dept. of Health Disease Control
(709) 576-3430

New Brunswick
New Brunswick Dept. of Health
(506) 453-2536
AIDS New Brunswick
(506) 459-7518
(800) 561-4009 (throughout NB)

Northwest Territories
AIDS Information Line
(403) 873-7017
(800) 661-0795 (throughout NWT)

Nova Scotia
Nova Scotia Dept. of Health, Epidemiology Div.
(902) 424-8698

Ontario
Ontario Ministry of Health, AIDS Section
(416) 668-6066
Throughout Ontario:
(800) 668-2437 (English and other languages)
(800) 267-7432 (French)

Prince Edward Island
P.E.I. Dept. of Health
(902) 368-4530

Quebec
Quebec Dept. of Health
(418) 643-9395
(800) 463-5656 (throughout Quebec)

Saskatchewan
Saskatchewan Health Education Line
(306) 787-3148
(800) 667-7766 (throughout Saskatchewan)

Yukon
Yukon Ministry of Health
(403) 668-9444 (Whitehorse)
(800) 661-0507 (throughout Yukon)

SOURCES: U.S. Department of Health and Human Services, Rockville, Maryland; Canadian Public Health Association, Ottawa, Ontario.

App. 22: Nursing Organizations

United States

American Academy of Ambulatory Nursing Administration
Box 56, N. Woodbury Rd., Pitman, NJ 08071; (609) 582–9617

American Academy of Nurse Practitioners
45 Foster St., Suite A, Lowell, MA 01851; (512) 442–4262

American Academy of Nursing
2420 Pershing Rd., Kansas City, MO 64108; (816) 474–5720

American Assembly for Men in Nursing
P.O. Box 31753, Independence, OH 44131

American Association of Neuroscience Nurses
218 N. Jefferson St., #204, Chicago, IL 60606; (312) 993–0043

American Association of Nurse Anesthetists
216 W. Higgins Rd., Park Ridge, IL 60068–5790; (708) 692–7050

American Association of Occupational Health Nurses, Inc.
50 Lenox Pointe, Atlanta, GA 30324; (404) 262–1162

American Association of Spinal Cord Injury Nurses
75–20 Astoria Blvd., Jackson Heights, NY 11370–1178; (718) 803–3782

American Board of Neuroscience Nursing
c/o Professional Examination Service, 475 Riverside Dr., New York, NY 10115; (212) 870–3248

American Board for Occupational Health Nurses
10448 N. Cedarbury Rd., Mequon, WI 53092; (414) 242–0704

American Board of Post Anesthesia Nursing Certification
c/o Examination Services, 475 Riverside Dr., New York, NY 10115; (212) 870–3169

American College of Nurse Midwives
1522 K St. NW, Suite 1000, Washington, DC 20005; (202) 289–0171

American Licensed Practical Nurses Association
1090 Vermont Ave. NW, Suite 1200, Washington, DC 20005; (202) 682–5800

American Nurses' Association
2420 Pershing Rd., Kansas City, MO 64108; (816) 474–5720

American Nurses' Foundation
1101 14th St. NW, Suite 200, Washington, DC 20005; (202) 789–1800

American Organization of Nurse Executives
AHA Bldg., 840 N. Lake Shore Dr., Chicago, IL 60611; (312) 280–4190

American Psychiatric Nurses' Association
c/o Christine Malin, 6900 Grove Rd., Thorofare, NJ 08086; (609) 848–7990

American Society of Ophthalmic Registered Nurses, Inc.
P.O. Box 193030, San Francisco, CA 94119; (415) 561–8513

American Society of Plastic and Reconstructive Surgical Nurses, Inc.
Box 56, N. Woodbury Rd., Pitman, NJ 08071; (609) 589–6247

American Society of Post Anesthesia Nurses
11512 Allecingie Pkwy., Richmond, VA 23235; (804) 379–5516

Assembly of Hospital Schools of Nursing
American Hospital Association, Center for Nursing, 840 N. Lake Shore Dr., Chicago, IL 60611; (312) 280–6432

Association of Operating Room Nurses
10170 E. Mississippi Ave., Denver, CO 80231; (303) 755–6300

Association of Pediatric Oncology Nurses
11512 Allecingie Pkwy., Richmond, VA 23235–4302; (804) 379–9150

Association of Rehabilitation Nurses
5700 Old Orchard Rd., 1st fl., Skokie, IL 60077; (708) 966–3433

Baromedical Nurses Association
P.O. Box 2727, Palm Desert, CA 92261; (619) 341–8033

Cassandra: Radical Feminist Nurses Network
P.O. Box 181039, Cleveland Heights, OH 44118.

Commission on Graduates of Foreign Nursing Schools
3600 Market St., Suite 400, Philadelphia, PA 19104–2651; (215) 222–8454

Council on Certification of Nurse Anesthetists
216 Higgins Rd., Park Ridge, IL 60068; (708) 692–7050

Dermatology Nurses Association
Box 56, N. Woodbury Rd., Pitman, NJ 08071; (609) 582–1915

Federation for Accessible Nursing Education and Licensure
2033 Sixth Ave., #804, Seattle, WA 98122; (206) 441–6020

Frontier Nursing Service
Wendover, KY 41775; (606) 672–2317

International Flying Nurses Association
c/o Terri A. Sinkowski, R.N., P.O. Box 561218, Harwood Heights, IL 60656

NAACOG: The Organization for Obstetric, Gynecologic, and Neonatal Nurses
409 12th St. SW, Washington, DC 20024; (202) 638–0026

NAACOG Certification Corporation
645 N. Michigan Ave., Suite 1058, Chicago, IL 60611; (312) 951–0207

National Association of Hispanic Nurses
2300 W. Commerce, Suite 304, San Antonio, TX 78207; (512) 226–9743

National Association of Orthopaedic Nurses, Inc.
Box 56, N. Woodbury Rd., Pitman, NJ 08071; (609) 582–0111

National Association of Pediatric Nurse Associates and Practitioners
1101 Kings Hwy. N., #206, Cherry Hill, NJ 08034; (609) 667–1773

National Association of Physician Nurses
900 S. Washington St., #G-13, Falls Church, VA 22046; (703) 237–8616

National Association of Registered Nurses
1520 Huguenot Rd., Suite 116, Midlothian, VA 23113; (804) 794–6513

National Association of School Nurses
Box 1300, Lamplighter Lane, Scarborough, ME 04074; (207) 883–2117

National Black Nurses Association, Inc.
P.O. Box 1823, Washington, DC 20013; (202) 393–6870

National Council of State Boards of Nursing, Inc.
676 N. St. Clair St., Suite 550, Chicago, IL 60611; (312) 787–6555

National Federation of Licensed Practical Nurses, Inc.
P.O. Box 18088, Raleigh, NC 27619; (919) 781–4791

National Federation of Specialty Nursing Organizations
875 Kings Hwy., Suite 200, West Deptford, NJ 08096; (609) 848–5932

National Flight Nurses Association
c/o Christine Malin, 6900 Grove Rd., Thorofare, NJ 08086; (609) 384–6725

National League for Nursing
350 Hudson St., New York, NY 10014; (212) 989–9393

National Nurses Society on Addictions
5700 Old Orchard Rd., 1st. fl., Skokie, IL 60077; (708) 966–0050

National Organization for the Advancement of Associate Degree Nursing
2033 Sixth Ave., Suite 804, Seattle, WA 98121; (206) 441–6020

North American Nursing Diagnosis Association
3525 Caroline St., St. Louis, MO 63104; (314) 577–8954

Nurse Consultants Association, Inc.
414 Plaza Dr., Suite 209, Westmont, IL 60559; (708) 655–0087

Nurses Educational Funds
555 W. 57th St., 13th fl., New York, NY 10019; (212) 582–8820

Nurses' House
350 Hudson St., New York, NY 10014; (212) 989–9393

Nurses Organization of Veterans Affairs
6728 Old McLean Village Dr., McLean, VA 22101; (202) 556–9222

Oncology Nursing Society
1016 Greentree Rd., 3rd fl., Pittsburgh, PA 15220; (412) 921–7373

Society for Advancement in Nursing
Box 307, Cooper Sta., 11th St. & 4th Ave., New York, NY 10003; (212) 998–5335

Society of Otorhinolaryngology and Head/Neck Nurses
439 N. Causeway, New Smyrna Beach, FL 32169; (904) 428–1695

Visiting Nurse Associations of America
3801 E. Florida Ave., Suite 806, Denver, CO 80210; (303) 753–0218

Canada

Academy of Chief Executive Nurses of Teaching Hospitals
Director of Nursing, Saint John Regional Hospital, P.O. Box 2100, Saint John, New Brunswick E2L 4L2; (506) 648–6369

Canadian Association of Addiction Nurses
c/o Royal Ottawa Hospital, Perley East, 1145 Carling Ave., Ottawa, Ontario K1Z 7K4; (613) 722–6521, ext. 6454

Canadian Association of Burn Nurses
11 May Ave; P.O. Box 359, Sharon, Ontario L0G 1V0; (416) 926–7021; (416) 926–7693, pager 1143

Canadian Association of Critical Care Nurses
P.O. Box 22006, London, Ontario N6C 4N0*; (519) 649–5284

Canadian Association for Enterostomal Therapy
Victorian Order of Nurses, Winnipeg Branch, 311–167 Lombard Ave., Winnipeg, Manitoba R3B 0T6; (204) 957–0650, ext. 37

Canadian Association for the History of Nursing
430 Hendon Dr. NW, Calgary, Alberta T2K 1Z7; (403) 289–3194

Canadian Association for Nursing Law
1 Evergreen Place, Winnipeg, Manitoba R3C 0E9

Canadian Association of Nurses in Independent Practice
55 McCaul St., P.O. Box 155, Toronto, Ontario M5T 2N7; (416) 683–3754

Canadian Association of Nurses in AIDS Care
Montreal General Hospital, 1650 Cedar Ave., Room 7112, Montreal, Quebec H3E 1A4; (514) 934–8070

Canadian Association for Nurse Administrators
c/o Medicine Hat Regional Hospital, Office of AEO-Patient Services, 666 Fifth St. SW, Medicine Hat, Alberta T1A 4H6; (403) 529–8018

Canadian Association of Nephrology Nurses and Technicians
6431 Seaforth St., Halifax, Nova Scotia B3L 1R4; (902) 428–5517

Canadian Association of Neuroscience Nurses
416 Preston Ave., Saskatoon, Saskatchewan S7H 2V2; (306) 966–1889

Canadian Association of Nurses in Oncology
c/o Manitoba Cancer Treatment and Research Foundation, 100 Olivia St., Winnipeg, Manitoba R3E 0V9; (204) 787–2233

Canadian Association of Pediatric Nurses
44 Dayfoot Dr., Georgetown, Ontario L7G 2L1; (416) 840–1440

Canadian Association of Quality Assurance Professionals
151 Bloor St. W., Suite 480, Toronto, Ontario M5S 1T3*

Canadian Association of Rehabilitation Nurses
1 Place Ville-Marie, Suite 3725, Montreal, Quebec H3B 3P4*; (514) 937–3661, ext. 119

Canadian Correctional Nurses Association
c/o New Brunswick Training School, R.R. #6, Fredericton, New Brunswick E3B 4X7; (506) 453–7800

Canadian Council of Cardiovascular Nurses
160 George St., Suite 200, Ottawa, Ontario K1N 9M2*; (613) 237–4361

Canadian Clinical Nurse Specialist Interest Group
80 Regina Ave., Toronto, Ontario M6A 1R6; (416) 789–5131, ext. 2620

Canadian Diabetes Association, Professional Health Workers Section
902–2060 Bellwood, Burnaby, British Columbia V5B 4V2; (416) 789–9551

Canadian Federation of Mental Health Nurses
331 Montgomery Ave., Winnipeg, Manitoba R3L 1T6; (204) 787–3345

Canadian Gerontological Nursing Association
Dean, Faculty of Nursing, University of New Brunswick, P.O. Box 4400, Fredericton, New Brunswick E3B 5A3; (506) 453–4642

Canadian Holistic Nurses Association
Box 1752, Kingston, Ontario K7L 5J6; (613) 549–6646

Canadian Intravenous Nurses Association
200–4433 Sheppard Ave. E., Agincourt, Ontario M1S 1V3*; (416) 292–0687

Canadian Nurse Educators Association
2280–15th Sideroad, R.R. #4, Thunder Bay, Ontario P7C 4Z2; (807) 475–6306

---

* Office and permanent mailing address

Nursing Organizations (*Continued*)

Canadian Nurses Association
50 The Driveway, Ottawa, Ontario K2P 1E2; (613) 237–2133

Canadian Nurses Respiratory Society
c/o Canadian Lung Association, 908–75 Albert St., Ottawa, Ontario K1P 5E7*; (613) 237–1208

Canadian Nursing Research Group
CSB-5-123, Faculty of Nursing, University of Alberta, Edmonton, Alberta T6G 2G3; (403) 492–2996

Canadian Obstetric Gynecologic and Neonatal Nurses
4375 Royal Ave., Montreal, Quebec H4A 2M7; (514) 934–4400, ext. 2389

Canadian Orthopaedic Nurses Association
410–9890 Manchester Dr., Burnaby, British Columbia V3N 4R4; (604) 875–4053

Canadian Society of Gastroenterology Nurses and Associates
GI Investigations Unit 4W1, Chedoke-McMaster Hospital, McMaster Div., 1200 Main St. W., Hamilton, Ontario L8N 3Z5

Community Health Nurses Association of Canada
1049 Flintlock Court, London, Ontario N6H 4M3; (519) 613–9900

Community and Hospital Infection Control Association-Canada
Senior Infection Control Nurse, Vancouver General Hospital, 855 12th Ave., Vancouver, British Columbia V5Z 1M9

Indian and Inuit Nurses of Canada
55 Murray St., 4th fl., Ottawa, Ontario K1N 5M3*; (613) 230–1864

National Association of Occupational Health Nurses
B. F. Goodrich Canada Inc., Scotford Chemical Group, P.O. Box 3418, Fort Saskatchewan, Alberta T8L 2T3; (403) 998–8780

National Emergency Nurses' Affiliation
55 Highland Park Dr., Apt. 101, Dartmouth, Nova Scotia B3A 4S4; (902) 463–6061

Nursing Sisters Association of Canada
52 Thorncliffe Dr., Suite 301, Toronto, Ontario M4N 1K5; (416) 424–1440

Operating Room Nurses Association of Canada
2864 W. 3rd Ave., Vancouver, British Columbia V6K 1M7; (604) 682–2344, ext. 2330

Provincial and Territorial Associations

Alberta Association of Registered Nurses
11620–168 St., Edmonton, Alberta T5M 4A6; (403) 451–0043

Registered Nurses Association of British Columbia
2855 Arbutus St., Vancouver, British Columbia V6J 3Y8; (604) 736–7331

Manitoba Association of Registered Nurses
647 Broadway, Winnipeg, Manitoba R3C 0X2; (204) 774–3477

Nurses Association of New Brunswick
165 Regent St., Fredericton, New Brunswick E3B 3W5; (506) 458–8731

Association of Registered Nurses of Newfoundland
55 Military Rd., Box 6116, St. John's, Newfoundland A1C 5X8; (709) 753–6040

Northwest Territories Registered Nurses Association
Box 2757, Yellowknife, Northwest Territories X1A 2R1; (403) 873–2745

Registered Nurses Association of Nova Scotia
120 Eileen Stubbs Ave., Suite 104, Dartmouth, Nova Scotia B3H 1Y1; (902) 468–9744

Registered Nurses Association of Ontario
33 Price St., Toronto, Ontario M4W 1Z2; (800) 268–7199; (416) 923–3523
For information on registration/licensure in Ontario, contact **College of Nurses of Ontario**†, 101 Davenport Rd., Toronto, Ontario M5R 3P1; (800) 387–5526; (416) 928–0900

Association of Registered Nurses of Prince Edward Island
P.O. Box 1838, Charlottetown, Prince Edward Island C1A 7N5; (902) 368–3764

For information on registration/licensure in Quebec, contact **l'Ordre des infirmières et infirmiers du Québec**†, 4200 ouest, boul. Dorchester, Montréal, Québec H3Z 1V4; (800) 363–6048; (514) 935–2501

Saskatchewan Registered Nurses Association
2066 Retallack St., Regina, Saskatchewan S4T 2K2; (306) 757–4643

Yukon Registered Nurses Association
Box 5371, Whitehorse, Yukon Y1A 4Z2; (403) 667–4062

* Office and permanent mailing address
† Not a provincial/territorial member of the Canadian Nurses Association
SOURCES: Encyclopedia of Associations, ed 26 (Gale Research Co., Detroit, 1992); Canadian Nurses Association, Ottawa, Ontario.

App. 23: Conceptual Models and Theories of Nursing

Jacqueline Fawcett, Ph.D., F.A.A.N.

THE FORERUNNERS

Florence Nightingale's Notes on Nursing

Overview

Nightingale equated knowledge of nursing with knowledge of sanitation. The focus of nursing knowledge was how to keep the body free from disease or in such a condition that it could recover from disease. According to Nightingale, nursing ought to signify the proper use of fresh air, light, warmth, cleanliness, quiet, and the proper selection and administration of diet—all at the least expense of vital power to the patient. That is, she maintained that the purpose of nursing was to put patients in the best condition for nature to act upon them.

Implications for Nursing Practice

Nursing practice encompassed both well and sick people. Nursing actions focused on both patients and their environments. Thirteen "hints" provided the boundaries of nursing practice:

1. *Ventilation and warming*—the nurse must be concerned first with keeping the air that patients breathe as pure as the external air, without chilling them.

2. *Health of houses*—attention to pure air, pure water, efficient drainage, cleanliness, and light will secure the health of houses.

3. *Petty management*—all the results of good nursing may be negated by one defect, which is not knowing how to manage what you do when you are there and what shall be done when you are not there.

4. *Noise*—unnecessary noise, or noise that creates an expectation in the mind, is that which hurts a patient. Anything that wakes a patient suddenly from sleep will invariably put the patient into a state of greater excitement and do more serious and lasting mischief than any continuous noise, however loud.

5. *Variety*—the nerves of the sick suffer from seeing the same walls, the same ceiling, the same surroundings during a long confinement to one or two rooms. The majority of cheerful cases can be found among patients who are not confined to one room, whatever their suffering, and the majority of depressed cases will be seen among those subjected to a long monotony of objects about them.

6. *Taking food*—the nurse should be conscious of the patient's diet and remember how much food that patient has had and ought to have each day.

7. *What food?*—to watch for the opinions the patient's stomach gives, rather than to read analyses of foods, is the business of all those who have to decide what the patient is to eat.

8. *Bed and bedding*—the patient should have a clean bed every 12 hours. The bed should be narrow so that the patient does not feel "out of humanity's reach." The bed should not be so high that the patient cannot easily get in and out of it. The bed should be in the brightest spot in the room, preferably near a window. Pillows should be used to support the back below the breathing apparatus, to allow shoulders room to fall back, and to support the head without throwing it forward.

9. *Light*—with the sick, second only to their need of fresh air is their need of light. Light, especially direct sunlight, has a purifying effect upon the air of a room.

10. *Cleanliness of rooms and walls*—the greater part of nursing consists in preserving cleanliness. The inside air can be kept clean only by excessive care to rid rooms and their furnishings of the organic matter and dust with which they become saturated. Without cleanliness, you cannot have all the effect of ventilation; without ventilation, you can

have no thorough cleanliness.

11. *Personal cleanliness* — nurses should always remember that if they allow patients to remain unwashed or to remain in clothing saturated with perspiration or other excretion, they are interfering injuriously with the natural processes of health just as much as if they were to give their patients a dose of slow poison.

12. *Chattering hopes and advices* — there is scarcely a greater worry that invalids have to endure than the incurable hopes of their friends. All friends, visitors, and attendants of the sick should avoid this practice of attempting to cheer the sick by making light of their danger and by exaggerating their probabilities of recovery.

13. *Observation of the sick* — the most important practical lesson nurses can learn is what to observe, how to observe, which symptoms indicate improvement, which indicate the reverse, which are important, which are not, which are the evidence of neglect and what kind of neglect.

Implications for Nursing Education

Nightingale's primary contribution to nursing education was her belief that nursing schools should be administratively and economically independent from hospitals, even though the training could take place in the hospital. The purpose of nursing education was to teach the theoretical and practical knowledge underlying the physician's orders. Knowledge of the 13 "hints" for nursing practice was considered an essential part of the training of every nurse.

Reference

Nightingale, F. (1859). *Notes on nursing: What it is, and what it is not.* London: Harrison and Sons. [Reprinted by J. B. Lippincott Co., Philadelphia]

Virginia Henderson's Definition of Nursing

Overview

The unique function of the nurse is to help individuals, sick or well, to perform those activities contributing to health or its recovery (or to peaceful death) that they would perform unaided if they had the necessary strength, will, or knowledge, and to do this in such a way as to help them gain independence as soon as possible.

Implications for Nursing Practice

As defined by Henderson, the practice of nursing requires nurses to know and understand patients by putting themselves in the place of the patients. Nurses should not take at face value everything that patients say, but rather should interact with patients to ascertain their true feelings. *Basic nursing care* involves helping the patient perform the following activities unaided: (1) breathe normally, (2) eat and drink adequately, (3) eliminate body wastes, (4) move and maintain desirable postures, (5) sleep and rest, (6) select suitable clothes, dress, and undress, (7) maintain body temperature within normal range by adjusting clothing and modifying the environment, (8) keep the body clean and well groomed and protect the integument, (9) avoid dangers in the environment and avoid injuring others, (10) communicate with others in expressing emotions, needs, fears, or opinions, (11) worship according to one's faith, (12) work in such a way that there is a sense of accomplishment, (13) play or participate in various forms of recreation, and (14) learn, discover, or satisfy the curiosity that leads to normal development and health and use the available health facilities.

Implications for Nursing Education

Henderson's definition identifies an area of health and human welfare in which the nurse is an expert and independent practitioner. This kind of nursing requires a liberal education within a college or university, with grounding in the physical, biological, and social sciences and ability to use analytical processes. The professional aspects of the curriculum should focus on the nurse's major function of supplementing patients when they need strength, will, or knowledge in performing daily activities or in carrying out prescribed therapy, with emphasis on the individualization of patient care.

Reference

Henderson, V. (1966). *The nature of nursing. A definition and its implications for practice, research, and education.* New York: Macmillan.

CONCEPTUAL MODELS

A *conceptual model* is defined as a set of abstract and general concepts and statements about those concepts. Conceptual models of nursing — also referred to as *conceptual frameworks, conceptual systems,* and *paradigms* — refer to global ideas about people, their environments and health, and nursing.

Dorothy Johnson's Behavioral System Model

Overview

Views the person as a behavioral system made up of all patterned, repetitive, and purposeful ways of behavior that characterize each person's life. Seven subsystems carry out specialized tasks or functions needed to maintain the integrity of the whole behavioral system and to manage its relationship to the environment.

1. *Affiliative:* Provides security needed for survival as well as social inclusion, intimacy, and formation and maintenance of social bonds.
2. *Dependency:* Succoring behavior that calls for a response of nurturance as well as approval, attention or recognition, and physical assistance.
3. *Ingestive:* Functions in appetite satisfaction, which is governed by social and psychological considerations as well as biological need for food and fluids.
4. *Eliminative:* Function is elimination, with regard to when, how, and under what conditions the individual eliminates wastes.
5. *Sexual:* Functions are procreation and gratification, with regard to behaviors dependent upon the individual's biological sex, including but not limited to courting and mating.
6. *Aggressive:* Function is protection and preservation of self and society.
7. *Achievement:* Function is mastery or control of some aspect of self or environment, with regard to intellectual, physical, creative, mechanical, social, and care-taking (of children, spouse, home) skills.

Structure of each subsystem includes four elements:

1. *Drive or goal:* Motivation for behavior. Cannot be observed directly but must be inferred from the individual's behavior and the consequences of that behavior.
2. *Set:* Individual's predisposition to act in certain ways to fulfill the function of the subsystem.
3. *Choice:* Individual's total behavioral repertoire for fulfilling subsystem functions. Behavioral repertoire encompasses the scope of action alternatives from which the person can choose.
4. *Action:* An individual's actual behavior in a situation. The only structural element that can be observed directly.

The functional requirements of subsystems are:

1. *Protection* from noxious influences with which the system cannot cope.
2. *Nurturance* through the input of appropriate supplies from the environment.
3. *Stimulation* to enhance growth and prevent stagnation.

Implications for Nursing Practice

Nursing practice is directed toward restoration, maintenance, or attainment of behavioral system balance and stability at the highest possible level for the individual. Assessment includes analysis of actions to determine if they are purposeful, orderly, and predictable. Nursing intervention includes *imposing temporary external regulatory or control mechanisms on behavior,* such as setting limits for behavior, inhibition of ineffective behavior, and helping patients to develop new behavior; *changing the structural elements of the subsystems* by altering set through instruction or counseling and adding choices by teaching new skills; and *fulfilling the subsystem functional requirements* by protecting the patient from overwhelming noxious influences, supplying adequate nurturance, and providing stimulation.

Implications for Nursing Education

Education based on this model requires a thorough grounding in the natural and social sciences, with emphasis on the genetic, neurological, and endocrine bases of behavior; psychological and social mechanisms for the regulation and control of behavior; social learning theories; and motivational structures and processes. The professional aspects of the curriculum focus on study of the behavioral system as a whole and as a composite of subsystems; pathophysiology; the clinical sciences of nursing and medicine; and the health care system.

Reference   Johnson, D. E. (1980). The behavioral system model for nursing. In J. P. Riehl & C. Roy, *Conceptual models for nursing practice* (2nd ed., pp. 207–216). New York: Appleton-Century-Crofts.

Imogene King's Interacting Systems Framework

Overview   Encompasses three open, dynamic, interacting systems.
1. *Personal systems* are individuals, who are regarded as rational, sentient, social beings. Concepts related to personal systems are:
   Perception—a process of organizing, interpreting, and transforming information from sense data and memory that gives meaning to one's experience, represents one's image of reality, and influences one's behavior.
   Self—a composite of thoughts and feelings that constitute a person's awareness of individual existence, of who and what he or she is.
   Growth and development—cellular, molecular, and behavioral changes in human beings that are a function of genetic endowment, meaningful and satisfying experiences, and an environment conducive to helping individuals move toward maturity.
   Body image—a person's perception of his or her body.
   Time—the duration between the occurrence of one event and the next.
   Space—the physical area called territory. Exists in all directions.
2. *Interpersonal systems* are composed of two or more individuals interacting in a given situation. Concepts related to interpersonal systems are:
   Interactions—the acts of two or more persons in mutual presence; a sequence of verbal and nonverbal behaviors that are goal directed.
   Communication—the vehicle by which human relations are developed and maintained. Includes intrapersonal, interpersonal, verbal, and nonverbal communication.
   Transaction—interaction in which human beings communicate with their environment to achieve valued goals.
   Role—a set of behaviors expected of a person occupying a position in a social system.
   Stress—a dynamic state whereby a human being interacts with the environment to maintain balance for growth, development, and performance, which involves an exchange of energy and information between the person and the environment for regulation and control of stressors.
3. *Social systems*—organized boundary systems of social roles, behaviors, and practices developed to maintain values and the mechanisms to regulate the practices and rules. Concepts related to social systems are:
   Organization—composed of human beings with prescribed roles and positions who use resources to accomplish personal and organizational goals.
   Authority—a transactional process characterized by active, reciprocal relations in which members' values, backgrounds, and perceptions play a role in defining, validating, and accepting the authority of individuals within an organization.
   Power—the process whereby one or more persons influence other persons in a situation.
   Status—the position of an individual in a group, or a group in relation to other groups, in an organization.
   Decision making—in organizations, a dynamic and systematic process by which goal-directed choice of perceived alternatives is made and acted upon by individuals or groups to answer a question and attain a goal.

Implications for Nursing Practice   The *theory of goal attainment* was derived from the personal and interpersonal systems of the Interacting Systems Framework. The theory proposes that nurse and client interactions are characterized by verbal and nonverbal communication in which information is exchanged and interpreted; by transactions, in which values, needs, and wants of each member of the dyad are shared; by perceptions of nurse and client and the situation; by self in role of client and self in role of nurse; and by stressors influencing each person and the situation in time and space. The theory of goal attainment is reflected in the nursing process of *perception, judgment, action, reaction, interaction, and transaction.* The process follows a sequence whereby nurse and client meet in some situation; perceive each other; make judgments about the other; take some mental action; react to each one's perceptions of the other; share information about their perceptions; identify special goals, problems, or concerns; explore means to achieve a goal and agree to means to the goal; and transact as goals are attained.

Implications for Nursing Education

The Interacting Systems Framework and the theory of goal attainment lead to a focus on the dynamic interaction of the nurse-client dyad. This focus, in turn, leads to emphasis on nursing student behavior as well as client behavior. The concepts related to the personal, interpersonal, and social systems serve as the theoretical content for nursing courses in associate and baccalaureate degree programs. The theoretical knowledge is used by students in learning experiences involving concrete nursing situations.

References

King, I. M. (1981). *A theory for nursing. Systems, concepts, process,* New York: Wiley.

King, I. M. (1986). *Curriculum and instruction in nursing.* Norwalk, CT: Appleton-Century-Crofts.

Myra Levine's Conservation Model

Overview

Focuses on conservation of the person's wholeness. Adaptation is the process by which people maintain their wholeness or integrity as they respond to the challenges of the perceptual, operational, and conceptual environments. The *perceptual environment* encompasses that part of the environment to which individuals respond with their sense organs. The *operational environment* includes those aspects of the environment that are not directly perceived, such as radiation, odorless and colorless pollutants, and microorganisms. The *conceptual environment* is the environment of language, ideas, symbols, concepts, and invention. Individuals respond to the environment by means of four integrated processes: fight-or-flight mechanism, inflammatory-immune response, stress response, and perceptual awareness.

Implications for Nursing Practice

The nursing process of this conceptual model is conservation, which is defined as "keeping together." Patients are participants in nursing care. They are regarded as temporarily dependent on the nurse. The goal of the nurse is to end the dependency as quickly as possible. Assessment of the patient's nursing requirements leads to development of a trophicognosis, defined as a nursing care judgment arrived at by the scientific method. Nursing intervention is structured according to four conservation principles:

1. *Conservation of energy*—a natural law that holds everywhere in the universe for all animate and inanimate entities. Nursing intervention is based on balancing the patient's energy input with energy output.
2. *Conservation of structural integrity*—focuses attention on healing. Nursing intervention is based on limiting the amount of tissue involvement in infection and disease.
3. *Conservation of personal integrity*—focuses attention on healing. Nursing intervention is based on helping the patient preserve his or her identity and selfhood.
4. *Conservation of social integrity*—focuses attention on the patient's place in family, community, and society. Nursing intervention is based on helping the patient to preserve his or her place in those groups.

Implications for Nursing Education

Education focuses on understanding of both the person and the environment, with emphasis on processes by which the person adapts to environmental challenges. Theoretical and clinical knowledge related to the four conservation principles provides the structure for nursing courses.

References

Levine, M. E. (1973). *Introduction to clinical nursing* (2nd ed.). Philadelphia: F. A. Davis.

Schaefer, K. M., & Pond, J. B. (Eds.). (1991). *Levine's conservation model: A framework for nursing practice.* Philadelphia: F. A. Davis.

Betty Neuman's Systems Model

Overview

Views the client as an open system in interaction with the environment. The client system is a composite of five interrelated variables: physiological, psychological, sociocultural, developmental, and spiritual. The client system is depicted as a central core surrounded by concentric rings. The *central core* is a basic structure of survival factors common to the species, such as variables contained within, innate or genetic features, and strength and weakness of the system parts, such as temperature range, genetic response patterns, ego structure, strengths and weaknesses of body organs, and cognitive ability. The *concentric rings* represent three mechanisms that protect the basic structure:

1. *Flexible line of defense* — outermost ring. Protective buffer for the client's normal or stable state. Ideally it prevents invasion of stressors and keeps the client system free from stressor reactions.
2. *Normal line of defense* — lies between the flexible line of defense and the lines of resistance and represents the client system's normal wellness state. It reflects what the client has become or evolved to over time and is the result of adjustment between client system variables and environmental stressors. Expansion of the normal line of defense reflects an enhanced state of wellness; contraction, a diminished state.
3. *Lines of resistance* — innermost concentric rings. Involuntarily activated when a stressor invades the normal line of defense. These lines contain internal factors that support the basic structure and the normal line of defense, such as mobilization of white blood cells. If the lines of resistance are effective, the system can reconstitute; if they are ineffective, death may ensue.

Environment is defined as "all internal and external factors or influences surrounding the client system."

1. *Internal environment* — "consists of all forces or interactive influences internal to or contained solely within the boundaries of the defined client system." It is the source of *intrapersonal stressors.*
2. *External environment* — consists of all forces or interaction influences external to or existing outside the defined client system. It is the source of *interpersonal and extrapersonal stressors.*
3. *Created environment* is subconsciously developed by the client as a symbolic expression of system wholeness. It supersedes and encompasses the internal and external environments.

Implications for Nursing Practice

The goal of nursing practice based on this model is "to facilitate optimal wellness through retention, attainment, or maintenance of client system stability." A *nursing diagnosis* is formulated on the basis of assessment of the variables and lines of defense and resistance making up the client system. *Nursing goals* are negotiated with the client and are achieved by means of primary, secondary, or tertiary prevention.

1. *Primary prevention* — action required to *retain* client system stability. Intervention involving primary prevention is selected when the risk of or hazard from a stressor is known but a reaction has not yet occurred. Interventions attempt to reduce the possibility of the client's encounter with the stressor or strengthen the flexible line of defense to decrease the possibility of a reaction when the stressor is encountered.
2. *Secondary prevention* — action required to *attain* system stability. Intervention involving secondary prevention is selected when a reaction to a stressor has already occurred. Interventions deal with existing symptoms and attempt to strengthen the lines of resistance through use of the client's internal and external resources.
3. *Tertiary prevention* — action required to *maintain* system stability.

2462

Intervention involving tertiary prevention is selected when some degree of client system stability has occurred following secondary prevention interventions.

Nursing outcomes are determined by means of evaluation of the results of prevention strategies.

Implications for Nursing Education

This model is an appropriate curriculum guide for all levels of nursing education. The components of the model serve as curriculum content, including the five variable areas (physiological, psychological, sociocultural, development, spiritual), the three categories of stressors (intrapersonal, interpersonal, extrapersonal), and the three prevention-as-intervention modalities (primary, secondary, tertiary).

Reference

Neuman, B. (1989). *The Neuman systems model. Application to nursing education and practice* (2nd ed.). Norwalk, CT: Appleton and Lange.

Dorothea Orem's Self-Care Framework

Overview

Central concepts:

1. *Self-care*—"action directed by individuals to themselves or their environments to regulate their own functioning and development in the interest of sustaining life, maintaining or restoring integrated functioning under stable or changing environmental conditions, and maintaining or bringing about a condition of well-being."

2. *Self-care agency*—"a complex capability of maturing and mature individuals to (1) determine the presence and characteristics of specific requirements for regulating their own functioning and development, (2) make judgments and decisions about what to do, and (3) perform care measures to meet specific self-care requisites."

3. *Therapeutic self-care demand*—"the action demand on individuals to meet some complex of universal, developmental, and health-deviation type self-care requisites." Universal self-care requisites are associated with life processes and maintenance of the integrity of human structure and function. Developmental self-care requisites are associated with human developmental processes and conditions and events that occur during various stages of the life cycle, as well as with events that may adversely affect development. Health-deviation self-care requisites are associated with genetic and constitutional defects and human structural and functional deviations and their effects, as well as with medical diagnostic and treatment measures prescribed or performed by physicians.

4. *Self-care deficit*—expression of a relationship of inadequacy between self-care agency and the therapeutic self-care demand.

5. *Nursing agency*—"a complex property or attribute of nurses developed through specialized education and training in the theoretical and practical nursing sciences and through their development of the art of nursing in reality situations."

6. *Nursing systems*—a dynamic action system produced by nurses as they engage in the diagnostic, prescriptive, and regulatory operations of the nursing practice. Nursing systems can be wholly compensatory, partly compensatory, or supportive-educative.

> *Wholly compensatory*—selected when the patient cannot or should not perform any self-care actions.
> *Partly compensatory*—selected when the patient can perform some but not all self-care actions.
> *Supportive-educative*—selected when the patient can and should perform all self-care actions.

Peripheral concept:

1. *Basic conditioning factors*—reflect features of individuals or their living situations, such as age, gender, health state, developmental stage, sociocultural orientation, health care system variables, family system elements, and patterns of living. Basic conditioning factors influence self-care and self-care agency.

2463

Theories derived from Self-Care Framework:

1. *Theory of self-care deficit*—"people can benefit from nursing because they are subject to health-related or health-derived limitations that render them incapable of continuous self-care . . . or that result in ineffective or incomplete care."

2. *Theory of self-care*—self-care is a "learned behavior that purposely regulates human structural integrity, functioning, and human development."

3. *Theory of nursing systems*—nursing systems are formed when nurses use their abilities to prescribe, design, and provide nursing for legitimate patients . . . by performing discrete actions and systems of actions that regulate the value of or the exercise of individuals' capabilities to engage in self-care and meet the self-care requisites of the individual therapeutically."

Implications for Nursing Practice

Nursing process encompasses *diagnosis* of self-care deficits and *prescription* for methods of assisting, including acting for or doing for another, guiding another, supporting another physically or psychologically, providing a developmental environment, and teaching another; *designing and planning* the required nursing system(s); and *producing care* to regulate therapeutic self-care demand and self-care agency.

Implications for Nursing Education

This framework and the theories derived from it provide a body of knowledge that can be used for curriculum development. The focus of both undergraduate and graduate nursing curricula is on components of self-care, self-care agency, self-care deficits, nursing agency, and nursing systems. Education for clinical skills emphasizes the methods of assisting.

Martha Rogers' Science of Unitary Human Beings

Overview

Focuses on the nature and direction of unitary human development. Four basic concepts:

1. *Energy fields*—"fundamental unit of both the living and the nonliving. Field is a unifying concept. Energy signifies the dynamic nature of the field." Two types of energy fields: human and environmental. These fields are in continuous motion and are infinite. They cannot be broken down into parts. Human beings and environment do not have energy fields, but rather *are* energy fields. Energy fields are open.

2. *Openness* is complete and continuous. Energy fields are not open a little or a lot, nor are they open just sometimes. The human and environmental fields are integral with one another.

3. *Pattern,* the distinguishing characteristic of an energy field, is perceived as a single wave that gives identity to the field. "Each human field pattern is unique and is integral with its own unique environmental field pattern." Pattern cannot be seen; what is seen or experienced are manifestations of field pattern. Energy fields are multidimensional.

4. *Pandimensionality* is a nonlinear domain without spatial or temporal attributes.

The nature and interaction of the human and environmental energy fields are described by three principles:

1. *Resonancy*—asserts that human and environmental fields are identified by wave patterns that manifest continuous change from lower to higher frequencies.

2. *Helicy*—asserts that human and environmental field patterns are continuous, innovative, and unpredictable, and are characterized by increasing diversity.

3. *Integrality*—emphasizes the continuous mutual human field and environmental field process.

Implications for Nursing Practice

The goal of nursing practice is to promote maximum well-being of the human and environmental energy fields. Guided by the principles of resonancy, helicy, and integrality. Emphasizes noninvasive modalities such as meditation, therapeutic touch, imagery, and relaxation, along with promotion of attitudes of hope, humor, and upbeat moods.

Nursing education based on this conceptual model requires a commitment to lifelong learning. Education for professional nursing occurs at the baccalaureate, master's, and doctoral levels. The purpose of professional nursing educational programs is to provide the knowledge and tools necessary for nursing practice. The liberal arts and sciences are a predominant component of the curriculum. The principles of resonancy, helicy, and integrality represent the major integrating concepts of the nursing courses.

Reference

Rogers, M. E. (1990). Nursing: Science of unitary, irreducible, human beings: Update 1990. In E. A. M. Barrett (Ed.), *Visions of Rogers' science-based nursing* (pp. 5–11). New York: National League for Nursing.

Callista Roy's Adaptation Model

Overview

Views the person as an adaptive system that is a biopsychosocial being required to adapt to environmental stimuli. Adaptation takes place in one biological and three psychosocial modes.
1. Biological, or *physiological,* mode: concerned with basic needs required to maintain the physical and physiological integrity of the human system.
2. Psychosocial modes:
   Self-concept mode — deals with people's conceptions of their physical and personal selves. The physical self deals with body sensation and body image. The personal self encompasses self-consistency, self-ideal, and the moral-ethical-spiritual self.
   Role function mode — concerned with people's performance of roles on the basis of their positions within society.
   Interdependence mode — deals with development and maintenance of satisfying affectional relationships with significant others.

The four modes are interrelated. Responses in any one mode may have an effect on or act as a stimulus in one or all of the other modes.

Types of environmental stimuli:
1. *Focal* — stimuli most immediately confronting the person.
2. *Contextual* — contributing factors in a situation.
3. *Residual* — other, unknown factors that may influence the situation. When the factors making up residual stimuli become known, they are considered focal or contextual stimuli.

Adaptation occurs through the regulator and cognator subsystems of the adaptive system, which are innate or acquired coping mechanisms used to respond to changing environmental stimuli.
1. *Regulator subsystem* — receives input from the external environment and from changes in the person's internal state and then processes the changes through neural-chemical-endocrine channels to produce responses.
2. *Cognator subsystem* — receives input from external and internal stimuli that involve psychological, social, physical, and physiological factors, including regulator subsystem outputs. These stimuli are then processed through cognitive/emotive pathways, including perceptual/information processing, learning, judgment, and emotion.

Responses of the adaptive system:
1. *Adaptive* — those that promote the integrity of the person in terms of the goals of the human adaptive system, including survival, growth, reproduction, and mastery.
2. *Ineffective* — those that do not contribute to the goals of the human adaptive system.

**Implications for
Nursing Practice**

Focus of nursing is promotion of adaptation. Six-step nursing process:
1. *First-level assessment* — collection of data regarding adaptive system behavior and determination of adaptive and ineffective responses.
2. *Second-level assessment* — assessment of influencing factors, i.e., identification of the focal and contextual stimuli that influence adaptive system behaviors.
3. *Nursing diagnosis* — nurse's interpretation of the assessment data.
4. *Goal setting* — statement of behavioral outcomes of nursing intervention.

5. *Nursing intervention* — management of environmental stimuli, which includes increasing, decreasing, maintaining, removing, or otherwise altering or changing relevant focal and/or contextual stimuli.
6. *Evaluation* — judgments regarding the effectiveness of nursing intervention.

Implications for Nursing Education

This model is an appropriate curriculum guide for diploma, associate degree, baccalaureate degree, and master's degree nursing education programs. Curriculum content is based on the components of the conceptual model. The vertical strands of the curriculum focus on theory and practice. The theory strand encompasses content on the adapting person, health/illness, and stress/disruption. The practice strand emphasizes nursing management of environmental stimuli. The horizontal strands include the nursing process and student adaptation and leadership.

References

Andrews, H. A., & Roy, C. (1986). *Essentials of the Roy adaptation model.* Norwalk, CT: Appleton-Century-Crofts.
Roy, C. (1984). *Introduction to nursing: An Adaptation model.* Englewood Cliffs, NJ: Prentice-Hall.

NURSING THEORY

A *theory* is defined as a set of relatively specific and concrete concepts and statements about those concepts. Nursing theories are derived from more abstract and general conceptual models and describe, explain, or predict phenomena of interest to nursing.

Madeleine Leininger's Theory of Cultural Care Diversity and Universality

Overview

Based on the assumptions that care is the central, dominant, and unifying feature of nursing and that care is a powerful means to help clients recover from illnesses or unfavorable human life conditions. Care and culture are inextricably linked together and cannot be separated into nursing care actions and decisions. People are born, live, become ill, and die within a cultural belief and practice system, but depend upon human care for growth and survival. The language usages, symbols, and meanings about care in diverse cultures have to be understood in order to derive the essences and patterns of cultural care. Knowledge of care values, meanings, expressions, symbols, and practices permits prediction of health (or well-being) of individuals, groups, and cultures.

Key concepts:
Culture — learned, shared, and transmitted values, beliefs, norms, and life practices of a particular group that guides thinking, decisions, and actions in patterned ways.
Care — as a noun, refers to phenomena related to assisting, supporting, or enabling behavior toward or for another individual or group with evident or anticipated needs to ameliorate or improve a human condition or lifeway.
Caring — as a verb, refers to action patterns.
Cultural care — subjective and cognitively known values, beliefs, and patterned expressions that assist, support, or enable another individual or group to maintain well-being, improve a human condition or lifeway, or face death and disabilities.
Cultural care diversity — variability of meanings, patterns, values, or symbols of care that are culturally derived by humans for their well-being or to improve a human condition and lifeway or to face death.
Cultural care universality — common, similar, or uniform meanings, patterns, values, or symbols of care that are culturally derived by humans for their well-being or to improve a human condition and lifeway or to face death.
Environmental context — the totality of an event, situation, or particular experience that gives meaning to human expressions, including social interactions and physical, ecological, emotional, and cultural dimensions.

2466

Health — a state of well-being that is culturally defined, valued, and practiced and which reflects the ability of individuals or groups to perform their daily role activities in a culturally satisfactory way.

Implications for Nursing Practice

This theory proposes that cultural care provides a means to study, explain, and predict nursing knowledge and nursing care practice. The theory can be used to study and practice nursing and human care in all cultures of the world. Includes three modalities of care that allow the nurse to provide culturally congruent care:

1. *Cultural care preservation or maintenance* — assistive, supportive, or enabling professional actions and decisions that help clients of a particular culture to preserve or maintain a state of health or to recover from illness and to face death.
2. *Cultural care accommodation or negotiation* — assistive, supportive, or enabling professional actions and decisions that help clients of a particular culture to adapt or to negotiate for a beneficial or satisfying health status or to face death.
3. *Cultural care repatterning or restructuring* — assistive, supportive, or enabling professional actions and decisions that help clients of a particular culture change their lifeways for new or different patterns that are culturally meaningful and satisfying or that support beneficial and healthy life patterns.

Implications for Nursing Education

The ultimate goal of this theory is to provide culturally congruent nursing care. Professional nursing care, learned in formal educational programs, builds upon the generic care given by naturalistic lay and folk care givers. The theory mandates a curricular emphasis on transcultural nursing knowledge, with formal study about different cultures in the world, as well as culture-universal and culture-specific health care needs of people and nursing care practices. Transcultural nurse generalists, who function with a broad and comparative perspective about diverse cultures, are prepared through baccalaureate nursing programs. Transcultural nurse specialists, who function with in-depth knowledge of care, health, and environmental factors related to specific cultures and with culture-specific skills, are prepared through master's and doctoral nursing programs.

References

Leininger, M. M. (1988). Leininger's theory of nursing: Cultural care diversity and universality. *Nursing Science Quarterly, 1,* 152–160.

Leininger, M. M. (1989). Transcultural nurse specialists and generalists: New practitioners in nursing. *Journal of Transcultural Nursing, 1,* 4–16.

Newman's Theory of Health as Expanding Consciousness

Overview

Health is the expansion of consciousness. The meaning of life and health is found in the evolving process of expanding consciousness.

Consciousness — The informational capacity of human beings, i.e., the ability of humans to interact with their environment. Includes interconnected cognitive and affective awareness, physiochemical maintenance, growth processes, and the immune system. Can be seen in the quantity and quality of the interaction between the human being and his or her environment. The process of life is toward higher levels of consciousness. Sometimes the process is smooth, pleasant, harmonious; other times it is difficult and disharmonious, as in disease.

Pattern — information that depicts the whole and represents the meaning of all the relationships of parts at once. Pattern is relatedness. Consciousness is a manifestation of an evolving pattern of person-environment interaction, and health and disease are manifestations of that evolving pattern. Recognition of that pattern is the key to the process of evolving to higher levels of consciousness. A person is identified by his or her pattern. Characteristics of patterning include movement, diversity, and rhythm. Patterns of evolving consciousness are seen as the relationships among the concepts of movement, space, and time.

Movement — central to understanding the nature of reality. People discover the world of *time-space* and establish personal territory through movement. When movement is restricted, the person becomes aware of personal limitations and the fact that old rules don't work anymore.

Implications for Nursing Practice

By applying this theory, nurses can help people understand the evolving pattern of their lives. The nurse and the person come together when old rules do not work and the person must make a choice. The choice involves learning how things work, discovering new rules, and moving on to a new level of being and understanding. The nurse facilitates the recognition of pattern by connecting with the person in an authentic way and by helping the person to discover new rules for a higher level of organization or consciousness.

Implications for Nursing Education

Within the context of this theory, research is regarded as praxis, or practice. Teaching the research methodology associated with the theory also teaches the student a practice methodology that is congruent with the theory. The components of the research methodology that facilitate elaboration of the pattern of expanding consciousness are: (1) establishing the mutuality of the process of inquiry, (2) focusing on the most meaningful persons and events in the interviewee's life, (3) organizing the data in narrative form and displaying it as sequential patterns over time, and (4) sharing the interviewer's perception of the pattern with the interviewee and seeking revision or confirmation.

References

Newman, M. A. (1986). *Health as expanding consciousness.* St Louis: Mosby.
Newman, M. A. (1990). Newman's theory of health as praxis. *Nursing Science Quarterly, 3,* 37–41.

Ida Jean Orlando's Theory of the Nursing Process Discipline

Overview

The focus of inquiry for professional nursing is the immediate experience of the person in a person-to-person contact that occurs in an automatic, sometimes instantaneous sequence made up of an internal, nonobservable reaction to the contact and an observable action. The reaction to the contact consists of the following:
1. The person perceives with a sense organ an object or objects.
2. The perceptions stimulate automatic thought.
3. Each thought stimulates an automatic feeling.
The observable action completes the sequence.
4. The person acts; i.e., the person responds to the contact.
Understanding of the person's immediate experience is obtained by exploring the meaning of the person's verbal and nonverbal behavior, which in turn is accomplished by use of the nursing process discipline. The requirements of the nursing process discipline are:
   a. What the nurse says to the patient must match (be consistent with) any or all of the items contained in the reaction.
   b. What the nurse does nonverbally must be expressed verbally.
   c. The expression must match one or all of the items contained in the reaction.
   d. The nurse must clearly communicate to the individual that the item being expressed belongs to the nurse.
   e. The nurse must ask the individual about the item expressed to obtain correction or verification from that individual.

Implications for Nursing Practice

The focus of encounters between nurses and patients is to learn what care is required by the patients, why the care is needed, and what to do about it. All of this is facilitated by application of the nursing process discipline, which is considered a disciplined professional response. This response is effective because when one individual in a person-to-person contact expresses his or her own immediate reaction, the other individual is more able to do likewise.

The nursing process discipline guides effectiveness in all person-to-person contacts of the nursing system, including the nurse's contacts with patients, other nurses, and other professional and nonprofessional people.

<table>
<tr><td>Implications for
Nursing Education</td><td>Focus is on training the student or graduate nurse to use a disciplined and professional response, rather than a personal and automatic one, in all person-to-person contacts. Training is facilitated by use of process recordings that include perceptions of or about the patient, thoughts and/ or feelings about the perception, and what was said and/or done to, with, or for the patient. Research has revealed that the process discipline can be successfully taught in 6 to 12 weeks.</td></tr>
<tr><td>References</td><td>Orlando, I. J. (1961). The dynamic nurse-patient relationship: Function, process and principles. New York: G. P. Putnam's Sons.
Orlando, I. J. (1972). The discipline and teaching of nursing process: An evaluative study. New York: G. P. Putnam's Sons.</td></tr>
</table>

Rosemarie Parse's Theory of Human Becoming

<table>
<tr><td>Overview</td><td>

Also called the theory of Man-Living-Health. Synthesizes Martha Rogers' concepts and principles about unitary human beings with the existential-phenomenological tenets of human subjectivity and intentionality and the concepts of coconstitution, coexistence, and situated freedom. The unity of Man-Living-Health is the focus of this theory. The term *man* is used in the generic sense of homo sapiens or mankind.

Man—an open being, more than and different from the sum of parts in mutual simultaneous interchange with the environment. Man chooses from options and bears responsibility for choices.

Health—a process of becoming experienced by the individual. It is man's *lived experiences*, a nonlinear entity that cannot be qualified as good, bad, more, or less. Unitary man's health is a synthesis of values, a way of living, a continuously changing process that man cocreates.

Three major principles of theory of human becoming:

1. *Structuring meaning multidimensionally is cocreating reality through the languaging of valuing and imaging.* Man constructs meaning from many levels of the universe, from the tacit and explicit, in the cocreating of what is real.
    Imaging—the picturing or making real of events, ideas, and people.
    Valuing—the living of cherished beliefs.
    Languaging—reflects images and values through speaking and moving.
2. *Cocreating rhythmical patterns of relating is living the paradoxical unity of revealing-concealing and enabling-limiting while connecting-separating.* Man and environment cocreate a rhythmical interchange.
    Connecting-separating—rhythmical pattern of distancing and relating, moving in one direction and away from others, yet always toward greater diversity.
    Enabling-limiting—rhythmical pattern of man's simultaneous choosing to enable movement in one direction and limit movement in another direction in a situation.
    Revealing-concealing—rhythmical pattern involving the simultaneous disclosing of some aspects of self and hiding of others.
3. *Cotranscending with the possibles is powering unique ways of originating in the process of transforming.* Man exists with others and in this interrelationship continues to cocreate self and chooses to make possibles actuals, which in turn creates other possibles.
    Originating—creating anew and generating unique ways of living.
    Powering—the pushing-resisting force in originating.
    Transforming—the changing of change, coconstituting anew in a deliberate way. Change is a continuous, ongoing process in the man-environment interrelationship that is recognized by increasing diversity and moving beyond where one is to the not-yet.

</td></tr>
<tr><td>Implications for
Nursing Education</td><td>Nursing curriculum would focus on the principles of the theory. Nursing course content flows from these three principles. Clinical courses emphasize the knowledge and skills needed in nursing practice. Graduate education builds on baccalaureate education and prepares specialists who concentrate on creating and testing concepts of the theory of human becoming.</td></tr>
</table>

References Parse, R. R. (1981). *Man-living-health. A theory of nursing.* New York: Wiley.

Parse, R. R. (1987). Parse's man-living-health theory of nursing. In R. R. Parse, *Nursing science. Major paradigms, theories, and critiques* (pp. 159–180). Philadelphia: Saunders.

Hildegard Peplau's Theory of Interpersonal Relations in Nursing

Overview

Nursing is a significant, therapeutic, and interpersonal process. It functions cooperatively with other human processes that make health possible for individuals in communities. The functions of interpersonal relations are being able to (1) understand one's own behavior, (2) help others to identify felt difficulties, and (3) apply principles of human relations to the problems that arise at all levels of experience.

Nurse-patient relationship consists of four phases:

1. *Phase of orientation*—the patient has a felt need signifying a health problem and seeks help to clarify the problem. The patient participates in the orienting process by asking questions, by trying to find out what needs to be known in order to feel secure, and by observing ways in which professional people respond. The nurse participates by helping the patient to recognize and understand the health problem and the extent of need for assistance, to understand what professional services can offer, to plan the use of professional services, and to harness energy from tension and anxiety connected with felt needs.

2. *Phase of identification*—the patient learns how to use the nurse-patient relationship as both come to know and respect each other as persons who have similarities and differences. The nurse uses professional education and skills to help the patient arrive at a point where full use can be made of the relationship in order to solve the health problem.

3. *Phase of exploitation*—the patient makes full use of available professional service.

4. *Phase of resolution*—the nurse helps the patient to organize actions so that the patient will want to be free for more productive social activities and relationships.

Implications for Nursing Practice

Nursing practice occurs within a relationship of nurses with patients. Throughout the four phases of this relationship, the nurse may function as a resource person, counselor, surrogate, and technical expert. As a *resource person*, the nurse gives specific, needed information that helps the patient understand the health problem and the new situation. As a *counselor*, the nurse listens to the patient review events that led up to hospitalization and feelings connected with these events. As a *surrogate* for mother, father, sibling, or other person, the nurse aids the patient by permitting re-enactment and examination of older feelings about prior relationships. As a *technical expert*, the nurse understands various professional devices and manipulates them with skill and discrimination in the interest of the patient.

Nurses *observe* the ways in which patients transform energy into patterns of action that bring satisfaction or security in the face of a recurring problem. Nurses and patients *communicate* with one another in terms of their views of themselves and their expectations of others. Nurses *record* the verbatim difficulties of patients and desymbolize the recordings to reveal hidden wishes and longings that may be the root of the problem.

Implications for Nursing Education

Nursing is an educative instrument, a maturing force, that aims to promote forward movement of personality in the direction of creative, constructive, productive, personal, and community living. The task of each school of nursing is to develop the nurse as a person who is aware of how he or she functions in a situation and as a person who wants to nurse patients in a helpful way. Nursing courses emphasize experiential teaching, whereby students participate in clinical experiences and formulate the principles and techniques of intervention in psychiatric situations through discussion of the experiences with classmates and faculty.

References

Peplau, H. E. (1951). Toward new concepts in nursing and nursing education. *American Journal of Nursing, 51*, 722–724.

Peplau, H. E. (1952). *Interpersonal relations in nursing.* New York: G. P. Putnam's Sons.

Reva Rubin's Theory of Clinical Nursing

Overview

Based on the premise that the proper study of nursing is not the nurse but the patient. Patients are persons undergoing subjectively involved experiences of varying degrees of tension or stress in a health problem situation. Nursing provides helping techniques whereby the patient endures, adjusts to, and usefully integrates the health problem in its many ramifications. Nursing care exists in a one-to-one relationship with the patient and depends on the best estimate available of the patient's situation, which is expressed as a fraction or ratio that reflects the level or intensity of nursing care required. If the situation is relatively insignificant, nursing care probably need not go beyond careful assessment. If the situation for the patient is overwhelming, nursing care may encompass a whole series of activities to lessen the effects on the patient or to reinforce the patient's ability to cope with the situation. The theory of clinical nursing has been used as a guide for nursing practice and nursing research. Studies guided by the relatively abstract theory of clinical nursing have led to the development of several more circumscribed theories of the maternal experience, including maternal touch, maternal role attachment, maternal tasks, body image and self-esteem in childbearing, and time and space in childbearing.

Implications for Nursing Practice

Nursing practice is guided through the phenomenon of *situational fluidity,* which characterizes nursing care in terms of time, definition or diagnostic sets, and actions. *Time:* Nursing operates within the present. Patient needs and behavior have an immediacy if not an urgency. *Definition* or *diagnostic sets:* Nursing diagnoses are based on the definition of capacities and limitations of the persons who are patients in relation to the situations in which they find themselves. *Actions:* Nursing actions are primarily directed toward helping the patient realign observations and expectations into a better "fit" with each other. All nursing conveys a message to patients about themselves in their immediate situations.

Implications for Nursing Education

The naturalistic method of observation is emphasized. Observation is of patients in action, involved in a natural situation and setting. The learners typically are graduate students in nursing. The nurse-observer is viewed as an identifiable and functional part of the setting, as well as a helpful adjunct in the situation. The student is trained to observe while providing nursing care for the patient and to record the entire nurse-patient interaction. The recorded observation serves as a data base for evaluating the quality and adequacy of nursing care as well as for generating new theories.

Reference

Rubin, R. (1984). *Maternal identity and the maternal experience.* New York: Springer.

Jean Watson's Theory of Human Caring

Overview

Deals with the caring actions taken by nurses as they interact with others. Values and assumptions that form the basis for the theory of human caring reflect a metaphysical, phenomenological-existential, and spiritual orientation that draws upon Eastern philosophy.

Values include (1) deep respect for the wonder and mysteries of life and the power of humans to change, (2) high regard and reverence for the spiritual-subjective center of the person with power to grow and change, and (3) a nonpaternalistic approach to helping a person gain more self-knowledge, self-control, and self-healing regardless of the presenting health-illness condition.

Assumptions deal with human life, nursing science, and the process of nursing. Watson's conception of *human life* is tied to notions that one's soul possesses a body that is not confined by objective space and time. The

2471

lived world of the experiencing person is not distinguished by external and internal notions of time and space, but shapes its own time and space, which is unconstrained by linearity. Nursing is a human science of persons and human health-illness experiences that are mediated by professional, personal, scientific, esthetic, and ethical human care transactions. The *process of nursing* is human care.

The main concept of this theory is *transpersonal human caring,* which is best understood within the context of three ancillary concepts:

1. *Human life:* spiritual-mental-physical being-in-the-world, which is continuous in time and space.
2. *Illness:* subjective turmoil or disharmony with a person's inner self or soul at some level or disharmony within the spheres of the person, either consciously or unconsciously. Not necessarily disease.
3. *Health:* unity and harmony within the mind, body, and soul. Transpersonal human caring and caring transactions are those scientific, professional, and ethical but also esthetic, creative, and personalized giving-receiving behaviors and responses between nurse and patient that allow for contact between the subjective world of the experiencing persons through physical, mental, or spiritual routes or some combination thereof.

Implications for Nursing Practice

The goal of nursing practice is to help persons gain a higher degree of harmony within the mind, body, and soul, which generates self-knowledge, self-reverence, self-healing, and self-care processes while increasing diversity. This goal is pursued through a human care process that involves *carative factors,* including (1) a humanistic-altruistic system of values; (2) faith-hope; (3) sensitivity to self and others; (4) a helping-trusting human care relationship; (5) expressing positive and negative feelings; (6) a creative problem-solving caring process; (7) transpersonal teaching and learning; (8) a supportive, protective, and/or corrective mental, physical, societal, and spiritual environment; (9) human needs assistance; and (10) existential-phenomenological-spiritual forces.

Implications for Nursing Education

Nursing education focuses on clarification of the values and views regarding human life, since Watson maintained that the nature of human life is the subject matter of nursing. A moral context for nursing education that emphasizes a way of being as a caring professional is required. A curriculum based on the theory of human caring acknowledges caring as a moral ideal and incorporates philosophical theories of human caring, health, and healing. The humanities, social-biomedical science, and human caring content and process are regarded as core areas of content. New approaches to study of concepts of caring are needed, such as courses using art, music, literature, poetry, drama, and movement to facilitate understanding of responses to health and illness as well as to new caring-healing modalities. Education for professional nursing should be at the postbaccalaureate level, with the award of the doctorate in nursing degree (N.D.).

References

Watson, J. (1985). *Nursing: Human science and human care. A theory of nursing.* Norwalk, CT: Appleton-Century-Crofts.
Watson, J. (1988). Human caring as moral context for nursing education. *Nursing and Health Care, 9,* 422–425.

SOURCE: Adapted from Fawcett, J. (1989). Analysis and evaluation of conceptual models of nursing (2nd ed.). Philadelphia: F.A. Davis.

App. 24: Diagnosis Related Groups (DRGs)

Major Diagnostic Category (MDC)

1 Diseases and disorders of the nervous system
2 Diseases and disorders of the eye
3 Diseases and disorders of the ear, nose, and throat
4 Diseases and disorders of the respiratory system
5 Diseases and disorders of the circulatory system
6 Diseases and disorders of the digestive system
7 Diseases and disorders of the hepatobiliary system and pancreas
8 Diseases and disorders of the musculoskeletal system and connective tissue
9 Diseases and disorders of the skin, subcutaneous tissue, and breast
10 Endocrine, nutritional, and metabolic diseases and disorders
11 Diseases and disorders of the kidney and urinary tract
12 Diseases and disorders of the male reproductive system
13 Diseases and disorders of the female reproductive system
14 Pregnancy, childbirth, and the puerperium
15 Newborns and other neonates with condition originating in perinatal period
16 Diseases and disorders of blood and blood-forming organs
17 Myeloproliferative disorders
18 Infectious and parasitic diseases
19 Mental diseases and disorders
20 Substance use and substance-induced organic mental disorders
21 Injuries, poisonings, and toxic effects of drugs
22 Burns
23 Factors influencing health status and other contacts with health services
24 No major diagnostic category

DRG	MDC		TITLE
1	1	S	Craniotomy, age > 17 except for trauma
2	1	S	Craniotomy for trauma, age > 17
3	1	S	Craniotomy, age < 18
4	1	S	Spinal procedures
5	1	S	Extracranial vascular procedures
6	1	S	Carpal tunnel release
7	1	S	Peripheral and cranial nerve and other nervous system procedures, age > 69 and/or C.C.
8	1	S	Peripheral and cranial nerve and other nervous system procedures, age < 70 without C.C.
9	1	M	Spinal disorders and injuries
10	1	M	Nervous system neoplasms, age > 69 and/or C.C.
11	1	M	Nervous system neoplasms, age < 70 without C.C.
12	1	M	Degenerative nervous system disorders
13	1	M	Multiple sclerosis and cerebellar ataxia
14	1	M	Specific cerebrovascular disorders except transient ischemic attack
15	1	M	Transient ischemic attack and precerebral occlusions
16	1	M	Nonspecific cerebrovascular disorders with C.C.
17	1	M	Nonspecific cerebrovascular disorders without C.C.
18	1	M	Cranial and peripheral nerve disorders, age > 69 and/or C.C.
19	1	M	Cranial and peripheral nerve disorders, age < 70 without C.C.
20	1	M	Nervous system infection except viral meningitis
21	1	M	Viral meningitis
22	1	M	Hypertensive encephalopathy
23	1	M	Nontraumatic stupor and coma
24	1	M	Seizure and headache, age > 69 and/or C.C.
25	1	M	Seizure and headache, age 18 to 69 without C.C.
26	1	M	Seizure and headache, age 0 to 17
27	1	M	Traumatic stupor and coma, coma > 1 hour

M = medical case; S = surgical case; C.C. = comorbidity or complication; O.R. = operating room

DRG	MDC		TITLE
28	1	M	Traumatic stupor and coma, coma <1 hour, age >69 and/or C.C.
29	1	M	Traumatic stupor and coma, coma <1 hour, age 18 to 69 without C.C.
30	1	M	Traumatic stupor and coma, coma <1 hour, age 0 to 17
31	1	M	Concussion, age >69 and/or C.C.
32	1	M	Concussion, age 18 to 69 without C.C.
33	1	M	Concussion, age 0 to 17
34	1	M	Other disorders of nervous system, age >69 and/or C.C.
35	1	M	Other disorders of nervous system, age <70 without C.C.
36	2	S	Retinal procedures
37	2	S	Orbital procedures
38	2	S	Primary iris procedures
39	2	S	Lens procedures with or without vitrectomy
40	2	S	Extraocular procedures except orbit, age >17
41	2	S	Extraocular procedures except orbit, age 0 to 17
42	2	S	Intraocular procedures except retina, iris, and lens
43	2	M	Hyphema
44	2	M	Acute major eye infections
45	2	M	Neurological eye disorders
46	2	M	Other disorders of the eye, age >17 with C.C.
47	2	M	Other disorders of the eye, age >17 without C.C.
48	2	M	Other disorders of the eye, age 0 to 17
49	3	S	Major head and neck procedures
50	3	S	Sialoadenectomy
51	3	S	Salivary gland procedures except sialoadenectomy
52	3	S	Cleft lip and palate repair
53	3	S	Sinus and mastoid procedures, age >17
54	3	S	Sinus and mastoid procedures, age 0 to 17
55	3	S	Miscellaneous ear, nose, and throat procedures
56	3	S	Rhinoplasty
57	3	S	Tonsil and adenoid procedures except tonsillectomy and/or adenoidectomy only, age >17
58	3	S	Tonsil and adenoid procedures except tonsillectomy and/or adenoidectomy only, age 0 to 17
59	3	S	Tonsillectomy and/or adenoidectomy only, age >17
60	3	S	Tonsillectomy and/or adenoidectomy only, age 0 to 17
61	3	S	Myringotomy with tube insertion, age >17
62	3	S	Myringotomy with tube insertion, age 0 to 17
63	3	S	Other ear, nose, and throat O.R. procedures
64	3	M	Ear, nose, and throat malignancy
65	3	M	Disequilibrium
66	3	M	Epistaxis
67	3	M	Epiglottitis
68	3	M	Otitis media and URI, age >69 and/or C.C.
69	3	M	Otitis media and URI, age 18 to 69 without C.C.
70	3	M	Otitis media and URI, age 0 to 17
71	3	M	Laryngotracheitis
72	3	M	Nasal trauma and deformity
73	3	M	Other ear, nose, and throat diagnoses, age >17
74	3	M	Other ear, nose, and throat diagnoses, age 0 to 17
75	4	S	Major chest procedures
76	4	S	Other respiratory system O.R. procedures with C.C.
77	4	S	Other respiratory system O.R. procedures without C.C.
78	4	M	Pulmonary embolism
79	4	M	Respiratory infections and inflammations, age >69 and/or C.C.
80	4	M	Respiratory infections and inflammations, age 18 to 69 without C.C.
81	4	M	Respiratory infections and inflammations, age 0 to 17
82	4	M	Respiratory neoplasms
83	4	M	Major chest trauma, age >69 and/or C.C.
84	4	M	Major chest trauma, age <70 without C.C.

DRG	MDC		TITLE
85	4	M	Pleural effusion, age >69 and/or C.C.
86	4	M	Pleural effusion, age <70 without C.C.
87	4	M	Pulmonary edema and respiratory failure
88	4	M	Chronic obstructive pulmonary disease
89	4	M	Simple pneumonia and pleurisy, age >69 and/or C.C.
90	4	M	Simple pneumonia and pleurisy, age 18 to 69 without C.C.
91	4	M	Simple pneumonia and pleurisy, age 0 to 17
92	4	M	Interstitial lung disease, age >69 and/or C.C.
93	4	M	Interstitial lung disease, age <70 without C.C.
94	4	M	Pneumothorax, age >69 and/or C.C.
95	4	M	Pneumothorax, age <70 without C.C.
96	4	M	Bronchitis and asthma, age >69 and/or C.C.
97	4	M	Bronchitis and asthma, age 18 to 69 without C.C.
98	4	M	Bronchitis and asthma, age 0 to 17
99	4	M	Respiratory signs and symptoms, age >69 and/or C.C.
100	4	M	Respiratory signs and symptoms, age <70 without C.C.
101	4	M	Other respiratory system diagnoses, age >69 and/or C.C.
102	4	M	Other respiratory system diagnoses, age <70 without C.C.
103	5	S	Heart transplant
104	5	S	Cardiac valve procedure with pump and with cardiac catheterization
105	5	S	Cardiac valve procedure with pump and without cardiac catheterization
106	5	S	Coronary bypass with cardiac catheterization
107	5	S	Coronary bypass without cardiac catheterization
108	5	S	Other cardiothoracic or vascular procedures with pump
109	5	S	Other cardiothoracic procedures without pump
110	5	S	Major reconstructive vascular procedures without pump, age >69 and/or C.C.
111	5	S	Major reconstructive vascular procedures without pump, age <70 without C.C.
112	5	S	Vascular procedures except major reconstruction without pump
113	5	S	Amputation for circulatory system disorders except upper limb and toe
114	5	S	Upper limb and toe amputation for circulatory system disorders
115	5	S	Permanent cardiac pacemaker implant with AMI, heart failure, or shock
116	5	S	Permanent cardiac pacemaker implant without AMI, heart failure, or shock
117	5	S	Cardiac pacemaker replacement and revision except pulse generator replacement
118	5	S	Cardiac pacemaker pulse generator replacement
119	5	S	Vein ligation and stripping
120	5	S	Other circulatory system O.R. procedures
121	5	M	Circulatory disorders with AMI and cardiovascular complications, discharged alive
122	5	M	Circulatory disorders with AMI without cardiovascular complications, discharged alive
123	5	M	Circulatory disorders with AMI, expired
124	5	M	Circulatory disorders except AMI, with cardiac catheterization and complex diagnosis
125	5	M	Circulatory disorders except AMI, with cardiac catheterization without complex diagnosis
126	5	M	Acute and subacute endocarditis
127	5	M	Heart failure and shock
128	5	M	Deep vein thrombophlebitis
129	5	M	Cardiac arrest, unexplained
130	5	M	Peripheral vascular disorders, age >69 and/or C.C.
131	5	M	Peripheral vascular disorders, age <70 without C.C.
132	5	M	Atherosclerosis, age >69 and/or C.C.
133	5	M	Atherosclerosis, age <70 without C.C.
134	5	M	Hypertension
135	5	M	Cardiac congenital and valvular disorders, age >69 and/or C.C.
136	5	M	Cardiac congenital and valvular disorders, age 18 to 69 without C.C.
137	5	M	Cardiac congenital and valvular disorders, age 0 to 17
138	5	M	Cardiac arrhythmia and conduction disorders, age >69 and/or C.C.
139	5	M	Cardiac arrhythmia and conduction disorders, age <70 without C.C.
140	5	M	Angina pectoris
141	5	M	Syncope and collapse, age >69 and/or C.C.

DRG	MDC		TITLE
142	5	M	Syncope and collapse, age <70 without C.C.
143	5	M	Chest pain
144	5	M	Other circulatory system diagnoses with C.C.
145	5	M	Other circulatory system diagnoses without C.C.
146	6	S	Rectal resection, age >69 and/or C.C.
147	6	S	Rectal resection, age <70 without C.C.
148	6	S	Major small and large bowel procedures, age >69 and/or C.C.
149	6	S	Major small and large bowel procedures, age <70 without C.C.
150	6	S	Peritoneal adhesiolysis, age >69 and/or C.C.
151	6	S	Peritoneal adhesiolysis, age <70 without C.C.
152	6	S	Minor small and large bowel procedures, age >69 and/or C.C.
153	6	S	Minor small and large bowel procedures, age <70 without C.C.
154	6	S	Stomach, esophageal, and duodenal procedures, age >69 and/or C.C.
155	6	S	Stomach, esophageal, and duodenal procedures, age 18 to 69 without C.C.
156	6	S	Stomach, esophageal, and duodenal procedures, age 0 to 17
157	6	S	Anal and stomal procedures, age >69 and/or C.C.
158	6	S	Anal and stomal procedures, age <70 without C.C.
159	6	S	Hernia procedures except inguinal and femoral, age >69 and/or C.C.
160	6	S	Hernia procedures except inguinal and femoral, age 18 to 69 without C.C.
161	6	S	Inguinal and femoral hernia procedures, age >69 and/or C.C.
162	6	S	Inguinal and femoral hernia procedures, age 18 to 69 without C.C.
163	6	S	Hernia procedures, age 0 to 17
164	6	S	Appendectomy with complicated principal diagnosis, age >69 and/or C.C.
165	6	S	Appendectomy with complicated principal diagnosis, age <70 without C.C.
166	6	S	Appendectomy without complicated principal diagnosis, age >69 and/or C.C.
167	6	S	Appendectomy without complicated principal diagnosis, age <70 without C.C.
168	6	S	Mouth procedures, age >69 and/or C.C.
169	6	S	Mouth procedures, age <70 without C.C.
170	6	S	Other digestive system O.R. procedures, age >69 and/or C.C.
171	6	S	Other digestive system O.R. procedures, age <70 without C.C.
172	6	M	Digestive malignancy, age >69 and/or C.C.
173	6	M	Digestive malignancy, age <70 without C.C.
174	6	M	G.I. hemorrhage, age >69 and/or C.C.
175	6	M	G.I. hemorrhage, age <70 without C.C.
176	6	M	Complicated peptic ulcer
177	6	M	Uncomplicated peptic ulcer, age >69 and/or C.C.
178	6	M	Uncomplicated peptic ulcer, age <70 without C.C.
179	6	M	Inflammatory bowel disease
180	6	M	G.I. obstruction, age >69 and/or C.C.
181	6	M	G.I. obstruction, age <70 without C.C.
182	6	M	Esophagitis, gastroenteritis, and miscellaneous digestive disorders, age >69 and/or C.C.
183	6	M	Esophagitis, gastroenteritis, and miscellaneous digestive disorders, age 18 to 69 without C.C.
184	6	M	Esophagitis, gastroenteritis, and miscellaneous digestive disorders, age 0 to 17
185	6	M	Dental and oral disorders except extractions and restorations, age >17
186	6	M	Dental and oral disorders except extractions and restorations, age 0 to 17
187	6	M	Dental extractions and restorations
188	6	M	Other digestive system diagnoses, age >69 and/or C.C.
189	6	M	Other digestive system diagnoses, age 18 to 69 without C.C.
190	6	M	Other digestive system diagnoses, age 0 to 17
191	7	S	Major pancreas, liver, and shunt procedures
192	7	S	Minor pancreas, liver, and shunt procedures
193	7	S	Biliary tract procedures except total cholecystectomy, age >69 and/or C.C.
194	7	S	Biliary tract procedures except total cholecystectomy, age <70 without C.C.
195	7	S	Total cholecystectomy with common duct exploration, age >69 and/or C.C.
196	7	S	Total cholecystectomy with common duct exploration, age <70 without C.C.
197	7	S	Total cholecystectomy without common duct exploration, age >69 and/or C.C.
198	7	S	Total cholecystectomy without common duct exploration, age <70 without C.C.

DRG	MDC		TITLE
199	7	S	Hepatobiliary diagnostic procedure for malignancy
200	7	S	Hepatobiliary diagnostic procedure for nonmalignancy
201	7	S	Other hepatobiliary or pancreas O.R. procedures
202	7	M	Cirrhosis and alcoholic hepatitis
203	7	M	Malignancy of hepatobiliary system or pancreas
204	7	M	Disorders of pancreas except malignancy
205	7	M	Disorders of liver except malignancy, cirrhosis, alcoholic hepatitis, age >69 and/or C.C.
206	7	M	Disorders of liver except malignancy, cirrhosis, alcoholic hepatitis, age <70 without C.C.
207	7	M	Disorders of the biliary tract, age >69 and/or C.C.
208	7	M	Disorders of the biliary tract, age <70 without C.C.
209	8	S	Major joint and limb reattachment procedure
210	8	S	Hip and femur procedures except major joint, age >69 and/or C.C.
211	8	S	Hip and femur procedures except major joint, age 18 to 69 without C.C.
212	8	S	Hip and femur procedures except major joint, age 0 to 17
213	8	S	Amputations for musculoskeletal system and connective tissue disorders
214	8	S	Back and neck procedures, age >69 and/or C.C.
215	8	S	Back and neck procedures, age <70 without C.C.
216	8	S	Biopsies of musculoskeletal system and connective tissue
217	8	S	Wound debridement and skin graft except hand for musculoskeletal and connective tissue disorders
218	8	S	Lower extremity and humerus procedures except hip, foot, femur, age >69 and/or C.C.
219	8	S	Lower extremity and humerus procedures except hip, foot, femur, age 18 to 69 without C.C.
220	8	S	Lower extremity and humerus procedures except hip, foot, femur, age 0 to 17
221	8	S	Knee procedures, age >69 and/or C.C.
222	8	S	Knee procedures, age <70 without C.C.
223	8	S	Major shoulder/elbow procedure or other upper extremity procedure with C.C.
224	8	S	Shoulder, elbow, or forearm procedure except major joint procedure without C.C.
225	8	S	Foot procedures
226	8	S	Soft tissue procedures, age >69 and/or C.C.
227	8	S	Soft tissue procedures, age <70 without C.C.
228	8	S	Major thumb or joint procedure or other hand or wrist procedure with C.C.
229	8	S	Hand or wrist procedure except major joint procedure without C.C.
230	8	S	Local excision and removal of internal fixation devices of hip and femur
231	8	S	Local excision and removal of internal fixation devices except hip and femur
232	8	S	Arthroscopy
233	8	S	Other musculoskeletal system and connective tissue O.R. procedures, age >69 and/or C.C.
234	8	S	Other musculoskeletal system and connective tissue O.R. procedures, age <70 without C.C.
235	8	M	Fractures of femur
236	8	M	Fractures of hip and pelvis
237	8	M	Sprains, strains, and dislocations of hip, pelvis, and thigh
238	8	M	Osteomyelitis
239	8	M	Pathological fractures and musculoskeletal and connective tissue malignancy
240	8	M	Connective tissue disorders, age >69 and/or C.C.
241	8	M	Connective tissue disorders, age <70 without C.C.
242	8	M	Septic arthritis
243	8	M	Medical back problems
244	8	M	Bone diseases and specific arthropathies, age >69 and/or C.C.
245	8	M	Bone diseases and specific arthropathies, age <70 without C.C.
246	8	M	Nonspecific arthropathies
247	8	M	Signs and symptoms of musculoskeletal system and connective tissue
248	8	M	Tendinitis, myositis, and bursitis
249	8	M	Aftercare, musculoskeletal system and connective tissue
250	8	M	Fractures, sprains, strains, and dislocations of forearm, hand, foot, age >69 and/or C.C.

DRG	MDC		TITLE
251	8	M	Fractures, sprains, strains, and dislocations of forearm, hand, foot, age 18 to 69 without C.C.
252	8	M	Fractures, sprains, strains, and dislocations of forearm, hand, foot, age 0 to 17
253	8	M	Fractures, sprains, strains, and dislocations of upper arm and lower leg except foot, age > 69 and/or C.C.
254	8	M	Fractures, sprains, strains, and dislocations of upper arm and lower leg except foot, age 18 to 69 without C.C.
255	8	M	Fractures, sprains, strains, and dislocations of upper arm and lower leg except foot, age 0 to 17
256	8	M	Other diagnoses of musculoskeletal system and connective tissue
257	9	S	Total mastectomy for malignancy, age > 69 and/or C.C.
258	9	S	Total mastectomy for malignancy, age < 70 without C.C.
259	9	S	Subtotal mastectomy for malignancy, age > 69 and/or C.C.
260	9	S	Subtotal mastectomy for malignancy, age < 70 without C.C.
261	9	S	Breast procedure for nonmalignancy except biopsy and local excision
262	9	S	Breast biopsy and local excision for nonmalignancy
263	9	S	Skin grafts and/or debridement for skin ulcer or cellulitis, age > 69 and/or C.C.
264	9	S	Skin grafts and/or debridement for skin ulcer or cellulitis, age < 70 without C.C.
265	9	S	Skin graft and/or debridement except for skin ulcer or cellulitis with C.C.
266	9	S	Skin graft and/or debridement except for skin ulcer or cellulitis without C.C.
267	9	S	Perianal and pilonidal procedures
268	9	S	Skin, subcutaneous tissue, and breast plastic procedures
269	9	S	Other skin, subcutaneous tissue, and breast O.R. procedures, age > 69 and/or C.C.
270	9	S	Other skin, subcutaneous tissue, and breast O.R. procedures, age < 70 without C.C.
271	9	M	Skin ulcers
272	9	M	Major skin disorders, age > 69 and/or C.C.
273	9	M	Major skin disorders, age < 70 without C.C.
274	9	M	Malignant breast disorders, age > 69 and/or C.C.
275	9	M	Malignant breast disorders, age < 70 without C.C.
276	9	M	Nonmalignant breast disorders
277	9	M	Cellulitis, age > 69 and/or C.C.
278	9	M	Cellulitis, age 18 to 69 without C.C.
279	9	M	Cellulitis, age 0 to 17
280	9	M	Trauma to the skin, subcutaneous tissue, and breast, age > 69 and/or C.C.
281	9	M	Trauma to the skin, subcutaneous tissue, and breast, age 18 to 69 without C.C.
282	9	M	Trauma to the skin, subcutaneous tissue, and breast age 0 to 17
283	9	M	Minor skin disorders, age > 69 and/or C.C.
284	9	M	Minor skin disorders, age < 70 without C.C.
285	10	S	Amputation of lower limb for endocrine, nutritional, and metabolic disorders
286	10	S	Adrenal and pituitary procedures
287	10	S	Skin grafts and wound debridement for endocrine, nutritional, and metabolic disorders
288	10	S	O.R. procedures for obesity
289	10	S	Parathyroid procedures
290	10	S	Thyroid procedures
291	10	S	Thyroglossal procedures
292	10	S	Other endocrine, nutritional, and metabolic O.R. procedures, age > 69 and/or C.C.
293	10	S	Other endocrine, nutritional, and metabolic O.R. procedures, age < 70 without C.C.
294	10	M	Diabetes, age > 35
295	10	M	Diabetes, age 0 to 35
296	10	M	Nutritional and miscellaneous metabolic disorders, age > 69 and/or C.C.
297	10	M	Nutritional and miscellaneous metabolic disorders, age 18 to 69 without C.C.
298	10	M	Nutritional and miscellaneous metabolic disorders, age 0 to 17
299	10	M	Inborn errors of metabolism
300	10	M	Endocrine disorders, age > 69 and/or C.C.
301	10	M	Endocrine disorders, age < 70 without C.C.
302	11	S	Kidney transplant
303	11	S	Kidney, ureter, and major bladder procedure for neoplasm
304	11	S	Kidney, ureter, and major bladder procedure for non-neoplasm, age > 69 and/or C.C.

DRG	MDC		TITLE
305	11	S	Kidney, ureter, and major bladder procedure for non-neoplasm, age <70 without C.C.
306	11	S	Prostatectomy, age >69 and/or C.C.
307	11	S	Prostatectomy, age <70 without C.C.
308	11	S	Minor bladder procedures, age >69 and/or C.C.
309	11	S	Minor bladder procedures, age <70 without C.C.
310	11	S	Transurethral procedures, age >69 and/or C.C.
311	11	S	Transurethral procedures, age <70 without C.C.
312	11	S	Urethral procedures, age >69 and/or C.C.
313	11	S	Urethral procedures, age 18 to 69 without C.C.
314	11	S	Urethral procedures, age 0 to 17
315	11	S	Other kidney and urinary tract O.R. procedures
316	11	M	Renal failure
317	11	M	Admit for renal dialysis
318	11	M	Kidney and urinary tract neoplasms, age >69 and/or C.C.
319	11	M	Kidney and urinary tract neoplasms, age <70 without C.C.
320	11	M	Kidney and urinary tract infections, age >69 and/or C.C.
321	11	M	Kidney and urinary tract infections, age 18 to 69 without C.C.
322	11	M	Kidney and urinary tract infections, age 0 to 17
323	11	M	Urinary stones, age >69 and/or C.C. and/or ESW lithotripsy
324	11	M	Urinary stones, age <70 without C.C.
325	11	M	Kidney and urinary tract signs and symptoms, age >69 and/or C.C.
326	11	M	Kidney and urinary tract signs and symptoms, age 18 to 69 without C.C.
327	11	M	Kidney and urinary tract signs and symptoms, age 0 to 17
328	11	M	Urethral stricture, age >69 and/or C.C.
329	11	M	Urethral stricture, age 18 to 69 without C.C.
330	11	M	Urethral stricture, age 0 to 17
331	11	M	Other kidney and urinary tract diagnoses, age >69 and/or C.C.
332	11	M	Other kidney and urinary tract diagnoses, age 18 to 69 without C.C.
333	11	M	Other kidney and urinary tract diagnoses, age 0 to 17
334	12	S	Major male pelvic procedures with C.C.
335	12	S	Major male pelvic procedures without C.C.
336	12	S	Transurethral prostatectomy, age >69 and/or C.C.
337	12	S	Transurethral prostatectomy, age <70 without C.C.
338	12	S	Testes procedures, for malignancy
339	12	S	Testes procedures, nonmalignancy, age >17
340	12	S	Testes procedures, nonmalignancy, age 0 to 17
341	12	S	Penis procedures
342	12	S	Circumcision, age >17
343	12	S	Circumcision, age 0 to 17
344	12	S	Other male reproductive system O.R. procedures for malignancy
345	12	S	Other male reproductive system O.R. procedures except for malignancy
346	12	M	Malignancy, male reproductive system, age >69 and/or C.C.
347	12	M	Malignancy, male reproductive system, age <70 without C.C.
348	12	M	Benign prostatic hypertrophy, age >69 and/or C.C.
349	12	M	Benign prostatic hypertrophy, age <70 without C.C.
350	12	M	Inflammation of the male reproductive system
351	12	M	Sterilization, male
352	12	M	Other male reproductive system diagnoses
353	13	S	Pelvic evisceration, radical hysterectomy, and radical vulvectomy
354	13	S	Uterine, adnexa procedures for non-ovarian/adnexal malignancy, age >69 and/or C.C.
355	13	S	Uterine, adnexa procedures for non-ovarian/adnexal malignancy, age <70 without C.C.
356	13	S	Female reproductive system reconstructive procedures
357	13	S	Uterine and adnexa procedures for ovarian or adnexal malignancy
358	13	S	Uterine and adnexa procedures for nonmalignancy, age >69 and/or C.C.
359	13	S	Uterine and adnexa procedures for nonmalignancy, age <70 without C.C.
360	13	S	Vagina, cervix, and vulva procedures
361	13	S	Laparoscopy and incisional tubal interruption

DRG	MDC		TITLE
362	13	S	Endoscopic tubal interruption
363	13	S	D&C, conization, and radio-implant for malignancy
364	13	S	D&C, conization except for malignancy
365	13	S	Other female reproductive system O.R. procedures
366	13	M	Malignancy, female reproductive system, age >69 and/or C.C.
367	13	M	Malignancy, female reproductive system, age <70 without C.C.
368	13	M	Infections, female reproductive system
369	13	M	Menstrual and other female reproductive system disorders
370	14	S	Cesarean section with C.C.
371	14	S	Cesarean section without C.C.
372	14	M	Vaginal delivery with complicating diagnoses
373	14	M	Vaginal delivery without complicating diagnoses
374	14	S	Vaginal delivery with sterilization and/or D&C
375	14	S	Vaginal delivery with O.R. procedure except sterilization and/or D&C
376	14	M	Postpartum and postabortion diagnoses without O.R. procedure
377	14	S	Postpartum and postabortion diagnoses with O.R. procedure
378	14	M	Ectopic pregnancy
379	14	M	Threatened abortion
380	14	M	Abortion without D&C
381	14	M	Abortion with D&C, aspiration curettage, or hysterotomy
382	14	M	False labor
383	14	M	Other antepartum diagnoses with medical complications
384	14	M	Other antepartum diagnoses without medical complications
385	15		Neonates, died or transferred to another acute care facility
386	15		Extreme immaturity or respiratory distress syndrome, neonate
387	15		Prematurity with major problems
388	15		Prematurity without major problems
389	15		Full-term neonate with major problems
390	15		Neonates with other significant problems
391	15		Normal newborns
392	16	S	Splenectomy, age >17
393	16	S	Splenectomy, age 0 to 17
394	16	S	Other O.R. procedures of the blood and blood-forming organs
395	16	M	Red blood cell disorders, age >17
396	16	M	Red blood cell disorders, age 0 to 17
397	16	M	Coagulation disorders
398	16	M	Reticuloendothelial and immunity disorders, age >69 and/or C.C.
399	16	M	Reticuloendothelial and immunity disorders, age <70 without C.C.
400	17	S	Lymphoma and leukemia with major O.R. procedure
401	17	S	Lymphoma and nonacute leukemia with other O.R. procedure with C.C.
402	17	S	Lymphoma and nonacute leukemia with other O.R. procedure without C.C.
403	17	M	Lymphoma and nonacute leukemia with C.C.
404	17	M	Lymphoma and nonacute leukemia without C.C.
405	17	M	Acute leukemia without major O.R. procedure, age 0 to 17
406	17	S	Myeloproliferative disorder or poorly differentiated neoplasm with major O.R. procedure and C.C.
407	17	S	Myeloproliferative disorder or poorly differentiated neoplasm with major O.R. procedure without C.C.
408	17	S	Myeloproliferative disorder or poorly differentiated neoplasm with other O.R. procedure
409	17	M	Radiotherapy
410	17	M	Chemotherapy
411	17	M	History of malignancy without endoscopy
412	17	M	History of malignancy with endoscopy
413	17	M	Other myeloproliferative disorder or poorly differentiated neoplasm diagnoses, age >69 and/or C.C.
414	17	M	Other myeloproliferative disorder or poorly differentiated neoplasm diagnoses, age <70 without C.C.
415	18	S	O.R. procedure for infectious and parasitic diseases

DRG	MDC		TITLE
416	18	M	Septicemia, age > 17
417	18	M	Septicemia, age 0 to 17
418	18	M	Postoperative and post-traumatic infections
419	18	M	Fever of unknown origin, age > 69 and/or C.C.
420	18	M	Fever of unknown origin, age 18 to 69 without C.C.
421	18	M	Viral illness, age > 17
422	18	M	Viral illness and fever of unknown origin, age 0 to 17
423	18	M	Other infectious and parasitic diseases diagnoses
424	19	S	O.R. procedures with principal diagnosis of mental illness
425	19	M	Acute adjustment reaction and disturbances of psychosocial dysfunction
426	19	M	Depressive neuroses
427	19	M	Neuroses except depressive
428	19	M	Disorders of personality and impulse control
429	19	M	Organic disturbances and mental retardation
430	19	M	Psychoses
431	19	M	Childhood mental disorders
432	19	M	Other diagnoses of mental disorders
433	20		Alcohol/drug use and induced organic mental disorders, left against medical advice
434	20		Alcohol/drug abuse, intoxicant-induced mental syndromes except dependency and/or other symptomatic treatment
435	20		Alcohol/drug dependence, detoxification, and/or other symptomatic treatment
436	20		Alcohol/drug dependence with rehabilitation therapy
437	20		Alcohol/drug dependence, combined rehabilitation and detoxification therapy
438			No longer valid
439	21	S	Skin grafts for injuries
440	21	S	Wound debridement for injuries
441	21	S	Hand procedures for injuries
442	21	S	Other O.R. procedures for injuries, age > 69 and/or C.C.
443	21	S	Other O.R. procedures for injuries, age < 70 without C.C.
444	21	M	Multiple trauma, age > 69 and/or C.C.
445	21	M	Multiple trauma, age 18 to 69 without C.C.
446	21	M	Multiple trauma, age 0 to 17
447	21	M	Allergic reactions, age > 17
448	21	M	Allergic reactions, age 0 to 17
449	21	M	Poisoning and toxic effects of drugs, age > 69 and/or C.C.
450	21	M	Poisoning and toxic effects of drugs, age 18 to 69 without C.C.
451	21	M	Poisoning and toxic effects of drugs, age 0 to 17
452	21	M	Complications of treatment, age > 69 and/or C.C.
453	21	M	Complications of treatment, age < 70 without C.C.
454	21	M	Other injuries, poisonings, and toxic effects diagnoses, age > 69 and/or C.C.
455	21	M	Other injuries, poisonings, and toxic effects diagnoses, age < 70 without C.C.
456	22		Burns, transferred to another acute care facility
457	22	M	Extensive burns without O.R. procedure
458	22	S	Nonextensive burns with skin grafts
459	22	S	Nonextensive burns with wound debridement or other O.R. procedure
460	22	M	Nonextensive burns without O.R. procedure
461	23	S	O.R. procedure with diagnoses of other contact with health services
462	23	M	Rehabilitation
463	23	M	Signs and symptoms with C.C.
464	23	M	Signs and symptoms without C.C.
465	23	M	Aftercare with history of malignancy as secondary diagnosis
466	23	M	Aftercare without history of malignancy as secondary diagnosis
467	23	M	Other factors influencing health status
468			Unrelated O.R. procedure
469			Primary diagnosis invalid as discharge diagnosis
470			Ungroupable
471	8	S	Bilateral or multiple major joint procedures of the lower extremity
472	22	S	Extensive burns with O.R. procedure
473	17	M	Acute leukemia without major O.R. procedure, age > 17

App. 25: Nursing Diagnoses

QUICK VIEW OF CONTENTS

Section 1: Organizes all approved NANDA nursing diagnoses by two nursing models: Gordon's Functional Health Patterns and Doenges & Moorhouse's Diagnostic Divisions. The use of a nursing model as a framework helps to organize the data needed to identify and validate nursing diagnoses.

Section 2: Provides a guide to choosing appropriate nursing diagnoses by alphabetically listing almost 300 diseases/disorders with their commonly associated nursing diagnoses. Each of the listed diseases/disorders has been cross referenced from its position in the body of the dictionary. The nursing diagnoses are written in the form of patient problem statements, also known as PES format (*Problem*, *Etiology*, *Signs/Symptoms*). The phrases "*may be* related to" and "*possibly* evidenced by" in the patient problem statements serve to help one individualize the care for the specific patient situations. A "high risk" diagnosis is not evidenced by signs and symptoms as the problem has not occurred and nursing interventions are directed at prevention. Since the patient's health status is perpetual and ongoing, other nursing diagnoses may be appropriate based on changing patient situations. To identify other applicable nursing diagnoses check with Section 1, then turn to Section 3 to test and validate your choices.

Section 3: Details all NANDA-approved diagnoses in alphabetical order with their associated etiology [Related Factors] and defining characteristics [Signs & Symptoms]. Here lies a specific focus on assessment data/evaluation criteria to help you complete the validation process.

SECTION 1

GORDON'S FUNCTIONAL HEALTH PATTERNS

HEALTH-PERCEPTION—HEALTH MANAGEMENT PATTERN
Health Maintenance, altered
Health-Seeking Behaviors (specify)
Infection, high risk for
Injury, high risk for
Noncompliance [compliance, altered] (specify)
Poisoning, high risk for
Protection, altered
Suffocation, high risk for
Trauma, high risk for

NUTRITIONAL—METABOLIC PATTERN
Aspiration, high risk for
Body Temperature, altered, high risk for
Breastfeeding, effective
Breastfeeding, ineffective
Fluid Volume Deficit [active loss]
Fluid Volume Deficit [regulatory failure]
Fluid Volume Deficit, high risk for
Fluid Volume Excess
Hyperthermia
Hypothermia
Nutrition, altered, less than body requirements
Nutrition, altered, more than body requirements
Nutrition, altered, high risk for more than body requirements
Oral Mucous Membrane, altered
Skin Integrity, impaired
Skin Integrity, impaired, high risk for
Swallowing, impaired
Thermoregulation, ineffective
Tissue Integrity, impaired

ELIMINATION PATTERN
Bowel Incontinence
Constipation
Constipation, colonic
Constipation, perceived
Diarrhea
Incontinence, functional
Incontinence, reflex
Incontinence, stress
Incontinence, total
Incontinence, urge
Urinary Elimination, altered patterns
Urinary Retention [acute/chronic]

ACTIVITY—EXERCISE PATTERN
Activity Intolerance
Activity Intolerance, high risk for
Airway Clearance, ineffective
Breathing Pattern, ineffective
Cardiac Output, decreased
Disuse Syndrome, high risk for
Diversional Activity Deficit
Dysreflexia
Fatigue
Gas Exchange, impaired

2483

Growth and Development, altered
Home Maintenance Management, impaired
Physical Mobility, impaired
Self-Care Deficit: feeding, bathing/hygiene, dressing/grooming, toileting
Tissue Perfusion, altered (specify): cerebral, cardiopulmonary, renal, gastrointestinal, peripheral

SLEEP—REST PATTERN
Sleep Pattern Disturbance

COGNITIVE—PERCEPTUAL PATTERN
Decisional Conflict (specify)
Knowledge Deficit [learning need] (specify)
Pain [acute]
Pain, chronic
Sensory-Perceptual Alterations (specify): visual, auditory, kinesthetic, gustatory, tactile, olfactory
Thought Processes, altered
Unilateral Neglect

SELF-PERCEPTION—SELF-CONCEPT PATTERN
Anxiety (specify level)
Body Image Disturbance
Fear
Hopelessness
Personal Identity Disturbance
Powerlessness
Self-Esteem, chronic low
Self-Esteem, disturbance
Self-Esteem, situational low

ROLE—RELATIONSHIP PATTERN
Communication, impaired verbal
Family processes, altered
Grieving, anticipatory
Grieving, dysfunctional
Parental Role Conflict
Parenting, altered
Parenting, altered, high risk for
Role Performance, altered
Social Interaction, impaired
Social Isolation
Violence, high risk for, directed at self/others

SEXUALITY—REPRODUCTIVE PATTERN
Rape-Trauma Syndrome
Rape-Trauma Syndrome: compound reaction
Rape-Trauma Syndrome: silent reaction
Sexual Dysfunction
Sexuality Patterns, altered

COPING—STRESS TOLERANCE PATTERN
Adjustment, impaired
Coping, defensive
Coping, ineffective, individual
Denial, ineffective
Family Coping, compromised
Family Coping, disabling
Family Coping, potential for growth
Post-Trauma Response

SOURCE: Adapted from Gordon, M: Manual of Nursing Diagnosis, 1991–1992. St. Louis, Mosby-Year Book, Inc., 1991.
NOTE: Information appearing in brackets has been added to clarify and facilitate the use of nursing diagnoses.

DOENGES & MOORHOUSE'S DIAGNOSTIC DIVISIONS

ACTIVITY/REST
Activity Intolerance
Activity Intolerance, high risk for
Disuse Syndrome, high risk for
Diversional Activity Deficit
Fatigue
Sleep Pattern Disturbance

CIRCULATION
Cardiac Output, decreased
Dysreflexia
Tissue Perfusion, altered (specify): cerebral, cardiopulmonary, renal, gastrointestinal, peripheral

EGO INTEGRITY
Adjustment, impaired
Anxiety (specify level)
Body Image Disturbance
Coping, defensive
Coping, ineffective individual
Decisional Conflict (specify)
Denial, ineffective
Fear
Grieving, anticipatory
Grieving, dysfunctional
Hopelessness
Personal Identity Disturbance
Post-Trauma Response
Powerlessness
Rape Trauma Syndrome
Rape Trauma Syndrome: compound reaction
Rape Trauma Syndrome: silent reaction
Self-Esteem, chronic low
Self-Esteem Disturbance
Self-Esteem, situational low
Spiritual Distress

ELIMINATION
Bowel Incontinence
Constipation
Constipation, colonic
Constipation, perceived
Diarrhea
Incontinence, functional
Incontinence, reflex
Incontinence, stress
Incontinence, total
Incontinence, urge
Urinary Elimination, altered patterns of
Urinary Retention [acute/chronic]

FOOD/FLUID

Breastfeeding, effective
Breastfeeding, ineffective
Fluid Volume Deficit [active loss]
Fluid Volume Deficit [regulatory failure]
Fluid Volume Deficit, high risk for
Fluid Volume Excess
Nutrition altered: less than body requirements
Nutrition altered: more than body requirements
Nutrition altered: high risk for more than body requirements
Oral Mucous Membrane, altered
Swallowing, impaired

HYGIENE

Self-Care Deficit: feeding, bathing/hygiene, dressing/grooming, toileting

NEUROSENSORY

Sensory-Perceptual Alterations (specify): visual, auditory, kinesthetic, gustatory, tactile, olfactory
Thought Processes, altered
Unilateral Neglect

PAIN/COMFORT

Pain [acute]
Pain, chronic

RESPIRATION

Airway Clearance, ineffective
Aspiration, high risk for
Breathing Pattern, ineffective
Gas Exchange, impaired

SAFETY

Body Temperature, altered, high risk for
Health Maintenance, altered
Home Maintenance Management, impaired
Hyperthermia
Hypothermia
Infection, high risk for
Injury, high risk for
Physical Mobility, impaired
Poisoning, high risk for
Protection, altered
Skin Integrity, impaired
Skin Integrity, impaired, high risk for
Suffocation, high risk for
Thermoregulation, ineffective
Tissue Integrity, impaired
Trauma, high risk for
Violence, high risk for: directed at self/others

SEXUALITY (Component of Ego Integrity and Social Interaction)

Sexual Dysfunction
Sexuality Patterns, altered

SOCIAL INTERACTION

Communication, impaired verbal
Family Coping, compromised
Family Coping, disabling
Family Coping, potential for growth
Family Processes, altered
Parental Role Conflict
Parenting, altered

            Parenting, altered, high risk for
            Role Performance, altered
            Social Interaction, impaired
            Social Isolation

TEACHING/LEARNING
            Growth and Development, altered
            Health-Seeking Behaviors (specify)
            Knowledge Deficit [learning need] (specify)
            Noncompliance [compliance, altered] (specify)

SOURCE: Adapted from Doenges and Moorhouse: Nurse's Pocket Guide: Nursing Diagnoses with
Interactions, ed. 3. F.A. Davis, Philadelphia, 1991, with permission.

NEWLY APPROVED NURSING DIAGNOSES
NANDA 10TH CONFERENCE, 1992

Caregiver Role Strain
Dysfunctional Ventilatory Weaning Response (DVWR)
High Risk for Caregiver Role Strain
High Risk for Peripheral Neurovascular Dysfunction
High Risk for Self-Mutilation
Interrupted Breastfeeding
Relocation Stress Syndrome
Inability to Sustain Spontaneous Ventilation
Ineffective Infant Feeding Pattern
Ineffective Management of Therapeutic Regimen (Individual)

SECTION 2

NURSING DIAGNOSES GROUPED BY
DISEASES/DISORDERS

abortion, spontaneous
Fluid volume deficit [active loss] may be related to excessive blood loss, possibly evidenced by hypoten-
    sion, decreased pulse volume and pressure, delayed capillary refill, or changes in sensorium.
Tissue perfusion, altered (specify) may be related to hypovolemia, possibly evidenced by: *peripheral:*
    hypotension, cool/pale skin, diminished pulses; *cerebral:* changes in sensorium; *renal:* decreased uri-
    nary output.
Anxiety (specify level) may be related to changes in health status of fetus/self, threat of death, possibly
    evidenced by restlessness, tremors, facial tension, focus on self, or feeling of uncertainty.
Infection, high risk for which may be related to altered myometrial integrity at site of placental attach-
    ment, surgically traumatized tissues, and/or decreased hemoglobin.
Knowledge deficit [learning need] may be related to lack of familiarity with new self/health-care needs,
    sources for support, possibly evidenced by requests for information, statement of concern/miscon-
    ceptions.
Grieving [expected] may be related to perinatal loss, possibly evidenced by crying, expressions of sorrow,
    or changes in eating habits/sleep patterns.

abruptio placentae
Fluid volume deficit [active loss] may be related to excessive blood loss, possibly evidenced by hypoten-
    sion, decreased pulse volume and pressure, delayed capillary refill, or changes in sensorium.

Anxiety (specify level) may be related to threat of death of fetus and/or self, possibly evidenced by focus on self, facial tension, restlessness, feeling of uncertainty, or expressions of concern.

Pain may be related to collection of blood between uterine wall and placenta, possibly evidenced by verbal complaints, abdominal guarding, muscle tension, or alterations in vital signs.

Gas exchange, impaired, fetal may be related to altered uteroplacental oxygen transfer, possibly evidenced by alterations in fetal heart rate and movement.

abscess, brain (acute)

Pain may be related to inflammation, edema of tissues, possibly evidenced by complaints of headache, restlessness, irritability, and moaning.

Body temperature, altered, high risk for may be related to inflammatory process/hypermetabolic state and dehydration.

Thought processes, altered may be related to physiologic changes (e.g., cerebral edema/altered perfusion, fever), possibly evidenced by inability to follow commands, altered attention span, or disorientation.

Suffocation/Trauma, high risk for which may be related to development of clonic/tonic muscle activity and changes in consciousness (seizure activity).

achalasia

Nutrition, altered: less than body requirements may be related to inability and/or reluctance to ingest adequate nutrients to meet metabolic demands, possibly evidenced by reported/observed inadequate intake, weight loss, pale conjunctiva and mucous membranes.

Pain may be related to spasm of the lower esophageal sphincter, possibly evidenced by complaints of substernal pressure, recurrent heartburn, or gastric fullness (gas pains).

Anxiety (specify level)/Fear may be related to recurrent pain, choking sensation, altered health status, possibly evidenced by verbalizations of distress, apprehension, restlessness, or insomnia.

Aspiration, high risk for which may be related to regurgitation/spillover of esophageal contents.

Knowledge deficit [learning need] may be related to lack of familiarity with pathology and treatment of condition, possibly evidenced by requests for information, statement of concern, or development of preventable complications.

Swallowing, impaired may be related to neuromuscular impairment, possibly evidenced by observed difficulty in swallowing or regurgitation.

acidosis, metabolic

Refer to diabetic ketoacidosis

Addison's disease

Fluid volume deficit [regulatory failure] may be related to vomiting, diarrhea, increased renal losses, possibly evidenced by delayed capillary refill, poor skin turgor, dry mucous membranes, or complaints of thirst.

Cardiac output, decreased may be related to hypovolemia and altered electrical conduction/dysrhythmias and/or diminished cardiac muscle mass, possibly evidenced by alterations in vital signs, changes in mentation, and irregular pulse or pulse deficit.

Fatigue may be related to decreased metabolic energy production, altered body chemistry (fluid, electrolyte, and glucose imbalance), possibly evidenced by unremitting/overwhelming lack of energy, inability to maintain usual routines, decreased performance, impaired ability to concentrate, lethargy, and disinterest in surroundings.

Body image disturbance may be related to changes in skin pigmentation, mucous membranes, loss of axillary/pubic hair, possibly evidenced by verbalization of negative feelings about body and decreased social involvement.

Physical mobility, impaired, high risk for which may be related to neuromuscular impairment (muscle wasting/weakness) and dizziness/syncope.

Nutrition, altered: less than body requirements may be related to glucocorticoid deficiency; abnormal fat, protein, and carbohydrate metabolism, nausea, vomiting, anorexia, possibly evidenced by weight loss, muscle wasting, abdominal cramps, diarrhea, and severe hypoglycemia.

Home maintenance management, impaired, high risk for which may be related to effects of disease process, impaired cognitive functioning, and inadequate support systems.

adenoidectomy

Anxiety (specify level)/Fear may be related to separation from supportive others, unfamiliar surroundings, and perceived threat of death, possibly evidenced by crying, apprehension, trembling, and sympathetic stimulation (pupil dilation, increased heart rate).

Airway clearance, ineffective, high risk for which may be related to sedation, collection of secretions/ blood in oropharynx, and vomiting.

Fluid volume deficit, high risk for which may be related to operative trauma to highly vascular site/ hemorrhage.

Pain may be related to physical trauma to oronasopharynx, presence of packing, possibly evidenced by restlessness, crying, and facial mask of pain.

adrenalectomy

Tissue perfusion, altered (specify) may be related to hypovolemia and vascular pooling (vasodilation), possibly evidenced by diminished pulses, pallor/cyanosis, hypotension, and changes in mentation.

Infection, high risk for which may be related to inadequate primary defenses (incision, traumatized tissues), suppressed inflammatory response, invasive procedures.

Knowledge deficit [learning need] may be related to unfamiliarity with long-term therapy requirements, possibly evidenced by request for information and statement of concern/misconception.

adult respiratory distress syndrome (ARDS)

Airway clearance, ineffective may be related to decreased ciliary action, increased amount and viscosity of secretions, and collapse of small airways, possibly evidenced by presence of rhonchi/rales, gurgling respirations, and recurrent cough.

Gas exchange, impaired may be related to changes in pulmonary capillary permeability with edema formation, alveolar collapse with intrapulmonary shunting, possibly evidenced by tachypnea, use of accessory muscles, retractions, cyanosis, and changes in mentation.

Fluid volume deficit, high risk for which may be related to active loss from diuretic use and restricted intake.

Fluid volume excess, high risk for which may be related to excessive sodium/fluid retention or administration.

Cardiac output, decreased, high risk for which may be related to alteration in preload (hypovolemia, vascular pooling, diuretic therapy, and increased intrathoracic pressure/use of PEEP).

Anxiety (specify level)/Fear may be related to situational crisis, change in health status/threat of death, possibly evidenced by increased tension, apprehension, restlessness, sympathetic stimulation, and focus on self.

affective disorder

Refer to bipolar disorders and depressive disorders, major

AIDS (acquired immune deficiency syndrome)

Infection, high risk for progression to sepsis/overgrowth which may be related to suppressed inflammatory response and immunosuppression in combination with inadequate primary defenses and malnutrition.

Fluid volume deficit, high risk for which may be related to excessive losses: copious diarrhea, profuse sweating, vomiting, hypermetabolic state, and fever; impaired intake: nausea and anorexia; lethargy.

Injury, high risk for, altered clotting factors which may be related to decreased vitamin K absorption, alteration in hepatic function, presence of autoimmune antiplatelet antibodies, and circulating endotoxins (sepsis).

Pain may be related to tissue inflammation/destruction: infections, internal/external cutaneous lesions, rectal excoriation, malignancies, necrosis, possibly evidenced by verbal complaints, self-focusing/narrowed focus, alteration in muscle tone, guarding behaviors, autonomic responses, and restlessness.

Skin integrity, impaired may be related to immunologic deficit (AIDS-related dermatitis, bacterial/ fungal infections, opportunistic disease processes/Kaposi's sarcoma), decreased level of activity, altered sensation, skeletal prominence, altered metabolic state, possibly evidenced by skin lesions, ulcerations, decubitus ulcer formation.

Fatigue may be related to decreased metabolic energy production, increased energy requirements (hypermetabolic state), overwhelming psychologic/emotional demands, altered body chemistry (side effects of medication, chemotherapy), possibly evidenced by unremitting/overwhelming lack of energy, inability to maintain usual routines, decreased performance; impaired ability to concentrate, lethargy/listlessness, and disinterest in surroundings.

Nutrition, altered: less than body requirements may by related to inability to ingest, digest, and/or absorb nutrients; nausea/vomiting, hyperactive gag reflex, intestinal disturbances, increased metabolic activity/nutritional needs (fever, infection), possibly evidenced by weight loss, decreased subcutaneous fat/muscle mass, lack of interest in food/aversion to eating, altered taste sensation, abdominal cramping, hyperactive bowel sounds, diarrhea, sore and inflamed buccal cavity.

Health maintenance, altered, high risk for which may be related to lack of material resources, impaired adjustment, and inadequate support systems.

Home maintenance management, impaired, high risk for which may be related to effects of disease process, insufficient finances, and inadequate support systems.

Social isolation may be related to alterations in physical appearance, state of wellness, phobic fear of others (transmission of disease), possibly evidenced by expressed feelings of rejection, absence of supportive significant others, and withdrawal from usual activities.

Thought processes, altered may be related to physiologic changes (hypoxemia, CNS infection by HIV, brain malignancies, and/or disseminated systemic opportunistic infection), alteration of drug metabolism/excretion, accumulation of toxic elements (renal failure, severe electrolyte imbalance, hepatic insufficiency), possibly evidenced by altered attention span, distractibility, memory deficit, disorientation, cognitive dissonance, delusional thinking, sleep disturbances, impaired ability to make decisions/problem solve, inability to follow complex commands/mental tasks, and loss of impulse control.

Powerlessness may be related to confirmed diagnosis of a terminal disease, incomplete grieving process, social ramifications of AIDS, alteration in body image, changes in desired lifestyle; progression of disease, possibly evidenced by feelings of loss of control over own life, depression over physical deterioration that occurs despite patient compliance with regimen, anger, apathy, withdrawal, passivity, dependence on others for care/decision making, resentment, and guilt.

aldosteronism, primary

Fluid volume deficit [regulatory failure] may be related to increased urinary losses, possibly evidenced by dry mucous membranes, poor skin turgor, dilute urine, excessive thirst, weight loss.

Physical mobility, impaired may be related to neuromuscular impairment, weakness, and pain, possibly evidenced by impaired coordination, decreased muscle strength, paralysis, and positive Chvostek's and Trousseau's signs.

Cardiac output, decreased, high risk for which may be related to hypovolemia and altered electrical conduction/dysrhythmias.

Alzheimer's disease

Trauma, high risk for which may be related to inability to recognize/identify danger in environment, disorientation, confusion, impaired judgment, weakness, and muscular incoordination.

Thought processes, altered may be related to physiologic changes (neuronal degeneration), sleep deprivation, possibly evidenced by memory deficit, impaired ability to make decisions/problem solve, distractibility, disorientation.

Sensory-perceptual alterations (specify) may be related to neurologic deficit (irreversible neuronal degeneration, sleep deprivation), environmental factors (socially restricted environment/homebound or institutionalization), possibly evidenced by memory loss, changes in usual response to stimuli, spatial disorientation, confusion, exaggerated emotional responses, anxiety, paranoia, hallucinations, inability to tell position of body parts, and diminished/altered sense of taste.

Self-care deficit (specify) may be related to perceptual/cognitive impairment, unstable gait, possibly evidenced by forgetfulness, disheveled appearance, body odor, incontinence, and decreased dietary intake.

Sleep pattern disturbance may be related to disorientation (day/night reversal), irritability, poor judgment potentiated by neurologic impairment, possibly evidenced by wakefulness and increased aimless wandering, inability to identify need/time for sleeping.

Fear may be related to decreasing functional ability, public disclosure of disabilities, progressive mental/physical deterioration, possibly evidenced by social isolation, aggressive behavior, apprehension, irritability, defensiveness, and suspiciousness.

Grieving, anticipatory may be related to perceived potential loss of self, possibly evidenced by expressions of sorrow and anger, altered sleep and/or eating patterns, changes in activity level, and libido.

Family coping, ineffective, compromised may be related to family disorganization, role changes, long-term illness exhausting supportive/financial capabilities of family member(s), possibly evidenced by verbalizations of frustrations in dealing with day-to-day care, expressed anger/guilt directed toward patient, and withdrawal from interaction with patient.

Home maintenance management, impaired may be related to progressive impaired cognitive functioning, insufficient family organization or planning, unfamiliarity with resources, inadequate support systems, possibly evidenced by household members expressing difficulty/requesting help in maintaining home in comfortable fashion, lack of necessary equipment or aids to care for patient, overtaxed family members, and disorderly surroundings.

Health maintenance, altered may be related to deterioration affecting ability in all areas, cognitive impairment, ineffective individual/family coping, dysfunctional grieving, possibly evidenced by reported or observed inability to take responsibility for meeting basic health practices, reported or observed lack of equipment/financial or other resources, and reported or observed impairment of personal support system.

amputation

Body image disturbance may be related to loss of a body part, possibly evidenced by verbalization of feelings of powerlessness, grief, preoccupation with loss, and unwillingness to look at/touch stump.

Fluid volume deficit, high risk for may be related to extensive surgical procedure interrupting vascular system.

Pain may be related to tissue trauma, severed nerves, possibly evidenced by complaints of incisional/phantom pain, guarding behavior, and narrowed focus.

Physical mobility, impaired may be related to loss of limb, altered sense of balance, possibly evidenced by impaired coordination, unsteady gait, and difficulty/inability to ambulate.

amyotrophic lateral sclerosis

Physical mobility, impaired may be related to muscle wasting/weakness, possibly evidenced by impaired coordination, limited range of motion, and impaired purposeful movement.

Breathing pattern, ineffective may be related to neuromuscular impairment, decreased energy, fatigue, tracheobronchial obstruction, possibly evidenced by shortness of breath, fremitus, respiratory depth changes, and reduced vital capacity.

Body image disturbance may be related to prolonged, debilitating illness with loss of ability to control body, possibly evidenced by verbalization of negative feelings about body, helplessness, observed decrease in social involvement.

Swallowing, impaired may be related to muscle wasting and fatigue, possibly evidenced by recurrent coughing/choking and signs of aspiration.

Powerlessness may be related to debilitating nature of illness, lack of control over outcome, possibly evidenced by expressions of frustration about inability to care for self and depression over physical deterioration.

Communication, impaired verbal may be related to physical barrier (neuromuscular impairment), possibly evidenced by impaired articulation, inability to speak in sentences, and use of nonverbal cues (changes in facial expression).

Self-care deficit (specify) may be related to neuromuscular impairment, decreased strength/endurance, depression, possibly evidenced by inability to perform tasks satisfactorily, disheveled appearance, body odor, and decreased dietary intake.

Grieving, anticipatory may be related to perceived potential loss of self, physio-psychosocial well-being, possibly evidenced by sorrow, choked feelings, expression of distress, changes in eating habits/sleeping patterns, and altered libido.

Home maintenance management, impaired may be related to effects of disease, inadequate support systems, change in financial status, possibly evidenced by lack of necessary equipment or aids, overtaxed family members.

anemia

Activity intolerance may be related to imbalance between oxygen supply and demand, possibly evidenced by reports of fatigue and weakness, abnormal heart rate with activity, and exertional dyspnea.

Knowledge deficit [learning need] may be related to inadequate understanding or misinterpretation of dietary/physiologic needs, possibly evidenced by inadequate dietary intake, request for information, and development of preventable complications.

anemia, sickle cell

Gas exchange, impaired may be related to altered oxygen-carrying capacity of blood, possibly evidenced by signs of hypoxia, changes in mentation, and restlessness.

Pain may be related to localized vascular stasis and occlusion, possibly evidenced by complaints of migratory joint and/or abdominal/back pain, and guarding/distraction behaviors (moaning, crying, restlessness).

Tissue perfusion, altered, (specify) may be related to stasis, occlusion of arterial/venous blood flow, possibly evidenced by signs and symptoms dependent on system involved, for example: *renal:* decreased specific gravity and pale urine in face of dehydration; *cerebral:* paralysis and decreased visual acuity; *peripheral:* distal ischemia and tissue infarctions.

Knowledge deficit [learning need] may be related to lack of exposure/recall regarding disease process, genetic factors, prognosis and treatment needs, misinterpretation of information, possibly evidenced by questions, statement of concern/misconceptions, exacerbation of condition, inadequate follow-through of therapy instructions, and development of preventable complications.

Growth and development, altered may be related to effects of physical condition, possibly evidenced by altered physical growth and delay/difficulty performing skills typical of age group.

Family coping, ineffective, compromised may be related to chronic nature of disease/disability, parent supervision, and lifestyle restrictions, possibly evidenced by protective behavior disproportionate to patient's ability or need for autonomy.

angina pectoris

Pain may be related to ischemia of cardiac muscle, possibly evidenced by verbal complaints, narrowed focus, distraction behaviors (restlessness, moaning), and autonomic responses (diaphoresis, elevation of vital signs).

Cardiac output, decreased may be related to inotropic changes (transient/prolonged myocardial ischemia, effects of medications), alterations in rate/rhythm and electrical conduction, possibly evidenced by changes in hemodynamic readings, dyspnea, restlessness, decreased tolerance for activity, fatigue, diminished peripheral pulses, cool/pale skin, changes in mental status, and continued chest pain.

Anxiety (specify level) may be related to change in health status and/or threat of death, possibly evidenced by verbalized apprehension, facial tension, extraneous movements, and focus on self.

Activity intolerance may be related to imbalance between oxygen supply and demand, possibly evidenced by exertional dyspnea, abnormal pulse/blood pressure response to activity, and ECG changes.

Knowledge deficit [learning need] may be related to lack of exposure, inaccurate/misinterpretation of information regarding disease process, prognosis and treatment needs, possibly evidenced by questions, request for information, statement of concern, and inaccurate follow-through of instructions.

Adjustment, impaired, high risk for which may be related to condition requiring long-term therapy/change in lifestyle, assault to self-esteem, and altered locus of control.

anorexia nervosa

Nutrition, altered: less than body requirements may be related to psychologic restrictions of food intake and/or excessive activity, possibly evidenced by weight loss, denial of hunger, and unusual hoarding or handling of food.

Fluid volume deficit, high risk for which may be related to inadequate intake of food and liquids, consistent self-induced vomiting, and laxative/diuretic use.

Body image disturbance may be related to altered perception of body, possibly evidenced by negative feelings about body, preoccupation with perceived image of self as fat, and change in social involvement.

Coping, ineffective individual may be related to maturational crisis and attempt to control environment, possibly evidenced by verbalization of poor self-esteem and difficulty meeting role-expectations, and poor problem-solving capabilities.

Family coping, ineffective, disabling may be related to ambivalent family relationships and ways of transacting issues of control, possibly evidenced by enmeshed family with lack of separation of individual members who may speak for one another.

anxiety disorders (dependent on degree)

Anxiety (specify level)/Powerlessness may be related to real or perceived threat to physical integrity or self-concept (may or may not be able to identify the threat), unconscious conflict about essential values/beliefs and goals of life, unmet needs, positive or negative self-talk, possibly evidenced by persistent feelings of apprehension and uneasiness, a general anxious feeling that patient has difficulty alleviating, sympathetic stimulation, extraneous movements (foot shuffling, hand/arm fidgeting, rocking movements, restlessness), poor eye contact, focus on self, impaired functioning, and free-floating anxiety.

Sleep pattern disturbance may be related to psychologic stress, repetitive thoughts, possibly evidenced by reports of difficulty in falling asleep/awakening earlier or later than desired, complaints of not feeling rested, dark circles under eyes, and frequent yawning.

Coping, ineffective individual may be related to unrealistic perceptions and inadequate coping methods, possibly evidenced by verbalization of inability to cope/problem solve, excessive compulsive behaviors (e.g., smoking, drinking), and emotional tension.

Fear may be related to phobic stimulus, possibly evidenced by response ranging from apprehension to panic, fight or flight response, and sympathetic stimulation (pupil dilation, increased heart rate).

2492

Social interaction, impaired may be related to low self-esteem and misinterpretation of internal/external stimuli, possibly evidenced by discomfort in social situations and withdrawal from or reported change in pattern of interactions.

aortic stenosis
Cardiac output, decreased may be related to structural changes of heart valve, possibly evidenced by fatigue, dyspnea, altered vital signs, and syncope.
Activity intolerance may be related to imbalance between oxygen supply and demand, possibly evidenced by exertional dyspnea, reported fatigue/weakness, and ECG changes/dysrhythmias.
Pain may be related to ischemia of cardiac muscle, possibly evidenced by verbal complaints, facial grimacing, narrowed focus, and autonomic responses (alterations in vital signs).

appendicitis
Pain may be related to inflammation, possibly evidenced by verbal complaints, guarding behavior, narrowed focus, and autonomic responses (diaphoresis, changes in vital signs).
Fluid volume deficit, high risk for which may be related to nausea, vomiting, and anorexia.
Infection, high risk for which may be related to release of pathogenic organisms into peritoneal cavity.

arrhythmia, cardiac
Refer to dysrhythmia, cardiac

arthritis, juvenile rheumatoid (also refer to arthritis, rheumatoid)
Growth and development, altered may be related to effects of physical disability and required therapy, possibly evidenced by lack of/delayed physical growth appropriate for age.
Social isolation, high risk for which may be related to delay in accomplishing developmental task, altered state of wellness, and changes in physical appearance.

arthritis, rheumatoid
Pain, chronic may be related to joint/muscle inflammation, degeneration, deformity, possibly evidenced by verbal complaints, narrowed focus, guarded movement, and physical and social withdrawal.
Physical mobility, impaired may be related to musculoskeletal impairment and pain, possibly evidenced by limited range of motion, reluctance to attempt movement, and decreased muscle strength.
Self-care deficit (specify) may be related to decreased strength/range of motion, pain, possibly evidenced by reported difficulties in performing tasks.
Body image disturbance may be related to change in body structure/function, possibly evidenced by negative feelings about body, feelings of helplessness, and preoccupation with change or loss.

arthroplasty
Infection, high risk for which may be related to breach of primary defenses (surgical incision), stasis of body fluids at operative site, and altered inflammatory response.
Fluid volume deficit, high risk for which may be related to surgical procedure/trauma to vascular area.
Physical mobility, impaired which may be related to decreased strength, pain, musculoskeletal changes, possibly evidenced by impaired coordination and reluctance to attempt movement.
Pain may be related to tissue trauma, local edema, surgical incision, possibly evidenced by verbal complaints, narrowed focus, guarded movement, and autonomic responses (diaphoresis, changes in vital signs).

arthroscopy
Knowledge deficit [learning need] may be related to unfamiliarity with procedure/outcomes and self-care needs, possibly evidenced by questions and requests for information.

asthma
Airway clearance, ineffective may be related to increased pulmonary secretions and bronchospasm, possibly evidenced by wheezing, tachypnea, and ineffective cough.
Gas exchange, impaired may be related to altered delivery of inspired oxygen, possibly evidenced by restlessness, irritability, cyanosis, and changes in ABGs.
Anxiety (specify level) may be related to perceived threat of death, possibly evidenced by apprehension, fearful expression, and extraneous movements.
Activity intolerance may be related to imbalance between oxygen supply and demand, possibly evidenced by fatigue and exertional dyspnea.

athlete's foot

Skin integrity, impaired may be related to fungal invasion, humidity, secretions, possibly evidenced by disruption of skin surface, complaints of painful itching.

Infection, high risk for spread which may be related to multiple breaks in skin, exposure to moist/warm environment.

autistic disorder

Social interaction, impaired may be related to organic brain dysfunction, disturbance in self-concept, lack of bonding and development of trust, inadequate sensory stimulation or abnormal response to sensory input, possibly evidenced by lack of responsiveness to others, lack of eye contact or facial responsiveness, treating persons as objects, lack of awareness of feelings in others, and indifference/aversion to comfort, affection, or physical contact.

Communication, impaired verbal may be related to organic brain dysfunction, psychologic barriers (inability to trust others, withdrawal into self, inadequate sensory stimulation, maternal deprivation) possibly evidenced by lack of interactive communication mode; does not use gestures or spoken language, absent or abnormal nonverbal communication; lack of eye contact or facial expression; peculiar patterns of speech (form, content, or speech production); and impaired ability to initiate or sustain conversation despite adequate speech.

Violence, high risk for: directed at self/others which may be related to organic brain dysfunction, inability to trust others, disturbance in self-concept, inadequate sensory stimulation or abnormal response to sensory input, maternal deprivation, and response to demands of therapy.

Family coping, ineffective, compromised/disabling may be related to chronic nature of condition and disability as well as parental supervision and lifestyle restrictions, possibly evidenced by expression of despair, denial, depression, distortion of reality regarding the patient's condition, and protective behavior disproportionate to patient's abilities or need for autonomy.

battered child syndrome

Self-esteem Disturbance may be related to deprivation and negative feedback of family members, possibly evidenced by lack of eye contact, withdrawal from social contacts, and discounting own needs.

Post-trauma response may be related to sustained/recurrent physical or emotional abuse, possibly evidenced by acting-out behavior, development of phobias, poor impulse control, and emotional numbness.

Parenting, altered may be related to poor role model/identity, unrealistic expectations, presence of stressors, and lack of support, possibly evidenced by verbalization of negative feelings, inappropriate caretaking behaviors, and evidence of physical/psychologic trauma to child.

Family coping, ineffective, compromised/disabled may be related to situational or developmental crisis and family disorganization, possibly evidenced by verbalized concern about ability to deal with current situation and display of disproportionate (too little or too much) protective behaviors.

benign prostatic hypertrophy

Urinary elimination, altered patterns of may be related to obstruction of bladder outlet, possibly evidenced by increasing urinary frequency, urgency, nocturia, incomplete bladder emptying, hesitancy, decrease in size/force of urinary stream, and post-void dribbling.

Pain may be related to mucosal irritation, bladder distension, renal colic, urinary infection, and radiation therapy, possibly evidenced by verbal complaints (bladder/rectal spasm), narrowed focus, altered muscle tone, grimacing, distraction behaviors, restlessness, and autonomic responses.

Sleep pattern disturbance may be related to urinary frequency and nocturia, possibly evidenced by complaints of interrupted sleep/not feeling well rested and irritability.

Infection, high risk for which may be related to urinary stasis.

Fear/anxiety (specify level) may be related to change in health status (possibility of surgical procedure/malignancy); embarrassment/loss of dignity associated with genital exposure before, during, and after treatment; and concern about sexual ability, possibly evidenced by increased tension, apprehension, worry, expressed concerns regarding perceived changes, and fear of unspecific consequences.

bipolar disorder

Violence, high risk for: directed at others/self which may be related to irritability and impulsive behavior and delusional thinking, angry response when ideas are refuted or wishes denied.

Nutrition, altered: less than body requirements may be related to inadequate intake in relation to metabolic expenditures, possibly evidenced by body weight 20 percent or more below ideal weight, observed inadequate intake, inattention to mealtimes, and distraction from task of eating.

Poisoning, high risk for (lithium toxicity) which may be related to narrow therapeutic range of drug, patient's ability/lack of ability to follow through with medication regimen and monitoring, and denial of need for information/therapy.

Sleep pattern disturbance may be related to lack of recognition of fatigue/need to sleep, hyperactivity, possibly evidenced by interrupted nighttime sleep, one or more nights without sleep, changes in behavior and performance, increasing irritability/restlessness, and dark circles under eyes.

Sensory-perceptual alterations (specify/overload) may be related to decrease in sensory threshold, endogenous chemical alteration, psychologic stress, sleep deprivation, possibly evidenced by increased distractibility and agitation, anxiety, disorientation, poor concentration, bizarre thinking, and motor incoordination.

Family processes, altered may be related to situational crises, illness, economics, change in roles, euphoric mood and grandiose ideas/actions, manipulative behavior and limit-testing, patient's refusal to accept responsibility for own actions, possibly evidenced by statements of difficulty coping with situation, lack of adaptation to change or not dealing constructively with illness, ineffective family decision-making process, failure to send and to receive clear messages, and inappropriate boundary maintenance.

borderline personality disorder

Violence, high risk for: directed at self/others which may be related to use of projection as a major defense mechanism, pervasive problems with negative transference, and feelings of guilt/need to "punish" self.

Thought processes, altered may be related to psychologic conflicts and brief psychotic episodes, delusional thinking, cognitive distortions, increasing anxiety/fear, and poor reality base, possibly evidenced by persecutory thoughts of "I am victim," perception of events as either grossly distorted or "did not happen at all," and interference with ability to think clearly and logically.

Self-Esteem Disturbance/Role Performance, altered may be related to lack of positive feedback, unmet dependency needs, retarded ego development, and fixation at an earlier level of development, possibly evidenced by difficulty identifying self or defining self-boundaries, extreme mood changes, lack of tolerance of rejection or being alone, unhappiness with self, striking out at others, performance of ritualistic self-damaging acts, and belief that punishing self is necessary.

Anxiety (severe to panic) may be related to unconscious conflicts, perceived threat to self-concept, unmet needs, possibly evidenced by transient psychotic symptoms, abuse of alcohol/other drugs, easy frustration and feelings of hurt, and performance of self-mutilating acts.

Social isolation may be related to immature interests, unaccepted social behavior, inadequate personal resources, and inability to engage in satisfying personal relationships, possibly evidenced by difficulty meeting expectations of others; experiences feelings of difference from others, expresses interests inappropriate to developmental age, and shows behavior unaccepted by dominant cultural group.

brain tumor

Pain may be related to pressure on brain tissues, possibly evidenced by complaints of headache, facial mask of pain, narrowed focus, and autonomic responses (changes in vital signs).

Thought processes, altered may be related to altered circulation to and/or destruction of brain tissue, possibly evidenced by memory loss, personality changes, and altered level of consciousness.

Sensory-perceptual alterations (specify) may be related to compression/displacement of brain tissue, disruption of neuronal conduction, possibly evidenced by changes in visual acuity, alterations in sense of balance/gait disturbance, and paresthesia.

Fluid volume deficit, high risk for which may be related to recurrent vomiting from irritation of vagal center in medulla, and decreased intake.

Self-care deficit (specify) may be related to sensory/neuromuscular impairment interfering with ability to perform tasks, possibly evidenced by unkempt/disheveled appearance, body odor, and verbalization/observation of inability to perform activities of daily living.

bronchitis

Airway clearance, ineffective may be related to excessive, thickened mucous secretions, possibly evidenced by presence of rhonchi, tachypnea, and ineffective cough.

Activity intolerance may be related to imbalance between oxygen supply and demand, possibly evidenced by complaints of fatigue, dypsnea, and abnormal vital sign response to activity.

Pain may be related to localized inflammation, persistent cough, aching associated with fever, possibly evidenced by complaints, distraction behavior, and facial mask of pain.

bronchopneumonia (also refer to bronchitis)

Gas exchange, impaired may be related to inflammatory process and collection of secretions affecting exchange across alveolar membrane, possibly evidenced by restlessness, dyspnea, cyanosis, and changes in mentation.

Hyperthermia may be related to infectious process and increased metabolic rate, possibly evidenced by flushed warm skin, diaphoresis, tachypnea/tachycardia, and increased body temperature.

burn (dependent on type, degree, and severity of the injury)

Pain may be related to destruction of/trauma to tissue and nerves and edema formation, possibly evidenced by verbal complaints, narrowed focus, distraction behavior, and autonomic responses (changes in vital signs).

Fluid volume deficit, high risk for which may be related to capillary damage and evaporation.

Infection, high risk for which may be related to loss of protective dermal barrier, presence of necrotic tissue, altered immune response, and stress.

Nutrition, altered: less than body requirements, high risk for which may be related to hypermetabolic state in response to burn injury/stress, inadequate intake.

Skin integrity, impaired may be related to tissue trauma, possibly evidenced by disruption of skin surface, destruction of skin layers (partial/full thickness burn).

Post-trauma response may be related to life-threatening event, possibly evidenced by re-experiencing the event, repetitive dreams/nightmares, psychic/emotional numbness, and sleep disturbance.

Diversional activity deficit may be related to long-term hospitalization, frequent lengthy treatments, and physical limitations, possibly evidenced by boredom, restlessness, withdrawal, and requests for something to do.

Growth and development, altered may be related to effects of physical disability, separation from significant others, and environmental deficiencies, possibly evidenced by loss of previously acquired skills and inability/reluctance to perform self-care.

bursitis

Pain may be related to inflammation of affected joint, possibly evidenced by verbal complaints, guarding behavior, and narrowed focus.

Physical mobility, impaired may be related to inflammation and swelling of joint and pain, possibly evidenced by diminished range of motion, reluctance to attempt movement, and imposed restriction of movement by medical treatment.

calculus, urinary

Pain may be related to tissue trauma and edema formation, possibly evidenced by complaints of sudden, severe, colicky pain; and guarding and distraction behaviors.

Urinary retention, high risk for which may be related to obstruction of urinary flow.

Infection, high risk for which may be related to stasis of urine.

Knowledge deficit [learning need] may be related to lack of exposure/recall and information misinterpretation regarding condition, prognosis, and treatment needs, possibly evidenced by requests for information, statements of concern, and recurrence/development of preventable complications.

cancer (also refer to chemotherapy)

Anxiety (specify level)/Fear may be related to change in health status, threat of death, threat to self-concept, and socioeconomic concerns, possibly evidenced by feelings of inadequacy, helplessness, and fear; insomnia; and focus on self.

Grieving, anticipatory may be related to potential loss (death) and perceived separation from significant others/lifestyle, possibly evidenced by anger, sadness, withdrawal, and changes in eating/sleep patterns and activities.

Pain may be related to the disease process (compression of nerve tissue, infiltration of nerves or their vascular supply, obstruction of a nerve pathway, inflammation), possibly evidenced by verbal complaints, self-focusing/narrowed focus, alteration in muscle tone, facial mask of pain, distraction/guarding behaviors, autonomic responses, and restlessness.

Family coping, ineffective, compromised/disabling may be related to chronic nature of disease and disability, ongoing treatment needs, and parental supervision and lifestyle restrictions, possibly evidenced by expression of denial/despair, depression, and protective behavior disproportionate to patient's abilities or need for autonomy.

Family coping, potential for growth may be related to the fact that the individual's needs are being sufficiently gratified and adaptive tasks effectively addressed, enabling goals of self-actualization to surface, possibly evidenced by verbalizations of impact of crisis on own values, priorities, goals, or relationships.

Fatigue may be related to decreased metabolic energy production, increased energy requirements (hypermetabolic state), overwhelming psychologic/emotional demands, and altered body chemistry (side effects of medications, chemotherapy), possibly evidenced by unremitting/overwhelming lack of energy, inability to maintain usual routines, decreased performance, impaired ability to concentrate, lethargy/listlessness, and disinterest in surroundings.

Family processes, altered, high risk for may be related to situational transition and/or crises, long-term illness, changes in roles/economic status, and developmental transition (anticipated loss of a family member).

2496

Home maintenance management, impaired may be related to debilitation, lack of resources, and/or inadequate support systems, possibly evidenced by verbalization of problem, request for assistance, and lack of necessary equipment or aids.

cardiac catheterization
Anxiety (specify level)/Fear may be related to change in health status and threat to self-concept/of death, possibly evidenced by sympathetic stimulation, increased tension, and apprehension.

Knowledge deficit [learning need] may be related to unfamiliarity with procedure, its outcomes, and disease process, possibly evidenced by verbalization of concern and request for information.

Tissue perfusion, altered cardiopulmonary and cerebral, high risk for may be related to interruption in arterial flow secondary to injection of dye, or emolization.

cardiac surgery
Anxiety (specify level)/Fear may be related to change in health status and threat to self-concept/of death, possibly evidenced by sympathetic stimulation, increased tension, and apprehension.

Knowledge deficit [learning need] may be related to lack of exposure/recall and misinterpretation of information, possibly evidenced by verbalization of concern and request for information.

Cardiac output, decreased, high risk for which may be related to decreased circulating fluid volume (preload), depressed myocardial contractility (pumping ability), changes in systemic vascular resistance (afterload), and alterations in electrical conduction.

Fluid volume deficit [active loss] may be related to intraoperative bleeding with inadequate blood replacement; bleeding related to insufficient heparin reversal, fibrinolysis, or platelet destruction; or volume depletion effects of intraoperative or postoperative diuretic therapy, possibly evidenced by increased pulse rate, decreased pulse volume/pressure, decreased urine output, hemoconcentration.

Gas exchange, impaired, high risk for which may be related to alveolar-capillary membrane changes (atelectasis), intestinal edema, inadequate function or premature discontinuation of chest tubes, and diminished oxygen-carrying capacity of the blood.

Pain may be related to tissue inflammation/trauma, edema formation, intraoperative nerve trauma, and myocardial ischemia, possibly evidenced by complaints of incisional discomfort/pain, paresthesia/pain in hand, arm, shoulder; anxiety; restlessness; irritability; distraction behaviors; and autonomic responses.

Skin/Tissue integrity, impaired related to mechanical trauma (surgical incisions, puncture wounds) and edema evidenced by disruption of skin surface.

carpal tunnel syndrome
Pain may be related to pressure on median nerve, possibly evidenced by complaints of pain, guarding behavior, and reluctance to use affected hand.

Physical mobility, impaired may be related to neuromuscular impairment and pain, possibly evidenced by decreased hand strength, limited range of motion, and reluctance to attempt movement.

Knowledge deficit [learning need] may be related to lack of exposure/recall and information misinterpretation regarding condition, prognosis, and treatment needs, possibly evidenced by questions, statements of concern, request for information, and inaccurate follow-through of instructions/development of preventable complications.

cast (upper extremity)
Trauma, high risk for additional injury which may be related to loss of skeletal integrity (fractures)/movement of skeletal fragments.

Pain may be related to movement of bone fragments, tissue trauma/edema, traction/immobility device, stress, and anxiety, possibly evidenced by verbal complaints, distraction behaviors, self-focusing/narrowed focus, facial mask of pain, guarding/protective behavior, alteration in muscle tone, and autonomic responses.

Tissue perfusion, altered, peripheral may be related to reduction/interruption of blood flow: direct vascular injury, tissue trauma, edema formation, thrombus formation, hypovolemia, possibly evidenced by cool, pale, or cyanotic fingers, delayed capillary refill; and complaints of numbness/tingling.

Skin integrity, impaired, high risk for which may be related to pressure of cast, moisture/debris under cast, and objects inserted under cast to relieve itching.

Self-care deficit (specify) may be related to impaired ability to perform self-care tasks, possibly evidenced by statements of need for assistance and observed difficulty in performing activities of daily living.

cataract

Sensory-perceptual alteration, visual may be related to altered sensory reception/status of sense organs, and therapeutically restricted environment, possibly evidenced by diminished acuity, visual distortions, and change in usual response to stimuli.

Trauma, high risk for which may be related to poor vision.

Anxiety (specify level)/Fear may be related to alteration in visual acuity and threat of permanent loss of vision/independence, possibly evidenced by feeling of uncertainty, apprehension, and expressed concerns.

Knowledge deficit [learning need] may be related to lack of information about ways of coping with altered abilities and therapy choices, possibly evidenced by requests for information and statement of concern.

cat scratch disease

Pain may be related to effects of circulating toxins (fever, headache, and lymphadenitis), possibly evidenced by complaints, guarding behavior, and autonomic response (changes in vital signs).

Hyperthermia may be related to inflammatory process, possibly evidenced by increased body temperature, flushed warm skin, tachypnea, and tachycardia.

cerebrovascular accident

Tissue perfusion, altered, cerebral may be related to interruption of blood flow (occlusive disorder, hemorrhage, cerebral vasospasm/edema), possibly evidenced by altered level of consciousness, memory loss, changes in motor/sensory responses, restlessness, language, intellectual and emotional deficits, and changes in vital signs.

Physical mobility, impaired may be related to neuromuscular impairment, decreased strength, and spasticity, possibly evidenced by inability to purposefully move involved body parts, limited range of motion, and impaired coordination.

Swallowing, impaired may be related to muscle paralysis and perceptual impairment, possibly evidenced by observed difficulty in swallowing, recurrent coughing, choking, and drooling.

Communication, impaired verbal may be related to motor and/or cognitive deficits, possibly evidenced by garbled speech, inability to find and/or use correct words and identify objects and/or written/spoken words.

Sensory-perceptual alterations (specify) may be related to altered sensory reception, transmission, integration (neurologic trauma or deficit), and psychologic stress (narrowed perceptual fields caused by anxiety), possibly evidenced by disorientation to time, place, and persons; changes in behavior pattern/usual response to stimuli; exaggerated emotional responses; poor concentration; bizarre thinking; reported/measured change in sensory acuity (hypoparethesia); altered sense of taste/smell; inability to tell position of body parts (proprioception); inability to recognize/attach meaning to objects (visual agnosia); altered communication patterns; and motor incoordination.

Neglect, unilateral, high risk for which may be related to sensory loss of part of visual field with perceptual loss of corresponding body segment.

Self-care deficit (specify) may be related to neuromuscular and/or cognitive impairment and depression, possibly evidenced by stated/observed inability to perform activities of daily living, requests for assistance, disheveled appearance, and incontinence.

Home maintenance management, impaired may be related to condition of individual family member, insufficient finances/family organization or planning, unfamiliarity with resources, and inadequate support systems, possibly evidenced by members expressing difficulty in managing home in a comfortable manner/requesting assistance with home maintenance, disorderly surroundings, and overtaxed family members.

Health maintenance, altered may be related to lack of ability to make deliberate and thoughtful judgments, perceptual or cognitive impairment, and ineffective individual/family coping, possibly evidenced by observed inability to take responsibility for meeting basic health practices/impairment of personal support system.

Body image disturbance/Role performance, altered may be related to biophysical, psychosocial, and cognitive/perceptual changes, possibly evidenced by actual change in structure and/or function, change in usual patterns of responsibility/physical capacity to resume role; and verbal/nonverbal response to actual or perceived change.

cesarean section

Knowledge deficit [learning need] may be related to incomplete/inadequate information regarding underlying procedure, pathophysiology, and care needs, possibly evidenced by verbalization of concerns/misconceptions and inappropriatre/exaggerated behavior.

Body image/Self-esteem disturbance may be related to required surgical intervention in an otherwise natural life event, possibly evidenced by expressions of disappointment and negative feelings about body/self.

Anxiety (specify level) may be related to actual/perceived threat to mother/fetus, emotional threat to self-esteem, and unmet needs/expectations, possibly evidenced by increased tension, restlessness, apprehension, uncertainty, fearfulness, feelings of inadequacy, sympathetic stimulation, trembling, and narrowed focus.

Pain may be related to tissue trauma and muscle contractions (afterpains), possibly evidenced by verbal complaints, guarding/distraction behaviors, and autonomic responses (changes in vital signs).

Infection, high risk for which may be related to interruption of skin barrier, invasive procedures, and delayed epithelialization at site of placental attachment.

chemotherapy

Fluid volume deficit, high risk for which may be related to gastrointestinal losses and interference with adequate intake (stomatitis/anorexia).

Nutrition, altered: less than body requirements may be related to inability to ingest adequate nutrients secondary to nausea, anorexia, and stomatitis, possibly evidenced by weight loss, aversion to eating, reported altered taste sensation, and sore, inflamed buccal cavity.

Oral mucous membranes, altered may be related to effects of therapeutic regimen, dehydration, and malnutrition, possibly evidenced by ulcerations, leukoplakia, decreased salivation, and complaints of pain.

Body image disturbance may be related to loss of hair and weight/body structure changes, possibly evidenced by negative feelings, preoccupation with change, and change in social involvement.

cholecystectomy

Pain may be related to interruption in skin/tissue layers with mechanical closure (sutures/staples) and invasive procedures (including NG tube), possibly evidenced by verbal complaints, guarding/distraction behaviors, and autonomic responses (changes in vital signs).

Oral mucous membrane, altered may be related to dehydration, mechanical trauma (NG tube), and mouth breathing, possibly evidenced by dry mouth, coated tongue, complaints of discomfort, and decreased salivation.

Breathing pattern, ineffective may be related to decreased lung expansion (pain and muscle weakness), ineffective cough, possibly evidenced by fremitus, tachypnea, and decreased respiratory depth.

cholelithiasis

Pain may be related to inflammation and distention of tissues, possibly evidenced by verbal complaints, guarding/distraction behaviors, and autonomic responses (changes in vital signs).

Nutrition, altered: less than body requirement may be related to inability to ingest/absorb adequate nutrients (food intolerance/pain, nausea/vomiting, anorexia), possibly evidenced by aversion to food/decreased intake and weight loss.

Knowledge deficit [learning need] may be related to lack of information about pathophysiology, therapy choices, and self-care needs, possibly evidenced by verbalization of concerns, questions, and recurrence of condition.

chronic obstructive lung disease

Airway clearance, ineffective may be related to increased production of tenacious secretions, retained secretions, decreased energy, and fatigue, possibly evidenced by presence of rhonchi, tachypnea, dyspnea, pallor or cyanosis, and chest x-ray findings.

Gas exchange, impaired may be related to altered oxygen delivery (obstruction of airways by secretions/bronchospasm, air-trapping) and alveoli destruction, possibly evidenced by dyspnea, confusion, restlessness, inability to move secretions, abnormal ABG values, changes in vital signs, and reduced tolerance for activity.

Activity intolerance may be related to imbalance between oxygen supply and demand, possibly evidenced by verbal reports of fatigue, exertional dyspnea, and abnormal vital sign response.

Nutrition, altered: less than body requirements may be related to inability to ingest adequate nutrients (dyspnea, fatigue, medication side effects, sputum production, anorexia, nausea/vomiting), possibly evidenced by weight loss, decreased muscle mass/subcutaneous fat, poor muscle tone, fatigue, reported altered taste sensation, aversion to eating, and lack of interest in food.

Infection, high risk for which may be related to decreased ciliary action, stasis of secretions, and debilitated state.

cirrhosis

Nutrition, altered: less than body requirements may be related to inability to ingest/absorb nutrients (anorexia, nausea, indigestion, impaired storage of vitamins), possibly evidenced by aversion to eating, observed lack of intake, muscle wasting, and weight loss.

Fluid volume excess may be related to compromised regulatory mechanism (e.g., SIADH, decreased plasma proteins/malnutrition) and excess sodium/fluid intake, possibly evidenced by edema/anasarca, weight gain, intake greater than output, changes in urine specific gravity, dyspnea, pleural effusion, and blood pressure changes.

Skin integrity, impaired, high risk for which may be related to altered circulation/metabolic state, accumulation of bile salts in skin, poor skin turgor, skeletal prominence, and presence of edema/ascites.

Thought processes, altered, high risk for which may be related to physiologic changes (increased serum ammonia level and inability of liver to detoxify certain enzymes/drugs).

Self-esteem/Body image disturbance may be related to biophysical changes/altered physical appearance, uncertainty of prognosis, changes in role function, self-destructive behavior (alcohol-induced disease), and need for behavior/lifestyle changes, possibly evidenced by verbalization of changes in lifestyle, fear of rejection or of reaction of others, negative feelings about body, and feelings of helplessness/hopelessness/powerlessness.

Knowledge deficit [learning need] may be related to lack of exposure/recall, information misinterpretation, and cognitive limitations, possibly evidenced by questions, request for information, statement of misconception, and inaccurate follow-through of instruction/development of preventable complications.

cocaine hydrochloride poisoning, acute

Thought processes, altered may be related to pharmacologic stimulation of the nervous system, possibly evidenced by altered attention span, disorientation, and hallucinations.

Breathing pattern, ineffective may be related to pharmacologic effects on respiratory center of the brain, possibly evidenced by tachypnea, altered depth of respiration, shortness of breath, and abnormal ABGs.

Coping, ineffective individual may be related to unwillingness to safely deal with actual/perceived stressors, possibly evidenced by use of potentially harmful substance.

coccidiodomycosis

Pain may be related to inflammation, possibly evidenced by verbal complaints, distraction behaviors, and narrowed focus.

Fatigue may be related to decreased energy production; states of discomfort, possibly evidenced by reports of overwhelming lack of energy, inability to maintain usual routine, emotional lability/irritability, impaired ability to concentrate, and decreased endurance/libido.

Knowledge deficit [learning need] may be related to lack of information about nature/course of disease and therapy needs, possibly evidenced by statements of concern and questions.

colitis, ulcerative (also refer to Crohn's disease)

Diarrhea may be related to inflammation, irritation or malabsorption of the bowel, toxins; segmental narrowing of the lumen, possibly evidenced by increased bowel sounds/peristalsis, urgency, frequent/watery stools (acute phase), changes in stool color, and abdominal pain.

Pain may be related to inflammation of the intestines/hyperperistalsis and anal/rectal irritation, possibly evidenced by verbal complaints, guarding/distraction behaviors, and autonomic responses (changes in vital signs).

Fluid volume deficit, high risk for which may be related to continued gastrointestinal losses (diarrhea, capillary plasma loss) and altered intake.

Nutrition, altered: less than body requirements may be related to altered intake/absorption of nutrients (medically restricted intake, fear that eating may cause diarrhea) and hypermetabolic state, possibly evidenced by weight loss, decreased subcutaneous fat/muscle mass, poor muscle tone, hyperactive bowel sounds, steatorrhea, pale conjunctiva and mucous membranes, and aversion to eating.

Coping, ineffective individual may be related to chronic nature and indefinite course of disease and inadequate handling of stressors, possibly evidenced by altered ability to problem solve, verbalization of inability to cope, and presence of anxiety, depression, and exacerbation of symptoms.

Powerlessness, high risk for which may be related to unresolved dependency conflicts, feelings of insecurity/resentment, repression of anger and aggressive feelings, lacking a sense of control in stressful situations, sacrificing own wishes for others, and retreat from aggression or frustration.

colostomy

Skin integrity, impaired may be related to absence of sphincter at stoma and chemical irritation from caustic bowel contents, possibly evidenced by erythema, excoriation of skin surrounding the stoma, and complaints of burning pain.

Diarrhea/Constipation (dependent on site) may be related to interruption/alteration of normal bowel function, changes in dietary/fluid intake, and effects of medication, possibly evidenced by symptoms dependent on problem identified.

Knowledge deficit [learning need] may be related to lack of exposure/recall, information misinterpretation regarding changes in physiologic function, and self-care/treatment needs, possibly evidenced by questions, statement of concern, and inaccurate follow-through of instruction/development of preventable complications.

Social interaction, impaired may be related to fear of embarrassing situation secondary to altered bowel control with loss of contents, odor, possibly evidenced by reduced participation and verbalized/observed discomfort in social situations.

Sexual dysfunction, high risk for which may be related to altered body structure/function, radical resection/treatment procedures, vulnerability/psychologic concern about response of significant other(s), and disruption of sexual response pattern (e.g., erection difficulty).

Body image disturbance may be related to biophysical changes (presence of stoma; loss of control of bowel elimination) and psychosocial factors (disease process/associated treatment regimen, i.e., cancer, colitis) possibly evidenced by verbalization of change in perception of self, negative feelings about body, fear of rejection/reaction of others, not touching/looking at stoma, and refusal to participate in care.

coma, diabetic

Fluid volume deficit [regulatory failure] may be related to hyperosmolar urinary losses and inadequate intake, possibly evidenced by dry mucous membranes, poor skin turgor, decreased pulse volume and pressure, and fever.

Nutrition, altered: less than body requirements may be related to inadequate utilization of nutrients, possibly evidenced by recent weight loss, reports of weakness, improper insulin therapy.

Breathing pattern, ineffective, high risk for may be related to neuromuscular or musculoskeletal impairment and decreased energy levels.

Infection, high risk for may be related to stasis of body fluids, invasive procedures, alteration in circulation and perfusion.

concussion of brain

Pain may be related to trauma to/edema of cerebral tissue, possibly evidenced by complaints of headache, guarding/distraction behaviors, and narrowed focus.

Fluid volume deficit, high risk for may be related to vomiting, decreased intake, and hypermetabolic state (fever).

congestive heart failure

Cardiac output, decreased may be related to altered myocardial contractility/inotropic changes; alterations in rate, rhythm, and electrical conduction; and structural changes, possibly evidenced by increased heart rate, changes in blood pressure, extra heart sounds, decreased urine output, diminished peripheral pulses, cool/ashen skin; diaphoresis, orthopnea, crackles, vascular distention, edema, and chest pain.

Activity intolerance may be related to imbalance between oxygen supply/demand, generalized weakness, and prolonged bedrest/immobility, possibly evidenced by weakness, fatigue, changes in vital signs, presence of dysrhythmias, dyspnea, pallor, and diaphoresis.

Fluid volume excess may be related to reduced glomerular filtration rate/increased ADH production, and sodium/water retention, possibly evidenced by orthopnea, S_3 heart sound, oliguria, edema, jugular vein distention, positive hepatojugular reflex, weight gain, hypertension, respiratory distress, and abnormal breath sounds.

Gas exchange, impaired, high risk for which may be related to alveolar-capillary membrane changes (fluid collection/shifts into interstitial space/alveoli).

Knowledge deficit [learning need] may be related to lack of understanding/misconceptions about interrelatedness of cardiac function/disease/failure, possibly evidenced by questions, statements of concern/misconceptions; and recurrent, preventable episodes of congestive heart failure.

Conn's syndrome

Refer to aldosteronism, primary

constipation

Pain may be related to abdominal fullness/pressure, straining to defecate, and trauma to delicate tissues, possibly evidenced by complaints, reluctance to defecate, and distraction behaviors.

Knowledge deficit [learning need] may be related to lack of understanding of dietary needs/bowel function, possibly evidenced by development of problem and verbalization of concerns/questions.

coronary artery bypass surgery

Cardiac output, decreased may be related to diminished circulating volume, alterations in electrical conduction, and increased systemic vascular resistance, possibly evidenced by changes in hemodynamic readings, presence of ECG changes/dysrhythmias, and diminished peripheral pulses.

Fluid volume deficit [active loss] may be related to blood loss and intraoperative use of diuretics, possibly evidenced by decreased right-sided filling pressures and blood pressure, concentrated urine with elevated specific gravity, dry mucous membranes, and decreased pulse volume/pressure.

Pain may be related to direct chest tissue/bone trauma, invasive tubes/lines, and donor site incision, possibly evidenced by verbal complaints, autonomic responses (changes in vital signs), and distraction behaviors.

Sensory-perceptual alterations (specify) may be related to restricted environment, sleep deprivation, continuous environmental sounds/activities, and psychologic stress of procedure, possibly evidenced by disorientation, alterations in behavior, exaggerated emotional responses, and visual/auditory distortions.

Crohn's disease (also refer to colitis, ulcerative)

Nutrition, altered: less than body requirements may be related to postprandial pain and decreased transit time through bowel, possibly evidenced by weight loss, aversion to eating, and observed lack of intake.

Diarrhea may be related to inflammation of small intestines, dietary intake, possibly evidenced by hyperactive bowel sounds, cramping, and loose liquid stools of increased frequency.

Knowledge deficit [learning need] may be related to insufficient information/misinterpretation regarding pathophysiology of nutritional needs, and prevention of recurrence, possibly evidenced by statements of concern, questions, and exacerbation of condition.

croup

Airway clearance, ineffective may be related to thick, tenacious mucus, and swelling/spasms of the epiglottis, possibly evidenced by harsh/brassy cough, tachypnea, use of accessory muscles, and presence of rhonchi.

Fluid volume deficit [active loss] may be related to decreased ability/aversion to swallowing, presence of fever, and increased respiratory losses, possibly evidenced by dry mucous membranes, poor skin turgor, and scanty/concentrated urine.

croup, membraneous (also refer to croup)

Suffocation, high risk for which may be related to inflammation of larynx with formation of false membrane.

Anxiety (specify level)/Fear may be related to change in environment, perceived threat to self (difficulty breathing), and perception of anxiety of adults, possibly evidenced by restlessness, facial tension, glancing about, and sympathetic stimulation.

Cushing's syndrome

Infection, high risk for which may be related to immunosuppressed inflammatory response, skin and capillary fragility, and negative nitrogen balance.

Nutrition, altered: less than body requirements may be related to inability to utilize nutrients (disturbance of carbohydrate metabolism), possibly evidenced by decreased muscle mass and increased resistance to insulin.

Self-care deficit (specify) may be related to muscle wasting, generalized weakness, fatigue, and demineralization of bones, possibly evidenced by statements of/observed inability to complete or perform activities of daily living.

Body image disturbance may be related to change in structure/appearance (effects of disease process, drug therapy), possibly evidenced by negative feelings about body, feelings of helplessness, and changes in social involvement.

Sexual dysfunction may be related to loss of libido, impotence, and cessation of menses, possibly evidenced by verbalization of concerns and/or dissatisfaction and alteration in relationship with significant other.

Trauma, high risk for (fractures) which may be related to increased protein breakdown and negative protein balance.

cystic fibrosis

Airway clearance, ineffective may be related to excessive production of thick mucus and decreased ciliary action, possibly evidenced by abnormal breath sounds, ineffective cough, cyanosis, and altered respiratory rate/depth.

Infection, high risk for which may be related to stasis of respiratory secretions and development of atelectasis.

Nutrition, altered: less than body requirements may be related to impaired digestive process and malabsorption of nutrients, possibly evidenced by failure to gain weight, muscle wasting, and retarded physical growth.

Knowledge deficit [learning need] may be related to insufficient information concerning pathophysiology of condition, medical management, and available community resources, possibly evidenced by statements of concern, questions, and misconceptions.

Family coping, ineffective, compromised may be related to chronic nature of disease and disability and parental supervision and lifestyle restrictions, possibly evidenced by protective behavior disproportionate to patient's abilities or need for autonomy.

cystitis

Pain may be related to inflammation and bladder spasms, possibly evidenced by verbal complaints, distraction behaviors, and narrowed focus.

Urinary elimination, altered patterns of may be related to inflammation/irritation of bladder, possibly evidenced by frequency, nocturia, and dysuria.

Knowledge deficit [learning need] may be related to inadequate information regarding pathophysiology, treatment, and prevention of recurrence, possibly evidenced by statements of concern and questions.

cytomegalic inclusion disease

Refer to herpes infections

dehiscence (abdominal)

Tissue integrity, impaired, high risk for which may be related to exposure of abdominal contents to external environment.

Skin integrity, impaired may be related to altered circulation, altered nutritional state (obesity/malnutrition), and physical stress on incision, possibly evidenced by poor/delayed wound healing and disruption of skin surface/wound closure.

Infection, high risk for which may be related to inadequate primary defenses (separation of incision, traumatized intestines, environmental exposure).

Fear/Anxiety, severe may be related to crises, perceived threat of death, possibly evidenced by fearfulness, restless behaviors, and sympathetic stimulation.

Knowledge deficit [learning need] may be related to lack of information/recall and misinterpretation of information, possibly evidenced by development of preventable complication, requests for information, and statement of concern.

dehydration

Fluid volume deficit (specify) may be related to etiology as defined by specific situation, possibly evidenced by dry mucous membranes, poor skin turgor, decreased pulse volume/pressure, and thirst.

Oral mucous membrane, altered, high risk for which may be related to dehydration and decreased salivation.

Knowledge deficit [learning need] may be related to lack of information, misinterpretation of fluid needs, possibly evidenced by questions, statement of concern/misconceptions, and inadequate follow-through of instructions/development of preventable complications.

delirium tremens

Sensory-perceptual alterations (specify) may be related to exogenous/endogenous chemical alterations, sleep deprivation, and psychologic stress, possibly evidenced by disorientation, restlessness, irritability, exaggerated emotional responses, and visual and auditory distortions/hallucinations.

Fluid volume deficit, high risk for which may be related to reduced intake, profuse diaphoresis, and agitation.

Trauma, high risk for which may be related to alterations in balance, reduced muscle coordination, and cognitive impairment.

Nutrition, altered: less than body requirements, high risk for which may be related to inability to absorb/utilize nutrients (depletion of liver glycogen stores, impaired gluconeogenesis), reduced intake, and debilitated state.

dementia, presenile (Alzheimer's disease)

Thought processes, altered may be related to cerebral neuronal degeneration, possibly evidenced by memory deficit, decreased ability to grasp ideas/problem solve and make decisions, altered attention span, disorientation, delusions, and inappropriate social behavior/affect.

Trauma, high risk for which may be related to changes in muscle coordination/balance and cognitive difficulties.

Fear may be related to sensory impairment, physical deterioration, separation from support systems, and public disclosure of disabilities, possibly evidenced by apprehension, irritability, defensiveness, suspiciousness, aggressive behavior, decreased self-assurance, and sympathetic stimulation.

Grieving, anticipatory may be related to early awareness of cognitive deficits and progressive permanent loss of abilities and self, possibly evidenced by expressions of distress, anger, sorrow, and alterations in sleep and activity.

Self-care deficit (specify) may be related to cognitive decline, physical limitations, frustration over loss of independence, and depression, possibly evidenced by impaired ability to perform activities of daily living.

Family processes, altered may be related to situational crisis; changing role responsibilities, relationships, and financial stability, possibly evidenced by difficulty expressing feelings and problem solving and adapting or dealing with situation constructively.

Home maintenance management, impaired may be related to progressively impaired cognitive functioning, insufficient family organization/planning, unfamiliarity with resources, and inadequate support systems, possibly evidenced by home surroundings appearing disorderly/unsafe, household members expressing difficulty and requesting help in maintaining home in safe/comfortable fashion, and overtaxed family members (e.g., exhausted/anxious).

Health maintenance, altered may be related to complete or partial lack of gross and/or fine motor skills, significant alteration in communication skills, and ineffective individual/family coping, possibly evidenced by reported or observed inability to take responsibility for meeting basic health practices.

depressive disorders, major depression, dysthymia

Violence, high risk for: directed at self/others which may be related to depressed mood and feelings of worthlessness and hopelessness.

Coping, ineffective individual may be related to personal vulnerability, inadequate supports systems, unrealistic perceptions, multiple life changes, inadequate coping method, unmet expectations, and actual/perceived loss, possibly evidenced by perception of events and stressors in a manner that precipitates depressive episode, perception of areas in life as unfulfilled or as losses, denial of loss, verbalization of inability to cope or ask for help, expression of guilt, crying/labile affect, and chronic anxiety/depression.

Sleep pattern disturbance may be related to biochemical alterations (decreased serotonin), unresolved fears and anxieties, and inactivity, possibly evidenced by difficulty in falling/remaining asleep, early morning awakening, complaints of not feeling rested, and dark circles under eyes.

Social isolation/Social interaction, impaired may be related to alterations in mental status/thought processes, inadequate personal resources, decreased energy/inertia, difficulty engaging in satisfying personal relationships, feelings of worthlessness/low self-concept, inadequacy in/absence of significant purpose in life, and knowledge/skill deficit about social interactions, possibly evidenced by decreased involvement with others, expressed feelings of difference from others, remaining in home/room/bed, refusing invitations/suggestions of social involvement, and dysfunctional interaction with peers, family, and/or others.

Family processes, altered may be related to situational crises of illness of family member, possibly evidenced by expressions of confusion, statements of difficulty coping with situation, family system not meeting needs of its members, difficulty accepting or receiving help appropriately, ineffective family decision-making process, and failure to send and to receive clear messages.

Injury, high risk for which may be related to electroconvulsive effects on the cardiovascular, respiratory, musculoskeletal, and nervous systems, and pharmacologic effects of anesthesia.

dermatitis seborrheica

Skin integrity, impaired may be related to chronic inflammatory condition of the skin, possibly evidenced by disruption of skin surface with dry or moist scales, yellowish crusts, erythema, and fissures.

diabetic ketoacidosis

Fluid volume deficit [regulatory failure] may be related to hyperosmolar urinary losses and inadequate intake, possibly evidenced by dry mucous membranes, poor skin turgor, decreased pulse volume/pressure, and elevated temperature.

Nutrition, altered: less than body requirements which may be related to inadequate utilization of nutrients, possibly evidenced by recent weight loss, reports of weakness, and imbalance between glucose/insulin levels.

Breathing pattern, ineffective, high risk for which may be related to neuromuscular/musculoskeletal impairment and decreased energy levels.

Infection, high risk for which may be related to stasis of body fluids, invasive procedures, and alteration in circulation/perfusion.

diabetes mellitus

Knowledge deficit [learning need] may be related to unfamiliarity with disease process/treatment and individual care needs, possibly evidenced by requests for information, statements of concern/misconceptions, inadequate follow-through of instructions, and development of preventable complications.

Nutrition, altered: less than body requirements may be related to inability to utilize nutrients (imbalance between intake and utilization of glucose) to meet metabolic needs, possibly evidenced by change in weight, weakness, increased thirst/urination, and hyperglycemia.

Adjustment, impaired, high risk for which may be related to all-encompassing change in lifestyle and self-concept requiring lifelong adherence to therapeutic regimen and altered locus of control.

Infection, high risk for which may be related to decreased leukocytic phagocytosis, circulatory changes, and impaired healing.

dialysis, peritoneal

Fluid volume excess may be related to excessive intake and/or fluid retention from dialysate drainage problems/inappropriate osmotic gradient of solution, possibly evidenced by weight gain, edema, intake greater than output, and changes in blood pressure and respiratory pattern.

Pain may be related to factors related to procedure as well as presence of edema and required activity restrictions, possibly evidenced by complaints (specify), distraction behaviors, and narrowed focus.

Infection, high risk for which may be related to compromised primary defenses, invasive procedures, and debilitated state.

Breathing pattern, ineffective, high risk for which may be related to increased abdominal pressure with decreased lung expansion, pain/discomfort, and anxiety.

Body image disturbance/Role performance, altered may be related to situational crisis and chronic illness with changes in usual roles, possibly evidenced by verbalization of changes in lifestyle, focus on past function, negative feelings about body, feelings of helplessness/powerlessness, extension of body boundary to incorporate environmental objects (e.g., dialysis machine), change in social involvement, overdependence on others for care, not taking responsibility for self-care/lack of follow-through, and self-destructive behavior.

Grieving, anticipatory may be related to actual or perceived loss, chronic and/or fatal illness, and thwarted grieving response to a loss, possibly evidenced by verbal expression of distress/unresolved issues, denial of loss; altered eating habits, sleep and dream patterns, activity levels, libido; crying, labile affect, feelings of sorrow, guilt, and anger.

Powerlessness may be related to illness-related regimen and health-care environment, possibly evidenced by verbal expression of having no control, depression over physical deterioration, nonparticipation in care, anger, and passivity.

diarrhea

Pain may be related to abdominal cramping and irritation/excoriation of skin, possibly evidenced by complaints (specify), facial grimacing, and autonomic responses.

Fluid volume deficit, high risk for which may be related to excessive losses through GI tract.

Knowledge deficit [learning need] may be related to lack of information regarding causative/contributing factors and therapeutic needs, possibly evidenced by statements of concern, questions, and development of preventable complications.

Skin integrity, impaired may be related to effects of excretions on delicate tissues, possibly evidenced by complaints of discomfort and disruption of skin surface/destruction of skin layers.

digitalis poisoning

Cardiac output, decreased may be related to chemical alterations/interference with myocardial electrical activity, possibly evidenced by changes in rate/rhythm/conduction (development/worsening of dysrthythmias).

Fluid volume deficit, high risk for which may be related to excessive losses from vomiting/diarrhea and decreased intake.

Knowledge deficit [learning need] may be related to information misinterpretation and lack of recall, possibly evidenced by inaccurate follow-through of instructions and development of preventable complications.

Thought processes, altered may be related to physiologic effects of toxicity/reduced cerebral perfusion and impaired judgment, possibly evidenced by disorientation and confusion.

dilation and curettage (also refer to abortion, spontaneous)

Knowledge deficit [learning need] may be related to unfamiliarity with surgical procedure, possible postprocedural complications, and therapeutic needs, possibly evidenced by requests for information and statements of concern/misconceptions.

disruptive behavior disorders (childhood, adolescence)

Coping, ineffective individual may be related to inadequate coping strategies, maturational crisis, multiple life changes, lack of control of impulsive actions, and personal vulnerability, possibly evidenced by inappropriate use of defense mechanisms, inability to meet role expectations, poor self-esteem, failure to assume responsibility for own actions, and excessive smoking/drinking/drug use.

Violence, high risk for: directed at self/others which may be related to dysfunctional family system and loss of significant relationships.

Adjustment, impaired may be related to nonexistent or unsuccessful ability to be involved in problem solving or goal setting, losses connected with current and/or past occurrences in individual situation (e.g., loss of self-esteem, family member/friends), poor school performance, relocation, lack of movement toward independence, and difficulty limiting expectations of self, possibly evidenced by ambivalence toward parent(s), anxiety, self-blame, anger, and feelings of rejection, assault to self-esteem, and altered locus of control.

Family coping, ineffective, compromised/disabling may be related to excessive guilt, anger, or blaming among family members regarding child's behavior; parental inconsistencies; disagreements regarding discipline, limit-setting; and approaches; and exhaustion of parental resources (prolonged coping with disruptive child), possibly evidenced by unrealistic parental expectations, rejection or overprotection of child; and exaggerated expressions of anger, disappointment, or despair regarding child's behavior or ability to improve or change.

Social interaction, impaired may be related to retarded ego-development, low self-esteem, dysfunctional family system, and neurolgic impairment, possibly evidenced by difficulty waiting turn in games or group situations, doesn't seem to listen to what is being said, has difficulty playing quietly and maintaining attention to task or play activity, often shifting from one activity to another and interrupting or intruding on others.

disseminated intravascular coagulation

Anxiety (specify level)/Fear may be related to sudden change in health status and threat of death, possibly evidenced by sympathetic stimulation, restlessness, focus on self, and apprehension.

Fluid volume deficit, high risk for which may be related to failure of regulatory mechanism (coagulation process) and active loss/hemorrhage.

Tissue perfusion, altered (specify) may be related to alteration of arterial/venous flow (microemboli throughout circulatory system and hypovolemia), possibly evidenced by changes in respiratory rate and depth, changes in mentation, decreased urinary output, and development of acral cyanosis/focal gangrene.

Gas exchange, impaired, high risk for which may be related to reduced oxygen-carrying capacity, development of acidosis, fibrin deposition in microcirculation, and ischemic damage of lung parenchyma.

Pain may be related to bleeding into joints/muscles, hematoma formation, and ischemic tissues with areas of acral cyanosis/focal gangrene, possibly evidenced by complaints (specify), narrowed focus, alteration in muscle tome, distraction behaviors, restlessness, autonomic responses, and guarding behavior.

dissociative disorders (including multiple personality)

Anxiety (severe/panic)/Fear may be related to maladaptation of ineffective coping continuing from early life, unconscious conflict(s), threat to self-concept, unmet needs, and phobic stimulus, possibly evidenced by fragmentation of the personality, maladaptive response to stress, increased tension, feelings of inadequacy, and focus on self/projection.

Violence, high risk for: directed at self/others which may be related to depressed mood, conflicting personalities, panic states, and suicidal/homicidal behaviors.

Personal identity disturbance may be related to psychologic conflicts (dissociative state), childhood trauma/abuse, threat to physical integrity/self-concept, and underdeveloped ego, possibly evidenced by confusion about sense of self, purpose or direction in life, memory loss, alteration in perception or experience of the self, loss of one's own sense of reality/the external world, poorly differentiated ego boundaries, and presence of more than one personality within the individual.

Family coping, ineffective, compromised may be related to multiple stressors repeated over period of time, prolonged progression of disorder that exhausts the supportive capacity of significant people, and temporary family disorganization and role changes, possibly evidenced by significant other describing inadequate understanding or knowledge base that interferes with effective assistive or supportive behaviors, and marital conflict.

diverticulitis

Pain may be related to inflammation of intestinal mucosa, abdominal cramping, and presence of fever/chills, possibly evidenced by complaints (specify), guarding/distraction behaviors, autonomic responses, and narrowed focus.

Diarrhea/Constipation (specify) may be related to altered structure/function and presence of inflammation, possibly evidenced by signs and symptoms dependent on specific problem, e.g., increase/decrease in frequency of stools and change in consistency.

Knowledge deficit [learning need] may be related to lack of information about disease process, potential complications, and therapeutic needs, possibly evidenced by statements of concern, request for information, and development of preventable complications.

Powerlessness, high risk for which may be related to chronic nature of disease process with recurrent episodes, in spite of cooperation with medical regimen.

Down syndrome (also refer to mental retardation)

Growth and development, altered may be related to effects of physical/mental disability, possibly evidenced by altered physical growth, delay/inability in performing skills and self-care/self-control activities appropriate for age.

Trauma, high risk for which may be related to poor muscle tone/coordination, weakness, and cognitive difficulties.

Nutrition, altered: less than body requirements may be related to poor muscle tone and protruding tongue, possibly evidenced by weak and ineffective sucking and observed lack of adequate intake with weight loss/failure to gain.

Family coping, potential for growth may be related to situational/maturational crisis requiring incorporation of new skills into family dynamics, possibly evidenced by expression of desire to establish support system, identifying health, promoting behaviors/experiences that optimize situation.

Grieving, dysfunctional, high risk for which may be related to loss of "the perfect child," chronic condition requiring long-term care, and unresolved feelings.

Parenting, altered, high risk for which may be related to interference/delayed development of parenting, and attachment behaviors.

Social isolation, high risk for which may be related to withdrawal from usual social interactions and activities, assumption of total child care, and becoming overindulgent/overprotective.

drug overdose

Breathing pattern, ineffective may be related to depressant effect on central nervous system with cognitive impairment, possibly evidenced by changes in respiratory depth, cyanosis, and abnormal ABGs.

Poisoning, high risk for which may be related to continued absorption and cumulative effects of ingested/injected drug(s).

Violence, high risk for: directed at self/others which may be related to suicidal behaviors and/or toxic reactions to drug(s).

Coping, ineffective individual may be related to personal vulnerability, difficulty handling new situations, and previous ineffective/inadequate coping skills with substitution of drug(s), possibly evidenced by denial, lack of acceptance that drug use is causing the present situation, altered social patterns/participation, impaired adaptive behavior and problem-solving skills, decreased ability to handle stress of illness/hospitalization, financial affairs in disarray, and employment difficulties.

Duchenne's muscular dystrophy

Physical mobility, impaired may be related to musculoskeletal impairment/weakness, possibly evidenced by decreased muscle strength, control, and mass; limited range of motion; and impaired coordination.

Growth and development, altered may be related to effects of physical disability, possibly evidenced by altered physical growth and altered ability to perform self-care/self-control activities appropriate to age.

Nutrition, altered: high risk for more than body requirements which may be related to sedentary lifestyle and dysfunctional eating patterns.

Family coping, compromised may be related to situational crisis/emotional conflicts around issues about hereditary nature of condition and prolonged disease/disability that exhausts supportive capacity of family members, possibly evidenced by preoccupation with personal reactions regarding disability and displaying protective behavior disproportionate (too little/too much) to patient's abilities/need for autonomy.

dysmenorrhea

Pain may be related to exaggerated uterine contractility, possibly evidenced by complaints (specify), guarding/distraction behaviors, narrowed focus, and autonomic responses (changes in vital signs).

Physical mobility, impaired, high risk for which may be related to severity of pain and presence of secondary symptoms (nausea, vomiting, syncope, chills).

Coping, ineffective individual may be related to chronic, recurrent nature of problem, anticipatory anxiety, and inadequate coping methods, possibly evidenced by muscular tension, headaches, general irritability, chronic depression, and verbalization of poor self-esteem.

dysrhythmia, cardiac

Cardiac output, decreased may be related to altered electrical conduction and reduced myocardial contractility, possibly evidenced by alterations in hemodynamic readings, ECG changes, fatigue, dyspnea, and syncope.

Anxiety (specify level) may be related to perceived threat of death, possibly evidenced by increased tension, apprehension, and expressed concerns.

Pain may be related to ischemic cardiac muscle, possibly evidenced by complaints of pain, narrowed focus, and autonomic responses (diaphoresis, changes in vital signs).

Knowledge deficit [learning need] may be related to lack of information/understanding of medical condition/therapy needs and unfamiliarity with information resources, possibly evidenced by questions, statement of misconception, failure to improve on previous regimen, and development of preventable complications.

Activity intolerance, high risk for which may be related to imbalance between myocardial oxygen supply and demand, and cardiac depressant effects of certain drugs (beta-blockers, antidysrhythmics).

eclampsia

Refer to pre-eclampsia

ectopic pregnancy (tubal)

Pain may be related to distention/rupture of fallopian tube, possibly evidenced by complaints (specify), guarding/distraction behaviors, facial mask of pain, and autonomic responses (diaphoresis, changes in vital signs).

Fluid volume deficit, high risk for which may be related to hemorrhagic losses and decreased/restricted intake.

Anxiety (specify level) may be related to threat of death and possible loss of ability to conceive, possibly evidenced by increased tension, apprehension, sympathetic stimulation, restlessness, and focus on self.

eczema (dermatitis)

Pain may be related to cutaneous inflammation and irritation, possibly evidenced by complaints (specify), irritability, and scratching.

Infection, high risk for which may be related to broken skin and tissue trauma.

Social isolation may be related to alterations in physical appearance, possibly evidenced by expressed feelings of rejection and decreased interaction with peers.

edema, pulmonary

Fluid volume excess may be related to excessive fluid/sodium intake and decreased cardiac functioning, possibly evidenced by dyspnea, presence of crackles (rales), pulmonary congestion on x-ray, restlessness, anxiety, and increased CVP.

Gas exchange, impaired may be related to altered blood flow and decreased alveolar-capillary exchange, possibly evidenced by hypoxia, restlessness, and confusion.

Anxiety (specify level)/Fear may be related to perceived threat of death (inability to breathe), possibly evidenced by responses ranging from apprehension to panic state, restlessness, and focus on self.

emphysema

Airway clearance, ineffective may be related to increased tenacious secretions, decreased energy level, and muscle wasting, possibly evidenced by abnormal breath sounds (rhonchi), ineffective cough, changes in rate/depth of respirations, and dyspnea.

Gas exchange, impaired may be related to alveolar capillary membrane changes, possibly evidenced by hypercapnea, hypoxia, restlessness, and changes in mentation.

Activity intolerance may be related to imbalance between oxygen supply and demand, possibly evidenced by reports of fatigue/weakness, exertional dyspnea, and abnormal vital sign response to activity.

Nutrition, altered: less than body requirements may be related to inability to ingest food because of shortness of breath, anorexia, and generalized weakness, possibly evidenced by lack of interest in food, reported altered taste, and observed inadequate intake and weight loss.

Infection, high risk for which may be related to inadequate primary defenses (stasis of body fluids, decrease of ciliary action), chronic disease process, and malnutrition.

Powerlessness may be related to illness-related regimen and health-care environment, possibly evidenced by verbal expression of having no control, depression over physical deterioration, and nonparticipation in care, anger, and passivity.

encephalitis

Pain may be related to inflammation/irritation of the brain and cerebral edema, possibly evidenced by complaints of headache, distraction behaviors, restlessness, and autonomic response (changes in vital signs).

Hyperthermia may be related to increased metabolic rate, illness, and dehydration, possibly evidenced by increased body temperature, flushed/warm skin, and increased pulse and respiratory rates.

Fluid volume deficit, high risk for which may be related to increased losses through diaphoresis, hypermetabolic state, and decreased fluid intake.

Trauma/Suffocation, high risk for which may be related to restlessness, clonic/tonic activity, altered sensorium, and cognitive impairment.

endocarditis

Cardiac output, decreased may be related to inflammation of lining of heart and structural change in valve leaflets, possibly evidenced by fatigue, changes in heart sounds, tachycardia, and variations in hemodynamic readings.

Anxiety (specify level) may be related to change in health status and threat of death, possibly evidenced by apprehension, expressed concerns, and focus on self.

Pain may be related to generalized inflammatory process and embolic phenomena, possibly evidenced by complaints, narrowed focus, distraction behaviors, and autonomic responses (changes in vital signs).

Tissue perfusion, altered (specify), high risk for which may be related to embolic interruption of arterial flow.

endometriosis

Pain may be related to pressure of concealed bleeding/formation of adhesions, possibly evidenced by complaints (specify), guarding/distraction behaviors, and narrowed focus.

Sexual dysfunction may be related to pain secondary to presence of adhesions, possibly evidenced by verbalization of problem, and alteration in relationship to significant other(s).

Knowledge deficit [learning need] may be related to lack of information regarding pathophysiology of condition and therapy needs, possibly evidenced by statements of concern and misconceptions.

enteritis

Refer to colitis, ulcerative and Crohn's disease

epididymitis

Pain may be related to inflammation, edema formation, and tension on the spermatic cord, possibly evidenced by complaints, guarding/distraction behaviors, and autonomic responses (changes in vital signs).

Infection, high risk for which may be related to inadequate primary defenses; insufficient knowledge to avoid spread of infection.

Knowledge deficit [learning need] may be related to lack of information about pathophysiology, outcome, and self-care needs, possibly evidenced by statements of concern, misconceptions, and questions.

epilepsy

Trauma/Suffocation, high risk for which may be related to tonic/clonic muscle activity and change in level of consciousness.

Fear may be related to unpredictable nature of condition and potential for harm, possibly evidenced by decreased self-assurance, verbalization of concern, and withdrawal from social contacts/activities.

Body image disturbance may be related to perceived neurologic functional change/weakness, possibly evidenced by negative feelings about "brain"/self, change in social involvement, feelings of helplessness, and preoccupation with perceived change or loss.

failure to thrive

Nutrition, altered: less than body requirements may be related to inability to ingest/digest/absorb nutrients (defects in organ function/metabolism, genetic factors), and physical deprivation/psychosocial factors), possibly evidenced by weight loss/lack of appropriate weight gain, laboratory tests reflecting nutritional deficiency, poor muscle tome, and pale conjunctiva.

Parenting, altered, high risk for may be related to lack of knowledge, inadequate bonding, unrealistic expectations for self/infant, and lack of appropriate response of child.

Knowledge deficit [learning need] may be related to lack of information about pathophysiology of condition, nutritional needs, growth expectations, and parenting skills, possibly evidenced by verbalization of concerns, questions, misconceptions, and development of preventable complications.

fetal alcohol syndrome

Injury, high risk for CNS damage which may be related to external chemical factors (alcohol intake by mother), placental insufficiency, fetal drug withdrawal in utero/postpartum, and prematurity.

Parenting, altered, high risk for which may be related to mental and/or physical illness, inability of mother to assume the overwhelming task of unselfish giving and nurturing, and presence of stressors (financial/legal problems).

Coping, ineffective individual (mother) may be related to personal vulnerability, low self-esteem, inadequate coping skills, and multiple stressors (repeated over period of time), possibly evidenced by inability to meet basic needs/role expectations/problem solving, and excessive use of drug(s).

Family coping, ineffective, disabling may be related to lack of/insufficient support from others, mother's drug problem and treatment status, together with poor coping skills, lack of family stability/overinvolvement of parents with children and multigenerational addictive behaviors, possibly evidenced by abandonment, rejection, neglectful relationships with family members, and decisions and actions by family that are detrimental.

fetal demise

Grieving, anticipatory may be related to loss of child and lack of resolution of previous grieving response, possibly evidenced by expressions of distress, changes in eating habits, alterations in sleep patterns, crying, anger, and denial.

Spiritual distress may be related to challenged belief and value system (birth is supposed to be the beginning of life, not of death) and intense suffering, possibly evidenced by questioning of religious beliefs, concern about purpose of life and death, and anger (may be directed at God for "letting this happen").

Role performance, altered may be related to situational crisis (perceived inadequacy in "normal" reproductive role), and unanticipated changes in parental roles, possibly evidenced by expressed concern about parenting abilities, feelings of failure/guilt, and sense of inadequacy.

fracture

Pain may be related to loss of skeletal integrity, soft-tissue trauma/swelling and muscle spasm, possibly evidenced by complaints (specify), guarding/distraction behaviors, and autonomic responses (changes in vital signs).

Tissue perfusion, altered, peripheral, high risk for which may be related to vascular injury, interruption of arterial/venous flow, secondary to swelling and/or thrombus formation.

Self-care deficit (specify), high risk for which may be related to loss of function and restrictive treatment modality.

Knowledge deficit [learning need] may be related to lack of information about healing process, therapy requirements, and potential complications, possibly evidenced by statements of concern, questions, and misconceptions.

Physical mobility, impaired may be related to neuromuscular skeletal impairment, pain/discomfort, and restrictive therapies, possibly evidenced by inability to purposefully move within the physical environment, imposed restrictions, reluctance to attempt movement, limited range of motion, and decreased muscle strength/control.

frostbite

Tissue integrity, impaired may be related to altered circulation and thermal injury, possibly evidenced by damaged/destroyed tissue.

Pain may be related to diminished circulation with tissue ischemia/necrosis and edema formation, possibly evidenced by complaints, guarding/distraction behaviors, narrowed focus, and autonomic responses (changes in vital signs).

Infection, high risk for which may be related to traumatized tissue/tissue destruction and compromised immune response in affected area.

gallstone

Refer to cholelithiasis

gangrene, dry

Tissue perfusion, altered, peripheral may be related to interruption in arterial flow, possibly evidenced by cool skin temperature, change in color (black), atrophy of affected part, and presence of pain.

Pain may be related to tissue hypoxia and necrotic process, possibly evidenced by complaints (specify), guarding/distraction behaviors, narrowed focus, and autonomic responses (changes in vital signs).

gas, lung irritant

Airway clearance, ineffective may be related to irritation/inflammation of airway, possibly evidenced by marked cough, abnormal breath sounds (wheezes), dyspnea, and tachypnea.

Gas exchange, impaired, high risk for which may be related to irritation/inflammation of alveolar membrane, dependent on type of agent and length of exposure.

Anxiety (specify level) may be related to change in health status and threat of death, possibly evidenced by increased tension, apprehension, and sympathetic stimulation.

gastritis, acute

Pain may be related to irritation/inflammation of gastric mucosa, possibly evidenced by complaints (specify), guarding/distraction behaviors, and autonomic responses (changes in vital signs).

Fluid volume deficit, high risk for may be related to excessive losses through vomiting and diarrhea, reluctance to ingest fluids, and continued bleeding.

gastritis, chronic

Nutrition, altered: less than body requirements, high risk for which may be related to inability to ingest adequate nutrients (prolonged nausea/vomiting, anorexia, epigastric pain).

Knowledge deficit [learning need] may be related to lack of information about pathophysiology, psychologic factors, therapy needs, and potential complications, possibly evidenced by verbalization of concerns, questions, misconceptions, and continuation of problem.

gastroenteritis

Refer to gastritis and enteritis

gender identity disorder

Anxiety, severe may be related to unconscious/conscious conflicts about essential values/beliefs (egodystonic gender identification), threat to self-concept, and unmet needs, possibly evidenced by increased tension, helplessness, hopelessness, feelings of inadequacy, uncertainty, insomnia, and focus on self.

Role performance, altered/Personal identity disturbance may be related to crisis in development in which person has difficulty knowing to which sex s/he belongs; sense of discomfort and inappropriateness about anatomic sex, possibly evidenced by confusion about sense of self, purpose or direction in life, sexual identification/preference, verbalization of desire to be/insistence that person is the opposite sex, change in self-perception of role, and conflict in roles.

Sexuality patterns, altered may be related to ineffective or absent role models and conflict with sexual orientation and/or preferences, possibly evidenced by verbalizations of discomfort with sexual orientation and/or role and lack of information about human sexuality.

Family coping, ineffective, compromised/disabling, high risk for which may be related to inadequate/incorrect information or understanding, temporary family disorganization and role changes, and patient providing little support in turn for primary person.

Family coping, potential for growth may be related to fact that individual's basic needs are sufficiently gratified and adaptive tasks effectively addressed to enable goals of self-actualization to surface, possibly evidenced by family member(s) attempt(s) to describe growth/impact of crisis on own values, priorities, goals, or relationships; family member(s) is/are moving in direction of health-promotion and enriching lifestyle that supports patient's search for self; and choosing experiences that optimize wellness.

glaucoma

Sensory-perceptual alterations, visual may be related to altered sensory reception and altered status of sense organ (increased intraocular pressure/atrophy of optic nerve head), possibly evidenced by progressive loss of visual field.

Anxiety (specify level) may be related to change in health status, presence of pain, possibility/reality of loss of vision, unmet needs, and negative self-talk, possibly evidenced by apprehension, uncertainty, and expressed concern regarding changes in life event.

glomerulonephritis

Fluid volume excess may be related to failure of regulatory mechanism (inflammation of glomerular membrane inhibiting filtration), possibly evidenced by weight gain, edema/anasarca, intake greater than output, and blood pressure changes.

Pain may be related to effects of circulating toxins and edema/distension of renal capsule, possibly evidenced by complaints (specify), guarding/distraction behaviors, and autonomic responses (changes in vital signs).

Nutrition, altered: less than body requirements may be related to anorexia and dietary restrictions, possibly evidenced by aversion to eating, reported altered taste, weight loss, and decreased intake.

Diversional activity deficit may be related to treatment modality, fatigue, and malaise, possibly evidenced by statements of boredom, restlessness, and irritability.

gonorrhea

Infection, high risk for dissemination/bacteremia which may be related to presence of infectious process in highly vascular area and lack of recognition of disease process.

Pain may be related to irritation/inflammation of mucosa and effects of circulating toxins, possibly evidenced by complaints (specify), guarding/distraction behaviors, and autonomic responses (changes in vital signs).

Knowledge deficit [learning need] may be related to lack of information about disease cause/transmission, therapy, and self-care needs, possibly evidenced by statements of concern, questions, misconceptions, and inaccurate follow-through of instruction/development of preventable complications.

gout

Pain may be related to inflammation of joint(s), possibly evidenced by complaints (specify), guarding/distraction behaviors, and autonomic responses (changes in vital signs).

Physical mobility, impaired may be related to joint pain/edema, possibly evidenced by reluctance to attempt movement, limited range of motion, and therapeutic restriction of movement.

Knowledge deficit [learning need] may be related to lack of information about cause, treatment, and prevention of condition, possibly evidenced by statements concern, questions, misconceptions, and inaccurate follow-through of instructions.

Guillain-Barré syndrome

Physical mobility, impaired may be related to neuromuscular impairment, possibly evidenced by decreased muscle strength/control, inability to purposefully move, and impaired coordination.

Anxiety (specify level) may be related to change in health status, threat to self-concept, and threat of death, possibly evidenced by apprehension, feelings of depression, powerlessness, insomnia, and focus on self.

Sensory-perceptual alterations (specify) may be related to neurologic disease, sleep deprivation, therapeutically restricted environment, endogenous chemical alterations (electrolyte imbalance, hypoxia), and psychologic stress, possibly evidenced by reported or observed change in usual response to stimuli, altered communication patterns, and measured change in sensory acuity and motor coordination.

Breathing pattern, ineffective, high risk for which may be related to neuromuscular impairment and decreased energy/lung expansion.

hay fever

Pain may be related to irritation/inflammation of upper airway mucous membranes and conjunctiva, possibly evidenced by complaints (specify), irritability, and restlessness.

Knowledge deficit [learning need] may be related to lack of information regarding underlying cause, appropriate therapy, and required lifestyle changes, possibly evidenced by statements of concern, questions, and misconceptions.

heatstroke

Hyperthermia may be related to prolonged exposure to hot environment/vigorous activity with failure of regulating mechanism of the body, possibly evidenced by high body temperature (above 105°F/ 40.6°C), flushed, hot skin, tachycardia, and seizures.

Cardiac output, decreased may be related to functional stress of hypermetabolic state, altered circulating volume/venous return, and direct myocardial damage secondary to hyperthermia, possibly evidenced by decreased peripheral pulses, dysrhythmias/tachycardia, and changes in mentation.

hemodialysis

Injury, high risk for which may be related to multiple factors causing loss of vascular access (e.g., thrombosis, infection, disconnection/hemorrhage).

Fluid volume deficit, high risk for which may be related to excessive fluid losses/shifts via ultrafiltration, hemorrhage from altered coagulation/disconnection of shunt, and fluid restrictions.

Body image disturbance may be related to change in function and dependence on mechanical support, possibly evidenced by negative feelings about body, feelings of helplessness and powerlessness, change in social involvement, preoccupation with change, and possible extension of body boundary to incorporate environmental object.

Nutrition, altered: less than body requirements, high risk for which may be related to inadequate ingestion of nutrients (dietary restrictions, anorexia, nausea/vomiting stomatitis).

Powerlessness may be related to illness-related regimen and health-care environment, possibly evidenced by verbal expression of having no control, depression over physical deterioration, nonparticipation in care, anger, and passivity.

Role performance, altered may be related to situational crisis and chronic illness with changes in usual roles, possibly evidenced by verbalization of changes in lifestyle/usual responsibilities, change in physical capacity to resume role, focus on past function, overdependence on others for care, not taking responsibility for self-care/lack of follow-through, and self-destructive behavior.

Coping, ineffective individual may be related to situational crises/personal vulnerability, multiple life changes, inadequate support systems, and severe pain/overwhelming threat to self, possibly evidenced by verbalization of inability to cope/asking for help, chronic worry, fatigue, insomnia, anxiety/depression, and inappropriate use of defense mechanisms.

Family coping, ineffective, compromised/disabling may be related to inadequate or incorrect information or understanding by a primary person, temporary family disorganization and role changes, patient providing little support in turn for the primary person, and prolonged disease/disability progression that exhausts the supportive capacity of significant persons, possibly evidenced by expressions of concern or complaints about significant other's/family's response to patient's health problem, preoccupation of significant other(s) with own personal reactions, display of intolerance/ rejection, and protective behavior disproportionate (too little or too much) to patient's abilities or need for autonomy.

hemophilia

Fluid volume deficit, high risk for which may be related to hemorrhagic losses.

Pain, chronic, high risk for which may be related to hemorrhage into joints.

Physical mobility, impaired, high risk for may be related to joint hemorrhage, swelling, degenerative changes, and muscle atrophy.

Family coping, ineffective, compromised may be related to prolonged nature of condition that exhausts the supportive capacity of significant people, possibly evidenced by protective behaviors disproportionate to patient's abilities/need for autonomy.

hemoptysis

Anxiety (specify level)/Fear may be related to perceived threat of death, possibly evidenced by apprehension, glancing about, facial tension, and statements of concern.

Airway clearance, ineffective, high risk for which may be related to collection of blood, mucus, and clot formation.

Fluid volume deficit, high risk for which may be related to excessive hemorrhagic losses.

hemorrhoid

Pain may be related to inflammation and edema of prolapsed varices, possibly evidenced by complaints (specify) and guarding/distraction behaviors.

Constipation may be related to pain on defecation and reluctance to defecate, possibly evidenced by frequency less than usual pattern and hard, formed stools.

hemorrhoidectomy

Pain may be related to edema/swelling and tissue trauma, possibly evidenced by complaints, guarding/distraction behaviors, focus on self, and autoimonic responses (changes in vital signs).

Urinary retention, high risk for which may be related to perineal trauma, edema/swelling, and pain.

Knowledge deficit [learning need] may be related to lack of information regarding therapeutic treatment and potential complications, possibly evidenced by statements of concern and questions.

hemothorax (also refer to pneumothorax)

Trauma/Suffocation, high risk for which may be related to concurrent disease/injury process, dependence on chest drainage system, and lack of safety education/precautions.

Anxiety (specify level) may be related to change in health status and threat of death, possibly evidenced by increased tension, restlessness, expressed concern, sympathetic stimulation, and focus on self.

hepatitis, acute viral

Fatigue may be related to decreased metabolic energy production and altered body chemistry, possibly evidenced by reports of lack of energy/inability to maintain usual routines, decreased performance, and increase in physical complaints.

Nutrition, altered: less than body requirements may be related to inability to ingest adequate nutrients (nausea, vomiting, anorexia), possibly evidenced by aversion to eating/lack of interest in food, observed lack of intake, and weight loss.

Pain may be related to inflammation and swelling of the liver, uticarial eruptions, arthralgia, and pruritus, possibly evidenced by complaints (specify), guarding/distraction behaviors, focus on self, and autonomic responses (changes in vital signs).

Home maintenance management, impaired, high risk for which may be related to effects of disease process and inadequate support systems.

Knowledge deficit [learning need] may be related to lack of understanding about disease process/transmission, treatment needs, and future expectations, possibly evidenced by questions, statement of concerns, inaccurate follow-through of instructions, and development of preventable complications.

hernia, hiatal

Pain may be related to regurgitation of acidic gastric contents, possibly evidenced by complaints (specify), facial grimacing, and focus on self.

Knowledge deficit [learning need] may be related to lack of information about pathophysiology and prevention of complications, possibly evidenced by statements of concern, questions, and recurrence of condition.

herniation of nucleus pulposus

Pain may be related to nerve compression/irritation and muscle spasms, possibly evidenced by complaints (specify), guarding/distraction behaviors, narrowed focus, and autonomic responses (changes in vital signs).

Physical mobility, impaired may be related to pain and therapeutic restrictions/traction, possibly evidenced by decreased muscle strength, limited range of motion, and reluctance to attempt movement.

Diversional activity deficit may be related to length of recuperation period and therapy restrictions, possibly evidenced by statements of boredom, disinterest, "nothing to do," and restlessness.

herpes, herpes simplex

Pain may be related to presence of localized inflammation and open lesions, possibly evidenced by complaints (specify), distraction behaviors, and restlessness.

Infection, high risk for secondary infection which may be related to broken, traumatized tissue and altered immune response.

Sexuality patterns, altered, high risk for which may be related to fear of transmitting the disease.

herpes zoster

Pain may be related to inflammation/local lesions along sensory nerve(s), possibly evidenced by complaints (specify), guarding/distraction behaviors, narrowed focus, and autonomic responses (changes in vital signs).

Knowledge deficit [learning need] may be related to lack of information about pathophysiology, therapeutic needs, and potential complications, possibly evidenced by statements of concern, questions, and misconceptions.

Hodgkin's disease (also refer to cancer/chemotherapy)

Knowledge deficit [learning need] may be related to lack of information about diagnosis, pathophysiology, treatment, and prognosis, possibly evidenced by statements of concern, questions, and misconceptions.

Pain may be related to manifestations of inflammatory response (fever, chills, night sweats) and pruritus, possibly evidenced by complaints (specify), distraction behaviors, and focus on self.

Anxiety (specify level)/Fear may be related to threat to self-concept and threat of death, possibly evidenced by apprehension, insomnia, focus on self, and increased tension.

Nutrition, altered: less than body requirements may be related to inability to ingest adequate nutrients (anorexia/dysphagia), possibly evidenced by weight loss, lack of interest in food, and observed decreased intake.

hydrocephalus

Tissue perfusion, altered, cerebral may be related to decreased arterial/venous blood flow (compression of brain tissue), possibly evidenced by changes in mentation, restlessness, irritability, complaints of headache, pupillary changes, and changes in vital signs.

Sensory-perceptual alterations, visual may be related to pressure on sensory/motor nerves, possibly evidenced by complaints of double vision, development of strabismus, nystagmus, pupillary changes, and optic atrophy.

Physical mobility, impaired, high risk for may be related to neuromuscular impairment, decreased muscle strength, and impaired coordination.

Infection, high risk for which may be related to invasive procedure/presence of shunt.

Knowledge deficit [learning need] may be related to lack of understanding of condition, prognosis, and long-term therapy needs/medical follow-up, possibly evidenced by questions, statement of concern, request for information, and inaccurate follow-through of instruction/development of preventable complications.

hyperbilirubinemia

Injury, high risk for effects of treatment which may be related to adverse effects of phototherapy/exchange transfusions.

Growth and development, altered, high risk for which may be related to effects of physical condition/collection of bilirubin in brain tissue (basal ganglia, brain stem nuclei).

Knowledge deficit [learning need] may be related to lack of exposure/recall and information misinterpretation, possibly evidenced by questions, statement of concern, and inaccurate follow-through of instruction/development of preventable complications.

hyperemesis gravidarum

Fluid volume deficit [active loss] may be relate to excessive gastric losses and reduced intake, possibly evidenced by dry mucous membranes, decreased/concentrated urine, decreased pulse volume and pressure, thirst, and hemoconcentration.

Nutrition, altered: less than body requirements may be related to inability to ingest/digest/absorb nutrients (prolonged vomiting), possibly evidenced by reported inadequate food intake, lack of interest in food/aversion to eating, and weight loss.

Coping, ineffective individual, high risk for which may be related to situational/maturational crisis (pregnancy, change in health status, projected role changes, concern about outcome).

hypertension

Cardiac output, decreased, high risk for may be related to increased afterload, (vasoconstriction), structural factors (increased systemic vascular resistance, myocardial ischemia, ventricular hypertrophy/rigidity).

Pain may be related to increased cerebral vascular pressure, possibly evidenced by reports of throbbing pain located in suboccipital region, present on awakening and disappearing spontaneously after being up and about; reluctance to move head; avoidance of bright lights and noise; increased muscle tension; reports of dizziness; blurred vision; nausea and vomiting.

Knowledge deficit [learning need] may be related to lack of information/misinterpretation regarding pathophysiology, therapeutic regimen, lifestyle changes, and potential complications, possibly evidenced by statements of concern/questions, inaccurate follow-through of instructions, and lack of control of condition.

Adjustment, impaired may be related to condition requiring change in lifestyle, altered locus of control, and absence of feelings of illness/denial, possibly evidenced by verbalization of nonacceptance of health status change and lack of movement toward independence.

Sexual dysfunction, high risk for which may be related to side effects of medication.

hyperthyroidism (also refer to thyrotoxicosis)

Fatigue may be related to hypermetabolic imbalance with increased energy requirements, irritability of central nervous system, and altered body chemistry, possibly evidenced by verbalization of overwhelming lack of energy to maintain usual routine, decreased performance, emotional lability/irritability, and impaired ability to concentrate.

Anxiety (specify level) may be related to increased stimulation of the central nervous system, possibly evidenced by increased nervous tension, apprehension, irritability, and emotional lability.

Nutrition, altered: less than body requirements, high risk for which may be related to inability to ingest adequate nutrients for increased metabolic rate/constant activity or impaired absorption of nutrients (vomiting/diarrhea).

Tissue integrity, impaired may be related to presence of periorbital edema and reduced ability to blink (protective mechanism), possibly evidenced by complaints of eye discomfort/dryness and development of corneal abrasion/ulceration.

hypoglycemia

Thought processes, altered may be related to inadequate glucose for cellular brain function and effects of endogenous hormone activity, possibly evidenced by irritability, changes in mentation, memory loss, altered attention span, and emotional lability.

Nutrition, altered: less than body requirements, high risk for which may be related to inadequate glucose metabolism and imbalance of glucose/insulin levels.

Knowledge deficit [learning need] may be related to lack of information/recall about pathophysiology of condition and therapy/self-care needs, possibly evidenced by development of hypoglycemia and statements of questions/misconceptions.

hypoparathyroidism (acute)

Injury, high risk for which may be related to neuromuscular excitability/tetany and formation of renal stones.

Pain may be related to recurrent muscle spasms and alteration in reflexes, possibly evidenced by complaints (specify), distraction behaviors, and narrowed focus.

Airway clearance, ineffective, high risk for which may be related to spasm of the laryngeal muscles.

hypothyroidism

Physical mobility, impaired may be related to weakness, fatigue, muscle aches, altered reflexes, and mucin deposits in joints and interstitial spaces, possibly evidenced by decreased muscle strength/control and impaired coordination.

Thought processes, altered may be related to actual physiologic changes with mucin deposits in interstitial spaces and decreased metabolic rate, possibly evidenced by forgetfulness, impaired ability to conceptualize/reason, and personality changes.

Sensory-perceptual alterations (specify) may be related to mucin deposits and nerve compression, possibly evidenced by paresthesias of hands and feet or decreased hearing.

Constipation may be related to decreased peristalsis/physical activity, possibly evidenced by frequency less than usual pattern; decreased bowel sounds; hard, dry stool; and development of fecal impaction.

hysterectomy

Pain may be related to tissue trauma/abdominal incision, possibly evidenced by complaints (specify), guarding/distraction behaviors, and autonomic responses (changes in vital signs).

Urinary retention, high risk for which may be related to localized edema and nerve trauma with temporary bladder atony.

Sexuality patterns, altered, high risk for which may be related to concerns regarding altered body function/structure.

ileocolitis
Refer to colitis

ileostomy
Refer to colostomy

ileus

Pain may be related to distension/edema and ischemia of intestinal tissue, possibly evidenced by complaints (specify), guarding/distraction behaviors, narrowed focus, and autonomic responses (changes in vital signs).

Diarrhea/Constipation may be related to presence of obstruction/changes in peristalsis, possibly evidenced by changes in frequency and consistency or absence of stool, alterations in bowel sounds, presence of pain, and cramping.

Fluid volume deficit, high risk for which may be related to increased intestinal losses (vomiting and diarrhea), and decreased intake.

impetigo

Skin integrity, impaired may be related to presence of infectious process and pruritus, possibly evidenced by open/crusted lesions.

Pain may be related to inflammation and pruritus, possibly evidenced by complaints (specify), distraction behaviors, and self-focusing.

Infection, high risk for secondary infection which may be related to broken skin, traumatized tissue, altered immune response, and virulence/contagious nature of causative organism.

Infection, high risk for transmission which may be related to virulent nature of causative organism.

influenza

Pain may be related to inflammation and effects of circulating toxins, possibly evidenced by complaints (specify), distraction behaviors, and narrowed focus.

Fluid volume deficit, high risk for which may be related to excessive gastric losses, hypermetabolic state, and altered intake.

Hyperthermia may be related to effects of circulating toxins and dehydration, possibly evidenced by increased body temperature, warm and flushed skin, and tachycardia.

insulin shock

Refer to hypoglycemia

intestinal obstruction

Refer to ileus

intra-aortic balloon counterpulsation

Physical mobility, impaired may be related to imposed restrictions for surgical procedure, abnormal cardiovascular response to activity, possibly evidenced by presence of restraints.

Tissue perfusion, altered, peripheral, high risk for may be related to arterial cannulation, necessity for limb restraints, formation of thrombi.

Anxiety (specify)/Fear may be related to change in health status, threat of death, situational crisis, possibly evidenced by apprehension and restlessness.

Sensory-perceptual alterations (specify), high risk for may be related to therapeutically and socially restricted environment, pain, sleep deprivation, psychologic stress, presence of continuous mechanical noise.

Kawasaki disease

Hyperthermia may be related to increased metabolic rate and dehydration, possibly evidenced by increased body temperature greater than normal range, flushed skin, increased respiratory rate, and tachycardia.

Pain may be related to inflammation and edema/swelling of tissues, possibly evidenced by complaints (specify), restlessness, guarding behavior, and narrowed focus.

Skin integrity, impaired may be related to inflammatory process, altered circulation, and edema, possibly evidenced by disruption of skin surface including macular rash and desquamation

Oral mucous membranes, altered may be related to inflammatory process, dehydration, and mouth breathing, possibly evidenced by pain, hyperemia, and fissures of lips.

Cardiac output, decreased, high risk for which may be related to structural changes/inflammation of coronary arteries and alterations in rate/rhythm or conduction.

labor, induced/augmented

Injury, high risk for maternal which may be related to deleterious effects of oxytocin administration, rapid labor, and delivery.

Injury, high risk for fetal which may be related to altered placental perfusion/cord prolapse and precipitous delivery.

Infection, high risk for which may be related to rupture of amniotic membranes.

Knowledge deficit [learning need] may be related to lack of exposure/recall, information misinterpretation, and unfamiliarity with information resources, possibly evidenced by questions, statement of concern/misconception, and inaccurate follow-through of instruction/development of preventable complications.

Pain may be related to rapid onset of strong, frequent contractions and level of anxiety, possibly evidenced by verbal complaints, distraction/guarding behaviors, and narrowed focus.

labor, stage I (active phase)

Pain may be related to contraction-related hypoxia, dilation of tissues, and pressure on adjacent structures combined with stimulation of both parasympathetic and sympathetic nerve endings, possibly evidenced by verbal complaints, distraction/guarding behaviors, and narrowed focus.

Urinary elimination, altered may be related to retention of fluid in the prenatal period, increased glomerular filtration rate, decreased adrenal stimulation, dehydration, hemorrhage, severe intrapartal hypertension, pressure of the presenting part, and regional anesthesia, possibly evidenced by increased/decreased output, decreased circulating blood volume, spasms of glomeruli and albuminuria, and reduced sensation.

Coping, ineffective individual/couple, high risk for which may be related to stressors accompanying labor, ineffective coping mechanisms, and pain.

Self-esteem disturbance, high risk for which may be related to use of medications to relieve intense contractions and inability to carry out wish for an unmedicated childbirth.

labor, stage II (expulsion)

Pain may be related to strong uterine contractions, tissue stretching/dilation and compression of nerves by presenting part of the fetus, diaphoresis, and bladder distention, possibly evidenced by complaints, facial grimacing, distraction/guarding behaviors, and narrowed focus.

Cardiac output, decreased may be related to repeated, prolonged Valsalva's maneuvers, effects of anesthesia/medications, and dorsal recumbent position occluding the inferior vena cava and partially obstructing the aorta, possibly evidenced by decreased venous return and changes in vital signs (blood pressure, pulse).

Gas exchange, impaired, fetal, high risk for which may be related to head compression with vagal stimulation (causing bradycardia and hypoxia), cord compression, maternal position/prolonged labor affecting placental perfusion, and effects of maternal anesthesia.

Skin integrity, impaired, high risk for which may be related to untoward stretching/lacerations of delicate tissues (precipitous labor, hypertonic contractile pattern, adolescence, large fetus) and application of forceps.

Breathing pattern, ineffective may be related to anxiety, pain, decreased energy, and fatigue, possibly evidenced by tachypnea, abnormal ABGs (maternal respiratory alkalosis), and changes in fetal heart rate/variability.

laminectomy

Tissue perfusion, altered (specify) may be related to diminished/interrupted blood flow, hypovolemia, possibly evidenced by paresthesia, numbness, decreased range of motion and muscle strength.

Pain may be related to traumatized tissues, localized inflammation, and edema, possibly evidenced by alteration in muscle tone, complaints (specify), and distraction/guarding behaviors.

Physical mobility, impaired may be related to imposed medical restrictions, decreased strength, and pain, possibly evidenced by limited range of motion, decreased muscle strength, and reluctance to attempt movement.

Sensory-perceptual alterations, kinesthetic, tactile may be related to inflammation/edema of compressed nerve or nerve root injury, possibly evidenced by changes in sensation, movement, color, or temperature of lower extremities.

Urinary retention, high risk for may be related to pain and swelling in operative area and reduced mobility.

laryngectomy

Airway clearance, ineffective may be related to surgical trauma, partial/total removal of the glottis, which results in temporary or permanent neck breathing, edema formation, and copious and thick secretions, possibly evidenced by dyspnea/difficulty breathing, changes in rate/depth of respiration, use of accessory respiratory muscles, weak/ineffective cough, abnormal breath sounds, and cyanosis.

Communication, impaired verbal may be related to anatomic deficit (removal of vocal cords), physical barrier (tracheostomy tube), and required voice rest, possibly evidenced by inability to speak, change in vocal characteristics, and impaired articulation.

Skin/Tissue integrity, impaired may be related to surgical removal of tissues/grafting, effects of radiation or chemotherapeutic agents, altered circulation/reduced blood supply, compromised nutritional status, edema formation, and pooling/continuous drainage of secretions, possibly evidenced by disruption of skin surface and destruction of skin layers.

2518

Oral mucous membrane, altered may be related to dehydration/absence of oral intake, poor/inadequate oral hygiene, pathologic condition (oral cancer), mechanical trauma (oral surgery), and nutritional deficits, possibly evidenced by xerostomia (dry mouth), oral discomfort, thick/mucoid saliva, decreased saliva production, dry and crusted/coated tongue, inflamed lips, absent teeth/gums, and halitosis.

laryngitis
Refer to croup

lead poisoning, acute (also refer to lead poisoning, chronic)
Trauma, high risk for which may be related to loss of coordination, altered level of consciousness, and clonic or tonic muscle activity. (Continuous exposure may lead to permanent neurologic damage.)
Fluid volume deficit, high risk for which may be related to excessive vomiting, diarrhea, or decreased intake.
Knowledge deficit [learning need] may be related to lack of information about sources of lead and prevention of poisoning, possibly evidenced by statements of concern, questions, and misconceptions.

lead poisoning, chronic (also refer to lead poisoning, acute)
Nutrition, altered: less than body requirements may be related to decreased intake (chemically induced changes in the gastrointestinal tract), possibly evidenced by anorexia, abdominal discomfort, reported metallic taste, and weight loss.
Thought processes, altered may be related to deposition of lead in central nervous system and brain tissue, possibly evidenced by personality changes, learning disabilities, and impaired ability to conceptualize and reason.
Pain may be related to deposition of lead in soft tissues and bone, possibly evidenced by complaints (specify), distraction behaviors, and focus on self.

leukemia
Infection, high risk for which may be related to inadequate secondary defenses (alterations in mature white blood cells, increased number of immature lymphocytes, immunosuppression and bone marrow suppression), invasive procedures, and malnutrition.
Anxiety (specify level)/Fear may be related to change in health status, threat of death, and situational crisis, possibly evidenced by apprehension, feelings of helplessness, and focus on self.
Activity intolerance may be related to imbalance between oxygen supply and demand, possibly evidenced by generalized weakness, report of fatigue, exertional dyspnea, and abnormal vital sign response activity.
Pain may be related to physical agents (infiltration of tissues/organs/central nervous system, expanding bone marrow) and chemical agents (antileukemic agents), possibly evidenced by complaints of abdominal discomfort, arthralgia, bone pain, headache, distraction behaviors, narrowed focus, and autonomic responses (changes in vital signs).

long-term care
Anxiety (specify level)/Fear may be related to change in health status, role functioning, interaction patterns, socioeconomic status, environment, unmet needs, recent life changes, and loss of friends/significant other(s), possibly evidenced by apprehension, restlessness, repetitive questioning, pacing, purposeless activity, and expressed concern regarding changes in life events.
Grieving, anticipatory may be related to perceived, actual, or potential loss of physiopsychosocial well-being, personal possessions, significant other(s), and cultural beliefs about aging, possibly evidenced by denial of feelings, depression, sorrow, guilt, alterations in activity level, sleep patterns, eating habits, and libido.
Poisoning, high risk for drug toxicity which may be related to reduced metabolism, impaired circulation, precarious physiologic balance, presence of multiple diseases/organ involvement, and use of multiple prescribed/OTC drugs.
Thought processes, altered may be related to physiologic changes of aging, loss of cells and brain atrophy, decreased blood supply, altered sensory input, pain, effects of medications, and psychologic conflicts (disrupted life pattern), possibly evidenced by slower reaction times, gradual memory loss, altered attention span, disorientation, and inability to follow.
Sleep pattern disturbance may be related to internal factors (illness, psychologic stress, inactivity), and external factors (environmental changes, facility routines), possibly evidenced by complaints of difficulty in falling asleep/not feeling well-rested, interrupted sleep, awakening earlier than desired, change in behavior/performance, increasing irritability, and listlessness.

Skin integrity, impaired, high risk for which may be related to general debilitation, reduced mobility, changes in skin turgor and muscle mass associated with aging, sensory/motor deficits, altered circulation (edema, poor nutrition), excretions/secretions, and problems with self-care.

Sexuality patterns, altered, high risk for which may be related to biopsychosocial alteration of sexuality, interference in psychologic/physical well-being, self-image, and lack of privacy/significant other(s).

lupus erythematosus, systemic

Pain may be related to widespread inflammatory process affecting connective tissues, blood vessels, serosal surfaces, and mucous membranes, possibly evidenced by multiple complaints (specify), guarding/distraction behaviors, self-focusing, and autonomic responses (changes in vital signs).

Skin/Tissue integrity, impaired may be related to chronic inflammation, edema formation, and altered circulation, possibly evidenced by presence of skin rash/lesions, ulcerations of mucous membranes, photosensitivity, and necrosis.

Fatigue may be related to increased energy requirements (chronic inflammation) and altered body chemistry (including effects of drug therapy), possibly evidenced by complaints of overwhelming lack of energy/inability to maintain usual routines, decreased performance, lethargy, and malaise.

Body image disturbance may be related to presence of chronic condition with rash, lesions, ulcers, purpura, mottled erythema of hands, alopecia, loss of strength, and altered body function, possibly evidenced by hiding body parts, negative feelings about body, feelings of helplessness, and change in social involvement.

Lyme disease

Pain may be related to systemic effects of toxins, presence of rash, urticaria, and joint swelling/inflammation, possibly evidenced by complaints (specify), guarding behavior, autonomic responses, and narrowed focus.

Fatigue may be related to increased energy requirements, altered body chemistry, and states of discomfort, possibly evidenced by complaints of overwhelming lack of energy/inability to maintain usual routines, decreased performance, lethargy, and malaise.

Cardiac output, decreased, high risk for which may be related to alteration in rate/rhythm/conduction.

Injury, high risk for complications which may be related to external biologic factors (presence of spirochete) and failure to initiate prompt treatment.

Mallory-Weiss syndrome

Fluid volume deficit, high risk for which may be related to excessive vascular losses, presence of vomiting, and reduced intake.

Knowledge deficit [learning need] may be related to lack of information regarding causes, treatment, and prevention of condition, possibly evidenced by statements of concern, questions, and recurrence of problem.

mastectomy

Skin/Tissue integrity, impaired may be related to tension on suture line (removal of large amount of tissue, edema formation), altered circulation, and changes in skin elasticity/sensation, tissue destruction (radiation), possibly evidenced by disruption of skin surface, and destruction of skin layers/subcutaneous tissues.

Physical mobility, impaired may be related to pain, alteration in normal musculature/tissue integrity, and edema formation, possibly evidenced by decreased muscle strength, limited range of motion, imposed medical restrictions, and reluctance to attempt movement.

Self-care deficit, bathing/dressing may be related to temporary loss/altered function of one or both arms, possibly evidenced by statements of inability to perform/complete self-care tasks.

Body image disturbance may be related to loss of body part denoting femininity, possibly evidenced by not looking at/touching area, negative feelings about body, preoccupation with loss, and change in social involvement/relationship.

mastitis

Pain may be related to erythema and edema of breast tissues, possibly evidenced by complaints (specify), guarding/distraction behaviors, self-focusing, and autonomic responses (changes in vital signs).

Infection, high risk for spread/abscess formation which may be related to traumatized tissues, stasis of body fluids, and insufficient knowledge to prevent complications.

Knowledge deficit [learning need] may be related to lack of information about pathophysiology, treatment, and prevention of complications, possibly evidenced by statements of concern, questions, and misconceptions.

mastoidectomy

Infection, high risk for spread which may be related to preexisting infection, surgical trauma, and stasis of body fluids in close proximity to brain.

Pain may be related to inflammation, tissue trauma, and edema formation, possibly evidenced by complaints (specify), distraction behaviors, restlessness, self-focusing, and autonomic responses (changes in vital signs).

Sensory-perceptual alterations, auditory may be related to presence of packing, edema, and surgical disturbance of middle ear structures, possibly evidenced by reported/tested hearing loss in affected ear.

measles

Pain may be related to inflammation of mucous membranes, conjunctiva, and presence of extensive skin rash with pruritus, possibly evidenced by complaints (specify), distraction behaviors, self-focusing, and autonomic responses (changes in vital signs).

Hyperthermia may be related to presence of viral toxins and inflammatory response, possibly evidenced by increased body temperature, flushed/warm skin, and tachycardia.

Infection, high risk for, secondary which may be related to altered immune response and traumatized dermal tissues.

Knowledge deficit [learning need] may be related to lack of information about pathophysiology, transmission, and prevention of disease, possibly evidenced by statements of concern, questions, misconceptions, and development of preventable complications.

meningitis, acute meningococcal

Pain may be related to inflammation/irritation of the meninges with spasm of extensor muscles (neck, shoulders, and back), possibly evidenced by complaints (specify), guarding/distraction behaviors, narrowed focus, and autonomic responses (changes in vital signs).

Hyperthermia may be related to infectious process (increased metabolic rate) and dehydration, possibly evidenced by increased body temperature, warm/flushed skin, and tachycardia.

Trauma/Suffocation, high risk for which may be related to alterations in level of consciousness, possible development of clonic/tonic muscle activity (seizures), and generalized weakness/prostration.

meniscectomy

Physical mobility, impaired may be related to pain, joint instability, and imposed medical restrictions of movement, possibly evidenced by decreased muscle strength/control, limited range of motion, and reluctance to attempt movement.

Knowledge deficit [learning need] may be related to lack of information about postoperative expectations, prevention of complications, and self-care needs, possibly evidenced by statements of concern, questions, and misconceptions.

mental retardation (also refer to Down syndrome)

Communication, impaired verbal may be related to developmental delay/impairment of cognitive and motor abilities, possibly evidenced by impaired articulation, difficulty with phonation, and inability to modulate speech/find appropriate words (dependent on degree of retardation).

Self-care deficit (specify), high risk for which may be related to impaired cognitive ability and motor skills.

Nutrition, altered: high risk for more than body requirements which may be related to decreased metabolic rate coupled with impaired cognitive development and dysfunctional eating patterns.

Social interaction, impaired may be related to impaired thought processes, communication barriers, and knowledge/skill deficit about ways to enhance mutuality, possibly evidenced by dysfunctional interactions with peers, family and/or significant other(s), and verbalized/observed discomfort in social situation.

Family coping, ineffective, compromised may be related to chronic nature of disease and disability, parental supervision, and lifestyle restrictions, possibly evidenced by protective behavior disproportionate to patient's abilities or need for autonomy.

Home maintenance management, impaired may be related to impaired cognitive functioning, insufficient finances/family organization or planning, lack of knowledge, and inadequate support systems, possibly evidenced by requests for assistance with home maintenance, expression of difficulty in maintaining home, disorderly surroundings, and overtaxed family members.

Sexual dysfunction, high risk for which may be related to biopsychosocial alteration of sexuality, ineffectual/absent role models, misinformation/lack of knowledge, and lack of significant other(s).

migraine

Pain may be related to functional disturbance of cranial circulation, possibly evidenced by complaints (specify), guarding/distraction behaviors, narrowed focus, and autonomic responses (changes in vital signs).

Physical mobility, impaired may be related to severe pain and intolerance to activity, possibly evidenced by reluctance to attempt movement, impaired coordination.

Knowledge deficit [learning need] may be related to lack of information regarding management of recurrent/temporarily debilitating condition, possibly evidenced by statements of concern, questions, and misconceptions.

mitral stenosis

Activity intolerance may be related to imbalance between oxygen supply and demand, possibly evidenced by reports of fatigue, weakness, exertional dyspnea, and tachycardia.

Gas exchange, impaired may be related to altered blood flow, possibly evidenced by restlessness, hypoxia, and cyanois (orthopnea/paroxysmal nocturnal dyspnea).

Knowledge deficit [learning need] may be related to lack of information regarding pathophysiology, therapeutic needs, and potential complications, possibly evidenced by statements of concern, questions, inaccurate follow-through of instructions, and development of preventable complications.

mononucleosis, infectious

Fatigue may be related to decreased energy production, states of discomfort, and increased energy requirements (inflammatory process), possibly evidenced by reports of overwhelming lack of energy, inability to maintain usual routines, lethargy, and malaise.

Pain may be related to inflammation of lymphoid and organ tissues, irritation of oropharyngeal mucous membranes, and effects of circulating toxins, possibly evidenced by complaints (specify), distraction behaviors, and self-focusing.

Hyperthermia may be related to inflammatory process, possibly evidenced by increased body temperature, warm/flushed skin, and tachycardia.

Knowledge deficit [learning need] may be related to lack of information regarding disease transmission, self-care needs, medical therapy, and potential complications, possibly evidenced by statements of concern, misconceptions, and inaccurate follow-through of instructions.

mood disorders

Refer to depressive disorders

multiple personality

Refer to dissociative disorders

multiple sclerosis

Physical mobility, impaired may be related to neuromuscular and perceptual impairment and decreased strength and endurance, possibly evidenced by impaired coordination, decreased muscle control and mass, and altered ability to move purposefully or perform routine tasks.

Sensory-perceptual alterations, visual, kinesthetic, tactile may be related to delayed/interrupted neuronal transmission, possibly evidenced by impaired vision, diplopia, disturbance of vibratory or position sense, parethesias, numbness, and blunting of sensation.

Urinary elimination, altered may be related to sensory-motor impairment, possibly evidenced by frequency, nocturia, and incontinence.

Thought processes, altered may be related to physiologic changes, involvement of pathways of emotional control, possibly evidenced by impaired judgment, emotional lability, and altered attention span.

Powerlessness/Hopelessness may be related to illness-related regimen and lifestyle of helplessness, possibly evidenced by verbal expressions of having no control or influence over the situation, depression over physical deterioration that occurs despite patient compliance with regimen, nonparticipation in care or decision making when opportunities are provided, passivity, decreased verbalization/affect, and lack of involvement in care/passively allowing care.

Home maintenance management, impaired may be related to effects of debilitating disease, impaired cognitive and/or emotional functioning, and inadequate support systems, possibly evidenced by reported difficulty, observed disorderly surroundings, and poor hygienic conditions.

2522

Family coping, compromised/disabling may be related to temporary family disorganization and role changes, situational crisis, patient providing little support in turn for significant other(s), prolonged disease/disability progression that exhausts that supportive capacity of significant other(s), feelings of guilt, anxiety, hostility, despair, and highly ambivalent family relationships, possibly evidenced by patient expressing/confirming concern or complaint about significant other(s) response to patient's illness, significant other(s) preoccupied with own personal reactions, intolerance, abandonment, neglectful care of the patient, and distortion of reality regarding patient's illness.

mumps

Pain may be related to presence of inflammation, circulating toxins, and enlargement of salivary glands, possibly evidenced by complaints (specify), guarding/distraction behaviors, self-focusing, and autonomic responses (changes in vital signs).

Hyperthermia may be related to inflammatory process, increased metabolic rate, and dehydration, possibly evidenced by increased body temperature, warm/flushed skin, and tachycardia.

Fluid volume deficit, high risk for which may be related to hypermetabolic state and painful swallowing with decreased intake.

myasthenia gravis

Breathing pattern/Airway clearance, ineffective may be related to neuromuscular weakness and decreased energy/fatigue, possibly evidenced by dyspnea, changes in rate/depth of respiration, ineffective cough, and adventitious breath sounds.

Communication, impaired verbal may be related to neuromuscular weakness, fatigue, and physical barrier (intubation), possibly evidenced by facial weakness, impaired articulation, hoarseness, and inability to speak.

Swallowing, impaired may be related to neuromuscular impairment of laryngeal/pharyngeal muscles and muscular fatigue, possibly evidenced by reported/observed difficulty swallowing, coughing/choking, and evidence of aspiration.

Anxiety (specify level)/Fear may be related to situational crisis, threat to self-concept, change in health/socioeconomic status, role function, separation from support systems, lack of knowledge, and inability to communicate, possibly evidenced by expressed concerns, increased tension, restlessness, apprehension, sympathetic stimulation, crying, focus on self, uncooperative behavior, withdrawal, anger, and noncommunication.

Sensory-perceptual alterations, visual may be related to neuromuscular impairment, possibly evidenced by visual distortions (diplopia) and motor incoordination.

Knowledge deficit [learning need] may be related to inadequate information regarding drug therapy, potential for crisis (myasthenic or cholinegic) and self-care management, possibly evidenced by statements of concern, questions, and misconceptions.

Physical mobility, impaired may be related to neuromuscular impairment, possibly evidenced by reports of progressive fatigability with repetitive/prolonged muscle use, impaired coordination, and decreased muscle strength/control.

myocardial infarction (also refer to myocarditis)

Pain may be related to ischemia of myocardial tissue, possibly evidenced by complaints (specify), guarding/distraction behaviors, facial mask of pain, self-focusing, and autonomic responses (diaphoresis, changes in vital signs).

Anxiety (specify level)/Fear may be related to threat of death, threat of change of health status, and role functioning and lifestyle, possibly evidenced by increased tension, apprehension, expressed concerns, restlessness, and sympathetic stimulation.

Cardiac output, decreased may be related to changes in preload, systemic vascular resistance, electrical conduction, and muscle contractility/depressant effects of some drugs, possibly evidenced by variations in hemodynamic readings, presence of ECG changes/dysrhythmias, cool/moist skin, and decreased peripheral pulses.

Activity intolerance may be related to imbalance between oxygen supply and demand and cardiac depressant effects of some drugs, possibly evidenced by generalized weakness, exertional angina, abnormal heart rate/blood pressure responses, and development of dysrhythmias.

myocarditis

Activity intolerance may be related to imbalance with oxygen supply and demand and enforced bedrest, possibly evidenced by reports of fatigue, exertional dyspnea, tachycardia/palpitations in response to activity, and ECG changes/dysrhythmias.

Knowledge deficit [learning need] may be related to lack of information regarding pathophysiology of condition and outcomes, medical therapy, and self-care needs/lifestyle changes, possibly evidenced by statements of concern, misconceptions, inaccurate follow-through of instructions, and development of preventable complications.

myringotomy
Refer to mastoidectomy

myxedema (also refer to hypothyroidism)
Body image disturbance may be related to change in structure/function (loss of hair/thickening of skin, mask-like facial expression, enlarged tongue, menstrual and reproductive disturbances), possibly evidenced by negative feelings about body, feelings of helplessness, and change in social involvement.
Nutrition, altered: more than body requirements may be related to decreased metabolic rate and activity level, possibly evidenced by weight gain greater than ideal for height and frame.
Cardiac output, decreased, high risk for which may be related to altered electrical conduction and myocardial contractility.

neonatal, normal newborn
Gas exchange, impaired, high risk for which may be related to prenatal or intrapartal stressors, excess production of mucus, or cold stress.
Body temperature, altered, high risk for which may be related to large body surface in relation to mass, limited amounts of insulating subcutaneous fat, nonrenewable sources of brown fat and few white fat stores, thin epidermis with close proximity of blood vessels to the skin, inability to shiver, and movement from a warm uterine environment to a much cooler environment.
Family processes, altered [bonding] may be related to developmental transition (gain of a family member), possibly evidenced by anxiety and excitement, expression of confusion/uncertainty, and difficulty accepting or receiving help appropriately.
Nutrition, altered: less than body requirements, high risk for which may be related to rapid metabolic rate, high caloric requirement, increased insensible water losses through pulmonary and cutaneous routes, and a potential for inadequate or depleted glucose stores.
Infection, high risk for which may be related to inadequate secondary defenses (deficiency of neutrophils and specific immunoglobulins), and inadequate primary defenses (traumatized tissues, decreased ciliary action).

neonatal, premature newborn
Gas exchange, impaired may be related to alveolar-capillary membrane changes (inadequate surfactant levels), altered blood flow (immaturity of pulmonary arteriole musculature), altered oxygen supply (immaturity of central nervous system and neuromuscular system, tracheobronchial obstruction), altered oxygen-carrying capacity of blood (anemia), and cold stress, possibly evidenced by respiratory difficulties, inadequate oxygenation of tissues, and acidemia.
Breathing pattern, ineffective may be related to decreased lung expansion/neuromuscular impairment (immaturity of the respiratory center, poor positioning, drug-related depression and metabolic imbalances), decreased energy/fatigue, inflammation process, and tracheobronchial obstruction, possibly evidenced by dyspnea, apneic spells, cyanosis, nasal flaring/use of accessory muscles, and abnormal ABGs.
Thermoregulation, ineffective, high risk for which may related to decreased ratio of body mass to surface area, decreased subcutaneous fat, inability to shiver or sweat, poor metabolic reserves, muted response to hypothermia, and frequent medical/nursing manipulations and interventions.
Fluid volume deficit, high risk for which may be related to increased susceptibility to fluid losses (urine, feces, and insensible losses through lungs and skin), thin skin and decreased insulating amounts of fat, immature kidney functioning, failure to conserve fluids during periods of dehydration, hypotension, and fluid shifts.

nephrectomy
Pain may be related to surgical tissue trauma with mechanical closure (suture), possibly evidenced by complaints (specify), guarding/distraction behaviors, self-focusing, and autonomic responses (changes in vital signs).
Fluid volume deficit, high risk for which may be related to excessive vascular losses and restricted intake.
Breathing pattern, ineffective may be related to incisional pain with decreased lung expansion, possibly evidenced by tachypnea, fremitus, changes in respiratory depth/chest expansion, and changes in ABGs.

2524

Constipation may be related to reduced dietary intake, decreased mobility, gastrointestinal obstructions (paralytic ileus), and incisional pain with defecation, possibly evidenced by decreased bowel sounds, reduced frequency/amount of stool, and hard/formed stool.

nephrotic syndrome

Fluid volume excess may be related to compromised regulatory mechanism with changes in hydrostatic/oncotic vascular pressure and increased activation of the renin-angiotensin-aldosterone system, possibly evidenced by edema/anasarca, effusions/ascites, weight gain, intake greater than output, and blood pressure changes.

Nutrition, altered: less than body requirements may be related to excessive protein losses and inability to ingest adequate nutrients (anorexia), possibly evidenced by weight loss/muscle wasting (may be difficult to assess due to edema), lack of interest in food, and observed inadequate intake.

Infection, high risk for which may be related to chronic disease and steroidal suppression of inflammatory responses.

Skin integrity, impaired, high risk for which may be related to presence of edema and activity restrictions.

neuralgia, trigeminal

Pain may be related to neuromuscular impairment with sudden violent muscle spasm, possibly evidenced by complaints (specify), guarding/distraction behaviors, self-focusing, and autonomic responses (changes in vital signs).

Knowledge deficit [learning need] may be related to lack of information regarding control of recurrent episodes, medical therapies, and self-care needs, possibly evidenced by statements of concern, questions, and exacerbation of condition.

neuritis

Pain may be related to nerve damage usually associated with a degenerative process, possibly evidenced by complaints (specify), guarding/distraction behaviors, self-focusing, and autonomic responses (changes in vital signs).

Knowledge deficit [learning need] may be related to lack of information regarding underlying causative factors, treatment, and prevention, possibly evidenced by statements of concern, questions, and misconceptions.

obesity

Nutrition, altered: more than body requirements may be related to excessive intake in relation to metabolic needs, possibly evidenced by weight 20 percent greater than ideal for height and frame, sedentary activity level, reported/observed dysfunctional eating patterns, and triceps skinfold greater than ideal for gender.

Body image disturbance may be related to mismatch between mental image and physical reality, possibly evidenced by negative feelings about body, feelings of helplessness, and change in social involvement.

Activity intolerance may be related to imbalance between oxygen supply and demand, and sedentary lifestyle, possibly evidenced by fatigue or weakness, exertional discomfort, and abnormal heart rate in response to activity.

Coping, ineffective individual may be related to personal vulnerability, unmet expectations, and inadequate coping methods, possibly evidenced by verbalization of difficulty dealing with anxiety and tension, overeating, and eating in response to stress.

osteoarthritis (degenerative joint disease)

Refer to arthritis, rheumatoid

(Although this is a degenerative process versus the inflammatory process of rheumatoid arthritis, nursing concerns are the same.)

osteomyelitis

Pain may be related to inflammation and tissue necrosis, possibly evidenced by complaints (specify), guarding/distraction behaviors, self-focus, and autonomic responses (changes in vital signs).

Hyperthermia may be related to increased metabolic rate and infectious process, possibly evidenced by increased body temperature and warm/flushed skin.

Tissue perfusion, altered (bone) may be related to inflammatory reaction with thrombosis of vessels, destruction of tissue, edema, and abscess formation, possibly evidenced by bone necrosis and continuation of infectious process and delayed healing.

Knowledge deficit [learning need] may be related to lack of information regarding pathophysiology of condition, long-term medical therapy, activity restriction, and prevention of complications, possibly evidenced by statements of concern, questions and misconceptions, and inaccurate follow-through of instructions.

osteoporosis
Pain may be related to movement of fractures and vertebral compression on spinal nerve/muscles/ligaments, possibly evidenced by complaints (specify), guarding/distraction behaviors, self-focus.
Trauma, high risk for which may be related to loss of bone integrity increasing risk of fracture with minimal or no stress.
Physical mobility, impaired may be related to pain and musculoskeletal impairment, possibly evidenced by limited range of motion, reluctance to attempt movement, and imposed restrictions/limitations.

palsy, cerebral (spastic hemiplegia)
Physical mobility, impaired may be related to muscular weakness/hypertonicity, increased deep tendon reflexes, tendency to contractures, and underdevelopment of affected limbs, possibly evidenced by decreased muscle strength/control/mass, limited range of motion, and impaired coordination.
Family coping, compromised may be related to permanent nature of condition, situational crisis, emotional conflicts/temporary family disorganization, and incomplete information/understanding of patient's needs, possibly evidenced by verbalized anxiety/guilt regarding patient's disability, inadequate understanding and knowledge base, and displaying protective behaviors disproportionate (too little/too much) to patient's abilities/need for autonomy.
Growth and development, altered may be related to effects of physical disability, possibly evidenced by altered physical growth, delay, or difficulty in performing skills (motor, social, expressive), and altered ability to perform self-care/self-control activities appropriate to age.

pancreatitis
Pain may be related to inflammation and edema of the pancreas with peritoneal irritation, possibly evidenced by complaints (specify), guarding/distraction behaviors, self-focus, autonomic responses (changes in vital signs), and alteration in muscle tone.
Fluid volume deficit, high risk for which may be related to excessive gastric losses (vomiting, nasogastric tube), hypermetabolic state, and hemorrhagic losses.
Breathing pattern, ineffective, high risk for which may be related to inflammatory process/pain with decreased lung expansion.
Nutrition, altered: less than body requirements may be related to medical restriction of intake as well as altered ability to digest nutrients, possibly evidenced by weight loss and reduced muscle mass.
Infection, high risk for which may be related to inadequate primary defenses: stasis of body fluids, altered peristalsis, change in pH secretions, immunosuppression, nutritional deficiencies, tissue destruction, and chronic disease.

paranoid disorders
Violence, high risk for, directed at self/others which may be related to perceived threats of danger and increased feelings of anxiety.
Anxiety, severe may be related to inability to trust (has not mastered tasks of trust versus mistrust), possibly evidenced by rigid delusional system (serves to provide relief from stress that justifies the delusion); frightened of other people and own hostility.
Powerlessness may be related to feelings of inadequacy, interpersonal interaction, sense of severely impaired self-esteem, and belief that individual has no control over situation(s), possibly evidenced by use of paranoid delusions, use of aggressive behavior to compensate, and expressions of recognition of damage paranoia has caused self and others.
Thought processes, altered may be related to psychologic conflicts, increasing anxiety, and fear, possibly evidenced by difficulties in the process and character of thought, interference with the ability to think clearly and logically, fragmentation and autistic thinking, and delusions.
Family coping, compromised may be related to temporary family disorganization/role changes, prolonged progression of condition that exhausts the supportive capacity of significant other(s), possibly evidenced by family system not meeting physical/emotional/spiritual needs of its members, inability to express or to accept wide range of feelings or feelings of members, and inappropriate boundary maintenance; significant other(s) describes preoccupation with personal reactions.

paraplegia (also refer to quadriplegia)
Physical mobility, impaired may be related to neuromuscular impairment (flaccid/spastic paralysis), possibly evidenced by loss of muscle control and coordination and inability to move purposefully.

Sensory-perceptual alterations, kinesthetic and tactile may be related to neurologic deficit with loss of sensory reception and transmission, possibly evidenced by reported/measured change in sensory acuity and loss of usual response to stimuli.

Incontinence, reflex may be related to loss of nerve conduction above the level of the reflex arc, possibly evidenced by lack of awareness of bladder filling/fullness, absence of urge to void, and uninhibited bladder contraction.

Body image disturbance/Role performance, altered may be related to loss of body functions, change in physical ability to resume role, perceived loss of self/identity, possibly evidenced by negative feelings about body/self, feelings of helplessness/powerlessness, delay in taking responsibility for self-care/participation in therapy, and change in social involvement.

Sexual dysfunction may be related to loss of sensation, altered function, possibly evidenced by seeking of confirmation of desirability, verbalization of concern, and alteration in relationship with significant other.

parathyroidectomy

Pain may be related to presence of surgical incision and effects of calcium imbalance (bone pain, tetany), possibly evidenced by complaints (specify), guarding/distraction behaviors, self-focus, and autonomic responses (changes in vital signs).

Fluid volume excess, high risk for which may be related to preoperative renal involvement, stress-induced release of ADH, and changing calcium/electrolyte levels.

Airway clearance, ineffective, high risk for which may be related to edema formation and laryngeal nerve damage.

Knowledge deficit [learning need] may be related to lack of information regarding postoperative care/complications and long-term needs, possibly evidenced by statements of concern, questions, and misconceptions.

Parkinson's disease

Physical mobility, impaired may be related to neuromuscular impairment (muscle weakness, tremors, bradykinesis) and musculoskeletal impairment (joint rigidity), possibly evidenced by decreased muscle strength/control, impaired coordination, and limited range of motion.

Swallowing impaired may be related to neuromuscular impairment/muscle weakness, possibly evidenced by reported/observed difficulty in swallowing, evidence of aspiration (choking, coughing, drooling).

Communication, impaired verbal may be related to muscle weakness and incoordination, possibly evidenced by impaired articulation, difficulty with phonation, and changes in rhythm and intonation.

pelvic inflammatory disease

Infection, high risk for spread which may be related to presence of infectious process in pelvic structures.

Pain may be related to inflammation, edema, and congestion of reproductive/pelvic tissues, possibly evidenced by complaints (specify), guarding/distraction behaviors, self-focus, and autonomic responses (changes in vital signs).

Hyperthermia may be related to inflammatory process/hypermetabolic state, possibly evidenced by increased body temperature, warm/flushed skin, and tachycardia.

Knowledge deficit [learning need] may be related to lack of information regarding cause/complications of condition, therapy needs, and transmission of disease to others, possibly evidenced by statements of concern, questions, and misconceptions.

periarteritis nodosa

Refer to polyarteritis (nodosa)

pericarditis

Pain may be related to inflammation and presence of effusion, possibly evidenced by complaints (specify), guarding/distraction behaviors, self-focus, and autonomic responses (changes in vital signs).

Activity intolerance may be related to imbalance between oxygen supply and demand, possibly evidenced by complaints of weakness/fatigue, exertional dyspnea, abnormal heart rate or blood pressure response, and signs of congestive heart failure.

Cardiac output, decreased, high risk for which may be related to accumulation of fluid (effusion) restricting cardiac filling/contractility.

Anxiety (specify level) may be related to change in health status and perceived threat of death, possibly evidenced by increased tension, apprehension, restlessness, and expressed concerns.

2527

peripheral vascular disease (atherosclerosis)

Tissue perfusion, altered, peripheral may be related to reductions or interruptions of arterial/venous blood flow, possibly evidenced by changes in skin temperature/color, lack of hair growth, blood pressure/pulse changes in extremity, presence of bruits, and complaints of claudication.

Activity intolerance may be related to imbalance between oxygen supply and demand, possibly evidenced by reports of muscle fatigue/weakness and exertional discomfort (claudication).

Tissue integrity, impaired, high risk for which may be related to altered circulation with decreased sensation and impaired healing.

peritonitis

Infection, high risk for spread/septicemia which may be related to inadequate primary defenses (broken skin, traumatized tissue, altered peristalsis), inadequate secondary defenses (immunosuppression), and invasive procedures.

Fluid volume deficit [active loss] may be related to excessive gastric losses (vomiting, diarrhea, nasogastric tube), hypermetabolic state, and restricted intake, possibly evidenced by dry mucous membranes, poor skin turgor, delayed capillary refill, weak peripheral pulses, diminished urinary output, dark/concentrated urine, hypotension, and tachycardia.

Pain may be related to inflammatory process and associated edema/distension of peritoneal tissues, possibly evidenced by complaints (specify), guarding/distraction behaviors, self-focus, autonomic responses (changes in vital signs), and alterations in muscle tone.

Hyperthermia may be related to inflammatory process/hypermetabolic state and dehydration, possibly evidenced by increased body temperature, warm/flushed skin, and tachycardia.

pheochromocytoma

Anxiety (specify level) may be related to excessive physiologic (hormonal) stimulation of the sympathetic nervous system, possibly evidenced by apprehension, shakiness, restlessness, focus on self, fearfulness, diaphoresis, and sense of impending doom.

Fluid volume deficit [active loss/regulatory failure] may be related to excessive gastric losses (vomiting/diarrhea), hypermetabolic state, diaphoresis, and hyperosmolar diuresis, possibly evidenced by hemoconcentration, dry mucous membranes, poor skin turgor, thirst, and weight loss.

Cardiac output, decreased/tissue perfusion, altered (specify) may be related to altered preload/decreased blood volume, altered systemic vascular resistance, and increased sympathetic activity from excessive secretion of catecholamines, possibly evidenced by cool/clammy skin, changes in blood pressure (hypertension/postural hypotension), visual disturbances, severe headache, and angina.

Knowledge deficit [learning need] may be related to lack of information regarding pathophysiology of condition, outcome, preoperative and postoperative care needs, possibly evidenced by statements of concern, questions, and misconceptions.

phlebitis

Refer to thrombophlebitis

phobia (also refer to anxiety disorders)

Fear may be related to learned irrational response to natural or innate origins (phobic stimulus), possibly evidenced by sympathetic stimulation and reactions ranging from apprehension to panic.

Social interaction, impaired may be related to intense fear of encountering feared object/activity or situation and anticipated loss of control, possibly evidenced by reported change of style/pattern of interaction, discomfort in social situations, and avoidance of phobic stimulus.

placenta previa

Fluid volume deficit, high risk for which may be related to excessive vascular losses.

Gas exchange, impaired, fetal may be related to altered blood flow, altered carrying capacity of blood (maternal anemia), and decreased surface area for gas exchange at site of placental attachment, possibly evidenced by changes in fetal heart rate and activity and release of meconium.

Anxiety (specify level) may be related to situational crisis, threat to/change in health status (potential for hemorrhage/fetal death), possibly evidenced by increased tension, apprehension, uncertainty, sympathetic stimulation, restlessness, and narrowed focus.

Diversional activity deficit, high risk for which may be related to imposed activity restrictions/bedrest.

pleurisy

Pain may be related to inflammation/irritation of the parietal pleura, possibly evidenced by complaints (specify), guarding/distraction behaviors, self-focus, and autonomic responses (changes in vital signs).

Breathing pattern, ineffective may be related to pain on inspiration, possibly evidenced by decreased respiratory depth, tachypnea, and dyspnea.

Infection, high risk for pneumonia which may be related to stasis of body fluids (pulmonary secretions), decreased lung expansion, and ineffective cough.

pneumonia
Refer to bronchitis, bronchopneumonia

pneumothorax (also refer to hemothorax)
Breathing pattern, ineffective may be related to decreased lung expansion, possibly evidenced by dyspnea, tachypnea, altered chest excursion, respiratory depth changes, cough, cyanosis, and abnormal ABGs.

Cardiac output, decreased, high risk for which may be related to compression/displacement of cardiac structures.

Pain may be related to irritation of nerve endings within pleural space by foreign object (chest tube), possibly evidenced by complaints (specify), guarding/distraction behaviors, self-focus, and autonomic responses (changes in vital signs).

polyarteritis (nodosa)
Tissue perfusion, altered (specify) may be related to reduction/interruption of blood flow, possibly evidenced by organ tissue infarctions, changes in organ function, and development of organic psychosis.

Hyperthermia may be related to widespread inflammatory process, possibly evidenced by increased body temperature and warm/flushed skin.

Pain may be related to inflammation, tissue ischemia, and necrosis of affected area, possibly evidenced by complaints (specify), guarding/distraction behaviors, self-focus, and autonomic responses (changes in vital signs).

Grieving, anticipatory may be related to perceived loss of self, possibly evidenced by expressions of sorrow and anger, altered sleep and/or eating patterns, changes in activity level, and libido.

polycythemia vera
Activity intolerance may be related to imbalance between oxygen supply and demand, possibly evidenced by reports of fatigue/weakness.

Tissue perfusion, altered (specify) may be related to reduction/interruption of arterial/venous blood flow (insufficiency, thrombosis, or hemorrhage), possibly evidenced by pain in affected area, impaired mental ability, visual disturbances, and color changes of skin/mucous membranes.

polyradiculitis
Refer to Guillain-Barré syndrome

postoperative recovery period
Breathing pattern, ineffective may be related to neuromuscular, perceptual/cognitive impairment, decreased lung expansion/energy, and tracheobrochial obstruction, possibly evidenced by changes in respiratory rate and depth, reduced vital capacity, apnea, cyanosis, and noisy respirations.

Body temperature, altered, high risk for which may be related to exposure to cool environment, effect of medications/anesthetic agents, extremes of age/weight, and dehydration.

Sensory-perceptual alteration (specify)/thought processes, altered may be related to chemical alteration: use of pharmaceutical agents, hypoxia; therapeutically restricted environment; excessive sensory stimuli and physiologic stress, possibly evidenced by changes in usual response to stimuli, motor incoordination, impaired ability to concentrate, reason, and make decisions; and disorientation to person, place, and time.

Pain may be related to disruption of skin, tissue, and muscle integrity, musculoskeletal/bone trauma, and presence of tubes and drains, possibly evidenced by verbal complaints, alteration in muscle tone, facial mask of pain, distraction/guarding behaviors, narrowed focus, and autonomic responses.

Skin/tissue integrity, impaired may be related to mechanical interruption of skin/tissues, altered circulation, effects of medication, accumulation of drainage, and altered metabolic state, possibly evidenced by disruption of skin surface/layers and tissues.

Infection, high risk for which may be related to broken skin, traumatized tissues, stasis of body fluids, presence of pathogens/contaminants, environmental exposure, and invasive procedures.

Fluid volume, deficit, high risk for which may be related to restriction of oral intake, loss of fluid through abnormal routes (indwelling tubes, drains), normal routes (vomiting, loss of vascular integrity, changes in clotting ability), and extremes of age and weight.

2529

postpartal period

Family processes, altered, high risk for which may be related to developmental transition (gain of a family member) and transient period of disequilibrium.

Fluid volume deficit, high risk for which may be related to excessive blood loss during delivery.

Pain may be related to tissue trauma/edema, muscle contractions, bladder fullness, and physical/psychologic exhaustion, possibly evidenced by verbal complaints, self-focusing, alteration in muscle tone, distraction behavior, and autonomic responses (changes in vital signs).

Urinary elimination, altered patterns of may be related to physiologic return to nonpregnant state (decrease in circulating blood volume, continued elevation in renal plasma flow), mechanical trauma/ tissue edema, and effects of medication/anesthesia, possibly evidenced by frequency, dysuria, urgency, incontinence, or retention.

Constipation may be related to decreased muscle tone associated with diastasis recti, prenatal effects of progesterone, dehydration, excess analgesia or anesthesia, pain (hemorrhoids, episiotomy, or perineal tenderness), prelabor diarrhea, and lack of intake, possibly evidenced by frequency less than usual pattern, hard-formed stool, straining at stool, decreased bowel sounds, and abdominal distension.

Sleep pattern disturbance may be related to discomfort, intense exhilaration/excitement, and anxiety, possibly evidenced by verbal complaints of difficulty in falling asleep/not feeling well-rested, interrupted sleep, frequent yawning, and irritability.

post-traumatic stress disorder

Anxiety (severe to panic)/fear may be related to current memory of past traumatic life event, threat to self-concept/death, change in environment, and negative self-talk, possibly evidenced by increased tension/wariness, sense of helplessness, apprehension, fearfulness, uncertainty/confusion, restlessness, somatic complaints, sense of impending doom, and sympathetic stimulation with cardiovascular excitement/palpitations.

Powerlessness may be related to being overwhelmed by symptoms of anxiety and lifestyle of helplessness/poor coping skills, possibly evidenced by verbal expression of lack of control over present situation/future outcome, reluctance to express true feelings, dependence on others, passivity and/or anger, and nonparticipation in care or decision making when opportunities are provided.

Violence, high risk for: directed at self/others which may be related to a startle reaction, an intrusive memory of an event causing a sudden acting-out of a feeling as if the event were occurring, use of alcohol/other drugs to ward off painful effects and produce psychic numbing, breaking through the rage that has been walled off, response to intense anxiety or panic state, and loss of control.

Coping, ineffective individual may be related to personal vulnerability, inadequate support system, unrealistic perceptions, unmet expectations, overwhelming threat to self, and multiple stressors repeated over period of time, possibly evidenced by verbalization of inability to cope or difficulty asking for help, muscular tension/headaches, chronic worry, and emotional tension.

Grieving, dysfunctional may be related to actual/perceived object loss (loss of self as seen before the traumatic incident occurred as well as other losses incurred in/after the incident), loss of physiopsychosocial well-being, thwarted grieving response to a loss, and lack of resolution of previous grieving response, possibly evidenced by verbal expression of distress at loss, anger, sadness, labile affect, alterations in eating habits/sleep and dream patterns/libido, reliving of past experiences, expression of guilt, and alterations in concentration.

Sleep pattern disturbance may be related to psychologic stress (anxiety, depression with recurring disruptive dreams), possibly evidenced by verbal complaints of difficulty in falling asleep/not feeling well-rested, insomnia, and reports of sleep disturbance (nightmares, dreams of personal death, disaster-related dreams, flashbacks, intrusive/trauma images, hypersomnia).

Family processes, altered may be related to situational crisis, possibly evidenced by expressions of confusion about what to do and that they are having difficulty coping, family system not meeting physical/emotional/spiritual needs of its members, not adapting to change or dealing with traumatic experience constructively, and ineffective family decision-making process.

pre-eclampsia

Fluid volume deficit [regulatory failure] may be related to a shift of circulating volume from the vascular bed to interstitial space, possibly evidenced by weight gain, edema formation, vasoconstriction, hemoconcentration, and altered serum sodium. (Note: Although signs of hypovolemia may be absent, the actual circulating volume is less than normal for pregnant state.)

Tissue perfusion, altered renal may be related to decreased blood flow (vasoconstriction) and relative hypovolemia, possibly evidenced by decreased urine output and abnormal laboratory values for renal function studies.

Gas exchange, impaired/nutrition, altered, less than body needs, fetal may be related to vasospasm of spiral arteries and relative hypovolemia, possibly evidenced by changes in fetal heart rate/activity, reduced weight gain, and premature delivery.

Knowledge deficit [learning need] may be related to lack of information regarding pathophysiology of condition, therapy, self-care/nutritional needs, and potential complications, possibly evidenced by statements of concern, questions, and misconceptions.

pregnancy

Nutrition, altered: less than body requirements, high risk for which may be related to insufficient intake to meet increased metabolic demands (nausea/vomiting, inadequate financial/nutritional knowledge, increased thyroid activity associated with the growth of fetal and maternal tissues).

Pain may be related to hormonal influences causing minor discomforts, possibly evidenced by complaints (nausea, breast changes, leg cramps, hemorrhoids, nasal stuffiness), alteration in muscle tone, restlessness, and autonomic responses (changes in vital signs).

Injury, high risk for, fetal which may be related to environmental/hereditary factors and problems of maternal well-being that directly affect the developing fetus.

Cardiac output, decreased, high risk for which may be related to increased fluid volume/cardiac output and hormonal effects of progesterone and relaxin that place the patient at risk for hypertension and/ or circulatory failure.

Family coping, potential for growth may be related to situational/maturational crisis with anticipated changes in family structure/roles, as evidenced by movement toward health promoting and enriching lifestyle, choosing experiences that optimize condition/pregnancy experience.

Constipation, high risk for which may be related to changes in dietary/fluid intake, decreased peristalsis, and effects of medications (iron).

Sleep pattern disturbance may be related to internal factors (discomfort, anxiety, inactivity), external factors (demands of daily life), possibly evidenced by complaints of difficulty falling asleep/not feeling well-rested, interrupted sleep, irritability, lethargy, and frequent yawning.

Role performance, altered, high risk for which may be related to difficulty adjusting to the overwhelming tasks associated with pregnancy/parenting, fear of injury to self/fetus, and weak ego.

Knowledge deficit [learning need] may be related to lack of information/recall of normal physiologic/ psychologic changes, and misinterpretation, possibly evidenced by questions, statement of concern, and inaccurate follow-through of instructions/development of preventable complications.

pregnancy, adolescent (also refer to pregnancy)

Family processes, altered may be related to situational/developmental transition (economic, change in roles/gain of a family member), possibly evidenced by family expressing confusion about what to do, unable to meet physical/emotional/spiritual needs of the members, family inability to adapt to change or to deal with traumatic experience constructively, does not demonstrate respect for individuality and autonomy of its members, ineffective family decision-making process, and inappropriate boundary maintenance.

Parenting, altered, high risk for which may be related to unmet social/emotional/maturational needs of parenting figures, unrealistic expectation of self/infant/partner, ineffective role model/social support, lack of role identity, and presence of stress (e.g., financial).

Social isolation may be related to restricted social sphere, stage of adolescence, and interference with accomplishing developmental tasks, possibly evidenced by expressions of feelings of aloneness/rejection/difference from others, uncommunicative, withdrawn, no eye contact, seeking to be alone, unacceptable behavior, and absence of supportive significant other(s).

Body image/self-esteem disturbance may be related to biophysical changes in body and change in life events, possibly evidenced by fear of rejection/reaction of others, negative feelings about body, difficulty accepting positive reinforcement, and nonparticipation in prenatal care.

Knowledge deficit [learning need] may be related to lack of exposure, information misinterpretation, unfamiliarity with information resources about pregnancy, and sense of vulnerability/denial of reality, possibly evidenced by questions, statement of concern/misconception, inaccurate follow-through of instruction, and development of preventable complications.

premenstrual tension syndrome

Pain may be related to vascular congestion/spasms, possibly evidenced by complaints (specify), distraction behaviors, and self-focusing.

Fluid volume excess may be related to abnormal alterations of hormonal levels, possibly evidenced by edema formation, weight gain, and changes in emotional status/irritability approximately one week before menstrual cycle.

Anxiety (specify level) may be related to cyclic changes in female hormones affecting other systems, possibly evidenced by feelings of inability to cope/loss of control, depersonalization, increased tension, apprehension, jitteriness, somatic complaints, and impaired functioning.

Knowledge deficit [learning need] may be related to lack of information regarding pathophysiology of condition and self-care/treatment needs, possibly evidenced by statements of concern, questions, misconceptions, and continuation of condition.

pressure ulcer or sore (also refer to ulcer, decubitus)

Tissue perfusion, altered, peripheral may be related to reduced/interrupted blood flow, possibly evidenced by presence of inflamed, necrotic lesion.

Knowledge deficit [learning need] may be related to lack of information regarding cause and prevention of condition and potential complications, possibly evidenced by statements of concern, questions, misconceptions, and inaccurate follow-through of instructions.

preterm labor

Activity intolerance may be related to imbalance between tissue oxygen supply/demand, possibly evidenced by increase in uterine irritability and cervical dilatation.

Poisoning, high risk for which may be related to toxic side effects of treatment and medications used to stop labor.

Injury, high risk for fetal which may be related to premature birth.

Anxiety (specify level) may be related to perceived or actual threats to self/fetus and inadequate time to prepare for labor, possibly evidenced by increased tension, restlessness, expressions of concern, and autonomic responses (changes in vital signs).

Knowledge deficit [learning need] may be related to lack of information about preterm labor and misconceptions/misinterpretation, possibly evidenced by questions, statement of concern, inaccurate follow-through of instruction, and development of preventable complications.

prostatectomy

Pain may be related to irritation of bladder mucosa and tissue trauma/edema, possibly evidenced by complaints (specify), distraction behaviors, self-focus, and autonomic responses (changes in vital signs).

Fluid volume deficit, high risk for which may be related to trauma to highly vascular area with excessive vascular losses.

Body image disturbance may be related to perceived threat of altered body/sexual function, possibly evidenced by preoccupation with change/loss, negative feelings about body, and statements of concern regarding functioning.

Urinary elimination, altered patterns of may be related to mechanical trauma, mucosal irritation, and neuromuscular impairment, possibly evidenced by dysuria, frequency, dribbling, and incontinence.

Sexual dysfunction, high risk for which may be related to situational crisis (incontinence, leakage of urine after catheter removal, involvement of genital area) and threat to self-concept/change in health status.

pruritus

Pain may be related to cutaneous hyperesthesia and inflammation, possibly evidenced by complaints (specify), distraction behaviors, and self-focus.

Skin integrity, impaired, high risk for which may be related to mechanical trauma (scratching) and development of vesicles/bullae that may rupture.

psoriasis

Skin integrity, impaired may be related to increased epidermal cell proliferation and absence of normal protective skin layers, possibly evidenced by scaling papules and plaques.

Body image disturbance may be related to cosmetically unsightly skin lesions, possibly evidenced by hiding affected body part, negative feelings about body, feelings of helplessness, and change in social involvement.

pulmonary embolus

Breathing pattern, ineffective may be related to tracheobrochial obstruction by inflammation, copious secretions or active bleeding; decreased lung expansion, possibly evidenced by changes in depth and/or rate of respiration, dyspnea/use of accessory muscles, altered chest excursion, abnormal breath sounds (crackles, wheezes), and cough (with or without sputum production).

Gas exchange, impaired may be related to altered blood flow to alveoli or to major portions of the lung, altered oxygen supply (atelectasis, airway/alveolar collapse), and exchange problems (pulmonary edema/effusion, excessive secretions/active bleeding), possibly evidenced by profound dyspnea, restlessness, apprehension, somnolence, cyanosis, and changes in ABGs (hypoxemia and hypercapnea).

Tissue perfusion, altered, cardiopulmonary may be related to interruption of blood flow (arterial/venous), exchange problems at alveolar level or at tissue level (acidotic shifting of the oxyhemoglobin curve), possibly evidenced by radiology/laboratory evidence of ventilation/perfusion mismatch, dyspnea, and central cyanosis.

Fear/anxiety (specify level) may be related to severe dyspnea/inability to breathe normally, perceived threat of death, threat to/change in health status, physiologic response to hypoxia/acidosis, and concern regarding unknown outcome of situation, possibly evidenced by restlessness, irritability, withdrawal or attack behavior, sympathetic stimulation (cardiovascular excitation, pupil dilation, sweating, vomiting, diarrhea), crying, voice quivering, and impending sense of doom.

purpura, idiopathic thrombocytopenic
Injury, high risk for which may be related to abnormal blood profile/risk of hemorrhage.

Activity intolerance may be related to decreased oxygen-carrying capacity/imbalance between oxygen supply and demand, possibly evidenced by reports of fatigue/weakness.

Knowledge deficit [learning need] may be related to lack of information regarding therapy choices, outcomes, and self-care needs, possibly evidenced by statements of concern, questions, and misconceptions.

pyelonephritis
Pain may be related to acute inflammation of renal tissues, possibly evidenced by complaints (specify), guarding/distraction behaviors, self-focus, and autonomic responses (changes in vital signs).

Hyperthermia may be related to inflammatory process/increased metabolic rate, possibly evidenced by increase in body temperature, warm/flushed skin, tachycardia, and chills.

Urinary elimination, altered patterns of may be related to inflammation/irritation of bladder mucosa, possibly evidenced by dysuria, urgency, and frequency.

Knowledge deficit [learning need] may be related to lack of information regarding therapy needs and prevention, possibly evidenced by statements of concern, questions, and recurrence of condition.

quadriplegia (also refer to paraplegia)
Breathing pattern, ineffective may be related to neuromuscular impairment, possibly evidenced by decreased respiratory depth, dyspnea, cyanosis, and abnormal ABGs.

Grieving, anticipatory may be related to perceived loss of self, anticipated alterations in lifestyle and expectations, and limitation of future options/choices, possibly evidenced by expressions of distress, anger, sorrow; choked feelings; and changes in eating habits, sleep, and communication patterns.

Self-care deficit, all areas related to neuromuscular impairment, evidenced by inability to perform self-care tasks.

Home maintenance management, impaired may be related to permanent effects of injury, inadequate/absent support systems and finances, and lack of familiarity with resources, possibly evidenced by expressions of difficulties, requests for information and assistance, outstanding debts/financial crisis, and lack of necessary aides and equipment.

rabies (exposure to)
Infection, high risk for which may be related to break in skin and exposure to rabies virus.

Knowledge deficit [learning need] may be related to lack of information regarding pathophysiology of infection, prophylaxis, and treatment needs, possibly evidenced by statements of concern, questions, and misconceptions.

Injury, high risk for community health which may be related to presence of transmissible infectious disease (rabies) in wild and/or domesticated animals.

rape
Knowledge deficit [learning need] may be related to lack of information regarding prophylactic treatment for individual concerns (sexually transmitted diseases, pregnancy, required medical/legal procedures, community resources/supports), possibly evidenced by statements of concern, questions, misconceptions, and exacerbation of symptoms.

Rape-trauma response (acute phase) related to actual or attempted sexual attack without consent, possibly evidenced by wide range of emotional reactions, including anxiety, fear, anger, embarrassment, and multisystem physical complaints.

Tissue integrity, impaired, high risk for which may be related to forceful sexual penetration and trauma to fragile tissues.

Raynaud's phenomenon

Pain may be related to vasospasm/altered perfusion of affected tissues and ischemia/destruction of tissues, possibly evidenced by verbal complaints, guarding of affected parts, self-focusing, and restlessness.

Tissue perfusion, altered, peripheral may be related to periodic reduction of arterial blood flow to affected areas, possibly evidenced by pallor, cyanosis, numbness, and paresthesia.

Knowledge deficit [learning need] may be related to lack of information regarding pathophysiology of the condition, potential for complications, therapy/self-care needs, possibly evidenced by statements of concern, questions, and misconceptions.

reflex sympathetic dystrophy (RSD)

Pain, (acute or chronic) may be related to continued nerve stimulation, possibly evidenced by complaints (specify), distraction/guarding behaviors, narrowed focus, changes in sleep patterns, and altered ability to continue previous activities.

Tissue perfusion, altered, peripheral may be related to reduction of arterial blood flow (arteriole vasoconstriction), possibly evidenced by complaints of pain, decreased skin temperature and pallor, diminished arterial pulsations, and swelling.

Sensory-perceptual alteration, tactile may be related to altered sensory reception, possibly evidenced by change in usual response to stimuli/abnormal sensitivity of touch, physiologic anxiety, and irritability.

Role performance, altered, high risk for which may be related to situational crisis and chronic disability.

Family coping, compromised, high risk for which may be related to temporary family disorganization and role changes and prolonged disability that exhausts the supportive capacity of significant other(s).

renal failure, acute

Fluid volume, excess may be related to compromised regulatory mechanisms (decreased kidney function), possibly evidenced by weight gain, edema/anasarca, intake greater than output, venous congestion, and altered electrolyte levels.

Nutrition, altered: less than body requirements may be related to inability to ingest/digest adequate nutrients (anorexia, nausea/vomiting, and ulcerations of oral mucosa) in addition to therapeutic dietary restrictions, possibly evidenced by weight loss/loss of muscle mass, lack of interest in food/aversion to eating, and observed inadequate intake.

Infection, high risk for which may be related to depression of immunologic defenses, invasive procedures, and malnutrition.

Thought processes, altered may be related to accumulation of toxic waste products and altered cerebral perfusion, possibly evidenced by disorientation, changes in recent memory, apathy, and episodic obtundation.

Fatigue may be related to decreased metabolic energy production/dietary restrictions, anemia, increased energy requirements, e.g., fever/inflammation and tissue regeneration, possibly evidenced by overwhelming lack of energy, inability to maintain usual activities, decreased performance, lethargy, and disinterest in surroundings.

Adjustment, impaired may be related to disability requiring change in lifestyle, inadequate support systems, and altered locus of control, possibly evidenced by verbalization of nonacceptance of health status change, lack of movement toward independence, extended period of shock, disbelief, or anger regarding health status change, and lack of future-oriented thinking.

renal transplantation

Fluid volume excess, high risk for which may be related to compromised regulatory mechanism (implantation of new kidney requiring adjustment period for optimal functioning).

Body image disturbance may be related to failure and subsequent replacement of body part and medication-induced changes in appearance, possibly evidenced by preoccupation with loss/change, hiding body part(s), negative feelings, and changes in social involvement.

Fear may be related to potential for transplant rejection/failure and threat of death, possibly evidenced by increased tension, apprehension, concentration on source and verbalizations of concern.

Infection, high risk for which may be related to broken skin/traumatized tissue, stasis of body fluids, immunosuppression, invasive procedures, and chronic disease.

respiratory distress syndrome of the premature infant (also refer to neonatal, premature newborn)

Gas exchange, impaired may be related to alveolar-capillary membrane changes (inadequate surfactant levels), altered oxygen supply (tracheobronchial obstruction, atelectasis), altered blood flow (immaturity of pulmonary arteriole musculature), altered oxygen-carrying capacity of blood (anemia), possibly evidenced by tachypnea, use of accessory muscles, retractions, expiratory grunting, pallor or cyanosis, abnormal ABGs, and tachycardia.

Infection, high risk for which may be related to inadequate primary defenses (decreased ciliary action, stasis of body fluids, traumatized tissues), inadequate secondary defenses (deficiency of neutrophils and specific immunoglobulins), invasive procedures, and malnutrition (absence of nutrient stores, increased metabolic demands).

Tissue perfusion, altered, gastrointestinal, high risk for which may be related to persistent fetal circulation and tissue hypoxia/ischemia.

Parenting, altered, actual or high risk for (bonding) which may be related to interruption/postponement of bonding process and separation from infant, possibly evidenced by lack of parental attachment behaviors.

retina, detachment of

Sensory-perceptual alterations, visual related to decreased sensory reception, possibly evidenced by visual distortions, decreased visual field, and changes in visual acuity.

Knowledge deficit [learning need] may be related to lack of information regarding therapy, prognosis, and self-care needs, possibly evidenced by statements of concern and questions.

Home maintenance management, impaired, high risk for which may be related to postoperative activity restrictions/limitations.

Reye's syndrome

Fluid volume deficit [active loss/regulatory failure] may be related to failure of regulatory mechanism (diabetes insipidus), excessive gastric losses (pernicious vomiting), and altered intake, possibly evidenced by increased/dilute urine output, sudden weight loss, decreased venous filling, dry mucous membranes, decreased skin turgor, hypotension, and tachycardia.

Tissue perfusion, decreased cerebral may be related to diminished arterial/venous blood flow and hypovolemia, possibly evidenced by memory loss, altered consciousness, and restlessness/agitation.

Trauma, high risk for which may be related to generalized weakness, reduced coordination, and cognitive deficits.

Breathing pattern, ineffective may be related to decreased energy and fatigue, cognitive impairment, tracheobronchial obstruction, and inflammatory process (aspiration pneumonia), possibly evidenced by tachypnea, abnormal ABGs, cough, and use of accessory muscles.

rheumatic fever

Pain may be related to migratory inflammation of joints, possibly evidenced by complaints (specify), guarding/distraction behaviors, self-focus, and autonomic responses (changes in vital signs).

Hyperthermia may be related to inflammatory process/hypermetabolic state, possibly evidenced by increased body temperature, warm/flushed skin, and tachycardia.

Activity intolerance may be related to generalized weakness, joint pain, and medical restrictions/bedrest, possibly evidenced by reports of fatigue, exertional discomfort, and abnormal heart rate in response to activity.

Cardiac output, decreased, high risk for which may be related to cardiac inflammation/enlargement and altered contractility.

rickets (osteomalacia)

Growth and development, altered may be related to dietary deficiencies/indiscretions, malabsorption syndrome, and lack of exposure to sunlight, possibly evidenced by altered physical growth and delay or difficulty in performing motor skills typical for age.

Knowledge deficit [learning need] may be related to lack of information regarding cause, pathophysiology, and therapy needs/prevention, possibly evidenced by statements of concern, questions, misconceptions, and inaccurate follow-through of instructions.

ringworm, tinea (also refer to athlete's foot)

Skin integrity, impaired may be related to fungal infection of the dermis, possibly evidenced by disruption of skin surfaces/presence of lesions.

Knowledge deficit [learning need] may be related to lack of information regarding infectious nature, therapy, and self-care needs, possibly evidenced by statements of concern, questions, and recurrence/spread.

rubella

Pain may be related to inflammatory effects of viral infection and presence of desquamating rash, possibly evidenced by complaints (specify), distraction behaviors/restlessness.

Knowledge deficit [learning need] may be related to lack of information regarding contagious nature, possible complications, and self-care needs, possibly evidenced by statements of concern, questions, and inaccurate follow-through of instructions.

scabies

Skin integrity, impaired may be related to presence of invasive parasite and development of pruritus, possibly evidenced by disruption of skin surface and inflammation.

Knowledge deficit [learning need] may be related to lack of information regarding communicable nature, possible complications, therapy, and self-care needs, possibly evidenced by questions and statements of concern about spread to others.

scarlet fever

Hyperthermia may be related to effects of circulating toxins, possibly evidenced by increased body temperature, warm/flushed skin, and tachycardia.

Pain (discomfort) may be related to inflammation of mucous membranes and effects of circulating toxins (malaise, fever), possibly evidenced by complaints (specify), distraction behaviors, guarding (decreased swallowing), and self-focus.

Fluid volume deficit, high risk for which may be related to hypermetabolic state (hyperthermia) and reduced intake.

schizophrenia (schizophrenic disorders)

Thought process, altered may be related to presence of psychologic conflicts, possibly evidenced by impaired ability to reason/problem solve, inappropriate affect, delusions, and auditory hallucinations.

Social isolation may be related to alterations in mental status, unacceptable social behaviors, inadequate personal resources, and inability to engage in satisfying personal relationships, possibly evidenced by dull affect, uncommunicative/withdrawn behavior, seeking to be alone, and inadequate/absent significant purpose in life.

Health maintenance management, altered may be related to altered ability to make deliberate and thoughtful judgments, altered communications, and possible lack of material resources, possibly evidenced by inability to take responsibility for meeting basic health practices in any or all functional areas and demonstrated lack of adaptive behaviors to internal or external environmental changes.

Violence, high risk for: directed at self/others which may be related to disturbances of thinking/feeling (depression, paranoia, suicidal ideation).

Coping, ineffective individual may be related to personal vulnerability, inadequate support system(s), unrealistic perceptions, inadequate coping methods, and disintegration of thought processes, possibly evidenced by impaired judgment/cognition and perception, diminished problem-solving/decision-making capacities, poor self-esteem, chronic anxiety, depression, inability to perform role expectations, and alteration in social participation.

Family coping, disabling may be related to ambivalent family system/relationships and difficulty of family members in coping effectively with patient's maladaptive behaviors, possibly evidenced by patient's expressions of despair at family's lack of reaction/involvement, neglectful relationships with patient, extreme distortion regarding patient's health problem including extreme denial about its existence/severity or prolonged overconcern, impaired restructuring of a meaningful life for individual family members, and impaired individuation.

Self-care deficit (specify) may be related to perceptual and cognitive impairment, immobility (withdrawal/isolation and decreased psychomotor activity), and side effects of psychotropic medications, possibly evidenced by inability or difficulty in areas of feeding self, keeping body clean, dressing appropriately and/or toileting self, and changes in bowel/bladder elimination.

sciatica

Pain may be related to peripheral nerve root compression, possibly evidenced by complaints (specify), guarding/distraction behaviors, and self-focus.

Physical mobility, impaired may be related to neurologic pain and muscular involvement, possibly evidenced by reluctance to attempt movement and decreased muscle strength/mass.

scleroderma (also refer to lupus erythematosus, systemic)

Physical mobility, impaired may be related to musculoskeletal impairment and associated pain, possibly evidenced by decreased strength, decreased range of motion, and reluctance to attempt movement.

Tissue perfusion, altered (specify) may be related to reduced arterial blood flow (arteriolar vasoconstriction), possibly evidenced by changes in skin temperature/color, ulcer formation, and changes in organ function (cardiopulmonary, gastrointestinal, renal).

Nutrition, altered: less than body requirements may be related to inability to ingest/digest/absorb adequate nutrients (sclerosis of the tissues rendering mouth immobile, decreased peristalsis of esophagus and small intestines, atrophy of smooth muscle of colon), possibly evidenced by weight loss, decreased intake, inability to ingest food, and reported/observed difficulty swallowing.

Adjustment, impaired may be related to disability requiring change in lifestyle, inadequate support systems, assault to self-esteem, and altered locus of control, possibly evidenced by verbalization of non-acceptance of health status change and lack of movement toward independence/future-oriented thinking.

Body image disturbance may be related to skin changes with induration, atrophy, and fibrosis, loss of hair, and skin and muscle contractures, possibly evidenced by verbalization of negative feelings about body, focus on past strength/function or appearance, fear of rejection or of reaction by others, hiding body part, and change in social involvement.

scoliosis

Body image disturbance may be related to altered body structure, use of therapeutic device(s), and activity restrictions, possibly evidenced by negative feelings about body, change in social involvement, and preoccupation with situation or refusal to acknowledge problem.

Knowledge deficit [learning need] may be related to lack of information regarding pathophysiology of condition and therapy needs and outcomes, possibly evidenced by statements of concern, questions, misconceptions, and inaccurate follow-through of instructions.

Adjustment, impaired may be related to lack of comprehension of long-term consequences of behavior, possibly evidenced by failure to adhere to treatment regimen/keep appointments and evidence of failure to improve.

sepsis, puerperal

Infection, high risk for spread/septic shock which may be related to broken skin, traumatized tissues, stasis of body fluids, invasive procedures, and altered immune response.

Hyperthermia may be related to inflammatory process/hypermetabolic state, possibly evidenced by increase in body temperature, warm/flushed skin, and tachycardia.

Parenting, altered, actual/high risk for may be related to presence of physical illness, medical/therapeutic interruption in bonding process, and threat to own survival, possibly evidenced by incomplete parental attachment behaviors and verbalized concern regarding role inadequacy.

Tissue perfusion, altered, peripheral, high risk for which may be related to interruption/reduction of blood flow (presence of infectious thrombi).

septicemia (also refer to sepsis, puerperal)

Tissue perfusion, altered (specify) may be related to changes in arterial/venous blood flow (selective vasoconstriction, presence of microemboli) and hypovolemia, possibly evidenced by changes in skin temperature/color, changes in blood pressure and pulse pressure, changes in sensorium, and decreased urinary output.

Fluid volume deficit, high risk for which may be related to presence of hypermetabolic state, vascular shifts to interstitial space, and reduced intake.

Cardiac output, decreased, high risk for which may be related to decreased preload (venous return and circulating volume), altered afterload (increased systemic vascular resistance), negative inotropic effects of hypoxia, complement activation, and lysosomal hydrolase.

serum sickness

Pain may be related to inflammation of the joints and skin eruptions, possibly evidenced by complaints (specify), guarding/distraction behaviors, and self-focus.

Knowledge deficit [learning need] may be related to lack of information regarding nature of condition, treatment needs, potential complications, and need to avoid causative agent, possibly evidenced by statements of concern, questions, and inaccurate follow-through of instructions.

sexually transmitted disease

Infection, high risk for transmission which may be related to contagious nature of infecting agent and insufficient knowledge to avoid exposure to/transmission of pathogens.

Skin/tissue integrity, impaired may be related to invasion of/irritation by pathogenic organism(s), possibly evidenced by disruptions of skin and inflammation of mucous membranes.

Knowledge deficit [learning need] may be related to lack of information regarding pathophysiology of condition, outcomes/complications, therapy needs, and transmission, possibly evidenced by statements of concern, questions, misconceptions, and inaccurate follow-through of instructions.

shock (also refer to shock, cardiogenic and shock, hemorrhagic)

Tissue perfusion, altered (specify) may be related to changes in circulating volume and/or vascular tone, possibly evidenced by changes in skin color/temperature and pulse pressure, reduced blood pressure, changes in mentation, and decreased urinary output.

Anxiety (specify level) may be related to change in health status and threat of death, possibly evidenced by increased tension, apprehension, sympathetic stimulation, restlessness, and expressions of concern.

shock, cardiogenic

Cardiac output, decreased may be related to structural damage, decreased myocardial contractility, and presence of dysrhythmias, possibly evidenced by ECG changes, variations in hemodynamic readings, jugular vein distention, cold/clammy skin, diminished peripheral pulses, and decreased urinary output.

shock, hemorrhagic

Fluid volume deficit [active loss] may be related to excessive vascular loss, possibly evidenced by hypotension, tachycardia, decreased pulse volume and pressure, change in mentation, and decreased/concentrated urine.

sick sinus syndrome

Cardiac output, decreased may be related to alterations in rate, rhythm, and electrical conduction, possibly evidenced by ECG evidence of dysrhythmias, complaints of palpitations/weakness, changes in mentation/consciousness, and syncope.

Trauma, high risk for which may be related to changes in cerebral perfusion with altered consciousness/loss of balance.

snow blindness

Sensory-perceptual alterations, visual may be related to altered status of sense organ (irritation of the conjunctiva, hyperemia), possibly evidenced by intolerance to light (photophobia) and decreased/loss of visual acuity.

Pain may be related to irritation/vascular congestion of the conjunctiva, possibly evidenced by complaints (specify), guarding/distraction behaviors, and self-focus.

Anxiety (specify level) may be related to situational crisis and threat to/change in health status, possibly evidenced by increased tension, apprehension, uncertainty, worry, restlessness, and focus on self.

somatoform disorders

Violence, high risk for: self-directed which may be related to depressed mood, feelings of powerlessness over physical condition, belief that s/he has serious illness, and hysterical response to chronic pain.

Pain, chronic may be related to severe level of anxiety, repressed/low self-esteem, unmet dependency needs, history of self or loved one having experienced a serious illness, fixation in earlier level of development, retarded ego development, and inadequate coping skills, possibly evidenced by multiple somatic complaints of several years' duration, absence of physiologic evidence for physical symptoms, narcissistic tendencies with total focus on self and physical symptoms, demanding behaviors, and denial of correlation between physical symptoms and psychologic problems.

Coping, ineffective individual may be related to severe level of anxiety that is repressed/low self-esteem, unmet dependency needs, fixation in earlier level of development, retarded ego development, and inadequate coping skills, possibly evidenced by multiple somatic complaints of several years' duration, demanding behaviors, and refusal to attend therapeutic activities.

Social isolation may be related to severe level of anxiety, low self-esteem, preoccupation with self and physical symptoms, chronic pain, and rejection by others due to focus on self/physical symptoms, possibly evidenced by sad/dull affect, absence of supportive significant other(s), uncommunicative/withdrawn behavior, lack of eye contact, and seeking to be alone.

sprain of ankle or foot

Pain may be related to trauma to/swelling in joint, possibly evidenced by complaints (specify), guarding/distraction behaviors, self-focusing, and autonomic responses (changes in vital signs).

Physical mobility, impaired may be related to musculoskeletal injury, pain, and therapeutic restrictions, possibly evidenced by reluctance to attempt movement and limited range of motion.

stapedectomy

Trauma, high risk for which may be related to increased middle-ear pressure with displacement of prosthesis and balancing difficulties/dizziness.

Infection, high risk for which may be related to surgically traumatized tissue, invasive procedures, and environmental exposure to upper respiratory infections.

Pain may be related to surgical trauma, edema formation, and presence of packing, possibly evidenced by complaints (specify), guarding/distraction behaviors, and self-focus.

substance dependency/abuse (also refer to drug overdose)

Coping, ineffective individual may be related to personal vulnerability, difficulty handling new situations, previous ineffective/inadequate coping skills with substitution of drug(s), and anxiety/fear, possibly evidenced by denial, lack of acceptance that drug use is causing the present situation, altered social patterns/participation, impaired adaptive behavior and problem-solving skills, and decreased ability to handle stress of illness/hospitalization.

Powerlessness may be related to substance addiction with/without periods of abstinence, episodic compulsive indulgence, attempts at recovery, and lifestyle of helplessness, possibly evidenced by ineffective recovery attempts, continuous/constant thinking about drug and/or obtaining drug, alteration in personal/occupational and social life.

Family coping, compromised/dysfunctional may be related to personal vulnerability of individual family members, codependency issues, situational crises, compromised social systems, family disorganization/role changes, and prolonged disease progression that exhausts supportive capability of family members, possibly evidenced by denial, lack of acceptance that drinking/drug use is causing the present situation, or belief that all problems are due to substance use, severely dysfunctional family (e.g., family violence, spouse/child abuse, separation/divorce), financial affairs in disarray, and employment difficulties.

Sexual dysfunction may be related to altered body function (neurologic damage and debilitating effects of drug use), possibly evidenced by progressive interference with sexual functioning; a significant degree of testicular atrophy, gynecomastia, impotence/decreased sperm counts in men; and loss of body hair, thin/soft skin, spider angiomas, and amenorrhea/increase in miscarriages in women.

surgery, general

Anxiety (specify level)/fear may be related to change in health status and threat of death and to self-concept, possibly evidenced by increased tension, apprehension, fear of unspecific consequences, sympathetic stimulation, and restlessness.

Knowledge deficit [learning need] may be related to lack of information regarding surgical procedure/expectation, postoperative routines/therapy, and self-care needs, possibly evidenced by statements of concern, questions, and misconceptions.

Breathing pattern, ineffective, high risk for which may be related to chemically induced muscular relaxation, perception/cognitive impairment, decreased energy, and incisional pain.

Fluid volume deficit, high risk for which may be related to preoperative/postoperative fluid deprivation, blood loss, and excessive GI losses (vomiting).

Pain may be related to intraoperative positioning, muscle retractions, and tissue trauma/presence of incision, possibly evidenced by complaints (specify), guarding/distraction behaviors, self-focus, and autonomic responses (changes in vital signs).

synovitis (knee)

Pain may be related to inflammation of synovial membrane of the joint with effusion, possibly evidenced by complaints (specify), guarding/distraction behaviors, self-focus, and autonomic responses (changes in vital signs).

Physical mobility, impaired may be related to pain and decreased strength of joint, possibly evidenced by limited range of motion and reluctance to attempt movement.

syphilis, congenital (also refer to sexually transmitted disease)

Pain may be related to inflammatory process, edema formation, and development of skin lesions, possibly evidenced by irritability/crying that may be increased with movement of extremities and autonomic responses (changes in vital signs).

Skin/Tissue integrity, impaired may be related to development of lesions/rash and irritation of mucous membranes, possibly evidenced by disruption of skin surfaces and rhinitis.

Growth and development, altered may be related to effects of infectious process, possibly evidenced by altered physical growth and delay or difficulty performing skills typical of age group.

Knowledge deficit [learning need] may be related to caretaker/parental lack of information regarding pathophysiology of condition, transmissibility, therapy needs, expected outcomes, and potential complications, possibly evidenced by statements of concern, questions, and misconceptions.

syringomyelia

Sensory-perceptual alterations (specify) may be related to neurologic lesion altering sensory reception, possibly evidenced by change in usual response to stimuli and motor incoordination.

Anxiety (specify level)/Fear may be related to change in health status, threat of change in role functioning and socioeconomic status, and threat to self-concept, possibly evidenced by increased tension, apprehension, uncertainty, focus on self, and expressed concerns.

Physical mobility, impaired may be related to neuromuscular and sensory impairment, possibly evidenced by decreased muscle strength, control and mass, and impaired coordination.

Self-care deficit (specify) may be related to neuromuscular and sensory impairments, possibly evidenced by statements of inability to perform care tasks.

Tay-Sachs disease

Growth and development, altered may be related to effects of physical condition, possibly evidenced by altered physical growth, loss of/failure to acquire skills typical of age, flat affect, and decreased responses.

Sensory-perceptual alterations, visual may be related to neurologic deterioration of optic nerve, possibly evidenced by loss of visual acuity.

Grieving, anticipatory (family) may be related to expected eventual loss of infant, possibly evidenced by expressions of distress, denial, guilt, anger, and sorrow; choked feelings; changes in sleep/eating habits; and altered libido.

Powerlessness (family) may be related to absence of therapeutic interventions for progressive/fatal disease, possibly evidenced by verbal expressions of having no control over situation/outcome and depression over physical/mental deterioration.

Spiritual distress, high risk for which may be related to challenged belief and value system by presence of fatal condition with racial/religious connotations and intense suffering.

Family coping, compromised may be related to situational crisis, temporary preoccupation with managing emotional conflicts and personal suffering, family disorganization, and prolonged/progressive disease, possibly evidenced by preoccupations with personal reactions, expressed concern about reactions of other family members, inadequate support of one another and altered communication patterns.

thrombophlebitis

Tissue perfusion, altered, peripheral may be related to interruption of venous blood flow, possibly evidenced by changes in skin color/temperature over affected area and development of edema.

Pain may be related to vascular inflammation/irritation and edema formation, possibly evidenced by complaints (specify), guarding/distraction behaviors, and self-focus.

Knowledge deficit [learning need] may be related to lack of information regarding pathophysiology of condition, therapy/self-care needs, and risk of embolization, possibly evidenced by statements of concern, questions, inaccurate follow-through of instructions, and development of preventable complications.

Physical mobility, impaired, high risk for which may be related to pain and discomfort and restrictive therapies/safety precautions.

thrombosis, venous
Refer to thrombophlebitis

thyroidectomy (also refer to hyperthyroidism, hypothyroidism, and hypoparathyroidism)

Airway clearance, ineffective, high risk for which may be related to hematoma/edema formation with tracheal obstruction.

Trauma, high risk for, to head/neck which may be related to loss of muscle control/support and position of suture line.

Pain may be related to presence of surgical incision and tissue trauma/edema, possibly evidenced by complaints (specify), guarding/distraction behaviors, self-focus, and autonomic responses (changes in vital signs).

Communication, impaired verbal may be related to tissue edema, pain/discomfort, and vocal cord injury/laryngeal nerve damage, possibly evidenced by impaired articulation, does not/cannot speak, and use of nonverbal cues.

thyrotoxicosis (also refer to hyperthyroidism)

Cardiac output, decreased, high risk for which may be related to uncontrolled hypermetabolic state increasing cardiac workload, changes in venous return and systemic vascular resistance, and alterations in rate, rhythm, and electrical conduction.

2540

Anxiety (specify level) may be related to physiologic factors: hypermetabolic state (central nervous system stimulation) and pseudocatecholamine effect of thyroid hormones, possibly evidenced by increased feelings of apprehension, shakiness, loss of control, panic, changes in cognition, distortion of environmental stimuli, extraneous movements, restlessness, and tremors.

Thought processes, altered, high risk for which may be related to physiologic changes (increased central nervous system stimulation/accelerated mental activity), and altered sleep patterns.

Knowledge deficit [learning need] may be related to lack of information regarding effects of condition and treatment needs and potential for complications/crisis situation, possibly evidenced by statements of concern, questions, misconceptions, and inaccurate follow-through of instructions.

tic douloureux
Refer to trigeminal neuralgia

tonsillectomy
Refer to adenoidectomy

tonsillitis
Pain may be related to inflammation of tonsils and effects of circulating toxins, possibly evidenced by complaints (specify), distraction behaviors, guarding (reluctance/refusal to swallow), self-focus, and autonomic responses (changes in vital signs).

Hyperthermia may be related to presence of inflammatory process/hypermetabolic state and dehydration, possibly evidenced by increased body temperature, warm/flushed skin, and tachycardia.

Knowledge deficit [learning need] may be related to lack of information regarding cause/transmission, treatment needs, and potential complications, possibly evidenced by statements of concern, questions, inaccurate follow-through of instructions, and recurrence of condition.

total joint replacement
Infection, high risk for which may be related to inadequate primary defenses (broken skin, exposure of joint), inadequate secondary defenses/immunosuppression (long-term corticosteroid use), invasive procedures, surgical manipulation, implantation of foreign body, and decreased mobility.

Physical mobility, impaired may be related to pain and discomfort, musculoskeletal impairment, and surgery/restrictive therapies, possibly evidenced by reluctance to attempt movement, difficulty purposefully moving within the physical environment, complaints of pain/discomfort on movement, limited range of motion, and decreased muscle strength/control.

Tissue perfusion, altered, peripheral, high risk for which may be related to reduced arterial/venous blood flow, direct trauma to blood vessels, tissue edema, improper location/dislocation of prosthesis, and hypovolemia.

Pain may be related to physical agents (traumatized tissues/surgical intervention, degeneration of joints) and psychologic factors (anxiety, advanced age), possibly evidenced by complaints (specify), distraction/guarding behaviors, self-focus, and autonomic responses (changes in vital signs).

toxemia of pregnancy
Refer to pregnancy-induced hypertension

toxic shock syndrome (also refer to septicemia)
Hyperthermia may be related to inflammatory process/hypermetabolic state and dehydration, possibly evidenced by increased body temperature, warm/flushed skin, and tachycardia.

Fluid volume deficit [active loss] may be related to increased gastric losses (diarrhea, vomiting), fever/hypermetabolic state, and decreased intake, possibly evidenced by dry mucous membranes, increased pulse, hypotension, delayed venous filling, decreased/concentrated urine, and hemoconcentration.

Pain may be related to inflammatory process, effects of circulating toxins, and skin disruptions, possibly evidenced by complaints (specify), guarding/distraction behaviors, self-focus, and autonomic responses (changes in vital signs).

Skin/Tissue integrity, impaired may be related to effects of circulating toxins and dehydration, possibly evidenced by development of desquamating rash, hyperemia and inflammation of mucous membranes.

traction
Pain may be related to direct trauma to tissue/bone and therapy restrictions, possibly evidenced by complaints (specify), guarding/distraction behaviors, self-focus, and autonomic responses (changes in vital signs).

Physical mobility, impaired may be related to skeletal impairment, pain, and therapeutic restrictions of movement, possibly evidenced by limited range of motion, inability to move purposefully in environment, and reluctance to attempt movement.

Infection, high risk for which may be related to invasive procedures including insertion of foreign body through skin/bone, presence of traumatized tissue, and reduced activity with stasis of body fluids.

Diversional activity deficit may be related to length of hospitalization and environmental lack of usual activity, possibly evidenced by statements of boredom, restlessness, and irritability.

trichinosis

Pain may be related to parasitic invasion of muscle tissues, edema of upper eyelids, small localized hemorrhages, and development of urticaria, possibly evidenced by complaints (specify), guarding, distraction behaviors/restlessness, and autonomic responses (changes in vital signs).

Fluid volume deficit [active loss] may be related to hypermetabolic state (fever, diaphoresis), excessive gastric losses (vomiting, diarrhea), and decreased intake/difficulty swallowing, possibly evidenced by dry mucous membranes, decreased skin turgor, hypotension, decreased venous filling, decreased/concentrated urine, and hemoconcentration.

Breathing pattern, ineffective may be related to myositis of the diaphragm and intercostal muscles, possibly evidenced by resulting changes in respiratory depth, tachypnea, dyspnea, and abnormal ABGs.

Knowledge deficit [learning need] may be related to lack of information regarding cause/prevention of condition, therapy needs, and possible complications, possibly evidenced by statements of concern, questions, and misconceptions.

tuberculosis (pulmonary)

Infection, high risk for spread/reactivation which may be related to inadequate primary defenses (decreased ciliary action/stasis of secretions, tissue destruction/extension of infection), lowered resistance/suppressed inflammatory response, malnutrition, environmental exposure, and insufficient knowledge to avoid exposure to pathogens.

Airway clearance, ineffective may be related to thick, viscous or bloody secretions, fatigue/poor cough effort, and tracheal/pharyngeal edema, possibly evidenced by abnormal respiratory rate, rhythm, and depth and abnormal breath sounds (rhonchi, wheezes), stridor and dyspnea.

Gas exchange, impaired, high risk for which may be related to decrease in effective lung surface, atelectasis, destruction of alveolar-capillary membrane and bronchial edema.

Activity intolerance may be related to imbalance between oxygen supply and demand, possibly evidenced by reports of fatigue, weakness, and exertional dyspnea.

Nutrition, altered: less than body requirements may be related to inability to ingest adequate nutrients (anorexia, effects of drug therapy, fatigue, insufficient financial resources), possibly evidenced by weight loss, reported lack of interest in food/altered taste sensation, and poor muscle tone.

Noncompliance (specify) [compliance, altered], high risk for which may be related to lengthy therapy requirements even after remission of symptoms as well as side effects of therapy.

tympanoplasty
Refer to stapedectomy

typhus (tick-borne/rocky mountain spotted fever)

Hyperthermia may be related to generalized inflammatory process (vasculitis), possibly evidenced by increased body temperature, warm/flushed skin, and tachycardia.

Pain may be related to generalized vasculitis and edema formation, possibly evidenced by complaints (specify), guarding/distraction behaviors, self-focus, and autonomic responses (changes in vital signs).

Tissue perfusion, altered (specify) may be related to reduction/interruption of blood flow (generalized vasculitis/thrombi formation), possibly evidenced by complaints of headache/abdominal pain, changes in mentation, and areas of peripheral ulceration/necrosis.

ulcer, decubitus

Skin/Tissue integrity, impaired may be related to altered circulation, nutritional deficit, fluid imbalance, impaired physical mobility, irritation of body excretions/secretions, and sensory impairments, evidenced by tissue damage/destruction.

Pain may be related to destruction of protective skin layers and exposure of nerves, possibly evidenced by complaints (specify), distraction behaviors, and self-focus.

Infection, high risk for which may be related to broken/traumatized tissue and increased environmental exposure, and nutritional deficits.

ulcer, peptic

Fluid volume deficit [active loss] may be related to vascular losses (hemorrhage), possibly evidenced by hypotension, tachycardia, delayed capillary refill, changes in mentation, restlessness, concentrated/decreased urine, pallor, and diaphoresis.

Tissue perfusion, altered (specify), high risk for which may be related to hypovolemia.

Fear/Anxiety (specify level) which may be related to change in health status and threat of death, possibly evidenced by increased tension, restlessness, irritability, fearfulness, trembling, tachycardia, diaphoresis, lack of eye contact, focus on self, withdrawal, and panic or attack behavior.

Pain may be related to caustic irritation/destruction of gastric tissues, possibly evidenced by complaints (specify), distraction behaviors, self-focus, and autonomic responses (changes in vital signs).

Knowledge deficit [learning need] may be related to lack of information regarding pathophysiology of condition, therapy/self-care needs, and potential complications, possibly evidenced by statements of concern, questions, inaccurate follow-through of instructions, and recurrence of condition.

unconsciousness (coma)

Suffocation, high risk for which may be related to cognitive impairment/loss of protective reflexes and purposeful movement.

Trauma, high risk for which may be related to cognitive impairment, generalized weakness/reduced coordination, and absence of purposeful movement.

Self-care deficit, total may be related to cognitive impairment and absence of purposeful activity, possibly evidenced by inability to perform tasks of care.

Tissue perfusion, altered, cerebral, high risk for which may be related to reduced/interrupted arterial/venous blood flow (direct injury, edema formation).

Infection, high risk for which may be related to stasis of body fluids (oral, pulmonary, urinary), invasive procedures, and nutritional deficits.

urinary diversion

Skin integrity, impaired, high risk for which may be related to absence of sphincter at stoma, character/flow of urine from stoma, reaction to product/chemicals, and improper fitting of appliance or removal of adhesive.

Body image/self-esteem disturbance, high risk for which may be related to biophysical factors: presence of stoma, loss of control of urine elimination; and psychosocial factors: altered body structure, disease process, and associated treatment regimen (cancer).

Pain may be related to physical factors: disruption of skin/tissues (incisions/drains); biologic: activity of disease process (cancer, trauma); psychologic factors: fear, anxiety, possibly evidenced by verbal complaints, self-focusing, guarding/distraction behaviors, restlessness, and autonomic responses (changes in vital signs).

Urinary elimination, altered patterns of may be related to surgical diversion, tissue trauma, and postoperative edema, possibly evidenced by loss of continence, changes in amount and character of urine, and urinary retention.

urolithiasis (urinary calculi)

Pain may be related to distention, trauma, and edema formation in sensitive tissue, possibly evidenced by complaints (specify), guarding/distraction behaviors, self-focus, and autonomic responses (changes in vital signs).

Urinary elimination, altered patterns of may be related to edema formation and irritation of ureteral and bladder tissues, possibly evidenced by urgency, frequency, retention, and hematuria.

Fluid volume deficit, high risk for may be related to stimulation of renal-intestinal reflexes causing nausea, vomiting, and diarrhea; changes in urinary output; and decreased intake.

uterine bleeding, abnormal

Anxiety (specify level) may be related to perceived change in health status and unknown etiology, possibly evidenced by apprehension, uncertainty, fear of unspecified consequences, expressed concerns, and focus on self.

Activity intolerance may be related to imbalance between oxygen supply and demand/decreased oxygen-carrying capacity of blood (anemia), possibly evidenced by reports of fatigue/weakness.

uterus, rupture of, in pregnancy

Fluid volume deficit [active loss] may be related to excessive vascular losses, possibly evidenced by hypotension, increased pulse rate, decreased venous filling, and decreased urine output.

Cardiac output, decreased may be related to decreased preload (hypovolemia), possibly evidenced by cold/clammy skin, decreased peripheral pulses, variations in hemodynamic readings, tachycardia, and cyanosis.

2543

Pain may be related to tissue trauma and irritation of accumulating blood, possibly evidenced by complaints (specify), guarding/distraction behaviors, self-focus, and autonomic responses (changes in vital signs).

Anxiety (specify level) may be related to threat of death of self/fetus, possibly evidenced by fearful/scared affect, sympathetic stimulation, stated fear of unspecified consequences, and expressed concerns.

vaginismus

Pain may be related to muscle spasm and hyperesthesia of the nerve supply to vaginal mucous membrane, possibly evidenced by complaints (specify), distraction behaviors, and self-focus.

Sexual dysfunction may be related to physical and/or psychologic alteration in function (severe spasms of vaginal muscles), possibly evidenced by verbalization of problem, inability to achieve desired satisfaction, and alteration in relationship with significant other.

vaginitis

Tissue integrity, impaired may be related to irritation/inflammation and mechanical trauma (scratching) of sensitive tissues, possibly evidenced by damaged/destroyed tissue, presence of lesions.

Pain may be related to localized inflammation and tissue trauma, possibly evidenced by complaints (specify), distraction behaviors, and self-focus.

Knowledge deficit [learning need] may be related to lack of information regarding hygienic and therapy needs and sexual behaviors/transmission of organisms, possibly evidenced by statements of concern, questions, and misconceptions.

varices, esophageal (also refer to ulcer, peptic)

Fluid volume deficit [active loss] may be related to excessive vascular loss, reduced intake, and gastric losses (vomiting), possibly evidenced by hypotension, tachycardia, decreased venous filling, and decreased/concentrated urine.

Anxiety (specify level)/Fear may be related to change in health status and threat of death, possibly evidenced by increased tension/apprehension, sympathetic stimulation, restlessness, focus on self, and expressed concerns.

varicose veins

Pain may be related to venous insufficiency and stasis, possibly evidenced by complaints (specify).

Body image disturbance may be related to change in structure (presence of enlarged, discolored tortuous superficial leg veins), possibly evidenced by hiding affected parts and negative feelings about body.

Skin/Tissue integrity, impaired, high risk for may be related to altered circulation/venous stasis and edema formation.

venereal disease

Refer to sexually transmitted disease

Wilm's tumor (also refer to cancer and chemotherapy)

Anxiety (specify level)/Fear may be related to change in environment and interaction patterns with family members and threat of death with family transmission and contagion of concerns, possibly evidenced by fearful/scared affect, distress, crying, insomnia, and sympathetic stimulation.

Injury, high risk for which may be related to nature of tumor (vascular, mushy with very thin covering) with increased danger of metastasis when manipulated.

Family processes, altered may be related to situational crisis of life-threatening illness, possibly evidenced by a family system that has difficulty meeting physical, emotional, and spiritual needs of its members, and inability in dealing with traumatic experience effectively.

Diversional activity, deficit may be related to environmental lack of age-appropriate activity (including activity restrictions) and length of hospitalization/treatment, possibly evidenced by restlessness, crying, lethargy, and acting-out behavior.

wound, bullet (depends on site and speed/character of bullet)

Fluid volume deficit, high risk for which may be related to excessive vascular losses, altered intake/restrictions.

Pain may be related to destruction of tissue (including organ and musculoskeletal), surgical repair, and therapeutic interventions, possibly evidenced by complaints (specify), guarding/distraction behaviors, self-focus, and autonomic responses (changes in vital signs).

Infection, high risk for which may be related to tissue destruction and increased environmental exposure, invasive procedures, and decreased hemoglobin.

Post-trauma response, high risk for which may be related to nature of incident (catastrophic accident, assault, suicide attempt) and possibly injury/death of other(s) involved.

2544

SECTION 3

NURSING DIAGNOSES THROUGH THE 9TH NATIONAL CONFERENCE IN ALPHABETICAL ORDER

NOTES:
1. Information appearing in brackets has been added by the authors to clarify and facilitate the use of nursing diagnoses.
2. A "HIGH RISK FOR" diagnosis is *not* evidenced by signs and symptoms, since the problem has not yet occurred, and nursing interventions are directed at prevention. Therefore, *risk* factors which are present are noted instead.
3. New approved nursing diagnoses (NANDA 10th Conference, 1992) appear on page 2584.

ACTIVITY INTOLERANCE

Diagnostic Division: Activity/Rest
   Definition: A state in which an individual has insufficient physiological or psychological energy to endure or complete required or desired daily activities.

RELATED FACTORS
Generalized weakness; Sedentary lifestyle; Imbalance between oxygen supply and demand; Bedrest or immobility; [Cognitive deficits/emotional status; underlying disease process/depression]

DEFINING CHARACTERISTICS

Subjective
Verbal report of fatigue or weakness; Exertional discomfort or dyspnea; [Pain]; [Verbalizes no desire and/or lack of interest in activity]

Objective
Abnormal heart rate or blood pressure response; Electrocardiographic changes reflecting arrhythmias or ischemia; [Pallor]; [Cyanosis]

ACTIVITY INTOLERANCE, HIGH RISK FOR

Diagnostic Division: Activity/Rest
   Definition: A state in which an individual is at risk of experiencing insufficient physiologic or psychologic energy to endure or complete required or desired daily activities.

RISK FACTORS
History of previous intolerance; Presence of circulatory/respiratory problems; Deconditioned status; Presence of circulatory/respiratory problems; Inexperience with the activity; [Early diagnosis of progressive disease state such as cancer, multiple sclerosis; extensive surgical procedures; Verbalized reluctance/inability to perform expected activity]

ADJUSTMENT, IMPAIRED

Diagnostic Division: Ego Integrity
   Definition: The state in which the individual is unable to modify his/her lifestyle or behavior in a manner consistent with a change in health status.

RELATED FACTORS
Disability requiring change in lifestyle; Inadequate support systems; Impaired cognition, sensory overload; Assault to self-esteem, altered locus of control; Incomplete grieving [severe emotional loss, physical and/or learning disability, life-threatening condition or disease].

DEFINING CHARACTERISTICS

Subjective
Verbalization of nonacceptance of health status change

Objective
Nonexistent or unsuccessful ability to be involved in problem-solving or goal setting; Lack of movement toward independence; Extended period of shock, disbelief, or anger regarding health status change; Lack of future-oriented thinking; [Lack of ability to limit expectations of self]

AIRWAY CLEARANCE, INEFFECTIVE

Diagnostic Division: Respiration
Definition: A state in which an individual is unable to clear secretions or obstructions from the respiratory tract to maintain airway patency.

RELATED FACTORS
Tracheobronchial infection, obstruction, secretion; Decreased energy and fatigue; Perceptual/cognitive impairment; Trauma; [Inhalation injury]

DEFINING CHARACTERISTICS

Subjective
[Statement of difficulty breathing]

Objective
Abnormal breath sounds; rales (crackles), rhonchi (wheezes)
Changes in rate or depth of respiration
Tachypnea
Cough, effective or ineffective, with or without sputum

Cyanosis
Dyspnea
[Apnea]
[Fear; anxiety; restlessness]
[Use of accessory muscles for breathing]
[Choking or noisy respirations]

ANXIETY [SPECIFY LEVEL]

Diagnostic Division: Ego Integrity
Definition: A vague uneasy feeling, the source of which is often nonspecific or unknown to the individual.

RELATED FACTORS
Unconscious conflict about essential values, [beliefs], and goals of life
Situational and [or] maturational crises
Interpersonal transmission and contagion
Threat to self-concept [perceived or actual], [unconscious conflict]
Threat of death [perceived or actual]

Threat to or change in health status [terminal illness], socioeconomic status, role functioning, environment, [safety], interaction patterns
Unmet needs
[Positive or negative self-talk]
[Physiologic factors, such as hyperthyroidism, pheochromocytoma, use of steroids]

DEFINING CHARACTERISTICS

Subjective
Increased tension
Painful and persistent increased helplessness
Scared
Shakiness
Regretful
Overexcited
Rattled
Distressed
Apprehension
Uncertainty
Fearful

Feelings of inadequacy
Fear of unspecific consequences
Expressed concern regarding changes in life events
Anxious
Worried
Jittery
[Somatic complaints]
[Sleeplessness]
[Sense of impending doom]
[Hopelessness]

Objective

Sympathetic stimulation: cardiovascular excitation, superficial vasoconstriction, pupil dilation

Increased wariness

Extraneous movements: foot shuffling; hand/arm movements

Increased perspiration

Restlessness

Insomnia

Glancing about; poor eye contact

Trembling; hand tremors

Facial tension

Voice quivering

Focus on self

[Urinary frequency]

[Repetitive questioning]

[Pacing; purposeless activity]

[Impaired functioning; immobility]

ASPIRATION, HIGH RISK FOR

Diagnostic Division: Respiration

Definition: The state in which an individual is at risk for entry of gastric secretions, oropharyngeal sections, [or exogenous food] or fluids into tracheobronchial passages solids due to dysfunction or absence of normal protective mechanisms].

RISK FACTORS

Reduced level of consciousness

Depressed cough and gag reflexes

Presence of tracheostomy or endotracheal tube

[Overinflated tracheostomy/endotracheal tube cuff]

[Inadequate tracheostomy/endotracheal tube cuff inflation]

Gastrointestinal tubes

Bolus tube feedings/medication administration

Situation hindering elevation of upper body

Increased intragastric pressure

Increased gastric residual

Decreased gastrointestinal motility

Delaying gastric emptying

Impaired swallowing [owing to inability of the epiglottis and true vocal cords to move to close off trachea]

Facial/oral/neck surgery or trauma

Wired jaws

BODY IMAGE DISTURBANCE

Diagnostic Division: Ego Integrity

Definition: Disruption in the way one perceives one's body image.

RELATED FACTORS

Biophysical [physical trauma/mutilation, pregnancy, physical change caused by biochemical agents (drugs), dependence on machine]; Psychosocial; Cultural or spiritual; [Cognitive/perceptual]; [Significance of body part or functioning with regard to age, sex, developmental level, or basic human needs]; [Maturational changes]

DEFINING CHARACTERISTICS

A or B must be present to justify the diagnosis of Body Image Disturbance. A = verbal response to actual or perceived change in structure and/or function; B = nonverbal response to actual or perceived change in structure and/or function.

The following clinical manifestations may be used to validate the presence of A or B:

Subjective

Verbalization of: Change in lifestyle; Fear of rejection or of reaction by others; Focus on past strength, function, or appearance; Negative feelings about body; Feelings of helplessness, hopelessness, or powerlessness; Preoccupation with change or loss; and/or [Feelings or depersonalization/grandiosity]

Refusal to verify actual change; Emphasis on remaining strengths, heightened achievement; Personalization of part or loss by name; Depersonalization of part or loss by impersonal pronouns; Extension of body boundary to incorporate environment objects

Objective

Missing body part; Actual change in structure and/or function; Not looking at/not touching body part; Trauma to nonfunctioning part; Change in ability to estimate spatial relationship of body to environment; Hiding or overexposing body part (intentional or unintentional); Change in social involvement; [Inability to differentiate internal/external stimuli/loss of ego boundaries]

BODY TEMPERATURE, ALTERED, HIGH RISK FOR

Diagnostic Division: Safety

Definition: The state in which the individual is at risk for failure to maintain body temperature within normal range.

RISK FACTORS

Extremes of age
Extremes of weight
Exposure to cold/cool or warm/hot environments
Dehydration
Inactivity or vigorous activity
Medications causing vasoconstriction/vasodilation, altered metabolic rate, sedation, [use or overdose of certain drugs or exposure to anesthesia]

Inappropriate clothing for environmental temperature
Illness or trauma affecting temperature regulation
[Infections, systemic or localized]
[Neoplasms, tumors, collagen vascular disease]

BOWEL INCONTINENCE

Diagnostic Division: Elimination

Definition: A state in which an individual experiences a change in normal bowel habits characterized by involuntary passage of stool.

RELATED FACTORS

To be developed by NANDA; (Neuromuscular/musculoskeletal involvement); (Perceptual or cognitive impairment); (Depression); (Severe anxiety); [Diarrhea and/or fecal impaction]

NOTE: These factors were identified when this diagnosis was originally accepted and have been retained here to assist the user until NANDA completes its work.

DEFINING CHARACTERISTICS

Objective

Involuntary passage of stool

BREASTFEEDING, EFFECTIVE

Diagnostic Division: Food/Fluid

Definition: The state in which a mother-infant dyad/family exhibits adequate proficiency and satisfaction with breastfeeding process.

RELATED FACTORS

Basic breastfeeding knowledge; Normal breast structure; Normal infant oral structure; Infant gestational age greater than 34 weeks; Support sources [available]; Maternal confidence

DEFINING CHARACTERISTICS

Subjective

Maternal verbalization of satisfaction with the breastfeeding process

Objective

Mother able to position infant at breast to promote a successful latch-on response; Infant is content after feedings; Regular and sustained sucking at the breast (8 to 10 times/24 hours); Adequate infant weight gain [appropriate infant weight patterns for age]; Signs and/or symptoms of oxytocin release (let down or milk ejection reflex); [Infant] Soft stools; over 6 wet diapers per day of unconcentrated urine; eagerness of infant to nurse

---

BREASTFEEDING, INEFFECTIVE

Diagnostic Division: Food/Fluid

Definition: The state in which a mother, infant, or child experiences dissatisfaction or difficulty with the breastfeeding process

RELATED FACTORS

Prematurity
Infant anomaly
Maternal breast anomaly
Previous breast surgery
Previous history of breastfeeding failure
Infant receiving [numerous or repeated] supplemental feedings with artificial nipple

Poor infant sucking reflex
Nonsupportive partner/family
Knowledge deficit
Interruption in breastfeeding
Maternal anxiety or ambivalence
Painful nipples/breast engorgement

DEFINING CHARACTERISTICS

Subjective

Unsatisfactory breastfeeding process; Persistence of sore nipples beyond the first week of breastfeeding; Insufficient emptying of each breast per feeding; Actual or perceived inadequate milk supply

Objective

Observable signs of inadequate infant intake [inappropriate weight loss or inadequate gain]; Nonsustained or insufficient opportunity for suckling at the breast; Infant inability [failure] to attach on to maternal breast correctly; Infant arching and crying at the breasts; Resisting latching on; Infant exhibiting fussiness and crying within the first hour after breastfeeding; Unresponsive to other comfort measures; No observable signs of oxytocin release

---

BREATHING PATTERN, INEFFECTIVE

Diagnostic Division: Respiration

Definition: The state in which an individual's inhalation and/or exhalation pattern does not enable adequate pulmonary inflation or emptying.

RELATED FACTORS

Neuromuscular/musculoskeletal impairment
Anxiety
Pain
Perception or cognitive impairment

Decreased energy and fatigue
[Alteration of patient's normal O_2/CO_2 ratio, e.g., O_2 therapy in presence of COPD]

DEFINING CHARACTERISTICS

Subjective
Shortness of breath

Objective

Dyspnea
Fremitus
Cyanosis
Nasal flaring
Assumption of 3-point position
Increased anteroposterior diameter
Tachypnea
Abnormal arterial blood gases

Cough
Respiratory depth changes
Pursed-lip breathing; prolonged expiratory phase
Use of accessory muscles
Altered chest excursion
[Reduced vital capacity]
[Tachycardia]

CARDIAC OUTPUT, DECREASED

Diagnostic Division: Circulation
Definition: A state in which the blood pumped by an individual's heart is sufficiently reduced so that it is inadequate to meet the needs of the body's tissues. (NOTE: In a hypermetabolic state, although cardiac output may be within normal range, it may still be inadequate to meet the needs of the body's tissues. Cardiac output and tissue perfusion are interrelated, although there are differences. When cardiac output is decreased, tissue perfusion problems will develop; however, tissue perfusion problems can exist without decreased cardiac output.)

RELATED FACTORS
To be developed by NANDA (Mechanical: alteration in preload [e.g., decreased venous return, altered myocardial contractility]; afterload [e.g., alteration in systemic vascular resistance]; inotropic changes in heart. Electrical: alterations in rate; rhythm; conduction. Structural [e.g., ventricular-septal rupture, ventricular aneurysm, papillary muscle rupture, valvular disease].)

NOTE: These factors were identified when this diagnosis was originally accepted and have been retained here to assist the user until NANDA completes its work.

DEFINING CHARACTERISTICS

Subjective
Fatigue; Dyspnea

Objective

Variations in blood pressure [hemodynamic] readings
Cyanosis; pallor of skin and mucous membranes
Cold, clammy skin
Orthopnea
Arrhythmias; [ECG changes]

Jugular vein distention
Oliguria; anuria
Decreased peripheral pulses
Rales
Restlessness

Other Possible Characteristics

Subjective
Syncope; Vertigo; Weakness; [Angina]

Objective
Edema; Change in mental status; Shortness of breath; Frothy sputum; Gallop rhythm, abnormal heart sounds; Cough; [Liver engorgement/ascites]

COMMUNICATION, IMPAIRED VERBAL

Diagnostic Division: Social Interaction
Definition: The state in which an individual experiences a decreased or absent ability to use or to understand language in human interaction

RELATED FACTORS
Decrease in circulation to brain; Brain tumor; Anatomic deficit, cleft palate; Developmental or age-related; Physical barrier (tracheostomy, intubation); Psychologic barriers, psychosis, lack of stimuli [depression, panic, anger]; Cultural difference; [Drug intake, chemical imbalance]

DEFINING CHARACTERISTICS

Subjective
[Reports of difficulty expressing self]

Objective
Unable to speak dominant language; Speaks or verbalizes with difficulty; Does not or cannot speak; Disorientation; Stuttering, slurring; Dyspnea; Difficulty forming words or sentences; Difficulty expressing thought verbally; Inappropriate verbalization [incessant, loose association of ideas, flight of ideas]; [Inability to modulate speech]; [Message inappropriate to content]; [Use of nonverbal cues, e.g., facial expression, gestures, pleading eyes, turning away]; [Frustration, anger, hostility]

CONSTIPATION

Diagnostic Division: Elimination
Definition: A state in which an individual experiences a change in normal bowel habits characterized by a decrease in frequency and/or passage of hard, dry stools.

RELATED FACTORS
To be developed by NANDA: (Neuromuscular/Musculoskeletal impairment, weak abdominal musculature); (Gastrointestinal obstructive lesions); (Pain on defecation); (Diagnostic procedures); (Pregnancy)

NOTE: These factors were identified when this diagnosis was originally accepted and have been retained here to assist the user until NANDA completes its work.

DEFINING CHARACTERISTICS
Subjective
Frequency less than usual pattern; Reported feeling of abdominal or rectal fullness or pressure; [Less than usual amount of stool]; [Nausea]

Objective
Hard-formed stools; Straining at stool; Palpable mass; Decreased activity level; [Decreased bowel sounds]; [Abdominal distention]

Other Possible Characteristics
Abdominal/back pain; Headache; Interference with daily living; Appetite impairment; and/or Use of laxatives

---

CONSTIPATION, COLONIC

Diagnostic Division: Elimination
Definition: The state in which an individual's pattern of elimination is characterized by hard, dry stool which results from a delay in passage of food residue.

RELATED FACTORS
Less than adequate fluid intake	Emotional disturbances
Less than adequate dietary intake	Chronic use of medication and enemas
Less than adequate fiber	Stress
Less than adequate physical activity	Change in daily routine
Immobility	Metabolic problems, e.g., hypothyroidism, hypocalcemia, hypokalemia
Lack of privacy	

DEFINING CHARACTERISTICS
Decreased frequency; Hard, dry stool; Straining at stool; Painful defecation; Abdominal distention; Palpable mass; Rectal pressure; Headache; Appetite impairment; Abdominal pain

---

CONSTIPATION, PERCEIVED

Diagnostic Division: Elimination
Definition: The state in which an individual makes a self-diagnosis of constipation and ensures a daily bowel movement through use of laxatives, enemas, and suppositories.

RELATED FACTORS
Cultural/family health beliefs; Faulty appraisal; Impaired thought processes

DEFINING CHARACTERISTICS
Major
Expectation of a daily bowel movement with the resulting overuse of laxatives, enemas, and suppositories; Expected passage of stool at same time every day

COPING, DEFENSIVE

Diagnostic Division: Ego Integrity
Definition: The state in which an individual repeatedly projects falsely positive self-evaluation based on a self-protective pattern which defends against underlying perceived threats to positive self-regard.

DEFINING CHARACTERISTICS

Subjective
Denial of obvious problems/weaknesses; Projection of blame/responsibility; Rationalizes failures; Hypersensitive to slight/criticism; Grandiosity

Objective
Superior attitude toward others; Difficulty establishing/maintaining relationships; Hostile laughter or ridicule of others; Difficulty in reality testing perceptions; Lack of followthrough or participation in treatment or therapy

COPING, INEFFECTIVE INDIVIDUAL

Diagnostic Division: Ego Integrity
Definition: Impairment of adaptive behaviors and problem-solving abilities of a person in meeting life's demands and roles.

RELATED FACTORS
Situational/maturational crises; Personal vulnerability; Inadequate support systems; Poor nutrition; Work overload, no vacations, [too many deadlines]; Unrealistic perceptions; [Multiple stressors, repeated over period of time]; [Multiple life changes, conflict]; Inadequate relaxation, little or no exercise]; [Unmet expectations]; [Inadequate coping method]; [Impairment of nervous system]; [Memory loss]; [Severe pain, overwhelming threat to self]

DEFINING CHARACTERISTICS

Subjective
Verbalization of inability to cope or inability to ask for help; Reports of chronic worry/anxiety/depression, poor self-esteem; [Complaints of muscular/emotional tension, lack of appetite, chronic fatigue, insomnia, general irritability]

Objective
Inability to problem-solve; Inability to meet role expectations/basic needs; Alteration in societal participation; Inappropriate use of defense mechanisms; Change in usual communication patterns; Verbal manipulation; High illness rate [including high blood pressure, ulcers, irritable bowel, frequent headaches/neckaches]; High rate of accidents; Destructive behavior toward self or others [including overeating, excessive smoking/drinking, overuse of prescribed tranquilizers, alcohol]; [Lack of assertive behaviors]

DECISIONAL CONFLICT (SPECIFY)

Diagnostic Division: Ego Integrity
Definition: The state of uncertainty about course of action to be taken when choice among competing actions involves risk, loss, or challenge to personal life values.

RELATED FACTORS
Unclear personal values/beliefs; Perceived threat to value system; Lack of experience or interference with decision making; Lack of relevant information; Support system deficit; Multiple or divergent sources of information

DEFINING CHARACTERISTICS

Subjective
Verbalized uncertainty about choices or of undesired consequences of alternative actions being considered; Verbalized feelings of distress or questioning personal values and beliefs while attempting a decision

Objective
Vacillation between alternative choices; Delayed decision-making; Self-focusing; Physical signs of distress or tension (increased heart rate, increased muscle tension, restlessness, etc.)

DENIAL, INEFFECTIVE

Diagnostic Division: Ego Integrity
   Definition: The state of a conscious or unconscious attempt to disavow the knowledge or meaning of an event to reduce anxiety/fear to the detriment of health.

RELATED FACTORS
To be developed by NANDA: [Personal vulnerability; unmet self-needs]; [Presence of overwhelming anxiety-producing feelings/situation; reality factors that are consciously intolerable]

DEFINING CHARACTERISTICS

Subjective
Minimizes symptoms; displaces source of symptoms to other organs; Unable to admit impact of disease on life pattern; Displaces fear of impact of the condition; Does not admit fear of death or invalidism

Objective
Delays seeking or refuses health care attention to the detriment of health; Does not perceive personal relevance of symptoms or danger; Makes dismissive gestures or comments when speaking of distressing events; Displays inappropriate affect; Uses home remedies (self-treatment) to relieve symptoms

---

DIARRHEA

Diagnostic Division: Elimination
   Definition: A state in which an individual experiences a change in normal bowel habits characterized by the frequent passage of loose, fluid, unformed stools.

RELATED FACTORS
To be developed by NANDA: (Stress and anxiety); (Medications, radiation, toxins, contaminants); (Dietary intake); (Inflammation, irritation, or malabsorption of bowel)
NOTE: These factors were identified when this diagnosis was originally accepted and have been retained here to assist the user until NANDA completes its work.

DEFINING CHARACTERISTICS

Subjective
Abdominal pain; Urgency; Cramping

Objective
Increased frequency; Increased frequency of bowel sounds; Loose, liquid stools

Other Possible Characteristics
Change in color

DISUSE SYNDROME, HIGH RISK FOR

Diagnostic Division: Activity/Rest
   Definition: A state in which an individual is at risk for deterioration of body systems as the result of prescribed or unavoidable musculoskeletal inactivity.

NOTE: NANDA identifies complications from immobility including pressure ulcer, constipation, stasis of pulmonary secretions, thrombosis, urinary tract infection/retention, decreased strength/endurance, orthostatic hypotension, decreased range of joint motion, disorientation, body image disturbance, and powerlessness.)

RISK FACTORS

Subjective
Severe pain, [chronic pain]

Objective
Paralysis; Mechanical or prescribed immobilization; Altered level of consciousness

DIVERSIONAL ACTIVITY DEFICIT

Diagnostic Division: Activity/Rest
**Definition: The state in which an individual experiences a decreased stimulation from or
interest or engagement in recreational or leisure activities (because of internal/external
factors that may or may not be beyond the individual's control).**

RELATED FACTORS

Environmental lack of diversional activity; Long-term hospitalization; Frequent, lengthy treatments;
[Physical limitations]; [Bedridden]; [Situational, developmental problem]; [Psychologic condition,
e.g., depression]

DEFINING CHARACTERISTICS

Subjective
Patient's statement regarding the following: Boredom; Wish there were something to do, to read, etc.;
Usual hobbies cannot be undertaken in hospital [or are restricted by physical limitations]

Objective
[Flat affect]; [Disinterested]; [Restless]; [Crying]; [Lethargy]; [Withdrawn]; [Hostile]

DYSREFLEXIA

Diagnostic Division: Circulation
**Definition: The state in which an individual with a spinal cord injury at T-7 or above ex-
periences a life-threatening uninhibited sympathetic response of the nervous system to a
noxious stimulus.**

RELATED FACTORS

Bladder or bowel distention; Skin irritation; Lack of patient and caregiver knowledge; [Sexual excita-
tion]

DEFINING CHARACTERISTICS

Individual with spinal cord injury (T7 or above) with:

Subjective
Headache (a diffuse pain in different portions of the head and not confined to any nerve distribution
area); Paresthesia; chilling; blurred vision; chest pain; metallic taste in mouth; nasal congestion; Pilomotor reflex (gooseflesh formation such as when skin is cooled)

Objective
Paroxysmal hypertension (sudden periodic elevated blood pressure where systolic pressure is over 140
mmHg and diastolic is above 90 mmHg); Bradycardia or tachycardia (pulse rate of less than 60 or over
100 beats per minute); Diaphoresis (above the injury); red splotches on skin (above the injury); pallor
(below the injury); Horner's syndrome (contraction of the pupil, partial ptosis of the eyelid, enophthalmos and sometimes loss of sweating over the affected side of the face); conjunctival congestion

FAMILY COPING, COMPROMISED

Diagnostic Division: Social Interaction
**Definition: [A usually supportive primary person (family member or close friend [signifi-
cant other]) is providing insufficient, ineffective, or compromised support, comfort, assistance, or encouragement that may be needed by the (patient) to manage or master adaptive tasks related to the (patient's) health challenge.]**

RELATED FACTORS

Inadequate or incorrect information or understanding by a primary person; Temporary preoccupation by a significant person who is trying to manage emotional conflicts and personal suffering and is unable to perceive or to act effectively in regard to [patient's] needs; Temporary family disorganization and role changes; Other situational or developmental crises or situations the significant person may be facing; [Patient] providing little support in turn for the primary person; Prolonged disease or disability progression that exhausts the supportive capacity of significant people

DEFINING CHARACTERISTICS

Subjective

[Patient] expresses or confirms a concern or complaint about significant other's response to [patient's] health problem; Significant person describes preoccupation with personal reactions, e.g., fear, anticipatory grief, guilt, anxiety, regarding [patient's] illness or disability, or to other situational or developmental crises; Significant person describes or confirms an inadequate understanding or knowledge base that interferes with effective assistive or supportive behaviors

Objective

Significant person attempts assistive or supportive behaviors with less than satisfactory results; Significant person withdraws or enters into limited or temporary personal communication with [patient] at time of need; Significant person displays protective behavior disproportionate (too little or too much) to [patient's] abilities or need for autonomy

FAMILY COPING, DISABLING

Diagnostic Division: Social Interaction

Definition: The behavior of a significant person (family member or other primary person) disables his or her own capacities and the (patient's) capacities to effectively address tasks essential to either person's adaptation to the health challenge.

RELATED FACTORS

Significant person with chronically unexpressed feelings of guilt, anxiety, hostility, despair, etc.; Dissonant discrepancy of coping styles being used to deal with the adaptive tasks by the significant person and [patient] or among significant people; Highly ambivalent family relationships; Arbitrary handling of a family's resistance to treatment, which tends to solidify defensiveness because it fails to deal adequately with underlying anxiety

DEFINING CHARACTERISTICS

Subjective

[Express despair regarding family reactions/lack of involvement]

Objective

Intolerance

Abandonment

Psychosomatic tendency

Agitation, depression, aggression, hostility

Rejection

Desertion

Taking on illness signs of [patient]

Neglectful relationships with other family members

Carrying on usual routines disregarding [patient's] needs

Neglectful care of the [patient] in regard to basic human needs and/or illness treatment

Distortion of reality regarding the [patient's] health problem, including extreme denial about its existence or severity

Decisions and actions by family that are detrimental to economic or social well-being

Impaired restructuring of a meaningful life for self; impaired individualization; prolonged overconcern for [patient]

[Patient's] development of helpless, inactive dependence

FAMILY COPING, POTENTIAL FOR GROWTH

Diagnostic Division: Social Interaction

Definition: The family member has effectively managed adaptive tasks involved with the (patient's) health challenge and is exhibiting desire and readiness for enhanced health and growth in regard to self and in relation to the (patient).

RELATED FACTORS

The person's basic needs are sufficiently gratified and adaptive tasks effectively addressed to enable goals of self-actualization to surface

DEFINING CHARACTERISTICS

Subjective

Family member attempting to describe growth impact of crisis on his/her own values, priorities, goals, or relationships; Individual expresses interest in making contact on a one-to-one basis or on a mutual-aid group basis with another person who has experienced a similar situation

Objective

Family member is moving in direction of health-promoting and enriching lifestyle that supports and monitors maturational processes, audits and negotiates treatment programs, and generally chooses experiences that optimize wellness

FAMILY PROCESSES, ALTERED

Diagnostic Division: Social Interaction

Definition: The state in which a family that normally functions effectively experiences a dysfunction.

RELATED FACTORS

Situational transition and/or crises [e.g., economic, change in roles, illness]; Development transition and/or crises [e.g., loss or gain of a family member]

DEFINING CHARACTERISTICS

Subjective

Family uninvolved in community activities; Unexamined family myths; [Family expresses confusion about what to do, verbalizes they are having difficulty coping with situation]

Objective

Family system unable to [does not] meet physical/emotional/spiritual needs of its members

Family unable to [does not] meet security needs of its members

Inability to accept or to receive help appropriately

Family inability to [does not] adapt to change or to deal with traumatic experience constructively

Parents do not demonstrate respect for each other's views on childrearing practices

Inability to express or to accept wide range of feelings/feelings of members

Inability of family members to relate to each other for mutual growth and maturation

Rigidity in function and roles

Family does not demonstrate respect for individuality and autonomy of its members

Family fails to accomplish current or past developmental task

Unhealthy family decision-making process

Failure to send and to receive clear messages

Inappropriate level and direction of energy

Inappropriate boundary maintenance

Inappropriate or poorly communicated family rules, rituals, symbols

FATIGUE

Diagnostic Division: Activity/Rest

Definition: An overwhelming sustained sense of exhaustion and decreased capacity for physical and mental work.

RELATED FACTORS

Decreased/increased metabolic energy production; Overwhelming psychological or emotional demands; Increased energy requirements to perform activities of daily living; Excessive social and/or role demands; States of discomfort; Altered body chemistry (e.g., medications, drug withdrawal, chemotherapy)

DEFINING CHARACTERISTICS

Subjective

Verbalization of an unremitting and overwhelming lack of energy; Inability to maintain usual routines; Perceived need for additional energy to accomplish routine tasks; Impaired ability to concentrate; Decreased libido

Objective

Increase in physical complaints; Emotionally labile or irritable; Lethargic or listless; Disinterest in surroundings/introspection; Decreased performance; Accident prone

FEAR

Diagnostic Division: Ego Integrity
   Definition: Feeling of dread related to an indentifiable source which the individual validates.

RELATED FACTORS

To be developed by NANDA: (Natural or innate origins; environmental stimuli (e.g., sudden noise), loss of physical support, heights, pain); (Learned response: conditioning, modeling from or identification with others); (Separation from support system in a potentially threatening situation such as hospitalization, treatments, etc.); (Knowledge deficit or unfamiliarity); (Phobic stimulus or phobia); (Language barrier) [or inability to communicate]; (Sensory impairment); [Threat of death, perceived or actual]

NOTE: These factors were identified when this diagnosis was originally accepted and have been retained here to assist the user until NANDA completes its work.

DEFINING CHARACTERISTICS

Subjective

Ability to identify object of fear; Panic; Scared; Jittery; [Increased tension; Apprehension; Frightened; Terrified]; [Impulsiveness]; [Decreased self-assurance]; [Associated physical symptoms: nausea, "heart beating fast," etc.]

Objective

[Attack/fight behavior — aggressive; flight behavior — withdrawal]; [Wide-eyed; Increased alertness; Concentration on source]; [Sympathetic stimulation: cardiovascular excitation, superficial vasoconstriction, pupil dilation, vomiting, diarrhea, diaphoresis, etc.]

FLUID VOLUME DEFICIT [ACTIVE LOSS]

Diagnostic Division: Food/Fluid
   Definition: The state in which an individual experiences vascular, cellular, or intracellular dehydration (in excess of needs or replacement capabilities owing to active loss).

RELATED FACTORS

Active loss [e.g., burns, abdominal cancer, hemorrhage, diarrhea, fistulas, use of hyperosmotic radiopaque contrast agents]

DEFINING CHARACTERISTICS

Objective

Decreased urine output; Output greater than intake; Decreased venous filling; Increased serum sodium; Concentrated urine; Sudden weight loss; Hemoconcentration

Other Defining Characteristics

Thirst	Dry mucous membranes
Hypotension [postural]	Increased body temperature
Decreased skin turgor	Weakness
Increased pulse rate	Decreased pulse volume and pressure
Dry skin	Change in mental state

FLUID VOLUME DEFICIT [REGULATORY FAILURE]

Diagnostic Division: Food/Fluid
   Definition: The state in which an individual experiences vascular, cellular, or intracellular dehydration [in excess of needs or replacement capabilities owing to failure of regulatory mechanisms].

RELATED FACTORS
Failure of regulatory mechanisms [e.g., adrenal disease, recovery phase of acute renal failure, uncontrolled diabetes mellitus/insipidus]

DEFINING CHARACTERISTICS

Subjective
[Complaints of fatigue, nervousness]

Objective
Increased urine output; Dilute urine; Sudden weight loss; Decreased venous filling; Hemoconcentration; Altered serum sodium

Other Defining Characteristics
Hypotension [postural]; Thirst; Increased pulse rate; Decreased skin turgor; Decreased pulse volume and pressure; Change in mental status; Increased body temperature; Dry skin/mucous membranes; Weakness; [Edema; possible weight gain]

FLUID VOLUME DEFICIT, HIGH RISK FOR

Diagnostic Division: Food/Fluid
Definition: The state in which an individual is at risk of experiencing vascular, cellular, or intracellular dehydration [due to active or regulatory losses of body water in excess of needs or replacement capability].

RISK FACTORS
Extremes of age and weight; Loss of fluid through abnormal routes, e.g., indwelling tubes; Knowledge deficiency related to fluid volume; Factors influencing fluid needs, e.g., hypermetabolic states; Medications, e.g., diuretics; Excessive losses through normal routes, e.g., diarrhea; Deviations affecting access to, intake of, or absorption of fluids, e.g., physical immobility

---

FLUID VOLUME EXCESS

Diagnostic Division: Food/Fluid
Definition: The state in which an individual experiences increased fluid retention and edema.

RELATED FACTORS
Compromised regulatory mechanism [e.g., SIADH or decreased plasma proteins — malnutrition, draining fistulas, burns, organ failure]; Excess fluid intake; Excess sodium intake; [Drug therapies, e.g., chlorpropamide, tolbutamide, vincristine, tryptyline, carbamazepine]

DEFINING CHARACTERISTICS

Subjective
Shortness of breath, orthopnea; Anxiety

Objective

Edema, anasarca	Altered electrolytes
Weight gain	Restlessness
Change in mental status	Central venous pressure changes
Intake greater than output	Pulmonary congestion on x-ray film
Oliguria	Abnormal breath sounds: crackles (rales)
Azotemia	Change in respiratory pattern
Effusion	Decreased hemoglobin, hematocrit
Third heart sound (53)	Pulmonary artery pressure changes
Blood pressure changes	Jugulovenous distention
Specific gravity changes	Positive hepatojugular reflux

GAS EXCHANGE, IMPAIRED

Diagnostic Division: Respiration
> **Definition: The state in which the individual experiences a decreased passage of oxygen and/or carbon dioxide between the alveoli of the lungs and the vascular system. [This may be an entity of its own, but it also may be an end result of other pathology with an interrelatedness between airway clearance and/or breathing pattern problems.]**

RELATED FACTORS
Ventilation perfusion imbalance; [Altered blood flow, e.g., pulmonary embolus, increased vascular resistance]; [Alveolar-capillary membrane changes, e.g., adult respiratory distress syndrome; chronic conditions, such as pneumoconiosis, asbestosis/silicosis]; [Altered oxygen supply, e.g., altitude sickness]; [Altered oxygen-carrying capacity of blood, e.g., sickle cell/other anemia, carbon monoxide poisoning]

DEFINING CHARACTERISTICS

Subjective
[Dyspnea]; [Sense of impending doom]

Objective

Confusion	Irritability
Restlessness	Hypercapnia
Inability to move secretions	[Cyanosis]
Hypoxia	[Tachycardia]
Somnolence	[Polycythemia]

GRIEVING, ANTICIPATORY

Diagnostic Division: Ego Integrity
> **Definition: [Response to loss before it actually occurs. *Note:* May be a healthy response requiring interventions of support and information-giving.]**

RELATED FACTORS
To be developed by NANDA: [Perceived potential loss of significant other, physiopsychosocial well-being, personal possessions]

DEFINING CHARACTERISTICS

Subjective
Sorrow; Guilt; Anger; Choked feelings; Denial of potential loss; Expression of distress at potential loss; Alterations in activity level; Sleep patterns; Changes in eating habits; Altered libido

Objective
Potential loss of significant object; Altered communication patterns; [Altered affect]; [Crying]

GRIEVING, DYSFUNCTIONAL

Diagnostic Division: Ego Integrity
> **Definition: [Delayed or exaggerated response to a perceived, actual, or potential loss.]**

RELATED FACTORS
Actual or perceived object loss (*object loss* is used in the broadest sense). Objects include people, possessions, a job, status, home, ideals, parts and processes of the body [e.g., amputation, paralysis, chronic/fatal illness]; [Thwarted grieving response to a loss]; [Lack of resolution of previous grieving response]; Absence of anticipatory grieving

DEFINING CHARACTERISTICS

Subjective
Verbal expression of distress at loss
Expression of unresolved issues
Idealization of lost object
Denial of loss
Anger
Sadness

Alterations in eating habits, sleep and dream patterns, activity levels, libido
Reliving of past experiences
Expression of guilt
[Hopelessness]

Objective
Crying; Difficulty in expressing loss; Interference with life functioning; Developmental regression; Labile affect; Alterations in concentration and/or pursuits of tasks; [Isolation]

GROWTH AND DEVELOPMENT, ALTERED

Diagnostic Division: Teaching/Learning
  Definition: [The state in which an individual demonstrates deviations in norms from his/her age group.]

RELATED FACTORS
Inadequate caretaking; Indifference, inconsistent responsiveness, multiple caretakers; Separation from significant others; Environmental and stimulation deficiencies; Effects of physical disability [handicapping condition]; Prescribed dependence [insufficient expectations for self-care]; [Physical/emotional neglect abuse]

DEFINING CHARACTERISTICS

Subjective
Delay or difficulty in performing skills (motor, social, or expressive) typical of age group; Altered physical growth; Inability to perform self-care or self-control activities appropriate for age; Loss of previously acquired skills; precocious or accelerated skill attainment

Objective
Flat affect; Listlessness, decreased responses

HEALTH MAINTENANCE, ALTERED

Diagnostic Division: Safety
  Definition: Inability to identify, manage, and/or seek out help to maintain health. [This diagnosis contains components of other nursing diagnoses. We recommend subsuming health maintenance interventions under the "basic" nursing diagnosis when a single causative factor is identified, e.g., Knowledge Deficit; Communication, impaired verbal; Thought Processes, altered; Individual/Family Coping, ineffective]

RELATED FACTORS
Lack of or significant alteration in communication skills (written, verbal, and/or gestural)
Complete or partial lack of gross and/or fine motor skills
Unachieved developmental tasks
Lack of ability to make deliberate and thoughtful judgments

Perceptual or cognitive impairment
Ineffective individual coping; dysfunctional grieving
Lack of material resource
Ineffective family coping: disabling spiritual distress

DEFINING CHARACTERISTICS

Subjective
Expressed interest in improving health behaviors; Reported or observed lack of equipment, financial, and/or other resources; Reported or observed impairment of personal support system

Objective

Demonstrated lack of knowledge regarding basic health practices; Reported or observed inability to take the responsibility for meeting basic health practices in any or all functional pattern areas; Demonstrated lack of adaptive behaviors to internal or external environmental changes; History of lack of health-seeking behavior

HEALTH-SEEKING BEHAVIORS (SPECIFY)

Diagnostic Division: Teaching/Learning
  Definition: A state in which an individual in stable health is actively seeking ways to alter personal health habits and/or the environment in order to move toward higher level of health. Stable health status is defined as age-appropriate illness prevention measures achieved, client reports good or excellent health, and signs and symptoms of disease, if present, are controlled

RELATED FACTORS

[Situation/maturation occurrence precipitating concern about current health status]

DEFINING CHARACTERISTICS

Subjective

Expressed desire to seek a higher level of wellness; Expressed desire to modify codependent behaviors; Expressed desire for increased control of health practice; Expression of concern about current environmental conditions on health status; Stated (or observed) unfamiliarity with wellness community resources

Objective

Observed desire to seek a higher level of wellness; Observed desire for increased control of health practice; Demonstrated or observed lack of knowledge in health promotion behaviors

HOME MAINTENANCE MANAGEMENT, IMPAIRED

Diagnostic Division: Safety
  Definition: Inability to independently maintain a safe, growth-promoting immediate environment.

RELATED FACTORS

Disease or injury of individual or family member
Insufficient finances
Impaired cognitive or emotional functioning
Lack of role modeling

Insufficient family organization or planning
Unfamiliarity with neighborhood resources
Lack of knowledge
Inadequate support systems

DEFINING CHARACTERISTICS

Subjective

Household members express difficulty in maintaining their home in a comfortable fashion; Household requests assistance with home maintenance; Household members describe outstanding debts or financial crises

Objective

Disorderly surroundings
Accumulation of dirt, food or hygienic wastes
Inappropriate household temperature
Lack of necessary equipment or aids
Presence of vermin or rodents
Unwashed or unavailable cooking equipment, clothes, or linen

Offensive odors
Overtaxed family members, e.g., exhausted, anxious
Repeated hygienic disorders, infestations, or infections

2561

HOPELESSNESS

Diagnostic Division: Ego Integrity
Definition: A subjective state in which an individual sees limited or no alternatives or personal choices available and is unable to mobilize energy on own behalf.

RELATED FACTORS
Prolonged activity restriction, creating isolation; Failing or deteriorating physiologic condition; Long-term stress; Abandonment; Lost belief in transcendent values/God

DEFINING CHARACTERISTICS

Subjective
Verbal cues (despondent content, "I can't," sighing)

Objective
Passivity, decreased verbalization; Decreased affect; Lack of initiative; Decreased response to stimuli; Turning away from speaker; Closing eyes; Shrugging in response to speaker; Decreased appetite, increased/decreased sleep; Lack of involvement in care/passively allowing care; Withdrawal from environs; [Lack of involvement/interest in significant other(s) (children, spouse)]

HYPERTHERMIA

Diagnostic Division: Safety
Definition: A state in which an individual's body temperature is elevated above his/her normal range.

RELATED FACTORS
Exposure to hot environment; Vigorous activity; Medications/anesthesia; Inappropriate clothing; Increased metabolic rate, illness or trauma; Dehydration; Inability or decreased ability to perspire

DEFINING CHARACTERISTICS

Subjective
Increase in body temperature above normal range; [Headache]

Objective
Flushed skin, warm to touch [Muscle rigidity]
Increased respiratory rate, tachycardia [Muscle fasciculations]
Seizures/convulsions [Confusion]
[Unstable blood pressure]

HYPOTHERMIA

Diagnostic Division: Safety
Definition: The state in which an individual's body temperature is reduced below normal range.

RELATED FACTORS
Exposure to cool or cold environment [prolonged exposure, immersion in cold water/near drowning, artificial hypothermia/cardiopulmonary bypass]; Inadequate clothing; Evaporation from skin in cool environment; Inability or decreased ability to shiver; Aging [or very young]; [Debilitating] illness or trauma, damage to hypothalamus; Malnutrition; Decreased metabolic rate, Inactivity; Consumption of alcohol; Medications causing vasodilation; [Vasodilation, e.g., sepsis, drug overdose]

DEFINING CHARACTERISTICS

Objective
Reduction in body temperature below normal range; Shivering (mild); Cool skin; Pallor (moderate); Slow capillary refill; Cyanotic nail beds; Hypertension; Tachycardia; Piloerection; [Core temperature 95 °F/35 °C: decreased pulse, increased respiration, poor judgment, memory loss]; [Core temperature 94 to 90 °F/34.4 to 32 °C: all vital signs decreased, myocardial irritability/dysrhythmias, muscle rigidity, no shivering, obtunded]; [Core temperature 85 °F/29.5 °C: no apparent vital signs, heart rate unresponsive to drug therapy, cyanotic, dilated pupils, appears dead]

INCONTINENCE, FUNCTIONAL

Diagnostic Division: Elimination
> **Definition: The state in which an individual experiences an involuntary, unpredictable passage of urine.**

RELATED FACTORS
Altered environment [e.g., poor lighting or inability to locate bathroom]; Sensory, cognitive [e.g., inattentiveness to urge to void, use of sedation], or mobility deficits [including difficulty in removing clothes]; [Increased urine production]; [Reluctance to use call light or bedpan]

DEFINING CHARACTERISTICS

Subjective
Urge to void or bladder contractions sufficiently strong to result in loss of urine before reaching an appropriate receptacle; [Voiding in large amounts]

INCONTINENCE, REFLEX

Diagnostic Division: Elimination
> **Definition: The state in which an individual experiences an involuntary loss of urine, occurring at somewhat predictable intervals when a specific bladder volume is reached.**

RELATED FACTORS
Neurologic impairment (e.g., spinal cord lesion that interferes with conduction of cerebral messages above the level of the reflex arc); [Cerebral lesion abolishing voluntary control]

DEFINING CHARACTERISTICS

Subjective
No [or only partial] awareness of bladder filling; No urge to void or feelings of bladder fullness; [Voids in large amounts]; [Unaware of being incontinent]

Objective
Uninhibited bladder contraction/spasm at regular intervals

INCONTINENCE, STRESS

Diagnostic Division: Elimination
> **Definition: The state in which an individual experiences a loss of urine of less than 50 ml occurring with increased abdominal pressure.**

RELATED FACTORS
Degenerative changes in pelvic muscles and structural supports associated with increased age; High intra-abdominal pressure (e.g., obesity, gravid uterus); Incompetent bladder outlet; Overdistention between voidings; Weak pelvic muscles and structural supports

DEFINING CHARACTERISTICS

Subjective

Reported or observed dribbling with increased abdominal pressure [e.g., coughing, sneezing, lifting, impact aerobics, changing position]; Urinary urgency, urinary frequency (more often than every 2 hours)

INCONTINENCE, TOTAL

Diagnostic Division: Elimination

Definition: The state in which an individual experiences a continuous and unpredictable loss of urine.

RELATED FACTORS

Neuropathy preventing transmission of reflex [signals to the reflex arc] indicating bladder fullness; Neurologic dysfunction causing triggering of micturition at unpredictable times [cerebral lesions]; Independent contraction of detrusor reflex owing to surgery; Trauma or disease affecting spinal cord nerves [destruction of sensory or motor neurons below the spinal cord level]; Anatomic (fistula)

DEFINING CHARACTERISTICS

Subjective

Constant flow of urine occurs at unpredictable times without distention or uninhibited bladder contractions/spasm; Nocturia; Lack of perineal or bladder filling awareness; Unawareness of incontinence

Objective

Unsuccessful incontinence refractory treatments

INCONTINENCE, URGE

Diagnostic Division: Elimination

Definition: The state in which an individual experiences involuntary passage of urine occurring soon after a strong sense of urgency to void.

RELATED FACTORS

Decreased bladder capacity (e.g., history of PID, abdominal surgeries, indwelling urinary catheter); Irritation of bladder stretch receptors causing spasm (e.g., bladder infection); alcohol; caffeine; increased fluids; increased urine concentration; overdistention of bladder

DEFINING CHARACTERISTICS

Subjective

Urinary urgency; Frequency (voiding more often than every 2 hours; Bladder contracture/spasm; Nocturia (more than two times per night)

Objective

Inability to reach toilet in time; Voiding in small amounts (less than 100 ml) or in large amounts (more than 550 ml)

INFECTION, HIGH RISK FOR

Diagnostic Division: Safety

Definition: The state in which an individual is at increased risk for being invaded by pathogenic organisms.

RISK FACTORS

Inadequate primary defenses (broken skin, traumatized tissue, decrease of ciliary action, stasis of body fluids, change in pH secretions, altered peristalsis)

Inadequate secondary defenses (e.g., decreased hemoglobin, leukopenia, suppressed inflammatory response) and immunosuppression

Inadequate acquired immunity; tissue destruction and increased environmental exposure

Chronic disease
Invasive procedures
Malnutrition
Pharmaceutical agents
Rupture of amniotic membranes
Insufficient knowledge to avoid exposure to pathogens

INJURY, HIGH RISK FOR

Diagnostic Division: Safety

Definition: A state in which the individual is at risk of injury as a result of environmental conditions interacting with the individual's adaptive and defensive resources. [Note: The potential for injury differs from individual to individual, and situation to situation. It is our belief that the environment is not safe, and there is no way to list everything that might present a danger to someone. Rather, we believe nurses have the responsibility to educate people throughout their life cycles to live safely in their environment.]

RISK FACTORS

Internal

Biochemical, regulatory function: (sensory, integrative, effector dysfunction; tissue hypoxia), immune-autoimmune; malnutrition; abnormal blood profile, (leukocytosis/leukopenia; altered clotting factors; thrombocytopenia; sickle cell, thalassemia; decreased hemoglobin); Physical: (broken skin, altered mobility); development age; (physiologic, psychosocial); Psychologic: (affective, orientation)

External

Biologic: (immunization level of community, microorganism); Chemical: (pollutants, poisons, drugs, pharmaceutical agents, alcohol, caffeine, nicotine, preservatives, cosmetics, and dyes), nutrients (vitamins, food types); Physical: (design, structure, and arrangement of community, building and/or equipment); move of transport/transportation; People-provider: (nosocomial agent; staffing patterns; cognitive, affective, and psychomotor factors)

KNOWLEDGE DEFICIT [LEARNING NEED] (SPECIFY)

Diagnostic Division: Teaching/Learning

Definition: [Lack of specific information necessary for patient/significant other(s) to make informed choices regarding condition/therapies/treatment plan.]

RELATED FACTORS

Lack of exposure
Information misinterpretation
Unfamiliarity with information resources
Lack of recall

Cognitive limitation
Lack of interest in learning
[Patient's request for no information]
[Inaccurate/incomplete information presented]

DEFINING CHARACTERISTICS

Subjective

Verbalization of the problem; [Statement of misconception]; [Request for information]

Objective

Inaccurate follow-through of instruction; Inadequate performance of test; Inappropriate or exaggerated behaviors, e.g., hysterical, hostile, agitated, apathetic; [Development of preventable complication]

NONCOMPLIANCE [COMPLIANCE, ALTERED] (SPECIFY)

Diagnostic Division: Teaching/Learning
   Definition: A person's informed decision not to adhere to a therapeutic recommendation.
   [Note: Noncompliance is a term that may create a negative situation for patient and caregiver that may foster difficulties in resolving the causative factors. Because patients have
   a right to refuse therapy, we see this as a situation in which the professional need is to
   accept the patient's point of view/behavior/choice(s) and to work together to find alternate means to meet original and/or revised goals.]

RELATED FACTORS
Patient value system: health beliefs, spiritual values, cultural influences; Patient and provider relationships; [Fear/anxiety]

DEFINING CHARACTERISTICS

Subjective
Statements by patient or significant others [e.g., unwillingness to follow treatment regimen]

Objective
Behavior indicative of failure to adhere by direct observation; Objective tests (physiologic measures,
   detection of markers); Evidence of development of complications; Failure to keep appointments; Evidence of exacerbation of symptoms; Failure to progress; [Inability to set or to attain mutual goals]

NUTRITION, ALTERED: LESS THAN BODY REQUIREMENTS

Diagnostic Division: Food/Fluid
   **Definition: The state in which an individual experiences an intake of nutrients insuffi-
   cient to meet metabolic needs.**

RELATED FACTORS
Inability to ingest or to digest food or to absorb nutrients because of biologic, psychologic, or economic
   factors; [Intake insufficient to meet metabolic demands]

DEFINING CHARACTERISTICS

Subjective
Reported inadequate food intake less than RDA	Lack of interest in food
Reported or evidence of lack of food	Perceived inability to ingest food
Aversion to eating	Satiety immediately after ingesting food
Reported altered taste sensation	Abdominal cramping
Abdominal pain with or without pathologic con-	Lack of information; misinformation; miscon-
ditions	ceptions

Objective
Body weight 20% or more under ideal for [height and frame]	Hyperactive bowel sounds
	Diarrhea and/or steatorrhea
Loss of weight with adequate food intake	Pale conjunctiva and mucous membranes
Poor muscle tone	Excessive loss of hair [or increased growth of hair
Weakness of muscles required for swallowing or	on body (lanugo)]
mastication	[Decreased subcutaneous fat/muscle mass]
Sore, inflamed buccal cavity	[Cessation of menses]
Capillary fragility	

NUTRITION, ALTERED: MORE THAN BODY REQUIREMENTS

Diagnostic Division: Food/Fluid
   **Definition: The state in which an individual is experiencing an intake of nutrients which
   exceeds metabolic needs.**

RELATED FACTORS

Excessive intake in relationship to metabolic need; [Underlying cause is often complex and may be difficult to diagnose/treat]

DEFINING CHARACTERISTICS

Subjective

Reported dysfunctional eating patterns: Pairing food with other activities; Eating in response to external cues such as time of day, social situation; Concentrating food intake at end of day; Eating in response to internal cues other than hunger, e.g., anxiety; Sedentary activity level

Objective

Weight 10% to 20% over ideal for height and frame; Triceps skinfold greater than 15 mm in men and 25 mm in women; Observed dysfunctional eating patterns [as noted in Subjective]; [Percentage of body fat greater than 18% to 20% for trim women; 10% to 12% for trim men]

NUTRITION, ALTERED: HIGH RISK FOR MORE THAN BODY REQUIREMENTS

Diagnostic Division: Food/Fluid

Definition: The state in which an individual is at risk of experiencing an intake of nutrients that exceeds metabolic needs.

RISK FACTORS

Reported/observed obesity in one or both parents [/spouse; hereditary predisposition]; Rapid transition across growth percentiles in infants or children [adolescence]; Reported use of solid food as major food source before 5 months of age; Reported/observed higher baseline weight at beginning of each pregnancy; Dysfunctional eating patterns: pairing food with other activities, eating in response to external cues such as time of day or social situation, concentrating food intake at end of day, eating in response to internal cues other than hunger, e.g., anxiety; Observed use of food as reward or comfort measure; [Socially/culturally isolated; lacking other outlets]; [Alteration in usual activity patterns/sedentary lifestyle]; [Alteration in usual coping patterns]; [Majority of foods consumed are concentrated, high-calorie sources]; [Significant/sudden decline in financial resources; lower socioeconomic status]

ORAL MUCOUS MEMBRANE, ALTERED

Diagnostic Division: Food/Fluid

Definition: The state in which the individual experiences disruptions in the tissue layers of the oral cavity.

RELATED FACTORS

Pathologic conditions: oral cavity (radiation to head and/or neck)

Trauma: Chemical, e.g., acidic foods, drugs, noxious agents, alcohol

Trauma: Mechanical, e.g., ill-fitting dentures, braces, tubes (endotracheal, nasogastric), surgery in oral cavity

Dehydration

NPO instructions for more than 24 hours

Malnutrition

Lack of or decreased salivation

Ineffective oral hygiene

Mouth breathing

Infection

Medication

DEFINING CHARACTERISTICS

Subjective

Xerostomia (dry mouth); Oral pain or discomfort

Objective	
Coated tongue	Oral lesions or ulcers
Stomatitis	Lack of or decreased salivation
Leukoplakia	Edema
Hyperemia	Oral plaque
Desquamation	Vesicles
Hemorrhagic gingivitis	Carious teeth
Halitosis	

PAIN [ACUTE]

Diagnostic Division: Pain/Comfort
> **Definition: [A state in which an individual experiences and reports the presence of severe discomfort or an uncomfortable sensation.]**

RELATED FACTORS
Injuring agents: biologic, chemical, physical, psychologic

DEFINING CHARACTERISTICS

Subjective
Communication (verbal or coded) of pain descriptors; [Expect fewer complaints from patients under 40, males, some cultural groups]; [Pain unrelieved and/or increased beyond tolerance]

Objective
Self-focusing

Narrowed focus (altered time perception, withdrawal from social contact, impaired thought process)

Alteration in muscle tone (may span from listless to rigid)

Facial mask of pain (eyes lack luster, "beaten look," fixed or scattered movement, grimace)

Distraction behavior (moaning, crying, pacing, seeking out other people and/or activities, restlessness)

Autonomic responses not seen in chronic, stable pain (diaphoresis, blood pressure and pulse rate changes, pupillary dilation, increased or decreased respiratory rate)

Guarding behavior; protective

[Fear/panic]

PAIN, CHRONIC

Diagnostic Division: Pain/Comfort
> **Definition: A state in which the individual experiences pain that continues for more than 6 months. [Pain is a signal that something is wrong and chronic pain is a learned form of behavior. It is a complex, separate entity, combining elements from other NDs: Powerlessness; Diversional Activity, altered; Family Processes, altered; Self-Care Deficit, etc.]**

RELATED FACTORS
Chronic physical/psychosocial disability

DEFINING CHARACTERISTICS

Subjective
Verbal report of pain experienced for more than 6 months; Fear of reinjury; Altered ability to continue previous activities; Anorexia, weight changes; Changes in sleep patterns; [Preoccupation with pain]; [Desperately seeks alternative solutions/therapies for relief/control of pain]

Objective
Observed evidence of pain experienced for more than 6 months; Physical and social withdrawal; Facial mask, guarded movement

PARENTAL ROLE CONFLICT

Diagnostic Division: Social Interaction
Definition: The state in which a parent experiences role confusion and conflict in response to crisis.

RELATED FACTORS

Separation from child due to chronic illness; Intimidation with invasive or restrictive modalities (e.g., isolation, intubation), specialized care centers, policies; Home care of a child with special needs (e.g., apnea monitoring, postural drainage, hyperalimentation); Change in marital status; Interruptions of family life due to home care regimen (treatments, caregiver's lack of respite)

DEFINING CHARACTERISTICS

Subjective

Parent(s) express concerns/feelings of inadequacy to provide for child's physical and emotional needs during hospitalization or in the home; Parent(s) express concerns about changes in parental role, family functioning, family communication, family health; Parent(s) express concern about perceived loss of control over decisions relating to their child; Parent(s) verbalize feelings of guilt, anger, fear, anxiety, and/or frustration about effect of child's illness on family process.

Objective

Demonstrated disruption in caretaking routines; Reluctance to participate in usual caretaking activities, even with encouragement and support; Demonstrated feelings of guilt, anger, fear, anxiety, and/or frustration about effect of child's illness on family process

---

PARENTING, ALTERED

Diagnostic Division: Social Interaction
Definition: The state in which a nurturing figure(s) experiences an inability to create an environment which promotes the optimum growth and development of another human being. (It is important to state as a preface to this diagnosis that adjustment to parenting in general is a normal maturational process that elicits nursing behaviors of prevention of potential problems and health promotion.)

RELATED FACTORS

Lack of available role model/ineffective role model; Lack of support between/from significant other(s); Interruption in bonding process, e.g., maternal, paternal, other; Mental and/or physical illness; Lack of knowledge; Limited cognitive functioning; Multiple pregnancies; Unrealistic expectation for self, infant, partner; Physical and psychosocial abuse of nurturing figure; Unmet social/emotional maturation needs of parenting figures; Perceived threat to own survival, physical and emotional; Presence of stress (financial, legal, recent crisis, cultural move [e.g., from another country, nationality]); Lack of role identity; Lack of appropriate response of child to relationship

DEFINING CHARACTERISTICS

Subjective

Verbalization cannot control child; Constant verbalization of disappointment in gender or physical characteristics of the infant/child; Verbalization of resentment toward the infant/child; Verbalization of role inadequacy [inability to care for/discipline child]; Verbal disgust at body functions of infant/child; Verbalizes desire to have child call him/her by first name versus traditional cultural tendencies

Objective

Abandonment; Runaway; Incidence of physical and psychologic trauma; Inattention to infant/child needs; Inappropriate caretaking behaviors (toilet training, sleep/rest, feeding); History of child abuse or abandonment by primary caretaker; Lack of parental attachment behaviors: inappropriate visual/tactile/auditory stimulation, negative identification of infant/child characteristics, negative attachment of meanings to infant/child characteristics, noncompliance with health appointments for self and/or infant/child; Inappropriate or inconsistent discipline practices; Frequent accidents/illness; Growth and development lag in the child; Child receives care from multiple caretakers without consideration for the needs of the infant/child; Compulsive seeking of role approval from others

PARENTING, ALTERED, HIGH RISK FOR

Diagnostic Division: Social Interaction
   Definition: The state in which a nurturing figure(s) is at risk to experience an inability to create an environment which promotes the optimum growth and development of another human being. (It is important to state as a preface to this diagnosis that adjustment to parenting in general is a normal maturational process that elicits nursing behaviors of prevention of potential problems and health promotion.)

RISK FACTORS
Lack of available model/ineffective role model; Lack of support between/from significant other(s); Interruption in bonding process, e.g., maternal, paternal, other; Mental and/or physical illness; Lack of knowledge; Limited cognitive functioning; Multiple pregnancies; Unrealistic expectation for self, infant, partner; Physical and psychosocial abuse of nurturing figure; Unmet social/emotional maturation needs of parenting figures; Perceived threat to own survival, physical and emotional; Presence of stress (financial, legal, recent crisis, culture move [e.g., from another country, nationality]); Lack of role identity; Lack of appropriate response of child to relationship

PERSONAL IDENTITY DISTURBANCE

Diagnostic Division: Ego Integrity
   Definition: Inability to distinguish between self and nonself.

RELATED FACTORS
To be developed by NANDA: [Organic brain syndrome]; [Poor ego differentiation, as in schizophrenia]; [Panic/dissociative states]; [Biochemical body change]

DEFINING CHARACTERISTICS (To be developed by NANDA)

Subjective
[Confusion about sense of self, purpose or direction in life, sexual identification/preference]

Objective
[Difficulty in making decisions]; [Poorly differentiated ego boundaries]

PHYSICAL MOBILITY, IMPAIRED

Diagnostic Division: Safety
   Definition: A state in which the individual experiences a limitation of ability for independent physical movement.

RELATED FACTORS
Intolerance to activity/decreased strength and endurance; Pain/discomfort; Neuromuscular/musculoskeletal impairment; Perceptual/cognitive impairment; Depression/severe anxiety; [Restrictive therapies/safety precautions, e.g., bed rest, limb immobilization]

DEFINING CHARACTERISTICS

Subjective
Reluctance to attempt movement; [Complaints of pain/discomfort on movement]

Objective
Inability to purposefully move within the physical environment, including bed mobility, transfer, and ambulation; Impaired coordination; Limited range of motion; Decreased muscle strength, control, and/or mass; Imposed restrictions of movement, including mechanical; medical protocol

POISONING, HIGH RISK FOR

Diagnostic Division: Safety
Definition: Accentuated risk of accidental exposure to or ingestion of drugs or dangerous products in doses sufficient to cause poisoning.

RISK FACTORS

Internal (individual)
Reduced vision; Lack of safety or drug education; Lack of proper precaution; Insufficient finances; Verbalization of occupational setting without adequate safeguards; Cognitive or emotional difficulties

External (environmental)
Large supplies of drugs in house

Dangerous products placed or stored within the reach of children or confused persons

Flaking, peeling paint or plaster in presence of young children

Paint, lacquer, etc., in poorly ventilated areas or without effective protection

Medicines stored in unlocked cabinets accessible to children or confused persons

Availability of illicit drugs potentially contaminated by poisonous additives

Chemical contamination of food and water

Unprotected contact with heavy metals or chemicals

Presence of poisonous vegetation

Presence of atmospheric pollutants

POST-TRAUMA RESPONSE

Diagnostic Division: Ego Integrity
Definition: The state of an individual's experiencing a sustained painful response to an overwhelming traumatic event.

RELATED FACTORS
Disasters [e.g., floods, earthquakes, tornadoes, airplane crashes], wars, epidemics, rape, assault, torture, catastrophic illness or accident, [being held hostage]

DEFINING CHARACTERISTICS

Subjective
Reexperience of the traumatic event which may be identified in cognitive, affective, and/or sensory motor activities (flashbacks, intrusive thoughts, repetitive dreams or nightmares, excessive verbalization of the traumatic event, verbalization of survival guilt or guilt about behavior required for survival); [Somatic reactions: chronic pains, nausea, changes in appetite, skeletal/muscle tension, exaggerated startle response, sensitivity to noise, insomnia, headaches, dizziness, unsteadiness, chronic fatigue and easy fatigability, sleep disturbance]

Objective
Psychic/emotional numbness (impaired interpretation of reality, confusion, dissociation or amnesia, vagueness about traumatic event, constricted affect); Altered lifestyle (self-destructiveness such as substance abuse, suicide attempt, or other acting-out behavior); difficulty with interpersonal relationships [loss of interest in usual activities, detachment, loss of feeling of intimacy/sexuality]; development of phobia regarding trauma; poor impulse control/irritability and explosiveness; [Disturbance of mood, e.g., depression, anxiety, embarrassment, fear, humiliation, self-blame, low self-esteem, fear of violence toward self or others]; [Cognitive disruption: confusion, loss of memory/concentration, indecisiveness]; [Social reactions: dependence on others, work/school failure, avoidance of close relationships, social isolation]

STAGES
Acute subtype: begins within 6 months and does not last longer than 6 months; Chronic subtype: lasts more than 6 months; Delayed subtype: period of latency of 6 months or more before onset of symptoms

POWERLESSNESS

Diagnostic Division: Ego Integrity
   Definition: Perception that one's own action will not significantly affect an outcome; a perceived lack of control over a current situation or immediate happening.

RELATED FACTORS
Health care environment; Interpersonal interaction; Illness-related regimen; Lifestyle of helplessness

DEFINING CHARACTERISTICS
Subjective

SEVERE
Verbal expressions of having no control or influence over situation, outcome, or self-care; Depression over physical deterioration that occurs despite patient compliance with regimens

MODERATE
Nonparticipation in care or decision making when opportunities are provided; Expressions of dissatisfaction and frustration over inability to perform previous tasks and/or activities; Expression of doubt regarding role performance; Reluctance to express true feelings, fearing alienation from caregivers

LOW
Expressions of uncertainty about fluctuating energy levels

Objective

SEVERE
Apathy; [Anger]; [Withdrawn]; [Resigned]; [Crying]

MODERATE
Does not monitor progress; Dependence on others that may result in irritability, resentment, anger, and guilt; Inability to seek information regarding care; Does not defend self-care practices when challenged; Passivity

LOW
Passivity

PROTECTION, ALTERED

Diagnostic Division: Safety
   Definition: The state in which an individual experiences a decrease in the ability to guard the self from internal or external threats such as illness or injury.

RELATED FACTORS
Extremes of age; Inadequate nutrition; Alcohol abuse; Abnormal blood profiles (leukopenia, thrombocytopenia, anemia, coagulation); Drug therapies (antineoplastic, corticosteroid, immune, anticoagulant, thrombolytic); Treatments (surgery, radiation); Diseases (e.g., cancer and immune disorders)

DEFINING CHARACTERISTICS
Subjective
Neurosensory alterations; Chilling; Itching; Insomnia; Fatigue; Weakness; Anorexia

Objective
Deficient immunity; Impaired healing; Altered clotting; Maladaptive stress response; Perspiring; Dyspnea; Cough; Restlessness; Immobility; Disorientation; Pressure sores

[*Note:* The purpose of this diagnosis seems to be to provide for the combining of multiple diagnoses under a single heading for ease of planning care when a number of variables may be present.]

RAPE TRAUMA SYNDROME

Diagnostic Division: Ego Integrity

Definition: Rape is forced and violent sexual penetration against the victim's will and without the victim's consent. The trauma syndrome that develops from an attack or attempted attack includes an acute phase of disorganization of the victim's lifestyle and a long-term process of reorganization of lifestyle. This syndrome includes the following three subcomponents: A, B, and C. [*NOTE:* While attacks are most often directed toward women, men also may be victims.]

DEFINING CHARACTERISTICS

A: Rape Trauma

ACUTE PHASE

Emotional reactions: anger, fear of physical violence and death, self-blame, embarrassment, humiliation, revenge; Multiple physical symptoms: muscle tension, sleep pattern disturbance

LONG-TERM PHASE

Changes in lifestyle (changes in residence; dealing with repetitive nightmares and phobias; seeking family support; seeking social network support)

B: Compound Reaction

All defining characteristics listed under A: Rape Trauma; Reactivated symptoms of previous conditions, e.g., physical illness, psychiatric illness; Reliance on alcohol and/or drugs

C: Silent Reaction

Abrupt changes in relationship with men; Increase in nightmares; Increasing anxiety during interview, e.g., blocking of associations, long periods of silence, minor stuttering, physical distress; Marked changes in sexual behavior; No verbalization of the occurrence of rape; Sudden onset of phobic reactions

ROLE PERFORMANCE, ALTERED

Diagnostic Division: Ego Integrity

Definition: Disruption in the way one perceives one's role performance.

RELATED FACTORS

To be developed by NANDA: [Crisis]; [Situational, e.g., male head of household is in a passive, dependent patient role]; [Developmental]; and/or [Health-illness, e.g., chronic illness]

DEFINING CHARACTERISTICS

Subjective

Change in self-perception of role; Denial of role; Lack of knowledge of role

Objective

Change in others' perception of role; Change in usual patterns of responsibility; Conflict in roles; Change in physical capacity to resume role; [Failure to assume role]

SELF-CARE DEFICIT: FEEDING, BATHING/HYGIENE, DRESSING/GROOMING, TOILETING

Diagnostic Division: Hygiene

Definition: A state in which the individual experiences an impaired ability to perform or to complete feeding, bathing, toileting, dressing, and grooming activities for oneself (on a temporary, permanent, or progressing basis). [*NOTE:* Self-care also may be expanded to include the practices used by the client to promote health, the individual responsibility for self, a way of thinking. Refer to Home Maintenance Management, impaired; Health Maintenance, altered.]

RELATED FACTORS

Intolerance to activity, decreased strength and endurance; Neuromuscular impairment; Depression; severe anxiety; Pain, discomfort; Perceptual or cognitive impairment; Musculoskeletal impairment

DEFINING CHARACTERISTICS

A. SELF-FEEDING DEFICIT

Inability to bring food from a receptacle to the mouth

B. SELF-BATHING/HYGIENE

Inability to wash body or body parts; to obtain or to get to water source; to regulate temperature or flow

C. SELF-DRESSING/GROOMING DEFICIT

Impaired ability to put on or to take off necessary items of clothing; to obtain or to replace articles of clothing; to fasten clothing; to maintain appearance at a satisfactory level

D. SELF-TOILETING DEFICIT

Related Factors (in addition to those previously noted): Impaired transfer ability; Intolerance to activity; decreased strength and endurance; Impaired mobility status

Defining Characteristics (Objective): Unable to get to toilet or commode; Unable to manipulate clothing for toileting; Unable to set on or rise from toilet or commode; Unable to carry out proper toilet hygiene; Unable to flush toilet or empty commode

---

SELF-ESTEEM, CHRONIC LOW

Diagnostic Division: Ego Integrity
Definition: Longstanding negative self-evaluation/feelings about self or self-capabilities.

RELATED FACTORS

[Continual negative evaluation of self/capabilities during childhood]; [Personal vulnerability]; [Life choices perpetuating failure]

DEFINING CHARACTERISTICS

Subjective

Longstanding or chronic: self-negating verbalization; Expressions of shame/guilt; Evaluates self as unable to deal with events; Rationalizes away/rejects positive feedback and exaggerates negative feedback about self

Objective

Hesitant to try new things/situations; Frequent lack of success in work or other life events; Overly conforming; Dependent on others' opinions; Lack of eye contact; Nonassertive/passive; Indecisive; Excessively seeks reassurance

---

SELF-ESTEEM DISTURBANCE

Diagnostic Division: Ego Integrity
Definition: Negative self-evaluation/feeling about self or self-capabilities which may be directly or indirectly expressed. [A human need for survival.]

RELATED FACTORS

["Failure" at life events, e.g., loss of job, divorce]; [Aging]

DEFINING CHARACTERISTICS

Subjective

Self-negating verbalization; Evaluates self as unable to deal with events; Expressions of shame/guilt; Rationalizes away/rejects positive feedback and exaggerates negative feedback about self; [Inability to accept positive reinforcement]

Objective

Hesitant to try new things/situations; Hypersensitive to slight or criticism; Grandiosity; Denial of problems obvious to others; Projection of blame/responsibility for problems; Rationalizing personal failures; [Not taking responsibility for self-care (self-neglect)]; [Lack of follow-through]; [Nonparticipation in therapy]; [Self-destructive behavior]; [Lack of eye contact]

SELF-ESTEEM, SITUATIONAL LOW

Diagnostic Division: Ego Integrity

Definition: Negative self-evaluation/feelings about self which develop in response to a loss or change in an individual who previously had a positive self-evaluation.

RELATED FACTORS

["Failure" at life events, e.g., loss of job, divorce]; [Aging]

DEFINING CHARACTERISTICS

Subjective

Episodic occurrence of negative self-appraisal in response to life events in a person with a previous positive self-evaluation; Verbalization of negative feelings about the self (helplessness, uselessness); Self-negating verbalizations; expressions of shame/guilt; Evaluates self as unable to handle situations/events

Objective

Difficulty making decisions

SENSORY-PERCEPTUAL ALTERATIONS (SPECIFY): VISUAL; AUDITORY; KINESTHETIC; GUSTATORY; TACTILE; OLFACTORY

Diagnostic Division: Neurosensory

Definition: A state in which an individual experiences a change in the amount or patterning of incoming stimuli accompanied by a diminished, exaggerated, distorted, or impaired response to such stimuli.

RELATED FACTORS

Altered environmental stimuli, excessive or insufficient; [Therapeutically restricted environments, e.g., isolation, intensive care, bed rest, traction, confining illnesses, incubator]; [Socially restricted environment (e.g., institutionalization, homebound, aging, chronic illness, dying, infant deprivation; stigmatized (e.g., mentally ill/retarded/handicapped); bereaved]; [Excessive noise level, e.g., work environment, patient's immediate environment (ICU with support machinery, etc.)]; Altered sensory reception, transmission, and/or integration: Neurologic disease/trauma/deficit, altered status of sense organs, inability to communicate/understand/speak/respond, sleep deprivation, and/or pain [phantom limb]; Chemical alterations: endogenous (electrolyte), [elevated BUN, elevated ammonia, hypoxia], and/or exogenous (drugs, etc.) [central nervous system stimulants or depressants, mind-altering drugs]; Psychologic stress [narrowed perceptual fields caused by anxiety]

DEFINING CHARACTERISTICS

Subjective

Anxiety [panic state]; Indication of body image alteration; Reported change in sensory acuity [e.g., photosensitivity, hypoesthesia/hyperesthesia, diminished/altered sense of taste, inability to tell position of body parts, proprioception]; [Pain]

Objective

Measured change in sensory acuity; Change in problem-solving abilities; [Lack of/poor concentration]; Altered abstraction/conceptualization; [Disordered thought sequencing]; Disoriented in time, in place, or with persons; Altered communication patterns; Change in usual response to stimuli; [Rapid mood swings, exaggerated emotional responses]; Change in behavior pattern; Apathy; Restlessness, irritability; [Bizarre thinking]; [Motor incoordination; altered sense of balance, e.g., Meniere's syndrome]

Other Possible Characteristics
Complaints of fatigue; Change in muscular tension; Hallucinations; Alteration in posture; Inappropriate responses

SEXUAL DYSFUNCTION

Diagnostic Division: Sexuality (Component of Social Interaction)
  Definition: The state in which an individual experiences a change in sexual function that is viewed as unsatisfying, unrewarding, or inadequate.

RELATED FACTORS
Biopsychosocial alteration of sexuality: Ineffectual or absent role models; Vulnerability; Misinformation or lack of knowledge; Physical abuse; Values conflict; Lack of privacy; Altered body structure or function: pregnancy, recent childbirth, drugs, surgery, anomalies, disease process, trauma, radiation; Psychosocial abuse, e.g., harmful relationships; Lack of significant other; [Loss of sexual desire]; [Disruption of sexual response pattern, e.g., premature ejaculation, dyspareunia]

DEFINING CHARACTERISTICS
Subjective
Verbalization of problem; Actual or perceived limitation imposed by disease and/or therapy; Inability to achieve desired satisfaction; Alterations in achieving perceived sex role; Conflicts involving values; Alterations in achieving sexual satisfaction; Seeking of confirmation of desirability

Objective
Alteration in relationship with significant other; Change of interest in self and others

SEXUALITY PATTERNS, ALTERED

Diagnostic Division: Sexuality (Component of Social Interaction)
  Definition: The state in which an individual expresses concern regarding his/her sexuality.

RELATED FACTORS
Knowledge/skill deficit about alternative responses to health-related transitions, altered body function or structure, illness or medical treatment; Lack of privacy; Lack of significant other; Ineffective or absent role models; Conflicts with sexual orientation or variant preferences; Fear of pregnancy or of acquiring a sexually transmitted disease; Impaired relationship with a significant other

DEFINING CHARACTERISTICS
Subjective
Reported difficulties, limitations, or changes in sexual behaviors or activities

SKIN INTEGRITY, IMPAIRED

Diagnostic Division: Safety
  Definition: A state in which the individual's skin is adversely altered. [An interruption in the integumentary system, the largest, multifunctional organ of the body.]

RELATED FACTORS
External (Environmental)
Hyperthermia or hypothermia; Chemical substance; Radiation; Physical immobilization; Humidity; Mechanical factors (shearing forces, pressure, restraint); [Excretions/secretions]; [Trauma: injury/surgery]

Internal (Somatic)

Medication; Altered nutritional state (obesity, emaciation); Metabolic state; Circulation; Sensation; Pigmentation; Skeletal prominence; Developmental factors; Alterations in turgor (change in elasticity); Immunologic deficit; [Excretions/secretions]; [Psychogenic]; [Presence of edema]

DEFINING CHARACTERISTICS

Subjective

[Complaints of itching/pain/numbness of affected/surrounding area]

Objective

Disruption of skin surface; Destruction of skin layers; Invasion of body structures

---

SKIN INTEGRITY, IMPAIRED, HIGH RISK FOR

Diagnostic Division: Safety

Definition: A state in which the individual's skin is at risk of being adversely altered.

RISK FACTORS

External (Environmental)

Chemical substance; Hypothermia or hyperthermia; Radiation; Physical immobilization; Excretions and secretions; Humidity; Mechanical factors (shearing forces, pressure, restraint)

Internal (Somatic)

Medication; Alterations in nutrition state (obesity, emaciation); Metabolic state; Circulation; Sensation; Pigmentation; Skeletal prominence; Developmental factors; Alterations in skin turgor (change in elasticity); Psychogenic; Immunologic; [Presence of edema]

SLEEP PATTERN DISTURBANCE

Diagnostic Division: Activity/Rest

Definition: Disruption of sleep time which causes patient discomfort or interferes with desired lifestyle.

RELATED FACTORS

Sensory alterations: Internal factors: illness, [pain]; psychologic stress [anxiety, depression]; [inactivity]; External factors: environmental changes, [including change of work shift] hospital routine; social cues; [demands of caring for others]

DEFINING CHARACTERISTICS

Subjective

Verbal complaints of difficulty in falling asleep; Verbal complaints of not feeling well rested; Awakening earlier or later than desired; Interrupted sleep; [Falls asleep during activities]

Objective

Changes in behavior and performance: Increasing irritability, Disorientation, Listlessness, Restlessness, Lethargy; Physical signs: Mild, fleeting nystagmus, Ptosis of eyelid, Slight hand tremor, Expressionless face; Thick speech with mispronunciation and incorrect words; Dark circles under eyes; Changes in posture; Frequent yawning

---

SOCIAL INTERACTION, IMPAIRED

Diagnostic Division: Social Interaction

Definition: The state in which an individual participates in an insufficient or excessive quantity or ineffective quality of social exchange

RELATED FACTORS

Knowledge/skill deficit about ways to enhance mutuality

Communication barriers [including head injury, stroke, other neurologic conditions affecting ability to communicate]

Self-concept disturbance

Absence of available significant others or peers

Limited physical mobility [e.g., neuromuscular disease]

Therapeutic isolation

Sociocultural dissonance

Environmental barriers

Altered thought processes

DEFINING CHARACTERISTICS

Subjective

Verbalized discomfort in social situations; Verbalized inability to receive or communicate a satisfying sense of belonging, caring, interest, or shared history; Family report of change of style or pattern of interaction

Objective

Observed discomfort in social situations; Observed inability to receive or communicate a satisfying sense of belonging, caring, interest, or shared history; Observed use of unsuccessful social interaction behaviors; Dysfunctional interaction with peers, family, and/or others

---

SOCIAL ISOLATION

Diagnostic Division: Social Interaction

Definition: Aloneness experienced by the individual and perceived as imposed by others and as a negative or threatened state.

RISK FACTORS

Factors contributing to the absence of satisfying personal relationships, such as the following:

Delay in accomplishing developmental tasks

Alterations in mental status

Altered state of wellness

Immature interests

Alterations in physical appearance

Unaccepted social behavior

Unaccepted social values

Inadequate personal resources

Inability to engage in satisfying personal relationships

[Traumatic incidents or events]

DEFINING CHARACTERISTICS

Subjective

Expresses feeling of aloneness imposed by others

Expresses values acceptable to subculture, but unable to accept values of dominant culture

Inability to meet expectations of others

Expresses feelings of rejection

Experiences feelings of difference from others

Inadequacy in or absence of significant purpose in life

Expresses interests inappropriate to developmental age or stage

Insecurity in public

Objective

Sad, dull affect

Absence of supportive significant other(s) — family, friends, group

Evidence of physical and/or mental handicap or altered state of wellness

Uncommunicative, withdrawn; no eye contact

Preoccupation with own thoughts; repetitive, meaningless actions

Inappropriate or immature interest and activities for developmental age or stage

Projects hostility in voice, behavior

Seeks to be alone or exists in subculture

Shows behavior unaccepted by dominant cultural group

SPIRITUAL DISTRESS (DISTRESS OF THE HUMAN SPIRIT)

Diagnostic Division: Ego Integrity

Definition: Disruption in the life principle that pervades a person's entire being and that integrates and transcends one's biologic and psychosocial nature.

2578

RELATED FACTORS

Separation from religious and cultural ties; Challenged belief and value system, e.g., result of moral or ethical implications of therapy or result of intense suffering

DEFINING CHARACTERISTICS

Subjective

Expresses concern with meaning of life and death and/or belief systems

Verbalizes inner conflict about beliefs; concern about relationship with deity

Questions moral and ethical implications of therapeutic regimen

Description of nightmares or sleep disturbances

[Unable to accept self]

Engages in self-blame

[Description of somatic complaints]

Anger toward God (as defined by the person)

Questions meaning of suffering

Questions meaning for own existence

Seeks spiritual assistance

Unable to choose [or chooses not] to participate in usual religious practices

Displacement of anger toward religious representatives

[Regards illness as punishment]

Does not experience that God is forgiving

Denies responsibilities for problems

Objective

Alteration in behavior or mood evidenced by anger, crying, withdrawal, preoccupation, anxiety, hostility, apathy, etc.; Gallows humor

---

SUFFOCATION, HIGH RISK FOR

Diagnostic Division: Safety

Definition: Accentuated risk of accidental suffocation (inadequate air available for inhalation).

RISK FACTORS

Internal (individual)

Reduced olfactory sensation; Reduced motor abilities; Lack of safety education, precautions; Cognitive or emotional difficulties [altered consciousness]; Disease or injury process

External (environmental)

Pillow placed in an infant's crib

Vehicle warming in closed garage

Children playing with plastic bags or inserting small objects into their mouths or noses

Discarded or unused refrigerators or freezers without removed doors

Children left unattended in bathtubs or pools

Household gas leaks

Smoking in bed

Use of fuel-burning heaters not vented to outside

Low-strung clothesline

Pacifier hung around infant's head

Eating of large mouthfuls of food

Propped bottle placed in an infant's crib

SWALLOWING, IMPAIRED

Diagnostic Division: Food/Fluid

Definition: The state in which an individual has decreased ability to voluntarily pass fluids and/or solids from the mouth to the stomach.

RELATED FACTORS

Neuromuscular impairment (e.g., decreased or absent gag reflex, decreased strength or excursion of muscles involved in mastication [and swallowing], perceptual impairment [decreased sensation in oral cavity], facial paralysis); Mechanical obstruction (e.g., edema, tracheostomy tube, tumor); Fatigue; Limited awareness; Reddened, irritated oropharyngeal cavity

DEFINING CHARACTERISTICS

Objective
Observed evidence of difficulty in swallowing (e.g., stasis of food in oral cavity [pocketing/squirreling of food, food sticking], coughing/choking); [drooling, stranding phlegm, swallowing incoordination — repeated swallows, nasal regurgitation, wet/hoarse voice]; Evidence of aspiration, [foamy phlegm]; [Facial droop, difficulty chewing]

THERMOREGULATION, INEFFECTIVE

Diagnostic Division: Safety
Definition: The state in which the individual's temperature fluctuates between hypothermia and hyperthermia.

RELATED FACTORS
Trauma or illness [e.g., cerebral edema, cerebrovascular accident, intracranial surgery, or head injury]; Immaturity, aging [e.g., loss/absence of brown adipose tissue]; Fluctuating environmental temperature; [Changes in temperature of hypothalamic tissue, causing alterations in emission of thermosensitive cells and regulation of heat loss/production]; [Changes in level/action of thyroxine and catecholamines]; [Changes in metabolic rate/activity]; [Chemical reactions in contracting muscles]

DEFINING CHARACTERISTICS

Objective
Fluctuations in body temperature above or below the normal range; See also defining characteristics present in hypothermia and hyperthermia

THOUGHT PROCESSES, ALTERED

Diagnostic Division: Neurosensory
Definition: A state in which an individual experiences a disruption in cognitive operations and activities.

RELATED FACTORS
To be developed by NANDA: [Physiologic changes]; [Sleep deprivation]; [Psychologic conflicts]

DEFINING CHARACTERISTICS

Subjective
[Ideas of reference, hallucinations, delusions]

Objective
Inaccurate interpretation of environment; Memory deficit/problems [disorientation to time, place, person, circumstances, and events]; Hypervigilance/hypovigilance; Cognitive dissonance, [Decreased ability to grasp ideas, make decisions, problem-solve, reason, abstract or conceptualize, calculate]; Distractibility [altered attention span]; Egocentricity; [Confabulation]; [Inappropriate social behavior]

Other Possible Characteristics
Inappropriate/nonreality-based thinking

TISSUE INTEGRITY, IMPAIRED

Diagnostic Division: Safety
Definition: A state in which an individual experiences damage to mucous membrane or corneal, integumentary, or subcutaneous tissue.

RELATED FACTORS

Altered circulation
Nutritional deficit/excess
Fluid deficit/excess
Knowledge deficit
Impaired physical mobility

Irritants, chemical (including body excretions, secretions, medications)
Thermal (temperature extremes)
Mechanical (pressure, shear, friction), radiation (including therapeutic radiation)

DEFINING CHARACTERISTICS

Objective
Damaged or destroyed tissue (cornea, mucous membrane, integumentary, or subcutaneous)

TISSUE PERFUSION, ALTERED (SPECIFY): CEREBRAL, CARDIOPULMONARY, RENAL, GASTROINTESTINAL, PERIPHERAL

Diagnostic Division: Circulation
Definition: The state in which an individual experiences a decrease in nutrition and oxygenation at the cellular level due to a deficit in capillary blood supply. [Tissue perfusion problems can exist without decreased cardiac output; however, there may be a relationship between cardiac output and tissue perfusion.]

RELATED FACTORS
Interruption of flow: arterial, venous; Hypervolemia; Exchange problems; Hypovolemia

DEFINING CHARACTERISTICS

Subjective
Claudication; [Angina]; [Palpitations]

Objective
Skin temperature, cold extremities
Slow-growing, dry thick brittle nails
Bruits
Slow healing of lesions
Blood pressure changes in extremities
Skin color: dependent, blue or purple [or mottled]; pale on elevation and color does not return on lowering leg
Diminished/[absent] arterial pulsations
Skin quality: shining, lack of lanugo

Round scars covered with atrophied skin
Gangrene
[Delayed capillary refill]
Subcomponents [cerebral, renal, gastrointestinal]: Cerebral: [Restlessness], [Altered consciousness], [Memory loss]; Renal: [Decreased urinary output], [Edema formation], [Hypertension]; Gastrointestinal: [Nausea/vomiting], [Abdominal distention], [Melena], [Pain]

TRAUMA, HIGH RISK FOR

Diagnostic Division: Safety
Definition: Accentuated risk of accidental tissue injury, e.g., wound, burn, fracture.

RISK FACTORS

Internal (individual)
Weakness
Balancing difficulties
Reduced large, or small, muscle coordination
Lack of safety education/precautions
Cognitive or emotional difficulties
Poor vision

Reduced temperature and/or tactile sensation
Reduced hand/eye coordination
Insufficient finances to purchase safety equipment or to effect repairs
History of previous trauma

External (environmental) [includes but is not limited to:]

Slippery floors, e.g., wet or highly waxed
Bathtub without hand grip or antislip equipment
Unsturdy or absent stair rails
High beds
Children playing without gates at top of stairs
Inappropriate call-for-aid mechanisms for bed-resting client
Snow or ice on stairs, walkways
Unanchored rugs
Use of unsteady ladder or chairs
Entering unlighted rooms
Unanchored electric wires
Litter or liquid spills on floors or stairways
Obstructed passageways
Unsafe window protection in homes with young children
Pot handles facing toward front of stove
Potential igniting of gas leaks
Bathing in very hot water, e.g., unsupervised bathing of young children
Experimenting with chemicals or gasoline
Children playing with matches, candles, cigarettes
Highly flammable children's toys or clothing
Overloaded fuse boxes
Sliding on coarse bed linen or struggling within bed restraints
Contact with acids or alkalis
Contact with intense cold
Overexposure to sun, sun lamps, radiotherapy
Guns or ammunition stored unlocked
Children playing with sharp-edged toys
Driving a mechanically unsafe vehicle

Driving at excessive speeds
Children riding in the front seat of car
Delayed lighting of gas burner or oven
Unscreened fires or heaters
Wearing of plastic aprons or flowing clothing around open flame
Inadequately stored combustibles or corrosives, e.g., matches, oily rags, lye
Contact with rapidly moving machinery, industrial belts, or pulleys
Faulty electrical plugs, frayed wires, or defective appliances
Playing with fireworks or gunpowder
Use of cracked dishware or glasses
Knives stored uncovered
Large icicles hanging from roof
Exposure to dangerous machinery
High-crime neighborhood and vulnerable individuals
Driving after partaking of alcoholic beverages or drugs
Driving without necessary visual aids
Smoking in bed or near oxygen
Grease waste collected on stoves
Unrestrained infants/children riding in car
Unsafe road or road-crossing conditions
Play or work near vehicle pathways, e.g., driveways, lanes, railroad tracks
Overloaded electrical outlets
Use of thin or worn pot holders or mitts
Nonuse or misuse of seat restraints
Nonuse or misuse of necessary headgear for motorized cyclists or young children carried on adult bicycles

---

UNILATERAL NEGLECT

Diagnostic Division: Neurosensory

Definition: The state in which an individual is perceptually unaware of and inattentive to one side of the body [and the immediate unilateral territory/space.]

RELATED FACTORS

Effects of disturbed perceptual abilities, e.g., [homonymous] hemianopsia [or visual inattention]; One-sided blindness, neurologic illness or trauma [Impaired cerebral blood flow]

DEFINING CHARACTERISTICS

Subjective

[Complaints of feeling that part does not belong to own self]

Objective

Consistent inattention to stimuli on an affective side; Inadequate self-care [inability to satisfactorily perform activities of daily living]; Positioning and/or safety precautions in regard to the affective side; Does not look toward affective side; Leaves food on plate on the affected side; [Does not touch affected side]; [Failure to use the affective side of the body without being reminded to do so]

URINARY ELIMINATION, ALTERED PATTERNS OF

Diagnostic Division: Elimination
Definition: The state in which an individual experiences a disturbance in urine elimination.

RELATED FACTORS
Multiple causality, including: Sensory motor impairment; Anatomical obstruction; Urinary tract infection; Mechanical trauma; [Surgical diversion]

DEFINING CHARACTERISTICS

Subjective
Frequency; Hesitance; Dysuria

Objective
Nocturia; Urgency; Incontinence; Retention

URINARY RETENTION [ACUTE/CHRONIC]

Diagnostic Division: Elimination
Definition: The state in which the individual experiences incomplete emptying of the bladder. [High urethral pressure inhibits voiding until increased abdominal pressure causes urine to be involuntarily lost, or high urethral pressure inhibits complete emptying of bladder.]

RELATED FACTORS
High urethral pressure caused by weak detrusor [absent detrusor]; Inhibition of reflex arc; Strong sphincter; Blockage [e.g., BPH, perineal swelling]; [Habituation of reflex arc]; [Use of medications with side effect of retention, e.g., atropine, belladonna, psychotropics, antihistamines, opiates]

DEFINING CHARACTERISTICS

Subjective
Sensation of bladder fullness; Dribbling; Dysuria

Objective
Bladder distention; Small, frequent voiding or absence of urine output; Residual urine [150 ml or more]; Overflow incontinence; [Reduced stream]

VIOLENCE, HIGH RISK FOR: DIRECTED AT SELF/OTHERS

Diagnostic Division: Safety
Definition: A state in which an individual experiences behaviors that can be physically harmful either to the self or to others. [The "harm" can range from neglect to abuse or even death and may be psychologic and/or physical.]

RISK FACTORS
Antisocial character
Catatonic excitement
Manic excitement
Panic states
Suicidal behavior
Toxic reactions to medication [illicit drugs/alcohol]
Battered women [spouse abuse]

Child abuse
Organic brain syndrome
Rage reactions
Temporal lobe epilepsy
[Negative role modeling]
[Developmental crisis]
[Hormonal imbalance, e.g., PMS, postpartal depression/psychosis]

DEFINING CHARACTERISTICS

Body language: clenched fists, facial expressions, rigid posture, tautness indicating intense effort to control

Overt and aggressive acts; goal-directed destruction of objects in environment

Self-destructive behavior and/or active aggressive suicidal acts

Hostile threatening verbalizations; boasting of prior abuse to others

Increased motor activity, pacing, excitement, irritability, agitation

Possession of destructive means: gun, knife, weapon

Suspicion of others, paranoid ideation, delusions, hallucinations

Substance abuse or withdrawal

Rage

[Expresses intent/desire to harm self or others, directly or indirectly]

Other Possible Characteristics

Inability to verbalize feelings

Provocative behavior: argumentative, dissatisfied, overreactive, hypersensitive

Fear of self or others

Vulnerable self-esteem

Anger

Repetition of verbalizations: continues complaints, requests, and demands

Increasing anxiety level

Depression (specifically active, aggressive, suicidal acts)

NEWLY APPROVED NURSING DIAGNOSES
NANDA 10TH CONFERENCE, 1992

CAREGIVER ROLE STRAIN

Definition: A caregiver's felt difficulty in performing the family caregiver role.

RELATED FACTORS

Pathophysiological

Illness severity of the care receiver

Addiction or codependency

Premature birth/congenital defect

Discharge of family member with significant home care needs

Caregiver health impairment

Unpredictable illness course or instability in the care receiver's health

Caregiver is female

Psychological or cognitive problems in care receiver

Developmental

Caregiver is not developmentally ready for caregiver role, e.g., young adult needing to provide care for a middle-aged parent

Developmental delay or retardation of the care receiver or caregiver

Psychosocial

Marginal family adaptation or dysfunction prior to the caregiving situation

Marginal caregiver's coping patterns

Past history of poor relationship between caregiver and care receiver

Caregiver is spouse

Care receiver exhibits deviant, bizarre behavior

Situational

Presence of abuse or violence

Presence of situational stressors which normally affect families, such as significant loss, disaster or crisis, poverty or economic vulnerability, major life events, e.g., birth, hospitalization, leaving home, returning home, marriage, divorce, employment, retirement, death

Duration of caregiving required
Inadequate physical environment for providing care, e.g., housing, transportation, community services, equipment
Family/caregiver isolation
Lack of respite and recreation for caregiver
Inexperience with caregiving
Caregiver's competing role commitments
Complexity/amount of caregiving tasks

DEFINING CHARACTERISTICS*

Caregivers report they:

Do not have enough resources (time, emotional strength, physical energy, help from others) to provide the care needed
Find it hard to do specific caregiving activities such as bathing, cleaning up after incontinence, having to manage behavior problems, and having to manage pain
Worry about such things as the care receiver's health and emotional state, having to put the care receiver in an institution, and who will care for the care receiver if something should happen to the caregiver
Feel that caregiving interferes with other important roles in their lives, such as being a worker, parent, spouse, or friend
Feel loss because the care receiver is like a different person compared to before caregiving began or, in the case of a child, that the care receiver was never the child the caregiver expected
Feel family conflict around issues of providing care, feeling that other family members do not do their share in providing care to the care receiver, or that not enough appreciation is shown for what the caregiver does
Feel stress or nervousness in their relationship with the care receiver
Feel depressed

*80% of caregivers report one or more of the above defining characteristics.

DYSFUNCTIONAL VENTILATORY WEANING RESPONSE (DVWR)

Definition: A state in which a patient cannot adjust to lowered levels of mechanical ventilator support, which interrupts and prolongs the weaning process.

RELATED FACTORS

Physical
Ineffective airway clearance
Sleep pattern disturbance
Inadequate nutrition
Uncontrolled pain or discomfort

Psychological
Knowledge deficit of the weaning process, patient role
Patient-perceived inefficacy about the ability to wean
Decreased motivation
Decreased self-esteem
Anxiety: moderate, severe
Fear
Hopelessness
Powerlessness
Insufficient trust in the nurse

Situational
Uncontrolled episodic energy demands or problems
Inappropriate pacing of diminished ventilator support
Inadequate social support
Adverse environment (noisy, active environment; negative events in the room; low nurse-patient ratio; extended nurse absence from bedside; unfamiliar nursing staff)
History of ventilator dependence greater than 1 week
History of multiple unsuccessful weaning attempts

DEFINING CHARACTERISTICS

Mild DVWR

Major
Restlessness
Slight increased respiratory rate from baseline

Minor
Responds to lowered levels of mechanical ventilator support with: expressed feelings of increased need for oxygen, breathing discomfort, fatigue, warmth; Queries about possible machine malfunction; Increased concentration on breathing

Moderate DVWR

Major
Responds to lowered levels of mechanical ventilator support with: Slight increase from baseline blood pressure less than 20 mm Hg; Slight increase from baseline heart rate less than 20 beats/minute; Baseline increase in respiratory rate less than 5 breaths/minute

Minor
Hypervigilence to activities
Inability to respond to coaching
Inability to cooperate
Apprehension
Diaphoresis
Eye widening "wide-eyed look"
Decreased air entry on auscultation
Color changes: pale, slight cyanosis
Slight respiratory accessory muscle use

Severe DVWR

Major
Responds to lowered levels of mechanical ventilator support with: Agitation; Deterioration in arterial blood gases from current baseline; Increase from baseline blood pressure more than 20 mm Hg; Increase from baseline heart rate more than 20 bears/minute; Respiratory rate increases significantly from baseline

Minor
Profuse diaphoresis
Full respiratory accessory muscle use
Shallow, gasping breaths
Paradoxical abdominal breathing
Discoordinated breathing with the ventilator
Decreased level of consciousness
Adventitious breath sounds, audible airway secretions
Cyanosis

HIGH RISK FOR CAREGIVER ROLE STRAIN

Definition: A caregiver is vulnerable for felt difficulty in performing the family caregiver role.

RISK FACTORS

Pathophysiological
Illness severity of the care receiver
Addiction or codependency
Premature birth/congenital defect
Discharge of family member with significant home care needs
Caregiver health impairment
Unpredictable illness course or instability in the care receiver's health
Caregiver is female
Psychological or cognitive problems in care receiver

Developmental
Caregiver is not developmentally ready for caregiver role, e.g., young adult needing to provide care for a middle-aged parent
Developmental delay or retardation of the care receiver or caregiver

Psychosocial
Marginal family adaptation or dysfunction prior to the caregiving situation
Marginal caregiver's coping patterns
Past history of poor relationship between caregiver and care receiver
Caregiver is spouse
Care receiver exhibits deviant, bizarre behavior

Situational
Presence of abuse or violence
Presence of situational stressors which normally affect families, such as significant loss, disaster or crisis, poverty or economic vulnerability, major life events, e.g., birth, hospitalization, leaving home, returning home, marriage, divorce, employment, retirement, death
Duration of caregiving required
Inadequate physical environment for providing care, e.g., housing, transportation, community services, equipment
Family/caregiver isolation
Lack of respite and recreation for caregiver
Inexperience with caregiving
Caregiver's competing role commitments
Complexity/amount of caregiving tasks

HIGH RISK FOR PERIPHERAL NEUROVASCULAR DYSFUNCTION

Definition: A state in which an individual is at risk of experiencing a disruption in circulation, sensation, or motion of an extremity.

RISK FACTORS
Fractures
Mechanical compression, e.g., tourniquet, cast, brace, dressing, or restraint
Orthopedic surgery
Trauma
Immobilization
Burns
Vascular obstruction

HIGH RISK FOR SELF-MUTILATION

Definition: A state in which an individual is at high risk to perform a deliberate act upon the self with the intent to injure, not kill, which produces immediate tissue damage to the body.

RISK FACTORS

Groups at Risk:
Clients with borderline personality disorder, especially females 16 to 25 years of age
Clients in psychotic state — frequently males in young adulthood
Emotionally disturbed and/or battered children
Mentally retarded and autistic children
Clients with a history of self-injury

Inability to cope with increased psychological-physiological tension in a healthy manner
Feelings of depression, rejection, self-hatred, separation anxiety, guilt, and depersonalization
Fluctuating emotions
Command hallucinations
Need for sensory stimuli
Parental emotional deprivation
Dysfunctional family

INTERRUPTED BREASTFEEDING

Definition: A break in the continuity of the breastfeeding process as a result of inability or inadvisability to put baby to breast for feeding.

RELATED FACTORS
Maternal or infant illness
Prematurity
Maternal employment
Contraindications to breastfeeding (e.g., drugs, true breastmilk jaundice)
Need to abruptly wean infant

DEFINING CHARACTERISTICS

Major
Infant does not receive nourishment at the breast for some or all of feedings

Minor
Maternal desire to maintain lactation and provide (or eventually provide) her breastmilk for her infant's nutritional needs
Separation of mother and infant
Lack of knowledge regarding expression and storage of breastmilk

---

RELOCATION STRESS SYNDROME

Definition: Physiological and/or psychosocial disturbances as a result of transfer from one environment to another.

RELATED FACTORS
Past, concurrent, and recent losses
Losses involved with decision to move
Feeling of powerlessness
Lack of adequate support system
Little or no preparation for the impending move
Moderate to high degree of environmental change
History and types of previous transfers
Impaired psychosocial health status
Decreased physical health status

DEFINING CHARACTERISTICS

Major
Anxiety
Apprehension
Increased confusion (elderly)
Depression
Loneliness

Minor
Verbalization of unwillingness to relocate
Sleep disturbance
Change in eating habits
Dependency
Gastrointestinal disturbances
Increased verbalization of needs
Insecurity
Lack of trust
Restlessness
Sad affect
Unfavorable comparison of post/pre-transfer staff

Verbalization of being concerned/upset about transfer
Vigilance
Weight change
Withdrawal

INABILITY TO SUSTAIN SPONTANEOUS VENTILATION

Definition: A state in which a patient is unable to maintain adequate breathing to support life. This is measured by deterioration of arterial blood gases, increased work of breathing and decreasing energy.

RELATED FACTORS
Metabolic factors
Respiratory muscle fatigue

DEFINING CHARACTERISTICS

Major
Dyspnea
Increased metabolic rate

Minor
Increased restlessness
Apprehension
Increased use of accessory muscles
Decreased tidal volume
Increased heart rate
Decreased pO2
Increased pcO2
Decreased cooperation
Decreased SaO2

INEFFECTIVE INFANT FEEDING PATTERN

Definition: A state in which an infant demonstrates an impaired ability to suck or coordinate the suck-swallow response.

RELATED FACTORS
Prematurity
Neurological impairment/delay
Oral hypersensitivity
Prolonged NPO

DEFINING CHARACTERISTICS
Inability to initiate or sustain an effective suck
Inability to coordinate sucking, swallowing, and breathing

INEFFECTIVE MANAGEMENT OF THERAPEUTIC REGIMEN (INDIVIDUAL)

Definition: A pattern of regulating and integrating into daily living a program for treatment of illness and the sequelae of illness that is unsatisfactory for meeting specific health goals.

RELATED FACTORS
Complexity of health care system
Complexity of therapeutic regimen
Decisional conflicts

Economic difficulties
Excessive demands made on individual or family
Family conflict
Family patterns of health care
Inadequate number and types of cues to action
Knowledge deficits
Mistrust of regimen and/or health care personnel
Perceived seriousness
Perceived susceptibility
Perceived barriers
Perceived benefits
Powerlessness
Social support deficits

DEFINING CHARACTERISTICS

Major

Inappropriate choices of daily living for meeting the goals of a treatment or prevention program

Minor

Acceleration (expected or unexpected) of illness symptoms
Verbalized desire to manage the treatment of illness and prevention of sequelae
Verbalized difficulty with regulation/integration of one or more prescribed regimens for treatment of illness and its effects or prevention of complications
Verbalized that did not take action to include treatment regimens in daily routines
Verbalized that did not take action to reduce risk factors for progression of illness and sequelae